SCHWARTZ'S
PRINCIPLES OF
SURGERY

SCHWARTZ'S PRINCIPLES OF SURGERY

EIGHTH EDITION

Editor-in-Chief

F. Charles Brunicardi, M.D., F.A.C.S.
DeBakey/Bard Professor and Chairman
Michael E. DeBakey Department of Surgery
Baylor College of Medicine
Houston, Texas

Associate Editors

Dana K. Andersen, M.D.
Harry M. Haidek Distinguished Professor and Chairman
Department of Surgery
University of Massachusetts Memorial Medical School
Worcester, Massachusetts

Timothy R. Billiar, M.D.
George Vance Foster Professor and Chairman of Surgery
Department of Surgery
University of Pittsburgh School of Medicine
Pittsburgh, Pennsylvania

David L. Dunn, M.D., Ph.D.
Jay Phillips Professor and Chairman
Department of Surgery
University of Minnesota Medical School
Minneapolis, Minnesota

John G. Hunter, M.D., F.A.C.S.
Professor and Chairman
Department of Surgery
Oregon Health & Science University
Portland, Oregon

Raphael E. Pollock, M.D., Ph.D., F.A.C.S.
Head, Division of Surgery
Professor and Chairman
Department of Surgical Oncology
Senator A.M. Aiken, Jr., Distinguished Chair
The University of Texas M.D. Anderson Cancer Center
Houston, Texas

Illustrations by Philip Ashley & Associates

McGRAW-HILL
MEDICAL PUBLISHING DIVISION

New York   Chicago   San Francisco   Lisbon   London   Madrid   Mexico City
Milan   New Delhi   San Juan   Seoul   Singapore   Sydney   Toronto

The McGraw·Hill Companies

Schwartz's Principles of Surgery, Eighth Edition

3 4 5 6 7 8 9 0   DOWDOW   0 9 8 7 6 5

ISBN: 0-07-141090-2

This book was set in Times Roman by TechBooks.
The editors were Marc Strauss, Michelle Watt, and Nicky Fernando.
The production supervisor was Catherine H. Saggese.
The cover designer was Aimee Nordin.
The index was prepared by Jerry Ralya.
RR Donnelley was the printer and binder.

This book is printed on acid-free paper.

Library of Congress Cataloging-in-Publication Data

   Schwartz's principles of surgery / edited by F. Charles
Brunicardi . . .
   [et al.]. – 8th ed.
      p. ;   cm.
   Rev. ed. of: Principles of surgery / editors, Seymour I.
Schwartz . . .
   [et al.]. 7th ed. 1999.
   Includes bibliographical references and index.
   ISBN 0-07-141090-2
   1. Surgery.   I. Title: Principles of surgery.   II. Brunicardi, F.
Charles.
   III. Schwartz, Seymour I., 1928-IV. Principles of surgery.
   [DNLM: 1. Surgery. 2. Surgical Procedures, Operative.
WO 100 S399 2005]
   RD31.P88 2005
   617–dc22   2003070716

To my wife, Melissa, my children, Isaac and Jackson, my mother, Rose, and my late father, Edward Brunicardi, for their love and support.
F.C.B.

To my wife, Cindy, and my children, Ashley, Lauren, Kathryn, Thomas, and Olivia.
D.K.A.

To my father, Robert R. Billiar, D.V.M., my first role model for professional excellence.
T.R.B.

To the outstanding students and teachers of the discipline of surgery at the University of Minnesota—past, present, and future.
D.L.D.

To my wife Laura, my children, Sarah, Sam, and Jillian, and the residents, fellows, and surgical faculty at OHSU who have created a community of health, collegiality, and open minded intellectual rigor.
J.G.H.

To my children, Samuel and Jessica Pollock, and my late father.
R.E.P.

Contents

Contributors

Vanita Ahuja, M.D. [CHAPTER 8]
Resident
Department of Surgery
Johns Hopkins Medical Institutions
Baltimore, Maryland

Louis H. Alarcon, M.D. [CHAPTER 12]
Assistant Professor
Departments of Surgery and Critical Care Medicine
University of Pittsburgh School of Medicine
Pittsburgh, Pennsylvania

Dana K. Andersen, M.D. [CHAPTER 32]
Harry M. Haidek Distinguished Professor and Chairman
Department of Surgery
University of Massachusetts Memorial Medical School
Worcester, Massachusetts

Peter B. Angood, M.D., F.A.C.S., F.C.C.M. [CHAPTER 11]
Professor of Surgery Anesthesia and
    Emergency Medicine
Chief, Division of Trauma & Critical Care
University of Massachusetts Medical School and
UMass-Memorial Health Care System
Worcester, Massachusetts

Chandrakanth Are, M.D. [CHAPTER 8]
Clinical Instructor and Assistant Chief of Service
Department of Surgery
Johns Hopkins Medical Institutions
Baltimore, Maryland

Stanley W. Ashley, M.D. [CHAPTER 27]
Professor and Vice Chairman
Department of Surgery
Brigham and Women's Hospital/Harvard
    Medical School
Boston, Massachusetts

Adrian Barbul, M.D., F.A.C.S. [CHAPTER 8]
Surgeon-in-Chief
Sinai Hospital of Baltimore
Professor and Vice-Chairman
Department of Surgery
Johns Hopkins Medical Institutions
Baltimore, Maryland

Samuel W. Beenken, M.D., F.R.C.S.(C.), F.A.C.S. [CHAPTER 16]
Professor of Surgery
University of Alabama at Birmingham
Birmingham, Alabama

Gregory J. Beilman, M.D., F.A.C.S. [CHAPTER 5]
Associate Professor of Surgery and Anesthesia
University of Minnesota Medical School
Minneapolis, Minnesota

Richard H. Bell, Jr., M.D., F.A.C.S. [CHAPTER 32]
Loyal and Edith Davis Professor and Chair
Department of Surgery
Feinberg School of Medicine
Northwestern University
Chicago, Illinois

Robert L. Bell, M.D., M.A. [CHAPTER 34]
Assistant Professor
Department of Surgery
Yale University School of Medicine
New Haven, Connecticut

Arie Belldegrun, M.D., F.A.C.S. [CHAPTER 39]
Roy and Carol Doumani Chair in Urologic Oncology
Professor of Urology
Chief, Division of Urologic Oncology
David Geffen School of Medicine at UCLA
Los Angeles, California

David H. Berger, M.D., F.A.C.S. [CHAPTER 29]
Associate Professor and Vice Chair
Michael E. DeBakey Department of Surgery
Baylor College of Medicine
Operative Care Line Executive
Chief, Surgical Services
Michael E. DeBakey Veterans Affairs Medical Center
Houston, Texas

Alan Bienstock, M.D., B.S. [CHAPTER 44]
Resident
Division of Plastic Surgery
Michael E. DeBakey Department of Surgery
Baylor College of Medicine
Houston, Texas

Timothy R. Billiar, M.D. *[CHAPTER 4]*
George Vance Foster Professor and Chairman
Department of Surgery
University of Pittsburgh School of Medicine
Pittsburgh, Pennsylvania

Kirby I. Bland, M.D., F.A.C.S. *[CHAPTER 16]*
Fay Fletcher Kerner Professor and Chairman
Deputy Director, UAB Comprehensive Cancer Center
Department of Surgery
University of Alabama at Birmingham
Birmingham, Alabama

F. Charles Brunicardi, M.D., F.A.C.S.
[CHAPTERS 14, 32]
DeBakey/Bard Professor and Chairman
Michael E. DeBakey Department of Surgery
Baylor College of Medicine
Houston, Texas

Kelli M. Bullard, M.D., F.A.C.S. *[CHAPTER 28]*
Assistant Professor of Surgery and Laboratory
    Medicine & Pathology
University of Minnesota
Minneapolis, Minnesota

Jon M. Burch, M.D. *[CHAPTER 6]*
Professor of Surgery
University of Colorado Health Sciences Center
Chief of General and Vascular Surgery
Denver Health Medical Center
Denver, Colorado

Ruth L. Bush, M.D. *[CHAPTER 22]*
Assistant Professor of Surgery
Division of Vascular Surgery and
    Endovascular Therapy
Michael E. DeBakey Department of Surgery
Baylor College of Medicine
Houston, Texas

Steven E. Calvano, Ph.D. *[CHAPTER 1]*
Associate Professor
Division of Surgical Sciences
Department of Surgery
UMDNJ–Robert Wood Johnson Medical School
New Brunswick, New Jersey

Rakesh K. Chandra, M.D. *[CHAPTER 17]*
Assistant Professor
Director, Division of Nasal and Sinus Disorders
Residency Program Director
Department of Otolaryngology–Head and Neck Surgery
University of Tennessee Health Science Center
Memphis, Tennessee

Changyi Chen, M.D., Ph.D. *[CHAPTER 22]*
Professor of Surgery
Division of Vascular Surgery and Endovascular Therapy
Michael E. DeBakey Department of Surgery
Baylor College of Medicine
Houston, Texas

Orlo H. Clark, M.D. *[CHAPTER 37]*
Professor of Surgery
Department of Surgery
University of California, San Francisco/Mt. Zion
    Medical Center
San Francisco, California

Stephen B. Colvin, M.D. *[CHAPTER 20]*
Chief, Cardiothoracic Surgery
New York University School of Medicine
New York, New York

Edward M. Copeland III, M.D. *[CHAPTER 16]*
Distinguished Professor of Surgery
University of Florida College of Medicine
Gainesville, Florida

Janice N. Cormier, M.D., M.P.H. *[CHAPTER 35]*
Assistant Professor of Surgery
Department of Surgical Oncology
The University of Texas M.D. Anderson
    Cancer Center
Houston, Texas

Joseph S. Coselli, M.D. *[CHAPTER 21]*
Professor and Chief
Division of Cardiothoracic Surgery
Michael E. DeBakey Department of Surgery
Baylor College of Medicine
Houston, Texas

Steven A. Curley, M.D., F.A.C.S. *[CHAPTER 30]*
Professor, Department of Surgical Oncology
Chief, Gastrointestinal Tumor Surgery
The University of Texas M.D. Anderson Cancer Center
Houston, Texas

Tom R. DeMeester, M.D. *[CHAPTER 24]*
The Jeffrey P. Smith Professor of General &
    Thoracic Surgery
Chairman, Department of Surgery
Keck School of Medicine
University of Southern California
Los Angeles, California

Daniel T. Dempsey, M.D., F.A.C.S. *[CHAPTER 25]*
Professor and Chairman of Surgery
Temple University School of Medicine
Philadelphia, Pennsylvania

Robert S. Dorian, M.D. *[CHAPTER 46]*
Chairman and Program Director
Department of Anesthesiology
Saint Barnabas Medical Center
Livingston, New Jersey

David L. Dunn, M.D., Ph.D. *[CHAPTERS 5, 10]*
Jay Phillips Professor and Chairman
Department of Surgery
University of Minnesota Medical School
Minneapolis, Minnesota

David E. Efron, M.D. *[CHAPTER 8]*
Assistant Professor
Department of Surgery
Johns Hopkins Medical Institutions
Baltimore, Maryland

Xin-Hua Feng, Ph.D. *[CHAPTER 14]*
Associate Professor of Surgery
Division of General Surgery
Michael E. DeBakey Department of Surgery
Baylor College of Medicine
Houston, Texas

Charles J. Filipi, M.D., F.A.C.S. *[CHAPTER 36]*
Professor of Surgery
Department of Surgery
Creighton University
Omaha, Nebraska

Mitchell P. Fink, M.D. *[CHAPTER 12]*
Professor and Chairman
Department of Critical Care Medicine
Watson Chair in Surgery
University of Pittsburgh
Pittsburgh, Pennsylvania

William E. Fisher, M.D., F.A.C.S. *[CHAPTER 32]*
Associate Professor of Surgery
Michael E. DeBakey Department of Surgery
Baylor College of Medicine
Houston, Texas

Robert J. Fitzgibbons, Jr., M.D. *[CHAPTER 36]*
Harry E. Stuckenhoff Professor of Surgery
Department of Surgery
Creighton University
Omaha, Nebraska

Henri R. Ford, M.D. *[CHAPTER 38]*
Benjamin R. Fisher Chair
Professor and Chief
Division of Pediatric Surgery
Children's Hospital of Pittsburgh
University of Pittsburgh School of Medicine
Pittsburgh, Pennsylvania

Reginald J. Franciose, M.D. *[CHAPTER 6]*
Assistant Professor of Surgery
University of Colorado Health Sciences Center
Attending Surgeon
Denver Health Medical Center
Denver, Colorado

Aubrey C. Galloway, M.D. *[CHAPTER 20]*
Professor of Surgery, Cardiothoracic Surgery
Director, Cardiac Surgical Research
New York University School of Medicine
New York, New York

Mary E. Giswold, M.D. *[CHAPTER 23]*
Surgical Resident
Department of Surgery
Oregon Health & Science University
Portland, Oregon

M. Sean Grady, M.D., F.A.C.S. *[CHAPTER 41]*
Charles Harrison Frazier Professor and Chairman
Department of Neurosurgery
University of Pennsylvania School of Medicine
Philadelphia, Pennsylvania

Eugene A. Grossi, M.D. *[CHAPTER 20]*
Professor of Surgery, Cardiothoracic Surgery
New York University School of Medicine
New York, New York

David J. Hackam, M.D., Ph.D. *[CHAPTER 38]*
Assistant Professor of Surgery, Cell Biology and
    Physiology
University of Pittsburgh School of Medicine
Attending Pediatric Surgeon
Co-Director, Fetal Diagnosis and Treatment Center
Children's Hospital of Pittsburgh
Pittsburgh, Pennsylvania

Scott L. Hansen, M.D. *[CHAPTER 15]*
Resident, Plastic and Reconstructive Surgery
University of California, San Francisco
San Francisco, California

Brian G. Harbrecht, M.D., F.A.C.S. *[CHAPTER 4]*
Associate Professor of Surgery
Department of Surgery
University of Pittsburgh
Pittsburgh, Pennsylvania

Rosemarie E. Hardin, M.D. *[CHAPTER 45]*
Resident
Department of Surgery
SUNY Health Science Medical Center
Brooklyn, New York

David M. Heimbach, M.D., F.A.C.S. *[CHAPTER 7]*
Professor of Surgery
University of Washington Burn Center
Harborview Medical Center
Seattle, Washington

James H. Holmes, M.D. *[CHAPTER 7]*
Burn Fellow & Acting Instructor in Surgery
Harborview Medical Center–University of Washington
Seattle, Washington

Abhinav Humar, M.D., F.R.C.S. (Can) *[CHAPTER 10]*
Associate Professor
Department of Surgery
University of Minnesota
Minneapolis, Minnesota

John G. Hunter, M.D., F.A.C.S. *[CHAPTERS 13, 31]*
Professor and Chairman
Department of Surgery
Oregon Health & Science University
Portland, Oregon

William W. Hurd, M.D., F.A.C.O.G., F.A.C.S. *[CHAPTER 40]*
Nicholas J. Thompson Professor and Chair
Department of Obstetrics and Gynecology
Wright State University School of Medicine
Dayton, Ohio

Bernard M. Jaffe, M.D. *[CHAPTER 29]*
Professor of Surgery
Tulane University School of Medicine
New Orleans, Louisiana

Blair A. Jobe, M.D. *[CHAPTER 13]*
Assistant Professor
Department of Surgery
Oregon Health & Science University
Portland, Oregon

Karen L. Kaplan, M.D. *[CHAPTER 3]*
Professor of Medicine (Hematology/Oncology)
University of Rochester School of Medicine
and Dentistry
Rochester, New York

Tara B. Karamlou, M.D. *[CHAPTER 19]*
Senior Research Fellow
Division of Cardiothoracic Surgery
Oregon Health & Science University
Portland, Oregon

Hyung L. Kim, M.D. *[CHAPTER 39]*
Assistant Professor
Department of Urology
Department of Cellular Stress Biology
Roswell Park Cancer Institute
Buffalo, New York

John Y.S. Kim, M.D. *[CHAPTER 44]*
Assistant Professor, Division of Plastic Surgery
Department of Surgery
Northwestern University School of Medicine
Chicago, Illinois

Rosemary A. Kozar, M.D., Ph.D. *[CHAPTER 2]*
Associate Professor of Surgery
University of Texas–Houston
Houston, Texas

Geeta Lal, M.D. *[CHAPTER 37]*
Assistant Professor
Surgical Oncology and Endocrine Surgery
Department of Surgery
University of Iowa Hospital and Clinics
Iowa City, Iowa

Everett Y. Lam, M.D. *[CHAPTER 23]*
Resident
Division of Vascular Surgery
Oregon Health & Science University
Portland, Oregon

Scott A. LeMaire, M.D. *[CHAPTER 21]*
Assistant Professor
Division of Cardiothoracic Surgery
Baylor College of Medicine
The Methodist DeBakey Heart Center
Houston, Texas

Edward Lin, D.O., C.N.S.P. *[CHAPTER 1]*
Assistant Professor of Surgery
Division of Gastrointestinal & General Surgery
Surgical Metabolism Laboratory
Emory University School of Medicine
Atlanta, Georgia

Peter H. Lin, M.D. *[CHAPTER 22]*
Associate Professor of Surgery
Division of Vascular Surgery and Endovascular Therapy
Michael E. DeBakey Department of Surgery
Baylor College of Medicine
Houston, Texas

Xia Lin, Ph.D. *[CHAPTER 14]*
Assistant Professor of Surgery
Division of General Surgery
Michael E. DeBakey Department of Surgery
Baylor College of Medicine
Houston, Texas

Stephen F. Lowry, M.D., F.A.C.S. *[CHAPTER 1]*
Professor and Chairman
Department of Surgery
UMDNJ-Robert Wood Johnson Medical School
New Brunswick, New Jersey

James D. Luketich, M.D. *[CHAPTER 18]*
Professor and Chief, Division of Thoracic and
    Foregut Surgery
University of Pittsburgh Medical Center
Pittsburgh, Pennsylvania

Alan B. Lumsden, M.D. *[CHAPTER 22]*
Professor of Surgery
Chief of Division of Vascular Surgery and
    Endovascular Therapy
Michael E. DeBakey Department of Surgery
Baylor College of Medicine
Houston, Texas

Michael A. Maddaus, M.D., F.A.C.S. *[CHAPTER 18]*
Professor and Head, Section of General Thoracic Surgery
Garamella-Lynch-Jensen Chair in Thoracic &
    Cardiovascular Surgery
Co-Director, Minimally Invasive Surgery Center
University of Minnesota
Minneapolis, Minnesota

Stephen J. Mathes, M.D. *[CHAPTER 15]*
Professor of Surgery
Chief, Division of Plastic and Reconstructive Surgery
University of California, San Francisco
San Francisco, California

Jeffrey B. Matthews, M.D., F.A.C.S. *[CHAPTER 15]*
Christian R. Holmes Professor and Chairman
Department of Surgery
University of Cincinnati
Cincinnati, Ohio

Rodrick McKinlay, M.D. *[CHAPTER 33]*
Gastrointestinal and Minimally Invasive Surgery
Rocky Mountain Associated Physicians
Salt Lake City, Utah

Funda Meric-Bernstam, M.D., F.A.C.S. *[CHAPTER 9]*
Assistant Professor
Department of Surgical Oncology
University of Texas M.D. Anderson Cancer Center
Houston, Texas

Gregory L. Moneta, M.D. *[CHAPTER 23]*
Professor and Chief Vascular Surgery
Oregon Health & Science University
Portland, Oregon

Ernest E. Moore, M.D., F.A.C.S. *[CHAPTER 6]*
Professor and Vice Chairman, Department of Surgery
University of Colorado Health Sciences Center
Chief of Surgery and Trauma Services
Denver Health Medical Center
Denver, Colorado

Frederick A. Moore, M.D. *[CHAPTER 2]*
James H. "Red" Duke, Jr. Professor & Vice Chairman
Department of Surgery
The University of Texas Houston Medical School
Houston, Texas

Martina F. Mutone, M.D. *[CHAPTER 40]*
Clinical Assistant Professor
Indiana University/Methodist Hospital
St. Vincent Hospitals and Health Services
Indianapolis, Indiana

Kurt Newman, M.D., F.A.C.S. *[CHAPTER 38]*
Executive Director and Surgeon-in-Chief
Joseph E. Robert, Jr. Center for Surgical Care
Children's National Medical Center
Professor of Surgery and Pediatrics
George Washington University School of Medicine
Washington, D.C.

Margrét Oddsdóttir, M.D. *[CHAPTER 31]*
Professor of Surgery
Chief of General Surgery
Landspitali–University Hospital
Reykjavik, Iceland

Adrian E. Park, M.D., F.R.C.S.(C), F.A.C.S. *[CHAPTER 33]*
Campbell and Jeanette Plugge Professor of Surgery
Professor and Head, Division of General Surgery
Department of Surgery
University of Maryland Medical Center
Baltimore, Maryland

Julie E. Park, M.D. *[CHAPTER 8]*
Resident
Department of Surgery
Johns Hopkins Medical Institutions
Baltimore, Maryland

Clayton A. Peimer, M.D. *[CHAPTER 43]*
Breech Chair of Orthopaedic Surgery
Henry Ford Health System
Detroit, Michigan

Andrew B. Peitzman, M.D., F.A.C.S. *[CHAPTER 4]*
Professor and Vice-Chairman, Department of Surgery
University of Pittsburgh Medical Center
Pittsburgh, Pennsylvania

Jeffrey H. Peters, M.D., F.A.C.S. *[CHAPTER 24]*
Professor and Chairman
University of Rochester School of Medicine and Dentistry
Surgeon-in-Chief
Strong Memorial Hospital
Department of Surgery
Rochester, New York

Raphael E. Pollock, M.D., Ph.D., F.A.C.S. *[CHAPTERS 9, 35]*
Head, Division of Surgery
Professor and Chairman
Department of Surgical Oncology
Senator A.M. Aiken, Jr., Distinguished Chair
The University of Texas M.D. Anderson Cancer Center
Houston, Texas

Thomas H. Quinn, Ph.D. *[CHAPTER 36]*
Professor of Anatomy and Surgery
Director of Clinical Anatomy
School of Medicine
Creighton University
Omaha, Nebraska

Robert E. Rogers, M.D. *[CHAPTER 40]*
Emeritus Professor, Obstetrics and Gynecology
Indiana University School of Medicine
Indianapolis, Indiana

David A. Rothenberger, M.D. *[CHAPTER 28]*
Professor of Surgery
Chief, Divisions of Colon and Rectal Surgery and
  Surgical Oncology
Department of Surgery
University of Minnesota
Minneapolis, Minnesota

Ashok K. Saluja, Ph.D. *[CHAPTER 32]*
Professor of Surgery, Medicine, and Cell Biology
University of Massachusetts Medical School
Worcester, Massachusetts

Paul C. Saunders, M.D. *[CHAPTER 20]*
Fellow
Division of Cardiothoracic Surgery
New York University School of Medicine
New York, New York

Philip R. Schauer, M.D. *[CHAPTER 26]*
Associate Professor of Surgery
Director of Bariatric Surgery
Chief, Minimally Invasive General Surgery
The University of Pittsburgh
Pittsburgh, Pennsylvania

Bruce D. Schirmer, M.D., F.A.C.S. *[CHAPTER 26]*
Stephen H. Watts Professor of Surgery
University of Virginia Health System
Charlottesville, Virginia

Charles F. Schwartz, M.D. *[CHAPTER 20]*
Assistant Professor of Surgery
Division of Cardiothoracic Surgery
New York University School of Medicine
New York, New York

David Schwartz, M.D., Ph.D., F.A.C.C. *[CHAPTER 3]*
Assistant Professor of Medicine
Cardiovascular Division
Washington University School of Medicine
Saint Louis, Missouri

Seymour I. Schwartz, M.D., F.A.C.S. *[CHAPTER 3]*
Distinguished Alumni Professor of Surgery
University of Rochester School of Medicine and
  Dentistry
Rochester, New York

Neal E. Seymour, M.D., F.A.C.S. *[CHAPTER 34]*
Associate Professor
Tufts University School of Medicine
Vice Chairman, Department of Surgery
Baystate Medical Center
Springfield, Massachusetts

Mark L. Shapiro, M.D. *[CHAPTER 11]*
Assistant Professor of Surgery
Department of Surgery
Division of Trauma and Critical Care
University of Massachusetts Medical School
Worcester, Massachusetts

Ram Sharony, M.D. *[CHAPTER 20]*
Minimally Invasive Cardiac Surgery Fellow
Division of Cardiothoracic Surgery
New York University Medical Center
New York, New York

Irving Shen, M.D. *[CHAPTER 19]*
Assistant Professor of Surgery
Division of Cardiothoracic Surgery
Oregon Health & Science University
Portland, Oregon

Saleh M. Shenaq, M.D. *[CHAPTER 44]*
Chief, Division of Plastic Surgery
Professor of Surgery
Michael E. DeBakey Department of Surgery
Baylor College of Medicine
Houston, Texas

Timothy D. Sielaff, M.D., Ph.D., F.A.C.S. *[CHAPTER 30]*
Associate Professor
Department of Surgery
University of Minnesota
Minneapolis, Minnesota

Michael L. Smith, M.D. *[CHAPTER 41]*
Resident
Department of Neurosurgery
University of Pennsylvania School of Medicine
Philadelphia, Pennsylvania

Dempsey Springfield, M.D. *[CHAPTER 42]*
Professor and Chairman
Department of Orthopaedics
The Mount Sinai School of Medicine
New York, New York

Gregory P. Sutton, M.D. *[CHAPTER 40]*
Director, Gynecologic Oncology
St. Vincent Oncology Center
St. Vincent Hospitals and Health Services
Indianapolis, Indiana

Ross M. Ungerleider, M.D. *[CHAPTER 19]*
Professor of Surgery
Chief, Division of Cardiothoracic Surgery
Oregon Health & Science University
Portland, Oregon

Randal S. Weber, M.D., F.A.C.S. *[CHAPTER 17]*
Hubert L. and Olive Stringer, Distinguished Professor and Chairman
Department of Head and Neck Surgery
University of Texas M.D. Anderson Cancer Center
Houston, Texas

Richard O. Wein, M.D. *[CHAPTER 17]*
Assistant Professor
Department of Otolaryngology and Communicative Sciences
University of Mississippi Medical Center
Jackson, Mississippi

Edward E. Whang, M.D. *[CHAPTER 27]*
Assistant Professor of Surgery
Brigham & Women's Hospital

Harvard Medical School
Boston, Massachusetts

David M. Young, M.D., F.A.C.S. *[CHAPTER 15]*
Associate Professor of Plastic Surgery
Department of Surgery
University of California, San Francisco
San Francisco, California

Michael E. Zenilman, M.D. *[CHAPTER 45]*
Clarence and Mary Dennis Professor and Chairman
Department of Surgery
SUNY Downstate Medical Center
Brooklyn, New York

Michael J. Zinner, M.D. *[CHAPTER 27]*
Moseley Professor of Surgery
Harvard Medical School
Surgeon-in-Chief and Chairman
Department of Surgery
Brigham & Women's Hospital
Boston, Massachusetts

Foreword

It began during the summer of 1967 when John DeCarville of McGraw-Hill convened David Hume, Richard Lillehei, G. Tom Shires, Frank Spencer, Edward Storer, and myself and proposed that we edit a new surgical textbook to serve as a companion to Harrison's *Principles of Internal Medicine*. We agreed, with the proviso that we could create a textbook that would differ from the previous and existing works in the field of surgery. We envisioned a truly modern textbook of surgery that would be panoramic in its scope by including all surgical specialties, and offer material directed at a sophisticated audience, consisting of medical students, who were regarded as graduate students, and that the text would also incorporate the knowledge sought after by surgeons in training, and as part of the continuing education of practicing surgeons. The narrative's attraction would be the presentation of the physiologic basis of the practices in addition to the pathology, diagnosis, and therapy, made readable as a consequence of consistency of style.

The first edition was published in 1969, and I have had the privilege of shepherding six subsequent editions. In each instance, as part of the credo of modernity, the material was brought up to date by effecting changes of between 30 and 40 percent in the subsequent edition. Now, the time has come to pass the mantle of responsibility to Dr. Brunicardi and his five associate editors, all of whom are actively engaged in clinical practice, research, and education.

As Sir William Osler wrote: "Everywhere the old order changes and happy they who can change with it." The editorship of the past seven editions of *Principles of Surgery* has generated much personal happiness and satisfaction. I am particularly appreciative of the reception that has been received from the readership. It is my hope that, over our tenure of 35 years, the needs of the audience have been fulfilled, and the current and future editors provide a continuum of the past.

Seymour I. Schwartz, M.D., F.A.C.S.

Preface

For the past 35 years, the *Principles of Surgery* has been edited by Dr. Seymour Schwartz and a group of outstanding co-editors. It has been considered the leading large textbook for general surgery worldwide. I was surprised and deeply honored to have been asked to assume the role of editor-in-chief and was determined to ensure that the reputation of this legendary book would carry on its tradition of excellence. In this effort, the first assigned task was to select a new group of co-editors. After careful deliberation, five departmental chairmen who are leading scholars in a variety of specialties were selected from universities around the country. Our first meeting to discuss the development of the eighth edition of *Schwartz's Principles of Surgery* defined our first goal: to preserve the style and structure of the classic *Principles of Surgery* with its basic and clinical sections and to preserve the titles of 95% of the chapters. However, it soon became apparent after a thorough review of each chapter that new authors, those who were leaders in their respective fields, would be selected to compose this extensively updated and modernized text. Upon completion, 76% of the chapters are from new authors. These chapters contain the latest in surgical science, surgical techniques, and therapy for students, residents, and surgeons. Six new chapters have been added to round out this eighth edition: Cell, Genomics, and Molecular Surgery, Soft Tissue Sarcomas, Anesthesia of the Surgical Patient, the Surgical Management of Obesity, Patient Safety, Errors, and Complications in Surgery, and Surgical Considerations in the Elderly. Another important component of this work identified by the editorial team was the artwork. A new artist (Philip Ashley & Associates) was selected to direct the art program, which provides clear and consistent learning aids throughout the text and visually reflects the comprehensive and updated nature of this book.

The editorial team is deeply honored to carry forward the tradition of this great textbook into the 21st century. As a team we have worked diligently to create a state-of-the-art textbook to help students, residents and surgeons study the craft of surgery and it is to students of surgery of all ages that we dedicate this book. It is your own devotion to learning the language of surgery that will translate into the best care of patients around the world. We hope the textbook will serve as the cornerstone of your own learning program as it has for the study of surgery for the past 35 years.

We wish to thank Katie Elsbury and Susie Lee for their exceptional skills in helping edit and coordinate all communication. We wish to thank Marc Strauss, Michelle Watt, and their team at McGraw-Hill for their willingness to work with us. We would also like to thank our families, whose love and support made this book possible.

F. Charles Brunicardi, M.D., F.A.C.S.
October 2004

Preface to the First Edition

The raison d'être for a new textbook in a discipline which has been served by standard works for many years was the Editorial Board's initial conviction that a distinct need for a modern approach in the dissemination of surgical knowledge existed. As incoming chapters were reviewed, both the need and satisfaction became increasingly apparent and, at the completion, we felt a sense of excitement at having the opportunity to contribute to the education of modern and future students concerned with the care of surgical patients.

The recent explosion of factual knowledge has emphasized the need for a presentation which would provide the student an opportunity to assimilate pertinent facts in a logical fashion. This would then permit correlation, synthesis of concepts, and eventual extrapolation to specific situations. The physiologic bases for diseases are therefore emphasized and the manifestations and diagnostic studies are considered as a reflection of pathophysiology. Therapy then becomes logical in this schema and the necessity to regurgitate facts is minimized. In appreciation of the impact which Harrison's *Principles of Internal Medicine* has had, the clinical manifestations of the disease processes are considered in detail for each area. Since the operative procedure represents the one element in the therapeutic armamentarium unique to the surgeon, the indications, important technical considerations, and complications receive appropriate emphasis. While we appreciate that a textbook cannot hope to incorporate an atlas of surgical procedures, we have provided the student a single book which will satisfy the sequential demands in the care and considerations of surgical patients.

The ultimate goal of the Editorial Board has been to collate a book which is deserving of the adjective "modern." We have therefore selected as authors dynamic and active contributors to their particular fields. The au courant concept is hopefully apparent throughout the entire work and is exemplified by appropriate emphasis on diseases of modern surgical interest, such as trauma, transplantation, and the recently appreciated importance of rehabilitation. Cardiovascular surgery is presented in keeping with the exponential strides recently achieved.

There are two major subdivisions to the next. In the first twelve chapters, subjects that transcend several organ systems are presented. The second portion of the book represents a consideration of specific organ systems and surgical specialties.

Throughout the text, the authors have addressed themselves to a sophisticated audience, regarding the medical student as a graduate student, incorporating material generally sought after by the surgeon in training and presenting information appropriate for the continuing education of the practicing surgeon. The need for a text such as we have envisioned is great and the goal admittedly high. It is our hope that this effort fulfills the expressed demands.

Seymour I. Schwartz, M.D., F.A.C.S.

SCHWARTZ'S
PRINCIPLES OF
SURGERY

PART I
BASIC CONSIDERATIONS

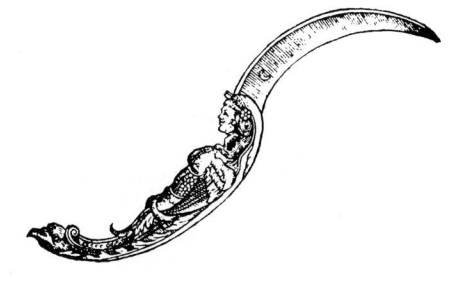

Systemic Response to Injury and Metabolic Support

Edward Lin, Steven E. Calvano, and Stephen F. Lowry

INTRODUCTION

The inflammatory response to injury and activation of cellular processes are inherently designed to restore tissue function and eradicate invading microorganisms. Local injuries of limited duration are usually followed by functional restoration with minimal intervention. By contrast, major insults to the host are associated with an overwhelming inflammatory response that, without appropriate and timely intervention, can lead to multiple organ failure and adversely impact patient survival. Therefore understanding how the inflammatory response is mobilized and ultimately controlled provides a functional framework upon which interventions and therapeutics are formulated for the surgical patient. The maturation of minimally invasive techniques for major surgery during the last decade has brought complementary perspectives to the injury response paradigm, and the immunologic benefits for these surgical approaches are undergoing validation. Furthermore, the sequencing of the human genome and available technology such as deoxyribonucleic acid (DNA) microarray analysis potentially affords surgeons additional tools to profile the genetic mechanisms governing the host response to injury.

This chapter addresses the hormonal, immunologic, and cellular responses to injury. The resultant metabolic and nutritional alterations of injury are discussed in continuum because the utilization of fuel substrates during injury also is subject to the influences of hormonal and inflammatory mediators.

THE SYSTEMIC INFLAMMATORY RESPONSE SYNDROME (SIRS)

Conceptually, the systemic response to injury can be broadly compartmentalized into two phases: (1) a proinflammatory phase characterized by activation of cellular processes designed to restore tissue function and eradicate invading microorganisms, and (2) an anti-inflammatory or *counterregulatory* phase that is important for preventing excessive proinflammatory activities as well as restoring homeostasis in the individual (Fig. 1-1). While the terminologies that describe the various facets of systemic inflammation are often used interchangeably, there are distinct criteria for each term (Table 1-1).

CENTRAL NERVOUS SYSTEM REGULATION OF INFLAMMATION

Reflex Inhibition of Inflammation

The central nervous system, operating through autonomic signaling, has an integral role in regulating the inflammatory response that is

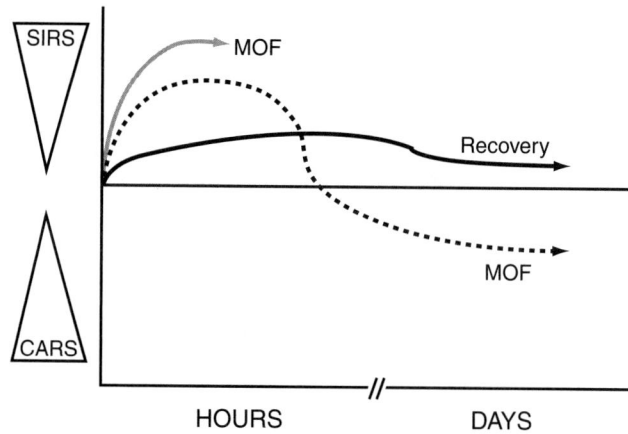

FIG. 1-1. *Schematic representation of the systemic inflammatory response syndrome (SIRS) to injury, followed by a period of convalescence mediated by the counterregulatory anti-inflammatory response syndrome (CARS). Severe inflammation may lead to acute multiple organ failure (MOF) and early death following injury (gray solid arrow). A lesser inflammatory response followed by excessive CARS may induce a prolonged immunosuppressed state that can also be deleterious to the host (broken arrow). Normal recovery after injury requires a period of systemic inflammation followed by a return to homeostasis (black solid arrow). (Concept adapted with permission from Guirao X, Lowry SF: Biologic control of injury and inflammation: Much more than too little or too late. World J Surg 20:437, 1996.)*

primarily involuntary. Classically, the autonomic system regulates heart rate, blood pressure, respiratory rate, gastrointestinal motility, and body temperature. An additional role of the autonomic nervous system is to regulate inflammation in a reflex manner, much like the patellar tendon reflex. Inflammation originating from a specific location sends afferent signals to the hypothalamus, which in turn rapidly relays opposing anti-inflammatory messages to the site of inflammation to reduce inflammatory mediator release by immunocytes (Fig. 1-2).

Afferent Signals to the Brain

The central nervous system (CNS) receives immunologic input from both the circulation and neural pathways. Indeed, areas of the CNS devoid of blood-brain barrier admit the passage of inflammatory mediators such as tumor necrosis factor (TNF-α). Fevers, anorexia, and depression in illness are attributed to the humoral (circulatory) route of inflammatory signaling. While the mechanism for vagal

Table 1-1

Clinical Spectrum of Infection and Systemic Inflammatory Response Syndrome (SIRS)

Term	Definition
Infection	Identifiable source of microbial insult
SIRS	Two or more of following criteria
	Temperature $\geq 38°C$ or $\leq 36°C$
	Heart rate ≥ 90 beats/min
	Respiratory rate ≥ 20 breaths/min or $Paco_2$ ≤ 32 mm Hg or mechanical ventilation
	White blood cell count $\geq 12,000/\mu L$ or $\leq 4000/\mu L$ or $\geq 10\%$ band forms
Sepsis	Identifiable source of infection + SIRS
Severe sepsis	Sepsis + organ dysfunction
Septic shock	Sepsis + cardiovascular collapse (requiring vasopressor support)

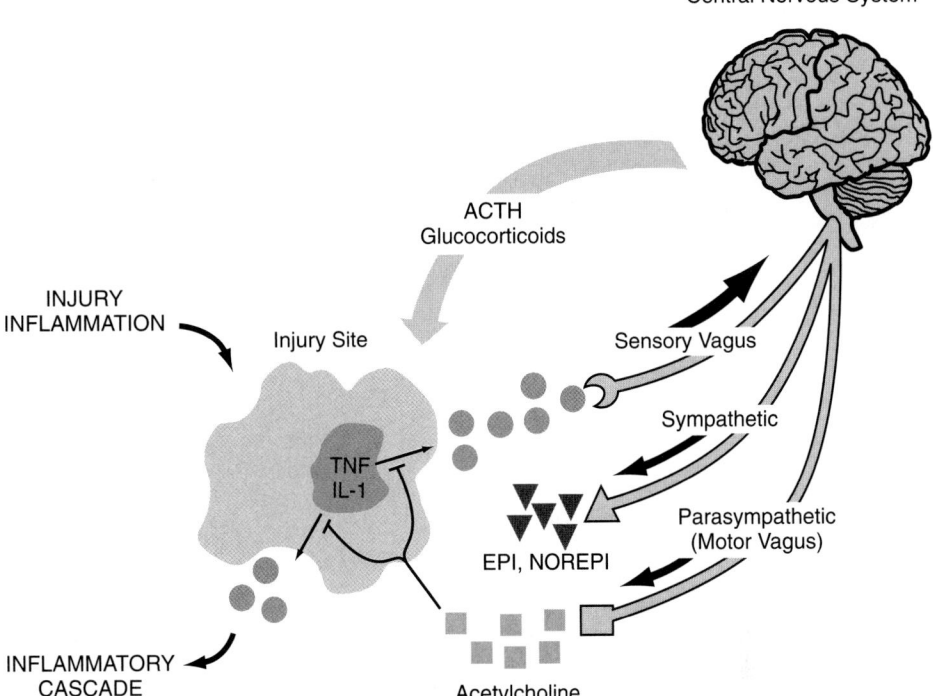

FIG. 1-2. Neural circuit relaying messages of localized injury to the brain (nucleus tractus solitarius). The brain follows with a hormonal response (ACTH, glucocorticoids) into the systemic circulation and by sympathetic release. The vagal response rapidly induces acetylcholine release directed at the site of injury to curtail the inflammatory response elicited by the activated immunocytes. This vagal response occurs in real time and is site specific. (*Concept adapted and recreated with permission from Tracey KJ: The inflammatory reflex. Nature 420:853, 2002.*)

sensory input is not fully understood, it has been demonstrated that afferent stimuli to the vagus nerve include cytokines (e.g., TNF-α and interleukin [IL]-1), baroreceptors, chemoreceptors, and thermoreceptors originating from the site of injury. This phenomenon is further demonstrated by blunting of fever response in animals after regional vagotomy at the site of injury.

Cholinergic Anti-Inflammatory Pathways

Tracey and colleagues have further linked reflex inhibition of inflammation to the parasympathetic signaling pathway whereby *acetylcholine,* the primary neurotransmitter of the parasympathetic system, reduces tissue macrophage activation. Furthermore, cholinergic stimulation directly reduces tissue macrophage release of the proinflammatory mediators TNF-α, IL-1, IL-18, and high mobility group protein (HMG-1), but not the anti-inflammatory cytokine IL-10. The attenuated inflammatory response induced by cholinergic stimuli was further validated by the identification of acetylcholine (nicotinic) receptors on tissue macrophages. In experimental models, direct electrical stimulation of the vagus nerve inhibits the tissue synthesis of inflammatory cytokines in the liver, spleen, and heart and reduces circulating levels as well. Complete vagotomy in mice significantly increases proinflammatory mediator release in response to injury.

In summary, vagal stimulation reduces heart rate, increases gut motility, dilates arterioles, and causes pupil constriction, as well as regulates inflammation. Unlike the humoral anti-inflammatory mediators that are released into the circulation and allowed to travel to a site of injury, signals discharged from the vagus nerve are precisely targeted at the site of injury or infection. Moreover, this cholinergic signaling occurs rapidly in real time. From the available preclinical studies, it can be proposed that impaired cholinergic activity from the vagus nerve portends a greater proinflammatory response in patients who are critically ill.

HORMONAL RESPONSE TO INJURY

Hormone Signaling Pathways

Hormones are chemically classified as *polypeptides* (e.g., cytokines, glucagon, and insulin), *amino acids* (e.g., epinephrine, serotonin, and histamine), or *fatty acids* (e.g., glucocorticoids, prostaglandins, and leukotrienes). Most hormone receptors generate signals by one of three major pathways, which overlap. Specifically, these receptor pathways are (1) *receptor kinases* such as insulin and insulin-like growth factor receptors, (2) *guanine nucleotide-binding* or *G-protein receptors* such as neurotransmitter and prostaglandin receptors, and (3) *ligand-gated ion channels* which permit ion transport when activated. Upon activation of membrane receptors, secondary signaling pathways are often utilized to amplify the initial stimuli. Hormone signals are further mediated by intracellular receptors with binding affinities for both the hormone itself, as well as for the targeted gene sequence on the DNA. These intracellular receptors may be located within the cytosol or may already be localized in the nucleus, bound to the DNA. The classic example of a cytosolic hormonal receptor is the glucocorticoid (GC) receptor (Fig. 1-3). Intracellular GC receptors are maintained in the cytosol by linking to the stress-induced protein, heat shock protein (HSP). When the glucocorticoid ligand binds to the GC receptor, the dissociation of HSP from the receptor activates the receptor-ligand complex and is transported to the nucleus.

Virtually every hormone of the hypothalamic-pituitary-adrenal (HPA) axis influences the physiologic response to injury and stress (Table 1-2), but some with direct influence on the inflammatory response or immediate clinical impact will be highlighted.

Adrenocorticotropic Hormone

Adrenocorticotropic hormone (ACTH) is synthesized and released by the anterior pituitary. In healthy humans, ACTH release

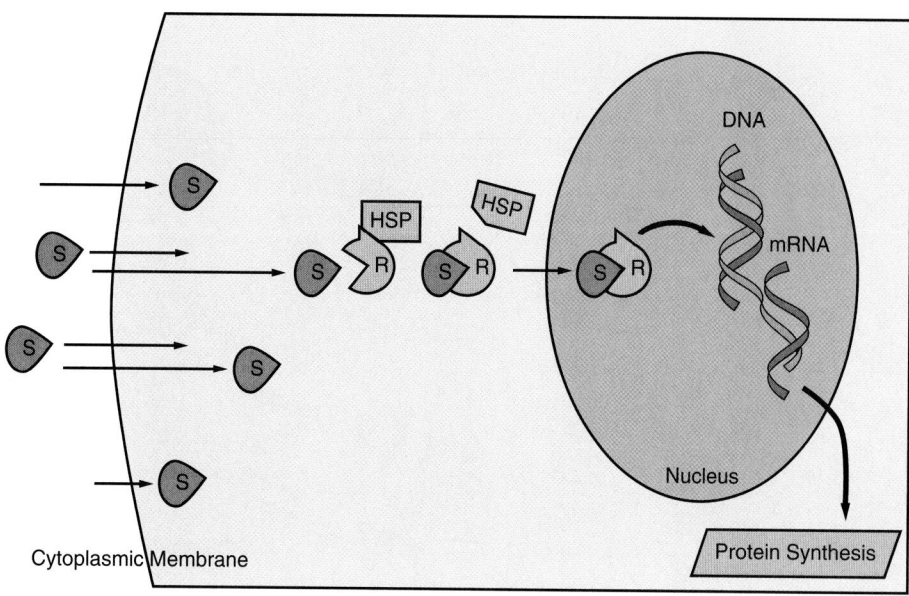

Cytoplasmic Membrane

FIG. 1-3. Simplified schematic of steroid transport into the nucleus. Steroid molecules (S) diffuse readily across cytoplasmic membranes. Intracellularly the receptors (R) are rendered inactive by being coupled to heat shock protein (HSP). When S and R bind, HSP dissociates, and the S-R complex enters the nucleus where the S-R complex induces DNA transcription, resulting in protein synthesis.

is regulated by circadian signals such that the greatest elevation of ACTH occurs late at night until the hours immediately before sunrise. This pattern is dramatically altered or obliterated in the injured subject. Most injury is characterized by elevations in corticotropin-releasing hormone and ACTH that are proportional to the severity of injury. Pain, anxiety, vasopressin, angiotensin II, cholecystokinin, vasoactive intestinal polypeptide (VIP), catecholamines, and proinflammatory cytokines are all prominent mediators of ACTH release in the injured patient.

Table 1-2
Hormones Regulated by the Hypothalamus, Pituitary, and Autonomic System

Hypothalamic Regulation
Corticotropin-releasing hormone
Thyrotropin-releasing hormone
Growth hormone-releasing hormone
Luteinizing hormone-releasing hormone

Anterior Pituitary Regulation
Adrenocorticotropic hormone
Cortisol
Thyroid-stimulating hormone
Thyroxine
Triiodothyronine
Growth hormone
Gonadotrophins
Sex hormones
Insulin-like growth factor
Somatostatin
Prolactin
Endorphins

Posterior Pituitary Regulation
Vasopressin
Oxytocin

Autonomic System
Norepinephrine
Epinephrine
Aldosterone
Renin-angiotensin system
Insulin
Glucagon
Enkephalins

Within the zona fasciculata of the adrenal gland, ACTH signaling activates intracellular pathways that lead to glucocorticoid production (Fig. 1-4). Conditions of excess ACTH stimulation will result in adrenal cortical hypertrophy.

Cortisol and Glucocorticoids

Cortisol is the major glucocorticoid in humans and is essential for survival during significant physiologic stress. Following injury, cortisol is elevated depending on the type of systemic stress. Burn patients have elevated circulating cortisol levels for up to 4 weeks, while soft tissue injury and hemorrhage may exhibit shorter periods of cortisol elevation.

Metabolically, cortisol potentiates the actions of glucagon and epinephrine that manifest as hyperglycemia. In the liver, cortisol stimulates the enzymatic activities favoring gluconeogenesis, but induces insulin resistance in muscles and adipose tissue. In skeletal muscle, cortisol induces protein degradation as well as the release of lactate that serve as substrates for hepatic gluconeogenesis. During injury, cortisol potentiates the release of free fatty acids, triglycerides, and glycerol from adipose tissue as a means of providing additional energy sources.

Acute adrenal insufficiency (AAI) can be a life-threatening complication most commonly seen in acutely ill patients with adrenal suppression from exogenously administered glucocorticoids with consequent atrophy of the adrenal glands. Clinically, these patients present with weakness, nausea, vomiting, fever, and hypotension. Objective findings include hypoglycemia from decreased gluconeogenesis, hyponatremia from impaired renal tubular sodium resorption, and hyperkalemia from diminished kaliuresis. In addition to cortisol deficiency, insufficient mineralocorticoid (aldosterone) activity also contributes to hyponatremia and hyperkalemia.

Glucocorticoids have long been employed as effective immunosuppressive agents. Immunologic changes associated with glucocorticoid administration include thymic involution, depressed cell-mediated immune responses reflected by decreases in T-killer and natural killer cell functions, T-lymphocyte blastogenesis, mixed lymphocyte responsiveness, graft-versus-host reactions, and delayed hypersensitivity responses. With glucocorticoid administration, monocytes lose the capacity for intracellular killing but appear

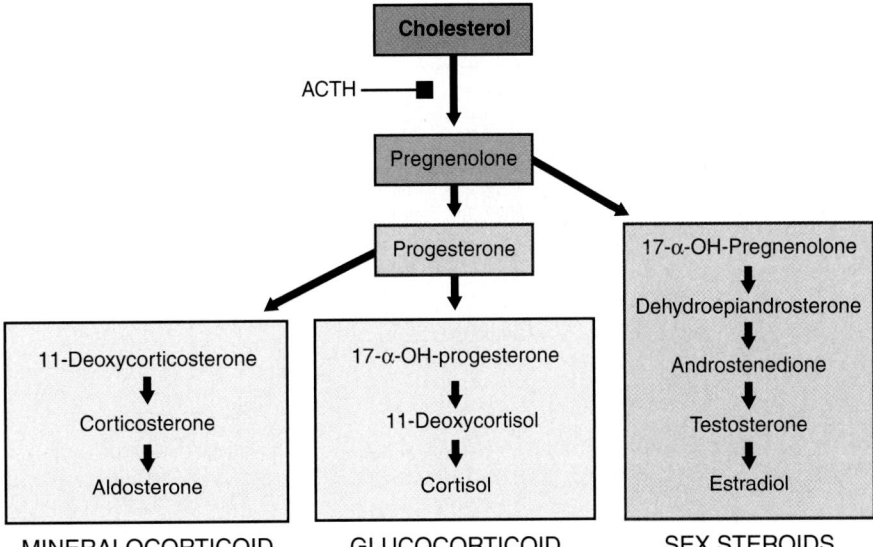

FIG. 1-4. Steroid synthesis from cholesterol. Adrenocorticotropic hormone (ACTH) is a principal regulator of steroid synthesis. The end products are mineralocorticoids, glucocorticoids, and sex steroids.

to maintain normal chemotactic and phagocytic properties. For neutrophils, glucocorticoids inhibit intracellular superoxide reactivity, suppress chemotaxis, and normalize apoptosis signaling mechanisms. However, neutrophil phagocytosis function remains unchanged. Finally, glucocorticoid infusion in human endotoxemia downregulates proinflammatory cytokine production (TNF-α, IL-1, and IL-6) and increases the production of the anti-inflammatory mediator IL-10. This glucocorticoid-induced downregulation of cytokine stimulation serves an important negative regulatory function in the inflammatory response. Clinically, the administration of pharmacologic doses of glucocorticoids has been associated with modest reductions in proinflammatory response in septic shock, surgical trauma, and coronary artery bypass surgery. However, the appropriate dosing, timing, and duration of glucocorticoid administration have not been validated.

Macrophage Inhibitory Factor

Macrophage inhibitory factor (MIF) is a glucocorticoid antagonist produced by the anterior pituitary that potentially reverses the immunosuppressive effects of glucocorticoids. MIF can be secreted systemically from the anterior pituitary and by T lymphocytes situated at the sites of inflammation. MIF is a proinflammatory mediator that potentiates gram-negative and gram-positive septic shock. In mice endotoxemia experiments, the administration of anti-MIF significantly improves survival.

Growth Hormones and Insulin-Like Growth Factors

During periods of stress, growth hormone (GH) promotes protein synthesis and also enhances the mobilization of fat stores. The protein synthesis properties of growth hormone in the recovering patient are mediated in part by the secondary release of insulin-like growth factor-1 (IGF-1). IGF, formerly called somatomedin C, circulates predominantly in bound form with several binding proteins and promotes amino acid incorporation and cellular proliferation and attenuates proteolysis. In the liver, IGFs are mediators of protein synthesis and glycogenesis. In adipose tissue, IGF increases glucose uptake and fat utilization. In skeletal muscles, IGF increases glucose uptake and protein synthesis. IGF also has a role in skeletal growth by promoting the incorporation of sulfate and proteoglycans into cartilage. The effects of IGF-1 can be inhibited by interleukin (IL)-1α, TNF-α, and IL-6. The decrease in protein synthesis and observed negative nitrogen balance following injury is attributed in large part to a reduction in IGF-1 levels. GH administration has been shown to improve the clinical course of pediatric burn patients. Its use in injured adult patients remains unproven. The liver is the predominant source of IGF-1, and pre-existing hepatic dysfunction (e.g., end-stage liver disease and protein-energy malnutrition) may further contribute to the negative nitrogen balance following injury. IGF binding proteins also are produced within the liver and are necessary for effective transport of IGF to the cell. IGF has the potential for attenuating the catabolic effects following surgical insults. Growth hormones also stimulate leukocyte function and cell proliferation, but the clinical benefits of such a response are unclear.

Catecholamines

The hypermetabolic state observed following severe injury is attributed to activation of the adrenergic system. Both norepinephrine (NE) and epinephrine (EPI) are increased three- to fourfold in plasma immediately following injury, with elevations lasting 24 to 48 hours before returning toward baseline levels.

In the liver, EPI promotes glycogenolysis, gluconeogenesis, lipolysis, and ketogenesis. It also causes decreased insulin release, but increases glucagon secretion. Peripherally, EPI increases lipolysis in adipose tissues and induces insulin resistance in skeletal muscle. These collectively manifest as stress-induced hyperglycemia, not unlike the effects of cortisol on blood sugar. Catecholamines also increase the secretion of thyroid and parathyroid hormones, T_4, T_3, and renin, but inhibit the release of aldosterone.

Like cortisol, EPI enhances leukocyte demargination with resultant neutrophilia and lymphocytosis. However, EPI occupation of β receptors present on leukocytes increases intracellular cyclic adenosine monophosphate (cAMP) and ultimately decreases lymphocyte responsiveness to mitogens.

There is strong evidence that blockade of β receptors in children with thermal injury reduces cardiac oxygen consumption and retention of lean muscle mass. In noncardiac surgical patients with heart disease, perioperative β-receptor blockade also reduced sympathetic activation and cardiac oxygen demand with significant reductions in cardiac-related deaths.

Table 1-3
Cytokines and Their Sources

Cytokine	Source	Comment
TNF-α	*Macrophages/monocytes* Kupffer cells Neutrophils NK cells Astrocytes Endothelial cells T lymphocytes Adrenal cortical cells Adipocytes Keratinocytes Osteoblasts Mast cells Dendritic cells	Among earliest responders following injury; half-life <20 min; activates TNF-receptor-1 and -2; induces significant shock and catabolism
IL-1	*Macrophages/monocytes* B and T lymphocytes NK cells Endothelial cells Epithelial cells Keratinocytes Fibroblasts Osteoblasts Dendritic cells Astrocytes Adrenal cortical cells Megakaryocytes Platelets Neutrophils Neuronal cells	Two forms (IL-α and IL-β); similar physiologic effects as TNF-α; induces fevers through prostaglandin activity in anterior hypothalamus; promotes β-endorphin release from pituitary; half-life <6 min
IL-2	*T lymphocytes*	Promotes lymphocyte proliferation, immunoglobulin production, gut barrier integrity; half-life <10 min; attenuated production following major blood loss leads to immunocompromise; regulates lymphocyte apoptosis
IL-3	*T lymphocytes* Macrophages Eosinophils Mast cells	
IL-4	*T lymphocytes* Mast cells Basophils Macrophages B lymphocytes Eosinophils Stromal cells	Induces B-lymphocyte production of IgG4 and IgE, mediators of allergic and anthelmintic response; downregulates TNF-α, IL-1, IL-6, IL-8
IL-5	*T lymphocytes* Eosinophils Mast cells Basophils	Promotes eosinophil proliferation and airway inflammation
IL-6	*Macrophages* B lymphocytes Neutrophils Basophils Mast cells Fibroblasts Endothelial cells Astrocytes Synovial cells Adipocytes Osteoblasts Megakaryocytes Chromaffin cells Keratinocytes	Elicited by virtually all immunogenic cells; long half-life; circulating levels proportional to injury severity; prolongs activated neutrophil survival
IL-8	*Macrophages/monocytes* T lymphocytes Basophils Mast cells Epithelial cells Platelets	Chemoattractant for neutrophils, basophils, eosinophils, lymphocytes

(Continued)

Table 1-3
Cytokines and Their Sources (*continued*)

Cytokine	Source	Comment
IL-10	*T lymphocytes* B lymphocytes Macrophages Basophils Mast cells Keratinocytes	Prominent anti-inflammatory cytokine; reduces mortality in animal sepsis and ARDS models
IL-12	*Macrophages/monocytes* Neutrophils Keratinocytes Dendritic cells B lymphocytes	Promotes T_H1 differentiation; synergistic activity with IL-2
IL-13	*T lymphocytes*	Promotes B-lymphocyte function; structurally similar to IL-4; inhibits nitric oxide and endothelial activation
IL-15	*Macrophages/monocytes* Epithelial cells	Anti-inflammatory effect; promotes lymphocyte activation; promotes neutrophil phagocytosis in fungal infections
IL-18	*Macrophages* Kupffer cells Keratinocytes Adrenal cortical cells Osteoblasts	Similar to IL-12 in function; elevated in sepsis, particularly gram-positive infections; high levels found in cardiac deaths
IFN-γ	*T lymphocytes* NK cells Macrophages	Mediates IL-12 and IL-18 function; half-life, days; found in wounds 5–7 days after injury; promotes ARDS
GM-CSF	*T lymphocytes* Fibroblasts Endothelial cells Stromal cells	Promotes wound healing and inflammation through activation of leukocytes
IL-21	*T lymphocytes*	Preferentially secreted by T_H2 cells; structurally similar to IL-2 and IL-15; activates NK cells, B and T lymphocytes; influences adaptive immunity
HMGB-I	*Monocytes/lymphocytes*	High mobility group box chromosomal protein; DNA transcription factor; late (downstream) mediator of inflammation (ARDS, gut barrier disruption); induces "sickness behavior"

ARDS = acute respiratory distress syndrome; GM-CSF = granulocyte-macrophage colony-stimulating factor; IFN = interferon; IgE = immunoglobulin E; IgG = immunoglobulin G; IL = interleukin; NK = natural killer; T_H1 = T helper subset cell 1; T_H2 = T helper subset cell 2; TNF = tumor necrosis factor.

Aldosterone

The mineralocorticoid aldosterone is synthesized, stored, and released in the adrenal zona glomerulosa. ACTH is the most potent stimulant of aldosterone release. The major function of aldosterone is to maintain intravascular volume by conserving sodium and eliminating potassium and hydrogen ions in the early distal convoluted tubules of the nephrons.

Patients with aldosterone deficiency develop hypotension and hyperkalemia, whereas patients with aldosterone excess develop edema, hypertension, hypokalemia, and metabolic alkalosis.

Insulin

Hormones and inflammatory mediators associated with stress response inhibit insulin release. Therefore, in conjunction with peripheral insulin resistance following injury, this results in stress-induced hyperglycemia and is in keeping with the general catabolic state immediately following major injury.

In the healthy individual, insulin exerts a global anabolic effect by promoting hepatic glycogenesis and glycolysis, glucose transport into cells, adipose tissue lipogenesis, and protein synthesis. In the injured patient, there are two phases to the pattern of insulin release. The first phase suppresses overall insulin release and occurs within a few hours after injury. The later phase is characterized by a return to normal or excessive insulin production, but with persistent hyperglycemia, consistent with peripheral resistance to insulin.

Activated lymphocytes express insulin receptors, and activation enhances T-cell proliferation and cytotoxicity. Institution of insulin therapy to newly diagnosed diabetics is associated with increased functional B- and T-lymphocyte populations. Recent evidence strongly suggests that tight control of glucose levels in the intensive care unit, particularly in diabetics, was associated with significant reductions in mortality.

Acute Phase Proteins

The acute phase proteins are nonspecific biochemical markers produced by hepatocytes in response to tissue injury, infection, or inflammation. Interleukin (IL)-6 is a potent inducer of acute phase proteins that can include proteinase inhibitors, coagulation and complement proteins, and transport proteins. Clinically, only C-reactive protein (CRP) has been consistently used as a marker of injury response due to its dynamic reflection of inflammation. Importantly, CRP levels do not show diurnal variations and are not affected by feeding. Only pre-existing liver failure will impair CRP production. Therefore it has become a useful biomarker of inflammation as well as response to treatment. Its accuracy surpasses that of the erythrocyte sedimentation rate.

MEDIATORS OF INFLAMMATION

Cytokines

Cytokines appear to be the most potent mediators of the inflammatory response. When functioning locally at the site of injury or infection, cytokines eradicate invading microorganisms and promote wound healing. However, overwhelming production of proinflammatory cytokines in response to injury can cause hemodynamic instability (i.e., septic shock) or metabolic derangements (i.e., muscle wasting). If uncontrolled, the outcome of these exaggerated responses is end-organ failure and death. The production of anti-inflammatory cytokines as part of the inflammation cascade serves to oppose the excessive actions of proinflammatory cytokines. However, inappropriate anti-inflammatory mediator release may render the patient immunocompromised and susceptible to overwhelming infections. To view cytokines merely as proinflammatory or anti-inflammatory oversimplifies their functions, and overlapping bioactivity is the rule (Table 1-3).

Heat Shock Proteins

Stimuli such as hypoxia, trauma, heavy metals, local trauma, and hemorrhage all induce the production of intracellular heat shock proteins (HSPs). HSPs are intracellular protein modifiers and transporters that are presumed to protect cells from the deleterious effects of traumatic stress. The classic example of HSP activity relates to the intracellular transport of steroid molecules. The formation of HSPs requires gene induction by the heat shock transcription factor. HSP expression is also ACTH-sensitive, and the production seems to decline with age.

Reactive Oxygen Metabolites

Reactive oxygen metabolites are short-lived, highly reactive molecular oxygen species with an unpaired outer orbit. They cause tissue injury by oxidation of unsaturated fatty acids within cell membranes.

Oxygen radicals are produced by complex processes that involve anaerobic glucose oxidation coupled with the reduction of oxygen to superoxide anion. Superoxide anion is an oxygen metabolite that is further metabolized to other reactive species such as hydrogen peroxide and hydroxyl radicals. Activated leukocytes are potent generators of reactive oxygen metabolites. Cells are not immune to damage by their own reactive oxygen metabolites, but are generally protected by oxygen scavengers that include glutathione and catalases. In ischemic tissues, the intracellular mechanisms for production of oxygen metabolites are fully activated, but remain nonfunctional due to a lack of oxygen supply. Upon restoration of blood flow and oxygen supply, large quantities of reactive oxygen metabolites are produced that lead to reperfusion injury.

Eicosanoids

The eicosanoid class of mediators, which encompasses prostaglandins (PG), thromboxanes (TX), leukotrienes (LT), hydroxyeicosatetraenoic acids (HETE), and lipoxins (LX), are oxidation derivatives of the membrane phospholipid arachidonic acid (eicosatetraenoic acid). Eicosanoids are secreted by virtually all nucleated cells except lymphocytes. The synthesis of arachidonic acid from phospholipids requires enzymatic activation of phospholipase A_2 (Fig. 1-5). Eicosanoids are generated either by the cyclooxygenase or the lipoxygenase pathways. Products of the cyclooxygenase pathway include all of the prostaglandins and thromboxanes. The lipoxygenase pathway generates the leukotrienes and HETE.

Eicosanoids are not stored within cells, but instead are synthesized rapidly upon stimulation by hypoxic injury, direct tissue injury, endotoxin, norepinephrine, vasopressin, angiotensin II, bradykinin, serotonin, acetylcholine, cytokines, and histamine. Many of these stimuli also induce the production of the second cyclooxygenase enzyme (COX-2), which converts arachidonate to prostaglandin E_2 (PGE_2). PGE_2 increases fluid leakage from blood vessels, but a rising PGE_2 level over several hours eventually feeds back to COX-2 and induces the formation of the anti-inflammatory lipoxin from neutrophils. Nonsteroidal anti-inflammatory drugs acetylate COX-2, which consequently reduces the PGE_2 levels and increases lipoxin production. COX-2 activity also can be inhibited by glucocorticoids.

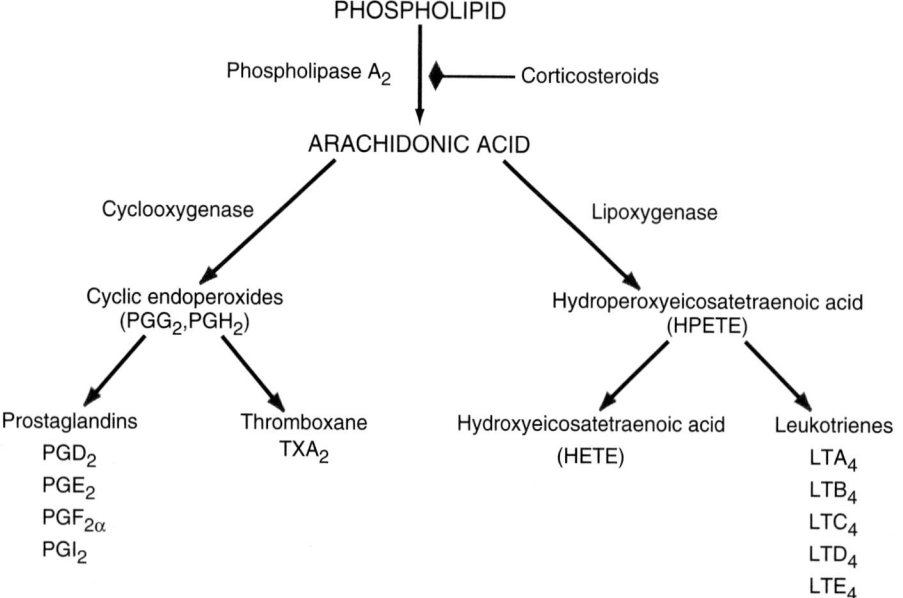

FIG. 1-5. Schematic diagram of arachidonic acid metabolism.

Table 1-4
Systemic Stimulatory and Inhibitory Actions of Eicosanoids

Organ/Function	Stimulator	Inhibitor
Pancreas		
Glucose-stimulated insulin secretion	12-HPETE	PGE_2
Glucagon secretion	PGD_2, PGE_2	
Liver		
Glucagon-stimulated glucose production	PGE_2	
Fat		
Hormone-stimulated lipolysis	PGE_2	
Bone		
Resorption	PGE_2, PGE-m, 6-K-PGE_1, $PGF_{1\alpha}$, PGI_2	
Pituitary		
Prolactin	PGE_1	
LH	PGE_1, PGE_2, 5-HETE	
TSH	PGA_1, PGB_1, PGE_1, $PGE_{1\alpha}$	
GH	PGE_1	
Parathyroid		
PTH	PGE_2	$PGF_{2\alpha}$
Pulmonary		
Bronchoconstriction	$PGF_{2\alpha}$, TXA_2, LTC_4, LTD_4, LTE_4	PGE_2
Renal		
Stimulate renin secretion	PGE_2, PGI_2	
Gastrointestinal		
Cytoprotective effect	PGE_2	
Immune Response		
Suppress lymphocyte activity	PGE_2	
Hematologic		
Platelet aggregation	TXA_2	PGI_2

GH = growth hormone; 5-HETE = 5-hydroxyeicosatetraenoic acid; 12-HETE = 12-hydroxyperoxy-eicosatetraenoic acid; 6-K-PGE_1 = 6-keto-prostaglandin E_1; LH = luteinizing hormone; LTC_4 = leukotriene C_4; LTD_4 = leukotriene D_4; LTE_4 = leukotriene E_4; PGA_1 = prostaglandin A_1; PGB_1 = prostaglandin B_1; PGD_2 = prostaglandin D_2; PGE_1 = prostaglandin E_1; $PGE_{1\alpha}$ = prostaglandin $E_{1\alpha}$; PGE_2 = prostaglandin E_2; PGE-m = 13,14-dihydro-15-keto-PGE_2 (major urine metabolite of PGE_2); PGF = prostaglandin F; $PGF_{1\alpha}$ = prostaglandin $F_{1\alpha}$; $PGF_{2\alpha}$ = prostaglandin $F_{2\alpha}$; PGI = prostaglandin I; PGI_2 = prostaglandin I_2; PTH = parathyroid hormone; TSH = thyroid-stimulating hormone; TXA_2 = thromboxane A_2.

Eicosanoids have diverse effects systemically on endocrine and immune function, neurotransmission, and vasomotor regulation (Table 1-4). Collectively, their deleterious effects are implicated in acute lung injury, pancreatitis, and renal failure. Leukotrienes are 1000 times more potent than histamines in promoting capillary leakage. They also are effective promoters of leukocyte adherence, neutrophil activation, bronchoconstriction, and vasoconstriction.

The metabolic effects of eicosanoids are well recognized. In the regulation of glucose, products of the cyclooxygenase pathway inhibit pancreatic β-cell release of insulin, while products of the lipoxygenase pathway promote β-cell activity. Hepatocytes also express specific receptors for PGE_2 that, when activated, inhibit gluconeogenesis. PGE_2 also can inhibit hormone-stimulated lipolysis.

Fatty Acid Metabolites

The role of fatty acid metabolism potentially has a role in the inflammatory response. Most commercially prepared enteral nutrition formulas contain omega-6 fatty acids as the primary source of lipids. Omega-6 fatty acids also serve as precursors of inflammatory mediators associated with injury and the stress response. Such mediators include leukotrienes, prostaglandins, and platelet-activating factor. By contrast, the anti-inflammatory effects of omega-3 fatty acids on chronic autoimmune diseases such as rheumatoid arthritis, psoriasis, and lupus have been documented in both animals and humans. Although the mechanisms are still unclear, animal studies substituting omega-3 for omega-6 fatty acids have demonstrated

attenuated inflammatory response in hepatic Kupffer cells as measured by TNF and IL-1 release and PGE_2 production. In animal injury studies, omega-3 reduces metabolic rate, normalizes glucose metabolism, attenuates weight loss, and improves nitrogen balance. Omega-3 fatty acid–supplemented feeding in animals minimizes ischemia/reperfusion injury in the myocardium, small intestine, and skeletal muscles. In rats, dietary omega-3 fatty acids, when compared to omega-6 fatty acids, ameliorates endotoxin-induced acute lung injury by suppressing the levels of proinflammatory eicosanoids in bronchoalveolar lavage fluid and reducing pulmonary neutrophil accumulation.

Kallikrein-Kinin System

Bradykinins are potent vasodilators that are produced through kininogen degradation by the serine protease kallikrein. Kallikrein exists in blood and tissues as inactive prekallikrein that is activated by various factors such as Hageman factor, trypsin, plasmin, factor XI, glass surfaces, kaolin, and collagen.

Kinins increase capillary permeability and tissue edema, evoke pain, inhibit gluconeogenesis, and increase bronchoconstriction. They also increase renal vasodilation and consequently reduce renal perfusion pressure. The resulting increase in renin formation activates sodium and water retention via the renin-angiotensin system.

Bradykinin release is stimulated by hypoxic and ischemic injury. Increased kallikrein activity and bradykinin levels are observed following hemorrhage, sepsis, endotoxemia, and tissue injury. Furthermore, these elevations are proportional to the magnitude of injury and mortality. Clinical trials utilizing bradykinin antagonists in attempts to reduce the deleterious sequelae of septic shock have only demonstrated modest reversal in gram-negative sepsis, but no overall improvement in survival.

Serotonin

The neurotransmitter serotonin (5-hydroxytryptamine, 5-HT) is a tryptophan derivative that is found in chromaffin cells of the intestine and in platelets. Patients with midgut carcinoid tumors often secrete 5-HT in excess. This neurotransmitter stimulates vasoconstriction, bronchoconstriction, and platelet aggregation. Serotonin is also a myocardial chronotrope and inotrope. Although serotonin is clearly released at sites of injury, its role in the inflammatory response is unclear.

Histamine

Histamine is derived from histidine and stored in neurons, skin, gastric mucosa, mast cells, basophils, and platelets. Histamine release is activated by increased calcium levels. There are two receptor types for histamine binding. H_1 binding stimulates bronchoconstriction, intestinal motility, and myocardial contractility. H_2 binding inhibits histamine release. Both H_1 and H_2 receptor activation induce hypotension, peripheral pooling of blood, increased capillary permeability, decreased venous return, and myocardial failure. The rise in histamine levels has been documented in hemorrhagic shock, trauma, thermal injury, endotoxemia, and sepsis.

CYTOKINE RESPONSE TO INJURY

Tumor Necrosis Factor

Following acute injury or during infections, TNF-α is among the earliest and most potent mediators of subsequent host responses. The primary sources of TNF-α synthesis include monocytes/ macrophages and T cells, which are abundant in the peritoneum and splanchnic tissues. Furthermore, Kupffer cells represent the single largest concentrated population of macrophages in the human body. Therefore, surgical or traumatic injuries to the abdominal viscera undoubtedly have profound influence on the generation of inflammatory mediators and homeostatic responses such as acute phase protein production. Although the half-life of TNF-α is less than 20 minutes, this brief appearance is sufficient to evoke marked metabolic and hemodynamic changes and activate mediators distally in the cytokine cascade. TNF-α is also a major inducer of muscle catabolism and cachexia during stress by shunting available amino acids to the hepatic circulation as fuel substrates. Other functions of TNF-α include coagulation activation, promoting the expression or release of adhesion molecules, prostaglandin E_2, platelet-activating factor (PAF), glucocorticoids, and eicosanoids.

Soluble (i.e., circulating) TNF receptors (sTNFRs) are proteolytically cleaved extracellular domains of membrane-associated TNFRs that are elevated and readily detectable in acute inflammation. sTNFRs retain their affinity for the binding of TNF-α and therefore compete with the cellular receptors for the binding of free TNF-α. This potentially represents an endogenous counterregulatory response to excessive systemic TNF-α activity. However, it should be noted that the functional biology of sTNFRs may not be limited to TNF-α antagonism, but may also serve as a carrier (e.g., transporter) or as a storage pool of bioactive TNF-α in the circulation.

Interleukin-1

IL-1 is primarily released by activated macrophages and endothelial cells. There are two known species of IL-1: IL-1α and IL-1β. IL-1α is predominantly cell membrane associated and exerts its influence via cellular contacts. IL-1β is more readily detectable in the circulation and capable of eliciting similar physiologic and metabolic alterations as TNF-α. With high doses of either IL-1 or TNF-α, these cytokines independently initiate a state of hemodynamic decompensation. At low doses, they can produce the same response only if administered simultaneously. These observations emphasize the synergistic roles of TNF-α and IL-1 in the inflammatory response. IL-1 is predominantly a local mediator with a half-life of approximately 6 minutes, making its ability to be detected in acute injury or illness even less likely than that of TNF-α. IL-1 induces the classic inflammatory febrile response to injury by stimulating local prostaglandin activity in the anterior hypothalamus. Attenuated pain perception after surgery can be mediated by IL-1 by promoting the release of β-endorphins from the pituitary gland and increasing the number of central opioid-like receptors.

Endogenous IL-1 receptor antagonists (IL-1ra) also are released during injury and serve as an endogenous autoregulator of IL-1 activity. This molecule effectively competes for binding to IL-1 receptors, yet exacts no overt signal transduction.

Interleukin-2

IL-2 is a primary promoter of T-lymphocyte proliferation, immunoglobulin production, and gut barrier integrity. Partly due to its circulation half-life of less than 10 minutes, IL-2 has not been readily detectable following acute injury. Attenuated IL-2 expression associated with major injuries or perioperative blood transfusions potentially contribute to the transient immunocompromised state of the surgical patient. There is evidence to suggest that accelerated lymphocyte apoptosis (i.e., lymphocyte depletion) exacerbates the injury-induced immunocompromise as a result of diminished IL-2 stimulation.

Interleukin-4

IL-4 is produced by activated type 2 T-helper (T_H2) lymphocytes and possesses diverse influence on hematopoietic cell proliferation. It is particularly important in antibody-mediated immunity and in antigen presentation. IL-4 also induces class switching in differentiating B lymphocytes to produce predominantly IgG4 and IgE, which are important immunoglobulins in allergic and anthelmintic responses. IL-4 has potent anti-inflammatory properties against activated macrophages by downregulating the effects of IL-1, TNF-α, IL-6, and IL-8, as well as oxygen radical production. IL-4 also appears to increase macrophage susceptibility to the anti-inflammatory effects of glucocorticoids.

Interleukin-6

TNF-α and IL-1 are potent inducers of IL-6 production from virtually all cells and tissues, including the gut. After injury, IL-6 levels in the circulation are detectable by 60 minutes, peak between 4 and 6 hours, and can persist for as long as 10 days. Circulating IL-6 levels appear to be proportional to the extent of tissue injury during an operation, more so than the duration of the surgical procedure itself. Recent evidence has demonstrated both a proinflammatory role and an anti-inflammatory role for IL-6. IL-6 is an important mediator of the hepatic acute phase response during injury and convalescence.

IL-6 not only induces neutrophil activation during injury and inflammation but also may delay the disposal of such neutrophils, thereby prolonging the injurious effects mediated by these cells. IL-6 also possesses anti-inflammatory properties during injury by attenuating TNF-α and IL-1 activity while promoting the release of soluble tumor necrosis factor receptors (sTNFRs) and IL-1 receptor antagonists.

Interleukin-8

IL-8 expression and activity is similar to that of IL-6 after injury and has been proposed as an additional biomarker for the risk of multiple organ failure. IL-8 does not produce the hemodynamic instability characteristic of TNF-α and IL-1, but is a chemoattractant and a potent activator of neutrophils.

Interleukin-10

IL-10 has emerged as a modulator of TNF-α activity. Experimental evidence has demonstrated that neutralization of IL-10 during endotoxemia increases monocyte TNF-α production and mortality, but restitution of IL-10 reduces TNF-α levels and the associated deleterious effects. IL-10 is also capable of attenuating IL-18 messenger ribonucleic acid (mRNA) expression in monocytes. In animal experiments, induction of IL-10 transcription has been shown to attenuate the systemic inflammatory response and reduce mortality during septic peritonitis. However, excessive rIL-10 administration in similar animal models has been associated with increased bacterial load and mortality.

Interleukin-12

IL-12 has a primary role in cell-mediated immunity and promotes the differentiation of T_H1 cells. In mice with fecal peritonitis as well as those with burn injury, survival increases with IL-12 administration, while IL-12 neutralization results in high mortality. IL-12 administration in nonhuman primates is capable of inducing an inflammatory response for up to 48 hours, independently of TNF-α and IL-1. IL-12 promotes neutrophil and coagulation activation, as well as the expression of both proinflammatory and anti-inflammatory mediators. Furthermore, IL-12 toxicity appears to be synergistic with IL-2. Although IL-12 detection following injury or severe infections is variable, most evidence would suggest that this cytokine contributes to the overall proinflammatory response.

Interleukin-13

IL-13 shares many structural and functional properties of IL-4. IL-4 and IL-13 modulate macrophage function, but unlike IL-4, IL-13 has no identifiable effect on T lymphocytes and only has influence on selected B-lymphocyte populations. IL-13 can inhibit nitric oxide production and the expression of proinflammatory cytokines and can enhance the production of IL-1ra. Furthermore, IL-13 attenuates leukocyte interaction with activated endothelial surfaces. The net effect of IL-13, along with IL-4 and IL-10, is anti-inflammatory.

Interleukin-15

IL-15 is a macrophage-derived cytokine with potent autocrine regulatory properties. As a result of shared receptor signaling components, both IL-15 and IL-2 possess similar bioactivity in promoting lymphocyte activation and proliferation. In neutrophils, IL-15 induces IL-8 production and nuclear factor-κB (NF-κB) activation and enhances phagocytic function against fungal infections.

Interleukin-18

IL-18, formerly interferon (IFN)-γ-inducing factor, is a proinflammatory cytokine product of activated macrophages. Structurally similar to IL-1β and functionally similar to IL-12, IL-18 promotes early resolution of bacterial infections in mice. Bacterial products IL-4 and IFN-γ can stimulate IL-18 production from monocytes. IL-18 signaling is associated with NF-κB and c-Jun N-terminal kinase (JNK) pathway activation, as well as the expression of functionally active intercellular adhesion molecule-1 (ICAM-1). Furthermore, murine endotoxemia models indicate that IL-18 is a downstream mediator of both TNF-α and Fas ligand–induced hepatotoxicity. Preliminary data have demonstrated significant elevations of circulating IL-18 during sepsis for as long as 21 days. This elevation in IL-18 is particularly pronounced in gram-positive sepsis.

Interferon-γ

Much of interleukin (IL)-12 and IL-18 biology is mediated via interferon (IFN)-γ. Human T helper lymphocytes activated by bacterial antigens, IL-2, IL-12, or IL-18 readily produce IFN-γ. Conversely, IFN-γ can induce the production of IL-2, IL-12, and IL-18. When released into the circulation, IFN-γ is detectable *in vivo* by 6 hours and may be persistently elevated for as long as 8 days. Injured tissues, such as operative wounds, also demonstrate the presence of IFN-γ production 5 to 7 days after injury. IFN-γ has important roles in activating circulating and tissue macrophages. Alveolar macrophage activation mediated by IFN-γ may induce acute lung inflammation after major surgery or trauma.

Granulocyte-Macrophage Colony-Stimulating Factor

In vitro studies have demonstrated a prominent role for granulocyte-macrophage colony-stimulating factor (GM-CSF) in delaying apoptosis (programmed cell death) of macrophages and neutrophils. This process may contribute to organ injury such as that found in acute respiratory distress syndrome (ARDS). This growth factor is effective in promoting the maturation and recruitment of functional leukocytes necessary for normal inflammatory cytokine response, and potentially in wound healing. Results of perioperative GM-CSF administration in patients undergoing major oncologic procedures and in patients with major burns have demonstrated enhanced neutrophil numbers and function.

High Mobility Group Box-1

High mobility group box-1 (HMGB-1) is a DNA transcription factor that is expressed 24 to 48 hours after the initial injurious event. Its peak has been associated with deleterious outcomes such as advanced ARDS and death. The appearance of this mediator is in contrast to the early appearances of TNF-α, IL-1, IL-6, and IL-8, which peak within minutes of injury and therefore are difficult to block. HMGB-1 is associated with weight loss, food aversion, shock, and the general "sickness behavior" seen in sepsis and the systemic inflammatory response syndrome. As a late mediator of the inflammatory response, anti-HMGB-1 strategies might be used in efforts to control the progression of the deleterious effects of inflammation and sepsis.

CELLULAR RESPONSE TO INJURY

Gene Expression and Regulation

A broad reiteration of terminology is used to characterize gene regulation. Identical DNA chains are found in every cell of the body; however, each of these cells expresses distinct structural and functional characteristics. By the activation and deactivation of certain genes in a stem cell, the highly organized process of *differentiation* leads to the ultimate function of the cell.

In humans, most genes are regulated at the stage of DNA transcription (i.e., intranuclear) (Fig. 1-6). Therefore, whether a gene is expressed or not in a disease is often determined by the production of corresponding messenger ribonucleic acid (mRNA). RNA from the original transcript can be further modified, termed *splicing,* to produce related but dissimilar mRNA and resultant proteins. In cytokine production in which RNA is required for rapid translation (i.e., protein synthesis) upon demand, protein caps at the 5′ and 3′ ends ensure RNA stability and prevent splicing. Once out of the nucleus, the mRNA can be inactivated or translated to form proteins. These proteins can further be modified for specific functions. In essence, these cytosolic modifications supplement the primary regulatory mechanisms within the nucleus.

How a particular gene is activated depends on the orderly assemblage of transcription factors (i.e., regulatory proteins) to specific DNA sequences immediately upstream to the target gene, known as the *promoter region.* The DNA binding sites are the *enhancer sequences,* and proteins that inhibit the initiation of transcription are *repressors.* Transcription factors become important during the inflammatory response because the ability to control the pathways leading to their activation means the ability to regulate the manner and magnitude by which a cell can respond to an injury stimulus.

Cell Signaling Pathways

Heat Shock Proteins

Heat shock proteins (HSPs), also known as stress proteins, are produced by cells in response to injury or tissue ischemia. HSPs are essential for the ability of cells to overcome stress. Cytosolic heat shock factors (HSFs) are the transcription factors that are activated by conformational changes upon injury, which translocate into the

nucleus and bind to the HSP promoter regions. The overarching role of HSPs is to attenuate the inflammatory response. Major mechanisms include reduction of oxygen metabolites, promoting T_H2 cell proliferation, and inhibiting NF-κB activation.

G-Protein Receptors

GTP-binding proteins (G-proteins) are the largest family of signaling receptors for cells and include many of the pathways associated with the inflammatory response. G-protein receptor activation turns on an adjacent effector protein, leading to downstream signaling. The two major second messengers of the G-protein pathway are (1) formation of cyclic adenosine monophosphate (cAMP), and (2) calcium, released from the endoplasmic reticulum (Fig. 1-7). An increase in cellular cAMP can activate gene transcription. For example, binding of epinephrine and norepinephrine activates the adrenergic receptor, leading to signaling through the G-protein/cAMP signaling pathways.

G-protein/calcium activation requires activation of the effector phospholipase C and phosphoinositols. When calcium is not needed, it is pumped into the mitochondria and the endoplasmic reticulum for storage. Further downstream in G-protein signaling is the activation of protein kinase C (PKC), which can activate NF-κB as well as other transcription factors.

Ligand-Gated Ion Channels

These receptor channels, when activated by a ligand, permit rapid flux of ions across the cell membrane. Neurotransmitters function by this pathway, and an example of such a receptor is the nicotinic acetylcholine receptor (Fig. 1-8).

Receptor Tyrosine Kinases

Receptor tyrosine kinases also are known as tyrosine kinase receptors because of their significant intracellular tyrosine kinase domains (Fig. 1-9). Examples of these receptors include insulin and various hormone growth factors (e.g., platelet-derived growth factor [PDGF], insulin-like growth factor [IGF]-1, epidermal growth factor [EGF], and vascular endothelial growth factor [VEGF]). Some cytokine-receptor activation also utilizes the tyrosine kinase pathway. When activated, the receptors dimerize, undergo

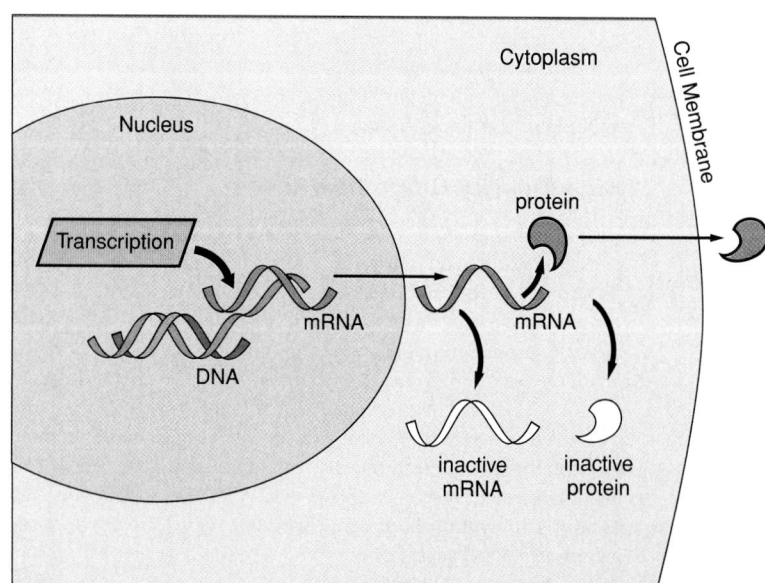

FIG. 1-6. Gene expression and protein synthesis can occur within a 24-hour period. The process can be regulated at various stages: transcription, mRNA processing, or protein packaging. At each stage, it is possible to inactivate the mRNA or protein, rendering these molecules nonfunctional.

G-PROTEIN RECEPTORS
(VASOACTIVE POLYPEPTIDES, MITOGENS, PHOSPHOLIPIDS,
NEUROTRANSMITTERS, PROSTAGLANDINS)

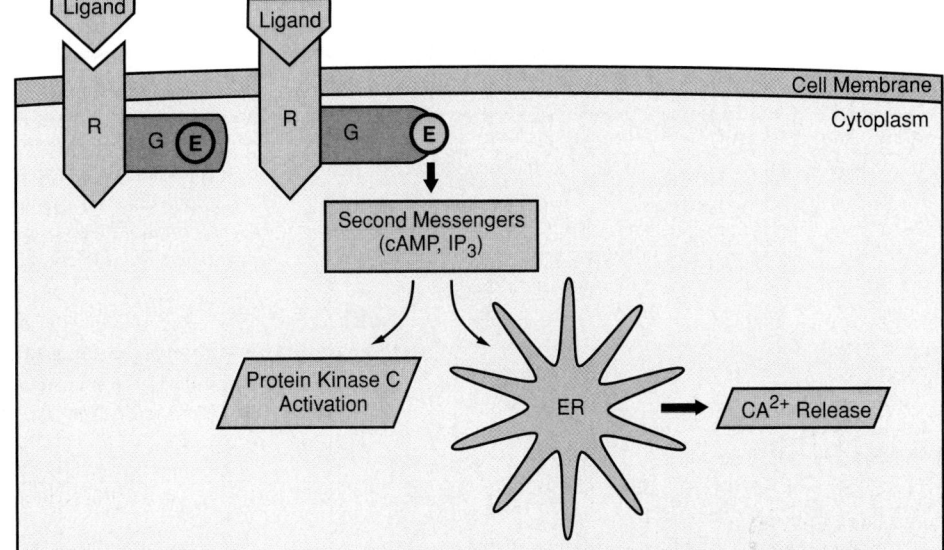

FIG. 1-7. G-protein–coupled receptors are transmembrane proteins. The G-protein receptors respond to ligands such as adrenaline and serotonin. Upon ligand binding to the receptor (R), the G-protein undergoes a conformational change through GTP-GDP conversion, and in turn activates the effector (E) component. The E component subsequently activates second messengers. The role of IP$_3$ is to induce release of calcium from the endoplasmic reticulum (ER).

phosphorylation, and recruit secondary signaling molecules. Activation of protein kinase receptors is important for gene transcription and cell proliferation.

Janus Kinase/Signal Transduction and Activator of Transcription (STAT) Signaling

Janus kinase (JAK) is the receptor for over 20 cytokines, including IFN-γ, IL-6, IL-10, IL-12, and IL-13. When ligands bind to the receptors, receptor dimerization occurs and enzymatic activation propagates through the JAK domains of the receptors (Fig. 1-10).

Activation occurs by phosphorylation, the common currency of most intracellular signal transduction, which then recruits STAT (*s*ignal *t*ransduction and *a*ctivator of *t*ranscription) proteins to the cytosolic portion of the receptors. Activated STAT proteins further dimerize and translocate into the nucleus as transcription factors. STAT-mediated transcription can activate different T-cell responses during injury and inflammation. For example, STAT4 activation promotes a T$_H$1 response, while STAT6 shifts towards a T$_H$2 response.

Suppressors of Cytokine Signaling

Suppressors of cytokine signaling (SOCS) specifically block JAK and STAT activation and ultimately regulate the signaling of

LIGAND-GATED ION CHANNELS
(NEUROTRANSMITTERS, AMINO ACIDS,
ACETYLCHOLINE)

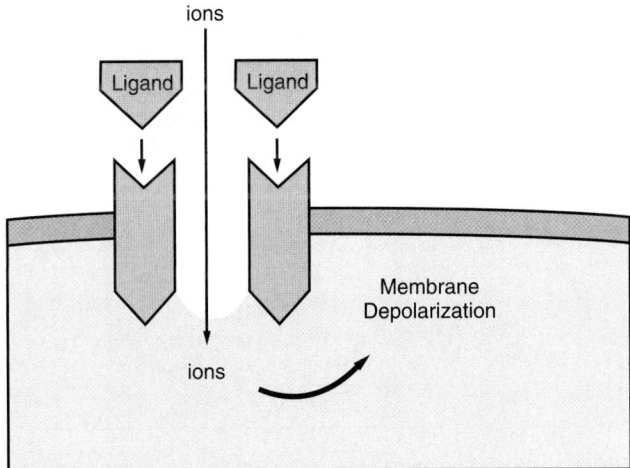

FIG. 1-8. Ligand-gated ion channels convert chemical signals into electrical signals, inducing a change in cell membrane potential. Upon activation of the channel, millions of ions per second influx into the cell. These channels are composed of many subunits, and the nicotinic acetylcholine receptor is one such example.

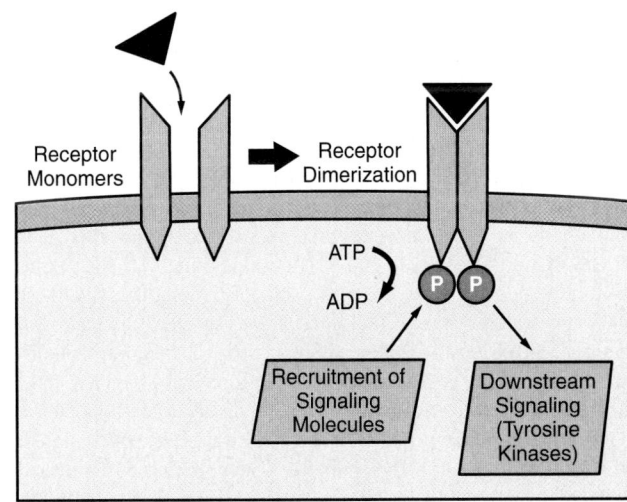

FIG. 1-9. The receptor tyrosine kinase requires dimerization of monomeric units. These receptors possess intrinsic enzymatic activity that requires multiple autophosphorylation steps to recruit and activate intracellular signaling molecules.

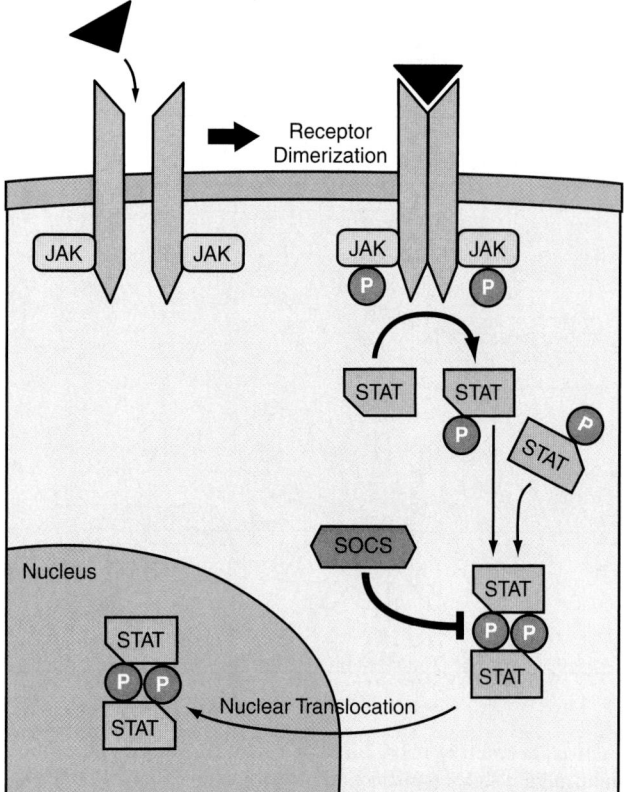

FIG. 1-10. The JAK/STAT signaling pathway also requires dimerization of monomeric units. STAT (signal transducers and activators of transcription) molecules possess "docking" sites that allow for STAT dimerization. The STAT complexes translocate into the nucleus and serve as gene transcription factors. JAK/STAT activation occurs in response to cytokines (e.g., IL-6) and cell stressors, and has been found to induce cell proliferation and inflammatory function. Intracellular molecules that inhibit STAT function, known as SOCS (suppressors of cytokine signaling), have been identified.

certain cytokines. A deficiency of SOCS activity may render a cell hypersensitive to certain stimuli such as inflammatory cytokines and growth hormones. One very clear association has been the specific attenuation of IL-6 signaling in macrophages by SOCS3 through the inhibition of STAT3.

Mitogen-Activated Protein Kinases

The mitogen-activated protein kinase (MAPK) pathway is a major cellular inflammatory signaling pathway with regulatory roles over cell proliferation and cell death (Fig. 1-11). There are over 20 MAPK isoforms, and the three major groups that alter gene expression are the JNK (c-Jun NH$_2$-terminal kinase), ERK (extracellular regulatory protein kinase), and p38 kinase. Broadly, these isoforms undergo several phosphorylations in order to reach final active forms. Conversely, removal of any phosphate groups significantly diminishes MAPK activity. The JNK pathway has clear links to the inflammatory response, with a regulatory role in apoptosis. TNF-α and IL-1 can activate the JNK pathway. Heat shock protein 72 is one example of a JNK inhibitor. The p38 kinase is activated in response to endotoxin, viruses, IL-1, IL-2, IL-7, IL-17, IL-18, TNF-α, and transforming growth factor (TGF)-β. The major role of p38-kinase activation is the recruitment and activation of leukocytes. These MAPK isoforms do not function independently, but exhibit appreciable "cross-talk," which can modulate the inflammatory response.

Nuclear Factor-κB

Nuclear factor (NF)-κB activates a wide spectrum of genes important for the activation of proinflammatory cytokines and acute phase proteins (Fig. 1-12). NF-κB is really a complex of smaller proteins, and the p50-p65 heterodimer complex is the most widely studied. In the cytosol, NF-κB is maintained by binding to the inhibitor protein I-κB. When a cell is exposed to an inflammatory stimulus (TNF-α or interleukin [IL]-β), a series of phosphorylation events leads to I-κB degradation. Interestingly, the rapid resynthesis of I-κB is one mechanism by which NF-κB activity is inhibited. Low intracellular I-κB concentration is a mechanism of prolonging the inflammatory response, because the enhanced activity of NF-κB appears to delay the apoptosis of activated immune cells.

Toll-Like Receptors and CD14

More than one half of the occurrences of sepsis syndrome is the result of gram-negative infections mediated by lipopolysaccharide (LPS), an endotoxin. Recognition of LPS and mounting the

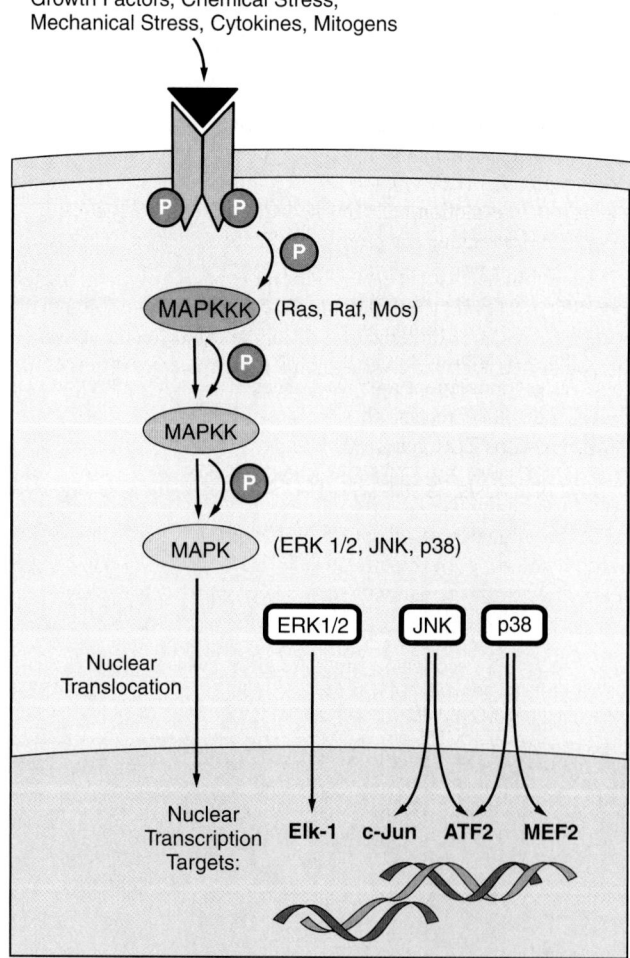

FIG. 1-11. The MAPK (mitogen-activated protein kinase) signaling pathway requires multiple phosphorylation steps. Ras, Raf, and Mos are examples of the MAP kinase kinase kinase (MAPKKK), which are upstream molecules. Well-characterized downstream kinases are ERK 1/2, JNK or SAPK (c-Jun NH$_2$-terminal kinases or stress-activated protein kinases), and p38 MAP kinases that target specific gene transcription sites in the nucleus. ATF = activating transcription factor; ERK = extracellular signal regulated kinase; MEF = myocyte-enhancing factor.

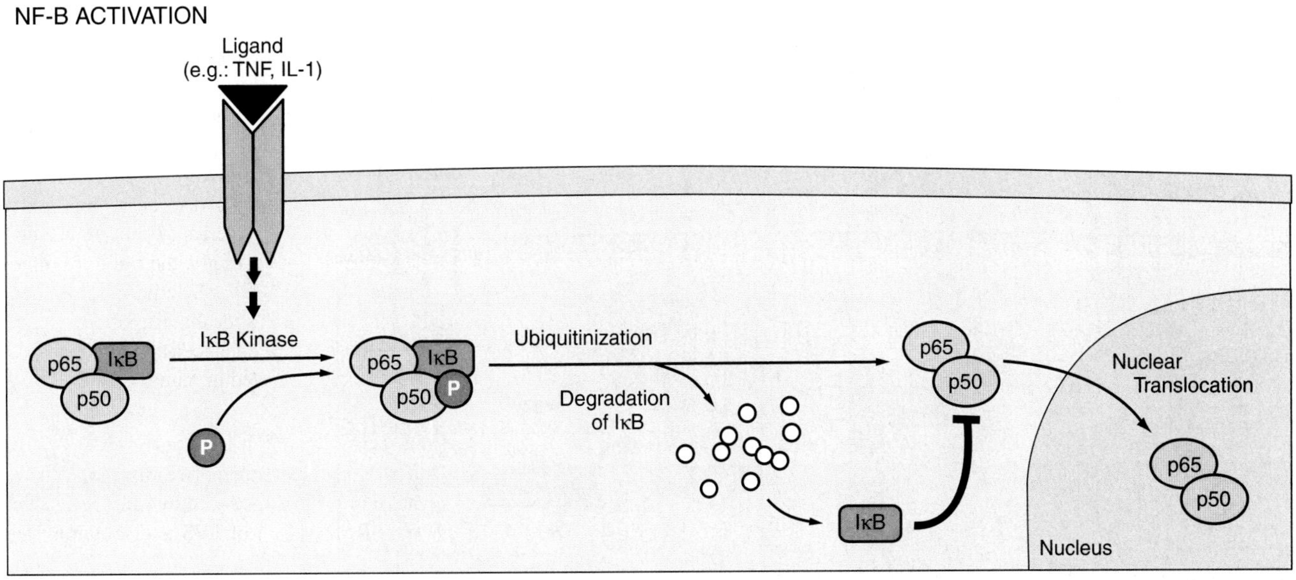

NF-B ACTIVATION

FIG. 1-12. I-κB binding to the p50-p65 subunits of NF-κB inactivates the molecule. Ligand binding to the receptor activates a series of downstream signaling molecules, of which I-κB kinase is one. The phosphorylated NF-κB complex further undergoes ubiquitinization and proteosome degradation of I-κB, activating NF-κB, which translocates into the nucleus. Rapid resynthesis of I-κB is one method of inactivating the p50-p65 complex.

appropriate inflammatory response by immune cells occurs primarily by the toll-like receptor-4 (TLR4) mechanism (Fig. 1-13). LPS-binding proteins (LBPs) carry LPS to the CD14/TLR4 complex, which sets into motion cellular mechanisms that activate MAPK, NF-κB, and cytokine gene promoters. TLR4 is primarily the receptor for gram-negative endotoxins and TLR2 is the counterpart for gram-positive sepsis. Receptors for IL-1 and IL-18 appear to share similar intracellular domains with toll-like receptors, and so there are significant similarities in signaling mechanisms. The fact that some patient populations are more susceptible to infectious complications than others recently has been associated with specific point mutations in the TLR gene.

Tumor Necrosis Factor and CD95-Induced Apoptosis

In the normal host, apoptosis is the principal mechanism by which senescent or dysfunctional cells, including macrophages and neutrophils, are systematically disposed of without activating other immunocytes or the release of proinflammatory contents. The cellular environment created by systemic inflammation disrupts the normal apoptotic machinery in activated immunocytes, consequently prolonging the inflammatory response.

Several proinflammatory cytokines (e.g., TNF-α, IL-1, IL-3, IL-6, GM-CSF, granulocyte colony-stimulating factor [G-CSF], and IFN-γ) and bacterial products (e.g., endotoxin) have been shown to delay macrophage and neutrophil apoptosis in vitro, while IL-4 and IL-10 accelerate apoptosis in activated monocytes.

In acute inflammation, the response of the immunocyte to TNF-α is perhaps the most widely investigated. This cytokine exerts its biologic effects by binding to specific cellular receptors, tumor necrosis factor receptor (TNFR)-1 (55 kDa) and TNFR-2 (75 kDa) (Fig. 1-14). Under physiologic conditions, TNFR-1 mediates most known biologic effects of soluble TNF-α, including inflammatory responses, NF-κB activation, and apoptosis. When TNFR-1 is exclusively activated, it precipitates circulatory shock reminiscent of

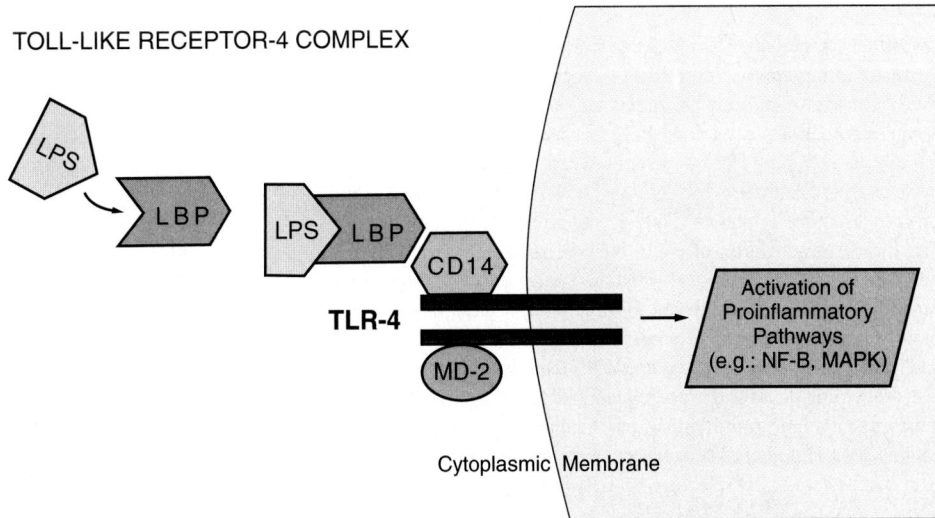

FIG. 1-13. LPS recognition by immune cells is primarily by the toll-like receptor-4/CD14/MD-2 complex. LPS is transported by LPS-binding protein (LBP) to the cell surface complex. Other cell surface LPS sensors include ion-gated channels, CD11b/CD18, and macrophage scavenger receptors.

TOLL-LIKE RECEPTOR-4 COMPLEX

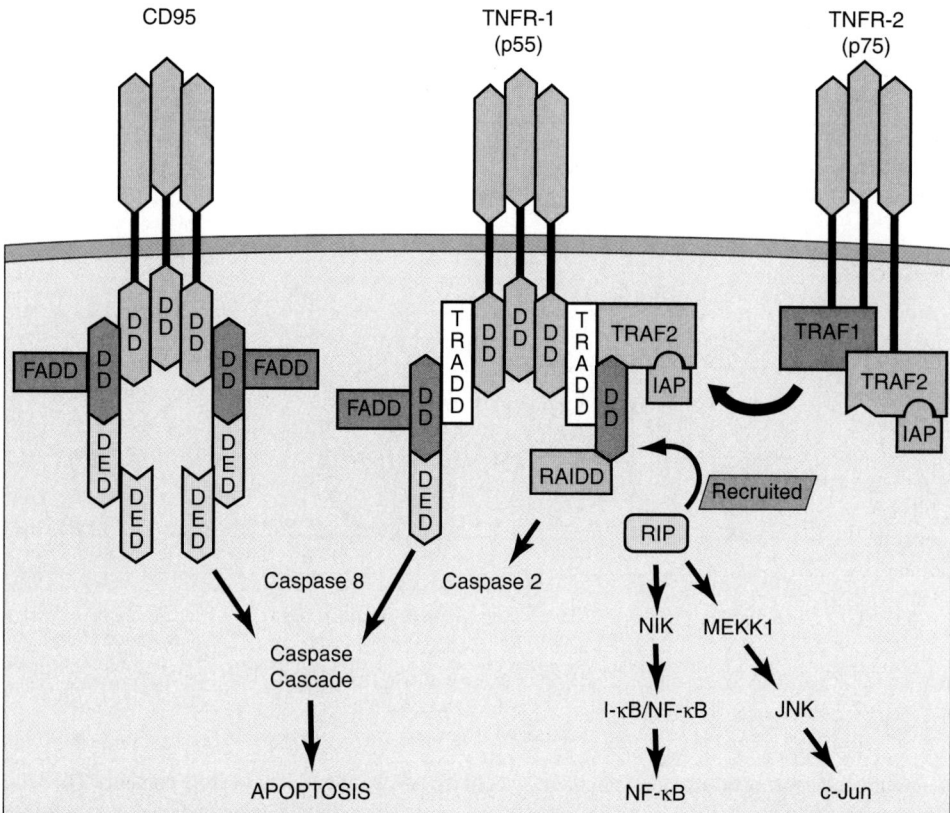

FIG. 1-14. Signaling pathway for tumor necrosis factor receptor (TNFR)-1 (55 kDa) and TNFR-2 (75 kDa) occurs by the recruitment of several adapter proteins to the intracellular receptor complex. Optimal signaling activity requires receptor trimerization. TNFR-1 initially recruits TNFR-associated death domain (TRADD) and induces apoptosis through the actions of proteolytic enzymes known as caspases, a pathway shared by another receptor known as CD95 (Fas). CD95 and TNFR-1 possess similar intracellular sequences known as death domains (DD), and both recruit the same adapter proteins known as Fas-associated death domains (FADD) prior to activating caspase-8. TNFR-1 also induces apoptosis by activating caspase-2 through the recruitment of RIP (receptor-interacting protein). RIP also has a functional component that can initiate NF-κB and c-Jun activation, both favoring cell survival and proinflammatory functions. TNFR-2 lacks a DD component, but recruits adapter proteins known as TRAF1 and TRAF2 (TNFR-associated factor) that interact with RIP to mediate NF-κB and c-Jun activation. TRAF2 also recruits additional proteins that are antiapoptotic, known as IAP (inhibitors of apoptosis protein). DED = death effector domain; RAIDD = RIP-associated ICH-1-like protein with death domain, which activates proapoptotic caspases; MEKK1 = mitogen-activated protein/ERK kinase kinase-1; JNK = c-Jun N-terminal kinase; NIK = NF-κB–inducing kinase; I-κB/NF-κB = inactive complex of NF-κB that becomes activated when the I-κB portion is cleaved. [Adapted with permission from Lin E, Calvano SE, Lowry SF: Tumor necrosis factor receptors in systemic inflammation, in Vincent JL (ed): Update in Intensive Care and Emergency Medicine: Immune Response in Critical Illness. Berlin: Springer-Verlag, 1999, p 365.]

severe sepsis. However, exclusive activation of TNFR-2 fails to induce any inflammatory responses or shock.

Signal transduction experiments and studies employing receptor gene-knockout technology have consistently demonstrated intracellular signaling "cross-talk" between TNFR-1 and TNFR-2 upon receptor activation by TNF-α. TNFR-1 mediates most of the proinflammatory effects of TNF-α, and it has been demonstrated that the early activation of c-Jun NH₂-terminal kinase (JNK) and p38 kinase prevents TNFR-1–mediated apoptosis. The activation of NF-κB and JNK is believed to be the major antiapoptotic, and therefore proinflammatory, factor; it is signal induced by TNFR-1 and TNFR-2. It is well-known that TNF-α–induced NF-κB activation delays cell death and is associated with the activation of diverse genes that include proinflammatory mediators. Inhibiting NF-κB activation in endothelial cells has been shown to reduce the expression of E-selectins, P-selectins, and IL-8. Exaggerated peripheral

blood monocyte NF-κB activation has been associated with higher mortality rates in patients with septic shock.

Members (i.e., homologues) of the intracellular human oncogene product Bcl-2 also are involved in regulating immunocyte survival during systemic inflammation. The intracellular expression of one such member, Bfl-1, is directly dependent upon NF-κB activity and is capable of suppressing TNF-α–induced apoptosis. Bfl-1 mRNA is inducible in neutrophils stimulated with agonists such as G-CSF, GM-CSF, and LPS. Inflammatory cytokines also can enhance neutrophil Mcl-1 expression, another antiapoptotic Bcl-2 homologue, which prolongs neutrophil survival and perpetuates inflammation. Monocytes activated by inflammatory stimuli such as TNF-α also can have prolonged survival as a result of upregulated Bfl-1 gene expression.

The CD95 (Fas) receptor shares much of its intracellular structure with TNFR-1. Unlike TNFR-1, the only known function of CD95 is to initiate programmed cell death. Neutrophils and macrophages express CD95, and this expression may have important implications in the cellular contribution to the inflammatory response. In fact, both clinical sepsis and experimental endotoxemia have demonstrated prolonged survival of neutrophils and diminished responsiveness to CD95 stimuli. Although the mechanisms are unclear, CD95 and TNFR activity may participate in organ injury during systemic inflammation.

Cell-Mediated Inflammatory Response

Platelets

Clot formation at the site of injury releases inflammatory mediators and serves as the principal chemoattractant for neutrophils and monocytes. The migration of platelets and neutrophils through the vascular endothelium occurs within 3 hours of injury and is mediated by serotonin release, platelet-activating factor, and prostaglandin E_2. Platelets can enhance or reduce neutrophil-mediated tissue injury by modulating neutrophil adherence to the endothelium and subsequent respiratory burst. Platelets are an important source of eicosanoids and vasoactive mediators. Nonsteroidal anti-inflammatory drugs irreversibly inhibit thromboxane production.

Lymphocytes and T-Cell Immunity

Injury, surgical or traumatic, is associated with acute impairment of cell-mediated immunity and macrophage function (Fig. 1-15).

T-helper lymphocytes are functionally divided into two subgroups, referred to as T_H1 and T_H2. While both T_H1 and T_H2 cells produce IL-3, TNF-α, and GM-CSF, T_H1 cell response is further characterized by the production of IFN-γ, IL-2, IL-12, and TNF-β

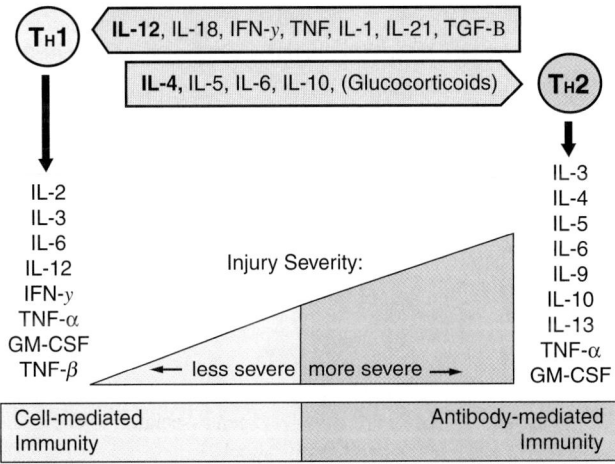

FIG. 1-15. *Specific immunity mediated by type I (T_H1) and type 2 (T_H2) T-helper lymphocytes following injury. A T_H1 response is favored in lesser injuries, with intact cell-mediated and opsonizing antibody immunity against microbial infections. This cell-mediated immunity includes activation of monocytes, B lymphocytes, and cytotoxic T lymphocytes. A shift toward the T_H2 response from naïve T-helper cells is associated with injuries of greater magnitude and is not as effective against microbial infections. A T_H2 response includes the activation of eosinophils, mast cells, and B-lymphocyte IgG4 and IgE production. (Primary stimulants and principal cytokine products of such responses are in* **bold** *characters.) IL-4 and IL-10 are known inhibitors of the T_H1 response. IFN-γ is a known inhibitor of the T_H2 response. Although not cytokines, glucocorticoids are potent stimulants of a T_H2 response, which may partly contribute to the immunosuppressive effects of cortisol. (Adapted with permission from Lin E, Calvano SE, Lowry SF: Inflammatory cytokines and cell response in surgery. Surgery 127:117, 2000.)*

(lymphotoxin), and T_H2 cell response is primarily characterized by IL-4, IL-5, IL-6, IL-9, IL-10, and IL-13 production. In severe infections and major injury, there appears to be a reduction in T_H1 (cell-mediated immunity) cytokine production, with a lymphocyte population shift toward the T_H2 response and its associated immunosuppressive effects. In patients with major burns, a shift to a T_H2 cytokine response has been a predictor of infectious complications. However, studies in patients undergoing major surgery have demonstrated a postoperative reduction in T_H1 cytokine production that is not necessarily associated with increased T_H2 response. Nevertheless, depressed T_H1 response and systemic immunosuppression following major insults to the host may be a useful paradigm in predicting the subset of patients who are prone to infectious complications and poor outcome. It should be noted that an excessive T_H1 response can conceivably lead to overwhelming inflammatory response and organ injury, but this phenomenon has not been well documented in surgical or trauma patients.

Eosinophils

Eosinophils are characteristically similar to neutrophils in that they migrate to inflamed endothelium and release cytoplasmic granules that are cytotoxic. As a result of different chemokine receptor expressions, eosinophils preferentially migrate to sites of parasitic infection and allergen challenge. Mature eosinophils reside in gastrointestinal, lung, and genitourinary tissues, but also can re-enter the circulation when needed. Major activators of eosinophils include IL-3, GM-CSF, IL-5, platelet-activating factor, and complement anaphylatoxins C3a and C5a.

Mast Cells

Mast cells are important as first-responders at sites of injury because they are pre-existent in tissues. In response to trauma or infection, activated mast cells produce histamine, cytokines, eicosanoids, proteases, and chemokines. The immediate results are vasodilation, recruitment of other immunocytes, and capillary leakage. TNF-α is secreted rapidly by mast cells because of the abundant stores within granules. Mast cells also can synthesize IL-3, IL-4, IL-5, IL-6, IL-10, IL-13, and IL-14, as well as migration-inhibitory factor (MIF).

Monocytes

In humans, downregulation in monocyte and neutrophil TNFR expression has been demonstrated experimentally and clinically (Fig. 1-16). In clinical sepsis, nonsurviving patients with severe sepsis have an immediate reduction in monocyte surface TNFR expression with failure to recover, while surviving patients have normal or near-normal receptor levels from the onset of clinically-defined sepsis (Fig. 1-17). In patients with congestive heart failure, there is also a significant decrease in the amount of monocyte surface TNFR expression when compared with control patients (Fig. 1-18). Thus, TNFR expression potentially can be used as a prognostic indicator of outcome in patients with systemic inflammation. There is also decreased CD95 expression following experimental endotoxemia in humans, which correlates with diminished CD95-mediated apoptosis. Taken together, the reduced receptor expression and delayed apoptosis may be a mechanism for prolonging the inflammatory response during injury or infection.

Neutrophils

Neutrophils mediate important functions in every form of acute inflammation, including acute lung injury, ischemia/reperfusion

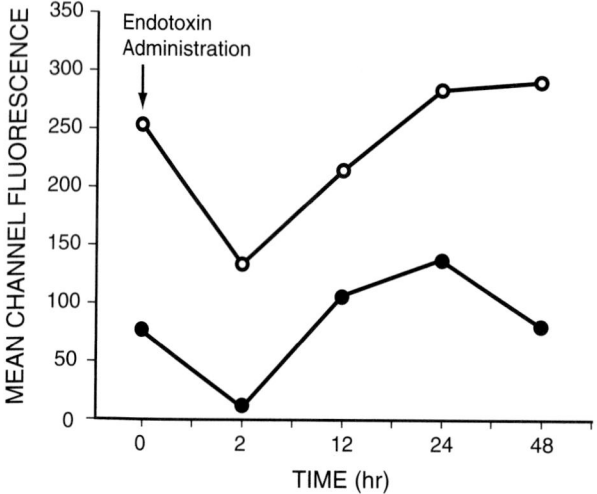

FIG. 1-16. Monocyte CD95 and TNFR expression in healthy adult subjects following intravenous endotoxin administration at time = 0 hours. A reduction in receptor expression is observed at time = 2 hours, corresponding to the time of maximal clinical response to the endotoxin. In the absence of further stimulus, receptor expression recovers to normal levels by 48 hours. (*Adapted with permission from Lin E, Katz JA, Calvano SE, et al: The influence of human endotoxemia on CD95-induced apoptosis. Arch Surg 133:1322, 1998.*)

injury, and inflammatory bowel disease. Within the bone marrow, G-CSF is the primary stimulus for neutrophil maturation. Inflammatory mediators from a site of injury induce neutrophil adherence to the vascular endothelium and promote eventual cell migration into the injured tissue. Neutrophil function is mediated by a vast array of intracellular granules that are chemotactic or cytotoxic to local tissue and invading microorganisms.

ENDOTHELIUM-MEDIATED INJURY

Neutrophil-Endothelium Interaction

Increased vascular permeability during inflammation is intended to facilitate oxygen delivery and immunocyte migration to the sites of injury. However, the accumulation and infiltration of inflammatory leukocytes, specifically neutrophils, at sites of injury contribute to the cytotoxicity of vital tissues and result in organ dysfunction. Ischemia/reperfusion (I/R) injury potentiates this response by unleashing oxygen metabolites, lysosomal enzymes that degrade tissue basal membranes, cause microvascular thrombosis, and activate myeloperoxidases. The recruitment of circulating neutrophils to endothelial surfaces is mediated by concerted actions of adhesion molecules referred to as selectins that are elaborated on cell surfaces (Table 1-5). Neutrophil rolling in the first 10 to 20 minutes following injury is mainly mediated by P-selectin expression (Fig. 1-19). This is consistent with the rapid expression of P-selectins from intracellular stores. Beyond 20 minutes, the influence of P-selectins diminishes secondary to internal degradation, and L-selectin becomes the principal mediator of leukocyte rolling. In conjunction with L-selectin, P-selectin glycoprotein ligand-1 (PSGL-1) is responsible for over 85% of monocyte-to-monocyte and monocyte-to-endothelium adhesion activity. Although there are distinguishable properties among individual selectins in leukocyte rolling, effective rolling most likely involves a significant degree of functional overlap. Similarly, L-selectin also initiates neutrophil-to-neutrophil interaction, in part by binding to leukocyte surface PSGL-1.

Nitric Oxide

Nitric oxide (NO) is derived from endothelial surfaces in response to acetylcholine stimulation, hypoxia, endotoxin, cellular injury, or mechanical shear stress from circulating blood. Normal vascular smooth muscle relaxation is maintained by a constant output of NO. NO also can reduce microthrombosis by reducing platelet adhesion

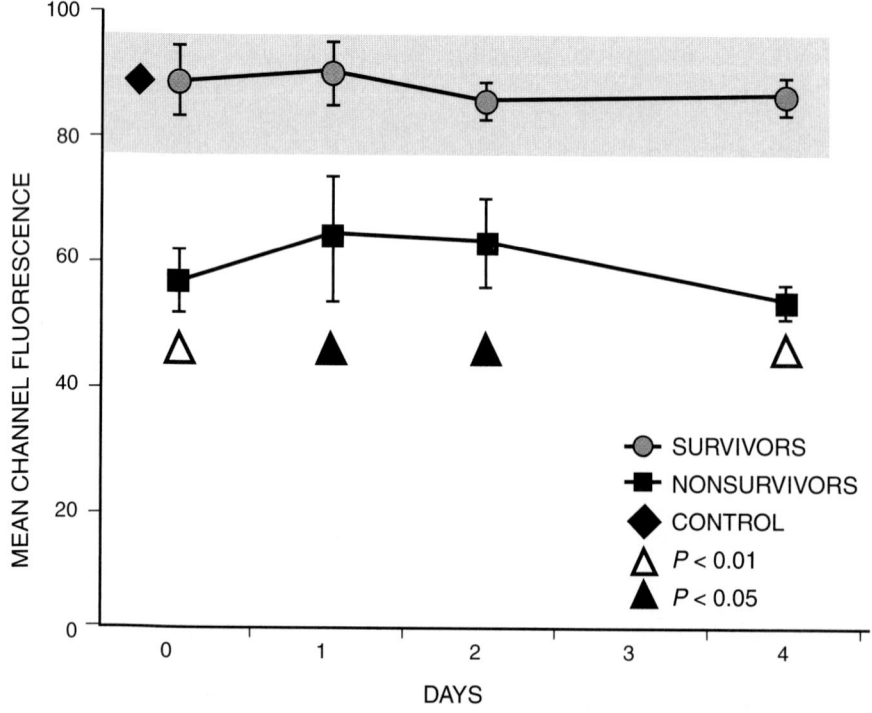

FIG. 1-17. Monocyte TNFR expression in healthy subjects, and in surviving and nonsurviving septic patients, on days 0 to 4. The gray box indicates the range of monocyte TNFR expression in surviving patients and healthy subjects. (*Adapted with permission from Calvano SE, van der Poll T, Coyle SM, et al: Monocyte tumor necrosis factor receptor levels as a predictor of risk in human sepsis. Arch Surg 131:434, 1996.*)

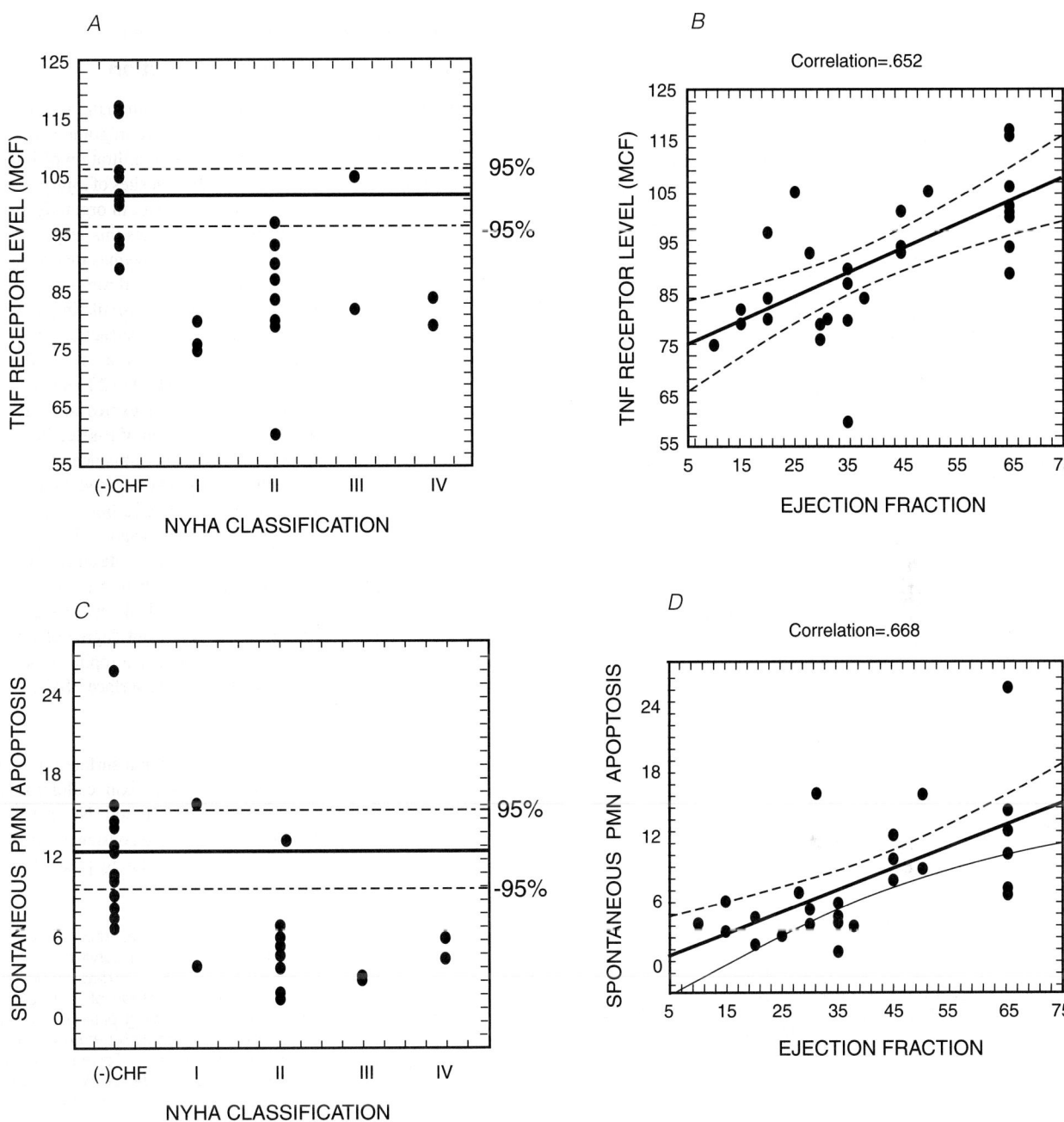

FIG. 1-18. *A.* Patients without congestive heart failure (CHF) expressed higher TNFR levels than patients with CHF stratified by New York Heart Association (NYHA) classification. Monocyte membrane-associated TNFR levels are expressed as mean channel fluorescence (MCF). *B.* Patients with higher monocyte TNFR expression also exhibited higher ejection fractions. *C.* Spontaneous apoptosis of polymorphonuclear cells (PMNs) was lower in patients with CHF, suggesting that the chronic inflammatory milieu of CHF patients contributes to the delay in PMN disposal. *D.* Patients with higher ejection fractions also exhibited higher spontaneous PMN apoptosis.

and aggregation (Fig. 1-20). NO also mediates protein synthesis in hepatocytes and electron transport in hepatocyte mitochondria. It is a readily diffusible substance with a half-life of a few seconds. NO spontaneously decomposes into nitrate and nitrite.

NO is formed from oxidation of L-arginine, a process catalyzed by nitric oxide synthase (NOS). Cofactors of NOS activity include calmodulin, ionized calcium, and reduced nicotinamide adenine dinucleotide phosphate (NADPH). In addition to the endothelium,

NO formation also occurs in neutrophils, monocytes, renal cells, Kupffer cells, and cerebellar neurons.

Prostacyclin

Although it is an arachidonate product, prostacyclin (PGI$_2$) is another important endothelium-derived vasodilator synthesized in response to vascular shear stress and hypoxia. PGI$_2$ shares similar

Table 1-5
Molecules That Mediate Leukocyte-Endothelial Adhesion, Categorized by Family

Adhesion Molecule	Action	Origin	Inducers of Expression	Target Cells
Selectins				
L-selectin	Fast rolling	Leukocytes	Native	Endothelium, platelets, eosinophils
P-selectin	Slow rolling	Platelets and endothelium	Thrombin, histamine	Neutrophils, monocytes
E-selectin	Very slow rolling	Endothelium	Cytokines	Neutrophils, monocytes, lymphocytes
Immunoglobulins				
ICAM-1	Firm adhesion/ transmigration	Endothelium, leukocytes, fibroblasts, epithelium	Cytokines	Leukocytes
ICAM-2	Firm adhesion	Endothelium, platelets	Native	Leukocytes
VCAM-1	Firm adhesion/ transmigration	Endothelium	Cytokines	Monocytes, lymphocytes
PECAM-1	Adhesion/ transmigration	Endothelium, platelets, leukocytes	Native	Endothelium, platelets, leukocytes
β_2-(CD18) Integrins				
CD18/11a	Firm adhesion/ transmigration	Leukocytes	Leukocyte activation	Endothelium
CD18/11b (Mac-1)	Firm adhesion/ transmigration	Neutrophils, monocytes, natural killer cells	Leukocyte activation	Endothelium
CD18/11c	Adhesion	Neutrophils, monocytes, natural killer cells	Leukocyte activation	Endothelium
β_1-(CD29) Integrins				
VLA-4	Firm Adhesion/ transmigration	Lymphocytes, monocytes	Leukocyte activation	Monocytes, endothelium, epithelium

ICAM = intercellular adhesion molecule; Mac = macrophage antigen; PECAM = platelet-endothelial cell adhesion molecule; VCAM = vascular cell adhesion molecule; VLA = very late antigen.

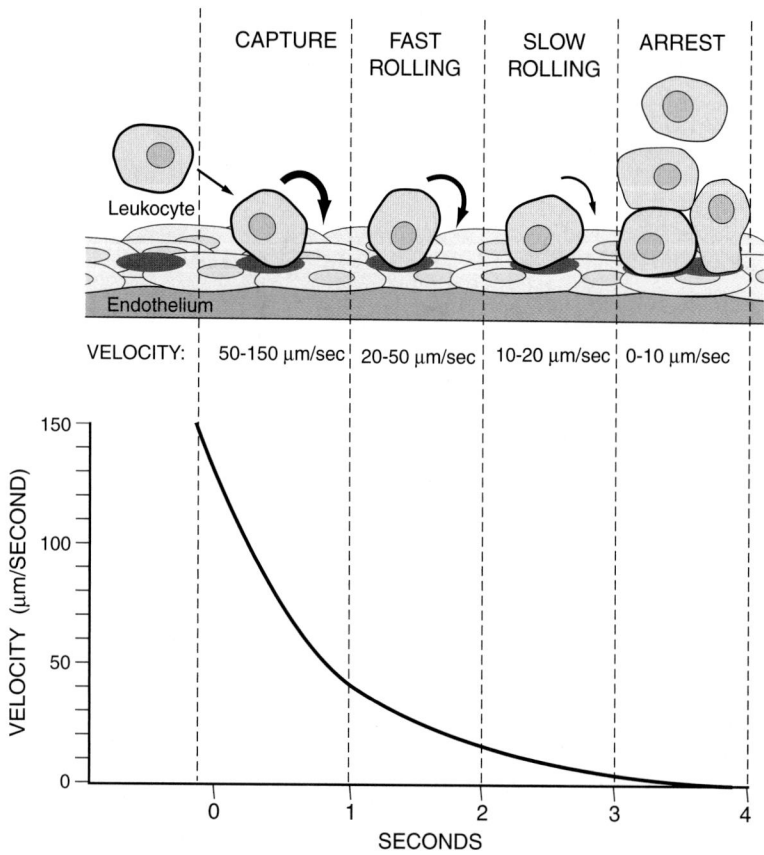

FIG. 1-19. Simplified sequence of selectin-mediated neutrophil-endothelium interaction following an inflammatory stimulus. *CAPTURE* (tethering), predominantly mediated by cell L-selectin with contribution from endothelial P-selectin, describes the initial recognition between leukocyte and endothelium, where circulating leukocytes marginate toward the endothelial surface. *FAST ROLLING* (50 to 150 μm/s) is a consequence of rapid L-selectin shedding from cell surfaces and formation of new downstream L-selectin to endothelium bonds, occurring in tandem. *SLOW ROLLING* (20 to 50 μm/s) is predominantly mediated by P-selectins. The slowest rolling (3 to 10 μm/s) prior to arrest is predominantly mediated by E-selectins, with contribution from P-selectins. *ARREST* (firm adhesion) leading to transmigration is mediated by β-integrins and the immunoglobulin family of adhesion molecules. In addition to interactions with the endothelium, activated leukocytes also recruit other leukocytes to the inflammatory site by direct interactions, which are mediated in part by selectins. (*Adapted with permission from Lin E, Calvano SE, Lowry SF: Selectin neutralization: Does it make biological sense? Crit Care Med 27:2050, 1999.*)

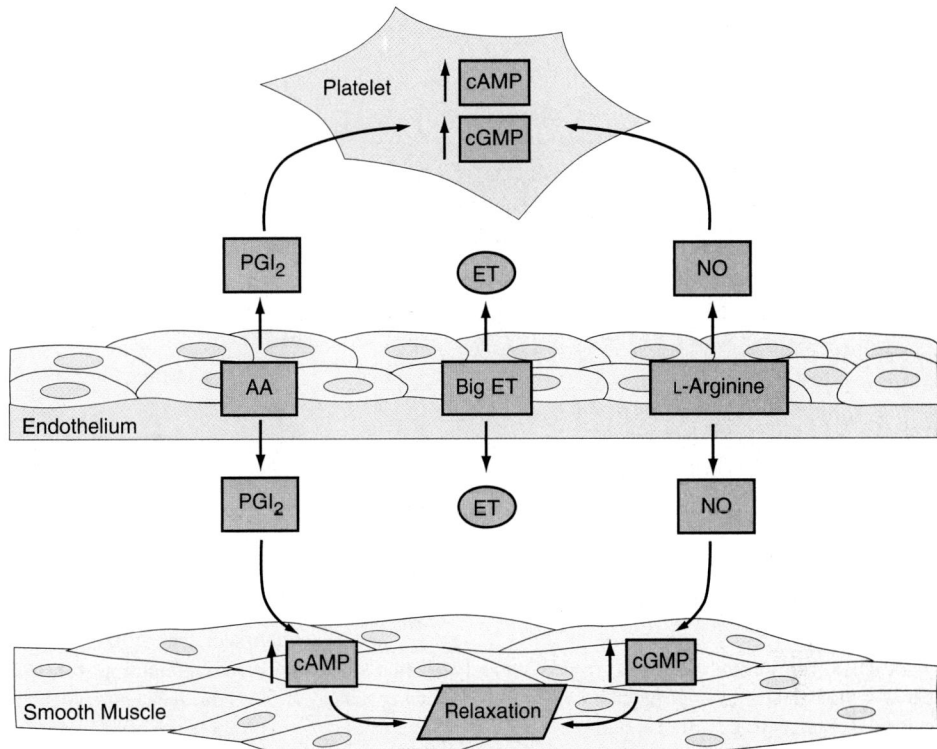

FIG. 1-20. Endothelial interaction with smooth muscle cells and with intraluminal platelets. Prostacyclin (PGI₂) is derived from arachidonic acid, and nitric oxide (NO) is derived from L-arginine. The increase in cyclic adenosine monophosphate (cAMP) and cyclic guanosine monophosphate (cGMP) results in smooth muscle relaxation and inhibition of platelet thrombus formation. Endothelins (ETs) are derived from "big ET," and they counter the effects of prostacyclin and nitric oxide.

functions with NO, inducing vasorelaxation and platelet deactivation by increasing cAMP. Clinically, it has been used to reduce pulmonary hypertension, particularly in the pediatric population.

Endothelins

Endothelins (ETs) are elaborated by vascular endothelial cells in response to injury, thrombin, transforming growth factor-β (TGF-β), IL-1, angiotensin II, vasopressin, catecholamines, and anoxia. Structurally formed from a 38-amino-acid precursor molecule, ET is a 21-amino-acid peptide with potent vasoconstricting properties. Of the peptides in this family (e.g., ET-1, ET-2, and ET-3), endothelial cells appear to exclusively produce ET-1. Moreover, ET-1 appears to be the most biologically active and the most potent known vasoconstrictor. It is estimated to be 10 times more potent than angiotensin II. Three endothelin receptors, referred to as ET_A, ET_B, and ET_C, have been identified and function by the G-protein-coupled receptor mechanism. ET_B receptors are linked to the formation of NO and prostacyclin (PGI₂), which serve as negative feedback mechanisms. The maintenance of physiologic tone in vascular smooth muscle depends on the balance between NO and ET production. The vasoconstrictor activity of ET can be reversed by the administration of acetylcholine, which stimulates NO production. Increased serum levels of ETs correlate with the severity of injury following major trauma, major surgical procedures, and in cardiogenic or septic shock.

Platelet-Activating Factor

Another endothelial-derived product is platelet-activating factor (PAF), a natural phospholipid constituent of cell membranes, which under normal physiologic conditions is minimally expressed. During acute inflammation, PAF is released by neutrophils, platelets, mast cells, and monocytes, and is expressed at the outer leaflet of endothelial cells. PAF can further activate neutrophils and platelets

and increase vascular permeability. Antagonists to PAF receptors have been experimentally shown to mitigate the effects of ischemia/reperfusion injury. Human sepsis is associated with a reduction in PAF-acetylhydrolase levels, which is the endogenous inactivator of PAF. Indeed, PAF-acetylhydrolase administration in patients with severe sepsis has shown some reduction in multiple organ dysfunction and mortality.

Atrial Natriuretic Peptides

Atrial natriuretic peptides (ANPs) are a family of peptides released primarily by atrial tissue, but are also synthesized by the gut, kidney, brain, adrenal glands, and endothelium. They induce vasodilation as well as fluid and electrolyte excretion. ANPs are potent inhibitors of aldosterone secretion and prevent reabsorption of sodium. There is some experimental evidence to suggest that ANP can reverse acute renal failure or early acute tubular necrosis.

SURGICAL METABOLISM

The initial hours following surgical or traumatic injury are metabolically associated with a reduced total body energy expenditure and urinary nitrogen wasting. Upon adequate resuscitation and stabilization of the injured patient, a reprioritization of substrate utilization ensues to preserve vital organ function and for the repair of injured tissue. This phase of recovery also is characterized by functions that all participate in the restoration of homeostasis, such as augmented metabolic rates and oxygen consumption, enzymatic preference for readily oxidizable substrates such as glucose, and stimulation of the immune system.

Understanding the collective alterations in amino acid (protein), carbohydrate, and lipid metabolism characteristic of the surgical patient lays the foundation upon which metabolic and nutritional support can be implemented.

FUEL UTILIZATION IN SHORT-TERM FASTING MAN (70 kg)

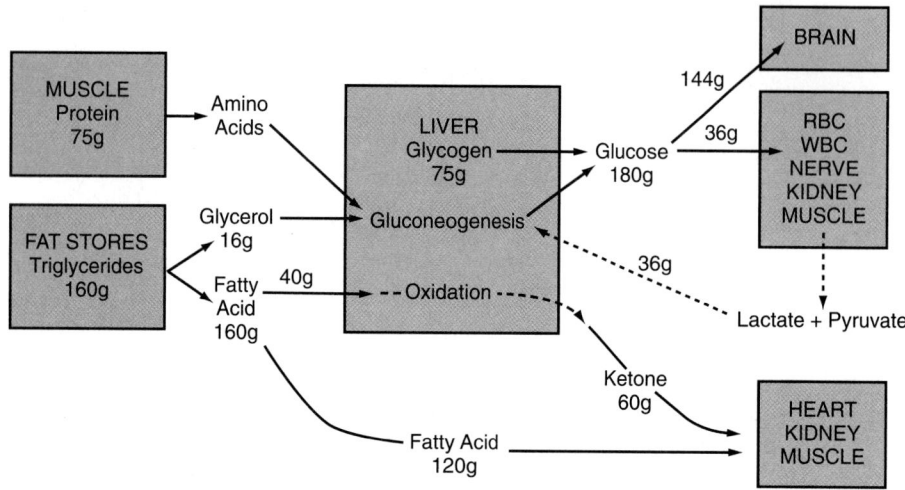

FIG. 1-21. Fuel utilization in a 70-kg man during short-term fasting with an approximate basal energy expenditure of 1800 calories. During starvation, muscle proteins and fat stores provide fuel for the host, with the latter being most abundant. (*Adapted with permission from Cahill GF: Starvation in man. N Engl J Med 282:668, 1970.*)

Metabolism During Fasting

Fuel metabolism during unstressed fasting states has historically served as the standard to which metabolic alterations following acute injury and critical illness are compared (Fig. 1-21). To maintain basal metabolic needs (i.e., at rest and fasting), a normal healthy adult requires approximately 25 kcal/kg per day drawn from carbohydrate, lipid, and protein sources. This requirement can be as high as 40 kcal/kg per day in severe stress states, such as those seen in patients with burn injuries.

In the healthy adult, principal sources of fuel during short-term fasting (<5 days) are derived from muscle protein and body fat, with fat being the most abundant source of energy (Table 1-6). The normal adult body contains 300 to 400 g of carbohydrates in the form of glycogen, of which 75 to 100 g are stored in the liver. Approximately 200 to 250 g of glycogen are stored within skeletal, cardiac, and smooth muscle cells. The greater glycogen stores within the muscle are not readily available for systemic use due to a deficiency in glucose-6-phosphatase, but are available for the energy needs of muscle cells. Therefore, in the fasting state, hepatic glycogen stores are rapidly and preferentially depleted, resulting in a fall of serum glucose concentration within hours (<16 hours).

During fasting, a healthy 70-kg adult will utilize 180 g of glucose per day to support the metabolism of obligate glycolytic cells such as neurons, leukocytes, erythrocytes, and the renal medullae. Other tissues that utilize glucose for fuel are skeletal muscle, intestinal mucosa, fetal tissues, and solid tumors.

Glucagon, norepinephrine, vasopressin, and angiotensin II can promote the utilization of glycogen stores (glycogenolysis) during fasting. While glucagon, epinephrine, and cortisol directly promote gluconeogenesis, epinephrine and cortisol also promote pyruvate shuttling to the liver for gluconeogenesis. Precursors for hepatic gluconeogenesis include lactate, glycerol, and amino acids such as alanine and glutamine. Lactate is released by glycolysis within skeletal muscles, as well as by erythrocytes and leukocytes. The recycling of lactate and pyruvate for gluconeogenesis is commonly referred to as the Cori cycle, which can provide up to 40% of plasma glucose during starvation (Fig. 1-22).

Lactate production from skeletal muscle is insufficient to maintain systemic glucose needs during short-term fasting (*simple starvation*). Therefore, significant amounts of protein must be degraded daily (75 g/d for a 70-kg adult) to provide the amino acid substrate for hepatic gluconeogenesis. Proteolysis during starvation, which results primarily from decreased insulin and increased cortisol release, is associated with elevated urinary nitrogen excretion from the normal 7 to 10 g per day up to 30 g or more per day. While proteolysis during starvation occurs mainly within skeletal muscles, protein degradation in solid organs also occurs.

Table 1-6

A. Body Fuel Reserves in a 70-kg Man and *B*. Energy Equivalent of Substrate Oxidation

A Component	Mass (kg)	Energy (kcal)	Days Available
Water and Minerals	49	0	0
Protein	6.0	24,000	13.0
Glycogen	0.2	800	0.4
Fat	15.0	140,000	78.0
Total	70.2	164,800	91.4

B Substrate	O$_2$ Consumed (L/g)	CO$_2$ Produced (L/g)	Respiratory Quotient	kcal/g	Recommended Daily Requirement
Glucose	0.75	0.75	1.0	4.0	7.2 g/kg per day
Dextrose	—	—	—	3.4	
Lipid	2.0	1.4	0.7	9.0	1.0 g/kg per day
Protein	1.0	0.8	0.8	4.0	0.8 g/kg per day

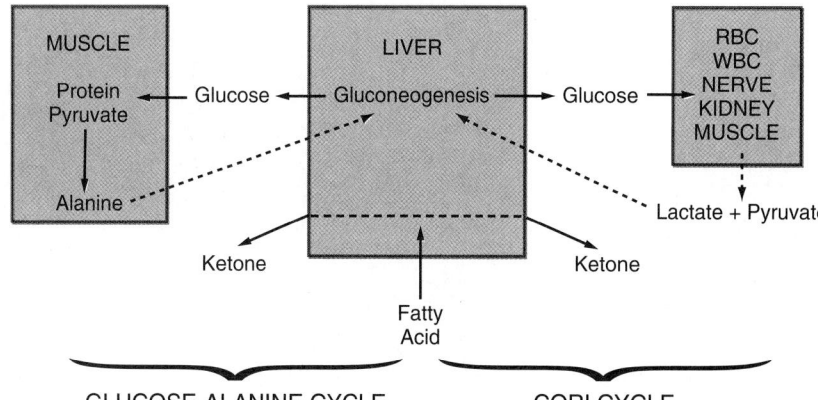

FIG. 1-22. The recycling of peripheral lactate and pyruvate for hepatic gluconeogenesis is accomplished by the Cori cycle. Alanine within skeletal muscles can also be utilized as a precursor for hepatic gluconeogenesis. During starvation, such fatty acid provides fuel sources for basal hepatic enzymatic function.

In *prolonged* starvation, systemic proteolysis is reduced to approximately 20 g per day and urinary nitrogen excretion stabilizes at 2 to 5 g per day (Fig. 1-23). This reduction in proteolysis reflects the adaptation by vital organs (e.g., myocardium, brain, renal cortex, and skeletal muscle) to using ketone bodies as their principal fuel source. In extended fasting, ketone bodies become an important fuel source for the brain after 2 days, and gradually become the principal fuel source by 24 days.

Enhanced deamination of amino acids for gluconeogenesis during starvation consequently increases renal excretion of ammonium ions. The kidneys also participate in gluconeogenesis by the utilization of glutamine and glutamate, and can become the primary source of gluconeogenesis during prolonged starvation, accounting for up to one half of systemic glucose production.

Lipid stores within adipose tissue provide up to 40% of caloric expenditure during starvation. Energy requirements for basal enzymatic and muscular functions (e.g., gluconeogenesis, neural transmission, and cardiac contraction) are met by the mobilization of triglycerides from adipose tissue. In a resting, fasting, 70-kg person, approximately 160 g of free fatty acids and glycerol can be mobilized from adipose tissue. Free fatty acid release is stimulated in part by a reduction in serum insulin levels and in part by the increase in circulating glucagon and catecholamine. Such free fatty acids, as with ketone bodies, are used as fuel by tissues such as the heart, kidney (renal cortex), muscle, and liver. The mobilization of lipid stores for energy importantly decreases the rate of glycolysis, gluconeogenesis, and proteolysis, as well as the overall glucose requirement to sustain the host. Furthermore, ketone bodies spare glucose utilization by inhibiting the enzyme pyruvate dehydrogenase.

Metabolism Following Injury

Injuries or infections induce unique neuroendocrine and immunologic responses that differentiate injury metabolism from that of unstressed fasting (Fig. 1-24). The magnitude of metabolic expenditure appears to be directly proportional to the severity of insult, with thermal injuries and severe infections having the highest energy demands (Fig. 1-25). The increase in energy expenditure is mediated in part by sympathetic activation and catecholamine release, which has been replicated by the administration of catecholamines to

FUEL UTILIZATION IN LONG-TERM FASTING MAN (70 kg)

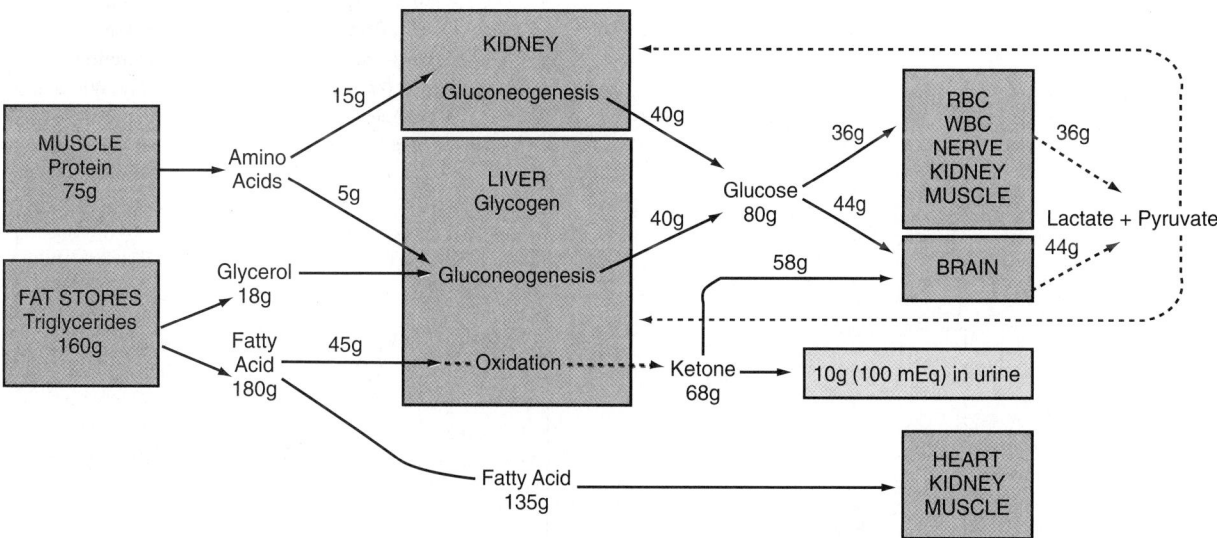

FIG. 1-23. Fuel utilization in extended starvation. Liver glycogen stores are depleted and there is adaptive reduction in proteolysis as a source of fuel. The brain utilizes ketones for fuel. The kidneys become important participants in gluconeogenesis. (*Adapted with permission from Cahill GF: Starvation in man. N Engl J Med 282:668, 1970.*)

FUEL UTILIZATION FOLLOWING TRAUMA

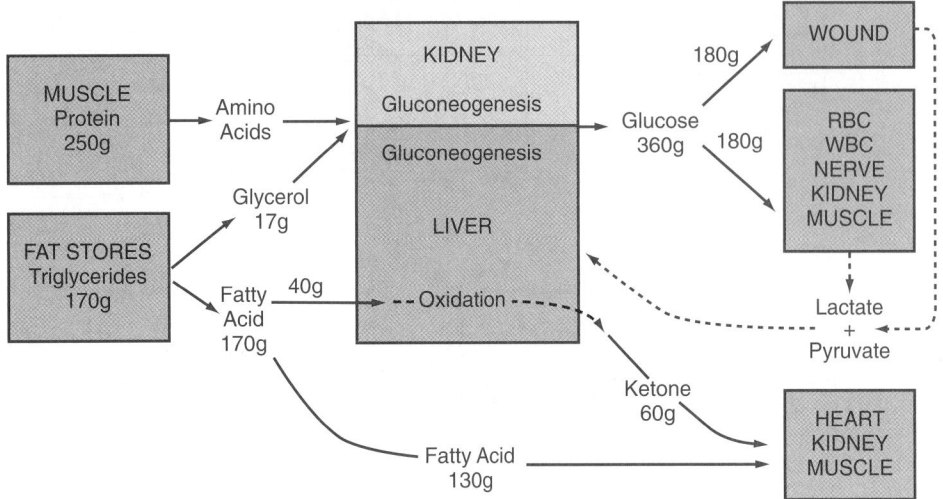

FIG. 1-24. Acute injury is associated with significant alterations in substrate utilization. There is enhanced nitrogen loss, indicative of catabolism. Fat remains the primary fuel source under these circumstances.

healthy human subjects. The discussion of lipid metabolism following injury is intentionally discussed first, because this macronutrient becomes the primary source of energy during stressed states.

Lipid Metabolism Following Injury

Lipids are not merely nonprotein, noncarbohydrate fuel sources that minimize protein catabolism in the injured patient, but lipid metabolism potentially influences the structural integrity of cell membranes as well as the immune response during systemic inflammation. Adipose stores within the body (triglycerides) are the predominant energy source (50 to 80%) during critical illness and following injury. Fat mobilization (lipolysis) occurs mainly in response to catecholamine stimulus of the hormone-sensitive triglyceride lipase. Other hormonal influences on lipolysis include adrenocorticotropic hormone, catecholamines, thyroid hormone, cortisol,

glucagon, growth hormone release, reduction in insulin levels, and increased sympathetic stimulus.

Lipid Absorption. Although poorly understood, adipose tissue provides fuel for the host in the form of free fatty acids and glycerol during critical illness and injury. Oxidation of 1 g of fat yields approximately 9 kcal of energy. Although the liver is capable of synthesizing triglycerides from carbohydrates and amino acids, dietary and exogenous sources provide the major source of triglycerides. Dietary lipids are not readily absorbable in the gut, but require pancreatic lipase and phospholipase within the duodenum to hydrolyze the triglycerides into free fatty acids and monoglycerides. The free fatty acids and monoglycerides are then readily absorbed by gut enterocytes, which resynthesize triglycerides by esterification of the monoglycerides with fatty acyl coenzyme A (acyl-CoA) (Fig. 1-26). Long-chain triglycerides (LCT), defined as those with 12 carbons or more, generally undergo this process of esterification and enter the circulation through the lymphatic system as chylomicrons. Shorter fatty acid chains directly enter the portal circulation and are transported to the liver by albumin carriers. Hepatocytes utilize free fatty acids as a fuel source during stress states, but can also synthesize phospholipids or triglycerides (i.e., very-low-density lipoproteins) during fed states. Systemic tissue (e.g., muscle and the heart) can utilize chylomicrons and triglycerides as fuel by hydrolysis with lipoprotein lipase at the luminal surface of capillary endothelium. Trauma or sepsis suppresses lipoprotein lipase activity in both adipose tissue and muscle, presumably mediated by TNF-α.

Lipolysis and Fatty Acid Oxidation. Periods of energy demand are accompanied by free fatty acid mobilization from adipose stores. This is mediated by hormonal influences (e.g., catecholamines, adrenocorticotropic hormone [ACTH], thyroid hormones, growth hormone, and glucagon) on triglyceride lipase through a cAMP pathway (Fig. 1-27). In adipose tissues, triglyceride lipase hydrolyzes triglycerides into free fatty acids and glycerol. Free fatty acids enter the capillary circulation and are transported by albumin to tissues requiring this fuel source (e.g., heart and skeletal muscle). Insulin inhibits lipolysis and favors triglyceride synthesis by augmenting lipoprotein lipase activity as well as intracellular levels of glycerol-3-phosphate. The use of glycerol for

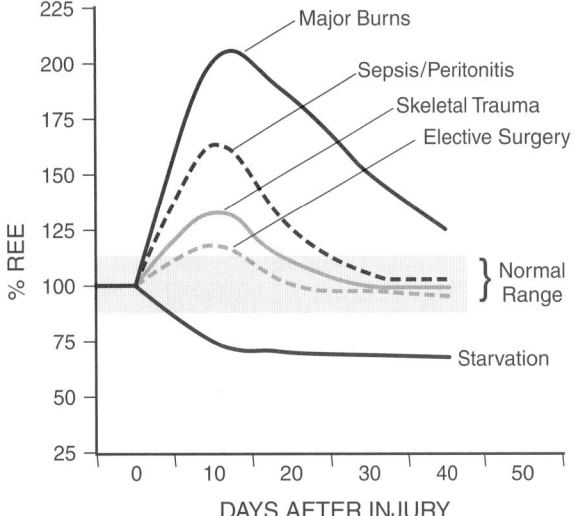

FIG. 1-25. The influence of injury severity on resting metabolism (resting energy expenditure, REE). The shaded area indicates normal REE. (*Adapted with permission from Long CL: Metabolic response to injury and illness: Estimation of energy and protein needs from indirect calorimetry and nitrogen balance. J Parenter Enteral Nutr 3:452, 1979.*)

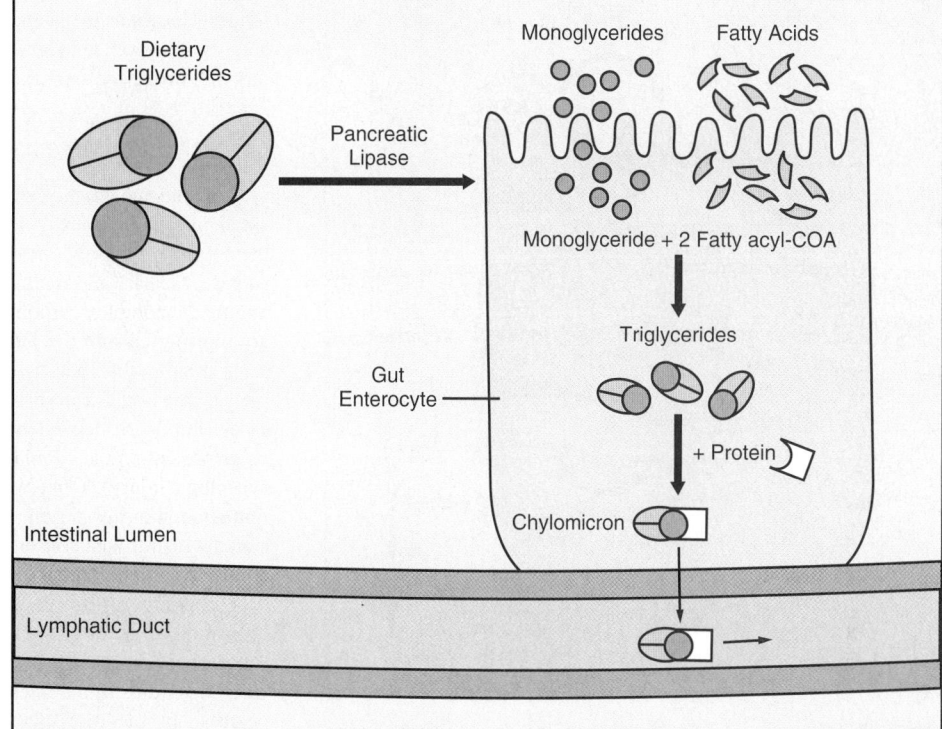

FIG. 1-26. Pancreatic lipase within the small intestinal brush borders hydrolyzes triglycerides into monoglycerides and fatty acids. These components readily diffuse into the gut enterocytes, where they are re-esterified into triglycerides. The resynthesized triglycerides bind carrier proteins to form chylomicrons, which are transported by the lymphatic system. Shorter triglycerides (those with less than 10 carbon atoms) can bypass this process and directly enter the portal circulation for transport to the liver.

fuel depends on the availability of tissue glycerokinase, which is abundant in the liver and kidneys.

Free fatty acids absorbed by cells conjugate with acyl-CoA within the cytoplasm. The transport of fatty acyl-CoA from the outer mitochondrial membrane across the inner mitochondrial membrane occurs via the carnitine shuttle (Fig. 1-28). Medium-chain

triglycerides (MCT), defined as those 6 to 12 carbons in length, bypass the carnitine shuttle and readily cross the mitochondrial membranes. This accounts in part for why MCTs are more efficiently oxidized than LCTs. Ideally, the rapid oxidation of MCTs makes them less prone to fat deposition, particularly within immune cells and the reticuloendothelial system—a common finding with lipid

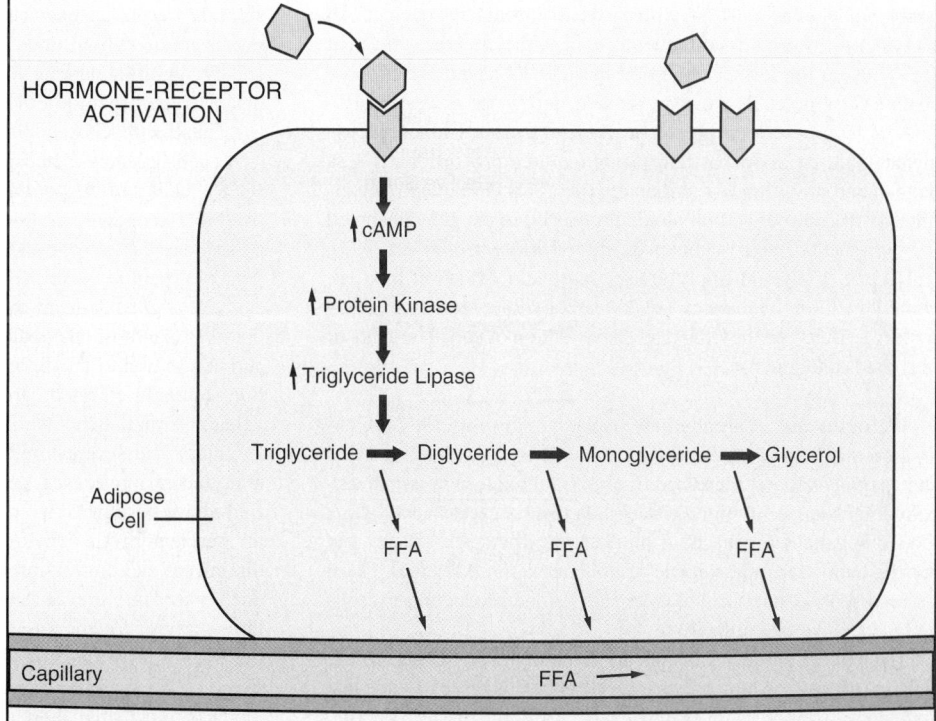

FIG. 1-27. Fat mobilization in adipose tissue. Triglyceride lipase activation by hormonal stimulation of adipose cells occurs through the cAMP pathway. Triglycerides are serially hydrolyzed with resultant free fatty acid (FFA) release at every step. The FFAs diffuse readily into the capillary bed for transport. Tissues with glycerokinase can utilize glycerol for fuel by forming glycerol-3-phosphate. Glycerol-3-phosphate can esterify with FFAs to form triglycerides, or can be used as a precursor for renal and hepatic gluconeogenesis. Skeletal muscle and adipose cells have little glycerokinase, and thus do not use glycerol for fuel.

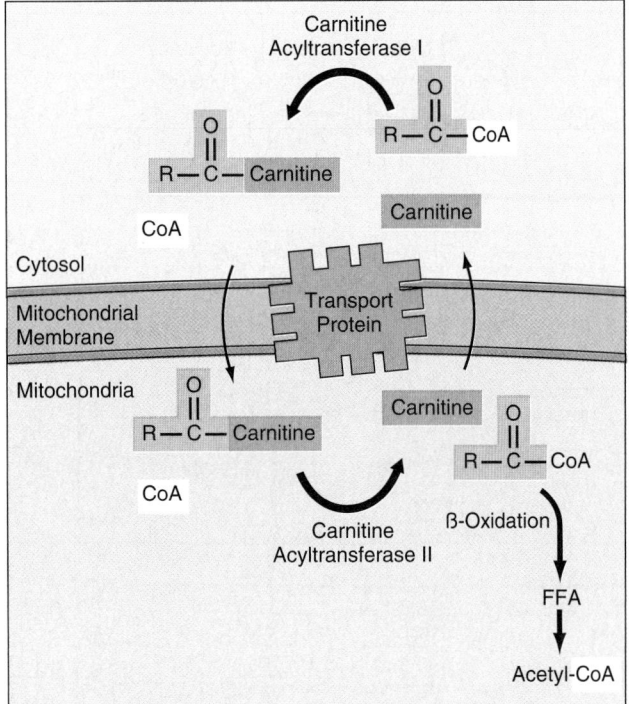

FIG. 1-28. Free fatty acids in the cells form fatty acyl-CoA with coenzyme A. Fatty acyl-CoA cannot enter the inner mitochondrial membrane and requires carnitine as a carrier protein (carnitine shuttle). Once inside the mitochondria, carnitine dissociates and fatty acyl-CoA is re-formed. The carnitine molecule is transported back into the cytosol for reuse. The fatty acyl-CoA undergoes β-oxidation to form acetyl-CoA for entry into the tricarboxylic acid cycle.

infusion in parenteral nutrition. However, exclusive use of MCTs as fuel in animal studies has been associated with higher metabolic demands and toxicity, as well as essential fatty acid deficiency.

Within the mitochondria, fatty acyl-CoA undergoes β-oxidation, which produces acetyl-CoA with each pass through the cycle. Each acetyl-CoA molecule subsequently enters the tricarboxylic acid (TCA) cycle for further oxidation to yield 12 adenosine triphosphate (ATP) molecules, carbon dioxide, and water. Excess acetyl-CoA molecules serve as precursors for ketogenesis. Unlike glucose metabolism, oxidation of fatty acids requires proportionally less oxygen and produces less carbon dioxide. This is frequently quantified as the ratio of carbon dioxide produced to oxygen consumed for the reaction, and is known as the *respiratory quotient* (RQ). An RQ of 0.7 would imply greater fatty acid oxidation for fuel, while an RQ of 1 indicates greater carbohydrate oxidation (*overfeeding*). An RQ of 0.85 suggests the oxidation of equal amounts of fatty acids and glucose.

Ketogenesis. Carbohydrate depletion slows acetyl-CoA entry into the TCA cycle secondary to depleted TCA intermediates and enzyme activity. Increased lipolysis and reduced systemic carbohydrate availability during starvation diverts excess acetyl-CoA toward hepatic ketogenesis. A number of extrahepatic tissues, but not the liver itself, are capable of utilizing ketones for fuel. Ketosis represents a state in which hepatic ketone production exceeds extrahepatic ketone utilization.

The rate of ketogenesis appears to be inversely related to the severity of injury. Major trauma, severe shock, and sepsis attenuate ketogenesis by increasing insulin levels and by rapid tissue oxidation

of free fatty acids. Minor injuries and infections are associated with modest elevations in plasma free fatty acid concentrations and ketogenesis. However, ketogenesis in minor stress states does not exceed that of nonstressed starvation.

Carbohydrate Metabolism

Ingested and enteral carbohydrates are primarily digested in the small intestine, where pancreatic and intestinal enzymes reduce the complex carbohydrates to dimeric units. Disaccharidases (e.g., sucrase, lactase, and maltase) within intestinal brush borders dismantle the complex carbohydrates into simple hexose units, which are transported into the intestinal mucosa. Glucose and galactose are primarily absorbed by energy-dependent active transport coupled to the sodium pump. Fructose absorption, however, occurs by concentration-dependent facilitated diffusion. Both fructose and galactose within the circulation as well as exogenous mannitol (for neurologic injury) do not evoke an insulin response. Intravenous administration of low-dose fructose in fasting humans has been associated with nitrogen conservation, but the clinical utility of fructose administration in human injury remains to be demonstrated.

Discussion of carbohydrate metabolism primarily refers to the utilization of glucose. The oxidation of 1 g of carbohydrate yields 4 kcal, but administered sugar solutions such as that found in intravenous fluids or parenteral nutrition provides only 3.4 kcal/g of dextrose. In starvation, glucose production occurs at the expense of protein stores (i.e., skeletal muscle). Hence, the primary goal for maintenance glucose administration in surgical patients serves to minimize muscle wasting. The exogenous administration of small amounts of glucose (approximately 50 g/d) facilitates fat entry into the TCA cycle and reduces ketosis. Unlike starvation in healthy subjects, studies providing exogenous glucose to septic and trauma patients never have been shown to fully suppress amino acid degradation for gluconeogenesis. This suggests that during periods of stress, other hormonal and proinflammatory mediators have profound influence on the rate of protein degradation and that some degree of muscle wasting is inevitable. The administration of insulin, however, has been shown to reverse protein catabolism during severe stress by stimulating protein synthesis in skeletal muscles and by inhibiting hepatocyte protein degradation. Insulin also stimulates the incorporation of elemental precursors into nucleic acids associated with RNA synthesis in muscle cells.

In cells, glucose is phosphorylated to form glucose-6-phosphate (G6P). G6P can be polymerized during glycogenesis or catabolized in glycogenolysis. Glucose catabolism occurs by cleavage to pyruvate or lactate (pyruvic acid pathway) or by decarboxylation to pentoses (pentose shunt) (Fig. 1-29).

Excess glucose from overfeeding, as reflected by RQs greater than 1.0, can result in conditions such as glucosuria, thermogenesis, and conversion to fat (lipogenesis). Excessive glucose administration results in elevated carbon dioxide production, which may be deleterious in patients with suboptimal pulmonary function.

Injury and severe infections acutely induce a state of peripheral glucose intolerance, despite ample insulin production several-fold above baseline. This may occur in part due to reduced skeletal muscle pyruvate dehydrogenase activity following injury, which diminishes the conversion of pyruvate to acetyl-CoA and subsequent entry into the TCA cycle. The consequent accumulation of three-carbon structures (e.g., pyruvate and lactate) are shunted to the liver as substrate for gluconeogenesis. Furthermore, regional tissue catheterization and isotope dilution studies have shown an increase in net splanchnic glucose production in septic patients by

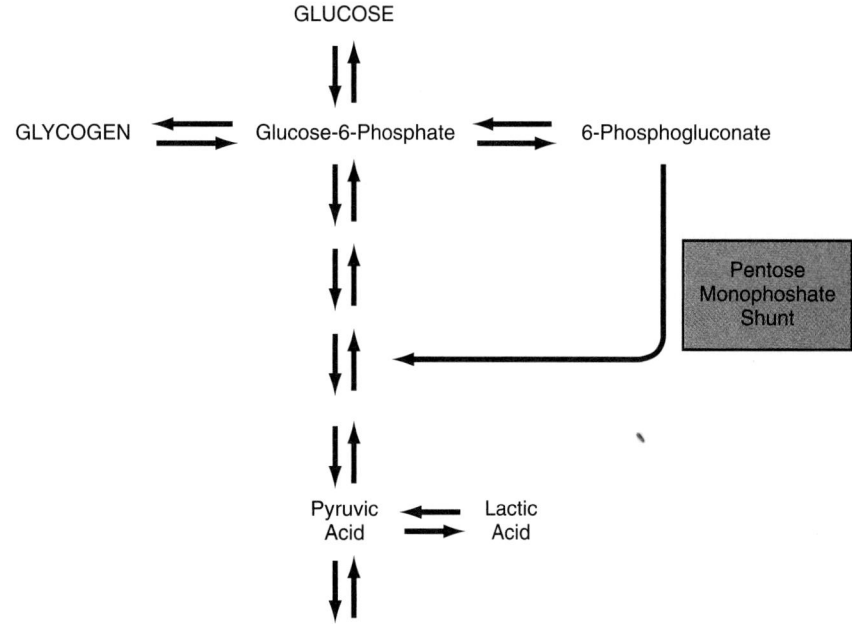

FIG. 1-29. Simplified schema of glucose catabolism through the pentose monophosphate pathway or by breakdown into pyruvate. Glucose-6-phosphate becomes an important "crossroad" for glucose metabolism.

50 to 60%, and a 50 to 100% increase in burn patients. The increase in plasma glucose levels is proportional to the severity of injury, and this net hepatic gluconeogenic response is believed to be under the influence of glucagon. Unlike the nonstressed subject, the hepatic gluconeogenic response to injury or sepsis cannot be suppressed by exogenous or excess glucose administration, but rather persists in the hypermetabolic, critically ill patient. Hepatic gluconeogenesis, arising primarily from alanine and glutamine catabolism, provides a ready fuel source for tissues such as those of the nervous system, wounds, and erythrocytes, which do not require insulin for glucose transport. The elevated glucose concentrations also provide a necessary energy source for leukocytes in inflamed tissues and in sites of microbial invasions.

The shunting of glucose away from nonessential organs such as skeletal muscle and adipose tissues is mediated by catecholamines. Experiments with infusing catecholamines and glucagon in animals have demonstrated elevated plasma glucose levels as a result of increased hepatic gluconeogenesis and peripheral insulin resistance. Interestingly, while glucocorticoid infusion alone does not increase glucose levels, it does prolong and augment the hyperglycemic effects of catecholamines and glucagon when infused concurrently.

Glycogen stores within skeletal muscles can be mobilized by epinephrine activation of β-adrenergic receptors, a GTP-binding protein (G-protein), which subsequently activates the second messenger, cAMP. cAMP activates phosphorylase kinase, which in turn leads to conversion of glycogen to glucose-1-phosphate. Phosphorylase kinase also can be activated by the second messenger, calcium, through the breakdown of phosphatidylinositol phosphate, which is the case in vasopressin-mediated hepatic glycogenolysis.

Glucose Transport and Signaling. Hydrophobic cell membranes are relatively impermeable to hydrophilic glucose molecules. There are two distinct classes of membrane glucose transporters in human systems. These are the facilitated diffusion glucose transporters (GLUT) that permit the transport of glucose down a concentration gradient (Table 1-7) and the Na^+/glucose transport system, which transports glucose molecules against concentration

gradients by active transport. The energy-dependent Na^+/glucose transport system is relatively prevalent on brush borders of small intestine enterocytes and the epithelium of proximal renal tubules.

More than five human facilitated diffusion glucose transporters have been cloned since 1985. GLUT 1 is the transporter in human erythrocytes. It is expressed on several other tissues, but little is found in the liver and skeletal muscle. Importantly, it is a constitutive part of the endothelium in the blood-brain barrier. GLUT 2 is predominantly expressed in the sinusoidal membranes of liver, renal tubules, enterocytes, and insulin-secreting β cells of the pancreas. GLUT 2 is important for rapid export of glucose resulting from gluconeogenesis. GLUT 3 is highly expressed in neuronal tissue of the brain, the kidney, and placenta, but GLUT 3 mRNA has been detected in almost every human tissue. GLUT 4 is significant to human metabolism because it is the *primary* glucose transporter of insulin-sensitive tissues, adipose tissue, and skeletal and cardiac muscle. These transporters are usually packaged as intracellular vesicles, but insulin induces rapid translocation of these vesicles to the cell surface. GLUT 4 function has important implications in the physiology of patients with insulin-resistant diabetes. GLUT 5 has been identified in several tissues, but is primarily expressed in the jejunum. Although it possesses some capacity for glucose transport, it is predominantly a fructose transporter.

Na^+/glucose transport systems are distinct glucose transport systems found in the intestinal epithelium and in the proximal renal

Table 1-7

Human Facilitated Diffusion Glucose Transporter Family

Type	Amino Acids	Major Expression Sites
GLUT 1	492	Placenta, brain, kidney, colon
GLUT 2	524	Liver, pancreatic β cells, kidney, small intestine
GLUT 3	496	Brain, testis
GLUT 4	509	Skeletal muscle, heart muscle, brown and white fat
GLUT 5	501	Small intestine, sperm

tubules. This system transports both sodium and glucose intracellularly, and glucose affinity for this transporter increases when sodium ions are attached. In addition, the Na⁺/glucose transport system within the intestinal lumen also enhances gut retention of water through osmotic absorption.

PROTEIN AND AMINO ACID METABOLISM

The average protein intake in healthy, young adults ranges from 80 to 120 g/d, and every 6 g of protein yields approximately 1 g of nitrogen. The degradation of 1 g of protein yields approximately 4 kcal of energy, almost the same as for carbohydrates.

Following injury the initial systemic proteolysis, mediated primarily by glucocorticoids, increases urinary nitrogen excretion to levels in excess of 30 g/d, which roughly corresponds to a loss in lean body mass of 1.5% per day. An injured individual who does not receive nutrition for 10 days can theoretically lose 15% lean body mass. Therefore amino acids cannot be considered a long-term fuel reserve, and indeed excessive protein depletion (i.e., 25 to 30% of lean body weight) is not compatible with sustaining life.

Protein catabolism following injury provides substrates for gluconeogenesis and for the synthesis of acute phase proteins. Radiolabeled amino acid incorporation studies and protein analyses confirm that skeletal muscles are preferentially depleted acutely following injury, while visceral tissues (e.g., the liver and kidney) remain relatively preserved. The accelerated urea excretion following injury is also associated with the excretion of intracellular elements such as sulfur, phosphorus, potassium, magnesium, and creatinine. Conversely, the rapid utilization of elements such as potassium and magnesium during recovery from major injury may indicate a period of tissue healing.

The net changes in protein catabolism and synthesis correspond to the severity and duration of injury (Fig. 1-30). Elective operations and minor injuries result in lower protein synthesis and moderate protein breakdown. Severe trauma, burns, and sepsis are associated with increased protein catabolism. The rise in urinary nitrogen and negative nitrogen balance can be detected early following injury and peak by 7 days. This state of protein catabolism may persist for as long as 3 to 7 weeks. The patient's prior physical status and age appear to influence the degree of proteolysis following injury or sepsis.

Activation of the ubiquitin-proteosome system in muscle cells is one of the major pathways for protein degradation during acute injury. This response is accentuated by tissue hypoxia, acidosis, insulin resistance, and elevated glucocorticoids.

NUTRITION IN THE SURGICAL PATIENT

The goal of nutritional support in the surgical patient is to prevent or reverse the catabolic effects of disease or injury. While several important biologic parameters have been used to measure the efficacy of nutrition regimens, the ultimate validation for nutritional support in surgical patients should be improvement in clinical outcome and restoration of function.

Estimating Energy Requirements

Overall nutritional assessment is undertaken to determine the severity of nutrient deficiencies or excess and to aid in predicting nutritional requirements. Pertinent information is obtained by determining the presence of weight loss, chronic illnesses, or dietary habits that influence the quantity and quality of food intake. Social habits predisposing to malnutrition and the use of medications that may influence food intake or urination should also be investigated. Physical examination seeks to assess loss of muscle and adipose tissues, organ dysfunction, and subtle changes in skin, hair, or neuromuscular function reflecting frank or impending nutritional deficiency. Anthropometric data (i.e., weight change, skinfold thickness, and arm circumference muscle area) and biochemical determinations (i.e., creatinine excretion, albumin, prealbumin, total lymphocyte count, and transferrin) may be used to substantiate the patient's history and physical findings. It is imprecise to rely on any single or fixed combination of the above findings to accurately assess nutritional status or morbidity. Appreciation for the stresses and natural history of the disease process, in combination with nutritional assessment, remains the basis for identifying patients in acute or anticipated need of nutritional support.

A fundamental goal of nutritional support is to meet the energy requirements for metabolic processes, core temperature

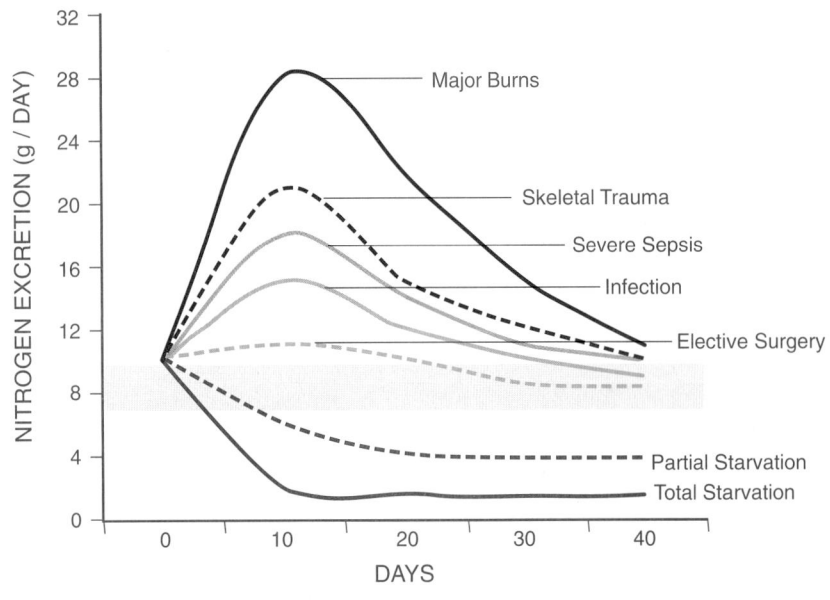

FIG. 1-30. The effect of injury severity on nitrogen wasting. (*Adapted with permission from Long CL: Metabolic response to injury and illness: Estimation of energy and protein needs from indirect calorimetry and nitrogen balance. J Parenter Enteral Nutr 3:452, 1979.*)

Table 1-8
Caloric Adjustments Above Basal Energy Expenditure (BEE) in Hypermetabolic Conditions

Condition	kcal/kg per day	Adjustment Above BEE	Grams of Protein/kg per day	Nonprotein Calories:Nitrogen
Normal/moderate malnutrition	25–30	1.1	1.0	150:1
Mild stress	25–30	1.2	1.2	150:1
Moderate stress	30	1.4	1.5	120:1
Severe stress	30–35	1.6	2.0	90–120:1
Burns	35–40	2.0	2.5	90–100:1

maintenance, and tissue repair. Failure to provide adequate nonprotein energy sources will lead to dissolution of lean tissue stores. The requirement for energy may be measured by indirect calorimetry or estimated from urinary nitrogen excretion, which is proportional to resting energy expenditure. However, the use of indirect calorimetry, particularly in the critically ill patient, is labor intensive and often leads to overestimation of caloric requirements.

Basal energy expenditure (BEE) may also be estimated using the Harris-Benedict equations:

$$BEE \text{ (men)} = 66.47 + 13.75 \text{ (W)} + 5.0 \text{ (H)} - 6.76 \text{ (A) kcal/d}$$

$$BEE \text{ (women)} = 655.1 + 9.56 \text{ (W)} + 1.85 \text{ (H)} - 4.68 \text{ (A) kcal/d}$$

where W = weight in kilograms,
H = height in centimeters, and
A = age in years.

These equations, adjusted for the type of surgical stress, are suitable for estimating energy requirements in over 80% of hospitalized patients. It has been demonstrated that the provision of 30 kcal/kg per day will adequately meet energy requirements in most postsurgical patients, with low risk of overfeeding. Following trauma or sepsis, energy substrate demands are increased, necessitating greater nonprotein calories beyond calculated energy expenditure (Table 1-8). These additional nonprotein calories provided after injury are usually 1.2 to 2.0 times greater than calculated resting energy expenditure (REE), depending on the type of injury. It is seldom appropriate to exceed this level of nonprotein energy intake during the height of the catabolic phase.

The second objective of nutritional support is to meet the substrate requirements for protein synthesis. An appropriate nonprotein calorie:nitrogen ratio of 150:1 (e.g., 1 g N = 6.25 g protein) should be maintained, which is the basal calorie requirement provided to prevent use of protein as an energy source. There is now greater evidence suggesting that increased protein intake, and a lower calorie:nitrogen ratio of 80:1 to 100:1, may benefit healing in selected hypermetabolic or critically ill patients. In the absence of severe renal or hepatic dysfunction precluding the use of standard nutritional regimens, approximately 0.25 to 0.35 g of nitrogen per kilogram of body weight should be provided daily.

Vitamins and Minerals

The requirements for vitamins and essential trace minerals usually can be easily met in the average patient with an uncomplicated postoperative course. Therefore vitamins are usually not given in the absence of preoperative deficiencies (Table 1-9). Patients maintained on elemental diets or parenteral hyperalimentation require complete vitamin and mineral supplementation. Commercial enteral diets contain varying amounts of essential minerals and vitamins. It is necessary to ensure that adequate replacement is available in the diet or by supplementation. Numerous commercial vitamin preparations are available for intravenous or intramuscular use, although most do not contain vitamin K and some do not contain vitamin B_{12} or folic acid. Supplemental trace minerals may be given intravenously by commercial preparations. Essential fatty acid supplementation may also be necessary, especially in patients with depletion of adipose stores.

Overfeeding

Overfeeding usually results from overestimation of caloric needs, as occurs when actual body weight is used to calculate the BEE in such patient populations as the critically ill with significant fluid overload and the obese. Indirect calorimetry can be used to quantify energy requirements, but frequently overestimates BEE by 10 to 15% in stressed patients, particularly if they are on a ventilator. In these instances, estimated dry weight should be obtained from preinjury records or family members. Adjusted lean body weight also can be calculated. Clinically, increased oxygen consumption, increased CO_2 production, fatty liver, suppression of leukocyte function, and increased infectious risks have all been documented with overfeeding.

ENTERAL NUTRITION

Rationale for Enteral Nutrition

Enteral nutrition generally is preferred over parenteral nutrition based on reduced cost and associated risks of the intravenous route. Laboratory models have long demonstrated that luminal nutrient contact reduces intestinal mucosal atrophy when compared with parenteral or no nutritional support. Studies comparing postoperative enteral and parenteral nutrition in patients undergoing gastrointestinal surgery have demonstrated reduced infection complications and acute phase protein production when fed by the enteral route. Yet, prospectively randomized studies for patients with adequate nutritional status (albumin ≥4 g/dL) undergoing gastrointestinal surgery demonstrate no differences in outcome and complications when administered enteral nutrition compared to maintenance intravenous fluids alone in the initial days following surgery. Furthermore, intestinal permeability studies in well-nourished patients undergoing upper gastrointestinal cancer surgery demonstrated normalization of intestinal permeability by the fifth postoperative day. At the other extreme, recent meta-analysis for critically ill patients demonstrates a 44% reduction in infectious complications in those receiving enteral nutritional support over those receiving parenteral nutrition. Most prospectively randomized studies for severe abdominal and thoracic trauma demonstrate significant reductions in infectious complications for patients given early enteral nutrition when compared with those who are unfed or receiving parenteral nutrition. The exception has been in studies for patients with closed-head injury, because no significant differences in outcome are demonstrated between early jejunal feeding compared with other nutritional support modalities.

Table 1-9
Common Manifestations of Vitamin and Mineral Deficiencies in Adults

	Major Manifestations of Deficiencies
Vitamins	
Vitamin A	Night blindness, corneal/conjunctiva drying
Vitamin D	Rickets, osteomalacia, bone pain
Vitamin E	Chronic cholestasis, spinocerebellar ataxia, hyporeflexia
Vitamin K	Hemorrhagic disorders
Thiamin (B_1)	Dry beriberi (mental status changes, peripheral neuropathy), wet beriberi (heart failure)
Riboflavin	Sebaceous gland inflammation
Niacin	Dermatosis, pellagra
Pyridoxine (B_6)	Peripheral neuropathy
Biotin	Dry and scaling skin, glossitis
Vitamin B_{12}	Pernicious anemia, neuropathy, myelopathy, glossitis
Folic acid	Similar to B_{12} deficiency
Pantothenic acid	Headache, insomnia, paresthesias
Vitamin C	Scurvy (weakness, listlessness, musculoskeletal pain), perifollicular hemorrhage
Essential fatty acids	Hair loss, dry skin, eczematoid dermatosis
Minerals	
Calcium	Dementia, encephalopathy, tetany
Phosphorus	Mental status changes, erythrocyte hemolysis, paresthesias
Potassium	Respiratory failure, paralytic ileus, tetany, arrhythmias
Magnesium	Hypocalcemia, hypokalemia, neuromuscular spasms, gut malabsorption
Iodine	Goiter
Iron	Microcytic anemia, fatigue, dyspnea
Copper	Hypochromic anemia (unresponsive to iron), neutropenia, osteoporosis
Zinc	Dermatosis, photophobia, night blindness, impaired wound healing, alopecia, diarrhea
Fluoride	No acute clinical signs
Selenium	Cardiomyopathy, myalgia, white nail beds
Chromium	Glucose intolerance
Cobalt	No acute clinical signs known
Molybdenum	Headache, night blindness, lethargy
Manganese	Hair thinning, weight loss, dermatitis

Moreover, early gastric feeding following closed-head injury was frequently associated with underfeeding and calorie deficiency due to difficulties overcoming gastroparesis and the high risk of aspiration.

The early initiation of enteral feeding in burn patients, while sensible and supported by retrospective analysis, is an empiric practice supported by limited prospective trials.

Recommendations for instituting early *enteral* nutrition to surgical patients with moderate malnutrition (albumin = 2.9 to 3.5 g/dL) can only be made by inferences due to a lack of data directly pertaining to this population. For these patients, it is prudent to offer enteral nutrition based on measured energy expenditure of the recovering patient, or if complications arise that may alter the anticipated course of recovery (e.g., anastomotic leaks, return to surgery, sepsis, or failure to wean from the ventilator). Other clinical scenarios with substantiated benefits from enteral nutritional support include permanent neurologic impairment, oropharyngeal dysfunction, short bowel syndrome, and bone marrow transplantation patients.

Collectively, the data support the use of early enteral nutritional support following major trauma and in patients who are anticipated to have prolonged recovery after surgery. Healthy patients without malnutrition undergoing uncomplicated surgery can tolerate 10 days of partial starvation (i.e., maintenance intravenous fluids only) before any significant protein catabolism occurs. Earlier intervention is likely indicated in patients with poorer preoperative nutritional status.

Initiation of enteral nutrition should occur immediately after adequate resuscitation, most readily determined by adequate urine output. Presence of bowel sounds and the passage of flatus or stool are not absolute requisites for initiating enteral nutrition, but feedings in the setting of gastroparesis should be administered distal to the pylorus. Gastric residuals of 200 mL or more in a 4- to 6-hour period or abdominal distention will require cessation of feeding and adjustment of the infusion rate. Concomitant gastric decompression with distal small bowel feedings may be appropriate in certain patients such as closed-head injury patients with gastroparesis. There is no evidence to support withholding enteric feedings for patients following bowel resection, or in those with low-output enterocutaneous fistulas of less than 500 mL/d, but low-residue formulations may be preferred. Enteral feeding should also be offered to patients with short-bowel syndrome or clinical malabsorption, but caloric needs, essential minerals, and vitamins should be supplemented with parenteral modalities.

Enteral Formulas

The functional status of the gastrointestinal tract determines the type of enteral solutions to be used. Patients with an intact gastrointestinal tract will tolerate complex solutions, but patients who have not been fed via the gastrointestinal tract for prolonged periods are less likely to tolerate complex carbohydrates such as lactose. In patients with malabsorption such as in inflammatory bowel diseases, absorption may be improved by provision of dipeptides, tripeptides, and medium-chain triglycerides (MCTs). However, MCTs are deficient in essential fatty acids, which necessitates supplementation with some long-chain triglycerides (LCT).

In general, factors that influence the choice of enteral formula include the extent of organ dysfunction (e.g., renal, pulmonary, hepatic, or gastrointestinal), the nutrient needs to restore optimal function and healing, and the cost of specific products. There are still no conclusive data to recommend one category of product over another, and nutritional support committees typically develop the most cost-efficient set of enteral formulary for the most commonly encountered disease categories within the institution.

Low-Residue Isotonic Formulas. Most provide a caloric density of 1.0 kcal/mL, and approximately 1500 to 1800 mL are required to meet daily requirements. These low-osmolarity compositions provide baseline carbohydrates, protein, electrolytes, water, fat, and fat-soluble vitamins (some do not have vitamin K) and typically have a nonprotein-calorie:nitrogen ratio of 150:1. These contain no fiber bulk and therefore leave minimum residue. These solutions are usually considered to be the standard or first-line formulas for stable patients with an intact gastrointestinal tract.

Isotonic Formulas with Fiber. These formulas contain soluble and insoluble fiber which are most often soy based. Physiologically, fiber-based solutions delay intestinal transit time and may reduce the incidence of diarrhea compared with nonfiber solutions. Fiber stimulates pancreatic lipase activity and are degraded by gut bacteria into short-chain fatty acids, an important fuel for colonocytes. There are no contraindications for using fiber-containing formulas in critically ill patients.

Immune-Enhancing Formulas. These formulas are fortified with special nutrients that are purported to enhance various aspects of immune or solid organ function. Such additives include glutamine, arginine, branched-chain amino acids, omega-3 fatty acids, nucleotides, and beta-carotene. While several trials have proposed that one or more of these additives reduce surgical complications and improve outcome, these results have not been uniformly corroborated by other trials. The addition of amino acids to these formulas generally doubles the amount of protein (nitrogen) found in standard formula; however, their use can be cost-prohibitive.

Calorie-Dense Formulas. The primary distinction of these formulas is a greater caloric value for the same volume. Most commercial products of this variety provide 1.5 to 2 kcal/mL, and therefore are suitable for patients requiring fluid restriction or those unable to tolerate large volume infusions. As expected, these solutions have higher osmolality than standard formulas and are suitable for intragastric feedings.

High-Protein Formulas. High-protein formulas are available in isotonic and nonisotonic mixtures and are proposed for critically ill or trauma patients with high protein requirements. These formulas comprise nonprotein calorie:nitrogen ratios between 80 and 120:1.

Elemental Formulas. These formulas contain predigested nutrients and provide proteins in the form of small peptides. Complex carbohydrates are limited, and fat content, in the form of MCTs and LCTs, is minimal. The primary advantage of such a formula is ease of absorption, but the inherent scarcity of fat, associated vitamins, and trace elements limits its long-term use as a primary source of nutrients. Due to its high osmolarity, dilution or slow infusion rates are usually necessary, particularly in critically ill patients. These formulas have been used frequently in patients with malabsorption, gut impairment, and pancreatitis, but their cost is significantly higher than that of standard formulas.

Renal-Failure Formulas. The primary benefits of the renal formula are the lower fluid volume and concentrations of potassium, phosphorus, and magnesium needed to meet daily calorie requirements. This formulation almost exclusively contains essential amino acids and has a high nonprotein:calorie ratio; however, it does not contain trace elements or vitamins.

Pulmonary-Failure Formulas. In these formulas, fat content is usually increased to 50% of the total calories, with a corresponding reduction in carbohydrate content. The goal is to reduce CO_2 production and alleviate ventilation burden for failing lungs.

Hepatic-Failure Formulas. Close to 50% of the proteins in this formula are branched-chain amino acids (e.g., leucine, isoleucine, and valine). The goal of such a formula is to reduce aromatic amino acid levels and increase branched-chain amino acids, which can potentially reverse encephalopathy in patients with hepatic failure. However, the use of this formula is controversial because no clear benefits have been proven by clinical trials. Protein restriction should be avoided in patients with end-stage liver disease, because they have significant protein energy malnutrition, predisposing them to additional morbidity and mortality.

Access for Enteral Nutritional Support

The available techniques and repertoire for enteral access have provided multiple options for feeding the gut. Presently utilized methods and preferred indications are summarized in Table 1-10.

Nasoenteric Tubes. Nasogastric feeding should be reserved for those with intact mental status and protective laryngeal reflexes to minimize risks of aspiration. Even in intubated patients, nasogastric feedings can often be recovered from tracheal suction. Nasojejunal feedings are associated with fewer pulmonary complications, but access past the pylorus requires greater effort to accomplish. Blind insertion of nasogastric feeding tubes is fraught with misplacement, and air instillation with auscultation is inaccurate for ascertaining proper positioning. Radiographic confirmation is usually required to verify the position of the nasogastric feeding tube.

Several methods have been recommended for the passage of nasoenteric feeding tubes into the small bowel, including prokinetic agents, right lateral decubitus positioning, gastric insufflation, tube angulation, and clockwise torque. However, the successful placement of feeding tubes by these methods is highly variable and operator dependent. Furthermore, it is time-consuming, and success rates for intubation past the duodenum into the jejunum by these methods are less than 20%. Fluoroscopy-guided intubation past the pylorus has a greater than 90% success rate, and more than half of these intubations result in jejunal placement. Similarly, endoscopy-guided placement past the pylorus has high success rates, but advancing the tube beyond the second portion of the duodenum using a standard gastroduodenoscope is unlikely to be successful.

Small bowel feeding is more reliable for delivering nutrition than nasogastric feeding. Furthermore, the risks of aspiration pneumonia can be reduced by 25% with small bowel feeding when compared with nasogastric feeding. The disadvantages of nasoenteric feeding tubes are clogging, kinking, inadvertent displacement or removal, and nasopharyngeal complications. If nasoenteric feeding will be required for longer than 30 days, access should be converted to a percutaneous one.

Percutaneous Endoscopic Gastrostomy. The most common indications for percutaneous endoscopic gastrostomy (PEG) placement include impaired swallowing mechanisms,

Table 1-10
Options for Enteral Feeding Access

Access Option	Comments
Nasogastric tube	Short-term use only; aspiration risks; nasopharyngeal trauma; frequent dislodgment
Nasoduodenal/nasojejunal	Short-term use; lower aspiration risks in jejunum; placement challenges (radiographic assistance often necessary)
Percutaneous endoscopic gastrostomy (PEG)	Endoscopy skills required; may be used for gastric decompression or bolus feeds; aspiration risks; can last 12–24 months; slightly higher complication rates with placement and site leaks
Surgical gastrostomy	Requires general anesthesia and small laparotomy; may allow placement of extended duodenal/jejunal feeding ports; laparoscopic placement possible
Fluoroscopic gastrostomy	Blind placement using needle and T-prongs to anchor to stomach; can thread smaller catheter through gastrostomy into duodenum/jejunum under fluoroscopy
PEG-jejunal tube	Jejunal placement with regular endoscope is operator dependent; jejunal tube often dislodges retrograde; two-stage procedure with PEG placement, followed by fluoroscopic conversion with jejunal feeding tube through PEG
Direct percutaneous endoscopic jejunostomy (DPEJ)	Direct endoscopic placement with enteroscope; placement challenges; greater injury risks
Surgical jejunostomy	Commonly applied during laparotomy; general anesthesia; laparoscopic placement usually requires assistant to thread catheter; laparoscopy offers direct visualization of catheter placement
Fluoroscopic jejunostomy	Difficult approach with injury risks; not commonly done

oropharyngeal or esophageal obstruction, and major facial trauma. It is frequently utilized for debilitated patients requiring caloric supplementation, hydration, or frequent medication dosing. It is also appropriate for patients requiring passive gastric decompression. Relative contraindications for PEG placement include ascites, coagulopathy, gastric varices, gastric neoplasm, and lack of a suitable abdominal site. Most tubes are 18F to 28F in size and may be used for 12 to 24 months.

Identification of the PEG site requires endoscopic transillumination of the anterior stomach against the abdominal wall. A 14-gauge angiocatheter is passed through the abdominal wall into the fully insufflated stomach. A guidewire is threaded through the angiocatheter, grasped by snares or forceps, and pulled out through the mouth. The tapered end of the PEG tube is secured to the guidewire and is pulled into position out of the abdominal wall. Once the PEG tube is secured without tension against the abdominal wall, many have reported using the tube within hours of placement. It has been the practice of some to connect the PEG tube to a drainage bag for passive decompression for 24 hours prior to use, allowing more time for the stomach to seal against the peritoneum.

If endoscopy is not available or technical obstacles preclude PEG placement, the interventional radiologist can attempt the procedure percutaneously under fluoroscopic guidance by first insufflating the stomach against the abdominal wall with a nasogastric tube. If this is also unsuccessful, surgical gastrostomy tube placement can be considered, particularly with minimally invasive methods. When surgery is consulted, it may be wise to consider directly accessing the small bowel for nutrition delivery.

While PEG tubes enhance nutritional delivery, facilitate nursing care, and are superior to nasogastric tubes, serious complications can occur in approximately 3% of patients. These complications include wound infection, necrotizing fasciitis, peritonitis, aspiration, leaks, dislodgment, bowel perforation, enteric fistulas, bleeding, and aspiration pneumonia. For patients with significant gastroparesis or gastric outlet obstruction, feedings through PEG tubes are hazardous. In this instance, the PEG tube can be used for decompression and to

allow access for converting the PEG tube to a transpyloric feeding tube.

Percutaneous Endoscopic Gastrostomy-Jejunostomy and Direct Percutaneous Endoscopic Jejunostomy. While gastric bolus feedings are more physiologic, patients who cannot tolerate gastric feedings or have significant aspiration risks should be fed directly past the pylorus. The percutaneous endoscopic gastrostomy-jejunostomy (PEG-J) method passes a 9F to 12F tube through an existing PEG tube, past the pylorus, and into the duodenum. This can be achieved by endoscopic or fluoroscopic guidance. With weighted catheter tips and guidewires, the tube can be further advanced past the ligament of Treitz. However, long-term PEG-J malfunction has been reported to be greater than 50% as a result of retrograde tube migration into the stomach, kinking, or clogging.

Direct percutaneous endoscopic jejunostomy (DPEJ) placement uses the same techniques as PEG tube placement, but requires an enteroscope or colonoscope to reach the jejunum. DPEJ malfunctions are probably less frequent than with PEG-J, and kinking or clogging is usually averted by placement of larger caliber catheters. The success rate of DPEJ placement is variable because of the complexity of endoscopic skills required to locate a suitable jejunal site. In such cases, surgical jejunostomy tube placement is more appropriate, especially when minimally invasive techniques are available.

Surgical Gastrostomy and Jejunostomy. In a patient undergoing complex abdominal or trauma surgery, thought should be given during surgery to the possible routes for subsequent nutritional support, because laparotomy affords direct access to the stomach or small bowel. The only absolute contraindication to feeding jejunostomy is distal intestinal obstruction. Relative contraindications include severe edema of the intestinal wall, radiation enteritis, inflammatory bowel disease, ascites, severe immunodeficiency, and bowel ischemia. Needle-catheter jejunostomies can also be done with a minimal learning curve. The biggest drawback is usually related to clogging and knotting of the 6F catheter.

Table 1-11
Incidence of Septic Morbidity in Parenterally and Enterally Fed Trauma Patients

Complication	Blunt Trauma		Penetrating Trauma		Total	
	TEN n = 48	TPN n = 44	TEN n = 38	TPN n = 48	TEN n = 44	TPN n = 84
Abdominal Abscess	2	1	2	6	4	7
Pneumonia	4	10	1	2	5	12
Wound Infection	0	2	3	1	3	3
Bacteremia	1	4	0	1	1	5
Urinary Tract	1	1	0	1	1	2
Other	5	4	1	1	6	5
Total Complications	**13**	**22**	**7**	**12**	**20**	**34**
% Complications per patient group	**27%**	**50%**	**18%**	**30%**	**23%**	**39%**

SOURCE: Adapted with permission from Katz JA, Lowry SF: Substrate utilization and hypermetabolism, in Bone RC (ed): *Sepsis and Multiorgan Failure.* Philadelphia: Williams & Wilkins, 1997, p 315.

Abdominal distention and cramps are common adverse effects of early enteral nutrition. Some have also reported impaired respiratory mechanics as a result of intolerance to enteral feedings. These are mostly correctable by temporarily discontinuing feeds and resuming at a lower infusion rate.

Pneumatosis intestinalis and small bowel necrosis are infrequent but significant problems associated with patients receiving jejunal tube feedings. Several contributing factors have been proposed, including the hyperosmolar consistency of enteral solutions, bacterial overgrowth, fermentation, and metabolic breakdown products. The common pathophysiology is believed to be bowel distention and consequent reduction in bowel wall perfusion. Risk factors for these complications include cardiogenic and circulatory shock, vasopressor use, diabetes mellitus, and chronic obstructive pulmonary disease. Therefore, enteral feedings in the critically ill patient should be delayed until adequate resuscitation has been achieved. Alternatively, dilution of standard enteral formula, delaying the progression to goal infusion rates, or using monomeric solutions with low osmolality requiring less digestion by the gastrointestinal tract have all been successfully employed.

PARENTERAL NUTRITION

Parenteral nutrition involves the continuous infusion of a hyperosmolar solution containing carbohydrates, proteins, fat, and other necessary nutrients through an indwelling catheter inserted into the superior vena cava. In order to obtain the maximum benefit, the ratio of calories to nitrogen must be adequate (at least 100 to 150 kcal/g nitrogen), and both carbohydrates and proteins must be infused simultaneously. When the sources of calories and nitrogen are given at different times, there is a significant decrease in nitrogen utilization. These nutrients can be given in quantities considerably greater than the basic caloric and nitrogen requirements, and this method has proved to be highly successful in achieving growth and development, positive nitrogen balance, and weight gain in a variety of clinical situations. Clinical trials and meta-analysis of parenteral feeding in the perioperative period have suggested that preoperative nutritional support may benefit some surgical patients, particularly those with extensive malnutrition. Short-term use of parenteral nutrition in critically ill patients (i.e., duration <7 days) when enteral nutrition may have been instituted is associated with higher rates of infectious complications. Following severe injury, parenteral nutrition is associated with higher rates of infectious risks when compared with enteral feeding (Table 1-11). Clinical studies have demonstrated that parenteral feeding with complete bowel rest results in augmented stress hormone and inflammatory mediator response to an antigenic challenge (Fig. 1-31). However, parenteral feeding still has fewer infectious complications compared with no feeding at all. In cancer patients, parenteral nutrition has not been shown to benefit clinical response, survival, or toxic effects of chemotherapy, while infectious complications increased.

Rationale for Parenteral Nutrition

The principal indications for parenteral nutrition are found in seriously ill patients suffering from malnutrition, sepsis, or surgical or accidental trauma, when use of the gastrointestinal tract for feedings is not possible. In some instances, intravenous nutrition may be used to supplement inadequate oral intake. The safe and successful use of parenteral nutrition requires proper selection of patients with specific nutritional needs, experience with the technique, and an awareness of the associated complications. As with enteral nutrition, the fundamental goals are to provide sufficient calories and nitrogen substrate to promote tissue repair and to maintain the integrity or growth of lean tissue mass. Listed below are situations in which parenteral nutrition has been used in an effort to achieve these goals:

1. Newborn infants with catastrophic gastrointestinal anomalies, such as tracheoesophageal fistula, gastroschisis, omphalocele, or massive intestinal atresia.
2. Infants who fail to thrive due to gastrointestinal insufficiency associated with short bowel syndrome, malabsorption, enzyme deficiency, meconium ileus, or idiopathic diarrhea.
3. Adult patients with short bowel syndrome secondary to massive small bowel resection (<100 cm without colon or ileocecal valve, or <50 cm with intact ileocecal valve and colon).
4. Enteroenteric, enterocolic, enterovesical, or high-output enterocutaneous fistulas (>500 mL/d).
5. Surgical patients with prolonged paralytic ileus following major operations (>7 to 10 days), multiple injuries, blunt or open abdominal trauma, or patients with reflex ileus complicating various medical diseases.
6. Patients with normal bowel length but with malabsorption secondary to sprue, hypoproteinemia, enzyme or pancreatic insufficiency, regional enteritis, or ulcerative colitis.
7. Adult patients with functional gastrointestinal disorders such as esophageal dyskinesia following cerebrovascular accident, idiopathic diarrhea, psychogenic vomiting, or anorexia nervosa.

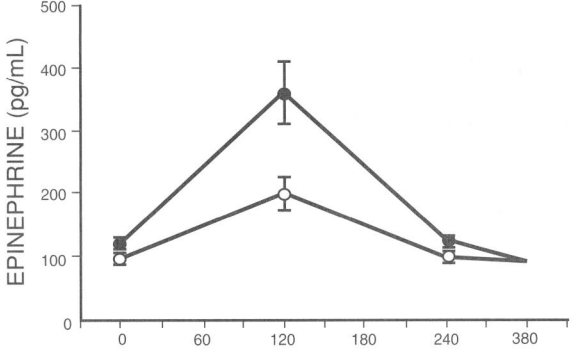

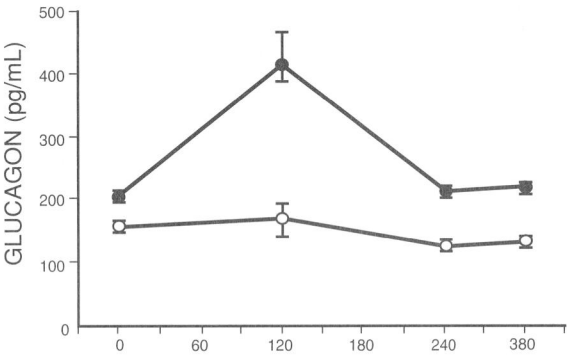

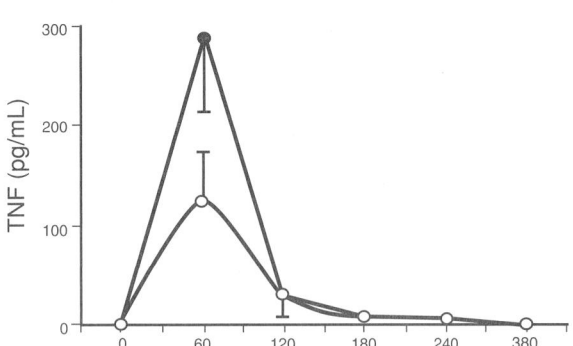

FIG. 1-31. The appearance of circulating epinephrine, glucagons, and tumor necrosis factor (TNF) after a bolus injection of endotoxin in subjects who received 7 days of parenteral nutrition and complete bowel rest (*closed circles*), as compared to subjects who received enteral feedings (*open circles*). Subjects receiving intravenous feedings and bowel rest had significantly exaggerated response to injury. (*Adapted with permission from Fong Y, Marano MA, Barber A, et al: Total parenteral nutrition and bowel rest modify the metabolic response to endotoxin in humans. Ann Surg 210:449, 1989.*)

8. Patients with granulomatous colitis, ulcerative colitis, and tuberculous enteritis, in which major portions of the absorptive mucosa are diseased.
9. Patients with malignancy, with or without cachexia, in whom malnutrition might jeopardize successful delivery of a therapeutic option.
10. Failed attempts to provide adequate calories by enteral tube feedings or high residuals.
11. Critically ill patients who are hypermetabolic for more than 5 days or when enteral nutrition is not feasible.

Conditions *contraindicating* hyperalimentation include the following:

1. Lack of a specific goal for patient management, or in cases in which instead of extending a meaningful life, inevitable dying is delayed.

2. Periods of hemodynamic instability or severe metabolic derangement (e.g., severe hyperglycemia, azotemia, encephalopathy, hyperosmolality, and fluid-electrolyte disturbances) requiring control or correction before attempting hypertonic intravenous feeding.
3. Feasible gastrointestinal tract feeding; in the vast majority of instances, this is the best route by which to provide nutrition.
4. Patients with good nutritional status.
5. Infants with less than 8 cm of small bowel, since virtually all have been unable to adapt sufficiently despite prolonged periods of parenteral nutrition.
6. Patients who are irreversibly decerebrate or otherwise dehumanized.

Total Parenteral Nutrition

Total parenteral nutrition (TPN), also referred to as central parenteral nutrition, requires access to a large-diameter vein to deliver the entire nutritional requirements of the individual. Dextrose content is high (15 to 25%) and all other macro- and micronutrients are deliverable by this route.

Peripheral Parenteral Nutrition

The lower osmolarity of the solution used for peripheral parenteral nutrition (PPN), secondary to reduced dextrose (5 to 10%) and protein (3%) levels, allows for its administration via peripheral veins. Some nutrients cannot be supplemented due to inability to concentrate them into small volumes. Therefore PPN is not appropriate for repleting patients with severe malnutrition. It can be considered if central routes are not available or if supplemental nutritional support is required. Typically, PPN is used for short periods (<2 weeks). Beyond this time, TPN should be instituted.

Initiating Parenteral Nutrition

The basic solution contains a final concentration of 15 to 25% dextrose and 3 to 5% crystalline amino acids. The solutions are usually prepared in sterile conditions in the pharmacy from commercially available kits containing the component solutions and transfer apparatus. Preparation in the pharmacy under laminar flow hoods reduces the incidence of bacterial contamination of the solution. Proper preparation with suitable quality control is absolutely essential to avoid septic complications.

The proper provision of electrolytes and amino acids is dependent on routes of fluid and electrolyte loss, renal function, metabolic rate, cardiac function, and the underlying disease state.

Intravenous vitamin preparations should also be added to parenteral formulas. Vitamin deficiencies are rare occurrences if such preparations are utilized. In addition, because vitamin K is not part of any commercially prepared vitamin solution, it should be supplemented on a weekly basis. During prolonged fat-free parenteral nutrition, essential fatty acid deficiency may become clinically apparent and manifests as dry, scaly dermatitis and loss of hair. The syndrome may be prevented by periodic infusion of a fat emulsion at a rate equivalent to 10 to 15% of total calories. Essential trace minerals may be required after prolonged total parenteral nutrition, and may be supplied by direct addition of commercial preparations. The most frequent presentation of trace mineral deficiencies is the eczematoid rash developing both diffusely and at intertriginous areas in zinc-deficient patients. Other rare trace mineral deficiencies include a microcytic anemia associated with copper deficiency, and glucose intolerance presumably related to chromium deficiency. The latter complications are seldom seen except in patients receiving parenteral nutrition for extended periods of time. The daily administration of commercially available trace mineral supplements will obviate most such problems.

Depending on fluid and nitrogen tolerance, parenteral nutrition solutions can generally be increased over 2 to 3 days to achieve the desired infusion rate. Insulin may be supplemented as necessary to ensure glucose tolerance. Additional intravenous fluids and electrolytes may occasionally be necessary with persistently high fluid losses. The patient should be carefully monitored for development of electrolyte, volume, acid-base, and septic complications. Vital signs and urinary output are regularly observed, and the patient should be weighed regularly. Frequent adjustments of the volume and composition of the solutions are necessary during the course of therapy. Electrolytes are drawn daily until stable and every 2 or 3 days thereafter. Blood counts, blood urea nitrogen, liver functions, and phosphate and magnesium levels are determined at least weekly.

The urine or capillary blood sugar level is checked every 6 hours and serum sugar concentration checked at least once daily during the first few days of the infusion and at frequent intervals thereafter. Relative glucose intolerance that often manifests as glycosuria may occur following initiation of parenteral nutrition. If blood sugar levels remain elevated or glycosuria persists, the dextrose concentration may be decreased, the infusion rate slowed, or regular insulin added to each bottle. The rise in blood glucose concentration observed after initiating parenteral nutrition may be temporary, as the normal pancreas increases its output of insulin in response to the continuous carbohydrate infusion. In patients with diabetes mellitus, additional insulin may be required.

Potassium is essential to achieve positive nitrogen balance and replace depleted intracellular stores. In addition, a significant shift of potassium ion from the extracellular to the intracellular space may take place because of the large glucose infusion, with resultant hypokalemia, metabolic alkalosis, and poor glucose utilization. In some cases as much as 240 mEq of potassium ion daily may be required. Hypokalemia may cause glycosuria, which would be treated with potassium, not insulin. Thus, before giving insulin, the serum potassium level must be checked to avoid exacerbating the hypokalemia.

Patients with insulin-dependent diabetes mellitus may exhibit wide fluctuations in blood glucose during parenteral nutrition. Partial replacement with lipid emulsions for dextrose calories may alleviate these problems in selected patients.

Lipid emulsions derived from soybean or safflower oils are widely used as an adjunctive nutrient to prevent the development of essential fatty acid deficiency. There is no evidence of enhanced metabolic benefit when greater than 10 to 15% of calories are provided as lipid emulsions. While the administration of 500 mL of 20% fat emulsion one to three times a week is sufficient to prevent essential fatty acid deficiency, it is common to provide fat emulsions on a daily basis to provide additional calories. The triple mix of carbohydrate, fat, and amino acids is infused at a constant rate during a 24-hour period. The theoretical advantages of a constant fat infusion rate include increased efficiency of lipid utilization and reduced impairment of reticuloendothelial function normally identified with bolus lipid infusions. The addition of lipids to an infusion bag may alter the stability of some micronutrients in a dextrose-amino acid preparation.

Intravenous Access Methods

Temporary or short-term access can be achieved with a 16-gauge, percutaneous catheter inserted into a subclavian or internal jugular vein and threaded into the superior vena cava. More permanent access, with the intention of providing long-term or home parenteral nutrition, can be achieved by placement of a catheter with a subcutaneous port for access, by tunneling a catheter with a substantial subcutaneous length, or threading a long catheter through the basilic or cephalic vein into the superior vena cava.

Complications of Parenteral Nutrition

Technical Complications

One of the more common and serious complications associated with long-term parenteral feeding is sepsis secondary to contamination of the central venous catheter. Contamination of solutions should be considered, but is rare when proper pharmacy protocols have been followed. This problem occurs more frequently in patients with systemic sepsis, and in many cases is due to hematogenous seeding of the catheter with bacteria. One of the earliest signs of systemic sepsis may be the sudden development of glucose intolerance (with or without temperature increase) in a patient who previously has been maintained on parenteral alimentation without difficulty. When this occurs or if high fever (>38.5°C) develops without obvious cause, a diligent search for a potential septic focus is indicated. Other causes of fever should also be investigated. If fever persists, the infusion catheter should be removed and cultured. If the catheter is the cause of fever, removal of the infectious source is usually followed by rapid defervescence. Some centers are now replacing catheters considered at low risk for infection over a guidewire. Should evidence of infection persist over 24 to 48 hours without a definable source, the catheter should be replaced in the opposite subclavian vein or into one of the internal jugular veins and the infusion restarted. It is prudent to delay reinserting the catheter by 12 to 24 hours, especially if bacteremia is present.

Other complications related to catheter placement include the development of pneumothorax, hemothorax, hydrothorax, subclavian artery injury, thoracic duct injury, cardiac arrhythmia, air embolism, catheter embolism, and cardiac perforation with tamponade. All of these complications may be avoided by strict adherence to proper techniques.

The use of multilumen catheters may be associated with a slightly increased risk of infection. This is most likely associated with greater catheter manipulation and intensive use. Catheter infections are highest when placed in the femoral vein, lower with jugular vein, and lowest for the subclavian vein. When catheters are indwelling for less than 3 days, infection risks are negligible. If indwelling time is 3 to 7 days, the infection risk is 3 to 5%. Greater than 7 days indwelling time is associated with a catheter infection risk of 5 to 10%.

Metabolic Complications

Hyperglycemia may develop with normal rates of infusion in patients with impaired glucose tolerance or in any patient if the hypertonic solutions are administered too rapidly. This is a particularly common complication in latent diabetics and in patients subjected to severe surgical stress or trauma. Treatment of the condition consists of volume replacement with correction of electrolyte abnormalities and the administration of insulin. This complication can be avoided with careful attention to daily fluid balance and frequent monitoring of blood sugar levels and serum electrolytes.

Increasing experience has emphasized the importance of not overfeeding the parenterally nourished patient. This is particularly true of the depleted patient in whom excess calorie infusion may result in carbon dioxide retention and respiratory insufficiency. In addition, excess feeding also has been related to the development of hepatic steatosis or marked glycogen deposition in selected patients. Cholestasis and formation of gallstones are common in patients receiving long-term parenteral nutrition. Mild but transient abnormalities of serum transaminase, alkaline phosphatase, and bilirubin may occur in many parenterally nourished patients. Failure of the liver enzymes to plateau or return to normal over 7 to 14 days should suggest another etiology.

Intestinal Atrophy

Lack of intestinal stimulation is associated with intestinal mucosal atrophy, diminished villous height, bacterial overgrowth, reduced lymphoid tissue size, reduced IgA production, and impaired gut immunity. The full clinical implications of these changes are not well realized, although bacterial translocation has been demonstrated in animal models. The most efficacious method to prevent these changes is to provide nutrients enterally. In patients requiring total parenteral nutrition, it may be feasible to infuse small amounts of trophic feedings via the gastrointestinal tract.

Special Formulations

Glutamine and Arginine

Glutamine is the most abundant amino acid in the human body, comprising nearly two thirds of the free intracellular amino acid pool. Of this, 75% is found within the skeletal muscles. In healthy individuals, glutamine is considered a nonessential amino acid because it is synthesized within the skeletal muscles and the lungs. Glutamine is a necessary substrate for nucleotide synthesis in most dividing cells, and hence provides a major fuel source for enterocytes. It also serves as an important fuel source for immunocytes such as lymphocytes and macrophages, as well as a precursor for glutathione, a major intracellular antioxidant. During stress states such as sepsis, or in tumor-bearing hosts, peripheral glutamine stores are rapidly depleted and the amino acid is preferentially shunted as a fuel source toward the visceral organs and tumors, respectively. These situations create, at least experimentally, a glutamine-depleted environment, with consequences including enterocyte and immunocyte starvation.

The beneficial effects of glutamine supplementation demonstrated experimentally are multifaceted (Table 1-12). However, glutamine metabolism during stress in humans may be more complex than in previously reported animal data. More advanced methods of detecting glutamine traffic in patients with gastrointestinal cancer

Table 1-12
Experimental Benefits of Glutamine and Arginine Supplementation

Glutamine
Enhances bowel absorptive capacity after intestinal resection
Decreases intestinal permeability
Early resolution of experimental pancreatitis
Maintains nitrogen balance
Promotes liver regeneration after hepatectomy
Restores mucosal immunoglobulin A function
Enhances bacterial clearance in peritonitis
Protects postradiation enterocyte viability
Restores intracellular glutathione levels
Facilitates tumor sensitivity to chemotherapy and radiation therapy
Enhances natural killer and lymphokine-activated killer cell function

Arginine
Minimizes hepatic ischemia/reperfusion injury
Reduces intestinal bacterial translocation
Enhances natural killer and lymphokine-activated killer cell function
Increases nitrogen retention and protein synthesis

have not demonstrated more tumor sequestration of glutamine than normal intestine. There are data demonstrating decreased dependency on TPN in severe cases of short bowel syndrome when glutamine therapy with modified diets and growth hormones are used. However, in patients with milder forms of short bowel syndrome and better nutritional status, glutamine supplementation did not demonstrate appreciable enhancement in intestinal absorption. In healthy subjects, glutamine-supplemented TPN did not attenuate endotoxin-induced symptoms or proinflammatory cytokine release compared to standard TPN. Although it is hypothesized that provision of glutamine may preserve immune cell and enterocyte function and enhance nitrogen balance during injury or sepsis, the clinical evidence in support of these phenomena in human subjects remains inconclusive.

Arginine, also a nonessential amino acid in healthy subjects, first attracted attention for its immunoenhancing properties, wound-healing benefits, and improved survival in animal models of sepsis and injury. As with glutamine, the benefits of experimental arginine supplementation during stress states are diverse. Clinical studies in which arginine was administered enterally have demonstrated net nitrogen retention and protein synthesis compared to isonitrogenous diets in critically ill and injured patients and following surgery for certain malignancies. Some of these studies also are associated with in vitro evidence of enhanced immunocyte function. The clinical utility of arginine in improving overall patient outcome remains an area of investigation.

Omega-3 Fatty Acids

The provision of omega-3 polyunsaturated fatty acids (canola oil or fish oil) displaces omega-6 fatty acids in cell membranes, which theoretically reduce the proinflammatory response from prostaglandin production.

Nucleotides

RNA supplementation in solutions is purported, at least experimentally, to increase cell proliferation, provide building blocks for DNA synthesis, and improve T-helper cell function.

Bibliography

Inflammatory Response
Abu-Soud HM, Hazen SL: Nitric oxide modulates the catalytic activity of myeloperoxidase. *J Biol Chem* 275:5425, 2000.
Agnese DM, Calvano JE, Hahm SJ, et al: Human toll-like receptor 4 mutations but not CD14 polymorphisms are associated with an increased risk of gram-negative infections. *J Infect Dis* 186:1522, 2002.
Agnese DM, Calvano JE, Hahm SJ, et al: Insulin-like growth factor binding protein-3 is upregulated in LPS-treated THP-1 cells. *Surg Infect* 3:119, 2002.
Aljada A, Ghanim H, Mohanty P, et al: Hydrocortisone suppresses intranuclear activator-protein-1 (AP-1) binding activity in mononuclear cells and plasma matrix metalloproteinase 2 and 9 (MMP-2 and MMP-9). *J Clin Endocrinol Metab* 86:5988, 2001.
Auerbach AD, Goldman L: Blockers and reduction of cardiac events in noncardiac surgery. *JAMA* 287:1445, 2002.
Bachetti T, Pasini E, Suzuki H, et al: Species-specific modulation of the nitric oxide pathway after acute experimentally induced endotoxemia. *Crit Care Med* 31:1509, 2003.
Bauhofer A, Stinner B, Kohlert F, et al: Granulocyte colony-stimulating factor but not peritoneal lavage increases survival rate after experimental abdominal contamination and infection. *Br J Surg* 89:1457, 2002.
Bergstrom M, Ivarsson M-L, Holmdahl L: Peritoneal response to pneumoperitoneum and laparoscopic surgery. *Br J Surg* 89:1465, 2002.

Bondestam J, Salven P, Jaaskela-Saari H, et al: Major surgery increases serum levels of vascular endothelial growth factor only temporarily. *Am J Surg* 179:57, 2000.

Briegel J, Jochum M, Gippner-Steppert C, et al: Immunomodulation in septic shock: Hydrocortisone differentially regulates cytokine responses. *J Am Soc Nephrol* 12:S70, 2001.

Calvano JE, Um JY, Agnese DM, et al: Influence of the TNF-alpha and TNF-beta polymorphisms upon infectious risk and outcome in surgical intensive care patients. *Surg Infect* 4:163, 2003.

Calvano SE, Coyle SM, Barbosa KS, Barie PS, Lowry SF: Multivariate analysis of 9 disease-associated variables for outcome prediction in patients with sepsis. *Arch Surg* 133:1347, 1998.

Carter Y, Liu G, Stephens WB, et al: Heat shock protein (HSP72) and p38 MAPK involvement in sublethal hemorrhage (SLH)-induced tolerance. *J Surg Res* 111:70, 2003.

Coopersmith CM, Stromberg PE, Dunne WM, et al: Inhibition of intestinal epithelial apoptosis and survival in a murine model of pneumonia-induced sepsis. *JAMA* 287:1716, 2002.

Daigle I, Yousefi S, Colonna M, et al: Death receptors bind SHP-1 and block cytokine-induced anti-apoptotic signaling in neutrophils. *Nat Med* 8:61, 2002.

Dinarello CA: Anti-cytokine therapies in response to systemic infection. *J Investig Dermatol Symp Proc* 6:244, 2001.

Fillinger MP, Rassias AJ, Guyre PM, et al: Glucocorticoid effects on the inflammatory and clinical responses to cardiac surgery. *J Cardiothorac Vasc Anesth* 16:163, 2002.

Grobmyer SR, Lin E, Lowry SF, et al: Elevation of IL-18 in human sepsis. *J Clin Immunol* 20:212, 2000.

Guicciardi ME, Gores GJ: AIP1: A new player in TNF signaling. *J Clin Invest* 111:1813, 20035.

Guicciardi ME, Miyoshi H, Bronk SF, et al: Cathepsin B knockout mice are resistant to tumor necrosis factor-alpha-mediated hepatocyte apoptosis and liver injury. *Am J Pathol* 159:2045, 2001.

Guirao X, Kumar A, Katz J, et al: Catecholamines increase monocyte TNF binding capacity by selective upregulation of the type-II (p75) receptor. *Am J Physiol* 273:E1203, 1997.

Gupta A, Watson DI: Effect of laparoscopy on immune infection. *Br J Surg* 88:1296, 2001.

Gutt CN, Kim Z-N, Schemmer P, et al: Impact of laparoscopic and conventional surgery on Kupffer cells, tumor-associated CD44 expression, and intrahepatic tumor spread. *Arch Surg* 137:1408, 2002.

Harlan JM, Winn RK: Leukocyte-endothelial interactions: Clinical trials of anti-adhesion therapy. *Crit Care Med* 30:S214, 2002.

Harris HW, Johnson JA, Wigmore SJ: Endogenous lipoproteins impact the response to endotoxin in humans. *Crit Care Med* 30:23, 2002.

Hazen SL, Chisolm GM: Oxidized phosphatidylcholines: Pattern recognition ligands for multiple pathways of the innate immune response. *Proc Natl Acad Sci USA* 99:12515, 2002.

Healy DP: New and emerging therapies for sepsis. *Ann Pharmacother* 36:648, 2002.

Henneke P, Golenbock DT: Innate immune recognition of lipopolysaccharide by endothelial cells. *Crit Care Med* 30:S207, 2002.

Hoefen RJ, Berk BC: The role of MAP kinases in endothelial activation. *Vasc Pharmacol* 38:271, 2002.

Hommes DW, Peppelenbosch MP, van Deventer SJH: Mitogen activated protein (MAP) kinase signal transduction pathways and novel anti-inflammatory targets. *Gut* 52:144, 2003.

Horng T, Barton GM, Flavell RA, et al: The adaptor molecule TIRAP provides signalling specificity for toll-like receptors. *Nature* 420:329, 2002.

Hotchkiss RS, Tinsley KW, Swanson PE, et al: Endothelial cell apoptosis in sepsis. *Crit Care Med* 30:S225, 2002.

Johnston JA, O'Shea JJ: Matching SOCS with function. *Nat Immunol* 4:507, 2003.

Kilger E, Weis F, Briegel J, et al: Stress doses of hydrocortisone reduce severe systemic inflammatory response syndrome and improve early outcome in a risk group of patients after cardiac surgery. *Crit Care Med* 31:1068, 2003.

Kim J-S, Qian T, Lemasters JJ: Mitochondrial permeability transition in the switch from necrotic to apoptotic cell death in ischemic rat hepatocytes. *Gastroenterology* 124:494, 2003.

Kirveskari J, Helinto M, Moilanen JAO, et al: Hydrocortisone reduced in vivo, inflammation-induced slow rolling of leukocytes and their extravasation into human conjunctiva. *Blood* 100:2203, 2002.

Knaus WA: APACHE 1978–2001: The development of a quality assurance system based on prognosis. *Arch Surg* 137:37, 2002.

Kotani J, Avallone NJ, Lin E, et al: Fas-mediated neutrophil apoptosis and associated A1 protein expression during systemic inflammation are regulated independently of both tumor necrosis factor receptors. *Shock* 19:201, 2003.

Kullo IJ, Hensrud DD, Allison TG: Comparison of numbers of circulating blood monocytes in men grouped by body mass index (<25, 25 to <30, >30). *Am J Cardiol* 89:1441, 2002.

Lauw FN, Pajkrt D, Hack CE, et al: Proinflammatory effects of IL-10 during human endotoxemia. *J Immunol* 165:2783, 2000.

Lemaire LC, van der Poll T, van Lanschot JJ, et al: Minimally invasive surgery induces endotoxin-tolerance in the absence of detectable endotoxemia. *J Clin Immunol* 18:414, 1998.

Le Roux CW, Chapman GA, Kong WM, et al: Free cortisol index is better than serum total cortisol in determining hypothalamic-pituitary-adrenal status in patients undergoing surgery. *J Clin Endocrinol Metab* 88:2045, 2003.

Lettinga KD, Florquin S, Speelman P, et al: Toll-like receptor 4 is not involved in host defense against pulmonary *Legionella pneumophila* infection in a mouse model. *J Infect Dis* 186:570, 2002.

Levi M, ten Cate H, van der Poll T: Endothelium: interface between coagulation and inflammation. *Crit Care Med* 30:S220, 2002.

Li X, Yang Y, Ashwell JD: TNF-RII and c-IAP1 mediate ubiquitination and degradation of TRAF2. *Nature* 416:345, 2002.

Lin E, Calvano SE, Lowry SF: Inflammatory cytokines and cell response in surgery. *Surgery* 127:117, 2000.

Lin E, Calvano SE, Lowry SF: Response of tumor necrosis factor receptors in systemic inflammation, in Vincent JL (ed): *1999 Yearbook of Intensive Care and Emergency Medicine.* Berlin: Springer-Verlag, 1999, p 384.

Lin E, Katz JA, Calvano SE, et al: The influence of human endotoxemia upon CD95-induced apoptosis. *Arch Surg* 133:1322, 1998.

Lin E, Lowry SF: Human response to endotoxin. *Sepsis* 2:255, 1999.

Lin E, Lowry SF: Inflammatory cytokines in major surgery: A functional perspective. *Intensive Care Med* 25:255, 1999.

Lin E, Lowry SF: Selectin neutralization: Does it make biological sense? *Crit Care Med* 27:2050, 1999.

Lyons A, Kelly JL, Rodrick ML, et al: Major injury induces increased production of interleukin-10 by cells of the immune system with a negative impact on resistance to infection. *Ann Surg* 226:450, 1997.

Madihally SV, Toner M, Yarmush ML, et al: Interferon gamma modulates trauma-induced muscle wasting and immune dysfunction. *Ann Surg* 236:649, 2002.

Marshall JC, Vincent J-L, Fink MP, et al: Measures, markers, and mediators: toward a staging system for clinical sepsis. A report of the Fifth Toronto Sepsis Roundtable, Toronto, Ontario, Canada, October 25–26, 2000. *Crit Care Med* 31:1560, 2003.

Marx C, Petros S, Bornstein SR, et al: Adrenocortical hormones in survivors and nonsurvivors of severe sepsis: Diverse time course of dehydroepiandrosterone, dehydroepiandrosterone-sulfate, and cortisol. *Crit Care Med* 31:1382, 2003.

Mokart D, Capo C, Blache JL, et al: Early postoperative compensatory anti-inflammatory response syndrome is associated with septic complications after major surgical trauma in patients with cancer. *Br J Surg* 89:1450, 2002.

Nathens AB, Neff MJ, Jurkovich GJ, et al: Randomized, prospective trial of antioxidant supplementation in critically ill surgical patients. *Ann Surg* 236:814, 2002.

Neudecker J, Sauerland S, Neugebauer E, et al: The European Association for Endoscopic Surgery clinical practice guideline on the pneumoperitoneum for laparoscopic surgery. *Surg Endosc* 16:1121, 2002.

Okajima K: Regulation of inflammatory responses by natural anticoagulants. *Immunol Rev* 184:258, 2001.

Pallua N, Low JFA, von Heimburg D: Pathogenic role of interleukin-6 in the development of sepsis. Part II: Significance of anti-interleukin-6 and anti-soluble interleukin-6 receptor-alpha antibodies in a standardized murine contact burn model. *Crit Care Med* 31:1495, 2003.

Pallua N, von Heimburg D: Pathogenic role of interleukin-6 in the development of sepsis. Part I: Study in a standardized contact burn murine model. *Crit Care Med* 31:1490, 2003.

Papanicolaou DA: The pathophysiologic roles of interleukin-6 in human disease. *Ann Intern Med* 128:127, 1998.

Pascual JL, Ferri LE, Seely AJE, et al: Hypertonic saline resuscitation of hemorrhagic shock diminishes neutrophil rolling and adherence to endothelium and reduces in vivo vascular leakage. *Ann Surg* 236:634, 2002.

Perretti M, Chiang N, La M, et al: Endogenous lipid- and peptide-derived anti-inflammatory pathways generated with glucocorticoid and aspirin treatment activate the lipoxin A4 receptor. *Nat Med* 8:1296, 2002.

Peters DL, Barber RC, Flood EM, et al: Methodologic quality and genotyping reproducibility in studies of tumor necrosis factor −308 G→A single nucleotide polymorphism and bacterial sepsis: Implications for studies of complex traits. *Crit Care Med* 31:1691, 2003.

Raeburn CD, Sheppard F, Barsness KA, et al: Cytokines for surgeons. *Am J Surg* 183:268, 2002.

Riedmann NC, Ward PA: Oxidized lipid protects against sepsis. *Nat Med* 8:1084, 2002.

Rowlands TE, Homer-Vanniasinkam S: Pro- and anti-inflammatory cytokine release in open versus endovascular repair of abdominal aortic aneurysm. *Br J Surg* 88:1335, 2001.

Rudiger HA, Clavien P-A: Tumor necrosis factor alpha, but not Fas, mediates hepatocellular apoptosis in the murine ischemic liver. *Gastroenterology* 122:202, 2002.

Rumalla VK, Calvano SE, Spotnitz AJ, et al: Alterations in immunocyte tumor necrosis factor receptor and apoptosis in patients with congestive heart failure. *Ann Surg* 236:254, 2002.

Rumalla V, Calvano SE, Spotnitz AJ, et al: The effects of glucocorticoid therapy on inflammatory responses to coronary artery bypass graft surgery. *Arch Surg* 136:1039, 2001.

Schuster DP, Metzler M, Opal S, et al: Recombinant platelet-activating factor acetylhydrolase to prevent acute respiratory distress syndrome and mortality in severe sepsis: Phase IIb, multicenter, randomized, placebo-controlled, clinical trial. *Crit Care Med* 31:1612, 2003.

Souza DG, Pinho V, Soares AC, et al: Role of PAF receptors during intestinal ischemia and reperfusion injury. A comparative study between PAF receptor-deficient mice and PAF receptor antagonist treatment. *Br J Pharmacol* 139:733, 2003.

Spark JI, Scott DJA: Role of the neutrophil in the development of systemic inflammatory response syndrome and sepsis following abdominal aortic surgery. *Br J Surg* 88:1583, 2001.

Straczkowski M, Dzienis-Straczkowska S, Stepien A, et al: Plasma interleukin-8 concentrations are increased in obese subjects and related to fat mass and tumor necrosis factor-alpha system. *J Clin Endocrinol Metab* 87:4602, 2002.

Szold O, Ben-Abraham R, Frolkis I, et al: Tumor necrosis factor as a mediator of cardiac toxicity following snake envenomation. *Crit Care Med* 31:1449, 2003.

Tadros T, Traber DL, Heggers JP, et al: Effects of interleukin-1 alpha administration on intestinal ischemia and reperfusion injury, mucosal permeability, and bacterial translocation in burn sepsis. *Ann Surg* 237:101, 2003.

Targarona EM, Balague C, Knook MM, et al: Laparoscopic surgery and surgical infection. *Br J Surg* 87:536, 2000.

Ure BM, Niewold TA, Bax NMA, et al: Peritoneal, systemic, and distant organ inflammatory responses are reduced by A laparoscopic approach and carbon dioxide vs air. *Surg Endosc* 16:836, 2002.

Utsugi M, Dobashi K, Ishizuka T, et al: C-jun N-terminal kinase negatively regulates lipopolysaccharide-induced IL-12 production in human macrophages: Role of mitogen-activated protein kinase in glutathione redox regulation of IL-12 production. *J Immunol* 171:628, 2003.

Van der Poll T, Endert E, Coyle SM, et al: Neutralization of TNF does not influence endotoxin induced changes in thyroid hormone metabolism in humans. *Am J Physiol* 276:R357, 1999.

Vesley DL: Natriuretic peptides and acute renal failure. *Am J Physiol Renal Physiol* 285:F167, 2003.

Vincent J-L, Sun Q, Dubois M-J: Clinical trials of immunomodulatory therapies in severe sepsis and septic shock. *Clin Infect Dis* 34:1084, 2002.

Vittimberga FJ Jr., Foley DP, Meyers WC, et al: Laparoscopic surgery and the systemic immune response. *Ann Surg* 227:326, 1998.

Vorchheimer DA, Fuster V: Inflammatory markers in coronary artery disease. *JAMA* 286:2154, 2001.

Williams DL, Ha T, Li C, et al: Modulation of tissue toll-like receptor 2 and 4 during the early phases of polymicrobial sepsis correlates with mortality. *Crit Care Med* 31:1808, 2003.

Wilmore DW: From Cuthbertson to fast-track surgery: 70 years of progress in reducing stress in surgical patients. *Ann Surg* 236:643, 2002.

Wong MM, Fish EN: Chemokines: attractive mediators of the immune response. *Semin Immunol* 15:5, 2003.

Xu N, Gao X-P, Minshall RD, et al: Time-dependent reversal of sepsis-induced PMN uptake and lung vascular injury by expression of CD18 antagonist. *Am J Physiol Lung Cell Mol Physiol* 282:L796, 2002.

Yamamoto M, Sato S, Hemmi H, et al: Essential role for TIRAP in activation of the signalling cascade shared by TLR2 and TLR4. *Nature* 420:324, 2002.

Yamaoka J, Kabashima K, Kawanishi M, et al: Cytotoxicity of IFN-gamma and TNF-alpha for vascular endothelial cell is mediated by nitric oxide. *Biochem Biophys Res Commun* 291:780, 2002.

Yang S, Zhou M, Chaudry IH, et al: Novel approach to prevent the transition from the hyperdynamic phase to the hypodynamic phase of sepsis. *Ann Surg* 236:625, 2002.

Zhang R, Brennan M-L, Fu X, et al: Association between myeloperoxidase levels and risk of coronary artery disease. *JAMA* 286:2136, 2001.

Zhang R, Brennan M-L, Shen Z, et al: Myeloperoxidase functions as a major enzymatic catalyst for initiation of lipid peroxidation at sites of inflammation. *J Biol Chem* 277:46116, 2002.

Zhang R, He X, Liu W, et al: AIP1 mediates TNF- alpha-induced ASK1 activation by facilitating dissociation of ASK1 from its inhibitor 14-3-3. *J Clin Invest* 111:1933, 2003.

Zhang R, Shen Z, Nauseef WM, et al: Defects in leukocyte-mediated initiation of lipid peroxidation in plasma as studied in myeloperoxidase-deficient subjects: Systematic identification of multiple endogenous diffusible substrates for myeloperoxidase in plasma. *Blood* 99:1802, 2002.

Nutritional Support

Bistrian BR: Clinical aspects of essential fatty acid metabolism: Jonathan Rhoads lecture. *J Parenter Enteral Nutr* 27:168, 2003.

Brooks AD, Hochwald SN, Heslin MJ, et al: Intestinal permeability after early postoperative enteral nutrition in patients with upper gastrointestinal malignancy. *J Parenter Enteral Nutr* 24:49, 2000.

Bruins MJ, Luiking YC, Soeters PB, et al: Effect of prolonged hyperdynamic endotoxemia on jejunal motility in fasted and enterally fed pigs. *Ann Surg* 237:44, 2003.

Btaiche IF: Branched-chain amino acids in patients with hepatic encephalopathy. *Nutr Clin Pract* 18:97, 2003.

Cerra FB, Benitez MR, Blackburn GL, et al: Applied nutrition in ICU patients: A consensus statement of the American College of Chest Physicians. *Chest* 111:769, 1997.

Chernoff R: Normal aging, nutrition assessment, and clinical practice. *Nutr Clin Pract* 18:12, 2003.

Exner R, Tamandl D, Goetzinger P, et al: Perioperative GLY-GLN infusion diminishes the surgery-induced period of immunosuppression. *Ann Surg* 237:110, 2003.

Fang JC, DiSario JA: Endoscopic approaches to enteral nutritional support. *Am Soc Gastrointest Endosc* 10:1, 2003.

Foitzik T, Eibl G, Schneider P, et al: T-3 fatty acid supplementation increases anti-inflammatory cytokines and attenuates systemic disease sequelae in experimental pancreatitis. *J Parenter Enteral Nutr* 26:351, 2002.

Gore DC, Wolfe RR: Glutamine supplementation fails to affect muscle protein kinetics in critically ill patients. *J Parenter Enteral Nutr* 26:342, 2002.

Guirao X: Impact of the inflammatory reaction on intermediary metabolism and nutrition status. *Nutrition* 18:949, 2002.

Heslin MJ, Brennan MF: Advances in perioperative nutrition: Cancer. *World J Surg* 24:1477, 2000.

Heslin MJ, Latkany L, Leung D, et al: A prospective, randomized trial of early enteral feeding after resection of upper gastrointestinal malignancy. *Ann Surg* 226:567, 1997.

Heyland DK: Immunonutrition in the critically ill patient: Putting the cart before the horse? *Nutr Clin Pract* 17:267, 2002.

Heyland DK, Drover JW, Dhaliwal R, et al: Optimizing the benefits and minimizing the risks of enteral nutrition in the critically ill: Role of small bowel feeding. *J Parenter Enteral Nutr* 26:S51, 2002.

Kono H, Fujii H, Asakawa M, et al: Protective effects of medium-chain triglycerides on the liver and gut in rats administered endotoxin. *Ann Surg* 237:246, 2003.

Kovacevich DS, Papke LF: Guidelines for the prevention of intravascular catheter-related infections: Centers for Disease Control and Prevention. *Nutr Clin Pract* 18:95, 2003.

Kudsk KA, Tolley EA, DeWitt RC, et al: Preoperative albumin and surgical site identify surgical risk for major postoperative complications. *J Parenter Enteral Nutr* 27:1, 2003.

Lin E, Goncalves JA, Lowry SF: Efficacy of nutritional pharmacology in surgical patients. *Curr Opin Clin Nutr Metab Care* 1:41, 1998.

Lin E, Kontani J, Lowry SF: Nutritional modulation of immunity and inflammatory response. *Nutrition* 14:545, 1998.

Lin E, Lowry SF: Substrate metabolism in surgery, in Norton JA (ed): *Surgery: Scientific Basis and Clinical Evidence*. New York: Springer-Verlag, 2000, p 95.

McClave SA, Lowen CC, Kleber MJ, et al: Clinical use of the respiratory quotient obtained from indirect calorimetry. *J Parenter Enteral Nutr* 27:21, 2003.

Mitch WE, Price SR: Mechanisms activating proteolysis to cause muscle atrophy in catabolic conditions. *J Ren Nutr* 13:149, 2003.

Ng ED, Panesar N, Longo WE, et al: Human intestinal epithelial and smooth muscle cells are potent producers of IL-6. *Mediators Inflamm* 12:3, 2003.

Parrish CR: Enteral feeding: The art and the science. *Nutr Clin Pract* 18:76, 2003.

Patton KM, Aranda-Michel J: Nutritional aspects in liver disease and liver transplantation. *Nutr Clin Pract* 17:332, 2002.

Polderman KH, Girbes ARJ: Central venous catheter use: Part 2. Infectious complications. *Intensive Care Med* 28:18, 2002.

Scolapio JS: Methods for decreasing risk of aspiration pneumonia in critically ill patients. *J Parenter Enteral Nutr* 26:S58, 2002.

Souba WW: Drug therapy: Nutritional support. *N Engl J Med* 336:41, 1997.

Spain DA: When is the seriously ill patient ready to be fed? *J Parenter Enteral Nutr* 26:S62, 2002.

Vanek VW: Ins and outs of enteral access: Part 2. Long-term access—esophagostomy and gastrostomy. *Nutr Clin Pract* 18:50, 2002.

Vanek VW: Ins and outs of enteral access: Part 3. Long-term access—jejunostomy. *Nutr Clin Pract* 18:201, 2003.

Vidal-Puig A, O'Rahilly S: Controlling the glucose factory. *Nature* 413:125, 2001.

Volpi E, Sheffield-Moore M, Rasmussen BB, et al: Basal muscle amino acid kinetics and protein synthesis in healthy young and older men. *JAMA* 286:1206, 2001.

Watters JM, Kirkpatrick SM, Norris SB, et al: Immediate postoperative enteral feeding results in impaired respiratory mechanics and decreased mobility. *Ann Surg* 226:369, 1997.

Zhou Y-P, Jiang Z-M, Sun Y-H, et al: The effect of supplemental enteral glutamine on plasma levels, gut function, and outcome in severe burns: A randomized, double-blind, controlled clinical trial. *J Parenter Enteral Nutr* 27:241, 2003.

CHAPTER 2

Fluid and Electrolyte Management of the Surgical Patient

Rosemary A. Kozar and Frederick A. Moore

INTRODUCTION

Fluid and electrolyte management are paramount to the care of the surgical patient. Changes in both fluid volume and electrolyte composition occur preoperatively, intraoperatively, and postoperatively, as well as in response to trauma and sepsis. The sections that follow review the normal anatomy of body fluids, electrolyte composition and concentration abnormalities and treatments, common metabolic derangements, and new alternative resuscitative fluids. These principles will then be discussed in relationship to management of specific surgical patients and their commonly encountered fluid and electrolyte abnormalities.

BODY FLUIDS

Total Body Water

Water constitutes approximately 50 to 60% of total body weight. The relationship between total body weight and total body water (TBW) is relatively constant for an individual and is primarily a reflection of body fat. Lean tissues such as muscle and solid organs have higher water content than fat and bone. As a result, young, lean males have a higher proportion of body weight as water than elderly or obese individuals. An average young adult male will have 60% of his total body weight as TBW, while an average young adult female's will be 50%. The lower percentage of TBW in females correlates with a higher percentage of adipose tissue and lower percentage of muscle mass in most. Estimates of TBW should be adjusted down approximately 10 to 20% in obese individuals and up by 10% in malnourished individuals. The highest percentage of TBW is found in newborns, with approximately 80% of their total body weight comprised of water. This decreases to about 65% by 1 year of age and thereafter remains fairly constant.

Fluid Compartments

TBW is divided into two functional fluid compartments, the extracellular and intracellular (Fig. 2-1). The extracellular fluid compartment comprises about one third of the TBW and the intracellular compartment the remaining two thirds. The extracellular water comprises 20% of the total body weight and is divided between plasma

% of Total Body Weight	Volume of TBW	Male (70 kg)	Female (60 kg)
Plasma 5%	Extracellular Volume	14,000 mL	10,000 mL
Interstitial Fluid 15%	Plasma	3500 mL	2500 mL
	Interstitial	10,500 mL	7500 mL
Intracellular Volume 40%	Intracellular volume	28,000 mL	20,000 mL
		42,000 mL	30,000 mL

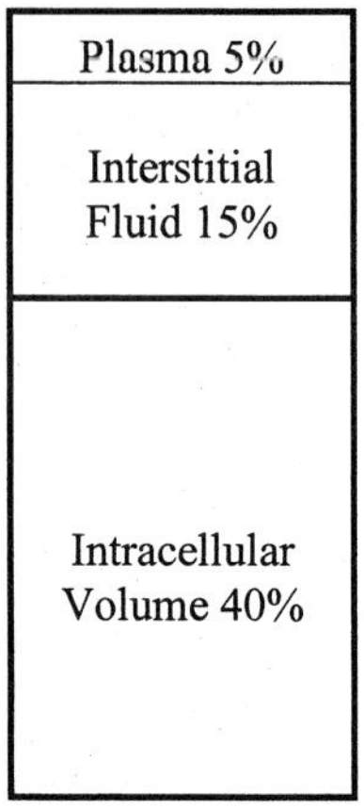

FIG. 2-1. Functional body fluid compartments. TBW = total body water.

(5% of body weight) and interstitial fluid (15% of body weight). Measurement of the intracellular compartment is determined indirectly by subtracting the measured extracellular fluid from the TBW. Intracellular water makes up approximately 40% of an individual's total body weight, with the largest proportion in the skeletal muscle mass.

Composition of Fluid Compartments

The chemical composition of the body fluid compartments is shown in Fig. 2-2. The extracellular fluid compartment is balanced between the principal cation—sodium and the principal anions—chloride and bicarbonate. The intracellular fluid compartment is comprised primarily of the cations, potassium and magnesium, and of the anions, phosphate and proteins. The concentration gradient between compartments is maintained by ATP-driven sodium-potassium pumps located within the cell membranes. The composition of the plasma and interstitial fluid differs only slightly in ionic composition, with the primary difference being the slightly higher protein composition in plasma. Proteins add to the osmolality of the plasma and contribute to the balance of forces that determine fluid balance across the capillary endothelium. Although the movement of ions and proteins between the various fluid compartments is restricted, water is freely diffusible. Water is distributed evenly throughout all fluid compartments of the body so that a given volume of water increases the volume of any one compartment relatively little. Sodium, however, is confined to the extracellular fluid compartment, and because of its osmotic and electrical properties, it remains associated with water. Therefore, sodium-containing fluids are distributed throughout the extracellular fluid and add to the volume of both the intravascular and interstitial spaces. While the administration of sodium-containing fluids will expand the intravascular volume, it also expands the interstitial space by approximately three times as much as the plasma.

Osmotic Pressure

The movement of water across a cell membrane depends primarily upon osmosis. To achieve osmotic equilibrium, water moves across a semipermeable membrane to equalize the concentration on both sides. This movement is determined by the concentration of the solutes on each side of the membrane. Osmotic pressure is measured in units of osmoles (osm) or milliosmoles (mOsm) that refer to the actual number of osmotically-active particles. For example, one

millimole (mmol) of sodium chloride contributes to 2 mOsm (one from sodium and one from chloride). The principal determinants of osmolality are the concentrations of sodium, glucose, and urea (blood urea nitrogen [BUN]):

$$\text{Calculated serum osmolality} = 2\text{ sodium} + \text{glucose}/18 + \text{BUN}/2.8$$

The osmolality of the intracellular and extracellular fluids is maintained between 290 and 310 mOsm in each compartment. Because cell membranes are permeable to water, any change in osmotic pressure in one compartment is accompanied by a redistribution of water until the effective osmotic pressure between compartments is equal. For example, if the extracellular fluid concentration of sodium increased, there would be a net movement of water from the intracellular to the extracellular compartment. Conversely, if the extracellular fluid concentration of sodium decreased, water would move into the cells. A change in volume in either one of the compartments, however, is not accompanied by the net movement of water as long as the concentration remains the same.

The concentration of electrolytes is usually expressed in terms of the chemical combining activity, or equivalents. An equivalent of an ion is its atomic weight expressed in grams divided by the valence:

$$\text{Equivalent} = \text{atomic weight (g)/valence}$$

For univalent ions such as sodium, 1 mEq is the same as 1 mmol. For divalent ions such as magnesium, 1 mmol equals 2 mEq. This is important in that the number of milliequivalents of cations must be balanced by the same number of milliequivalents of anions.

CLASSIFICATION OF BODY FLUID CHANGES

Normal Exchange of Fluid and Electrolytes

The normal person consumes an average of 2000 mL of water per day, approximately 75% from oral intake and the rest is extracted from solid foods. Daily water losses include about 1 L in urine, 250 mL in stool, and 600 mL as insensible losses. Insensible losses occur through both the skin (75%) and lungs (25%) and by definition is pure water. Insensible losses can be increased by such factors as fever, hypermetabolism, and hyperventilation. Sweating, on the other hand, is an active process and involves loss of (hypotonic) electrolytes and water. To clear the products of metabolism, the

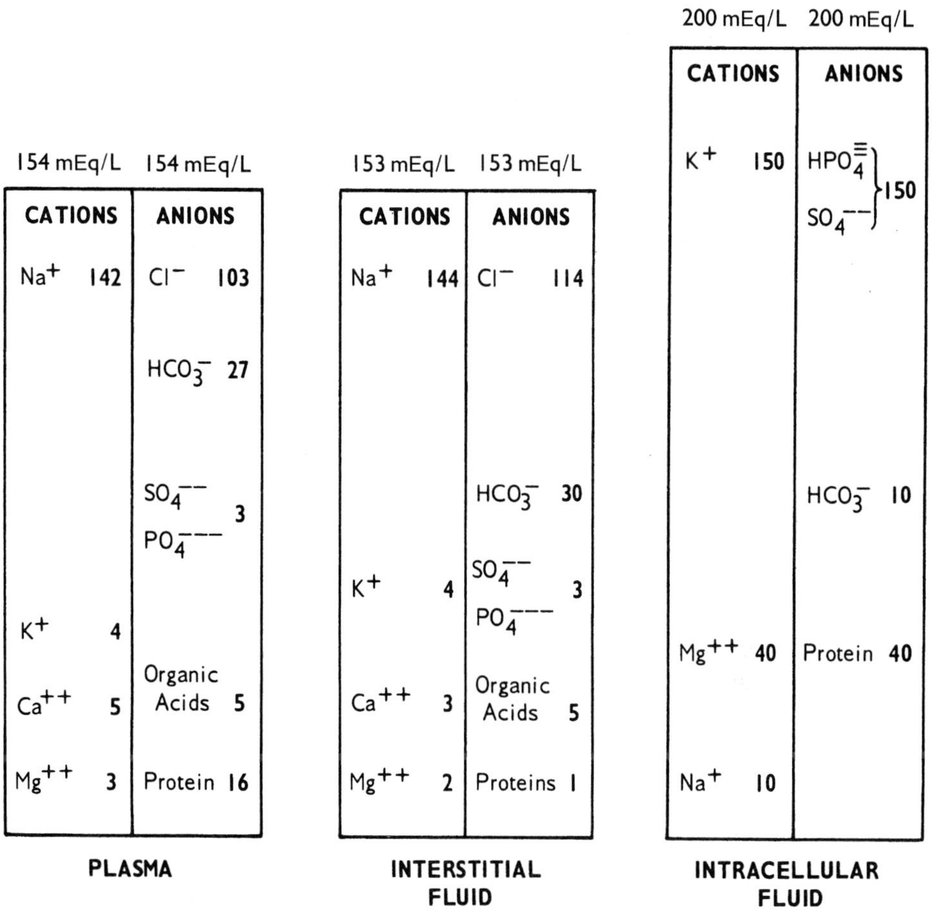

FIG. 2-2. Chemical composition of body fluid compartments.

kidneys must excrete a minimum of 500 to 800 mL of urine per day, regardless of the amount of oral intake.

The normal person also consumes about 3 to 5 g of salt per day, with the balance maintained by the kidneys. With hyponatremia, sodium excretion can be reduced to as little as 1 mEq/d or maximized up to 5000 mEq/d to achieve balance in lieu of salt-wasting kidneys.

Disturbances in Fluid Balance

Extracellular volume deficit is the most common fluid disorder in surgical patients and can be either acute or chronic. Acute volume deficit is associated with cardiovascular and central nervous system signs, while chronic deficits display tissue signs, such as a decrease in skin turgor and sunken eyes, in addition to cardiovascular and central nervous system signs (Table 2-1). Laboratory examination may reveal an elevated blood urea nitrogen level if the deficit is severe enough to reduce glomerular filtration and hemoconcentration. Urine osmolality will usually be higher than serum osmolality, and urine sodium will be low, typically less than 20 mEq/L. Sodium concentration does not necessarily reflect volume status, and therefore may be high, normal, or low when a volume deficit is present. The most common etiology of volume deficit in surgical patients is a loss of gastrointestinal fluids (Table 2-2) from nasogastric suction, vomiting, diarrhea, or fistula. Additionally, sequestration secondary to soft-tissue injuries, burns, and intra-abdominal processes such as peritonitis, obstruction, or prolonged surgery can also lead to volume deficits.

Extracellular volume excess may be iatrogenic or secondary to renal dysfunction, congestive heart failure, or cirrhosis. Both plasma and interstitial volumes are increased. Symptoms are primarily pulmonary and cardiovascular (see Table 2-1).

Volume Control

Volume changes are sensed by both osmoreceptors and baroreceptors. Osmoreceptors are specialized sensors that detect even small changes in fluid osmolality through osmoreceptor-driven changes in thirst and diuresis through the kidneys.[1] For example, when plasma osmolality is increased, thirst is stimulated and water consumption increases.[2] Additionally, the hypothalamus is stimulated to secrete vasopressin, which increases water reabsorption in the kidneys. Together, these two mechanisms return the plasma osmolality

Table 2-1
Signs and Symptoms of Volume Disturbances

System	Volume Deficit	Volume Excess
Generalized	Weight loss Decreased skin turgor	Weight gain Peripheral edema
Cardiac	Tachycardia Orthostasis/hypotension Collapsed neck veins	Increased cardiac output Increased central venous pressure Distended neck veins Murmur
Renal	Oliguria Azotemia	
Gastrointestinal Pulmonary	Ileus	Bowel edema Pulmonary edema

Table 2-2
Composition of Gastrointestinal Secretions

Type of Secretion	Volume (mL/24 h)	Na (mEq/L)	K (mEq/L)	Cl (mEq/L)	HCO₃⁻ (mEq/L)
Stomach	1000–2000	60–90	10–30	100–130	0
Small intestine	2000–3000	120–140	5–10	90–120	30–40
Colon		60	30	40	0
Pancreas	600–800	135–145	5–10	70–90	95–115
Bile	300–800	135–145	5–10	90–110	30–40

to normal. Baroreceptors also modulate volume in response to changes in pressure and circulating volume through specialized pressure sensors located in the aortic arch and carotid sinuses.[3] Baroreceptor responses are both neural, through sympathetic and parasympathetic parts, and hormonal, including renin-angiotensin, aldosterone, atrial natriuretic peptide, and renal prostaglandins. The net result is alterations in renal sodium levels and water reabsorption in order to restore the volume to normal.

Concentration Changes

Changes in serum sodium are inversely proportional to TBW. Therefore, abnormalities in TBW are reflected by abnormalities in serum sodium.

Hyponatremia

A low serum sodium level occurs when there is an excess of extracellular water relative to sodium. Extracellular volume can be high, normal, or low (Fig. 2-3). For most cases of hyponatremia, sodium concentration is decreased as a consequence of either sodium depletion or dilution.[4] Dilutional hyponatremia frequently results from excess extracellular water and therefore is associated with a high extracellular volume status. Either intentional (excessive oral water intake) or iatrogenic (intravenous) excess free water administration can cause hyponatremia. Postoperative patients are particularly prone to increased secretion of antidiuretic hormone, which increases reabsorption of free water from the kidneys with subsequent volume expansion and hyponatremia. This is usually self-limiting in that both hyponatremia and volume expansion decrease antidiuretic hormone secretion. Additionally, a number of drugs can cause water retention and subsequent hyponatremia, such as the antipsychotics and tricyclic antidepressants as well as angiotensin-converting enzyme inhibitors. The elderly are particularly susceptible to drug-induced hyponatremia. Physical signs of volume overload are usually absent and laboratory evaluation reveals hemodilution. Depletional causes of hyponatremia result from either a decreased intake or increased loss of sodium-containing fluids. Etiologies include decreased sodium intake, such as that from a low-sodium diet or enteral feeds that are typically low in sodium, gastrointestinal losses (vomiting, prolonged nasogastric suctioning, or diarrhea), or renal losses (diuretics or primary renal disease). Depletional hyponatremia is often accompanied by extracellular volume deficit.

Hyponatremia can also be seen with an excess of solute relative to free water, such as with untreated hyperglycemia or mannitol administration. Glucose exerts an osmotic force in the extracellular compartment, causing a shift of water from the intracellular to the extracellular space and subsequent dilutional hyponatremia. Hyponatremia can therefore be seen when the effective osmotic pressure of

the extracellular compartment is normal or even high. When evaluating hyponatremia in the presence of hyperglycemia, the corrected sodium concentration should be calculated:

> For every 100-mg/dL increment in plasma glucose above
> normal, the plasma sodium should decrease by 1.6 mEq/L.

Lastly, extreme elevations in plasma lipids and proteins can cause pseudohyponatremia, since there is no true decrease in extracellular sodium relative to water.

Signs and symptoms of hyponatremia (Table 2-3) are dependent upon the degree of hyponatremia and the rapidity with which it occurred. Clinical manifestations are primarily central nervous system in etiology and are related to cellular water intoxication and associated increases in intracranial pressure.

To help differentiate the etiology of hyponatremia, a systematic review of the causes of hyponatremia should be undertaken. First, exclude hyperosmolar causes (hyperglycemia or mannitol) and pseudohyponatremia. Next, consider depletional versus dilutional causes of hyponatremia. Depletional causes are usually associated with dehydration. When sodium losses are extrarenal as from gastrointestinal losses, urine sodium levels are usually low (<20 mEq/L), whereas with renal causes of sodium loss, urine sodium levels are usually high (>20 mEq/L). Dilutional causes of hyponatremia are usually associated with a high effective circulating volume. A normal volume status in the case of hyponatremia should prompt an evaluation for a syndrome of inappropriate secretion of antidiuretic hormone.

Hypernatremia

Hypernatremia results from either a loss of free water or a gain of sodium in excess of water. Like hyponatremia, it can be associated with an increased, normal, or decreased extracellular volume (see Fig. 2-3). Hypervolemic hypernatremia is usually caused either by iatrogenic administration of sodium-containing fluids (including sodium bicarbonate) or mineralocorticoid excess as seen in hyperaldosteronism, Cushing's syndrome, and congenital adrenal hyperplasia. Urine sodium is typically greater than 20 mEq/L and urine osmolarity is greater than 300 mOsm/L. Normovolemic hypernatremia can be associated with renal (diabetes insipidus, diuretics, renal disease) or nonrenal (gastrointestinal or skin) causes of water loss.

Lastly, hypovolemic hypernatremia can be due to either renal or nonrenal water loss. Renal causes include diabetes insipidus, osmotic diuretics, adrenal failure, and renal tubular diseases. The urine sodium concentration is less than 20 mEq/L and urine osmolarity is less than 300 to 400 mOsm/L. Nonrenal water loss can occur secondary to gastrointestinal fluid losses such as diarrhea, or skin fluid losses such as fever or tracheotomies. Additionally, thyrotoxicosis can cause water loss as can the use of hypertonic glucose solutions for peritoneal dialysis. With nonrenal water loss, the urine sodium concentration is less than 15 mEq/L and the urine osmolarity is greater than 400 mOsm/L.

Symptomatic hypernatremia usually results only in patients with impaired thirst or restricted access to fluid, as thirst will result in increased water intake. Symptoms are rare until the serum sodium concentration exceeds 160 mEq/L but, once present, are associated with significant morbidity and mortality. As symptoms are related to hyperosmolarity, central nervous system effects predominate (see Table 2-3). Water shifts from the intracellular to the extracellular space in response to a hyperosmolar extracellular space, resulting in cellular dehydration. This can put traction on the cerebral vessels and

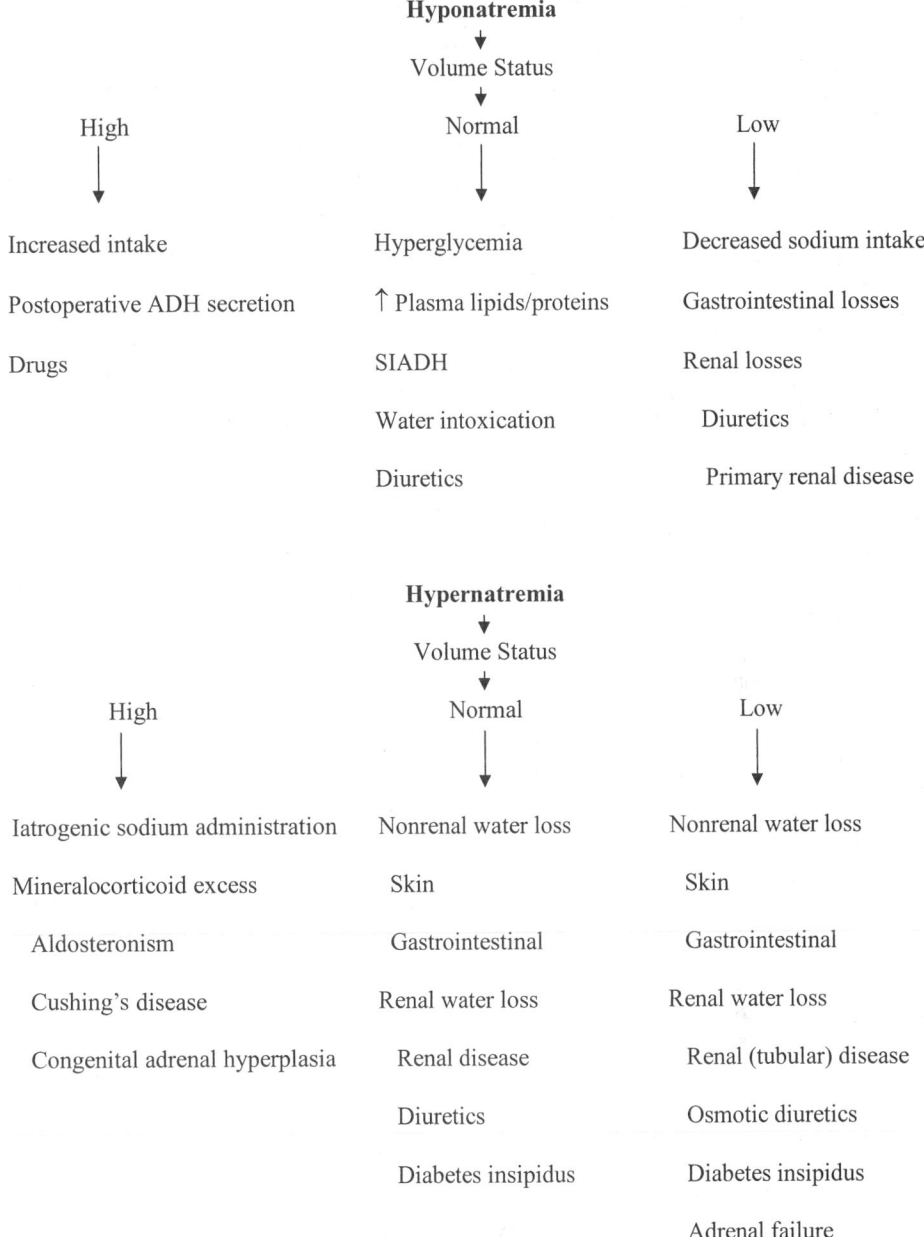

FIG. 2-3. Evaluation of sodium abnormalities.

lead to subarachnoid hemorrhage. Central nervous system symptoms can range from restlessness and irritability to seizures, coma, and death. The classic signs of hypovolemic hypernatremia (tachycardia, orthostasis, and hypotension) may be present, as can dry, sticky mucous membranes.

Composition Changes: Etiology and Diagnosis

Potassium Abnormalities

The average dietary intake of potassium is approximately 50 to 100 mEq/d, which in the absence of hypokalemia is excreted primarily in the urine. Extracellular potassium is maintained within a narrow range, principally by renal excretion of potassium, which can range from 10 to 700 mEq/d. Although only 2% of the total body potassium (4.5 mEq/L × 14 L = 63 mEq) is located within the extracellular compartment, this small amount is critical to cardiac and neuromuscular function; thus even minor changes can

have major effects on cardiac activity. The intracellular and extracellular distribution of potassium is influenced by a number of factors, including surgical stress, injury, acidosis, and tissue catabolism.

Hyperkalemia. Hyperkalemia is defined as a serum potassium concentration above the normal range of 3.5 to 5.0 mEq/L. It is caused by an excessive potassium intake, increased release of potassium from cells, or impaired excretion by the kidneys (Table 2-4).[5] Increased intake can be either from oral or intravenous supplementation, as well as from blood transfusions. Cell destruction or breakdown can release potassium in association with hemolysis, rhabdomyolysis, crush injuries, and gastrointestinal hemorrhage. Acidosis and a rapid increase of extracellular osmolality (hyperglycemia or mannitol administration) can raise serum potassium levels by causing a shift of potassium ions to the extracellular compartment.[6] Since the majority of total body potassium is intracellular, even small shifts of intracellular potassium out of the intracellular

Table 2-3
Clinical Manifestations of Abnormalities in Serum Sodium

Body System	Hyponatremia
Central nervous system	Headache, confusion, hyper- or hypoactive deep tendon reflexes, seizures, coma, increased intracranial pressure
Musculoskeletal	Weakness, fatigue, muscle cramps/twitching
Gastrointestinal	Anorexia, nausea, vomiting, watery diarrhea
Cardiovascular	Hypertension and bradycardia if significant increases in intracranial pressure
Tissue	Lacrimation, salivation
Renal	Oliguria

Body System	Hypernatremia
Central nervous system	Restlessness, lethargy, ataxia, irritability, tonic spasms, delirium, seizures, coma
Musculoskeletal	Weakness
Cardiovascular	Tachycardia, hypotension, syncope
Tissue	Dry sticky mucous membranes, red swollen tongue, decreased saliva and tears
Renal	Oliguria
Metabolic	Fever

fluid compartment can lead to a significant rise in extracellular potassium. A number of medications can contribute to hyperkalemia, particularly in the presence of renal insufficiency, including potassium-sparing diuretics, angiotensin-converting enzyme inhibitors, and nonsteroidal anti-inflammatories. Since aldosterone plays an important role in stimulating potassium secretion from the collecting ducts, any drug (like spironolactone and angiotensin-converting enzyme inhibitors) that interferes with aldosterone activity inhibits potassium secretion. Impaired potassium excretion also occurs with renal insufficiency and renal failure.

Symptoms of hyperkalemia are primarily gastrointestinal, neuromuscular, and cardiovascular (Table 2-5). Gastrointestinal symptoms include nausea, vomiting, intestinal colic, and diarrhea;

Table 2-4
Etiology of Potassium Abnormalities

Hyperkalemia
Increased intake
  Potassium supplementation
  Blood transfusions
  Endogenous load/destruction: hemolysis, rhabdomyolysis, crush injury, gastrointestinal hemorrhage
Increased release
  Acidosis
  Rapid rise of extracellular osmolality (hyperglycemia or mannitol)
Impaired excretion
  Potassium-sparing diuretics
  Renal insufficiency/failure

Hypokalemia
Inadequate intake
  Dietary, potassium-free intravenous fluids, potassium-deficient total parenteral nutrition
Excessive potassium excretion
  Hyperaldosteronism
  Medications
Gastrointestinal losses
  Direct loss of potassium from gastrointestinal fluid (diarrhea)
  Renal loss of potassium (gastric fluid, either as vomiting or high nasogastric output)

neuromuscular symptoms range from weakness to ascending paralysis to respiratory failure; while cardiovascular manifestations range from electrocardiogram (ECG) changes to cardiac arrhythmias and arrest. ECG changes that may be seen with hyperkalemia include:

Peaked T waves (early change)
Flattened P wave
Prolonged PR interval (first-degree block)
Widened QRS complex
Sine wave formation
Ventricular fibrillation

Hypokalemia. Hypokalemia is more commonly seen in the surgical patient. It may be caused by inadequate intake (dietary, potassium-free intravenous fluids, or total parenteral nutrition with inadequate potassium replacement), excessive renal excretion (hyperaldosteronism, medications such as diuretics that increase potassium excretion, or drugs such as penicillin that promote renal tubular loss of potassium), loss in gastrointestinal secretions (direct loss of potassium in stool or renal potassium loss from vomiting or high nasogastric output), or intracellular shifts (as seen with metabolic alkalosis or insulin therapy) (see Table 2-4). The change in potassium associated with alkalosis can be calculated by the following formula:

Potassium decreases by 0.3 mEq/L for every
0.1 increase in pH above normal.

Additionally, drugs such as amphotericin, aminoglycosides, foscarnet, cisplatin, and ifosfamide that induce magnesium depletion will cause renal potassium wastage.[7,8] In cases in which potassium deficiency is due to magnesium depletion,[9] potassium repletion is difficult unless hypomagnesemia is first corrected.

The symptoms of hypokalemia (see Table 2-5), like that of hyperkalemia, are primarily related to gastrointestinal, neuromuscular, and cardiac causes and include ileus, constipation, weakness, fatigue, diminished tendon reflexes, paralysis, and cardiac arrest (pulseless electrical activity or asystole). ECG changes suggestive of hypokalemia include:

U waves
T-wave flattening

Table 2-5
Clinical Manifestations of Abnormalities in Potassium, Magnesium, and Calcium

	Increased Serum Levels		
System	Potassium	Magnesium	Calcium
Gastrointestinal	Nausea/vomiting, colic, diarrhea	Nausea/vomiting	Anorexia, nausea/vomiting, abdominal pain
Neuromuscular	Weakness, paralysis, respiratory failure	Weakness, lethargy, decreased reflexes	Weakness, confusion, coma, bone pain
Cardiovascular	Arrhythmia, arrest	Hypotension, arrest	Hypertension, arrhythmia, polyuria
Renal			Polydipsia

	Decreased Serum Levels		
System	Potassium	Magnesium	Calcium
Gastrointestinal	Ileus, constipation		
Neuromuscular	Decreased reflexes, fatigue, weakness, paralysis	Hyperactive reflexes, muscle tremors, tetany, seizures	Hyperactive reflexes, paresthesias, carpopedal spasm, seizures
Cardiovascular	Arrest	Arrhythmia	Heart failure

ST-segment changes
Arrhythmias (especially if patient is taking digitalis)

Magnesium Abnormalities

Magnesium is the fourth most common mineral in the body and is found primarily in the intracellular compartment, as is potassium. Of the fraction found in the extracellular space, one third is bound to serum albumin. Therefore the plasma level of magnesium may be a poor indicator of total body stores in the presence of hypoalbuminemia. Magnesium should be replaced until levels are in the upper limit of normal. The normal dietary intake is approximately 20 mEq (240 mg) daily and is excreted in both the feces and urine. The kidneys have a remarkable ability to conserve magnesium, as well as sodium.

Hypermagnesemia. Hypermagnesemia is rare but can be seen with impaired renal function and excess intake in the form of total parenteral nutrition or magnesium-containing laxatives and antacids. Symptoms (see Table 2-5) may be gastrointestinal (nausea and vomiting), neuromuscular (weakness, lethargy, and decreased reflexes), or cardiovascular (hypotension and arrest). ECG changes are similar to those seen with hyperkalemia and include:

Increased PR interval
Widened QRS complex
Elevated T waves

Hypomagnesemia. Magnesium depletion is a common problem in hospitalized patients, particularly in the ICU.[10] The kidney is primarily responsible for magnesium homeostasis through regulation by calcium/magnesium receptors on renal tubular cells that sense serum magnesium levels.[11] Hypomagnesemia results from a variety of etiologies ranging from poor intake (starvation, alcoholism, prolonged use of intravenous fluids, and total parenteral nutrition with inadequate supplementation of magnesium), increased renal excretion (alcohol, most diuretics, and amphotericin B), gastrointestinal losses (diarrhea), malabsorption, acute pancreatitis, diabetic ketoacidosis, and primary aldosteronism.

Magnesium depletion is characterized by neuromuscular and central nervous system hyperactivity, and symptoms are similar to those of calcium deficiency, including hyperactive reflexes, muscle tremors, and tetany with a positive Chvostek's sign (see Table 2-5).

Severe deficiencies can lead to delirium and seizures. A number of ECG changes can also occur and include:

Prolonged QT and PR intervals
ST-segment depression
Flattening or inversion of P waves
Torsades de pointes
Arrhythmias

Hypomagnesemia is important not only for its direct effects on the nervous system but also because it can produce hypocalcemia and lead to persistent hypokalemia. When hypokalemia or hypocalcemia coexist with hypomagnesemia, magnesium should be aggressively replaced to assist in restoring potassium or calcium homeostasis.

Calcium Abnormalities

The vast majority of the body's calcium is contained within the bone matrix with only less than 1% found in the extracellular fluid. Serum calcium is distributed among three forms: protein-bound (40%), complexed to phosphate and other anions (10%), and ionized (50%). It is the ionized fraction that is responsible for neuromuscular stability and can be measured directly. When measuring total serum calcium levels, the albumin concentration must be taken into consideration:

Adjust total serum calcium down by 0.8 mg/dL

for every 1-g/dL decrease in albumin.

Unlike changes in albumin, changes in pH will affect the ionized calcium concentration. Acidosis decreases protein binding, thereby increasing the ionized fraction of calcium.

Hypercalcemia. Hypercalcemia is defined as a serum calcium level above the normal range of 8.5 to 10.5 mEq/L, or an increase in the ionized calcium level above 4.2 to 4.8 mg/dL. Primary hyperparathyroidism in the outpatient setting and malignancy (associated bony metastasis or due to secretion of parathyroid hormone–related protein) in hospitalized patients account for most cases of symptomatic hypercalcemia.[12] Symptoms of hypercalcemia (see Table 2-5), which vary with the degree of severity, include neurologic (depression, confusion, stupor, or coma), musculoskeletal (weakness and back and extremity pain), renal (polyuria and polydipsia as kidneys lose their ability to concentrate), and gastrointestinal (anorexia, nausea, vomiting, constipation, abdominal pain, and weight loss). Cardiac symptoms also are present and can include hypertension, cardiac arrhythmias, and a worsening of digitalis toxicity. ECG changes of hypercalcemia include:

Shortened QT interval
Prolonged PR and QRS intervals
Increased QRS voltage
T-wave flattening and widening
AV block (can progress to complete heart block, then cardiac arrest with severe hypercalcemia)

Hypocalcemia. Hypocalcemia is defined as a serum calcium level below the normal range of 8.5 to 10.5 mEq/L, or a decrease in the ionized calcium level below the range of 4.2 to 4.8 mg/dL. The etiologies of hypocalcemia include pancreatitis, massive soft tissue infections such as necrotizing fasciitis, renal failure, pancreatic and small bowel fistulas, hypoparathyroidism, toxic shock syndrome, abnormalities in magnesium, and tumor lysis syndrome. In addition, transient hypocalcemia commonly occurs following removal of a parathyroid adenoma as atrophy of the remaining glands and avid bone uptake of calcium occurs. Hungry bone syndrome can develop postoperatively in secondary or tertiary hyperparathyroidism as bone is being rapidly remineralized, requiring high-dose calcium supplementation.[13] Additionally, malignancies associated with increased osteoclastic activity such as breast and prostate cancer can lead to hypocalcemia from increased bone formation.[14] Calcium precipitation with organic anions is also a cause of hypocalcemia, such as that seen with hyperphosphatemia (tumor lysis syndrome or rhabdomyolysis), pancreatitis (chelation with free fatty acids), or massive blood transfusion (citrate).[15,16] Hypocalcemia rarely results from decreased intake, as bone reabsorption can maintain normal levels for prolonged periods of time.

Asymptomatic hypocalcemia may occur with hypoproteinemia (normal ionized calcium), but symptoms can develop with alkalosis (decreased ionized calcium). In general, symptoms do not occur until the ionized fraction falls below 2.5 mg/dL, and are neuromuscular and cardiac in origin (see Table 2-5), including paresthesias of the face and extremities, muscle cramps, carpopedal spasm, stridor, tetany, and seizures. Patients will demonstrate hyperreflexia and positive Chvostek's sign (spasm resulting from tapping over the facial nerve) and Trousseau's sign (spasm resulting from pressure applied to the nerves and vessels of the upper extremity, as when obtaining a blood pressure). Decreased cardiac contractility and heart failure can also accompany hypocalcemia, as do the following ECG changes:

Prolonged QT interval
T-wave inversion
Heart blocks
Ventricular fibrillation

Phosphorus Abnormalities

Phosphorus is the primary intracellular divalent anion and is abundant in metabolically active cells. Phosphorus is responsible for maintaining energy production in the form of glycolysis or high-energy phosphate products such as adenosine triphosphate (ATP), and levels are tightly controlled by renal excretion.

Hyperphosphatemia. Hyperphosphatemia can be due to decreased urinary excretion or increased intake or production of phosphorus. Most cases of hyperphosphatemia are seen in patients with impaired renal function. Hypoparathyroidism or hyperthyroidism also can decrease urinary excretion of phosphorus and

thus lead to hyperphosphatemia. Increased release of endogenous phosphorus can be seen in association with cell destruction, such as with rhabdomyolysis, tumor lysis syndrome, hemolysis, sepsis, severe hypothermia, or malignant hyperthermia. Excessive phosphate administration (phosphorus-containing laxatives) may also lead to elevated phosphate levels. Most cases of hyperphosphatemia are asymptomatic, but significant hyperphosphatemia can lead to metastatic soft tissue calcium-phosphorus complexes.

Hypophosphatemia. Hypophosphatemia can be due to a decrease in phosphorus intake, an intracellular shift of phosphorus, or an increase in phosphorus excretion. Decreased intake can occur with malnutrition or if decreased gastrointestinal absorption is present (malabsorption or phosphate binders). Most cases are due to an intracellular shift of phosphorus as occurs in association with respiratory alkalosis, insulin therapy, the refeeding syndrome, and hungry bone syndrome. Clinical manifestations of hypophosphatemia are usually absent until levels fall significantly. In general, symptoms are related to adverse effects on the oxygen availability of tissue and to a decrease in high-energy phosphates and can be manifested as cardiac dysfunction or muscle weakness.

Acid-Base Balance

Acid-Base Homeostasis

The pH of body fluids is maintained within a narrow range despite the ability of the kidneys to generate large amounts of HCO_3^- and the normal large acid load produced as by-products of metabolism. Important buffers include:

Intracellular proteins and phosphates
Extracellular bicarbonate-carbonic acid system

Compensation for acid-base derangements is either respiratory (for metabolic derangements) or metabolic (for respiratory derangements). Changes in ventilation in response to metabolic abnormalities are mediated by hydrogen-sensitive chemoreceptors found in the carotid body and brain stem. Acidosis stimulates the chemoreceptors to increase ventilation while alkalosis decreases the activity of the chemoreceptors and thus decreases ventilation. The kidneys provide compensation for respiratory abnormalities by either increasing or decreasing bicarbonate reabsorption for respiratory acidosis or alkalosis, respectively. Unlike the prompt change in ventilation that occurs with metabolic abnormalities, the compensatory response in the kidneys to respiratory abnormalities is delayed. Compensation does not begin for at least 6 hours and continues for several days. Because of this delayed compensatory response, respiratory acid-base derangements are classified as acute (before renal compensation) or chronic (after renal compensation). The predicted compensatory changes in response to metabolic or respiratory derangements are listed in Table 2-6.[17] If the expected change in pH is exceeded, then a mixed acid-base abnormality may be present (Table 2-7).

Metabolic Derangements

Metabolic Acidosis. Metabolic acidosis results from an increased intake of acids, an increased generation of acids, or an increased loss of bicarbonate (Table 2-8). The body responds by:

Producing buffers (extracellular bicarbonate and intracellular from bone and muscle)
Increasing ventilation (Kussmaul respirations)
Increasing renal reabsorption and generation of bicarbonate

Table 2-6
Predicted Changes in Acid-Base Disorders

Disorder	Predicted Change
Metabolic	
Metabolic acidosis	$Pco_2 = 1.5 \times HCO_3^- + 8$
Metabolic alkalosis	$Pco_2 = 0.7 \times HCO_3^- + 21$
Respiratory	
Acute respiratory acidosis	$\Delta pH = (Pco_2 - 40) \times 0.008$
Chronic respiratory acidosis	$\Delta pH = (Pco_2 - 40) \times 0.003$
Acute respiratory alkalosis	$\Delta pH = (40 - Pco_2) \times 0.008$
Chronic respiratory alkalosis	$\Delta pH = (40 - Pco_2) \times 0.017$

The kidney will also increase secretion of hydrogen and thus increase urinary excretion of NH_4^+ ($H^+ + NH_3^+ = NH_4^+$). In evaluating a patient with a low serum bicarbonate level and metabolic acidosis, first measure the anion gap (AG), an index of unmeasured anions.

$$AG = [Na] - [Cl + HCO_3]$$

The normal AG is less than 12 mmol/L and is due primarily to albumin, so that the estimated AG must be adjusted for albumin (hypoalbuminemia reduces the AG).[18]

$$\text{corrected AG} = \text{actual AG} - \{2.5(4.5 - \text{albumin})\}$$

Metabolic acidosis with an increased AG occurs from either exogenous acid ingestion (ethylene glycol, salicylate, or methanol) or endogenous acid production of:

β-Hydroxybutyrate and acetoacetate in ketoacidosis
Lactate in lactic acidosis
Organic acids in renal insufficiency

One of the most common causes of severe metabolic acidosis in surgical patients is lactic acidosis. With shock, lactate is produced as a by-product of inadequate tissue perfusion. The treatment is to restore perfusion with volume resuscitation rather than to attempt to correct the abnormality with exogenous bicarbonate. With adequate perfusion, the lactic acid is metabolized and the pH level returns to normal. The administration of bicarbonate for the treatment of metabolic acidosis is controversial as it is not clear that acidosis is deleterious.[19] The overzealous administration of bicarbonate can lead to metabolic alkalosis, which shifts the oxyhemoglobin dissociation curve to the left, interfering with oxygen unloading at the tissue level, and can be associated with arrhythmias that are

difficult to treat. An additional disadvantage is that sodium bicarbonate can actually exacerbate intracellular acidosis. Administered bicarbonate can combine with the excess hydrogen ions to form carbonic acid, which is then converted to CO_2 and water, thus raising the Pco_2. This would be undesirable in most situations and could compound ventilation abnormalities in patients with underlying acute respiratory distress syndrome. This CO_2 can diffuse into cells, but bicarbonate remains extracellular, thereby worsening intracellular acidosis. There are commercially available buffers that do not increase CO_2 production and avoid intracellular acidosis, including carbicarb and tromethamine. Carbicarb is an eqimolar mixture of sodium bicarbonate and sodium carbonate. Carbonate combines with hydrogen ions, producing bicarbonate rather than CO_2. However, this buffer is not yet available for use in humans. An alternative buffer that also does not generate CO_2 and is available for clinical use is tris-hydroxymethyl aminomethane (THAM). THAM is excreted by the kidneys and therefore should be used with caution in patients with renal insufficiency. Side effects include hyperkalemia and hypoglycemia.

Metabolic acidosis with a normal anion gap results from either acid administration (HCl or NH_4^+) or a loss of bicarbonate from gastrointestinal sources such as diarrhea, fistulas (enteric, pancreatic, or biliary), ureterosigmoidostomy, or from renal loss. The bicarbonate loss is accompanied by a gain of chloride, thus the AG remains unchanged. To determine if the loss of bicarbonate is renal in etiology, the urinary $[NH_4^+]$ can be measured. A low urinary $[NH_4^+]$ in the face of hyperchloremic acidosis would indicate the kidney as the site of loss, and evaluation for renal tubular acidosis should be undertaken. A proximal renal tubular acidosis results from decreased tubular reabsorption of HCO_3^-, while distal renal tubular acidosis results from decreased acid excretion. The carbonic anhydrase inhibitor acetazolamide also causes bicarbonate loss from the kidneys.

Metabolic Alkalosis. Normal acid-base homeostasis prevents metabolic alkalosis from developing unless both an increase in bicarbonate generation and impaired renal excretion of bicarbonate occurs (Table 2-9). The majority of patients will also have hypokalemia (extracellular potassium ions exchange with intracellular hydrogen ions, allowing the hydrogen ions to buffer excess HCO_3^-). A problem that may be encountered in surgical patients with pyloric obstruction (seen in infants with pyloric stenosis or adults with duodenal ulcer disease) is hypochloremic, hypokalemic, or metabolic alkalosis. Unlike vomiting associated with an open pylorus that involves a loss of gastric as well as pancreatic, biliary, and intestinal

Table 2-7
Respiratory and Metabolic Components of Acid-Base Disorders

Type of Acid-Base Disorder	Acute (Uncompensated)			Chronic (Partially Compensated)		
	pH	Pco2 (Respiratory Component)	Plasma HCO3−[a] (Metabolic Component)	pH	Pco2 (Respiratory Component)	Plasma HCO3−[a] (Metabolic Component)
Respiratory acidosis	↓↓	↑↑	N	↓	↑↑	↑
Respiratory alkalosis	↑↑	↓↓	N	↑	↓↓	↓
Metabolic acidosis	↓↓	N	↓↓	↓	↓	↓
Metabolic alkalosis	↑↑	N	↑↑	↑	↑?	↑

[a]Measured as standard bicarbonate, whole blood buffer base, CO_2 content, or CO_2 combining power. The *base excess value* is positive when the standard bicarbonate is above normal and negative when the standard bicarbonate is below normal.

Table 2-8
Etiology of Metabolic Acidosis

Increased Anion Gap Metabolic Acidosis
Exogenous acid ingestion
Ethylene glycol
Salicylate
Methanol
Endogenous acid production
Ketoacidosis
Lactic acidosis
Renal insufficiency
Normal Anion Gap
Acid administration (HCl)
Loss of bicarbonate
Gastrointestinal losses (diarrhea, fistulas)
Ureterosigmoidoscopy
Renal tubular acidosis
Carbonic anhydrase inhibitor

secretions, vomiting with an obstructed pylorus results only in the loss of gastric fluid, which is high in chloride and hydrogen, and thus a hypochloremic alkalosis. Initially the urinary bicarbonate level is high to compensate for the alkalosis. Hydrogen ion reabsorption also ensues with an accompanied potassium ion excretion. Additionally, in response to the volume deficit, aldosterone-mediated sodium reabsorption is accompanied by potassium excretion. The resulting hypokalemia leads to the excretion of hydrogen ions in the face of alkalosis, a paradoxic aciduria. Treatment includes replacement of the volume deficit with isotonic saline and potassium once adequate urine output is ensured.

Respiratory Derangements

Under normal circumstances blood P_{CO_2} is tightly maintained by alveolar ventilation, controlled by the respiratory centers in the pons and medulla oblongata.

Respiratory Acidosis. This condition is associated with the retention of CO_2 secondary to decreased alveolar ventilation. The principal causes are listed in Table 2-10. As compensation is primarily renal, it is a delayed response. Treatment is directed at the underlying cause and at measures to ensure adequate ventilation. This may entail patient-initiated volume expansion or noninvasive (bilevel positive airway pressure; BIPAP) or invasive (endotracheal intubation) ventilation strategies.

Table 2-9
Etiology of Metabolic Alkalosis

Increased Bicarbonate Generation
1. Chloride losing (urinary chloride greater than 20 mEq/L)
Mineralocorticoid excess
Profound potassium depletion
2. Chloride sparing (urinary chloride less than 20 mEq/L)
Loss from gastric secretions (emesis or nasogastric suction)
Diuretics
3. Excess administration of alkali
Acetate in parenteral nutrition
Citrate in blood transfusions
Antacids
Bicarbonate
Milk-alkali syndrome
Impaired Bicarbonate Excretion
1. Decreased glomerular filtration
2. Increased bicarbonate reabsorption (hypercarbia or potassium depletion)

Table 2-10
Etiology of Respiratory Acidosis: Hypoventilation

Narcotics
CNS injury
Pulmonary: significant
Secretions
Atelectasis
Mucus plug
Pneumonia
Pleural effusion
Pain from abdominal or thoracic injuries or incisions
Limited diaphragmatic excursion from intra-abdominal pathology
Abdominal distention
Abdominal compartment syndrome
Ascites

Respiratory Alkalosis. Most cases of respiratory alkalosis are acute in nature and secondary to alveolar hyperventilation. Etiologies include pain or anxiety, neurologic disorders (meningitis, trauma), drugs (such as salicylates), fever or gram-negative bacteremia, thyrotoxicosis, or hypoxemia. Acute hypocapnia can cause an uptake of potassium and phosphate into cells and increased binding of calcium to albumin, leading to symptomatic hypokalemia, hypophosphatemia, and hypocalcemia, with subsequent arrhythmias, paresthesias, muscle cramps, and seizures. Treatment should be directed at the underlying cause, but may also require direct treatment of the hyperventilation.

FLUID AND ELECTROLYTE THERAPY

Parenteral Solutions

There are a number of commercially available electrolyte solutions for parenteral administration. The most common solutions are listed in Table 2-11. The type of fluid administered depends on the patient's volume status and the type of concentration or compositional abnormality present. Both lactated Ringer's and normal saline are considered isotonic and are useful in replacing gastrointestinal losses and extracellular volume deficits. Lactated Ringer's is slightly hypotonic in that it contains 130 mEq of sodium, which is balanced by 109 mEq of chloride and 28 mEq of lactate. Lactate is used rather than bicarbonate because it is more stable in intravenous fluids during storage. It is converted into bicarbonate in the liver following infusion, even in the face of hemorrhagic shock. Recent evidence has suggested that resuscitation using lactated Ringer's may be deleterious because it activates the inflammatory response and induces apoptosis. The component that has been implicated is the D isomer of lactate, which unlike the D isomer is not a normal intermediary in mammalian metabolism. Traditionally, solutions contain a 50:50 mixture of the D and D isomer. In vitro studies show that only the D isomer does not activate neutrophils.[20]

Sodium chloride is mildly hypertonic, containing 154 mEq of sodium that is balanced by 154 mEq of chloride. The high chloride concentration imposes a significant chloride load upon the kidneys and may lead to a hyperchloremic metabolic acidosis. It is an ideal solution, however, for correcting volume deficits associated with hyponatremia, hypochloremia, and metabolic alkalosis.

The less concentrated sodium solutions, such as 0.45% sodium chloride, are useful to replace ongoing gastrointestinal losses as well as for maintenance fluid therapy in the postoperative period. This solution provides sufficient free water for insensible losses and enough sodium to aid the kidneys in adjustment of serum sodium

Table 2-11
Electrolyte Solutions for Parenteral Administration

Solution	Electrolyte Composition (mEq/L)						
	Na	CL	K	HCO$_3^-$	Ca	Mg	mOsm
Extracellular fluid	142	103	4	27	5	3	280–310
Lactated Ringer's	130	109	4	28	3		273
0.9% Sodium chloride	154	154					308
D$_5$ 0.45% Sodium chloride	77	77					407
D$_5$ W							253
3% Sodium chloride	513	513					1026

levels. The addition of 5% dextrose (50 g of dextrose per liter) supplies 200 kcal/L, and it is always added to solutions containing less than 0.45% sodium chloride to maintain osmolality and thus prevent lysis of red blood cells that may occur with rapid infusion of hypotonic fluids. The addition of potassium is useful once adequate renal function and urine output are established.

Alternative Resuscitative Fluids

A number of alternative solutions for volume expansion and resuscitation are now available and are listed in Table 2-12.[21] Hypertonic saline solutions (3.5% and 5%) are used for correction of severe sodium deficits and are discussed elsewhere in this chapter. Hypertonic saline (7.5%) has been used as a treatment modality in patients with closed head injuries.[22] It has been shown to increase cerebral perfusion and decrease intracranial pressure, thus decreasing brain edema.[23] Small-volume hypertonic saline, compared to large-volume isotonic saline, has also been shown to be an effective volume expander in models of hemorrhagic shock.[24] However, there also have been concerns of increased bleeding, as hypertonic saline is an arteriolar vasodilator. A meta-analysis of prospective randomized controlled trials in trauma patients suggests that hypertonic saline may be no better than standard-of-care isotonic saline.[25] In subgroup analysis, however, patients with shock and a concomitant closed head injury did demonstrate benefit. Renewed interest in this solution has occurred with recent evidence of its anti-inflammatory and immunomodulatory properties.[26–28]

Colloids are also used in surgical patients and have long been debated as effective volume expanders compared to isotonic crystalloids. Due to their molecular weight, they are confined to the intravascular space and their infusion results in more efficient plasma volume expansion. However, under conditions of severe hemorrhagic shock, capillary membrane permeability increases, permitting colloids to enter the interstitial space, which can worsen edema and impair tissue oxygenation. The theory that these high molecular

weight agents "plug" capillary leaks that occur during neutrophil-mediated organ injury has not been established.[29,30] There are four major types of colloids available—albumin, dextrans, hetastarch, and gelatins—that are described by their molecular weight and size in Table 2-12. Colloid solutions with smaller size particles and lower molecular weights exert a greater oncotic effect, but are retained within the circulation for a shorter period of time than larger and higher molecular weight colloids.

Albumin (molecular weight 70,000) is prepared from pooled human plasma, then heat sterilized. It is typically available as either a 5% (osmolality 300 mOsm/L) or 25% (osmolality 1500 mOsm/L) solution. Because it is a derivative of blood, it can be associated with allergic reactions. Albumin has been shown to induce renal failure and impair pulmonary function when used for resuscitation of hemorrhagic shock.[31,32]

Dextrans are glucose polymers produced by bacteria grown on sucrose media and are available as either 40,000 (dextran 40) or 70,000 (dextran 70) molecular-weight solutions. They lead to initial volume expansion due to their osmotic effect, but are associated with alterations in blood viscosity. Thus dextrans are used primarily to lower blood viscosity rather than as volume expanders. Dextrans have, however, been used in association with hypertonic saline to help maintain intravascular volume.

Hydroxyethyl starch solutions are another group of alternative plasma expanders and volume replacement solutions. Hetastarches are produced by the hydrolysis of insoluble amylopectin, followed by a varying number of substitutions of hydroxyl groups for carbon groups on glucose molecules. The molecular weights can range from 1000 to 3,000,000. The high molecular weight hydroxyethyl starch, hetastarch (average molecular weight 480,000), which comes as a 6% solution, is the only hydroxyethyl starch approved for use in the United States. Hemostatic derangements have been related to decreases in von Willebrand factor and factor VIII:c, and its use has been associated with postoperative bleeding in cardiac and

Table 2-12
Alternative Resuscitative Fluids

Solution	Molecular Weight	Osmolality (mOsm/L)	Sodium (mEq/L)
Hypertonic saline (7.5%)		2565	1283
Albumin 5%	70,000	300	130–160
Albumin 25%	70,000	1500	130–160
Dextran 40	40,000	308	154
Dextran 70	70,000	308	154
Hetastarch	450,000	310	154
Hextend	670,000	307	143
Gelofusine	30,000	NA	154

neurosurgery patients.[33,34] Hetastarch also can induce renal dysfunction in patients with septic shock and in recipients of kidneys procured from brain-dead donors.[35,36] Currently, hetastarch has a limited role in massive resuscitation because of its associated coagulopathy and hyperchloremic acidosis (due to its high chloride content). Hextend is a modified, balanced, high molecular weight hydroxyethyl starch that is suspended in a lactate-buffered solution, rather than in saline. A phase III clinical study comparing Hextend to a similar 6% hydroxyethyl starch in patients undergoing major abdominal surgery demonstrated no adverse effects on coagulation with Hextend other than the known effects of hemodilution.[37] Hextend has not been tested in massive resuscitation, and not all clinical studies show consistent results.[38]

Gelatins are the fourth group of colloids and are produced from bovine collagen. The two major types are urea-linked gelatin and succinylated gelatin (modified fluid gelatin, Gelofusine). Gelofusine has been used abroad with mixed results[39,40] and is currently not approved for use in the United States.

Correction of Life-Threatening Electrolyte Abnormalities[41]

Sodium

Hypernatremia. Treatment of hypernatremia usually consists of treatment of the associated water deficit. In hypovolemic patients, volume should be restored with normal saline. Once adequate volume status has been achieved, the water deficit is replaced using a hypotonic fluid such as 5% dextrose, 5% dextrose in 1/4 normal saline, or enteral water. This is the formula used to estimate the amount of water required to correct hypernatremia:

$$\text{Water deficit (L)} = \frac{\text{serum sodium} - 140}{140} \times \text{TBW}$$

Estimate TBW as 50% of lean body mass in men and 40% in women

The rate of fluid administered should be titrated to achieve a decrease in serum sodium of no more than 1 mEq/h and 12 mEq/d for treatment of acute hypernatremia. Even slower correction should be undertaken with chronic hypernatremia (0.7 mEq/L/h), as overly rapid correction can lead to cerebral edema and herniation. The type of fluid depends on the severity and ease of correction. Oral or enteral replacement is acceptable in most cases, or intravenous replacement with half- or quarter-normal saline can be used. Caution should also be exercised when using 5% dextrose in water in order to avoid overly rapid correction. Frequent neurologic evaluation as well as frequent evaluation of serum sodium levels also should be performed.

Hyponatremia. Most cases of hyponatremia can be treated by free water restriction and, if severe, the administration of sodium. In patients with normal renal function, symptomatic hyponatremia does not occur until the serum sodium level is greater than or equal to 120 mEq/L. If neurologic symptoms are present, then 3% normal saline should be used to increase the sodium by no more than 1 mEq/L per hour until the serum sodium level reaches 130 mEq/L or neurologic symptoms are improved. Correction of asymptomatic hyponatremia should increase the sodium level by no more than 0.5 mEq/L to a maximum increase of 12 mEq/L per day, and even slower in chronic hyponatremia. The rapid correction of hyponatremia can lead to pontine myelinolysis,[42] with seizures, weakness/paresis, akinetic movements, and unresponsiveness, and may

result in permanent brain damage and death. Magnetic resonance imaging (MRI) may assist in the diagnosis.[43]

Potassium

Hyperkalemia. Treatment options for symptomatic hyperkalemia are listed in Table 2-13. The goal of therapy is to reduce the total body potassium, shift potassium from extracellular to intracellular, and to protect the cells from the effects of increased potassium. All patients should have exogenous sources of potassium discontinued, including potassium supplementation in intravenous fluids and enteral and parenteral solutions. Potassium can be removed from the body with a cation-exchange resin, such as Kayexalate, which binds potassium in exchange for sodium. It can be administered either orally (preferred) or rectally. Measures should also include attempts to shift potassium intracellularly with glucose and bicarbonate. Nebulized albuterol (10 to 20 mg) may also be used. Glucose alone will cause a rise in insulin secretion, but in the acutely ill this response may be blunted and therefore both glucose and insulin are recommended. Circulatory overload and hypernatremia may result from the administration of Kayexalate and bicarbonate, so care should be exercised when administering these agents. When ECG changes are present, calcium chloride or calcium gluconate (5 to 10 mL of 10% solution) should also be administered to counteract the myocardial effects of hyperkalemia. It should be used cautiously in patients on digitalis as digitalis toxicity may occur. All of the above measures are temporary (lasting from 1 to approximately 4 hours). Dialysis should be considered when conservative measures fail.

Hypokalemia. Treatment for hypokalemia consists of potassium repletion, the rate of which is determined by the symptoms (Table 2-14). Oral repletion is adequate for mild and asymptomatic hypokalemia. If intravenous repletion is required, usually no more than 10 to 20 mEq/h is advisable in an unmonitored setting. This amount can be increased to 40 mEq/h when accompanied by ECG monitoring, and even more so in the case of imminent cardiac arrest from a malignant arrhythmia associated with hypokalemia. Caution should be exercised when oliguria or impaired renal function is coexistent.

Magnesium

Hypermagnesemia. Treatment for hypermagnesemia consists of measures to withhold exogenous sources of magnesium, correct volume deficit, and correct acidosis if present. To manage acute symptoms, calcium chloride (5 to 10 mL) should be administered to antagonize the cardiovascular effects. If elevated levels or symptoms persist, dialysis is indicated.

Table 2-13
Treatment of Symptomatic Hyperkalemia

Potassium removal
  Kayexalate
    Oral administration is 15–30 g in 50–100 mL of 20% sorbitol
    Rectal administration is 50 g in 200 mL 20% sorbitol
  Dialysis
Shift potassium
  Glucose 1 ampule of D_{50} and regular insulin 5–10 units intravenous
  Bicarbonate 1 ampule intravenous
Counteract cardiac effects
  Calcium gluconate 5–10 mL of 10% solution

Table 2-14
Electrolyte Replacement Therapy Protocol

Potassium
Serum potassium level <4.0 mEq/L:
    Asymptomatic, tolerating enteral nutrition: KCl 40 mEq per enteral access × 1 dose
    Asymptomatic, not tolerating enteral nutrition: KCl 20 mEq IV q2h × 2 doses
    Symptomatic: KCl 20 mEq IV q1h × 4 doses
    Recheck potassium level 2 hours after end of infusion; if <3.5 mEq/L and asymptomatic, replace as per
      above protocol

Magnesium
Magnesium level 1.0–1.8 mEq/L:
    Magnesium sulfate 0.5 mEq/kg in normal saline 250 mL infused IV over 24 h × 3 days
    Recheck magnesium level in 3 days
Magnesium level <1.0 mEq/L:
    Magnesium sulfate 1 mEq/kg in normal saline 250 mL infused IV over 24 h × 1 day, then 0.5 mEq/kg in
      normal saline 250 mL infused IV over 24 h × 2 days
    Recheck magnesium level in 3 days
If patient has gastric access and needs a bowel regimen:
    Milk of magnesia 15 mL (approximately 49 mEq magnesium) q24h per gastric tube; hold for diarrhea

Calcium
Normalized calcium level <4.0 mg/dL:
    With gastric access and tolerating enteral nutrition: Calcium carbonate suspension 1250 mg/5 mL q6h per
      gastric access; recheck ionized calcium level in 3 days
    Without gastric access or not tolerating enteral nutrition: Calcium gluconate 2 g IV over 1 h × 1 dose;
      recheck ionized calcium level in 3 days

Phosphate
Phosphate level 1.0–2.5 mg/dL:
    Tolerating enteral nutrition: Neutra-Phos 2 packets q6h per gastric tube or feeding tube
    No enteral nutrition: $KPHO_4$ or $NaPO_4$ 0.15 mmol/kg IV over 6 h × 1 dose
    Recheck phosphate level in 3 days
Phosphate level <1.0 mg/dL:
    Tolerating enteral nutrition: $KPHO_4$ or $NaPO_4$ 0.25 mmol/kg over 6 h × 1 dose
    Recheck phosphate level 4 hours after end of infusion; if <2.5 mg/dL, begin Neutra-Phos 2 packets q6h
    Not tolerating enteral nutrition: $KPHO_4$ or $NaPO_4$ 0.25 mmol/kg (LBW) over 6 h × 1 dose; recheck
      phosphate level 4 hours after end of infusion; if <2.5 mg/dL, then $KPHO_4$ or $NaPO_4$ 0.15 mmol/kg
      (LBW) IV over 6 h × 1 dose

3 mmol $KPHO_4$ = 3 mmol Phos and 4.4 mEq K^+ = 1 mL
3 mmol $NaPHO_4$ = 3 mmol Phos and 4 mEq Na^+ = 1 mL
Neutra-Phos 1 packet = 8 mmol Phos, 7 mEq K^+, 7 mEq Na^+
Use patient's lean body weight (LBW) in kilograms for all calculations.
Disregard protocol if patient has renal failure, is on dialysis, or has a creatinine clearance <30 mL/min.

Hypomagnesemia. Correction of magnesium depletion can be oral if asymptomatic and mild. Otherwise, intravenous repletion is indicated and depends on severity (see Table 2-14) and symptoms. For those with severe deficits (<1.0 mEq/L) or those who are symptomatic, administer 1 to 2 g of magnesium sulfate intravenously over 15 minutes or over 2 minutes if secondary to torsades de pointes (irregular ventricular arrhythmia). Caution should be exerted when giving large amounts of magnesium as magnesium toxicity may develop. The administration of simultaneous calcium gluconate will counteract the adverse side effects of a rapidly rising magnesium level and correct hypocalcemia, which is frequently associated with hypomagnesemia.

Calcium

Hypercalcemia. Treatment is required when hypercalcemia is symptomatic, which usually occurs when the serum level exceeds 12 mg/dL. The initial treatment is aimed at repleting the associated volume deficit and then inducing a brisk diuresis with normal saline. Treatment of hypercalcemia associated with malignancies is discussed later in this chapter.

Hypocalcemia. Asymptomatic hypocalcemia can be treated with oral or intravenous calcium (see Table 2-14). Acute symptomatic hypocalcemia should be treated intravenously with 10% calcium gluconate to achieve a serum concentration of 7 to 9 mg/dL. Associated deficits in magnesium, potassium, and pH must also be corrected. In fact, hypocalcemia will be refractory to treatment if hypomagnesemia is not first corrected. Routine calcium supplementation is no longer recommended in association with massive blood transfusions.[44]

Phosphorus

Hyperphosphatemia. Phosphate binders such as sucralfate or aluminum-containing antacids can be used to lower serum phosphorus levels. Calcium acetate tablets are also useful when hypocalcemia is simultaneously present. Dialysis is usually reserved for patients with renal failure.

Hypophosphatemia. Depending on the level of depletion and tolerance to oral supplementation, a number of repletion strategies are available (see Table 2-14).

Preoperative Fluid Therapy

The administration of maintenance fluid should be all that is required in an otherwise healthy individual prior to the time of surgery. This does not, however, include replacement of a pre-existing deficit or ongoing fluid losses. A frequently utilized formula for calculating maintenance fluids is as follows:

For the first 0 to 10 kg	Give 100 mL/kg per day
For the next 10 to 20 kg	Give an additional 50 mL/kg per day
For weight >20 kg	Give 20 mL/kg per day

For example, a 60-kg female would receive a total of 2400 mL of fluid daily: 1000 mL for the first 10 kg of body weight (10 kg × 100 mL/kg per day), 1000 mL for the next 20 kg of body weight (20 kg × 50 mL/kg per day), and 400 mL for the last 40 kg of body weight (20 kg × 20 mL/kg per day).

However, many surgical patients have volume and/or electrolyte abnormalities associated with their surgical disease. Preoperative evaluation of a patient's volume status and pre-existing electrolyte abnormalities are an important part of preoperative assessment and care. Volume deficits should be considered in patients presenting with obvious gastrointestinal loss such as emesis or diarrhea, as well as in patients with poor oral intake secondary to their disease. Less obvious are those fluid losses known as third-space or nonfunctional losses that occur with gastrointestinal obstruction, peritoneal or bowel inflammation, ascites, crush injuries, burns, and severe soft tissue infections (such as necrotizing fasciitis). The diagnosis of volume deficit is primarily clinical (see Table 2-1), though the physical signs may vary with the chronicity of the deficit. Cardiovascular signs (tachycardia and orthostasis) predominate with acute volume loss and are accompanied by oliguria and hemoconcentration. In general, acute volume deficits should be corrected prior to the time of operation.

Once a volume deficit is diagnosed, prompt fluid replacement should be instituted, usually with an isotonic crystalloid, depending on the particular electrolyte profile. Patients with cardiovascular signs of volume deficit should receive a bolus of 1 to 2 L of isotonic fluid followed by a continuous infusion. Close monitoring during this period is imperative. Resuscitation should be guided by the reversal of the signs of volume deficit such as restoration of vital signs, maintenance of adequate urine output ($1/2$ to 1 mL/kg per hour in an adult), and correction of base deficit. Patients who fail to correct their volume deficit, those with impaired renal function, and the elderly should be considered for more intense monitoring in an ICU setting for measurement of central venous pressure or cardiac output.

If symptomatic electrolyte abnormalities accompany volume deficit, the abnormality should be corrected to the extent that the acute symptom is relieved prior to surgical intervention. For correction of severe hypernatremia associated with a volume deficit, it is safer to slowly correct the hypernatremia with 0.45% saline or even lactated Ringer's rather than 5% dextrose alone. This will safely and slowly correct the hypernatremia and correct the associated volume deficit.

Intraoperative Fluid Therapy

With the induction of anesthesia, compensatory mechanisms are lost and hypotension will develop if volume deficits are not appropriately corrected prior to the time of surgery. Hemodynamic instability can be avoided by correcting known fluid losses, replacing ongoing losses, and providing adequate maintenance fluid therapy preoperatively. In addition to measured blood loss during surgery, open abdominal surgeries are associated with continued third-space losses due not only to the pre-existing conditions but also to exposed bowel during the time of surgery. Large soft tissue wounds, complex fractures with associated soft tissue injury, and burns all have additional third-space losses that must be considered in the operating room.

Postoperative Fluid Therapy

Postoperative fluid therapy should be based on the patient's current estimated volume status and projected ongoing fluid losses. Any deficits from either preoperative or intraoperative losses should be corrected and ongoing requirements should be included along with maintenance fluids. Third-space losses, though difficult to quantitate, should be included in fluid replacement strategies. In the initial postoperative period, an isotonic solution should be administered. The adequacy of resuscitation should be guided by the restoration of vital signs and urine output and, in more complicated cases, by the correction of base deficit or lactate. If uncertainty exists, a central venous catheter or Swan-Ganz catheter can be inserted to help guide fluid therapy. After the initial 24 to 48 hours, fluids can be changed to 0.45% saline with added dextrose in patients unable to tolerate enteral nutrition. If normal renal function and adequate urine output are present, potassium may be added to the intravenous fluids. Daily fluid orders should begin with assessment of the patient's volume status and assessment of electrolyte abnormalities. In general, there is no need to check electrolyte levels in the first few days of an uncomplicated postoperative course. All known losses (gastrointestinal, drains, and urine output) as well as insensible losses are replaced with the appropriate parenteral solution.

Special Considerations in the Postoperative Patient

Volume excess is a common disorder in the postoperative period. The administration of isotonic fluids in excess of actual need may result in volume expansion. This may be due to the overestimation of third-space losses or ongoing gastrointestinal losses that are difficult to quantitate, such as diarrhea. The earliest sign of volume overload is weight gain. The average postoperative patient who is not receiving nutritional support should lose approximately $1/4$ to $1/2$ pound per day. Additional signs of volume excess may also be present as listed in Table 2-1. Peripheral edema may not necessarily be associated with volume overload, as overexpansion of total extracellular fluid may exist in association with a deficit in the circulating plasma volume.

Volume deficits also can be encountered in surgical patients if preoperative losses were not completely corrected, intraoperative losses were underestimated, or postoperative losses were greater than appreciated. The clinical manifestations are described in Table 2-1 and include tachycardia, orthostasis, and oliguria. Hemoconcentration also may be present. Treatment will depend on the amount and composition of fluid lost. In most cases of volume deficit, replacement with an isotonic fluid will be sufficient.

ELECTROLYTE ABNORMALITIES IN SPECIFIC SURGICAL PATIENTS

Neurologic Patients

Syndrome of Inappropriate Secretion of Antidiuretic Hormone (SIADH)

The syndrome of inappropriate secretion of antidiuretic hormone (SIADH) can occur following head injury or surgery to the central nervous system, but it also is seen in association with drugs (such as morphine, nonsteroidals, and oxytocin) and in a number of pulmonary (pneumonia, abscess, and tuberculosis) and endocrine disease states (hypothyroidism and glucocorticoid deficiency). Additionally, it can be seen in association with a number of malignancies (most notably small-cell cancer of the lung, but also pancreatic carcinoma, thymoma, and Hodgkin's disease).[45] It should be considered in patients who are euvolemic and hyponatremic with elevated urine sodium (usually greater than 20 mEq/L) and urine osmolality. Antidiuretic hormone (ADH) stimulation is considered inappropriate in that it is not caused by osmotic or volume-related conditions. Correction of the underlying problem should be attempted when possible. In most cases, restriction of free water will correct the problem. The goal is to achieve net water balance, but to avoid volume depletion that compromises renal function. Furosemide also can be used to induce free water loss. If hyponatremia persists, the addition of isotonic or hypertonic fluids should be tried next. The administration of isotonic saline can sometimes worsen the problem if the urinary sodium concentration is higher than the infused sodium concentration. Loop diuretics may be helpful in this situation by preventing the urine from concentrating further. In chronic conditions of SIADH, when long-term fluid restriction is difficult to maintain or is ineffective, demeclocycline and lithium can be used to induce free water loss.

Diabetes Insipidus

Diabetes insipidus (DI) is a disorder of antidiuretic hormone stimulation and is manifested by dilute (free of solute) urine in the case of hypernatremia. Central DI results from a defect in antidiuretic hormone secretion, and nephrogenic DI from a defect in end-organ responsiveness to ADH. Central DI is frequently seen in association with pituitary surgery or injury (closed head injury or anoxic encephalopathy).[46] Nephrogenic DI occurs in association with hypokalemia, radiocontrast dye, and certain drugs such as aminoglycosides and amphotericin. In patients tolerating oral intake, volume status is usually normal as thirst stimulates increased intake. Volume depletion can occur in patients incapable of oral intake. The diagnosis can be confirmed by documenting an increase in urine osmolality in response to a period of water deprivation. If mild, free water replacement is all that is needed. In more severe cases, vasopressin can be added. The usual dose of vasopressin is 5 U subcutaneously every 6 to 8 hours. Caution should be utilized, however, in that excess vasopressin can cause SIADH.

Cerebral Salt Wasting

Cerebral salt wasting is a diagnosis of exclusion that occurs in patients with a cerebral lesion and renal wasting of sodium and chloride with no other identifiable cause (i.e., a diagnosis of exclusion).[47] Natriuresis in a patient with a contracted extracellular volume should prompt the possible diagnosis of cerebral salt wasting. Hyponatremia is frequently observed but is nonspecific and occurs as a secondary event, differentiating it from SIADH.

Malnourished Patients: Refeeding Syndrome

Refeeding syndrome is a potentially lethal condition that can occur with rapid and excessive feeding of patients with severe underlying malnutrition due to starvation, alcoholism, delayed enteral or parenteral support, anorexia nervosa, or massive weight loss in obese patients.[48] With refeeding, a shift in metabolism from fat to carbohydrate stimulates insulin release, resulting in the cellular uptake of electrolytes, particularly phosphate, magnesium, potassium, and calcium. Due to blunted basal insulin secretion, severe hyperglycemia may also arise. The refeeding syndrome can be associated with oral, enteral, or parenteral refeeding, and symptoms

include cardiac arrhythmias, confusion, respiratory failure, and even death. To prevent the development of refeeding syndrome, underlying electrolyte and volume deficits should be corrected. Additionally, thiamine should be administered prior to the initiation of feeding. Caloric repletion should be instituted slowly, at 20 kcal/kg per day and should gradually increase over the first week.[49] Vital signs, fluid balance, and electrolytes should be closely monitored and any deficits corrected.

Acute Renal Failure Patients

There are a number of fluid and electrolyte abnormalities specific to patients with acute renal failure. With the onset of renal failure, an accurate assessment of volume status must be made. If prerenal azotemia is present, then correction of the underlying volume deficit is mandatory. On the other hand, once acute tubular necrosis is established, measures should be taken to restrict daily fluid intake to match urine output and insensible and gastrointestinal losses. Oliguric renal failure requires close monitoring of serum potassium. Temporizing measures to correct hyperkalemia are reviewed in Table 2-13 and should be instituted early, with consideration of dialysis. Hyponatremia is common in established renal failure and derives from the breakdown of proteins, carbohydrates, and fats, as well as administered free water. Dialysis is required for severe hyponatremia. Hypocalcemia, hypermagnesemia, and hyperphosphatemia also are associated with acute renal failure. Hypocalcemia should be verified by measuring ionized calcium, as many patients also are hypoalbuminemic. Phosphate binders can be used to control hyperphosphatemia, but dialysis may be required in more severe cases. Metabolic acidosis is commonly seen with renal failure, as the kidneys lose their ability to clear acid byproducts. Bicarbonate can be used, but dialysis is frequently required as well. Dialysis may be by either intermittent or continuous therapy. However, normalization of sodium, potassium, and bicarbonate may be achieved more frequently if continuous therapy is used.[50]

Cancer Patients

Fluid and electrolyte abnormalities are common in patients with cancer. The etiology may be common to all patient populations or be specific to cancer patients.[51] Hyponatremia is frequently hypovolemic due to renal loss of sodium from diuretics or salt-wasting nephropathy as seen with some chemotherapeutic agents such as cisplatin. Cerebral salt wasting also can occur in patients with intracerebral lesions. Normovolemic hyponatremia may occur in association with SIADH from cervical cancer, lymphoma, and leukemia, or from certain chemotherapeutic agents. Hypernatremia in cancer patients is most often due to poor oral intake or gastrointestinal volume loss (ileus, obstruction). Central DI can also lead to hypernatremia in patients with central nervous system lesions.

Hypokalemia can develop from gastrointestinal losses associated with diarrhea due to radiation enteritis or chemotherapy, or directly from tumors such as villous adenomas of the colon. Tumor lysis syndrome can precipitate severe hyperkalemia from massive cell destruction.

Hypocalcemia can be seen following removal of a thyroid or parathyroid tumor or following a central neck dissection by damage to the parathyroid glands. Hungry bone syndrome produces acute and profound hypocalcemia following parathyroid surgery for secondary or tertiary hyperparathyroidism when calcium is rapidly taken up by bones. Prostate and breast cancer can result in increased osteoblastic activity that increases bone formation thereby decreasing serum calcium. Acute hypocalcemia also can occur with hyperphosphatemia as phosphorus complexes with calcium. Hypomagnesemia is a side effect of ifosfamide and cisplatin therapy. Hypophosphatemia can be seen with hyperparathyroidism as phosphorus reabsorption is decreased, while oncogenic osteomalacia increases urinary excretion of phosphorus. Other causes of hypophosphatemia in cancer patients include renal tubular dysfunction from multiple myeloma, Bence Jones proteins, and certain chemotherapeutic agents. Acute hypophosphatemia can occur as rapidly proliferating malignant cells take up phosphorus in acute leukemia or from hungry bone syndrome following parathyroidectomy. Tumor lysis syndrome or bisphosphonates (used in the treatment of increased calcium) can also cause hyperphosphatemia.

Malignancy is the most common etiology of hypercalcemia in hospitalized patients and is due to increased bone resorption or decreased renal excretion. Bone destruction occurs from bony metastasis as seen with breast or renal cell cancer, but also can occur with multiple myeloma. With Hodgkin's and non-Hodgkin's lymphoma, hypercalcemia results from increased calcitriol formation, which in turn increases absorption of calcium from both the gastrointestinal tract and bone. Humoral hypercalcemia of malignancy is a common cause of hypercalcemia in cancer patients. As parathyroid-related protein is secreted, it binds to parathyroid receptors, stimulating calcium resorption from bone and decreasing renal excretion of calcium. The treatment of hypercalcemia of malignancy should begin with saline volume expansion. This alone will decrease renal reabsorption of calcium as the associated volume deficit is corrected. Once an adequate volume status has been achieved, a loop diuretic may be added. Unfortunately, these measures are only temporary and additional measures need to be taken. A variety of drugs are available with varying times of onset, duration of action, and side effects.[52] Bisphosphonates (etidronate and pamidronate) inhibit bone resorption and osteoclastic activity. They act slowly (within 48 hours) but last for up to 15 days. Calcitonin also is effective by inhibiting bone resorption and increasing renal excretion of calcium. It acts quickly (within 2 to 4 hours), but its use is limited by the development of tachyphylaxis. Corticosteroids may decrease tachyphylaxis and can be used alone to treat hypercalcemia. Gallium nitrates are potent inhibitors of bone resorption. They display a long duration of action but can cause nephrotoxicity. Mithramycin is an antibiotic that blocks osteoclastic activity but can be associated with liver, renal, and hematologic abnormalities, and therefore its use is limited to the treatment of Paget's disease of the bone. For patients in whom hypercalcemia is severe and refractory, or who are unable to tolerate volume expansion (due to pulmonary edema or congestive heart failure), dialysis is an option.

Tumor lysis syndrome results when the release of intracellular metabolites is greater than the kidneys' excretory capacity. A rapid release of uric acid, potassium, and phosphorus occurs and is associated with marked hyperuricemia, hyperkalemia, hyperphosphatemia, hypocalcemia, and acute renal failure. It is typically seen with poorly differentiated lymphomas and leukemias, but also can be seen with a number of solid tumor malignancies. Tumor lysis syndrome most commonly develops following treatment with chemotherapy or radiotherapy. Once it develops, volume expansion should be undertaken, as should correction of electrolyte abnormalities. Associated hypocalcemia should not be treated unless it is symptomatic, to avoid metastatic calcifications. Dialysis may be required for impaired renal function or for correction of electrolyte abnormalities.

References

1. Bourque CW, Oliet SHR: Osmoreceptors in the central nervous system. *Annu Rev Physiol* 59:601, 1997.
2. Sticker EM, Huang W, Sved AF: Early osmoregulatory signals in the control of water intake and neurohypophyseal hormone secretion. *Physiol Behavior* 76:415, 2002.
3. Stauss HM: Baroreceptor reflex function. *Am J Physiol Regul Integr Comp Physiol* 283:R284, 2002.
4. Miller M: Syndromes of excess antidiuretic hormone release. *Crit Care Clin* 17:11, 2001.
5. Kapoor M, Chan G: Fluid and electrolyte abnormalities. *Crit Care Clin* 17:571, 2001.
6. Adrogue HJ, Lederer ED, Suki WN, et al: Determinants of plasma potassium in diabetic ketoacidosis. *Medicine* 65:163, 1986.
7. Swan S: Aminoglycoside nephrotoxicity. *Semin Nephrol* 17:27, 1997.
8. Cobos E, Hall RR: Effects of chemotherapy on the kidney. *Semin Nephrol* 13:297, 1993.
9. Kobrin SM, Goldfarb S: Magnesium deficiency. *Semin Nephrol* 10:525, 1990.
10. Wong ET, Rude RK, Singer FR, et al: A high prevalence of hypomagnesemia and hypermagnesemia in hospitalized patients. *Am J Clin Pathol* 79:348, 1983.
11. Quamme GA: Renal magnesium handling: New insights in understanding old problems. *Kidney Int* 52:1180, 1997.
12. Fisken FA, Heath DA, Somers S, et al: Hypercalcemia in hospital patients: Clinical and diagnostic aspects. *Lancet* 1:202, 1981.
13. Cruz DN, Perazella MA: Biochemical aberrations in a dialysis patient following parathyroidectomy. *Am J Kidney Dis* 29:759, 1997.
14. Bushinsky DA, Monk RD: Calcium. *Lancet* 352:306, 1998.
15. Dunlay RW, Camp MA, Allon M, et al: Calcitriol in prolonged hypocalcemia due to tumor lysis syndrome. *Ann Intern Med* 110:162, 1989.
16. Reber PM, Heath H: Hypocalcemic emergencies. *Med Clin North Am* 19:93, 1995.
17. Marino PL: Acid-base interpretations, in Marino PL (ed): *The ICU Book*, 2nd ed. Baltimore: Williams & Wilkins, 1998, p 581.
18. Gluck SL: Acid-base. *Lancet* 352:474, 1998.
19. Gauthier PM, Szerlip HM: Metabolic acidosis in the intensive care unit. *Crit Care Clin* 18:289, 2002.
20. Koustova E, Standon K, Gushchin V, et al: Effects of lactated Ringer's solution on human leukocytes. *J Trauma* 53:872, 2002.
21. Roberts JS, Bratton SL: Colloid volume expanders. Problems, pitfalls, and possibilities. *Drugs* 55:621, 1998.
22. Moore FA, McKinley BA, Moore EE: The next generation in shock resuscitation. *Lancet* (In press).
23. Shackford SR: Effects of small-volume resuscitation on intracranial pressure and related cerebral variables. *J Trauma* 42:S48, 1997.
24. Moore EE: Hypertonic saline dextran for post-injury resuscitation: Experimental background and clinical experience. *Aust NZ J Surg* 61:L732, 1991.
25. Wade CE, Kramer GC, Grady JJ, et al: Efficacy of 7.5% saline and 6% dextran-70 in treating trauma. A meta-analysis of controlled clinical studies. *Surgery* 122:609, 1997.
26. Coimbra R, Hoyt DB, Junger WG, et al: Hypertonic saline resuscitation decreases susceptibility to sepsis after hemorrhagic shock. *J Trauma* 42:602, 1997.
27. Zallen G, Moore EE, Tamura DY, et al: Hypertonic saline resuscitation abrogates neutrophil priming by mesenteric lymph. *J Trauma* 48:45, 2000.
28. Rotstein OD: Novel strategies for immunomodulation after trauma: Revisiting hypertonic saline as a resuscitative strategy for hemorrhagic shock. *J Trauma* 49:580, 2000.
29. Ley K: Plugging the leaks. *Nat Med* 7:1105, 2001.
30. Conhaim RL, Watson KE, Potenza BM, et al: Pulmonary capillary sieving of hetastarch is not altered by LPS-induced sepsis. *J Trauma* 46:800, 1999.
31. Lucas CE: The water of life: A century of confusion. *J Am Coll Surg* 192:86, 2001.

32. Lucas CE, Ledgerwood AM, Higgins RF, et al: Impaired pulmonary function after albumin resuscitation from shock. *J Trauma* 20:446, 1980.

33. Jonge E, Levi M: Effects of different plasma substitutes on blood coagulation: A comparative review. *Crit Care Med* 291:1261, 2001.

34. Cope JT, Banks D, Mauney MC, et al: Intraoperative hetastarch infusion impairs hemostasis after cardiac operations. *Ann Thorac Surg* 63:78, 1997.

35. Schortgen F, Lacherade JC, Bruneel F, et al: Effects of hydroxyethyl-starch and gelatin on renal function in severe sepsis: A multicenter randomized study. *Lancet* 357:911, 2001.

36. Cittanova ML, Leblance I, Legendre C, et al: Effect of hydroxyethyl-starch in brain-dead kidney donors on renal function in kidney-transplant recipients. *Lancet* 348:1620, 1996.

37. Gan TJ, Bennett-Guerrero E, Phillips-Bute B, et al: Hextend, a physiologically balanced plasma expander for large volume use in major surgery: A randomized phase III clinical trial. *Anesth Analg* 88:992, 1999.

38. Boldt J, Haisch G, Suttner S, et al: Effects of a new modified, balanced hydroxyethyl starch preparation (Hextend) on measures of coagulation. *Br J Anaesth* 89:772, 2002.

39. Wu JJ, Huang MS, Tang GJ, et al: Hemodynamic response of modified fluid gelatin compared with lactated Ringer's solution for volume expansion in emergency resuscitation of hypovolemic shock patients: Preliminary report of a prospective, randomized trial. *World J Surg* 25:598, 2001.

40. Rittoo D, Gosling P, Bonnici C, et al: Splanchnic oxygenation in patients undergoing abdominal aortic aneurysm repair and volume expansion with eloHAES. *Cardiovascular Surg* 10:128, 2002.

41. European Resuscitation Council: Part 8. Advanced challenges in resuscitation. Section 1: Life-threatening electrolyte abnormalities. *Resuscitation* 46:253, 2000.

42. Laureno R, Karp BI: Myelinolysis after correction of hyponatremia. *Ann Med* 126:67, 1997.

43. Chua GC, Sitoh YY, Lim CC, et al: MRI findings in osmotic myelinolysis. *Clin Radiol* 57:800, 2002.

44. American College of Surgeons: Shock, in the *American College of Surgeons Advanced Trauma Life Support Manual*, 6th ed. Chicago: American College of Surgeons, 1997.

45. Miller M: Syndromes of excess antidiuretic hormone release. *Crit Care Clin* 17:11, 2001.

46. Ober KP: Endocrine crises. Diabetes insipidus. *Crit Care Clin* 7:109, 1991.

47. Singh S, Bohn D, Carlotti APCP: Cerebral salt wasting: Truths, fallacies, theories, and challenges. *Crit Care Med* 30:2575, 2002.

48. Kozar RA, McQuiggan MM, Moore FA: Nutritional support in trauma patients, in Shikora SA, Martindale RG, Schwaitzberg SD (eds): *Nutritional Considerations in the Intensive Care Unit*, 1st ed. Dubuque, IA: Kendall/Hunt Publishing, 2002, p 229.

49. Crook MA, Hally V, Panteli JV: The importance of the refeeding syndrome. *Nutrition* 17:632, 2001.

50. Uchino S, Bellomo R, Ronco C: Intermittent versus continuous renal replacement therapy in the ICU: Impact on electrolyte and acid-base balance. *Intensive Care Med* 27:1037, 2001.

51. Kapoor M, Chan GZ: Fluid and electrolyte abnormalities. *Crit Care Clin* 17:503, 2002.

52. Barri YM, Knochel JP: Hypercalcemia and electrolyte disturbances in malignancy. *Hematol Oncol Clin North Am* 10:775, 1996.

CHAPTER 3

Hemostasis, Surgical Bleeding, and Transfusion

David Schwartz, Karen L. Kaplan, and Seymour I. Schwartz

BIOLOGY OF HEMOSTASIS

Hemostasis is a complex process that prevents or terminates blood loss from a disrupted intravascular space. Four major physiologic events participate, both in sequence and interdependently, in the hemostatic process. Vascular constriction, platelet plug formation, fibrin formation, and fibrinolysis occur in that general order, but the products of each of these four processes are interrelated in such a way that there is a continuum and multiple reinforcements. The process is shown schematically in Fig. 3-1. In the normal blood vessel, endothelial cells function to prevent clotting (Table 3-1). They interfere with platelet recruitment by inactivating adenosine diphosphate (ADP). Endothelial cells also release several products that inhibit the coagulation process. Heparan sulfate acts to catalyze the inhibition of thrombin by antithrombin. Thrombomodulin down-modulates the coagulation process through the activation of protein C. Prostaglandin I_2 (prostacyclin) inhibits platelet aggregation, as does nitric oxide (in addition to its vasodilator effects).

Vascular Constriction

When a vessel is injured, several processes are initiated. Vasoconstriction is the initial vascular response to injury. It is more pronounced in vessels with medial smooth muscles, but occurs even at the capillary level. It is dependent upon local contraction of smooth muscle that has a reflex response to various stimuli. The initial vascular constriction occurs before any platelet adherence to the site of injury. Adherence of endothelial cells to adjacent endothelial cells may be sufficient to cause cessation of blood loss from the intravascular space. Vasoconstriction is subsequently linked to platelet plug formation. Thromboxane A_2 (TXA_2), which is derived from the release of arachidonic acid from platelet membranes during aggregation, is a powerful vasoconstrictor. Endothelin synthesized by injured endothelium is also a vasoconstrictor. Serotonin, 5-hydroxytryptamine (5-HT), released during platelet aggregation, is another vasoconstrictor, but it has been shown that when platelets have been depleted of serotonin in vivo, constriction is not inhibited. Bradykinin and fibrinopeptides in the coagulation schema also are capable of contracting vascular smooth muscle. Some patients with mild bleeding disorders and a prolonged bleeding time have, as their only abnormality, capillary loops that fail to constrict in response to injury.

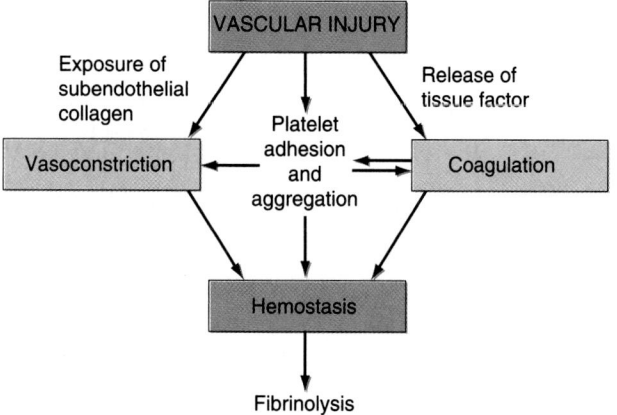

FIG. 3-1. Schematic of processes initiated by vascular injury.

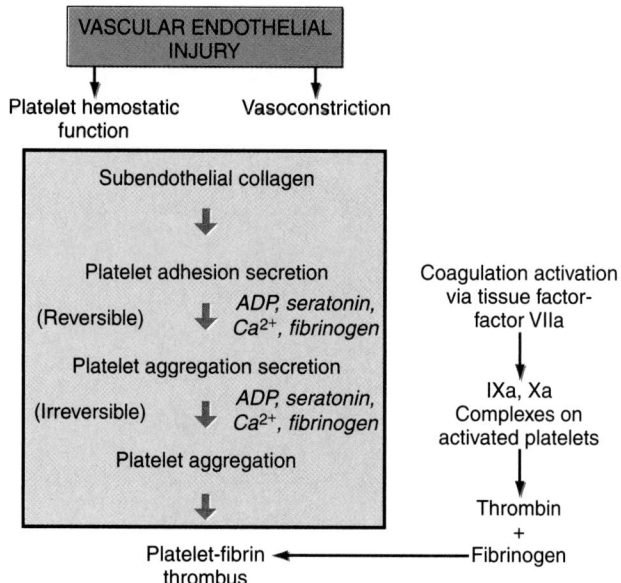

FIG. 3-2. Schematic of platelet activation and thrombus formation.

A lateral incision in a small artery may remain open because of physical forces, whereas a similarly sized vessel that is completely transected may contract to the extent that bleeding ceases spontaneously. The vascular response to injury also is affected by the contribution of pressure provided by surrounding tissues. Bleeding from a small venule ruptured by trauma in the thigh of an athlete may be negligible because of the compressive effect of the surrounding muscle. In the same individual, bleeding from a similar vessel in the nasal mucosa may be significant. When there is low perivascular pressure, as seen in patients with muscle atrophy accompanying aging, in patients on prolonged steroid therapy, and in patients with Ehlers-Danlos syndrome, bleeding tends to be more persistent. Vascular abnormalities, such as hereditary hemorrhagic telangiectasia, may predispose the patient to bleeding from the involved region.

Platelet Function

Platelets are 2 to 4 μm in diameter anucleate fragments of megakaryocytes with normal circulating numbers falling between 150,000 and 400,000/μL. Thrombopoietin is the predominant mediator of platelet production, although other inflammatory mediators, such as interleukin (IL)-6 and IL-11, may play a role. Up to 30% of circulating platelets may be sequestered in the spleen and can be released in response to catecholamines. If not consumed in a clotting reaction, platelets are normally removed by the spleen with an average life span of 7 to 10 days.

Platelets play an integral role in hemostasis along two pathways: by forming a hemostatic plug and by contributing to thrombin formation (Fig. 3-2). Platelets, which normally do not adhere to each other or to the vessel wall, form a plug that stops bleeding when vascular disruption occurs. Injury to the intimal layer in the vascular wall exposes subendothelial collagen to which platelets adhere within 15 seconds of the traumatic event. This requires von Willebrand factor (vWF), a protein in the subendothelium that is lacking in patients with von Willebrand's disease. vWF binds to glycoprotein (GP) I/IX/V on the platelet membrane. Platelet adhesion also is mediated by an interaction between collagen in the subendothelium and GP IaIIa on the platelet surface. Following adhesion, the platelets expand and develop pseudopodal processes and also initiate a release reaction that recruits other platelets from the circulating blood to seal the disrupted vessel. Up to this point, this process is known as *primary hemostasis,* and the aggregation is reversible and is not associated with secretion. Heparin does not interfere with this reaction, which is why hemostasis can occur in the heparinized patient. ADP and serotonin are the principal mediators in this process of aggregation. Various prostaglandins have opposing activities. Arachidonic acid released from platelet membranes is converted by cyclooxygenase to prostaglandin G_2 (PGG$_2$) and then to prostaglandin H_2 (PGH$_2$), which, in turn, is converted to TXA$_2$. TXA$_2$ has potent vasoconstriction and platelet aggregation effects. The arachidonic acid may also be shuttled to adjacent endothelial cells and converted to prostacyclin (PGI$_2$), which is a vasodilator and

Table 3-1
Properties of the Endothelium Related to Hemostasis and Thrombosis

Antithrombotic	*Hemostatic/Prothrombotic*
Antiplatelet activities	Platelet-activating properties
Prostacyclin production	Endothelin production
Nitric oxide production	von Willebrand factor production
Ecto-ADPases	Procoagulant properties
Anticoagulant activities	Tissue factor production
Thrombomodulin—protein C	Binding of clotting factors
Heparan sulfate—antithrombin	Fibrinolysis inhibition
Fibrinolytic activation	Plasminogen activator inhibitor-1 production
Plasminogen activator production	Endothelial-mediated vasoconstriction
tPA	Endothelin production
uPA	Endothelial barrier function

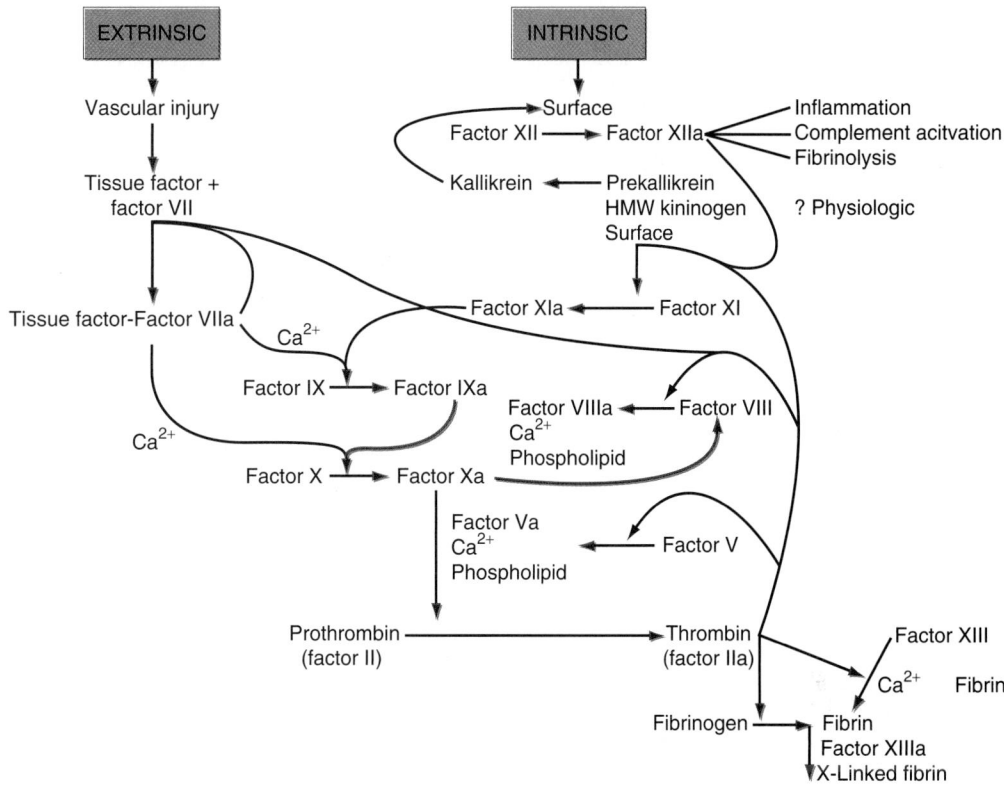

FIG. 3-3. Schematic of the coagulation system showing the many feedback loops that occur.

acts to inhibit platelet aggregation. Platelet cyclooxygenase is irreversibly inhibited by aspirin and reversibly blocked by nonsteroidal anti-inflammatory agents, but is not affected by COX-2 inhibitors.

In the second wave of platelet aggregation, a release reaction occurs in which several substances including ADP, Ca^{2+}, serotonin, TXA_2, and α-granule proteins are discharged. Fibrinogen is a required cofactor for this process, acting as a bridge for the GP IIbIIIa receptor on the activated platelets during formation of a platelet plug. The release reaction results in compaction of the platelets into an "amorphous" plug, in a process that is no longer reversible. Thrombospondin, another protein secreted by the α-granule, stabilizes fibrinogen binding to the activated platelet surface and strengthens the platelet–platelet interactions. Platelet factor 4 (PF4) and β-thromboglobulin are also secreted during the release reaction, as is an inhibitor of plasminogen activation. PF4 is a potent heparin antagonist and it blocks angiogenesis.

The second wave of platelet aggregation is inhibited by aspirin and nonsteroidal anti-inflammatory drugs (NSAIDs)(through the inhibition of cyclooxygenase), by cyclic adenosine monophosphate (cAMP), and nitric oxide. As a consequence of the release reaction, alterations occur in the phospholipids of the platelet membrane that allow calcium and clotting factors to bind to the platelet surface, forming enzymatically active complexes. The altered lipoprotein surface (sometimes referred to as platelet factor 3) catalyzes reactions that are involved in the conversion of prothrombin (factor II) to thrombin (factor IIa, Fig. 3-3) by activated factor X (Xa) in the presence of factor V and calcium, and it is involved in the reaction by which activated factor IX (IXa), factor VIII, and calcium activate factor X. Platelets may also play a role in the initial activation of factors XI and XII.

If congenital abnormalities exist, they can result in abnormal aggregation, as a result of effects on either the "first wave" of

aggregation (the intrinsic ability of platelets to aggregate) or the "second wave" of the process (granule release).

Coagulation

Under physiologic conditions, hemostasis is accomplished by a complex sequence of interactions between platelets, the vascular wall, and multiple circulating or membrane-bound coagulation factors. Historically, the coagulation cascade has been depicted as two intersecting pathways (see Fig. 3-3). The intrinsic pathway begins with factor XII and through a cascade of enzymatic reactions, activates factors XI, IX, and VII in sequence. This pathway is referred to as "intrinsic" because all of the components leading ultimately to fibrin clot formation are intrinsic to the circulating plasma and no surface is required to initiate the process. In contrast, the extrinsic pathway requires exposure of tissue factor on the surface of the injured vessel wall to initiate the arm of the cascade beginning with factor VII. The two arms of the coagulation cascade merge to a common pathway at factor X, and activation proceeds in sequence of factors II (prothrombin) and I (fibrinogen). Clot formation occurs after proteolytic conversion of fibrinogen to fibrin.

One useful feature of the "Y diagram" of the coagulation cascade with two merging arms is that commonly used laboratory tests can segregate abnormalities of clotting to one of the two arms (Table 3-2). An elevated activated partial thromboplastin time (aPTT) is associated with abnormal function of the intrinsic arm of the cascade, while the prothrombin time (PT) is associated with the extrinsic arm. Prolongation of the aPTT or PT occurs when the amount of one or more factors involved is low (usually less than 50% of normal). Vitamin K deficiency or warfarin use affect factors II, VII, IX, X. High levels of factor VIII can sometime cause normalization of the aPTT in patients with liver disease. Fibrinogen levels usually

Table 3-2
Coagulation Factors Tested by the PT and the aPTT

PT	aPTT
VII	XII
X	High molecular weight kininogen
V	Prekallikrein
II (prothrombin)	XI
Fibrinogen	IX
	VIII
	X
	V
	II
	Fibrinogen

aPTT = activated partial thromboplastin time; PT = prothrombin time.

need to be less than 50 mg/dL to cause prolongation of the PT and aPTT. By looking at the PT and aPTT one can decide which specific factors need to be assayed. The aPTT (and less often the PT) may be prolonged in the presence of an inhibitor, either directed against a specific factor or else against phospholipids (the so-called lupus anticoagulant). Mixing patient plasma 1:1 with normal plasma, with and without incubation for 1 hour at 37°C (98.6°F), can distinguish between factor deficiency and the presence of an inhibitor. While convenient from the perspective of laboratory testing, the concept of the intrinsic and extrinsic pathways does not account for some important clinical observations. For example, the paradigm suggests that deficiency of factor XII or other contact factors should lead to bleeding as is seen with deficiencies in factors IX and VIII. Patients deficient in factor XII, however, do not bleed abnormally.

Recently, efforts have been made to present the coagulation cascade in a more physiologically relevant format. The primary physiologic pathway for coagulation is initiated by the exposure of tissue factor (TF) when the luminal surface of a vessel is breached and blood comes in contact with TF exposed in the subendothelium. Propagation of the clotting reaction then ensues with a sequence of four enzymatic reactions, each of which is characterized by the following features.

- A proteolytic enzyme generates the next enzyme in the cascade by cleavage of a proenzyme.
- The reactions occur on a phospholipid surface, such as a platelet membrane, in the presence of γ-carboxyglutamyl residues on the proteins and calcium ions.
- Each reaction requires a helper protein to bring the enzyme and substrate together.

One to 2% of factor VII in the plasma exists as factor VIIa which binds to TF upon exposure of the latter molecule by injury to the vascular wall. The TF-VIIa (extrinsic Xase) complex catalyzes the activation of factor X to factor Xa. The reaction takes place on the phospholipid surface provided by platelets that have adhered to and been activated at the site of injury. The Xase complex is four orders of magnitude more active at converting factor X than is factor VIIa alone. The Xase complex also activates factor IX to factor IXa. Factor Xa, together with Va and Ca^{2+} and phospholipid, comprises the prothrombinase complex that converts prothrombin to thrombin. Thrombin has multiple functions in the clotting process, including conversion of fibrinogen to fibrin and activation of factors V, VII, VIII, XI, and XIII, as well as activation of platelets.

Factor VIIIa combines with factor IXa (generated by the extrinsic Xase as above or by factor XIa formed by thrombin or factor XIIa

action on factor XI on the activated platelet membrane) to form the intrinsic factor Xase, which is responsible for the bulk of the conversion of factor X to Xa. Intrinsic Xase (the VIIIa–IXa complex) is about 50 times more effective at catalyzing factor X activation than is the extrinsic (TF-VIIa) Xase complex and five to six orders of magnitude more effective than is factor IXa alone.

Factor Xa combines with factor Va, also on the activated platelet membrane surface to form the prothrombinase complex, which is responsible for converting prothrombin to thrombin. As with the Xase complex, the prothrombinase is significantly more effective at catalyzing its substrate than is factor Xa alone. Once formed, thrombin leaves the membrane surface and converts fibrinogen by two cleavage steps into fibrin and two small peptides termed fibrinopeptides A and B. Removal of fibrinopeptide A permits end-to-end polymerization of the fibrin molecules, whereas cleavage of fibrinopeptide B allows side-to-side polymerization of the fibrin clot. This latter step is facilitated by thrombin-activatable fibrinolysis inhibitor (TAFI), which acts to stabilize the resultant clot.

The coagulation system is exquisitely regulated. In addition to clot formation that must occur to prevent bleeding at the time of vascular injury, two related processes must exist to balance propagation of the clot before the entire vascular bed is thrombosed in response to a local insult. First, there is a feedback inhibition on the coagulation cascade, which deactivates the enzyme complexes leading to thrombin formation. Second, mechanisms of fibrinolysis allow for breakdown of the fibrin clot and subsequent repair of the injured vessel with deposition of connective tissue.

Tissue factor pathway inhibitor (TFPI) blocks the extrinsic factor Xase complex (TF-VIIa), eliminating this catalyst's production of factors Xa and IXa. TFPI is normally present in the circulation at low concentrations (~2.5 nmol/L), and additional inhibitor is present on the endothelium and can be released in response to heparin. Antithrombin III (AT-III) effectively neutralizes all of the procoagulant serine proteases and only weakly inhibits the TF-VIIa complex. The primary effect is to quench the production of thrombin. A third major mechanism of inhibition of thrombin formation is the protein C system. Upon its formation, thrombin binds constitutively to thrombomodulin and activates protein C to activated protein C (APC), which then forms a complex with its cofactor, protein S, on a phospholipid surface. The APC–protein S complex cleaves factors Va and VIIIa so they are no longer able to participate in the formation of Xase or prothrombinase complexes. Of interest is an inherited form of factor V that carries a genetic mutation, called factor V Leiden, that is resistant to cleavage by APC, thereby remaining active (procoagulant). Patients with factor V Leiden are predisposed to venous thromboembolic events. As a result of the three systems described above, feedback inhibition of thrombin formation exists at upstream, intermediate, and downstream portions of the coagulation cascade to "turn off" thrombin formation once the procoagulant sequence is initially activated.

The same thrombin–thrombomodulin complex that leads to formation of activated protein C also activates TAFI. In addition to clot stabilization, removal of the terminal lysine on the fibrin molecule by TAFI also renders the clot more susceptible to lysis by plasmin. Degradation of fibrin clot is accomplished by plasmin, a serine protease derived from the proenzyme plasminogen. Plasmin formation occurs as a result of one of several plasminogen activators. Tissue plasminogen activator (tPA) is made by the endothelium and other cells of the vascular wall and is the main circulating form of this family of enzymes. tPA is selective for fibrin-bound plasminogen so that endogenous fibrinolytic activity occurs predominantly at the site of clot formation. The other major plasminogen activator, urokinase

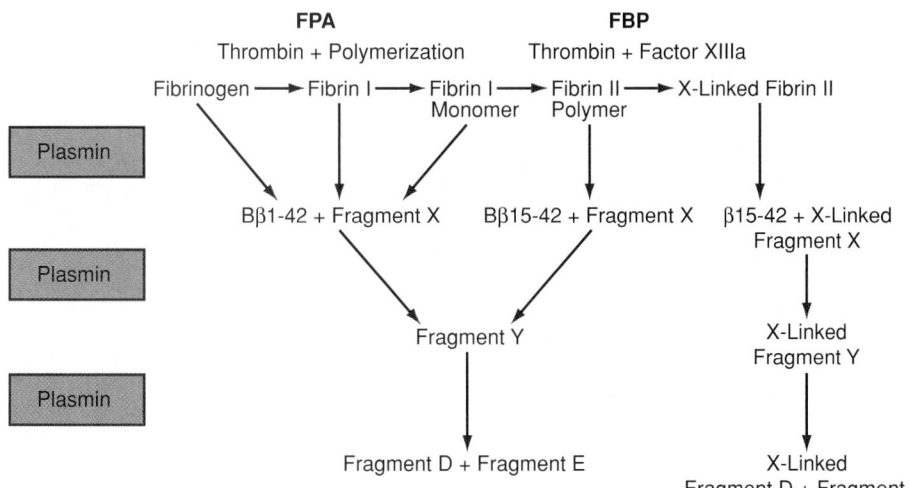

FIG. 3-4. *Schematic of fibrin formation and dissolution.*

plasminogen activator (uPA), also produced by endothelial cells as well as by urothelium, is not selective for fibrin-bound plasminogen.

Because of the complex nature of hemostasis, potential interference in the process can occur at many levels. Platelet number or function can be insufficient to adequately support coagulation. Abnormalities in platelet function may be caused by either endogenous (e.g., uremia) or exogenous (e.g., aspirin or other antiplatelet agents) factors. Alternatively, abnormalities in the clotting factors may underlie a problem of abnormal bleeding. As with platelet dysfunction, the cause may be an intrinsic defect in one of the factors (detailed later in this chapter) or may result from pharmacotherapy.

Fibrinolysis

As part of the wound-healing process, the fibrin clot undergoes lysis. Breakdown of the clot within the lumen of the vessel permits restoration of blood flow, and fibrin clot in the vessel wall may be replaced with connective tissue. Fibrinolysis is initiated at the same time as the clotting mechanism under the influence of circulating kinases, tissue activators, and kallikrein that are present in many organs, including the vascular endothelium. Fibrin is degraded by plasmin, a serine protease derived from the proenzyme plasminogen. Plasminogen levels are known to rise as a consequence of exercise, venous occlusion, and anoxia. Plasminogen may be converted by one of several plasminogen activators including tPA and uPA. tPA is synthesized by endothelial cells and is released by the cells on thrombin stimulation as single-chain tPA and is then cleaved by plasmin to form two-chain tPA. Bradykinin, cleaved from high molecular weight kininogen by kallikrein, enhances release of tPA. Both tPA and plasminogen bind to fibrin as it forms, and this trimolecular complex cleaves fibrin very efficiently. Endothelial cells also synthesize uPA. A pro-form of this enzyme binds to the uPA receptor and autoactivates. Kallikrein can also activate prourokinase to uPA. After plasmin is generated it cleaves fibrin, and somewhat less efficiently, it will also degrade fibrinogen. Fully cross-linked fibrin is also a relatively poor substrate for plasmin. Plasminogen activation may also be initiated by activation of factor XII, which leads to the generation of kallikrein from prekallikrein and cleavage of high molecular weight kininogen by kallikrein.

Several characteristics of the enzymatic reactions ensure that fibrinolysis occurs at a controlled rate and preferentially at the site of the clot. tPA activates plasminogen more efficiently when it is bound to fibrin, so that plasmin is formed selectively on the clot.

Plasmin is inhibited by α_2-antiplasmin, a protein which is crosslinked to fibrin by factor XIII, which helps to ensure that clot lysis does not occur too quickly. Any circulating plasmin also is inhibited by α_2-antiplasmin and circulating tPA or urokinase, and is rapidly inhibited by circulating plasminogen activator inhibitors (e.g., PAI-1). Clot lysis yields fibrin degradation products including E-nodules and D-dimers. The smaller fragments interfere with normal platelet aggregation and the larger fragments may be incorporated into the clot in lieu of normal fibrin monomers, resulting in an unstable clot. The presence of D-dimers in the circulation may be used as a marker of thrombosis or other conditions in which a significant activation of the fibrinolytic system is present. The final inhibitor for the fibrinolytic system is TAFI, a procarboxypeptidase that is activated by the thrombin–thrombomodulin complex. The active enzyme removes lysine residues from fibrin that are essential for binding plasminogen. The sequence of fibrin formation and its dissolution by plasmin is presented in schematic form in Fig. 3-4.

CONGENITAL HEMOSTATIC DEFECTS

Coagulation Factor Deficiencies

Factor VIII and Factor IX

Hemophilia. Inherited deficiencies of all of the coagulation factors are seen, but the three most frequent are factor VIII deficiency (hemophilia A and von Willebrand's disease), factor IX deficiency (hemophilia B or Christmas disease), and factor XI deficiency. Both hemophilia A and hemophilia B are inherited as sex-linked recessive disorders. The first historical mention of an inherited bleeding disorder that affected male children was in the Talmud in the second century, relating to circumcision of subsequent male children after prolonged bleeding in one. The clinical severity of both hemophilia A and hemophilia B depends on the measurable level of factor VIII or factor IX in the patient's plasma. Severe disease has factor levels less than 1% of normal, moderately severe disease has levels of 1 to 5%, and mild disease has levels of 5 to 30%. Patients with severe hemophilia have severe spontaneous bleeds, frequently into joints, leading to crippling arthropathies, but these patients also develop intramuscular hematomas, retroperitoneal hematomas, and gastrointestinal and genitourinary bleeding. Intracranial bleeding, retropharyngeal bleeding, and bleeding from the tongue or lingual

Table 3-3
Types of Factor VIII and Factor IX Products

Purification Method	Specific Activity	Examples
Factor VIII		
Conventional fractionation		
Intermediate purity	1–10 U/mg	Humate-P, Profilate-OSD
High purity	50–100 U/mg	Alphanate SD, Koate-HP
Monoclonal antibody purification		
Ultrahigh purity	>3000 U/mg	AHF-M, Hemofil-M, Monoclate-P
Recombinant		
Ultrahigh purity	>3000 U/mg	Bioclate, Helixate, Kogenate, Recombinate
Factor IX		
Factor IX complex concentrates		
Intermediate purity	<50 U/mg	Bebulin, Konyne-80, Profilnine SD, Proplex-T
Monoclonal antibody purification		
High purity	>160 U/mg	Mononine
Affinity chromatography purification		
High purity	>160 U/mg	AlphaNine SD
Recombinant		
Ultrahigh purity	270 U/mg	BeneFIX

frenulum may be life-threatening. Patients with moderately severe hemophilia have much less spontaneous bleeding but are likely to bleed severely after trauma or surgery. Retroperitoneal hematomas have been seen after lifting a heavy object. Mild hemophiliacs do not bleed spontaneously. They are likely to have mild bleeding after major trauma or surgery. Because platelet function is normal and the initial response to an injury is platelet activation and formation of a platelet plug, patients with hemophilia may not bleed immediately after an injury or minor surgery but will begin to bleed several hours later. This is especially common in mild hemophiliacs after tooth extractions or tonsillectomy. Hemophilia may not have been diagnosed in these patients prior to their first minor procedure.

Treatment of patients with hemophilia A or B is with factor VIII or factor IX concentrate, respectively. As Table 3-3 shows, for both factors there are various types of concentrate. Recombinant factor VIII is strongly recommended for patients who have not been treated previously and is generally recommended for patients who are both

HIV-and hepatitis C virus (HCV)-seronegative. The need for recombinant factor VIII is less clear for HIV-negative, HCV-positive, and HIV-positive patients. There has been concern that intermediate purity products might impair the immune response, but using ultrahigh purity factor VIII products has not affected survival of HIV-positive hemophilic patients. For factor IX replacement the preferred products are recombinant or high purity factor IX because of the risk of thrombosis with the intermediate purity factor IX (prothrombin complex) concentrates. These concentrates contain varying amounts of factors II, VII, and X and are reported to induce thrombosis when used in high doses. The cost of concentrates increases with the specific activity of factor VIII or factor IX. Table 3-4 shows the desired factor VIII and factor IX levels and doses for management of various clinical situations. Recent work shows that at least in some situations, constant infusion of factors VIII or IX is preferable to intermittent bolus injections. Another option for patients with mild to moderate hemophilia A with minor bleeds is administration of

Table 3-4
Guidelines for Factors VIII and IX Replacement in Hemophilia

Type of Bleeding	Hemostatic Factor Level Desired	Factor VIII Dose (U/kg)	Factor IX Dose (U/kg)
Central nervous system	100% initially, then 50–100% for 10–14 days	50 q12h or continuous infusion	100, then 50 q12h or continuous infusion
Trauma or surgery	100% initially, then 50% until wound healing begins, then 30% until wound healing complete	50 q12h or continuous infusion	100, then q24h
Retroperitoneal	100% initially, then 50% until complete resolution	50 q12h for 6 days	40 q12h for 6 days
Retropharyngeal	50–70%	50 q12h for 4 days	40 qd for 4 days
Gastrointestinal	50–100%	50 q12h for 3 days or until bleeding subsides	40 qd for 3 days or until bleeding subsides
Hematuria	40%	40 qd for 3–5 days	40 qd for 3 days
Tooth extraction	50%	40 once, then EACA 100 mg/kg daily for 7–10 days	30 once, then EACA 100 mg/kg daily for 6 days
Mouth	30–40%	40 once, then EACA 100 mg/kg daily for 6 days	20 once, then EACA 100 mg/kg daily for 6 days
Intramuscular	40–50%	20–30 q12h	40–60 qod as needed
Acute hemarthrosis	30–50%	10–20 qd as needed	15 qod as needed

EACA = ϵ-aminocaproic acid.

Table 3-5
Products for Treatment of Patients with Factor VIII Inhibitors

Factor IX complex concentrates Intermediate purity	Bebulin, Konyne-80, Profilnine SD, Proplex-T	<50 U/mg
Factor IX complex concentrates—activated	Autoplex-T, FEIBA VH	<50 U/mg
Porcine factor VIII concentrate	Hyate C	>150 U/mg
Recombinant factor VIIa	NovoSeven	

1-deamino-D-arginine vasopressin (DDAVP, desmopressin), which induces the release of vWF from endothelial cells, raising the levels of vWF and associated factor VIII. DDAVP can be given intravenously at a dose of 0.3 μg/kg daily or by nasal spray (Stimate) at one puff in each nostril daily.

Hemophilia patients with inhibitors are a particular problem to treat. Up to 20% of factor VIII–deficient hemophiliacs develop inhibitors. Some of these are low titer (<5 Bethesda units/mL) and can be treated with higher-than-usual doses of factor VIII to achieve the desired plasma level of factor VIII. For patients with high titer inhibitors it is not possible to achieve adequate factor VIII levels with factor VIII preparations. Table 3-5 lists alternatives for treatment. These include porcine factor VIII if it can be shown that the inhibitor does not cross-react with the porcine material, prothrombin complex concentrates or activated prothrombin complex concentrates, or recombinant factor VIIa. The last is probably the most effective but, because it must be given every 2 hours in situations with active bleeding, can be very expensive. Recombinant factor VIIa is likely to be useful in factor IX–deficient patients with inhibitors as well.

ε-Aminocaproic acid (EACA), or Amicar, an inhibitor of fibrinolysis, is frequently a useful adjunct to factor VIII or IX or DDAVP in treatment of bleeding in patients with hemophilia, especially for bleeding because of tooth extraction or other oral bleeding and for urinary tract bleeding, because both saliva and urine contain high concentrations of plasminogen activator activity. Excess EACA can lead to thrombosis, so the drug should be used with some caution. Dosing is usually 1 to 2 g every 4 to 6 hours, and it can be given orally or intravenously.

Consultation with a hematologist is indicated prior to surgery for any hemophilia patient, but is essential for patients with inhibitors.

von Willebrand's Disease. von Willebrand's disease (vWD) is another disorder with low factor VIII. It is an autosomal dominant disorder, and the primary defect is a low level of the vWF, a large glycoprotein with two functions. One function is to serve as a carrier for factor VIII; thus when vWF levels are low, factor VIII levels are variably decreased because of loss of the carrier protein. More importantly, in most patients, vWF is necessary for normal platelet adhesion to exposed subendothelium and for normal aggregation under high shear conditions, so patients with vWD have bleeding that is characteristic of platelet disorders—typically easy bruising and mucosal bleeding. Menorrhagia is common in women with vWD. von Willebrand's disease is classified into three types. Type I is a partial quantitative deficiency, type II is a qualitative defect, and type III is total deficiency. There are two options for treatment of vWD. One is to use an intermediate purity factor VIII concentrate such as Humate-P that contains vWF as well as factor VIII. The product is labeled with vWF units as well as with factor VIII units, and the dosing should be by the vWF units for vWD. The monoclonal antibody–purified and recombinant products do

not contain recombinant factor VIII and should not be used in this setting. The second option is use of DDAVP, which raises endogenous vWF levels by release of the factor from endothelial cells. DDAVP can be used once a day, but not more often, because time is needed for synthesis of a new store of vWF within the endothelial cells. In general, type I patients respond well to DDAVP. Type II patients may respond, depending on the particular defect. Type III patients usually do not respond. Before using DDAVP to treat bleeding in vWD, the patient must be given a trial dose of 0.3 μg/kg over 15 minutes and the levels of factor VIII, von Willebrand antigen, and von Willebrand ristocetin cofactor activity should be measured 1 to 2 hours later to determine whether there has been an adequate response. Table 3-6 shows recommended schedules for various types of bleeding for patients with vWD. Again, DDAVP should only be used if the patient has been shown to be responsive to it. EACA is a useful adjunct, as for hemophilia.

Factor XI Deficiency

Factor XI deficiency, sometimes referred to as hemophilia C, is prevalent in the Ashkenazi Jewish population (heterozygote frequency about 1:8) and occurs sporadically in other populations. It is generally a mild bleeding disorder, inherited as an autosomal recessive trait. Spontaneous bleeding is rare, but bleeding may occur after surgery or trauma. Treatment of patients with factor XI deficiency who present with bleeding or in whom surgery is planned and who are known to have bled previously is with fresh-frozen plasma (FFP). Each milliliter of plasma contains 1 unit of factor XI activity so the number of milliliters needed depends on the patient's baseline level, the desired level, and the plasma volume. Daily infusion is usually adequate because the half-life is approximately 48 hours. Factor XI concentrates are available in Europe, but caution is necessary because of activation of coagulation. DDAVP may also be useful in the prevention of surgical bleeding in patients with factor XI deficiency.

Deficiency of Factors II (Prothrombin), V, and X

Inherited deficiencies of these proteins are rare. All three are inherited as autosomal recessive traits, with significant bleeding in homozygotes with less than 1% of normal activity, although surgical bleeding has been reported with heterozygous factor X deficiency. Bleeding in any of these deficiencies is treated with FFP. For factors X and II, FFP contains one unit of activity of each of these per milliliter, but factor V activity of plasma is somewhat less because of less stability of factor V. The half-life of prothrombin (factor II) is long (approximately 72 hours) and only about a 25% level is needed for hemostasis, therefore a single infusion of FFP is usually sufficient. For factor X deficiency, a level of 10 to 20% is usually adequate, except for complicated surgical procedures. The half-life of factor X is approximately 48 hours. Prothrombin complex

Table 3-6
Guidelines for Replacement Therapy in von Willebrand's Disease

vWD Type	Severity of Hemorrhage	Dose and Duration
Type I, moderate/severe (<30% ristocetin cofactor)	Minor	DDAVP 0.3μg/kg daily for 1–2 doses or Humate-P 15–20 U/kg daily for 1–2 doses
	Major/surgical	Humate-P, 50–75 U/kg first dose, then 40–60 U/kg every 8–12 hours to maintain level >50% for 3 days, then 40–50 U/kg daily for up to 7 days
Type I, mild	Minor	DDAVP 0.3 μg/kg daily for 1–2 doses
	Major/surgical	DDAVP 0.3 μg/kg daily for 2–3 doses or Humate-P, 40–50 U/kg first dose, then 20–30 U/kg every 12 hours for 3 days
Type IIa	Minor	Humate-P, 15–20 U/kg first dose, then 15–20 U/kg every 24 hours if needed or DDAVP 0.3 μg/kg daily for 1–2 doses
	Major/surgical	Humate-P, 50–75 U/kg first dose, then 40–60 U/kg every 8–12 hours to maintain level >50% for 3 days, then 40–50 U/kg daily for up to 7 days
Type IIb	Minor	Humate-P, 15–20 U/kg first dose, then 15–20 U/kg every 24 hours if needed
	Major/surgical	Humate-P, 50–75 U/kg first dose, then 40–60 U/kg every 8–12 hours to maintain level >50% for 3 days, then 40–50 U/kg daily for up to 7 days
Type III	Minor	Humate-P, 40–50 U/kg for 1–2 doses
	Major	Humate-P, 60–80 U/kg first dose, then 40–60 U/kg every 8–12 hours to maintain level >50% for 3 days, then 40–60 U/kg for up to 7 days

concentrates also can be used to treat deficiencies of prothrombin or factor X. Daily infusions of FFP are used to treat bleeding in factor V deficiency, with a goal of 20 to 25% activity. Factor V deficiency may be coinherited with factor VIII deficiency. In those patients, the genetic defect is in a gene responsible for a common biosynthetic step in the synthesis of the two proteins, which are structurally and evolutionarily related. Treatment of bleeding in individuals with the combined deficiency requires factor VIII concentrate and FFP. Some patients with factor V deficiency are also lacking the factor V normally present in platelets and may need platelet transfusions as well as FFP.

Factor VII Deficiency

Congenital factor VII deficiency is another rare disorder. Bleeding is uncommon unless the level is less than 3%. Treatment is with FFP or with recombinant factor VIIa. The half-life of recombinant factor VIIa is very short (approximately 2 hours), but excellent hemostasis can be achieved with frequent infusions. The half-life of factor VII in FFP is longer, approximately 4 hours.

Factor XIII Deficiency

Congenital factor XIII deficiency also is rare. It is inherited as an autosomal recessive trait. Bleeding is typically delayed because clots form normally but are susceptible to fibrinolysis. Umbilical stump bleeding is characteristic, and there is a high risk of intracranial bleeding. Spontaneous abortion is usual in women with factor XIII deficiency unless they receive replacement therapy. The half-life of factor XIII is quite long, approximately 9 to 14 days. Replacement can be accomplished with FFP, cryoprecipitate, or a factor XIII concentrate. Levels of 1 to 2% are usually adequate for hemostasis.

Platelet Functional Defects

Inherited Defects

Inherited platelet functional defects include abnormalities of platelet surface proteins, abnormalities of platelet granules, and enzyme defects. The major surface protein abnormalities are

thrombasthenia and Bernard-Soulier syndrome. Thrombasthenia (Glanzmann's disease) is caused by an absence of functional glycoprotein IIb IIIa, the receptor for fibrinogen and also a receptor for vWF. Because platelets must bind fibrinogen or vWF to expose the ADP receptor so they can bind ADP and aggregate, platelets of thrombasthenic patients do not aggregate. Bleeding in thrombasthenic patients must be treated with platelet transfusions. The Bernard-Soulier syndrome is caused by a defect in the GP Ib/IX/V receptor for vWF that is necessary for platelet adhesion to the subendothelium. Again, transfusion of normal platelets is required for bleeding in these patients. Both thrombasthenia and Bernard-Soulier syndrome are rare diseases.

The most common intrinsic platelet defect is known as storage pool disease. It may involve loss of dense granules (storage sites for ADP, ATP, Ca^{2+}, and inorganic phosphate) and α-granules (storage sites for a large number of proteins, some of which are specific to platelets [e.g, PF4 and β-thromboglobulin], while others are present in both platelet α-granules and plasma [e.g., fibrinogen, vWF, and albumin]). Dense granule deficiency is the most prevalent of these. It may be an isolated defect or occur with partial albinism in the Hermansky-Pudlak syndrome. Bleeding is variable, depending on how severe the granule defect is. Bleeding is primarily caused by the decreased release of ADP from these platelets. An isolated defect of the α-granules is known as gray platelet syndrome because of the appearance of the platelets on Wright's stain. Bleeding is usually mild with this syndrome. A few patients have been reported who have decreased numbers of both dense and α-granules. These patients have a more severe bleeding disorder. Patients with mild bleeding as a consequence of a form of storage pool disease may have decreased bleeding if given DDAVP. It is likely that the high levels of vWF in the plasma after DDAVP somehow compensate for the intrinsic platelet defect. With more severe bleeding, platelet transfusion is required.

A number of other intrinsic platelet defects are described, including deficiency of cyclooxygenase and abnormalities in platelet actin, myosin, cytoskeletal proteins, and enzymes involved in various aspects of platelet metabolism. If the bleeding is mild, DDAVP may be helpful, but otherwise platelet transfusion is required. For surgery in any of these platelet disorders, if the patient is not known to respond to DDAVP, platelet transfusion should be given.

Quantitative Platelet Defects

Inherited thrombocytopenia is rare and, if significant, should be treated with platelet transfusion.

ACQUIRED HEMOSTATIC DEFECTS

Platelet Abnormalities

Acquired abnormalities of platelets may be quantitative or qualitative, although some patients have both types of defects. Quantitative defects may be a result of failure of production, shortened survival, or sequestration. Failure of production is generally a result of a more general marrow disorder (leukemia, myelodysplastic syndrome, severe vitamin B_{12} or folate deficiency, chemotherapeutic drugs, radiation, acute ethanol intoxication, or viral infection). If the platelet count needs to be raised for surgery or because of spontaneous bleeding, platelet transfusion is used, sometimes with the addition of EACA. Patients who become refractory to random donor platelets may get a better increment in the count with human leukocyte antigen (HLA)-matched platelets.

Shortened platelet survival is seen in immune thrombocytopenia, disseminated intravascular coagulation (see below), or disorders characterized by platelet thrombi such as thrombotic thrombocytopenic purpura and hemolytic uremic syndrome. Immune thrombocytopenia may be idiopathic or associated with other autoimmune disorders or low-grade B-cell malignancies, and it may also be secondary to viral infections (including HIV) or drugs. Idiopathic or secondary immune thrombocytopenia often presents with a very low platelet count, petechiae and purpura, and epistaxis and gum bleeding. Large platelets are seen on peripheral smear. Initial treatment is with corticosteroids (1 mg/kg per day), intravenous gamma globulin (2 g/kg over 2 to 5 days), or anti-D immunoglobulin (75 μg/kg) in patients who are Rh-positive. Intravenous gamma globulin acts approximately 12 hours faster than steroids; anti-D also acts rapidly. Platelet transfusions are not usually needed, but if there is central nervous system bleeding or active bleeding from other sites, they may be given. Survival of the transfused platelets is usually short. Because the circulating platelets in immune thrombocytopenia (ITP) are young and functional, bleeding is less for a given platelet count than when there is failure of platelet production. If the platelet count cannot be maintained medically with these or second-line agents, splenectomy is indicated and leads to complete or partial remission in approximately 80% of patients. Platelet transfusion is not usually needed for splenectomy in patients with ITP. Treatment of drug-induced immune thrombocytopenia may be simply withdrawal of the offending drug, but corticosteroids or IVIg or anti-D immunoglobulin may hasten recovery of the count. Drugs that should be suspected are heparin, quinidine and quinine, gold salts, sulfonamides, valproic acid, and chlorothiazide, but a large number of other drugs have also been reported to cause ITP.

Heparin-induced thrombocytopenia (HIT) is a special case of drug-induced immune thrombocytopenia. The platelet count typically begins to fall 5 to 7 days after heparin has been started, but if it is a re-exposure, the decrease in count may occur within 1 to 2 days. Thrombocytopenia is not usually severe. HIT should be suspected if the platelet count falls to less than 100,000 or if it drops by 50% from baseline in a patient receiving heparin. While HIT is more common with full-dose unfractionated heparin (1 to 3%),

it can occur with prophylactic doses or with low molecular weight heparins. If it develops with unfractionated heparin, the antibody is likely to cross-react with low molecular weight heparin. In addition to the mild to moderate thrombocytopenia, this disorder is characterized by a high incidence of thrombosis that may be arterial or venous. When thrombosis occurs, the disorder is sometimes referred to as heparin-induced thrombocytopenia-thrombosis syndrome (HITTS). If HIT is suspected clinically, heparin should be stopped promptly and an alternative anticoagulant should be instituted, because stopping heparin without addition of another anticoagulant is not adequate to prevent thrombosis in this setting. The alternative anticoagulants available in the United States are lepirudin and argatroban. In Canada and Europe, danaparoid also is available. This is a heparinoid that has about 20% cross-reactivity with HIT antibodies in vitro, but a much lower cross-reactivity in vivo. Warfarin should not be started in patients with HIT until the platelet count has recovered to greater than 100,000. Platelet transfusion is rarely needed in HIT because the count is usually only moderately decreased and the clinical issue is thrombosis rather than bleeding.

These are also disorders in which thrombocytopenia is a result of platelet activation and formation of platelet thrombi. Thrombin is not usually involved. In thrombotic thrombocytopenic purpura (TTP), it is thought that ultralarge vWF molecules interact with platelets, leading to activation. These ultralarge molecules result from inhibition of the metalloproteinase that normally cleaves von Willebrand factor by an antibody against the enzyme. TTP is classically characterized by thrombocytopenia, microangiopathic hemolytic anemia, renal abnormalities, fever, and neurologic signs or symptoms. The most effective treatment for TTP is plasmapheresis. Platelet transfusion should not be used in TTP unless necessary, and may be required for placement of a large-bore catheter to allow plasmapheresis. Most patients survive their initial episode of TTP with plasmapheresis, but chronic or relapsing cases have been seen with increasing frequency.

Hemolytic uremic syndrome (HUS) often occurs secondary to infection by *Escherichia coli* 0157:H7 or other Shiga toxin–producing bacteria. The metalloproteinase is normal in these cases. HUS is usually associated with some degree of renal failure, with many patients requiring renal-replacement therapy. Neurologic symptoms are less frequent with HUS.

A number of patients have a syndrome that has features of both TTP and HUS. This may occur with autoimmune diseases, especially systemic lupus erythematosus; with HIV infection; or secondary to drugs, including ticlopidine, mitomycin C, gemcitabine, and immunosuppressive agents used in organ transplantation (cyclosporine and tacrolimus). The most important point in treating these patients is discontinuation of the involved drug. Plasmapheresis is usually used, but it is not clear what etiologic factor is being removed by the pheresis.

Thrombocytopenia is the most common abnormality of hemostasis that results in bleeding in the surgical patient. The patient may have a reduced platelet count as a result of a variety of disease processes, such as idiopathic thrombocytopenic purpura, thrombotic thrombocytopenic purpura, and systemic lupus erythematosus, or secondary hypersplenism and splenomegaly of sarcoid, Gaucher's disease, lymphoma, and portal hypertension. In these circumstances, the marrow usually demonstrates a normal or increased number of megakaryocytes. By contrast, when thrombocytopenia occurs in patients with leukemia or uremia and in patients on cytotoxic therapy, there is generally a reduced number of megakaryocytes in the marrow.

Thrombocytopenia may occur acutely as a result of massive blood loss followed by replacement with stored blood. Exchange of 1 blood volume (~11 units in a 75-kg man) decreases the platelet count from approximately 250,000/μL to approximately 80,000/μL. Thrombocytopenia may also be induced by the administration of heparin (HIT) and may be associated with thrombotic and hemorrhagic complications. HIT should be suspected if the platelet count falls to less than 100,000 or if it drops by 50% from baseline in a patient receiving heparin. While HIT is more common with therapeutic dosing of unfractionated heparin, it can occur with prophylactic doses or with use of the low molecular weight heparins. The most common form of this response is thought to have an immunologic basis and has been reported in 0.6% of patients receiving heparin. The lowest platelet counts usually occur after 4 to 15 days of treatment in patients given heparin for the first time, and 2 to 9 days in those patients given subsequent courses of heparin. The thrombocytopenia may be associated with coincidental thrombosis. The thrombocytopenia is reversible upon discontinuation of heparin use.

Thrombocytopenia is often accompanied by impaired platelet function. Impaired ADP-stimulated aggregation has been demonstrated in patients receiving a blood transfusion of more than 10 units. Uremia may be associated with increased bleeding time and impaired aggregation, which can be corrected by hemodialysis or peritoneal dialysis. Defective aggregation and platelet secretion can occur in patients with thrombocythemia, polycythemia vera, or myelofibrosis.

Several commonly used drugs interfere with platelet function as part of their intended mechanism of action, including aspirin, clopidogrel, dipyridamole, and the glycoprotein IIb IIIa (GP IIb IIIa) inhibitors. Aspirin irreversibly inhibits platelet function. Clopidogrel and abciximab have sufficiently long half-lives, therefore platelet transfusions may be required if surgery is indicated within a few days of discontinuing therapy. A variety of other drugs may also interfere with platelet function, including indomethacin, ibuprofen, phenothiazines, penicillins, chelating agents, lidocaine, dextran, beta-adrenergic blockers, nitroglycerin, furosemide, and antihistamines (Table 3-7).

The presence and extent of thrombocytopenia can be defined rapidly by a platelet count. In general, 50,000 platelets/μL is adequate for normal hemostasis, but if there is associated platelet dysfunction, there may be a poor correlation between the platelet count and the extent of bleeding. The template bleeding time is the most reliable in vivo test of hemostatic function.

When thrombocytopenia is present in a patient for whom an elective operation is being considered, it is managed on the basis of how much the platelet count is reduced and the cause of the reduction. A count of greater than 50,000/μL requires no specific therapy. If thrombocytopenia is caused by acute alcoholism, drug effect, or viral infection, the platelet level will return to near normal within 1 to 3 weeks. Occasionally, severe thrombocytopenia may be secondary to vitamin B_{12} or folic acid deficiency, in which case it is associated with a megaloblastic bone marrow. This condition generally occurs 2 to 3 years after total gastrectomy or in association with severe intestinal malabsorption. In either case, supplying the appropriate nutrient will correct the thrombocytopenia in 2 to 3 days.

If the patient has idiopathic thrombocytopenia or lupus erythematosus, and a platelet count of less than 50,000/μL, an attempt to raise the platelet count with steroid therapy or plasmapheresis may prove successful. The administration of platelet transfusions in these patients with the spleen in place is generally ineffective. The administration of gamma globulin may temporarily increase the platelet

Table 3-7
Other Classes of Drugs that Affect Platelet Function

*Drugs that increase platelet cyclic adenosine monophosphate or
   cyclic guanosine monophosphate*
   Adenylate cyclase activators
   Phosphodiesterase inhibitors
   Nitric oxide and nitric oxide donors
Antimicrobials
   Penicillins
   Cephalosporins
Cardiovascular drugs
   Beta-adrenergic blockers
   Vasodilators
   Calcium channel blockers
Psychotropics and anesthetics
   Tricyclic antidepressants
   Phenothiazines
   Local anesthetics
   Some general anesthetics (halothane)
Miscellaneous
   Dextrans
   Lipid-lowering agents
   Antihistamines
   Ethanol
   Vitamin E
   Radiographic contrast agents
   Foods (e.g., garlic, onion, ginger, clove, turmeric)

count. Splenectomy alone should not be performed to correct the thrombocytopenia associated with splenectomy secondary to portal hypertension.

Sequestration is another important cause of thrombocytopenia and usually involves sequestration of platelets in an enlarged spleen from any cause (portal hypertension, sarcoid, lymphoma, Gaucher's disease). The total body platelet mass is essentially normal in patients with hypersplenism, but a much larger fraction of the platelets than normal are in the enlarged spleen. Platelet survival is mildly decreased. Bleeding is less than anticipated from the count because sequestered platelets can be mobilized to some extent and enter the circulation. Platelet transfusion does not increase the platelet count as much as it would in a normal person because the transfused platelets will end up in the spleen. Splenectomy is not indicated to correct the thrombocytopenia of hypersplenism caused by portal hypertension.

Other disorders associated with abnormal platelet function include uremia, myeloproliferative disorders, monoclonal gammopathies, and liver disease. The platelet dysfunction of uremia can often be corrected by dialysis, administration of DDAVP, or chronic low-dose estrogen therapy. Platelet transfusion may not be helpful if the patient is uremic when the platelets are given. Platelet dysfunction in myeloproliferative disorders is intrinsic to the platelets and usually improves if the platelet count can be reduced to normal with chemotherapy. If possible, surgery should be delayed until the count has been decreased. These patients are at risk for both bleeding and thrombosis. Platelet dysfunction in patients with monoclonal gammopathies is a result of interaction of the monoclonal protein with platelets. Treatment with chemotherapy, or occasionally plasmapheresis, to lower the amount of monoclonal protein improves hemostasis.

Prophylactic platelet administration as a routine accompaniment to massive blood transfusion is not required or indicated to prevent a hemostatic defect. Platelet packs are administered preoperatively to rapidly increase the platelet count in surgical patients with thrombocytopenia caused by marrow suppression or in association with massive bleeding and replacement with banked red blood cells. Special platelet transfusion sets are used to reduce the loss of platelets as a result of adherence. One unit of platelet concentrate contains approximately 5.5×10^{10} platelets and would be expected to increase the circulating platelet count by about $10,000/\mu L$ in the average 70-kg person. Hence a transfusion of 4 to 8 pool platelet concentrates should raise the count by 40,000 to $80,000/\mu L$ and should provide adequate hemostasis, as documented by bleeding time and control of the hemorrhagic manifestations. Fever, infection, hepatosplenomegaly, and the presence of antiplatelet alloantibodies decrease the effectiveness of platelet transfusions. In patients refractory to standard platelet transfusion, the use of HLA-compatible platelets coupled with special processors has proved effective. Platelet aggregometry has been applied to screening for potential donors.

Acquired Hypofibrinogenemia

Defibrination Syndrome

The largest proportion of patients with fibrinogen-related problems of surgical concern are in this group. The fibrinogen deficiency rarely is an isolated defect, because thrombocytopenia and factors II, V, VII, VIII, and X deficiencies of variable severity usually accompany this state.

The majority of patients with acquired hypofibrinogenemia suffer from intravascular coagulation, more properly known as *defibrination syndrome* or *consumptive coagulopathy,* and it is to this group of patients that the term *disseminated intravascular coagulation* (DIC) has been applied. Systemic bleeding, however, dominates the clinical manifestations; thrombi are rarely found at autopsy. The syndrome, now recognized with increasing frequency, is caused by the introduction of thromboplastic materials into the circulation. Because this material is found in most tissues, many disease processes may activate the coagulation system. Evidence of the thrombotic process includes patchy necrosis of the skin, hematuria and oliguria, confusion caused by cerebral ischemia, gastrointestinal bleeding, and hemorrhage into the adrenal cortex causing acute onset of hypotension. The hemorrhagic disasters of the perinatal period, e.g., retained dead fetus, premature separation of the placenta, and amniotic fluid embolus, are caused primarily by this pathophysiologic mechanism. The hemorrhagic state that follows hemolytic transfusion reactions also is related to this process. Defibrination has been observed as a complication of extracorporeal circulation, head trauma, mucin-producing and disseminated carcinoma, lymphomas, HUS, rickettsial infection, snakebite, burns, aortic surgery, and shock from any cause. Release of thromboplastic material has long been a recognized complication of gram-negative sepsis and has been attributed to the effects of circulating endotoxin on platelets. Septicemia caused by gram-positive organisms may also be associated with DIC.

The differentiation of DIC with secondary protective fibrinolysis from primary fibrinolytic states can be extremely difficult because the thrombin time (TT) is prolonged in both cases, as is the prothrombin time (PT) and activated partial thromboplastin time (aPTT). There is no laboratory test to confirm or exclude the diagnosis. The combination of a low platelet count, a positive plasma protamine test indicating the presence of fibrin monomer–fibrinogen complexes in the plasma, and reduced fibrinogen accompanied by increased fibrin degradation products, viewed in the context of the patient's underlying disease, is highly suggestive of the diagnosis. The fibrinogen level is generally below 100 mg/dL when there is significant diffuse bleeding.

Treatment. The most important facets of treatment are relieving the patient's causative primary medical or surgical problem and maintaining adequate capillary flow. The use of intravenous fluids to maintain volume, and sometimes vasodilators to open the arterioles, is indicated. If insufficient blood flow is related to the inability of a damaged heart to pump, the use of drugs such as dobutamine may be indicated. Viscosity may be affected by an increased hematocrit concentration, and therefore a plasma expander may be beneficial.

If there is active bleeding, hemostatic factors should be replaced with FFP, which is usually sufficient to correct the hypofibrinogenemia; cryoprecipitate, which also provides fibrinogen (250 mg/10 mL); and platelet concentrates. There is little evidence that this replacement therapy will "fuel the fire" and accelerate the pathophysiologic process. Most studies show that heparin is not helpful in acute forms of DIC, but the drug is indicated for purpura fulminans or venous thromboembolism. Fibrinolytic inhibitors such as EACA may be used to block the accumulation of degradation products but are dangerous if the thrombotic process is still active. They should not be used without prior effective antithrombotic treatment with heparin.

Primary Fibrinolysis

The acquired hypofibrinogenic state in the surgical patient also can be a result of pathologic fibrinolysis. This may occur in patients with metastatic prostate carcinoma, shock, sepsis, hypoxia, neoplasia, cirrhosis, and portal hypertension, and in those patients on extracorporeal bypass.

The pathogenesis of this bleeding disorder is complex. Secondary to shock or hypoxia, a release of excessive plasminogen activator into the circulation occurs. This is thought to consist of endogenous kinases that can be released from vascular endothelium and other tissues. Pharmacologic activation of plasminogen also occurs with pyrogens, epinephrine, nicotinic acid, and acetylcholine. Electric shock and pneumoencephalography also have been reported to cause activation. Patients with cirrhosis and portal hypertension have a diminished ability to clear normal amounts of plasminogen activator from the blood. Sufficient urokinase to cause fibrinolysis can be released during operations on the prostate. The administration of therapeutic thrombolytic agents also can result in diffuse bleeding.

In addition to the reduction in levels of plasma fibrinogen, diminution of factors V and VIII occurs, because they also serve as substrates for the enzyme plasmin. Thrombocytopenia is not an accompaniment of the purely fibrinolytic state, but platelet dysfunction is seen secondary to proteolysis of surface receptors. Polymerization of fibrin monomers, a step in normal fibrin formation, is interfered with by the proteolytic residue of fibrinogen and fibrin. The fibrin and fibrinogen breakdown products usually disappear from the circulation in a matter of hours. The whole blood clot lysis time defines increased fibrinolytic activity if a non-anticoagulated blood sample lyses in a test tube in less than 8 hours. A euglobulin lysis time of 20 minutes or less provides a more rapid assessment.

Treatment. The successful treatment of the underlying disorder usually is followed by rapid spontaneous recovery, because the severity of fibrinolytic bleeding is dependent upon the concentration of breakdown products in the circulation. EACA, which is a synthetic amino acid, interferes with fibrinolysis by inhibiting plasminogen activation. The drug may be administered intravenously or orally. An initial dose of 5 g for the average-sized adult is followed by another 1 g every 1 to 2 hours until the hemorrhagic state subsides. Treatment rarely is required for more than 2 to 3 days. Just as the administration of EACA in a patient with consumptive coagulopathy is potentially dangerous, the administration of heparin in the patient who has a primary pathologic fibrinolysis is fraught with danger. Thus, fine clinical judgment and reliable laboratories are needed to avoid therapeutic complications. Restraint is recommended in definitive treatment of fibrinolysis and consumptive coagulopathy, and measures designed to reverse the shock and stabilize the patient are emphasized.

Myeloproliferative Diseases

The polycythemic patient, particularly with marked thrombocytosis, is a major surgical risk. Operations should be considered only for the most grave surgical emergencies. If possible, the operation should be deferred until medical management has effected normal blood volume, hematocrit level, and platelet count. Spontaneous thrombosis is a complication of polycythemia vera and can be explained in part by increased blood viscosity, increased platelet count, and an increased tendency toward stasis. Paradoxically, a significant tendency toward spontaneous hemorrhage also is noted in these patients.

Myeloid metaplasia frequently represents part of the natural history of polycythemia vera. Approximately 50% of patients with myeloid metaplasia are postpolycythemic. There is evidence suggesting qualitative platelet abnormalities in these patients. Abnormalities in platelet aggregation and release have been demonstrated in these patients.

Treatment. Thrombocytosis can be reduced by the administration of hydroxyurea or anagrelide. Elective surgical procedures should be delayed weeks to months after institution of treatment. Ideally, the hematocrit level should be kept below 48% and the platelet count under 400,000/μL. Before operation, a thorough laboratory examination of hemostatic function should be conducted. When an emergency procedure is required, the erythremic and thrombocytotic states should be reduced by phlebotomy and replacement of the blood removed with lactated Ringer's solution. The operation, at all times, must be performed fastidiously.

Coagulopathy of Liver Disease

Patients with liver disease may have bleeding for several reasons. All of the coagulation factors are synthesized by hepatocytes, although factor VIII levels behave differently from those of other factors with hepatic insufficiency. Levels of the vitamin K–dependent factors and factor V decrease progressively with decreasing hepatocyte function. Fibrinogen and factor VIII levels tend to be elevated with mild liver disease. Fibrinogen levels decrease with progression from Cook's class A to B to C cirrhosis. Factor VIII is low only with very severe liver disease. Because hepatic function is progressively impaired, the ability of hepatocytes to degrade activated clotting factors decreases; consequently, low-grade DIC may develop. Primary fibrinolysis also is seen in acute hepatic failure and in chronic liver disease. Also, fibrinogen synthesis, although normal in amount, may be qualitatively abnormal, with increased sialic acid content, correlating with prolongation of the thrombin time. In addition to these coagulation factor abnormalities, thrombocytopenia is seen in patients with cirrhosis who have hypersplenism. Platelet dysfunction may be present as well, as a consequence of interaction of fibrinogen/fibrin degradation products with the platelet fibrinogen receptor and of plasmin degradation of platelet surface receptors.

Treatment of bleeding in patients with coagulopathy caused by liver disease is usually done with FFP, but because the coagulopathy is usually not a result of decreased levels of factor V as discussed previously, it is not usually possible to completely correct the patient's PT. Prothrombin complex concentrates do not contain factor V, and there are no factor V concentrates available. If the fibrinogen is less than 100 mg/dL, administration of cryoprecipitate (8 to 10 bags) may be helpful. Cryoprecipitate is also a source of factor VIII for the occasional liver disease patient with a low factor VIII level. If significant thrombocytopenia is present, platelet transfusions may be helpful, but if there is marked splenomegaly, the rise in platelet count will be much less than would otherwise be expected.

Acquired Coagulation Inhibitors

The most common acquired coagulation inhibitor is the lupus anticoagulant. Although the antibody of the lupus anticoagulant prolongs the aPTT in vitro, it increases the risk of thrombosis in vivo. The antibody interacts in vivo with β_2-microglobulin and phospholipid, and interferes with the ability of proteins C and S to complex with phospholipid to exert their anticoagulant effect. In vitro it also binds phospholipid and it depletes the phospholipid necessary for the formation of the factor VIII-IX-phospholipid complex that cleaves factor X and the factor V-X-phospholipid complex that cleaves prothrombin. Various laboratory tests can be done to identify lupus anticoagulants, but the simplest is a 1:1 mix, in which the patient plasma is mixed with an equal volume of normal plasma. If the patient's prolonged aPTT is caused by factor deficiency, it should correct with normal plasma, but if there is an inhibitor, the aPTT of the mixture will be prolonged. A frequently used test for lupus anticoagulants is the Russell's viper venom time, which is highly sensitive to phospholipid.

Specific inhibitors of individual coagulation factors may also be seen, but, fortunately, these are rare. It is recommended that a hematologist be consulted to help with management of patients with specific factor inhibitors. Factor VIII inhibitors are seen most often. They occur in 15 to 20% of hemophiliacs as a result of immunization by transfused factor VIII. Depending on the titer of the inhibitor, the bleeding patient can be treated with high-dose factor VIII, porcine factor VIII if the antibody does not cross-react, or with unactivated or activated prothrombin complex concentrates. Recently, these patients were treated with recombinant factor VIIa, which, with tissue factor, directly activates factor X and leads to thrombin generation and hemostasis. Immunoaffinity plasmapheresis has been used to specifically remove anti-factor VIII antibodies.

Factor VIII inhibitors also occur in patients who do not have hemophilia. The most common clinical settings are the postpartum period or in individuals with autoimmune disorders such as systemic lupus erythematosus or rheumatoid arthritis. They are also sometimes seen in elderly men without other disease. Bleeding may be severe in patients with acquired factor VIII inhibitors. Active bleeding may be treated with porcine factor VIII, prothrombin complex concentrates, or recombinant factor VIIa. Additionally, immunosuppressive therapy with corticosteroids, cyclophosphamide, azathioprine, or cyclosporine may decrease the titer of the antibody or even eliminate it. Plasmapheresis, along with immunosuppression, has been used in patients with very high titer anticoagulants. Because the antibodies are usually IgG, several plasmaphereses are usually necessary to lower the titer.

Other Diseases

Paraprotein Disorders

Paraprotein disorders are characterized by production of an abnormal globulin or fibrinogen that interferes with clotting or platelet function. This may be an IgM in Waldenström's macroglobulinemia, an IgG or IgA in multiple myeloma, a cryoglobulin in liver disease (especially hepatitis C) or autoimmune diseases, or a cryofibrinogen. Cryoglobulins and cryofibrinogens often are associated with thrombosis of small vessels in the skin, leading to severe ulceration. Chemotherapy is usually effective in lowering the paraproteins of macroglobulinemia and myeloma, although for rapid removal presurgery, plasmapheresis may be needed. Cryoglobulins and cryofibrinogens are usually removed by plasmapheresis.

Hypersplenism

Hypersplenism is associated with platelet sequestration. The total body platelet mass is essentially normal in patients with hypersplenism, but a much larger fraction of the platelets than normal are in the enlarged spleen. Platelet survival is mildly decreased. Bleeding is less than anticipated from the count because sequestered platelets can be mobilized to some extent and enter the circulation. Platelet transfusion does not increase the platelet count as much as it would in a normal person because the transfused platelets will end up in the spleen.

Anticoagulation and Bleeding

Spontaneous bleeding may be a complication of anticoagulant therapy with either heparin, warfarin, or one of the newer anticoagulants, including the low molecular weight heparins and the factor Xa inhibitors. The incidence of bleeding complications related to heparin is reduced with a continuous infusion technique, regulating the aPTT between 1.5 and 2.5 times the upper limit of normal. Bleeding complications for patients administered therapeutic dosing of the low molecular weight heparins are roughly comparable to those seen with therapeutic dosing of unfractionated heparin. Therapeutic anticoagulation is more reliably achieved with low molecular weight heparin, and laboratory testing is not routinely used to monitor dosing of these agents. If monitoring is needed for low molecular weight heparins (e.g., in the presence of renal insufficiency or severe obesity), the drug effect should be determined with an assay for anti-Xa activity. An exaggerated response to oral anticoagulants may occur if dietary vitamin K is inadequate. The anticoagulant effect of the warfarin is consistently reduced in patients receiving barbiturates, and increased warfarin requirements have also been documented in patients taking contraceptives, other estrogen-containing compounds, corticosteroids, and adrenocorticotropic hormone (ACTH). Therefore, reduced anticoagulant dosage should be instituted after discontinuance of any of these drugs. Medications known to increase the effect of oral anticoagulants include phenylbutazone, the cholesterol-lowering agent clofibrate, anabolic steroids (norethandrolone), L-thyroxine, glucagons, amiodarone, quinidine, and a variety of antibiotics (particularly the cephalosporins).

Unexplained bleeding in medical and paramedical personnel occasionally is caused by self-administered anticoagulants. The onset of hematuria or melena in the patient receiving anticoagulants should be investigated, because it has been shown that anticoagulants may unmask underlying tumors. Patients with bleeding secondary to anticoagulation may present only with epistaxis, gastrointestinal hemorrhage, or hematuria. Physical examination, however, almost always reveals other signs of bleeding, such as ecchymoses, petechiae, or hematoma. Bleeding secondary to anticoagulation therapy is not an uncommon cause of rectus sheath hematoma, simulating appendicitis, and intramural intestinal or retroperitoneal hematoma.

Surgical intervention may prove necessary in patients receiving anticoagulation therapy. Increasing experience suggests that

surgical treatment can be undertaken without discontinuing the anticoagulant program. The risk of thrombotic complications reportedly is increased when anticoagulation therapy is discontinued suddenly. If so, this may not be related to what has been called the "rebound phenomenon," but may represent an event in a patient who has an underlying thrombotic tendency. When the aPTT is less than 1.3 times control in a heparinized patient, or when the International Normalized Ratio (INR) is less than 1.5 in a patient on warfarin, reversal of anticoagulation therapy may not be necessary. Meticulous surgical technique is mandatory, and the patient must be observed closely.

Certain surgical procedures should not be performed in the face of anticoagulation. In sites where even minor bleeding can cause great morbidity, e.g., the central nervous system and the eye, anticoagulants should be discontinued, and, if necessary, reversed. Because of the added problem of local fibrinolysis, prostatic surgical treatment should not be carried out in a patient on anticoagulants. Procedures requiring blind needle introduction should be avoided. Deaths have been reported after sympathetic block for peripheral vascular disease in patients receiving anticoagulation.

Emergency operations are occasionally necessary in patients who have been heparinized as treatment for deep venous thrombosis. The first step in managing these patients is discontinuation of heparin; this may be sufficient if the operation can be delayed for several hours. For more rapid reversal, 1 mg of protamine sulfate for every 100 units of heparin most recently administered is immediately effective. For each hour that has elapsed since the last heparin dose, the amount of protamine should be halved. The formation of both extrinsic and intrinsic prothrombinase can be retarded, prolonging the PT and aPTT tests. Some patients exhibit the phenomenon of "heparin rebound" after apparently adequate heparin neutralization with protamine; prolongation of the clotting time recurs after adequate postoperative antagonism of the heparin, which can contribute to postoperative bleeding. In one of the author's experience, this is a major cause of "unexplained" postoperative bleeding after cardiac and vascular surgical procedures. Some of the prolongation of the aPTT after heparin neutralization with protamine may also be a result of the anticoagulant effect of protamine. Activation of fibrinolysis and thrombocytopenia may also contribute to the problem of postoperative bleeding.

Bleeding infrequently is related to hypoprothrombinemia if the prothrombin concentration is greater than 15%. In the elective surgical patient who is receiving coumarin-derivative therapy sufficient to effect anticoagulation, the drug can be discontinued several days before operation and the prothrombin concentration then checked. A level greater than 50% is considered safe. If emergency surgical treatment is required, parenteral injection of vitamin K can be used. Because the reversal of warfarin may take several hours, more rapid reversal can be accomplished with fresh-frozen plasma or prothrombin complex concentrate (Konyne or Proplex). Parenteral administration of vitamin K also is indicated in elective surgical treatment of patients with biliary obstruction or malabsorption who may be vitamin K–deficient. The drug should result in a normal PT or INR. By contrast, if low levels of factors II, VII, IX, and X are a result of hepatocellular dysfunction, vitamin K administration is ineffective. Vitamin K therapy should not be prolonged over 1 week if no response is noted. Vitamin K is an oxidant, and one must be aware that patients with red cell enzyme deficiencies may sustain hemolysis after its administration. For patients on warfarin who would be at high risk for thrombosis with no anticoagulation, low molecular weight heparin should be administered while the INR is decreasing and restarted at prophylactic doses as soon as possible after surgery, with escalation to full therapeutic levels as tolerated and while warfarin is restarted.

Cardiopulmonary Bypass

Overheparinization, heparin rebound, inadequate protamine neutralization, protamine excess, and thrombocytopenia all have been indicated as causes of excessive bleeding in patients undergoing cardiopulmonary bypass. DIC is difficult to document in most patients. The predisposing factors that seem to be associated with excessive bleeding are prolonged perfusion times, prior use of oral anticoagulants, cyanotic heart disease, hypothermia, and prior use of antiplatelet drugs. It is currently believed that the two factors most important in triggering excessive bleeding associated with cardiopulmonary bypass are excessive fibrinolysis and platelet function defects, with the latter the more important element.

The laboratory evaluation of patients with bleeding should include INR, aPTT, complete blood count (CBC), platelet count, peripheral blood smear examination, and measurement of fibrin degradation products. A heparin assay can indicate the heparin level. Plasminogen and plasmin assays also are available, although not routinely performed in most laboratories.

The management of cardiopulmonary bypass hemorrhage should include the empiric administration of 6 to 8 units of platelet concentrates as rapidly as possible. If hyperheparinemia is believed to be the major factor, 25% of the calculated dose of protamine should be administered and repeated every 30 to 60 minutes until the bleeding ceases. If there is laboratory evidence of excess fibrinolysis, EACA should be given at an initial dose of 5 to 10 g followed by 1 to 2 g/h until bleeding ceases. EACA may be associated with ventricular arrhythmia, hypotension, and hypokalemia. Aprotinin, a protease inhibitor that acts as an antifibrinolytic agent, has been shown to reduce transfusion requirements associated with cardiac surgery and orthotopic liver transplantation. Desmopressin acetate also is effective in reducing blood loss during cardiac surgery. Laboratory evidence of HIT is often found after cardiopulmonary bypass; however, clinically significant HIT is rare unless the patient has had previous heparin exposure or is continued on heparin in the postoperative period.

Local Hemostasis

Significant surgical bleeding is usually caused by ineffective local hemostasis. The goal of local hemostasis is to prevent or interrupt the flow of blood from a disrupted vessel that has been incised or transected. Hemostasis may be accomplished by interrupting the flow of blood to the involved area or by direct closure of the blood vessel wall defect. The techniques are classified as mechanical, thermal, or chemical.

Mechanical Procedures

The oldest mechanical method of effecting closure of a bleeding point, or of preventing blood from entering the area of disruption, is digital pressure. When pressure is applied to an artery proximal to an area of bleeding, profuse bleeding may be reduced, permitting more definitive action. A tourniquet that occludes a major vessel proximal to the bleeding site in an extremity is an example, as is the Pringle maneuver, which occludes the hepatic artery and portal vein in the hepatoduodenal ligament as a method of controlling bleeding from a transected cystic artery or the raw surface of the liver.

Direct digital pressure over a bleeding site often is effective and has the advantage of being less traumatic than any hemostatic clamp. All clamps, including the so-called atraumatic vascular clamps,

result in damage to the intimal wall of a blood vessel. The most obvious disadvantage of digital pressure is that it cannot be used permanently. The hemostat represents a temporary mechanical device to stem bleeding. For smaller and noncritical vessels, the trauma to adjacent tissue produced by the hemostat is of little consequence. When bleeding occurs from a vessel that should be preserved, relatively atraumatic hemostasis limiting the extent of intimal damage and subsequent thrombosis is optimal.

Generally, a ligature or a hemoclip replaces the hemostat as a permanent method of effecting hemostasis of a single disrupted vessel. When a small vessel was transected, a simple ligature is sufficient. For large arteries with pulsation and longitudinal motion, a transfixion suture to prevent slipping is indicated. When the bleeding is from a lateral defect in a large vessel, sutures are required. The adventitia and media constitute the major holding forces in a vessel wall, and multiple fine sutures or small hemoclips are preferable.

Aulus Cornelius Celsus devised the use of the ligature in the first century. Because of the strong influence of Galen, who was inclined to cautery, ligature did not gain popularity. Paré, in 1552, rediscovered the principle of ligature. In 1800, Philip Syng Physick of Philadelphia was the first to employ an absorbable suture made from buckskin and parchment. In 1858, Simpson introduced fine-wire suture; Lister used catgut (made from sheep intestine) in 1881. Halsted, in the early 1900s, indicated the advantages of nonabsorbable silk and emphasized the importance of incorporating as little tissue as possible in the suture. In 1911, Cushing reported on the use of silver clips to effect hemostasis in areas that are hard to reach. Historically, a wide variety of inert materials has been used for staples.

All sutures represent foreign material, and selection is based on their intrinsic characteristics and the state of the wound. Nonabsorbable sutures, such as silk, polyethylene, and wire, evoke less tissue reaction than absorbable material such as catgut, polyglycolic (Dexon), and polyglactin (Vicryl). The latter are preferable for grossly infected wounds because the nonabsorbable material can lead to extrusion or sinus formation. Monofilament wire and coated sutures have an advantage over multifilament material in the presence of infection because the latter tends to fragment and permit sinus formation.

Diffuse bleeding from multiple small vessels can be controlled by pressure applied directly over the bleeding area, and this is now deemed preferable to the prolonged use of a proximally placed tourniquet because the latter is associated with a greater danger of tissue necrosis. Direct pressure applied by means of packs affords the best method of controlling diffuse bleeding from large areas. Rarely is it necessary to leave a pack at the bleeding site and remove it at a second sitting. If this is done, several days should elapse before removal, and recurrent bleeding is a possibility. The question of whether hot wet packs or cold wet packs are preferable has been investigated. Unless the heat is so great as to denature protein, it can actually increase bleeding, whereas cold packs promote hemostasis by inducing vascular spasm and increasing endothelial adhesiveness. Bleeding from cut bone can be controlled by packing beeswax on the raw surface to effect pressure. Gravity suits have been used to create generalized pressure and to temporarily decrease intra-abdominal bleeding.

The recently introduced Harmonic Scalpel is an instrument that cuts and coagulates tissue via vibration at 55 kHz. The device converts electrical energy into mechanical motion. The motion of the blade causes collagen molecules within the tissue to become denatured forming a coagulum. There is no significant electrical current that flows through the patient. The instrument has proved advantageous in performing thyroidectomy, hemorrhoidectomy, transsection of the short gastric veins during splenectomy, and in transecting hepatic parenchyma.

Thermal Agents

Heat achieves hemostasis by denaturation of protein that results in coagulation of large areas of tissue. With actual cautery, heat is transmitted from the instrument by conduction directly to the tissue; with electrocautery, heating occurs by induction from an alternating current source. When electrocautery is employed, the amplitude setting should be high enough to produce prompt coagulation, but not so high as to set up an arc between the tissue and the cautery tip. This avoids burns outside the operative field and prevents the exit of current through electrocardiographic leads, other monitoring devices, or permanent pacemakers or defibrillators, if present. A negative plate should be placed beneath the patient to avoid severe skin burns. The advantage of the cautery is that it saves time; the disadvantage is that more tissue is necrosed than with precise ligature. Certain anesthetic agents cannot be used with electrocautery because of the hazard of explosion.

A direct current also can result in hemostasis. Because the protein moieties and cellular elements of blood have a negative surface charge, they are attracted to a positive pole where a thrombus is formed. Direct currents in the 20- to 100-mA range have successfully controlled diffuse bleeding from a raw surface. Argon gas is particularly effective in the control of bleeding from a transected raw surface.

Local cooling has been applied to control bleeding from the eroded mucosa of the esophagus and stomach. Direct cooling with iced saline is effective and acts by increasing the local intravascular hematocrit and by causing vasoconstriction of the arterioles. Generalized hypothermia is of little value, because to reduce blood flow to a visceral organ, the systemic temperature must be reduced to the level of $35°C$ ($95°F$). At this point, shivering, ventricular fibrillation, and profound thrombocytopenia may occur.

Extreme cooling, i.e., cryogenic procedures, have been applicable in gynecology and as a method of destroying hepatic metastases. Temperatures ranging between -20 and $-180°C$ (-4 and $-292°F$) are used to induce freezing around the tip of a cannula. At temperatures of $-20°C$ ($-4°F$), tissue, capillaries, and arterioles undergo necrosis caused by dehydration and destruction of lipid molecules.

Chemical Agents

Epinephrine, injected locally or applied topically, induces vasoconstriction and can reduce bleeding. The drug is generally used for an oozing site such as the tonsillar bed or for a bleeding duodenal ulcer that is concurrently cauterized. Skeletal muscle was used by Cushing, in 1911, for its hemostatic property. Shortly thereafter, hemostatic fibrin was introduced. The properties required for local hemostatic material include handling ease, rapid absorption, and hemostatic action independent of generalized clotting. The most widely used of the commercially available materials are gelatin (Gelfoam), oxidized cellulose (Oxycel), oxidized regenerated cellulose (Surgicel), and micronized collagen (Avitene). All these act, in part, by transmitting pressure against the wound surface, and the interstices provide a scaffold on which the clot can organize (Table 3-8).

Gelfoam is made from denatured animal skin gelatin. Gelfoam has no intrinsic hemostatic action, but it can be used in combination with topical thrombin, for which it serves as an absorbable carrier. Its main hemostatic activity is related to the contact between blood and the large surface area of the sponge transmitting pressure. Oxycel

and Surgicel are both capable of reacting with blood and producing a sticky mass that functions as an artificial clot. These substances are relatively inert and are liquefied in 1 to 4 weeks. Surgicel has a small antibacterial effect.

Fibrin sealant is made up of human sealer protein concentrate, bovine fibrinolysis inhibitor, human thrombin, and calcium chloride. It has been used successfully on bleeding surfaces of the spleen and liver and in the treatment of bleeding encountered when managing abdominal trauma and during cardiovascular procedures. Thrombin preparations have also been used for hemostasis, but carry a small risk of antibody formation and subsequent disturbances in coagulation.

TRANSFUSION

Background

In 1667, Jean-Baptiste Denis and a surgeon, Emmerez, transfused blood from a sheep into a 15-year-old boy who had been bled many times as treatment for fever. The patient apparently improved, and a successful experience was reported simultaneously for another patient. Because of two subsequent deaths associated with transfusion from animals to humans, criminal charges were brought against Denis. In 1668, transfusions in humans were forbidden unless approved by the Faculty of Medicine in Paris. Human blood replacement was accepted in the latter half of the nineteenth century. In 1900, Landsteiner introduced the concept of blood grouping and identified the major A, B, and O groups. In 1939, the Rh group was recognized by Levine and Stetson. The introduction of preservative solutions, such as acid-citrate-dextrose (ACD), citrate-phosphate-dextrose (CPD), and citrate-phosphate-double dextrose-adenine (CP2D-A), have extended the shelf life of blood to up to 6 weeks. Preservation of blood and its constituents has been successful and emphasis has been placed on component therapy. The most recent advance has been the development of a hemoglobin substitute to provide oxygen-carrying capacity.

Characteristics of Blood and Replacement Therapy

Blood

Blood has been described as a vehicular organ that perfuses all other organs. It provides transportation of oxygen to satisfy the body's metabolic demands and removes the by-product carbon dioxide. Hemostatic governors, including hormones, coagulation factors, and antibodies, are carried to and from the appropriate site by the fluid portion of the blood. Red blood cells with their oxygen-carrying capacity, white blood cells that function in body defense processes, and platelets that contribute to the hemostatic process comprise the formed elements of blood.

Replacement Therapy

Typing and Cross-Matching. In selecting blood for transfusion, serologic compatibility is established routinely for the recipients' and donors' A, B, O, and Rh groups. Cross-matching between the donors' red blood cells and the recipients' sera (the major cross-match) is performed. As a rule, Rh-negative recipients should be transfused only with Rh-negative blood. Because this group represents only 15% of the population, the supply is limited. If the recipient is an elderly male who has not been transfused previously, the administration of Rh-positive blood is acceptable if Rh-negative blood is not available. Anti-Rh antibodies form within several weeks of transfusion. If additional transfusions are needed

Table 3-8
Topical Absorbable Hemostatic Agents

	Oxidized Cellulose	*Collagen*	*Thrombin*	*Gelatin Sponge*

Material	Oxidized gauze (OG)
	Oxidized regenerated
	   cellulose knit (ORC)
		Purified bovine
		   collagen sponge
		Microfibrillar
		   Powder
		   Web
		Nonwoven web
			Protein of bovine origin;
			   powder
				Purified gelatin

Time to hemostasis	Average 2–8 min	Average 1–5 min	Concentration-dependent Usually less than 1 min	Not specified on label
Absorption time	OG = 3–4 weeks ORC = 1–2 weeks	Approximately 8–12 weeks	Absorbed immediately	4–6 weeks

Handling
   characteristics
	Conforms well
	Easy to wrap
	Packs easily
	Good suture base
		Sponges
		   Easy to apply and remove
		   Conform wet or dry
		   Hold suture
		Microfibrillar
		   Packs well
		   Difficult to apply and
		      remove
		   Sticks to gloves and
		      instruments
			May be used as
			   Powder
			   Liquid
			   With gelatin sponge
			Requires preparation and/or
			   special storage
				Friable sponge, may be
				   used wet or dry
				Conforms only if
				   premoistened
				Poor suture base

Special features	ORC—Bactericidal	Sponges Good wet integrity	Fast acting	

within several days, more Rh-positive blood can be used. Anti-Rh antiserum (RhoGAM) should be given if Rh-positive products have been given to an Rhnegative patient. Rh-positive blood should not be transfused to Rh-negative females who are capable of child-bearing. Administration of hyperimmune anti-Rh globulin to Rh-negative women shortly before or after childbirth largely eliminates Rh disease in subsequent offspring.

In the patient who is receiving repeated transfusions, serum drawn not more than 72 hours before cross-matching should be used for matching with cells of the donor. Emergency transfusion can be accomplished with type O blood. O-negative and type-specific red blood cells are equally safe for emergency transfusion. Problems are associated with the administration of four or more units of O-negative blood because there is a significant increase in the risk of hemolysis.

In patients with clinically significant cold agglutinins, blood should be administered through a blood warmer. If these antibodies are present in high titer, hypothermia is contraindicated.

In patients who have been multiply transfused and who have developed alloantibodies, or who have autoimmune hemolytic anemia with pan-red blood cell antibodies, typing and cross-matching is often difficult, and sufficient time should be allotted preoperatively to accumulate blood that might be required during the operation. Cross-matching should always be performed before the administration of dextran because it interferes with the typing procedure.

The use of autologous predeposit transfusion is growing. Up to 5 units can be collected for subsequent use during elective procedures. Patients can donate blood if their hemoglobin concentration exceeds 11 g/dL or if the hematocrit is greater than 34%. The first procurement is performed 40 days before the planned operation and the last one is performed 3 days before the operation. Donations can be scheduled at intervals of 3 to 4 days. Recombinant human erythropoietin (rHuEPO) accelerates generation of red blood cells and allows for more frequent harvesting of blood.

Banked Whole Blood. This is now rarely indicated and rarely available. With the new preservatives, the shelf life has been

extended to 40 ± 5 days. At least 70% of the transfused erythrocytes remain in the circulation for 24 hours after transfusion and are viable. The changes in the red blood cells that occur during storage include reduction of intracellular ADP and 2,3-diphosphoglycerate (2,3-DPG), which alters the curve of oxygen dissociation from hemoglobin, decreasing the function of oxygen transport. Banked blood is a poor source of platelets because they lose their ability to survive transfusion after 24 hours of storage. Among the clotting factors, all but factor V and VIII are stable in banked blood. Within 21 days of storage, the pH decreases from 7.00 to 6.68, and the lactic acid level increases from 20 to 150 mg/dL. The potassium concentration rises steadily to 32 mEq/dL, and the ammonia concentration rises from 50 to 680 mg/dL at the end of 21 days. The hemolysis that occurs during storage is insignificant.

Fresh Whole Blood. This refers to blood that is administered within 24 hours of its donation and is rarely indicated. Because of the time required for testing for infectious disease, it must be administered untested. One unit of platelet concentrate has more viable platelets than 1 unit of fresh blood. Fresh whole blood is a poor source of platelets and factor VIII.

Packed Red Blood Cells and Frozen Red Blood Cells. Packed red blood cells is the product of choice for most clinical situations. Concentrated suspensions of red blood cells can be prepared by removing most of the supernatant plasma after centrifugation. The preparation reduces but does not eliminate reaction caused by plasma components. It also reduces the amount of sodium, potassium, lactic acid, and citrate administered. Essentially, it provides oxygen-carrying capacity.

Frozen red blood cells are not available for use in emergencies. They are used for patients who are known to have been previously sensitized. The red blood cell viability is improved, and the ATP and 2,3-DPG concentrations are maintained.

Leukocyte-Reduced and Leukocyte-Reduced/Washed Red Blood Cells. These products are prepared by filtration that removes about 99.9% of the white blood cells and most of the platelets (leukocyte-reduced red blood cells), and, if necessary, by additional saline washing (leukocyte-reduced/washed red blood cells). Leukocyte-reduction prevents almost all febrile, nonhemolytic transfusion reactions (fever and/or rigors), alloimmunization to HLA class I antigens, and platelet transfusion refractoriness and cytomegalovirus transmission. In most western nations, it is the standard red blood cell transfusion product. In the United States, controversy over "universal leukoreduction" has led to some centers restricting leukoreduction to those patients with a history of febrile, nonhemolytic transfusion reactions and to those patients who will require ongoing chronic red blood cell transfusion therapy. Opponents of universal leukoreduction believe that additional costs are not justified because they are of the opinion that transfused allogenic white blood cells have no significant immunomodulatory effects. Supporters of universal leukocyte reduction argue that allogenic transfusion of white cells predisposes to postoperative bacterial infection and multiorgan failure. Of eight randomized trials in surgical patients, six demonstrate reduced postoperative infections in patients transfused with leukocyte-reduced red blood cells. Washed, leukocyte-reduced red blood cells are usually given only to patients who have had reactions (rash, urticaria, anaphylaxis) to unwashed red blood cells.

Platelet Concentrates. The indications for platelet transfusion include thrombocytopenia caused by massive blood loss and replacement with platelet-poor products, thrombocytopenia caused by inadequate production, and qualitative platelet disorders. The preparations should be used within 120 hours of donation. One unit of platelet concentrate has a volume of approximately 50 mL. Platelet preparations can transmit infectious diseases and account for allergic reactions similar to those caused by blood transfusion. When treating bleeding caused by thrombocytopenia or preparing some thrombocytopenic patients for an operation, it is advisable to elevate the platelet count to the range of 50,000 to 100,000/μL. Prevention of HLA alloimmunization can be achieved by leukocyte reduction through filtration. In rare cases, patients who become alloimmunized through previous transfusion, or those patients who are refractory from sensitization through prior pregnancies, HLA-matched platelets can be used. There is a growing body of information suggesting that platelet transfusion thresholds can safely be lowered in patients without signs of hemostatic deficiency and who have no history of poor tolerance to low platelet counts. For example, prophylactic platelet transfusions were traditionally employed at counts below 20,000/μL in nonbleeding patients with leukemia, but it is now clear that a threshold of 10,000/μL is equally effective. Bleeding that occurs with counts over 40,000/μL is almost never a result of thrombocytopenia per se. This is of particular importance because preliminary data suggest that multiple platelet transfusions predispose to multiorgan failure and mortality is dose-dependent.

Frozen Plasma and Volume Expanders. Frozen plasma prepared from freshly donated blood is the usual source of the vitamin K–dependent factors and is the only source of factor V, although factor V is less stable than the vitamin K–dependent factors. FFP is the source of factors II and X, and is also the only source of factor XI in the United States. The risk of infectious disease is the same whether FFP, whole blood, or red blood cells is administered. Lactated Ringer's solution or buffered saline solution administered in amounts two to three times the estimated blood loss is effective and associated with fewer complications. Dextran or a combination of lactated Ringer's solution and normal serum albumin are preferred for rapid volume expansion. Commercially available dextran

probably should not be administered in amounts exceeding 1 L/d because prolongation of the bleeding time and consequent hemorrhage can occur. Low molecular weight dextran (30–40,000 Da) possesses a higher colloidal pressure than plasma and effects some reversal of erythrocyte agglutination.

Concentrates and Recombinant DNA Technology. Antihemophilic concentrates are prepared from plasma and are available for treatment of factor VIII or factor IX deficiency. Table 3–3 lists the preparations of plasma-derived and recombinant factors VIII and IX. Some of the concentrates are 20 to 30 times as potent as an equal volume of FFP. Albumin also has been concentrated, so 25 g can be administered to provide the equivalent of 500 mL of plasma and has the advantage of being hepatitis-free.

Human Polymerized Hemoglobin (PolyHeme). This is a universally compatible, immediately available, disease-free, oxygen-carrying resuscitative fluid that has been successfully used in massively bleeding patients when red blood cells were not transfused.

Indications for Replacement of Blood and Its Elements

General Indications

Improvement in Oxygen-Carrying Capacity. Oxygen-carrying capacity is primarily a function of the red blood cells. When anemia can be treated by specific therapy, such as erythropoietin, transfusion should be withheld. Acute anemias are more disabling than chronic anemia because patients with chronic anemia have undergone an adjustment to the deficiency. In pregnancy, there is a moderate drop in the hematocrit level, and transfusions are not indicated to correct the physiologic anemia of pregnancy if an operation is required. The correction of chronic anemia before surgical intervention is often not necessary. A 1988 National Institutes of Health Consensus Report challenged the dictum that a hemoglobin value of less than 10 g/dL or a hematocrit level less than 30% indicates a need for preoperative red blood cell transfusion. It is suggested that cardiac output does not increase significantly in healthy individuals until the hemoglobin value decreases to approximately 7 g/dL. Patients with chronic anemia and a hemoglobin value of less than 7 g/dL in whom intraoperative bleeding is not anticipated do not require a transfusion preoperatively. There is no correlation between anemia and dehiscence or severity of postoperative infection.

Blood volume can be replaced with dextran solution or lactated Ringer's solution with a reduction of the hemoglobin value to levels below 10 g/dL and little demonstrable change in the oxygen-carrying capacity or the ability to remove carbon dioxide. Human polymerized hemoglobin can be used to increase oxygen-carrying capacity. A whole blood substitute, Fluosol-DA, also has been proposed as a solution with increased oxygen-handling capability.

Volume Replacement. The most common indication for blood transfusion in surgical patients is the replenishment of the blood volume, a deficit of which is difficult to evaluate. Values for "normal blood volume" are variable, and the techniques of measurement are relatively inaccurate, particularly when there is a rapidly changing situation, such as hemorrhage. Chronically ill and elderly patients might have a diminution of blood volume. Many of these patients are well accommodated to the condition. In patients with cardiac decompensation, the blood volume is often greater than "normal."

Table 3-9
Replacement of Clotting Factors

Factors	Normal Level	Life Span In Vivo (Half-Life)	Fate During Coagulation	Level Required for Safe Hemostasis	Stability in ACD Bank Blood (4°C)	Ideal Agent for Replacing Deficit
I (fibrinogen)	200–400 mg/ 100 mL	72 h	Consumed	60–100 mg/ 100 mL	Very stable	Bank blood; concentrated fibrinogen
II (prothrombin)	20 mg/100 mL (100%)	72 h	Consumed	15–20%	Stable	Bank blood; concentrated preparation
V (proaccelerin, accelerator globulin labile factor)	100%	36 h	Consumed	5–20%	Labile (40% at 1 week)	Fresh-frozen plasma; blood under 7 days
VII (proconvertin, serum prothrombin conversion accelerator [SPCA] stable factor)	100%	5 h	Survives	5–30%	Stable	Bank blood; concentrated preparation
VIII (antihemophilic factor [AHF], antihemophilic globulin [AHG])	100% (50–150%)	6–12 h	Consumed	30%	Labile (20–40% at 1 week)	Fresh-frozen plasma; concentrated antihemophilic factor; cryoprecipitate
IX (Christmas factor, plasma thromboplastin component [PTC])	100%	24 h	Survives	20–30%	Stable	Fresh-frozen plasma; bank blood; concentrated preparation
X (Stuart-Prower factor)	100%	40 h	Survives	15–20%	Stable	Bank blood; concentrated preparation
XI (plasma thromboplasma antecedent [PTA])	100%	Probably 40–80 h	Survives	10%	Probably stable	Bank blood
XII (Hageman factor)	100%	Unknown	Survives	Deficit produces no bleeding tendency	Stable	Replacement not required
XIII (fibrinase, fibrin-stabilizing factor [FSF])	100%	4–7 days	Survives	Probably less than 1%	Stable	Bank blood
Platelets	150,000– 400,000/μL	8–11 days	Consumed	60,000– 100,000/μL	Very labile (40% at 20 h; 0 at 48 h)	Fresh blood or plasma fresh platelet concentrate (not frozen plasma)

SOURCE: Salzman EW: Hemorrhagic disorders, in Kinney JM, Egdahl RH, Zuidema GD (eds): *Manual of Preoperative and Postoperative Care,* 2d ed., Philadelphia, WB Saunders, 1971, p 157, with permission.

Measurements of hemoglobin or hematocrit levels are used to assess blood loss. These measurements can be misleading in the face of acute blood loss because the levels can be normal in spite of severely contracted blood volume. After a healthy adult rapidly loses about 1000 mL of blood, the venous hematocrit falls only 3% during the first hour, 5% at 24 hours, 6% at 48 hours, and 8% at 72 hours. Both the amount and the rate of bleeding are factors in the development of signs and symptoms of blood loss. A healthy adult can lose 500 mL in 15 minutes with only minor effects on the circulation and little change in pulse or blood pressure. Loss of 15 to 30% of blood volume (class II hemorrhage) is associated with tachycardia and decreased pulse pressure. Loss of 30 to 40% (class III hemorrhage) results in tachycardia, tachypnea, hypotension, oliguria, and changes in mental status.

Loss of blood in the operating room can be evaluated by estimating the amount of blood in the wound and on the drapes and weighing the sponges. The loss determined by weighing the sponges is only 70% of the true loss. In patients with normal preoperative values, blood loss up to 20% of total blood volume (TBV) is replaced with crystalloid solution. Blood loss of up to 50% of TBV is replaced with crystalloid solutions and packed red blood cells. Blood loss above 50% of TBV is replaced with crystalloids, red blood cells, and albumin or plasma. Continued bleeding above 50% should receive the same components plus FFP to overcome the chelating effect of citrate in the blood products on the circulating coagulation factors.

If electrolyte solutions are used to replace blood volume, an amount three to four times the lost volume is required because of diffusion into the interstitial space.

Replacement of Clotting Factors. Transfusion of platelets and/or proteins contributing to coagulation may be indicated in specific patients before or during an operative procedure (Table 3-9). The clotting defects are often multiple.

Specific Indications

Massive Transfusion. The term *massive transfusion* implies a single transfusion greater than 2500 mL or 5000 mL transfused over a period of 24 hours. Table 3-10 shows the approximate percentages of original blood volume remaining after varying degrees of hemorrhage and transfusion. A variety of problems can attend the use of massive transfusion. Circulatory overload or DIC might occur. Dilutional thrombocytopenia, impaired platelet function, and deficiencies of factors V, VIII, and XI result. Routine alkalization is not advisable because this could have an adverse effect on the hemoglobin dissociation curve and also is accompanied by an increased sodium load.

Citrate toxicity from the use of stored blood may result in young children, in patients with severe hypotension, or in patients with liver disease. The toxicity is related to an excessive binding of ionized

Table 3-10
Percentage of Original Blood Volume Remaining in a Patient with a 5-L Blood Volume Transfused with 500-mL Units

Situation[a]	Magnitude of Hemorrhage and Transfusion		
	1 Blood Volume (10 Units)	2 Blood Volumes (20 Units)	3 Blood Volumes (30 Units)
Best	37	14	5
Usual	25–30	10	2–4
Worst	18	3	0.4

[a]The "best" situation requires simultaneous and equal replacement during hemorrhage; the "worst" situation means initial loss of one-half blood volume not replaced until the hemorrhage has stopped.
SOURCE: From Collins JA: Massive blood transfusions, in *Clinics in Hematology,* Philadelphia, WB Saunders, 1976.

calcium. The use of stored blood also provides a potassium load, but there are no effects in the face of normal renal function.

When large volume transfusions are administered, a heat exchanger should be used because hypothermia can cause a decrease in cardiac rate and output and also a decrease in blood pH.

The use of blood from multiple donors increases the risk of hemolytic reaction as a consequence of incompatibility.

When massive transfusions are administered, the pH, blood gases, and potassium should be measured regularly and abnormalities corrected immediately. If diffuse bleeding is noted, coagulation tests and platelet counts should be measured and deficiencies corrected.

Methods of Administering Blood

Routine Administration. The rate of transfusion depends upon the patient's status. Usually 5 mL/min is administered for the first minute, after which 10 to 20 mL/min is given. When there is marked oligemia, 500 mL can be given within 10 minutes and a second 500 mL also can be given within 10 minutes. As much as 1500 mL/min can be administered through two 7.5-F catheters.

Other Methods. Blood can be instilled intraperitoneally or into the medullary cavity of long bones and the sternum. Approximately 90% of red blood cells injected intraperitoneally enter the circulation, but uptake is not complete for at least a week. Intraoperative autotransfusion is a potentially life-saving adjunct. Approximately 250 mL of blood can be retrieved, washed or filtered, and returned to the patient over a 5-minute period. Another approach to anticipated intraoperative large blood losses is hemodilution. At the onset of the procedure, red blood cells are removed while the intravascular volume is maintained with crystalloid or colloid. The reduced blood viscosity improves the microcirculatory perfusion. The removed blood can then be retransfused during the operation to replace lost blood.

Complications

Hemolytic Reactions. The incidence of nonfatal hemolytic transfusion reactions is approximately 1 per 6000 units of blood administered. Fatal hemolytic reactions occur once for every 100,000 units administered. Hemolytic reactions because of incompatibility of A, B, O, and Rh groups or many other independent systems can result from errors in the laboratory of a technical or clerical nature, or from the administration of the wrong blood type. Immediate hemolytic reactions occur during transfusion of mismatched blood (usually ABO mismatch) and are characterized by intravascular destruction of red blood cells and consequent hemoglobinemia and hemoglobinuria. Circulating haptoglobin is capable of binding 100 mg hemoglobin/dL plasma, and the complex is cleared by a specific hemoglobin-haptoglobin scavenger receptor on macrophages. When the binding capacity is exceeded, free hemoglobin circulates, and the heme is released and combines with albumin to form methem-albumin. When the free hemoglobin exceeds 25 mg/dL some is excreted in the urine, but in most individuals, hemoglobinuria occurs when the plasma level exceeds 150 mg/dL. Renal toxicity from free hemoglobin in the plasma consists of tubular necrosis and precipitation of hemoglobin within the tubules. Within the circulating blood, DIC can be initiated by antibody–antigen complexes activating factor XII and complement, leading to activation of the coagulation cascade.

Delayed hemolytic transfusions occur 2 to 10 days after transfusion and are characterized by extravascular hemolysis, mild anemia, and indirect (unconjugated) hyperbilirubinemia. They occur when an individual has a low antibody titer at the time of transfusion, but the titer increases after transfusion as a result of an anamnestic response. Antibodies to Jk[a] or Rh antigens are most frequent, with anti-K and anti-Fy[a] next in frequency.

Clinical Manifestations. If the patient is awake, the most common symptoms of immediate transfusion reactions are heat and pain along the vein into which the blood is being transfused, flushing of the face, pain in the lumbar region, and constricting chest pain. The patient might experience chills, fever, respiratory distress, hypotension, and tachycardia. In patients who are anesthetized and have an open wound, the two dominant signs are diffuse bleeding and hypotension. There is a sudden fall in the platelet count, an increase in fibrinolytic activity, and consumption of coagulation factors, especially factors V and VIII. The mortality and morbidity rates are very high if the patient has received a full unit of incompatible blood.

The incidences reported in a large series of patients with immediate hemolytic transfusion reactions were as follows: oliguria 58%, hemoglobinuria 56%, hypotension 50%, jaundice 40%, nausea and vomiting 30%, flank pain 25%, cyanosis and hypothermia 22%, dyspnea 20%, chills 18%, diffuse bleeding 16%, and abnormal neurologic signs 10%. The laboratory criteria for a transfusion reaction are hemoglobinuria with a concentration of free hemoglobin over 5 mg/dL, a serum haptoglobin level below 50 mg/dL, and serologic criteria that show incompatibility of the donor and recipient blood. A positive Coombs' test indicates transfused cells coated with patient antibody and is diagnostic.

Delayed hemolytic transfusions may also be manifest by fever and recurrent anemia. Jaundice and decreased haptoglobin usually occur, and low-grade hemoglobinemia and hemoglobinuria may be seen. The Coombs' test is usually positive, and the blood bank must identify the antigen to prevent subsequent reactions to it.

Treatment. If an immediate hemolytic transfusion reaction is suspected, the transfusion should be stopped immediately, and a sample of the recipient's blood should be drawn and sent along with the suspected unit to the blood bank for comparison with the pretransfusion samples. A Foley catheter should be inserted and the hourly urine output measured. Because renal toxicity is affected by the rate of urinary excretion and pH, and because alkalinizing the urine prevents precipitation of hemoglobin within the tubules, attempts are made to initiate diuresis and alkalinize the urine. This can be accomplished by mannitol or furosemide plus 45 mEq bicarbonate. If marked oliguria or anuria develops, the fluid intake and potassium are restricted and the patient is treated as one with renal shutdown. In some instances, dialysis is required. Delayed hemolytic transfusion reactions do not usually require specific intervention.

Febrile and Allergic Reactions. These are relatively frequent, occurring in about 1% of transfusions. Reactions are usually mild and consist of urticaria and fever occurring within 60 to 90 minutes of the start of the transfusion. In rare instances, anaphylactic shock develops. Allergic reactions are caused by the transfusion of antibodies from hypersensitive donors or the transfusion of antigens to which the recipient is hypersensitive. Allergic reactions can occur after the administration of any blood product. Treatment consists of the administration of antihistamines, epinephrine, or steroids, depending on the severity of reaction. Repeated reactions can be prevented by the use of leukocyte-depleted or washed red blood cells.

Bacterial Sepsis. Bacterial contamination of infused blood is rare and can be acquired from contaminated collection bags or poor cleaning of the donor's skin. Gram-negative organisms, especially coliform and *Pseudomonas* species, which are capable of growth at 4°C (39.2°F), are the most common cause. Clinical manifestations include fever, chills, abdominal cramps, vomiting, and diarrhea. There may be hemorrhagic manifestations and increased bleeding. If the diagnosis is suspected, the transfusion should be discontinued and the blood cultured. Emergency treatment includes oxygen, adrenergic blocking agents, and antibiotics.

Embolism. Although air embolism has been reported as a complication, healthy individuals can tolerate large amounts of air injected intravenously at a rapid rate. The normal adult can tolerate an embolism of 200 mL of air. Smaller amounts, however, can cause alarming signs. Manifestations of venous air embolism include a rise in venous pressure, cyanosis, a "mill wheel murmur" over the precordium, tachycardia, hypotension, and syncope. Treatment consist of placing the patient on the left side in a head down position with the feet up. Arterial air embolism may be visible in the retinal vessels or as blood flows from transected vessels. Plastic tubes used for transfusion can break off within a vein and embolize into the right atrium or pulmonary artery. Embolized catheters have been successfully removed.

Superficial Thrombophlebitis. Prolonged infusions into a peripheral vein are associated with venous thrombosis. Intravenous infusions that last more than 8 hours are more likely to be followed by thrombophlebitis, with an increased incidence in the lower limbs. Treatment consists of discontinuation of the infusion and the application locally of warm moist compresses. Embolization from superficial thrombophlebitis or venous thrombosis is extremely rare.

Overtransfusion and Pulmonary Edema. Overloading the circulation is an avoidable complication. It can occur with rapid infusion of blood, plasma expanders, and other fluids, particularly in patients with heart disease. To prevent the complication, the central venous pressure should be measured whenever large amounts of fluid are administered. Circulatory overload is manifest by a rise in venous pressure, dyspnea, and cough. Rales can generally be heard at the lung bases. Treatment consists of diuresis, placing the patient in a sitting position, and, occasionally, venesection.

A syndrome of transfusion-related acute lung injury (TRALI) is sometimes seen after transfusion and is characterized as mild to life-threatening. Noncardiogenic pulmonary edema is often accompanied by fever, rigors, and a "white out" chest x-ray. Treatment

is discontinuation of any transfusion, notification of the transfusion service, and intensive pulmonary support, sometimes including intubation. This type of pulmonary edema does not respond to diuretics and is thought to be caused by infused donor antigranulocyte or anticlass I or II MHC antibodies.

Transmission of Disease. Malaria, Chagas' disease, brucellosis, and, very rarely, syphilis are among the diseases that have been transmitted by transfusion. Malaria can be transmitted by all blood components. The species most commonly implicated is *Plasmodium malariae*. The incubation period ranges from 8 to 100 days; the initial manifestations are shaking chills and spiking fever. Cytomegalovirus (CMV) infection resembling infectious mononucleosis also has occurred.

Transmission of hepatitis C and HIV-1 has been dramatically minimized by the introduction of better antibody and nucleic acid screening for these pathogens. The infection rate for these pathogens is now estimated to be less than 1 per 1,000,000 units transfused. Hepatitis B may still occur in about 1 in 100,000 transfusions in nonimmune recipients. Hepatitis A is very rarely transmitted because there is no asymptomatic carrier state. Recent concerns about the rare transmission of these and other pathogens, such as West Nile virus, are being addressed by current trials of "pathogen inactivation systems" that reduce infectious levels of all viruses and bacteria known to be transmittable by transfusion. Prion disorders, e.g., Creutzfeldt-Jakob disease, also are transmissible by transfusion, but there is currently no information on inactivation of prions in blood products for transfusion.

TESTS OF HEMOSTASIS AND BLOOD COAGULATION (TABLE 3-11)

Abnormalities in hemostasis can result in bleeding complications ranging from a benign local hematoma to life-threatening exsanguinations. Given the complicated cascade of cellular and enzymatic processes required for normal hemostasis to occur, it is possible for one or more of several different abnormalities within the cascade to contribute to a bleeding disorder. The abnormality may be the result of a primary deficiency or defect in one component of the clotting cascade. Alternatively, hemostasis may be impaired either intentionally as a consequence of pharmacologic therapy with an anticoagulant or antiplatelet agent, or unintentionally as a result of comorbid conditions such as thrombocytopenia, hepatic congestion, pharmacotherapy, or sepsis. The initial approach to assessing hemostatic function is a careful review of the patient's clinical history (including previous experiences with abnormal bleeding or bruising), drug use, and basic laboratory testing.

Congenital disorders in platelet function and of clotting factors are discussed elsewhere in this chapter. Common screening laboratory testing includes platelet count, PT or INR, aPTT, and bleeding time. Less commonly used studies include the TT and an examination of the peripheral blood smear.

Platelet dysfunction can occur at either extreme of platelet count. The normal platelet count ranges from 150,000 to 400,000/μL. Platelet counts greater than 1,000,000/μL may be associated with bleeding or thrombotic complications. Clinical signs and symptoms of thrombocytopenia are usually not observed until the platelet count falls below 100,000/μL. Increased bleeding complications may be seen with major surgical procedures when the platelets are below 100,000/μL and with minor surgical procedures when the counts

Table 3-11
Screening Tests in Adults, Healthy Term Infants, and Premature Infants

	Adults	Term Infants	Premature Infants (32–35 Weeks' Gestation)
Platelet count (per μL)[a]	$300,000 \pm 50,000$	$259,000 \pm 35,000$	$239,000 \pm 50,000$
Bleeding time (min)[a]	4 ± 1.5	4 ± 1.5	4 ± 1.5
Prothrombin time (PT) (s)[a]	12–14	13–17	18
International Normalized Ratio (INR)	1.0	1.0	1.0
Partial thromboplastin time (PTT) (s)[a]	45	71	100
Thrombin time (TT) (s)	10	14	14
Fibrinogen (mg/dL)[b]	200–350	117–225	–

[a]Values published by Hathaway and Bonnar.
[b]Values obtained in this laboratory.
Values for infants 35 to 39 weeks' gestation lie between those of term and 32- to 35-week infants. Values for older children (>3 months) are the same as those for adults.
SOURCE: Karpatkin M: Screening tests in hemostasis *Pediatr Clin North Am* 27:831, 1980, with permission.

are below 50,000/μL. Spontaneous hemorrhage can occur when the counts fall below 20,000/μL.

The PT and aPTT are variations of plasma recalcification times initiated by the addition of a thromboplastic agent. The PT reagent contains thromboplastin and calcium that, when added to plasma, leads to the formation of a fibrin clot. The PT test measures the function of factors I, II, V, VII, and X. Factor VII is part of the extrinsic pathway and the remaining factors are part of the common pathway. Factor VII has the shortest half-life of the coagulation factors, and its synthesis is vitamin K–dependent. The PT test is best suited to detect abnormal coagulation caused by vitamin K deficiencies, including that seen in response to warfarin therapy (Fig. 3-5).

Variations in thromboplastin activity can lead to differences in PT measured for a given plasma sample. For this reason, it can be difficult to accurately assess the degree of anticoagulation on the basis of the PT alone. To account for these variations, the INR is now the method of choice for PT reporting. The PT value obtained for a given specimen is adjusted to account for differences in sensitivity of different thromboplastin sources. The International Sensitivity Index (ISI) is unique to each batch of thromboplastin, and its value is furnished by the manufacturer to the hematology laboratory. Human

brain thromboplastin has an ISI of 1, and the optimal reagent has an ISI between 1.3 and 1.5. The INR is a calculated number derived from the following equation:

$$INR = (PT_{patient}/PT_{normal})^{ISI}$$

The aPTT reagent contains a phospholipid substitute, activator, and calcium, which, in the presence of plasma, leads to fibrin clot formation. The aPTT measures function of factors I, II, and V of the common pathway and factors VIII, IX, X, and XII of the intrinsic pathway Heparin therapy is often monitored by following aPTT values with a therapeutic target range of 1.5 to 2.5 times the control value (approximately 50 to 80 seconds). Low molecular weight heparins are selective Xa inhibitors that may mildly elevate the aPTT, but therapeutic monitoring is not routinely recommended.

The bleeding time is used to evaluate platelet and vascular dysfunction. Several standard methods have been described; however, the Ivy bleeding time is most commonly used. The upper limit or normal bleeding time with the Ivy test is 7 minutes. A template aids in administering a uniform test and adds to the reproducibility of the results. An abnormal bleeding time suggests either platelet dysfunction (intrinsic or drug-induced), vWD, or certain vascular defects. Many laboratories are replacing the template bleeding time with an in vitro test in which blood is sucked through a capillary and the platelets adhere to the walls of the capillary and aggregate. The closure time in this system appears to be more reproducible than the bleeding time and also correlates with bleeding in vWD, primary platelet function disorders, aspirin use, and other platelet dysfunction disorders.

Additional medications may significantly impair hemostatic function, such as antiplatelet agents (clopidogrel and glycoprotein IIb IIIa inhibitors), anticoagulant agents (hirudin, chondroitin sulfate, dermatan sulfate), and thrombolytic agents (streptokinase, tPA). Laboratory testing is not routinely used to follow the therapeutic efficacy of these agents. Knowledge of the pharmacokinetics of these agents is usually sufficient to predict the time course of hemostatic abnormalities in patients receiving these medications. If abnormalities in any of the coagulation studies cannot be explained by known medications used, congenital abnormalities of coagulation, or comorbid disease(s), further investigation of the underlying etiology is warranted, as outlined in Table 3-12.

VITAMIN K CYCLE

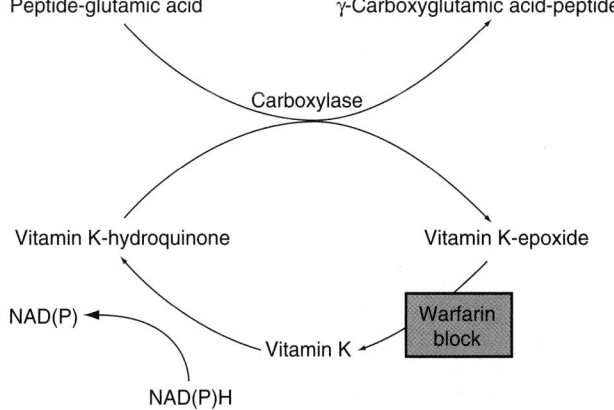

FIG. 3-5. Schematic of the vitamin K cycle and warfarin effects.

Table 3-12
Evaluation of Abnormal Screening Coagulation Tests

Abnormal Test	Additional Test Results	Clinical Conditions
Isolated prolonged PT	Low factor VII alone	Factor VII deficiency
	Factors II, VII, IX, X assays all low; factor VIII high	Warfarin with acute phase reaction
	Factors II, V, VII, IX, X assays all low; factor VIII high	Liver disease with acute phase reaction
Isolated prolonged aPTT	Mixing study positive	Inhibitor
	Lupus anticoagulant positive	Lupus anticoagulant
	Low factor VIII	vWD or factor VIII inhibitor in a female; vWD or hemophilia A in a male
	Low factor IX	Hemophilia B in a male
	Low factor XI	Factor XI deficiency
	Low factor XII, prekallikrein, or high molecular weight kininogen	No bleeding associated with these; thrombotic tendency possible
Prolonged PT and aPTT	Low factors II, VII, IX, X; normal factor V	Warfarin
	Low factors II, V, VII, IX, X	Liver disease
	Low factors V and VIII, low factor II, low fibrinogen, low platelets, high D-dimer fibrinogen degradation product	DIC
	Prolonged thrombin time, normal fibrinogen and platelets	Heparin likely
Low fibrinogen	Factors, platelets normal	Congenital hypo/afibrinogenemia
	Elevated fibrinogen degradation product, prolonged PT, aPTT, platelets normal	Primary fibrinolysis
Prolonged bleeding time or PFA-100 closure time	Normal platelet count	Primary platelet dysfunction or vWD or uremic platelet dysfunction

EVALUATION OF THE SURGICAL PATIENT AS A HEMOSTATIC RISK

Preoperative Evaluation of Hemostasis

The patient's history provides meaningful clues to the presence of a bleeding tendency. It is reasonable to use a questionnaire on which the patient indicates (1) prolonged bleeding or swelling after biting the lip or tongue, (2) bruises without apparent injury, (3) prolonged bleeding after dental extraction, (4) excessive menstrual bleeding, (5) bleeding problems associated with major and minor operations, (6) medical problems receiving a physician's attention within the past 5 years, (7) medications including aspirin or remedies for headache taken within the past 10 days, and (8) a relative with a bleeding problem.

Four levels of concern have been proposed on the basis of the history and surgical procedure being considered. At level I, the history is negative and the procedure contemplated is relatively minor, e.g., breast biopsy or hernia repair; no screening tests are recommended. At level II, the history is negative, screening tests may have been performed in the past, and a major operation is planned, but the procedure usually is not attended by significant bleeding: a platelet count and blood smear and aPTT are recommended to detect any thrombocytopenia, circulating anticoagulant, or intravascular coagulation. Level III pertains to the patient whose history is suggestive of defective hemostasis and to the patient who is to undergo an operative procedure in which hemostasis may be impaired, e.g., operating using pump oxygenation or cell savers, or procedures in which a large, raw surface is anticipated. Level III also pertains to situations in which minimal postoperative bleeding could be injurious, such as intracranial operations. At this level, a platelet count and bleeding time test should be performed to assess platelet function; an aPTT and INR should be used to assess coagulation and the fibrin clot should be incubated to screen for abnormal fibrinolysis. Level IV pertains to patients who present with a history highly suggestive of

a hemostatic defect. A hematologist should be consulted, and, in addition to the tests prescribed for level III patients, the bleeding time test should be repeated 4 hours after the ingestion of 600 mg of aspirin, provided that the operation is scheduled to take place 10 or more days after this study. In the case of an emergency procedure, platelet aggregation tests using ADP, collagen, epinephrine, and ristocetin should be performed, and a TT is indicated to detect any dysfibrinogenemia or a circulating, weak, heparin-like anticoagulant. Patients with liver disease, renal failure, obstructive jaundice, and the possibility of disseminated malignant disease should have a platelet count, INR, and aPTT performed preoperatively. In uremic patients, the most common deficit is a qualitative platelet abnormality. This is best detected by the bleeding time test.

Evaluation of Excessive Intraoperative or Postoperative Bleeding

Excessive bleeding during or shortly after a surgical procedure may be the result of one or more of the following factors: (1) ineffective local hemostasis, (2) complications of blood transfusion, (3) a previously undetected hemostatic defect, (4) consumptive coagulopathy, and/or (5) fibrinolysis. Excessive bleeding from the field of the procedure unassociated with bleeding from other sites, e.g., central venous pressure line, intravenous line, or tracheostomy, usually suggests inadequate mechanical hemostasis rather than a defect in the biologic process. An exception to this rule applies to operations on the prostate, pancreas, and liver because operative trauma may stimulate local plasminogen activation and lead to increased fibrinolysis on the raw surface. In these circumstances 24- to 48-hour interruption of plasminogen activation by the administration of EACA may prove effective.

Although one may be reasonably certain on clinical grounds that surgical bleeding is related to local problems, laboratory investigation must be confirmatory. Prompt examination should be made of the blood smear to determine the number of platelets, and an actual platelet count should be done if the smear is equivocal. An aPTT, a one-stage PT, and a TT all can be determined within minutes. Correct interpretation of the results should confirm the clinical impression or identify the problem.

As pointed out previously, massive blood transfusion is a well-documented cause of thrombocytopenia. Although most patients who receive 10 units or more of banked blood within a period of 24 hours will be measurably thrombocytopenic, this is usually *not* associated with hemostatic failure. Therefore, prophylactic administration of platelets is not indicated, but if there is evidence of diffuse bleeding, 8 to 10 packs of fresh platelet concentrates should be given empirically, because no clear association has been documented between the platelet count, bleeding time, and the occurrence of profuse bleeding.

Another cause of hemostatic failure related to the administration of blood is a hemolytic transfusion reaction. The first hint of a transfusion reaction in an anesthetized patient may be diffuse bleeding in an operative field that had previously been dry. The pathogenesis of this bleeding is thought to be related to the release of ADP from hemolyzed red blood cells, resulting in diffuse platelet aggregation, after which the platelet clumps are swept out of the circulation. Release of procoagulants may result in progression of the clotting mechanism and intravascular defibrination. In addition, the fibrinolytic mechanism may be triggered.

Transfusion purpura is an uncommon cause of thrombocytopenia and associated bleeding after transfusion. When this occurs the donor platelets are of the uncommon Pl^{A1} group. The platelets sensitize the recipient, who makes antibody to the foreign platelet antigen. The foreign platelet antigen does not completely disappear from the recipient circulation but seems to attach to the recipient's own platelets. The antibody, which attains a sufficient titer within 6 or 7 days after the sensitizing transfusion, then destroys the recipient's own platelets. The resultant thrombocytopenia and bleeding may continue for several weeks. This uncommon cause of thrombocytopenia should be considered if bleeding follows transfusion by 5 or 6 days. Platelet transfusions are of little help in the management of this syndrome because the new donor platelets usually are subject to the binding of antigen and damage from the antibody. Corticosteroids may be of some help in reducing the bleeding tendency. Posttransfusion purpura is self-limited, and the passage of several weeks inevitably leads to subsidence of the problem.

DIC and disseminated fibrinolysis occur intraoperatively or postoperatively when control mechanisms fail to restrain the hemostatic process to the area of tissue damage. Either process can cause diffuse bleeding and can be caused by trauma, incompatible transfused blood, sepsis, necrotic tissue, fat emboli, retained products of conception, toxemia of pregnancy, large aneurysms, and liver diseases. It is important to distinguish between the two processes or the dominant element causing intraoperative or postoperative bleeding. No single test can confirm or exclude the diagnosis or distinguish between the two disorders. The combination of thrombocytopenia, defined by smear or platelet count, positive plasma protamine test for fibrin monomers, a low fibrinogen level, and an elevated level of fibrinogen degradation product provides strong indications for DIC. The euglobulin lysis time provides a method of detecting diffuse fibrinolysis.

Diffuse intraoperative and postoperative bleeding is a complication of biliary tract surgery in cirrhotic patients. This has been related to portal hypertension and coagulopathy associated with chronic liver disease. The tests used to distinguish DIC from fibrinolysis pertain. The therapeutic approach includes the intravenous

administration of vasopressin to effect a temporary reduction in portal hypertension and EACA to correct the increased fibrinolysis.

An operation performed in a patient with sepsis sometimes is attended by continued bleeding. Severe hemorrhagic disorders due to thrombocytopenia have occurred as a result of gram-negative sepsis. The pathogenesis of endotoxin-induced thrombocytopenia has been studied in detail, and it has been suggested that a labile factor, possibly factor V, is necessary for this interaction. Defibrination and hemostatic failure also may occur with meningococcemia, *Clostridium perfringens* sepsis, and staphylococcal sepsis. Hemolysis appears to be one mechanism in sepsis leading to defibrination. Evaluation of these patients includes a platelet count, INR, aPTT, and TT.

Bibliography

General
Colman RW, Hirsh J, Marder VJ, et al (eds): *Hemostasis and Thrombosis, Basic Principles and Clinical Practice*, 4th ed. Philadelphia: Lippincott Williams and Wilkins, 2001.
Goodnight SH Jr., Hathaway WE (eds): *Disorders of Hemostasis and Thrombosis, a Clinical Guide*, 2nd ed. New York: McGraw Hill, 2001.
Ratnoff OD, Forbes CD (eds): *Disorders of Hemostasis*. Philadelphia: WB Saunders, 1991.

Biology of Hemostasis
Kristiansen M, Graversen JH, Jacobsen C, et al: Identification of the haemoglobin scavenger receptor. *Nature* 409:198, 2001.
MacKinney AA Jr. (ed): *Hematology for Students*. New York: Taylor and Francis, 2002.
Mann KG, Butenas S, Brummel K: The dynamics of thrombin formation. *Arterioscler Thromb Vasc Biol* 23:17, 2003.
Shattil AJ, Bennett JS: Platelets and their membranes in hemostasis: Physiology and pathophysiology. *Ann Intern Med* 94:108, 1980.
Weiss HJ: Platelet physiology and abnormalities of platelet function (Part I). *N Engl J Med* 293:531, 1975.
Weiss HJ: Platelet physiology and abnormalities of platelet function (Part II). *N Engl J Med* 293:580, 1975.

Congenital Hemostatic Defects
Brown B, Steed DL, Webster MW, et al: General surgery in adult hemophiliacs. *Surgery* 99:154, 1986.
Curtiss PH Jr: Orthopedic management of patients with hereditary disorders of blood coagulation. *Mod Treat* 5:84, 1968.
Kasper CK, Boylen AL, Ewing NP, et al: Hematologic management of hemophilia A for surgery. *JAMA* 253:1279, 1985.
Nilsson IM, Larsson SA, Bergentz SE, et al: The use of blood components in the treatment of congenital coagulation disorders. *World J Surg* 11:14, 1987.
Rudowski WJ: Major surgery in haemophilia. *Annu Rev Coll Surg Engl* 63:111, 1981.

Acquired Hemostatic Defects
Bechstein WO, Riess H, Blumhardt G, et al: Aprotinin in orthotopic liver transplantation. *Semin Thromb Hemost* 19:262, 1993.
Bell WR: Disseminated intravascular coagulation. *Johns Hopkins Med J* 146:289, 1980.
Bick RL: Disseminated intravascular coagulation and related syndromes: A clinical review. *Semin Thromb Hemost* 14:299, 1988.
Bijsterveld NR, Moons AH, Boekholdt SM, et al: Ability of recombinant factor VIIa to reverse the anticoagulant effect of the pentasaccharide fondaparinux in healthy volunteers. *Circulation* 106:2550, 2002.
Feinstein DI: Treatment of disseminated intravascular coagulation. *Semin Thromb Hemost* 14:351, 1988.

Francis CW, Davidson BL, Berkowitz SD, et al: Ximelagatran versus warfarin for the prevention of venous thromboembolism after total knee arthroplasty. A randomized double-blind trial. *Ann Intern Med* 137:648, 2002.

George JN, Raskob GE, Shah SR, et al: Drug-induced thrombocytopenia: A systematic review of published cases. *Ann Intern Med* 129:886, 1998.

Hoak JC, Koepke JA: Platelet transfusions. *Clin Haematol* 5:69, 1976.

Kaplan KL, Francis CW: Heparin-induced thrombocytopenia. *Blood Rev* 13:1, 1999.

Kaplan KL, Francis CW: Direct thrombin inhibitors. *Semin Hematol* 39:187, 2002.

Kappa JR, Fisher CA, Berkowitz HD, et al: Heparin-induced platelet activation in sixteen surgical patients: Diagnosis and management. *J Vasc Surg* 5:101, 1987.

Livio M, Mannucci PM, Vigano G, et al: Conjugated estrogens for the management of bleeding associated with renal failure. *N Engl J Med* 315:731, 1986.

Martinez J, Palascak JE, Kwasniak D: Abnormal sialic acid content of the dysfibrinogenemia with liver disease. *J Clin Invest* 61:535, 1978.

Murkin JM, Lux J, Shannon NA, et al: Aprotinin significantly decreases bleeding and transfusion requirements in patients receiving aspirin and undergoing cardiac operations. *J Thorac Cardiovasc Surg* 107:554, 1994.

Salzman EW, Weinstein MJ, Reilly D, et al: Adventures in hemostasis. *Arch Surg* 128:212, 1993.

Schwartz SI: Myeloproliferative disorders. *Ann Surg* 182:464, 1975.

Schwartz SI, Hoepp LM, Sachs S, et al: Splenectomy for thrombocytopenia. *Surgery* 88:497, 1980.

Silver D, Kapsch DN, Tsoi EK, et al: Heparin-induced thrombocytopenia, thrombosis and hemorrhage. *Ann Surg* 198:301, 1983.

Slichter SJ: Identification and management of defects in platelet hemostasis in massively transfused patients. *Prog Clin Biol Res* 108:225, 1982.

Turpie AG, Bauer KA, Eriksson BI, et al: Fondaparinux vs. enoxaparin for the prevention of venous thromboembolism in major orthopedic surgery: A meta-analysis of 4 randomized double-blind studies. *Arch Intern Med* 162:1833, 2002.

Tests of Hemostasis and Blood Coagulation

Bowie EJ, Owen CA Jr: The significance of abnormal preoperative hemostatic tests. *Prog Hemost Thromb* 5:179, 1980.

Hathaway WE, Bonnar J: *Perinatal Coagulation.* New York, Grune and Stratton, 1978.

Karpatkin M: Screening tests in hemostasis. *Pediatr Clin North Am* 27:831, 1980.

Rapaport SI: Preoperative hemostatic evaluation: Which tests, if any? *Blood* 61:229, 1983.

Local Hemostasis

Abbott W, Austen WG: The effectiveness and mechanism of collagenin-duced topical hemostasis. *Surgery* 78:723, 1975.

Chung CC, Ha JP, Tsang WW: Double-blind randomized trial comparing Harmonic Scalpel hemorrhoidectomy, bipolar scissors hemorrhoidectomy, and scissors excision: Ligation technique. *Dis Colon Rectum* 45:789, 2002.

Codispoti M, Mankad PS: Significant merits of a fibrin sealant in the presence of a coagulopathy following pediatric cardiac surgery: Randomized controlled trial. *Eur J Cardiothorac Surg* 22:200, 2002.

Cushing H: The control of bleeding in operations for brain tumor. *Ann Surg* 54:1, 1911.

Evans BE: Local hemostatic agents (and techniques). *Scand J Haematol* 33(Suppl 40):417, 1984.

Gertsch P, Pellone A, Guerra A, et al: Initial experience with the Harmonic Scalpel in liver surgery. *Hepatogastroenterology* 47:763, 2000.

Jackson MR, Alving BM: Fibrin sealant in preclinical and clinical studies. *Curr Opin Hematol* 6:415, 1999.

Matthew TL, Spotnitz WD, et al: Four years' experience with fibrin sealant in thoracic and cardiovascular surgery. *Ann Thorac Surg* 50:40, 1990.

Schenk WG 3rd, Goldthwaite CA Jr., Burks S, et al: Fibrin sealant facilitates hemostasis in arteriovenous polytetrafluoroethylene grafts for renal dialysis. *Am Surg* 68:728, 2002.

Siperstein AE, Berber E, Morkoyun E: The use of the Harmonic Scalpel vs. conventional knot tying vessel ligation in thyroid surgery. *Arch Surg.* 137:137, 2002.

Streiff MB, Ness PM: Acquired FV inhibitors: A needless iatrogenic complication of bovine thrombin exposure. *Transfusion* 42:18, 2002.

Transfusion

Allen JB, Allen FB: The minimum acceptable level of hemoglobin. *Int Anesthesiol Clin* 20:1, 1982.

Amberson WR: Blood substitutes. *Biol Rev* 12:48, 1987.

Anderson KC, Ness PM (eds): *Scientific Basis of Transfusion Medicine—Implications for Clinical Practice,* 2nd ed. Philadelphia: WB Saunders, 2000.

Blumberg N, Heal JM: Transfusion immunomodulation and leukoreduction. *Probl Gen Surg* 17:7, 2000.

Busch MP, Eble BE, Khayam-Bashi H, et al: Evaluation of screened blood donations for human immunodeficiency virus type 1 infection by culture and DNA amplification of pooled cells. *N Engl J Med* 325:1, 1991.

Carson JL, Poses RM, Spence RK, et al: Severity of anaemia and operative mortality and morbidity. *Lancet* 1:727, 1988.

Collins JA: Massive blood transfusions, in *Clinics in Hematology.* Philadelphia, WB Saunders, 1976.

Council on Scientific Affairs: Autologous blood transfusions. *JAMA* 256:2378, 1986.

Eschbach JW, Egrie JC, Downing MR, et al: Correction of the anemia of end-stage renal disease with recombinant human erythropoietin. *N Engl J Med* 316:73, 1987.

Glover JL, Broadie TA: Intraoperative autotransfusion. *World J Surg* 11:60, 1987.

Goodnough LT, Vizmeg K, et al: The impact of autologous blood ordering and blood procurement practices on allogeneic blood exposure in elective orthopedic surgery patients. *Am J Clin Pathol* 101:354, 1994.

Harrigan C, Lucas CE, et al: Serial changes in primary hemostasis after massive transfusion. *Surgery* 98:836, 1985.

Hoff HE, Guillemin R: The tercentenary of transfusion in man. *Cardiovasc Res Cent Bull* 6:47, 1967.

Hogman CF, Bagge L, et al: The use of blood components in surgical transfusion therapy. *World J Surg* 11:2, 1987.

Keeling MM, Gray LA, et al: Intraoperative autotransfusion: Experience in 725 consecutive cases. *Ann Surg* 197:536, 1983.

Martin E, Hansen E, et al: Acute limited normovolemic hemodilution: A method for avoiding homologous transfusion. *World J Surg* 11:53, 1987.

Messmer KFW: Acceptable hematocrit levels in surgical patients. *World J Surg* 11:41, 1987.

Perioperative Red Cell Transfusion: National Institutes of Health Consensus Development Conference Statement, vol 7, no 4, June 27–29, 1988. US Department of Health and Human Services, Bethesda, MD.

Peterman T: Transfusion-associated acquired immunodeficiency syndrome. *World J Surg* 11:38, 1987.

Reed RL, Ciavarella D, et al: Prophylactic platelet administration during massive transfusion. *Ann Surg* 203:40, 1986.

Rizza CR: Coagulation factor therapy. *Clin Haematol* 5:113, 1976.

Seidl S, Kuhnl P: Transmission of diseases by blood transfusion. *World J Surg* 11:30, 1987.

Seyfried H, Walewska I: Immune hemolytic transfusion reactions. *World J Surg* 11:25, 1987.

Snyder EL (ed): *Blood Transfusion Therapy: A Physician's Handbook.* Arlington, VA, American Association of Blood Banks, 1983.

Trubel W, Gunen E, et al: Recovery of intraoperatively shed blood in aortoiliac surgery: Comparison of cell washing with simple filtration. *Thorac Cardiovasc Surg* 43:165, 1995.

Vanderlinde ES, Heal JM, Blumberg N: Clinical review: Autologous transfusion. *BMJ* 324:772, 2002.

Waxman K, Tremper KK, et al: Perfluorocarbon infusion in bleeding patients refusing blood transfusions. *Arch Surg* 119:721, 1984.

CHAPTER 4

Shock

Andrew B. Peitzman, Brian G. Harbrecht, and Timothy R. Billiar

INTRODUCTION AND HISTORICAL BACKGROUND

Shock may be defined as inadequate delivery of oxygen and nutrients to maintain normal tissue and cellular function. The resultant cellular injury is initially reversible; if the hypoperfusion is severe enough and prolonged, the cellular injury becomes irreversible. The clinical manifestations of shock are the result of stimulation of the sympathetic and neuroendocrine stress responses, inadequate oxygen delivery, and end-organ dysfunction. Gross defined shock as a "rude unhinging of the machinery of life."[1] Blood pressure alone is an insensitive measure of shock; significant hypoperfusion and cellular death may be ongoing, despite normal blood pressure. Inadequate oxygen delivery is presumed to be the pathologic defect in shock. The management of the patient in shock is empiric; securing the airway and restoration of vascular volume and tissue perfusion often occur prior to definitive diagnosis.[2]

Claude Bernard suggested that the organism attempts to maintain constancy in the internal environment against external forces that attempted to disrupt the *milieu interieur*.[3] Walter B. Cannon carried Bernard's observations further and introduced the term "homeostasis," emphasizing that an organism's ability to survive was related to maintenance of homeostasis.[4] The failure of physiologic systems to buffer the organism against external forces results in organ and cellular dysfunction, what is clinically recognized as shock. Cannon made several significant contributions in the early twentieth century to the understanding of shock.[4,5] He first described the "fight or flight response," generated by elevated levels of catecholamines in the bloodstream. Cannon's observations on the battlefields of World War I led him to propose that the initiation of shock was due to a disturbance of the nervous system that resulted in vasodilatation and hypotension. He proposed that secondary shock, with its attendant capillary permeability leak, was caused by a "toxic factor" released from the tissues.[4,5]

In a series of critical experiments, Alfred Blalock documented that the shock state in hemorrhage was associated with reduced cardiac output and due to volume loss, not a "toxic factor."[6] In 1934, Blalock proposed four categories of shock: hypovolemic, vasogenic, cardiogenic, and neurogenic.[6] *Hypovolemic shock,* the most common type, results from loss of circulating blood volume. This may result from loss of whole blood (hemorrhagic shock), plasma, interstitial fluid (bowel obstruction), or a combination. *Vasogenic shock* results from decreased resistance within capacitance vessels, usually seen in sepsis. *Neurogenic shock* is a form of vasogenic shock in which spinal cord injury or spinal anesthesia causes vasodilatation due to acute loss of sympathetic vascular tone. *Cardiogenic shock* results from failure of the heart as a pump, as in arrhythmias or acute heart failure. In recent clinical practice, six types of shock have been described: hypovolemic, septic (vasodilatory), neurogenic, cardiogenic, obstructive, and traumatic shock. *Obstructive shock,* caused by pulmonary embolism or tension pneumothorax, results in depressed cardiac output, which results from mechanical impediment to circulation rather than a primary cardiac failure. In *traumatic shock,* the soft tissue injury and long bone fractures that occur in association with blood loss yield an upregulation of proinflammatory mediators that is more complex than simple hemorrhagic shock. The clinical dilemma faced in a patient with shock is that the etiology may not be immediately apparent. Inadequate treatment results in ongoing hypoperfusion and activation of inflammatory mediators.[2,7] Thus, treatment of the patient in shock is initially empiric, while the underlying etiology of the shock state is investigated.

In 1947, Wiggers developed a sustainable, irreversible model of hemorrhagic shock based on uptake of shed blood in a reservoir to maintain a set level of hypotension.[8] G. Tom Shires added further understanding of hemorrhagic shock with a series of laboratory and clinical studies demonstrating that a large extracellular fluid (ECF) deficit, greater than could be attributed to vascular refilling alone, occurred in severe hemorrhagic shock. These seminal studies form the scientific basis for the current treatment of hemorrhagic shock with red blood cells and lactated Ringer's solution or isotonic saline.[9-11]

As resuscitation strategies evolved, additional consequences of sustained shock became apparent. During the Vietnam War, aggressive fluid resuscitation with red blood cells and crystalloid solution or plasma resulted in survival of patients who previously would have succumbed to hemorrhagic shock. Renal failure became a less frequent clinical problem; however, a new disease process, acute fulminant pulmonary failure, appeared as an early cause of death after seemingly successful surgery to control hemorrhage. Initially called "shock lung" or "DaNang lung," the clinical problem became recognized as adult respiratory distress syndrome (ARDS), now more widely known as acute respiratory distress syndrome. This led to new methods of prolonged mechanical ventilation. Our current concept of ARDS is as a component in the spectrum of multiple organ system failure.

Much of the understanding of the pathophysiology of hemorrhagic shock is based on laboratory studies using modified Wiggers' models of hemorrhagic shock. In these models, blood pressure is kept constant via either the withdrawal or reinfusion of blood during progressive physiologic decompensation. Recent studies have challenged the relevance of the Wiggers model to the clinical scenario in which early treatment occurs in the setting of ongoing blood loss (e.g., ruptured abdominal aortic aneurysm or gunshot wound to a great vessel).[5,12] Studies over the past decade have extended the 1918 observations of Cannon, that "restoration of blood pressure prior to control of active bleeding may result in loss of blood that is sorely needed," and challenged the appropriate endpoints in resuscitation of uncontrolled hemorrhage.[13,14] Core principles in the early management of the critically-ill or injured patient include: (1) definitive control of the airway must be secured, (2) control of active hemorrhage must occur promptly (generally in the operating room, as delay in control of ongoing bleeding increases mortality), (3) volume resuscitation with red blood cells and crystalloid solution must occur while operative control of bleeding is achieved (operating room resuscitation), (4) unrecognized or inadequately corrected hypoperfusion increases morbidity and mortality (i.e., inadequate resuscitation results in avoidable early deaths from shock), and (5) excessive fluid resuscitation may exacerbate bleeding (i.e., uncontrolled resuscitation is harmful). Thus, both inadequate and uncontrolled volume resuscitation are harmful.[15]

PATHOPHYSIOLOGY

Shock is defined as tissue hypoperfusion that is insufficient to maintain normal aerobic metabolism. Simply stated, this represents an imbalance between substrate delivery (supply) and cellular substrate requirements (demand). The initial insult, whether hemorrhage, injury, or infection, initiates both a neuroendocrine and inflammatory mediator response. The magnitude of the physiologic response is proportional to both the degree and the duration of the shock. While the quantitative nature of the physiologic response in shock will vary with the etiology of shock, the qualitative nature of the response to shock is similar, with common pathways in all types of shock. Persistent hypoperfusion will result in hemodynamic derangements, end-organ dysfunction, cell death, and death of the patient if treated late or inadequately. Hemorrhagic shock is seen most often clinically; bleeding and resuscitation produce a "whole body" ischemia-reperfusion injury. The physiologic responses to

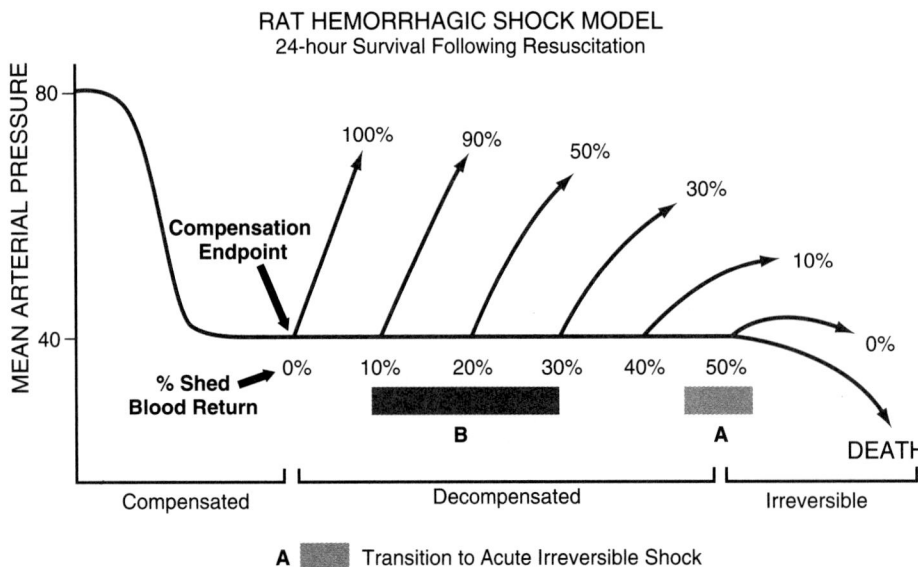

RAT HEMORRHAGIC SHOCK MODEL
24-hour Survival Following Resuscitation

FIG. 4-1. Rat model of hemorrhagic shock through the phases of compensation, decompensation, and irreversibility. The percentages shown above the curve represent survival rates. (*Reproduced with permission from Shah N, Kelly E, Billiar TR, et al: Utility of clinical parameters in a quantitative model of irreversible hemorrhagic shock. Shock 10:343, 1998.*)

A ▢ Transition to Acute Irreversible Shock
B ▮ Transition to Subacute Lethal Shock

hypovolemia are directed at preservation of perfusion to the heart and brain. To this end, vasoconstriction occurs, fluid excretion is curtailed, and fluid is shifted into the intravascular space. The major mechanisms achieving this response are: (1) prompt increase in cardiac contractility and peripheral vascular tone via the autonomic nervous system, (2) hormonal response to preserve salt and intravascular volume, and (3) changes in the local microcirculation to regulate regional blood flow. With substantial physiologic compensatory mechanisms for small volume blood loss, predominantly through the neuroendocrine response, hemodynamics may be maintained. This represents the *compensated phase* of shock. With continued hypoperfusion often not apparent clinically, cell death and tissue injury are ongoing and the *decompensation phase* of shock evolves. At this point in treatment, the cellular dysfunction can be reversed with appropriate volume resuscitation. If volume loss continues or volume resuscitation is insufficient, a vicious physiologic cycle will develop. With persistent hypoperfusion with low cardiac output, regional tissue hypoperfusion and progressive tissue and microcirculatory changes induce cardiovascular decompensation. This progression to the *irreversible phase* of shock is often insidious and recognized only in retrospect. Sufficient tissue injury and cell death have occurred to this point that continued volume resuscitation fails to reverse the process. In the laboratory, this condition represents the "uptake phase" of Wigger's model of hemorrhagic shock, when shed blood must be returned to the animal to sustain the blood pressure at the set point[8] (Fig. 4-1). Ultimately, even massive quantities of fluid resuscitation and vasopressors fail to maintain adequate blood pressure. As discussed later in this chapter, this vasodilatory response probably represents the common late phase of all forms of shock, regardless of etiology.[16,17]

NEUROENDOCRINE RESPONSE

The goal of the neuroendocrine response to hemorrhage is to maintain perfusion to the heart and the brain, even at the expense of other organ systems. Peripheral vasoconstriction occurs and fluid excretion is inhibited. The mechanisms include autonomic control of peripheral vascular tone and cardiac contractility, hormonal response to stress and volume depletion, and local microcirculatory mechanisms that are organ specific and regulate regional blood flow. The initial stimulus is loss of circulating blood volume in hemorrhagic shock. The magnitude of the neuroendocrine response is based on both the volume of blood lost and the rate at which it is lost.

Afferent Signals

Afferent impulses transmitted from the periphery are processed within the central nervous system (CNS) and activate the reflexive effector responses or efferent impulses. These effector responses are designed to expand plasma volume, maintain peripheral perfusion and tissue oxygen delivery, and restore homeostasis. The afferent impulses that initiate the body's intrinsic adaptive responses and converge in the CNS originate from a variety of sources. The initial inciting event is usually loss of circulating blood volume. Other stimuli that can produce the neuroendocrine response include pain, hypoxemia, hypercarbia, acidosis, infection, changes in temperature, emotional arousal, or hypoglycemia. The sensation of pain from injured tissue is transmitted via the spinothalamic tracts, resulting in activation of the hypothalamic-pituitary-adrenal axis, as well as activation of the autonomic nervous system (ANS) to induce direct sympathetic stimulation of the adrenal medulla to release catecholamines.

Baroreceptors also are an important afferent pathway in initiation of adaptive responses to shock. Volume receptors, sensitive to changes in both chamber pressure and wall stretch, are present within the atria of the heart. They become activated with low volume hemorrhage or mild reductions in right atrial pressure. Receptors in the aortic arch and carotid bodies respond to alterations in pressure or stretch of the arterial wall, responding to larger reductions in intravascular volume or pressure. These receptors normally inhibit induction of the ANS. When activated, these baroreceptors diminish their output, thus disinhibiting the effect of the ANS. The autonomic nervous system then increases its output, principally via sympathetic activation at the vasomotor centers of the brain stem, producing centrally-mediated constriction of peripheral vessels.

Chemoreceptors in the aorta and carotid bodies are sensitive to changes in oxygen tension, H^+ ion concentration, and CO_2 levels. Stimulation of the chemoreceptors results in vasodilatation of the coronary arteries, slowing of the heart rate, and vasoconstriction of the splanchnic and skeletal circulation. In addition, a variety of protein and nonprotein mediators are produced at the site of injury as part of the inflammatory response, and they act as afferent impulses and induce a host response. These mediators include histamine, cytokines, eicosanoids, and endothelins, among others that are discussed in greater detail later in this chapter.

Efferent Signals

Cardiovascular Response

Changes in cardiovascular function are a result of the neuroendocrine response and ANS response to shock, and constitute a prominent feature of both the body's adaptive response mechanism, and the clinical signs and symptoms of the patient in shock. Hemorrhage results in diminished venous return to the heart and decreased cardiac output. This is compensated by increased cardiac heart rate and contractility, as well as venous and arterial vasoconstriction. Stimulation of sympathetic fibers innervating the heart leads to activation of β_1-adrenergic receptors that increase heart rate and contractility in this attempt to increase cardiac output. Increased myocardial oxygen consumption occurs as a result of the increased workload; thus, myocardial oxygen supply must be maintained or myocardial dysfunction will develop.

Direct sympathetic stimulation of the peripheral circulation via the activation of α_1-adrenergic receptors on arterioles induces vasoconstriction and causes a compensatory increase in systemic vascular resistance and blood pressure. The arterial vasoconstriction is not uniform; marked redistribution of blood flow results. Selective perfusion to tissues occurs due to regional variations in arteriolar resistance, with blood shunted away from less essential organ beds such as the intestine, kidney, and skin. In contrast, the brain and heart have autoregulatory mechanisms that attempt to preserve their blood flow despite a global decrease in cardiac output. Direct sympathetic stimulation also induces constriction of venous vessels, decreasing the capacitance of the circulatory system and accelerating blood return to the central circulation.

Increased sympathetic output induces catecholamine release from the adrenal medulla. Catecholamine levels peak within 24 to 48 hours of injury, and then return to baseline. Persistent elevation of catecholamine levels beyond this time suggests ongoing noxious afferent stimuli. The majority of the circulating epinephrine is produced by the adrenal medulla, while norepinephrine is derived from synapses of the sympathetic nervous system. Catecholamine effects on peripheral tissues include stimulation of hepatic glycogenolysis and gluconeogenesis to increase circulating glucose availability to peripheral tissues, an increase in skeletal muscle glycogenolysis, suppression of insulin release, and increased glucagon release.

Hormonal Response

The stress response includes activation of the autonomic nervous system as discussed above, as well as activation of the hypothalamic-pituitary-adrenal axis. Shock stimulates the hypothalamus to release corticotropin-releasing hormone, that results in the release of adrenocorticotropic hormone (ACTH) by the pituitary. ACTH subsequently stimulates the adrenal cortex to release cortisol. Cortisol acts synergistically with epinephrine and glucagon to induce a catabolic state. Cortisol stimulates gluconeogenesis and insulin resistance, resulting in hyperglycemia as well as muscle cell protein breakdown and lipolysis to provide substrates for hepatic gluconeogenesis. Cortisol causes retention of sodium and water by the nephrons of the kidney. In the setting of severe hypovolemia, ACTH secretion occurs independently of cortisol negative feedback inhibition.

The renin-angiotensin system is activated in shock. Decreased renal artery perfusion, β-adrenergic stimulation, and increased renal tubular sodium concentration cause the release of renin from the juxtaglomerular cells. Renin catalyzes the conversion of angiotensinogen (produced by the liver) to angiotensin I, which is then converted to angiotensin II by angiotensin-converting enzyme (ACE) produced in the lung. While angiotensin I has no significant functional activity, angiotensin II is a potent vasoconstrictor of both splanchnic and peripheral vascular beds, and also stimulates the secretion of aldosterone, ACTH, and antidiuretic hormone (ADH). Aldosterone, a mineralocorticoid, acts on the nephron to promote reabsorption of sodium, and as a consequence, water. Potassium and hydrogen ions are lost in the urine in exchange for sodium.

The pituitary also releases vasopressin or ADH in response to hypovolemia, changes in circulating blood volume sensed by baroreceptors and left atrial stretch receptors, and increased plasma osmolality detected by hypothalamic osmoreceptors. Epinephrine, angiotensin II, pain, and hyperglycemia increase production of ADH. ADH levels remain elevated for about 1 week after the initial insult, depending on the severity and persistence of the hemodynamic abnormalities. ADH acts on the distal tubule and collecting duct of the nephron to increase water permeability, decrease water and sodium losses, and preserve intravascular volume. Also known as arginine vasopressin, ADH acts as a potent mesenteric vasoconstrictor, shunting circulating blood away from the splanchnic organs during hypovolemia.[18] This may contribute to intestinal ischemia and predispose to intestinal mucosal barrier dysfunction in shock states. Vasopressin also increases hepatic gluconeogenesis and increases hepatic glycolysis.

In septic states, endotoxin directly stimulates arginine vasopressin secretion independently of blood pressure, osmotic, or intravascular volume changes. Proinflammatory cytokines also contribute to arginine vasopressin release. Interestingly, patients on chronic therapy with ACE inhibitors are more at risk of developing hypotension and vasodilatory shock with open heart surgery. Low plasma levels of arginine vasopressin were confirmed in these patients.[19]

Circulatory Homeostasis

Preload

At rest, the majority of the blood volume is within the venous system. Venous return to the heart generates ventricular end-diastolic wall tension, a major determinant of cardiac output. Gravitational shifts in blood volume distribution are quickly corrected by alterations in venous capacity. With decreased arteriolar inflow, there is active contraction of the venous smooth muscle and passive elastic recoil in the thin-walled systemic veins. This increases venous return to the heart, thus maintaining ventricular filling.

Most alterations in cardiac output in the normal heart are related to changes in preload. Increases in sympathetic tone have a minor effect on skeletal muscle beds, but produce a dramatic reduction in splanchnic blood volume, which normally holds 20% of the blood volume.

The normal circulating blood volume is maintained within narrow limits by the kidney's ability to manage salt and water balance with external losses via systemic and local hemodynamic changes and hormonal effects of renin, angiotensin, and antidiuretic hormone. These relatively slow responses maintain preload by altering circulating blood volume. Acute responses to intravascular volume include changes in venous tone, systemic vascular resistance, and intrathoracic pressure, with the slower hormonal changes less important in the early response to volume loss. Furthermore, the net effect of preload on cardiac output is influenced by cardiac determinants of ventricular function, which include coordinated atrial activity and tachycardia.

Ventricular Contraction

The Frank-Starling curve describes the force of ventricular contraction as a function of its preload. This relationship is based on force of contraction being determined by initial muscle length. Intrinsic cardiac disease will shift the Frank-Starling curve and alter mechanical performance of the heart. In addition, cardiac dysfunction has been demonstrated experimentally in burns and in hemorrhagic, traumatic, and septic shock.

Afterload

Afterload is the force that resists myocardial work during contraction. Arterial pressure is the major component of afterload influencing the ejection fraction. This vascular resistance is determined by precapillary smooth muscle sphincters. Blood viscosity will also increase vascular resistance. As afterload increases in the normal heart, stroke volume can be maintained by increases in preload. In shock, with decreased circulating volume and therefore diminished preload, this compensatory mechanism to sustain cardiac output is impeded. The stress response with acute release of catecholamines and sympathetic nerve activity in the heart increases contractility and heart rate.

Microcirculation

Shock induces profound changes in tissue microcirculation that are thought to contribute to organ function, organ dysfunction, and the systemic consequences of severe shock. These changes have been studied most extensively in models of sepsis and hemorrhage. After hemorrhage, larger arterioles vasoconstrict, most likely due to sympathetic stimulation, while smaller, distal arterioles dilate, presumably due to local mechanisms.[20] Furthermore, flow at the capillary level is heterogeneous, with endothelial cell swelling and the aggregation of leukocytes producing diminished capillary perfusion in some vessels both during shock and following resuscitation[21] (Fig. 4-2). In sepsis, similar changes in microcirculatory function can also be demonstrated. Regional differences in blood flow can be demonstrated after proinflammatory stimuli, and the microcirculation in many organs is heterogeneous; blood flow is heterogenous between and within organ systems. In hemorrhagic shock, correction

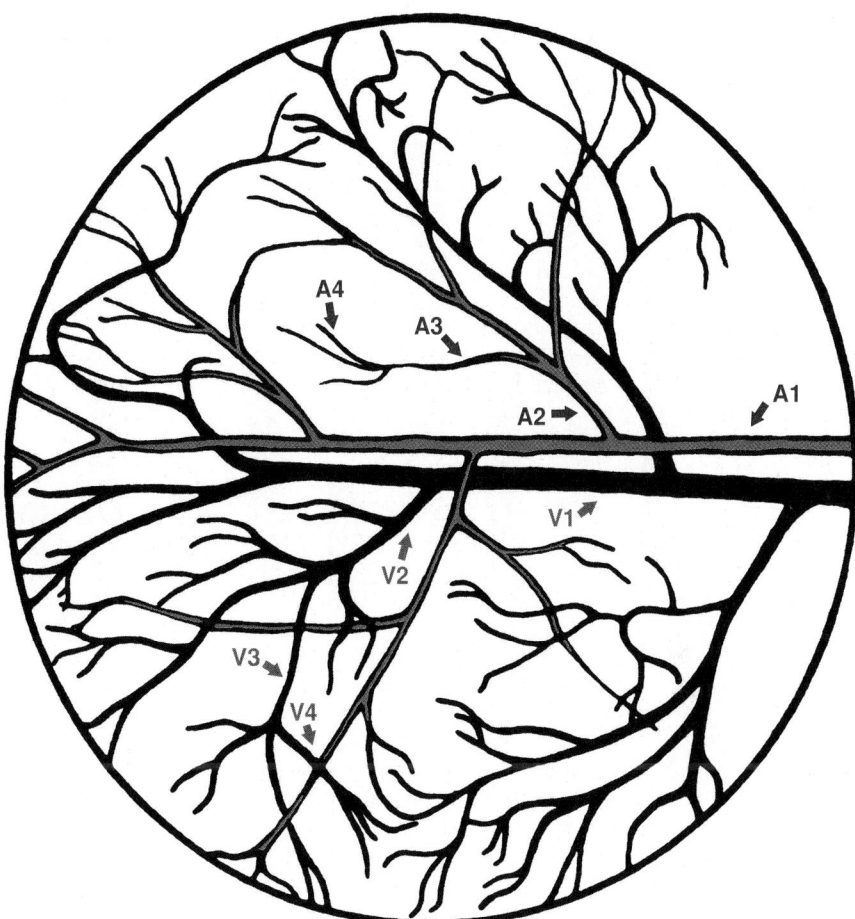

FIG. 4-2. Anatomic nomenclature of cremaster muscles. Progressively smaller arteriolar branches emanate from the major inflow arteriole (A_1). The first-order arteriole is accompanied by a parallel and adjacent first-order venule (V_1). A_2 vessels (arcade arterioles) and accompanying veins (V_e) arise as perpendicular branches of the first-order vessels. Successive arteriolar branches originate from the second-order vessels as A_3 and A_4 arterioles without accompanying veins. (Reproduced with permission from Flint et al.[20])

of hemodynamic parameters and oxygen delivery and consumption generally restores tissue oxygenation. In contrast, regional tissue dysoxia often persists in sepsis, despite restoration of oxygen delivery and consumption variables.[22] Whether this defect in oxygen extraction is the result of regional hypoxia or a defect in the pathways of mitochondrial respirations is not resolved.[23] Shunting of oxygen from the microcirculation has been proposed as a possible etiology of the regional dysoxia seen in sepsis, despite adequate oxygen delivery.[23]

With transition to decompensated shock, further vasodilation of the small arterioles increases, with progressive loss of vasomotor tone of the entire vascular bed as shock deepens. The manifestation of this loss of peripheral tone is observed clinically as ongoing volume requirements and nonresponsiveness to catecholamine infusion.

The decreases in capillary perfusion and blood flow result in diminished capillary hydrostatic pressure. The changes in hydrostatic pressure promote an influx of fluid from the extravascular or extracellular space into the capillaries to increase circulating volume. However, these changes are associated with further loss of intracellular fluid volume due to increased cellular swelling. Resuscitation with volumes of fluid sufficient to restore the extracellular fluid deficit are associated with improved outcome after shock.

This observation is based on seminal experiments performed by Dr. G. Tom Shires.[9–11] These studies confirmed deficits in the red blood cell mass, plasma volume, and ECF space following hemorrhagic shock in dogs by measurement with a triple isotope technique. Furthermore, this ECF deficit persisted when shed blood or shed

blood plus plasma was used in resuscitation. Only infusion of both shed blood plus lactated Ringer's (LR) solution (similar in composition to ECF) repleted the red blood cell mass, plasma volume, and ECF space. The long-term survivorship reflected the importance of this physiologic observation in hemorrhagic shock: blood alone (20%), blood plus plasma (30%), and blood plus LR (70%) (Fig. 4-3). This ECF deficit was confirmed in humans. Additional studies by this group demonstrated significant dysfunction of the cellular membrane in prolonged hemorrhagic shock. Depolarization of the cell membrane resulted in uptake of water and sodium by the cell (cell swelling), and loss of potassium from the cell with loss of membrane integrity. Depolarization of the cell membrane was proportional to the degree and duration of hypotension (Fig. 4-4). Thus, the loss of extracellular fluid volume during prolonged hemorrhagic shock is due to transcapillary influx of interstitial fluid into the vascular space due to decreased capillary hydrostatic pressures and cellular uptake of the fluid. This uptake of fluid by the intracellular compartment is a major site of fluid sequestration following prolonged hemorrhagic shock (Fig. 4-5). Studies in red blood cells, hepatocytes, and skeletal muscle suggested that inhibition or dysfunction of membrane active transport (Na-K-ATPase pump) was the basis of the membrane dysfunction (Fig. 4-6). These changes were reversible with appropriate resuscitation[9–11] (Fig. 4-7).

Capillary occlusion from endothelial cell swelling and neutrophil sludging and adherence may prevent restoration of capillary flow after adequate resuscitation, and is termed *no-reflow*. The nonperfused capillary beds further compound the ischemic injury. Neutrophil

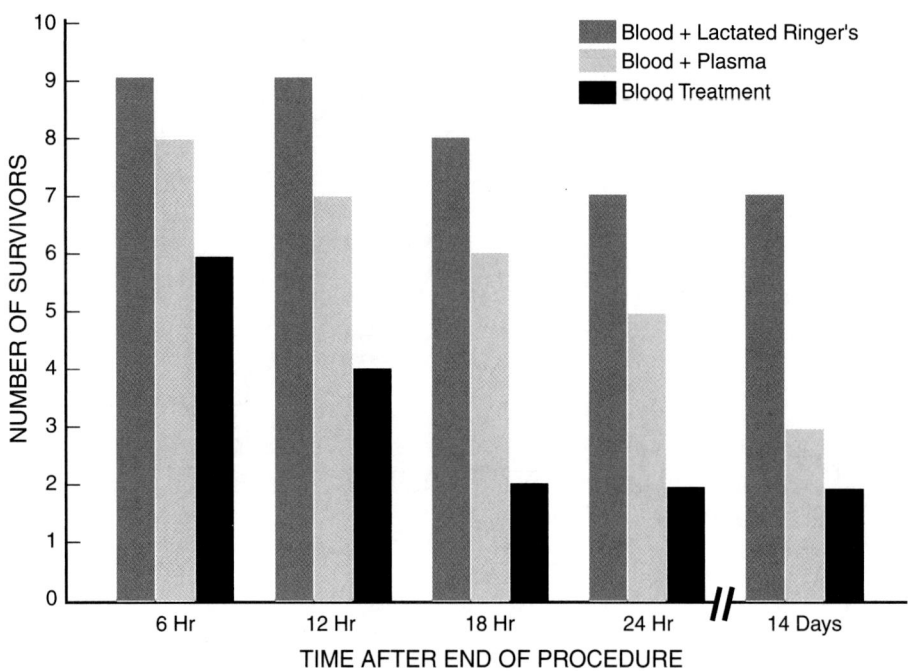

FIG. 4-3. Survival in acute hemorrhagic shock in dogs. Resuscitation with shed blood only, shed blood plus plasma, or shed blood plus lactated Ringer's (LR) solution. The long-term survival rate in the groups resuscitated with shed blood only (20%) or shed blood plus plasma (30%) was no different than in untreated, hemorrhaged animals. Resuscitation with shed blood plus LR solution yielded a 70% long-term survival rate.*(Reproduced with permission from Shires et al.[11])*

sludging in the capillaries with adherence to endothelial cells results in release of proinflammatory mediators by these cells. Neutrophil depletion in animals subjected to hemorrhagic shock produces fewer capillaries with no-reflow and lower mortality.[21]

CELLULAR EFFECTS

Depending on the magnitude of the insult and the compensatory ability of the cells, the response at the cellular level may be one of

compensation, dysfunction, or death. The aerobic respiration apparatus of the cell (i.e., oxidative phosphorylation by mitochondria), is the most susceptible to inadequate oxygen delivery to the tissues. As oxygen tension within cells decreases, there is a decrease in oxidative phosphorylation and the generation of adenosine triphosphate (ATP) slows or stops. When oxygen delivery is impaired so severely that mitochondrial respiration cannot be sustained, the state is called "dysoxia."[24] The loss of ATP has widespread effects on cellular function and morphology. As oxidative phosphorylation slows,

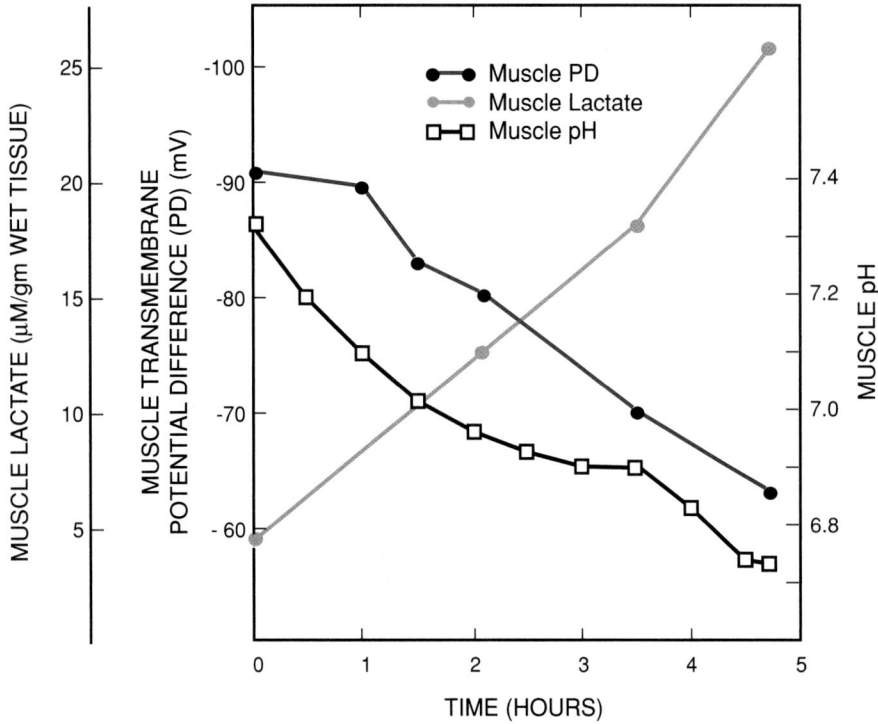

FIG. 4-4. Progressive decline in skeletal muscle membrane potential (PD) and muscle pH associated with increase in muscle lactate in hemorrhagic shock in primates. *(Reproduced with permission from Peitzman et al.[10])*

NORMAL

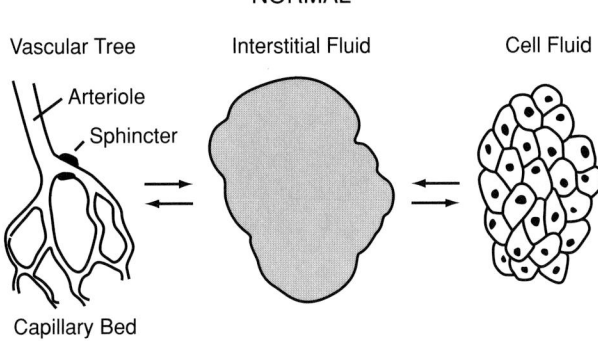

HEMORRHAGIC SHOCK

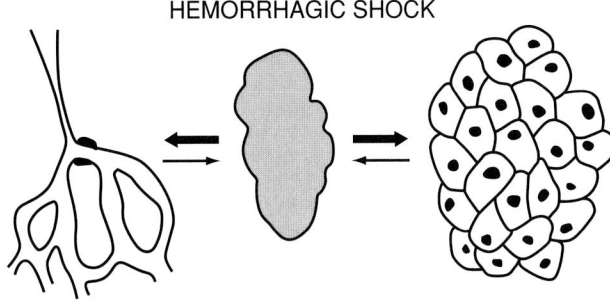

FIG. 4-5. *Interstitial fluid volume falls in hemorrhagic shock, in part because of the uptake of fluid by the intracellular compartment. [Reproduced with permission from Shires GT III, Canizaro PC, Carrico CJ, et al: Shock, in Schwartz SI, Shires GT, Spencer FC (eds): Principles of Surgery. New York: McGraw Hill, 1989, p 137.]*

the cells shift to anaerobic glycolysis that allows for the production of ATP from the breakdown of cellular glycogen. Unfortunately, anaerobic glycolysis is much less efficient than oxygen-dependent mitochondrial pathways. Under aerobic conditions, pyruvate, the end-product of glycolysis, is fed into the Krebs cycle for further oxidative metabolism. Under hypoxic conditions, the mitochondrial pathways of oxidative catabolism are impaired, and pyruvate is

instead converted into lactate. The accumulation of lactic acid and inorganic phosphates is accompanied by a reduction in pH, resulting in intracellular metabolic acidosis.

Decreased intracellular pH (intracellular acidosis) can alter the activity of cellular enzymes, lead to changes in cellular gene expression, impair cellular metabolic pathways, and impede cell membrane ion exchange.[25] Acidosis also leads to changes in cellular calcium (Ca^{2+}) metabolism and Ca^{2+}-mediated cellular signaling which alone can interfere with the activity of specific enzymes and cell function. These changes in the normal cell function may progress to cellular injury or cell death.

As cellular ATP is depleted under hypoxic conditions, the activity of the membrane Na^+,K^+-ATPase slows, and thus the maintenance of cellular membrane potential and cell volume is impaired.[9,11] Na^+ accumulates intracellularly, while K^+ leaks into the extracellular space. The net gain of intracellular sodium is accompanied by a gain in intracellular water and the development of cellular swelling. This influx is associated with a reduction in extracellular fluid volume. Endoplasmic reticulum swelling is the first ultrastructural change seen in hypoxic cell injury. Eventually, mitochondrial and cell swelling is observed. The changes in cellular membrane potential impair a number of cellular physiologic processes that are dependent on the membrane potential, such as myocyte contractility, cell signaling, and the regulation of intracellular Ca^{2+} concentrations. Once intracellular organelles such as lysosomes or cell membranes rupture, the cell will undergo death by necrosis.

Hypoperfusion and hypoxia can induce cell death by apoptosis as well. Animal models of shock and ischemia-reperfusion have demonstrated apoptotic cell death in lymphocytes, intestinal epithelial cells, hepatocytes, and other cells.[26] Apoptosis has been detected in trauma patients with ischemia-reperfusion injury, where both lymphocyte and intestinal epithelial cell apoptosis occur in the first 3 hours of injury. The intestinal mucosal cell apoptosis may compromise bowel integrity and lead to translocation of bacteria and endotoxins into the portal circulation during shock. Lymphocyte apoptosis also has been hypothesized to contribute to the immune suppression that is observed in trauma patients.

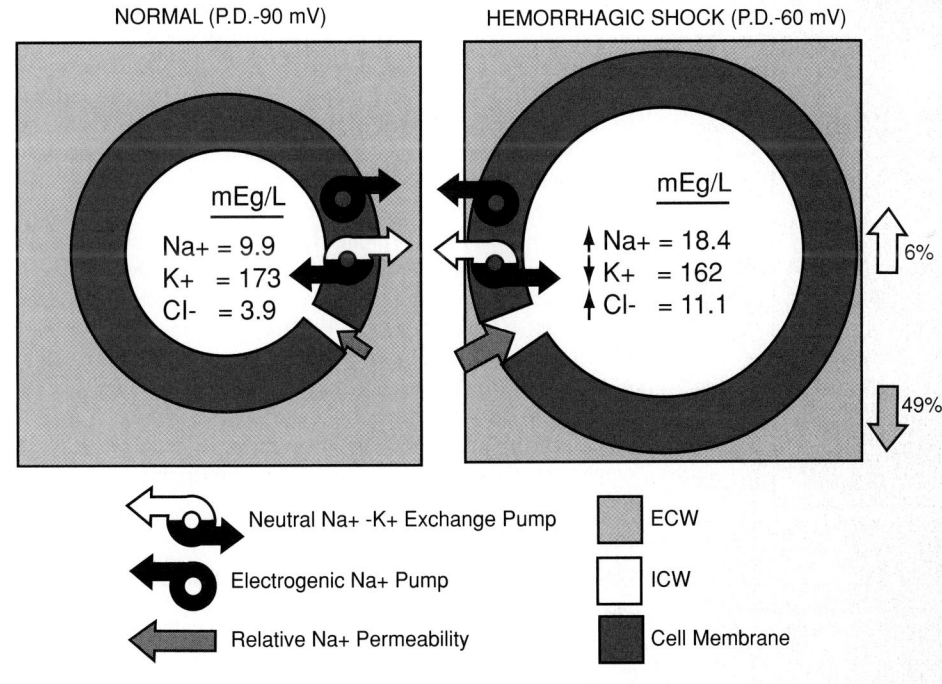

FIG. 4-6. *Changes from normal electrolyte and water distribution to that seen in late hemorrhagic shock. In late hemorrhagic shock, the cell membrane depolarizes, the cell takes up sodium, chloride, and water, and loses potassium. The extracellular fluid volume declined 49% in late hemorrhagic shock. [Reproduced with permission from Shires GT III, Canizaro PC, Carrico CJ, et al: Shock, in Schwartz SI, Shires GT, Spencer FC (eds): Principles of Surgery. New York: McGraw Hill, 1989, p 137.]*

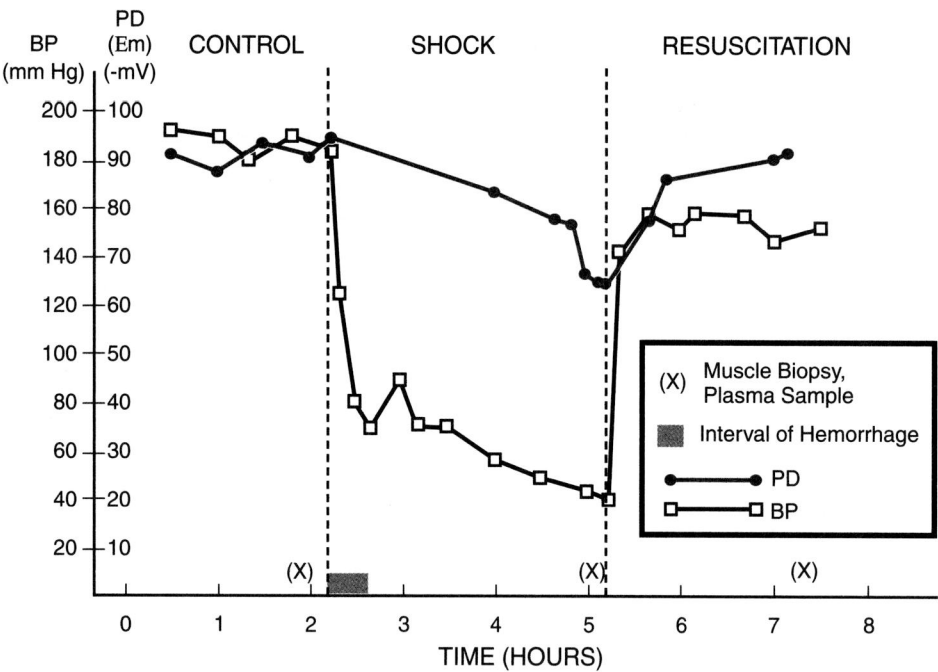

FIG. 4-7. Changes in membrane potential (PD) and systolic blood pressure (BP) during extended hemorrhagic shock and resuscitation. The changes in membrane potential and fluid and electrolyte shifts were reversed with adequate fluid resuscitation. [Reproduced with permission from Shires GT III, Canizaro PC, Carrico CJ, et al: Shock, in Schwartz SI, Shires GT, Spencer FC (eds): Principles of Surgery. New York: McGraw Hill, 1989, p 137.]

As cells become hypoxic and ATP-depleted, other ATP-dependent cell processes are affected, such as synthesis of enzymes and structural proteins, repair of DNA damage, and intercellular signal transduction. Tissue hypoperfusion also results in decreased availability of metabolic substrates and the accumulation of metabolic by-products, some of which may be toxic to cells.

Tissue hypoperfusion and cellular hypoxia result not only in intracellular acidosis, but also in systemic metabolic acidosis as metabolic by-products of anaerobic glycolysis exit the cells. The systemic changes in acid/base status may lag behind changes at the tissue level (Fig. 4-8). In the setting of acidosis, the oxyhemoglobin dissociation curve is shifted toward the right. The decreased affinity of hemoglobin in erythrocytes for oxygen results in increased O_2 release and increased tissue extraction of oxygen. In addition, hypoxia stimulates the production of erythrocyte 2, 3-diphosphoglycerate (2, 3-DPG), further contributing to the right shift of the oxyhemoglobin dissociation curve, promoting O_2 availability to the tissues during shock.

Epinephrine and norepinephrine have a profound impact on cellular metabolism. Hepatic glycogenolysis, gluconeogenesis, ketogenesis, skeletal muscle protein breakdown, and adipose tissue lipolysis are increased by catecholamines. Cortisol, glucagon, and ADH also contribute to the catabolism during shock. Epinephrine induces further release of glucagon, while inhibiting the pancreatic β-cell release of insulin. The result is a catabolic state with glucose mobilization, hyperglycemia, protein breakdown, negative nitrogen balance, lipolysis, and insulin resistance during shock and injury. The relative underutilization of glucose by peripheral tissues preserves it for the glucose-dependent organs such as the heart and brain.

In addition to induction of changes in cellular metabolic pathways, shock also induces changes in cellular gene expression. The DNA binding activity of a number of nuclear transcription factors is altered by hypoxia and the production of oxygen radicals or nitrogen radicals that are produced at the cellular level by shock. Expression of other gene products such as heat-shock proteins, vascular endothelial growth factor (VEGF), inducible nitric oxide synthase (iNOS), and cytokines also is clearly increased by shock. Many of these shock-induced gene products, such as cytokines, have the ability themselves to subsequently alter gene expression in specific target cells and tissues.[27] The involvement of multiple pathways emphasizes the complex, integrated, and overlapping nature of the response to shock.

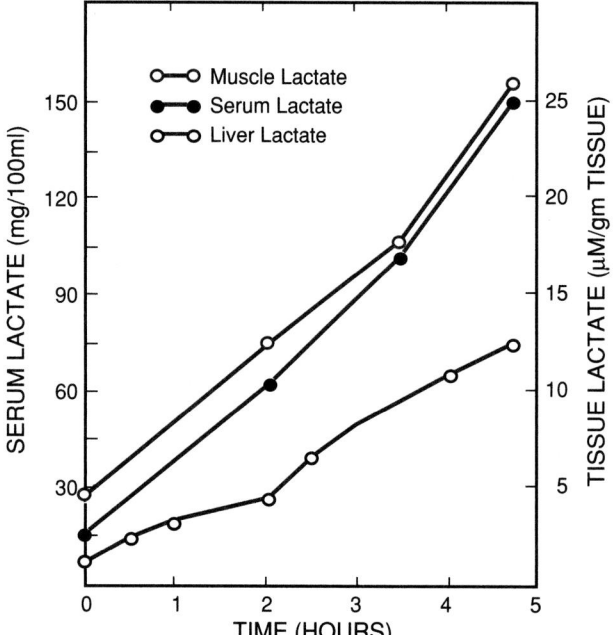

FIG. 4-8. Progressive increases in serum lactate, muscle lactate, and liver lactate in a baboon model of hemorrhagic shock. (Reproduced with permission from Peitzman et al.[10])

IMMUNE AND INFLAMMATORY RESPONSE

Alterations in the activity of the innate host immune system can be responsible for both the development of shock (i.e., distributive

Table 4-1
Inflammatory Mediators in Shock

Proinflammatory	Anti-Inflammatory
IL-1α/β	IL-4
	IL-10
IL-2	IL-13
IL-6	IL-1ra
IL-8	PGE$_2$
IFN	TGFβ
TNF	
PAF	
TNFR I/TNFR II	

IL-1α = interleukin 1α; IL-1β = interleukin 1β; IL-1ra = interleukin 1ra; IL-2 = interleukin 2; IL-4 = interleukin 4; IL-6 = interleukin 6; IL-8 = interleukin 8; IL-10 = interleukin 10; IL-13 = interleukin 13; IFN = interferon; PAF = platelet-activating factor; PGE$_2$ = prostaglandin E$_2$; TGF-β = transforming growth factor-β; TNF = tumor necrosis factor; TNFR I = tumor necrosis factor receptor I; TNFR II = tumor necrosis factor receptor II.

or septic shock following severe infection), and the pathophysiologic sequelae of shock such as the proinflammatory changes seen following hemorrhage or multisystem trauma. When these predominantly paracrine mediators gain access to the systemic circulation, they can induce a variety of metabolic changes that are collectively referred to as the *host inflammatory response*. Understanding of the intricate, redundant, and interrelated pathways that comprise the inflammatory response to shock continues to expand. Despite limited understanding of how many therapeutic interventions impact the host response to illness, inappropriate or excessive inflammation appears to be an essential event in the development of ARDS, multiple organ dysfunction syndrome (MODS), and posttraumatic immunosuppression that can prolong recovery.[28]

The immune response to shock encompasses the elaboration of mediators with both proinflammatory and anti-inflammatory properties (Table 4-1). Furthermore, new mediators, new relationships between mediators, and new functions of known mediators are continually being identified. As new pathways are uncovered, understanding of the immune response to injury and the potential for therapeutic intervention by manipulating the immune response following shock will expand. What seems clear at present, however, is that the innate immune response can help restore homeostasis, or if it is excessive, promote cellular and organ dysfunction.

Multiple mediators have been implicated in the host immune response to shock. It is likely that some of the most important mediators have yet to be discovered, and the roles of many known mediators have not been defined. A comprehensive description of all of the mediators and their complex interactions is beyond the scope of this chapter. For a general overview, a brief description of the more extensively studied mediators, as well as some of the known effects of these substances, are discussed below. A more comprehensive review can be found in Chapter 1, "The Systemic Response to Injury and Metabolic Support."

Tumor necrosis factor-α (TNF-α) was one of the first cytokines to be described, and is one of the earliest cytokines released in response to injurious stimuli. Monocytes, macrophages, and T cells release this potent proinflammatory cytokine. TNF-α levels peak within 90 minutes of stimulation and return frequently to baseline levels within 4 hours. Release of TNF-α may be induced by bacteria or endotoxin, and leads to the development of shock and hypoperfusion, most commonly observed in septic shock. Production of TNF-α may also be induced following other insults, such as hemorrhage and ischemia. TNF-α levels correlate with mortality in animal

models of hemorrhage.[29] In contrast, the increase in serum TNF-α levels reported in trauma patients is far less than that seen in septic patients.[30] Once released, TNF-α can produce peripheral vasodilation, activate the release of other cytokines, induce procoagulant activity, and stimulate a wide array of cellular metabolic changes. During the stress response, TNF-α contributes to the muscle protein breakdown and cachexia.

Interleukin-1β (IL-1β) has actions that are similar to those of TNF-α. IL-1β has a very short half-life (6 minutes) and primarily acts in a paracrine fashion to modulate local cellular responses. Systemically, IL-1β produces a febrile response to injury by activating prostaglandins in the posterior hypothalamus, and causes anorexia by activating the satiety center. This cytokine also augments the secretion of ACTH, glucocorticoids, and beta-endorphins. In conjunction with TNF-α, IL-1β can stimulate the release of other cytokines such as interleukin-2 (IL-2), interleukin-4 (IL-4), interleukin-6 (IL-6), interleukin-8 (IL-8), granulocyte-macrophage colony-stimulating factor (GM-CSF), and interferon-γ (INF-γ).

IL-2 is produced by activated T cells in response to a variety of stimuli and activates other lymphocyte subpopulations and natural killer (NK) cells. The lack of clarity regarding the role of IL-2 in the response to shock is intimately associated with that of understanding immune function after injury. Some investigators have postulated that increased IL-2 secretion promotes shock-induced tissue injury and the development of shock.[31] Others have demonstrated that depressed IL-2 production is associated with, and perhaps contributes to, the depression in immune function after hemorrhage that may increase the susceptibility of patients who develop shock to suffer infections.[32–35] It has been postulated that overly exuberant proinflammatory activation promotes tissue injury, organ dysfunction, and the subsequent immune dysfunction/suppression that may be evident later.[28] Emphasizing the importance of temporal changes in the production of mediators, both the initial excessive production of IL-2 and later depressed IL-2 production are probably important in the progression of shock.

IL-6 is elevated in response to hemorrhagic shock, major operative procedures, or trauma. Elevated IL-6 levels correlate with mortality in shock states. IL-6 contributes to lung, liver, and gut injury after hemorrhagic shock.[36–38] Thus, IL-6 may play a role in the development of diffuse alveolar damage and ARDS. IL-6 and IL-1β are mediators of the hepatic acute phase response to injury, and enhance the expression and activity of complement, C-reactive protein, fibrinogen, haptoglobin, amyloid A, and α-antitrypsin, and promote neutrophil activation.[39]

IL-10 is considered an anti-inflammatory cytokine that may have immunosuppressive properties. Its production is increased after shock and trauma, and it has been associated with depressed immune function clinically, as well as an increased susceptibility to infection.[40] IL-10 is secreted by T cells, monocytes, and macrophages, and inhibits proinflammatory cytokine secretion, oxygen radical production by phagocytes, adhesion molecule expression, and lymphocyte activation.[40–42] Administration of IL-10 depresses cytokine production and improves some aspects of immune function in experimental models of shock and sepsis.[43,44]

The complement cascade can be activated by injury, shock, and severe infection, and contributes to host defense and proflammatory activation. Significant complement consumption occurs after hemorrhagic shock.[45] In trauma patients, the degree of complement activation is proportional to the magnitude of injury and may serve as a marker for severity of injury. Patients in septic shock also demonstrate activation of the complement pathway, with elevations of the activated complement proteins C3a and C5a. Activation of

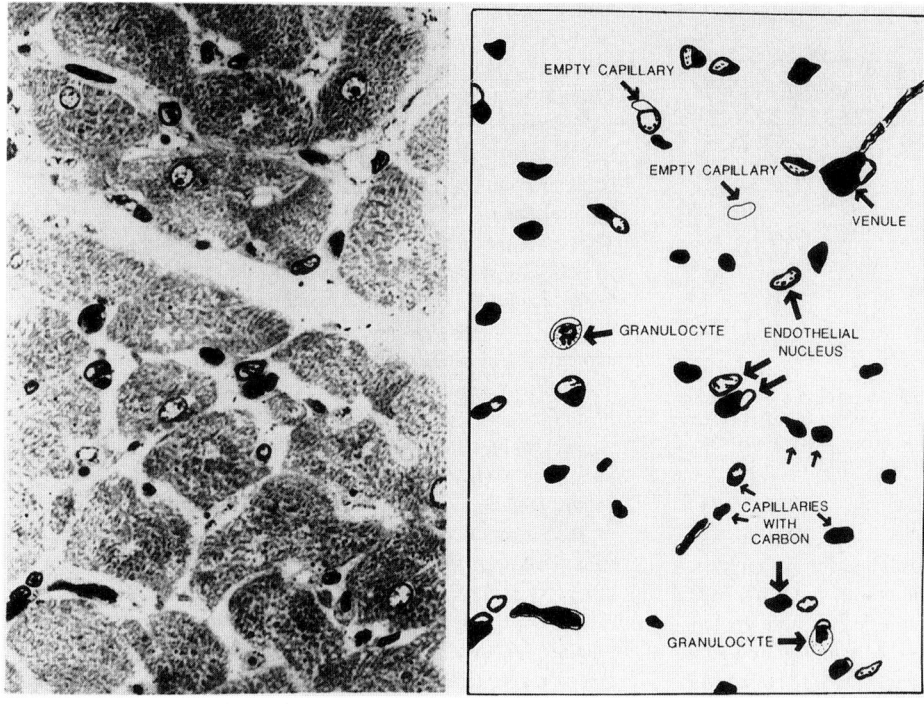

FIG. 4-9. Photomicrograph of myocardium cross-section after 7 hours of hemorrhagic shock and 2 hours of reperfusion in a conventional rat. Approximately 80% of the capillaries show reflow (contain carbon). Capillaries that are filled with carbon and capillaries without carbon are distributed in a random fashion. (*Reproduced with permission from Barroso-Aranda et al.[21]*)

the complement cascade can contribute to the development of organ dysfunction. Activated complement factors C3a, C4a, and C5a are potent mediators of increased vascular permeability, smooth muscle cell contraction, histamine and arachidonic acid by-product release, and adherence of neutrophils to vascular endothelium. Activated complement acts synergistically with endotoxin to induce the release of TNF-α and IL-1β. The development of ARDS and MODS in trauma patients correlates with the intensity of complement activation.[46] Complement and neutrophil activation may correlate with mortality in multiply-injured patients.

Neutrophil activation is an early event in the upregulation of the inflammatory response; neutrophils are the first cells to be recruited to the site of injury. Neutrophils (PMNs) remove infectious agents, foreign substances that have penetrated host barrier defenses, and nonviable tissue through phagocytosis. However, activated PMNs and their products may also produce cell injury and organ dysfunction. Activated PMNs generate and release a number of substances that may induce cell or tissue injury such as reactive oxygen species, lipid-peroxidation products, proteolytic enzymes (elastase, cathepsin G), and vasoactive mediators (leukotrienes, eicosanoids, and platelet-activating factor). Oxygen free radicals such as superoxide anion, hydrogen peroxide, and hydroxyl radical are released and induce lipid peroxidation, inactivate enzymes, and consume antioxidants (such as glutathione and tocopherol). Ischemia-reperfusion activates PMNs and causes PMN-induced organ injury. In animal models of hemorrhagic shock, activation of PMNs correlates with irreversibility of shock and mortality, and neutrophil depletion prevents the pathophysiologic sequelae of hemorrhagic and septic shock[25] (Figs. 4-9 and 4-10). Human data corroborate the activation of neutrophils in trauma and shock and suggest a role in the development of MODS.[47] Plasma markers of PMN activation, such as elastase, correlate with severity of injury in humans.

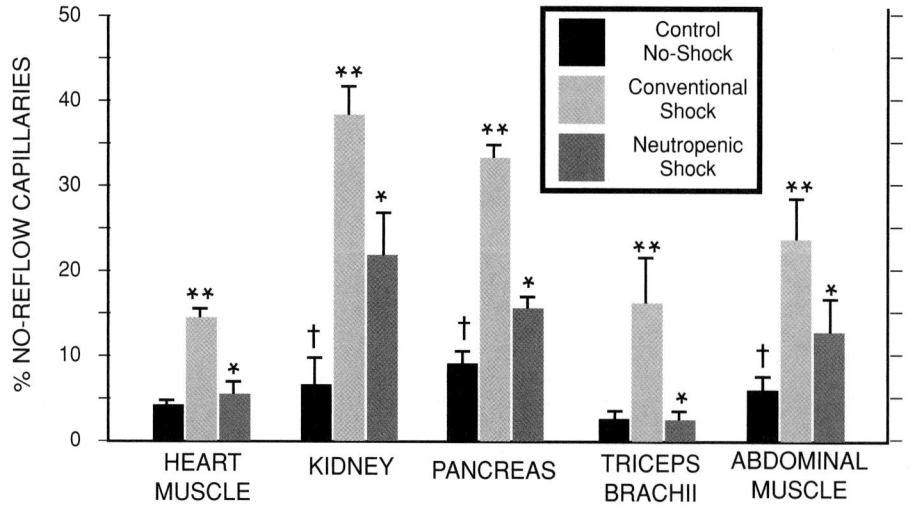

FIG. 4-10. Histogram of percentage of capillaries with no-reflow (without carbon) from heart muscle, kidney, pancreas, triceps brachii, and abdominal muscle in three experimental groups of rats: control or no shock (*black bars*), hemorrhagic shock in conventional rats (*light brown bars*), and hemorrhagic shock in neutropenic rats (*dark brown bars*). * p <0.005 conventional versus neutropenic shock, ** p <0.005 conventional versus control, † p <0.01 neutropenic shock versus control. (*Reproduced with permission from Barroso-Aranda et al.[21]*)

Interactions between endothelial cells and leukocytes are important in the inflammatory process. The vascular endothelium contributes to regulation of blood flow, leukocyte adherence, and the coagulation cascade. Extracellular ligands such as intercellular adhesion molecules (ICAMs), vascular cell adhesion molecules (VCAMs), and the selectins (E-selectin, P-selectin) are expressed on the surface of endothelial cells, and are responsible for leukocyte adhesion to the endothelium. This interaction allows activated neutrophils to migrate into the tissues to combat infection, but can also lead to PMN-mediated cytotoxicity and microvascular and tissue injury.

A host of cellular changes occur following shock. While many of the intracellular and intercellular pathways that are important in shock are being elucidated; undoubtedly there are many more that have yet to be identified. Many of the mediators produced during shock interact with cell surface receptors on target cells to alter target cell metabolism. These signaling pathways may be altered by changes in cellular oxygenation, redox state, high-energy phosphate concentration, gene expression, or intracellular electrolyte concentration induced by shock. Cells communicate with their external environment through the use of cell surface membrane receptors, which once bound by a ligand, transmit their information to the interior of the cell through a variety of signaling cascades. These signaling pathways may subsequently alter the activity of specific enzymes, the expression or breakdown of important proteins, or affect intracellular energy metabolism. Intracellular calcium (Ca^{2+}) homeostasis and regulation represents one such pathway. Intracellular Ca^{2+} concentrations regulate many aspects of cellular metabolism; many important enzyme systems require Ca^{2+} for full activity. Profound changes in intracellular Ca^{2+} levels and Ca^{2+} transport are seen in models of shock.[48–50] Alterations in Ca^{2+} regulation may lead to direct cell injury, changes in transcription factor activation, alterations in the expression of genes important in homeostasis, and the modulation of the activation of cells by other shock-induced hormones or mediators.[51–54]

A proximal portion of the intracellular signaling cascade consists of a series of kinases that transmit and amplify the signal through the phosphorylation of target proteins. The oxygen radicals produced during shock and the intracellular redox state are known to influence the activity of components of this cascade such as protein tyrosine kinases, mitogen activated kinases (MAPKs), protein kinase C, extracellular signal-regulated kinases (ERKs), and p21[ras].[55–60] Either through changes in these signaling pathways, changes in the activation of enzyme systems through Ca^{2+}-mediated events, or direct conformational changes to oxygen-sensitive proteins, oxygen radicals also regulate the activity of a number of transcription factors that are important in gene expression such as nuclear factor kappa B (NF-κB), APETALA1 (AP-1), and hypoxia-inducible factor 1 (HIF-1).[55,56,61,62] It is therefore becoming increasingly clear that oxidant-mediated direct cell injury is merely one consequence of the production of oxygen radicals during shock.

The study of the effects of shock on the regulation of gene expression as an important biologic effect was stimulated by the work of Buchman and colleagues.[63] The effects of shock on the expression and regulation of numerous genes and gene products has been studied in both experimental animal models and human patients. The study of single genes of interest remains the most common method of investigation. However, recent technical advances in the field of molecular biology have led to the development of techniques for the assessment of changes in gene expression at the mRNA and protein levels (e.g., genomic and proteomic analysis).[64–66] These techniques are beginning to be applied to the study of many forms of shock and undoubtedly will produce interesting findings in the future.

Despite extensive research into the physiologic response to shock, a great deal of individual patient variability in the response to relatively similar disease processes is seen clinically. The inability to distinguish which patient will have an uneventful recovery and which will suffer complications, infectious episodes, and organ dysfunction has driven the search for biologic mechanisms to the level of genetic makeup of the individual. Genetic variants called polymorphisms have been described that are normal genetic variants that exist in the population and can account for variations in the individual response to a number of diseases.[67–69] Clarifying the role of these differences in genetic makeup and responsiveness to account for the differences in the individual's unique response to shock will be critical to understanding shock.[70–73]

CELLULAR HYPOPERFUSION

Hypoperfused cells and tissues experience what has been termed *oxygen debt,* a concept first proposed by Crowell in 1961.[74] The oxygen debt is the deficit in tissue oxygenation over time that occurs during shock. When oxygen delivery is limited, oxygen consumption can be inadequate to match the metabolic needs of cellular respiration, creating a deficit in oxygen requirements at the cellular level. The measurement of oxygen deficit utilizes calculation of the difference between the estimated oxygen demand and the actual value obtained for oxygen consumption. Under normal circumstances, cells can "repay" the oxygen debt during reperfusion. The magnitude of the oxygen debt correlates with the severity and duration of hypoperfusion. Surrogate values for measuring oxygen debt include base deficit and lactate levels, and are discussed later in this chapter.

FORMS OF SHOCK

Hemorrhagic or Hypovolemic Shock

The most common cause of shock in the surgical or trauma patient is loss of circulating volume from hemorrhage. Acute blood loss results in reflexive decreased baroreceptor stimulation from stretch receptors in the large arteries, resulting in decreased inhibition of vasoconstrictor centers in the brain stem, increased chemoreceptor stimulation of vasomotor centers, and diminished output from atrial stretch receptors. These changes increase vasoconstriction and peripheral arterial resistance. Hypovolemia also induces sympathetic stimulation, leading to epinephrine and norepinephrine release, activation of the renin-angiotensin cascade, and increased vasopressin release. Peripheral vasoconstriction is prominent, while lack of sympathetic effects on cerebral and coronary vessels and local autoregulation promote maintenance of cardiac and CNS blood flow.

Diagnosis

Treatment of shock is initially empiric. The airway must be secured and volume infusion for restoration of blood pressure initiated while the search for the cause of the hypotension is pursued. Shock in a trauma patient and postoperative patient should be presumed to be due to hemorrhage until proven otherwise. The clinical signs of shock may be evident with an agitated patient, including cool clammy extremities, tachycardia, weak or absent peripheral pulses, and hypotension. Such apparent clinical shock results from at least 25 to 30% loss of the blood volume. However, substantial volumes of blood may be lost before the classic clinical manifestations of shock are evident. Thus when a patient is significantly tachycardiac or hypotensive, this represents both significant blood loss and physiologic decompensation. The clinical and physiologic response to hemorrhage has been classified according to the magnitude of volume loss.[75] Loss of up to 15% of the circulating volume (700 to 750 mL for a 70-kg patient) may produce little in terms of obvious symptoms, while loss of up to 30% of the circulating volume (1.5 L) may result in mild tachycardia, tachypnea, and anxiety. Hypotension, marked tachycardia [i.e., pulse >110 to 120 beats per minute (bpm)], and confusion may not be evident until more than 30% of the blood volume has been lost; loss of 40% of circulating volume (2 L) is immediately life threatening, and generally requires operative control of bleeding. Young healthy patients with vigorous compensatory mechanisms may tolerate larger volumes of blood loss while manifesting fewer clinical signs despite the presence of significant peripheral hypoperfusion. These patients may maintain a near-normal blood pressure until a precipitous cardiovascular collapse occurs. Elderly patients may be taking medications that either promote bleeding (e.g., warfarin or aspirin), or mask the compensatory responses to bleeding (e.g., beta blockers). In addition, atherosclerotic vascular disease, diminishing cardiac compliance with age, inability to elevate heart rate or cardiac contractility in response to hemorrhage, and overall decline in physiologic reserve decrease the elderly patient's ability to tolerate hemorrhage.

In addressing the sensitivity of vital signs and identifying major thoracoabdominal hemorrhage, a study retrospectively identified patients with injury to the trunk and with an abbreviated injury score of 3 or greater who required immediate surgical intervention and transfusion of at least 5 units of blood within the first 24 hours. Ninety-five percent of patients had a heart rate greater than 80 bpm at some point during their postinjury course. However, only 59% of patients achieved a heart rate greater than 120 bpm. Ninety-nine percent of all patients had a recorded blood pressure of less than 120 mm Hg at some point. Ninety-three percent of all patients had a recorded systolic blood pressure (SBP) of less than 100 mm Hg.[76] A more recent study corroborated that tachycardia was not a reliable sign of hypotension following trauma.[77] Tachycardia was present in only 65% of hypotensive patients.

In management of trauma patients, understanding the patterns of injury of the patient in shock will help direct the evaluation and management. Identifying the sources of blood loss in patients with penetrating wounds is relatively simple since potential bleeding sources will be located along the known or suspected path of the wounding object. Patients with penetrating injuries who are in shock usually require operative intervention. Patients who suffer multisystem injuries from blunt trauma have multiple sources of potential hemorrhage. Blood loss sufficient to cause shock is generally of a large volume, and there are a limited number of sites that can harbor sufficient extravascular blood volume to induce hypotension (e.g., external, intrathoracic, intra-abdominal, retroperitoneal, and long bone fractures). In the nontrauma patient, the gastrointestinal tract must always be considered as a site for blood loss. Substantial blood loss externally may be suspected from prehospital medical reports documenting a substantial blood loss at the scene of an accident, history of massive blood loss from wounds, visible brisk bleeding, or presence of a large hematoma adjacent to an open wound. Injuries to major arteries or veins with associated open wounds may cause massive blood loss rapidly. Direct pressure must be applied and sustained to minimize ongoing blood loss. Persistent bleeding from uncontrolled smaller vessels can, over time, precipitate shock if inadequately treated.

When major blood loss is not immediately visible, internal (intracavitary) blood loss should be suspected. Each pleural cavity can hold 2 to 3 L of blood and can therefore be a site of significant blood loss. Diagnostic and therapeutic tube thoracostomy may be indicated in unstable patients based on clinical findings and clinical suspicion. In a more stable patient, a chest radiograph may be obtained to look for evidence of hemothorax. Major retroperitoneal hemorrhage typically occurs in association with pelvic fractures, which is confirmed by pelvic radiography in the resuscitation bay. Intraperitoneal hemorrhage is probably the most common source of blood loss inducing shock. The physical exam for detection of substantial blood loss or injury is insensitive and unreliable; large volumes of intraperitoneal blood may be present before physical exam findings are apparent. Findings with intra-abdominal hemorrhage include abdominal distension, abdominal tenderness, or visible abdominal wounds. Hemodynamic abnormalities generally stimulate a search for blood loss prior to the appearance of obvious abdominal findings. Adjunctive tests are essential in the diagnosis of intraperitoneal bleeding; intraperitoneal blood may be rapidly identified by diagnostic ultrasound or diagnostic peritoneal lavage.

Treatment

Control of ongoing hemorrhage is an essential component of the resuscitation of the patient in shock. As mentioned above, treatment of hemorrhagic shock is instituted concurrently with diagnostic evaluation to identify a source. Patients who fail to respond to initial resuscitative efforts should be assumed to have ongoing active hemorrhage from large vessels and require prompt operative intervention. The appropriate priorities in these patients are (1) secure the airway, (2) control the source of blood loss, and (3) intravenous volume resuscitation. Identifying the body cavity harboring active hemorrhage will help focus operative efforts; however, because time is of the essence, rapid treatment is essential and diagnostic laparotomy or thoracotomy may be indicated. The actively bleeding patient cannot be resuscitated until control of ongoing hemorrhage is achieved.

Patients who respond to initial resuscitative efforts, but then deteriorate hemodynamically, frequently have injuries that require operative intervention. The magnitude and duration of their response will dictate whether diagnostic maneuvers can be performed to identify the site of bleeding. However, hemodynamic deterioration generally denotes ongoing bleeding for which some form of intervention (i.e., operation or interventional radiology) is required. Patients who have lost significant intravascular volume, but hemorrhage is controlled or abated, will often respond to resuscitative efforts if the depth and duration of shock have been limited.

A subset of patients exists who fail to respond to resuscitative efforts despite adequate control of ongoing hemorrhage. These patients have ongoing fluid requirements despite adequate control of hemorrhage, have persistent hypotension despite restoration of intravascular volume necessitating vasopressor support, and may exhibit a futile cycle of uncorrectable hypothermia, hypoperfusion, acidosis, and coagulopathy that cannot be interrupted despite maximum therapy. These patients have deteriorated to decompensated or irreversible shock with peripheral vasodilation and resistance to vasopressor infusion. Mortality is inevitable once the patient manifests shock in its terminal stages.

Cardiogenic Shock

Cardiogenic shock is defined clinically as circulatory pump failure leading to diminished forward flow and subsequent tissue hypoxia, in the setting of adequate intravascular volume. Hemodynamic criteria include sustained hypotension (i.e., SBP <90 mm Hg for at least 30 minutes), reduced cardiac index (<2.2 L/min per square meter), and elevated pulmonary artery wedge pressure (>15 mm Hg).[78]

Mortality rates for cardiogenic shock are 50 to 80%. Acute, extensive myocardial infarction (MI) is the most common cause of cardiogenic shock; a smaller infarction in a patient with existing left ventricular dysfunction may also precipitate shock. Cardiogenic shock complicates 5 to 10% of acute MIs. Conversely, cardiogenic shock is the most common cause of death in patients hospitalized with acute MI. Although shock may develop early after myocardial infarction, it is typically not found on admission. Seventy-five percent of patients who have cardiogenic shock complicating acute MIs develop signs of cardiogenic shock within 24 hours after onset of infarction (average 7 hours). Recognition of the patient with occult hypoperfusion is critical to prevent progression to obvious cardiogenic shock with its high mortality rate; early initiation of therapy to maintain blood pressure and cardiac output is vital. Rapid assessment, adequate resuscitation, and reversal of the myocardial ischemia are essential in optimizing outcome in patients with acute MI. Prevention of infarct extension is a critical component. Large segments of nonfunctional but viable myocardium contribute to the development of cardiogenic shock after MI. In the setting of acute MI, expeditious restoration of cardiac output is mandatory to minimize mortality; the extent of myocardial salvage possible decreases exponentially with increased time to restoration of coronary blood flow. The degree of coronary flow after percutaneous transluminal coronary angioplasty (PTCA) correlates with in-hospital mortality (i.e., 33% mortality with complete reperfusion, 50% mortality with incomplete reperfusion, and 85% mortality with absent reperfusion).[79] Inadequate cardiac function can be a direct result of cardiac injury, including profound myocardial contusion, blunt cardiac valvular injury, or direct myocardial damage[78–80] (Table 4-2). The pathophysiology of cardiogenic shock involves a vicious cycle of myocardial ischemia which causes myocardial dysfunction, which results in more myocardial ischemia.[78] When sufficient mass of the left ventricular wall is necrotic or ischemic and fails to pump, the stroke volume decreases. Autopsy series of patients dying from cardiogenic shock have found damage to 40% of the left ventricle.[81] Ischemia distant from the infarct zone may contribute to the systolic dysfunction in patients with cardiogenic shock. The majority of these patients have multivessel disease, with limited vasodilator

Table 4-2
Causes of Cardiogenic Shock

Acute myocardial infarction
 Pump failure
 Mechanical complications
  Acute mitral regurgitation from papillary muscle rupture
  Ventricular septal defect
  Free-wall rupture
  Pericardial tamponade
 Right ventricular infarction
Other causes of cardiogenic shock
 End-stage cardiomyopathy
 Myocarditis
 Severe myocardial contusion
 Prolonged cardiopulmonary bypass
 Septic shock with severe myocardial depression
 Left ventricular outflow obstruction
  Aortic stenosis
  Hypertrophic obstructive cardiomyopathy
 Obstruction to left ventricular filling
  Mitral stenosis
  Left atrial myxoma
 Acute mitral regurgitation
 Acute aortic insufficiency

SOURCE: Adapted with permission from Hollenberg et al.[78]

reserve and pressure-dependent coronary flow in multiple areas of the heart. Myocardial diastolic function is impaired in cardiogenic shock as well. Decreased compliance results from myocardial ischemia, and compensatory increases in left ventricular filling pressures progressively occur.

Diminished cardiac output or contractility in the face of adequate intravascular volume (preload) may lead to underperfused vascular beds and reflexive sympathetic discharge. Increased sympathetic stimulation of the heart, either through direct neural input or from circulating catecholamines, increases heart rate, myocardial contraction, and myocardial oxygen consumption, that may not be relieved by increases in coronary artery blood flow in patients with fixed stenoses of the coronary arteries. Diminished cardiac output may also decrease coronary artery blood flow, resulting in a scenario of increased myocardial oxygen demand at a time when myocardial oxygen supply may be limited. Acute heart failure may also result in fluid accumulation in the pulmonary microcirculatory bed, decreasing myocardial oxygen delivery even further.

Diagnosis

Rapid identification of the patient with pump failure and institution of corrective action are essential in preventing the ongoing spiral of decreased cardiac output from injury causing increased myocardial oxygen needs that cannot be met, leading to progressive and unremitting cardiac dysfunction. In evaluation of possible cardiogenic shock, other causes of hypotension must be excluded, including hemorrhage, sepsis, pulmonary embolism, and aortic dissection. Signs of circulatory shock include hypotension, cool and mottled skin, depressed mental status, tachycardia, and diminished pulses. Cardiac exam may include dysrhythmia, precordial heave, or distal heart tones. Confirmation of a cardiac source for the shock requires electrocardiogram and urgent echocardiography. Other useful diagnostic tests include chest radiograph, arterial blood gases, electrolytes, complete blood count, and cardiac enzymes. Invasive cardiac monitoring, which is generally not necessary, can be useful to exclude right ventricular infarction, hypovolemia, and possible mechanical complications.

Making the diagnosis of cardiogenic shock involves the identification of cardiac dysfunction or acute heart failure in a susceptible patient. Since patients with blunt cardiac injury typically have multisystem injury, hemorrhagic shock from intra-abdominal bleeding, intrathoracic bleeding, and bleeding from fractures must be excluded. Relatively few patients with blunt cardiac injury will develop cardiac pump dysfunction. Those who do generally exhibit cardiogenic shock early in their evaluation. Therefore, establishing the diagnosis of blunt cardiac injury is secondary to excluding other etiologies for shock and establishing that cardiac dysfunction is present. Invasive hemodynamic monitoring with a pulmonary artery catheter may uncover evidence of diminished cardiac output and elevated pulmonary artery pressure.

Treatment

After ensuring that an adequate airway is present and ventilation is sufficient, attention should be focused on support of the circulation. Intubation and mechanical ventilation are often required, if only to decrease work of breathing and facilitate sedation of the patient. Rapidly excluding hypovolemia and establishing the presence of cardiac dysfunction is essential. Treatment of cardiac dysfunction includes maintenance of adequate oxygenation to ensure adequate myocardial oxygen delivery and judicious fluid administration to avoid fluid overload and development of cardiogenic pulmonary edema. Electrolyte abnormalities, commonly hypokalemia and hypomagnesemia, should be corrected. Pain is treated with intravenous morphine sulfate or fentanyl. Significant dysrhythmias and heart block must be treated with antiarrhythmic drugs, pacing, or cardioversion if necessary. Early consultation with cardiology is essential in current management of cardiogenic shock, particularly in the setting of acute myocardial infarction.[78]

When profound cardiac dysfunction exists, inotropic support may be indicated to improve cardiac contractility and cardiac output. Dobutamine primarily stimulates cardiac β_1 receptors to increase cardiac output, but may also vasodilate peripheral vascular beds, lower total peripheral resistance, and lower systemic blood pressure through effects on β_2 receptors. Ensuring adequate preload and intravascular volume is therefore essential prior to instituting therapy with dobutamine. Dopamine stimulates α receptors (vasoconstriction), β_1 receptors (cardiac stimulation), and β_2 receptors (vasodilation), with its effects on β receptors predominating at lower doses. Dopamine may be preferable to dobutamine in treatment of cardiac dysfunction in hypotensive patients. Tachycardia and increased peripheral resistance from dopamine infusion may worsen myocardial ischemia. Titration of both dopamine and dobutamine infusions may be required in some patients.

Epinephrine stimulates α and β receptors and may increase cardiac contractility and heart rate; however, it also may have intense peripheral vasoconstrictor effects that impair further cardiac performance. Catecholamine infusions must be carefully controlled to maximize coronary perfusion, while minimizing myocardial oxygen demand. Balancing the beneficial effects of impaired cardiac performance with the potential side effects of excessive reflex tachycardia and peripheral vasoconstriction requires serial assessment of tissue perfusion using indices such as capillary refill, character of peripheral pulses, adequacy of urine output, or improvement in laboratory parameters of resuscitation such as pH, base deficit, and lactate. Invasive monitoring is generally necessary in these unstable patients. The phosphodiesterase inhibitors amrinone and milrinone may be required on occasion in patients with resistant cardiogenic shock. These agents have long half-lives and induce thrombocytopenia and hypotension, and use is reserved for patients unresponsive to other treatment.

Patients whose cardiac dysfunction is refractory to cardiotonics may require mechanical circulatory support with an intra-aortic balloon pump (IABP).[82] Intra-aortic balloon pumping increases cardiac output and improves coronary blood flow by reduction of systolic afterload and augmentation of diastolic perfusion pressure. Unlike vasopressor agents, these beneficial effects occur without an increase in myocardial oxygen demand. IABP can be inserted at the bedside in the ICU via the femoral artery through either a cutdown or using the percutaneous approach. Aggressive circulatory support of patients with cardiac dysfunction from intrinsic cardiac disease has led to more widespread application of these devices and more familiarity with their operation by both physicians and critical care nurses.

Preservation of existing myocardium and preservation of cardiac function are priorities of therapy for patients who have suffered an acute myocardial infarction. Ensuring adequate oxygenation and oxygen delivery, maintaining adequate preload with judicious volume restoration, minimizing sympathetic discharge through adequate relief of pain, and correcting electrolyte imbalances are all straightforward nonspecific maneuvers that may improve existing cardiac function or prevent future cardiac complications. Anticoagulation and aspirin are given for acute myocardial infarction. Although thrombolytic therapy reduces mortality in patients with acute myocardial infarction, its role in cardiogenic shock is less clear.

Patients in cardiac failure from an acute MI may benefit from pharmacologic or mechanical circulatory support in a manner similar to that of patients with cardiac failure related to blunt cardiac injury. Additional pharmacologic tools may include the use of β-blockers to control heart rate and myocardial oxygen consumption, nitrates to promote coronary blood flow through vasodilatation, and ACE inhibitors to reduce ACE-mediated vasoconstrictive effects that increase myocardial workload and myocardial oxygen consumption.

Current guidelines of the American Heart Association recommend percutaneous transluminal coronary angiography for patients with cardiogenic shock, ST elevation, left bundle-branch block, and age less than 75 years.[83] Early definition of coronary anatomy and revascularization is the pivotal step in treatment of patients with cardiogenic shock from acute MI.[80] When feasible, PTCA (generally with stent placement) is the treatment of choice. Coronary artery bypass grafting seems to be more appropriate for patients with multiple vessel disease or left main coronary artery disease.

Vasodilatory Shock (Septic Shock)

In the peripheral circulation, profound vasoconstriction is the typical physiologic response to arterial pressure that is insufficient for tissue perfusion, usually causing cardiogenic or hemorrhagic shock. In vasodilatory shock, hypotension results from failure of the vascular smooth muscle to constrict appropriately. Vasodilatory shock is characterized by both peripheral vasodilatation with resultant hypotension, and resistance to treatment with vasopressors. Despite the hypotension, plasma catecholamine levels are elevated and the renin-angiotensin system is activated in vasodilatory shock.[84,85] The most frequently encountered form of vasodilatory shock is *septic shock*. Other causes of vasodilatory shock include hypoxic lactic acidosis, carbon monoxide poisoning, decompensated and irreversible hemorrhagic shock, terminal cardiogenic shock, and postcardiotomy shock (Table 4-3). Thus, vasodilatory shock seems to represent the final common pathway for profound and prolonged shock of any etiology.[17]

Despite advances in intensive care, the mortality rate for severe sepsis remains 30 to 50%.[86,87] In the United States, 750,000 cases of sepsis occur annually, one-third of which are fatal.[88] Sepsis accounts for 9.3% of deaths in the United States, as many yearly as myocardial infarction. Septic shock is a by-product of the body's response to invasive or severe localized infection, typically from bacterial or fungal pathogens. In the attempt to eradicate the pathogens, the immune and other cell types (e.g., endothelial cells) elaborate soluble mediators that enhance macrophage and neutrophil killing effector mechanisms, increase procoagulant activity and fibroblast activity to localize the invaders, and increase microvascular blood flow to enhance delivery of killing forces to the area of invasion. When this response is overly exuberant or becomes systemic rather than localized, manifestations of sepsis may be evident. These

Table 4-3
Causes of Vasodilatory Shock

Sepsis
Prolonged and severe hypotension
Hemorrhagic shock
Cardiogenic shock
Cardiopulmonary bypass
Inadequate tissue oxygenation
Hypoxic lactic acidosis
Carbon monoxide poisoning

SOURCE: Modified with permission from Landry et al.[17]

findings include enhanced cardiac output, peripheral vasodilation, fever, leukocytosis, hyperglycemia, and tachycardia. In septic shock, the vasodilatory effects are due in part to the upregulation of the inducible isoform of nitric oxide synthase (iNOS or NOS 2) in the vessel wall. iNOS produces large quantities of nitric oxide for sustained periods of time. This potent vasodilator suppresses vascular tone and renders the vasculature resistant to the effects of vasoconstricting agents.[89]

Diagnosis

Attempts to standardize terminology have led to the establishment of criteria for the diagnosis of sepsis in the hospitalized adult. These criteria include manifestations of the host response to infection, in addition to identification of an offending organism. The terms *sepsis, severe sepsis,* and *septic shock* are used to quantify the magnitude of the systemic inflammatory reaction. Patients with *sepsis* have evidence of an infection, as well as systemic signs of inflammation (e.g., fever, leukocytosis, and tachycardia). Hypoperfusion with signs of organ dysfunction is termed *severe sepsis. Septic shock* requires the presence of the above, associated with more significant evidence of tissue hypoperfusion and systemic hypotension. Beyond the hypotension, maldistribution of blood flow and shunting in the microcirculation further compromise delivery of nutrients to the tissue beds.[90]

Recognizing septic shock begins with defining the patient at risk. The clinical manifestations of septic shock will usually become evident and prompt the initiation of treatment before bacteriologic confirmation of an organism or the source of an organism is identified. In addition to fever, tachycardia, and tachypnea, signs of hypoperfusion such as confusion, malaise, oliguria, or hypotension may be present. These should prompt an aggressive search for infection including a thorough physical exam, inspection of all wounds, evaluation of intravascular catheters or other foreign bodies, obtaining appropriate cultures, and adjunctive imaging studies as needed.

Treatment

Evaluation of the patient in septic shock begins with an assessment of the adequacy of their airway and ventilation. Severely obtunded patients and patients whose work of breathing is excessive require intubation and ventilation to prevent respiratory collapse. Since vasodilation and decrease in total peripheral resistance may produce hypotension, fluid resuscitation and restoration of circulatory volume with balanced salt solutions is essential. Empiric antibiotics must be chosen carefully based on the most likely pathogens (gram-negative rods, gram-positive cocci, and anaerobes), since the portal of entry of the offending organism and its identity may not be evident until culture data return or imaging studies are completed. Knowledge of the bacteriologic profile of infections in an individual unit can be obtained from most hospital infection control departments and will suggest potential responsible organisms. Antibiotics should be tailored to cover the responsible organisms once culture data are available, and if appropriate, the spectrum of coverage narrowed. Long-term empiric broad-spectrum antibiotic use should be minimized to reduce the development of resistant organisms, and to avoid the potential complications of fungal overgrowth and antibiotic-associated colitis from overgrowth of *Clostridium difficile*. Intravenous antibiotics will be insufficient to adequately treat the infectious episode in the settings of infected fluid collections, infected foreign bodies, and devitalized tissue. These situations may require multiple operations to ensure proper wound hygiene and healing.

The majority of septic patients have hyperdynamic physiology with supranormal cardiac output and low systemic vascular resistance. On occasion, septic patients may have low cardiac output despite volume resuscitation and even vasopressor support. Mortality in this group is high. Despite the increasing incidence of septic shock over the past several decades, the overall mortality rates have changed little. Studies of interventions including immunotherapy, resuscitation to pulmonary artery endpoints with hemodynamic optimization (cardiac output and oxygen delivery, even to supranormal values), and optimization of mixed venous oxygen measurements up to 72 hours after admission to the intensive care unit have not changed mortality. Negative results from these studies have led to the suggestion that earlier interventions directed at improving global tissue oxygenation may be of benefit. To this end, Rivers and colleagues reported that goal-directed therapy of septic shock and severe sepsis initiated in the emergency department and continued for 6 hours significantly improved outcome.[91] This approach involved adjustment of cardiac preload, afterload, and contractility to balance oxygen delivery with oxygen demand. They found that goal-directed therapy during the first 6 hours of hospital stay (initiated in the emergency department) had significant effects, such as higher mean venous oxygen saturation, lower lactate levels, lower base deficit, higher pH, and decreased 28-day mortality (49.2 vs. 33.3%) compared to the standard therapy group. The frequency of sudden cardiovascular collapse was also significantly less in the group managed with goal-directed therapy (21.0 vs. 10.3%). Interestingly, the goal-directed therapy group received more intravenous fluids during the initial 6 hours, but the standard therapy group required more intravenous fluid by 72 hours. The authors emphasize that continued cellular and tissue decompensation is subclinical and often irreversible when obvious clinically. Goal-directed therapy allowed identification and treatment of these patients with insidious illness (global tissue hypoxia in the setting of normal vital signs).

After first-line therapy of the septic patient with antibiotics, intravenous fluids, and intubation if necessary, vasopressors may be necessary to treat patients with septic shock. Catecholamines are the vasopressors used most often. Occasionally, patients with septic shock will develop arterial resistance to catecholamines. Arginine vasopressin, a potent vasoconstrictor, is often efficacious in this setting.[18]

Hyperglycemia and insulin resistance are typical in critically-ill and septic patients, including patients without underlying diabetes mellitus. A recent study reported significant positive impact of tight glucose management on outcome in critically-ill patients.[92] The two treatment groups in this randomized, prospective study were assigned to receive intensive insulin therapy (maintenance of blood glucose between 80 and 110 mg/dL) or conventional treatment (infusion of insulin only if the blood glucose level exceeded 215 mg/dL, with a goal between 180 and 200 mg/dL). The mean morning glucose level was significantly higher in the conventional treatment as compared to the intensive insulin therapy group (153 vs. 103 mg/dL). Mortality in the intensive insulin treatment group (4.6%) was significantly lower than in the conventional treatment group (8.0%), representing a 42% reduction in mortality. This reduction in mortality was most notable in the patients requiring longer than 5 days in the ICU. Furthermore, intensive insulin therapy reduced episodes of septicemia by 46%, reduced duration of antibiotic therapy, and decreased the need for prolonged ventilatory support and renal replacement therapy.

Additional adjunctive immune modulation strategies have been developed for the treatment of septic shock. These include the use of antiendotoxin antibodies, anticytokine antibodies, cytokine receptor antagonists, immune enhancers, a non–isoform-specific nitric oxide synthase inhibitor, and oxygen radical scavengers. These compounds are each designed to alter some aspect of the host immune response to shock that is hypothesized to play a key role in its pathophysiology. However, most of these strategies have failed to demonstrate efficacy in human patients despite utility in well-controlled animal experiments. It is unclear whether the failure of these compounds is due to poorly designed clinical trials, inadequate understanding of the interactions of the complex host immune response to injury and infection, or animal models of shock that poorly represent the human disease. A recent study reported benefit from intravenous infusion of recombinant human activated protein C for severe sepsis.[93] Activated protein C is an endogenous protein that promotes fibrinolysis and inhibits thrombosis and inflammation. The authors conducted a randomized, prospective, multicenter trial assessing the efficacy of activated protein C in patients with systemic inflammation and organ failure due to acute infection. Treatment with activated protein C reduced the 28-day mortality rate from 31 to 25%; the reduction in relative risk of death was 19.4%.

The use of corticosteroids in the treatment of sepsis and septic shock has been controversial for decades. The observation that severe sepsis is often associated with adrenal insufficiency or glucocorticoid receptor resistance has generated renewed interest in therapy for septic shock with corticosteroids.[87,94,95] A single intravenous dose of 50 mg of hydrocortisone improved mean arterial blood pressure response relationships to norepinephrine and phenylephrine in patients with septic shock, and was most notable in patients with relative adrenal insufficiency. A more recent study evaluated therapy with hydrocortisone (50 mg intravenously every 6 hours) and fludrocortisone (50 μg orally once daily) versus placebo for 1 week in patients with septic shock.[95] As in earlier studies, the authors performed corticotropin tests on these patients to document and stratify patients by relative adrenal insufficiency. In this study, 7-day treatment with low doses of hydrocortisone and fludrocortisone significantly and safely lowered the risk of death in patients with septic shock and relative adrenal insufficiency.

Neurogenic Shock

Neurogenic shock refers to diminished tissue perfusion as a result of loss of vasomotor tone to peripheral arterial beds. Loss of vasoconstrictor impulses results in increased vascular capacitance, decreased venous return, and decreased cardiac output. Neurogenic shock is usually secondary to spinal cord injuries from vertebral body fractures of the cervical or high thoracic region that disrupt sympathetic regulation of peripheral vascular tone. Rarely, a spinal cord injury without bony fracture, such as an epidural hematoma impinging on the spinal cord, can produce neurogenic shock. Sympathetic input to the heart, which normally increases heart rate and cardiac contractility, and input to the adrenal medulla, which increases catecholamine release, may also be disrupted, preventing the typical reflex tachycardia that occurs with hypovolemia. Acute spinal cord injury results in activation of multiple secondary injury mechanisms: (1) vascular compromise to the spinal cord with loss of autoregulation, vasospasm, and thrombosis, (2) loss of cellular membrane integrity and impaired energy metabolism, and (3) neurotransmitter accumulation and release of free radicals. Importantly, hypotension contributes to the worsening of acute spinal cord injury as the result of further reduction in blood flow to the spinal cord. Management of acute spinal cord injury with attention to blood pressure control,

oxygenation, and hemodynamics, essentially optimizing perfusion of an already ischemic spinal cord, seems to result in improved neurologic outcome. Patients with hypotension from spinal cord injury are best monitored in an intensive care unit, and carefully followed for evidence of cardiac or respiratory dysfunction.

Diagnosis

Acute spinal cord injury may result in bradycardia, hypotension, cardiac dysrhythmias, reduced cardiac output, and decreased peripheral vascular resistance. The severity of the spinal cord injury seems to correlate with the magnitude of cardiovascular dysfunction. Patients with complete motor injuries are over five times more likely to require vasopressors for neurogenic shock, as compared to those with incomplete lesions.[96] The classic description of neurogenic shock consists of decreased blood pressure associated with bradycardia (absence of reflexive tachycardia due to disrupted sympathetic discharge), warm extremities (loss of peripheral vasoconstriction), motor and sensory deficits indicative of a spinal cord injury, and radiographic evidence of a vertebral column fracture. Patients with multisystem trauma that includes spinal cord injuries often have head injuries that may make identification of motor and sensory deficits difficult in the initial evaluation. Furthermore, associated injuries may occur that result in hypovolemia, further complicating the clinical presentation. In a subset of patients with spinal cord injuries from penetrating wounds, most of the patients with hypotension had blood loss as the etiology (74%) rather than neurogenic causes, and few (7%) had the classic findings of neurogenic shock.[97] In the multiply-injured patient, other causes of hypotension including hemorrhage, tension pneumothorax, and cardiogenic shock must be sought and excluded.

Treatment

After the airway is secured and ventilation is adequate, fluid resuscitation and restoration of intravascular volume will often improve perfusion in neurogenic shock. Most patients with neurogenic shock will respond to restoration of intravascular volume alone, with satisfactory improvement in perfusion and resolution of hypotension. Administration of vasoconstrictors will improve peripheral vascular tone, decrease vascular capacitance, and increase venous return, but should only be considered once hypovolemia is excluded as the cause of the hypotension, and the diagnosis of neurogenic shock established. If the patient's blood pressure has not responded to what is felt to be adequate volume resuscitation, dopamine may be utilized first. A pure α-agonist, such as phenylephrine may be used primarily or in patients unresponsive to dopamine. Specific treatment for the hypotension is often of brief duration, as the need to administer vasoconstrictors typically lasts 24 to 48 hours. On the other hand, life-threatening cardiac dysrhythmias and hypotension may occur up to 14 days after spinal cord injury.

The duration of the need for vasopressor support for neurogenic shock may correlate with the overall prognosis or chances of improvement in neurologic function. As mentioned, appropriate rapid restoration of blood pressure and circulatory perfusion may improve perfusion to the spinal cord, prevent progressive spinal cord ischemia, and minimize secondary cord injury. Restoration of normal blood pressure and adequate tissue perfusion should precede any operative attempts to stabilize the vertebral fracture.

Obstructive Shock

Commonly, mechanical obstruction of venous return in trauma patients is due to the presence of tension pneumothorax. Cardiac tamponade occurs when sufficient fluid has accumulated in the pericardial sac to obstruct blood flow to the ventricles. The hemodynamic abnormalities in pericardial tamponade are due to elevation of intracardiac pressures with limitation of ventricular filling in diastole with resultant decrease in cardiac output. Acutely, the pericardium does not distend; thus small volumes of blood may produce cardiac tamponade. If the effusion accumulates slowly (e.g., in the setting of uremia, heart failure, or malignant effusion), the quantity of fluid producing cardiac tamponade may reach 2000 mL. The major determinant of the degree of hypotension is the pericardial pressure. With either cardiac tamponade or tension pneumothorax, reduced filling of the right side of the heart from either increased intrapleural pressure secondary to air accumulation (tension pneumothorax), or increased intrapericardial pressure precluding atrial filling secondary to blood accumulation (cardiac tamponade) results in decreased cardiac output associated with increased central venous pressure.

Diagnosis and Treatment

The diagnosis of tension pneumothorax should be made on clinical examination. The classic findings include respiratory distress (in an awake patient), hypotension, diminished breath sounds over one hemithorax, hyperresonance to percussion, jugular venous distention, and shift of mediastinal structures to the unaffected side with tracheal deviation. In most instances, empiric treatment with pleural decompression is indicated rather than delaying to wait for radiographic confirmation. When a chest tube cannot be immediately inserted, such as in the prehospital setting, the pleural space can be decompressed with a large caliber needle. Immediate return of air should be encountered with rapid resolution of hypotension. Unfortunately, not all of the clinical manifestations of tension pneumothorax may be evident on physical exam. Hyperresonance may be difficult to appreciate in a noisy resuscitation area. Jugular venous distention may be absent in a hypovolemic patient. Tracheal deviation is a late finding and often not apparent on clinical examination. Practically, three findings are sufficient to make the diagnosis of tension pneumothorax: respiratory distress or hypotension, decreased lung sounds, and hypertympany to percussion. Chest x-ray findings that may be visualized include deviation of mediastinal structures, depression of the hemidiaphragm, and hypo-opacification with absent lung markings. As discussed above, definitive treatment of a tension pneumothorax is immediate tube thoracostomy. The chest tube should be inserted rapidly, but carefully, and should be large enough to evacuate any blood that may be present in the pleural space. Our preference is via the fourth intercostal space (nipple level) at the anterior axillary line.

Cardiac tamponade results from the accumulation of blood within the pericardial sac, usually from penetrating trauma or chronic medical conditions such as heart failure or uremia. While precordial wounds are most likely to injure the heart and produce tamponade, any projectile or wounding agent that passes in proximity to the mediastinum can potentially produce tamponade. Blunt cardiac rupture, a rare event in trauma victims who survive long enough to reach the hospital, can produce refractory shock and tamponade in the multiply-injured patient. The manifestations of cardiac tamponade may be catastrophic such as total circulatory collapse and cardiac arrest, or they may be more subtle. A high index of suspicion is warranted to make a rapid diagnosis. Patients who present with circulatory arrest from cardiac tamponade require emergency pericardial decompression, usually through a left thoracotomy. The indications for this maneuver are discussed in Chap. 6. Cardiac tamponade may also be associated with dyspnea, orthopnea, cough, peripheral edema, chest pain, tachycardia, muffled heart tones, jugular venous distention, and elevated central venous pressure. Beck's triad consists of hypotension, muffled heart tones, and neck vein distention. Unfortunately, absence of these clinical findings may not be sufficient to exclude cardiac injury and cardiac tamponade. Muffled heart tones may be difficult to appreciate in a busy trauma center and jugular venous distention and central venous pressure may be diminished by coexistent bleeding. Therefore, patients at risk for cardiac tamponade whose hemodynamic status permits additional diagnostic tests frequently require additional diagnostic maneuvers to confirm cardiac injury or tamponade.

Invasive hemodynamic monitoring may support the diagnosis of cardiac tamponade if elevated central venous pressure, pulsus paradoxus (i.e., decreased systemic arterial pressure with inspiration), or elevated right atrial and right ventricular pressure by pulmonary artery catheter are present. These hemodynamic profiles suffer from lack of specificity, the duration of time required to obtain them in critically-injured patients, and their inability to exclude cardiac injury in the absence of tamponade. Chest radiographs may provide information on the possible trajectory of a projectile, but rarely are diagnostic since the acutely filled pericardium distends poorly. Echocardiography has become the preferred test for the diagnosis of cardiac tamponade. Good results in detecting pericardial fluid have been reported, but the yield in detecting pericardial fluid depends on the skill and experience of the ultrasonographer, body habitus of the patient, and absence of wounds that preclude visualization of the pericardium. Standard two-dimensional or transesophageal echocardiography are sensitive techniques to evaluate the pericardium for fluid, and are typically performed by examiners skilled at evaluating ventricular function, valvular abnormalities, and integrity of the proximal thoracic aorta. Unfortunately, these skilled examiners are rarely immediately available at all hours of the night, when many trauma patients present; therefore waiting for this test may result in inordinate delays. In addition, while both ultrasound techniques may demonstrate the presence of fluid or characteristic findings of tamponade (large volume of fluid, right atrial collapse, poor distensibility of the right ventricle), they do not exclude cardiac injury per se. Pericardiocentesis to diagnose pericardial blood and potentially relieve tamponade may be utilized. Performing pericardiocentesis under ultrasound guidance has made the procedure safer and more reliable. An indwelling catheter may be placed for several days in patients with chronic pericardial effusions. Needle pericardiocentesis may not evacuate clotted blood and has the potential to produce cardiac injury, making it a poor alternative in busy trauma centers.

Diagnostic pericardial window represents the most direct method to determine the presence of blood within the pericardium. The procedure is best performed in the operating room under general anesthesia. It can be performed through either the subxiphoid or transdiaphragmatic approach. Adequate equipment and personnel to rapidly decompress the pericardium, explore the injury, and repair the heart should be present. Once the pericardium is opened and tamponade relieved, hemodynamics usually improve dramatically and formal pericardial exploration can ensue. Exposure of the heart can be achieved by extending the incision to a median sternotomy, performing a left anterior thoracotomy, or performing bilateral anterior thoracotomies ("clamshell").

Traumatic Shock

The systemic response after trauma, combining the effects of soft tissue injury, long bone fractures, and blood loss, is clearly a different physiologic insult than simple hemorrhagic shock. Multiple organ failure, including acute respiratory distress syndrome (ARDS), develops relatively often in the blunt trauma patient, but rarely after pure hemorrhagic shock (such as a gastrointestinal bleed). The hypoperfusion deficit in traumatic shock is magnified by the proinflammatory activation that occurs following the induction of shock. In addition to ischemia or ischemia-reperfusion, accumulating evidence demonstrates that even simple hemorrhage induces proinflammatory activation that results in many of the cellular changes typically ascribed only to septic shock.[98,99] Examples of traumatic shock include small volume hemorrhage accompanied by soft tissue injury (femur fracture, crush injury), or any combination of hypovolemic, neurogenic, cardiogenic, and obstructive shock that precipitate rapidly progressive proinflammatory activation. In laboratory models of traumatic shock, the addition of a soft tissue or long bone injury to hemorrhage produces lethality with significantly less blood loss when the animals are stressed by hemorrhage. Treatment of traumatic shock is focused on correction of the individual elements in order to diminish the cascade of proinflammatory activation, and includes prompt control of hemorrhage, adequate volume resuscitation to correct oxygen debt, débridement of nonviable tissue, stabilization of bony injuries, and appropriate treatment of soft tissue injuries.

ENDPOINTS IN RESUSCITATION

Shock is defined as inadequate perfusion to maintain normal organ function. With prolonged anaerobic metabolism, tissue acidosis and oxygen debt accumulate. Thus the goal in the treatment of shock is restoration of adequate organ perfusion and tissue oxygenation. Resuscitation is complete when oxygen debt is repaid, tissue acidosis is corrected, and aerobic metabolism restored. Clinical confirmation of this endpoint remains a challenge.

Resuscitation of the patient in shock requires simultaneous evaluation and treatment; the etiology of the shock often is not initially apparent. Hemorrhagic shock, septic shock, and traumatic shock are the most common types of shock encountered on surgical services. To optimize outcome in bleeding patients, early control of the hemorrhage and adequate volume resuscitation, including both red blood cells and crystalloid solutions, are necessary. Expedient operative resuscitation is mandatory to limit the magnitude of activation of multiple mediator systems and to abort the microcirculatory changes, which may evolve insidiously into the cascade that ends in irreversible hemorrhagic shock. Attempts to stabilize an actively bleeding patient anywhere but in the operating room are inappropriate. Any intervention that delays the patient's arrival in the operating room for control of hemorrhage increases mortality thus the important concept of *operating room resuscitation* of the critically-injured patient.

Recognition by care providers of the patient who is in the compensated phase of shock is equally important, but more difficult based on clinical criteria. Compensated shock exists when inadequate tissue perfusion persists, despite normalization of blood pressure and heart rate. Even with normalization of blood pressure, heart rate, and urine output, 80 to 85% of trauma patients have inadequate tissue perfusion as evidenced by increased lactate or decreased mixed venous oxygen saturation.[100,101] Persistent, occult hypoperfusion is frequent in the intensive care unit, with resultant significant increase in infection rate and mortality in major trauma patients. Patients failing to reverse their lactic acidosis within 12 hours of admission (acidosis that was persistent despite normal

Table 4-4
Endpoints in Resuscitation

Systemic/global
    Lactate
    Base deficit
    Cardiac output
    Oxygen delivery and consumption
Tissue-specific
    Gastric tonometry
    Tissue pH, oxygen, carbon dioxide levels
    Near infrared spectroscopy
Cellular
    Membrane potential
    Adenosine triphosphate (ATP)

heart rate, blood pressure, and urine output), developed an infection three times as often as those who normalized their lactate levels within 12 hours of admission. In addition, mortality was fourfold higher in patients who developed infections. Both injury severity score and occult hypotension (lactic acidosis) longer than 12 hours were independent predictors of infection.[102,103] Thus recognition of subclinical hypoperfusion requires information beyond vital signs and urinary output.

Endpoints in resuscitation can be divided into *systemic* or *global parameters, tissue-specific parameters,* and *cellular parameters.* Global endpoints include vital signs, cardiac output, pulmonary artery wedge pressure, oxygen delivery and consumption, lactate, and base deficit (Table 4-4).

Assessment of Endpoints in Resuscitation

Oxygen Transport

Attaining supranormal oxygen transport variables has been proposed as a means to correct oxygen debt. Shoemaker and associates published the first randomized study examining supranormal oxygen consumption and delivery as endpoints in resuscitation.[104] The supranormal oxygen transport variables include oxygen delivery greater than 600 mL/min per square meter, cardiac index greater than 4.5 L/min per square meter, and oxygen consumption index greater than 170 mL/min per square meter. These authors reported a significant reduction in mortality in the patients achieving supranormal endpoints. More recent publications suggest that patients unable to increase oxygen delivery have a higher mortality, as opposed to it being a true benefit of the therapy.[105–107] This observation strongly correlates with age of the patient, with older patients less able to generate supranormal oxygen delivery. Gattinoni and colleagues reported effects of hemodynamic therapy in critically-ill patients on 10,726 patients in 56 intensive care units. Seven hundred sixty-two patients met the predefined diagnostic categories and were assigned to one of three groups: control group, supranormal cardiac index group, and oxygen saturation group (with a goal of achieving normal venous oxygen saturation). The authors found that hemodynamic therapy aimed at reaching supranormal values for cardiac index or normal values for mixed venous oxygen saturation did not reduce morbidity or mortality among critically-ill patients.[108] In this paper's accompanying editorial, it was noted that failure to achieve both values is a relatively common problem, particularly among older or more severely-ill patients. These results emphasize the importance of adequate volume replacement, maintenance of normal blood pressure, and the use of minor doses of inotropic drugs to maintain a normal cardiac output. In a recent paper from Shoemaker's group, supranormal values were achieved intentionally in 70% of the treatment group and spontaneously by 40% of the control group.[107] Mortality, incidence of organ failure and sepsis, and length of stay were no different between the treatment and control groups. Patients in each group who attained supranormal values had better outcomes than those who could not, and mortality was 30% in patients unable to reach supranormal values and 0% in patients with supranormal indices. Age younger than 40 years was the sole independent variable that predicted ability to reach these supraphysiologic endpoints. Thus, the evidence is insufficient to support the routine use of a strategy to maximize oxygen delivery in a group of unselected patients.

Inability to repay oxygen debt is a predictor of mortality and organ failure; the probability of death has been directly correlated to the calculated oxygen debt in hemorrhagic shock. Direct measurement of the oxygen debt in the resuscitation of patients is difficult. The easily obtainable parameters of arterial blood pressure, heart rate, urine output, central venous pressure, and pulmonary artery occlusion pressure are poor indicators of the adequacy of tissue perfusion. Therefore, surrogate parameters have been sought to estimate the oxygen debt; serum lactate and base deficit have been shown to correlate with oxygen debt.

Lactate

Lactate is generated by conversion of pyruvate to lactate by lactate dehydrogenase in the setting of insufficient oxygen. Lactate is released into the circulation and is predominantly taken up and metabolized by the liver and kidneys. The liver accounts for approximately 50% and the kidney for about 30% of whole body lactate uptake. Elevated serum lactate is an indirect measure of the oxygen debt, and therefore an approximation of the magnitude and duration of the severity of shock. The admission lactate level, highest lactate level, and time interval to normalize the serum lactate are important prognostic indicators for survival. For example, in a study of 76 consecutive patients, 100% survival was observed among the patients with normalization of lactate within 24 hours, 78% survival when lactate normalized between 24 and 48 hours, and only 14%

survivorship if it took longer than 48 hours to normalize the serum lactate.[101] In contrast, individual variability of lactate may be too great to permit accurate prediction of outcome in any individual case. Base deficit and volume of blood transfusion required in the first 24 hours of resuscitation may be better predictors of mortality than the plasma lactate alone.

Base Deficit

Base deficit is the amount of base in millimoles that is required to titrate 1 L of whole blood to a pH of 7.40 with the sample fully saturated with O_2 at 37°C and a $Paco_2$ of 40 mm Hg. It is usually measured by arterial blood gas analysis in clinical practice as it is readily and quickly available. The mortality of trauma patients can be stratified according to the magnitude of base deficit measured in the first 24 hours after admission.[109] In a retrospective study of over 3000 trauma admissions, patients with a base deficit worse than 15 mmol/L had a mortality of 70%. Base deficit can be stratified into mild (3 to 5), moderate (6 to 14) and severe (≥15) categories, with a trend toward higher mortality with worsening base deficit in patients with trauma. Both the magnitude of the perfusion deficit as indicated by the base deficit and the time required to correct it are major factors determining outcome in shock. (Fig. 4-11).

Indeed, when elevated base deficit persists (or lactic acidosis) in the trauma patient, ongoing bleeding is often the etiology. Trauma patients admitted with a base deficit greater than 15 mmol/L required twice the volume of fluid infusion and 6 times more blood transfusion in the first 24 hours, as compared to patients with mild acidosis. Transfusion requirements increased as base deficit worsened and ICU and hospital lengths of stay increased. Mortality increased as base deficit worsened; the frequency of organ failure increased with greater base deficit.[110] The probability of trauma patients developing ARDS has been reported to correlate with severity of admission base deficit and lowest base deficit within the first 24 hours postinjury.[111] Persistently high base deficit is associated with abnormal oxygen utilization and higher mortality. Monitoring base

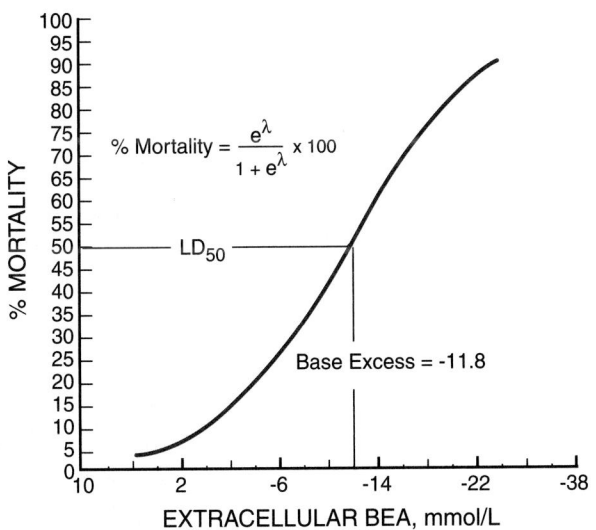

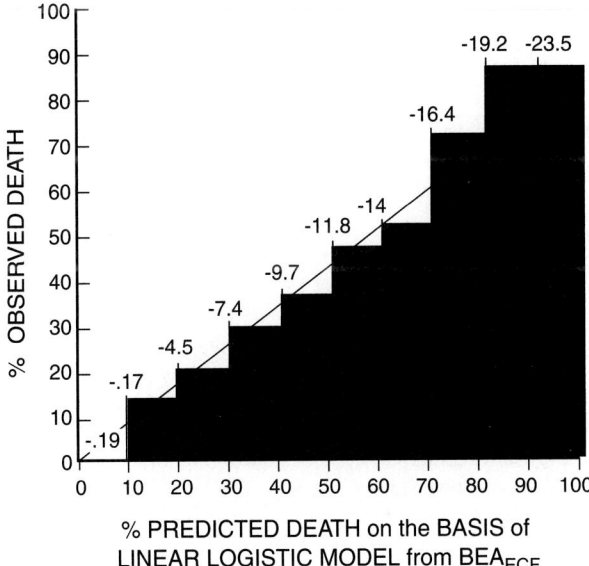

FIG. 4-11. The relationship between base deficit (negative base excess) and mortality in trauma patients. (Reproduced with permission from Siegel JH, Rivkind AI, Dalal S, et al: Early physiologic predictors of injury severity and death in blunt multiple trauma. Arch Surg 125:498, 1990.)

deficit in the resuscitation of trauma patients assists in assessment of oxygen transport and efficacy of resuscitation.[112]

Factors that may compromise the utility of the base deficit in estimating oxygen debt are the administration of bicarbonate, hypothermia, hypocapnia (overventilation), heparin, ethanol, and ketoacidosis. However, the base deficit remains one of the most widely used estimates of oxygen debt for its clinical relevance, accuracy, and availability.

Gastric Tonometry

Lactate and base deficit indicate global tissue acidosis. Several authors have suggested that tissue-specific endpoints, rather than systemic endpoints, are more predictive of outcome and adequate resuscitation in trauma patients. With heterogeneity of blood flow, regional tissue beds may be hypoperfused. Gastric tonometry has been used to assess perfusion of the gastrointestinal tract. The concentration of carbon dioxide accumulating in the gastric mucosa can be sampled with a specially designed nasogastric tube. With the assumption that gastric bicarbonate is equal to serum levels, gastric mucosal pH (pHi) is calculated by applying the Henderson-Hasselbalch equation. pHi should be greater than 7.3; pHi will be lower in the setting of decreased oxygen delivery to the tissues. pHi is a good prognostic indicator; patients with normal pHi have better outcomes than those patients with pHi less than 7.3.[113–115] Goal-directed human studies, with pHi as an endpoint in resuscitation, have shown normalization of pHi to correlate with improved outcome in several studies, and with contradictory findings in other studies. Utility of pHi as a singular endpoint in the resuscitation of critically-ill patients remains controversial.[113–117]

Near Infrared Spectroscopy

Near infrared (NIR) spectroscopy can measure tissue oxygenation and redox state of cytochrome a,a₃ on a continuous, noninvasive basis. The NIR probe emits multiple wavelengths of light in the near infrared spectrum (650 to 1100 nm). Photons are then either absorbed by the tissue or reflected back to the probe. Maximal exercise in laboratory studies resulted in reduction of cytochrome a,a₃; this correlated with tissue lactate elevation. NIR spectroscopy can be used to compare tissue oxyhemoglobin levels (indicating tissue oxygen supply to cytochrome a,a₃ with mitochondrial oxygen consumption), thus demonstrating flow-independent mitochondrial oxidative dysfunction and the need for further resuscitation. Trauma patients with decoupled oxyhemoglobin and cytochrome a,a₃ have redox dysfunction and have been shown to have a higher incidence of organ failure (89 vs. 13%).[7,118]

Tissue pH, Oxygen, and Carbon Dioxide Concentration

Tissue probes with optical sensors have been used to measure tissue pH and partial pressure of oxygen and carbon dioxide in subcutaneous sites, muscle, and the bladder. These probes may utilize transcutaneous methodology with Clark electrodes or direct percutaneous probes.[119,120] The percutaneous probes can be inserted through an 18-gauge catheter and hold promise as continuous monitors of tissue perfusion.

Right Ventricular End-Diastolic Volume Index

Right ventricular end-diastolic volume index (RVEDVI) seems to more accurately predict preload for cardiac index than does pulmonary artery wedge pressure.[121] Chang and colleagues reported that 50% of trauma patients had persistent splanchnic ischemia that was reversed by increasing RVEDVI.[121] RVEDVI is a parameter which seems to correlate with preload-related increases in cardiac output. More recently, these authors have described left ventricular power output as an endpoint (LVP >320 mm Hg·L/min per square meter), which is associated with improved clearance of base deficit and a lower rate of organ dysfunction following injury.[122]

Controversies about Fluids Used for Resuscitation

As mentioned earlier, the debate comparing crystalloid to colloid solutions has continued for decades. Several recent review papers and meta-analyses have confirmed that either fluid can be used to adequately volume resuscitate the trauma patient.[123,124] No difference in overall mortality, length of stay, or incidence of pulmonary edema was noted in comparison of crystalloid to colloids in fluid resuscitation of critically-ill patients. Subgroup analysis suggested a significant survival advantage in trauma patients in favor of crystalloid resuscitation. A systematic review of 30 randomized trials of human albumin administration in 1419 critically-ill patients similarly noted an increased risk of mortality with the use of albumin infusion in treatment of hypovolemia, burns, and hypoalbuminemia.[124] In addition, albumin is several times more expensive than crystalloid solutions. The expense of the infusion of albumin-containing solution cannot be justified.

Several papers have suggested improved outcome with the use of hypertonic saline in the treatment of hemorrhagic shock. The clinical trials have shown marginal benefit with the infusion of hypertonic saline (7.5% sodium chloride).[125] The benefit of hypertonic saline solutions may be immunomodulatory, in addition to shifting of fluids from intracellular compartments.

Use of Blood in Transfusion

Volume resuscitation in the trauma patient requires restoration of intravascular volume and repletion of sufficient oxygen-carrying capacity with red blood cell transfusion. Delay of transfusion of red blood cells in the actively-bleeding trauma patient would be expected to increase mortality.[126] In contrast, blood transfusion carries inherent risks including transfusion reaction, infection, and immunosuppression. Several recent papers have helped clarify what levels of hemoglobin and hematocrit are appropriate in the treatment of critically-ill patients.[127,128] A prospective, randomized trial in 838 ICU patients demonstrated that Hgb levels as low as 7.0 to 9.0 g/dL did not increase mortality in critically-ill patients, compared to a group transfused to Hgb levels of 10.0 to 12.0 g/dL.[127] A subgroup analysis from this study of patients specifically evaluating patients with cardiac disease, suggested that patients with unstable angina or acute myocardial infarction require a higher hemoglobin and hematocrit.[128] Thus, in stable ICU patients, Hgb of 7.0 to 9.0 g/dL is tolerated without apparent increase in mortality. Patients with active cardiac disease require hematocrits greater than 30%. Based on the data by Wu and associates, patients with acute myocardial infarction have lower mortality with hematocrit levels over 33%.[129]

Hypotensive Resuscitation

Cannon and colleagues first made the observation that attempts to increase blood pressure in soldiers with uncontrolled sources of hemorrhage is counterproductive, with increased bleeding and higher mortality.[5] Several laboratory studies confirmed the observation that attempts to restore normal blood pressure with fluid infusion or vasopressors was rarely achievable and resulted in more bleeding and higher mortality.[14] A prospective, randomized clinical study compared delayed fluid resuscitation (upon arrival in the operating room) with standard fluid resuscitation (with arrival by the paramedics) in hypotensive patients with penetrating torso injury. The authors reported that delayed fluid resuscitation resulted in lower patient mortality.[13] Further laboratory studies demonstrated that fluid restriction in the setting of profound hypotension resulted in early deaths from severe hypoperfusion. These studies also showed that aggressive crystalloid resuscitation attempting to normalize blood pressure resulted in marked hemodilution, with hematocrits of 5%.[14] Reasonable conclusions in the setting of uncontrolled hemorrhage include: any delay in surgery for control of hemorrhage increases mortality; with uncontrolled hemorrhage attempting to achieve normal blood pressure may increase mortality, particularly with penetrating injuries and short transport times; a goal of systolic blood pressure of 80 to 90 mm Hg may be adequate in the patient with penetrating injury; and profound hemodilution should be avoided by early transfusion of red blood cells. For the patient with blunt injury, where the major cause of death is a closed head injury, the increase in mortality with hypotension in the setting of brain injury must be avoided. In this setting, a systolic blood pressure of 110 mm Hg would seem to be more appropriate.

References

1. Gross SA: *A System of Surgery: Pathologic, Diagnostic, Therapeutic and Operative.* Philadelphia: Lea and Febiger, 1872.
2. Chambers NK, Buchman TG: Shock at the Millennium. Walter B. Cannon and Alfred Blalock. *Shock* 13:497, 2000.
3. Bernard C: Lecons sur les phenomenes de la vie communs aux animaux et aux vegetaux. Paris: JB Ballieve, 1879, p. 4.
4. Cannon WB: *Traumatic Shock.* New York: D. Appleton and Co., 1923, p. 1.
5. Cannon WB, Fraser J, Cowell EM: The preventive treatment of wound shock. *JAMA* 70:618, 1918.
6. Blalock A: Principles of surgical care, shock and other problems. St. Louis: CV Mosby, 1940, p. 1.
7. Cairns BC, Moore FA, Haenel JB, et al: Evidence for early supply independent mitochondrial dysfunction in patients developing multiple organ failure after trauma. *J Trauma* 42:532, 1997.
8. Wiggers CJ: Experimental hemorrhagic shock, in *Physiology of Shock.* New York: Commonwealth, 1950, p. 121.
9. Carrico CJ, Canizaro PC, Shires GT: Fluid resuscitation following injury: Rationale for the use of balanced salt solutions. *Crit Care Med* 4:46, 1976.
10. Peitzman AB, Corbett WA, Shires GT III, et al: Cellular function in liver and muscle during hemorrhagic shock in primates. *Surg Gynecol Obstet* 161:419, 1985.
11. Shires GT, Coln D, Carrico CJ, et al: Fluid therapy in hemorrhagic shock. *Arch Surg* 88:688, 1964.
12. Shaftan GW, Chiu CJ, Dennis C, et al: Fundamentals of physiologic control of arterial hemorrhage. *Surgery* 58:851, 1965.
13. Bickell WH, Wall MJ, Pepe PE, et al: Immediate versus delayed resuscitation for hypotensive patients with penetrating torso injuries. *N Engl J Med* 331:1105, 1994.
14. Marshall HP, Capone A, Courcoulas AP, et al : Effects of hemodilution on long-term survival in an uncontrolled hemorrhagic shock model in rats. *J Trauma* 43:673, 1997.
15. Peitzman AB, Billiar TR, Harbrecht BG, et al: Hemorrhagic shock. *Curr Prob Surg* 32:925, 1995.
16. Robin JK, Oliver JA, Landry DW: Vasopressin deficiency in the syndrome of irreversible shock. *J Trauma* 54:S149, 2003.
17. Landry DW, Oliver JA: Mechanisms of disease: The pathogenesis of vasodilatory shock. *N Engl J Med* 345:588, 2001.
18. Dunser MW, Wenzel V, Mayr AJ, et al: Management of vasodilatory shock. Defining the role of arginine vasopressin. *Drugs* 63:237, 2003.
19. Argenziano M, Chen JM, Choudhri AF, et al: Management of vasodilatory shock after cardiac surgery: Identification of predisposing factors and use of a novel pressor agent. *J Thorac Cardiovasc Surg* 116:973, 1998.
20. Flint LM, Cryer HM, Simpson CJ, et al: Microcirculatory norepinephrine constrictor response in hemorrhagic shock. *Surgery* 96:240, 1984.
21. Barroso-Aranda J, Schmid-Schonbein GW, Zweifach BW, et al: Granulocytes and no-reflow phenomenon in irreversible hemorrhagic shock. *Circ Res* 63:437, 1988.
22. Nelson DP, Samsel RW, Wood LDH, et al: Pathologic supply dependency of systemic and intestinal oxygen uptake during endotoxemia. *J Appl Physiol* 64:2410, 1988.
23. Ince C, Sinaasappel M: Microcirculatory oxygenation and shunting in sepsis and shock. *Crit Care Med* 27:1369, 1999.
24. Robin ED: Of men and mitochondria: Coping with hypoxic dysoxia. *Am Rev Resp Dis* 122:517, 1980.
25. Stacpoole PW: Lactic acidosis and other mitochondrial disorders. *Metabolism* 46:306, 1997.
26. Xu YX, Ayala A, Monfils B, et al: Mechanism of intestinal mucosal immune dysfunction following trauma-hemorrhage: Increased apoptosis associated with elevated Fas expression in Peyer's patches. *J Surg Res* 70:55, 1997.
27. Kelly E, Shah NS, Morgan NN, et al: Physiologic and molecular characterization of the role of nitric oxide in hemorrhagic shock: Evidence that type II nitric oxide synthase does not regulate vascular decompensation. *Shock* 7:157, 1997.
28. Sauaia A, Moore FA, Moore EE, et al: Early predictors of post-injury multiple organ failure. *Arch Surg* 129:39, 1994.
29. Jiang J, Bahrami S, Leichtfried G, et al: Kinetics of endotoxin and tumor necrosis factor appearance in portal and systemic circulation after hemorrhagic shock in rats. *Ann Surg* 221:100, 1995.
30. Endo S, Inada K, Yamada Y, et al: Plasma endotoxin and cytokine concentrations in patients with hemorrhagic shock. *Crit Care Med* 22:949, 1994.
31. Kell MR, Kavanagh EG, Goebel A, et al: Injury primes the immune system for an enhanced and lethal T-cell response against bacterial superantigen. *Shock* 12:139, 1999.
32. Abraham E, Regan RF: The effects of hemorrhage and trauma on interleukin 2 production. *Arch Surg* 120:1341, 1985.
33. Faist E, Schinkel C, Zimmer S, et al: Inadequate interleukin-2 synthesis and interleukin-2 messenger expression following thermal and mechanical trauma in humans is caused by defective transmembrane signaling. *J Trauma* 34:846, 1993.
34. Wichmann MW, Zellweger R, DeMaso CM, et al: Melatonin administration attenuates depressed immune functions after trauma-hemorrhage. *J Surg Res* 63:256, 1996.
35. Puyana JC, Pellegrini JD, De AK, et al: Both T-helper-1 and T-helper-2-type lymphokines are depressed in posttrauma anergy. *J Trauma* 44:1037, 1998.
36. Fink MP: Intestinal epithelial hyperpermeability: Update on the pathogenesis of gut mucosal barrier dysfunction in critical illness. *Curr Opin Crit Care* 9:143, 2003.
37. Yang R, Han X, Uchiyama T, et al: IL-6 is essential for the development of gut barrier dysfunction after hemorrhagic shock and resuscitation in mice. *Am J Physiol* 285:G621, 2003.
38. Meng ZH, Dyer K, Billiar TR, et al: Essential role for IL-6 in postresuscitation inflammation in hemorrhagic shock. *Am J Physiol* 280:C343, 2001.
39. Meng ZH, Dyer K, Billiar TR, et al: Distinct effects of systemic infusion of G-CSF vs IL-6 on lung and liver inflammation and injury in hemorrhagic shock. *Shock* 14:41, 2000.
40. Neidhardt R, Kell M, Steckholzer U, et al: Relationship of interleukin-10 plasma levels to severity of injury and clinical outcome in injured patients. *J Trauma* 42:863, 1997.
41. Lyons A, Kelly JL, Rodrick ML, et al: Major injury induces increased production of interleukin-10 by cells of the immune system with a negative impact on resistance to infection. *Ann Surg* 226:450, 1997.

42. Kasai T, Inada K, Takakuwa T, et al: Anti-inflammatory cytokine levels in patients with septic shock. *Res Commun Mol Path Pharm* 98:34, 1997.

43. Karakozis S, Hinds M, Cook JW, et al: The effects of interleukin-10 in hemorrhagic shock. *J Surg Res* 90:109, 2000.

44. Kahlke V, Dohn C, Meis T, et al: Early interleukin-10 treatment improves survival and enhances immune function only in males after hemorrhage and subsequent sepsis. *Shock* 18:24, 2002.

45. Younger JG, Sasaki N, Waite MD, et al: Detrimental effects of complement activation in hemorrhagic shock. *J Appl Physiol* 90:441, 2001.

46. Moore EE, Moore FA, Franciose RJ, et al: The postischemic gut serves as a priming bed for circulating neutrophils that provoke multiple organ failure. *J Trauma* 37:881, 1994.

47. Adams JM, Hauser CJ, Livingston DH, et al: Early trauma polymorphonuclear neutrophil responses to chemokines are associated with development of sepsis, pneumonia and organ failure. *J Trauma* 51:452, 2001.

48. Lau YT, Hwang TL, Chen MF, et al: Calcium transport by rat liver plasma membranes during sepsis. *Circ Shock* 38:238, 1992.

49. Gasbarrini A, Borle AB, Farghali H, et al: Effect of anoxia on intracellular ATP, Na$^+$, Ca^{2+}, Mg^{2+}, and cytotoxicity in rat hepatocytes. *J Biol Chem* 267:6654, 1992.

50. Herman B, Gores GJ, Nieminen AL, et al: Calcium and pH in anoxic and toxic injury. *Crit Rev Toxicol* 21:127, 1990.

51. Trump BF, Berezesky IK: Calcium-mediated cell injury and death. *FASEB J* 9:219, 1995.

52. Maki A, Berezesky IK, Fargnoli J, et al: Role of [Ca^{2+}] in induction of c-fos, c-jun, and c-myc mRNA in rat PTE after oxidative stress. *FASEB J* 6:919, 1992.

53. Mauger J-P, Poggioli J, Claret M: Synergistic stimulation of the Ca^{2+} influx in rat hepatocytes by glucagon and the Ca^{2+}- linked hormones vasopressin and angiotensin II. *J Biol Chem* 260:11635, 1985.

54. Somogyi R, Zhao M, Stucki JW: Modulation of cytosolic [Ca^{2+}] oscillations in hepatocytes results from cross-talk among second messengers. *Biochem J* 286:869, 1992.

55. Sen CK, Packer L: Anti-oxidant and redox regulation of gene transcription. *FASEB J* 10:709, 1996.

56. Suzuki YJ, Forman HJ, Sevanian A: Oxidants as stimulators of signal transduction. *Free Rad Mol Biol* 22:269, 1997.

57. Wang X, Martindale JL, Liu Y, et al: The cellular response to oxidative stress: Influences of mitogen-activated protein kinase signaling pathways on cell survival. *Biochem J* 333:291, 1998.

58. Khadaroo RG, Lu Z, Powers KA, et al: Impaired activation of mitogen-activated protein kinases after hemorrhagic shock. *Surgery* 132:360, 2002.

59. McCloskey CA, Zuckerbraun BS, Gallo DJ, et al: A role for angiotensin II in the activation of extracellular signal-related kinases in the liver during hemorrhagic shock. *Shock* 20:316, 2003.

60. Lander HM, Ogiste JS, Teng KK, et al: p21^{ras} as a common signaling target of reactive free radicals and cellular redox stress. *J Biol Chem* 270:21195, 1995.

61. Guillemin K, Krasnow M: The hypoxic response: Huffing and HIFing. *Cell* 89:9, 1997.

62. Bertges DJ, Fink MP, Delude RL: Hypoxic signal transduction in critical illness. *Crit Care Med* 28:N78, 2000.

63. Buchman TG, Cabin DE, Vickers S, et al: Molecular biology of circulatory shock. Part II. Expression of four groups of hepatic genes is enhanced after resuscitation from cardiogenic shock. *Surgery* 108:559, 1990.

64. Wiegand G, Selleng K, Grundling M, et al: Gene expression pattern in human monocytes as a surrogate marker for systemic inflammatory response syndrome (SIRS). *Mol Med* 5:192, 1999.

65. Zamora R, Vodovotz Y, Aulak KS: A DNA microassay study of nitric oxide–induced genes in mouse hepatocytes: Implications for hepatic heme oxygenase-1 expression in ischemia/reperfusion. *Nitric Oxide* 7:165, 2002.

66. Cobb JP, Laramie JM, Stormo GD, et al: Sepsis gene expression profiling: Murine splenic compared with hepatic responses determined by using complementary DNA microarrays. *Crit Care Med* 30:2711, 2002.

67. Burt RA: Genetics of host response to malaria. *Int J Parasitol* 29:973, 1999.

68. Lin MT, Storer B, Martin PJ, et al: Relation of interleukin-10 promoter polymorphism to graft-versus-host disease and survival after hematopoietic-cell transplantation. *N Engl J Med* 349:2201, 2003.

69. Gray IC, Campbell DA, Spun NK: Single nucleotide polymorphisms as tools in human genetics. *Hum Mol Genet* 9:2403, 2000.

70. Mira JP, Cariou A, Grall F, et al: Association of TNF2, a TNF-α promoter polymorphism, with septic shock susceptibility and mortality. *JAMA* 282:561, 1999.

71. O'Keefe GE, Hybki DL, Munford RS: The G-A single nucleotide polymorphism at the −308 position in the tumor necrosis factor-α promoter increases the risk for severe sepsis after trauma. *J Trauma* 52:817, 2002.

72. Holmes CL, Russell JA, Walley KR: Genetic polymorphisms in sepsis and septic shock: Role in prognosis and potential for therapy. *Chest* 124:1103, 2003.

73. Barber RC, O'Keefe GE: Characterization of a single nucleotide polymorphism in the lipopolysaccharide binding protein and its association with sepsis. *Am J Respir Crit Care Med* 167:1316, 2003.

74. Crowell JW: Oxygen debt and irreversible hemorrhagic shock. *Fed Proc* 20:116, 1961.

75. American College of Surgeons Committee on Trauma: Advanced Trauma Life Support Course. Chicago: American College of Surgeons, 1997, p. 1.

76. Luna GK, Eddy AC, Copass M: The sensitivity of vital signs in identifying major thoraco-abdominal hemorrhage. *Am J Surg* 157:512, 1989.

77. Victorino GP, Battistella FD, Wisner DH: Does tachycardia correlate with hypotension after trauma? *J Am Coll Surg* 196:679, 2003.

78. Hollenberg SM, Kavinsky CJ, Parillo JE: Cardiogenic shock. *Ann Intern Med* 131:47, 1999.

79. Webb JG, Sanborn TA, Sleeper LA, et al: Percutaneous coronary intervention for cardiogenic shock in the SHOCK trial registry. *Am Heart J* 141:964, 2001.

80. Menon V, Hochman JS: Management of cardiogenic shock complicating acute myocardial infarction. *Heart* 88:531, 2002.

81. Alonso DR, Scheidt S, Post M, et al: Pathophysiology of cardiogenic shock: Quantification of myocardial necrosis, clinical, pathologic, and electrocardiographic correlations. *Circulation* 48:588, 1973.

82. Goldstein DJ, Oz MC: Mechanical support for postcardiotomy cardiogenic shock. *Semin Thorac Cardiovasc Surg* 12:220, 2000.

83. Gibbons RJ, Smith SC Jr., Antman E: American College of Cardiology/American Heart Association Clinical Practice Guidelines: Part II: Evolutionary changes in a continuous quality improvement project. *Circulation* 107:3101, 2003.

84. Benedict CR, Rose RA: Arterial norepinephrine changes in patients with septic shock. *Circ Shock* 38:165, 1992.

85. Cumming AD, Driedger A, McDonald JWD, et al: Vasoactive hormones in the renal response to systemic sepsis. *Am J Kidney Dis* 11:23, 1988.

86. Angus DC, Birmingham MC, Balk RA, et al: E5 murine monoclonal antiendotoxin antibody in gram-negative sepsis: A randomized controlled trial. *JAMA* 283:1723, 2000.

87. Annane D, Sebille V, Troche G, et al: A 3-level prognostic classification in septic shock based on cortisol levels and cortisol response to corticotrophin. *JAMA* 283:1038, 2000.

88. Linde-Zwirble WT, Angus DC, Carcillo J, et al: Age-specific incidence and outcome of sepsis in the U.S. *Crit Care Med* 27:A33, 1999.

89. McCloskey CA, Billiar TR: Nitric oxide in shock: Sepsis and hemorrhage, in Salvemini D, Billiar TR, Vodovotz Y (eds): *Nitric Oxide and Inflammation*. Basel: Birkhauser Verlag, 2001, p. 225.

90. Bogolioubov A, Keefe DL, Groeger JS: Circulatory shock. *Crit Care Clinics* 17:697, 2001.

91. Rivers E, Nguyen B, Harstad S, et al: Early goal-directed therapy in the treatment of severe sepsis and septic shock. *N Engl J Med* 345:1368, 2001.

92. Van der Berghe G, Wouters P, Weekers F, et al: Intensive insulin therapy in critically-ill patients. *N Engl J Med* 345:1359, 2001.

93. Bernard GF, Vincent J-L, Laterre P-F, et al: Efficacy and safety of recombinant human activated protein C for severe sepsis. *N Engl J Med* 344:699, 2001.

94. Annane D, Bellissant E, Sebille V, et al: Impaired pressor sensitivity to noradrenaline in septic shock patients with and without impaired renal function reserve. *Br J Clin Pharmacol* 46:589, 1998.

95. Annane D, Sebille V, Charpentier C, et al: Effect of treatment with low doses of hydrocortisone and fludrocortisone on mortality in patients with septic shock. *JAMA* 288:862, 2002.

96. Levi L, Wolf A, Belzberg H: Hemodynamic parameters in patients with acute spinal cord trauma. *Neurosurgery* 33:1007, 1993.

97. Zipnick RI, Scalea TM, Trooskin SZ, et al: Hemodynamic responses to penetrating spinal cord injuries. *J Trauma* 35:578, 1993.

98. Leone M, Boutiere B, Camoin-Jau L, et al: Systemic endothelial activation is greater in septic than in traumatic-hemorrhagic shock but does not correlate with endothelial activation in skin biopsies. *J Trauma* 30:808, 2002.

99. Roumen RM, Redl H, Schlag G, et al: Inflammatory mediators in relation to the development of multiple organ failure in patients after severe blunt trauma. *Crit Care Med* 23:886, 1986.

100. Abou-Khalil B, Scalea TM, Trooskin SZ, et al: Hemodynamic responses to shock in young trauma patients: Need for invasive monitoring. *Crit Care Med* 22:633, 1994.

101. Abramson D, Scalea TM, Hitchcock R, et al: Lactate clearance and survival following injury. *J Trauma* 35:584, 1993.

102. Blow O, Magliere L, Claridge JA, et al: The golden hour and the silver day: Detection and correction of occult hypoperfusion within 24 hours improves outcome from major trauma. *J Trauma* 47:964, 1999.

103. Claridge JA, Crabtree TD, Pelletier SJ, et al: Persistent occult hypoperfusion is associated with a significant increase in infection rate and mortality in major trauma patients. *J Trauma* 48:8, 2000.

104. Shoemaker WC, Appel PL, Kram HB, et al: Prospective trial of supranormal values of survivors as therapeutic goals in high-risk surgical patients. *Chest* 94:1176, 1988.

105. McKinley BA, Kozar RA, Cocanour CS, et al: Normal versus supranormal oxygen delivery goals in shock resuscitation: The response is the same. *J Trauma* 53:825, 2003.

106. Heyland DK, Cook DJ, King D, et al: Maximizing oxygen delivery in critically-ill patients: A methodologic appraisal of the evidence. *Crit Care Med* 24:517, 1996.

107. Velmahos GC, Demetriades D, Shoemaker WC, et al: Endpoints of resuscitation of critically injured patients: Normal or supranormal? *Ann Surg* 232:409, 2000.

108. Gattinoni L, Brazzi L, Pelosi P, et al: A trial of goal-oriented hemodynamic therapy in critically-ill patients. *N Engl J Med* 333:1025, 1995.

109. Rutherford EJ, Morris JA Jr., Reed GW, et al: Base deficit stratifies mortality and determines therapy. *J Trauma* 33:417, 1992.

110. Davis JW, Parks SN, Kaups KL, et al: Admission base deficit predicts transfusion requirements and risk of complications. *J Trauma* 41:769, 1996.

111. Rixen D, Raum M, Bouillon B, et al: Base deficit development and its prognostic significance in post-trauma critical illness. *Shock* 15:83, 2001.

112. Kincaid EH, Miller PR, Meredith JW, et al: Elevated arterial base deficit in trauma patients: A marker of impaired oxygen utilization. *J Am Coll Surg* 187:384, 1998.

113. Ivatury RR, Simon RJ, Havriliak D, et al: Gastric mucosal pH and oxygen delivery and oxygen consumption indices in the assessment of adequacy of resuscitation after trauma: A prospective, randomized study. *J Trauma* 39:128, 1995.

114. Maynard N, Bihari D, Beale R, et al: Assessment of splanchnic oxygenation by gastric tonometry in patients with acute circulatory failure. *JAMA* 270:1203, 1993.

115. Chang MC, Cheatham ML, Nelson LD, et al: Gastric tonometry supplements information provided by systemic indicators of oxygen transport. *J Trauma* 37:488, 1994.

116. Gutierrez G, Bismar H, Dantzker DR, et al: Comparison of gastric intramucosal pH with measures of oxygen transport and consumption in critically-ill patients. *Crit Care Med* 20:451, 1992.

117. Gomersall CD, Joynt GM, Freebairn RC, et al: Resuscitation of critically-ill patients based on the results of gastric tonometry: A prospective, randomized, controlled trial. *Crit Care Med* 28:607, 2000.

118. Cohn SM, Crookes BA, Proctor KG: Near-infrared spectroscopy in resuscitation. *J Trauma* 54:S199, 2003.

119. McKinley BA, Marvin RG, Cocanour CS, et al: Tissue hemoglobin O_2 saturation during resuscitation of traumatic shock monitored using near infrared spectrometry. *J Trauma* 48:637, 2000.

120. Knudson MM, Bermudez KM, Doyle CA, et al: Use of tissue oxygen tension measurements during resuscitation from hemorrhagic shock. *J Trauma* 42:608, 1997.

121. Cheatham ML, Nelson LD, Chang MC, et al: Right ventricular end diastolic volume index as a predictor of positive end-expiratory pressure. *Crit Care Med* 26:1801, 1998.

122. Chang MC, Meredith JW, Kincaid EH, et al: Maintaining survivors' values of left ventricular power output during shock resuscitation: A prospective pilot study. *J Trauma* 49:26, 2000.

123. Choi PT-L, Yip G, Quinonez LG, et al: Crystalloids vs. colloids in fluid resuscitation: A systematic review. *Crit Care Med* 27:200, 1999.

124. Cochrane Injuries Group albumin reviewers: Human albumin administration in critically-ill patients: A systematic review of randomized controlled trials. *Br Med J* 317:235, 1998.

125. Vassar MJ, Fischer RP, O'Brien PE, et al: A multicenter trial for resuscitation of injured patients with 7.5% sodium chloride. *Arch Surg* 128:1003, 1993.

126. Mann DV, Robinson MK, Rounds ID, et al: Superiority of blood over saline resuscitation from hemorrhagic shock. *Ann Surg* 226:653, 1997.

127. Hebert PC, Wells G, Blajchman MA, et al: A multicenter, randomized controlled clinical trial of transfusion requirements in critical care. *N Engl J Med* 340:409, 1999.

128. Hebert PC, Yetisir E, Martin C, et al: Is a low transfusion threshold safe in critically-ill patients with cardiovascular disease? *Crit Care Med* 29:227, 2001.

129. Wu W-C, Rathore SS, Wang Y, et al: Blood transfusion in elderly patients with acute myocardial infarction. *N Engl J Med* 345:1230, 2001.

CHAPTER 5

Surgical Infections

David L. Dunn and Gregory J. Beilman

HISTORICAL BACKGROUND

Although treatment of infection has been an integral part of the surgeon's practice since the dawn of time, the body of knowledge that led to the present field of surgical infectious disease was derived from the evolution of germ theory and antisepsis. Application of the latter to clinical practice, concurrent with the development of anesthesia, was pivotal in allowing surgeons to expand their repertoire to encompass complex procedures that previously were associated with extremely high rates of morbidity and mortality due to postoperative infections. However, until recently the occurrence of infection related to the surgical wound was the rule rather than the exception. In fact, the development of modalities to effectively prevent and treat infection has occurred only within the last several decades.

A number of observations by nineteenth-century physicians and investigators were critical to our current understanding of the pathogenesis, prevention, and treatment of surgical infections. In 1846, Ignaz Semmelweis, a Magyar physician, took a post at the Allgemein Krankenhaus in Vienna. He noticed that the mortality from puerperal ("childbed") fever was much higher in the teaching ward (1:11) than in the ward where patients were delivered by midwives (1:29). He also made the interesting observation that women who delivered prior to arrival on the teaching ward had a negligible mortality rate. The tragic death of a colleague due to overwhelming infection after a knife scratch received during an autopsy of a woman who had died of puerperal fever led Semmelweis to observe that pathologic changes in his friend were identical to those of women dying from this postpartum disease. He then hypothesized that puerperal fever was caused by putrid material transmitted from patients dying of this disease by carriage on the examining fingers of the medical students and physicians who frequently went from the autopsy room to the wards. The low mortality noted in the midwives' ward, Semmelweis realized, was due to the fact that midwives did not participate in autopsies. Fired with the zeal of his revelation, he posted a notice on the door to the ward requiring all caregivers to rinse their hands thoroughly in chlorine water prior to entering the area. This simple intervention reduced mortality from puerperal fever to 1.5%, surpassing the record of the midwives. In 1861, he published his classic work on childbed fever based on records from his practice. Unfortunately, Semmelweis' ideas were not well accepted by the authorities of the time.[1] Despondent, he committed suicide in 1865 by intentionally cutting his finger during the autopsy of a woman who died of puerperal fever, presumably as the ultimate proof of his tenets.

Louis Pasteur performed a body of work during the latter part of the nineteenth century that provided the underpinnings of modern microbiology, at the time known as "germ theory." His work in humans followed experiments identifying infectious agents in silkworms. He was able to elucidate the principle that contagious diseases are caused by specific microbes and that these microbes are foreign to the infected organism. Using this principle he developed techniques of sterilization critical to oenology, and identified several bacteria responsible for human illnesses, including *Staphylococcus, Streptococcus,* and pneumococcus.

Joseph Lister, the son of a wine merchant, was appointed professor of surgery at the Glasgow Royal Infirmary in 1859. In his early practice, he noted that over 50% of his patients undergoing amputation died due to postoperative infection. After hearing of Pasteur's theory, Lister experimented with the use of a solution of carbolic acid, which he knew was being used to treat sewage. He first reported his findings to the British Medical Association in 1867 using dressings saturated with carbolic acid on 12 patients with compound fractures; 10 recovered without amputation, one survived with amputation, and one died of causes unrelated to the wound. In spite of initial resistance, his methods were quickly adopted throughout Europe.

From 1878 until 1880, Robert Koch was the District Medical Officer for Wollstein, which was an area in which anthrax was endemic. Performing experiments in his home, without the benefit of scientific equipment and academic contact, Koch developed techniques for culture of *Bacillus anthracis* and proved the ability of this organism to cause anthrax in healthy animals. He developed the following four postulates to identify the association of organisms with specific diseases: (1) the suspected pathogenic organism should be present in all cases of the disease and absent from healthy animals, (2) the suspected pathogen should be isolated from a diseased host and grown in a pure culture in vitro, (3) cells from a pure culture of the suspected organism should cause disease in a healthy animal, and (4) the organism should be reisolated from the newly diseased animal and shown to be the same as the original. He used these same techniques to identify the organisms responsible for cholera and tuberculosis. During the next century, Koch's postulates, as they came to be called, became critical to our understanding of surgical infections and remain so today.[2]

The first intra-abdominal operation to treat infection via "source control" (i.e., surgical intervention to eliminate the source of infection) was appendectomy. This operation was pioneered by Charles McBurney at the New York College of Physicians and Surgeons, among others.[3] McBurney's classic report on early operative intervention for appendicitis was presented before the New York Surgical Society in 1889. Appendectomy for the treatment of appendicitis, previously an often fatal disease, was popularized after the 1902 coronation of King Edward VII of England was delayed due to his need for an appendectomy, which was performed by Sir Frederick Treves. The king desperately needed an appendectomy but strongly opposed going into the hospital, protesting, "I have a coronation on hand." However, Treves was adamant, stating, "It will be a funeral, if you don't have the operation." Treves carried the debate, and the king lived.

During the twentieth century the discovery of effective antimicrobials added another tool to the armamentarium of modern surgeons. Sir Alexander Fleming, after serving in the British Army Medical Corps during World War I, continued work on the natural antibacterial action of the blood and antiseptics. In 1928, while studying influenza virus, he noted a zone of inhibition around a mold colony (*Penicillium notatum*) that serendipitously grew on a plate of *Staphylococcus,* and he named the active substance penicillin. This first effective antibacterial agent subsequently led to the development of hundreds of potent antimicrobials, set the stage for their use as prophylaxis against postoperative infection, and became a critical component of the armamentarium to treat aggressive, lethal surgical infections.

Concurrent with the development of numerous antimicrobial agents were advances in the field of clinical microbiology. Many new microbes were identified, including numerous anaerobes; the autochthonous microflora of the skin, gastrointestinal tract, and other parts of the body that the surgeon encountered in the process of an operation were characterized in great detail. However, it remained unclear whether these organisms, anaerobes in particular, were commensals or pathogens. Subsequently, the initial clinical observations of surgeons such as Frank Meleney, William Altemeier, and others provided the key, when they observed that aerobes and anaerobes could synergize to cause serious soft tissue and severe intra-abdominal infection.[4,5] Thus, the concepts that resident microbes were nonpathogenic until they entered a sterile body cavity at the time of surgery, and that many, if not most, surgical infections were polymicrobial in nature, became critical ideas and were promulgated by a number of clinician-scientists over the last several decades.[6,7] These tenets became firmly established after microbiology laboratories demonstrated the invariable presence of aerobes and anaerobes in peritoneal cultures obtained at the time of

surgery for intra-abdominal infection due to a perforated viscus or gangrenous appendicitis. Clinical trials provided evidence that optimal therapy for these infections required effective source control, plus the administration of antimicrobial agents directed against both types of pathogens.

William Osler, a prolific writer and one of the fathers of American medicine, made an observation in 1904 in his treatise *The Evolution of Modern Medicine* that was to have profound implications for the future of treatment of infection: "Except on few occasions, the patient appears to die from the body's response to infection rather than from it."[8] The discovery of the first cytokines began to allow insight into the organism's response to infection, and led to an explosion in our understanding of the host inflammatory response. Expanding knowledge of the multiple pathways activated during the response to invasion by infectious organisms has permitted the design of new therapies targeted at modifying the inflammatory response to infection, which seems to cause much of the end-organ dysfunction and failure. Preventing and treating this process of multiple organ failure during infection is one of the major challenges of modern critical care and surgical infectious disease.

PATHOGENESIS OF INFECTION
Host Defenses

The mammalian host possesses several layers of endogenous defense mechanisms that serve to prevent microbial invasion, limit proliferation of microbes within the host, and contain or eradicate invading microbes. These defenses are integrated and redundant so that the various components function as a complex, highly regulated system that is extremely effective in coping with microbial invaders. They include site-specific defenses that function at the tissue level, as well as components that freely circulate throughout the body in both blood and lymph. Systemic host defenses invariably are recruited to a site of infection, a process that begins immediately upon introduction of microbes into a sterile area of the body. Perturbation of one or more components of these defenses (e.g., via immunosuppressants, chronic illness, and burns) may have substantial negative impact on resistance to infection.

Entry of microbes into the mammalian host is precluded by the presence of a number of barriers that possess either an epithelial (integument) or mucosal (respiratory, gut, and urogenital) surface. However, barrier function is not solely limited to physical characteristics: host barrier cells may secrete substances that limit microbial proliferation or prevent invasion. Also, resident or commensal microbes (endogenous or autochthonous host microflora) adherent to the physical surface and to each other may preclude invasion, particularly of virulent organisms (colonization resistance).[9]

The most extensive physical barrier is the integument or skin. In addition to the physical barrier posed by the epithelial surface, the skin harbors its own resident microflora that may block the attachment and invasion of noncommensal microbes. Microbes also are held in check by chemicals that sebaceous glands secrete and by the constant shedding of epithelial cells. The endogenous microflora of the integument primarily comprises gram-positive aerobic microbes belonging to the genera *Staphylococcus* and *Streptococcus,* as well as *Corynebacterium* and *Propionibacterium* species. These organisms plus *Enterococcus faecalis* and *faecium, Escherichia coli* and other Enterobacteriaceae, and yeast such as *Candida albicans* can be isolated from the infraumbilical regions of the body. Diseases of the skin (e.g., eczema and dermatitis) are associated with overgrowth of skin commensal organisms, and barrier breaches invariably lead to the introduction of these microbes.

The respiratory tract possesses several host defense mechanisms that facilitate the maintenance of sterility in the distal bronchi and alveoli under normal circumstances. In the upper respiratory tract, respiratory mucus traps larger particles including microbes. This mucus is then passed into the upper airways and oropharynx by ciliated epithelial cells, where the mucus is cleared via coughing. Smaller particles arriving in the lower respiratory tract are cleared via phagocytosis by pulmonary alveolar macrophages. Any process that diminishes these host defenses can lead to development of bronchitis or pneumonia.

The urogenital, biliary, pancreatic ductal, and distal respiratory tracts do not possess resident microflora in healthy individuals, although microbes may be present if these barriers are affected by disease (e.g., malignancy, inflammation, calculi, or foreign body), or if microorganisms are introduced from an external source (e.g., urinary catheter or pulmonary aspiration). In contrast, significant numbers of microbes are encountered in many portions of the gastrointestinal tract, with vast numbers being found within the oropharynx and distal colorectum, although the specific organisms differ.

One would suppose that the entire gastrointestinal tract would be populated via those microbes found in the oropharynx, but this is not the case. This is because after ingestion these organisms routinely are killed in the highly acidic, low-motility environment of the stomach during the initial phases of digestion. Thus, small numbers of microbes populate the gastric mucosa [$\sim 10^2$ to 10^3 colony-forming units (CFU)/mL]; this population expands in the presence of drugs or disease states that diminish gastric acidity. Microbes that are not destroyed within the stomach enter the small intestine, in which a certain amount of microbial proliferation takes place, such that approximately 10^5 to 10^8 CFU/mL are present in the terminal ileum.

The relatively low-oxygen, static environment of the colon is accompanied by the exponential growth of microbes that comprise the most extensive host endogenous microflora. Anaerobic microbes outnumber aerobic species approximately 100:1 in the distal colorectum, and approximately 10^{11} to 10^{12} CFU/g are present in feces. Large numbers of facultative and strict anaerobes (*Bacteroides fragilis, distasonis,* and *thetaiotaomicron, Bifidobacterium, Clostridium, Eubacterium, Fusobacterium, Lactobacillus,* and *Peptostreptococcus* species) as well as several orders of magnitude fewer aerobic microbes (*Escherichia coli* and other Enterobacteriaceae, *Enterococcus faecalis* and *faecium, Candida albicans* and other *Candida* spp.) are present. Intriguingly, although colonization resistance on the part of this extensive, well-characterized host microflora effectively prevents invasion of enteric pathogens such as *Salmonella, Shigella, Vibrio,* and other enteropathogenic bacterial species, these same organisms provide the initial inoculum for infection should perforation of the gastrointestinal tract occur. It is of great interest that only some of these microbial species predominate in established intra-abdominal infection.

Once microbes enter a sterile body compartment (e.g., pleural or peritoneal cavity) or tissue, additional host defenses act to limit and/or eliminate these pathogens. Initially, several primitive and relatively nonspecific host defenses act to contain the nidus of infection, which may include microbes as well as debris, devitalized tissue, and foreign bodies, depending on the nature of the injury. These defenses include the physical barrier of the tissue itself, as well as the capacity of proteins such as lactoferrin and transferrin to sequester the critical microbial growth factor iron, thereby limiting microbial growth. In addition, fibrinogen within the inflammatory fluid has the ability to trap large numbers of microbes during the process in

which it polymerizes into fibrin. Within the peritoneal cavity, unique host defenses exist, including a diaphragmatic pumping mechanism whereby particles including microbes within peritoneal fluid are expunged from the abdominal cavity via specialized structures on the undersurface of the diaphragm. Concurrently, containment by the omentum, the so-called "gatekeeper" of the abdomen and intestinal ileus, serves to wall off infection. However, the latter processes and fibrin trapping have a high likelihood of contributing to the formation of an intra-abdominal abscess.

Microbes also immediately encounter a series of host defense mechanisms that reside within the vast majority of tissues of the body. These include resident macrophages and low levels of complement (C) proteins and immunoglobulins (Ig, antibodies).[10] Resident macrophages secrete a wide array of substances in response to the above-mentioned processes, some of which appear to regulate the cellular components of the host defense response. Macrophage cytokine synthesis is upregulated. Secretion of tumor necrosis factor-α (TNF-α), of interleukins (IL)-1β, 6, and 8; and of interferon-γ (INF-γ) occurs within the tissue milieu, and, depending on the magnitude of the host defense response, the systemic circulation.[11] Concurrently, a counterregulatory response is initiated consisting of binding proteins (TNF-BP), cytokine receptor antagonists (IL-1ra), and anti-inflammatory cytokines (IL-4 and IL-10).

The interaction of microbes with these first-line host defenses leads to microbial opsonization (C1q, C3bi, and IgFc), phagocytosis, and both extracellular (C5b6-9 membrane attack complex) and intracellular microbial destruction (phagocytic vacuoles). Concurrently, the classical and alternate complement pathways are activated both via direct contact with and via IgM>IgG binding to microbes, leading to the release of a number of different complement protein fragments (C3a, C4a, C5a) that are biologically active, acting to markedly enhance vascular permeability. Bacterial cell wall components and a variety of enzymes that are expelled from leukocyte phagocytic vacuoles during microbial phagocytosis and killing act in this capacity as well.

Simultaneously, the release of substances to which polymorphonuclear leukocytes (PMNs) in the bloodstream are attracted takes place. These consist of C5a, microbial cell wall peptides containing N-formyl-methionine, and macrophage secretion of cytokines such as IL-8. This process of host defense recruitment leads to further influx of inflammatory fluid into the area of incipient infection, and is accompanied by diapedesis of large numbers of PMNs, a process that begins within several minutes and may peak within hours or days. The magnitude of the response and eventual outcome generally are related to several factors: (1) the initial number of microbes, (2) the rate of microbial proliferation in relation to containment and killing by host defenses, (3) microbial virulence, and (4) the potency of host defenses. In regard to the latter, drugs or disease states that diminish any or multiple components of host defenses are associated with higher rates and potentially more grave infections.

Definitions

Several possible outcomes can occur subsequent to microbial invasion and the interaction of microbes with resident and recruited host defenses: (1) eradication, (2) containment, often leading to the presence of purulence—the hallmark of chronic infection (e.g., a furuncle in the skin and soft tissue or abscess within the parenchyma of an organ or potential space), (3) locoregional infection (cellulitis, lymphangitis, and aggressive soft tissue infection) with or without

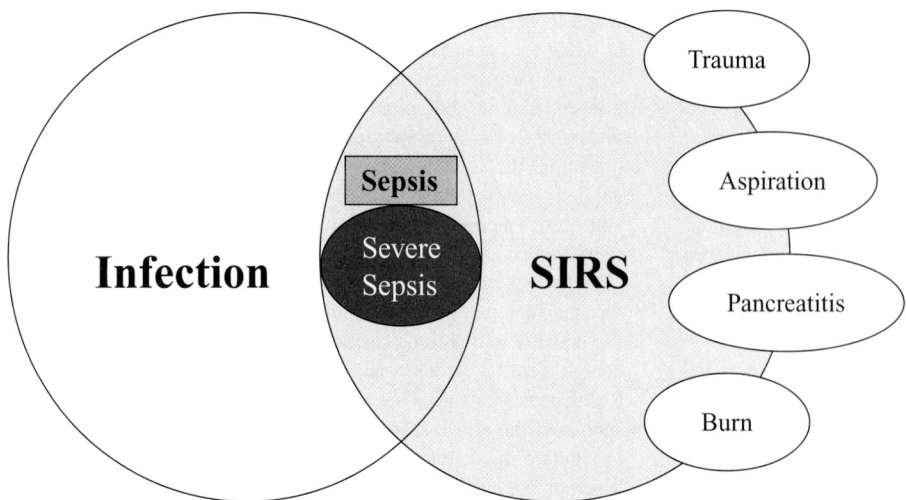

FIG. 5-1. Relationship between sepsis and systemic response. A number of clinical conditions can cause a systemic inflammatory response, including infection. Sepsis is infection plus this response. Severe sepsis is a subset of sepsis characterized by end-organ dysfunction.

distant spread of infection (metastatic abscess), or (4) systemic infection (bacteremia or fungemia). Obviously, the latter represents the failure of resident and recruited host defenses at the local level, and is associated with significant morbidity and mortality in the clinical setting. In addition, it is not uncommon that disease progression occurs such that serious locoregional infection is associated with concurrent systemic infection. A chronic abscess also may intermittently drain and/or be associated with bacteremia.

Infection is defined by identification of microorganisms in host tissue or the bloodstream, plus an inflammatory response to their presence. At the site of infection the classic findings of rubor, calor, and dolor in areas such as the skin or subcutaneous tissue are common. Most infections in normal individuals with intact host defenses are associated with these local manifestations, plus systemic manifestations such as elevated temperature, elevated white blood cell (WBC) count, tachycardia, or tachypnea. The systemic manifestations noted above comprise the *systemic inflammatory response syndrome* (SIRS).

SIRS can be caused by a variety of disease processes, including pancreatitis, polytrauma, malignancy, and transfusion reaction, as well as infection (Fig. 5-1). Strict criteria for SIRS (tachycardia, tachypnea, fever, and elevated WBC count) recently have been broadened to include additional clinical indicators noted in Table 5-1.[12] SIRS caused by infection is termed *sepsis*, and is mediated by the production of a cascade of proinflammatory mediators produced in response to exposure to microbial products. These products include lipopolysaccharide (endotoxin, LPS) derived from gram-negative organisms; peptidoglycans and teichoic acids from gram-positive organisms; multiple cell wall components such as mannan from yeast and fungi; and many others. Patients have developed sepsis if they have met clinical criteria for SIRS and have evidence of a local or systemic source of infection.

Severe sepsis is characterized as sepsis (defined above) combined with the presence of new-onset organ failure. Severe sepsis is the most common cause of death in noncoronary critical care units, with more than 200,000 deaths occurring annually in the United States.[13] A number of organ dysfunction scoring systems have been described.[14,15] With respect to clinical criteria, a patient with sepsis and the need for ventilatory support, with oliguria unresponsive to aggressive fluid resuscitation, or with hypotension requiring vasopressors should be considered to have developed severe sepsis. *Septic shock* is a state of acute circulatory failure identified by the presence of persistent arterial hypotension (systolic blood pressure <90 mm Hg) despite adequate fluid resuscitation, without other

identifiable causes. Septic shock is the most severe manifestation of infection, occurring in approximately 40% of patients with severe sepsis; it has an attendant mortality rate of 60 to 80%.[16]

Clinicians dedicated to improving the treatment of sepsis have recently developed a new classification scheme for this entity.[12] This scheme has borrowed from the tumor-node-metastasis (TNM) staging scheme developed for oncology. The impetus for development of this scheme was related to the heterogeneity of the patient population developing sepsis, an example of which would include two patients, both in the intensive care unit (ICU), who develop criteria

Table 5-1
Criteria for Systemic Inflammatory Response Syndrome (SIRS)

General variables
    Fever (core temp >38.3°C)
    Hypothermia (core temp <36°C)
    Heart rate >90 bpm
    Tachypnea
    Altered mental status
    Significant edema or positive fluid balance (>20 mL/kg over 24 hours)
    Hyperglycemia in the absence of diabetes
Inflammatory variables
    Leukocytosis (WBC >12,000)
    Leukopenia (WBC <4000)
    Bandemia (>10% band forms)
    Plasma C-reactive protein >2 s.d. above normal value
    Plasma procalcitonin >2 s.d. above normal value
Hemodynamic variables
    Arterial hypotension (SBP <90 mm Hg, MAP <70, or SBP decrease >40 mm Hg)
    Svo_2 >70%
    Cardiac index >3.5 L/min per square meter
Organ dysfunction variables
    Arterial hypoxemia
    Acute oliguria
    Creatinine increase
    Coagulation abnormalities
    Ileus
    Thrombocytopenia
    Hyperbilirubinemia
Tissue perfusion variables
    Hyperlactatemia
    Decreased capillary filling

bpm = beats per minute; MAP = mean arterial pressure; SBP = systolic blood pressure; s.d. = standard deviations; Svo_2 = venous oxygen saturation; WBC = white blood cell count.

Table 5-2
PIRO Classification Scheme

Domain	Means of Classification
Predisposition	Premorbid illness that affects probability of survival (e.g., immunosuppression, age, genetics)
Insult (infection)	Type of infecting organisms, location of disease, intervention (source control)
Response	SIRS, other signs of sepsis, presence of shock, tissue markers (e.g., C-reactive protein, IL-6)
Organ dysfunction	Organ dysfunction as a number of failing organs or composite score

IL-6 = interleukin-6; SIRS = systemic inflammatory response syndrome.

consistent with septic shock. While both have infection and sepsis-associated hypotension, one might expect a different outcome in a young, healthy patient who develops urosepsis than in an elderly, immunosuppressed lung transplant recipient who develops invasive fungal infection. The PIRO Staging System stratifies patients based on their *p*redisposing conditions (P), the nature and extent of the *i*nfection (I), the nature and magnitude of the host *r*esponse (R), and the degree of concomitant *o*rgan dysfunction (O). Current definitions using this system are listed in Table 5-2. Clinical trials evaluating the utility of this scoring system for prognostication and for examination of the impact of adjuvant therapies are underway.

MICROBIOLOGY OF INFECTIOUS AGENTS

A partial list of common pathogens that cause infections in surgical patients is provided in Table 5-3.

Bacteria

Bacteria are responsible for the majority of surgical infections. Specific species are identified using Gram's stain and growth characteristics on specific media. The Gram's stain is an important evaluation that allows rapid classification of bacteria by color. This color is related to the staining characteristics of the bacterial cell wall: gram-positive bacteria stain blue and gram-negative bacteria stain red. Bacteria are classified based upon a number of additional characteristics including morphology (cocci and bacilli), the pattern of division [e.g., single organisms, groups of organisms in pairs (diplococci), clusters (staphylococci), and chains (streptococci)], and the presence and location of spores.

Gram-positive bacteria that frequently cause infections in surgical patients include aerobic skin commensals (*Staphylococcus aureus* and *epidermidis* and *Streptococcus pyogenes*) and enteric organisms such as *Enterococcus faecalis* and *faecium*. Aerobic skin commensals cause a large percentage of surgical site infections (SSIs), either alone or in conjunction with other pathogens; enterococci can cause nosocomial infections [urinary tract infections (UTIs) and bacteremia] in immunocompromised or chronically-ill patients, but are of relatively low virulence in healthy individuals.

There are many pathogenic gram-negative bacterial species that are capable of causing infection in surgical patients. Most gram-negative organisms of interest to the surgeon are bacilli belonging to the family Enterobacteriaceae, including *Escherichia coli*, *Klebsiella pneumoniae*, *Serratia marcescens*, and *Enterobacter*, *Citrobacter*, and *Acinetobacter* spp. Other gram-negative bacilli of note include *Pseudomonas* spp., including *Pseudomonas aeruginosa* and *fluorescens* and *Xanthomonas* spp.

Table 5-3
Common Pathogens in Surgical Patients

Gram-positive aerobic cocci
   Staphylococcus aureus
   Staphylococcus epidermidis
   Streptococcus pyogenes
   Streptococcus pneumoniae
   Enterococcus faecium, E. faecalis
Gram-negative aerobic bacilli
   Escherichia coli
   Haemophilus influenzae
   Klebsiella pneumoniae
   Proteus mirabilis
   Enterobacter cloacae, E. aerogenes
   Serratia marcescens
   Acinetobacter calcoaceticus
   Citrobacter freundii
   Pseudomonas aeruginosa
   Xanthomonas maltophilia
Anaerobes
   Gram-positive
      Clostridium perfringens, C. tetani, C. septicum
      Clostridium difficile
      Peptostreptococcus spp.
   Gram-negative
      Bacteroides fragilis
      Fusobacterium spp.
Other bacteria
   Mycobacterium avium-intracellulare
   Mycobacterium tuberculosis
   Nocardia asteroides
   Legionella pneumophila
   Listeria monocytogenes
Fungi
   Aspergillus fumigatus, A. niger, A. terreus, A. flavus
   Blastomyces dermatitidis
   Candida albicans
   Candida glabrata, C. paropsilosis, C. krusei
   Coccidiodes immitis
   Cryptococcus neoformans
   Histoplasma capsulatum
   Mucor/Rhizopus
Viruses
   Cytomegalovirus
   Epstein-Barr virus
   Hepatitis B, C viruses
   Herpes simplex virus
   Human immunodeficiency virus
   Varicella zoster virus

Anaerobic organisms are unable to grow or divide poorly in air, as most do not possess the enzyme catalase, which allows for metabolism of reactive oxygen species. Anaerobes are the predominant indigenous flora in many areas of the human body, with the particular species dependent on the site. For example, *Propionibacterium acnes* and other species are a major component of the skin microflora and cause the infectious manifestation of acne. As noted above, large numbers of anaerobes contribute to the microflora of the oropharynx and colorectum.

Infection due to *Mycobacterium tuberculosis* was once one of the most common causes of death in Europe, causing one in four deaths in the seventeenth and eighteenth centuries. In the nineteenth and twentieth centuries, thoracic surgical intervention was often required for severe pulmonary disease, now an increasingly uncommon occurrence in developed countries. This organism and other related organisms (*M. avium-intracellulare* and *M. leprae*) are known as acid-fast bacilli. Other acid-fast bacilli include *Nocardia* spp. These organisms typically are slow-growing, sometimes necessitating observation in culture for weeks to months prior to final

Table 5-4
Antifungal Agents and Their Characteristics

Antifungal	Advantages	Disadvantages	Approximate Daily Cost
Amphotericin B	Broad-spectrum, inexpensive	Renal toxicity, premeds, IV only	$16
Liposomal amphotericin B	Broad-spectrum	Expensive, IV only, renal toxicity	$333
Fluconazole	IV and PO availability	Narrow-spectrum, drug interactions (class)	$104
Itraconazole	IV and PO availability	Narrow-spectrum, no CSF penetration	$151
Voriconazole	IV and PO availability, broad-spectrum	IV diluent accumulation in renal failure, visual disturbances	$272
Caspofungin	Broad-spectrum	IV only, poor CSF penetration	$280

CSF = cerebrospinal fluid.

identification, although DNA-based analysis can provide a means for preliminary, rapid detection.

Fungi

Fungi typically are identified by use of special stains [e.g., potassium hydroxide (KOH), India ink, methenamine silver, or Giemsa]. Initial identification is assisted by observation of the form of branching and septation in stained specimens or in culture. Final identification is based on growth characteristics in special media, similar to bacteria, as well as on the capacity for growth at a different temperature (25 vs. 37°C). Fungi of relevance to surgeons include those that cause nosocomial infections in surgical patients as part of polymicrobial infections or fungemia (e.g., *Candida albicans* and related species), rare causes of aggressive soft tissue infections (e.g., *Mucor, Rhizopus,* and *Absidia* spp.), and so-called opportunistic pathogens that cause infection in the immunocompromised host (e.g., *Aspergillus fumigatus, niger, terreus,* and other spp., *Blastomyces dermatitidis, Coccidioides immitis,* and *Cryptococcus neoformans*). Agents currently available for antifungal therapy are described in Table 5-4.

Viruses

Due to their small size and necessity for growth within cells, viruses are difficult to culture, requiring a longer time than is typically optimal for clinical decision making. Previously, viral infection was identified by indirect means (i.e., the host antibody response). Recent advances in technology have allowed for the identification of the presence of viral deoxyribonucleic acid (DNA) or ribonucleic acid (RNA) using methods such as polymerase chain reaction. Similarly to many fungal infections, most viral infections in surgical patients occur in the immunocompromised host, particularly those receiving immunosuppression to prevent rejection of a solid organ allograft. Relevant viruses include adenoviruses, cytomegalovirus, Epstein-Barr virus, herpes simplex virus, and varicella-zoster virus. Surgeons must be aware of the manifestations of hepatitis B and C virus, as well as human immunodeficiency virus infections, including their capacity to be transmitted to health care workers (see below). Prophylactic and therapeutic use of antiviral agents is discussed in Chap. 10.

PREVENTION AND TREATMENT OF SURGICAL INFECTIONS

General Principles

Maneuvers to diminish the presence of exogenous (surgeon and operating room environment) and endogenous (patient) microbes are termed *prophylaxis,* and consist of the use of mechanical, chemical, and antimicrobial modalities, or a combination of these methods.

As described above, the host resident microflora of the skin (patient and surgeon) and other barrier surfaces represent a potential source of microbes that can invade the body during trauma, thermal injury, or elective or emergent surgical intervention. For this reason, operating room personnel are versed in mild mechanical exfoliation of the skin of the hands and forearms using antibacterial preparations, and intraoperatively sterile technique is employed. Similarly, application of an antibacterial agent to the skin of the patient at the proposed operative site takes place prior to creating an incision. Also, if necessary, hair removal should take place using a clipper rather than a razor; the latter promotes overgrowth of skin microbes in small nicks and cuts. Dedicated use of these modalities clearly has been shown to diminish the quantity of skin microflora, and although a direct correlation between praxis and reduced infection rates has not been demonstrated, comparison to infection rates prior to the use of antisepsis and sterile technique makes clear their utility and importance.

Additional maneuvers are prudent when undertaking bowel surgery. Preparation of areas of the body such as the distal colorectum requires that body waste in the form of bacteria-laden feces be removed to the greatest extent possible. Current practice has the patient ingesting a clear liquid diet for 12 to 24 hours prior to colonic resection, concurrent with using a cathartic preparation (saline laxative or polyethylene glycol) and ingesting large amounts of fluid to flush the contents of the colon.

The aforementioned modalities are not capable of sterilizing the hands of the surgeon or the skin or epithelial surfaces of the patient, although the inoculum can be reduced considerably. Thus, entry through the skin, into the soft tissue, and into a body cavity or hollow viscus invariably is associated with the introduction of some degree of microbial contamination. For that reason, patients who undergo procedures that may be associated with the ingress of significant numbers of microbes (e.g., colonic resection) or in whom the consequences of any type of infection due to said process would be dire (e.g., prosthetic vascular graft infection) should receive an antimicrobial agent. For example, oral antimicrobial agents typically are administered during mechanical preparation of the colon, after which an intravenous antimicrobial agent is administered immediately prior to creating the skin incision.

Source Control

The primary precept of surgical infectious disease therapy consists of drainage of all purulent material, débridement of all infected, devitalized tissue, and debris, and/or removal of foreign bodies at the site of infection, plus remediation of the underlying cause of infection.[17] A discrete, walled-off purulent fluid collection (i.e., an abscess) requires drainage via percutaneous drain insertion or an operative approach in which incision and drainage take place.

An ongoing source of contamination (e.g., bowel perforation) or the presence of an aggressive, rapidly-spreading infection (e.g., necrotizing soft tissue infection) invariably requires expedient, aggressive operative intervention, both to remove contaminated material and infected tissue (e.g., radical débridement or amputation) and to remove the initial cause of infection (e.g., bowel resection). Other treatment modalities such as antimicrobial agents, albeit critical, are of secondary importance to effective surgery with regard to treatment of surgical infections and overall outcome. Rarely, if ever, can an aggressive surgical infection be cured only by the administration of antibiotics, and never in the face of an ongoing source of contamination. Also, it has been repeatedly demonstrated that delay in operative intervention, whether due to misdiagnosis or the need for additional diagnostic studies, is associated with increased morbidity and occasional mortality.[18-20]

Appropriate Use of Antimicrobial Agents

A classification of antimicrobial agents, mechanisms of action, and spectrum of activity is shown in Table 5-5. *Prophylaxis* consists of the administration of an antimicrobial agent or agents prior to initiation of certain specific types of surgical procedures in order to reduce the number of microbes that enter the tissue or body cavity. Agents are selected according to their activity against microbes likely to be present at the surgical site, based on knowledge of host microflora. For example, patients undergoing elective colon resection should undergo mechanical preparation of the bowel plus receive intraluminal agents directed against aerobes and anaerobes (e.g., neomycin + metronidazole); immediately prior to creating the incision, the patient should receive a single dose of any one of a large number of intravenous agents with a similar spectrum of activity (e.g., cefoxitin, cefotetan, or ampicillin-sulbactam). Use of these prophylactic measures constitutes the current standard of care in North America, leading to SSI rates of approximately 4% subsequent to elective colorectal surgery.[21,22]

By definition, prophylaxis is limited to the time prior to and during the operative procedure; in the vast majority of cases only a single dose of antibiotic is required, and only for certain types of procedures (see below). However, patients who undergo complex, prolonged procedures in which the duration of the operation exceeds the serum drug half-life should receive an additional dose or doses of the antimicrobial agent. Nota bene: There is no evidence that administration of postoperative doses of an antimicrobial agent provides additional benefit, and this practice should be discouraged, as it is costly and is associated with increased rates of microbial drug resistance. Guidelines for prophylaxis are provided in Table 5-6.

Empiric therapy comprises the use of an antimicrobial agent or agents when the risk of a surgical infection is high, based on the underlying disease process (e.g., ruptured appendicitis), or when significant contamination during surgery has occurred (e.g., inadequate bowel preparation or considerable spillage of colon contents). Obviously, prophylaxis merges into empiric therapy in situations in which the risk of infection increases markedly because of intraoperative findings. Empiric therapy also often is employed in critically-ill patients in whom a potential site of infection has been identified and severe sepsis or septic shock occurs. Invariably, empiric therapy should be limited to a short course of drug (3 to 5 days), and should be curtailed as soon as possible based on microbiologic data (i.e., absence of positive cultures) coupled with improvements in the clinical course of the patient.

Similarly, empiric therapy merges into therapy of established infection in some patients as well. However, among surgical patients, the manner in which therapy is employed, particularly in relation to the use of microbiologic data (culture and antibiotic sensitivity patterns), differs depending on whether the infection is monomicrobial or polymicrobial. Monomicrobial infections frequently are nosocomial infections occurring in postoperative patients, such as UTIs, pneumonia, or bacteremia. Evidence of sepsis syndrome (e.g., positive urine esterase plus a Gram's stain indicating the presence of microbes) in such individuals, coupled with evidence of local infection (e.g., an infiltrate on chest roentgenogram plus a positive Gram's stain in bronchoalveolar lavage samples) should lead the surgeon to initiate empiric antibiotic therapy. Drug selection must be based on initial evidence (gram-positive vs. gram-negative microbes, yeast), coupled with institutional and unit-specific drug sensitivity patterns. Within 24 to 72 hours, culture and sensitivity reports will allow refinement of the antibiotic regimen to select the most efficacious agent. The clinical course of the patient is monitored closely, and in some cases (e.g., UTI) follow-up studies (urine culture) should be obtained after completion of therapy.

Although the primary therapeutic modality to treat polymicrobial surgical infections is source control as delineated above, antimicrobial agents play an important role as well. Culture results are of lesser importance in managing these types of infections, as it has been repeatedly demonstrated that only a limited cadre of microbes predominate in the established infection, selected from a large number present at the time of initial contamination. Invariably it is difficult to identify all microbes that comprise the initial polymicrobial inoculum. For this reason, the antibiotic regimen should not be modified solely on the basis of culture information, as it is less important than the clinical course of the patient. For example, patients who undergo appendectomy for gangrenous, perforated appendicitis, or bowel resection for intestinal perforation, should receive an antimicrobial agent or agents directed against aerobes and anaerobes for 3 to 5 days, occasionally longer. A survey of several decades of clinical trials examining the effect of antimicrobial agent selection on the treatment of intra-abdominal infection revealed striking similarities in outcome among regimens that possessed aerobic and anaerobic activity (~10 to 30% failure rates): most failures could not be attributed to antibiotic selection, but rather were due to the inability to achieve effective source control.[23]

Duration of antibiotic administration should be decided at the time the drug regimen is prescribed. As noted above, prophylaxis is limited to a single dose administered immediately prior to creating the incision. Empiric therapy should be limited to 3 to 5 days or less, and should be curtailed if the presence of a local site or systemic infection is not revealed.[24] This precept is highlighted by a study in which patients in whom SIRS was identified were closely monitored for the presence of infection: less than half of them were found to harbor infection.[25]

Therapy for monomicrobial infections follows standard guidelines: 7 to 10 days for UTIs, and 14 to 21 days for pneumonia and bacteremia. Antibiotic therapy for osteomyelitis, endocarditis, or prosthetic infections in which it is hazardous to remove the device consists of prolonged courses of an antibiotic or several agents in combination for 6 to 12 weeks. The specific agents are selected based on analysis of the degree to which the organism is killed in vitro using the minimum inhibitory concentration (MIC) of a standard pure inoculum of 10^5 CFU/mL of the organism isolated from the site of infection or bloodstream. Sensitivities are reported in relation to the achievable blood level of each antibiotic in a panel of agents. The least toxic, least expensive agent to which the organism is most sensitive should be selected, although the latter parameter is of paramount importance. Serious or recrudescent infection may

Table 5-5
Antimicrobial Agents

Antibiotic Class, Generic Name	Trade Name	Mechanism of Action	Organism								
			S. pyogenes	MSSA	MRSA	S. epidermidis	Enterococcus	VRE	E. coli	P. aeruginosa	Anaerobes
Penicillins		Cell wall synthesis inhibitors (bind penicillin-binding protein)									
Penicillin G			1	0	0	0	+/−	0	0	0	1
Nafcillin	Nallpen, Unipen		1	1	0	+/−	0	0	0	0	0
Piperacillin	Pipracil		1	0	0	0	+/−	0	1	1	+/−
Penicillin/beta lactamase inhibitor combinations		Cell wall synthesis inhibitors/beta lactamase inhibitors									
Ampicillin-sulbactam	Unasyn		1	1	0	+/−	1	+/−	1	0	1
Ticarcillin-clavulanate	Timentin		1	1	0	+/−	+/−	0	1	1	1
Piperacillin-tazobactam	Zosyn		1	1	0	1	+/−	0	1	1	1
First-generation cephalosporins		Cell wall synthesis inhibitors (bind penicillin-binding protein)									
Cephazolin, cephalexin	Ancef, Keflex		1	1	0	+/−	0	0	1	0	0
Second-generation cephalosporins		Cell wall synthesis inhibitors (bind penicillin-binding protein)									
Cefoxitin	Mefoxin		1	1	0	+/−	0	0	1	0	1
Cefotetan	Cefotan		1	1	0	+/−	0	0	1	0	1
Cefuroxime	Ceftin		1	1	0	+/−	0	0	1	0	0
Third- and fourth-generation cephalosporins		Cell wall synthesis inhibitors (bind penicillin-binding protein)									
Ceftriaxone	Rocefin		1	1	0	+/−	0	0	1	0	0
Ceftazidime	Fortaz		1	+/−	0	+/−	0	0	1	1	0
Cefepime	Maxipime		1	1	0	+/−	0	0	1	1	0
Cefotaxime	Cefotaxime		1	1	0	+/−	0	0	1	+/−	0
Carbapenems		Cell wall synthesis inhibitors (bind penicillin-binding protein)									
Imipenem-cilastatin	Primaxin		1	1	0	1	+/−	0	1	1	1
Meropenem	Merrem		1	1	0	1	0	0	1	1	1
Ertapenem	Invanz		1	1	0	1	0	0	1	1	1
Aztreonam	Azactam	Cell wall synthesis inhibitor (bind penicillin-binding protein)	0	0	0	0	0	0	1	1	0
Aminoglycosides		Alteration of cell membrane, binding and inhibition of 30S ribosomal unit									
Gentamicin			0	1	0	+/−	1	0	1	1	0
Tobramycin, amikacin			0	1	0	+/−	0	0	1	1	0

Fluoroquinolones

Generic	Trade	Mechanism								
Ciprofloxacin	Cipro	Inhibit topoisomerase II and IV (DNA synthesis inhibition)	+/-	0	1	0	0	1	1	0
Gatifloxacin	Tequin		1	+/-	1	+/-	0	1	+/-	+/-
Levofloxacin	Levaquin		1	0	1	0	0	1	+/-	0

Glycopeptides

Generic	Trade	Mechanism								
Vancomycin	Vancocin	Cell wall synthesis inhibition (peptidoglycan synthesis inhibition)	1	1	1	1	0	0	0	0
Quinupristin-Dalfopristin	Synercid	Inhibits 2 sites on 50S ribosome (protein synthesis inhibition)	1	1	1	1	1	0	0	+/-

Generic	Trade	Mechanism								
Linezolid	Zyvox	Inhibits 50S ribosomal activity (protein synthesis inhibition)	1	1	1	1	1	0	0	+/-
Daptomycin	Cubicin	Binds bacterial membrane, results in depolarization, lysis	1	1	1	1	1	0	0	0
Rifampin		Inhibits DNA-dependent RNA polymerase	1	1	1	+/-	0	0	0	0
Clindamycin	Cleocin	Inhibits 50S ribosomal activity (protein synthesis inhibition)	1	0	0	0	0	1	0	1
Metronidazole	Flagyl	Production of toxic intermediates (free radical production)	0	0	0	0	0	0	0	1

Macrolides

Generic	Trade	Mechanism								
Erythromycin		Inhibit 50S ribosomal activity (protein synthesis inhibition)	1	0	+/-	0	0	0	0	0
Azithromycin	Zithromax		1	0	0	0	0	0	0	0
Clarithromycin	Biaxin		1	0	+/-	0	0	1	0	0
Trimethoprim-sulfamethoxazole	Bactrim, Septra	Inhibits sequential steps of folate metabolism	+/-	0	+/-	0	0	1	0	0

Tetracyclines

Generic	Trade	Mechanism								
Minocycline	Minocin	Bind 30S ribosomal unit (protein synthesis inhibition)	1	0	0	0	0	0	0	+/-
Doxycycline	Vibromycin		1	+/-	0	0	0	1	0	+/-

E. coli = Escherichia coli; MRSA = methicillin-resistant *Staphylococcus aureus;* MSSA = methicillin-sensitive *Staphylococcus aureus; P. aeruginosa = Pseudomonas aeruginosa; S. epidermidis = Staphylococcus epidermidis; S. pyogenes = Streptococcus pyogenes;* VRE = vancomycin-resistant enterococcus.

1 = Reliable activity; +/- = variable activity; 0 = no activity.

The sensitivities presented are generalizations. The clinician should confirm sensitivity patterns at the locale where the patient is being treated since these patterns may vary widely depending on location.

Table 5-6
Prophylactic Use of Antibiotics

Site	Antibiotic	Alternative (e.g., penicillin allergic)
Cardiovascular surgery	Cefazolin	Vancomycin
Gastroduodenal area	Cefazolin, cefotetan, cefoxitin, ampicillin-sulbactam	Fluoroquinolone
Biliary tract with active infection (e.g., cholecystitis)	Cefotetan, cefoxitin	Fluoroquinolone plus clindamycin or metronidazole
Obstructed small bowel	Ampicillin-sulbactam	
Colorectal area	Ticarcillin-clavulanate, piperacillin-tazobactam, carbapenem	
Head and neck	Cefazolin	Aminoglycoside plus clindamycin
Neurosurgical procedures	Cefazolin	Vancomycin
Orthopedic surgery	Cefazolin	Vancomycin
Breast	Cefazolin	Vancomycin

require therapy with two or more agents, particularly if a multidrug-resistant pathogen is causative, limiting therapeutic options to drugs to which the organism is only moderately sensitive. Commonly an agent may be administered intravenously for 1 to 2 weeks, following which the treatment course is completed with oral drug. However, this should only be undertaken in patients who demonstrate progressive clinical improvement, and the oral agent should be capable of achieving high serum levels as well (e.g., fluoroquinolones).

The majority of studies examining the optimal duration of antibiotic therapy for the treatment of polymicrobial infection have focused on patients who develop peritonitis. Cogent data exist to support the contention that satisfactory outcomes are achieved with 12 to 24 hours of therapy for penetrating gastrointestinal trauma in the absence of extensive contamination, 3 to 5 days of therapy for perforated or gangrenous appendicitis, 5 to 7 days of therapy for treatment of peritoneal soilage due to a perforated viscus with moderate degrees of contamination, and 7 to 14 days of therapy to adjunctively treat extensive peritoneal soilage (e.g., feculent peritonitis) or that occurring in the immunosuppressed host.[26] It bears repeating that the eventual outcome is more closely linked to the ability of the surgeon to achieve effective source control than to the duration of antibiotic administration.

In the later phases of postoperative antibiotic treatment of serious intra-abdominal infection, the absence of an elevated WBC count, lack of band forms of PMNs on peripheral smear, and lack of fever ($<100.5°F$) provide close to complete assurance that infection has been eradicated.[27] Under these circumstances, antibiotics can be discontinued with impunity. However, the presence of one or more of these indicators does not mandate continuing antibiotics or altering the antibiotic(s) administered. Rather, a search for an extra-abdominal source of infection or a residual or ongoing source of intra-abdominal infection (e.g., abscess or leaking anastomosis) should be sought, the latter mandating maneuvers to effect source control.

Allergy to antimicrobial agents must be considered prior to prescribing them. First, it is important to ascertain whether a patient has had any type of allergic reaction in association with administration of a particular antibiotic. However, one should take care to ensure that the purported reaction consists of true allergic symptoms and signs, such as urticaria, bronchospasm, or other similar manifestations, rather than indigestion or nausea. Penicillin allergy is quite common, the reported incidence ranging from 0.7 to 10%. Although avoiding the use of any beta-lactam drug is appropriate in patients who manifest significant allergic reactions to penicillins, the incidence of cross-reactivity appears highest for carbapenems, much lower for cephalosporins (~5 to 7%), and extremely small or nonexistent for monobactams.

Severe allergic manifestations to a specific class of agents, such as anaphylaxis, generally preclude the use of any agents in that class, except under circumstances in which use of a certain drug represents a lifesaving measure. In some centers, patients undergo intradermal testing using a dilute solution of a particular antibiotic to determine whether a severe allergic reaction would be elicited by parenteral administration, although this type of testing is rarely employed because it is simpler to select an alternative class of agent. Should administration of a specific agent to which the patient is allergic become necessary, desensitization using progressively higher doses of antibiotic can be undertaken, providing the initial testing does not cause severe allergic manifestations.

Misuse of antimicrobial agents is rampant in the inpatient and outpatient setting, and is associated with an enormous financial impact on health care costs, adverse reactions due to drug toxicity and allergy, the occurrence of new infections such as *Clostridium difficile* colitis, and the development of multiagent drug resistance among nosocomial pathogens. Each of these factors has been directly correlated with overall drug administration. It has been estimated that in the United States, in excess of $20 billion is spent on antibiotics each year, and the appearance of so-called "super bugs"—microbes sensitive to few if any agents—has been sobering.[28] The responsible practitioner limits prophylaxis to the period during the operative procedure, does not convert prophylaxis into empiric therapy except under well-defined conditions, sets the duration of antibiotic therapy from the outset, curtails antibiotic administration when clinical and microbiologic evidence does not support the presence of an infection, and limits therapy to a short course in every possible instance. The utility of prophylactic antibiotics to prevent infections related to thoracostomy tube insertion has been demonstrated,[29,30] but prolonged treatment while a thoracostomy tube remains in situ, or prolonged therapy of biliary, intra-abdominal, or abscess drain cultures is not to be condoned.

INFECTIONS OF SIGNIFICANCE IN SURGICAL PATIENTS

Surgical Site Infections

SSIs are infections of the tissues, organs, or spaces exposed by surgeons during performance of an invasive procedure. SSIs are classified into incisional and organ/space infections, and the former are further subclassified into superficial (limited to skin and subcutaneous tissue) and deep incisional categories.[31] The development of SSIs is related to three factors: (1) the degree of microbial contamination of the wound during surgery, (2) the duration of the procedure, and (3) host factors such as diabetes, malnutrition,

Table 5-7
Risk Factors for Development of Surgical Site Infections

Patient factors
    Older age
    Immunosuppression
    Obesity
    Diabetes mellitus
    Chronic inflammatory process
    Malnutrition
    Peripheral vascular disease
    Anemia
    Radiation
    Chronic skin disease
    Carrier state (e.g., chronic *Staphylococcus* carriage)
    Recent operation
Local factors
    Poor skin preparation
    Contamination of instruments
    Inadequate antibiotic prophylaxis
    Prolonged procedure
    Local tissue necrosis
    Hypoxia, hypothermia
Microbial factors
    Prolonged hospitalization (leading to nosocomial organisms)
    Toxin secretion
    Resistance to clearance (e.g., capsule formation)

obesity, immune suppression, and a number of other underlying disease states. Table 5-7 lists risk factors for development of SSIs. By definition, an incisional SSI has occurred if a surgical wound drains purulent material or if the surgeon judges it to be infected and opens it.

Surgical wounds are classified based on the presumed magnitude of the bacterial load at the time of surgery[32] (Table 5-8). *Clean wounds* (class I) include those in which no infection is present; only skin microflora potentially contaminate the wound, and no hollow viscus that contains microbes is entered. Class ID wounds are similar except that a prosthetic device (e.g., mesh or valve) is inserted. *Clean/contaminated wounds* (class II) include those in which a hollow viscus such as the respiratory, alimentary, or genitourinary tracts with indigenous bacterial flora is opened under controlled circumstances without significant spillage of contents. *Contaminated wounds* (class III) include open accidental wounds encountered early after injury, those with extensive introduction of bacteria into a normally sterile area of the body due to major breaks in sterile technique (e.g., open cardiac massage), gross spillage of viscus contents such as from the intestine, or incision through inflamed,

Table 5-8
Wound Class, Representative Procedures, and Expected Infection Rates

Wound Class	Examples of Cases	Expected Infection Rates
Clean (class I)	Hernia repair, breast biopsy	1.0–5.4%
Clean/contaminated (class II)	Cholecystectomy, elective GI surgery	2.1–9.5%
Contaminated (class III)	Penetrating abdominal trauma, large tissue injury, enterotomy during bowel obstruction	3.4–13.2%
Dirty (class IV)	Perforated diverticulitis, necrotizing soft tissue infections	3.1–12.8%

albeit nonpurulent, tissue. *Dirty wounds* (class IV) include traumatic wounds in which a significant delay in treatment has occurred and in which necrotic tissue is present, those created in the presence of overt infection as evidenced by the presence of purulent material, and those created to access a perforated viscus accompanied by a high degree of contamination. The microbiology of SSIs is reflective of the initial host microflora such that SSIs following creation of a class I wound are invariable, due solely to skin microbes found on that portion of the body, while SSIs subsequent to a class II wound created for the purpose of elective colon resection may be caused by either skin microbes or colonic microflora, or both.

In the United States, hospitals are required to conduct surveillance for the development of SSIs for a period of 30 days after the operative procedure.[33] Such surveillance has been associated with greater awareness and a reduction in SSI rates, probably in large part based upon the impact of observation and promotion of adherence to appropriate care standards. Several different SSI risk stratification schemes have been developed via retrospective, multivariate analysis of large surveillance data sets. The National Nosocomial Infection Surveillance (NNIS) risk index is commonly used and assesses three factors: (1) American Society of Anesthesiologists (ASA) Physical Status score >2, (2) class III/IV wound, and (3) duration of operation greater than the 75th percentile for that particular procedure, to refine the risk of infection beyond that achieved by use of wound classification alone. Intriguingly, the risk of SSIs for class I wounds varies from approximately 1 to 2% for patients with low NNIS scores, to approximately 15% for patients with high NNIS scores (e.g., long operations and/or high ASA scores), and it seems clear that additional refinements are required.[34]

SSIs are associated with considerable morbidity and occasional lethality, as well as substantial health care costs and patient inconvenience and dissatisfaction.[35] For that reason, surgeons strive to avoid SSIs by using the maneuvers described in the previous section. Also, the use of prophylactic antibiotics may serve to reduce the incidence of SSI rates during certain types of procedures. For example, it is well accepted that a single dose of an antimicrobial agent should be administered immediately prior to commencing surgery for class ID, II, III, and IV types of wounds.[36] It seems reasonable that this practice should be extended to patients in any category with high NNIS scores, although this remains to be proven. Thus the utility of prophylactic antibiotics in reducing the rate of wound infection subsequent to clean surgery remains controversial, and these agents should not be employed under routine circumstances (e.g., in healthy young patients). However, because of the potential dire consequences of a wound infection after clean surgery in which prosthetic material is implanted into tissue, patients who undergo such procedures should receive a single preoperative dose of an antibiotic. Administration guidelines for prophylactic antibiotics are noted above.

Surgical management of the wound is also a critical determinant of the propensity to develop an SSI. In healthy individuals, class I and II wounds may be closed primarily, while skin closure of class III and IV wounds is associated with high rates of incisional SSIs (~25 to 50%). The superficial aspects of these latter types of wounds should be packed open and allowed to heal by secondary intention, although selective use of delayed primary closure has been associated with a reduction in incisional SSI rates.[37] It remains to be determined whether NNIS-type stratification schemes can be employed prospectively in order to target specific subgroups of patients who will benefit from the use of prophylactic antibiotic and/or specific wound management techniques. One clear example based on cogent data from clinical trials is that class III wounds in healthy patients undergoing appendectomy for perforated or gangrenous appendicitis can be primarily closed as long as antibiotic therapy directed against aerobes and anaerobes is administered. This practice leads to SSI rates of approximately 3 to 4%.[38]

Recent investigations have studied the effect of additional maneuvers in an attempt to further reduce the rate of SSIs. The adverse effects of hyperglycemia on white blood cell function have been well described.[39] A number of recent studies have reported the effects of hyperglycemia in vivo in diabetic patients, with increased SSI rates being associated with hyperglycemia in cardiac surgery patients undergoing bypass.[40,41] On this basis, it is recommended that clinicians maintain appropriate blood sugar control in diabetic patients in the perioperative period to minimize the occurrence of SSIs.

The effects of the level of inhaled oxygen and prewarming of the wound on SSI rates also have been studied. Although an initial study provided evidence that patients who received high levels of inhaled oxygen during colorectal surgery developed fewer SSIs,[42] data to the contrary recently have been reported.[43] In another study, preoperative warming of the wound site for 30 minutes prior to surgery among patients undergoing clean surgery was associated with a decrease in SSIs (5% with warmed wounds vs. 14% without).[44] Unfortunately, several of the aforementioned studies report SSI rates among study patients that are higher than those reported and expected among similar groups of patients, making comparison difficult. Of note, stratification using the NNIS classification methodology was not employed. Further evaluation via multicenter studies is needed prior to implementation of these modalities as standard therapies.

Effective therapy for incisional SSIs consists solely of incision and drainage without the addition of antibiotics. Antibiotic therapy is reserved for patients in whom evidence of severe cellulitis is present, or who manifest concurrent sepsis syndrome. The open wound often is allowed to heal by secondary intention, with dressings being changed twice a day. The use of topical antibiotics and antiseptics to further wound healing remains unproven, although anecdotal studies indicate their potential utility in complex wounds that do not heal with routine measures.[45] Although culture results are of epidemiologic interest, they rarely serve to direct therapy because antibiotics are not routinely withheld until results are known. The treatment of organ/space infections is discussed in the following section.

Intra-Abdominal Infections

Microbial contamination of the peritoneal cavity is termed *peritonitis* or *intra-abdominal infection,* and is classified according to etiology. *Primary microbial peritonitis* occurs when microbes invade the normally sterile confines of the peritoneal cavity via hematogenous dissemination from a distant source of infection or direct inoculation. This process is more common among patients who retain large amounts of peritoneal fluid due to ascites, and in those individuals who are being treated for renal failure via peritoneal dialysis. These infections invariably are monomicrobial and rarely require surgical intervention. The diagnosis is established based on identification of risk factors as noted above, physical examination that reveals diffuse tenderness and guarding without localized findings, absence of pneumoperitoneum on abdominal flat plate and upright roentgenograms, the presence of more than 100 WBCs/mL, and microbes with a single morphology on Gram's stain performed on fluid obtained via paracentesis. Subsequent cultures will demonstrate the presence of *E. coli, K. pneumoniae,* pneumococci, streptococci, enterococci, or *C. albicans,* although many different pathogens can be causative. Treatment consists of administration of an antibiotic to which the organism is sensitive; often 14 to 21 days of therapy

are required. Removal of indwelling devices (e.g., peritoneal dialysis catheter or peritoneovenous shunt) may be required for effective therapy of recurrent infections.

Secondary microbial peritonitis occurs subsequent to contamination of the peritoneal cavity due to perforation or severe inflammation and infection of an intra-abdominal organ. Examples include appendicitis, perforation of any portion of the gastrointestinal tract, or diverticulitis. As noted previously, effective therapy requires source control to resect the diseased organ; débridement of necrotic, infected tissue and debris; and administration of antimicrobial agents directed against aerobes and anaerobes.[46] This type of antibiotic regimen should be chosen because in most patients the precise diagnosis cannot be established until exploratory laparotomy is performed, and the most morbid form of this disease process is colonic perforation, due to the large number of microbes present. A combination of agents or single agents with a broad spectrum of activity can be used for this purpose; conversion of a parenteral to an oral regimen when the patient's ileus resolves provides results similar to those achieved with intravenous antibiotics.[47] Effective source control and antibiotic therapy is associated with low failure rates and a mortality rate of approximately 5 to 6%; inability to control the source of infection leads to mortality greater than 40%.[48]

The response rate to effective source control and use of appropriate antibiotics has remained approximately 70 to 90% over the past several decades.[23,49,50] Patients in whom standard therapy fails develop an intra-abdominal abscess, leakage from a gastrointestinal anastomosis leading to postoperative peritonitis, or *tertiary (persistent) peritonitis.* The latter is a poorly understood entity that is more common in immunosuppressed patients in whom peritoneal host defenses do not effectively clear or sequester the initial secondary microbial peritoneal infection. Microbes such as *Enterococcus faecalis* and *faecium, Staphylococcus epidermidis, C. albicans,* and *Pseudomonas aeruginosa* can be identified, typically in combination, and may be selected based on their lack of responsiveness to the initial antibiotic regimen, coupled with diminished activity of host defenses. Unfortunately, even with effective antimicrobial agent therapy, this disease process is associated with mortality rates in excess of 50%.[51,52]

Formerly, the presence of an intra-abdominal abscess mandated surgical reexploration and drainage. Today, the vast majority of such abscesses can be effectively diagnosed via abdominal computed tomographic (CT) imaging techniques and drained percutaneously. Surgical intervention is reserved for those individuals who harbor multiple abscesses, those with abscesses in proximity to vital structures such that percutaneous drainage would be hazardous, and those in whom an ongoing source of contamination (e.g., enteric leak) is identified. The necessity of antimicrobial agent therapy and precise guidelines that dictate duration of catheter drainage have not been established. A short course (3 to 7 days) of antibiotics that possess aerobic and anaerobic activity seems reasonable, and most practitioners leave the drainage catheter in situ until it is clear that cavity collapse has occurred, output is less than 10 to 20 mL/d, no evidence of an ongoing source of contamination is present, and the patient's clinical condition has improved.

Organ-Specific Infections

Hepatic abscesses are rare, currently accounting for approximately 15 per 100,000 hospital admissions in the United States. Pyogenic abscesses account for approximately 80% of cases, the remaining 20% being equally divided among parasitic and fungal forms.[53] Formerly, pyogenic liver abscesses were caused by pylephlebitis due to neglected appendicitis or diverticulitis. Today, manipulation of the biliary tract to treat a variety of diseases has become a more common cause, although in nearly 50% of patients no cause is identified. The most common aerobic bacteria identified in recent series include *E. coli, K. pneumoniae,* and other enteric bacilli, enterococci, and *Pseudomonas* spp., while the most common anaerobic bacteria are *Bacteroides* spp., anaerobic streptococci, and *Fusobacterium* spp. *Candida albicans* and other similar yeasts cause the majority of fungal hepatic abscesses. Small (<1 cm), multiple abscesses should be sampled and treated with a 4- to 6-week course of antibiotics. Larger abscesses invariably are amenable to percutaneous drainage, with parameters for antibiotic therapy and drain removal similar to those mentioned above. Splenic abscesses are extremely rare and are treated in a similar fashion. Recurrent hepatic or splenic abscesses may require operative intervention—unroofing and marsupialization or splenectomy, respectively.

Secondary pancreatic infections (e.g., infected pancreatic necrosis or pancreatic abscess) occur in approximately 10 to 15% of patients who develop severe hemorrhagic pancreatitis. The surgical treatment of this disorder was pioneered by Bradley and Allen, who noted significant improvements in outcome for patients undergoing repeated pancreatic débridement of infected pancreatic necrosis.[54] Current care of patients with severe acute pancreatitis includes staging with dynamic, contrast-enhanced helical CT scan with 3-mm tomographs to determine the extent of pancreatic necrosis, coupled with the use of one of several prognostic scoring systems. Patients who exhibit significant pancreatic necrosis (grade >C, Fig. 5-2) should be carefully monitored in the ICU and undergo follow-up

CT examination. The weight of current evidence also favors administration of empiric antibiotic therapy to reduce the incidence and severity of secondary pancreatic infection, which typically occurs several weeks after the initial episode of pancreatitis.[55] Several randomized, prospective trials have demonstrated a decrease in the rate of infection and mortality using agents such as carbapenems or fluoroquinolones that achieve high pancreatic tissue levels.[56–58]

In two small studies, enteral feedings initiated early, using nasojejunal feeding tubes placed past the ligament of Treitz, have also been associated with decreased development of infected pancreatic necrosis, possibly due to a decrease in gut translocation of bacteria.[59,60] Recent guidelines support the practice of enteral alimentation in these patients, with the addition of parenteral nutrition if nutritional goals cannot be met by tube feedings alone.[61]

The presence of secondary pancreatic infection should be suspected in patients whose systemic inflammatory response (fever, elevated WBC count, or organ dysfunction) fails to resolve, or in those individuals who initially recuperate, only to develop sepsis syndrome 2 to 3 weeks later. CT-guided aspiration of fluid from the pancreatic bed for performance of Gram's stain and culture analysis is of critical importance. A positive Gram's stain or culture from CT-guided aspiration, or identification of gas within the pancreas on CT scan, mandate operative intervention.

Surgery for secondary pancreatic infection is designed to remove the infected inflammatory focus. It is the practice of the authors to expose the pancreatic bed through a transverse incision in the abdominal wall and lesser sac. A jejunal feeding tube, gastrostomy tube, and cholecystectomy (if indicated) are all performed at the index

FIG. 5-2. Contrast-enhanced CT scan of pancreas with severe pancreatic necrosis. Note the lack of intravenous contrast in the boggy pancreatic bed (*large black arrow*).

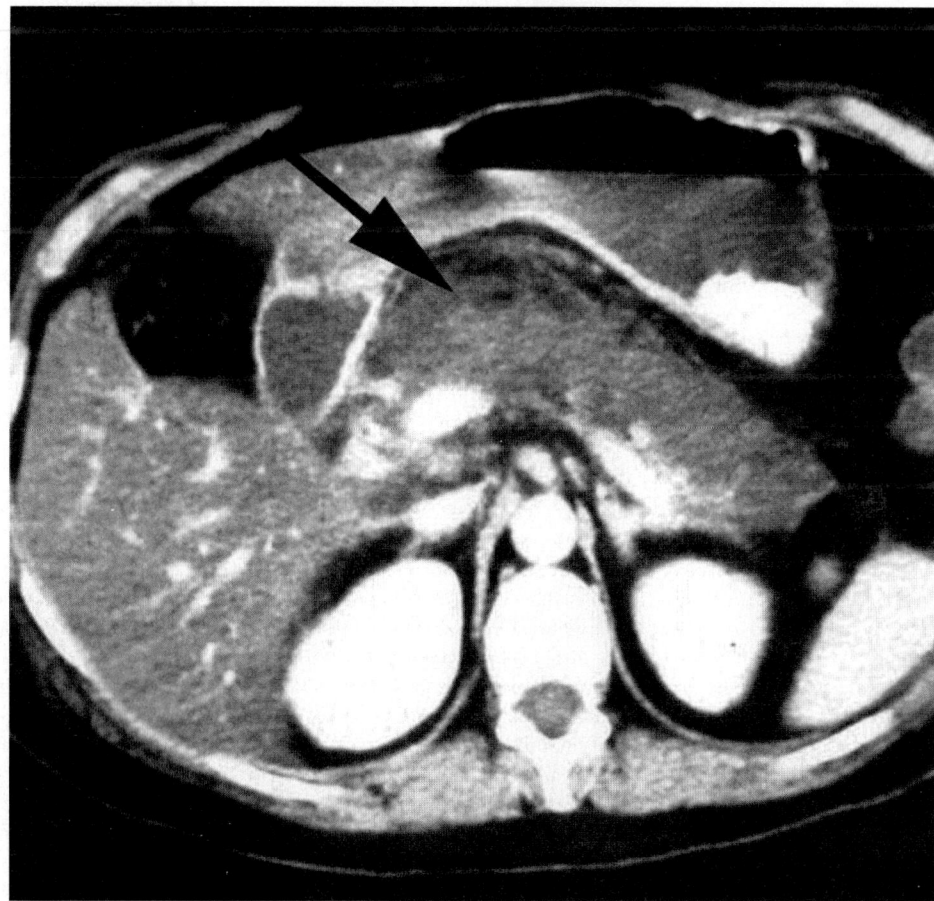

operation if patient condition permits. The gastrocolic omentum is tacked to the abdominal wall on the peritoneal edges of the wound in order to sequester the intestines from the inflammatory process. After initial gentle débridement of necrotic tissue, the pancreatic bed is packed with gauze dressings and the abdomen closed temporarily with a permanent mesh or packed open. This mesh allows repeated reoperations without damage to the remaining fascia. In a similar fashion to surgery for necrotizing soft tissue infection, the surgeon should plan on scheduled relaparotomy and undertake débridement until necrotic tissue and purulence are absent and granulation tissue forms. Approximately 20 to 25% of patients will develop a gastrointestinal fistula, which either heals or is amenable to surgical repair after resolution of the pancreatic infection.

Infections of the Skin and Soft Tissue

These infections can be classified according to whether or not surgical intervention is required. For example, superficial skin and skin structure infections such as cellulitis, erysipelas, and lymphangitis invariably are effectively treated with antibiotics alone, although a search for a local source of infection should be undertaken. Generally, drugs that possess activity against the gram-positive skin microflora that are causative are selected. Furuncles or boils may drain spontaneously or require surgical incision and drainage. Antibiotics are prescribed if significant cellulitis is present or if cellulitis does not rapidly resolve after surgical drainage.

Aggressive soft tissue infections are rare, difficult to diagnose, and require immediate surgical intervention plus administration of antimicrobial agents. Failure to do so results in an extremely high mortality rate (~80 to 100%), and even with rapid recognition and intervention, current mortality rates remain approximately 30 to 50%.[62,63] Eponyms and classification in the past have been a hodgepodge of terminology, such as Meleney's synergist gangrene, rapidly spreading cellulitis, gas gangrene, and necrotizing fasciitis, among others. Today it seems best to delineate these serious infections based on the soft tissue layer(s) of involvement (e.g., skin and superficial soft tissue, deep soft tissue, and muscle) and the pathogen(s) that cause them.[64]

Patients at risk for these types of infections include those who are elderly, immunosuppressed, or diabetic; those who suffer from peripheral vascular disease; or those with a combination of these factors. The common thread among these host factors appears to be compromise of the fascial blood supply to some degree, and if this is coupled with the introduction of exogenous microbes, the result can be devastating. However, it is of note that over the last decade, extremely aggressive necrotizing soft tissue infections among healthy individuals due to streptococci have been described as well.

Initially, the diagnosis is established solely upon a constellation of clinical findings, not all of which are present in every patient. Not surprisingly, patients often develop sepsis syndrome or septic shock without an obvious cause. The extremities, perineum, trunk, and torso are most commonly affected, in that order. Careful examination should be undertaken for an entry site such as a small break or sinus in the skin from which grayish, turbid semipurulent material ("dishwater pus") can be expressed, as well as for the presence of skin changes (bronze hue or brawny induration), blebs, or crepitus. The patient often develops pain at the site of infection that appears to be out of proportion to any of the physical manifestations. Any of these findings mandates immediate surgical intervention, which should consist of exposure and direct visualization of potentially infected tissue (including deep soft tissue, fascia, and underlying muscle) and radical resection of affected areas. Radiologic studies

should be undertaken only in patients in whom the diagnosis is not seriously considered, as they delay surgical intervention and frequently provide confusing information. Unfortunately, surgical extirpation of infected tissue frequently entails amputation and/or disfiguring procedures; however, incomplete procedures are associated with higher rates of morbidity and mortality (Fig. 5-3).

During the procedure a Gram's stain should be performed on tissue fluid. Antimicrobial agents directed against gram-positive and gram-negative aerobes and anaerobes (e.g., vancomycin plus a carbapenem), as well as high-dose aqueous penicillin G (16,000 to 20,000 U/d), the latter to treat clostridial pathogens, should be administered. Approximately 70 to 80% of such infections are polymicrobial, the remainder being caused by a single organism such as *Pseudomonas aeruginosa, Clostridium perfringens,* or *Streptococcus pyogenes.* The microbiology of these polymicrobial infections is similar to that of secondary microbial peritonitis, with the exception that gram-positive cocci are more commonly encountered. Most patients should be returned to the operating room on a scheduled basis to determine if disease progression has occurred. If so, additional resection of infected tissue and débridement should take place. Antibiotic therapy can be refined based on culture and sensitivity results, particularly in the case of monomicrobial soft tissue infections.

Postoperative Nosocomial Infections

Surgical patients are prone to develop a wide variety of nosocomial infections during the postoperative period, which include SSIs, UTIs, pneumonia, and bacteremic episodes.[65] SSIs are discussed above, and the latter types of nosocomial infections are related to prolonged use of indwelling tubes and catheters for the purpose of urinary drainage, ventilation, and venous and arterial access, respectively.

The presence of a postoperative UTI should be considered based on urinalysis demonstrating WBCs or bacteria, a positive test for leukocyte esterase, or a combination of these elements. The diagnosis is established after $>10^4$ CFU/mL of microbes are identified by culture techniques in symptomatic patients, or $>10^5$ CFU/mL in asymptomatic individuals. Treatment for 10 to 14 days with a single antibiotic that achieves high levels in the urine is appropriate. Postoperative surgical patients should have indwelling urinary catheters removed as quickly as possible, typically within 1 to 2 days, as long as they are mobile.

Prolonged mechanical ventilation is associated with an increased incidence of pneumonia, and is frequently due to pathogens common in the nosocomial environment.[66] Frequently these organisms are highly resistant to many different agents.[67] The diagnosis is established based on roentgenographic evidence of one or more areas of pulmonary consolidation. Consideration should be given to performing bronchoalveolar lavage to obtain samples to assess by Gram's stain and to performing a culture to assess for the presence of microbes. Surgical patients should be weaned from mechanical ventilation as soon as feasible, based on oxygenation and inspiratory effort.

Infection associated with indwelling intravascular catheters has become a common problem among hospitalized patients. Because of the complexity of many surgical procedures, these devices are increasingly used for physiologic monitoring, vascular access, drug delivery, and hyperalimentation. Among the several million catheters inserted each year in the United States, approximately 25% will become colonized, and approximately 5% will be associated with bacteremia. Prolonged insertion, insertion under emergency

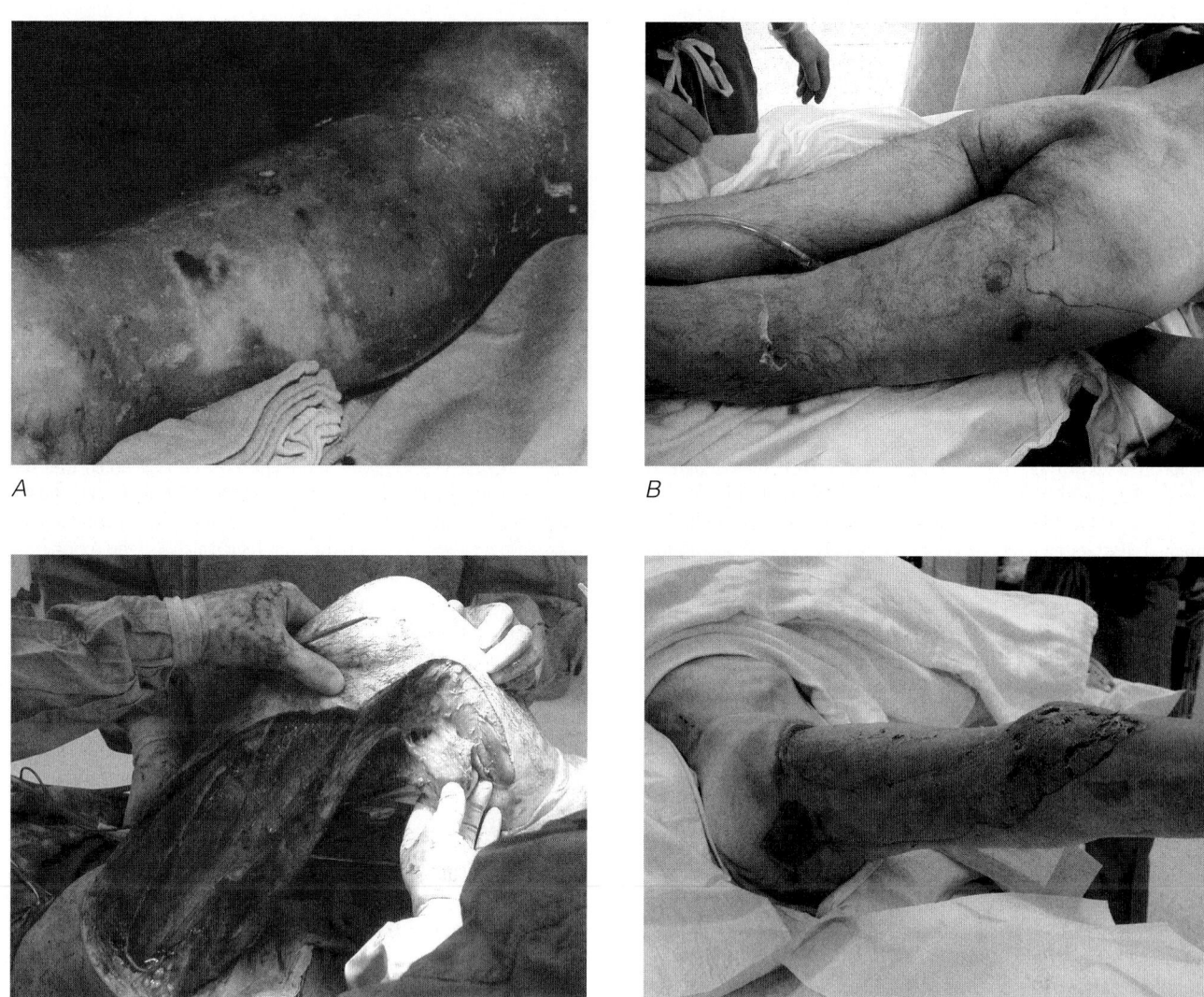

FIG. 5-3. Necrotizing soft tissue infection. *A. This patient has severe late necrotizing fasciitis and myositis due to beta-hemolytic streptococcal infection. The patient died 16 hours after the operation due to overwhelming infection despite aggressive débridement. B. This patient has necrotizing soft tissue infection involving the fascia secondary to E. coli infection prior to débridement. Note subtle skin changes involving the posterior thigh. C. This shows patient B during initial débridement, demonstrating the need to débride all involved tissue. In this patient, débridement was carried down to viable muscle. D. This shows patient B several weeks later after skin grafting.*

conditions, manipulation under nonsterile conditions, and perhaps the use of multilumen catheters increase the risk of infection.[68]

Many patients who develop intravascular catheter infections are asymptomatic, often exhibiting an elevation in the blood WBC count. Blood cultures obtained from a peripheral site and drawn through the catheter that reveal the presence of the same organism increase the index of suspicion for the presence of a catheter infection. Obvious purulence at the exit site of the skin tunnel, severe sepsis syndrome due to any type of organism when other potential causes have been excluded, or bacteremia due to gram-negative aerobes or fungi should lead to catheter removal. Selected catheter infections due to low-virulence microbes such as *Staphylococcus epidermidis* can be effectively treated in approximately 50 to 60% of patients with a 14- to 21-day course of an antibiotic, which should be considered when no other vascular access site exists.[69] The use of antibiotic-bonded catheters is associated with lower rates of

colonization, but their expense has precluded widespread use.[70–72] Routine, scheduled catheter changes over a guidewire are associated with slightly lower rates of infection, but an increase in the insertion-related complication rate.[73] The surgeon should carefully consider the need for any type of vascular access device, rigorously attend to their maintenance to prevent infection, and remove them as quickly as possible. Use of antibacterial or antifungal agents to prevent catheter infection is of no utility and is contraindicated.

Sepsis Syndrome

A number of studies have demonstrated the importance of empiric antimicrobial agent therapy in patients who develop severe sepsis syndrome and subsequently are found to have developed bacteremia, concurrent with fluid resuscitation, metabolic support, and control of any site-specific source of infection, leading to secondary bacteremic events. Use of institutional and unit-specific sensitivity patterns and knowledge of likely pathogens are critical in selecting an appropriate agent for the treatment of presumed bacteremia. Retrospective reviews demonstrate that appropriate therapy is associated with a two- to threefold reduction in mortality.[74–77] A number of new therapies for treatment of patients with severe sepsis have recently been demonstrated to be of significant benefit in patients with severe sepsis or septic shock.

Over the past several decades, a series of clinical trials have examined the effect of a number of different agents [e.g., antiendotoxin monoclonal antibodies (MABs), IL-1ra, and anti-TNF-α MABs] upon outcome during severe sepsis. Until recently, no agent has shown efficacy. Drotracogin alpha (activated), also known as Xigris, is a recombinant form of human-activated protein C. The use of this agent in a series of patients with sepsis syndrome has been associated with a 6% overall reduction in mortality (31 to 25%, $p = 0.005$).[78] This agent has been demonstrated to have antithrombotic, profibrinolytic, and anti-inflammatory properties, although the specific mechanism of action remains to be established. Further analysis of the surgical cohort of patients in this study has demonstrated the benefit of this agent without incurring an increased risk of hemorrhage.[79] The use of this agent should be considered in patients with severe infection who have completed their source control procedure, and who develop severe sepsis with at least one organ failing. Current recommendations are a dose of 24 μg/kg per hour given for 96 hours. The infusion should be interrupted for procedures or surgery, or for significant life-threatening bleeding.

A number of investigators have revisited the issue of corticosteroids for the treatment of septic shock. High-dose corticosteroid therapy had been previously investigated in the late 1980s and early 1990s with no evidence of benefit for septic patients. Recent interest has arisen for the use of corticosteroids in patients presenting to the ICU in septic shock subsequent to the observation that many patients in this state harbor adrenal insufficiency.[80] A number of randomized, controlled trials have demonstrated the benefit of replacement doses of corticosteroids in patients with severe shock states.[81,82] In patients who develop septic shock, currently we initiate low-dose hydrocortisone (100 mg/8 h) after performing a corticotropin stimulation test (baseline cortisol level, corticotropin 250 μg intravenously, cortisol level 1 hour later). Adrenal insufficiency is identified if the baseline cortisol level is less than 30 μg/dL, or if an increase of less than 9 μg/dL occurs after corticotropin stimulation. Low-dose steroid therapy should be discontinued in patients with normal adrenal function.

Blood-Borne Pathogens

While alarming to contemplate, the risk of human immunodeficiency virus (HIV) transmission from patient to surgeon is low. By December 31, 2001, there had been six cases of surgeons with HIV seroconversion from a possible occupational exposure, from a total of 469,850 HIV cases to that date reported to the Centers for Disease Control and Prevention (CDC). Of the groups of health care workers with likely occupationally acquired HIV infection (n = 195), surgeons were one of the lower risk groups (compared to nurses at 59 cases and nonsurgeon physicians at 18 cases).[83] Transmission of HIV (and other infections spread by blood and body fluid) from patient to health care worker can be minimized by observation of universal precautions, which include the following: (1) routine use of barriers (such as gloves and/or goggles) when anticipating contact with blood or body fluids, (2) washing of hands and other skin surfaces immediately after contact with blood or body fluids, and

(3) careful handling and disposal of sharp instruments during and after use.

Postexposure prophylaxis for HIV has significantly decreased the risk of seroconversion for health care workers with occupational exposure to HIV. Steps to initiate postexposure prophylaxis should be initiated within hours rather than days for the most effective preventive therapy. Postexposure prophylaxis with a two- or three-drug regimen should be initiated for health care workers with significant exposure to patients with an HIV-positive status. If a patient's HIV status is unknown, it may be advisable to begin postexposure prophylaxis while testing is carried out, particularly if the patient is at high risk for infection due to HIV (e.g., intravenous narcotic use). Generally, postexposure prophylaxis is not warranted for exposure to sources with unknown status, such as deceased persons or needles from a sharps container.

The risks for surgeons of acquiring HIV infection have recently been evaluated by Goldberg and coauthors.[84] They noted that the risks are related to the prevalence of HIV infection in the population being cared for, the probability of transmission from a percutaneous injury suffered while caring for an infected patient, the number of such injuries sustained, and the use of postexposure prophylaxis. Annual calculated risks in Glasgow, Scotland, ranged from one in 200,000 for general surgeons not utilizing postexposure prophylaxis to as low as one in 10,000,000 with use of routine postexposure prophylaxis after significant exposures.

Hepatitis B virus (HBV) is a DNA virus that only affects humans. Primary infection with HBV generally is self-limited ($\sim$6% of those infected are over 5 years of age), but can progress to a chronic carrier state. Death from chronic liver disease or hepatocellular cancer occurs in roughly 30% of chronically infected persons. Surgeons and other health care workers are at high risk for this blood-borne infection and should receive the HBV vaccine; children are routinely vaccinated in the United States.[85] This vaccine has contributed to a significant decline in the number of new cases of HBV per year in the United States, from approximately 250,000 in the 1980s to approximately 78,000 in 2001.[86] In the postexposure setting, hepatitis B immune globulin (HBIG) confers approximately 75% protection from HBV infection.[87]

Hepatitis C virus (HCV), previously known as non-A, non-B hepatitis, is a RNA flavivirus first identified specifically in the late 1980s. This virus is confined to humans and chimpanzees. A chronic carrier state develops in 75 to 80% of patients with the infection, with chronic liver disease occurring in three-fourths of patients developing chronic infection. The number of new infections per year has declined since the 1980s due to the incorporation of testing of the blood supply for this virus. Fortunately, HCV virus is not transmitted efficiently through occupational exposures to blood, with the seroconversion rate after accidental needlestick reported to be approximately 2%.[88]

To date, a vaccine to prevent HCV infection has not been developed. Experimental studies in chimpanzees with HCV immunoglobulin using a model of needlestick injury have failed to demonstrate a protective effect of this treatment in seroconversion after exposure, and no effective antiviral agents for postexposure prophylaxis are available. Early treatment of infection with interferon-α has been considered; however, this exposes patients who may not develop HCV infection–related sequelae to the side effects of this drug.[89]

Biologic Warfare Agents

Several infectious organisms have been studied by the United States and the former Soviet Union and presumably other entities for potential use as biologic weapons. Programs involving biologic agents in the United States were halted by presidential decree in 1971. However, concern remains that these agents could be used by rogue states or terrorist organizations as alternatives to nuclear weapons as weapons of mass destruction, as they are relatively inexpensive to make in terms of infrastructure development. If so, all physicians including surgeons would need to familiarize themselves with the manifestations of infection due to these pathogens. The typical agent is selected for the ability to be spread via the inhalational route, as this is the most efficient mode of mass exposure. Some potential agents are discussed in the following sections.

Bacillus Anthracis (Anthrax)

Anthrax is a zoonotic disease occurring in domesticated and wild herbivores. The first identification of inhalational anthrax as a disease occurred among woolsorters in England in the late 1800s. The largest recent epidemic of inhalational anthrax occurred in Sverdlovsk, Russia, in 1979 after accidental release of anthrax spores from a military facility. Inhalational anthrax develops after a 1- to 6-day incubation period, with nonspecific symptoms including malaise, myalgia, and fever. Over a short period of time, these symptoms worsen, with development of respiratory distress, chest pain, and diaphoresis. Characteristic chest roentgenographic findings include a widened mediastinum and pleural effusions. A key aspect in establishing the diagnosis is eliciting an exposure history. Rapid antigen tests are currently under development for identification of this gram-positive rod. Drugs such as cephalosporins and trimethoprim-sulfamethoxazole are not active against this agent. Postexposure prophylaxis consists of administration of either ciprofloxacin or doxycycline.[90] If an isolate is demonstrated to be penicillin-sensitive, the patient should be switched to amoxicillin. Inhalational exposure followed by the development of symptoms is associated with a high mortality rate. Treatment options include combination therapy with ciprofloxacin, clindamycin, and rifampin, with clindamycin added to block production of toxin, and rifampin for its ability to penetrate the central nervous system and intracellular locations.

Yersinia Pestis (Plague)

Plague is caused by the gram-negative organism Yersinia pestis. The naturally occurring disease in humans is transmitted via flea bites from rodents. It was the first biologic warfare agent, and was used in the Crimean city of Caffa by the Tartar army, whose soldiers catapulted bodies of plague victims at the Genoese. When plague is used as a biologic warfare agent, clinical manifestations include epidemic pneumonia with blood-tinged sputum if aerosolized bacteria were used, or bubonic plague if fleas were used as carriers. Individuals who develop a painful lesion termed a "bubo" associated with fever, severe malaise, and exposure to fleas should be suspected to have plague. Diagnosis is confirmed via aspirate of the bubo and a direct antibody stain to detect plague bacillus. Typical morphology for this organism is that of a bipolar safety-pin–shaped gram-negative organism. Postexposure prophylaxis for patients exposed to plague consists of doxycycline. Treatment of the pneumonic or bubonic/septicemic form includes administration of aminoglycosides, doxycycline, ciprofloxacin, and chloramphenicol.[91]

Smallpox

Variola, the causative agent of smallpox, was a major cause of infectious morbidity and mortality until its eradication in the late 1970s. During the European colonization of North America, British commanders may have used it against native inhabitants and the colonists by distribution of blankets from smallpox victims. Even in the absence of laboratory-preserved virus, the prolonged viability of variola virus has been demonstrated in scabs up to 13 years after collection; the potential for reverse genetic engineering using the known sequence of smallpox also makes it a potential biologic weapon.[92] This has resulted in the United States undertaking a vaccination program for key health care workers. Variola virus is highly infectious in the aerosolized form: after an incubation period of 10 to 12 days, clinical manifestations of malaise, fever, vomiting, and headache appear, followed by development of a characteristic centripetal rash (which is found to predominate on the face and extremities). The fatality rate may reach 30%. Postexposure prophylaxis with smallpox vaccine has been noted to be effective for up to 4 days postexposure. Cidofovir, an acyclic nucleoside phosphonate analogue, has demonstrated activity in animal models of poxvirus infections and may offer promise for the treatment of smallpox.[93]

Francisella Tularensis (Tularemia)

The principal reservoir of this gram-negative aerobic organism is the tick. After inoculation, this organism proliferates within macrophages. This organism has been considered a potential bioterrorist threat due to a very high infectivity rate after aerosolization. Patients with tularemia pneumonia develop a cough and demonstrate pneumonia on chest roentgenogram. Enlarged lymph nodes are seen in approximately 85% of patients. The organism can be cultured from tissue samples, but this is difficult. Alternative diagnosis is based on acute-phase agglutination tests. Treatment of inhalational tularemia consists of administration of aminoglycosides or second-line agents such as doxycycline and ciprofloxacin.

References

1. Nuland SB: *The Doctors' Plague: Germs, Childbed Fever, and the Strange Story of Ignaz Semmelweis.* New York: WW Norton & Co., 2003, p 1.
2. Wangensteen OH, Wangensteen SD: Germ theory of infection and disease, in Wangensteen OH, Wangensteen SD: *The Rise of Surgery. From Empiric Craft to Scientific Discipline.* Minneapolis: University of Minnesota Press, 1978, p 387.
3. Rutkow E: Appendicitis: The quintessential American surgical disease. *Arch Surg* 133:1024, 1998.
4. Meleney F: Bacterial synergism in disease processes with confirmation of synergistic bacterial etiology of certain types of progressive gangrene of the abdominal wall. *Ann Surg* 94:961, 1931.
5. Altemeier WA: *Manual of Control of Infection in Surgical Patients.* Chicago: American College of Surgeons Press, 1976, p 1.
6. Bartlett JG: Intra-abdominal sepsis. *Med Clin North Am* 79:599, 1995.
7. Dunn DL, Simmons RL: The role of anaerobic bacteria in intra-abdominal infections. *Rev Infect Dis* 6:S139, 1984.
8. Osler W: *The Evolution of Modern Medicine.* New Haven, CT: Yale University Press, 1913, p 1.
9. Dunn DL: Autochthonous microflora of the gastrointestinal tract. *Perspect Colon Rectal Surg* 2:105, 1990.
10. Dunn DL, Meakins JL: Humoral immunity to infection and the complement system, in: Howard RJ, Simmons RL, (eds): *Surgical Infectious Diseases,* 3rd ed. Norwalk, CT: Appleton & Lange, 1995, p 295.
11. Hack C, Aarden LA, Thijs LG: Role of cytokines in sepsis. *Adv Immunol* 66:101, 1997.
12. Levy MM, Fink MP, Marshall JC, et al: 2001 SCCM/ESICM/ACCP/ ATS/SIS International Sepsis Definitions Conference. *Crit Care Med* 31:1250, 2003.
13. Angus DC, Linde-Zwirble WT, Lidicer J, et al: Epidemiology of severe sepsis in the United States. *Crit Care Med* 29:1303, 2001.
14. Marshall JC, Cook DJ, Christou NV, et al: Multiple organ dysfunction score: A reliable descriptor of a complex clinical outcome. *Crit Care Med* 23:1638, 1995.

15. Ferreira FL, Bota DP, Bross A, et al: Serial evaluation of the SOFA score to predict outcome in critically ill patients. *JAMA* 286:1754, 2002.

16. Valles J, Rello J, Ochagavia A, et al : Community-acquired bloodstream infection in critically ill patients. *Chest* 123:1615, 2003.

17. Dunn DL: The biological rationale, in Schein M, Marshall JC (eds): *Source Control. A Guide to the Management of Surgical Infections.* New York: Springer-Verlag, 2003, p 9.

18. Rozycki GS, Tremblay L, Feliciano DV, et al: Three hundred consecutive emergent celiotomies in general surgery patients: Influence of advanced diagnostic imaging techniques and procedures on diagnosis. *Ann Surg* 235:681, 2002.

19. Cappendijk VC, Hazebroek FW: The impact of diagnostic delay on the course of acute appendicitis. *Arch Dis Child* 83:64, 2000.

20. Lee SL, Walsh AJ, Ho HS: Computed tomography and ultrasonography do not improve and may delay the diagnosis and treatment of acute appendicitis. *Arch Surg* 136:556, 2001.

21. Nichols RL, Smith JW, Garcia RY, et al: Current practices of preoperative bowel preparation among North American colorectal surgeons. *Clin Infect Dis* 24:609, 1997.

22. Tang R, Chen HH, Wang YL, et al : Risk factors for surgical site infection after elective resection of the colon and rectum: A single-center prospective study of 2809 consecutive patients. *Ann Surg* 234:181, 2001.

23. Solomkin JS, Meakins JL Jr., Allo MD, et al: Antibiotic trials in intra-abdominal infections. A critical evaluation of study design and outcome reporting. *Ann Surg* 200:29, 1984.

24. Barie PS: Modern surgical antibiotic prophylaxis and therapy—less is more. *Surg Infect* 1:23, 2000.

25. Bossink AW, Groeneveld J, Hack CE, et al: Prediction of mortality in febrile medical patients: How useful are systemic inflammatory response syndrome and sepsis criteria? *Chest* 113:1533, 1998.

26. Bohnen JM: Duration of antibiotic treatment in surgical infections of the abdomen. Postoperative peritonitis. *Eur J Surg* 576:50, 1996.

27. Stone HH, Bourneuf AA, Stinson LD: Reliability of criteria for predicting persistent or recurrent sepsis. *Arch Surg* 120:17, 1985.

28. Turnidge J: Impact of antibiotic resistance on the treatment of sepsis. *Scand J Infect Dis* 35:677, 2003.

29. Nichols RL, Smith JW, Muzik AC, et al: Preventive antibiotic usage in traumatic thoracic injuries requiring closed tube thoracostomy. *Chest* 106:1493, 1994.

30. Gonzalez RP, Holevar MR: Role of prophylactic antibiotics for tube thoracostomy in chest trauma. *Am Surg* 64:617, 1998.

31. Mangram AJ, Horan TC, Pearson ML, et al: Guideline for prevention of surgical site infection, 1999. Hospital Infection Control Practices Advisory Committee. *Infect Control Hosp Epidemiol* 20:250, 1999.

32. Martone WJ, Nichols RL: Recognition, prevention, surveillance, and management of surgical site infections. *Clin Infect Dis* 33:S67, 2001.

33. Weiss CA 3rd, Statz CL, Dahms RA, et al: Six years of surgical wound infection surveillance at a tertiary care center: Review of the microbiologic and epidemiological aspects of 20,007 wounds. *Arch Surg* 134:1041, 1999.

34. Roy MC, Herwaldt LA, Embrey R, et al: Does the Centers for Disease Control's NNIS system risk index stratify patients undergoing cardiothoracic operations by their risk of surgical-site infection? *Infect Control Hosp Epidemiol* 21:186, 2000.

35. Perencevich EN, Sands KE, Cosgrove SE, et al: Health and economic impact of surgical site infections diagnosed after hospital discharge. *Emerg Infect Dis* 9:196, 2003.

36. Page CP, Bohnen JM, Fletcher JR, et al: Antimicrobial prophylaxis for surgical wounds. Guidelines for clinical care. *Arch Surg* 128:79, 1993.

37. Cohn SM, Giannotti G, Ong AW, et al: Prospective randomized trial of two wound management strategies for dirty abdominal wounds. *Ann Surg* 233:409, 2001.

38. Margenthaler JA, Longo WE, Virgo KS, et al: Risk factors for adverse outcomes after the surgical treatment of appendicitis in adults. *Ann Surg* 238:59, 2003.

39. McManus LM, Bloodworth RC, Prihoda TJ, et al: Agonist-dependent failure of neutrophil function in diabetes correlates with extent of hyperglycemia. *J Leukoc Biol* 70:395, 2001.

40. Trick WE, Scheckler WE, Tokars JI, et al: Modifiable risk factors associated with deep sternal site infection after coronary artery bypass grafting. *J Thorac Cardiovasc Surg* 119:108, 2000.

41. Russo PL, Spellman DW: A new surgical-site infection risk index using risk factors identified by multivariate analysis for patients undergoing coronary artery bypass graft surgery. *Infect Control Hosp Epidemiol* 23:372, 2002.

42. Greif R, Akca O, Horn EP, et al: Supplemental perioperative oxygen to reduce the incidence of wound infection. *N Engl J Med* 342:161, 2000.

43. Pryor KO, Fahey TJ 3rd, Lien CA, et al: Surgical site infection and the routine use of perioperative hyperoxia in a general surgical population: A randomized controlled trial. *JAMA* 291:79, 2004.

44. Melling AC, Ali B, Scott EM, et al: Effects of preoperative warming on the incidence of wound infection after clean surgery: A randomized controlled trial. *Lancet* 358:876, 2001.

45. Grubbs BC, Statz CL, Johnson EM, et al: Salvage therapy of open, infected surgical wounds: A retrospective review using Techni-Care. *Surg Infect* 1:109, 2000.

46. Solomkin JS, Mazuski JE, Baron EJ, et al: Infectious Diseases Society of America. Guidelines for the selection of anti-infective agents for complicated intra-abdominal infections. *Clin Infect Dis* 37:997, 2003.

47. Solomkin JS, Reinhart HH, Dellinger EP, et al: Results of a randomized trial comparing sequential intravenous/oral treatment with ciprofloxacin plus metronidazole to imipenem/cilastatin for intra-abdominal infections. The Intra-Abdominal Infection Study Group. *Ann Surg* 223:303, 1996.

48. Solomkin JS, Dellinger EP, Christou NV, et al: Results of a multicenter trial comparing imipenem/cilastatin to tobramycin/clindamycin for intra-abdominal infections. *Ann Surg* 212:58, 1990.

49. Solomkin JS, Yellin AE, Rotstein OD, et al: Protocol 017 Study Group. Ertapenem versus piperacillin/tazobactam in the treatment of complicated intra-abdominal infections: Results of a double-blind, randomized comparative phase III trial. *Ann Surg* 237:235, 2003.

50. Solomkin JS, Wilson SE, Christou NV, et al: Results of a clinical trial of clinafloxacin versus imipenem/cilastatin for intra-abdominal infections. *Ann Surg* 233:79, 2001.

51. Malangoni MA: Evaluation and management of tertiary peritonitis. *Am Surg* 66:157, 2000.

52. Evans HL, Raymond DP, Pelletier SJ, et al: Tertiary peritonitis is not an independent predictor of mortality in surgical patients with intra-abdominal infection. *Surg Infect* 2:255, 2001.

53. Leslie DB, Dunn DL: Hepatic abscess, in Cameron JL (ed): *Current Surgical Therapy,* 8th ed (In press).

54. Bradley EL III, Allen K: A prospective longitudinal study of observation versus surgical intervention in the management of necrotizing pancreatitis. *Am J Surg* 161:19, 1991.

55. Golub R, Siddiqi F, Pohl D: Role of antibiotics in acute pancreatitis: A metaanalysis. *J Gastrointest Surg* 2:496, 1998.

56. Pederzoli P, Bassi C, Vesentini S, et al: A randomized multicenter clinical trial of antibiotic prophylaxis of septic complications in acute necrotizing pancreatitis with imipenem. *Surg Gynecol Obstet* 176:480, 1993.

57. Delcenserie R, Yzet T, Ducroix JP: Prophylactic antibiotics in treatment of severe acute alcoholic pancreatitis. *Pancreas* 13:198, 1996.

58. Sainio V, Kemppainen E, Puolakkainen P, et al: Early antibiotic treatment in acute necrotising pancreatitis. *Lancet* 346:663, 1995.

59. Kalfarentzos F, Kehagias J, Mead N, et al: Enteral nutrition is superior to parenteral nutrition in severe acute pancreatitis: Results of a randomized prospective trial. *Br J Surg* 84:1665, 1997.

60. Windsor AC, Kanwar S, Li AG, et al: Compared with parenteral nutrition, enteral feeding attenuates the acute phase response and improves disease severity in acute pancreatitis. *Gut* 42:431, 1998.

61. Meier R, Beglinger C, Layer P, et al: ESPEN guidelines on nutrition in acute pancreatitis. European Society of Parenteral and Enteral Nutrition. *Clin Nutr* 21:173, 2002.

62. Bilton BD, Zibari GB, McMillan RW, et al: Aggressive surgical management of necrotizing fasciitis serves to decrease mortality: A retrospective study. *Am Surg* 64:397, 1998.

63. Malangoni MA: Necrotizing soft tissue infections: Are we making any progress? *Surg Infect* 2:145, 2001.

64. Sawyer MD, Dunn DL: Serious bacterial infections of the skin and soft tissues. *Curr Opin Infect Dis* 8:293, 1995.

65. National Nosocomial Infections Surveillance System: National Nosocomial Infections Surveillance (NNIS) System Report, data summary from January 1992 to June 2002. *Am J Infect Control* 30:458, 2002.

66. Kollef MH: Treatment of ventilator-associated pneumonia: Get it right from the start. *Crit Care Med* 31:969, 2003.

67. Hoffken G, Niederman MS: Nosocomial pneumonia: The importance of a de-escalating strategy for antibiotic treatment of pneumonia in the ICU. *Chest* 122:2183, 2002.

68. Bullard KM, Dunn DL: Diagnosis and treatment of bacteremia and intravascular catheter infections. *Am J Surg* 172:S13, 1996.

69. Marr KA, Sexton DJ, Conlon PJ, et al: Catheter-related bacteremia and outcome of attempted catheter salvage in patients undergoing hemodialysis. *Ann Intern Med* 127:275, 1997.

70. Maki DG, Stolz SM, Wheeler S, et al: Prevention of central venous catheter-related bloodstream infection by use of an antiseptic-impregnated catheter. A randomized, controlled trial. *Ann Intern Med* 127:257, 1997.

71. Raad I, Darouiche R, Dupuis J, et al: Central venous catheters coated with minocycline and rifampin for the prevention of catheter-related colonization and bloodstream infections. A randomized, double-blind trial. *Ann Intern Med* 127:267, 1997.

72. Darouiche RO, Raad II, Heard SO, et al: A comparison of two antimicrobial-impregnated central venous catheters. *N Engl J Med* 340:1, 1999.

73. Cobb D, High KP, Sawyer RG, et al: A controlled trial of scheduled replacement of central venous and pulmonary-artery catheters. *N Engl J Med* 327:1062, 1992.

74. McCue JD: Improved mortality in gram-negative bacillary bacteremia. *Arch Intern Med* 145:1212, 1985.

75. Rello J, Ricart M, Mirelis B, et al: Nosocomial bacteremia in a medical-surgical intensive care unit: Epidemiologic characteristics and factors influencing mortality in 111 episodes. *Intensive Care Med* 20:94, 1994.

76. Hurley JC: Reappraisal with meta-analysis of bacteremia, endotoxemia, and mortality in gram-negative sepsis. *J Clin Microbiol* 33:1278, 1995.

77. Menashe G, Borer A, Yagupsky P, et al: Clinical significance and impact on mortality of extended-spectrum beta lactamase-producing Enterobacteriaceae isolates in nosocomial bacteremia. *Scand J Infect Dis* 33:188, 2001.

78. Bernard GR, Vincent JL, Laterre PF, et al: Efficacy and safety of recombinant human activated protein C for severe sepsis. *N Engl J Med* 344:699, 2001.

79. Ely EW, Laterre PF, Angus DC, et al: PROWESS Investigators. Drotrecogin alfa (activated) administration across clinically important subgroups of patients with severe sepsis. *Crit Care Med* 31:12, 2003.

80. Annane D, Sebille V, Troche G, et al: A 3-level prognostic classification in septic shock based on cortisol levels and cortisol response to corticotropin. *JAMA* 283:1038, 2000.

81. Annane D, Sebille V, Charpentier C, et al: Effect of treatment with low doses of hydrocortisone and fludrocortisone on mortality in septic shock. *JAMA* 288:862, 2002.

82. Keh D, Boehnke T, Weber-Cartens S, et al: Immunologic and hemodynamic effects of "low-dose" hydrocortisone in septic shock. *Am J Respir Crit Care Med* 167:512, 2003.

83. Centers for Disease Control and Prevention: Updated U.S. Public Health Service guidelines for the management of occupational exposures to HBV, HCV, and HIV and recommendations for post-exposure prophylaxis. *MMWR* 50:23, 2001.

84. Goldberg D, Johnston J, Cameron S, et al: Risk of HIV transmission from patients to surgeons in the era of post-exposure prophylaxis. *J Hosp Infect* 44:99, 2000.

85. http://www.cdc.gov/mmwr/preview/mmwrhtml/mm5140a5.htm. Recommended Adult Immunization Schedule-United States, 2002–2003, October 11, 2002/51(40); 904–908.

86. Centers for Disease Control: Hepatitis B vaccination—United States, 1982–2002. *MMWR* 51:549, 2002.

87. ACIP: Immune globulins for protection against viral hepatitis. *MMWR* 30:423, 1981.

88. Puro V, Petrosillo N, Ippolito G, et al: Risk of hepatitis C seroconversion after occupational exposure in health care workers. *Am J Infect Control* 23:273, 1995.

89. Centers for Disease Control: Recommendations for the prevention and control of hepatitis C virus (HCV) infection and HCV-related chronic disease. *MMWR* 47:19, 1998.

90. Inglesby TV, O'Toole T, Henderson DA, et al: Anthrax as a biological weapon. *JAMA* 287:2236, 2002.

91. Inglesby TV, Dennis DT, Henderson DA, et al: Plague as a biological weapon. *JAMA* 283:2281, 2000.

92. Tucker JB: *Scourge: The Once and Future Threat of Smallpox.* New York: Grove Press, 2001, p 1.

93. DeClercq E: Cidofovir in the treatment of poxvirus infections. *Antiviral Res* 55:1, 2002.

CHAPTER 6

Trauma

Jon M. Burch, Reginald J. Franciose, and Ernest E. Moore

INTRODUCTION

Trauma or injury has been defined as damage to the body caused by an exchange with environmental energy that is beyond the body's resilience.* Trauma remains the most common cause of death for all individuals between the ages of 1 and 44 years and is the third most common cause of death regardless of age.[1] The United States government classifies accidental death under the following categories: accidents and adverse effects; suicide, homicide, and legal intervention; and all other external causes. Accidents and adverse effects account for approximately 100,000 deaths per year, with motor vehicle accidents accounting for nearly 50%. Homicides, suicides, and other causes are responsible for another 50,000 deaths each year. However, death is a poor indicator of the magnitude of the problem since most injured patients survive. For example, in 2000 there were approximately 148,209 trauma-related deaths, but 29,549,711 patients

---

*William Haddon, Jr., first director of the National Highway Traffic Safety Administration

with nonfatal injuries required hospital treatment. The aggregate lifetime costs for all injured patients was estimated to be in excess of $260 trillion. For these reasons, trauma must be considered a major public health issue. The American College of Surgeons Committee on Trauma addresses this issue by assisting in the development of trauma centers and systems. These institutions have been shown to have a significant positive impact on outcomes.[1–3]

INITIAL EVALUATION AND RESUSCITATION OF THE INJURED PATIENT

Primary Survey

Treatment of trauma patients begins in the field by emergency medical services (EMS) personnel and is completed by rehabilitation specialists. This chapter describes the surgeon's vital role in the continuum of treatment of injured patients. Although the Advanced Trauma Life Support (ATLS) course of the American College of Surgeons Committee on Trauma is directed at primary care physicians in rural communities, its format and basic tenets are sound for all physicians and will be followed closely throughout this chapter. The initial treatment of seriously injured patients consists of a primary survey, resuscitation, secondary survey, diagnostic evaluation, and definitive care. Although the concepts are presented in a sequential fashion, in reality they often proceed simultaneously. The process begins with the identification and treatment of conditions that constitute an immediate threat to life. The ATLS course refers to this as the primary survey or "ABCs" (*A*irway, with cervical spine protection, *B*reathing, and *C*irculation). Any life-threatening problem identified in the initial survey must be treated before advancing to the next step.

Airway Management

Ensuring an adequate airway is the first priority in the primary survey. This is essential since efforts to restore cardiovascular integrity will be futile unless the oxygen content of the blood is adequate. Simultaneously, all blunt trauma patients require cervical spine immobilization until injury is ruled out. This can be accomplished with a hard (Philadelphia) collar or the placement of sandbags on both sides of the head taped to the back board. Soft collars do not immobilize the cervical spine.

In general, patients who are conscious and have a normal voice do not require further evaluation or early attention to their airway. Exceptions to this principle include patients with penetrating injuries to the neck and an expanding hematoma; evidence of chemical or thermal injury to the mouth, nares or, hypopharynx; extensive subcutaneous air in the neck; complex maxillofacial trauma; or airway bleeding. Although these patients may initially have a satisfactory airway, it may become obstructed if soft-tissue swelling or edema progresses. In these cases, elective intubation should be performed prior to evidence of airway compromise.

Patients who have an abnormal voice or altered mental status require further airway evaluation. Direct laryngoscopic inspection will often reveal blood, vomit, the tongue, foreign objects, or soft-tissue swelling as sources of airway obstruction. Suctioning may afford immediate relief in many patients. Altered mental status is the most common indication for intubation because of the patient's inability to protect the airway. Options for airway access include nasotracheal, orotracheal, or surgical. Nasotracheal intubation can only be accomplished in patients who are breathing spontaneously and is contraindicated in the apneic patient. Although nasotracheal intubation is frequently employed by paramedics in the field, the

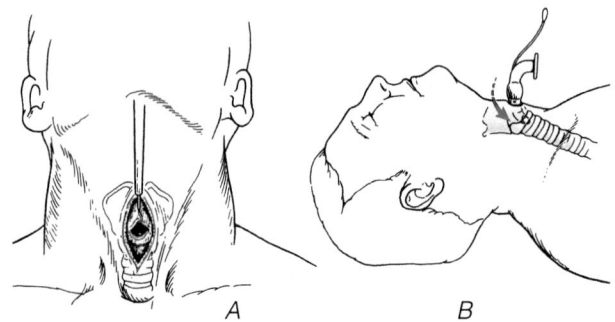

FIG. 6-1. *Cricothyroidotomy is recommended for an emergency surgical airway. Vertical incisions are preferred to avoid injury to the anterior jugular veins, which are located just lateral to the midline. Hemorrhage from these vessels will obscure vision and prolong the procedure. When making an incision in the cricothyroid membrane, the blade of the knife should be angled inferiorly to avoid injury to the vocal cords. A. Heavy silk suture for traction on the thyroid cartilage. B. Insertion of the cricothyroid tube.*

primary use for this technique in the emergency department (ED) is becoming limited to those few patients requiring emergent airway support who are prohibitive candidates for paralyzation. The use of prehospital intubation has not been shown to be superior to using a bag and mask in children.[4]

Orotracheal intubation also can be performed in patients with potential cervical spine injuries, provided that manual in-line cervical immobilization is maintained.[5] The advantages of orotracheal intubation are the direct visualization of the vocal cords, the ability to use larger-diameter endotracheal tubes, applicability to apneic patients, and its familiarity to most physicians. The disadvantage of orotracheal intubation is that conscious patients usually require neuromuscular blockade or deep sedation. To a large extent, rapid sequence induction with orotracheal intubation has become the standard in experienced trauma centers with the availability of pulse oximetry. The major advantage is rapid, definitive airway control. The disadvantages include inability to intubate, aspiration, and complications of the required medications. Those who attempt rapid sequence induction must be thoroughly familiar with the details and contraindications of the procedure (see Chap. 12).

Patients in whom attempts at intubation have failed or are precluded from intubation due to extensive facial injuries require a surgical airway. Cricothyroidotomy (Fig. 6-1) and percutaneous transtracheal ventilation are preferred over tracheostomy in most emergency situations because of their simplicity and safety. One disadvantage of cricothyroidotomy is the inability to place a tube greater than 6 mm in diameter due to the limited aperture of the cricothyroid space. Cricothyroidotomy is also relatively contraindicated in patients under the age of 12 because of the risk of damage to the cricoid cartilage and the subsequent risk of subglottic stenosis.

Percutaneous transtracheal ventilation is accomplished by inserting a large-bore, intravenous catheter through the cricothyroid membrane and into the trachea, and attaching it with tubing to an oxygen source capable of delivering 50 pounds per square inch (psi) or greater. A hole cut in the tubing allows for intermittent ventilation by occluding and releasing the hole. Adequate oxygenation can be maintained for more than 30 minutes. However, since exhalation occurs passively, ventilation is limited and carbon dioxide retention may occur. Although emergent tracheostomy has fallen into disfavor because of its technical difficulties, it may still be necessary in cases of laryngotracheal separation or laryngeal fractures, where cricothyroidotomy may cause further damage or result in the complete loss of the airway.

Breathing

Once a secure airway is obtained, adequate oxygenation and ventilation must be assured. All injured patients should receive supplemental oxygen therapy and be monitored by pulse oximetry. The following conditions may constitute an immediate threat to life due to inadequate ventilation: tension pneumothorax, open pneumothorax, or flail chest/pulmonary contusion. All of these diagnoses can be made with a combination of physical examination and chest x-ray.

The diagnosis of tension pneumothorax is implied by the finding of respiratory distress in combination with any of the following physical signs: tracheal deviation away from the affected side, lack of or decreased breath sounds on the affected side, distended neck veins or systemic hypotension, or subcutaneous emphysema on the affected side. Immediate tube thoracostomy is indicated without awaiting chest x-ray confirmation (Fig. 6-2). In tension pneumothorax the collapsed lung acts as a one-way valve, and each inhalation allows additional air to accumulate in the pleural space. The normal negative intrapleural pressure becomes positive, depressing the ipsilateral hemidiaphragm and forcing the mediastinal structures into the contralateral chest. The contralateral lung is then compressed, and the heart is rotated about the superior and inferior vena cava, decreasing venous return and cardiac output while distending the neck veins. An unrecognized simple pneumothorax can be converted to a tension pneumothorax if the patient is placed on a positive-pressure mechanical ventilator. A tension pneumothorax also can develop in a patient breathing spontaneously.

An open pneumothorax or sucking chest wound occurs with full-thickness loss of the chest wall, permitting free communication between the pleural space and the atmosphere. This compromises ventilation by two mechanisms. In addition to collapse of the lung on the injured side, if the diameter of the injury is greater than the narrowest portion of the upper airway, air will preferentially move through the injury site rather than the trachea and impair ventilation on the contralateral side. Occlusion of the injury may result in converting an open pneumothorax into a tension pneumothorax. Proper treatment in the field involves placing an occlusive dressing, which is taped on three sides over the wound. The occlusive dressing permits effective ventilation on inspiration, while the untaped side allows accumulated air to escape from the pleural space, preventing a tension pneumothorax. Definitive treatment requires wound closure and tube thoracostomy.

Flail chest occurs when four or more ribs are fractured in at least two locations. Paradoxical movement of this free-floating segment of chest wall may occasionally be sufficient to compromise ventilation. However, it is of greater physiologic importance that patients with flail chest frequently have an underlying pulmonary contusion. Pulmonary contusion with or without rib fractures may compromise oxygenation or ventilation to the extent that intubation and mechanical ventilation is required. Respiratory failure in these patients may not be immediate, and frequent re-evaluation is warranted. The initial chest x-ray usually underestimates the degree of pulmonary contusion, and the lesion tends to evolve with time and fluid resuscitation.

Circulation

With a secure airway and adequate ventilation established, circulatory status is addressed next. A rough first approximation of the patient's cardiovascular status is obtained by palpating peripheral pulses. In general, a systolic blood pressure (SBP) of 60 mm Hg is required for the carotid pulse to be palpable, 70 mm Hg for the femoral pulse, and 80 mm Hg for the radial pulse. At this point in the patient's treatment, hypotension is assumed to be caused by hemorrhage. Blood pressure and pulse should be measured at least every 15 minutes.

External control of hemorrhage should be obtained before restoring circulating volume. Manual compression and splints will frequently control extremity hemorrhage as effectively as tourniquets, with less tissue damage. Blind clamping should be avoided because of the risk to adjacent structures, particularly nerves. The importance of digital control of hemorrhage for penetrating injuries of the head, neck, thoracic outlet, groin, and extremities cannot be overemphasized. This should be done with a gloved finger placed through the wound directly on the bleeding vessel, applying only enough pressure to control active bleeding. The surgeon performing this maneuver must then walk with the patient to the operating room for definitive treatment. Maintaining hemostasis with the usual flurry of activity and walking with the patient requires considerable concentration. Scalp lacerations through the galea aponeurotica tend to bleed profusely. These can be temporarily controlled with Rainey clips or a full-thickness, large nylon continuous stitch.

Intravenous access for fluid resuscitation is begun with two peripheral catheters, 16-gauge or larger in an adult. Blood should be drawn simultaneously and sent for typing and hematocrit. Since the flow of liquid through a tube is proportional to the diameter and inversely proportional to length, venous lines for volume resuscitation should be short with a large diameter. For patients requiring vigorous fluid resuscitation, saphenous vein cutdowns at the ankle (Fig. 6-3)

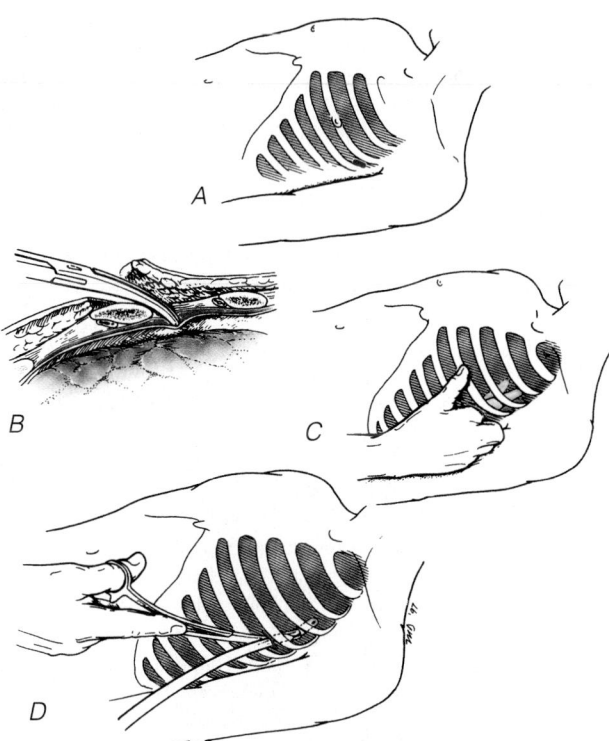

FIG. 6-2. *A.* Tube thoracostomy for trauma is performed in the fourth or fifth intercostal space at the anterior axillary line to avoid iatrogenic injury to the liver or spleen. *B.* A curved clamp is used to enter the pleural space. It is directed over the top of the rib to avoid injury to the intercostal bundle located just beneath the rib. *C.* The incision should be digitally explored to identify pleural adhesions. *D.* 36F to 40F chest tubes are employed. The tube is directed superiorly and posteriorly with the aid of a large clamp.

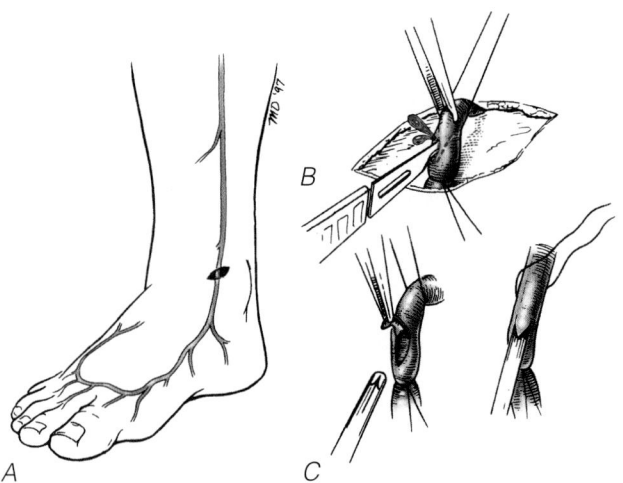

FIG. 6-3. Saphenous vein cutdowns are excellent sites for fluid resuscitation access. *A.* The vein is consistently found 1 to 1.5 cm anterior to the medial malleolus. *B.* Proximal and distal traction sutures are placed. Distal suture is ligated. *C.* Short 10- to 14-gauge intravenous catheters should be used, and they should be secured with both sutures and tape to prevent dislodgment.

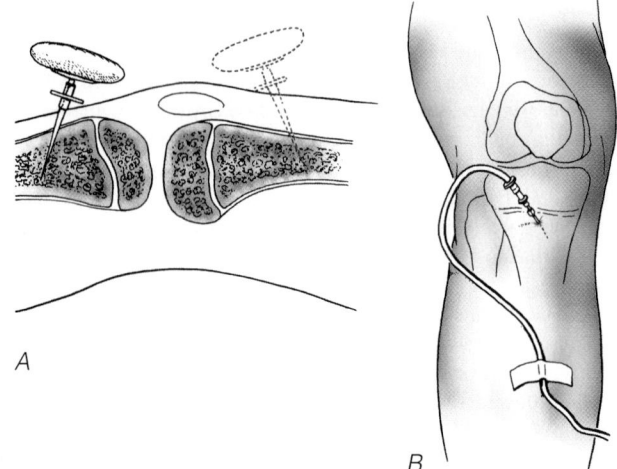

FIG. 6-4. Intraosseous infusions are indicated for children <6 years of age in whom one or two attempts at intravenous access have failed. *A.* The proximal tibia is the preferred location. Alternatively, the distal femur can be used if the tibia is fractured. *B.* The needle should be directed away from the epiphyseal plate to avoid injury. The position is satisfactory if bone marrow can be aspirated or if saline can be easily infused without evidence of extravasation. Several different proprietary devices are available for intraosseous infusion, and the surgeon should be familiar with their design.

or percutaneous femoral vein catheter introducers are preferred. The saphenous vein is reliably found 1 cm anterior and 1 cm superior to the medial malleolus. Short 10-gauge catheters can be quickly placed, even in an exsanguinating patient with collapsed veins. Venous access in the lower extremities provides effective volume resuscitation in cases of abdominal venous injury, including the vena cava. In general, jugular and subclavian central venous introducers are less desirable for initial access in trauma patients because placement may interfere with individuals performing other life-saving procedures. Secondary central venous introducers should be placed in the operating room (OR) in the event vena caval cross-clamping is performed.

In hypovolemic pediatric patients less than 6 years of age, percutaneous femoral vein cannulation is relatively contraindicated because of the risk of venous thrombosis. If two attempts at percutaneous peripheral access are unsuccessful, interosseous cannulation should be performed in the proximal tibia or distal femur if the tibia is fractured (Fig. 6-4). This is a safe emergency technique; however, once alternative access has been established, the cannula should be removed because of the risk of osteomyelitis.

Initial Fluid Resuscitation

Initial fluid resuscitation is a 1-L intravenous (IV) bolus of normal saline, Ringer's lactate, or other isotonic crystalloid in an adult, or 20 mL/kg Ringer's lactate in a child. In the U. S. crystalloid alone is employed, while in other parts of the world colloid is often added. This is repeated one time in an adult and twice in a child prior to administering red blood cells (RBC). The goal of fluid resuscitation is to re-establish tissue perfusion. Classic signs and symptoms of shock are tachycardia, hypotension, tachypnea, mental status changes, diaphoresis, and pallor. None of these signs or symptoms taken alone can predict the patient's organ perfusion status. When viewed as a constellation, they can help to evaluate the patient's response to treatment. Patients who have a good response to fluid infusion (i.e., normalization of vital signs, clearing of the sensorium) and evidence of good peripheral perfusion (warm fingers and toes with normal capillary refill) are presumed to have adequate overall perfusion.

There are several caveats that must be considered when making this presumption. Although tachycardia may be the earliest sign of ongoing blood loss, individuals in good physical condition, particularly trained athletes with a low resting pulse rate, may manifest only a relative tachycardia. Patients on beta-blocking medications may not be able to increase their heart rate in response to stress. In children, bradycardia or relative bradycardia can occur with severe blood loss, and is an ominous sign often heralding cardiovascular collapse. On the other hand, hypoxia, pain, apprehension, and stimulant drugs (cocaine, amphetamines) will produce a tachycardia unrelated to physiologic demands. Hypotension is not a reliable early sign of hypovolemia. In healthy patients blood volume must decrease by 30 to 40% before hypotension occurs (Table 6-1). Younger patients with good sympathetic tone can maintain systemic blood pressure with severe intravascular deficits until they are on the verge of cardiac arrest. In contrast, pregnancy increases circulating blood volume and a relatively larger volume of blood loss must occur before signs and symptoms become apparent.

Acute changes in mental status can be caused by hypoxia, hypercarbia, or hypovolemia, or may be an early sign of increasing intracranial pressure (ICP). An abnormal mental status should prompt an immediate re-evaluation of the ABCs and consideration of an evolving central nervous system (CNS) injury. A deterioration in mental status may be subtle and may not progress in a predictable fashion. For example, previously calm, cooperative patients may become anxious and combative as they become hypoxic. However, a patient who is agitated and combative from drugs or alcohol may become somnolent if hypovolemic shock develops. Urine output is a quantitative and relatively reliable indicator of organ perfusion. Adequate urine output is .5 mL/kg per hour in an adult, 1 mL/kg per hour in a child, and 2 mL/kg per hour in an infant less than 1 year of age.

Based on the initial response to fluid resuscitation, hypovolemic injured patients can be separated into three broad categories: responders, transient responders, and nonresponders. Individuals who are

Table 6-1
Signs and Symptoms for Different Classes of Shock

	Class I	*Class II*	*Class III*	*Class IV*
Blood loss (mL)	Up to 750	750–1500	1500–2000	>2000
Blood loss (%BV)	Up to 15%	15–30%	30–40%	>40%
Pulse rate	<100	>100	>120	>140
Blood pressure	Normal	Normal	Decreased	Decreased
Pulse pressure (mm Hg)	Normal or increased	Decreased	Decreased	Decreased
Respiratory rate	14–20	20–30	30–40	>35
Urine output (mL/h)	>30	20–30	5–15	Negligible
CNS/mental status	Slightly anxious	Mildly anxious	Anxious and confused	Confused and lethargic

BV = blood volume; CNS = central nervous system.

stable or have a good response to their initial fluid therapy as evidenced by normalization of their vital signs, mental status, and urine output are unlikely to have significant continuing hemorrhage, and further diagnostic evaluation for occult injuries can proceed in an orderly fashion (see Secondary Survey section below). At the other end of the spectrum are nonresponders with persistent hypotension. This group requires immediate diagnosis and treatment to prevent a fatal outcome. Patients who respond transiently and then deteriorate comprise the most complex group with regard to decision making. In general, they are either underresuscitated or have ongoing hemorrhage. In such patients with penetrating trauma, the need for operative intervention for the control of hemorrhage is usually evident. Blunt trauma patients with multisystem injury, however, require careful planning. It is in this group that the greatest number of preventable deaths is likely to occur.

Persistent Hypotension

Nonresponders. The spectrum of disease in this category ranges from nonsurvivable multisystem injury to problems as simple as a tension pneumothorax. Persistent hypotension in these patients is usually cardiogenic or due to uncontrolled hemorrhage. An evaluation of the patient's neck veins and central venous pressure (CVP) will usually distinguish between these two categories. CVP determines right ventricular preload, and in otherwise healthy trauma patients, its measurement yields objective information regarding the patient's overall volume status. Although central venous catheters are inappropriate for administering large volumes of fluid, they are valuable for measuring CVP. A hypotensive patient with flat neck veins and a CVP less than 5 cm H_2O is hypovolemic and is likely to have ongoing hemorrhage. A hypotensive patient with distended neck veins or a CVP greater than 15 cm H_2O is likely to be in cardiogenic shock. The CVP, however, may be falsely elevated if the patient is agitated and straining or fluid administration is overzealous; isolated readings must be interpreted with caution.

In trauma patients the differential diagnosis of cardiogenic shock is a short list: (1) tension pneumothorax, (2) pericardial tamponade, (3) myocardial contusion or infarction, and (4) air embolism. Tension pneumothorax is the most frequent cause of cardiac failure and has been discussed above. Traumatic pericardial tamponade is most often associated with penetrating injury to the heart. As blood leaks out of the injured heart, it accumulates in the pericardial sac. Because the pericardium is not acutely distensible, the pressure in the pericardial sac will rise to match that of the injured chamber. Since this pressure is usually greater than that of the right atrium, right atrial filling is impaired and right ventricular preload is reduced. This leads to decreased right ventricular output and increased CVP. Increased intrapericardial pressure also impedes myocardial blood flow, which

leads to subendocardial ischemia and a further reduction in cardiac output. This vicious cycle may progress insidiously with injury of the vena cava or atria, or precipitously with injury of either ventricle. With acute tamponade, as little as 100 mL of blood within the pericardial sac can produce life-threatening hemodynamic compromise. Patients usually present with a penetrating injury in proximity to the heart, and they are hypotensive and have distended neck veins or an elevated CVP. The classic findings of Beck's triad (hypotension, distended neck, and muffled heart sounds) and pulsus paradoxus are not reliable indicators of acute tamponade. Ultrasonography (US) in the ED using a subxiphoid or parasternal view is extremely helpful if the findings are clearly positive (Fig. 6-5); however, equivocal findings are common. Early in the course of tamponade, blood pressure and cardiac output will transiently improve with fluid administration. This may lead the surgeon to question the diagnosis or be lulled into a false sense of security.

Once the diagnosis of cardiac tamponade is established, pericardiocentesis should be performed (Fig. 6-6). Evacuation of as little as 15 to 25 mL of blood may dramatically improve the patient's hemodynamic profile. Pericardiocentesis should be done even if the patient appears to stabilize with volume loading since subclinical myocardial ischemia can lead to sudden lethal arrhythmias, and

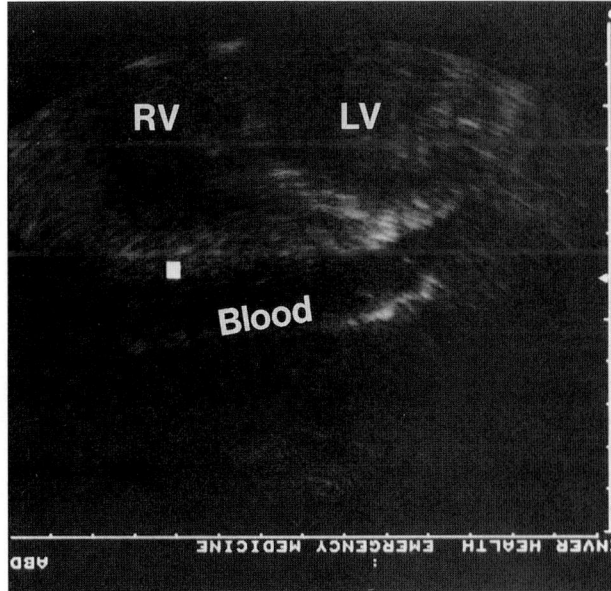

FIG. 6-5. Subxiphoid pericardial ultrasound reveals a large pericardial tamponade.

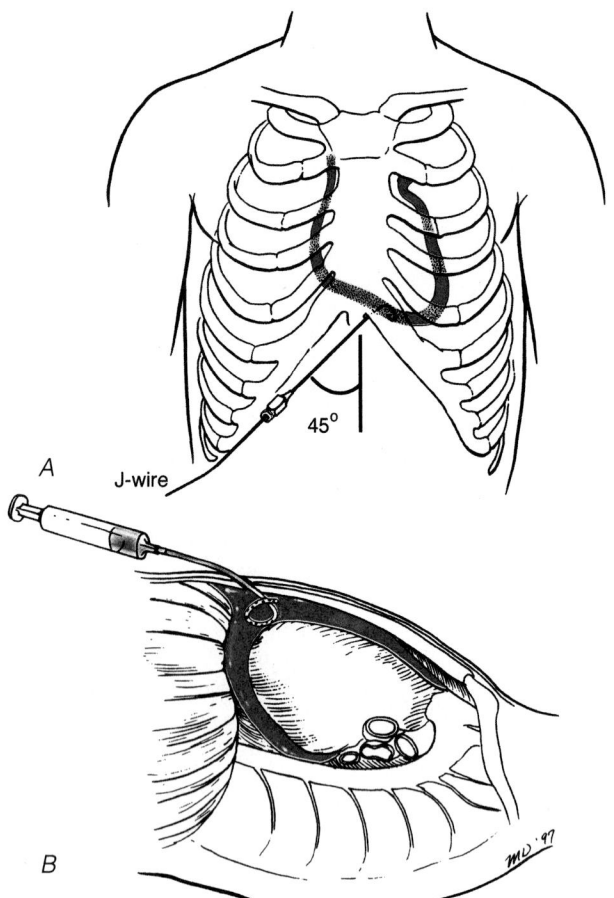

FIG. 6-6. Pericardiocentesis is indicated for patients with evidence of pericardial tamponade. *A.* Kits are available which utilize the Seldinger technique. *B.* With the J-wire in position, a pigtail catheter with multiple holes is placed. Blood can be repeatedly aspirated until the patient undergoes surgery.

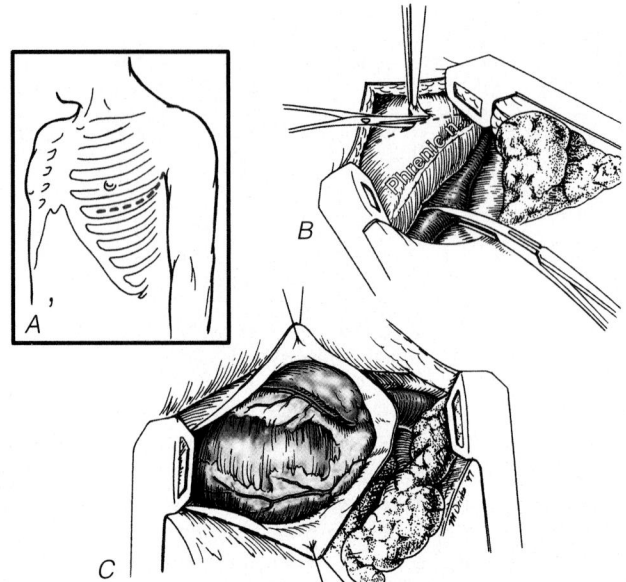

FIG. 6-7. *A.* Emergency department (ED) thoracotomies are performed through the fourth or fifth intercostal space using the anterolateral approach. *B.* If the thoracotomy is performed for abdominal injury, the descending thoracic aorta is clamped. If the patient's blood pressure improves to >70 mm Hg, he or she is transported to the OR for laparotomy. For patients who fail to generate this pressure, further treatment is futile. If the thoracotomy is performed for a cardiac injury, the pericardium is opened longitudinally and anterior to the phrenic nerve. *C.* The heart can then be rotated out of the pericardium for repair.

patients with tamponade may decompensate unpredictably. While pericardiocentesis is being performed, preparation should be made for emergent transport to the OR. Emergent pericardiocentesis is successful in decompressing the tamponade in approximately 80% of cases; most failures are due to clotted blood within the pericardium. If pericardiocentesis is unsuccessful and the patient remains severely hypotensive (SBP <70 mm Hg) or shows other signs of hemodynamic instability, ED thoracotomy should be performed (Fig. 6-7). This is best accomplished using a left anterolateral thoracotomy and a longitudinal pericardiotomy anterior to the phrenic nerve, followed by evacuation of the pericardial sac and temporary control of the cardiac injury. The patient is then transported to the OR for definitive repair (Fig. 6-8).

Myocardial contusion from direct myocardial impact occurs in approximately one third of patients sustaining significant blunt chest trauma. The diagnostic criteria for myocardial contusion include some specific electrocardiographic abnormalities (i.e., ventricular dysrhythmias, atrial fibrillation, sinus bradycardia, and bundle-branch block). Transient sinus tachycardia is not indicative of contusion. Serial cardiac enzyme determinations (CPK-MB fraction) lack sensitivity, are not predictive of complications under these conditions, and are not recommended. While the diagnosis is common, acute, life-threatening complications of ventricular arrhythmias and cardiac pump failure occur in less than 5% and less than 1% of

patients sustaining major blunt chest trauma, respectively. Arrhythmias are treated by pharmacologic suppression. The management of cardiogenic shock from cardiac pump failure includes early placement of a Swan-Ganz pulmonary artery catheter to optimize fluid administration; inotropic support; and urgent echocardiography to rule out septal or free wall rupture, valvular disruption, or pericardial tamponade. Patients with refractory cardiogenic shock may require placement of an intra-aortic balloon pump to decrease myocardial work and enhance coronary perfusion.

Acute myocardial infarction is frequently the cause of motor vehicle accidents or other trauma in older patients. While the ideal initial management would be to provide optimal treatment for the evolving infarction, decisions regarding lytic therapy and emergent angioplasty must be individualized according to the patient's other injuries.

Air embolism is a frequently overlooked lethal complication of pulmonary injury. It occurs when air from an injured bronchus enters an adjacent injured pulmonary vein and returns to the left heart. Air accumulation in the left ventricle impedes diastolic filling, and during systole it is pumped into the coronary arteries, disrupting coronary perfusion. A typical scenario is a patient with a penetrating chest injury who appears hemodynamically stable but suddenly arrests after being intubated and placed on positive pressure ventilation. Air emboli also have been described in conjunction with blunt thoracic trauma and can occur at any time when manipulating a pulmonary venous injury. The patient should be placed in the Trendelenburg position to trap the air in the apex of the left ventricle. Emergency thoracotomy is followed by cross-clamping the pulmonary hilum on the side of the injury to prevent further introduction of air. Air is aspirated from the apex of the left ventricle with an 18-gauge needle and 50-mL syringe. Vigorous open cardiac

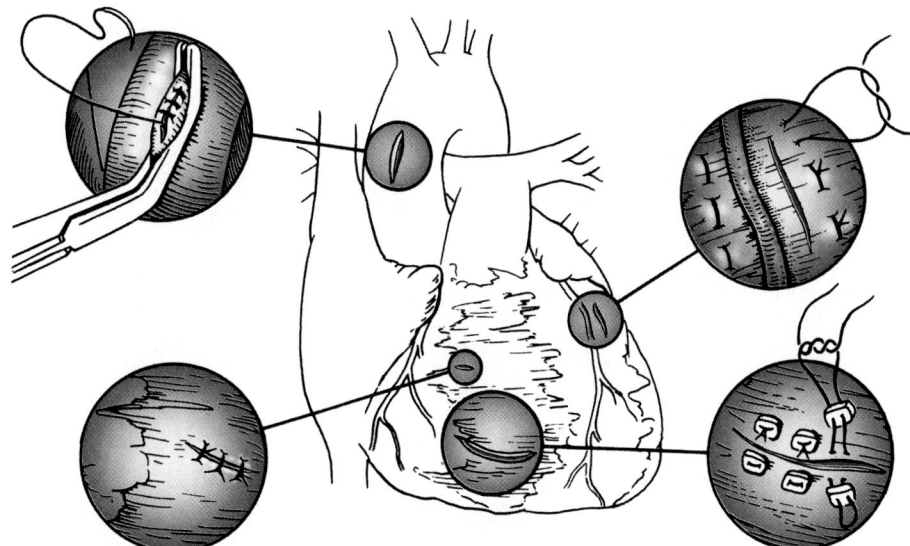

FIG. 6-8. A variety of techniques may be necessary to repair cardiac injuries. Wounds in proximity to coronary arteries must be repaired with horizontal mattress sutures placed under the artery to avoid infarctions distal to the repair. Pledgeted sutures may be necessary to prevent the sutures from pulling through the myocardium, particularly in the right ventricle.

massage is used to force the air bubbles through the coronary arteries. The highest point of the aortic root is also aspirated to prevent air from entering the coronaries or embolizing to the brain. The patient should be kept in the Trendelenburg position and the hilum clamped until the pulmonary venous injury is controlled.

Persistent hypotension and flat neck veins due to uncontrolled hemorrhage are associated with a high mortality. A rapid search for the source or sources of hemorrhage, including visual inspection with knowledge of the injury mechanism, abdominal ultrasound, and anteroposterior (AP) chest and pelvic x-rays will usually indicate the regions of the body responsible for the blood loss. Type O RBC (O-negative for women of childbearing age) or type-specific RBC should be administered and the patient taken directly to the OR for exploration. For patients with a sustained SBP of less than 70 mm Hg in spite of crystalloid and blood administration, ED thoracotomy should be considered.[6] The clearest indication for this procedure is penetrating chest trauma; survival is reported to be as high as 30%. A small percentage of patients with penetrating abdominal trauma survive, but the role of ED thoracotomy in blunt abdominal trauma remains controversial. The goal of ED thoracotomy for thoracic injuries is control of hemorrhage; for abdominal injuries the goal is to sustain central circulation and limit abdominal blood loss by clamping the descending thoracic aorta. Every effort should be made to replace the aortic clamp to below the renal arteries within 30 minutes. Longer clamping times proximal to the abdominal viscera are seldom associated with survival. Because the decision to perform an ED thoracotomy can be intimidating, the algorithm in Fig. 6-9 is used by these authors to assist in this decision.

Transient Responders. Hypotensive patients who transiently respond to fluid administration usually have some degree of active hemorrhage. Those with penetrating injuries should be taken to the OR for exploration. Those with multiple blunt injuries constitute a diagnostic and therapeutic dilemma. These patients often require sophisticated evaluation such as computed tomography (CT) and angiography. It is during these diagnostic evaluations and the necessary transportation of the patient where the greatest hazard exists since monitoring is compromised and the environment is suboptimal to deal with acute problems. Therefore the surgeon must accompany the patient and be prepared to abort the examination if hypotension recurs. If operation is necessary, the patient should be

given type-specific RBC and be taken immediately to the OR to localize the hemorrhage as described in the scenario of the patient with persistent hypotension above. An operating room should be immediately available when these patients arrive in the ED.

Recently, the traditional volume resuscitation (described above) of patients sustaining penetrating torso trauma has been questioned. The concept of volume resuscitation is based on canine laboratory experiments performed by Wiggers, who carefully controlled the removal and replacement of blood. These experiments proved that the depth and duration of hypotension determined whether the animal lived or died. It has therefore been assumed that any hypotension is dangerous and must be treated, preferably with blood or crystalloid. Others argue that the body's hemostatic mechanisms frequently control hemorrhage initially and that increased venous and subsequent arterial pressure from fluid resuscitation may disrupt tenuous hemostasis. Furthermore, active bleeding increases as venous and arterial pressure increases. Laboratory studies support these concepts. A prospective randomized study of hypotensive patients who sustained penetrating torso trauma and required operative treatment has recently been completed.[7,8] One half of the patients received volume resuscitation, while fluid was withheld in the others until the operation was begun. As is common with clinical studies, methodologic imperfections existed; however, there was no survival advantage for those resuscitated in the traditional fashion. In fact, subgroup analysis suggested a survival disadvantage for pericardial tamponade. However, it must be emphasized that patients with profound hypotension (SBP <70 mm Hg) are at risk for sudden death. Ultimately it may well be that controlled hypotension is the optimal middle ground. Clinical research is ongoing to determine the optimal material and endpoints for resuscitation of shock.[9–11]

Secondary Survey

Once the conditions that constitute an immediate threat to life have been addressed or excluded, the patient is examined in a systematic fashion, literally head to toe, to identify all occult injuries. Seriously injured patients must have all of their clothing removed to accomplish this objective. Special attention should be given to the patient's back, axillae, and perineum, since injuries in these areas are easily overlooked. All patients should undergo digital rectal examination

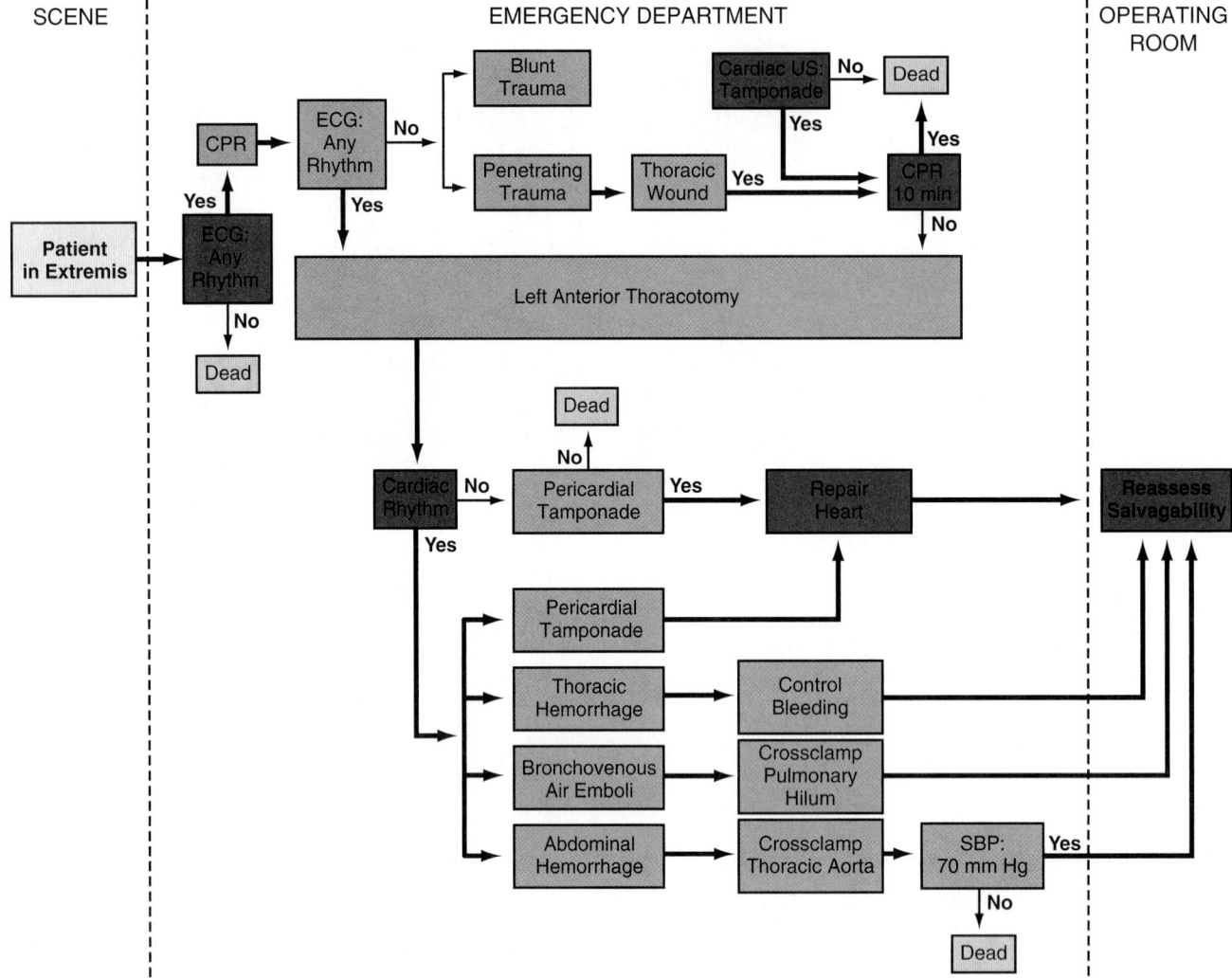

FIG. 6-9. Algorithm for ED thoracotomy.

to evaluate sphincter tone and to look for blood, perforation, or a high-riding prostate. A Foley catheter should be inserted to decompress the bladder, obtain a urine specimen, and monitor urine output. Stable patients at risk for urethral injury should undergo urethrography before catheterization. Signs of urethral injury include blood at the meatus, perineal or scrotal hematomas, or a high-riding prostate. However, in the case of persistent hypovolemic shock, an initial attempt at a Foley catheterization should be made; if this is unsuccessful, a percutaneous suprapubic cystostomy should be placed. A nasogastric tube should be inserted to decrease the risk of gastric aspiration and to allow inspection of stomach contents for blood suggestive of occult gastroduodenal injury.

Selective radiographs are obtained early in the ED evaluation. For patients with severe blunt trauma, anterior and posterior chest and pelvic radiographs should be obtained as soon as possible. For patients with truncal gunshot wounds, posteroanterior and lateral radiographs of the chest and abdomen are warranted. It also is helpful to mark the entrance and exit sites of penetrating wounds with metallic clips or staples so that the trajectory of the missile or blade can be estimated.

Many trauma patients cannot provide specific information about the nature of their injury mechanism. EMS personnel and police are trained to evaluate an injury scene and should be questioned. For automobile accidents, the speed of the vehicles involved in the accident, the angle of impact (if any), the use of restraints, airbag deployment, the condition of the steering wheel and windshield, the amount of intrusion, whether the patient was ejected from the vehicle, and whether anyone was dead at the scene should all be ascertained. The patient's physiologic condition in the field is also important. Vital signs and mental status in the ED can be compared with those at the scene; improvement or deterioration provides critical prognostic information.

Mechanisms and Patterns of Injury

Evaluation and decision making are far more difficult in blunt than in penetrating trauma. In general, more energy is transferred over a wider area during blunt trauma than from a gunshot wound (GSW) or stab wound (SW). As a result, blunt trauma is associated with multiple widely distributed injuries, whereas in penetrating wounds the damage is localized to the path of the bullet or knife. Trauma surgeons often separate patients who have sustained blunt trauma into categories according to their risk for multiple injuries: high-energy transfer and low-energy transfer. Injuries involving high-energy

Table 6-2
Glasgow Coma Scale[a]

		Adults	Infants/Children
Eye opening	4	Spontaneous	Spontaneous
	3	To voice	To voice
	2	To pain	To pain
	1	None	None
Verbal	5	Oriented	Alert, normal vocalization
	4	Confused	Cries but consolable
	3	Inappropriate words	Persistently irritable
	2	Incomprehensible words	Restless, agitated, moaning
	1	None	None
Motor response	6	Obeys commands	Spontaneous, purposeful
	5	Localizes pain	Localizes pain
	4	Withdraws	Withdraws
	3	Abnormal flexion	Abnormal flexion
	2	Abnormal extension	Abnormal extension
	1	None	None

[a] Score is calculated by adding the scores of the best motor response, best verbal response, and eye opening. Scores range from 3 (the lowest) to 15 (normal).

transfer include auto-pedestrian accidents, motor vehicle accidents in which the car's change of speed exceeds 20 mph or in which the patient has been ejected, motorcycle accidents, and falls from heights greater than 20 feet. In fact, the greatest risk factors reflecting magnitude of injury that are strongly associated with life-threatening injuries are death of another occupant in the vehicle and an extrication time greater than 20 minutes.

Patients who have sustained high-energy transfer trauma have certain patterns of injury related to the mechanism. For example, when unrestrained drivers suffer frontal impacts, their heads strike the windshield, their chests and upper abdomens hit the steering column, and their legs or knees contact the dashboard. The resultant injuries frequently include facial fractures, cervical spine fractures, laceration of the thoracic aorta, myocardial contusion, injury to the spleen and liver, and fractures of the pelvis and lower extremities. When evaluating such patients, the discovery of one of these injuries should prompt a search for others.

Low-energy trauma, such as being struck with a club or falling from a bicycle, usually does not result in widely distributed injuries. However, potentially lethal lacerations of internal organs can still occur because the net energy transfer to any given location may be substantial.

Penetrating injuries are classified according to the wounding agent (i.e., SWs, GSWs, or shotgun wounds [SGWs]). GSWs are subdivided further into high- and low-velocity injuries, because the speed of the bullet is much more important than its weight in determining kinetic energy. Experience in urban trauma centers indicates that high-velocity GSWs (bullet speed greater than 2000 ft/s) are rare in the civilian setting. Shotgun injuries are divided into close-range (<7 m) and long-range wounds. Close-range SGWs are tantamount to high-velocity wounds because the entire energy of the load is delivered to a small area, often with devastating results. Long-range SGWs result in a diffuse pellet pattern in which many pellets miss the victim, and those that do strike are dispersed and of comparatively low energy.

Regional Assessment and Special Diagnostic Tests

Based upon mechanism, location of injuries identified on physical examination, screening x-rays, and the patient's overall condition, additional diagnostic studies are often indicated. It must again be emphasized that the patient is in constant jeopardy when undergoing special diagnostic testing, and the surgeon should be in attendance and be prepared to alter plans as circumstances demand. Hemodynamic, respiratory, and mental status will determine the most appropriate course of action. With these issues in mind, additional diagnostic tests will be discussed on an anatomic basis.

Head

The Glasgow Coma Scale (GCS) score should be determined for all injured patients (Table 6-2). It is calculated by adding the scores of the best motor response, best verbal response, and eye opening. Scores range from 3 (the lowest) to 15 (normal). Scores of 13 to 15 indicate mild head injury, 9 to 12 moderate injury, and less than 9 severe injury. The GCS is useful for both triage and prognosis.

Examination of the head should focus on potentially treatable neurologic injuries. Of great importance is that the presence of lateralizing findings (e.g., a unilateral dilated pupil unreactive to light, asymmetric movement of the extremities either spontaneously or in response to noxious stimuli, or a unilateral Babinski sign) suggests a treatable intracranial mass lesion or major structural damage. Stroke syndromes should prompt a search for carotid dissection or thrombosis using duplex scanning or angiography. Otorrhea, rhinorrhea, raccoon eyes, and Battle's sign (ecchymosis behind the ear) can be seen with basilar skull fractures. While not necessarily requiring treatment, these fractures increase the risk of meningitis in the postinjury period. Finally, the head and face should be systematically palpated for fractures. All patients with a significant closed-head injury (GCS <14) should have a CT scan performed. For penetrating injuries, plain skull films should be obtained. They may provide information that either adds to or supplants CT.

Cerebral pathologic lesions from blunt trauma include hematomas, contusions, hemorrhage into ventricular and subarachnoid spaces, and diffuse axonal injury (DAI). Hematomas are further classified according to location. Epidural hematomas occur when blood accumulates between the skull and dura, and are caused by disruption of the middle meningeal artery or other small arteries in that potential space from a skull fracture (Fig. 6-10). Subdural hematomas occur between the dura and cortex, and are caused by venous disruption or laceration of the parenchyma of the brain (Fig. 6-11). Because of the underlying brain injury, prognosis

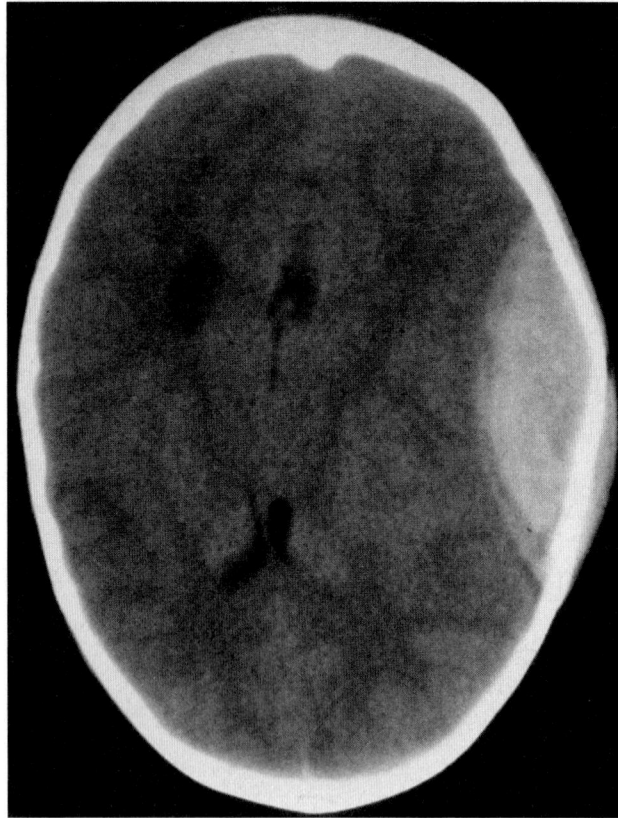

FIG. 6-10. Large epidural hematoma with midline shift. This is an obvious indication for operative decompression.

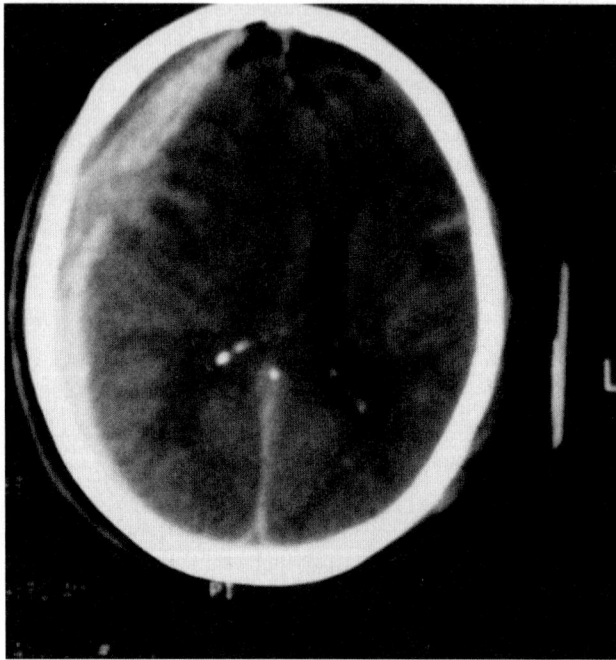

FIG. 6-11. CT scan of a patient with a subdural hematoma. In addition, there is air in the subarachnoid space and the ventricles. In comparing the complexity of the pathology in this figure with that in Fig. 6-10, it becomes apparent why decision making is more complex with subdural hematomas and outcomes less predictable.

is much worse with subdural hematomas. Intraparenchymal hematomas and contusions can occur anywhere within the brain. Hemorrhage may occur into the ventricles, and while usually not massive, this blood may cause postinjury hydrocephalus. Diffuse hemorrhage into the subarachnoid space may cause vasospasm and reduce cerebral blood flow. DAI results from high-speed deceleration injury and represents direct axonal damage. On CT, a blurring of the gray-white matter interface may be seen, along with multiple small punctate hemorrhages. While prognosis is difficult to predict and extremely variable, early evidence of DAI on CT scan is associated with a poor outcome. Magnetic resonance imaging (MRI) can often identify DAI with greater precision than CT.

Significant penetrating injuries are usually produced by bullets from hand guns, but an array of other weapons or instruments can injure the cerebrum via the orbit or through the thinner temporal region of the skull. While the diagnosis is usually obvious, in some instances wounds in the auditory canal, mouth, and nose can be elusive. Prognosis is variable, but most supratentorial wounds that injure both hemispheres are fatal.

Neck

In evaluating the neck of blunt trauma victims, attention should be focused on signs and symptoms of an occult cervical spine injury. Because of the devastating consequences of quadriplegia, all patients should be assumed to have cervical spine injuries until proven otherwise. The presence of posterior midline pain or tenderness should provoke a thorough radiologic evaluation. Unfortunately there is no perfect test to detect all injuries. The three-view cervical spine series includes lateral view with visualization of C7 through T1, anteroposterior, and transoral odontoid views, and will detect most significant fractures and subluxations. If pain or tenderness persists in spite of normal plain x-rays, a CT should be performed. CT will identify almost all fractures but can miss some subluxations. A combination of both can identify virtually all injuries. An exception to this is a pure ligamentous injury. These rare and dangerous injuries may not be visible with standard imaging techniques. Flexion and extension views can be performed and may reveal opening of the intervertebral space. However, this should only be done in the presence of an experienced surgeon, since in the past patients have been rendered permanently quadriplegic when flexed and extended by inexperienced individuals (Fig. 6-12). A safer method may be to instruct the patient to carefully move the head without touching them, since it is commonly believed that patients will not injure themselves.

Spinal cord injuries can be complete or partial. Complete injuries cause either permanent quadriplegia or paraplegia, depending on the level of injury. These patients have a complete loss of motor function and sensation two or more levels below the bony injury. Patients with high spinal cord disruption are at risk for spinal shock due to physiologic disruption of sympathetic fibers. Significant neurologic recovery is rare. There are several partial or incomplete spinal cord injury syndromes. Central cord syndrome usually occurs in older persons who suffer hyperextension injuries. Motor function and pain and temperature sensation are preserved in the lower extremities but diminished in the upper extremities. Some functional recovery usually occurs, but is seldom a return to normal. Anterior cord syndrome is characterized by diminished motor function and pain and temperature sensation below the level of the injury. Position, vibratory sensation, and crude touch are maintained. Prognosis for recovery is poor. Brown-Sequard syndrome is usually the result of a penetrating injury in which the right or left half of the spinal cord

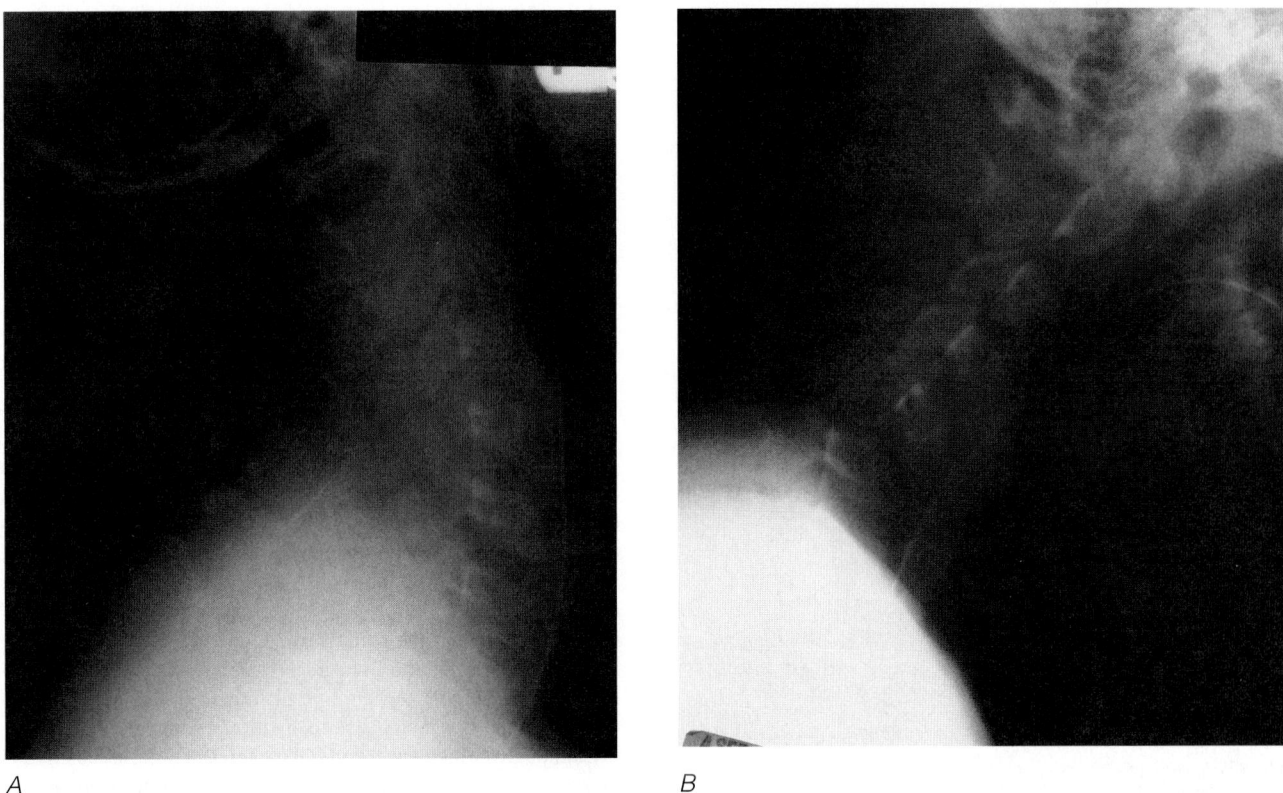

FIG. 6-12. *This patient was struck by a motor vehicle. He complained of persistent neck pain in spite of normal screening x-rays. Flexion and extension radiographs were ordered, but were performed by an inexperienced operator. A. The extension film was normal. B. The patient became acutely and permanently quadriplegic when actively flexed by the examiner. In spite of the angulation of the upper neck and head, the radiograph was taken in the upright position.*

is transected. This rare lesion is characterized by the ipsilateral loss of motor function, proprioception, and vibratory sensation, whereas pain and temperature sensation are lost on the contralateral side.

Penetrating injuries of the anterior neck that violate the platysma are considered significant because of the density of critical structures in this region. While mandatory exploration may be appropriate in some circumstances, patients are now managed selectively in most centers (Fig. 6-13).[12–14] Selective management is based on the neck and is divided into three zones (Fig. 6-14). Zone I is between the clavicles and cricoid cartilage and is also referred to as the thoracic outlet. Zone II is between the cricoid cartilage and the

angle of the mandible. Zone III is above the angle of the mandible. The evaluation and management of visceral and vascular injuries in the thoracic outlet (zone I) are complicated by the overlying ribs, sternum, and clavicles. Since the incision may be different depending on the injured structures, a precise preoperative diagnosis is desirable. Patients with zone I injuries should undergo angiography of the great vessels, soluble contrast esophagram followed by barium esophagram, esophagoscopy, and bronchoscopy. However, as outlined above, hemodynamically unstable patients should not undergo this extensive evaluation, but rather should be taken directly to the OR.

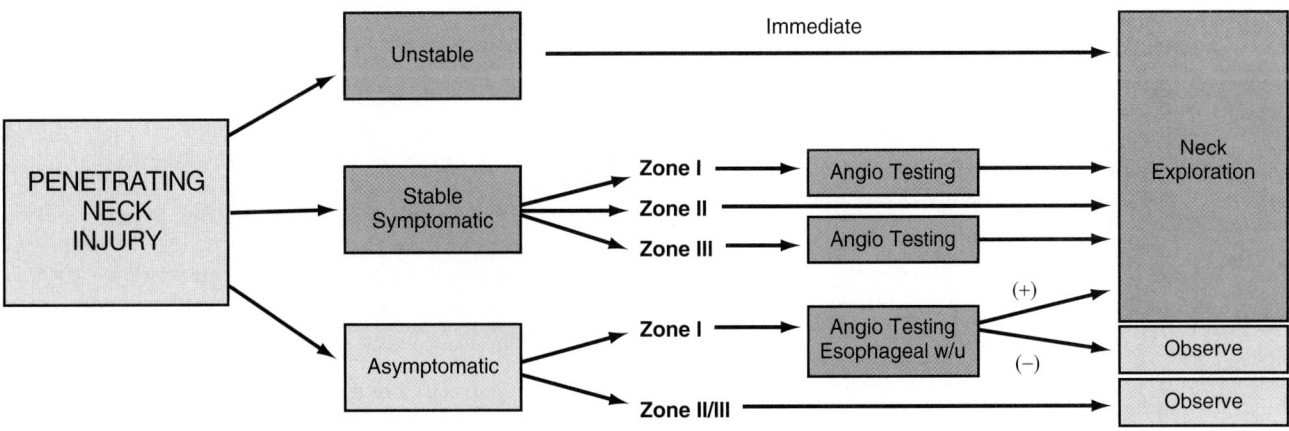

FIG. 6-13. *Algorithm for the selective management of penetrating neck injuries.*

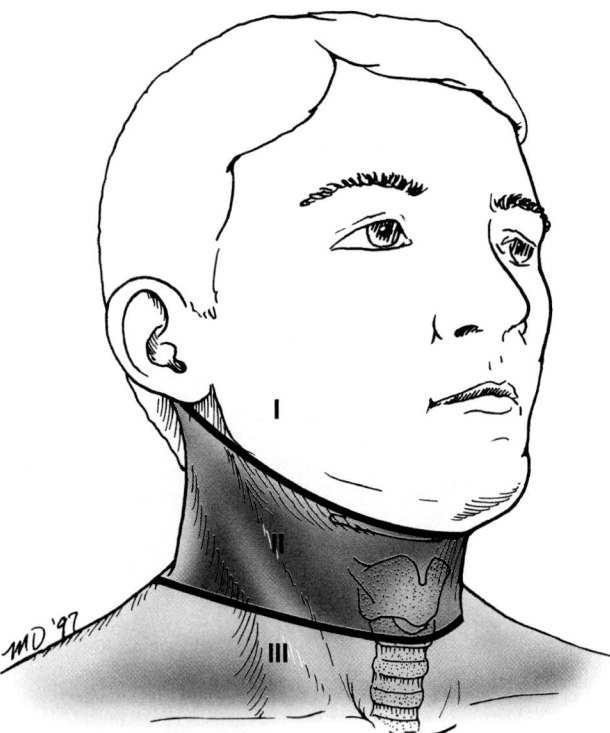

FIG. 6-14. For the purpose of evaluating penetrating injuries, the neck is divided into three zones. Zone I is below the clavicles and is also known as the thoracic outlet. Zone II is located between the clavicles and hyoid bone, and zone III is above the hyoid.

Patients with zone II injuries are the easiest to evaluate. Unstable patients or those with evidence of airway compromise, an expanding hematoma, or significant external hemorrhage (including hemorrhage into the mouth) should be explored promptly. Stable patients without the above findings can be evaluated selectively. Penetrating neck wounds in stable patients should be locally explored to determine the depth of penetration. Those that do not penetrate the platysma are insignificant and should be closed; these patients can be sent home. The vast majority of the remaining zone II penetrating wounds are observed for 12 hours. However, patients with right to left transcervical GSWs may warrant diagnostic evaluation. Carotid and vertebral angiography, direct laryngoscopy, tracheoscopy, esophagoscopy, and esophagram may be necessary, depending on the trajectory.

Patients with zone III penetrating injuries require carotid and vertebral angiography if there is evidence of arterial bleeding. This is important for three reasons: (1) exposure of the distal internal carotid and vertebral arteries is difficult, (2) the internal carotid artery may have to be ligated, a maneuver associated with a high risk of stroke, and (3) active hemorrhage from the external carotid and vertebral arteries can be controlled by selective embolization. Associated injuries of the pharynx are of little consequence and require no special evaluation.

Chest

Blunt trauma to the chest may involve the chest wall, thoracic spine, heart, lungs, thoracic aorta and great vessels, and rarely the esophagus. Most of these injuries can be evaluated by physical examination and chest x-ray.[15] Patients with large air leaks following tube thoracostomy and those who are difficult to ventilate should

Table 6-3
Findings on Chest X-Ray Suggestive of an Aortic Tear[a]

1. Widened mediastinum
2. Abnormal aortic contour
3. Tracheal shift
4. Nasogastric tube shift
5. Left apical cap
6. Left or right paraspinal stripe thickening
7. Depression of the left main bronchus
8. Obliteration of the aorticopulmonary window
9. Left pulmonary hilar hematoma

[a]Findings are listed in the order of decreasing sensitivity.

undergo fiber-optic bronchoscopy to search for bronchial tears or foreign bodies.

Perhaps the most feared occult injury in trauma surgery is a tear of the descending thoracic aorta.[16] Widening of the mediastinum on AP chest x-ray strongly suggests this injury. The widening is caused by the formation of a hematoma around the injured aorta, which is temporarily contained by the mediastinal pleura. Posterior rib fractures and laceration of small vessels also can produce similar hematomas. Should the hematoma rupture into the chest with an aortic injury, the patient will exsanguinate in seconds. Other findings suggestive of an aortic tear are noted in Table 6-3. However, it is well established that this injury can occur with an entirely normal chest x-ray, although the incidence is approximately 2%. Because of this and the dire consequences of missing the diagnosis, CT and angiography are frequently performed based on the mechanism of injury.[17] Aortic tears occur when shearing forces are created in the chest. This is most often seen in high-energy transfer deceleration motor vehicle injuries with frontal or lateral impact. However, it may also occur following an ejection injury or fall. The tear usually occurs just distal to the left subclavian artery, where the aorta is tethered by the ligamentum arteriosum (Fig. 6-15). In 2 to 5% of cases the tear occurs in the ascending aorta, transverse arch, or at the diaphragm.

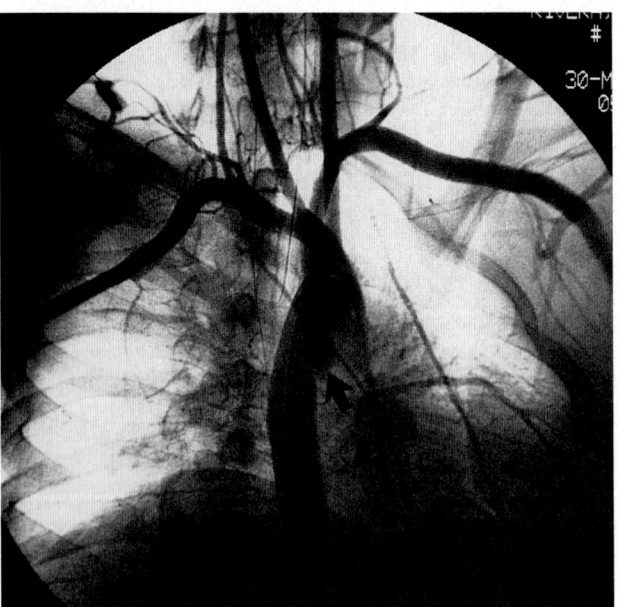

FIG. 6-15. Tears of the descending thoracic aorta can be subtle, even with angiography. Multiple views are often necessary to identify the lesion. The arrow indicates the pseudoaneurysm.

Dynamic spiral CT is an excellent screening test. Positive findings are a hematoma around the aorta or injury of the aorta. This test appears to be highly sensitive, but its specificity is unknown. A clearly widened mediastinum on chest x-ray or abnormalities on CT are an absolute indication for emergent aortography.

Penetrating thoracic trauma is considerably easier to evaluate. Physical examination, plain PA and lateral chest x-rays with metallic markings of entrance and exit wounds, and CVP measurement will disclose the vast majority of injuries. Injuries of the esophagus and trachea are exceptions. Based on the estimated trajectory of the missile or blade, bronchoscopy should be performed to evaluate the trachea. Esophagoscopy can be performed to evaluate the esophagus, but injuries have been missed with this technique alone.[18] Therefore patients at risk should also undergo a soluble contrast esophagram looking for extravasation of contrast. If no extravasation is seen, a barium esophagram should be performed for greater detail. Failure to identify esophageal injuries leads to fulminant mediastinitis that is often fatal. As in the neck, right to left transmediastinal GSWs frequently cause visceral or vascular injuries. Stable patients should be carefully evaluated for tracheal and esophageal injuries as outlined above. Angiography is occasionally indicated.

Abdomen

The abdomen is a diagnostic black box. Fortunately, with few exceptions it is not necessary to determine which intra-abdominal organs are injured, only whether an exploratory laparotomy is necessary. Physical examination of the abdomen is unreliable in making this determination. However, most authorities agree that the presence of abdominal rigidity or gross abdominal distention in a patient with truncal trauma is an indication for prompt surgical exploration. For the majority of patients suffering blunt abdominal trauma, it is not clear whether exploration is needed. Serial examinations by the same surgeon can detect early peritoneal inflammation and the need for laparotomy before serious infections and hemorrhagic complications occur. Drugs, alcohol, and head and spinal cord injuries complicate physical examination. It may also be impractical in patients who require general anesthesia for the treatment of other injuries. These patients will all require further diagnostic testing.

The diagnostic approach to penetrating and blunt abdominal trauma differs substantially. As a rule, little preoperative evaluation is required for firearm injuries that penetrate the peritoneal cavity, because the chance of internal injury is over 90% and laparotomy is mandatory. Anterior truncal GSWs between the fourth intercostal space and the pubic symphysis, whose trajectory by x-ray or entrance/exit wound suggests peritoneal penetration, should be operated on. GSWs to the back or flank are somewhat more difficult to evaluate because of the greater thickness of tissue between the skin and the abdominal organs. If in doubt, it is always safer to explore the abdomen than to equivocate when the depth of penetration is uncertain.

In contrast to GSWs, SWs that penetrate the peritoneal cavity are less likely to injure intra-abdominal organs. Anterior and lateral SWs to the trunk should be explored under local anesthesia in the ED to determine whether the peritoneum has been violated. Injuries that do not penetrate the peritoneal cavity do not require further evaluation. As with GSWs, SWs to the flank and back are more difficult to evaluate. Some authorities have recommended a triple-contrast CT to detect occult retroperitoneal injuries of the colon, duodenum, and urinary tract. However, since CT does not always identify enteric injuries, the authors have employed soluble contrast radiographs of

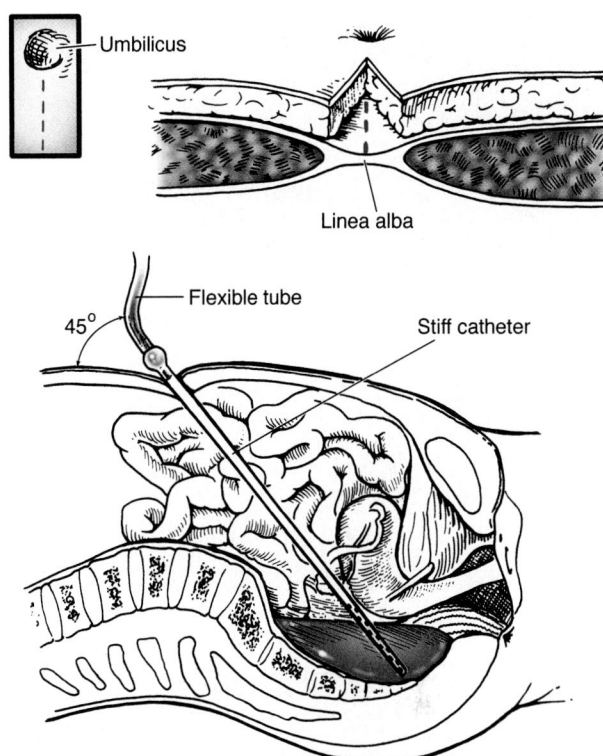

FIG. 6-16. *Diagnostic peritoneal lavage is performed through an infraumbilical incision. The linea alba is sharply incised. The catheter pierces the peritoneum with the aid of the trocar and is directed into the pelvis.*

the colon and duodenum followed by barium if necessary. The larger final images may improve sensitivity. Diagnostic peritoneal lavage (DPL) remains the most sensitive test available for determining the presence of intra-abdominal injury (Fig. 6-16).[19] For SWs to the abdomen, its sensitivity for detecting intra-abdominal injury exceeds 95%. The results of DPL are considered to be grossly positive if more than 10 mL of free blood can be aspirated after insertion of the catheter. If less than 10 mL is withdrawn, a liter of normal saline is instilled and the patient is gently rocked from side to side and up and down. The effluent is withdrawn and sent to the laboratory for red blood cell count and amylase and alkaline phosphatase levels. A red blood cell count greater than $100,000/\mu L$ is considered positive. The detection of bile, vegetable or fecal material, or the observation of effluent draining through a chest tube, a nasogastric tube, or a Foley catheter also constitutes a positive result. In equivocal cases, measurement of amylase and alkaline phosphatase levels can be helpful in identifying hollow visceral perforation.[20] White blood cell counts of the lavage effluent are not considered valid indicators of intraperitoneal injury.

SWs to the lower chest present a unique diagnostic opportunity. After the administration of adequate local anesthesia and extension of the wound as necessary, a finger is placed into the thoracic cavity to palpate the diaphragm. Confirmation of diaphragm penetration is an indication for laparotomy. For similar cases when a hole is not palpable, but risk of a diaphragmatic injury exists, a DPL should be performed. A red blood cell count in the effluent of more than 10,000 is considered positive when evaluating for a diaphragmatic injury. For red blood cell counts between 1000 and 10,000, thoracoscopy should be considered.

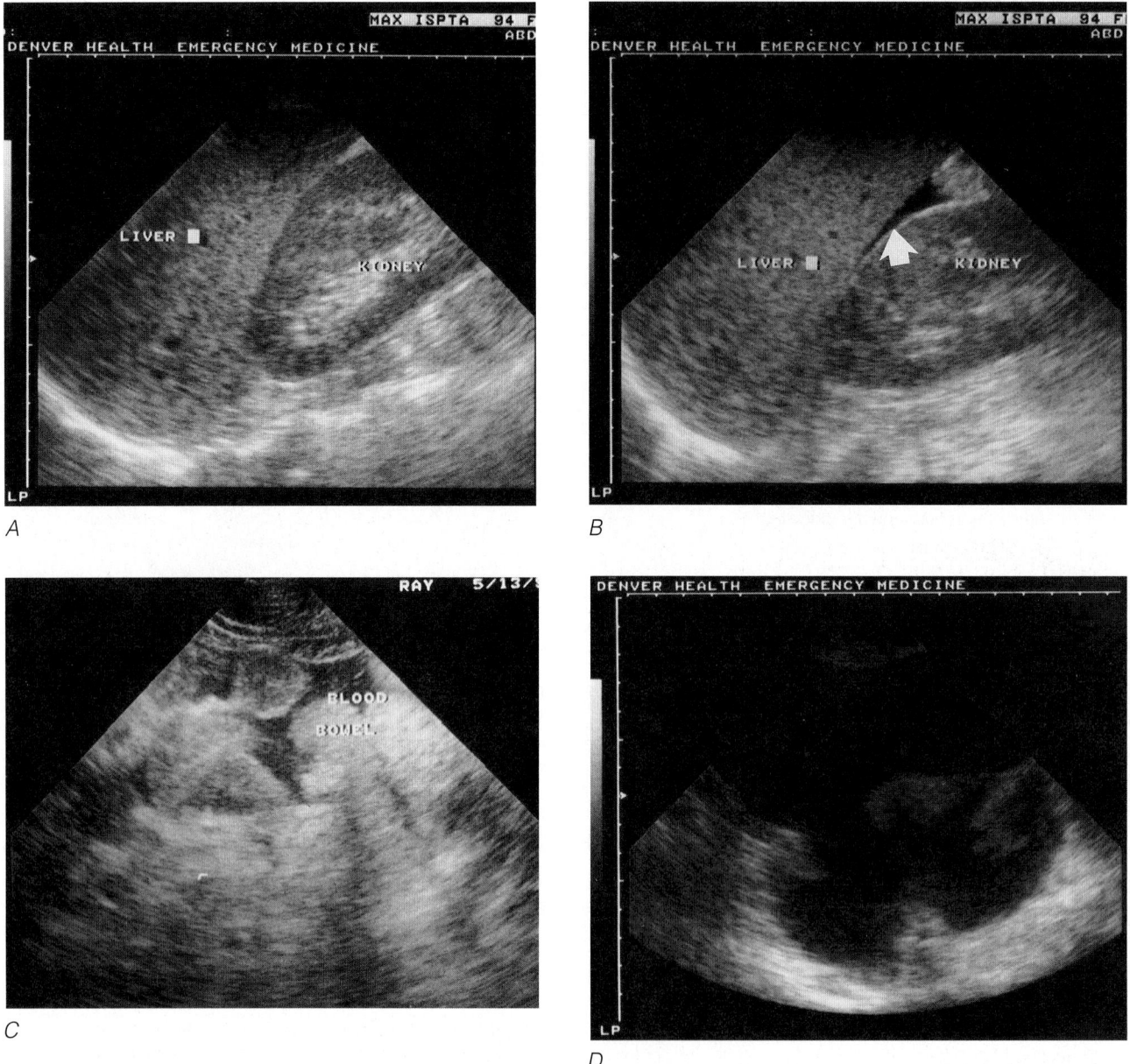

FIG. 6-17.   Ultrasonic imaging for fluid in Morison's pouch has proven to be a reliable method for detecting intra-abdominal hemorrhage. *A.* normal image. *B.* This image demonstrates a fluid stripe between the right kidney and liver; this is considered a positive study. Fluid may also be detected between loops of bowel, as in *C*, or in the pelvis, as in *D*.

Blunt abdominal trauma is currently evaluated by US in most major trauma centers, with CT in selected cases to refine the diagnosis. US performed by a surgeon or an emergency physician in the ED has largely replaced DPL.[21] Evaluation of the entire abdomen is not the goal, but ultrasound is used in specific anatomic regions (e.g., Morison's pouch, the left upper quadrant, and the pelvis) to identify free intraperitoneal fluid (Fig. 6-17). Although this method is exquisitely sensitive for detecting intraperitoneal fluid collections larger than 250 mL, it is relatively poor for staging solid organ injuries. DPL is still appropriate for patients whose condition cannot be explained by US.

The use of CT for the diagnosis of blunt abdominal trauma gained considerable popularity in the early 1980s. It was reported that injuries of the liver, spleen, and kidneys could be diagnosed

with great precision using this method. However, much of the initial enthusiasm has been tempered by the recognition of several limitations: (1) the need for high-quality radiographs, (2) the need for radiologists skilled in the interpretation of postinjury CT images, (3) the need for proper patient preparation, (4) poor sensitivity for intestinal injuries and acute pancreatic injuries, and (5) relatively poor correlation between splenic and hepatic CT images and the subsequent risk of bleeding requiring an operation.

Despite these limitations, CT remains an important diagnostic tool because of its specificity for hepatic, splenic, and renal injuries (Fig. 6-18). CT is indicated primarily for hemodynamically stable patients who are candidates for nonoperative therapy. CT is also indicated for hemodynamically stable patients who have unreliable physical examinations or other conditions (i.e., intracranial injury)

A

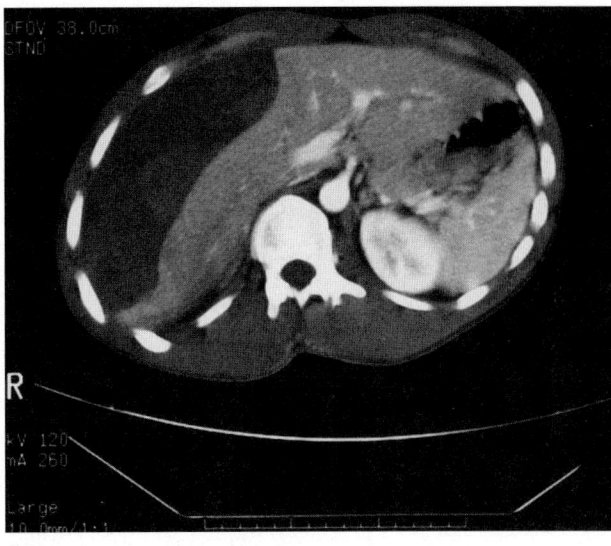

B

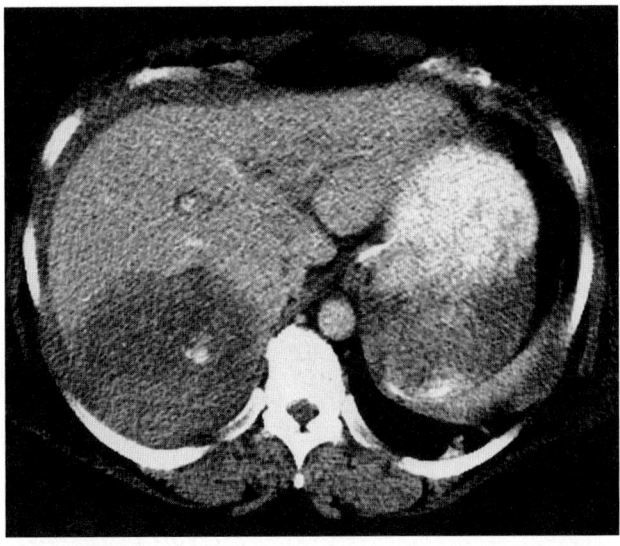

C

FIG. 6-18. *A.* Parenchymal destruction of the posterior aspect of the right hepatic lobe with extravasation of blood. The image in *B* reveals a large subcapsular hematoma. Both patients were successfully treated nonoperatively. *C.* A blunt splenic injury with parenchymal disruption and extravasation.

that require CT evaluation. The algorithm the authors use to evaluate blunt abdominal trauma is outlined in Fig. 6-19.

As laparoscopic cholecystectomy has gained widespread popularity, surgeons have become comfortable with this technology. Because of the excellent view provided of the liver and anterior diaphragm, laparoscopy seems to be an ideal diagnostic tool for stable patients with possible anterior, upper abdominal injuries.[22] One potential concern is carbon dioxide gas embolism through injuries of the hepatic veins. However, this complication can be eliminated with gasless laparoscopy. The role of laparoscopy remains to be clarified, but it may expand with the availability of smaller laparoscopes that can be inserted under local anesthesia.

Pelvis

Blunt injury to the pelvis frequently produces complex fractures (Fig. 6-20). Plain x-rays will reveal gross abnormalities, but CT scans may be necessary to assess the pelvic for stability. Sharp

spicules of bone can lacerate the rectum or vagina. The finding of gross blood on digital examination strongly suggests injury to these organs. Proctoscopy or speculum examination may reveal the injury. In questionable cases, soluble contrast x-rays are diagnostic. The bladder can be lacerated by sharp fracture fragments; or if the bladder is full, a direct blow to the hypogastrium can generate sufficient intravesicular pressure to cause rupture. Gross blood on urinalysis may not always occur, and a cystogram should be performed if more than a few red blood cells are seen on urinalysis. Urethral injuries are suspected by the findings of blood at the meatus, scrotal or perineal hematomas, and a high-riding prostate on rectal exam.

Urethrograms should be done in stable patients prior to placing the Foley catheter to avoid false passage and subsequent stricture. Major vascular injuries are uncommon in blunt pelvic trauma; however, thrombosis or disruption of both the arteries and veins in the iliofemoral system may occur. Angiography is indicated if thrombosis of the arterial system is suspected. Evaluation of penetrating injuries of the pelvis is similar to that for blunt injuries in stable patients.

Management of Blunt Abdominal Trauma
Adult and Pediatric (Age > 12)

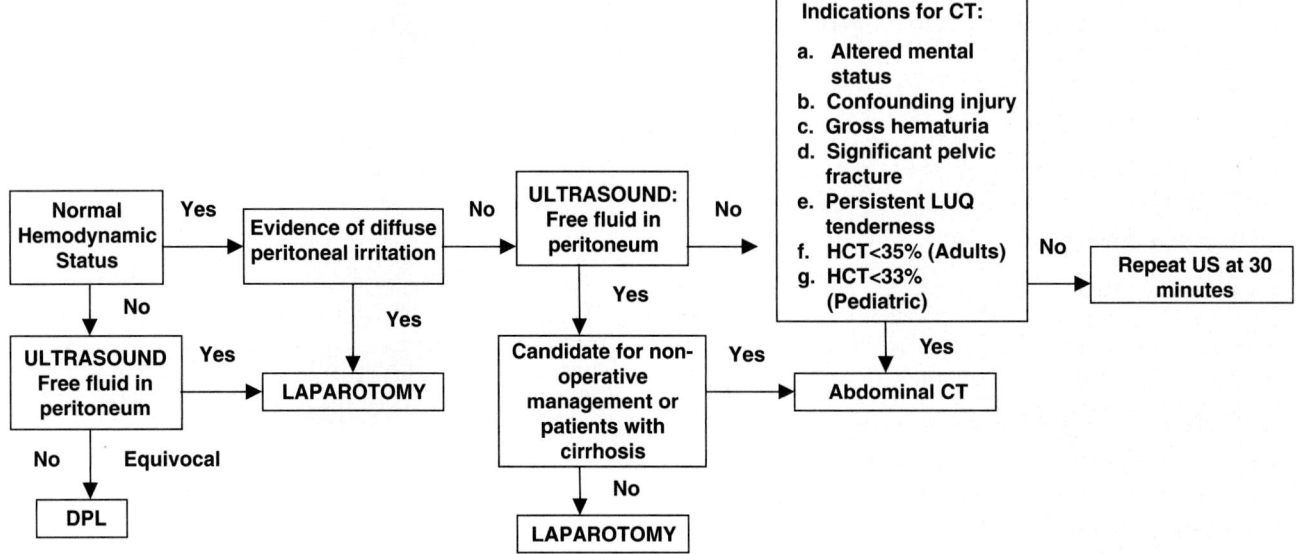

FIG. 6-19. *Algorithm for the initial evaluation of blunt abdominal trauma. DPL = diagnostic peritoneal lavage; LUQ = left lower quadrant; US = ultrasound.*

However, visceral and vascular injuries are much more common, and laparotomy is often required. Surgeons should be aware that life-threatening hemorrhage can be associated with pelvic fractures. The source may be the lower lumbar arteries and veins or branches of the internal iliac arteries and veins. These injuries are frequently not amenable to surgical repair and usually occur with disruption of the posterior elements of the pelvis.

Extremities

Injury of the extremities from any cause requires plain x-rays to evaluate fractures. Ligamentous injuries, particularly those of the knee and shoulder when related to sports activities, can be imaged

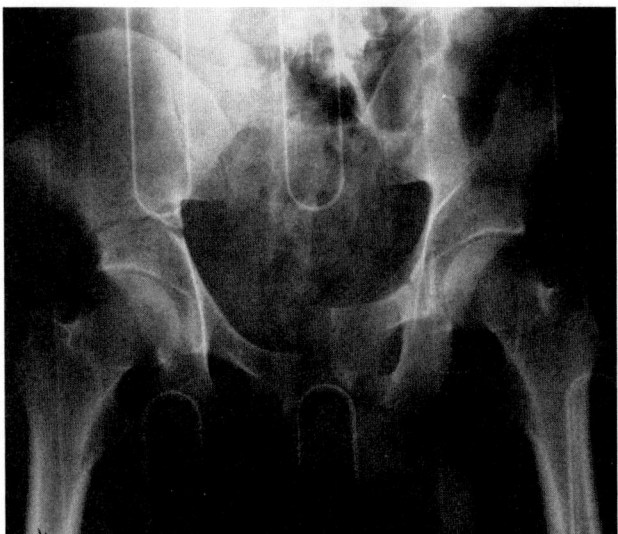

FIG. 6-20. *This is a biomechanically unstable pelvic fracture. There is disruption of the pubic symphysis and sacroiliac joints with vertical displacement. Fractures which involve the posterior elements can cause life-threatening hemorrhage.*

with MRI. The assessment of vascular injuries is somewhat controversial. In general, vascular diagnosis is limited to the arterial system unless there is uncontrolled external venous hemorrhage or venous injuries are uncovered during operative exploration. It is distinctly uncommon to see a patient with a venous complication related to trauma that was not identified and treated while evaluating an arterial injury. Therefore the preoperative diagnosis of venous injury is not pursued.

Physical diagnosis will serve to identify and localize arterial injuries in many instances. Physical findings are classified as either hard signs or soft signs (Table 6-4). In general, hard signs constitute indications for operative exploration, whereas soft signs are indications for observation or further testing. Arteriography may be helpful to localize the injury in some patients with penetrating injuries and hard signs. For example, a bullet which enters the lateral hip and exits below the knee medially and is associated with a femoral shaft fracture and absent popliteal pulse could have injured either the femoral or popliteal artery almost anywhere. Arteriography would be useful to localize the injury and limit the dissection.

In vascular trauma, controversy exists regarding the management of patients with soft signs of injury, particularly in those with injuries in proximity to major vessels. It is known that some of these patients will have arterial injuries that require repair. One approach has been to measure SBP using Doppler US and compare the injured side with the uninjured side.[23] If the pressures are within 10% of each other, a significant injury is excluded and no further evaluation is performed.

Table 6-4
Signs and Symptoms of Arterial Injury

Hard Signs *(Operation Mandatory)*	*Soft Signs* *(Further Evaluation Desirable)*
Pulsatile hemorrhage	Proximity
Significant hemorrhage	Minor hemorrhage
Thrill or bruit	Small hematoma
Acute ischemia	Associated nerve injury

If the difference is greater than 10%, an arteriogram is indicated. Others argue that there are occult injuries, such as pseudoaneurysms or injuries of the profunda femoris or peroneal arteries, which may not be detected with this technique. If hemorrhage occurs from these injuries, compartment syndrome and limb loss may occur. While busy trauma centers continue to debate this issue, the surgeon who is obliged to treat the occasional injured patient may be better served by performing angiography in selected patients with soft signs.

TREATMENT

General Considerations

Seriously injured patients are more fragile than their age and physical condition imply. Procedures that are well tolerated in older patients, such as hepatic lobectomy for hepatoma, are usually lethal in the multiply injured patient. As a result there has been a remarkable change in operative approach over the past 20 years. In general, faster techniques are employed, and shorter, more frequent operations have become common. For example, at the authors' institution, virtually all suture lines are created with a running single layer. There is no evidence that this method is less secure than interrupted multilayer techniques, and it is faster. Drains, once considered mandatory for many parenchymal injuries and some anastomoses, have virtually disappeared. Fluid collections that accumulate in a delayed fashion are now effectively managed by interventional radiologists. Injuries once thought to mandate resection, such as splenic injuries, are now managed with suture repair or even nonoperatively. The treatment of colonic injuries by primary repair is another example. The authors believe these conceptual changes have significantly improved survival in our patients, and all have been developed through the extensive experience of major urban trauma centers and the forums for the free exchange of ideas provided by the American College of Surgeons Committee on Trauma, the American Association for the Surgery of Trauma, the International Association of Trauma and Surgical Intensive Care, the Pan-American Trauma Congress, and other surgical organizations. Trauma surgery is no longer the sole product of its military forbears.

The management of patients with multiple injuries requires the early establishment of therapeutic priorities. While the concept of life over limb and limb over cosmesis seems obvious, decision making can be as subtle as the following common scenarios demonstrate. A patient in a frontal-impact motor vehicle accident presents with a blood pressure of 80 mm Hg systolic and a pulse of 120 bpm. The patient responds to the initial fluid challenge with normalization of the vital signs. Evaluation reveals left lower rib fractures and a wide mediastinum on chest x-ray. US demonstrates free intraperitoneal fluid. Hypotension recurs. The patient probably has a tear of the thoracic aorta and a splenic injury, and recurrent hypotension suggests ongoing hemorrhage. The correct decision is to perform emergency laparotomy and treat the splenic injury first. Even though an aortic tear is a more lethal injury, hypotension is usually not from a torn aorta. If it is from the aorta, the injury is not survivable in most instances due to the complexity of the operation and the length of time required for preparation. Furthermore, both procedures are difficult to perform simultaneously due to positioning problems and lack of space. Therefore the patient's best chance for survival is for the surgeon to assume the injured spleen is the source of recurrent hypotension. Laparotomy for splenectomy can be set up and performed very quickly, and intraoperative transesophageal echo or intravascular US can be used to confirm a tear in the thoracic aorta.

Closed-head injuries are common with both abdominal and thoracic trauma. One scenario of this is a patient who hits a tree while skiing. Evaluation reveals an epidural hematoma with an 8-mm midline shift and hypotension with free intraperitoneal fluid. Fortunately, a craniotomy and laparotomy can and should be done simultaneously. In fact, craniotomy for trauma can be performed concurrent with almost any procedure.

Another dilemma is a serious fracture (e.g., an open comminuted femoral fracture) in a patient who has just undergone a major thoracoabdominal procedure. These operations cannot be performed simultaneously because treatment of the femoral fracture requires a fracture table. Patients are commonly in poor metabolic condition following extensive truncal operations due to hypothermia, metabolic acidosis, and the coagulopathy that inevitably accompany hemorrhagic shock and massive transfusion (see Staged Operations below). Patients in this condition do not tolerate additional blood or thermal energy loss well and are at risk for sudden death. In this situation the open femoral fracture will have to be deferred until the patient's metabolic situation improves, in spite of increasing the risk of osteomyelitis and even limb loss. Many other combinations of injuries and physiologic states can be anticipated that impact decision making. It is the trauma surgeon's responsibility to assess the probable outcomes of different therapeutic strategies and choose which is in the patient's best interest.

Transfusion Practices and the Blood Bank

Component therapy is a fact of life in all hospitals. Fresh whole blood, arguably the optimal replacement material for shed blood, is no longer available. Therefore whole blood must be re-created from its component parts: packed red blood cells (PRBCs), fresh-frozen plasma (FFP), and platelet packs. This is not to imply that all trauma patients requiring transfusions receive all three. To the contrary, most trauma patients receive between one and five units of PRBCs and no other components. However, major trauma centers and their associated blood banks have the capability of transfusing tremendous quantities of blood components. It is not unusual to see 100 component units transfused during one procedure and have the patient survive. Red blood cell transfusion rates (a seldom-used figure) of 20 to 40 units of packed red cells per hour are not uncommon in severely injured patients. Often hospitals and blood banks that do not treat large numbers of trauma patients have difficulty comprehending these figures and are more concerned about avoiding unnecessary elective transfusions. The appropriate administrative shortcuts should be in place that permit transfusion at these rates should a crisis occur. The medical directors of blood banks can only understand the trauma surgeon's dilemma if they witness such events first-hand in the OR. Then the administrative controls can be established that allow them to alter their usual, but appropriate, parsimonious practices. A special understanding of trust must exist between surgeons, anesthesiologists, and blood bank directors who frequently deal with severely injured patients.

Contemporary transfusion practices in trauma require the surgeon to identify the insidious signs of coagulopathy, such as excessive bleeding from the cut edges of skin, fascia, and peritoneum, which were previously controlled. While the local volume of coagulopathic hemorrhage in one visual field may seem small compared to a hole in the aorta or vena cava, blood loss from the entire area of dissection can lead to exsanguination. The usual measurements of coagulation capability (i.e., prothrombin time [PT], partial thromboplastin time [PTT], and platelet count) have a turnaround time of more than 30 minutes in most institutions. As a result these tests are of limited value in patients who have lost two or three blood volumes while waiting for the test to return. Under such conditions, transfusion must be empiric and based on the surgeon's observations. In general, at the first sign of coagulopathic hemorrhage, the previously lost plasma proteins and platelets must be restored with FFP and platelet packs. Additional transfusions should be administered with equal ratios of PRBCs, FFP, and platelets.

The causal relationship of core hypothermia, metabolic acidosis, and postinjury coagulopathy has been observed in a number of studies. The pathophysiology is multifactorial and includes inhibition of temperature-dependent enzyme-activated coagulation cascades, platelet dysfunction, endothelial abnormalities, and a poorly understood fibrinolytic activity. The role of metabolic acidosis in the pathogenesis of a coagulopathy is less clear. Animal work has demonstrated impaired hemostasis at a pH of 7.20, while others have suggested that pH directly affects platelet function. Another series of experiments implicated acidosis in the propagation of disseminated intravascular coagulation with the secondary consumption of clotting factors. In addition, both hypothermia and metabolic acidosis have adverse effects on both myocardial performance and tissue perfusion.

Primary hemostasis relies on platelet adherence and aggregation to injured endothelium, resulting in the formation of the platelet plug. A platelet count of 50,000/μL is considered adequate for tissue hemostasis if they are normal. However, platelet dysfunction is a well-documented complication of massive transfusion, which is clearly aggravated by associated hypothermia. Consequently, the recommended target of more than 100,000 cells/μL for platelet transfusion in other high-risk patients should be extended to severely injured patients.

Blood typing, and to a lesser extent cross-matching, is essential to avoid life-threatening intravascular hemolytic transfusion reactions. A complete type and cross-match requires from 20 to 45 minutes to complete and reduces the risk of an intravascular hemolysis to approximately 0.004%. However, if 20 units of PRBCs are needed within 1 hour, an army of technicians would be required to perform this service. Furthermore, 20 to 45 minutes is far too long for a patient with exsanguinating hemorrhage to wait. Therefore, trauma patients requiring emergency transfusions are given type O, type-specific, or biologically compatible red blood cells. As a cross-check for ABO compatibility, one of the many steps of the cross-match (e.g., a saline cross-match) is often performed. The administrative and laboratory time required is approximately 5 minutes, and the risk of intravascular hemolysis is about 0.05%. The risk increases to 1.0% with a history of previous transfusions or pregnancy and up to 3.0% with both. This increased risk of transfusion reaction is due to the presence of irregular antibodies (i.e., Kell, Duffy, and Kidd blood groups) in the patient's plasma, which occurs in about 1 in 1000 patients. Intravascular hemolysis can occur with ABO-compatible PRBCs if the patient has an irregular antibody. However, they are usually not as severe as ABO-incompatible hemolytic reactions, and the time required to detect the antibodies biochemically or by cross-match (25 to 45 minutes) makes the slight increased risk of hemolytic reaction a reasonable trade-off for rapid availability. It should also be noted that preformed antibodies are rapidly depleted by hemorrhage and that they are produced slowly. This also diminishes the severity of intravascular hemolysis should it occur. An alternative strategy for those patients who are consistently stable and do not appear to have serious injuries is to perform a type and screen as a cost-saving measure. If blood is subsequently needed urgently, low-titer, type-specific red blood cells can be administered with the same risk of intravascular hemolysis as with fully-typed and cross-matched blood, provided the screen for irregular antibodies is negative. Unstable patients should receive O⁻, O⁺, or type-specific red blood cells depending on age, sex, and availability. Other components should be type-specific or biologically compatible.

Prophylactic Measures

Numerous prospective randomized studies have demonstrated lower infection rates and improved survival for patients receiving one preoperative antibiotic compared to another. The comparison of an antibiotic to placebo has been attempted but abandoned and will likely never be performed. Therefore all injured patients undergoing an operation should receive presumptive antibiotics. Presently, the authors use second-generation cephalosporins for laparotomies and first-generation cephalosporins for all other operations. Additional doses should be administered during the procedure based on blood loss and the half-life of the antibiotic. The role of postoperative antibiotics in trauma patients remains to be defined, but the trend has been to reduce the duration. Tetanus prophylaxis is administered to all patients according to published guidelines.

Deep venous thrombosis and other venous complications occur more often in injured patients than generally believed. This is particularly true for patients with major fractures of the pelvis and lower extremities, those with coma or spinal cord injury, and probably in those with injury of the large veins in the abdomen and lower extremities. The authors employ pulsatile compression stockings in all injured patients and also selectively place inferior vena caval filters for those at very high risk. The role of inferior vena caval filters may expand in the future when removable devices become commercially available. Low molecular weight heparin has been demonstrated to be safe and effective in patients with orthopedic injuries. Its utility in patients with other injuries remains to be elucidated.

A final prophylactic measure that is not usually considered in this context is thermal protection. Hemorrhagic shock impairs perfusion and metabolic activity throughout the body. With declining metabolism, heat production and body temperature decrease. The injured patient receives a second thermal insult with the removal of insulating clothes. As a result, trauma patients can become seriously hypothermic with temperatures as low as 34°C by the time they reach the OR. Hypothermia impairs coagulation and myocardial contractility and increases myocardial irritability. Although it can be argued that intentional hypothermia has protective features for patients with massive head injuries, most authorities agree that the deleterious effects outweigh the potential benefits. Injured patients whose intraoperative core temperature drops below 32°C are at risk for fatal arrhythmias as well as defective coagulation. Thermal prophylaxis should begin in the ED by maintaining an ambient temperature that is comfortable for an exposed patient. Fluids should be stored at body temperature, and blood products should be administered through rapid warming devices. Once visualization of the patient is no longer necessary, he or she should be kept scrupulously covered with warm blankets or other devices until the temperature returns to normal.

Principles and Techniques of Vascular Repair

A knowledge of vascular surgical techniques is essential for surgeons caring for injured patients. Life- or limb-threatening injuries occur everywhere in the body; bullets, knives, fractures, and shearing forces do not discriminate between visceral and vascular structures. Whether vascular experience is obtained by performing elective vascular procedures or a fellowship in vascular surgery is irrelevant; the concepts are the same. General surgery requires precision on a scale of millimeters; vascular surgery requires precision on a scale of tenths of millimeters. Visual magnification is necessary for many repairs. A complete set of instruments specifically designed for vascular surgery should always be available. These sets must contain the clamps, tissue forceps, scissors, and needle-holders necessary to control and repair vessels ranging from the thoracic aorto to the tibial arteries, using sutures ranging in size from 3-0 to 7-0.

The initial control of vascular injuries should be accomplished digitally by applying just enough pressure directly on the bleeding site to stop the hemorrhage. Some bleeding vessels may need to be gently pinched between the thumb and index finger. These maneuvers, along with suction, usually create a dry enough field to safely permit the dissection necessary to define the injury. In general, sharp dissection with fine scissors is preferable to blunt dissection, since the latter may aggravate the injury. Once a sufficient length of vessel is available, a vascular thumb forceps is used to grasp the vessel. If the vessel is not transected, forceps can be placed directly across the injury. This will minimize or eliminate bleeding while the dissection necessary for clamping is completed. If the vessel is transected (or nearly so), digital control is maintained on one side while the other is occluded with a thumb forceps. The vessel is then sharply mobilized to allow an appropriate vascular clamp to be applied. When definitive control of all injuries is achieved, heparinized saline (50 U/mL) is injected into the proximal and distal ends of the injured vessel to prevent thrombosis. The exposed intima and media at the site of the injury are highly thrombogenic, and small clots often form. These clots should be carefully removed to prevent thrombosis or embolism when the clamps are removed. Due to the frequency with which embolism occurs, routine balloon catheter exploration of the distal vessel has been recommended. Ragged edges of the injury site should be judiciously débrided using sharp dissection.

Injuries of the large veins such as the vena cava and innominate and iliac veins pose a special problem for hemostasis. Numerous large tributaries make adequate hemostasis difficult to achieve, and their thin walls render them susceptible to further or additional iatrogenic injury. When such an injury is encountered, tamponade with a folded laparotomy pad held directly over the bleeding site will usually establish hemostasis sufficient to prevent exsanguination. If hemostasis is not adequate to expose the vessel proximal and distal to the injury, sponge sticks can be strategically placed on either side of the injury and carefully adjusted to improve hemostasis. This maneuver requires both skill and discipline to maintain a dry field. On occasion the operative field will be sufficient to delineate and repair the injury. However, it is often difficult or impossible for the assistant or assistants to maintain complete control of hemorrhage with sponge sticks. In this situation, the vessel can be exposed on either side of the sponge stick and a vascular clamp applied. The clamp can then be sequentially advanced toward the injury until hemostasis is complete.

Options for the treatment of vascular injuries are listed in Table 6-5. Some arteries and most veins can be ligated without significant sequelae. Arteries for which repair should always be

attempted include the carotid, innominate, brachial, superior mesenteric, proper hepatic, renal, iliac, femoral, popliteal, and the aorta. In the forearm and lower leg, at least one of the two palpable vessels should be salvaged. The list of veins for which repair should be attempted is short: the superior vena cava, the inferior vena cava proximal to the renal veins, and the portal vein. There are notable vessels not listed for which repair is not necessary (e.g., the subclavian artery and the superior mesenteric vein). The surgeon must keep in mind that there are few absolutes when discussing the treatment of vascular injuries. The portal vein can be ligated successfully, provided adequate fluid is administered to compensate for the dramatic but transient edema which occurs in the bowel. If the alternative to ligation is exsanguination, the correct decision is obvious. On the other hand, ligation of some vessels such as the popliteal vein and left or right branch of the portal vein may result in morbidity for the patient which is not life-threatening. Therefore the authors attempt to repair all arteries larger than 3 mm and all veins larger than 10 mm in diameter, depending on the patient's physiologic condition.

Within the last decade, some arterial injuries have been treated by observation without subsequent complications. These include small pseudoaneurysms, intimal dissections, small intimal flaps, and arteriovenous fistulas in the extremities, and occlusions of small (<2 mm) arteries. Follow-up angiography is obtained within 2 to 4 weeks to ensure that healing has occurred.

Lateral suture is appropriate for small arterial injuries with little or no loss of tissue. End-to-end anastomosis is used if the vessel is transected or nearly so. The severed ends of the vessel are mobilized, and small branches are ligated and divided as necessary to obtain the desired length. Arterial defects of 1 to 2 cm can usually be bridged. The surgeon should not be reluctant to divide small branches to obtain additional length since most injured patients have normal vasculature and the preservation of potential collateral flow is not as important as in atherosclerotic surgery. To avoid postoperative stenosis, particularly in smaller arteries, some techniques such as beveling or spatulation should be used so that the completed anastomosis is slightly larger in diameter than the native artery (Fig. 6-21).

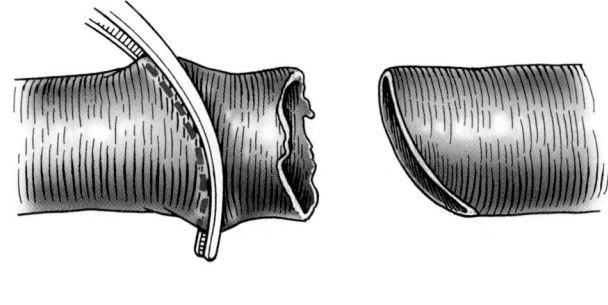
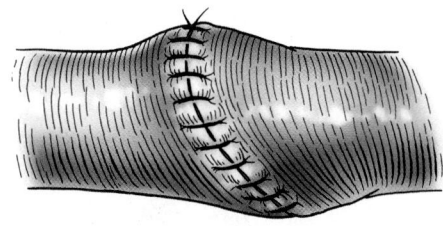

FIG. 6-21. Small arteries that are repaired with an end-to-end anastomosis are prone to thrombosis. Enlarging the anastomosis by beveling the cut ends of the injured vessel can minimize this problem. A hemostat is a useful adjunct to cut the curve.

Table 6-5
Options for the Treatment of Vascular Injuries

Observation
Ligation
Lateral suture
End-to-end anastomosis
Interposition grafts
    Autogenous vein
    Autogenous artery
    PTFE
    Dacron
Transpositions
Extra-anatomic bypass
Interventional radiology

PTFE = polytetrafluoroethylene.

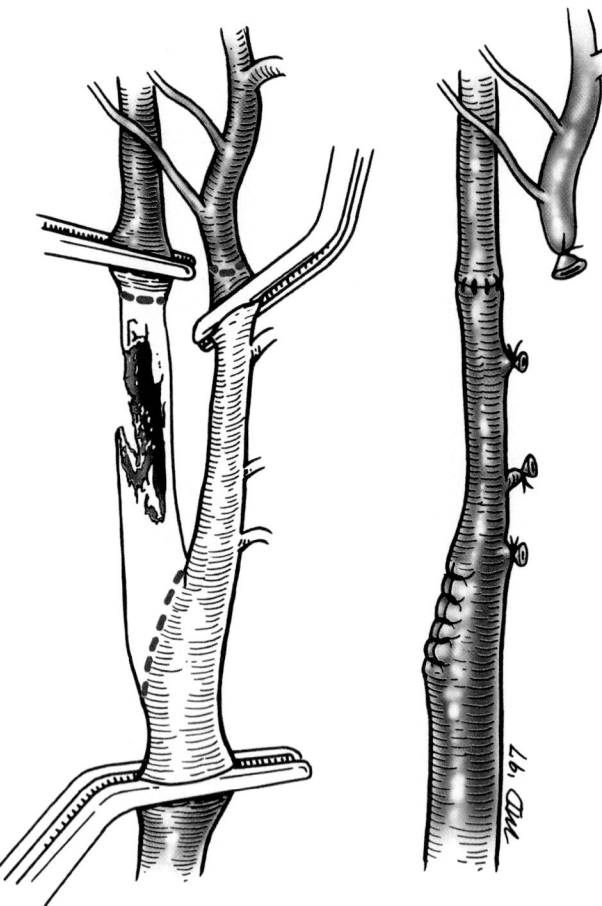

FIG. 6-22. Carotid transposition is an effective approach for treating proximal injuries of the internal carotid artery.

Interposition grafts are employed when end-to-end anastomosis cannot be accomplished without tension and in spite of mobilization. For vessels less than 6 mm in diameter, autogenous saphenous vein from the groin should be used since polytetrafluoroethylene (PTFE) grafts less than 6 mm in diameter have a prohibitive rate of

thrombosis. In practice, injuries of the brachial, popliteal, and internal carotid arteries require the saphenous vein for interposition grafting. When the saphenous vein is harvested for treating an arterial injury in the lower extremity, it should be taken from the contralateral extremity. Since the status of the ipsilateral venous system is unknown, the saphenous vein on that side may become an important tributary. Larger arteries must be bridged by artificial grafts. Some authorities have advocated the use of free internal iliac arterial grafts because of the greater thickness and strength of its wall compared to that of the saphenous vein. The authors believe that this vessel is unnecessarily tedious to remove and has no advantage over the saphenous vein.

Transposition procedures can be used when an artery has a bifurcation of which one vessel can safely be ligated. Injuries of the proximal internal carotid can be treated by mobilizing the adjacent external carotid, dividing it distal to the internal injury, and performing an end-to-end anastomosis between it and the distal internal carotid (Fig. 6-22). The proximal stump of the internal carotid is oversewn in such a way as to avoid a blind pocket where a clot may form. Injuries of the ipsilateral external and contralateral common iliac arteries can be handled in a similar fashion, provided flow is maintained in at least one internal iliac artery (Fig. 6-23).

Arterial injuries are often grossly contaminated from enteric or external sources. Many surgeons are naturally reluctant to place artificial grafts in situ in this circumstance. The situation arises most often with aortic or iliac arterial injuries when the colon is also injured. For the aorta there are few options. Ligation of the aorta with unilateral or bilateral axillofemoral bypass can be performed. However, these are lengthy procedures which are prone to thrombosis and infection. Furthermore, most patients who require an aortic graft will not tolerate the time required to perform an axillofemoral bypass. Therefore, even in the presence of fecal contamination, it has been common practice to use PTFE or Dacron in situ for aortic injuries. Every effort is made to remove and control contamination following the control of hemorrhage, but before the graft is brought into the operative field. This includes copious irrigation of the abdominal cavity and changing of drapes, gowns, gloves, and instruments. Following placement of the graft, it is covered with peritoneum or omentum prior to definitive treatment of the enteric injuries. Curiously, graft infection has been rare in these instances.

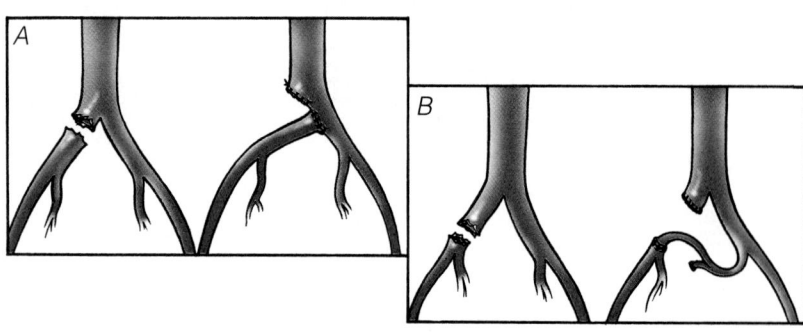

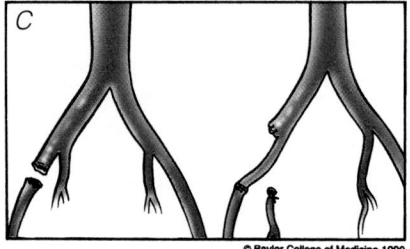

FIG. 6-23. Transposition procedures can be used with iliac arterial injuries to eliminate the dilemma of placing an interposition graft in the presence of enteric or fecal contamination. *A.* Right common iliac artery transposed to left common iliac artery. *B.* Left internal iliac artery transposed to distal right common iliac artery. *C.* Right internal iliac artery transposed to right external iliac artery.

© Baylor College of Medicine 1990

Table 6-6
Suture Selection for Repair of Vascular Injuries

Aorta	3-0
Iliac and innominate arteries	4-0
Femoral, subclavian, axillary, common carotid, renal, superior mesenteric, common and proper hepatic arteries	5-0
Popliteal and brachial arteries	6-0
Radial, ulnar, and tibial arteries	7-0
Large veins	5-0
Smaller veins	6-0

A similar approach can be used for iliac arterial injuries, but in most cases this can be avoided by the innovative use of transposition procedures.

Suture selection for arterial injuries is based on the diameter of the vessel being repaired (Table 6-6). The use of progressively finer suture for smaller-diameter vessels encourages the inclusion of less tissue with more closely placed sutures, which is necessary for success. When performing anastomoses where the vessels are tethered (e.g., the thoracic and abdominal aorta), the authors employ the parachute technique to ensure precision placement of the posterior suture line (Fig. 6-24). If this technique is used, traction on both ends of the suture must be maintained, or leakage from the posterior aspect of the suture line is probable. A single temporary suture 180° from the posterior row is often used to maintain alignment.

Venous injuries are inherently more difficult to repair successfully due to their propensity to thrombose. Small injuries without loss of tissue can be treated with lateral suture. More complex repairs often fail. It should be noted that thrombosis does not occur acutely, but rather gradually over 1 to 2 weeks. Advantage can be taken of this fact because adequate collateral circulation, sufficient

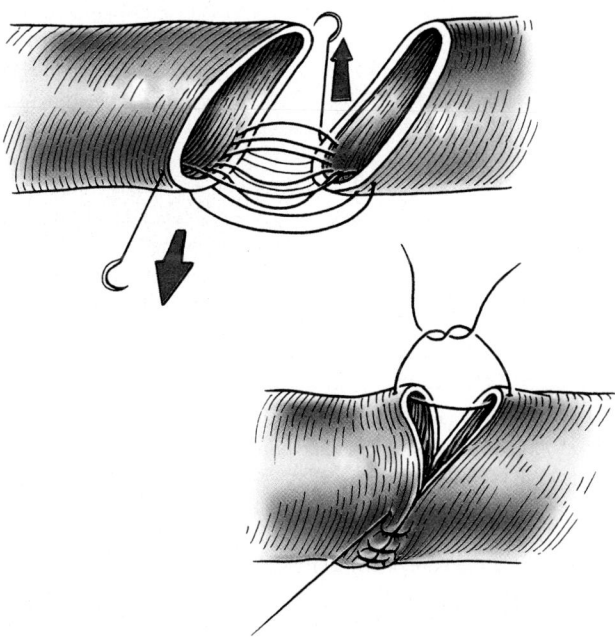

FIG. 6-24. The parachute technique is helpful for accurate placement of posterior sutures of an anastomosis when the arterial end is fixed and an interposition graft is necessary. Traction must be maintained on both ends of the suture to prevent loosening and leakage of blood. Only six stitches can be placed before the graft must be pulled down to the artery.

to avoid acute venous hypertensive complications, usually develops within several days. Therefore it is reasonable to use PTFE for venous interposition grafting and accept a gradual but eventual thrombosis while buying time for collateral circulation to develop. On the other hand, chronic venous hypertensive complications in the lower extremities can often be avoided with any level of ligation by: (1) elastic bandages carefully applied in the OR at the end of the procedure, and (2) continuous elevation of the lower extremities to 30°. These measures should be maintained for 1 week. The patient is then ambulated. If no edema occurs with the bandages removed, elevation is no longer necessary. It is a reasonable precaution to have the patient wear compressive stockings up to the knee for a few months afterwards.

There are several circumstances in which a more aggressive approach should be considered. Ligation of the superior vena cava has been associated with sudden blindness due to compression of the optic nerve from venous hypertension. Ligation of the suprarenal vena cava is believed to be associated with acute renal failure from venous hypertension. Chronic venous insufficiency of the lower extremities may be caused by ligation of the infrarenal vena cava or any in-line vein below that level, particularly the popliteal vein. Interposition grafting can be considered in these situations, but the choice of material is problematic. One option is to use artificial material since it is rapidly available in hemodynamically correct sizes. The drawback is that thrombosis is inevitable when these are placed below the renal veins. Artificial grafts have performed satisfactorily in cases of suprarenal vena caval and superior vena caval replacement. The jugular vein can be used to replace similar-sized vessels (e.g., the portal or femoral veins). The saphenous vein is too small to replace any important vein. Panel grafts and spiral grafts constructed around a chest tube using saphenous vein have occasionally been performed. These procedures are extremely tedious and have no apparent advantage over ligation in most instances.

The technology employed by interventional radiologists is advancing at an incredible pace. They have the ability to cannulate virtually any artery in the body and either dilate it, place an intraluminal filter, stent or graft it, or occlude it. At present their services are most valuable for treating arterial or venous injuries that are surgically inaccessible, such as stent placement in the internal carotid artery near or in the base of the skull, controlling hemorrhage in hepatic injuries, or pelvic fractures (Figs. 6-25, 6-26, and 6-27).

Staged Operations, Abdominal Compartment Syndrome, and Nonoperative Management

The most common causes of death for trauma patients are head injury, exsanguination from cardiovascular injuries, and sepsis with multiple organ failure. Another cause of death has become apparent as the capability of delivering massive quantities of red blood cells and other components developed. Surgeons are now able to continue to operate on the most severely injured patients until a constellation of metabolic derangements develop. These are characterized by the triad of an obvious coagulopathy, profound hypothermia, and metabolic acidosis. Hypothermia from evaporative and conductive heat loss and diminished heat production occurs in spite of warming blankets and blood warmers. The metabolic acidosis of shock is exacerbated by aortic clamping, vasopressors, massive transfusions, and impaired myocardial performance. Coagulopathy is caused by dilution, hypothermia, and acidosis. Each of these factors reinforces the others, resulting in a critically ill patient who is at high risk for a fatal arrhythmia. This downward spiral has been referred to as the *bloody vicious cycle* (Fig. 6-28).

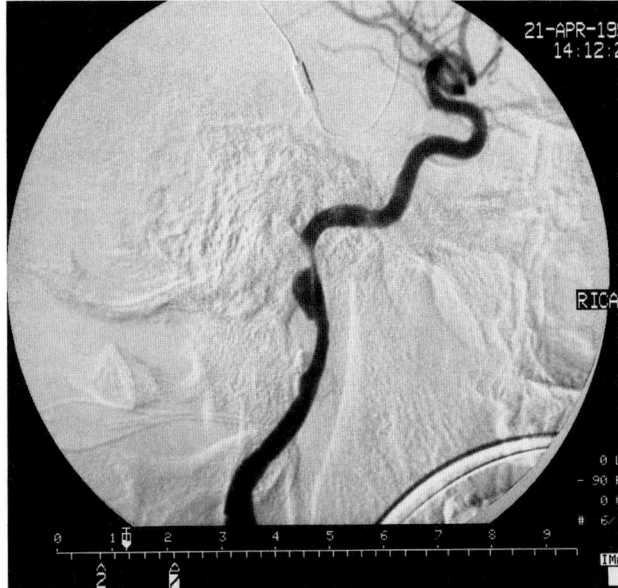

A

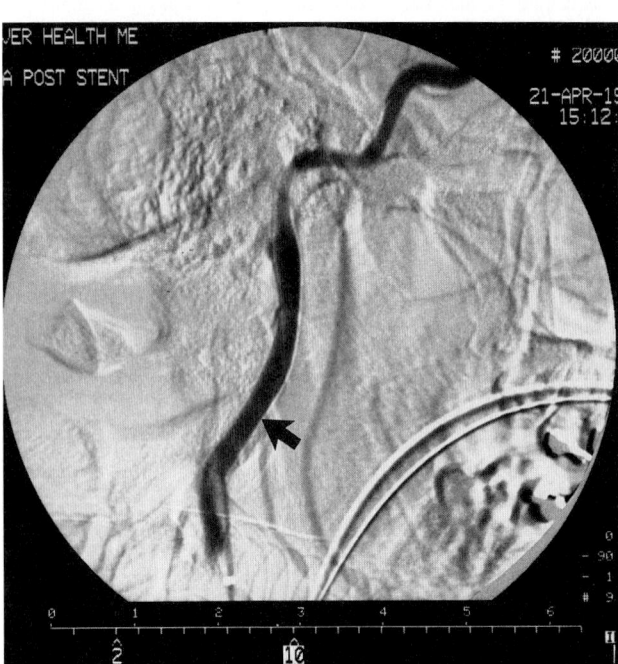

B

FIG. 6-25. Carotid dissection and pseudoaneurysm due to blunt trauma are being recognized with increasing frequency. The image in *A* shows both a pseudoaneurysm and a dissection. The image in *B* shows an intravascular stent placed by an interventional radiologist.

Heat loss appears to be the central event since neither of the other components can be corrected until core temperature returns toward normal. Laboratory and mathematical heat exchange models have demonstrated that evaporative heat loss from an open abdomen is by far the greatest source. A concomitant open thoracic cavity greatly accelerates the rate of the patient's deterioration and can cause the syndrome by itself. This is the rationale for the immediate abdominal closure and the reason it has been successful.[24,25]

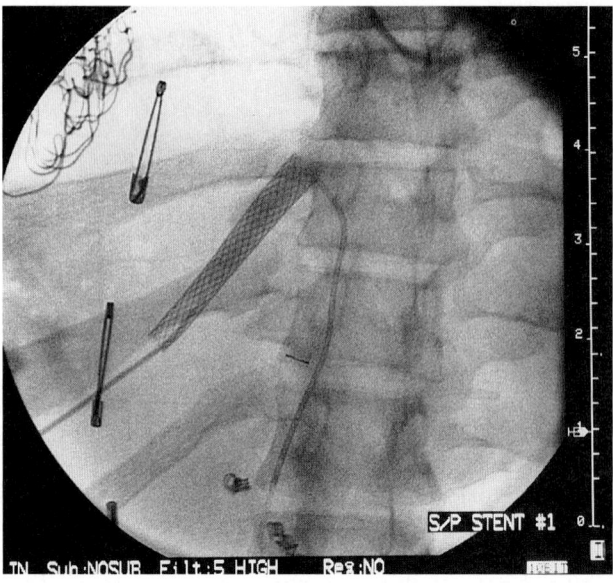

FIG. 6-26. This patient has an extensive hepatic parenchymal injury associated with a laceration of the right hepatic vein. The surgeon was able to control the venous hemorrhage with packs. The patient was then transported to the interventional radiology suite, where the hepatic venous injury was treated with a stent and several arterial injuries were embolized with coils (visible at the bottom of the image). Radiopaque markers of laparotomy pads are visible in the upper left of the image.

Staged operations are indicated when a coagulopathy develops and core temperature drops below 34°C. A refractory acidosis almost always exists. Several unorthodox techniques can be used to expedite wound closure. Bleeding raw surfaces, often of the liver, are packed with laparotomy pads. Small enteric injuries are closed with staples, and large ones are stapled on both sides with the GIA stapler and the damaged segment removed. Clamps may be left on unrepaired vascular injuries, or the vessels are ligated. Injuries of the pancreas and kidneys are not treated if they are not bleeding. No drains are placed, and the abdomen is closed with sharp towel clips that include only the skin, placed 2 cm apart (Fig. 6-29). Towel clips are used because they do not cause bleeding as needles do and they can be applied very rapidly, usually in 60 to 90 seconds. The closure of just the skin allows for the abdominal or thoracic cavities to accommodate a greater volume without increased pressure. The clips are covered with a towel, and a plastic adhesive sheet is placed over the towel to prevent excessive fluid from draining onto the patient's bedding. Cold, wet drapes are removed, and the patient is covered from head to toe with layers of warm blankets. It should be noted that many of these unorthodox treatments, including the creation of closed-loop bowel obstructions and unrepaired renal injuries, are not compatible with survival. However, reoperation is planned within 2 to 24 hours, and the treatments are tolerated well within that time frame. Furthermore, the goal is to complete the procedure as soon as possible or the patient will certainly die. If the surgeon believes that the patient's metabolic problems can be corrected in a short time (2 hours or less), the patient may remain in the operating room while additional blood products are administered and rewarming measures are instituted. Patients who are in very poor condition and will require several hours for metabolic corrections should be transferred to the surgical intensive care unit (SICU). If the patient's condition improves as evidenced by normalization of coagulation studies, the

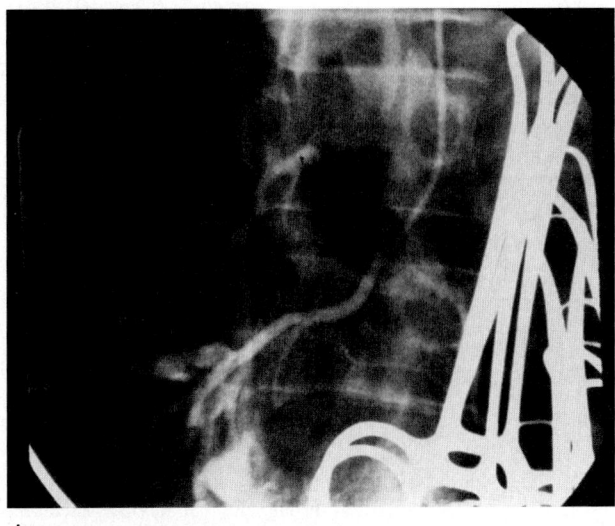

A

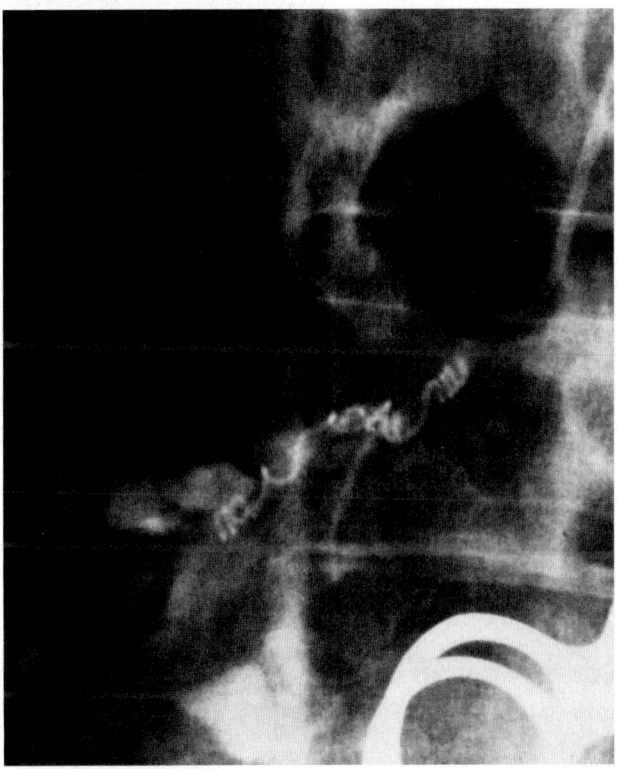

B

FIG. 6-27. This patient has life-threatening hemorrhage due to a pelvic fracture. *A.* Angiography revealed extravasation from the right fifth lumbar artery. *B.* The hemorrhage was controlled with coil embolization.

correction of acid-base balance, and a core temperature of at least 36°C, they should be returned to the operating room for removal of packs and definitive treatment of injuries.

There are several complications associated with this treatment. Failure to identify noncoagulopathic hemorrhage can lead to exsanguination. Most patients with coagulopathic hemorrhage will have a gradual decrease in the need for PRBCs, FFP, and platelets, and an improvement in coagulation studies as temperature rises. Patients

"THE BLOODY VICIOUS CYCLE"

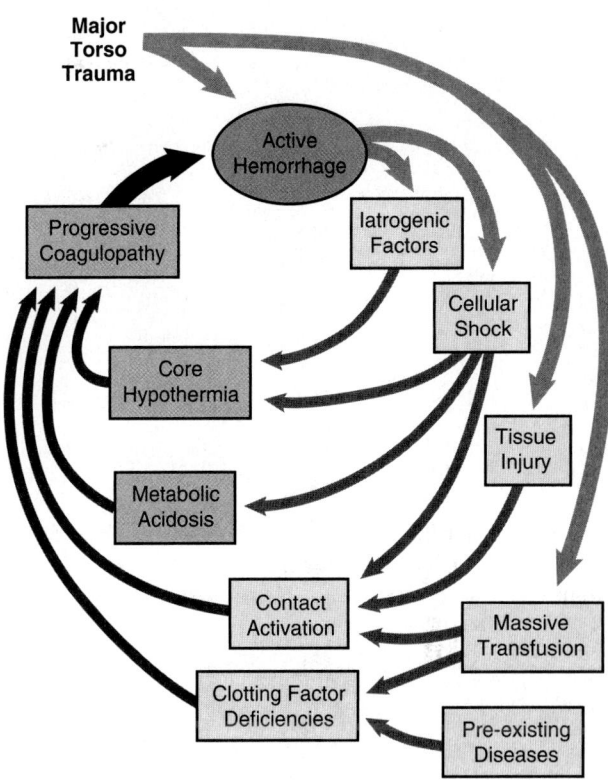

FIG. 6-28. The bloody vicious cycle.

with vascular hemorrhage will not, and they must be returned to the OR for re-exploration.

A second complication is referred to as the abdominal or thoracic compartment syndrome. These entities are caused by an acute increase in intracavitary pressure. In the abdomen, the compliance of the abdominal wall and the diaphragm permit the accumulation of many liters of fluid before intra-abdominal pressure (IAP) increases. There are primarily two sources for this fluid: blood and edema. Blood accumulates due to the coagulopathy or missed vascular injury described above. The cause of edema is multifactorial. Ischemia and reperfusion cause capillary leakage; loss of oncotic pressure occurs; and in the case of the small bowel, which is often

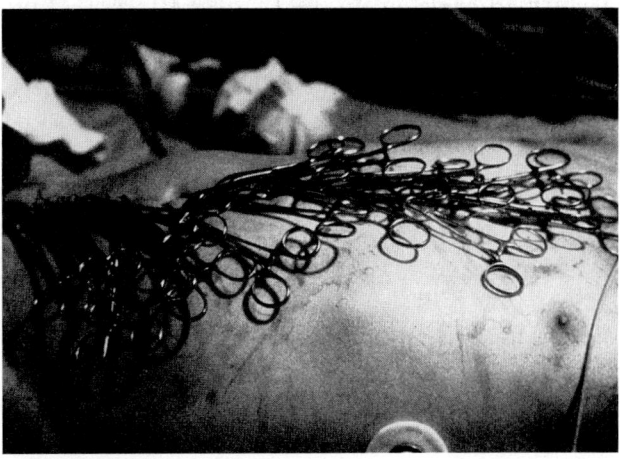

FIG. 6-29. The towel-clip closure.

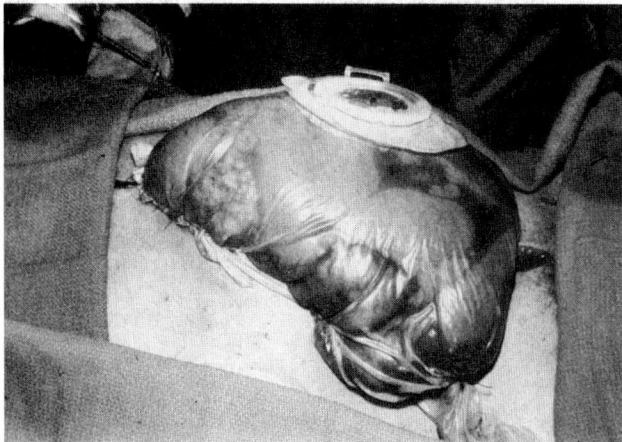

FIG. 6-30. Massive intestinal edema precludes routine abdominal closure.

Table 6-7
Recommended Treatment for Abdominal Compartment Syndrome According to Intra-Abdominal Pressure (IAP)

IAP in cm H_2O	Treatment
<15	Normal
15–25	Volume expansion; may need decompression
26–35	Watch Po_2, Sao_2, urine output; decompression is likely
>35	Decompress in OR

eviscerated, prolongation and narrowing of veins and lymphatics caused by traction impairs venous and lymphatic drainage. The resulting edema may be dramatic (Fig. 6-30). Similar phenomena occur in the chest. As fluid continues to accumulate, the compliant limit of the abdominal cavity is eventually exceeded, and IAP increases. When IAP exceeds 15 mm Hg, serious physiologic changes begin to occur. The lungs are compressed by the upward displacement of the diaphragm. This causes a decrease in functional residual capacity, increased airway pressure, and ultimately hypoxia. Cardiac output decreases due to diminished venous return to the heart and increased afterload. Blood flow to every intra-abdominal organ is reduced due to increased venous resistance. As IAP exceeds 25 to 30 mm Hg, life-threatening hypoxia and anuric renal failure occur. Cardiac output is further reduced, but can be returned toward normal with volume expansion and inotropic support.[26] However, the only method for treating hypoxia and renal failure is to decompress the abdominal cavity by opening the incision. This results in an immediate diuresis and a resolution of hypoxia. Failure to decompress the abdominal cavity will eventually cause lethal hypoxia and/or organ failure. There have been a few reports of sudden hypotension when the abdomen is opened. However, volume loading to enhance cardiac output has largely eliminated this problem. IAP is measured using the Foley catheter. Since the bladder is a passive reservoir at low volumes (50 to 100 mL), it imparts no intrinsic pressure but can transmit IAP. Fifty milliliters of saline are injected into the aspiration port of the urinary drainage tube with an occlusive clamp placed across the tube just distal to the port. The saline is used to create a standing column of fluid between the bladder and port that can transmit IAP to a recording device. The needle in the port is connected to a CVP manometer using a three-way stopcock. The manometer is filled with saline and opened to the drainage tube. IAP is read at the meniscus with the manometer zeroed at the pubic symphysis. Bladder pressures measured in this fashion are both reliable and consistent. Pressures less than 15 mm Hg do not require decompression. Table 6-7 lists the authors' recommendations according to IAP.

In the chest similar phenomena occur. Edema of the heart and lungs develops and the heart may also dilate. Blood accumulation is rarely a problem because of the use of chest tubes. However, the diagnosis is usually apparent in the OR since the heart tolerates compression poorly. Attempts to close the chest in this setting are associated with profound hypotension, and it becomes obvious that an alternative method of closure is necessary. At present the most popular material used to accommodate the addition of volume in

the chest or abdomen is a 3-L plastic urologic irrigation bag, which has been cut open and sterilized. The bag is sewn to the skin or fascia using no. 2 nylon suture with a simple running technique (Fig. 6-31). As many as four bags may need to be sewn together to cover a large defect. Closed suction drains are placed beneath the plastic to remove the blood and serous fluid that inevitably accumulate. The entire closure is covered with an iodinated plastic adhesive sheet to simplify nursing care. Patients whose renal function has not been impaired will have a remarkable diuresis. Exogenous fluids are held to a minimum to facilitate the resolution of edema. Definitive wound closure can usually be performed in 48 to 72 hours.

Patients who develop sepsis and multiple organ failure (MOF) are problematic and do not resolve their edema until sepsis and MOF resolve. This may require several weeks. The bags have been left in place up to 3 weeks with the patient surviving. However, the authors make every effort to at least close the skin over the viscera to decrease protein and heat loss and to inhibit infection. If these attempts are unsuccessful and the abdomen remains open with granulating tissue exposed, lateral traction forces of the abdominal wall will eventually cause an enteric fistula. The risk of developing a fistula increases rapidly after 2 weeks with an open abdomen. These problems are extremely difficult to treat. Several approaches have been used to avoid this catastrophic complication, including polyglycolic acid or polypropylene mesh sewn to the fascia, split-thickness skin grafts placed directly on the bowel, musculocutaneous flaps, and traction devices.[27] Of these options, skin grafts appear to have the greatest success, although the abdominal wall hernia will eventually require reconstruction.

Nonoperative treatment for blunt injuries of the liver, spleen, and kidneys is now the rule rather than the exception.[28] Up to 90% of

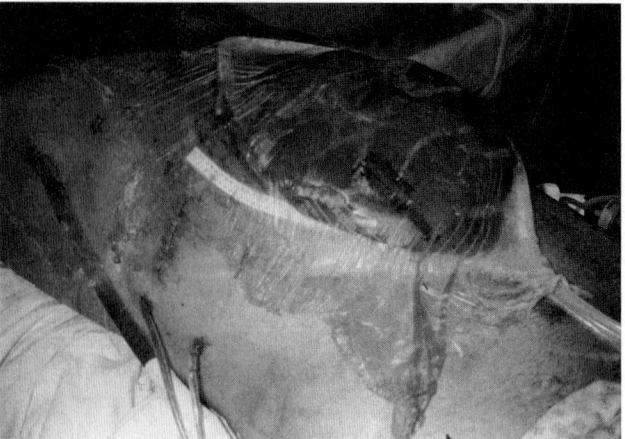

FIG. 6-31. Sterilized and opened 3-L urologic irrigation bags are an inexpensive method for abdominal closure and prevent dangerous increases in intra-abdominal pressure.

children and 50% of adults are treated in this manner.[29] As interventional radiology continues to advance, these numbers will certainly increase. The primary requirement for this therapy is hemodynamic stability. The extent of the patient's injuries should be delineated by CT. Recurrent hemorrhage from the liver and kidneys has been uncommon, but delayed hemorrhage or rupture of the spleen is an important consideration in the decision to pursue nonoperative management. The patient should be monitored in the intensive care unit for at least the first 24 hours. Since CT will miss some enteric injuries, frequent abdominal examination should be performed. Usually the fall in hematocrit will stabilize within 24 hours. If the hematocrit continues to fall, angiography with embolization of bleeding sites should be considered, particularly for hepatic and renal injuries. CT is usually repeated at least once during the hospitalization to assess major hepatic or splenic lesions requiring transfusion. Gradually increasing activity is permitted following discharge. Patients involved in contact or high-impact sports such as football should have complete healing of the injury documented radiographically before resuming participation. This can take several months.

Complications of nonoperative treatment include continuing hemorrhage; delayed hemorrhage; necrosis of liver, spleen, or kidney from embolization; abscess; biloma; and urinoma. Hemorrhage may be treated by interventional radiology, although open operative control is often necessary. Most infectious complications can be treated by percutaneous drainage. Bilomas are usually resorbed.

Head

Injuries of the Brain

General principles of the management of cerebral injuries have changed in recent years. Attention is now focused on maintaining or enhancing cerebral perfusion rather than merely lowering intracranial pressure (ICP). For example, it has been found that hyperventilation to a PCO_2 less than 30 mm Hg to induce cerebral vasoconstriction actually exacerbates cerebral ischemia in spite of decreasing ICP. These secondary iatrogenic cerebral injuries cause more harm than previously appreciated. Other treatments or conditions that must be avoided include decreased cardiac output due to the excessive use of osmotic diuretics, sedatives, or barbiturates, and hypoxia. Nevertheless, the measurement of ICP is still important and is efficiently accomplished with a ventriculostomy tube. The tube also permits the withdrawal of cerebrospinal fluid, which is the safest method for lowering ICP. Although an ICP of 10 mm Hg is believed to be the upper limit of normal, therapy is not usually initiated until the ICP reaches 20 mm Hg. Cerebral perfusion pressure (CPP) is an important measurement which is used to monitor therapy. CPP is equal to the mean arterial pressure (MAP) minus the ICP, and 60 mm Hg is the lowest acceptable pressure. This figure can be adjusted by either lowering ICP or raising MAP. In practice, both are manipulated. Paralysis, sedation, osmotic diuresis, and barbiturate coma are all still used, with coma being the last resort. The goal of fluid therapy is to achieve a euvolemic state, and arbitrary fluid restriction is avoided. Whether boosting MAP with pressors or inotropes in patients with an elevated ICP resistant to treatment improves outcome is unclear, although recent data suggest it does. Moderate hypothermia may also be helpful by decreasing metabolic requirements.[30]

Indications for operative intervention for space-occupying hematomas are based on the amount of midline shift, the location of the clot, and the patient's ICP.[31] A shift of more than 5 mm is usually considered an indication for evacuation. However, this is not an absolute rule. Smaller hematomas causing less shift that are in treacherous locations such as the posterior fossa may require

drainage due to the threat of brain stem compression or herniation. Removal of small hematomas may also improve ICP and CPP in patients with an elevated ICP that is refractory to medical therapy. The treatment of diffuse axonal injury (DAI) includes the control of cerebral edema and general supportive care. The authors frequently employ percutaneous tracheostomy for airway control and percutaneous endoscopic gastrostomy for enteral access in head injured patients whose recovery is unlikely or prolonged. Prognosis is related to the GCS. Serious head injuries, with GCS scores of 3 to 8, have a poor prognosis, and an institutional existence is almost a certainty. Mild brain injury, with GCS scores of 13 to 15, have a good prognosis; independent living is likely. However, neuropsychiatric testing often reveals significant abnormalities.

General surgeons in small or rural communities without emergency neurosurgical coverage may be required to drill a burr hole as a life-saving measure.[32] This may be needed in a patient with an epidural hematoma. As blood from a torn vessel (usually the middle meningeal artery) accumulates, the temporal lobe, if forced medially, will compress the third cranial nerve and eventually the brain stem. This sequence of events results in this typical clinical course: (1) initial loss of consciousness, (2) awakening and a lucid interval, (3) recurrent loss of consciousness with a unilaterally fixed and dilated pupil, and (4) cardiac arrest. Since these patients do not usually have a serious underlying cortical injury, their chance for a complete recovery is often good. The burr hole should be made on the same side as the dilated pupil, as shown in Fig. 6-32. The goal of the

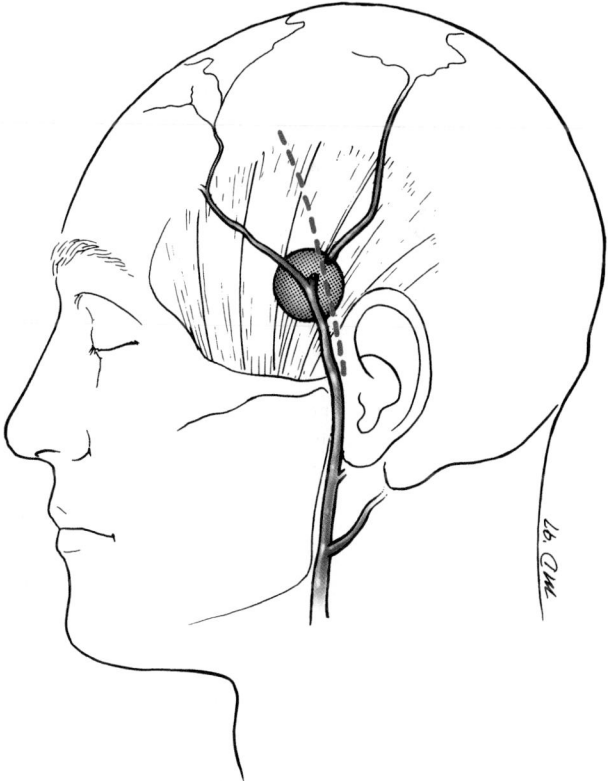

FIG. 6-32. This figure indicates the optimal position for a decompressive burr hole for a presumed epidural hematoma when preoperative localization studies cannot be performed. One or more branches of the external carotid artery must usually be ligated to gain access to the skull. No attempt should be made to control intracranial hemorrhage through the burr hole. Rather, the patient's head should be wrapped with a bulky absorbent dressing and the patient then transferred to a neurosurgeon for definitive care.

procedure is not to control the hemorrhage, but to decompress the intracranial space. Since a craniotomy is required for the control of hemorrhage, the patient's head should be loosely wrapped with a thick layer of gauze to absorb the bleeding and the patient then transferred to a facility with emergency neurosurgical capability for a craniotomy.

Neck

Blunt Injury

Cervical Spine. Blunt trauma may involve the cervical spine, spinal cord, larynx, carotid and vertebral arteries, and the jugular veins. Treatment of injuries to the cervical spine is based on the level of injury, the stability of the spine, the presence of subluxation, the extent of angulation, and the extent of neurologic deficit. In general, cautious axial traction in line with the mastoid process is used to reduce subluxations. A halo-vest combination can accomplish this and also provide rigid external fixation for definitive treatment when left in place for 3 to 6 months. Today this device is the treatment of choice for many cervical spine injuries. Surgical fusion is usually reserved for those with neurologic deficit, those who demonstrate angulation greater than 11° on flexion and extension x-rays, or those who remain unstable after external fixation.

Spinal Cord. Injuries of the spinal cord, particularly complete injuries, remain essentially untreatable. Approximately 3% of patients who present with flaccid quadriplegia actually have concussive injuries, and these patients represent the very few who seem to have miraculous recoveries. A recent prospective randomized study comparing methylprednisolone with placebo demonstrated a significant improvement in outcome (usually one or two spinal levels) for those who received the corticosteroid within 8 hours of injury.[33] The standard dosage is 30 mg/kg given as an IV bolus, followed by a 5.4-mg/kg infusion administered over the next 23 hours. Patients with spinal cord injuries are also at high risk for deep venous thrombosis and pulmonary embolus. Prophylactic anticoagulation is essential.[34]

Larynx. The larynx may be fractured by a direct blow, which can result in airway compromise. A hoarse voice is highly suggestive. A cricothyroidotomy, or tracheostomy if time permits, should be done to protect the airway in cases of severe fracture. The larynx is anatomically repaired with fine wires and sutures. If direct repair of internal laryngeal structures is necessary, the thyroid cartilage is split longitudinally in the midline and opened like a book. This is referred to as a laryngeal fissure.

Carotid and Vertebral Arteries. Blunt injury to the carotid or vertebral arteries may cause dissection, thrombosis, or pseudoaneurysm. More than one half of patients have a delayed diagnosis. Facial contact resulting in hypertension and rotation appears to be the mechanism. To reduce delayed recognition, the authors employ CT angiography in patients at risk, to identify these injuries before neurologic symptoms develop.[35,36] The injuries frequently occur at or extend into the base of the skull and are usually not surgically accessible. Currently accepted treatment for thrombosis and dissection is anticoagulation with heparin followed by warfarin for 3 months. Pseudoaneurysms also occur near the base of the skull. If they are small, they can be followed with repeat angiography. If enlargement occurs, consideration should be given to the placement by an interventional radiologist of a stent across the aneurysm. Another possibility is to approach the intracranial portion of the carotid by

removing the overlying bone and performing a direct repair. This method has only recently been described and has been performed in a limited number of patients.

Thrombosis of the internal jugular veins caused by blunt trauma can occur unilaterally or bilaterally. These injuries are usually discovered incidentally and are generally asymptomatic. Bilateral thrombosis can aggravate cerebral edema in patients with serious head injuries. Stent placement should be considered in such patients if their ICP remains elevated. Laryngeal edema resulting in airway compromise also can occur.

Penetrating Injuries

Penetrating injuries in zones II or III that require operative intervention are explored using an incision along the anterior border of the sternocleidomastoid muscle. If bilateral exploration is necessary, the inferior end of the incision can be extended to the opposite side. Midline wounds or significant bilateral injuries can be exposed via a large collar incision at the appropriate level. Alternatively, bilateral anterior sternocleidomastoid incisions can be employed.

Carotid and Vertebral Arteries. Exposure of the distal carotid artery in zone III is difficult (Fig. 6-33). The first step is to divide the ansa cervicalis and mobilize the hypoglossal nerve. Next, the portion of the posterior belly of the digastric muscle that overlies the internal carotid is resected. The glossopharyngeal and vagus nerves are mobilized and retracted as necessary. If accessible, the styloid process and attached muscles are removed. At this point anterior displacement of the mandible may be helpful, and various methods for accomplishing this have been devised. Some authorities have advocated division and elevation of the vertical ramus. However, two remaining structures still prevent exposure of the internal carotid to the base of the skull: the parotid gland and facial nerve. Excessive anterior traction on the mandible or parotid may damage the facial nerve, particularly the mandibular branch. Unless the surgeon is willing to resect the parotid and divide the facial nerve, division of the ramus is seldom helpful.

While it would seem obvious that all penetrating carotid injuries should be repaired, this may not be the case. During the 1960s surgeons attempted to revascularize patients who suffered acute strokes due to atherosclerotic carotid artery disease. It quickly became apparent that these patients fared worse than those who were treated nonoperatively. This unfortunate outcome was believed to be due to the conversion of an ischemic infarct to a hemorrhagic infarct that was associated with a higher mortality rate. The same phenomenon is believed by some to occur in patients with carotid injuries. In fact, subsequent studies have rarely identified this complication. This has led to a more aggressive approach of repairing all penetrating carotid injuries regardless of the patient's neurologic status, or repairing all except those in comatose patients. Inaccessible carotid injuries near the base of the skull can be treated by interventional radiologists with a stent if the anatomy of the injury is favorable. Otherwise the artery will need to be thrombosed or ligated. If ligation is necessary, the patient should be anticoagulated with heparin followed by warfarin for 3 months. This treatment may prevent a stroke by inhibiting the generation of thrombi from the surface of the clot at the circle of Willis while the endothelium heals. Without anticoagulation the risk of stroke with ligation has been approximately 20 to 30%, and most strokes occur a few days after ligation. Tangential wounds of the internal jugular vein should be repaired by lateral venorrhaphy, but extensive wounds are efficiently addressed by ligation.

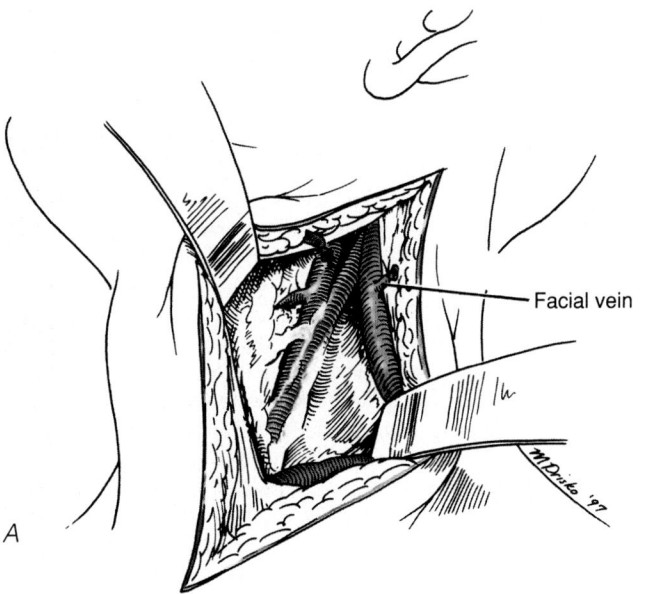

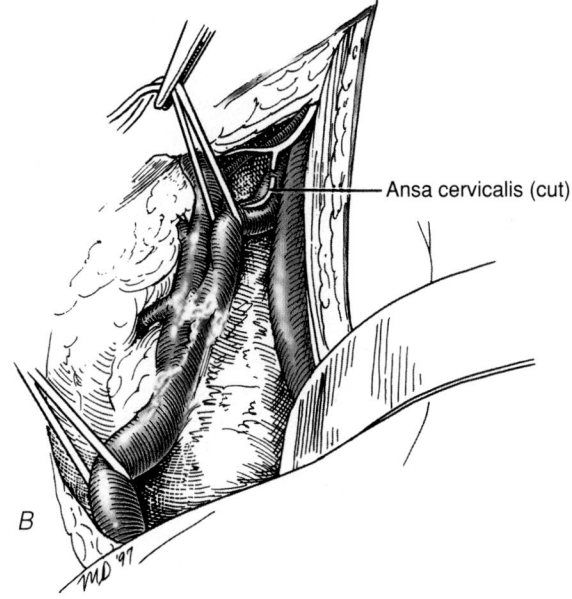

Facial vein

Ansa cervicalis (cut)

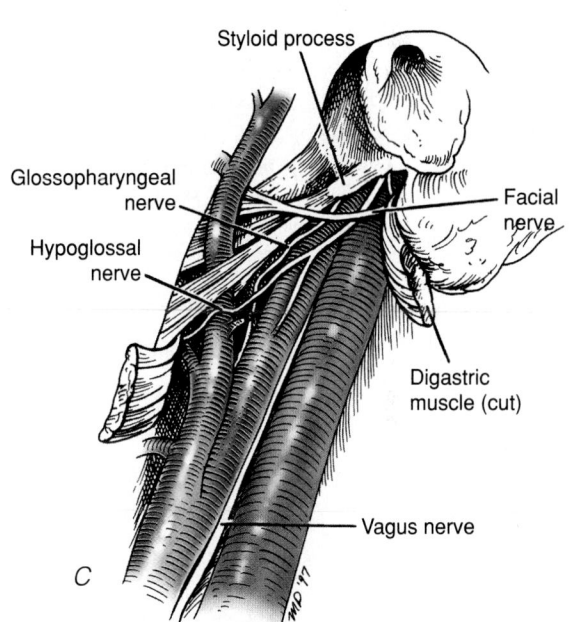

Styloid process

Glossopharyngeal
nerve

Hypoglossal
nerve

Facial
nerve

Digastric
muscle (cut)

Vagus nerve

FIG. 6-33. Exposure of the internal carotid artery requires division of the facial vein (A). Division of the ansa cervicalis (B) permits mobilization of the hypoglossal nerve, which enhances exposure of the internal carotid. Exposure of the distal internal carotid artery is facilitated by resection of the posterior belly of the digastric muscle (C). Further measures are seldom helpful because of the overlying parotid gland and facial nerve.

Vertebral artery injuries usually result from penetrating trauma, although thrombosis and pseudoaneurysms can occur from blunt injury. The diagnosis is made by angiography or when significant hemorrhage is noted posterior to the carotid sheath during neck exploration. Exposure of the vertebral artery above C6 where it enters its bony canal is complicated by the overlying anterior elements of the canal and the tough fascia covering the artery between the elements. The artery is approached through an anterior neck incision by retracting the contents of the carotid sheath medially (Fig. 6-34). The muscular attachments to the elements are removed. Care must be taken to avoid injury to the cervical spinal nerves, which are located directly behind and lateral to the bony canal. Some authorities have recommended using a high-speed burr to remove the anterior element of the canal, thereby avoiding the venous plexus between the elements. The authors have not found this to be a problem, and

have often carefully excised the fascia between the elements and lifted the artery out of its canal with a tissue forceps. The treatment for vertebral artery injuries is ligation both proximal and distal to the injury. There is rarely, if ever, an indication for repair. Neurologic complications are uncommon. Exposure of the vertebral artery above C2 is extremely difficult. Rather than using a direct operative approach, the authors expose the vessel below C5, outside the bony canal, clamp the artery proximally, and insert a no. 3 balloon-tipped catheter.[37] The catheter is advanced to the level of the injury or distal to it, and the balloon is inflated with saline until back-bleeding stops. The tube to the catheter is crimped over onto itself and secured in this position with several heavy silk sutures. The catheter is trimmed so it can be left in the wound under the skin. The proximal end of the artery is ligated. One week later the catheter is removed under local anesthesia. Rebleeding has not occurred in the authors'

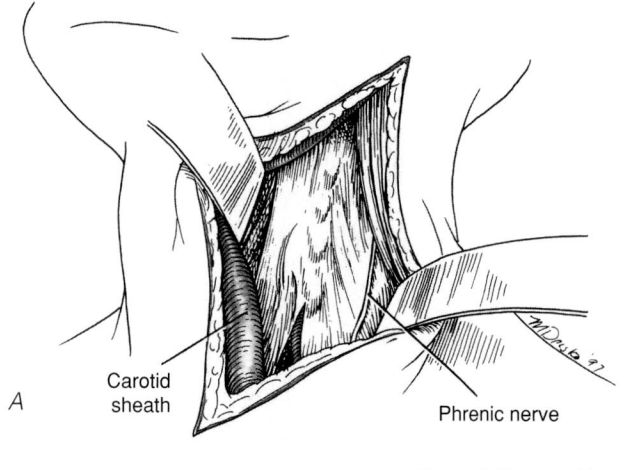

A

Carotid sheath

Phrenic nerve

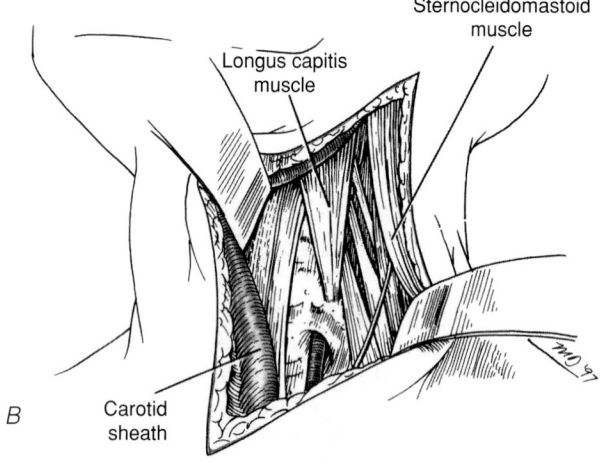

Sternocleidomastoid muscle

Longus capitis muscle

B

Carotid sheath

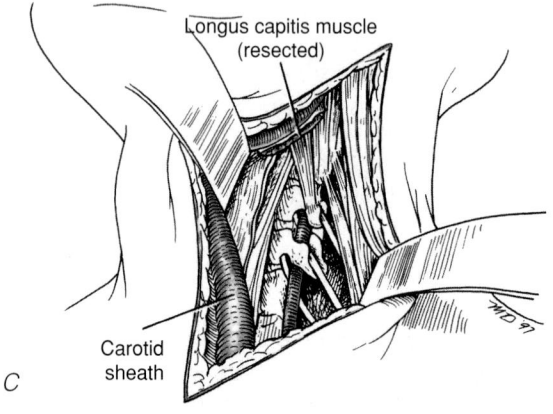

Longus capitis muscle (resected)

C

Carotid sheath

FIG. 6-34. *A. Exposure of the vertebral artery is begun by retracting the contents of the carotid sheath medially. B. Muscles that insert on the lateral elements of the cervical spine are removed. C. The vertebral artery is exposed by removing the tough fascia between the lateral elements or by removing the elements themselves. Note that the cervical nerve roots exit immediately lateral and posterior to the lateral element. They are easily injured if care is not taken.*

experience. The same approach can be used for the distal internal carotid. An alternative approach is to have the interventional radiologist place coils to induce thrombosis proximal and distal to the injury if the lesion is diagnosed by angiography. However, not all vertebral injuries can be treated by this method. Injuries of the

proximal vertebrae can be exposed by a median sternotomy with a neck extension.

Trachea and Esophagus. Injuries of the trachea are repaired with a running 3-0 absorbable monofilament suture. Tracheostomy is not required in most patients. Esophageal injuries are repaired in a similar fashion. If an esophageal wound is large or if tissue is missing, a sternocleidomastoid muscle pedicle flap is warranted, and a closed suction drain is a reasonable precaution. The drain should be near but not in contact with the esophageal or any other suture line. It can be removed in 7 to 10 days if the suture line remains secure. Care must be taken when exploring the trachea and esophagus to avoid iatrogenic injury to the recurrent laryngeal nerve.

Penetrating injuries of the neck often create wounds in adjacent hollow structures (e.g., the trachea and esophagus or carotid artery and esophagus). If following repair these adjacent suture lines are in contact, the stage is set for devastating postoperative fistulous complications. To avoid these complications, viable tissue should routinely be interposed between adjacent suture lines. Viable strips of the sternocleidomastoid muscle or strap muscles are useful for this purpose.

Thoracic Outlet

Great Vessels

Most injuries of the great vessels of the thoracic outlet (zone I) are caused by penetrating trauma, although the innominate and subclavian arteries are occasionally injured from blunt trauma.[38–40] As mentioned previously, angiography is desirable for planning the incision. If this is not possible due to hemodynamic instability, a reasonable approach can be inferred from the chest x-ray and the location of the wounds. If the patient has a left hemothorax, a left third or fourth interspace anterolateral thoracotomy should be performed because the proximal left subclavian artery may be injured. Hemorrhage can be controlled digitally until the vascular injury is delineated. Additional incisions or extensions are often required. A third or fourth interspace right anterolateral thoracotomy may be used for thoracic outlet injury presenting with hemodynamic instability and a right hemothorax. A median sternotomy with a right clavicular extension also can be used. Unstable patients with injuries near the sternal notch may have a large mediastinal hematoma or have lost blood directly to the outside. These patients should be explored via a median sternotomy.

If angiography has identified an arterial injury, a more direct approach can be employed. Figure 6-35 shows the various incisions that are used depending on the location of the arterial injury. A median sternotomy is used for exposure of the innominate, proximal right carotid and subclavian, and the proximal left carotid arteries. The proximal left subclavian artery presents a unique challenge. Because it arises from the aortic arch far posteriorly, it is not readily approached via median sternotomy. A posterolateral thoracotomy provides excellent exposure but severely limits access to other structures and is not recommended. The best option is to create a full-thickness flap of the upper chest wall. This is accomplished with a third or fourth interspace anterolateral thoracotomy for proximal control, a supraclavicular incision with a resection of the medial third of the clavicle, and a median sternotomy, which links the two horizontal incisions. The ribs can be cut laterally for additional exposure, which allows the flap to be folded laterally with little effort. This incision has been referred to as a book or trap-door thoracotomy for obvious reasons (Fig. 6-36). The mid-portion of the subclavian artery is accessible by removing the proximal third of either clavicle,

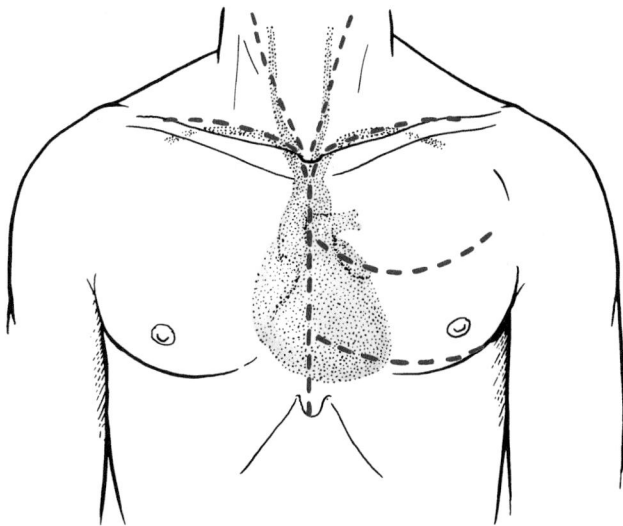

FIG. 6-35. *Incisions for thoracic outlet arterial injuries. The choice of the incision is based on the underlying injured vessel. Since this information is not always available, the surgeon must be prepared to extend the initial incision or perform additional incisions.*

with the skin incision made directly over the clavicle. Muscular attachments are stripped away, and the clavicle is divided with a Gigli saw. The medial remnant of the clavicle is forcefully elevated. The periosteum is dissected from the posterior aspect of the bone until the sternoclavicular joint is reached. The capsular attachments are cut with a heavy scissors or knife and the bone is discarded. The periosteum and underlying fascia are very tough and must be sharply incised along the direction of the vessel. The subclavian vein is mobilized and the artery is directly underneath. The anterior scalene is divided for injuries just proximal to the thyrocervical trunk; the

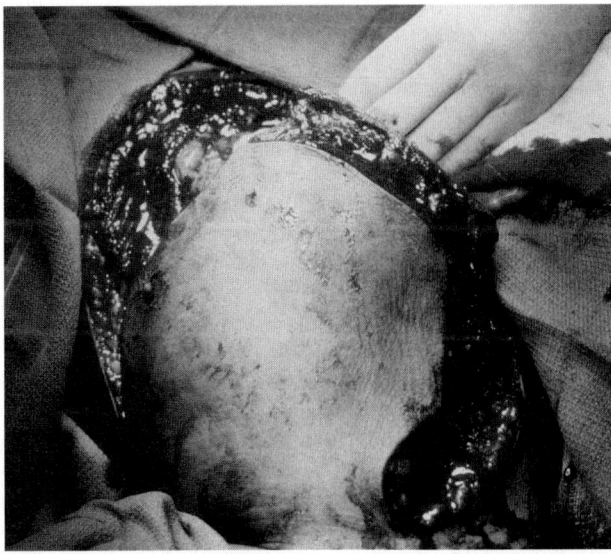

FIG. 6-36. *This left anterolateral thoracotomy incision is referred to as a book or trap-door thoracotomy. Usually the lower incision (to the left of the picture) is performed through the third or fourth interspace; however, this patient suffered a cardiac arrest, which necessitated a fifth interspace resuscitative thoracotomy. The proximal left subclavian artery was injured. The addition of a supraclavicular incision and median sternotomy permitted exposure and control of this problematic vessel.*

relatively small phrenic nerve should be identified on its anterior aspect and spared. Iatrogenic injury to cords of the brachial plexus can occur.

The great vessels are rather fragile and are easily torn during dissection or crushed with a clamp. For this reason some advocate oversewing proximal injuries of the artery on the side of the aortic arch and sewing a graft onto a new location on the arch. The graft is then sewn to the artery without tension. These authors have not found this necessary, provided the vessels are handled with care. Technical details of the repair are similar to those described in the Principles and Techniques of Vascular Repair section of this chapter.

Trachea and Esophagus

The trachea and esophagus are difficult to approach at the thoracic outlet. The combination of a neck incision and a high anterolateral thoracotomy may be used. Alternatively, these structures can be approached via a median sternotomy, provided the left innominate vein and artery are divided. Temporary division of the innominate artery is tolerated well in otherwise healthy people, but the vessel should be repaired following treatment of the tracheal or esophageal injury. The vein does not need to be repaired. As in the neck, adjacent suture lines should be separated by viable tissue. A portion of the sternocleidomastoid can be rotated down for this purpose.

Chest

The most common life-threatening complications from both blunt and penetrating thoracic injury are hemothorax, pneumothorax, or a combination of both. Approximately 85% of these patients can be treated definitively with a chest tube. Because of the viscosity of blood at various stages of coagulation, a 36F or larger chest tube should be used. If one tube fails to completely evacuate the hemothorax (a "caked hemothorax"), a second tube should be placed (Fig. 6-37). If the second chest tube does not remove the blood, a thoracotomy should be performed because of the risk of life-threatening hemorrhage. Common sources of blood loss include intercostal vessels, internal thoracic artery, pulmonary parenchyma, and the heart. Less common sources are the great vessels, aortic arch, azygos vein, superior vena cava, and inferior vena cava. Blood may also enter the chest from an abdominal injury through a perforation or tear in the

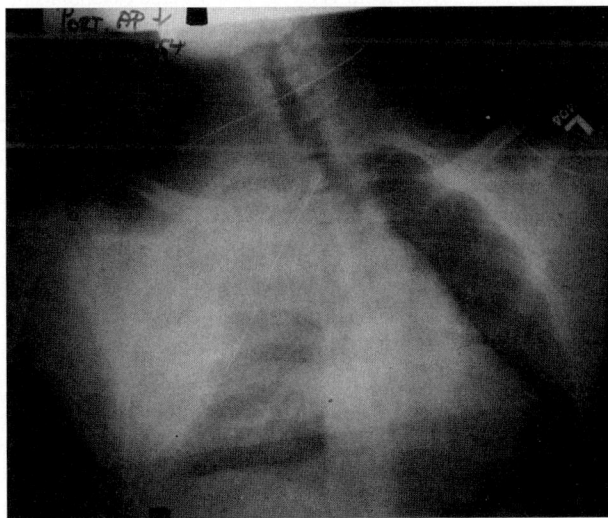

FIG. 6-37. A caked hemothorax.

Table 6-8

Indications for Operative Treatment of Penetrating Thoracic Injuries

Caked hemothorax
Large air leak with inadequate ventilation or persistent collapse of the lung
Drainage of more than 1500 mL of blood when chest tube is first inserted
Continuous hemorrhage of more than 200 mL/h for ≥3 consecutive h
Esophageal perforation
Pericardial tamponade

diaphragm. Indications for operative treatment of penetrating thoracic injuries are listed in Table 6-8.

The indications for thoracotomy in blunt trauma are based on specific preoperative diagnoses.[41] These include pericardial tamponade, tear of the descending thoracic aorta, rupture of a mainstem bronchus, and rupture of the esophagus. Thoracotomy for hemothorax in the absence of the above diagnoses is rarely indicated. A shattered chest wall that produces a hemothorax is better treated by the interventional radiologist with embolization.

Thoracic Incisions

The selection of incisions is important and depends on the organs being treated. For exploratory thoracotomy for hemorrhage, the patient is supine and an anterolateral thoracotomy is performed. Depending on findings, the incision can be extended across the sternum or even further for a bilateral anterolateral thoracotomy. The fifth interspace is usually preferred unless the surgeon has a precise knowledge of which organs are injured and that exposure would be enhanced by selecting a different interspace. The heart, lungs, aortic arch, great vessels, and esophagus are accessible with these incisions. Although it may seem obvious, care should be taken to ligate the internal thoracic artery and veins if they are transected. It is remarkable how often this step is overlooked, resulting in continuous blood loss, which obscures the field and endangers the patient.

The heart also can be approached via a median sternotomy. Since little else can be done in the chest through this incision, it is usually reserved for stab wounds of the anterior chest in patients who present with pericardial tamponade. Posterolateral thoracotomies are rarely used, since ventilation is impaired in the dependent lung and the incision cannot be extended. There are two specific exceptions. Injuries of the posterior aspect of the trachea or mainstem bronchi near the carina are inaccessible from the left or from the front. The only possible approach is through the right chest using a posterolateral thoracotomy. A tear of the descending thoracic aorta can only be repaired through a left posterolateral thoracotomy. These authors utilize left heart bypass for these procedures, therefore the patient's hips and legs are rotated toward the supine position to gain access to the left groin for femoral artery cannulation. It also is helpful for optimal exposure to resect the fourth rib and enter the chest through its bed.

Heart

Most cardiac injuries are the result of penetrating trauma, and any part of the heart is susceptible. Control of hemorrhage while the heart is being repaired is crucial and several techniques can be used. The atria can be clamped with a Satinsky vascular clamp. Digital control and suturing beneath the finger is possible anywhere in the heart, though the technique requires skill and a long, curved cardiovascular needle. The reality of blood-borne viral infections raises the question of whether this method should ever be used

today. If the hole is small, a peanut sponge clamped in the tip of a hemostat can be placed into the wound, or the blood loss may be accepted while sutures are being placed. For larger holes a 16F Foley catheter with a 30-mL balloon can be inflated with 10 mL of saline. Gentle traction on the catheter will control hemorrhage from any cardiac wound since wounds too large for balloon tamponade are incompatible with survival. Suture placement with the balloon inflated is problematic. Usually the ends of the wound are closed progressively toward the middle until the amount of blood loss is acceptable with the balloon removed. The use of skin staples for the temporary control of hemorrhage has become popular, particularly when ED thoracotomy has been performed. It has the advantages of reducing the risk of needle-stick injury to the surgeon or assistant, and does not mandate the attention required by a balloon catheter. In most instances, however, hemostasis is neither perfect or definitive. Inflow occlusion of the heart, by clamping the superior and inferior vena cava can be performed for short periods, and this may be essential for the treatment of extensive or multiple wounds, as well as for those that are difficult to expose. These factors necessitate that the surgeon work very quickly.

Trauma surgeons accept the fact that interior structures of the heart may be damaged, impairing cardiac output. However, immediate repair of valvular damage or acute septal defects is rarely necessary and requires total cardiopulmonary bypass, which has a high mortality in this situation.[42] Most patients who survive to make it to the hospital do well with only external repair. Following recovery, the heart can be thoroughly evaluated, and if necessary, secondary repair can be performed under more controlled conditions. Coronary artery injuries also pose difficult problems. Ligation leads to acute infarction distal to the tie; but again, reconstruction requires bypass. The right coronary artery can probably be ligated anywhere, but the resultant arrhythmias may be extremely resistant to treatment. The left anterior descending and circumflex cannot be ligated proximally without causing a large infarct. Fortunately, such injuries are extremely rare as they usually produce death in the field.

Blunt cardiac injury can present in several ways. A sharp blow to the pericardium can provoke ventricular fibrillation.[43] This is referred to as a commotio cordis and is inevitably fatal unless it is recognized immediately and resuscitation implemented. The heart also can be contused. Most of these patients present with new arrhythmias (e.g., a bundle-branch block or premature ventricular contractions). Cardiac enzymes have not been helpful in making the diagnosis.[44] Finally, the heart can rupture; the right atrium and right ventricle are most susceptible, but survival is possible provided the diagnosis is suspected.[45]

Lungs, Trachea, and Bronchi

Pulmonary injuries requiring operative intervention usually result from penetrating injury. Formerly the entrance and exit wounds were oversewn to control hemorrhage. This set the stage for air embolism which occasionally caused sudden death in the operating room or in the immediate postoperative period.[46] A recent development, pulmonary tractotomy, has been employed to reduce this problem as well as the need for pulmonary resection (Fig. 6-38).[47] Linear stapling devices are inserted directly into the injury tract and positioned to cause the least degree of devascularization. Two staple lines are created and the lung is divided between. This allows direct access to the bleeding vessels and leaking bronchi. No effort is made to close the defect. Lobectomy or pneumonectomy is rarely necessary. Lobectomy is only indicated for a completely devascularized or destroyed lobe. Parenchymal injuries severe enough to require pneumonectomy are rarely survivable, and

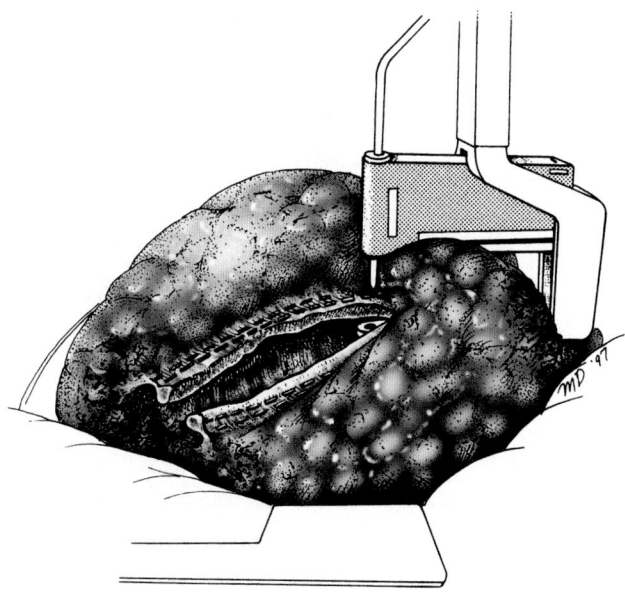

FIG. 6-38. Pulmonary tractotomy. Dividing the pulmonary paren-chyma between adjacent staple lines permits rapid direct access to injured vessels or bronchi along the tract of a penetrating injury.

major pulmonary hilar injuries necessitating pneumonectomy are usually lethal in the field.[48]

Injuries of the trachea are managed in the same fashion described above. Since exposure can be difficult, provisions should be made to deflate the lung on the operative side by using a double-lumen endotracheal tube (a double-lumen tube is seldom needed for cardiac or pulmonary injury). Repair of mainstem bronchial injuries and tracheal injuries near the carina may result in a complete loss of ventilation when the overlying pleura is opened, even if a double-lumen tube is used. Gases from the ventilator will preferentially escape from the injury, and neither lung will be ventilated. Digital occlusion of the injury can control air loss if the injury is small. Larger injuries are an imminent threat to life. To avoid this catastrophe, a 6- or 7-mm endotracheal tube can be inserted through the injury into the opposite bronchus to permit single lung ventilation while the injury is being repaired. If ventilation is inadequate, the surgeon can insert and inflate the endotracheal tube into the main bronchus on the opposite side through the injury to permit ventilation of one lung while the injury is repaired. Eventually the tube will have to be removed to close the defect, but the remaining hole can be controlled digitally. Alternatively, it may be possible for the anesthesiologist to cannulate the opposite bronchus, though little time is available.

Trachea and Esophagus

The majority of esophageal injuries are caused by penetrating trauma through blunt disruption.[49] Because of their proximity, combined tracheoesophageal injuries do occur. Many authors recommend the interposition of viable muscle between the repairs to prevent tracheoesophageal fistulas.[50]

Descending Thoracic Aorta

Repair of injuries to the descending thoracic aorta have been highly controversial, both with respect to whom should repair them and how it should be accomplished.[51–54] At present, both thoracic and general surgeons are treating them, with an emerging trend moving toward general surgeons managing them with greater frequency. With respect to methodology, the concern has been the occurrence

of paraplegia from ischemic injury of the spinal cord. Conceptually, two techniques have been advocated. The simpler technique, often referred to as "clamp-and-sew," is accomplished with the application of vascular clamps proximal and distal to the injury and repairing or replacing the damaged portion of the aorta. This method results in transient hypoperfusion of the spinal cord distal to the clamps as well as in all abdominal organs. Large doses of vasodilators are also required to reduce afterload and avoid acute left heart failure. If the clamping time is short, less than 30 minutes, paraplegia has been uncommon. Longer clamping times have been associated with paraplegia in approximately 10% of patients. Unfortunately, clamping times of less than 30 minutes have been difficult to achieve for many tears requiring complex repair. The alternative approach has been to provide some method for maintaining a reasonable degree of perfusion for organs distal to the clamps. Two techniques have been used to accomplish this goal. The first is with the use of a shunt, a temporary extra-anatomic route around the clamps. A heparin-impregnated tube, the Gott shunt, has been specifically designed for this purpose. However, the volume of blood flow to the distal aorta is marginal. The second method has been to employ left heart bypass. With this method a volume of oxygenated blood is siphoned from the left heart and pumped into the distal aorta. Flow rates of 2 to 3 L/min appear to provide adequate protection by maintaining a distal perfusion pressure greater than 65 mm Hg. The authors prefer this method. The left superior pulmonary vein is cannulated to remove blood from the heart rather than the left atrium because the vein is tougher and less prone to tearing (Fig. 6-39). The left femoral artery is cannulated to return the blood to the distal aorta. A centrifugal

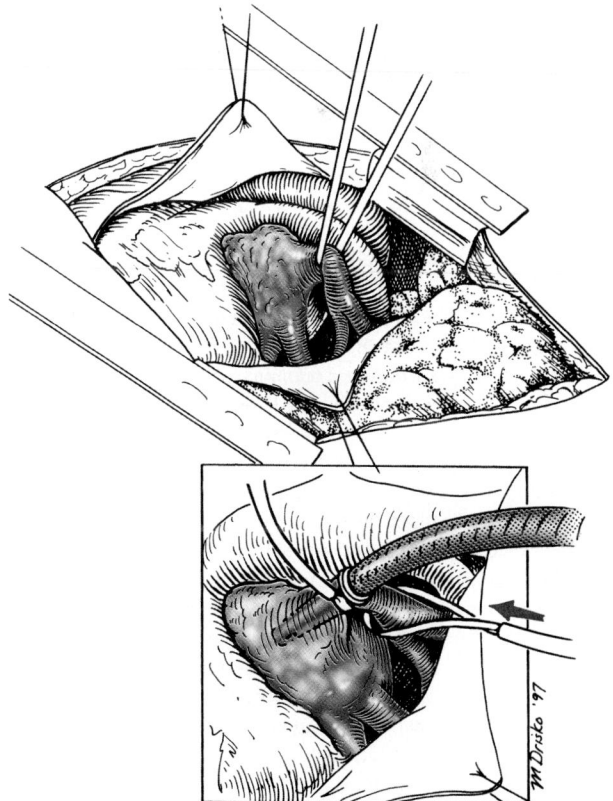

FIG. 6-39. When repairing a tear of the descending thoracic aorta, perfusion of the spinal cord while the aorta is clamped is achieved by using left heart bypass. The arterial cannula is inserted in the left femoral artery, and the left superior pulmonary vein is used as a source for oxygenated blood. The vein is preferable to the left atrium because it is less prone to tearing.

pump is employed because it is not as thrombogenic as a roller pump and heparinization is not required. This can be a significant benefit in a patient with multiple injuries, particularly in those with intracranial hemorrhage. However, occasional small cerebral infarcts have occurred, and 5000 to 10,000 units of heparin are usually administered unless contraindicated by associated injuries.

Once bypass is initiated, the proximal vascular clamp is applied between the left common carotid and left subclavian arteries, and the distal clamp is placed distal to the injury. The left subclavian is clamped separately. The hematoma is entered and the injury evaluated. In most patients a short, gelatin-sealed Dacron graft (usually 18 to 22 mm in diameter) is placed. Primary repair without a graft is possible in some patients. A 3-0 polypropylene suture is used for the anastomoses or suture lines. Air and clot are flushed from the aorta between two clamps and the subclavian artery prior to tying the final suture. Following completion of the repair, the clamps are removed and the patient is weaned from the pump. The cannulae are then removed and the vessels are repaired. A recent meta-analysis comparing clamp-and-sew with left heart bypass revealed a significantly lower incidence of paraplegia when the pump was used.

Injuries of the transverse arch do occur from blunt trauma. The proximal clamp can usually be placed between the innominate and left carotid arteries without cerebral infarction. However, the proximal clamp cannot be placed proximal to the innominate artery. A possible approach to injuries in which the clamps completely exclude the cerebral circulation is with profound hypothermia and circulatory arrest (see Chapter 21).

Small intimal flaps of the thoracic aorta without hematomas can be treated nonoperatively. Intraluminal mediastinal stents may also provide a solution, but their role remains to be defined. Penetrating injuries of the thoracic aorta are rare and do not afford enough time to set up the pump; therefore there is no choice but to use the clamp-and-sew technique. Partially occluding clamps should be used if possible.

Abdomen

Emergent Abdominal Exploration

All abdominal explorations in adults are performed using a long midline incision because of its versatility. For children under the age of 6, a transverse incision may be advantageous. If the patient has been in shock or is currently unstable, no attempt should be made to control bleeding from the abdominal wall until major sources of hemorrhage have been identified and controlled. The incision should be made with a scalpel rather than with an electrosurgical unit because it is faster. Liquid and clotted blood is rapidly evacuated with multiple laparotomy pads and suction. Additional pads are then placed in each quadrant to localize hemorrhage, and the aorta is palpated to estimate blood pressure.

If exsanguinating hemorrhage is encountered upon opening the abdomen, it is usually caused by injury to the liver, aorta, inferior vena cava, or iliac vessels. If the liver is the source, the hepatic pedicle should be immediately clamped (a Pringle maneuver) and the liver compressed posteriorly by tightly packing several laparotomy pads between the hepatic injury and the underside of the right anterior chest wall (Figs. 6-40 and 6-41). This combination of maneuvers will temporarily control the hemorrhage from virtually all survivable hepatic injuries.

If exsanguinating hemorrhage originates near the midline in the retroperitoneum, direct manual pressure is applied with a laparotomy pad and the aorta is exposed at the diaphragmatic hiatus and clamped. The same approach is used in the pelvis except that the

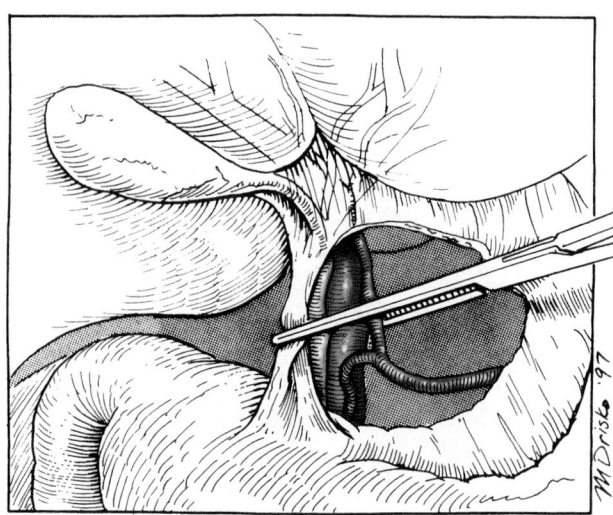

FIG. 6-40. The Pringle maneuver.

infrarenal aorta can be clamped, which is both easier and safer because splanchnic and renal ischemia are avoided. Injuries of the iliac vessels pose a unique problem for emergency vascular control. Because there are so many large vessels in proximity, multiple vascular injuries are common. Furthermore, venous injuries are not controlled with aortic clamping. A helpful maneuver in these instances is pelvic vascular isolation (Fig. 6-42). For stable patients with large midline hematomas, clamping the aorta proximal to the hematoma is also a wise precaution. Many surgeons take a few moments, once overt hemorrhage has been controlled, to identify obvious sources of enteric contamination and minimize further spillage. This can be accomplished with a running suture or with Babcock clamps.

Any organ can be injured by either blunt or penetrating trauma; however, certain organs are injured more often depending on the

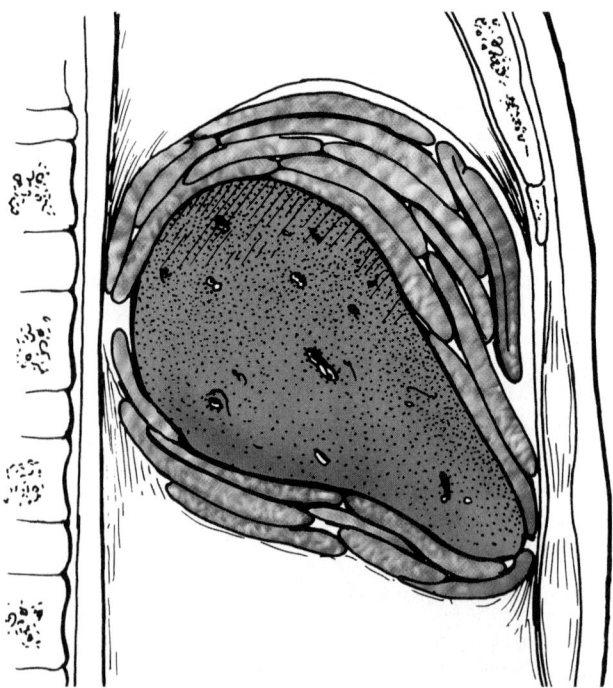

FIG. 6-41. A sagittal view of packs placed to control hepatic hemorrhage.

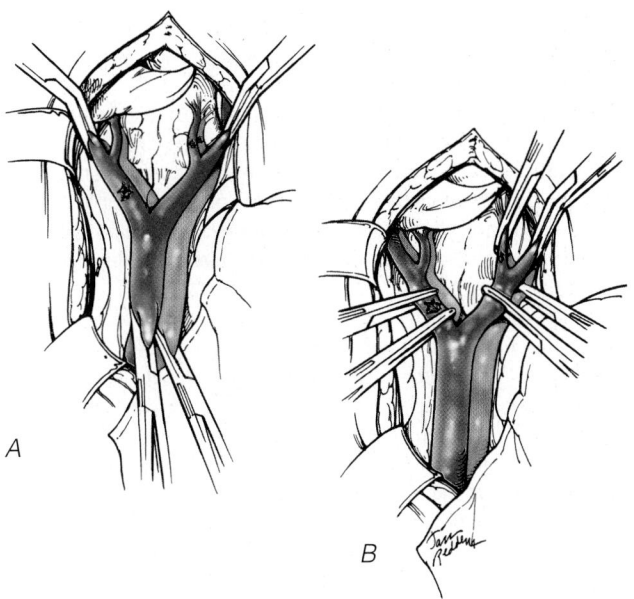

FIG. 6-42. Pelvic vascular isolation. A. The initial position of the clamps. B. As the dissection continues, the clamps are moved progressively closer to the vascular injuries until definitive control of hemorrhage is achieved.

mechanism. In blunt trauma, organs that cannot yield to impact by elastic deformation are most likely to be injured. The solid organs, liver, spleen, and kidneys, are representative of this group. For penetrating trauma, organs with the largest surface area when viewed from the front are most prone to injury (i.e., the small bowel, liver, and colon). Since bullets and knives usually follow straight lines, adjacent structures are commonly injured (e.g., the pancreas and duodenum). Penetrating trauma is not limited by the elastic properties of the tissue, and vascular injuries are far more common. While these concepts simplify the localization of injuries, unless the patient has exsanguinating hemorrhage, a methodical exploration should always be carried out.

All abdominal organs are systematically examined by visualization, palpation, or both. Missed injuries are a serious problem with often fatal results. In penetrating trauma missed injuries can occur if wound tracks are not followed their entire distance. A second common reason for missed injuries is failure to explore retroperitoneal structures such as the ascending and descending colons, the second and third portion of the duodenum, and ureters. Furthermore, injuries of the aorta or vena cava may be temporarily tamponaded by overlying structures. If the retroperitoneum is opened and the injury overlooked, delayed massive hemorrhage may occur following abdominal closure. Blunt abdominal injuries are usually obvious, but injuries of the pancreas, duodenum, bladder, and even the aorta can be overlooked.

Vascular Injuries

Injury to the major arteries and veins in the abdomen are a technical challenge to the surgeon and are often fatal.[55–62] All vessels are susceptible to injury with penetrating trauma. Vascular injuries in blunt trauma are far less common and usually involve the renal arteries and veins, though all other vessels, including the aorta, can be injured. Several vessels are notoriously difficult to expose. These include the retrohepatic vena cava; suprarenal aorta; the celiac axis; the proximal superior mesenteric artery; the junction of the superior mesenteric, splenic, and portal veins; and the bifurcation of the

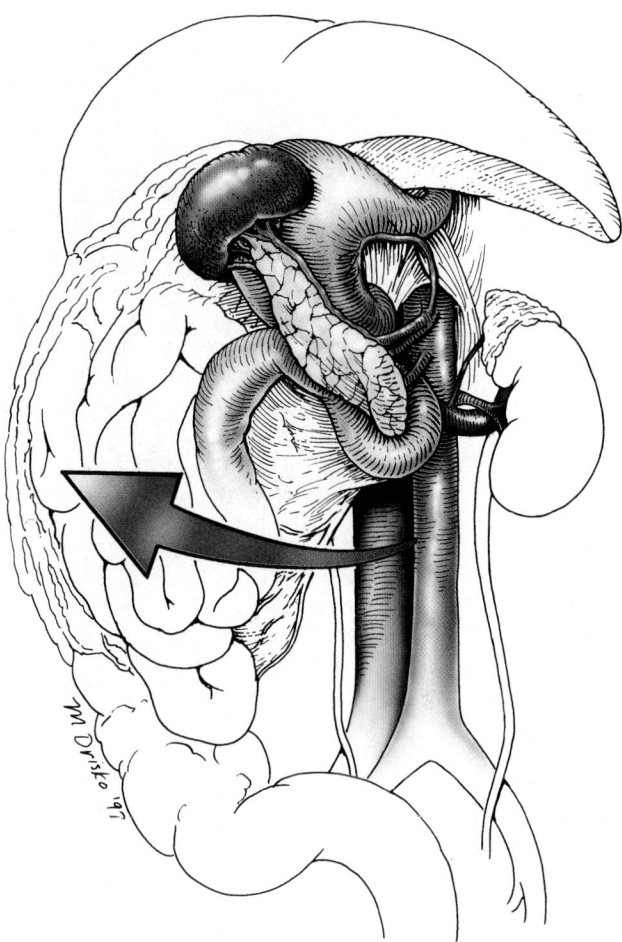

FIG. 6-43. Left medial visceral rotation is used to expose the upper abdominal aorta.

vena cava. Maneuvers have been described to aid in the exposure of all of these vessels. The suprarenal aorta, celiac axis, proximal superior mesenteric, and left renal arteries can all be exposed by left medial visceral rotation (Fig. 6-43). This is accomplished by incising the left lateral peritoneal reflection beginning at the distal descending colon and extending the incision past the splenic flexure, around the posterior aspect of the spleen, behind the gastric fundus, and ending at the esophagus. This incision permits the left colon, spleen, pancreas, and stomach to be rotated toward the midline. Division of the left crus of the diaphragm will permit access to the aorta above the celiac axis. The maneuver is much more difficult and time-consuming than it first appears. In contrast, mobilization of the right colon and a Kocher maneuver will expose the entire vena cava except the retrohepatic portion, and it is technically simple. This is referred to as a right medial visceral rotation (Fig. 6-44). The kidney can be left in situ or mobilized with the remaining viscera with both right and left medial rotations.

The junction of the superior mesenteric, splenic, and portal veins can be exposed in elective surgery by dissecting the vessels from the pancreas as required when performing a distal splenorenal shunt. However, in the presence of massive bleeding from a venous injury, this may be impossible. Therefore in trauma surgery, the neck of the pancreas is divided without hesitation. This provides excellent exposure of this difficult area. Management of the transected pancreas will be discussed below.

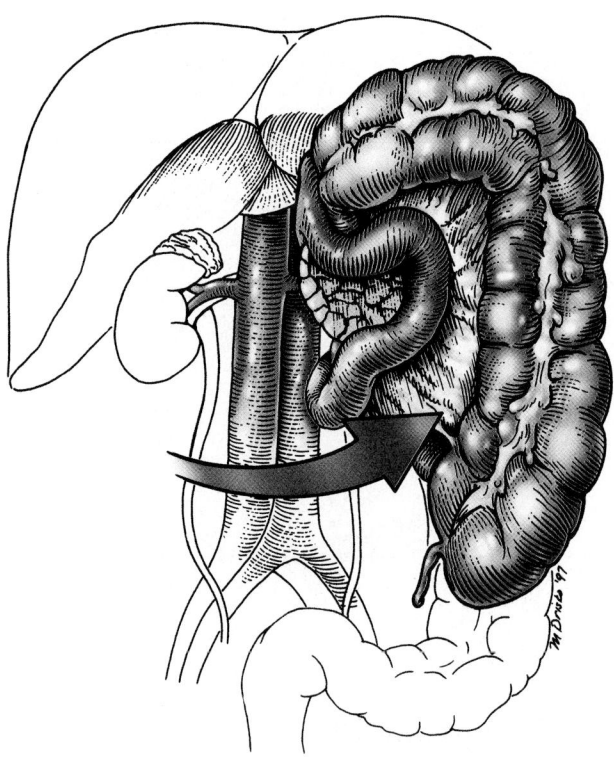

FIG. 6-44. Right medial visceral rotation is used to expose the infrahepatic vena cava.

The bifurcation of the vena cava is obscured by the right common iliac artery. This vessel should be divided to expose extensive vena caval injuries of this area (Fig. 6-45). The artery must be repaired after the venous injury is treated or amputation occurs in as many as 50% of patients.

Liver

The lower costal margins impair visualization and a direct approach to the liver. Exposure of the right lobe can be improved by elevating the right costal margin with a large Richardson retractor. The right lobe can be mobilized by dividing the right triangular and coronary ligaments. Following division of the right triangular ligament, the dissection is continued medially, dividing the superior and inferior coronary ligaments. The right lobe can then be rotated

medially into the surgical field. Mobilization of the left lobe is accomplished in the same fashion. Care must be taken when dividing any of the coronary ligaments due to their proximity to the hepatic veins and retrohepatic vena cava. On occasion it may be necessary to extend the midline abdominal incision into the chest. This is best accomplished with a median sternotomy. The pericardium and diaphragm can be divided toward the center of the inferior vena cava. The combination of incisions provides outstanding exposure of the hepatic veins and retrohepatic vena cava while avoiding injury to the phrenic nerves.

The Pringle maneuver is one of the most useful techniques for evaluating the extent of hepatic injuries (see Fig. 6-40). In patients with extensive hepatic injuries, the Pringle maneuver will differentiate between hemorrhage of the hepatic artery and portal vein, which ceases when the clamp is applied, and that from the hepatic veins and retrohepatic vena cava, which will not. The authors prefer to manually tear the lesser omentum and place the clamp from the left side while guiding the posterior blade of the clamp through the foramen of Winslow with the aid of the left index finger. This approach has the advantages of avoiding injury to the structures within the hepatic pedicle, assuring that the clamp will be placed properly the first time, and including any aberrant or accessory left hepatic arteries between the blades of the clamp.

Techniques for the temporary control of hemorrhage from the liver are necessary when dealing with an extensive injury to provide the anesthesiologist with sufficient time to restore circulating blood volume before proceeding, and because it is not possible to control hemorrhage from more than one location in the abdomen simultaneously. The temporary hemostatic techniques which have proven most useful are hepatic compression, the Pringle maneuver, and perihepatic packing. Manual compression of a bleeding hepatic injury may be a life-saving maneuver (Fig. 6-46). The addition of laparotomy pads on the surface of the liver distributes digital forces and lessens the chance of aggravating the injury. If the lacerated edges of the liver are carefully opposed and the proper forces applied, hemorrhage from almost any hepatic injury can be controlled. The obvious drawback is that considerable skill is required and that little else can be done while the liver is being compressed. Manual compression is best suited for immediate attempts to prevent exsanguination and for periodic control during a complex procedure.

Perihepatic packing also is capable of controlling hemorrhage from most hepatic injuries, and it has the advantage of freeing the surgeon's hands.[63] The laparotomy pads should remain folded, with

FIG. 6-45. Division of the right common iliac artery to expose the bifurcation of the inferior vena cava.

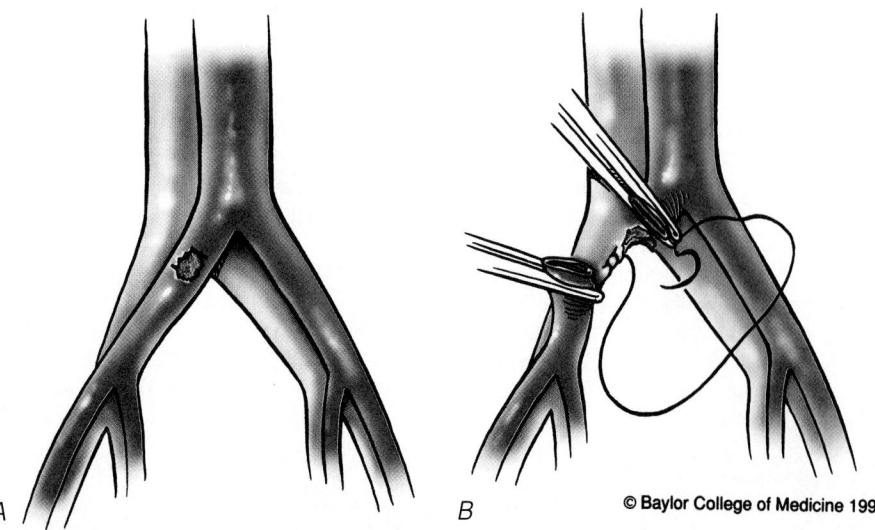

A

B

© Baylor College of Medicine 1990

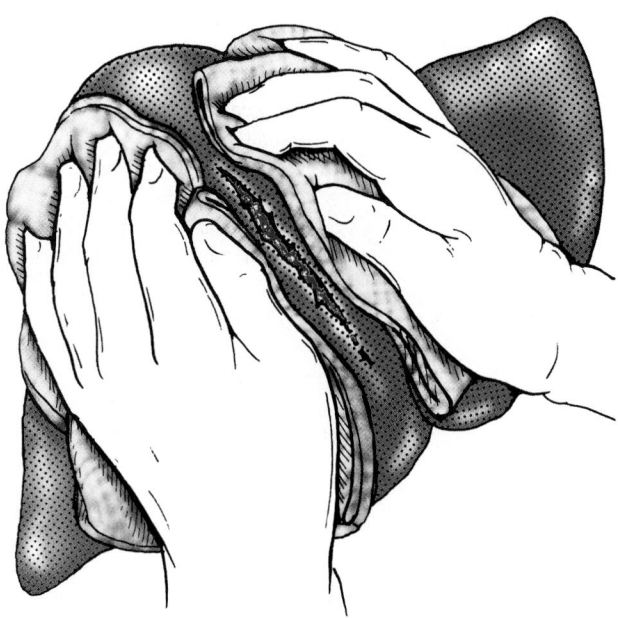

FIG. 6-46. Manual compression of the liver.

two or three stacked together. The right costal margin is elevated, and the pads are strategically placed over and around the bleeding site (see Fig. 6-41). Additional pads should be placed between the liver, diaphragm, and anterior chest wall until the bleeding has been controlled. Ten to fifteen pads may be required to control the hemorrhage from an extensive right lobar injury. The effectiveness of packing may be enhanced by downward pressure on the right costal margin by an assistant. Packing of injuries of the left lobe is not as effective since there is insufficient abdominal and thoracic wall anterior to the left lobe to provide adequate compression with the abdomen open. Fortunately, hemorrhage from the left lobe can usually be controlled by mobilizing the lobe and compressing it between the surgeon's hands.

Two complications may be caused by packing hepatic injuries. Tight packing can compress the inferior vena cava and reduce cardiac filling, and the right diaphragm will be forced cephalad, increasing airway pressures and decreasing tidal volume and functional residual capacity. Depending on the patient's condition, the surgeon must decide whether these complications outweigh the risk of additional blood loss.

Perihepatic packing will not reliably control hemorrhage from larger branches of the hepatic artery. The Pringle maneuver is often used as an adjunct to packing for the temporary control of the arterial hemorrhage. Properly applied, a Pringle maneuver will eliminate all hepatopedal flow. The length of time that a Pringle maneuver can remain in place without causing irreversible ischemic damage to the liver is unknown. Several authors have documented a Pringle maneuver applied for over 1 hour without appreciable hepatic damage; this seems a reasonable figure. Another option for temporary control of hepatic hemorrhage is with a tourniquet. Following mobilization of the bleeding lobe, a 1-inch Penrose drain is wrapped around the liver near the anatomic division between the left and right lobes. The drain is cinched until hemorrhage ceases; tension is maintained by placing a clamp on the drain. Unfortunately, tourniquets are difficult to use because they often slip off or even tear through the parenchyma. An alternative is the use of the Lin liver clamp, though it also suffers the same shortcomings as the tourniquet. If successful, the occluding device is removed in 24 hours and nonviable tissue is resected.

Special techniques have been developed for controlling hemorrhage from juxtahepatic venous injuries. These formidable procedures include hepatic vascular isolation with clamps, the atriocaval shunt, and the Moore-Pilcher balloon. Hepatic vascular isolation with clamps is accomplished by the application of a Pringle maneuver, clamping the aorta at the diaphragm, and clamping the suprarenal and suprahepatic vena cava. While this technique has enjoyed success in elective procedures, its use in trauma patients has had mixed results because patients in profound hemorrhagic shock do not tolerate the precipitous loss of venous return to the heart.

The atriocaval shunt was designed to achieve hepatic vascular isolation while permitting venous blood to enter the heart from below the diaphragm. After a few early successes, enthusiasm for the shunt declined as mortality rates with its use ranged from 50 to 80%. The shunt must be precisely constructed and properly positioned on the first attempt since patients with juxtahepatic venous injuries do not tolerate the continuing blood loss associated with repeated unsuccessful attempts to position the shunt correctly. A variation of the original atriocaval shunt has been the substitution of a 9-mm endotracheal tube for the usual large chest tube (Fig. 6-47). While this change may seem trivial, surrounding the suprarenal vena cava with a snare tourniquet is extremely difficult since exsanguinating hemorrhage must be controlled by posterior compression of the liver, which severely restricts access to that segment of the vena cava.

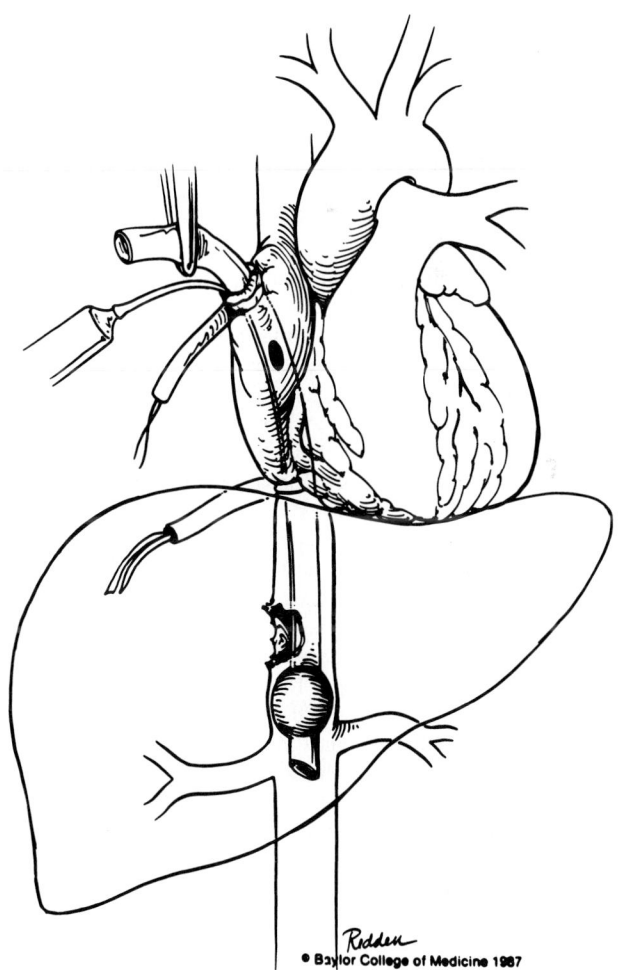

FIG. 6-47. Atriocaval shunt using a 9-mm endotracheal tube. A hole must be cut in the tube to allow blood to flow into the right atrium from the inferior vena cava.

An alternative to the atriocaval shunt is the Moore-Pilcher balloon. This device is inserted through the femoral vein and advanced into the retrohepatic vena cava. When the balloon is inflated, the hepatic veins and vena cava are occluded, thereby achieving vascular isolation. The catheter itself is hollow, and holes placed below the balloon permit blood to flow into the right atrium from the inferior vena cava.

Surgeons who attempt hepatic vascular isolation should be aware that none of the techniques provide complete hemostasis. The residual bleeding following successful vascular isolation can be readily removed with suction. Regardless of the technique employed, a Pringle maneuver should always be used. Because of the technical challenge and high mortality associated with hepatic vascular isolation, there has been a recent trend to avoid a direct operative approach to the injured vessels. If massive venous hemorrhage is seen from behind the liver, and if reasonable hemostasis can be achieved with perihepatic packing, the patient can be transferred to the interventional radiology suite, where hemorrhage from arterial sources are embolized and stents are placed to bridge venous injuries (see Fig. 6-26). The patient is then treated as described in the Staged Operations section, above.

Numerous methods for the definitive control of hepatic hemorrhage have been developed. Minor lacerations may be controlled with manual compression applied directly to the injury site. For similar injuries which do not respond to compression, topical hemostatic techniques have been successful. Small bleeding vessels may be controlled with electrocautery, although the power output of the machine may have to be increased. Bleeding surfaces immune to electrocautery may respond to the argon beam coagulator. Microcrystalline collagen can be used. The powder is placed on a clean 4 × 4 sponge and applied directly to the oozing surface. Pressure is maintained for 5 to 10 minutes. Topical thrombin also can be applied to minor bleeding injuries by saturating either a gelatin foam sponge or a microcrystalline collagen pad and applying it to the bleeding site.

Fibrin glue has been used for both superficial and deep lacerations and appears to be an effective topical agent. Fibrin glue is made by mixing concentrated human fibrinogen (cryoprecipitate) with bovine thrombin and calcium. Since the coagulum forms quickly, the fibrinogen and thrombin-calcium solution are placed in separate syringes joined with a Y connector. Spray-on applicators have also been used. However, enthusiasm has been tempered by reports of fatal anaphylactic reactions and idiopathic hypotension related to an antigenic response to the bovine component.

Suturing of the hepatic parenchyma remains an effective hemostatic technique. Although this treatment has been maligned as a cause of hepatic necrosis, hepatic sutures are often used for persistently bleeding lacerations less than 3 cm in depth. It is also an appropriate alternative for deeper lacerations if the patient will not tolerate further hemorrhage. The preferred suture is 2-0 or 0 chromic attached to a large, curved, blunt needle. The large diameter of the suture helps prevent it from pulling through Glisson's capsule. A simple running technique is used to approximate the edges of shallow lacerations. Deeper lacerations may be managed with interrupted horizontal mattress sutures placed parallel to the edge of the laceration. When tying the suture, the tension is adequate when visible hemorrhage ceases or the liver blanches around the suture.

Most sources of venous hemorrhage within the liver can be managed with parenchymal sutures, and even injuries of the retrohepatic vena cava and hepatic veins have been successfully tamponaded by closing the hepatic parenchyma over the bleeding vessel.

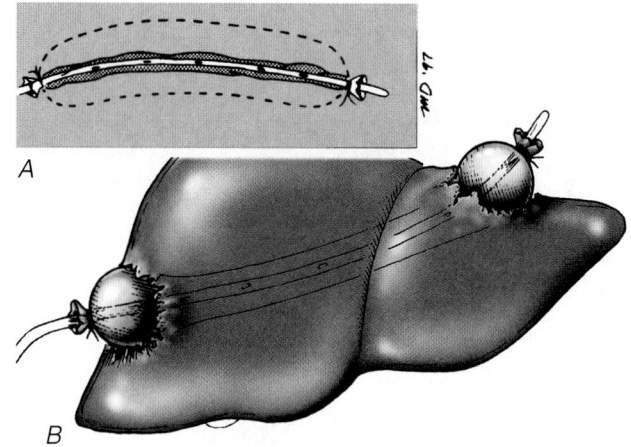

FIG. 6-48. *A. Intrahepatic balloon used to tamponade hemorrhage form transhepatic penetrating injuries. B. Intrahepatic balloon in situ.*

Venous hemorrhage due to penetrating wounds that traverse the central portion of the liver can be managed by suturing the entrance and exit wounds with horizontal mattress sutures. Although intrahepatic hematomas may form that can become infected, this may be preferable to an intracaval shunt or deep hepatotomy. Suturing of the hepatic parenchyma is not always successful in controlling the hemorrhage, particularly if it is of arterial origin.

Hepatotomy with selective ligation of bleeding vessels is an important technique usually reserved for transhepatic penetrating wounds. Hepatotomy is performed using the finger fracture technique. The dissection continues until the bleeding vessels are identified and controlled. It should be remembered that considerable blood loss may be incurred since the division of additional viable hepatic tissue is often required to reach the bleeding vessels. An alternative to suturing the entrance and exit wounds of a transhepatic injury or extensive hepatotomy is the use of an intrahepatic balloon.[64] Tying a large Penrose drain to a hollow catheter and ligating the opposite end of the drain (Fig. 6-48) is the method preferred by these authors. The balloon is then inserted into the bleeding wound and inflated with soluble contrast media. If control of the hemorrhage is successful, a stopcock or clamp is used to occlude the catheter and maintain the inflation. The catheter is left in the abdomen and removed at a subsequent operation 24 to 48 hours later. Recurrent hemorrhage may occur when the balloon is deflated, but is usually amenable to selective embolization.

Hepatic arterial ligation may be appropriate for patients with recalcitrant arterial hemorrhage from deep within the liver. However, its utility is limited since hemorrhage from the portal and hepatic venous systems will continue. Its primary role is in transhepatic injuries when application of the Pringle maneuver results in the cessation of arterial hemorrhage. Arterial ligation is a reasonable alternative to a deep hepatotomy, particularly in unstable patients. While ligation of the right or left hepatic artery is well tolerated in humans, ligation of the proper hepatic artery (distal to the origin of the gastroduodenal artery) is not necessarily associated with survival. The fate of the dearterialized lobe is unpredictable. The authors have seen lobar necrosis requiring anatomic lobectomy following arterial ligation.

An uncommon but perplexing hepatic injury is the subcapsular hematoma. This lesion occurs when the parenchyma of the liver is disrupted by blunt trauma, but Glisson's capsule remains intact. The hematoma may be recognized either at the time of the surgery or preoperatively if a CT scan is performed. Regardless of how the lesion is diagnosed, subsequent decision making is often difficult. Subcapsular hematomas involving less than 50% of the surface of the liver that are not expanding or ruptured should be left alone or packed if discovered on exploratory laparotomy. Hematomas that are expanding during an operation may require exploration. These lesions are often caused by uncontrolled arterial hemorrhage, and packing alone may not be successful. An alternative strategy would be to pack the liver close to the abdomen to control venous hemorrhage and to transport the patient to the angiographic suite for hepatic arteriography and embolization of the bleeding vessel. Ruptured hematomas require exploration and selective ligation, with or without packing.

Resectional débridement is indicated for the removal of peripheral portions of nonviable hepatic parenchyma. The mass of tissue removed should rarely exceed 25% of the liver. Since additional blood loss may occur, it should be reserved for patients who are in good metabolic condition and who will tolerate additional blood loss. Resectional débridement is performed by finger fracture. An alternative for patients with extensive unilobar injuries is anatomic hepatic resection; however, the mortality rate for trauma patients exceeds 50% in most series. It has largely been replaced by perihepatic packing, resectional débridement, and hepatotomy with selective ligation, and is probably never indicated in the acute setting. There are two circumstances, however, where anatomic resections are appropriate. The first is with extensive injuries of the lateral segment of the left lobe. Since hemorrhage can be easily controlled with bimanual compression, uncontrolled blood loss is not as problematic as with the left or right anatomic lobectomies. Another indication for anatomic lobectomy occurs in patients whose hemorrhage has been controlled by perihepatic packing and/or arterial ligation, but whose left or right lobe is nonviable. Since the mass of the remaining necrotic liver is large and the risk of subsequent infection is high, it should be removed as soon as the patient's condition permits.

Several centers have reported patients with devastating hepatic injuries or necrosis of the entire liver who have undergone successful hepatic transplantation. Clearly this dramatic therapy requires the best judgment possible. The patient must have all other injuries delineated (particularly those to the central nervous system) and have an excellent chance of survival excluding the hepatic injury. Cost and donor availability will limit such procedures, but it seems probable that hepatic transplantation for trauma will continue to be performed in rare and extraordinary circumstances.

Omentum has been used to fill large defects in the liver. The rationale for this is that it provides an excellent source of macrophages and that it fills a potential dead space with viable tissue. The omentum can also provide a little additional support for parenchymal sutures and is often strong enough to prevent them from cutting through Glisson's capsule.

Several prospective and retrospective studies have clearly demonstrated that the use of Penrose or sump drains is associated with a greater risk of intra-abdominal sepsis when compared to those treated with closed suction drains or no drains. Drains are not necessary for minor lacerations. However, they should be used if bile is seen oozing from the liver and in most patients with deep central injuries.

The complications following significant hepatic trauma include hemorrhage, infections, and various fistulas. Postoperative hemorrhage can be expected in a considerable percentage of patients treated with perihepatic packing. The source may be either persistent coagulopathy or a missed vascular injury. In most instances where postoperative hemorrhage is suspected, the patient is best served by a return to the operating room. Arteriography with embolization may be considered in selected patients.

Infections within and around the liver occur in about 3% of injured patients. Perihepatic infections develop more often in victims of penetrating trauma than blunt trauma, presumably due to the greater frequency of enteric contamination of the former. Persistent elevation of temperature and white blood cell count after the third or fourth postoperative day should prompt a search for intra-abdominal infection. In the absence of pneumonia, line sepsis, or urinary tract infection, an abdominal CT scan with intravenous and upper gastrointestinal contrast should be obtained. Many perihepatic infections can be treated with CT-guided drainage. However, infected hematomas and infected necrotic liver cannot be expected to respond to percutaneous drainage. Right twelfth rib resection remains an excellent approach for posterior infections and provides superior drainage.

Bilomas are loculated collections of bile, which may or may not be infected. If infected, the biloma is essentially an abscess and should be treated as such. If sterile, it will eventually be reabsorbed. Biliary ascites is caused by disruption of a major bile duct. Reoperation with the establishment of appropriate drainage is the prudent course. Even if the source of bile leakage can be identified, primary repair of the injured duct is unlikely to be successful. It is best to wait until a firm fistulous communication is established with adequate drainage.

Biliary fistulas occur in approximately 3% of patients with hepatic injuries. They are usually of little consequence, and most will close without specific treatment. Rarely, a fistulous communication will form with intrathoracic structures in patients with associated diaphragm injuries and result in a bronchobiliary or pleurobiliary fistula. Due to the pressure differential between the biliary tract and the thoracic cavity, most of these fistulas have required operative closure. However, the authors have treated a pleurobiliary fistula by endoscopic sphincterotomy with stent placement, which then closed spontaneously.

Since hemorrhage from hepatic injuries is often treated without identifying and controlling each individual bleeding vessel, arterial pseudoaneurysms may develop. If the pseudoaneurysm enlarges, it will eventually rupture into the parenchyma of the liver, a bile duct, or into an adjacent portal venous branch. Rupture into a bile duct results in hemobilia, which is characterized by intermittent episodes of right upper quadrant pain, upper gastrointestinal hemorrhage, and jaundice. If the aneurysm ruptures into a portal vein, portal venous hypertension with bleeding esophageal varices may occur. Each of these complications is exceedingly rare, and both are best managed with hepatic arteriography and embolization. Biliovenous fistulas have also been reported. Serum bilirubin rises very rapidly and extremely high values are common. Sphincterotomy of the papilla of Vater may hasten closure.

Gallbladder and Extrahepatic Bile Ducts

Injuries of the gallbladder are treated by lateral suture or cholecystectomy, whichever is easier. If lateral suture is performed, absorbable suture should be used to prevent the formation of calculi. Injuries of the extrahepatic bile ducts are a challenge. Because of the proximity of the portal vein, hepatic artery, and vena cava, associated vascular injuries are common and the patient's physiologic status is often poor (see Staged Operations section, above). Furthermore, the ducts are of normal size and texture (i.e., small in diameter and thin walled). These factors usually preclude primary repairs except for the smallest lacerations with no loss of tissue. These injuries

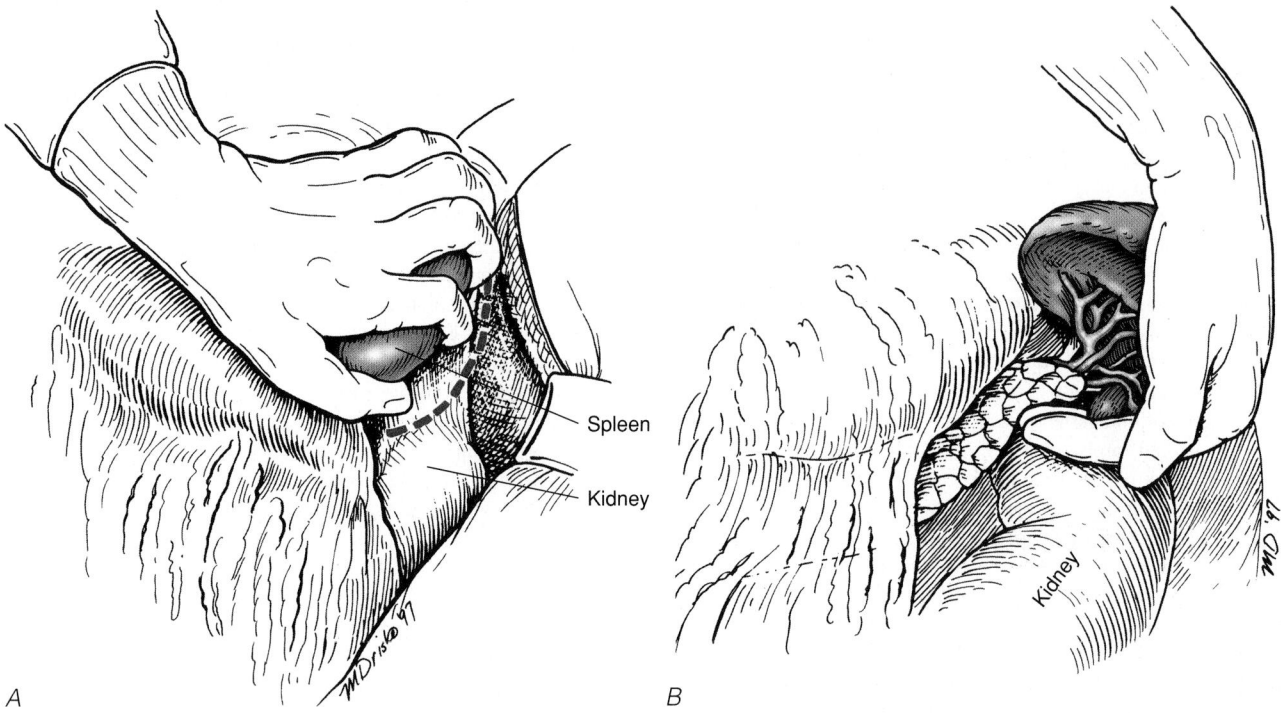

FIG. 6-49. When mobilizing the spleen for repair or removal, the peritoneum and endoabdominal fascia behind the spleen must be incised. The incision should be made about 1 cm lateral to the reflection of the peritoneum onto the spleen. Traction must not be applied to the spleen or the peritoneal reflection will tear, which often results in splenectomy. Instead, the peritoneal reflection is exposed by applying posterior pressure and rotating the spleen medially (A). The plane between the pancreas and left kidney is then developed (B). When completed, the spleen should be able to reach the level of the abdominal incision.

can be treated by the insertion of a T tube through the wound, or by lateral suture using 4-0 to 6-0 monofilament absorbable suture. Virtually all transections and any injury associated with significant tissue loss will require a Roux-en-Y choledochojejunostomy.[65] The anastomosis is performed using a single-layer interrupted technique (because it is almost impossible to do a running stitch) using 4-0 or 5-0 monofilament absorbable suture. A round patch of seromuscular tissue the size of the common duct is removed from the jejunum at the site of the anastomosis to inhibit wound contraction. The mucosa and submucosa are punctured but not resected. Full-thickness bites of the duct and jejunum are taken. Because of the small size of the duct, only 6 to 8 stitches can be used. T tubes are not placed. The jejunum is then sutured to the areolar tissue of the hepatic pedicle or porta hepatis to take any tension off the anastomosis.

Injuries of the hepatic ducts are almost impossible to satisfactorily repair under emergency circumstances. One approach is to intubate the duct for external drainage and attempt a repair when the patient recovers. Alternatively, the duct can be ligated if the opposite lobe is normal and uninjured. For patients who are critically ill, the common duct also can be treated by intubation with external drainage.

Spleen

Splenic injuries are treated nonoperatively, by splenic repair (splenorrhaphy), partial splenectomy, or resection, depending on the extent of the injury and the condition of the patient.[66–68] Enthusiasm for splenic salvage has been driven by the evolving trend toward nonoperative management of solid organ injuries and the rare but often fatal complication of overwhelming postsplenectomy

infection (OPSI).[69] These infections are caused by encapsulated bacteria (i.e., *Streptococcus pneumoniae*, *Haemophilus influenzae*, and *Neisseria meningitidis*) and are very resistant to treatment. OPSI occurs most often in young children and immunocompromised adults. It is uncommon in otherwise healthy adults. For this reason attempts to salvage the spleen are more vigorous in children.

In order to safely remove or repair the spleen it should be mobilized to the extent that it can be brought to the surface of the abdominal wall without tension. This requires division of the attachments between the spleen and splenic flexure of the colon. Next, an incision is made in the peritoneum and endoabdominal fascia beginning at the inferior pole, a centimeter or two away from the spleen, and continuing posteriorly and superiorly until the esophagus is encountered, similarly to a left medial visceral rotation (Fig. 6-49). Care must be taken not to pull on the posterior aspect of the spleen or it will tear at the peritoneal reflection, causing significant hemorrhage. Rather, the spleen should be rotated counterclockwise with posterior pressure applied to expose the peritoneal reflection. It is often helpful to rotate the operating table 20° to the patient's right, so the weight of abdominal viscera aids in the retraction. A plane can then be established between the spleen and pancreas and Gerota's fascia, which can be extended to the aorta. This will complete mobilization and permit the spleen to be repaired or removed without struggling for exposure.

Hilar injuries or a pulverized splenic parenchyma are usually treated by splenectomy. These authors have selectively reimplanted six pieces of the spleen (40 × 40 × 3 mm) within the leafs of the omentum. Technetium scans have confirmed their viability, and immunoglobulin M (IgM) levels have normalized. However, the patient's response to an antigenic challenge has not been evaluated.

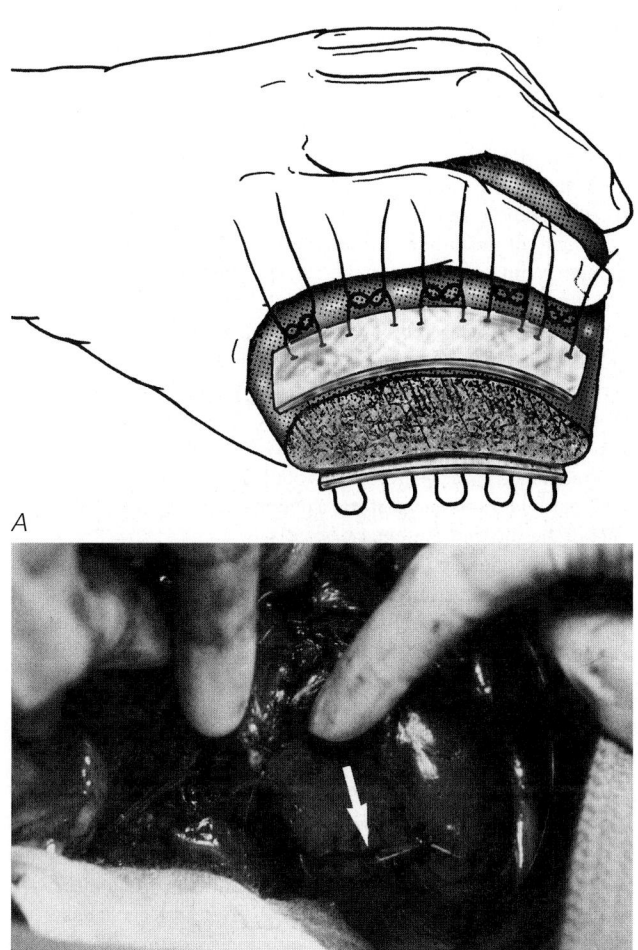

A

B

FIG. 6-50. *A. This method can be used to control hemorrhage from the spleen, liver, or kidney. Dacron, omentum, and absorbable artificial materials have been used to support the sutures. B. The arrow indicates a splenorrhaphy performed with a running simple suture.*

Splenectomy is also indicated for lesser splenic injuries in patients who have developed a coagulopathy and have multiple abdominal injuries, and it is usually necessary in patients with failed splenic salvage attempts. Partial splenectomy can be used in patients in whom only a portion of the spleen has been destroyed, usually the superior or inferior half. Following removal of the damaged portion, the same methods used to control hemorrhage from hepatic parenchyma can be used for the spleen (see Liver section, above). When placing horizontal mattress sutures across a raw edge, gentle compression of the parenchyma by an assistant will facilitate hemostasis (Fig. 6-50). Following ligation of the sutures and releasing compression, the spleen will expand slightly and further tighten the sutures. Drains are never used after completion of the repair or resection. If splenectomy is performed, vaccines against the encapsulated bacteria are administered. The pneumococcal vaccine is routinely given, and vaccines effective against *Haemophilus influenzae* and *Neisseria meningitidis* should be used if available.

Diaphragm

In blunt trauma the diaphragm is injured on the left in 75% of cases, presumably because the liver diffuses some of the energy on the right side.[70] For both blunt and penetrating trauma, the diagnosis

is suggested by an abnormality of the diaphragmatic shadow on chest x-ray. Many of these are subtle, particularly with penetrating injuries, and further diagnostic evaluation may be warranted (see Chest section, above). The typical injury from blunt trauma is a tear in the central tendon, which may be large. Regardless of the etiology, acute injuries are repaired through an abdominal incision. The laceration is closed with a no. 1 monofilament permanent suture, using a simple running technique. Occasionally, large avulsions or SGWs with extensive tissue loss will require polypropylene mesh to bridge the defect.[71]

Duodenum

Duodenal hematomas are caused by a direct blow to the abdomen and occur more often in children than adults. Blood accumulates between the seromuscular and submucosal layers, eventually causing obstruction. The diagnosis is suspected by the onset of vomiting following blunt abdominal trauma; barium examination of the duodenum reveals either the coiled spring sign or obstruction. Most duodenal hematomas in children can be managed nonoperatively with nasogastric suction and parenteral nutrition. Resolution of the obstruction occurs in the majority of patients if this therapy is continued for 7 to 14 days. If surgical intervention becomes necessary, evacuation of the hematoma is associated with equal success but fewer complications than bypass procedures. Despite few existing data on adults, there is no reason to believe that their hematomas should be treated differently from those of children. A new approach is laparoscopic evacuation if the obstruction persists more than 7 days.

Duodenal perforations can be caused by both blunt and penetrating trauma (Fig. 6-51). Blunt injuries are difficult to diagnose because the contents of the duodenum have a neutral pH, few bacteria, and are often contained by the retroperitoneum. Mortality may exceed 30% if the lesion is not identified and treated within 24 hours. The perforations are not reliably identified by initial oral contrast CT examinations, therefore the authors often obtain contrast x-rays with soluble contrast followed with barium if necessary. Most

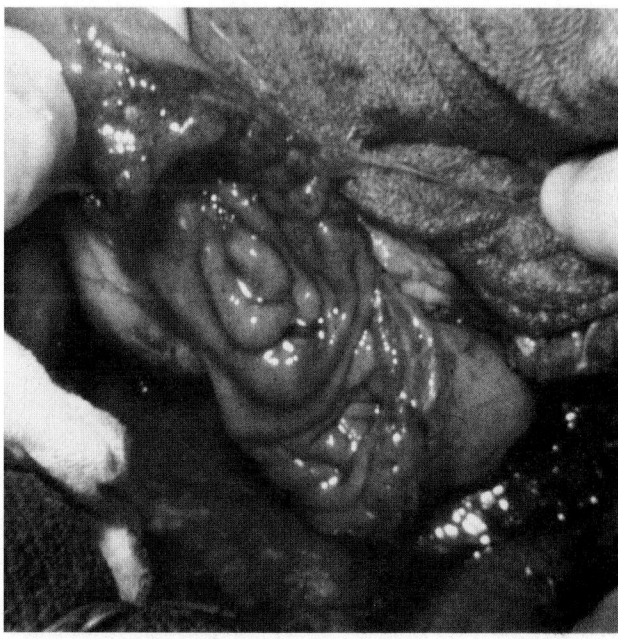

FIG. 6-51. *Blunt perforation of the duodenum at the junction of the third and fourth portions.*

perforations of the duodenum can be treated by primary repair. The authors prefer to use a running single-layer suture of 3-0 monofilament. The wound should be closed in a direction that results in the largest residual lumen. Occasionally, penetrating injuries will damage only the pancreatic aspect of the second or third portion. Because the duodenum cannot be adequately mobilized to repair the injury directly, the wound should be extended laterally or the duodenum divided so the pancreatic aspect can be sutured from the inside. As with other intestinal suture lines, duodenal repairs or anastomoses do not benefit from adjunctive external drainage.

Challenges arise when there is a substantial loss of duodenal tissue. Extensive injuries of the first portion of the duodenum can be repaired by débridement and anastomosis because of the mobility and rich blood supply of the distal gastric atrium and pylorus. In contrast, the second portion is tethered to the head of the pancreas by its blood supply and the ducts of Wirsung and Santorini, so the length of duodenum that can be mobilized from the pancreas is limited to approximately 1 cm. Unlike the jejunum, ileum, or colon, this mobilization will yield little additional tissue to alleviate tension on the suture line. As a result, suture repair of the second portion when tissue is lost often results in an unacceptably narrow lumen, and end-to-end anastomosis is virtually impossible; therefore more sophisticated repairs are required. For extensive injuries proximal to the accessory papilla, débridement and end-to-end anastomosis is appropriate. For lesions between the accessory papilla and the papilla of Vater, a vascularized jejunal graft, either a patch or tubular interposition graft, may be required. Experience with these procedures is limited. Duodenal injuries with tissue loss distal to the papilla of Vater and proximal to the superior mesenteric vessels are best treated by Roux-en-Y duodenojejunostomy (Fig. 6-52). The distal portion of the duodenum is oversewn, the jejunum is sutured end-to-end to the proximal duodenum, and the

defunctionalized distal duodenum and proximal jejunum are drained into the jejunum. Alternatively, the short defunctionalized duodenum can be resected; however, this is a rather tedious dissection behind the superior mesenteric vessels that may not be tolerated by a patient who has been in protracted shock.

Injuries to the third and fourth portions of the duodenum with tissue loss pose other problems. Owing to the notoriously short mesentery of the third and fourth portions of the duodenum, mobilization is limited because of the risk of ischemia. While end-to-end duodenojejunal anastomoses are possible in these regions, the technique used must resemble that of a hand-sewn, low anterior rectal anastomosis, with a posterior row of interrupted sutures placed while the ends of the bowel are far apart. The jejunum is then parachuted down to the duodenum, and the anterior row is completed. In the experience of these authors, duodenal fistulas are common when this method is used. Therefore it is our preference to resect the third and fourth portions and perform a duodenojejunostomy on the right side of the superior mesenteric vessels.

An important adjunct for high-risk or complex duodenal repairs is the pyloric exclusion technique (Fig. 6-53).[72] By occluding the pylorus and performing a gastrojejunostomy, the gastrointestinal stream can be diverted away from the duodenal repair. If a fistula does develop, it is functionally an end fistula, which is easier to manage and more likely to close than a lateral fistula, and the patient can take food by mouth to maintain nutritional status. To perform a pyloric exclusion, a gastrostomy is first made on the greater curvature as close to the pylorus as possible. The pylorus is then grasped with a Babcock clamp via the gastrostomy and oversewn with a 0 polypropylene suture. A gastrojejunostomy restores gastrointestinal continuity. Vagotomy is not necessary because marginal ulceration occurs at the same frequency (approximately 3%) as duodenal ulceration occurs in the same patient population. Experience has shown that the absorbable sutures do not last long enough to be effective, and even heavy polypropylene will give way in 3 to 4 weeks in most patients. A linear staple line across the outside of the pylorus provides the most permanent pyloric closure.

Pancreas

Blunt pancreatic transection at the neck of the pancreas can occur with a direct blow to the abdomen. As an isolated injury it is more difficult to detect than blunt duodenal rupture; however, a missed pancreatic injury is more benign. Since the main pancreatic duct is transected, the patient will develop a pseudocyst or pancreatic ascites, but there is little inflammation since the pancreatic enzymes remain inactivated. The diagnosis can occasionally be made with CT using fine cuts through the pancreas. However, CT will not identify a significant number of transections if performed within 6 hours of injury.[73,74]

Optimal management of pancreatic trauma is determined by the location of the injury and whether or not the main pancreatic duct is injured. Pancreatic injuries in which the pancreatic duct is not injured may be treated by drainage or left alone. In contrast, pancreatic injuries associated with a ductal injury always require treatment to prevent pancreatic ascites or a major external fistula. Direct exploration of perforations or lacerations will confirm the diagnosis of a ductal injury in most instances. This leaves a small but significant percentage of patients in whom the diagnosis is in doubt, and more invasive investigations may be required. One recommendation has been to perform operative pancreatography. This procedure requires direct access to the duct either by way of a duodenotomy or following resection of the tail of the pancreas. Five French pediatric feeding

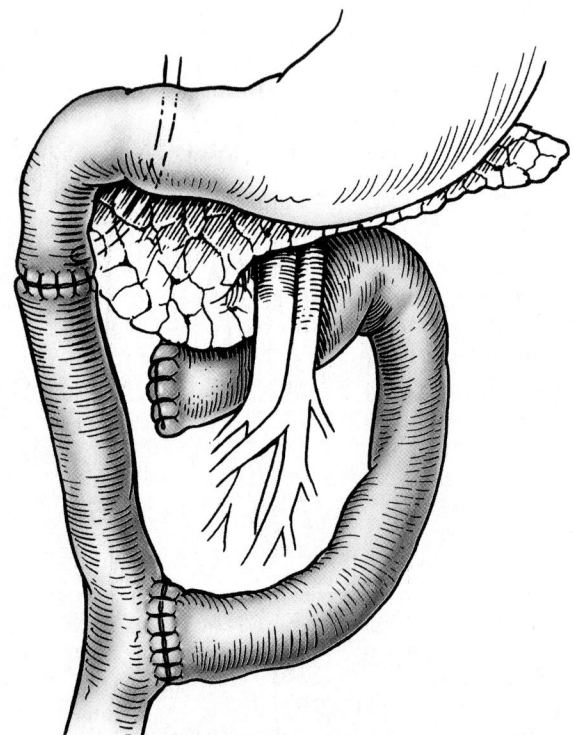

FIG. 6-52. Roux-en-Y duodenojejunostomy is used to treat duodenal injuries between the papilla of Vater and superior mesenteric vessel when tissue loss precludes primary repair.

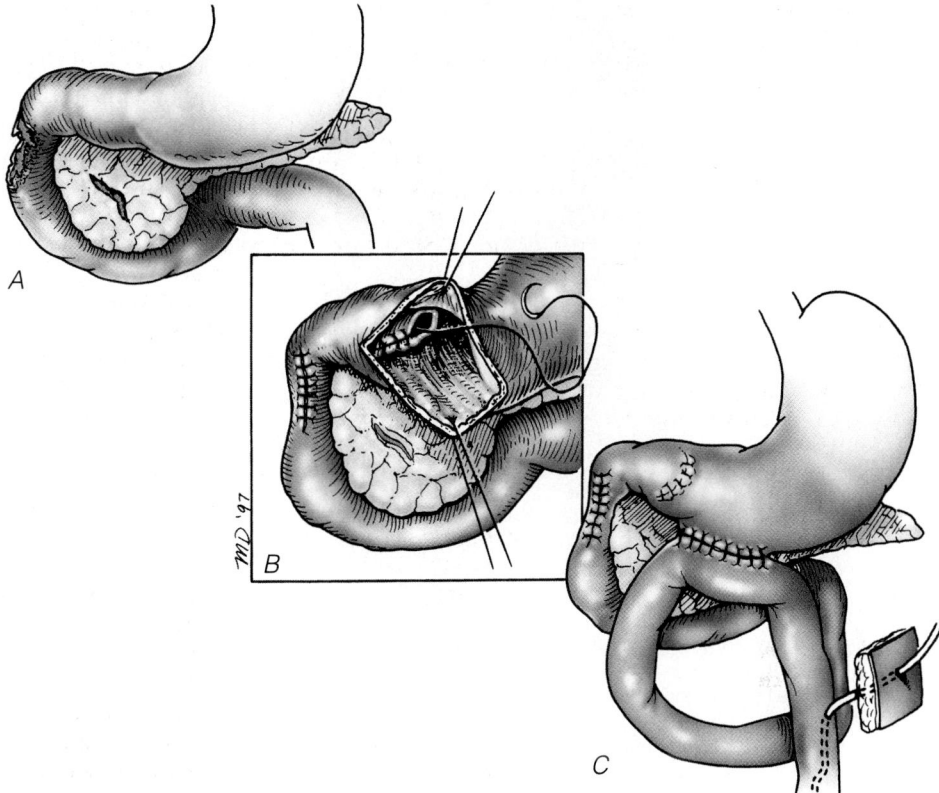

FIG. 6-53. *A.* Pyloric exclusion is used to treat combined injuries of the duodenum and the head of the pancreas, as well as isolated duodenal injuries when the duodenal repair is less than optimal. *B.* The pylorus is oversewn through a gastrotomy. The gastrotomy will subsequently be used to create a gastrojejunostomy. *C.* These authors frequently employ needle-catheter jejunostomy tube feedings for these patients.

tubes are used for cannulating the duct. Two to four milliliters of full-strength contrast material is slowly injected; injuries are identified by obstruction or extravasation. Great care must be taken to avoid overdistention of the duct with contrast, which can produce pancreatitis. The obvious shortcoming of this approach is the creation of a duodenal wound that must heal in a less-than-optimal environment. While those who advocate transduodenal pancreatography have had few duodenal fistulas, some have occurred. The problems associated with lateral duodenal fistulas are sufficient to dampen any surgeon's enthusiasm for this approach. If the patient already has a duodenal wound in the second portion, the above objections to pancreatography are mitigated.

An expeditious alternative to pancreatography is to pass a 1.5- to 2.0-mm coronary artery dilator into the main duct via the papilla and observe the pancreatic wound. If the dilator is seen in the wound, a ductal injury is confirmed. When inserted through the papilla of Vater, care must be taken to ensure that the dilator enters the pancreatic duct and not the bile duct. This can be determined by palpation of the hepatic pedicle. The limitations of this approach are the same as those for pancreatography.

A third method for identifying pancreatic ductal injuries is the use of endoscopic retrograde pancreatography (ERP). This technique may be difficult to perform in an anesthetized patient in the operating room, but the surgeon can assist by manipulating the duodenum or occluding the distal portion to facilitate air insufflation. ERP is very helpful in the delayed diagnosis of a ductal injury or in those patients who are too sick to explore adequately during the initial operation.

It is apparent based on the above options that no ideal method exists for identifying pancreatic ductal injuries that cannot be ruled out by direct exploration. This dilemma tends to encourage aggressive local exploration, which may create a ductal injury where none existed. For injuries involving the neck, body, or tail of the pancreas,

this is of minor consequence because a simple resection distal to the injury cures the lesion. However, this is not the case for injuries to the head of the pancreas, which cannot be treated with a simple resection. Rather than accepting the risks of pancreatography or aggressive local exploration, a final option for identifying ductal injuries in the head of the pancreas is to do nothing other than drain the pancreas (Fig. 6-54). If pancreatic fistula or pseudocyst develops, the diagnosis is confirmed. While this approach may not seem rational, the alternatives are also uninspiring. Fortunately, the majority of pancreatic fistulas will close spontaneously with only supportive care. The authors prefer this approach over operative pancreatography when the diagnosis of ductal injury in the head of the pancreas is not apparent and ERP is not promptly available.

Several options are available for treating injuries of the neck, body, and tail of the pancreas when the main duct is transected. Historically, distal pancreatectomy with splenectomy has been the preferred approach.[75] However, during the past 15 years, increasing interest in splenic preservation has stimulated the use of the splenic-preserving distal pancreatectomy. This procedure is performed by dissecting the pancreas from the splenic vein. Another method for splenic preservation is to bury the distal transected end of the pancreas in a Roux-en-Y limb. This technique also conserves the distal pancreas, but is seldom performed because of the added complexity of the Roux-en-Y and the risks of pancreatojejunostomy.

For injuries to the head of the pancreas that involve the main pancreatic duct but not the intrapancreatic bile duct, there are few options. Distal pancreatectomy alone is rarely indicated because the risk of pancreatic insufficiency is significant if more than 85 to 90% of the gland is resected. A more limited resection from the site of the injury to the neck of the pancreas, with preservation of the pancreaticoduodenal vessels and common duct, will allow for closure of the injured proximal pancreatic duct. Pancreatic function

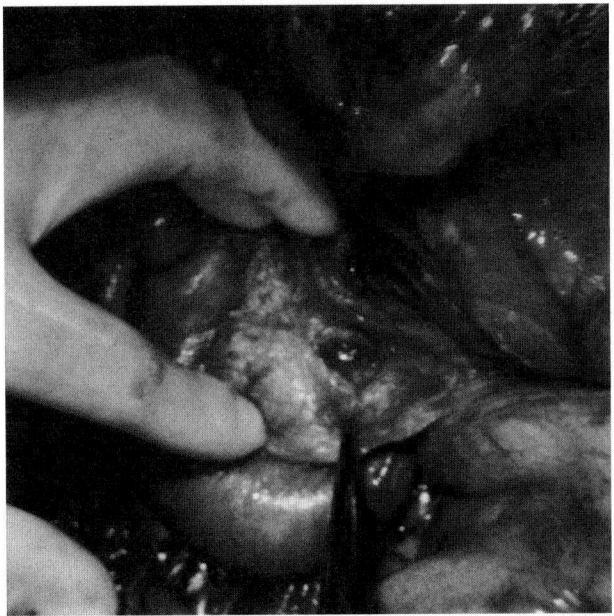

FIG. 6-54. Stab wound through the head of the pancreas. No injury of the main pancreatic duct could be identified upon exploration. The patient was treated with closed-suction drainage alone and never developed a pancreatic fistula.

can then be preserved by a Roux-en-Y pancreatojejunostomy with the distal pancreas (Fig. 6-55).

In contrast to injuries of the pancreatic duct, the diagnosis of injuries to the intrapancreatic common bile duct is simple. The first method is to squeeze the gallbladder and observe the pancreatic

wound. If bile is seen leaking from the pancreatic wound, the presence of an injury is established. Operative cholangiography is diagnostic in questionable cases. If a patient with an intrapancreatic bile duct injury is critically ill from hemorrhage, external drainage can be utilized until the patient is fit for definitive treatment. Small tangential perforations of the intrapancreatic bile duct may heal with this treatment alone, although it is seldom recommended. Most authorities advocate division of the common bile duct superior to the first portion of the duodenum, ligation of the distal common duct, and reconstruction with a Roux-en-Y choledochojejunostomy.

The use of drains has played an important role in the management of pancreatic injuries. While many authorities advocate routine drainage of all pancreatic injuries, it is not the practice of these authors to drain contusions, lacerations in which the probability of a major ductal injury is small, or pancreatic anastomoses. However, draining pancreatic injuries is recommended when there is a possible major ductal injury, though it cannot be identified. If a drain is desirable, prospective studies have demonstrated that closed-suction devices are associated with fewer infectious complications than sump or Penrose drains. Almost all pancreatic fistulas will close spontaneously. Nutritional support is important and electrolyte replacement may be necessary.

Pancreatoduodenal Injuries

Because the pancreas and duodenum are in physical contact, combined pancreaticoduodenal injuries are common, particularly following penetrating trauma. These lesions are dangerous because of the risk of duodenal suture line dehiscence and the development of a lateral duodenal fistula. Each injury should be assessed as previously outlined. The simplest treatment is to repair the duodenal injury and drain the pancreatic injury. This method is appropriate for combined injuries without major duodenal tissue loss and without

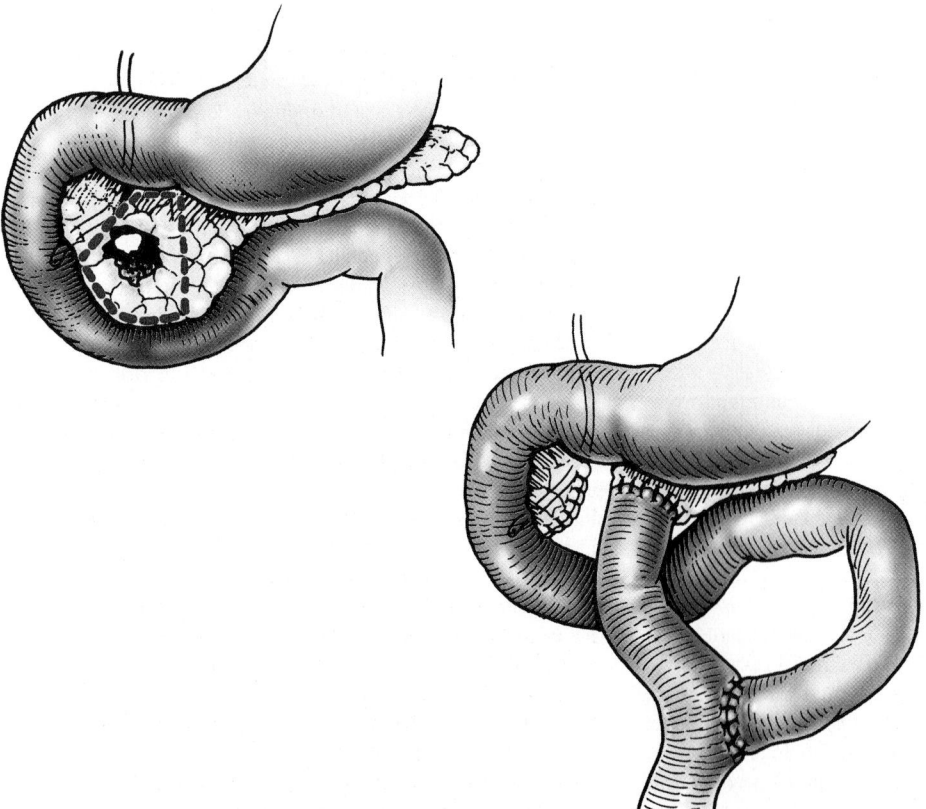

FIG. 6-55. Roux-en-Y pancreatojejunostomy is used to treat pancreatic injuries when the main duct is injured and distal pancreatectomy may result in pancreatic insufficiency. The pancreas between the common bile duct and neck is resected, but the body and tail are preserved.

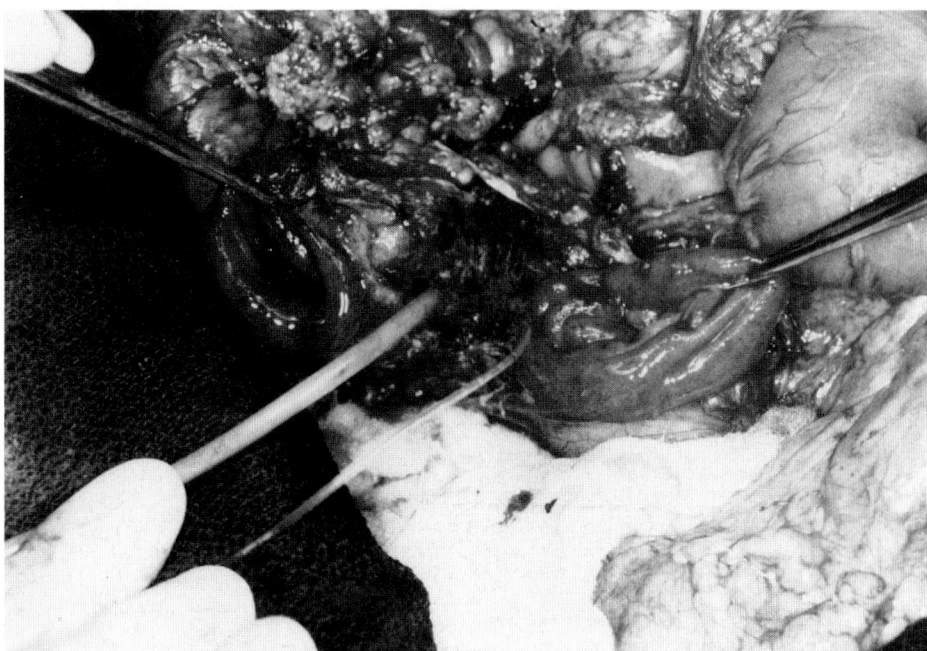

FIG. 6-56. Although a pancreatoduo-denectomy is a formidable procedure, there are circumstances in which it is clearly the best option. This patient suf-fered a stab wound, which transected the second portion of the duodenum and extended into the head of the pancreas. Local exploration revealed transection of both the intrapancreatic common bile duct (large tube) and the main pancreatic duct (small tube). He recovered uneventfully following the resection.

pancreatic or biliary ductal injuries. With more extensive injuries, consideration should be given to providing additional protection for the duodenal suture line. The authors prefer pyloric exclusion to other alternatives.

While most pancreatic and duodenal injuries can be treated with relatively simple procedures, a few will require extensive operations such as pancreatoduodenectomy (Fig. 6-56). Examples of such injuries include transection of both the intrapancreatic bile duct and the main pancreatic duct in the head of the pancreas, avulsion of the papilla of Vater from the duodenum, and destruction of the entire second portion of the duodenum. Most injuries of this nature are caused by high-energy gunshot wounds. In patients with a pancreatoduo-denal injury who also have an intrapancreatic bile duct injury, it is possible to use the combination of pyloric exclusion and Roux-en-Y choledochojejunostomy to avoid a pancreatoduodenectomy. How-ever, the complexity and unpredictable physiology of the combined procedures makes the pancreatoduodenectomy more attractive.

Colon

The treatment of injuries of the colon has been debated for nearly a century. Finally, during the past decade, something resembling a consensus has been reached.[76,77] There are three conceptually differ-ent methods for treating colonic injuries: primary repair, colostomy, and exteriorized repair. Primary repairs include lateral suture of per-forations and resection of the damaged colon with reconstruction by ileocolostomy or colocolostomy. The advantage of primary repairs is that definitive treatment is carried out at the initial operation. The disadvantage is that suture lines are created in suboptimal conditions and leakage may occur. Several different styles of colostomies have been used to manage colonic injuries. In some instances the injured colon can be exteriorized like a loop colostomy. The injured area can be resected and an end colostomy or ileostomy performed, and the distal colon can be brought to the abdominal wall as a mucous fistula or oversewn and left in the abdominal cavity. Finally, a loop colostomy can be created proximal to a suture line, which is left in the abdominal cavity. The advantage of colostomy is avoiding

an unprotected suture line in the abdomen. The disadvantage is that a second operation is required to close the colostomy. Often overlooked disadvantages are the complications associated with the creation of a colostomy, some of which may be fatal. Exteriorized repairs are created by suspending a repaired perforation or anas-tomosis on the abdominal wall with an appliance after the fashion of a loop colostomy. If after 10 days the suture line does not leak, it can be returned to the abdominal cavity under local anesthesia without subsequent risk of leakage. If the repair breaks down before 10 days, it is treated as a loop colostomy. Healing is successful in 50 to 60% of cases. The advantage is avoidance of an intraperitoneal suture line when it is at risk of leakage, and the disadvantage is that 40 to 50% of patients will require colostomy closure. Stomal complications similar to those of colostomies also can occur with the exteriorization.

Numerous large retrospective and several prospective studies have now clearly demonstrated that primary repair is safe and effec-tive in the majority of patients with penetrating injuries. Colostomy is still appropriate in a few patients, but the current dilemma is how to select them. Exteriorized repair is probably no longer indicated since most patients who were once candidates for this treatment are now successfully managed by primary repair. Two methods have been advocated that result in 75 to 90% of penetrating colonic in-juries being safely treated by primary repair. The first is to repair all perforations not requiring resection. If resection is required due to the local extent of the injury, and it is proximal to the middle colic artery, the proximal portion of the right colon up to and including the injury is resected and an ileocolostomy performed. If resection is required distal to the middle colic artery, an end colostomy is created and the distal colon oversewn and left within the abdomen. The theory behind this approach is that an ileocolostomy heals more reliably than colocolostomy, because in the trauma patient who has suffered shock and may be hypovolemic, assessing the adequacy of the blood supply of the colon is much less reliable than in elec-tive procedures. The blood supply of the terminal ileum is never a problem. The other approach is to repair all injuries regardless of the extent and location (including colocolostomy), and reserve

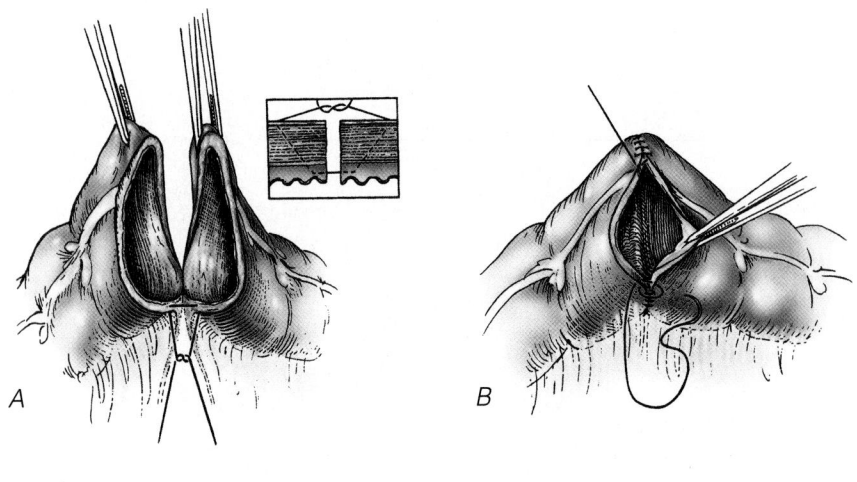

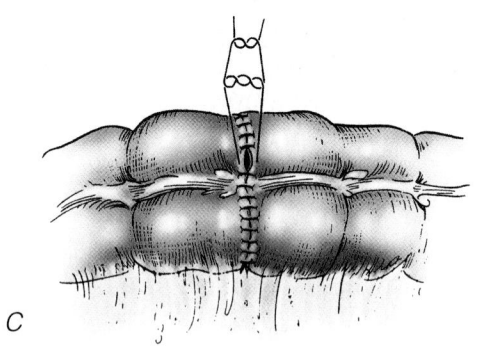

FIG. 6-57. A single-layer running suture technique is used for gastrointestinal repairs and anastomoses whenever possible. The authors do not recommend use of this method on the stomach because of the risk of postoperative hemorrhage. *A.* For an anastomosis the suture line is started at the mesenteric border. The stitches are placed 3 to 4 mm from the edge of the bowel and include all layers except the mucosa (see insert in *A*). *B.* To ensure a secure suture line on the mesenteric border, both limbs of the suture are brought out from the mesenteric border. *C.* Each stitch is advanced 3 to 4 mm, and the suture is tied near the antimesenteric border.

colostomy for patients with protracted shock and extensive contamination. The theory used to support this approach is that systemic factors are more important than local factors in determining whether a suture line will heal. Both of these approaches are reasonable and result in the majority of patients being treated by primary repairs. When a colostomy is required, regardless of the theory used to reach that conclusion, performing a loop colostomy proximal to a distal repair should be avoided because a proximal colostomy does not protect a distal suture line. All suture lines and anastomoses are performed with the running single-layer technique described in Fig. 6-57.[78]

Complications related to the colonic injury and its treatment may include intra-abdominal abscess, fecal fistula, wound infection, and stomal complications. Intra-abdominal abscess occurs in approximately 10% of patients, and most are managed with percutaneous drainage. Fistulas occur in 1 to 3% of patients and usually present as an abscess or wound infection, which after drainage is followed by continuous fecal output. Most colonic fistulas will heal spontaneously. Wound infection can be effectively avoided by leaving the skin and subcutaneous tissue open and relying on healing by secondary intention. The skin can be closed primarily in approximately 60% of patients without developing an infection. However, this treatment should be reserved for injuries with little contamination and in patients with minimal blood loss and little subcutaneous fat.

Stomal complications include necrosis, stenosis, obstruction, and prolapse. Taken together they occur in approximately 5% of patients, and most require reoperation. Necrosis is a particularly serious complication which must be recognized and treated promptly. Failure to do so can result in life-threatening septic complications including necrotizing fasciitis.

Rectum

Rectal injuries are similar to colonic injuries with respect to the ecology of the luminal contents, the structures and blood supply of the wall, and the nature and frequency of complications. They differ in two important ways: mechanisms of injury and accessibility. The rectum is often injured by GSWs, rarely by SWs, and frequently by acts of auto-eroticism and sexual misadventure. The rectum is also subject to high-pressure injuries which can be caused by air guns or water under high pressure as used in golf course irrigation systems. Access to the rectum is limited because of the surrounding bony pelvis.

The diagnosis is suggested by the course of projectiles, the presence of blood on digital examination of the rectum, and history. Patients in whom a rectal injury is suspected should undergo proctoscopy. Hematomas, contusions, lacerations, and gross blood may be seen. If the diagnosis is still in question, x-ray examinations with soluble contrast enemas are indicated. At times it may be difficult to determine whether an injury is present. These authors believe that these patients should be treated as if they do have an injury.

The portion of the rectum proximal to the peritoneal reflection is referred to as the intraperitoneal segment and that distal to the reflection as the extraperitoneal segment. This distinction is blurred somewhat because the broad posterior aspect of the intraperitoneal portion could be considered as either. Injuries of the intraperitoneal portion (including its posterior aspect) are treated as previously outlined in the section on colonic injuries. Access to extraperitoneal injuries is so restricted, especially in the narrow male pelvis, that indirect treatment is usually required. While colostomies proximal to a suture line are avoided in patients with colonic injuries, there

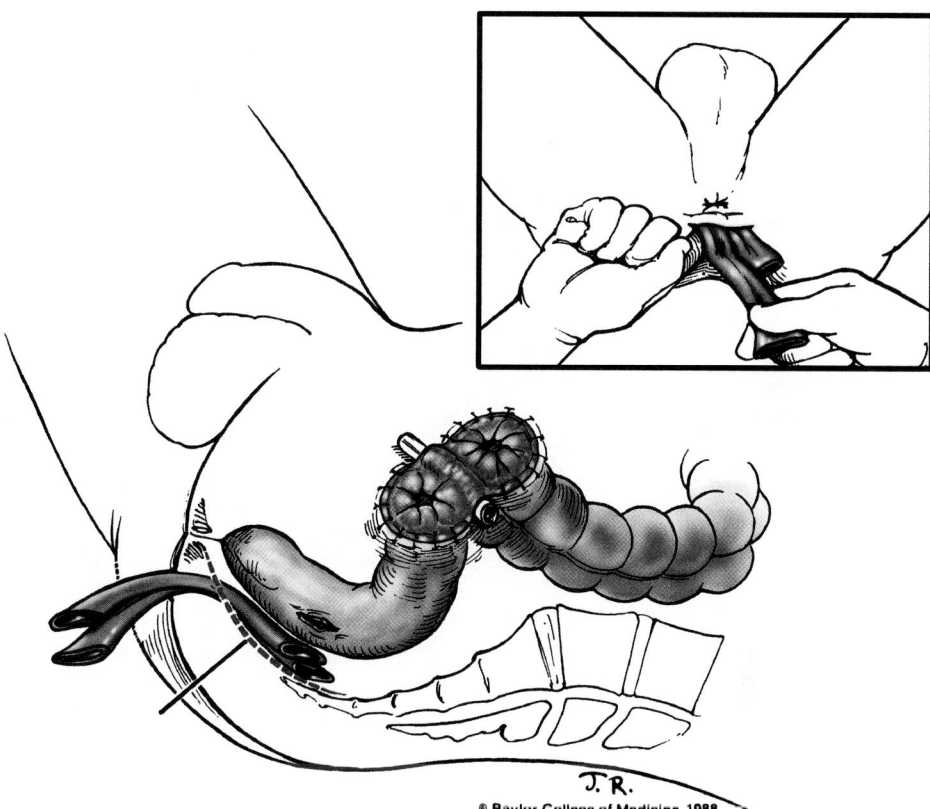

FIG. 6-58. A properly constructed loop colostomy will completely divert the fecal stream. The essential elements include maintaining the spur of the colostomy above the level of the skin, a longitudinal colotomy, and immediate maturation. The drains are placed through a retroanal incision. The fascia of Waldeyer is often very tough and may need to be incised. The drains are then advanced to the level of the rectal injury.

© Baylor College of Medicine 1988

is often no option in patients with extraperitoneal injuries, and sigmoid colostomies are appropriate for most patients.[79] Properly constructed loop colostomies are preferred because they are quick and easy to fashion and provide total fecal diversion. Essential elements include: (1) adequate mobilization of the sigmoid colon so the loop will rest on the abdominal wall without tension, (2) maintenance of the spur of the colostomy (the common wall of the proximal and distal limbs after maturation) above the level of the skin with a one-half-inch nylon rod or similar device, (3) longitudinal incision in the tenia coli, and (4) immediate maturation in the OR using 3-0 braided absorbable suture (Fig. 6-58). A staple line can be applied across the distal limit to ensure complete diversion, but it is not necessary and does complicate closure of the colostomy. A mucous fistula is never required and should be avoided because of the risk of necrosis if the inferior mesenteric or superior rectal arteries were injured or otherwise ligated.

If a perforation is inadvertently uncovered during dissection, it should be repaired as described above. Otherwise it is not necessary to explore the extraperitoneal rectum to repair perforation. Furthermore, it may be extremely difficult or impossible to accomplish this task. If the injury is so extensive that the surgeon feels it must be repaired, the patient is better off treated by dividing the rectum at the level of injury, oversewing or stapling the distal rectum, and creating an end colostomy (Hartmann's procedure). In rare instances in which the anal sphincters have been destroyed, an abdominoperineal resection may be necessary.

Extraperitoneal injuries of the rectum should be drained via a retroanal incision (see Fig. 6-58). Waldeyer's fascia is particularly tough at this level and may need to be sharply incised. The drains, either Penrose or closed suction, should be placed close to the perforation or suture line and should be left in until they fall out spontaneously or drainage diminishes, which usually occurs within 7 to

10 days. Irrigation of the distal rectum with various solutions is advocated by some authorities. It does not appear to be either helpful or harmful in retrospective studies. It may be of benefit in a patient whose rectum is loaded with feces. If it is done, the irrigation solution should be isotonic and the anus should be mechanically dilated to avoid building up pressure that might force feces out of an unrepaired perforation. If the patient has a concomitant bladder injury and adjacent suture lines are created, a flap of viable omentum should be placed between them to reduce the risk of a rectovesical fistula.

There have been a few reports of treating small extraperitoneal rectal injuries by suture or drainage alone. The outcomes have been acceptable and colostomies have been avoided. However, there has not been sufficient experience to recommend this approach since pelvic sepsis associated with rectal injury is highly lethal.

Complications are similar in frequency and nature to colonic injuries. Pelvic osteomyelitis may also occur. Bone biopsy should be performed to secure the diagnosis and bacteriology. Culture-specific intravenous antibiotics should be administered for 2 to 3 months. Débridement may be necessary.

Stomach and Small Intestine

Injuries of the stomach and small bowel pose no special problems or controversies. Gastric injuries can occasionally be missed if a wound is located within the mesentery of the lesser curvature or high in the posterior fundus. The stomach should be clamped at the pylorus and inflated with air or methylene blue–colored saline if there is any question. Patients with injuries that damage both nerves of Latarjet or both vagi should have a drainage procedure (see Chap. 25). If the distal antrum or pylorus is severely damaged, it can be reconstructed with a Billroth I or II procedure. Although the authors emphasize the single-layer running suture line, a running

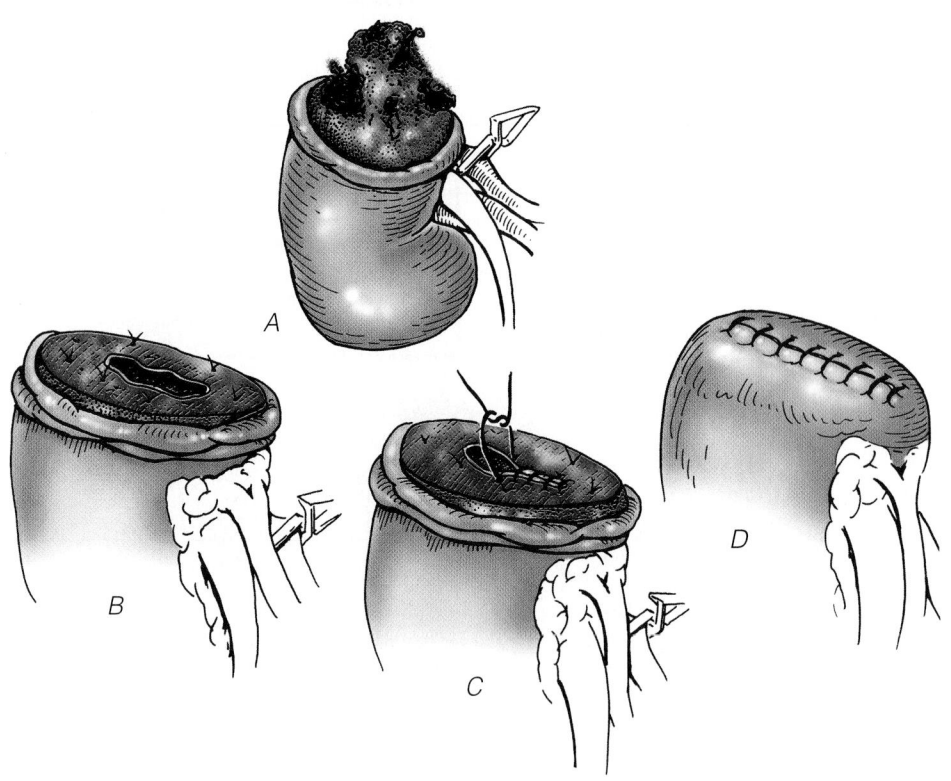

FIG. 6-59. Renal parenchymal injuries can sometimes be repaired by partial nephrectomy. The need for repair depends on the patient's condition and the status of the other kidney. *A.* Intermittent vascular control permits precise control of bleeding vessels. *B.* The renal capsule is carefully preserved. *C.* and *D.* The collecting system is closed with absorbable suture, and the remaining capsule is closed over the collecting system repair.

two-layer suture line is preferred for the stomach due to its rich blood supply and because postoperative hemorrhage has occurred when the single-layer technique has been used in the stomach.

With the almost universal use of CT for the diagnosis of blunt abdominal injury, injury to the small intestine can be missed.[80] Wounds of the mesenteric border also can be missed if the exploration is not comprehensive. Most injuries are treated with a lateral single-layer running suture. Multiple penetrating injuries often occur close together. Rather than performing many lateral repairs, judicious resections with end-to-end anastomosis may save considerable time.

Kidneys

There are several unique aspects to the diagnosis and treatment of renal injuries. Three imaging techniques, CT, intravenous pyelography (IVP), and arteriography, can be used to accurately evaluate the extent of a renal injury. However, the contrast material required for each is nephrotoxic and limits the number of studies that can be performed. The fact that there are two identical organs makes the sacrifice of one a viable therapeutic option. Nearly 95% of all blunt renal injuries are treated nonoperatively. The diagnosis is suspected by the finding of microscopic or gross hematuria and confirmed by CT or IVP. Most cases of urinary extravasation and hematuria will resolve in a few days with bed rest. Persistent gross hematuria can be treated by embolization. Persistent urinomas can be drained percutaneously. Operative treatment is occasionally necessary for similar lesions that do not respond to these less invasive measures.

If a perinephric hematoma is encountered during laparotomy from blunt trauma, exploration is indicated if it is expanding or pulsatile. Very large hematomas should be explored because of the risk of a major vascular injury. Much has been written about the need for vascular control at the junction of the renal vessels with

the aorta and vena cava prior to entering the hematoma. The authors have not found this necessary or desirable. If emergent vascular control is necessary, a large curved vascular clamp can easily be placed across the hilum from below, with the clamp parallel to the vena cava and aorta.

Hemostatic and reconstructive techniques used to treat blunt renal injuries are similar to those used to treat the liver and spleen, although two additional concepts are employed: the collecting system should be closed separately, and the renal capsule preserved to close over the repair of the collecting system (Fig. 6-59). Permanent sutures should be avoided because of the risk of calculus formation. The authors prefer absorbable monofilament sutures because of their lack of abrasiveness. If nephrectomy is being considered and the status of the opposite kidney is unknown, it should be palpated. The presence of a palpably normal opposite kidney is assurance that the patient will not be rendered anephric by a unilateral nephrectomy. Unilateral renal agenesis occurs in 1 in 1000 patients.

The renal arteries and veins are uniquely susceptible to traction injury caused by blunt trauma. As the artery is stretched, the inelastic intima and media may rupture. This causes thrombus formation, resulting in high-grade stenosis or thrombosis. The injury can be detected by CT, IVP, or duplex scanning. If the patient does not have more urgent injuries and treatment and repair can be accomplished within 3 hours of admission, it should be attempted. Successful renal artery repair in a patient who presents with complete thrombosis is rare. If repair is not possible within this time frame, leaving the kidney in situ to resorb does not necessarily lead to hypertension or abscess formation. Isolated renal vein injuries can occur from blunt trauma. The vein may either be torn or avulsed from the vena cava. In either case a large hematoma develops, which often leads to an operation and nephrectomy.

All penetrating wounds to kidneys are explored. Bleeding perforations and lacerations are treated using the same hemostatic

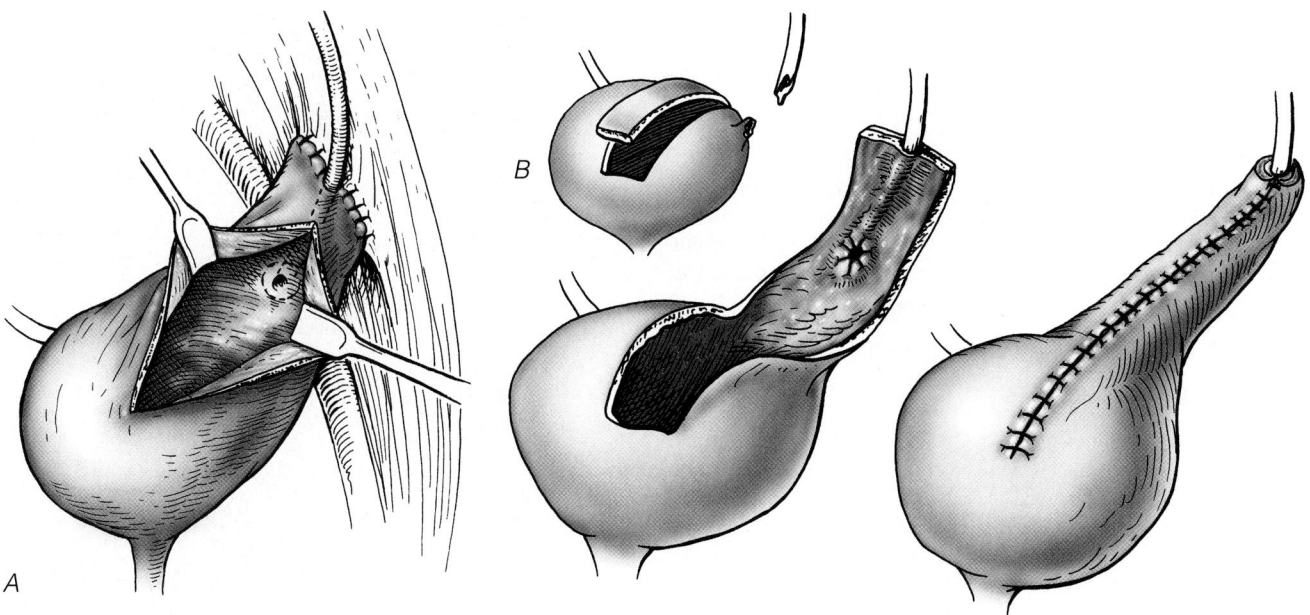

FIG. 6-60. *A. The psoas hitch is used for distal ureteral injuries when only minimal additional length is needed. This is accomplished by mobilizing the bladder and suturing the dome to the psoas muscle. A submucosal ureteral tunnel helps prevent reflux. B. A Boari flap can be constructed when more length is required.*

techniques as described above. Renal vascular injuries are common following penetrating trauma, and they may be deceptively tamponaded and result in delayed hemorrhage. Injuries involving the collecting system should be closed separately if they are large. Small perforations that penetrate the collecting system can be controlled by suture of the capsule and parenchyma. Perforations of the renal pelvis should be meticulously repaired with fine sutures. While drains have been routinely employed by urologists for all urologic injuries, the authors believe they should be used more selectively. The same concept applies to the use of ureteral stents.

Ureters

Injuries to the ureters from external trauma are rare. They occur in a few patients with pelvic fractures and are uncommon in penetrating trauma because the silhouette they present is so small. The diagnosis in blunt trauma may be made by CT, IVP, or retrograde ureterography. More often the injury is not identified until a complication (e.g., a urinoma) becomes apparent. In penetrating trauma, ureteral injuries are discovered during the exploration of the retroperitoneum, although missed injuries are not unusual in this setting as well. If an injury is suspected but not identified, methylene blue or indigo carmine is administered intravenously. Staining of the tissue by the dye may facilitate identification of the injury. Most injuries can be repaired primarily using the same technique described above for small arteries. The suture the authors use is 5-0 absorbable monofilament. When the ureter is mobilized, the dissection should be at least 1 cm away from the ureter to avoid injury to its delicate vascular plexus. The kidney also can be mobilized to gain length. Injuries of the distal ureter can be treated by reimplantation. The psoas hitch and Boari flap may be helpful in selected distal ureteral injuries (Fig. 6-60). If the patient is critically ill and being considered for a staged laparotomy, or if the surgeon is uncomfortable with ureteral repair, the ureter can be ligated on both sides of the injury and a nephrostomy performed (Fig. 6-61).

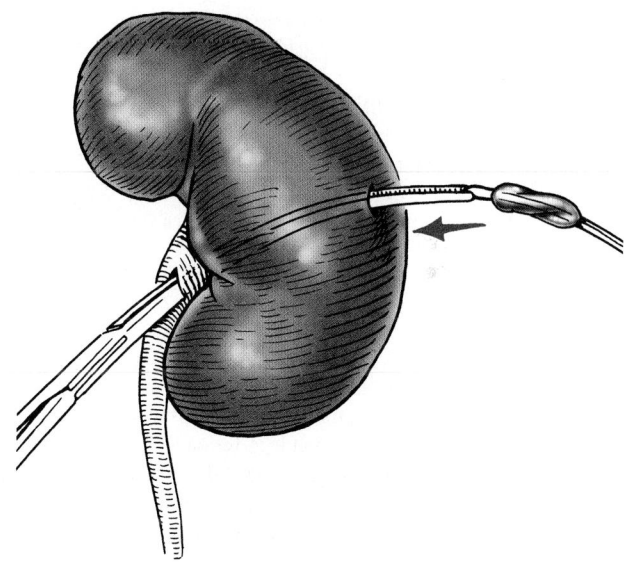

FIG. 6-61. *Nephrostomy is a valuable technique in the management of proximal ureteral injuries when renal function must be preserved and the patient will not tolerate the time required for ureteral repair, or the complexity of the repair is beyond the surgeon's skill.*

Bladder

Bladder injuries are diagnosed by cystography, CT, or during laparotomy. A postvoid view enhances the accuracy of cystography.[81] Blunt ruptures of the intraperitoneal portion are closed with a running single-layer closure using 3-0 absorbable monofilament suture. Blunt extraperitoneal rupture is treated with a Foley catheter; direct operative repair is not necessary. Cystograms can be used to determine when the Foley catheter can be removed, usually in 10 to 14 days. Penetrating bladder injuries are treated in the same fashion, although injuries near the trigone should be repaired through an incision in the dome so that iatrogenic injury to the intravesicular ureter is avoided by direct visualization.

Urethra

Blunt disruption of the posterior urethra is managed by bridging the defect with a Foley catheter. This usually requires passing catheters through the urethral meatus and through an incision in the bladder. Once the catheter bridges the defect, healing occurs as the intervening hematoma resorbs. Strictures are not uncommon, but can be managed electively. Penetrating injuries are treated by direct repair.

Gynecologic Injuries

Gynecologic injuries are rare. Occasionally the vagina will be lacerated by a sharp bone fragment from a pelvic fracture. Penetrating injuries to the vagina, uterus, fallopian tubes, and ovaries are also uncommon. The usual hemostatic techniques are used to control bleeding, and suture repair is used to close defects that communicate with a lumen. Repair of a transected fallopian tube can be attempted but probably is unjustified. A suboptimal repair will increase the risk of tubal pregnancy. Transection at the injury site with proximal ligation and distal salpingectomy is a more prudent approach.

Trauma in pregnancy also is rare. Blunt trauma can cause uterine rupture, which almost always results in fetal demise. The outcomes of penetrating uterine injuries are more variable and are dependent on penetration of the uterine cavity, damage to the placenta, and fetal injury. Spontaneous abortion is a frequent outcome. On occasion a mother will present with life-threatening injuries including severe head injury or cardiac arrest from hemorrhagic shock. If the fetus is viable by dates or examination, an emergency cesarean section should be considered even if the mother is not salvageable. This occurs more often with severe head injury than cardiac arrest from hemorrhagic shock.

Completion of the Laparotomy and Postoperative Considerations

Following repair of all injuries, the abdomen is irrigated with saline warmed to body temperature. Although this will not eliminate all bacteria, an effort should be made to remove blood clots, food particles, and gross enteric and fecal contamination.

Patients with moderate to severe injuries are at risk for multiple organ failure (MOF) and nosocomial infection. The authors are of the opinion that the integrity of the gut plays a pivotal role in the severity and outcome of these complications. Needle-catheter jejunostomies are placed in all such patients prior to abdominal closure (Fig. 6-62). Enteric feedings are initiated as soon as the patient arrives in the surgical intensive care unit (SICU) and are advanced to full strength within 72 hours. Total parenteral nutrition may be necessary in some patients, but does cause mucosal atrophy, which may impair the barrier function of the mucosa.

The abdominal incision is closed with a running no. 2 nylon suture that includes at least 1.5 cm of fascia. Tension of the suture should be sufficient to just approximate the fascia but no more. Subcutaneous sutures are never used. The skin is closed selectively depending on the amount of contamination and subcutaneous tissue. Patients with more contamination and subcutaneous fat should have the skin and subcutaneous tissue left open. All patients initially treated with staged laparotomy should have the skin and subcutaneous tissue left open.

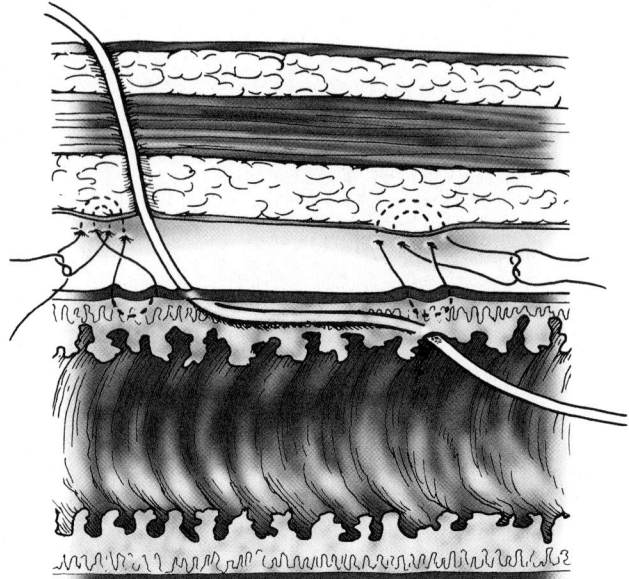

FIG. 6-62. Needle-catheter jejunostomies are frequently used to provide enteral nutrition to seriously injured patients. Seven French catheters are placed through a submucosal tunnel in the proximal jejunum. Soluble dietary formulas can be started within 24 hours and advanced to full caloric and nitrogen requirements within a few days.

Pelvis

Pelvic fractures can cause exsanguinating retroperitoneal hemorrhage without associated major vascular injury; branches of the internal iliac vessels and the lower lumbar arteries are often responsible. Hemorrhage also comes from small veins and from the cancellous portion of the fractured bones. A direct surgical approach is rarely effective since many of the sources of hemorrhage are outside of the surgical field. Most pelvic fractures that cause life-threatening hemorrhage involve disruption of the posterior elements (i.e., the sacroiliac joints and associated ligaments) and are often biomechanically unstable.[82,83]

A hemodynamically unstable patient with an unstable pelvic fracture may be bleeding from sources other than the pelvis (e.g., the spleen). However, large retroperitoneal hematomas can also cause a hemoperitoneum, particularly if overlying peritoneum ruptures. Determining the source of hemorrhage is a dilemma since it is desirable not to operate for a retroperitoneal hematoma, whereas a laparotomy may be essential to deal with hemorrhage from the spleen or liver. The authors have employed diagnostic peritoneal lavage (DPL), and more recently US, to aid in this decision. If ten or more milliliters of free blood can be aspirated from the peritoneal cavity, or if US is unequivocally positive, the blood is assumed to be coming from an injury unrelated to the pelvic fracture and a laparotomy is performed. If the DPL is positive by laboratory analysis or if it is negative, attention is directed toward treating the pelvic fracture. Clearly the decision to operate or not may be wrong, and the plan may need to be altered accordingly.

Several methods have been employed to control hemorrhage associated with pelvic fractures. These include immediate external fixation, military antishock trousers (MAST), angiography with embolization, and pelvic packing. No single technique is effective for treating all fractures and there is little agreement among specialists as to which should be used. Anterior external fixation is not intended to provide definitive fracture stabilization in most instances. Its

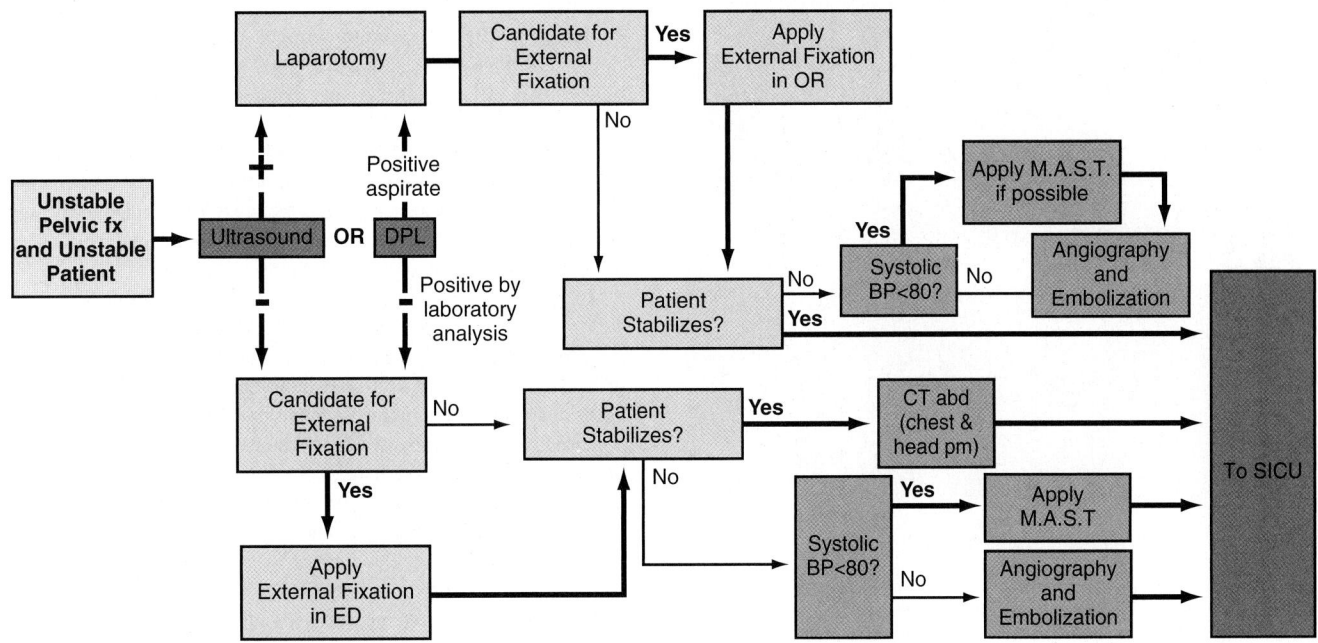

FIG. 6-63. Algorithm for the management of mechanically unstable pelvic fractures in hemodynamically unstable patients. MAST = military antishock trousers, SICU = surgical intensive care unit.

advocates intend for the device to decrease pelvic volume, tamponade bleeding, and to prevent secondary hemorrhage which may occur if the fractured bones shift. Many orthopedic surgeons remain unconvinced of the efficacy of external fixation for grossly unstable posterior fractures. MAST can provide some stability for the fracture and probably tamponade venous hemorrhage. The disadvantages are the loss of access to the abdomen and the risk of lower extremity compartment syndrome. Angiography with embolization is very effective for controlling arterial hemorrhage, but arterial hemorrhage occurs in only 10 to 20% of patients with active hemorrhage from pelvic fractures. Pelvic packing may control venous hemorrhage. The only reason to consider its use is when a pelvic hematoma is inadvertently entered or if it has ruptured.

Because of the options available and differences of opinions regarding treatment, the authors have found it desirable to reach agreements with the other specialists involved, including orthopedic surgeons, interventional radiologists, the director of the blood bank, and anesthesiologists.[84,85] These agreements avoid the loss of time due to unnecessary debate. The algorithm used to decide which option to use is depicted in Fig. 6-63.

Another clinical challenge is the open pelvic fracture. In many instances the wounds are located in the perineum and the risk of pelvic sepsis and osteomyelitis is high. To reduce the risk of infection, a sigmoid colostomy is recommended. The pelvic wound is manually débrided and then irrigated daily with a high-pressure, pulsatile irrigation system until granulation tissue covers the wound. The wound is then left to heal by secondary intention. This approach has been remarkably successful with these difficult wounds.

Extremities

For the most part, injuries of the extremities are within the domain of the orthopedic and plastic surgeons, except for isolated vascular injuries which have been discussed above. However, there are two extremity injuries which need to be emphasized: vascular injuries associated with fractures and compartment syndromes.

Vascular Injuries with Fractures

Vascular injuries associated with fractures are rare, occurring in only 0.5 to 3% of all patients with extremity fractures. They are also more severe than isolated vascular injuries or fractures, and amputation rates of more than 50% have been noted. These injuries can be caused by both blunt and penetrating trauma. Certain fractures and dislocations are more likely to be associated with vascular injury than others. In the upper extremity, a fracture of the clavicle or first rib may lacerate the distal subclavian artery. The axillary artery may be injured in patients with dislocations of the shoulder or proximal humeral fractures. Supracondylar fractures of the distal humerus and dislocations of the elbow are known for their association with brachial arterial injuries. In all the above fractures and dislocations, vascular injuries are uncommon and occur in only a small fraction of patients.

In the lower extremity, the orthopedic injury most commonly associated with vascular injury is dislocation of the knee, where the popliteal artery and/or vein may be injured in as many as 30% of patients. The popliteal vessels may also be injured in patients with supracondylar fractures of the femur or tibial plateau fractures. Vascular injury can occur in patients with combined fractures of the tibia and fibula.

The importance of a careful neurologic examination in these patients cannot be overemphasized. Three distinctly different mechanisms can produce paralysis and numbness in an injured extremity: ischemia, nerve injury, and compartment syndrome. As a result, failure to accurately document the neuromuscular function of the injured extremity can and will lead to missed injuries, improper treatment, and unrealistic expectations on the part of the patient.

Perhaps the greatest controversy in the treatment of patients with combined orthopedic and vascular injuries is the order in which the procedures are to be performed. Advocates of initial fracture treatment argue that it is difficult to judge the length of a vascular graft (or whether one is required) when the ends of the fractured bone are overriding or if angulation exists. Also, extensive orthopedic

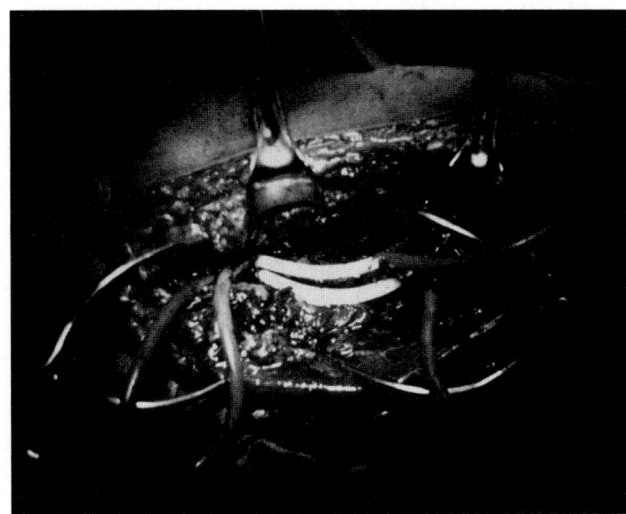

FIG. 6-64. Temporary arterial and venous shunts used to bridge large defects in the popliteal artery and vein in a patient with a comminuted supracondylar femur fracture. The shunts were used because the extremity was ischemic and extensive manipulation was necessary to treat the fracture. This manipulation would have risked disruption of a delicate vascular repair if the latter were performed first.

manipulation may easily disrupt delicate vascular repairs. Opponents of this approach argue that the length of time required to stabilize the fracture may cause further ischemic damage to the limb. Recently, the use of temporary intravascular shunts has been recommended as a compromise to avoid ischemia during fracture treatment.

A rational approach would be to consider all the above options based on the condition of the patient's extremity. If the extremity is clearly viable and there is no hemorrhage from the vascular injury, the fracture should be treated first. If the limb is at risk from ischemia, prompt revascularization is required. When little or no fracture manipulation is anticipated, definitive vascular repair is performed first. If extensive manipulation is required in a ischemic extremity, temporary shunts can be placed followed by vascular repair after the fracture has been treated (Fig. 6-64).

The extent of injury required for combined orthopedic and vascular injuries frequently results in open fractures, and the use of external fixation devices for these injuries has become common. Unfortunately, these devices may significantly hinder vascular repair because of their location and bulk. Preoperative planning between the vascular and orthopedic surgeon should avoid this technical problem.

Because of the severity of combined orthopedic and vascular injuries, the need for immediate amputation may arise. When the primary nerve is transected in addition to a fracture and arterial injury, such as the popliteal nerve, popliteal artery, and distal femur, primary amputation should be strongly considered.[86-88] This difficult clinical decision is best reached through a collaborative effort involving the trauma surgeon, orthopedic surgeon, and in certain cases, the neurosurgeon. Prolonged rehabilitation resulting in a paralyzed, anesthetic extremity prone to ulceration is hardly better than the prompt fitting of a good prosthesis.

Compartment Syndrome

Compartment syndromes can occur anywhere in the extremities, including the thighs, buttocks, arms, and hands. As in the abdomen, the pathophysiology is an acute increase in pressure in a closed space, which impairs blood flow to the structures within. The etiologies of extremity compartment syndromes include arterial hemorrhage into a compartment, venous ligation or thrombosis, crush injuries, infections, crotalid envenomation, and ischemia/reperfusion. In conscious patients, pain is the prominent symptom. Active or passive motion of involved muscles increases the pain. Progression to paralysis can occur. The most prone site is in the anterior compartment of the leg; a well-described early sign is paresthesia or numbness between the first and second toes caused by pressure on the deep peroneal nerve.

In comatose or obtunded patients, the diagnosis is more difficult to secure. A compatible history, firmness of the compartment to palpation, and diminished mobility of the joint are suggestive. The presence or absence of a pulse distal to the affected compartment is notoriously unreliable in the diagnosis of a compartment syndrome. A frozen joint and myoglobinuria are late signs and suggest a poor prognosis. As in the abdomen, compartment pressure can be measured. The small, hand-held Stryker device is a convenient tool for this purpose. Pressures greater than 45 mm Hg usually require operative intervention. Patients with pressures between 30 and 45 mm Hg should be carefully evaluated and closely watched.

Treatment consists of measures to reduce compartment pressure and include elevation of the extremity, evacuation of hematomas, and fasciotomy. As long as neurologic and muscular functions are intact, elevation and observation are sufficient. The evacuation of hematomas due to arterial injury almost always results in a fasciotomy since the compartment must be opened to treat the vascular injury. Since the lower extremity is most frequently involved, the two-incision, four-compartment fasciotomy is shown in Fig. 6-65. Note that the soleus must be detached from the tibia to decompress the deep flexor compartment.

Prognosis is related to the severity, duration, and etiology of the compartment syndrome. The best results are obtained in patients with arterial hemorrhage and venous ligation or thrombosis who undergo early fasciotomy. Those who develop compartment syndrome from crush injuries, crotalid envenomation, and particularly ischemia/reperfusion have a poor prognosis because of the pre-existing muscle and nerve damage caused by the original insult. Fasciotomy should still be attempted, although infection and amputation are a frequent outcome.

Prognosis and Outcome Evaluation

Prognosis and outcome evaluation for various injuries began during World War I. At that time mortality was calculated according to the organ injured. For example, all patients who suffered an injury to the colon were determined to have lived or died. Accordingly, frequency of death was then assigned to that particular organ, and it was assumed that any patient with a colonic injury had the same probability of dying. Since no other factors such as associated injuries or physiologic condition were considered, it is not surprising that any abdominal visceral injury was associated with a mortality rate of 50 to 60%. This practice continued during World War II and resulted in some remarkable conclusions, which have subsequently been shown to be incorrect. Perhaps the best example of this was the conclusion that performing colostomies for all colonic injuries during WWII resulted in a reduction of mortality for patients so treated from 60% during WWI to 30% in WWII. Civilian literature in the second half of this century indicated that the number of injured organs, major fractures, blood loss, and the presence of shock were all predictive of outcome, but only in the crudest fashion. The quality of the local EMS system is another confounding factor. Regions with rapid response and transport are more likely to bring

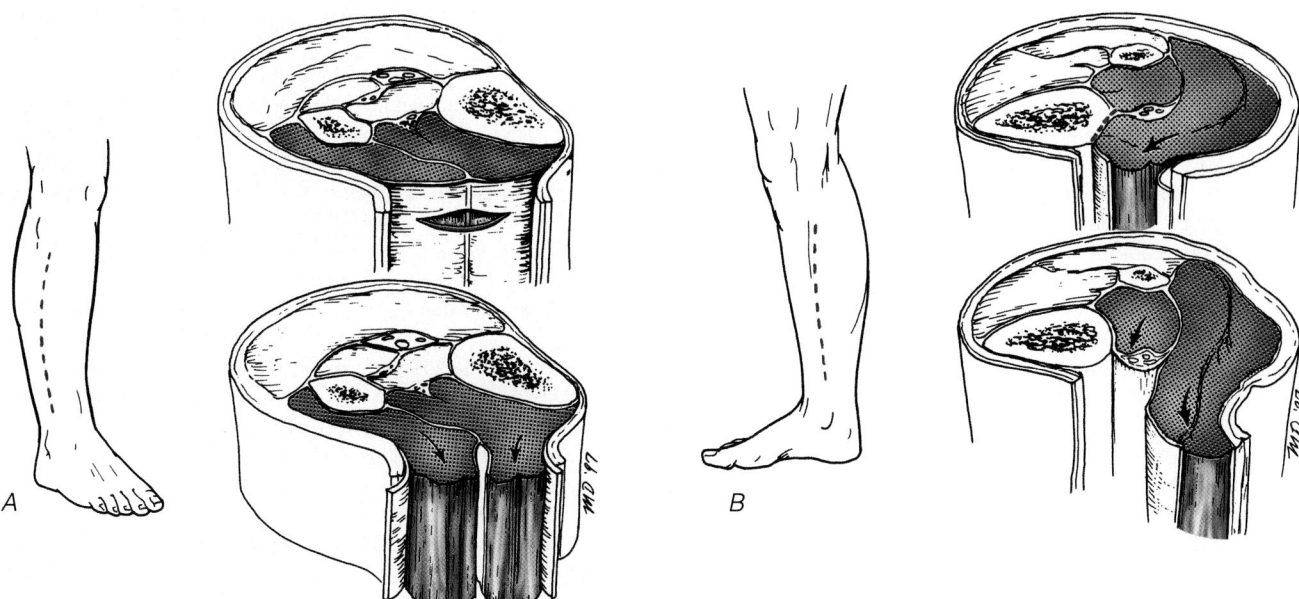

FIG. 6-65. The two-incision, four-compartment fasciotomy. For trauma patients, both the skin and fascia should be incised for the entire length of the compartment. *A.* To facilitate identification of both the anterior and lateral compartments, a small transverse incision is used to find the fascial raphe between the two compartments. *B.* In order to decompress the deep flexor compartment, the soleus muscle must be detached from the tibia. Care must be taken not to injure the distal popliteal neuromuscular bundle, which lies immediately beneath the soleus muscle in the proximal leg.

severely injured patients to the ED with signs of life than those with less-efficient systems. As a result, mortality is paradoxically greater in regions with better EMS systems.

At present there are both anatomic and physiologic grading systems. The anatomic systems are derived from the Abbreviated Injury Scale (AIS) which was developed during the 1950s. The AIS is a list which assigns a number from 1 (minor injury) to 6 (always fatal) for the various spectrum of organ injuries. However, since the AIS only evaluates solitary injuries, it cannot reflect the additional impact of multiple injuries. The Injury Severity Score (ISS) was devised to address this concern. The ISS is calculated by squaring the AIS from the three worst injured of six body compartments (head and neck, face, chest, abdomen and pelvis, extremities, and external) and adding them together. Scores can range from 0 to 75. The ISS is further characterized according to the mechanism of injury (blunt vs. penetrating) and age (less than 55 years vs. 55 years or older). However, the ISS suffers from the inability to consider multiple injuries in one compartment, the assumption that all compartments are of equal significance, and the lack of recognition of the patient's physiologic status. Several physiologic scoring systems have been developed. The Revised Trauma Score (RTS) is most commonly used today. It is calculated from the GCS, blood pressure, and respiratory rate, with the GCS being most heavily weighted. The RTS is a purely physiologic score which is compromised by the relative insensitivity of these common clinical measurements. More recently, the TRISS method (Trauma and Injury Severity Score) was developed to incorporate both the RTS and ISS, thereby combining physiologic and anatomic scores, as well as enhancing the importance of head injury. Unfortunately, TRISS remains fundamentally flawed because of the limitations of RTS and ISS. Newer versions of the TRISS concept, such as ASCOT (A Severity Characterization of Trauma), have also failed to improve the prediction of postinjury mortality. Perhaps more important than mortality, outcome assessment must include the critical issues of total medical resource consumption (e.g., complications, hospital length of stay, and cost for medical care) and capacity to return to preinjury functional status. Several functional outcome scales have been developed, but a standard has yet to be established.

BITES AND STINGS OF ANIMALS AND INSECTS

Rabies

In 1950, approximately 5000 cases of rabies were reported among dogs and 18 were reported in humans. In comparison, only 160 cases of rabies in dogs were reported in 1989. In 1991, there were three patients who died from rabies in the United States. Wild animals now constitute the most important potential source of infection for both humans and domestic animals in the United States. However, the many possible exposures that result from frequent contact between domestic dogs and humans continue to be the basis of most antirabies treatment.

Approximately 10,000 patients receive postexposure prophylaxis for rabies annually.[89] Rabies among wild animals, especially skunks, foxes, raccoons, and bats, accounts for more than 85% of cases. Any mammal may carry rabies. Rodents are almost never found to be infected with rabies and have not been known to cause rabies among humans in the United States. Woodchucks accounted for 70% of rabies cases among rodents reported to the Centers for Disease Control and Prevention. In all cases involving rodents, the state or local health department should be consulted before a decision is made to initiate postexposure antirabies prophylaxis. Many of the cases of human rabies reported in the past 10 years have resulted in exposure outside of the United States. The dog remains the major animal with rabies and the major source of rabies among humans in the rest of the world.

Circumstances surrounding the attack frequently furnish vital information as to whether or not vaccine is indicated. Most domestic animal bites are provoked attacks, and if this history is obtained, rabies vaccine can usually be withheld if the animal appears healthy.

Children are frequently bitten while attempting to separate fighting animals or while teasing or accidentally hurting the animal. Bites during attempts to feed or handle an apparently healthy animal are generally regarded as provoked. Postexposure prophylaxis combining local wound treatment, passive immunization, and vaccination is over 90% effective when appropriately applied. An unprovoked attack by a domestic animal is more likely than a provoked attack to indicate that the animal is rabid. A fully vaccinated dog or cat is unlikely to become infected with rabies, although rare cases have been reported.

Any penetration of the skin by teeth constitutes a bite exposure. Bites to the face and hands carry the highest risk, but the site of the bite should not influence the decision to begin treatment. Nonbites include scratches, abrasions, open wounds, or mucous membranes contaminated with saliva. If the material containing the virus is dry, the virus can be considered noninfectious. Other contact by itself, such as petting a rabid animal and contact with the blood, urine, or feces, does not constitute an exposure and is not an indication for prophylaxis.

Most animal bites sustained by human beings are caused by dogs and cats, and in most instances it is possible to observe the biting animal for the development of rabies. Domestic animals that bite a person should be captured and observed for symptoms of rabies for 10 days. If none develop, the animal may be assumed to be nonrabid. If the animal dies or is killed, the head is sent promptly to a public health laboratory for examination. The tissue requires refrigeration, but not freezing, and transportation to the laboratory following death of the animal must be rapid. Clinical signs of rabies in wild animals cannot be interpreted reliably; therefore any wild animal that bites or scratches a person should be killed at once (without unnecessary damage to the head) and the brain examined for evidence of rabies. Travelers to Asia, Africa, and Central and South America should be aware that greater than 50% of the rabies cases among humans in the United States result from exposure to dogs outside the United States (Table 6-9).

It is generally accepted that the incubation period for rabies in human beings ranges from 10 days to 1 year, with most cases occurring 20 to 90 days from exposure. In cases of exposure of the head, neck, or upper extremities, the incubation period is potentially less than 30 days. Local care of the animal bite should consist of thorough irrigation, cleansing with soap solution, and débridement.

Administration of tetanus toxoid and an antibiotic might be indicated.

Postexposure prophylaxis in addition to local wound treatment consists of both human rabies immune globulin (HRIG) (Imogam Rabies) and vaccine. There are two rabies vaccines currently available in the United States: human diploid cell rabies vaccine (HDCV) and rabies vaccine adsorbed (RVA) (Imovax). Either is administered in conjunction with HRIG at the beginning of postexposure therapy. A regimen of five 1-mL doses of HDCV or RVA is given intramuscularly. The first dose of the five-dose course is given as soon as possible after exposure. Additional doses are given on days 3, 7, 14, and 28 after the first vaccination. For adults, the vaccine is always administered intramuscularly in the deltoid area. For children, the anterolateral aspect of the thigh is also acceptable. The gluteal area should never be used for HDCV or RVA injections since administration in this area results in lower neutralizing antibody titers.

Postexposure antirabies vaccinations should always include administration of both passive antibody and vaccine, with the exception of persons who have previously received complete vaccine regimens with a cell culture vaccine, or persons who have been vaccinated with other types of vaccines and have had documented rabies antibody titers. These persons should receive only vaccine. Because the antibody response after the recommended postexposure vaccination regimen has been satisfactory, routine postvaccination serologic testing is not recommended, unless the patient is known to be immunosuppressed. The state health department may be contacted for recommendations on this matter.

HRIG is administered only once to provide immediate antibodies until the patient responds to the vaccine by actively producing antibodies. If HRIG was not given when vaccination was begun, it can be given through the seventh day after administration of the first dose of vaccine. Beyond the seventh day, HRIG is not indicated since the antibody response to cell culture vaccine is presumed to have occurred. The recommended dosage of HRIG is 20 IU/kg. This formula is applicable for all age groups, including children. If anatomically feasible, up to one half the dose of HRIG should be thoroughly infiltrated in the area around the wound, and the rest should be administered intramuscularly in the gluteal area. HRIG should never be administered in the same syringe or into the same anatomic site as vaccine. Because HRIG may partially suppress active production of

Table 6-9
Rabies Postexposure Prophylaxis Guide, United States, 1991

Animal Type	Evaluation and Disposition of Animal	Postexposure Prophylaxis Recommendations
Dogs and cats	Healthy and available	Should not begin prophylaxis for 10 days observation unless animal develops symptoms of rabies[a]
	Rabid or suspected rabid	Immediate vaccination
	Unknown (escaped)	Consult public health officials
Skunks, raccoons, bats, foxes, and most other carnivores; woodchucks	Regarded as rabid unless geographic area is known to be free of rabies or until animal proven negative by laboratory tests[b]	Immediate vaccination
Livestock, rodents, and lagomorphs (rabbits and hares)	Consider individually	Consult public health officials; bites of squirrels, hamsters, guinea pigs, gerbils, chipmunks, rats, mice, other rodents, rabbits, and hares almost never require antirabies treatment

[a]During the 10-day holding period, begin treatment with human rabies immune globulin and human diploid cell rabies vaccine or rabies vaccine adsorbed at first sign of rabies in a dog or cat that has bitten someone. The symptomatic animal should be killed immediately and tested.
[b]The animal should be killed and tested as soon as possible. Holding for observation is not recommended. Discontinue vaccine if immunofluorescence test results of the animal are negative.
SOURCE: Rabies Prevention—United States 1991. *MMWR* 40 (RR-3):1, 1991.

Table 6-10
Rabies Postexposure Prophylaxis Schedule, United States, 1991

Vaccination Status	Treatment	Regimen[a]
Not previously vaccinated	Local wound cleansing	All postexposure treatment should begin with immediate thorough cleansing of all wounds with soap and water
	HRIG	20 IU/kg body weight; if anatomically feasible, up to one half the dose should be infiltrated around the wound(s) and the rest should be administered IM in the gluteal area; HRIG should not be administered in the same syringe or into the same anatomic site as vaccine; because HRIG may partially suppress active production of antibody, no more than the recommended dose should be given
	Vaccine	HDCV or RVA, 1.0 mL, IM (deltoid area[b]) one each on days 0, 3, 7, 14, and 28
Previously vaccinated[c]	Local wound cleansing	All postexposure treatment should begin with immediate thorough cleansing of all wounds with soap and water
	HRIG	HRIG should not be administered
	Vaccine	HDCV or RVA, 1.0 mL, IM (deltoid area[b]), one each on days 0 and 3

[a] These regimens are applicable for all age groups, including children.
[b] The deltoid area is the only acceptable site of vaccination for adults and older children. For younger children, the outer aspect of the thigh may be used. Vaccine should never be administered in the gluteal area.
[c] Any person with a history of pre-exposure vaccination with HDCV or RVA, prior postexposure prophylaxis with HDCV or RVA, or previous vaccination with any other type of rabies vaccine and a documented history of antibody response to the prior vaccination.
HDCV = human diploid cell rabies vaccine; HRIG = human rabies immune globulin; RVC = rabies vaccine adsorbed.
SOURCE: Rabies Prevention—United States 1991. *MMWR* 40 (RR-3):1, 1991.

antibody, no more than the recommended dose should be given (Table 6-10).

Local reaction such as pain, erythema, and swelling or itching at the injection site has been reported in 30 to 75% of recipients. Headache, nausea, abdominal pain, muscle aches, and dizziness have been reported in from 5 to 40% of recipients. Cases of neurologic illness resembling Guillain-Barré syndrome that resolved have been reported. Local pain and low-grade fever may follow injections of HRIG. There is no evidence that hepatitis B virus, human immunodeficiency virus, or other viruses have ever been transmitted by commercially available HRIG in the United States. Corticosteroids can interfere with the development of active immunity after vaccination and may predispose the patient to rabies. When rabies postexposure prophylaxis is administered to persons receiving steroids or other immunosuppressive therapy, it is especially important that a serum sample be tested for rabies antibody to ensure that an acceptable antibody response has developed. Because of the potential consequences of inadequately treated rabies exposure, and because there is no indication that fetal abnormalities have been associated with rabies vaccination, pregnancy is not considered a contraindication to postexposure prophylaxis.

Manifestations and Treatment of Rabies

Symptoms of rabies include a 2- to 4-day prodromal period in which the patient reaches the excited stage. Paresthesia in the region of the bite is an important early symptom. Other symptoms include headaches, vertigo, stiff neck, malaise, lethargy, and severe pulmonary symptoms including wheezing, hyperventilation, and dyspnea. The patient may have spasm of the throat muscles with dysphagia. The outstanding clinical symptom of rabies is related to swallowing. Drooling, maniacal behavior, and convulsions ensue and are followed by coma, paralysis, and death. Intensive respiratory supportive care is essentially the only treatment to offer. Phenytoin can be used for seizures.

Snakebites

Pit Vipers

In North America all the poisonous snakes of medical importance are members of the family Crotalidae, or pit vipers, and the coral snake of the Elapidae family. The pit vipers include rattlesnakes, the cottonmouth moccasin, and the copperhead. Approximately 8000 persons are bitten each year by poisonous snakes, with over 98% of bites occurring on the extremities. Rattlesnakes are responsible for approximately 70% of all deaths due to snakebites, while death from the bite of a copperhead is extremely rare.

Pit vipers are named for their characteristic pit, an incredibly sensitive heat-sensing organ that is located between the eye and the nostril on each side of the head. As a rule, these snakes may be identified by their elliptical pupil, as opposed to the round pupil of harmless snakes. Nonpoisonous snakes do not have pits. However, the coral snake does have a round pupil and lacks the facial pit. Pit vipers have two well-developed fangs that protrude from the maxillae, whereas most nonpoisonous snakes have rows of teeth without fangs. Pit vipers also may be identified by turning the snake's belly upward and noting the single row of subcaudal plates (Fig. 6-66). The coral snake is a brightly colored small snake with red, yellow, and black rings. This color combination occurs also in nonpoisonous snakes, but the alternating colors are different. Only the coral snake has a red ring next to a yellow ring; when red touches yellow, it is a coral snake. The nose of the coral snake is black.

The venom of poisonous snakes consists of enzymatic, complex proteins that affect all soft tissues. Venoms have been shown to have neurotoxic, hemorrhagic, thrombogenic, hemolytic, cytotoxic, antifibrinolytic, and anticoagulant effects. Most venoms contain

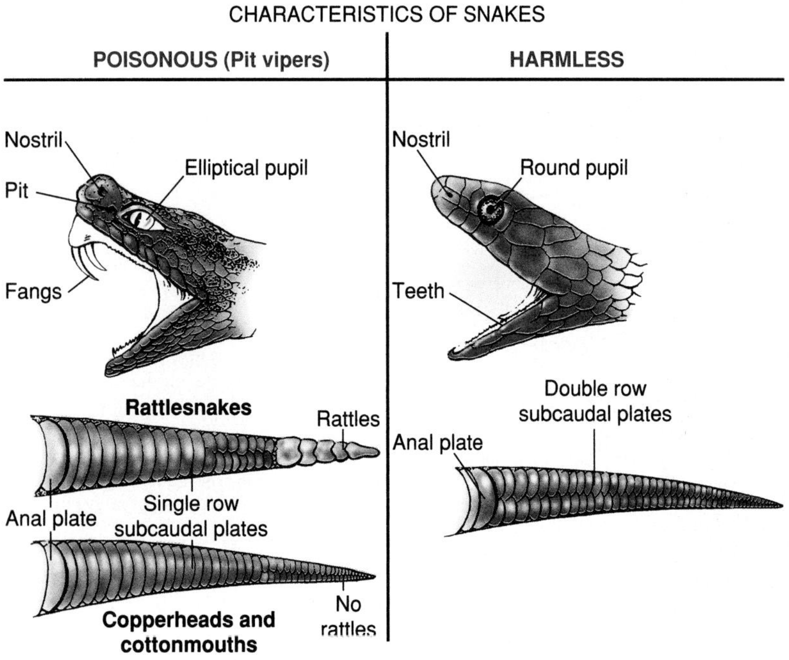

CHARACTERISTICS OF SNAKES

FIG. 6-66. Characteristics of poisonous and non-poisonous snakes. *(From Parrish HM: Texas snakebite statistics. Tex State J Med 60:592, 1964, with permission.)*

hyaluronidase, which enhances the rapid spread of venom by way of the superficial lymphatics. There may be considerable variation in the venom effect. Either neurotoxic features such as muscle cramping, fasciculation, weakness, and respiratory paralysis occur, or hemolytic characteristics may predominate, depending on the snake.

Clinical Manifestations of Crotalid Envenomation. Crotalid envenomation is graded on a scale from 0 to IV (Table 6-11). Pain from the bite of a pit viper is excruciating and probably the symptom that most easily differentiates poisonous from nonpoisonous snakebites. Pit vipers characteristically produce one or two fang marks. Hypotension, weakness, sweating and chills, dizziness, nausea, and vomiting are other systemic symptoms. Local signs and symptoms may include swelling, tenderness, pain, and ecchymosis, and may appear within minutes at the site of venom injection. If no edema or pain is present within 30 minutes following injury, the pit viper probably did not inject any venom. Swelling may continue to increase for 24 hours. Hemorrhage vesiculations, bullae, and petechiae may appear between 8 and 36 hours postbite, with thrombosis of superficial vessels and eventual sloughing of tissues. Systemic symptoms include paresthesias and muscle fasciculations. Muscle fasciculations are most common following a rattlesnake bite and often affect the perioral region. Fasciculations almost never follow a copperhead bite and rarely follow a cottonmouth bite. They are often seen in the face muscles and over the neck, back, and the involved extremity, and can occur within 10 minutes.

Table 6-11
Grading of Crotalid Envenomation

Grade	Signs and Symptoms
0: No envenomation	One or more fang marks, minimal pain, less than 1 inch of surrounding edema and erythema at 12 h, systemic involvement
I: Minimal envenomation	Fang marks, moderate to severe pain, 1 to 5 inches of surrounding edema and erythema in the first 12 h after bite, systemic involvement usually not present
II: Moderate envenomation	Fang marks; severe pain; 6 to 12 inches of surrounding edema and erythema in first 12 h after bite; possible systemic involvement including nausea, vomiting, giddiness, shock, or neurotoxic symptoms
III: Severe envenomation	Fang marks, severe pain, more than 12 inches of surrounding edema and erythema usually present and may include generalized petechiae and ecchymosis
IV: Very severe envenomation	Systemic involvement is always present, and symptoms may include renal failure, blood-tinged secretions, coma, and death; local edema may extend beyond the involved extremity to the ipsilateral trunk

The venom from rattlesnakes produces deleterious changes in the blood cells, defects in blood coagulation, injuries to the intimal linings of vessels, damage to the heart muscles, alterations in respiration, and to a lesser extent, changes in neuromuscular conduction. Pulmonary edema is common in severe poisoning, and hemorrhage into the lungs, kidneys, heart, and peritoneum may occur. Hematemesis, melena, changes in salivation, and muscle fasciculations may be seen. Urinalysis may reveal hematuria, glycosuria, and proteinuria. Red blood cells and platelets can decrease, and bleeding and clotting times are usually prolonged. Total afibrinogenemia is a hallmark of severe envenomation.

Blood should be immediately drawn for typing and crossmatching because hemolysis may later make this difficult. Since hemolysis and injury to kidneys and liver may occur, it is important to follow alterations in the clotting mechanism and renal and liver function, as well as electrolyte status.

Coral Snakes

The coral snake contributes to only 3% of all snake bites and 1.5% of all deaths from poisonous snakes. Bites by the coral snake occasionally provoke blurred vision, ptosis, drowsiness, increased salivation, and sweating. The patient may notice paresthesias about the mouth and throat, sometimes slurring of speech, and nausea and vomiting. Pain is not a constant complaint nor is edema a constant finding. Coral snake venom causes more extensive changes in the nervous system, and death may occur from inadequate ventilation.

Management of Snakebites

Application of a tourniquet, and incision and suction are appropriate if done within 1 hour from the time of the bite. The snake injects venom into the subcutaneous tissue which is absorbed by capillaries and lymphatics. The tourniquet should be applied loosely to obstruct only venous and lymphatic flow. The tourniquet is not released once applied and may be left in place during the 30 minutes that suction is being applied. The tourniquet may be removed after definitive treatment has been instituted and the patient is not in shock.

Incision and suction for 30 minutes may be of benefit if accomplished within 30 minutes after snakebite. The incision should be longitudinal and not cruciate. When two fang marks are seen, the depth of the venom injection is generally considered to be one third of the distance between the fang marks. Severe bites may result in envenomations deep to the fascia, and surgical exploration may be indicated. Incisions made proximal to the bite are contraindicated.

The average snakebite does not require surgical excision. This procedure is reserved for the most severe envenomations. It has been shown that wide excision of the entire area around the snakebite within 1 hour from the time of injection can remove most of the venom. Excision of the fang marks, including skin and subcutaneous tissue, should be considered in severe bites and in patients known to be allergic to horse serum that are seen within 1 hour following the bite. Most fatalities from snakebites do not occur for 6 to 48 hours following the bite, giving time to institute other measures.

The most important treatment for snakebite is antivenin, although many patients will not require it.[90] Copperhead envenomation rarely necessitates antivenin. Most snakebite fatalities in the United States during the past 20 years have involved either delay in obtaining treatment, no antivenin treatment, or inadequate dosage. The formerly available Antivenin (Crotalidae) Polyvalent was a horse serum product and was plagued by serum sickness and allergic reactions. Recently a new antivenin has been approved by the FDA, and is available, Crotalidae Polyvalent Immune Fab.[91,92] This is an ovine serum product which is five times as potent as the original product and has fewer allergic reactions. It is indicated for systemic crotalid envenomation. Four to six vials are administered intravenously. Additional 4- to 6-vial infusions are given until control of symptoms is achieved. Symptoms can recur after control is achieved. Therefore additional 2-vial infusions are required at 6, 12, and 18 hours following initial control. The incidence of serum sickness with the new antivenin is 16%. The original crotalid antivenin is no longer manufactured, nor is coral snake antivenin. However, in the case of the latter, sufficient stores are available to last several years.[93,94]

Information concerning identification of a snake or the proper antivenin frequently can be obtained from the nearest zoo herpetarium. A major problem with bites by exotic poisonous snakes is the choice and availability of suitable antivenin. Physicians confronted with this situation may obtain advice from the local poison center or the national hotline at 800-222-1222.

Intravenous fluids are frequently required to replace the decreased extracellular fluid volume resulting from edema formation. Fascial planes may become very tense with obstruction of venous and later arterial flow, requiring fasciotomy. Adequate antivenin treatment usually makes surgical intervention unnecessary. These patients may need blood, since anemia can develop from the hematologic effects. As afibrinogenemia has been reported, fibrinogen may be required. Vitamin K may also be required. Bleeding and clotting abnormalities are treated with antivenin in addition to blood components. Antibiotics are recommended to prevent secondary infection, although their benefit is unproven. Tetanus toxoid is administered. The most common species of organisms isolated from rattlesnake venom are *Pseudomonas aeruginosa*, *Proteus* spp., *Clostridium* spp., and *Bacteroides fragilis*.

Stinging Insects and Animals

Hymenoptera

The most important insects that produce serious and possibly fatal anaphylactic reactions are arthropods of the order Hymenoptera.[95] This group includes the honeybee, bumblebee, wasp, yellow and black hornets, and the fire ant. The venom of these stinging insects is just as potent as that of snakes and causes more deaths in the United States yearly than are caused by snakebites.

All insects of the order Hymenoptera except the bee retain their stinger and are in a position to sting repeatedly, each time injecting some portion of the venom sac contents. The worker honeybee sinks its barbed sting into the skin and it cannot be withdrawn. As the bee attempts to escape, it is disemboweled. The stinger with the bowel, muscles, and venom sac attached is left behind. The muscles controlling the venom sac, although separated from the bee, rhythmically contract for as long as 20 minutes, driving the stinger deeper and deeper into the skin and continuing to inject the venom.

Symptoms consist of one or more of the following: localized pain, swelling, generalized erythema, a feeling of intense heat throughout the body, headache, blurred vision, injected conjunctivae, swollen and tender joints, itching, apprehension, urticaria, petechial hemorrhages of the skin and mucous membranes, dizziness, weakness, sweating, severe nausea, abdominal cramps, dyspnea, constriction of the chest, asthma, angioneurotic edema, vascular collapse, and possible death from anaphylaxis. Fatal cases may manifest glottal and laryngeal edema, pulmonary and cerebral edema, visceral congestion, meningeal hyperemia, and intraventricular hemorrhage. Death apparently results from a combination of shock, respiratory failure, and central nervous system changes. Most deaths from insect stings occur within 15 to 30 minutes.

Early application of a tourniquet may prevent rapid spread of the venom. Affected persons should be taught to remove the venom sac if present, being careful not to squeeze the sac. It may be necessary for some patients to carry an emergency kit, which is commercially available. Patients should be taught to give themselves an epinephrine injection. Patients having severe reactions should first receive 0.3 to 0.5 mL of a 1:1000 solution of epinephrine intravenously.

Stingrays

Approximately 750 persons each year are stung by stingrays. As the spine, which is curved and has serrated edges, enters the flesh, the sheath surrounding the spine ruptures, and venom is released.[96] As the spine is withdrawn, fragments of the sheath may remain in the wound. The wound edges are often jagged and bleed freely. Pain is usually immediate and severe, increasing to maximum intensity in 1 to 2 hours and lasting for 12 to 48 hours. Treatment consists of copious irrigation with water to wash out any toxin and fragments of the spine's integumentary sheath. It has been noted that the venom is inactivated when exposed to heat. Therefore the area of the bite should be placed in water as hot as the patient can stand without injury for 30 minutes to 1 hour. After soaking, the wound may be further débrided and treated appropriately. Patients treated in this manner were shown to have rapid and uncomplicated healing of the wound. Patients not treated with heat had tissue necrosis with prolonged drainage and chronically infected wounds.

Portuguese Man-of-War

Following a severe sting there may be almost immediate severe nausea, gastric cramping, and constriction and tightness of throat and chest with severe muscle spasm. There is intense burning pain with weakness and perhaps respiratory distress. The most important emergency treatment is to inactivate the nematocysts immediately, to prevent their continuous firing of toxins.[97] This is accomplished by applications of a substance of high alcohol content, such as rubbing alcohol, followed by application of a drying agent, such as flour, baking soda, talc, or shaving cream. The tentacles may then be removed by shaving. Alkaline agents such as baking soda are then applied in order to neutralize the toxins, which are acidic. Meperidine and diphenhydramine may dramatically relieve the pain and symptoms. Aerosol corticosteroid-analgesic balm is helpful.

Spider Bites

Black Widow Spider. The most common biting spider in the United States is the black widow (*Latrodectus mactans*) (Fig. 6-67). The female spider has a reddish-orange hourglass-shaped marking on its ventral surface. *Latrodectus* venom is primarily neurotoxic in action and appears to center on the spinal cord. Following a bite by the black widow spider, the majority of patients experience pain within 30 minutes and a small wheal with an area of erythema appears. Nausea and vomiting occur in approximately one third of patients, headache in one fourth, and dyspnea may develop. The time of onset of symptoms following the bite is from 30 minutes to 6 hours. The severe symptoms last from 24 to 48 hours. Generalized muscle spasm is the most prominent physical finding. Cramping muscle spasms occur in the thighs, lumbar region, abdomen, or thorax. Priapism and ejaculation have been reported. Most patients recover within 24 hours.

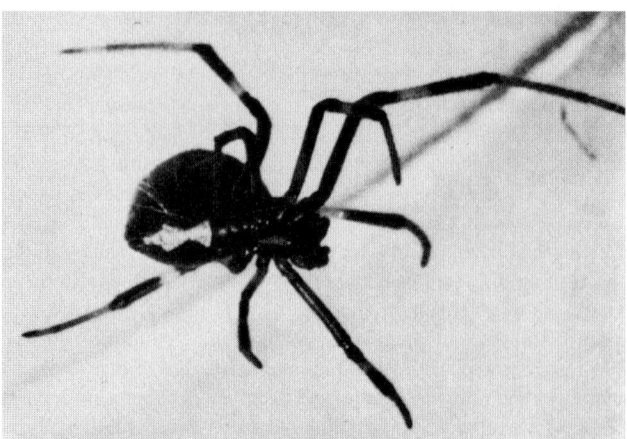

FIG. 6-67. Abdominal view of a female black widow spider showing the hourglass marking. (*From Paton BC: Bites: Human, dog, spider, and snake. Surg Clin North Am 43:537, 1963, with permission.*)

Treatment consists of narcotics for the relief of pain and a muscle relaxant for relief of spasm. Either methocarbamol (Robaxin) or 10 mL of a 10% solution of calcium gluconate relieves the symptoms. It is believed that calcium acts by depressing the threshold for depolarization at the neuromuscular junctions. Calcium gluconate may give instant relief of muscular pain and methocarbamol can be administered intravenously, 10 mL over a 5-minute period with a second ampule started in a saline solution drip. Although *Latrodectus mactans* antivenin is available, it is rarely required.[98] The manufacturer recommends its use for patients with underlying cardiovascular disease. The antivenin is prepared from horse serum and is administered intramuscularly after appropriate skin tests. Hospitalization may be required for the young, elderly, and patients with significant chronic diseases or with severe signs and symptoms of envenomation.

Brown Recluse Spider. The distinguishing mark of the *Loxosceles reclusa* is the darker violin-shaped band over the dorsal cephalothorax (Fig. 6-68). The spider is native to the south-central United States. The body ranges from 7 mm to 1.2 cm and including the legs ranges from 2 to 3 cm.

The initial bite may go unnoticed or be accompanied by a mild stinging sensation. Pain may recur 6 to 8 hours afterward. A mild envenomation is associated with local urticaria and erythema, which usually resolves spontaneously. More severe bites result in progression to necrosis and sloughing of skin with residual ulcer formation. A generalized macular and erythematous rash may appear in 12 to 24 hours. Erythema develops, with bleb or blister formation surrounded by an irregular area of ischemia. A zone of hemorrhage and induration and a surrounding halo of erythema may develop peripherally. The central ischemia turns dark, and eschar forms by the seventh day. By the fourteenth day the area sloughs, leaving an open ulcer. Approximately 3 weeks is required for the lesion to heal. The pain may be out of proportion for the size of the area involved. The progression from blue to black gives the bite a necrotic appearance, and the more severe ones develop within a few hours to 2 days. Systemically, the patient may have fever, nausea, vomiting, weakness, arthralgia, malaise, and even petechiae. The two principal systemic effects, hemolysis and thrombocytopenia, have been responsible for deaths. Hemoglobinemia, hemoglobinuria, leukocytosis, and proteinuria may also occur, and there may be eventual

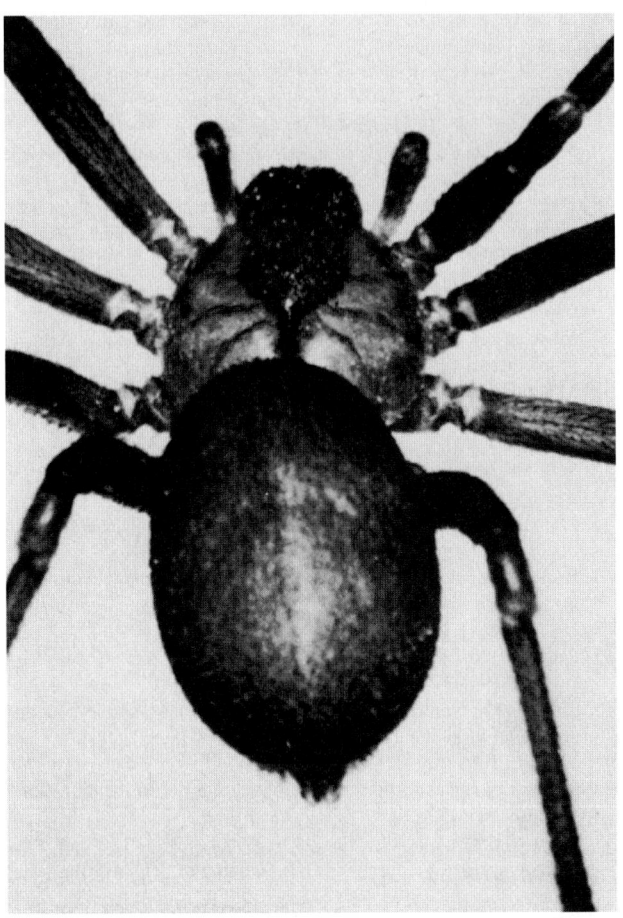

FIG. 6-68. The distinguishing mark of the *Loxosceles reclusa* is the darker violin-shaped band over the dorsal cephalothorax. (*From Dillaha CJ, Jansen GT, et al: North American loxocelism. JAMA 188:33, 1964, with permission.*)

renal failure. *Loxosceles* venom is chiefly cytotoxic in action. Laboratory studies are obtained in patients with severe envenomation including prothrombin time, partial thromboplastin time, platelet count, and urinalysis. The pathophysiology of the bite is that intravascular coagulation and the formation of microthrombi within the capillary occur, leading to capillary occlusion, hemorrhage, and necrosis.

Treatment is conservative because of the difficulty in predicting the severity of the bite. Various treatments have been advocated in addition to early excision, including corticosteroids, heparin, phentolamine, dextran, and infusion, but clinical studies have failed to identify the benefit of these agents. The dose for steroids has varied from 30 to 80 mg of methylprednisolone daily tapered over a period of several days. A leukocyte inhibitor, dapsone, which is used in leprosy, appears to be effective in reducing inflammation at the site of the brown recluse venom injection.[99] Treatment with dapsone is 100 mg daily for 14 days before surgical excision, if required. The incidence of scarring and deformity was much less in the dapsone-treated group than with observation and subsequent surgical excision. However, there are significant side effects associated with dapsone treatment, including dose-dependent hemolytic anemia, methemoglobinemia, and rash. Whether or not dapsone improves morbidity following brown recluse spider bites awaits further clinical evaluation. Conservative therapy seems to be the preferred treatment. Excision of the necrotic area with skin grafting may be required at a later date.

Scorpion Stings

Of the numerous species of scorpions in the United States, only one, *Centruroides exilicauda* or the bark scorpion, is medically significant. It is found primarily in the dessert Southwest. Ranging in length form 1 to 7 cm, it is usually yellowish brown in color and may have vertical bands on its dorsum. A tubercle at the base of the stinger distinguishes the bark scorpion from other species. The venom is neurotoxic and causes the release of neurotransmitters from the autonomic nervous system and adrenal gland. It also causes the depolarization of neuromuscular junctions.

The sting causes intense pain with few other local symptoms. Hyperesthesia persists at the site so that a light tap will reproduce the intense pain. The tap test reinforces the diagnosis. In addition to pain, other symptoms reflect the neurotoxic nature of the venom and include anxiety, blurred vision or temporary blindness, wandering eye movements, dyspnea, wheezing, dysphagia, involuntary urination and defecation, and opisthotonos. Somatic muscular contractions resembling seizures, hypertension, supraventricular tachyarrhythmias, and fever are also seen.

In general these stings have been of little significance in adults and are satisfactorily treated with cold compresses. In contrast, infants and small children have died from scorpion envenomations, though not since 1968. Small children with signs of envenomation should be admitted to the hospital and monitored. No special diagnostic tests are indicated. Treatment consists of airway management for excessive secretions, sedation, and treatment of arrhythmias and hypertension if indicated.[100] Calcium gluconate has been used to treat muscle spasms. Narcotics should not be used since they appear to aggravate the neurotoxic effects of the venom. A goat-derived antivenin is available, but only in the state of Arizona.

References

1. Sauaia A, Moore FA, Moore EE, et al: Epidemiology of trauma deaths: a reassessment. *J Trauma* 38:185, 1995.
2. Nathens AB, Jurkovich J, Maier RV, et al: Relationship between trauma center volume and outcomes. *JAMA* 285:1164, 2001.
3. MacKenzie EJ, Hoyt DB, Sacra JC, et al: National inventory of hospital trauma centers. *JAMA* 289:1515, 2003.
4. Gaushe M, Lewis RJ, Stratton SJ, et al: Effect of out-of-hospital pediatric endotracheal intubation on survival and neurological outcome. *JAMA* 283:783, 2000.
5. Shatney CH, Brunner RD, Nguyen TQ: The safety of orotracheal intubation in patients with unstable cervical spine fracture or high spinal cord injury. *Am J Surg* 170:676, 1995.
6. Branney S, Moore E, Feldhaus K, et al: Critical analysis of two decades of experience with postinjury emergency department thoracotomy. *J Trauma* 45:87, 1998.
7. Bickell WH, Wall MJ, Pepe PE, et al: Immediate versus delayed fluid resuscitation for hypotensive patients with penetrating torso injuries. *N Engl J Med* 331:1105, 1994.
8. Capone AC, Safar P, Stezoski W, et al: Improved outcome with fluid restriction in treatment of uncontrolled hemorrhagic shock. *J Am Coll Surg* 180:49, 1995.
9. Mattox KL, Maningas PA, Moore EE, et al: Prehospital hypertonic saline/dextran infusion for post-traumatic hypotension. *Ann Surg* 213:482, 1991.
10. Velmahos GC, Demetriades D, Shoemaker WC, et al: Endpoints of resuscitation of critically injured patients: Normal or supranormal. *Ann Surg* 232:409, 2000.

11. Moore EE: Blood substitutes—the future is now. *J Am Coll Surg* 196:1, 2003.

12. Atteberry LR, Dennis JW, Menawat SS, et al: Physical examination alone is safe and accurate for evaluation of vascular injuries in penetrating zone II neck trauma. *J Am Coll Surg* 179:657, 1994.

13. Biffl WL, Moore EE, Rehse DH, et al: Selective management of penetrating neck trauma based on cervical level of injury. *Am J Surg* 174:678, 1997.

14. Demetriades D, Theodorou D, Cornwell E, et al: Evaluation of penetrating injuries of the neck: a prospective study of 223 patients. *World J Surg* 21:41, 1997.

15. Meldon SW, Moettus LN: Thoracolumbar spine fractures: clinical presentation and the effect of altered sensorium and major injury. *J Trauma* 39:1110, 1995.

16. Parmley LF, Mattingly TW, Marian WC, et al: Nonpenetrating traumatic injury of the aorta. *Circulation* 17:1086, 1953.

17. Richardson P, Mirvis SE, Scorpio R, et al: Value of CT in determining the need for angiography when findings of mediastinal hemorrhage on chest radiographs are equivocal. *AJR* 156:273, 1991.

18. Flowers JL, Graham SM, Ugarte MA, et al: Flexible endoscopy for the diagnosis of esophageal trauma. *J Trauma* 40:261, 1996.

19. Henneman PL, Marx JA, Moore EE, et al: Diagnostic peritoneal lavage: accuracy in predicting necessary laparotomy following blunt and penetrating trauma. *J Trauma* 30:1345, 1990.

20. McAnena OJ, Marx JA, Moore EE, et al: Peritoneal lavage enzyme determinations following blunt and penetrating abdominal trauma. *J Trauma* 31:1161, 1991.

21. Rozycki GS, Ochsner MG, Schmidt JA, et al: A prospective study of surgeon-performed ultrasound as the primary adjuvant modality for injured patient assessment. *J Trauma* 39:492, 1995.

22. Ivatury RR, Simon RJ, Weksler B, et al: Laparoscopy in the evaluation of the intrathoracic abdomen after penetrating injury. *J Trauma* 33:101, 1992.

23. Johansen K, Lynch K, Paun M, et al: Noninvasive vascular tests reliably exclude occult arterial trauma in injured extremities. *J Trauma* 31:515, 1991.

24. Burch JM, Ortiz VB, Richardson RJ, et al: Abbreviated laparotomy and planned reoperation for critically injured patients. *Ann Surg* 215:476, 1992.

25. Moore EE: Staged laparotomy for the hypothermia, acidosis, and coagulopathy syndrome. *Am J Surg* 172:405, 1996.

26. Ridings PC, Bloomfield GL, Blocher CR, et al: Cardiopulmonary effects of raised intra-abdominal pressure before and after intravascular volume expansion. *J Trauma* 39:1071, 1995.

27. Shestak KC, Edington HJD, Johnson RR: The separation of anatomic components technique for the reconstruction of massive midline abdominal wall defects: Anatomy, surgical technique, applications, and limitations revisited. *Plast Reconstr Surg* 105:731, 2000.

28. Malhotra AK, Fabian TC, Croce MA, et al: Blunt hepatic injury: A paradigm shift from operative to nonoperative management in the 1990s. *Ann Surg* 231:804, 2000.

29. Tepas JJ III, Frykberg ER, Schinco MA, et al: Pediatric trauma is very much a surgical disease. *Ann Surg* 237:775, 2003.

30. Marion DW, Penrod LE, Kelsey SF, et al: Treatment of traumatic brain injury with moderate hypothermia. *N Engl J Med* 336:540, 1997.

31. Guidelines for the management of severe traumatic brain injury. *J Neurotrauma* 17:451, 2000.

32. Rinker C, McMurry F, Groeneweg V, et al: Emergency craniotomy in a rural level III trauma center. *J Trauma* 44:984, 1998.

33. Bracken MB, Shepard MJ, Collins WF, et al: A randomized, controlled trial of methylprednisolone or nalozone in the treatment of acute spinal-cord injury. Results of the second National Acute Spinal Cord Injury Study. *N Engl J Med* 322:1405, 1990.

34. Wing P, Merli G, Feuer H, et al: Prevention of venous thromboembolism in the acute treatment phase after spinal cord injury: A randomized, multicenter trial comparing low-dose heparin plus intermittent pneumatic compression with enoxaparin. *J Trauma* 54:1116, 2003.

35. Miller PR, Fabian TC, Croce MA, et al: Prospective screening for blunt cerebrovascular injuries. *Ann Surg* 236:386, 2002.

36. Biffl W, Moore E, Ryu R, et al: The unrecognized epidemic of blunt carotid arterial injuries—early diagnosis improves neurologic outcome. *Ann Surg* 228:462, 1998.

37. Feliciano DV, Burch JM, Mattox KL, et al: Balloon catheter tamponade in cardiovascular wounds. *Am J Surg* 160:583, 1990.

38. Cox CS, Allen GS, Fischer RP, et al: Blunt versus penetrating subclavian artery injury: Presentation, injury pattern, and outcome. *J Trauma* 46:445, 1999.

39. Bladergroen M, Brockman R, Luna G, et al: A twelve-year study of cervicothoracic vascular injuries. *Am J Surg* 157:483, 1989.

40. Johnston RH, Wall MJ, Mattox KL: Innominate artery trauma: A thirty-year experience. *J Vasc Surg* 17:134, 1993.

41. Mansour MA, Moore EE, Moore FA, et al: Exigent postinjury thoracotomy analysis of blunt versus penetrating trauma. *Surg Gynecol Obstet* 175:97, 1992.

42. Wall MJ, Mattox KL, Chen C, et al: Acute management of complex cardiac injuries. *J Trauma* 42:905, 1997.

43. Maron BJ, Gohman TE, Kyle SB, et al: Clinical profile and spectrum of commotio cordis. *JAMA* 287:9, 2002.

44. Biffl WL, Moore FA, Moore EE, et al: Cardiac enzymes are irrelevant in the patient with suspected myocardial contusion. *Am J Surg* 169:523, 1994.

45. Perchinsky MJ, Long WB, Hill JG: Blunt cardiac rupture. *Arch Surg* 130:852, 1995.

46. Thomas AN, Stephens BG: Air embolism: A cause of morbidity and death after penetrating chest trauma. *J Trauma* 14:633, 1974.

47. Wall MJ, Hirshberg A, Mattox KL, et al: Pulmonary tractotomy with selective vascular ligation for penetrating injuries to the lung. *Am J Surg* 168:665, 1994.

48. Cryer HG, Mavroudis C, Yu J, et al: Shock, transfusion, and pneumonectomy. Death is due to right heart failure and increased pulmonary vascular resistance. *Ann Surg* 212:197, 1990.

49. Beal SL, Pottmeyer EW, Spisso JM: Esophageal perforation following external blunt trauma. *J Trauma* 28:1425, 1988.

50. Weiman DS, Pate JW, Walker WA, et al: Combined gunshot injuries of the trachea and esophagus. *World J Surg* 20:1096, 1996.

51. Kim FJ, Moore EE, Moore FA, et al: Trauma surgeons can render definitive surgical care for major thoracic injuries. *J Trauma* 36:871, 1994.

52. Mattox KL, Holzman M, Pickard LR, et al: Clamp/repair: A safe technique for treatment of blunt injury to the descending thoracic aorta. *Ann Thoracic Surg* 40:456, 1985.

53. Von Oppell UO, Dunne TT, De Groot MK, et al: Traumatic aortic rupture: Twenty-year metaanalysis of mortality and risk of paraplegia. *Ann Thoracic Surg* 58:585, 1994.

54. Fabian TC, Richardson JD, Croce MA, et al: Prospective study of blunt aortic injury: Multicenter trial of the American Association for the Surgery of Trauma. *J Trauma* 42:374, 1997.

55. Accola KD, Feliciano DV, Mattox KL, et al: Management of injuries to the superior mesenteric artery. *J Trauma* 26:313, 1986.

56. Asensio JA, Britt LD, Borzotta A, et al: Multi-institutional experience with the management of superior mesenteric artery injuries. *J Am Coll Surg* 193:354, 2001.

57. Burch JM, Richardson RJ, Martin RR, et al: Penetrating iliac vascular injuries: Experience with 233 consecutive patients. *J Trauma* 30:1450, 1990.

58. Mullins RJ, Lucas CE, Ledgerwood AM: The natural history following venous ligation for civilian injuries. *J Trauma* 20:737, 1980.

59. Pachter HL, Drager S, Godfrey N, et al: Traumatic injuries of the portal vein. *Ann Surg* 189:383, 1979.

60. Roth SM, Wheeler JR, Gregory RT, et al: Blunt injury of the abdominal aorta: A review. *J Trauma* 42:748, 1997.

61. Jurkovich GJ, Hoyt DB, Moore FA, et al: Portal triad injuries. *J Trauma* 39:426, 1995.

62. Prager M, Polterauer P, Bohmig HJ, et al: Collagen versus gelatin-coated Dacron versus stretch polytetrafluoroethylene in abdominal

aortic bifurcation graft surgery: Results of a seven-year prospective, randomized multicenter trial. *Surgery* 130:408, 2001.

63. Asensio JA, Roldan G, Petrone P, et al: Operative management and outcomes in 103 AAST-OIS grades IV and V complex hepatic injuries: Trauma surgeons still need to operate, but angioembolization helps. *J Trauma* 54:647, 2003.

64. Poggetti RS, Moore EE, Moore FA, et al: Balloon tamponade for bilobar transfixing hepatic gunshot wounds. *J Trauma* 33:694, 1992.

65. Lillemoe KD, Melton GB, Cameron JL, et al: Postoperative bile duct strictures: Management and outcome in the 1990s. *Ann Surg* 232:430, 2000.

66. Sclafani SJ, Shaftan GW, Scalea TM, et al: Nonoperative salvage of computed tomography-diagnosed splenic injuries: Utilizations of angiography for triage and embolization for hemostasis. *J Trauma* 39:818, 1995.

67. Cocanour CS, Moore FA, Ware DN, et al: Age should not be a consideration for nonoperative management of blunt splenic injury. *J Trauma* 48:606, 2000.

68. Haan J, Scott J, Boyd-Kranis RL, et al: Admission angiography for blunt splenic injury: Advantages and pitfalls. *J Trauma* 51:1161, 2001.

69. Peitzman AB, Heil B, Rivera L, et al: Blunt splenic injury in adults: Multi-institutional study of the Eastern Association for the Surgery of Trauma. *J Trauma* 49:177, 2000.

70. Boulanger BR, Milzman DP, Rosati C, et al: A comparison of right and left blunt traumatic diaphragmatic rupture. *J Trauma* 35:255, 1993.

71. Bender JS, Lucas CE: Management of close-range shotgun injuries to the chest by diaphragmatic transposition: Case reports. *J Trauma* 30:1581, 1990.

72. Vaughn GD, Frazier OH, Graham D, et al: The use of pyloric exclusion in the management of severe duodenal injuries. *Am J Surg* 134:785, 1977.

73. Bradley EL, Young PR, Chang MC, et al: Diagnosis and initial management of blunt pancreatic trauma. *Ann Surg* 227:861, 1998.

74. Fulcher AS, Turner MA, Yelon JA, et al: Magnetic resonance cholangiopancreatography (MRCP) in the assessment of pancreatic duct trauma and its sequelae: Preliminary findings. *J Trauma* 48:1001, 2000.

75. Cogbill TH, Moore EE, Voeller GR, et al: Distal pancreatectomy for trauma: a multicenter experience. *J Trauma* 31:1600, 1991.

76. George SM, Fabian TC, Voeller GR, et al: Primary repair of colon wounds: A prospective trial in nonselected patients. *Ann Surg* 209:728, 1989.

77. Demetriades D, Murray JA, Chan L, et al: Penetrating colon injuries requiring resection: Diversion or primary anastomosis? An AAST prospective multicenter study. *J Trauma* 50:765, 2001.

78. Burch JM, Franciose RJ, Moore EE, et al: Single-layer continuous versus two-layer interrupted intestinal anastomosis—A prospective randomized study. *Ann Surg* 231:832, 2000.

79. Renz BM, Feliciano DV, Sherman R: Same admission colostomy closure (SACC). A new approach to rectal wounds: A prospective study. *Ann Surg* 218:279, 1993.

80. Fakhry SM, Watts DD, Luchette FA: Current diagnostic approaches lack sensitivity in the diagnosis of perforated blunt small bowel injury: Analysis from 275,557 trauma admissions from the EAST multi-institutional HVI trial. *J Trauma* 54:295, 2003.

81. Deck AJ, Shaves S, Talner L, et al: Current experience with computed tomographic cystography and blunt trauma. *World J Surg* 25:1592, 2001.

82. Burgess AR, Eastridge BJ, Young JWR, et al: Pelvic ring disruptions: Effective classification system and treatment protocols. *J Trauma* 30:848, 1990.

83. Eastridge BJ, Starr A, Minei JP, et al: The importance of fracture pattern in guiding therapeutic decision-making in patients with hemorrhagic shock and pelvic ring disruptions. *J Trauma* 53:446, 2002.

84. Biffl WL, Smith WR, Moore EE, et al: Evolution of a multidisciplinary clinical pathway for the management of unstable patients with pelvic fractures. *Ann Surg* 233:843, 2001.

85. Lawless MW, Laughlin RT, Wright DG, et al: Massive pelvis injuries treated with amputations: Case reports and literature review. *J Trauma* 42:1169, 1997.

86. Bosse MJ, MacKenzie EJ, Kellam JF, et al: An analysis of outcomes of reconstruction or amputation of leg-threatening injuries. *N Engl J Med* 347:1924, 2002.

87. Melton SM, Croce MA, Patton JH, et al: Popliteal artery trauma. Systemic anticoagulation and intraoperative thrombolysis improves limb salvage. *Ann Surg* 225:518, 1997.

88. Pape HC, Grimme K, van Griensven M, et al: Impact of intramedullary instrumentation versus damage control for femoral fractures on immunoinflammatory parameters: Prospective randomized analysis by the EPOFF Study Group. *J Trauma* 55:7, 2003.

89. Fishbein D, Robinson L: Rabies. *N Engl J Med* 329:1632, 1993.

90. Burch JM, Agarwal R, Mattox KL, et al: The treatment of crotalid envenomation without antivenin. *J Trauma* 28:35, 1988.

91. Gold BS, Dart RC, Barish RA: Bites of venomous snakes. *N Engl J Med* 347:347, 2002.

92. Dart RC, Seifert SA, Boyer LV: A randomized multicenter trial of crotaline polyvalent immune Fab (ovine) antivenom for the treatment for crotaline snakebite in the United States. *Arch Intern Med* 161:2030, 2001.

93. Gaar GG: Assessment and management of coral and other exotic snake envenomations. *J Fla Med Assoc* 83:178, 1996.

94. Rawat S, Laing G, Smith DC, et al: A new antivenom to treat eastern coral snake (*Micrurus fulvius fulvius*) envenoming. *Toxicon* 32:185, 1994.

95. Ditto AM: Hymenoptera sensitivity: diagnosis and treatment. *Allergy Asthma Proc* 23:381, 2002.

96. Meyer PK: Stingray injuries. *Wilderness Environ Med* 8:24, 1997.

97. Auerbach PS: Marine envenomation, in Auerbach PS (ed): *Wilderness Medicine: Management of Wilderness and Environmental Emergencies*, 3rd ed. St. Louis: Mosby-Year Book, 1995.

98. Clark RF: The safety and efficacy of antivenin *Latrodectus mactans*. *Annu Rev Neurosci* 24:933, 2001.

99. Rees RS, Altebern DP, Lynch JB, et al: Brown recluse spider bites: A comparison of early surgical excision vs. dapsone and delayed surgical excision. *Ann Surg* 202:659, 1985.

100. Gibley R, Williams M, Walter F, et al: Continuous intravenous midazolam infusion for *Centruroides exilicauda* scorpion envenomation. *Ann Emerg Med* 34:620, 1999.

Burns

James H. Holmes and David M. Heimbach

Pain Control

Chronic Problems

Hypertrophic Scar Formation
Marjolin's Ulcer
Heterotopic Ossification

INTRODUCTION

Thermal burns and related injuries are a major cause of death and disability in the United States. The introduction of burn centers in the 1960s and 1970s provided the basis for regional specialty-treatment centers, which were the first to provide a truly multidisciplinary approach to care. The interactive multidisciplinary team has proven to be the least expensive and most efficient method of treating major burn injury, of which the initial acute care is only a small part of the total treatment. Burn patients often require years of supervised rehabilitation, reconstruction, and psychosocial support. Omission of any step in the treatment regimen by any of the burn team members, including the burn surgeon, nurses, therapists, nutritionists, or psychosocial support staff, can result in less than optimal outcomes.

EPIDEMIOLOGY

In the United States, approximately 1.1 million individuals annually are burned seriously enough to seek health care; about 45,000 of these require hospitalization, and about 4500 die. More than 90% of burns are preventable; nearly one half are smoking related or due to substance abuse.[1,2] While prevention of burns is still the long-term solution to burn care, advances in the care of burned patients during the past 30 years are among the most dramatic in medicine.

The annual federal expenditure for research on cancer, heart disease, and stroke vastly exceeds that for trauma and burns, despite the fact that trauma and burns account for a loss of productive person-years from injury that is greater than that of cancer, heart disease, and stroke combined. The annual number of burn deaths in the United States has decreased from approximately 15,000 in 1970 to around 4500 currently. Over the same period, the burn size associated with a 50% mortality rate (i.e., the LD_{50}) has increased from 30% of the total body surface area (TBSA) to greater than 80% TBSA in otherwise healthy young adults.[3,4] The duration of hospital stay has been cut in half. Almost 95% of the patients admitted to burn centers in the U.S. now survive, and over one half of them return to preburn levels of physical and social functioning within 12 to 24 months following injury.[5,6]

The quality of burn care is no longer measured only by survival, but also by long-term function and appearance. Although small burns are not usually life threatening, they need the same attention as larger burns to achieve optimal outcomes. Even in the largest burn centers, the average burn size requiring admission is less than 15% TBSA. The surgeon's goal for any burn is well-healed, durable skin with normal function and near-normal appearance. Scarring, a virtual certainty with deep burns, can be minimized by appropriate early surgical intervention and long-term scar management. These goals require individualized patient care plans based on burn characteristics and host factors.

As with other forms of trauma, burns frequently affect children and young adults. In children under 8 years of age, the most common burns are scalds, usually from the spilling of hot liquids.[7] In older children and adults, the most common burns are flame-related, usually the result of house fires, the ill-advised use of flammable

liquids as accelerants, or are smoking- or alcohol-related.[8] Chemicals or hot liquids, followed by electricity, and then molten or hot metals most often cause work-related burns.[9] The hospital expenses and the societal costs related to time away from work or school are staggering.[10] Most burns are limited in extent, but a significant burn of the hand or foot may keep manual workers away from work for a year or more, or even permanently. The eventual outcome for the burned patient is related to injury severity, individual physical characteristics of the patient, motivation of the patient, quality of the treatment, and after-care support.

Etiology

Cutaneous burns are caused by the application of heat, cold, or caustic chemicals to the skin. When heat is applied to the skin, the depth of injury is proportional to the temperature applied, duration of contact, and thickness of the skin.

Scald Burns

Scalds, usually from hot water, are the most common cause of burns in civilian practice. Water at 140°F (60°C) creates a deep partial-thickness or full-thickness burn in 3 seconds. At 156°F (69°C), the same burn occurs in 1 second.[11] As a reference point, freshly brewed coffee generally is about 180°F (82°C). Boiling water always causes deep burns; likewise, thick soups and sauces, which remain in contact with the skin longer, invariably cause deep burns. Exposed areas of skin tend to be burned less deeply than clothed areas, as the clothing retains the heat and keeps the hot liquid in contact with the skin for a longer period of time. Immersion scalds are always deep, severe burns.[12] The liquid causing an immersion scald may not be as hot as with a spill scald; however, the duration of contact with the skin is longer during immersion, and these burns frequently occur in small children or elderly patients who have thinner skin.

Deliberate scalds are a common form of reported child abuse and are responsible for about 5% of the pediatric admissions to burn centers. The physician should note any discrepancy between the history provided by the caregiver and the distribution or probable cause of a burn.[13] Any suspicious burn requires in-patient admission and must be reported promptly to the appropriate authorities.

Scald burns from grease or hot oil are usually deep partial-thickness or full-thickness burns, as the oil or grease may be in the range of 400°F (200°C).[14] Tar and asphalt burns are a special kind of scald.[15] The "mother pot" at the back of a roofing truck maintains tar at a temperature of 400 to 500°F (200 to 260°C). Burns caused by tar directly from the mother pot are invariably full-thickness burns. However, by the time the tar has been spread on a roof or street, its temperature has been lowered to the point where most burns caused by it are partial-thickness in depth. The tar should be removed by application of a petroleum-based ointment or a nontoxic solvent (e.g., Medisol or sunflower oil) under a dressing. The dressing may be removed and the ointment or solvent reapplied frequently until the tar has dissolved. Only then can the extent of the injury and the depth of the burn be estimated accurately.[16,17]

Flame Burns

Flame burns are the second most common mechanism of thermal injury. Although the incidence of injuries caused by house fires has decreased with the use of smoke detectors, smoking-related fires, improper use of flammable liquids, motor vehicle collisions, and ignition of clothing by stoves or space heaters also are responsible for flame burns. Patients whose bedding or clothes have been on fire rarely escape without some full-thickness burns.

Flash Burns

Flash burns are next in frequency. Explosions of natural gas, propane, butane, petroleum distillates, alcohols, and other combustible liquids, as well as electrical arcs cause intense heat for a brief time period.[18,19] Clothing, unless it ignites, is protective against flash burns. Flash burns generally have a distribution over all exposed skin, with the deepest areas facing the source of ignition.[20] Flash burns are typically epidermal or partial thickness, their depth depending on the amount and kind of fuel that explodes. However, electrical arc burns and those from gasoline are often full-thickness and require grafting. At least some areas of flash burns often heal without requiring extensive skin grafting, but the burns generally cover a large TBSA, and in an explosive environment may be associated with significant thermal damage to the upper airway.

Contact Burns

Contact burns result from contact with hot metals, plastic, glass, or hot coals. They are usually limited in extent, but are invariably deep. Toddlers who touch or fall with outstretched hands against irons, ovens, and wood-burning stoves are likely to suffer deep burns of the palms.[21–23] It is common for patients involved in industrial accidents to have associated crush injuries because these accidents are commonly caused by contact with presses or other hot, heavy objects.[24] Motor vehicle and motorcycle collisions may leave victims in contact with hot engine parts.[25] The exhaust pipes of motorcycles cause a characteristic burn of the medial lower leg, that although small, usually requires excision and grafting. Contact burns are often fourth-degree burns, especially those in unconscious or postictal patients, and those caused by molten materials.[26–28]

Burn Prevention

More than 90% of all burns are preventable, and ongoing prevention and education efforts seem to be the most effective means to impact burn incidence. Over the past 20 years several critical legislative actions, such as that mandating flame-resistant sleepwear for children, have decreased burns and burn mortality.[29] Smoke detectors, required in all residential rental units and new construction, have likely contributed to decreased burn severity and mortality.[30] Many states have initiated legislation mandating that the maximum temperature for home and public hot water heaters be set to below 140°F (60°C), with positive results.[31] Individual burn centers, the American Burn Association (ABA), and the International Society for Burn Injury (ISBI) have all produced multiple public service announcements regarding hot water, carburetor flashes, grilling-related burns, scalds, and other kinds of burn injury. Numerous programs are directed at school-aged children; for example, the "Stop, Drop, and Roll" sequence. A national program aimed at keeping smoke detector batteries fresh uses the slogan "Change your clock, change your smoke detector battery".

HOSPITAL ADMISSION AND BURN CENTER REFERRAL

The severity of symptoms from smoke inhalation and the magnitude of associated burns dictate the need for hospital admission and specialized care. Any patient who has a symptomatic inhalation injury or more than trivial burns should be admitted to a hospital.

As a rule of thumb, if the burns cover more than 5 to 10% TBSA, the patient should be referred to a designated burn center. In the absence of burns, admission depends on the severity of respiratory symptoms, presence of premorbid medical problems, and the social circumstances of the patient. Otherwise healthy patients with mild respiratory symptoms [i.e., only a few expiratory wheezes with minimal sputum production, normal carboxyhemoglobin (COHb), and normal blood gas values] who have a place to go and someone to stay with them can be observed for 1 to 2 hours and then discharged from the emergency department. Patients with premorbid cardiovascular or pulmonary disease who have any symptoms related to smoke inhalation should be admitted for observation. Patients with moderate symptoms (i.e., generalized wheezing with mild hoarseness and moderate sputum production, but normal COHb and blood gas values) are admitted to a medical-surgical unit for close observation and symptomatic treatment. Patients with severe symptoms (e.g., air hunger, severe wheezing, and copious sputum production with typically abnormal blood gas values, regardless of COHb levels) should be intubated and admitted to an intensive care unit, or preferably a burn unit.

Burn Center Referral Criteria

The ABA has identified the following injuries as those requiring referral to a burn center after initial assessment and stabilization at an emergency department:

1. Partial-thickness and full-thickness burns totaling greater than 10% TBSA in patients under 10 or over 50 years of age.
2. Partial-thickness and full-thickness burns totaling greater than 20% TBSA in other age groups.
3. Partial-thickness and full-thickness burns involving the face, hands, feet, genitalia, perineum, or major joints.
4. Full-thickness burns greater than 5% TBSA in any age group.
5. Electrical burns, including lightning injury.
6. Chemical burns.
7. Inhalation injury.
8. Burn injury in patients with preexisting medical disorders that could complicate management, prolong the recovery period, or affect mortality.
9. Any burn with concomitant trauma (e.g., fractures) in which the burn injury poses the greatest risk of morbidity or mortality. If the trauma poses the greater immediate risk, the patient may be treated initially in a trauma center until stable, before being transferred to a burn center. The physician's decisions should be made with the regional medical control plan and triage protocols in mind.
10. Burn injury in children admitted to a hospital without qualified personnel or equipment for pediatric care.
11. Burn injury in patients requiring special social, emotional, and/or long-term rehabilitative support, including cases involving suspected child abuse.

Burn Center Verification and a National Burn Registry

In 1995, in conjunction with the American College of Surgeons Committee on Trauma (ACS-COT), the ABA initiated a program of Burn Center Verification. A detailed document outlines the resources and processes necessary to provide optimal care of the burn patient.[32] The program is voluntary, and burn centers may be reviewed to verify that they provide state-of-the-art care for burn patients. This process involves a lengthy questionnaire, a site visit, a written report, and approval by the joint verification committees. By 2003, about 60 centers had undergone this verification process. A national burn registry is kept by U.S. and Canadian burn centers to provide national statistics regarding incidence, epidemiology, and outcome of burn cases.

EMERGENCY CARE

Care at the Scene

Airway

Once flames are extinguished, initial attention must be directed to the airway. Immediate cardiopulmonary resuscitation is rarely necessary, except in electrical injuries or in patients with severe carbon monoxide poisoning. For these unfortunate patients, cardiopulmonary resuscitation (CPR) should be performed per Advanced Cardiac Life Support (ACLS) guidelines. Any patient rescued from a burning building or exposed to a smoky fire should be placed on 100% oxygen via a nonrebreather mask if there is any suspicion of smoke inhalation. If the patient is unconscious or in respiratory distress, endotracheal intubation should be performed by appropriately trained personnel.

Other Injuries and Transport

Once an airway is secured, the patient is assessed for other injuries and then transported to the nearest hospital. If a burn center is within a 30-minute transport time and the burn is severe without associated trauma, the patient may be taken directly to that facility. Patients should be kept flat and warm and be given nothing by mouth. The emergency medical personnel should place an intravenous line and begin fluid administration with lactated Ringer's (LR) solution at a rate of approximately 1 L/h in the case of a severe burn; otherwise, a maintenance rate is appropriate assuming no concomitant, nonthermal trauma. For transport, the patient should be wrapped in a clean sheet and blanket. Sterility is not required. Before or during transport, constricting clothing and jewelry should be removed from burned parts, because local swelling begins almost immediately.

Cold Application

Small burns, particularly scalds, may be treated with immediate application of cool water. It has been mathematically demonstrated that cooling cannot reduce skin temperature enough to prevent further tissue damage, but there is evidence in animals that cooling delays edema formation, probably by reducing initial thromboxane production.[33-35] After several minutes have elapsed, further cooling does not alter the pathologic process. Iced water should never be used, even on the smallest of burns.[36] If ice or cold water is used on larger burns, systemic hypothermia often follows, and the associated cutaneous vasoconstriction can extend the thermal damage.

Emergency Room Care

The primary rule for the emergency physician is to ignore the burn. As with any form of trauma, the airway, breathing, and circulation protocol (ABC) must be strictly followed. Although a burn is a dramatic injury, a careful search for other life-threatening injuries is the first priority. Only after making an overall assessment of the patient's condition should attention be directed to the burn.

Emergency Assessment of Inhalation Injury

The patient's history is an important part of assessing the extent of their injuries. Inhalation injury should be suspected in anyone with a flame burn, and assumed until proven otherwise in anyone burned in an enclosed space. The acrid smell of smoke on a victim's clothes should raise suspicion. The rescuers are the most important historians and should be questioned carefully before they leave the receiving facility.

Careful inspection of the mouth and pharynx should be done early. Hoarseness and expiratory wheezes are signs of potentially serious airway edema or inhalation injury. Copious mucus production and carbonaceous sputum (i.e., expectorated sputum and not just black flecks in the saliva) are positive signs, but their absence does not rule out airway injury. Carboxyhemoglobin levels should be obtained, and elevated levels or any symptoms of CO poisoning are presumptive evidence of associated inhalation injury.

A decreased P:F ratio, the ratio of arterial oxygen pressure (Pao_2) to the percentage of inspired oxygen (Fio_2), is one of the earliest indicators of smoke inhalation. A ratio of 400 to 500 is normal; patients with impending pulmonary problems have a ratio of less than 300. A ratio of less than 250 is an indication for endotracheal intubation rather than for increasing the inspired oxygen concentration.

Fiberoptic bronchoscopy is inexpensive, is quickly performed in experienced hands, and is useful for accurately assessing edema of the upper airway. Although bronchoscopy documents tracheal erythema, it does not materially influence the treatment of pulmonary injury.[37]

Fluid Resuscitation in the Emergency Room

As burns approach 20% TBSA, local proinflammatory cytokines enter the circulation and result in a systemic inflammatory response.[38] The microvascular leak, permitting loss of fluid and protein from the intravascular compartment into the extravascular compartment, becomes generalized. Cardiac output decreases as a result of burn shock and myocardial injury.[39] The resulting intense sympathetic response leads to increased systemic vascular resistance and decreased perfusion to the skin and viscera. Decreased flow to the skin may convert a zone of stasis to one of coagulation, thereby increasing the depth of burn. Decreased cardiac output may depress central nervous system (CNS) function, and in extreme cases, ultimately lead to cardiac failure in healthy patients or to myocardial infarction in patients with premorbid coronary artery atherosclerosis. Impairment in CNS function manifests as restlessness, followed by lethargy, and finally by coma. If resuscitation is inadequate, burns of 30% TBSA frequently lead to acute renal failure, which in the case of a severe burn almost invariably results in a fatal outcome.

Resuscitation begins by starting intravenous LR solution at a rate of 1000 mL/h in adults and 20 mL/kg per hour in young children. Burn patients requiring intravenous resuscitation (i.e., generally those with burns greater than 20% TBSA) should have a Foley catheter placed and urine output monitored hourly, the goal being 30 mL/h in adults and 1.0 mL/kg per hour in young children. Once the extent of the burn is ascertained, resuscitation should be tailored to the injury using the Parkland formula (Table 7-1), as both over- and underresuscitation are deleterious.

Patients with burns covering less than 50% TBSA usually can begin resuscitation via two large-bore peripheral intravenous lines. Because of the high incidence of septic thrombophlebitis, lower extremities should not be used as portals for peripheral intravenous lines. Upper extremities are preferable, even if the intravenous line must pass through burned skin or eschar. Patients with burns greater than 50% TBSA, or those who have associated medical problems, are at the extremes of age, or have concomitant inhalation injuries should have additional central venous access established with invasive hemodynamic monitoring. Because of the hemodynamic instability in patients with burns greater than 65% TBSA, these patients

Table 7-1
Formulas for Estimating Adult Burn Patient Resuscitation Fluid Needs

	Electrolyte	*Colloid*	*D_5W*
Colloid formulas			
Evans	Normal saline 1.0 mL/kg/% burn	1.0 mL/kg/% burn	2000 mL
Brooke	Lactated Ringer's 1.5 mL/kg/% burn	0.5 mL/kg	2000 mL
Slater	Lactated Ringer's 2 L/24 h	Fresh frozen plasma 75 mL/kg/24 h	
Crystalloid formulas			
Parkland	Lactated Ringer's	4 mL/kg/% burn	
Modified Brooke	Lactated Ringer's	2 mL/kg/% burn	
Hypertonic saline formulas			
Hypertonic saline solution (Monafo)—Volume to maintain urine output at 30 mL/h; fluid contains 25 mEq Na/L			
Modified hypertonic (Warden)—Lactated Ringer's + 50 mEq NaHCO₃ (180 mEq Na/L) for 8 h to maintain urine output at 30–50 mL/h; lactated Ringer's to maintain urine output at 30–50 mL/h beginning 8 h postburn			
Dextran formula (Demling)— Dextran 40 in saline: 2 mL/kg/h for 8 h; lactated Ringer's: volume to maintain output at 30 mL/h; fresh frozen plasma: 0.5 mL/kg/h for 18 h beginning 8 h postburn			

SOURCE: Reproduced with permission from Warden GD: Burn shock resuscitation. *World J Surg* 16:16, 1992.

should be transferred as quickly as possible to a burn center so they can be monitored in an intensive care setting.

Tetanus Prophylaxis

Burns are tetanus-prone wounds. The need for tetanus prophylaxis is determined by the patient's current immunization status. Previous immunization within 5 years requires no treatment, immunization within 10 years requires a tetanus toxoid booster, and unknown immunization status requires hyperimmune serum (i.e., Hyper-Tet).

Gastric Decompression

Many burn centers begin enteral feeding on admission to reduce the risk of gastric ulceration (Curling's ulcer), prevent ileus, and blunt catabolism.[40] If patient transport is via air ambulance or is going to take more than a few hours, the safest course is usually to decompress the stomach with a nasogastric tube.

Pain Control

During the shock phase of burn care, medications should be given intravenously. Subcutaneous and intramuscular injections are variably absorbed depending on perfusion and should be avoided. Pain control is best managed with small intravenous doses of an opiate until analgesia is adequate without inducing hypotension.

Psychosocial Care

Psychosocial care should begin immediately. The patient and family must be comforted and given a realistic assessment regarding the prognosis of the burns. In house fires, patients' loved ones, pets, and possessions may have been lost. If the family is not available, some member of the team, usually the social worker, should determine the extent of personal loss. If the patient is a child, and if the circumstances of the burn are suspicious, physicians in all states are required by law to report any suspected case of child abuse to local authorities.

Care of the Burn Wound

After all other assessments have been completed, attention should be directed to the burn. If the patient is to be transferred during the first postburn day, which is almost always the case, the burn wounds can be minimally dressed in gauze. However, the size of the burn should be calculated to establish the proper level of fluid resuscitation, and pulses distal to circumferential deep burns should be monitored. The patient can be wrapped in a clean sheet and kept warm until arriving at the definitive care center.

Escharotomy

Thoracic Escharotomy. The adequacy of respiration must be monitored continuously throughout the resuscitation period. Early respiratory distress may be due to the compromise of ventilation caused by chest wall inelasticity related to a deep circumferential burn wound of the thorax. Pressures required for ventilation increase and arterial P_{CO_2} rises. Inhalation injury, pneumothorax, or other causes can also result in respiratory distress and should be appropriately treated.

Thoracic escharotomy is seldom required, even with a circumferential chest wall burn. When required, escharotomies are performed bilaterally in the anterior axillary lines. If there is significant extension of the burn onto the adjacent abdominal wall, the escharotomy incisions should be extended to this area by a transverse incision along the costal margins (Fig. 7-1).

Escharotomy of the Extremities. Edema formation in the tissues under the tight, unyielding eschar of a circumferential burn on an extremity may produce significant vascular compromise that, if left unrecognized and untreated, will lead to permanent, serious neuromuscular and vascular deficits. All jewelry must be removed from the extremities to avoid distal ischemia. Skin color, sensation, capillary refill, and peripheral pulses must be assessed hourly in any extremity with a circumferential burn. The occurrence of any of the following signs or symptoms may indicate poor perfusion of a distal extremity warranting escharotomy: cyanosis, deep tissue pain, progressive paresthesia, progressive decrease or absence of pulses, or the sensation of cold extremities. An ultrasonic flowmeter (Doppler) is a reliable means for assessing arterial blood flow, the need for an escharotomy, and also can be used to assess adequacy of circulation after an escharotomy.[41]

Transfers to a burn center within 6 hours of injury should not require escharotomy at the referring hospital. When necessary, escharotomies may be done as bedside procedures with a sterile field and scalpel or electrocautery. Local anesthesia is unnecessary because full-thickness eschar is insensate; however, intravenous opiates or anxiolytics should be utilized. The incision, which must avoid major neurovascular and musculotendinous structures, should be placed along the mid-medial or mid-lateral aspect of the extremity.

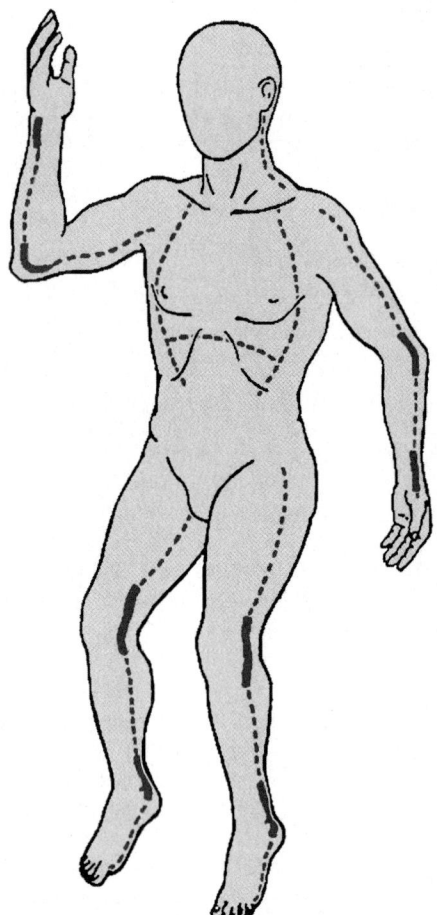

FIG. 7-1. Locations for escharotomies. The incisions are placed along the mid-medial and mid-lateral lines of the extremities and the thorax (*dashed lines*). The skin is especially tight along major joints, and decompression at these sites must be complete (*solid lines*). Neck and digital escharotomies are rarely necessary.

To permit adequate separation of the cut edges for decompression, the incision should be carried down through the eschar, which includes devitalized dermis, to the subcutaneous fat. The incision should extend the length of the constricting full-thickness burn and across involved joints (see Fig. 7-1). When a single escharotomy incision does not result in restoring adequate distal perfusion, a second escharotomy incision on the contralateral aspect of the extremity should be performed. A digital escharotomy is never required.

Because burn patients are at risk for developing a compartment syndrome up to 72 hours following injury, any involved extremity should be continually reassessed for signs of increased compartment pressures that can occur after initial decompression. A compartment syndrome following initially adequate escharotomy, albeit rare, requires urgent operative fasciotomy. As primary release or decompression maneuvers, fasciotomies are virtually never indicated except with major electrical burns.

BURN SEVERITY

The severity of any burn injury is related to the size and depth of the burn, and to the part of the body that has been burned. Burns are the only truly quantifiable form of trauma. The single most important factor in predicting burn-related mortality, need for specialized care, and the type and likelihood of complications is the overall size of the

burn as a proportion of the patient's TBSA. Treatment plans, including initial resuscitation and subsequent nutritional requirements, are directly related to the size of burn.

Burn Size

A general idea of the burn size can be made by using the *rule of nines*. Each upper extremity accounts for 9% of the TBSA, each lower extremity accounts for 18%, the anterior and posterior trunk each account for 18%, the head and neck account for 9%, and the perineum accounts for 1%. Although the rule of nines is reasonably accurate for adults, a number of more precise charts have been developed that are particularly helpful in assessing pediatric burns. Most emergency rooms have such a chart. A diagram of the burn can be drawn on the chart, and more precise calculations of the burn size made from the accompanying TBSA estimates given.

Children under 4 years of age have much larger heads and smaller thighs in proportion to total body size than do adults. In infants the head accounts for nearly 20% of the TBSA; a child's body proportions do not fully reach adult percentages until adolescence. Even when using precise diagrams, interobserver variation may vary by as much as ±20%.[42] An observer's experience with burned patients, rather than educational level, appears to be the best predictor of the accuracy of burn size estimation. For smaller burns, an accurate assessment of size can be made by using the patient's palmar hand surface, including the digits, which amounts to approximately 1% of TBSA.

Burn Depth

Along with burn size and patient age, the depth of the burn is a primary determinant of mortality. Burn depth is also the primary determinant of the patient's long-term appearance and functional outcome.

Burns not extending all the way through the dermis leave behind epithelium-lined skin appendages, including sweat glands and hair follicles with attached sebaceous glands. When dead dermal tissue is removed, epithelial cells swarm from the surface of each appendage to meet swarming cells from neighboring appendages, forming a new, fragile epidermis on top of a thinned and scarred dermal bed. Skin appendages vary in depth, and the deeper the burn, the fewer the appendages that contribute to healing, and the longer the burn takes to heal. The longer the burn takes to heal, the less dermis remains, the greater the inflammatory response, and the more severe the scarring.

When nonoperative treatment is the norm, as it is in many developing countries, an accurate assessment of burn depth is of little importance except for predicting mortality. On the other hand, with aggressive surgical treatment, an accurate estimation of burn depth is crucial. Burns that heal within 3 weeks usually do so without hypertrophic scarring or functional impairment, although long-term pigmentary changes are common. Burns that take longer than 3 weeks to heal often produce unsightly hypertrophic scars, frequently lead to functional impairment, and provide only a thin, fragile epithelial covering for many weeks or months. State-of-the-art burn care involves early excision and grafting of all burns that will not heal within 3 weeks. The challenge is to determine which burns *will* heal within 3 weeks, and are thus better treated by nonoperative wound care.

An understanding of burn depth requires an understanding of skin thickness. The deepest layer of epidermal cells (basal layer) is an intensely active layer of epithelial cells under layers of dead keratinized cells, and is superficial to the active structural framework of the skin, the dermis. The thickness of skin varies with the age and sex of the individual and the area of the body. The thickness of the living epidermis is relatively constant, but keratinized (dead and cornified) epidermal cells may reach a thickness of 0.5 cm on the palms and soles. The thickness of the dermis varies from less than 1 mm on the eyelids and genitalia to more than 5 mm on the posterior trunk. The proportional thickness of skin in each body area in children is similar to that in adults, but infant skin thickness in each specific area may be less than one half that of adult skin. The skin does not reach adult thickness until puberty. Similarly, in patients over 50 years of age, dermal atrophy has begun; all areas of skin become thin in elderly patients, and the skin appendages are far less active.

Burn depth is dependent upon the temperature of the burn source, the thickness of the skin, the duration of contact, and the heat-dissipating capability of the skin (i.e., blood flow). A scald in an infant or elderly patient will be deeper than an identical scald in a young adult. A diabetic with impaired sensation or an intoxicated patient with an impaired sensorium who lies on a heating pad all night may sustain full-thickness burns, because of the long duration of contact with the pad and the pressure of the body weight that occludes cutaneous blood flow and prevents heat dissipation.

Burns are classified according to increasing depth as epidermal (first-degree), superficial and deep partial-thickness (second-degree), full-thickness (third-degree), and fourth-degree. Because most deep burns are excised and grafted, such a precise characterization is not necessary for non–life-threatening burns. A more pertinent classification might be "shallow burns" and "deep burns." Nevertheless, distinguishing between deep burns that are best treated by early excision and grafting, and shallow burns that heal spontaneously, is not always straightforward, and many burns have a mixture of clinical characteristics, making precise classification difficult.

Shallow Burns

Epidermal Burns (First-Degree). As implied, these burns involve only the epidermis. They do not blister, but become erythematous because of dermal vasodilation, and are quite painful. Over 2 to 3 days the erythema and pain subside. By about the fourth day, the injured epithelium desquamates in the phenomenon of peeling, which is well known after sunburn.

Superficial Partial-Thickness (Second-Degree). Superficial partial-thickness burns include the upper layers of dermis, and characteristically form blisters with fluid collection at the interface of the epidermis and dermis. Blistering may not occur until some hours after injury, and burns originally appearing to be epidermal may subsequently be diagnosed as superficial partial-thickness burns after 12 to 24 hours. When blisters are removed, the wound is pink and wet; currents of air passing over it cause pain. The wound is hypersensitive, and the burns blanch with pressure. If infection is prevented, superficial partial-thickness burns heal spontaneously in less than 3 weeks, and do so without functional impairment. They rarely cause hypertrophic scarring, but in pigmented individuals the healed burn may never completely match the color of the surrounding normal skin.

Deep Burns

Deep Partial-Thickness (Second-Degree). Deep partial-thickness burns extend into the reticular layers of the dermis. They also blister, but the wound surface is usually a mottled pink-and-white color immediately after the injury because of the varying blood supply to the dermis (white areas have little to no blood flow and pink areas have some blood flow). The patient complains of discomfort rather than pain. When pressure is applied to the burn, capillary refill occurs slowly or may be absent. The wound is often less sensitive to pinprick than the surrounding normal skin. By the second day, the wound may be white and is usually fairly dry. If not excised and grafted, and if infection is prevented, these burns will heal in 3 to 9 weeks, but invariably do so with considerable scar formation. Unless active physical therapy is continued throughout the healing process, joint function can be impaired, and hypertrophic scarring is common.

Full-Thickness (Third-Degree). Full-thickness burns involve all layers of the dermis and can heal only by wound contracture, epithelialization from the wound margin, or skin grafting. They appear white, cherry red, or black, and may or may not have deep blisters. Full-thickness burns are described as being leathery, firm, and depressed when compared with adjoining normal skin, and they are insensate. The difference in depth between a deep partial-thickness burn and a full-thickness burn may be less than 1 mm. The clinical appearance of full-thickness burns can resemble that of deep partial-thickness burns. They may be mottled in appearance, rarely blanch on pressure, and may have a dry, white appearance. In some cases, the burn is translucent, with clotted vessels visible in the depths. Some full-thickness burns, particularly immersion scalds, have a red appearance and initially may be confused with superficial partial-thickness burns. However, they can be distinguished because they do not blanch with pressure. Full-thickness burns develop a classic burn eschar, a structurally intact but dead and denatured dermis that if left in situ over days and weeks, separates from the underlying viable tissue.

Fourth-Degree. Fourth-degree burns involve not only all layers of the skin, but also subcutaneous fat and deeper structures. These burns almost always have a charred appearance, and frequently only the cause of the burn gives a clue to the amount of underlying tissue destruction. Electrical burns, contact burns, some immersion burns, and burns sustained by patients who are unconscious at the time of burning may all be fourth-degree.

Assessment of Burn Depth

The standard technique for determining burn depth has been clinical observation of the wound. The difference in depth between a shallow burn that heals in 3 weeks, a deep partial-thickness burn that heals only after many weeks, and a full-thickness burn that will not heal at all, may be only a matter of a few tenths of a millimeter. A burn is a dynamic process for the first few days; a burn appearing shallow on day 1 may appear considerably deeper by day 3. Furthermore, the kind of topical wound care used can dramatically change the appearance of the burn. For these reasons, and because of the increasing importance of an accurate assessment of burn depth for planning definitive care of burn wounds, there is considerable interest in technology that will help determine burn depth more precisely and more quickly than clinical observation.

Evaluation by an experienced surgeon as to whether a partial-thickness burn will heal in 3 weeks is about 70% accurate.[43] In experienced hands, however, early excision and grafting provides better results than nonoperative care for such indeterminate burns.[44] Other techniques to quantify burn depth involve (1) the ability to detect dead cells or denatured collagen (e.g., biopsy, ultrasound, and vital dyes), (2) assessment of changes in blood flow (e.g., fluorometry, laser Doppler, and thermography), (3) analysis of the color of the wound (e.g., light reflectance methods), and (4) evaluation of physical changes, such as edema (e.g., nuclear magnetic resonance imaging).[45–55]

Nonetheless, the most common modality of burn depth estimation used in state-of-the-art burn care today is still clinical observation. To date, machines have proven to be significantly more cumbersome and only slightly more accurate than humans in assessing burn depth, and so remain only research instruments.

THE PHYSIOLOGIC RESPONSE TO BURN INJURY

Burn patients with or without inhalation injury commonly manifest an inflammatory process involving the entire organism; the term *systemic inflammatory response syndrome* (SIRS) summarizes that condition. SIRS with infection (i.e., sepsis syndrome) is a major factor determining morbidity and mortality in thermally injured patients. Pathologic alterations of the metabolic, cardiovascular, gastrointestinal, and coagulation systems occur, with resulting hypermetabolism; increased cellular, endothelial, and epithelial permeability; classic hemodynamic alterations; and often extensive microthrombosis. The cardiovascular manifestations of SIRS largely disappear within 24 to 72 hours, but the patient remains in a hypermetabolic state until wound coverage is achieved.

Burn Shock

Burn shock is a complex process of circulatory and microcirculatory dysfunction that is not easily or fully repaired by fluid resuscitation. Tissue trauma and hypovolemic shock result in the formation and release of local and systemic mediators, which produce an increase in vascular permeability and microvascular hydrostatic pressure.[56] Most mediators act to increase permeability by altering venular endothelial integrity. The early phase of burn edema, lasting from minutes to an hour, is attributed to mediators such as histamine, products of platelet activation, eicosanoids, and proteolytic products of the coagulation, fibrinolytic, and kinin cascades. Vasoactive amines may also act by increasing microvascular blood flow or vascular pressures, accentuating the burn edema.

Histamine is probably responsible for the early phase of increased vascular permeability after burn injury, because it is released in large quantities from mast cells in burned skin immediately after injury.[57] It predominantly disrupts venular endothelial tight junctions, permitting egress of fluid and proteins. Serum histamine peaks in the first several hours following a burn, suggesting that histamine is involved only in the very early increase in microvascular permeability.

Serotonin is released immediately postburn via platelet aggregation, and acts directly to increase pulmonary vascular resistance, and indirectly to amplify the vasoconstrictive effects of norepinephrine, histamine, angiotensin II, and select eicosanoids at the microvascular level.[58]

Eicosanoids, vasoactive products of arachidonic acid metabolism, are released in burn tissue and contribute to the formation of burn edema. These substances do not directly alter vascular permeability, but increased levels of the vasodilator prostaglandins (PG), such as PGE_2, and prostacyclin (PGI_2), result in arterial dilatation in burn tissue that increases blood flow and hydrostatic pressure in the injured microcirculation and accentuates edema formation. Increased concentrations of PGI_2 and the vasoconstrictor thromboxane (TX) A_2 have been demonstrated in burn tissue, burn blister fluid, lymph, and wound sera.[59]

The activation of multiple proteolytic cascades occurs immediately after burn injury. Kinins, specifically the bradykinins,

increase vascular permeability, primarily in the venule.[60] Platelet-activating factor is released after burn injury and increases capillary permeability.[61] Concomitant with the systemic microvascular leak early after a burn, a hypercoagulable and hyperfibrinolytic state exists. As hematologically measured, it resembles disseminated intravascular coagulation (DIC) and may correlate with organ failure and outcome.[62]

In addition to the loss of microvascular integrity, thermal injury also causes changes at the cellular level. The reduction in cardiac output after burn injury is a result of cellular shock, hypovolemic shock, and increased systemic vascular resistance (SVR) due to sympathetic stimulation from the release of multiple mediators. The cardiac myocyte shock state is a result of impaired calcium homeostasis and subsequent intracellular signaling dysregulation.[63,64] Effective pharmacologic interventions to reverse this burn-specific form of cardiogenic shock are still in the experimental stages. Following successful resuscitation, cardiac output normalizes within 24 to 72 hours, and then increases to supranormal levels during the wound healing phase of burn management.

Metabolic Response to Burn Injury

Hypermetabolism

Resting energy expenditure (REE) after burn injury can be as much as 100% above predictions based on standard calculations for size, age, sex, and weight. Some debate persists regarding the genesis of this phenomenon, but increased heat loss from the burn wound and increased beta-adrenergic stimulation are probably primary factors.[65,66] Radiant heat loss is increased from the burn wound secondary to increased blood flow and integumentary loss. Measurement of REE is helpful in assessing nutritional status. On average, the REE is approximately 1.3 times the predicted basal metabolic rate (BMR) obtained using the Harris-Benedict equation.

Glucose metabolism is elevated in almost all critically-ill patients, including those with burn injuries. Studies have focused particularly on burn patients because their relatively stable physiologic condition allows reproducible experimental conditions. Gluconeogenesis and glycogenolysis are increased in burn patients. In addition, plasma insulin levels typically are elevated in burn patients. The basal rate of glucose production is elevated despite this hyperinsulinemic state, which can be defined as hepatic insulin resistance. Hence, hyperglycemia complicates the acute management of many significant burns and may be related to poor outcomes, specifically increased mortality and decreased graft take.[67] Further, hyperglycemia may exacerbate muscle catabolism in burn patients while not influencing REE.[68] Exogenous insulin administration to achieve euglycemia has been shown to decrease donor site healing time and decrease length of stay, while ameliorating skeletal muscle catabolism.[69,70]

Lipolysis occurs at a rate in excess of the requirements for fatty acids as an energy source due to alterations in substrate cycling. In burn patients, the majority of released fatty acids are not oxidized, but rather re-esterified into triglycerides, resulting in fat accumulation in the liver. The acute and long-term consequences of this hepatic steatosis are unclear. However, in a pediatric autopsy study, 80% of the fatalities over 10 years had hepatic steatosis, and it appeared to correlate with sepsis.[71] Beta-blockade using propranolol appears promising as a means to manipulate peripheral lipolysis and potentially prevent hepatic steatosis, although clinical outcome data with respect to fatty acid metabolism are still lacking.[72]

Proteolysis is increased in burn patients as compared to normal individuals who are fed isonitrogenous, isocaloric diets. Following utilization, protein is excreted primarily in the urine as urea. This results in an increased efflux of amino acids from the skeletal muscle pool, including gluconeogenic amino acids. In particular, alanine and glutamine (Gln) are released at an increased rate. Muscle protein breakdown is accelerated while acute phase proteins are produced at an increased rate in the liver. Wound healing requires enhanced protein synthesis and increased immunologic activity. Protein intake greater than 1 g/kg per day has been recommended for all thermally injured patients, and for burn patients with normal renal function, the recommended protein intake is 2 g/kg per day. The importance of Gln intake or its metabolic precursors has been investigated in critically-ill burn patients. Current standard nutritional formulations have largely omitted Gln or its precursors; however, beneficial effects have been found with Gln and ornithine α-ketoglutarate (OKG) supplementation. In particular, gram-negative bacteremia and possibly mortality were reduced with parenteral Gln supplementation, while inflammation was blunted and nutritional parameters were improved.[73] Similarly, enteral OKG supplementation was associated with increased plasma Gln levels, enhanced wound healing, and improved nitrogen metabolism.[74,75] The precise mechanisms by which direct and indirect Gln supplementation improves outcome remain unclear and are a fertile area of metabolism research. The anabolic steroid oxandrolone also has been shown to improve donor-site healing time, diminish weight loss, and blunt protein catabolism during the acute phase of burn wound healing.[76]

Neuroendocrine Response

Catecholamines are massively elevated following burn injury, and appear to be the major endocrine mediators of the hypermetabolic response in thermally injured patients. Pharmacologic beta-blockade utilizing propranolol diminishes the intensity of postburn hypermetabolism in pediatric patients as demonstrated by improved skeletal muscle protein kinetics with diminished REE and oxygen consumption; however, clinical outcome data are still lacking, and these results have yet to be demonstrated in adult burn patients.[77] Conversely, growth hormone (GH) levels are attenuated following thermal injury. Although early studies of exogenous GH as an anticatabolic agent were promising in the pediatric population, ultimately its use has been supplanted by less expensive, safer, and equally effective pharmacotherapies.[78] Propranolol has been shown to be superior to GH, while oxandrolone is equally as effective as GH in ameliorating catabolism.[79, 80] Both propranolol and oxandrolone have fewer significant side effects than GH, and oxandrolone appears to be equally effective in adults and children.

Thyroid hormone serum concentrations are altered in patients with large burns. Total thyronine (T_3) and thyroxine (T_4) concentrations are reduced, and reverse T_3 concentrations are elevated, while cellular concentrations are likely normal. Concentrations of free T_3 and T_4 fall markedly in the presence of sepsis in burned patients.[81] Burn injuries abolish the normal diurnal variation in glucocorticoid secretion, producing persistent hypercortisolemia. Although catabolic, cortisol does not appear to appreciably influence metabolic activity alone, but acts additively and synergistically with the catecholamines and glucagon. Glucagon concentrations are related directly to metabolic rate and appear to exert effects via insulin and insulin-like growth factor-1 modulation.[82]

Immunologic Response to Burn Injury

The immune status of the burn patient has a profound impact on outcome in terms of survival and major morbidity. Many mediators are released from both injured and uninjured tissues at the wound site where they exert local and systemic effects. The timetable of induction/suppression and physiologic sequela are similar in patients suffering thermal and non-thermal trauma (see Chap. 1, "The Systemic Response to Injury and Metabolic Support"). The greatest difficulty in attempting to decipher the body's response to injury is the complex interaction between the multiple, redundant inflammatory cascades and the immune system.

FLUID MANAGEMENT

Proper fluid management is critical to survival following major thermal injury. Prior to World War II, hypovolemic shock with consequent acute renal failure was the leading cause of death from burns. Mortality related to burn-induced hypovolemia has decreased considerably with increased understanding of the massive fluid shifts and hemodynamic changes that occur during burn shock. Much of the early knowledge about burn shock resuscitation dates to two U.S. disasters: the Rialto Theater fire in New Haven, Connecticut, in 1921, and the Coconut Grove fire in Boston, Massachusetts, in 1942. An aggressive approach to fluid therapy has subsequently led to reduced mortality rates in the first 48 hours postburn; nonetheless, approximately 50% of the deaths still occur within the first 10 days after burn injury, owing to multiple organ failure syndrome (MOFS) and overwhelming sepsis. One of the principal causes, particularly of MOFS, is inadequate fluid resuscitation and maintenance. Fluid management following successful resuscitation from burn shock is equally as important.

Pathophysiology of Burn Shock

Burn shock is both hypovolemic and cellular in etiology. It is characterized by specific hemodynamic changes including decreased cardiac output, increased extracellular fluid, decreased plasma volume, and oliguria. As with treating other forms of shock, the primary goal is to restore and preserve tissue and end-organ perfusion. In burn shock, resuscitation is complicated by obligatory burn edema. The voluminous extravascular fluid shifts that result from a major burn are unique to thermal trauma.

A major component of burn shock is the increase in systemic microvascular permeability. Direct thermal injury results in significant changes in the microcirculation, both systemically and locally. Maximal edema formation occurs between 8 and 12 hours following injury in smaller burns, and between 12 and 24 hours in major thermal injuries. The rate of progression of tissue edema is dependent on the adequacy of resuscitation. As previously described, multiple mediators have been implicated in causing the microvascular changes via a direct increase in vascular permeability or an increase in intravascular hydrostatic pressure. The end result of these changes in the microvasculature due to thermal injury is disruption of the normal barriers separating the intravascular and interstitial compartments, with rapid equilibrium between the two compartments. Hence, plasma volume is severely depleted (hypovolemia), while there is a marked increase in extracellular fluid (edema).

Thermal injury also causes changes at the cellular level. Baxter originally demonstrated that in burns covering more than 30% TBSA, there is a systemic decrease in cell transmembrane potential. This decrease in potential, defined by the Nernst equation, results from an increase in intracellular Na^+ concentrations secondary to a decrease in Na^+-K^+-ATPase activity responsible for maintaining the transcellular ionic gradient. This has subsequently been confirmed in modern animal models.[83] Resuscitation only partially restores the transmembrane potential and intracellular Na^+ concentrations to normal, implying that hypovolemia is not solely responsible for the cellular defects seen with burn shock. The aforementioned animal models have also implicated defective adenosine triphosphate (ATP) metabolism as a cause. Membrane potential may not return to normal for many days following thermal injury, despite adequate resuscitation. If resuscitation is inadequate, cellular transmembrane potential progressively decreases, and ultimately results in cell death.

Burn Shock Resuscitation

The primary goal of fluid resuscitation is to ensure end-organ perfusion by replacing fluid that is sequestered as a result of the thermal injury. Support of the burned patient in this manner is principally aimed at the first 24 to 48 hours after injury, when the rate of development of hypovolemia is maximal. A critical concept to understanding burn shock is that massive fluid shifts occur even though total body water initially remains unchanged. What actually changes is the volume of each fluid compartment, with intracellular and interstitial volumes increasing at the expense of intravascular volume. Edema formation is inevitable and is undoubtedly accentuated by the resuscitation process.[84]

Many careers and lifetimes have been devoted to studying burn shock resuscitation, resulting in unquestionably significant advancements in burn care. Multiple resuscitation formulas, employing various solutions at different volumes and rates, have evolved from that research (see Table 7-1). However, neither the National Institutes of Health (NIH) in 1978 nor ABA in 2001 has been able to provide consensus or evidence-based guidelines demonstrating the superiority of one formula over another for burn shock resuscitation. Nonetheless, accepted recommendations continue to be that resuscitation should proceed in a manner sufficient to maintain end-organ perfusion and abrogate electrolyte disturbances, while being flexible and amenable to individual patient differences, regardless of the composition, volume, or infusion rate of the solution employed.[85]

Crystalloid Resuscitation

Crystalloid, in particular lactated Ringer's solution (LR) with a sodium concentration of 130 mEq/L, is by far the most extensively used resuscitation fluid.[86] It is the recommended resuscitation solution of both the ACS-COT and the ABA. Proponents of crystalloid resuscitation argue that colloids are no better, and are certainly more expensive, than crystalloid for maintaining intravascular volume initially after thermal injury. This argument is predicated upon the observation that even large proteins, on the order of 300 kd, leak from capillaries for approximately 24 hours after thermal injury;[87] hence any theoretical advantage of colloids is negated. This is supported by the lack of clinical effect, and potential detriment, found when using colloid in the only prospective randomized clinical trial of crystalloid vs. colloid in burn resuscitation.[88]

The quantity of crystalloid needed for adequate resuscitation is dependent on the monitoring parameters. If a urinary output of 0.5 mL/kg of body weight per hour represents adequate end-organ perfusion, approximately 3 mL/kg for each percent TBSA burned will be needed in the first 24 hours. However, if 1 mL/kg or more body weight per hour is optimal, considerably more fluid will be needed, with more edema resulting. The Parkland formula recommends 4 mL LR/kg for each percent TBSA burned over the first 24 hours, with one half of that amount administered in the first 8 hours, and the remaining half over the next 16 hours[89] (see Table 7-1). The modified Brooke Army Hospital formula recommends 2 mL LR/kg per percent TBSA burned over the first 24 hours (see

Table 7-1). In major burns, hypoproteinemia, and in particular hypoalbuminemia, invariably develops as a consequence of the acute phase response. Whether crystalloid resuscitation exacerbates hypoalbuminemia, and the clinical relevance thereof, remains to be elucidated. Nonetheless, it appears that crystalloid resuscitation may lead to greater edema formation than other regimens, but again the clinical relevance of this is uncertain.

Colloid Resuscitation

Plasma proteins generate the inward oncotic force that counteracts the outward intravascular hydrostatic force, as dictated by Starling's law of the capillaries. Without protein, intravascular volume could not be maintained. Protein replacement was an integral component of early formulas for burn resuscitation. The Evans formula uses 1 mL/kg body weight per percent TBSA burned each for colloid and crystalloid over the first 24 hours (see Table 7-1). In the original Brooke Army Hospital formula, 0.5 mL/kg per percent TBSA burned was administered as colloid and 1.5 mL/kg per percent TBSA burned as crystalloid (see Table 7-1). Considerable confusion and some controversy exist concerning the role of protein, specifically albumin, in burn shock resuscitation. There are three approaches:

1. Protein solutions are not given in the first 24 hours because during this period they are no more effective than crystalloid in maintaining intravascular volume.
2. Proteins, specifically albumin, should be given from the beginning of resuscitation with crystalloid.
3. Protein should not be given between 8 to 12 hours postburn because of the massive fluid shifts during this period, after which they should be used.

Multiple colloid solutions are available, each with specific effects, risks, and benefits. Heat-fixed plasma protein solutions (e.g., Plasmanate) contain denatured and aggregated protein fractions, which diminish their overall oncotic effect. Albumin solutions and hetastarch, a synthetic polysaccharide colloid, are similar in their oncotic activity. Fresh frozen plasma (FFP) contains all the protein fractions that exert oncotic and nononcotic functions. The optimal amount of protein/colloid for burn shock resuscitation, if any, remains undefined.

Albumin is the principal colloid used clinically and reported in studies. More recently, FFP (75 mL/kg per 24 hours) combined with LR solution (2 L/24 h) was studied during burn shock[90] (see Table 7-1). The estimated volume of FFP is calculated, but the actual volume infused is titrated to maintain an adequate urine output. The authors espouse the use of FFP to decrease resuscitation volumes, limit weight gain, and reduce edema; however, no clinically meaningful benefit or difference was realized with the use of FFP.

Many burn centers use some form of colloid at some point during burn shock resuscitation, but without supporting level I data. In fact, as mentioned previously, level I data exist to the contrary. Nonetheless, it does appear that albumin is not associated with increased mortality when used in burn resuscitation.[91]

Hypertonic Saline

The resuscitation of burn patients with a salt solution of 240 to 300 mEq/L of sodium, rather than LR, was conceived as a means to reduce edema (owing to the smaller total fluid requirements) while ensuring perfusion. Various approaches using hypertonic solutions have been proposed (see Table 7-1). Physiologically, a shift of intracellular water into the extracellular space occurs as the result of the hypertonic-hyperosmolar solution. Thus, extracellular fluid increases as intracellular fluid decreases, giving the appearance of less edema. Several studies have reported that this intracellular water depletion is apparently not detrimental, but the concept remains controversial. Current recommendations are that the serum sodium levels should not exceed 160 mEq/dL. Initial animal models and nonrandomized clinical trials appeared to substantiate this approach. However, two recent prospective randomized clinical trials and a systematic review failed to demonstrate any benefit to hypertonic saline resuscitation.[92–94] In fact, Bortolani and Barisoni found increased mortality with hypertonic saline in the more severely burned patients they studied.[93] Hypertonic resuscitation may prove beneficial to selected burn patients; however, this subset of patients has not been defined, and currently hypertonic saline resuscitation remains experimental.

Dextran

Dextran is a colloid consisting of glucose molecules that have been polymerized into chains to form high-molecular-weight polysaccharides. This compound is available commercially in a number of molecular sizes. Dextran with an average molecular weight of 40 kd is referred to as low molecular weight dextran (LMWD). Dextran is excreted by the kidneys, with approximately 40% being removed within 24 hours and the remainder slowly metabolized. Demling and associates used dextran 70 and LMWD in ovine models to limit edema in nonburned tissues.[95,96] Dextran 70 prevented edema formation, but was associated with increased protein losses from burned tissue. LMWD improved microcirculatory flow by decreasing red blood cell aggregation, and the net fluid requirements with LMWD were about half those noted with LR solution alone. Thus, they proposed a resuscitation formula employing LMWD in saline, LR, and FFP as outlined in Table 7-1. Finally, in a prospective randomized trial, dextran 70 offered no benefit over crystalloid resuscitation with LR.[97] Dextran is not currently used for burn resuscitation.

Special Considerations in Burn Shock Resuscitation

Pediatric Fluid Resuscitation. The burned child represents a special challenge, as resuscitation must be much more precise than that for an adult with a similar burn.[98] Children weighing less than 20 kg have limited physiologic reserves, especially with respect to glucose. As such, most smaller children, and particularly those weighing less than 20 kg, require the addition of glucose-based maintenance fluids to the calculated resuscitation volumes, or profound hypoglycemia will ensue owing to minimal glycogen reserves. Maintenance fluids may be administered intravenously using a dextrose-balanced salt solution or as enteral feeds. Children require relatively more fluid on a per kilogram basis for burn shock resuscitation than adults, with resuscitation fluid requirements for children averaging approximately 6 mL/kg per percent TBSA of burn.[99] This is most likely reflective of the near twofold increase in urine output (1.0 to 1.5 mL/kg body weight per hour) required to ensure adequate end-organ perfusion in children. Nonetheless, general resuscitation formulas, excluding maintenance fluid therapy, are similar for children and adults, but children commonly require formal resuscitation for relatively small burns of 10 to 20% TBSA. Thus, the TBSA threshold for burn center referral of children is lower than that for adults.

Inhalation Injury. Inhalation injury undoubtedly increases the fluid requirements for successful resuscitation following thermal injury. Patients with documented inhalation injury require approximately 1.5 times the resuscitation volumes compared to patients without inhalation injury.[100] Inhalation injury accompanying thermal trauma increases the magnitude of the total body injury via disproportionate increases in systemic inflammation.

Invasive Hemodynamic Monitoring. The use of pulmonary artery catheters (PACs), with or without goal-directed therapy, has not typically been part of burn shock resuscitation. Nonetheless, certain patients may benefit from invasive hemodynamic monitoring to try and precisely direct their resuscitation. It is generally accepted that patients with known significant premorbid cardiac or pulmonary disease, associated inhalation injury, or concomitant nonthermal trauma, as well as the elderly might require PAC monitoring during burn resuscitation. Goal-directed, hemodynamic resuscitation in burn patients has met with mixed results.[101,102] As in trauma and surgical critical care patients, it is likely that attainment of hemodynamic goals merely represents sufficient physiologic reserve to survive the injury, and not specific salutary effects of the therapy.[103] In fact, hemodynamic resuscitation of burn shock is universally associated with substantially increased fluid volumes and predisposes to complications of overresuscitation.

Overresuscitation. Failure to institute appropriate early fluid resuscitation following thermal injury is associated with substantially worse outcomes. With modern burn care in the United States, this has become the rare exception, excluding international transfers from developing countries. In fact, many burn patients may actually be overresuscitated.[104] Specific complications have emerged that appear to only be attributable to excessive resuscitation. Prior to the early 1990s, abdominal compartment syndrome (ACS) was virtually unheard of following thermal injury. Reports and studies of ACS have increasingly appeared in the literature since that time, and it is now discussed as if it is an uncommon, but well recognized, and accepted, consequence of thermal trauma.[105–108] However, this begs the question, "If ACS is a typical consequence of major thermal injury resuscitation, then why was it not described prior to the 1990s?" ACS is preventable and iatrogenic in the vast majority of patients, owing to injudicious resuscitation. However, there is a small minority of patients in whom overwhelming volumes (>1.5 times predicted volume) are required, for as yet unclear reasons, to ensure successful resuscitation. In our experience with these select patients, plasmapheresis (i.e., plasma exchange therapy) has emerged as a useful resuscitation adjunct to minimize further fluid requirements once a patient has demonstrated refractoriness to standard resuscitation. Tanaka and colleagues reported the successful use of high-dose (66 mg/kg per hour for 24 hours) intravenous vitamin C to reduce resuscitation volumes in patients sustaining major burns, with an apparent decrease in edema-related complications and mechanical ventilation times.[109] Early and *appropriate* resuscitation following major thermal injury is of paramount importance to ensure a good outcome; however, overresuscitation may produce complications that nullify the gains.

Choice of Fluids and Rate of Administration

All of the solutions reviewed are effective in restoring tissue perfusion. Most patients can be resuscitated with crystalloid, specifically lactated Ringer's solution. Normal saline should be avoided, as the volumes required for resuscitation invariably lead to a complicating hyperchloremic metabolic acidosis. In patients with massive burns, young children, and burns complicated by severe inhalation injury, a combination of fluids can be used to achieve the desired goal of end-organ perfusion while minimizing edema.

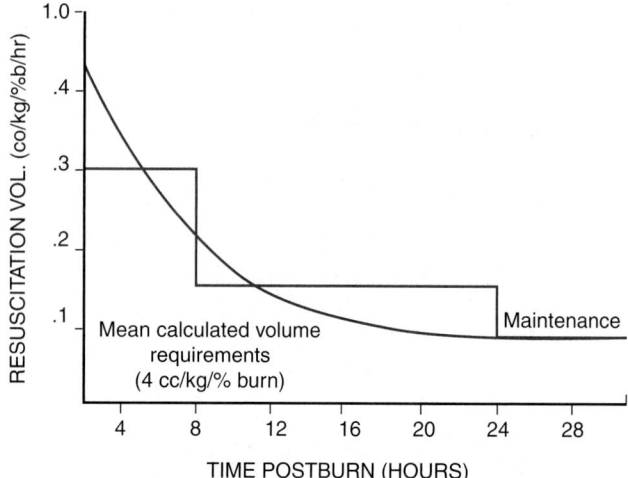

FIG. 7-2. Physiologic curve of fluid requirements compared with the Parkland formula for calculating postburn fluid replacement.

Resuscitation formulas should only be considered general guidelines for burn shock resuscitation. The Parkland formula, for instance, decreases the volume administered by 50% at 8 hours postburn. The relationship between volume required and time postburn, depicted by the smooth curve in Fig.7-2, represents the influence of temporal changes in microvascular permeability and edema formation on fluid requirements. The gentle changes depicted by the curve are in sharp contrast with the abrupt changes in the fluid infusion rate prescribed by the Parkland formula. Ultimately, the volume and rate of infused fluid should maintain a urine output of 30 mL/h in adults (~0.5 mL/kg per hour), with lower limits acceptable in the face of known renal insufficiency, and 1.0 to 1.5 mL/kg per hour in children.

Resuscitation is considered successful when there is no further accumulation of edema, usually between 18 and 24 hours postburn, and the volume of infused fluid required to maintain adequate urine output approximates the patient's maintenance fluid volume, which is normal maintenance volume plus evaporative water loss.

Fluid Replacement Following Burn Shock Resuscitation

The injured microvasculature may manifest increased permeability for several days following successful resuscitation, but the rate of fluid loss is considerably less than that seen in the first 24 hours.[110] Burn edema formation at 24 hours postburn is nearly maximal, and the interstitial space may well be saturated. Additional fluid requirements depend on the type of fluid used during the initial resuscitation. If hypertonic saline resuscitation was used, a hyperosmolar state results, and the addition of free water is required to restore isosmolarity.

If colloid was not used during resuscitation and the serum oncotic pressure is low because of intravascular protein depletion/dilution, supplementation may be needed. Protein supplementation requirements vary with the resuscitation used. The Brooke formula proposes 0.3 to 0.5 mL/kg per percent TBSA burned of 5% albumin during the second 24 hours postburn. The Parkland formula replaces the remaining plasma volume deficit, which varies from 20 to 60% of the total circulating plasma volume, with colloid. Colloid replacement should be used sparingly, in the form of albumin, and only after 24 hours postburn.

Regardless of whether colloid is used or not, patients should receive appropriate maintenance fluids. The total daily maintenance fluid requirement in the adult patient is calculated by the following formula, where m^2 is square meters of TBSA:

Total maintenance fluid $= (1500 \text{ mL/m}^2)$
$+$ evaporative water loss $[(25 + \% \text{ TBSA burn}) \times m^2 \times 24]$

This fluid may be given intravenously or enterally. A general guideline is that a patient will require approximately 1.5 times their normal maintenance fluids following successful resuscitation from a major thermal injury. The solution infused intravenously should be one half normal saline with potassium supplements. Because of the loss of intracellular potassium during burn shock, the potassium requirement in adults with normal renal function is approximately 120 mEq/d.

After initial resuscitation, urine output alone is an unreliable guide to sufficient hydration. Respiratory water losses, osmotic diuresis secondary to hyperglycemia, high-protein/high-calorie enteral nutrition, and derangements in antidiuretic hormone (ADH) mechanisms contribute to increased fluid losses despite apparently adequate urine output. Adult patients with major thermal injuries require a urine output of approximately 1000 to 1500 mL/24 h; children require approximately 3 to 4 mL/kg per hour averaged over 24 hours. The measurement of serum sodium concentration is not only a means of diagnosing dehydration, but is a good guide for estimating and managing ongoing fluid replacement. Other useful indices of the state of hydration include body weight change, fractional excretion of sodium (FENa), serum and urine nitrogen concentrations, serum and urine glucose concentrations, the intake and output record, and clinical examination. Serum electrolytes, calcium, magnesium, and phosphate levels should also be monitored and maintained within normal limits.

INHALATION INJURY

Of some 45,000 fire victims admitted to hospitals each year, approximately 30% sustain smoke or thermal damage to the respiratory tree. Carbon monoxide (CO) poisoning, thermal injury, and smoke inhalation are three distinct aspects of clinical inhalation injury. Although the symptoms and treatment of each vary, the distinct injuries may coexist and require concomitant treatment.

Carbon Monoxide Poisoning

The majority of house fire deaths can be attributed to CO poisoning. CO is a colorless, odorless, and tasteless gas with an affinity for hemoglobin (Hb) approximately 200 times that of oxygen. When inhaled and absorbed, CO binds to Hb to form carboxyhemoglobin (COHb). COHb interferes with oxygen delivery to the tissues by at least five mechanisms. First, it prevents reversible displacement of oxygen on the Hb molecule. Second, COHb shifts the oxygen-Hb dissociation curve to the left, thereby decreasing oxygen unloading from normal hemoglobin at the tissue level.[111] Third, CO binds to reduced cytochrome a_3, resulting in less effective intracellular respiration.[112] Fourth, CO can bind to cardiac and skeletal muscle, resulting in direct toxicity.[113] Finally, CO can act in the central nervous system in a poorly understood fashion, causing demyelination and associated neurologic symptoms.[114]

Levels of COHb are easily measured, but the degree of impairment may not directly correlate with blood levels of COHb.[115] Levels less than 10% typically do not cause symptoms. At a COHb level of approximately 20%, healthy persons complain of headache, nausea, vomiting, and loss of manual dexterity. At approximately 30%, patients become weak, confused, and lethargic. In a fire, this level can be fatal because the victim loses the desire and ability to flee. At levels of 40 to 60%, the patient lapses into a coma, and levels greater than 60% are usually fatal. In very smoky fires, COHb levels of 40 to 50% can be reached after only a few minutes of exposure.

CO is reversibly bound to the heme molecules of Hb, and despite intense affinity, readily dissociates according to the laws of mass action. The half-life ($t_{1/2}$) of COHb when breathing room air is approximately 4 hours. On 100% oxygen, the $t_{1/2}$ is reduced to 45 to 60 minutes.[116] In a hyperbaric oxygen chamber at 2 atm, it is approximately 30 minutes, and at 3 atm it is about 15 to 20 minutes.

The importance of CO poisoning in victims of inhalation injury was dramatically demonstrated in the 1979 MGM Grand Hotel and 1981 Hilton Hotel fires in Las Vegas, Nevada. Although only a small number of thermal injuries occurred, 123 people died at the scene, primarily from CO poisoning. At the same time, the efficacy of prompt assessment and treatment of inhalation injury was demonstrated. Of more than 400 individuals who received hospital evaluation for inhalation injury, mortality was less than 1%, while the rate of significant complications including myocardial infarction, respiratory failure, and pneumonia was 1% each.

Diagnosis and Treatment

Patients burned in an enclosed space or having any signs or symptoms of neurologic impairment should be placed on 100% oxygen via a nonrebreather face mask while waiting for measurement of COHb levels. The use of pulse oximetry (SpO_2) to assess arterial oxygenation in the CO-poisoned patient is contraindicated, as the COHb results in erroneously elevated SpO_2 measurements.[117] If intubation is required, then hyperventilation with 100% oxygen should be instituted. The use of hyperbaric oxygen (HBO) therapy remains controversial. Early human studies of HBO therapy in acute CO poisoning produced mixed results.[118] Two recent well-designed, prospective, randomized clinical trials compared normobaric oxygen therapy to HBO therapy in patients suffering CO poisoning *without concomitant burns*.[119,120] Scheinkestel and associates from Australia demonstrated no benefit, and possible adverse consequences, of HBO on neuropsychologic outcomes following acute, severe CO poisoning.[119] Conversely, Weaver and colleagues from Salt Lake City, Utah, showed a significant improvement in cognitive outcomes with the use of HBO. It should be noted that the inclusion criteria, and particularly the HBO protocols, were different between these two studies, making comparison difficult. The question remains as to who warrants HBO therapy, under what protocol, and what will be the anticipated outcome.[121]

While HBO therapy may be innocuous in isolated CO poisoning, in the presence of concomitant burns and smoke inhalation, the rate of catastrophic complications during treatment in the hyperbaric chamber is potentially quite high.[122] Resuscitation and early enteral nutrition efforts with close monitoring, so instrumental to a good outcome with modern burn care, can be severely hampered or impossible while a patient is in the chamber. Furthermore, interfacility transport of a critically burned patient subjects them to many potential compromises in care. To date, no prospective randomized trial in patients with CO poisoning *and* thermal injury has been conducted. Thus, HBO therapy in burn patients with CO poisoning is of unknown therapeutic value or efficacy, and should only be utilized when: (1) the COHb is greater than 25%, (2) a neurologic deficit exists, (3) no formal burn resuscitation is required (typically TBSA

<10 to 15%), (4) pulmonary function is stable with an intact airway, and (5) interfacility transfer does not compromise burn care.[123]

Thermal Airway Injury

The term "pulmonary burn" is a misnomer. True thermal damage to the lower respiratory tact and pulmonary parenchyma is extremely rare, unless live steam or exploding gases are inhaled. The air temperature near the ceiling of a burning room may reach 540°C (1000°F) or more, but air has such poor heat-carrying capacity that most of the heat is dissipated in the oropharynx, nasopharynx, and upper airway. Thus the heat dissipation in the upper airway can cause significant thermal injury to the proximal tracheobronchial tree.

Thermal injury to the respiratory tract is usually immediate and manifests as mucosal and submucosal erythema, edema, hemorrhage, and ulceration.[124] Thermal injury is usually limited to the upper airway (above the vocal cords) and proximal trachea for two reasons: (1) the oropharynx and nasopharynx provide an effective mechanism for heat exchange because of their relatively large surface area, associated air turbulence, and mucosal fluid lining that acts as a heat reservoir; and (2) sudden exposure to hot air typically triggers reflex closure of the vocal cords, reducing the potential for lower airway injury. Animal models have demonstrated that significant heat exchange also occurs in the subglottic airway between the vocal cords and the tracheal bifurcation, with protection and sparing of the distal airways. Thus the lower tracheobronchial tree is rarely exposed to hot, ambient gas at a fire scene. An exception is the inhalation of super heated steam, where because of heat dissipation in the respiratory tract as the steam condenses into water, severe injury has been reported in the distal airways with measurable injury in the alveoli. In these patients the lower tracheobronchial tree is rapidly obstructed, and they usually die from untreatable asphyxiation.

Patients with the greatest risk of upper airway obstruction are those injured in an explosion, with burns of the face and upper thorax, and those who have been unconscious in a fire. Mucosal burns of the mouth, oropharynx, nasopharynx, and larynx result in edema formation and may lead to upper airway obstruction at any time following the injury, but particularly during the first 24 hours postburn. Any patient with burns of the face should have a careful examination of the mouth and pharynx, and if these are abnormal, the larynx should also be visualized immediately. Red, dry mucosa or small mucosal blisters raise the possibility of direct thermal injury and potential airway obstruction. The presence of significant intraoral and pharyngeal burns is a clear indication for immediate endotracheal intubation, as progressive edema can make later intubation extremely hazardous, if not impossible. Mucosal burns are rarely full-thickness, and can be successfully managed with good oral hygiene. Once the patient is intubated, the tube should remain in place until the edema subsides, as manifested by a vigorous cuff leak upon deflation in adults. Steroids have no place in the management of upper airway edema resulting from thermal injury.

Smoke Inhalation

A nightclub fire in Dublin, Ireland, in 1981 added a great deal to the understanding of smoke inhalation injury because the disaster site was meticulously reconstructed and the event reenacted for scientific analysis. Within minutes, visibility was reduced to less than 1 m and ambient temperatures reached 1160°C. Near the fire, dramatic changes in inhaled gas concentrations were noted: oxygen was reduced to less than 2%, CO increased to greater than 3%, hydrogen cyanide was measured at 250 ppm (it is lethal at >100 ppm), and hydrogen chloride was measured at 8500 ppm.

Hydrogen cyanide, a common product of the combustion of polyurethane and nitrogen-containing polymers, is an even more effective inhibitor of cellular respiration than CO, and also interferes with oxygen utilization at the tissue level. By inhibiting the final step of oxidative phosphorylation via reversible inhibition of cytochrome oxidase, cyanide halts aerobic metabolism, inducing lactic acidosis and cellular anoxia. Cyanide is exquisitely injurious to tissues with minimal anaerobic reserve e.g., the CNS. Combined exposure to cyanide and CO results in a rapidly fatal synergistic decrease in tissue oxygen utilization.

Hundreds of toxic products are released during combustion (flaming) or pyrolysis (smoldering), depending on the type of fuel burned, the oxygen content of the environment, and the actual temperature of burning. Some 280 toxic substances have been identified in wood smoke alone. Petrochemical science has produced a wealth of plastic materials used in homes and automobiles, that when burned, produce nearly all of these substances, and many other products not yet characterized. Prominent by-products of incomplete combustion are oxides and hydrogenated moieties of sulfur and nitrogen, as well as numerous aldehydes. One aldehyde, acrolein (from acrylics, polypropylene, and cellulose), causes severe pulmonary edema in atmospheric concentrations of 10 ppm or less.

After inhalation, highly soluble acidic and basic compounds rapidly dissolve in the water lining the mucosa of the respiratory tract, causing direct epithelial injury, manifested as epithelial edema, submucosal hemorrhage, and necrosis. Epithelial injury can occur at all levels of the respiratory tract, from oropharynx to alveolus. The anatomic level at which the damage occurs is dependent on the ventilatory pattern, the smoke composition (i.e., particulate concentration, particle size, and chemical components), and the distribution of particle deposition. Fat-soluble compounds tend to do more damage in the distal airway and alveolus. Although the chemical mechanisms of injury may be different among toxic products, the overall end-organ response is relatively homogeneous and reasonably well defined.[125,126] There is an immediate loss of bronchial epithelial cilia and decreased alveolar surfactant levels. Atelectasis results, compounded by small-airway edema, and is only slowly reversed by normal ventilation. This regional hypoventilation results in worsening atelectasis, intrapulmonary shunt, and subsequent hypoxemia.

Chemical irritation of the respiratory tract incites a localized acute inflammatory response. The initial response is an approximate 10-fold increase in bronchial blood flow. Concurrently, alveolar macrophages are stimulated and release cytokines, which activate circulating neutrophils that localize to the site of injury and release reactive oxygen species and proteases, resulting in increased pulmonary microvascular permeability. The development of airway edema, combined with the sloughing of necrotic epithelium and impairment of the mucociliary clearance of secretions, produces airway obstruction in small and large airways. The result is heterogeneous ventilation, and the mismatch between ventilation and perfusion leads to hypoxemia.

Wheezing and air hunger are common early manifestations of inhalation injury. The pulmonary parenchymal damage associated with inhalation injury appears to be dose dependent.[127] Within a few hours, tracheobronchial epithelium sloughs, and a hemorrhagic tracheobronchitis develops. Ongoing neutrophil activation leads to further pulmonary endothelial disruption; concomitantly, pulmonary lymph flow increases, with both enhancing pulmonary edema. In severe cases, the hemorrhagic tracheobronchitis and airway plugging result in extreme ventilation deficits, and patients succumb to a severe respiratory acidosis because of their inability to clear CO_2. In other cases, particularly those associated with thermal injury, interstitial edema becomes most prominent, resulting in acute respiratory distress syndrome (ARDS) and oxygenation difficulties.

Concomitant cutaneous thermal injury results in the systemic release of inflammatory mediators, including prostaglandins and reactive oxygen intermediates (ROIs) that can aggravate pulmonary injury independent of smoke inhalation.[128] In particular, thromboxane-A_2 released from burned tissue causes a variety of changes in the lung, including pulmonary hypertension, reduced dynamic compliance, and increased lipid peroxidation. ROIs generated as a consequence of neutrophil activation and increases in xanthine oxidase contribute to lung injury. Decreased plasma oncotic pressure, from the loss of plasma proteins via increased microvascular permeability in both burned and unburned tissue, creates an abnormal pressure gradient in the pulmonary circulation that results in pulmonary edema. These changes help explain the degree of synergy in cases of combined inhalation and burn injuries.

Early in the course of inhalation injury, pulmonary function is variable.[129] Classically, decreased functional residual capacity (FRC), decreased vital capacity, and evidence of obstructive disease with reduction in flow rates, an increase in dead space, and a rapid decrease in compliance occur. Much of the variability in pulmonary response appears to be related more to the severity of the associated cutaneous burn than to the degree of smoke inhalation.

Without associated cutaneous thermal injury, the mortality from isolated inhalation injury is quite low. The disease rarely progresses to ARDS, and symptomatic treatment usually leads to complete resolution of symptoms in a few days. However, in the presence of burns, inhalation injury approximately doubles the mortality rate from burns of any size. Pulmonary symptoms are usually present on admission, but they may be delayed for 12 to 24 hours following injury.

Diagnosis

The incidence of smoke inhalation injury in victims of fire varies with diagnostic criteria.[130] The incidence may be as low as 2 to 15% when single or restrictive criteria based on history and physical examination are used, but as high as 30% when based on objective tests such as fiberoptic bronchoscopy (FOB). The overall incidence of smoke inhalation in the United States has fallen over the past 3 decades, primarily because of the use of home smoke detectors.

Anyone with a flame burn sustained in an enclosed space should be assumed to have an inhalation injury until proved otherwise. The acrid smell of smoke on the victim's clothes should raise immediate suspicion. In obtaining a history, emphasis should be placed on findings specific to the smoke exposure and to the type of therapy instituted prior to hospitalization. When exposure occurs in a closed space, such as a building or an automobile, the smoke is less diluted by ambient air, resulting in greater pulmonary exposure to CO and other smoke constituents than in an open-space exposure. The duration of exposure correlates with the severity of lung injury.

A thorough examination should be performed and include evaluation of the face and oropharyngeal airway for hoarseness, stridor, edema, or soot impaction suggesting injury; chest auscultation for wheezing or rhonchi suggesting injury to distal airways; level of consciousness associated with decreased with hypoxemia, CO poisoning, or cyanide poisoning; and testing for the presence of neurologic deficits associated with CO. Copious mucus production and carbonaceous *expectorated* sputum are hard signs of inhalation injury, but their absence does not rule out injury. COHb levels should be obtained; an elevated COHb or any symptoms of CO poisoning are presumptive evidence of associated smoke inhalation.

Anyone suspected of smoke inhalation should have an arterial blood gas drawn. One of the earliest indicators of injury is a decreased P:F ratio, the ratio of arterial oxygen pressure (Pao_2) to inspired oxygen as assessed by pulse oximetry (Fio_2). A ratio of about 400 is normal; patients with impending pulmonary problems have a ratio of less than 300 (e.g., a Pao_2 of <150 with an Fio_2 of 0.50). A P:F ratio less than 250 is an indication for vigorous pulmonary therapy and intubation, not an indication for merely increasing the Fio_2. A P:F ratio less than 200 defines ARDS.

The early need for bronchoscopic evaluation and diagnosis remains controversial. Some recommend the routine use of FOB, noting that it is inexpensive, quickly performed in experienced hands, and is highly useful in assessing airway injury, if not the gold standard.[130–132] However, aside from documenting the presence of edema, tracheal erythema, and/or carbon deposits, FOB does not materially influence the treatment of smoke inhalation. It is operator-dependent and not risk-free. In addition, yield with FOB appears to be strongly dependent upon clinical suspicion (i.e., pretest probability) of inhalation injury. Given these limitations, it is recommended that a history, physical examination, and laboratory studies be used to make the diagnosis of inhalation injury, and the use of FOB be reserved for exceptional cases requiring therapeutic FOB (e.g., expansion of lobar collapse or removal of obstructing intrabronchial secretions or casts).

Treatment

Upper Airway. No standard treatment has evolved to ensure survival after smoke inhalation. In the presence of increasing oropharyngeal and laryngeal edema, rapid endotracheal intubation is indicated. A tracheostomy is never an emergency procedure and should not be used as the initial step in airway management, especially in patients with burns to the face and neck. Instead, a soft-cuffed endotracheal tube should be inserted and left in place until the edema subsides. An adult patient's ability to breathe around the tube with the cuff deflated is an indication for removal of the tube. This assessment is difficult in children due to their smaller anatomy, the use of uncuffed endotracheal tubes, the increased incidence of postextubation stridor, and the frequent need for reintubation.[133] The incidence of postextubation stridor in burn victims is as high as 47%, compared to 4% in elective surgical patients. The treatment of postextubation stridor includes the administration of nebulized racemic epinephrine and helium-oxygen (heliox) mixtures.[134] Steroids are never used.

Lower Airway and Alveoli. Tracheobronchitis, commonly seen with inhalation injury, produces wheezing, coughing, and retained secretions. The ventilation-perfusion mismatch present in these patients can result in mild to moderate hypoxemia, varying with the degree of premorbid lung disease; therefore supplemental oxygen should be administered routinely. Increased airway resistance is more often the result of edema and retained secretions than true bronchospasm. Although a trial of bronchodilators is indicated in those patients with premorbid bronchospastic disease, the overall efficacy is questionable. Inhaled beta$_2$ agonists, racemic epinephrine, terbutaline, or theophylline are used most commonly.

The usual presenting sign of distal airway injury is hypoxemia, diagnosed by pulse oximetry or arterial blood gas. Because most inhalation victims receive supplemental oxygen, significant alveolar-arterial oxygen gradients can be missed by pulse oximetry; an Spo_2 less than 95% does not occur until the Pao_2 is less than 80 mm Hg. Arterial blood gas analysis is the monitoring modality of choice in assessing oxygenation after inhalation injury. Remember

that COHb can erroneously elevate Spo_2. Initial therapy should always include the administration of high-flow oxygen, to augment systemic oxygenation and reduce COHb in cases of CO poisoning. Upper airway patency absolutely must be assured, and airway resistance minimized with chest physiotherapy and/or bronchodilators. Central hypoventilation caused by CO or cyanide poisoning should be treated immediately as previously described.

Overall treatment for smoke inhalation is supportive, with the goal being maintenance of adequate oxygenation and ventilation until the lungs heal. Mild cases are treated with humidified oxygen, vigorous pulmonary toilet, and bronchodilators as needed. The need for mechanical ventilation is determined by repeated blood gas measurements demonstrating refractory hypoxemia. Because of the frequent presence of atelectasis after alveolar exposure to smoke, positive end-expiratory pressure (PEEP) can be quite useful in recruiting atelectatic regions and increasing FRC, thus increasing oxygenation. Ventilator tidal volumes should be chosen so that plateau pressures are consistently less than 35 cm H_2O, typically achieved with about 6 mL/kg ideal body weight, in order to limit barotrauma. The precise mode of initial mechanical ventilation appears less important than ensuring a lung protective strategy.

High-frequency percussive ventilation (HFPV) has been utilized in burn patients with inhalation injury. HFPV appears to provide superior oxygenation at a lower Fio_2, with lower airway pressures than conventional mechanical ventilation (CMV). Initial small cohort studies of HFPV in both adults and children appeared promising, with decreased pneumonia and mortality rates, improved gas exchange and pulmonary mechanics, and minimal barotrauma with virtually no reported adverse effects.[131,135–138] Many hypothesized that the benefits of HFPV were apparently due to enhanced clearance of bronchial secretions. However, in the only prospective randomized controlled trial of HFPV compared to CMV in inhalation injury, HFPV only improved the P:F ratio during the first 3 days, without any difference in the other variables measured, including pneumonia and mortality.[139] The management and outcome of inhalation injury need to be prospectively examined using modern lung protective ventilation strategies; where HFPV will fit into a modern approach remains to be seen.

Other reported adjuncts to appropriate mechanical ventilation for inhalation injury are: intrabronchial surfactant administration, aerosolized heparin/acetylcysteine, and extracorporeal membrane oxygenation when all else fails.[140–144] Results are encouraging, but the treatments remain experimental at this time.

Elective tracheostomy in burn patients remains controversial. Nonetheless, if the upper airway is in danger of imminent obstruction and endotracheal intubation attempts are unsuccessful, emergent cricothyroidotomy is indicated, with conversion to a formal tracheostomy soon thereafter. The indications for nonemergent tracheostomy have changed over the last 2 decades. After a period in the 1970s, when tracheostomy was the standard method of securing the upper airway after severe burn injury, several reports associated the procedure with mortality rates ranging from 50 to 100%, due to a greater incidence of overwhelming pulmonary infection. Improvements in endotracheal tube construction resulted in specific efforts to avoid tracheostomy in burn patients during the 1980s. Currently, mortality rates, infectious complications, and airway sequelae in adult and pediatric burn patients with tracheostomy are no different from patients treated with long-term endotracheal tubes.[145–149] For patients requiring prolonged endotracheal intubation, tracheostomy should be performed at the discretion of the managing burn surgeon. There is no outcome benefit to early tracheostomy in burn patients.[150] Patients with anterior neck burns who require tracheostomy should undergo successful excision and grafting of the area prior to creation of the stoma. This minimizes pulmonary and burn wound infectious complications associated with the tracheostomy.

Prophylactic antibiotics are *not* indicated with inhalation injury, which is a chemical pneumonitis.[130] Subsequent burn wound management and treatment of eventual bacterial pneumonia may be made more difficult with the early use of antibiotics, as it rapidly leads to the selection of resistant organisms.[151] Likewise, steroids are *contraindicated* with inhalation injury, although their anti-inflammatory actions were originally thought to be helpful. In a prospective, randomized, controlled, blinded study of patients with inhalation injury and major burns, those treated with steroids experienced a higher mortality rate and more septic complications than controls not treated with steroids.[152]

WOUND MANAGEMENT

Early Excision and Grafting

For many years, burns were treated by daily washing (tanking), removal of loose dead tissue, and topical application of saline-soaked dressings until the burns healed primarily or granulation tissue appeared in the base of the wound. Epidermal and superficial partial-thickness burns healed within 3 weeks, and full-thickness burns healed over many weeks if infection was prevented. Full-thickness burns lost their eschar in 2 to 6 weeks via bacterial collagenase production and daily mechanical débridements. When the granulating bed became free of debris and relatively uninfected, split-thickness skin grafts (STSGs) were applied, usually some 3 to 8 weeks after injury. A 50% graft take was considered acceptable. Repeated graftings eventually closed the wound. The prolonged and intense inflammatory response with this method made hypertrophic scarring and contractures part of normal burn treatment. Vigorous physical therapy, nutritional support, psychologic support, and pain management were required daily for many weeks to yield a satisfactory result.

Fortunately, this is no longer standard procedure. For deeper burns (i.e., deep partial-thickness and full-thickness burns), rather than waiting for spontaneous separation, the eschar is surgically removed and the wound closed via grafting techniques and/or immediate flap procedures tailored to the individual patient. This aggressive surgical approach to burn wound management has become known as early excision and grafting (E&G). Several technical advances have made this possible, including a safer autologous blood supply, better monitoring equipment and methods, and a better understanding of the deranged physiology of patients with major burns. The ability to stabilize the patient within a few days of the injury has enabled the surgeon to remove deep burn wounds before invasive infection occurs. The optimal timing of early E&G has yet to be definitively determined; however, E&G within 3 to 7 days, and certainly by 10 days, following injury appears prudent. An aggressive surgical approach to large and small burns has produced a number of major advancements. In fact, early E&G has reduced burn mortality more than any other intervention (Fig. 7-3). Early wound closure also reduces hospital stay, duration of illness, septic complications, and the need for major reconstruction, while decreasing hospital costs.[44,153–155] Early studies did not demonstrate dramatic differences in cosmetic or functional results, but as surgeons have become more experienced with early E&G, both improved function and appearance have resulted. This is particularly true with burns of the face, hands, and feet.[156–165]

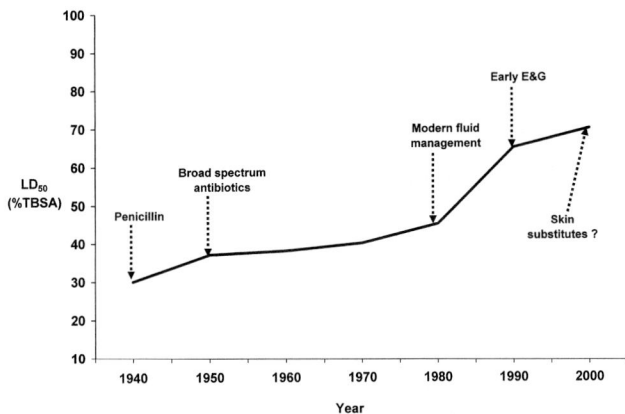

FIG. 7-3. Effects of various interventions upon 50% mortality rate (LD$_{50}$) in burn patients over time.

Current Status of Wound Care

Solid clinical and experimental evidence support the following conclusions:

1. Small (i.e., <20%) full-thickness burns and burns of indeterminate depth, if treated by an experienced surgeon, can be safely excised and grafted with a decrease in hospital stay, costs, and time away from work or school.
2. Early E&G dramatically decreases the number of painful débridements required.
3. Patients with burns of 20 to 40% TBSA will have fewer infectious wound complications if treated with early E&G.
4. In animal models, the immunosuppression and hypermetabolism associated with burns can be ameliorated by early burn wound removal.

Clinical impressions, without hard data supporting them, include the following:

1. Scarring is less severe in wounds closed early, leading to better appearance and fewer reconstructive procedures. There is no good measure of "acceptable" cosmetic appearance, and comparative studies await a consistent scale to measure results.
2. Mortality from wound infection is lower in patients with major burns after early excision. Because wounds exceeding donor skin availability cannot be closed completely until donor sites can be reharvested, definitive proof will come only when a durable permanent covering (i.e., skin substitute) can be applied in a timely fashion.
3. Mortality from other complications of major burns may be lower with early E&G. Ameliorating the stress, hypermetabolism, and overall bacterial load of the patients enables them to resist other complications. The only data to support this conclusion come from animal studies.

Technical Considerations

Excision of greater than 10% of TBSA should be done in a highly structured environment, preferably a dedicated burn center. Without tourniquets and/or topical hemostatic agents, blood loss can be massive, and graft loss can be catastrophic. Excellent monitoring, nursing, physical therapy, nutritional support, anesthesia, and 24-hour physician coverage are mandatory. Smaller burns in important areas (e.g., hands, face, and feet) also require considerable experience.

Excisional procedures should be performed as early as possible after the patient is stabilized, usually within a week of injury. This allows the wound to be closed before infection occurs, and in extensive burns, allows donor sites to be re-cropped as soon as possible. Cosmetic results are better if the wound can be excised and grafted before the intense inflammatory response becomes well established. Any burn projected to take longer than 3 weeks to heal is a candidate for excision within the first postburn week. Wound excision is adaptable to all age groups, but infants, small children, and elderly patients require close perioperative monitoring.

Excision can be performed to include the burn and subcutaneous fat to the level of the investing fascia (fascial excision), or by tangentially removing thin slices of burned tissue until a viable bed remains (tangential excision). Fascial excision assures a viable bed for grafting, but takes longer, sacrifices potentially viable tissue, and leaves a permanent cosmetic defect. Tangential excision can create massive blood loss and risks grafting on a bed of uncertain viability, but sacrifices minimal living tissue, and leads to a superior cosmetic result. Fascial excisions are typically reserved for deeper burns; however, they can be useful in selected patients with large full-thickness burns involving only the superficial subcutaneous fat. Subcutaneous fat in older burn patients (i.e., age >60 years) does not readily support skin grafts well. Therefore, in these authors' experience, more fascial excisions are being performed with the immediate application of INTEGRA and subsequent grafting in such patients.[166]

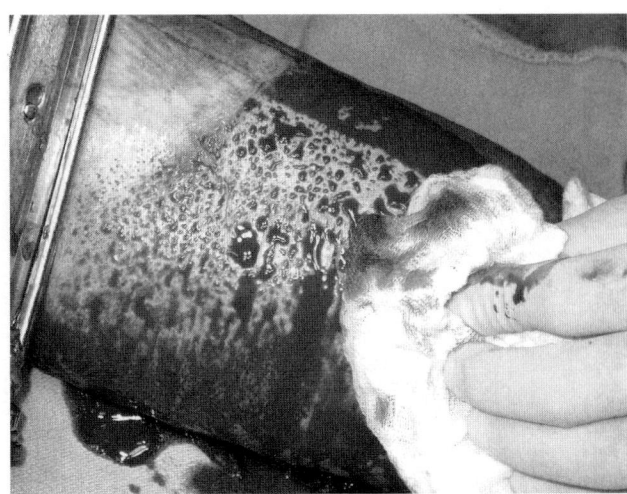

FIG. 7-5. *Healthy, viable wound bed with brisk bleeding following tangential excision.*

Tangential (Sequential) Excision

The principle of tangential excision is to excise layers of eschar at a tangential angle to the surface until viable tissue is reached. The burn can be removed with a variety of instruments, usually hand dermatomes (Fig. 7-4). Relatively shallow burns and some burns of moderate depth will bleed briskly from thousands of capillaries after one slice. If the bed does not bleed briskly, another slice of the same depth is taken until a viable bed of dermis or subcutaneous fat is reached with resultant brisk bleeding (Fig. 7-5). If inspection of the dermal bed reveals a surface that appears gray or dull rather than white and shiny, or if there are thrombosed vessels, the excision should be carried deeper. Any fat that has a brownish discoloration, petechial appearance, or contains thrombosed blood vessels will not support a graft, and must be excised until the bed contains uniformly yellow fat with briskly bleeding vessels. Bleeding is controlled with sponges soaked in 1:10,000 epinephrine solution applied to the excision bed. Continued bleeding is then controlled with judicious electrocautery. Major bleeding is rare, and when it occurs, it invariably is associated with inadequate cauterization of a vessel with pulsatile flow.

Areas on the extremities may be excised under tourniquet; however, this requires experience. The cadaveric appearance of the dermis and the lack of brisk bleeding with the tourniquet inflated can easily mislead the surgeon into sacrificing normal tissue by carrying the excision deeper than necessary.

Fascial Excision

Fascial excision is typically reserved for patients with deep full-thickness burns, or with large, life-threatening full-thickness burns (Fig. 7-6). The most common technique uses electrocautery with cutting and coagulating capabilities.

The advantages of fascial excision include:

1. It results in a reliable bed of known viability.
2. Tourniquets can routinely be used for extremities.
3. Operative blood loss is less than with tangential excision.
4. Less experience is required to ensure an optimal bed.

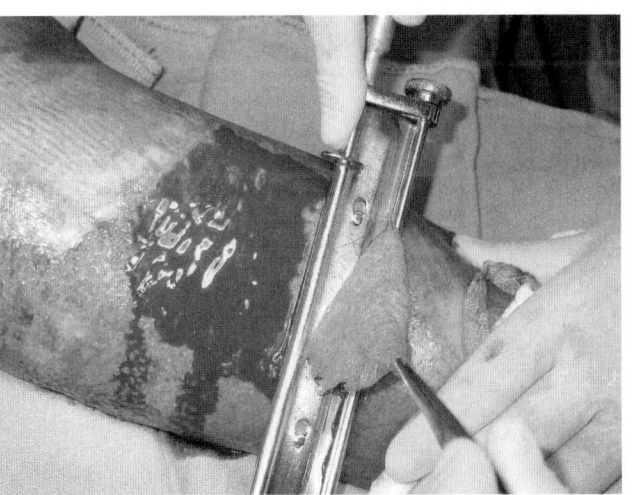

A

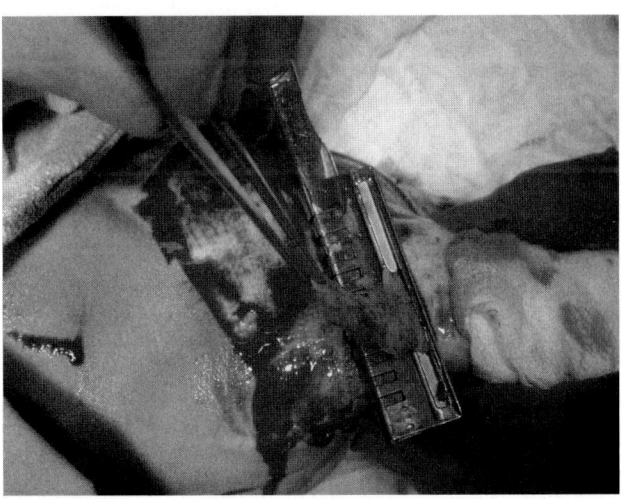

B

FIG. 7-4. *Tangential excisions using (A) Watson, and (B) Goulian knives.*

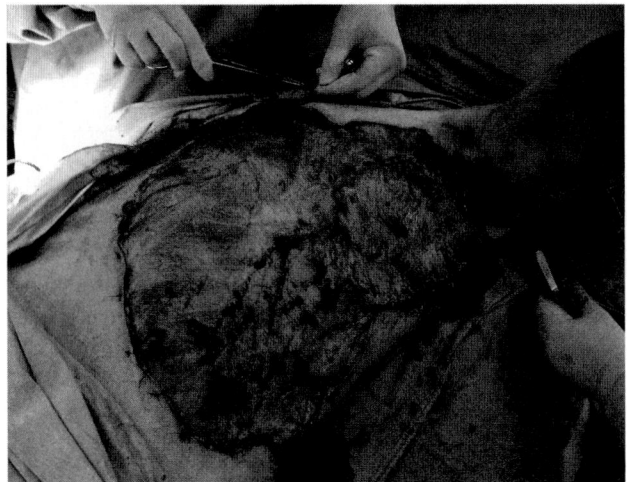

FIG. 7-6. *Fascial excision wound bed. Note tacking sutures along the edges to minimize the appearance of the defect.*

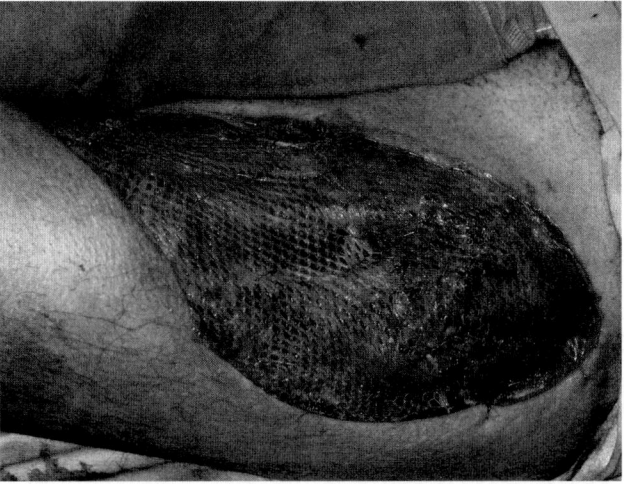

FIG. 7-7. *Typical appearance of meshed split-thickness skin graft secured with staples.*

The disadvantages include:

1. Longer operative times.
2. The possibility of severe cosmetic deformity, especially in obese patients.
3. There is a higher incidence of distal edema when the excision is circumferential.
4. There is greater danger of damage to superficial neuromuscular structures.
5. Cutaneous denervation, which may or may not be permanent, occurs.
6. Skin graft loss from the relatively less vascular fascia over joints (especially the elbow, knee, or ankle) can lead to an ungraftable bed and require eventual flap coverage.

Early Reconstruction

A potential advantage to E&G is to provide a closed wound before the localized intense cutaneous, and subsequently systemic, inflammatory response is maximal. If careful attention is given to sound principles of plastic surgery, the risk that there will be a need for subsequent reconstruction can be decreased. Graft junctures should be avoided over joints, and grafts should be placed transversely when possible. Thick STSGs (e.g., >0.015 inch) typically yield a better appearance than do thin grafts (e.g., ≤0.010 inch). If the burn is well excised, and the skin can be spared, thick grafts should be used on the face, neck, and other cosmetically important areas, with hands being an exception.[160] The resultant donor sites from the thick STSGs can be overgrafted with very thin STSGs (e.g., ≤0.008 inch) if needed, to minimize hypertrophic scarring of the donor site. Typically in larger burns (>20% TBSA), STSGs are meshed to allow greater wound coverage per graft (Fig. 7-7). This is particularly important when donor sites are limited. However, if at all possible, cosmetically important areas should be grafted with a single sheet of STSG (Fig. 7-8). Although meshed STSGs provide coverage with excellent function, the meshed pattern will persist as a permanent reminder of the burn (Fig. 7-9).

Adjacent pieces of STSG should be approximated carefully with a small amount of overlap. While staples are adequate for securing most grafts, cosmetically critical areas, such as the face, should be sutured. Hypafix, a porous, elastic, and adherent dressing material, is another option for securing STSGs (Fig. 7-10). Commercially-available fibrin glues are another atraumatic means to affix STSGs. Initial studies are promising, and the possibility for enhanced healing with improved cosmesis awaits validation in an ongoing multicenter

trial. If the wound can be left open or placed in a dry dressing after sheet grafting, Steri-Strips can be used effectively. They will not remain in place if the wound is covered with moist dressings.

Keeping these early reconstructive principles in mind during the first operations may avert the need for later procedures entirely, and will help convert what could be major reconstructive efforts into minor ones.

Donor Sites

In the past, when only full-thickness burns were grafted and patients endured many weeks of daily débridements, donor sites were treated cavalierly. They were covered with either dry fine mesh gauze, or gauze impregnated with a dye or other antimicrobial agent. They were left to desiccate, and the gauze usually separated from the wound in 2 to 3 weeks. As aggressive programs of early E&G developed, care and healing of donor sites became a priority. With early excision, the patient was spared the painful daily débridement, and with burn pain diminished, patients focused on donor site pain. Donor sites are quite painful as they are a superficial partial-thickness injury. Appropriate dressings diminish donor site pain.

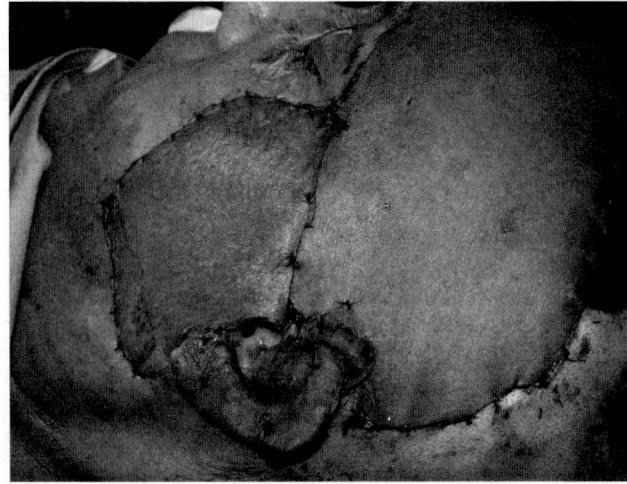

FIG. 7-8. *Excised face burn with single sheet split-thickness skin graft secured with sutures.*

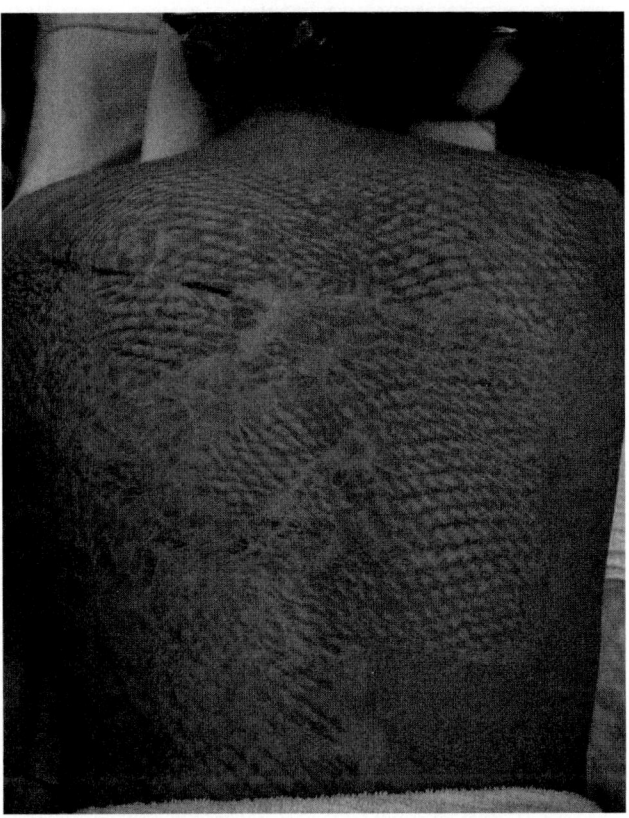

FIG. 7-9. Typical scarring associated with widely meshed split-thickness skin grafts prior to the availability of dermal substitutes.

There are numerous dressings available for donor site wound care. Reports indicate that there is no optimal donor site dressing; however, moist wound healing is superior to dry wound healing. All dressings seem to work, and differences in healing times are minimal among the moist wound healing modalities. Comfort levels and ease of care are the most significant determinants.

Healed donor sites are still not free of complications. In addition to hypertrophic scarring and pigmentation changes, blistering for several weeks may trouble patients. Blisters are self-limiting

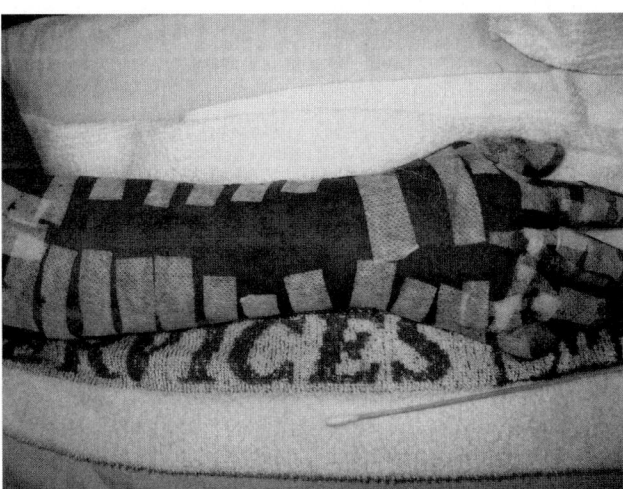

FIG. 7-10. Sheet split-thickness skin graft of right arm secured with Hypafix.

and treated with bandages or ointments until they re-epithelialize. Donor site infections occur in approximately 5% of patients and can be devastating, with conversion of a partial-thickness to a full-thickness wound requiring a STSG for closure. Infection is treated aggressively with systemic and topical antibiotics.[167]

Skin Substitutes

The next major step in burn care is likely to be an artificial skin that will be readily available, perform a barrier function (epidermis), and provide the structural durability and flexibility of the dermis. It must be permanent, affordable, resist hypertrophic scarring, provide normal pigmentation, and grow with developing children. Progress toward this goal has been substantial over the past decade; however, the ideal artificial skin has yet to be developed.[168]

Dermal Substitutes

The development of dermal substitutes has added greatly to the capabilities of the burn surgeon, especially when faced with a large burn and limited donor sites. They readily facilitate complete excision of the entire burn with wound closure. Depending on the product, grafting with STSG may be immediate or delayed until the dermal substitute has engrafted. Currently three dermal substitutes are available in the United States: INTEGRA, AlloDerm, and Dermagraft. These products are fundamentally similar in that they allow for the creation of a "neo-dermis" populated by the patient's own mesenchymal cells upon which a thin STSG is placed. The use of thinner STSG allows for earlier re-cropping of donor sites, quicker closure of the complete burn, and less donor site scarring. Successful use of any one of the available dermal substitutes is technique-dependent and associated with a learning curve.

AlloDerm is a cryopreserved allogeneic dermis from which the epithelial elements have been removed with hypertonic saline prior to freeze-drying. It is treated in a detergent to kill any viruses. The result is a theoretically antigen-free, complete dermal scaffolding with intact epidermal basement membrane proteins. Immediately following excision to viable tissue, AlloDerm is rehydrated, treated according to the manufacturer's specifications, and applied to the wound bed. It is designed to be immediately autografted with a thin STSG (e.g., <0.010 inch). Early results of clinical trials appear favorable compared to standard grafting techniques.[169,170]

Dermagraft consists of human neonatal fibroblasts cultured on Biobrane. Biobrane is a biosynthetic dressing composed of a silicone membrane coated on one side with porcine collagen and imbedded with nylon mesh. The neonatal fibroblasts are seeded into the nylon mesh. Following excision, Dermagraft is prepared according to the manufacturer's recommendations and affixed to the wound. Approximately 2 weeks after application, the silicone membrane is removed and the wound bed grafted with a STSG. Early clinical trials also appear encouraging.[171,172] Dermagraft, however, is a dressing, and does not provide full dermal scaffolding, thus requiring standard thickness skin grafts.

INTEGRA was developed by Burke and Yannas in the 1980s and became commercially available in 1996.[173] Of all the dermal substitutes, the greatest experience has been gained with INTEGRA, both worldwide and in the United States It is a bilaminate membrane consisting of a porous collagen-chondroitin 6-sulfate fibrillar layer (dermal analogue) bonded to a thin silicone layer (temporary epidermis). INTEGRA is applied to a freshly excised burn wound and allowed to vascularize for 14 days or longer (Fig. 7-11). An ultra-thin (0.006 to 0.008 inch) STSG is placed after removal of the silicone layer from the vascularized "neo-dermis" (see Fig. 7-11C).

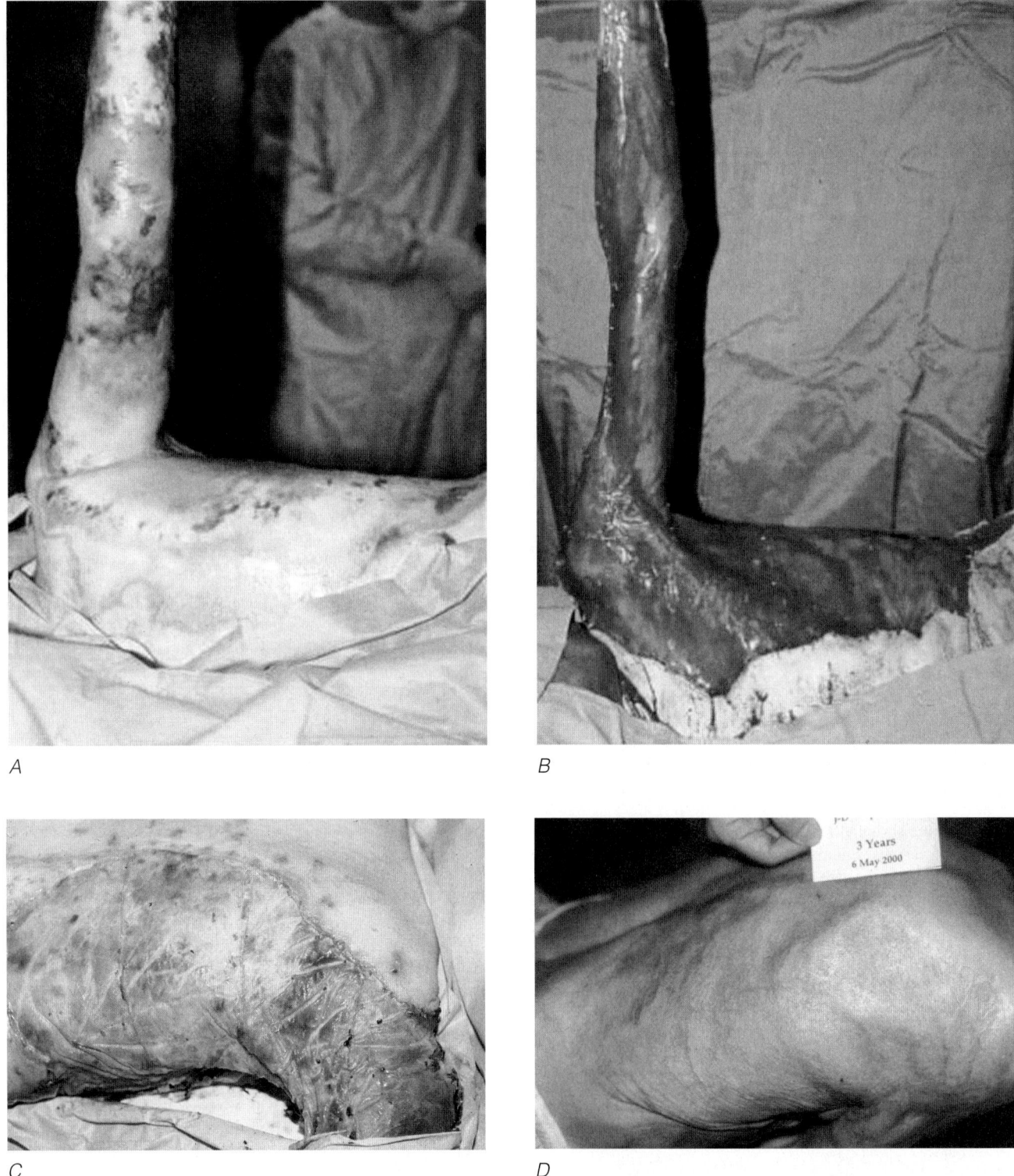

FIG. 7-11. INTEGRA. (*A*) Full-thickness burn prepared for fascial excision. (*B*) Integra applied to the freshly excised wound bed and secured with staples. (*C*) Healthy, vascularized INTEGRA "neo-dermis" which is ready for grafting following silicone membrane removal. (*D*) Results at 3 years with full range of motion of the right shoulder. Note superior cosmesis obtained with INTEGRA.

The ultra-thin donor sites allow for faster total wound closure by early re-cropping of donor sites and more rapid donor site healing, while cosmesis is improved.[174]

INTEGRA is prepared in the operating room according to the manufacturer's specifications, including 1:1 meshing, and affixed with staples to freshly excised burn wounds (see Fig. 7-11B). An integral aspect of INTEGRA wound coverage is the widely expanded elastic net dressing that must be stapled over the INTEGRA to prevent shearing. After at least 14 days in topical antibiotic–soaked dressings, a 0.006-inch STSG is applied to the extent that available donor sites allow. The grafts are dressed appropriately and kept moist with topical antibiotic solution until acceptable take is evident.

Donor sites can be re-cropped until complete coverage of the INTEGRA is obtained. Of note, the silicone layer should not be removed until the time of grafting, regardless of the time since initial application. Premature removal of the silicone layer leads to growth of granulation tissue that increases the risk of hypertrophic scar formation. However, fluid collections in or below the INTEGRA should be drained or "windowed" if they appear purulent or are large enough to threaten engraftment.

A recent review of these authors' experience with INTEGRA from 1996 to 2001 at the University of Washington Burn Center indicates that outcomes correlate with experience with the product and meticulous attention to details.[174a] For comparison and to assess technical improvement, patients were divided into two groups: 1996 to 1999 (group I) and 2000 to 2001 (group II). Group I had 57 patients with burns averaging 39% TBSA and an average age of 40 years. The average percentage take of INTEGRA was 76%. Group II consisted of 39 patients with burns averaging 37% TBSA and an average age of 35 years. In stark contrast, the average percentage take of INTEGRA was 97%. No differences were observed between the groups with respect to number of operations required, length of stay, or mortality. The outcomes improved with increasing experience, underscoring the learning curve associated with the use of dermal substitutes. While no change in mortality associated with use of INTEGRA has been observed, there has been less hypertrophic scarring (see Fig. 7-11D).

The safety and efficacy of INTEGRA has been further validated in a multicenter, postapproval, clinical trial.[175] INTEGRA and STSG takes were excellent, and associated infectious complications were minimal.

Cultured Skin

Apligraf is an FDA-approved biologic dressing composed of cultured neonatal keratinocytes and fibroblasts. This allograft bioengineered product has been approved for use in chronic nonhealing ulcers, but has not yet been widely marketed for the burn patient. One indication for use of this product might be in an elderly patient at significant risk for a nonhealing donor site, who has a small deep burn that has started to granulate. It can be used as a biologic dressing to enhance primary healing, or even as a STSG substitute, but only in small burns.[176] Apligraf may also improve the cosmetic outcome of meshed STSGs when it is used as an overlay dressing on the STSG.[177]

Advances in tissue culture techniques have led to the development, and ultimate commercial availability, of cultured epithelial autografts (CEAs). Epicel is currently the only FDA-approved CEA product available. These grafts are created from a full-thickness biopsy of the patient's own skin and require 3 weeks to grow. They are quite expensive at approximately $14,500 for 750 cm². Early

small series and case reports of massively burned patients were promising. However, this enthusiasm was tempered by subsequent concerns about CEA durability and graft take.[178] Cost also has limited the use of CEAs by many burn centers. Nonetheless, when coupled with standard burn therapy, CEAs may be potentially life saving for the massively burned patient. CEA combined with a dermal substitute is a logical extension of these advancements, and initial results are encouraging.[179] Further investigation of this next step is underway.

NUTRITIONAL SUPPORT

The nutritional effects of the hypermetabolic response to thermal injury are manifested as exaggerated energy expenditure and massive nitrogen loss. Nutritional support is aimed at provision of calories to match energy expenditure, while providing enough nitrogen to replace or support body protein stores.

The changes in metabolism are triggered by drastic alterations in the neuroendocrine and cytokine profiles, resulting in protein catabolism, gluconeogenesis, and lipolysis. Plasma insulin levels are normal to elevated, but are low relative to increased glucagon concentrations. Catecholamines and glucocorticoids also antagonize the action of insulin. These metabolic and hormonal derangements have important consequences for nutritional status.

Caloric Requirements

Hypermetabolism and catabolism are universal consequences of injury, regardless of the etiology. The magnitude of increase in the metabolic rate following thermal injury is directly proportional to the TBSA of the burn. The total energy expenditure may be elevated anywhere from 15 to 100% above basal needs, significantly exceeding the metabolic increases of other injuries. Energy needs must be evaluated carefully in formulating a nutritional plan. If the regimen is deficient in calories, anabolism will be suboptimal, and the nitrogen balance will continue to be negative. Mathematical formulas exist for the calculation of daily caloric requirements in burn patients. The formula most widely used is Long's modification of the Harris-Benedict equation. (Table 7-2) The original Harris-Benedict equation estimates BMR with reasonable accuracy. Long proposed that the BMR be multiplied by various stress factors depending upon the type of injury. The modification for burn patients uses a factor of 1.5. The more severely ill the patient, the less accurate standard formulas are for estimating calorie expenditure.

Table 7-2
Long Modification of the Harris-Benedict Equation

Men
  BMR = $(66.47 \pm 13.75 \text{ weight} \pm 5.0 \text{ height} = 6.76 \text{ age})$
    × (activity factor) × (injury factor)
Women
  BMR = $(655.10 \pm 9.56 \text{ weight} + 1.85 \text{ height} = 4.68 \text{ age})$
    × (activity factor) × (injury factor)
Activity factor
  Confined to bed: 1.2
  Out of bed: 1.3
Injury factor
  Minor operation: 1.20
  Skeletal trauma: 1.35
  Major sepsis: 1.60
  Severe thermal burn: 1.5

BMR = basal metabolic rate.

Periodic determination of REE via indirect calorimetry may be utilized to allow more accurate adjustments of caloric provision. REE determinations should not be construed as equivalent to the 24-hour calorie requirement. Compensations must be made for daily energy fluctuations that occur with physical therapy, stress, temperature elevations, dressing changes, and other influences on metabolic rate.[180] Total urine nitrogen (TUN) excretion is easy to measure, and accurately reflects the degree of catabolism; whereas calculated nitrogen excretion using the urine urea nitrogen (UUN) underestimates catabolism and nitrogen losses in burned patients.[181] The TUN should be monitored regularly, with the goal being a persistently positive nitrogen balance. Various visceral proteins are commonly measured, typically as part of a "nutrition panel," to assess ongoing nutritional status. Analysis of these values is precarious, and instead of periodic static assessment, positive trends over time should be sought.[182,183]

Carbohydrates

Carbohydrates, in the form of glucose, appear to be the best source of nonprotein calories in the thermally-injured patient.[184] Certain tissues, including the burn wound, neural tissues, and the formed elements of the blood, utilize glucose in an obligatory fashion. Provision of glucose to these tissues occurs at the expense of lean body mass (i.e., skeletal muscle) if adequate nutrition is not provided. In the unfed state, the major sources for hepatic gluconeogenesis are the burn wound and skeletal muscle. The wound utilizes glucose by anaerobic glycolytic pathways, producing large amounts of lactate as an end product. The wound meets its high glucose requirements via increased glucose delivery, which is made possible by the enhanced circulation to the wound.

In the liver, lactate is extracted and utilized for gluconeogenesis via the Cori cycle. Concomitantly, alanine, glutamine (Gln), and other amino acids contribute to the increased gluconeogenesis. Increased ureagenesis, with urea derived from body protein stores, parallels the rise in hepatic glucose production. Peripheral amino acids and wound lactate account for approximately 50 to 60% of the new glucose produced by the liver. The hyperglycemia observed in hypermetabolic burn patients is a consequence of accelerated glucose flux, not decreased peripheral utilization.

Because glucose that is obtained via gluconeogenic pathways ultimately derives from protein stores, depletion of body protein during burn hypermetabolism leads to energy deficits, malfunctioning of glucose-dependent energetic processes, and skeletal muscle wasting. High-carbohydrate enteral nutrition formulations appear to blunt the catabolism, resulting in skeletal muscle sparing.[185] Optimal glucose oxidation during burn hypermetabolism occurs at intakes of approximately 5 mg/kg per minute; exogenous supply at rates above this result in its use by nonoxidative pathways, without contributing to energy balance.[186]

Protein

Combining glucose and protein-containing nutrients improves nitrogen balance and allows more calories to be used for the restoration of nitrogen balance than would be possible if either nutrient were used alone. After thermal injury, carbohydrate and protein nutrients cooperatively contribute to the improvement in nitrogen equilibrium by at least two distinct mechanisms. Protein administration promotes synthesis of visceral and muscle protein, without appreciably affecting the rate of catabolism.[187] Exogenous glucose retards catabolism, but exerts little effect on protein synthesis. Both mechanisms improve nitrogen balance, and sufficient glucose (i.e.,

$\sim$7 g/kg per day) and protein (i.e., $\sim$2 g/kg per day) should be components of the nutritional regimen for the severely-burned catabolic patient.

The importance of Gln as a metabolic fuel source has been recognized, and it is considered a conditionally-essential amino acid.[188] The gastrointestinal tract preferentially uses Gln as an energy source, and disposes of the majority of it as ammonia, urea, and citrulline. The alanine generated from Gln is used for gluconeogenesis. During critical illness, circulating concentrations of Gln fall, and supplemental exogenous Gln is necessary to meet requirements. As noted earlier, Gln supplementation has been associated with improved outcomes following thermal injury.

Fat

The role of fat as a source of nonprotein calories is dependent on the extent of injury and associated hypermetabolism. Recall that following significant thermal injury, there are alterations in substrate cycling and fatty acid oxidation that favor re-esterification and hepatic deposition of triglycerides. Fat appears to be a poor caloric source overall, and especially for the maintenance of nitrogen equilibrium and lean body mass, in burn-induced hypermetabolism.[189] Patients with only moderate elevations in metabolic rate can use lipid calories efficiently, but these patients rarely require nutritional support.

Even more important than their energy inefficiency, fats appear to affect outcome following thermal injury. Not only the total volume of fat administered, but also the particular fatty acid moiety, is important. Patients fed low-fat enteral diets ($\leq$15% of nonprotein calories as fat) had fewer infectious complications, improved wound healing, shorter lengths of stay, and apparently reduced mortality compared to controls fed standard, relatively high-fat, enteral diets.[190,191] Omega-3 fatty acid supplementation appears to confer some outcome benefit; however, this is more definitive in animal models than in humans.

Vitamins and Minerals

Vitamin requirements in critically-ill, hypermetabolic burn patients remain poorly defined. The fat-soluble vitamins (A, D, E, and K) are extensively stored in fat depots and are only slowly depleted during prolonged feeding of vitamin-free solutions. The water-soluble vitamins (B complex and C) are not stored in appreciable amounts, and are rapidly depleted. All vitamins should be supplemented. The dosage guidelines of the National Advisory Group/American Medical Association (NAG/AMA) are reasonable for burn patients unless symptoms of deficiency occur. Of note, all commercially-available enteral feeding formulations meet NAG/AMA recommendations for vitamins and minerals. Vitamin C (ascorbic acid) has an essential role in wound repair via participation in collagen synthesis, and plasma levels are frequently low in burn patients. It is prudent to supplement the NAG/AMA recommended dose with approximately 1000 mg of vitamin C daily. Larger doses may cause diarrhea or nephrolithiasis, will interfere with laboratory studies, and are excreted unchanged. Excessive doses of vitamins A and D produce toxicity; monitoring of serum levels is often misleading in burn patients, since the concentrations of the vitamin carrier proteins are commonly decreased.

Minerals and trace elements are essential because of their role in metabolic processes. Frequent determinations of serum sodium, potassium, chloride, calcium, magnesium, and phosphorus are the best guides to electrolyte replacement. Less is known about trace element requirements after thermal injury. Zinc is an important cofactor in enzymatic function and wound repair, and zinc deficiency has been documented in burn patients.[192] Thus, empiric zinc supplementation is warranted following major burns. Periodic measurements of serum and plasma zinc, copper, manganese, and chromium are the best way to determine replacement dosages. Nonetheless, a recent study demonstrated reduced pneumonia rates when trace elements were administered as supplemental doses above the NAG/AMA recommendations, raising the possibility of overall increased requirements in the thermally injured.[193]

Route of Administration

The route of nutritional support is important because it directly influences outcome. Total enteral nutrition (TEN) is the overwhelmingly favored mode of alimentation in the severely burned. Total parenteral nutrition (TPN) is used only when complete enteral failure is encountered, as TPN is associated with increased mortality.[194]

Patients with burns covering less than 20% of their TBSA who are not complicated by facial injury, inhalation injury, malnutrition, or psychologic disturbances can typically be maintained on high-calorie, high-protein, oral diets. However, the oral route alone cannot meet the nutritional requirements of patients with major burns, and these patients should be fed enterally via a gastric or duodenal feeding tube regardless of their motivation to eat. A functioning gastrointestinal (GI) tract should always be used.

In severely-burned patients, gastroparesis may limit intragastric nutritional support, particularly in the early postburn period. However, immediate intragastric feeding appears to limit gastroparesis and is unquestionably safe.[195,196] Even in the face of intragastric feeding intolerance, TEN should not be abandoned. Postpyloric feeding tends to work well in the burn patient with gastroparesis.[197] Prokinetics should be used as needed. The precise GI tract location (i.e., intragastric vs. postpyloric) for optimal TEN provision is controversial and a matter of preference; the location is probably less important than simply ensuring adequate TEN.

TEN has significant advantages over TPN that translate into reduced morbidity and improved mortality.[40] Enteral nutrients maintain the integrity of the GI tract via preservation of gut mucosal mass and immunity, which appears to reduce bacterial translocation and the incidence of gut-derived infection.[198] Conversely, the absence of intraluminal nutrients leads to increased apoptosis and decreased mucosal mass.[199] TEN enhances splanchnic perfusion with an improvement in gut oxygen balance, even during resuscitation from burn shock.[200] Historically, Curling's ulcers and GI hemorrhage were common burn-related complications, which prompted aggressive pharmacologic gastric acid suppression. Aggressive, early, intragastric TEN alone has proven to be adequate ulcer prophylaxis, and virtually eliminated Curling's ulcers.[201] TEN is also less expensive than TPN.

Studies have shown that institution of TEN immediately upon admission is safe and beneficial.[202,203] This early nutritional regimen appears to blunt the intensity of hypermetabolism and more effectively maintains preinjury weight without significant complications. However, the optimal timing of early TEN has yet to be defined.[204] TEN should not be withheld during perioperative periods, as this only leads to energy deficits and increased catabolism; perioperative TEN, including intraoperative infusion, has been proven to be safe.[205]

TPN should be instituted only upon complete enteral failure. Protracted ileus and the overuse of narcotics with resultant constipation are frequent causes of TEN failures. Sepsis is associated with ileus and hyperglycemia; these signs may be the only evidence of this complication.[206] Aggressive bowel regimens with laxatives and fiber supplements, not just stool softeners, should be routine proactive measures to avert constipation. If TPN has to be administered, it is useful to continue some enteral nutrition, particularly Gln supplementation. The benefits of enteral nutrition are realized, even with low volumes.

Composition of Enteral Nutrition

Numerous commercially available formulations exist to choose from today. The ultimate goal is to provide nutritional support tailored to meet the needs of critically-ill burn patients. Standard meal replacement products or supplements formulated for nonstressed or minimally-stressed patients do not meet the unique nutritional requirements of moderately- or severely-stressed burn patients. Numerous studies indicate that specialized feeding regimens improve burn-related metabolic derangements while enhancing nutritional status.

In burn patients, a high-protein, high-carbohydrate, low-fat diet with fiber is optimal. As noted earlier, appropriate supplements to include Gln, vitamins, minerals, and trace elements are indicated, and add to the benefits of TEN. Immune-enhancing diets (e.g., IMPACT) offer no clear advantage over standard high-protein formulas in the burn population.[207] Monitoring of TEN to assess tolerance and effectiveness is as important as the selection of the formula or timing of initiation. Careful nutrition and metabolic assessment can help ensure optimal support with minimal complications. Although superior to TPN, TEN still has associated complications, and any evidence of feeding intolerance should be actively investigated.[208]

INFECTION

Infectious mortality following thermal injury has significantly declined over the past 2 decades, with the greatest reduction attributed to early E&G. However, following successful resuscitation, most acute morbidity and virtually all mortality in severely burned patients are still related to infection. Thermal injury causes profound immunosuppression that is proportional to the TBSA of the burn wound. A direct relationship between specific immunologic defects and infection has yet to be definitively established in humans; nonetheless, the resultant invariable, global immunosuppression makes the burn patient exquisitely susceptible to infection. Sepsis develops when the balance between host factors and pathogenic or opportunistic organisms is unfavorably altered. Nonetheless, prophylactic systemic antibiotics are *not* part of modern burn care, as they do not reduce septic complications and only lead to increased bacterial resistance.

Risk Factors for Infection

The extent of burn injury (i.e., TBSA) is one of the major determinants of overall outcome, and the incidence of infection correlates with burn severity.[209] Children appear to be more susceptible to systemic infection than adults for any given size burn.[210] However, burns involving less than 20% TBSA in otherwise healthy individuals are rarely associated with life-threatening infection. The presence of an inhalation injury strongly correlates with infection, particularly pneumonia. Premorbid diabetes significantly increases infection rates following thermal injury, especially when coupled with poor glycemic control.[211] Age per se is not an independent risk factor for infection following thermal injury, although it has a significant impact on overall outcome.

Clinical Manifestations and Diagnosis

Many of the physiologic criteria defining sepsis are noninfectious sequelae of postinjury hypermetabolism. Hyperthermia, tachycardia, increased ventilation, and high cardiac output, indicative of sepsis as well as a hyperdynamic-hypermetabolic state, are part of the normal response to major burns in otherwise healthy patients.

Body temperature regulation is altered in burn patients, and is partially dependent upon environmental conditions. Hyperthermia ($\geq 38.5°C$) is routinely present following thermal injury, particularly in children, and is a poor indicator of infection.[212,213] Conversely, hypothermia commonly heralds sepsis, usually due to gram-negative organisms. Leukocytosis in the burn patient is also nonspecific. As long as large wounds remain open, variable elevations in leukocyte counts are common. Thrombocytosis is invariable following major thermal injury, whereas thrombocytopenia is a fairly reliable manifestation of sepsis. Likewise, sudden feeding intolerance is commonly associated with significant infection.

Other traditional manifestations of sepsis are potentially even more nonspecific in the burn patient. An altered mental status can be caused by various medications commonly used in modern burn care, particularly opioids. Hyperglycemia may be precipitated by administration of the necessary high-calorie, high-carbohydrate diet, as well as being a consequence of the neuroendocrine response to thermal injury. Increased fluid requirements, hypotension, and oliguria may be related to inadequate ongoing fluid replacement following successful resuscitation.

The most important observations are related to the temporal association of the aforementioned physiologic events. Abrupt onset of hyperglycemia, fall in blood pressure, and decrease in urinary output should suggest the possibility that the patient is becoming unstable. If these findings are associated with development of hypothermia, feeding intolerance, and/or a falling platelet count, the patient is probably developing sepsis. It is important to do an immediate infection work-up and administer the appropriate antimicrobials.

Even with firm clinical evidence of sepsis, a definitive microbiologic diagnosis of infection can sometimes be difficult to obtain. Blood cultures have a relatively low yield in the burn population, and other anatomic sites of potential infection (e.g., wounds, respiratory tract, and urine) should preferentially be cultured.[214] Recently, serum procalcitonin has been shown to be a sensitive marker of significant infection in burn patients.[215,216] However, further validation is required prior to its widespread clinical use in the diagnosis of infection. A thorough physical exam and awareness of the infections commonly encountered in burn patients allows an orderly evaluation of the potentially infected patient.

Specific Infections

Wound Infection

A change in the flora of burn wound infections over the past few decades is probably related to the proliferation of broad-spectrum parenteral and topical antibiotics. Before the availability of penicillin, streptococci and staphylococci were the predominant infecting organisms. By the late 1950s, gram-negative bacteria, especially *Pseudomonas* species, had emerged as the dominant organisms causing fatal wound infections in burn patients.[217]

All burn wounds become colonized by 72 hours after injury with the patient's own flora or with endemic organisms from the treatment facility. Bacteria colonize the surface of the wound and may penetrate the avascular eschar. This colonization is invariable and without clinical significance; hence, routine early wound cultures

are not efficacious and only increase costs.[218] Bacterial proliferation may occur beneath the eschar at the viable-nonviable tissue interface, leading to eschar separation if early E&G is not practiced. In a few patients, microorganisms may breach this barrier and invade the deeper underlying viable tissue, producing wound sepsis.

The essential pathologic feature of burn wound sepsis is invasion of organisms into viable tissue, which is diagnosed via biopsy and quantitative tissue culture demonstrating greater than 10^5 organisms per gram of tissue. The organisms spread to the perivascular structures, with direct vessel wall invasion, causing a vasculitis and thrombosis. Hemorrhagic necrosis follows. Subsequently, organisms invade the bloodstream, producing sepsis with potential metastatic lesions. Any organisms capable of invading tissue can produce burn wound sepsis. The predominant organisms causing burn wound infection vary depending on the treatment facility flora. Burn wound infection can be focal, multifocal, or generalized. The likelihood of sepsis increases in proportion to the size of the wound. Superficial wound swab cultures should never be used to evaluate potential invasive burn wound infection. Once the diagnosis of burn wound sepsis is confirmed, appropriate parenteral antibiotics should be administered and the wound promptly excised.

Before the introduction of effective topical antimicrobial agents, up to 60% of the deaths in burn centers were caused by burn wound sepsis. The three agents with proven broad-spectrum antimicrobial activity when applied to the burn wound are silver sulfadiazine (SSD), mafenide acetate, and silver nitrate (Table 7-3). SSD is the most common agent used in burn centers and has antifungal properties in addition to good bacterial coverage. However, SSD does not penetrate eschar. Only mafenide acetate is able to penetrate eschar, and it is the only agent capable of suppressing dense subeschar bacterial proliferation. The main disadvantage of mafenide acetate is its carbonic anhydrase inhibition, which may interfere with renal buffering mechanisms. Bicarbonate is consumed, chloride is retained, and the resulting hyperchloremic metabolic acidosis is compensated for by an increase in ventilation and subsequent respiratory alkalosis. However, this is typically of little clinical consequence. Silver nitrate must be used before bacteria have penetrated the wound. Its disadvantages are the associated electrolyte imbalances (e.g., hyponatremia), which are common, and methemoglobinemia, which is unusual. Since the introduction of effective topical therapy, fungal burn wound infections, primarily involving highly invasive Phycomycetes and *Aspergillus* organisms, has increased.

A newly emerging variant of burn wound infection, the "melting graft-wound syndrome," was recently reported from the authors' burn center, and involves progressive epithelial loss (melting) from a previously well-taken graft, healed burn wound, or healed donor site. Historically, such epithelial loss was attributed to the growth of *Streptococcus* species; however, "melting" without significant streptococcal colonization or infection was encountered. Wound cultures from affected patients mainly grew *Staphylococcus aureus* (including methicillin-resistant *S. aureus*), and none grew *Streptococcus* species. These infections have potentially devastating consequences. As such, appropriate systemic antibiotics, topical antibiotics, and aggressive wound care are mandatory for effective treatment. Reexcision and grafting rarely are required for salvage.

Pneumonia

One result of the prolonged and improved survival of severely burned patients is that the respiratory tract has become the most common source of infection. It is generally agreed that inhalation injury

Table 7-3
Topical Antimicrobial Agents for Burn Wound Care

	Silver Nitrate	*Mafenide Acetate*	*Silver Sulfadiazine*
Active component	0.5% in aqueous solution	11.1% in water-miscible base	1.0% in water-miscible base
Spectrum of antimicrobial activity	Gram-negative—good	Gram-negative—good	Gram-negative—variable
	Gram-positive—good	Gram-positive—good	Gram-positive—good
	Yeast—good	Yeast—poor	Yeast—good
Method of Wound care	Occlusive dressings	Exposure	Exposure or single-layer dressings
Advantages	Painless	Penetrates eschar	Painless
	No hypersensitivity reaction	Wound appearance readily monitored	Wound appearance readily monitored when exposure method used
	No gram-negative resistance	Joint motion unrestricted	Easily applied
	Dressings reduce evaporative heat loss	No gram-negative resistance	Joint motion unrestricted when exposure method used
	Greater effectiveness against yeasts		Greater effectiveness against yeast
Disadvantages	Deficits of sodium, potassium, calcium, and chloride	Painful on partial-thickness burns	Neutropenia and thrombocytopenia
	No eschar penetration	Susceptibility to acidosis as a result of carbonic anhydrase inhibition	Hypersensitivity—infrequent
	Limitation of joint motion by dressings	Hypersensitivity reactions in 7% of patients	Limited eschar penetration
	Methemoglobinemia—rare		
	Argyria—rare		
	Staining of environment and equipment		

increases the risk of developing pneumonia. However, this may be more related to endotracheal intubation than the actual inhalation injury.[219]

The diagnosis of pneumonia is confirmed by the presence of characteristic infiltrates on chest radiographs and positive sputum cultures. Following inhalation injury, early infiltrates usually represent chemical pneumonitis and not infection, although this injured pulmonary tissue may become infected. The most efficacious and sensitive method of obtaining tracheobronchial specimens for microbiologic analysis remains controversial. Regardless of specimen collection methodology, colonization of the upper airway in patients requiring mechanical ventilation should not be confused with a respiratory tract infection.

When pneumonia is clinically suspected, broad-spectrum antibiotics appropriate for the endemic bacterial flora should be promptly instituted, and subsequently narrowed according to culture results. Single-agent therapy is generally appropriate and efficacious regardless of the pathogen, including *Pseudomonas aeruginosa*. Pneumonia still carries a significant mortality rate of approximately 25% in mechanically-ventilated burn patients.[220] Prophylactic antibiotics should not be used, as they only select for resistant organisms and do not reduce the incidence of pneumonia. Likewise, early tracheostomy does not lower pneumonia rates in either children or adults suffering major thermal injury.[146,147] Consistent infection control practices and timely extubation seem to be the only effective means to lower the incidence of pneumonia.

Vascular Catheter-Related Infections

With evolving technology and a trend toward invasive hemodynamic monitoring, central venous catheterization is commonplace in many burn centers. This practice is quite appropriate in patients with cardiopulmonary pathology or concomitant nonthermal trauma, which mandate central monitoring. However, burn shock resuscitation does not require central venous access, and can be quite successfully accomplished employing only peripheral access. All vascular access modalities carry risk, in particular infectious complications, and central line complications can be life threatening.

The incidence of peripheral suppurative thrombophlebitis following thermal injury is miniscule in the modern era, as saphenous venous cutdowns have been abandoned and standard line care is routine.[220] The true incidence of central line sepsis in burn patients is unknown. Technologic advancements and various interventions have been directed at reducing catheter-related bloodstream infections (CRBSIs) in at-risk patient populations.[221] Antimicrobial-impregnated central lines are quite efficacious in reducing CRBSIs in surgical patients, and in all likelihood are also effective in burn patients, although they have not been thoroughly studied in the burned population. Likewise, routine central venous catheter changes without evidence of infection are probably unwarranted and only increase complication rates; there are no conclusive data in the burn literature to support routine catheter changes. Contrary to popular belief, the specific central line site does not appear to influence infection rates in the burn patient.[222] However, the distance from the burn wound does appear to correlate inversely with CRBSI, and every effort should be made to place intravenous lines as far from the burn as possible.[223] As with pneumonia, the most effective measures to reduce CRBSIs are infection control practices and timely removal of the device. When diagnosed, CRBSI should be appropriately treated with systemic antimicrobials and immediate removal of the catheter.

ELECTRICAL INJURY AND BURNS

Electrical injuries are particularly dangerous, as they can be instantaneously fatal and also put rescuers in significant danger. Injury severity depends on the amperage of the current (determined by the voltage of the source and the resistance of the victim), the pathway of current through the victim's body, and the duration of contact with the source. Electrical current sources are typically classified as either low- or high-voltage, with 1000 volts (V) being the dividing line, and distinct injuries are associated with each type.[224] Over 95% of all electrical injuries and electrical burns are caused by low-voltage commercial alternating current in the range of 0 to 220 V. An electrical burn potentially has three different components: (1) the true electrical injury from current flow, (2) an arc or flash flame injury produced by current arcing at a temperature of approximately 4000°C from its source to ground, and (3) a flame injury from the ignition of clothing or surroundings.

Care at the Scene

If the victim remains in contact with the electrical source, the rescuer must absolutely avoid touching the victim until the current is shut off. Once away from the source of current, the standard ABCs (airway, breathing, and circulation) must be rapidly evaluated and supported if necessary. Respiratory arrest secondary to paralysis of the central respiratory control system or due to paralysis of the respiratory muscles can occur; thus an airway should always be established and maintained. Ventricular fibrillation or asystole are not uncommon, and cardiopulmonary resuscitation according to Basic Life Support/Advanced Cardiac Life Support/Advanced Trauma Life Support protocols should be instituted if pulses are not palpable. Once an airway is established and pulses return, a careful search must be made for associated life-threatening injuries. Electrically injured patients frequently fall from heights and may have serious head or spine injuries, as well as long bone fractures. The intense tetanic contractions associated with electrical injury alone can cause fractures or joint dislocations. All significant electrical burns should be referred to a dedicated burn center.

Acute Management and Multisystem Involvement

Electrical burns are thermal injuries from very intense heat and from electrical disruption of cell membranes.[225] As electrical current meets tissue, it is converted to heat in direct proportion to the amperage of the current and the resistance of the tissues through which it passes. The smaller the size of the body part through which the electricity passes, the more intense the heat and the less the heat is dissipated into surrounding tissue. Fingers, hands, forearms, feet, and lower legs are frequently totally destroyed by high-voltage injuries. Areas of larger volume, like the trunk, usually dissipate enough current to prevent extensive damage to viscera unless the contact point(s) are on the abdomen or chest.[226] While cutaneous manifestations of electrical burns may appear limited, burned skin should not be considered the only injury, as massive underlying tissue destruction may be present. Resuscitation needs are usually far in excess of what would be expected on the basis of the cutaneous burn size, and associated flame and/or flash burns often compound the problem.

Myoglobinuria frequently accompanies electrical burns, but the clinical significance appears to be trivial.[227] Disruption of muscle cells releases cellular debris and myoglobin into the circulation to be filtered by the kidney. If this condition is untreated, the consequence can be irreversible renal failure. However, modern burn resuscitation protocols alone appear to be sufficient treatment for myoglobinuria.

Cardiac damage, such as myocardial contusion or infarction, may be present. More likely, the conduction system may be deranged. Household current at 110 V either does no damage or induces ventricular fibrillation. If there are no electrocardiographic rhythm abnormalities present upon initial emergency department evaluation, the likelihood that they will appear later is minuscule.

Even with high-voltage injuries, a normal cardiac rhythm on admission generally means that subsequent dysrhythmia is unlikely. Studies confirm that commonly measured cardiac enzymes bear little correlation to cardiac dysfunction, and elevated enzymes may be from skeletal muscle damage.[228,229] Mandatory electrocardiogram (ECG) monitoring and cardiac enzyme analysis in an ICU setting for 24 hours following injury is unnecessary in patients with electrical burns, even those resulting from high-voltage current, in patients who have stable cardiac rhythms on admission.[230]

The nervous system is exquisitely sensitive to electricity. The most devastating injury with frequent brain damage occurs when current passes through the head, but spinal cord damage is possible whenever current has passed from one side of the body to the other. Schwann cells are quite susceptible, and delayed transverse myelitis can occur days or weeks after injury.[231,232] Conduction initially remains normal through existing myelin, but as myelin wears out, it is not replaced and conduction ceases. Anterior spinal artery syndrome from vascular dysregulation can also precipitate spinal cord dysfunction. Damage to peripheral nerves is common and may cause permanent functional impairment.[233,234] Every patient with an electrical injury must have a thorough neurologic exam as part of the initial assessment. Persistent neurologic symptoms may lead to chronic pain syndromes, and posttraumatic stress disorders are apparently more common after electrical burns than thermal burns.

Cataracts are a well-recognized sequela of high-voltage electrical burns.[235,236] They occur in 5 to 7% of patients, frequently are bilateral, occur even in the absence of contact points on the head, and typically manifest within 1 to 2 years of injury. Electrically injured patients should undergo a thorough ophthalmologic examination early during their acute care.

Wound Management

There are two unique situations in which immediate surgical treatment is indicated for patients with electrical burns. Rarely, massive deep tissue necrosis will lead to acidosis or myoglobinuria that will not resolve with standard resuscitation techniques; major débridement and/or amputation may be necessary as an emergency procedure. More commonly, injured deep tissues undergo significant swelling, increasing the risk of compartment syndrome, and potentially leading to further tissue loss. Careful monitoring as previously described, including measurement of compartment pressures, is mandatory. Escharotomies and fasciotomies should be performed at compartment pressures of 30 mm Hg or more, or with clinical indications of compartment syndrome. Any progression of median or ulnar nerve deficit in a hand that has been electrically burned is an indication for immediate median and ulnar nerve release at the wrist. It appears that selective decompression of electrically burned upper extremities, as guided by clinical findings, is superior to mandatory decompression in preserving overall tissue viability.[237] If immediate decompression or débridement is not required, definitive surgical procedures can be done in the usual time frame, between days 3 and 5. This prevents invasive bacterial infection and allows for clear delineation of tissue viability.

CHEMICAL BURNS

Strong acids or alkalis cause most chemical burns. They typically are associated with industrial accidents, assaults, or the improper use of harsh household solvents and cleaners. In contrast to thermal injury, chemical burns cause progressive damage and injury until the chemicals are inactivated by reaction with tissues or diluted by therapeutic irrigation. Individual circumstances can vary, but acid burns typically are more self-limiting than alkali burns. Acids tend to "tan" the skin, creating an impermeable barrier of coagulation necrosis debris along the leading edge of the chemical burn that limits further penetration. Alkalis combine with cutaneous lipids to create a soap, and are thus able to continue dissolving the skin until they are neutralized.

Initial Care

All involved clothing should be removed, and unlike thermal injury, the burns should be irrigated with copious amounts of tepid water at the accident scene following chemical exposures. Chemicals will continue to burn until physically removed. Irrigating for at least 15 minutes under a running stream of tepid water may limit the overall severity of the burn; however, care should be taken to avoid hypothermia. Neutralizing agents or antidotes are contraindicated, except with hydrofluoric acid burns. Delay deepens the chemical burn, and neutralizing agents may even produce thermal burns, as they frequently generate substantial heat upon neutralization of the offending agent.[238] Powdered chemicals should be brushed off skin and clothing. All significant chemical burns should be referred to a dedicated burn center.

Wound Management

A full-thickness chemical burn may appear deceptively superficial, causing only a mild brownish discoloration of the skin. The skin may remain intact during the first few days postburn, and only then begin to slough spontaneously. Chemical burns should be considered deep partial-thickness or full-thickness until proven otherwise. As such, they are best treated by early E&G after full demarcation of injury.

Some chemicals, such as phenol, cause severe systemic effects, while hydrofluoric acid may cause death from hypocalcemia even after moderate exposure. Hydrofluoric acid burns are unique chemical burns in that they should be acutely treated with an antidote, calcium. Calcium gluconate should be administered intra-arterially as well as topically, and all electrolyte abnormalities aggressively corrected.[239]

PAIN CONTROL

All burn injuries are painful, whether the injury is simply sunburn or an extensive partial-thickness or full-thickness burn covering a large portion of the body. Attempts to manage pain in the thermally injured are frequently frustrating because of the unpredictable physiologic and psychologic reactions to the burn.[240] An epidermal burn damages the outer layers of skin, the epidermis, producing mild pain and discomfort. Without the protective covering of the epidermis, nerve endings are sensitized and exposed to stimulation. The pain associated with partial-thickness burns varies depending on the extent of dermal destruction. Superficial partial-thickness burns initially are the most painful; even the slightest air current blowing across the exposed dermis causes the patient excruciating pain. Areas of deep partial-thickness or full-thickness injury show little or no response to sharp stimuli, yet a patient may complain of a deep aching pain, which is related to the inflammatory response. The physiologic effects of pain are primarily responses to catecholamines, and include increased heart rate, blood pressure, and respiration; decreased O_2 saturation; palmar sweating; facial flushing; and pupillary dilation.

Total elimination of pain in burn patients is not possible, short of general anesthesia. The burn patient may experience acute pain from dressing changes, operative procedures, and rehabilitation therapy exercises. Patients may also have chronic background pain associated with the wound maturation process. There is a wide degree of intra- and interindividual variation with respect to the experience of burn-related pain.[241] Pain management involves both pharmacologic and nonpharmacologic modalities. The mainstays of pharmacologic pain control are analgesics, principally opioids and nonsteroidal anti-inflammatory drugs. Anesthetic agents, namely ketamine and nitrous oxide, are quite useful for extremely painful procedures such as dressing changes. Psychotropic drugs (e.g., anxiolytics, tranquilizers, and/or antidepressants) also can be useful in the management of burn wounds. The concomitant use of benzodiazepines with opioids appears to be additive and reduces opiate requirements.[242] Nonpharmacologic methods have become more prevalent over the past decade, as efficacious techniques have evolved.[243,244] Virtual reality therapy as an adjunct to analgesics appears particularly promising.[245]

CHRONIC PROBLEMS

Hypertrophic Scar Formation

Hypertrophic scarring is a potentially devastating consequence of thermal injuries and is unfortunately all too common. The etiology and pathophysiology of hypertrophic scars are still incompletely understood. Burn scar hypertrophy classically develops in deeper partial-thickness and full-thickness injuries that are allowed to heal by primary intention. Hypertrophy of excised and grafted burn wounds occurs less frequently, and is partly dependent on the time from injury to excision, the site of the wound, and the patient's race or ethnicity.[246,247] Delayed excision is more likely to result in hypertrophic scarring, and pigmented individuals are at an increased risk. Donor sites also can become hypertrophic, and this propensity appears to be related to graft thickness, donor site infection, and patient characteristics.

Numerous etiologies for hypertrophic scarring, ranging from cellular and histologic to biochemical, have been proposed. Upregulation and overproduction of transforming growth factor-β (TGF-β) appears to be a promising possibility, with potential therapies already clinically available.[248] However, gene array technology has shown that the etiology is likely quite complex, with multiple gene alterations being involved.[249]

Hypertrophic scarring should be distinguished from a keloid. Both exhibit excessive collagen formation; however, a keloid grows beyond the original dimensions of the injury, while a hypertrophic scar is confined to its original anatomic boundaries. Hypertrophic scars frequently flatten with time and pressure, whereas keloids do not.

Numerous treatments have been postulated for hypertrophic scarring; however, few have proven to be efficacious.[250–252] Pressure applied directly to a hypertrophic scar via various vehicles has been the most widely used treatment modality. Elasticized, custom-fitted, compression garments and silicone dressings are the most widely used and accepted pressure therapies. Long-term controlled trials have not clearly demonstrated *permanent* benefits from compression therapy, but compression garments quickly reduce the mass of hypertrophic immature scars, and provide patients with tangible evidence of the benefits of conscientious follow-up. The mechanism by which compression/pressure reduces scar mass is not well defined, but histologic remodeling occurs.[253] The most successful approach to residual hypertrophic burn scars is initial pressure therapy until the wound matures, followed by subsequent excision and grafting if necessary. Intralesional injection of corticosteroids may reduce the bulk of the hypertrophic scar mass, and may be used in combination with other treatment modalities. It is believed that triamcinolone, the most commonly used steroid, acts by decreasing collagen synthesis and increasing collagen degradation.

Classically, approximately 20% of the patients treated in burn facilities were readmitted for reconstructive procedures. The most common areas of reconstruction involve the hand and wrist, arm and forearm, face, and neck. Improved inpatient burn treatment and scar management have reduced the need for subsequent reconstructive surgery to around 5 to 10% in the authors' burn center.

Marjolin's Ulcer

Chronic ulceration of old burn scars was noted by Marjolin to predispose to malignant degeneration. Squamous cell carcinoma is most common, although basal cell carcinomas occasionally occur, and rare tumors such as malignant fibrous histiocytoma, sarcoma, and melanoma have been reported. Chronic breakdown of a healed burn scar should lead to the suspicion of malignant degeneration.[254] These lesions typically appear decades after the original injury in wounds that healed primarily, but acute cases arising within a year of injury have been reported. They also can arise in grafted areas and appear to have an even longer time to occurrence when they do.[255] The precise incidence of burn scar carcinoma is unknown, but appears to be lower in countries where early excision and grafting have been adopted.

Malignancy mandates wide excision, with potential amputation if the lesion is on an extremity. Burn scar carcinomas can metastasize, typically to regional nodal basins. Prophylactic regional lymph node dissection has not improved survival, but sentinel lymph node biopsy is a promising modality to direct therapeutic node dissection and awaits validation in this population. On a selected basis, adjuvant radiation may be warranted. Generally, outcome is good with prompt diagnosis and resection.

Heterotopic Ossification

Heterotopic ossification (HO) is a rare complication of thermal injury, but is associated with significant morbidity.[256] It most commonly occurs in patients with major full-thickness burns and is found adjacent to an involved joint 1 to 3 months after injury. The upper extremity is most commonly affected. The therapist, who discovers increased pain and decreased range of motion of involved joints, usually makes the diagnosis. Limitation of physical activity usually precedes radiographic evidence of calcification, which is located in the muscle and surrounding soft tissue of the joint. Although the mechanism causing HO is not known, it has been suggested that bleeding into the soft tissue due to aggressive physical therapy is the culprit.[257] Prolonged immobilization of a joint encompassed by a burn also appears to promote HO.[258] Restricted activity promotes mobilization of body calcium stores and may lead to deposition of calcium in the soft tissues.

Some propose resection of all ossified soft tissue, but others recommend modification of rehabilitation therapy regimens and allowing the reabsorption of ossified tissue. Surgical intervention is certainly warranted with evidence of neuromuscular compromise. Bisphosphonates and external beam radiation have been advocated as prophylactic measures in high-risk patients; however, solid prospective data supporting these recommendations is lacking.

References

1. Grobmyer SR, Maniscalco SP, Purdue GF, et al: Alcohol, drug intoxication, or both at the time of burn injury as a predictor of complications and mortality in hospitalized patients with burns. *J Burn Care Rehabil* 17:532, 1996.
2. Barillo DJ, Brigham PA, Kayden DA, et al: The fire-safe cigarette: A burn prevention tool. *J Burn Care Rehabil* 21:162, 2000; discussion 164.
3. Saffle JR, Davis B, Williams P: Recent outcomes in the treatment of burn injury in the United States: A report from the American Burn Association Patient Registry. *J Burn Care Rehabil* 16:219, 1995; discussion 288.
4. Pruitt BA Jr.: Centennial changes in surgical care and research. *Ann Surg* 232:287, 2000.
5. Wrigley M, Trotman BK, Dimick A, et al: Factors relating to return to work after burn injury. *J Burn Care Rehabil* 16:445, 1995; discussion 444.
6. Brych SB, Engrav LH, Rivara FP, et al: Time off work and return to work rates after burns: Systematic review of the literature and a large two-center series. *J Burn Care Rehabil* 22:401, 2001.
7. Herndon DN, Spies M: Modern burn care. *Semin Pediatr Surg* 10:28, 2001.
8. Munster AM: Burns of the world. *J Burn Care Rehabil* 17:477, 1996.
9. Islam SS, Nambiar AM, Doyle EJ, et al: Epidemiology of work-related burn injuries: Experience of a state-managed workers' compensation system. *J Trauma* 49:1045, 2000.
10. Keswani MH: The 1996 Everett Idris Evans Memorial Lecture. The cost of burns and the relevance of prevention. *J Burn Care Rehabil* 17:485, 1996.
11. Moritz A, Henriques F: Studies of thermal injury II. The relative importance of time and surface temperature in the causation of cutaneous burns. *Am J Pathol* 23:695, 1947.
12. Yeoh C, Nixon JW, Dickson W, et al: Patterns of scald injuries [see comments]. *Arch Dis Child* 71:156, 1994.
13. Peck MD, Priolo-Kapel D: Child abuse by burning: A review of the literature and an algorithm for medical investigations. *J Trauma* 53:1013, 2002.
14. Whitaker IS, Oliver DW: A 5-year retrospective study: Burn injuries due to hot cooking oil. *Burns* 28:401, 2002.
15. Baruchin AM, Schraf S, Rosenberg L, et al: Hot bitumen burns: 92 hospitalized patients. *Burns* 23:438, 1997.
16. Renz BM, Sherman R: Hot tar burns: Twenty-seven hospitalized cases. *J Burn Care Rehabil* 15:341, 1994.
17. Turegun M, Ozturk S, Selmanpakoglu N: Sunflower oil in the treatment of hot tar burns. *Burns* 23:442, 1997.
18. Yarbrough DR III: Burns due to aerosol can explosions. *Burns* 24:270, 1998.
19. Still J, Law E, Orlet HK, et al: An unusual mechanism of burn injury due to flaming drinks. *Am Surg* 63:252, 1997.
20. Barnes SJ, Mercer DM, Cochrane TD: Flash burns to the face. *Burns* 15:250, 1989.
21. Datubo-Brown DD, Gowar JP: Contact burns in children. *Burns* 15:285, 1989.
22. Sheridan RL, Baryza MJ, Pessina MA, et al: Acute hand burns in children: Management and long-term outcome based on a 10-year experience with 698 injured hands. *Ann Surg* 229:558, 1999.
23. Yen KL, Bank DE, O'Neill AM, et al: Household oven doors: A burn hazard in children. *Arch Pediatr Adolesc Med* 155:84, 2001.
24. Sagi A, Amir A, Fliss DM, et al: Combined thermal and crush injury to the hand and fingers. *Burns* 23:176, 1997.
25. Gibran NS, Engrav LH, Heimbach DM, et al: Engine block burns: Dupuytren's fourth-, fifth-, and sixth-degree burns. *J Trauma* 37:176, 1994.
26. Karacaoglan N, Uysal A: Deep burns following epileptic seizures. *Burns* 21:546, 1995.
27. Grube BJ, Heimbach DM, Engrav LH: Molten metal burns to the lower extremity. *J Burn Care Rehabil* 8:403, 1987.
28. Margulies DR, Navarro RA, Kahn AM: Molten metal burns: Early treatment improves outcome. *Am Surg* 64:947, 1998.
29. Liao CC, Rossignol AM: Landmarks in burn prevention. *Burns* 26:422, 2000.

30. Warda L, Tenenbein M, Moffatt ME: House fire injury prevention update. Part II. A review of the effectiveness of preventive interventions. *Inj Prev* 5:217, 1999.

31. Erdmann T, Feldman K, Rivara F, et al: Tap water burn prevention: The effect of legislation. *Pediatrics* 88:572, 1991.

32. No authors listed: Hospital and prehospital resources for optimal care of patients with burn injury: Guidelines for development and operation of burn centers. American Burn Association. *J Burn Care Rehabil* 11:98, 1990.

33. Diller K, Hayes L, Baxter C: A mathematical model for the thermal efficacy of cooling therapy for burns. *J Burn Care Rehabil* 4:81, 1983.

34. Blomgren I, Eriksson E, Bagge U: The effect of different cooling temperatures and immersion fluids on post-burn oedema and survival of the partially scalded hairy mouse ear. *Burns Incl Therm Inj* 11:161, 1985.

35. Heggers J, Robson M, London M: Cooling and the prostaglandin effect in the thermal injury. *J Burn Care Rehabil* 3:350, 1982.

36. Sawada Y, Urushidate S, Yotsuyanagi T, Ishita K: Is prolonged and excessive cooling of a scalded wound effective? *Burns* 23:55, 1997.

37. Masanes MJ, Legendre C, Lioret N, et al: Fiberoptic bronchoscopy for the early diagnosis of subglottal inhalation injury: Comparative value in the assessment of prognosis. *J Trauma* 36:59, 1994.

38. Arturson G: Forty years in burns research—the postburn inflammatory response. *Burns* 26:599, 2002.

39. Huang YS, Yang ZC, Yan BG, et al: Pathogenesis of early cardiac myocyte damage after severe burns. *J Trauma* 46:428, 1999.

40. Hansbrough JF: Enteral nutritional support in burn patients. *Gastrointest Endosc Clin North Am* 8:645, 1998.

41. Moylan JA Jr., Inge WW Jr., Pruitt BA Jr.: Circulatory changes following circumferential extremity burns evaluated by the ultrasonic flowmeter: An analysis of 60 thermally injured limbs. *J Trauma* 11:763, 1971.

42. Hammond JS, Ward CG: Transfers from emergency room to burn center: Errors in burn size estimate. *J Trauma* 27:1161, 1987.

43. Heimbach D, Engrav L, Grube B, et al: Burn depth: A review. *World J Surg* 16:10, 1992.

44. Engrav L, Heimbach D, Reus J, et al: Early excision and grafting vs. nonoperative treatment of burns of indeterminant depth: A randomized prospective study. *J Trauma* 23:1001, 1983.

45. Ho-Asjoe M, Chronnell CM, Frame JD, et al: Immunohistochemical analysis of burn depth. *J Burn Care Rehabil* 20:207, 1999.

46. Watts AM, Tyler MP, Perry ME, et al: Burn depth and its histological measurement. *Burns* 27:154, 2001.

47. Wachtel TL, Leopold GR, Frank HA, et al: B-mode ultrasonic echo determination of depth of thermal injury. *Burns Incl Therm Inj* 12:432, 1986.

48. Davies M, Adendorff D, Rode H, Vandereit LS, et al: Colouring the damaged tissues on the burn wound surface. *Burns* 6:156, 1980.

49. Sheridan RL, Schomaker KT, Lucchina LC, et al: Burn depth estimation by use of indocyanine green fluorescence: Initial human trial. *J Burn Care Rehabil* 16:602, 1995.

50. Still JM, Law EJ, Klavuhn KG, et al: Diagnosis of burn depth using laser-induced indocyanine green fluorescence: A preliminary clinical trial. *Burns* 27:364, 2001.

51. Yeong EK, Mann R, Goldberg M, et al: Improved accuracy of burn wound assessment using laser Doppler. *J Trauma* 40:956, 1996.

52. Pape SA, Skouras CA, Byrne PO: An audit of the use of laser Doppler imaging (LDI) in the assessment of burns of intermediate depth. *Burns* 27:233, 2001.

53. Cole R, Jones S, Shakespeare P: Thermographic assessment of hand burns. *Burns* 16:60, 1990.

54. Heimbach D, Afromowitz M, Engrav L, et al: Burn depth estimation—man or machine. *J Trauma* 24:373, 1984.

55. Schweizer MP, Olsen JI, Shelby J, et al: Noninvasive assessment of metabolism in wounded skin by 31P-NMR in vivo. [published erratum appears in *J Trauma* 34:following table of contents.] *J Trauma* 33:828, 1992.

56. Gibran NS, Heimbach DM: Mediators in thermal injury. *Semin Nephrol* 13:344, 1993.

57. Santos FX, Arroyo C, Garcia I, et al: Role of mast cells in the pathogenesis of postburn inflammatory response: Reactive oxygen species as mast cell stimulators. *Burns* 26:145, 2000.

58. Zhang XJ, Irtun O, Zheng Y, et al: Methysergide reduces nonnutritive blood flow in normal and scalded skin. *Am J Physiol Endocrinol Metab* 278:E452, 2000.

59. Hahn EL, Gamelli RL: Prostaglandin E2 synthesis and metabolism in burn injury and trauma. *J Trauma* 49:1147, 2000.

60. Nwariaku FE, Sikes PJ, Lightfoot E, et al: Effect of a bradykinin antagonist on the local inflammatory response following thermal injury. *Burns* 22:324, 1996.

61. Ono I, Gunji H, Hasegawa T, et al: Effects of a platelet activating factor antagonist on oedema formation following burns. *Burns* 19:202, 1993.

62. Garcia-Avello A, Lorente JA, Cesar-Perez J, et al: Degree of hypercoagulability and hyperfibrinolysis is related to organ failure and prognosis after burn trauma. *Thromb Res* 89:59, 1998.

63. White DJ, Maass DL, Sanders B, et al: Cardiomyocyte intracellular calcium and cardiac dysfunction after burn trauma. *Crit Care Med* 30:14, 2002.

64. Thomas JA, Tsen MF, White DJ, et al: IRAK contributes to burn-triggered myocardial contractile dysfunction. *Am J Physiol Heart Circ Physiol* 283:H829, 2002.

65. Kelemen JJ III, Cioffi WG Jr., Mason AD Jr., et al: Effect of ambient temperature on metabolic rate after thermal injury. *Ann Surg* 223:406, 1996.

66. Yu YM, Tompkins RG, Ryan CM, et al: The metabolic basis of the increase in energy expenditure in severely burned patients. *J Parenter Enteral Nutr* 23:160, 1999.

67. Gore DC, Chinkes D, Heggers J, et al: Association of hyperglycemia with increased mortality after severe burn injury. *J Trauma* 51:540, 2001.

68. Gore DC, Chinkes DL, Hart DW, et al: Hyperglycemia exacerbates muscle protein catabolism in burn-injured patients. *Crit Care Med* 30:2438, 2002.

69. Pierre EJ, Barrow RE, Hawkins HK, et al: Effects of insulin on wound healing. *J Trauma* 44:342, 1998.

70. Thomas SJ, Morimoto K, Herndon DN, et al: The effect of prolonged euglycemic hyperinsulinemia on lean body mass after severe burn. *Surgery* 132:341, 2002.

71. Barret JP, Jeschke MG, Herndon DN: Fatty infiltration of the liver in severely burned pediatric patients: Autopsy findings and clinical implications. *J Trauma* 51:736, 2001.

72. Morio B, Irtun O, Herndon DN, et al: Propranolol decreases splanchnic triacylglycerol storage in burn patients receiving a high-carbohydrate diet. *Ann Surg* 236:218, 2002.

73. Wischmeyer PE, Lynch J, Liedel J, et al: Glutamine administration reduces Gram-negative bacteremia in severely burned patients: A prospective, randomized, double-blind trial versus isonitrogenous control. *Crit Care Med* 29:2075, 2001.

74. De Bandt JP, Coudray-Lucas C, Lioret N, et al: A randomized controlled trial of the influence of the mode of enteral ornithine alpha-ketoglutarate administration in burn patients. *J Nutr* 128:563, 1998.

75. Coudray-Lucas C, Le Bever H, Cynober L, et al: Ornithine alpha-ketoglutarate improves wound healing in severe burn patients: A prospective randomized double-blind trial versus isonitrogenous controls. *Crit Care Med* 28:1772, 2000.

76. Demling RH, Orgill DP: The anticatabolic and wound healing effects of the testosterone analog oxandrolone after severe burn injury. *J Crit Care* 15:12, 2000.

77. Herndon DN, Hart DW, Wolf SE, et al: Reversal of catabolism by beta-blockade after severe burns. *N Engl J Med* 345:1223, 2001.

78. Murphy KD, Lee JO, Herndon DN: Current pharmacotherapy for the treatment of severe burns. *Expert Opin Pharmacother* 4:369, 2003.

79. Hart DW, Wolf SE, Chinkes DL, et al: Beta-blockade and growth hormone after burn. *Ann Surg* 236:450, 2002; discussion 456.

80. Demling RH: Comparison of the anabolic effects and complications of human growth hormone and the testosterone analog, oxandrolone, after severe burn injury. *Burns* 25:215, 1999.

81. Vaughan GM, Pruitt BAJ: Thyroid function in critical illness and burn injury. *Semin Nephrol* 13:359, 1993.

82. Nygren J, Sammann M, Malm M, et al: Distributed anabolic hormonal patterns in burned patients: The relation to glucagon. *Clin Endocrinol Oxf* 43:491, 1995.

83. Xia ZF, Horton JW, Zhao PY, et al: In vivo studies of cellular energy state, pH, and sodium in rat liver after thermal injury. *J Appl Physiol* 76:1507, 1994.

84. Kinsky MP, Guha SC, Button BM, Kramer GC: The role of interstitial starling forces in the pathogenesis of burn edema. *J Burn Care Rehabil* 19:1, 1998.

85. Yowler CJ, Fratianne RB: Current status of burn resuscitation. *Clin Plast Surg* 27:1, 2000.

86. Fakhry SM, Alexander J, Smith D, et al: Regional and institutional variation in burn care. *J Burn Care Rehabil* 16:86, 1995; discussion 85.

87. Zikria BA, King TC, Stanford J, et al: A biophysical approach to capillary permeability. *Surgery* 105:625, 1989.

88. Goodwin C, Dorethy J, Lam V, et al: Randomized trial of efficacy of crystalloid and colloid resuscitation on hemodynamic response and lung water following thermal injury. *Ann Surg* 197:520, 1983.

89. Baxter C: Fluid volume and electrolyte changes in the early post-burn period. *Clin Plast Surg* 1:693, 1974.

90. Du G, Slater H, Goldfarb I: Influences of different resuscitation regimens on acute early weight gain in extensively burned patients. *Burns* 17:147, 1991.

91. Wilkes MM, Navickis RJ: Patient survival after human albumin administration. A meta-analysis of randomized, controlled trials. *Ann Intern Med* 135:149, 2001.

92. Gunn M, Hansbrough J, Davis J, et al: Prospective, randomized trial of hypertonic sodium lactate versus lactated Ringer's solution for burn shock resuscitation. *J Trauma* 29:1261, 1989.

93. Bortolani A Governa M, Barisoni D: Fluid replacement in burned patients. *Acta Chir Plast* 38:132, 1996.

94. Bunn F, Roberts I, Tasker R, et al: Hypertonic versus isotonic crystalloid for fluid resuscitation in critically ill patients. *Cochrane Database Syst Rev* 4:CD002045, 2000.

95. Kramer G, Gunther R, Nerlich M, et al: Effect of dextran-70 on increased microvascular fluid and protein flux after thermal injury. *Circ Shock* 9:529, 1982.

96. Demling RH, Kramer G, Gunther R, et al: Effect of nonprotein colloid on postburn edema formation in soft tissues and lung. *Surgery* 95:593, 1984.

97. Hall K, Sorenson B: The treatment of burn shock: Results of a 5-year randomized controlled clinical trial of Dextran 70 vs. Ringer lactate solution. *Burns* 5:107, 1978.

98. Barrow RE, Jeschke MG, Herndon DN: Early fluid resuscitation improves outcomes in severely burned children. *Resuscitation* 45:91, 2000.

99. Graves TA, Cioffi WG, McManus WF, et al: Fluid resuscitation of infants and children with massive thermal injury. *J Trauma* 28:1656, 1988.

100. Dai NT, Chen TM, Cheng TY, et al: The comparison of early fluid therapy in extensive flame burns between inhalation and noninhalation injuries. *Burns* 24:671, 1998.

101. Schiller WR, Bay RC: Hemodynamic and oxygen transport monitoring in management of burns. *S Afr Med J* 86:475, 1996.

102. Holm C, Melcer B, Horbrand F, et al: Haemodynamic and oxygen transport responses in survivors and non-survivors following thermal injury. *Burns* 26:25, 2000.

103. Lorente JA, Ezpeleta A, Esteban A, et al: Systemic hemodynamics, gastric intramucosal PCO2 changes, and outcome in critically ill burn patients. *Crit Care Med* 28:1728, 2000.

104. Engrav LH, Colescott PL, Kemalyan N, et al: A biopsy of the use of the Baxter formula to resuscitate burns or do we do it like Charlie did it? *J Burn Care Rehabil* 21:91, 2000.

105. Greenhalgh DG, Warden GD: The importance of intra-abdominal pressure measurements in burned children. *J Trauma* 36:685, 1994.

106. Ivy ME, Atweh NA, Palmer J, et al: Intra-abdominal hypertension and abdominal compartment syndrome in burn patients [see comments]. *J Trauma* 49:387, 2000.

107. Hobson KG, Young KM, Ciraulo A, et al: Release of abdominal compartment syndrome improves survival in patients with burn injury. *J Trauma* 53:1129, 2002; discussion 1133.

108. Latenser BA, Kowal-Vern A, Kimball D, et al: A pilot study comparing percutaneous decompression with decompressive laparotomy for acute abdominal compartment syndrome in thermal injury. *J Burn Care Rehabil* 23:190, 2002.

109. Tanaka H, Matsuda T, Miyagantani Y, et al: Reduction of resuscitation fluid volumes in severely burned patients using ascorbic acid administration: A randomized, prospective study. *Arch Surg* 135:326, 2000.

110. Lund T: The 1999 Everett Idris Evans memorial lecture. Edema generation following thermal injury: An update. *J Burn Care Rehabil* 20:445, 1999.

111. Jackson D, Menges H: Accidental carbon monoxide poisoning. *JAMA* 243:772, 1980.

112. Brown SD, Piantadosi CA: Reversal of carbon monoxide-cytochrome c oxidase binding by hyperbaric oxygen in vivo. *Adv Exp Med Biol* 248:747, 1989.

113. Coburn R: Mechanisms of carbon monoxide toxicity. *Prevent Med* 8:310, 1979.

114. Hardy KR, Thom SR: Pathophysiology and treatment of carbon monoxide poisoning. *J Toxicol Clin Toxicol* 32:613, 1994.

115. Thom SR, Keim LW: Carbon monoxide poisoning: A review of epidemiology, pathophysiology, clinical findings, and treatment options including hyperbaric oxygen therapy. *J Toxicol Clin Toxicol* 27:141, 1989.

116. Weaver LK, Howe S, Hopkins R, et al: Carboxyhemoglobin half-life in carbon monoxide-poisoned patients treated with 100% oxygen at atmospheric pressure. *Chest* 117:801, 2000.

117. Hampson NB: Pulse oximetry in severe carbon monoxide poisoning. *Chest* 114:1036, 1998.

118. Tibbles PM, Perrotta PL: Treatment of carbon monoxide poisoning: A critical review of human outcome studies comparing normobaric oxygen with hyperbaric oxygen [see comments]. *Ann Emerg Med* 24:269, 1994.

119. Scheinkestel CD, Bailey M, Myles PS, et al: Hyperbaric or normobaric oxygen for acute carbon monoxide poisoning: A randomised controlled clinical trial [see comments]. *Med J Aust* 170:203, 1999.

120. Weaver L, Hopkins R, Chan K, et al: Hyperbaric oxygen for acute carbon monoxide poisoning. *N Engl J Med* 347:1057, 2002.

121. Hampson NB, Dunford RG, Kramer CC, et al: Selection criteria utilized for hyperbaric oxygen treatment of carbon monoxide poisoning. *J Emerg Med* 13:227, 1995.

122. Grube B, Marvin J, Heimbach D: Therapeutic hyperbaric oxygen: Help or hindrance in burn patients with carbon monoxide poisoning? *J Burn Care Rehab* 9:249, 1988.

123. ABA, Care guidelines Chapter four: Management of carbon monoxide and cyanide poisoning. *J Burn Care Rehabil* 23:14s, 2000.

124. Stone H, Rhame D, Corbitt J: Respiratory burns: A correlation of clinical and laboratory results. *Ann Surg* 165:157, 1967.

125. Herndon DN, Traber LD, Linares H, et al: Etiology of the pulmonary pathophysiology associated with inhalation injury. *Resuscitation* 14:43, 1986.

126. Demling RH: Smoke inhalation injury. *New Horiz* 1:422, 1993.

127. Kimura R, Traber LD, Herndon DN, et al: Increasing duration of smoke exposure induces more severe lung injury in sheep. *J Appl Physiol* 64:1107, 1988.

128. Jin LJ, Lalonde C, Demling RH: Lung dysfunction after thermal injury in relation to prostanoid and oxygen radical release. *J Appl Physiol* 61:103, 1986.

129. Demling RH, Chen C: Pulmonary function in the burn patient. *Semin Nephrol* 13:371, 1993.

130. Herndon DN, Thompson PB, Traber DL: Pulmonary injury in burned patients. *Crit Care Clin* 1:79, 1985.

131. Pruitt BJ, Cioffi W, Shimazu T, et al: Evaluation and management of patients with inhalation injury. *J Trauma* 30:S63, 1990.

132. Masanes MJ, Legendre C, Lioret N, et al: Fiberoptic bronchoscopy for the early diagnosis of subglottal inhalation injury: Comparative value in the assessment of prognosis. *J Trauma* 36:59, 1994.

133. Kemper K, Benson M, Bishop M: Predictors of postextubation stridor in pediatric trauma patients. *Crit Care Med* 19:352, 1991.

134. Rodeberg DA, Easter AJ, Washam MA, et al: Use of a helium-oxygen mixture in the treatment of postextubation stridor in pediatric patients with burns. *J Burn Care Rehabil* 16:476, 1995.

135. Cioffi WG, Graves TA, McManus WF, et al: High-frequency percussive ventilation in patients with inhalation injury. *J Trauma* 29:350, 1989.

136. Rue LW III, Cioffi WG, Mason AD, et al: Improved survival of burned patients with inhalation injury. *Arch Surg* 128:772, 1993.

137. Reper P, Dankaert R, van Hille F, et al: The usefulness of combined high-frequency percussive ventilation during acute respiratory failure after smoke inhalation. *Burns* 24:34, 1998.

138. Cortiella J, Mlcak R, Herndon D: High frequency percussive ventilation in pediatric patients with inhalation injury. *J Burn Care Rehabil* 20:232, 1999.

139. Reper P, Wibaux O, Van Laeke P, et al: High frequency percussive ventilation and conventional ventilation after smoke inhalation: A randomised study. *Burns* 28:503, 2002.

140. Pallua N, Warbanow K, Noah EM, et al: Intrabronchial surfactant application in cases of inhalation injury: First results from patients with severe burns and ARDS. *Burns* 24:197, 1998.

141. Tortorolo L, Chiaretti A, Piastra M, et al: Surfactant treatment in a pediatric burn patient with respiratory failure. *Pediatr Emerg Care* 15:410, 1999.

142. Desai MH, Mlcak R, Richardson J, et al: Reduction in mortality in pediatric patients with inhalation injury with aerosolized heparin/acetylcystine therapy. *J Burn Care Rehabil* 19:210, 1998.

143. Chou NK, Chen YS, Ko WJ, et al: Application of extracorporeal membrane oxygenation in adult burn patients. *Artif Organs* 25:622, 2001.

144. Pierre EJ, Zwischenberger JB, Angel C, et al: Extracorporeal membrane oxygenation in the treatment of respiratory failure in pediatric patients with burns. *J Burn Care Rehabil* 19:131, 1998.

145. Palmieri TL, Jackson W, Greenhalgh DG: Benefits of early tracheostomy in severely burned children. *Crit Care Med* 30:922, 2002.

146. Barret JP, Desai MH, Herndon DN: Effects of tracheostomies on infection and airway complications in pediatric burn patients. *Burns* 26:190, 2000.

147. Coln CE, Purdue GF, Hunt JL: Tracheostomy in the young pediatric burn patient. *Arch Surg* 133:537, 1998; discussion 539.

148. Caruso DM, al-Kasspooles MF, Matthews MR, et al: Rationale for "early" percutaneous dilatational tracheostomy in patients with burn injuries. *J Burn Care Rehabil* 18:424, 1997.

149. Jones WG, Madden M, Finkelstein J, et al: Tracheostomies in burn patients. *Ann Surg* 209:471, 1989.

150. Saffle JR, Morris SE, Edelman L: Early tracheostomy does not improve outcome in burn patients. *J Burn Care Rehabil* 23:431, 2002.

151. Mayhall C, Polk R, Haynes B: Infections in burned patients. *Infect Control* 4:454, 1983.

152. Moylan J: Supportive therapy in burn care. Smoke inhalation. Diagnostic techniques and steroids. *J Trauma* 19(11 Suppl):917, 1979.

153. Burke J, Quinby W, Bondoc C: Primary excision and prompt grafting as routine therapy for the treatment of thermal burns in children. *Surg Clin North Am* 56:477, 1976.

154. Gray D, Pine R, Harner T: Early excision versus conventional therapy in patients with 20 to 40 percent burns. *Am J Surg* 144:76, 1982.

155. Herndon DN, Barrow RE, Rutan RL, et al: A comparison of conservative versus early excision. Therapies in severely burned patients. *Ann Surg* 209:547, 1989; discussion 552.

156. Engrav L, Heimbach D: Early reconstruction of facial burns. *West J Med* 154:203, 1991.

157. Hunt JL, Purdue GF, Spicer T, et al: Face burn reconstruction—does early excision and autografting improve aesthetic appearance? *Burns Incl Therm Inj* 13:39, 1987.

158. Cole J, Engrav L, Heimbach D, et al: Early excision and grafting of face and neck burns in patients over 20 years. *Plast Reconstr Surg* 109:1266, 2002.

159. Covey MH, Dutcher K, Heimbach DM, et al: Return of hand function following major burns. *J Burn Care Rehabil* 8:224, 1987.

160. Mann R, Gibran NS, Engrav LH, et al: Prospective trial of thick vs. standard split-thickness skin grafts in burns of the hand. *J Burn Care Rehabil* 22:390, 2001.

161. Matsumura H, Engrav LH, Nakamura DY, et al: The use of the Millard "crane" flap for deep hand burns with exposed tendons and joints. *J Burn Care Rehabil* 20:316, 1999.

162. Sheridan RL, Hurley J, Smith MA, et al: The acutely burned hand: Management and outcome based on a ten-year experience with 1047 acute hand burns. *J Trauma* 38:406, 1995.

163. Grube BJ, Engrav LH, Heimbach DM: Early ambulation and discharge in 100 patients with burns of the foot treated by grafts. *J Trauma* 33:662, 1992.

164. Gore D, Desai M, Herndon DN, et al: Comparison of complications during rehabilitation between conservative and early surgical management in thermal burns involving the feet of children and adolescents. *J Burn Care Rehabil* 9:92, 1988.

165. Goldberg DP, Kucan JO, Bash D: Reconstruction of the burned foot. *Clin Plast Surg* 27:145, 2000.

166. Holmes JH, Honari S, Gibran N: Excision and grafting of the large burn wound. *Prob Gen Surg* 20:47, 2003.

167. Matsumura H, Meyer NA, Mann R, et al: Melting graft-wound syndrome. *J Burn Care Rehabil* 19:292, 1988.

168. Sheridan RL, Tompkins RG: Skin substitutes in burns. *Burns* 25:97, 1999.

169. Wainwright D, Madden M, Luterman A, et al: Clinical evaluation of an acellular allograft dermal matrix in full-thickness burns. *J Burn Care Rehabil* 17:124, 1996.

170. Sheridan R, Choucair R, Donelan M, et al: Acellular allodermis in burns surgery: 1-year results of a pilot trial. *J Burn Care Rehabil* 19:528, 1998.

171. Hansbrough JF, Mozingo DW, Kealey GP, et al: Clinical trials of a biosynthetic temporary skin replacement, Dermagraft-Transitional Covering, compared with cryopreserved human cadaver skin for temporary coverage of excised burn wounds. *J Burn Care Rehabil* 18:43, 1997.

172. Purdue GF, Hunt JL, Still JJ, et al: A multicenter clinical trial of a biosynthetic skin replacement, Dermagraft-TC, compared with cryopreserved human cadaver skin for temporary coverage of excised burn wounds. *J Burn Care Rehabil* 18:52, 1997.

173. Burke J, Yannas I, Quinby WJ, et al: Successful use of a physiologically acceptable artificial skin in the treatment of extensive burn injury. *Ann Surg* 194:413, 1981.

174. Heimbach D, Luterman A, Burke J, et al: Artificial dermis for major burns. A multicenter randomized controlled trial. *Ann Surg* 208:313, 1988.

174a. Unpublished data presented in abstract form at the International Society of Burn Injury Quadrennial Congress, August 2002, Seattle, Washington.

175. Heimbach DM, Warden GD, Luterman A, et al: Multicenter postapproval clinical trial of Integra dermal regeneration template for burn treatment. *J Burn Care Rehabil* 24:42, 2003.

176. Kirsner RS: The use of Apligraf in acute wounds. *J Dermatol* 25:805, 1998.

177. Waymack P, Duff RG, Sabolinski M: The effect of a tissue engineered bilayered living skin analog, over meshed split-thickness autografts on the healing of excised burn wounds. The Apligraf Burn Study Group. *Burns* 26:609, 2000.

178. Munster AM: Cultured skin for massive burns. A prospective, controlled trial. *Ann Surg* 224:372, 1996.

179. Boyce S, Kagan R, Yakuboff K, et al: Cultured skin substitutes reduce donor skin harvesting for closure of excised, full-thickness burns. *Ann Surg* 235:269, 2002.

180. Wall-Alonso E, Schoeller DA, Schechter L, Gottlieb LJ: Measured total energy requirements of adult patients with burns. *J Burn Care Rehabil* 20:329, 1999; discussion 328.

181. Konstantinides FN, Radmer WJ, Becker WK, et al: Inaccuracy of nitrogen balance determinations in thermal injury with calculated total urinary nitrogen. *J Burn Care Rehabil* 13:254, 1992.

182. Rettmer RL, Williamson JC, Labbe RF, Heimbach DM: Laboratory monitoring of nutritional status in burn patients. *Clin Chem* 38:334, 1992.

183. Manelli JC, Badetti C, Botti G, et al: A reference standard for plasma proteins is required for nutritional assessment of adult burn patients. *Burns* 24:337, 1998.

184. Wolfe RR: Herman Award Lecture, 1996: Relation of metabolic studies to clinical nutrition—the example of burn injury. *Am J Emerg Med* 14:629, 1996.

185. Hart DW, Wolf SE, Zhang XJ, et al: Efficacy of a high-carbohydrate diet in catabolic illness. *Crit Care Med* 29:1318, 2001.

186. Sheridan RL, Yu YM, Prelack K, et al: Maximal parenteral glucose oxidation in hypermetabolic young children: A stable isotope study [see comments]. *J Parenter Enteral Nutr* 22:212, 1998.

187. Wolfe R, Goodenough R, Burke J, et al: Response of protein and urea kinetics in burn patients to different levels of protein intake. *Ann Surg* 197:163, 1983.

188. Wilmore DW: The effect of glutamine supplementation in patients following elective surgery and accidental injury. *J Nutr* 131 (9 Suppl):2543S, 2001; discussion 2550S.

189. Goodenough R, Wolfe R: Effect of total parenteral nutrition on free fatty acid metabolism in burned patients. *J Parenter Enteral Nutr* 8:357, 1984.

190. Gottschlich M, Jenkins M, Warden G, et al: Differential effects of three enteral dietary regimens on selected outcome variables in burn patients. *J Parenter Enteral Nutr* 14:225, 1990.

191. Garrel DR, Razi M, Lariviere F, et al: Improved clinical status and length of care with low-fat nutrition support in burn patients. *J Parenter Enteral Nutr* 19:482, 1995.

192. Selmanpakoglu AN, Cetin C, Sayal A, et al: Trace element (Al, Se, Zn, Cu) levels in serum, urine and tissues of burn patients. *Burns* 20:99, 1994.

193. Berger MM, Spertini F, Shenkin A, et al: Trace element supplementation modulates pulmonary infection rates after major burns: A double-blind, placebo-controlled trial. *Am J Clin Nutr* 68:365, 1998.

194. Herndon D, Barrow R, Stein M, et al: Increased mortality with intravenous supplemental feeding in severely burned patients. *J Burn Care Rehabil* 10:309, 1989.

195. Hansbrough WB, Hansbrough JF: Success of immediate intragastric feeding of patients with burns. *J Burn Care Rehabil* 14:512, 1993.

196. Raff T, Hartmann B, Germann G: Early intragastric feeding of seriously burned and long-term ventilated patients: A review of 55 patients. *Burns* 23:32, 1997.

197. Sefton EJ, Boulton-Jones JR, Anderton D, et al: Enteral feeding in patients with major burn injury: The use of nasojejunal feeding after the failure of nasogastric feeding. *Burns* 28:386, 2002.

198. Peng YZ, Yuan ZQ, Xiao GX: Effects of early enteral feeding on the prevention of enterogenic infection in severely burned patients. *Burns* 27:145, 2001.

199. Jeschke MG, Debroy MA, Wolf SE, et al: Burn and starvation increase programmed cell death in small bowel epithelial cells. *Dig Dis Sci* 45:415, 2000.

200. Andel H, Rab M, Andel D, et al: Impact of early high caloric duodenal feeding on the oxygen balance of the splanchnic region after severe burn injury. *Burns* 27:389, 2001.

201. Raff T, Germann G, Hartmann B: The value of early enteral nutrition in the prophylaxis of stress ulceration in the severely burned patient. *Burns* 23:319, 1997.

202. Koller J, Kvalteni K: Early enteral nutrition in severe burns. *Acta Chir Plast* 36:57, 1994.

203. Chiarelli A, Enzi G, Casadei A, et al: Very early nutrition supplementation in burned patients. *Am J Clin Nutr* 51:1035, 1990.

204. Gottschlich MM, Jenkins ME, Mayes T, et al: The 2002 Clinical Research Award. An evaluation of the safety of early vs. delayed enteral support and effects on clinical, nutritional, and endocrine outcomes after severe burns. *J Burn Care Rehabil* 23:401, 2002.

205. Jenkins ME, Gottschlich MM, Warden GD: Enteral feeding during operative procedures in thermal injuries. *J Burn Care Rehabil* 15:199, 1994.

206. Wolf SE, Jeschke MG, Rose JK, et al: Enteral feeding intolerance: An indicator of sepsis-associated mortality in burned children. *Arch Surg* 132:1310, 1997; discussion 1313.

207. Saffle JR, Wiebke G, Jennings K, et al: Randomized trial of immune-enhancing enteral nutrition in burn patients. *J Trauma* 42:793, 1997; discussion 800.

208. Scaife CL, Saffle JR, Morris SE: Intestinal obstruction secondary to enteral feedings in burn trauma patients. *J Trauma* 47:859, 1999.

209. Merrell S, Saffle J, Larson C, et al: The declining incidence of fatal sepsis following thermal injury. *J Trauma* 29:1362, 1989.

210. Rodgers GL, Mortensen J, Fisher MC, et al: Predictors of infectious complications after burn injuries in children. *Pediatr Infect Dis J* 19:990, 2000.

211. McCampbell B, Wasif N, Rabbitts A, et al: Diabetes and burns: Retrospective cohort study. *J Burn Care Rehabil* 23:157, 2002.

212. Rodgers GL, Kim J, Long SS: Fever in burned children and its association with infectious complications. *Clin Pediatr (Phila)* 39:553, 2000.

213. Parish RA, Novack AH, Heimbach DM, et al: Fever as a predictor of infection in burned children. *J Trauma* 27:69, 1987.

214. Keen A, Knoblock L, Edelman L, et al: Effective limitation of blood culture use in the burn unit. *J Burn Care Rehabil* 23:183, 2002.

215. Sachse C, Machens HG, Felmerer G, et al: Procalcitonin as a marker for the early diagnosis of severe infection after thermal injury. *J Burn Care Rehabil* 20:354, 1999.

216. von Heimburg D, Stieghorst W, Khorram-Sefat R, et al: Procalcitonin—a sepsis parameter in severe burn injuries. *Burns* 24:745, 1998.

217. Smith DJ Jr., Thomson PD: Changing flora in burn and trauma units: Historical perspective—experience in the United States. *J Burn Care Rehabil* 13:276, 1992.

218. Miller PL, Matthey FC: A cost-benefit analysis of initial burn cultures in the management of acute burns. *J Burn Care Rehabil* 21:300, 2000.

219. Rue LW III, Cioffi WG, Mason AD Jr., et al: The risk of pneumonia in thermally injured patients requiring ventilatory support. *J Burn Care Rehabil* 16(3 Pt 1):262, 1995.

220. Still J, Newton T, Friedman B, et al: Experience with pneumonia in acutely burned patients requiring ventilator support. *Am Surg* 66:206, 2000.

221. Gillespie P, Siddiqui H, Clarke J: Cannula related suppurative thrombophlebitis in the burned patient. *Burns* 26:200, 2000.

222. Still JM, Law E, Thiruvaiyaru D, et al: Central line-related sepsis in acute burn patients. *Am Surg* 64:165, 1998.

223. Ramos GE, Bolgiani AN, Patino O, et al: Catheter infection risk related to the distance between insertion site and burned area. *J Burn Care Rehabil* 23:266, 2002.

224. Garcia-Sanchez V, Gomez Morell P: Electric burns: High- and low-tension injuries. *Burns* 25:357, 1999.

225. Lee RC: Injury by electrical forces: Pathophysiology, manifestations, and therapy. *Curr Probl Surg* 34:677, 1997.

226. Haberal M, Ucar N, Bayraktar U, et al. Visceral injuries, wound infection and sepsis following electrical injuries. *Burns* 22:158, 1996.

227. Rosen CL, Adler JN, Rabban JT, et al: Early predictors of myoglobinuria and acute renal failure following electrical injury. *J Emerg Med* 17:783, 1999.

228. Hammond J, Ward CG: Myocardial damage and electrical injuries: Significance of early elevation of CPK-MB isoenzymes. *South Med J* 79:414, 1986.

229. Housinger T, Green L, Shahangian S, et al: A prospective study of myocardial damage in electrical injuries. [published erratum appears in *J Trauma* 26:659, 1986.] *J Trauma* 25:122, 1985.

230. Purdue GF, Hunt JL: Electrocardiographic monitoring after electrical injury: Necessity or luxury. *J Trauma* 26:166, 1986.

231. Grossman AR, Tempereau CE, Brones MF, et al: Auditory and neuropsychiatric behavior patterns after electrical injury. *J Burn Care Rehabil* 14:169, 1993.

232. Koller J, Orsagh J: Delayed neurological sequelae of high-tension electrical burns. *Burns* 15:175, 1989.

233. Grube B, Heimbach D, Engrav L, et al: Neurologic consequences of electrical burns. *J Trauma* 30:254, 1990.

234. Lynch CD, Pollock M: Nerve thermal injury. *Prog Brain Res* 115:453, 1998.

235. Boozalis GT, Purdue GF, Hunt JL, et al: Ocular changes from electrical burn injuries. A literature review and report of cases. *J Burn Care Rehabil* 12:458, 1991.

236. Saffle J, Crandall A, Warden G: Cataracts: A long-term complication of electrical injury. *J Trauma* 25:17, 1985.

237. Mann R, Gibran N, Engrav L, et al: Is immediate decompression of high voltage electrical injuries to the upper extremity always necessary? *J Trauma* 40:584, 1996; discussion 587.

238. Yano K, Hata Y, Matsuka K, et al: Effects of washing with a neutralizing agent on alkaline skin injuries in an experimental model. *Burns* 20:36, 1994.

239. Lin TM, Tsai CC, Lin SD, et al: Continuous intra-arterial infusion therapy in hydrofluoric acid burns. *J Occup Environ Med* 42:892, 2000.

240. Latarjet J, Choinére M: Pain in burn patients. *Burns* 21:344, 1995.

241. Choiniére M, Melzack R, Rondeau J, et al: The pain of burns: Characteristics and correlates. *J Trauma* 29:1531, 1989.

242. Patterson DR, Ptacek JT, Carrougher GJ, et al: Lorazepam as an adjunct to opioid analgesics in the treatment of burn pain. *Pain* 72:367, 1997.

243. Patterson DR, Adcock RJ, Bombardier CH: Factors predicting hypnotic analgesia in clinical burn pain. *Int J Clin Exp Hypn* 45:377, 1997.

244. Hoffman HG, Patterson DR, Carrougher GJ: Use of virtual reality for adjunctive treatment of adult burn pain during physical therapy: A controlled study. *Clin J Pain* 16:244, 2000.

245. Hoffman HG, Patterson DR, Carrougher GJ, et al: Effectiveness of virtual reality-based pain control with multiple treatments. *Clin J Pain* 17:229, 2001.

246. Deitch E, Wheelahan T, Rose M, et al: Hypertrophic burn scars: Analysis of variables. *J Trauma* 23:895, 1983.

247. Matsumura H, Engrav LH, Gibran NS, et al: Cones of skin occur where hypertrophic scar occurs. *Wound Repair Regen* 9:269, 2001.

248. Wang R, Ghahary A, Shen Q, et al: Hypertrophic scar tissues and fibroblasts produce more transforming growth factor-beta1 mRNA and protein than normal skin and cells. *Wound Repair Regen* 8:128, 2000.

249. Tsou R, Cole JK, Nathens AB, et al: Analysis of hypertrophic and normal scar gene expression with cDNA microarrays. *J Burn Care Rehabil* 21:541, 2000.

250. Roques C: Massage applied to scars. *Wound Repair Regen* 10:126, 2002.

251. Van den Kerckhove E, Stappaerts K, Boeckx W, et al: Silicones in the rehabilitation of burns: A review and overview. *Burns* 27:205, 2001.

252. Judge J, May R, DeClement F: Control of hypertrophic scarring in burn patients using tubular support bandages. *J Burn Care Rehab* 5:221, 1984.

253. Costa AM, Peyrol S, Porto LC, et al: Mechanical forces induce scar remodeling. Study in non-pressure-treated versus pressure-treated hypertrophic scars. *Am J Pathol* 155:1671, 1999.

254. Copcu E, Aktas A, Sisman N, et al: Thirty-one cases of Marjolin's ulcer. *Clin Exp Dermatol* 28:138, 2003.

255. Turegun M, Nisanci M, Guler M: Burn scar carcinoma with longer lag period arising in previously grafted area. *Burns* 23:496, 1997.

256. Richards AM, Klaassen MF: Heterotopic ossification after severe burns: A report of three cases and review of the literature. *Burns* 23:64, 1997.

257. Crawford C, Varghese G, Mani M, et al: Heterotopic ossification: Are range of motion exercises contraindicated? *J Burn Care Rehab* 7:323, 1986.

258. Elledge ES, Smith AA, McManus WF, et al: Heterotopic bone formation in burned patients. *J Trauma* 28:684, 1988.

CHAPTER 8

Wound Healing

Adrian Barbul[1]

HISTORY OF WOUND HEALING

The earliest accounts of wound healing date back to about 2000 B.C., when the Sumerians employed two modes of treatment: a spiritual method consisting of incantations, and a physical method of applying poultice-like materials to the wound. The Egyptians were the first to differentiate between infected and diseased wounds compared to noninfected wounds. The 1650 B.C. Edwin Smith Surgical Papyrus, a copy of a much older document, describes at least 48 different types of wounds. A later document (Ebers Papyrus, 1550 B.C.) relates the use of concoctions containing honey (antibacterial properties), lint (absorbent properties), and grease (barrier) for treating wounds. These same properties are still considered essential in contemporary daily wound management.

The Greeks, equipped with the knowledge bequeathed by the Egyptians, went even further and classified wounds as acute or chronic in nature. Galen of Pergamum (120–201 A.D.), appointed as the doctor to the Roman gladiators, had an enormous number of wounds to deal with following[1] gladiatorial combats. He emphasized the importance of maintaining a moist environment to ensure adequate healing. It took almost 19 centuries for this important concept to be proven scientifically, when it was shown that the epithelialization rate increases by 50% in a moist wound environment when compared to a dry wound environment.[1]

The next major stride in the history of wound healing was the discovery of antiseptics and their importance in reducing wound infections. Ignaz Philipp Semmelweis, a Hungarian obstetrician (1818–1865), noted that the incidence of puerperal fever was much

---

[1]With assistance from David E. Efron, MD; Chandrakanth Are, MD; Julie E. Park, MD; and Vanita Ahuja, MD.

lower if medical students, following cadaver-dissection class and prior to attending childbirth, washed their hands with soap and hypochlorite. Louis Pasteur (1822–1895) was instrumental in dispelling the theory of spontaneous generation of germs and proving that germs were always introduced into the wound from the environment. Joseph Lister probably made one of the most significant contributions to wound healing. On a visit to Glasgow, Scotland, Lister noted that some areas of the city's sewer system were less murky than the rest. He discovered that the water from pipes that were dumping waste containing carbolic acid (phenol) was clear. In 1865, Lister began soaking his instruments in phenol and spraying the operating rooms, reducing the mortality rates from 50 to 15%. This practice led to the suspension of Lister, although subsequent confirmation of his results paved the way for his triumphant return to Edinburgh.

After attending an impressive lecture by Lister in 1876, Robert Wood Johnson left the meeting and began 10 years of research that would ultimately result in the production of an antiseptic dressing in the form of cotton gauze impregnated with iodoform. Since then, several other materials have been used to impregnate cotton gauze to achieve antisepsis.

The 1960s and 1970s led to the development of polymeric dressings. These polymeric dressings can be custom made to specific parameters, such as permeability to gases (occlusive vs. semiocclusive), varying degrees of absorbency, and different physical forms. Due to the ability to customize, the available range of materials that aid in wound care has grown exponentially to include an ever expanding variety. Currently, the practice of wound healing encompasses manipulation and/or use of, among others, inflammatory cytokines, growth factors, and bioengineered tissue. It is the combination of all these modalities that enables optimal wound healing.

PHASES OF WOUND HEALING

As noted by John Hunter (1728–1793), a keen observer of biologic phenomena, "... the injury alone has in all cases a tendency to produce the disposition and the means of a cure."[1a] Normal wound healing follows a predictable pattern that can be divided into overlapping phases defined by the cellular populations and biochemical activities: (a) hemostasis and inflammation, (b) proliferation, and (c) maturation and remodeling. An approximate timeline of these events is depicted in Fig. 8-1. This sequence of events is fluid and overlapping, and in most circumstances spans the time from injury to resolution of acute wounds. All wounds need to progress through this series of cellular and biochemical events that characterizes the phases of healing in order to successfully re-establish tissue integrity.

Hemostasis and Inflammation

Hemostasis precedes and initiates inflammation with the ensuing release of chemotactic factors from the wound site (Fig. 8-2A). Wounding by definition disrupts tissue integrity, leading to division of blood vessels and direct exposure of extracellular matrix to platelets. Exposure of subendothelial collagen to platelets results in platelet aggregation, degranulation, and activation of the coagulation cascade. Platelet α granules release a number of wound-active substances, such as platelet-derived growth factor (PDGF), transforming growth factor-β (TGF-β), platelet-activating factor (PAF), fibronectin, and serotonin. In addition to achieving hemostasis, the fibrin clot serves as scaffolding for the migration into the wound of

inflammatory cells such as polymorphonuclear leukocytes (PMNs, neutrophils) and monocytes.

Cellular infiltration after injury follows a characteristic, predetermined sequence (see Fig. 8-1). PMNs are the first infiltrating cells to enter the wound site, peaking at 24 to 48 hours. Increased vascular permeability, local prostaglandin release, and the presence of chemotactic substances such as complement factors, interleukin-1 (IL-1), tumor necrosis factor-α (TNF-α), TGF-β, platelet factor 4, or bacterial products all stimulate neutrophil migration.

The postulated primary role of neutrophils is phagocytosis of bacteria and tissue debris. PMNs are also a major source of cytokines early during inflammation, especially TNF-α,[2] which may have a significant influence on subsequent angiogenesis and collagen synthesis (see Fig. 8-2B). PMNs also release proteases such as collagenases, which participate in matrix and ground substance degradation in the early phase of wound healing. Other than their role in limiting infections, these cells do not appear to play a role in collagen deposition or acquisition of mechanical wound strength. On the contrary, neutrophil factors have been implicated in delaying the epithelial closure of wounds.[3]

The second population of inflammatory cells that invades the wound consists of macrophages, which are recognized as being essential to successful healing.[4] Derived from circulating monocytes, macrophages achieve significant numbers in the wound by 48 to 96 hours postinjury and remain present until wound healing is complete.

Macrophages, like neutrophils, participate in wound débridement via phagocytosis and contribute to microbial stasis via oxygen radical and nitric oxide synthesis (see Fig. 8-2B). The macrophage's most pivotal function is activation and recruitment of other cells via mediators such as cytokines and growth factors, as well as directly by cell-cell interaction and intercellular adhesion molecules (ICAM). By releasing such mediators as TGF-β, vascular endothelial growth factor (VEGF), insulin-like growth factor (IGF), epithelial growth factor (EGF), and lactate, macrophages regulate cell proliferation, matrix synthesis, and angiogenesis.[5,6] Macrophages also play a significant role in regulating angiogenesis and matrix deposition and remodeling (Table 8-1).

T lymphocytes comprise another population of inflammatory/immune cells that routinely invades the wound. Less numerous than macrophages, T-lymphocyte numbers peak at about 1 week postinjury and truly bridge the transition from the inflammatory to the proliferative phase of healing. Though known to be essential to wound healing, the lymphocytes' role in wound healing is not fully defined.[7] A significant body of data supports the hypothesis that T lymphocytes play an active role in the modulation of the wound environment. Depletion of most wound T lymphocytes decreases wound strength and collagen content,[8] while selective depletion of the CD8+ suppressor subset of T lymphocytes enhances wound healing. However, depletion of the CD4+ helper subset has no effect.[9] Lymphocytes also exert a downregulating effect on fibroblast collagen synthesis by cell-associated interferon (IFN)-γ, TNF-α, and IL-1. This effect is lost if the cells are physically separated, suggesting that extracellular matrix synthesis is regulated not only via soluble factors but also by direct cell-cell contact between lymphocytes and fibroblasts.[10]

Proliferation

The proliferative phase is the second phase of wound healing and roughly spans days 4 through 12 (see Fig. 8-2C). It is during this phase that tissue continuity is re-established. Fibroblasts and endothelial cells are the last cell populations to infiltrate the healing

PHASES OF HEALING

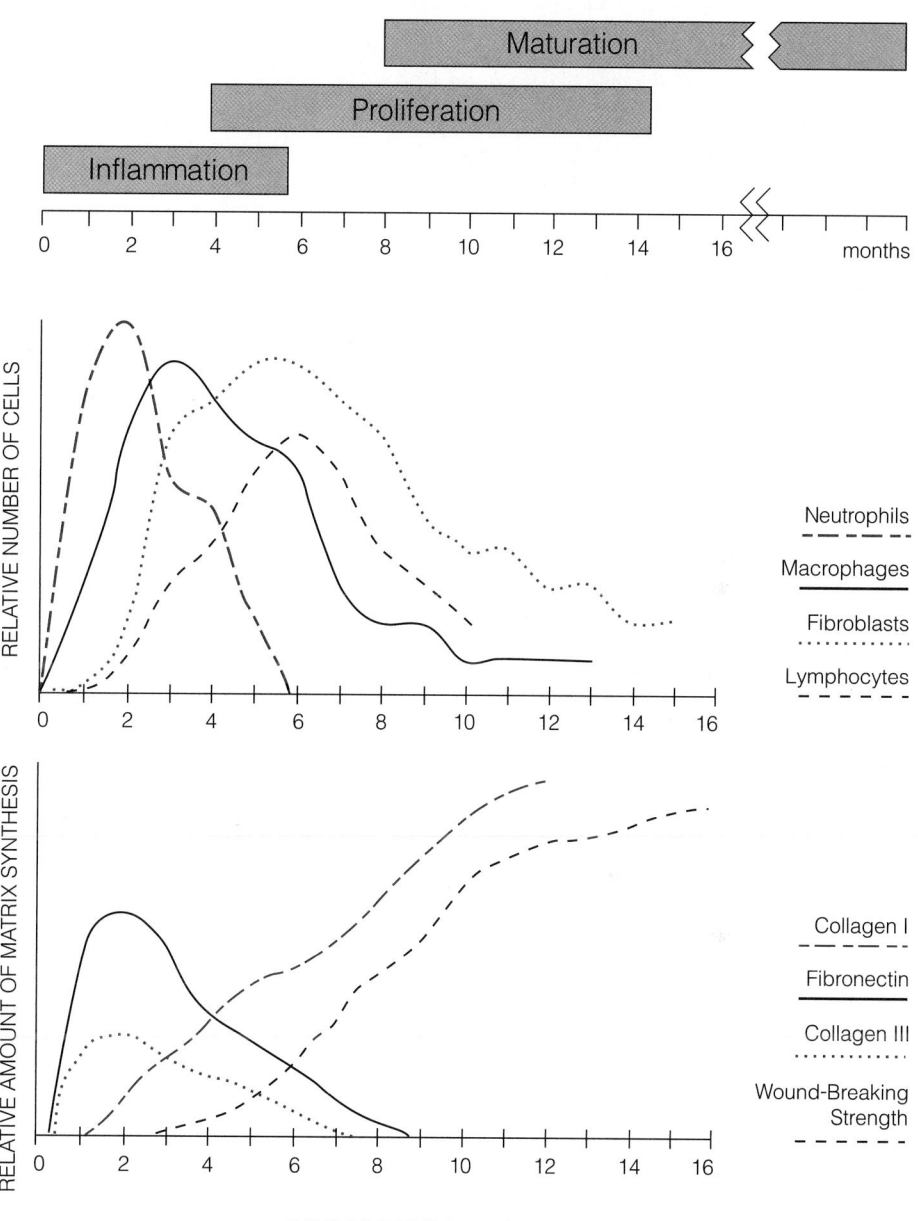

FIG. 8-1. *The cellular, biochemical, and mechanical phases of wound healing.*

wound, and the strongest chemotactic factor for fibroblasts is PDGF.[11,12] Upon entering the wound environment, recruited fibroblasts first need to proliferate, and then become activated, to carry out their primary function of matrix synthesis and remodeling. This activation is mediated mainly by the cytokines and growth factors released from wound macrophages.

Fibroblasts isolated from wounds synthesize more collagen than nonwound fibroblasts, they proliferate less, and they actively carry out matrix contraction. Although it is clear that the cytokine-rich wound environment plays a significant role in this phenotypic alteration and activation, the exact mediators are only partially characterized.[13,14] Additionally, lactate, which accumulates in significant amounts in the wound environment over time (~10 mmol), is a potent regulator of collagen synthesis through a mechanism involving ADP-ribosylation.[15,16]

Endothelial cells also proliferate extensively during this phase of healing. These cells participate in the formation of new capillaries (angiogenesis), a process essential to successful wound healing. Endothelial cells migrate from intact venules close to the wound. Their migration, replication, and new capillary tubule formation is under the influence of such cytokines and growth factors as TNF-α, TGF-β, and VEGF. Although many cells produce VEGF, macrophages represent a major source in the healing wound, and VEGF receptors are located specifically on endothelial cells.[17,18]

Matrix Synthesis

Biochemistry of Collagen

Collagen, the most abundant protein in the body, plays a critical role in the successful completion of adult wound healing. Its

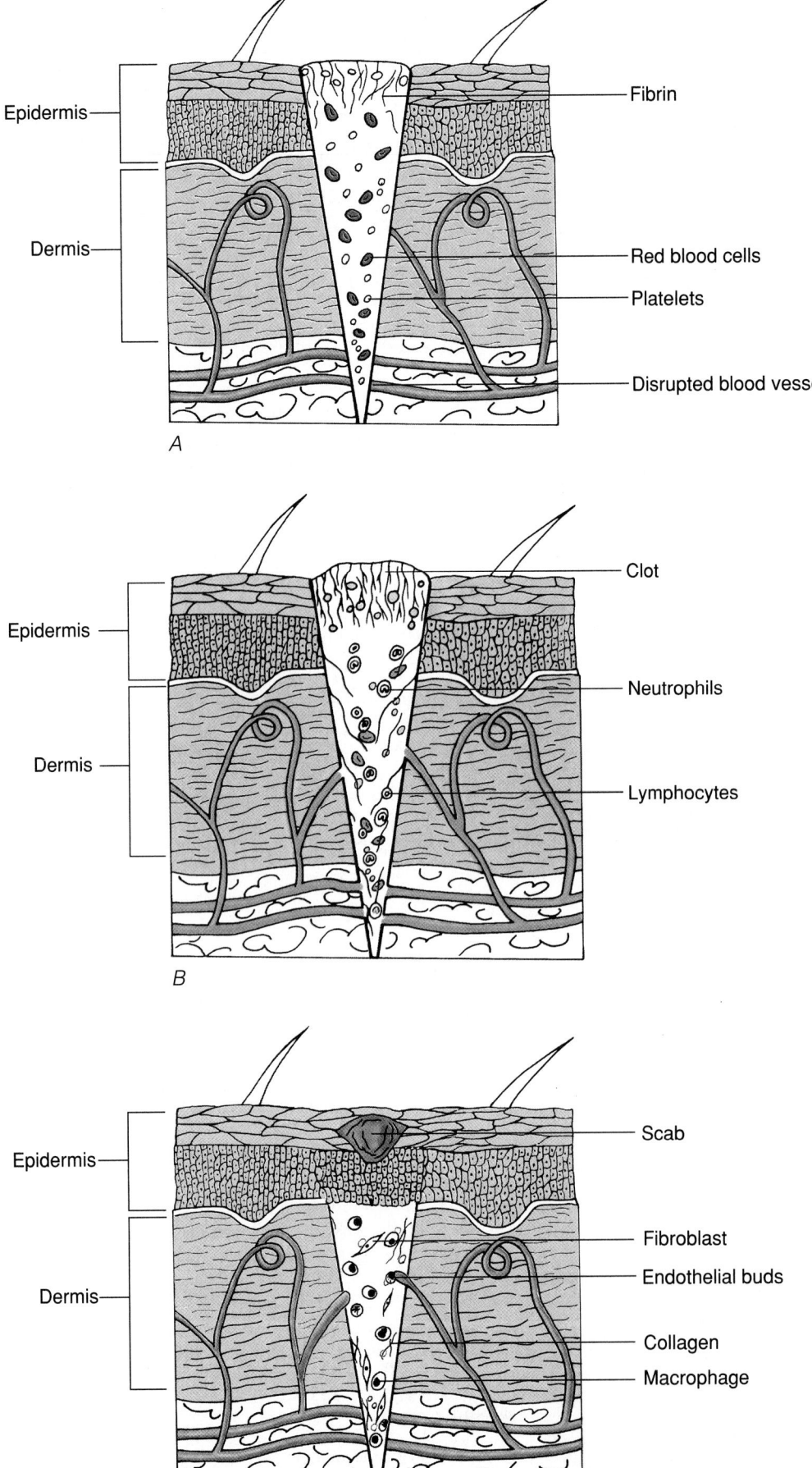

Epidermis

Dermis

Fibrin

Red blood cells

Platelets

Disrupted blood vessel

A

Epidermis

Dermis

Clot

Neutrophils

Lymphocytes

B

Epidermis

Dermis

Scab

Fibroblast

Endothelial buds

Collagen

Macrophage

C

FIG. 8-2. The phases of wound healing viewed histologically. *A.* The hemostatic/inflammatory phase. *B.* Latter inflammatory phases reflecting infiltration by mononuclear cells and lymphocytes. *C.* The proliferative phase with associated angiogenesis and collagen synthesis.

Table 8-1
Macrophage Activities During Wound Healing

Activity	Mediators
Phagocytosis	Reactive oxygen species
	Nitric oxide
Débridement	Collagenase, elastase
Cell recruitment and activation	Growth factors: PDGF, TGF-β, EGF, IGF
	Cytokines: TNF-α, IL-1, IL-6
	Fibronectin
Matrix synthesis	Growth factors: TGF-β, EGF, PDGF
	Cytokines: TNF-α, IL-1, IFN-γ
	Enzymes: arginase, collagenase
	Prostaglandins
	Nitric oxide
Angiogenesis	Growth factors: FGF, VEGF
	Cytokines: TNF-α
	Nitric oxide

EGF = epithelial growth factor; FGF = fibroblast growth factor; IGF = insulin-like growth factor; IFN-γ = interferon-γ; IL-1 = interleukin-1; IL-6 = interleukin-6; PDGF = platelet-derived growth factor; TGF-β = transforming growth factor-β; TNF-α = tumor necrosis factor-α; TNF-β = tumor necrosis factor-β; VEGF = vascular endothelial growth factor.

deposition, maturation, and subsequent remodeling are essential to the functional integrity of the wound.

Although there are at least 18 types of collagen described, the main ones of interest to wound repair are types I and III. Type I collagen is the major component of extracellular matrix in skin. Type III, which is also normally present in skin, becomes more prominent and important during the repair process.

Biochemically, each chain of collagen is composed of a glycine residue in every third position. The second position in the triplet is made up of proline or lysine during the translation process. The polypeptide chain that is translated from mRNA contains approximately 1000 amino acid residues and is called *protocollagen*. Release of protocollagen into the endoplasmic reticulum results in the hydroxylation of proline to hydroxyproline and of lysine to hydroxylysine by specific hydroxylases (Fig. 8-3). Prolyl hydroxylase requires oxygen and iron as cofactors, α-ketoglutarate as cosubstrate, and ascorbic acid (vitamin C) as an electron donor. In the endoplasmic reticulum, the protocollagen chain is also glycosylated by the linking of galactose and glucose at specific hydroxylysine residues. These steps of hydroxylation and glycosylation alter the hydrogen bonding forces within the chain, imposing steric changes that force the protocollagen chain to assume an α-helical configuration. Three α-helical chains entwine to form a right-handed superhelical structure called *procollagen*. At both ends, this structure contains nonhelical peptide domains called *registration peptides*. Although initially joined by weak, ionic bonds, the procollagen molecule becomes much stronger by the covalent cross-linking of lysine residues.

Extracellularly, the nonhelical registration peptides are cleaved by a procollagen peptidase, and the procollagen strands undergo further polymerization and cross-linking. The resulting collagen monomer is further polymerized and cross-linked by the formation of intra- and intermolecular covalent bonds.

Collagen synthesis, as well as posttranslational modifications, are highly dependent on systemic factors such as an adequate oxygen supply; the presence of sufficient nutrients (amino acids and carbohydrates) and cofactors (vitamins and trace metals); and the local wound environment (vascular supply and lack of infection).

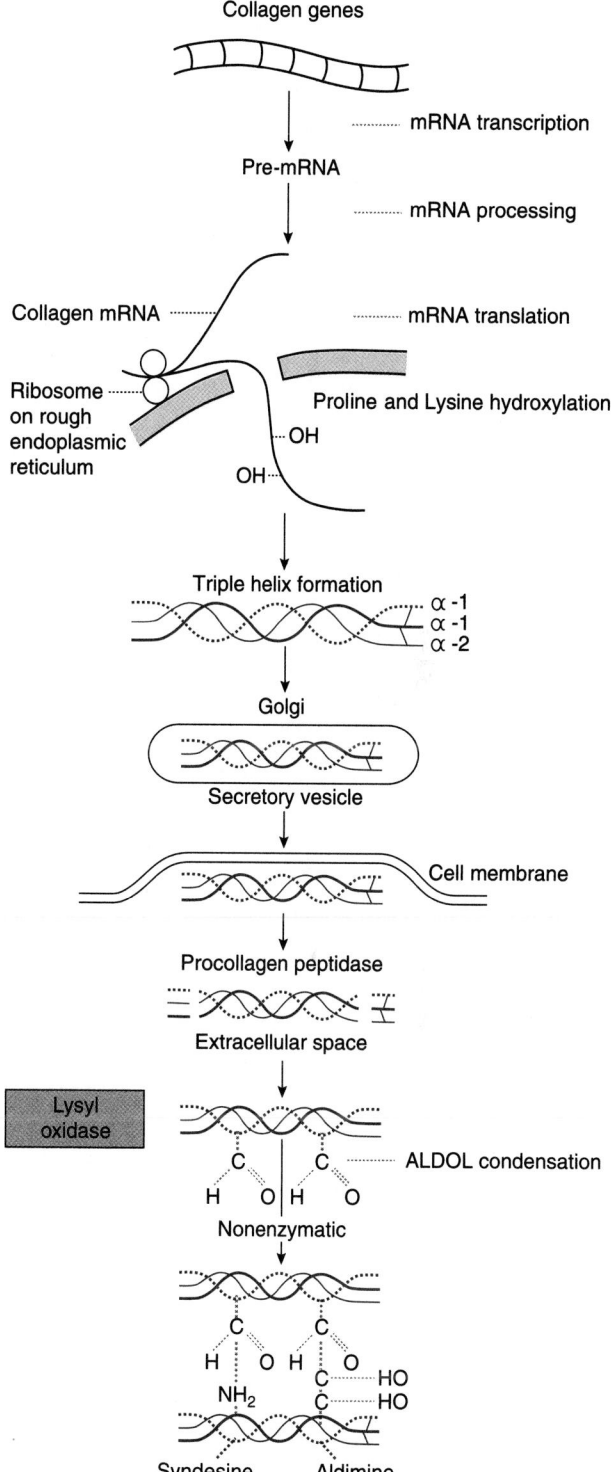

FIG. 8-3. The steps of collagen synthesis.

Addressing these factors and reversing nutritional deficiencies can optimize collagen synthesis and deposition.

Proteoglycan Synthesis

Glycosaminoglycans comprise a large portion of the "ground substance" that makes up granulation tissue. Rarely found free, they couple with proteins to form *proteoglycans*. The polysaccharide chain is made up of repeating disaccharide units composed of glucuronic or iduronic acid and a hexosamine, which is usually sulfated. The disaccharide composition of proteoglycans varies from about 10 units in the case of heparan sulfate to as much as 2000 units in the case of hyaluronic acid.

The major glycosaminoglycans present in wounds are dermatan and chondroitin sulfate. Fibroblasts synthesize these compounds, increasing their concentration greatly during the first 3 weeks of healing. The interaction between collagen and proteoglycans is being actively studied. It is thought that the assembly of collagen subunits into fibrils and fibers is dependent upon the lattice provided by the sulfated proteoglycans. Furthermore, it appears that the extent of sulfation is critical in determining the configuration of the collagen fibrils. As scar collagen is deposited, the proteoglycans are incorporated into the collagen scaffolding. However, with scar maturation and collagen remodeling, the content of proteoglycans gradually diminishes.

Maturation and Remodeling

The maturation and remodeling of the scar begins during the fibroplastic phase, and is characterized by a reorganization of previously synthesized collagen. Collagen is broken down by matrix metalloproteinases (MMPs), and the net wound collagen content is the result of a balance between collagenolysis and collagen synthesis. There is a net shift toward collagen synthesis and eventually the re-establishment of extracellular matrix composed of a relatively acellular collagen-rich scar.

Wound strength and mechanical integrity in the fresh wound are determined by both the quantity and quality of the newly deposited collagen. The deposition of matrix at the wound site follows a characteristic pattern: fibronectin and collagen type III constitute the early matrix scaffolding; glycosaminoglycans and proteoglycans represent the next significant matrix components; and collagen type I is the final matrix. By several weeks postinjury the amount of collagen in the wound reaches a plateau, but the tensile strength continues to increase for several more months.[19] Fibril formation and fibril cross-linking result in decreased collagen solubility, increased strength, and increased resistance to enzymatic degradation of the collagen matrix. Scar remodeling continues for many (6 to 12) months postinjury, gradually resulting in a mature, avascular, and acellular scar. The mechanical strength of the scar never achieves that of the uninjured tissue.

There is a constant turnover of collagen in the extracellular matrix, both in the healing wound, as well as during normal tissue homeostasis. Collagenolysis is the result of collagenase activity, a class of matrix metalloproteinases that require activation. Both collagen synthesis and lysis are strictly controlled by cytokines and growth factors. Some factors affect both aspects of collagen remodeling. For example, TGF-β increases new collagen transcription and also decreases collagen breakdown by stimulating synthesis of tissue inhibitors of metalloproteinase.[20] This balance of collagen deposition and degradation is the ultimate determinant of wound strength and integrity.

Epithelialization

While tissue integrity and strength are being re-established, the external barrier must also be restored. This process is characterized primarily by proliferation and migration of epithelial cells adjacent to the wound (Fig. 8-4). The process begins within 1 day of injury and is seen as thickening of the epidermis at the wound

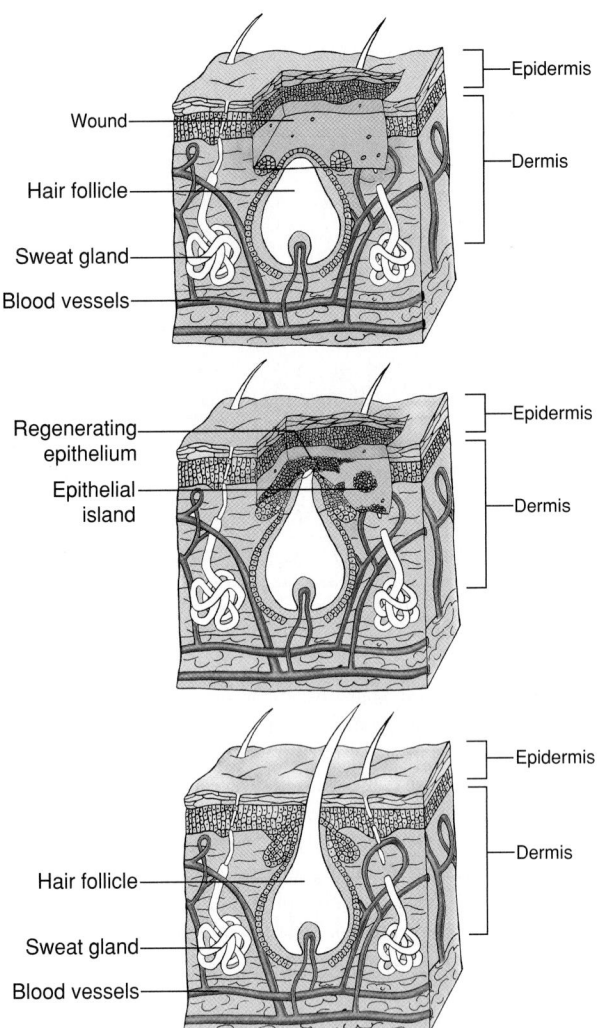

FIG. 8-4. The healing by epithelialization of superficial cutaneous wounds.

edge. Marginal basal cells at the edge of the wound lose their firm attachment to the underlying dermis, enlarge, and begin to migrate across the surface of the provisional matrix. Fixed basal cells in a zone near the cut edge undergo a series of rapid mitotic divisions, and these cells appear to migrate by moving over one another in a leapfrog fashion until the defect is covered.[21] Once the defect is bridged, the migrating epithelial cells lose their flattened appearance, become more columnar in shape, and increase their mitotic activity. Layering of the epithelium is re-established, and the surface layer eventually keratinizes.[22]

Re-epithelialization is complete in less than 48 hours in the case of approximated incised wounds, but may take substantially longer in the case of larger wounds, where there is a significant epidermal/dermal defect. If only the epithelium and superficial dermis are damaged, such as occurs in split-thickness skin graft donor sites or in superficial second-degree burns, then repair consists primarily of re-epithelialization with minimal or no fibroplasia and granulation tissue formation. The stimuli for re-epithelialization remain incompletely defined; however, it appears that the process is mediated by a combination of a loss of contact inhibition; exposure to constituents of the extracellular matrix, particularly fibronectin; and cytokines produced by immune mononuclear cells.[23,24] In particular

Table 8-2
Growth Factors Participating in Wound Healing

Growth Factor	Wound Cell Origin	Cellular and Biological Effects
Platelet-derived growth factor (PDGF)	Platelets, macrophages, monocytes, smooth muscle cells, endothelial cells	Chemotaxis: fibroblasts, smooth muscle, monocytes, neutrophils Mitogenesis: fibroblasts, smooth muscle cells Stimulation of angiogenesis Stimulation of collagen synthesis
Fibroblast growth factor (FGF)	Fibroblasts, endothelial cells, smooth muscle cells, chondrocytes	Stimulation of angiogenesis (by stimulation of endothelial cell proliferation and migration) Mitogenesis: mesoderm and neuroectoderm Stimulates fibroblasts, keratinocytes, chondrocytes, myoblasts
Keratinocyte growth factor (KGF)	Keratinocytes, fibroblasts	Significant homology with FGF; stimulates keratinocytes
Epidermal growth factor (EGF)	Platelets, macrophages, monocytes (also identified in salivary glands, duodenal glands, kidney, and lacrimal glands)	Stimulates proliferation and migration of all epithelial cell types
Transforming growth factor-α (TGF-α)	Keratinocytes, platelets, macrophages	Homology with EGF; binds to EGF receptor Mitogenic and chemotactic for epidermal and endothelial cells
Transforming growth factor-β (TGF-β) (3 isoforms: β_1, β_2, β_3)	Platelets, T lymphocytes, macrophages, monocytes, neutrophils	Stimulates angiogenesis TGF-β_1 stimulates wound matrix production (fibronectin, collagen glycosaminoglycans); regulation of inflammation TGF-β_3 inhibits scar formation
Insulin-like growth factors (IGF-1, IGF-2)	Platelets (IGF-1 in high concentrations in liver; IGF-2 in high concentrations in fetal growth)	Likely the effector of growth hormone action Promotes protein/extracellular matrix synthesis Increase membrane glucose transport
Vascular endothelial growth factor (VEGF)	Macrophages, fibroblasts, keratinocytes	Similar to PDGF Mitogen for endothelial cells (not fibroblasts) Stimulates angiogenesis
Granulocyte-macrophage colony-stimulating factor (GM-CSF)	Macrophage/monocytes, endothelial cells, fibroblasts	Stimulates macrophage differentiation/proliferation

EGF, TGF-β, basic fibroblast growth factor (bFGF), PDGF, and IGF-1 have been shown to promote epithelialization.

Role of Growth Factors in Normal Healing

Growth factors and cytokines are polypeptides produced in normal and wounded tissue that stimulate cellular migration, proliferation, and function. They are often named for the cells from which they were first derived (e.g., platelet-derived growth factor, PDGF) or for their initially identified function (e.g., fibroblast growth factor, FGF). These names are often misleading because growth factors have been demonstrated to have multiple functions. Most growth factors are extremely potent and produce significant effects in nanomolar concentrations.

They may act in an autocrine manner (where the growth factor acts on the cell producing it), a paracrine manner (by release into the extracellular environment, where it acts on the immediately neighboring cells), or in an endocrine manner (where the effect of the substance is distant to the site of release, and the substance is carried to the effector site through the blood stream). The timing of release may be as important as concentration in determining the effectiveness of growth factors. As these polypeptides exert their effects by cell-surface receptor binding, the appropriate receptor on the responding cells must be present at the time of release in order for the biologic effect to occur. Table 8-2 summarizes the principal growth factors found in healing wounds and their known effects on cells participating in the healing process. Growth factors have divergent actions on different cells; they can be chemoattractive to one cell type while stimulating replication of a different cell type. Little is known about the ratio of growth factor concentrations, which may be as important as the absolute concentration of individual growth factors.

Growth factors act on cells via surface receptor binding. Various receptor types have been described, such as ion channels, G-protein linked, or enzyme linked. The response elicited in the cell is usually one of phosphorylation or dephosphorylation of second-messenger molecules through the action of phosphatases or kinases, resulting in activation or deactivation of proteins in the cytosol or nucleus of the target cell. Phosphorylation of nuclear proteins is followed by the initiation of transcription of target genes.[25] The signal is stopped by internalization of the receptor-ligand complex.

Wound Contraction

All wounds undergo some degree of contraction. For wounds that do not have surgically approximated edges, the area of the wound will be decreased by this action (healing by secondary intention); the shortening of the scar itself results in contracture. The myofibroblast has been postulated as being the major cell responsible for contraction, and it differs from the normal fibroblast in that it possesses a cytoskeletal structure. Typically this cell contains α-smooth muscle actin in thick bundles called *stress fibers,* giving myofibroblasts contractile capability.[26] The α-smooth muscle actin is undetectable until day 6, and then is increasingly expressed for the next 15 days of wound healing.[27] After 4 weeks this expression fades and the cells are believed to undergo apoptosis.[28] A puzzling point is that the identification of myofibroblasts in the wound does not correspond directly to the initiation of wound contraction, which starts almost immediately after injury.

Fibroblasts placed in a collagen lattice in vitro actively move in the lattice and contract it without expressing stress fibers. It is postulated that the movement of cells with concomitant reorganization of the cytoskeleton is responsible for contraction.[29]

HERITABLE DISEASES OF CONNECTIVE TISSUE

Heritable diseases of connective tissue consist of a group of generalized, genetically determined, primary disorders of one of the elements of connective tissue: collagen, elastin, or mucopolysaccharide. Five major types, Ehlers-Danlos syndrome, Marfan syndrome, osteogenesis imperfecta, epidermolysis bullosa, and acrodermatitis enteropathica, will be discussed, as they provide a unique challenge to the surgeon.

Ehlers-Danlos Syndrome

Ehlers-Danlos syndrome (EDS) is a group of 10 disorders that present as a defect in collagen formation. Characteristics include thin, friable skin with prominent veins, easy bruising, poor wound healing, abnormal scar formation, recurrent hernias, and hyperextensible joints. Gastrointestinal problems include bleeding, hiatal hernia, intestinal diverticulae, and rectal prolapse. Small blood vessels are fragile, making suturing difficult during surgery. Large vessels may develop aneurysms, varicosities, arteriovenous fistulas, or may spontaneously rupture.[30-32] EDS must be considered in every child with recurrent hernias and coagulopathy, especially when accompanied by platelet abnormalities and low coagulation factor levels. Inguinal hernias in these children resemble those seen in adults. Great care should be taken to avoid tearing the skin and fascia. The transversalis fascia is thin and the internal ring is greatly dilated. An adult-type repair with the use of mesh or felt may result in a lower incidence of recurrence.[33] Table 8-3 presents a description of EDS subtypes.

Table 8-3
Clinical, Genetic, and Biochemical Aspects of Ehlers-Danlos Subtypes

Type	Clinical Features	Inheritance	Biochemical Defect
I	Skin: soft, hyperextensible, easy bruising, fragile, atrophic scars; hypermobile joints; varicose veins; premature births	AD	Not known
II	Similar to type I, except less severe	AD	Not known
III	Skin: soft, not hyperextensible, normal scars; small and large joint hypermobility	AD	Not known
IV	Skin: thin, translucent, visible veins, normal scarring, no hyperextensibility; no joint hypermobility; arterial, bowel, and uterine rupture	AD	Type III collagen defect
V	Similar to type II	XLR	Not known
VI	Skin: hyperextensible, fragile, easy bruising; hypermobile joints; hypotonia; kyphoscoliosis	AR	Lysyl hydroxylase deficiency
VII	Skin: soft, mild hyperextensibility, no increased fragility; extremely lax joints with dislocations	AD	Type I collagen gene defect
VIII	Skin: soft, hyperextensible, easy bruising, abnormal scars with purple discoloration; hypermobile joints; generalized periodontitis	AD	Not known
IX	Skin: soft, lax; bladder diverticula and rupture; limited pronation and supination; broad clavicle; occipital horns	XLR	Lysyl oxidase defect with abnormal copper use
X	Similar to type II with abnormal clotting studies	AR	Fibronectin defect

AD = autosomal dominant; AR = autosomal recessive; XLR = X-linked recessive.
SOURCE: Reproduced with permission from Phillips et al.[30]

Marfan Syndrome

Patients with Marfan syndrome have tall stature, arachnodactyly, lax ligaments, myopia, scoliosis, pectus excavatum, and aneurysm of the ascending aorta. The genetic defect is in an extracellular protein, fibrillin, that is associated with elastic fibers. Patients who suffer from this syndrome also are prone to hernias. Surgical repair of a dissecting aneurysm is difficult, as the soft connective tissue fails to hold sutures. Skin may be hyperextensible, but shows no delay in wound healing.[34,35]

Osteogenesis Imperfecta

Patients with osteogenesis imperfecta (OI) have brittle bones, osteopenia, low muscle mass, hernias, and ligament and joint laxity. OI is a result of a mutation in type I collagen. There are four major OI subtypes with mild to lethal manifestations. Patients experience dermal thinning and increased bruisability. Scarring is normal and the skin is not hyperextensible. Surgery can be successful but difficult in these patients, as the bones fracture easily under minimal stress.[30,33] Table 8-4 lists the various features associated with the clinical subtypes of OI.

Epidermolysis Bullosa

Epidermolysis bullosa (EB) is classified into three major subtypes: EB simplex, junctional EB, and dystrophic EB. The genetic defect involves impairment in tissue adhesion within the epidermis, basement membrane, or dermis, resulting in tissue separation and blistering with minimal trauma. Characteristic features of EB are blistering and ulceration. Management of nonhealing wounds in patients with EB is a challenge, as their nutritional status is compromised because of oral erosions and esophageal obstruction. Surgical interventions include esophageal dilatation and gastrostomy tube placement. Dermal incisions must be meticulously placed to avoid further trauma to skin.[33,36] The skin requires nonadhesive pads covered by "bulky" dressing to avoid blistering.

Acrodermatitis Enteropathica

Acrodermatitis enteropathica (AE) is an autosomal recessive disease of children that causes an inability to absorb sufficient zinc from breast milk or food. The AE mutation affects zinc uptake in the intestine by preventing zinc from binding to the cell surface and its translocation into the cell. Zinc deficiency is associated with impaired granulation tissue formation, as zinc is a necessary cofactor for DNA polymerase and reverse transcriptase, and its deficiency may impair healing due to inhibition of cell proliferation.

AE is characterized by impaired wound healing as well as erythematous pustular dermatitis involving the extremities and the areas around the bodily orifices. Diagnosis is confirmed by the presence of an abnormally low blood zinc level ($<100~\mu$g/dL). Oral supplementation with 100 to 400 mg zinc sulfate orally per day is curative for impaired healing.[37,38]

HEALING IN SPECIFIC TISSUES

Gastrointestinal Tract

Healing of full-thickness injury to the gastrointestinal tract remains an unresolved clinical issue. Healing of full-thickness GI wounds begins with a surgical or mechanical reapposition of the bowel ends, which is most often the initial step in the repair process. Sutures or staples are principally used, although various other means such as buttons, plastic tubes, and various wrappings have been attempted with variable success. Failure of healing results in dehiscence, leaks, and fistulas, which carry significant morbidity and mortality. Conversely, excessive healing can be just as troublesome, resulting in stricture formation and stenosis of the lumen. Repair of the gastrointestinal tract is vital to restoring the integrity of the luminal structure, and to the resumption of motor, absorptive, and barrier functions.

The gross anatomic features of the GI tract are remarkably constant throughout most of its length. Within the lumen, the epithelium is supported by the lamina propria and underlying muscularis mucosa. The submucosa lies radially and circumferentially outside of these layers, is comprised of abundant collagenous and elastic fibers, and supports neural and vascular structures. Further toward the peritoneal surface of the bowel are the inner and outer muscle layers and ultimately a peritoneal extension, the serosa. The submucosa is the layer that imparts the greatest tensile strength and greatest suture-holding capacity, a characteristic that should be kept in mind during surgical repair of the GI tract. Additionally, serosal healing is essential for quickly achieving a watertight seal from the luminal side of the bowel. The importance of the serosa is underscored by the significantly higher rates of anastomotic failure observed clinically in segments of bowel that are extraperitoneal and lack serosa (i.e., the esophagus and rectum).

Injuries to all parts of the gastrointestinal tract undergo the same sequence of healing as cutaneous wounds. However, there are some significant differences (Table 8-5). Mesothelial (serosal) and mucosal healing can occur without scarring. The early integrity of the anastomosis is dependent on formation of a fibrin seal on the serosal side, which achieves watertightness, and on the suture-holding capacity of the intestinal wall, particularly the submucosal layer. There is a significant decrease in marginal strength during the first week due to an early and marked collagenolysis. The lysis of collagen is carried out by collagenase derived from neutrophils, macrophages, and intraluminal bacteria. Collagenase activity occurs early in the healing process, and during the first 3 to 5 days collagen breakdown far exceeds collagen synthesis. The integrity of the anastomosis represents equilibrium between collagen lysis, which occurs early, and collagen synthesis, which takes a few days to initiate (Fig. 8-5). Collagenase is expressed postinjury in all segments of the gastrointestinal tract, but it is much more marked in the colon compared to the small bowel. Collagen synthesis in the gastrointestinal tract is carried out by both fibroblasts and smooth muscle cells. Colon fibroblasts produce greater amounts of collagen than skin fibroblasts, reflecting different phenotypic features, as well as different responses to cytokines and growth factors among these different fibroblast populations. Ultimate anastomotic strength is not always related to the absolute amount of collagen, and the structure and arrangement of the collagen matrix may be more important.[39]

Table 8-4
Osteogenesis Imperfecta: Clinical and Genetic Features

Type	Clinical Features	Inheritance
I	Mild bone fragility, blue sclera	Dominant
II	"Prenatal lethal"; crumpled long bones, thin ribs, dark blue sclera	Dominant
III	Progressively deforming; multiple fractures; early loss of ambulation	Dominant/recessive
IV	Mild to moderate bone fragility; normal or gray sclera; mild short stature	Dominant

SOURCE: Reproduced with permission from Phillips et al.[30]

Table 8-5
Comparison of Wound Healing in the Gastrointestinal Tract and Skin

		GI Tract	*Skin*
Wound Environment	pH	Varies throughout GI tract in accordance with local exocrine secretions	Usually constant except during sepsis or local infection
	Microorganisms	Aerobic and anaerobic, especially in the colon and rectum; problematic if they contaminate the peritoneal cavity	Skin commensals rarely cause problems; infection usually results from exogenous contamination or hematogenous spread
	Shear stress	Intraluminal bulk transit and peristalsis exert distracting forces on the anastomosis	Skeletal movements may stress the suture line but pain usually acts as a protective mechanism preventing excess movement
	Tissue oxygenation	Dependent on intact vascular supply and neocapillary formation	Circulatory transport of oxygen as well as diffusion
Collagen Synthesis	Cell type	Fibroblasts and smooth muscle cells	Fibroblasts
	Lathyrogens	D-Penicillamine has no effect on collagen cross-linking	Significant inhibition of cross-linking with decreased wound strength
	Steroids	Contradictory evidence exists concerning their negative effect on GI healing; increased abscess in the anastomotic line may play a significant role	Significant decrease in collagen accumulation
Collagenase Activity		Increased presence throughout GI tract after transection and reanastomosis; during sepsis excess enzyme may promote dehiscence by decreasing suture-holding capacity of tissue	Not as significant a role in cutaneous wounds
Wound Strength		Rapid recovery to preoperative level	Less rapid than GI tissue
Scar Formation	Age	Definite scarring seen in fetal wound sites	Usually heals without scar formation in the fetus

Technical Considerations

Traditional teaching holds that in order for an anastomosis to heal without complications it must be tension-free, have an adequate blood supply, receive adequate nutrition, and be free of sepsis. Although sound principles for all wound healing, there are several considerations unique to anastomotic healing. From a technical viewpoint, the ideal method of suturing two ends of bowel together has not yet been identified. Although debate exists concerning methods of creating an anastomosis, clinically there has been no convincing evidence that a given technique has any advantage over another (i.e., hand-sutured versus stapled, continuous versus interrupted sutures, absorbable versus nonabsorbable sutures, or single- versus two-layer closure). It is known, however, that hand-sutured everting anastomoses are at greater risk of leakage and cause greater adhesion formation, but have a lower incidence of stenosis. As no definite superiority of any one method exists, it is recommended that surgeons be familiar with several techniques and apply them as circumstances dictate.

Bone

Following any type of injury to bone, several changes take place at the site of injury to restore structural and functional integrity. Most

of the phases of healing resemble those observed in dermal healing, but some notable individual characteristics apply to bone injuries. The initial stage of hematoma formation consists of an accumulation of blood at the fracture site, which also contains devitalized soft tissue, dead bone, and necrotic marrow. The next stage accomplishes the liquefaction and degradation of nonviable products at the fracture site. The normal bone adjacent to the injury site can then undergo revascularization, with new blood vessels growing into the fracture site. This is similar to the formation of granulation tissue in soft tissue. The symptoms associated with this stage are characteristic of inflammation, with clinical evidence of swelling and erythema.

Three to four days following injury, soft tissue forms a bridge between the fractured bone segments in the next stage (soft callus stage). This soft tissue is deposited where neovascularization has taken place and serves as an internal splint, preventing damage to the newly laid blood vessels and achieving a fibrocartilaginous union. The soft callus is formed externally along the bone shaft and internally within the marrow cavity. Clinically, this phase is characterized by the end of pain and inflammatory signs.

The next phase (hard callus stage) consists of mineralization of the soft callus and conversion to bone. This may take up to 2 to 3 months and leads to complete bony union. The bone is now

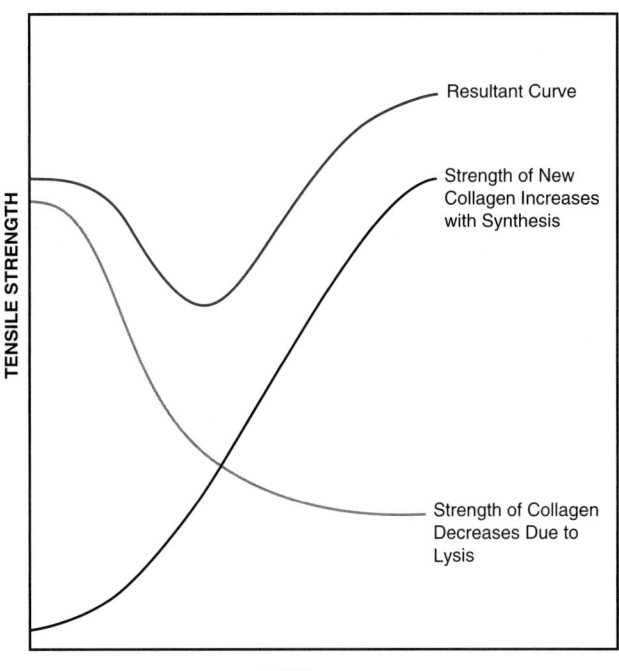

FIG. 8-5. *Diagrammatic representation of the concept of gastrointestinal wound healing as a fine balance between collagen synthesis and collagenolysis. The "weak" period, where collagenolysis exceeds collagen synthesis, can be prolonged or exacerbated by any factors that upset the equilibrium. (Reproduced with permission from Hunt TK, Van Winkle W Jr.: Wound healing: Normal repair, in Fundamentals of Wound Management in Surgery. New York: Chirurgecom, 1976, p 29.)*

considered strong enough to allow weight bearing and will appear healed on radiographs. This stage is followed by the remodeling phase, in which the excessive callus is reabsorbed and the marrow cavity is recanalized. This remodeling allows for the correct transmission of forces and restores the contours of the bone.

As in dermal healing, the process of osseous union is mediated by soluble growth factors and cytokines. The most extensively studied group is the bone morphogenic proteins (BMPs), which belong to the TGF-β superfamily. By stimulating the differentiation of mesenchymal cells into chondroblasts and osteoblasts, BMPs directly affect bone and cartilage repair. Other growth factors such as PDGF, TGF-β, TNF-α, and bFGF also participate in bony repair by mediating the inflammatory and proliferative phases of healing.

Cartilage

Cartilage consists of cells (chondrocytes) surrounded by an extracellular matrix made up of several proteoglycans, collagen fibers, and water. Unlike bone, cartilage is very avascular and depends on diffusion for transmittal of nutrients across the matrix. Additionally, the hypervascular perichondrium contributes substantially to the nutrition of the cartilage. Therefore, injuries to cartilage may be associated with permanent defects due to the meager and tenuous blood supply.

The healing response of cartilage depends on the depth of injury. In a superficial injury, there is disruption of the proteoglycan matrix and injury to the chondrocytes. There is no inflammatory response, but an increase in synthesis of proteoglycan and collagen dependent entirely on the chondrocyte. Unfortunately, the healing power of cartilage is often inadequate and overall regeneration is incomplete.

Therefore, superficial cartilage injuries are slow to heal and often result in persistent structural defects.

In contrast to superficial injuries, deep injuries involve the underlying bone and soft tissue. This leads to the exposure of vascular channels of the surrounding damaged tissue that may help in the formation of granulation tissue. Hemorrhage allows for the initiation of the inflammatory response and the subsequent mediator activation of cellular function for repair. As the granulation tissue is laid down, fibroblasts migrate toward the wound and synthesize fibrous tissue that undergoes chondrification. Gradually, hyaline cartilage is formed, which restores the structural and functional integrity of the injured site.

Tendon

Tendons and ligaments are specialized structures that link muscle and bone, and bone and bone, respectively. They consist of parallel bundles of collagen interspersed with spindle cells. Tendons and ligaments can be subjected to a variety of injuries, such as laceration, rupture, and contusion. Due to the mobility of the underlying bone or muscles, the damaged ends usually separate. Tendon and ligament healing progresses in a similar fashion as in other areas of the body (i.e., through hematoma formation, organization, laying down of reparative tissue, and scar formation). Matrix is characterized by accumulation of type I and III collagen along with increased water, DNA, and glycosaminoglycan content. As the collagen fibers are organized, transmission of forces across the damaged portion can occur. Restoration of the mechanical integrity may never be equal to that of the undamaged tendon.

Tendon vasculature has a clear effect on healing. Hypovascular tendons tend to heal with less motion and more scar formation than tendons with better blood supply. The specialized cells, tenocytes, are very metabolically active and retain a large regenerative potential, even in the absence of vascularity. Cells on the tendon surface are identical to those within the sheath, and play a role in tendon healing as well.

Nerve

Nerve injuries are very common, with an estimated 200,000 repairs performed every year in the United States. Peripheral nerves are a complex arrangement of axons, non-neuronal cells, and extracellular elements. There are three types of nerve injuries: neurapraxia (focal demyelination), axonotmesis (interruption of axonal continuity but preservation of Schwann cell basal lamina), and neurotmesis (complete transection). Following all types of injury, the nerve ends progress through a predictable pattern of changes involving three crucial steps: (1) survival of axonal cell bodies; (2) regeneration of axons that grow across the transected nerve to reach the distal stump; and (3) migration and connection of the regenerating nerve ends to the appropriate nerve ends or organ targets.

Phagocytes remove the degenerating axons and myelin sheath from the distal stump (Wallerian degeneration). Regenerating axonal sprouts extend from the proximal stump and probe the distal stump and the surrounding tissues. Schwann cells ensheathe and help in remyelinating the regenerating axons. Functional units are formed when the regenerating axons connect with the appropriate end targets. Several factors play a role in nerve healing, such as growth factors, cell adhesion molecules, and non-neuronal cells and receptors. Growth factors include nerve growth factor, brain-derived neurotropic factor, basic and acidic fibroblastic growth factors, and neuroleukin. Cell-adhesion molecules involved in nerve healing include nerve-adhesion molecule, neuron-glia adhesion molecule, myelin adhesion glycoprotein, and N-cadherin. This complex interplay of growth factors and adhesion molecules helps in nerve regeneration.

Fetal Wound Healing

The main characteristic that distinguishes the healing of fetal wounds from that of adult wounds is the apparent lack of scar formation. Understanding how fetal wounds achieve integrity without evidence of scarring holds promise for the possible manipulation of unwanted fibrosis or excessive scar formation in adults. Although early fetal healing is characterized by the absence of scarring and resembles tissue regeneration, there is a phase of transition during gestational life when a more adult-like healing pattern emerges. This so-called "transition wound" occurs at the beginning of the third trimester, and during this period there is scarless healing; however, there is a loss of the ability to regenerate skin appendages.[40] Eventually a classic, adult-patterned healing with scar formation occurs exclusively, although overall healing continues to be faster than in adults.

There are a number of characteristics that may influence the differences between fetal and adult wounds. These include wound environment, inflammatory responses, differential growth factor profiles, and wound matrix.

Wound Environment

The fetus is bathed in a sterile, temperature-stable fluid environment, though this alone does not explain the observed differences. Experiments have demonstrated that scarless healing may occur outside of the amniotic fluid environment, and conversely, scars can form in utero.[41,42]

Inflammation

The extent and robustness of the inflammatory response correlates directly with the amount of scar formation in all healing wounds. Reduced fetal inflammation due to the immaturity of the fetal immune system may partially explain the lack of scarring observed. Not only is the fetus neutropenic, but fetal wounds contain lower numbers of PMNs and macrophages.[43]

Growth Factors

Fetal wounds are notable for the absence of TGF-β, which may have a significant role in scarring. Conversely, blocking TGF-β1 or TGF-β2 using neutralizing antibodies considerably reduces scar formation in adult wounds. Exogenous application of TGF-β3 downregulates TGF-β1 and TGF-β2 levels at the wound site with a resultant reduction in scarring.[44] Thus, the balance between the concentration and/or activity of TGF-β isoforms may be important for regulating scar production.

Wound Matrix

The fetal wound is characterized by excessive and extended hyaluronic acid production, a high-molecular-weight glycosaminoglycan that is produced primarily by fibroblasts. Although adult wounds also produce hyaluronic acid, its synthesis is sustained only in the fetal wound. Components of amniotic fluid, most specifically fetal urine, have a unique ability to stimulate hyaluronic acid production.[45] Fetal fibroblasts produce more collagen than adult fibroblasts, and the increased level of hyaluronic acid may aid in the orderly organization of collagen. As a result of these findings, hyaluronic acid is used topically to enhance healing and to inhibit postoperative adhesion formation.[46]

CLASSIFICATION OF WOUNDS

Wounds are classified as either acute or chronic. Acute wounds heal in a predictable manner and time frame. The process occurs with few, if any, complications, and the end result is a well-healed wound. Surgical wounds can heal in several ways. An incised wound that is clean and sutured closed is said to heal by primary intention. Often, because of bacterial contamination or tissue loss, a wound will be left open to heal by granulation tissue formation and contraction; this constitutes healing by secondary intention. Delayed primary closure, or healing by tertiary intention, represents a combination of the first two, consisting of the placement of sutures, allowing the wound to stay open for a few days, and the subsequent closure of the sutures (Fig. 8-6).

The healing spectrum of acute wounds is broad (Fig. 8-7). In examining the acquisition of mechanical integrity and strength during healing, the normal process is characterized by a constant and continual increase that reaches a plateau at some point postinjury. Wounds with delayed healing are characterized by decreased wound-breaking strength in comparison to wounds that heal at a normal rate; however, they eventually achieve the same integrity and strength as wounds that heal normally. Conditions such as nutritional deficiencies, infections, or severe trauma cause delayed healing, which reverts to normal with correction of the underlying pathophysiology. Impaired healing is characterized by a failure to achieve mechanical strength equivalent to normally healed wounds. Patients with compromised immune systems such as those with diabetes, chronic steroid usage, or tissues damaged by radiotherapy are prone to this type of impaired healing. The surgeon must be aware of these situations and exercise great care in the placement of incision and suture selection, postoperative care, and adjunctive

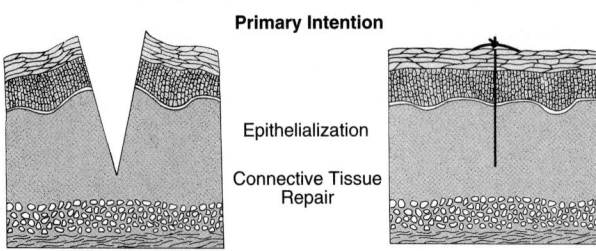

Primary Intention

Epithelialization

Connective Tissue Repair

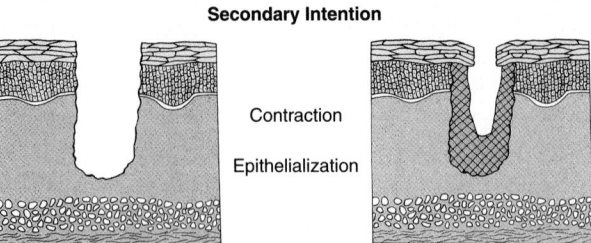

Secondary Intention

Contraction

Epithelialization

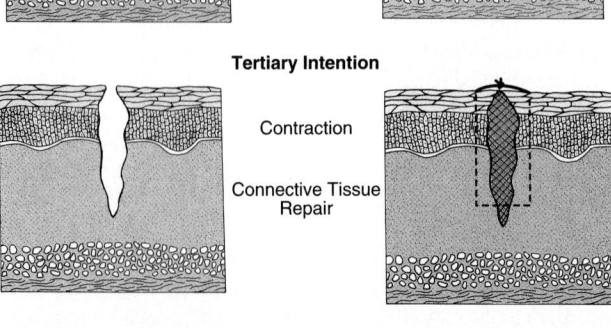

Tertiary Intention

Contraction

Connective Tissue Repair

FIG. 8-6. *Different clinical approaches to the closure and healing of acute wounds.*

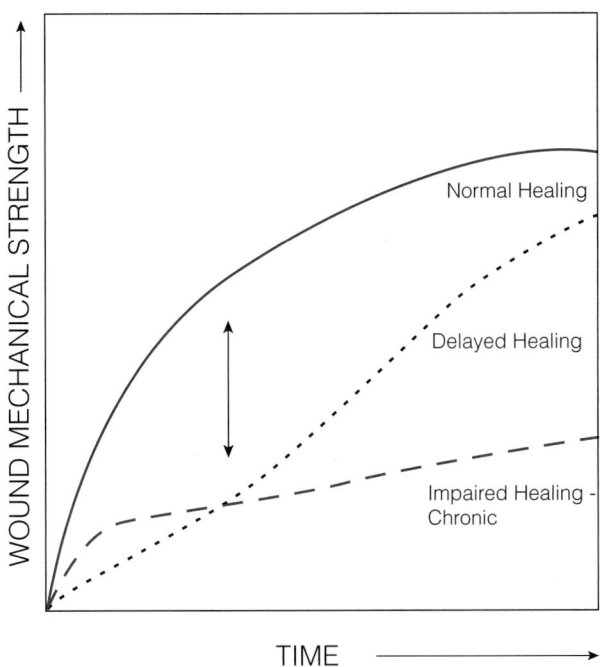

FIG. 8-7. *The acquisition of wound mechanical strength over time in normal, delayed, and impaired healing.*

therapy to maximize the chances of healing without supervening complications.

Normal healing is affected by both systemic and local factors (Table 8-6). The clinician must be familiar with these factors and should attempt to counteract their deleterious effects. Complications occurring in wounds with higher risk can lead to failure of healing or the development of chronic, nonhealing wounds.

Factors Affecting Wound Healing

Advanced Age

Most surgeons believe that aging produces intrinsic physiologic changes that result in delayed or impaired wound healing. Clinical experience with elderly patients tends to support this belief. Studies of hospitalized surgical patients show a direct correlation between older age and poor wound healing outcomes such as dehiscence

Table 8-6
Factors Affecting Wound Healing

Systemic
    Age
    Nutrition
    Trauma
    Metabolic diseases
    Immunosuppression
    Connective tissue disorders
    Smoking
Local
    Mechanical injury
    Infection
    Edema
    Ischemia/necrotic tissue
    Topical agents
    Ionizing radiation
    Low oxygen tension
    Foreign bodies

and incisional hernia.[47,48] However, these statistics fail to take into account underlying illnesses or diseases as a possible source of impaired wound healing in the elderly. The increased incidence of cardiovascular disease, metabolic diseases (diabetes mellitus, malnutrition, and vitamin deficiencies), cancer, and the prevalent use of drugs that impair wound healing may all contribute to the higher incidence of wound problems in the elderly. However, more recent clinical experience suggests that major operative interventions can be accomplished safely in the elderly.

The results of animal studies regarding the effects of aging on wound healing have yielded contradictory results. In healthy human volunteers there was a significant delay of 1.9 days in the epithelialization of superficial skin defects in those older than 70 years of age when compared to younger volunteers.[49] In the same volunteers, using a micro-model of fibroplasia, no difference in DNA or hydroxyproline wound accumulation could be demonstrated between the young and elderly groups; however, the young volunteers had a significantly higher amount of total α-amino nitrogen in their wounds, a reflection of total protein content of the wound. Thus, although wound collagen synthesis does not seem to be impaired with advanced age, noncollagenous protein accumulation at wounded sites is decreased with aging, which may impair the mechanical properties of scarring in elderly patients.

Hypoxia, Anemia, and Hypoperfusion

Low oxygen tension has a profoundly deleterious effect on all aspects of wound healing. Fibroplasia, although stimulated initially by the hypoxic wound environment, is significantly impaired by local hypoxia. Optimal collagen synthesis requires oxygen as a cofactor, particularly for the hydroxylation steps. Increasing subcutaneous oxygen tension levels by increasing the fraction of inspired oxygen (FIO_2) of inspired air for brief periods during and immediately following surgery results in enhanced collagen deposition and in decreased rates of wound infection after elective surgery.[50–52]

Major factors affecting local oxygen delivery include hypoperfusion either for systemic reasons (low volume or cardiac failure) or due to local causes (arterial insufficiency, local vasoconstriction, or excessive tension on tissues). The level of vasoconstriction of the subcutaneous capillary bed is exquisitely responsive to fluid status, temperature, and hyperactive sympathetic tone as is often induced by postoperative pain. Correction of these factors can have a remarkable influence on wound outcome, particularly on decreasing wound infection rates.[51–53] Mild to moderate normovolemic anemia does not appear to adversely affect wound oxygen tension and collagen synthesis, unless the hematocrit falls below 15%.[53]

Steroids and Chemotherapeutic Drugs

Large doses or chronic usage of glucocorticoids reduce collagen synthesis and wound strength.[54] The major effect of steroids is to inhibit the inflammatory phase of wound healing (angiogenesis, neutrophil and macrophage migration, and fibroblast proliferation) and the release of lysosomal enzymes. The stronger the anti-inflammatory effect of the steroid compound used, the greater the inhibitory effect on wound healing. Steroids used after the first 3 to 4 days postinjury do not affect wound healing as severely as when they are used in the immediate postoperative period. Therefore if possible, their use should be delayed or, alternatively, forms with lesser anti-inflammatory effects should be administered.

In addition to their effect on collagen synthesis, steroids also inhibit epithelialization and contraction and contribute to increased rates of wound infection, regardless of the time of administration.[55]

Steroid-delayed healing of cutaneous wounds can be stimulated to epithelialize by topical application of vitamin A.[54,55] Collagen synthesis of steroid-treated wounds also can be stimulated by vitamin A.

All chemotherapeutic antimetabolite drugs adversely affect wound healing by inhibiting early cell proliferation and wound DNA and protein synthesis, all of which are critical to successful repair. Delay in the use of such drugs for about 2 weeks postinjury appears to lessen the wound healing impairment.[56] Extravasation of most chemotherapeutic agents is associated with tissue necrosis, marked ulceration, and protracted healing at the affected site.[57]

Metabolic Disorders

Diabetes mellitus is the best known of the metabolic disorders contributing to increased rates of wound infection and failure.[58] Uncontrolled diabetes results in reduced inflammation, angiogenesis, and collagen synthesis. Additionally, the large and small vessel disease that is the hallmark of advanced diabetes contributes to local hypoxemia. Defects in granulocyte function, capillary ingrowth, and fibroblast proliferation all have been described in diabetes. Obesity, insulin resistance, hyperglycemia, and diabetic renal failure all contribute significantly and independently to the impaired wound healing observed in diabetics.[59] In wound studies on experimental diabetic animals, insulin restores collagen synthesis and granulation tissue formation to normal levels if given during the early phases of healing.[60] In clean, noninfected, and well-perfused experimental wounds in human diabetic volunteers, type I diabetes mellitus was noted to decrease wound collagen accumulation in the wound, independent of the degree of glycemic control. Type II diabetic patients showed no effect on collagen accretion when compared to healthy, age-matched controls.[61] Furthermore, the diabetic wound appears to be lacking in sufficient growth factor levels, which signal normal healing. It remains unclear whether decreased collagen synthesis or an increased breakdown due to an abnormally high proteolytic wound environment is responsible.

Careful preoperative correction of blood sugar levels improves the outcome of wounds in diabetic patients. Increasing the inspired oxygen tension, judicious use of antibiotics, and correction of other coexisting metabolic abnormalities all can result in improved wound healing.

Uremia also has been associated with disordered wound healing. Experimentally, uremic animals demonstrate decreased wound collagen synthesis and breaking strength. The contribution of uremia alone to this impairment, rather than that of associated malnutrition, is difficult to assess.[59] The clinical use of dialysis to correct the metabolic abnormalities and nutritional restoration should impact greatly on the wound outcome of such patients.

Nutrition

The important role of nutrition in the recovery from traumatic or surgical injury has been recognized by clinicians since the time of Hippocrates. Poor nutritional intake or lack of individual nutrients significantly alters many aspects of wound healing. The clinician must pay close attention to the nutritional status of patients with wounds, since wound failure or wound infections may be no more than a reflection of poor nutrition. Although the full interaction of nutrition and wound healing is still not fully understood, efforts are being made to develop wound-specific nutritional interventions and the pharmacologic use of individual nutrients as modulators of wound outcomes.

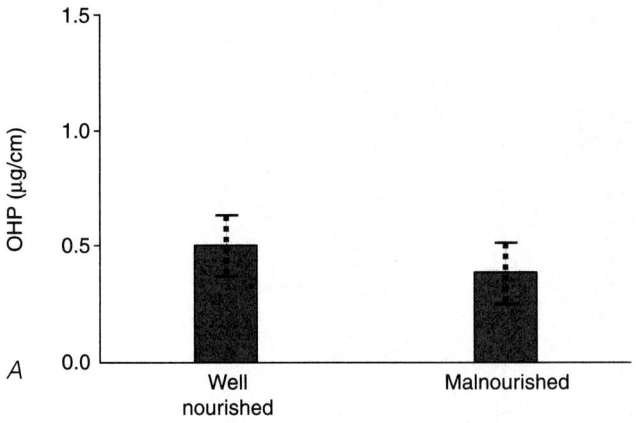

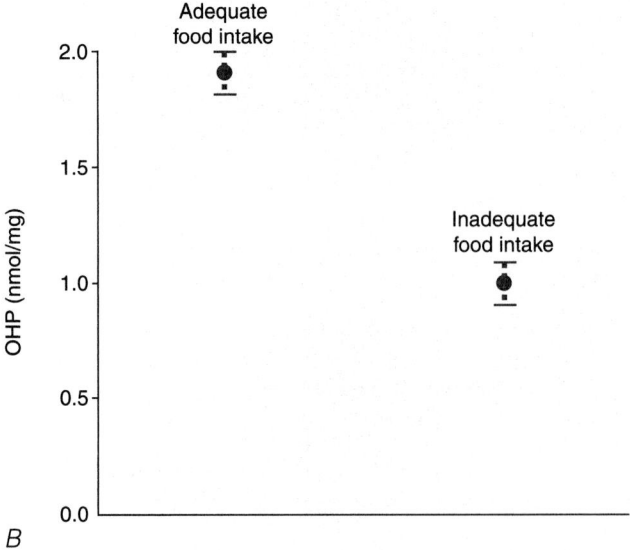

FIG. 8-8. *Effect of malnutrition on collagen deposition in experimental human wounds. OHP = hydroxyproline.*

Experimental rodents fed either a 0 or 4% protein diet have impaired collagen deposition with a secondary decrease in skin and fascial wound-breaking strength and increased wound infection rates. Induction of energy-deficient states by providing only 50% of the normal caloric requirement leads to decreased granulation tissue formation and matrix protein deposition in rats. Acute fasting in rats markedly impairs collagen synthesis while decreasing procollagen mRNA.[62]

Clinically, it is extremely rare to encounter pure energy or protein malnutrition, and the vast majority of patients exhibit combined protein-energy malnutrition. Such patients have diminished hydroxyproline accumulation (an index of collagen deposition) into subcutaneously implanted polytetrafluoroethylene tubes when compared to normally nourished patients (Fig. 8-8). Furthermore, malnutrition correlates clinically with enhanced rates of wound complications and increased wound failure following diverse surgical procedures. This reflects impaired healing response as well as reduced cell-mediated immunity, phagocytosis, and intracellular killing of bacteria by macrophages and neutrophils during protein-calorie malnutrition.[62]

Two additional nutrition-related factors warrant discussion. First, the degree of nutritional impairment need not be long-standing in humans, as opposed to the experimental situation. Thus patients with brief preoperative illnesses or reduced nutrient intake in the period immediately preceding the injury or operative intervention will demonstrate impaired fibroplasia.[63,64] Second, brief and not necessarily intensive nutritional intervention, either via the parenteral or enteral route, can reverse or prevent the decreased collagen deposition noted with malnutrition or with postoperative starvation.[65]

The possible role of single amino acids in enhanced wound healing has been studied for the last several decades. Arginine appears most active in terms of enhancing wound fibroplasia. Arginine deficiency results in decreased wound-breaking strength and wound-collagen accumulation in chow-fed rats. Rats that are given 1% arginine HCl supplementation, and are therefore not arginine-deficient, have enhanced wound-breaking strength and collagen synthesis when compared to chow-fed controls.[66] Studies have been carried out in healthy human volunteers to examine the effect of arginine supplementation on collagen accumulation. Young, healthy, human volunteers (aged 25 to 35 years) were found to have significantly increased wound collagen deposition following oral supplementation with either 30 g of arginine aspartate (17 g of free arginine) or 30 g of arginine HCl (24.8 g of free arginine) daily for 14 days.[67] In a study of healthy older humans (aged 67 to 82 years), daily supplements of 30 g of arginine aspartate for 14 days resulted in significantly enhanced collagen and total protein deposition at the wound site when compared to controls given placebos. There was no enhanced DNA synthesis present in the wounds of the arginine-supplemented subjects, suggesting that the effect of arginine is not mediated by an inflammatory mode of action.[68] In this study, arginine supplementation had no effect on the rate of epithelialization of a superficial skin defect. This further suggests that the main effect of arginine on wound healing is to enhance wound collagen deposition. Recently, a dietary supplemental regimen of arginine, β-hydroxy-β-methyl butyrate, and glutamine was found to significantly and specifically enhance collagen deposition in elderly, healthy human volunteers when compared to an isocaloric, isonitrogenous supplement[69] (Fig. 8-9). As increases in breaking strength during the first weeks of healing are directly related to new collagen synthesis, arginine supplementation may result in an improvement in wound strength as a consequence of enhanced collagen deposition.

The vitamins most closely involved with wound healing are vitamin C and vitamin A. Scurvy or vitamin C deficiency leads to a defect in wound healing, particularly via a failure in collagen synthesis and cross-linking. Biochemically, vitamin C is required for the conversion of proline and lysine to hydroxyproline and hydroxylysine, respectively. Vitamin C deficiency has also been associated with an increased incidence of wound infection, and if wound infection does occur, it tends to be more severe. These effects are believed to be due to an associated impairment in neutrophil function, decreased complement activity, and decreased walling-off of bacteria secondary to insufficient collagen deposition. The recommended dietary allowance is 60 mg daily. This provides a considerable safety margin for most healthy nonsmokers. In severely injured or extensively burned patients this requirement may increase to as high as 2 g daily. There is no evidence that excess vitamin C is toxic; however, there is no evidence that supertherapeutic doses of vitamin C are of any benefit.[70]

Vitamin A deficiency impairs wound healing, while supplemental vitamin A benefits wound healing in nondeficient humans and animals. Vitamin A increases the inflammatory response in wound healing, probably by increasing the lability of lysosomal membranes. There is an increased influx of macrophages, with an increase in their activation and increased collagen synthesis. Vitamin A

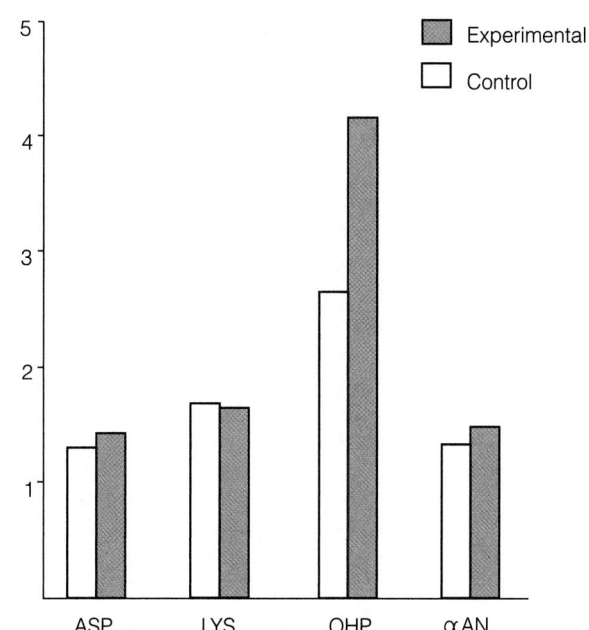

FIG. 8-9. *Ratios of 14- to 7-day values for aspartate (ASP), hydroxyproline (OHP), lysine (LYS), and alpha-amino nitrogen (α-AN) in volunteers given dietary supplements of arginine, β-hydroxy-β-methylbutyrate, and glutamine. *P <0.05. (Reproduced with permission from Yue et al.[59])*

directly increases collagen production and epidermal growth factor receptors when it is added in vitro to cultured fibroblasts. As mentioned before, supplemental vitamin A can reverse the inhibitory effects of corticosteroids on wound healing. Vitamin A also can restore wound healing that has been impaired by diabetes, tumor formation, cyclophosphamide, and radiation. Serious injury or stress leads to increased vitamin A requirements. In the severely injured patient, supplemental doses of vitamin A have been recommended. Doses ranging from 25,000 to 100,000 IU per day have been advocated.

The connections between specific minerals and trace elements and deficits in wound healing are complex. Frequently, deficiencies are multiple and include macronutrient deficiencies. As with some of the vitamins described above, the specific trace element may function as a cofactor or part of an enzyme that is essential for homeostasis and wound healing. Clinically, preventing deficiencies is often easier to accomplish than diagnosing them.

Zinc is the most well-known element in wound healing and has been used empirically in dermatologic conditions for centuries. It is essential for wound healing in animals and humans. There are over 150 known enzymes for which zinc is either an integral part or an essential cofactor, and many of these enzymes are critical to wound healing.[71] With zinc deficiency there is decreased fibroblast proliferation, decreased collagen synthesis, impaired overall wound strength, and delayed epithelialization. These defects are reversed by zinc supplementation. To date, no study has shown improved wound healing with zinc supplementation in patients who are not zinc deficient.[72]

Infections

Wound infections continue to represent a major medical problem, both in terms of how they affect the outcome of surgical procedures, and for their impact on the length of hospital stay and medical costs.[73] Many otherwise successful surgical operations fail because of the development of wound infections. The occurrence of infections is of major concern when implants are used, and their occurrence may lead to the removal of the prosthetic material, thus subjecting the patient to further operations and severe risk of morbidity and mortality. Infections can weaken an abdominal closure or hernia repair and result in wound dehiscence or recurrence of the hernia. Cosmetically, infections can lead to disfiguring, unsightly, or delayed closures.

Exhaustive studies have been undertaken that examine the appropriate prophylactic treatment of operative wounds. Bacterial contaminants normally present on skin are prevented from entry into deep tissues by intact epithelium. Surgery breaches the intact epithelium, allowing bacteria access to these tissues and the bloodstream. Antibiotic prophylaxis is most effective when adequate concentrations of antibiotic are present in the tissues at the time of incision. Addition of antibiotics after operative contamination has occurred is clearly ineffective in preventing postoperative wound infections.

Studies that compare operations performed with and without antibiotic prophylaxis demonstrate that class II, III, and IV procedures (see below) treated with appropriate prophylactic antibiotics have only one third the wound infection rate of previously reported untreated series. More recently, repeat dosing of antibiotics has been shown to be essential in decreasing postoperative wound infections in operations with durations exceeding the biochemical half-life ($t_{1/2}$) of the antibiotic, or in which there is large-volume blood loss and fluid replacement. In lengthy cases, those in which prosthetic implants are used, or when unexpected contamination is encountered, additional doses of antibiotic may be administered for 24 hours postoperatively.

Selection of antibiotics for use in prophylaxis should be tailored to the type of surgery to be performed, operative contaminants that might be encountered during the procedure, and the profile of resistant organisms present at the institution where the surgery is performed. The continuing widespread appearance of methicillin-resistant *Staphylococcus aureus* (MRSA), and vancomycin-resistant enterococci (VRE), has significantly restricted the selection of these agents for routine use.

Patients with prosthetic heart valves or any implanted vascular or orthopedic prostheses should receive antibiotic prophylaxis prior to any procedure in which significant bacteremia is anticipated. Dental procedures require prophylaxis with broad-spectrum penicillins or amoxicillin, while urologic instrumentation should be pretreated with a second-generation cephalosporin. Patients with prostheses who undergo gastrointestinal surgery should receive anaerobic coverage combined with a cephalosporin.

The incidence of wound infection is about 5 to 10% nationwide and has not changed during the last few decades. Quantitatively, it has been shown that if the wound is contaminated with $>10^5$ microorganisms, the risk of wound infection is markedly increased, but this threshold may be much lower in the presence of foreign materials. The source of pathogens for the infection is usually the endogenous flora of the patient's skin, mucous membranes, or from hollow organs. The most common organisms responsible for wound infections in order of frequency are *Staphylococcus* species, coagulase-negative *Streptococcus*, enterococci, and *Escherichia coli*. The incidence of wound infection bears a direct relationship to the degree of contamination that occurs during the operation from the disease process itself (clean—class I, clean contaminated—class II, contaminated—class III, and dirty—class IV). Many factors contribute to the development of postoperative wound infections. Most surgical wound infections become apparent within 7 to 10 days postoperatively, although a small number manifest only years after the original operative intervention. With the hospital stay becoming shorter and shorter, many infections are detected in the outpatient

setting, leading to underreporting of the true incidence of wound infections. There has been much debate about the actual definition of wound infection. The narrowest definition would include wounds that drain purulent material with bacteria identified on culture. The more broad definition would include all wounds draining pus, whether or not the bacteriologic studies are positive; wounds that are opened by the surgeon; and wounds that the surgeon considers infected.

Anatomically, wound infections can be classified as superficial or suprafascial and deep, involving fascia, muscle, or the abdominal cavity. About three fourths of all wound infections are superficial, involving skin and subcutaneous tissue only. Clinical diagnosis is easy when a postoperative wound looks edematous and erythematous and is tender. Often the presentation is more subtle, and development of postoperative fever, usually low-grade; development of a mild and unexplained leukocytosis; or the presence of undue incisional pain should direct attention to the wound. Inspection of the wound is most useful in detecting subtle edema around the suture or staple line, manifested as a waxy appearance of the skin, which characterizes the early phase of infection. If a wound infection is suspected, several stitches or staples around the most suspicious area should be removed with insertion of a cotton-tipped applicator into the subcutaneous area to open a small segment of the incision. This causes minimal if any discomfort to the patient. Presence of pus mandates further opening of the subcutaneous and skin layers to the full extent of the infected pocket. Samples should be taken for aerobic and anaerobic cultures, with very few patients requiring antibiotic therapy. Patients who are immunosuppressed (diabetics and those on steroids or chemotherapeutic agents), who have evidence of tissue penetration or systemic toxicity, or who have had prosthetic devices inserted (vascular grafts, heart valves, artificial joints, or mesh) should be treated with systemic antibiotics.

Deep wound infections arise immediately adjacent to the fascia, either above or below it, and often have an intra-abdominal component. Most intra-abdominal infections do not, however, communicate with the wound. Deep infections present with fever and leukocytosis. The incision may drain pus spontaneously or the intra-abdominal extension may be recognized following the drainage of what was thought to be a superficial wound infection, but pus draining between the fascial sutures will be noted. Sometimes wound dehiscence will occur. The most dangerous of the deep infections is necrotizing fasciitis. It results in high mortality, particularly in the elderly. This is an invasive process that involves the fascia and leads to secondary skin necrosis. Pathophysiologically, it is a septic thrombosis of the vessels between the skin and the deep layers. The skin demonstrates hemorrhagic bullae and subsequent frank necrosis, with surrounding areas of inflammation and edema. The fascial necrosis is usually wider than the skin involvement or than the surgeon estimates on clinical grounds. The patient is toxic, has high fever, tachycardia, and marked hypovolemia, which if uncorrected, progresses to cardiovascular collapse. Bacteriologically, this is a mixed infection, and samples should be obtained for Gram's stain smears and cultures to aid in diagnosis and treatment. As soon as bacteriologic studies have been sent, high-dose penicillin treatment needs to be started (20 to 40 million U/d intravenously). Cardiovascular resuscitation with electrolyte solutions, blood, and/or plasma is carried out as expeditiously as possible prior to induction of anesthesia. The aim of surgical treatment is thorough removal of all necrosed skin and fascia. If viable skin overlies necrotic fascia, multiple longitudinal skin incisions can be made to allow for excision of the devitalized fascia. Although removal of all necrotic tissue is the goal of the first surgical intervention, the distinction between necrotic and simply edematous tissue often is difficult. Careful inspection every 12 to 24 hours will reveal any new necrotic areas, and these need further débridement and excision. When all necrotic tissue has been removed and the infection has been controlled, the wounds may be covered with homo- or xenografts until definitive reconstruction and autografting can take place.

The mere presence of bacteria in an open wound, either acute or chronic, does not constitute an infection, because large numbers of bacteria can be present in the normal situation. Secondly, the bacteria grown may not be representative of the bacteria causing the actual wound infection. There seems to be confusion as to what exactly constitutes wound infection. For purposes of clarity, we have to differentiate between contamination, colonization, and infection. *Contamination* is the presence of bacteria without multiplication, *colonization* is multiplication without host response, and *infection* is the presence of host response in reaction to deposition and multiplication of bacteria. The presence of a host response helps to differentiate between infection and colonization as seen in chronic wounds. The host response that helps in diagnosing wound infection comprises cellulitis, abnormal discharge, delayed healing, change in pain, abnormal granulation tissue, bridging, and abnormal color and odor.

As discussed previously, neutrophils play a major role in preventing wound infections. Chronic granulomatous disease (CGD) comprises a genetically heterogeneous group of diseases in which the reduced nicotinamide adenine dinucleotide phosphate (NADPH)-dependent oxide enzyme is deficient. This defect impairs the intracellular killing of microorganisms, leaving the patient liable to infection by bacteria and fungi. Afflicted patients have recurrent infections and form granulomas, which can lead to obstruction of the gastric antrum and genitourinary tracts and poor wound healing. Surgeons become involved when the patient develops infectious or obstructive complications.

The nitroblue tetrazolium (NBT) reduction test is used to diagnose CGD. Normal neutrophils can reduce this compound, while neutrophils from affected patients do not, facilitating the diagnosis via a colorimetric test. Clinically, patients develop recurrent infections such as pneumonia, lymphadenitis, hepatic abscess, and osteomyelitis. Organisms most commonly responsible are *Staphylococcus aureus*, *Aspergillus*, *Klebsiella*, *Serratia*, or *Candida*. When CGD patients require surgery, a preoperative pulmonary function test should be considered since they are predisposed to obstructive and restrictive lung disease. Wound complications, mainly infection, are common. Sutures should be removed as late as possible since the wounds heal slowly. Abscess drains should be left in place for a prolonged period until the infection is completely resolved.[74]

Chronic Wounds

Chronic wounds are defined as wounds that have failed to proceed through the orderly process that produces satisfactory anatomic and functional integrity or that have proceeded through the repair process without producing an adequate anatomic and functional result. The majority of wounds that have not healed in 3 months are considered chronic. *Skin ulcers*, which usually occur in traumatized or vascularly compromised soft tissue, are also considered chronic in nature, and proportionately are the major component of chronic wounds. In addition to the factors discussed above that can delay wound healing, other causative mechanisms may also play a role in the etiology of chronic wounds. Repeated trauma, poor perfusion or oxygenation, and/or excessive inflammation contribute to the causation and the perpetuation of the chronicity of wounds.

Unresponsiveness to normal regulatory signals also has been implicated as a predictive factor of chronic wounds. This may come about as a failure of normal growth factor synthesis,[75] and thus an increased breakdown of growth factors within a wound environment that is markedly proteolytic because of overexpression of protease activity or a failure of the normal antiprotease inhibitor mechanisms.[76] Fibroblasts from chronic wounds also have been found to have decreased proliferative potential, perhaps because of senescence[77] or decreased expression of growth factor receptors.[78] Chronic wounds occur due to various etiologic factors, and several of the most common are discussed below.

Malignant transformation of chronic ulcers can occur in any long-standing wound (Marjolin's ulcer). Any wound that does not heal for a prolonged period of time is prone to malignant transformation. Malignant wounds are differentiated clinically from nonmalignant wounds by the presence of overturned wound edges. In patients with suspected malignant transformations, biopsy of the wound edges must be performed to rule out malignancy. Cancers arising de novo in chronic wounds include both squamous and basal cell carcinomas.

Ischemic Arterial Ulcers

These wounds occur due to a lack of blood supply and are painful at presentation. They are usually associated with other symptoms of peripheral vascular disease, such as intermittent claudication, rest pain, night pain, and color changes. These wounds commonly are present at the most distal portions of the extremities such as the interdigital clefts, although more proximal locations are also encountered. On examination, there may be diminished or absent pulses with decreased ankle-brachial index and poor formation of granulation tissue. Other signs of peripheral ischemia, such as dryness of skin, hair loss, scaling, and pallor can be present. The wound itself is usually shallow with smooth margins, and a pale base and surrounding skin may be present. The management of these wounds is two-pronged and includes revascularization and wound care. Nonhealing of these wounds is the norm unless successful revascularization is performed. After establishing adequate blood supply, most such wounds progress to heal satisfactorily.

Venous Stasis Ulcers

Although there is unanimous agreement that venous ulcers are due to venous stasis and back pressure, there is less consensus as to what are the exact pathophysiologic pathways that lead to ulceration and impaired healing. On the microvascular level, there is alteration and distention of the dermal capillaries with leakage of fibrinogen into the tissues; polymerization of fibrinogen into fibrin cuffs leads to perivascular cuffing that can impede oxygen exchange, thus contributing to ulceration. These same fibrin cuffs and the leakage of macromolecules such as fibrinogen and α_2-macroglobulin trap growth factors and impede wound healing. Another hypothesis suggests that neutrophils adhere to the capillary endothelium and cause plugging with diminished dermal blood flow. Venous hypertension and capillary damage lead to extravasation of hemoglobin. The products of this breakdown are irritating and cause pruritus and skin damage. The resulting brownish pigmentation of skin combined with the loss of subcutaneous fat produces characteristic changes called lipodermatosclerosis. Regardless of the pathophysiologic mechanisms, the clinically characteristic picture is that of an ulcer that fails to re-epithelialize despite the presence of adequate granulation tissue.

Venous stasis occurs due to the incompetence of either the superficial or deep venous systems. Chronic venous ulcers are usually due to the incompetence of the deep venous system and are commonly painless. Stasis ulcers tend to occur at the sites of incompetent perforators, the most common being above the medial malleolus, over Cockett's perforator. Upon examination, the typical location combined with a history of venous incompetence and other skin changes is diagnostic. The wound is usually shallow with irregular margins and pigmented surrounding skin.

The cornerstone of treatment of venous ulcers is compression therapy, although the best method to achieve it remains controversial. Compression can be accomplished via rigid or flexible means. The most commonly used method is the rigid, zinc oxide–impregnated, nonelastic bandage. Others have proposed a four-layered bandage approach as a more optimal method of obtaining graduated compression. Wound care in these patients focuses on maintaining a moist wound environment, which can be achieved with hydrocolloids. Other, more modern approaches include use of vasoactive substances and growth factor application, as well as the use of skin substitutes. Most venous ulcers can be healed with perseverance and by addressing the venous hypertension. Unfortunately, recurrences are frequent.[79]

Diabetic Wounds

Ten to 15% of diabetic patients run the risk of developing ulcers. There are approximately 50,000 to 60,000 amputations performed in diabetic patients each year in the United States. The major contributors to the formation of diabetic ulcers include neuropathy, foot deformity, and ischemia. It is estimated that 60 to 70% of diabetic ulcers are due to neuropathy, 15 to 20% are due to ischemia, and another 15 to 20% are due to a combination of both. The neuropathy is both sensory and motor, and is secondary to persistently elevated glucose levels. The loss of sensory function allows unrecognized injury to occur from ill-fitting shoes, foreign bodies, or other trauma. The motor neuropathy or Charcot's foot leads to collapse or dislocation of the interphalangeal or metatarsophalangeal joints, causing pressure on areas with little protection. There is also severe micro- and macrovascular circulatory impairment.

Once ulceration occurs, the chances of healing are poor. The management of diabetic wounds involves local and systemic measures. Achievement of adequate blood sugar levels is very important. Most diabetic wounds are infected, and eradication of the infectious source is paramount to the success of healing. Treatment should address the possible presence of osteomyelitis, and should employ antibiotics that achieve adequate levels both in soft tissue and bone. Wide débridement of all necrotic or infected tissue is another cornerstone of treatment. Off-loading of the ulcerated area by using specialized orthotic shoes or casts allows for ambulation while protecting the fragile wound environment. Topical application of PDGF and granulocyte-macrophage colony-stimulating factor has met with limited but significant success in achieving closure. The application of engineered skin allograft substitutes, although expensive, has also shown some significant success.[80]

Decubitus or Pressure Ulcers

The incidence of pressure ulcers ranges from 2.7 to 9% in the acute care setting, in comparison to 2.4 to 23% in long-term care facilities. The expense of pressure sore management in the United States is approximately $1.3 billion annually, with an average cost of $50,000 to $60,000 per ulcer. A pressure ulcer is a localized area of tissue necrosis that develops when a soft tissue is compressed between a bony prominence and an external surface. Excessive pressure causes capillary collapse and impedes the delivery of nutrients to body tissues. Pressure ulcer formation is accelerated in the presence of friction, shear forces, and moisture. Other contributory factors in the pathogenesis of pressure ulcers include immobility, altered activity levels, altered mental status, chronic conditions, and

altered nutritional status. The four stages of pressure ulcer formation are as follows: stage I, nonblanchable erythema of intact skin; stage II, partial-thickness skin loss involving epidermis or dermis or both; stage III, full-thickness skin loss, but not through the fascia; and stage IV, full-thickness skin loss with extensive involvement of muscle and bone.

The treatment of established pressure ulcers is most successful when carried out in a multidisciplinary manner by involving wound care teams consisting of physicians, nurses, dietitians, physical therapists, and nutritionists. Care of the ulcer itself comprises débridement of all necrotic tissue, maintenance of a favorable moist wound environment that will facilitate healing, relief of pressure, and addressing host issues such as nutritional, metabolic, and circulatory status. Débridement is most efficiently carried out surgically, but enzymatic proteolytic preparations and hydrotherapy also are used. The wound bed should be kept moist by employing dressings that absorb secretions but do not desiccate the wound. Operative repair, usually involving flap rotation, has been found to be useful in obtaining closure. Unfortunately, recurrence rates are extremely high, owing to the population at risk and the inability to fully address the causative mechanisms.[81]

EXCESS HEALING

Clinically, excess healing can be as significant as wound failure. It is likely that more operative interventions are required for correction of the morbidity associated with excessive healing than are required for wound failure. The clinical manifestations of exuberant healing are protean and differ in the skin (mutilating or debilitating scars, burn contractions), tendons (frozen repairs), the GI tract (strictures or stenoses), solid organs (cirrhosis, pulmonary fibrosis), or the peritoneal cavity (adhesive disease).

Excess Dermal Scarring

Hypertrophic scars (HTS) and keloids represent an overabundance of fibroplasia in the dermal healing process. HTS rise above the skin level but stay within the confines of the original wound and often regress over time. Keloids rise above the skin level as well, but extend beyond the border of the original wound and rarely regress spontaneously (Fig. 8-10). Both HTS and keloids occur after trauma to the skin, and may be tender, pruritic, and cause a burning sensation. Keloids are fifteen times more common in darker-pigmented ethnicities, with individuals of African, Spanish, and Asian ethnicities being especially susceptible. Men and women are equally affected. Genetically, the predilection to keloid formation appears to be autosomal dominant with incomplete penetration and variable expression.[82,83]

HTS usually develop within 4 weeks after trauma. The risk of HTS increases if epithelialization takes longer than 21 days, independent of site, age, and race. Rarely elevated more than 4 mm above the skin level, HTS stay within the boundaries of the wound. They usually occur across areas of tension and flexor surfaces, which tend to be at right angles to joints or skin creases. The lesions are initially erythematous and raised, and over time may evolve into pale, flatter scars.

Keloids can result from surgery, burns, skin inflammation, acne, chickenpox, zoster, folliculitis, lacerations, abrasions, tattoos, vaccinations, injections, insect bites, ear piercing, or may arise spontaneously. Keloids tend to occur 3 months to years after the initial insult, and even minor injuries can result in large lesions. They vary in size from a few millimeters to large, pedunculated lesions

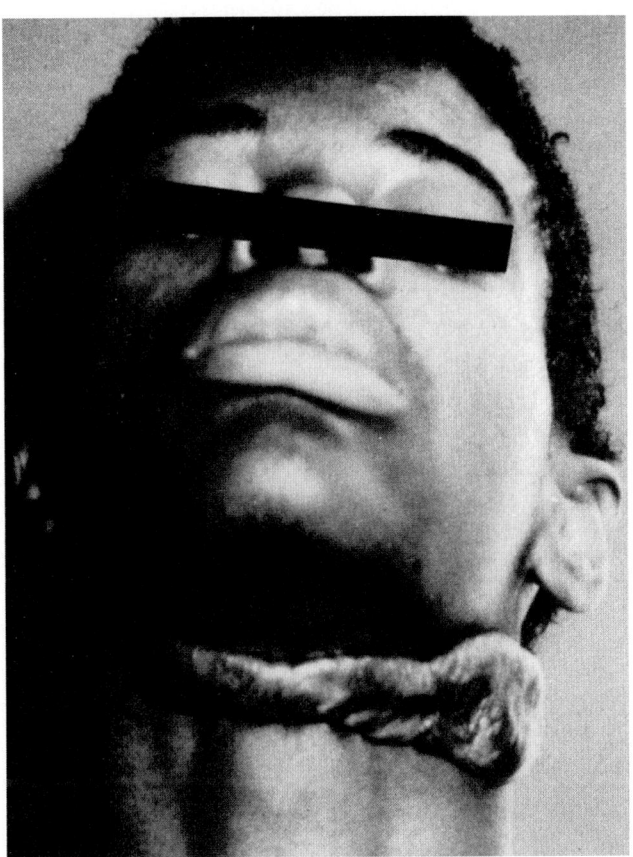

FIG. 8-10. Recurrent keloid on the neck of a 17-year-old patient that had been revised several times. [*Reproduced with permission from Murray JC, Pinnell SR: Keloids and excessive dermal scarring, in Cohen IK, Diegalmann RF, Lindblad WJ (eds): Wound Healing: Biochemical and Clinical Aspects. Philadelphia: WB Saunders, 1993.*]

with a soft to rubbery or hard consistency. While they project above surrounding skin, they rarely extend into underlying subcutaneous tissues. Certain body sites have a higher incidence of keloid formation, including the skin of the earlobe as well as the deltoid, presternal, and upper back regions. They rarely occur on eyelids, genitalia, palms, soles, or across joints. Keloids rarely involute spontaneously, while surgical intervention can lead to recurrence, often with a worse result.

Histologically, both HTS and keloids demonstrate increased thickness of the epidermis with an absence of rete ridges. There is an abundance of collagen and glycoprotein deposition. Normal skin has distinct collagen bundles, mostly parallel to the epithelial surface, with random connections between bundles by fine fibrillar strands of collagen. In HTS, the collagen bundles are flatter, more random, and the fibers are in a wavy pattern. In keloids, the collagen bundles are virtually nonexistent, and the fibers are connected haphazardly in loose sheets with a random orientation to the epithelium. The collagen fibers are larger and thicker and myofibroblasts are generally absent.[84]

Keloidal fibroblasts have normal proliferation parameters, but synthesize collagen at a rate 20 times greater than that observed in normal dermal fibroblasts, and 3 times higher than fibroblasts derived from HTS. Abnormal amounts of extracellular matrix such as fibronectin, elastin, and proteoglycans also are produced. The synthesis of fibronectin, which promotes clot generation, granulation tissue formation, and re-epithelialization, decreases during the normal healing process; however, production continues at high levels

for months to years in HTS and keloids. This perturbed synthetic activity is mediated by altered growth factor expression. TGF-β expression is higher in HTS, and both HTS- and keloid-derived fibroblasts respond to lower concentrations of TGF-β than do normal dermal fibroblasts. HTS also express increased levels of insulin-like growth factor-1, which reduces collagenase mRNA activity and increases mRNA for types I and II procollagen.

The underlying mechanisms that cause HTS and keloids are not known. The immune system appears to be involved in the formation of both HTS and keloids, although the exact relationship is unknown. Much is inferred from the presence of various immune cells in HTS and keloids. For example, in both HTS and keloids, keratinocytes express human leukocyte antigen (HLA)-2 and ICAM-1 receptors, which are absent in normal scar keratinocytes. Keloids also have increased deposition of immunoglobulins IgG, IgA, and IgM, and their formation correlates with serum levels of IgE. Antinuclear antibodies against fibroblasts, epithelial cells, and endothelial cells are found in keloids, but not HTS. HTS have higher T-lymphocyte and Langerhans' cell contents. There is also a larger number of mast cells present in both HTS and keloids compared to normal scars. Other mechanisms that may cause abnormal scarring include mechanical tension (although keloids often occur in areas of minimal tension) and prolonged irritation and/or inflammation that may lead to the generation of abnormal concentrations of profibrotic cytokines.

Treatment goals include restoration of function to the area, relief of symptoms, and prevention of recurrence. Many patients seek intervention due to cosmetic concerns. Because the underlying mechanisms causing keloids and HTS remain unknown, many different modalities of treatment have been used without consistent success.

Excision alone of keloids is subject to a high recurrence rate, ranging from 45 to 100%. There are fewer recurrences when surgical excision is combined with other modalities such as intralesional corticosteroid injection, topical application of silicone sheets, or the use of radiation or pressure. Surgery is recommended for debulking large lesions or as second-line therapy when other modalities have failed. Silicone application is relatively painless and should be maintained for 24 hours a day for about 3 months to prevent rebound hypertrophy. It may be secured with tape or worn beneath a pressure garment. The mechanism of action is not understood, but increased hydration of the skin, which decreases capillary activity, inflammation, hyperemia, and collagen deposition, may be involved. Silicone is more effective than other occlusive dressings and is an especially good treatment for children and others who cannot tolerate the pain involved in other modalities.[82]

Intralesional corticosteroid injections decrease fibroblast proliferation, collagen and glycosaminoglycan synthesis, the inflammatory process, and TGF-β levels. When used alone, however, there is a variable rate of response and recurrence, therefore steroids are recommended as first-line treatment for keloids and second-line treatment for HTS if topical therapies have failed. Intralesional injections are more effective on younger scars. They may soften, flatten, and give symptomatic relief to keloids, but they cannot make the lesions disappear nor can they narrow wide HTS. Success is enhanced when used in combination with surgical excision. Serial injections every 2 to 3 weeks are required. Complications include skin atrophy, hypopigmentation, telangiectasias, necrosis, and ulceration.

Although radiation destroys fibroblasts, it has variable, unreliable results and produces poor results with 10 to 100% recurrence when used alone. It is more effective when combined with surgical excision. The timing, duration, and dosage for radiation therapy is still controversial, but doses ranging from 1500 to 2000 rads appear effective. Given the risks of hyperpigmentation, pruritus, erythema, paresthesias, pain, and possible secondary malignancies, radiation should be reserved for adults with scars resistant to other modalities.

Pressure aids collagen maturation, flattens scars, and improves thinning and pliability. It reduces the number of cells in a given area, possibly by creating ischemia, which decreases tissue metabolism and increases collagenase activity. External compression is used to treat HTS, especially after burns. Therapy must begin early, and a pressure between 24 and 30 mm Hg must be achieved in order to exceed capillary pressure, yet preserve peripheral blood circulation. Garments should be worn for 23 to 24 hours a day for up to 1 or more years to avoid rebound hypertrophy. Scars older than 6 to 12 months respond poorly.

Topical retinoids also have been used as treatment for both HTS and keloids, with reported responses of 50 to 100%. Intralesional injections of INF-γ, a cytokine released by T lymphocytes, reduce collagen types I, II, and III by decreasing mRNA and possibly by reducing levels of TGF-β. This treatment is experimental, and complications are frequent and dose-dependent. Intralesional injections of chemotherapeutic agents such as 5-fluorouracil have been used both alone and in combination with steroids. The use of bleomycin has been reported to achieve some success in older scars resistant to steroids.

Peritoneal Scarring

Peritoneal adhesions are fibrous bands of tissues formed between organs that are normally separated and/or between organs and the internal body wall. Most intra-abdominal adhesions are a result of peritoneal injury, either by a prior surgical procedure or due to

intra-abdominal infection. Postmortem examinations demonstrate adhesions in 67% of patients with prior surgical procedures and in 28% with a history of intra-abdominal infection. Intra-abdominal adhesions are the most common cause (65 to 75%) of small bowel obstruction, especially in the ileum. Operations in the lower abdomen have a higher chance of producing small bowel obstruction. Following rectal surgery, left colectomy, or total colectomy, there is an 11% chance of developing small bowel obstruction within 1 year, and this rate increases to 30% by 10 years. Adhesions also are a leading cause of secondary infertility in women and can cause substantial abdominal and pelvic pain. Adhesions account for 2% of all surgical admissions and 3% of all laparotomies in general surgery.[85]

Adhesions form when the peritoneal surface is damaged due to surgery, thermal or ischemic injury, inflammation, or foreign body reaction. The injury disrupts the protective mesothelial cell layer lining the peritoneal cavity and the underlying connective tissue. The injury elicits an inflammatory response consisting of hyperemia, fluid exudation, release and activation of white blood cells and platelets in the peritoneal cavity, activation of inflammatory cytokines, and the onset of the coagulation and complement cascades. Fibrin deposition occurs between the damaged but opposed serosal surfaces. These filmy adhesions are often transient and degraded by proteases of the fibrinolytic system, with restoration of the normal peritoneal surface. If insufficient fibrinolytic activity is present, permanent fibrous adhesions will form by collagen deposition within 1 week of the injury (Fig. 8-11).

Extensive research has been done on the effect of surgery and peritonitis on the fibrinolytic and inflammatory cascades within the peritoneal cavity. During normal repair, fibrin is principally

FIG. 8-11. Fibrin formation and degradation in peritoneal tissue repair and adhesion formation.

PERITONEAL INJURY

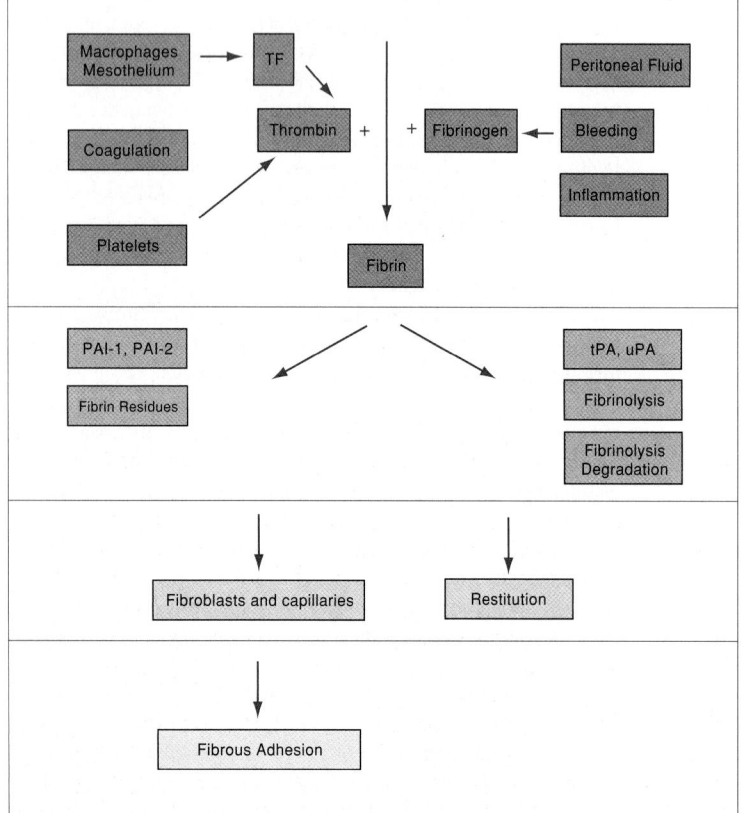

degraded by the fibrinolytic protease plasmin, which is derived from inactive plasminogen through the action of two plasminogen activators (PA): tissue-type plasminogen activator (tPA) and urokinase-type plasminogen activator (uPA). Fibrinolytic activity in peritoneal fluid is reduced after abdominal surgery due to initial decreases in tPA levels and later to increases in plasminogen activator inhibitor-1 (PAI-1), which are induced by various cytokines, including TNF-α, IL-1, and interleukin-6 (IL-6).[86]

There are two major strategies for adhesion prevention or reduction. Surgical trauma is minimized within the peritoneum by careful tissue handling, avoiding desiccation and ischemia, and spare use of cautery, laser, and retractors. Fewer adhesions form with laparoscopic surgical techniques due to reduced tissue trauma. The second major advance in adhesion prevention has been the introduction of barrier membranes and gels, which separate and create barriers between damaged surfaces, allowing for adhesion-free healing. Modified oxidized regenerated cellulose and hyaluronic acid membranes or solutions have been shown to reduce adhesions in gynecologic patients, and are being investigated for their ability to prevent adhesion formation in general surgical patients.

TREATMENT OF WOUNDS

Local Care

Management of acute wounds begins with obtaining a careful history of the events surrounding the injury. The history is followed by a meticulous examination of the wound. Examination should assess the depth and configuration of the wound, the extent of nonviable tissue, and the presence of foreign bodies and other contaminants. Examination of the wound may require irrigation and débridement of the edges of the wound, and is facilitated by use of local anesthesia. Antibiotic administration and tetanus prophylaxis may be needed, and planning the type and timing of wound repair should take place.

After completion of the history, examination, and administration of tetanus prophylaxis, the wound should be meticulously anesthetized. Lidocaine (0.5 to 1%) or bupivacaine (0.25 to 0.5%) combined with a 1:100,000 to 1:200,000 dilution of epinephrine provides satisfactory anesthesia and hemostasis. Epinephrine should not be used in wounds of the fingers, toes, ears, nose, or penis, due to the risk of tissue necrosis secondary to terminal arteriole vasospasm in these structures. Injection of these anesthetics can result in significant initial patient discomfort, and this can be minimized by slow injection, infiltration of the subcutaneous tissues, and buffering the solution with sodium bicarbonate. Care must be observed in calculating the maximum dosages of lidocaine or bupivacaine in order to avoid toxicity-related side effects.

Irrigation to visualize all areas of the wound and remove foreign material is best accomplished with normal saline (without additives). High-pressure wound irrigation is more effective in achieving complete débridement of foreign material and nonviable tissues. Iodine, povidone-iodine, hydrogen peroxide, and organically based antibacterial preparations have all been shown to impair wound healing due to injury to wound neutrophils and macrophages, and thus should not be used. All hematomas present within wounds should be carefully evacuated and any remaining bleeding sources controlled with ligature or cautery. If the injury has resulted in the formation of a marginally viable flap of skin or tissue, these should be resected or revascularized prior to further wound repair and closure.

After the wound has been anesthetized, explored, irrigated, and débrided, the area surrounding the wound should be cleaned, inspected, and the surrounding hair clipped. The area surrounding the wound should be prepared with povidone-iodine or similar solution and draped with sterile towels. Having ensured hemostasis and adequate débridement of nonviable tissues and removal of any remaining foreign bodies, irregular, macerated, or beveled wound edges should be débrided in order to provide a fresh edge for reapproximation. Although plastic surgical techniques such as W- or Z-plasty are seldom recommended for acute wounds, great care must be taken to realign wound edges properly. This is particularly important for wounds that cross the vermilion border, eyebrow, or hairline. Initial sutures that realign the edges of these different tissue types will speed and greatly enhance the aesthetic outcome of the wound repair.

In general, the smallest suture required to hold the various layers of the wound in approximation should be selected in order to minimize suture-related inflammation. Nonabsorbable or slowly absorbing monofilament sutures are most suitable for approximating deep fascial layers, particularly in the abdominal wall. Subcutaneous tissues should be closed with braided absorbable sutures, with care to avoid placement of sutures in fat. Although traditional teaching in wound closure has emphasized multiple-layer closures, additional layers of suture closure are associated with increased risk of wound infection, especially when placed in fat. Drains may be placed in areas at risk of forming fluid collections.

In areas of significant tissue loss, rotation of adjacent musculocutaneous flaps may be required to provide sufficient tissue mass for closure. These musculocutaneous flaps may be based upon intrinsic blood supply, or may be moved from distant sites as free flaps and anastomosed into the local vascular bed. In areas with significant superficial tissue loss, split-thickness skin grafting may be required and will speed formation of an intact epithelial barrier to fluid loss and infection. Split-thickness skin grafts are readily obtained using manual or mechanical dermatomes, and the grafts may be "meshed" in order to increase the surface area of their coverage. It is essential to ensure hemostasis of the underlying tissue bed prior to placement of split-thickness skin grafts, as the presence of a hematoma below the graft will prevent the graft from taking, resulting in sloughing of the graft. In acute, contaminated wounds with skin loss, use of porcine xenografts or cadaveric allografts is prudent until the danger of infection passes.

After closing deep tissues and replacing significant tissue deficits, skin edges should be reapproximated for cosmesis and to aid in rapid wound healing. Skin edges may be quickly reapproximated with stainless steel staples or nonabsorbable monofilament sutures. Care must be taken to remove these from the wound prior to epithelialization of the skin tracts where sutures or staples penetrate the dermal layer. Failure to remove the sutures or staples prior to 7 to 10 days after repair will result in a cosmetically inferior wound. Where wound cosmesis is important, the above problems may be avoided by placement of buried dermal sutures using absorbable braided sutures. This method of wound closure allows for a precise reapproximation of wound edges, and may be enhanced by application of wound closure tapes to the surface of the wound. Intradermal absorbable sutures do not require removal. Use of skin tapes alone is only recommended for closure of the smallest superficial wounds. Larger wounds generate sufficient lateral tension that the epithelial edges either separate or curl upward under the tapes, resulting in inadequate epithelial apposition and poor cosmesis.

Recently, development and testing of octyl-cyanoacrylate tissue glues have shown new promise for the management of simple, linear wounds with viable skin edges. These new glues are less prone to brittleness and have superior burst-strength characteristics. Studies have shown them to be suitable for use in contaminated situations without significant risk of infection. When used in the above types of wounds, these glues appear to provide superb cosmetic results and result in significantly less trauma than sutured repair, particularly when used in pediatric patients.

Antibiotics

Antibiotics should be used only when there is an obvious wound infection. Most wounds are contaminated or colonized with bacteria. The presence of a host response constitutes an infection and justifies the use of antibiotics. Signs of infection to look for include erythema, cellulitis, swelling, and purulent discharge. Indiscriminate use of antibiotics should be avoided to prevent emergence of multidrug-resistant bacteria.

Antibiotic treatment of acute wounds must be based upon organisms suspected to be found within the infected wound and the patient's overall immune status. When a single specific organism is suspected, treatment may be commenced using a single antibiotic. Conversely, when multiple organisms are suspected, as with enteric contamination or when a patient's immune function is impaired by diabetes, chronic disease, or medication, treatment should commence with a broad-spectrum antibiotic or several agents in combination. Lastly, the location of the wound and the quality of tissue perfusion to that region will significantly impact wound performance after injury. Antibiotics can also be delivered topically as part of irrigations or dressings, although their efficacy is questionable.

Dressings

The main purpose of wound dressings is to provide the ideal environment for wound healing. The dressing should facilitate the major changes taking place during healing to produce an optimally healed wound. Although the ideal dressing is still not a clinical reality, technological advances are promising (Table 8-7).

Covering a wound with a dressing mimics the barrier role of epithelium and prevents further damage. In addition, application of compression provides hemostasis and limits edema. Occlusion of a wound with dressing material helps healing by controlling the level of hydration and oxygen tension within the wound. It also allows transfer of gases and water vapor from the wound surface to the atmosphere. Occlusion affects both the dermis and epidermis, and it has been shown that exposed wounds are more inflamed and develop more necrosis than covered wounds. Occlusion also helps in dermal collagen synthesis and epithelial cell migration and limits tissue desiccation. Since it may enhance bacterial growth, occlusion is contraindicated in infected and highly exudative wounds.

Dressings can be classified as primary or secondary. A primary dressing is placed directly on the wound and may provide absorption of fluids and prevent desiccation, infection, and adhesion of a

Table 8-7
Desired Characteristics of Wound Dressings

Promote wound healing (maintain moist environment)
Conformability
Pain control
Odor control
Nonallergenic and nonirritating
Permeability to gas
Safety
Nontraumatic removal
Cost-effectiveness
Convenience

secondary dressing. A secondary dressing is one that is placed on the primary dressing for further protection, absorption, compression, and occlusion. Many types of dressings exist and are designed to achieve certain clinically desired endpoints.

Absorbent Dressings

Accumulation of wound fluid can lead to maceration and bacterial overgrowth. Ideally, the dressing should absorb without getting soaked through, as this would permit bacteria from the outside to enter the wound. The dressing must be designed to match the exudative properties of the wound and may include cotton, wool, and sponge.

Nonadherent Dressings

Nonadherent dressings are impregnated with paraffin, petroleum jelly, or water-soluble jelly for use as nonadherent coverage. A secondary dressing must be placed on top to seal the edges and prevent desiccation and infection.

Occlusive and Semiocclusive Dressings

Occlusive and semiocclusive dressings provide a good environment for clean, minimally exudative wounds. These film dressings are waterproof and impervious to microbes, but permeable to water vapor and oxygen.

Hydrophilic and Hydrophobic Dressings

These dressings are components of a composite dressing. Hydrophilic dressing aids in absorption, whereas a hydrophobic dressing is waterproof and prevents absorption.

Hydrocolloid and Hydrogel Dressings

Hydrocolloid and hydrogel dressings attempt to combine the benefits of occlusion and absorbency. Hydrocolloids and hydrogels form complex structures with water, and fluid absorption occurs with particle swelling, which aids in atraumatic removal of the dressing. Absorption of exudates by the hydrocolloid dressing leaves a yellowish-brown gelatinous mass after dressing removal that can be washed off. Hydrogel is a cross-linked polymer that has high water content. Hydrogels allow a high rate of evaporation without compromising wound hydration, which makes them useful in burn treatment.

Alginates

Alginates are derived from brown algae and contain long chains of polysaccharides containing mannuronic and glucuronic acid. The ratios of these sugars vary with the species of algae used, as well as the season of harvest. Processed as the calcium form, alginates turn into soluble sodium alginate through ion exchange in the presence of wound exudates. The polymers gel, swell, and absorb a great deal of fluid. Alginates are being used when there is skin loss, in open surgical wounds with medium exudation, and on full-thickness chronic wounds.

Absorbable Materials

Absorbable materials are mainly used within wounds as hemostats and include collagen, gelatin, oxidized cellulose, and oxidized regenerated cellulose.

Medicated Dressings

Medicated dressings have long been used as a drug-delivery system. Agents delivered in the dressings include benzoyl peroxide, zinc oxide, neomycin, and bacitracin-zinc. These agents have been shown to increase epithelialization by 28%.

The type of dressing to be used depends on the amount of wound drainage. A nondraining wound can be covered with semiocclusive dressing. Drainage of less than 1 to 2 mL/d may require a semiocclusive or absorbent nonadherent dressing. Moderately draining wounds (3 to 5 mL/d) can be dressed with a nonadherent primary layer plus an absorbent secondary layer plus an occlusive dressing to protect normal tissue. Heavily draining wounds (>5 mL/d) require a similar dressing as moderately draining wounds, but with the addition of a highly absorbent secondary layer.

Mechanical Devices

Mechanical therapy augments and improves on certain functions of dressings, in particular the absorption of exudates and control of odor. The V.A.C. (vacuum-assisted closure) system assists in wound closure by applying localized negative pressure to the surface and margins of the wound. This negative pressure therapy is applied to a special foam dressing cut to the dimensions of the wound and positioned in the wound cavity or over a flap or graft. The continuous negative pressure is very effective in removing exudates from the wound. This form of therapy has been found to be effective for chronic open wounds (diabetic ulcers and stages 3 and 4 pressure ulcers), acute and traumatic wounds, flaps and grafts, and subacute wounds (i.e., dehisced incisions).

Skin Replacements

All wounds require coverage in order to prevent evaporative losses and infection and to provide an environment that promotes healing. Both acute and chronic wounds may demand use of skin replacement, and several options are available.

Conventional Skin Grafts

Skin grafts have long been used to treat both acute and chronic wounds. Split- or partial-thickness grafts consist of the epidermis plus part of the dermis, while full-thickness grafts retain the entire epidermis and dermis. Autologous grafts (autografts) are transplants from one site on the body to another; allogeneic grafts (allografts, homografts) are transplants from a living nonidentical donor or cadaver to the host; and xenogeneic grafts (heterografts) are taken from another species (e.g., porcine). Split-thickness grafts require less blood supply to restore skin function. The dermal component of full-thickness grafts lends mechanical strength and resists wound contraction better, resulting in improved cosmesis. Allogeneic and xenogeneic grafts require the availability of tissue, are subject to rejection, and may contain pathogens.

The use of skin grafts or bioengineered skin substitutes and other innovative treatments (e.g., topically applied growth factors, systemic agents, and gene therapy) cannot be effective unless the wound bed is adequately prepared. This may include débridement to remove necrotic or fibrinous tissue, control of edema, revascularization of the wound bed, decreasing the bacterial burden, and minimizing or eliminating exudate. Temporary placement of allografts or xenografts may be used to prepare the wound bed.

Skin Substitutes

Originally devised to provide coverage of extensive wounds with limited availability of autografts, skin substitutes also have gained acceptance as natural dressings. Manufactured by tissue engineering, they combine novel materials with living cells to provide functional skin substitutes, providing a bridge between dressings and skin grafts.

Skin substitutes have theoretical advantages of being readily available, not requiring painful harvest, and they may be applied freely or with surgical suturing. In addition, they promote healing, either by stimulating host cytokine generation or by providing cells that may also produce growth factors locally. Their disadvantages include limited survival, high cost, and the need for multiple applications (Table 8-8). Allografting, albeit with a very thin graft, may at times be required to accomplish complete coverage.

A variety of skin substitutes are available, each with its own set of advantages and disadvantages; however, the ideal skin substitute has yet to be developed (Table 8-9). The development of the newer composite substitutes, which provide both the dermal and epidermal components essential for permanent skin replacement, may represent an advance toward that goal. The acellular (e.g., native collagen or synthetic material) component acts as a scaffold, promotes cell migration and growth, and activates tissue regeneration and remodeling. The cellular elements re-establish lost tissue and associated function, synthesize extracellular matrix components, produce essential mediators such as cytokines and growth factors, and promote proliferation and migration.

Cultured epithelial autografts (CEAs) represent expanded autologous or homologous keratinocytes. CEAs are expanded from a biopsy of the patient's own skin, will not be rejected, and can stimulate re-epithelialization as well as the growth of underlying connective tissue. Keratinocytes harvested from a biopsy roughly

Table 8-8
Desired Features of Tissue-Engineered Skin

Rapid re-establishment of functional skin (epidermis/dermis)
Receptive to body's own cells (e.g., rapid "take" and integration)
Graftable by a single, simple procedure
Graftable on chronic or acute wounds
Engraftment without use of extraordinary clinical intervention (i.e., immunosuppression)

Table 8-9
Advantages and Disadvantages of Various Bioengineered Skin Substitutes

Skin Substitute	Advantages	Disadvantages
Cultured allogeneic keratinocyte grafts	No biopsy needed "Off the shelf" availability Provides wound coverage Promotes healing	Unstable Does not prevent wound contracture Inadequate cosmesis Possibility of disease transmission Fragile
Bioengineered dermal replacements	Prevents contracture Good prep for graft application	Limited ability to drive re-epithelialization Largely serve as temporary dressings
Cultured bilayer skin equivalents	More closely mimics normal anatomy Does not need secondary procedure Easily handled Can be sutured, meshed, etc	Cost Short shelf life True engraftment questionable

the size of a postage stamp are cultured with fibroblasts and growth factors and grown into sheets that can cover large areas and give the appearance of normal skin. Until the epithelial sheets are sufficiently expanded, the wound must be covered with an occlusive dressing or a temporary allograft or xenograft. The dermis regenerates very slowly, if at all, for full-thickness wounds, because the sheets are very fragile, difficult to work with, are susceptible to infection, and do not resist contracture well, leading to poor cosmetic results.

CEAs are available from cadavers, unrelated adult donors, or from neonatal foreskins. Fresh or cryopreserved cultured allogeneic keratinocytes can be left in place long enough to be superseded by multiplying endogenous skin cells because, unlike allografts containing epidermal Langerhans' cells, they do not express major histocompatibility antigens. Cryopreserved CEAs are readily available "off the shelf," and provide growth factors that may aid healing. However, like autologous keratinocyte sheets, the grafts lack the strength provided by a dermal component and pose a risk of disease transmission.

Viable fibroblasts can be grown on bioabsorbable or nonbioabsorbable meshes to yield living dermal tissue that can act as a scaffold for epidermal growth. Fibroblasts stimulated by growth factors can produce type I collagen and glycosaminoglycans (e.g., chondroitin sulfates), which adhere to the wound surface to permit epithelial cell migration, as well as adhesive ligands (e.g., the matrix protein fibronectin), which promote cell adhesion. This approach has the virtue of being less time-consuming and expensive than culturing keratinocyte sheets. There are a number of commercially available, bioengineered dermal replacements approved for use in burn treatment as well as other indications.

Bioengineered skin substitutes have evolved from keratinocyte monolayers to dermal equivalents to split-thickness products with a pseudo-epidermis, and most recently, to products containing both epidermal and dermal components that resemble the three-dimensional structure and function of normal skin (see Table 8-9). Indicated for use with standard compression therapy in the treatment of venous insufficiency ulcers and for the treatment of neuropathic diabetic foot ulcers, these bilayered skin equivalents also are being used in a variety of wound care settings.

Growth Factor Therapy

As discussed previously, it is believed that nonhealing wounds result from insufficient or inadequate growth factors in the wound environment. A simplistic solution would be to flood the wound with single or multiple growth factors in order to "jump-start" healing and re-epithelialization. Although there is a large body of work demonstrating the effects of growth factors in animals, translation of these data into clinical practice has met with limited success. Growth factors for clinical use may be either recombinant or homologous/autologous. Autologous growth factors are harvested from the patient's own platelets, yielding an unpredictable combination and concentration of factors, which are then applied to the wound. This approach allows treatment with patient-specific factors at an apparently physiologic ratio of growth factor concentrations. Recombinant molecular biologic means permit the purification of high concentrations of individual growth factors. Current FDA-approved formulations, as well as those used experimentally, deliver concentrations approximately 10^3 times higher than those observed physiologically.

At present, only platelet-derived growth factor BB (PDGF-BB) is currently approved by the FDA for treatment of diabetic foot ulcers. Application of recombinant human PDGF-BB in a gel

suspension to these wounds increases the incidence of total healing and decreases healing time. Several other growth factors have been tested clinically and show some promise, but currently none are approved for use. A great deal more needs to be discovered about the concentration, temporal release, and receptor cell population before growth factor therapy is to make a consistent impact on wound healing.

References

1. Winter GD: Formation of the scab and the rate of epithelialisation of superficial wounds in the skin of the young domestic pig. *Nature* 193:293, 1962.
1a. Gulliver G (ed): *The Works of John Hunter.* London: Longman, 1837.
2. Feiken E, Romer J, Eriksen J, et al: Neutrophils express tumor necrosis factor-alpha during mouse skin wound healing. *J Invest Dermatol* 105:120, 1995.
3. Dovi JV, He L-K, DiPietro LA: Accelerated wound closure in neutrophil-depleted mice. *J Leukoc Biol* 73:448, 2003.
4. Leibovich SJ, Ross R: The role of the macrophage in wound repair. A study with hydrocortisone and antimacrophage serum. *Am J Pathol* 78:71, 1975.
5. DiPietro LA: Wound healing: The role of the macrophage and other immune cells. *Shock* 4:233, 1995.
6. Zabel DD, Feng JJ, Scheuenstuhl H, et al: Lactate stimulation of macrophage-derived angiogenic activity is associated with inhibition of Poly(ADP-ribose) synthesis. *Lab Invest* 74:644, 1996.
7. Schäffer MR, Barbul A: Lymphocyte function in wound healing and following injury. *Br J Surg* 85:444, 1998.
8. Efron JE, Frankel HL, Lazarou SA, et al: Wound healing and T-lymphocytes. *J Surg Res* 48:460, 1990.
9. Barbul A, Breslin RJ, Woodyard JP, et al: The effect of in vivo T helper and T suppressor lymphocyte depletion on wound healing. *Ann Surg* 209:479, 1989.
10. Rezzonico R, Burger D, Dayer JM: Direct contact between T lymphocytes and human dermal fibroblasts or synoviocytes down-regulates types I and III collagen production via cell-associated cytokines. *J Biol Chem* 273:18720, 1998.
11. Grotendorst GR: Chemoattractants and growth factors, in Cohen K, Diegelmann RF, Lindblad WJ (eds): *Wound Healing, Biochemical and Clinical Aspects.* Philadelphia: WB Saunders, 1992, p 237.
12. Bonner JC, Osornio-Vargas AR, et al: Differential proliferation of rat lung fibroblasts induced by the platelet-derived growth factor-AA, -AB, and -BB isoforms secreted by rat alveolar macrophages. *Am J Respir Cell Mol Biol* 5:539, 1991.
13. Pricolo VE, Caldwell MD, Mastrofrancesco B, et al: Modulatory activities of wound fluid on fibroblast proliferation and collagen synthesis. *J Surg Res* 48:534, 1990.
14. Regan MC, Kirk SJ, Wasserkrug HL, et al: The wound environment as a regulator of fibroblast phenotype. *J Surg Res* 50:442, 1991.
15. Gimbel ML, Hunt TK, Hussain MZ: Lactate controls collagen gene promoter activity through poly-ADP-ribosylation. *Surg Forum* 51:26, 2000.
16. Ghani QP, Hussain MZ, Hunt TK: Control of procollagen gene transcription and prolyl hydroxylase activity by poly(ADP-ribose), in Poirier G, Moreaer A (eds): *ADP-Ribosylation Reactions.* New York: Springer-Verlag, 1992, p 111.
17. Xiong M, Elson G, Legarda D, et al: Production of vascular endothelial growth factor by murine macrophages: Regulation by hypoxia, lactate, and the inducible nitric oxide synthase pathway. *Am J Pathol* 153:587, 1998.
18. Ferrara N, Davis-Smith T: The biology of vascular endothelial growth factor. *Endocrine Rev* 18:4, 1997.
19. Levenson SM, Geever EF, Crowley LV, et al: The healing of rat skin wounds. *Ann Surg* 161:293, 1965.

20. Zhou LJ, Ono I, Kaneko F: Role of transforming growth factor-beta 1 in fibroblasts derived from normal and hypertrophic scarred skin. *Arch Dermatol Res* 289:645, 1997.

21. Stenn KS, Depalma L: Re-epithelialization, in Clark RAF, Hensen PM (eds): *The Molecular and Cellular Biology of Wound Repair*. New York: Plenum, 1988, p 321.

22. Johnson FR, McMinn RMH: The cytology of wound healing of the body surface in mammals. *Biol Rev* 35:364, 1960.

23. Woodley DT, Bachman PM, O'Keefe EJ: The role of matrix components in human keratinocyte re-epithelialization, in Barbul A, Caldwell MD, Eaglstein WH, et al (eds): *Clinical and Experimental Approaches to Dermal and Epidermal Repair. Normal and Chronic Wounds*. New York: Wiley-Liss, 1991, p 129.

24. Lynch SE: Interaction of growth factors in tissue repair, in Barbul A, Caldwell MD, Eaglstein WH, et al (eds): *Clinical and Experimental Approaches to Dermal and Epidermal Repair. Normal and Chronic Wounds*. New York: Wiley-Liss, 1991, p 341.

25. Jans DA, Hassan G: Nuclear targeting by growth factors, cytokines, and their receptors: A role in signaling? *Bioassays* 20:400, 1998.

26. Schmitt-Graff A, Desmouliere A, Gabbiani G: Heterogeneity of myofibroblast phenotypic features: An example of fibroblastic cell plasticity. *Virchows Arch* 425:3, 1994.

27. Darby I, Skalli O, Gabbiani G: Alpha-smooth muscle actin is transiently expressed by myofibroblasts during experimental wound healing. *Lab Invest* 63:21, 1990.

28. Desmouliere A, Redard M, Darby I, et al: Apoptosis mediates the decrease in cellularity during the transition between granulation tissue and scar. *Am J Pathol* 146:56, 1995.

29. Ehrlich HP: Wound closure: Evidence of cooperation between fibroblasts and collagen matrix. *Eye* 2:149, 1988.

30. Phillips C, Wenstrup RJ: Biosynthetic and genetic disorders of collagen, in Cohen IK, Diegelman RF, Linbald WJ (eds): *Wound Healing Biochemical and Clinical Aspects*. Philadelphia: WB Saunders, 1992, p 152.

31. Sidhu-Malik NK, Wenstrup RJ: The Ehlers-Danlos syndromes and Marfan syndrome: Inherited diseases of connective tissue with overlapping clinical features. *Semin Dermatol* 14:40, 1995.

32. Woolley MM, Morgan S, Hays DM: Heritable disorders of connective tissue. Surgical and anesthetic problems. *J Pediatr Surg* 2:325, 1967.

33. McEntyre RL, Raffensperger JG: Surgical complications of Ehlers-Danlos syndrome in children. *J Pediatr Surg* 13:531, 1977.

34. Hunt TK: Disorders of wound healing. *World J Surg* 4:271, 1980.

35. Anonymous: Heritable disorders of connective tissue. *JAMA* 224 (5 Suppl):774, 1973.

36. Carter DM, Lin AN: Wound healing and epidermolysis bullosa. *Arch Dermatol* 124:732, 1988.

37. Kruse-Jarres JD: Pathogenesis and symptoms of zinc deficiency. *Am Clin Lab* 20:17, 2001.

38. Okada A, Takagi Y, Nezu R, et al: Zinc in clinical surgery—a research review. *Jpn J Surg* 20:635, 1990.

39. Thornton FJ, Barbul A: Healing in the gastrointestinal tract. *Surg Clin North Am* 77:549, 1997.

40. Lorenz PH, Whitby DJ, Longaker MT, et al: Fetal wound healing. The ontogeny of scar formation in the non-human primate. *Ann Surg* 217:391, 1993.

41. Longaker MT, Whitby DJ, Ferguson MWJ, et al: Adult skin wounds in the fetal environment heal with scar formation. *Ann Surg* 219:65, 1994.

42. Lorenz HP, Longaker MT, Perkocha LA, et al: Scarless wound repair: A human fetal skin model. *Development* 114:253, 1992.

43. Adzick NS, Harrison MR, Glick PL, et al: Comparison of fetal, newborn and adult rabbit wound healing by histologic, enzyme-histochemical and hydroxyproline determinations. *J Pediatr Surg* 20:315, 1991.

44. Shah M, Foreman DM, Ferguson MWJ: Neutralizing antibody to TGF-β1,2 reduces cutaneous scarring in adult rodents. *J Cell Sci* 107:1137, 1994.

45. Longaker MT, Adzick NS: The biology of fetal wound healing: A review. *Plast Reconstr Surg* 87:788, 1990.

46. Seeger JM, Kaelin LD, Staples EM, et al: Prevention of postoperative pericardial adhesions using tissue-protective solutions. *J Surg Res* 68:63, 1997.

47. Halasz NA: Dehiscence of laparotomy wounds. *Am J Surg* 116:210, 1968.

48. Mendoza CB, Postlethwait RW, Johnson WD: Incidence of wound disruption following operation. *Arch Surg* 101:396, 1970.

49. Holt D, Kirk SJ, Regan MC, et al: Effect of age on wound healing in healthy humans. *Surgery* 112:293, 1992.

50. Jonson K, Jensen JA, Goodson WH III, et al: Tissue oxygenation, anemia and perfusion in relation to wound healing in surgical patients. *Ann Surg* 214:605, 1991.

51. Hopf HW, Hunt TK, West JM, et al: Wound tissue oxygen tension predicts the risk of wound infection in surgical patients. *Arch Surg* 132:997, 1997.

52. Greif R, Akca O, Horn EP, et al: Supplemental perioperative oxygen to reduce the incidence of surgical-wound infection. Outcomes Research Group. *N Engl J Med* 342:161, 2000.

53. Kurz A, Sessler D, Leonhardt R: Perioperative normothermia to reduce the incidence of surgical-wound infection and shorten hospitalization. *N Engl J Med* 334:1209, 1996.

54. Ehrlich HP, Hunt TK: Effects of cortisone and vitamin A on wound healing. *Ann Surg* 167:324, 1968.

55. Anstead GM: Steroids, retinoids, and wound healing. *Adv Wound Care* 11:277, 1998.

56. Ferguson MK: The effect of antineoplastic agents on wound healing. *Surg Gynecol Obstet* 154:421, 1982.

57. Larson DL: Alterations in wound healing secondary to infusion injury. *Clin Plast Surg* 17:509, 1990.

58. Cruse PJE, Foord RA: A prospective study of 23,649 surgical wounds. *Arch Surg* 107:206, 1973.

59. Yue DK, McLennan S, Marsh M, et al: Effects of experimental diabetes, uremia, and malnutrition on wound healing. *Diabetes* 36:295, 1987.

60. Goodson WH III, Hunt TK: Studies of wound healing in experimental diabetes mellitus. *J Surg Res* 22:221, 1977.

61. Black E, Vibe-Petersen J, Jorgensen LN, et al: Decrease in collagen deposition in wound repair in type I diabetes independent of glycemic control. *Arch Surg* 138:34, 2003.

62. Williams JZ, Barbul A: Nutrition and wound healing. *Surg Clin North Am* 83:571, 2003.

63. Goodson WH, Jensen JA, Gramja-Mena L, et al: The influence of a brief preoperative illness on postoperative healing. *Ann Surg* 205:250, 1987.

64. Winsor JA, Knight GS, Hill GL: Wound healing in surgical patients: Recent food intake is more important than nutritional status. *Br J Surg* 75:135, 1988.

65. Haydock DA, Hill GL: Improved wound healing response in surgical patients receiving intravenous nutrition. *Br J Surg* 74:320, 1987.

66. Seifter E, Rettura G, Barbul A, et al: Arginine: An essential amino acid for injured rats. *Surgery* 84:224, 1978.

67. Barbul A, Lazarou S, Efron DT, et al: Arginine enhances wound healing in humans. *Surgery* 108:331, 1990.

68. Kirk SJ, Regan MC, Holt D, et al: Arginine stimulates wound healing and immune function in aged humans. *Surgery* 114:155, 1993.

69. Williams JZ, Abumrad NN, Barbul A: Effect of a specialized amino acid mixture on human collagen deposition. *Ann Surg* 236:369, 2002.

70. Levenson SM, Seifter E, VanWinkle W: Nutrition, in Hunt TK, Dunphy JE (eds): *Fundamentals of Wound Management in Surgery*. New York: Appleton-Century-Crofts, 1979, p 286.

71. Jeejeebhoy KN, Cheong WK: Essential trace metals: Deficiencies and requirements, in Fischer JE (ed): *Nutrition and Metabolism in the Surgical Patient*. Boston: Little, Brown and Company, 1996, p 295.

72. Wilkinson EAJ, Hawke CI: Oral zinc for arterial and venous ulcers (Cochrane Review), in *The Cochrane Library*, 1:2002. Oxford: Update Software.

73. Robson MC: Wound infection: A failure of wound healing caused by an imbalance of bacteria. *Surg Clin North Am* 77:637, 1997.

74. Liese JG, Jenrossek V, Jannson A, et al: Chronic granulomatous disease in adults. *Lancet* 347:220, 1996.

75. Falanga V, Eaglstein WH: The "trap" hypothesis of venous ulceration. *Lancet* 341:1006, 1993.

76. Lobmann R, Ambrosch A, Schultz G, et al: Expression of matrix-metalloproteinases and their inhibitors in the wounds of diabetic and non-diabetic patients. *Diabetologia* 45:1011, 2002.

77. Stanley A, Osler T: Senescence and the healing rates of venous ulcers. *J Vasc Surg* 33:1206, 2001.

78. Kim BC, Kim HT, Park SH, et al: Fibroblasts from chronic wounds show altered TGF-β-signaling and decreased TGF-β type II receptor expression. *J Cell Physiol* 195:331, 2003.

79. Flour M: Venous ulcer management: Has research led to improved healing for the patient? in *The Oxford European Wound Healing Course Handbook*. Oxford: Positif Press, 2002, p 33.

80. Jeffcoate WJ, Harding KG: Diabetic foot ulcers. *Lancet* 361:1545, 2003.

81. Eaglstein WH, Falanga V: Chronic wounds. *Surg Clin North Am* 77:689, 1997.

82. Niessen FB, Spauwen PH, Schalkwijk J, et al: On the nature of hypertrophic scars and keloids: A review. *Plast Reconstr Surg* 104:1435, 1999.

83. Marneros AG, Norris JE, Olsen BR, et al: Clinical genetics of familial keloids. *Arch Dermatol* 137:1429, 2001.

84. Tredget EE, Nedelec B, Scott PG, et al: Hypertrophic scars, keloids, and contractures. *Surg Clin North Am* 77:701, 1997.

85. Dijkstra FR, Nieuwenhuijzen M, Reijnen MM, et al: Recent clinical developments in pathophysiology, epidemiology, diagnosis and treatment of intra-abdominal adhesions. *Scand J Gastroenterol Suppl* 232:52, 2000.

86. Cheong YC, Laird SM, Shellton JB, et al: The correlation of adhesions and peritoneal fluid cytokine concentrations: A pilot study. *Hum Reprod* 17:1039, 2002.

CHAPTER 9

Oncology

Funda Meric-Bernstam and Raphael E. Pollock

Cancer Screening and Diagnosis
Surgical Therapy
Systemic Therapy

INTRODUCTION

As the population ages, oncology is becoming a larger portion of surgical practice. The surgeon often is responsible for the initial diagnosis and management of solid tumors. Knowledge of cancer epidemiology, etiology, staging, and natural history is required for initial patient assessment, as well as to determine the optimal surgical therapy.

Modern cancer therapy is multidisciplinary, involving the coordinated care of surgeons, medical oncologists, radiation oncologists, reconstructive surgeons, pathologists, radiologists, and primary care physicians. *Primary* (or *definitive*) *therapy* refers to en bloc resection of tumor with adequate margins of normal tissues and in some cases regional lymph nodes. *Adjuvant therapy* refers to radiation therapy and systemic therapies, including chemotherapy, immunotherapy, hormonal therapy, and increasingly, biologic therapy. The primary goal of surgical and radiation therapy is local and regional control. On the other hand, the primary goal of systemic therapies is systemic control by treating distant foci of subclinical disease to prevent recurrence. Surgeons must be familiar with adjuvant therapies to coordinate multidisciplinary care and to determine the best sequence of therapy.

Recent advances in molecular biology are revolutionizing medicine. Nowhere has basic biology had a greater and more immediate impact than in oncology. New information is being translated rapidly into clinical use, with the development of new prognostic and predictive markers and new biologic therapies. It is therefore essential that surgeons understand the principles of molecular oncology in order to appropriately interpret these new contributions and incorporate them into practice.

Table 9-1
Estimated New Cancer Cases and Deaths, United States, 2003[a]

	Estimated New Cases Both Sexes	Estimated Deaths Both Sexes
All cancers	**1,334,100**	**556,500**
Oral cavity and pharynx	**27,700**	**7200**
Digestive system	**252,400**	**133,600**
Esophagus	13,900	13,000
Stomach	22,400	12,100
Small intestine	5300	1100
Colon and rectum	147,500	57,100
Anus, anal canal, and anorectum	4000	500
Liver and intrahepatic bile duct	17,300	14,400
Gallbladder and other biliary	6800	3500
Pancreas	30,700	30,000
Other digestive organs	4500	1900
Respiratory system	**185,800**	**163,700**
Larynx	9500	3800
Lung and bronchus	171,900	157,200
Other respiratory organs	4400	2700
Bones and joints	**2400**	**1300**
Soft tissue (including heart)	**8300**	**3900**
Skin (excluding basal and squamous)	**58,800**	**9800**
Melanoma–skin	54,200	7600
Other nonepithelial–skin	4600	2200
Breast	**212,600**	**40,200**
Genital system	**313,600**	**56,300**
Uterine cervix	12,200	4100
Uterine corpus	40,100	6800
Ovary	25,400	14,300
Vulva	4000	800
Vagina and other genital, female	2000	800
Prostate	220,900	28,900
Testis	7600	400
Penis and other genital, male	1400	200
Urinary system	**91,700**	**25,100**
Urinary bladder	57,400	12,500
Kidney and renal pelvis	31,900	11,900
Ureter and other urinary organs	2400	700
Eye and orbit	**2200**	**200**
Brain and other nervous system	**18,300**	**13,100**
Endocrine system	**23,800**	**2300**
Thyroid	22,000	1400
Other endocrine	1800	900
Lymphoma	**61,000**	**24,700**
Multiple myeloma	**14,600**	**10,900**
Leukemia	**30,600**	**21,900**
Other and unspecified primary sites[b]	**30,300**	**42,300**

[a]Excludes basal and squamous cell skin cancers and in situ carcinomas except those of urinary bladder.
[b]More deaths than cases suggest lack of specificity in recording underlying causes of death on death certificate.
SOURCE: Modified with permission from Jemal et al.[1]

EPIDEMIOLOGY

Basic Principles of Cancer Epidemiology

The term *incidence* refers to the number of new cases occurring; incidence usually is expressed as the number of new cases per 100,000 persons per year. *Mortality* refers to the number of deaths occurring and is expressed as the number of deaths per 100,000 persons per year. Incidence and mortality data are usually available through cancer registries. Mortality data are also available as public records in many countries where deaths are registered as vital statistics, often with the cause of death. In areas where cancer registries do not exist, mortality data are used to extrapolate incidence rates; these numbers are likely to be less accurate than registry data, however, as the relationship between incidence and cause-specific death is likely to vary significantly among countries owing to the variation in health care delivery.

The incidence of cancer is variable by geography. This is due in part to genetic differences and in part to differences in environmental and dietary exposures. Epidemiologic studies that monitor trends in cancer incidence and mortality have tremendously enhanced our understanding of the etiology of cancer. Furthermore, analysis of trends in cancer incidence and mortality allows us to monitor the effects of different preventive and screening measures, as well as the evolution of therapies for specific cancers.

The two types of epidemiologic studies that are conducted most often to investigate the etiology of cancer and the effect of prevention modalities are cohort studies and case-control studies. Cohort studies follow a group of people who initially do not have a disease over time and measure the rate of development of a disease. In cohort studies, a group that is exposed to a certain environmental factor or intervention usually is compared to a group that has not been exposed (e.g., smokers versus nonsmokers). Case-control studies compare a group of patients affected with a disease to a group of individuals without the disease for a given exposure. The results are expressed in terms of an odds ratio, or relative risk. A relative risk less than 1 indicates a protective effect, while a relative risk greater than 1 indicates an increased risk of developing the disease with exposure.

Cancer Incidence and Mortality in the United States

In the year 2003, an estimated 1,334,100 new cases of invasive cancer will be diagnosed in the United States.[1] In addition, over a million cases of basal and squamous cell carcinomas of the skin, 37,700 cases of melanoma in situ, and 55,700 cases of carcinoma in situ of the breast are predicted.[1] Furthermore, an estimated 556,500 people will die from cancer in the United States in the same year.[1] The estimated new cancer cases and deaths by cancer type are shown in Table 9-1. The most common causes of cancer death in men are cancers of the lung and bronchus, prostate, and colon and rectum; in women, the most common cancers are of the lung and bronchus, breast, and colon and rectum (Fig. 9-1).

Trends in Cancer Incidence and Mortality

Cancer deaths accounted for 23% of all deaths in the United States in 2000, second only to deaths from heart disease, which accounted for 29.6% of total deaths.[1] As the life expectancy of the human population increases because of reductions in other causes of death such as infections and cardiovascular disease, cancer is becoming the leading cause of death. Cancer is already the leading cause of death among women aged 40 to 79 and among men aged 60 to 79.[1]

ESTIMATED NEW CASES

MEN:		WOMEN:	
Prostate	33%	Breast	32%
Lung and Bronchus	14%	Lung and Bronchus	12%
Colon and Rectum	11%	Colon and Rectum	11%
Urinary Bladder	6%	Uterine Corpus	6%
Melanoma of the Skin	4%	Ovary	4%
Non-Hodgkin's Lymphoma	4%	Non-Hodgkin's Lymphoma	3%
Kidney	3%	Melanoma of the Skin	3%
Oral Cavity	3%	Thyroid	3%
Leukemia	3%	Pancreas	2%
Pancreas	2%	Urinary Bladder	2%
All Other Sites	17%	All Other Sites	20%

ESTIMATED DEATHS

MEN:		WOMEN:	
Lung and Bronchus	31%	Lung and Bronchus	25%
Prostate	10%	Breast	15%
Colon and Rectum	10%	Colon and Rectum	11%
Pancreas	5%	Pancreas	6%
Non-Hodgkin's Lymphoma	4%	Ovary	5%
Leukemia	4%	Non-Hodgkin's Lymphoma	4%
Esophagus	4%	Leukemia	4%
Liver	3%	Uterine Corpus	3%
Urinary Bladder	3%	Brain	2%
Kidney	3%	Multiple Myeloma	2%
All Other Sites	22%	All Other Sites	23%

FIG. 9-1. Ten leading cancer types for the estimated new cancer cases and deaths, by sex, United States, 2003. Excludes basal and squamous cell skin cancers and in situ carcinomas except urinary bladder. Percentages may not total 100% due to rounding. (*Modified from Jemal et al,*[1] *with permission.*)

Cancer incidence increased by 0.3% per year in females during the period from 1987 to 1999, but it stabilized in males between 1995 and 1999.[1] The annual age-adjusted cancer incidence rates among males and females for selected cancer types are shown in Fig. 9-2. Interestingly, prostate cancer rates increased dramatically between 1988 and 1992, and declined between 1992 and 1995. These trends are thought to reflect the extensive use of prostate-specific antigen (PSA) screening, leading to the earlier diagnosis of prostate cancers.[1]

From 1992 to 1999, for all cancer types combined, cancer death rates decreased by 1.5% per year in males and by 0.6% per year in females. In fact, the 5-year survival rates from 1974 to 1998 reveal improvement in relative 5-year survival rates for cancers in almost all sites (Table 9-2). How much of this improvement reflects actual improvement of cancer therapy and how much simply reflects earlier diagnosis of tumors with stage-for-stage outcome remaining unchanged, is not yet known.

Global Statistics on Cancer Incidence and Mortality

It has been estimated that there were a total of 8.1 million new cancer cases around the world in 1990, a number 37% higher than estimates for 1975; this represents a growth rate of 2.1% per year, faster than the 1.7% per year growth of the world population.[2] Lung cancer is the leading cancer in the world, accounting for 1.04 million new cases and 921,000 deaths per year.[2] Second is stomach cancer, which accounts for 789,000 new cases and 628,000 deaths per year.[2] Breast cancer is the third most common cancer (796,000 cases per year)

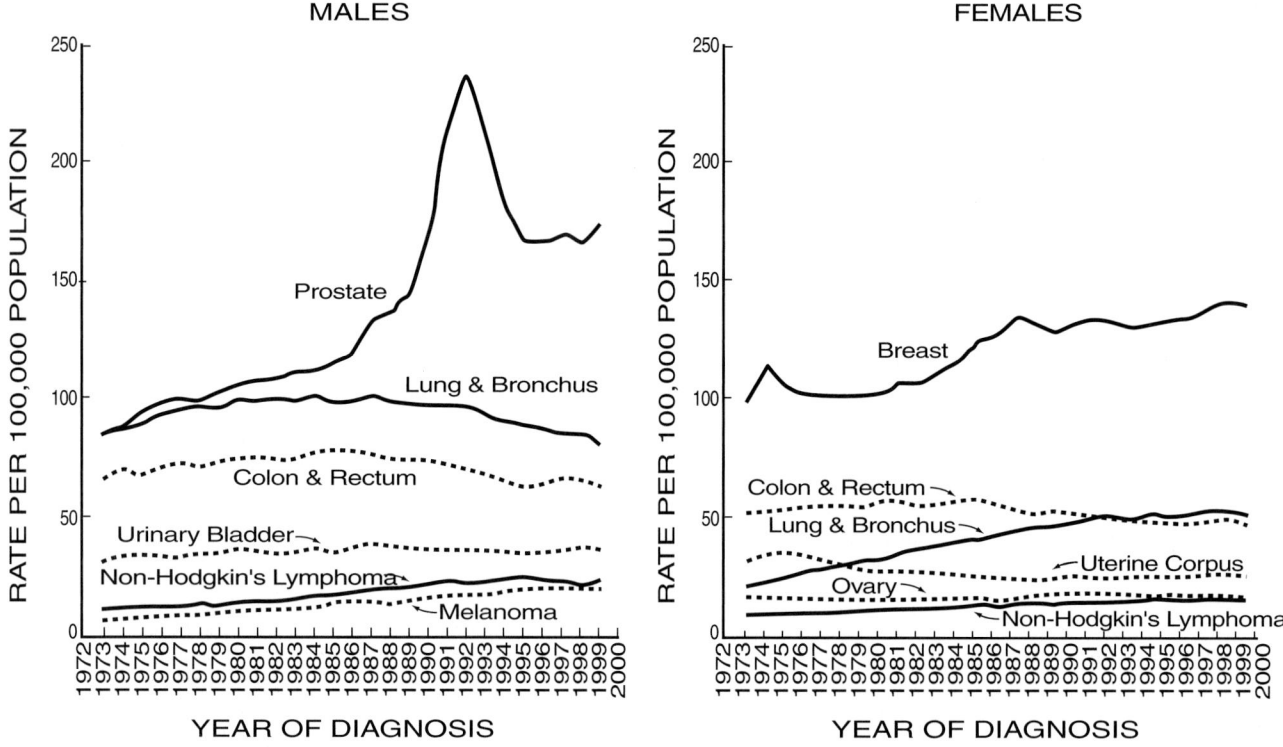

FIG. 9-2. *Annual age-adjusted cancer incidence rates among males and females for selected cancer types, United States, 1973 to 1999. Rates are age adjusted to the 2000 U.S. standard population. (Modified from Jemal et al,[1] with permission.)*

Table 9-2

Five-Year Relative Survival Rates Adjusted to Normal Life Expectancy by Year of Diagnosis, United States 1974 to 1998

Cancer Type	Relative Five-Year Survival Rates (%)		
	1974–1976	1983–1985	1992–1998
All cancers	50	52	62
Brain	22	27	32
Breast (female)	75	78	86
Uterine cervix	69	69	71
Colon	50	58	62
Uterine corpus	88	83	84
Esophagus	5	8	13
Hodgkin's disease	71	79	84
Kidney	52	56	62
Larynx	66	67	64
Leukemia	34	41	46
Liver	4	6	7
Lung and bronchus	12	14	15
Melanoma of the skin	80	85	89
Multiple myeloma	24	28	30
Non-Hodgkin's lymphoma	47	54	55
Oral cavity	53	53	56
Ovary	37	41	53
Pancreas	3	3	4
Prostate	67	75	97
Rectum	49	55	62
Stomach	15	17	22
Testis	79	91	95
Thyroid	92	93	96
Urinary bladder	73	78	82

SOURCE: Modified with permission from Jemal et al.[1]

and the fifth most common cause of cancer death, following colorectal cancer (783,000 cases, 437,000 deaths) and liver cancer (437,000 cases, 427,000 deaths).[2]

Stomach Cancer

The incidence of stomach cancer varies significantly among different regions of the world. The age-adjusted incidence is highest in Japan (77.9 per 100,000 men, 33.3 per 100,000 women). In comparison, the rates are much lower in North America, eastern and northern Africa, and South and Southeast Asia (5.9 to 9.0 per 100,000 men, 2.6 to 5.3 per 100,000 women).[2] The difference in risk by country is presumed to be due to differences in dietary factors and in the incidence of infection with *Helicobacter pylori*, which is known to play a major role in gastric cancer development.[2] Fortunately, a steady decline is being observed in the incidence and mortality rates of gastric cancer. This may be related to improvements in preservation and storage of foods.[2]

Breast Cancer

The incidence of breast cancer is high in all of the most highly developed regions except Japan, including the United States and Canada, Australia, and Northern and Western Europe, ranging from 67.3 to 86.3 per 100,000 women per year.[2] In comparison, the rates are relatively low (less than 30 per 100,000 women) in sub-Saharan Africa (except South Africa) and Asia. The highest breast cancer incidence is in the United States and the lowest is in China. Although breast cancer has been linked to cancer susceptibility genes, mutations in these genes account for only 5 to 10% of breast tumors, suggesting that the wide geographic variations in breast cancer incidence are not due to geographic variations in the prevalence of these

Table 9-3
Estimated Five-Year Survival Rates (%) for Selected Cancer Sites by Region of the World

Region	Oral Cavity & Pharynx	Stomach	Colon & Rectum	Pancreas	Larynx	Lung	Melanoma	Breast (Female)	Uterine Cervix	Uterine Corpus	Ovary	Prostate	Testis	Bladder	Non-Hodgkin's Lymphoma	Hodgkin's Disease	Leukemias
Australia/New Zealand	76	29	54	2	62	13	85	68	62	80	40	63	90	68	56	74	44
North America	70	34	61	7	71	20	78	73	54	87	45	79	91	80	61	76	39
Northwestern Europe	60	21	46	0	52	7	74	63	54	75	32	49	89	57	56	67	32
Southern Europe	61	17	45	0	44	8	70	57	57	73	43	22	69	61	57	65	32
Eastern Europe	42	10	30	12	34	12	55	63	41	50	43	40	82	46	43	53	24
Japan	56	53	57	7	74	21	40	74	65	62	38	52	46	70	50	79	21

SOURCE: Modified with permission from Parkin et al.[2]

genes. Most of the differences, therefore, are attributed to differences in reproductive factors, diet, and other environmental differences. Indeed, breast cancer risk increases significantly in females who have migrated from Asia to America.[3] Overall, the incidence of breast cancer is rising in most countries.

Colon and Rectal Cancer

The incidence of colon and rectal cancer is higher in developed countries than developing countries. The incidence rates are highest in Australia/New Zealand, North America, and Northern and Western Europe (26.11 to 45.81 cases per 100,000 population).[2] In contrast, the incidence is relatively low in North Africa, South America, and Eastern, Southeastern, and Western Asia (2.26 to 8.75 per 100,000 population). These geographic differences are thought to reflect environmental exposures and are presumed to be mainly dietary differences.

Liver Cancer

In contrast to colon cancer, 80% of liver cancers occur in developing countries.[2] The incidence of liver cancer is especially high in China and other countries in Eastern Asia (32.19 to 35.84 per 100,000 men), while it is relatively low in North and South America and Europe (2.74 to 5.23 per 100,000 men).[2] Worldwide, the major risk factors for liver cancer are infection with hepatitis viruses and consumption of foods contaminated with aflatoxin. Hepatitis B immunization in children has recently been shown to reduce the incidence of hepatitis infection in China, Korea, and West Africa.[4] Whether this will translate into a reduction in the incidence in liver cancer in these regions will soon be determined.

Prostate Cancer

The incidence of prostate cancer is dramatically higher in North America (92.39 per 100,000 men) than in China, Japan, and the rest of Asia (1.08 to 8.51 per 100,000), and even in Northern and Western Europe (34.70 to 39.55 per 100,000).[2] A considerable part of the international differences in prostate cancer incidence is thought to reflect differences in diagnostic practices. As previously mentioned, the introduction of PSA screening has led to a significant increase in the diagnosis of prostate cancer in the United States (see Fig. 9-2).

Esophageal Cancer

Geographic variations in the incidence of esophageal cancer are also striking. The highest incidence of this cancer is in Southern Africa and China (21.58 to 32.60 per 100,000 men, and 9.91 to 11.93 per 100,000 women).[2] The risk is 15-fold lower in men in North, Middle, and West Africa and 5-fold lower in men in Europe and North America. These geographic differences are attributed to nutritional deficiencies and exposures to exogenous carcinogens. Esophageal cancer in North America and Europe is attributed to tobacco and alcohol use.

The mortality rates of different cancers also vary significantly among countries. This is attributable not only to variations in incidence but also to variations in survival after a cancer diagnosis. The estimated 5-year survival rates for selected cancer sites in different regions of the world are presented in Table 9-3. These 5-year survival rates are influenced not only by treatment patterns but also by variations in cancer screening practices, which affect the stage of cancer at diagnosis. For example, the 5-year survival rate of stomach cancer is much higher in Japan, where the cancer incidence is high enough to warrant mass screening and is presumed to lead to earlier diagnosis. In the case of prostate cancer, the mortality rates diverge much less than the incidence rates among countries. Survival rates for prostate cancer are much higher in North America than in developing countries (88 versus 41%).[2] It is possible that the extensive screening practices in the United States allow discovery of cancers at an earlier, more curable stage; however, it is also possible that this screening leads to discovery of more latent, less biologicallyaggressive cancers, which may not have caused death even if they had not been identified.

In summary, the incidence rates of many common cancers vary widely by geography. This is due in part to genetic differences, including racial and ethnic differences. It is due also in part to differences in environmental and dietary exposures, factors that can potentially be altered. Therefore, establishment of regional and international databases is critical to improving our understanding of the etiology of cancer, and will ultimately assist in the initiation of targeted strategies for global cancer prevention. Furthermore, the monitoring of cancer mortality rates and 5-year, cancer-specific survival rates will identify regions where there are inequities of health care, so that access to health care can be facilitated and guidelines for treatment can be established.

CANCER BIOLOGY

Cell Proliferation and Transformation

In normal cells, cell growth and proliferation are under strict control. In cancer cells, cells become unresponsive to normal growth controls, leading to uncontrolled growth and proliferation. Abnormally proliferating, transformed cells outgrow normal cells in the culture dish (i.e., in vitro) and commonly display several abnormal characteristics.[5] These include loss of contact inhibition (i.e., cells continue to proliferate after a confluent monolayer is formed); an altered appearance and poor adherence to other cells or the substratum; loss of anchorage-dependence for growth; immortalization; and gain of tumorigenicity (i.e., the ability to give rise to tumors when injected into an appropriate host).

Cancer Initiation

Tumorigenesis is proposed to have three steps: initiation, promotion, and progression. Initiating events may lead a single cell to acquire a distinct growth advantage, such as gain of function of genes known as oncogenes, or loss of function of genes known as tumor suppressor genes. Although tumors usually arise from a single cell or clone, it is thought that sometimes not a single cell but rather a large number of cells in a target organ may have undergone the initiating genetic event, thus many normal-appearing cells may have an elevated malignant potential. This is referred to as a *field effect*. The initiating events are usually genetic and occur as deletions of tumor suppressor genes or amplification of oncogenes. Subsequent events can lead to accumulations of additional deleterious mutations in the clone.

Cancer is a disease of clonal progression as tumors arise from a single cell and accumulate mutations that confer on the tumor an increasingly aggressive behavior. Most tumors are thought to go through a progression from benign lesions to in situ tumors to invasive cancers (e.g., atypical ductal hyperplasia to ductal carcinoma in situ to invasive ductal carcinoma of the breast). Fearon and Vogelstein proposed the model for colorectal tumorigenesis seen in Fig. 9-3.[6] Colorectal tumors arise from the mutational activation of oncogenes coupled with mutational inactivation of tumor

suppressor genes, the latter being the predominant change.[6] Mutations in at least four or five genes are required for formation of a malignant tumor, while fewer changes suffice for a benign tumor. Although genetic mutations often occur in a preferred sequence, a tumor's biologic properties are determined by the total accumulation of its genetic changes.

Gene expression is a multistep process that starts from transcription of a gene into messenger ribonucleic acid (mRNA) and then translation of this sequence into the functional protein. There are several controls at each level. In addition to alterations at the genome level, alterations at the transcription level (e.g., methylation of the DNA leading to transcriptional silencing), or at the mRNA processing, mRNA stability, mRNA translation, or protein stability levels, can alter critical proteins and thus contribute to tumorigenesis. For example, cyclin D1 protein expression is regulated at several levels, including cyclin D1 mRNA transcription (via the Ras/Raf signaling pathway discussed below), cyclin D1 mRNA stability (via the phosphoinositide-13 kinase PI3-K/Akt pathway), cyclin D1 translation (via overexpression of eIF4E), and cyclin D1 protein stability (via glycogen synthase kinase-3β activity). Alteration in any of these pathways can lead to overexpression of cyclin D1 and facilitate passage through the G_1 phase of the cell cycle, promoting cell proliferation.

Cell-Cycle Dysregulation in Cancer

Tumors often arise from adult tissues that are quiescent. The proliferative advantage of tumor cells is a direct result of their ability to bypass quiescence.[7] Cancer cells often show alterations in signal transduction pathways that lead to proliferation in response to external signals. Mutations or alterations in the expression of cell-cycle proteins, growth factors, growth factor receptors, intracellular signal transduction proteins, and nuclear transcription factors all can lead to disturbance of the basic regulatory mechanisms that control the cell cycle, allowing unregulated cell growth and proliferation.

The cell cycle is divided into four phases (Fig. 9-4).[8] During the synthetic or S phase, the cell generates a single copy of its genetic material, while in the mitotic or M phase, the cellular components

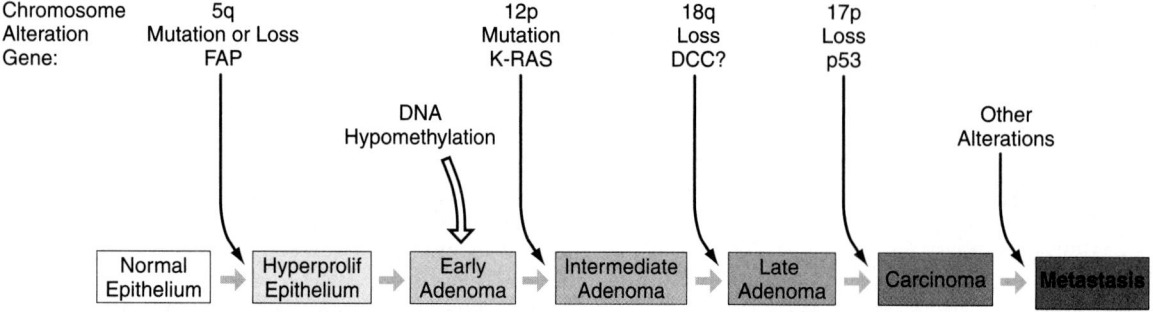

FIG. 9-3. A genetic model for colorectal tumorigenesis. Tumorigenesis proceeds through a series of genetic alterations involving oncogenes and tumor suppressor genes. In general, the three stages of adenomas represent tumors of increasing size, dysplasia, and villous content. Individuals with familial adenomatous polyposis (FAP) inherit a mutation on chromosome 5q. In tumors arising in individuals without polyposis, the same region may be lost or mutated at a relatively early stage of tumorigenesis. A ras gene mutation (usually K-ras) occurs in one cell of a pre-existing small adenoma, which, through clonal expansion, produces a larger and more dysplastic tumor. The chromosomes most frequently deleted include 5q, 17p, and 18q. Allelic deletions of chromosome 17p and 18q usually occur at a later stage of tumorigenesis than do deletions of chromosome 5q or ras gene mutations. The order of these changes varies, however, and accumulation of these changes, rather than their order of appearance, seems most important. Tumors continue to progress once carcinomas have formed, and the accumulated chromosomal alterations correlate with the ability of the carcinomas to metastasize and cause death. (Modified from Fearon et al,[6] with permission.)

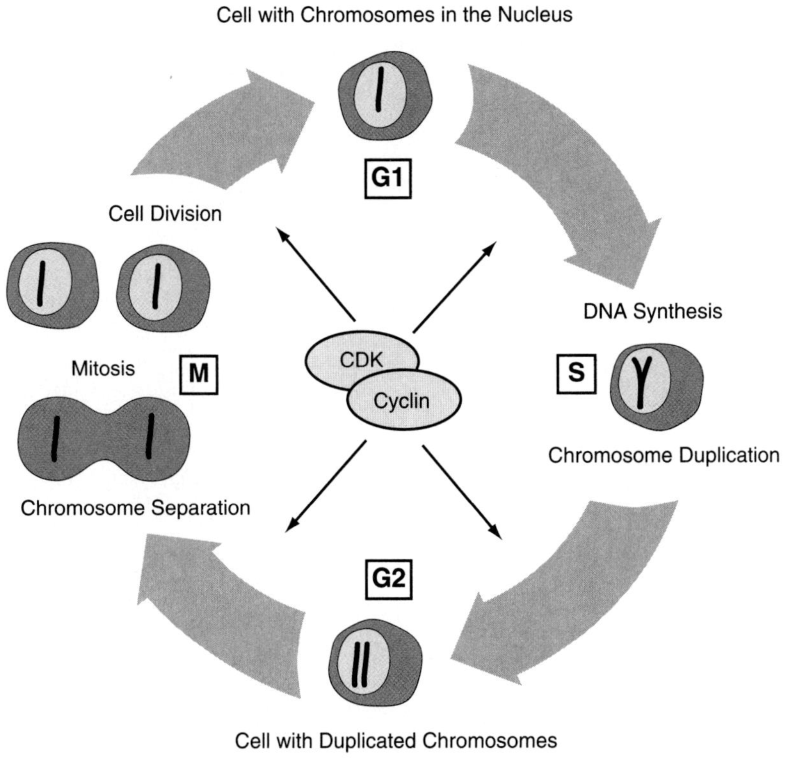

Cell with Chromosomes in the Nucleus

FIG. 9-4. Schematic representation of the phases of the cell cycle. Mitogenic growth factors can drive a quiescent cell from G_0 into the cell cycle. Once the cell cycle passes beyond the restriction point, mitogens are no longer required for progression into and through S phase. The DNA is replicated in S phase, and the chromosomes are condensed and segregated in mitosis. In early G_1 phase, certain signals can drive a cell to exit the cell cycle and enter a quiescent phase. Cell-cycle checkpoints have been identified in G_1, S, G_2, and M. (*Modified from Kastan et al,*[8] *with permission.*)

are partitioned between the two identical daughter cells.[7] The G_1 and G_2 phases represent gap phases during which the cells prepare themselves for completion of the S and M phases, respectively. When cells cease proliferation, they exit the cell cycle and enter the quiescent state referred to as G_0.

Cell-cycle progression is regulated by a series of checkpoints that prevent cells from entering a new phase without completing the previous phase. The central regulators are serine-threonine kinases referred to as the cyclin-dependent kinases (CDKs). CDK4 and CDK6 are thought to be involved in the early G_1 phase, whereas CDK2 is required to complete G_1 and initiate S phase.[7] CDK4 and CDK6 form active complexes with the D-type cyclins, cyclins D1, D2, and D3. CDK2 is activated by the E-type cyclins, cyclins E1 and E2, during the G_1/S transition and by the A-type cyclins, cyclins A1 and A2, during the S phase.

The principal downstream target of the activated complex of cyclin D and CDK4 or CDK6 is the retinoblastoma protein (Rb). In its hypophosphorylated form, Rb suppresses cellular growth by binding the E2F family of transcription factors. Furthermore, Rb binding to the promoter as a complex with E2F can actively repress transcription through chromatin remodeling, by recruiting proteins such as histone diacetylases and SWI/SNF complexes.[9] Following cyclin/CDK-mediated phosphorylation, Rb releases E2F transcription factors that then activate downstream transcriptional targets involved in S phase, such as DNA polymerase alpha, cyclin A, cyclin E, and CDK1 (Fig. 9-5).[9]

Regulators of CDKs can affect cell-cycle progression. CDKs are phosphorylated and activated by CDK-activating kinase. CDKs are phosphorylated on other residues that have an inhibitory effect by WEE1 and MYT1.[7] This inhibition is relieved by CDC25 phosphatases, CDC25A, CDC25B, and CDC25C, which dephosphorylate these residues, triggering entry into mitosis. CDK inhibitors (CKIs) comprise two classes, the INK4 family and the WAF/Kip family. The INK4 family has four members: INK4A (p16), INK4B (p15), INK4C (p18), and INK4D (p19). The INK4 proteins bind CDK4 and CDK6 and prevent their association with D-type cyclins and cyclin D activation. The WAF/Kip family members include WAF1 (p21), KIP1 (p27), and KIP2 (p57). These CKIs bind and inactivate cyclin/CDK2 complexes.[10] CKIs are believed to regulate the cell cycle in response to growth-inhibitory stimuli such as DNA damage, hypoxia, serum starvation, and transforming growth factor beta (TGF-β).[9]

Molecular alterations of human tumors have demonstrated that cell-cycle regulators are frequently mutated.[7] Other alterations include overexpression of cyclins D1 and E, and CDK4 and CDK6, and loss of CKIs INK4A, INK4B, and KIP1.[7] These alterations underscore the importance of cell-cycle regulation in the prevention of human cancers.

Oncogenes

Normal cellular genes that contribute to cancer when abnormal are called *oncogenes*. The normal counterpart of such a gene is referred to as a *protooncogene*. Oncogenes are usually designated by three-letter abbreviations, such as *myc* or *ras*. Oncogenes are further designated by the prefix of "v-" for virus or "c-" for cell or chromosome, corresponding to the origin of the oncogene when it was first detected. Protooncogenes can be activated (have increased activity) or overexpressed (expressed at increased protein levels) by translocation (e.g., *abl*), promoter insertion (e.g., c-*myc*), mutations (e.g., *ras*), or amplification (e.g., HER2/*neu*). More than 100 oncogenes have been identified.[11]

Oncogenes may be growth factors (e.g., platelet-derived growth factor), growth factor receptors (e.g., HER2/*neu*), intracellular signal transduction molecules (e.g., *ras*), nuclear transcription factors (e.g., c-*myc*), or other molecules involved in the regulation of cell growth and proliferation. Growth factors are ubiquitous proteins that are produced and secreted by cells locally and that stimulate

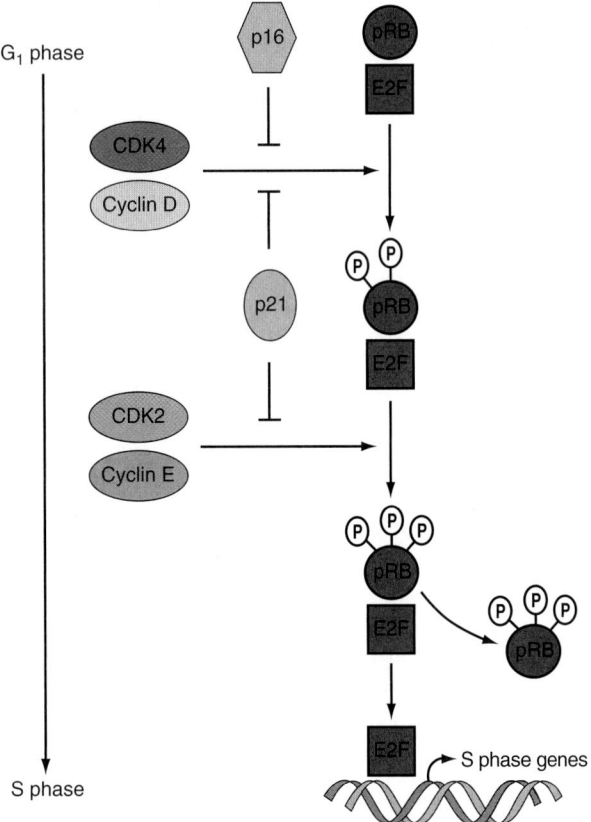

FIG. 9-5. The G$_1$-S phase transition. Cyclin-D–CDK4 and cyclin-E–CDK2 complexes are activated. These sequentially phosphorylate the retinoblastoma protein (pRB) transcription factor. Binding of hypophosphorylated pRB to E2F transcription factors inhibits entry into S phase. However, hyperphosphorylated pRB releases E2F, which results in activation of genes required for S-phase entry. Members of the INK4A and Cip/Kip CDKI families (represented by p16 and p21, respectively) can inhibit cyclin–CDK complexes and mediate G$_1$–S cell-cycle arrest. CDK = cyclin-dependent kinase; CDKI = CDK inhibitor. (*Modified from Stewart et al,*[267] *with permission.*)

cell proliferation by binding specific cell-surface receptors on the same cells (autocrine stimulation) or on neighboring cells (paracrine stimulation). Persistent overexpression of growth factors can lead to uncontrolled autostimulation and neoplastic transformation. Alternatively, growth factor receptors can be aberrantly activated (turned on) through mutations, or overexpressed (continually presenting cells with growth-stimulatory signals, even in the absence of growth factors), leading cells to respond as if growth factor levels are altered. The growth-stimulating effect of growth factors and other mitogens is mediated through postreceptor signal transduction molecules. These molecules mediate the passage of growth signals from the outside to the inside of the cell and then to the cell nucleus, initiating the cell cycle and DNA transcription. Aberrant activation or expression of cell-signaling molecules, cell-cycle molecules, or transcription factors may play an important role in neoplastic transformation. Three of the best-studied oncogenes are discussed here.

ras

The *ras* family of genes encodes small GTP-binding proteins that regulate several cellular processes. The H- and K-*ras* genes were first identified as the cellular counterparts of the oncogenes of the Harvey and Kirsten rat sarcoma viruses, while N-*ras* was isolated from a neuroblastoma.[12] The N-, H-, and K-*ras* genes are located on chromosomes 1, 11, and 12, respectively, and encode for 21-kDa

proteins that are nearly identical in amino acid sequence, but appear not to be redundant in function.[12]

ras cycles between active GTP-bound and inactive GDP-bound states. Various extracellular stimuli can promote *ras* activation, including various receptor and nonreceptor tyrosine kinases, G protein–coupled receptors, and integrins.[13] Guanine nucleotide exchange factors (GEFs) stimulate formation of *ras*-GTP. *ras* has an intrinsic ability to hydrolyze GTP, but this hydrolysis is slow. GTPase-activating proteins (GAPs) stimulate hydrolysis of the bound GTP to return *ras* to its inactive form. Missense mutations of *ras* at amino acid positions 12, 13, or 61 render *ras* insensitive to GAPs, resulting in mutant proteins that are persistently activated.[14] Approximately 20% of all tumors have activating mutations in one of the *ras* genes.[15] The frequency of *ras* mutations varies widely by cancer type (e.g., 90% of pancreatic cancers, but less than 5% of breast cancers).[12,15] Tumors that lack *ras* mutations, however, may undergo activation of the *ras* signaling pathway by other mechanisms, such as growth factor receptor activation, loss of GAP, or activation of *ras* effectors.[15]

The Ras proteins require posttranslational modification by farnesyltransferase. After association with the intracellular membrane via its farnesyl group, GTP-bound Ras then binds and activates several downstream pathways. The best characterized downstream signaling pathway is that initiated by the serine-threonine kinase Raf. Activated Raf phosphorylates and activates mitogen-activated protein kinases (MAPKs) 1 and 2 (MEK1 and MEK2).[15] MEK1 and 2 phosphorylate and activate MAPKs extracellular signal-regulated kinases 1 and 2 (ERK1 and ERK2). ERK phosphorylates the ETS family of transcriptional factors, leading to expression of cell-cycle regulatory proteins such as D-type cyclins, enabling the cell to progress through the G$_1$ phase of the cell cycle. A second pathway activated by Ras is PI3-K, an important component of the survival signaling induced by Ras. A third pathway is the Ras-related Ral proteins, which along with the PI3-K/Akt pathway, contributes to inhibition of the forkhead transcription factors that promote cell-cycle arrest by inducing p27. Further, Ras also associates with phospholipase Cε, linking Ras to activation of protein kinase C (PKC) and calcium mobilization. Together, the Ras signaling pathways promote malignant transformation by increasing proliferation, which is accomplished by inducing cell-cycle regulators such as cyclin D1, suppressing cell-cycle inhibitors such as p27, and enhancing survival signaling through the PI3-K/Akt pathway.

c-myc

The c-*myc* protooncogene encoding the c-Myc nuclear transcription factor was first identified as the cellular homologue of the viral oncogene (v-*myc*) of the avian myelocytomatosis retrovirus.[16] The *myc* gene is located on the region of chromosome 8 that is translocated in Burkitt's lymphoma.[17] Elevated or deregulated expression of c-*myc* has been detected in a wide range of tumors, including breast, colon, cervical, and small-cell lung carcinomas, osteosarcomas, melanomas, glioblastomas, and myeloid leukemias.[5] c-*myc* mediates transcriptional regulation of a diverse group of genes as part of a dimeric complex with a partner protein termed Max,[18,19] which is thought to be due to chromatin remodeling. One of the key biologic functions of c-Myc is to promote cell-cycle progression. After mitogenic or serum stimulation, c-*myc* levels are rapidly increased, and cells enter the cell cycle. Activation of c-*myc* often allows cell-cycle progression even in the absence of external growth factors.[20] c-*myc* also enhances cell growth, which may be achieved at least in part through activating pathways of protein synthesis by inducing the transcription of a variety of translation initiation factors and ribosomal proteins.[18,19] c-*myc* also inhibits differentiation of many cell types. Interestingly, c-*myc* sensitizes cells to a wide range of apoptotic stimuli. It is possible that c-*myc* functions predominate in different genetic backgrounds, explaining why in some studies c-Myc expression has been found to be a poor prognostic factor, while in others high c-Myc levels correlate with a better outcome.[21]

HER2/*neu*

Protein tyrosine kinases account for a large portion of known oncogenes. HER2/*neu,* also known as c-*erb*B-2, is a member of the epidermal growth factor (EGF) receptor (EGFR) family and is one of the best characterized tyrosine kinases. Unlike other receptor tyrosine kinases, HER2/*neu* does not have a direct soluble ligand. It plays a key role in signaling, however, as it is the preferred partner in heterodimer formation with all the other EGFR family members (EGFR/c-*erb*B-1, HER2/c-*erb*B-3, and HER3/c-*erb*B-4), which bind at least 30 ligands including EGF, transforming growth factor alpha (TGF-α), heparin-binding EGF-like growth factor, amphiregulin, and heregulin.[22] Heterodimerization with HER2/*neu* potentiates recycling of receptors rather than degradation, enhances signal potency and duration, increases affinity for ligands, and increases catalytic activity.[22]

The specificity and potency of the intracellular signals are affected by the identity of the ligand, the composition of the receptors, and the phosphotyrosine-binding proteins associated with the erbB molecules. The Ras- and Shc-activated MAPK pathway is a target of all erbB ligands, which increase the transcriptional activity of early response genes such as c-*myc,* c-*fos,* and c-*jun*.[23] MAPK-independent pathways such as the PI3K pathway also are activated by most erbB dimers, although the potency and kinetics of activation may differ.[24] Stimulation of the PI3K pathway through HER2 signaling can lead to activation of survival molecule Akt, which suppresses apoptosis by phosphorylating Bad and modulating caspase-9, Raf, and the forkhead transcription factors. Further, HER2 signaling may also lead to Akt-mediated activation of IκB kinases, which phosphorylate and thus trigger the degradation of NF-κB inhibitor IκBα. This allows release of IκBα-sequestered NF-κB and its nuclear translocation.[23]

The mutant rat *neu* gene was first recognized as an oncogene in neuroblastomas from carcinogen-treated rats.[25] Although HER2/*neu* mutations are rare in human cancer, the HER2/*neu* gene is frequently amplified and the protein overexpressed in many cancers, including breast, ovarian, lung, gastric, and oral cancers.[26] Overexpression of HER2/*neu* results in ligand-independent activation of HER2/*neu* kinase, leading to mitogenic signaling. HER2/*neu* overexpression is associated with increased cell proliferation and anchorage-independent growth as well as resistance to proapoptotic stimuli. Further, overexpression of HER2/*neu* increases cell migration and upregulates the activities of matrix metalloproteinases and in vitro invasiveness. In animal models, HER2/*neu* increases tumorigenicity, angiogenesis, and metastasis. These results all suggest that HER2/*neu* plays a key role in cancer biology.

Alterations in Apoptosis in Cancer Cells

Apoptosis (programmed cell death) is a genetically-regulated program to dispose of cells. Cancer cells must avoid apoptosis if tumors are to arise. The growth of a tumor mass is dependent not only on an increase of proliferation of tumor cells but also on a decrease in their apoptotic rate. Apoptosis is distinguished from necrosis because it leads to several characteristic changes. In early apoptosis, the changes in membrane composition lead to extracellular exposure of phosphatidylserine residues, which avidly bind annexin, a

characteristic used to discriminate apoptotic cells in laboratory studies. Late in apoptosis there are characteristic changes in nuclear morphology, such as chromatin condensation, nuclear fragmentation, and DNA laddering, as well as membrane blebbing. Apoptotic cells are then engulfed and degraded by phagocytic cells. The effectors of apoptosis are a family of proteases called caspases (cysteine-dependent and aspartate-directed proteases). The initiator caspases (e.g., 8, 9, and 10), which are upstream, cleave the downstream executioner caspases (e.g., 3, 6, and 7) that carry out the destructive functions of apoptosis.[9]

Two principal molecular pathways signal apoptosis by cleaving the initiator caspases with the potential for cross-talk: the mitochondrial pathway and the death receptor pathway. In the mitochondrial pathway, sometimes referred to as the intrinsic pathway, death results from the release of cytochrome c from the mitochondria. Cytochrome c, procaspase-9, and apoptotic protease-activating factor-1 (Apaf-1) form an enzyme complex, referred to as the *apoptosome,* which activates the effector caspases.[9] In addition to these proteins, the mitochondria contain other proapoptotic proteins such as SMAC/DIABLO. The mitochondrial pathway can be stimulated by many factors, including DNA damage, reactive oxygen species, or withdrawal of survival factors. The mitochondrial membrane permeability determines whether the apoptotic pathway will proceed.[9] The Bcl-2 family of regulatory proteins includes proapoptotic proteins (e.g., Bax, Bad, and Bak) and antiapoptotic proteins (e.g., Bcl-2 and Bcl-xL); the activity of the Bcl-2 proteins is centered on the mitochondria, where they regulate membrane permeability.[9] Growth factors promote survival signaling through the PI3-K/Akt pathway, which phosphorylates and inactivates proapoptotic Bad. In contrast, growth factor withdrawal may promote apoptosis through signaling by unphosphorylated Bad. The heat shock proteins, including Hsp70 and Hsp27, are also involved in inhibition of downstream apoptotic pathways by blocking formation of the apoptosome complex and inhibiting release of cytochrome c from the mitochondria.[27]

The second principal apoptotic pathway is the death receptor pathway, sometimes referred to as the extrinsic pathway. Cell-surface death receptors include Fas/APO1/CD95, tumor necrosis factor receptor 1 (TNFR1), and KILL-ER/DR5, which bind their ligands FasL, TNF, and TRAIL, respectively.[9] When the receptors are bound by their ligands, they form a death-inducing signaling complex (DISC). At the DISC, procaspase-8 and procaspase-10 are cleaved, yielding active initiator caspases.[28] The death receptor pathway may be regulated at the cell surface by the expression of "decoy" receptors for Fas (DcR3) and TRAIL (TRID and TRUNDD). The decoy receptors are closely related to the death receptors but lack a functional death domain, therefore they bind death ligands, but do not transmit a death signal.[9] Another regulatory group is the FADD-like interleukin-1 protease-inhibitory proteins (FLIPs). FLIPs have homology to caspase-8; they bind to the DISC and inhibit the activation of caspase-8. Finally, inhibitors of apoptosis proteins (IAPs) block caspase-3 activation and have the ability to regulate both the death receptor and the mitochondrial pathway. The IAP family includes XIAP (hILP, MIHA, and ILP-1), cIAP1 (MIHB and HIAP2), cIAP2 (HIAP1, MIHC, and API2), NAIP, ML-IAP, ILP2, livin (KIAP), apollon, and survivin. NF-κB also induces cellular resistance to apoptosis by transcriptionally activating cIAP1 and cIAP2, as well as other specific antiapoptotic proteins such as A20 and Mn-SOD.[27]

In human cancers, aberrations in the apoptotic program include increased expression of Fas and TRAIL decoy receptors; increased expression of antiapoptotic Bcl-2; increased expression of IAP-related protein survivin; increased expression of c-FLIP; mutations or downregulation of proapoptotic Bax, caspase-8, APAF1,

XAF1, and death receptors CD95, TRAIL-R1, and TRAIL-R2; alterations of the *p53* pathway; overexpression of growth factors and growth factor receptors; and activation of the PI3-K/Akt survival pathway.[9,28]

Cancer Invasion

A feature of malignant cells is their ability to invade the surrounding normal tissue. Tumors in which the malignant cells appear to lie exclusively above the basement membrane are referred to as *in situ cancer,* while tumors in which the malignant cells are demonstrated to breach the basement membrane, penetrating into surrounding stroma, are termed *invasive cancer.* The ability to invade involves changes in adhesion, initiation of motility, and proteolysis of the extracellular matrix (ECM).

Cell-to-cell adhesion in normal cells involves interactions between cell-surface proteins. Calcium adhesion molecules of the cadherin family (E-cadherin, P-cadherin, and N-cadherin) are thought to enhance the cells' ability to bind to one another and suppress invasion. Migration occurs when cancer cells penetrate and attach to the basal matrix of the tissue being invaded; this allows the cancer cell to pull itself forward within the tissue. Attachment to glycoproteins of the ECM such as fibronectin, laminin, and collagen is mediated by tumor cell integrin receptors. Integrins are a family of glycoproteins that form heterodimeric receptors for ECM molecules. The integrins can form at least 25 distinct pairings of its alpha and beta subunits, and each pairing is specific for a unique set of ligands. For example, $\alpha v \beta 1$ selectively binds fibronectin.[29] In addition to regulating cell adhesion to the ECM, integrins relay molecular signals regarding the cellular environment that influence shape, survival, proliferation, gene transcription, and migration.[29]

Cell motility has been linked to motility factors that convert the cell to a motile status, which is characterized by the appearance of membrane ruffling, lamellae, and pseudopodia. Factors that are thought to play a role in cancer cell motility include autocrine motility factor, autotaxin, scatter factor (also known as hepatocyte growth factor), TGF-α, EGF, and insulin-like growth factors.[30]

Serine, cysteine, and aspartic proteinases and matrix metalloproteinases (MMPs) have all been implicated in cancer invasion. Urokinase and tissue plasminogen activators (uPA and tPA) are serine proteases that convert plasminogen into plasmin. Plasmin, in return, can degrade several ECM components, including fibrin, fibronectin, laminin, and proteoglycans.[31] Plasmin also may activate several MMPs, such as MMP-1, MMP-3, and MMP-9.[31] uPA has been more closely correlated with tissue invasion and metastasis than tPA. Plasminogen activator inhibitors (PAI-1 and PAI-2) are produced in tissues and counteract the activity of plasminogen activators.

MMPs comprise a family of metal-dependent endopeptidases that includes more than 21 types. Upon activation, MMPs degrade a variety of ECM components. Although MMPs are often referred to by their common names, which reflect the ECM component they have specificity for, a sequential numbering system has been adopted for standardization. For example, collagenase-1 is now referred to as MMP-1. The MMPs are further classified as secreted and membrane-type MMPs. Most of the MMPs are synthesized as inactive zymogens (pro-MMP) and are activated by proteolytic removal of the propeptide domain outside the cell by other active MMPs or serine proteinases.

MMPs are upregulated in almost every type of cancer. Some of the MMPs are expressed by cancer cells, while others are expressed by the tumor stromal cells. Experimental models have demonstrated that MMPs promote cancer progression by increasing cancer cell growth, migration, invasion, angiogenesis, and metastasis. MMPs exert these effects by cleaving not only structural components of the

ECM but also growth factor–binding proteins, growth factor precursors, cell adhesion molecules, and other proteinases.[32] The activity of MMPs is regulated by their endogenous inhibitors, including α_2-macroglobulin, membrane-bound inhibitors RECK (reversion-inducing cysteine-rich protein with kazal domains), and tissue inhibitors of MMPs (TIMP-1, -2,- 3, and -4).[32] Of these, the best studied are the TIMPS. TIMPs reversibly inhibit MMPs in a 1:1 stoichiometric fashion, thus regulation of MMPs occurs at three levels: alterations of gene expression, activation of latent zymogens, and inhibition by endogenous inhibitors.[33] Alterations of all three levels of control have been associated with tumor progression.

Angiogenesis

Angiogenesis is the establishment of new blood vessels from a preexisting vascular bed. This neovascularization is essential for tumor growth and metastasis. Tumors develop an angiogenic phenotype as a result of accumulated genetic alterations and in response to local selection pressures such as hypoxia. Many of the common oncogenes and tumor suppressor genes have been shown to play a role in inducing angiogenesis, including *ras, myc,* HER2/*neu,* and mutations in *p53*.[34]

In response to the angiogenic switch, pericytes retract and the endothelium secretes several growth factors such as basic fibroblast growth factor (FGF), platelet-derived growth factor (PDGF), and insulin-like growth factor (IGF).[34] The basement membrane and stroma around the capillary are proteolytically degraded, which is mediated in most part by uPA. The endothelium then migrates through the degraded matrix, initially as a solid cord, then forming lumina. Finally, sprouting tips anastomose to form a vascular network surrounded by a basement membrane.

Angiogenesis is mediated by factors produced by various cells including tumor cells, endothelial cells, stromal cells, and inflammatory cells. The first proangiogenic factor was identified by Folkman and colleagues in 1971.[35] Since then, several other factors have been shown to be proangiogenic or antiangiogenic (Table 9-4). Of the angiogenic stimulators, the best studied are the vascular endothelial growth factors (VEGF). The VEGF family consists of six growth factors (VEGF-A, VEGF-B, VEGF-C, VEGF-D, VEGF-E, and placental growth factor) and three receptors (VEGFR1 or Flt-1, VEGFR2 or KDR/FLK-1, and VEGFR3 or FLT4).[36] Neuropilin 1 and 2 also may act as receptors for VEGF.[37] VEGF is induced by hypoxia and by different growth factors and cytokines, including EGF, PDGF, TNF-α, TGF-β, and interleukin 1β (IL-1β).[31] VEGF has various functions including increasing vascular permeability, inducing endothelial cell proliferation and tube formation, and inducing

Table 9-4
Proangiogenic and Antiangiogenic Factors

Proangiogenic	*Antiangiogenic*
Fibroblast growth factors 1 and 2	Angioarrestin
Angiogenin	Angiostatin
Hepatocyte growth factor	Antiangiogenic antithrombin
Interleukin-8	Endostatin
Placental growth factor	Interferons-α,-β,-γ
Platelet-derived growth factor	Platelet factor 4
Platelet-derived endothelial-cell growth factor	Thrombospondins 1 and 2
Transforming growth factors-α, -β	Tissue inhibitors of metalloproteinase-1, -2, -3
Tumor necrosis factor-α	Tumstatin
Vascular endothelial growth factor	Vasculostatin
Others	Others

SOURCE: Modified with permission from McCarty et al.[36]

endothelial cell synthesis of proteolytic enzymes such as uPA, PAI-1, UPAR, and MMP-1.[31,34,38] Furthermore, VEGF may mediate blood flow by its effects on the vasodilator nitric oxide[38] and act as an endothelial survival factor, thus protecting the integrity of the vasculature.[39] The proliferation of new lymphatic vessels, lymphangiogenesis, is also thought to be controlled by the VEGF family. Signaling in lymphatic cells is thought to be modulated by VEGFR3.[40] Experimental studies with VEGF-C and VEGF-D have shown that they can induce tumor lymphangiogenesis and direct metastasis via the lymphatic vessels and lymph nodes.[40,41]

PDGFs A, B, C, and D also play important roles in angiogenesis. PDGFs can not only enhance endothelial cell proliferation directly but also upregulate VEGF expression in vascular smooth muscle cells, promoting endothelial cell survival via a paracrine effect.[36] The angiopoietins, angiopoietin 1 (Ang-1) and angiopoietin 2 (Ang-2), in return, are thought to regulate blood vessel maturation. Ang-1 and Ang-2 both bind endothelial cell receptor Tie-2, but only the binding of Ang-1 activates signal transduction; thus Ang-2 is an Ang-1 antagonist.[31] Ang-1, via the Tie-2 receptor, induces remodeling and stabilization of blood vessels. Upregulation of Ang-2 by hypoxic induction of VEGF inhibits Ang-1–induced Tie-2 signaling, resulting in destabilization of vessels and making endothelial cells responsive to angiogenic signals, thus promoting angiogenesis in the presence of VEGF. Therefore the balance between these factors determines the angiogenetic capacity of a tumor.[42,43]

Tumor angiogenesis is regulated by several factors in a coordinated fashion. In addition to upregulation of proangiogenic molecules, angiogenesis also can be encouraged by suppression of naturally occurring inhibitors. Such inhibitors of angiogenesis include thrombospondin 1 and angiostatin. It has been proposed that the generation of inhibitors of angiogenesis by primary tumors results in the accumulation of inhibitors at distant sites, suppressing metastasis, and with resection of the primary tumor, the source of the inhibitors is removed, occasionally leading to growth of metastases.[34]

Indeed, angiogenesis is a prerequisite not only for primary tumor growth but also for metastasis. Angiogenesis in the primary tumor, as determined by microvessel density, has been demonstrated to be an independent predictor of distant metastatic disease and survival in several cancers.[34,44] Expression of angiogenic factors such as VEGFs has had prognostic value in many studies.[34] These findings further emphasize the importance of angiogenesis in cancer biology.

Metastasis

Metastases arise from the spread of cancer cells from the primary site and the formation of new tumors in distant sites. The metastatic process consists of a series of steps that need to be successfully completed (Fig. 9-6). First, the primary cancer must develop access to the circulation through either the blood circulatory system or the lymphatic system. After the cancer cells are shed into the circulation, they must survive. Next, the circulating cells lodge in a new organ and extravasate into the new tissue. Next, the cells need to initiate growth in the new tissue and eventually establish vascularization to

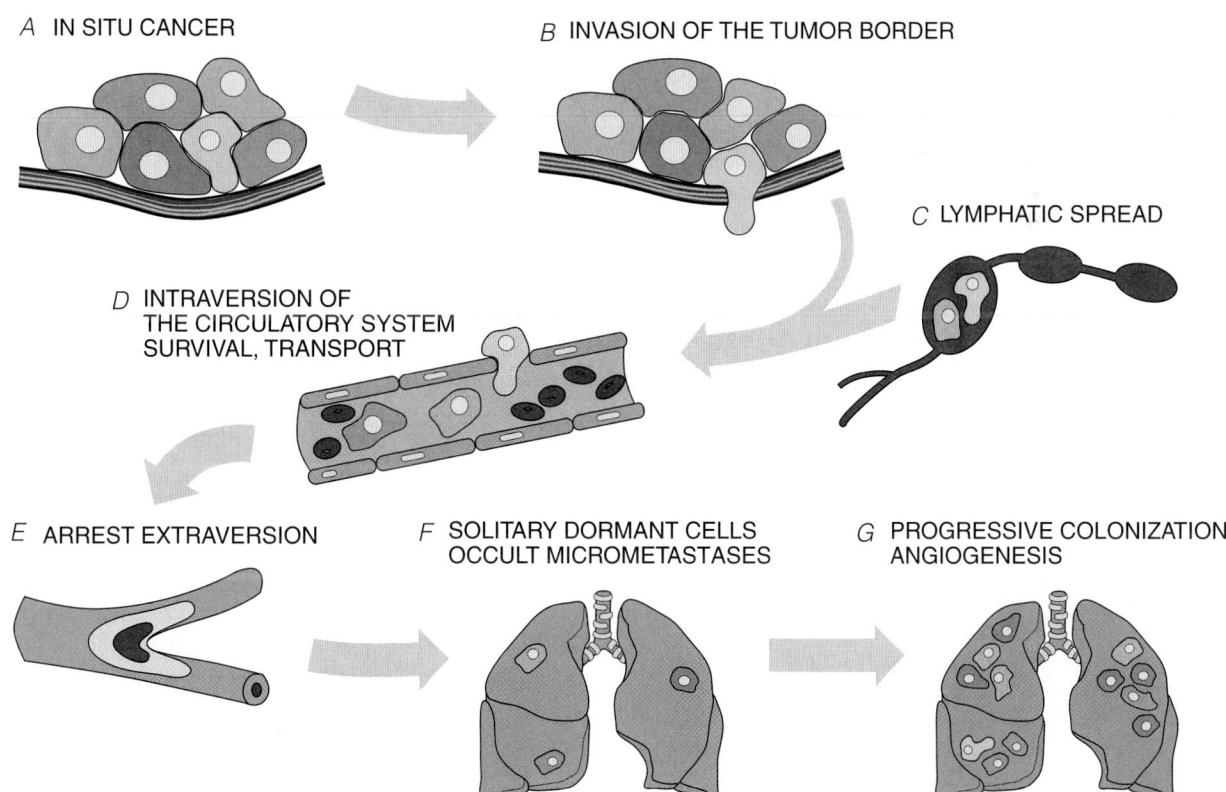

FIG. 9-6. *The metastatic process. A schematic representation of the metastatic process, beginning with A. an in situ cancer surrounded by an intact basement membrane. B. Invasion requires reversible changes in cell–cell and cell–extracellular matrix adherence, destruction of proteins in the matrix and stroma, and motility. C. Metastasizing cells can enter the circulation via the lymphatics, or D. directly enter the circulation. E. Intravascular survival of the tumor cells and extravasation of the circulatory system follows. F. Metastatic single cells can colonize sites and remain dormant for years as occult micrometastases. G. Subsequent progression and neovascularization leads to clinically detectable metastases and progressively growing, angiogenic metastases. (Modified from Steeg,[50] with permission.)*

sustain the new tumor. Overall, metastasis is an inefficient process, although the initial steps of hematogenous metastasis (the arrest of tumor cells in the organ and extravasation) are believed to be performed efficiently.[45] Only a small subset of cancer cells is then able to initiate micrometastases, while an even smaller portion go on to grow into macrometastases.

Metastases can sometimes arise several years after the treatment of primary tumors. For example, although most breast cancer recurrences occur within the first 10 years after the initial treatment, and recurrences are rare after 20 years,[46] breast cancer recurrences have been reported as late as 50 years after the original tumor.[47] This phenomenon is referred to as *dormancy,* and it remains one of the biggest challenges in cancer biology. Persistence of solitary cancer cells in a secondary site such as the liver or bone marrow is one possible contributor to dormancy.[48] Another explanation of dormancy is that cells remain viable in a quiescent state and then get reactivated by a physiologically perturbing event.[47] Interestingly, primary tumor removal has been proposed to be a potentially perturbing factor.[49] An alternate explanation is that cells establish preangiogenic metastases in which they continue to proliferate but that the proliferative rate is balanced by the apoptotic rate.[45] Therefore, when these small metastases acquire the ability to be vascularized, substantial tumor growth can be achieved at the metastatic site, leading to clinical detection.

Several types of tumors metastasize in an organ-specific pattern. One explanation for this is mechanical and is based on the different circulatory drainage patterns of the tumors. When different tumor types and their preferred metastasis sites were compared, 66% of organ-specific metastases were explained on the basis of blood flow alone.[45] The other explanation for preferential metastasis is what is referred to as the "seed and soil" theory, the dependence of the seed (the cancer cell) on the soil (the secondary organ). According to this theory, once cells have reached a secondary organ, their growth efficiency in that organ is based on the compatibility of the cancer cell's biology with its new microenvironment. For example, breast cancer cells may grow more efficiently in bone than in some other organs because of favorable molecular interactions that occur in the bone microenvironment. The ability of cancer cells to grow in a specific site likely depends on features inherent to the cancer cell, features inherent to the organ, and the interplay between the cancer cell and its microenvironment.[45]

Many of the oncogenes discovered to date, such as HER2/*neu,* *ras,* and *myc,* are thought to potentiate not only malignant transformation but also one or more of the steps required in the metastatic process. Metastasis also may involve the loss of metastasis suppressor genes.[50] Metastasis suppressor genes such as the ones listed in Table 9-5 can decrease metastatic potential when reintroduced into a metastatically competent cell line without altering primary tumor growth.[50] Laboratory work involving cancer cell lines that have been selected to have a higher metastatic potential have led to the realization that these more highly metastatic cells have a different gene expression profile than their less metastatic parental counterparts. This in turn has led to the currently held belief that the ability of a primary tumor to metastasize may be predictable by analysis of its gene expression profile. Indeed, several studies have recently focused on identifying a gene expression profile or a "molecular signature" that is associated with metastasis.[51] It has been shown that such a gene expression profile can be used to predict the probability of remaining free of distant metastasis.[52] Notably, this hypothesis differs from the multistep tumorigenesis theory in that the ability to metastasize is considered an inherent quality of the tumor from the beginning. It is assumed that metastasis develops not from a few

Table 9-5
Metastasis-Suppressing Genes

Gene	Cancer Cell Type	Gene Function
NM23	Melanoma Breast Colon Oral squamous cell	Histidine kinase; phosphorylates KSR, which might reduce ERK 1 and 2 activation
MKK4	Prostate Ovarian	MAPKK; phosphorylates and activates p38 and JNK kinases
KAI1	Prostate Breast	Integrin interaction EGFR desensitization
BRMS1	Breast Melanoma	Gap-junctional communication
KiSS1	Melanoma Breast	G-protein-coupled-receptor ligand
RHOGDI2	Bladder	Regulates RHO and RAC function
CRSP3	Melanoma	Transcriptional coactivator
VDUP1	Melanoma	Thioredoxin inhibitor

EGFR = epidermal growth factor receptor; ERK = extracellular signal-regulated kinase; JNK = JUN-terminal kinase; KSR = kinase suppressor of RAS; MAPKK = mitogen-activated protein kinase kinase.

SOURCE: Modified with permission from Steeg.[50]

rare cells in the primary tumor that develop the ability to metastasize but that all cells in tumors with such molecular signatures develop the ability to metastasize.[53] The reality probably lies in between in that some early genetic changes detectable in the entire tumor can give tumors an advantage in the metastatic process, while additional genetic changes can give a clone of cells additional advantages, thus allowing them to succeed in metastasis.

CANCER ETIOLOGY

Cancer Genetics

One widely held opinion is that cancer is a genetic disease that arises from an accumulation of mutations that leads to the selection of cells with increasingly aggressive behavior. These mutations may lead either to a gain of function by oncogenes or to a loss of function by tumor suppressor genes. Most mutations in cancer are somatic and are found only in the cancer cells. Most of our information on human cancer genes has been gained from hereditary cancers. In the case of hereditary cancers, the individual carries a particular germline mutation in every cell. In the past decade, more than 30 genes for autosomal dominant hereditary cancers have been identified (Table 9-6). A few of these hereditary cancer genes are oncogenes, but most are tumor suppressor genes. Though hereditary cancer syndromes are rare, somatic mutations that occur in sporadic cancer have been found to disrupt the cellular pathways altered in hereditary cancer syndromes, suggesting that these pathways are critical to normal cell growth, cell cycle, and proliferation.

The following criteria may suggest the presence of a hereditary cancer[54]:

1. Tumor development at a much younger age than usual
2. Presence of bilateral disease
3. Presence of multiple primary malignancies
4. Presentation of a cancer in the less affected sex (e.g., male breast cancer)
5. Clustering of the same cancer type in relatives
6. Cancer associated with other conditions such as mental retardation or pathognomonic skin lesions

It is crucial that all surgeons taking care of cancer patients be aware of hereditary cancer syndromes, since a patient's genetic

Table 9-6
Genes Associated with Hereditary Cancer

Genes	Location	Syndrome	Cancer Sites and Associated Traits
APC	17q21	Familial adenomatous polyposis (FAP)	Colorectal adenomas and carcinomas, duodenal and gastric tumors, desmoids, medullablastomas, osteomas
BMPRIA	10q21-q22	Juvenile polyposis coli	Juvenile polyps of the gastrointestinal tract, gastrointestinal and colorectal malignancy
BRCA1	17q21	Breast/ovarian syndrome	Breast cancer, ovarian cancer, colon cancer, prostate cancer
BRCA2	13q12.3	Breast/ovarian syndrome	Breast cancer, ovarian cancer, colon cancer, prostate cancer, cancer of the gallbladder and bile duct, pancreatic cancer, gastric cancer, melanoma
p16; CDK4	9p21; 12q14	Familial melanoma	Melanoma, pancreatic cancer, dysplastic nevi, atypical moles
CDH1	16q22	Hereditary diffuse gastric cancer	Gastric cancer
hCHK2	22q12.1	Li-Fraumeni and hereditary breast cancer	Breast cancer, soft-tissue sarcoma, brain tumors
hMLH1; hMSH2; hMSH6; hPMS1; hPMS2	3p21; 2p22-21; 2p16; 2q31-33; 7p22	Hereditary nonpolyposis colorectal cancer	Colorectal cancer, endometrial cancer, transitional cell carcinoma of the ureter and renal pelvis, and carcinomas of the stomach, small bowel, ovary, and pancreas
MEN1	11q13	Multiple endocrine neoplasia type 1	Pancreatic islet cell cancer, parathyroid hyperplasia, pituitary adenomas
MET	7q31	Hereditary papillary renal cell carcinoma	Renal cancer
NF1	17q11	Neurofibromatosis type 1	Neurofibroma, neurofibrosarcoma, acute myelogenous leukemia, brain tumors
NF2	22q12	Neurofibromatosis type 2	Acoustic neuromas, meningiomas, gliomas, ependymomas
PTC	9q22.3	Nevoid basal cell carcinoma	Basal cell carcinoma
PTEN	10q23.3	Cowden disease	Breast cancer, thyroid cancer, endometrial cancer
rb	13q14	Retinoblastoma	Retinoblastoma, sarcomas, melanoma, and malignant neoplasms of brain and meninges
RET	10q11.2	Multiple endocrine neoplasia type 2	Medullary thyroid cancer, pheochromocytoma, parathyroid hyperplasia
SDHB; SDHC; SDHD	1p363.1-p35; 1q21; 11q23	Hereditary paraganglioma and pheochromocytoma	Paraganglioma, pheochromocytoma
SMAD4/DPC4	18q21.1	Juvenile polyposis coli	Juvenile polyps of the gastrointestinal tract, gastrointestinal and colorectal malignancy
STK11	19p13.3	Peutz-Jeghers syndrome	Gastrointestinal tract carcinoma, breast carcinoma, testicular cancer, pancreatic cancer, benign pigmentation of the skin and mucosa
p53	17p13	Li-Fraumeni syndrome	Breast cancer, soft-tissue sarcoma, osteosarcoma, brain tumors, adrenocortical carcinoma, Wilms tumor, phyllodes tumor of the breast, pancreatic cancer, leukemia, neuroblastoma
TSC1; TSC2	9q34;16p13	Tuberous sclerosis	Multiple hamartomas, renal cell carcinoma, astrocytoma
VHL	3p25	von Hippel-Lindau disease	Renal cell carcinoma, hemangioblastomas of retina and central nervous system, pheochromocytoma
WT	11p13	Wilms' tumor	Wilms' tumor, aniridia, genitourinary abnormalities, mental retardation

SOURCE: Modified with permission from Marsh et al.[251]

background has significant implications for patient counseling, planning of surgical therapy, and cancer screening and prevention. Some of the more commonly encountered hereditary cancer syndromes are discussed here.

rb1 Gene and Hereditary Retinoblastoma

The *rb1* gene was the first tumor suppressor to be cloned.[55] Retinoblastoma has long been known to occur in hereditary and nonhereditary forms. In approximately 40% of cases of retinoblastoma in the United States, the individual has a predispostion conferred by a germline mutation.[56] Interestingly, although most children with an affected parent develop bilateral retinoblastoma, some develop unilateral retinoblastoma. Furthermore, some children with an affected parent are not affected themselves, but then have an affected child, indicating that they are *rb1* mutation carriers. These findings

led to the theory that a single mutation is not sufficient for tumorigenesis. Dr. Alfred Knudson hypothesized that hereditary retinoblastoma involves two mutations, one of which is germline, while the other, nonhereditary retinoblastoma, is due to two somatic mutations (Fig. 9-7).[57] Thus both hereditary and nonhereditary forms of retinoblastoma involve the same number of mutations, a hypothesis known as Knudson's "two-hit" hypothesis. A "hit" may be a point mutation, a chromosomal deletion referred to as allelic loss, or a loss of heterozygosity (LOH), or silencing of an existing gene.

Retinoblastoma is a pediatric retinal tumor. Most of these tumors are detected within the first 7 years of life. Bilateral disease is usually diagnosed earlier, at an average age of 12 months. The outcome for tumors contained within the eye are good, with cure rates of greater than 95%. However, once the tumor extends outside the eye, the mortality rate is high.[58] A higher incidence of second extraocular primary tumors, especially sarcomas, malignant melanomas, and

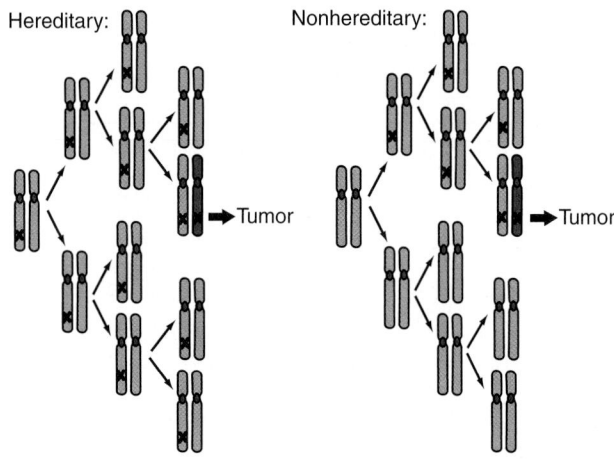

FIG. 9-7. *"Two-hit" tumor formation in both hereditary and nonhereditary cancers. A "one-hit" clone is a precursor to the tumor in nonhereditary cancers, whereas all cells are one-hit clones in hereditary cancer. (Modified from Knudson,[57] with permission.)*

malignant neoplasms of the brain and meninges have been reported in patients with germline mutations.[59,60]

The *rb1* gene product, the Rb protein, is a regulator of transcription that controls the cell cycle, differentiation, and apoptosis in normal development (see Fig. 9-5).[61] The E2F transcription factor regulates the expression of genes that are involved in transition from G_1 to S phase of the cell cycle. E2F-mediated transcription is negatively regulated by the Rb protein.[62] Rb can repress transcription by at least two different mechanisms:[63] it can directly bind the transactivation domain of E2F, blocking its ability to activate transcription, or it can bind to the promoter as a complex with E2F and actively repress transcription through chromatin remodeling. The ability of Rb to repress E2F-mediated transcription is regulated by the phosphorylation of Rb by CDK4 and CDK6, which disrupts the association between Rb and E2F. The activities of the CDKs are in turn regulated by their activator D-type cyclins (D1, D2, and D3) and their inhibitors, the INK4 family of CDK inhibitors (p15, p16, p18, and p19). Besides hereditary retinoblastoma, Rb protein is commonly inactivated directly by mutation in many sporadic tumors.[64] Moreover, other molecules in the Rb pathway, such as p16, CDK4, and CDK6, have been identified in a number of sporadic tumors, suggesting that the Rb pathway is critical in malignant transformation.[65,66]

p53 and Li-Fraumeni Syndrome

Li-Fraumeni syndrome (LFS) was first defined on the basis of observations of clustering of malignancies, including early-onset breast cancer, soft-tissue sarcomas, brain tumors, adrenocortical tumors, and leukemia.[67] Criteria for classic LFS in an individual (the proband) include: (1) a bone or soft-tissue sarcoma when younger than 45 years, (2) a first-degree relative with cancer before age 45 years, and (3) another first- or second-degree relative with either a sarcoma diagnosed at any age or any cancer diagnosed before age 45 years.[68] Approximately 70% of LFS families have been shown to have germline mutations in the tumor suppressor *p53* gene.[69,70] Breast carcinoma, soft-tissue sarcoma, osteosarcoma, brain tumors, adrenocortical carcinoma, Wilms' tumor, and phyllodes tumor of the breast are strongly associated; pancreatic cancer is moderately associated; and leukemia and neuroblastoma are weakly associated with germline *p53* mutations.[71] Mutations of *p53* have not been detected in approximately 30% of LFS families,[72] and it is

hypothesized that genetic alterations in other proteins interacting with *p53* function may play a role in these families.

p53 is the most commonly mutated known gene in human cancer. The *p53* protein regulates cell-cycle progression as well as apoptotic cell death as part of stress response pathways following ionizing or ultraviolet (UV) irradiation, chemotherapy, acidosis, growth factor deprivation, or hypoxia. When cells are exposed to stressors, *p53* acts as a transcription factor for genes that induce cell-cycle arrest or apoptosis. The transcriptional targets of *p53* include p21/WAF1, mdm2, IGF-binding protein 3, GADD45, and 14-3-3 sigma factor.[73] A majority of *p53* mutations are found within a central DNA recognition motif and disrupt DNA binding by *p53*. Families with germline missense mutations in the DNA-binding domain show a more highly penetrant phenotype than families with other *p53* mutations.[74] Furthermore, proband cancers are linked with significantly younger ages at diagnosis in patients with missense mutations in the DNA-binding domain.[74]

hCHK2, Li-Fraumeni Syndrome, and Hereditary Breast Cancer

Germline mutations in the *hCHK2* gene have recently been identified as another susceptibility gene for LFS.[75] *hCHK2* encodes for the human homologue of the yeast Cds1 and the RAD53 G_2 checkpoint, whose activation by DNA damage prevents entry into mitosis. CHK2 directly phosphorylates *p53*, suggesting that CHK2 may be involved in *p53* regulation after DNA damage. CHK2 also regulates *BRCA1* function after DNA damage.[76] The protein truncation mutation *1100delC* in exon 10 identified in LFS and breast cancer abolishes the kinase function of CHK2. Another reported mutation in *hCHK2* is a missense mutation (*R145W*) that destabilizes the protein, shortening its half-life.[77]

While some investigators found *hCHK2* mutations in classic LFS families, others have reported that the phenotypes of CHK2 families are not typical for LFS and involve no sarcomas or childhood cancers.[54,75] The CHK2 mutation originally reported in LFS (*1100delC*) is found in 1.4% of population controls, but is found at an increased frequency (3.1%) among breast cancer patients with a family history.[78] Patients with bilateral breast cancers are six times more likely to have the mutation than patients with unilateral breast cancer.[78] Thus *hCHK2* mutations may play a role in hereditary breast cancer families as well as LFS families, but the extent of this is unclear. *hCHK2* mutations are rare in sporadic breast tumors.[79]

BRCA1, BRCA2, and Hereditary Breast-Ovarian Cancer Syndrome

It is estimated that 5 to 10% of breast cancers are hereditary. Of women with early-onset breast cancer (aged 40 years or younger), nearly 10% have a germline mutation in *BRCA1* or *BRCA2*.[80] Mutation carriers are more prevalent among women who have a first- or second-degree relative with premenopausal breast cancer or ovarian cancer at any age. The likelihood of a *BRCA* mutation is higher in patients who belong to a population in which founder mutations may be prevalent, such as in the Ashkenazi Jewish population.[81] The cumulative risks for a female *BRCA1* mutation carrier of developing breast cancer and ovarian cancer by age 70 have been estimated to be 87 and 44%, respectively.[82] The cumulative risks of breast cancer and ovarian cancer by age 70 in *BRCA2* families were estimated to be 84 and 27%, respectively.[83] Although male breast cancer can occur with either *BRCA1* or *BRCA2*, the majority of families (76%) with both male and female breast cancer are *BRCA2*.[83] Besides breast and ovarian cancer, *BRCA1* and *BRCA2* may be associated with increased risks for several other cancers. *BRCA1* confers a fourfold increased risk for colon cancer and three-fold increased risk for prostate cancer.[82] *BRCA2* confers a fivefold increased risk for prostate cancer, sevenfold in men younger than 65 years.[84] Furthermore, *BRCA2* confers a fivefold increased risk for gallbladder and bile duct cancers, fourfold increased risk for pancreatic cancer, and threefold increased risk for gastric cancer and malignant melanoma.[84]

BRCA1 was the first breast cancer susceptibility gene identified, and has been mapped to 17q21. *BRCA2,* mapped to 13q12.3, was reported shortly afterward. *BRCA1* and *BRCA2* encode for large nuclear proteins, 208 kDa and 384 kDa, respectively, that have been implicated in processes fundamental to all cells, including DNA repair and recombination, checkpoint control of the cell cycle, and transcription.[85] Although early studies suggested that the two proteins function together as a complex, subsequent data demonstrated that they have distinct functions.[86,87] In fact, breast cancers arising in *BRCA1* or *BRCA2* mutations are different at the molecular level and have been found to have distinct gene expression profiles.[88] Breast cancers associated with *BRCA1* are more likely to exhibit higher mitotic counts, have a pushing border, and have more lymphocytic infiltration than sporadic cancers.[89] Breast cancers associated with *BRCA2* are more likely to have a pushing border and lower mitotic count than sporadic tumors.[89] *BRCA1*-associated tumors are more likely to be estrogen receptor–negative, while *BRCA2*-associated tumors are more likely to be estrogen receptor–positive.[90] Currently, data are inadequate to support the use of *BRCA1* and *BRCA2* status to counsel prognosis and systemic therapy for breast cancer. However, the differences in estrogen-receptor status in *BRCA1* and *BRCA2* mutation carriers may have implications for chemoprevention strategies and need further study.

APC Gene and Familial Adenomatous Polyposis

Patients affected with familial adenomatous polyposis (FAP) characteristically develop hundreds to thousand of polyps in the colon and rectum. The polyps usually appear in adolescence and, if left untreated, progress to colorectal cancer. FAP is associated with benign extracolonic manifestations that may be useful in identifying new cases, including congenital hypertrophy of the retinal pigment epithelium, epidermoid cysts, and osteomas. In addition to colorectal cancer, patients with FAP are at risk for upper intestinal neoplasms (gastric and duodenal polyps, duodenal and periampullary cancer), hepatobiliary tumors (hepatoblastoma, pancreatic cancer, and cholangiocarcinoma), thyroid carcinoma, desmoid tumors, and medulloblastomas.

The adenomatous polyposis coli (*APC*) tumor suppressor gene product is widely expressed in many tissues and plays an important role in cell-cell interactions, cell adhesion, regulation of β-catenin, and maintenance of cytoskeletal microtubules. Alterations in *APC* lead to dysregulation of several physiologic processes that govern colonic epithelial cell homeostasis, including cell-cycle progression, migration, differentiation, and apoptosis.[91] Mutations in the *APC* gene have been identified in FAP and in 80% of sporadic colorectal cancers.[92] Furthermore, *APC* mutations are the earliest known genetic alterations in colorectal cancer progression,[93] emphasizing its importance in cancer initiation. The germline mutations in *APC* may arise from point mutations, insertions, or deletions that lead to a premature stop codon and a truncated, functionally inactive protein.[94,95] The risk of developing specific manifestations of FAP is correlated with the position of the FAP mutations, a phenomenon referred to as genotype-phenotype correlation.[96] For example, desmoids usually are associated with mutations between codons 1403 and 1578.[97,98] Mutations in the extreme 5′ or 3′ ends of *APC,* or in the alternatively spliced region of exon 9, are associated with an attenuated version of FAP.[96] Better understanding of the genotype-phenotype correlations may assist in patient counseling and therapeutic planning.

Mismatch Repair Genes and Hereditary Nonpolyposis Colorectal Cancer

Hereditary nonpolyposis colorectal cancer (HNPCC), also referred to as Lynch syndrome, is an autosomal dominant hereditary cancer syndrome that predisposes to a wide spectrum of cancers, including colorectal cancer without polyposis. Some have proposed that HNPCC consists of at least two syndromes: Lynch syndrome I, which entails hereditary predisposition for colorectal cancer with early age of onset (approximately age 44 years) and an excess of synchronous and metachronous colonic cancers; and Lynch syndrome II, featuring a similar colonic phenotype accompanied by a high risk for carcinoma of the endometrium, transitional cell carcinoma of the ureter and renal pelvis, and carcinomas of the stomach, small bowel, ovary, and pancreas.[99] The diagnostic criteria for HNPCC are referred to as the Amsterdam criteria, or the "3-2-1-0 rule." The classic Amsterdam criteria were recently revised to include other HNPCC-related cancers (Table 9-7).[100] These criteria are met when three or more family members have histologically verified, HNPCC-associated cancers (one of whom is a first-degree relative of the other two), two or more generations are involved, at least one individual was diagnosed before age 50 years, and no individuals have FAP (see Table 9-7).

During DNA replication, DNA polymerases may introduce single nucleotide mismatches or small insertion or deletion loops. These errors are corrected through a process referred to as *mismatch repair.* When mismatch repair genes are inactivated, DNA mutations in other genes that are critical to cell growth and proliferation accumulate rapidly. In HNPCC, germline mutations have been identified in several genes that play a key role in DNA nucleotide mismatch repair: *hMLH1* (human mutL homologue 1), *hMSH2* (human mutS homologue 2), *hMSH6,* and *hPMS1* and *hPMS2* (human postmeiotic segretation 1 and 2), of which *hMLH1* and *hMSH2* are the most common.[101–106] The hallmark of HNPCC is microsatellite instability, which occurs on the basis of unrepaired mismatches and small insertion or deletion loops. Microsatellite instability can be tested by comparing the DNA of a patient's tumor with DNA from adjacent normal epithelium, amplifying the DNA with polymerase chain reaction (PCR) using a standard set of markers (BAT25, BAT26, D2S123, D5S346, and D17S250), comparing the amplified genomic DNA sequences, and classifying the degree of microsatellite instability as high, low, or stable.[107] Such microsatellite instability

Table 9-7

Revised Criteria for Hereditary Nonpolyposis Colon Cancer (Amsterdam Criteria II)

Three or more relatives with an HNPCC-associated cancer (colorectal cancer, endometrial cancer, cancer of the small bowel, ureter, or renal pelvis), one of whom is a first-degree relative of the other two
At least two successive generations affected
At least one diagnosed before age 50 years
Familial adenomatous polyposis excluded
Tumors verified by pathologic examination

SOURCE: Modified with permission from Vasen et al.[100]

testing may help select patients who are more likely to have germline mutations.

PTEN and Cowden Disease

Somatic deletions or mutations in the tumor suppressor gene *PTEN* (phosphatase and tensin homologue deleted on chromosome 10) have been observed in a number of glioma and breast, prostate, and renal carcinoma cell lines and several primary tumor specimens.[108] *PTEN* also is referred to as the gene mutated in multiple advanced cancers 1 (MMAC1). *PTEN* was identified as the susceptibility gene for the autosomal dominant syndrome Cowden disease (CD) or multiple hamartoma syndrome.[109,110] Trichilemmomas, benign tumors of the hair follicle infundibulum, and mucocutaneous papillomatosis are pathognomonic of CD. Other common features include thyroid adenomas and multinodular goiters, breast fibroadenomas, and hamartomatous gastrointestinal polyps. The diagnosis of CD is made when an individual or family has a combination of pathognomonic major and/or minor criteria proposed by the International Cowden Consortium (Table 9-8). CD is associated with an increased risk of breast and thyroid cancers. Breast cancer develops in 25 to 50% of affected women, and thyroid cancer develops in 3 to 10% of all affected individuals.[111,112] *PTEN* mutations have been identified in 81% of CD families tested, and identification of a *PTEN* mutation has been correlated with the presence of malignant breast disease.[113]

PTEN encodes a 403-amino-acid protein, tyrosine phosphatase (PTPase). *PTEN* negatively controls the PI3K signaling pathway for the regulation of cell growth and survival by dephosphorylating phosphoinositol 3,4,5-triphosphate; thus mutation of *PTEN* leads to

Table 9-8
Cowden Disease Diagnostic Criteria

Pathognomonic criteria
Mucocutaneous lesions
    Trichilemmomas, facial
    Acral keratoses
    Papillomatous lesions
    Mucosal lesions

Major criteria
Breast cancer
Thyroid cancer, especially follicular thyroid carcinoma type
Macrocephaly (≥97th percentile)
Lhermitte-Duclos disease
Endometrial carcinoma

Minor criteria
Other thyroid lesions (e.g., goiter)
Mental retardation (IQ ≤75)
Gastrointestinal hamartomas
Fibrocystic disease of the breast
Lipomas
Fibromas
Genitourinary tumors (e.g., uterine fibroids) or malformation

Operational diagnosis in an individual
Mucocutaneous lesions alone if there are:
    Six or more facial papules, of which three or more must be
      trichilemmoma, or
    Cutaneous facial papules and oral mucosal papillomatosis, or
    Oral mucosal papillomatosis and acral keratoses, or
    Palmoplantar keratoses, six or more
Two major criteria, but one must be macrocephaly or Lhermitte-Duclos
    disease
One major and three minor criteria
Four minor criteria

SOURCE: Modified with permission from Eng.[111]

constitutive activation of the PI3K/AKT signaling pathway.[114] The "hot spot" for *PTEN* mutations has been identified in exon 5. Forty-three percent of CD mutations have been identified in this exon, which contains the PTPase core domain.[113] This suggests that the *PTEN* catalytic activity is vital for its biologic function.

p16 and Hereditary Malignant Melanoma

p16, also known as INK4A, CDKN1, CDKN2A, or MTS-1, is a tumor suppressor that acts by binding CDK4 and CDK6 and inhibiting the catalytic activity of the CDK4-6/cyclin D complex that is required for phosphorylation of Rb and subsequent cell-cycle progression (see Fig. 9-5). *p16* was found to have germline mutations in 13 of 18 (72%) of familial melanoma kindreds studied in initial reports.[115] Subsequent studies suggest that germline mutations in *p16* account for 20% of melanoma-prone families.[116] *p16* mutations that alter its ability to inhibit the catalytic activity of the CDK4-6/cyclin D complex not only increase the risk of melanoma by 75-fold but also increase the risk of pancreatic cancer by 22-fold.[117,118] Interestingly, *p16* mutations that do not appear to alter its function increase the risk of melanoma by 38-fold and do not increase the risk of pancreatic cancer.[117] Genetic evaluation of primary tumors has revealed that *p16* is inactivated in a significant portion of sporadic tumors, including cancer of the pancreas, esophagus, head and neck, stomach, breast, and colon, as well as melanomas, through point mutation, promoter methylation, or deletion.[119]

E-Cadherin and Hereditary Diffuse Gastric Cancer

E-cadherin is a cell adhesion molecule that plays an important role in normal architecture and function of epithelial cells. The adhesive function of E-cadherin is dependent on interaction of its cytoplasmic domain with β- and γ-catenins and may be regulated by phosphorylation of β-catenin.

Hereditary diffuse gastric carcinoma is a newly identified, autosomal dominant cancer syndrome that results from germline mutations in the E-cadherin gene, *CDH1*. Carriers of *CDH1* mutations have a 70 to 80% chance of developing gastric cancer.[120] Furthermore, mutations of *CDH1* have been described in sporadic cancers of the ovary, endometrium, breast, and thyroid.[121] However, frequent mutations have been identified in only two particular tumors: diffuse gastric carcinomas and lobular breast carcinomas. Invasive lobular breast carcinomas often show inactivating mutations in combination with an LOH of the wild-type *CDH1* allele.[122] Interestingly, in gastric carcinomas the predominant mutations are exon skipping, causing in-frame deletions, while most mutations identified in lobular breast cancers are premature stop codons,[121] suggesting a genotype-phenotype correlation.

RET Protooncogene and Multiple Endocrine Neoplasia Type 2

The *RET* gene encodes for a transmembrane receptor tyrosine kinase that plays a role in proliferation, migration, and differentiation of cells derived from the neural crest. Gain-of-function mutations in the *RET* gene are associated with medullary thyroid carcinoma in isolation or multiple endocrine neoplasia type 2 (MEN2) syndromes. MEN2A is associated with medullary thyroid carcinoma and pheochromocytoma (in 50%) or parathyroid adenoma (in 20%), while MEN2B is associated with medullary thyroid carcinoma, marfanoid habitus, mucosal neuromas, and ganglioneuromatosis.[123] *RET* mutations lead to uncontrolled growth of the thyroid c cells, and in familial medullary cancer, c-cell hyperplasia progresses to bilateral, multicentric medullary thyroid cancer. Mutations in the *RET* gene have also been identified in 40 to 60% of sporadic medullary thyroid cancers.[124]

Tissue Specificity of Hereditary Cancer

In spite of our increasing understanding of hereditary cancer genes, the tissue specificity of the hereditary cancers remains poorly understood. For example, while mutations in genes such as *rb* and *p53* are encountered frequently in sporadic cancers arising in a variety of tissues, it is unclear why germline mutations in these genes would lead to tumors predominantly in selected tissues. However, mutations in tumor suppressor genes are insufficient to produce tumors, and usually the development of cancer involves accumulation of multiple genetic alterations. The rate at which these changes occur in different tissues after inactivation of different tumor suppressor genes may account for some of the tissue distribution seen with hereditary cancer syndromes.

Genetic Modifiers of Risk

Individuals carrying identical germline mutations vary in regard to cancer penetrance (whether cancer will develop or not) and cancer phenotype (the tissues involved). It is thought that this variability may be due to environmental influences or, if genetic, to genetic modifiers of risk. Similarly, genetic modifiers of risk also can play a role in determining whether an individual will develop cancer after exposure to carcinogens.

Chemical Carcinogens

The first report that cancer could be caused by environmental factors was by John Hill in 1761, who reported the association between nasal cancer and excessive use of tobacco snuff.[125] Currently, approximately 60 to 90% of cancers are thought to be due to environmental factors.[126] Any agent that can contribute to tumor formation is referred to as a *carcinogen* and can be chemical, physical, or viral agents. Chemicals are classified into three groups based on how they contribute to tumor formation.[126] The first group of chemical agents, the genotoxins, can initiate carcinogenesis by causing a mutation. The second group, the co-carcinogens, by themselves cannot cause cancer, but potentiate carcinogenesis by enhancing the potency of genotoxins. The third group, tumor promoters, enhance tumor formation when given after exposure to genotoxins.

The International Agency for Research on Cancer (IARC) maintains a registry of human carcinogens that is available through the World Wide Web (www.iarc.fr). The compounds are categorized into five groups based on an analysis of epidemiologic studies, animal models, and short-term mutagenesis tests. Group 1 contains what are considered to be proven human carcinogens, based on formal epidemiologic studies among workers who were exposed for long periods (several years) to the chemicals. Group 2A contains what are considered to be probable human carcinogens. This group has shown suggestive epidemiologic evidence, but the data are insufficient to establish causality. There is evidence of carcinogenicity, however, from animal studies carried out under conditions relevant to human exposure. Group 2B contains what are considered to be possible carcinogens, since these substances show a clear statistically and biologically significant increase in the incidence of malignant tumors in more than one animal species or strain. Group 3 agents are not classifiable as to carcinogenicity in humans. Group 4 agents are probably not carcinogenic to humans. Selected substances that have been classified as proven carcinogens (group 1) by the IARC are listed in Table 9-9.

Table 9-9
Selected IARC Group 1 Chemical Carcinogens[a]

Chemical	*Predominant Tumor Type*[b]
Aflatoxins	Liver cancer
Arsenic	Skin cancer
Benzene	Leukemia
Benzidine	Bladder cancer
Beryllium	Lung cancer
Cadmium	Lung cancer
Chinese-style salted fish	Nasopharyngeal carcinoma
Chlorambucil	Leukemia
Chromium [VI] compounds	Lung cancer
Coal tar	Skin cancer, scrotal cancer
Cyclophosphamide	Bladder cancer, leukemia
Diethylstilbestrol (DES)	Vaginal and cervical clear cell adenocarcinomas
Ethylene oxide	Leukemia, lymphoma
Estrogen replacement therapy	Endometrial cancer, breast cancer
Nickel	Lung cancer, nasal cancer
Tamoxifen[c]	Endometrial cancer
Vinyl chloride	Angiosarcoma of the liver, hepatocellular carcinoma, brain tumors, lung cancer, malignancies of lymphatic and hematopoietic system
TCDD (2,3,7,8-tetrachlorodibenzo-para-dioxin)	Soft-tissue sarcoma
Tobacco products, smokeless	Oral cancer
Tobacco smoke	Lung cancer, oral cancer, pharyngeal cancer, laryngeal cancer, esophageal cancer (squamous cell, pancreatic cancer, bladder cancer, liver cancer, renal cell carcinoma, cervical cancer, leukemia)

[a] Based on information in the IARC monographs.[137]

[b] Only tumor types for which causal relationships are established are listed. Other cancer types may be linked to the agents with a lower frequency or with insufficient data to prove causality.

[c] Tamoxifen has been shown to prevent contralateral breast cancer.

IARC = The International Agency for Research on Cancer.

Physical Carcinogens

Physical carcinogenesis can occur through induction of inflammation and cell proliferation over a period of time or through exposure to physical agents that induce DNA damage. Foreign bodies can cause chronic irritation that can expose cells to carcinogenesis by other environmental agents. In animal models, for example, subcutaneous implantation of a foreign body can lead to tumors that have been attributed to chronic irritation from the foreign objects. In humans, clinical scenarios associated with chronic irritation and inflammation such as chronic nonhealing wounds, burns, and inflammatory bowel syndrome have all been associated with an increased risk of cancer. *Helicobacter pylori* is associated with gastritis and gastric cancer, and thus its carcinogenicity may be considered physical carcinogenesis. The liver fluke *Opisthorchis viverrini* similarly leads to local inflammation and cholangiocarcinoma.

The induction of lung and mesothelial cancers from asbestos fibers and nonfibrous particles such as silica are other examples of foreign-body–induced physical carcinogenesis.[127] Animal experiments have demonstrated that the dimensions and durability of the asbestos and other fibrous minerals are the key determinants of their carcinogenicity.[128] Short fibers can be inactivated by phagocytosis, while long fibers ($>10\ \mu m$) are cleared less effectively and are encompassed by proliferating epithelial cells. The long fibers support cell proliferation and have been shown to preferentially induce tumors. Asbestos-associated biologic effects also may be mediated through reactive oxygen and nitrogen species. Furthermore, an interaction occurs between asbestos and silica and components of cigarette smoke. Polycyclic aromatic hydrocarbons (PAH) in cigarette smoke are metabolized by epithelial cells and form DNA adducts. If PAH is coated on asbestos, PAH uptake is increased.[127] Both PAH and asbestos impair lung clearance, potentially increasing uptake further. Therefore, physical carcinogens may be synergistic with chemical carcinogens.

Radiation is the best known agent of physical carcinogenesis and is classified as ionizing radiation (x-rays, gamma rays, and alpha and beta particles) or nonionizing radiation (UV). The carcinogenic potential of ionizing radiation was recognized soon after Roentgen's discovery of x-rays in 1895. Within the next 20 years, a large number of radiation-related skin cancers were reported, and leukemia was reported in five radiation workers.[129] Long-term follow-up of survivors of the Hiroshima and Nagasaki atom bombs revealed that virtually all tissues exposed to radiation are at risk for cancer.

Radiation can induce a spectrum of DNA lesions that includes damage to the nucleotide bases, cross-linking, and DNA single- and double-strand breaks (DSBs).[130] Misrepaired DSBs are the principal lesions of importance in the induction of chromosomal abnormalities and gene mutations.[130] DSBs in irradiated cells are repaired primarily by a nonhomologous end-joining process, which is error prone, thus DSBs facilitate the production of chromosomal rearrangements and other large-scale changes such as chromosomal deletions. It is thought that radiation may initiate cancer by inactivating tumor suppressor genes. Activation of oncogenes appears to play a lesser role in radiation carcinogenesis.[130]

Although it has been assumed that the initial genetic events induced by radiation are direct mutagenesis from radiation, other indirect effects may contribute to carcinogenesis. For example, radiation induces genomic instability in cells that persists for at least 30 generations after irradiation.[130] Therefore, even if cells do not acquire mutations at initial irradiation, they remain at risk for developing new mutations for several generations. Moreover, even cells that have not been directly irradiated appear to be at risk, a phenomenon referred to as the "bystander effect."[130] Irradiated cells may secrete cytokines or other factors that increase production of reactive oxygen species in bystander cells, or alternatively, the bystander effect may involve cell-cell communication via gap junctions.[131,132]

Nonionizing UV radiation is a potent DNA-damaging agent and is known to induce skin cancer in experimental animals. Most nonmelanoma human skin cancers are thought to be induced by repeated exposure to sunlight, leading to a series of mutations that allow the cells to escape normal growth control. For example, mutations in the *ras* oncogene and in the tumor suppressors *p53* and *PTCH* have been identified in human skin cancers.[133] In most cases, the mutations induced by the UVB spectrum have been localized to pyrimidine-rich sequences, which indicate that these sites are probably the targets for UV-induced DNA damage and subsequent mutation and transformation.[134] Patients with inherited xeroderma pigmentosum lack one or more DNA-repair pathways, conferring susceptibility to UV-induced cancers, especially on sun-exposed body parts. Patients with ataxia telangiectasia mutated syndrome also have a radiation-sensitive phenotype.[135]

Viral Carcinogens

One of the first observations that cancer may be caused by transmissible agents was by Peyton Rous in 1911 when he demonstrated that

Table 9-10
Selected Viral Carcinogens[a]

Virus	Predominant Tumor Type[b]
Epstein-Barr virus	Burkitt's lymphoma
	Hodgkin's disease
	Immunosuppression-related lymphoma
	Sinonasal angiocentric T-cell lymphoma
	Nasopharyngeal carcinoma
Hepatitis B	Hepatocellular carcinoma
Hepatitis C	Hepatocellular carcinoma
Human immunodeficiency virus-1	Kaposi's sarcoma
	Non-Hodgkin's lymphoma
Human papillomavirus types 16 and 18	Cervical cancer
	Anal cancer
Human T-cell lymphotropic viruses	Adult T-cell leukemia/lymphoma

[a]Based on information in the International Agency for Research on Cancer Monographs.[137]

[b]Only tumor types for which causal relationships are established are listed. Other cancer types may be linked to the agents with a lower frequency or with insufficient data to prove causality.

cell-free extracts from sarcomas in chickens could transmit sarcomas to other animals injected with these extracts.[136] This was subsequently discovered to represent viral transmission of cancer by the Rous sarcoma virus (RSV). At present, several human viruses are known to have oncogenic properties, and several have been causally linked to human cancers (Table 9-10).[137] It is estimated that 15% of all human tumors worldwide are caused by viruses.[138]

Viruses may cause or increase the risk of malignancy through several mechanisms, including direct transformation, expression of oncogenes that interfere with cell-cycle checkpoints or DNA repair, expression of cytokines or other growth factors, and alteration of the immune system. Oncogenic viruses may be RNA or DNA viruses. Oncogenic RNA viruses are retroviruses and contain a reverse transcriptase. After the viral infection, the single-stranded RNA viral genome is transcribed into a double-stranded DNA copy, which is then integrated into the chromosomal DNA of the cell. Retroviral infection of the cell is permanent, thus integrated DNA sequences remain in the host chromosome. Oncogenic transforming retroviruses carry oncogenes derived from cellular genes. These cellular genes, referred to as protooncogenes, usually are involved in mitogenic signaling and growth control, and include protein kinases, G proteins, growth factors, and transcription factors (Table 9-11).[138]

Integration of the provirus upstream of a protooncogene may produce chimeric virus-cell transcripts and recombination during the next round of replication that could lead to incorporation of the cellular gene into the viral genome.[138] On the other hand, many retroviruses do not possess oncogenes, but can cause tumors in animals regardless. This occurs by integration of the provirus near a normal cellular protooncogene and activation of the expression of these genes by the strong promoter and enhancer sequences in the integrated viral sequence.

Unlike the oncogenes of the RNA viruses, those of the DNA tumor viruses are viral, not cellular in origin. These genes are required for viral replication utilizing the host cell machinery. In permissive hosts, infection with an oncogenic DNA virus may result in a productive lytic infection, leading to cell death and the release of newly formed viruses. In nonpermissive cells, the viral DNA can be integrated into the cellular chromosomal DNA, and some of the early viral genes can be synthesized persistently, leading to transformation

Table 9-11
Retroviruses Containing Cellular Oncogenes

Oncogene	Virus Name	Origin	Protein Product
abl	Abelson murine leukemia virus	Mouse	Tyrosine kinase
fes	ST feline sarcoma virus	Cat	Tyrosine kinase
fps	Fujinami sarcoma virus	Chicken	Tyrosine kinase
src	Rous sarcoma virus	Chicken	Tyrosine kinase
erbB	Avian erythroblastosis virus	Chicken	Epidermal growth factor receptor
fms	McDonough feline sarcoma virus	Cat	Colony-stimulating factor receptor
kit	Hardy-Zuckerman-4 feline sarcoma virus	Cat	Stem cell factor receptor
mil	Avian myelocytoma virus	Chicken	Serine/threonine kinase
mos	Moloney murine sarcoma virus	Mouse	Serine/threonine kinase
raf	Murine sarcoma virus 3611	Mouse	Serine/threonine kinase
sis	Simian sarcoma virus	Monkey	Platelet-derived growth factor
H-ras	Harvey murine sarcoma virus	Rat	GDP/GTP binding
K-ras	Kirsten murine sarcoma virus	Rat	GDP/GTP binding
erbA	Avian erythroblastosis virus	Chicken	Transcription factor (thyroid hormone receptor)
ets	Avian myeloblastosis virus E26	Chicken	Transcription factor
fos	FBJ osteosarcoma virus	Mouse	Transcription factor (AP1 component)
jun	Avian sarcoma virus-17	Chicken	Transcription factor (AP1 component)
myb	Avian myeloblastosis virus	Chicken	Transcription factor
myc	MC29 myelocytoma virus	Chicken	Transcription factor (NP-κB family)

GDP = guanosine diphosphate; GTP = guanosine triphosphate.

SOURCE: Modified with permission from Butel.[138]

of cells to a neoplastic state. The binding of viral oncoproteins to cellular tumor suppressor proteins *p53* and Rb is fundamental to the carcinogenesis induced by most DNA viruses, while others target different cellular proteins. DNA viruses have been shown to transactivate several cellular genes, including IL-6, c-*myc,* c-*jun,* c-*fos,* c-H-*ras,* inducible nitric oxide synthase, AP-1, AP-2, NF-κB, and SP1.[139]

Like other types of carcinogenesis, viral carcinogenesis is a multistep process. Some retroviruses contain two, rather than one, cellular oncogenes in their genome and are more rapidly tumorigenic than single-gene transforming retroviruses,[138] emphasizing the cooperation between transforming genes. Furthermore, some viruses encode genes that suppress or delay apoptosis, such as the adenovirus E1B-19K protein that is functionally similar to the Bcl-2 family of antiapoptotic proteins,[138,140] which may also play a critical role in transformation.

Although immunocompromised individuals are at elevated risk, most patients infected with oncogenic viruses do not develop cancer. When cancer does develop, it usually occurs several years after the viral infection. It is estimated, for example, that the risk of hepatocelluar carcinoma among hepatitis C virus–infected individuals is 1 to 3% after 30 years.[141] There may be synergy between various environmental factors and viruses in carcinogenesis. Factors that predispose to hepatocellular carcinoma among hepatitis C virus–infected patients include heavy alcohol intake, hepatitis B co-infection, and possibly diabetes.[141]

CANCER RISK ASSESSMENT

Cancer risk assessment is an important part of the initial evaluation of any patient. A patient's cancer risk is not only an important determinant of cancer screening recommendations but also may alter how aggressively an indeterminant finding will be pursued for diagnosis. A "probably benign" mammographic lesion, for example, defined as those with less than a 2% probability of malignancy (American College of Radiology category III), is usually managed with a 6-month follow-up mammogram in a patient at baseline cancer risk,[142] but

obtaining a tissue diagnosis may be preferable in a patient at high risk for breast cancer.

Cancer risk assessment starts with a complete history that includes history of environmental exposures to potential carcinogens and a detailed family history. Risk assessment for breast cancer, for example, includes a family history to determine whether another member of the family is known to carry a breast cancer susceptibility gene; whether there is familial clustering of breast cancer, ovarian cancer, thyroid cancer, sarcoma, adrenocortical carcinoma, endometrial cancer, brain tumors, dermatologic manifestations, leukemia, or lymphoma; and whether the patient is from a population at increased risk such as individuals of Ashkenazi Jewish descent.[143] Patients who have a family history suggestive of a cancer susceptibility syndrome such as hereditary breast ovarian syndrome, LFS, or CD would benefit from genetic counseling and possibly genetic testing.

Patients who do not seem to have a strong hereditary component of risk can be evaluated on the basis of their age, race, personal history, and exposures. One of the most commonly used models for risk assessment in breast cancer is the Gail model.[144] Gail and colleagues analyzed the data from 2852 breast cancer cases and 3146 controls from the Breast Cancer Detection and Demonstration Project, a mammography screening project conducted in the 1970s, and developed a model for projecting breast cancer incidence. The model uses risk factors such as an individual's age, age at menarche, age at first live birth, number of first-degree relatives with breast cancer, number of previous breast biopsies, and whether the biopsies revealed atypical ductal hyperplasia (Table 9-12). The National Cancer Institute (NCI) and the National Surgical Adjuvant Breast and Bowel Project (NSABP) Biostatistics Center developed a breast cancer risk assessment tool, which is available on the World Wide Web, that is based on the Gail model.[145] This tool incorporates the risk factors utilized in the Gail model, as well as race and ethnicity, and allows a health professional to project a woman's individualized estimated risk for invasive breast cancer over a 5-year period and over her lifetime (to age 90 years). Notably, these risk projections assume that the woman is undergoing regular clinical

Table 9-12
Assessment of Risk for Invasive Breast Cancer

Risk Factor	Relative Risk
Age at menarche (years)	
>14	1.00
12–13	1.10
<12	1.21
Age at first live birth (years)	
Patients with no first-degree relatives with cancer	
<20	1.00
20–24	1.24
25–29 or nulliparous	1.55
≥30	1.93
Patients with one first degree-relative with cancer	
<20	1.00
20–24	2.64
25–29 or nulliparous	2.76
≥30	2.83
Patients with ≥2 first-degree relatives with cancer	
<20	6.80
20–24	5.78
25–29 or nulliparous	4.91
≥30	4.17
Breast biopsies (n)	
Patients aged <50 years at counseling	
0	1.00
1	1.70
≥2	2.88
Patients aged ≥50 years at counseling	
0	1.00
1	1.27
≥2	1.62
Atypical hyperplasia	
No biopsies	1.00
At least 1 biopsy, no atypical hyperplasia	0.93
No atypical hyperplasia, hyperplasia status unknown for at least 1 biopsy	1.00
Atypical hyperplasia in at least 1 biopsy	1.82

SOURCE: Modified with permission from Gail et al.[144]

breast exams and screening mammograms. Also of note is that this program underestimates the risk for women who have already had a diagnosis of invasive or noninvasive breast cancer, and does not take into account specific genetic predispositions such as mutations in *BRCA1* or *BRCA2*. However, these risk assessment tools have been validated[146,147] and are now in widespread clinical use. Similar models are in development or being validated for other cancers. For example, a lung cancer risk prediction model, which includes age, sex, asbestos exposure history, and smoking history, has been found to predict risk of lung cancer.[148]

CANCER SCREENING

Early detection is the key to success in cancer therapy. Screening for common cancers using relatively noninvasive tests is expected to lead to early diagnosis, allow more conservative surgical therapies with decreased morbidity, and potentially improve surgical cure rates and overall survival rates. Key factors that influence screening guidelines are the prevalence of the cancer in the population, the risk associated with the screening measure, and whether early diagnosis actually affects outcome. The value of a widespread screening measure is likely to go up with the prevalence of the cancer in a population, often determining the age cutoffs for screening, and explaining

why only common cancers are screened for. The risks involved with the screening measure are a significant consideration, especially with more invasive screening measures such as colonoscopy. The consequences of a false-positive screening test also need to be considered. For example, when 1000 screening mammograms are performed, only two to four new incidences of cancer will be identified[149]; this number is slightly higher (six to 10 prevalent cancers per 1000 mammograms) in the initial screening mammograms performed. However, as many as 10% of screening mammograms may be potentially suggestive of abnormality, requiring further imaging (i.e., a 10% recall rate). Of those women with abnormal mammograms, only 5 to 10% will be determined to have a breast cancer. Among women for whom biopsy is recommended, 25 to 40% will have a breast cancer. A false-positive screen is likely to induce significant emotional distress in patients, leads to unnecessary biopsies, and has cost implications for the health care system.

The 2003 American Cancer Society guidelines for the early detection of cancer are listed in Table 9-13.[150] These guidelines are updated periodically to incorporate emerging technologies and new data on the efficacy of screening measures. For example, the 2003 guidelines incorporated immunochemical fecal occult blood tests (FOBT), as it was felt that the lack of dietary restrictions associated with the test made it more acceptable to the subjects than the guaiac-based tests, and the FOBT is likely to have equal or better sensitivity and specificity.[150] In contrast, evidence was insufficient to support the use of highly publicized emerging technologies such as CT colonography for routine screening.

Besides the American Cancer Society, several other professional bodies make recommendations for screening. For example, clinical guidelines for colorectal cancer screening have been developed by the American College of Gastroenterology, U.S. Preventive Services Task Force, and a Multidisciplinary Expert Panel.[151] Although these screening guidelines differ somewhat, most organizations do not emphasize one screening strategy as superior to another, but all emphasize the importance of screening for individuals aged 50 years and older.

Screening guidelines are developed for the general baseline-risk population. These guidelines need to be modified for patients who are at high risk. For example, more intensive colorectal cancer screening is recommended for individuals at increased risk because of a history of adenomatous polyps, a personal history of colorectal cancer, a family history of either colorectal cancer or colorectal adenomas diagnosed in a first-degree relative before age 60 years, personal history of inflammatory bowel disease of significant duration, or family history of FAP or HNPCC.[150]

CANCER DIAGNOSIS

The definitive diagnosis of solid tumors is usually obtained with a biopsy of the lesion. Biopsy determines the tumor histology and grade and thus assists in definitive therapeutic planning. When a biopsy has been obtained at an outside institution, the slides should be reviewed to confirm the outside diagnosis.

Biopsies of mucosal lesions usually are obtained endoscopically (e.g., via colonoscope, bronchoscope, or cystoscope). Lesions that are easily palpable, such as those of the skin, can either be excised or sampled by punch biopsy. Deep-seated lesions can be localized with CT scan or ultrasound guidance for biopsy.

A sample of a lesion can be obtained with a needle or with an open incisional or excisional biopsy. Fine-needle aspiration is easy and relatively safe, but has the disadvantage of not giving information

Table 9-13

American Cancer Society Recommendations for Early Detection of Cancer in Average-Risk, Asymptomatic People

Cancer Site	Population	Test or Procedure	Frequency
Breast	Women, age 20+	Breast self-examination	Monthly, starting at age 20
		Clinical breast examination	Every 3 years, ages 20–39
			Annual, starting at age 40
		Mammography	Annual, starting at age 40
Colorectal	Men and women, age 50+	Fecal occult blood test (FOBT) *or*	Annual, starting at age 20
		Flexible sigmoidoscopy *or*	Every 5 years, starting at age 50
		Fecal occult blood test and flexible sigmoidoscopy *or*	Annual FOBT and flexible sigmoidoscopy every 5 years, starting at age 50
		Double-contrast barium enema (DCBE) *or*	DCBE every 5 years, starting at age 50
		Colonoscopy	Colonoscopy every 10 years, starting at age 50
Prostate	Men, age 50+	Digital rectal examination (DRE) and prostate-specific antigen test (PSA)	Offer PSA and DRE annually, starting at age 50, for men who have life expectancy of at least 10 years
Cervix	Women	Pap test	Cervical cancer screening beginning 3 years after first vaginal intercourse, but no later than 21 years of age; screening every year with conventional Pap tests or every 2 years using liquid-based Pap tests; at or after age 30, women who have had three or more normal Pap tests and no abnormal Pap tests in the last 10 years, and women who have had a total hysterectomy, may choose to stop cervical cancer screening
Cancer-related check-up	Men and women, age 20+	On the occasion of a periodic health examination, the cancer-related check-up should include examination of the thyroid, testicles, ovaries, lymph nodes, oral cavity, and skin, as well as health counseling about tobacco, sun exposure, diet and nutrition, risk factors, sexual practices, and environmental and occupational exposures.	

SOURCE: Modified with permission from Smith et al.[150]

on tissue architecture. For example, fine-needle aspiration biopsy of a breast mass can make the diagnosis of malignancy, but cannot differentiate between an invasive and noninvasive tumor. Therefore core-needle biopsy is more advantageous when the histology will affect the recommended therapy. Core biopsy, like fine-needle aspiration, is relatively safe and can be performed either by direct palpation (e.g., a breast mass or a soft-tissue mass) or can be guided by an imaging study (e.g., stereotactic core biopsy of the breast). Core biopsies, like fine-needle aspirations, have the disadvantage of introducing sampling error. For example, 19 to 44% of patients with a diagnosis of atypical ductal hyperplasia on core biopsy of a mammographic abnormality are found to have carcinoma upon excision of the lesion.[152] It is crucial to ensure that the histologic findings are consistent with the clinical scenario, and to know the appropriate interpretation of each histologic finding. A needle biopsy in which the report is inconsistent with the clinical scenario should be either repeated or followed by an open biopsy.

Open biopsies have the advantage of providing more tissue for histologic evaluation and the disadvantage of being an operative procedure. Incisional biopsies are reserved for very large lesions in which a definitive diagnosis cannot be made with needle biopsy. Excisional biopsies are performed for lesions in which core biopsy is either not possible or is nondiagnostic. Excisional biopsies should be performed with curative intent, that is, by obtaining adequate tissue around the lesion to ensure negative surgical margins. Orientation of the margins by sutures or clips by the surgeon and inking of the specimen margins by the pathologist will allow for determination of the surgical margins and will guide surgical re-excision if one or more of the margins are positive for microscopic tumor or close. The biopsy incision should be oriented to allow for excision of the biopsy scar if repeat operation is necessary. Furthermore, the biopsy incision should directly overlie the area to be removed rather than tunneling from another site, which runs the risk of contaminating a larger field. Finally, meticulous hemostasis during a biopsy is essential, since a hematoma can lead to contamination of the tissue planes and can make subsequent follow-up with physical examinations much more challenging.

CANCER STAGING

Cancer staging is a system used to describe the anatomic extent of a malignant process in an individual patient. Staging systems may incorporate relevant clinical prognostic factors such as tumor size, location, extent, grade, and dissemination to regional lymph nodes or distant sites. Accurate staging is essential in designing an appropriate treatment regimen for an individual patient. Staging of the lymph node basin is considered a standard part of primary surgical therapy for most surgical procedures, and is discussed later in this chapter. Cancer patients who are considered to be at high risk for distant metastasis usually undergo a preoperative staging work-up. This involves a set of imaging studies of sites of preferential metastasis for a given cancer type. For example, for a patient with breast cancer, a staging work-up would include a chest x-ray, bone scan, and liver ultrasound or CT scan of the abdomen to evaluate for lung, bone, and liver metastases, respectively. A staging work-up is usually performed only for patients likely to have metastasis on the basis of their primary tumor characteristics; for example, a staging work-up in a patient with ductal carcinoma in situ of the breast or a small invasive breast tumor is likely to be low yield and not cost-effective.

Standardization of staging systems is essential to allow for comparison of different studies from different institutions and worldwide. The staging systems proposed by the American Joint

Table 9-14
Melanoma Staging Sites

Primary Tumor (T)

TX	Primary tumor cannot be assessed (e.g., shave biopsy or regressed melanoma)
T0	No evidence of primary tumor
Tis	Melanoma in situ
T1	Melanoma ≤ 1.0 mm in thickness with or without ulceration
T1a	Melanoma ≤ 1.0 mm in thickness and level II or III, no ulceration
T1b	Melanoma ≤ 1.0 mm in thickness and level IV or with ulceration
T2	Melanoma 1.01–2 mm in thickness with or without ulceration
T2a	Melanoma 1.01–2.0 mm in thickness, no ulceration
T2b	Melanoma 1.01–2.0 mm in thickness, with ulceration
T3	Melanoma 2.01–4 mm in thickness with or without ulceration
T3a	Melanoma 2.01–4.0 mm in thickness, no ulceration
T3b	Melanoma 2.01–4.0 mm in thickness, with ulceration
T4	Melanoma greater than 4.0 mm in thickness with or without ulceration
T4a	Melanoma >4.0 mm in thickness, no ulceration
T4b	Melanoma >4.0 mm in thickness, with ulceration

Regional Lymph Nodes (N)

NX	Regional lymph nodes cannot be assessed
N0	No regional lymph node metastasis
N1	Metastasis in one lymph node
N1a	Clinically occult (microscopic) metastasis
N1b	Clinically apparent (macroscopic) metastasis
N2	Metastasis in two to three regional nodes or intralymphatic regional metastasis without nodal metastases
N2a	Clinically occult (microscopic) metastasis
N2b	Clinically apparent (macroscopic) metastasis
N2c	Satellite or in-transit metastasis *without* nodal metastasis
N3	Metastasis in four or more regional nodes, or matted metastatic nodes, or satellite(s) *with* metastasis in regional node(s)

Distant Metastasis (M)

MX	Distant metastasis cannot be assessed
M0	No distant metastasis
M1	Distant metastasis
M1a	Metastasis to skin, subcutaneous tissues, or distant lymph nodes
M1b	Metastasis to lung
M1c	Metastasis to all other visceral sites or distant metastasis at any site associated with an elevated serum lactate dehydrogenase (LDH)

Clinical Stage Grouping

Stage 0	Tis	N0	M0
Stage IA	T1a	N0	M0
Stage IB	T1b	N0	M0
	T2a	N0	M0
Stage IIA	T2b	N0	M0
	T3a	N0	M0
Stage IIB	T3b	N0	M0
	T4a	N0	M0
Stage IIC	T4b	N0	M0
Stage III	Any T	N1	M0
	Any T	N2	M0
	Any T	N3	M0
Stage IV	Any T	Any N	M1

Pathologic Stage Grouping

Stage 0	Tis	N0	M0
Stage IA	T1a	N0	M0
Stage IB	T1b	N0	M0
	T2a	N0	M0
Stage IIA	T2b	N0	M0
	T3a	N0	M0
Stage IIB	T3b	N0	M0
	T4a	N0	M0
Stage IIC	T4b	N0	M0
Stage IIIA	T1-4a	N1a	M0
	T1-4a	N2a	M0
Stage IIIB	T1-4b	N1a	M0
	T1-4b	N2a	M0
	T1-4a	N1b	M0
	T1-4a	N2b	M0
	T1-4a/b	N2c	M0
Stage IIIC	T1-4b	N1b	M0
	T1-4b	N2b	M0
	Any T	N3	M0
Stage IV	Any T	Any N	M1

SOURCE: Modified with permission from Greene et al.[153]

Committee on Cancer (AJCC) and the Union Internationale Contre Cancer (International Union Against Cancer, UICC) are among the most widely accepted staging systems. Both the AJCC and the UICC have adopted a shared TNM staging system that defines the cancer in terms of the anatomic extent of disease and is based on assessment of three components: the primary tumor (T), the presence (or absence) and extent of nodal metastases (N), and the presence (or absence) and extent of distant metastases (M). The TNM staging system implemented in the sixth edition of the AJCC Staging System, which took effect in January 2003, is shared by the AJCC and UICC.

The TNM staging applies only to cases that have been microscopically confirmed to be malignant. Standard TNM staging (clinical and pathologic) is completed at initial diagnosis. The timeline for staging is through the first course of surgery or 4 months, whichever is longer.[153] Clinical staging (cTNM or TNM) is based on information gained up until the initial definitive treatment. Pathologic staging (pTNM) includes clinical information and information obtained from pathologic examination of the resected primary tumor and regional lymph nodes. Other classifications, such as re-treatment (rTNM) or autopsy staging (aTNM), should be clearly identified as such.

The clinical measurement of tumor size (T) is the one judged to be the most accurate for each individual case based on physical examination and imaging studies. For example, in breast cancer the size of the tumor could be obtained from a physical exam, mammogram, or ultrasound. The tumor size is based only on the invasive component; therefore if a patient has a 0.4-cm invasive breast cancer with 5 cm of associated ductal carcinoma in situ, the tumor is still classified as a T1a tumor, which refers to a tumor more than 0.1 cm but not more than 0.5 cm in greatest dimension.[153]

If even one lymph node is involved by tumor, the N component is at least N1. For many solid tumor types, simply the absence or presence of lymph node involvement is recorded and the tumor is categorized either as N0 or N1. For other tumor types, the number of lymph nodes involved, the size of the lymph nodes or the lymph node metastasis, or the regional lymph node basin involved also has been shown to have prognostic value. In these cancers, N1, N2, N3, or N4 suggests an increasing abnormality of lymph nodes based on size, characteristics, and location. NX indicates that the lymph nodes cannot be fully assessed.

Cases in which there is no distant metastasis are designated M0, cases in which one or more distant metastases are detected are designated M1, and cases in which the presence of distant metastasis cannot be assessed are designated MX. In clinical practice, negative findings on clinical history and examination are sufficient to designate a case as M0. However, in clinical trials, routine follow-up staging work-ups often are performed to standardize the detection of distant metastases.

The practice of dividing cancer cases into groups according to stage is based on the observation that the survival rates are higher for localized (lower stage) tumors than for tumors that have extended beyond the organ of origin. Therefore staging is used to analyze and compare groups of patients. Such staging assists in (1) selection of therapy, (2) estimation of prognosis, (3) evaluation of treatments, (4) exchange of information among treatment centers, and (5) continued investigation of human cancers.[153] As an example, the melanoma staging system is shown in Table 9-14. This staging system can distinguish different prognostic groups on the basis of 15-year survival curves (Fig. 9-8). Notably, the AJCC regularly updates its staging system to incorporate advances in prognostic technology in order to improve the predictive accuracy of the TNM

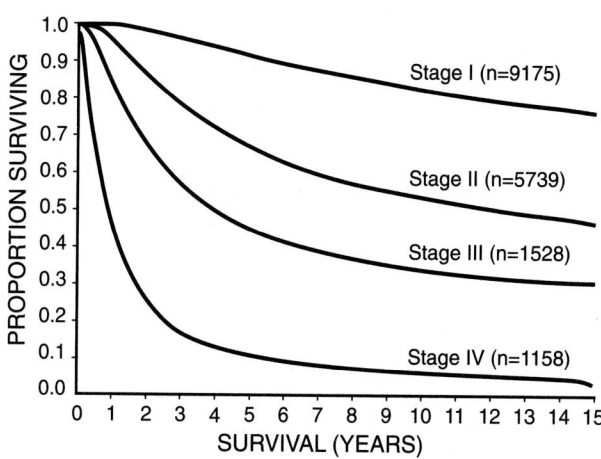

FIG. 9-8. Fifteen-year survival curves for the melanoma staging system, comparing survival rates for localized melanoma (stages I and II), regional metastases (stage III), and distant metastases (stage IV). The numbers in parentheses are the numbers of patients from the American Joint Committee on Cancer (AJCC) melanoma staging database used to calculate the survival rates. The differences between the curves are highly significant (p < 0.0001). (Modified from Greene et al,[153] with permission.)

system. Therefore it is important to know which revision of a staging system is being used when evaluating studies.

TUMOR MARKERS

Prognostic and Predictive Tissue Markers

Tumor markers are substances that can be detected in higher than normal amounts in the serum, urine, nipple aspirate fluid, or tissues of patients with certain types of cancer. Tumors markers are produced either by the cancer cells themselves or by the body as a response to the cancer.

Over the past decade, there has been an especially large interest in identifying tissue tumor markers that can be used as prognostic or predictive markers. Although the terms *prognostic marker* and *predictive marker* are sometimes used interchangeably, the term prognostic marker usually is used to describe molecular markers that predict disease-free survival, disease-specific survival, and overall survival, while the term predictive marker is often used in the context of predicting response to certain therapies.

The goal is to identify prognostic markers that can give information on prognosis independent of other clinical characteristics, and therefore can provide information in addition to what can be projected on the basis of clinical presentation. This would allow us to further classify patients as being at higher or lower risk within clinical subgroups and to identify patients who may benefit most from adjuvant therapy. Ideally, prognostic tumor markers would be able to help determine which group of patients with node-negative breast cancer is at higher risk of relapse and thus provide adjuvant systemic therapy only to that group. Thousands of papers have been published regarding potential prognostic tumor markers for breast cancer. Some of these proposed markers are listed in Table 9-15. Unfortunately, most of the studies are retrospective, have small sample sizes and differing endpoints, and use different methods of marker detection. In a review of studies with sample sizes greater than 200 and follow-up more than 5 years, Mirza and colleagues concluded that tumor grade, Ki-67, S-phase fraction, mitotic index, cathepsin-D, and vascular invasion showed a significant association with survival

Table 9-15
Potential Prognostic Markers for Breast Cancer

Tumor characteristics
  Tumor grade
  Tumor histology
  Lymphovascular invasion
Hormone receptors
  Estrogen receptor
  Progesterone receptor
Cell-cycle and proliferation markers
  Ki-67
  Proliferating cell nuclear antigen
  Ploidy
  Thymidine-labeling index
  S-phase fraction
  Cyclin D1
  Cyclin E
  Cyclin A
  p21
Proteases and their inhibitors
  Cathepsin-D
  Urokinase-type plasminogen activator
  PAI-1
  Matrix metalloproteinases
Angiogenesis
  Microvessel density
  Vascular endothelial growth factor
Growth factors and signal transduction molecules
  HER2/*neu*
  Epidermal growth factor receptor
  Transforming growth factor-α
  Insulin-like growth factor
  Insulin-like growth factor binding protein
  Phosphorylated Akt
Tumor suppressor genes
  p53
  Rb
  PTEN
Apoptosis-related factors
  Apoptotic index
  Bcl-2

Table 9-16
Sensitivity and Specificity of Some Common Tumor Markers

Marker	Cancer	Sensitivity	Specificity
Prostate-specific antigen (4 μg/L)	Prostate	57–93%	55–68%
Carcinoembryonic antigen	Colorectal	40–47%	90%
	Breast	45%	81%
	Recurrent disease	84%	100%
Alpha-fetoprotein	Hepatocellular	98%	65%
CA 19.9	Pancreatic	78–90%	95%
CA 27.29	Breast	62%	83%
CA 15.3	Breast	57%	87%

SOURCE: Adapted from Laboratory Medicine Newsletter.[156]

Serum Markers

Serum markers are under active investigation as they may allow early diagnosis of a new cancer or may be used to follow a cancer's response to therapy or monitor for recurrence. Unfortunately, identification of serum markers of clinical value has been challenging. Many of the tumor markers proposed so far have had low sensitivities and specificities (Table 9-16).[156] Tumor markers may not be elevated in all patients with cancer, especially in the early stages, when a serum marker would be most useful for diagnosis. Therefore when using a tumor marker to monitor recurrence, it is important to be certain that the tumor marker was elevated prior to primary therapy. Moreover, tumor markers can be elevated in benign conditions. Many tumor markers are not specific for a certain type of cancer and can be elevated with more than one type of tumor. Because there may be significant laboratory variability, it is important to obtain serial results from the same laboratory.[157] In spite of these many clinical limitations, several serum markers are in clinical use. A few of the commonly measured serum tumor markers are discussed below.

Prostate-Specific Antigen

Prostate-specific antigen (PSA) is potentially the best serum marker now available. PSA is an androgen-regulated serine protease produced by the prostate epithelium. PSA is normally present in low concentrations in the blood of all adult males. PSA levels may be elevated in the blood of men with benign prostate conditions such as prostatitis and benign prostatic hyperplasia, as well as in men with prostate cancer.[158] PSA levels have been shown to be useful in monitoring the effectiveness of prostate cancer treatment and for recurrence after therapy. In monitoring for recurrence, a trend of increasing levels is considered more significant than a single absolute elevated value.

Although PSA is widely used for prostate cancer screening in the United States,[159] and the American Urologic Association and the American Cancer Society both recommend yearly PSA levels for men aged 50 years and older with a life expectancy of greater than 10 years, a specified indication level to initiate a work-up, an interval at which to obtain PSA levels, and the utility of PSA screening all remain controversial. Results of a large, multicenter study suggested that a serum total PSA level of 4 ng/mL should be used as a threshold for prostate biopsies,[160] but 20 to 50% of clinically significant prostate cancers occur in men with total serum PSA levels less than 4 ng/mL.[161] Others have suggested that biennial PSA screening is sufficient to detect almost all prostate cancers while curable and that the screening interval can be altered on the basis of PSA level.[162] Finally, although the use of serum

outcomes. However, HER2/*neu* status and DNA ploidy showed no association. Estrogen receptor status and *p53* status yielded mixed results.[154] The 2000 update of the American Society of Clinical Oncology (ASCO) Clinical Practice Guidelines state that the data were insufficient to recommend the routine use of DNA flow cytometry-derived parameters, *p53* status, and cathepsin-D.[155] However, the same publication recommended that estrogen and progesterone receptors and HER2/*neu* be measured in every patient with primary breast cancer. Interestingly, the data were deemed insufficient to allow recommendation that HER2/*neu* be used as a prognostic marker. Thus these recommendations were made not only on the basis of the prognostic value of these markers but also on their value as predictive markers.

Predictive markers are markers that can prospectively identify patients who will benefit from a certain therapy. Some of the best predictive markers are estrogen receptor and HER2/*neu*, which can identify patients who can benefit from antiestrogen therapies (e.g., tamoxifen) and anti-HER2/*neu* therapies (e.g., trastuzumab), respectively. There is increasing interest in identifying predictive markers for chemotherapy so that patients can be given the regimens they are most likely to benefit from, while those who are not likely to benefit from existing conventional therapies can be spared the toxicity of the therapy and be offered investigational therapies.

PSA screening does lead to earlier prostate cancer detection,[161] it remains to be demonstrated that this translates into a survival benefit.[163,164] In fact, the European Committee of Cancer Screening has concluded that the evidence does not support the introduction of population-based PSA screening in Europe.[165] The efficacy of PSA as a screening tool is being evaluated in two randomized controlled trials,[163] and it is hoped that these will answer this question.

Carcinoembryonic Antigen

Carcinoembryonic antigen (CEA) is a glycoprotein found in the embryonic endodermal epithelium. Elevated CEA levels have been detected in patients with primary colorectal cancer, as well as patients with breast, lung, ovarian, prostate, liver, or pancreatic cancer. Levels of CEA also may be elevated in benign conditions such as diverticulitis, peptic ulcer disease, bronchitis, liver abscess, and alcoholic cirrhosis, especially in smokers and in elderly persons.

CEA is most commonly used for the management of colorectal cancer. However, the appropriate use of CEA in patients with colorectal cancer has been debated.[166,167] Use of CEA levels as a screening test for colorectal cancer is not recommended.[155] CEA levels may be useful if obtained preoperatively and postoperatively in patients with a diagnosis of colorectal cancer. Preoperative elevation of CEA is an indicator of poor prognosis. Patients with CEA levels greater than 5 ng/mL before surgery have been found to have an almost fourfold relative risk of recurrence.[167] However, the ASCO Clinical Practice Guidelines state that the data are insufficient to support the use of CEA to determine whether to give a patient adjuvant therapy,[155] but the data are stronger for the use of CEA for monitoring for postoperative recurrence. Serial CEA measurements can detect recurrent colorectal cancer with a sensitivity of 80% and specificity of 70% and provide a lead time of 5 months.[168] CEA is the most cost-effective approach to detecting metastasis, with 64% of recurrences being detected first by an elevation in CEA level.[155] Therefore, if resection of recurrent colorectal cancer would be clinically indicated, ASCO guidelines recommend that postoperative CEA testing be performed every 2 to 3 months in patients with stage II or III disease for 2 or more years after diagnosis.[155]

There is interest in using CEA levels for monitoring patients with breast cancer. Incidence of elevated CEA level increases with increasing stage of breast cancer. CEA levels are elevated in 10% of women with stage I breast cancer, 19% of women with stage II disease, 31% of women with stage III disease, and 64% of women with stage IV disease.[155] Elevated CEA levels have been reported before breast cancer relapse in 46% of patients, with a lead time of 4.9 months.[169] However, elevated CEA levels have a 12% false-positive rate. The ASCO guidelines state that the routine use of CEA for screening, diagnosis, staging, or surveillance of breast cancer is not recommended because available data are insufficient.[155]

Alpha-Fetoprotein

Alpha-fetoprotein (AFP) is a glycoprotein normally produced by a developing fetus. AFP levels decrease soon after birth to around 10 ng/mL in healthy adults.[170] An elevated level of AFP suggests the presence of either primary liver cancer or a germ cell tumor of the ovary or testicle. Rarely, other types of cancer such as gastric cancer are associated with an elevated AFP level.[158] Benign conditions that can cause elevations of AFP include cirrhosis, hepatic necrosis, acute hepatitis, chronic active hepatitis, ataxia-telangiectasia, Wiskott-Aldrich syndrome, and pregnancy.[158,171]

AFP is considered to be sensitive and specific enough to be used for screening for hepatocellular carcinoma (HCC) in high-risk populations. Current consensus recommendations are to screen healthy hepatitis B virus carriers with annual or semiannual AFP levels, and to screen carriers with cirrhosis or chronic hepatitis and patients with cirrhosis of any etiology with twice-yearly AFP levels and liver ultrasounds.[172] Although AFP has been used widely for a long time, its efficacy in early diagnosis of HCC is limited. With improvements in imaging technology, a larger proportion of patients diagnosed with HCC are now AFP-seronegative. For example, 64.6% of patients diagnosed with HCC in Japan in 1996 and 1997 had a serum AFP level greater than 20 ng/mL, compared with 81.1% of the patients diagnosed in 1980 and 1981.[170]

Cancer Antigen 15-3

Cancer antigen 15-3 (CA 15-3) is an epitope of a large membrane glycoprotein, encoded by the *MUC1* gene, which tumor cells shed into the bloodstream. The CA 15-3 epitope is recognized by two monoclonal antibodies in a sandwich radioimmunoassay. CA 15-3 levels are most useful in following the course of treatment in women diagnosed with advanced breast cancer. The CA 15-3 levels are infrequently elevated in early breast cancer. Only 9% of patients with stage I breast cancer and 19% of women with stage II cancer have elevated CA 15-3 levels.[155] The predictive value of a positive test result is calculated to be 0.7% for stage I disease and 1.5% for stage II disease[155] emphasizing that CA 15-3 is not an appropriate screening tool. CA 15-3 levels can be elevated in benign conditions such as chronic hepatitis, tuberculosis, sarcoidosis, pelvic inflammatory disease, endometriosis, systemic lupus erythematosus, pregnancy and lactation, and in other types of cancer such as lung, ovarian, endometrial, and gastrointestinal cancers.

The sensitivity of CA 15-3 is higher for metastatic disease, and studies have shown it to be between 54 and 87%, with specificity as high as 96%. This has led to interest in using CA 15-3 for monitoring patients with advanced breast cancer for recurrence. Elevated CA 15-3 levels have been reported before relapse in 54% of patients, with a lead time of 4.2 months.[169] Therefore, detection of elevated CA 15-3 levels during follow-up should prompt evaluation for recurrent disease. However, 6 to 8% of patients without recurrence will have elevated CA 15-3 levels that require evaluation. Moreover, monitoring with CA 15-3 has had no demonstrated impact on survival. Therefore, the ASCO guidelines state that the routine use of CA 15-3 for screening, diagnosis, staging, or surveillance of breast cancer is not recommended because available data are insufficient.[155]

Cancer Antigen 27-29

The *MUC-1* gene product in the serum may be quantitated by using radioimmunoassay with a monoclonal antibody against the cancer antigen 27-29 (CA 27-29). CA 27-29 levels can be elevated in breast cancer as well as in cancers of the colon, stomach, kidney, lung, ovary, pancreas, uterus, and liver.[158] First-trimester pregnancy, endometriosis, benign breast disease, kidney disease, and liver disease also may be associated with elevated CA 27-29 levels.

CA 27-29 has been reported to have a sensitivity of 57%, a specificity of 98%, a positive predictive value of 83%, and a negative predictive value of 93% in detecting breast cancer recurrences.[173] Although CA 27-29 was found to predict recurrence an average of 5.3 months before other symptoms or tests,[173] no effect on disease-free and overall survival rates has been demonstrated.[174] Therefore, the ASCO guidelines state that, like CA 15-3, the routine use of CA

27-29 for screening, diagnosis, staging, or surveillance of breast cancer is not recommended because available data are insufficient.[155]

Circulating HER2/neu Extracellular Domain

The extracellular domain (ECD) of the HER2/*neu* oncogene can be measured in the circulation. Because of the known role of HER2/neu overexpression in breast cancer biology, there has been a large amount of interest in determining the utility of circulating HER2/neu ECD as a prognostic and predictive marker. Levels of HER2/neu ECD were elevated in 35 to 40% of patients with metastatic breast cancer in one study, and elevated levels have been associated with a poor prognosis.[175] The predictive role of HER2/neu ECD has been controversial.[175–177] Elevated HER2/neu ECD levels are associated with overexpression of HER2/neu in the tumor.[177] Thus HER2/neu ECD monitoring is likely to be helpful only in HER2/neu-overexpressing tumors, if at all. As a prognostic or predictive marker, the added value of measuring HER2/neu ECD in addition to HER2/neu in the primary tumor is unclear. Furthermore, data supporting the use of HER2/neu ECD to monitor for recurrence of HER2/neu-overexpressing tumors are limited.[178] Therefore, at this time the data are limited to support the routine use of HER2/neu ECD for cancer screening, diagnosis, staging, or surveillance.[155]

Circulating Cancer Cells

It has been suggested that circulating cancer cells can be an effective tool in selecting patients who have a high risk of relapse. One methodology widely used to detect cancer cells in the peripheral blood is reverse transcriptase (RT)-PCR. The use of this methodology to detect circulating cancer cells as a prognostic marker is under active investigation by many groups; however, its high sensitivity and potential for contamination leading to false-positive results has made investigation especially challenging. Data to support its use clinically are limited. In a recent study semiquantitative RT-PCR for three melanoma markers (tyrosinase, p97, and MelanA/MAET1) was used to detect circulating melanoma cells. Investigators concluded that detection of circulating melanoma cells has no additional prognostic value.[179]

SURGICAL APPROACHES TO CANCER THERAPY

Multidisciplinary Approach to Cancer

Although surgery is the most effective therapy for most solid tumors, most patients die of metastatic disease. Therefore to improve patient survival rates, a multimodality approach with systemic therapy and radiation therapy is key for most tumors. It is important that surgeons involved in cancer care know not only how to perform a cancer operation but also the alternatives to surgery and be well versed in reconstructive options. It is also crucial that the surgeon be familiar with the indications for and complications of preoperative and postoperative chemotherapy and radiation therapy. Although the surgeon will not be delivering these other therapies, as the first physician to see a patient with a cancer diagnosis, he or she is ultimately responsible for initiating the appropriate consultations. As such, the surgeon often is responsible for determining the most appropriate adjuvant therapy for a given patient, as well as the best sequence for therapy. In most instances, a multidisciplinary approach beginning at the patient's initial presentation is likely to yield the best result.

Surgical Management of Primary Tumors

The goal of surgical therapy for cancer is to achieve oncologic cure. A curative operation presupposes that the tumor is confined to the organ of origin, or to the organ and the regional lymph node basin. Patients in whom the primary tumor is not resectable with negative surgical margins are considered to have inoperable disease. The operability of primary tumors is best determined before surgery with appropriate imaging studies that can define the extent of local-regional disease. For example, a preoperative thin-section CT scan is obtained to determine resectability for pancreatic cancer, which is based on the absence of extrapancreatic disease, the absence of tumor extension to the superior mesenteric artery and celiac axis, and a patent superior mesenteric vein–portal vein confluence.[180] Disease involving multiple distant metastases is deemed inoperable since it is usually not curable with surgery of the primary tumor. Therefore patients who are at high risk of having distant metastasis should have a staging work-up prior to surgery for their primary tumor. On occasion, primary tumors are resected in these patients for palliative reasons, such as improving the quality of life by alleviating pain, infection, or bleeding. An example of this is toilet mastectomies for large ulcerated breast tumors. Patients with limited metastases from a primary tumor on occasion are considered surgical candidates if the natural history of isolated distant metastases for that cancer type is favorable, or the potential complications associated with leaving the primary tumor intact are significant.

In the past it was presumed that the more radical the surgery, the better the oncologic outcome would be. Over the past 20 years, this has been recognized as not necessarily being true, leading to more conservative operations, with wide local excisions replacing compartmental resections of sarcomas; and partial mastectomies, skin-sparing mastectomies, and breast-conserving therapies replacing radical mastectomies for breast cancer. The uniform goal for all successful oncologic operations seems to be achieving widely negative margins with no evidence of macroscopic or microscopic tumor at the surgical margins. For example, positive surgical margins have been shown to be a predictor of systemic recurrence and poor disease-specific survival rates after breast-conserving therapy for invasive breast cancer (Fig. 9-9).[181] This may be because the residual tumor at the primary tumor site is a source for systemic

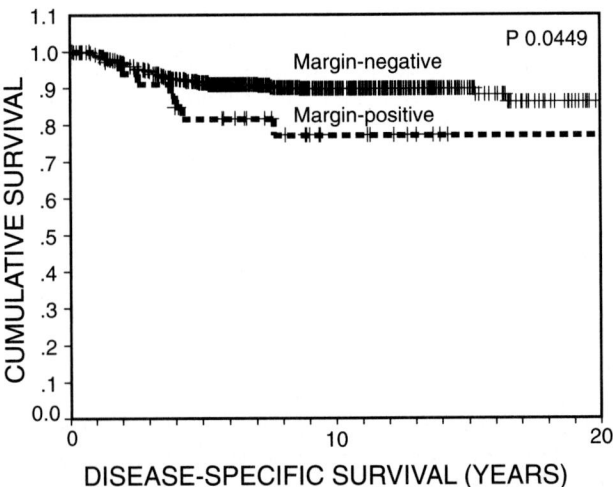

FIG. 9-9. Disease-specific survival in patients who had negative surgical margins and patients who had positive margins with breast-conserving surgery. (*Modified from Meric et al,*[181] *with permission.*)

spread of the tumor besides increasing the risk of local recurrence of the tumor. The importance of negative surgical margins for local tumor control and/or survival has been documented repeatedly for several other tumor types, including sarcoma, pancreatic cancer, and rectal cancer.[182–186] Thus it is clear that every effort should be made to achieve microscopically negative surgical margins. Inking of the margins, orientation of the specimen by the surgeon, and immediate gross evaluation of the margins by the pathologist with frozen section analysis where necessary may assist in achieving negative margins at the first operation. In the end, although radiation therapy and systemic therapy can assist in decreasing local recurrence rates in the setting of positive margins, adjuvant therapy cannot substitute for adequate surgery.

Although it is clear that the surgical gold standard is negative surgical margins, the appropriate surgical margins for optimal local control are controversial for most cancer types. In most tumors, cancer cells are thought to extend several millimeters beyond the gross tumor. Furthermore, histologic margin analysis is thought to be susceptible to some sampling error. For some cancer types such as breast cancer, patients who have "close surgical margins" have been demonstrated to have a higher local recurrence rate than patients who had "widely negative margins."[187] Even in breast cancer, however, the optimal margin width remains controversial. This may be in part because endorsing a certain clear margin distance would suggest that mastectomy should be performed in patients in whom that width could not be achieved with breast-conserving surgery, even though negative margins were achieved. In contrast, in melanoma the optimal margin width for any tumor depth has been defined, owing to the systematic study of this question in randomized clinical trials.[188,189] Although such randomized studies may not be possible in all tumor types, it is important to determine optimum surgical margins for each cancer type so that adjuvant radiation and systemic therapy can be offered to patients deemed to be at increased risk for local failure.

Surgical Management of the Regional Lymph Node Basin

Most neoplasms metastasize via the lymphatics. Therefore, most oncologic operations have been designed to remove the primary tumor and draining lymphatics en bloc. This type of operative approach is usually undertaken when the lymph nodes draining the primary tumor site lie adjacent to the tumor bed, as is the case for colorectal cancers and gastric cancers. For tumors where the regional lymph node basin is not immediately adjacent to the tumor (e.g., melanomas), lymph node surgery can be performed through a separate incision. Unlike most carcinomas, soft-tissue sarcomas rarely metastasize (<5%) to the lymph nodes, therefore lymph node surgery is usually not necessary.

It is generally accepted that a formal lymphadenectomy is likely to minimize the risk of regional recurrence of most cancers. For example, the introduction of total mesorectal excision of rectal cancer has been associated with a large decline in local-regional recurrence, and this procedure has become the new standard of operative management.[190] On the other hand, there have been two opposing views regarding the role of lymphadenectomy on survival of cancer patients.[191] The traditional Halsted view states that lymphadenectomy is important for staging and survival. The opposing view counters that cancer is systemic at inception and that lymphadenectomy, although useful for staging, does not affect survival. For most cancers, involvement of the lymph nodes is one of the most significant prognostic factors. Interestingly, the number of lymph nodes removed has been found to have an inverse relationship with overall survival rate in many solid tumors, including breast cancer, colon cancer, and lung cancer.[191–193] Although this seems to support the Halsted theory that more extensive lymphadenectomy yielding more nodes reduces the risk of regional recurrence, there may be alternate explanations for the same finding. For example, the surgeon who performs a more extensive lymphadenectomy may obtain wider margins around the tumor, or even provide better overall care such as ensuring that patients receive the appropriate adjuvant therapy or undergo a more thorough staging work-up. Alternatively, the pathologist may perform a more thorough examination, identifying more nodes and more accurately staging the nodes. The effect of appropriate staging on survival is twofold. Patients with nodal metastases may be offered adjuvant therapy, improving their survival chances. Further, the improved staging can improve perceived survival rates through a "Will Rogers effect," meaning identification of metastases that had formerly been silent and unidentified leads to a stage migration and thus to a perceived improvement in chances of survival. Clearly the impact of lymphadenectomy on survival will not be easily resolved. Since minimizing regional recurrences as much as possible is a goal of cancer treatment, the standard of care remains lymphadenectomy for most tumors.

A relatively new development in the surgical management of the clinically negative regional lymph node basin is the introduction of lymphatic mapping technology (Fig. 9-10). Lymphatic mapping and sentinel lymph node biopsy were first reported in 1977 by Cabanas for penile cancer.[194] Morton and colleagues implemented this approach for the treatment of melanoma,[195] and Giuliano and colleagues further adapted the technology to breast cancer.[196] Now sentinel node biopsy is the standard of care for the management of melanoma and is rapidly becoming the standard of care in breast cancer. Moreover, the utility of sentinel node biopsy is being explored in other cancers such as esophageal, gastric, colon, and head and neck cancers.[197–201]

The first node to receive drainage from the tumor site is termed the *sentinel node*. This node is the node most likely to contain metastases, if metastases to that regional lymph node basin are present. The goal of lymphatic mapping and sentinel lymph node biopsy is to identify and remove the lymph node most likely to contain metastases in the least invasive fashion. The practice of sentinel lymph node biopsy followed by selective regional lymph node dissection for patients with a positive sentinel lymph node avoids the morbidity of lymph node dissections in patients with negative nodes. An additional advantage of the sentinel lymph node technique is that it directs attention to a single node, allowing more careful analysis of the lymph node most likely to have a positive yield and increasing the accuracy of nodal staging.[202]

Two criteria are used to assess the efficacy of a sentinel lymph node biopsy: the sentinel lymph node identification rate and the false-negative rate. The sentinel lymph node identification rate is the proportion of patients in whom a sentinel lymph node was identified and removed among all patients undergoing an attempted sentinel lymph node biopsy. The false-negative rate is the proportion of patients with regional lymph node metastases in whom the sentinel lymph node was found to be negative. False-negative biopsies may be due to identification of the wrong node or to missing the sentinel node (i.e., surgical error), or they may be due to the cancer cells establishing metastases not in the first encountered node, but in a second echelon node (i.e., biologic variation). Alternatively, false-negative biopsies may be due to inadequate histologic evaluation of the lymph node. A sentinel lymph node can be identified

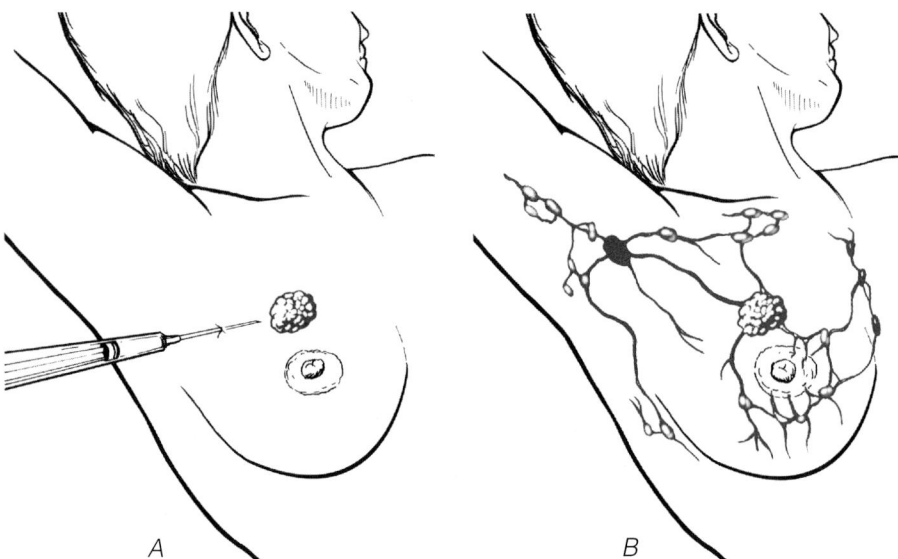

FIG. 9-10. Lymphatic mapping and sentinel lymph node biopsy for breast cancer. *A.* Peritumoral injection of blue dye. *B.* Blue dye draining into the sentinel lymph node. [*Modified from Meric F, Hunt KK: Surgical options for breast cancer, in Hunt KK, Robb GL, Strom EA, et al (eds): M. D. Anderson Cancer Care Series—Breast Cancer. New York, NY, Springer, 2001; p. 187.*]

in almost 100% of melanoma patients and in 94% of breast cancer patients.[203–207] The false-negative rates for sentinel lymph node biopsy in larger series range between 0 and 11%.[202,206,208,209] Both increases in the identification rate and decreases in the false-negative rate have been observed as surgeons gain experience with the technique. For breast cancer, therefore, it is recommended that until a surgeon documents an identification rate of greater than 90% and a false-negative rate of less than 5%, he or she should continue to perform concomitant axillary dissections.[210]

Lymphatic mapping is performed by using isosulfan blue dye,[196] technetium-labeled sulfur colloid or albumin,[211] or a combination of both techniques to detect sentinel nodes. The combination of blue dye and technetium has been reported to improve the capability of detecting sentinel lymph nodes.[212] The nodal drainage pattern usually is determined with a preoperative lymphoscintogram, and the "hot" and/or blue nodes are identified with the assistance of a gamma probe and careful nodal basin exploration. Careful manual palpation is a crucial part of the procedure to minimize the false-negative rate. The nodes are evaluated with serial sectioning, hematoxylin and eosin staining, and immunohistochemical staining with S-100 and HMB-45 for melanoma and cytokeratin for breast cancer.

In spite of widespread use of lymphatic mapping, there are still controversies about some technical aspects such as how many nodes should be removed.[213,214] Other controversies that remain in lymphatic mapping for breast cancer include the roles of lymphoscintigraphy, internal mammary nodal mapping, and immunohistochemistry, and the indications for completion of node dissection. The uses of sentinel node biopsy after an excisional biopsy in patients with large breast tumors, in patients who have received preoperative chemotherapy, and in patients with multicentric disease also have been controversial. However, it is increasingly apparent that, although these patients may have a higher risk for a false-negative sentinel node, the accuracy is still high enough to justify sentinel node biopsy in most patients.[215–217]

Surgical Management of Distant Metastases

The treatment of a patient with distant metastases depends on the number and sites of metastases, the cancer type, the rate of tumor growth, the previous treatments delivered and the responses to these treatments, and the patient's age, physical condition, and desires.

Although once a tumor has metastasized it is usually not curable with surgical therapy, such therapy has resulted in cure in selected cases with isolated metastases to the liver, lung, or brain.

Patient selection is the key to success of surgical therapy for distant metastases. The cancer type is a major determinant in surgical decision making. A liver metastasis from a colon cancer is much more likely to be an isolated, and thus resectable, lesion than a liver metastasis from a breast carcinoma. The growth rate of the tumor also plays an important role and can be determined in part by the disease-free interval and the time between treatment of the primary tumor and detection of the distant recurrence. Patients with longer disease-free intervals have a higher survival rate after surgical metastasectomy than those with a short disease-free interval. Similarly, patients who have synchronous metastases (metastases diagnosed at the initial cancer diagnosis) do worse after metastasectomy than patients who develop metachronous metastases (metastasis diagnosed after a disease-free interval). The natural history of metastatic disease is so poor in some tumors (e.g., pancreatic cancer) that there is no role at this time for surgical metastasectomy. In cancers with more favorable outlooks, observation for several weeks or months, potentially with initial treatment with systemic therapy, can allow the surgeon to monitor for metastases at other sites.

In curative surgery for distant metastases, as with surgery for primary tumors, the goal is to resect the metastases with negative margins. In patients with hepatic metastases that are unresectable because their location near intrahepatic blood vessels precludes a margin-negative resection, or because of multifocality or inadequate hepatic function, tumor ablation with cryotherapy or radiofrequency ablation is an alternative.[218,219] Curative resections or ablative procedures should be attempted only if the lesions are accessible and the procedure can be performed safely.

CHEMOTHERAPY

Clinical Use of Chemotherapy

In patients with documented distant metastatic disease, chemotherapy is usually the primary modality of therapy. The goal of therapy in this setting is to decrease the tumor burden, thus prolonging survival. It is rare to achieve cure with chemotherapy for metastatic disease in most solid tumors. Chemotherapy administered to a patient who is at high risk for distant recurrence, but has no evidence of distant disease, is referred to as *adjuvant chemotherapy*.

The goal of adjuvant chemotherapy is eradication of micrometastatic disease, with the intent of decreasing relapse rates and improving survival rates. An overview of 69 randomized trials of adjuvant combination chemotherapy performed by the Early Breast Cancer Trialists' Collaborative Group determined that adjuvant chemotherapy in women younger than 50 years at randomization changed the 10-year survival rate for those with node-negative disease from 71 to 78% (an absolute benefit of 7%), and for those with node-positive disease from 42 to 53% (an absolute benefit of 11%).[220]

Adjuvant therapy can be given after surgery (postoperative chemotherapy) or before surgery (preoperative chemotherapy, neoadjuvant chemotherapy, or induction therapy). A portion or all of the planned adjuvant chemotherapy can be administered prior to the surgical removal of the primary tumor. Preoperative chemotherapy has three potential advantages. The first is that preoperative regression of tumor can facilitate resection of tumors that were initially inoperable or allow more conservative surgery for patients whose cancer was operable to begin with. In the NSABP B-18 project, for example, women were randomly assigned to receive either preoperative or postoperative adjuvant doxorubicin and cyclophosphamide. More patients treated before surgery than after surgery underwent breast conservation (68 versus 60%).[221] The second advantage of preoperative chemotherapy is the treatment of micrometastases without the delay of postoperative recovery. Although it was initially assumed that this would translate into a survival advantage, most studies have not demonstrated such.[221] The third goal is the ability to assess a cancer's response to treatment clinically, after a number of courses of chemotherapy, and pathologically, after surgical resection. This is especially important if alternative treatment regimens are available to be offered to patients whose disease responded inadequately.

However, there are some potential disadvantages to preoperative chemotherapy. Although disease progression while receiving preoperative chemotherapy is rare in chemotherapy-sensitive tumors such as breast cancer, it is more frequent in relatively chemotherapy-resistant tumors such as sarcomas.[222,223] Thus patient selection is critical to ensure that the opportunity to treat disease surgically is not lost by giving preoperative chemotherapy. Often, rates of postoperative wound infection, flap necrosis, and delays in postoperative adjuvant therapy do not differ between patients who are treated with preoperative chemotherapy and patients who are treated with surgery first.[223,224] However, preoperative chemotherapy can introduce special challenges to tumor localization, margin analysis, lymphatic mapping, and pathologic staging.

Response to chemotherapy is monitored clinically with imaging studies as well as physical examinations. Response usually is defined as complete response, partial response, minimal response or stable disease, or progression. Complete response is defined as the disappearance of all evidence of disease and no evidence of new disease for a specified interval, usually 4 weeks. Partial response is defined as a 50% or more decrease of the product of the two largest perpendicular tumor diameters (relative to the initial product), determined by two observations not less than 4 weeks apart. In addition, there can be no appearance of new lesions or progression of any lesion. Stable disease refers to the situation in which neither complete or partial response nor progression has been demonstrated. Progressive disease refers to a 25% or greater increase in the product of one or more measurable lesions (relative to the smallest size measured since treatment start) or the appearance of new lesions.

Cancer is usually not detectable until 10^9 cancer cells (1 g) are present.[225] A 3-log increase in cancer cells produces 10^{12} cells (1 kg), which can be fatal. A clinical "complete response" (i.e., disappearance of all clinically detectable disease) can be achieved with millions of cancer cells still remaining.

Principles of Chemotherapy

Chemotherapy destroys cells by first-order kinetics, meaning that with the administration of a drug a constant percentage of cells are killed, not a constant number of cells. If a patient with 10^{12} tumor cells is treated with a dose that results in 99.9% cell kill (3-log cell kill), the tumor burden will be reduced from 10^{12} to 10^9 cells (or 1 kg to 1 g). If the patient is retreated with the same drug, which theoretically could result in another 3-log cell kill, the number of cells would decrease from 10^9 to 10^6 (1 g to 1 mg) rather than being eliminated totally.

Chemotherapeutic agents can be classified according to the phase of the cell cycle they are effective in. Cell-cycle phase–nonspecific agents (e.g., alkylating agents) have a linear dose-response curve, such that the fraction of cells killed increases with dose of the drug.[226] In contrast, the cell-cycle phase–specific drugs have a plateau with respect to cell killing ability, and cell kill will not increase with further increases in drug dose.

Anticancer Agents

Alkylating Agents

Alkylating agents are cell-cycle–nonspecific agents, meaning that they are able to kill cells in any phase of the cell cycle. They act by cross-linking the two strands of the DNA helix or by other direct damage to the DNA.[225] The damage to the DNA prevents cell division and, if severe enough, leads to apoptosis. The alkylating agents comprise three main subgroups: classic alkylators, nitrosoureas, and miscellaneous DNA-binding agents (Table 9-17).

Antitumor Antibiotics

Antitumor antibiotics are the products of fermentation of microbial organisms. Like the alkylating agents, these agents are cell-cycle nonspecific. Antitumor antibiotics damage the cell by interfering with DNA or RNA synthesis, although the exact mechanism of action may differ by agent.

Antimetabolites

Antimetabolites are generally cell-cycle–specific agents that have their major activity during the S phase of the cell cycle and have little effect on cells in G_0. These drugs are most effective, therefore, in tumors that have a high growth fraction. Antimetabolites are structural analogues of naturally occurring metabolites involved in DNA and RNA synthesis. Therefore, they interfere with normal synthesis of nucleic acids by substituting for purines or pyrimidines in the metabolic pathway to inhibit critical enzymes in nucleic acid synthesis. The antimetabolites include folate antagonists, purine antagonists, and pyrimidine antagonists (see Table 9-17).

Plant Alkaloids

Plant alkaloids are derived from plants such as the periwinkle plant, *Vinca rosea* (e.g., vincristine, a vinca alkaloid), or the root of mandrake, *Podophyllum peltatum* (e.g., etoposide, a podophyllotoxin).[226] Vinca alkaloids affect the cell by binding to tubulin in the S phase. This blocks microtubule polymerization,

Table 9-17
Classification of Chemotherapeutic Agents

Alkylating agents
  Classic alkylating agents
    Busulfan
    Chlorambucil
    Cyclophosphamide
    Ifosfamide
    Mechlorethamine (nitrogen mustard)
    Melphalan
    Mitomycin C
    Triethylene thiophosphoramide (thiotepa)
  Nitrosoureas
    Carmustine (BCNU)
    Lomustine (CCNU)
    Semustine (Me CCNU)
    Streptozocin
  Miscellaneous DNA-binding agents
    Carboplatin
    Cisplatin
    Dacarbazine (DTIC)
    Hexamethylmelamine
    Procarbazine
Antitumor Antibiotics
  Antibiotics
    Bleomycin
    Dactinomycin (actinomycin D)
    Daunorubicin
    Doxorubicin
    Idarubicin
    Plicamycin (mithramycin)
Antimetabolites
  Folate analogues
    Methotrexate
  Purine analogues
    Azathioprine
    Mercaptopurine
    Thioguanine
    Cladribine (2 CdA)
    Fludarabine
    Pentostatin
  Pyrimidine analogues
    Capocitabine
    Cytarabine
    Floxuridine
    Gemcitabine
  Ribonucleotide reductase inhibitors
    Hydroxyurea
Plant Alkaloids
  Vinca alkaloids
    Vinblastine
    Vincristine
    Vindesine
    Vinorelbine
  Epipodophyllotoxins
    Etoposide
    Teniposide
  Taxanes
    Paclitaxel
    Docetaxel
Miscellaneous Agents
    Asparaginase
    Estramustine
    Milotane

resulting in impaired mitotic spindle formation in the M phase. Taxanes such a paclitaxel, on the other hand, cause excess polymerization and stability of microtubules, blocking the cell cycle in mitosis. The epipodophyllotoxins act to inhibit a DNA enzyme called topoisomerase II by stabilizing the DNA–topoisomerase II

complex. This results in an inability to synthesize DNA, thus the cell cycle is stopped in G_1 phase.[226]

Combination Chemotherapy

Combination chemotherapy may provide greater efficacy than single-agent therapy by three mechanisms: (1) it provides maximum cell kill within the range of toxicity for each drug that can be tolerated by the host, (2) it offers a broader range of coverage of resistant cell lines in a heterogeneous population, and (3) it prevents or delays the emergence of drug-resistant cell lines.[226] In selecting combination regimens, drugs known to be active as single agents are usually selected. Drugs with different mechanisms of action are combined to allow for additive or synergistic effects. Combining cell-cycle–specific and cell-cycle–nonspecific agents may be especially advantageous. Drugs with differing dose-limiting toxic effects are combined to allow for each drug to be given at therapeutic doses. Drugs with different patterns of resistance are combined whenever possible to minimize cross-resistance. The treatment-free interval between cycles is kept at the shortest possible time that will allow for recovery of the most sensitive normal tissue.

Drug Resistance

Several tumor factors influence tumor cell kill. Tumors are heterogenous, and, according to the Goldie Coldman hypothesis, tumor cells are genetically unstable and tend to mutate to form different cell clones. This has been used as an argument for giving chemotherapy as soon as possible in treatment, in order to reduce the likelihood of resistant clones emerging. Tumor size is another important variable. The greater the tumor, the larger the heterogeneity. Moreover, according to the Gompertzian model, cancer cells initially grow rapidly (exponential growth phase), then the growth slows down owing to hypoxia and decreased nutrient supply. Because of the larger proportion of cells dividing, smaller tumors may be more chemosensitive.

Multiple mechanisms of chemotherapy resistance have been identified (Table 9-18). Cells may exhibit reduced sensitivity to drugs by virtue of their cell-cycle distribution. For example, cells in G_0 phase are resistant to drugs active in the S phase. This phenomenon of "kinetic resistance" is usually temporary, and if the drug level can be maintained, all cells will eventually pass through the vulnerable phase of the cell cycle.[226] Alternatively, tumor cells may exhibit "pharmacologic resistance," when the failure to kill cells is due to insufficient drug concentration. This may occur when tumor cells are located in sites where effective drug concentrations are difficult to achieve (such as the central nervous system), or can be due to enhanced metabolism of the drug after its administration, decreased conversion of the drug to active form, or a decrease in the intracellular drug level due to increased removal of the drug from the cell associated with enhanced expression of P-glycoprotein, the protein product of the multidrug resistance gene 1 (*MDR-1*). Other mechanisms of resistance include decreased affinity of the target enzyme for the drug, altered amount of the target enzyme, or enhanced repair of the drug-induced defect.

For drug-sensitive cancers, another factor limiting optimum killing is proper dosing. A dose reduction of 20% because of drug toxicity can lead to a decline in the cure rate by as much as 50%.[226] On the other hand, a twofold increase in dose can be associated with a tenfold (1 log) increase in tumor cell kill.

Table 9-18
General Mechanisms of Drug Resistance

Cellular and biochemical mechanisms
  Decreased drug accumulation
    Decreased drug influx
    Increased drug efflux
    Altered intracellular trafficking of drug
  Decreased drug activation
  Increased inactivation of drug or toxic intermediate
  Increased repair of drug-induced damage to
    DNA
    Protein
    Membranes
  Drug targets altered (quantitatively or qualitatively)
  Altered cofactor or metabolite levels
  Altered gene expression
    DNA mutation, amplification, or deletion
    Altered transcription, posttranscription processing, or translation
    Altered stability of macromolecules
  Mechanisms relevant in vivo
    Pharmacologic and anatomic drug barriers (tumor sanctuaries)
    Host-drug interactions
      Increased drug inactivation by normal tissues
      Decreased drug activation by normal tissues
      Relative increase in normal tissue drug sensitivity (toxicity)
    Host-tumor interactions

SOURCE: Modified with permission from Morrow et al.[252]

Drug Toxicity

Tumors are more susceptible than normal tissue to chemotherapeutic agents, in part because they have a higher proportion of dividing cells. Normal tissues with a high growth fraction, such as the bone marrow, oral and intestinal mucosa, and hair follicles are also sensitive to chemotherapeutic effects. Therefore, treatment with chemotherapeutic agents can produce toxic effects such as bone marrow suppression, stomatitis, ulceration of the gastrointestinal tract, and alopecia. Organ-specific toxic effects of selected anticancer agents are listed in Table 9-19.[227] Toxic effects are usually graded from 0 to 4 on the basis of World Health Organization standard criteria.[228] Significant drug toxicity may necessitate a dose reduction. A toxic effect requiring a dose modification or change in dose intensity is referred to as a *dose-limiting toxic effect.* As maintaining dose intensity is important to maintaining as high a tumor cell kill as possible, several supportive strategies have been developed, such as administration of colony-stimulating factors and erythropoietin for poor bone marrow reserve and administration of cytoprotectants such as MESNA and amifostine to prevent renal dysfunction.

Administration of Chemotherapy

Chemotherapy usually is administered systemically (intravenously, intramuscularly, subcutaneously, or orally). Systemic administration treats micrometastases at widespread sites and prevents systemic recurrence. However, it increases the drug's toxicity to a wide range of organs throughout the body. One method to minimize systemic toxicity while enhancing target organ delivery of chemotherapy is regional administration of chemotherapy. Many of these approaches require surgical access, such as intrahepatic delivery of chemotherapy for hepatic carcinomas or metastatic colorectal cancer with a hepatic artery infusion pump, limb perfusion for extremity melanoma and sarcoma, or intraperitoneal hyperthermic perfusion for pseudomyxoma peritonei.

HORMONAL THERAPY

Some tumors, most notably breast and prostate cancers, originate from tissues whose growth is under hormonal control. The first attempts at hormonal therapy were through surgical ablation of the organ producing the hormones of interest, such as oophorectomy for breast cancer. Currently, hormonal manipulation is accomplished by several different modes (Table 9-20). Hormones or hormone-like agents can be administered to inhibit tumor growth by blocking or antagonizing the naturally occurring substance, such as estrogen antagonist tamoxifen. Other substances that block the synthesis of the natural hormone can be administered as alternatives. Aromatase inhibitors, for example, block the peripheral conversion of endogenous androgens to estrogens in postmenopausal women.

Hormonal therapy provides a highly tumor-specific form of therapy in sensitive tissues. In breast cancer, estrogen and progesterone receptor status is used to predict the success of hormonal therapy. Recently, several other biologic variables have been found to have an impact on the success of hormonal therapy, and these variables are likely to be incorporated into clinical practice in the near future.

BIOLOGIC THERAPY

Over the past decade, increasing understanding of cancer biology has fostered the emerging field of molecular therapeutics. The basic principle of molecular therapeutics is to exploit the molecular differences between normal cells and cancer cells to develop targeted therapies. The ideal molecular target would be exclusively expressed in the cancer cells, be the driving force of the proliferation of the cancer cells, and be critical to their survival. A large number of molecular targets are currently being explored, both preclinically and in clinical trials. The major groups of targeted therapies include inhibitors of growth factor receptors, inhibitors of intracellular signal transduction, cell-cycle inhibitors, apoptosis-based therapies, and antiangiogenic compounds.

Protein kinases have come to the forefront as attractive therapeutic targets with the success of STI571 (imitanib mesylate, Gleevec) in chronic myelogenous leukemia and gastrointestinal stromal tumors and trastuzumab (Herceptin) in breast cancer, which work by targeting bcr-*abl*, c-*kit*, and HER2/*neu,* respectively. Sequencing the human genome has revealed about 500 protein kinases.[229] Several tyrosine kinases have been shown to have oncogenic properties (see Table 9-11), and many other protein kinases have been shown to be aberrantly activated in cancer cells. Therefore, protein kinases involving these aberrantly activated pathways are being aggressively pursued in molecular therapeutics. Potential targets such as HER2/*neu* can be targeted via different strategies such as transcriptional downregulation, targeting of mRNA RNA inhibition, antisense strategies, direct inhibition of protein activity, and induction of immunity against the protein (Table 9-21). Most of the compounds in development are monoclonal antibodies like trastuzumab or small-molecule kinase inhibitors like STI-571. Some of the kinase inhibitors in clinical development include inhibitors of EGFR, Ras, Raf, MEK, mammalian target of rapamycin (mTOR), CDK, PKC, and 3-phosphoinositide-dependent protein kinase 1 (PDK-1) (Fig. 9-11).[229]

Development of molecularly targeted agents for clinical use has several unique challenges.[229] Once an appropriate compound is identified and confirmed to have preclinical activity, predictive markers for activity in the preclinical setting must be defined. Expression of a target may not be sufficient to predict response, since

Table 9-19
Toxic Effects of Some Common Chemotherapeutic Agents

Drug	Toxic Effects
Alkylating agents	
Busulfan	Myelosuppression, pulmonary fibrosis, gonadal dysfunction, marrow failure
Chlorambucil	Myelosuppression, gonadal dysfunction, secondary leukemia
Cyclophosphamide	Leukopenia, cystitis, nausea and vomiting, alopecia, cardiac necrosis, gonadal dysfunction, SIADH
Ifosfamide	Myelosuppression, cystitis, nephrotoxicity, hepatotoxicity, lethargy, and confusion
Dacarbazine	Nausea and vomiting, flu-like syndrome, myelosuppression, hepatotoxicity
Cisplatin	Nausea and vomiting, nephrotoxicity, neurotoxicity, hearing loss, electrolyte imbalance
Carboplatin	Myelosuppression, nausea and vomiting
Melphalan	Myelosuppression, anorexia, nausea and vomiting
Mechlorethamine	Myelosuppression, secondary leukemia, severe vesicant, nausea and vomiting, alopecia, rash, gonadal dysfunction, neurotoxicity
Nitrosoureas (carmustine, BCNU; lomustine, CCNU)	Myelosuppression, secondary leukemia, hepatotoxicity, pulmonary fibrosis, nausea and vomiting, nephrotoxicity, confusion
Streptozocin	Nephrotoxicity, nausea and vomiting, myelosuppression, hepatotoxicity, hypoglycemia
Procarbazine	Myelosuppression, monoamine oxidase inhibition, nausea and vomiting, lethargy, myalgias, arthralgias, neurotoxicity, dermatitis
Mitomycin C	Myelosuppression, severe vesicant, weakness, anorexia, hemolytic anemia, renal insufficiency, nausea and vomiting
Antitumor antibiotics	
Anthracyclines	
Doxorubicin, daunorubicin, idarubcin	Myelosuppression, cardiomyopathy, alopecia, nausea and vomiting, mucositis, radiation recall, severe vesicant
Bleomycin	Pneumonitis, pulmonary fibrosis, fever and chills, anaphylaxis, dermatitis, mild myelosuppression
Actinomycin D	Myelosuppression, nausea and vomiting, mucositis, dermatitis, alopecia, diarrhea, severe vesicant, radiation recall
Antimetabolites	
Cytosine arabinoside	Myelosuppression, ischemic bowel, stomatitis, nausea and vomiting, hepatotoxicity, cerebellar toxicity
5-Fluorouracil	Mucositis, diarrhea, myelosuppression, dermatitis, hepatotoxicity (intra-arterial therapy), nausea and vomiting
Floxuridine	Mucositis, biliary sclerosis, nausea and vomiting, abdominal pain
6-Mercaptopurine	Myelosuppression, cholestasis, rash, anorexia, nausea and vomiting
Methotrexate	Myelosuppression, stomatitis, diarrhea, intestinal bleeding and perforation, arachnoiditis, hepatic dysfunction, cirrhosis, radiation recall, pneumonitis, renal dysfunction
Gemcitabine	Myelosuppression, weakness
Pentostatin	Nephrotoxicity, risk of severe infections without neutropenia, lethargy, hepatotoxicity, mild myelosuppression
Fludarabine	Myelosuppression, tumor lysis syndrome, weakness, neurotoxicity, edema, pneumonitis, nausea and vomiting, anorexia, gastrointestinal bleeding, stomatitis, diarrhea
Plant alkaloids	
Epipodophyllotoxins	
Etoposide (VP-16)	Myelosuppression, nausea and vomiting, alopecia, ileus, hypotension
Teniposide (VM-26)	Same as etoposide
Taxanes	
Paclitaxel (Taxol)	Myelosuppression, alopecia, cardiac arrhythmias, neurotoxicity, abdominal pain, muscular cramps, and myalgias
Docetaxel (Taxotere)	Same as paclitaxel, fluid third-spacing (vascular leak syndrome)
Vinca alkaloids	
Vincristine	Mild myelosuppression, neuropathy, ileus, SIADH
Vinblastine	Myelosuppression, mild neuropathy, ileus, abdominal pain, nausea and vomiting
Vinorelbine	Myelosuppression, neuropathy, ileus, diarrhea
Camptothecins	
Topotecan, innotecan (CPT-11) 9-Aminocamptothecin	Myelosuppression, diarrhea (CPT-11), nausea and vomiting, pulmonary toxicity, weakness
Miscellaneous agents	
Mitoxantrone	Myelosuppression, nausea and vomiting (mild), minimal cardiotoxicity, alopecia (mild), blue sclera and nails
Mitotane	Nausea and vomiting, depression, dermatitis, lethargy
Hydroxyurea reductase	Myelosuppression, nausea and vomiting, increased blood urea nitrogen, headaches, dermatitis
Amsacrine	Myelosuppression, vesicant, phlebitis, alopecia, stomatitis, hepatotoxicity, neurotoxicity
L-Asparaginase	Allergic reactions, nausea and vomiting, anorexia, hepatitis, pancreatitis, coagulopathy (usually subclinical), lethargy, depression, glucose intolerance

SIADH = syndrome of inappropriate secretion of antidiuretic hormone.

SOURCE: Modified with permission from Ellis et al.[227]

the pathway of interest may not be activated or be critical to the cancer's survival. Although in traditional phase I trials the goal is to identify the maximum tolerated dose, the maximum dose of biologic agents may not be necessary to achieve the desired biologic effect. Thus assays to verify modulation of the target need to be developed to determine at what dose the desired effect is achieved. When phase II and III clinical trials are initiated, biomarker modulation studies should be integrated into the trial in order to determine

Table 9-20
Hormonal Anticancer Agents

Pharmacologic Category and Products Available	Clinical Applications
Androgens	
Testosterone propionate	Breast cancer
Fluoxymesterone	
Antiandrogens	
Flutamide	Prostate cancer
Finasteride	
Antiestrogens	
Tamoxifen	Breast cancer
Estrogens	
Diethylstilbestrol	Prostate cancer
Ethinyl estradiol	Breast cancer
Glucocorticoids	
Hydrocortisone	Leukemia, lymphoma
Prednisone	Breast cancer
Dexamethasone	Multiple myeloma
Gonadotropin inhibitors	
Leuprolide	Prostate cancer
Goserelin acetate	Breast cancer
Progestins	
Hydroxyprogesterone caproate	Endometrial cancer
Medroxyprogesterone	Breast cancer
Aromatase inhibitors	
Aminoglutethimide	Prostate cancer
	Breast cancer
Somatostatin analogues	
Octreotide acetate	Neuroendocrine tumor of the gut, carcinoid vipoma, APUD tumors[a]

[a] APUD = amine precursor update (and) decarboxylation.

SOURCE: Modified with permission from Section 10 Systemic Chemotherapy.[225]

whether clinical response correlates with target modulation, and thus to identify additional parameters that impact response. Rational dose selection and limiting study populations to patients most likely to respond to the molecular therapy as determined by predictive markers are most likely to lead to successful clinical translation of a product. Finally, most biologic agents are cytostatic, not cytotoxic. Thus rational combination therapy of new biologic agents with either established chemotherapeutic agents that have synergy or with other biologic agents is more likely to lead to cancer cures.

IMMUNOTHERAPY

The aim of immunotherapy is to induce or potentiate inherent antitumor immunity that can destroy cancer cells. Central to the process of antitumor immunity is the ability of the immune system to recognize tumor-associated antigens present on human cancers and to direct cytotoxic responses through humoral or T-cell–mediated immunity. Overall, T-cell–mediated immunity appears to have the greater potential of the two for eradicating tumor cells. T cells recognize antigens on the surfaces of target cells as small peptides presented by class I and class II major histocompatibility complex (MHC) molecules.

Antitumor strategies that have been investigated are summarized in Table 9-22. One approach to antitumor immunity is nonspecific immunotherapy, which stimulates the immune system as a whole by administering bacterial agents or their products, such as bacille Calmette-Guérin (BCG). This approach is thought to activate the effectors of antitumor response such as natural killer cells and macrophages, as well as polyclonal lymphocytes.[230] Another approach to nonspecific immunotherapy is systemic administration of cytokines such as IL-2, interferon alpha, and interferon gamma. IL-2 stimulates proliferation of cytotoxic T lymphocytes and maturation of effectors such as natural killer cells into lymphokine-activated killer cells. Interferons, on the hand, exert antitumor effects directly (by inhibiting tumor cell proliferation), indirectly (by activating host immune cells including macrophages, dendritic cells, and natural killer cells), and by enhancing human leukocyte antigen (HLA) class I expression on tumor cells.[230]

Antigen-specific immunotherapy can be active, achieved through antitumor vaccines, or passive. In passive immunotherapy, antibodies to specific tumor-associated antigens can be produced by hybridoma technique and then administered to patients whose cancers express these antigens, inducing antibody-dependent cellular cytotoxicity.

The early attempts at vaccination against cancers utilized allogeneic cultured cancer cells, including irradiated cells, cell lysates, or shed antigens isolated from tissue culture supernatants.[231] An alternate strategy is the use of autologous tumor vaccines, which have the potential advantage of being more likely to contain antigens relevant for the individual patient, but have the disadvantage of needing a large amount of tumor tissue for preparation, which restricts eligibility of patients for this modality. Strategies to enhance immunogenicity of tumor cells include the introduction of genes encoding cytokines or chemokines, or fusion of the tumor cells to allogeneic

Table 9-21
Strategies Targeting HER2/*neu*

Her2/neu Targeting Agents	Mechanism of Action
Anti-HER2/*neu* antibodies (trastuzumab)	Downregulation of cell surface HER2/*neu* expression
Tyrosine kinase inhibitors	Inhibition of HER2/*neu* tyrosine kinase activity
Anti-HER2/*neu* peptides[253]	Peptides based on the binding motifs of the anti-HER2/*neu* antibodies
Adenovirus 5 E1 A[254]	Repression of HER2/*neu* mRNA transcription
PEA3[255]	Repression of HER2/*neu* mRNA transcription
HER2/*neu* antisense oligonucleotides[256–258]	Downregulation of HER2/*neu* mRNA levels
HER2/*neu* hammerhead ribozymes[259,260]	Downregulation of HER2/*neu* mRNA levels
HER2/*neu* small inhibitor RNA	Downregulation of HER2/*neu* mRNA levels
Retinoids[261,262]	Downregulation of HER2/*neu* mRNA and protein expression
HER2/*neu* vaccines[263,264]	Induction of immunity against HER2/*neu*-overexpressing cells
HER2/*neu* promoter-driven suicide genes (e.g., deaminase, cytosine deaminase gene)[265]	Targeted expression of toxic genes in HER2/*neu*-overexpressing cells

SOURCE: Modified with permission from Meric et al.[26]

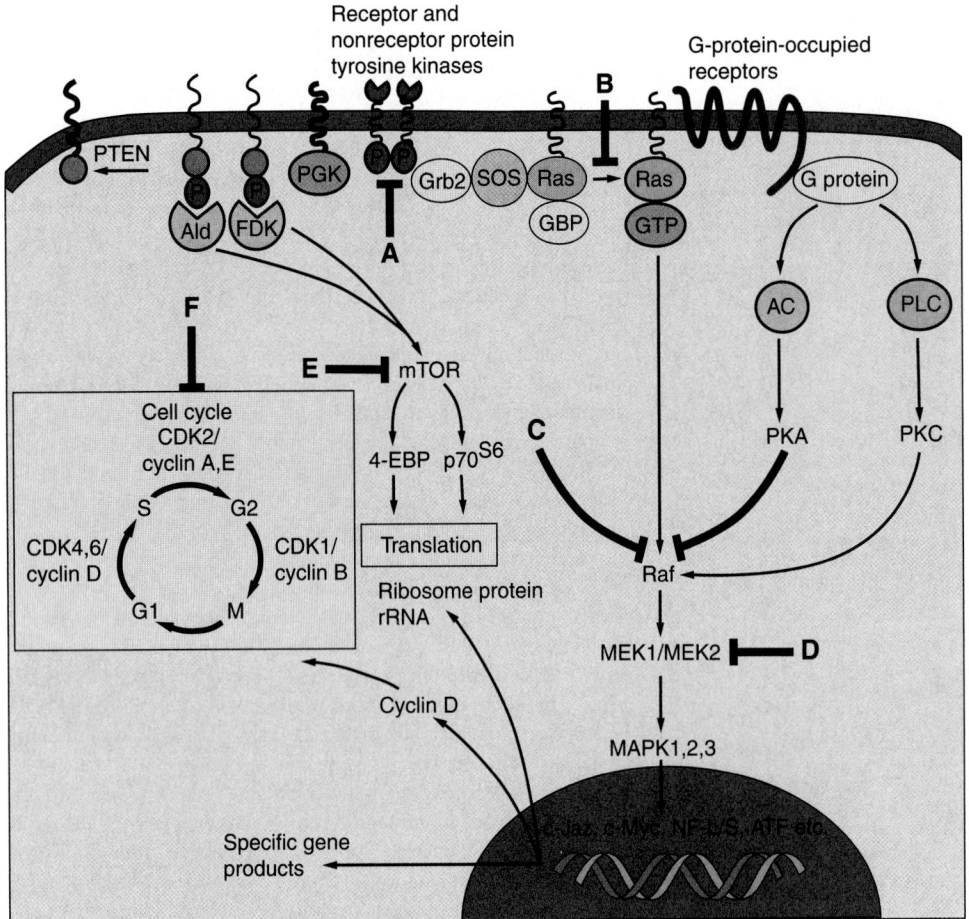

FIG. 9-11. A schematic illustration of some of the principal pathways that are affected by biologic therapies. Growth factors increase tyrosine kinase activity. Downstream events include the recruitment of adaptor molecules such as growth factor receptor bound (Grb), which binds to phosphorylated tyrosines to recruit effectors such as the scaffold protein son of sevenless (SOS), which alters the affinity of Ras isoforms for guanosine diphosphate (GDP), allowing exchange for guanosine triphosphate (GTP), which activates Ras. Activated GTP-bound Ras activates Raf, which in turn activates mitogen-activated protein kinase kinases (MEKs) to phosphorylate mitogen-activated protein kinases (MAPKs) that then influence gene expression. Activated tyrosine kinase receptors also can activate phosphatidylinositol 3-kinase (PI3K), which phosphorylates inositol-containing lipids. These in turn recruit molecules such as phosphoinositide-dependent kinase-1 (PDK1) and protein kinase B (Akt). PDK1 contributes to the activation of Akt, which then phosphorylates numerous substrates, leading to activation of the mammalian target of rapamycin (mTOR), which in turn increases the translation efficiency of growth-regulatory gene products through its effects on the eukaryotic inhibition factor 4E-binding protein (4E-BP) and $p70^{S6}$ kinase ($p70^{S6}$K). Increased translational efficiency complements the output from MAPK-influenced gene transcription, which includes elaboration of increased ribosomal RNA (rRNA) and ribonucleoprotein synthesis and elaboration of cyclin D homologues. The D-type cyclins cause an increase in cell proliferation through activation of cyclin-dependent kinases (CDKs). Seven transmembrane G-protein-coupled receptors can activate protein kinases A (PKA) and C (PKC), which modulate the activity of Raf and hence input into the MAPK pathway. The letters A–F in the figure refer to the sites of action of classes of biologic therapy, including: A. epidermal growth factor (EGF)–receptor directed agents; B. Ras antagonists, including farnesyl transferase antagonists; C. Raf antagonists; D. MEK-directed approaches; E. mTOR inhibitors; and F. CDK antagonists. AC = adenylate cyclase; PTEN = phosphatase and tensin homologue deleted on chromosome 10. (Modified from Dancey et al,[229] with permission.)

MHC II–bearing cells.[231] Alternatively, heat shock proteins derived from a patient's tumor can be utilized, as heat shock protein peptide complexes are readily taken up by dendritic cells for presentation to T cells.[231]

Identification of tumor antigens has made it possible to perform antigen-specific vaccination. Tumor antigens recognized by T cells fall into several categories as presented in Table 9-23. Vaccines directed at defined tumor antigens aim to combine selected

tumor antigens and appropriate routes for delivering these antigens to the immune system to optimize antitumor immunity.[232] Several different vaccination approaches are under study including tumor cell–based vaccines, peptide-based vaccines, recombinant virus–based vaccines, DNA-based vaccines, and dendritic cell vaccines (Table 9-24).

In adoptive transfer, antigen-specific (i.e., cytotoxic T lymphocytes) or antigen-nonspecific (i.e., natural killer cells) effector cells

Table 9-22
Antitumor Immunotherapy Strategies

Nonspecific immunotherapy	Exogenous immunostimulants	BCG, OK-432
	Cytokines	IL-2, IFN-α, IFN-γ[a]
Antigen-specific immunotherapy	Passive	Monoclonal antibodies to TAA
	Active (vaccination)	Undefined TAA
		Whole tumor cells
		Modified tumor cells[a]
		Shed antigens
		Heat shock proteins
		Defined TAA
		Recombinant protein
		Ganglioside
		Ab idiotype
		Anti-TAA (antibody)
		Peptide ($\pm$ IL-2)
		DNA[b]
		Viral vector
Adoptive transfer	CTL ($\pm$ IL-2)	
Dendritic cells	NK cells ($\pm$ IL-2)	
	Pulsed with peptides/tumor cells	
	Transfected (modified viruses)	
	Fused with tumor cells (hybrid)	

[a]Tumor cells can be genetically engineered to secrete cytokines such as IL-2 and IFN-α.

[b]Coding for TAA $\pm$ cytokines.

Ab = antibody; BCG = bacille Calmette-Guérin; CTL = cytotoxic T lymphocytes; IFN-α = interferon alpha; IFN-γ = interferon gamma; IL-2 = interleukin-2; NK = natural killer; TAA = tumor-associated antigen.

SOURCE: Modified with permission from Mocellin.[230]

Table 9-23
Categories and Examples of Tumor-Associated Antigens Recognized by Human T Cells

Category	Tumor Antigens	Cancers Expressing the Antigen
Cancer testis antigens	MAGE-1	Melanoma, breast, head and neck, bladder,
	MAGE-2	gastric, and lung cancers
	MAGE-3	
	MAGE-12	
	BAGE	
	GAGE	
	NY-ESO-1	
Differentiation antigens	Tyrosinase	Melanoma[a]
	TRP-1	
	TRP-2	
	gp 100	
	MART-1	
	MC1R	
Tumor-specific antigens	Immunoglobulin idiotype	B-cell NHL, MM
	CDK4	
	Caspase-8	Melanoma
	β-Catenin	Head and neck cancers
	CIA 0205	Melanoma
	BCR/ABL	Bladder cancer
	Mutated p21/*ras*	CML
	Mutated *p53*	Pancreatic, colon, lung cancers
		Colorectal, lung, bladder, head and neck cancers
Overexpressed self antigen	Proteinase 3	CML
	WT 1	CML, ALL, AML
	MUC-1	Breast adenocarcinoma
	CEA	Colon, breast, pancreatic cancers
	Normal *p53*	Breast, colon, and other cancers
	Her2/neu	Breast and ovary and lung cancers
	PAP	Prostate cancer
	PSA	Prostate cancer
	PSMA	Prostate cancer
	α-fetoprotein	Liver cancer
	G250	Renal cell carcinoma
Viral antigens	HPV E6/E7	Cervical and penile cancers
	EBV LMP2a	EBV (+) Hodgkin's disease
	HCV	Liver cancer
	HHV-8	Kaposi's sarcoma

[a]Some of these tumours express all of the tumor antigens in this category.

ALL = acute lymphoblastic leukemia; AML = acute myeloid leukemia; CEA = carcinoembryonic antigens; CML = chronic myeloid leukemia; EBV = Epstein-Barr virus; HCV = hepatitis C virus; HHV = human herpes virus; HPV = human papilloma virus; NHL = non-Hodgkin's lymphoma; MM = multiple myeloma.

SOURCE: Modified with permission from Dermime et al.[232]

Table 9-24
Types of Vaccines

Type of Vaccine	Relative Advantage(s)	Relative Disadvantage(s)
Allogeneic cellular	Simple to prepare, broad spectrum of potential antigens	Irrelevant "allo" antigens, difficult to precisely characterize component, requires adjuvant
Autologous cellular	Patient-specific unique antigens, presents numerous antigens	Custom-made individual vaccine production, requires adjuvant
Autologous heat shock proteins	Patient-specific unique antigens, presents numerous antigens	Custom-made individual vaccine production, production can be difficult, few clinical data to date
Purified protein or carbohydrate	Well-defined components, safety and immunogenicity established (carbohydrates) in mature clinical trials	Production can be difficult, requires adjuvant
Peptide	Simple to prepare, safety established in early trials	Single epitope, HLA-restricted, requires adjuvant
Dendritic cell	Inherently immunogenic, potentially numerous epitopes	Production can be difficult, limited epitopes, and HLA restriction when used with peptides
Recombinant virus	Inherently immunogenic, numerous epitopes	Neutralizing immunity to vector
DNA	Simple to prepare, numerous epitopes, immunostimulatory sequences in vector	Few clinical data to date

HLA = human leukocyte antigen.

SOURCE: Modified with permission from Perales et al.[231]

can be transferred to a patient.[230] These effector cells can be obtained from the tumor (tumor-infiltrating lymphocytes) or the peripheral blood.

Clinical experience in patients with metastatic disease has shown objective tumor responses to a variety of immunotherapeutic modalities.[230] It is thought, however, that the immune system is overwhelmed with the tumor burden in this setting, and thus adjuvant therapy may be preferable, reserving immunotherapy for decreasing tumor recurrences. Trials to date suggest that immunotherapy is a potentially useful approach in the adjuvant setting.[230] How to best select patients for this approach and how to integrate immunotherapy with other therapies are not well understood for most cancer types.

GENE THERAPY

Gene therapy is being pursued as a possible approach to modifying the genetic program of cancer cells as well as for treatment of

metabolic diseases. The field of cancer gene therapy utilizes a variety of strategies, ranging from replacement of mutated or deleted tumor suppressor genes to enhancement of immune responses to cancer cells (Fig. 9-12).[233] Indeed, in preclinical models, approaches such as replacement of tumor suppressor genes leads to growth arrest or apoptosis (Table 9-25). However, the translation of these findings into clinically useful tools presents special challenges.

One of the main difficulties in getting gene therapy technology from the laboratory to the clinic is the lack of a perfect delivery system.[234] An ideal vector would be administered through a noninvasive route and would transduce all of the cancer cells and none of the normal cells. Furthermore, the ideal vector would have a high degree of activity, that is, it would produce an adequate amount of the desired gene product to achieve target cell kill. Unlike genetic diseases in which delivery of the gene of interest into only a portion of the cells may be sufficient to achieve clinical effect, cancer requires either that the therapeutic gene is delivered to all of the cancer cells, or that a therapeutic effect is achieved on nontransfected

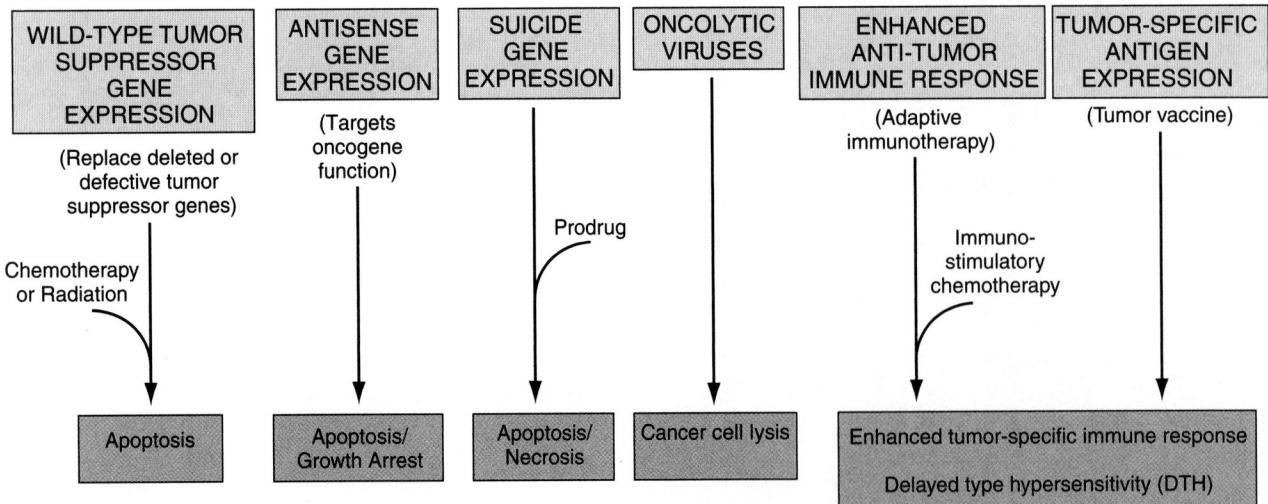

FIG. 9-12. Different strategies for gene therapy. (Modified from Cusack et al,[233] with permission.)

Table 9-25
Vectors for Cancer Gene Therapy

Vector	Advantages	Disadvantages
Retrovirus	Small genome Stable colinear integration Efficient gene transfer Nontoxic to host cells Infects dividing cells	Requires actively dividing cells Carries small DNA sequences only Low titer Transient expression Insertional mutagenesis Random integration Labile in vivo
Adenovirus	High viral titers Highly efficient gene transfer Nontoxic to host cells Infects dividing and nondividing cells	Transient expression Carries small DNA sequences only Immunogenic
Adeno-associated virus	Small genome Integrates into chromosome 19 Efficient gene transfer Nonpathogenic to humans Infects dividing and nondividing cells Weakly immunogenic	Carries small DNA sequences only Safety questionable Loss of nonrandom integration over time Low viral titers
Poxvirus (vaccinia virus)	Transient gene expression Highly efficient gene transfer and expression	Strongly immunogenic Safe for immunosuppressed patients
Herpes simplex virus	Infects dividing and nondividing cells Neurotropic High viral titers Large insert size Potential for prolonged gene expression	Toxicity related to lytic infection Safety questionable
Protein/DNA complexes	Cell-specific targeting Unlimited size	Inefficient gene transfer Safety questionable
Liposomes	Synthetic Unlimited size	Inefficient gene transfer
Nonviral plasmid	Transient gene expression Few safety concerns	Inefficient gene transfer

SOURCE: Modified with permission from Smith et al.[150]

cells as well as transfected cells through a "bystander effect." On the other hand, treatment of a metabolic disease requires prolonged gene expression, while transient expression may be sufficient for cancer therapy.

Several vector systems are under study for gene therapy and are summarized in Table 9-26; however, none are considered ideal. One of the promising approaches to increase the number of tumor cells transduced is the use of a replication-competent virus, such as a parvovirus, human reovirus, or vesicular stomatitis virus, that selectively replicates within malignant cells and lyses them more efficiently than it does normal cells.[234] Another strategy to kill tumor cells with suicide genes exploits tumor-specific expression elements, such as the MUC-1, PSA, CEA, or VEGF promoters, that can be utilized to achieve tissue-specific or tumor-specific expression of the desired gene.[235]

As the goal in cancer therapy is to eradicate systemic disease, optimization of delivery systems is the key to success for gene therapy strategies. Gene therapy is likely to be most successful when combined with standard therapies, but it will provide the advantage of customization of therapy based on the molecular status of an individual's tumor.

RADIATION THERAPY

Physical Basis of Radiation Therapy

Ionizing radiation is energy strong enough to remove an orbital electron from an atom.[236] This radiation can be electromagnetic, such

as a high-energy photon, or particulate, such as an electron, proton, neutron, or alpha particle. Radiation therapy is delivered primarily as high-energy photons (gamma rays and x-rays) and charged particles (electrons). Gamma rays are photons that are released from the nucleus of a radioactive atom. X-rays are photons that are created electronically, such as with a clinical linear accelerator. Currently, high-energy radiation is delivered to tumors primarily with linear accelerators. X-rays traverse the tissue, depositing the maximum dose beneath the surface, and thus spare the skin. Electrons are used to treat superficial skin lesions, superficial tumors, or surgical beds to a depth of 5 cm. Gamma rays typically are produced by radioactive sources used in brachytherapy.

The dose of radiation absorbed correlates with the energy of the beam. The basic unit is the amount of energy absorbed per unit of mass (joules per kilogram) and is known as a gray (Gy). One gray is equivalent to 100 rads, the unit of radiation measurement used in the past.

Biologic Basis of Radiation Therapy

Radiation deposition results in DNA damage manifested by single- and double-strand breaks in the sugar phosphate backbone of the DNA molecule.[237] Cross-linking between the DNA strands and chromosomal proteins also occurs. The mechanism of DNA damage differs by the type of radiation delivered. Electromagnetic radiation is indirectly ionizing through short-lived hydroxyl radicals produced primarily by the ionization of cellular hydrogen peroxide (H_2O_2).[237]

Table 9-26
Effects of Expressing Tumor Suppressors in Tissue Culture and in Mouse Models

Gene Product	Function	Expression in Cell Lines	Expression in Mouse Models
INK4A	Blocks cell cycle by inhibiting CDK4	Growth arrest (some evidence of resistance)	Tumor suppression
INK4A-KIP1 fusion	Blocks cell cycle by repressing E2F	Apoptosis	Regression
rb	Blocks cell cycle by repressing E2F	Growth arrest	Tumor suppression
p130	Blocks cell cycle by repressing E2F	Growth arrest	Regression
ARF	Protects *p53* by inhibiting MDM2	Growth arrest	Not done
p53	Promotes cell-cycle arrest and apoptosis	Growth arrest; increased radiosensitivity	Tumor suppression; reduced metastasis
PTEN	Degrades 3-phosphorylated phosphoinositides, which activate growth and survival pathways	Growth arrest; apoptosis; increased radiosensitivity	Tumor suppression or no effect
APC	Targets β-catenin for degradation	Apoptosis	Not done
BRCA1	Genome integrity	Growth arrest or apoptosis	Tumor suppression

SOURCE: Modified with permission from McCormick.[266]

Protons and other heavy particles are directly ionizing and directly damage DNA.

Radiation damage is manifested primarily by the loss of cellular reproductive integrity. Most cell types do not show signs of radiation damage until they attempt to divide, so slowly proliferating tumors may persist for months and appear viable. Some cell types, however, undergo apoptosis.

The extent of DNA damage following radiation is dependent on several factors. The most important of these is cellular oxygen. Hypoxic cells are significantly less radiosensitive than aerated cells. Since oxygen is thought to prolong the half-life of free radicals produced by the interaction of x-rays and cellular H_2O_2, indirectly ionizing radiation is less efficacious in tumors with areas of hypoxia.[237] In contrast, radiation damage from directly ionizing radiation is independent of cellular oxygen levels.

The extent of DNA damage from indirectly ionizing radiation is dependent on the phase of the cell cycle. The most radiation-sensitive phases are G_2 and M, while G_1 and late S phases are less sensitive.[238] Thus irradiation of a population of tumor cells results in killing of a greater proportion of cells in G_2 and M phases. However, delivery of radiation in divided doses, a concept referred to as *fractionation,* allows the surviving G_1 and S phase cells to progress to more sensitive phases, a process referred to as *reassortment.* In contrast to DNA damage following indirectly ionizing radiation, that following exposure to directly ionizing radiation is less dependent on the cell-cycle phase.[239]

Several chemicals can modify the effects of ionizing radiation. These include hypoxic cell sensitizers such as metronidazole and misonidazole, which mimic oxygen and increase cell kill of hypoxic cells.[237] A second category of radiation sensitizers are thymidine analogues iododeoxyuridine and bromodeoxyuridine. These molecules are incorporated into the DNA in place of thymidine and render the cells more susceptible to radiation damage; however, they are associated with considerable acute toxicity. Furthermore, several chemotherapeutic agents sensitize cells to radiation through various mechanisms, including 5-fluorouracil, actinomycin D, gemcitabine, paclitaxel, topotecan, doxorubicin, and vinorelbine.[237]

Radiation Therapy Planning

Radiation therapy is delivered in a homogeneous dose to a well-defined region that includes tumor and/or surrounding tissue at risk for subclinical disease. The first step in planning is to define the target to be irradiated as well as the dose-limiting organs in the vicinity.[240] Treatment planning includes evaluation of alternative treatment techniques, which is done through a process referred to as *simulation.* Once the beam distribution is determined that will best achieve homogenous delivery to the target volume and minimize the dose to the normal tissue, immobilization devices and markings or tattoos on the patient's skin are used to ensure that each daily treatment is given in the same way. Conventional fractionation is 1.8 to 2 Gy per day, administered 5 days each week for 3 to 7 weeks.

Radiation therapy may be used as the primary modality for palliation in certain patients with metastatic disease, mostly patients with bony metastases. In this scenario, radiation is recommended for symptomatic metastases only.[240] However, lytic metastases in weight-bearing bones such as the femur, tibia, or humerus also are considered for irradiation. Another scenario in which radiation might be appropriate is spinal cord compression due to metastases to the vertebral body extending posteriorly to the spinal canal.

The goal of adjuvant radiation therapy is to decrease local-regional recurrence rates. Adjuvant radiation therapy can be given before surgery, after surgery, or in selected cases, during surgery. Preoperative radiation therapy has several advantages. It may minimize seeding of the tumor during surgery and it allows for smaller treatment fields because the operative bed has not been contaminated with tumor cells. Finally, radiation therapy for inoperable tumors may achieve adequate reduction to make them operable. The disadvantages of preoperative therapy are an increased risk of postoperative wound healing problems and the difficulty in planning subsequent radiation therapy in patients who have positive surgical margins. If radiation therapy is given postoperatively, it is usually given 3 to 4 weeks after surgery to allow for wound healing. The advantage of postoperative radiation therapy is that the surgical specimen can be evaluated histologically and radiation therapy can be reserved for patients who are most likely to benefit from it. Further, the radiation therapy can be modified on the basis of margin status. The disadvantages of postoperative radiation therapy are that the volume of normal tissue requiring irradiation may be larger owing to surgical contamination of the tissue planes and that the tumor may be less sensitive to radiation owing to poor oxygenation. Postlaparotomy adhesions may decrease the mobility of the small bowel loops, increasing the risk for radiation injury in abdominal or pelvic irradiation. Given the potential advantages and disadvantages of both approaches, the roles of preoperative and postoperative radiation therapy are being actively evaluated and compared for many cancer types.

Another mode of postoperative radiation therapy is brachytherapy. In brachytherapy, unlike external beam therapy, the radiation source is in contact with the tissue being irradiated. The radiation source may be cesium, gold, iridium, or radium.[236] Brachytherapy is administered with temporary or permanent implants such as needles, seeds, or catheters. Temporary brachytherapy catheters are placed either during open surgery or percutaneously soon after surgery. The implants are loaded interstitially and treatment usually is given postoperatively for a short duration such as 1 to 3 days.[236] Although brachytherapy has the advantage of patient convenience owing to the shorter treatment duration, it has the disadvantages of leaving scars at the catheter insertion site and requiring special facilities for inpatient brachytherapy therapy. Furthermore, oncologic consequences of the limited treatment volume and duration are not well understood.

Chemotherapy can be given before or concurrently with radiation. Chemotherapy before radiation has the advantage of reducing the tumor burden, facilitating radiation therapy. On the other hand, some chemotherapy regimens given concurrently with radiation may sensitize the cells to radiation therapy.

Side Effects

Both tumor and normal tissue have radiation dose-response relationships that can be plotted on a sigmoidal curve (Fig. 9-13). A minimum dose of radiation must be given before any response is seen. The response to radiation then increases slowly with an increase in dose. At a certain dose level the curves become exponential, with increases in tumor response and normal tissue toxicity with each incremental dose increase. The side effects of radiation therapy can be acute, occurring during or 2 to 3 weeks after therapy, or chronic, occurring weeks to years after therapy. The side effects depend on the tissue included in the target volume. Some of the

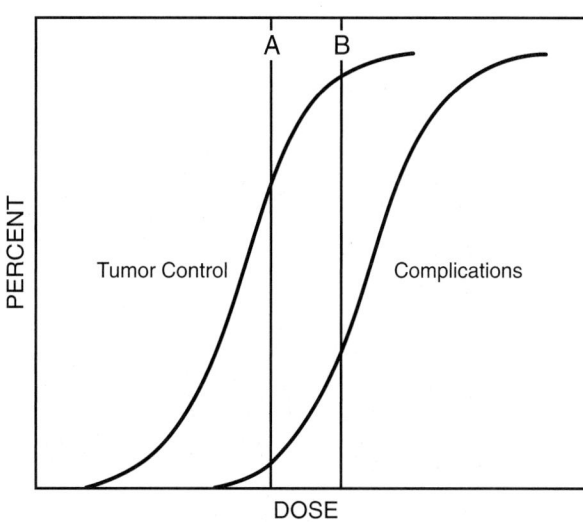

FIG. 9-13. The probabilities of tumor control and of complications at different doses. *A.* At lower doses, the probability of complications is low, with a moderate chance of tumor control. *B.* Increasing the dose may gain a higher chance of tumor control at the price of significantly higher complication risks. (*Modified from Eisbruch et al,[240] with permission.*)

major acute and chronic sequelae of radiation are summarized in Table 9-27.[240,241] In addition to these, a small increase in the risk of secondary malignancies is attributable to radiation therapy.

CANCER PREVENTION

The old axiom "an ounce of prevention is worth a pound of cure" is being increasingly recognized in oncology. Cancer prevention can be divided into three categories: (1) primary prevention (i.e., preventing initial cancers in healthy individuals); (2) secondary prevention (i.e., preventing cancer in individuals with premalignant conditions); and (3) tertiary prevention (i.e., preventing second primary cancers in patients cured of their initial disease).[242]

The administration of systemic or local therapies to prevent the development of cancer, called *chemoprevention,* is being actively explored for several cancer types. In breast cancer, the NSABP Breast Cancer Prevention Trial demonstrated that tamoxifen reduces the risk of breast cancer by one half and reduces the risk of estrogen-receptor–positive tumors by 69% in high-risk

Table 9-27
Local Effects of Radiation

Organ	Acute Changes	Chronic Changes
Skin	Erythema, wet or dry desquamation, epilation	Telangiectasia, subcutaneous fibrosis, ulceration
Gastrointestinal tract	Nausea, diarrhea, edema, ulceration, hepatitis	Stricture, ulceration, perforation, hematochezia
Kidney		Nephropathy, renal insufficiency
Bladder	Dysuria	Hematuria, ulceration, perforation
Gonads	Sterility	Atrophy, ovarian failure
Hematopoietic tissue	Lymphopenia, neutropenia, thrombocytopenia	Pancytopenia
Bone	Epiphyseal growth arrest	Necrosis
Lung	Pneumonitis	Pulmonary fibrosis
Heart		Pericarditis, vascular damage
Upper aerodigestive tract	Mucositis, xerostomia, anosmia	Xerostomia, dental caries
Eye	Conjunctivitis	Cataract, keratitis, optic nerve atrophy
Nervous system	Cerebral edema	Necrosis, myelitis

SOURCE: Modified with permission from Daly et al.[241]

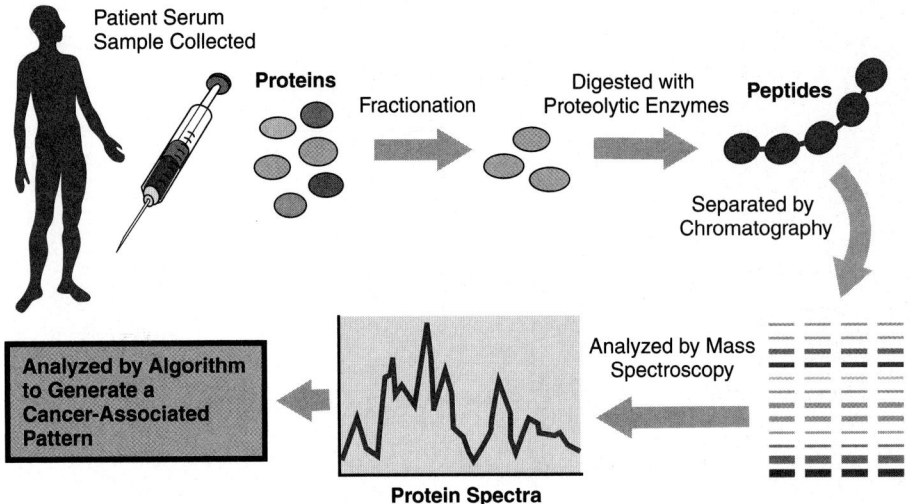

FIG. 9-14. Proteomic detection of cancer. Protein-pattern analysis can be used to detect cancer cells in samples of tissues and fluids such as blood. Proteins can be isolated from samples, fractionated, and digested with proteolytic enzymes. The resulting peptides are separated by chromatography, and the resulting pattern is analyzed by techniques such as mass spectroscopy. Bioinformatic tools can then be used to identify cancer-specific proteomic patterns and to detect cancer in other patients based on similarities between the individual's proteomic patterns and the cancer-associated pattern. (*Modified from Sidransky,[247] with permission.*)

patients.[243] Therefore tamoxifen has been approved by the Food and Drug Administration (FDA) for breast cancer chemoprevention. Several other agents, including raloxifene and fenretinide, also show promise for breast cancer prevention and are under active investigation.[244] Celecoxib has been shown to reduce polyp number and polyp burden in patients with familial adenomatous polyposis (FAP), leading to its approval by the FDA for these patients. In head and neck cancer, 13-*cis*-retinoic acid was shown to both reverse oral leukoplakia and reduce second primary tumor development.[245,246] Thus the chemoprevention trials completed so far have demonstrated success in primary, secondary, and tertiary prevention. Although the successes of these chemoprevention studies are impressive, much remains to be done over the next few years to improve patient selection and decrease therapy-related toxic effects. It is important for surgeons to be aware of these preventive options since they are likely to be involved in the diagnosis of premalignant and malignant conditions, and will be the ones to counsel patients about their chemopreventive options.

In selected scenarios, the risk of cancer is high enough to justify surgical prevention. These high-risk scenarios include hereditary cancer syndromes such as hereditary breast ovarian cancer syndrome, hereditary diffuse gastric cancer, multiple endocrine neoplasia type 2, FAP, and HNPCC, as well as some nonhereditary scenarios such as chronic ulcerative colitis. Most prophylactic surgeries are large ablative surgeries (e.g., bilateral risk-reducing mastectomy or total proctocolectomy). Therefore it is important that the patient be completely informed about potential surgical complications as well as long-term lifestyle consequences. Further, the conservative options of close surveillance and chemoprevention need to be discussed. The patient's cancer risk needs to be assessed accurately and implications for survival discussed. Ultimately, the decision to proceed with surgical prevention should be individualized and made with caution.

TRENDS AND EVOLVING TECHNOLOGIES IN ONCOLOGY

Cancer Screening and Diagnosis

It is clear that the practice of oncology will change dramatically over the next few decades as our understanding of the molecular basis of cancer and available technologies are evolving rapidly. One of the critical changes expected is earlier detection of cancers. With improvements in available imaging modalities and development of newer functional imaging technologies, it is likely that many tumors may be detected at earlier, more curable stages in the near future.

Another area of rapid development is the identification of serum markers. High-throughput technologies such as matrix-assisted laser-desorption-ionization time of flight (MALDI-TOF) mass spectroscopy and liquid chromatography-ion-spray tandem mass spectroscopy (LC-MS/MS) have revolutionized the field of proteomics and are now being used to compare serum protein profiles between patients with cancer and individuals without cancer (Fig. 9-14).[247] Recently, investigators have compared the proteomic profiles of patients with prostate cancer and ovarian cancer to those of controls, identifying unique proteins in the sera of cancer patients.[248,249] Identification of unique proteins as well as unique proteomic profiles for most cancer types is being pursued actively by many researchers, which if successful, could dramatically enhance our ability to detect cancers early.

Surgical Therapy

The current trend in surgery is moving toward more conservative resections. With earlier identification of tumors, more conservative surgeries may be possible. The goal, however, is always to remove the tumor en bloc with wide negative margins. Another interesting area being explored is the destruction of tumors by such techniques as radiofrequency ablation, cryoablation, and heat-producing technologies such as lasers, microwaves, or focused ultrasound.[250] Three pilot studies have demonstrated that radiofrequency ablation is effective for destruction of small primary breast cancers.[250] Although this approach remains experimental and potentially of limited applicability because of the need for expertise in breast imaging, with the development of imaging technologies that can accurately map the extent of cancer cells, these types of noninvasive interventions are likely to come to the forefront. However, these techniques will be limited to cancers not involving hollow viscera.

The debate over how to manage the regional lymph node basins for certain cancer types continues. With an increasing understanding of the metastatic process, surgeons may be able to stratify patients on the basis of the likelihood of their disease to spread metastatically, based on the gene expression profile of their primary tumors, and offer regional therapy accordingly.

Systemic Therapy

The current trend in systemic therapy is moving toward individualized therapy. It now is presumed that all cancers of a certain cell origin are the same, thus all patients are offered the same systemic therapy. Not all patients respond to these therapies, however, emphasizing the biologic variability within the groups. Therefore the intent is to determine the underlying biology of each tumor in order to tailor therapy accordingly. The approaches utilized include high-throughput techniques such as proteomics, or more frequently, transcriptional profiling in which the relative mRNA levels for thousands of genes can be determined simultaneously in a given tumor by using microarray technology. The transcriptional profiling approach is being used to identify molecular signatures that correlate with response to certain agents. It is likely that in the near future tumors can be tested and treatments individualized. Patients who will respond to conventional therapies can be given these regimens, while patients who will not respond are not, sparing them the toxicity. Instead, these patients can be offered novel therapies. Furthermore, with emerging biologic therapies, it is likely that patients may be given a combination of biologic therapies specifically targeting the alterations in their own tumors. Finally, stratification of patients by gene expression profile for prognosis may assist in determining which patients are at higher risk of relapse, sparing patients whose tumors have less aggressive biologic characteristics further therapy.

References

1. Jemal A, Murray T, Samuels A, et al: Cancer statistics, 2003. *CA Cancer J Clin* 53:5, 2003.
2. Parkin DM, Pisani P, Ferlay J: Global cancer statistics. *CA Cancer J Clin* 49:33, 1999.
3. Ziegler RG, Hoover RN, Pike MC, et al: Migration patterns and breast cancer risk in Asian-American women. *J Natl Cancer Inst* 85:1819, 1993.
4. Sikora K: Developing a global strategy for cancer. *Eur J Cancer* 35:1870, 1999.
5. Pelengaris S, Khan M, Evan G: c-MYC: More than just a matter of life and death. *Nat Rev Cancer* 2:764, 2002.
6. Fearon ER, Vogelstein B: A genetic model for colorectal tumorigenesis. *Cell* 61:759, 1990.
7. Malumbres M, Barbacid M: To cycle or not to cycle: A critical decision in cancer. *Nat Rev Cancer* 1:222, 2001.
8. Kastan MB, Skapek SX: Molecular biology of cancer: the cell cycle, in DeVita VT, Hellman S, Rosenberg SA (eds): *Cancer: Principles and Practice of Oncology.* Philadelphia: Lippincott Williams & Wilkins, 2001, p 91.
9. Corn PG, El-Deiry WS: Derangement of growth and differentiation control in oncogenesis. *Bioessays* 24:83, 2002.
10. Ho A, Dowdy SF: Regulation of G(1) cell-cycle progression by oncogenes and tumor suppressor genes. *Curr Opin Genet Dev* 12:47, 2002.
11. Blume-Jensen P, Hunter T: Oncogenic kinase signalling. *Nature* 411:355, 2001.
12. Malaney S, Daly RJ: The ras signaling pathway in mammary tumorigenesis and metastasis. *J Mammary Gland Biol Neoplasia* 6:101, 2001.
13. Shields JM, Pruitt K, McFall A, et al: Understanding Ras: "It ain't over 'til it's over." *Trends Cell Biol* 10:147, 2000.
14. Cox AD, Der CJ: Ras family signaling: Therapeutic targeting. *Cancer Biol Ther* 1:599, 2002.
15. Downward J: Targeting RAS signalling pathways in cancer therapy. *Nat Rev Cancer* 3:11, 2003.
16. Vennstrom B, Sheiness D, Zabielski J, et al: Isolation and characterization of c-myc, a cellular homolog of the oncogene (v-myc) of avian myelocytomatosis virus strain 29. *J Virol* 42:773, 1982.
17. Dalla-Favera R, Bregni M, Erikson J, et al: Human c-myc oncogene is located on the region of chromosome 8 that is translocated in Burkitt lymphoma cells. *Proc Natl Acad Sci USA* 79:7824, 1982.
18. Guo QM, Malek RL, Kim S, et al: Identification of c-myc responsive genes using rat cDNA microarray. *Cancer Res* 60:5922, 2000.
19. Coller HA, Grandori C, Tamayo P, et al: Expression analysis with oligonucleotide microarrays reveals that MYC regulates genes involved in growth, cell cycle, signaling, and adhesion. *Proc Natl Acad Sci USA* 97:3260, 2000.
20. Lutz W, Leon J, Eilers M: Contributions of Myc to tumorigenesis. *Biochim Biophys Acta* 1602:61, 2002.
21. Liao DJ, Dickson RB: c-Myc in breast cancer. *Endocr Relat Cancer* 7:143, 2000.
22. Eccles SA: The role of c-erbB-2/HER2/neu in breast cancer progression and metastasis. *J Mammary Gland Biol Neoplasia* 6:393, 2001.
23. Wang SC, Hung MC: HER2 overexpression and cancer targeting. *Semin Oncol* 28:115, 2001.
24. Yarden Y, Sliwkowski MX: Untangling the ErbB signalling network. *Nat Rev Mol Cell Biol* 2:127, 2001.
25. Schechter AL, Stern DF, Vaidyanathan L, et al: The neu oncogene: An erb-B-related gene encoding a 185,000-Mr tumour antigen. *Nature* 312:513, 1984.
26. Meric F, Hung MC, Hortobagyi GN, et al: HER2/neu in the management of invasive breast cancer. *J Am Coll Surg* 194:488, 2002.
27. Kim R, Tanabe K, Uchida Y, et al: Current status of the molecular mechanisms of anticancer drug-induced apoptosis. The contribution of molecular-level analysis to cancer chemotherapy. *Cancer Chemother Pharmacol* 50:343, 2002.
28. Igney FH, Krammer PH: Death and anti-death: Tumour resistance to apoptosis. *Nat Rev Cancer* 2:277, 2002.
29. Hood JD, Cheresh DA: Role of integrins in cell invasion and migration. *Nat Rev Cancer* 2:91, 2002.
30. http://www.path.sunysb.edu/courses/im/: Cancer Invasion and Metastasis, 2001, State University of New York Pathology Department.
31. Liekens S, De Clercq E, Neyts J: Angiogenesis: Regulators and clinical applications. *Biochem Pharmacol* 61:253, 2001.
32. Egeblad M, Werb Z: New functions for the matrix metalloproteinases in cancer progression. *Nat Rev Cancer* 2:161, 2002.
33. John A, Tuszynski G: The role of matrix metalloproteinases in tumor angiogenesis and tumor metastasis. *Pathol Oncol Res* 7:14, 2001.
34. Fox SB, Gasparini G, Harris AL: Angiogenesis: Pathological, prognostic, and growth-factor pathways and their link to trial design and anticancer drugs. *Lancet Oncol* 2:278, 2001.
35. Folkman J, Merler E, Abernathy C, et al: Isolation of a tumor factor responsible for angiogenesis. *J Exp Med* 133:275, 1971.
36. McCarty MF, Liu W, Fan F, et al: Promises and pitfalls of anti-angiogenic therapy in clinical trials. *Trends Mol Med* 9:53, 2003.
37. Soker S, Takashima S, Miao HQ, et al: Neuropilin-1 is expressed by endothelial and tumor cells as an isoform-specific receptor for vascular endothelial growth factor. *Cell* 92:735, 1998.
38. Reinmuth N, Parikh AA, Ahmad SA, et al: Biology of angiogenesis in tumors of the gastrointestinal tract. *Microsc Res Tech* 60:199, 2003.
39. Nor JE, Christensen J, Mooney DJ, et al: Vascular endothelial growth factor (VEGF)-mediated angiogenesis is associated with enhanced endothelial cell survival and induction of Bcl-2 expression. *Am J Pathol* 154:375, 1999.
40. Stacker SA, Achen MG, Jussila L, et al: Lymphangiogenesis and cancer metastasis. *Nat Rev Cancer* 2:573, 2002.
41. He Y, Kozaki K, Karpanen T, et al: Suppression of tumor lymphangiogenesis and lymph node metastasis by blocking vascular endothelial growth factor receptor 3 signaling. *J Natl Cancer Inst* 94:819, 2002.
42. Ahmad SA, Liu W, Jung YD, et al: Differential expression of angiopoietin-1 and angiopoietin-2 in colon carcinoma. A possible mechanism for the initiation of angiogenesis. *Cancer* 92:1138, 2001.

43. Ahmad SA, Liu W, Jung YD, et al: The effects of angiopoietin-1 and -2 on tumor growth and angiogenesis in human colon cancer. *Cancer Res* 61:1255, 2001.

44. Weidner N, Semple JP, Welch WR, et al: Tumor angiogenesis and metastasis—correlation in invasive breast carcinoma. *N Engl J Med* 324:1, 1991.

45. Chambers AF, Groom AC, MacDonald IC: Dissemination and growth of cancer cells in metastatic sites. *Nat Rev Cancer* 2:563, 2002.

46. Karrison TG, Ferguson DJ, Meier P: Dormancy of mammary carcinoma after mastectomy. *J Natl Cancer Inst* 91:80, 1999.

47. Meltzer A: Dormancy and breast cancer. *J Surg Oncol* 43:181, 1990.

48. Naumov GN, MacDonald IC, Weinmeister PM, et al: Persistence of solitary mammary carcinoma cells in a secondary site: A possible contributor to dormancy. *Cancer Res* 62:2162, 2002.

49. Demicheli R: Tumour dormancy: findings and hypotheses from clinical research on breast cancer. *Semin Cancer Biol* 11:297, 2001.

50. Steeg PS: Metastasis suppressors alter the signal transduction of cancer cells. *Nat Rev Cancer* 3:55, 2003.

51. Ramaswamy S, Ross KN, Lander ES, et al: A molecular signature of metastasis in primary solid tumors. *Nat Genet* 33:49, 2003.

52. van de Vijver MJ, He YD, van't Veer LJ, et al: A gene-expression signature as a predictor of survival in breast cancer. *N Engl J Med* 347:1999, 2002.

53. Webb T: Microarray studies challenge theories of metastasis. *J Natl Cancer Inst* 95:350, 2003.

54. Vahteristo P, Tamminen A, Karvinen P, et al: p53, CHK2, and CHK1 genes in Finnish families with Li-Fraumeni syndrome: Further evidence of CHK2 in inherited cancer predisposition. *Cancer Res* 61:5718, 2001.

55. Friend SH, Bernards R, Rogelj S, et al: A human DNA segment with properties of the gene that predisposes to retinoblastoma and osteosarcoma. *Nature* 323:643, 1986.

56. Knudson AG Jr.: Mutation and cancer: Statistical study of retinoblastoma. *Proc Natl Acad Sci USA* 68:820, 1971.

57. Knudson AG: Two genetic hits (more or less) to cancer. *Nat Rev Cancer* 1:157, 2001.

58. de Sutter E, Havers W, Hopping W, et al: The prognosis of retinoblastoma in terms of survival. A computer assisted study. Part II. *Ophthalmic Paediatr Genet* 8:85, 1987.

59. Francois J, de Sutter E, Coppieters R, et al: Late extraocular tumours in retinoblastoma survivors. *Ophthalmologica* 181:93, 1980.

60. Eng C, Li FP, Abramson DH, et al: Mortality from second tumors among long-term survivors of retinoblastoma. *J Natl Cancer Inst* 85:1121, 1993.

61. DiCiommo D, Gallie BL, Bremner R: Retinoblastoma: The disease, gene and protein provide critical leads to understand cancer. *Semin Cancer Biol* 10:255, 2000.

62. Chellappan SP, Hiebert S, Mudryj M, et al: The E2F transcription factor is a cellular target for the RB protein. *Cell* 65:1053, 1991.

63. Harbour JW, Dean DC: Rb function in cell-cycle regulation and apoptosis. *Nat Cell Biol* 2:E65, 2000.

64. Harbour JW, Lai SL, Whang-Peng J, et al: Abnormalities in structure and expression of the human retinoblastoma gene in SCLC. *Science* 241:353, 1988.

65. Classon M, Harlow E: The retinoblastoma tumour suppressor in development and cancer. *Nat Rev Cancer* 2:910, 2002.

66. Nevins JR: The Rb/E2F pathway and cancer. *Hum Mol Genet* 10:699, 2001.

67. Li FP, Fraumeni JF Jr.: Soft-tissue sarcomas, breast cancer, and other neoplasms. A familial syndrome? *Ann Intern Med* 71:747, 1969.

68. Li FP, Fraumeni JF Jr., Mulvihill JJ, et al: A cancer family syndrome in twenty-four kindreds. *Cancer Res* 48:5358, 1988.

69. Birch JM, Hartley AL, Tricker KJ, et al: Prevalence and diversity of constitutional mutations in the p53 gene among 21 Li-Fraumeni families. *Cancer Res* 54:1298, 1994.

70. Frebourg T, Barbier N, Yan YX, et al: Germ-line p53 mutations in 15 families with Li-Fraumeni syndrome. *Am J Hum Genet* 56:608, 1995.

71. Birch JM, Alston RD, McNally RJ, et al: Relative frequency and morphology of cancers in carriers of germline TP53 mutations. *Oncogene* 20:4621, 2001.

72. Evans SC, Mims B, McMasters KM, et al: Exclusion of a p53 germline mutation in a classic Li-Fraumeni syndrome family. *Hum Genet* 102:681, 1998.

73. Fisher DE: The p53 tumor suppressor: Critical regulator of life and death in cancer. *Apoptosis* 6:7, 2001.

74. Birch JM, Blair V, Kelsey AM, et al: Cancer phenotype correlates with constitutional TP53 genotype in families with the Li-Fraumeni syndrome. *Oncogene* 17:1061, 1998.

75. Bell DW, Varley JM, Szydlo TE, et al: Heterozygous germ line hCHK2 mutations in Li-Fraumeni syndrome. *Science* 286:2528, 1999.

76. Lee JS, Collins KM, Brown AL, et al: hCds1-mediated phosphorylation of BRCA1 regulates the DNA damage response. *Nature* 404:201, 2000.

77. Lee SB, Kim SH, Bell DW, et al: Destabilization of CHK2 by a missense mutation associated with Li-Fraumeni syndrome. *Cancer Res* 61:8062, 2001.

78. Vahteristo P, Bartkova J, Eerola H, et al: A CHEK2 genetic variant contributing to a substantial fraction of familial breast cancer. *Am J Hum Genet* 71:432, 2002.

79. Ingvarsson S, Sigbjornsdottir BI, Huiping C, et al: Mutation analysis of the CHK2 gene in breast carcinoma and other cancers. *Breast Cancer Res* 4:R4, 2002.

80. Loman N, Johannsson O, Kristoffersson U, et al: Family history of breast and ovarian cancers and BRCA1 and BRCA2 mutations in a population-based series of early-onset breast cancer. *J Natl Cancer Inst* 93:1215, 2001.

81. Tobias DH, Eng C, McCurdy LD, et al: Founder BRCA 1 and 2 mutations among a consecutive series of Ashkenazi Jewish ovarian cancer patients. *Gynecol Oncol* 78:148, 2000.

82. Ford D, Easton DF, Bishop DT, et al: Risks of cancer in BRCA1-mutation carriers. Breast Cancer Linkage Consortium. *Lancet* 343:692, 1994.

83. Ford D, Easton DF, Stratton M, et al: Genetic heterogeneity and penetrance analysis of the BRCA1 and BRCA2 genes in breast cancer families. The Breast Cancer Linkage Consortium. *Am J Hum Genet* 62:676, 1998.

84. Cancer risks in BRCA2 mutation carriers. The Breast Cancer Linkage Consortium. *J Natl Cancer Inst* 91:1310, 1999.

85. Venkitaraman AR: Cancer susceptibility and the functions of BRCA1 and BRCA2. *Cell* 108:171, 2002.

86. Liu Y, West SC: Distinct functions of BRCA1 and BRCA2 in double-strand break repair. *Breast Cancer Res* 4:9, 2002.

87. Venkitaraman AR: Functions of BRCA1 and BRCA2 in the biological response to DNA damage. *J Cell Sci* 114:3591, 2001.

88. Hedenfalk I, Duggan D, Chen Y, et al: Gene-expression profiles in hereditary breast cancer. *N Engl J Med* 344:539, 2001.

89. Lakhani SR, Jacquemier J, Sloane JP, et al: Multifactorial analysis of differences between sporadic breast cancers and cancers involving BRCA1 and BRCA2 mutations. *J Natl Cancer Inst* 90:1138, 1998.

90. King MC, Wieand S, Hale K, et al: Tamoxifen and breast cancer incidence among women with inherited mutations in BRCA1 and BRCA2: National Surgical Adjuvant Breast and Bowel Project (NSABP-P1) Breast Cancer Prevention Trial. *JAMA* 286:2251, 2001.

91. Goss KH, Groden J: Biology of the adenomatous polyposis coli tumor suppressor. *J Clin Oncol* 18:1967, 2000.

92. Sieber OM, Tomlinson IP, Lamlum H: The adenomatous polyposis coli (APC) tumour suppressor—genetics, function and disease. *Mol Med Today* 6:462, 2000.

93. Jen J, Powell SM, Papadopoulos N, et al: Molecular determinants of dysplasia in colorectal lesions. *Cancer Res* 54:5523, 1994.

94. Nishisho I, Nakamura Y, Miyoshi Y, et al: Mutations of chromosome 5q21 genes in FAP and colorectal cancer patients. *Science* 253:665, 1991.

95. Groden J, Thliveris A, Samowitz W, et al: Identification and characterization of the familial adenomatous polyposis coli gene. *Cell* 66:589, 1991.

96. Fearnhead NS, Britton MP, Bodmer WF: The ABC of APC. *Hum Mol Genet* 10:721, 2001.

97. Caspari R, Olschwang S, Friedl W, et al: Familial adenomatous polyposis: desmoid tumours and lack of ophthalmic lesions (CHRPE) associated with APC mutations beyond codon 1444. *Hum Mol Genet* 4:337, 1995.

98. Davies DR, Armstrong JG, Thakker N, et al: Severe Gardner syndrome in families with mutations restricted to a specific region of the APC gene. *Am J Hum Genet* 57:1151, 1995.

99. Lynch HT, Smyrk TC, Watson P, et al: Genetics, natural history, tumor spectrum, and pathology of hereditary nonpolyposis colorectal cancer: An updated review. *Gastroenterology* 104:1535, 1993.

100. Vasen HF, Watson P, Mecklin JP, et al: New clinical criteria for hereditary nonpolyposis colorectal cancer (HNPCC, Lynch syndrome) proposed by the International Collaborative group on HNPCC. *Gastroenterology* 116:1453, 1999.

101. Leach FS, Nicolaides NC, Papadopoulos N, et al: Mutations of a mutS homolog in hereditary nonpolyposis colorectal cancer. *Cell* 75:1215, 1993.

102. Fishel R, Lescoe MK, Rao MR, et al: The human mutator gene homolog MSH2 and its association with hereditary nonpolyposis colon cancer. *Cell* 75:1027, 1993.

103. Miyaki M, Konishi M, Tanaka K, et al: Germline mutation of MSH6 as the cause of hereditary nonpolyposis colorectal cancer. *Nat Genet* 17:271, 1997.

104. Bronner CE, Baker SM, Morrison PT, et al: Mutation in the DNA mismatch repair gene homologue hMLH1 is associated with hereditary non-polyposis colon cancer. *Nature* 368:258, 1994.

105. Papadopoulos N, Nicolaides NC, Wei YF, et al: Mutation of a mutL homolog in hereditary colon cancer. *Science* 263:1625, 1994.

106. Nicolaides NC, Papadopoulos N, Liu B, et al: Mutations of two PMS homologues in hereditary nonpolyposis colon cancer. *Nature* 371:75, 1994.

107. Gruber SB, Kohlmann W: The genetics of hereditary non-polyposis colorectal cancer. *J Natl Comprehensive Cancer Network* 1:137, 2003.

108. Steck PA, Pershouse MA, Jasser SA, et al: Identification of a candidate tumour suppressor gene, MMAC1, at chromosome 10q23.3 that is mutated in multiple advanced cancers. *Nat Genet* 15:356, 1997.

109. Liaw D, Marsh DJ, Li J, et al: Germline mutations of the PTEN gene in Cowden disease, an inherited breast and thyroid cancer syndrome. *Nat Genet* 16:64, 1997.

110. Nelen MR, van Staveren WC, Peeters EA, et al: Germline mutations in the PTEN/MMAC1 gene in patients with Cowden disease. *Hum Mol Genet* 6:1383, 1997.

111. Eng C: Will the real Cowden syndrome please stand up: Revised diagnostic criteria. *J Med Genet* 37:828, 2000.

112. Starink TM, van der Veen JP, Arwert F, et al: The Cowden syndrome: A clinical and genetic study in 21 patients. *Clin Genet* 29:222, 1986.

113. Marsh DJ, Coulon V, Lunetta KL, et al: Mutation spectrum and genotype-phenotype analyses in Cowden disease and Bannayan-Zonana syndrome, two hamartoma syndromes with germline PTEN mutation. *Hum Mol Genet* 7:507, 1998.

114. Cantley LC, Neel BG: New insights into tumor suppression: PTEN suppresses tumor formation by restraining the phosphoinositide 3-kinase/AKT pathway. *Proc Natl Acad Sci USA* 96:4240, 1999.

115. Hussussian CJ, Struewing JP, Goldstein AM, et al: Germline p16 mutations in familial melanoma. *Nat Genet* 8:15, 1994.

116. Greene MH: The genetics of hereditary melanoma and nevi. 1998 update. *Cancer* 86:2464, 1999.

117. Goldstein AM, Fraser MC, Struewing JP, et al: Increased risk of pancreatic cancer in melanoma-prone kindreds with p16INK4 mutations. *N Engl J Med* 333:970, 1995.

118. Ranade K, Hussussian CJ, Sikorski RS, et al: Mutations associated with familial melanoma impair p16INK4 function. *Nat Genet* 10:114, 1995.

119. Rocco JW, Sidransky D: p16(MTS-1/CDKN2/INK4a) in cancer progression. *Exp Cell Res* 264:42, 2001.

120. Fitzgerald RC, Caldas C: E-cadherin mutations and hereditary gastric cancer: prevention by resection? *Dig Dis* 20:23, 2002.

121. Berx G, Becker KF, Hofler H, et al: Mutations of the human E-cadherin (CDH1) gene. *Hum Mutat* 12:226, 1998.

122. Berx G, Van Roy F: The E-cadherin/catenin complex: An important gatekeeper in breast cancer tumorigenesis and malignant progression. *Breast Cancer Res* 3:289, 2001.

123. Alsanea O, Clark OH: Familial thyroid cancer. *Curr Opin Oncol* 13:44, 2001.

124. van der Harst E, de Krijger RR, Bruining HA, et al: Prognostic value of RET proto-oncogene point mutations in malignant and benign, sporadic phaeochromocytomas. *Int J Cancer* 79:537, 1998.

125. Redmond DE Jr.: Tobacco and cancer: the first clinical report, 1761. *N Engl J Med* 282:18, 1970.

126. Loechler EL, Henry B, Seo K-Y: Cellular responses to chemical carcinogens, in Coleman WB, Tsongalis GJ (eds): *The Molecular Basis of Human Cancer*. Totowa, NJ: Humana Press, 2002, p 203.

127. Timblin CR, Jannsen-Heininger Y, Mossman BT: Physical agents in human carcinogenesis, in Coleman WB, Tsongalis GJ (eds): *The Molecular Basis of Human Cancer*. Totowa, NJ: Humana Press, 2002, p 223.

128. Stanton MF, Layard M, Tegeris A, et al: Relation of particle dimension to carcinogenicity in amphibole asbestoses and other fibrous minerals. *J Natl Cancer Inst* 67:965, 1981.

129. Upton AC: Historical perspectives on radiation carcinogenesis, in Upton AC, Albert RE, Burns FJ, et al (eds): *Radiation Carcinogenesis*. New York: Elsevier, 1986, p 1.

130. Little JB: Radiation carcinogenesis. *Carcinogenesis* 21:397, 2000.

131. Lehnert BE, Goodwin EH, Deshpande A: Extracellular factor(s) following exposure to alpha particles can cause sister chromatid exchanges in normal human cells. *Cancer Res* 57:2164, 1997.

132. Azzam EI, de Toledo SM, Gooding T, et al: Intercellular communication is involved in the bystander regulation of gene expression in human cells exposed to very low fluences of alpha particles. *Radiat Res* 150:497, 1998.

133. Sarasin A: The molecular pathways of ultraviolet-induced carcinogenesis. *Mutat Res* 428:5, 1999.

134. Ananthaswamy HN, Pierceall WE: Molecular mechanisms of ultraviolet radiation carcinogenesis. *Photochem Photobiol* 52:1119, 1990.

135. Hall J, Angele S: Radiation, DNA damage and cancer. *Mol Med Today* 5:157, 1999.

136. Rous P: A sarcoma of the fowl transmissible by an agent separable from the tumor cells. *J Exp Med* 13:397, 1911.

137. http://monographs.iarc.fr/monoeval/grlist.html: Lists of IARC Evaluations, 2002, International Agency for Research on Cancer (IARC).

138. Butel JS: Viral carcinogenesis: Revelation of molecular mechanisms and etiology of human disease. *Carcinogenesis* 21:405, 2000.

139. Rabe C, Cheng B, Caselmann WH: Molecular mechanisms of hepatitis B virus-associated liver cancer. *Dig Dis* 19:279, 2001.

140. White E: Regulation of p53-dependent apoptosis by E1A and E1B. *Curr Top Microbiol Immunol* 199(Pt 3):34, 1995.

141. El-Serag HB: Hepatocellular carcinoma and hepatitis C in the United States. *Hepatology* 36:S74, 2002.

142. Whitman GJ, Stelling CB: Stereotactic core needle biopsy of breast lesions: Experience at The University of Texas M. D. Anderson Cancer Center, in Singletary SE (ed): *Breast Cancer*. New York: Springer-Verlag, 1999, p 4.

143. http://www.nccn.org/physician_gls/f_guidelines.html: National Comprehensive Cancer Network—Practice Guidelines, 2003, NCCN.

144. Gail MH, Brinton LA, Byar DP, et al: Projecting individualized probabilities of developing breast cancer for white females who are being examined annually. *J Natl Cancer Inst* 81:1879, 1989.

145. http://bcra.nci.nih.gov/brc/q1.htm: Breast Cancer Risk Assessment Tool, 2000, National Cancer Institute.

146. Costantino JP, Gail MH, Pee D, et al: Validation studies for models projecting the risk of invasive and total breast cancer incidence. *J Natl Cancer Inst* 91:1541, 1999.

147. Rockhill B, Spiegelman D, Byrne C, et al: Validation of the Gail et al. model of breast cancer risk prediction and implications for chemoprevention. *J Natl Cancer Inst* 93:358, 2001.

148. Bach PB, Kattan MW, Thornquist MD, et al: Variations in lung cancer risk among smokers. *J Natl Cancer Inst* 95:470, 2003.

149. Bassett LW, Hendrick RE, Bassford TL: Quality determinants of mammography. Clinical Practice Guideline No. 13. AHCPR Publication No. 95-0632. Rockville, MD: Agency for Health Care Policy and Research, Public Health Services, U.S., HHS, October 1994.

150. Smith RA, Cokkinides V, Eyre HJ: American Cancer Society guidelines for the early detection of cancer, 2003. *CA Cancer J Clin* 53:27, 2003.

151. Walsh JM, Terdiman JP: Colorectal cancer screening: Scientific review. *JAMA* 289:1288, 2003.

152. Jacobs TW, Connolly JL, Schnitt SJ: Nonmalignant lesions in breast core needle biopsies: To excise or not to excise? *Am J Surg Pathol* 26:1095, 2002.

153. Greene FL, Page DL, Fleming ID, et al (eds): *AJCC Cancer Staging Manual*, 6th ed. New York: Springer-Verlag, 2002, p 484.

154. Mirza AN, Mirza NQ, Vlastos G, et al: Prognostic factors in node-negative breast cancer: A review of studies with sample size more than 200 and follow-up more than 5 years. *Ann Surg* 235:10, 2002.

155. Bast RC Jr., Ravdin P, Hayes DF, et al: 2000 update of recommendations for the use of tumor markers in breast and colorectal cancer: Clinical practice guidelines of the American Society of Clinical Oncology. *J Clin Oncol* 19:1865, 2001.

156. http://medicine.wustl.edu/~labmed/1996vol4no9.html:Tumor Marker Overview, 1996, Laboratory Medicine Newsletter.

157. http://www.vh.org/adult/patient/cancercenter/tumormarker/: Tumor Marker Tests, 1997, Virtual Hospital.

158. http://cis.nci.nih.gov/fact/5_18.htm: Cancer Facts, 1998, National Cancer Institute.

159. Sirovich BE, Schwartz LM, Woloshin S: Screening men for prostate and colorectal cancer in the United States: Does practice reflect the evidence? *JAMA* 289:1414, 2003.

160. Catalona WJ, Richie JP, deKernion JB, et al: Comparison of prostate specific antigen concentration versus prostate specific antigen density in the early detection of prostate cancer: Receiver operating characteristic curves. *J Urol* 152:2031, 1994.

161. Balk SP, Ko YJ, Bubley GJ: Biology of prostate-specific antigen. *J Clin Oncol* 21:383, 2003.

162. Hugosson J, Aus G, Lilja H, et al: Prostate specific antigen based biennial screening is sufficient to detect almost all prostate cancers while still curable. *J Urol* 169:1720, 2003.

163. Harris R, Lohr KN: Screening for prostate cancer: an update of the evidence for the U.S. Preventive Services Task Force. *Ann Intern Med* 137:917, 2002.

164. Coldman AJ, Phillips N, Pickles TA: Trends in prostate cancer incidence and mortality: An analysis of mortality change by screening intensity. *CMAJ* 168:31, 2003.

165. Ito K, Schrder FH: Informed consent for prostate-specific antigen-based screening—European view. *Urology* 61:20, 2003.

166. Macdonald JS: Oral fluoropyrimidines: A closer look at their toxicities. *Am J Clin Oncol* 22:475, 1999.

167. Carriquiry LA, Pineyro A: Should carcinoembryonic antigen be used in the management of patients with colorectal cancer? *Dis Colon Rectum* 42:921, 1999.

168. Duffy MJ: Carcinoembryonic antigen as a marker for colorectal cancer: is it clinically useful? *Clin Chem* 47:624, 2001.

169. Molina R, Zanon G, Filella X, et al: Use of serial carcinoembryonic antigen and CA 15.3 assays in detecting relapses in breast cancer patients. *Breast Cancer Res Treat* 36:41, 1995.

170. Fujiyama S, Tanaka M, Maeda S, et al: Tumor markers in early diagnosis, follow-up and management of patients with hepatocellular carcinoma. *Oncology* 62(Suppl 1):57, 2002.

171. http://www.labcorp.com/datasets/labcorp/html/chapter/mono/ri019500.htm: Alpha-Fetoprotein (AFP), Serum, Tumor Marker (Serial Monitor) (480012), 2001, Laboratory Corporation of America Holdings and Lexi-Comp Inc.

172. Nguyen MH, Keeffe EB: Screening for hepatocellular carcinoma. *J Clin Gastroenterol* 35:S86, 2002.

173. Chan DW, Beveridge RA, Muss H, et al: Use of Truquant BR radioimmunoassay for early detection of breast cancer recurrence in patients with stage II and stage III disease. *J Clin Oncol* 15:2322, 1997.

174. Outcomes of cancer treatment for technology assessment and cancer treatment guidelines. American Society of Clinical Oncology. *J Clin Oncol* 14:671, 1996.

175. Hayes DF, Yamauchi H, Broadwater G, et al: Circulating HER-2/erbB-2/c-neu (HER-2) extracellular domain as a prognostic factor in patients with metastatic breast cancer: Cancer and Leukemia Group B Study 8662. *Clin Cancer Res* 7:2703, 2001.

176. Lipton A, Ali SM, Leitzel K, et al: Elevated serum Her-2/neu level predicts decreased response to hormone therapy in metastatic breast cancer. *J Clin Oncol* 20:1467, 2002.

177. Colomer R, Montero S, Lluch A, et al: Circulating HER2 extracellular domain and resistance to chemotherapy in advanced breast cancer. *Clin Cancer Res* 6:2356, 2000.

178. Molina R, Jo J, Zanon G, et al: Utility of C-erbB-2 in tissue and in serum in the early diagnosis of recurrence in breast cancer patients: Comparison with carcinoembryonic antigen and CA 15.3. *Br J Cancer* 74:1126, 1996.

179. Palmieri G, Ascierto PA, Perrone F, et al: Prognostic value of circulating melanoma cells detected by reverse transcriptase-polymerase chain reaction. *J Clin Oncol* 21:767, 2003.

180. Grau AM, Spitz FR, Bouvet M, et al: Pancreatic adenocarcinoma, in Feig BW, Berger DH, Fuhrman GM (eds): *The M. D. Anderson Surgical Oncology Handbook*. Philadelphia: Lippincott Williams & Wilkins, 2003, p 303.

181. Meric F, Mirza NQ, Vlastos G, et al: Positive surgical margins and ipsilateral breast tumor recurrence predict disease-specific survival after breast-conserving therapy. *Cancer* 97:926, 2003.

182. Stocchi L, Nelson H, Sargent DJ, et al: Impact of surgical and pathologic variables in rectal cancer: A United States community and cooperative group report. *J Clin Oncol* 19:3895, 2001.

183. Kuvshinoff B, Maghfoor I, Miedema B, et al: Distal margin requirements after preoperative chemoradiotherapy for distal rectal carcinomas: Are < or = 1 cm distal margins sufficient? *Ann Surg Oncol* 8:163, 2001.

184. Youssef E, Fontanesi J, Mott M, et al: Long-term outcome of combined modality therapy in retroperitoneal and deep-trunk soft-tissue sarcoma: Analysis of prognostic factors. *Int J Radiat Oncol Biol Phys* 54:514, 2002.

185. Stojadinovic A, Leung DH, Hoos A, et al: Analysis of the prognostic significance of microscopic margins in 2084 localized primary adult soft tissue sarcomas. *Ann Surg* 235:424, 2002.

186. Yeo CJ, Abrams RA, Grochow LB, et al: Pancreaticoduodenectomy for pancreatic adenocarcinoma: postoperative adjuvant chemoradiation improves survival. A prospective, single-institution experience. *Ann Surg* 225:621, 1997.

187. Chan KC, Knox WF, Sinha G, et al: Extent of excision margin width required in breast conserving surgery for ductal carcinoma in situ. *Cancer* 91:9, 2001.

188. Balch CM, Soong SJ, Smith T, et al: Long-term results of a prospective surgical trial comparing 2 cm vs. 4 cm excision margins for 740 patients with 1–4 mm melanomas. *Ann Surg Oncol* 8:101, 2001.

189. Moore HG, Riedel E, Minsky BD, et al: Adequacy of 1-cm distal margin after restorative rectal cancer resection with sharp mesorectal excision and preoperative combined-modality therapy. *Ann Surg Oncol* 10:80, 2003.

190. Kapiteijn E, van de Velde CJ: The role of total mesorectal excision in the management of rectal cancer. *Surg Clin North Am* 82:995, 2002.

191. Sigurdson ER: Lymph node dissection: Is it diagnostic or therapeutic? *J Clin Oncol* 21:965, 2003.

192. Gajra A, Newman N, Gamble GP, et al: Effect of number of lymph nodes sampled on outcome in patients with stage I non-small-cell lung cancer. *J Clin Oncol* 21:1029, 2003.

193. Fisher B, Slack NH: Number of lymph nodes examined and the prognosis of breast carcinoma. *Surg Gynecol Obstet* 131:79, 1970.

194. Cabanas RM: An approach for the treatment of penile carcinoma. *Cancer* 39:456, 1977.

195. Morton DL, Wen DR, Wong JH, et al: Technical details of intraoperative lymphatic mapping for early stage melanoma. *Arch Surg* 127:392, 1992.

196. Giuliano AE, Kirgan DM, Guenther JM, et al: Lymphatic mapping and sentinel lymphadenectomy for breast cancer. *Ann Surg* 220:391, 1994.

197. Kitagawa Y, Fujii H, Mukai M, et al: Intraoperative lymphatic mapping and sentinel lymph node sampling in esophageal and gastric cancer. *Surg Oncol Clin North Am* 11:293, 2002.

198. Pitman KT, Johnson JT, Brown ML, et al: Sentinel lymph node biopsy in head and neck squamous cell carcinoma. *Laryngoscope* 112:2101, 2002.

199. Stein HJ, Sendler A, Siewert JR: Site-dependent resection techniques for gastric cancer. *Surg Oncol Clin North Am* 11:405, 2002.

200. Wexner SD, Sands DR: What's new in colon and rectal surgery. *J Am Coll Surg* 196:95, 2003.

201. Feig BW, Curley S, Lucci A, et al: A caution regarding lymphatic mapping in patients with colon cancer. *Am J Surg* 182:707, 2001.

202. Giuliano AE, Dale PS, Turner RR, et al: Improved axillary staging of breast cancer with sentinel lymphadenectomy. *Ann Surg* 222:394, 1995.

203. Gershenwald JE, Thompson W, Mansfield PF, et al: Multi-institutional melanoma lymphatic mapping experience: The prognostic value of sentinel lymph node status in 612 stage I or II melanoma patients. *J Clin Oncol* 17:976, 1999.

204. Giuliano AE, Jones RC, Brennan M, et al: Sentinel lymphadenectomy in breast cancer. *J Clin Oncol* 15:2345, 1997.

205. Krag D, Weaver D, Ashikaga T, et al: The sentinel node in breast cancer—a multicenter validation study. *N Engl J Med* 339:941, 1998.

206. Hill AD, Tran KN, Akhurst T, et al: Lessons learned from 500 cases of lymphatic mapping for breast cancer. *Ann Surg* 229:528, 1999.

207. Cox CE, Bass SS, Boulware D, et al: Implementation of new surgical technology: Outcome measures for lymphatic mapping of breast carcinoma. *Ann Surg Oncol* 6:553, 1999.

208. Bass SS, Cox CE, Ku NN, et al: The role of sentinel lymph node biopsy in breast cancer. *J Am Coll Surg* 189:183, 1999.

209. McMasters KM, Wong SL, Tuttle TM, et al: Preoperative lymphoscintigraphy for breast cancer does not improve the ability to identify axillary sentinel lymph nodes. *Ann Surg* 231:724, 2000.

210. Schwartz GF, Giuliano AE, Veronesi U: Proceedings of the consensus conference on the role of sentinel lymph node biopsy in carcinoma of the breast, April 19–22, 2001, Philadelphia, Pennsylvania. *Cancer* 94:2542, 2002.

211. Krag DN, Weaver DL, Alex JC, et al: Surgical resection and radiolocalization of the sentinel lymph node in breast cancer using a gamma probe. *Surg Oncol* 2:335, 1993.

212. Albertini JJ, Lyman GH, Cox C, et al: Lymphatic mapping and sentinel node biopsy in the patient with breast cancer. *JAMA* 276:1818, 1996.

213. Porter GA, Ross MI, Berman RS, et al: How many lymph nodes are enough during sentinel lymphadenectomy for primary melanoma? *Surgery* 128:306, 2000.

214. McMasters KM, Reintgen DS, Ross MI, et al: Sentinel lymph node biopsy for melanoma: How many radioactive nodes should be removed? *Ann Surg Oncol* 8:192, 2001.

215. Breslin TM, Cohen L, Sahin A, et al: Sentinel lymph node biopsy is accurate after neoadjuvant chemotherapy for breast cancer. *J Clin Oncol* 18:3480, 2000.

216. Bedrosian I, Reynolds C, Mick R, et al: Accuracy of sentinel lymph node biopsy in patients with large primary breast tumors. *Cancer* 88:2540, 2000.

217. Haigh PI, Hansen NM, Qi K, et al: Biopsy method and excision volume do not affect success rate of subsequent sentinel lymph node dissection in breast cancer. *Ann Surg Oncol* 7:21, 2000.

218. Pearson AS, Izzo F, Fleming RY, et al: Intraoperative radiofrequency ablation or cryoablation for hepatic malignancies. *Am J Surg* 178:592, 1999.

219. Curley SA, Izzo F: Radiofrequency ablation of primary and metastatic hepatic malignancies. *Int J Clin Oncol* 7:72, 2002.

220. Polychemotherapy for early breast cancer: an overview of the randomised trials. Early Breast Cancer Trialists' Collaborative Group. *Lancet* 352:930, 1998.

221. Fisher B, Bryant J, Wolmark N, et al: Effect of preoperative chemotherapy on the outcome of women with operable breast cancer. *J Clin Oncol* 16:2672, 1998.

222. Meric F, Hess KR, Varma DG, et al: Radiographic response to neoadjuvant chemotherapy is a predictor of local control and survival in soft tissue sarcomas. *Cancer* 95:1120, 2002.

223. Meric F, Mirza NQ, Buzdar AU, et al: Prognostic implications of pathological lymph node status after preoperative chemotherapy for operable T3N0M0 breast cancer. *Ann Surg Oncol* 7:435, 2000.

224. Broadwater JR, Edwards MJ, Kuglen C, et al: Mastectomy following preoperative chemotherapy. Strict operative criteria control operative morbidity. *Ann Surg* 213:126, 1991.

225. http://reach.ucf.edu/~OncEduc1/PDF/sec10.pdf: Section 10 Systemic Chemotherapy, University of Central Florida.

226. Page R: Principles of chemotherapy, in Pazdur R, Hoskins WJ, Coia LR, et al (eds): *Cancer Management: A Multidisciplinary Approach.* Melville, NY: PRR, Inc., 2001, p 21.

227. Ellis LM, Jones DV, Chiao PJ, et al: Tumor biology, in Greenfield LJ, Mulholland MW, Oldham KT, et al (eds): *Surgery: Scientific Principles and Practice.* Philadelphia: Lippincott-Williams & Wilkins, 1997, p 455.

228. Miller AB, Hoogstraten B, Staquet M, et al: Reporting results of cancer treatment. *Cancer* 47:207, 1981.

229. Dancey J, Sausville EA: Issues and progress with protein kinase inhibitors for cancer treatment. *Nat Rev Drug Discov* 2:296, 2003.

230. Mocellin S, Rossi CR, Lise M, et al: Adjuvant immunotherapy for solid tumors: from promise to clinical application. *Cancer Immunol Immunother* 51:583, 2002.

231. Perales MA, Wolchok JD: Melanoma vaccines. *Cancer Invest* 20:1012, 2002.

232. Dermime S, Armstrong A, Hawkins RE, et al: Cancer vaccines and immunotherapy. *Br Med Bull* 62:149, 2002.

233. Cusack JC Jr., Tanabe KK: Introduction to cancer gene therapy. *Surg Oncol Clin North Am* 11:497, 2002.

234. Hunt KK, Vorburger SA: Tech. Sight. Gene therapy. Hurdles and hopes for cancer treatment. *Science* 297:415, 2002.

235. McCormick F: New-age drug meets resistance. *Nature* 412:281, 2001.

236. Gazda MJ, Coia LR: Principles of radiation therapy, in Pazdur R, Hoskins WJ, Coia LR, et al (eds): *Cancer Management: A Multidisciplinary Approach.* Melville, NY: PRR, Inc, 2001, p 9.

237. Mundt AJ, Roeske JC, Weichelbaum RR: Principles of radiation oncology, in Bast RC Jr., Kuff DW, Pollock RE, et al (eds): *Cancer Medicine,* 5th ed. Hamilton, Ontario: B. C. Decker Inc., 2000, p 465.

238. Terasima T, Tolmach LJ: Variation in several responses of HeLa cells to x-irradiation during the division cycle. *Biophysics J* 3:11, 1963.

239. Raju MR, Amols HI, Bain E, et al: A heavy particle comparative study. Part III: OER and RBE. *Br J Radiol* 51:712, 1978.

240. Eisbruch A, Lichter AS: What a surgeon needs to know about radiation. *Ann Surg Oncol* 4:516, 1997.

241. Daly JM, Bertagnolli M, DeCosse JJ, et al: Oncology, in Schwartz S, Spencer F, Galloway A, et al (eds): *Principles of Surgery.* New York: McGraw-Hill, 1999, p 297.

242. Hong WK: General keynote: the impact of cancer chemoprevention. *Gynecol Oncol* 88:S56, 2003.

243. Fisher B, Costantino JP, Wickerham DL, et al: Tamoxifen for prevention of breast cancer: report of the National Surgical Adjuvant Breast and Bowel Project P-1 Study. *J Natl Cancer Inst* 90:1371, 1998.

244. Arun B, Hortobagyi GN: Progress in breast cancer chemoprevention. *Endocr Relat Cancer* 9:15, 2002.

245. Lippman SM, Batsakis JG, Toth BB, et al: Comparison of low-dose isotretinoin with beta carotene to prevent oral carcinogenesis. *N Engl J Med* 328:15, 1993.

246. Hong WK, Lippman SM, Itri LM, et al: Prevention of second primary tumors with isotretinoin in squamous-cell carcinoma of the head and neck. *N Engl J Med* 323:795, 1990.

247. Sidransky D: Emerging molecular markers of cancer. *Nat Rev Cancer* 2:210, 2002.

248. Paweletz CP, Liotta LA, Petricoin EF 3rd: New technologies for biomarker analysis of prostate cancer progression: Laser capture microdissection and tissue proteomics. *Urology* 57:160, 2001.

249. Petricoin EF, Ardekani AM, Hitt BA, et al: Use of proteomic patterns in serum to identify ovarian cancer. *Lancet* 359:572, 2002.

250. Singletary SE, Fornage BD, Sneige N, et al: Radiofrequency ablation of early-stage invasive breast tumors: an overview. *Cancer J* 8:177, 2002.

251. Marsh D, Zori R: Genetic insights into familial cancers—update and recent discoveries. *Cancer Lett* 181:125, 2002.

252. Morrow CS, Cowan KH: Drug resistance and its clinical circumvention, in Bast RC Jr., Kufe DW, Pollock RE, et al (eds): *Cancer Medicine*, 5th ed. Hamilton, Ontario: B. C. Decker, 2000, p 539.

253. Houimel M, Schneider P, Terskikh A, et al: Selection of peptides and synthesis of pentameric peptabody molecules reacting specifically with ErbB-2 receptor. *Int J Cancer* 92:748, 2001.

254. Yu D, Suen TC, Yan DH, et al: Transcriptional repression of the neu protooncogene by the adenovirus 5 E1A gene products. *Proc Natl Acad Sci USA* 87:4499, 1990.

255. Xing X, Wang SC, Xia W, et al: The ets protein PEA3 suppresses HER-2/neu overexpression and inhibits tumorigenesis. *Nat Med* 6:189, 2000.

256. Ro JS, el-Naggar A, Ro JY, et al: c-erbB-2 amplification in node-negative human breast cancer. *Cancer Res* 49:6941, 1989.

257. Vaughn JP, Iglehart JD, Demirdji S, et al: Antisense DNA downregulation of the ERBB2 oncogene measured by a flow cytometric assay. *Proc Natl Acad Sci USA* 92:8338, 1995.

258. Funato T, Kozawa K, Fujimaki S, et al: Increased sensitivity to cisplatin in gastric cancer by antisense inhibition of the her-2/neu (c-erbB-2) gene. *Chemotherapy* 47:297, 2001.

259. Lui VW, He Y, Huang L: Specific down-regulation of HER-2/neu mediated by a chimeric U6 hammerhead ribozyme results in growth inhibition of human ovarian carcinoma. *Mol Ther* 3:169, 2001.

260. Juhl H, Downing SG, Wellstein A, et al: HER-2/neu is rate-limiting for ovarian cancer growth. Conditional depletion of HER-2/neu by ribozyme targeting. *J Biol Chem* 272:29482, 1997.

261. Offterdinger M, Schneider SM, Huber H, et al: Retinoids control the expression of c-erbB receptors in breast cancer cells. *Biochem Biophys Res Commun* 251:907, 1998.

262. Grunt Th W, Dittrich E, Offterdinger M, et al: Effects of retinoic acid and fenretinide on the c-erbB-2 expression, growth and cisplatin sensitivity of breast cancer cells. *Br J Cancer* 78:79, 1998.

263. Murray JL, Przepiorka D, Ioannides CG: Clinical trials of HER-2/neu-specific vaccines. *Semin Oncol* 27:71, 2000.

264. Knutson KL, Schiffman K, Disis ML: Immunization with a HER-2/neu helper peptide vaccine generates HER-2/neu CD8 T-cell immunity in cancer patients. *J Clin Invest* 107:477, 2001.

265. Pandha HS, Martin LA, Rigg A, et al: Genetic prodrug activation therapy for breast cancer: A phase I clinical trial of erbB-2-directed suicide gene expression. *J Clin Oncol* 17:2180, 1999.

266. McCormick F: Cancer gene therapy: fringe or cutting edge? *Nat Rev Cancer* 1:130, 2001.

267. Stewart ZA, Westfall MD, Pietenpol JA: Cell-cycle dysregulation and anticancer therapy. *Trends Pharmacol Sci* 24:139, 2003.

CHAPTER 10

Transplantation

Abhinav Humar and David L. Dunn

INTRODUCTION

References to transplantation have existed in the scientific literature for centuries, yet the field of modern transplantation did not come into being until the latter half of the twentieth century. Thus, given its short history, it is truly remarkable how far this area of medicine has advanced. From an experimental procedure just 50 years ago,

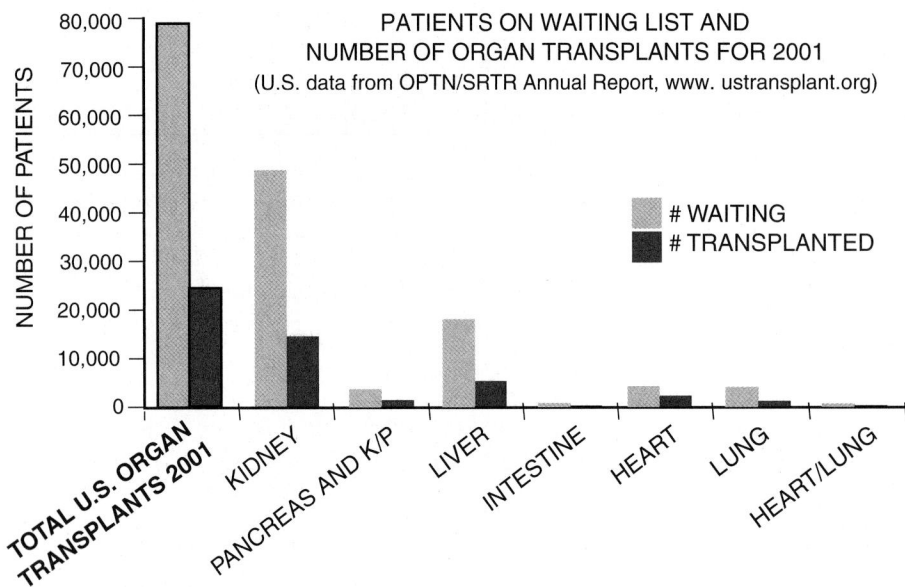

FIG. 10-1. Patients on a waiting list and number of organ transplants performed for 2001. *(Reprinted from U.S. data from the Organ Procurement and Transplant Network/Scientific Registry of Transplant Recipients Annual Report, www.ustransplant.org.)*

transplantation has evolved to become the treatment of choice for end-stage organ failure resulting from almost any of a wide variety of causes. Transplantation of the kidney, liver, pancreas, intestine, heart, and lungs has now become commonplace in all parts of the world.

In fact, transplantation is now so widely accepted and successful that the main problem facing the field today is not surgical technique, rejection, or management of complications, but rather supply of organs. An increasing number of diseases and patients are now potentially treatable with transplants; however, this increase, coupled with the decrease in contraindications to transplants, has meant an increasing number of patients are now awaiting organ replacement therapy. The number of transplants performed yearly has increased over the last decade, but has not kept pace with the exponentially growing waiting list. The gap is ever-widening between the number of transplants performed and the number of waiting patients (Fig. 10-1).

Transplantation statistics in the United States are tracked by the United Network for Organ Sharing (UNOS). In 2001, 78,265 patients were awaiting a transplant, while the number of transplants performed in that year was 23,848.

Definitions

Transplantation is the act of transferring an organ, tissue, or cell from one place to another. Broadly speaking, transplants are divided into three categories based on the similarity between the donor and the recipient: autotransplants, allotransplants, and xenotransplants. *Autotransplants* involve the transfer of tissue or organs from one part of an individual to another part of the same individual. They are the most common type of transplants and include skin grafts, vein grafts for bypasses, bone and cartilage transplants, and nerve transplants. Since the donor and the recipient are the same person and no immunologic disparity exists, no immunosuppression is required. *Allotransplants* involve transfer from one individual to a different individual of the same species—the most common scenario for most solid organ transplants performed today. Immunosuppression is required for allograft recipients in order to prevent rejection. Finally, *xenotransplants* involve transfer across species barriers. Currently, xenotransplants are largely relegated to the laboratory, given the complex, potent immunologic barriers to success.

This chapter deals mainly with allotransplantation. The first part discusses immunobiology, mechanisms of the rejection process, and medications currently used to achieve immunosuppression. The second part focuses on the various transplants, including kidney, pancreas, islet cell, liver, intestine, heart, and lungs. Clinical indications, surgical care, and posttransplant follow-up of these abdominal and thoracic organ recipients are described.

History

Attempts at transplantation have been documented since ancient times, but they are largely of only historic interest. They had no lasting impact on the field of modern transplantation, which did not originate until the latter half of the twentieth century. Important events in the first half of the twentieth century included the development of the surgical techniques for vascular anastomosis by Alexis Carrel; the first human-to-human kidney transplants by Yu Yu Voronoy in the 1930s (which were unsuccessful because of failure to address the immunologic barriers); and the studies of skin transplantation in animal models by Sir Peter Medawar in the 1940s.[1–3] Medawar's work was especially crucial: it provided scientific evidence for the role of the immune system in the failure of allografts to function long-term, through a process later termed *rejection*. His work and observations formed the basis for modern transplant immunobiology.

The first human kidney transplant with long-term success was performed in Boston by Joseph Murray in 1954.[4] Since it was a living-donor transplant between identical twin brothers, the recipient required no immunosuppression and lived for more than 20 years, eventually dying of coronary artery disease. Soon, other centers performed similar transplants, which then led to attempts at kidney transplants between nonidentical individuals, using total body radiation and agents such as 6-mercaptopurine for immunosuppression. By the late 1950s to early 1960s, the combination of azathioprine with corticosteroids allowed kidney allotransplantation to advance out of the realm of experimental therapy.[5,6]

Along with azathioprine and corticosteroids, the development of antilymphocyte serum (antibodies against human lymphoid tissue) gave clinicians reliable, adequate immunosuppression, allowing the birth of extrarenal transplants.[7] In 1963, the first liver transplant was performed by Thomas Starzl in Denver. The first pancreas transplant was performed in 1966 in Minneapolis by William Kelly and Richard Lillehei. Christiaan Barnard performed the first heart transplant in 1967 in Cape Town, South Africa. The 1970s saw other firsts with intestine, lung, and islet transplants.

Kidney transplants flourished during the 1970s, but extrarenal transplants remained largely experimental. One major reason was that rejection remained a major obstacle to the success of these transplanted organs. A dramatic change occurred, however, with the introduction in the early 1980s of cyclosporine. At that time, it was the most specific immunosuppressive agent available. It improved graft survival after kidney transplants by 30% and allowed extrarenal transplants to develop as viable therapies. Since that time, and especially in the 1990s, many new agents have been developed and approved for use in clinical transplantation; scores of others are currently being tested in clinical trials. These agents have allowed for progressively more specific targeting of the immune system pathways involved in the rejection process. As a result, rejection rates have substantially declined for all types of transplants and graft survival rates have increased.

A large part of the recent success of transplants is due to the developments in clinical immunosuppression. But other discoveries also have played a role. More powerful immunosuppression has often meant more risk of infection with opportunistic viral, fungal, and bacterial pathogens. The development of powerful and effective antimicrobial, antifungal, and antiviral therapy (in parallel with immunosuppressive agents) has been crucial to successful solid organ transplantation.

Surgical innovations, beyond the first successful attempts at the various transplants, have continued. In the late 1980s and early 1990s, the development of cadaveric split-liver transplant techniques and of living-donor liver transplants have expanded the donor pool and helped alleviate the significant shortage of donors. The development of laparoscopic donor nephrectomy enabled faster recovery of living kidney donors, thereby increasing their numbers. The 1990s ushered in innovations with thoracic, pancreatic, and cellular transplants.

TRANSPLANT IMMUNOBIOLOGY

The technical advances and techniques that made transplants possible were described almost a hundred years ago. Yet it was only after a basic understanding of transplant immunobiology was obtained could the obstacle of rejection be overcome, thus making clinical transplants possible. The success of transplants today is due in large part to control of the rejection process, thanks to an ever-deepening understanding of the immune process triggered by a transplant.[8]

The immune system is important not only in graft rejection, but also in the body's defense system against viral, bacterial, fungal, and other pathogens. It also helps prevent tumor growth and helps the body respond to shock and trauma. As with the body's reaction to an infection, graft rejection is triggered when specific cells of the transplant recipient, namely T and B lymphocytes, recognize foreign antigens.

Transplant Antigens

The main antigens involved in triggering rejection are coded for by a group of genes known as the major histocompatibility complex (MHC). These antigens and hence genes define the "foreign" nature of one individual to another within the same species. In humans, the MHC complex is known as the human leukocyte antigen (HLA) system. It comprises a series of genes located on chromosome 6. The HLA antigens are grouped into two classes, which differ in their structure and cellular distribution. Class I molecules (named HLA-A, -B, and -C) are found on the membrane of all nucleated cells. Class II molecules (named HLA-DR, -DP, and -DQ) are generally expressed by antigen-presenting cells (APCs) such as B lymphocytes, monocytes, and dendritic cells.

In a nontransplant setting, the function of the HLA gene product is to present antigens as fragments of foreign proteins that can be recognized by T lymphocytes. In the transplant setting, HLA molecules can initiate rejection and graft damage, via either humoral or cellular mechanisms. Humoral rejection occurs if the recipient has circulating antibodies specific to the donor's HLA from prior exposure (i.e., blood transfusion, previous transplant, or pregnancy), or if posttransplant, the recipient develops antibodies specific to the donor's HLA. The antibodies then bind to the donor's recognized foreign antigens, activating the complement cascade and leading to cell lysis. The blood group antigens of the ABO system, though not part of the HLA system, may also trigger this form of humoral rejection.

Cellular rejection is the more common type of rejection after organ transplants. Mediated by T lymphocytes, it results from their activation and proliferation after exposure to donor MHC molecules.

Allorecognition and Destruction

The recognition of foreign HLA antigens by the recipient T cells is referred to as *allorecognition*.[9] This process may occur by either a direct or an indirect pathway. In the direct pathway, the recipient's T cells directly interact with donor HLA molecules, leading to the generation of activated cytotoxic T cells. In the indirect pathway, the recipient's own APCs first process the donor's antigens (which may be shed from the parenchymal cells of the graft into the recipient's circulation, or alternatively may be encountered by the recipient's APCs in the graft itself); then the recipient's APCs present the donor's antigens to the recipient T cells, leading to the activation of those T cells.

Regardless of the method of presentation of foreign MHC, the subsequent steps are similar. Binding of the T cell to the foreign molecule occurs at the T-cell receptor (TCR)-CD3 complex on the surface of the lymphocyte. This binding leads to transduction of a signal to the cell, named signal 1. This signal by itself, however, is not sufficient to result in T-cell activation. Full activation requires transduction of a second signal that is not antigen-dependent. Signal 2 is provided by the binding of accessory molecules on the T cell to corresponding molecules (ligands) on the APC. An example is CD25 on the T lymphocytes binding with its ligand B7 on the surface of the APC. Transmission of signal 1 and 2 to the cell nucleus leads to interleukin-2 (IL-2) gene expression and to production of this important cytokine. IL-2 then permits the entire cascade of T-cell activation to proceed, leading to proliferation and differentiation of these cells into cells capable of causing damage to the graft.

T-cell activation is key in initiating the rejection process, but B-cell activation and antibody production also play a role. Foreign antigens are acquired by immunoglobulin receptors on the surface of B cells. These antigens are then processed similarly to the way that APCs process the donor's antigens. The antigen-presenting B cells can then interact with activated T-helper cells. This interaction leads to B-cell proliferation, differentiation into plasma cells, and to antibody production.

Clinical Rejection

Graft rejection is a complex process involving several components, including T lymphocytes, B lymphocytes, macrophages, and cytokines, with resultant local inflammatory injury and graft damage.[10–12] Rejection can be classified into four types, based on timing and pathogenesis: hyperacute, accelerated acute, acute, and chronic.

Hyperacute

This type of rejection, which usually occurs within minutes after the transplanted organ is reperfused, is due to the presence of preformed antibodies in the recipient, antibodies that are specific to the donor. These antibodies may be directed against the donor's HLA antigens or they may be anti-ABO blood group antibodies. Either way, they bind to the vascular endothelium in the graft and activate the complement cascade, leading to platelet activation and to diffuse intravascular coagulation. The result is a swollen, darkened graft, which undergoes ischemic necrosis. This type of rejection is generally not reversible, so prevention is key.

Prevention is best done by making sure the graft is ABO-compatible and by performing a pretransplant cross-match. The cross-match is an in vitro test that involves mixing the donor's cells with the recipient's serum to look for evidence of donor cell destruction by recipient antibodies. A positive cross-match indicates the presence of preformed antibodies in the recipient that are specific to the donor, thus a high risk of hyperacute rejection if the transplant is performed.

Accelerated Acute

This type of rejection, seen within the first few days posttransplant, involves both cellular and antibody-mediated injury. It is likely when a recipient has been sensitized by previous exposure to antigens present in the donor, resulting in an immunologic memory response.

Acute

This used to be the most common type of rejection, but with modern immunosuppression it is becoming less and less common. Acute rejection is usually seen within days to a few months posttransplant. It is predominantly a cell-mediated process, with lymphocytes being the main cells involved. Biopsy of the affected organ demonstrates a cellular infiltrate, with membrane damage and apoptosis of graft cells. The process may be associated with systemic symptoms such as fever, chills, malaise, and arthralgias. However, with current immunosuppressive drugs, most acute rejection episodes are generally asymptomatic. They usually manifest with abnormal laboratory values (e.g., elevated creatinine in kidney transplant recipients, and elevated transaminase levels in liver transplant recipients).

Acute rejection episodes may also be mediated by a humoral, rather than cellular, immune response. B cells may generate anti-donor antibodies, which can damage the graft. Establishing the diagnosis may be difficult, as biopsy may not demonstrate a significant cellular infiltrate; special immunologic stains may be necessary.

Chronic

This form of rejection occurs months to years posttransplant. Now that short-term graft survival rates have improved so markedly, chronic rejection is an increasingly common problem. Histologically, the process is characterized by atrophy, fibrosis, and arteriosclerosis. Both immune and nonimmune mechanisms are likely involved. Clinically, graft function slowly deteriorates over months to years.

CLINICAL IMMUNOSUPPRESSION

The success of modern transplantation is in large part due to the successful development of effective immunosuppressive agents. Without these agents, only transplants between genetically identical individuals would be possible. In the 1960s, just two immunosuppressive agents were available, but over 15 agents are now approved in the United States by the Food and Drug Administration (FDA) for clinical immunosuppression, with scores of others in various stages of clinical trials (Table 10-1). Thus the therapeutic armamentarium for transplant patients has broadened significantly, with a variety of drug combinations and protocols. Characteristics of some common immunosuppressive agents are shown in Table 10-2.

Immunosuppressive drugs are generally used in combination with others rather than alone. *Induction immunosuppression* refers to the drugs administered immediately posttransplant to induce immunosuppression. *Maintenance immunosuppression* refers to the drugs administered to maintain immunosuppression once recipients have recovered from the operative procedure.

Individual drugs can be categorized as either biologic or nonbiologic agents. *Biologic agents* consist of antibody preparations directed at various cells or receptors involved in the rejection process; they are generally used in induction (rather than maintenance) protocols. *Nonbiologic agents* form the mainstay of maintenance protocols.

Nonbiologic Agents

Corticosteroids

Historically, corticosteroids represent the first family of drugs used for clinical immunosuppression. Today steroids remain an integral component of most immunosuppressive protocols, and often are the first-line agents in the treatment of acute rejection. Despite

Table 10-1
Immunosuppressive Drugs by Classification

Immunophilin binders
Calcineurin inhibitors
Cyclosporine
Tacrolimus (FK506)
Noninhibitors of calcineurin
Sirolimus (rapamycin)
Antimetabolites
Inhibitors of de novo purine synthesis
Azathioprine
Mycophenolate mofetil (MMF)
Inhibitors of de novo pyrimidine synthesis
Leflunomide
Biologic immunosuppression
Polyclonal antibodies
ATGAM
Thymoglobulin
Monoclonal antibodies
OKT3
IL-2R (humanized)
Others
Deoxyspergualin
Corticosteroids
FTY720

ATGAM = antithymocyte gamma-globulin; OKT3 = anti-CD3 monoclonal antibody; IL-2R = interleukin-2 receptor.

Table 10-2
Characteristics of Common Immunosuppressive Drugs

Drug	Mechanism of Action	Adverse Effects	Clinical Uses	Dosage
Cyclosporine	Binds to cyclophilin; inhibits calcineurin and IL-2 synthesis	Nephrotoxicity; tremor; hypertension; hirsutism	Improved bioavailability of microemulsion form; used as mainstay of maintenance protocols	Oral dose is 8 to 10 mg/kg/d (given in 2 divided doses)
Tacrolimus (FK506)	Binds to FKBPs; inhibits calcineurin and IL-2 synthesis	Nephrotoxicity; hypertension; neurotoxicity; GI toxicity (nausea, diarrhea)	Improved patient and graft survival in (liver) primary and rescue therapy; used as mainstay of maintenance, like cyclosporine	IV 0.05 to 0.1 mg/kg/d; PO 0.15 to 0.3 mg/kg/d (given q12h)
Mycophenolate mofetil (MMF)	Antimetabolite; inhibits enzyme necessary for de novo purine synthesis	Leukopenia; GI toxicity	Effective for primary and rescue therapy in kidney transplants; may replace azathioprine	1.0 g bid PO (may need 1.5 g in black recipients)
Sirolimus (rapamycin)	Inhibits lymphocyte effects driven by IL-2 receptor	Thrombocytopenia; increased serum cholesterol/LDL; vasculitis (animal studies)	May allow early withdrawal of steroids and decreased calcineurin doses	3 to 5 mg/d, adjusted to trough drug levels
Corticosteroids	Multiple actions; anti-inflammatory; inhibit lympokine production	Cushingoid state; glucose intolerance; osteoporosis	Used in induction, maintenance, and treatment of acute rejection	Varies from milligrams to several grams per day; maintenance doses, 5 to 10 mg/d
Azathioprine (AZA)	Antimetabolite; interferes with DNA and RNA synthesis	Thrombocytopenia; neutropenia; liver dysfunction	Used in maintenance protocols	1 to 3 mg/kg/d for maintenance

FKBPs = FK506-binding proteins; IL-2 = interleukin-2; LDL = low-density lipoproteins.

their proven benefit, steroids have significant side effects, especially with long-term use. Hence there has been considerable interest recently in withdrawing steroids from long-term maintenance protocols. The newer immunosuppressive agents may make doing so possible.

Steroids have both anti-inflammatory and immunosuppressive properties as the two are closely related. Their effects on the immune system are complex. Although they have been used clinically for years, their exact mechanism of action is not fully understood. Primarily, they inhibit the production of T-cell lymphokines, which are needed to amplify macrophage and lymphocyte responses. Steroids also have a number of other immunosuppressive effects that are not as specific. For example, they cause lymphopenia secondary to the redistribution of lymphocytes from the vascular compartment back to lymphoid tissue, inhibit migration of monocytes, and function as anti-inflammatory agents by blocking various permeability-increasing agents and vasodilators.

Steroids in high doses are the first-line choice of many clinicians for the initial treatment of acute cellular rejection. Steroids also are an integral part of most maintenance immunosuppressive regimens. High-dose intravenous (IV) steroids are usually administered immediately posttransplant as induction therapy, followed by relatively high-dose oral steroids (e.g., prednisone at 30 mg/d in adults), tapering to the maintenance dose of 5 to 15 mg/d over 3 to 6 months.

Adverse effects of steroid therapy are numerous and contribute significantly to morbidity in transplant recipients.[13] Individual response varies markedly, but many of the side effects are dose-dependent. Common side effects include mild cushingoid facies and habitus, acne, increased appetite, mood changes, hypertension, proximal muscle weakness, glucose intolerance, and impaired wound healing. Less common are posterior subcapsular cataracts, glaucoma, and aseptic necrosis of the femoral heads. High-dose steroid use, such as bolus therapy for treatment of acute rejection,

increases the risk of opportunistic infections, osteoporosis, and in children, growth retardation. These serious side effects have fueled the current interest in withdrawing patients from steroids within a few months posttransplant, or avoiding steroids altogether. Promising results with steroid withdrawal and avoidance protocols have been reported by several centers. Steroids will likely no longer play a large part in maintenance immunosuppression in the near future.

Azathioprine

An antimetabolite, azathioprine (AZA) is a derivative of 6-mercaptopurine, the active agent. It was first introduced for clinical immunosuppression in 1962; in combination with corticosteroids, it became the standard agent worldwide for the next two decades. Until the introduction of cyclosporine, it was the most widely used immunosuppressive drug, but now has become an adjunctive component of immunosuppressive drug regimens. With the introduction of newer agents, the use of AZA may be discontinued altogether.

AZA acts late in the immune process, affecting the cell cycle by interfering with DNA synthesis, thus suppressing proliferation of activated B and T lymphocytes. AZA is valuable in preventing the onset of acute rejection, but is not effective in the treatment of rejection episodes themselves.

The most significant side effect of AZA is bone marrow suppression. All three hematopoietic cell lines can be affected, leading to leukopenia, thrombocytopenia, and anemia. Suppression is often dose-related; it is usually reversible with dose reduction or temporary cessation of the drug. Other significant side effects include hepatotoxicity, gastrointestinal disturbances (nausea and vomiting), pancreatitis, and alopecia. Of note is its reaction with allopurinol, a drug commonly used to treat gout. Allopurinol inhibits the breakdown of AZA and its metabolites, resulting in excessive accumulation of AZA and toxicity. Severe, prolonged neutropenia has been reported in patients treated with both drugs at standard doses. Patients who require allopurinol should receive half the standard dose of AZA and undergo careful hematologic monitoring.

Cyclosporine

The introduction of cyclosporine in the early 1980s dramatically altered the field of transplantation.[14–16] It significantly improved results after kidney transplants, but its greatest impact was on extrarenal transplants. When it was introduced, cyclosporine was the most specific immunosuppressive agent available. Compared with steroids or AZA, it much more selectively inhibits the immune response. Currently, cyclosporine plays a central role in maintenance immunosuppression in almost all types of organ transplants.

Cyclosporine binds with its cytoplasmic receptor protein, cyclophilin, which subsequently inhibits the activity of calcineurin. Doing so impairs expression of several critical T-cell activation genes, the most important being for IL-2. As a result, T-cell activation is suppressed. The metabolism of cyclosporine is via the cytochrome P450 system, therefore several drug interactions are possible. Inducers of P450 such as phenytoin decrease blood levels; drugs such as erythromycin, cimetidine, ketoconazole, and fluconazole increase them.

Adverse effects of cyclosporine can be classified as renal or nonrenal. Nephrotoxicity is the most important and troubling adverse effect of cyclosporine. Cyclosporine has a vasoconstrictor effect on the renal vasculature. This vasoconstriction (likely a transient, reversible, and dose-dependent phenomenon) may cause early posttransplant graft dysfunction or may exaggerate existing poor graft function. Also, long-term cyclosporine use may result in interstitial fibrosis of the renal parenchyma, coupled with arteriolar lesions. The exact mechanism is unknown, but renal failure may eventually result.

A number of nonrenal side effects may also be seen with the use of cyclosporine. Cosmetic complications, most commonly hirsutism and gingival hyperplasia, may result in considerable distress, possibly leading to noncompliant behavior, especially in adolescents and women. Several neurologic complications, including headaches, tremor, and seizures, also have been reported. Other nonrenal side effects include hyperlipidemia, hepatotoxicity, and hyperuricemia.

Tacrolimus

Tacrolimus (FK506) is a metabolite of the soil fungus *Streptomyces tsukubaensi,* found in Japan. Released in the United States in April 1994 for use in liver transplantation, it is currently used in a fashion similar to cyclosporine. Tacrolimus, like cyclosporine, is a calcineurin inhibitor and has a very similar mechanism of action. Cyclosporine acts by binding cyclophilins, while tacrolimus acts by binding FK506-binding proteins (FKBPs). The tacrolimus-FKBP complex inhibits the enzyme calcineurin, which is essential for activating transcription factors in response to the rise in intracellular calcium seen with stimulation of the TCR. The net effect of tacrolimus is to inhibit T-cell function by preventing synthesis of IL-2 and other important cytokines. The main difference between tacrolimus and cyclosporine, other than the actual immunophilin each binds to, is in relative potency: tacrolimus is 100 times more potent than cyclosporine on a molar basis. Similarly to cyclosporine, tacrolimus is primarily metabolized by the P450 enzyme system of the liver; therefore similar drug interactions occur.

Adverse effects of tacrolimus and cyclosporine are similar. The most common problems include nephrotoxicity, neurotoxicity, impaired glucose metabolism, hypertension, infection, and gastrointestinal (GI) disturbances. Nephrotoxicity is dose-related and reversible with dose reduction. Neurotoxicity seen with tacrolimus ranges from mild symptoms (tremors, insomnia, and headaches) to more severe events (seizures and coma); it is usually related to high levels and resolves with dose reduction. These side effects are most common early posttransplant and subsequently tend to decrease in incidence.

The hyperglycemic effect of tacrolimus does not appear to be dose-related. Its cause is unknown. However, in most studies, its incidence is significantly higher with tacrolimus than with cyclosporine. Other common side effects involve the GI tract, ranging from mild cramps to severe diarrhea. Hypertension, hypercholesterolemia, and hypomagnesemia occur with equal frequency with tacrolimus. As with other immunosuppressive drugs, infection and malignancy remain the most serious long-term adverse events.

Sirolimus

A macrolide antibiotic derived from a soil actinomycete originally found on Easter Island (Rapa Nui), sirolimus (previously known as rapamycin) is structurally similar to tacrolimus and binds to the same immunophilin (FKBP). Unlike tacrolimus, it does not affect calcineurin activity, and therefore does not block the calcium-dependent activation of cytokine genes. Rather, the active complex binds so-called target of rapamycin (TOR) proteins (Fig. 10-2), resulting in inhibition of P7056 kinase (an enzyme linked to cell division). The net result is to prevent progression from the G_1 to the S phase of the cell cycle, halting cell division.

To date, sirolimus has been used in a variety of combinations and situations. It is most commonly used in conjunction with one of the calcineurin inhibitors. In such combinations, sirolimus is usually used to help withdraw or avoid the use of steroids completely in maintenance immunosuppressive regimens. It has also been used as an alternative to tacrolimus or cyclosporine, as part of a calcineurin-sparing protocol. The advantage of this type of protocol is that it is not associated with long-term nephrotoxicity (as may be seen with the calcineurin agents). Hence, sirolimus may prove to be better for long-term preservation of renal function in transplant recipients.

The major side effects of sirolimus include neutropenia, thrombocytopenia, and a significant elevation of the serum triglyceride and cholesterol levels. It has also been associated with impaired wound healing, leading to a higher incidence of wound-related complications.

Mycophenolate Mofetil

Mycophenolate mofetil (MMF) was approved in May 1995 by the FDA for use in the prevention of acute rejection after kidney transplants. It has since been rapidly incorporated into routine clinical practice at many centers as part of maintenance regimens. A semisynthetic derivative of mycophenolate acid (MPA), it is isolated from the mold *Penicillium glaucum.* It works by inhibiting inosine monophosphate dehydrogenase, which is a crucial, rate-limiting enzyme in de novo synthesis of purines. Specifically, this enzyme catalyzes the formation of guanosine nucleotides from inosine. Many cells have a salvage pathway and therefore can bypass this need for guanosine nucleotide synthesis by the de novo pathway. Activated lymphocytes, however, do not possess this salvage pathway and require de novo synthesis for clonal expansion. The

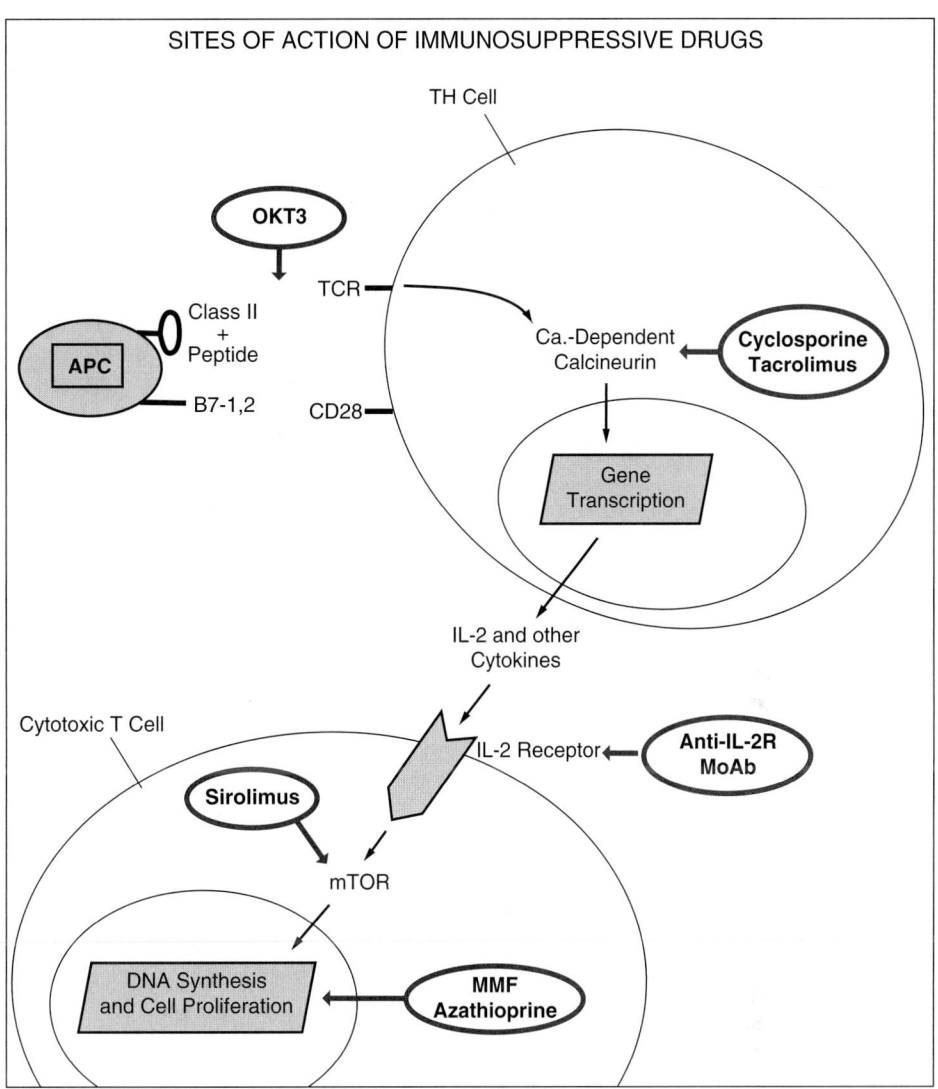

SITES OF ACTION OF IMMUNOSUPPRESSIVE DRUGS

FIG. 10-2. Sites of action of immunosuppressive drugs.

net result is a selective, reversible antiproliferative effect on T and
B lymphocytes.

MMF differs from cyclosporine, tacrolimus, and sirolimus in that
it does not affect cytokine production or the events immediately after
antigen recognition. Rather, MMF works further distally in the chain
of activation events to prevent proliferation of the stimulated T cell
(see Fig. 10-2). Like AZA, it is an antimetabolite; unlike AZA, its
impact is selective: it only affects lymphocytes, not neutrophils or
platelets. In several clinical trials, it has proven to be more effective
than AZA, and has largely replaced it.

The incidence and types of adverse events with MMF are similar to those seen with AZA. Notable exceptions are GI side effects (diarrhea, gastritis, and vomiting), which are more common
with MMF. Clinically significant leukopenia also is more common, affecting about one third of recipients. Dose reduction or
temporary drug cessation usually is adequate to treat leukopenia
(Table 10-3).

Biologic Agents

Polyclonal antibodies directed against lymphocytes have been used
in clinical transplantation since the 1960s. Monoclonal antibody
techniques, developed later, allowed in turn for the development

of biologic agents (such as OKT3) targeted to specific subsets of
cells. A number of different monoclonal antibodies (MABs) are
currently under development or have been recently approved for use
in clinical transplantation.[18] Many are directed against functional
secreted molecules of the immune system or their receptors, rather
than against actual groups of cells.

Polyclonal Antibodies

Polyclonal antibodies are produced by immunizing animals
(such as horses, goats, or rabbits) with human lymphoid tissue, allowing for an immune response, removing the resultant immune
sera, and purifying the sera in an effort to remove unwanted antibodies. What remain are antibodies that will recognize human
lymphocytes.

After administration of these antibodies into a transplant recipient, the total lymphocyte count should fall. Lymphocytes, especially
T cells, are either lysed after antibody binding and complement deposition at the cell surface, inactivated by binding to T-cell receptors,
or are cleared from the circulation and deposited into the reticuloendothelial system. Polyclonal antibodies have been successfully
used to prevent rejection and to treat acute rejection episodes.[17]
Currently available polyclonal preparations include antithymocyte

Table 10-3
Side Effects and Drug Interactions of Immunosuppressive Drugs

	Common Side Effects	*Medications That Increase Blood Levels*	*Medications That Decrease Blood Levels*	*Medications That Potentiate Toxicity*
Cyclosporine	Hypertension, nephrotoxicity, hirsutism, neurotoxicity, gingival hyperplasia	Verapamil, clarithromycin, doxycycline, azithromycin, erythromycin, fluconazole, itraconazole, ketoconazole	Isoniazid, carbamazepine, phenobarbital, phenytoin, rifampin	Nephrotoxicity: acyclovir, ganciclovir, aminoglycosides, nonsteroidal anti-inflammatories
Tacrolimus (FK506)	Hypertension, nephrotoxicity, hyperglycemia, neurotoxicity	Verapamil, clarithromycin, doxycycline, azithromycin, erythromycin, fluconazole, itraconazole, ketoconazole	Isoniazid, carbamazepine, phenobarbital, phenytoin, rifampin	Nephrotoxicity: acyclovir, ganciclovir, aminoglycosides, nonsteroidal anti-inflammatories
Azathioprine (AZA)	Leukopenia, anemia, thrombocytopenia, GI upset			Bone marrow suppression: allopurinol, sulfonamides
Mycophenolate mofetil (MMF)	Leukopenia, thrombocytopenia, GI upset		Cholestyramine, antacids	
Prednisone	Hyperglycemia, osteoporosis, cataracts, myopathy, weight gain			

globulin (obtained by immunizing horses with human thymocytes) and Thymoglobulin (obtained by immunizing rabbits with human thymocytes).

Monoclonal Antibodies

MABs are produced by the hybridization of murine antibody-secreting B lymphocytes with a nonantibody-secreting myeloma cell line. A number of MABs have been produced that are active against different stages of the immune response. OKT3 remains the most commonly used MAB, but the last few years have seen the introduction of a number of "humanized" MABs (genetically engineered to possess large domains of human antibody while retaining the murine antigen binding site), which have a significantly lower potential for toxicity than OKT3.

OKT3 is directed against the CD3 antigen complex found on all mature human T cells. The CD3 complex is an integral part of the TCR. Inactivation of CD3 by OKT3 causes the TCR to be lost from the cell surface. The T cells are then ineffective and are rapidly cleared from the circulation and deposited into the reticuloendothelial system. Efficacy of OKT3 can be measured by monitoring levels of CD3-positive cells in the circulation. If it is effective, the percentage of CD3-positive cells should fall to and stay below 5%. Failure to reach this level indicates an inadequate OKT3 dose or the presence of recipient antibodies directed against OKT3, the latter scenario being more common after repeated administration of the drug.

OKT3 is highly effective and versatile. Most commonly, it is used to treat severe acute rejection episodes (i.e., those resistant to steroids). OKT3 also has been used as prophylaxis against rejection, as induction therapy, and as primary rejection treatment.

Significant, even life-threatening adverse effects may be seen after OKT3 administration, most commonly immediately after one of the first several doses. Such effects may occur when cytokines (such as tumor necrosis factor, IL-2, and γ-interferon) are released by T cells from the circulation. The most common symptoms are fever, chills, and headaches. The most serious side effect of OKT3 is a rapidly developing, noncardiogenic pulmonary edema; the risk of this side effect significantly increases if the patient is fluid-overloaded at the time of OKT3 treatment. Other serious side effects include encephalopathy, aseptic meningitis, and nephrotoxicity.

Several other MABs targeting different steps of the immune process are available for clinical use. As noted, IL-2 is an important cytokine necessary for the proliferation of cytotoxic T cells. Two MABs are currently approved to target the IL-2 receptor (IL-2R): basiliximab and dacluzimab. Both are humanized products and therefore are not associated with significant first-dose reactions or drug-specific adverse events. They have been proven effective as induction agents, decreasing the incidence of acute rejection in kidney transplant recipients when compared to placebo in clinical trials. They have not been used to treat established acute rejection. More recently, alemtuzumab, a MAB directed against the CD52 antigen found on B and T cells, has been used, usually as an induction agent.

Organ Procurement and Preservation

The biggest problem facing transplant centers today is the shortage of organ donors. Mechanisms that might increase the number of available organs include: (1) optimizing the current donor pool (e.g., the use of multiple organ donors or marginal donors); (2) increasing the number of living-donor transplants (e.g., the use of living unrelated donors); (3) using unconventional and controversial donor sources (e.g., using deceased donors without cardiac activity or anencephalic donors); and (4) performing xenotransplants. The largest potential increase in the number of available organs would result from improving donation rates from suitable deceased donors. By recent estimates, over 10,000 brain-dead donors are potentially available in the United States annually. Currently, however, only about one half of them are actually used. The single most important reason for the lack of deceased donor organ retrieval is the inability to obtain consent from the surviving next-of-kin. The need for public education is crucial, including more effective educational campaigns to increase awareness of the importance of organ transplants.

Deceased Donors

Most extrarenal transplants performed today, and roughly one half of all renal transplants, are from deceased donors. These donors are deceased individuals who meet the criteria for brain death, but whose organs are being perfused by life-support measures, allowing adequate time for referral to an organ procurement organization. A member of that organization can then ascertain whether donation is possible, and if so, approach the potential donor's family and possibly obtain consent to procure suitable organs.

Crucial to the concept of deceased donor organ donation is the concept of brain death. Brain death means that all brain and brain stem function has irreversibly ceased, while circulatory and ventilatory functions are maintained temporarily. The clinical diagnosis of brain death rests on three criteria: (1) irreversibility of the neurologic insult; (2) absence of clinical evidence of cerebral function; and most important, (3) absence of clinical evidence of brain stem function. When testing for brain death, hypothermia, medication side effects, drug overdose, and intoxication must be excluded. Brain death can be diagnosed by routine neurologic examinations (including cold caloric and apnea testing on two separate occasions at least 6 hours apart), coupled with prior establishment of the underlying diagnosis. Confirmatory tests must verify the absence of intracranial blood flow on brain flow studies or the presence of an isoelectric electroencephalogram (EEG) reading.

Once the diagnosis of brain death has been established, the process of organ donation can be initiated.[19,20] The focus then switches from the treatment of elevated intracranial pressure to preserving organ function and optimizing peripheral oxygen delivery.[21] It is important to keep in mind that management of the deceased organ donor is an active process, requiring aggressive monitoring and intervention to ensure that perfusion to the organs of interest is not compromised. For all organ donors, core temperature, systemic arterial blood pressure, arterial oxygen saturation, and urine output must be determined routinely and frequently. Arterial blood gases, serum electrolytes, blood urea nitrogen, serum creatinine, liver enzymes, hemoglobin, and coagulation tests also need to be monitored regularly. Hemodynamic instability can be marked after brain death, with wide swings between the extremes of hypotension and hypertension. Hypotension is usually secondary to hypovolemia, due to a combination of vasomotor collapse after brain death and the effects of treatment protocols to decrease intracranial pressure. Hypertension may also be seen, often secondary to raised intracranial pressure. It can be treated with short-acting vasodilatory agents or with rapidly reversible beta blockers.

Respiratory maintenance with vigorous tracheobronchial toilet is important, with frequent suctioning using aseptic precautions. Maintaining adequate systemic arterial perfusion pressure and brisk urine output (>1 to 2 mL/kg per hour), while minimizing the use of vasopressors, contributes to good kidney allograft function and reduces the rate of acute tubular necrosis (ATN) posttransplant. Polyuria is frequent in brain-dead donors, usually secondary to diabetes insipidus. It should be suspected when urine volumes exceed 300 mL/h in conjunction with hypernatremia, elevated serum osmolality, and a low urinary sodium concentration and osmolality. Once urine output due to diabetes insipidus exceeds 300 mL/h, desmopressin (a synthetic analogue of vasopressin) should be administered.

After brain death, hypothermia usually ensues. Adverse effects of hypothermia include decreased myocardial contractility, hypotension, cardiac dysrhythmias, cardiac arrest, hepatic and renal dysfunction, acidosis, and coagulopathy. Therefore donor core temperature must be maintained in the normal range.

Living Donors

Living-donor transplantation is unique in that surgeons commonly operate on a healthy individual (i.e., a living donor) who has no medical disorders and does not require an operation. The use of living donors is an integral and important part of the field of transplantation today. The first transplants ever performed used living donors. Today living donors are commonly used for every type of transplant except heart transplants. The number of such transplants continues to increase on a yearly basis. But living-donor transplants pose a unique set of medical, ethical, financial, and psychosocial problems that must be dealt with by the transplant team.

The use of living donors offers numerous advantages. Primary is the availability of a life-saving organ. A certain percentage of transplant candidates die while waiting for a deceased donor organ as a direct result of a complication, or of progression of their underlying disease. For such ill candidates, the advantage of a living donor is obvious. Even for candidates who would receive a deceased donor organ, a living-donor transplant may significantly shorten the waiting time. A shorter waiting time generally implies a healthier candidate—one whose body has not been ravaged by prolonged end-stage organ failure. Moreover, living-donor transplants are planned (rather than emergency) procedures, allowing for better preoperative preparation of the potential recipient. Receiving an organ from a closely matched relative may also have immunologic benefits. Lastly, long-term results may be superior with living-donor transplants, which is certainly the case with kidney transplants.

The disadvantages of a living-donor transplant for the potential recipient are minimal. With some organ transplants (e.g., living donor liver or lung) the procedure may be more technically complex, resulting in an increased incidence of surgical complications. However, this disadvantage is offset by numerous advantages.

The major disadvantage of living-donor transplants is to the donor. Medically, there is no possibility of benefit for the donor, only potential for harm. The risk of death associated with donation depends on the organ being removed. For nephrectomy, the mortality risk is estimated to be less than 0.05%. However, for partial hepatectomy, it is about 0.5%. Risks for surgical and medical complications also depend on the procedure being performed. In addition, long-term complications or problems may be associated with partial loss of organ function through donation. The guiding principle of all living-donor transplants should be the minimization of risk to the donor. What risk there is must be carefully explained to the potential donor, and written informed consent should be obtained.

The kidney, the first organ to be used for living-donor transplants, is the most common type of organ donated by living donors today. Potential donors are first evaluated to ensure that they have normal renal function with two equally functioning kidneys and that they do not have any significant risk factors for developing renal disease (e.g., hypertension or diabetes). The anatomy of their kidneys and the vasculature can be determined by using various radiologic imaging techniques, including an intravenous pyelogram (IVP), arteriogram, or computed tomographic angiogram (CTA). Which kidney is removed depends on the anatomy. If there is any minor abnormality in one kidney, that kidney should be removed. If both kidneys are the same, the left kidney is preferred because of

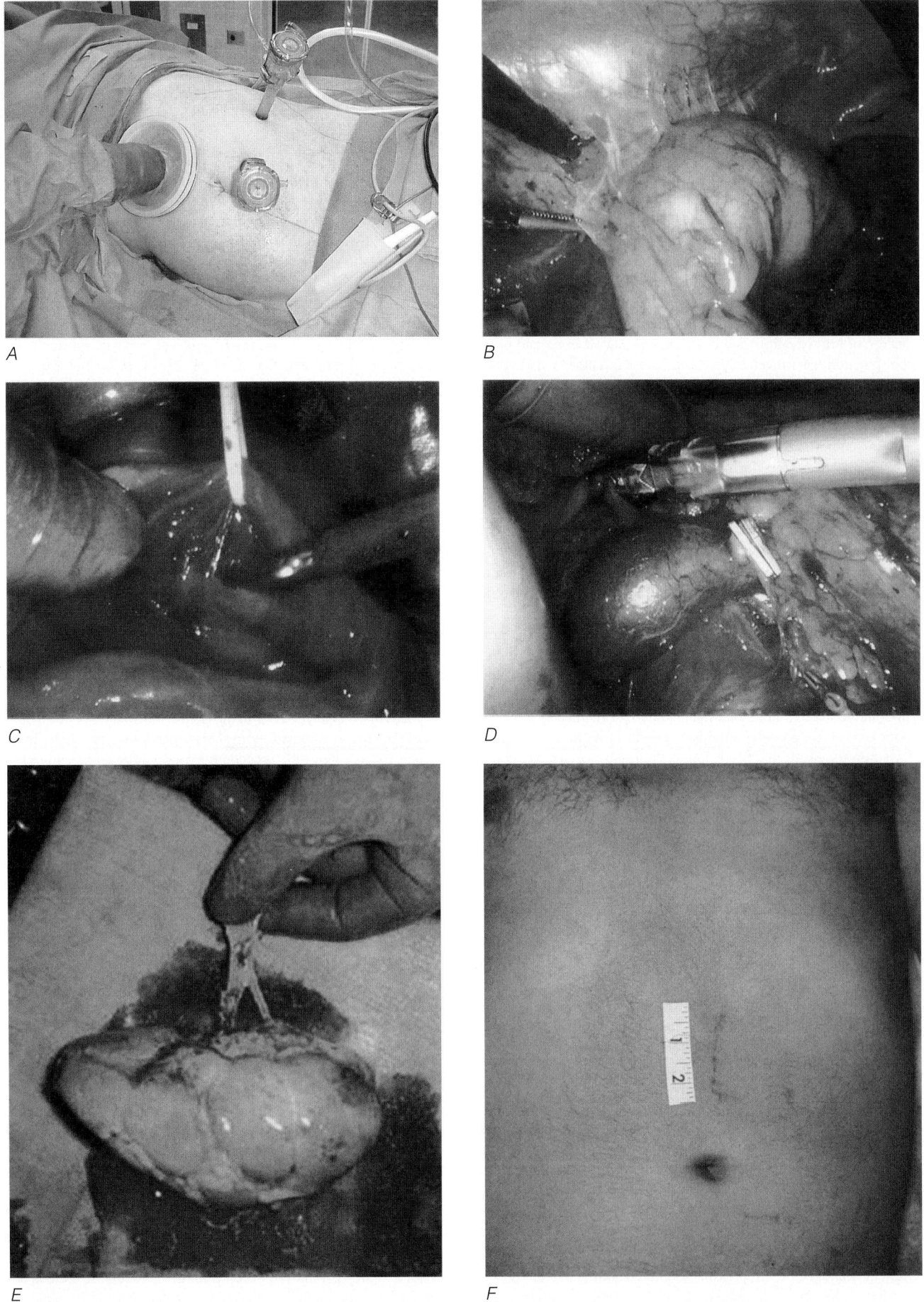

FIG. 10-3. Hand-assisted laparoscopic donor nephrectomy for living-donor kidney transplant. *A.* Placement of hand port and other ports for hand-assisted technique. *B.* Mobilization of colon to expose kidney. *C.* Isolation and mobilization of the ureter into the pelvis. *D.* Mobilization of the renal vein with division of branches. *E.* Removal of kidney after division of vascular structures and ureter. *F.* Incisions in donor 2 weeks postdonation.

the longer left renal vein. Nephrectomy can be performed through a flank incision, by an anterior retroperitoneal approach, or by a laparoscopic technique. With the laparoscopic technique, an intraperitoneal approach is used. This involves mobilization of the colon, isolation of the ureter and renal vessels, mobilization of the kidney, division of the renal vessels, and removal of the kidney (Fig. 10-3A to F).

Living-donor liver transplants have been performed for almost 15 years. Initially, they involved adult donors and pediatric recipients. In such cases, the left lateral segment of the donor's liver is resected (Fig. 10-4A). Inflow to the graft occurs via the donor's left hepatic artery and left portal vein; outflow is via the left hepatic vein. For adult recipients, a larger piece of the liver is required; usually the right lobe is chosen (Fig. 10-4B). The liver has a remarkable ability to regenerate, and the remnant piece in the donor will achieve close to the original liver volume within 4 to 6 weeks after donation. As mentioned, the risks for living liver donors are higher than those for living kidney donors. The risks are also generally higher for right lobe donors than for left lateral segment donors. The most worrisome complication for living liver donors is a bile leak, either from the cut surface of the liver or from the bile duct stump.

Living-donor transplants with organs besides the kidney and liver are not as common, but are performed at various centers. Living-donor pancreas transplants involve a distal pancreatectomy, with the graft consisting of the body and tail of the pancreas; vascular inflow and outflow are provided by the splenic artery and splenic vein. Living-donor intestinal transplants usually involve removal of about 200 cm of the donor's ileum, with inflow and outflow provided by the ileocolic vessels. Living-donor lung transplants involve removal of one lobe of one lung from each of two donors; both grafts are then transplanted into the recipient.

Preservation

Organ preservation methods have played an important role in the success of cadaver donor transplants. They have resulted in improved graft function immediately posttransplant and have diminished the incidence of primary nonfunction of organs. By prolonging the allowable cold ischemia times, they have also allowed for better organ allocation and for safer transplants.[22,23]

The most common methods involve the use of hypothermia and pharmacologic inhibition to slow down metabolic processes in the organ once it has been removed from the deceased donor. Hypothermia very effectively slows down enzymatic reactions and metabolic activity, allowing the cell to make its limited energy reserves last much longer. A temperature decrease from 37°C to 4°C (the temperature of most preservation solutions) slows metabolism about 12-fold. However, in the absence of any energy inflow into the cell, degradative reactions begin to provide the cell with an energy source. The result can be destruction of important structural elements and, eventually, structural damage to the cells and the organ. So while hypothermia greatly slows enzymatic reactions, they continue nonetheless, leading to an accumulation of potentially detrimental end products within the cell. Hypothermia also contributes to the development of cellular swelling because the membrane ion pumps are slow to function.

Cold storage solutions have been developed to improve organ preservation by ameliorating some of the detrimental effects of hypothermia alone. Essentially, these solutions suppress hypothermia-induced cellular swelling and minimize the loss of potassium from the cell. Agents that do not readily permeate the cell membrane and that have an electrolyte composition resembling the intracellular

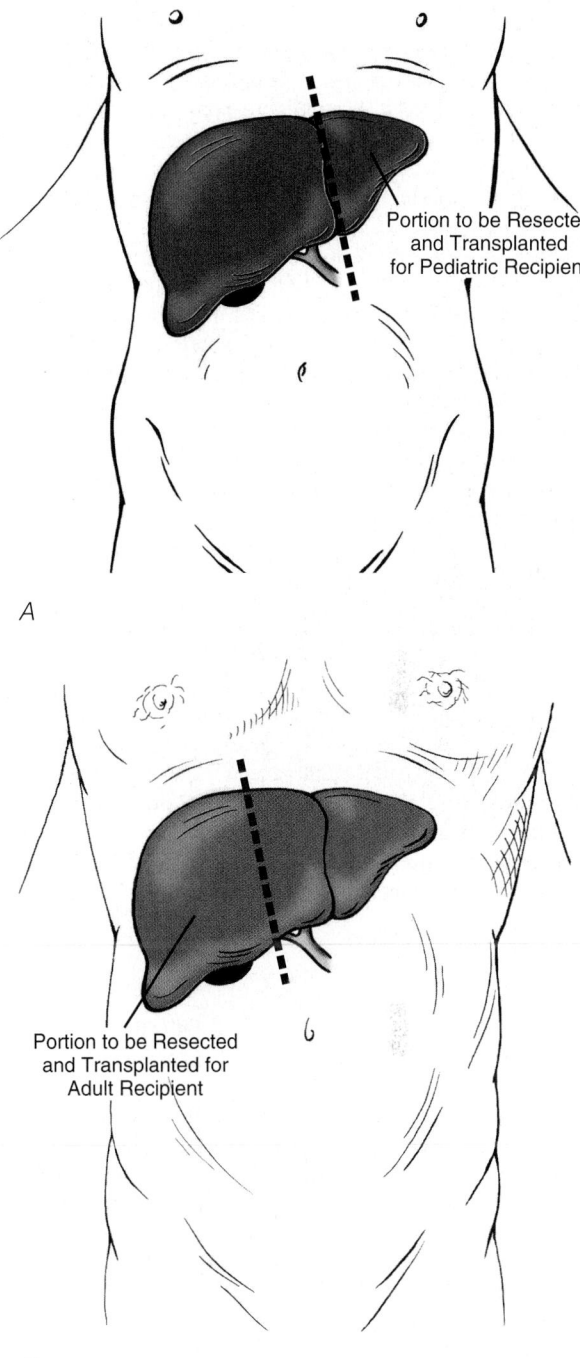

A

B

FIG. 10-4. *A. Resection for an adult-to-child living-donor liver transplant. B. Resection for an adult-to-adult living-donor liver transplant.*

environment (low sodium, high potassium) are used, thus preventing the loss of cellular potassium.

The most commonly used fluid worldwide is the University of Wisconsin (UW) solution.[24] It contains lactobionate, raffinose, and hydroxyethyl starch. Lactobionate is impermeable and prevents intracellular swelling; it also lowers the concentration of intracellular calcineurin and free iron, which may be beneficial in reducing reperfusion injury. Hydroxyethyl starch, a synthetic colloid, may help decrease hypothermia-induced cell swelling of endothelial cells and reduce interstitial edema.

Although cold preservation has improved cadaver donor transplant results, the amount of time that an organ can be safely preserved is limited. After that, the incidence of organ nonfunction starts to increase. With kidneys, exceeding the preservation time limit results in delayed graft function, requiring dialysis support for the recipient until function improves. With livers, the result is primary nonfunction, requiring an urgent retransplant. How long an organ can be safely preserved depends on the type of organ and on the condition of the donor. With kidneys, cold ischemic times should be kept below 36 to 40 hours; after that, delayed graft function significantly increases. With pancreata, more than 24 hours of ischemia increases problems due to pancreatitis and duodenal leaks. With livers, more than 16 hours of ischemia increases the risk for primary nonfunction and biliary complications. Hearts and lungs tolerate preservation poorly; ideally, ischemia times should be below 6 hours. With marginal donors, all of these times should be adjusted further downward.

KIDNEY TRANSPLANTATION

A kidney transplant now represents the treatment of choice for patients with end-stage renal disease (ESRD). It offers the greatest potential for restoring a healthy, productive life in most such patients. Compared with dialysis, it is associated with better patient survival and superior quality of life, and is more cost-effective.[25,26] Currently, there are nearly 60,000 patients in the United States awaiting a kidney transplant. Because of the success of the procedure, the waiting list has grown dramatically since the 1990s. Unfortunately, the number of available organs has not kept pace, resulting in an ever-increasing waiting period.

History

The history of kidney transplantation is in many ways the history of transplantation itself. The kidney was the first organ to be transplanted regularly, and it remains the most common organ transplanted today. The first clinical cadaver donor kidney transplant was performed in 1933 by Voronoy, a Ukrainian surgeon, with unsuccessful results secondary to rejection. In the 1950s, this immunologic barrier was circumvented by performing the kidney transplants between identical twins. The era of modern kidney transplantation began with the introduction of azathioprine to suppress the immune system. With the demonstration of the synergistic affect of glucocorticoids, renal transplantation was established as a viable option for the treatment of ESRD. Polyclonal antilymphocyte agents, such as antilymphocyte globulin, were soon developed, significantly contributing to the treatment of acute rejection. The introduction of cyclosporine in the 1980s significantly improved graft and patient survival rates, allowing for a dramatic increase in the number of kidney transplants.

Preoperative Evaluation

Very few absolute contraindications to kidney transplants exist. Therefore, most patients with ESRD should be considered as potential transplant candidates. However, the surgery and general anesthesia impose a significant cardiovascular stress. Subsequent lifelong immunosuppression also is associated with some risk. Pretransplant evaluation should identify any factors that would contraindicate a transplant or any risk factors that could be minimized pretransplant.[27]

The preoperative evaluation can be divided into four parts: medical, surgical, immunologic, and psychosocial. The purpose of the medical evaluation is to identify risk factors for the surgical procedure. Mortality posttransplant usually is due to underlying cardiovascular disease, so a detailed cardiac evaluation is necessary. Any history of congestive heart failure, angina, myocardial infarction, or stroke should be elicited. Patients with symptoms suggestive of cardiovascular disease or with significant risk factors (e.g., diabetes, age over 50, previous myocardial infarction) should undergo further cardiac evaluation with stress testing or angiography. Any problems identified should be treated appropriately (medically or surgically) before proceeding with the transplant.

Untreated malignancy and active infection are absolute contraindications to a transplant, because of the requisite lifelong immunosuppression. After curative treatment of malignancy, an interval of 2 to 5 years is recommended pretransplant. This recommendation is influenced by the type of malignancy, with longer observation periods for neoplasms such as melanoma or breast cancer and shorter periods for carcinoma in situ or low-grade malignancies such as basal cell carcinoma of the skin. Chronic infections such as osteomyelitis or endocarditis must be fully treated and a suitable waiting period must occur to ensure lack of recrudescence.

The medical evaluation also should concentrate on GI problems such as peptic ulcer disease, symptomatic cholelithiasis, and hepatitis. Patients who demonstrate serologic evidence of hepatitis C or B, but without evidence of active hepatic inflammation or cirrhosis, are acceptable transplant candidates. A biopsy may be helpful to determine the extent of the underlying liver disease. These patients are at increased risk for progression of their underlying liver disease after receiving immunosuppression, but exhibit excellent long-term survival rates and improved quality of life posttransplant, as compared with patients undergoing chronic dialysis.

The surgical evaluation should identify vascular or urologic abnormalities that may contraindicate or complicate a transplant. Evidence of vascular disease that is revealed by the history (claudication or rest pain) or the physical examination (diminished or absent pulse or bruit) should be evaluated further by Doppler studies or angiography. Severe aortoiliac disease may make a transplant technically impossible; an option in such patients is a revascularization procedure such as aortobifemoral graft placement pretransplant. Areas of significant arterial stenosis proximal to the planned site of implantation may need preoperative balloon angioplasty. Urologic evaluation should exclude chronic infection in the native kidney, which may require nephrectomy pretransplant. Other indications for nephrectomy include huge polycystic kidneys, significant vesicoureteral reflux, or uncontrollable renovascular hypertension. Children especially require a complete urologic examination to evaluate reflux and bladder outlet obstruction.

The immunologic evaluation involves determining blood type, tissue type (HLA-A, -B, or -DR antigens), and presence of any cytotoxic antibodies against HLA antigens (because of prior transplants, blood transfusions, or pregnancies). If a living-donor transplant is planned, a cross-match should be performed early on during the initial evaluation.

The psychosocial evaluation is necessary to ensure that transplant candidates understand the nature of the transplant procedure and its attendant risk. They must be capable of rigorously adhering to the medical regimen posttransplant. Patients who have not been compliant with their medical regimen in the past must demonstrate a willingness and capability to do so before they undergo the transplant.

One important aspect of the preoperative evaluation is the search for and evaluation of potential living donors. Living-donor kidney recipients enjoy improved long-term success, avoid a prolonged wait, and are able to plan the timing of their transplant in advance. Moreover, they have a significantly decreased incidence of ATN and increased potential for HLA matching. As a result, living-donor transplants generally have better short- and long-term results, as compared with cadaver donor transplants. Of course, the risks to the living donor must be acceptably low. The donor must be fully aware of potential risks and must freely give informed consent. The search for a living donor should not be restricted to immediate family members. Results with living, unrelated donors are comparable to those with living, related (non-HLA-identical) donors.[28]

Surgical Procedure

The surgical technique for kidney transplantation has changed very little from the original pelvic operation described in the 1950s. The transplanted kidney is usually placed in a heterotopic position, with no need for native nephrectomy except in select circumstances. Retroperitoneal placement is preferred, to allow for easy access for percutaneous renal biopsy. Usually, the right iliac fossa is chosen because of the more superficial location of the iliac vein on this side (Fig. 10-5). However, the left iliac fossa should be used if the recipient may be a candidate for a future pancreas transplant, if it is a second transplant, or if there is significant arterial disease on the right side.

With the standard approach, the dissection is extraperitoneal. The iliac vessels are identified and assessed for suitability for anastomosis. The internal iliac artery can be used as the inflow vessel, with an end-to-end anastomosis, or the external iliac artery can be used with an end-to-side anastomosis. To minimize the risk of lymphocele formation after surgery, only a modest length of artery is dissected free and the lymphatics overlying the artery are ligated. The donor renal vein is anastomosed end to side to the external iliac vein.

After the vascular anastomosis is completed and the kidney perfused, urinary continuity can be restored by a number of well-described techniques. The important principles are to attach the ureter to the bladder mucosa in a tension-free manner and to cover the distal 1 cm of the ureter with a submucosal tunnel, thus protecting against reflux during voiding.

Intraoperative care of kidney transplant recipients is not unlike that of other patients undergoing major surgical procedures. To decrease the incidence of ATN posttransplant, a liberal hydration policy is employed intraoperatively. Adequate perfusion of the transplanted kidney is important to ensure postoperative diuresis. Central venous pressure (CVP) should be maintained around 10 mm Hg, and systolic blood pressure should be greater than 120 mm Hg. Maintaining adequate CVP is especially important in smaller, pediatric recipients, because reperfusion of an adult-sized kidney graft may divert a significant amount of their own blood volume. Administering mannitol and furosemide just before reperfusion usually is helpful in maximizing perfusion to the kidney graft.

Early Postoperative Care

The immediate postoperative care of all recipients involves (1) stabilizing the major organ systems (e.g., cardiovascular, pulmonary, and renal); (2) evaluating graft function; (3) achieving adequate immunosuppression; and (4) monitoring and treating complications directly and indirectly related to the transplant. Initially, hemodynamic stability is assessed, as with all postsurgical patients. Blood pressure, heart rate, and urine output are measured. CVP monitoring may be useful in guiding fluid replacement therapy. Achieving hemodynamic stability is important for the recipient's overall status, but it is also necessary to optimize graft function; hemodynamically unstable recipients experience poor perfusion of their kidney graft.

Careful attention to fluid and electrolyte management is crucial. In general, recipients should be kept euvolemic or slightly hypervolemic. If initial graft function is good, fluid replacement can be regulated by hourly replacement of urine. Half-normal saline is a good solution to use for urine replacement. Aggressive replacement of electrolytes, including calcium, magnesium, and potassium, may be necessary, especially for recipients undergoing brisk diuresis. Those with ATN and fluid overload or hyperkalemia may need fluid restriction and even hemodialysis. Magnesium levels should be kept above 2 mEq/L to prevent seizures, and phosphate levels kept between 2 and 5 mEq/L for proper support of the respiratory and alimentary tracts. Marked hyperglycemia, which may be secondary to steroids, should be treated with insulin.

Hypotension is unusual early after a kidney transplant. When it occurs, it is usually related to hypovolemia. The treatment is to optimize preload and afterload and, only if necessary, to use inotropic agents such as dopamine or dobutamine. Systemic hypertension is more common early posttransplant. If hypertension is catecholamine-mediated or an effect of immunosuppressive agents, it usually responds well to treatment with calcium channel blockers. However, if it is secondary to fluid overload, and if the recipient has poor kidney function, dialysis may be necessary.

A critical aspect of postoperative care is the repeated evaluation of graft function, which in fact begins intraoperatively, soon after the kidney is reperfused. Signs of good kidney function include appropriate color and texture, along with evidence of urine production. Postoperatively, urine output is the most readily available and easily measured indicator of graft function. Urine volume may range from none (anuria) to large quantities (polyuria). When using posttransplant urine volume to monitor graft function, the clinician must have at least some knowledge of the recipient's pretransplant urine volume, if any. If an individual was relatively anuric pretransplant, but then has normal urine output posttransplant, graft function is evident. However, if urine volume was significantly high pretransplant, normal urine output posttransplant does not necessarily mean good graft function; the urine may be from the native kidneys rather than from the graft. Laboratory values of obvious use in assessing graft function include serum blood urea nitrogen (BUN) and creatinine levels.

Recipients can be divided into three groups (by initial graft function as indicated by their urine output and serum creatinine) as those with: (1) immediate graft function (IGF), characterized by a brisk diuresis posttransplant and rapidly falling serum creatinine level; (2) slow graft function (SGF), characterized by a moderate degree of kidney dysfunction posttransplant, with modest amounts of urine and a slowly falling creatinine level, but no need for dialysis at any time posttransplant; and (3) delayed graft function (DGF), which represents the far end of the spectrum of posttransplant graft dysfunction and is defined by the need for dialysis posttransplant.[29]

Decreased or minimal urine output is a frequent concern posttransplant. Most commonly, it is due to an alteration in volume

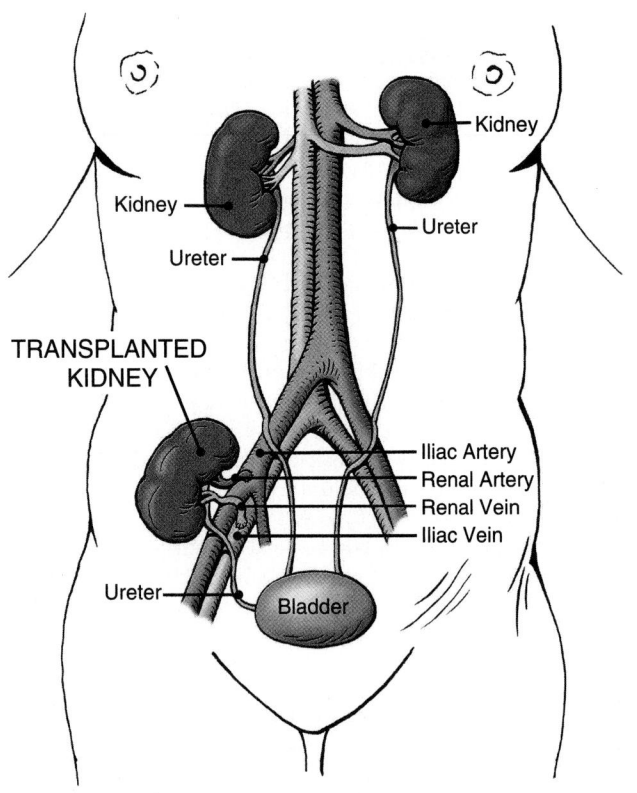

A

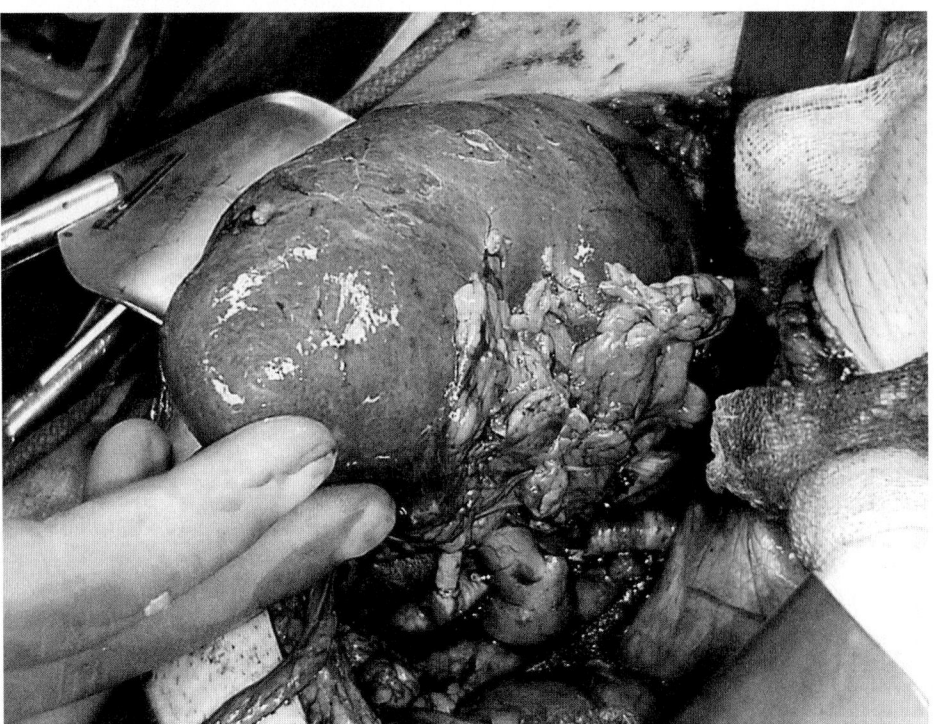

B

FIG. 10-5. Kidney graft in a heterotopic position in the right iliac fossa.

status. Other causes include a blocked urinary catheter, vascular thrombosis, a urinary leak or obstruction, early acute rejection, drug toxicity, or DGF (Table 10-4). Early diagnosis is important, and begins with an assessment of the recipient's volume status. The urinary catheter is checked to exclude the presence of occlusion with clots or debris. Other diagnostic tests that may be warranted, depending on

the suspected cause, include a Doppler ultrasound, nuclear medicine scan, or a biopsy.

Complications

Monitoring for potential surgical and medical complications is important. Early diagnosis and appropriate intervention can minimize

Table 10-4
Causes of Increased Serum Creatinine Early After Kidney Transplant

Cause	Characteristics	Diagnosis	Treatment
Hypovolemia	Decreased CVP Decreasing urine output Low blood pressure Low Hgb if due to bleeding	Check Hgb and CVP	Rehydrate with appropriate fluids
Vascular thrombosis	Sudden drop in urine output Dark hematuria Tender, swollen graft	Ultrasound with Doppler	Re-explore for thrombectomy or nephrectomy
Bladder outlet obstruction	Clots in urinary catheter Sudden drop in urine output	Distended bladder on examination or by ultrasound	Irrigate or change bladder catheter
Ureteral obstruction		Euvolemic Ultrasound showing hydroureter Possible lymphocele on ultrasound	Do percutaneous nephrostogram Drainage of lymphocele (if it is the cause of ureter obstruction)
Drug toxicity	High CSA or FK506 level	Check drug levels	Decrease dosage of drugs
Acute rejection	May have risk factors such as low drug levels, high PRA	Kidney biopsy	Administer bolus steroid or antilymphocyte treatment Begin plasmapheresis and IVIG if humoral rejection

CSA = cyclosporine; CVP = central venous pressure; FK506 = tacrolimus; Hgb = hemoglobin; IVIG = intravenous immuneglobulin; PRA = panel-reactive antibodies.

the detrimental impact on the graft and recipient. Potential complications that may occur early after surgery include hemorrhage, vascular complications, urologic complications, lymphocele, and several others.

Hemorrhage

Bleeding is uncommon after a kidney transplant; it usually occurs from unligated vessels in the graft hilum or from the retroperitoneum of the recipient. A falling hematocrit level, hypotension, or tachycardia should all raise the possibility of bleeding. Surgical exploration is seldom required because bleeding often tamponades. However, ongoing transfusion requirements, hemodynamic instability, and compression of the kidney by hematoma are all indications for surgical re-exploration.

Vascular Complications

Vascular complications can involve the donor vessels (renal artery thrombosis or stenosis, renal vein thrombosis), the recipient vessels (iliac artery thrombosis, pseudoaneurysms, and deep venous thrombosis), or both. Renal artery thrombosis usually occurs early posttransplant; it is uncommon, with an incidence of less than 1%. However, it is a devastating complication, usually resulting in graft loss. Typically, it occurs secondary to a technical problem such as intimal dissection or torsion of the vessels. Risk factors for thrombosis include hypotension, multiple renal arteries, unidentified injury to the intima of the artery, hyperacute rejection, unrelenting acute rejection, and a hypercoagulable state. Under these circumstances there is a sudden cessation of urine output. Diagnosis is easily made with color flow Doppler studies. Urgent thrombectomy is indicated, but most such grafts cannot be salvaged and require removal. Stenosis of the renal artery is a late complication and presents with evidence of graft dysfunction or hypertension. First-line treatment is with interventional radiologic techniques; surgery is reserved for stenosis that does not respond.

Renal vein thrombosis is not as common as its arterial counterpart, but again, graft loss is the usual end result. Causes include angulation or torsion of the vein, compression by hematomas or lymphoceles, anastomotic stenosis, and extension of an underlying deep venous thrombosis. Again, Doppler studies are the best diagnostic

test. Urgent thrombectomy is rarely successful, and nephrectomy is usually required. Venous thromboembolic complications that affect the recipient vessels (deep venous thrombosis and pulmonary embolism) are not uncommon. The incidence of deep venous thrombosis is close to 5%; the incidence of pulmonary embolism 1%. Identified risk factors include recipient age over 40, hypercoagulable states, diabetes, and a history of deep venous thrombosis. For recipients with these risk factors, prophylaxis with low-dose heparin is recommended.

Urologic Complications

Urinary tract complications, manifesting as leakage or obstruction, generally occur in 2 to 10% of kidney recipients. The underlying cause is often related to poor blood supply and ischemia of the transplant ureter. Leakage most commonly occurs from the anastomotic site. Causes other than ischemia include undue tension created by a short ureter, and direct surgical injury. Presentation is usually early (before the fifth posttransplant week); symptoms include fever, pain, swelling at the graft site, increased creatinine level, decreased urine output, and cutaneous urinary drainage. Diagnosis can be confirmed initially with a hippurate renal scan, although a percutaneous nephrostogram is required for precise definition. Early surgical exploration with ureteral re-implantation is usually indicated, although small leaks may be managed by percutaneous nephrostomy and stent placement with good results.

Ureteral obstruction may develop early or late. Early obstruction may be due to edema, blood clots, hematomas, or torsion of the ureter. Late obstruction generally is due to scarring and fibrosis from chronic ischemia. Patients develop an elevated serum creatinine level. An ultrasound to look for hydronephrosis is a good initial test. Percutaneous transluminal dilatation, followed by placement of an internal or external stent, is a good initial treatment. If repeated dilatations and stenting are required, surgical intervention (e.g., ureteral reimplantation or ureteropyelostomy using native ureter) should be undertaken.

Lymphocele

The reported incidence of lymphoceles (fluid collections of lymph that generally result from cut lymphatic vessels in the

Table 10-5
Patient Survival Rates (%) After Various Transplants

	Time Posttransplant				
	3 months	1 year	3 years	5 years	10 years
Kidney					
Deceased donor	97.3	94.0	88.4	79.9	59.4
Living donor	99.0	97.7	94.7	89.7	79.4
SPK	97.1	95.1	89.2	82.6	60.8
PAK	97.9	95.5	89.3	77.3	64.7
PTA	100.0	98.6	86.0	77.8	68.2
Liver					
Deceased donor	91.1	86.4	79.5	72.4	59.4
Living donor	91.0	85.2	80.2	85.6	85.2
Intestine	92.3	84.6	72.9	48.6	50.0
Heart	89.5	85.1	78.6	69.8	50.0
Lung	88.2	77.4	59.3	42.5	22.7
Heart-Lung	73.4	59.6	44.8	48.6	29.7

SPK = simultaneous pancreas-kidney transplant; PAK = pancreas after kidney transplant; PTA = pancreas transplant alone.

SOURCE: Data from the Organ Procurement and Transplant Network/Scientific Registry of Transplant Recipients 2002 Annual Report, www.ustransplant.org.

recipient) is 0.6 to 18%. Lymphoceles usually do not occur until at least two weeks posttransplant. Symptoms are generally related to the mass effect and compression of nearby structures (e.g., ureter, iliac vein, allograft renal artery), and patients develop hypertension, unilateral leg swelling on the side of the transplant, and elevated serum creatinine. Ultrasound is used to confirm a fluid collection, although percutaneous aspiration may be necessary to exclude presence of other collections such as urinomas, hematomas, or abscesses. The standard surgical treatment is creation of a peritoneal window to allow for drainage of the lymphatic fluid into the peritoneal cavity where it can be absorbed. Either a laparoscopic or an open approach may be used. Another option is percutaneous insertion of a drainage catheter, with or without sclerotherapy; however, it is associated with some risk of recurrence or infection.

Other Complications

A wide variety of medical complications can be seen after a kidney transplant. Infections are probably the most common, but the incidence has declined significantly in recent years, due to improvements in prophylaxis regimens. Common sites for infection include the urinary tract, the pulmonary system, and the wound. Noninfectious medical complications affecting the cardiac, gastrointestinal, and neurologic systems have also been well described posttransplant.[30] Such complications are often related to the administration of immunosuppressive drugs, thereby facilitating the occurrence of infections due to opportunistic microbes.

Late Posttransplant Care

The goal of late posttransplant care of the kidney transplant recipient is to optimize immunosuppression, carefully monitor graft function, and screen and monitor for complications that are directly or indirectly related to immunosuppressive medications. Optimizing immunosuppression entails fitting it to the individual recipient's needs. Recipients at low risk for rejection should have their immunosuppression lowered to minimize side effects and complications. Careful attention should be paid to compliance; it is often easy for recipients to become less attentive to their medications as they progress through the posttransplant period. Monitoring kidney

function may help detect noncompliance, but is also important to detect late rejection episodes, recurrence of disease, or late technical problems (such as renal artery stenosis or ureteric stricture). Other potential problems in these recipients include hypercholesterolemia, hypertriglyceridemia, and increased blood pressure, which may or may not be related to the immunosuppressive drugs. Screening for malignancy (especially skin, colorectal, breast, cervical, and prostate) is important, although the incidence of many of these malignancies is equivalent to those seen in the general population. Patients should be immunized, ideally pretransplant, for *Haemophilus influenzae, Streptococcus pneumoniae,* and *Neisseria meningitidis,* as this is important to minimize infectious complications due to these pathogens.

Results

Posttransplant outcomes have steadily improved over the past three decades due to improvements in immunosuppression, antirejection therapy, organ retrieval techniques, perioperative care, and treatment of infectious posttransplant complications.[31–33] Since the late 1980s, the use of modern immunosuppressive drugs has been a primary factor, especially in those previously considered to be at high-risk, such as diabetic, pediatric, and older recipients.

Most centers now report patient survival rates exceeding 95% during the first posttransplant year for all kidney recipients (Table 10-5). Living-donor transplants still have an advantage over cadaver donor transplant, but even this difference is diminishing with modern immunosuppression. The survival advantage after a transplant, as compared with dialysis, is probably greatest for diabetic patients. Without a transplant, their overall survival is 26% at 5 years; with a transplant, it jumps to about 80%. The major cause of death in all kidney recipients is cardiovascular (myocardial infarction or stroke); sepsis accounts for less than 3%, while malignancy accounts for 2%.

The incidence of acute rejection has declined steadily since the early 1990s. Most centers now report acute rejection rates of 10 to 20% at 1 year posttransplant. This decline has been a major factor in the improvement in graft survival rates, which are now about 75 to 80% at 5 years and 60 to 65% at 10 years posttransplant for all kidney recipients[34] (Table 10-6). Currently, the most common cause of graft loss is recipient death (usually from cardiovascular

Table 10-6
Graft Survival Rates (%) After Various Transplants

	Time Posttransplant				
	3 months	1 year	3 years	5 years	10 years
Kidney					
Deceased donor	93.5	88.4	78.5	63.3	36.4
Living donor	96.8	94.4	88.3	76.5	55.5
SPK	97.0	95.1	89.8	83.9	64.0
PAK	86.5	78.3	60.2	45.5	16.4
PTA	87.4	81.2	57.1	32.4	16.2
Liver					
Deceased donor	85.8	80.2	71.4	63.5	45.1
Living donor	83.0	76.3	72.4	73.0	42.7
Intestine	78.3	67.2	44.9	19.7	0
Heart	89.0	84.4	77.5	68.1	46.4
Lung	87.3	76.2	57.5	40.5	17.5
Heart-Lung	73.9	60.1	46.9	41.8	28.1

SPK = simultaneous pancreas-kidney transplant; PAK = pancreas after kidney transplant; PTA = pancreas transplant alone.
SOURCE: Data from the Organ Procurement and Transplant Network/Scientific Registry of Transplant Recipients 2002 Annual Report, www.ustransplant.org.

causes) with a functioning graft. The second most common cause is chronic allograft nephropathy. Characterized by a slow, unrelenting deterioration of graft function, it likely has multiple causes (both immunologic and nonimmunologic).[35,36] The graft failure rate due to surgical technique has remained at about 2%.

PANCREAS TRANSPLANTATION

Diabetes mellitus is a very common medical condition with immense medical, social, and financial costs. In North America, it is the leading cause of kidney failure, blindness, nontraumatic amputations, and impotence. The discovery of insulin in 1922 by Banting and Best changed diabetes from a lethal disease to a chronic illness. However, even though exogenous insulin can prevent the acute metabolic complications and decrease the incidence of secondary complications associated with diabetes, it cannot provide a homeostatic environment comparable to that afforded by a functioning pancreas. Only a functioning pancreas can provide immediate insulin responses to the moment-to-moment changes in glucose levels.

A successful pancreas transplant can establish normoglycemia and insulin independence in diabetic recipients, with glucose control similar to that seen with a functioning native pancreas. A pancreas transplant also has the potential to halt progression of some secondary complications of diabetes. No current method of exogenous insulin administration can produce a euglycemic, insulin-independent state akin to that achievable with a technically successful pancreas graft. In addition to improved metabolic control and beneficial effects on secondary complications, a pancreas transplant can substantially enhance quality of life, more than that achieved by exogenous insulin administration. Indeed, the modern management of diabetes by exogenous insulin may be as burdensome as dialysis is for kidney failure, as it consists of four blood glucose determinations daily, coupled with four insulin injections or a constantly present needle. A successful pancreas transplant obviates the need for such constant invasive monitoring.

Currently, the main drawback of a pancreas transplant is the need for immunosuppression. Pancreas transplants are now preferentially performed in diabetic patients with kidney failure who also are candidates for a kidney transplant, as they already require immunosuppression to prevent kidney rejection. However, a pancreas transplant alone (PTA) is appropriate for nonuremic diabetics if their day-to-day quality of life is so poor (e.g., labile serum glucose with ketoacidosis and/or hypoglycemic episodes, or progression of severe diabetic retinopathy, nephropathy, neuropathy, and/or enteropathy) that chronic immunosuppression is justified to achieve insulin independence.[37] As immunosuppressive agents become safer, it is likely that PTA will become increasingly common.

History

The first human pancreas transplant was performed in 1966; however, the procedure was not performed with any frequency until many years later. During the 1970s, a small number of institutions performed a few pancreas transplants, and their success rates were low, mainly because of problems with rejection. A dramatic improvement in outcome occurred in the 1980s, after advances in surgical techniques and the introduction of cyclosporine for immunosuppression. In the United States, the inception of UNOS in 1987 facilitated nationwide organ procurement and allocation. A steady growth in the application of pancreas transplants soon followed. By the mid-1990s, more than 1000 pancreas transplants were being performed annually in the United States, with improved results paralleling the introduction of even newer immunosuppressive drugs such as tacrolimus and MMF.

Results also improved because of refinements in surgical technique. By the mid-1970s, the following three techniques were in use: enteric drainage (ED), urinary drainage (first into the ureter, and later modified by direct implantation into the bladder), and duct injection. During the 1980s, bladder drainage (BD) was shown to be safe, and it became the predominant technique in all pancreas recipient categories, as it facilitated allograft monitoring via measurement of urine amylase levels (Fig. 10-6). The 1990s saw a shift back to ED, especially in patients who underwent a simultaneous kidney transplant (Fig. 10-7). In such recipients, the serum creatinine level can be used as a surrogate marker for pancreas rejection when both organs come from the same donor.

Management of vascularization of the pancreas graft has also evolved. Venous drainage of the graft venous effluent can be into

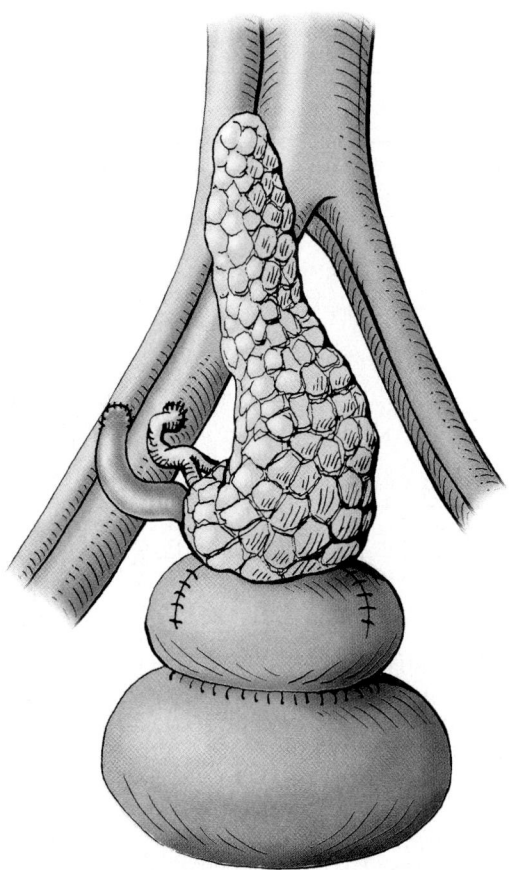

FIG. 10-6. *Isolated pancreas transplant with bladder drainage of the pancreatic secretions.*

either the systemic or the portal circulation. Portal drainage is more physiologic and may even lower the incidence of rejection.

Preoperative Evaluation

The preoperative evaluation for pancreas transplant recipients does not differ substantially from that for diabetic kidney transplant recipients. Examination of the cardiovascular system is most important because significant coronary artery disease may be present without angina.[38] Noninvasive testing may not identify coronary artery disease, so coronary angiography is routinely performed. Detailed neurologic, ophthalmologic, metabolic, and kidney function testing may be needed to assess the degree of progression of secondary complications. Any contraindications to a transplant, such as active malignancy or infection, must be ruled out. A thorough evaluation of the peripheral vascular system is essential, given the high incidence of peripheral vascular disease in diabetics. The patency of the iliac system needs to be determined, because the iliac vessels will serve as the inflow source for the pancreas.

Once a patient is determined to be a good candidate for a pancreas transplant, with no obvious contraindications, it is important to decide which type of pancreas transplant is best for that individual. First, the degree of kidney dysfunction and the need for a kidney transplant must be determined. Patients with stable kidney function (creatinine less than 2.0 mg/dL and minimal protein in the urine) are candidates for a PTA. However, patients with moderate kidney insufficiency will likely require a kidney transplant as well; further deterioration of kidney function often occurs once calcineurin inhibitors are started for immunosuppression.

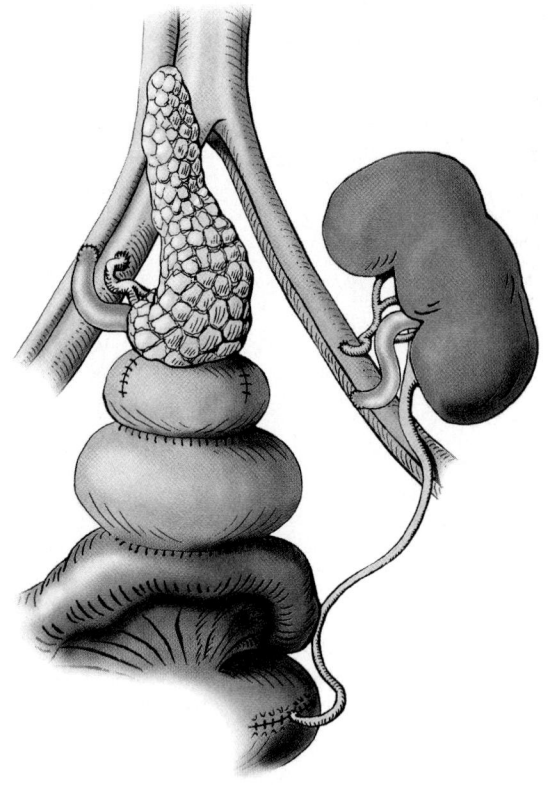

FIG. 10-7. *Combined kidney-pancreas transplant with enteric drainage of the pancreatic secretions.*

For patients requiring both a kidney and a pancreas transplant, various options are available. The two transplants can be performed either simultaneously or sequentially. A living donor or a deceased donor can be used, or both. Which option is best for the individual patient depends on the degree of kidney dysfunction, the availability of donors, and personal preference. The following options are currently possible:

1. Deceased-donor, simultaneous pancreas-kidney transplant (SPK): The most common option worldwide, deceased-donor SPK transplants have well-documented long-term survival results for both the kidney and the pancreas grafts. The recipient has the advantage of undergoing both transplants at the same time, and therefore may potentially become dialysis-free and insulin-independent at the same time. There is also an immunologic advantage, as acute rejection rates are significantly lower for SPK (versus PTA) recipients.

2. Living-donor kidney transplant, followed weeks to months later by a deceased-donor pancreas transplant (pancreas after kidney [PAK] transplant): If a living donor is available for the kidney transplant, then this is a good option for uremic diabetic patients. It offers the possibility of performing the kidney transplant as soon as the living-donor evaluation is complete, rendering the recipient dialysis-free within a short period. A living-donor (vs. deceased-donor) kidney transplant has superior long-term results. By performing the two operations sequentially instead of simultaneously, the overall surgical complication rate may be decreased, perhaps because by the time of the pancreas transplant, the effects of uremia have resolved and patients are in better metabolic and nutritional condition.[39] The disadvantage is that the long-term pancreas graft survival rates for PAK recipients are still somewhat inferior to those of individuals receiving SPK transplants.

3. Simultaneous deceased-donor pancreas and living-donor kidney transplant (SPLK): Candidates with a suitable living donor for the kidney transplant who have not yet progressed to dialysis can be placed on the

deceased-donor pancreas transplant waiting list. When a deceased-donor pancreas becomes available, the living donor for the kidney is called in at the same time, and both procedures are performed simultaneously. Advantages include use of a living donor for the kidney, shorter waiting times, and a single operation.[40] Technically, this option may be more difficult to organize, as it requires using two full surgical teams and two full operating rooms, and at times the donor and the recipient will need to be called in from different locations. It also may create difficult timing issues for the living donor, who must come in quickly for an emergent operation.

4. Living-donor, simultaneous pancreas-kidney transplant: If a single individual is suitable to donate both a kidney and a hemipancreas, then another potential option exists. It is especially useful for candidates with a high level of preformed antibodies, or those who have difficulty acquiring a deceased donor organ. The main disadvantage of this approach is to the living donor, who has to undergo a surgical procedure of substantial magnitude with its attendant risks and morbidity.

Surgical Procedure

The initial preparation of the donor pancreas is a crucial component of a successful transplant. Direct physical examination of the pancreas often is the best or only way to confirm its suitability. If it is sclerotic, calcific, or markedly discolored, it should not be used. Before implantation, a surgical procedure is undertaken to remove the spleen and any excess duodenum and to ligate blood vessels at the root of the mesentery (Fig. 10-8). The inflow vessels to the graft are the splenic and superior mesenteric arteries; outflow is via the portal vein. Arterial reconstruction is performed before implanting the graft in the recipient. The donor superior mesenteric and splenic arteries are connected, most commonly using a reversed segment of donor iliac artery as a Y-graft (Fig. 10-9); doing so allows for a single arterial anastomosis in the recipient.

The pancreas graft is then implanted via an anastomosis of the aforementioned arterial graft to the recipient common iliac artery or distal aorta, and, via a venous anastomosis of the donor portal vein to the recipient iliac vein (for systemic drainage), or to the superior mesenteric vein (for portal drainage).[41] If both a kidney and a pancreas are transplanted, they are placed in an intraperitoneal position, with the kidney usually in the left iliac fossa and the pancreas in the right iliac fossa. If the pancreas is drained via the portal route, then it usually sits higher in the mid-abdomen.

Once the pancreas is revascularized, a drainage procedure must be performed to handle the pancreatic exocrine secretions. Options include anastomosing the donor duodenum to the recipient bladder or to the small bowel, with the small bowel either in continuity or connected to a Roux-en-Y limb. Some centers always use enteric drainage, others always use bladder drainage, and others tailor the approach according to the recipient category. Both enteric drainage and bladder drainage now have a relatively low surgical risk. The main advantage of bladder drainage is the ability to directly measure enzyme activity in the pancreatic graft exocrine secretions by measuring the amount of amylase in the urine. A decrease in urine amylase is a sensitive marker for rejection, even though it is not entirely specific. Urine amylase always decreases before hyperglycemia ensues. A rise in serum amylase may precede a decrease in urine amylase, but serum amylase by itself is less sensitive (it does not always rise, but urine amylase always decreases), and is no more specific for the diagnosis of rejection. The leak rate is the same whether the pancreas is drained to the bladder or to the bowel, but the consequences of a bladder leak are much less severe than those associated with a bowel leak. The disadvantages of bladder drainage include complications such as dehydration and acidosis

(from loss of alkalotic pancreatic secretions in the urine), and local problems with the bladder such as infection, hematuria, stones, and urethritis. Because of these chronic complications, between 10 and 20% of bladder-drained graft recipients are ultimately converted to enteric drainage.

Enteric drainage is more physiologic and has fewer long-term complications. However, the ability to monitor for rejection is decreased, given the absence of urinary amylase. Rejection in SPK transplant recipients almost always affects both the kidney and the pancreas; therefore, the serum creatinine level can be used as a marker for rejection of the pancreas. Hence, most centers now use enteric drainage for SPK transplants. If the kidney and the pancreas are from different donors, or if a PTA is performed, then bladder drainage is preferred, so rejection of the pancreas can be detected earlier.

Postoperative Care

In general, pancreas recipients do not require intensive care monitoring in the postoperative period. Laboratory values—serum glucose, hemoglobin, electrolytes, and amylase—are monitored daily. The serum glucose level is monitored even more frequently if normoglycemia is not immediately achieved. Nasogastric suction and IV fluids are continued for the first several days until bowel function returns. In the early postoperative period, regular insulin is infused to maintain plasma glucose levels less than 150 mg/dL, because chronic hyperglycemia may be detrimental to beta cells. In recipients who undergo bladder drainage, a Foley catheter is left in place for 10 to 14 days. At most centers, some form of prophylaxis is instituted against bacterial, fungal, and viral infections. In addition, many centers routinely institute some form of prophylaxis against thrombosis of the allograft; options include low-dose heparin, low molecular weight heparin, or oral antiplatelet agents for the first week posttransplant.

Complications

One crucial aspect of posttransplant care is monitoring for rejection and complications (both surgical and medical). Rejection episodes may be identified by an increase in serum creatinine (in SPK recipients), a decrease in urinary amylase (in recipients with bladder drainage), an increase in serum amylase, or by an increase in serum glucose levels. Unfortunately, complications are common after pancreas transplants. The pancreas graft is susceptible to a unique set of complications because of its exocrine secretions and low blood flow. However, the incidence of graft-related complications has decreased significantly since the early 1990s due to better preservation techniques, better surgical methods, improved prophylaxis regimens, and improved immunosuppression.[42] Potential complications are described below.

Thrombosis

The incidence of thrombosis is approximately 6% for pancreas transplants reported to the UNOS registry. Low-dose heparin, dextran, or antiplatelet agents are administered routinely in the early postoperative period at many centers, although these agents slightly increase the risk of postoperative bleeding. Arterial or venous thrombosis is most common within the first several days posttransplant, heralded by an increase in blood glucose levels, an increase in insulin requirements, or a decrease in urine amylase levels. Venous thrombosis also is characteristically accompanied by hematuria, tenderness and swelling of the graft, and ipsilateral lower extremity edema. Treatment consists of graft removal.

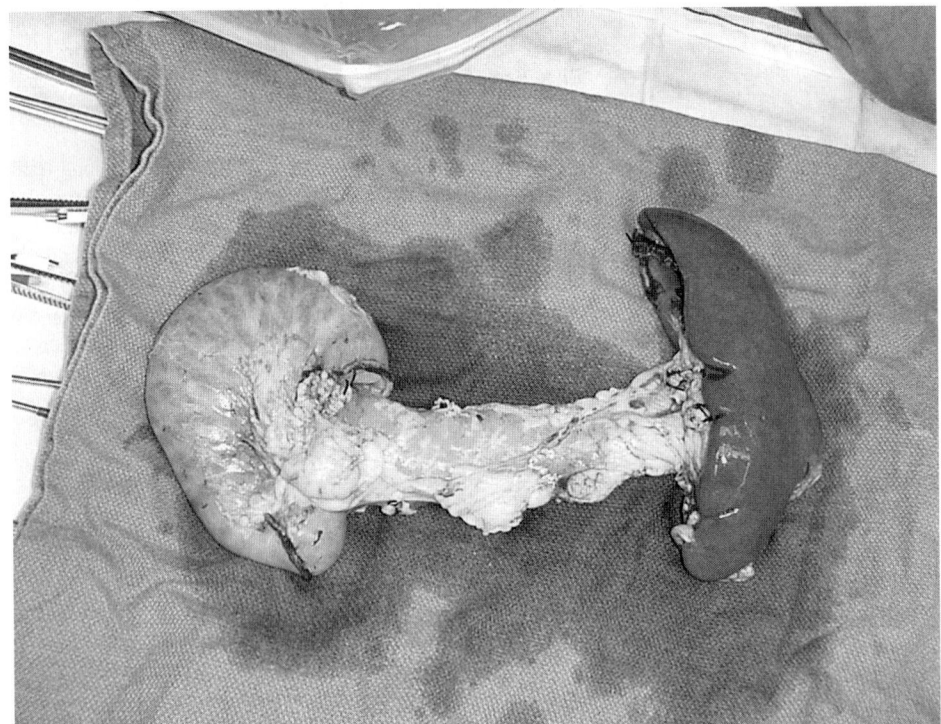

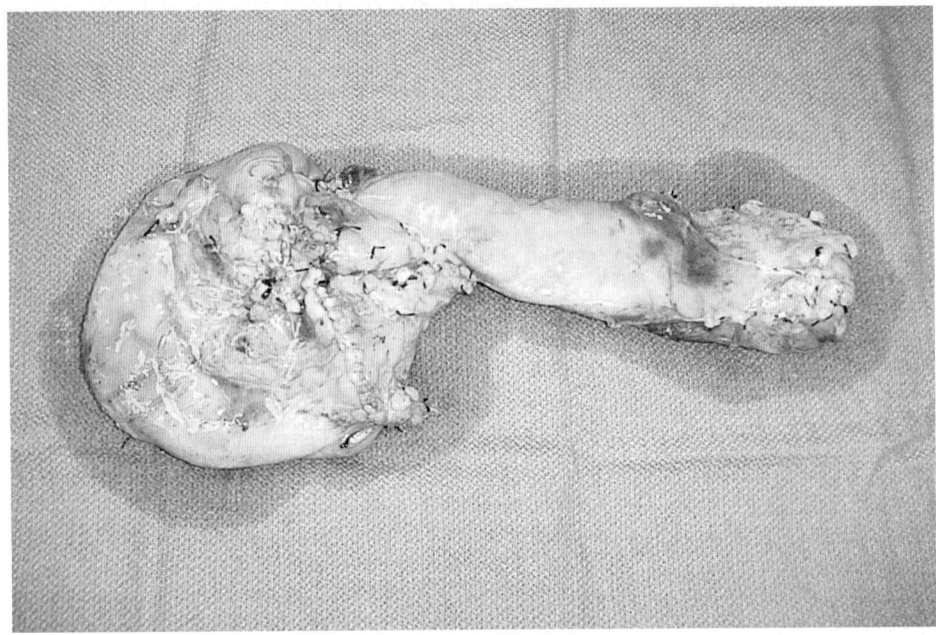

FIG. 10-8. Pancreas graft before (*above*) and after (*below*) bench preparation.

Hemorrhage

Postoperative bleeding may be minimized by meticulous intraoperative control of bleeding sites. Hemorrhage may be exacerbated by anticoagulants and antiplatelet drugs, but their benefits seem to outweigh the risks. Bleeding is a much less significant cause (<1%) of graft loss than is thrombosis, according to UNOS registry data. Significant bleeding is treated by immediate re-exploration.

Pancreatitis

Most cases of graft pancreatitis occur early, tend to be self-limited, and are probably due to ischemic preservation injury. Clinical manifestations may include graft tenderness and fever, in

addition to hyperamylasemia. Treatment consists of IV fluid replacement and keeping the recipient fasting. Later episodes of graft pancreatitis may be caused by reflux into the allograft duct (in recipients who undergo bladder drainage) or by cytomegalovirus (CMV) infection. Reflux is treated by urinary catheter drainage, and occasionally by conversion to enteric drainage. CMV infections are treated with appropriate antiviral agents.

Urologic Complications

Urologic complications are almost exclusively limited to recipients with bladder drainage. Hematuria is not uncommon in the first several months posttransplant, but it is usually transient and

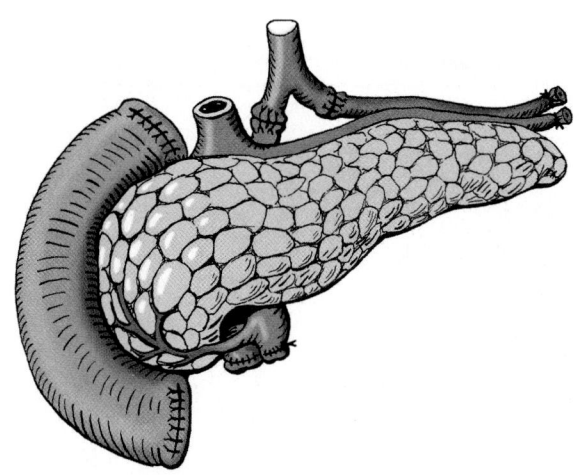

FIG. 10-9. *Bench preparation of the pancreas demonstrating an iliac artery Y-graft to reconstruct the arterial blood supply.*

self-limiting. Bladder calculi may develop because exposed sutures or staples along the duodenocystostomy serve as a nidus for stone formation. Recurrent urinary tract infections commonly occur concurrently. Treatment consists of cystoscopy with removal of the sutures or staples. Urinary leaks, most commonly from the proximal duodenal cuff or from the duodenal anastomosis to the bladder, typically occur during the first several weeks posttransplant. Small leaks can be successfully managed by prolonged (at least 2 weeks) urinary catheter drainage; larger leaks require surgical intervention.

Other urinary complications include chronic, refractory, metabolic acidosis because of bicarbonate loss, persistent and recurrent urinary tract infections, and urethritis. Along with recurrent hematuria, these complications are the major indications for converting recipients from bladder drainage to enteric drainage. Because 10 to 20% of recipients with initial bladder drainage will require conversion to enteric drainage, a recent trend has been to perform enteric drainage at the time of the transplant. Enteric drainage is associated with significantly fewer urinary tract infections and urologic complications, but it obviates the use of urinary amylase determinations.

Infections

Infections remain a significant problem after pancreas transplants.[43] Most common are superficial wound infections and intra-abdominal infections, often related to graft complications such as leaks. Thanks to appropriate perioperative antimicrobial regimens (for prophylaxis against gram-positive bacteria, gram-negative bacteria, and yeast) the incidence of significant infections has decreased. Still, it remains about 10% and is associated with significant morbidity and mortality. Thus, if serious intra-abdominal infections occur (whether or not associated with the above complications), re-exploration and graft removal must be strongly considered, along with concurrent reduction in immunosuppression.

Results

The International Pancreas Transplant Registry (IPTR) maintains data on pancreas transplants. Analyses of IPTR data have been published yearly since the mid-1980s. The results (particularly as measured by long-term insulin independence) have continually improved over time. Patient survival rates are not significantly different between the three main recipient categories and are greater than 90%

at 3 years posttransplant. Most deaths are due to pre-existing cardiovascular disease; the mortality risk of a pancreas transplant per se is extremely low (e.g., patient survival at 1 year for PTA recipients is >95%). Pancreas graft survival rates at 1 year remain higher in the SPK (~90%) than in the PAK (~85%) and PTA (~75%) categories, according to IPTR data. The differences are due in part to the decreased ability to monitor for rejection episodes in enteric-drained, solitary pancreas transplant recipients. With improving immunosuppressive protocols and the decreasing incidence of acute rejection, the difference between the three categories has been steadily decreasing since the late 1990s.[44,45]

Islet Cell Transplantation

The pancreas consists of two separate functional systems (endocrine and exocrine), but it is only the endocrine component that is of use in the transplant process. However, many of the complications seen with whole-organ pancreas transplants are due to the exocrine component. Therefore, the concept of transplanting simply the cells responsible for the production of insulin is very logical and attractive.

Islet cell transplantation involves extracting islets of Langerhans from a donor's pancreas and then injecting them into a diabetic recipient. These islet cells then engraft into the recipient and secrete insulin, providing excellent moment-to-moment control of blood glucose, as is seen with a whole-organ pancreas transplant. Compared with exogenous insulin injections, an islet cell transplant offers advantages similar to those of a whole-organ pancreas transplant. A successful islet transplant provides perfect glucose homeostasis, freeing the diabetic patient from the burden of frequent glucose monitoring and insulin injections. It potentially prevents secondary complications of diabetes and significantly improves quality of life.

Unlike a whole-organ pancreas transplant, an islet cell transplant is not a major surgical procedure. It can generally be performed as an outpatient procedure, with minimal recovery time for the recipient. It avoids a major surgical procedure, with its associated mortality and morbidity. Given this significantly lower surgical risk, islet cell transplants could theoretically have much wider application than whole-organ transplants.

Typically, a pancreas is procured from a suitable deceased donor. Isolating the islets is a complex process, which generally involves digesting the pancreas with a collagenase solution to separate the islet cells. The islets may then be purified (i.e., separated from the acinar cells). The purified islets can then be injected into the recipient, most commonly into the portal vein. The islet cells then engraft in the hepatic parenchyma and secrete insulin, which drains into the circulation. Potential complications associated with the injection include portal hypertension, hepatic abscesses, and bacteremia.

One major disadvantage of an islet cell transplant (similar to that of a whole-organ transplant) is the need for long-term immunosuppression. This disadvantage has limited the use of islet cell transplants to patients with kidney failure who require immunosuppression because of a kidney transplant.

This immunologic problem is compounded by the fact that islet cell rejection can be difficult to monitor and diagnose. One possible method of avoiding the need for immunosuppression is to surround the islets with a semipermeable membrane, a process called *microencapsulation*. This process would allow small molecules such as oxygen and glucose to reach the islet cells and would allow insulin to reach the systemic circulation. But microencapsulation would prevent immune cells and large molecules such as antibodies from reaching the islet cells. The islet cells would then survive and function well inside the membranes, while being protected from immunologic damage.

Islet cell transplants have been a possibility for many years, but the results have generally been poor. In 1995, a report of the International Islet Transplant Registry indicated that of 270 recipients, only 5% were insulin-independent at 1 year posttransplant. Recently, however, significantly improved results have been reported by using steroid-free immunosuppression and islet injections from multiple donors. These recent successes have stimulated a flurry of islet transplant activity at centers across the world. As results are likely to continue to improve, it is possible that islet cell transplants may come to replace whole-organ pancreas transplants.

LIVER TRANSPLANTATION

The field of liver transplantation has undergone remarkable advances in the last two decades. An essentially experimental procedure in the early 1980s, a liver transplant is now the treatment of choice for patients with acute and chronic liver failure. Patient survival at 1 year posttransplant has increased from 30% in the early 1980s to more than 85% at present. The major reasons for this dramatic increase include refined surgical and preservation techniques, better immunosuppressive protocols, more effective treatment of infections, and improved care during the critical perioperative period. However, a liver transplant remains a major undertaking, with the potential for complications affecting every major organ system.

History

The history of liver transplantation began with experimental transplants performed in dogs in the late 1950s. The first liver transplant attempted in humans was in 1963 by Thomas Starzl. The recipient was a 3-year-old boy with biliary atresia who unfortunately died of hemorrhage. The first successful liver transplant was in 1967, again by Starzl. Yet, for the next 10 years, liver transplants remained essentially experimental, with survival rates well below 50%. Still, advances in the surgical procedure and in anesthetic management continued to be made during that time.

The major breakthrough for the field came in the early 1980s, with the introduction and clinical use of the immunosuppressive agent cyclosporine. Patient survival dramatically improved, and liver transplantation was soon being recognized as a viable therapeutic option. Results continued to improve through the 1980s, due to ongoing improvements in immunosuppression, critical care management, surgical technique, and preservation solutions. The late 1980s and 1990s saw a dramatic increase in the number of liver transplants, and an even greater increase in the number of patients waiting for a transplant. This in turn increased waiting times as well as mortality rates for those waiting.

The longer waiting time and higher mortality rates for patients on the deceased-donor liver transplant waiting list led to the development of innovative surgical techniques such as split-liver transplants and living-donor liver transplants. Initially these new techniques were mainly applied to pediatric patients because of the difficulty associated with finding appropriate size-matched organs for them. However, as the number of adults on the waiting list grew, these techniques began to be applied for adult recipients as well. The use of living-donor liver transplants progressed at an even more rapid pace in countries such as Japan, where the concept of deceased-donor organ donation was not widely accepted.

Table 10-7
Diseases Amenable to Treatment by a Liver Transplant

Cholestatic liver diseases
    Primary biliary cirrhosis
    Primary sclerosing cholangitis
    Biliary atresia
    Alagille syndrome
Chronic hepatitis
    Hepatitis B
    Hepatitis C
    Autoimmune hepatitis
Alcoholic liver disease
Metabolic diseases
    Hemochromatosis
    Wilson's disease
    Alpha$_1$-antitrypsin deficiency
    Tyrosinemia
    Cystic fibrosis
Hepatic malignancy
    Hepatocellular carcinoma
    Neuroendocrine tumor metastatic to liver
Fulminant hepatic failure
Others
    Cryptogenic cirrhosis
    Polycystic liver disease
    Budd-Chiari syndrome
    Amyloidosis

Preoperative Evaluation

A liver transplant is indicated for liver failure, whether acute or chronic.[46] Liver failure is signaled by a number of clinical symptoms (e.g., ascites, variceal bleeding, hepatic encephalopathy, and malnutrition), and by biochemical liver test results that suggest impaired hepatic synthetic function (e.g., hypoalbuminemia, hyperbilirubinemia, and coagulopathy). The cause of liver failure often influences its presentation. For example, patients with acute liver failure generally have hepatic encephalopathy and coagulopathy, whereas patients with chronic liver disease most commonly have ascites, GI bleeding, and malnutrition.

Diseases Treatable by Transplant

A host of diseases are potentially treatable by a liver transplant (Table 10-7). Broadly, they can be categorized as acute or chronic, and then subdivided by the cause of the liver disease. Chronic liver diseases account for the majority of liver transplants today. The most common cause in North America is chronic hepatitis, usually due to hepatitis C and less commonly to hepatitis B. Chronic alcohol abuse accelerates the process, especially with hepatitis C. Progression from chronic infection to cirrhosis is generally slow, usually occurring over a period of 10 to 20 years. Chronic hepatitis may also result from autoimmune causes, primarily in women. It can present either acutely over months or insidiously over years. Alcohol often plays a role in end-stage liver disease (ESLD) secondary to hepatitis C, but it may also lead to liver failure in the absence of viral infection. In fact, alcohol is the most common cause of ESLD in the United States. Such patients are generally suitable candidates for a transplant as long as an adequate period of sobriety can be documented.

Cholestatic disorders also account for a significant percentage of transplant candidates with chronic liver disease. In adults, the most common causes are primary biliary cirrhosis (PBC) and primary sclerosing cholangitis (PSC). PBC, a destructive disorder of interlobular bile ducts, can progress to cirrhosis and liver failure over several decades. It most commonly affects middle-aged women.

Table 10-8
Indications for a Liver Transplant in Patients with Acute Liver Failure

Acetaminophen toxicity
pH <7.30
Prothrombin time >100 seconds (INR >6.5)
Serum creatinine >300 μmol/L (>3.4 mg/dL)

No acetaminophen toxicity
Prothrombin time >100 seconds (INR >6.5)
Age <10 or >40 years
Non-A, non-B hepatitis
Duration of jaundice before onset of encephalopathy >7 days
Serum creatinine >300 μmol/L (>3.4 mg/dL)

INR = International Normalized Ratio.

PSC, a disease characterized by inflammatory injury of the bile duct, occurs mostly in young men, 70% of whom have inflammatory bowel disease. In children, biliary atresia is the most common cholestatic disorder. It is a destructive, inflammatory condition of the bile ducts, and if left untreated, it usually results in death within the first 1 to 2 years of life.

A variety of metabolic diseases can result in progressive, chronic liver injury and cirrhosis, including hereditary hemochromatosis (an autosomal recessive disorder characterized by chronic iron accumulation, which may result in cirrhosis, cardiomyopathy, and endocrine disorders including diabetes), alpha$_1$-antitrypsin deficiency (which may result in cirrhosis at any age, most commonly in the first or second decade of life), and Wilson's disease (an autosomal recessive disorder of copper excretion, which may present as either fulminant hepatic failure or chronic hepatitis and cirrhosis).

Hepatocellular carcinoma (HCC) may be a complication of cirrhosis from any cause, most commonly with hepatitis B, hepatitis C, hemochromatosis, and tyrosinemia. HCC patients may have stable liver disease, but are not candidates for hepatic resection because of the underlying cirrhosis; they are best treated with a liver transplant. The best transplant candidates are those with a single lesion less than 5 cm in size or with no more than three lesions, the largest no greater than 3 cm in size. Otherwise, recurrence rates posttransplant are exceedingly high. Exceptions include patients with a large fibrolamellar hepatoma, who generally do well posttransplant.

A host of other diseases may lead to chronic liver failure and are potentially amenable to treatment with a transplant, including Budd-Chiari syndrome (obstruction of the hepatic veins secondary to thrombus, which leads to hepatic congestion, ascites, and eventually liver damage) and polycystic liver disease (in which a large number of cysts, depending on their size, can lead to debilitating symptoms).

Acute liver disease, more commonly termed *fulminant hepatic failure* (FHF), is defined as the development of hepatic encephalopathy and profound coagulopathy shortly after the onset of symptoms, such as jaundice, in patients without pre-existing liver disease. The most common causes include acetaminophen overdose, acute hepatitis B infection, various drugs and hepatotoxins, and Wilson's disease; often, however, no cause is identified. Treatment consists of appropriate critical care support, giving patients time for spontaneous recovery. The prognosis for spontaneous recovery depends on the patient's age (those younger than 10 and older than 40 years have a poor prognosis), the underlying cause, and the severity of liver injury (as indicated by degree of hepatic encephalopathy, coagulopathy, and kidney dysfunction; Table 10-8). A subset of patients may have delayed onset of hepatic decompensation that occurs 8 weeks to 6 months after the onset of symptoms. This condition is often referred to as subacute hepatic failure; these patients rarely recover without a transplant.

Indications for Transplant

The presence of chronic liver disease alone with established cirrhosis is not an indication for a transplant. Some patients have well-compensated cirrhosis with a low expectant mortality. Patients with decompensated cirrhosis, however, have a poor prognosis without transplant. The signs and symptoms of decompensated cirrhosis include:

1. Hepatic encephalopathy (HE): In its early stages, HE may begin with subtle sleep disturbances, depression, and emotional lability. Increasing severity of HE is indicated by increasing somnolence, altered speech, and in extreme cases, coma. Physical examination shows the typical flapping tremor of asterixis. Blood tests often reveal an elevated serum ammonia level. HE may occur spontaneously, but is more commonly triggered by a precipitating factor such as spontaneous bacterial peritonitis (SBP), GI bleeding, use of sedatives, constipation, or excessive dietary protein intake.

2. Ascites: Ascites is generally associated with portal hypertension. The initial approach to the management of ascites is sodium restriction and diuretics. If this approach is not successful, patients may require repeated large-volume (4 to 6 L) paracentesis. A better option to diuretic-resistant ascites requiring frequent paracentesis is transjugular intrahepatic portosystemic shunting (TIPS). A potential complication of TIPS is progression of liver failure or disabling encephalopathy. Patients with signs of far-advanced liver disease such as hyperbilirubinemia, HE, and renal dysfunction generally are not good candidates for TIPS.

3. Spontaneous bacterial peritonitis (SBP): This complication of chronic liver failure generally signals advanced disease. It often tends to be recurrent. Anaerobic gram-negative bacteria account for 60% of the cultured organisms; gram-positive cocci account for the remainder. Diagnosis is confirmed if percutaneous sampling of the abdominal fluid shows a neutrophil count of greater than 250 cells/mL. Treatment with a third-generation cephalosporin is generally effective.

4. Portal hypertensive bleeding: The likelihood of patients with cirrhosis developing varices ranges from 35 to 80%. About one third of those with varices will experience bleeding. The risk of recurrent bleeding approaches 70% by 2 years after the index bleeding episode. Each episode of bleeding is associated with a 30% mortality rate. Thus, urgent treatment of the acute episode and steps to prevent rebleeding are essential. Endoscopy is indicated to diagnose and treat the acute bleed with either band ligation or sclerotherapy. Other therapies include vasoactive drugs such as octreotide or vasopressin, balloon tamponade, TIPS, and emergency surgical procedures (such as a portosystemic shunt or transection of the esophagus). Generally, patients whose endoscopic procedure fails should undergo emergency TIPS, if feasible, to control bleeding. Beta blockers have been shown to be of value in preventing the first bleeding episode in patients with varices and in preventing rebleeding.

5. Hepatorenal syndrome (HRS): In patients with advanced liver disease and ascites, HRS is characterized by oliguria (<500 mL of urine/day) in association with low urine sodium (<10 mEq/L). It is a functional disorder; the kidneys have no structural abnormalities, and the urine sediment is normal. The differential diagnosis includes acute tubular necrosis, drug nephrotoxicity, and chronic intrinsic renal disease. HRS may be precipitated by volume depletion from diuresis, SBP, or agents such as nonsteroidal anti-inflammatory drugs. Patients may require dialysis support, but the only effective treatment is a liver transplant.

6. Others: Other signs and symptoms of decompensated cirrhosis include severe weakness and fatigue, which may sometimes be the primary symptoms. Such weakness can be debilitating, leading to the inability to work or even to carry out daily functions. It may be associated with malnutrition and muscle wasting, which at times may be quite severe. Biochemical abnormalities, advanced liver disease, and loss of synthetic function are associated with a low serum albumin, a high serum bilirubin, and a rise in the serum International Normalized Ratio (INR).

Generally, FHF patients are more acutely ill than chronic liver failure patients, and thus require more intensive care pretransplant. FHF patients have more severe hepatic parenchymal dysfunction, as manifested by coagulopathy, hypoglycemia, and lactic acidosis. Infectious complications also are more common, as is the incidence of kidney failure and neurologic complications, especially cerebral edema.

Coagulopathy usually is secondary to the impaired hepatic synthesis of clotting factors. Necrosis, as a result of disseminated intravascular coagulation (DIC), may also be associated with FHF. Close attention should be given to the serum glucose level, which is more likely to be decreased in FHF patients. Intravenous glucose should be administered at a sufficient rate to maintain euglycemia.

The prevalence of bacterial infection in FHF patients is very high, a reflection of the loss of the immunologic functions of the liver. The respiratory and urinary systems are the most common sources. In addition, almost one third of FHF patients develop some form of fungal infection, usually secondary to *Candida* species. Sepsis is generally a contraindication to a liver transplant; if it is unrecognized pretransplant, the outcome posttransplant is poor.

Multiple organ dysfunction syndrome, characterized by respiratory distress, kidney failure, increased cardiac output, and decreased systemic vascular resistance, is a well-described complication of FHF. It may be due to impaired clearance of vasoactive substances by the liver. Mechanical ventilation and dialysis support may become necessary pretransplant. Hemodynamic abnormalities may manifest as hypotension and worsening tissue oxygenation.

Cerebral edema is substantially more common in FHF patients. As many as 80% of the patients who die secondary to FHF have evidence of cerebral edema. The pathogenesis is unclear, but it may be due to potential neurotoxins that are normally cleared by the liver. Establishing the diagnosis may be problematic; patients are often sedated and ventilated, making clinical examination difficult. Radiologic imaging is neither sensitive nor specific. Several centers have tried intracranial pressure (ICP) monitoring; therapy (e.g., mannitol, hyperventilation, and thiopental) can then be directed to achieve an adequate cerebral perfusion pressure (above 50 mm Hg). ICP monitoring also helps predict the likelihood of neurologic recovery posttransplant. Sustained cerebral perfusion pressures of less than 40 mm Hg have been associated with postoperative neurologic death. Disadvantages of ICP monitoring include the risks of performing it in patients with severe coagulopathy; it is also a possible source of infection and may precipitate an intracranial hemorrhage.

The indications for a liver transplant are numerous (and increasing), with the number of absolute contraindications few (and decreasing with time).[46] There are no specific age limits for recipients; their mean age is steadily increasing. Patients must have adequate cardiac and pulmonary function. Coronary artery disease is uncommon in liver transplant candidates, but those with cirrhosis may develop significant hypoxia and pulmonary hypertension. Those with severe hypoxemia or with right atrial pressures greater than 60 mm Hg rarely survive a liver transplant. Other contraindications, as with other types of transplants, include uncontrolled systemic infection and malignancy. HCC patients with metastatic disease, obvious vascular invasion, or significant tumor burden are not suitable transplant candidates. Patients with other types of extrahepatic malignancy should be deferred for at least 2 years after completing curative therapy before a transplant is attempted.

Currently, the most common contraindication to a liver transplant is ongoing substance abuse. Before considering patients for a transplant, most centers require a documented period of abstinence, demonstration of compliant behavior, and willingness to pursue a chemical dependency program.

Once the indications for a transplant and the absence of contraindications have been established, a careful search for underlying medical disorders of the cardiovascular, pulmonary, neurologic, genitourinary, and gastrointestinal systems must be made. Serologic evaluation to screen for the presence of underlying viral infections is important. Unique to patients with chronic liver disease, the pretransplant evaluation must assess for any evidence of hepatopulmonary syndrome, pulmonary hypertension, and hepatorenal syndrome.

Hepatopulmonary syndrome is characterized by impaired gas exchange, resulting from intrapulmonary arteriovenous shunts. These shunts may lead to severe hypoxemia, especially when patients are in the upright position (orthodeoxia). A transplant may be contraindicated if intrapulmonary shunting is severe, as manifested by hypoxemia that is only partially improved with high inspired oxygen concentrations.

Pulmonary hypertension is seen in a small proportion of patients with established cirrhosis. Its exact cause is unknown. Diagnosing pulmonary hypertension pretransplant is critical, because major surgical procedures in the presence of nonreversible pulmonary hypertension are associated with a very high risk of mortality.

The development of hepatorenal syndrome indicates rapid hepatic deterioration. It is a clear indication for a liver transplant. Patients with hepatorenal syndrome or with kidney failure from any cause have worse outcomes posttransplant, as compared to patients with no kidney dysfunction. Therefore, all attempts must be made to avoid or reverse any kidney dysfunction pretransplant. Once the cause of kidney dysfunction is established, appropriate therapy should be initiated, including optimization of volume status with invasive monitoring techniques, large-volume paracentesis, cessation of nephrotoxic drugs, nonpressor doses of dopamine, or judicious use of diuretics, as indicated. If such therapy is unsuccessful, dialysis support may be required until a liver transplant becomes available.

Surgical Procedure

The surgical procedure is divided into three phases: pre-anhepatic, anhepatic, and post-anhepatic. The pre-anhepatic phase involves mobilizing the recipient's diseased liver in preparation for its removal. The basic steps include isolating the supra- and infrahepatic vena cava, portal vein, and hepatic artery, and then dividing the bile duct. Given existing coagulopathy and portal hypertension, the recipient hepatectomy may be the most difficult aspect of the transplant procedure. The anesthesia team must be prepared to deal with excessive blood loss.

Once the above structures have been isolated, vascular clamps are applied. The recipient's liver is removed, thus beginning the anhepatic phase. This phase is characterized by decreased venous return to the heart because of occlusion of the inferior vena cava and portal vein. Some centers routinely employ a venovenous bypass (VVB) system during this time, in which blood is drawn from the lower body and bowels via a cannula in the common femoral vein and portal vein, and returned through a central venous cannula in the upper body. Potential advantages of bypass include improved hemodynamic stability, reduction of bleeding from an engorged portal system, and avoidance of elevated venous pressure in the renal

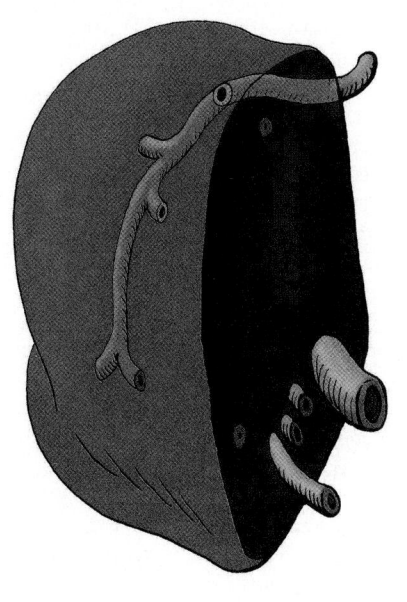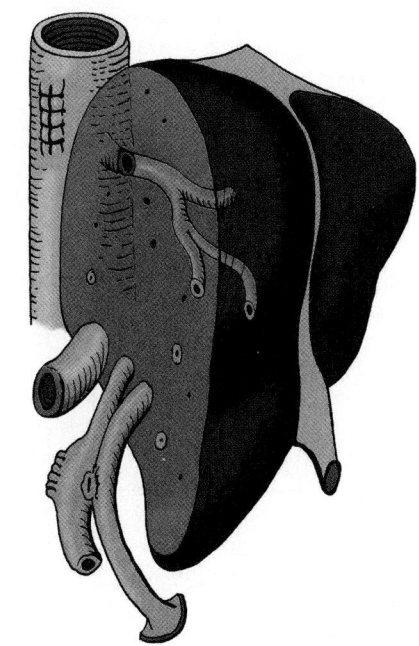

FIG. 10-10. Plane of transection used for adult-to-adult living-donor liver transplants or for a cadaver split-liver transplant for two adult recipients.

veins. However, many centers do not routinely use VVB. VVB does have potential complications such as air embolism, thromboembolism, hypothermia, and trauma to vessels. Some centers use VVB selectively, reserving it for patients who demonstrate hemodynamic instability with a trial of caval clamping. Few randomized trials have measured specific clinical outcomes with or without VVB.

With the recipient liver removed, the donor liver is anastomosed to the appropriate structures to place it in an orthotopic position. The suprahepatic caval anastomosis is performed first, followed by the infrahepatic cava and the portal vein. The portal and caval clamps may be removed at this time. The new liver is then allowed to reperfuse. Either before or after this step, the hepatic artery may be anastomosed.

With the clamps removed and the new liver reperfused, the postanhepatic phase begins, often characterized by marked changes in the recipient's status. The most dramatic changes in hemodynamic parameters usually occur on reperfusion, namely hypotension and the potential for serious cardiac arrhythmias. Severe coagulopathy may also develop because of the release of natural anticoagulants from the ischemic liver or because of active fibrinolysis. Both ε-aminocaproic acid and aprotinin have been used prophylactically to prevent fibrinolysis and decrease transfusion requirements. Electrolyte abnormalities, most commonly hyperkalemia and hypercalcemia, are often seen after reperfusion, but they usually are transient and respond well to treatment with calcium chloride and sodium bicarbonate. After reperfusion, the final anastomosis is performed, establishing biliary drainage. The recipient's remaining common bile duct (choledochoduodenostomy) or a loop of bowel (choledochojejunostomy) may be used.

Variations on the Standard Procedure

Several variations of the standard operation have been described. With the "piggyback technique," the recipient's inferior vena cava is preserved, the infrahepatic donor cava is oversewn, and the suprahepatic cava is anastomosed to the confluence of the recipient hepatic veins. With this technique, the recipient's vena cava does not have to be completely cross-clamped during anastomosis, thus

allowing blood from the lower body to return to the heart uninterrupted, without the need for VVB. The piggyback technique has many advantages, including improved hemodynamic stability, improved kidney perfusion, and avoidance of the complications possible with VVB. However, no randomized studies have demonstrated the superiority of one technique over the other.

Another important variation of the standard operation is a partial transplant, either a living-donor transplant or a deceased-donor split-liver transplant. Both have developed in response to the donor shortage and are gaining in popularity. Usually, in living-donor liver transplants for pediatric recipients, the left lateral segment or left lobe is used; for adult recipients, the right lobe is used. Split-liver transplants from deceased donors involve dividing the donor liver into two segments, each of which is subsequently transplanted (Fig. 10-10).

Living-Donor Liver Transplant

The greatest advantage of a living-donor liver transplant is that it avoids the often lengthy waiting period experienced with deceased-donor organ transplants. Over 15,000 people are now waiting for liver transplants in the United States, but only 4500 transplants are performed every year.[47] Roughly 25% of the candidates will die of their liver disease before having the chance to undergo a transplant. For those who do receive a transplant from a deceased donor, the waiting time can be significant, resulting in severe debilitation. With a living-donor liver transplant, this waiting time can be avoided, allowing the transplant to be performed before the recipient's health deteriorates further.

A partial hepatectomy in an otherwise healthy donor is a significant undertaking, so all potential donors must be carefully evaluated. Detailed medical screening must ensure that the donor is medically healthy, radiologic evaluation must ensure that the anatomy of the donor's liver is suitable, and a psychosocial evaluation must ensure that the donor is mentally fit and not being coerced in any way. The decision to donate should be made entirely by the potential donor after careful consideration of the risks and of the potential complications.

If the recipient is a child, the lateral segment of the donor's liver (about 25% of the total liver) is removed[48] (see Fig. 10-4A). If the recipient is an adult, a larger portion of the liver needs to be removed. Usually the right lobe of the liver, which comprises ~60% of the total liver, is used (see Fig. 10-4B). The operative procedure involves isolating the blood vessels supplying the portion of the liver to be removed, transecting the hepatic parenchyma, and then removing the portion to be transplanted.

The overall incidence of complications after living-donor liver donation ranges from 10 to 15%. There is also a small risk (<0.5%) of death.[49] Bile duct problems are the most worrisome complication after donor surgery. Bile may leak from the cut surface of the liver or from the site where the bile duct is divided. That site may later become strictured. Generally, bile leaks resolve spontaneously with simple drainage. Strictures and sometimes bile leaks may require endoscopic retrograde cholangiopancreatography (ERCP) and stenting. If the above measures fail, a reoperation may be required. Intra-abdominal infections developing in donors are usually related to a biliary problem. Other complications after donor surgery may include incisional problems such as infections and hernias. The risk of deep venous thrombosis (DVT) and pulmonary embolism (PE) is the same as for other major abdominal procedures.

The recipient operation with living-donor liver transplants is not greatly different from whole-organ deceased-donor liver transplants. The hepatectomy is performed in a similar fashion; the vena cava should be preserved in all such cases because the graft will generally only have a single hepatic vein for outflow. This is then anastomosed directly to the recipient's preserved vena cava. Outflow problems tend to be more common with partial vs. whole transplants, especially with right lobe transplants. Various methods have been described to improve the outflow of the graft, such as including the middle hepatic vein with the graft, reimplanting accessory hepatic veins, and reimplanting large tributaries that drain the right lobe into the middle hepatic vein.[50–53] Inflow to the graft can be re-established by anastomosing the donor organ hepatic artery and portal vein branch to the corresponding structures in the recipient.

Split-Liver Transplants

Another method to increase the number of liver transplants is to split the liver from a deceased donor into two grafts, which are then transplanted into two recipients.[54] Thus, a whole adult liver from such a donor can be divided into two functioning grafts. The vast majority of split-liver transplants have been between one adult and one pediatric recipient. Usually the liver is split into a smaller portion (the left lateral segment, which can be transplanted into a pediatric recipient) and a larger portion (the extended right lobe, which can be transplanted into a normal-sized adult recipient). The benefits for pediatric recipients have been tremendous, including an expansion of the donor pool and a significant decrease in waiting times and mortality rates.

Splitting the liver as described above has no negative impact on the adult waiting list; however, it does not improve it. Adults now account for the majority of patients awaiting a transplant, and therefore the majority of patients dying on the waiting list. Therefore, if split-liver transplants are to have a significant impact on waiting list time and mortality, they must be performed so the resulting two grafts can be used in two adult recipients.[55] The concern is that the smaller of the two pieces would not be of sufficient size to sustain life in a normal-sized adult. However, with appropriate donor and recipient selection criteria, a small percentage of livers from deceased donors could be split and transplanted into two adult recipients (see Fig. 10-10).

Postoperative Care

The immediate postoperative care for liver recipients involves: (1) stabilizing the major organ systems (e.g., cardiovascular, pulmonary, and renal); (2) evaluating graft function and achieving adequate immunosuppression; and (3) monitoring and treating complications directly and indirectly related to the transplant.[56,57] This initial care should generally be performed in an intensive care unit (ICU) setting because recipients usually require mechanical ventilatory support for the first 12 to 24 hours. The goal is to maintain adequate oxygen saturation, acid-base equilibrium, and stable hemodynamics. Continuous hemodynamic monitoring is important to ensure adequate perfusion of the graft and vital organs. Hemodynamic instability occurring early posttransplant is usually due to fluid imbalance, but the presence of ongoing bleeding must first be excluded. Instability also may be secondary to the myocardial dysfunction that is often seen early in the reperfusion phase, but which may persist into the early postoperative period. Such dysfunction is characterized by decreased compliance and contractility of the ventricles. The usual treatment is to optimize preload and afterload, and to use inotropic agents such as dopamine or dobutamine if necessary.

Fluid management, electrolyte status, and kidney function require frequent evaluation. Most liver recipients have an increased extravascular volume but a reduced intravascular volume. Attention should be given to the potassium, calcium, magnesium, phosphate, and glucose levels. Potassium may be elevated because of poor kidney function, a residual perfusion effect, or medications. Diuretics may be required to remove excess fluid acquired intraoperatively, but they may result in hypokalemia. Magnesium levels should be kept above 2 mEq/L to prevent seizures, and phosphate levels between 2 and 5 mEq/L for proper support of the respiratory and alimentary tracts. Marked hypoglycemia, which may be secondary to steroids, should be treated with insulin. Hypoglycemia is often an indication of poor hepatic function.

A crucial aspect of postoperative care is to repeatedly evaluate graft function. In fact, doing so begins intraoperatively, soon after the liver is reperfused. Signs of hepatic function include good texture and good color of the graft, evidence of bile production, and restoration of hemodynamic stability. Postoperatively, hepatic function can be assessed using clinical signs and laboratory values. Patients who rapidly awaken from anesthesia and whose mental status progressively improves likely have a well-functioning graft. Laboratory indicators of good graft function include normalization of the coagulation profile, resolution of hypoglycemia and hyperbilirubinemia, and clearance of serum lactate. Adequate urine production and good output of bile through the biliary tube (if present) are also indicators of good graft function. Serum transaminase levels will usually rise during the first 48 to 72 hours posttransplant secondary to preservation injury, and then should fall rapidly over the next 24 to 48 hours.

Another important aspect of postoperative care is to monitor for any surgical and medical complications. The incidence of complications tends to be high after liver transplants, especially in patients who were severely debilitated pretransplant. Surgical complications related directly to the operation include postoperative hemorrhage and anastomotic problems.

Postoperative bleeding is common. Usually multifactorial, it may be compounded by an underlying coagulopathy resulting from deficits in coagulation, fibrinolysis, and platelet function. Blood loss should be monitored via the abdominal drains; hemoglobin levels and CVP should be measured serially. If bleeding persists despite correction of coagulation deficiencies, an exploratory laparotomy should be performed.

The incidence of vascular complications after liver transplants ranges from 8 to 12%. Thrombosis is the most common early event, with stenosis and pseudoaneurysm formation occurring later. Hepatic artery thrombosis (HAT) has a reported incidence of about 3 to 5% in adults and about 5 to 10% in children. The incidence tends to be higher in partial liver transplant recipients. After HAT, liver recipients may be asymptomatic or may develop severe liver failure secondary to extensive necrosis. Doppler ultrasound evaluation is the initial investigative method of choice, with more than 90% sensitivity and specificity. If HAT is suggested by radiologic imaging, urgent re-exploration is indicated, with thrombectomy and revision of the anastomosis. If hepatic necrosis is extensive, a retransplant is indicated. However, HAT also may present in a less dramatic fashion. Thrombosis may render the common bile duct ischemic, resulting in a localized or diffuse bile leak from the anastomosis or in a more chronic, diffuse biliary stricture.

Thrombosis of the portal vein is less common. Signs include liver dysfunction, tense ascites, and variceal bleeding. Doppler evaluation should be used to establish the diagnosis. If thrombosis is diagnosed early, operative thrombectomy and revision of the anastomosis may be successful. If thrombosis occurs late, liver function is usually preserved due to the presence of collaterals; a retransplant is then unnecessary and attention is directed toward relieving the left-sided portal hypertension.

Biliary complications remain a significant problem after liver transplants, affecting 10 to 35% of all recipients. A higher incidence generally is seen after partial liver transplants, in which bile leaks may occur from the anastomoses or from the cut surface of the liver. Biliary complications manifest either as leaks or as obstructions. Leaks tend to occur early postoperatively and often require surgical repair; obstructions usually occur later and can be managed with radiologic or endoscopic techniques. Clinical symptoms of a bile leak include fever, abdominal pain, and peritoneal irritation. Ultrasound may demonstrate a fluid collection; however, cholangiography is required for diagnosis. Some leaks may be successfully managed by endoscopic placement of a biliary stent. If the leak does not respond to stent placement or if the liver recipient is systemically ill, a laparotomy is warranted. Biliary strictures occur later postoperatively and manifest as cholangitis or cholestasis, or both. Initial treatment involves balloon dilatation or stent placement across the stricture site, or both. If these initial options fail, surgical revision is required.

One devastating complication posttransplant is primary nonfunction of the hepatic allograft, with an attendant mortality rate of greater than 80% without a retransplant. By definition, primary nonfunction results from poor or no hepatic function from the time of the transplant procedure. The incidence in most centers is about 3 to 5%. Factors associated with primary nonfunction include advanced donor age, increased fat content of the donor liver, prolonged donor hospitalization prior to organ procurement, prolonged cold ischemia time, and partial liver donation. Intravenous prostaglandin E_1 may have some useful effects and can be administered to recipients with suspected primary nonfunction. Ultimately, however, they should be listed for an urgent retransplant.

Medical complications (both infectious and noninfectious) are common posttransplant, especially in patients who were debilitated pretransplant. Almost any organ system may be involved. The neurologic, respiratory, and renal systems are commonly affected. Neurologic complications generally manifest as a decreased level of consciousness, seizures, or focal neurologic deficits. The most common cause of a decreased level of consciousness is sedation from drugs that have accumulated in the bloodstream over a period of days. Another cause is a poorly functioning or nonfunctioning graft with resulting liver failure and hepatic encephalopathy. Central pontine myelinolysis, which may result from marked fluctuations in serum sodium levels and osmolality, is an uncommon cause of a patient not regaining consciousness posttransplant. Recipients who developed FHF, especially those with severe hepatic encephalopathy and evidence of cerebral edema preoperatively, invariably have a period of diminished consciousness posttransplant. Postoperative seizures usually occur de novo and tend to be of the generalized tonic-clonic variety. Causes can include electrolyte abnormalities, effects of drugs such as cyclosporine and tacrolimus, structural abnormalities such as intracranial hemorrhage and cerebral infarctions, and infectious processes such as encephalitis or brain abscesses.

The pulmonary system is one of the most common sites of complications posttransplant. Infectious and noninfectious pulmonary complications can occur in up to 75% of liver recipients. Noninfectious complications such as pulmonary edema, pleural effusion, atelectasis, and acute respiratory distress syndrome predominate during the first week, and generally manifest with respiratory distress and hypoxemia. The lungs are a very common site of posttransplant infections, which predominate after the first posttransplant week. Organisms may be bacterial, fungal, or viral, with different pathogens predominating at different times posttransplant. Early infections posttransplant are generally secondary to gram-negative organisms or fungi. Risk factors include mechanical ventilation, atelectasis, and aspiration.

Some degree of kidney dysfunction is very common posttransplant, affecting almost all liver recipients. About 10% develop kidney failure severe enough to require dialysis. Postoperative kidney problems that may have been present pretransplant are most commonly due to HRS or ATN. Usually, such problems will improve posttransplant, but recipients with severe pretransplant kidney dysfunction are at greater risk for persistent kidney impairment posttransplant, and some patients will require renal transplantation. Other causes of postoperative renal dysfunction include systemic hypovolemia, drug nephrotoxicity, or pre-existing kidney disease.

Infectious complications after liver transplant are common and can be devastating. Early infections (within the first month posttransplant) usually are related to surgical complications, initial graft function, or pre-existing comorbid conditions. Risk factors include prolonged surgery, large-volume blood transfusions, primary nonfunction requiring a retransplant, and reoperations for bleeding or bile leaks. The most common early infections are intra-abdominal and wound infections. Intra-abdominal infections should always lead the surgeon to consider the possibility of a bile leak. If an intra-abdominal infection is suspected, a CT scan should be performed, with aspiration and culture of any fluid collections that are identified. The biliary tree should be evaluated to exclude the presence of a bile leak. Patients with FHF are at high risk for fungal infections, usually secondary to *Candida* or *Aspergillus* species. Common sites include the abdomen, lungs, and central nervous system.

Late postoperative infections (generally occurring after the first month posttransplant) are usually a reflection of the recipient's overall immunosuppressed state. Immunosuppressive drugs depress cell-mediated immunity, leading to opportunistic infections with viral, fungal, and parasitic pathogens. The risk increases with the level and length of immunosuppression, especially when acute rejection episodes are treated with bolus high-dose steroids or antilymphocyte agents. Viral infections generally are not seen until after the first month posttransplant. CMV is the most common pathogen involved. Its presentation ranges from asymptomatic infection to tissue-invasive disease. Epstein-Barr virus (EBV), another member of the herpesvirus family, also may be seen posttransplant. A wide spectrum of clinical presentations is possible, including an asymptomatic rise in antibody titers, a mononucleosis syndrome, hepatitis, and posttransplant lymphoproliferative disorder (PTLD). The most severe form of infection, PTLD can present as a localized tumor of the lymph nodes or GI tract, or rarely as a rapidly progressive, diffuse, often fatal lymphomatous infiltration.

Other aspects of postoperative care, especially in the later posttransplant period, involve careful monitoring of the recipient for any evidence of graft rejection, complications related to immunosuppression, and recurrence of the original disease.[58] After the recipient is discharged from the hospital, use of routine blood tests, including liver function tests, is important in order to monitor for acute rejection. The incidence of acute rejection is now about 30%; most episodes are asymptomatic and occur relatively early posttransplant. Most commonly, the serum bilirubin or transaminase levels are elevated. A percutaneous liver biopsy is then performed to confirm the diagnosis. Treatment is with high-dose corticosteroids; however, if there is no significant response, antilymphocyte therapy should be initiated.

Immunosuppressive drugs are important to prevent rejection, but they are associated with a host of potential complications that recipients should be regularly evaluated for, including nephrotoxicity (especially prevalent with use of calcineurin inhibitors), cardiovascular and metabolic complications (such as hypertension, hyperlipidemia, diabetes, osteoporosis, and obesity), and malignancy (often related to long-term suppression of the immune system).

Disease recurrence is a significantly more important problem after liver transplants than with other solid organ transplants. Recurrence of hepatitis C is almost universal after transplants for this condition. Fortunately, only a minority of recipients experience aggressive recurrence leading to cirrhosis and liver failure. Ribavirin and α-interferon therapy should be considered in recipients with evidence of significant recurrence, as indicated by liver biopsy findings. Recurrence of hepatitis B has been significantly decreased by the routine use of hepatitis B immune globulin and the antiviral agent lamivudine posttransplant, but recurrence may still be seen with resistant viral strains. Other diseases that may recur posttransplant are primary sclerosing cholangitis, primary hepatic malignancy, and autoimmune hepatitis.

Pediatric Liver Transplants

Liver transplants have become a well-established procedure to treat liver failure in pediatric patients. As a result of refinements in surgical technique, the advent of new immunosuppressive agents, and improvements in critical care, patient survival at 1 year has improved from 20% in the 1970s to 90% currently. In several ways, liver transplants for pediatric patients are quite similar to those for adults; however, several features make pediatric patients unique.

The clinical indications for a pediatric liver transplant are similar to those already mentioned for adults. Endpoints that require a transplant include evidence of portal hypertension as manifested by variceal bleeding and ascites, significant jaundice, intractable pruritus, encephalopathy, failing synthetic function (e.g., hypoalbuminemia or coagulopathy), poor quality of life, and failure to thrive (as manifested by poor weight gain or poor height increase).

Biliary atresia is the most common indication for a pediatric liver transplant. The incidence of biliary atresia is about 1 in 10,000 infant births. Once the diagnosis is established, a portoenterostomy, or Kasai procedure, is indicated to drain microscopic ducts within the porta hepatis. Successful bile flow can be achieved in 40 to 60% of patients whose Kasai procedure takes place early in their life. However, even with a Kasai procedure, 75% of children with biliary atresia eventually require a liver transplant because of progressive cholestasis followed by cirrhosis. Other cholestatic disorders that may eventually require a transplant include sclerosing cholangitis, familial cholestasis syndromes, and paucity of intrahepatic bile ducts (as seen with Alagille syndrome).

Metabolic disorders probably account for the next largest group of disorders that may require a liver transplant. Such disorders may directly result in liver failure or may have mainly extrahepatic manifestations. Alpha$_1$-antitrypsin deficiency is the most common metabolic disorder that may require a liver transplant. Such patients may present with jaundice in the neonatal period, but this usually resolves. Subsequently, they may present in late childhood or early adolescence with cirrhosis and portal hypertension. Another metabolic disorder resulting in liver failure is tyrosinemia, a hereditary disorder characterized by deficiency of an enzyme that degrades the metabolic products of tyrosine, resulting in cirrhosis and a greatly increased risk for hepatocellular carcinoma. Still another is Wilson's disease, an autosomal recessive disorder characterized by copper accumulation in the liver, central nervous system, kidneys, eyes, and other organs, that may present as fulminant, subfulminant, or chronic liver failure. Metabolic disorders that do not affect liver function, but are treatable by a liver transplant, include urea cycle defects, most commonly ornithine transcarbamoylase deficiency (which may result in profound neurologic damage if not corrected early). Primary oxalosis, which results in kidney failure due to hyperoxaluria, can be treated by a kidney transplant to correct the kidney failure and by a liver transplant to correct the enzymatic defect so renal failure does not recur.

FHF may be seen in children from similar causes as seen in adults. Of note, younger children (<10 years old) with FHF have a poor prognosis for spontaneous recovery of liver function without a transplant. Other conditions that may require a transplant include chronic hepatitis (usually due to autoimmune or viral causes), and malignancy (most commonly a hepatoblastoma).

The surgical procedure for children does not differ significantly from that used in adults. The recipient's size is a more important variable in pediatric transplants, and it has an impact on both the donor and the recipient operations. For pediatric patients (especially infants and small children), the chance of finding a size-matched graft from a deceased donor may be very small, as the vast majority of such donors are adults. With adult grafts for pediatric patients, options include reduced-size liver transplants, in which a portion of the liver, such as the right lobe or extended right lobe, is resected and discarded; split-liver transplants in which a whole liver is divided into two functional grafts; and living-donor liver transplants in which a portion, usually the left lateral segment, is resected from a living donor. Graft implantation may be more demanding in pediatric patients, given the small caliber and delicate nature of the vessels. Use of venovenous bypass is usually not technically possible because of the small size of the vessels. For that reason, and given the increasing use of partial transplants, vena cava–sparing procedures are generally performed in children.

Surgical complications, especially those related to the vascular anastomoses, tend to be more frequent in pediatric recipients. HAT is three to four times more common in children. Factors associated with this increased risk include small recipient weight (less than 10 kg), use of just the left lateral segment (rather than the whole liver), and complex arterial reconstructions.

Patient survival rates have improved dramatically for pediatric liver recipients since the early 1990s. Most centers now report patient survival of close to 90% at 1 year posttransplant. Even for small recipients, patient survival rates at 1 year are 80 to 85%. Also, pediatric recipients enjoy close to normal growth and development posttransplant. Usually, growth accelerates immediately posttransplant.

Results

Patient and graft survival rates after liver transplants have improved significantly since the mid-1990s, with most centers now reporting graft survival rates of 85 to 90% at 1 year. The main factors affecting short-term (within the first year posttransplant) patient and graft survival are the medical condition of the patient at the time of transplant and the development of early postoperative surgical complications. Severely debilitated patients with numerous comorbid conditions such as kidney dysfunction, coagulopathy, and malnutrition, have a significantly higher risk of early posttransplant mortality. Such patients are more likely to develop surgical and medical complications (especially infections) and are unable to tolerate them. The national U.S. data show that for 2001, patient survival at 1 year was 86.4%, while graft survival was 80.2%.

Long-term survival rates (after the first year posttransplant) depend more on the cause of the underlying liver disease and on the presence or absence in the recipient of risk factors for other medical problems (especially cardiovascular disease). Generally, from 1 to 10 years posttransplant, survival curves slowly decline. Roughly half of the deaths in this time period are due to events not related to the underlying liver disease (e.g., myocardial infarctions, cerebrovascular accidents, and trauma). The other half of the deaths, however, are related to complications either of the underlying liver disease (e.g., recurrence) or of immunosuppression (e.g., infection or malignancy).

The original cause of liver failure has an impact on long-term survival rates as well. Primary biliary cirrhosis in adults and biliary atresia in children generally are associated with a better long-term outcome, because recurrence of these diseases in the transplanted liver is rare. However, recipients with HCC or hepatitis C usually have poorer long-term outcomes, because these diseases often recur posttransplant.

INTESTINAL TRANSPLANTATION

Intestinal transplants have been performed in the laboratory for years. The first human intestinal transplant was performed in 1966, but it remained essentially an experimental procedure, producing dismal results well into the 1980s. Newer immunosuppressive drugs have played a significant role in the success with the procedure since the mid-1990s. However, intestinal transplants remain the least frequently performed of all transplants, with the highest rejection rates and the lowest graft survival rates.

There are several reasons why the number of intestinal transplants has not increased dramatically. As with kidney failure

patients, a medical alternative exists for patients with intestinal failure, namely, long-term total parenteral nutrition (TPN). Unlike kidney failure patients, however, patients with intestinal failure have no survival advantage with a transplant vs. medical therapy. Immunologically, the small intestine is the most difficult organ to transplant. It is populated with highly immunocompetent cells, perhaps explaining the reason for the high rejection rates and the need for higher levels of immunosuppression. Moreover, monitoring for rejection in intestinal transplant recipients is difficult, as there is no good blood or urine laboratory test to indicate it. Lastly, the intestinal lumen is filled with potential infective pathogens that can gain access to the recipient's circulation if there is any breakdown of the mucosal barrier (which can occur during an acute rejection episode).

Preoperative Evaluation

Currently an intestinal transplant is indicated for irreversible intestinal failure that is not successfully managed by TPN (because of malnutrition and failure to thrive) or that has life-threatening complications (e.g., hepatic dysfunction, repeated episodes of sepsis secondary to central access, loss of central venous access sites).[59] Currently, patients who are stable while receiving TPN without such complications generally are not considered to be suitable transplant candidates because their estimated annual survival rate is higher with TPN.

The causes of intestinal failure are different in adult than in pediatric patients. Most commonly, though, the underlying disease results in extensive resection of the small bowel with resultant short bowel syndrome.[60] The development of short bowel syndrome depends not only on the length of bowel resected, but also on the location of the resection, on the presence or absence of the ileocecal valve, and on the presence or absence of the colon. As a rough guideline, most patients can tolerate resection of 50% of their intestine with subsequent adaptation, avoiding the need for long-term parenteral nutritional support. Loss of greater than 75% of the intestine, however, usually necessitates some type of parenteral nutritional support. The most common causes of intestinal failure in children are necrotizing enterocolitis, gastroschisis, and volvulus. In adults, Crohn's disease, massive resection of ischemic bowel due to mesenteric vascular thrombosis, and trauma are the most common causes.

The pretransplant evaluation does not differ greatly from that for other transplants. Absolute contraindications such as malignancy and active infection must be ruled out, and hepatic function should be evaluated carefully. If there is evidence of significant liver dysfunction and cirrhosis, a combined liver and intestinal transplant is indicated. The serologic status of the potential recipient should also be evaluated carefully—especially regarding CMV status. Transplant candidates who are CMV-seronegative should not receive an organ from a donor who is seropositive, because of a very high incidence of highly morbid and occasionally lethal invasive CMV disease posttransplant in such recipients.

Surgical Procedure

The operative procedure varies, depending on whether or not a liver transplant is also performed.[61,62] In the case of an isolated intestinal transplant, the graft may be from a living or deceased donor. With a living donor, about 200 cm of the distal small bowel is used; inflow to the graft is via the ileocolic artery, and outflow via the ileocolic vein. With a deceased donor, the graft is based on the superior mesenteric artery for inflow and on the superior mesenteric vein for outflow. For a combined liver and intestinal transplant, the

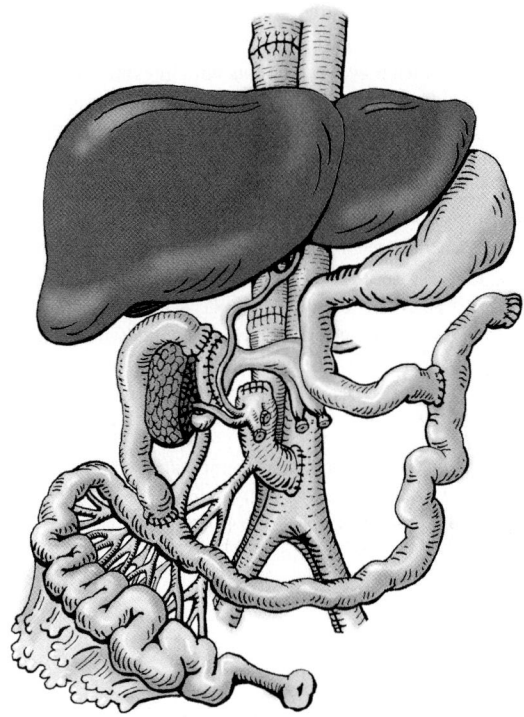

FIG. 10-11. Combined liver, pancreas, and intestine transplant.

graft is usually procured intact with an aortic conduit that contains both the celiac and superior mesenteric arteries. The common bile duct can be maintained intact in the hepatoduodenal ligament along with the first part of the duodenum and a small rim of the head of the pancreas (Fig. 10-11). Doing so avoids a biliary reconstruction in the recipient.

The recipient operation varies, depending on the graft being implanted. Generally, arterial inflow to the graft is achieved using the recipient's infrarenal aorta to perform an end-to-side anastomosis. Venous drainage of the graft can be performed to the systemic or portal circulation. Systemic drainage will lead to certain metabolic abnormalities, but there is no firm evidence to suggest that such abnormalities are of any obvious detriment to the recipient. GI continuity can be achieved by a number of different methods. A stoma is useful for ready endoscopic access to the transplanted bowel to perform a biopsy, which is the only reliable method to monitor for and diagnose acute rejection.

Postoperative Care

The early posttransplant care for intestinal transplant patients is in many ways similar to that of other transplant recipients. Initial care should take place in an ICU so that fluid, electrolytes, and blood product replacement can be carefully monitored. Broad-spectrum antibiotics are routinely administered, given the high risk for infectious complications.

A number of different immunosuppressive protocols have been described. Many involve some form of induction therapy, followed by tacrolimus-based maintenance immunosuppression. Regardless of the protocol, intestinal transplants clearly have a high risk of rejection. Therefore, careful monitoring for rejection is imperative and involves endoscopy with biopsy of the graft mucosa. Acute rejection episodes are often associated with infections. Rejection results in damage to the intestinal mucosa, leading to impaired barrier

function and bacterial translocation. Therefore, advanced rejection can be very difficult to treat as concurrent infection invariably is present.

Short-term results after intestinal transplantation have improved dramatically, mainly due to improvements in surgical technique and in immunosuppression.[63,64] Nonetheless, intestinal transplants are still associated with a high complication rate. Potential complications include enteric leaks with generalized peritonitis or localized intra-abdominal abscesses, graft thrombosis, respiratory infections, and life-threatening hemorrhage. Long-term results also have improved, but remain inferior to all other types of abdominal transplants.

HEART AND LUNG TRANSPLANTATION

Heart transplantation is a well-established therapy for end-stage heart failure, and is performed in age groups from neonates to senior citizens.[65] About 3500 heart transplants are performed each year, with roughly 10% taking place in pediatric recipients. The major limitation, as with almost all other types of transplants, is the inability to meet the demand with sufficient numbers of suitable donor organs.

Lung transplantation is a newer field than heart transplantation, and far fewer lung transplants (about 1000) are performed each year. Results have improved since the early 1990s, mainly due to improvements in immunosuppression and refinements in surgical techniques, in particular with modification of the airway anastomosis.[66] A combined heart-lung transplant is usually reserved for patients who have pulmonary hypertension and obvious right-sided heart failure.[67]

Preoperative Evaluation

A heart transplant is generally indicated in the presence of end-stage heart failure. The most common cause is ischemic or dilated cardiomyopathy, followed by intractable angina, valvular disease, congenital heart disease, life-threatening recurrent ventricular arrhythmias, and isolated intracardiac tumors.

Contraindications to a heart transplant are similar to those for other types of transplants, including active malignancy or infection, numerous or advanced comorbid conditions, and obvious noncompliance with medical care recommendations. Specific to heart transplantation is the need to exclude the presence of severe, nonreversible pulmonary hypertension, which could cause acute right-sided heart failure posttransplant.

Isolated lung transplants are performed for a number of indications, including chronic obstructive pulmonary disease, idiopathic pulmonary fibrosis, cystic fibrosis, and pulmonary hypertension (without right-sided heart failure).[68–70] Patients with chronic obstructive pulmonary disease or idiopathic pulmonary fibrosis generally are treated with a single-lung transplant; those with cystic fibrosis or pulmonary hypertension (without right-sided heart failure) usually require a bilateral single-lung transplant. Patients with pulmonary hypertension with significant right-sided heart failure, or those with Eisenmenger's syndrome, usually require a combined heart-lung transplant.

Surgical Procedure

Donor Selection

As with other organ transplants, donor selection criteria are important to ensure posttransplant success. The vast majority of lung transplants are performed with organs from deceased donors. A small number of lung transplants have used living-donor organs; in such cases, two living donors each contribute a lobe of a lung, and both lobes are then implanted into the appropriate hemithorax of a single recipient.

Numerous tests can be done to try to assess the suitability of hearts and lungs from deceased donors. Ultimately, however, physical examination at the time of procurement is likely the best method. The blood group, height, and weight of the donor must be compatible with the potential recipient. A heart donor should have a normal echocardiogram and must not currently require high doses of inotropes to maintain blood pressure. The presence of significant coronary artery disease can be excluded using coronary angiography if necessary.

Lung donor criteria are usually more restrictive than heart donor criteria, but have been liberalized over the past several years. The best tests of lung donor suitability are arterial blood gas analysis, chest roentgenogram, bronchoscopy, and physical examination of the lungs at the time of procurement. Bronchoscopy is especially important, and any findings of significant secretions or evidence of bacterial or fungal infection in the donor should preclude the recovery of the lungs.

Recipient Operation

A heart transplant is an orthotopic procedure. Therefore the first step of the procedure for heart or heart-lung recipients is removal of their corresponding thoracic organs. The recipient's aorta and vena cava are cannulated, an aortic cross-clamp is applied, and the diseased heart is excised along the atrioventricular groove. The recipient is maintained on cardiopulmonary bypass during this time. The new heart is then placed in an orthotopic position, with anastomoses performed in the following order: left atrium, right atrium, pulmonary artery, and aorta. Several variations to the original technique have been described, such as performing the aortic anastomosis before the pulmonary artery anastomosis to allow reperfusion of the heart and to minimize the ischemic time. Another variation is to perform selective anastomoses of the inferior and superior vena cava (rather than just of the right atrium); doing so is believed to allow for better geometry of the right atrium and to decrease the incidence of posttransplant atrial arrhythmias.

In heart-lung transplants, the new organs are implanted en bloc. Right and left pneumonectomies are carried out, with isolation and division of the trachea just above the carina. Anastomoses are then performed between the donor and recipient trachea, right atrium, and aorta.

Single-lung transplants are performed through a standard posterolateral thoracotomy. The superior and inferior pulmonary veins, pulmonary artery, and main stem bronchus are dissected. The pulmonary artery is then clamped to assess the recipient's hemodynamic status; cardiopulmonary bypass is used if necessary, although most recipients do not require bypass support. The bronchus and appropriate vascular structures are then clamped and the pneumonectomy completed. The bronchial anastomosis is performed first, followed by the pulmonary arterial and left atrial anastomoses. A telescoped bronchial anastomosis reduces the incidence of complications, most notably leaks. A pedicle of vascularized omentum can also be wrapped around the anastomosis for further reinforcement. Bilateral single-lung transplants are performed in a similar fashion, each side sequentially.

Postoperative Care

The immediate postoperative care does not differ significantly from any other major cardiac or pulmonary procedure. However, heart or lung recipients are at greater risk for infections than their nontransplant counterparts, and require appropriate precautions and prophylaxis regimens. As with other transplant recipients, maintenance immunosuppressive therapy is started immediately posttransplant.

After heart or heart-lung transplants, cardiac output is sustained by establishing a heart rate of 90 to 110 beats per minute, using either temporary epicardial atrial pacing or low-dose isoproterenol. For recipients who may suffer transient right-sided heart failure, adequate preload is important. Use of an oximetric Swan-Ganz catheter can be helpful to monitor pulmonary artery pressure and measure cardiac output. Urine output and arterial blood gases must be carefully monitored. Hypotension and a low cardiac output usually respond to an infusion of volume and to minor adjustments in inotropic support.

Cardiac tamponade can occur in heart recipients. It should be suspected in those who become hypotensive with concurrent increases in central venous pressure and whose mediastinal chest tube output decreases suddenly. Serious ventricular failure posttransplant is unusual and can be related to poor donor organ selection, poor graft preservation, long ischemic time, or rarely, hyperacute rejection. Inotropes and pulmonary vasodilators can be used to manage ventricular failure; if it seems likely that the graft will recover, an intra-aortic balloon pump or a ventricular assist device can be added. In the case of a very severe rejection episode, the only option is to list the recipient for a retransplant.

Lung or heart recipients are initially cared for in the ICU.[71] Attempts should be made to wean them early from the ventilator. Acute failure of a transplanted lung may be seen early posttransplant. Reasons include the inherent difficulty of lung preservation, unrecognized injury or trauma to the donor lung, and reperfusion edema. Lung graft failure can manifest as hypoxemia, infiltrates on radiographic examination, or copious secretions in the presence of reperfusion edema. Care of such recipients involves active diuresis and high levels of positive end-expiratory pressure (PEEP) to maintain small airway patency. They should be kept intubated as necessary and extubated as the acute injury resolves. The diagnosis of a failing lung graft should be made using transbronchial biopsy (to exclude the presence of rejection) and bronchoalveolar lavage (to exclude the presence of early infection). Extracorporeal membrane oxygenation (ECMO) can be used as a last resort to maintain function while a diagnosis is being established and appropriate therapy initiated.

Complications can be surgical or medical, and may occur early or late posttransplant. Many of the complications, especially those occurring late, are medical in nature and are similar to those seen after other types of transplants. Generally, they are related to the medications and to the immunosuppressed state. Examples include hypertension, hyperglycemia, osteoporosis, and malignancy. Certain complications, such as airway problems, are unique to lung and heart recipients. Rejection, both acute and chronic, can occur, but manifests in very different ways as compared with abdominal organ transplants.

Early attempts at lung transplantation were severely hampered by a high incidence of airway complications. This anastomosis is at high risk for problems because of the poor blood supply. However, increased experience and refinements in surgical technique have dramatically reduced airway complications. Nonetheless, about

10 to 15% of lung recipients develop some airway complication, often resulting in significant morbidity and occasional mortality. Airway complications can occur after heart-lung or lung transplants, but are much less common after heart-lung transplants because a good blood supply is maintained to the tracheal anastomosis. After solitary and double-lung transplants, the bronchial anastomosis is at much greater risk for partial dehiscence, airway stenosis, or both. Hypotension, poor lung preservation, rejection, and infection can compromise blood flow to the anastomoses. The result can be ischemic necrosis and poor healing of the airway, leading to partial or total dehiscence or chronic narrowing of the bronchus.

Postoperative surveillance of the bronchial anastomosis is important. In the operating room, bronchoscopy is performed to establish the baseline appearance of the anastomosis. Frequent routine bronchoscopy is useful to survey the anastomosis for early signs of dehiscence, as well as to monitor for rejection and infection. Dehiscence usually occurs within 3 to 6 weeks posttransplant. Early signs on bronchoscopy include abnormal appearance of the mucosa at the suture line, loosened sutures or knots within the airway, and herniation of tissue into the airway in case of an omental wrap. If the recipient is clinically stable and the area of dehiscence is small, conservative treatment with antibiotics and serial evaluation via bronchoscopy is appropriate. Development of a bronchopleural or bronchovascular fistula requires reoperation.

Chronic airway stenosis may develop after initial healing. It may be managed in a variety of ways, including repeated dilations of the airway with a rigid bronchoscope, use of a metallic stent, or laser photocoagulation to débride granulation tissue.

Lung or heart organ transplant recipients are susceptible to bacterial, fungal, and viral infections. Infections are particularly problematic in lung recipients, with as many as 15 to 20% likely to develop some type of significant infectious disease. Fungal infections due to *Candida* and *Aspergillus* are generally more serious than bacterial infections.[72] Most *Aspergillus* infections, which are caused by the inhalation of aerosolized fungal spores, generally occur within the first 3 months posttransplant. Among lung transplant recipients who have underlying cystic fibrosis, infections due to *Pseudomonas aeruginosa* are common. The most morbid viral infection is caused by CMV.

Rejection can be acute or chronic. Acute rejection tends to be characterized by the presence of an inflammatory infiltrate (mostly lymphocytes) in the organ parenchyma, and is usually seen early posttransplant. Chronic rejection tends to be a later phenomenon; it is characterized by obliteration of small vessels and fibrosis.[73,74] For both lung or heart recipients, rejection usually does not have clinical symptoms until the rejection episode is advanced. Therefore, routine monitoring with transbronchial biopsy (for lung recipients) and with endomyocardial biopsy (for heart recipients) is important for early diagnosis. For heart-lung recipients, rejection of the lungs may occur without rejection of the heart, so biopsy of both organs may be necessary.

Fortunately, most acute rejection episodes can be effectively reversed. Much more difficult to treat is the process of chronic rejection, which has been a major obstacle to long-term survival. In heart recipients, chronic rejection manifests as graft arteriosclerosis, which is seen in 30 to 40% of recipients by 3 years posttransplant, and in 40 to 60% of recipients by 5 years. In lung transplant recipients, chronic rejection manifests as bronchiolitis obliterans, characterized clinically by a decreased forced expiratory volume in 1 second (FEV_1) and histologically by inflammation and fibrosis of small airways.

INFECTION AND MALIGNANCY

Immunosuppressive therapy has played an essential role in the success of clinical transplants. However, it is a double-edged sword, because suppression of the immune system prevents or decreases the risk of rejection while concomitantly predisposing the transplant recipient to a wide variety of complications, including infections and malignancies.[75] Infections in transplant recipients may be caused by so-called opportunistic microbes, organisms that would not be harmful to a normal, nonimmunosuppressed host, as well as more common pathogens.

Infections

Transplant recipients exhibit an increased risk for infectious complications posttransplant, which can lead to significant morbidity and mortality. Numerous risk factors include long-standing end-stage organ failure (which can lead to an immunosuppressed state even before any immunosuppressive drugs are begun), impaired tissue healing, and poor vascular flow due to coexisting illnesses such as diabetes. The transplant surgery itself, which may involve opening nonsterile viscera such as the bladder or bowel, and the posttransplant need for powerful immunosuppressive agents further increase the risk for infections.

The spectrum of possible infections in transplant recipients is wide. Infections may occur early or late posttransplant. They may be related directly to the surgical procedure, to some complication that develops afterward, or to the recipient's overall immunosuppressed state (i.e., opportunistic). Infections are classified by the type of pathogen involved into bacterial, viral, or fungal infections. However, more than one type of pathogen may be involved in several different types of infections (e.g., pneumonia may be caused by a viral, bacterial, or fungal pathogen). Moreover, a number of different pathogens may be involved in a single infection (e.g., an intra-abdominal abscess can be due to several different bacterial and fungal pathogens).

Infections can also be classified by the primary method of treatment into surgical or medical infections. Surgical infections require some surgical intervention as an integral part of their treatment. They generally occur soon after the transplant operation and are usually related directly to it, or to some complication occurring as a result of it. Surgical infections are less likely to be related to the recipient's overall immunosuppressed state, though obviously this plays some role. Typical examples of surgical infections include generalized peritonitis, intra-abdominal abscesses, and wound infections. In contrast, medical infections do not generally require an invasive intervention for treatment, but rather are primarily treated with antiviral, antibacterial, or antifungal agents. They tend to occur later posttransplant and are usually related to the recipient's overall immunosuppressive state. Typical examples of medical infections include those secondary to CMV, polyomavirus-induced nephropathy, pneumonias, and EBV-related problems.

Risk factors for posttransplant infections are classified into those present in the recipient pretransplant, those related to the donor, those related to the recipient intraoperatively, and those that occur posttransplant. Pretransplant latent infections can reactivate or worsen early posttransplant, once high-dose immunosuppression is initiated. Pretransplant immunity, or lack of immunity, to certain viral pathogens can be an especially important risk factor for post-transplant infections. For example, recipients seronegative for CMV or EBV have a high incidence of posttransplant infections with these viruses, especially if their donor was seropositive. The recipient's overall medical status may be a factor in posttransplant infections. Poor nutritional status, advanced peripheral vascular disease, frequent hospitalizations pretransplant, and recipient obesity are all well-described risk factors for posttransplant infectious complications, especially involving the wound. Donor factors may also play an important role. Although transmission of bacterial infections from the donor are uncommon, viruses such as CMV, EBV, hepatitis B or C, and human immunodeficiency virus (HIV) can certainly be transmitted to any recipient who has not had previous exposure to them.

Intraoperative risk factors for infections include a longer operative procedure with significant bleeding, prolonged cold and warm ischemia of the graft, and certain types of transplants (e.g., pancreas and intestinal transplants are associated with a significantly higher risk of infections vs. kidney transplants). Posttransplant risk factors for infection are generally related either to the development of posttransplant complications or to the level of immunosuppression. Leaks from anastomoses with spillage of contaminated fluid (e.g., bile, urine, and enteric contents) will lead to a localized and possibly generalized infection. The level of immunosuppression is an important risk factor posttransplant, especially for opportunistic infections. The higher the level of immunosuppression, the greater the risk. Long induction protocols involving powerful antilymphocyte agents or bolus antirejection treatment, particularly several treatments in sequence, have been clearly identified as risk factors for a variety of infections.

The most common surgical infections, especially in liver and pancreas transplant recipients, are intra-abdominal infections. They are also the most likely to be life-threatening. They may range from diffuse peritonitis to localized abscesses. Their presentation, management, and clinical course will in part depend on their underlying cause, their location, and on the recipient's overall medical condition.

The incidence of intra-abdominal infections in transplant recipients has steadily decreased over time. Nonetheless, intra-abdominal infections continue to be a major problem. Among pancreas recipients, they are the second most common technical reason for graft loss (after vascular thrombosis). Leaks from anastomoses with spillage of contaminated fluid are probably the most significant risk factor for intra-abdominal infections. Other risk factors include increased donor age (especially in pancreas transplants), recipient obesity, donor obesity, and prolonged pretransplant dialysis, especially peritoneal dialysis.

The clinical presentation of intra-abdominal infections will depend on their severity and location. Generalized peritonitis is usually associated with some catastrophic event such as biliary disruption or graft duodenal leak with spillage of enteric contents or urine into the peritoneal cavity. It may also occur as a result of perforation of some other viscus, unrelated to the transplant (e.g., perforated gastric ulcer or perforated cecum). Generalized peritonitis is diagnosed clinically; the physical examination is the most helpful tool. Such patients appear ill, with tachycardia, elevated temperature, falling blood pressure, and diffuse tenderness with guarding on palpation of the abdomen, although immunosuppression may mask many of the usual signs and symptoms. A plain film or CT scan of the abdomen is not usually necessary, but may demonstrate free air. Treatment involves prompt return of the recipient to the operating room to determine the reason for the peritonitis; the next step will often depend on the degree of contamination.

Fortunately, most intra-abdominal infections do not fall into the generalized peritonitis category. Instead, most of them consist of localized fluid collections in and around the graft. Patients usually develop symptoms such as fever, nausea, vomiting, and abdominal distention, with localized pain and guarding over the region of the fluid collection. A CT scan with contrast is the best diagnostic tool in this clinical situation. In pancreas recipients, about one half of these localized abscesses are monomicrobial; common isolates include enterococcus, *Escherichia coli, Klebsiella,* and *Pseudomonas* species. The other one half of such abscesses tend to be polymicrobial, containing two or more bacteria or both bacterial and fungal species. The most common fungal species isolated is *Candida albicans,* but recently *Candida krusei* and *Candida glabrata* have been increasing in incidence. Treatment of localized intra-abdominal infections involves adequate drainage and administration of appropriate antibacterial or antifungal agents. These infections often can be drained percutaneously under radiologic guidance, at least as an initial approach. However, if the infected fluid is not adequately drained or if the recipient does not improve clinically, a laparotomy should be performed to achieve adequate drainage of all infected fluid.

Medical infections posttransplant tend to be more varied compared to surgical infections, and can involve bacterial, viral, or fungal pathogens. Bacterial infections primarily occur in the first few weeks posttransplant. The major sites are the incisional wound, respiratory tract, urinary tract, and bloodstream. Administration of perioperative systemic antibiotics decreases the risk and incidence of some infections. Viral infections in transplant recipients often involve the herpesvirus group; CMV is clinically the most important.[76–78] CMV establishes latent infection in its host and persists throughout life, and infection has been correlated with the overall degree of immunosuppression. CMV infection usually occurs 4 to 12 weeks posttransplant or after treatment of rejection. A wide spectrum of disease manifestations may be seen during CMV infection. The infection may be subclinical, or it may present with a mild flu-like syndrome. Leukopenia, myalgia, and malaise are usual. CMV may also present as tissue-invasive disease, resulting in interstitial pneumonitis, hepatitis, or gastrointestinal ulcerations. CMV-seronegative recipients of organs from CMV-seropositive donors are at highest risk. The incidence of CMV disease is reduced by use of prophylactic ganciclovir for 12 weeks posttransplant. Symptomatic disease is generally treated with IV ganciclovir or valganciclovir, and if severe or life-threatening, by a reduction in immunosuppression.

Fungal infections are most commonly caused by *Candida* species; *Aspergillus, Cryptococcus, Blastomyces, Mucor, Rhizopus,* and other species account for a much smaller percentage of fungal infections, but are more serious.[79] Among patients who develop invasive *Candida* or *Aspergillus* infections, the mortality rate usually exceeds 20%. The standard treatment of serious posttransplant fungal infections has been with amphotericin B, along with overall reduction in immunosuppression. However, newer antifungal agents that are less toxic are showing promise.

Malignancy

Transplant recipients are at increased risk for developing certain types of de novo malignancies, including nonmelanomatous skin cancers (three- to sevenfold increased risk), lymphoproliferative disease (two- to threefold increased risk), gynecologic and urologic cancers, and Kaposi's sarcoma. The risk ranges from 1% among renal allograft recipients to approximately 5 to 6% among recipients of small bowel and multivisceral transplants.[80]

Skin Cancers

The most common malignancies in transplant recipients are skin cancers.[81] They tend to be located on sun-exposed areas and are usually squamous or basal cell carcinomas. Often they are multiple and have an increased predilection to metastasize. Human papillomavirus DNA has been detected in these tumors, suggesting that immunosuppression may have a permissive effect on viral proliferation. Diagnosis and treatment are the same as for the general population. Patients are encouraged to use sunscreen liberally and avoid significant sun exposure.

Posttransplant Lymphoproliferative Disorder

Lymphomas constitute the largest group of noncutaneous neoplasms in transplant recipients.[82–84] The vast majority (>95%) of these lymphomas consist of a spectrum of B-cell proliferation disorders associated with EBV, known collectively as PTLD. Risk factors include a high degree of immunosuppression, anti–T-cell antibody therapy, tacrolimus, and primary EBV infection posttransplant. A wide variety of clinical manifestations may be seen. Symptoms may be systemic and include fever, fatigue, weight loss, or progressive encephalopathy. Lymphadenopathy may be localized, diffuse, or absent. Intrathoracic PTLD may present with well-circumscribed pulmonary nodules, with or without mediastinal adenopathy. Abdominal pain, rectal bleeding, or bowel perforation may occur with intra-abdominal involvement. Allograft involvement may occur and cause organ dysfunction. Central nervous system involvement is much more common (~15 to 20%), as compared with lymphomas in the nontransplant patient population.

Diagnosis is confirmed by histologic examination of tissue specimens, including in situ DNA hybridization studies to detect the EBV genome. Treatment includes reduction of immunosuppression, use of IV ganciclovir, surgical extirpative therapy, or chemotherapy or newer agents such as monoclonal antibodies targeted to B cells (anti-CD20 MAB), the latter limited to patients whose tumors express the CD20 cell surface marker. Often a combination of these modalities is used. Mortality can exceed 80% with aggressive tumors.

Other Malignancies

A variety of other malignancies occur with increased incidence in transplant recipients. Conventional treatment is appropriate for most malignancies posttransplant. Immunosuppression should be reduced, particularly if bone marrow suppressive chemotherapeutic agents are administered. However, allograft function should be maintained for those organs that are critical to survival, such as the heart, liver, and lung. For other types of transplants with alternative therapies to fall back on if necessary (e.g., hemodialysis for kidney transplants, exogenous insulin for pancreas or islet cell transplants, and TPN for intestinal transplants), the risks of ongoing immunosuppression must be weighed against the benefits of organ function compared to the alternative therapies.

THE FUTURE OF TRANSPLANTATION

Dramatic advances have been made in the field of transplantation since the late 1970s, but it remains fraught with problems. A major disadvantage is the need for long-term, indeed lifelong, immunosuppression. Associated with immunosuppression is an increased risk for malignancies and infections, as well as a host of other potential side effects not related to the immune system. That is why tolerance, or the ability to maintain the allograft without the need for long-term immunosuppression, remains the goal for all transplant recipients. *Tolerance* is defined as a state of donor-specific hyporeactivity in the absence of immunosuppressive medications (i.e., the recipient's immune system does not attack the transplanted organ, but is intact and able to mount a response to an organ from a different donor). Many different therapeutic approaches have been tested to induce tolerance; however, none have yet shown significant promise.

Perhaps even greater than the problems of long-term immunosuppression is the significant discrepancy between the demand for, and the supply of, organs. The increase in the number of transplants being performed has not kept pace with the increase in the number of patients being placed on the waiting list. The result has been longer waiting times and sicker patients once the transplant finally takes place, if it does at all. Several methods have been proposed to increase the number of transplants being performed. The increasing use of living donors has led to the greatest increase in the number of transplants. However, further increasing the living donor pool by including higher-risk procedures and higher-risk donors will quickly reach a limit if donor morbidity and donor mortality increase. The use of xenografts may prove to be the solution to the organ shortage problem, but difficult immunologic hurdles remain. Mechanical devices may represent another solution and would also have the advantage of not requiring immunosuppression.[85,86] However, completely implantable, long-lasting biomechanical devices offer their own set of unique problems, which may be worse than those associated with long-term immunosuppression.

Xenotransplantation

Clinical xenotransplants (i.e., transplants of organs between different species) have offered great hope for solving the problem of the expanding waiting list, but the primary hurdle is the formidable immunologic barrier between species.[87] Other problems include the potential risk of transmission of infections (zoonoses) and the ethical problems involved with using animals for widespread human transplants.

It is generally accepted that successful xenotransplants for humans would probably involve the use of the pig, which would likely be much more readily accepted by the general population than, for example, a primate donor.[88] Pigs would also be easier to raise on a large-scale basis and likely would be less expensive to manage, compared to primates.

The immunologic barrier in pig-to-human xenotransplants is complex, but generally involves three components. The first is hyperacute rejection (HAR), which is mediated by the presence of natural xenoantibodies in humans. These antibodies bind to antigens found mainly on vascular endothelial cells of porcine donor organs, leading to complement activation, intravascular coagulation, and rapid graft ischemia soon after the transplant. After HAR, the next barrier is delayed xenograft rejection, which occurs later than HAR, but is likely still mediated by the presence of xenoreactive antibodies combined with platelet aggregation and activation of the coagulation cascade. The third barrier is a process similar to classic T-cell–mediated acute rejection in allografts. Many different options are being tested to overcome these barriers, including the genetic engineering of pigs to express human genes, use of agents to inhibit platelet aggregation and complement activation, and administration of powerful immunosuppressive drugs.[88,89]

Besides the immunologic issues, the potential infectious risks also need to be more clearly defined.[90] The risks associated with the transmission of porcine viruses into human transplant recipients and then potentially into the entire human population are not fully known and must be studied in detail.

Other Therapies

Xenotransplantation is not the only therapeutic approach currently being investigated for organ replacement therapy. Other possible approaches include cellular transplants, organogenesis, and artificial and bioartificial devices.[91,92]

Cellular transplants involve the injection of cells that have the potential to replace cells in an organ that has been damaged by disease, thereby augmenting the function of that organ. An example of a cellular transplant would be the injection of stem cells or isolated hepatocytes into a failing liver. Such a procedure would most likely work best in patients with enzymatic or genetic defects. For patients with well-established chronic liver disease with cirrhosis, a cellular transplant would have limitations, because the underlying problem of portal hypertension would not be addressed. Another example of a cellular transplant would be the transplantation of stem cells or primitive muscle cells into a damaged heart. After healing, the cells could potentially function as cardiac muscle cells, thereby augmenting cardiac function. Considerable research has already been done in this area. Cellular transplants show promise, but overall have several limitations. Primary is the inability of cellular transplants to improve the function of structurally complex organs such as the kidney, which consists of several different cell types, all arranged in a specific pattern to allow for proper function.

One potential approach to overcoming this limitation is organogenesis, which essentially involves growing organs de novo from primitive cells or stem cells. However, this form of therapy is still in the theoretical phase and is unlikely to be a clinically viable option in the near future.

Much further along in the clinical realm of organ replacement therapies is the use of bioartificial and artificial mechanical devices. Considerable investigative work has been undertaken to develop a bioreactor using artificial elements and hepatocytes to treat liver failure as a bridge to liver transplantation. However, consistent results have yet to be achieved in the clinical setting. The heart model is in the most advanced stage of development. Various implantable assist devices are already in routine clinical use. Currently, these are usually temporary devices that serve as a bridge to a transplant. Several different models of a totally implantable artificial heart are also currently under development and have been used occasionally. Thromboembolic complications and infections remain the primary problems with these devices.

The future of transplantation is certainly exciting. Continued active research will focus on newer immunosuppressive drugs, tolerance, xenotransplants, cellular transplants, and artificial devices. Most transplant centers in the next decade will probably offer some combination of these new therapies to potential transplant recipients.

References

1. Carrel A: The transplantation of organs. *NY Med J* 99:839, 1914.
2. Guthrie CC: *Blood Vessel Surgery and Its Applications.* New York: Longmans Green, 1912.
3. Hamilton DNH, Reid WA: Yu Yu Voronoy and the first human kidney allograft. *Surg Gynecol Obstet* 159:289, 1984.
4. Merrill JP, Murray JE, Harrison JH: Successful homotransplantation of the human kidney between identical twins. *JAMA* 160:277, 1956.
5. Calne RY, Alexandre GP, Murray JE: A study of the effects of drugs in prolonged survival of homologous renal transplants in dogs. *Ann NY Acad Sci* 99:743, 1962.
6. Murray JE, Merrill JP, Harrison JH, et al: Prolonged survival of human-kidney homografts by immunosuppressive drug therapy. *N Engl J Med* 268:1315, 1963.
7. Starzl TE, Marchioro TL, Waddell WR: The reversal of rejection in human renal homografts with subsequent development of homograft tolerance. *Surg Gynecol Obstet* 117:385, 1963.
8. Valente JF, Alexander JW: Immunobiology of renal transplantation. *Surg Clin North Am* 78:1, 1998.
9. Krensky AM: Molecular basis of transplant rejection and acceptance. *Pediatr Nephrol* 5:422, 1991.
10. Ball ST, Dallman MJ: Transplantation immunology. *Curr Opin Nephrol Hypertens* 4:465, 1995.
11. Hancock WW: Current trends in transplant immunology. *Curr Opin Nephrol Hypertens* 8:317, 1999.
12. Cuturi MC, Blancho G, Josien R, et al: The biology of allograft rejection. *Curr Opin Nephrol Hypertens* 3:578, 1994.
13. Fryer JP, Granger DK, Leventhal JR, et al: Steroid-related complications in the cyclosporine era. *Clin Transplantation* 8:224, 1994.
14. Burke JF, Pirsch JD, Ramos EL, et al: Long-term efficacy and safety of cyclosporine in renal transplant recipients. *N Engl J Med* 331:358, 1994.
15. Calne RY, Rolles K, White DJG, et al: Cyclosporin A initially as the only immunosuppressant in 34 recipients of cadaveric organs. *Lancet* 2:1033, 1979.
16. Sweny P, Farrington K, Younis F, et al: Sixteen months experience with cyclosporin A in human kidney transplantation. *Transplant Proc* 13:365, 1981.
17. Matas AJ, Tellis VA, Quinn T, et al: ALG treatment of steroid-resistant rejection in patients receiving cyclosporine. *Transplantation* 41:579, 1986.
18. Rose SM, Turka L, Kerr L, et al: Advances in immune-based therapies to improve solid organ graft survival. *Adv Intern Med* 47:293, 2001.
19. Van Buren CT, Barakat O: Organ donation and retrieval. *Surg Clin North Am* 74:1055, 1994.
20. Kootstra G, Kievit J, Nederstigt A: Organ donors: Heartbeating and non-heartbeating. *World J Surg* 26:181, 2002.
21. Delgado DH, Rao V, Ross HJ: Donor management in cardiac transplantation. *Can J Cardiol* 18:1217, 2002.
22. St Peter SD, Imber CJ, Friend PJ: Liver and kidney preservation by perfusion. *Lancet* 359:604, 2002.
23. Van der Werf WJ, D'Alessandro AM, Hoffmann RM, et al: Procurement, preservation, and transport of cadaver kidneys. *Surg Clin North Am* 78:41, 1998.
24. D'Alessandro AM, Southard JH, Love RB, et al: Organ preservation. *Surg Clin North Am* 74:1083, 1994.
25. Schaubel D, Desmeules M, Mao Y, et al: Survival experience among elderly end-stage renal disease patients. A controlled comparison of transplantation and dialysis. *Transplantation* 60:1389, 1995.
26. Wolfe RA, Ashby VB, Milford EL, et al: Comparison of mortality in all patients on dialysis, patients on dialysis awaiting transplantation, and recipients of a first cadaveric transplant. *N Engl J Med* 341:1725, 1990.
27. Kasiske BL, Ramos EL, Gaston RS, et al: The evaluation of renal transplant candidates: clinical practice guidelines. *J Am Soc Nephrol* 6:1, 1995.
28. Terasaki PI, Cecka JM, Gjertson DW, et al: High survival rates of kidney transplants from spousal and living unrelated donors. *N Engl J Med* 333:333, 1995.
29. Humar A, Ramcharan T, Kandaswamy R, et al: Risk factors for slow graft function after kidney transplant: A multivariate analysis. *Clin Transplant* 16:425, 2002.

30. Sells RA: Cardiovascular complications following renal transplantation. *Transplantation Rev* 11:111, 1997.

31. Cosio F, Alamir A, Yim S, et al: Patient survival after renal transplantation: I. The impact of dialysis pretransplant. *Kidney Int* 53:767, 1998.

32. Asderakis A, Augustine T, Dyer P, et al: Pre-emptive kidney transplantation: The attractive alternative. *Nephrol Dial Transplant* 13:1799, 1998.

33. Friedman A: Strategies to improve outcomes after renal transplantation. *N Engl J Med* 346:2089, 2002.

34. Matas AJ, Humar A, Payne WD, et al : Decreased acute rejection in kidney transplant recipients is associated with decreased chronic rejection. *Ann Surg* 230:493, discussion 498, 1999.

35. Massy ZA, Guijarro C, Wiederkehr MR, et al: Chronic renal allograft rejection: Immunologic and nonimmunologic risk factors. *Kidney Int* 49:518, 1996.

36. Schweitzer EJ, Matas AJ, Gillingham K, et al: Causes of renal allograft loss: Progress in the '80s, challenges for the '90s. *Ann Surg* 214:679, 1991.

37. Sutherland DE, Gruessner RW, Najarian JS, et al: Solitary pancreas transplants: A new era. *Transplant Proc* 30:280, 1998.

38. Manske CL, Wang Y, Rector T, et al: Coronary revascularisation in insulin-dependent diabetic patients with chronic renal failure. *Lancet* 340:998, 1992.

39. Humar A, Ramcharan T, Kandaswamy R, et al: Pancreas after kidney transplant. *Am J Surg* 182:155, 2001.

40. Farney AC, Cho E, Schweitzer E, et al: Simultaneous cadaver pancreas living-donor kidney transplantation: A new approach for the type 1 diabetic uremic patient. *Ann Surg* 232:696, 2000.

41. Krishnamurthi V, Philosophe B, Bartlett ST: Pancreas transplantation: Contemporary surgical techniques. *Urol Clin North Am* 28:833, 2001.

42. Humar A, Kandaswamy R, Granger D, et al: Decreased surgical risks of pancreas transplantation in the modern era. *Ann Surg* 231:269, 2000.

43. Lumbreras C, Fernandez I, Velosa J, et al: Infectious complications following pancreatic transplantation: Incidence, microbiological and clinical characteristics, and outcome. *Clin Infect Dis* 20:514, 1995.

44. Sutherland DE, Gruessner RW, Dunn DL, et al: Lessons learned from more than 1000 pancreas transplants at a single institution. *Am Surg* 233:463, 2001.

45. McChesney LP: Advances in pancreas transplantation for the treatment of diabetes. *Dis Mon* 45:88, 1999.

46. Wiesner RH: Current indications, contraindications, and timing for liver transplantation, in Busutill RW, Klintmalm GB (eds): *Transplantation of the Liver*. Philadelphia: WB Saunders, 1996, p 71.

47. Ferguson ME, Ferguson RM: Rescuing Prometheus: A policy proposal to alleviate excess demand for liver transplantation. *Clin Transplant* 11:49, 1997.

48. Strong RW, Lynch SV, Ong TN, et al: Successful liver transplantation from a living donor to her son. *N Engl J Med* 322:1505, 1990.

49. Trotter JF, Wachs M, Everson GT, et al: Adult-to-adult transplantation of the right hepatic lobe from a living donor. *N Engl J Med* 346:1074, 2002.

50. Wachs ME, Bak TE, Karrer FM, et al: Adult living donor liver transplantation using a right hepatic lobe. *Transplantation* 66:1313, 1998.

51. Kiuchi T, Inomata Y, Uemoto S, et al: Living-donor liver transplantation in Kyoto, 1997. *Clin Transpl* 191, 1997.

52. Marcos A, Fisher RA, Ham JM, et al: Right lobe living donor liver transplantation. *Transplantation* 68:798, 1999.

53. Fan ST, Lo CM, Liu CL: Technical refinement in adult-to-adult living donor liver transplantation using right lobe graft. *Ann Surg* 231:126, 2000.

54. Rogiers X, Malago M, Gawad K, et al: In situ splitting of cadaveric livers. The ultimate expansion of a limited donor pool. *Ann Surg* 224:331, 1996.

55. Humar A, Ramcharan T, Sielaff T, et al: Split liver transplantation for 2 adult recipients: An initial experience. *Am J Transplant* 1:366, 2001.

56. Everson GT, Kam I: Immediate postoperative care, in Maddrey WC, Schiff ER, Sorrell MF (eds): *Transplantation of the Liver*. Baltimore: Lippincott Williams & Wilkins, 2001, p 131.

57. Humar A, Gruessner R: Critical care of the liver transplant recipient, in Rippe I, Fink C (eds): *Intensive Care Medicine,* 4th ed. CITY: Lippincott-Raven, 1998, p 2219.

58. Brown A, Williams R: Long-term postoperative care, in Maddrey WC, Schiff ER, Sorrell MF (eds): *Transplantation of the Liver*. Baltimore: Lippincott Williams & Wilkins. 2001, p 163.

59. Buchman AL, Scolapio J, Fryer J: AGA technical review on short bowel syndrome and intestinal transplantation. *Gastroenterology* 124:1111, 2003.

60. Westergaard H: Short bowel syndrome. *Semin Gastrointest Dis* 13:210, 2002.

61. Sokal EM, Cleghorn G, Goulet O, et al: Liver and intestinal transplantation in children: Working Group Report of the First World Congress of Pediatric Gastroenterology, Hepatology, and Nutrition. *J Pediatr Gastroenterol Nutr* 35(Suppl 2):S159, 2002.

62. Kato T, Ruiz P, Thompson JF, et al: Intestinal and multivisceral transplantation. *World J Surg* 26:226, 2002.

63. Abu-Elmagd K, Bond G, Reyes J, et al: Intestinal transplantation: A coming of age. *Adv Surg* 36:65, 2002.

64. Reyes J, Mazariegos GV, Bond GM, et al: Pediatric intestinal transplantation: Historical notes, principles and controversies. *Pediatr Transplant* 6:193, 2002.

65. Miniati DN, Robbins RC: Heart transplantation: A thirty-year perspective. *Annu Rev Med* 53:189, 2002.

66. Kesten S: Advances in lung transplantation. *Dis Mon* 45:101, 1999.

67. Reichart B, Gulbins H, Meiser BM, et al: Improved results after heart-lung transplantation: A 17-year experience. *Transplantation* 75:127, 2003.

68. Cassivi SD, Meyers BF, Battafarano RJ, et al: Thirteen-year experience in lung transplantation for emphysema. *Ann Thorac Surg* 74:1663, 2002.

69. Egan TM, Detterbeck FC, Mill MR, et al: Long-term results of lung transplantation for cystic fibrosis. *Eur J Cardiothorac Surg* 22:602, 2002.

70. Egan TM, Detterbeck FC: The ABCs of LTX for BAC. *J Thorac Cardiovasc Surg* 125:20, 2003.

71. Goudarzi BM, Bonvino S: Critical care issues in lung and heart transplantation. *Crit Care Clin* 19:209, 2003.

72. Kubak BM: Fungal infection in lung transplantation. *Transpl Infect Dis* 4(Suppl 3):24, 2002.

73. Boucek RJ Jr., Boucek MM: Pediatric heart transplantation. *Curr Opin Pediatr* 14:611, 2002.

74. Marelli D, Laks H, Kobashigawa JA, et al: Seventeen-year experience with 1083 heart transplants at a single institution. *Ann Thorac Surg* 74:1558, 2002.

75. Penn I: The effect of immunosuppression on pre-existing cancers. *Transplantation* 55:742, 1993.

76. Hibberd PL, Snydman DR: Cytomegalovirus infection in organ transplant recipients. *Infect Dis Clin North Am* 9:863, 1995.

77. Kaufman DB, Leventhal JR, Gallon LG, et al: Risk factors and impact of cytomegalovirus disease in simultaneous pancreas-kidney transplantation. *Transplantation* 72:1940, 2001.

78. Dunn DL, Mayoral JL, Gillingham KJ, et al: Treatment of invasive CMV disease in solid organ transplant patients with ganciclovir. *Transplantation* 51:98, 1991.

79. Patel R, Paya CV: Infections in solid-organ transplant recipients. *Clin Microbiol Rev* 10:86, 1997.

80. Lutz J, Heemann U: Tumours after kidney transplantation. *Curr Opin Urol* 13:105, 2003.

81. Euvrard S, Kanitakis J, Claudy A: Skin cancers after organ transplantation. *N Engl J Med* 348:1681, 2003.

82. Green M: Management of Epstein-Barr virus induced post-transplant lymphoproliferative disease in recipients of solid organ transplantation. *Am J Transplant* 1:103, 2001.

83. Cockfield SM: Identifying the patient at risk for post-transplant lymphoproliferative disorder. *Transpl Infect Dis* 3:70, 2001.

84. Preiksaitis JK, Keay S: Diagnosis and management of post-transplant lymphoproliferative disorder in solid-organ transplant recipients. *Clin Infect Dis* 33(Suppl 1):S38, 2001.

85. Boehmer JP: Device therapy for heart failure. *Am J Cardiol* 91:53D, 2003.

86. Deng MC, Naka Y: Mechanical circulatory support devices—state of the art. *Heart Fail Monit* 2:120, 2002.

87. Dooldeniya MD, Warrens AN: Xenotransplantation: Where are we today? *J R Soc Med* 96:111, 2003.

88. Dorling A: Clinical xenotransplantation: Pigs might fly? *Am J Transplant* 2:695, 2002.

89. Einsiedel EF, Ross H: Animal spare parts? A Canadian public consultation on xenotransplantation. *Sci Eng Ethics* 8:579, 2002.

90. Valdes Gonzalez R: Xenotransplantation's benefits outweigh risks. *Nature* 420:268, 2002.

91. Elliott RB, Garkavenko O, Escobar L, et al: Concerns expressed about the virological risks of xenotransplantation. *Xenotransplantation* 9:422, 2002.

92. O'Connell P: Pancreatic islet xenotransplantation. *Xenotransplantation* 9:367, 2002.

CHAPTER 11

Patient Safety, Errors, and Complications in Surgery

Mark L. Shapiro and Peter B. Angood

INTRODUCTION

The term "medical errors" has become a commonly-used industry term that has become prevalent in the quality improvement (QI) dialogue in the United States in the past few years. This concept of medical errors has received an abundance of attention, primarily due to the Institute of Medicine's (IOM) 2000 report on the subject.[1] It was the first of several reports produced by the Institute as part of a broad initiative to focus attention on the current status of the American health care system, and to precipitate change in the practice of health care. According to this report, approximately 98,000 medical error–related deaths occur annually—a figure that quickly received the attention of the lay public, health care payors, governmental representatives, and non-health care industry business leaders.

However, complications in surgery have been an issue for centuries and are not a new concept. Surgeons fear any form of complication in their patients and do their utmost to prevent any that may be related to surgical diseases or to surgical treatments. It has been well recognized for decades that the onset of a complication will prolong the course of illness and lengthen hospital stay, as well as increase morbidity and mortality rates. Therefore the prevention of complications is of the utmost importance for surgeons.

Traditionally, surgical textbooks have focused on complications and less on the processes that may initially have led to the complications. The dialogue that has arisen around medical errors now more reasonably provides the surgical community an opportunity and an improved environment to focus on processes of care that can lead to a decrease in complications. Although complications do occur that are related specifically to a surgical disease, it also is important to analyze the processes of care in an effort to decrease complications related to the treatment of disease. It is these processes of care that are increasingly being recognized as the etiology for error—not the diseases or treatments themselves.

This chapter provides an overview of medical errors, patient safety, processes of care, reporting of complications, and the infrastructure related to the improvement process, in an attempt to minimize errors and complications for health care systems. Additionally, this chapter addresses several of the more common complications seen in surgery, and offers insight on the management strategies that are examples of current best practices. More information related to the specific variety of surgical diseases and their treatment are covered Chap. 5.

ISSUES PERTINENT TO ERRORS AND COMPLICATIONS

Patient Safety Initiatives

As a result of the Institute of Medicine reports, as well as the natural evolution of QI initiatives in health care, the focus for many QI efforts has now begun to shift toward patient safety and medical errors. Previously, most efforts in surgical QI programs have been oriented toward patient diseases and their complications (e.g., postoperative abscesses following perforated viscus repair), provider decisions (e.g., a delay in diagnosis or errors in decision making), and to a lesser extent, the system processes related to patient care. Now that the awareness of patient safety concerns has moved beyond organized health care system enterprises and a few professional organizations, the focus for QI programs on many levels also has appropriately begun to shift toward patient safety.

As a collective term, "patient safety" can have a predominantly negative connotation if it is interpreted in a way that implies that if the patient is left unprotected, harm will occur during interactions with current health care systems. This is not necessarily the correct interpretation. Health care is a complex industry, and the processes of providing integrated patient care have become more complex in recent decades for a multitude of reasons. With this complexity comes an inherent risk that system failures may occur. It is an improvement in patient safety, accomplished through stronger vigilance and refinement of the processes for care, that is the primary thrust for current patient safety initiatives. When systems do not have enough oversight and attention focused on the integration of the myriad processes necessary for providing care, failures can occur and patients may have adverse outcomes as a result. The current focus on patient safety is a healthy development for the industry, as it has provided the impetus for organizations and individual practitioners to review processes of care in such a way that patient safety becomes a priority in patient management. This can be viewed as a natural evolution of any industry in which ongoing change and adaptation to change are necessary components for the ultimate improvement, refinement, and survival of the industry. These changes promise to bring a marked improvement to the health care industry by instituting a more patient-friendly and safe environment; with-

out these changes, patients become increasingly at risk of harm and medical errors.

Processes of Care

The simplicity of the phrase "processes of care" does not adequately reflect the intricacy of the highly complex set of systems involved. Those familiar with health care quality improvement or process improvement initiatives recognize that even the simplest of processes, when broken into component parts and analyzed, becomes complex. The root causes of process failures are notoriously difficult to identify, and the ability to develop tangible solutions for the root causes is equally difficult to initiate on a long-term basis. Despite the millions of dollars and extensive expenditure of human resources during the past decade, the direct application of non-health care industry quality improvement and process improvement practice models continues to be problematic in providing successful solutions for the health care industry.

Recognizing the inherent complexity that characterizes all health care processes is necessary before alternative quality improvement solutions can be sought. Recently, groups such as The Joint Commission for Accreditation of Healthcare Organizations (JCAHO), The Leapfrog Group, and The Institute for Healthcare Improvement (IHI) have begun offering alternative quality improvement solutions specific to health care. As awareness concerning the need for change and the mechanisms by which it can be successfully instituted are emerging, it has begun to culminate in the waves of change that are now being witnessed.

Quality Improvement Processes

Fortunately, quality improvement (QI) systems are now an integral part of health care. While there are a variety of QI models and organizational structures that have been adapted to health care, the majority of programs focus on recognition of problems, errors, system inefficiency, or patient safety concerns. The net result is that most QI programs remain relatively reactive and less proactive in the analysis and management of issues that are identified. Additionally, a shift toward a forward-thinking system of QI also needs to occur in order for ongoing improvements in care efficiencies to become an inherent goal for practitioners in the various health care systems and environments. By redirecting the focus of QI improvements in this manner, the current mentality in health care would move from one of complacence to one of continued betterment.

A strong QI program should have the following components: (1) an expectation that all levels of employees can provide ongoing identification of problems and issues, (2) that reporting of problems can occur in an environment where employee job security is not threatened, (3) there is recognition and tabulation of identified problems with objective feedback to the reporting employee and those potentially affected by the reporting, (4) all problems are processed after they are evaluated for significance and prioritized, (5) objective clarification of the issues related to the identified problems are solicited, (6) clinical and administrative databases are maintained to provide comparative reference data for evaluating the identified problems, (7) organized discussion forums are maintained for refinement of the evaluation process and for the development of proposed solutions to identified problems, (8) a system for soliciting more detailed information when complex problems require further analysis prior to initiating change, (9) a respected reporting system within an organizational hierarchy that is recognized internally and externally as a valid QI program, (10) the reporting system is integrated with other QI programs and process improvement initiatives within the health care system, (11) there is an oversight committee for institutional QI programs and/or a reporting mechanism directly to an institution's board of governors, (12) an ability to mobilize institutional resources when significant problems have been identified and the proposed solutions are beyond simple restructuring or behavior change, (13) monitoring and tracking of success or failure when solutions are initiated in response to completely processed problems, (14) documentation of the entire QI process in a record system that is easily obtained and reviewed at all times, (15) ongoing communication to the employees who are affected by the changes (or planned lack of change) instituted by the QI program, (16) reassessment of the changes after an appropriate length of time to ensure that long-term change has occurred, (17) forums for repeat discussions when difficult problems remain resistant to significant change or improvements, and (18) as needed, an incentive or reward system to facilitate change in human behavior. While this is a detailed set of components, there is a need to maintain this continuum of activities so that ongoing change can occur.

Regardless of how a QI program is structured, resources are required for their management. These resources include trained QI employees within an organizational hierarchy, the development and maintenance of appropriate databases, ongoing education programs for employees and physicians, reasonable incentive and reward strategies to stimulate change, and recognition by the institution that QI is an essential component for the viability of the organization's operation. The current QI system for health care is reactionary and does not promote an environment for learning how to manage processes more efficiently, nor does it foster the cultural mentality of ongoing quality improvement. This paradigm shift to a proactive expectation of ongoing QI is essential to the emergence of the next generation of health care.

Communication Strategies

Communication failures or losses are the most important component when errors and complications occur in health care. Similarly, for improvements and refinements to take place, maintaining an integrated process of communication is essential for high quality care to exist and flourish.

Surgeons rely heavily on institutional resources in order to practice patient care. Traditionally, the individual surgeon has been able to set the tone and expectations for their individual practice preferences, while institutions attempted to cater to all surgeons on an individual basis. In this type of system, the more organized surgeons often have preferential treatment because of their ability to work within the system, while less organized surgeons often have a somewhat frustrating experience when trying to effectively manage the system. This often leads to a chaotic organizational environment within institutions in terms of how to best manage surgical patients as an overall group. Facile institutions evolved complex processes in order to maintain institution-specific systems whereby individual surgeon preferences are managed efficiently (but inconsistently). Less facile institutions have not been able to maintain this type of environment. The basic premise of catering to all individual surgeons has not altered for many years, and yet it is clearly not the most efficient organizational strategy for health care systems.

Simultaneously, the evolution for other health care professionals is such that there are now numerous health care disciplines that offer training and credentialing. These individual training programs currently function in relative isolation from other health care disciplines and medical schools in terms of how they provide integrated services within a health care institution. To date, individual institutions

have been unable to recognize that employees and health care professionals are not trained to function as an integrated team within a culture that has patient care and institutional priorities as the ultimate goal. Surgeons expect to retain their individual preferences, while all groups of practitioners remain untrained regarding how to work within an integrated structure. Therefore it is not surprising that the net result is poor communication and subsequent system failures. The failure of communication is therefore a common etiology for medical error.

One of the basic future tenets for health care system improvement will be the development of improved models of refined communication infrastructures, so that all health care disciplines become aware of the importance of efficient team communication. With this knowledge, health care professionals will be able to contribute to a communication infrastructure in such a way that the patient and institutional needs are placed ahead of individual practitioner or surgeon preferences. In the interim, professionals from each discipline must make concerted efforts to develop communication practices that reflect efforts to place patient care as the priority, and to recognize that interactions as a team will ultimately provide improved outcomes with a lower potential for complications and medical errors. These communication strategies should be instituted in verbal practices as well as included as written documentation within medical records.

Documentation of Care and Evolving Issues

There should be no doubt that documentation is now considered the essence of high-quality patient care. While at times documentation remains an arduous task, the practice of relying on the documentation contained within the medical record must be rigorously maintained, meaning procedures should never be presumed to have been performed if they have not been documented properly. The medical record is the only legal document that maintains a long-term transcription of patient care activity, and as such its maintenance should be considered a priority.

The confidentiality of all medical information for patients is also now recognized as a priority in health care. While individual practitioners and institutions are still struggling with the ramifications of recent federal regulations to protect confidentiality of medical information, these new regulations have not yet been fully tested with legal challenges to clarify their boundaries. However, their essence should still be respected.

In order to provide optimal documentation in a medical record, patient contacts for all types of interactions should be recorded. For outpatient care, the office charts need to show thorough documentation of all patient visits and correspondence, examination results, laboratory and radiology investigations, and assessment of the medical problems with a proposed plan of care, as well as records of procedures, pathology results, and any complications encountered. Inpatient medical records need to be equally thorough, but are more complicated because of the need for all health care providers to document their interactions with patients. The essence of this level of documentation should be focused on identifying patient care problems, assessing their severity, and proposing plans for how to manage them. As care standards evolve, so should those of documentation (i.e., including the results of tests and the impact the care plan may have on patient care). Patient preferences and the results of family discussions should be noted in the records, while all complications should be explained with an objective description of the issues. Orders written for care plans need to be promptly and clearly written in order to minimize confusion. Any unclear orders should not be interpreted or carried out without further clarification, as this only creates the opportunity for errors.

Medical records are not the forum for open discussion, inflammatory remarks on care, or denigrating comments on the patient, their family, friends and/or other health care providers. The records should always be clearly stated, objective, and maintained in an up-to-date manner. All entries must be dated and timed, and should not be back-dated at a later review of the record. Discussions related to ethically-sensitive issues must also be clearly stated, but not filled with innuendo or open-ended statements. Redundancy and regurgitation of results from tests and investigations within medical progress notes should be minimized, and notations oriented primarily to the identification of problems and the plan to manage them.

The development of information systems technology and electronic recording of medical data have been relatively slow in progress and adoption in the health care industry. This refinement and ongoing adoption of technology will ultimately occur, but the essential need for succinct, confidential, and objective record entries will remain constant, regardless of the maintenance method employed.

Complications Related to Surgery and Anesthesia Systems

The relationships between surgeons and anesthesiologists are an important component of providing surgical care for patients. Historically, these departments have functioned independently and autonomously; however, current changes in health care are providing an opportunity for these relationships to be reassessed for improvement.

The surgeon is typically the primary physician provider for surgical patients during management of their disease processes. Surgeons rely heavily on consultants and hospital systems for this disease management, yet many of these processes are not under the direct control of the surgeons. Specifically, the fund of knowledge and practices for anesthesia has dramatically changed in recent decades, but the interrelationship between surgeons and the anesthesia teams often remains misconceived, or even ill-conceived, in many medical centers. The overlapping responsibilities between surgeons and anesthesiologists require better definition and clarification so that improvements in quality and system efficiencies can occur.

Perioperative care should therefore involve a continuous, linear knowledge of a patient's surgical and comorbid conditions such that all medical providers are cognizant of the various issues throughout the management of a patient's surgical disease state. To this end, an improved flow of information between surgeons and anesthesiologists needs to occur during the preoperative, intraoperative, and postoperative management of patients. When issues, errors, or complications are developing for any particular patient, the communication and decision making can be simplified so a minimum of redundant discussion or relearning of data occurs. Surgeons need to remain aware of the anesthesia-related developments in this perioperative period so that changes in surgical care can be adjusted as needed.

An exceedingly important aspect of this perioperative care paradigm is the intraoperative component of care. Open and continuous dialogue between the surgical and anesthesia teams is essential for optimal intraoperative management. A constant awareness between the two teams should exist regarding the physiologic status of the patient and the effects that surgical or anesthetic interventions may create for that patient. This is well recognized for vascular, pulmonary, and cardiac operations, but has been less well recognized for operative cases that are performed emergently (i.e., unstable trauma cases, septic shock cases, and patients with metabolic or intravascular volume abnormalities). Even though surgeons often remain the dominant health care provider in the postoperative period, the anesthesia team can clearly help to optimize the postoperative physiologic status of the patient by maximizing intraoperative care and thereby anticipating the surgical team's concerns for the postoperative period. This intraoperative dialogue remains underutilized in many circumstances.

Ethics of Reporting and Communication with Complications

Due to the very personal nature of medical care, patients enter into a trust relationship and an implied informal contract (or covenant) with a surgeon and the associated institutions when soliciting care for their medical problems. The expectation should be that open communication will occur between providers and patients in such a fashion that this trust relationship and contract are not violated at any time during the relationship. Should problems or complications in care occur, then open communication necessarily must be maintained as part of that relationship and contract, as this is morally, ethically, and legally the correct action. The reporting of complications is an important component of peer review and quality improvement initiatives to facilitate improvements in care; however, it is equally important that the patient and their family members are included in the dialogue related to complications. Similarly, the institution(s) involved in the care of a patient who develops complications must also be kept informed of potential problems and complications, so that an institutional response to the family may also be constructed in a timely fashion. This latter point is especially important for those situations in which the patient and/or family members choose to respond in a potentially angry or hostile fashion when a complication or error in care has developed, because the institution may often be able to offer resources to the patients, families, and health care providers with a more balanced perspective than individual practitioners.

Any time a procedure is performed, the potential for unforeseen difficulties or complications exists. The problems may arise as a result of a patient's primary surgical disease and their comorbid conditions, or may arise due to technical problems, medication delivery errors, system process errors, communication errors, or a myriad of other unexpected developments.

During the process of obtaining informed consent for any procedure, it is always prudent to describe for the patient and their significant others the potential complications that may occur. While it is not necessary to detail all of the possible problems or difficulties that may arise in a procedure, it is important to introduce the concept that no procedure should be assumed to be simple or straightforward. Reassurance that all diligent efforts will be made to minimize the potential for problems should be effectively conveyed to the patient

In general, patients and families are fairly accepting of a medical error when they have been informed ahead of time that the possibility for errors and complications exists. Similarly, patients often are accepting of errors when open and direct communication is made to them shortly after the recognition of a procedural complication or error. Open, honest, and direct communication between the responsible surgeon and the patient or the designated health care proxy, as soon as is practical usually aids in minimizing misunderstanding or animosity surrounding the development of a procedure-related complication. Noncommunicative actions such as denial and avoidance breed a sense of distrust and are therefore counterproductive. Again, it is imperative that objective and honest documentation of the causes and discussions surrounding procedural complications be of the utmost importance.

COMPLICATIONS IN MINOR PROCEDURES

Central Venous Access Lines

The decision to obtain central venous access must be a thoughtful one, and the data regarding the risk and cost of complications must be underscored. Steps to decrease complications include the following:

1. Ensure that the patient's condition indeed warrants central venous access. Experienced personnel should insert the line with proper positioning and sterile technique. Controversy exists as to whether or not placing the patient in Trendelenburg position facilitates access.
2. Antibiotic-coated catheters may decrease the rate of central line sepsis, although they initially are more expensive.
3. Routine central line changes should not be performed, and the lines should be removed as soon as adequate peripheral intravenous access can be established for medications that do not require central access.

One of the most common complications of central venous access is pneumothorax. It is not just inexperienced clinicians that create these iatrogenic injuries, but pneumothorax rates appear to be higher among the inexperienced. Pneumothorax occurrence rates from both subclavian and internal jugular vein approaches are on the order of 1 to 6%. The first step in prevention is proper positioning of the patient during the procedure. Even if a pneumothorax is not suspected to have occurred during the procedure, a chest x-ray is still needed to confirm the presence or absence of a pneumothorax following the line insertion. The decision regarding the need for a thoracostomy tube is similar to that described for bronchoscopy; if the patient is stable, then expectant observation may be adequate, but if any concerns about the patient's clinical condition exist, a thoracostomy tube should be placed. Occasionally, a delayed presentation of pneumothorax will manifest as late as 48 to 72 hours after central venous access attempts. This usually creates significant clinical compromise such that a tube thoracostomy is required.

Other complications that bear mentioning for both central venous and pulmonary artery catheters include transient arrhythmias during catheter insertion, arterial puncture with hematoma formation or persistent bleeding, and occasionally loss of a guidewire in the vena cava. Arrhythmias (the most common complication) result from myocardial irritability secondary to the guidewire placement, and usually will resolve when the catheter or guidewire is withdrawn from the right heart. Arterial puncture with bleeding can be troublesome, but the majority will resolve with direct pressure on or near the arterial injury site. It is only the rare case that will require angiography, stent placement, or surgery to repair the puncture site, but these patients usually will do well following the procedure, and have no significant arterial abnormalities over the long term. A lost guidewire or catheter now can be readily retrieved with interventional angiography techniques, and no longer represents an automatic need for surgical exploration to retrieve the lost material.

Another error with central access lines involving either a venous line or a pulmonary artery line is that of air embolus. These are estimated to occur in 0.2 to 1% of patients. However, when an air embolism does occur, the results often can be dramatic and mortality can reach 50%. Treatment may prove futile if the diagnosis is ignored, especially if the air embolism bolus is larger than 50 mL. Clinical auscultation over the precordium often is nonspecific, so

a portable chest x-ray may be required if the patient will tolerate the procedure. Nonetheless, aspiration via a central venous line accessing the heart may assist in decreasing the volume of gas in the right side of the heart, and minimize the amount traversing into the pulmonary circulation. Maneuvers to entrap the air in the right heart include placing the patient in the left lateral decubitus position and in Trendelenburg position, so the entrapped air can then be aspirated or anatomically stabilized within the right ventricle. If the patient survives these initial maneuvers, then consideration should be given as to whether the patient goes to the operating room for controlled surgical removal of the air, or if an angiographic approach is undertaken. The advantage of the operative approach is that the resources needed to salvage the patient are more readily available in the operating suite, should there be an acute deterioration in the patient's condition.

Perhaps the most dreaded complication of the pulmonary artery catheter is a pulmonary artery rupture. There usually is a sentinel bleed noted when a pulmonary artery catheter balloon is inflated, and then the patient begins to have uncontrolled coughing with hemoptysis. Reinflation of the catheter balloon is the initial step in management, followed by immediate airway intubation with mechanical ventilation, an urgent portable chest x-ray, and notification of the operating room that an emergent thoracotomy may be required. If there is no further bleeding after the balloon is reinflated, and the x-ray shows no significant consolidation of lung fields from ongoing bleeding and the patient is easily ventilated, then a conservative nonoperative approach may be considered. This approach might include observation alone if the patient has no signs of bleeding or hemodynamic compromise; however, more typically today a pulmonary angiogram with angioembolization or vascular stenting is the next step in treatment. For hemodynamically unstable patients after pulmonary artery rupture, unless the patient is already in the operating room having thoracic surgery, attempts at salvaging these catastrophic situations often is unsuccessful because of the time needed to perform the thoracotomy and identify the branch of the pulmonary artery that has ruptured.

Another complication that may well be underreported is central venous line infections.[1-4] The Centers for Disease Control and Prevention (CDC) reports mortality rates of 12 to 25% when a central venous line infection becomes systemic, and this carries a cost of approximately $25,000 per episode. The CDC does not recommend routine central line changes, but when the clinical suspicion is high, the site of venous access must be changed. Additionally, nearly 15% of hospitalized patients will acquire central venous line sepsis (defined as >15 colony-forming units [CFU] on an agar roll plate, or $>10^3$ CFU on sonication). In many instances, once an infection is recognized as central line sepsis, removing the line is adequate. *Staphylococcus aureus* infections, however, present a unique problem because of the potential for metastatic seeding of bacterial emboli. The treatment for this situation is 4 to 6 weeks of tailored antibiotic therapy.

Arterial Lines

Arterial lines are placed to facilitate arterial blood gas draws and to optimize hemodynamic monitoring. They often are *not* removed when central venous access is not in place so ongoing phlebotomy can easily be performed, a practice that may lead to higher complication rates.

Arterial access is preferably obtained via a sterile Seldinger technique, and a variety of arteries are utilized, such as the radial, femoral, brachial, axillary, dorsal pedis, and superficial temporal arteries. Although complications generally occur less than 1% of the time, when present they can be catastrophic. Complications include arterial spasm, bacteremia, thrombosis (the most common complication), bleeding (second most common), hematoma, pulselessness, and infection (0 to 10%). One could argue that should thrombosis or distal embolization occur, a hand is more precious than a foot, yet the literature suggests that the risk is nearly the same for both femoral and radial cannulation. This also is true for infection rates between the two sites as well. For complications related to thrombosis, bleeding, and infected catheters with bacteremia, the catheters should all be removed and direct pressure placed for 5 to 10 minutes following removal. Thrombosis with distal tissue ischemia often can be treated with anticoagulation, but occasionally a surgical intervention is required to reestablish adequate inflow. The occurrence of pseudo-aneurysms and arteriovenous fistulae is remarkably low for these catheters.

Endoscopy and Bronchoscopy

For gastrointestinal endoscopy, the most dreaded risk is perforation. Perforation may occur for 1:10,000 patients with endoscopy alone, but carries a higher incidence rate when performed with biopsy (0 to 30%). This increased risk often occurs due to complications of intubating a gastrointestinal diverticulum (either esophageal or colonic), and also from the presence of weakened tissue in the wall of the intestine related to an inflammatory response secondary to infection (e.g., diverticulitis) or glucocorticoid use (e.g., inflammatory bowel disease).

Recognition that a perforation has occurred often is straightforward, but on occasion may be difficult. Patients will usually complain of diffuse abdominal pain shortly after the procedure, and then will quickly progress with worsening abdominal discomfort on examination. For patients that are difficult to evaluate, a change in clinical status may take several hours, and occasionally as long as 24 to 48 hours, to become manifest. When concern for a perforation exists, the patient should immediately have radiologic studies to assess for free intraperitoneal air, retroperitoneal air, or a pneumothorax. A delay in diagnosis of an endoscopic perforation creates the potential for ongoing gastrointestinal contamination and systemic sepsis.

Treatment for a gastrointestinal endoscopy perforation is usually surgical exploration to locate the perforation, decontaminate the surrounding tissues, and then to surgically close the perforation site. The exact type of surgery depends on the site of perforation and the degree of contamination or sepsis that is found at surgery. There are some patients in whom surgical exploration is not required; however, these are the exception rather than the rule. The patient who may be a candidate for nonoperative management usually is one for whom suspicions for perforation arise during an elective, bowel-prepped, endoscopy, and yet the patient does not have significant pain or clinical signs of perforation. With the concern for perforation, an x-ray is usually performed that then shows free air. If the patient remains without significant pain and with a benign abdominal exam, then this type of patient may be observed in a monitored setting, kept on strict dietary restriction, placed on broad-spectrum antibiotics, and closely observed for 48 to 72 hours to detect any deterioration in clinical status. If the patient remains with an uneventful course, a diet is gradually increased and the antibiotics discontinued after 3 to 7 days. If the patient clinically deteriorates at any time, immediate surgery is required.

Bronchoscopy, however, has several indications but relatively less-severe complications compared with perforation. Indications for bronchoscopy include removal of foreign bodies, biopsy for cancer, difficult intubations, diagnosis for pneumonia, and delivery of

medications. The contraindications are relatively few and include a partial arterial pressure of oxygen (Po_2) less than 60 mm Hg on 100% supplemental oxygen, an evolving myocardial infarction, and therapeutic anticoagulation. The complications of bronchoscopy include bronchial plugging (the most common complication), hypoxemia, pneumothorax, lobar collapse, and bleeding. When each of these is diagnosed appropriately and in a timely fashion, they are rarely life-threatening. Bleeding is usually quick to resolve and rarely requires surgery, but occasionally may require repeat endoscopy for thermocoagulation or fibrin glue application. The presence of a pneumothorax necessitates placement of a thoracostomy tube only when significant oxygenation deterioration occurs or the pulmonary mechanics are significantly compromised; otherwise expectant observation is adequate. The presence of a lobar collapse or mucous plugging usually will respond to aggressive pulmonary toilet, but occasionally requires repeat bronchoscopy.

Tracheostomy

One of the oldest operations performed is that of the tracheostomy, and when performed correctly, it leads to decreased ventilator days, decreased length of intensive care unit (ICU) or hospital stay, and improved pulmonary toilet. Tracheostomies are now performed open, percutaneously, with or without bronchoscopy, and with or without Doppler guidance, and yet complications still arise. Some of the complications tend to be minor and include changes in levels of partial pressure of arterial carbon dioxide (Pco_2), radiographic changes in the postprocedure x-rays, and minor fluctuation in the pulse oximetry saturation levels.

The indications for tracheostomy are important when deciding how and when to commit to a surgical airway. Historically, those patients on a moderate to high level of positive end-expiratory pressure (PEEP) have been considered not to be the best candidates for early tracheostomy for various reasons. A recent study examined PEEP and hypoxemia at 1 and 24 hours postprocedure. The study concluded that it was safe to perform percutaneous dilatational tracheostomy on patients with high PEEP settings because the patients did not have adverse oxygenation at 1 and 24 hours status postprocedure.[5]

Hypercarbia is known to contribute to intracranial hypertension for traumatic brain injury patients. Using fiberoptic bronchoscopy (FOB) in percutaneous tracheostomy will contribute to hypercapnia if the endotracheal tube (ET) is small (<7.5 mm), or if the minute ventilation is such that adequate ventilation is not administered during the procedure. Croce and colleagues examined FOB performed on patients with closed head injury when evaluating for pneumonia, and were able to confirm that intracranial pressure (ICP) did rise with a concomitant decrease in the cerebral perfusion pressure (CPP).[6]

Recent studies evaluating the incidence of pneumothorax and the need for routine posttracheostomy chest x-ray do not support their routine use after either percutaneous or open tracheostomy.[7,8] However, one reason for continuing to perform routine chest x-ray after a tracheostomy is for identifying and resolving significant lobar collapse that occurs from copious tracheal secretions or mechanical obstruction from any number of etiologies.

The most dramatic complication involving the tracheostomy is a tracheoinnominate artery fistula (TIAF).[9,10] These fistulas rarely occur (~0.3%), but when present, carry a 50 to 80% mortality rate. TIAFs can occur as quickly as 2 days after tracheostomy, but also as late as 2 months postprocedure. The prototypical patient at risk for a TIAF is a thin woman with a long, gracile neck. The patient may have a sentinel bleed, which occurs in 50% of TIAF cases, followed by a most spectacular bleed. Should a sentinel bleed be suspected,

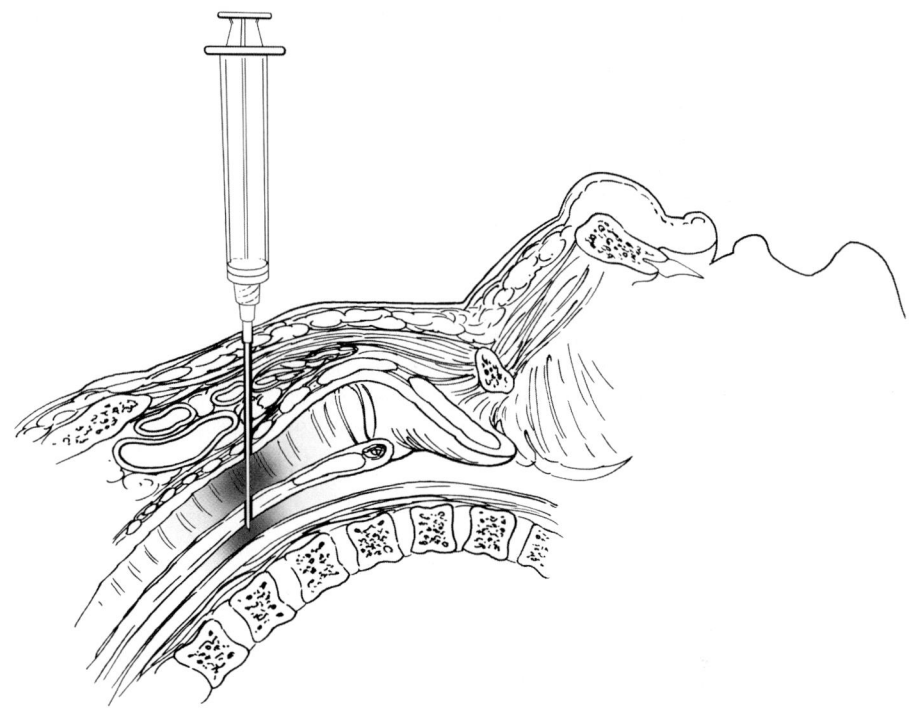

FIG. 11-1. This illustration depicts hyper-extension of the neck. In an effort to gain improved exposure to the tracheal rings (2 and 3), and to bring the trachea into a more anterior position, the surgeon may be misguided into a more inferiorly placed tracheostomy. This is a potential mechanism for a tracheoesophageal fistula (TEF).

the patient should be transported immediately to the operating room for fiberoptic evaluation. Although survival to this level is rare, for patients who are initially surviving, the conduct of the team identifying a TIAF during exsanguination is as follows (Figs. 11-1 and 11-2):

1. Inflate the tracheostomy balloon cuff to high pressure in order to attempt compression of the innominate artery.
2. Reintubate the patient with an endotracheal tube via the orotracheal or nasotracheal route.
3. If needed, remove the tracheostomy, and place a finger through the tracheostomy site in order to apply direct pressure anteriorly for compression of the innominate artery.
4. Sterile preparation of the patient for a median sternotomy should include the assistant's hand in the operative field.
5. Once exposed, surgically ligate the innominate artery proximally and distally to the injury.

FIG. 11-2. This illustration depicts improper positioning (attitude) of the percutaneous needle. It is possible to access the innominate artery via the trachea, thus placing the patient at risk for early tracheoinnominate artery fistula (TIAF).

6. Mobilize a soft tissue flap to protect the injured tracheal site from recurrent fistula.

Percutaneous Endogastrostomy

Technical errors usually are to blame for endoscopically-misplaced feeding tubes. Although it is not absolutely imperative to transilluminate the abdomen, doing so may decrease the margin for error and prevent inadvertent colotomies. While an unplanned colotomy is potentially catastrophic, other frustrating common errors include the overzealous retrograde pulling of the wire lasso through the abdominal wall and out the oropharynx, the antegrade pulling of the percutaneous endogastrostomy (PEG) tube disc out of the anterior gastric wall during placement, and progressive erosion of the PEG tube through the anterior abdominal wall over the first few weeks following PEG placement. A misplaced PEG that is still being utilized for administration of tube feeds may create intra-abdominal

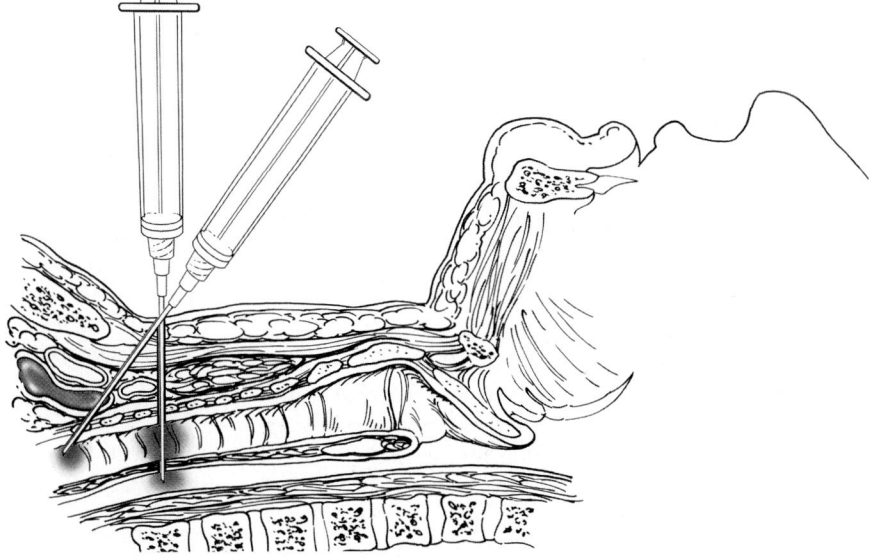

sepsis with peritonitis and/or an abdominal wall abscess with necrotizing fasciitis. As in other minor procedures, the initial placement
techniques must be fastidious in order to avoid these complications. Usually the colotomies, intraperitoneal leakage of tube feeds
with peritonitis, and abdominal wall abscesses manifest slowly over
time, but once present require surgery to correct the complications
and to replace the PEG with an alternate feeding tube, usually a
jejunostomy.

Other issues are more related to direct patient management, such
as wrist restraints for the confused and combative, sedation and/or
anxiolysis, or unexplained removal. There should be timely replacement of the tube with an alternative tube within 6 to 8 hours of
dislodgment, because the gastrostomy site closes rapidly. Once replaced, the new tube should not be utilized until a simple contrast
x-ray has been performed to confirm the new tube's intragastric
position.

Tube Thoracostomy

Tube thoracostomy is performed for pneumothorax, hemothorax,
and pleural effusions or empyemas. The aforementioned diagnoses
are commonly found on chest x-ray, but also can be seen on ultrasound and computed tomographic (CT) scans. A chest tube can be
easily placed with a combination of local analgesia and light conscious sedation. Common complications include inadequate analgesia or sedation, incomplete penetration of the pleura with formation
of a subcutaneous track for the tube, lacerations to the lung or
diaphragm, intraperitoneal placement of the tube through the diaphragm, and bleeding related to these various lacerations or injury
to pleural adhesions. Additional problems are related to maintenance
of the tubes, with slippage of the tubes out of position, or mechanical
problems related to the drainage system. All of these complications
can be avoided with proper initial insertion techniques, plus a daily
review of the drainage system and follow-up radiographs. Occasionally these tubes will need replacement due to malfunctions or
clogging of the tubes, but the replacement techniques are the same
as for the original insertion. Removal of these tubes occasionally
will create a residual pneumothorax if the patient does not maintain
positive intrapleural pressure during tube removal and initial dressing application. Replacement of a tube in this setting depends on the
clinical status of the patient, but expectant observation of the residual pneumothorax is acceptable. The development of an empyema
related specifically to the presence of the thoracostomy tube itself is
a debatable topic, but some centers now are moving to a protocol of
antibiotics for the duration of the chest tube placement as an attempt
to decrease empyema rates.

Diagnostic Peritoneal Lavage

Diagnostic peritoneal lavage (DPL) is less commonly performed in
the emergent trauma setting, but the indications are chiefly for the
hemodynamically-unstable patient who arrives in the emergency
department with neurologic impairment and an uncertain etiology
for blood loss. Should such a patient have life-threatening hemodynamic lability and an obvious source is yet to be found after initial resuscitation measures, then an emergent DPL is performed—
especially when an abdominal trauma ultrasound is not available or
is not reliable in a particular institution. It is imperative that the stomach and bladder be decompressed via nasogastric tube and bladder
catheterization prior to DPL, as both of these organs can be lacerated during the procedure (Fig. 11-3). It also has been recognized
that the small or large bowel and the major vessels of the retroperitoneum can be punctured inadvertently. While the renal system is

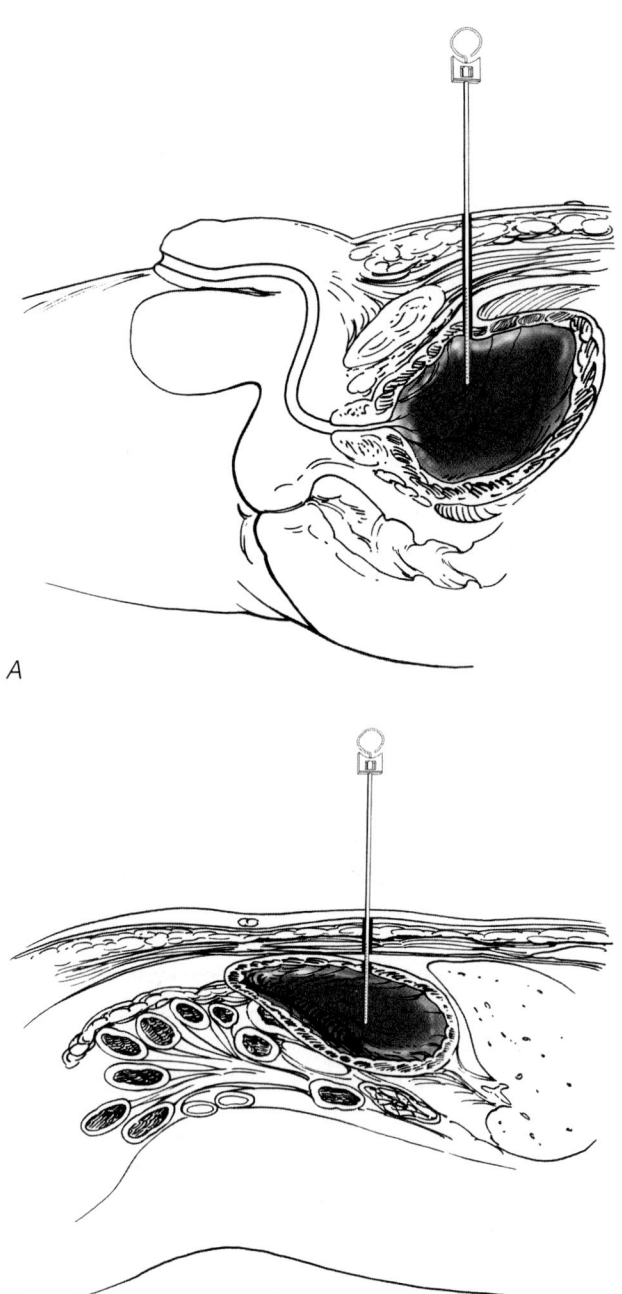

A

B

FIG. 11-3. This illustration depicts improper positioning of the DPL
catheter, with overdistention of the urinary bladder (*A*) and the stomach (*B*). This error in technique clearly demonstrates the importance of
decompressing hollow viscus before embarking on a diagnostic peritoneal lavage.

not usually involved, the occasional horseshoe or pelvic kidney may
become lacerated. All of these injuries usually will require surgical
exploration and repair, because of the difficulty of making an accurate diagnosis, as well as the potential for confounding a trauma
resuscitation with untreated iatrogenic injuries.

Complications with Angiography

As vascular stent strategies evolve and the use of angiography by surgeons increases beyond intraoperative studies or for trauma cases,
the complications related to angiography are becoming more readily

recognized. Dissection of a cannulated artery can lead to a variety of vascular malperfusion findings that include (but are not limited to) ischemic stroke from a carotid artery dissection or occlusion, mesenteric ischemia from dissection of the superior mesenteric artery, or a more innocuous finding of "blue toe syndrome" from a dissected artery in a peripheral limb with thromboembolic disease. The important initial step is for recognition of the ischemic tissue bed, and confirmation of the diagnosis with clinical findings and/or a combination of invasive or noninvasive imaging studies. The severity of the ischemia and the extent of the dissection will then determine if full anticoagulation and aspirin would be adequate therapy, or whether the patient shall require urgent surgical exploration to repair the dissection.

Bleeding secondary to angiography usually is related to bleeding at the vascular access site, but also may be related to a ruptured vessel at the distal portion of the angiography catheter. Local access site bleeding usually is readily detected, but may not be visible when the blood loss is tracking into the retroperitoneal tissue planes. These patients can present with hemorrhagic shock of an undetermined etiology, and so the angiography site needs to be closely inspected, and an abdominopelvic CT scan done to delineate the extent of bleeding into the retroperitoneum. The initial management is direct compression at the access site and clinical observation with resuscitation as indicated. For those patients that do not respond to resuscitation measures and continue to have decreasing hematocrit levels with evidence of hemodynamic compromise, there should be plans for urgent surgical exploration to control the bleeding site. Patients with a similar clinical picture that likely have bleeding at the more distal portions of the original angiography study path should have repeat angiography in order to define the bleeding source so that angioembolization techniques can be utilized to control the bleeding. However, surgery is needed for those cases where angio-embolization is unsuccessful.

Renal-related complications of angiography occur in approximately 1 to 2% of patients. Contrast nephropathy often is a temporary and possibly a preventable complication of radiologic workups utilizing contrast dye for CT, angiography, and/or venography. The research results have been mixed regarding the prevention of acute tubular necrosis from intravenous contrast with administration of n-acetylcysteine. There are some studies that suggest an overall improvement of renal function with n-acetylcysteine use, and other studies that report that its use has no overall benefit. If n-acetylcysteine is to provide benefit, twice-daily dosing 24 hours before and on the day of the radiographic study is suggested. It also is suggested that the greatest benefit with n-acetylcysteine is derived from improved intravenous hydration before and after the procedure. Nonionic contrast also may be of benefit in higher-risk patients. The contemporary literature does not support the use of other adjuncts such as administration of furosemide or mannitol prior to angiography, and these practices may add to overall morbidity rather than salvage renal function. As a current minimum, improved intravenous hydration before and after the procedure is still likely the simplest and most efficient method for providing renal protection from dye contrast.

Complications with Biopsies

Biopsies are performed for multiple reasons, including cosmesis, pathologic diagnosis, and prognostic evaluation. Lymph node biopsies have direct and indirect complications. Direct complications include bleeding, infection, lymph leakage, and seromas. Measures to prevent direct complications include proper surgical hemostasis,

proper wound preparation with chlorhexidine, gluconate/isopropyl alcohol, or a similar preparation, and possibly a single preoperative dose of antibiotic to cover skin flora 30 to 60 minutes before incision. Bleeding at a biopsy site usually will manifest shortly after the procedure, but often can be controlled with direct pressure. Infection at a biopsy site will generally not manifest for 5 to 10 days postoperatively, and will usually require opening of the wound to drain the necrotic infected tissue in order to facilitate wound healing. Seromas or lymphatic leaks may be difficult to manage at times. Depending on the volume and duration of leakage, control of a leak may take up to a few weeks to resolve with aspiration of seromas and the application of pressure dressings. If a seroma or leak does not resolve, it may be necessary to take the patient back to the operating room in order to place some form of closed suction drain into the wound. This usually is not necessary, and conservative management prevails.

Some surgeons prefer to place a closed suction drain in the vicinity of the dissection at the time of biopsy. At the time of drain placement and for the duration of the indwelling drain, antibiotics may be given, depending on the location of the drain, patient allergies, or the available formulary. Should a patient suffer an adverse event related to the antibiotics, this would exemplify an indirect complication.

ORGAN SYSTEM COMPLICATIONS

Neurologic System

Neurologic complications that arise for surgical patients include motor or sensory deficits and mental status changes. Motor and sensory deficits without direct neurologic injury via surgery are often detected in patients as neurapraxia secondary to improper positioning and/or padding during operations. Many operating rooms now have a gelatinous mattress that ensures even distribution of body weight so that pressure points on the otherwise unprotected body are attenuated. The motor and sensory nerves affected largely dictate the manifestation of neurapraxia. The anesthesiologist, the surgeon, and entire operating team must work together to provide adequate assurance that the patient will not develop these types of postoperative neurapraxia. Treatment is largely clinical observation, and the majority will resolve spontaneously within 1 to 3 months. Documentation of the extent of neurologic deficit with nerve conduction studies may offer some prognostic outlook for the patient, but does not change overall management.

Direct injury to nerves during a surgical intervention is a well-known complication of several specific operations, including superficial parotidectomy (facial nerve), carotid endarterectomy (hypoglossal nerve), prostatectomy (nervi erigentes) and inguinal herniorraphy (ilioinguinal nerve). It is possible that the nerve injury may simply be a stretch injury, or in a more severe scenario, an unintentionally severed nerve. In addition to loss of function, severed nerves also run the risk of developing a traumatic neuroma. Rarely does this specific injury require a subsequent surgery, but if the pain is intractable, operative intervention is an option. If nerve severance has occurred, then decisions regarding the choice of ongoing clinical observation versus an elective nerve graft repair are not made until several weeks of observation, so that delineation of the persistent deficit can be obtained. Success with nerve grafts remains less than optimal.

Mental status changes in the postoperative patient can have numerous causes (Table 11-1). Some of the possibilities are reasonably easy to diagnose if other clinical factors are obvious (e.g., sepsis plus bacteremia, leukocytosis, fever, and purulence from a wound), but others may not be so obvious and are diagnoses of exclusion.

Table 11-1
Common Causes of Mental Status Changes

Electrolyte Imbalance	Toxins	Trauma	Metabolic	Medications
Sodium	Ethanol	Closed head injury	Thyrotoxicosis	Aspirin
Magnesium	Methanol	Pain	Adrenal insufficiency	Beta blockers
Calcium	Venoms and poisons	Shock	Hypoxemia	Narcotics
Inflammation	Ethylene glycol	Psychiatric	Acidosis	Antiemetics
Sepsis	Carbon monoxide	Dementia	Severe Anemia	MAOIs
AIDS		Depression	Hyperammonemia	TCAs
Cerebral abscess		ICU psychosis	Poor glycemic control	Amphetamines
Meningitis		Schizophrenia	Hypothermia	Antiarrhythmics
Fever/hyperpyrexia			Hyperthermia	Corticosteroids
				Anabolic steroids

AIDS = acquired immunodeficiency syndrome; ICU = intensive care unit; MAOI = monoamine oxidase inhibitor; TCA = tricyclic antidepressant.

Nonetheless, mental status changes must be vigilantly followed and continually assessed. CT scanning should be employed early in the patient's diagnostic course if all other reasonable diagnoses have been ruled out.

Atherosclerotic disease plays a role in the risk for intraoperative and postoperative stroke (i.e., cerebrovascular accidents or CVAs), and usually is an extension of preexisting disease. When this tragic event occurs, other comorbidities should be assessed, since other events or problems may have contributed to the patient's condition such that they became susceptible to a CVA. Possibilities include technical issues related to intraoperative handling of a calcified central artery, arterial dissection, introducing air (embolism) into an artery, and intraoperative hypotension. Postoperatively, hypotension and hypoxemia are the most likely causes of CVA.

The diagnosis is most often confirmed by head CT scan, and cerebral angiography is usually reserved for those patients who have had direct manipulation of either the carotid or vertebral arteries, or for patients with symptoms that cannot be explained by the clinical scenario. Management of postoperative surgical patients with a fresh CVA is largely supportive once the diagnosis is made, and includes adequate intravascular volume replacement plus optimal oxygen delivery. Neurologic consultation is important to obtain so that decisions regarding the possible need for thrombolysis and anticoagulation can be made in a timely fashion.

Ears, Eyes, and Nose

The general surgeon typically has little direct involvement with the eyes. On occasion there might be forgotten contact lenses in a trauma patient with the appearance of conjunctivitis. Perioperatively, patients may also develop or acquire corneal abrasions.

Persistent epistaxis can be troublesome following nasogastric tube placement or removal, and when this occurs, nasal packing is the best treatment option if prolonged persistent direct pressure on the external nares fails. Anterior and posterior nasal gauze packing with balloon tamponade, angioembolization, and even fibrin glue placement may be required, but another option is angioembolization for refractory cases. The use of antibiotics for posterior packing is controversial, but the incidence of toxic shock syndrome is documented at approximately 17:100,000 cases of nasal surgery. First-generation cephalosporins usually are initiated at the same time as the nasal packing; however, no data exist that prove antibiotics provide improved outcome or prevent infection. One small (n = 22) study showed that when antibiotic-impregnated gauze was used with cefazolin, the gauze was not as foul smelling and was only lightly colonized with gram-negative bacteria.[11] This is

in comparison to the placebo group, which demonstrated a higher incidence of foul-smelling packing colonized with gram-negative organisms. Interestingly, neither group suffered from significant infectious complications.

Other than sacrificing some of the superficial cervical nerves or incidentally damaging the greater auricular nerve during neck or facial surgery, errors committed in the care of patients with surgery involving the ear are limited. External otitis and otitis media occasionally are noticed postoperatively if a patient complains of ear pain, but these are not common problems. Treatment is focused on topical antibiotics and nasal decongestion for symptomatic improvement.

Ototoxicity due to aminoglycoside administration occurs at rates of less than 0.002% (in a study of >2100 patients) to about 10% in humans. Studies of aminoglycosides in animals (mostly guinea pigs) demonstrate that ototoxicity occurs much more often in these animals compared to humans. Perhaps the most important issue regarding ototoxicity due to aminoglycoside use is that it is often irreversible. Recent data show that iron chelating agents, as well as alpha-tocopherol, may be protective against ototoxicity. More studies are needed to confirm these findings, even though the practice is being implemented in some centers as an investigational agent. Vancomycin-related ototoxicity occurs about 3% of the time when used alone, and as high as 6% when used with other ototoxic agents. The promising finding associated with vancomycin is that the ototoxicity due to vancomycin is self-limiting.[12,13]

Vascular Problems of the Neck

Vascular surgery errors in the carotid vessels of the neck are fairly straightforward. Technical errors from carotid endarterectomy presenting after surgery manifest themselves as a neurologic deficit (e.g., hemiplegia or aphasia) or bleeding with an expanding neck hematoma. These complications warrant immediate return to the operating room since often there is either a stenotic lesion with thrombus or an arterial dissection, and both of these require emergent operative intervention. An expanding hematoma in the postoperative care area also warrants emergent airway intubation and subsequent transfer to the operating room. Intraoperative anticoagulation with heparin during carotid surgery makes bleeding a postoperative risk, especially when the high-risk patient is not reversed. Contemporary data do not support the concept that a postoperative hematoma should be blamed on the use of low molecular weight dextran for carotid surgery.

Infection after carotid endarterectomy is rare, but when present, is usually due to an infected synthetic graft. Several complications can arise, such as arteriovenous fistulae, pseudoaneurysms, and hematomas, all of which are treated surgically.

It is important to have good communication with the anesthesia team when working at the carotid bifurcation, because intraoperative hypotension can be related to increased tone from the baroreceptors, or hypertension can be due to stimulation of the carotid sinus. Should a patient become hypotensive when manipulating the carotid bifurcation, an injection of 1% lidocaine solution into this structure should attenuate this reflexive response. In the immediate postoperative period, persistent hemodynamic lability occasionally can be difficult to control, and reasons for this largely arise from pain control issues. If adequate analgesia is provided and labile blood pressures persist, the use of vasoactive agents is warranted to control blood pressure in order to minimize the potential for bleeding and/or ischemia. The requirement for these agents is usually for less than 24 hours.

The most common late complication following carotid endarterectomy is myocardial infarction; death rates from 20 to 100% have been seen after this complication. The possibility of a postoperative myocardial infarction should be considered as a cause of labile blood pressure and arrhythmias in high-risk patients. An electrocardiogram and echocardiogram are especially helpful, in addition to the measurement of cardiac enzymes. Treatment should follow standard acute coronary syndrome protocols.

Thyroid and Parathyroid Glands

Surgery of the thyroid and parathyroid glands can lend itself to various complications. Bleeding should be obvious, but specific electrolyte abnormalities will also contribute to postoperative morbidity, and possibly mortality, if not followed closely.

Electrolyte abnormalities largely involve calcium and to a lesser extent phosphate. During thyroidectomy—whether subtotal or total—close follow-up of serum calcium levels (preferably ionized calcium) is warranted. Acutely, patients can have frank manifestations of hypocalcemia in the immediate postoperative period. These include electrocardiogram changes (shortened P-R interval), muscle spasm (tetany, Chvostek's sign, and Trousseau's sign), paresthesias, and laryngospasm. Treatment includes calcium gluconate infusion, and if tetany ensues, chemical paralysis with intubation. Maintenance treatment is thyroid hormone replacement in addition to calcium carbonate and vitamin D.

A recurrent laryngeal nerve injury occurs in less than 5% of patients. Of those with injury, approximately 10% are permanent. As the thyroid gland is dissected from lateral to medial, the dissection near the inferior thyroid artery is a common area for injury. At the conclusion of the operation many surgeons choose to perform direct laryngoscopy to assess vocal cord apposition. The cord on the affected side will be in the paramedian position. Where a total thyroidectomy is performed and bilateral cords have been injured, the chance of a successful extubation is poor. The cords are found to be in the midline, and an early sign of respiratory distress is stridor with labored breathing. If paralysis of the cords is not permanent, function may return 1 to 2 months after injury. Permanent injury to the cords can be treated by various techniques to stent the cords in a position of function; however, there are differing rates of success, and these procedures are only performed several months after the surgery.

Superior laryngeal nerve injury is less debilitating, providing the patient's profession is not related to their vocal performance, as the common symptom is loss of projection of the voice. The glottic aperture is asymmetrical on direct laryngoscopy and management is based on clinical observation.

Respiratory System

Errors in surgery that put the respiratory system in jeopardy are not always confined to technical errors yielding pneumothoraces. These include malnutrition, inadequate pain control, inadequate mechanical ventilation, inadequate pulmonary toilet, and all phases of pneumonia (i.e., prevention, diagnosis, and management).

Pneumothoraces can have an insidious presentation or a more dramatic manifestation. The tension pneumothorax may have the clinical presentation of hypotension, hypoxemia, and tracheal deviation away from the affected side. If severe enough, the patient appears toxic and nears complete cardiovascular collapse. Treatment is by needle thoracostomy, followed by tube thoracostomy. Placement of the needle is often described as the midclavicular line in the second rib interspace, but it also may be placed where the chest tube will be inserted, the fifth intercostal space in the anterior axillary line. Tension pneumothorax is an emergency and warrants tube thoracostomy in all occurrences.

Hemothorax rarely is due to an operative error, and is most commonly the result of trauma. Other benign reasons for hemothorax include ruptured pulmonary cysts, rupture of pulmonary arteriovenous fistulae, ruptures of aneurysmal disease within the subclavian, and rupture of the innominate and aortic vessels. Trauma patients usually require tube thoracotomy for hemothorax. Should there be a delay in evacuation of the hemothorax, the patient is at significant risk for empyema and entrapped lung. If evacuation of the hemothorax is incomplete with tube thoracostomy, the patient should undergo video-assisted thoracoscopy, because of the advantages related to pain control, length of hospital stay, and a more rapid return to normal function.

Pulmonary atelectasis is not always thought of as a complication. Nonetheless, the loss of functional residual capacity (FRC) of the lung has clinical as well as cellular implications. Many postoperative surgery patients—especially those with poor pain control—can be found lying in bed watching television or reading. An increase of the lungs' FRC by 700 mL or more can be accomplished by sitting these patients up to greater than 45°, which improves spontaneous ventilation remarkably. For mechanically-ventilated patients it recently has been accepted that simply placing the head of the patient's bed at 30 to 45 degrees in elevation improves pulmonary outcomes. The prevention of atelectasis is facilitated by delivering adequate tidal volumes (8 to 10 mL/kg), preventing the abdominal domain from impinging on the thoracic cavity, and by sitting the patient up in bed as much as possible. This includes having the ventilated patient out of bed and sitting in a chair if possible. Should the patient develop acute respiratory distress syndrome, then lower tidal volumes are recommended, and the functional alveoli would then be supported with positive end-expiratory pressure.

Pulmonary aspiration occurs daily in everyone to a small degree, but this microaspiration is not significant or injurious, because healthy individuals have adequate defense mechanisms in place to avoid the development of serious complications such as pneumonitis or pneumonia. These defenses include the upper digestive system where secretions are rendered relatively free from harmful organisms due to gastric acidity. Furthermore, the tracheobronchial tree is lined with active cilia that mobilize secretions cephalad, and when combined with a productive, unrestricted cough, keeps the healthy individual safe from aspirated material.

Aspiration complications include pneumonitis and pneumonia. The treatment of pneumonitis is similar to that for acute lung injury (see below), and includes oxygenation with general supportive care. Antibiotics are usually contraindicated unless known organisms are

detected with bacteriologic analysis. Hospitalized patients who develop aspiration pneumonia carry a mortality rate as high as 70 to
80%. Early, aggressive, and repeated bronchoscopy for suctioning
of aspirated material from the tracheobronchial tree will help to
minimize the inflammatory reaction of pneumonitis and facilitate
improved pulmonary toilet.

Patients with inadequate pulmonary toilet, for whatever reason,
are at increased risk for bronchial plugging and lobar collapse. Patients with copious and tenacious secretions tend to develop these
plugs most often, but foreign bodies in the bronchus can be the
cause of lobar collapse as well. The diagnosis of bronchial plugging is suspected by chest x-ray and clinical suspicion when there is
acute pulmonary decompensation with increased work of breathing
and hypoxemia. Fiberoptic bronchoscopy can be useful in diagnosis, but its utility for assisting with pulmonary toilet when other
routine bedside physical therapy maneuvers fail is debatable regarding its benefit to relieve this complication. Only a few studies exist
on the utility of bronchoscopy for pulmonary toilet, and they have
variable results, but when the resources are readily available, the
cost-effectiveness of performing bronchoscopy may be worthwhile.

Pneumonia

Pneumonia is the second most common nosocomial infection and
it is the most common nosocomial infection in ventilated patients.[13]
Pneumonia may be a difficult diagnosis to make in a patient with
acute lung injury or the systemic inflammatory response syndrome.
Trauma patients with pulmonary contusions are also difficult for
making the diagnosis of pneumonia.

The significance of pneumonia cannot be overstated. Ventilator-
associated pneumonia (VAP) occurs in 15 to 40% of ventilated ICU
patients, and accrues at a daily probability rate of 5% per day, up to
70% at 30 days. In fact, transporting the ventilated patient out of the
ICU to radiology or other hospital areas increases the risk of VAP
by 15%. The 30-day mortality rate of nosocomial pneumonia can
be as high as 40%, and depends on the microorganisms involved
and the timeliness of initiating appropriate treatment.

Once the diagnosis of pneumonia is suspected (an abnormal chest
x-ray, fever, productive cough with purulent sputum, and no other
obvious fever sources), it is invariably necessary to initially begin
treatment with broad-spectrum antibiotics until proper identification, colony count ($\geq$100,000 CFU), and sensitivity of the microorganisms are determined.[14] Current data suggest that a single-agent
antibiotic may be better than a double-agent, and it is imperative
that the spectrum of antibiotic coverage be narrowed as soon as the
culture sensitivities have been identified. However, initial double-
coverage antibiotic strategy for the two pathogens, *Pseudomonas*
and *Acinetobacter* spp., may outweigh the risks of not providing
double-coverage for these particularly virulent organisms.

A higher number of antibiotic changes before the specific treatment of pneumonia can occur has been demonstrated to increase
mortality. One of the most helpful tools in treating pneumonia and
other infections is the tracking of a medical center's antibiogram
every 6 to 12 months.[15] Some institutions will rotate the availability
and usage of their formulary antibiotics according to their antibiogram, but the efficacy of this practice remains controversial.

An adjunct to decrease the opportunity for perioperative pneumonia has been the more widespread implementation of epidural
anesthesia. This method of pain control improves pulmonary toilet and the early return of bowel function; both have a significant
impact on the potential for aspiration and for acquiring pneumonia. This is in contrast to a recent study of 515 patients using

patient-controlled analgesia, where the infectious risks for pneumonia were higher than with epidural anesthesia.[16]

Acute Lung Injury and Acute Respiratory Distress Syndrome

Acute lung injury (ALI) is a diagnosis applied to patients with
similar findings to those with acute respiratory distress syndrome
(ARDS). These should be considered a spectrum of the same disease process, with the difference being in the degree of oxygenation
deficits of patients. The pathology, pathophysiology, and the mechanism of lung injury for ALI are the same as for ARDS, except that
the arterial oxygen to inspired oxygen (PaO_2:FIO_2) ratio is >200
but <300 for ALI and <200 for ARDS. Both types of patients
will require some form of positive pressure ventilatory assistance
in order to improve the oxygenation deficits, while simultaneously
treating the primary etiology of the initiating disease. The definition
of ARDS includes the following (Table 11-2):

1. A known etiology or disease exists that would predispose to ARDS
2. Pulmonary artery occlusion pressures are less than 18 mm Hg
3. No clinical evidence exists for right heart failure, subsequent to left heart
   failure
4. Diffuse bilateral pulmonary infiltrates are found on chest x-ray
5. The PaO_2:FIO_2 ratio is less than 200

The recent multicenter ARDS Research Network (ARDSnet)
research trial demonstrated improved clinical outcomes for ARDS
patients ventilated at tidal volumes of 5 to 7 mL/kg.[17] This was a
complex research initiative, but it is important to note that these
ventilator settings are for patients with ARDS, and caution should
be exercised about extrapolating the data to otherwise healthy patients requiring ventilatory support for a variety of other reasons.
The beneficial effects of PEEP for ARDS were confirmed in this
study as well. In general, the maintenance of PEEP during ventilatory support is managed based on blood gas analysis, pulmonary
mechanics, and requirements for supplemental oxygen. As gas exchange improves with resolving ARDS, the initial step in decreasing
ventilatory support should be to decrease the levels of supplemental
oxygen first, and then to slowly bring the PEEP levels back down to
minimal levels.[18] This is done in order to minimize the potential for
recurrent alveolar collapse and a worsening gas exchange, if there
are still some areas of the lungs involved with the ARDS process
and weaning is premature.

The practice of placing patients prone for mechanical ventilation in ARDS has produced interesting controversy. The risks
involved with turning patients prone include hypotension, extubation, accidental central venous access removal but oxygenation
and ventilation arguably improves. Since the landmark paper[19] by
Gattinoni was published describing prone ventilation for ARDS,
which was only practiced once per 24-hour period for 6 to 8
hours, several variations have produced interesting results that need

Table 11-2

Inclusion Criteria for the Acute Respiratory Distress Syndrome (ARDS)

Acute onset
Predisposing condition
PaO_2:FIO_2 ratio <200 (regardless of positive end-expiratory pressure)
Bilateral infiltrates
Pulmonary artery occlusion pressure <18 mm Hg
No clinical evidence of right heart failure

further investigation before claiming that this labor-intensive therapy should be a standard of care.[20,21]

For those not suffering from ARDS, underventilation of patients' lungs may create iatrogenic injury by producing an atelectatic lung with progressive alveolar collapse, or derecruitment. This can make ventilator weaning, or liberation from the ventilator, more difficult than might be expected, while also subjecting patients to the additional risks of pneumonia, tracheostomy, or superinfection. A ventilatory recruitment process with mechanical ventilation also has its price. As the loss of functional alveoli increases (atelectasis), the production of surfactant from the type II pneumocytes decreases and makes alveolar recruitment more difficult. When these alveoli are then reexpanded with PEEP or larger tidal volumes, the alveoli may have significant airway shearing forces exerted on them by the ventilatory pressure.[22,23] This process can then injure the alveolar cell membrane, creating the stimulus for a subsequent release of local and systemic cytokines, which then further increases the inflammatory mediator response throughout the pulmonary tissue and the body as a whole. Several studies are currently examining the efficacy of recruitment maneuvers, and the data show that more prospective, randomized, controlled studies need to be performed to make a proper conclusion.

Failure to Wean from Ventilation

Not all patients can be liberated easily from mechanical ventilation. When the respiratory muscle energy demands are not balanced, or there is an ongoing active disease state external to the lungs, patients may require prolonged ventilatory support. An acceptance that protocol-driven ventilator weaning strategies are successful has become gradually but progressively more popular. The use of a weaning protocol for patients on mechanical ventilation greater than 48 hours reduces the incidence of VAP and the overall length of time on mechanical ventilation, when compared with non-protocol managed ventilator weaning. This use of ventilator weaning protocols should continue to be initiated on a widespread basis.

Unfortunately there is still no truly reliable way of predicting which patient will be successfully extubated after a weaning program, and the decision for extubation is based on a combination of clinical parameters and measured pulmonary mechanics.[23] The Tobin Index (frequency:tidal volume ratio), also known as the rapid shallow breathing index (RSBI), is perhaps the best negative predictive instrument when performed as Yang and Tobin originally described.[24] If the result equals <105, then there is nearly a 70% chance the patient will pass extubation. If the score is >105, the patient has an approximately 80% chance of failing extubation. Other parameters such as the negative inspiratory force, minute ventilation, and respiratory rate are important to assess, but individually have no better predictive value than the RSBI.[25]

Malnutrition and poor nutritional support may adversely affect the respiratory system. The respiratory quotient (RQ), or respiratory exchange ratio (RER), is the ratio of the rate of carbon dioxide produced to the rate of oxygen uptake ($RQ = Vco_2/Vo_2$). Briefly, lipids, carbohydrates, and protein, when used as fuel, have differing effects on energy. Patients consuming a diet consisting mostly of carbohydrates would have an RQ of 1 or greater. A diet mostly of lipids would be closer to 0.7, and a diet of mostly protein would be closer to 0.8. Ideally, an RQ of 0.75 to 0.85 would suggest that a patient's nutritional intake was of adequate balance and composition. An excess of carbohydrate in nutritional therapy occasionally may negatively affect ventilator weaning because of the abnormal RQ and altered pulmonary gas exchange.

The administration of recombinant human growth hormone (hGH) to optimize a patient's respiratory status has received critical review. In the septic patient it should not be used, as this may worsen clinical outcomes, but patients who are not infected but who require a prolonged ventilator wean may benefit from recombinant hGH. The research data on pediatric populations tend to be stronger, and investigational studies are ongoing in the adult population. An anabolic steroid that is under investigational clinical use is oxandrolone, and its use is primarily for its anabolic properties in the nutritionally replete patient who has significant ongoing nitrogen losses.

The decisions and timing for performing a tracheostomy in order to facilitate weaning remains controversial. Although not without risk, tracheostomy will decrease the pulmonary dead space and provides for improved pulmonary toilet. When performed prior to 7 to 10 days of ventilatory support, tracheostomy may decrease the incidence of VAP, the overall length of ventilator time, and the number of ICU patient days.

Pulmonary Embolism

The occurrence of pulmonary embolism (PE) is probably underdiagnosed. Its etiology stems from deep vein thrombosis (DVT). Virchow's triad of venous stasis, a propensity to form thrombus, and a local vascular injury are the cardinal findings in those patients who develop a DVT. The diagnosis of PE usually is made with a high degree of clinical suspicion for PE and by utilizing corroborating imaging techniques such as ventilation:perfusion nuclear scans (VQ scans) or CT pulmonary angiogram. Clinical findings include elevated central venous pressure, hypoxemia, shortness of breath, hypocarbia secondary to tachypnea, and right heart strain noted on electrocardiogram. The VQ scans often are unhelpful because of the indeterminate nature for the study with patients who have been lying in bed for a prolonged period, and have subsequently developed significant atelectasis.

The pulmonary angiogram remains the gold standard for diagnosing PE, but several centers have shifted to using spiral CT angiogram as the study of choice because of its relative ease of use and reasonable rates of diagnostic accuracy. There still needs to be more definitive studies completed to confirm the adequacy and predictive capabilities of spiral CT in the diagnosis of PE. For cases without clinical contraindications to therapeutic anticoagulation, a pulmonary angiogram is not an emergent procedure in the acute setting, and patients should be empirically started on heparin infusion until the imaging studies are completed if the suspicion of a PE is strong.

Although many institutions provide sequential compression devices on the lower extremities, no study exists to date that proves these devices actually decrease the incidence of PE. However, these devices have been shown to decrease the incidence of DVT. Neurosurgical and orthopedic patients have higher rates than general surgery patients, but other patients with a high propensity to form thrombosis and are at risk for PE include trauma patients and obstetric patients.

Typically, venous clots will form in the lower extremities and propagate to the pelvic veins. CT scanning will often detect pelvic vein clots, but lower extremity duplex imaging cannot reliably image the pelvic veins. The relevant literature is not clear as to the best way to manage patients for DVT screening or prophylaxis. The use of lower extremity duplex screening, subcutaneous heparin (either twice or three times daily), and low molecular weight heparins that have better bioavailability are hot topics for debate. Outpatient therapy for DVT and PE is not only the standard of care, but is cost effective. Treatment is ambulation and low molecular weight heparin or warfarin administration for a total of 3 to 6 months. The use of either agent is not without complications, only one of which is bleeding. Heparin-induced thrombocytopenia II (HIT II) is a difficult diagnosis to document, and has a thrombosis complication rate as high as 40%. When the diagnosis of HIT is made, it is important to anticoagulate patients for 2 weeks using synthetic substances such as argatroban or lepirudin, depending on the patient's renal or hepatic function.

Finally, a discussion of DVT and PE would not be complete without including caval interruption devices. The Greenfield filter has been most widely studied, and it has a failure rate of about 2 to 4%. Newer devices include those with nitinol wire that expands with body temperature, and retrievable filters. The newer retrievable filters can be deployed and then retrieved as long as 4 to 6 weeks later. The indications for caval filters generally fall into three categories: a failure or complication with anticoagulation, a known free-floating venous clot, and a prior history of PE. Patients with spinal cord injury and multiple long-bone or pelvic fractures frequently receive caval filters, and there appears to be a low long-term complication rate with the use of caval filters in younger trauma patients.

Cardiac System

Cardiac abnormalities can manifest themselves in a variety of forms. For instance, systolic dysfunction with dilated ventricular size, decreased contractility, and decreased cardiac output is often treated with diuresis, afterload reduction, and inotropic support. Diastolic dysfunction with ventricular hypertrophy that has increased contractility and decreased cardiac output is often treated with beta blockade or calcium channel blockers. Coronary insufficiency and myocardial ischemia also can create unpredictable difficulties with an acute coronary syndrome. Anticipation of these factors can prevent the morbidity and possible mortality associated with perioperative cardiac problems.

When evaluating the potential candidacy of elderly patients for surgery, in addition to a careful history and physical examination, the preoperative ECG remains important. If these indicators raise any suspicion for cardiac disease, a more extensive cardiac or cardiopulmonary work-up is required before surgery.

Arrhythmias

Chronic and acute arrhythmias often are seen preoperatively in elderly patients. Atrial fibrillation commonly occurs between postoperative days 3 to 5 in high-risk patients. These are typically the days in which patients begin to mobilize their interstitial fluid into the vascular fluid space, with a presumed rise in the oncotic pressure so that the fluid in the interstitial space flows back into the vascular space, and thereby increases the cardiac preload. The heart is then exposed to more volume than a marginally-functioning heart can manage.

The most common form of perioperative arrhythmia is atrial fibrillation.[26] Difficulties for surgical patients with atrial arrhythmias include the arrhythmia itself, anticoagulation that is often associated with atrial fibrillation, and the other cardiac or blood pressure medications that the patients are currently prescribed. Contemporary, evidence-based practice suggests that rate control is more important than rhythm control for atrial fibrillation.[27,28] The first-line strategy for this includes beta blockade and/or calcium channel blockade. Beta blockade must be utilized judiciously, because hypotension, as well as withdrawal from beta blockade with rebound

hypertension, are primary drawbacks to these agents. Calcium channel blockers are a viable option if beta blockers are not tolerated by the patient, but caution must be exercised in those with a history of congestive heart failure. There also is an increased risk for conduction abnormalities and heart block when using both types of agents concomitantly.[29–31] While digoxin is still a faithful standby medication, it has limitations due to the need for optimal dosing levels. Additionally, patients with renal insufficiency are difficult to manage. The therapeutic window for digoxin is highly variable and renders serum digoxin levels fairly useless except for documenting digoxin toxicity. Cardioversion may be required if patients become hemodynamically unstable and the rhythm cannot be controlled.

Ventricular arrhythmias and other tachyarrhythmias may occur in surgical patients as well. Similar to atrial rhythm problems, these may best be controlled with beta blockade, but the use of other antiarrhythmics or cardioversion may be required if patients become hemodynamically unstable and the rhythm cannot be controlled. There must also be close monitoring of electrolyte abnormalities and other potential causative etiologies for the ventricular arrhythmias. Occasionally, formal cardiac electrophysiology studies will be needed to clarify the etiology of the arrhythmias so that medical or surgical treatment can be tailored, including the possible surgical ablation of ventricular foci. Sudden cardiac death in hospital may still occur with these arrhythmias and is a distressing event.

Ischemia

Cardiac ischemia is always a concern. Acute myocardial infarction (AMI) can present as insidiously as worsening diabetes mellitus (DM), or it can be more dramatic with the classic presentation of shortness of breath (SOB), chest pain or jaw pain with radiation of pain to the left arm, and as rapid-onset cardiogenic shock. The work-up for any of these presentations begins with clinical suspicion and a laboratory investigation to rule out AMI. The work-up may also begin on the surgical floor with a chest x-ray and ECG, but the AMI patient should be transferred to a monitored (telemetry) floor as soon as a bed is available. *M*orphine, supplemental *o*xygen, *n*itroglycerine, and *a*spirin (MONA) are the initial therapeutic maneuvers for those who are being investigated for AMI.

Hypertension in the immediate postoperative period may be merely a failure of adequate pain control, but other causes include hypoxia, volume overload, and rebound hypertension from not resuming beta blockade and/or clonidine. Perioperative hypertension carries significant morbidity and aggressive control with medication(s) is warranted. Patients with chronic atherosclerotic disease present with hypertension 20 to 50% of the time, and reasons for perioperative hypertension include cerebrovascular disease, renal artery stenosis, and aorto-occlusive disease. Pheochromocytoma is an uncommon finding that causes hypertension, but should be considered if there are imaging studies suggestive for an adrenal mass.

With the concerns for arrhythmias, myocardial ischemia, and hypertension that may exacerbate perfusion abnormalities, the concept of routine perioperative cardiac protective strategies with beta blockade is rapidly becoming adopted. The success of cardiac protection in acute coronary syndromes makes this an appealing concept, but further studies are still required before cardiac protective protocols in routine perioperative care are accepted.

Gastrointestinal System

Surgery of the esophagus is potentially complicated because of its anatomic location and blood supply. The two primary types of esophageal resection performed are the transhiatal resection and the transthoracic (Ivor-Lewis) resection.[32] Each carries its own risks and benefits, but they can have successful outcomes with minimal 28-day morbidity and mortality rates.

The transhiatal resection has the advantage that a formal thoracotomy incision is avoided. The dissection of the esophagus is blind, however, and the blood supply from the aortoesophageal arteries may lend itself to moderate blood loss if not controlled properly. Furthermore, a proper mediastinal lymph node dissection for staging is not conducted, and the cervical anastomosis tends to leak more than with other resections. However, when a leak does occur, simple opening of the cervical incision and draining the leak is all that is usually required. When compared with the Ivor-Lewis resection, survival and recurrence data, and morbidity and mortality rates all seem to be equal.

The transthoracic Ivor-Lewis resection includes an esophageal anastomosis performed in the chest near the level of the azygos vein. These resections tend not to leak as often, but when they do, they can be difficult to control if not managed properly. The reported mortality is about 50% with an anastomotic leak, and the overall mortality is about 5%. Nutritional support strategies must be addressed early for these patients in order to maximize the potential for survival.

Nissen fundoplication is an operation that is fraught with possibilities for error. Bleeding is always a potential hazard, so dissection of the short gastric vessels must be done with care. Laparoscopic port site bleeding, injury to the aorta, and liver lacerations can also contribute to significant blood loss. The fundoplication may be too tightly wrapped or become unwrapped postoperatively. The use of a bougie dilator intraoperatively depends on the size of the patient, but it is usually between 54 and 60F, and is used to facilitate the proper tension for the Nissen wrap. Postoperative edema and patient noncompliance will produce immediate postoperative symptoms of odynophagia and dysphagia. Failure of wrap integrity is well described in the literature. The reasons for failure usually include wrap dehiscence, gastric herniation, too short a wrap, and a loosened wrap. Studies examining repair of the esophageal hiatus are controversial. The prevailing principle was that a posterior repair was better, but newer studies have called this into question. Reoperative failure rates in the contemporary literature are around 3 to 5%.[33,34]

Postoperative ileus is related to dysfunction of the neural reflex axis of the intestine. Early return to ambulation may be one of the most beneficial maneuvers patients can perform, but there is no clear data that this initiates a return of GI function, but there are no clear data that this is actually the case. Exacerbation of an ileus due to excess perioperative narcotic use may delay return of bowel function. Epidural anesthesia in abdominal surgery is becoming more popular, and the data show that pain control is improved, there is an earlier return of bowel function, and length of hospital stay is shortened. Although still not generally accepted, the limited use of nasogastric tubes and the initiation of early postoperative feeding before the full return of bowel function can both contribute significantly to a shorter time for postoperative ileus.

The method of bowel surgery likely plays a role in postoperative bowel function as well. Numerous studies have shown a decreased length of stay and improved pain control when bowel surgery is performed laparoscopically. This has been challenged recently in at least one study, in which patients with open colon resection were fed at the same time as the laparoscopically treated patients and the study showed no difference in hospital length of stay.[35]

Pharmacologic agents commonly used to stimulate bowel function include metoclopramide and erythromycin. Metoclopramide's efficacy is limited to the stomach, and it may help primarily with gastroparesis. Erythromycin is a motilin-agonist that works throughout the stomach and bowel. Several studies demonstrate significant benefit from the administration of erythromycin in those suffering from an ileus. Several recent small studies have examined the role of cyclooxygenase-2 (COX-2) inhibitors and chewing gum, but larger controlled studies will be needed to support the findings that COX-2 inhibitors for analgesia and the use of chewing gum can lead to an earlier return of bowel function and decreased length of stay.[36]

Early postoperative small bowel obstruction is a rare finding and occurs less than 1% of the time. When it does occur, adhesions are largely to blame, and are the nidus of obstruction about 90% of the time. Internal and external hernias make up nearly 7% of obstructions, while technical errors, infections, or abscesses make up the remainder. No one can accurately predict which patients will form obstructive postoperative adhesions, because all patients who undergo surgery likely form adhesions to some extent, and there is very little that surgeons can do to limit this natural healing process. Hyaluronidase is a mucolytic enzyme that degrades connective tissue (chiefly hyaluronic acid), and this agent has many uses in surgery. The manufacturer of a methylcellulose form of hyaluronidase, Seprafilm, maintains that patients treated with this agent have a 50% decrease in adhesion formation. This should translate into a lower occurrence of postoperative bowel obstruction, but this has not been shown. In one study of 183 patients operated on for benign disease with colectomy and subsequent ileoanal pouch construction, 9% developed a bowel obstruction in the treatment group, and 10% developed an obstruction in the control group.[37] Other studies suggest that Seprafilm prevents postoperative bowel obstructions.[38,39]

Gastrointestinal fistulae of any sort—enterocutaneous (>20% in Crohn's disease), colovesicular, rectovaginal, aortoenteric (~0.3 to 2% with aortic reconstructive surgery), or pancreatic (10 to 29% of pancreatic resections)—are associated with extensive morbidity and mortality. Common causes for fistula formation include: distal obstruction, external beam radiation, inadequate nutrition, inflammation, neoplastic disease, foreign body reaction, and trauma. The original cause of the fistula must be recognized early so that definitive management can be undertaken in a timely fashion. This may mean nonoperative management with observation and nutritional support, or a delayed operative management strategy that also includes nutritional support and wound care.

Gastrointestinal bleeding as a complication of surgery can occur perioperatively (Table 11-3). Intraoperatively, a poorly tied suture, a technically poor staple line, or a missed injury can all lead to postoperative intestinal bleeding.[40,41] Postoperative intestinal bleeding is most often an upper intestinal bleed. In the ICU, the upper intestinal tract is the source of bleeding about 85% of the time. Surgical control of intestinal bleeding is required in 30 to 40% of patients. The diagnostic accuracy of upper endoscopy in upper gastrointestinal bleeding is 90%.[42] In addition, in those patients whose bleeding has stopped, clear evidence does not exist, nor support emergent endoscopy in order to decrease the morbidity of recurrent bleeding. The most common causes of upper gastrointestinal bleeding are esophageal varices, gastric varices, and duodenal ulcers.

When patients in the ICU have a major bleed from stress gastritis, the mortality risk is as high as 50%. Thus it remains important to keep the gastric pH greater than 4 in order to decrease the overall risk for stress gastritis to 6 or 7%. Stress gastritis prophylaxis was addressed recently in 2002 by Cash.[43] In short, there are only two populations that require stress gastritis prophylaxis: patients mechanically ventilated for 48 hours or greater and patients who

Table 11-3
Common Causes of Upper and Lower Gastrointestinal Hemorrhage

Upper GI Bleed	Lower GI Bleed
Erosive esophagitis	Angiodysplasia
Gastric varices	Radiation proctitis
Esophageal varices	Hemangioma
Dieulafoy's lesion	Diverticulosis
Aortoduodenal fistula	Neoplastic diseases
Mallory-Weiss tear	Trauma
Peptic ulcer disease	Vasculitis
Trauma	Hemorrhoids
Neoplastic disease	Aortoenteric fistula
	Intussusception
	Ischemic colitis
	Inflammatory bowel disease
	Postprocedure bleeding

are coagulopathic. The benefits of proton pump inhibitors over H_2 antagonists were not clear, although other studies suggest that proton pump inhibitors may be more effective.

Hepatobiliary-Pancreatic System

Errors in surgery involving the hepatobiliary tree are most always technical. Laparoscopic cholecystectomy has become the standard of care for cholecystectomy, but laparoscopic cholecystectomy still has complications that can be devastating. Common bile duct injury is a primary concern for all who perform these operations. Intraoperative cholangiography has not been shown to decrease the incidence of common bile duct injuries, and often these errors have occurred prior to the cholangiogram because the surgical dissection was done under difficult conditions.[44,45] When they do occur it is important, if possible, to identify the injury early because delayed bile duct leaks often lead to a more complex repair and a more severely ill patient.

The repair of common bile duct injuries depends on the mechanism of injury. Ischemic injury is largely due to devascularization of the common bile duct. Frequently this has a delayed presentation in which the patient complains of chronic abdominal pain days to weeks after an operation. Ultrasonography and/or endoscopic retrograde cholangiopancreatography (ERCP) demonstrate a stenotic, smooth common bile duct. Liver function studies are elevated. The recommended treatment is a Roux-en-Y hepaticojejunostomy. The other injury that may present itself in a delayed fashion after cholecystectomy is that of a biloma. These patients may present with diffuse abdominal pain that may be severe or moderate, with or without peritonitis. Liver function tests usually demonstrate hyperbilirubinemia, and the diagnosis of a biliary leak can be confirmed with a combination of CT scan, ERCP, or dimethyl iminodiacetic acid (HIDA) scan. Once a leak is confirmed, then a retrograde biliary stent and external drainage is the treatment of choice and surgery is not required. The leak may take several weeks to stop, and repeat laparotomy is only needed if the patient develops sepsis or peritonitis.

Hyperbilirubinemia in the surgical patient can be a complex problem. A careful history and physical exam is of paramount importance in order to be able to quickly diagnose its etiology and form a cost-effective treatment plan. Cholestasis makes up the majority of causes for hyperbilirubinemia, but other mechanisms of hyperbilirubinemia include reabsorption of blood (e.g., hematoma from trauma), decreased excretion (e.g., sepsis), increased unconjugated

bilirubin (e.g., hemolytic anemia), hyperthyroidism, and impaired excretion due to congenital abnormalities or acquired disease. Errors in surgery that cause hyperbilirubinemia largely involve technical problems, such as missed or iatrogenic injuries.

Although cirrhosis is largely a medical problem, surgeons are often asked to help manage and to operate on the cirrhotic patient. Hernias, a perforated viscus from peptic ulcer disease or diverticulitis, or acute cholecystitis with or without cholangitis often present a surgical management challenge in the cirrhotic patient. Ascites leak in the postoperative period can be an issue when any abdominal operation has been performed, because fluid management is complex. Maintaining proper intravascular oncotic pressure in the immediate postoperative period can be very difficult, and resuscitation should be maintained with crystalloid solutions. Although it may be tempting to replace fluid losses with albumin, anecdotal data do not support this practice. Prevention of renal failure and the management of the hepatorenal syndrome can be difficult, as the demands of fluid resuscitation and altered glomerular filtration become competitive. It is not unreasonable for the patient to be placed on their outpatient doses of spironolactone and other diuretic agents in the resuscitative phase of postoperative care. These patients often have a labile course and close attention is required by the surgical team to ensure a safe recovery. The operative mortality in cirrhotic patients is 10% for Child class A, 30% for Child class B, and 82% for Child class C patients.[46]

Pyogenic liver abscesses occur in less than 0.5% of adult admissions, but can be problematic. They are due to retained necrotic liver tissue, perforated appendix (rarely seen today), benign or malignant hepatobiliary obstruction, and hepatic arterial occlusion. The treatment is long-term antibiotics with percutaneous drainage of large abscesses. Smaller abscesses will often resolve with antibiotics alone.

Pancreatitis can occur following injection of contrast during cholangiography and ERCP. These episodes range from a mild elevation in amylase and lipase with abdominal pain, to a fulminant course of pancreatitis with necrosis requiring surgical débridement. Traumatic injuries to the pancreas during surgical procedures, as well as during elective or nonelective splenectomy, comprise the most common cases that can be complicated by pancreatitis and pancreatic fistulae. Management of the pancreatitis will depend on whether drains were placed at the time of the initial operation. The usual course of treatment will involve serial CT scans and percutaneous drainage to manage infected fluid and abscess collections. The utility of somatostatin for control of pancreatic fistulae is arguable. Management of these fistulae initially includes ERCP with or without pancreatic stenting, percutaneous drainage of any fistula fluid collections, total parenteral nutrition with bowel rest, and repeated CT scans. The majority of pancreatic fistulae will eventually heal spontaneously.

Renal System

Renal failure can be classified as prerenal failure, intrinsic renal failure, and postrenal failure. Postrenal failure, or obstructive renal failure, should always be considered when oliguria or anuria occurs. While this is an uncommon cause of renal failure, the possibility must be ruled out before embarking on a course of investigation for acute-onset oliguria. The most common cause is a misplaced or clogged urinary catheter. Other, less-common causes to consider are unintentional ligation or transection of ureters during a difficult surgical dissection (e.g., colon resection for diverticular disease), or a large retroperitoneal hematoma (e.g., ruptured aortic aneurysm).

Table 11-4
Urinary Electrolytes Associated with Acute Renal Failure and Their Possible Etiologies

	FE_{Na}	Osmolarity	UR_{Na}	Etiology
Prerenal	<1	>500	<20	CHF, cirrhosis
Intrinsic failure	>1	<350	>40	Sepsis, shock

CHF = congestive heart failure; FE_{Na} = fractional excretion of sodium; UR_{Na} = urinary excretion of sodium.

Low urine output (oliguria) is initially evaluated by examining the patient and flushing the Foley catheter using sterile technique. When this fails to produce the desired response, it is reasonable to administer an intravenous fluid challenge with a crystalloid fluid bolus of 500 to 1000 mL. However, the immediate postoperative patient must be examined and have recent vital signs recorded with total intake and output tabulated, as well as urinary electrolytes measured (Table 11-4). A hemoglobin and hematocrit level should be checked immediately. Patients in compensated shock from acute blood loss may manifest anemia and end-organ malperfusion as oliguria alone. It is the responsibility of the clinician to identify the cause early and to treat it aggressively.

Acute tubular necrosis (ATN) carries a mortality risk of 25 to 50%. This broad range in mortality reflects the myriad complications that can cause this insult. When ATN is due to poor inflow (prerenal), the remedy begins with intravenous administration of crystalloid or colloid fluids as needed. If cardiac insufficiency is the problem, the optimization of vascular volume is achieved first, followed by inotropic agents as needed. These types of patients should be managed in a monitored setting with close observation of hemodynamic parameters.

Intrinsic renal failure and subsequent ATN are often the result of direct renal toxins. Aminoglycosides, vancomycin, and furosemide are well known agents that contribute directly to nephrotoxicity. Contrast-induced nephropathy usually leads to a subtle or transient rise in creatinine. In patients who are not adequately resuscitated or have poor cardiac function, a contrast nephropathy may have permanent effects on renal function.[47–50]

Several medications have been used for preservation of renal function, and two deserve mention for historic purposes only: fenoldopam and dopamine. A review of the recent literature demonstrates that these agonists do not change mortality or preserve renal function when used for declining renal performance, and their use should now be discouraged.[51,52] The use of n-acetylcysteine has had mixed results for preserving or improving renal function with contrast nephropathy, and recent studies suggest that it has limited value.

The treatment of renal failure related to myoglobinuria has also shifted away from the use of sodium bicarbonate for alkalinizing the urine, to merely maintaining brisk urine output of 100 mL/h with crystalloid fluid infusion. Mannitol and furosemide are not recommended as long as the intravenous fluid achieves the goal rate of urinary output.

Musculoskeletal System

Compartment Syndrome

A compartment syndrome can develop in any compartment of the body. This problem is often the domain of the orthopedic surgeon, but other surgeons must be aware of this phenomenon and be able to recognize it expeditiously in order to treat it appropriately.

Compartment syndrome of the extremities generally occurs after a closed fracture. The injury alone may predispose the patient to compartment syndrome, but aggressive fluid resuscitation can exacerbate the problem. Pain with passive motion is the hallmark of compartment syndrome, and the anterior compartment of the leg is usually the first compartment to be involved in the lower extremity. In this instance, once the diagnosis is suspected, confirmation is sought by doing direct pressure measurement of the individual compartments. If the pressures are elevated greater than 20 to 25 mm Hg in any of the compartments, then consideration to perform a four-compartment fasciotomy is required. Similarly, in the upper extremity a fasciotomy with a lazy S incision extending from wrist to brachium is performed after the diagnosis is confirmed. The vascular surgeon is familiar with compartment syndrome due to ischemia-reperfusion injury. These patients often have an ischemic time lasting around 4 to 6 hours. The morbidity of a fasciotomy is not zero, yet the complications of a missed diagnosis or undertreatment of a compartment syndrome has significant long-term impact on patients. Renal failure, foot drop, tissue loss, and a permanent loss of function are the most severe complications. Judicious fluid resuscitation, early fasciotomy, and elevation of the extremity all play a role helping to resolve the tissue edema in those patients at risk.

Decubitus Ulcers

Decubitus ulcers are preventable complications. All patients confined to bedrest due to traumatic paralysis, dementia, chemical paralysis, or patients unable to care for themselves are at high risk for decubitus pressure ulcers. Ischemic changes in the microcirculation of the skin can be seen early on and are clinically significant after approximately 2 hours of sustained pressure. Routine skin care and turning of the patient helps ensure a reduction in skin ulceration. This can be labor intensive and may not always be reliably performed. Special mattresses and beds with air or sand are available to help with this ubiquitous problem. The treatment of a decubitus ulcer in the noncoagulopathic patient is surgical débridement. Once the wound bed has a viable granulation base without an excess of fibrinous debris, a vacuum-assisted closure (VAC) dressing (see below) can be applied. Wet to moist dressings with frequent dressing changes is the alternative, and is labor intensive. Expensive topical enzyme preparations that are seemingly effective are also available, but not all insurance companies reimburse for these creams and lotions. If the wounds do not heal over time, then consideration for surgical soft tissue coverage must be given.

Contractures

Muscle contractures are the products of disuse. Whether from trauma, amputation, or from vascular insufficiency, contractures can be prevented with routine physical therapy and splinting. Adequate padding will be needed to prevent skin breakdown, but if not attended to early, the contractures will prolong rehabilitation and may lead to further wounds and wound healing issues. Sometimes it is better to commit the patient to a more proximal amputation so the sequelae of contractures with subsequent ulceration does not take place. Depending on the functional status of the patient, contracture releases may be required for long-term care.

Hematologic System

The surgical dogma to maintain hematocrit levels in all patients at >30% at all times is no longer valid. Patients requiring a hematocrit of >30% are only those who have *symptomatic* anemia, or those who have significant cardiac disease, or the critically-ill patient who requires increased oxygen-carrying capacity in order to adequately perfuse end-organs within 72 hours of initial presentation. Indeed, these patients may require hemoglobin much higher than 10 to 12 mg/dL. Other than these select patients, the decision to provide transfusion of packed red blood cells should generally not occur until the hemoglobin level reaches 7.0 mg/dL or the hematocrit reaches 21%.

Much of the stored blood available for transfusion at busier hospitals is old blood. This means that centers with a relatively high demand for blood (e.g., high-volume tertiary care centers and level 1 trauma centers) do not generally receive freshly donated blood. When blood is stored for several days, the compound 2,3-diphosphoglycerate (2,3-DPG) is broken down. It is the presence of 2,3-DPG that unloads the oxygen from the hemoglobin and delivers the oxygen to the tissues, so if this compound is not present, effective oxygen delivery is compromised.

Transfusion reactions are common complications of blood transfusion. This can be attenuated with a leukocyte filter, but not completely prevented. The manifestations of a transfusion reaction include simple fever, pruritus, chills, muscle rigidity, and renal failure from myoglobinuria. Discontinuing the transfusion and returning the blood products to the blood bank is an important first step, but symptomatic care of the patients is essential. Administration of antihistamine and possibly steroids may be required to control the reaction symptoms. Severe transfusion reactions are rare but can be life-threatening, so aggressive supportive care is required.

Infectious complications in blood transfusion can be deadly. These range from cytomegalovirus (more or less benign in the non-transplant patient), to human immunodeficiency virus (HIV), to the hepatitis viruses, which can lead to the subsequent complication of hepatocellular carcinoma. While the efficiency of infectious agent screening in blood products has improved, there are still considerable risks and universal precautions should be rigidly maintained for all patients (Table 11-5).

EPO II, a recent study published in *JAMA*, reviewed transfusion practices and compared them with the cost of treatment with

Table 11-5
Rate of Viral Transmission in Blood Product Transfusions[a]

HIV	1:1.9 million
HBV[b]	1:137,000
HCV	1:1 million

HBV = hepatitis B virus; HCV = hepatitis C virus; HIV = human immunodeficiency virus.

[a]Post-nucleic acid amplification technology (1999). Earlier rates were erroneously reported higher due to lack of contemporary technology.

[b]HBV is reported with pre-nucleic acid amplification technology. Statistical information is unavailable in post-nucleic acid amplification technology at this writing.

Note that bacterial transmission is 50 to 250 times higher than viral transmission per transfusion.

synthetic erythropoietin.[53] The study showed a decreased need for blood transfusion by 0.6 of a unit of blood after erythropoietin treatment. The high cost of the drug as well as all the other risks previously mentioned must be carefully considered before administering a transfusion. Furthermore, mature red cells are not mobilized into the circulation for 10 to 14 days after drug treatment, and exogenous iron must also be supplemented along with the drug. This makes the argument for erythropoietin poor in a patient suffering from acute blood loss, but patients with anemia from chronic disease may benefit from this agent with iron supplementation.

The vicious cycle of acidosis, coagulopathy, and hypothermia is a common occurrence for surgeons involved with septic or hemodynamically unstable patients. In such situations every effort should be made to get the patient stabilized as rapidly as possible, which should include "damage-control" surgical strategies and transfer of patients to the ICU for active ongoing resuscitation with rewarming. The intra- and postoperative vigilance of resuscitation parameters cannot be overstated when patients are prone to these often preventable complications of resuscitation and shock. Correction of the coagulation abnormalities with fresh frozen plasma and platelet administration is usually required to facilitate the correction of the bleeding abnormalities.

A potentially correctable error in surgery is the performance of elective procedures on therapeutically anticoagulated patients. Those patients on heparin or warfarin can have their anticoagulation profile normalized by administration of fresh frozen plasma (FFP). Each unit of FFP contains 200 to 250 mL of plasma and includes 1 unit of coagulation factor per milliliter of plasma.

Patients who are thrombocytopenic rarely need to be transfused with platelets. It is most important to delineate why the patient has a low platelet count. Usually there is a self-limiting or reversible condition such as sepsis. Rarely it is due to heparin-induced thrombocytopenia (HIT I and HIT II). Complications secondary to HIT II can be extremely morbid because of the thrombogenic nature of the complication. Simple precautions to limit this hypercoagulable state are to use saline solution flushes instead of heparin solutions, and to limit the use of heparin-coated catheters. The treatment is anticoagulation with synthetic agents such as argatroban. Thrombocytopenia actually develops in about 10% of patients treated with heparin. Transfusion of platelets during this diathesis only stimulates further degranulation of the platelets and promotes thrombosis.

The surgical dogma that platelet transfusions should be initiated for platelet counts less than 20,000, and that invasive procedures should not be performed with platelet counts less than 50,000 are largely unproven. Transfusions are recommended when platelet counts are low and ongoing bleeding from raw surface areas persists. When transfusion is indicated, it is important to know as a guide that 1 unit of platelets will increase the platelet count by 5000 to 7500 per μL in adults.

For patients with uncontrollable bleeding due to disseminated intravascular coagulopathy (DIC), an expensive but useful drug is factor VIIa.[54–56] Largely used in hepatic trauma and obstetric emergencies, this agent may mean the difference between life or death in some circumstances, but if after two or three doses there is no improvement, factor VIIa is unlikely to work at all. The combination of ongoing, nonsurgical bleeding and renal failure can sometimes be successfully treated with desmopressin (DDAVP).

In addition to classic hemophilia, other coagulation factor deficiencies can be difficult to manage in surgery. When required, transfusion of appropriate replacement products is coordinated with the regional blood bank center prior to surgery. Other blood dyscrasias seen by surgeons include hypercoagulopathic patients. Those who carry congenital anomalies such as the most common, factor V Leiden deficiency, as well as protein C and S deficiencies, are likely to form thromboses if inadequately anticoagulated. These conditions are often diagnosed after spontaneous arterial clotting; nonetheless, early postsurgical clotting not due to a technical error should prompt investigation of these conditions.

ABDOMINAL COMPARTMENT SYNDROME

Abdominal compartment syndrome (ACS) and intra-abdominal hypertension are now well recognized entities that represent a clinical spectrum of the same problem. Multiple trauma, thermal burns, retroperitoneal injuries, and surgery related to the retroperitoneum are the major initial causative factors that may lead to an ACS. Ruptured abdominal aortic aneurysm, major pancreatic injury and resection, or multiple intestinal injuries are also examples of clinical situations in which there is often a large volume of IV fluid resuscitation required that puts these patients at risk for developing intra-abdominal hypertension and abdominal compartment syndrome. Manifestations of ACS typically include progressive abdominal distention followed by increased peak airway ventilator pressures, oliguria followed by anuria, and then an insidious development of intracranial hypertension.[57] These findings are related to elevation of the diaphragm and inadequate venous return from the vena cava or renal veins secondary to the transmitted pressure on the venous system, not compression of the renal parenchyma or ureters.

Measurement of abdominal pressures was shown to be a useful technique by Kron et al, and is easily accomplished by transducing bladder pressures from the urinary catheter after instilling 100 mL of sterile saline into the urinary bladder.[58] This method is more accurate and minimally invasive compared to the measurement of intra-gastric or intra-colonic pressures. Pressures greater than 20 mm Hg are considered to constitute intra-abdominal hypertension, but intra-abdominal pressure greater than 25 to 30 mm Hg, with at least one of the following—compromised respiratory mechanics and ventilation, oliguria or anuria, or increasing intracranial pressures—is recognized as ACS.[59–61]

The treatment of symptomatic ACS is to open any recent abdominal incision in order to release the abdominal fascia, or to open the fascia directly if no abdominal incision is present. Immediate improvement in mechanical ventilation pressures, intracranial pressures, and renal output is usually noted. When expectant management for ACS is considered in the operating room, the abdominal fascia should be left open and covered under sterile conditions with plans for a second-look operation and delayed fascial closure. The more difficult decision for surgical management is when intra-abdominal hypertension is present, but the various manifestations of ACS are not yet seen. Patients in this situation should be monitored closely with repeated examinations and measurements of bladder pressure, so that any further deterioration is detected and operative management can be initiated. Left untreated, ACS may lead to multiple system end-organ dysfunction or failure, and has a high mortality.

The consequences of an open abdomen are small but they are not negligible. Attempts to close the abdomen wall should therefore occur every 48 to 72 hours until the fascia can be reapproximated. It is unclear whether a forced fluid diuresis to decrease soft tissue and bowel wall edema is of value, but if the patient is able to tolerate a diuresis, this strategy should be attempted, because if the patient cannot be safely closed within 5 to 7 days following release of the abdominal fascia, a large incisional hernia is the net result. If unable

to be closed, these patients should have some type of absorbable mesh closure to cover the viscera, followed by a split-thickness skin graft to cover the hernia defect. After the wound has healed, reduction and closure of the ventral hernia is performed with lateral releases of the fascia about 9 months to 1 year after the initial surgery. The optimal timing of the hernia repair surgery may be confirmed preoperatively when the skin graft overlying the ventral hernia freely tents up off the underlying viscera. Occasionally soft tissue expansion is required in the preoperative period to facilitate the hernia closure without undue tension.

WOUNDS, DRAINS, AND INFECTION

Wound Infection

The indiscriminate use of antibiotics is a universal problem that continues to plague intensive care units and hospitals across the country.[62] Beginning with prophylactic antibiotics, there exist no prospective, randomized, double-blind, controlled studies that demonstrate that antibiotics used beyond 24 hours in the perioperative period prevent infections. There is a general trend toward providing a single preoperative dose, as antibiotic prophylaxis may not impart any benefit at all beyond the initial dosing. Serial irrigation of the operative field and the surgical wound with saline solution has shown benefit in controlling wound inoculum.[63] Irrigation with an antibiotic-based solution has not demonstrated significant benefit in controlling postoperative infection.

The practice of having iodophor-impregnated polyvinyl placed over the operative wound area for the duration of the surgical procedure has not shown a significant decrease in the rate of wound infection.[64–68] In fact, skin preparation with 70% isopropyl alcohol still has the best bacteria killing ratio, but it is flammable, and could be hazardous when electrocautery is utilized. The contemporary formulae of chlorhexadine gluconate with isopropyl alcohol or povidone-iodine and iodophor with alcohol are more advantageous.[69–71]

There is a difference between wound colonization and infection. Overtreating colonization is just as injurious as undertreating infection (Table 11-6). The true diagnosis of a wound infection is confirmed by sending at least 1 g of tissue to microbiology, and if the culture returns with more than 10^5 colony-forming units (CFU) per gram of tissue, a diagnosis of wound infection may be rendered. This warrants expeditious and proper antibiotic/antifungal treatment.[15,72] Often, however, the clinical signs raise enough suspicion that the patient is treated before a confirmatory culture is undertaken. The clinical signs of wound infection include *rubor, tumor, calor,* and *dolor* (redness, swelling, heat, and pain), and once the diagnosis of wound infection has been established, the most definitive treatment remains open drainage of the wound in order to facilitate wound dressing care. The use of antibiotics for wound infection treatment should be limited.[73–76]

Table 11-6
Common Causes of Leukocytosis

Infection
Systemic inflammatory response syndrome
Glucocorticoid administration
Splenectomy
Leukemia
Medications
Physiologic stress
Increases in interleukin-1 and tumor necrosis factor

One type of wound dressing/drainage system that is rapidly gaining popularity is the VAC dressing. The principle of the system is to decrease local wound edema and to promote healing through the application of a sterile dressing that is then covered and placed under controlled suction for a period of 2 to 4 days at a time. Although a costly dressing, the benefits are frequently dramatic and may offset the costs of nursing care, frequent dressing changes, wound infection, and operative wound débridement. However, further studies are still needed to fully investigate the various claims related to the use of this dressing system.

Drain Management

The often-cited reasons for applying a surgical drain are:

1. To collapse surgical dead space in areas of redundant tissue (e.g., neck and axilla).
2. To provide focused drainage of an abscess or infected surgical site.
3. To provide early warning notice of a surgical leak—either bowel contents, secretions, urine, air, or blood.
4. To control an established fistula leak.

There are several types of drains available and they have a variety of uses, but researchers have recently studied the benefits and alternatives to operative drainage. Open drains have often been used for large contaminated wounds such as perirectal or perianal fistulas and subcutaneous abscess cavities. There are two varieties—the Penrose drain and the wick gauze drain. Inarguably, they prevent premature closure of an abscess cavity in a contaminated wound, but they do not address the fact that bacteria are free to travel in either direction along the drain tract. Drains such as Penrose drains are therefore potentially harmful when used in cases in which a synthetic graft is in proximity to the wound, or the operative site has not been previously contaminated or infected. Similarly, when used for several days, wick gauze drains can do more harm than good, because they are bathed in bacteria within the warm, moist confines of the wound, and do not provide an egress to the surface for harmful bacteria. Toxic shock syndrome, an overwhelming infection most often caused by *Staphylococcus aureus* and occasionally by *Streptococcus* spp., can occur in this setting, and patients can quickly succumb if not treated emergently. The use of both of these open drains is to be discouraged in the majority of procedures.

The use of closed suction drains also remains controversial, but a wide variety of surgical sites are commonly drained by closed suction drainage systems. The contemporary literature does not support closed suction drainage to "protect an anastomosis," or to "control a leak" when placed at the time of surgery. These closed suction devices can exert a negative pressure of 70 to 170 mm Hg at the level of the drain, therefore the presence of this excess suction may call into question whether an anastomosis breaks down on its own, or if the drain creates a suction injury that promotes leakage (Fig. 11-4).[77] Furthermore, patients with these drains in place often have higher infection rates and the drains clog early, so they may not provide their claimed benefits. Studies are ongoing, but there does not appear to be any benefit to the early use of closed suction drains.[78]

This is not to say that all drains are bad. CT- or ultrasound-guided placement of percutaneous drains is now the standard of care for abscesses, loculated infections, and other isolated fluid collections such as pancreatic leaks. The risk of surgery for these patients is often greater in the acute setting, and the risk can often be reduced in these instances by percutaneous drainage and a brief course of antibiotics.[79,80]

The use of antibiotics when drains are placed should be examined from a cost-benefit perspective. There are good data to suggest that

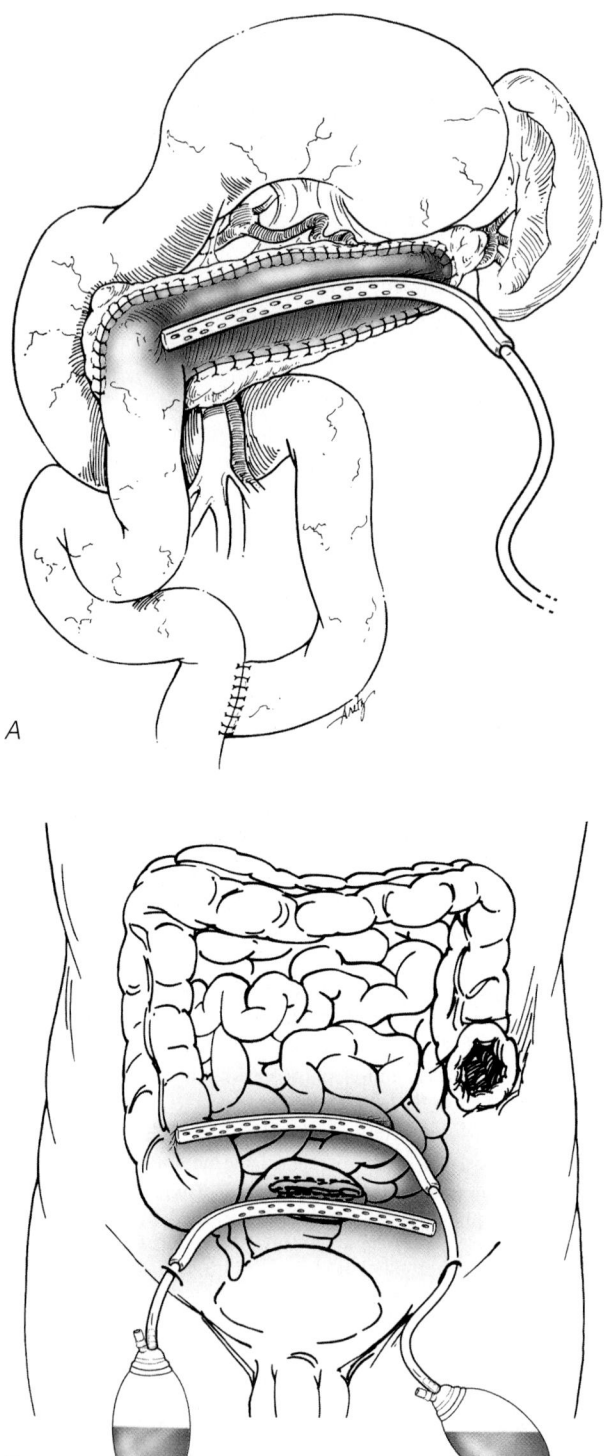

A

B

FIG. 11-4. This illustration demonstrates typical intraoperative placement of closed suction devices in pancreatic or small bowel surgery, where there may be an anastomosis. At negative pressures of 70 to 170 mm Hg, these devices may actually encourage anastomotic leaks and not prevent them, or become clogged prematurely.

antibiotics are not necessary when a wound is drained. Twenty-four to 48 hours of antibiotic use after drain placement is prophylactic, and after this period only specific treatment of positive cultures should be performed, to avoid increased drug resistance and superinfection.

Urinary Catheters

The placement of a urinary drainage (Foley) catheter is usually a simple and benign procedure. Nonetheless, several complications can occur that lead to an increased length of hospital stay and morbidity. It is recommended that the catheter be inserted its full length up to the hub, and that urine flow is established before the balloon is inflated, because misplacement of the catheter in the urethra with premature inflation of the balloon can lead to tears and disruption of the urethra.

Elderly males with enlarged prostatic tissue can make catheter insertion difficult, so an attempt with a catheter coudé is warranted. If this attempt is also unsuccessful, then a consult to a urologist for endoscopic placement of the catheter may be required to prevent harm to the urethra. For patients with urethral strictures, filiform-tipped catheters and followers may be used, but these can potentially injure the bladder as well. If endoscopic attempts fail, the patient may require a percutaneously placed suprapubic catheter in order to obtain decompression of the bladder. Follow-up investigations of these patients are recommended so definitive care of the urethral abnormalities can be pursued.

The number one nosocomial infection is urinary tract infection (UTI). These infections are classified into complicated and uncomplicated forms. The uncomplicated type is most often a UTI that can be treated with trimethoprim-sulfamethoxazole for 3 days. The complicated UTI usually involves the hospitalized patient with an indwelling catheter whose UTI is diagnosed as part of a fever work-up. There is controversy over the interpretation of urine culture results of less than 100,000 CFU/ml. Before treating such a patient, one should change the catheter and then repeat the culture to see if the catheter was simply colonized with organisms. On the other hand, as with other surgical infections, an argument can be made that until the foreign body (catheter) is removed, the bladder will continue to be the nidus of infection, and antibiotics should be started. Cultures with more than 100,000 CFU/ml should be treated with the appropriate antibiotics and the catheter removed as soon as possible. Undertreatment or misdiagnosis of a UTI can lead to urosepsis and septic shock. This can be diagnosed during a sepsis work-up, and the treatment is as for any septic patient—control of the infectious source and resuscitation with optimization of end-organ perfusion and oxygen delivery.

The opinions of researchers are mixed over the proper way to treat *Candida albicans* fungal bladder infections. Continuous bladder washings with fungicidal solution for 72 hours have been recommended, but this is not always effective. Replacement of the urinary catheter and a course of fluconazole are appropriate treatments, but some infectious disease specialists claim that *C. albicans* in the urine may serve as an indication of fungal infection elsewhere in the body. If this is the case, then screening cultures for other sources of fungal infection should be performed whenever a fungal UTI is found.

Empyema

One of the most debilitating infections is an empyema, or infection of the pleural space. Frequently, an overwhelming pneumonia is the source of an empyema, but a retained hemothorax, systemic sepsis, esophageal perforation from any cause, and infections with a predilection for the lung (e.g., tuberculosis) are potential etiologies as well. The diagnosis is confirmed by chest x-ray or CT scan, followed by aspiration of pleural fluid for bacteriologic analysis. Gram's stain, lactate dehydrogenase, protein, pH, and cell count are ordered, and broad-spectrum antibiotics are initiated while the laboratory analyzes the tissue or fluid. Once the specific organisms are confirmed, anti-infective agents are tailored appropriately. Placement of a thoracostomy tube is needed to evacuate and drain the infected pleural fluid, but depending on the specific nidus of infection, video-assisted thoracoscopy (VATS) may also be helpful for irrigation and drainage of the infection.

Three stages of empyema are recognized: acute, fibropurulent, and chronic. The acute phase is best managed as described above. VATS is now recognized as being superior for providing effective pleural decortication for the second stage of empyema, and is superior to an open thoracotomy in terms of recovery time, narcotic utilization, and length of hospital stay. Rarely, an empyema will advance to the chronic phase. Should this occur, marsupialization of the pleura to the pleural surface should be done in order to drain the chronically infected pleural space.

Abdominal Abscesses

Postsurgical intra-abdominal abscesses can present with vague complaints of intermittent abdominal pain, fever, leukocytosis, and the occasional change in bowel habits. Depending on the type and timing of the original procedure, the clinical assessment of these complaints is sometimes difficult, and more often than not a CT scan will be required. When a fluid collection within the peritoneal cavity is found on CT scan, antibiotics and percutaneous drainage of the collection is the treatment of choice. Even when drainage is established, there must still be a determination as to what the cause of the infection was, so tailored antibiotic therapy can be initiated. Initial antibiotic treatment is usually with broad-spectrum antibiotics such as piperacillin-tazobactam or imipenem. Should the patient exhibit signs of peritonitis and/or have free air on x-ray or CT scan, then reexploration should be considered. For patients who present primarily (i.e., not postoperatively) with the clinical and radiologic findings of an abscess but are clinically stable, the etiology of the abscess must be determined. A plan for drainage of the abscess and decisions about further diagnostic studies with consideration of the timing of any definitive surgery all need to be balanced. This can be a complex set of decisions, depending on the etiology (e.g., appendicitis or diverticulitis); but if the patient exhibit signs of peritonitis, urgent surgical exploration should be considered.

Necrotizing Fasciitis

Postoperative infections that progress to the fulminant soft tissue infection known as necrotizing fasciitis are uncommon but do occur. Group A streptococcal (M types 1, 3, 12, and 28) soft tissue infections, as well as infections with *Clostridium perfringens* and *C. septicum* carry a mortality of 30 to 70%. Septic shock can be present because of the rapidity with which a patient becomes hypotensive—less than 6 hours following inoculation. Manifestations of a group A *Streptococcus pyogenes* infection in its most severe form include hypotension, renal insufficiency, coagulopathy, hepatic insufficiency, ARDS, tissue necrosis, and erythematous rash.

These findings constitute a surgical emergency and the mainstay of treatment remains wide débridement of the necrotic tissue to the level of bleeding, viable tissue. A grey serous fluid at the level of the necrotic tissue is usually noted, and as the infection spreads, thrombosed blood vessels are noted along the tissue planes involved with the infection. Typically, the patient requires serial trips to the operating room for wide débridement until the infection is under control. Antibiotics are an important adjunct to surgical débridement and broad-spectrum coverage should be used because these infections may be polymicrobial (i.e., so-called mixed-synergistic infections).

Table 11-7
Mortality Associated with Patients Exhibiting Two or More Criteria for Systemic Inflammatory Response Syndrome (SIRS)

Prognosis	Mortality
2 SIRS criteria	5%
3 SIRS criteria	10%
4 SIRS criteria	15–20%

S. pyogenes is eradicated with penicillin, and it should still be used as the initial drug of choice.

Systemic Inflammatory Response Syndrome, Sepsis, and Multiple-Organ Dysfunction Syndrome

The continuum of the systemic inflammatory response syndrome (SIRS) and the multiple-organ dysfunction syndrome (MODS) continues to carry significant mortality risks (Table 11-7). Specific criteria have been established for the diagnosis of SIRS (Table 11-8), but are in the process of being revised through consensus among several professional organizations.

Of note, two criteria are not required for the diagnosis of SIRS: lowered blood pressure and blood cultures positive for infection. Patients can be systemically ill without being hypotensive, and if the patient has developed bacteremia and/or fungemia, they are diagnosed as having sepsis. This raises the question of how one acquires SIRS without infection. The key to understanding this disease is to appreciate the competing release of anti-inflammatory and proinflammatory cytokines related to tissue malperfusion or injury. The dominant cytokines currently implicated in this process include interleukin (IL)-1, IL-6, and tissue necrosis factor (TNF). Other mediators include nitric oxide, inducible macrophage-type nitric oxide synthase (iNOS), and prostaglandin I_2 (PGI_2). The precise delineation of all the mediators involved and the interactions of these mediators is still under active research, and a complete understanding of the etiology for SIRS/MODS has yet to be elucidated.

Sepsis is categorized as sepsis, severe sepsis, and septic shock. An oversimplification of sepsis would be to define it as SIRS plus infection. Severe sepsis is defined as sepsis plus signs of cellular hypoperfusion or end-organ dysfunction. Septic shock would then be sepsis associated with hypotension after adequate fluid resuscitation. Although each stage has its own definition, it is easy to understand the confusion among clinicians when discussing a patient's disease course in relation to their level of illness. Furthermore, such classification may not result in any change in treatment. However, it does predict mortality.

MODS is the culmination of septic shock and multiple end-organ failure. Usually there is an inciting event (e.g., perforated sigmoid diverticulitis), and as the patient undergoes resuscitation, he or she develops cardiac hypokinesis and oliguric or anuric renal failure,

Table 11-8
Inclusion Criteria for the Systemic Inflammatory Response Syndrome (SIRS)

Temperature >38 or <36°C
Heart rate >90 beats/min
Respiratory rate >20 breaths/min or $Paco_2$ <32 mm Hg
White blood cell count <4000 or >12,000 cells/mm³ or > 10% immature forms

followed by the development of ARDS and eventually septic shock with death.[52]

Management of SIRS/MODS includes aggressive global resuscitation and support of end-organ perfusion, correction of the inciting etiology, control of infectious complications, and management of iatrogenic complications.[81–83] Despite several research initiatives over the past two decades, there is still no specific focused treatment that can be considered reliable in the management of SIRS/MODS. The only agent showing potential benefit is drotrecogin α, or recombinant activated protein C, but its use is restricted to monitored phase 3 clinical research trials at this time.[84,85] Other adjuncts for supportive therapy include tight glucose control, low tidal volumes in ARDS, vasopressin in septic shock, and steroid replacement therapy.

NUTRITIONAL AND METABOLIC SUPPORT COMPLICATIONS

Nutrition-Related Complications

Patients with malnutrition can be divided into two groups: those who are underfed and those who are overfed. Both overfeeding and underfeeding can be detrimental. The calculated respiratory quotient (RQ) can provide insight into the nutritional status of the patient, but other nutritional parameters should be evaluated as well. It is easiest to measure RQ in intubated patients, but there are also ways to test nonintubated patients. Under a steady state, it may only take 2 to 4 hours to complete RQ testing, and this would be more cost-effective than the traditional 24-hour RQ tests. Calculating metabolic demands is also complicated in septic patients, such that the resting energy expenditure (REE) is increased by 40 to 50%, and for every degree of fever above 37.5°C, the REE increases by 10 to 15%. Even the medications that are associated with sepsis management may play a role in increasing the REE, for example dopamine (4% increase), dobutamine (5% increase), and norepinephrine (25% increase).

A basic principle for managing septic or hypermetabolic patients is to use enteral feeding whenever possible, but there are concerns with enteral feeding about aspiration, ileus (see above), and to a lesser extent, sinusitis. There is no difference in aspiration rates when a small-caliber feeding tube is placed transpylorically into the duodenum or if it remains in the stomach. Feeding tubes placed in the jejunum place the patient at lower risk for pneumonia, but patients who are fed via nasogastric tubes are at risk for aspiration pneumonia, because these relatively large-bore tubes stent open the esophagus, creating the possibility of gastric reflux. The use of enteric and gastric feeding tubes obviates complications of total parenteral nutrition (TPN), such as pneumothorax, line sepsis, upper extremity deep venous thrombosis, and the related expense. There are still no data demonstrating that starting TPN early is of any benefit for surgical patients if it is discontinued before 10 to 14 days, but data do suggest that in the severely malnourished, it is appropriate to prescribe TPN perioperatively. There is growing evidence to support the initiation of enteral feeding in the early postoperative period, prior to the return of bowel function, and that it is well tolerated and is associated with fewer intestinal problems such as prolonged ileus or constipation.

There are no consistent data which prove the hypothesis of bacterial translocation in human subjects, yet this is one of the primary reasons cited for beginning "trophic" enteral feeding. Although enteral feeding should still be encouraged, this definition of trophic feeding has yet to be widely accepted. Surgical nutritionists claim that the benefits of less-than-goal enteric feeds (trophic feeds) are similar to that of goal feeds. This concept is important because many patients receive enteral tube feeds at 10, 15, or 20 mL per hour as a measure to prevent translocation. Unfortunately, this rationale is still not of proven value in humans.

In patients who have had any type of nasal intubation that are having high, unexplained fevers, sinusitis must be entertained as a diagnosis. CT scan of the sinuses is warranted, followed by aspiration of sinus contents so the organism(s) are appropriately treated, and the patient does not remain on unnecessary broad-spectrum antibiotics for a prolonged period.

Patients who have not been enterally fed for prolonged periods secondary to multiple operations, those who have had enteral feeds interrupted for any other reason, or those with poor enteral access are at risk for the refeeding syndrome, which is characterized by severe hypophosphatemia and respiratory failure. Slow progression of the enteral feeding administration rate can avoid this complication.

Common TPN problems are mostly related to electrolyte abnormalities that may develop. These electrolyte errors include deficits or excesses in sodium, potassium, calcium, magnesium, and phosphate. Acid-base abnormalities can also occur with the improper administration of acetate or bicarbonate solutions. Each of these electrolytes needs to be monitored in the acute hospital setting initially, and all abnormalities corrected in a timely fashion in order to avoid the related complications. A careful daily review of the patient's laboratory results and the ordering of the TPN mixture will usually avoid these problems, but complacency and automatic ordering of solutions without assessing lab results will lead to problems. When abnormalities occur, it is important to calculate any electrolyte and free water excess or deficits before beginning corrective treatment, because this will help to avoid further problems related to improper correction of the original abnormality.

As one example, the most common cause for hypernatremia in hospitalized patients is underresuscitation, and conversely, hyponatremia is most often caused by fluid overload. Treatment for hyponatremia is fluid restriction in mild or moderate cases and the administration of hypertonic saline for severe cases. An overly rapid correction of the sodium abnormality may result in central pontine myelinolysis, which then results in a severe neurologic deficit. Treatment for hyponatremic patients includes fluid restriction and/or administration of free water boluses to correct the free water deficit by 50% in the first 24 hours. After the first 24 hours, the deficit is reevaluated and the remaining deficit is then corrected over the next 24 to 48 hours. An overcorrection of hyponatremia can result in severe cerebral edema and a significant neurologic deficit or seizures.

Another potential problem with TPN is its use in anticoagulated patients. Patients who are anticoagulated with warfarin may not reach their anticoagulation goals because the TPN solution may contain vitamin K.

Glycemic Control

In 2001, an important study by van den Berghe demonstrated that tight glycemic control (insulin therapy; IT) is associated with an improvement in mortality in the critical care setting. This study has called attention to the benefits of controlling blood sugar via insulin management, and demonstrates that significantly improved patient outcomes can be attained using a relatively simple protocol of care. Interestingly, this trial was terminated early when an interim analysis demonstrated a clear mortality benefit to tight glucose control.[86]

Briefly, this prospective, randomized, controlled trial of 2500 patients had two study arms: the intensive-control arm, where patient serum glucose was maintained between 80 and 110 mg/dL with insulin infusion; and the control arm, where patients received an insulin infusion only if blood glucose was >215 mg/dL, but serum glucose was then maintained at 180 to 200 mg/dL. The primary measured outcome was mortality from any cause for surgical intensive care unit patients. Secondary outcomes included days on mechanical ventilation, bloodstream infections, use of antibiotics, markers of inflammation, renal replacement therapy, and the use of vasopressors.

The results were as follows: The tight glycemic control group had an average serum glucose level of 103 mg/dL, and the average glucose level in the control group was 153 mg/dL, with insulin infusions maintained in 40% of the treated patients. Hypoglycemic episodes (glucose <40 mg/dL) occurred in 39 patients in the IT group, while the control group had episodes in 6 patients. Mortality of the IT group was 4.6%, but the control group had 8% mortality, a 42% relative risk reduction. Secondary findings in the IT group included an improvement in overall morbidity, a decreased percentage of ventilator days, less renal impairment, decreased hyperbilirubinemia, a lower incidence of bloodstream infections, fewer patients on antibiotics for >10 days, and less evidence of polyneuropathy. Limitations of this study are that it included primarily a surgical population (63% cardiac surgery, 37% other surgery), and it is not known whether it was truly the tight control of glucose that contributed to the improvement in mortality, or whether it was the anabolic properties of increased insulin levels that made the difference.[86–88]

Metabolism-Related Complications

Despite contemporary criticism of the use and abuse of "stress-dosed steroids" for patients with even a remote history of glucocorticoid use, many still receive potentially harmful doses of hydrocortisone or its equivalent in the perioperative period. Many times the patient's primary care physician or the anesthesiologist administers steroids unbeknownst to the surgeon, and the patient does not receive subsequent doses. The original two case reports on steroid deficiency are from the 1950s; they described patients who were on steroids, underwent surgery, and also received blood transfusions.[89,90] Each patient suffered cardiovascular collapse postoperatively, one in the recovery room and the other on the floor. It was never definitively determined why these patients deteriorated so quickly, but the conclusion of each case report was that the collapse was attributed to adrenal insufficiency, and this became the impetus for using "stress-dosed steroids."

Since that time several studies, including those by Chernow and others, strongly discourage the use of supraphysiologic doses of steroids when patients are on low or maintenance doses (e.g., 5 to 15 mg of prednisone daily), and suggest providing no more than physiologic replacement steroids in the perioperative period. When patients are on steroid replacement doses equal to or greater than 20 mg per day of prednisone, it may be appropriate to administer a scheduled dose of additional glucocorticoid for no more than two perioperative days. The dosing of glucocorticoid replacement in this setting is dependent on the length of surgery and the severity of the original steroid-deficient disease state.[91–93]

Annane and colleagues recently provided the best trial to date of the utility of physiologic replacement of steroids in septic patients. After a cosyntropin stimulation test, the trial was divided into responders and nonresponders. The nonresponders (n = 229) were separated into a placebo group and a group that received physiologic replacement of 50 mg hydrocortisone intravenously every 6 hours for 7 days, as well as 50 μg of oral fludrocortisone daily for 7 days. The study reported a 28-day mortality of 63% in the nonresponder placebo group and 53% mortality in the nonresponder, physiologic replacement group. Furthermore, vasopressin was discontinued for more patients in the treatment group (57%) than the placebo group (40%). The complication/adverse effect profiles in each group were similar.[83]

Methods of checking for adrenal insufficiency are varied and no single method is standard. Some suggest that a baseline serum cortisol level is all that is warranted, with the absolutely lowest acceptable level being 20 μg/dL. Others suggest performing a rapid adrenocorticotropic hormone (ACTH) assay, which gives three points of reference on which to base a treatment decision. With this method, a baseline serum cortisol level is drawn, and then followed by the administration of 250 μg of cosyntropin. At exactly 30 and 60 minutes following the dose of cosyntropin, serum cortisol levels are obtained. Theoretically, the results should return within 1 hour, and there should be an incremental increase in the cortisol level of between 7 and 10 μg/dL for each half hour. If the patient is below these levels, a diagnosis of adrenal insufficiency is made, and glucocorticoid and mineralocorticoid administration is then warranted. Mixed results are common, and in such cases the clinical picture is unclear. Checking for other signs and symptoms to confirm the diagnosis (i.e., high fevers, prolonged use of vasoactive agents, hyperkalemia, and hyponatremia, among others) is often helpful for decision making regarding replacement therapy in these cases.[81]

Thyroid hormone abnormalities can also occur in surgical patients with previously undiagnosed thyroid abnormalities. Thyrotoxicosis is mentioned later, but hypothyroidism and the so-called "sick-euthyroid syndrome" are more commonly recognized in the critical care setting. When surgical patients are not progressing satisfactorily in the perioperative period, either in the ICU or on the floor, screening for thyroid abnormalities should be performed. These are often patients that have vague, nonspecific symptoms, and demonstrate a slow progression to recovery. If the results of thyroid function screening tests show mild to moderate hypothyroidism, then thyroid replacement should be begun immediately and thyroid function studies monitored closely. Occasionally, patients with low normal or marginally abnormal results may also benefit from replacement therapy. All patients should be reassessed after the acute illness has subsided regarding the need for chronic thyroid replacement therapy. Parenthetically, it should always be remembered that patients who are already on thyroid replacement medication must have their medication maintained during a surgical illness, and that thyroid hormone levels should be assessed if the patient exhibits poor progression with their surgical disease.

PROBLEMS WITH THERMOREGULATION

Hypothermia

Hypothermia is defined as a core temperature less than 95°F (35°C), and can be divided into subsets of mild (35 to 32°C), moderate (32 to 28°C), and severe (< 28°C) hypothermia. Shivering, the body's attempt to reverse the effects of hypothermia, occurs between 37 and 31°C, but ceases at temperatures below 31°C. Individual variation exists as to how the body responds to the etiology and onset of hypothermia, the duration of hypothermia, and the degree of hypothermia. Interestingly, patients who are borderline to moderately hypothermic are at higher risk for complications of hypothermia than are those who are more profoundly hypothermic.

Hypothermia creates a coagulopathy that is related to platelet and clotting cascade enzyme dysfunction. This triad of metabolic acidosis, coagulopathy, and hypothermia is commonly found with unstable trauma patients, but can also occur during long operative cases, and in patients with blood dyscrasias. The enzymes that contribute to the clotting cascade and platelet activity are most efficient at normal body temperatures; therefore when patients are developing hypothermia in the operating room, all measures must be utilized to reduce heat loss and to actively warm the patient.[94]

Other anatomic and physiologic concerns are related to the cardiac, respiratory, and renal systems. The most common cardiac abnormality is the development of arrhythmias when body temperature drops below 35°C, and these are usually related to ventricular dysfunction with the abnormal acid-base environment. Bradycardia begins to occur with temperatures below 30°C. It is well known that hypothermia may induce carbon dioxide retention until the body's production of CO_2 decreases significantly from the hypothermia, resulting in respiratory acidosis. Renal dysfunction of hypothermia manifests itself as a paradoxic polyuria, and is related to an increased glomerular filtration rate, as peripheral vascular constriction creates central shunting of blood. This is potentially perplexing for patients that are undergoing resuscitation for hemodynamic instability, because the brisk urine output provides a false sense of an adequate intravascular fluid volume.

Changes in neurologic function are inconsistent in hypothermia, but at a body temperature somewhere between 20 and 30°C an electroencephalogram will demonstrate a flat waveform. Clinical deterioration in reasoning and decision-making skills decline inconsistently as body temperature falls, and will result in profound coma as the temperature drops below 30°C. The debate regarding the benefits of planned hypothermia for improving outcomes with traumatic brain injury and for cardiac arrest resuscitation are continuing, and no consensus has been clarified to date.

Diagnosis of hypothermia is most important, so accurate measurement techniques are required to get a true core temperature before making the diagnosis. Once diagnosed, ongoing efforts to prevent heat loss are essential and should include removal of all wet clothing or bedding and also maintaining the patient in a warm, dry environment. If these efforts are unsuccessful, then active rewarming of the patient must occur. Methods used to warm patients include warm air forced over the patient, heated intravenous fluids given via a countercurrent mechanism, and more aggressive measures such as bilateral chest tubes with warm solution lavage, intraperitoneal rewarming lavage, femoral artery–femoral vein vascular perfusion bypass, and possibly extracorporeal membrane oxygenation. Adding a heated circuit to mechanical ventilation does not increase core temperatures, but it does prevent secondary heat loss. The rate of rise of the measured core temperature will determine the sequence and timing for active rewarming interventions. A rate of rise of 2 to 4°C/h is considered adequate, but the most consistent complication for nonbypass rewarming is arrhythmia with ventricular arrest. The use of antiarrhythmics and early use of vascular bypass for patients rewarming too slowly is therefore often the preferred treatment.

Hyperthermia

Hyperthermia is the diagnosis for a core temperature greater than 38.6° C, and has a host of etiologies (Table 11-9) which are treated in a variety of ways.[95] Hyperpyrexia differs from hyperthermia in that an elevated core temperature due to SIRS is mediated by cytokine activation. Similarly to trauma, age plays a major role in tolerance and mortality of hyperthermia.

Hyperthermia can be environmentally induced (e.g., summer heat with inability to dissipate heat or control exposure), iatrogenically induced (e.g., heat lamps and medications), endocrine in origin (e.g., pheochromocytoma and thyroid storm), or neurologically

Table 11-9
Common Causes of Elevated Temperature in Surgical Patients

Hyperthermia	Hyperpyrexia
Environmental	Sepsis
Malignant hyperthermia	Infection
Neuroleptic malignant syndrome	Drug reaction
Thyrotoxicosis	Transfusion reaction
Pheochromocytoma	Collagen disorders
Carcinoid syndrome	Factitious syndrome
Iatrogenic	Neoplastic disorders
Central/hypothalamic responses	
Pulmonary embolism	
Adrenal insufficiency	

induced (i.e., hypothalamic). Hyperthermia complications in surgery largely stem from adverse effects of medications or occasionally the undiagnosed endocrinopathy or head-injured patient.

Malignant hyperthermia (MH) occurs after exposure to agents such as succinylcholine and some halothane-based inhalational anesthetics. The presentation is dramatic, with rapid onset of increased temperature, rigors, and myoglobinuria related to myonecrosis. Medications must be discontinued immediately and dantrolene administered (2.5 mg/kg every 5 minutes) until symptoms subside. Other supportive measures and aggressive active cooling are also implemented, such as alcohol baths, packing in ice, or the use of fans. For cases of severe malignant hyperthermia, the mortality rate is nearly 30%.

Neuroleptic malignant syndrome (NMS) is different than MH. All classes of neuroleptics [dopamine (D_2)-receptor antagonists] are associated with NMS, and dopamine receptor blockade is considered to be the cause of NMS. NMS is more likely to develop following initiation of neuroleptic therapy or an increase in the dose. The onset can be within hours, but on average it is 4 to 14 days after initiation of therapy. However, NMS can occur at any time during neuroleptic use, even years after initiating therapy. Symptoms include muscle rigidity, tachycardia, urinary incontinence, hemodynamic lability, respiratory distress, and changes in mental status. As with MH, treatment begins with discontinuing the offending medication and initiation of active cooling measures. In retrospective studies, dopamine agonists appear to decrease mortality and shorten the course of NMS, so the administration of medications such as bromocriptine or amantadine is used to control the syndrome's manifestations. The use of dantrolene in this setting is controversial. Despite aggressive treatment, mortality reaches 5%. Patients should avoid future use of the same medications that caused the initial NMS episode.[96]

Thyrotoxicosis can occur after surgery, as well as with childbirth, severe infections, and undiagnosed Graves' disease. Hyperthermia (>40°C), anxiety, copious diaphoresis, congestive heart failure (present in about one fourth of episodes), tachycardia (most commonly atrial fibrillation), and hypokalemia (up to 50% of patients), are hallmarks of the disease. The treatment of thyrotoxicosis is to control the crisis itself. Glucocorticoids, propylthiouracil, beta blockade, and iodide are delivered in an emergent fashion. As the name suggests, these patients are usually toxic and require supportive measures as well. Acetaminophen, cooling using the modalities noted above, and vasoactive agents are often indicated and utilized.

Central neurologic causes of hyperthermia are diagnosed largely by exclusion. The etiology of central hyperthermia is unclear, but the hyperthermia related to blood clotting within brain tissue is well documented. Treatment usually involves controlling the symptoms using conservative measures, but clonidine has been used for central hyperthermia with good results. The length of time that the crisis persists is unpredictable, so care is focused on providing general support until it ends.

ISSUES IN CARING FOR OBESE PATIENTS AND PATIENTS AT THE EXTREMES OF AGE

Now well recognized, obesity is a serious problem in the United States. Obesity begins when patients are young, and by adulthood the consequences cost millions of dollars and thousands of lost workdays. The rapid growth of bariatric surgery and the opening of bariatric surgery centers are indicative of an awareness of this growing national health care crisis.

Surgery in the obese patient has multiple risks, and it is important to optimize these patients before, during, and after surgery in order to minimize these risks. Optimization begins preoperatively with teaching, not only about dietary modifications, but about exercise and pulmonary toilet issues as well. Some patients will require a full cardiovascular work-up as well, since obese patients often have eccentric left ventricular hypertrophy, right ventricular hypertrophy, and congestive heart failure. Sleep studies and patient history may also reveal significant sleep apnea and gastroesophageal reflux disease. Glycemic control is often poor and contributes significantly to infection and diabetes. Also noted is the higher risk for DVT in obese patients. The obese patient has a decrease in antithrombin III levels, and since the volume of distribution is increased in obese patients compared with those with a normal body mass index, medication dosages must be adjusted appropriately.

Measures to optimize physiologic function in obese patients include keeping the head of the bed elevated at all times. This can improve the functional residual capacity of the lungs by almost a liter, thereby decreasing complications associated with atelectasis and pneumonia. Proper glycemic control via a tight insulin sliding scale is also recommended. Finally, the risk of DVT may be attenuated by immediate use of prophylactic doses of low molecular weight heparin and early ambulation. Low molecular weight heparins are encouraged because the volume of distribution is more reliable than with unfractionated heparin.

Issues for surgery in the very young and the very old have many similarities when it comes to potential errors and complications. Perhaps the most notable similarity is the lack of physiologic reserve. The elderly may have end-organ insufficiency, while the young can have underdeveloped or anomalous organ function that may not yet have become manifest. Similarly, the immune responses at the extremes of age are often compromised. This makes diagnosing an infection difficult; elderly adults may not be capable of mounting a febrile response, and young children can often resolve fevers overnight, and the cause may remain undiagnosed.

Other alterations in these groups include the amount and distribution of total body water and total body fat. This is important to consider because some medications are predominantly distributed to fat stores, and this deposition may lead to altered drug clearance. Similarly, total body water is decreased and serum concentrations of medications may be higher than anticipated. In both groups there is a lower lean body mass, which may potentiate the adverse effects of some anesthetic agents. Metabolism of various analgesic and anesthetic agents can be protracted, leading to postoperative problems such as prolonged intubation and the need for the administration of reversal agents.

Other issues that can lead to complex decision making include those related to communication. Whether due to neurologic impairments, agitation, confusion, or an inability to comprehend a language, these factors associated with the extremes of age increase the potential for medical errors. Open and direct communication with the supporting family members is critical for optimal outcomes in these patient groups.

References

1. Kohn LT, Corrigan JM, Donaldson MS (eds): *To Err Is Human: Building a Safer Health System.* Committee on Quality of Health Care in America, Institute of Medicine. Washington, DC: National Academy Press, 2000.

2. Veenstra DL, Saint S, Sullivan SD: Cost-effectiveness of antiseptic-impregnated central venous catheters for the prevention of catheter-related bloodstream infection. *JAMA* 282:554, 1999.

3. O'Grady NP, Alexander M, Dellinger EP, et al: Guidelines for the prevention of intravascular catheter-related infections. *Am J Infect Control* 30:476, 2002.

4. Stoiser B, Kofler J, Staudinger T, et al: Contamination of central venous catheters in immunocompromised patients: A comparison between two different types of central venous catheters. *J Hosp Infect* 50:202, 2002.

5. Beiderlinden M, Groeben H, Peters J: Safety of percutaneous dilational tracheostomy in patients ventilated with high positive end-expiratory pressure (PEEP). *Intensive Care Med* 29:944, 2003.

6. Kerwin AJ, Croce MA, Timmons SD, et al: Effects of fiberoptic bronchoscopy on intracranial pressure in patients with brain injury: A prospective clinical study. *J Trauma* 48:878, 2000; discussion 882.

7. Tyroch AH, Kaups K, Lorenzo M, et al: Routine chest radiograph is not indicated after open tracheostomy: A multicenter perspective. *Am Surg* 68:80, 2002.

8. Datta D, Onyirimba F, McNamee MJ: The utility of chest radiographs following percutaneous dilatational tracheostomy. *Chest* 123:1603, 2003.

9. Gelman JJ, Aro M, Weiss SM: Tracheo-innominate artery fistula. *J Am Coll Surg* 179:626, 1994.

10. Keceligil HT, Erk MK, Kolbakir F, et al: Tracheoinnominate artery fistula following tracheostomy. *Cardiovasc Surg* 3:509, 1995.

11. Bandhauer F, Buhl D, Grossenbacher R: Antibiotic prophylaxis in rhinosurgery. *Am J Rhinol* 16:135, 2002.

12. Rybak MJ, Abate BJ, Kang SL, et al: Prospective evaluation of the effect of an aminoglycoside dosing regimen on rates of observed nephrotoxicity and ototoxicity. *Antimicrob Agents Chemother* 43:1549, 1999.

13. Sandur S, Stoller JK: Pulmonary complications of mechanical ventilation. *Clin Chest Med* 20:223, 1999.

14. Salem M, Tainsh RE, Bromberg J, et al: Perioperative glucocorticoid coverage: A reassessment 42 years after emergence of a problem. *Ann Surg* 219:416, 1994.

15. Hughes MG, Evans HL, Chong TW, et al: Effect of an intensive care unit rotating empiric antibiotic schedule on the development of hospital-acquired infections on the non-intensive care unit ward. *Crit Care Med* 32:53, 2004.

16. Horn SD, Wright HL, Couperus JJ, et al: Association between patient-controlled analgesia pump use and postoperative surgical site infection in intestinal surgery patients. *Surg Infect (Larchmt)* 3:109, 2002.

17. The Acute Respiratory Distress Syndrome Network: Ventilation with lower tidal volumes as compared with traditional tidal volumes for acute lung injury and the acute respiratory distress syndrome. *N Engl J Med* 342:1301, 2000.

18. Valente Barbas CS: Lung recruitment maneuvers in acute respiratory distress syndrome and facilitating resolution. *Crit Care Med* 31 (4 Suppl):S265, 2003.

19. Gattinoni L, Tognoni G, Pesenti A, et al: Effect of prone positioning on the survival of patients with acute respiratory failure. *N Engl J Med* 315:568, 2001.

20. Fridrich P, Krafft P, Hochleuthner H, et al: The effects of long-term prone positioning in patients with trauma-induced adult respiratory distress syndrome. *Anesth Analg* 83:1206, 1996.

21. Langer M, Mascheroni D, Marcolin R, et al: The prone position in ARDS patients. A clinical study. *Chest* 94:103, 1988.

22. Gronski T Jr., Lum E, Campbell J, et al: A murine model of volutrauma: Potential contribution of inflammatory cell proteases to lung injury. *Chest* 116(1 Suppl):28S, 1999.

23. Singh JM, Stewart TE: High-frequency mechanical ventilation principles and practices in the era of lung-protective ventilation strategies. *Respir Care Clin North Am* 8:247, 2002.

24. Yang KL, Tobin MJ: A prospective study of indexes predicting the outcome of trials of weaning from mechanical ventilation. *N Engl J Med* 324:1445, 1991.

25. Epstein SK: Etiology of extubation failure and the predictive value of the rapid shallow breathing index. *Am J Respir Crit Care Med* 152:545, 1995.

26. Falk RH: Atrial fibrillation. *N Engl J Med* 344:24, 2001.

27. Van Gelder IC, Hagens VE, Bosker HA, et al: A comparison of rate control and rhythm control in patients with recurrent persistent atrial fibrillation. *N Engl J Med* 347:1834, 2001.

28. A comparison of rate control and rhythm control in patients with atrial fibrillation. The atrial fibrillation follow-up investigation of rhythm management (AFFIRM) investigators. *N Engl J Med* 347:1825, 2002.

29. Gottlieb SS, McCarter RJ, Vogel RA: Effect of beta-blockade on mortality among high-risk and low-risk patients after myocardial infarction. *N Engl J Med* 339:489, 1998.

30. Hjalmarson A, Herlitz J, Malek I, et al: Effect on mortality of metoprolol in acute myocardial infarction. (A double-blind randomized trial.) *Lancet* 318:823, 1981.

31. Poldermans D, Boersma E, Bax JJ: The effect of bisoprolol on perioperative mortality and myocardial infarction in high-risk patients undergoing vascular surgery. *N Engl J Med* 341:1789, 1999.

32. Franklin RH: Ivor Lewis Lecture, 1975. The advancing frontiers of oesophageal surgery. *Ann R Coll Surg Engl* 59:284, 1977.

33. Hagedorn C, Jonson C, Lonroth H, et al: Efficacy of an anterior as compared with a posterior laparoscopic partial fundoplication: Results of a randomized, controlled clinical trial. *Ann Surg* 238:189, 2003.

34. Watson DI, Jamieson GG, Devitt PG, et al: A prospective randomized trial of laparoscopic Nissen fundoplication with anterior vs. posterior hiatal repair. *Arch Surg* 136:745, 2001.

35. Stewart BT, Woods RJ, Collopy BT, et al: Early feeding after elective open colorectal resections: A prospective randomized trial. *Aust N Z J Surg* 68:125, 1998.

36. Asao T, Kuwano H, Nakamura J, et al: Gum chewing enhances early recovery from postoperative ileus after laparoscopic colectomy. *J Am Coll Surg* 195:30, 2002.

37. Beck DE, Cohen Z, Fleshman JW, et al: A prospective, randomized, multicenter, controlled study of the safety of Seprafilm adhesion barrier in abdominopelvic surgery of the intestine. *Dis Colon Rectum* 46:1310, 2003.

38. Tang CL, Seow-Choen F, Fook-Chong S, et al: Bioresorbable adhesion barrier facilitates early closure of the defunctioning ileostomy after rectal excision: A prospective, randomized trial. *Dis Colon Rectum* 46:1200, 2003.

39. Beck DE, Cohen Z, Fleshman JW, et al: A prospective, randomized, multicenter, controlled study of the safety of Seprafilm adhesion barrier in abdominopelvic surgery of the intestine. *Dis Colon Rectum* 46:1310, 2003.

40. Smoot RL, Gostout CJ, Rajan E, et al: Is early colonoscopy after admission for acute diverticular bleeding needed? *Am J Gastroenterol* 98:1996, 2003.

41. Sorbi D, Gostout CJ, Peura D, et al: An assessment of the management of acute bleeding varices: A multicenter prospective member-based study. *Am J Gastroenterol* 98:2424, 2003.

42. Domschke W, Lederer P, Lux G: The value of emergency endoscopy in upper gastrointestinal bleeding: Review and analysis of 2014 cases. *Endoscopy* 15:126, 1983.

43. Cash BD: Evidence-based medicine as it applies to acid suppression in the hospitalized patient. *Crit Care Med* 30(6 Suppl):S373, 2002.

44. Lidwig K, Bernhardt J, Steffen H, et al: Contribution of intraoperative cholangiography to incidence and outcome of common bile duct injuries during laparoscopic cholecystectomy. *Surg Endosc* 16:1098, 2002.

45. Flum DR, Dellinger EP, Cheadle A, et al: Intraoperative cholangiography and risk of common bile duct injury during cholecystectomy. *JAMA* 289:1639, 2003.

46. Yoon YH, Yi H, Grant BF, et al: Liver cirrhosis mortality in the United States, 1970–98. Bethesda, MD: National Institute on Alcohol Abuse and Alcoholism, Surveillance Report #57, 2001.

47. Solomon R, Werner C, Mann D, et al: Effects of saline, mannitol, and furosemide to prevent acute decreases in renal function induced by radiocontrast agents. *N Engl J Med* 24:331:1416, 1994.

48. Stevens MA, McCullough PA, Tobin KJ, et al: A prospective randomized trial of prevention measures in patients at high risk for contrast nephropathy: Results of the P.R.I.N.C.E. study. Prevention of radiocontrast induced nephropathy clinical evaluation. *J Am Coll Cardiol* 33:403, 1999.

49. Birck R, Krzossok S, Markowetz F, et al: Acetylcysteine for prevention of contrast nephropathy: Meta-analysis. *Lancet* 362:598, 2003.

50. Baker CS, Wragg A, Kumar S, et al: A rapid protocol for the prevention of contrast-induced renal dysfunction: The RAPPID study. *J Am Coll Cardiol* 41:2114, 2003.

51. Kellum JA, Decker J: Use of dopamine in acute renal failure: A meta-analysis. *Crit Care Med* 29:1526, 2001.

52. Power DA, Duggan J, Brady HR: Renal-dose (low-dose) dopamine for the treatment of sepsis-related and other forms of acute renal failure: Ineffective and probably dangerous. *Clin Exp Pharmacol Physiol Suppl* 26:S23, 1999.

53. Corwin HL, Gettinger A, Pearl RG, et al: Efficacy of recombinant human erythropoietin in critically ill patients: A randomized controlled trial. *JAMA* 288:2827, 2002.

54. Laffan M, O'Connell NM, Perry DJ, et al: Analysis and results of the recombinant factor VIIa extended-use registry. *Blood Coagul Fibrinolysis* 14(Suppl 1):S35, 2003.

55. Hedner U: Dosing with recombinant factor VIIa based on current evidence. *Semin Hematol* 41(1 Suppl):35, 2004.

56. Midathada MV, Mehta P, Waner M, et al: Recombinant factor VIIa in the treatment of bleeding. *Am J Clin Pathol* 121:124, 2004.

57. Bloomfield GL, Dalton JM, Sugerman HJ, et al: Treatment of increasing intracranial pressure secondary to the acute abdominal compartment syndrome in a patient with combined abdominal and head trauma. *J Trauma* 39:1168, 1995.

58. Kron I, Harman PK, Nolan SP: The measurement of intra-abdominal pressure as a criterion for abdominal re-exploration. *Ann Surg* 199:28, 1984.

59. Ivatury RR, Porter JM, Simon RJ, et al: Intra-abdominal hypertension after life-threatening penetrating abdominal trauma: Prophylaxis, incidence, and clinical relevance to gastric mucosal pH and abdominal compartment syndrome. *J Trauma* 44:1016, 1998.

60. Ivatury RR, Sugerman HJ, Peitzman AB: Abdominal compartment syndrome: Recognition and management. *Adv Surg* 35:251, 2001.

61. Saggi BH, Sugerman HJ, Ivatury RR, et al: Abdominal compartment syndrome. *J Trauma* 45:597, 1998.

62. Gorecki PJ, Schein M, Mehta V, et al: Surgeons and infectious disease specialists: Different attitudes towards antibiotic treatment and prophylaxis in common abdominal surgical infections. *Surg Infect (Larchmt)* 1:115, 2000; discussion 125.

63. Anglen J, Apostoles PS, Christensen G, et al: Removal of surface bacteria by irrigation. *J Orthop Res* 14:251, 1966.

64. Lewis DA, Leaper DJ, Speller DC: Prevention of bacterial colonization of wounds at operation: Comparison of iodine-impregnated ("Ioban") drapes with conventional methods. *J Hosp Infect* 5:431, 1984.

65. O'Rourke E, Runyan D, O'Leary J, et al: Contaminated iodophor in the operating room. *Am J Infect Control* 31:255, 2003.

66. Ostrander RV, Brage ME, Botte MJ: Bacterial skin contamination after surgical preparation in foot and ankle surgery. *Clin Orthop* 406:246, 2003.

67. Ghogawala Z, Furtado D: In vitro and in vivo bactericidal activities of 10%, 2.5%, and 1% povidone-iodine solution. *Am J Hosp Pharm* 47:1562, 1990.

68. Anderson RL, Vess RW, Carr JH: Investigations of intrinsic *Pseudomonas cepacia* contamination in commercially manufactured povidone-iodine. *Infect Control Hosp Epidemiol* 12:297, 1991.

69. Birnbach DJ, Meadows W, Stein DJ, et al: Comparison of povidone iodine and DuraPrep, an iodophor-in-isopropyl alcohol solution, for skin disinfection prior to epidural catheter insertion in parturients. *Anesthesiology* 98:164, 2003.

70. Moen MD, Noone MG, Kirson I: Povidone-iodine spray technique versus traditional scrub-paint technique for preoperative abdominal wall preparation. *Am J Obstet Gynecol* 187:1434, 2002; discussion 1436.

71. Strand CL, Wajsbort RR, Sturmann K: Effect of iodophor vs. iodine tincture skin preparation on blood culture contamination rate. *JAMA* 269:1004, 1993.

72. Paterson DL, Ko WC, Von Gottberg A, et al: International prospective study of *Klebsiella pneumoniae* bacteremia: Implications of extended-spectrum beta-lactamase production in nosocomial infections. *Ann Intern Med* 140:26, 2004.

73. Wittmann DH, Schein M: Let us shorten antibiotic prophylaxis and therapy in surgery. *Am J Surg* 172:26S, 1966.

74. Dellinger EP: Duration of antibiotic treatment in surgical infections of the abdomen. Undesired effects of antibiotics and future studies. *Eur J Surg Suppl* 576:29, 1996; discussion 31.

75. Fry DE: Basic aspects of and general problems in surgical infections. *Surg Infect (Larchmt)* 2(Suppl 1):S3, 2001.

76. Barie PS: Modern surgical antibiotic prophylaxis and therapy—less is more. *Surg Infect (Larchmt)* 1:23, 2000.

77. Grobmyer SR, Graham D, Brennan MF, et al: High-pressure gradients generated by closed-suction surgical drainage systems. *Surg Infect (Larchmt)* 3:245, 2002.

78. Williams J, Toews D, Prince M: Survey of the use of suction drains in head and neck surgery and analysis of their biomechanical properties. *J Otolaryngol* 32:16, 2003.

79. Harisinghani MG, Gervais DA, Maher MM, et al: Transgluteal approach for percutaneous drainage of deep pelvic abscesses: 154 Cases. *Radiology* 228:701, 2003.

80. Cantasdemir M, Kara B, Cebi D, et al: Computed tomography-guided percutaneous catheter drainage of primary and secondary iliopsoas abscesses. *Clin Radiol* 58:811, 2003.

81. Vincent JL, Abraham E, Annane D, et al: Reducing mortality in sepsis: New directions. *Crit Care* 6(Suppl 3):S1, 2002.

82. Malay MB, Ashton RC Jr., Landry DW, et al: Low-dose vasopressin in the treatment of vasodilatory septic shock. *J Trauma* 47:699, 1999; discussion 703.

83. Annane D, Sebille V, Charpentier C, et al: Effect of treatment with low doses of hydrocortisone and fludrocortisone on mortality in patients with septic shock. *JAMA* 288:862, 2002.

84. Dhainaut JF, Laterre PF, LaRosa SP, et al: The clinical evaluation committee in a large multicenter phase 3 trial of drotrecogin alfa (activated) in patients with severe sepsis (PROWESS): Role, methodology, and results. *Crit Care Med* 31:2291, 2003; see also p 2405.

85. Betancourt M, McKinnon PS, Massanari RM, et al: An evaluation of the cost effectiveness of drotrecogin alfa (activated) relative to the number of organ system failures. *Pharmacoeconomics* 21:1331, 2003.

86. van den Berghe G, Wouters P, Weekers F, et al: Intensive insulin therapy in the critically ill patients. *N Engl J Med* 345:1359, 2001.

87. Finney SJ, Zekveld C, Elia A, et al: Glucose control and mortality in critically ill patients. *JAMA* 290:2041, 2003.

88. Furnary AP, Gao G, Grunkemeier GL, et al: Continuous insulin infusion reduces mortality in patients with diabetes undergoing coronary artery bypass grafting. *J Thorac Cardiovasc Surg* 125:1007, 2003.

89. Salem M, Tainsh RE, Bromberg J, et al: Perioperative glucocorticoid coverage: A reassessment 42 years after emergence of a problem. *Ann Surg* 219:416, 1994.

90. Fraser CG, Preuss FS, Bigford WD: Adrenal atrophy and irreversible shock associated with cortisone therapy. *JAMA* 149:1542, 1952.

91. La Rochelle GE Jr., La Rochelle AG, Ratner RE, et al: Recovery of the hypothalamic-pituitary-adrenal axis in patients with rheumatic diseases receiving low-dose prednisone. *Am J Med* 95:258, 1993.

92. Bromberg JS, Alfrey EJ, Barker CF, et al: Adrenal suppression and steroid supplementation in renal transplant recipients. *Transplantation* 51:385, 1991.

93. Freidman RJ, Schiff CF, Bromberg JS: Use of supplemental steroids in patients having orthopaedic operations. *J Bone Joint Surg* 77A:1801, 1995.

94. Kempainen RR, Brunette DD: The evaluation and management of accidental hypothermia. *Respir Care* 49:192, 2004.

95. O'Donnell J, Axelrod P, Fisher C, et al: Use and effectiveness of hypothermia blankets for febrile patients in the intensive care unit. *Clin Infect Dis* 24:1208, 1977.

96. Bond WS: Detection and management of the neuroleptic malignant syndrome. *Clin Pharm* 3:302, 1984.

Suggested Reading

Angel LF, Simpson CB: Comparison of surgical and percutaneous dilational tracheostomy. *Clin Chest Med* 24:423, 2003.

Arom KV, Richardson JD, Webb G, et al: Subxiphoid pericardial window in patients with suspected traumatic pericardial tamponade. *Ann Thorac Surg* 23:545, 1977.

Black FO, Gianna-Poulin C, Pesznecker SC: Recovery from vestibular ototoxicity. *Otol Neurotol* 22:662, 2001.

Chastre J, Wolff M, Fagon JY, et al: Comparison of 8 vs. 15 days of antibiotic therapy for ventilator-associated pneumonia in adults: A randomized trial. *JAMA* 290:2588, 2003.

Demling RH, DeSanti L: Oxandrolone induced lean mass gain during recovery from severe burns is maintained after discontinuation of the anabolic steroid. *Burns* 29:793, 2003.

Derkay CS, Hirsch BE, Johnson JT, et al: Posterior nasal packing. Are intravenous antibiotics really necessary? *Arch Otolaryngol Head Neck Surg* 115:439, 1989.

Erkut ZA, Klooker T, Endert E, et al: Stress of dying is not suppressed by high-dose morphone or by dementia. *Neuropsychopharmacology* 29:152, 2004.

Kazmers A, Ramnauth S, Williams M: Intraoperative insertion of Greenfield filters: Lessons learned in a personal series of 152 cases. *Am Surg* 68:877, 2002.

Rougier F, Claude D, Maurin M, et al: Aminoglycoside nephrotoxicity: Modeling, simulation, and control. *Antimicrob Agents Chemother* 47:1010, 2003.

Schroeder ET, Zheng L, Yarasheski KE, et al: Treatment with oxandrolone and the durability of effects in older men. *J Appl Physiol* 96:1055, 2004.

Zannetti S, Cao P, De Rango P, et al: Intraoperative assessment of technical perfection in carotid endarterectomy: A prospective analysis of 1305 completion procedures. Collaborators of the EVEREST study group. Eversion versus standard carotid endarterectomy. *Eur J Vasc Endovasc Surg* 18:52, 1999.

CHAPTER 12

Physiologic Monitoring of the Surgical Patient

Louis H. Alarcon and Mitchell P. Fink

INTRODUCTION

The Latin verb *monere*, which means "to warn," is the origin for the English word *monitor*. In modern medical practice, patients are monitored in order to detect alterations in various physiologic parameters, providing advanced warning of impending deterioration in the status of one or more organ systems. With this knowledge, appropriate actions may be taken in a timely fashion to prevent or ameliorate the physiologic derangement. Physiologic monitoring is used, however, not only to warn, but also to titrate fluid resuscitation or the infusion of vasoactive or inotropic drugs. Monitoring tools also can be valuable for diagnostic evaluation and assessment of prognosis. The intensive care unit (ICU) and operating room are the two locations where the most advanced monitoring capabilities are routinely employed in the care of critically-ill patients.

In the broadest sense, physiologic monitoring encompasses a spectrum of endeavors, ranging in complexity from the routine and intermittent measurement of the classic "vital signs" (i.e., temperature, pulse, arterial blood pressure, and respiratory rate) to the continuous recording of the oxidation state of cytochrome oxidase, the terminal element in the mitochondrial electron transport chain. The ability to assess clinically relevant parameters of tissue and organ status and employ this knowledge to improve patient outcomes represents the goal of critical care medicine. Unfortunately, consensus is lacking regarding the most appropriate parameters to monitor in order to achieve this goal. Taking the wrong therapeutic action because of bad data or misinterpretation of good data can lead to a worse outcome than having no data at all. Of the highest importance is the integration of physiologic data obtained from monitoring into a coherent treatment plan. Current technologies available to assist the clinician in this endeavor are summarized in the following sections of this chapter, as well as a brief look at emerging techniques that may soon enter into clinical practice.

Mammalian cells generally cannot store oxygen for subsequent use in oxidative metabolism, although a relatively tiny amount is stored in muscle tissue as oxidized myoglobin. Thus aerobic synthesis of adenosine triphosphate (ATP), the energy "currency" of cells, requires the continuous delivery of oxygen by diffusion from hemoglobin in red blood cells to the oxidative machinery within mitochondria. In essence, the goal of hemodynamic monitoring is to ensure that the flow of oxygenated blood through the microcirculation is sufficient to support aerobic metabolism at the cellular level. Delivery of oxygen to mitochondria can be inadequate for several reasons. For example, cardiac output, hemoglobin, or the oxygen content of arterial blood can each be inadequate for independent reasons. Alternatively, despite adequate cardiac output, perfusion of capillary networks can be impaired as a consequence of dysregulation of arteriolar tone, microvascular thrombosis, or obstruction of nutritive vessels by sequestered leukocytes or platelets. Hemodynamic monitoring that does not take into account all of these factors will portray an incomplete and perhaps misleading picture of cellular physiology.

Under normal conditions when the supply of oxygen is plentiful, aerobic metabolism is determined by factors other than the availability of oxygen. These factors include the hormonal milieu and mechanical workload of contractile tissue. However, in pathologic circumstances when oxygen availability is inadequate, oxygen utilization ($\dot{V}o_2$) becomes dependent upon oxygen delivery ($\dot{D}o_2$). The relationship of $\dot{V}o_2$ to $\dot{D}o_2$ over a broad range of $\dot{D}o_2$ values is commonly represented as two intersecting straight lines. In the region of higher $\dot{D}o_2$ values, the slope of the line is approximately equal to zero, indicating that $\dot{V}o_2$ is largely independent of $\dot{D}o_2$. In contrast, in the region of low $\dot{D}o_2$ values, the slope of the line is nonzero and positive, indicating that $\dot{V}o_2$ is supply-dependent. The region where the two lines intersect is called the point of critical oxygen delivery ($\dot{D}o_{2crit}$), and represents the transition from supply-independent to supply-dependent oxygen uptake. In anesthetized humans undergoing cardiac surgery, systemic $\dot{D}o_{2crit}$ is approximately 300 to 330 mL/min per square meter.[1,2] The slope of the supply-dependent region of the plot reflects the maximal oxygen extraction capability of the vascular bed being evaluated.

The dual-line representation for depicting $\dot{D}o_2$-$\dot{V}o_2$ relationships has proven useful and informative. Nevertheless, other approaches for depicting $\dot{D}o_2$-$\dot{V}o_2$ relationships may be equally or even more relevant. For example, some investigators believe that experimentally derived $\dot{D}o_2$-$\dot{V}o_2$ data are optimally characterized by using the classic Michaelis-Menten relationship for describing the kinetics of an enzymatic reaction, a view that is prompted by the recognition that the oxygen-consuming reaction in mitochondria is catalyzed by an enzyme, cytochrome oxidase.[3]

ARTERIAL BLOOD PRESSURE

The pressure exerted by blood in the systemic arterial system, commonly referred to simply as "blood pressure," is a cardinal parameter measured as part of the hemodynamic monitoring of patients. Extremes in blood pressure are either intrinsically deleterious or are indicative of a serious perturbation in normal physiology. In an earlier era, blood pressure served as a proxy for cardiac output; the term "shock" was used more or less as a synonym for arterial hypotension. Although it is now known that arterial blood pressure is a complex function of both cardiac output and vascular input impedance, clinicians, especially inexperienced ones, tend to assume that the presence of a normal blood pressure is evidence that cardiac output and tissue perfusion are adequate. This assumption is frequently incorrect and is the reason why some critically ill patients may benefit from forms of hemodynamic monitoring in addition to measurement of arterial pressure.

Blood pressure can be determined directly by measuring the pressure within the arterial lumen or indirectly using a cuff around an extremity. When the equipment is properly set up and calibrated, direct intra-arterial monitoring of blood pressure provides accurate and continuous data. Additionally, intra-arterial catheters provide a convenient way to obtain samples of blood for measurements of arterial blood gases and other laboratory studies. Despite these advantages, intra-arterial catheters are invasive devices and occasionally are associated with serious complications. Noninvasive monitoring of blood pressure is desirable in many circumstances.

Noninvasive Measurement of Arterial Blood Pressure

Both manual and automated means for the noninvasive determination of blood pressure use an inflatable cuff to increase pressure around an extremity. If the cuff is too narrow (relative to the extremity), the measured pressure will be artifactually elevated. Therefore, the width of the cuff should be approximately 40% of its circumference.

In addition to using a cuff to cause vascular compression and thereby cessation of blood flow, noninvasive means for measuring blood pressure also require some means for detecting the presence or absence of arterial pulsations. Several methods exist for this purpose. The time-honored approach is the auscultation of the Korotkoff sounds, which are heard over an artery distal to the cuff as the cuff is deflated from a pressure higher than systolic pressure to one less than diastolic pressure. *Systolic pressure* is defined as the pressure in the cuff when tapping sounds are first audible. *Diastolic pressure* is the pressure in the cuff when audible pulsations first disappear.

Another means for pulse detection when measuring blood pressure noninvasively depends upon the detection of oscillations in the pressure within the bladder of the cuff. This approach is simple, and unlike auscultation, can be performed even in a noisy environment (e.g., a busy emergency room). Unfortunately, this approach is neither accurate nor reliable. Other methods, however, can be used to reliably detect the reappearance of a pulse distal to the cuff and thereby estimate systolic blood pressure. Two excellent and widely available approaches for pulse detection are use of a Doppler stethoscope (reappearance of the pulse produces an audible amplified signal) or a pulse oximeter (reappearance of the pulse is indicated by flashing of a light-emitting diode).

A number of automated devices are capable of repetitively measuring blood pressure noninvasively. Some of these devices measure pressure oscillations in the inflatable bladder encircling the extremity to detect arterial pulsations as pressure in the cuff is gradually lowered from greater than systolic to less than diastolic pressure.[4] Another automated noninvasive device uses a piezoelectric crystal positioned over the brachial artery as a pulse detector.[4] According to one clinical study of these approaches, the most accurate is oscillometry combined with stepped deflation of the sphygmomanometric cuff. Using this approach and comparing the results of oscillometry to those obtained by invasive intra-arterial monitoring, errors in the measurement of mean blood pressure greater than 10 or 20 mm Hg occur in 0 and 8.5% of readings, respectively.[4]

Another noninvasive approach for measuring blood pressure relies on a technique called photoplethysmography. This method is capable of providing continuous information, since systolic and diastolic blood pressures are recorded on a beat-to-beat basis. Photoplethysmography uses the transmission of infrared light to estimate the amount of hemoglobin (directly related to the volume of blood) in a finger placed under a servo-controlled inflatable cuff. A feedback loop controlled by a microprocessor continually adjusts the pressure in the cuff to maintain the blood volume of the finger constant. Under these conditions, the pressure in the cuff reflects the pressure in the digital artery. Although results obtained using photoplethysmography generally agree closely with those obtained by invasive monitoring of blood pressure, the difference between the two methods occasionally can be large (20 to 40 mm Hg) in some patients.[5] This problem limits the usefulness of photoplethysmography as a stand-alone method for monitoring arterial blood pressure, particularly in high-risk situations.

However, if initial photoplethysmographic readings are corrected by comparison with measurements obtained noninvasively by an oscillometric device, then photoplethysmography is sufficiently accurate to be used for continuous monitoring in most situations.[5]

Invasive Monitoring of Arterial Blood Pressure

Direct monitoring of arterial pressure almost always is performed by using fluid-filled tubing to connect an intra-arterial catheter to an external strain-gauge transducer. The signal generated by the transducer is electronically amplified and displayed as a continuous waveform by an oscilloscope. Digital values for systolic and diastolic pressure also are displayed. Mean pressure, calculated by electronically averaging the amplitude of the pressure waveform, also can be displayed.

The fidelity of the catheter-tubing-transducer system is determined by numerous factors, including the compliance of the tubing, the surface area of the transducer diaphragm, and the compliance of the diaphragm. If the system is underdamped, then the inertia of the system, which is a function of the mass of the fluid in the tubing and the mass of the diaphragm, causes overshoot of the points of maximum positive and negative displacement of the diaphragm during systole and diastole, respectively. Thus in an underdamped system, systolic pressure will be overestimated and diastolic pressure will be underestimated. In an overdamped system, displacement of the diaphragm fails to track the rapidly changing pressure waveform, and systolic pressure will be underestimated and diastolic pressure will be overestimated. It is important to note that even in an underdamped or overdamped system, mean pressure will be accurately recorded, provided the system has been properly calibrated. When using direct measurement of intra-arterial pressure to monitor patients, physicians and nurses should be in the habit of using mean pressure for making clinical decisions.

The degree of ringing (i.e., overshoot and undershoot) in a minimally damped system is determined by its resonant frequency. Ideally, the resonant frequency of the system should be at least five times greater than the highest frequency component of the pressure waveform. The resonant frequency can be too low for optimal performance if the connector tubing is too compliant or there are air bubbles in the fluid column between the arterial pressure source and the diaphragm of the transducer. For arterial pressure monitoring, the optimal resonance frequency is higher than is practically obtainable. Therefore, to prevent excessive ringing, some degree of damping is essential. To determine if the combination of resonance frequency and damping is adequate, one can pressurize the system to approximately 300 mg Hg by pulling the tab that controls the valve between the monitoring system and the high-pressure bag of flush solution. When the valve is abruptly closed by allowing the tab to snap back into its normal position, a sharp pressure transient will be introduced into the system. The resulting pressure tracing can be observed on a strip chart recording. Damping is optimal if at least two oscillations are observed, and there is at least a threefold decrease in the amplitude of successive oscillations.

The radial artery at the wrist is the site most commonly used for intra-arterial pressure monitoring. It is important to recognize, however, that measured arterial pressure is determined in part by the site where the pressure is monitored. Central (i.e., aortic) and peripheral (e.g., radial artery) pressures typically are different as a result of the impedance and inductance of the arterial tree.[6] Systolic pressures typically are higher and diastolic pressures are lower in the periphery, whereas mean pressure is approximately the same in the aorta and more distal sites.

Distal ischemia is an uncommon complication of intra-arterial catheterization. The incidence of thrombosis is increased when larger-caliber catheters are employed and when catheters are left in place for an extended period of time. The incidence of thrombosis can be minimized by using a 20-gauge (or smaller) catheter in the radial position and leaving the catheter in place for as short a duration as feasible, preferably less than 4 days. The risk of distal ischemic injury can be minimized by ensuring that adequate collateral flow is present. At the wrist, adequate collateral flow can be documented by performing a modified version of the Allen test, wherein the artery to be cannulated is digitally compressed while using a Doppler stethoscope to listen for perfusion in the palmar arch vessels.

Another potential complication of intra-arterial monitoring is retrograde embolization of air bubbles or thrombi into the intracranial circulation. In order to minimize the risk of this rare but potentially devastating complication, great care should be taken to avoid flushing arterial lines when air is present in the system, and only small volumes of fluid (less than 5 mL) should be employed for this purpose. Catheter-related infections can occur with any intravascular monitoring device. However, catheter-related bloodstream infection is a relatively uncommon complication of intra-arterial lines used for monitoring, typically accounting for only approximately 1% of all cases of bacteremia attributable to an intravascular catheter.[7]

ELECTROCARDIOGRAPHIC MONITORING

The electrocardiogram (ECG) records the electrical activity associated with cardiac contraction by detecting voltages on the body surface. A standard 3-lead ECG is obtained by placing electrodes that correspond to the left arm (LA), right arm (RA), and left leg (LL). The limb leads are defined as lead I (LA-RA), lead II (LL-RA), and lead III (LL-LA). The ECG waveforms can be continuously displayed on a monitor, and the devices can be set to sound an alarm if an abnormality of rate or rhythm is detected. Continuous ECG monitoring is widely available and applied to critically ill and perioperative patients. Monitoring of the ECG waveform is essential in patients with acute coronary syndromes or blunt myocardial injury, because dysrhythmias are the most common lethal complication. In patients with shock or sepsis, dysrhythmias can occur as a consequence of inadequate myocardial oxygen delivery or as a complication of vasoactive or inotropic drugs used to support blood pressure and cardiac output. Dysrhythmias can be detected by continuously monitoring the ECG tracing, and timely intervention may prevent serious complications. With appropriate computing hardware and software, continuous ST-segment analysis also can be performed to detect ischemia or infarction. This approach has proven useful to detect silent myocardial ischemia in patients undergoing weaning from mechanical ventilation.[8,9]

Additional information can be obtained from a 12-lead ECG, which is essential for patients with potential myocardial ischemia or to rule out cardiac complications in other acutely ill patients. Continuous monitoring of the 12-lead ECG is now available and is proving to be beneficial in certain patient populations. In a study of 185 vascular surgical patients, continuous 12-lead ECG monitoring was able to detect transient myocardial ischemic episodes in 20.5% of the patients.[9] This study demonstrated that the precordial lead V_4, which is not routinely monitored on a standard 3-lead ECG, is the most sensitive for detecting perioperative ischemia and infarction. To detect 95% of the ischemic episodes, two or more precordial leads were necessary. Thus, continuous 12-lead ECG monitoring may provide greater sensitivity than 3-lead ECG for the detection of perioperative myocardial ischemia, and is likely to become standard for monitoring high-risk surgical patients.

CARDIAC OUTPUT AND RELATED PARAMETERS

Bedside catheterization of the pulmonary artery was introduced into clinical practice in 1970.[10] Although the Swan-Ganz catheter initially was used primarily to manage patients with cardiogenic shock and other acute cardiac diseases, indications for this form of invasive hemodynamic monitoring gradually expanded to encompass a wide variety of clinical conditions.[10] By 1996, more than 2 million balloon-tipped pulmonary artery catheters were being sold worldwide.[11] Clearly, many clinicians must believe that information valuable for the management of critically ill patients is afforded by having a pulmonary artery catheter (PAC) in place. However, unambiguous data in support of this view are scarce, and several studies suggest that bedside pulmonary artery catheterization actually is associated with poorer outcomes in selected populations of patients.

Determinants of Cardiac Performance

Preload

Starling's law of the heart states that the force of muscle contraction depends on the initial length of the cardiac fibers. Using terminology that derives from early experiments using isolated cardiac muscle preparations, preload is the stretch of ventricular myocardial tissue just prior to the next contraction. Preload is determined by end-diastolic volume (EDV). For the right ventricle, central venous pressure (CVP) approximates right ventricular end-diastolic pressure (EDP). For the left ventricle, pulmonary artery occlusion pressure (PAOP), which is measured by transiently inflating a balloon at the end of a pressure monitoring catheter positioned in a small branch of the pulmonary artery, approximates left ventricular end-diastolic pressure. The presence of atrioventricular valvular stenosis will alter this relationship.

Clinicians frequently use EDP as a surrogate for EDV, but EDP is determined not only by volume but also by the diastolic compliance of the ventricular chamber. Ventricular compliance is altered by various pharmacologic agents and pathologic conditions. Furthermore, the relationship between EDP and true preload is not linear, but rather is exponential.

Afterload

Afterload is another term derived from in vitro experiments using isolated strips of cardiac muscle, and is defined as the force resisting fiber shortening once systole begins. Several factors comprise the in vivo correlate of ventricular afterload, including ventricular intracavitary pressure, wall thickness, chamber radius, and chamber geometry. Since these factors are difficult to assess clinically, afterload is commonly approximated by calculating systemic vascular resistance, defined as mean arterial pressure (MAP) divided by cardiac output.

Contractility

Contractility is defined as the inotropic state of the myocardium. Contractility is said to increase when the force of ventricular contraction increases at constant preload and afterload. Clinically, contractility is difficult to quantify, because virtually all of the available measures are dependent to a certain degree on preload and afterload. If pressure-volume loops are constructed for each cardiac cycle, small changes in preload and/or afterload will result in shifts of the

point defining the end of diastole. These end-systolic points on the pressure-versus-volume diagram describe a straight line, known as the isovolumic pressure line. A steeper slope of this line indicates greater contractility.

Placement of Central Venous and/or Pulmonary Artery Catheters

In its simplest form, the PAC has four channels. One channel terminates in a balloon at the tip of the catheter. The proximal end of this channel is connected to a syringe to permit inflation of the balloon with air. Prior to insertion of the PAC, the integrity of the balloon should be verified by inflating it. In order to minimize the risk of vascular or ventricular perforation by the relatively inflexible catheter, it also is important to verify that the inflated balloon extends just beyond the tip of the device. A second channel in the catheter contains wires that are connected to a thermistor located near the tip of the catheter. At the proximal end of the PAC, the wires terminate in a fitting that permits connection to appropriate hardware for the calculation of cardiac output using the thermodilution technique (see below). The final two channels are used for pressure monitoring and the injection of the thermal indicator for determinations of cardiac output. One of these channels terminates at the tip of the catheter; the other terminates 20 cm proximal to the tip.

Placement of a PAC requires access to the central venous circulation. Such access can be obtained at a variety of sites, including the antecubital, femoral, jugular, and subclavian veins. Percutaneous placement through either the jugular or subclavian vein generally is preferred. Right internal jugular vein cannulation carries the lowest risk of complications, and the path of the catheter from this site into the right atrium is straight. In the event of inadvertent arterial puncture, local pressure is significantly more effective in controlling bleeding from the carotid artery as compared to the subclavian artery. Nevertheless, it is more difficult to keep occlusive dressings in place on the neck than in the subclavian fossa. Furthermore, the anatomic landmarks in the subclavian position are quite constant, even in patients with anasarca or massive obesity; the subclavian vein is always attached to the deep (concave) surface of the clavicle. In contrast, the appropriate landmarks to guide jugular venous cannulation are sometimes difficult to discern in obese or very edematous patients. However, ultrasonic imaging can facilitate jugular venipuncture.[12–14]

Cannulation of the vein is normally performed percutaneously, using the Seldinger technique. A small-bore needle is inserted through the skin and subcutaneous tissue into the vein. After documenting return of venous blood, a guidewire with a flexible tip is inserted through the needle into the vein and the needle is withdrawn. A dilator/introducer sheath is passed over the wire, and the wire and the dilator are removed. The introducer sheath is equipped with a side port, which can be used for administering fluid. The introducer sheath also is equipped with a diaphragm that permits insertion of the PAC while preventing the backflow of venous blood. The proximal terminus of the distal port of the PAC is connected through low-compliance tubing to a strain-gauge transducer, and the tubing-catheter system is flushed with fluid. While constantly observing the pressure tracing on an oscilloscope, the PAC is advanced with the balloon deflated until respiratory excursions are observed. The balloon is then inflated, and the catheter advanced further, while monitoring pressures sequentially in the right atrium and right ventricle en route to the pulmonary artery. The pressure waveforms for the right atrium, right ventricle, and pulmonary artery are each characteristic and easy to recognize. The catheter is advanced out the

Table 12-1

Directly Measured and Derived Hemodynamic Data Obtainable by Bedside Pulmonary Artery Catheterization

Standard PAC	PAC with Additional Feature(s)	Derived Parameters
CVP	$S\bar{v}O_2$ (continuous)	SV (or SVI)
PAP	Q_T or Q_T^* (continuous)	SVR (or SVRI)
PAOP	RVEF	PVR (or PVRI)
$S\bar{v}O_2$ (intermittent)		RVEDV
Q_T or Q_T^* (intermittent)		$\dot{D}O_2$
		$\dot{V}O_2$
		ER
		Q_S/Q_T

CVP = mean central venous pressure; $\dot{D}O_2$ = systemic oxygen delivery; ER = systemic oxygen extraction ratio; PAOP = pulmonary artery occlusion (wedge) pressure; PAP = pulmonary artery pressure; PVR = pulmonary vascular resistance; PVRI = pulmonary vascular resistance index; Q_S/Q_T = fractional pulmonary venous admixture (shunt fraction); Q_T = cardiac output; Q_T^* = cardiac output indexed to body surface area (cardiac index); RVEDV = right ventricular end-diastolic volume; RVEF = right ventricular ejection fraction; SV = stroke volume; SVI = stroke volume index; $S\bar{v}O_2$ = fractional mixed venous (pulmonary artery) hemoglobin saturation; SVR = systemic vascular resistance; SVRI = systemic vascular resistance index; $\dot{V}O_2$ = systemic oxygen utilization.

pulmonary artery until a damped tracing indicative of the "wedged" position is obtained. The balloon is then deflated, taking care to ensure that a normal pulmonary arterial tracing is again observed on the monitor; leaving the balloon inflated can increase the risk of pulmonary infarction or perforation of the pulmonary artery. Unnecessary measurements of the pulmonary artery occlusion pressure are discouraged as rupture of the pulmonary artery may occur.

Hemodynamic Measurements

Even in its simplest embodiment, the PAC is capable of providing clinicians with a remarkable amount of information about the hemodynamic status of patients. Additional information may be obtained if various modifications of the standard PAC are employed. By combining data obtained through use of the PAC with results obtained by other means (i.e., blood hemoglobin concentration and oxyhemoglobin saturation), derived estimates of systemic oxygen transport and utilization can be calculated. Direct and derived parameters obtainable by bedside pulmonary arterial catheterization are summarized in Table 12-1. The equations used to calculate the derived parameters are summarized in Table 12-2. The approximate normal ranges for a number of these hemodynamic parameters (in adults) are shown in Table 12-3.

Measurement of Cardiac Output by Thermodilution

Before the development of the PAC, determining cardiac output (Q_T) at the bedside required careful measurements of oxygen consumption (Fick method) or spectrophotometric determination of indocyanine green dye dilution curves. Measurements of Q_T using the thermodilution technique are simple and reasonably accurate. The measurements can be performed repetitively and the principle is straightforward. If a bolus of an indicator is rapidly and thoroughly mixed with a moving fluid upstream from a detector, then the concentration of the indicator at the detector will increase sharply and then exponentially diminish back to zero. The area under the resulting time-concentration curve is a function of the volume of indicator injected and the flow rate of the moving stream of fluid. Larger volumes of indicator result in greater areas under the curve, and faster flow rates of the mixing fluid result in smaller areas under the curve. When Q_T is measured by thermodilution, the indicator is heat and the detector is a temperature-sensing thermistor at the distal end

of the PAC. The relationship used for calculating Q_T is called the Stewart-Hamilton equation:

$$Q_T = [V \times (T_B - T_I) \times K_1 \times K_2] \times \int T_B(t)dt$$

Table 12-2

Formulas for Calculation of Hemodynamic Parameters That Can Be Derived by Using Data Obtained by Pulmonary Artery Catheterization

Q_T^* (L·min^{-1}·m^{-2}) = Q_T/BSA, where BSA is body surface area (m^2)

SV (mL) = Q_T/HR, where HR is heart rate (min^{-1})

SVR (dyne·sec·cm^{-5}) = [(MAP – CVP) × 80] /Q_T, where MAP is mean arterial pressure (mm Hg)

SVRI (dyne·sec·cm^{-5}·m^{-2}) = [(MAP – CVP) × 80] /Q_T^*

PVR (dyne·sec·cm^{-5}) = [(PAP – PAOP) × 80] /QT, where PPA is mean pulmonary artery pressure

PVRI (dyne.sec.cm^{-5}m^{-2}) = [(PAP – PAOP) × 80] /Q_T^*

RVEDV (mL) = SV/RVEF

$\dot{D}O_2$ (mL·min^{-1}·m^{-2}) = Q_T^* × CaO_2 × 10, where CaO_2 is arterial oxygen content (mL/dL)

$\dot{V}O_2$(mL·min^{-1}·m^{-2}) = Q_T^* × (CaO_2 – $C\bar{v}O_2$) × 10, where $C\bar{v}O_2$ is mixed venous oxygen content (mL/dL)

CaO_2 = (1.36 × Hgb × SaO_2) + (0.003 + PaO_2), where Hgb is hemoglobin concentration (g/dL), SaO_2 is fractional arterial hemoglobin saturation, and PaO_2 is the partial pressure of oxygen in arterial blood

$C\bar{v}O_2$ = (1.36 × Hgb × $S\bar{v}O_2$) + (0.003 + $P\bar{v}O_2$), where $P\bar{v}O_2$ is the partial pressure of oxygen in pulmonary arterial (mixed venous) blood

Q_S/Q_T = (CcO_2 – CaO_2)/(CcO_2 – $C\bar{v}O_2$), where CcO_2 (mL/dL) is the content of oxygen in pulmonary end capillary blood

CcO_2 = (1.36 × Hgb) + (0.003 + PAO_2), where PAO_2 is the alveolar partial pressure of oxygen

PAO_2 = [FIO_2 × (P_B – P_{H_2O})] – $PacO_2$/RQ, where FIO_2 is the fractional concentration of inspired oxygen, P_B is the barometric pressure (mm Hg), P_{H_2O} is the water vapor pressure (usually 47 mm Hg), $PacO_2$ is the partial pressure of carbon dioxide in arterial blood (mm Hg), and RQ is respiratory quotient (usually assumed to be 0.8)

$C\bar{v}O_2$ = central venous oxygen pressure; CVP = mean central venous pressure; $\dot{D}O_2$ = systemic oxygen delivery; PAOP = pulmonary artery occlusion (wedge) pressure; PVR = pulmonary vascular resistance; PVRI = pulmonary vascular resistance index; Q_S /Q_T = fractional pulmonary venous admixture (shunt fraction); Q_T = cardiac output; Q_T^* = cardiac output indexed to body surface area (cardiac index); RVEDV = right ventricular end-diastolic volume; RVEF = right ventricular ejection fraction; SV = stroke volume; SVI = stroke volume index; $S\bar{v}O_2$ = fractional mixed venous (pulmonary artery) hemoglobin saturation; SVR = systemic vascular resistance; SVRI = systemic vascular resistance index; $\dot{V}O_2$ = systemic oxygen utilization.

Table 12-3

Approximate Normal Ranges for Selected Hemodynamic Parameters in Adults

Parameter	Normal Range
CVP	0–6 mm Hg
Right ventricular systolic pressure	20–30 mm Hg
Right ventricular diastolic pressure	0–6 mm Hg
PAOP	6–12 mm Hg
Systolic arterial pressure	100–130 mm Hg
Diastolic arterial pressure	60–90 mm Hg
MAP	75–100 mm Hg
Q_T	4–6 L/min
Q_T*	2.5–3.5 L·min^{-1}·m^{-2}
SV	40–80 mL
SVR	800–1400 dyne·sec·cm^{-5}
SVRI	1500–2400 dyne·sec·cm^{-5}·m^{-2}
PVR	100–150 dyne·sec·cm^{-5}
PVRI	200–400 dyne·sec·cm^{-5}·m^{-2}
Cao_2	16–22 mL/dL
Cvo_2	~15 mL O_2 dL blood
Do_2	400–660 mL·min^{-1}·m^{-2}
Vo_2	115–165 mL·min^{-1}·m^{-2}

Cao_2 = arterial oxygen content; Cvo_2 = central venous oxygen pressure; CVP = mean central venous pressure; Do_2 = systemic oxygen delivery; MAP = mean arterial pressure; PAOP = pulmonary artery occlusion (wedge) pressure; PVR = pulmonary vascular resistance; PVRI = pulmonary vascular resistance index; Q_T = cardiac output; Q_T* = cardiac output indexed to body surface area (cardiac index); SV = stroke volume; SVI = stroke volume index; SVR = systemic vascular resistance; SVRI = systemic vascular resistance index; Vo_2 = systemic oxygen utilization.

where V is the volume of the indicator injected, T_B is the temperature of blood (i.e., core body temperature), T_I is the temperature of the indicator, K_1 is a constant that is the function of the specific heats of blood and the indicator, K_2 is an empirically derived constant that accounts for several factors (the dead space volume of the catheter, heat lost from the indicator as it traverses the catheter, and the injection rate of the indicator), and $\int T_B(t)dt$ is the area under the time-temperature curve. In clinical practice, the Stewart-Hamilton equation is solved by a microprocessor.

Determination of cardiac output by the thermodilution method is generally quite accurate, although it tends to systematically overestimate Q_T at low values.[15] Changes in blood temperature and Q_T during the respiratory cycle can influence the measurement. Therefore, results generally should be recorded as the mean of two or three determinations obtained at random points in the respiratory cycle. Using cold injectate widens the difference between T_B and T_I and thereby increases signal-to-noise ratio. Nevertheless, most authorities recommend using room temperature injectate (normal saline or 5% dextrose in water) to minimize errors resulting from warming of the fluid as it transferred from its reservoir to a syringe for injection.

Technologic innovations have been introduced that permit continuous measurement of Q_T by thermodilution. In this approach, thermal transients are not generated by injecting a bolus of a cold indicator, but rather by heating the blood with a tiny filament located on the PAC upstream from the thermistor. By correlating the amount of current supplied to the heating element with the downstream temperature of the blood, it is possible to estimate the average blood flow across the filament and thereby calculate Q_T. Based upon the results of several studies, continuous determinations of Q_T using this approach agree well with data generated by conventional measurements using bolus injections of a cold indicator.[16–18] Information is lacking regarding the clinical value of being able to

monitor Q_T continuously, and since this technology is relatively expensive, it has not been widely adopted.

Mixed Venous Oximetry

The Fick equation can be written as $Q_T = \dot{V}o_2/(Cao_2 - C\bar{v}o_2)$, where Cao_2 is the content of oxygen in arterial blood and $C\bar{v}o_2$ is the content of oxygen in mixed venous blood. The Fick equation can be rearranged as follows: $C\bar{v}o_2 = Cao_2 - \dot{V}o_2/Q_T$. If the small contribution of dissolved oxygen to $C\bar{v}o_2$ and Cao_2 is ignored, the rearranged equation can be rewritten as $S\bar{v}o_2 = Sao_2 - \dot{V}o_2/(Q_T \times Hgb \times 1.36)$, where $S\bar{v}o_2$ is the fractional saturation of hemoglobin in mixed venous blood, Sao_2 is the fractional saturation of hemoglobin in arterial blood, and Hgb is the concentration of hemoglobin in blood. Thus it can be seen that $S\bar{v}o_2$ is a function of $\dot{V}o_2$ (i.e., metabolic rate), Q_T, Sao_2, and Hgb. Accordingly, subnormal values of $S\bar{v}o_2$ can be caused by a decrease in Q_T (due, for example, to heart failure or hypovolemia), a decrease in Sao_2 (due, for example, to intrinsic pulmonary disease), a decrease in Hgb (i.e., anemia), or an increase in metabolic rate (due, for example, to seizures or fever). With a conventional PAC, measurements of $S\bar{v}o_2$ require aspirating a sample of blood from the distal (i.e., pulmonary arterial) port of the catheter and injecting the sample into a blood gas analyzer. Therefore for practical purposes, measurements of $S\bar{v}o_2$ can be performed only intermittently.

By adding a fifth channel to the PAC, it has become possible to monitor $S\bar{v}o_2$ continuously. The fifth channel contains two fiber-optic bundles, which are used to transmit and receive light of the appropriate wavelengths to permit measurements of hemoglobin saturation by reflectance spectrophotometry. A clinical study of the Abbott Oximetrix PAC has documented that the device provides measurements of $S\bar{v}o_2$ that agree quite closely with those obtained by conventional analyses of blood aspirated from the pulmonary artery.[19] Despite the theoretical value of being able to monitor $S\bar{v}o_2$ continuously, data are lacking to show that this capability favorably improves outcome. Indeed, in several studies, the ability to monitor $S\bar{v}o_2$ was not shown to affect the management of critically ill patients.[20–22] Moreover, in another large study, titrating the resuscitation of critically ill patients to maintain $S\bar{v}o_2$ greater than 69% (i.e., in the normal range) failed to improve mortality or change length of ICU stay.[23] In a recent prospective, observational study of 3265 patients undergoing cardiac surgery with either a standard PAC or a PAC with continuous $S\bar{v}o_2$ monitoring, the oximetric catheter was associated with fewer arterial blood gases and thermodilution cardiac output determinations, but no difference in patient outcome.[24] Since pulmonary artery catheters that permit continuous monitoring of $S\bar{v}o_2$ are much more expensive than conventional PACs, the routine use of these devices cannot be recommended.

The saturation of oxygen in the right atrium or superior vena cava ($Sc\bar{v}o_2$) correlates closely with $S\bar{v}o_2$ over a wide range of conditions.[25] Since measurement of $Sc\bar{v}o_2$ requires placement of a central venous catheter rather than a PAC, it is somewhat less invasive and easier to carry out. By using a central venous catheter equipped to permit fiber-optic monitoring of $Sc\bar{v}o_2$, it may be possible to improve the resuscitation of patients with shock during the first few critical hours after presentation to the hospital.[25,26]

Right Ventricular Ejection Fraction

Ejection fraction (EF) is calculated as (EDV – ESV)/EDV, where ESV is end-systolic volume. EF is an ejection-phase measure of myocardial contractility. By equipping a PAC with a thermistor with a short time constant, the thermodilution method can be used to estimate right ventricular (RV) EF. Measurements of RVEF by thermodilution agree reasonably well with those obtained by other means, although values obtained by thermodilution typically are lower than those obtained by radionuclide cardiography.[27,28] Stroke volume (SV) is calculated as EDV − ESV. Left ventricular (LV) SV also equals Q_T/HR, where HR is heart rate. Since LVSV is equal to RVSV, it is possible to estimate right ventricular end-diastolic volume (RVEDV) by measuring RVEF, Q_T, and HR.

Several studies have attempted to assess the clinical value of RVEF measurements using these catheters. In one study, use of an RVEF catheter did not alter therapy in 93% of patients with sepsis, hemorrhagic shock, or acute respiratory distress syndrome (ARDS), but was useful in cases of abdominal compartment syndrome with high pulmonary artery occlusion pressure despite low preload.[29] In a series of 46 trauma patients who required more than 10 L of fluid in the first 24 hours of resuscitation, there was a better correlation between RV volume and Q_T than there was with pulmonary artery occlusion pressure.[30] However, data are lacking to show that outcomes are improved by making measurements of RVEF in addition to Q_T and other parameters measured by the conventional PAC. Accordingly, the use of pulmonary artery catheters that permit RVEF measurements cannot be recommended at this time.

Effect of Pulmonary Artery Catheterization on Outcome

In 1996, Connors and colleagues reported surprising results in a major observational study evaluating the value of pulmonary artery catheterization in critically ill patients.[31] They took advantage of an enormous data set, which had been previously (and prospectively) collected for another purpose at five major teaching hospitals in the United States. These researchers compared two groups of patients: those who did and those who did not undergo placement of a PAC during their first 24 hours of ICU care. The investigators recognized that the value of their intended analysis was completely dependent on the robustness of their methodology for case-matching, because sicker patients (i.e., those at greater risk of mortality based upon the severity of their illness) were presumably more likely to undergo pulmonary artery catheterization. Accordingly, the authors used sophisticated statistical methods for generating a cohort of study (i.e., PAC) patients, each one having a paired control matched carefully for severity of illness. A critical assessment of their published findings supports the view that the cases and their controls were indeed remarkably well-matched with respect to a large number of pertinent clinical parameters. Connors and associates concluded that placement of a pulmonary artery catheter during the first 24 hours of stay in an ICU is associated with a significant increase in the risk of mortality, even when statistical methods are used to account for severity of illness.

Although the report by Connors and coworkers generated an enormous amount of controversy in the medical community, the results reported actually confirmed the results of two prior similar observational studies. The first of these studies used as a database 3263 patients with acute myocardial infarction treated in central Massachusetts in 1975, 1978, 1981, and 1984 as part of the Worcester Heart Attack Study.[32] For all patients, hospital mortality was significantly greater for patients treated using a PAC, even when multivariate statistical methods were employed to control for key potential confounding factors such as age, peak circulating creatine kinase concentration, and presence or absence of new Q waves on the electrocardiogram. The second large observational study of patients with acute myocardial infarction also found that hospital mortality

was significantly greater for patients managed with the assistance of a PAC, even when the presence or absence of "pump failure" was considered in the statistical analysis.[33] In neither of these earlier reports did the authors conclude that placement of a PAC was truly the cause of worsened survival after myocardial infarction. As a result of the study by Connors and colleagues, experts in the field questioned the value of bedside pulmonary artery catheterization, and some even called for a moratorium on the use of the PAC.[34]

Since publication of the Connors study, a large observational study of patients admitted to a medical ICU concluded that patients who underwent placement of a PAC were sicker than those who did not receive this type of monitoring.[31,35] However, risk-adjusted mortality was similar for patients treated with or without the use of a PAC.

Relatively few prospective, randomized controlled trials of pulmonary artery catheterization have been performed. These trials are summarized in Table 12-4. All of these studies are flawed in one or more ways. The study by Pearson and associates was underpowered with only 226 patients enrolled.[36] In addition, the attending anesthesiologists were permitted to exclude patients from the CVP group at their discretion; thus randomization was compromised. The study by Tuman and coworkers was large (1094 patients were enrolled), but different anesthesiologists were assigned to the different groups.[37] Furthermore, 39 patients in the CVP group underwent placement of a PAC because of hemodynamic complications. All of the individual single-institution studies of vascular surgery patients were relatively underpowered, and all excluded at least certain categories of patients (e.g., those with a history of recent myocardial infarction).[38–41]

In the largest randomized controlled trial of the PAC, Sandham and associates randomized 1994 American Society of Anesthesiologists (ASA) class III and IV patients undergoing major thoracic, abdominal, or orthopedic surgery to placement of a PAC or CVP catheter.[42] In the patients assigned to receive a PAC, physiologic goal-directed therapy was implemented by protocol. There were no differences in mortality at 30 days, 6 months, or 12 months between the two groups, and ICU length of stay was similar. There was a significantly higher rate of pulmonary emboli in the PAC group (0.9 vs. 0%). This study has been criticized because most of the patients enrolled were not in the highest risk category.

The limitations of these studies notwithstanding, the weight of current evidence suggests that routine pulmonary artery catheterization is not useful for the vast majority of patients undergoing cardiac, major peripheral vascular, or ablative surgical procedures. Based upon the exclusion criteria used in two recent prospective randomized trials, reasonable criteria for perioperative monitoring without use of a PAC are presented in Table 12-5.

One of the reasons for using a PAC to monitor critically ill patients is to optimize cardiac output and systemic oxygen delivery. Defining what constitutes the optimum cardiac output, however, has proven to be difficult. Based upon an extensive observational database and comparisons of the hemodynamic and oxygen transport values recorded in survivors and nonsurvivors, Bland and colleagues proposed that "goal-directed" hemodynamic resuscitation should aim to achieve a Q_T greater than 4.5 L/min per square meter and $\dot{D}o_2$ greater than 600 mL/min per square meter.[43] Prompted by these observational findings, a number of investigators have conducted randomized trials designed to evaluate the effect on outcome of goal-directed as compared to conventional hemodynamic resuscitation. Some studies provide support for the notion that interventions designed to achieve supraphysiologic goals for $\dot{D}o_2$, $\dot{V}o_2$,

Table 12-4

Summary of Randomized, Prospective Clinical Trials Comparing Pulmonary Artery Catheter (PAC) with Central Venous Pressure (CVP) Monitoring

Author	Study Population	Groups	Outcomes
Pearson et al [36]	"Low risk" patients undergoing cardiac or vascular surgery	CVP catheter (group 1); PAC (group 2); PAC with continuous $S\bar{v}o_2$ readout (group 3)	No differences among groups for mortality or length of ICU stay; significant differences in costs (group 1 < group 2 < group 3)
Tuman et al [37]	Cardiac surgical patients	PAC; CVP	No differences between groups for mortality, length of ICU stay, or significant noncardiac complications
Isaakson et al [38]	Aortic surgery patients	PAC; CVP	No differences between groups for mortality, length of ICU stay, or length of hospital stay
Joyce et al [39]	Aortic surgery patients	PAC; CVP	No differences between groups for mortality or postoperative cardiac complications
Bender et al [40]	Vascular surgery patients	PAC; CVP	No differences between groups for mortality, length of ICU stay, or length of hospital stay
Valentine et al [41]	Aortic surgery patients	PAC + hemodynamic optimization in ICU night before surgery; CVP	No difference between groups for mortality or length of ICU stay; significantly higher incidence of postoperative complications in PAC group
Sandham et al [42]	"High risk" major surgery	PAC; CVP	No differences between groups for mortality, length of ICU stay; increased incidence of pulmonary embolism in PAC group

ICU = intensive care unit; $S\bar{v}o_2$ = fractional mixed venous (pulmonary artery) hemoglobin saturation.

and Q_T improve outcome.[44–48] However, other published studies do not support this view, and a meta-analysis concluded that interventions designed to achieve supraphysiologic goals for oxygen transport do not significantly reduce mortality rates in critically ill patients.[29,49–53] At this time, supraphysiologic resuscitation of patients in shock cannot be endorsed.

Intuitively, invasive monitoring using a PAC should improve outcome, particularly in subgroups of patients at high risk for major derangements in cardiac performance and perfusion of vital organs. As summarized above, convincing evidence that such monitoring is beneficial is lacking. There is no explanation for the apparent lack of effectiveness of pulmonary artery catheterization. Although no firm answer to this question can be provided, Connors has offered several suggestions.[54] First, even though bedside pulmonary artery catheterization is quite safe, the procedure is associated with a finite incidence of serious complications, including ventricular arrhythmias, catheter-related sepsis, central venous thrombosis, pulmonary arterial perforation, and as noted above, pulmonary embolism.[42,54–59] The adverse effects of these complications on outcome may equal or even outweigh any benefits associated with using a PAC to guide therapy. Second, the data generated by the PAC may be inaccurate, leading to inappropriate therapeutic interventions. Third, the measurements, even if accurate, are often misinterpreted in practice. A study by Iberti and associates showed that 47% of 496 clinicians were unable to accurately

interpret a straightforward recording of a tracing obtained with a PAC, and 44% could not correctly identify the determinants of systemic $\dot{D}o_2$.[60] A more recent study has confirmed that even well-trained intensivists are capable of misinterpreting results provided by pulmonary artery catheterization.[61] Furthermore, the current state of understanding is primitive when it comes to deciding what is the best management for certain hemodynamic disturbances, particularly those associated with sepsis or septic shock. Taking all of this into consideration, it may be that interventions prompted by measurements obtained with a PAC are actually harmful to patients. It also should be remembered that the PAC has been available for about 30 years, and during this period, clinicians using pulmonary artery catheterization have learned a great deal about the kinds of hemodynamic perturbations that are commonly encountered in a variety of clinical situations. As a result, the marginal benefit now available by placing a PAC may be quite small. Less invasive modalities are available that can provide clinically useful hemodynamic information.

It may be true that aggressive hemodynamic resuscitation of patients, guided by various forms of monitoring, is valuable only during certain critical periods, such as the first few hours after presentation with septic shock or during operations. For example, Rivers and colleagues reported that survival of patients with septic shock is significantly improved when resuscitation in the emergency department is guided by a protocol that seeks to keep $Scvo_2$ greater than 70%.[26] Similarly, a study using an ultrasound-based device (see below) to assess cardiac filling and SV showed that maximizing SV intraoperatively results in fewer postoperative complications and shorter hospital length of stay.[62]

Minimally Invasive Alternatives to the Pulmonary Artery Catheter

Because of the questionable benefits and risks and costs associated with bedside pulmonary artery catheterization, there has been interest for many years in the development of practical means for less invasive monitoring of hemodynamic parameters. Several approaches have been developed, which have achieved variable

Table 12-5

Suggested Criteria for Perioperative Monitoring Without Use of a Pulmonary Artery Catheter in Patients Undergoing Cardiac or Major Vascular Surgical Procedures

No anticipated need for suprarenal or supraceliac aortic cross-clamping
No history of myocardial infarction during 3 months prior to operation
No history of poorly compensated congestive heart failure
No history of coronary artery bypass graft surgery during 6 weeks prior to operation
No history of ongoing symptomatic mitral or aortic valvular heart disease
No history of ongoing unstable angina pectoris

degrees of success. None of these methods render the standard thermodilution technique of the pulmonary artery catheter obsolete. However, these strategies may contribute to improvements in the hemodynamic monitoring of critically ill patients.

Doppler Ultrasonography

When ultrasonic sound waves are reflected by moving erythrocytes in the bloodstream, the frequency of the reflected signal is increased or decreased, depending on whether the cells are moving toward or away from the ultrasonic source. This change in frequency is called the Doppler shift, and its magnitude is determined by the velocity of the moving red blood cells. Therefore, measurements of the Doppler shift can be used to calculate red blood cell velocity. With knowledge of both the cross-sectional area of a vessel and the mean red blood cell velocity of the blood flowing through it, one can calculate blood flow rate. If the vessel in question is the aorta, then Q_T can be calculated as:

$$Q_T = HR \times A \times \int V(t)dt$$

where A is the cross-sectional area of the aorta and $\int V(t)dt$ is the red blood cell velocity integrated over the cardiac cycle.

Two approaches have been developed for using Doppler ultrasonography to estimate Q_T. The first approach uses an ultrasonic transducer, which is manually positioned in the suprasternal notch and focused on the root of the aorta. Aortic cross-sectional area can be estimated using a nomogram, which factors in age, height, and weight, back-calculated if an independent measure of Q_T is available, or by using two-dimensional transthoracic or transesophageal ultrasonography. While this approach is completely noninvasive, it requires a highly-skilled operator in order to obtain meaningful results, and is labor-intensive. Moreover, unless Q_T measured using thermodilution is used to back-calculate aortic diameter, accuracy using the suprasternal notch approach is not acceptable.[63,64] Accordingly, the method is useful only for obtaining very intermittent estimates of Q_T, and has not been widely adopted by clinicians.

A more promising approach has been introduced. In this method, which was originally described by Daigle and colleagues, blood flow velocity is continuously monitored in the descending thoracic aorta using a transducer introduced into the esophagus in sedated or anesthetized patients.[65] The current embodiment of this concept is called the CardioQ, which is manufactured by Deltex Medical Limited (Chichester, UK). The device consists of a continuous-wave Doppler transducer mounted at the tip of a transesophageal probe. The probe is advanced into the esophagus to about 35 cm from the incisors (in adults) and connected to a monitor, which continuously displays the blood flow velocity profile in the descending aorta as well as the calculated Q_T. In order to maximize the accuracy of the device, the probe position must be adjusted to obtain the peak velocity in the aorta. In order to transform blood flow in the descending aorta into Q_T, a correction factor is applied that is based on the assumption that only 70% of the flow at the root of the aorta is still present in the descending thoracic aorta. Aortic cross-sectional area is estimated using a nomogram based on the patient's age, weight, and height. Results using these methods appear to be reasonably accurate across a broad spectrum of patients and are clinically useful because, unlike a conventional PAC, the Deltex device provides a continuous readout of Q_T.[66] In this multicenter study, good correlation was found between esophageal Doppler and thermodilution (r = 0.95), with a small systematic underestimation (bias 0.24 L/min) using esophageal Doppler. The ultrasonic device

also calculates a derived parameter termed *flow time corrected* (FTc), which is the systolic flow time in the descending aorta corrected for heart rate. FTc is a function of preload, contractility, and vascular input impedance. Although it is not a pure measure of preload, Doppler-based estimates of SV and FTc have been used successfully to guide volume resuscitation in high-risk surgical patients undergoing major operations.[62]

Impedance Cardiography

The impedance to flow of alternating electrical current in regions of the body is commonly called *bioimpedance*. In the thorax, changes in the volume and velocity of blood in the thoracic aorta lead to detectable changes in bioimpedance. The first derivative of the oscillating component of thoracic bioimpedance (dZ/dt) is linearly related to aortic blood flow. On the basis of this relationship, empirically derived formulas have been developed to estimate SV, and subsequently Q_T, noninvasively. This methodology is called *impedance cardiography*. The approach is attractive because it is completely noninvasive, provides a continuous readout of Q_T, and does not require extensive training for use. Despite these advantages, a number of studies suggest that measurements of Q_T obtained by impedance cardiography are not sufficiently reliable to be used for clinical decision making and have poor correlation with standard methods such as thermodilution and ventricular angiography.[67-69] Impedance cardiography also has been proposed as a way to estimate left ventricular EF, but the results obtained show poor agreement with those obtained by radionuclide ventriculography.[69,70] Based upon these data, impedance cardiography cannot be recommended at the present time for hemodynamic monitoring of critically ill patients.

Pulse Contour Analysis

Perhaps one of the least invasive and most appealing methods for determining cardiac output is an approach called *pulse contour analysis*, originally described by Wesseling and colleagues for estimating SV on a beat-to-beat basis.[71] The mechanical properties of the arterial tree and SV determine the shape of the arterial pulse waveform. The pulse contour method of estimating Q_T uses the arterial pressure waveform as an input for a model of the systemic circulation in order to determine beat-to-beat flow through the circulatory system. The parameters of resistance, compliance, and impedance are initially estimated based on the patient's age and sex, and can be subsequently refined by using a reference standard measurement of Q_T. A commercially available device, the PulseCO Hemodynamic Monitor (LiDCO, Ltd., London, UK) utilizes this technology. In the LiDCO system, the reference standard estimation of Q_T is obtained periodically using the indicator dilution approach by injecting the indicator (a dilute solution of lithium ion) into a central venous catheter and detecting the transient increase in lithium ion concentration in the blood using an arterial catheter equipped with a lithium-sensitive sensor that is placed in a femoral artery.

Measurements of Q_T based on pulse contour monitoring are comparable in accuracy to standard pulmonary artery catheter (PAC)-thermodilution methods, but it uses an approach that is much less invasive since arterial and central venous, but not transcardiac, catheterization is needed.[72] Using on-line pressure waveform analysis, the computerized algorithms can calculate SV, Q_T, systemic vascular resistance, and an estimate of myocardial contractility, the rate of rise of the arterial systolic pressure (dP/dT).

The use of pulse contour analysis has been applied using an even less invasive technology based on totally noninvasive photo-plethysmographic measurements of arterial pressure.[73] However, the accuracy of this technique has been questioned and its clinical utility remains to be determined.[74]

Partial Carbon Dioxide Rebreathing

Partial carbon dioxide (CO_2) rebreathing uses the Fick principle to estimate Q_T noninvasively. By intermittently altering the dead space within the ventilator circuit via a rebreathing valve, changes in CO_2 production (Vco_2) and end-tidal CO_2 ($ETCO_2$) are used to determine cardiac output using a modified Fick equation ($Q_T = \Delta Vco_2/\Delta ETCO_2$).[75] A commercially available device, the NICO monitor, uses this Fick principle to calculate Q_T using intermittent partial CO_2 rebreathing through a disposable rebreathing loop. The device consists of a CO_2 sensor based on infrared light absorption, an airflow sensor, and a pulse oximeter. Changes in intrapulmonary shunt and hemodynamic instability impair the accuracy of Q_T estimated by partial CO_2 rebreathing. Continuous in-line pulse oximetry and inspired fraction of inspired O_2 (FIO_2) are used to estimate shunt fraction to correct Q_T.

Some studies of the partial CO_2 rebreathing approach suggest that the NICO system is not accurate when thermodilution is used as the gold standard for measuring Q_T.[72,76] However, other studies suggest that the partial CO_2 rebreathing method for determination of Q_T compares favorably to measurements made using a PAC in critically ill patients.[77]

Transesophageal Echocardiography

Transesophageal echocardiography (TEE) has made the transition from operating room to intensive care unit. TEE requires that the patient be sedated and usually intubated for airway protection. Using this powerful technology, global assessments of LV and RV function can be made, including determinations of ventricular volume, EF, and Q_T. Segmental wall motion abnormalities, pericardial effusions, and tamponade can be readily identified with TEE. Doppler techniques allow estimation of atrial filling pressures. The technique is somewhat cumbersome and requires considerable training and skill in order to obtain reliable results.

Assessing Preload Responsiveness

Although pulse contour analysis using the somewhat invasive PulseCO approach or partial CO_2 rebreathing may be able to provide fairly reliable estimates regarding SV and Q_T, these approaches alone can offer little or no information about the adequacy of preload. Thus, if Q_T is low, some other means must be employed to estimate preload. Most clinicians assess the adequacy of cardiac preload by determining CVP or PAOP. However, neither CVP nor PAOP correlate well with the true parameter of interest, left ventricular end-diastolic volume (LVEDV).[78] Extremely high or low CVP or PAOP results are informative, but readings in a large middle zone (i.e., 5 to 20 mm Hg) are not very useful. Furthermore, changes in CVP or PAOP fail to correlate well with changes in stroke volume.[79] Echocardiography can be used to estimate LVEDV, but this approach is dependent on the skill and training of the individual using it, and isolated measurements of LVEDV fail to predict the hemodynamic response to alterations in preload.[80-84]

When intrathoracic pressure increases during the application of positive airway pressure in mechanically ventilated patients, venous return decreases, and as a consequence, left ventricular stroke volume (LVSV) also decreases. Therefore, pulse pressure variation (PPV) during a positive pressure episode can be used to predict the responsiveness of cardiac output to changes in preload.[85] PPV is defined as the difference between the maximal pulse pressure and the minimum pulse pressure divided by the average of these two pressures.[85] Michard and colleagues validated this approach by comparing PPV, CVP, PAOP, and systolic pressure variation as predictors of preload responsiveness in a cohort of critically ill patients. They classified patients as being preload responsive if their cardiac index increased by at least 15% after rapid infusion of a standard volume of intravenous fluid.[86] Receiver-operating characteristic (ROC) curves demonstrated that PPV was the best predictor of preload responsiveness. Although atrial arrhythmias can interfere with the usefulness of this technique, PPV remains a useful approach for assessing preload responsiveness in most patients because of its simplicity and reliability.[84]

Tissue Capnometry

Global indices of Q_T, oxygen delivery ($\dot{D}o_2$), or oxygen utilization ($\dot{V}o_2$) provide little useful information regarding the adequacy of cellular oxygenation and mitochondrial function. On theoretical grounds, measuring tissue pH to assess the adequacy of perfusion is an extremely attractive concept. As a consequence of the stoichiometry of the reactions responsible for the substrate level phosphorylation of adenosine diphosphate (ADP) to form ATP, anaerobiosis is inevitably associated with the net accumulation of protons.[87] Accordingly, knowing that tissue pH is not in the acid range should be enough information to conclude that global perfusion as well as arterial oxygen content are sufficient to meet the metabolic demands of the cells, even without knowledge of the actual values for tissue blood flow or oxygen delivery. The detection of tissue acidosis should alert the clinician to the possibility that perfusion is inadequate. Prompted by this reasoning, Fiddian-Green and colleagues promulgated the idea that tonometric measurements of tissue Pco_2 in the stomach or sigmoid colon could be used to estimate mucosal pH (pH_i) and thereby monitor visceral perfusion in critically ill patients.[88-90]

Unfortunately, the notion of using tonometric estimates of gastrointestinal mucosal pH_i for monitoring perfusion is predicated on a number of assumptions, some of which may be partially or completely invalid. Furthermore, currently available methods for performing measurements of gastric mucosal Pco_2 in the clinical setting remain rather cumbersome and expensive. It is perhaps for these reasons that gastric tonometry for monitoring critically ill patients has primarily been utilized as a research tool. Some recent developments in the field may change this situation, and monitoring tissue Pco_2 seems likely to become common in emergency departments, intensive care units, and operating rooms in the relatively near future.

As originally proposed by Fiddian-Green and associates, tonometric determination of mucosal carbon dioxide tension, Pco_{2muc}, can be used to calculate pH_i by using the Henderson-Hasselbalch equation as follows: $pH_i = \log ([HCO_3^-]_{muc}/0.03 \times Pco_{2muc})$, where $[HCO_3^-]_{muc}$ is the concentration of bicarbonate anion in the mucosa.[91] Whereas Pco_{2muc} can be measured with reasonable accuracy and precision using tonometric methods, $[HCO_3^-]_{muc}$ cannot be measured directly, but must be estimated by assuming that the concentration of bicarbonate anion in arterial blood, $[HCO_3^-]_{art}$, is approximately equal to $[HCO_3^-]_{muc}$. Under normal conditions, the assumption that $[HCO_3^-]_{art} \cong [HCO_3^-]_{muc}$ is probably valid. Under pathologic conditions, however, the assumption that $[HCO_3^-]_{art} \cong [HCO_3^-]_{muc}$ is almost certainly invalid. For example, when blood flow to the ileal mucosa is very low, HCO_3^- in the tissue is titrated by hydrogen ions produced as a result of anaerobic metabolism, and replenishment of tissue HCO_3^- stores from arterial blood is impeded by stagnant perfusion. Thus under such conditions, $[HCO_3^-]_{muc}$ is less than $[HCO_3^-]_{art}$, and tonometric estimates of pH_i based on the Henderson-Hasselbalch equation underestimate the degree of tissue acidosis present.[92]

There is another inherent problem in using pH_i as an index of perfusion. As noted above, pH_i calculated using the Henderson-Hasselbalch equation is a function of both PCO_{2muc} and $[HCO_3^-]_{art}$. Under steady-state conditions, the first of these parameters, PCO_{2muc}, reflects the balance between inflow of CO_2 into the interstitial space and outflow of CO_2 from the interstitial space. CO_2 can enter the interstitial compartment via three mechanisms: diffusion of CO_2 from arterial blood, production as a result of aerobic metabolism of carbon-containing fuels, and production as a result of titration of HCO_3^- by protons liberated during anaerobic metabolism. CO_2 leaves the interstitial compartment by diffusing into venous blood. If blood flow to the mucosa decreases, then PCO_{2muc} increases as a result of decreased extraction of CO_2 into venous blood. If mucosal perfusion decreases sufficiently, (i.e., to less than the anaerobic threshold for the tissue), then PCO_{2muc} also increases as a result of increased production due to titration of HCO_3^-.[76] Clearly, therefore, an increase in PCO_{2muc} *can* reflect a decrease in mucosal perfusion. However, as documented experimentally by Salzman and colleagues, an increase in PCO_{2muc} also can be caused by arterial hypercarbia, leading to increased diffusion of CO_2 from arterial blood into the interstitium.[93] Similarly, changes in $[HCO_3^-]_{art}$ can occur as a result of factors unrelated to either tissue perfusion or the adequacy of aerobic metabolism (e.g., diabetic ketoacidosis, iatrogenic alkalinization due to administration of sodium bicarbonate solution). For these reasons, tonometrically derived estimates of pH_i are not a reliable way to assess mucosal perfusion.

Although PCO_2 and pH are affected by changes in perfusion in all tissues, efforts to monitor these parameters in patients using tonometric methods have focused on the mucosa of the gastrointestinal tract, particularly the stomach, for both practical and theoretical reasons. From a practical standpoint, the stomach is already commonly intubated in clinical practice for purposes of decompression and drainage or feeding. Placement of a nasogastric or orogastric tube is generally regarded as minimally invasive. Thus the psychologic barrier to using the lumen of the stomach as a monitoring site is low. However, there are theoretical reasons why monitoring gastrointestinal mucosal perfusion might be more desirable than monitoring perfusion in other sites. First, when global perfusion is compromised, blood flow to the splanchnic viscera decreases to a greater extent than does perfusion to the body as a whole.[94] Thus, a marker of compromised splanchnic perfusion should be a leading indicator of impending adverse changes in blood flow to other organs.[95] Second, the gut has been hypothesized to be the "motor" of the multiple organ system dysfunction syndrome, and in experimental models, intestinal mucosal acidosis, whether due to inadequate perfusion or other causes, has been associated with hyperpermeability to hydrophilic solutes.[80,96] Therefore, ensuring adequate splanchnic perfusion might be expected to minimize derangements in gut barrier function and, on this basis, improve outcome for patients.

The stomach, however, may not be an ideal location for monitoring tissue PCO_2. First, CO_2 can be formed in the lumen of the stomach when hydrogen ions secreted by parietal cells in the mucosa titrate luminal bicarbonate anions, which are present either as a result of backwash of duodenal secretions or secretion by gastric mucosal cells. Measurements of gastric PCO_2 and pH_i can be confounded by gastric acid secretion, as documented in a study of normal volunteers by Heard and associates and subsequently confirmed by others.[97–100] Consequently, accurate measurements of gastric PCO_2 and pH_i depend on pharmacologic blockade of luminal proton secretion using histamine receptor antagonists or proton pump inhibitors. The need for using pharmacologic therapy adds to the cost and complexity of the monitoring strategy. Second, enteral feeding can interfere with measurements of gastric mucosal PCO_2, necessitating temporary cessation of the administration of nutritional support or the placement of a postpyloric tube.[101]

Despite the problems noted above, measurements of gastric pH_i and/or mucosal-arterial PCO_2 gap have been proven to be a remarkably reliable predictor of outcome in a wide variety of critically ill individuals, including general medical intensive care unit patients, victims of multiple trauma, patients with sepsis, and patients undergoing major surgical procedures.[89,102–108] In studies using endoscopic measurements of gastric mucosal blood flow by laser Doppler flowmetry, the development of gastric mucosal acidosis has been shown to correlate with mucosal hypoperfusion.[109] The development of low pH_i in the colon has been shown to correlate with an exaggerated host inflammatory response in patients undergoing aortic surgery.[110] Moreover, in a landmark prospective, randomized, multicentric clinical trial of monitoring in medical intensive care unit patients, titrating resuscitation to a gastric pH_i endpoint rather than conventional hemodynamic indices resulted in higher 30-day survival rate.[111] In another study, Ivatury and associates randomized 57 trauma patients into two groups.[112] In the first group, the administration of fluids and vasoactive drugs was titrated to achieve a gastric pH_i greater than 7.30. In the second group, resuscitation was titrated to achieve a calculated systemic oxygen delivery index greater than 600 mL/min per square meter or systemic oxygen utilization greater than 150 mL/min per square meter. Although survival was not significantly different in the two arms of the study, failure to normalize gastric pH_i within 24 hours was associated with a high mortality rate (54%), whereas normalization of pH_i was associated with a significantly lower mortality rate (7%).

It seems likely that monitoring tissue PCO_2 (tissue capnometry) will play an increasingly important role in the management of critically ill patients because of two important insights. First, the directly measured parameter, namely tissue PCO_2, provides more reliable information about perfusion than does the derived parameter, pH_i.[113–115] By eliminating the potentially confounding effects of systemic hypocarbia or hypercarbia, calculating and monitoring the gap between tissue PCO_2 and arterial PCO_2 may prove to be even more valuable than simply following changes in tissue PCO_2. The second recent insight is that it may not be necessary, or even desirable, to monitor tissue PCO_2 in the stomach or other portions of the gastrointestinal tract. For example, Sato and colleagues showed that changes in gastric wall and esophageal tissue PCO_2 track each other closely in rats subjected to hemorrhagic shock.[116] Similar results were reported by Guzman and coworkers in a study of dogs infused with lipopolysaccharide.[117] It appears probable that monitoring tissue PCO_2 in other nongastric sites such as the space under the tongue may require even less invasion of the patient, and yet be as informative as measuring PCO_2 in the wall of the esophagus or the gut.[118,119]

Results from some preliminary clinical studies support the view that the monitoring of tissue PCO_2 in the sublingual mucosa may provide valuable clinical information. Increased sublingual PCO_2 ($PslCO_2$) was associated with decreases in arterial blood pressure and Q_T in patients with shock due to hemorrhage or sepsis.[120] In a study of critically ill patients with septic or cardiogenic shock, the $Pslco_2$-$Paco_2$ gradient was found to be a good prognostic indicator, being 9.2 ± 5.0 mm Hg in the survivors and 17.8 ± 11.5 mm Hg in nonsurvivors.[121] This study also demonstrated that sublingual capnography was superior to gastric tonometry in predicting patient survival. The $Pslco_2$-$Paco_2$ gradient also correlated with the mixed venous-arterial Pco_2 gradient, but failed to correlate with blood lactate level, mixed venous O_2 saturation ($S\bar{v}o_2$), or systemic $\dot{D}o_2$. These latter findings suggest that the $Pslco_2$-$Paco_2$ gradient may be a better marker of tissue hypoxia than are these other parameters.

RESPIRATORY MONITORING

The requirement for mechanical ventilation is a hallmark for many intensive care patients. The ability to monitor various parameters of respiratory function is critically important in these patients, in order to assess the adequacy of oxygenation and ventilation, guide weaning and liberation from mechanical ventilation, and detect adverse events associated with respiratory failure and mechanical ventilation. These parameters include gas exchange, neuromuscular activity, respiratory mechanics, and patient effort.

Arterial Blood Gases

The standard for respiratory monitoring has been to carry out intermittent measurements of arterial blood gases. Blood gas analysis provides useful information when caring for patients with respiratory failure. However, even in the absence of respiratory failure or the need for mechanical ventilation, blood gas determinations also can be valuable to detect alterations in acid-base balance due to low Q_T, sepsis, renal failure, severe trauma, medication or drug overdose, or altered mental status. Arterial blood can be analyzed for pH, Po_2, Pco_2, HCO_3^- concentration and calculated base deficit. When indicated, carboxyhemoglobin and methemoglobin levels also can be measured. In recent years, efforts have been made to decrease the unnecessary use of arterial blood gas analysis. Serial arterial blood gas determinations are not necessary for routine weaning from mechanical ventilation in the majority of postoperative patients.

Most bedside blood gas analyses still involve removal of an aliquot of blood from the patient, although continuous bedside arterial blood gas determinations are now possible without sampling via an indwelling arterial catheter that contains a biosensor. In studies comparing the accuracy of continuous arterial blood gas and pH monitoring with a conventional laboratory blood gas analyzer, excellent agreement between the two methods has been demonstrated.[122] Continuous monitoring can reduce the volume of blood loss due to phlebotomy and dramatically decrease the time necessary to obtain blood gas results. Continuous monitoring, however, is expensive and is not widely employed.

Determinants of Oxygen Delivery

The primary goal of the cardiovascular and respiratory systems is to deliver oxygenated blood to the tissues. $\dot{D}o_2$ is dependent to a greater degree on the oxygen saturation of hemoglobin (Hgb) in arterial blood (Sao_2) than on the partial pressure of oxygen in arterial blood (Pao_2). $\dot{D}o_2$ also is dependent on Q_T and Hgb. Dissolved oxygen in blood, which is proportional to the Pao_2, makes only a negligible contribution to $\dot{D}o_2$, as is apparent from the equation: $\dot{D}o_2 = Q_T \times [(Hgb \times Sao_2 \times 1.36) + (Pao_2 \times 0.0031)]$.

Sao_2 in mechanically ventilated patients depends on the mean airway pressure, the fraction of inspired oxygen (Fio_2), and $S\bar{v}o_2$.

Thus, when Sao_2 is too low, the clinician has only a limited number of ways to improve this parameter. The clinician can increase mean airway pressure by increasing positive-end expiratory pressure (PEEP) or inspiratory time. Fio_2 can be increased to a maximum of 1.0 by decreasing the amount of room air mixed with the oxygen supplied to the ventilator. $S\bar{v}o_2$ can be increased by increasing Hgb or Q_T or decreasing oxygen utilization (e.g., by administering a muscle relaxant and sedation).

Peak and Plateau Airway Pressure

Airway pressures are routinely monitored in mechanically ventilated patients. The peak airway pressure measured at the end of inspiration (P_{peak}) is a function of the tidal volume, the resistance of the airways, lung/chest wall compliance, and peak inspiratory flow. The airway pressure measured at the end of inspiration when the inhaled volume is held in the lungs by briefly closing the expiratory valve is termed *the plateau airway pressure* ($P_{plateau}$). Plateau airway pressure is independent of the airways resistance, and is related to the lung/chest wall compliance and tidal volume. Mechanical ventilators monitor P_{peak} with each breath and can be set to trigger an alarm if the P_{peak} exceeds a predetermined threshold. $P_{plateau}$ is not measured routinely with each delivered tidal volume, but rather is measured intermittently by setting the ventilator to close the exhalation circuit briefly at the end of inspiration and record the airway pressure when airflow is zero.

If both P_{peak} and $P_{plateau}$ are increased (and tidal volume is not excessive), then the problem is a decrease in the compliance in the lung/chest wall unit. Common causes of this problem include pneumothorax, lobar atelectasis, pulmonary edema, pneumonia, acute respiratory distress syndrome (ARDS), active contraction of the chest wall or diaphragmatic muscles, abdominal distention, and intrinsic PEEP, such as occurs in patients with bronchospasm and insufficient expiratory times. When P_{peak} is increased but $P_{plateau}$ is relatively normal, the primary problem is an increase in airway resistance, such as occurs with bronchospasm, use of a small-caliber endotracheal tube, or kinking or obstruction of the endotracheal tube. A low P_{peak} also should trigger an alarm, as it suggests a discontinuity in the airway circuit involving the patient and the ventilator.

Ventilator-induced lung injury (VILI) is now an established clinical entity of great relevance to the care of critically ill patients. Excessive airway pressure and tidal volume adversely affect pulmonary and possibly systemic responses to critical illness. Subjecting the lung parenchyma to excessive pressure, known as barotrauma, can result in parenchymal lung injury, diffuse alveolar damage similar to ARDS, and pneumothorax, and can impair venous return and therefore limit cardiac output. Lung-protective ventilation strategies have been developed to prevent the development of VILI and improve patient outcomes. In a large, multicenter randomized trial of patients with ARDS from a variety of etiologies, limiting plateau airway pressure to less than 30 cm H_2O and tidal volume to less than 6 mL/kg of ideal body weight reduced 28-day mortality by 22% relative to a ventilator strategy that used a tidal volume of 12 mL/kg.[123] For this reason, monitoring of plateau pressure and using a low tidal volume strategy in patients with ARDS is now the standard of care.

Pulse Oximetry

Continuous, noninvasive monitoring of arterial oxygen saturation is possible using light-emitting diodes and sensors placed on the skin. Pulse oximetry employs two wavelengths of light (i.e., 660 nm and

940 nm) to analyze the pulsatile component of blood flow between the light source and sensor. Because oxyhemoglobin and deoxyhemoglobin have different absorption spectra, differential absorption of light at these two wavelengths can be used to calculate the fraction of oxygen saturation of hemoglobin. Under normal circumstances, the contributions of carboxyhemoglobin and methemoglobin are minimal. However, if carboxyhemoglobin levels are elevated, the pulse oximeter will incorrectly interpret carboxyhemoglobin as oxyhemoglobin and the arterial saturation displayed will be falsely elevated. When the concentration of methemoglobin is markedly increased, the SaO_2 will be displayed as 85%, regardless of the true arterial saturation.[124] The accuracy of pulse oximetry begins to decline at SaO_2 values less than 92%, and tends to be unreliable for values less than 85%.[125]

Several studies have assessed the frequency of arterial oxygen desaturation in hospitalized patients and its effect on outcome. For example, in a study of general medical patients, Bowton and associates found that patients who had an episode of hypoxemia (SaO_2 <90% for 5 minutes) in the first 24 hours of hospital admission had a mortality rate three times higher than that of patients who did not have an episode of arterial desaturation.[126] Because of its clinical relevance, ease of use, noninvasive nature, and cost-effectiveness, pulse oximetry has become a routine monitoring strategy in patients with respiratory disease, intubated patients, and those undergoing surgical intervention under sedation or general anesthesia. Pulse oximetry is especially useful in the titration of FIO_2 and PEEP for patients receiving mechanical ventilation, and during weaning from mechanical ventilation. The widespread use of pulse oximetry has decreased the need for arterial blood gas determinations in critically ill patients.

Capnometry

Capnometry is the measurement of PCO_2 in the airway throughout the respiratory cycle. In healthy subjects, end-tidal PCO_2 ($PETCO_2$) is about 1 to 5 mm Hg less than $PaCO_2$.[127] Thus, $PETCO_2$ can be used to estimate $PaCO_2$ without the need for blood gas determination. However, changes in $PETCO_2$ may not correlate with changes in $PaCO_2$ during a number of pathologic conditions (see below).

Capnography allows the confirmation of endotracheal intubation and continuous assessment of ventilation, integrity of the airway, operation of the ventilator, and cardiopulmonary function. Capnometers are configured with either an in-line sensor or a sidestream sensor. The sidestream systems are lighter and easy to use, but the thin tubing that samples the gas from the ventilator circuit can become clogged with secretions or condensed water, preventing accurate measurements. The in-line devices are bulky and heavier, but are less likely to become clogged. Continuous monitoring with capnography has become routine during surgery under general anesthesia and for some intensive care patients. A number of situations can be promptly detected with continuous capnography. A sudden reduction in $PETCO_2$ suggests either obstruction of the sampling tubing with water or secretions, or a catastrophic event such as loss of the airway, airway disconnection or obstruction, ventilator malfunction, or a marked decrease in Q_T. If the airway is connected and patent and the ventilator is functioning properly, then a sudden decrease in $PETCO_2$ should prompt efforts to rule out cardiac arrest, massive pulmonary embolism, or cardiogenic shock. $PETCO_2$ can be persistently low during hyperventilation or with an increase in dead space such as occurs with pulmonary embolization (even in the absence of a change in Q_T). Causes of an increase in $PETCO_2$ include reduced minute ventilation or increased metabolic rate.

Indices of Readiness for Liberation from Mechanical Ventilation

Patients are intubated and receive mechanical ventilation when their ability to oxygenate and ventilate are exceeded by the demands of their disease process. A number of complications can occur while patients are on mechanical ventilation. For this reason, patients should be liberated from the mechanical ventilator promptly when this form of support is no longer necessary. To minimize the time a patient is subjected to the perils of mechanical ventilation, the physician should identify and reverse the cause of respiratory failure and recognize when the patient is ready for liberation from the ventilator. In the past, the emphasis was placed on gradually weaning the patient through progressively lower levels of ventilatory support.

Numerous investigators have tried to identify parameters that can indicate readiness for liberation from mechanical ventilation.[128] There is no perfect indicator to identify the patient who is ready for discontinuation of ventilatory support. The work of breathing is a major determinant of a patient's ability to breathe spontaneously; if the workload exceeds the physiologic capacity of the patient, spontaneous breathing will ultimately fail. The work of breathing on mechanical ventilation has two components: physiologic and imposed. The imposed work of breathing is the component that is determined by the resistance of the endotracheal tube and ventilator circuit. The physiologic workload is imposed by the resistance to movement of the lung/chest wall and the resistance of the airways. Work of breathing can be quantified using a portable device in intubated patients. An esophageal balloon catheter is used to estimate intrapleural pressure. Pressure and flow transducers are placed in the ventilator circuit and provide data for calculation of work of breathing. Physiologic work of breathing is normally about 0.5 to 0.6 J/L, and successful liberation from mechanical ventilation is likely when the physiologic work of breathing is less than 0.8 J/L.[129] Work of breathing is rarely used today to assess readiness for liberation from mechanical ventilation.

Another standard measure used to estimate readiness for liberation from mechanical ventilation is the maximal inspiratory airway pressure (PI_{max}), also known as negative inspired force (NIF). This parameter assesses global inspiratory muscle strength and neuromuscular integrity. This maneuver is performed while the patient performs a maximum inspiratory effort against an occluded airway, preceded by complete exhalation to residual volume. Values that are more negative than −30 cm H_2O are thought by many to be predictive of weaning success, whereas values less negative than −20 cm H_2O are thought to predict weaning failure. However, in a study of 100 medical patients recovering from respiratory failure, the predictive value of this test alone was low.[130] This parameter should be regarded as relatively worthless.

A measure of respiratory drive can be obtained by measuring the mouth occlusion pressure at 0.1 second after onset of inspiratory effort against an occluded airway ($P_{0.1}$). In intubated patients, $P_{0.1}$ has been shown to correlate with work of breathing during pressure support ventilation (r = 0.87).[131] One study suggested that an elevated $P_{0.1}$ value predicts failure to wean from mechanical ventilation, but because measurement of $P_{0.1}$ requires instrumentation that is not present on most ventilators, the practical utility of this parameter is limited.[132]

Rapid, shallow breathing is a common finding in patients who fail to wean from mechanical ventilation. This finding can be quantified using the rapid, shallow breathing index during spontaneous breathing defined as the ratio of respiratory rate (f) to tidal volume (V_T). If $f:V_T$ is between 60 and 105 during a 1-minute T-piece trial, weaning from mechanical ventilation is likely to be successful.[130,133] Other data suggest that f:V_T has low negative predictive value (i.e., f:V_T greater than 105 does not necessarily preclude successful weaning).[134] Sedation, which lowers respiratory drive, may lower the respiratory rate, thereby producing a misleadingly low f:V_T. The accuracy of this index in patients who have been ventilated for prolonged periods of time has not been evaluated.

One integrative index combines four indices of readiness for liberation: compliance (Crs), rate, oxygenation, and pressure (PI$_{max}$), known as the CROP index. It is calculated by the following equation: CROP = dynamic Crs × PI$_{max}$ × (PaO_2 / PAO_2)/f, where PAO_2 is the calculated alveolar partial pressure of oxygen. The CROP index offers a reasonable assessment of ability to liberate from mechanical ventilation. A CROP index greater than 13 has a sensitivity of 0.81, specificity 0.57, positive predictive value 0.71, and a negative predictive value of 0.7 in predicting successful liberation from the ventilator.[130] While no single index of readiness for liberation from mechanical ventilation is perfect, using a combination of these parameters along with correcting the underlying cause of respiratory failure and ensuring hemodynamic stability remains the best strategy for determining the ability of a patient to successfully breathe spontaneously without positive airway pressure.

RENAL MONITORING

Urine Output

Bladder catheterization with an indwelling catheter allows the monitoring of urine output, usually recorded hourly by the nursing staff. With a patent Foley catheter, urine output is a gross indicator of renal perfusion. The generally accepted normal urine output is 0.5 mL/kg per hour for adults and 1 to 2 mL/kg per hour for neonates and infants. Oliguria may reflect inadequate renal artery perfusion due to hypotension, hypovolemia, or low Q_T. Low urine flow also can be a sign of intrinsic renal dysfunction. It is important to recognize that normal urine output does not exclude the possibility of impending renal failure.

Bladder Pressure

The triad of oliguria, elevated peak airway pressures, and elevated intra-abdominal pressure is known as the abdominal compartment syndrome (ACS). This syndrome, first described in patients after repair of ruptured abdominal aortic aneurysm, is associated with interstitial edema of the abdominal organs, resulting in elevated intra-abdominal pressure.[135] When intra-abdominal pressure exceeds venous or capillary pressures, perfusion of the kidneys and other intra-abdominal viscera is impaired. Oliguria is a cardinal sign. While the diagnosis of ACS is a clinical one, measuring intra-abdominal pressure is useful to confirm the diagnosis. Ideally, a catheter inserted into the peritoneal cavity could measure intra-abdominal pressure to substantiate the diagnosis. In practice, transurethral bladder pressure measurement reflects intra-abdominal pressure and is most often used to confirm the presence of ACS. After instilling 50 to 100 mL of sterile saline into the bladder via a Foley catheter, the tubing is connected to a transducing system to measure bladder pressure. Most authorities recommend that a bladder pressure greater than 20 to 25 mm Hg confirms the diagnosis of ACS.[136] Less commonly, gastric or inferior vena cava pressures can be monitored with appropriate catheters to detect elevated intra-abdominal pressures.

NEUROLOGIC MONITORING

Intracranial Pressure

Because the brain is rigidly confined within the bony skull, cerebral edema or mass lesions increase intracranial pressure (ICP). Monitoring of ICP is currently recommended in patients with severe traumatic brain injury (TBI), defined as a Glasgow Coma Scale (GCS) score less than or equal to 8 with an abnormal CT scan, and in patients with severe TBI and a normal CT scan if two or more of the following are present: age greater than 40 years, unilateral or bilateral motor posturing, or systolic blood pressure less than 90 mm Hg.[137] ICP monitoring also is indicated in patients with acute subarachnoid hemorrhage with coma or neurologic deterioration, intracranial hemorrhage with intraventricular blood, ischemic middle cerebral artery stroke, fulminant hepatic failure with coma and cerebral edema on CT scan, and global cerebral ischemia or anoxia with cerebral edema on CT scan. The goal of ICP monitoring is to ensure that cerebral perfusion pressure (CPP) is adequate to support perfusion of the brain. CPP is equal to the difference between MAP and ICP: CPP = MAP – ICP.

One type of ICP measuring device consists of a fluid-filled catheter inserted into a ventricle and connected to an external pressure transducer. This device permits measurement of ICP, but also allows drainage of cerebrospinal fluid (CSF) as a means to lower ICP and sample CSF for laboratory studies. Other devices locate the pressure transducer within the central nervous system and are used only to monitor ICP. These devices can be placed in the intraventricular, parenchymal, subdural, or epidural spaces. Ventriculostomy catheters are the accepted standard for monitoring ICP in patients with TBI due to their accuracy, ability to drain CSF, and low complication rate. The associated complications include infection (5%), hemorrhage (1.4%), catheter malfunction or obstruction (6.3 to 10.5%), and malposition with injury to cerebral tissue.[138]

The purpose of ICP monitoring is to detect and treat abnormal elevations of ICP that may be detrimental to cerebral perfusion and function. In TBI patients, ICP greater than 20 mm Hg is associated with unfavorable outcomes.[139] However, few studies have shown that treatment of elevated ICP improves clinical outcomes in human trauma patients. In a randomized, controlled, double-blind trial, Eisenberg and colleagues demonstrated that maintaining ICP less than 25 mm Hg in patients without craniectomy and less than 15 mm Hg in patients with craniectomy is associated with improved outcome.[140] In patients with low CPP, therapeutic strategies to correct CPP can be directed at increasing MAP or decreasing ICP. While it often has been recommended that CPP be maintained above 70 mm Hg, data to support this recommendation are not convincing.[141]

Electroencephalogram and Evoked Potentials

Electroencephalography offers the capacity to monitor global neurologic electrical activity, while evoked potential monitoring can assess pathways not detected by the conventional EEG. Continuous EEG (CEEG) monitoring in the intensive care unit permits ongoing evaluation of cerebral cortical activity. It is especially useful in obtunded and comatose patients. CEEG also is useful for monitoring of therapy for status epilepticus and detecting early changes associated with cerebral ischemia. CEEG can be used to adjust the level of sedation, especially if high-dose barbiturate therapy is being used to manage elevated ICP. Somatosensory and brain stem evoked potentials are less affected by the administration of sedatives than is the EEG. Evoked potentials are useful for localizing brain stem lesions or proving the absence of such structural lesions in cases of metabolic or toxic coma. They also can provide prognostic data in posttraumatic coma.

A recent advance in EEG monitoring is the use of the bispectral index (BIS) to titrate the level of sedative medications. While sedative drugs are usually titrated to the clinical neurologic examination, the BIS device has been used in the operating room to continuously monitor the depth of anesthesia. The BIS is an empiric measurement statistically derived from a database of over 5000 EEGs.[142] The BIS is derived from bifrontal EEG recordings and analyzed for burst suppression ratio, relative alpha:beta ratio, and bicoherence. Using a multivariate regression model, a linear numeric index (BIS) is calculated, ranging from 0 (isoelectric EEG) to 100 (fully awake). Its use has been associated with lower consumption of anesthetics during surgery and earlier awakening and faster recovery from anesthesia.[143] The BIS also has been validated as a useful approach for monitoring the level of sedation for ICU patients, using the revised Sedation-Agitation Scale as a gold standard.[144]

Transcranial Doppler Ultrasonography

This modality provides a noninvasive method for evaluating cerebral hemodynamics. Transcranial Doppler (TCD) measurements of middle and anterior cerebral artery blood flow velocity are useful for the diagnosis of cerebral vasospasm after subarachnoid hemorrhage. Qureshi and associates demonstrated that a decrease in mean flow velocity as assessed by TCD is an independent predictor of symptomatic vasospasm in a prospective study of patients with aneurysmal subarachnoid hemorrhage.[145] TCD does not measure cerebral blood flow, and as such can be used to estimate cerebral blood flow if vessel diameter is constant. In addition, while some have proposed using TCD to estimate ICP, studies have shown that TCD is not a reliable method for estimating ICP and CPP, and currently cannot be endorsed for this purpose.[146] TCD also is useful to confirm the clinical examination for determining brain death in patients with confounding factors such as the presence of CNS depressants or metabolic encephalopathy.

Jugular Venous Oximetry

When the arterial oxygen content, hemoglobin concentration, and the oxyhemoglobin dissociation curve are constant, changes in jugular venous oxygen saturation (SjO_2) reflect changes in the difference between cerebral oxygen delivery and demand. Generally, a decrease in SjO_2 reflects cerebral hypoperfusion, whereas an increase in SjO_2 indicates the presence of hyperemia. SjO_2 monitoring cannot detect decreases in regional cerebral blood flow if overall perfusion is normal or above normal. This technique requires the placement of a catheter in the jugular bulb, usually via the internal jugular vein. Catheters that permit intermittent aspiration of jugular venous blood for analysis or continuous oximetry catheters are available.

Low SjO_2 is associated with poor outcomes after TBI.[147] Nevertheless, the value of monitoring SjO_2 remains unproven. If it is employed, it should not be the sole monitoring technique, but rather should be used in conjunction with ICP and CPP monitoring. By monitoring ICP, CPP, and SjO_2, early intervention with volume, vasopressors, and hyperventilation has been shown to prevent ischemic events in patients with TBI.[148]

Transcranial Near-Infrared Spectroscopy

Transcranial near-infrared spectroscopy is a noninvasive continuous monitoring method to determine cerebral oxygenation. It employs technology similar to that of pulse oximetry to determine the concentrations of oxy- and deoxyhemoglobin with near-infrared light and sensors, and takes advantage of the relative transparency of the skull to light in the near-infrared region of the spectrum. McCormick and associates demonstrated that cerebral desaturation can occur more than 2 hours prior to any clinical deterioration in neurologic status.[149] Nevertheless, this form of monitoring remains largely a research tool at the present time.

References

1. Komatsu T, Shibutani K, Okamoto K, et al: Critical level of oxygen delivery after cardiopulmonary bypass. *Crit Care Med* 15:194, 1987.
2. Shibutani K, Komatsu T, Kubal K, et al: Critical level of oxygen delivery in anesthetized man. *Crit Care Med* 11:640, 1983.
3. Lubarsky DA, Smith LR, Sladen RN, et al: Defining the relationship of oxygen delivery and consumption: Use of biologic system models. *J Surg Res* 58:503, 1995.
4. Lehmann KG, Gelman JA, Weber MA, et al: Comparative accuracy of three automated techniques in the noninvasive measurement of central blood pressure in men. *Am J Cardiol* 81:1004, 1998.
5. Epstein RH, Bartkowski RR, Huffnagle S: Continuous noninvasive finger blood pressure during controlled hypotension. *Anesthesiology* 75:796, 1991.
6. Remington JW, Wood EH: Formation of peripheral pulse contour in man. *J Appl Physiol* 9:433, 1956.
7. Siegman-Igra Y, Golan H, Schwartz D, et al: Epidemiology of vascular catheter-related bloodstream infections in a large university hospital in Israel. *Scand J Infect Dis* 32:411, 2000.
8. Chatila W, Ani S, Guaglianone D, et al: Cardiac ischemia during weaning from mechanical ventilation. *Chest* 109:1577, 1996.
9. Landensberg G, Mosseri M, Wolf Y, et al: Perioperative myocardial ischemia and infarction: Identification by continuous 12-lead electrocardiogram with online ST-segment monitoring. *Anesthesiology* 96:264, 2002.
10. Swan HJC, Ganz W, Forrester J, et al: Catheterization of the heart in man with use of a flow-directed balloon-tipped catheter. *N Engl J Med* 283:447, 1970.
11. Ginosar Y, Sprung CL: The Swan-Ganz catheter: Twenty-five years of monitoring. *Crit Care Clin* 12:771, 1996.
12. Mallory DL, McGee WT, Shawker TH, et al: Ultrasound guidance improves the success rate of internal jugular vein cannulation. A prospective, randomized trial. *Chest* 98:157, 1990.
13. Denys BG, Uretsky BF, Reddy PS: Ultrasound-assisted cannulation of the internal jugular vein. A prospective comparison to the external landmark-guided technique. *Circulation* 87:1557, 1993.
14. Hayashi H, Amano M: Does ultrasound imaging before puncture facilitate internal jugular vein cannulation? Prospective randomized comparison with landmark-guided puncture in ventilated patients. *J Cardiothorac Vasc Anesth* 16:572, 2002.
15. van Grondelle A, Ditchey RV, Groves BM, et al: Thermodilution method overestimates low cardiac output in humans. *Am J Physiol* 245:H690, 1983.
16. Mihaljevic T, von Segesser LK, Tonz M, et al: Continuous versus bolus thermodilution cardiac output measurements—a comparative study. *Crit Care Med* 23:944, 1995.
17. Haller M, Zollner C, Briegel J, et al: Evaluation of a new continuous thermodilution cardiac output monitor in critically-ill patients: A prospective criterion standard study. *Crit Care Med* 23:860, 1995.
18. Mihm FG, Gettinger A, Hanson CW, et al: A multicenter evaluation of a new continuous cardiac output pulmonary artery catheter system. *Crit Care Med* 26:1346, 1998.
19. Rouby J-J, Poete P, Bodin L, et al: Three mixed venous saturation catheters in patients with circulatory shock and respiratory failure. *Chest* 98:954, 1991.
20. Boutros AR, Lee C: Value of continuous monitoring of mixed venous blood oxygen saturation in the management of critically-ill patients. *Crit Care Med* 14:132, 1986.

21. Jastremski MS, Chelluri L, Beney KM, et al: Analysis of the effects of continuous on-line monitoring of mixed venous oxygen saturation on patient outcomes and cost-effectiveness. *Crit Care Med* 17:148, 1989.

22. Kyff JV, Vaughn S, Yang SC, et al: Continuous monitoring of mixed venous oxygen saturation in patients with acute myocardial infarction. *Chest* 95:607, 1989.

23. Gattinoni L, Brazzi L, Pelosi P, et al: A trial of goal-oriented hemodynamic therapy in critically-ill patients. *N Engl J Med* 333:1025, 1995.

24. London MJ, Moritz TE, Henderson WG, et al: Standard versus fiberoptic pulmonary artery catheterization for cardiac surgery in the Department of Veterans Affairs: A prospective, observational, multicenter analysis. *Anesthesiology* 96:860, 2003.

25. Rivers EP, Anders DS, Powell D: Central venous oxygen saturation monitoring in the critically-ill patient. *Curr Opin Crit Care* 7:204, 2003.

26. Rivers E, Nguyen B, Havstad S, et al: Early goal-directed therapy in the treatment of severe sepsis and septic shock. *N Engl J Med* 345:1368, 2001.

27. Dhainaut J-F, Brunet F, Monsallier JF, et al: Bedside evaluation of right ventricular performance using a rapid computerized thermodilution method. *Crit Care Med* 15:148, 1987.

28. Jardin F, Gueret P, Dubourg O, et al: Right ventricular volumes by thermodilution in the adult respiratory distress syndrome: A comparative study using two-dimensional echocardiography as a reference method. *Chest* 88:34, 1985.

29. Yu M, Takigushi S, Takanishi D, et al: Evaluation of the clinical usefulness of thermodilution volumetric catheters. *Crit Care Med* 23:681, 1995.

30. Chang MC, Blinman TA, Rutherford EJ, et al: Preload assessment in trauma patients during large-volume shock resuscitation. *Arch Surg* 131:728, 1996.

31. Connors AF Jr., Speroff T, Dawson NV, et al: The effectiveness of right heart catheterization in the initial care of critically-ill patients. *JAMA* 276:889, 1996.

32. Gore JM, Goldberg RJ, Spodick DH, et al: A community-wide assessment of the use of pulmonary artery catheters in patients with acute myocardial infarction. *Chest* 92:721, 1987.

33. Zion MM, Balkin J, Rosenmann D, et al: Use of pulmonary artery catheters in patients with acute myocardial infarction. Analysis of experience in 5841 patients in the SPRINT Registry. *Chest* 98:1331, 1990.

34. Dalen JE, Bone RC: Is it time to pull the pulmonary artery catheter? *JAMA* 276:916, 1997.

35. Afessa B, Spencer S, Khan W, et al: Association of pulmonary artery catheter use with in-hospital mortality. *Crit Care Med* 29:1145, 2001.

36. Pearson KS, Gomez MN, Moyers JR, et al: A cost/benefit analysis of randomized invasive monitoring for patients undergoing cardiac surgery. *Anesth Analg* 69:336, 1989.

37. Tuman KJ, McCarthy RJ, Spiess BD, et al: Effect of pulmonary artery catheterization on outcome in patients undergoing coronary artery surgery. *Anesthesiology* 70:199, 1989.

38. Isaakson IJ, Lowdon JD, Berry AJ, et al: The value of pulmonary artery and central venous monitoring in patients undergoing abdominal aortic reconstructive surgery: A comparative study of two selected, randomized groups. *J Vasc Surg* 12:754, 1990.

39. Joyce WP, Provan JL, Ameli FM, et al: The role of central haemodynamic monitoring in abdominal aortic surgery. A prospective randomised study. *Eur J Vasc Surg* 4:633, 1990.

40. Bender JS, Smith-Meek MA, Jones CE: Routine pulmonary artery catheterization does not reduce morbidity and mortality of elective vascular surgery: Results of a prospective, randomized trial. *Ann Surg* 226:229, 1997.

41. Valentine RJ, Duke ML, Inman MH, et al: Effectiveness of pulmonary artery catheters in aortic surgery: A randomized trial. *J Vasc Surg* 27:203, 1998.

42. Sandham JD, Hull RD, Brant RF, et al: A randomized, controlled trial of the use of pulmonary-artery catheters in high-risk surgical patients. *N Engl J Med* 348:5, 2003.

43. Bland RD, Shoemaker WC, Abraham E, et al: Hemodynamic and oxygen transport patterns in surviving and nonsurviving postoperative patients. *Crit Care Med* 13:85, 1985.

44. Shoemaker WC, Appel PL, Kram HB, et al: Prospective trial of supranormal values of survivors as therapeutic goals in high-risk surgical patients. *Chest* 94:1176, 1988.

45. Bishop MH, Shoemaker WC, Appel PL, et al: Prospective, randomized trial of survivor values of cardiac index, oxygen delivery, and oxygen consumption as resuscitative endpoints in severe trauma. *J Trauma* 38:780, 1995.

46. Boyd O, Grounds RM, Bennett ED: A randomized clinical trial of the effect of deliberate perioperative increase of oxygen delivery on mortality in high-risk surgical patients. *JAMA* 270:2699, 1993.

47. Fleming A, Bishop M, Shoemaker W, et al: Prospective trial of supranormal values as goals of resuscitation in severe trauma. *Arch Surg* 127:1175, 1992.

48. Yu M, Burchell S, Hasaniya NWMA, et al: Relationship of mortality to increasing oxygen delivery in patients >50 years of age: A prospective, randomized trial. *Crit Care Med* 26:1011, 1998.

49. Yu M, Levy MH, Smith P, et al: Effect of maximizing oxygen delivery on morbidity and mortality rates in critically-ill patients: A prospective, randomized, controlled study. *Crit Care Med* 21:830, 1993.

50. Tuchschmidt J, Fried J, Astiz M, et al: Elevation of cardiac output and oxygen improves outcome in septic shock. *Chest* 102:216, 1992.

51. Hayes MA, Timmins AC, Yau EHS, et al: Elevation of systemic oxygen delivery in the treatment of critically-ill patients. *N Engl J Med* 330:1717, 1994.

52. Alia I, Esteban A, Gordo F, et al: A randomized and controlled trial of the effect of treatment aimed at maximizing oxygen delivery in patients with severe sepsis or septic shock. *Chest* 115:453, 1999.

53. Heyland DK, Cook DJ, King D, et al: Maximizing of oxygen delivery in critically-ill patients: A methodologic appraisal of the evidence. *Crit Care Med* 24:517, 1996.

54. Connors AF Jr.: Right heart catheterization: Is it effective? *New Horiz* 5:195, 1997.

55. Sprung CL, Pozen RG, Rozanski JJ, et al: Advanced ventricular arrhythmias during bedside pulmonary artery catheterization. *Am J Med* 72:203, 1982.

56. Iberti TJ, Benjamin E, Gruppi L, et al: Ventricular arrhythmias during pulmonary artery catheterization in the intensive care unit. Prospective study. *Am J Med* 78:451, 1985.

57. Mermel LA, Maki DG: Infectious complications of Swan-Ganz pulmonary artery catheters. Pathogenesis, epidemiology, prevention, and management. *Am J Respir Crit Care Med* 149:1020, 1994.

58. Connors AF Jr., Castele RJ, Farhat NZ, et al: Complications of right heart catheterization. A prospective autopsy study. *Chest* 88:567, 1985.

59. Urschel JD, Myerowitz PD: Catheter-induced pulmonary artery rupture in the setting of cardiopulmonary bypass. *Ann Thorac Surg* 56:585, 1993.

60. Iberti TJ, Fischer EP, Leibowitz AB, et al: A multicenter study of physicians' knowledge of the pulmonary artery catheter. *JAMA* 264:2928, 1990.

61. Gnaegi A, Feihl F, Perret C: Intensive care physicians' insufficient knowledge of right-heart catheterization at the bedside: Time to act? *Crit Care Med* 25:213, 1997.

62. Gan TJ, Soppitt A, Maroof M, et al: Goal-directed intraoperative fluid administration reduces length of hospital stay after major surgery. *Anesthesiology* 97:820, 2002.

63. Cerny JC, Ketslakh M, Poulos CL, et al: Evaluation of the Velcom-100 pulse Doppler cardiac output computer. *Chest* 100:143, 1991.

64. Donovan KD, Dobb GJ, Newman MA, et al: Comparison of pulsed Doppler and thermodilution methods for measuring cardiac output in critically-ill patients. *Crit Care Med* 15:853, 1987.

65. Daigle RE, Miller CW, Histand MB, et al: Nontraumatic aortic blood flow sensing by use of an ultrasonic esophageal probe. *J Appl Physiol* 38:1153, 1975.

66. Valtier B, Cholley BP, Belot J-P, et al: Noninvasive monitoring of cardiac output in critically-ill patients using transesophageal Doppler. *Am J Respir Crit Care Med* 158:77, 1998.

67. Imhoff M, Lehner JH, Lohlein D: Noninvasive whole-body electrical bioimpedance cardiac output and invasive thermodilution cardiac output in high-risk surgical patients. *Crit Care Med* 28:2812, 2000.

68. Genoni M, Pelosi P, Romand JA, et al: Determination of cardiac output during mechanical ventilation by electrical bioimpedance or thermodilution in patients with acute lung injury: Effects of positive end-expiratory pressure. *Crit Care Med* 26:1441, 1998.

69. Marik PE, Pendelton JE, Smith R: A comparison of hemodynamic parameters derived from transthoracic electrical bioimpedance with those parameters obtained by thermodilution and ventricular angiography. *Crit Care Med* 25:1545, 1997.

70. Miles DS, Gotshall RW, Quinones JD, et al: Impedance cardiography fails to measure accurately left ventricular ejection fraction. *Crit Care Med* 18:221, 1990.

71. Wesseling KH, Purschke R, Smith NT, et al: A computer module for the continuous monitoring of cardiac output in the operating theatre and the ICU. *Acta Anaesethesiol Belg* 27(Suppl):327, 1976.

72. Mielck F, Fuhre W, Hanekop G, et al: Comparison of continuous cardiac output measurements in patients after cardiac surgery. *J Cardiothorac Vasc Anesth* 17:211, 2003.

73. Hirschl MM, Binder M, Gwechenberger M, et al: Noninvasive assessment of cardiac output in critically-ill patients by analysis of the finger blood pressure waveform. *Crit Care Med* 25:1909, 1997.

74. Remmen JJ, Aengevaeren RM, Verheugt WA, et al: Finapres arterial pulse wave analysis with Modeflow is not a reliable non-invasive method for assessment of cardiac output. *Clin Sci* 103:143, 2002.

75. Gedeon A, Forslund L, Hedenstierna G, et al: A new method for noninvasive bedside determination of pulmonary flow. *Med Biol Eng Comput* 18:411, 1980.

76. van Heerden PV, Baker S, Lim SI, et al: Clinical evaluation of the non-invasive cardiac output (NICO) monitor in the intensive care unit. *Anaesth Intensive Care* 28:427, 2000.

77. Odenstedt H, Stenquist O, Lundin S: Clinical evaluation of a partial CO_2 rebreathing technique for cardiac output monitoring in critically-ill patients. *Acta Anaesthesiol Scand* 46:152, 2002.

78. Godje O, Peyerl M, Seebauer T, et al: Central venous pressure, pulmonary capillary wedge pressure and intrathoracic blood volumes as preload indicators in cardiac surgery patients. *Eur J Cardiothorac Surg* 13:533, 1998.

79. Lichtwarck-Aschoff M, Zeravik J, Pfeiffer UJ: Intrathoracic blood volume accurately reflects circulatory volume status in critically-ill patients with mechanical ventilation. *Intensive Care Med* 18:142, 1992.

80. Konstadt SN, Thys D, Mindich BP, et al: Validation of quantitative intraoperative transesophageal echocardiography. *Anesthesiology* 65:418, 1986.

81. Clements FM, Harpole DH, Quill T, et al: Estimation of left ventricular volume and ejection fraction by two-dimensional transoesophageal echocardiography: Comparison of short axis imaging and simultaneous radionuclide angiography. *Br J Anaesth* 64:331, 1990.

82. Urbanowicz JH, Shaaban MJ, Cohen NH, et al: Comparison of transesophageal echocardiographic and scintigraphic estimates of left ventricular end-diastolic volume index and ejection fraction in patients following coronary artery bypass grafting. *Anesthesiology* 72:607, 1990.

83. Smith MD, MacPhail B, Harrison MR, et al: Value and limitations of transesophageal echocardiography in determination of left ventricular volumes and ejection fraction. *J Am Coll Cardiol* 19:1213, 1992.

84. Gunn SR, Pinsky MR: Implications of arterial pressure variation in patients in the intensive care unit. *Curr Opin Crit Care* 7:212, 2001.

85. Michard F, Chemla D, Richard C, et al: Clinical use of respiratory changes in arterial pulse pressure to monitor the hemodynamic effects of PEEP. *Am J Respir Crit Care Med* 159:935, 1999.

86. Michard F, Boussat S, Chemla D, et al: Relation between respiratory changes in arterial pulse pressure and fluid responsiveness in septic patients with acute circulatory failure. *Am J Respir Crit Care Med* 162:134, 2000.

87. Mommsen TP, Hochachka PW: Protons and anaerobiosis. *Science* 219:1391, 1983.

88. Schiedler MG, Cutler BS, Fiddian-Green RG: Sigmoid intramural pH for prediction of ischemic colitis during aortic surgery. A comparison with risk factors and inferior mesenteric artery stump pressures. *Arch Surg* 122:881, 1987.

89. Fiddian-Green RG, Baker S: Predictive value of the stomach wall pH for complications after cardiac operations. Comparison with other monitoring. *Crit Care Med* 15:153, 1987.

90. Fiddian-Green RG, McGough E, Pittenger G, et al: Predictive value of intramural pH and other risk factors for massive bleeding from stress ulceration. *Gastroenterology* 85:613, 1983.

91. Fiddian-Green RG, Pittenger G, Whitehouse WM: Back-diffusion of CO_2 and its influence on the intramural pH in gastric mucosa. *J Surg Res* 33:39, 1982.

92. Antonsson JB, Boyle CC, Kruithoff KL, et al: Validation of tonometric measurement of gut intramural pH during endotoxemia and mesenteric occlusion in pigs. *Am J Physiol* 259:G519, 1990.

93. Salzman AL, Strong KE, Wang H, et al: Intraluminal "balloonless" air tonometry: A new method for determination of gastrointestinal mucosal P_{CO_2}. *Crit Care Med* 22:126, 1994.

94. Reilly PM, Wilkins KB, Fuh KC, et al: The mesenteric hemodynamic response to circulatory shock: An overview. *Shock* 15:329, 2001.

95. Dantzker DR: The gastrointestinal tract: The canary of the body? *JAMA* 270:1247, 1993.

96. Fink MP: Intestinal epithelial hyperpermeability: Update on the pathogenesis of gut mucosal barrier dysfunction in critical illness. *Curr Opin Crit Care* 9:143, 2003.

97. Heard SO, Helsmoortel CM, Kent JC, et al: Gastric tonometry in healthy volunteers: Effect of ranitidine on calculated intramural pH. *Crit Care Med* 19:271, 1989.

98. Kolkman JJ, Groeneveld AB, Meuwissen SG: Effect of ranitidine on basal and bicarbonate enhanced intragastric P_{CO_2}: A tonometric study. *Gut* 35:737, 1994.

99. Kolkman JJ, Groeneveld AB, Meuwissen SG: Gastric P_{CO_2} tonometry is independent of carbonic anhydrase inhibition. *Dig Dis Sci* 42:99, 1997.

100. Parviainen I, Vaisanen O, Ruokonen E, et al: Effect of nasogastric suction and ranitidine on the calculated gastric intramucosal pH. *Intensive Care Med* 22:319, 1996.

101. Levy B, Perrigault P-F, Gawalkiewicz P, et al: Gastric versus duodenal feeding and gastric tonometric measurements. *Crit Care Med* 26:1991, 1998.

102. Doglio GR, Pusajo JF, Egurrola MA, et al: Gastric mucosal pH as a prognostic index of mortality in critically-ill patients. *Crit Care Med* 19:1037, 1991.

103. Maynard N, Bihari D, Beale R, et al: Assessment of splanchnic oxygenation by gastric tonometry in patients with acute circulatory failure. *JAMA* 270:1203, 1993.

104. Roumen RMH, Vreugde JPC, Goris RJA: Gastric tonometry in multiple trauma patients. *J Trauma* 36:313, 1994.

105. Chang MC, Cheatham ML, Nelson LD, et al: Gastric tonometry supplements information provided by systemic indicators of oxygen transport. *J Trauma* 37:488, 1994.

106. Miller PR, Kincaid EH, Meredith JW, et al: Threshold values of intramucosal pH and mucosal-arterial CO_2 gap during shock resuscitation. *J Trauma* 45:868, 1998.

107. Marik PE: Gastric intramucosal pH: A better predictor of multiorgan dysfunction syndrome and death than oxygen-derived variables in patients with sepsis. *Chest* 104:225, 1993.

108. Bjork M, Hedberg B: Early detection of major complications after abdominal aortic surgery: Predictive value of sigmoid colon and gastric intramucosal pH monitoring. *Br J Surg* 81:25, 1994.

109. Elizalde JI, Hernández C, Llach J, et al: Gastric intramucosal acidosis in mechanically ventilated patients: Role of mucosal blood flow. *Crit Care Med* 26:827, 1998.

110. Soong CV, Halliday MI, Barclay GR, et al: Intramucosal acidosis and systemic host response in abdominal aortic aneurysm surgery. *Crit Care Med* 25:1472, 1997.

111. Gutierrez G, Palizas F, Doglio G, et al: Gastric intramucosal pH as a therapeutic index of tissue oxygenation in critically-ill patients. *Lancet* 339:195, 1992.

112. Ivatury RR, Simon RJ, Islam S, et al: A prospective randomized study of end points of resuscitation after major trauma: Global oxygen transport indices versus organ-specific gastric mucosal pH. *J Am Coll Surg* 183:145, 1996.

113. Russell JA: Gastric tonometry: Does it work? *Intensive Care Med* 23:3, 1997.

114. Groeneveld AB, Kolkman JJ: Splanchnic tonometry: A review of physiology, methodology, and clinical applications. *J Crit Care* 9:198, 1994.

115. Schlichtig R, Mehta N, Gayowski TJP: Tissue-arterial Pco$_2$ difference is a better marker of ischemia than intramural pH (pHi). *J Crit Care* 11:51, 1996.

116. Sato Y, Weil MH, Tang W, et al: Esophageal Pco$_2$ as a monitor of perfusion failure during hemorrhagic shock. *J Appl Physiol* 82:558, 1997.

117. Guzman JA, Lacoma FJ, Kruse JA: Gastric and esophageal intramucosal Pco$_2$ (Pico$_2$) during endotoxemia. Assessment of raw Pico$_2$ and Pco$_2$ gradients as indicators of hypoperfusion in a canine model of septic shock. *Chest* 113:1078, 1998.

118. Povoas HP, Weil MH, Tang W, et al: Decreases in mesenteric blood flow associated with increases in sublingual Pco$_2$ during hemorrhagic shock. *Shock* 15:398, 2001.

119. Nakagawa Y, Weil MH, Tang W, et al: Sublingual capnometry for diagnosis and quantitation of circulatory shock. *Am J Resp Crit Care Med* 157:1838, 1998.

120. Weil MH, Nakagawa Y, Tang W, et al: Sublingual capnometry: A new noninvasive measurement for diagnosis and quantitation of severity of circulatory shock. *Crit Care Med* 27:1225, 1999.

121. Marik PE: Sublingual capnography: A clinical validation study. *Chest* 120:923, 2001.

122. Haller M, Kilger E, Briegel J, et al: Continuous intra-arterial blood gas and pH monitoring in critically-ill patients with severe respiratory failure: A prospective, criterion standard study. *Crit Care Med* 22:580, 1994.

123. The Acute Respiratory Distress Syndrome Network: Ventilation with lower tidal volumes as compared with traditional tidal volumes for acute lung injury and the acute respiratory distress syndrome. The Acute Respiratory Distress Syndrome Network. *N Engl J Med* 342:1301, 2000.

124. Tremper K: Pulse oximetry. *Chest* 95:713, 1989.

125. Shoemaker WC, Belzberg H, Wo CC, et al: Multicenter study of noninvasive monitoring systems as alternatives to invasive monitoring of acutely ill emergency patients. *Chest* 114:1643, 1998.

126. Bowton DL, Scuderi PE, Haponik EF: The incidence and effect on outcome of hypoxemia in hospitalized medical patients. *Am J Med* 97:38, 1994.

127. Jubran A, Tobin MJ: Monitoring during mechanical ventilation. *Clin Chest Med* 17:453, 1996.

128. MacIntyre NR, Cook DJ, Guyatt GH: Evidence-based guidelines for weaning and discontinuing ventilatory support: A collective task force facilitated by the American College of Chest Physicians; the American Association for Respiratory Care; and the American College of Critical Care Medicine. *Chest* 120:375S, 2001.

129. Kirton OC, DeHaven CB, Morgan JP, et al: Elevated imposed work of breathing masquerading as ventilator weaning intolerance. *Chest* 108:1021, 1995.

130. Yang KL, Tobin MJ: A prospective study of indexes predicting the outcome of trials of weaning from mechanical ventilation. *N Engl J Med* 324:1445, 1991.

131. Alberti A, Gallo F, Fongaro A, et al: P$_{0.1}$ is a useful parameter in setting the level of pressure support ventilation. *Intensive Care Med* 21:547, 1995.

132. Capdevila XJ, Perrigault PF, Perey PJ, et al: Occlusion pressure and its ratio to maximum inspiratory pressure are useful predictors for successful extubation following T-piece weaning trial. *Chest* 108:482, 1995.

133. Jacob B, Chatilla W, Manthous CA: The unassisted respiratory rate: tidal volume ratio accurately predicts weaning outcome in postoperative patients. *Crit Care Med* 25:253, 1996.

134. Lee KH, Hui KP, Chan TB, et al: Rapid shallow breathing (frequency-tidal volume ratio) did not predict extubation outcome. *Chest* 105:540, 1994.

135. Kron IL, Harman PK, Nolan SP: The measurement of intra-abdominal pressure as a criterion for abdominal reexploration. *Ann Surg* 199:28, 1984.

136. Ivatury RR, Porter JM, Simon RJ, et al: Intra-abdominal hypertension after life-threatening penetrating abdominal trauma: Prophylaxis, incidence, and clinical relevance to gastric mucosal pH and abdominal compartment syndrome. *J Trauma* 44:1016, 1998.

137. The Brain Trauma Foundation. The American Association of Neurological Surgeons. The Joint Section on Neurotrauma and Critical Care: Indications for intracranial pressure monitoring. *J Neurotrauma* 17:479, 2000.

138. The Brain Trauma Foundation. The American Association of Neurological Surgeons. The Joint Section on Neurotrauma and Critical Care: Recommendations for intracranial pressure monitoring technology. *J Neurotrauma* 17:497, 2000.

139. Juul N, Morris GF, Marshall SB, et al: Intracranial hypertension and cerebral perfusion pressure: Influence on neurological deterioration and outcome in severe head injury. The Executive Committee of the International Selfote. *J Neurosurg* 92:1, 2000.

140. Eisenberg HM, Frankowski RF, Contant CF, et al: High-dose barbiturate control of elevated intracranial pressure in patients with severe head injury. *J Neurosurg* 69:15, 1988.

141. The Brain Trauma Foundation. The American Association of Neurological Surgeons. The Joint Section on Neurotrauma and Critical Care: Guidelines for cerebral perfusion pressure. *J Neurotrauma* 17:507, 2000.

142. Sigl JC, Chamoun NG: An introduction to bispectral analysis for the electroencephalogram. *J Clin Monit* 10:392, 1994.

143. Gan TJ, Glass PS, Windsor A, et al: Bispectral index monitoring allows faster emergence and improved recovery from propofol, alfentanil, and nitrous oxide anesthesia. BIS Utility Study Group. *Anesthesiology* 87:808, 1997.

144. Simmons LE, Riker RR, Prato BS, et al: Assessing sedation during intensive care unit mechanical ventilation with the Bispectral Index and the Sedation-Agitation Scale. *Crit Care Med* 27:1499, 1999.

145. Qureshi AI, Sung GY, Razumovsky AY, et al: Early identification of patients at risk for symptomatic vasospasm after aneurysmal subarachnoid hemorrhage. *Crit Care Med* 28:984, 2000.

146. Czosnyka M, Matta BF, Smielewski P, et al: Cerebral perfusion pressure in head-injured patients: A noninvasive assessment using transcranial Doppler ultrasonography. *J Neurosurg* 88:802, 1998.

147. Feldman Z, Robertson CS: Monitoring of cerebral hemodynamics with jugular bulb catheters. *Crit Care Clin* 13:51, 1997.

148. Vigue B, Ract C, Benayed M, et al: Early SjvO$_2$ monitoring in patients with severe brain trauma. *Intensive Care Med* 25:445, 1999.

149. McCormick P, Stewart M, Goetting M, et al: Noninvasive cerebral optical spectroscopy for monitoring cerebral oxygen delivery and hemodynamics. *Crit Care Med* 19:89, 1999.

CHAPTER 13

Minimally-Invasive Surgery

Blair A. Jobe and John G. Hunter

Minimally-invasive surgery describes an area of surgery that crosses all traditional disciplines, from general surgery to neurosurgery. It is not a discipline unto itself, but more a philosophy of surgery, a way of thinking. Minimally-invasive surgery is a means of performing major operations through small incisions, often using miniaturized, high-tech imaging systems, to minimize the trauma of surgical exposure. Some believe that *minimal access surgery* more accurately describes the small incisions generally necessary to gain access to surgical sites in high-tech surgery, but John Wickham's term *minimally-invasive surgery* (MIS) is widely used because it describes the paradox of postmodern high-tech surgery—small holes, big operations—and the "minimalness" of the access and invasiveness of the procedures, captured in three words.

HISTORICAL BACKGROUND

While the term *minimally-invasive surgery* is relatively recent, the history of its component parts is nearly 100 years old. What is considered the newest and most popular variety of MIS, laparoscopy, is in fact the oldest. Primitive laparoscopy, placing a cystoscope within an inflated abdomen, was first performed by Kelling in 1901.[1] Illumination of the abdomen required hot elements at the tip of the scope and was dangerous. In the late 1950s Hopkins described the rod lens, a method of transmitting light through a solid quartz rod with no heat and little light loss.[1] Around the same time, thin quartz fibers were discovered to be capable of trapping light internally and conducting it around corners, opening the field of fiberoptics and allowing the rapid development of flexible endoscopes.[2,3] In the 1970s the application of flexible endoscopy grew faster than that of rigid endoscopy except in a few fields such as gynecology and orthopedics.[4] By the mid-1970s rigid and flexible endoscopes made a rapid transition from diagnostic instruments to therapeutic ones. The explosion of video-assisted surgery in the past 10 years was a result of the development of compact, high-resolution charge-coupled devices which could be mounted on the internal end of flexible endoscopes or on the external end of a Hopkins telescope. Coupled with bright light sources, fiberoptic cables, and high-resolution video monitors, the videoendoscope has changed our understanding of surgical anatomy and reshaped surgical practice.

While optical imaging produced the majority of MIS procedures, other (traditionally radiologic) imaging technologies allowed the development of innovative procedures in the 1970s. Fluoroscopic imaging allowed the adoption of percutaneous vascular procedures, the most revolutionary of which was balloon angioplasty. Balloon-based procedures spread into all fields of medicine, assisting in a minimally-invasive manner to open up clogged lumens. Stents were then developed that were used in many disciplines to keep the newly ballooned segment open. The culmination of fluoroscopic balloon and stent proficiency is exemplified by the transvenous intrahepatic portosystemic shunt (TIPS) (Fig. 13-1).

MIS procedures using ultrasound imaging have been limited to fairly crude exercises, such as fragmenting kidney stones and freezing liver tumors, because of the relatively low resolution of ultrasound devices. Newer, high-resolution ultrasound methods with high-frequency crystals may act as a guide while performing minimally-invasive resections of individual layers of the intestinal wall.

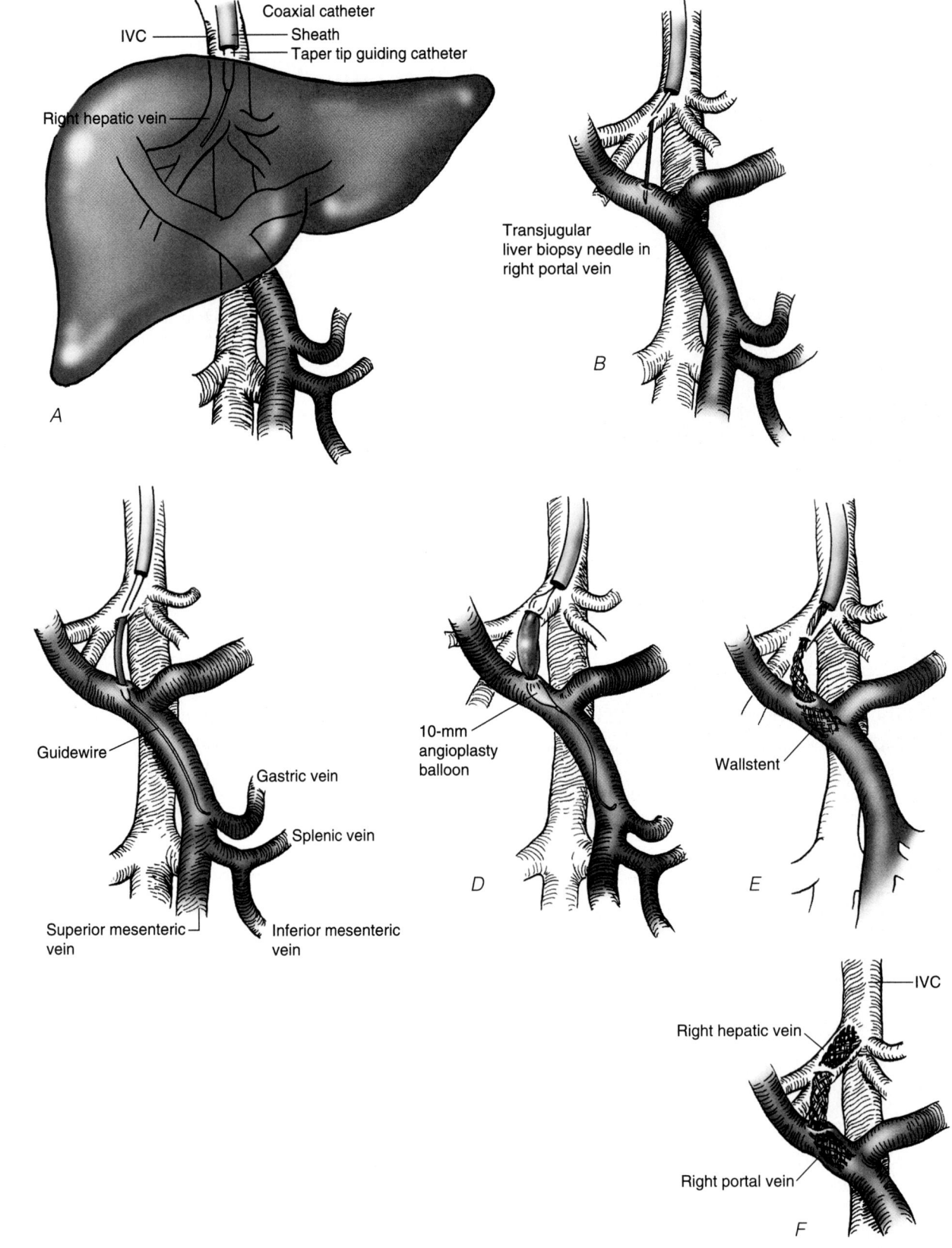

FIG. 13-1. With the transvenous intrahepatic portosystemic shunt (TIPS), percutaneous access to the superior vena cava is followed by the retrograde cannulation of the hepatic veins. Next a needle is advanced through the hepatic parenchyma until the portal venous radicle is located. A guidewire is passed across this connection, and after dilation a metallic stent is expanded with a balloon. While not often performed by surgeons, TIPS represents a particularly creative example of minimally-invasive surgery. *(Reproduced with permission from Hunter JG, Sackier JM (eds): Minimally-Invasive Surgery. New York: McGraw-Hill, 1993, p 271.)*

Axial imaging, such as computed tomography (CT), has allowed the development of an area of MIS that is not often recognized because it requires only a CT scanner and a long needle. CT-guided drainage of abdominal fluid collections and percutaneous biopsy of abnormal tissues are minimally-invasive means of performing procedures that previously required a celiotomy. Recently, CT-guided percutaneous radiofrequency ablation has emerged as a useful treatment for primary and metastatic liver tumors. This procedure has also been performed laparoscopically under ultrasound guidance.[5]

A powerful, noninvasive method of imaging that will allow the development of the least invasive—and potentially noninvasive—surgery is magnetic resonance imaging (MRI).

MRI is an extremely valuable diagnostic tool, but it is only slowly coming to be of therapeutic value. One obstacle to the use of MRI for MIS is that image production and refreshment of the image as a procedure progresses are slow. Another is that all instrumentation must be nonmetallic when working with the powerful magnets of an MRI scanner. Moreover, MRI magnets are bulky and limit the surgeon's access to the patient. Open magnets have been developed that allow the surgeon to stand between two large MRI coils, obtaining access to the portion of the patient being scanned. The advantage of MRI, in addition to the superb images produced, is that there is no radiation exposure to patient or surgeon. Some neurosurgeons are accumulating experience using MRI to perform frameless stereotactic surgery.

THE MINIMALLY-INVASIVE TEAM

From the beginning, the tremendous success of minimally-invasive surgery has been founded on the understanding that a team approach is necessary. The numerous laparoscopic procedures range from basic to advanced complexity, and require that the surgical team have an intimate understanding of the operative conduct (Table 13-1). Minimally-invasive procedures require complicated and fragile equipment that demands constant maintenance. In addition, multiple intraoperative adjustments to the equipment, camera, insufflator, monitors, and patient/surgeon position are made during these procedures. As such, a coordinated team approach is mandated in order to ensure patient safety and excellent outcomes.

A typical MIS team may consist of a laparoscopic surgeon and an operating room nurse with an interest in laparoscopic surgery.

Table 13-1
Laparoscopic Surgical Procedures

	Today		Tomorrow
Basic	**Advanced**		**Tomorrow**
Appendectomy	Nissen fundoplication		Intracorporeal anastomosis
Cholecystectomy	Heller myotomy		Cancer surgery
Hernia repair	Gastrectomy		Telepresence surgery
	Esophagectomy		
	Enteral access		
	Bile duct exploration		
	Pancreatectomy		
	Colectomy		
	Splenectomy		
	Adrenalectomy		
	Nephrectomy		
	Lymph node dissection		
	Robotics		
	Stereo imaging		
	Telemedicine		
	Laparoscopy-assisted		
	procedures		

Adding dedicated laparoscopic assistants and circulating staff with an intimate knowledge of the equipment will add to and enhance the team nucleus. Studies have demonstrated that having a designated laparoscopic team reduces the conversion rate and overall operative time, which is translated into a cost savings for patient and hospital.[6]

PHYSIOLOGY

Even with the least invasive of the MIS procedures, physiologic changes occur. Many minimally-invasive procedures require minimal or no sedation, and there are few alterations to the cardiovascular, endocrinologic, or immunologic systems. The least invasive of such procedures include stereotactic biopsy of breast lesions and flexible gastrointestinal endoscopy. Minimally-invasive procedures that require general anesthesia have a greater physiologic impact because of the anesthetic agent, the incision (even if small), and the induced pneumoperitoneum.

Laparoscopy

The unique feature of endoscopic surgery in the peritoneal cavity is the need to lift the abdominal wall from the abdominal organs. Two methods have been devised for achieving this.[7] The first, used by most surgeons, is the induction of a pneumoperitoneum. Throughout the early twentieth century intraperitoneal visualization was achieved by inflating the abdominal cavity with air, using a sphygmomanometer bulb.[8] The problem with using air insufflation is that nitrogen is poorly soluble in blood and is slowly absorbed across the peritoneal surfaces. Air pneumoperitoneum was believed to be more painful than nitrous oxide pneumoperitoneum but less painful than carbon dioxide pneumoperitoneum. Subsequently, carbon dioxide and nitrous oxide were used for inflating the abdomen. N_2O had the advantage of being physiologically inert and rapidly absorbed. It also provided better analgesia for laparoscopy performed under local anesthesia when compared with CO_2 or air.[9] Despite initial concerns that N_2O would not suppress combustion, controlled clinical trials have established its safety within the peritoneal cavity.[10] In addition, nitrous oxide has recently been shown to reduce the intraoperative end-tidal CO_2 and minute ventilation required to maintain homeostasis when compared to CO_2 pneumoperitoneum.[10] The effect of N_2O on tumor biology and the development of port site metastasis are unknown. As such, caution should be exercised when performing laparoscopic cancer surgery with this agent. Finally, the safety of N_2O pneumoperitoneum in pregnancy has yet to be elucidated.

The physiologic effects of CO_2 pneumoperitoneum can be divided into two areas: (1) gas-specific effects and (2) pressure-specific effects (Fig. 13-2). CO_2 is rapidly absorbed across the peritoneal membrane into the circulation. In the circulation, CO_2 creates a respiratory acidosis by the generation of carbonic acid.[11] Body buffers, the largest reserve of which lies in bone, absorb CO_2 (up to 120 L) and minimize the development of hypercarbia or respiratory acidosis during brief endoscopic procedures.[11] Once the body buffers are saturated, respiratory acidosis develops rapidly, and the respiratory system assumes the burden of keeping up with the absorption of CO_2 and its release from these buffers.

In patients with normal respiratory function this is not difficult; the anesthesiologist increases the ventilatory rate or vital capacity on the ventilator. If the respiratory rate required exceeds 20 breaths per minute, there may be less efficient gas exchange and increasing hypercarbia.[12] Conversely, if vital capacity is increased substantially, there is a greater opportunity for barotrauma and greater respiratory motion–induced disruption of the upper abdominal

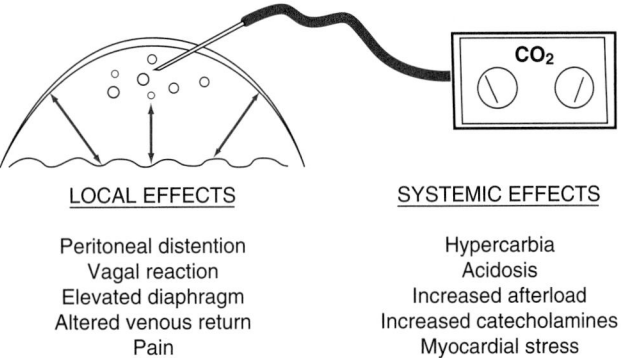

LOCAL EFFECTS

Peritoneal distention
Vagal reaction
Elevated diaphragm
Altered venous return
Pain

SYSTEMIC EFFECTS

Hypercarbia
Acidosis
Increased afterload
Increased catecholamines
Myocardial stress

FIG. 13-2. *Carbon dioxide gas insufflated into the peritoneal cavity has both local and systemic effects that cause a complex set of hemodynamic and metabolic alterations. [Reproduced with permission from Hunter JG (ed): Baillière's Clinical Gastroenterology Laparoscopic Surgery. London/Philadelphia: Baillière Tindall, 1993, p 758.]*

operative field. In some situations it is advisable to evacuate the pneumoperitoneum or reduce the intra-abdominal pressure to allow time for the anesthesiologist to adjust for hypercarbia.[13] While mild respiratory acidosis probably is an insignificant problem, more severe respiratory acidosis leading to cardiac arrhythmias has been reported.[14] Hypercarbia also causes tachycardia and increased systemic vascular resistance, which elevates blood pressure and increases myocardial oxygen demand.[11,14]

The pressure effects of the pneumoperitoneum on cardiovascular physiology also have been studied. In the hypovolemic individual, excessive pressure on the inferior vena cava and a reverse Trendelenburg position with loss of lower extremity muscle tone may cause decreased venous return and cardiac output.[11,15] This is not seen in the normovolemic patient. The most common arrhythmia created by laparoscopy is bradycardia. A rapid stretch of the peritoneal membrane often causes a vagovagal response with bradycardia and occasionally hypotension.[16] The appropriate management of this event is desufflation of the abdomen, administration of vagolytic agents (e.g., atropine), and adequate volume replacement.[17]

With the increased intra-abdominal pressure compressing the inferior vena cava, there is diminished venous return from the lower extremities. This has been well documented in the patient placed in the reverse Trendelenburg position for upper abdominal operations. Venous engorgement and decreased venous return promote venous thrombosis.[18,19] Many series of advanced laparoscopic procedures in which deep venous thrombosis (DVT) prophylaxis was not used demonstrate the frequency of pulmonary embolus. This usually is an avoidable complication with the use of sequential compression stockings, subcutaneous heparin, or low-molecular-weight heparin.[20] In short-duration laparoscopic procedures, such as appendectomy, hernia repair, or cholecystectomy, the risk of DVT may not be sufficient to warrant extensive DVT prophylaxis.

The increased pressure of the pneumoperitoneum is transmitted directly across the paralyzed diaphragm to the thoracic cavity, creating increased central venous pressure and increased filling pressures of the right and left sides of the heart. If the intra-abdominal pressures are kept under 20 mm Hg, the cardiac output usually is well maintained.[19,20,21] The direct effect of the pneumoperitoneum on increasing intrathoracic pressure increases peak inspiratory pressure, pressure across the chest wall, and also the likelihood of barotrauma. Despite these concerns, disruption of blebs and consequent pneumothoraces are rare after uncomplicated laparoscopic surgery.[21]

Increased intra-abdominal pressure decreases renal blood flow, glomerular filtration rate, and urine output. These effects may be mediated by direct pressure on the kidney and the renal vein.[22,23] The secondary effect of decreased renal blood flow is to increase plasma renin release, thereby increasing sodium retention. Increased circulating antidiuretic hormone (ADH) levels also are found during the pneumoperitoneum, increasing free water reabsorption in the distal tubules.[24] Although the effects of the pneumoperitoneum on renal blood flow are immediately reversible, the hormonally mediated changes, such as elevated ADH levels, decrease urine output for up to 1 hour after the procedure has ended. Intraoperative oliguria is common during laparoscopy, but the urine output is not a reflection of intravascular volume status; intravenous fluid administration during an uncomplicated laparoscopic procedure should not be linked to urine output. Because fluid losses through the open abdomen are eliminated with laparoscopy, the need for supplemental fluid during a laparoscopic surgical procedure is rare.

The hemodynamic and metabolic consequences of pneumoperitoneum are well tolerated by healthy individuals for a prolonged period and by most individuals for at least a short period. Difficulties can occur when a patient with compromised cardiovascular function is subjected to a long laparoscopic procedure. It is during these procedures that alternative approaches should be considered or insufflation pressure reduced. Alternative gases that have been suggested for laparoscopy include the inert gases helium, neon, and argon. These gases are appealing because they cause no metabolic effects, but are poorly soluble in blood (unlike CO_2 and N_2O) and are prone to create gas emboli if the gas has direct access to the venous system.[19] Gas emboli are rare but serious complications of laparoscopic surgery.[20,25] They should be suspected if hypotension develops during insufflation. Diagnosis may be made by listening (with an esophageal stethoscope) for the characteristic "mill wheel" murmur. The treatment of gas embolism is to place the patient in a left lateral decubitus position with the head down to trap the gas in the apex of the right ventricle.[20] A rapidly placed central venous catheter then can be used to aspirate the gas out of the right ventricle.

In some situations minimally-invasive abdominal surgery should be performed without insufflation. This has led to the development of an abdominal lift device that can be placed through a 10- to 12-mm trocar at the umbilicus.[26] These devices have the advantage of creating little physiologic derangement, but they are bulky and intrusive. The exposure and working room offered by lift devices also are inferior to those accomplished by pneumoperitoneum. Lifting the anterior abdominal wall causes a "pinching in" of the lateral flank walls, displacing the bowel medially and anteriorly into the operative field. A pneumoperitoneum, with its well-distributed intra-abdominal pressure, provides better exposure. Abdominal lift devices also cause more postoperative pain, but they do allow the performance of MIS with standard (nonlaparoscopic) surgical instruments.

Early it was predicted that the surgical stress response would be significantly lessened with laparoscopic surgery, but this is not always the case. Serum cortisol levels after laparoscopic operations are often higher than after the equivalent operation performed through an open incision.[27] In terms of endocrine balance, the greatest difference between open and laparoscopic surgery is the more rapid equilibration of most stress-mediated hormone levels after laparoscopic surgery. Immune suppression also is less after laparoscopy than after open surgery. There is a trend toward more rapid normalization of cytokine levels after a laparoscopic procedure than after the equivalent procedure performed by celiotomy.[28]

Transhiatal mobilization of the thoracic esophagus is commonly performed as a component of many laparoscopic upper abdominal procedures. Entering the posterior mediastinum transhiatally exposes the thoracic organs to positive insufflation pressure and may result in decreased venous return and a resultant decrease in cardiac output. If there is compromise of the mediastinal pleura with resultant CO_2 pneumothorax, the defect should be enlarged so as to prevent a tension pneumothorax.

Thoracoscopy

The physiology of thoracic MIS (thoracoscopy) is different from that of laparoscopy. Because of the bony confines of the thorax it is unnecessary to use positive pressure when working in the thorax.[29] The disadvantages of positive pressure in the chest include decreased venous return, mediastinal shift, and the need to keep a firm seal at all trocar sites. Without positive pressure, it is necessary to place a double-lumen endotracheal tube so that the ipsilateral lung can be deflated when the operation starts. By collapsing the ipsilateral lung, working space within the thorax is obtained. Because insufflation is unnecessary in thoracoscopic surgery, it can be beneficial to utilize standard instruments via extended port sites in conjunction with thoracoscopic instruments. This approach is particularly useful when performing advanced procedures such as thoracoscopic anatomic pulmonary resection.

Extracavitary Minimally-Invasive Surgery

Many new MIS procedures are creating working spaces in extrathoracic and extraperitoneal locations. Laparoscopic inguinal hernia repair usually is performed in the anterior extraperitoneal Retzius space.[30,31] Laparoscopic nephrectomy often is performed with retroperitoneal laparoscopy. Recently, an endoscopic retroperitoneal approach to pancreatic necrosectomy has been introduced.[32] Lower extremity vascular procedures and plastic surgical endoscopic procedures require the development of working space in unconventional planes, often at the level of the fascia, sometimes below the fascia, and occasionally in nonanatomic regions.[33] Some of these techniques use insufflation of gas, but many use balloon inflation to develop the space, followed by low-pressure gas insufflation or lift devices to maintain the space (Fig. 13-3). These techniques produce fewer and less severe adverse physiologic consequences than does the pneumoperitoneum, but the insufflation of gas into extraperitoneal locations can spread widely, causing subcutaneous emphysema and metabolic acidosis.

Anesthesia

The most important factors in appropriate anesthesia management are related to CO_2 pneumoperitoneum.[17] The laparoscopic surgeon can influence cardiovascular performance by releasing intraabdominal retraction and dropping the pneumoperitoneum. Insensible fluid losses are negligible, and therefore intravenous fluid administration should not exceed a maintenance rate. MIS procedures usually are outpatient procedures, and short-acting anesthetic agents are preferable. Because the factors that require hospitalization after laparoscopic procedures include the management of nausea, pain, and urinary retention, the anesthesiologist should minimize the use of agents that provoke these conditions and maximize the use of medications that prevent such problems. Critical to the anesthesia management of these patients is the use of nonnarcotic analgesics (e.g., ketorolac) and the liberal use of antiemetic agents.

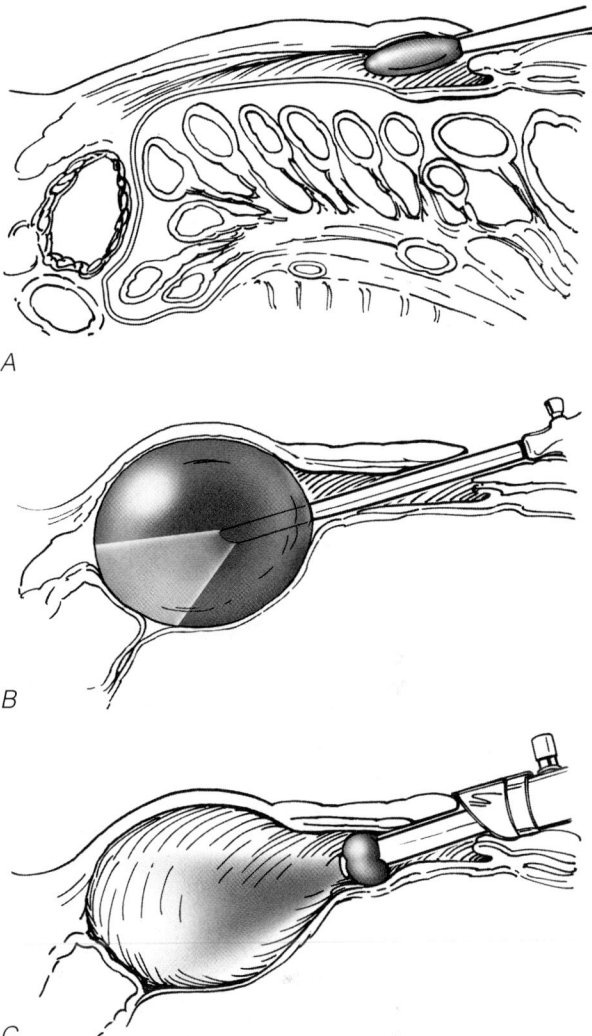

A

B

C

FIG. 13-3. Balloons are used to create extra-anatomic working spaces. In this example a balloon is introduced into the space between the posterior rectus sheath and the rectus abdominis muscle. The balloon is inflated in the preperitoneal space to create working room for extraperitoneal endoscopic hernia repair.

GENERAL PRINCIPLES OF ACCESS AND EQUIPMENT

The most natural ports of access for MIS are the anatomic portals of entry and exit. The nares, mouth, urethra, and anus are used to access the respiratory, gastrointestinal, and urinary systems. The advantage of using these points of access is that no incision is required. The disadvantages lie in the long distances between the orifice and the region of interest.

Access to the vascular system may be accomplished under local anesthesia by cutting down and exposing the desired vessel, usually in the groin. Increasingly, vascular access is obtained with percutaneous techniques using a small incision, a needle, and a guidewire, over which are passed a variety of different sized access devices. This approach, known as the Seldinger technique, is most frequently used by general surgeons for placement of Hickman catheters, but also is used to gain access to the arterial and venous system for performance of minimally-invasive procedures. Guidewire-assisted, Seldinger-type techniques also are helpful for gaining access to the gut for procedures such as percutaneous endoscopic gastrostomy, for gaining access to the biliary system through the liver, and for gaining access to the upper urinary tract.

In thoracoscopic surgery, the access technique is similar to that used for placement of a chest tube. In these procedures general anesthesia and split-lung ventilation are essential. A small incision is made over the top of a rib and, under direct vision, carried down through the pleura. The lung is collapsed, and a trocar is inserted across the chest wall to allow access with a telescope. Once the lung is completely collapsed, subsequent access may be obtained with direct puncture, viewing all entry sites through the videoendoscope. Because insufflation of the chest is unnecessary, simple ports that keep the small incisions open are all that is required to allow repeated access to the thorax.

Laparoscopic Access

The requirements for laparoscopy are more involved, because the creation of a pneumoperitoneum requires that instruments of access (trocars) contain valves to maintain abdominal inflation.

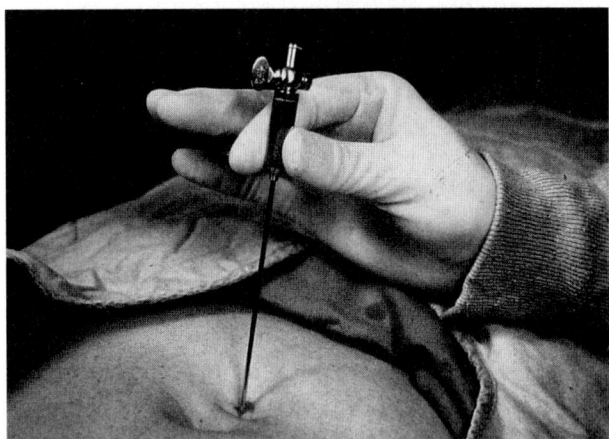

A

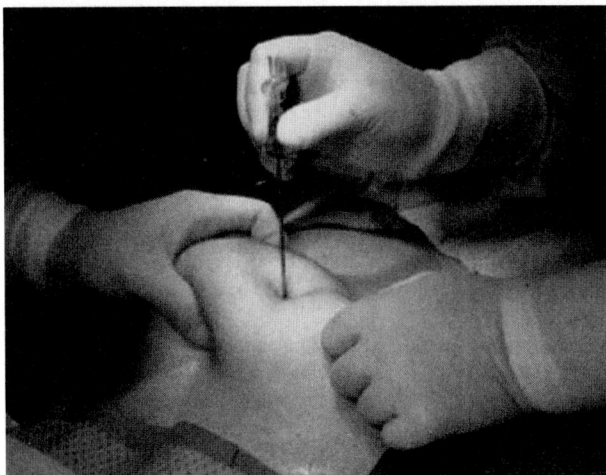

B

FIG. 13-4. *A. Insufflation of the abdomen is accomplished with a Veress needle held at its serrated collar with a thumb and forefinger. B. Because linea alba is fused to the umbilicus, the abdominal wall is grasped with fingers or penetrating towel clip in order to elevate the abdominal wall away from the underlying structures.*

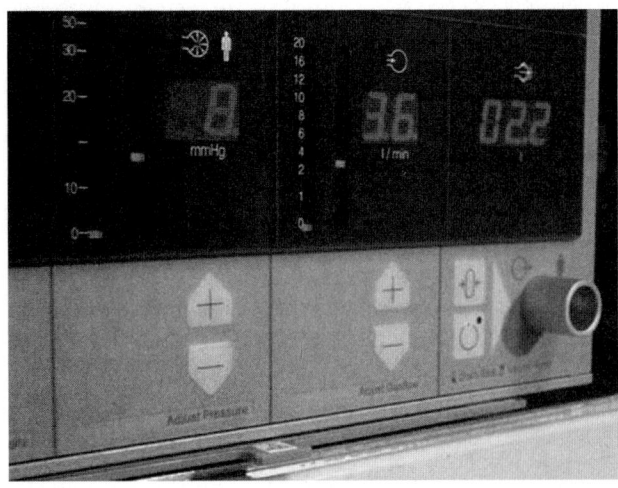

FIG. 13-5. *It is essential to be able to interpret the insufflator pressure readings and flow rates. These readings indicate proper intraperitoneal placement of the Veress needle.*

Two methods are used for establishing abdominal access during laparoscopic procedures.[34,35] The first, direct puncture laparoscopy, begins with the elevation of the relaxed abdominal wall with two towel clips or a well-placed hand. A small incision is made in the umbilicus, and a specialized spring-loaded (Veress) needle is placed in the abdominal cavity (Fig. 13-4A and B). With the Veress needle, two distinct pops are felt as the surgeon passes the needle through the abdominal wall fascia and the peritoneum. The umbilicus usually is selected as the preferred point of access because in this location the abdominal wall is quite thin, even in obese patients. The abdomen is inflated with a pressure-limited insufflator. CO_2 gas is usually used, with maximal pressures in the range of 14 to 15 mm Hg. During the process of insufflation it is essential that the surgeon observe the pressure and flow readings on the monitor to confirm an intraperitoneal location of the Veress needle tip (Fig. 13-5). Laparoscopic surgery can be performed under local anesthesia, but general anesthesia is preferable. Under local anesthesia, N_2O is used as the insufflating agent, and insufflation is stopped after 2 L of gas is insufflated or when a pressure of 10 mm Hg is reached.

After peritoneal insufflation, direct access to the abdomen is obtained with a 5- or 10-mm trocar. The critical issues for safe direct-puncture laparoscopy include the use of a vented stylet for the trocar, or a trocar with a safety shield or dilating tip. The trocar must be pointed away from the sacral promontory and the great vessels.[36] Patient position should be surveyed prior to trocar placement to ensure a proper trajectory. For performance of laparoscopic cholecystectomy, the trocar is angled toward the right upper quadrant.

Occasionally the direct peritoneal access (Hasson) technique is advisable.[37] With this technique, the surgeon makes a small incision just below the umbilicus and under direct vision locates the abdominal fascia. Two Kocher clamps are placed on the fascia, and with a curved Mayo scissors a small incision is made through the fascia and underlying peritoneum. A finger is placed into the abdomen to make sure that there is no adherent bowel. A sturdy suture is placed on each side of the fascia and secured to the wings of a specialized trocar, which is then passed directly into the abdominal cavity (Fig. 13-6). Rapid insufflation can make up for some of the time lost with the initial dissection. This technique is preferable for the abdomen of patients who have undergone previous operations in which small bowel may be adherent to the undersurface of the abdominal

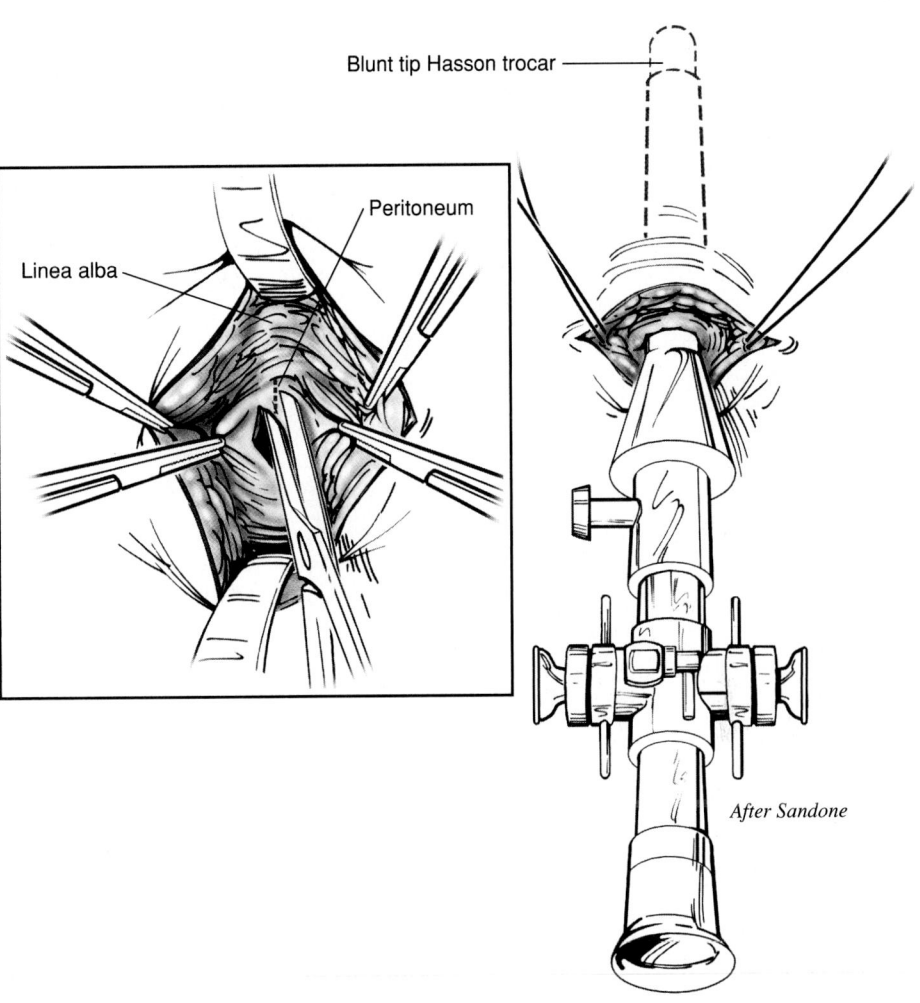

Blunt tip Hasson trocar

Peritoneum

Linea alba

After Sandone

FIG. 13-6. The open laparoscopy technique involves identification and incision of the peritoneum, followed by the placement of a specialized trocar with a conical sleeve to maintain a gas seal. Specialized wings on the trocar are attached to sutures placed through the fascia to prevent loss of the gas seal.

wound. The close adherence of bowel to the peritoneum in the previously operated abdomen does not eliminate the possibility of intestinal injury, but should make great vessel injury extremely unlikely. Because of the difficulties in visualizing the abdominal region immediately adjacent to the primary trocar, it is recommended that the telescope be passed through a secondary trocar in order to inspect the site of initial abdominal access.[35] Secondary punctures are made with 5- and 10-mm trocars. For safe access to the abdominal cavity, it is critical to visualize all sites of trocar entry.[35,36] At the completion of the operation, all trocars are removed under direct vision and the insertion sites are inspected for bleeding. If bleeding occurs, direct pressure with an instrument from another trocar site or balloon tamponade with a Foley catheter placed through the trocar site generally stops the bleeding within 3 to 5 minutes. When this is not successful, a full-thickness abdominal wall suture has been used successfully to tamponade trocar site bleeding.

It is generally agreed that 5-mm trocars need no site suturing. Ten-millimeter trocars placed off the midline and above the transverse mesocolon do not require repair. Conversely, if the fascia has been dilated to allow the passage of the gallbladder, all midline 10-mm trocar sites should be repaired at the fascial level with interrupted sutures. Specialized suture delivery systems similar to crochet needles have been developed for mass closure of the abdominal wall in obese patients, in whom it is difficult to visualize the fascia through a small skin incision. Failure to close lower abdominal trocar

sites that are 10 mm in diameter or larger can lead to an incarcerated hernia.

Access for Subcutaneous and Extraperitoneal Surgery

There are two methods for gaining access to nonanatomic spaces. For retroperitoneal locations, balloon dissection is effective. This access technique is appropriate for the extraperitoneal repair of inguinal hernias and for retroperitoneal surgery for adrenalectomy, nephrectomy, lumbar discectomy, pancreatic necrosectomy, or para-aortic lymph node dissection.[38,39] The initial access to the extraperitoneal space is performed in a way similar to direct puncture laparoscopy, except that the last layer (the peritoneum) is not traversed. Once the transversalis fascia has been punctured, a specialized trocar with a balloon on the end is introduced. The balloon is inflated in the extraperitoneal space to create a working chamber. The balloon then is deflated and a Hasson trocar is placed. An insufflation pressure of 10 mm Hg usually is adequate to keep the extraperitoneal space open for dissection and will limit subcutaneous emphysema. Higher gas pressures force CO_2 into the soft tissues and may contribute to hypercarbia. Extraperitoneal endosurgery provides less working space than laparoscopy, but eliminates the possibility of intestinal injury, intestinal adhesion, herniation at the trocar sites, and ileus. These issues are important for laparoscopic hernia repair

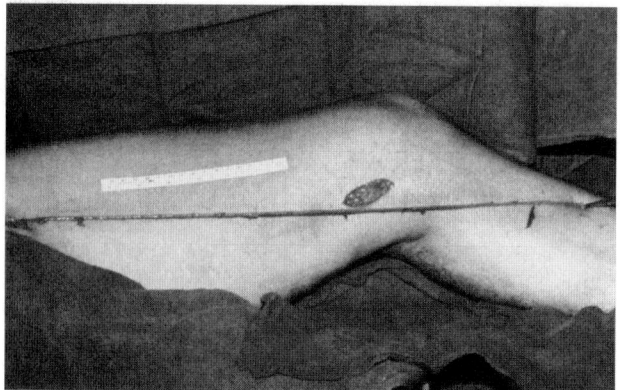

A

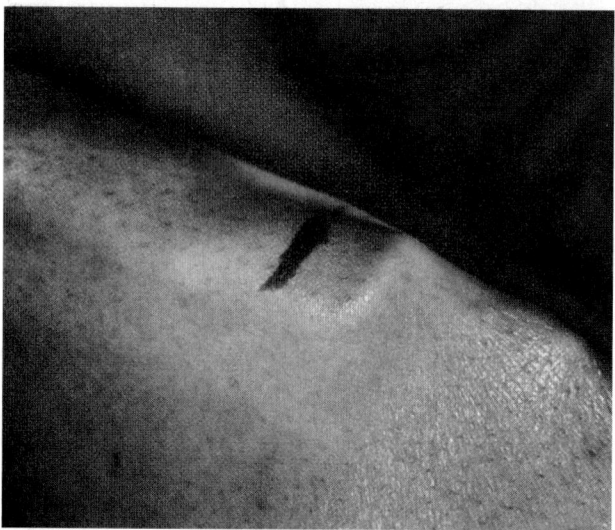

B

FIG. 13-7. *A. With two small incisions, virtually the entire saphenous vein can be harvested for bypass grafting. B. The lighted retractor in the subcutaneous space during saphenous vein harvest is seen illuminating the skin. (Reproduced with permission from Bostwick J III, Eaves F III, Nahai F: Endoscopic Plastic Surgery. St Louis: Quality Medical Publishers, 1995, p 542.)*

because extraperitoneal approaches prevent the small bowel from sticking to the prosthetic mesh.[31]

Subcutaneous surgery, the newest method of access in minimally-invasive surgery, uses the creation of working room in nonanatomic spaces. This technique has been most widely used in cardiac, vascular, and plastic surgery.[33] In cardiac surgery, subcutaneous access has been used for saphenous vein harvesting, and in vascular surgery for ligation of subfascial perforating veins (Linton procedure). With minimally-invasive techniques the entire saphenous vein above the knee may be harvested through a single incision[40,41] (Fig. 13-7). Once the saphenous vein is located, a long retractor that holds a 5-mm laparoscope allows the coaxial dissection of the vein and coagulation or clipping of each side branch. A small incision above the knee also can be used to ligate perforating veins in the lower leg.

Subcutaneous access is also used for plastic surgical procedures.[41] Minimally-invasive approaches are especially well suited to cosmetic surgery, in which attempts are made to hide the incision. It is easier to hide several 5-mm incisions than one long incision. The technique of blunt dissection along fascial planes combined with

lighted retractors and endoscope-holding retractors is most successful for extensive subcutaneous surgery. Some prefer gas insufflation of these soft tissue planes. The primary disadvantage of soft tissue insufflation is that subcutaneous emphysema can be created.

Hand-Assisted Laparoscopic Access

Hand-assisted laparoscopic surgery (HALS) is thought to combine the tactile advantages of open surgery with the minimal access of laparoscopy and thoracoscopy. This approach is commonly used to assist with difficult cases before conversion to celiotomy is necessary. Additionally, HALS is employed to help surgeons negotiate the steep learning curve associated with advanced laparoscopic procedures.[42] This technology employs a "port" for the hand which preserves the pneumoperitoneum and enables endoscopic visualization in combination with the use of minimally-invasive instruments (Fig. 13-8). Formal investigation of this modality has been limited primarily to case reports and small series, and has focused primarily on solid organ and colon surgery.

Port Placement

Trocars for the surgeon's left and right hand should be placed at least 10 cm apart. For most operations it is possible to orient the telescope between these two trocars and slightly retract from them. The ideal trocar orientation creates an equilateral triangle between the surgeon's right hand, left hand, and the telescope, with 10 to 15 cm on each leg. If one imagines the target of the operation (e.g., the gallbladder or gastroesophageal junction) oriented at the apex of a second equilateral triangle built on the first, these four points of reference create a diamond (Fig. 13-9). The surgeon stands behind the telescope, which provides optimal ergonomic orientation but frequently requires that a camera operator (or robotic arm) reach between the surgeon's hands to guide the telescope.

The position of the operating table should permit the surgeon to work with both elbows in at the sides, with arms bent 90° at the elbow.[43] It usually is necessary to alter the operating table position with left or right tilt with the patient in the Trendelenburg or reverse Trendelenburg position, depending on the operative field.[44,45]

Imaging Systems

Two methods of videoendoscopic imaging are widely used. Both methods use a camera with a charge-coupled device (CCD), which is an array of photosensitive sensor elements (pixels) that convert the incoming light intensity to an electric charge. The electric charge is subsequently converted into a black-and-white image.[46] The first of these is flexible videoendoscopy, where the CCD camera is placed on the internal end of a long, flexible endoscope. In the second method, thin quartz fibers are packed together in a bundle, and the CCD camera is mounted on the external end of the endoscope. Most standard gastrointestinal endoscopes have the CCD chip at the distal end, but small, delicate choledochoscopes and nephroscopes are equipped with fiberoptic bundles.[47] Distally-mounted CCD chips were developed for laparoscopy, but are unpopular.

Video cameras come in two basic designs. The one-chip camera has a black-and-white video chip that has an internal processor capable of converting gray scales to approximate colors. Perfect color representation is not possible with a one-chip camera, but perfect color representation is rarely necessary for endosurgery. The most accurate color representation is obtained using a three-chip video camera. A three-chip camera has red, green, and blue (RGB) input, and is identical to the color cameras used for television production.[46] RGB imaging provides the highest fidelity, but is

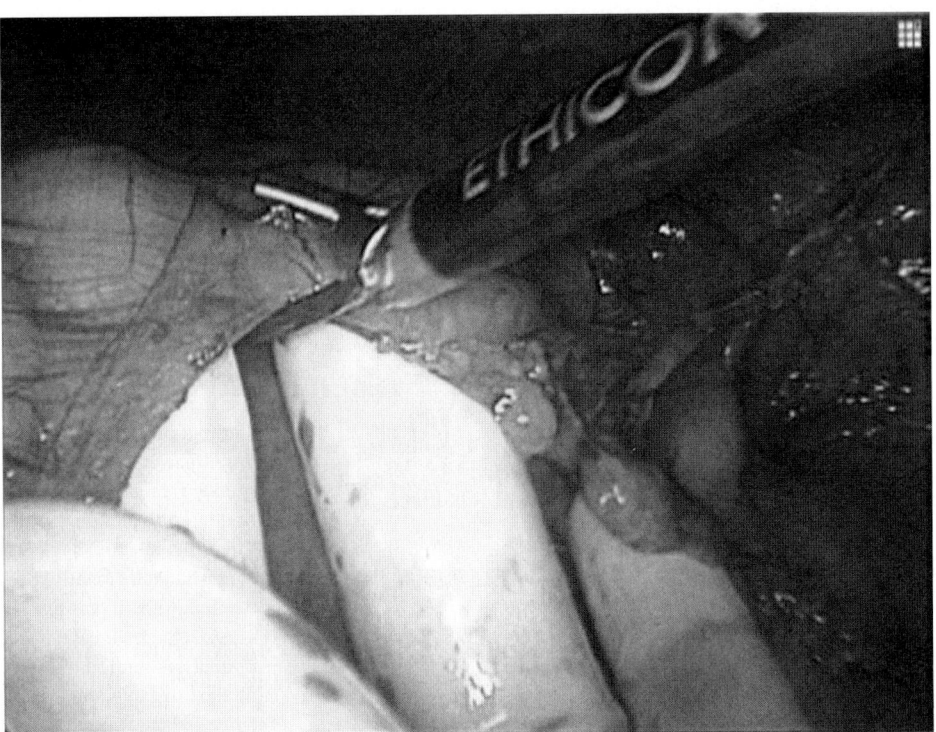

A

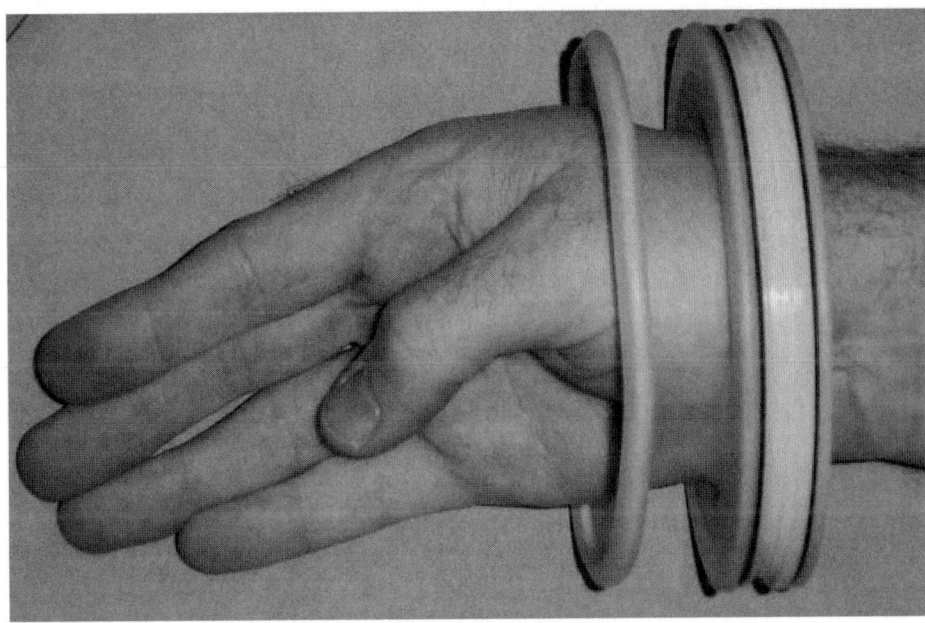

FIG. 13-8. This is an example of hand-assisted laparoscopic surgery during left colectomy. The surgeon uses a hand to provide retraction and counter tension during mobilization of the colon from its retroperitoneal attachments, as well as during division of the mesocolon. This technique is particularly useful in the region of the transverse colon.

B

probably not necessary for everyday use. An additional feature of newer video cameras is digital enhancement. Digital enhancement detects edges, areas where there are drastic color or light changes between two adjacent pixels.[48] By enhancing this difference, the image appears sharper and surgical resolution is improved. Digital enhancement is available on one- and three-chip cameras. Priorities in a video system for MIS are illumination first, resolution second, and color third. Without the first two attributes, video surgery is unsafe. Imaging for laparoscopy, thoracoscopy, and subcutaneous surgery uses a rigid metal telescope, usually 30 cm in length. This telescope contains a series of quartz optical rods with

differing optical characteristics that provide a specific character to each telescope.[49] These metal telescopes vary in size from 2 to 10 mm in diameter. Since light transmission is dependent on the cross-sectional area of the quartz rod, when the diameter of a rod/lens system is doubled, the illumination is quadrupled. Little illumination is needed in highly-reflective, small spaces such as the knee, and a very small telescope will suffice. When working in the abdominal cavity, especially if blood is present, the full illumination of a 10-mm telescope usually is necessary.

Rigid telescopes may have a flat or angled end. The flat end provides a straight view (0°), and the angled end provides an oblique

THE DIAMOND OF SUCCESS

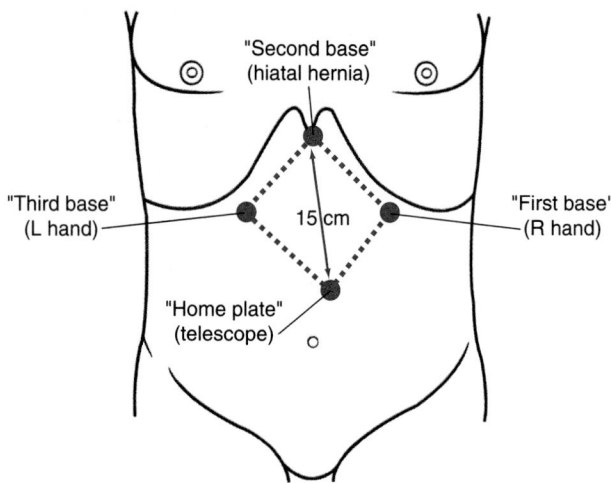

FIG. 13-9. The diamond configuration created by placing the telescope between the left and the right hand, recessed from the target by about 15 cm. The distance between the left and the right hand is also ideally 10 to 15 cm. In this "baseball diamond" configuration, the surgical target occupies the second base position.

view (30 or 45°).[46] Angled scopes allow greater flexibility in viewing a wider operative field through a single trocar site (Fig. 13-10); rotating an angled telescope changes the field of view. The use of an angled telescope has distinct advantages for most videoendoscopic procedures, particularly in visualizing the common bile duct during laparoscopic cholecystectomy or visualizing the posterior esophagus or the tip of the spleen during laparoscopic fundoplication.

Light is delivered to the endoscope through a fiberoptic light cable. These light cables are highly inefficient, losing more than 90% of the light delivered from the light source. Extremely bright light sources (300 watts) are necessary to provide adequate illumination for video endosurgery.

The quality of the videoendoscopic image is only as good as the weakest component in the imaging chain (Fig. 13-11). Therefore it is important to use a video monitor that has a resolution equal to or greater than the camera being used.[49] *Resolution* is the ability of

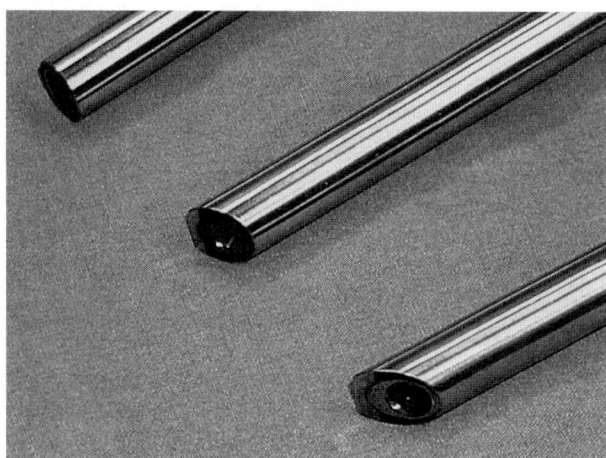

FIG. 13-10. The laparoscope tips come in a variety of angled configurations. All laparoscopes have a 70° field of view. A 30° angled scope enables the surgeon to view this field at a 30° angle to the long axis of the scope.

the optical system to distinguish between line pairs. The larger the number of line pairs per millimeter, the sharper and more detailed the image. Most high-resolution monitors have up to 700 horizontal lines. High definition television (HDTV) can deliver up to eight times more resolution than the standard NTSC/PAL monitors; when combined with digital enhancement, a very sharp and well-defined image can be achieved.[46,49] A heads-up display (HUD) is a high-resolution liquid crystal monitor that is built into eyewear worn by the surgeon.[50] This technology allows the surgeon to view the endoscopic image and operative field simultaneously. The proposed advantages of HUD include a high-resolution monocular image, which affords the surgeon mobility and reduces vertigo and eyestrain. However, this technology has not yet been widely adopted.

There has been recent interest in three-dimensional endoscopy. Three-dimensional laparoscopy provides the additional depth of field that is lost with two-dimensional endosurgery and allows greater facility for novice laparoscopists performing complex tasks of dexterity, including suturing and knot tying.[51] The advantages of three-dimensional systems are less obvious to experienced laparoscopists. Additionally, because three-dimensional systems require the flickering of two similar images, which are resolved with special glasses, the images' edges become fuzzy and resolution is lost. The optical accommodation necessary to rectify these slightly differing images negates any advantage offered by the additional depth of field.

Energy Sources for Endoscopic and Endoluminal Surgery

MIS uses conventional energy sources, but the requirement of bloodless surgery to maintain optimal visualization has spawned new ways of applying energy. The most common energy source is radiofrequency (RF) electrosurgery using an alternating current with a frequency of 500,000 cycles/s (Hz). Tissue heating progresses through the well-known phases of coagulation (60°C), vaporization and desiccation (100°C), and carbonization (>200°C).[52]

The two most common methods of delivering RF electrosurgery are with monopolar and bipolar electrodes. With monopolar electrosurgery a remote ground plate on the patient's leg or back receives the flow of electrons that originate at a point source, the surgical electrode. A fine-tipped electrode causes a high current density at the site of application and rapid tissue heating. Monopolar electrosurgery is inexpensive and easy to modulate to achieve different tissue effects.[53] A short-duration, high-voltage discharge of current (coagulation current) provides extremely rapid tissue heating. Lower-voltage, higher-wattage current (cutting current) is better for tissue desiccation and vaporization. When the surgeon desires tissue division with the least amount of thermal injury and least coagulation necrosis, a cutting current is used.

With bipolar electrosurgery the electrons flow between two adjacent electrodes. The tissue between the two electrodes is heated and desiccated. There is little opportunity for tissue cutting when bipolar current is used, but the ability to coapt the electrodes across a vessel provides the best method of small-vessel coagulation without thermal injury to adjacent tissues[54] (Fig. 13-12).

In order to avoid thermal injury to adjacent structures, the laparoscopic field of view must include all uninsulated portions of the electrosurgical electrode. In addition, the integrity of the insulation must be maintained and assured. Capacitive coupling occurs when a plastic trocar insulates the abdominal wall from the current; in turn the current is bled off of a metal sleeve or laparoscope into the viscera[52] (Fig. 13-13A). This may result in thermal necrosis and a

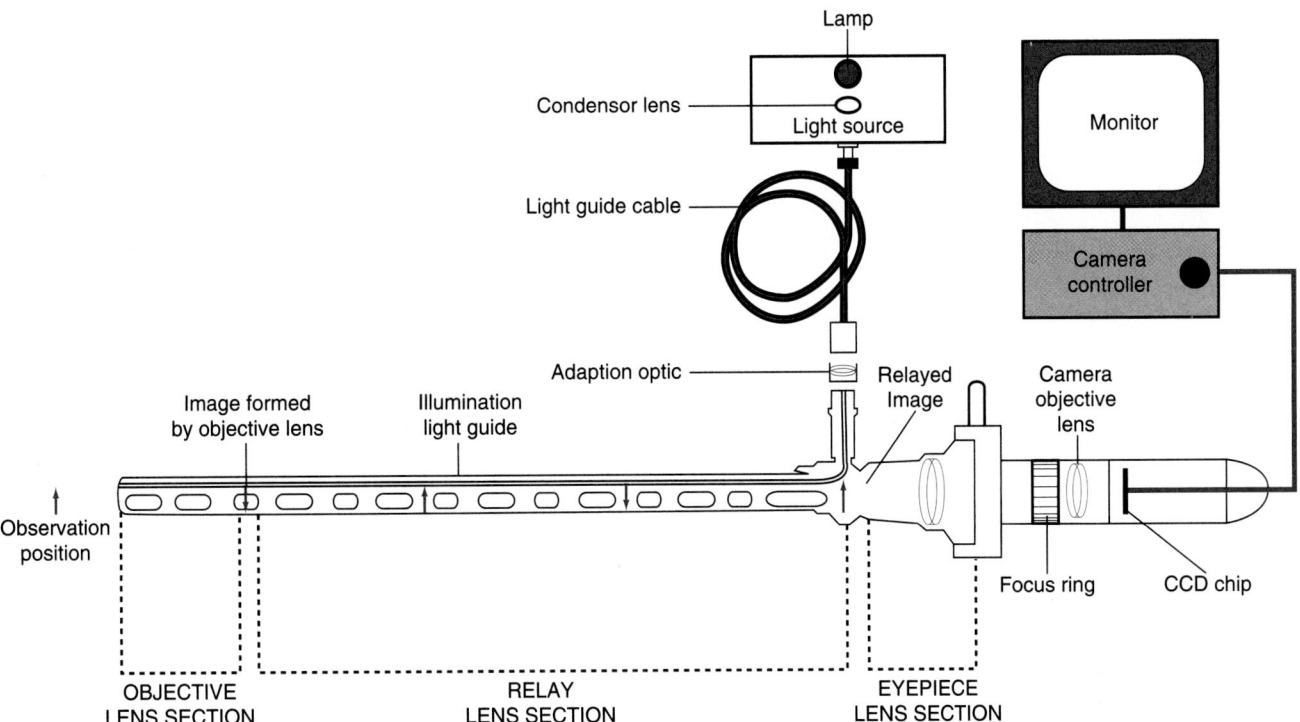

FIG. 13-11. The Hopkins rod lens telescope includes a series of optical rods that effectively transmit light to the eyepiece. The video camera is placed on the eyepiece to provide the working image. The image is only as clear as the weakest link in the image chain. (*Reproduced with permission from Prescher et al.[46]*)

delayed fecal fistula. Another potential mechanism for unrecognized visceral injury may occur with the direct coupling of current to the laparoscope and adjacent bowel[52] (Fig. 13-13B).

Another method of delivering radiofrequency electrosurgery is argon beam coagulation. This is a type of monopolar electrosurgery in which a uniform field of electrons is distributed across a tissue surface by the use of a jet of argon gas. The argon gas jet distributes electrons more evenly across the surface than does spray

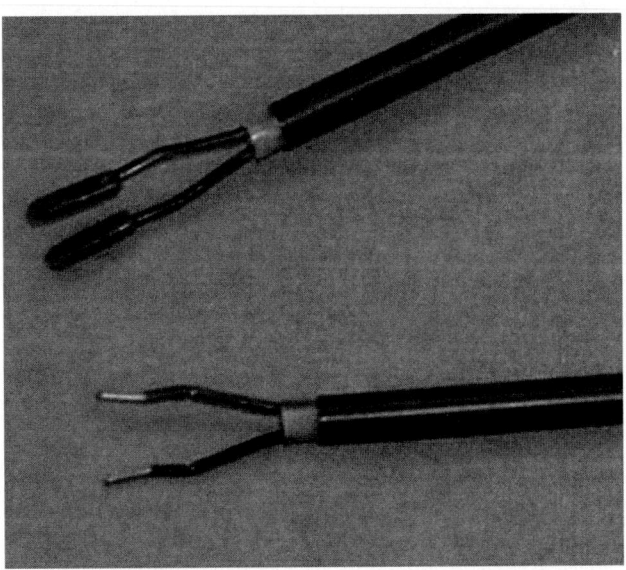

FIG. 13-12. An example of bipolar coagulation devices. The flow of electrons passes from one electrode to the other and the intervening tissue is heated and desiccated.

electrofulguration. This technology has its greatest application for coagulation of diffusely bleeding surfaces such as the cut edge of liver or spleen. It is of less use in laparoscopic procedures because the increased intra-abdominal pressures created by the argon gas jet can increase the chances of a gas embolus. It is paramount to vent the ports and closely monitor insufflation pressure when using this source of energy within the context of laparoscopy.

With endoscopic endoluminal surgery, radiofrequency alternating current in the form of a monopolar circuit represents the mainstay for procedures such as snare polypectomy, sphincterotomy, lower esophageal sphincter ablation, and "hot" biopsy.[55,56] A grounding ("return") electrode is necessary for this form of energy. Bipolar electrocoagulation is used primarily for thermal hemostasis. The electrosurgical generator is activated by a foot pedal so the endoscopist may keep both hands free during the endoscopic procedure.

Gas, liquid, and solid-state lasers have been available for medical application since the mid-1960s.[57] The CO_2 laser (wavelength 10.6 μm) is most appropriately used for cutting and superficial ablation of tissues. It is most helpful in locations unreachable with a scalpel such as excision of vocal cord granulomas. The CO_2 laser beam must be delivered with a series of mirrors and is therefore somewhat cumbersome to use. The next most popular laser is the neodymium yttrium-aluminum-garnet (Nd:YAG) laser. Nd:YAG laser light is 1.064 μm (1064 nm) in wavelength. It is in the near-infrared portion of the spectrum, and, like CO_2 laser light, is invisible to the naked eye. A unique feature of the Nd:YAG laser is that 1064-nm light is poorly absorbed by most tissue pigments and therefore travels deep into tissue.[58] Deep tissue penetration provides deep tissue heating (Fig. 13-14). For this reason the Nd:YAG laser is capable of the greatest amount of tissue destruction with a single application.[57] Such capabilities make it the ideal laser for destruction of large fungating tumors of the rectosigmoid, tracheobronchial tree, or esophagus.

CAPACITIVE COUPLED FAULT CONDITION   CONDUCTION THROUGH UNGROUNDED TELESCOPE

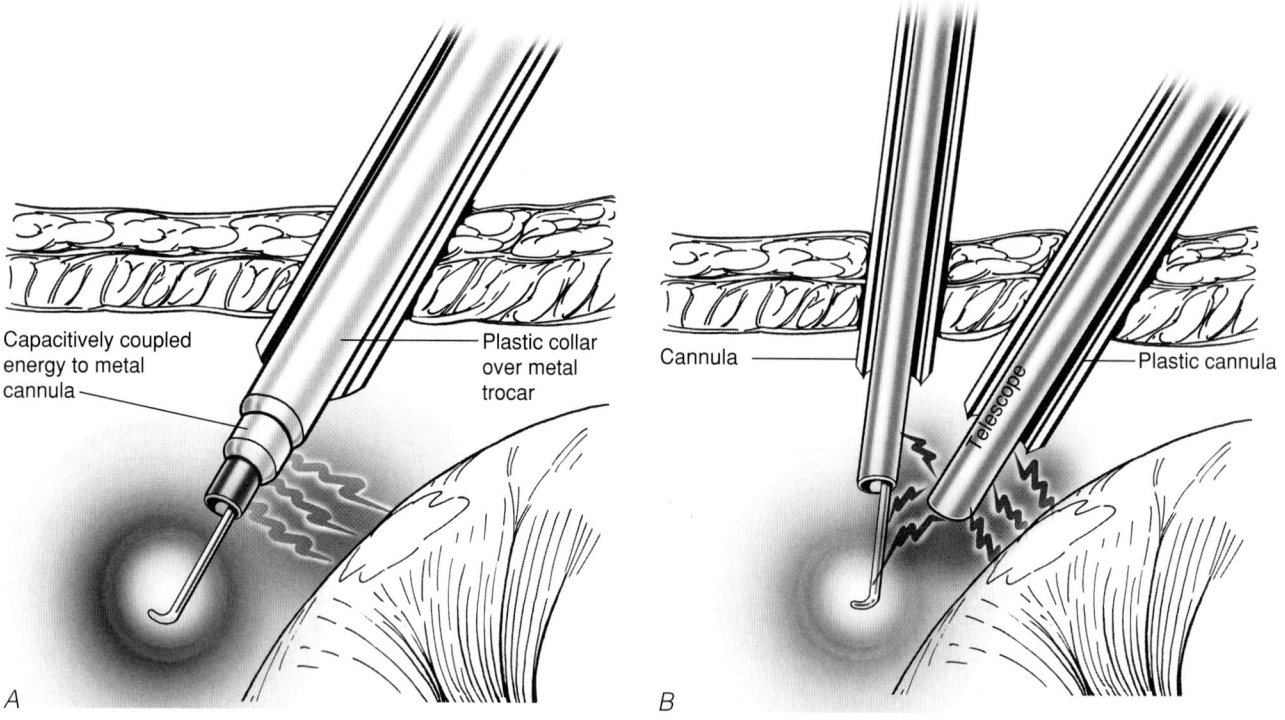

FIG. 13-13. *A.* Capacitive coupling occurs as a result of high current density bleeding from a port sleeve or laparoscope into adjacent bowel. *B.* Direct coupling occurs when current is transmitted directly from the electrode to a metal instrument or laparoscope, and then into adjacent tissue. *(Reproduced with permission from Odell.[52])*

A disadvantage is that the deep tissue heating may cause perforation of a hollow viscus.

When it is desirable to coagulate flat lesions in the cecum, a different laser should be chosen. The frequency-doubled Nd:YAG laser, also known as the KTP laser (potassium thionyl phosphate crystal

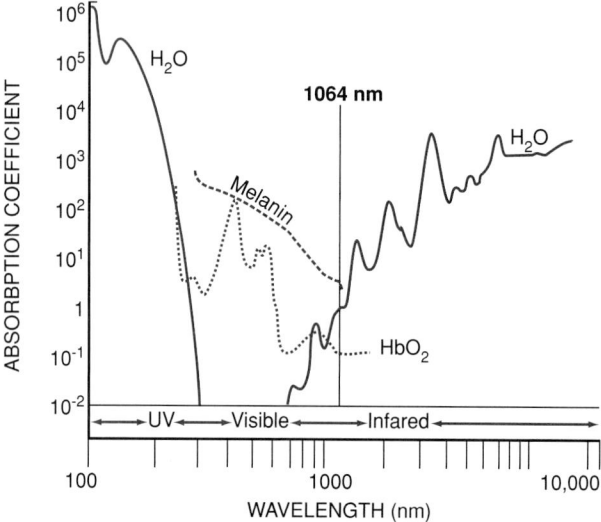

FIG. 13-14. This graph shows the absorption of light by various tissue compounds (water, melanin, and oxyhemoglobin) as a function of the wavelength of the light. The nadir of the oxyhemoglobin and melanin curves is close to 1064 nm, the wavelength of the neodymium yttrium-aluminum-garnet laser. *[Reproduced with permission from Hunter JG, Sackier JM (eds): Minimally-Invasive Surgery. New York: McGraw-Hill, 1993, p 28.]*

is used to double the Nd:YAG frequency), provides 532-nm light. This is in the green portion of the spectrum, and at this wavelength, selective absorption by red pigments in tissue (such as hemangiomas and arteriovenous malformations) is optimal. The depth of tissue heating is intermediate, between those of the CO_2 and the Nd:YAG lasers. Coagulation (without vaporization) of superficial vascular lesions can be obtained without intestinal perforation.[58]

In flexible gastrointestinal endoscopy, the CO_2 and Nd:YAG lasers have largely been replaced by heater probes and endoluminal stents. The heater probe is a metal ball that is heated to a temperature (60 to 100°C) that allows coagulation of bleeding lesions without perforation.

Photodynamic therapy (PDT) is a palliative treatment for obstructing cancers of the gastrointestinal tract.[59] Patients are given an intravenous dose of porfimer sodium, which is a photosensitizing agent that is taken up by malignant cells. Two days after administration, the drug is endoscopically activated using a laser. The activated porfimer sodium generates oxygen free radicals, which kills the tumor cells. The tumor is later endoscopically débrided. The use of this modality for definitive treatment of early cancers is in experimental phases and has yet to become established.

A unique application of laser technology provides extremely rapid discharge ($<10^{-6}$ s) of large amounts of energy ($>10^3$ volts). These high-energy lasers, of which the pulsed dye laser has seen the most clinical use, allow the conversion of light energy to mechanical disruptive energy in the form of a shock wave. Such energy can be delivered through a quartz fiber, and with rapid repetitive discharges, can provide sufficient shock-wave energy to fragment kidney stones and gallstones.[60] Shock waves also may be created with miniature electric spark-plug discharge systems known as electrohydraulic lithotriptors. These devices also are inserted through thin probes for

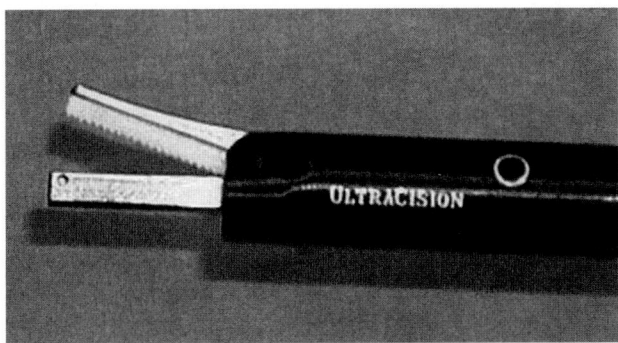

FIG. 13-15. The Harmonic Scalpel has revolutionized hemostasis and dissection in minimally-invasive surgery and has significantly facilitated the performance of advanced laparoscopic and thoracoscopic procedures. Ultrasonic energy is used to create a rapidly oscillating "working arm" which serves to heat intervening tissue with friction, which fuses the cell membranes together.

endoscopic application. Lasers have the advantage of pigment selectivity, but electrohydraulic lithotriptors are more popular because they are substantially less expensive and are more compact.

Methods of producing shock waves or heat with ultrasonic energy are also of interest. Extracorporeal shockwave lithotripsy creates focused shock waves that intensify as the focal point of the discharge is approached. When the focal point is within the body, large amounts of energy are capable of fragmenting stones. Slightly different configurations of this energy can be used to provide focused internal heating of tissues. Potential applications of this technology include the ability to noninvasively produce sufficient internal heating to destroy tissue without an incision.

A third means of using ultrasonic energy is to create rapidly-oscillating instruments that are capable of heating tissue with friction; this technology represents a major step forward in energy technology.[61] An example of its application is the laparoscopic coagulation shears (LCS) device (Harmonic Scalpel), which is capable of coagulating and dividing blood vessels by first occluding them and then providing sufficient heat to weld the blood vessel walls together and to divide the vessel (Fig. 13-15). This nonelectric method of coagulating and dividing tissue with a minimal amount of collateral damage has facilitated the performance of numerous endosurgical procedures.[62] It is especially useful in the control of bleeding from medium-sized vessels that are too big to manage with monopolar electrocautery and require bipolar desiccation followed by cutting.

Instrumentation

Hand instruments for MIS usually are duplications of conventional surgical instruments made longer, thinner, and smaller at the tip. It is important to remember that when grasping tissue with laparoscopic instruments, a greater force is applied over a smaller surface area, which increases the risk for perforation or injury.[63]

Certain conventional instruments such as scissors are easy to reproduce with a diameter of 3 to 5 mm and a length of 20 to 45 cm, but other instruments, such as forceps and clamps, cannot provide remote access. Different configurations of graspers were developed to replace the various configurations of surgical forceps and clamps. Standard hand instruments are 5 mm in diameter and 30 cm in length, but smaller and shorter hand instruments are now available for pediatric surgery, for microlaparoscopic surgery, and for arthroscopic procedures.[63] A unique laparoscopic hand instrument is the monopolar electrical hook. This device is usually configured with a suction and irrigation apparatus to eliminate smoke and blood from the operative field. The monopolar hook allows tenting of tissue

over a bare metal wire with subsequent coagulation and division of the tissue.

Robotic Assistance

The term "robot" defines a device that has been programmed to perform specific tasks in place of those usually performed by people. The equipment that has been introduced under the heading of robotic assistance would perhaps be more aptly termed *computer-assisted surgery*, as it is controlled entirely by the surgeon for the purpose of improving team performance. An example of computer-assisted surgery includes laparoscopic camera holders, which enable the surgeon to maneuver the laparoscope either with head movements or voice activation (Fig. 13-16). Randomized studies with such camera holders have demonstrated a reduction in operative time, steadier image, and a reduction in the number of required laparoscope cleanings.[64] This device has the advantage of eliminating the need for a human camera holder, which serves to free valuable operating room personnel for other duties.

Another form of computer assistance involves the use of voice-activated system controls for the camera, light source, insufflators, and telephone. Studies have demonstrated a reduction in the time required to perform these tasks when compared to human intervention.[65]

Room Setup and the Minimally-Invasive Suite

Nearly all MIS, whether using fluoroscopic, ultrasound, or optical imaging, incorporates a video monitor as a guide. Occasionally two images are necessary to adequately guide the operation, as in procedures such as endoscopic retrograde cholangiopancreatography (ERCP), laparoscopic common bile duct exploration, and laparoscopic ultrasonography. When two images are necessary, the images should be displayed on two adjacent video monitors or projected on a single screen with a picture-in-picture effect. The video monitor(s) should be set across the operating table from the surgeon. The patient should be interposed between the surgeon and the video monitor; ideally, the operative field also lies between the surgeon and the monitor. In pelviscopic surgery it is best to place the video monitor at the patient's feet, and in laparoscopic cholecystectomy, the monitor is placed at the 10 o'clock position (relative to the patient) while the surgeon stands on the patient's left at the 4 o'clock position. The insufflating and patient-monitoring equipment ideally also is placed across the table from the surgeon, so that the insufflating pressure and the patient's vital signs and end-tidal CO_2 tension can be monitored.

The development of the minimally-invasive surgical suite has been a tremendous contribution to the field of laparoscopy in that it has facilitated the performance of advanced procedures and techniques (Fig. 13-17). By having the core equipment (monitors, insufflators, and imaging equipment) located within mobile, ceiling-mounted consoles, the surgery team is able to accommodate and make small adjustments rapidly and continuously throughout the procedure. The specifically designed minimally-invasive surgical suite serves to decrease equipment and cable disorganization, ease the movements of operative personnel around the room, improve ergonomics, and facilitate the use of advanced imaging equipment such laparoscopic ultrasound.[66] While having a minimally-invasive surgical suite available is very useful, it is not essential to successfully carry out advanced laparoscopic procedures.

Patient Positioning

Patients usually are placed in the supine position for laparoscopic surgery. When the operative field is the gastroesophageal junction or

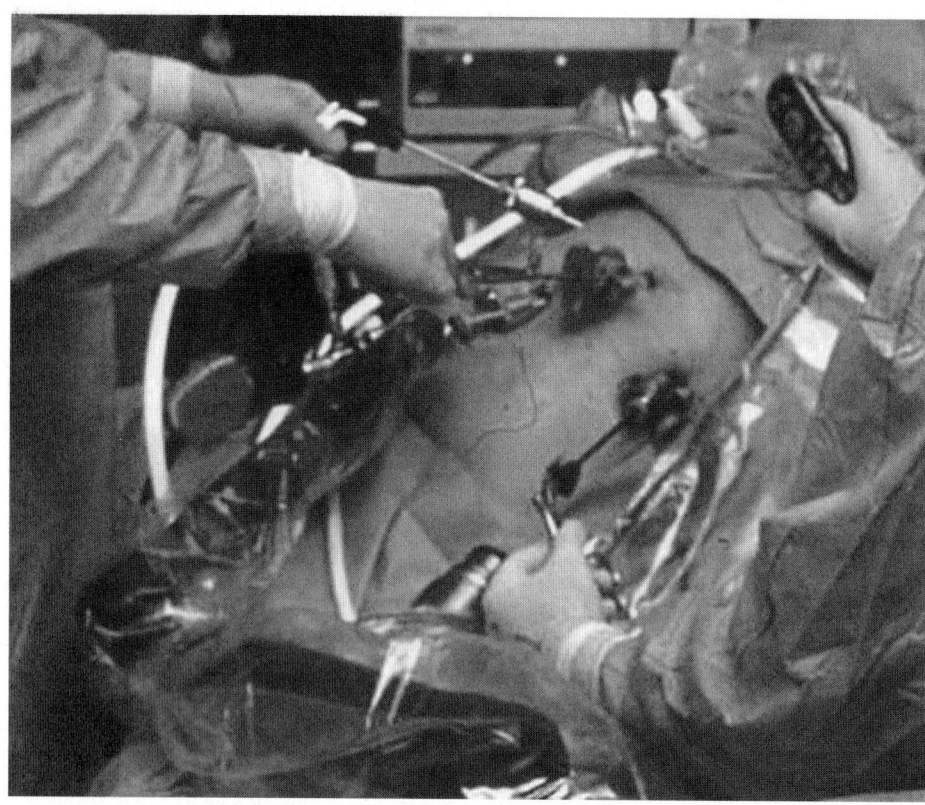

FIG. 13-16. The surgeon controlled computer-assisted camera holder obviates the need for an additional assistant. This device may reduce operative times and provide a steadier image.

the left lobe of the liver, it is easiest to operate from between the legs. The legs may be elevated in Allen stirrups or abducted on leg boards to achieve this position. When pelvic procedures are performed, it usually is necessary to place the legs in Allen stirrups to gain access to the perineum. A lateral decubitus position with the table flexed provides the best access to the retroperitoneum when performing nephrectomy or adrenalectomy. For laparoscopic splenectomy, a 45°-tilt of the patient provides excellent access to the lesser sac and the lateral peritoneal attachments to the spleen. For thoracoscopic surgery, the patient is placed in the lateral position with table flexion in order to open the intercostal spaces and the distance between the iliac crest and costal margin (Fig. 13-18).

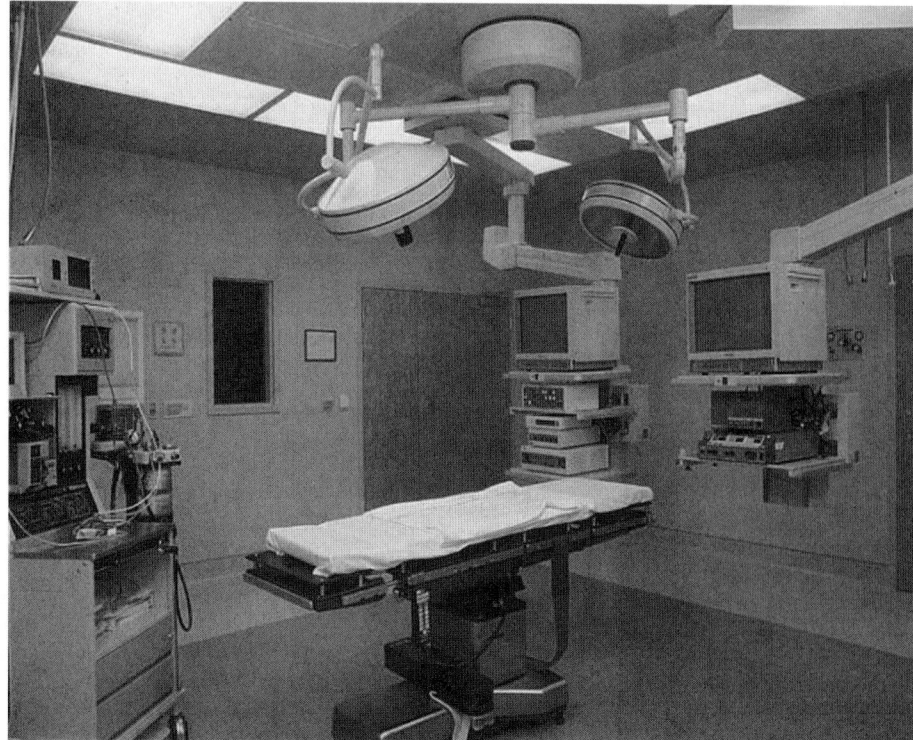

FIG. 13-17. An example of a typical minimally-invasive surgery suite. All core equipment is located on easily movable consoles. These operating rooms tend to be larger in size because of the need for multiple types of equipment.

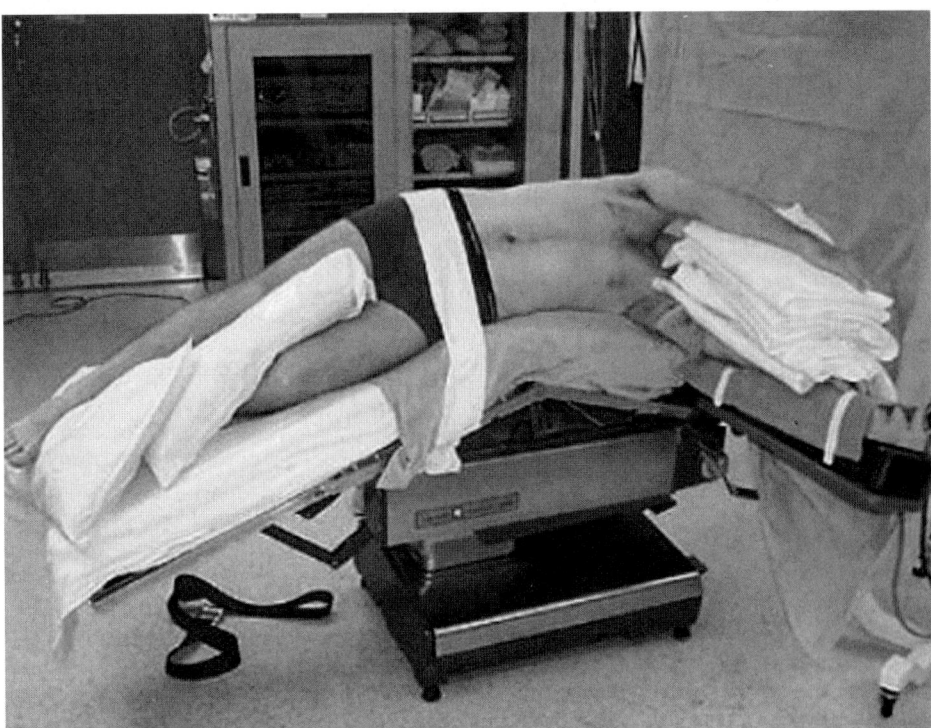

FIG. 13-18. Proper padding and protection of pressure points is an essential consideration in laparoscopic and thoracoscopic approaches. In preparation for thoracoscopy, this patient is placed in left lateral decubitus position with the table flexed, which serves to open the intercostal spaces and increase the distance between the iliac crest and inferior costal margin. Sequential compression devices should also be placed.

When the patient's knees are to be bent for extended periods or the patient is going to be placed in a reverse Trendelenburg position for more than a few minutes, deep venous thrombosis prophylaxis should be used. Sequential compression of the lower extremities during prolonged (more than 90 min) laparoscopic procedures increases venous return and provides inhibition of thromboplastin activation.

SPECIAL CONSIDERATIONS

Pediatric Considerations

The advantages of MIS in children may be more significant than in the adult population.[67] MIS in the adolescent is little different from that in the adult, and standard instrumentation and trocar positions can usually be used. However, laparoscopy in the infant and young child requires specialized instrumentation. The instruments are shorter (15 to 20 cm), and many are 3 mm in diameter rather than 5 mm.[68] Because the abdomen of the child is much smaller than that of the adult, a 5-mm telescope provides sufficient illumination for most operations. The development of 5-mm clippers and bipolar devices has obviated the need for 10-mm trocars in pediatric laparoscopy.[68] Because the abdominal wall is much thinner in infants, a pneumoperitoneum pressure of 8 mm Hg can provide adequate exposure. Deep venous thrombosis is rare in children, and prophylaxis against thrombosis is probably unnecessary.

Pregnancy

Concerns about the safety of laparoscopic cholecystectomy or appendectomy in the pregnant patient have been eliminated. The pH of the fetus follows the pH of the mother linearly, and therefore fetal acidosis may be prevented by avoiding a respiratory acidosis in the mother.[69] A second concern was that of increased intra-abdominal pressure, but it has been proved that midpregnancy uterine contractions provide a much greater pressure in utero than a pneumoperitoneum. Experience in well over 100 cases of laparoscopic cholecystectomy in pregnancy have been reported with uniformly good results.[70] The operation should be performed during the second trimester if possible. Protection of the fetus against intraoperative x-rays is imperative. Some believe it advisable to track fetal pulse rates with a transvaginal ultrasound probe. Access to the abdomen in the pregnant patient should take into consideration the height of the uterine fundus, which reaches the umbilicus at 20 weeks. In order not to damage the uterus or its blood supply, most surgeons feel that the open (Hasson) approach should be used in favor of direct puncture laparoscopy. The patient should be positioned slightly on the left side in order to avoid compression of the vena cava by the uterus. Because pregnancy poses a risk for thromboembolism, sequential compression devices are essential for all procedures.

Cancer

MIS techniques have been used for many decades to provide palliation for the patient with an obstructive cancer. Laser treatment, intracavitary radiation, stenting, and dilation are outpatient techniques that can be used to reestablish the continuity of an obstructed esophagus, bile duct, ureter, or airway. MIS techniques also have been used in the staging of cancer. Mediastinoscopy is still used occasionally before thoracotomy to assess the status of the mediastinal lymph nodes. Laparoscopy also is used to assess the liver in patients being evaluated for pancreatic, gastric, or hepatic resection. New technology and greater surgical skills allow for accurate minimally-invasive staging of cancer.[71] Occasionally it is appropriate to perform palliative measures (e.g., laparoscopic gastrojejunostomy to bypass a pancreatic cancer) at the time of diagnostic laparoscopy if diagnostic findings preclude attempts at curative resection.[72]

The most controversial role of MIS techniques is that of providing potentially curative surgery to the patient with cancer. It is possible to perform laparoscopy-assisted colectomy, gastrectomy, pancreatectomy, and hepatectomy in patients with intra-abdominal malignant disease, as well as thoracoscopic esophagectomy and pneumonectomy in patients with intrathoracic malignant disease. There are not yet enough data to indicate whether minimally-invasive surgical techniques provide survival rates or disease-free intervals comparable to those of conventional surgical techniques. It has been proven that in laparoscopy-assisted colectomy and gastrectomy a number of lymph nodes equal to that of an open procedure can be removed without any compromise of resection margins. A second concern centers on excessive tumor manipulation and the possibility that cancer cells would be shed during the dissection. Alarming reports of trocar site implantation with viable cancer cells have appeared in the literature.

Considerations in the Elderly and Infirm

Laparoscopic cholecystectomy has made possible the removal of a symptomatic gallbladder in many patients previously thought to be too elderly or too ill to undergo a laparotomy. Older patients are more likely to require conversion to celiotomy because of disease chronicity.[73]

Operations on these patients require close monitoring of anesthesia. The intraoperative management of these patients may be more difficult with laparoscopic access than with open access. The advantage of MIS lies in what happens after the operation. Much of the morbidity of surgery in the elderly is a result of impaired mobility.[73] In addition, pulmonary complications, urinary tract sepsis, deep venous thrombosis, pulmonary embolism, congestive heart failure, and myocardial infarction often are the result of improper fluid management and decreased mobility. By allowing rapid and early mobilization, laparoscopic surgery has made possible the safe performance of procedures in the elderly and infirm.

Cirrhosis and Portal Hypertension

Patients with hepatic insufficiency pose a significant challenge for any type of surgical intervention.[74] The ultimate surgical outcome in this population relates directly to the degree of underlying hepatic dysfunction.[75] Often, this group of patients has minimal reserve, and the stress of an operation will trigger complete hepatic failure or hepatorenal syndrome. These patients are at risk for major hemorrhage at all levels, including trocar insertion, operative dissection in a field of dilated veins, and secondary to an underlying coagulopathy.[75] Additionally, ascitic leak from a port site may occur, leading to bacterial peritonitis. Therefore a watertight port site closure should be carried out in all patients.

It is essential that the surgeon be aware of the Child class of severity of cirrhosis of the patient prior to intervening so that appropriate preoperative optimization can be completed. For example, if a patient has an eroding umbilical hernia and ascites, a preoperative paracentesis or transjugular intrahepatic portosystemic shunt (TIPS) procedure in conjunction with aggressive diuresis may be considered. Because these patients commonly are intravascularly depleted, insufflation pressures should be reduced in order to prevent a decrease in cardiac output and minimal amounts of low-salt intravenous fluids should be given.

Economics of Minimally-Invasive Surgery

Minimally-invasive surgical procedures reduce the costs of surgery most when length of hospital stay can be shortened. For example, shorter hospital stays can be demonstrated in laparoscopic cholecystectomy, fundoplication, splenectomy, and adrenalectomy.

Procedures such as inguinal herniorrhaphy that are already performed as outpatient procedures are less likely to provide cost advantage. Procedures that still require a 4- to 7-day hospitalization, such as laparoscopy-assisted colectomy, are even less likely to deliver a lower bottom line than their open-surgery counterparts. Nonetheless, with responsible use of disposable instrumentation and a commitment to the most effective use of the inpatient setting, most laparoscopic procedures can be made less expensive than their conventional equivalents.

ROBOTIC SURGERY

With the development of advanced laparoscopic procedures, the limitations of minimally-invasive surgical techniques and instrumentation have become accentuated. For example, the mobility and positioning of a laparoscopic instrument is limited by the placement of the port site on the abdominal wall. This may prevent the surgeon from obtaining the desired instrument angle and position to perform a complex maneuver. In addition, the fine motor movements required to perform complex minimally-invasive surgical procedures may be difficult to perform with standard laparoscopic instruments and imaging. Computer-enhanced ("robotic") surgery was developed with the intent of circumventing the limitations of laparoscopy and thoracoscopy, and to make minimally-invasive surgical techniques accessible to those without a laparoscopic background.[76] In addition, remote site surgery (telesurgery), in which the surgeon is a great distance from the patient (e.g., combat or space), has potential future applications. This was recently exemplified when a team of surgeons located in New York performed a cholecystectomy on a patient located in France.[77]

These devices offer a three-dimensional view with hand- and wrist-controlled instruments that possess multiple degrees of freedom, thereby facilitating surgery with a one-to-one movement ratio that mimics open surgery (Fig. 13-19). Additionally, computer-enhanced surgery also offers tremor control. The surgeon is physically separated from the operating table and the working arms of the device are placed over the patient (Fig. 13-20). An assistant remains at the bedside and changes the instruments as needed.

Because this equipment is very costly, a primary limitation to its uniform acceptance has been attempting to achieve increased value in the form of improved clinical outcomes. There have been two randomized controlled trials that compared robotic and conventional laparoscopic approaches to Nissen fundoplication.[78,79] While there was a reduction in operative time, there was no difference in ultimate outcome. Similar results have been achieved for laparoscopic cholecystectomy.[80] Finally, it may be too early in its development (due to bulky equipment, difficulty in accessing patients, and limited instrumentation) for widespread adoption of this technology.

ENDOLUMINAL SURGERY

The fields of vascular surgery, interventional radiology, neuroradiology, gastroenterology, general surgery, pulmonology, and urology all encounter clinical scenarios that require the urgent restoration of luminal patency of a "biologic cylinder."[81] Based on this need, fundamental techniques have been pioneered that are applicable to all specialties and virtually every organ system. As a result, all minimally-invasive surgical procedures, from coronary artery angioplasty to palliation of pancreatic malignancy, involve the use of an endoluminal balloon, dilator, prostheses, biopsy forceps, chemical agent, or thermal technique[81] (Table 13-2). Endoluminal balloon

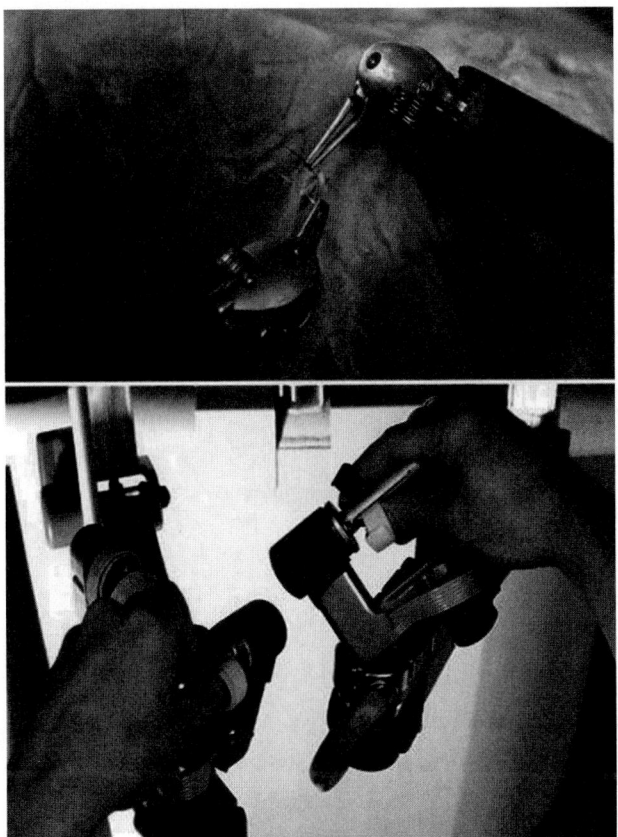

FIG. 13-19. Robotic instruments and hand controls. The surgeon is in a sitting position and the arms and wrists are in an ergonomic and relaxed position.

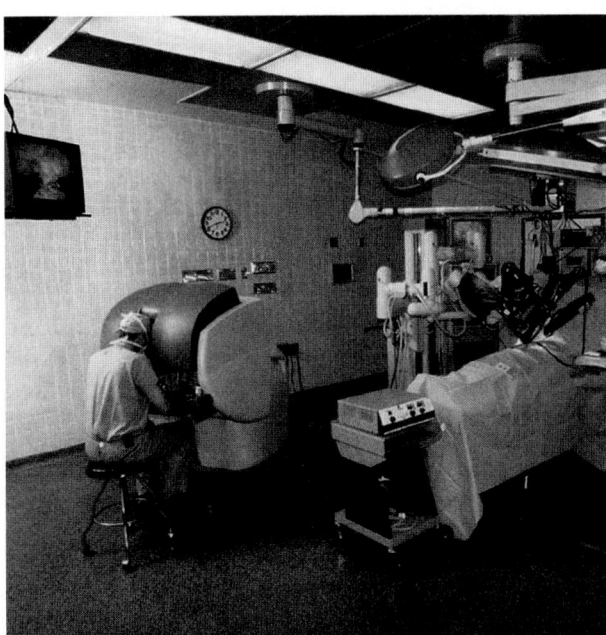

FIG. 13-20. Room set-up and position of surgeon and assistant for robotic surgery.

dilators may be inserted through an endoscope, or they may be fluoroscopically guided. Balloon dilators all have low compliance—that is, the balloons do not stretch as the pressure within the balloon is increased. The high pressures achievable in the balloon create radial expansion of the narrowed vessel or orifice, usually disrupting the atherosclerotic plaque, the fibrotic stricture, or the muscular band (e.g., esophageal achalasia).[82]

Once the dilation has been attained, it is frequently beneficial to hold the lumen open with a stent.[83] Stenting is particularly valuable in treating malignant lesions and in endovascular procedures (Fig. 13-21). Stenting usually is not applicable for long-term management of benign gastrointestinal strictures except in patients with limited life expectancy[83,84,85] (Fig. 13-22A and B).

A variety of stents are available that are divided into two basic categories, plastic stents and expandable metal stents[84] (Fig. 13-23). Plastic stents came first and are used widely as endoprostheses for temporary bypass of obstructions in the biliary or urinary systems. Metal stents generally are delivered over a balloon and expanded with the balloon to the desired size. These metal stents usually are made of titanium or nitinol. Although great progress has been made with expandable metal stents, two problems remain: propensity for tissue ingrowth through the interstices of the stent and stent migration. Ingrowth may be an advantage in preventing stent migration, but such tissue ingrowth may occlude the lumen and cause obstruction anew. This is a particular problem when stents are used for palliation of gastrointestinal malignant growth, and may be a problem for the long-term use of stents in vascular disease. Filling the interstices

with Silastic or other materials may prevent tumor ingrowth, but also makes stent migration more likely. In an effort to minimize stent migration, stents have been incorporated with hooks and barbs.

Most recently, anticoagulant-eluding coronary artery stents have been placed in specialized centers.[86] This exciting technological advance may dramatically increase the long-term patency rates of stents placed in patients with coronary artery disease and peripheral atherosclerosis.

Intraluminal Surgery

The successful application of minimally-invasive surgical techniques to the lumen of the gastrointestinal tract has hinged upon the development of a port that maintains access to the gastrointestinal lumen while preventing intraperitoneal leakage of intestinal contents and facilitating adequate insufflation[87] (Fig. 13-24).

Table 13-2
Modalities and Techniques of Restoring Luminal Patency

Modality	Technique
Core out	Photodynamic Therapy
	Laser
	Coagulation
	Endoscopic biopsy forceps
	Chemical
	Ultrasound
Fracture	Ultrasound
	Endoscopic biopsy
	Balloon
Dilate	Balloon
	Bougie
	Angioplasty
	Endoscope
Bypass	Transvenous intrahepatic portosystemic shunt
	Surgical (synthetic or autologous conduit)
Stent	Self-expanding metal stent
	Plastic stent

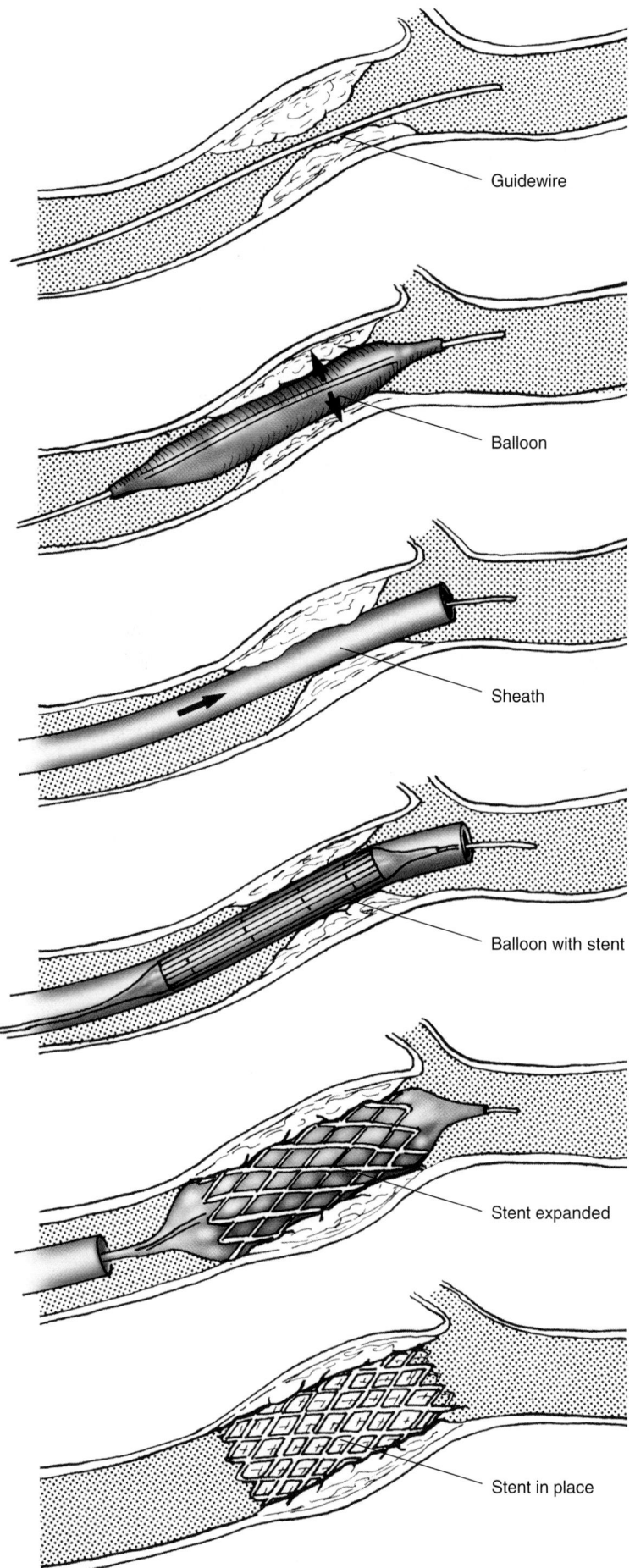

Guidewire

Balloon

Sheath

Balloon with stent

Stent expanded

Stent in place

FIG. 13-21. The deployment of a metal stent across an isolated vessel stenosis is illustrated. [*Reproduced with permission from Hunter JG, Sackier JM (eds): Minimally-Invasive Surgery. New York: McGraw-Hill, 1993, p 325.*]

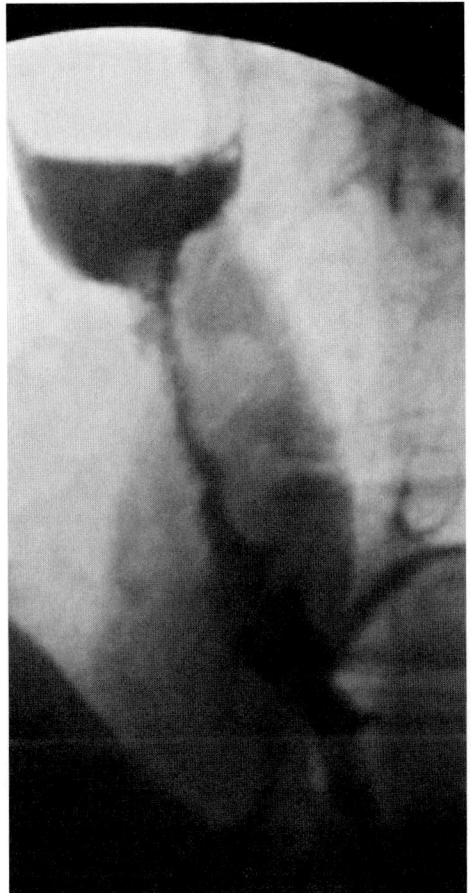 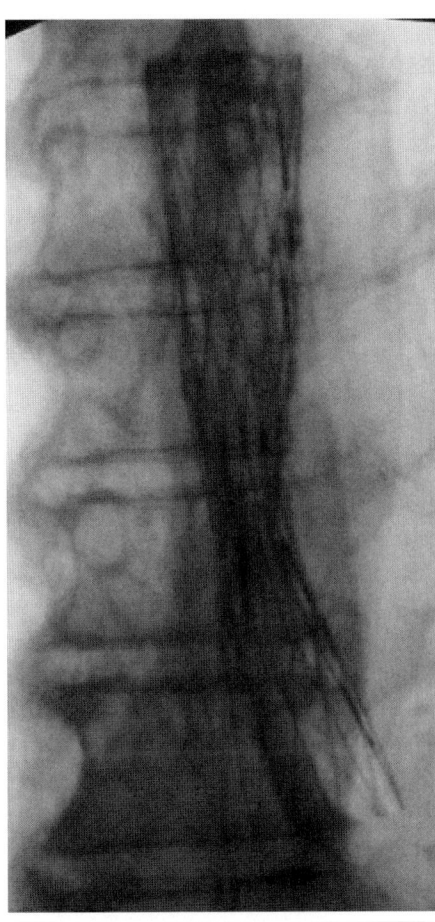

FIG. 13-22. This is an esophagram in a patient with severe dysphagia secondary to advanced esophageal cancer (A) before and (B) after placement of a covered self-expanding metal stent.

A   *B*

Procedures that are gaining acceptance include resection of benign and early malignant gastric tumors, transanal resection of polyps (transanal endoscopic microsurgery), pancreatic cyst gastrostomy, and biliary sphincterotomy.

The location of the lesion within the gastrointestinal tract is of utmost importance when considering an intraluminal approach. For example, a leiomyoma that is located on the anterior gastric wall may not be amenable to intraluminal resection because the working ports must also penetrate the anterior surface of the stomach. Preoperative endoscopy and endoscopic ultrasound should be routinely employed in order to determine resectability.[87]

EDUCATION AND SKILL ACQUISITION

Surgeons in Training and Skill Acquisition

Surgeons in training acquire their skills in minimally-invasive techniques through a series of operative experiences of graded complexity. This training occurs on patients. With the recent constraints placed on resident work hours, providing adequate minimally-invasive training to future surgeons within a relatively brief time frame has become of paramount importance.

Laparoscopic surgery demands a unique set of skills that require the surgeon to function at the limit of his or her psychomotor abilities. The introduction of virtual reality training devices presents a unique opportunity to improve and enhance experiential learning in endoscopy and laparoscopy for all surgeons. This technology has the advantage of enabling objective measurement of psychomotor skills, which can be used to determine progress in skill acquisition, and ultimately technical competency.[88,89] This technology will most likely be used to create benchmarks for the performance of future minimally-invasive techniques. In addition, virtual reality training enables the surgeon to build an experience base prior to venturing into the operating room.[90] Be that as it may, no studies have demonstrated that simulator training improves overall patient outcome.

Some hospitals and training programs have established virtual reality and laparoscopic training centers that are accessible at all hours for surgeons' use.

Telementoring

In response to the Institute of Medicine's call for the development of unique technologic solutions to deliver health care to rural and underserved areas, surgeons are beginning to explore the feasibility of telementoring. Teleconsultation or telementoring is two-way audio and visual communication between two geographically separated providers. This communication can take place in the office setting, or directly in the operating room when complex scenarios are encountered. Although local communication channels may limit its performance in rural areas, the technology is available and currently being employed (Fig. 13-25).

INNOVATION AND INTRODUCTION OF NEW PROCEDURES

The revolution in minimally-invasive general surgery, which occurred in 1990, created ethical challenges for the profession. The

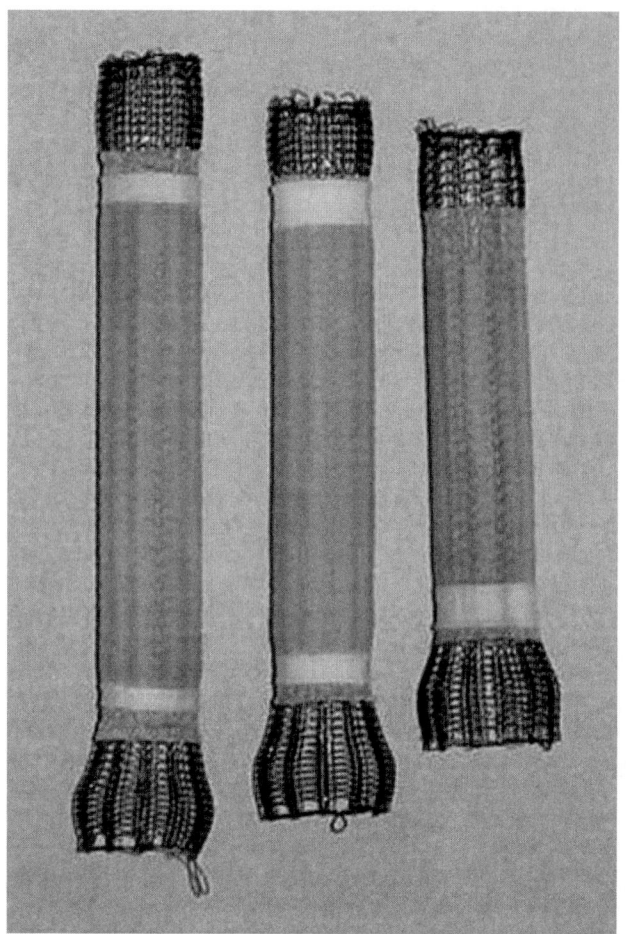

FIG. 13-23. Covered self-expanding metal stents. These devices can be placed fluoroscopically or endoscopically.

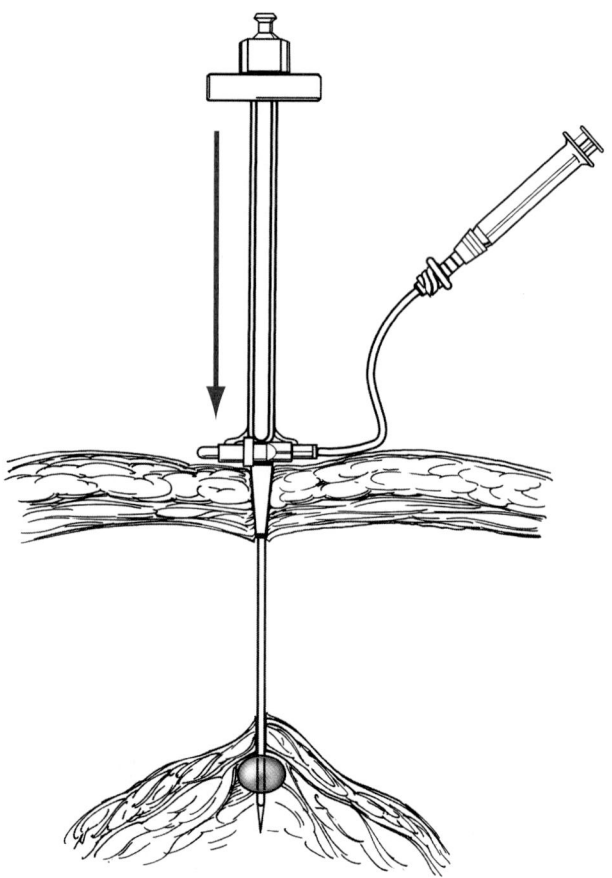

FIG. 13-24. An illustration of a radially expanding trocar used for intraluminal surgery. The stomach is insufflated using a nasogastric tube, and the anterior gastric wall is pierced with the trocar under laparoscopic guidance. A balloon is inflated and used to draw the stomach up to the anterior abdominal wall. [*Reproduced with permission from Eubanks WS, Swanstrom LL, Soper NJ (eds): Mastery of Endoscopic and Laparoscopic Surgery. Philadelphia: Lippincott Williams & Wilkins, 1999, p 215.*]

problem was this: If competence is gained from experience, how was the surgeon to climb the competence curve (otherwise known as the learning curve) without injuring patients? If it was indeed impossible to achieve competence without making mistakes along the way, how should one effectively communicate this to patients such that they understand the weight of their decisions? Even more fundamentally important is determining the path that should be followed before one recruits the first patient for a new procedure.

Although procedure development is fundamentally different than drug development (i.e., there is great individual variation in the performance of procedures, but no difference between one tablet and the next), adherence to a process similar to that used to develop a new drug is a reasonable path for a surgical innovator. At the outset the surgeon must identify the problem that is not solved with current surgical procedures. For example, while the removal of a gallbladder through a Kocher incision is certainly effective, it creates a great deal of disability, pain, and scarification. As a result of those issues, many patients with very symptomatic biliary colic delayed operation until life-threatening complications occurred. Clearly there was a need for developing a less invasive approach (Fig. 13-26).

Once the opportunity has been established, the next step involves a search through other disciplines for technologies and techniques that might be applied. Again, this is analogous to the drug industry, where secondary drug indications have often turned out to be more therapeutically important than the primary indication for drug

development. The third step is in vivo studies in the most appropriate animal model. Certainly these types of studies are controversial because of the resistance to animal experimentation, and yet without such studies many humans would be injured or killed during the developmental phase of medical drugs, devices, and techniques. These steps are often called the preclinical phase of procedure development.

The decision as to when such procedures are ready to come out of the lab is a difficult one. Put simply, the procedure should be reproducible, provide the desired effect, and not have serious side effects. Once these three criteria are reached, the time for human application has arrived. Before the surgeon discusses the new procedure with his patient, it is important to achieve full institutional support. Clearly, involvement of the medical board, the chief of the medical staff, and the institutional review board are essential before commencing on a new procedure. These bodies are responsible for the use of safe, high quality medical practices within their institution, and they will demand that great caution and all possible safeguards are in place before proceeding.

The dialogue with the patient who is to be first must be thorough, brutally honest, and well documented. The psychology that allows a patient to decide to be first is quite interesting, and may under certain circumstances require psychiatric evaluation. Certainly

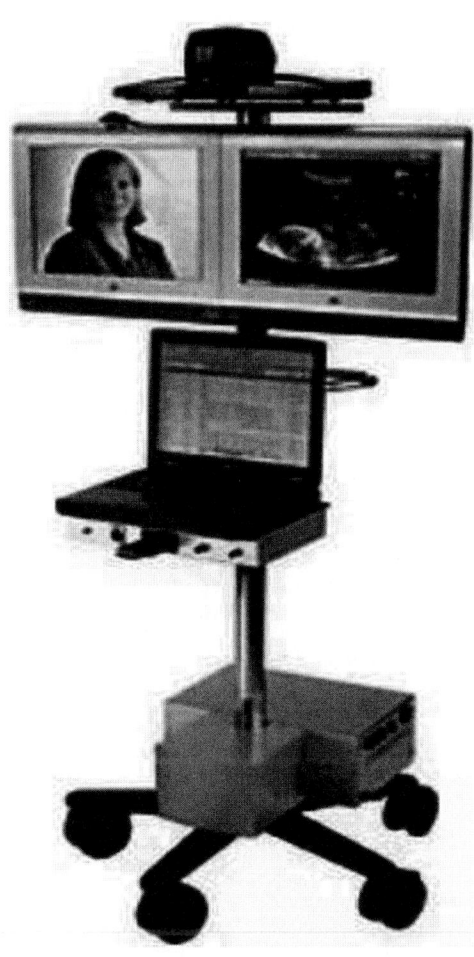

FIG. 13-25. Teleconsultation and telementoring are carried out between two providers who are geographically separated. The console has a video camera, microphone, and flat screen display which can be positioned at the operating room table or in the clinic.

hand, when the benefits of the new approach are small and the risks are largely unknown, a more complete psychological profile may be necessary before proceeding.

For new surgical procedures, it is generally wise to assemble the best possible operative team, including a surgeon experienced with the old technique, and assistants who have participated in the earlier animal work. This initial team of experienced physicians and nurses should remain together until full competence with the procedure is attained. This may take 10 procedures, or it may take 50 procedures. The team will know that it has achieved competence when the majority of procedures take the same length of time, and the team is relaxed and sure of the flow of the operation. This will complete phase I of the procedure development.

In phase II, the efficacy of the procedure is tested in a nonrandomized fashion. Ideally, the outcome of new techniques must be as good or better than the procedure that is being replaced. This phase should occur at several medical centers to prove that good outcomes are achievable outside of the pioneering institution. These same requirements may be applied to the introduction of new technology into the operating room. The value equation requires that the additional measurable procedure quality exceeds the additional measurable cost to the patient or health care system. In phase III, a randomized trial pits the new procedure against the old.

Once the competence curve has been climbed, it is appropriate for the team to engage in the education of others. During the ascension of the competence curve, other learners in the institution (i.e., surgical residents) may not have the opportunity to participate in the first case series. While this may be difficult for them to swallow, the best interest of the patient must be put before the education of the resident.

The second stage of learning occurs when the new procedure has proven its value and a handful of experts exist, but the majority of surgeons have not been trained to perform the new procedure. In this setting, it is relatively unethical for surgeons to forge ahead with a new procedure in humans as if they had spent the same amount of time in intensive study that the first team did. The fact that one or several surgical teams were able to perform an operation does not ensure that all others with the same medical degrees can perform the operation with equal skill. It behooves the learners to contact the experts and request their assistance to ensure an optimal outcome at the new center. While it is important that the learners contact

if a dying cancer patient has a chance with a new drug, this makes sense. Similarly, if the standard surgical procedure has a high attendant morbidity and the new procedure offers a substantially better outcome, the decision to be first is understandable. On the other

FIG. 13-26. The progress of general surgery can be reflected by a series of performance curves. General anesthesia and sterile technique allowed the development of maximally invasive open surgery over the last 125 years. Video optics allowed the development of minimally invasive surgery over the last 25 years. Non invasive (seamless) surgery will result when a yet undiscovered transformational event allows surgery to occur without an incision, and perhaps without anesthesia.

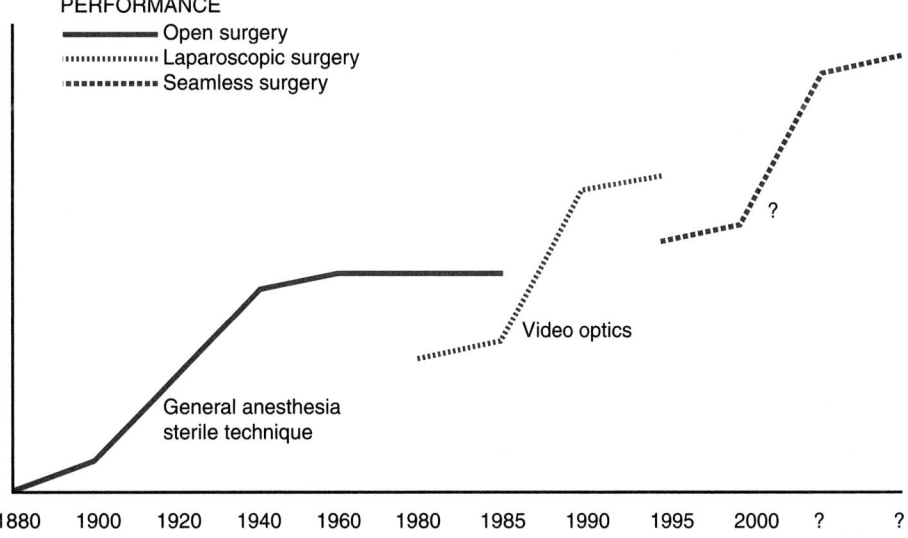

the experts, it is equally important that the experts be willing to share their experience with their fellow professionals. As well, the experts should provide feedback to the learners as to whether they feel the learners are equipped to forge ahead on their own. If not, further observation and assistance from the experts are required. While this approach may sound obvious, it is fraught with difficulties. In many situations ego, competitiveness, and monetary concerns have short-circuited this process and led to poor patient outcomes. To a large extent, MIS has recovered from the black eye that it received early in development, when inadequately trained surgeons caused an excessive number of significant complications.

If innovative procedures and technologies are to be developed and applied without the mistakes of the past, surgeons must be honest when they answer these questions: Is this procedure safe? Would I consider undergoing this procedure if I developed a surgical indication? Is the procedure as good or better than the procedure it is replacing? Do I have the skills to apply this procedure safely and with equivalent results to the more experienced surgeon? If the answer to any of these questions is "no," or "I don't know," there is a professional obligation to seek another procedure or outside assistance before subjecting a patient to the new procedure.

References

1. Hopkins HH: Optical principles of the endoscope, in Berci G (ed): *Endoscopy.* New York: Appleton-Century-Crofts, 1976, p 3.
2. Katzir A: Optical fibers in medicine. *Sci Am* 260:120, 1989.
3. Hisschowitz BI: A personal history of the fiberscope. *Gastroenterology* 76:864, 1979.
4. Veritas TF: Coelioscopy: A synthesis of Georg Kelling's work with insufflation, endoscopy, and lufttamponade, in Litynski GS (ed): *Highlights in the History of Laparoscopy.* Frankfurt/Main: Barbara Bernert Verlag, 1996, p 3.
5. Wood BJ, Ramkaransingh JR, Fogo T, et al: Percutaneous tumor ablation with radiofrequency. *Cancer* 94:443, 2002.
6. Kenyon TA, Lenker MP, Bax TW, Swanstrom LL: Cost and benefit of the trained laparoscopic team. A comparative study of a designated nursing team vs a nontrained team. *Surg Endosc* 11:812, 1997.
7. Smith RS, Fry WR, et al: Gasless laparoscopy and conventional instruments: The next phase of minimally-invasive surgery. *Arch Surg* 128:1102, 1993.
8. Litynski GS: Highlights in the history of laparoscopy. *Frankfurt am main*, Germany: Barbara Bernet, Verlag, 1996, p 78.
9. Hunter JG, Staheli J, et al: Nitrous oxide pneumoperitoneum revisited: Is there a risk of combustion? *Surg Endosc* 9:501, 1995.
10. Tsereteli Z, Terry ML, et al: Prospective randomized clinical trial comparing nitrous oxide and carbon dioxide pneumoperitoneum for laparoscopic surgery. *J Am Coll Surg* 195:173, 2002.
11. Callery MP, Soper NJ: Physiology of the pneumoperitoneum, in Hunter (ed): *Baillière's Clinical Gastroenterology: Laparoscopic Surgery.* London/Philadelphia: Baillière Tindall, 1993, p 757.
12. Ho HS, Gunther RA, et al: Intraperitoneal carbon dioxide insufflation and cardiopulmonary functions. *Arch Surg* 127:928, 1992.
13. Wittgen CM, Andrus CH, et al: Analysis of the hemodynamic and ventilatory effects of laparoscopic cholecystectomy. *Arch Surg* 126:997, 1991.
14. Cullen DJ, Eger EI: Cardiovascular effects of carbon dioxide in man. *Anesthesiol* 41:345, 1974.
15. Cunningham AJ, Turner J, et al: Transoesophageal echocardiographic assessment of haemodynamic function during laparoscopic cholecystectomy. *Br J Anaesth* 70:621, 1993.
16. Harris MNE, Plantevin OM, Crowther A, et al: Cardiac arrhythmias during anaesthesia for laparoscopy. *Br J Anaesth* 56:1213, 1984.
17. Borten M, Friedman EA: Choice of anaesthesia, in *Laparoscopic Complications: Prevention and Management.* Toronto: BC Decker, 1986, p 173.
18. Jorgenson JO, Hanel K, Lalak NJ, et al: Thromboembolic complications of laparoscopic cholecystectomy (Letter). *Br Med J* 306:518, 1993.
19. Ho HS, Wolfe BM: The physiology and immunology of endosurgery, in Toouli JG, Gossot D, Hunter JG (eds): *Endosurgery.* New York/London: Churchill-Livingstone, 1996, p 163.
20. Sackier JM, Nibhanupudy B: The pneumoperitoneum-physiology and complications, in Toouli JG, Gossot D, Hunter JG (eds): *Endosurgery.* New York/London: Churchill-Livingstone, 1996, p 155.
21. Kashtan J, Green JF, Parsons EQ, et al: Hemodynamic effects of increased abdominal pressure. *J Surg Res* 30:249, 1981.
22. McDougall EM, Monk TG, Wolf JS Jr., et al: The effect of prolonged pneumoperitoneum on renal function in an animal model. *J Am Coll Surg* 182:317, 1996.
23. Lindberg F, Bergqvist D, Bjorck M, Rasmussen I: Renal hemodynamics during carbon dioxide pneumoperitoneum: An experimental study in pigs. *Surg Endosc* 17:480, 2003.
24. Hazebroek EJ, de Vos tot Nederveen Cappel R, Gommers D, et al: Antidiuretic hormone release during laparoscopic donor nephrectomy. *Arch Surg* 137:600, 2002; discussion 605.
25. Ostman PL, Pantle-Fisher FH, Fanre EA, et al: Circulatory collapse during laparoscopy. *J Clin Anesth* 2:129, 1990.
26. Alijani A, Cuschieri A: Abdominal wall lift systems in laparoscopic surgery: Gasless and low-pressure systems. *Semin Laparosc Surg* 8:53, 2001.
27. Ozawa A, Konishi F, Nagai H, et al: Cytokine and hormonal responses in laparoscopic-assisted colectomy and conventional open colectomy. *Surg Today* 30:107, 2000.
28. Burpee SE, Kurian M, Murakame Y, et al: The metabolic and immune response to laparoscopic versus open liver resection. *Surg Endosc* 16:899, 2002.
29. Gossot D: Access modalities for thoracoscopic surgery, in Toouli JG, Gossot D, Hunter JG (eds): *Endosurgery.* New York/London: Churchill-Livingstone, 1996, p 743.
30. Memon MA, Cooper NJ, Memon B, et al: Meta-analysis of randomized clinical trials comparing open and laparoscopic inguinal hernia repair. *Br J Surg* 90:1479, 2003.
31. Himpens J: Laparoscopic preperitoneal approach to the inguinal hernia, in Toouli JG, Gossot D, Hunter JG (eds): *Endosurgery.* New York/London: Churchill-Livingstone, 1996, p 949.
32. Horvath KD, Kao LS, Wherry KL, et al: A technique for laparoscopic-assisted percutaneous drainage of infected pancreatic necrosis and pancreatic abscess. *Surg Endosc* 15:1221, 2001.
33. Eaves FF: Basics of endoscopic plastic surgery, in Bostwick J, Eaves FF, Nahai F (eds): *Endoscopic Plastic Surgery.* St Louis: Quality Medical Publishing, 1995, p 59.
34. Byron JW, Markenson G, et al: A randomised comparison of Veress needle and direct insertion for laparoscopy. *Surg Gynecol Obstet* 177:259, 1993.
35. Fletcher DR: Laparoscopic access, in Toouli JG, Gossot D, Hunter JG (eds): *Endosurgery.* New York/London: Churchill-Livingstone, 1996, p 189.
36. Hanney RM, Alle KM, Cregan PC: Major vascular injury and laparoscopy. *Aust N Z J Surg* 65:533, 1995.
37. Catarci M, Carlini M, Gentileschi P, Santoro E: Major and minor injuries during the creation of pneumoperitoneum. A multicenter study on 12,919 cases. *Surg Endosc* 15:566, 2001.
38. Siperstein AE, Berber E, Engle KL, et al: Laparoscopic posterior adrenalectomy: Technical considerations. *Arch Surg* 135:967, 2000.
39. Vasilev SA, McGonigle KF: Extraperitoneal laparoscopic para-aortic lymph node dissection. *Gynecol Oncol* 61:315, 1996.
40. Schurr UP, Lachat ML, Reuthebuch O, et al: Endoscopic saphenous vein harvesting for CABG—a randomized prospective trial. *Thorac Cardiovasc Surg* 50:160, 2002.
41. Lumsden AB, Eaves FF: Vein harvest, in Bostwick J, Eaves FF, Nahai F (eds): *Endoscopic Plastic Surgery.* St. Louis: Quality Medical Publishing, 1995, p 535.
42. Targarona EM, Gracia E, Rodriguez M, et al: Hand-assisted laparoscopic surgery. *Arch Surg* 138:138, 1003.

43. Berquer R, Smith WD, Davis S: An ergonomic study of the optimum operating table height for laparoscopic surgery. *Surg Endosc* 16:416, 2002.

44. Berguer R, Smith WD, Chung YH: Performing laparoscopic surgery is significantly more stressful for the surgeon than open surgery. *Surg Endosc* 15:1204, 2001.

45. Emam TA, Hanna G, Cuschieri A: Ergonomic principles of task alignment, visual display, and direction of execution of laparoscopic bowel suturing. *Surg Endosc* 16:267, 2002.

46. Prescher T: Video imaging, in Toouli JG, Gossot D, Hunter JG (eds): *Endosurgery*. New York/London: Churchill-Livingstone, 1996, p 41.

47. Margulies DR, Shabot MM: Fiberoptic imaging and measurement, in Hunter JG, Sackier JM (eds): *Minimally-Invasive Surgery*. New York: McGraw-Hill, 1993, p 7.

48. Wenzl R, Lehner R, Holzer A, et al: Improved laparoscopic operating techniques using a digital enhancement video system. *J Am Assoc Gynecol Laparosc* 5:175, 1998.

49. Berci G, Paz-Partlow M: Videoendoscopic technology, in Toouli JG, Gossot D, Hunter JG (eds): *Endosurgery*. New York/London: Churchill-Livingstone, 1996, p 33.

50. Levy ML, Day JD, Albuquerque F, et al: Heads-up intraoperative endoscopic imaging: A prospective evaluation of techniques and limitations. *Neurosurgery* 40:526, 1997.

51. Taffinder N, Smith SG, Huber J, et al: The effect of a second-generation 3D endoscope on the laparoscopic precision of novices and experienced surgeons. *Surg Endosc* 13:1087, 1999.

52. Odell RC: Laparoscopic electrosurgery, in Hunter JG, Sackier JM (eds): *Minimally-Invasive Surgery*. New York: McGraw-Hill, 1993, p 33.

53. Voyels CR, et al: Education and engineering solutions for potential problems with laparoscopic monopolar electrosurgery. *Am J Surg* 164:57, 1992.

54. Blanc B, d'Ercole C, Gaiato ML, Boubli L: Cause and prevention of electrosurgical injuries in laparoscopy. *J Am Coll Surg* 179:161, 1994.

55. Tucker RD: Principles of electrosurgery, in Sivak MV (ed): *Gastroenterologic Endoscopy*, 2nd ed. Philadelphia: WB Saunders, 2000, p 125.

56. Barlow DE: Endoscopic application of electrosurgery: A review of basic principles. *Gastrointest Endosc* 28:73, 1982.

57. Trus TL, Hunter JG: Principles of laser physics and tissue interaction, in Toouli JG, Gossot D, Hunter JG (eds): *Endosurgery*. New York/London: Churchill-Livingstone, 1996, p 103.

58. Bass LS, Oz MC, Trokel SL, et al: Alternative lasers for endoscopic surgery: Comparison of pulsed thulium-holmium-chromium:YAG with continuous-wave neodymium:YAG laser for ablation of colonic mucosa. *Lasers Surg Med* 11:545, 1991.

59. Greenwald BD: Photodynamic therapy for esophageal cancer. *Chest Surg Clin North Am* 10:625, 2000.

60. Hunter JG, Bruhn E, Godman G, et al: Reflectance spectroscopy predicts safer wavelengths for pulsed laser lithotripsy of gallstones (abstract). *Gastrointest Endosc* 37:273, 1991.

61. Amaral JF, Chrostek C: Comparison of the ultrasonically activated scalpel to electrosurgery and laser for laparoscopic surgery. *Surg Endosc* 7:141, 1993.

62. Huscher CG, Liriei MM, Di Paola M, et al: Laparoscopic cholecystectomy by ultrasonic dissection without cystic duct and artery ligature. *Surg Endosc* 17:442, 2003.

63. Jobe BA, Kenyon T, Hansen PD, Swanstrom LL: Mini-laparoscopy: Current status, technology and future applications. *Minim Invasive Ther Allied Technol* 7:201, 1998.

64. Aiono S, Gilbert JM, Soin B, et al: Controlled trial of the introduction of a robotic camera assistant (EndoAssist) for laparoscopic cholecystectomy. *Surg Endosc* 16:1267, 2002.

65. Luketich JD, Fernando HC, Buenaventura PO, et al: Results of a randomized trial of HERMES-assisted versus non-HERMES-assisted laparoscopic antireflux surgery. *Surg Endosc* 16:1264, 2002.

66. Herron DM, Gagner M, Kenyon TL, Swanstrom LL: The minimally-invasive surgical suite enters the 21st century. A discussion of critical design elements. *Surg Endosc* 15:415, 2001.

67. Georgeson KE: Pediatric laparoscopy, in Toouli JG, Gossot D, Hunter JG (eds): *Endosurgery*. New York/London: Churchill-Livingstone, 1996, p 929.

68. Holcomb GW: Diagnostic laparoscopy: Equipment, technique, and special concerns in children, in Holcomb GW (ed): *Pediatric Endoscopic Surgery*. Norwalk, CT: Appleton & Lange, p 9.

69. Hunter JG, Swanstrom LL, et al: Carbon dioxide pneumoperitoneum induces fetal acidosis in a pregnant ewe model. *Surg Endosc* 9:272, 1995.

70. Morrell DG, Mullins JR, et al: Laparoscopic cholecystectomy during pregnancy in symptomatic patients. *Surgery* 112:856, 1992.

71. Callery MP, Strasberg SM, Doherty GM, et al: Staging laparoscopy with laparoscopic ultrasonography: Optimizing resectability in hepatobiliary and pancreatic malignancy. *J Am Coll Surg* 185:33, 1997.

72. Parekh D: Minimal access surgery for cancer of the foregut and pancreas, in Peters JH, DeMeester TR (eds): *Minimally-Invasive Surgery of the Foregut*. St. Louis: Quality Medical Publishing, 1995, p 262.

73. Fried GM, Clas D, Meakins JL: Minimally-invasive surgery in the elderly patient. *Surg Clin North Am* 74:375, 1994.

74. Borman PC, Terblanche J: Subtotal cholecystectomy: For the difficult gallbladder in portal hypertension and cholecystitis. *Surgery* 98:1, 1985.

75. Litwin DWM, Pham Q: Laparoscopic surgery in the complicated patient, in Eubanks WS, Swanstrom LJ, Soper NJ (eds): *Mastery of Endoscopic and Laparoscopic Surgery*. Philadelphia: Lippincott Williams & Wilkins, 2000, p 57.

76. Birkett DH: Robotics. *Surg Endosc* 16:1257, 2002.

77. Marescaux J, Leroy J, Gagner M, et al: Transatlantic robot-assisted telesurgery. *Nature* 413:379, 2001.

78. Melvin WS, Needleman BJ, Krause KR, et al: Computer-enhanced vs. standard laparoscopic antireflux surgery. *J Gastrointest Surg* 6:11, 2002.

79. Costi R, Himpens J, Bruyns J, Cadiere GB: Robotic fundoplication: from theoretic advantages to real problems. *J Am Coll Surg* 197:500, 2003.

80. Ruurda JP, Broeders IA, Simmermacher RP, et al: Feasibility of robot-assisted laparoscopic surgery: An evaluation of 35 robot-assisted laparoscopic cholecystectomies. *Surg Laparosc Endosc Percutan Tech* 12:41, 2002.

81. Fleischer DE: Stents, cloggology, and esophageal cancer. *Gastrointest Endosc* 43:258, 1996.

82. Foutch P, Sivak M: Therapeutic endoscopic balloon dilatation of the extrahepatic biliary ducts. *Am J Gastroenterol* 80:575, 1985.

83. Hoepffner N, Foerster EC, et al: Long-term experience in wall stent therapy for malignant choledochostenosis. *Endoscopy* 26:597, 1994.

84. Kozarek RA, Ball TJ, et al: Metallic self-expanding stent application in the upper gastrointestinal tract: Caveats and concerns. *Gastrointest Endosc* 38:1, 1992.

85. Anderson JR, Sorenson SM, Kruse A, et al: Randomized trial of endoscopic endoprosthesis versus operative bypass in malignant obstructive jaundice. *Gut* 30:1132, 1989.

86. Ruygrok PN, Sim KH, Chan C, Rachman OJ, et al: Coronary intervention with a heparin-coated stent and aspirin only. *J Invasive Cardiol* 15:439, 2003.

87. Bhoyrul S, Way LW: Intraluminal gastric surgery, in Duh Q-Y (ed): *Laparoscopic Surgery: Laparoscopic Access to the Gastrointestinal Tract*. New York: Decker Medical, 1995, p 189.

88. Gallagher AG, Smith CD, Bowers SP, et al: Psychomotor skills assessment in practicing surgeons experienced in performing advanced laparoscopic procedures. *J Am Coll Surg* 197:479, 2003.

89. Cuschieri A: Visual displays and visual perception in minimal access surgery. *Semin Laparosc Surg* 2:209, 1995.

90. Gallagher AG, Hughs C, Reinhardt-Rutland AH, et al: Transfer of skill from "virtual reality" (VR): A case control comparison of traditional and VR training in laparoscopic skill acquisition. *MITAT* 9:347, 2000.

CHAPTER 14

Cell, Genomics, and Molecular Surgery

Xin-Hua Feng, Jeffrey B. Matthews, Xia Lin, and F. Charles Brunicardi

OVERVIEW OF MOLECULAR BIOLOGY

One of the goals of modern biology is to analyze the molecular structure and gain a fuller understanding of how cells, organs, and entire organisms function, both in a normal state and under pathologic conditions. Significant progress has been made in molecular studies of metabolism pathways, gene expression, cellular signaling, and organ development in humans. The advent of recombinant DNA technology, polymerase chain reaction (PCR) techniques, and completion of the Human Genome Project are positively affecting human society by not only broadening our knowledge and understanding of disease development but also by bringing about necessary changes in disease treatment.

Today's practicing surgeons are becoming increasingly aware that many modern surgical procedures rely on the information gained through molecular research. Genomic information, such as BRCA and RET-protooncogene, is being used to help direct prophylactic procedures to remove potentially harmful tissues before they do damage to patients. Molecular engineering has led to cancer-specific gene therapy that could serve in the near future as a more effective adjunct to surgical debulking of tumors than radiation or chemotherapy, so surgeons will benefit from a clear introduction to how basic biochemical and biologic principles relate to the developing area of molecular biology.

This chapter will review the current information on modern molecular biology in the surgical community. It is written with the intent of serving two functions. First, to introduce or update the readers about the general concepts of molecular cell biology, which are essential for comprehending the real power and potential of modern molecular technology. The second aim is to inform the reader about the modern molecular techniques that are commonly used for surgical research and to provide a fundamental introduction on the background of how these techniques are developed and applied to benefit patients.

Basic Concepts of Molecular Research

The modern era of molecular biology, which has been mainly concerned with how genes govern cell activity, began in 1953 when James D. Watson and Francis H. C. Crick discovered the secret of life by deducing the double-helical structure of deoxyribonucleic acid, or DNA.[1,2] The year 2003 marked the 50th anniversary of this great discovery. Prior to 1953, one of the most mysterious aspects of biology was how genetic material was precisely duplicated from one generation to the next. Although DNA had been implicated as genetic material, it was the base-paired structure of DNA that provided a logical interpretation of how a double helix could "unzip" to make copies of itself. This DNA synthesis, termed *replication,* immediately gave rise to the notion that a template was involved in the transfer of information between generations, and thus confirmed the suspicion that DNA carried an organism's hereditary information.

Within cells DNA is packed into chromosomes. One important feature of DNA as genetic material is its ability to encode important information for all of a cell's functions (Fig. 14-1). Based on the principles of base complementarity, scientists also discovered how information in DNA is accurately transferred into the protein structure.

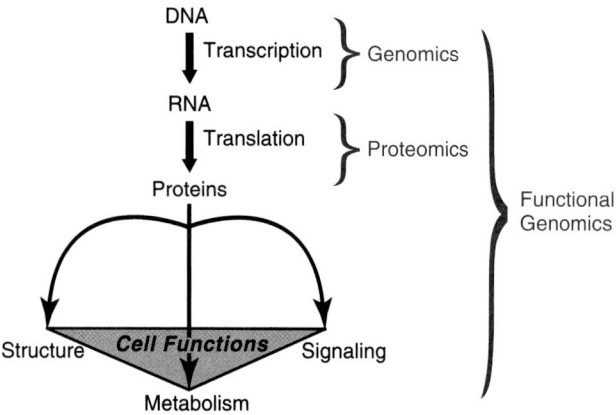

FIG. 14-1. *The flow of genetic information from DNA to protein to cell functions. The process of transmission of genetic information from DNA to RNA is called* transcription, *and the process of transmission from RNA to protein is called* translation. *Proteins are the essential controlling components for cell structure, cell signaling, and metabolism.* Genomics *and* proteomics *are the study of the genetic composition of a living organism at the DNA and protein level, respectively. The study of the relationship between genes and their cellular functions is called* functional genomics.

DNA serves as a template for RNA synthesis, termed *transcription,* including messenger RNA (mRNA, or the protein-encoding RNA), ribosomal RNA (rRNA), and transfer RNA (tRNA). mRNA carries the information from DNA to make proteins, termed *translation,* with the assistance of rRNA and tRNA. Each of these steps is precisely controlled in such a way that genes are properly expressed in each cell at a specific time and location. Thus the differential gene activity in a cell determines its actions, properties, and functions.

Molecular Approaches to Surgical Research

Rapid advances in molecular and cellular biology over the past half century have revolutionized the understanding of disease and will radically transform the practice of surgery. In the future, molecular techniques will be increasingly applied to surgical disease and will lead to new strategies for the selection and implementation of operative therapy. Surgeons should be familiar with the fundamental principles of molecular and cellular biology so that emerging scientific breakthroughs can be translated into improved care of the surgical patient.

The greatest advances in the field of molecular biology have been in the areas of analysis and manipulation of DNA.[1] Since Watson and Crick's discovery of DNA structure, an intensive effort has been made to unlock the deepest biologic secrets of DNA. Among the avalanche of technical advances, one discovery in particular has drastically changed the world of molecular biology: the uncovering of the enzymatic and microbiologic techniques that produce recombinant DNA. Recombinant DNA technology involves the enzymatic manipulation of DNA and, subsequently, the cloning of DNA. DNA molecules are cloned for a variety of purposes including safeguarding DNA samples, facilitating sequencing, generating probes, and expressing recombinant proteins in one or more host organisms. DNA can be produced by a number of means including restricted digestion of an existing vector, PCR, and cDNA synthesis. As DNA cloning techniques have developed over the past 25 years, researchers have moved from studying DNA to studying the functions of proteins, and from cell and animal models to molecular therapies in humans. Expression of recombinant proteins provides

a method for analyzing gene regulation, structure, and function. In recent years the uses for recombinant proteins have expanded to include a variety of new applications, including gene therapy and biopharmaceuticals. The basic molecular approaches for modern surgical research include DNA cloning, cell manipulation, disease modeling in animals, and clinical trials in human patients.

FUNDAMENTALS OF MOLECULAR AND CELL BIOLOGY

DNA and Heredity

DNA forms a right-handed, double-helical structure that is composed of two antiparallel strands of unbranched polymeric deoxyribonucleotides linked by phosphodiesterase bonds between the 5′ carbon of one deoxyribose moiety to the 3′ carbon of the next (Fig. 14-2). DNA is composed of four types of

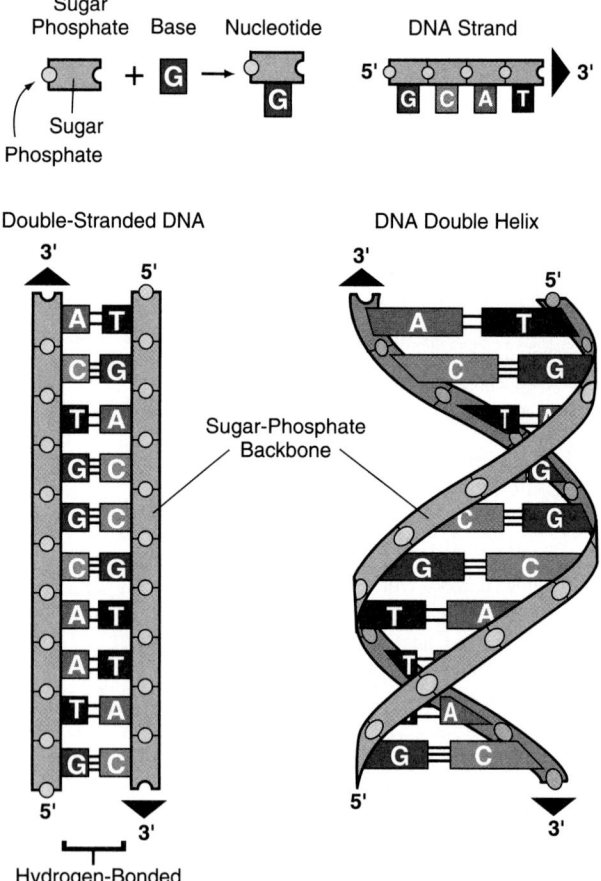

FIG. 14-2. *Schematic representation of a DNA molecule forming a double helix. DNA is made of four types of nucleotides, which are linked covalently into a DNA strand. A DNA molecule is composed of two DNA strands held together by hydrogen bonds between the pair bases. The arrowheads at the ends of the DNA strands indicate the polarities of the two strands, which run antiparallel to each other in the DNA molecule. The diagram at the bottom left of the figure shows the DNA molecule straightened out. In reality, the DNA molecule is twisted into a double helix, of which each turn of DNA is made up of 10.4 nucleotide pairs, as shown on the right. (Reproduced with permission from Alberts et al.[1])*

deoxyribonucleotides: adenine (A), cytosine (C), guanine (G), and thymine (T). The nucleotides are joined together by phosphodiester bonds. In the double-helical structure deduced by Watson and Crick, the two strands of DNA are complementary to each other. Because of size, shape, and chemical composition, A always pairs with T, and C with G, through the formation of hydrogen bonds between complementary bases that stabilize the double helix.

Recognition of the hereditary transmission of genetic information is attributed to the Austrian monk, Gregor Mendel. His seminal work, ignored upon publication until its rediscovery in 1900, established the laws of segregation and of independent assortment. These two principles established the existence of paired elementary units of heredity and defined the statistical laws that govern them.[3] DNA was isolated in 1869, and a number of important observations of the inherited basis of certain diseases were made in the early part of the 20th century. Although today it appears easy to understand how DNA replicates, prior to the 1950s, the idea of DNA as the primary genetic material was not appreciated. The modern era of molecular biology began in 1944 with the demonstration that DNA was the substance that carried genetic information. The first experimental evidence that DNA was genetic material came from simple transformation experiments conducted in the 1940s using *Streptococcus pneumoniae*. One strain of the bacteria could be converted into another by incubating it with DNA from the other, just as the treatment of the DNA with DNase would inactivate the transforming activity of the DNA. Similarly, in the early 1950s, before the discovery of the double-helical structure of DNA, the entry of viral DNA and not the protein into the host bacterium was believed to be necessary in order to initiate infection by the bacterial virus or bacteriophage. Key historical events concerning genetics are outlined in Table 14-1.

For cells to pass on the genetic material (DNA) to each progeny, the amount of DNA must be doubled. Watson and Crick recognized that the complementary base-pair structure of DNA implied the existence of a template-like mechanism for the copying of genetic material.[2] The transfer of DNA material from the mother cell to a daughter cell takes place during somatic cell division (also called *mitosis*). Before a cell divides, DNA must be precisely duplicated. During replication, the two strands of DNA separate and each strand creates a new complementary strand by precise base-pair matching (Fig. 14-3). The two new double-stranded DNAs carry the same genetic information, which can then be passed on to two daughter cells. Proofreading mechanisms ensure that the replication process occurs in a highly accurate manner. The fidelity of DNA replication is absolutely crucial to maintaining the integrity of the genome from generation to generation. However, mistakes can still occur during this process, resulting in *mutations,* which may lead to a change of the DNA's encoded protein and, consequently, a change of the cell's behavior. For example, there are many mutations present in the genome of a cancer cell.

Gene Regulation

Living cells have the necessary machinery to enzymatically transcribe DNA into RNA and translate the mRNA into protein. This machinery accomplishes the two major steps required for gene expression in all organisms: transcription and translation (Fig. 14-4). However, gene regulation is far more complex, particularly in eukaryotic organisms. For example, many gene transcripts must be spliced to remove the intervening sequences. The sequences that are spliced off are called *introns,* which appear to be useless, but in fact may carry some regulatory information. The sequences that are joined together, and are eventually translated into protein, are called *exons.* Additional regulation of gene expression includes modification of mRNA, control of mRNA stability, and its nuclear export into cytoplasm (where it is assembled into ribosomes for translation). After mRNA is translated into protein, the levels and functions of the proteins can be further regulated posttranslationally. However, the

Table 14-1
Historical Events in Genetics and Molecular Biology

Year	Investigator	Event
1865	Mendel	Laws of genetics established
1869	Miescher	DNA isolated
1905	Garrod	Human inborn errors of metabolism
1913	Sturtevant	Linear map of genes
1927	Muller	X-rays cause inheritable genetic damage
1928	Griffith	Transformation discovered
1941	Beadle and Tatum	"One gene, one enzyme" concept
1944	Avery, MacLeod, McCarty	DNA as material of heredity
1950	McKlintock	Existence of transposons confirmed
1953	Watson and Crick	Double-helical structure of DNA
1957	Benzer and Kornberg	Recombination and DNA polymerase
1966	Nirenberg, Khorana, Holley	Genetic code determined
1970	Temin and Baltimore	Reverse transcriptase
1972	Cohen, Boyer, Berg	Recombinant DNA technology
1975	Southern	Transfer of DNA fragments from sizing gel to nitrocellulose (Southern blot)
1977	Sanger, Maxim, Gilbert	DNA sequencing methods
1982		GenBank database established
1985	Mullis	Polymerase chain reaction
1986		Automated DNA sequencing
1989	Collins	Cystic fibrosis gene identified by positional cloning and linkage analysis
1990		Human Genome Project initiated
1997	Roslin Institute	Mammalian cloning (Dolly)
2001	IHGSC and Celera Genomics	Draft versions of human genome sequence published
2003		Human Genome Project completed

DNA IS A TEMPLATE FOR ITS OWN DUPLICATION

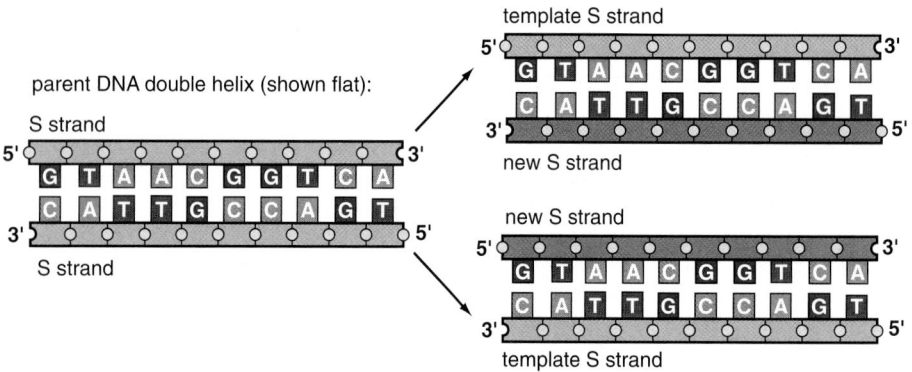

FIG. 14-3. DNA replication. As the nucleotide A only pairs with T, and G with C, each strand of DNA can determine the nucleotide sequence in its complementary strand. In this way, double-helical DNA can be copied precisely. (Reproduced with permission from Alberts et al.[1])

following sections will mainly focus on gene regulation at transcriptional and translational levels.

Transcription

Transcription is the enzymatic process of RNA synthesis from DNA.[4] In bacteria, a single RNA polymerase carries out all RNA synthesis, including that of mRNA, rRNA, and tRNA. Transcription often is coupled with translation in such a way that an mRNA molecule is completely accessible to ribosomes, and bacterial protein synthesis begins on an mRNA molecule even while it is still being synthesized. Therefore, a discussion of gene regulation with a look at the simpler prokaryotic system precedes that of the more complex transcription and posttranscriptional regulation of eukaryotic genes.

Transcription in Bacteria. Initiation of transcription in prokaryotes begins with the recognition of DNA sequences by RNA polymerase. First, the bacterial RNA polymerase catalyzes RNA synthesis through loose binding to any region in the double-stranded DNA and then through specific binding to the *promoter* region with the assistance of accessory proteins called *σ factors* (sigma factors). A promoter region is the DNA region upstream of the transcription initiation site. RNA polymerase binds tightly at the promoter sites and causes the double-stranded DNA structure to unwind.

Consequently, few nucleotides can be base-paired with the DNA template to begin transcription. Once transcription begins, the σ factor is released. The growing RNA chain may begin to peel off as the chain elongates. This occurs in such a way that there are always about 10 to 12 nucleotides of the growing RNA chains that are base-paired with the DNA template.

The bacterial promoter contains a region of about 40 bases that include two conserved elements called *−35 region* and *−10 region*. The numbering system begins at the initiation site, which is designated +1 position, and counts backwards (in negative numbers) on the promoter and forward on the transcribed region. Although both regions on different promoters are not the same sequences, they are fairly conserved and very similar. This conservation provides the accurate and rapid initiation of transcription for most bacterial genes. It is also common in bacteria that one promoter serves to transcribe a series of clustered genes, called an *operon*. A single transcribed mRNA contains a series of coding regions, each of which is later independently translated. In this way, the protein products are synthesized in a coordinated manner. Most of the time these proteins are involved in the same metabolic pathway, thus demonstrating that the control by one operon is an efficient system. After initiation of transcription, the polymerase moves along the DNA to elongate the chain of RNA, although at a certain point it will stop. Each step of RNA synthesis, including initiation, elongation, and termination,

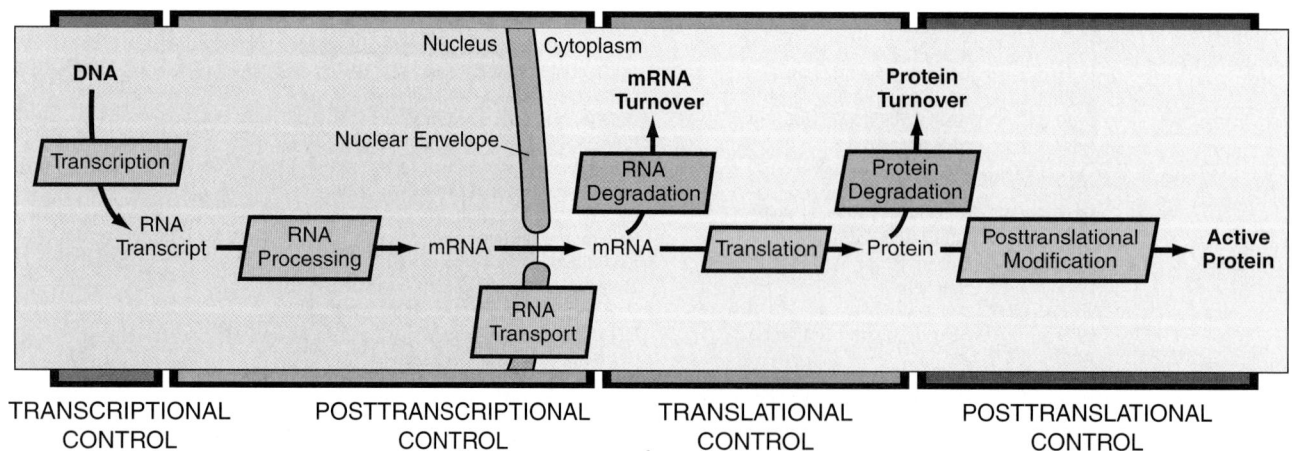

FIG. 14-4. Four major steps in the control of eukaryotic gene expression. Transcriptional and posttranscriptional control determine the level of mRNA that is available to make a protein, while translational and posttranslational control determine the final outcome of functional proteins. Note that posttranscriptional and posttranslational controls consist of several steps.

will require the integral functions of RNA polymerase as well as the interactions of the polymerase with regulatory proteins.

Transcription in Eukaryotes. Transcription mechanisms in eukaryotes differ from those in prokaryotes. The unique features of eukaryotic transcription are as follows: (1) Three separate RNA polymerases are involved in eukaryotes: RNA polymerase I transcribes the precursor of 5.8S, 18S, and 28S rRNAs; RNA polymerase II synthesizes the precursors of mRNA; RNA polymerase III makes tRNAs and 5S rRNAs. (2) In eukaryotes, the initial transcript is often the precursor to final mRNAs, tRNAs, and rRNAs. The precursor is then modified and/or processed into its final functional form. RNA splicing is one type of processing to remove the noncoding introns (the region between coding exons) on an mRNA. (3) In contrast to bacterial DNA, eukaryotic DNA often is packaged with histone and nonhistone proteins into chromatins. Transcription will only occur when the chromatin structure changes in such a way that DNA is accessible to the polymerase. (4) RNA is made in the nucleus and transported into cytoplasm, where translation occurs. Therefore, unlike bacteria, eukaryotes undergo uncoupled transcription and translation.

Eukaryotic gene transcription also involves the recognition and binding of RNA polymerase to the promoter DNA. However, the interaction between the polymerase and DNA is far more complex in eukaryotes than in prokaryotes. Because the majority of studies have been focused on the regulation and functions of proteins, this chapter primarily focuses on how protein-encoding mRNA is made by RNA polymerase II.

Translation

DNA directs the synthesis of RNA; RNA in turn directs the synthesis of proteins. Proteins are variable-length polypeptide polymers composed of various combinations of 20 different amino acids and are the working molecules of the cell. The process of decoding information on mRNA to synthesize proteins is called *translation* (see Fig. 14-1). Translation takes place in ribosomes composed of rRNA and ribosomal proteins. The numerous discoveries made during the 1950s made it easy to understand how DNA replication and transcription involves base-pairing between DNA and DNA, or DNA and RNA. However, at that time it was still impossible to comprehend how mRNA transfers the information to the protein-synthesizing machinery. The genetic information on mRNA is composed of arranged sequences of four bases that are transferred to the linear arrangement of 20 amino acids on a protein. Amino acids are characterized by a central carbon unit linked to four side chains: an amino group ($-NH_2$), a carboxy group ($-COOH$), a hydrogen, and a variable ($-R$) group. The amino acid chain is assembled via peptide bonds between the amino group of one amino acid and the carboxy group of the next. Because of this decoding, the information carried on mRNA relies on tRNA. Translation involves all three RNAs. The precise transfer of information from mRNA to protein is governed by *genetic code*; the set of rules by which codons are translated into an amino acid (Table 14-2). A *codon*, a triplet of three bases, codes for one amino acid. In this case, random combinations of the four bases form $4 \times 4 \times 4$, or 64 codes. Since 64 codes are more than enough for 20 amino acids, most amino acids are coded by more than one codon. The start codon is AUG, which also corresponds to methionine; therefore, almost all proteins begin with this amino acid. The sequence of nucleotide triplets that follows the start codon signal is termed the *reading frame*. The codons on mRNA are sequentially recognized by tRNA adaptor proteins. Specific enzymes termed *aminoacyl-tRNA synthetases* link a specific amino acid to a specific tRNA. The translation of mRNA to protein requires the ribosomal complex to move stepwise along the mRNA until the initiator methionine sequence is identified. In concert with various protein initiator factors, the met-tRNA is positioned on the mRNA and protein synthesis begins. Each new amino acid is added sequentially by the appropriate tRNA in conjunction with proteins called *elongation factors*. Protein synthesis proceeds in the amino-to-carboxy-terminus direction.

The biologic versatility of proteins is astounding. Among many other functions, proteins serve as enzymes that catalyze critical biochemical reactions, carry signals to and from the extracellular environment, and mediate diverse signaling and regulatory functions in the intracellular environment. They also transport ions and various small molecules across plasma membranes. Proteins make up the

Table 14-2
The Genetic Code

First Base in Codon		Second Base in Codon											Third Base in Codon
		U			C			A			G		
U		UUU	Phe	[F]	UCU	Ser	[S]	UAU	Tyr	[Y]	UGU	Cys	[C]	U
		UUC	Phe	[F]	UCC	Ser	[S]	UAC	Tyr	[Y]	UGC	Cys	[C]	C
		UUA	Leu	[L]	UCA	Ser	[S]	UAA	*STOP*		UGA	*STOP*		A
		UUG	Leu	[L]	UCG	Ser	[S]	UAG	*STOP*		UGG	Trp	[W]	G
C		CUU	Leu	[L]	CCU	Pro	[P]	CAU	His	[H]	CGU	Arg	[R]	U
		CUC	Leu	[L]	CCC	Pro	[P]	CAC	His	[H]	CGC	Arg	[R]	C
		CUA	Leu	[L]	CCA	Pro	[P]	CAA	Gln	[Q]	CGA	Arg	[R]	A
		CUG	Leu	[L]	CCG	Pro	[P]	CAG	Gln	[Q]	CGG	Arg	[R]	G
A		AUU	Ile	[I]	ACU	Thr	[T]	AAU	Asn	[N]	AGU	Ser	[S]	U
		AUC	Ile	[I]	ACC	Thr	[T]	AAC	Asn	[N]	AGC	Ser	[S]	C
		AUA	Ile	[I]	ACA	Thr	[T]	AAA	Lys	[K]	AGA	Arg	[R]	A
		AUG	Met	[M]	ACG	Thr	[T]	AAG	Lys	[K]	AGG	Arg	[R]	G
G		GUU	Val	[V]	GCU	Ala	[A]	GAU	Asp	[D]	GGU	Gly	[G]	U
		GUC	Val	[V]	GCC	Ala	[A]	GAC	Asp	[D]	GGC	Gly	[G]	C
		GUA	Val	[V]	GCA	Ala	[A]	GAA	Glu	[E]	GGA	Gly	[G]	A
		GUG	Val	[V]	GCG	Ala	[A]	GAG	Glu	[E]	GGG	Gly	[G]	G

A = adenine; C = cytosine; G = guanine; U = uracil; Ala = alanine; Arg = arginine; Asn = asparagine; Asp = aspartic acid; Cys = cysteine; Glu = glutamic acid; Gln = glutamine; Gly = glycine; His = histidine; Ile = isoleucine; Leu = leucine; Lys = lysine; Met = methionine; Phe = phenylalanine; Pro = proline; Ser = serine; Thr = threonine; Trp = tryptophan; Tyr = tyrosine; Val = valine. Letter in [ ] indicates single lettercode for amino acid.

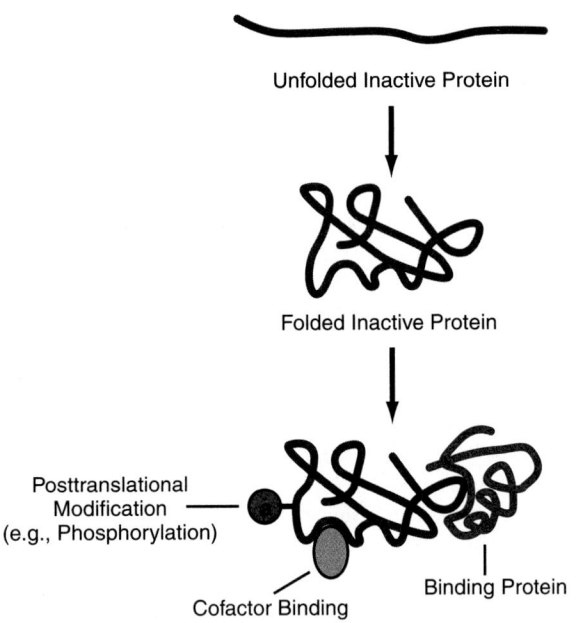

FIG. 14-5. *Maturation of a functional protein. Although the linear amino acid sequence of a protein is often shown, the function of a protein is also controlled by its correctly folded three-dimensional structure. In addition, many proteins also have covalent posttranslational modifications such as phosphorylation or noncovalent binding to a small molecule or a protein.*

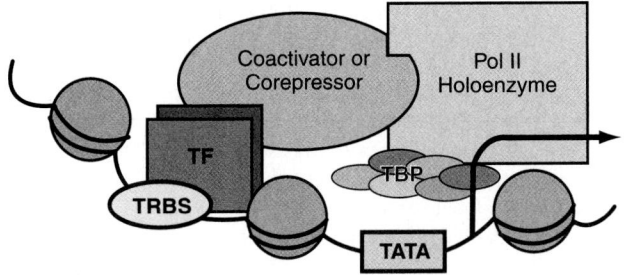

FIG. 14-6. *Transcriptional control by RNA polymerase. DNA is packaged into a chromatin structure. TATA = the common sequence on the promoter recognized by TBP and polymerase II holoenzyme; TBP = TATA-binding protein and associated factors; TF = hypothetical transcription factor; TFBS = transcription factor binding site; ball-shaped structures = nucleosomes. Coactivator or corepressor are factors linking the TF with the Pol II complex.*

key structural components of cells and the extracellular matrix and are responsible for cell motility. The unique functional properties of proteins are largely determined by their structure (Fig. 14-5).

Regulation of Gene Expression

The human organism is made up of a myriad of different cell types that, despite their vastly different characteristics, contain the same genetic material. This cellular diversity is controlled by the *genome* and accomplished by tight regulation of gene expression. This leads to the synthesis and accumulation of different complements of RNA and, ultimately, to the proteins found in different cell types. For example, muscle and bone express different genes or the same genes at different times. Moreover, the choice of which genes are expressed in a given cell at a given time depends on signals received from its environment. There are multiple levels at which gene expression can be controlled along the pathway from DNA to RNA to protein (see Fig. 14-4). *Transcriptional control* refers to the mechanism for regulating when and how often a gene is transcribed. Splicing of the primary RNA transcript (*RNA processing control*) and selection of which completed mRNAs undergo nuclear export (*RNA transport control*) represent additional potential regulatory steps. The mRNAs in the cytoplasm can be selectively translated by ribosomes (*translational control*), or selectively stabilized or degraded (*mRNA degradation control*). Finally, the resulting proteins can undergo selective activation, inactivation, or compartmentalization (*protein activity control*).

Because a large number of genes are regulated at the transcriptional level, regulation of gene transcripts (i.e., mRNA) is often referred to as *gene regulation* in a narrow definition. Each of the steps during transcription is properly regulated in eukaryotic cells. Because genes are differentially regulated from one another, one

gene can be differentially regulated in different cell types or at different developmental stages. Therefore, gene regulation at the level of transcription is largely context-dependent. However, there is a common scheme that applies to transcription at the molecular level (Fig. 14-6). Each gene promoter possesses unique sequences called *TATA boxes* that can be recognized and bound by a large complex containing RNA polymerase II, forming the basal transcription machinery. Usually located upstream of the TATA box (but sometimes longer distances) are a number of regulatory sequences referred to as *enhancers* that are recognized by regulatory proteins called *transcription factors*. These transcription factors specifically bind to the enhancers, often in response to environmental or developmental cues, and cooperate with each other and with basal transcription factors to initiate transcription. Regulatory sequences that negatively regulate the initiation of transcription also are present on the promoter DNA. The transcription factors that bind to these sites are called *repressors,* in contrast to the *activators* that activate transcription. The molecular interactions between transcription factors and promoter DNA, as well as between the cooperative transcription factors, are highly regulated. Specifically, the recruitment of transcription factors to the promoter DNA occurs in response to physiologic signals. A number of structural motifs in these DNA-binding transcription factors facilitate this recognition and interaction. These include the helix-turn-helix, the homeodomain motif, the zinc finger, the leucine zipper, and the helix-loop-helix motifs.

Human Genome

Genome is a collective term for all genes present in one organism. The human genome contains DNA sequences of 3 billion base pairs, carried by 23 pairs of chromosomes. The human genome has an estimated 25,000 to 30,000 genes, and overall it is 99.9 percent identical in all people.[5,6] Approximately 3 million locations where single-base DNA differences exist have been identified and termed *single nucleotide polymorphisms* (SNPs). SNPs may be critical determinants of human variation in disease susceptibility and responses to environmental factors.

The completion of the human genome sequence in 2003 represented another great milestone in modern science. The human genome project created the field of *genomics*, which is the study of genetic material in detail (see Fig. 14-1). The medical field is building upon the knowledge, resources, and technologies emanating from the human genome to further the understanding of the relationship of the genes and their mutations to human health and disease. This expansion of genomics into human health applications resulted in the field of genomic medicine.

The emergence of genomics as a science will transform the practice of medicine and surgery in this century. This breakthrough has allowed scientists the opportunity to gain remarkable insights into the lives of humans. Ultimately, the goal is to use this information to develop new ways to treat, cure, or even prevent the thousands of diseases that afflict humankind. In the 21st century, work will begin to incorporate the information embedded in the human genome sequence into surgical practices. By doing so, the genomic information can be used for diagnosing and predicting disease and disease susceptibility. Diagnostic tests can be designed to detect errant genes in patients suspected of having particular diseases or of being at risk for developing them. Furthermore, exploration into the function of each human gene is now possible, which will shed light on how faulty genes play a role in disease causation. This knowledge also makes possible the development of a new generation of therapeutics based on genes. Drug design is being revolutionized as researchers create new classes of medicines based on a reasoned approach to the use of information on gene sequence and protein structure function rather than the traditional trial-and-error method. Drugs targeted to specific sites in the body promise to have fewer side effects than many of today's medicines. Finally, other applications of genomics will involve the transfer of genes to replace defective versions or the use of gene therapy to enhance normal functions such as immunity.

Proteomics refers to the study of the structure and expression of proteins as well as the interactions among proteins encoded by a human genome (see Fig. 14-1).[7] A number of Internet-based repositories for protein sequences exist, including Swiss-Prot (http://www.expasy.ch). These databases allow comparisons of newly identified proteins with previously characterized sequences to allow prediction of similarities, identification of splice variants, and prediction of membrane topology and posttranslational modifications. Tools for proteomic profiling include two-dimensional gel electrophoresis, time-of-flight mass spectrometry, matrix-assisted laser desorption/ionization, and protein microarrays. *Structural proteomics* aims to describe the three-dimensional structure of proteins that is critical to understanding function. *Functional genomics* seeks to assign a biochemical, physiologic, cell biologic, and/or developmental function to each predicted gene. An ever-increasing arsenal of approaches including transgenic animals, RNA interference, and various systematic mutational strategies will allow dissection of functions associated with newly discovered genes. While the potential of this field of study is vast, it is in its early stages.

It is anticipated that a genomic and proteomic approach to human disease will lead to a new understanding of pathogenesis that will aid in the development of effective strategies for early diagnosis and treatment.[8] For example, identification of altered protein expression in organs, cells, subcellular structures, or protein complexes may lead to development of new biomarkers for disease detection. Moreover, improved understanding of how protein structure determines function will allow rational identification of therapeutic targets, and thereby not only accelerate drug development, but also lead to new strategies to evaluate therapeutic efficacy and potential toxicity.[7]

Cell Cycle and Apoptosis

Every organism has many different cell types. Many cells grow, while some cells such as nerve cells and striated muscle cells do not. All growing cells have the ability to duplicate their genomic DNA and pass along identical copies of this genetic information to every daughter cell. Thus the cell cycle is the fundamental mechanism to maintain tissue homeostasis. A cell cycle comprises four periods: G_1 (first gap phase before DNA synthesis), S (synthesis phase when DNA replication occurs), G_2 (the gap phase before mitosis), and M (mitosis, the phase when two daughter cells with identical DNA are generated) (Fig. 14-7). After a full cycle, the daughter cells enter G_1 again, and when they receive appropriate signals, undergo another cycle, and so on. The machinery that drives cell cycle progression is made up of a group of enzymes called cyclin-dependent kinases (CDK). Cyclin expression fluctuates during the cell cycle, and cyclins are essential for CDK activities and form complexes with CDK. The cyclin A/CDK1 and cyclin B/CDK1 drive the progression for the M phase, while cyclin A/CDK2 is the primary S phase complex. Early G_1 cyclin D/CDK4/6 or late G_1 cyclin E/CDK2 controls the G_1-S transition. There also are negative regulators for CDK termed *CDK inhibitors* (CKIs), which inhibit the assembly or activity of the cyclin-CDK complex. Expression of cyclins and CKIs often are regulated by developmental and environmental factors.

The cell cycle is connected with signal transduction pathways as well as gene expression. While the S and M phases are rarely subjected to changes imposed by extracellular signals, the G_1 and G_2 phases are the primary periods when cells decide whether to move on to the next phase or not. During the G_1 phase, cells receive green- or red-light signals, S phase entry or G_1 arrest, respectively. Growing cells proliferate only when supplied with appropriate mitogenic growth factors. Cells become committed to entry of the cell cycle only toward the end of G_1. Mitogenic signals stimulate the activity of early G_1 cyclin-dependent kinases (e.g., cyclin D/CDK4) that inhibit the activity of pRb protein and activate the transcription factor called E2F to induce the expression of batteries of genes essential for G_1-S progression. Meanwhile, cells also receive antiproliferative signals such as those from tumor suppressors. These antiproliferative signals also act in the G_1 phase to stop cells' progress into the S phase by inducing CKI production. For example, when DNA is damaged, cells will repair the damage before entering the S phase. Therefore, G_1 contains one of the most important checkpoints for cell cycle progression. If the analogy is made that CDK is to a cell as an engine is to a car, then cyclins and CKI are the gas pedal and brake, respectively. Accelerated proliferation or improper cell cycle progression with damaged DNA would be disastrous. Genetic gain-of-function mutations in oncogenes (that often promote expression or activity of the cyclin/CDK complex) or loss-of-function mutations in tumor suppressor (that stimulate production of CKI) are causal factors for malignant transformation.

In addition to cell cycle control, cells use genetically programmed mechanisms to kill cells. This cellular process, called *apoptosis* or *programmed cell death,* is essential for the maintenance of tissue homeostasis (Fig. 14-8). Normal tissues undergo proper apoptosis to remove unwanted cells, those that have completed their jobs or have been damaged or improperly proliferated. Apoptosis can be activated by many physiologic stimuli such as death receptor signals (e.g., Fas or cytokine tumor necrosis factor [TNF]), growth factor deprivation, DNA damage, and stress signals. Two major pathways control the biochemical mechanisms governing apoptosis: the death receptor and mitochondrial. However, recent advances in apoptosis research suggest an interconnect of the two pathways. What is central to the apoptotic machinery is the activation of a cascade of proteinases called caspases. Similarly to CDK in the cell cycle, activities and expression of caspases are well controlled by positive and negative regulators. The complex machinery of apoptosis must be tightly controlled. Perturbations of this process can cause neoplastic transformation or other diseases.

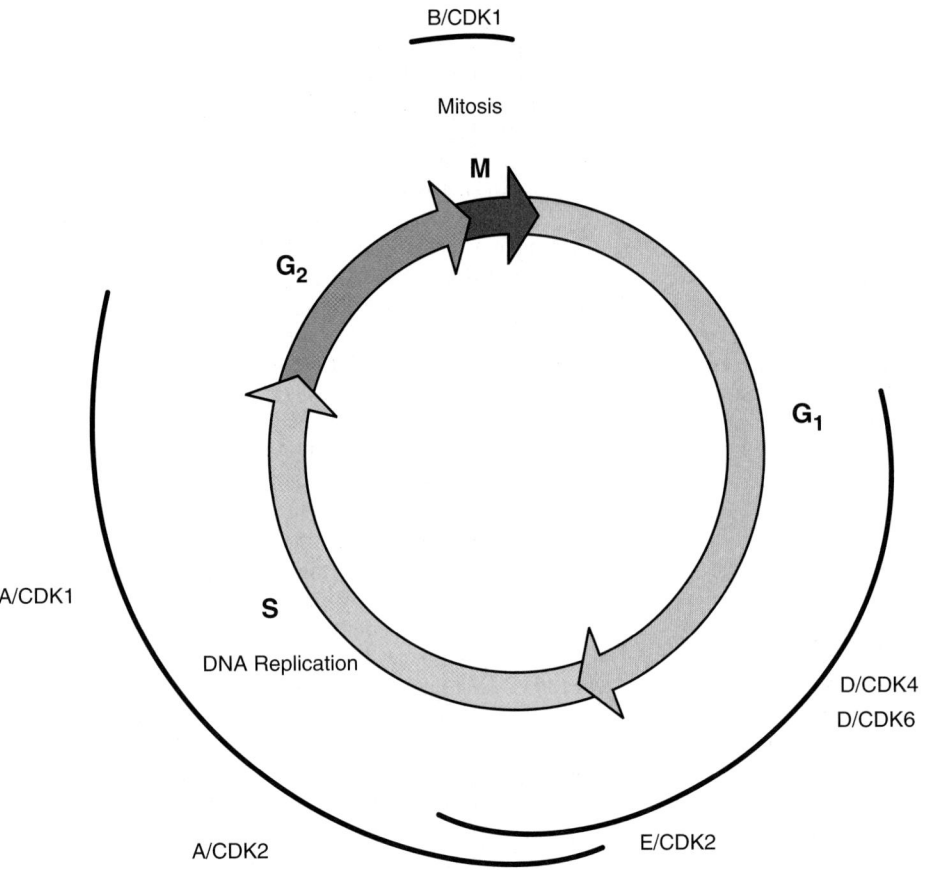

FIG. 14-7. The cell cycle and its control system. M is the mitosis phase, when the nucleus and the cytoplasm divide; S is the phase when DNA is duplicated; G_1 is the gap between M and S; G_2 is the gap between S and M. A complex of cyclin and cyclin-dependent kinase (CDK) controls specific events of each phase. Without cyclin, CDK is inactive. Different cyclin/CDK complexes are shown around the cell cycle. A, B, D, and E stand for cyclin A, cyclin B, cyclin D, and cyclin E, respectively.

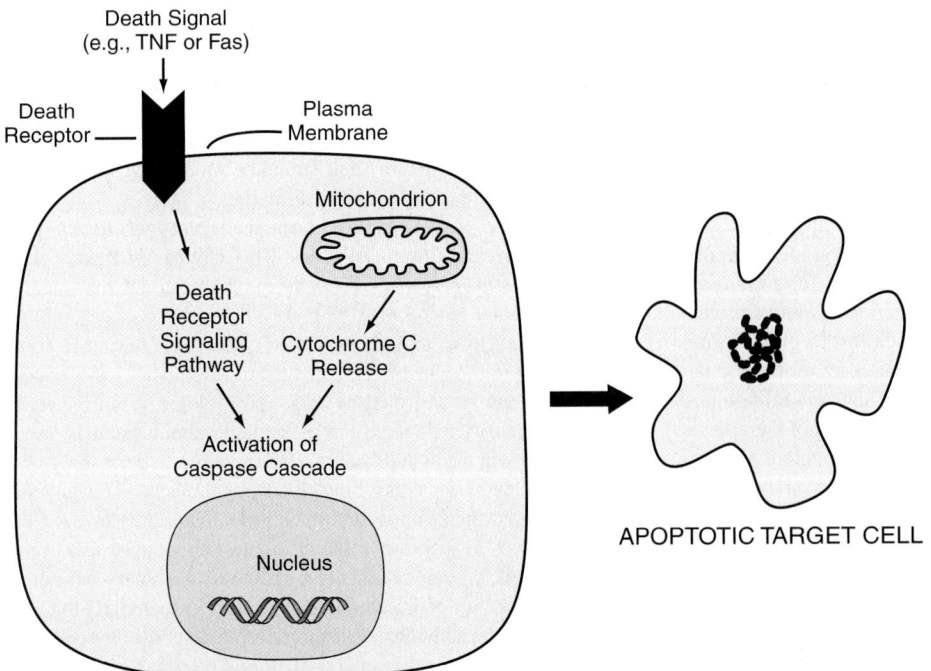

FIG. 14-8. A simplified view of the apoptosis pathways. Extracellular death receptor pathways include the activation of Fas and TNF receptors, and consequent activation of the caspase pathway. Intracellular death pathway indicates the release of cytochrome c from mitochondria, which also triggers the activation of the caspase cascade. During apoptosis, cells undergo DNA fragmentation, nuclear and cell membrane breakdown, and are eventually digested by other cells.

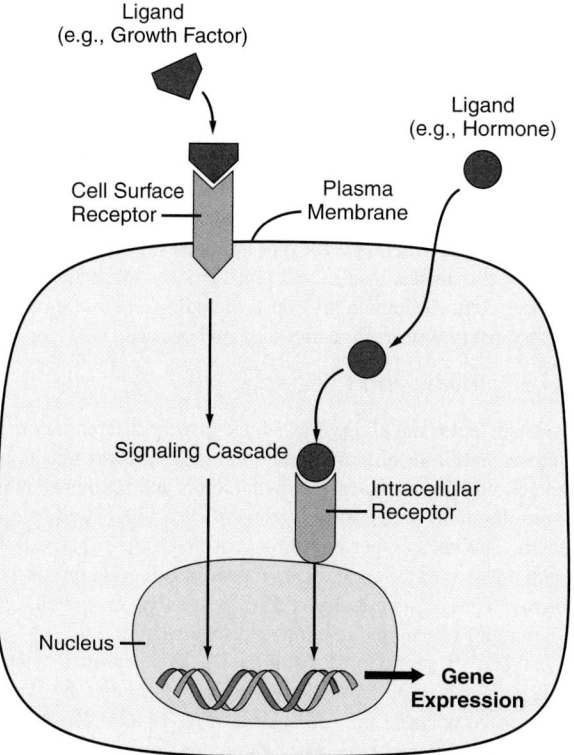

FIG. 14-9. *Cell-surface and intracellular receptor pathways. Extracellular signaling pathway: Most growth factors and other hydrophilic signaling molecules are unable to move across the plasma membrane and directly activate cell-surface receptors such as G-protein–coupled receptors and enzyme-linked receptors. The receptor serves as the receiver, and in turn activates the downstream signals in the cell. Intracellular signaling pathway: Hormones or other diffusible molecules enter the cell and bind to the intracellular receptor in the cytoplasm or in the nucleus. Either extracellular or intracellular signals often reach the nucleus to control gene expression.*

Signal Transduction Pathways

Gene expression in a genome is controlled in a temporal and spatial manner, at least in part by signaling pathways.[9] A signaling pathway generally begins at the cell surface and, after a signaling relay by a cascade of intracellular effectors, ends up in the nucleus (Fig. 14-9). All cells have the ability to sense changes in their external environment. The bioactive substances to which cells can respond are many and include proteins, short peptides, amino acids, nucleotides/nucleosides, steroids, retinoids, fatty acids, and dissolved gases. Some of these substances are lipophilic and thereby can cross the plasma membrane by diffusion to bind with a specific target protein within the cytoplasm (intracellular receptor). Other substances bind directly with a transmembrane protein (cell-surface receptor). Binding of ligand to receptor initiates a series of biochemical reactions (*signal transduction*) typically involving protein-protein interactions and the transfer of high-energy phosphate groups, leading to various cellular end responses.

Control and specificity through simple protein-protein interactions—referred to as *adhesive interactions*—is a common feature of signal transduction pathways in cells.[10] Signaling also involves catalytic activities of signaling molecules such as protein kinases/phosphatases that modify the structures of key signaling proteins. Upon binding and/or modification by upstream signaling molecules, downstream effectors undergo a conformational (allosteric) change and, consequently, a change in function. The signal that originates at the cell surface and is relayed by the cytoplasmic proteins often ultimately reaches the transcriptional apparatus in the nucleus. It alters the DNA binding and activities of transcription factors that directly turn genes on or off in response to the stimuli. Abnormal alterations in signaling activities and capacities in otherwise normal cells can lead to diseases such as cancer.

Advances in biology in the last two decades have dramatically expanded the view on how cells are wired with signaling pathways. In a given cell, many signaling pathways operate simultaneously and cross-talk with one another. A cell generally may react to a hormonal signal in a variety of ways: (1) by changing its metabolite or protein, (2) by generating an electric current, or (3) by contracting. Cells are continually subject to multiple input signals that simultaneously and sequentially activate multiple receptor and non–receptor-mediated signal transduction pathways. While the regulators responsible for cell behavior are rapidly identified as a result of genomic and proteomic techniques, the specific functions of the individual proteins, how they assemble, and the networks that control cellular behavior remain to be defined. An increased understanding of cell regulatory pathways—and how they are disrupted in disease—will likely reveal common themes based on protein interaction domains that direct associations of proteins with other polypeptides, phospholipids, nucleic acids, and other regulatory molecules. Advances in the understanding of signaling networks will require methods of investigation that move beyond traditional "linear" approaches into medical informatics and computational biology. The bewildering biocomplexity of such networks mandates multidisciplinary and transdisciplinary research collaboration. The vast amount of information that is rapidly emerging from genomic and proteomic data mining will require the development of new modeling methodologies within the emerging disciplines of medical mathematics and physics.

Signaling pathways often are grouped according to the properties of signaling receptors. Many hydrophobic signaling molecules are able to diffuse across plasma membranes and directly reach specific cytoplasmic targets. Steroid hormones, thyroid hormones, retinoids, and vitamin D are examples that exert their activity upon binding to structurally related receptor proteins that are members of the *nuclear hormone receptor superfamily*. Ligand binding induces a conformational change that enhances transcriptional activity of these receptors. Most extracellular signaling molecules interact with transmembrane protein receptors that couple ligand binding to intracellular signals, leading to biologic actions.

There are three major classes of cell-surface receptors: *transmitter-gated ion channels, seven-transmembrane (G-protein coupled) receptors (7TM/GPCRs),* and *enzyme-linked receptors.* The superfamily of 7TM/GPCRs is one of the largest families of proteins, representing over 800 genes of the human genome. Members of this superfamily share a characteristic seven-transmembrane configuration. The ligands for these receptors are diverse and include hormones, chemokines, neurotransmitters, proteinases, inflammatory mediators, and even sensory signals such as odorants and photons. Most 7TM/GPCRs signal through *heterotrimeric G-proteins,* which are guanine-nucleotide regulatory complexes. Thus the receptor serves as the receiver, the G-protein serves as the transducer, and the enzyme serves as the effector arm. *Enyzme-linked receptors* possess an extracellular ligand-recognition domain and a cytosolic domain that either has intrinsic enzymatic activity or directly links with an enzyme. Structurally, these receptors usually have only one transmembrane-spanning domain. Of at least five forms of enzyme-linked receptors classified by the nature of the enzyme activity to which they are coupled, the growth factor receptors such as tyrosine kinase receptor or serine/threonine kinase receptors mediate diverse cellular events including cell growth, differentiation, metabolism, and survival/apoptosis. Dysregulation (particularly mutations) of these receptors is thought to underlie conditions of abnormal cellular proliferation in the context of cancer. The following sections will further review two examples of growth factor signaling pathways and their connection with human diseases.

Insulin Pathway and Diabetes[11]

The discovery of insulin in the early 1920s is one of the most dramatic events in the treatment of human disease. *Insulin* is a peptide hormone that is secreted by the beta cell of the pancreas. Insulin is required for the growth and metabolism of most mammalian cells, which contain cell-surface insulin receptors (InsR). Insulin binding to InsR activates the kinase activity of InsR. InsR then adds phosphoryl groups, a process referred to as *phosphorylation,* and subsequently activates its immediate intracellular effector, called *insulin receptor substrate* (IRS). IRS plays a central role in coordinating the signaling of insulin by activating distinct signaling pathways, the PI3K-Akt pathway and MAPK pathway, both of which possess multiple protein kinases that can control transcription, protein synthesis, and glycolysis (Fig. 14-10).

The primary physiologic role of insulin is in glucose homeostasis, which is accomplished through the stimulation of glucose uptake into insulin-sensitive tissues such as fat and skeletal muscle. Defects in insulin synthesis/secretion and/or responsiveness are major causal factors in diabetes, one of the leading causes of death and disability in the United States, affecting an estimated 16 million Americans. Type 2 diabetes accounts for about 90% of all cases of diabetes. Clustering of type 2 diabetes in certain families and ethnic populations points to a strong genetic background for the disease. More than 90% of affected individuals have insulin resistance, which develops when the body is no longer able to respond correctly to insulin circulating in the blood. Although relatively little is known about the biochemical basis of this metabolic disorder, it is clear

that the insulin-signaling pathways malfunction in this disease. It also is known that genetic mutations in the InsR or IRS cause type 2 diabetes, although which one is not certain. The majority of type 2 diabetes cases may result from defects in downstream-signaling components in the insulin-signaling pathway. Type 2 diabetes also is associated with declining beta-cell function, resulting in reduced insulin secretion; these pathways are under intense study. A full understanding of the basis of insulin resistance is crucial for the development of new therapies for type 2 diabetes. Furthermore, apart from type 2 diabetes, insulin resistance is a central feature of several other common human disorders, including atherosclerosis and coronary artery disease, hypertension, and obesity.

TGF-β Pathway and Cancers[12]

Growth factor signaling controls cell growth, differentiation, and apoptosis. While insulin and many mitogenic growth factors promote cell proliferation, some growth factors and hormones inhibit cell proliferation. Transforming growth factor-beta (TGF-β) is one of them. The balance between mitogens and TGF-β plays an important role in controlling the proper pace of cell cycle progression. The growth inhibition function of TGF-β signaling in epithelial cells plays a major role in maintaining tissue homeostasis.

The TGF-β superfamily comprises a large number of structurally related growth and differentiation factors that act through a receptor complex at the cell surface (Fig. 14-11). The complex consists of transmembrane serine/threonine kinases. The receptor signals through activation of heterotrimeric complexes of intracellular effectors called SMADs (which is contracted from homologous *Caenorhabditis elegans* Sma and *Drosophila* Mad, two evolutionarily conserved genes for TGF-β signaling). Upon phosphorylation by the receptors, SMAD complexes translocate into the nucleus,

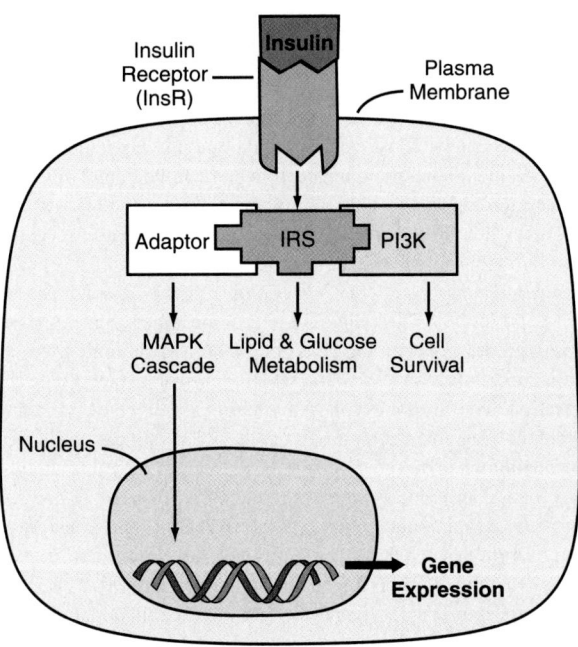

FIG. 14-10. Insulin signaling pathway. Insulin is a peptide growth factor that binds to and activates the heterotetrameric receptor complex (InsR). InsR possesses protein tyrosine kinase activity and is able to phosphorylate the downstream insulin receptor substrate (IRS). Phosphorylated IRS serves as a scaffold and controls the activation of multiple downstream pathways for gene expression, cell survival, and glucose metabolism. Inactivation of the insulin pathway can lead to type 2 diabetes.

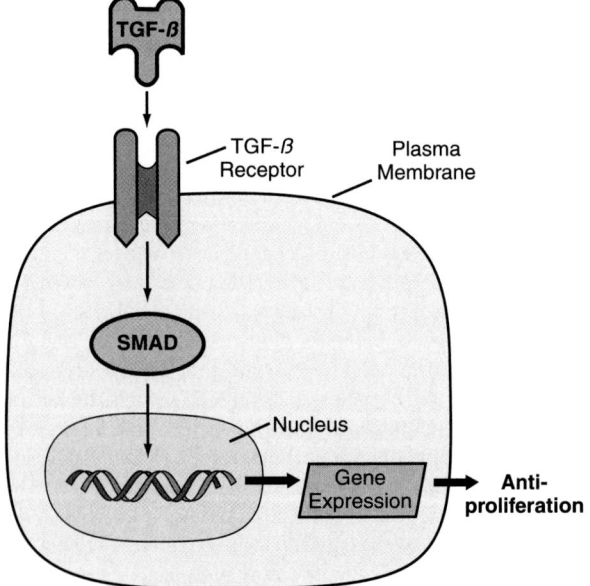

FIG. 14-11. TGF-β signaling pathway. The TGF-β family has at least 29 members encoded in the human genome. They are also peptide growth factors. Each member binds to a heterotetrameric complex consisting of a distinct set of type I and type II receptors. TGF-β receptors are protein serine/threonine kinases and can phosphorylate the downstream substrates called SMAD proteins. Phosphorylated SMADs are directly transported into the nucleus, where they bind to the DNA and regulate gene expression that is responsible for inhibition of cell proliferation. Inactivation of the TGF-β pathway through genetic mutations in the TGF-β receptors or SMADs is frequent in human cancer, leading to the uncontrolled proliferation of cancer cells.

where they bind to gene promoters and cooperate with specific transcription factors to regulate the expression of genes that control cell proliferation and differentiation. For example, TGF-β strongly induces the transcription of a gene called $p15^{INK4B}$ (a type of CKI) and, at the same time, reduces the expression of many oncogenes such as c-Myc. The outcome of the altered gene expression leads to the inhibition of cell cycle progression. Therefore, activation of TGF-β signaling is an intrinsic mechanism for cells to ensure controlled proliferation.

Resistance to TGF-β's anticancer action is one hallmark of human cancer cells. TGF-β receptors and SMADs are identified as tumor suppressors. The TGF-β signaling circuit can be disrupted in a variety of ways and in different types of human tumors. Some lose TGF-β responsiveness through downregulation or mutations of their TGF-β receptors. The cytoplasmic SMAD4 protein, which transduces signals from ligand-activated TGF-β receptors to downstream targets, may be eliminated through mutation of its encoding gene. The locus encoding cell cycle inhibitor p15^{INK4B} may be deleted. Alternatively, the immediate downstream target of its actions, cyclin-dependent kinase 4 (CDK4), may become unresponsive to the inhibitory actions of p15^{INK4B} because of mutations that block p15 binding. The resulting cyclin D/CDK4 complexes constitutively inactivate tumor suppressor pRb by hyperphosphorylation. Finally, functional pRb, the end target of this pathway, may be lost through mutation of its gene. For example, in pancreatic and colorectal cancers 100% of cells derived from these cancers carry genetic defects in the TGF-β signaling pathway. Therefore, the antiproliferative pathway converging onto pRb and the cell division cycle is, in one way or another, disrupted in a majority of human cancer cells.

Gene Therapy and Molecular Drugs in Cancer

Modern advances in the use of molecular biology to manipulate genomes have greatly contributed to the understanding of the molecular basis for how cells live, die, or differentiate. Given the fact that human diseases arise from improper changes in the genome, the continuous understanding of how the genome functions will make it possible to tailor medicine on an individual basis. Although significant hurdles remain, the course toward therapeutic application of molecular biology has already been mapped out by many proof-of-principle studies in the literature. In this section, cancer is used as an example to elaborate some therapeutic applications of molecular biology. Modern molecular medicine includes gene therapy and molecular drugs that target genes or gene products that wire human cells.

Cancer is a complex disease, involving uncontrolled growth and spread of tumor cells (Fig. 14-12). Cancer development depends on the acquisition and selection of specific characteristics that set the tumor cell apart from normal somatic cells. Cancer cells have defects in regulatory circuits that govern normal cell proliferation and homeostasis. Many lines of evidence indicate that tumorigenesis in humans is a multistep process and that these steps reflect genetic alterations that drive the progressive transformation of normal human cells into highly malignant derivatives. The genomes of tumor cells are invariably altered at multiple sites, having suffered disruption through lesions as subtle as point mutations and as obvious as changes in chromosome complement. A succession of genetic changes, each conferring one or another type of growth advantage, leads to the progressive conversion of normal human cells into cancer cells.

Cancer research in the past 20 years has generated a rich and complex body of knowledge, revealing cancer to be a disease involving dynamic changes in the genome. The causes of cancer include genetic predisposition, environmental influences, infectious

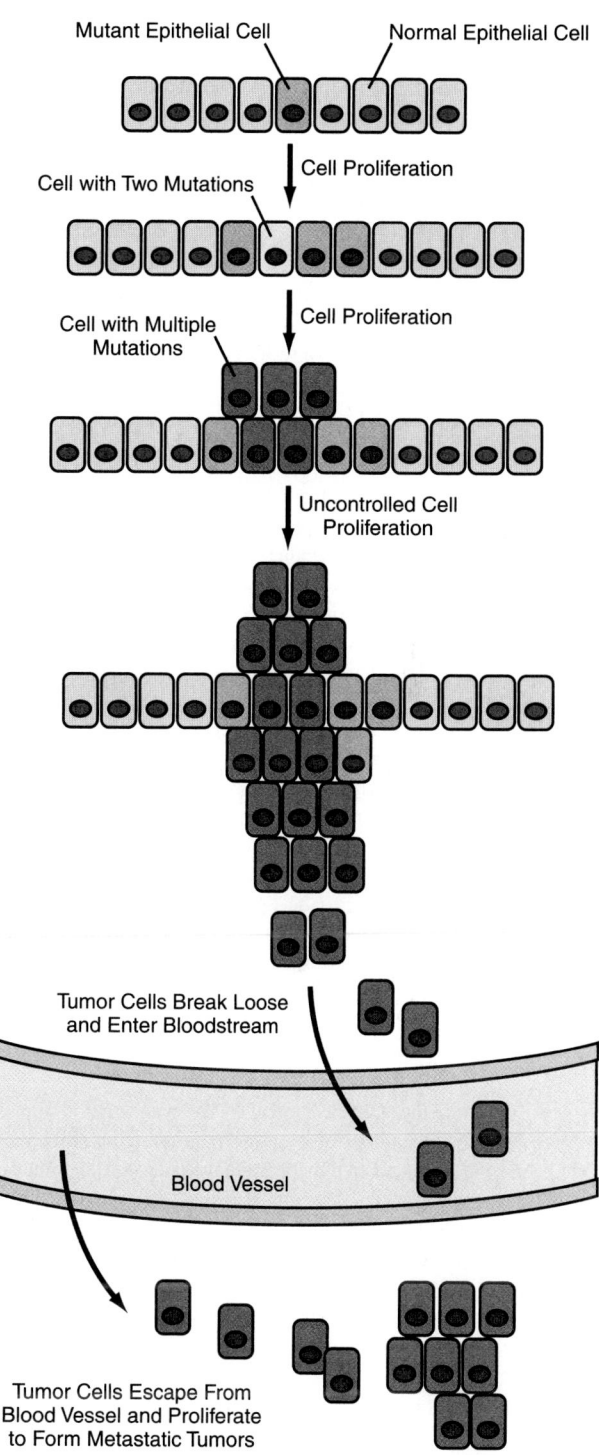

FIG. 14-12. *Tumor clonal evolution and metastasis. A tumor develops from mutant cells with multiple genetic mutations. Through repeated alterations in the genome, mutant epithelial cells are able to develop into a cluster of cells (called a tumor clone) that proliferates in an uncontrollable fashion. Further changes in the tumor cells can transform the tumor cells into a population of cells that can enter the blood vessels and repopulate in a new location.*

agents, and aging. These transform normal cells into cancerous ones by derailing a wide spectrum of regulatory pathways including signal transduction pathways, cell cycle machinery, or apoptotic pathways.[13] The early notion that cancer was caused by mutations in genes critical for the control of cell growth implied that genome stability is important for preventing oncogenesis. There are two classes of cancer genes in which alteration has been identified in human and animal cancer cells: oncogenes, with dominant gain-of-function mutations, and tumor suppressor genes, with recessive loss-of-function mutations. In normal cells, oncogenes promote cell growth by activating cell cycle progression, while tumor suppressors counteract oncogenes' functions. Therefore, the balance between oncogenes and tumor suppressors maintains a well-controlled state of cell growth.

During the development of most types of human cancer, cancer cells can break away from primary tumor masses, invade adjacent tissues, and hence travel to distant sites where they form new colonies. This spreading process of tumor cells, called *metastasis,* is the cause of 90% of human cancer deaths. Metastatic cancer cells that enter the bloodstream can reach virtually all tissues of the body. Bones are one of the most common places for these cells to settle and start growing again. Bone metastasis is one of the most frequent causes of pain in people with cancer. It can also cause bones to break and create other symptoms and problems for patients.

The progression in the knowledge of cancer biology has been accelerating in recent years. All of the scientific knowledge acquired through hard work and discovery has made it possible for cancer treatment and prevention. As a result of explosive new discoveries, some modern treatments were developed. The success of these therapies, together with traditional treatments such as surgical procedures, is further underscored by the fact that in 2002 the cancer rate was reduced in the United States. Current approaches to the treatment of cancer involve killing cancer cells with toxic chemicals, radiation, or surgery. Alternatively, several new biologic- and gene-based therapies are aimed at enhancing the body's natural defenses against invading cancers. Understanding the biology of cancer cells has led to the development of designer therapies for cancer prevention and treatment. Gene therapy, immune system modulation, genetically engineered antibodies, and molecularly designed chemical drugs, are all promising fronts in the war against cancer.

Immunotherapy

The growth of the body is controlled by many natural signals through complex signaling pathways. Some of these natural agents have been used in cancer treatment and have been proven effective for fighting several cancers through the clinical trial process. These naturally occurring biologic agents such as interferons, interleukins, and other cytokines can now be produced in the laboratory. These agents, as well as the synthetic agents that mimic the natural signals, are given to patients to influence the natural immune response agents either by directly altering the cancer cell growth, or by acting indirectly to help healthy cells control the cancer. One of the most exciting applications of immunotherapy has come from the identification of certain tumor targets called *antigens* and the aiming of an antibody at these targets. This was first used as a means of localizing tumors in the body for diagnosis, and was more recently used to attack cancer cells. Trastuzumab (Herceptin) is an example of such a drug.[15] Trastuzumab is a monoclonal antibody that neutralizes the mitogenic activity of cell-surface growth factor receptor HER-2. Approximately 25% of breast cancers overexpress HER-2. These tumors tend to grow faster and are generally more likely to recur than tumors that do not overproduce HER-2. Trastuzumab is designed to attack cancer cells that overexpress HER-2. Trastuzumab slows or stops the growth of these cells and increases the survival of HER-2–positive breast cancer patients. Another significant example is the administration of interleukin-2 (IL-2) to patients with metastatic melanoma or kidney cancer, which has been shown to mediate the durable regression of metastatic

cancer. IL-2, a cytokine produced by human T-helper lymphocytes, has a wide range of immune regulatory effects, including the expansion of lymphocytes following activation by a specific antigen. IL-2 has no direct impact on cancer cells. The impact of IL-2 on cancers in vivo derives from its ability to expand lymphocytes with antitumor activity. The expanded lymphocytes somehow recognize the antigen on cancer cells. Thus, the molecular identification of cancer antigens has opened new possibilities for the development of effective immunotherapies for patients with cancer. Clinical studies using immunization with peptides derived from cancer antigens have shown that high levels of lymphocytes with antitumor activity can be produced in cancer-bearing patients. Highly avid antitumor lymphocytes can be isolated from immunized patients and grown in vitro for use in cell-transfer therapies.

Chemotherapy

The primary function of anticancer chemicals is to block different steps involved in cell growth and replication. These chemicals often block a critical chemical reaction in a signal transduction pathway or during DNA replication or gene expression. For example, STI571, also known as Gleevec, is one of the first molecularly targeted drugs based on the changes that cancer causes in cells.[16] STI571 offers promise for the treatment of chronic myeloid leukemia (CML) and may soon surpass interferon-α as the standard treatment for the disease. In CML, STI571 is targeted at the Bcr-Abl kinase, an activated oncogene product in CML (Fig. 14-13). Bcr-Abl is an overly activated protein kinase resulting from a specific genetic abnormality generated by chromosomal translocation that is found in the cells of patients with CML. STI571-mediated inhibition of Bcr-Abl-kinase activity not only prevents cell growth of Bcr-Abl–transformed leukemic cells, but also induces apoptosis. Clinically, the drug quickly corrects the blood cell abnormalities caused by the leukemia in a majority of patients, achieving a complete disappearance of the leukemic blood cells and the return of normal blood cells. Additionally, the drug appears to have some effect on other cancers including certain brain tumors and gastrointestinal stromal tumors (GISTs), a very rare type of stomach cancer.

Gene Therapy

Gene therapy is an experimental treatment that involves genetically altering a patient's own tumor cells or lymphocytes (cells of the immune system, some of which can attack cancer cells). For years, the concept of gene therapy has held promise as a new, potentially potent weapon to attack cancer. Although a rapid progression in the understanding of the molecular and clinical aspects of gene therapy has been witnessed in the past decade, gene therapy treatment has not yet been shown to be superior to standard treatments in humans.

Several problems must be resolved in order to transform it into a clinically relevant form of therapy. The major issues that limit its translation to the clinic are improving the selectivity of tumor targeting, improving the delivery to the tumor, and the enhancement of the transduction rate of the cells of interest. In most gene therapy trials for malignant diseases, tumors can be accessed and directly injected (in situ gene therapy). The in situ gene therapy also offers a better distribution of the vector virus throughout the tumor. Finally, a combination of gene therapy strategies will be more effective than the use of a single gene therapy system. An important aspect of effective gene therapy involves the choice of appropriate genes for manipulation. Genes that promote the production of messenger chemicals or other immune-active substances can be transferred into the patient's cells. These include genes that inhibit cell cycle progression, induce apoptosis, enhance host immunity against cancer cells, and block the ability of cancer cells to metastasize. Gene therapy is still

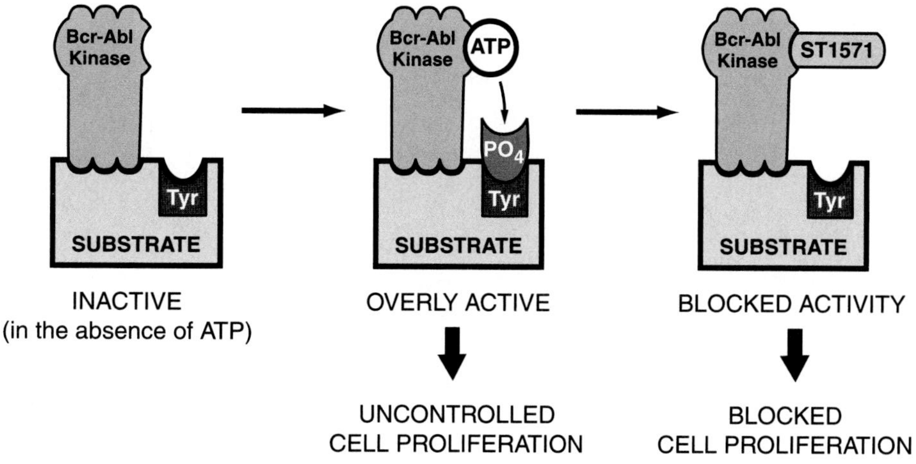

FIG. 14-13. Mechanism of STI571 as a molecular drug. Bcr-Abl is an overly activated oncogene product resulting from a specific genetic abnormality generated by chromosomal translocation that is found in cells of patients with chronic myeloid leukemia (CML). Bcr-Abl is an activated protein kinase and thus requires ATP to phosphorylate substrates, which in turn promote cell proliferation. STI571 is a small molecule that competes with the ATP-binding site and thus blocks the transfer of phosphoryl group to substrate.

experimental and is being studied in clinical trials for many different types of cancer. The mapping of genes responsible for human cancer is likely to provide new targets for gene therapy in the future. The preliminary results of gene therapy for cancer are encouraging, and as advancements are made in the understanding of the molecular biology of human cancer, the future of this rapidly developing field holds great potential for treating cancer.

It is noteworthy that the use of multiple therapeutic methods has proven more powerful than a single method. The use of chemotherapy after surgery to destroy the few remaining cancerous cells in the body is called *adjuvant* therapy. Adjuvant therapy was first tested and found to be effective in breast cancer. It was later adopted for use in other cancers. A major discovery in chemotherapy is the advantage of multiple chemotherapeutic agents (known as combination or cocktail chemotherapy) over single agents. Some types of fast-growing leukemias and lymphomas (tumors involving the cells of the bone marrow and lymph nodes) responded extremely well to combination chemotherapy, and clinical trials led to gradual improvement of the drug combinations used. Many of these tumors can be cured today by combination chemotherapy. As cancer cells carry multiple genetic defects, the use of combination chemotherapy, immunotherapy, and gene therapies may be more effective in treating cancers.

Stem Cell Research

Stem cell biology represents a cutting-edge scientific research field with potential clinical applications.[17] It may have an enormous impact on human health by offering hope for curing human diseases such as diabetes mellitus, Parkinson's disease, neurologic degeneration, and congenital heart disease. Stem cells are endowed with two remarkable properties (Fig. 14-14). First, stem cells can proliferate in an undifferentiated but pluripotent state, and as a result can self-renew. Second, they have the ability to differentiate into many specialized cell types. There are two groups of stem cells: embryonic stem (ES) cells and adult stem cells. Human ES cells are derived from early preimplantation embryos called *blastocysts* (5 days postfertilization), and are capable of generating all differentiated cell types in the body. Adult stem cells are present in and can be isolated from adult tissues. They are often tissue-specific and can only generate the cell types comprising a particular tissue in the body; however, in some cases they can transdifferentiate into cell types found in other tissues. Hematopoietic stem cells are adult stem cells. They reside in bone marrow and are capable of generating all cell types of the blood and immune system.

Stem cells can be grown in culture and be induced to differentiate into a particular cell type, either in vitro or in vivo. With the recent and continually increasing improvement in culturing stem cells, scientists are beginning to understand the molecular mechanisms of stem cell self-renewal and differentiation in response to environmental cues. It is believed that discovery of the signals that control self-renewal versus differentiation will be extremely important for the therapeutic use of stem cells in treating disease. It is possible that success in the study of the changes in signal transduction pathways in stem cells will lead to the development of therapies to specifically differentiate stem cells into a particular cell type to replace diseased or damaged cells in the body.

TECHNOLOGIES OF MOLECULAR AND CELL BIOLOGY

DNA Cloning

Since the advent of recombinant DNA technology three decades ago, hundreds of thousands of genes have been identified. Recombinant DNA technology is the technology that uses advanced enzymatic and microbiologic techniques to manipulate DNA.[18] Pure pieces of any DNA can be inserted into bacteriophage DNA or other carrier DNA such as plasmids to produce recombinant DNA in bacteria. In this way, DNA can be reconstructed, amplified, and used to manipulate the functions of individual cells or even organisms. This technology, often referred to as *DNA cloning,* is the basis of all other DNA analysis methods. It is only with the awesome power of recombinant DNA technology that the completion of the Human Genome Project was possible. It has also led to the identification of

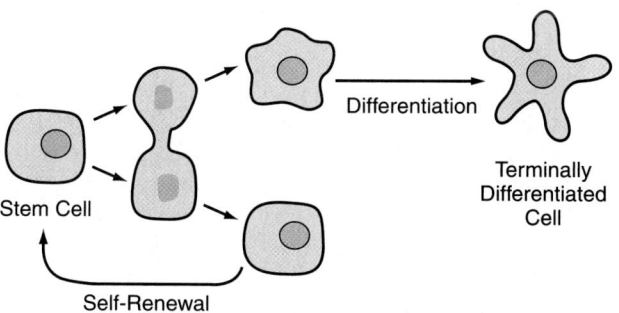

FIG. 14-14. Stem cells. A stem cell is capable of self-renewal (unlimited cell cycle) and differentiation (becoming nondividing cells with specialized functions). Differentiating stem cells often undergo additional cell divisions before they become fully mature cells that carry out specific tissue functions.

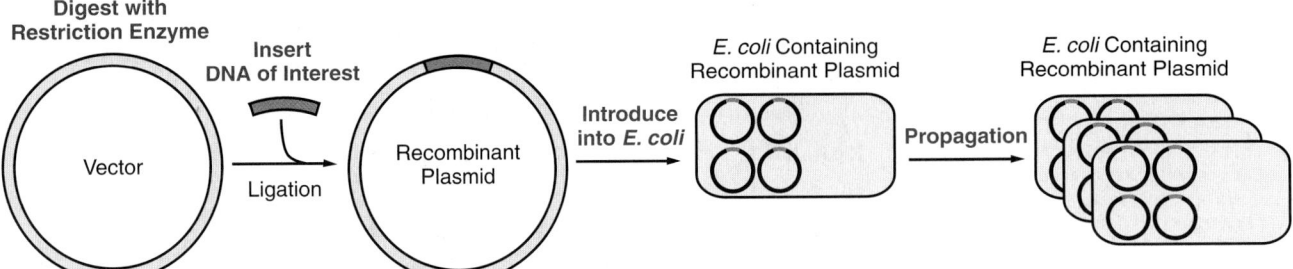

FIG. 14-15. Generation of recombinant DNA. The vector is a circular DNA molecule that is capable of replicating in *Escherichia coli* cells. Insert DNA (often your favorite gene) is ligated to the vector, after ends of both DNA are properly treated with restriction enzymes. Ligated DNA (i.e., the recombinant plasmid DNA) is then transformed into *E. coli* cells, where it replicates to produce recombinant progenies. *E. coli* cells carrying the recombinant plasmid can be propagated to yield large quantities of plasmid DNA.

the entire gene complements of organisms such as viruses, bacteria, worms, flies, and plants.

Molecular cloning refers to the process of cloning a DNA fragment of interest into a DNA vector that is ultimately delivered into bacterial or mammalian cells or tissues[19,20] (Fig. 14-15). This represents a very basic technique that is widely used in almost all areas of biomedical research. DNA vectors are often called *plasmids,* which are extrachromosomal molecules of DNA that vary in size and can replicate and be transmitted from bacterial cell to cell. Plasmids can be propagated either in the cytoplasm, or after insertion, as part of the bacterial chromosome in *Escherichia coli*. The process of molecular cloning involves several steps of manipulation of DNA. First, the vector plasmid DNA is cleaved with a restriction enzyme to create compatible ends with the foreign DNA fragment to be cloned. The vector and the DNA fragment are then joined in vitro by a DNA ligase. Finally, the ligation product is introduced into competent host bacteria; this procedure is called *transformation,* which can be done by either calcium/heat shock or electroporation. Precautions must be taken in every step of cloning in order to generate the desired DNA construct. The vector must be correctly prepared to maximize the creation of recombinants; for example, it must be enzymatically treated to prevent self-ligation. Host bacteria must be made sufficiently competent to permit the entry of recombinant plasmids into cells. The selection of desired recombinant plasmid-bearing *E. coli* is normally achieved by the property of drug resistance conferred by the plasmid vectors. The plasmids encoding markers provide specific resistance to (i.e., the ability to grow in the presence of) antibiotics such as ampicillin, kanamycin, and tetracycline. The foreign component in the plasmid vector can be a mammalian expression cassette, which can direct expression of foreign genes in mammalian cells. The resulting plasmid vector can be amplified in *E. coli* to prepare large quantities of DNA for its subsequent applications such as transfection, gene therapy, transgenics, and knockout mice.

Detection of Nucleic Acids and Proteins

Southern Blot Hybridization

Southern blotting refers to the technique of transferring DNA fragments from an electrophoresis gel to a membrane support, and the subsequent analysis of the fragments by hybridization with a radioactively labeled probe (Fig. 14-16).[21] Southern blotting is named after E. M. Southern, who in 1975 first described the technique of DNA analysis. It enables reliable and efficient analysis of size-fractionated DNA fragments in an immobilized membrane support.

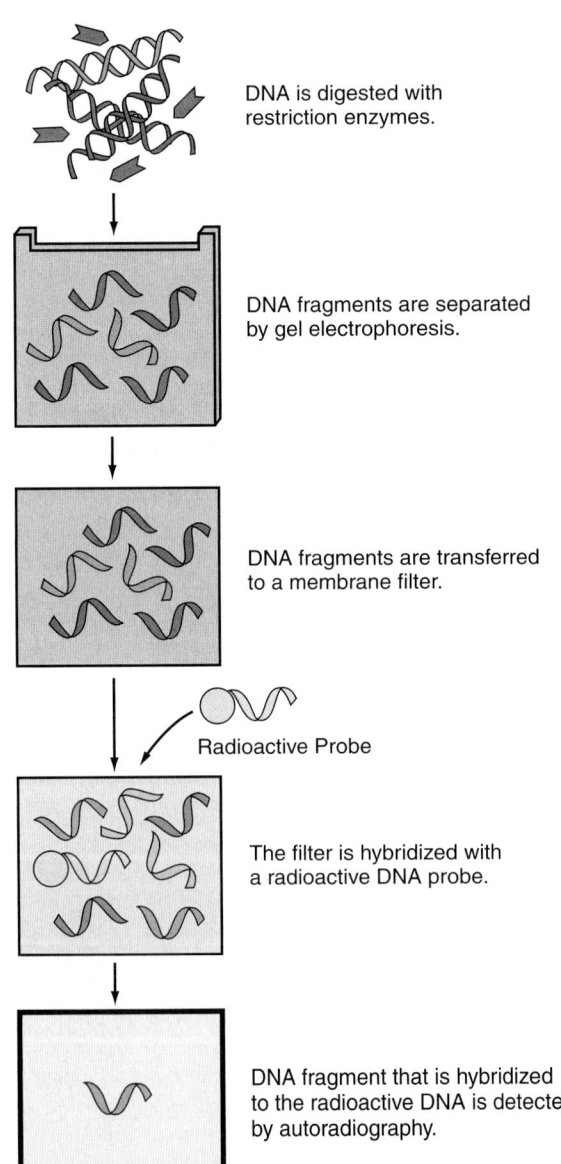

DNA is digested with restriction enzymes.

DNA fragments are separated by gel electrophoresis.

DNA fragments are transferred to a membrane filter.

Radioactive Probe

The filter is hybridized with a radioactive DNA probe.

DNA fragment that is hybridized to the radioactive DNA is detected by autoradiography.

FIG. 14-16. Southern blotting. Restriction enzymatic fragments of DNA are separated by agarose gel electrophoresis, transferred to a membrane filter, and then hybridized to a radioactive probe.

Southern blotting is composed of several steps. It normally begins with the digestion of the DNA samples with appropriate restriction enzymes(s) and the separation of DNA samples in an agarose gel with appropriate DNA size markers. The DNA gel is stained with ethidium bromide and photographed with a ruler laid alongside the gel so that band positions can later be identified on the membrane. The DNA gel is then treated so the DNA fragments are denatured (i.e., strand separation). The DNA is then transferred onto a nitrocellulose membrane by capillary diffusion or under electricity. After immobilization, the DNA can be subjected to hybridization analysis, enabling bands with sequence similarity to a radioactively labeled probe to be identified.

The development of Southern transfer and the associated hybridization techniques made it possible for the first time to obtain information about the physical organization of single and multicopy sequences in complex genomes. The later application of Southern blotting hybridization to the study of restriction fragment length polymorphisms (RFLPs) opened up new possibilities such as genetic fingerprinting and prenatal diagnosis of genetic diseases.

Northern Blot Hybridization

Northern blotting refers to the technique of size fractionation of RNA in a gel and the transferring of an RNA sample to a solid support (membrane) in such a manner that the relative positions of the RNA molecules are maintained. The resulting membrane is then hybridized with a labeled probe complementary to the mRNA of interest. Signals generated from detection of the membrane can be used to determine the size and abundance of the target RNA. In principle, Northern blot hybridization is similar to Southern blot hybridization (and hence its name), with the exception that RNA, not DNA, is on the membrane. Although RT-PCR has been used in many applications (described below), Northern analysis is the only method that provides information regarding mRNA size and has remained a standard method for detection and quantitation of mRNA. The process of Northern hybridization involves several steps, as does Southern hybridization, including electrophoresis of RNA samples in an agarose-formaldehyde gel, transfer to a membrane support, and hybridization to a radioactively labeled DNA probe. Data from hybridization allows quantification of steady-state mRNA levels, and at the same time, provides information related to the presence, size, and integrity of discrete mRNA species. Thus, Northern blot analysis, also termed *RNA gel blot analysis,* is commonly used in molecular biology studies relating to gene expression.

Polymerase Chain Reaction

PCR is an in vitro method for the polymerase-directed amplification of specific DNA sequences using two oligonucleotide primers that hybridize to opposite strands and flank the region of interest in the target DNA (Fig. 14-17).[22] One cycle of PCR reaction involves template denaturation, primer annealing, and the extension of the annealed primers by DNA polymerase. Because the primer extension products synthesized in one cycle can serve as a template in the next, the number of target DNA copies nearly doubles at each cycle. Thus a repeated series of cycles result in the exponential accumulation of a specific fragment in which the termini are sharply defined by the 5' ends of the primers. The introduction of the thermostable DNA polymerase (e.g., Taq polymerase) transforms the PCR into a simple and robust reaction. The reaction components (e.g., template, primers, Taq polymerase, 2'-deoxynucleoside 5'-triphosphates [dNTPs], and buffer) could all be assembled and the amplification reaction carried out by simply cycling the temperatures within the reaction tube. The specificity and yield in amplifying a particular DNA fragment by PCR reaction is affected by the proper setting of the reaction parameters (e.g., enzyme, primer, and Mg^{2+} concentration, as well as the temperature cycling profile). Modifying various PCR parameters to optimize the specificity of amplification yields more homogenous products, even in rare template reactions.

The emergence of the PCR technique has dramatically altered the approach to both fundamental and applied biologic problems. The capability of amplifying a specific DNA fragment from a gene or the whole genome greatly advances the study of the gene and its function. It is simple, yet robust, speedy, and most of all, flexible. As a recombinant DNA tool, it underlies almost all of molecular biology. This revolutionary technique enabled the modern methods for the isolation of genes, construction of a DNA vector, introduction of alterations into DNA, and quantitation of gene expression, making it a fundamental cornerstone of genetic and molecular analysis.

Immunoblotting and Immunoprecipitation

Analyses of proteins are primarily carried out by antibody-directed immunologic techniques. For example, Western blotting, also called immunoblotting, is performed to detect protein levels in a population of cells or tissues, whereas immunoprecipitation is used to concentrate proteins from a larger pool. Using specific antibodies, microscopic analysis called *immunofluorescence* and *immunohistochemistry* is possible for the subcellular localization and expression of proteins in cells or tissues, respectively.

Immunoblotting refers to the process of identifying a protein from a mixture of proteins (Fig. 14-18). It consists of five steps: (1) sample preparation; (2) electrophoresis (separation of a protein mixture by sodium dodecyl sulfate-polyacrylamide gel electrophoresis, or SDS-PAGE); (3) transfer (the electrophoretic transfer of proteins from gel onto membrane support, e.g., nitrocellulose, nylon, or polyvinylidene difluoride [PVDF]); (4) staining (the subsequent immunodetection of target proteins with specific antibody); and (5) development (colorimetric or chemiluminescent visualization of the antibody-recognized protein). Thus, immunoblotting combines the resolution of gel electrophoresis with the specificity of immunochemical detection. Immunoblotting is a powerful tool used to determine a number of important characteristics of proteins. For example, immunoblotting analysis will determine the presence and the quantity of a protein in a given cellular condition and its relative molecular weight. Immunoblotting also can be used to determine whether posttranslational modification such as phosphorylation has occurred on a protein. Importantly, through immunoblotting analysis a comparison of the protein levels and modification states in normal versus diseased tissues is possible.

Immunoprecipitation, another widely used immunochemical technique, is a method which uses antibody to enrich a protein of interest and any other proteins that are associated with it (Fig. 14-19). The principle of the technique lies in the property of a strong and specific affinity between antibodies and their antigens to locate and pull down target proteins in solution. Once the antibody-antigen (target protein) complexes are formed in the solution, they are collected and purified using small agarose beads with covalently attached protein A or protein G. Both protein A and protein G specifically interact with the antibodies, thus forming a large immobilized complex of antibody-antigen bound to beads. The purified protein can then be analyzed by a number of biochemical methods. When immunoprecipitation is combined with immunoblotting, it can be used for the sensitive detection of proteins in low concentrations,

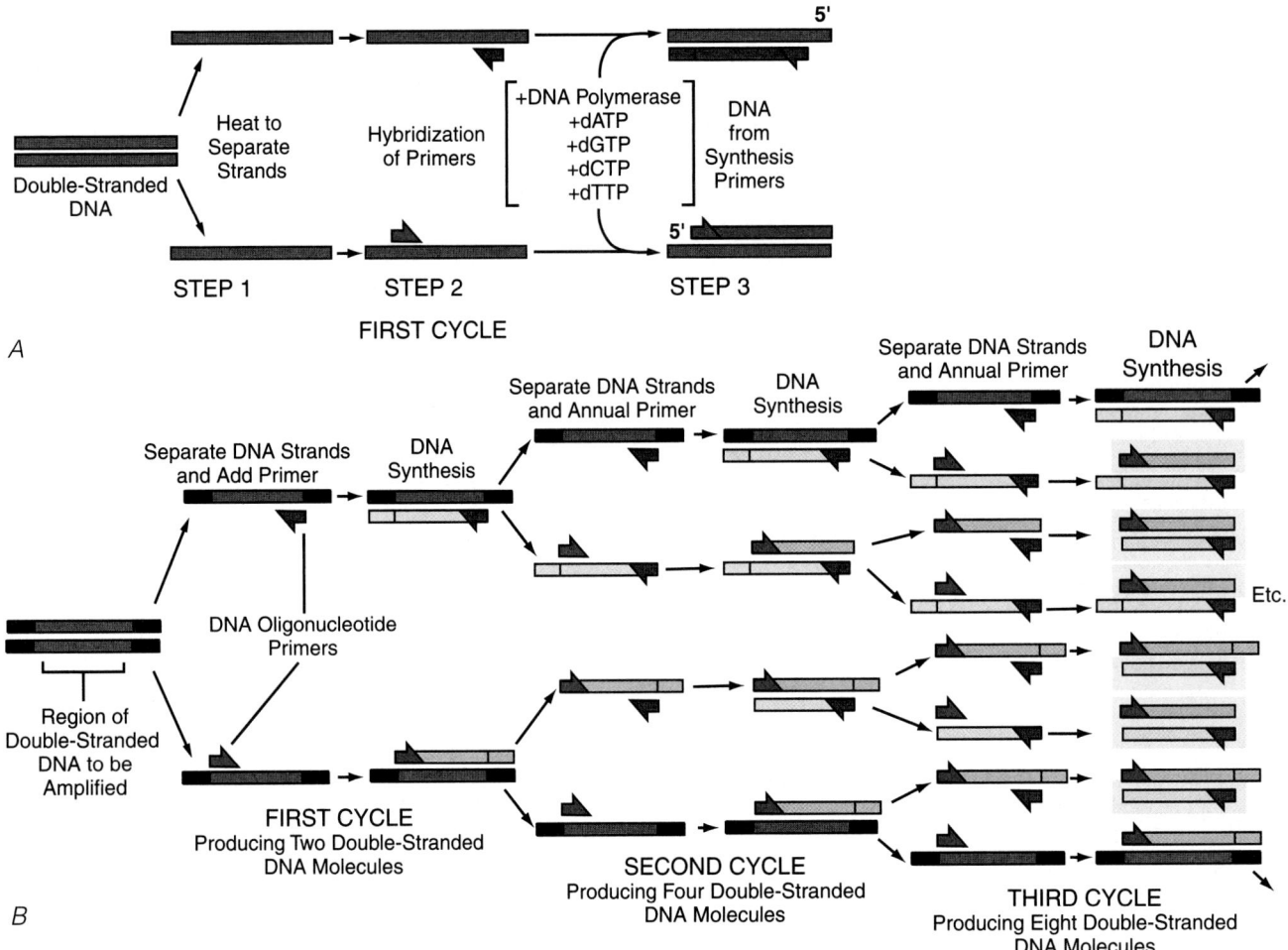

FIG. 14-17. *Amplification of DNA using the PCR technique. Knowledge of the DNA sequence to be amplified is used to design two synthetic DNA oligonucleotides, each complementary to the sequence on one strand of the DNA double helix at opposite ends of the region to be amplified. These oligonucleotides serve as primers for in vitro DNA synthesis, which is performed by a DNA polymerase, and they determine the segment of the DNA that is amplified. A. PCR starts with a double-stranded DNA, and each cycle of the reaction begins with a brief heat treatment to separate the two strands (Step 1). After strand separation, cooling of the DNA in the presence of a large excess of the two primer DNA oligonucleotides allows these primers to hybridize to complementary sequences in the two DNA strands (Step 2). This mixture is then incubated with DNA polymerase and the four deoxyribonucleoside triphosphates so that DNA is synthesized, starting from the two primers (Step 3). The entire cycle is then begun again by a heat treatment to separate the newly synthesized DNA strands. B. As the procedure is performed over and over again, the newly synthesized fragments serve as templates in their turn, and within a few cycles the predominant DNA is identical to the sequence bracketed by and including the two primers in the original template. Of the DNA put into the original reaction, only the sequence bracketed by the two primers is amplified because there are no primers attached anywhere else. In the example illustrated in (B), three cycles of reaction produce 16 DNA chains, 8 of which (boxed in brown) are the same length as and correspond exactly to one or the other strand of the original bracketed sequence shown at the far left; the other strands contain extra DNA downstream of the original sequence, which is replicated in the first few cycles. After three more cycles, 240 of the 256 DNA chains correspond exactly to the original bracketed sequence, and after several more cycles, essentially all of the DNA strands have this unique length. (Reproduced with permission from Alberts et al.[1])*

which would otherwise be difficult to detect. Combined immunoprecipitation and immunoblotting analysis is very efficient in analyzing the protein-protein interactions or determining the posttranslational modifications of proteins. In addition, immunoprecipitated proteins can be used as preparative steps for assays such as intrinsic or associated enzymatic activities. The success of immunoprecipitation is influenced by two major factors: the abundance of the protein in the original preparation and the specificity and affinity of the antibody for this protein.

DNA Microarray

Now that the human genome sequence is completed, the primary focus of biologists is rapidly shifting toward gaining an understanding of how genes function. One of the interesting findings about the human genome is that there are only approximately 25,000 to 30,000 protein-encoding genes. However, it is known that genes and their products function in a complicated and yet orchestrated fashion and that the surprisingly small number of genes from the genome sequence is sufficient to make a human being. Nonetheless, with the

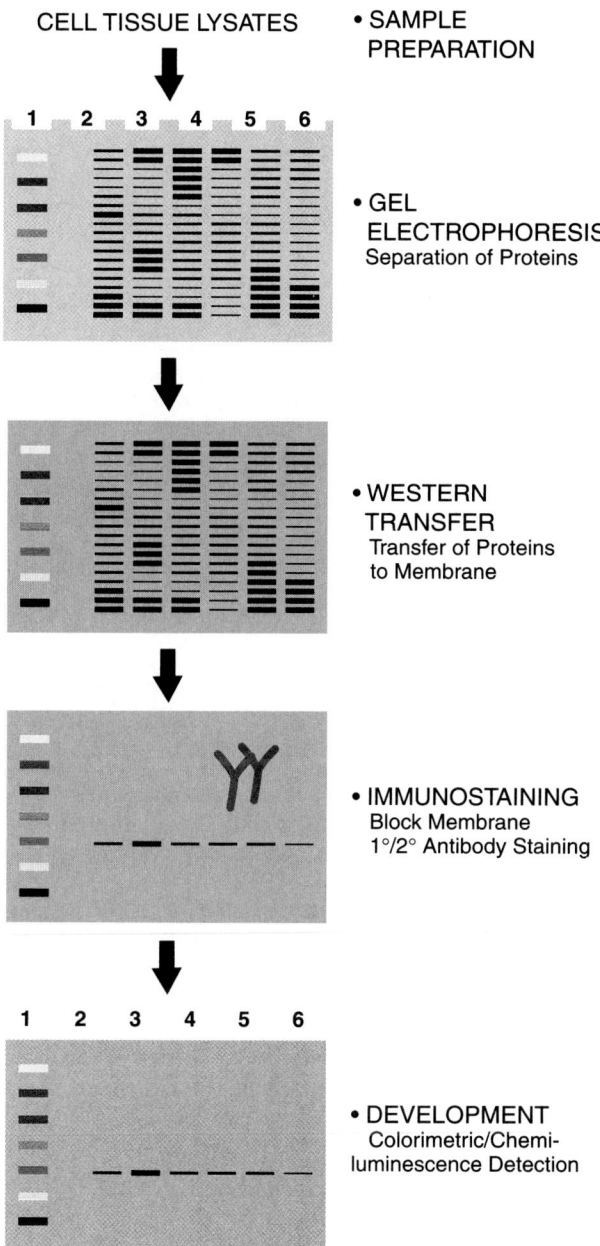

CELL TISSUE LYSATES

- SAMPLE PREPARATION

1 2 3 4 5 6

- GEL ELECTROPHORESIS
Separation of Proteins

- WESTERN TRANSFER
Transfer of Proteins to Membrane

- IMMUNOSTAINING
Block Membrane
1°/2° Antibody Staining

1 2 3 4 5 6

- DEVELOPMENT
Colorimetric/Chemi-luminescence Detection

FIG. 14-18. Immunoblotting. Proteins are prepared from cells or tissues, separated according to size by SDS-polyacrylamide gel electrophoresis, and transferred to a membrane filter. Detection of a protein of interest can be done by sequential incubation with a primary antibody directed against the protein, and then with an enzyme-conjugated secondary antibody that recognizes the primary antibody. Visualization of the protein is carried out by using colorimetric or luminescent substrates for the conjugated enzyme.

tens of thousands of genes present in the genome, traditional methods in molecular biology, which generally work on a one-gene-in-one-experiment basis, cannot generate the whole picture of genome function. In the past several years, a new technology called *DNA microarray* has attracted tremendous interest among biologists as well as clinicians. This technology promises to monitor the whole genome on a single chip so researchers can have a better picture of the interactions among thousands of genes simultaneously.

DNA microarray, also called gene chip, DNA chip, and gene array, refers to large sets of probes of known sequences orderly arranged on a small chip, enabling many hybridization reactions to be carried out in parallel in a small device (Fig. 14-20).[23] Like Southern and Northern hybridization, the underlying principle of this technology is the remarkable ability of nucleic acids to form a duplex between two strands with complementary base sequences. DNA microarray provides a medium for matching known and unknown DNA samples based on base-pairing rules, and automating the process of identifying the unknowns. Microarrays require specialized robotics and imaging equipment that spot the samples on a glass or nylon substrate, carry out the hybridization, and analyze the data generated. DNA microarrays containing different sets of genes from a variety of organisms are now commercially available, allowing biologists to simply purchase the chips and perform hybridization and data collection. The massive scale of microarray experiments requires the aid of computers. They are used during the capturing of the image of the hybridized target, the conversion of the image into usable measures of the extent of hybridization, and the interpretation of the extent of hybridization into a meaningful measure of the amount of the complementary sequence in the target. Some data-analysis packages are available commercially or can be found in the core facility of certain institutions.

DNA microarray technology has produced many significant results in quite different areas of application. There are two major application forms for the technology: identification of sequence (gene/gene mutation) and determination of expression level (abundance) of genes. For example, analysis of genomic DNA detects amplifications and deletions found in human tumors. Differential gene expression analysis has also uncovered networks of genes differentially present in cancers that cannot be distinguished by conventional means.

Cell Manipulations

Cell Culture

Cell culture has become one of the most powerful techniques, as cultured cells are being used in a diversity of biologic fields ranging from biochemistry to molecular and cellular biology.[24] Through their ability to be maintained in vitro, cells can be manipulated by the introduction of genes of interest (cell transfection) and be transferred into in vivo biologic receivers (cell transplantation) to study the biologic effect of the interested genes (Fig. 14-21). In general, cell culture procedures are simple and straightforward. In the laboratory, cells are cultured either as a monolayer (in which cells grow as one layer on culture dishes) or in suspension.

It is important to know the wealth of information concerning cell culturing before attempting the procedure. For example, conditions of culture will depend on the cell types to be cultured (e.g., origins of the cells such as epithelial or fibroblasts, or primary versus immortalized/transformed cells). It is also necessary to use special culture medium that has been used to establish the cell line (if it is a cell line), including the type and concentration of serum used to maintain the growth of cells in vitro. If primary cells are derived from human patients or animals, some commercial resources have a variety of culture media available for testing. Generally, cells are manipulated in a sterile hood and the working surfaces are wiped with 80% EtOH solution. Cultured cells are maintained in a humidified CO_2 incubator at 37°C and need to be examined daily under an inverted microscope to check for possible contamination and confluency (the area cells occupy on the dish). As a general rule, cells should be fed with fresh medium every 2 to 3 days and split when they reach confluency. Depending upon the growth rate of cells, the actual time and number of plates required to split cells in

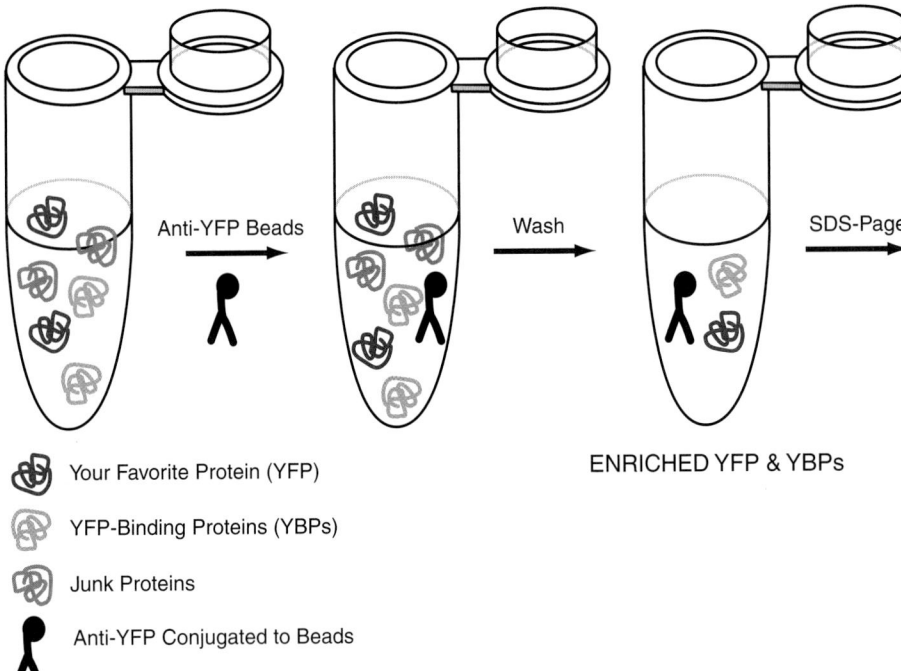

Your Favorite Protein (YFP)

YFP-Binding Proteins (YBPs)

Junk Proteins

Anti-YFP Conjugated to Beads

ENRICHED YFP & YBPs

FIG. 14-19. Immunoprecipitation. Proteins prepared from cells or tissues can be enriched using an antibody directed against them. The antibody is first conjugated to agarose beads and then incubated with protein mixture. Owing to the specific high-affinity interaction between antibody and its antigen (the protein), the antigen-antibody complex can be collected on beads by centrifugation. The immunoprecipitated protein can then be analyzed by immunoblotting. Alternatively, if proteins are radiolabeled in cells or tissues, detection of immunoprecipitated proteins can be achieved by simple SDS-PAGE electrophoresis followed by autoradiography.

two varies from cell line to cell line. Splitting a monolayer requires the detachment of cells from plates by using a trypsin treatment, of which concentration and time period vary depending on cell lines. If cultured cells grow continuously in suspension, they are split or subcultured by dilution.

Because cell lines may change their properties when cultured, it is not possible to maintain cell lines in culture indefinitely. Therefore it is essential to store cells at various time passages for future use. The common procedure is to use cryopreservation. The solution for cryopreservation is fetal calf serum (FCS) containing 10% dimethyl sulfoxide (DMSO) or glycerol, stored in liquid nitrogen ($-196°C$). Cells can be stored for many years using this method.

Cell Transfection

Cells are cultured for two reasons: to maintain and to manipulate them (see Fig. 14-21). The transfer of foreign macromolecules, such as nucleic acid, into living cells provides an efficient method for studying a variety of cellular processes and functions at the molecular level. DNA transfection has become an important tool for studying the regulation and function of genes. The cDNA to be expressed should be in a plasmid vector, behind an appropriate promoter working in mammalian cells (e.g., the constitutively active cytomegalovirus promoter or inducible promoter). Depending on the cell type, many ways of introducing DNA into mammalian cells have been developed. Commonly used approaches include calcium phosphate, electroporation, liposome-mediated transfection, the nonliposomal formulation, and the use of viral vectors. These methods have shown variable success when attempting to transfect a wide variety of cells. Transfection can be performed in the presence or absence of serum. It is suggested to test the transfection efficiency of cell lines of interest by comparing transfection with several different approaches. For a detailed transfection protocol, it is best to follow the manufacturer's instructions for the particular reagent. General considerations for a successful transfection depend on several parameters, such as the quality and quantity of DNA and cell culture (type of cell and growth phase). To minimize variations

in both of these in transfection experiments, it is best to use cells that are healthy, proliferate well, and are plated at a constant density. After DNA is introduced into the cells, it is normally maintained epitopically in cells and will be diluted while host cells undergo cell division. Therefore, functional assays should be performed 24 to 72 hours after transfection, also termed *transient transfection*. In many applications, it is important to study the long-term effects of DNA in cells by stable transfection. Stable cell clones can be selected for DNA integration into the host cell genome, when plasmids carry an antibiotic-resistant marker. In the presence of antibiotics, only those cells that continuously carry the antibiotic-resistant marker (after generations of cell division) can survive. One application of stable transfection is the generation of transgenic or knockout mouse models, in which the transgene has to be integrated in the mouse genome. Stable cells can also be transplanted into host organs.

Genetic Manipulations

Understanding how genes control the growth and differentiation of the mammalian organism has been the most challenging topic of modern research. This challenge derives from the curiosity to know how a human being is generated and how it has evolved from simpler organisms. It is also essential for us to understand how genetic mutations and chemicals lead to the pathologic condition of human bodies. The knowledge and ability to change the genetic program will inevitably make a great impact on society and have far-reaching effects on how we think of ourselves.

The mouse has become firmly established as the primary experimental model for studying how genes control mammalian development. Genetically altered mice are powerful model systems in which to study the function and regulation of genes.[25] The gene function can be studied by creating mutant mice through homologous recombination (gene knockout). A gene of interest can also be introduced into the mouse (transgenic mouse) in order to study its effect on development or diseases. As mouse models do not precisely represent human biology, genetic manipulations of human somatic or embryonic stem cells provide a great means for the understanding

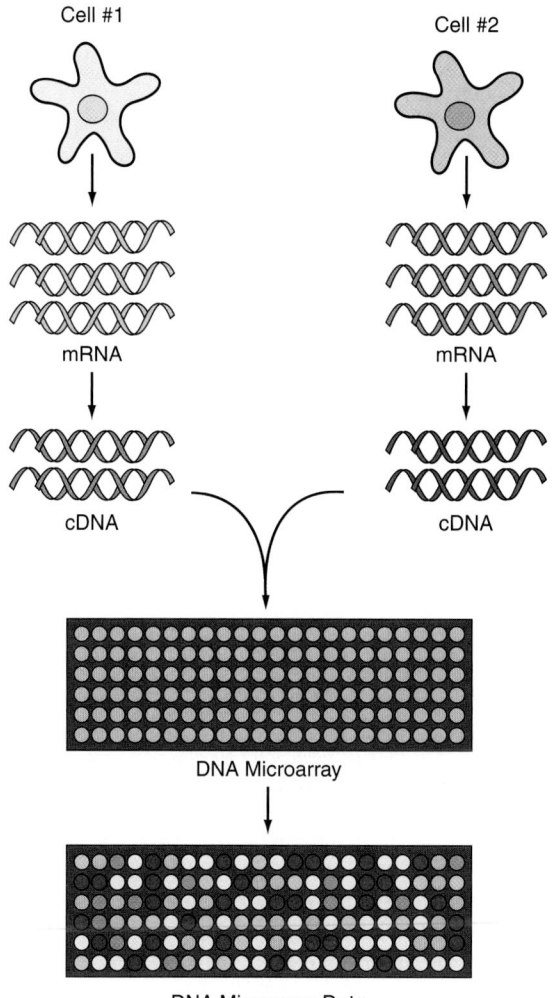

Cell #1   Cell #2

mRNA   mRNA

cDNA   cDNA

DNA Microarray

DNA Microarray Data

FIG. 14-20. DNA microarrays. DNA microarrays, also referred to as gene chips, have arrayed oligonucleotides or cDNAs corresponding to tens or hundreds of distinct genes. DNA microarray is used to comparatively analyze gene expression in different cells or tissues. mRNAs extracted from different sources are converted into cDNAs, which are then labeled with different fluorescent dyes. The two fluorescent cDNA probes are mixed and hybridized to the same DNA microarrays. The ratio of dark brown to light brown fluorescence at each spot on the chip represents the relative expression of levels of that gene between two different cells. In the example shown in the figure, cDNA from cell #1 is labeled with dark brown fluorescence and the cell #2 light brown fluorescence. On the microarray, dark brown spots demonstrate that the gene in cell sample #1 is expressed at a higher level than the corresponding gene in cell sample #2. The light brown spots indicate that the gene in cell sample #1 is also expressed at a higher level than the corresponding gene in cell sample #2. Beige spots represent equal expression of the gene in both cell samples.

of the molecular networks in human cells. In all cases, the gene to be manipulated must first be cloned. Gene cloning has been made easy by recombinant DNA technology and the availability of human and mouse genomes (see the section on the human genome, above). The following section briefly describes the technologies and the principles behind them.

Transgenic Mice

During the past 20 years, DNA cloning and other techniques have allowed the introduction of new genetic material into the mouse germline. As early as 1980, the first genetic material was

successfully introduced into the mouse germline by using pronuclear microinjection of DNA (Fig. 14-22). These animals, called *transgenic,* contain foreign DNA within their genomes. In simple terms, a transgenic mouse is created by the microinjection of DNA into the one-celled mouse embryo, allowing the efficient introduction of cloned genes into the developing mouse somatic tissues, as well as into the germline.

Designs of a Transgene. The transgenic technique has proven to be extremely important for basic investigations of gene regulation, creation of animal models of human disease, and genetic engineering of livestock. The design of a transgene construct is a simple task. Like constructs used in cell transfection, a simple transgene construct consists of a protein-encoding gene and a promoter which precedes it. The most common applications for the use of transgenic mice are similar to those in the cell culture system: (1) to study the functions of proteins encoded by the transgene, and (2) to analyze the tissue-specific and developmental-stage–specific activity of a gene promoter. Examples of the first application include overexpression of oncogenes, growth factors, hormones, and other key regulatory genes, as well as genes of viral origins. Overexpression of the transgene normally represents gain-of-function mutations. The tissue distribution or expression of a transgene is determined primarily by *cis*-acting promoter enhancer elements within or in the immediate vicinity of the genes themselves. Thus, controlled expression of the transgene can be made possible by using an inducible or tissue-specific promoter. Furthermore, transgenic mice carrying dominant negative mutations of a regulatory gene also have been generated. For example, a truncated growth factor receptor that can bind to the ligand, but loses its catalytic activity when expressed in mice, can block the growth factor binding to the endogenous protein. In this way, the transgenic mice exhibit a loss of function of phenotype, possibly resembling the knockout of the endogenous gene. The second application of the transgenic expression is to analyze the gene promoter of interest. The gene promoter of interest is normally fused to a reporter gene that encodes β-galactosidase (also called LacZ), luciferase, or green fluorescence protein (GFP). Chemical staining of LacZ activity or detection of chemiluminescence/fluorescence can easily visualize the expression of the reporter gene. The amount of the reporter gene activity represents the activity of the promoter, and thus reporter activities are tightly correlated to expression of the gene in which the promoter is used to drive the reporter gene expression.

Production of Transgenic Mice. The success of generating transgenic mice is largely dependent on the proper quality and concentration of the DNA supplied for microinjection. For DNA to be microinjected into mouse embryos it should be linearized by restriction digestion to increase the chance of proper transgene integration. Concentration of DNA should be accurately determined. Mice that develop from injected eggs are often termed *founder* mice.

Genotyping of Transgenic Mice. The screening of founder mice and the transgenic lines derived from the founders is accomplished by determining the integration of the injected gene into the genome. This is normally achieved by performing PCR or Southern blot analysis with a small amount of DNA extracted from the mouse tail. Once a given founder mouse is identified to be transgenic, it will be mated to begin establishing a transgenic line.

Analysis of Phenotype of Transgenic Mice. Phenotypes of transgenic mice are dictated by both the expression pattern and biologic functions of the transgene. Depending on the promoter

A

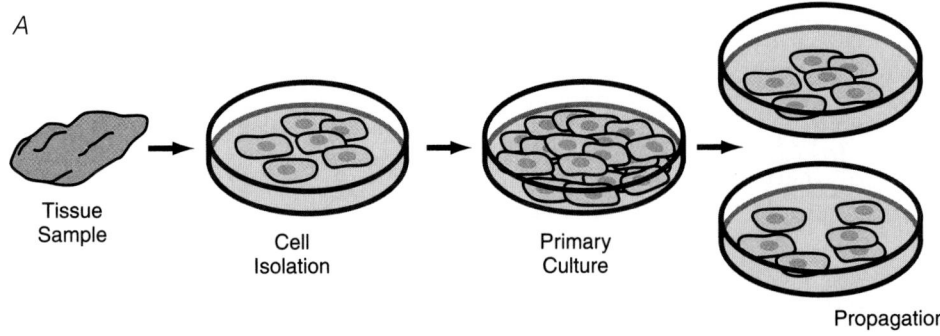

B

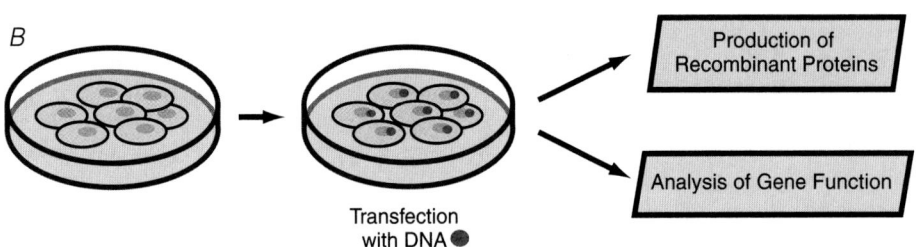

FIG. 14-21. *Cell culture and transfection. A. Primary cells can be isolated from tissues and cultured in medium for a limited period of time. After genetic manipulations to overcome the cell aging process, primary cells can be immortalized into cell lines for long-term culture. B. DNA can be introduced into cells to produce recombinant gene products or to analyze the biologic functions of the gene.*

and the transgene, phenotypes can be predictable or unpredictable. Elucidation of the functions of the transgene-encoded protein in vitro often offers some clue to what the protein might do in vivo. When a constitutively active promoter is used to drive the expression of transgenes, mice should express the gene in every tissue; however, this mouse model may not allow the identification and study of the earliest events in disease pathogenesis. Ideally, the use of tissue-specific or inducible promoter allows one to determine if the pathogenic protein leads to a reversible or irreversible disease process. For example, rat insulin promoter can target transgene expression exclusively in the beta cells of pancreatic islets. The phenotype of insulin promoter-mediated transgenic mice is projected to affect the function of human beta cells.

Gene Knockout in Mice

The isolation and genetic manipulation of embryonic stem (ES) cells represents one of the most important milestones for modern genetic technologies. Several unique properties of these ES cells, such as the pluripotency to differentiate into different tissues in an embryo, make them an efficient vehicle for introducing genetic alterations into this species. Thus, this technology provides an important breakthrough, making it possible to genetically manipulate

ES cells in a controlled way in the culture dish and then introduce the mutation into the germline (Fig. 14-23). This not only makes mouse genetics a powerful approach for addressing important gene functions but also identifies the mouse as a great system to model human disease.

Targeting Vector. The basic concept in building a target vector to knock out a gene is to use two segments of homologous sequence to a gene of interest that flank a part of the gene essential for functions (e.g., the coding region). In the target vector, a positive selectable marker (e.g., the *neo* gene) is placed between the homology arms. Upon the homologous recombination between the arms of the vector and the corresponding genomic regions of the gene of interest in ES cells, the positive selectable marker will replace the essential segment of the target gene, thus creating a null allele. In addition, a negative selectable marker also can be used alone or in combination with the positive selectable marker, but must be placed outside of the homologous arms to enrich for homologous recombination. To create a conditional knockout (i.e., gene knockout in a spatiotemporal fashion), site-specific recombinases such as the popular cre-loxP system are used. If the consensus loxP sequences that are recognized by cre recombinases are properly designed into targeting loci, controlled expression of the recombinase as a transgene

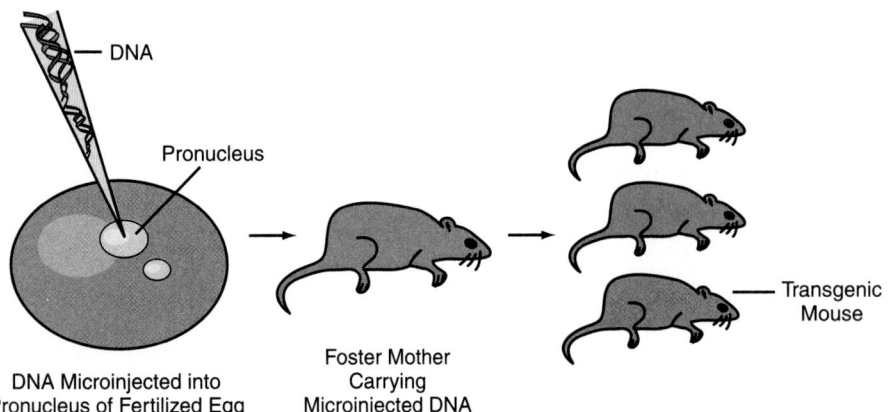

FIG. 14-22. *Transgenic mouse technology. DNA is microinjected into a pronucleus of a fertilized egg, which is then transplanted into a foster mother. The microinjected egg develops offspring mice. Incorporation of the injected DNA into offspring is indicated by the different coat color of offspring mice.*

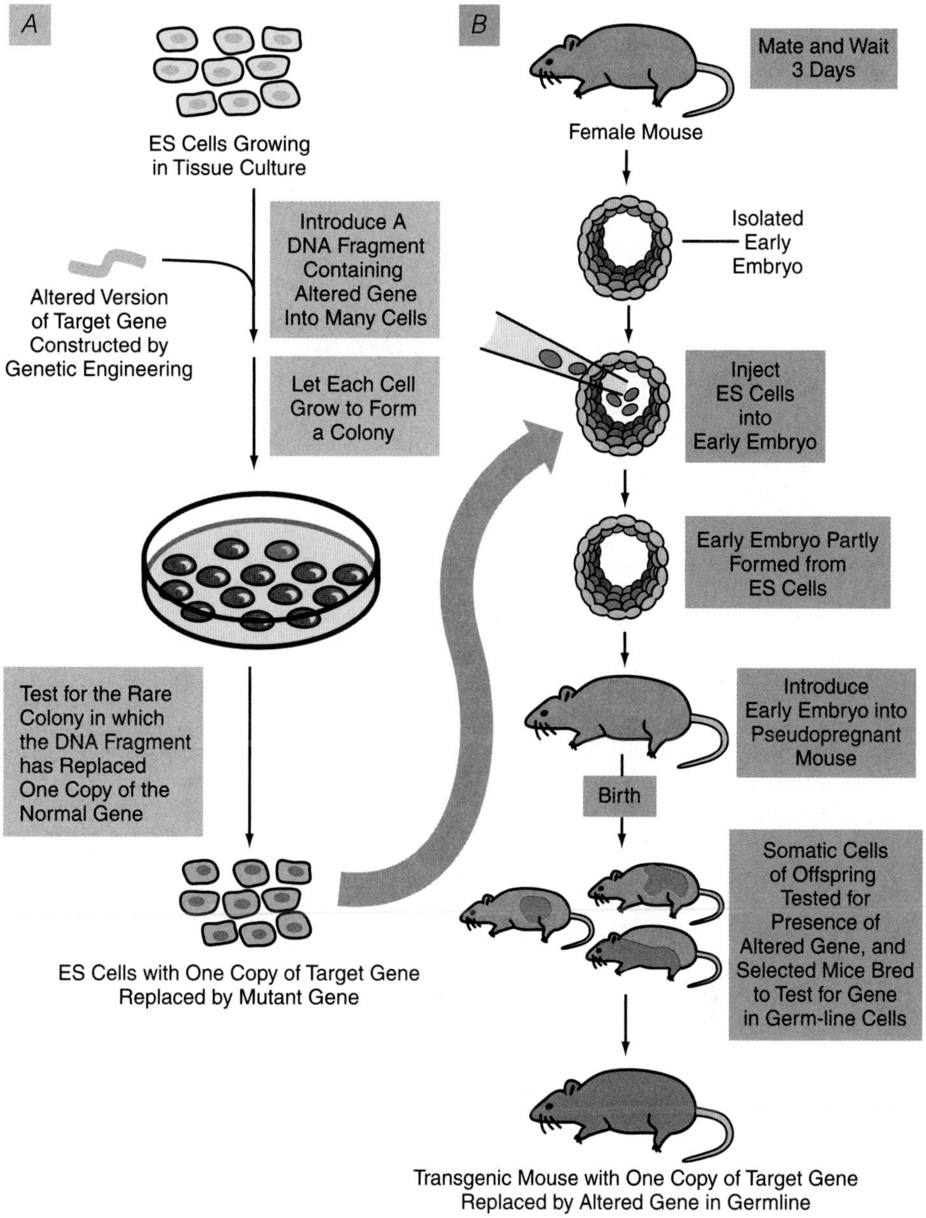

FIG. 14-23. Knockout mouse technology. Summary of the procedures used for making gene replacements in mice. In the first step (A), an altered version of the gene is introduced into cultured ES (embryonic stem) cells. Only a few rare ES cells will have their corresponding normal genes replaced by the altered gene through a homologous recombination event. Although the procedure is often laborious, these rare cells can be identified and cultured to produce many descendants, each of which carries an altered gene in place of one of its two normal corresponding genes. In the next step of the procedure (B), these altered ES cells are injected into a very early mouse embryo; the cells are incorporated into the growing embryo, and a mouse produced by such an embryo will contain some somatic cells that carry the altered gene. Some of these mice will also contain germline cells that contain the altered gene. When bred with a normal mouse, some of the progeny of these mice will contain the altered gene in all of their cells. If two such mice are in turn bred (not shown), some of the progeny will contain two altered genes (one on each chromosome) in all of their cells. If the original gene alteration completely inactivates the function of the gene, these mice are known as knockout mice. When such mice are missing genes that function during development, they often die with specific defects long before they reach adulthood. These defects are carefully analyzed to help decipher the normal function of the missing gene. (Reproduced with permission from Alberts et al.[1])

can result in the site-specific recombination at the right time and in the right place (i.e., cell type or tissue). This method is markedly useful to prevent developmental compensations and to introduce null mutations in the adult mouse that would otherwise be lethal. Overall, this cre-loxP system allows for spatial and temporal control over transgene expression and takes advantage of inducers with minimal pleiotropic effects.

Introduction of the Targeting Vector into ES Cells. ES cell lines can be obtained from other investigators, commercial sources, or established from blastocyst-stage embryos. To maintain ES cells at their full developmental potential, optimal growth conditions should be provided in culture. If culture conditions are inappropriate or inadequate, ES cells may acquire genetic lesions or alter their gene expression patterns, and consequently decrease their pluripotency. Excellent protocols are available in public domains or in mouse facilities in most institutions.

To alter the genome of ES cells, the targeting vector DNA is then transfected into ES cells. Electroporation is the most widely used and the most efficient transfection method for ES cells. Similar procedures for stable cell transfection are used for selecting ES cells that carry the targeting vector. High-quality, targeting-vector DNA free of contaminating chemicals is first linearized and then electroporated into ES cells. Stable ES cells are selected in the presence of a positive selectable antibiotic drug. After a certain period of time and depending on the type of antibiotics, all sensitive cells die and the resistant cells grow into individual colonies of the appropriate size for subcloning by picking. It is extremely important to minimize the time during which ES cells are in culture between selection and injection into blastocysts. Before injecting the ES cells, DNA is prepared from ES colonies to screen for positive ES cells that exhibit the correct integration or homologous recombination of the targeting vector. Positive ES colonies are then expanded and used for creation of chimeras.

Creation of the Chimera. A chimeric organism is one in which cells originate from more than one embryo. Here, chimeric mice are denoted as those that contain some tissues from the ES cells

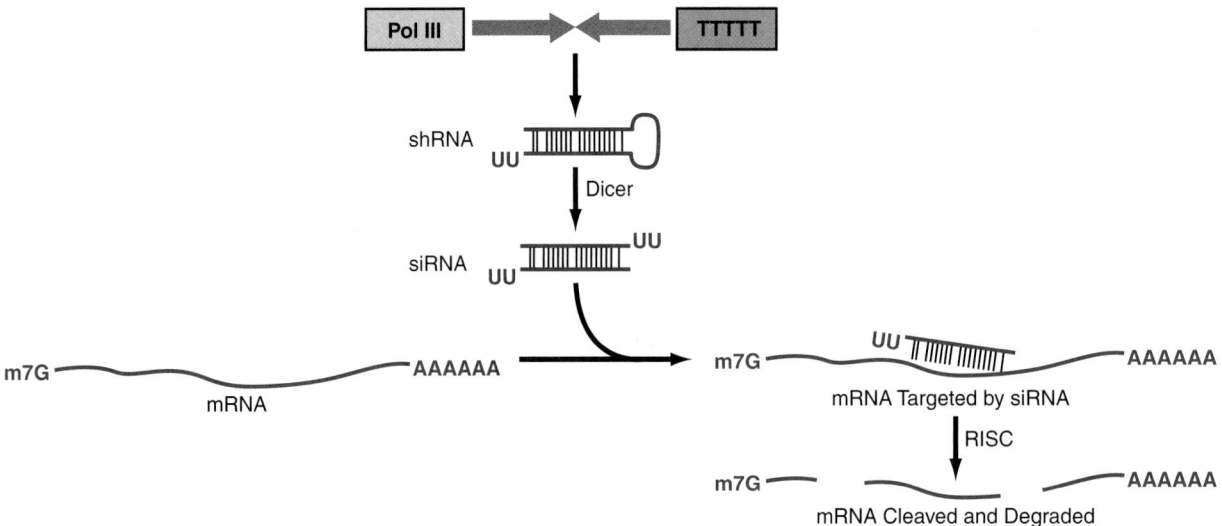

FIG. 14-24. RNA inference in mammalian cells. Small interfering RNA (siRNA) can be produced from a polymerase III–driven expression vector. Such a vector first synthesizes a 19–29 nt dsRNA stem and a loop (labeled as shRNA in the figure), and then the RNase complex called *Dicer* processes the hairpin RNA into a small dsRNA (labeled as siRNA in the figure). siRNA can be chemically synthesized and directly introduced into the target cell. In the cell, through RNA-induced silencing complex (RISC), siRNA recognizes and degrades target mRNAs.

with an altered genome. When these ES cells give rise to the lineage of the germ layer, the germ cells carrying the altered genome can be passed on to the offspring, thus creating the germline transmission from ES cells. There are two methods for introducing ES cells into preimplantation-stage embryos: injection and aggregation. The injection of embryonic cells directly into the cavity of blastocysts is one of the fundamental methods for generating chimeras, but aggregation chimeras also have become an important alternative for transmitting the ES cell genome into mice. The mixture of recognizable markers (e.g., coat color) that are specific for the donor mouse and ES cells can be used to identify chimeric mice. However, most experimenters probably use existing mouse core facilities already established in some institutions, or contract a commercial vendor for the creation of a chimera.

Genotyping and Phenotyping of Knockout Animals. The next step is to analyze whether germline transmission of targeted mutation occurs in mice. DNA from a small amount of tissue from offspring of the chimera is extracted and subjected to genomic PCR or Southern blot DNA hybridization. Positive mice (i.e., those with properly integrated targeting vector into the genome) will be used for the propagation of more knockout mice for phenotype analysis. When the knockout genes are crucial for early embryogenesis, mice often die in utero, an occurrence called *embryonic lethality*. When this happens, only the phenotype of the homozygous (both alleles ablated) knockout mouse embryos and the phenotype of the heterozygous (only one allele ablated) adult mice can be studied. Since most are interested in the phenotype of adult mice, in particular when using mice as disease models, it is recommended to create the conditional knockout using the cre-loxP system so that the gene of interest can be knocked out at will.

To date, more than 5000 genes have been disrupted by homologous recombination and transmitted through the germline. The phenotypic studies of these mice provide ample information on the functions of these genes in growth and differentiation of organisms, and during development of human diseases.

RNA Interference

While gene ablation in animal models provides an important means to understand the in vivo functions of genes of interest, animal models may not adequately represent human biology. Alternatively, gene targeting can be used to knock out genes in human cells, including human embryonic stem cells. A number of recent advances have made gene targeting in somatic cells as easy as in murine embryonic stem cells.[25] However, gene targeting (knocking out both alleles) in somatic cells is a time-consuming process.

Development of RNA interference (RNAi) technology in the past few years has provided a more promising approach to understanding the biologic functions of human genes in human cells.[26] RNAi is an ancient natural mechanism by which small, double-stranded RNA (dsRNA) acts as a guide for an enzyme complex that destroys complementary RNA and downregulates gene expression in a sequence-specific manner. Although the mechanism by which dsRNA suppresses gene expression is not entirely understood, experimental data provide important insights. In nonmammalian systems such as *Drosophila,* it appears that longer dsRNA is processed into 21–23 nt dsRNA (called *small interfering RNA* or siRNA) by an enzyme called *Dicer* containing RNase III motifs. The siRNA apparently then acts as a guide sequence within a multicomponent nuclease complex to target complementary mRNA for degradation. Since long dsRNA induces a potent antiviral response pathway in mammalian cells, short siRNAs are used to perform gene silencing experiments in mammalian cells (Fig. 14-24).

For siRNA studies in mammalian cells, researchers have used two 21-mer RNAs with 19 complementary nucleotides and 3′ terminal noncomplementary dimers of thymidine or uridine. The antisense siRNA strand is fully complementary to the mRNA target sequence. Target sequences for an siRNA are identified visually or by software. The target 19 nucleotides should be compared to an appropriate genome database to eliminate any sequences with significant homology to other genes. Those sequences that appear to be specific to the gene of interest are the potential siRNA target sites. A few of these target sites are selected for siRNA design. The antisense siRNA strand is the reverse complement of the target sequence. The sense strand of the siRNA is the same sequence as the target mRNA sequence. A deoxythymidine dimer is routinely incorporated at the 3' end of the sense strand siRNA, though it is unknown whether this noncomplementary dinucleotide is important for the activity of siRNAs.

There are two ways to introduce siRNA to knock down gene expression in human cells:

1. RNA transfection: siRNA can be made chemically or using an in vitro transcription method. Like DNA oligos, chemically synthesized siRNA oligos can be commercially ordered. However, synthetic siRNA is expensive and several siRNAs may have to be tried before a particular gene is successfully silenced. In vitro transcription provides a more economic approach. Both short and long RNA can be synthesized using bacteriophage RNA polymerase T7, T3, or SP6. In the case of long dsRNAs, RNase such as recombinant Dicers will be used to process the long dsRNA into a mixture of 21–23 nt siRNA. siRNA oligos or mixtures can be transfected into a few characterized cell lines such as HeLa (human cervical carcinoma) and 293T cells (human kidney carcinoma). Transfection of siRNA directly into primary cells may be difficult.
2. DNA transfection: Expression vectors for expressing siRNA have been made using RNA polymerase III promoters such as U6 and H1. These promoters precisely transcribe a hairpin structure of dsRNA, which will be processed into siRNA in the cell (see Fig. 14-24). Therefore, properly-designed DNA oligos corresponding to the desired siRNA will be inserted downstream of the U6 or H1 promoter. There are two advantages of the siRNA expression vectors over siRNA oligos. First, it is easier to transfect DNA into cells. Second, stable populations of cells can be generated that maintain the long-term silencing of target genes. Furthermore, the siRNA expression cassette can be incorporated into a retroviral or adenoviral vector to provide a wide spectrum of applications in gene therapy.

There has been a fast and fruitful development of RNAi tools for in vitro and in vivo use in mammals. These novel approaches, together with future developments, will be crucial to put RNAi technology to use for effective disease therapy or to exert the awesome power of mammalian genetics. Therefore, the applications of RNAi to human health are enormous. siRNA can be applied as a new tool for sequence-specific regulation of gene expression in functional genomics and biomedical studies. With the availability of the human genome sequences, RNAi approaches hold tremendous promise for unleashing the dormant potential of sequenced genomes.

Practical applications of RNAi will possibly result in new therapeutic interventions. In 2002, the concept of using siRNA in battling infectious diseases and carcinogenesis was proven effective. These include notable successes in blocking replication of viruses, such as human immunodeficiency virus (HIV), hepatitis B virus (HBV), and hepatitis C virus (HCV), in cultured cells using siRNA targeted at the viral genome or the human gene encoding viral receptors. RNAi has been shown to antagonize the effects of HCV in mouse models. In cancers, silencing of oncogenes such as c-Myc or Ras can slow down the proliferation rate of cancer cells. Finally, siRNA also has potential applications for some dominant genetic disorders.

The 21st century, already heralded as the "century of the gene," carries great promise for alleviating suffering from disease and improving human health. On the whole, completion of the human genome blueprint, the promise of gene therapy, and the existence of stem cells has captured the imagination of the public and the biomedical community for good reason. Aside from their potential in curing human diseases, these emerging technologies have also provoked many political, economic, religious, and ethical discussions. As more is discerned about the technological advances, more

attention must also be paid to concerns for their inherent risks and social implications. Surgeons must take the opportunity to participate together with scientists to make realistic promises and to face the new era of modern medicine.

References

1. Alberts B, Johnson A, Lewis J, et al: *Molecular Biology of the Cell,* 4th ed. New York: Garland Science, 2002.
2. Watson JD, Crick FH: Molecular structure of nucleic acids; a structure for deoxyribose nucleic acid. *Nature* 171:737, 1953.
3. Mendel G: Versuche über Planzen-Hybriden. *Verhandlungen des naturforschenden Vereines, Abhandlungen.* Brünn: 4, 3, 1866.
4. Carey M, Smale ST: *Transcriptional Regulation in Eukaryotes.* New York: Cold Spring Harbor Laboratory Press, 2000.
5. Wolfsberg TG, Wetterstrand KA, Guyer MS, et al: A User's Guide to the Human Genome. *Nature Genetics* Supplement, 2002. (also see the Nature website: http://www.nature.com/nature/focus/humangenome/)
6. U.S. Department of Energy: Genomics and its impact on science and society: The human genome project and beyond. Published online by Human Genome Management Information System (HGMIS): http://www.ornl.gov/hgmis/publicat/primer, March 2003.
7. Simpson RJ: *Protein and Proteomics.* New York: Cold Spring Harbor Laboratory Press, 2003.
8. Hanash S: Disease proteomics. *Nature* 422:226, 2003.
9. Ptashne M, Gann A: *Genes & Signals.* New York: Cold Spring Harbor Laboratory Press, 2002.
10. Pawson T, Nash P: Assembly of cell regulatory systems through protein interaction domains. *Science* 300:445, 2003.
11. Lizcano JM, Alessi DR: The insulin signalling pathway. *Curr Biol* 12:R236, 2002.
12. Derynck R, Feng XH: TGF-β receptor signaling. *Biochim Biophys Acta* 1333:F105, 1997.
13. Hanahan D, Weinberg RA: The hallmarks of cancer. *Cell* 100:57, 2000.
14. Zwick E, Bange J, Ullrich A: Receptor tyrosine kinases as targets for anticancer drugs. *Trends Mol Med* 8:17, 2002.
15. McNeil C: Heceptin raises its sights beyond advanced breast cancer. *J Natl Cancer Inst* 90:882, 1998.
16. Druker BJ, Tamura S, Buchdunger E, et al: Effects of a selective inhibitor of the Abl tyrosine kinase on the growth of Bcr-Abl positive cells. *Nat Med* 2:561, 1996.
17. Kiessling AA, Anderson SC: *Human Embryonic Stem Cells: An Introduction to the Science and Therapeutic Potential.* Boston: Jones & Bartlett Pub, 2003.
18. Cohen SN, Chang AC, Boyer HW, et al: Construction of biologically functional bacterial plasmids in vitro. *Proc Natl Acad Sci USA* 70:3240, 1973.
19. Sambrook J: *Molecular Cloning, A Laboratory Manual,* 3rd ed. New York: Cold Spring Harbor Laboratory Press, 2001.
20. Ausubel FM, Brent R, Kingston RE, et al: *Current Protocols in Molecular Biology.* New York: John Wiley & Sons, 2003.
21. Southern EM: Detection of specific sequences among DNA fragments separated by gel electrophoresis. *J Mol Biol* 98:503, 1975.
22. Mullis K, Faloona F, Scharf S, et al: Specific enzymatic amplification of DNA in vitro: The polymerase chain reaction. *Cold Spring Harb Symp Quant Biol* 51:263, 1986.
23. Bowtell D, Sambrook J: *DNA Microarrays, A Molecular Cloning Manual.* New York: Cold Spring Harbor Laboratory Press, 2003.
24. Bonifacino JS, Dasso M, Harford JB, et al: *Current Protocols in Cell Biology.* New York: John Wiley & Sons, 2003.
25. Nagy A, Gertsenstein M, Vintersten K, et al: *Manipulating The Mouse Embryo, A Laboratory Manual,* 3rd ed. New York: Cold Spring Harbor Laboratory Press, 2003.
26. Hannon GJ: *RNAi, A Guide To Gene Silencing.* New York: Cold Spring Harbor Laboratory Press, 2003.

PART II
SPECIFIC CONSIDERATIONS

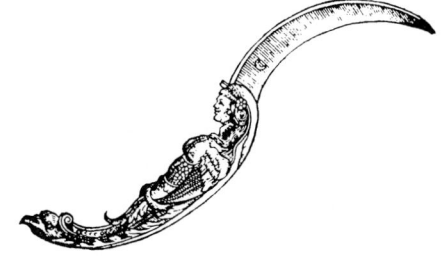

CHAPTER 15

Skin and Subcutaneous Tissue

Scott L. Hansen, Stephen J. Mathes, and David M. Young

The skin is the largest and among the most complex organs of the body. Its uniform appearance belies its great variation from region to region of the body and the complex organization and interaction of the many different cells and matrices of the skin. Although the skin functions simply as a protective barrier to interface with our environment, its structure and physiology are complex.[1]

In its role as an environmental buffer, the skin protects against most noxious agents, such as chemicals (by the impermeability of the epidermis), solar radiation (by means of pigmentation), infectious agents (through efficient immunosurveillance), and physically deforming forces (by the durability of the dermis). Its efficient ability to conserve or disperse heat makes the skin the major organ responsible for thermoregulation. To direct all these functions, the skin has a highly specialized nervous structure.

These various functions are better served by different components of skin, so that teleologically regional variation develops. The palms and soles are particularly thick, to bear weight. The fingertips have the highest density of sensory innervation and allow for intricate tasks. Even the lines of the skin, first described by Langer, are oriented perpendicularly to the long axis of muscles to allow the greatest degree of stretching and contraction without deformity.

The relative ease of observing and obtaining skin specimens for examination and experiments has made the skin one of the best-studied tissues of the human body. Thus, the study of skin is not just the subject of the field of dermatology, but also has launched the fields of immunology, transplantation, and wound healing.[2,3] Although this chapter emphasizes surgically treated diseases of the skin, it is important for students of surgery to be familiar with the basic physiology and structure of skin because many of the future advances in medicine will come from these studies.

ANATOMY AND PHYSIOLOGY

Traditionally the skin has been divided into three layers: the epidermis, the basement membrane, and the dermis (Fig. 15-1). The

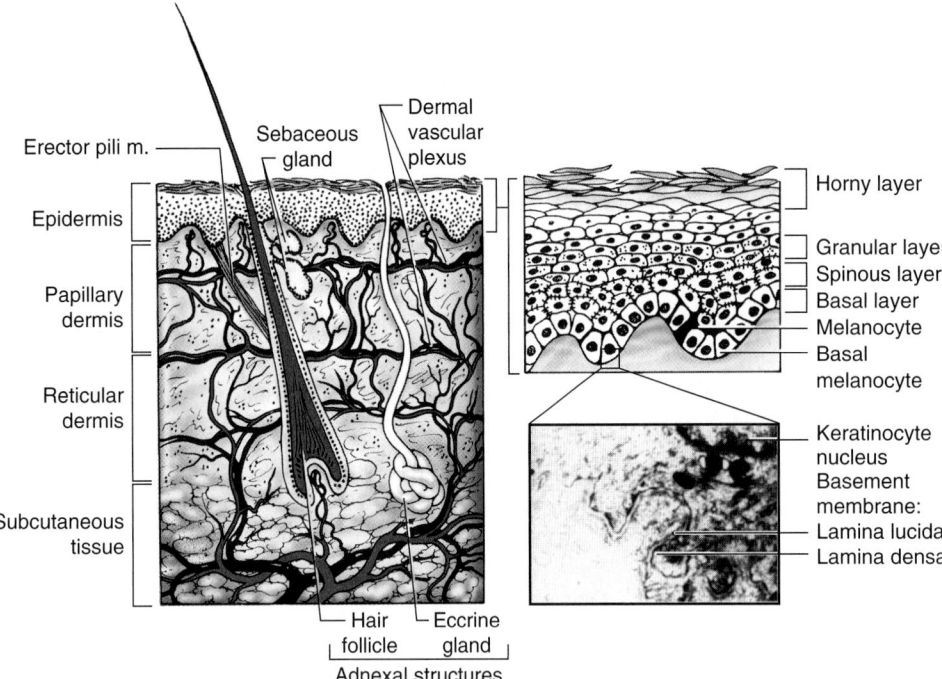

FIG. 15-1. *The histologic section of skin (left) demonstrates a complex organization of cells, connective tissue, blood vessels, and adnexal structures. The drawing (upper right) depicts the orderly maturation of keratinocytes in the epidermis. The electron micrograph (lower right) shows details of the basement membrane, which is the interface between the epidermis and the dermis.*

epidermis is composed mainly of cells, with very little extracellular matrix. Each cell type serves a specific barrier function. Keratinocytes provide a mechanical barrier, melanocytes provide a barrier to radiation, and Langerhans' cells provide an immunologic barrier.[4] The dermis contains mostly extracellular matrix, providing support for nerves, vasculature, and adnexal structures. The dermis allows skin to resist deforming forces and return to its resting state, thus providing durability. The basement membrane is a specialized structure that anchors the epidermis to the dermis.[5]

The main cell type in the epidermis is the keratinocyte. The deep, mitotically active, basal cells are a single-cell layer of the least-differentiated keratinocytes. Some multiplying cells leave the basal layer and begin to travel upward. In the spinous layer, they lose the ability to undergo mitosis. These differentiated cells start to accumulate keratohyalin granules in the granular layer. Finally, in the horny layer, the keratinocytes age, the once-numerous intercellular connections disappear, and the dead cells are shed. Using radioactive and fluorescence labeling, experiments show the keratinocyte transit time to be between 40 and 56 days. The control of keratinocyte multiplication and subsequent maturation is an area of active study and may clarify the complex mechanism of cellular differentiation. Melanocytes migrate to the epidermis from precursor cells in the neural crest.[6] They lie scattered beneath basal cells and have dendritic processes that reach out to surrounding keratinocytes. They number approximately 1 for every 35 keratinocytes. The melanocytes produce the pigment melanin from tyrosine and cysteine. The pigment is packaged in melanosomes and transported to the tips of the dendritic processes. The tips are sheared off (apocopation) and then phagocytized by the keratinocyte, thus transferring the pigment to the keratinocyte. Once in the keratinocyte, they aggregate on the superficial side of the nucleus in an umbrella shape. The density of melanocytes is constant among individuals of different skin color. The rate of melanin production, transfer

to keratinocytes, and melanosome degradation determine the degree of skin pigmentation.[7] Genetically activated factors, as well as ultraviolet radiation, hormones such as estrogen, adrenocorticotropic hormone, and melanocyte-stimulating hormone, influence these activities.[8]

The internal skeleton of cells (intermediate filaments), called *keratins* in epithelial cells, play an important role in the function of the epidermis. Intermediate filaments provide flexible scaffolding that enables the cell to resist external stress. The importance of these structures was revealed when mice expressing genetically mutated keratins developed blistering diseases similar to those found in humans.[9] Different keratins are expressed at different stages of keratinocyte maturation. In the mitotically active inner layer of the epidermis, the keratinocytes mainly express keratins 5 and 14. Patients with epidermolysis bullosa simplex, a blistering disease, were found to have a point mutation in one or the other keratin gene, thus revealing the etiology of one of the more baffling skin diseases.[10] Furthermore, because intermediate filaments play an important role in many epithelial cells and also in neurons, several genetic diseases of the gastrointestinal tract, liver, and peripheral nervous system have been traced to mutations in these genes.[11]

The Langerhans' cells migrate from the bone marrow and function as the skin's macrophages. The Langerhans' cells constitutively express class II major histocompatibility antigens and have antigen-presenting capabilities. These cells play a crucial role in immunosurveillance against viral infections and neoplasms of the skin, and may initiate skin allograft rejection.[12]

The dermis is mostly comprised of several structural proteins. Collagen constitutes 70 percent of the dry weight of dermis and is responsible for its remarkable tensile strength. Tropocollagen consists of three polypeptide chains (formed mainly of hydroxyproline, hydroxylysine, and glycine) wrapped in a helix. These long molecules are then cross-linked to one another to form collagen fibers. Of the seven structurally distinct collagens, the skin contains mostly type I. Early fetal dermis contains mostly type III (reticulin fibers) collagen, but this remains only in the basement membrane zone and the perivascular regions in postnatal skin. Elastic fibers are highly branching proteins that are capable of being reversibly stretched to twice their resting length.[13] This allows skin to return to its original form after stretching. Ground substance, consisting of various polysaccharide–polypeptide (glycosaminoglycans) complexes, is an amorphous material that fills the remaining spaces. The nonsulfated form is mostly hyaluronic acid, and the sulfated forms are heparin sulfate, dermatan sulfate, and chondroitin-6-sulfate. Glycosaminoglycans, which can hold up to 1000 times their own volume in water, constitute most of the volume of dermis.[14]

Fibroblasts are scattered throughout the dermis and are responsible for production and maintenance of the protein matrix. Recently, proteins that control the proliferation and migration of fibroblasts have been isolated. The study of fibroblast activity by these growth factor interactions is crucial to understanding wound healing and organogenesis.

The basement membrane zone of the dermoepidermal junction is a highly organized structure of proteins that anchors the epidermis to the dermis. Mechanical disruption or a genetic defect in the synthesis of this structure results in separation of the epidermis from the dermis.

The remaining structures of the skin are situated in the dermis. An intricate network of blood vessels regulates body temperature. Vertical vascular channels interconnect two horizontal plexuses, one at the dermal–subcutaneous junction and one in the papillary dermis. Glomus bodies are tortuous arteriovenous shunts that allow a tremendous increase in blood flow to the skin when open. This ability not only provides for the nutritional needs of the skin, but enables it to dissipate a vast amount of body heat when needed.[15]

Thermoregulation is carried out by autonomic fibers that synapse to sweat glands, hair erector muscles, and control points in the vasculature. Sensory innervation follows a dermatomal distribution from segments of the spinal cord. These fibers connect to corpuscular receptors (pacinian, Meissner's, and Ruffini's) that respond to pressure, vibration, and touch, as well as to "unspecialized" free nerve endings associated with Merkel cells of the basal epidermis, and to hair follicles. These nerves are stimulated by temperature, touch, pain, and itch. The skin has three main adnexal structures. The eccrine glands, which produce sweat, are located over the entire body but are concentrated on the palms, soles, axillae, and forehead. Hair follicles consist of a mitotically active germinal center that produces a cylinder of tightly packed, cornified epithelial cells. Control of the growth cycle of the hair is poorly understood. The sebaceous glands produce an oily substance that coats the skin. Together these two structures form a pilosebaceous unit. The apocrine glands are found primarily in the axillae and the anogenital region. In lower mammals, these glands produce scent hormones (pheromones).

Hair follicles have more important functions than merely the production of the hair structure. The hair follicle contains a reservoir of pluripotential cells that serve many functions. These stem cells have been shown to be critical in maintaining the reproductive ability of the epidermis.[16] These cells are capable of near limitless expansion to replace the cells shed in normal epidermal turnover and to restore epidermal continuity after wounding. In the example of a skin graft donor site, the residual hair follicle left after the upper (split-thickness) layer of skin is removed supplies all of the new keratinocytes needed to regenerate the epidermis. Hair follicle cells appear to be able to regenerate themselves, participate in wound healing, and even in hematopoiesis.[17,18]

INJURIES TO SKIN AND SUBCUTANEOUS TISSUE

Injuries that violate the continuity of the skin and subcutaneous tissue can occur as a result of trauma or from various environmental exposures. Environmental exposures that damage the skin and subcutaneous tissues include caustic substances, exposure to extreme temperatures, prolonged or excessive pressure, and exposure to radiation. Disruption of the continuity of the skin allows the entry of organisms that can lead to local or systemic infection.

Traumatic Injuries

Traumatic wounds include penetrating, blunt, and shear forces (sliding against a fixed surface), bite, and degloving injuries. Sharp lacerations, bullet wounds, "road rash" (injury from scraping against road pavement), and degloving injuries should be treated by gentle cleansing, débridement of all foreign debris and necrotic tissue, and application of a proper dressing. Dirty or infected wounds should be left open to heal by secondary intention or delayed primary closure. Clean lacerations may be closed primarily. Road rash injuries are treated as second-degree burns and degloving injuries as third-degree or full-thickness burns. The degloved skin can be placed back on the wound like a skin graft and assessed daily for survival. If the skin becomes necrotic, it is débrided and the wound is covered with split-thickness skin grafts.

Special consideration should be given to bite wounds. It is estimated that 4.5 million bites occur annually, accounting for 2% of all visits to emergency rooms.[19] Common bite wounds include those delivered by either a human or canine. The most serious human bite is that of a clenched fist injury. This occurs when the closed fist hits a person's teeth, often during a fight, termed "fight bite." These small wounds may seem innocuous but can lead to significant morbidity if not recognized early and treated, given that the human oral flora contains multiple species of aerobic and anaerobic bacteria. The most common infectious organisms found with human bites are *Viridans streptococci, Staphylococcus aureus, Eikenella corrodens, Haemophilus influenzae,* and beta-lactamase-producing bacteria.[20] The underlying metacarpophalangeal joint is susceptible to injury because it can be penetrated and inoculated with organisms, as can the underlying bone or tendon. The management of these wounds includes drainage, copious irrigation, antibiotic therapy, extremity immobilization, and elevation. Dog bites account for the most common animal bite wound. Dog bites differ from human bites in that they are a more crushing-type injury because of the animal's round teeth and strong jaws. The dog's jaw can exert more than 450 pounds of pressure per square inch.[21] This pressure has a greater potential to disrupt structures deep to the skin and subcutaneous tissues such as bones, vessels, tendons, muscles, and nerves. Mixed organisms, both aerobic and anaerobic, have been cultured from dog bite wounds. The most common organisms include *Pasteurella multocida, Staphylococcus* species, alpha-hemolytic streptococci, *Eikenella corrodens, Actinomyces,* and *Fusobacterium.*[20] The management of these wounds includes copious irrigation, débridement of devitalized tissue, and antibiotic therapy.

Exposure to Caustic Substances

Many substances can disrupt the integrity of the skin. Injuries commonly seen by physicians are those caused by environmental chemicals, either alkali or acidic solutions, or may occur iatrogenically as a complication of intravenous fluid administration.

Alkaline agents, which are often used as industrial-grade cleaning solvents and household cleaning agents, are responsible for more than 15,000 skin burns in the United States annually.[22] After penetrating the skin, alkaline substances cause saponification of fat, which allows for deeper penetration and increased tissue damage.[23,24] Management of these injuries should be rapid as the tissue damage produced by alkaline agents is progressive once penetration is achieved. Current management of alkaline burn injury is immediate irrigation of the affected area with a continuous flow of water, which should be maintained for at least 2 hours or longer if needed for symptomatic relief.[23,25] Large wounds, or wounds associated with damage to underlying structures such as tendons or nerves, require additional reconstructive surgery. Recently, it was found experimentally that neutralization of alkaline wounds demonstrated a more rapid return to physiologic pH, less-severe tissue damage, and improved wound healing in comparison to those wounds treated with water.[26]

Hydrofluoric and sulfuric acid are common agents that cause skin injury from acidic solution exposure. The effect an acid has on the skin is determined by the concentration, duration of contact, amount, and penetrability. Hydrofluoric acid is a colorless, fuming liquid that has a highly corrosive effect on skin, causing extensive liquefactive necrosis and severe pain.[27] Deep tissue injury may result, damaging nerves, blood vessels, tendons, and bone. The initial treatment after contact with the skin is copious irrigation, which must be continued for at least 15 to 30 minutes with either water or normal saline.[28] The second aspect of treatment aims to inactivate the free fluoride ion by promoting the formation of an insoluble fluoride salt. Many topical therapies have been advocated and their role in treatment largely anecdotal. Topical quaternary ammonium compounds are still widely used.[29] Topical calcium carbonate gel has been shown to detoxify the fluoride ion and relieve pain.[30,31] The treatment involves massage of a 2.5% calcium carbonate gel into the area of exposure for at least 30 minutes.[32] Some investigators advocate continuing this treatment six times per day for 4 days.[33]

Sulfuric acid exposure can cause full-thickness tissue necrosis. Treatment after exposure is immediate copious irrigation of the affected area. This dilutes and removes the sulfuric acid while returning the skin to a normal pH.[34,35]

Intravenous fluid that extravasates into the peripheral tissues during a venous infusion is a common problem. Intravenous fluid (IVF) extravasation is defined as leakage of injectable fluids out of the vein into the interstitial space. This problem may be the result of a displacement of the IV line or from increased vascular permeability. Depending on the solution being injected, surrounding tissue may be injured to varying degrees. The most common substances that extravasate are cationic solutions (e.g., potassium ion, calcium ion, bicarbonate), osmotically active chemicals (e.g., total parenteral nutrition or hypertonic dextrose solutions), and antibiotics and cytotoxic drugs. Patients undergoing chemotherapy have a 4.7% risk for developing extravasation.[36] In children, the incidence is increased to 11 to 58%.[37] The dorsum of the hand is the most common site of extravasation in the adult, which may result in exposed extensor tendons and loss of function. Other common sites include the antecubital fossa and dorsum of foot and scalp in neonates. The most common intravenous fluid extravasations causing necrosis in the infant are high-concentration dextrose solutions, calcium, bicarbonate, and parenteral nutrition. Newborn babies are at risk because of the fragility and small caliber of their veins, their poor ability to verbalize their pain, and the system of delivery, which pumps the intravenous fluid under pressure.[38]

Extravasation causes tissue necrosis either from chemical toxicity, osmotic toxicity, or from the effects of pressure in a closed environment. In most instances, the tissue necrosis is underestimated. Commonly infused drugs that extravasate in adult patients are the chemotherapeutic agents doxorubicin (Adriamycin) and

paclitaxel.[39] The direct toxic effects of doxorubicin on living cells cause cellular death that is perpetuated by the release of doxorubicin-DNA complexes from dead cells. This cellular death prevents the release of cytokines and growth factors, which results in the failure of activation of the cells important in wound healing.[40,41] Following extravasation, edema, erythema, and induration are usually present with variable amounts of necrotic tissue, the extent of which is not readily apparent. Along with the soft-tissue defect, the limb is also subject to an alteration in function. Injury to underlying nerves, muscles, tendons, and blood vessels must be taken into account. When the extravasation is in proximity to a major artery in the forearm or leg, that extremity is at great risk for amputation. Treatment options vary from early débridement to observation.[42] Gault described a percutaneous saline flush-out technique for both neonates and cancer patients. This involves vigorous liposuction with a small cannula introduced through a small incision adjacent to the area of extravasation. The area is then flushed thoroughly with saline, which is allowed to egress through small stab wounds.[43] This has proved to be useful in acute exacerbations, while patients who present more than 24 hour after extravasation do not benefit from flush-out. Although many options of treatment are available, many investigators have found that an expectant approach is successful in treating the vast majority of patients with extravasation injuries.[39,44] Surgery is limited to those patients with necrotic tissue, pain, or damage of underlying structures such as tendons or nerves.

Temperature

Skin exposed to extremes of temperature is at risk of injury. These include hypo- or hyperthermic injuries.

Hyperthermic injury (burns) cause varying degrees of tissue injury, depending on the temperature and length of exposure. Tissue is damaged from heat coagulation in the zone of coagulation, which becomes necrotic tissue. Surrounding the zone of coagulation is the zone of stasis, which has marginal tissue perfusion and questionable viability. The zone of hyperemia is closest to the normal tissue and represents the tissue's response to injury with an increase in blood flow. Burn wounds are covered in greater detail in Chap. 7.

Hypothermia is defined as a core body temperature of less than 35°C (95°F).[45] Frostbite is defined as the acute freezing of tissues. Frostbite severity is related to the duration of exposure and to the temperature gradient at the skin surface.[46] It has been shown experimentally that the tensile strength of a healing wound decreases by 20% in a cold (12°C [53.6°F]) wound environment. Severe hypothermia primarily affects the vasculature as the blood vessels become severely injured by a combination of direct cellular injury and microvascular thrombosis. McCauley and coworkers have outlined the treatment protocol for frostbite, which includes rapid rewarming, close observation, elevation and splinting, daily hydrotherapy, and serial débridements.[47]

Pressure Ulcers (Decubitus Ulcers)

Pressure ulcers, as the name implies, are caused by excessive, unrelieved pressure. In animal studies, 60 mm Hg of pressure applied to the skin for 1 hour produces histologically identifiable injuries such as venous thrombosis, muscle degeneration, and tissue necrosis.[48] Normal arteriole, capillary, and venule pressures are 32, 20, and 12 mm Hg, respectively.[49] Pressure generated under the ischial tuberosities while a person is seated can reach 300 mm Hg, and sacral pressure can range from 100 to 150 mm Hg while a person lies on a standard hospital mattress.[50] Healthy individuals regularly shift their body weight, even while asleep. Sitting in one position for extended periods of time causes pain via increased pressure in certain

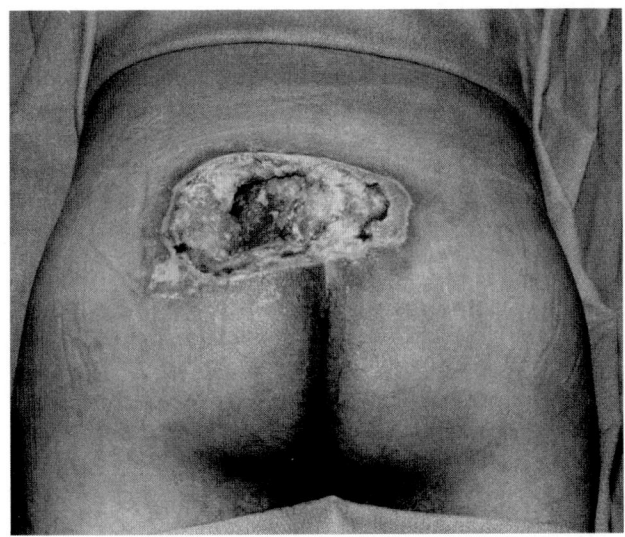

A

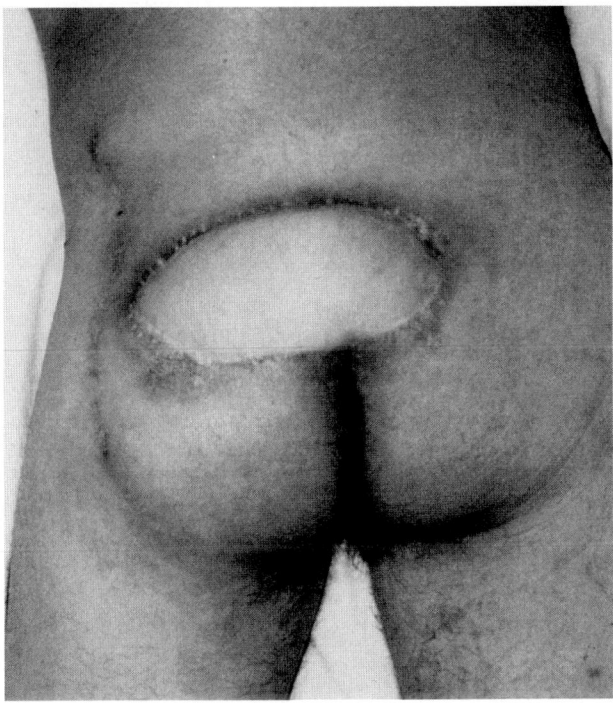

B

FIG. 15-2. Sacral decubitus ulcer is (A) débrided and (B) covered with a flap.

areas; this, in turn, stimulates the initiation of movement. Patients unable to sense pain or to shift their body weight, such as paraplegics or bedridden individuals, develop prolonged elevated tissue pressures, and, eventually, necrosis. Muscle tissue is more sensitive to ischemia than the overlying skin. Therefore, the necrotic area is usually wider and deeper than it appears on first inspection (Fig. 15-2).

Treatment of pressure sores requires relief of pressure with special cushions and beds and nutritional support to promote healing. The necrotic tissue should be removed, often along with the underlying bony prominence. Shallow ulcers may close by secondary intention, but deeper wounds with involvement of the underlying bone require surgical débridement and coverage. To prevent future breakdown of the area, stable coverage should be obtained with local

musculocutaneous or fasciocutaneous flaps. Prevention of ulcers is best achieved by close attention to susceptible areas and frequent repositioning of paralyzed patients. Air flotation mattresses and gel seat cushions redistribute pressure, decrease the incidence of pressure ulcers, and are cost-effective in the care of patients at high risk. The addition of growth factors to these wounds has been found to increase healing and offers promising future therapeutic uses.[51]

Radiation Exposure

The source of radiation includes an industrial accident that results in an acute injury, therapeutic radiation for the treatment of malignancy, and chronic radiation injury such as solar (ultraviolet) and occupational exposure.

Acute radiation injuries such as those that occur in an industrial accident are devastating. The dose of radiation exposure is oftentimes lethal. In addition to the development of skin lesions (cutaneous radiation syndrome), patients suffer from gastrointestinal hemorrhage, bone marrow suppression, and multiorgan system failure. The most notable industrial radiation exposure accident occurred in 1986 at the Chernobyl nuclear power plant. Of the 237 individuals initially suspected of being exposed, 54 suffered from cutaneous radiation syndrome. The severity of symptoms ranged widely and included xerosis (dry skin), cutaneous telangiectasias and subungual splinter hemorrhages, hemangiomas and lymphangiomas, epidermal atrophy, disseminated keratoses, extensive dermal and subcutaneous fibrosis with partial ulcerations, and pigment changes (radiation lentigo). To date, no cutaneous malignancies have been noted.[52]

Solar or ultraviolet (UV) radiation represents the most common form of radiation exposure. The ultraviolet spectrum is divided into UVA (400 to 315 nm), UVB (315 to 290 nm), and UVC (290 to 200 nm).[53] With regard to skin damage and development of skin cancers, the only significant wavelengths are in the ultraviolet spectrum. The ozone layer absorbs UV wavelengths below 290 nm, thus allowing only UVA and UVB to reach the earth. UVB is responsible for the acute sunburns and for the chronic skin damage leading to malignant degeneration, although it makes up less than 5% of the solar UV radiation that hits the earth.

The treatment of various malignancies oftentimes includes radiation therapy. Given the basis of this therapy to act upon rapidly dividing cell types, the skin and subcutaneous tissue are significantly affected. The extent of cellular damage is dependent on the radiation dose, its timing, and the cell type being treated. Acute radiation changes include erythema and basal epithelial cellular death. Dry desquamation may proceed to moist desquamation. With cellular repair, permanent hyperpigmentation is observed in the field of radiation. Chronic radiation changes begin at 4 to 6 months and are characterized by a loss of capillaries as a result of thrombosis and fibrinoid necrosis of vessel walls. This fibrosis and hypovascularity are generally progressive, which eventually may lead to ulceration because of poor tissue perfusion.

INFECTION

Bacterial Infections

Simple

Cellulitis is a superficial spreading infection of the skin and subcutaneous tissue. This infection is heralded by erythema, warmth, tenderness, and edema. The most common organism associated with cellulitis is group A streptococci or *Staphylococcus aureus*.

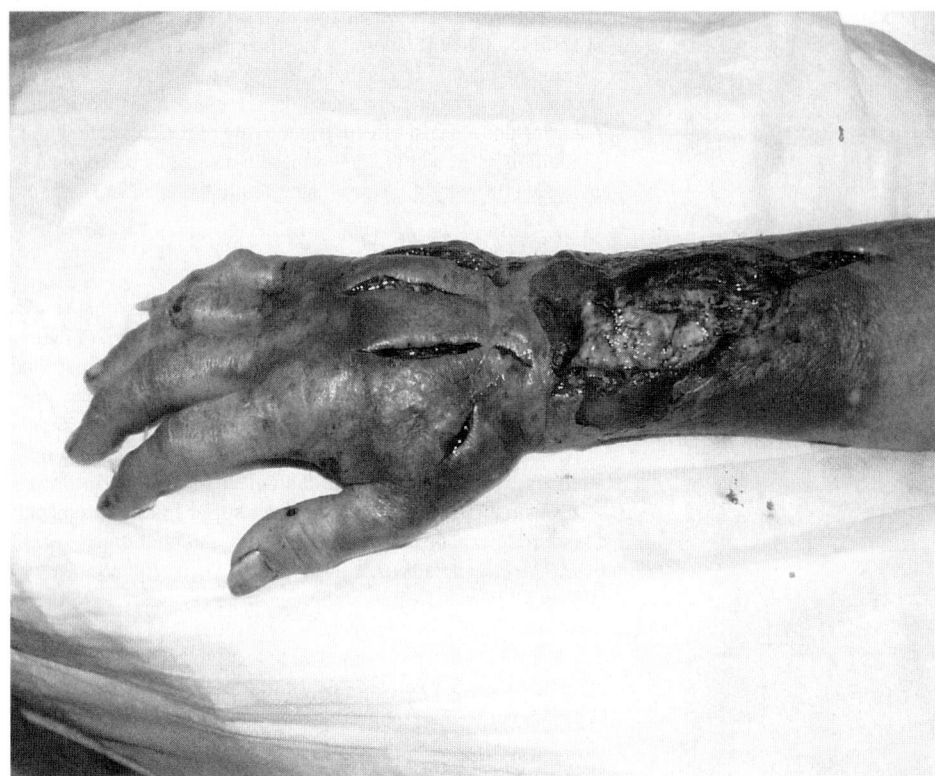

FIG. 15-3. Necrotizing soft-tissue infection of the hand.

Folliculitis, Furuncles, and Carbuncles

Folliculitis is infection and inflammation of a hair follicle. The causative organism is usually the gram-positive organism *Staphylococcus*, but occasionally involves gram-negative organisms. A furuncle (boil) begins as folliculitis but progresses to form a nodule that eventually becomes fluctuant. The abscess eventually ruptures and usually resolves. Deep-seated infections that result in multiple draining cutaneous sinuses are called carbuncles.

Folliculitis usually resolves with time and adequate hygiene. Warm soaks to a furuncle may hasten liquefaction, speed drainage, and encourage healing. Occasionally antibiotics are used to manage surrounding cellulitis. Carbuncles are more difficult to treat and require incision and drainage or wide excision of the infected tissue and sinuses.

An abscess is a localized accumulation of pus with an associated superficial cellulitis. The body's response is to isolate this accumulation, necessitating drainage.

Extensive Soft-Tissue Infection

Necrotizing Soft-Tissue Infections. Certain infections progress rapidly with severe soft-tissue destruction. These infections are referred to as necrotizing, denoting rapid spread associated with septic shock. In 1883, Fournier termed a specific necrotizing infection (*Fournier's gangrene*) involving the perineum.[54] Fournier's gangrene is now defined as an abrupt, rapidly progressive, gangrenous infection of the external genitalia, perineum, or abdominal wall. In 1924, Meleney described a lethal and rapidly progressing soft-tissue infection caused by a microaerophilic streptococcus termed *Meleney's gangrene*.[55] He also coined the term *synergistic gangrene*, which is characterized by a symbiosis of anaerobic streptococci and staphylococci.[56] The eponyms given to these necrotizing soft-tissue infections through the years, although of historical importance, describe the same problem. Currently, the classification is based on (1) the tissue plane affected and extent of invasion, (2) the anatomic site, and (3) the causative pathogen(s). Deep soft-tissue infections are classified as either necrotizing fasciitis or necrotizing myositis. Necrotizing fasciitis represents a rapid, extensive infection of the fascia deep to the adipose tissue (Fig. 15-3). Necrotizing myositis is less common and primarily involves the muscles and spreads to the adjacent soft tissues. The most common organisms isolated from patients presenting with necrotizing soft-tissue infections include the gram-positive organisms: group A streptococci, enterococci, coagulase-negative staphylococci, *S. aureus, S. epidermidis,* and *Clostridium* species; the gram-negative organisms: *Escherichia coli, Enterobacter, Pseudomonas* species, *Proteus* species, *Serratia* species, and bacteroides.[57] Infections with *Vibrio* also have been documented.[58] Polymicrobial infections tend to be a more common finding in necrotizing infections than a single organism.[59] Recently, bacteriology reports indicate an increasing incidence of methicillin-resistant *S. aureus* (MRSA). The risk factors for development of necrotizing soft-tissue infection include diabetes mellitus, malnutrition, obesity, chronic alcoholism, peripheral vascular disease, chronic lymphocytic leukemia, steroid use, renal failure, cirrhosis, and autoimmune deficiency syndrome.[60]

Necrotizing soft-tissue infections require early recognition and intervention. Broad-spectrum antibiotics, aggressive surgical débridement, and intensive care unit support are essential. The patient generally requires aggressive fluid replacement to offset acute renal failure from ongoing sepsis and shock. Débridement should be extensive, including all skin, subcutaneous tissue, and muscle, until there is no further evidence of infected tissue. This is followed by frequent return to the operating room for additional débridement as needed. Some authors advocate the use of hyperbaric oxygen, although the benefit remains controversial.[61]

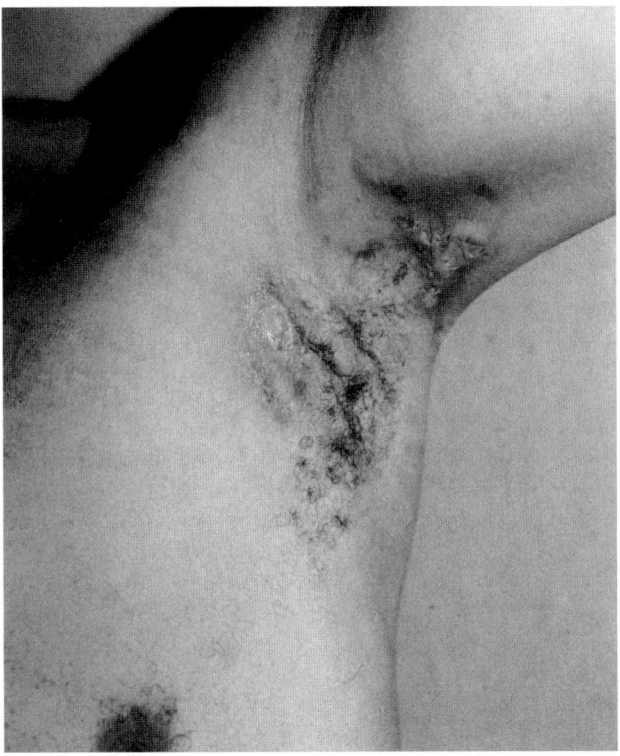

FIG. 15-4. *Active hidradenitis suppurativa of the axilla.*

Hidradenitis Suppurativa

Once considered to be "apocrine acne," hidradenitis suppurativa is actually a defect of terminal follicular epithelium.[62] This follicular defect leads to a blockage of the apocrine glands, which secondarily become infected. This disease arises most commonly in the apocrine gland–bearing skin, namely the axilla, inguinal, and perianal regions. There is a genetic component with probable hormonal influence on gene expression.[63] An abscess forms with subsequent drainage and sinus formation. Repeated infections create a wide area of inflamed and scarred tissue that is foul-smelling and painful (Fig. 15-4). Treatment of acute infections includes application of warm compresses, antibiotics, and open drainage.[64] Proper hygiene and discontinuation of deodorants may prevent recurrence. Chronic hidradenitis requires wide excision and closure with skin grafts.

Pilonidal Disease

Infected pilonidal cysts of the sacrococcygeal region occur primarily in young adults and are four times more common in males.[65] The pathogenesis of the disease is much debated, but heavy activity inducing sweat and buttock friction, such as occurred in jeep drivers in World War II (jeep driver's disease), is associated with a higher incidence of pilonidal disease. The infection likely begins in a pilosebaceous unit in the natal cleft. Recurrent trauma causes obstruction of a hair follicle and leads to infection. The localized folliculitis spreads into the surrounding soft tissue and produces an abscess.[66] This eventually drains to the surface and produces a sinus that is usually located lateral to the midline. The sinus is lined with granulation tissue but over time can epithelialize. Constant movement and friction of the buttocks causes hair and loose debris to enter the tract, inciting a foreign-body reaction.

Acute pilonidal abscesses should be incised and drained.[67] Without further therapy, many will recur. Use of perioperative antibiotics

does not affect the outcome of the disease.[68] There are many different ways of treating the chronic sinus tract, including tract curettage, local excision and closure, wide excision and marsupialization, and wide excision and flap closure.[69–71] Each method has benefits and drawbacks. Patients undergoing primary closure stay in the hospital longer but return to work sooner than patients with the wound left open after excision. Nonsurgical treatment of a pilonidal lesion by natal-cleft shaving and perineal hygiene requires the least amount of hospitalization, but may have a higher recurrence rate. Squamous cell carcinoma arising from pilonidal sinus is a rare complication and should be considered when managing these wounds.[72,73]

Actinomycosis

Actinomycosis is a granulomatous suppurative bacterial disease caused by actinomyces. Forty to 60% of the actinomycotic infections occur in the craniofacial skeleton, and the mandible is the site of predilection.[74,75] Actinomycotic infection is usually caused by tooth extraction, odontogenic infection, or trauma.[76] *Actinomyces* is an organism of the Actinomycetaceae family in the Actinomycetales order. Other actinomycetes, including *Nocardia, Actinomadura,* and *Streptomyces* cause mycetomas, which are deep cutaneous infections that present as nodules and spread to form draining tracts to the skin and surrounding soft tissue. Chronic disease causes fibrosis and contractures. The most common site for infection is the foot (Madura foot).[77]

The anaerobic gram-positive bacteria that cause these infections were once believed to be fungi because they grow slowly as branched filaments and chains. Diagnosis depends on the presence of characteristic sulfur granules on microscopic examination.[78] Special stains should be used to exclude fungal infection. Penicillin and sulfonamides are effective against these infections.[76,79] Abscesses and areas of chronic scarring may require surgical therapy.

Lymphogranuloma Venereum

Chlamydia trachomatis is a sexually transmitted, intracellular, gram-negative bacterium. After infection and a 2-week incubation period, an inconspicuous ulcer appears on the penis or labia, although in more than half of the cases, this lesion is not noticed or does not appear. A few weeks later, inguinal lymphadenopathy is apparent.[80] The nodes become very large and painful (buboes) and are occasionally confused with an incarcerated inguinal hernia. Adenopathy can occur above and below the inguinal ligament, forming a characteristic groove.[81] The matted nodes may suppurate, and occasionally rupture. Surgical drainage of unruptured abscesses is not recommended because a chronic draining sinus often develops. Active infection is treated with doxycycline for 1 week or azithromycin in one dose for uncomplicated disease and 14 days of treatment with doxycycline for complicated disease.[82,83] Inflammation from infection can lead to lymphatic obstruction and chronic lower extremity edema. Rectal strictures also can occur.

Atypical *Mycobacterium*

There has been an increase in the incidence of nontuberculous mycobacteria over the past two decades.[84] Acid-fast bacilli are common in the environment, and have been found in 27% of surgical samples of skin.[85] Varieties of mycobacteria known to cause cutaneous disease are the *Mycobacterium fortuitum* complex, *Mycobacterium ulcerans,* and *Mycobacterium marinum.*[86,87] Cutaneous lesions caused by atypical mycobacterium are often associated with immunosuppression.[88] *Mycobacterium ulcerans* manifests as a skin ulcer, termed *Buruli's ulcer. Mycobacterium marinum* is usually acquired through minor skin lesions associated with aquatic activity, such as the handling of fish tanks.[89,90] Refractory cutaneous lesions caused by atypical mycobacteria are often misdiagnosed because clinicians fail to recognize this type of skin infection.

Viral

Human Papillomavirus

Warts are epidermal growths associated with human papillomavirus (HPV) infection. Histologically they are characterized by hyperkeratosis (hypertrophy of the horny layer), acanthosis (hypertrophy of the spinous layer), and papillomatosis. Koilocytes, which are large keratinocytes with eccentric nuclei, are present. Different morphologic types have a propensity to occur on different parts of the body. The common wart (verruca vulgaris) is found on the fingers and toes, and has a rough, gray-brown surface. Plantar warts (verruca plantaris) occur on the soles and palms, and may look like a callus. Flat warts (verruca plana), which are flat but slightly raised, appear on the face, legs, and hands. Venereal warts (condylomata acuminata) grow in the moist areas around the vulva, anus, and scrotum.

Warts can be removed by a number of chemicals, including formalin, podophyllum, and phenol-nitric acid. Curettage with electrodesiccation also can be used for scattered lesions. Treatment of extensive areas of skin requires surgical excision under general anesthesia.[91] Because of the infectious etiology, recurrences are common, and repeated excisions often are necessary to eliminate lesions. Some warts (especially human papillomavirus types 5, 8, and 10) are associated with squamous cell cancers, therefore lesions that grow rapidly or ulcerate should be biopsied.[92]

Condylomata acuminata is now one of the most common sexually transmitted viral infections and is largely HPV types 6 and 11.[93,94] Patients with human immunodeficiency virus (HIV) infection are more likely to develop clinically significant venereal warts. The lesions often are multiple and can grow large in size (Buschke-Löwenstein tumor).[95] Small lesions can be treated with podophyllotoxin cream. Larger lesions have a significant risk of malignant transformation and should be excised. The lesions often recur. Adjuvant therapy with interferon, isotretinoin, or autologous tumor vaccine decreases recurrence rates. Immune response modifiers, such as imiquimod, currently show the greatest promise in treating HPV-induced anogenital lesions, both with respect to complete response and in preventing recurrence.[91,93]

Human Immunodeficiency Virus

Patients infected with HIV commonly display skin manifestations of their disease. Immune deficiency can occur as a result of infectious processes such as HIV, which causes acquired immunodeficiency syndrome (AIDS), or secondary to immunosuppressive medications, as is the case for transplant recipients. Frequently, people with HIV develop chronic wounds, which become problem wounds given their intrinsic wound-healing deficiencies. The risk of surgical wound complications increases with the progression of the disease. Many studies have shown a greater incidence of poor wound healing following laparotomy, anorectal surgery, and orthopedic surgery.[96–98] The cause for delayed wound healing is unknown but is thought to be secondary to a decreasing T-cell CD4$^+$ count, presence of an opportunistic infection, low serum albumin, and poor nutrition.[99] Davis and Wastell showed that when comparing biomechanical parameters in the wounds of 11 patients with HIV to those of 11 patients with age-matched control wounds, the wounds of the HIV patients had a lower resilience, toughness, and

maximum extension than did the wounds of the control group. These parameters describe the properties of tissues using a tensiometer to determine how the wounds responded to load and deformation. *Resilience* describes the ability of tissue to endure loads without inducing a tension exceeding the elastic limit; *toughness* is the property of tissue that enables it to endure loads; and *maximum extension* is the displacement of the tissue at the point of wound rupture. The overall weakened ability of wound healing in the HIV patient is a consequence of an impairment of the underlying healing process that results in collagen deposition and cross-linking.[100]

Inflammatory Diseases

Pyoderma Gangrenosum

Pyoderma gangrenosum (PG) is a relatively uncommon destructive cutaneous lesion that was first described in 1930 by Brunsting and associates.[101] A rapidly enlarging, necrotic lesion with an undermined border and surrounding erythema characterize this disease. This cutaneous skin lesion is associated with an underlying systemic disease in 50% of cases. Common underlying disorders include inflammatory bowel disease, rheumatoid arthritis, hematologic malignancy, and monoclonal immunoglobulin A (IgA) gammapathy.[102] Recognition of the underlying disease is of paramount importance in the management of skin ulceration because surgical treatment without medical management is fraught with complication. The majority of patients are treated with systemic steroids and cyclosporine.[103] In some instances, medical management alone results in a protracted course with a slowly healing wound. Thus, some clinicians believe that in addition to control of the inflammatory phase, local wound care and coverage with a skin graft is efficacious.[104]

Staphylococcal Scalded Skin Syndrome and Toxic Epidermal Necrolysis

Staphylococcal scalded skin syndrome and toxic epidermal necrolysis create a similar clinical picture, which includes erythema of the skin, bullae formation, and, eventually, wide areas of skin loss. Staphylococcal scalded skin syndrome (SSSS) is caused by an exotoxin produced during a staphylococcal infection of the nasopharynx or middle ear in the pediatric population.[105] Toxic epidermal necrolysis (TEN) is thought to be an immunologic reaction to certain drugs, such as sulfonamides, phenytoin, barbiturates, and tetracycline.[106] Diagnosis can be made with a skin biopsy examination because SSSS produces a cleavage plane in the granular layer of the epidermis, whereas TEN occurs at the dermoepidermal junction.[107] The injury is similar to a second-degree burn. Treatment involves fluid and electrolyte replacement and wound care as in a burn injury. Patients with less than 10% of epidermal detachment are classified as Stevens-Johnson syndrome, whereas those with more than 30% of total body surface area involvement are classified as TEN.[108] In Stevens-Johnson syndrome, epithelial sloughing of the respiratory and alimentary tracts occurs with resultant respiratory failure and intestinal malabsorption. Patients with TEN should be treated in burn units to decrease the morbidity from the wounds.[109] The skin slough has been successfully treated with cadaveric or porcine skin or semisynthetic biologic dressings (Biobrane).[110,111] Temporary coverage with a biologic dressing allows the underlying epidermis to regenerate spontaneously. Corticosteroid therapy has not been efficacious.

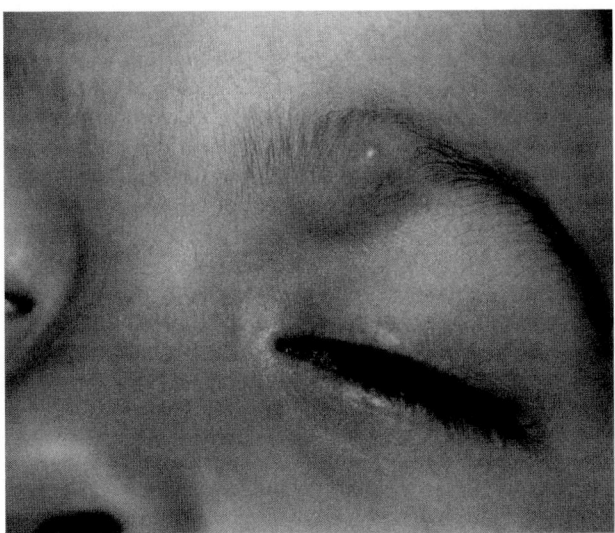

FIG. 15-5. *Dermoid cysts are commonly found on the eyebrow.*

BENIGN TUMORS

Cysts (Epidermal, Dermoid, Trichilemmal)

Epidermal cysts are the most common type of cutaneous cyst and can occur anywhere on the body as a single, firm nodule.[112] On the scrotum they are often multiple and can calcify. Trichilemmal (pilar) cysts, the next most common, occur more often in females and usually on the scalp. When ruptured, these cysts have a characteristic strong odor. Dermoid cysts are present at birth and may result from epithelium trapped during midline closure in fetal development. Dermoid cysts are most often found in the midline of the face (e.g., on the nose or forehead) and are also common on the eyebrow (Fig. 15-5).[113]

On gross examination, it is difficult to distinguish one type of cyst from another. They are all subcutaneous, thin-walled nodules containing a white, creamy center. Histologic examination is needed to differentiate them. The walls of all these cysts consist of a layer of epidermis oriented with the basal layer superficial and the more mature layers deep (i.e., with the epidermis growing into the center of the cyst). The desquamated cells (keratin) collect in the center and form the creamy substance of the cyst. Epidermal cysts have a completely mature epidermis containing a granular layer. Trichilemmal cyst walls do not contain a granular layer but do have a distinctive outer layer resembling the outer root sheath of the hair follicle (trichilemmoma). Dermoid cysts have a squamous epithelium, eccrine glands, pilosebaceous units, and, occasionally, bone, tooth, or nerve tissue. Surgeons often refer to cutaneous cysts as sebaceous cysts because they appear to contain sebum; however, this is a misnomer because the substance is actually keratin.

Cysts usually are asymptomatic and ignored until they rupture and cause local inflammation. The area becomes infected and an abscess forms. Incision and drainage is recommended for an acutely infected cyst. After resolution of the abscess the cyst wall must be excised or the cyst will recur. Similarly, when excising an unruptured cyst, care must be taken to remove the entire wall in order to prevent recurrence.

Keratoses (Seborrheic, Solar)

Seborrheic keratoses commonly occur on the chest, back, and abdomen of older individuals. The lesions are light brown or yellow and have a velvety, greasy texture. They are rarely mistaken for other lesions, so biopsy and treatment are seldom needed.[114] Sudden eruptions of multiple lesions in elderly patients may be associated with internal malignancies.

Solar (or actinic) keratoses also are found in the older age group. They arise in sun-exposed areas of the body, such as the face, the forearms, and the back of the hands. Histologically they contain atypical-appearing keratinocytes and evidence of solar damage in the dermis.[115] These are thought to be premalignant lesions, and squamous cell carcinoma may develop over time.[116] Treatment is by local removal or application of topical 5-fluorouracil.[117] Malignancies that do develop rarely metastasize.

Nevi (Acquired, Congenital)

Acquired melanocytic nevi are classified as junctional, compound, or dermal, depending on the location of the nevus cells. This classification does not represent different types of nevi but rather different stages in the maturation of nevi. Initially, nevus cells accumulate in the epidermis (junctional), migrate partially into the dermis (compound), and finally rest completely in the dermis (dermal). Eventually most lesions undergo involution.

Congenital nevi are much rarer, occurring in only 1% of neonates.[118] These lesions are larger and may contain hair. Histologically they appear similar to acquired nevi. Congenital giant lesions (giant hairy nevus) most often occur in a bathing trunk distribution or on the chest and back (Fig. 15-6). These lesions are cosmetically unpleasant. In addition, they develop malignant melanoma in

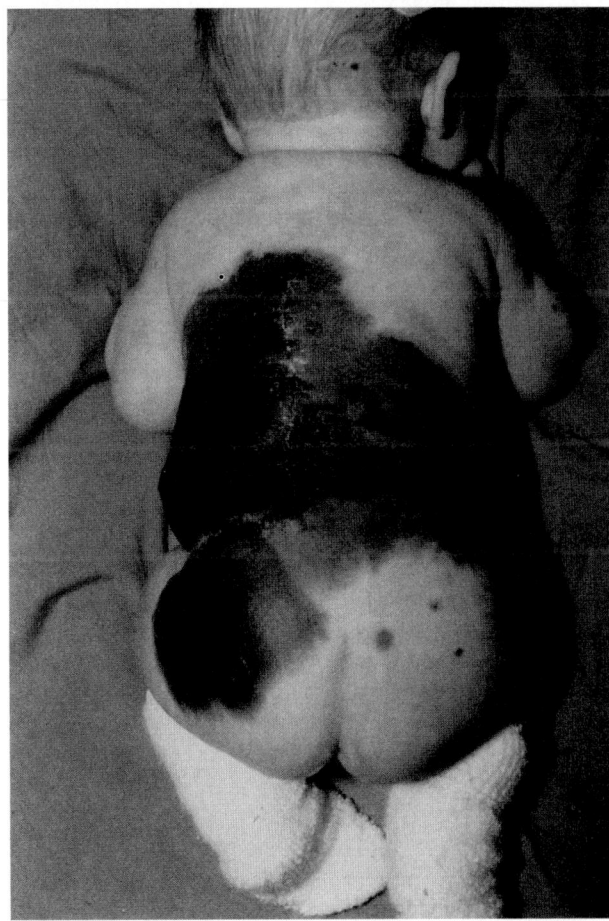

FIG. 15-6. *Giant hairy nevus in an infant.*

1 to 5% of the cases.[119] Excision of the nevus is the treatment of choice, but often the lesion is so large that closure of the wound with autologous skin grafts is not possible because of the lack of adequate donor sites. Serial excisions over several years with either primary closure or skin grafting and tissue expansion of the normal surrounding skin are the present modes of therapy.

Vascular Tumors

Hemangiomas (Capillary, Cavernous)

Hemangiomas are benign vascular neoplasms that arise soon after birth. They initially undergo rapid cellular proliferation and slowly involute through early childhood.[120] Capillary (strawberry) hemangiomas are soft, compressible papular lesions with sharp borders located mostly on the shoulders, face, and scalp.[121] Cavernous hemangiomas are bright red or purple and have a spongy consistency. Histologically, capillary hemangiomas are composed of endothelial cells seen primarily in fetal veins. Cavernous lesions contain large, blood-filled spaces lined by normal-appearing endothelial cells.

Hemangiomas can enlarge during the first year of life, and more than 90% of them involute over time. Allowing lesions to regress spontaneously usually gives optimal cosmetic results (Fig. 15-7). Acute treatment is limited to lesions that interfere with function, such as vision, feeding, and urination, or those that lead to systemic problems, such as thrombocytopenia and high-output cardiac

failure. The growth of rapidly enlarging lesions can be stopped with prednisone or interferon alpha-2a treatment.[122] Hemangiomas that remain after early adolescence will generally not involute, therefore surgical excision is recommended.

Vascular Malformations (Port-Wine Stains, Arteriovenous Malformations, Glomus Tumors)

Vascular malformations are a result of structural abnormalities formed during fetal development and hence are not neoplasms. Unlike hemangiomas, vascular malformations do not undergo rapid growth and involution but rather grow in proportion to the body. Histologically they contain enlarged vascular spaces lined by non-proliferating endothelium, and not the mitotically active endothelial cells of a hemangioma.

The port-wine stain (nevus flammeus) is a flat, dull-red capillary malformation that can be located on the trunk, extremities, and, most commonly, along a trigeminal distribution on the face. Histologically these nevi are composed of ectatic capillaries lined by mature endothelium. They may be part of the Sturge-Weber syndrome (leptomeningeal angiomatosis, epilepsy, and glaucoma). Unsightly lesions can be covered with cosmetics, treated with pulsed dye laser, or surgically excised.

Arteriovenous malformations are high-flow lesions. They appear as a mass under the skin, with locally elevated temperature, a dermal stain, and a thrill and bruit. Overlying ischemic ulcers, adjacent bone

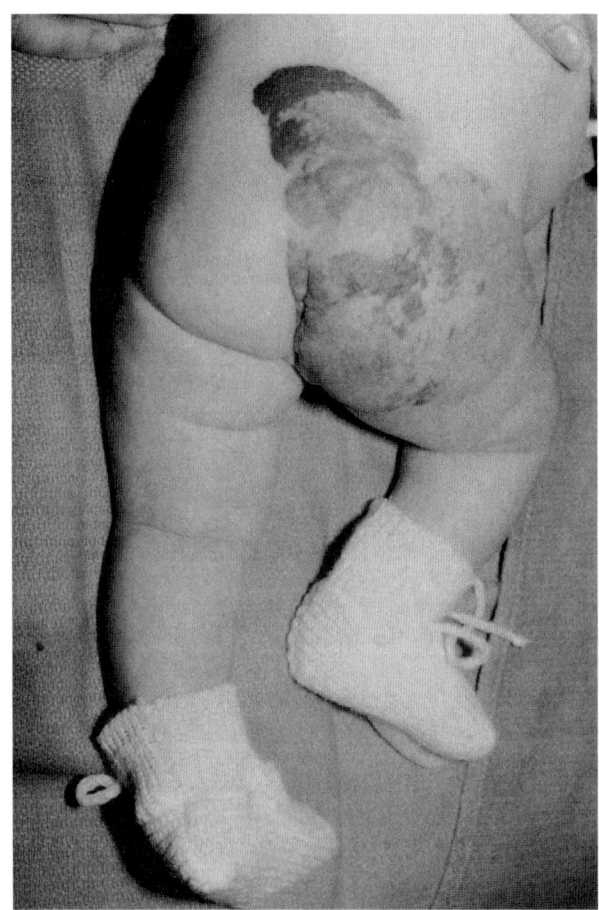

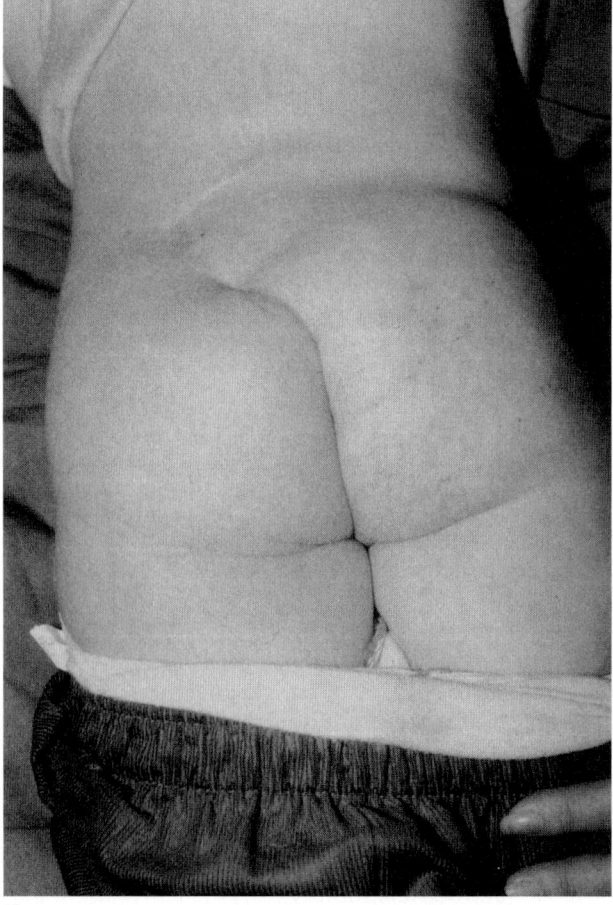

A   *B*

FIG. 15-7. *A. Large hemangioma. B. Regression without therapy.*

destruction, or local hypertrophy may occur. Large malformations can cause cardiac enlargement and congestive heart failure.

Complications of arteriovenous malformations, such as pain, hemorrhage, ulceration, cardiac effects, and destruction of surrounding structures, should be treated by elimination of the lesion. Therapy consists of angiography with selective embolization or complete surgical resection.[123] Embolization is particularly useful for lesions not accessible to surgery or in patients in which resection would cause a significant deformity. Embolization also can be used preoperatively to reduce blood loss during surgery. Occasionally, hypothermia and cardiac bypass are required in order to minimize blood loss during surgical excision of large lesions.

Glomus tumors are blue-gray nodules that are extremely tender. They can occur anywhere on the body, but the most common location is subungual. The tumor arises from a glomus body and histologically resembles the arterial portion of the glomus. Excision of the tumor relieves the pain.

Soft-Tissue Tumors (Acrochordons, Dermatofibromas, Lipomas)

Acrochordons (skin tags) are fleshy, pedunculated masses located on the axillae, trunk, and eyelids. They are composed of hyperplastic epidermis over a fibrous connective tissue stalk. These lesions are usually small and are always benign.

Dermatofibromas are usually solitary nodules measuring approximately 1 to 2 cm in diameter. They are found primarily on the legs and sides of the trunk. The lesions are composed of whorls of connective tissue containing fibroblasts. The mass is not encapsulated and vascularization is variable. Dermatofibromas can be diagnosed by clinical examination. When lesions enlarge to 2 to 3 cm, excisional biopsy is recommended to assess for malignancy. Lipomas are the most common subcutaneous neoplasm. They are found mostly on the trunk but may appear anywhere. They may sometimes grow to a large size. Microscopic examination reveals a lobulated tumor containing normal fat cells. Excision is performed for diagnosis and to restore normal skin contour.

Neural Tumors (Neurofibromas, Neurilemomas, Granular Cell Tumors)

Benign cutaneous neural tumors arise primarily from the nerve sheath. Neurofibromas can be sporadic and solitary but are more commonly noted in multiple formations associated with café-au-lait spots and an autosomal dominant inheritance (von Recklinghausen's disease). The lesions are firm, discrete nodules attached to a nerve. Histologically there is proliferation of perineurial and endoneurial fibroblasts and Schwann cells embedded in collagen. Neurilemomas are solitary tumors found along peripheral nerves of the head and extremities. They are discrete nodules that may be locally painful or radiate along the distribution of the nerve. Microscopically, the tumor contains Schwann cells with nuclei packed in palisading rows.

Granular cell tumors are usually solitary lesions of the skin or, more commonly, the tongue. They consist of granular cells derived from Schwann cells that often infiltrate the surrounding striated muscle.

MALIGNANT TUMORS

The most common cancers of the skin arise from the cells of the epidermis and are, in order of frequency, basal cell carcinoma,

squamous cell carcinoma, and melanoma.[124] Malignancies arising from cells of the dermis or adnexal structures are much less common.

Environmental influences and concomitant diseases are associated with an increased incidence of epidermal malignancies. These factors have been extensively studied and form some of our best understanding about the causes of cancer.

Epidemiology

Increased exposure to ultraviolet radiation is associated with an increased development of all three of the common skin malignancies.[125] Epidemiologic studies have shown that people with outdoor occupations have skin malignancies more often than people who work indoors. Squamous cell cancer is much more common on the lower lip than the upper. People with fair complexions are more prone to skin cancer.[126] These same people also are more likely to develop malignancies if they live in areas of the world that receive more sunlight, such as New Zealand, as compared to Great Britain. Albino individuals of dark-skinned races are prone to develop cutaneous neoplasms that usually are rare in the nonalbino members, suggesting that melanin has a large role in protection from carcinogenesis.[127]

Other factors associated with skin malignancies also have been identified. Chemical carcinogens have long been known. In the eighteenth century, Sir Percival Pott noted the association of soot and scrotal cancer in chimney sweeps. Tar, arsenic, and nitrogen mustard are known carcinogens.[128] Human papillomavirus has been found in certain squamous cell cancers and may be linked with oncogenesis.[129] Radiation therapy in the past for skin lesions such as acne vulgaris, when it resulted in radiation dermatitis, is associated with an increased incidence of basal and squamous cell cancers in the treated areas. Any area of skin subjected to chronic irritation, such as burn scars (Marjolin's ulcers), repeated sloughing of skin from bullous diseases, and decubitus ulcers, all have an increased chance of developing squamous cell cancer.[130,131] A variant of this type of lesion develops on skin that has suffered repeated burns.

Systemic immunologic dysfunction is related to an increase in cutaneous malignancies. Immunosuppressed patients receiving chemotherapy for other malignancies or immunosuppressants for organ transplants have an increased incidence of basal cell and squamous cell cancers and malignant melanoma. AIDS is associated with an increased risk of developing skin neoplasms.[132] Patients with HIV should be monitored vigilantly for signs of skin cancer.

Basal Cell Carcinoma

Basal cell carcinomas contain cells that resemble the basal cells of the epidermis. It is the most common type of skin cancer and is subdivided into several types by gross and histologic morphology.[133] The nodulocystic or noduloulcerative type accounts for 70% of basal cell carcinomas. It is a waxy, cream-colored lesion with rolled, pearly borders (Fig. 15-8). It often contains a central ulcer. When these lesions are large they are called "rodent ulcers." Pigmented basal cell carcinomas are tan to black in color and should be distinguished by biopsy examination from melanoma. Superficial basal cell cancers occur more commonly on the trunk and form a red, scaling lesion that is sometimes difficult to distinguish grossly from Bowen's disease. A rare form of basal cell carcinoma is the basosquamous type, which contains elements of basal cell and squamous cell cancer. These lesions can metastasize more like a squamous cell carcinoma and should be treated aggressively. Other types include morpheaform, adenoid, and infiltrative carcinomas.[134]

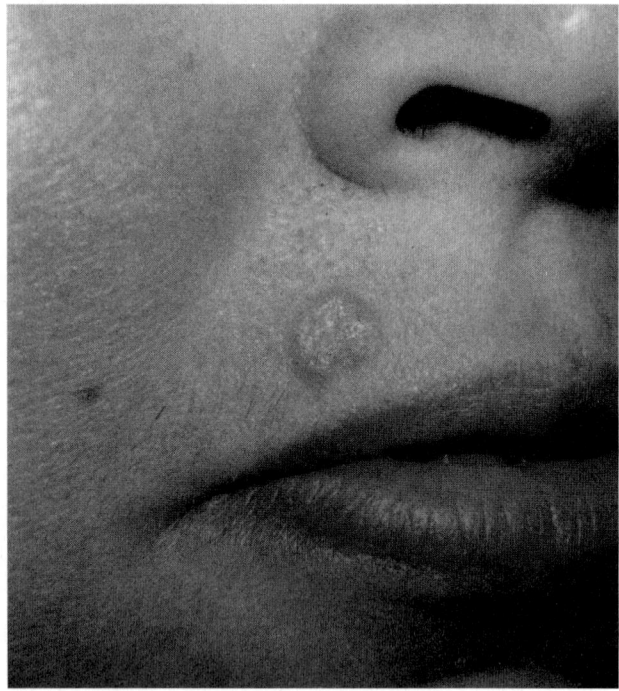

FIG. 15-8. *Basal cell carcinoma with rolled, pearly borders.*

Basal cell carcinomas usually are slow growing, and patients often neglect these lesions for years. Metastasis and death from this disease are extremely rare, but these lesions can cause extensive local destruction. The majority of small (less than 2 mm), nodular lesions may be treated by dermatologists with curettage and electrodesiccation or laser vaporization.[135] A drawback to these procedures is that no pathologic specimen is obtained to confirm the diagnosis or evaluate the tumor margins. Larger tumors, lesions that invade bone or surrounding structures, and more aggressive histologic types (morpheaform, infiltrative, and basosquamous) are best treated by surgical excision with a 2- to 4-mm margin of normal tissue.[136] Histologic confirmation that the margins of resection do not contain tumor is required. Because nodular lesions are less likely to recur, the smaller margin may be used, whereas other types need a wider margin of resection. Alternative methods of treatment, such as radiation therapy and Mohs' surgery, are discussed later under "Alternative Therapy."

Squamous Cell Carcinoma

Squamous cell carcinomas arise from keratinocytes of the epidermis. It is less common than basal cell carcinoma but is more devastating because it can invade surrounding tissue and metastasize more readily. In situ lesions have the eponym of Bowen's disease, and in situ squamous cell carcinomas of the penis are referred to as erythroplasia of Queyrat. Contrary to previous reports, Bowen's disease is not a marker for other systemic malignancies.

Tumor thickness correlates well with its biologic behavior. Lesions that recur locally are more than 4 mm thick and lesions that metastasize are 10 mm or more.[137] The location of the lesion also is important. Tumors arising in burn scars (Marjolin's ulcer), areas of chronic osteomyelitis, and areas of previous injury metastasize early.[138] Lesions on the external ear frequently recur and involve regional lymph node basins early.[139] Squamous cell cancers in

areas with solar damage behave less aggressively and usually require only local excision.

Although small lesions can be treated with curettage and electrodesiccation, most surgeons recommend excision of the tumor. Lesions should be excised with a 1-cm margin if possible, and histologic confirmation that the margins are tumor-free is mandatory. Tumor-invading bone should be excised if recurrence is to be avoided. Regional lymph node excision is indicated for clinically palpable nodes (therapeutic lymph node dissection). Lesions arising in chronic wounds behave aggressively and are more likely to spread to regional lymph nodes. For these lesions lymphadenectomy before the development of palpable nodes is indicated (prophylactic lymph node dissection). Metastatic disease is a poor prognostic sign, with only 13% of patients surviving after 10 years.

Alternative Therapy

Alternatives to surgical therapy for squamous and basal cell cancers consist of radiation therapy or topical 5-fluorouracil for patients unable or unwilling to undergo surgery. Radiation therapy for small and superficial lesions obtains cure rates comparable to surgical excision. Radiation damage to surrounding normal skin with inflammation and scarring can be a problem. Also the development of cutaneous malignancies in irradiated skin is a serious long-term risk with this treatment modality.

For lesions on the face or near the nose or eye, resection of a wide rim of normal tissue to remove the entire tumor can cause significant functional and cosmetic problems. These lesions can be removed by Mohs' micrographic surgery. Mohs' technique, developed in 1932, is a method to serially excise a tumor by taking small increments of tissue until the entire tumor is removed.[140] Each piece of tissue removed is frozen and immediately examined microscopically to determine whether the entire lesion has been resected. The advantage of the Mohs' technique is that the entire margin of resection is evaluated, while with wide excision and traditional histologic examination, only selected samples of the surgical margin are examined. The major benefit of Mohs' technique is the ability to remove a tumor with the least sacrifice of uninvolved tissue. This technique is effective for treating carcinomas around the eyelids and nose, where tissue loss is most conspicuous. However, one major drawback is that the procedure can be extremely lengthy (up to several days) since complete excision may require multiple attempts. Cure rates are comparable to those of wide excision.

Patients with basal cell carcinomas have been treated with intralesional injection of interferon.[141] The majority of the lesions were eliminated or controlled by the injections. The lesions that did not respond required surgical excision. When lesions respond to injections, operation is avoided and no reconstruction of the defect is required. The major disadvantages of this treatment are the need for multiple office visits over several weeks for injections, the systemic side effects of interferon, and a potential need for surgery if the lesions do not respond to injections. Clinical trials with combinations of retinoids (vitamin A derivatives) and interferon have demonstrated good response rates in patients with advanced, inoperable squamous cell carcinomas.[142] These results suggest that interferon is likely to have a greater role in therapy of cutaneous neoplasms in the future.

Malignant Melanoma

What was a relatively rare disease 50 years ago has now become alarmingly more common. The rise in the rate of melanoma is the highest of any cancer in the United States. In 1935, the annual incidence of the disease was 1 per 100,000 people. By 1991, the incidence had risen to 12.9 per 100,000 people. The 1998 age-adjusted rate for invasive melanoma is 18.3 per 100,000 for white males and 13.0 per 100,000 for white females in the United States.[143,144] The increasing rate of melanoma incidents is not associated with a corresponding increase in melanoma death. Since 1980 there has been no evidence of a linear trend in melanoma deaths, probably as the result of earlier detection and treatment.[145]

Because melanoma is becoming so common, it is important for all physicians to be familiar with this disease. The important clinical features of a melanoma include a pigmented lesion with an irregular, raised surface and irregular borders. Approximately 5 to 10% of melanomas are not pigmented. Lesions that change in color and size and ulcerate over a few months' time are considered suspicious and should be biopsied. Surgery remains the mainstay of therapy for melanoma, so it is imperative that surgeons be aware of the latest methods of diagnosis, staging, and therapy.

Pathogenesis

Melanoma arises from transformed melanocytes and can arise anywhere that melanocytes have migrated during embryogenesis. The eye, central nervous system, gastrointestinal tract, and even the gallbladder have been reported as primary sites of the disease. More than 90% of melanomas are found on the skin; however, 4% are discovered as metastases without an identifiable primary site. Many melanomas, especially in the early phases of growth, are found to contain areas of tumor regression on histologic examination. Regression represents a host immune response to the tumor. Metastatic melanomas with unknown primary sites probably arise from completely regressed lesions that are difficult to locate.

Nevi are benign melanocytic neoplasms found on the skin of most people. Dysplastic nevi are less common and contain a histologically identifiable focus of atypical melanocytes. This type of nevus may represent an intermediate between a benign nevus and a true malignant melanoma. It is well documented that patients with melanoma have significantly more nevi and dysplastic nevi than matched controls.[146] The relative risk of developing melanoma increases with the number of dysplastic nevi that a patient develops.[147] The relationship is similar to that between the number of colonic polyps and the development of colon cancer. Patients with dysplastic nevi and family members with dysplastic nevi and melanoma are at increased risk for developing melanoma, suggesting that in these patients there is a genetic component to the risk of developing the malignancy. Between 6 and 14% of malignant melanomas have been reported to occur in a familial pattern.[148]

Once the melanocyte has transformed into the malignant phenotype, the growth of the lesion is radial in the plane of the epidermis. Even though microinvasion of the dermis can be observed during this radial growth phase, metastases do not occur. Only when the melanoma cells form nests in the dermis are metastases observed. The transformed cells in the vertical growth phase are morphologically different and express different cell-surface antigens than those in the radial phase or cells of the dysplastic nevus. In addition, these cells behave differently in cell culture. They can grow in a less enriched media and have a longer life span.

Types

There are four common types of melanoma. These are, in order of decreasing frequency, superficial spreading, nodular, lentigo

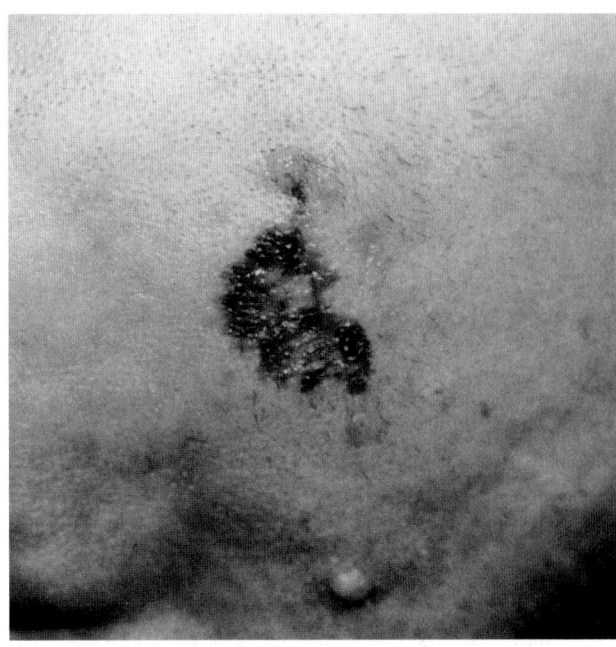

FIG. 15-9. This is the typical appearance of a superficial spreading melanoma. Note the area of regression in the center of the lesion.

maligna, and acral lentiginous. Each has distinct characteristics and behaviors.

The most common type, representing up to 70% of melanomas, is the superficial spreading type.[149] These lesions occur anywhere on the skin except the hands and feet. They are flat, commonly contain areas of regression, and measure 1 to 2 cm in diameter at the time of diagnosis (Fig. 15-9). There is a relatively long radial growth phase before vertical growth begins.[150,151]

The nodular type accounts for 15 to 30% of melanomas.[149] These lesions are darker and raised. The histologic criterion for a nodular melanoma is the lack of radial growth peripheral to the area of vertical growth; hence, all nodular melanomas are in the vertical growth phase at the time of diagnosis.[152] Although it is an aggressive lesion, the prognosis for a patient with a nodular-type lesion is the same as that for a patient with a superficial spreading lesion of the same depth of invasion.

The lentigo maligna type, accounting for 4 to 15% of melanomas, occurs mostly on the neck, the face, and the back of the hands of elderly people.[149] These lesions are always surrounded by dermis with heavy solar degeneration.[153] They tend to become quite large before a diagnosis is made, but also have the best prognosis because invasive growth occurs late. Only 5 to 8% of lentigo malignas are estimated to evolve to invasive melanoma.[154]

Acral lentiginous type is the least-common subtype, representing only 2 to 8% of melanoma in whites. It occurs on the palms and soles and in the subungual regions. Although melanoma among dark-skinned people is relatively rare, the acral lentiginous type accounts for 29 to 72% of all melanomas in dark-skinned people (African Americans, Asians, and Hispanics) than in people with less-pigmented skin.[149,155] Subungual lesions appear as blue-black discolorations of the posterior nail fold and are most common on the great toe or thumb. The additional presence of pigmentation in the proximal or lateral nail folds (Hutchinson's sign) is diagnostic of subungual melanoma.

Table 15-1
TNM Classification of Melanoma of the Skin

Primary tumor (T)	
T1	1.0 mm in thickness or less
T1a	Without ulceration and Clark level II/III
T1b	With ulceration or level IV/V
T2	1.01–2.0 mm in thickness
T2a	Without ulceration
T2b	With ulceration
T3	2.01–4.0 mm in thickness
T3a	Without ulceration
T3b	With ulceration
T4	4.01 mm or greater in thickness
T4a	Without ulceration
T4b	With ulceration
Nodal status (N)	
N1	1 node
N1a	Micrometastasis (as diagnoses after sentinel lymph node or lymphadenectomy)
N1b	Macrometastasis (clinically detectable, confirmed by pathology)
N2	2–3 nodes
N2a	Micrometastasis
N2b	Macrometastasis
N2c	In-transit met(s) without metastatic nodes
N3	4 or more metastatic nodes, or matted nodes, or in-transit met(s)/satellite(s) with metastatic node(s)
Metastasis (M)	
M1	Distant skin, subcutaneous or nodal matastasis, serum LDH normal
M2	Lung metastasis, normal LDH
M3	All other visceral metastasis with normal LDH or any distant mets with elevated LDH

LDH = lactic dehydrogenase.

Prognostic Factors

The original staging system classified melanoma into local (stage I), regional lymph node (stage II), and metastatic (stage III) disease. This staging system was not advantageous given that most patients were categorized into stage I disease, therefore limiting its usefulness in prognostic studies. The most current staging system, from the American Joint Committee on Cancer (AJCC), contains the best method of interpreting clinical information in regard to prognosis of this disease (Table 15-1).[156] Historically, the vertical thickness of the primary tumor (Breslow thickness) and the anatomic depth of invasion (Clark level) have represented the dominant factors in the T classification the melanoma staging system.

The T classification of lesions comes from the original observation by Clark that prognosis is directly related to the level of invasion of the skin by the melanoma. Whereas Clark used the histologic level (I, superficial to basement membrane [in situ]; II, papillary dermis; III, papillary/reticular dermal junction; IV, reticular dermis; and V, subcutaneous fat), Breslow modified the approach to obtain a more reproducible measure of invasion by the use of an ocular micrometer. The lesions were measured from the granular layer of the epidermis or the base of the ulcer to the greatest depth of the tumor (I, 0.75 mm or less; II, 0.76 to 1.5 mm; III, 1.51 to 4.0 mm; IV, 4.0 mm or more).[157] These levels of invasion have been subsequently modified and incorporated in the AJCC staging system (Fig. 15-10). The new staging system has largely replaced the Clark level with another histologic feature, ulceration, based on analysis of large databases available to the AJCC Melanoma Committee.[158]

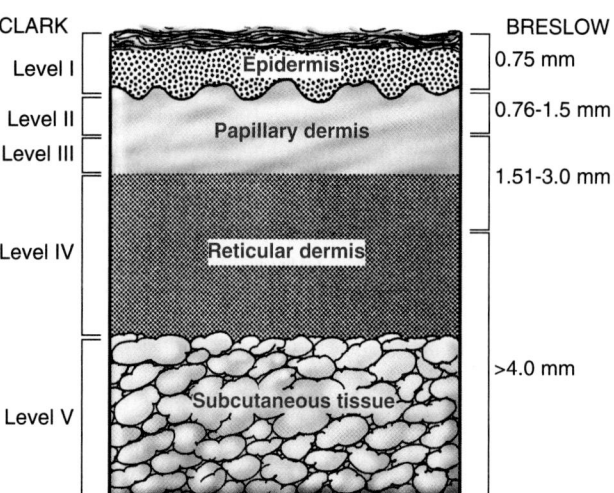

FIG. 15-10. The primary melanoma is classified according to its depth of invasion in the skin. The criteria for Clark's and Breslow's levels are illustrated. The current T classification adopted by the AJCC is a modification of these classifications.

Evidence of tumor in regional lymph nodes is a poor prognostic sign. This is accounted for in the staging system by advancing any T classifications from stage I or II to stage III (Table 15-2). The 15-year survival rate drops precipitously with the presence of lymph node metastasis (Fig. 15-11). The number of positive lymph nodes also is correlated with survival rates.

The presence of distant metastasis is a grave prognostic sign (stage IV). The median survival ranges from 2 to 7 months, depending on the number and site of metastases, but survival up to a few years has been reported.

Other independent prognostic factors have been identified:

Anatomic Location. Independent of histologic type and depth of invasion, people with lesions of the extremities have a better prognosis than people with melanomas of the head and neck or trunk (82% 10-year survival rate for localized disease of the extremity, compared to a 68% survival rate with a lesion of the face).[159] Most melanomas in men are located on the trunk (45%), and the majority of melanomas in women are located on the lower extremities (42%).[160]

Ulceration. Presence of ulceration in a lesion carries a worse prognosis. For unknown reasons these melanomas are more

Table 15-2
Stage Grouping

Stage IA	T1a	N0	M0
IB	T1b	N0	M0
	T2a	N0	M0
IIA	T2b	N0	M0
	T3a	N0	M0
IIB	T3b	N0	M0
	T4a	N0	M0
IIC	T4b	N0	M0
III	Any T	N1	M0
		N2	
		N3	
IV	Any T	Any N	Any M1

SOURCE: From the American Joint Committee on Cancer Staging.

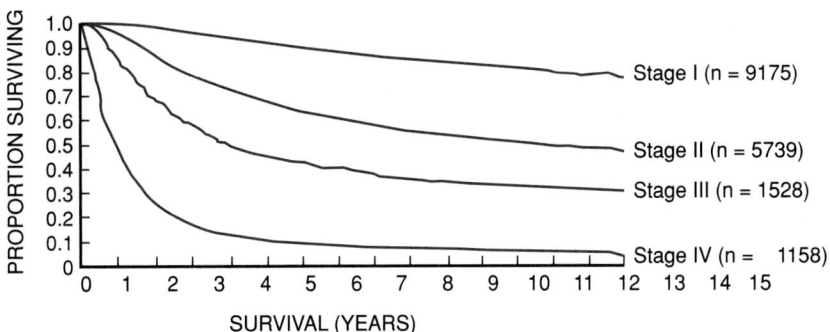

FIG. 15-11. The graph summarizes the data for 15-year survival rates of patients with melanoma grouped according to stage. (*From Balch et al,*[158] *with permission.*)

aggressive than those without ulceration. The 10-year survival rate for patients with local disease (stage I) and an ulcerated melanoma was 50%, compared to 78% for the same stage lesion without ulceration. Early studies identified that the incidence of ulceration increases with increasing thickness, from 12.5% in melanomas less than 0.75 mm to 72.5% in melanomas greater than 4.0 mm.[161] Recent evidence suggests that tumors ulcerate as the result of increased angiogenesis.[162]

Gender. Numerous studies demonstrate that females have an improved survival compared to males.[159] Women tend to acquire melanomas in more favorable anatomic sites, and these lesions are less likely to contain ulceration. After correcting for thickness, age, and location, females continue to have a higher survival rate than men (80% 10-year survival for women vs. 61% 10-year survival rate for men with stage I disease).[163]

Histologic Type. In general, there is no significant difference between different histologic tumor types in terms of prognosis, when matched for tumor thickness, gender, age, or other.[160] Nodular melanomas have the same prognosis as superficial spreading types when lesions are matched for depth of invasion. Lentigo maligna types, however, have a better prognosis even after correcting for thickness, and acral lentiginous lesions have a worse prognosis. Even though the various types of melanoma have similar prognoses when controlled for the other prognostic factors, acral lentiginous melanoma has a shorter interval to recurrence.[164,165]

Treatment

The treatment of melanoma is primarily surgical. The indication for procedures such as lymph node dissection, sentinel lymphadenectomy, superficial parotidectomy, and resection of distant metastases have changed somewhat over time, but the only hope for cure and the best treatment for regional control and palliation remains surgery (Fig. 15-12). Most cases of cutaneous melanoma are cured by excision of the primary tumor alone. Radiation therapy, regional and systemic chemotherapy, and immunotherapy are effective in a limited set of circumstances, but none are a first-line option.

All suspicious lesions should undergo excisional biopsy. A 1-mm margin of normal skin is taken if the wound can be closed primarily. If removal of the entire lesion creates too large a defect, then an incisional biopsy of a representative part is recommended. Biopsy incisions should be made with the expectation that a subsequent wide excision of the biopsy site may be done. Once a diagnosis of melanoma is made, the biopsy scar and any remains of the lesion need to be removed to eradicate any remaining tumor. Four

randomized prospective trials have been completed to address the issue of resection margins.[166] The results of these trials suggest that lesions 1 mm or less in thickness can be treated with a 1-cm margin. For lesions 1 mm to 4 mm thick, a 2-cm margin is recommended. There is little data to support the use of margins wider than 2 cm.[167] The surrounding tissue should be removed down to the fascia to remove all lymphatic channels. If the deep fascia is not involved by the tumor, removing it does not affect recurrence or survival rates, so the fascia is left intact. If the defect cannot be closed primarily, a skin graft or local flap is used.

All clinically positive lymph nodes should be removed by regional nodal dissection. If possible, the lymphatics between the lesion and the regional nodes are removed in continuity. Leaving tumor behind results in recurrence of lesions that cause great morbidity. When groin lymph nodes are removed, the deep (iliac) nodes must be removed along with the superficial (inguinal) nodes, or disease will recur in that region. For axillary dissections the nodes medial to the pectoralis minor muscle must also be resected. For lesions on the face, anterior scalp, and ear, a superficial parotidectomy to remove parotid nodes and a modified neck dissection is recommended. Disruption of the lymphatic outflow does cause significant problems with chronic edema, especially of the lower extremity.

Treatment of regional lymph nodes that do not obviously contain tumor in patients without evidence of metastasis (stages I and II) is determined by considering the possible benefits of the procedure as weighed against the risks. In patients with thin lesions (less than 0.75 mm), the tumor cells are still localized in the surrounding tissue, and the cure rate is excellent with wide excision of the primary lesion; therefore treatment of regional lymph nodes is not beneficial. With very thick lesions (more than 4 mm), it is highly likely that the tumor cells have already spread to the regional lymph nodes and distant sites. Removal of the lymph nodes has no effect on survival. Most of these patients die of metastatic disease before developing problems in regional nodes. Because there are significant morbid effects of lymphadenectomy, most surgeons defer the procedure until clinically evident disease appears. Approximately 40% of these patients eventually develop disease in the lymph nodes and require a second palliative operation. Elective lymphadenectomy is sometimes performed in these patients as a staging procedure before entry into clinical trials.

In patients with intermediate-thickness tumors (T2 and T3, 0.76 to 4.0 mm) and no clinical evidence of nodal or metastatic disease, the use of prophylactic dissection (elective lymph node dissection on clinically negative nodes) is controversial. Numerous retrospective studies suggested that patients with primary melanoma who underwent elective lymph node dissection had improved survival.[168]

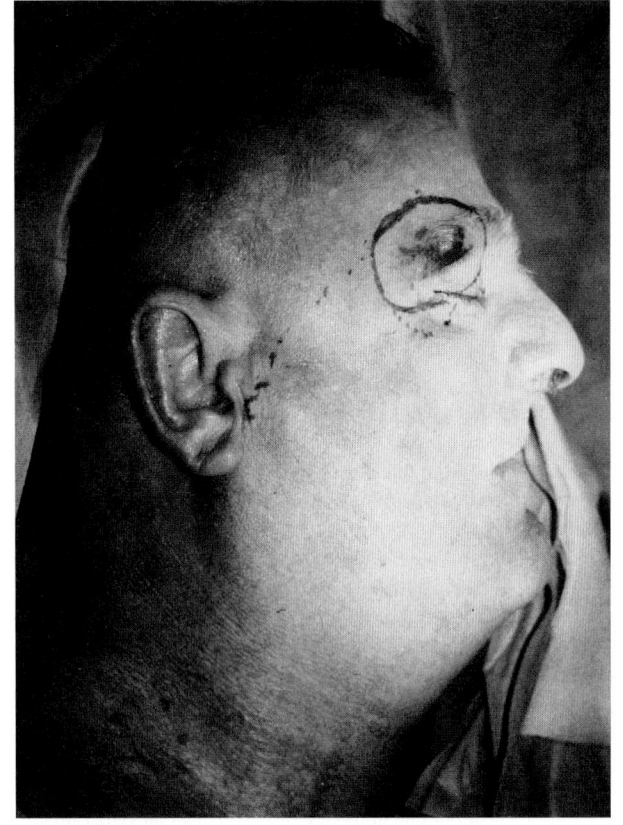

A

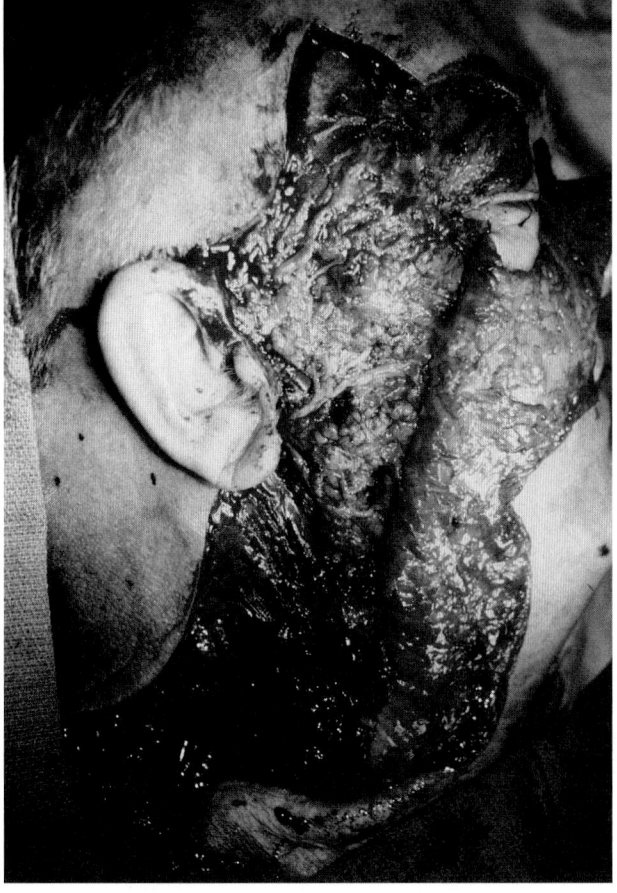

B

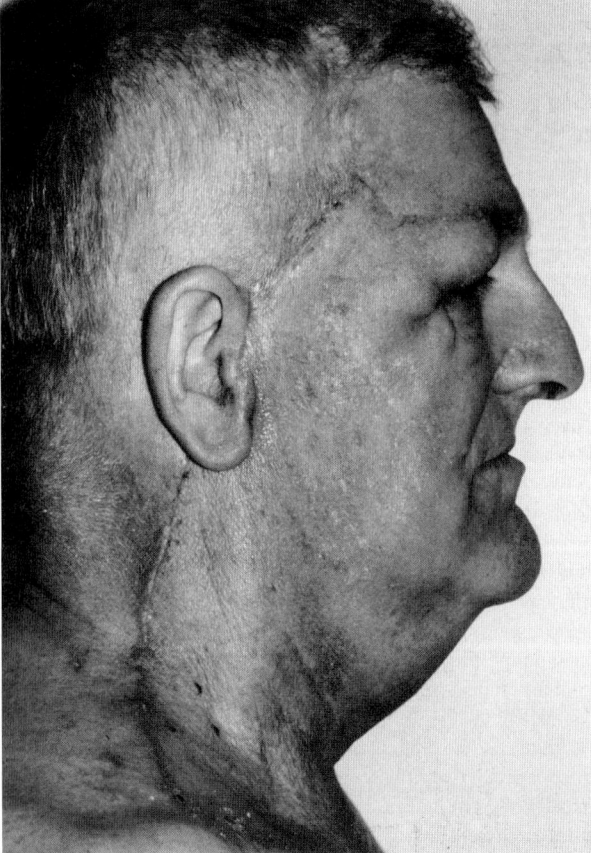

C

FIG. 15-12. *A.* A patient with a deep melanoma (T4) over the right eyebrow. He also had a palpable 1.5-cm preauricular lymph node (N1). *B.* He was treated by wide excision of the primary lesion, superficial parotidectomy, and modified radical neck dissection. *C.* Reconstruction of the forehead defect was done with a cervicofacial advancement flap.

However, prospective, randomized studies have not demonstrated that elective lymph node dissection improves survival in patients with intermediate-thickness melanomas.[169] Careful examination of specimens in patients undergoing elective lymph node dissection have found that, in 25 to 50% of the cases, specimens contain micrometastases. Among patients who do not have an elective lymph node dissection, 20 to 25% eventually develop clinically evident disease and require lymphadenectomy. More evidence suggests that there may be improved survival with elective lymph node dissection in patients with a higher risk of developing metastasis (i.e., lesions with ulceration or those located on the trunk, head, and neck). The most compelling argument for the potential benefits of elective lymph node dissection comes from evidence in large clinical trials; patients with intermediate-thickness melanomas without elective node dissection continue to die of the disease 10 years later, whereas patients who had an elective lymph node dissection do not. Although not yet statistically significant, these differences may become statistically viable in the future.

Sentinel lymphadenectomy for malignant melanoma is a surgical modality gaining acceptance. The sentinel node may be preoperatively located with the use of a gamma camera, which identifies the radioisotope injected into the primary lesion. Some investigators suggest that preoperative identification provides the surgeon greater reliability in localizing the lymph node.[170] Others map intraoperatively, with the injection of 1% isosulfan blue dye into the site of the primary melanoma.[166] These techniques enable the surgeon to identify the lymphatic drainage from the primary lesion and determine the first (sentinel) lymph node draining the tumor. The node is removed, and if micrometastases are identified in frozen-section examination, a complete lymph node dissection is performed.

When the sentinel node can be identified, it serves as an accurate indication of the status of the rest of the nodes in the region. This method may be used to identify patients who would benefit from lymph node dissection, while sparing others an unnecessary operation. Whether this procedure actually improves survival in these patients awaits the results of clinical trials.

When patients develop distant metastases, surgical therapy may be indicated. Once melanoma has spread to a distant site, median survival is 7 to 8 months and the 5-year survival rate is less than 5%.[171] Solitary lesions in the brain, gastrointestinal tract, or skin that are symptomatic should be excised when possible. Although cure is extremely rare, the degree of palliation can be high and asymptomatic survival prolonged.[172] A decision to operate on metastatic lesions must be made after careful deliberation with the patient.

A promising area in the nonsurgical treatment of melanoma is the use of immunologic manipulation. Interferon-α (INF-α) 2b is the only FDA-approved adjuvant treatment for AJCC stages IIB/III melanoma.[173] Several randomized trials of INF-α adjuvant therapy have been conducted.[174,175] In these patients, both the relapse-free interval and overall survival were improved with use of INF-α.[176] Side effects were common and frequently severe; the majority of the patients required modification of the initial dosage and 24% discontinued treatment. These recent findings are encouraging because past trials of adjuvant therapy have never demonstrated a beneficial effect.

Vaccines have been developed with the hope of stimulating the body's own immune system against the tumor. Melanoma cells contain a number of distinctly different cell-surface antigens. Monoclonal antibodies have been raised against these antigens. These antibodies have been used alone or linked to a radioisotope or cytotoxic agent in an effort to selectively kill tumor cells. All treatments are currently investigational. One defined-antigen vaccine has entered clinical testing, the ganglioside G_{M2}. Gangliosides are carbohydrate antigens found on the surface of melanomas as well as many other tumors.[177]

Although initially thought to be ineffective in the treatment of melanoma, radiation therapy has been shown to be useful. High-dose-per-fraction radiation produces a better response rate than low-dose large-fraction therapy. It has been found that postoperative radiation to the neck or axilla after radical lymph node dissections decreases regional recurrence rates in node-positive patients.[178,179] Radiation therapy is the treatment of choice for patients with symptomatic multiple brain metastases. Up to 70% of treated patients show measurable improvement in tumor size, symptomatology, or performance status.[180]

Hyperthermic regional perfusion of the limb with a chemotherapeutic agent (e.g., melphalan) is the treatment of choice for patients with local recurrence or in-transit lesions (local disease in lymphatics) on an extremity that is not amenable to excision. In-transit metastases develop in 5 to 8% of melanoma patients with a high-risk primary melanoma (>1.5 mm).[181] The goal of regional perfusion therapy is to increase the dosage of the chemotherapeutic agent to maximize tumor response while limiting systemic toxic effects. Melphalan is generally heated to an elevated temperature (up to 41.5°C [106.7°F]) and perfused for 60 to 90 minutes.[182] While difficult to perform and associated with complications (neutropenia, amputation, death), it does produce a high response rate (greater than 50%).[183] The introduction of tumor necrosis factor alpha or interferon-γ with melphalan results in the regression of more than 90% of cutaneous in-transit metastasis.[184,185] Prospective clinical trials are under way to evaluate the use of regional perfusion for melanoma of the limbs as adjuvant therapy for patients with stage I disease. In addition, regional perfusion therapy for metastatic disease to the liver is under investigation.

OTHER MALIGNANCIES

Merkel Cell Carcinoma (Primary Neuroendocrine Carcinoma of the Skin)

Originally thought to be a variant of squamous cell carcinoma, it was only recently demonstrated by immunohistochemical markers that Merkel cell carcinomas are of neuroepithelial differentiation.[186] These tumors are associated with a synchronous or metasynchronous squamous cell carcinoma 25% of the time. These tumors are very aggressive, and wide local resection with 3-cm margins is recommended. Local recurrence rates are high, and distant metastases occur in one-third of patients. Prophylactic regional lymph node dissection and adjuvant radiation therapy are recommended. Overall, the prognosis is worse than for malignant melanoma.

Extramammary Paget's Disease

This tumor is histologically similar to the mammary type. It is a cutaneous lesion that appears as a pruritic red patch that does not resolve.[187] Biopsy demonstrates classic Paget's cells. Paget's disease is thought to be a cutaneous extension of an underlying adenocarcinoma, although an associated tumor cannot always be demonstrated.

Adnexal Carcinomas

This group includes the rare-type tumors apocrine, eccrine, and sebaceous carcinomas. They are locally destructive and can cause death by distant metastasis.

Angiosarcomas

Angiosarcomas may arise spontaneously, mostly on the scalp, face, and neck. They usually appear as a bruise that spontaneously bleeds or enlarges without trauma.[188] Tumors also may arise in areas of prior radiation therapy or in the setting of chronic lymphedema of the arm, such as after mastectomy (Stewart-Treves syndrome). The angiosarcomas that arise in these areas of chronic change occur decades later. The tumors consist of anaplastic endothelial cells surrounding vascular channels. While total excision of early lesions can provide occasional cure, the prognosis usually is poor, with 5-year survival rates of less than 20%. Chemotherapy and radiation therapy are used for palliation.

Kaposi's Sarcoma

Kaposi's sarcoma (KS) appears as rubbery bluish nodules that occur primarily on the extremities but may appear anywhere on the skin and viscera. These lesions are usually multifocal rather than metastatic. Histologically the lesions are composed of capillaries lined by atypical endothelial cells. Early lesions may resemble hemangiomas, while older lesions contain more spindle cells and resemble sarcomas.[189]

Classic KS is seen in people of Eastern Europe or sub-Saharan Africa. The lesions are locally aggressive but undergo periods of remission. Visceral spread of the lesions is rare, but a subtype of the African variety has a predilection for spreading to lymph nodes. A different variety of KS has been described for people with AIDS or with immunosuppression from chemotherapy. For reasons not yet understood, AIDS-related KS occurs primarily in male homosexuals and not in intravenous drug abusers or hemophiliacs. In this form of the disease, the lesions spread rapidly to the nodes, and the gastrointestinal and respiratory tract often are involved. Development of AIDS-related KS may be associated with concurrent infection with a herpes-like virus.[190]

Treatment for all types of KS consists of radiation to the lesions. Combination chemotherapy is effective in controlling the disease, although most patients develop an opportunistic infection during or shortly after treatment. Surgical treatment is reserved for lesions that interfere with vital functions, such as bowel obstruction or airway compromise.

Dermatofibrosarcoma Protuberans

Dermatofibrosarcoma protuberans consists of large nodular lesions located mainly on the trunk. They often ulcerate and become infected. With enlargement, the lesions become painful. Histologically, the lesions contain atypical spindle cells, probably of fibroblast origin, located around a core of collagen tissue. Sometimes they are mistaken for an infected keloid. Metastases are rare and surgical excision can be curative. Excision must be complete because local recurrences are common.

Fibrosarcoma

Fibrosarcomas are hard, irregular masses found in the subcutaneous fat. The fibroblasts appear markedly anaplastic with disorganized growth. If they are not excised completely, metastases usually develop. The 5-year survival rate after excision is approximately 60%.

Liposarcoma

Liposarcomas arise in the deep muscle planes and, rarely, from the subcutaneous tissue. They occur most commonly on the thigh. An enlarging lipoma should be excised and inspected to distinguish it from a liposarcoma. Wide excision is the treatment of choice, with radiation therapy reserved for metastatic disease.

SKIN MALIGNANCIES ASSOCIATED WITH GENETIC SYNDROMES

There are several well-recognized diseases associated with an increased incidence of skin malignancies. Some are associated with a specific neoplasm, whereas others appear to have the less specific effect of leaving the patient susceptible to a variety of neoplasms. Many of these syndromes are linked to specific chromosome mutations that give rise to the increased risk of malignant transformation of the skin lesions, offering hope for better diagnostic and therapeutic interventions.[191]

Diseases linked with basal cell carcinoma include the basal cell nevus (Gorlin's) syndrome[192] and nevus sebaceus of Jadassohn. Basal cell nevus syndrome is an autosomal dominant disorder characterized by the growth of hundreds of basal cell carcinomas during young adulthood. Palmar and plantar pits are a common physical finding and represent foci of neoplasms. Treatment is limited to excision of only aggressive and symptomatic lesions. Nevus sebaceus of Jadassohn is a lesion containing several cutaneous tissue elements that develops during childhood. This lesion is associated with a variety of neoplasms of the epidermis, but most commonly basal cell carcinoma.

Diseases associated with squamous cell carcinoma may have a causative role in the development of carcinoma. Skin diseases that cause chronic wounds, such as epidermolysis bullosus and lupus erythematosus, are associated with a high incidence of squamous cell carcinoma. Epidermodysplasia verruciformis is a rare autosomal recessive disease associated with infection with human papillomavirus. Large verrucous lesions develop early in life and often progress to invasive squamous cell carcinoma in middle age.

Xeroderma pigmentosum is an autosomal recessive disease associated with a defect in cellular repair of DNA damage. The inability of the skin to correct DNA damage from ultraviolet radiation leaves these patients prone to cutaneous malignancies. Squamous cell carcinomas are most frequent, but basal cell carcinomas, melanomas, and even acute leukemias are seen.[193]

Dysplastic nevi represent a precursor to melanoma. Familial dysplastic nevus syndrome is an autosomal dominant disorder. Patients develop multiple dysplastic nevi, and longitudinal studies have demonstrated an almost 100% incidence of melanoma. Gene mapping of the defects found in familial dysplastic nevus syndrome have identified several candidate "melanoma" genes.[194] It remains to be determined whether these germline mutations are also found in sporadic cases of melanoma. Much like other familial malignancy syndromes, genetic analysis of the hereditary defect may shed much needed light on the molecular mechanisms that lead to malignant transformation. Much like familial polyposis coli and the association with colon cancer, familial dysplastic nevus syndrome is treated by close surveillance and frequent biopsy of all suspicious lesions. Similarly, the development of colon cancer can be arrested with total proctocolectomy; unfortunately, a similar solution is not possible in patients with familial dysplastic nevi.

FUTURE DEVELOPMENTS IN SKIN SURGERY

Despite three decades of effort, the major challenge in surgical therapy for diseases of the skin remains the lack of an optimum replacement for diseased or damaged tissue. Autologous skin grafts

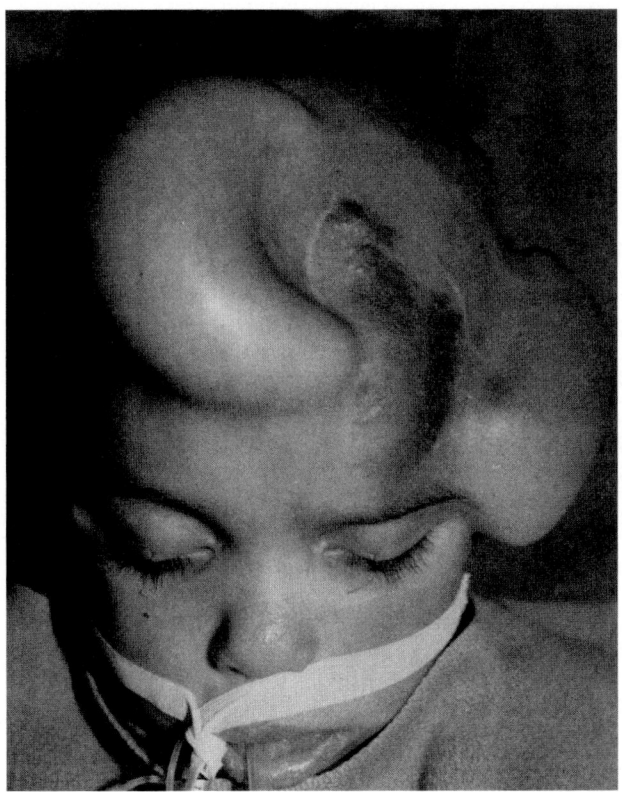

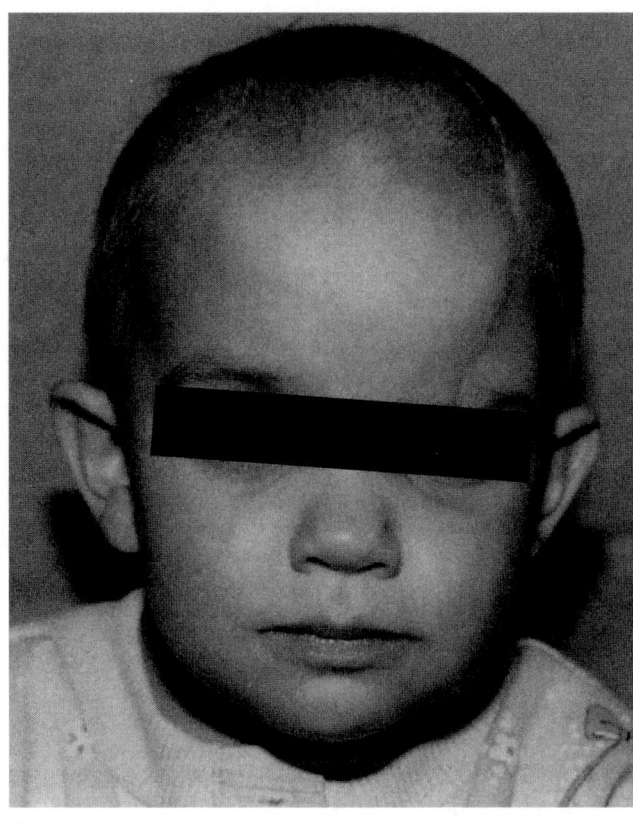

A   B

FIG. 15-13. *A. Tissue expanders are used in the scalp of an infant for excision of a neurofibroma. B. After excision and closure of scalp defect.*

are still the best method to treat skin defects, but donor-site problems and limited availability of autologous skin remain problematic. Tissue expansion with subcutaneous balloon implants (Fig. 15–13) produces new epidermis; however, much of this tissue is rearrangement of the old tissue. Expansion of skin produces a limited amount of useful tissue.[195–197] The future of surgical therapy for diseases of the skin lies in the development of engineered skin replacements. Current research is directed at identifying different materials and cells that can be used to replace both epidermis and dermis.

The expansion of epidermis by the growth and maturation of keratinocytes in culture is readily performed.[198,199] A small skin biopsy specimen can produce enough autologous epithelium to cover the entire body surface (Fig. 15-14). However, on the body, the cultured epidermis often blisters and sloughs as a consequence of slow restoration of the basement membrane.[200] Additionally, replacing epidermis without the underlying dermis leads to severe wound contractures and hypertrophic scars. Restoration of damaged dermis remains a critical unsolved problem.

Several dermal replacements based on synthetic materials or cadaveric sources are in clinical use.[201] A bovine-collagen and shark-proteoglycan–based dermis (Integra) has been used primarily in burn patients for more than a decade. This prosthetic dermis, available in ready-to-use form, can cover large surface areas.[202] Vascularization of this dermis takes 2 to 3 weeks, and final epidermal coverage of the wound requires a thin skin graft. The final result is functionally and aesthetically good, but in the setting of acute burn coverage, the engraftment rate of the material and high cost has been problematic. Despite its limitations, it is the first promising dermal replacement to be widely used and has a proven record of safety and efficacy.[203] Cadaveric dermis, with all of the cellular elements

removed, is not antigenic and is not rejected by the recipient patient. This human dermal matrix is commercially available (AlloDerm) and functions much like Integra, with similar limitations of engraftment and high cost. Both forms of dermal replacements are more frequently used in delayed reconstruction of burn patients than in the acute setting.[204,205] The third type of skin replacements use dermal matrix material combined with mesenchymal cells (fibroblasts) from an allogenic source (TransCyte), typically discarded neonatal foreskin specimens.[206,207] These products have the advantage of a matrix containing cells that secrete growth factors and cytokines to accelerate wound healing, but have a disadvantage in that the recipient patient ultimately rejects the cells. Whether these products are actual skin replacements or biologic dressings remains an issue because a biologic dressing would have limited use in patients in need of large amounts of skin tissue.

The main issue still confounding investigators in the field of soft-tissue replacement is the need to find a wider source of autologous skin cells that can be manipulated to repopulate natural or synthetic matrices for use as permanent skin replacements. Identifying sources of mesenchymal stem cells may be one promising solution. Stem cells in hair follicles have been used for some time to grow keratinocyte cultures for replacement of the epidermis.[208] Recent studies have identified bone marrow–derived stem cells, which traffic between the marrow and skin, that mature into endothelial cells and fibroblasts in the skin. Identifying methods to collect and culture these cells may lead to a source of autologous cells for future skin replacement.[209] In addition, as more is learned about the protein factors that control wound healing and tissue growth, the replacement for damaged skin will eventually come from complete organogenesis of tissue. Characterization of these growth factors on

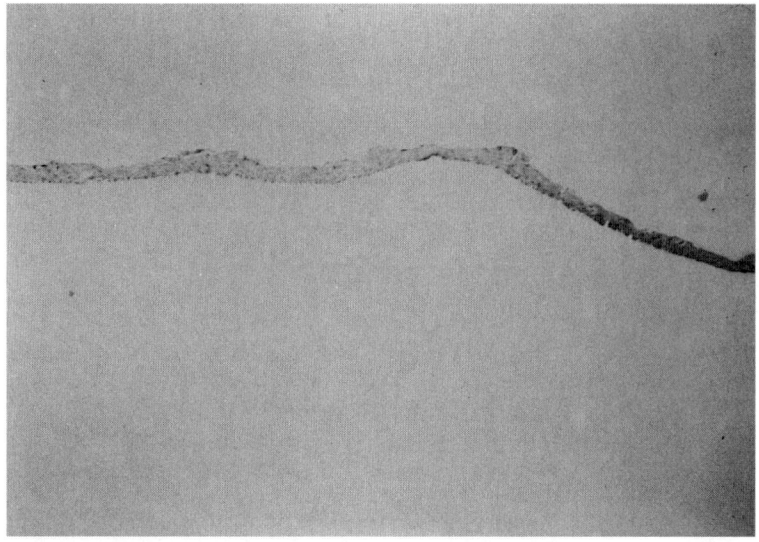

A

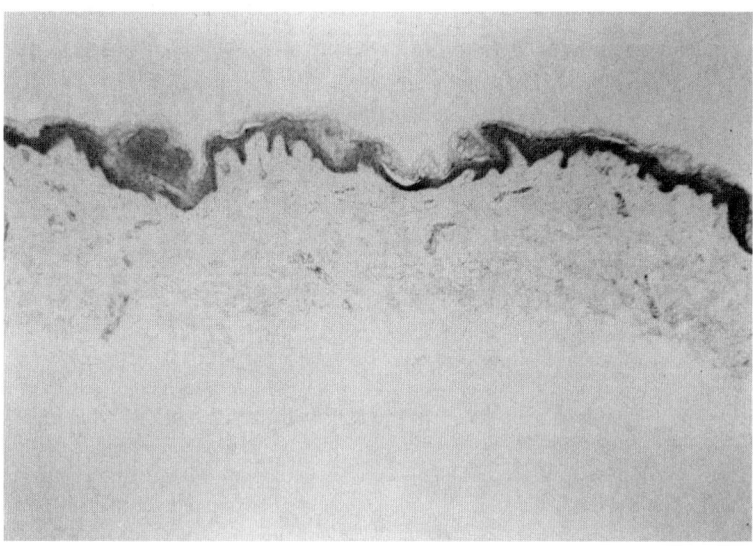

B

FIG. 15-14. *A.* Photomicrograph of mature cultured epithelium; it lacks a dermal matrix. *B.* Photomicrograph of split-thickness skin graft for comparison of thickness with the thin cultured epithelium.

a structural and functional level is progressing rapidly. Factors have been isolated that cause specific mesenchymal cells to proliferate, migrate, and organize into structures such as capillaries or even rudimentary organoid tissue.[210–212] This may allow generation of new tissue in situ for skin replacement.

References

1. Byrne C, Hardman M, Nield K: Covering the limb—Formation of the integument. *J Anat* 202:113, 2003.
2. Medawar P: The behavior and fate of skin autografts and skin homografts in rabbits. *J Anat* 78:176, 1944.
3. Ballantyne D, Converse J: *Experimental Skin Grafts and Transplantation Immunity.* New York: Springer-Verlag, 1979.
4. Nemes Z, Steinert PM: Bricks and mortar of the epidermal barrier. *Exp Mol Med* 31:5, 1999.
5. Andriani F, Margulis A, Lin N, et al: Analysis of microenvironmental factors contributing to basement membrane assembly and normalized epidermal phenotype. *J Invest Dermatol* 120:923, 2003.
6. Dupin E, Le Douarin NM: Development of melanocyte precursors from the vertebrate neural crest. *Oncogene* 22:3016, 2003.
7. Flaxman BA, Sosio AC, Van Scott EJ: Changes in melanosome distribution in caucasoid skin following topical application of *N*-mustard. *J Invest Dermatol* 60:321, 1973.
8. Halaban R: The regulation of normal melanocyte proliferation. *Pigment Cell Res* 13:4, 2000.
9. Vassar R, Coulombe PA, Degenstein L, et al: Mutant keratin expression in transgenic mice causes marked abnormalities resembling a human genetic skin disease. *Cell* 64:365, 1991.
10. Bonifas JM, Rothman AL, Epstein EH Jr: Epidermolysis bullosa simplex: Evidence in two families for keratin gene abnormalities. *Science* 254:1202, 1991.
11. Fuchs E, Cleveland DW: A structural scaffolding of intermediate filaments in health and disease. *Science* 279:514, 1998.
12. Tamaki K, Stingl G, Katz SI: The origin of the Langerhans cells. *J Invest Dermatol* 74:309, 1980.
13. Meigel WN, Gay S, Weber L: Dermal architecture and collagen type distribution. *Arch Dermatol Res* 259:1, 1977.
14. Johnson WC, Helwig EB: Histochemistry of the acid mucopolysaccharides of the skin in normal and in certain pathologic conditions. *Am J Clin Pathol* 40:123, 1961.
15. Braverman IM: The cutaneous microcirculation. *J Investig Dermatol Symp Proc* 5:3, 2000.

16. Akiyama M, Dale BA, Sun TT, et al: Characterization of hair follicle bulge in human fetal skin: The human fetal bulge is a pool of undifferentiated keratinocytes. *J Invest Dermatol* 105:844, 1995.

17. Oshima H, Rochat A, Kedzia C, et al: Morphogenesis and renewal of hair follicles from adult multipotent stem cells. *Cell* 104:233, 2001.

18. Lako M, Armstrong L, Cairns PM, et al: Hair follicle dermal cells repopulate the mouse haematopoietic system. *J Cell Sci* 115:3967, 2002.

19. Smith PF, Meadowcroft AM, May DB: Treating mammalian bite wounds. *J Clin Pharm Ther* 25:85, 2000.

20. Madoff LC: Infectious complications of bites and burns, in Braunwald E, Fauci AS, Kasper DL, et al (eds): *Harrison's Principles of Internal Medicine,* 15th ed. New York, NY: McGraw Hill, 2001; p 817.

21. Presutti RJ: Bite wounds: Early treatment and prophylaxis against infectious complications. *Postgrad Med* 101:243, 1997.

22. Lorette JJ, Wilkinson JA: Alkaline chemical burn to the face requiring full-thickness skin grafting. *Ann Emerg Med* 17:739, 1998.

23. Herbert K, Lawrence JC: Chemical burns. *Burns* 15:381, 1989.

24. Lee KAP, Opeskin K: Fatal alkali burns. *Forensic Sci Int* 72:219, 1995.

25. Yano K, Hata Y, Matsuka K, et al: Effects of washing with a neutralizing agent on alkaline skin injuries in an experimental model. *Burns* 20:36, 1994.

26. Andrews K, Mowlavi A, Milner SM: The treatment of alkaline burns of the skin by neutralization. *Plast Reconstr Surg* 111:1918, 2003.

27. Kirkpatrick JJR, Enion DS, Burd DAR: Hydrofluoric acid burns: A review. *Burns* 21:483, 1995.

28. Upfal M, Doyle C: Medical management of hydrofluoric acid exposure. *J Occup Med* 32:726, 1990.

29. MacKinnon MA: Hydrofluoric acid burns. *Dermatol Clin* 6:67, 1988.

30. Caravatti EM: Acute hydrofluoric acid exposure. *Am J Emerg Med* 6:143, 1988.

31. Matsuno K: The treatment of hydrofluoric acid burns. *Occup Med* 46:313, 1996.

32. Anderson WJ, Anderson JR: Hydrofluoric acid burns of the hand: Mechanism of injury and treatment. *J Hand Surg* 13:52, 1988.

33. Trevino MA, Herrmann GH, Sprout WL: Treatment of severe hydrofluoric acid exposures. *J Occup Med* 25:861, 1983.

34. Leonard LG, Scheulen JJ, Munster AM: Chemical burns: Effect of prompt first aid. *J Trauma* 22:420, 1982.

35. Bond SJ, Schnier GC, Sundine MJ, et al: Cutaneous burns caused by sulfuric acid drain cleaner. *J Trauma* 44:523, 1998.

36. Wang J, Cortes E, Sinks LF, et al: Therapeutic effect and toxicity of Adriamycin in patients with neoplastic disease. *Cancer* 28:837, 1971.

37. Yosowitz P, Ekland DA, Shaw RC, et al: Peripheral intravenous infiltration necrosis. *Am J Surg* 182:553, 1975.

38. Flemmer L, Chan JSL: A pediatric protocol for management of extravasation injuries. *Pediatr Nurs* 19:355, 1993.

39. Langstein HN, Duman H, Seelig D, et al: Retrospective study of the management of chemotherapeutic extravasation injury. *Ann Plast Surg* 49:369, 2002.

40. Cox RF: Managing skin damage induced by doxorubicin hydrochloride and daunorubicin hydrochloride. *Am J Hosp Pharm* 41:2410, 1984.

41. Dorr RT, Alberts DS, Stone A: Cold protection and heat enhancement of doxorubicin skin toxicity in the mouse. *Cancer Treat Rep* 69:431, 1985.

42. Linder RM, Upton J, Osteen R: Management of extensive doxorubicin hydrochloride extravasation injuries. *J Hand Surg* 8:32, 1983.

43. Gault DT: Extravasation injury. *Br J Plast Surg* 46:91, 1993.

44. Kumar RJ, Pegg SP, Kimble RM: Management of extravasation injuries. *ANZ J Surg* 71:285, 2001.

45. Biem J, Koehncke N, Classen D, et al: Out of the cold: Management of hypothermia and frostbite. *CMAJ* 168:305, 2003.

46. Murphy JV, Banwell PE, Roberts AHN, et al: Frostbite: Pathogenesis and treatment. *J Trauma* 48:171, 2000.

47. McCauley RL, Hing DN, Robson MC, et al: Frostbite injuries: A rational approach based on pathophysiology. *J Trauma* 23:143, 1983.

48. Nola GT, Vistnes LM: Differential response of skin and muscle in the experimental production of pressure sores. *Plast Reconstr Surg* 66:728, 1980.

49. Thomas DR: Pressure ulcers, in Cassel CK, Cohen HJ, Larson EB, et al (eds): *Geriatric Medicine,* 3rd ed. New York: Springer, 1997, p 767.

50. Goode PS, Allman RM: Pressure ulcers, in Duthie EH Jr, Katz PR (eds): *Practice of Geriatrics,* 3rd ed. Philadelphia: WB Saunders, 1998, p 228.

51. Robson MC, Hill DP, Smith PD, et al: Sequential cytokine therapy for pressure ulcers: Clinical and mechanistic response. *Ann Surg* 231:600, 2000.

52. Gottlober P, Steinert M, Weiss M, et al: The outcome of local radiation injuries: 14 years of follow-up after the Chernobyl accident. *Radiat Res* 155:409, 2001.

53. Poh-Fitzpatrick MB: The biologic actions of solar radiation on skin, with a note on sunscreens. *J Dermatol Surg* 3:199, 1977.

54. Fournier A: Gangréne foudroyante de la verge. *Semaine Med* 3:345, 1883.

55. Meleney FL: Hemolytic streptococcus gangrene. *Arch Surg* 9:317, 1924.

56. Meleney FL: Bacterial synergism in disease processes with confirmation of the synergistic bacterial etiology of a certain type of progressive gangrene of the abdominal wall. *Ann Surg* 94:961, 1931.

57. Cunningham JD, Silver L, Rudikoff D: Necrotizing fasciitis: A plea for early diagnosis and treatment. *Mt Sinai J Med* 68:253, 2001.

58. Yuen KY, Ma L, Wong SSY, et al: Fatal necrotizing fasciitis due to *Vibrio damsela. Scand J Infect Dis* 25:659, 1993.

59. Elliot D, Kufera JA, Myers RAM: The microbiology of necrotizing soft tissue infections. *Am J Surg* 179:361, 2000.

60. Elliot DC, Kufera JA, Myers RAM: Necrotizing soft tissue infections. Risk factors for mortality and strategies for management. *Ann Surg* 224:672, 1996.

61. Riseman JA, Zamboni WA, Curtis A, et al: Hyperbaric oxygen therapy for necrotizing fasciitis reduces mortality and the need for débridements. *Surgery* 108:847, 1990.

62. Brown TJ, Rosen T, Orengo IF: Hidradenitis suppurativa. *South Med J* 91:1107, 1998.

63. Slade DE, Powell BW, Mortimer PS: Hidradenitis suppurativa: Pathogenesis and management. *Br J Plast Surg* 56:451, 2003.

64. Mitchell KM, Beck DE: Hidradenitis suppurativa. *Surg Clin North Am* 82:1187, 2002.

65. Hull TL, Wu J: Pilonidal disease. *Surg Clin North Am* 82:1169, 2002.

66. Aydede H, Erhan Y, Sakarya S, et al: Comparison of three methods in surgical treatment of pilonidal disease. *ANZ J Surg* 71:362, 2001.

67. da Silva JH: Pilonidal cyst: Cause and treatment. *Dis Colon Rectum* 43:1146, 2000.

68. Sondenaa K, Diab R, Nesvik I, et al: Influence of failure of primary wound healing on subsequent recurrence of pilonidal sinus. Combined prospective study and randomized controlled trial. *Eur J Surg* 168:614, 2002.

69. Petersen S, Koch R, Stelzner S, et al: Primary closure techniques in chronic pilonidal sinus: a survey of the results of different surgical procedures. *Dis Colon Rectum* 45:1458, 2002.

70. Oncel M, Kurt N, Kement M, et al: Excision and marsupialization versus sinus excision for the treatment of limited chronic pilonidal disease: A prospective, randomized trial. *Tech Coloproctol* 6:165, 2002.

71. Chintapatla S, Safarani N, Kumar S, et al: Sacrococcygeal pilonidal sinus: Historical review, pathological insight and surgical options. *Tech Coloproctol* 7:3, 2003.

72. Williamson JD, Silverman JF, Tafra L: Fine-needle aspiration cytology of metastatic squamous-cell carcinoma arising in a pilonidal sinus, with literature review. *Diagn Cytopathol* 20:367, 1999.

73. Abboud B, Ingea H: Recurrent squamous-cell carcinoma arising in sacrococcygeal pilonidal sinus tract: Report of a case and review of the literature. *Dis Colon Rectum* 42:525, 1999.

74. Bennhoff DF: Actinomycosis: Diagnostic and therapeutic considerations and review of 32 cases. *Laryngoscope* 94:1198, 1984.

75. Nagler R, Peled M, Laufer D: Cervicofacial actinomycosis. *Oral Surg Oral Med Oral Pathol Oral Radiol Endod* 83:652, 1997.

76. Miller M, Haddad AJ: Cervicofacial actinomycosis. *Oral Surg Oral Med Oral Pathol Oral Radiol Endod* 83:496, 1998.

77. Queiroz-Telles F, McGinnis MR, Salkin I, et al: Subcutaneous mycoses. *Infect Dis Clin North Am* 17:59, 2003.

78. Regezi JA, Sciubba J: *Oral pathology,* 2nd ed. Philadelphia: WB Saunders, 1993, p 45.

79. Nielsen PM, Novak A: Acute cervicofacial actinomycosis. *Int J Oral Maxillofac Surg* 16:440, 1987.

80. Mabey D, Peeling RW: Lymphogranuloma venereum. *Sex Transm Infect* 78:90, 2002.

81. Schachter J, Osoba AO: Lymphogranuloma venereum. *Br Med Bull* 39:151, 1983.

82. Clinical Effectiveness Group: National guideline for the management of lymphogranuloma venereum. *Sex Transm Inf* 75:S40, 1999.

83. Martin DH, Mroczkowski TF, Dalu ZA, et al: A controlled trial of single dose of azithromycin for the treatment of chlamydial urethritis and cervicitis. The Azithromycin for Chlamydial Infections Study Group. *N Engl J Med* 327:921, 1992.

84. Weitzul S, Eichhorn PJ, Pandya AG: Nontuberculous mycobacterial infections of the skin. *Dermatol Clin* 18:359, 2000.

85. Mori T: Acid-fast bacilli detected in umbilical cords and skins of humans in cases of surgical operation. *Nippon Rai Gakkai Zasshi* 59:98, 1990.

86. Escalonilla P, Esteban J, Soriano ML, et al: Cutaneous manifestations of infection by nontuberculous mycobacteria. *Clin Exp Dermatol* 23:214, 1998.

87. Palenque E: Skin disease and nontuberculous atypical mycobacteria. *Int J Dermatol* 39:659, 2000.

88. Chemlal K, Portaels: Molecular diagnosis of nontuberculous mycobacteria. *Curr Opin Infect Dis* 16:77, 2003.

89. Jernigan JA, Farr BM: Incubation period and sources of exposure for cutaneous *Mycobacterium marinum* infection: Case report and review of the literature. *Clin Infect Dis* 31:439, 2000.

90. Kullavanijaya P: Atypical mycobacterial cutaneous infection. *Clin Dermatol* 17:153, 1999.

91. Brentjens MH, Yeung-Yue KA, Lee PC, et al: Human papillomavirus: A review. *Dermatol Clin* 20:315, 2002.

92. Harwood CA, Proby CM: Human papillomaviruses and non-melanoma skin cancer. *Infect Dis* 15:101, 2002.

93. Tyring S, Conant M, Marini M, et al: Imiquimod: An international update on therapeutic uses in dermatology. *Int J Dermatol* 41:810, 2002.

94. Koutsky L: Epidemiology of genital human papillomavirus infection. *Am J Med* 102:3, 1997.

95. Frega A, Stentella P, Tinari A, et al: Giant condyloma acuminatum or Buschke- Löwenstein tumor: Review of the literature and report of three cases treated by CO_2 laser surgery. A long-term follow-up. *Anticancer Res* 22:1201, 2002.

96. Davis PA, Corless DJ, Gazzard BG, et al: Increased risk of wound complications and poor wound healing following laparotomy in HIV-seropositive and AIDS patients. *Dis Surg* 16:60, 1999.

97. Eriguchi M, Takeda Y, Yoshizaki I, et al: Surgery in patients with HIV infection: Indications and outcome. *Biomed Pharmacother* 51:474, 1997.

98. Morandi E, Merlini D, Salvaggio A, et al: Prospective study of healing time after hemorrhoidectomy: Influence of HIV infection, acquired immunodeficiency syndrome, and anal wound infection. *Dis Colon Rectum* 42:1140, 1999.

99. Luck JV Jr: Orthopaedic surgery on the HIV-positive patient: Complications and outcome. *Instr Course Lect* 43:543, 1994.

100. Davis PA, Wastell C: A comparison of biomechanical properties of excised mature scars from HIV patients and non-HIV controls. *Am J Surg* 180:217, 2000.

101. Brunsting LA, Goeckerman WH, O'Leary PA: Pyoderma (ecthyma) gangrenosum—clinical and experimental observations in five cases occurring in adults. *Arch Dermatol* 22:655, 1930.

102. Von Den Driesch P: Pyoderma gangrenosum: A report of 44 cases with follow-up. *Br J Dermatol* 137:1000, 1997.

103. Wollina U: Clinical management of pyoderma gangrenosum. *Am J Clin Dermatol* 3:149, 2002.

104. Cliff S, Holden CA, Thomas PRS, et al: Split skin grafts in the treatment of pyoderma gangrenosum. *Dermatol Surg* 25:299, 1999.

105. Patel GK, Finlay AY: Staphylococcal scalded skin syndrome: Diagnosis and management. *Am J Clin Dermatol* 4:165, 2003.

106. Atiyeh BS, Dham R, Yassin MF, et al: Treatment of toxic epidermal necrolysis with moisture-retentive ointment: A case report and review of the literature. *Dermatol Surg* 29:185, 2003.

107. Ladhani S, Joannou CL, Lochrie DP, et al: Clinical, microbial, and biochemical aspects of the exfoliative toxins causing staphylococcal scalded-skin syndrome. *Clin Microbiol Rev* 12:224, 1999.

108. Roujeau JC, Stern RS: Severe cutaneous reactions to drugs. *N Engl J Med* 331:1272, 1994.

109. Spies M, Sanford AP, Aili Low JF, et al: Treatment of extensive toxic epidermal necrolysis in children. *Pediatrics* 108:1162, 2001.

110. Arevalo JM, Lorente JA: Skin coverage with Biobrane biomaterial for the treatment of patients with toxic epidermal necrolysis. *J Burn Care Rehabil* 20:406, 1999.

111. Bradley T, Brown RE, Kucan JO, et al: Toxic epidermal necrolysis: A review and report of the successful use of Biobrane for early wound coverage. *Ann Plast Surg* 35:124, 1995.

112. Mackie RM: Epidermoid cyst, in Champion RH, Burton JL, Burns DA, et al (eds): *Rook/Wilkinson/Ebling Textbook of Dermatology,* vol. 2, 6th ed. Oxford: Blackwell Science, 1998, p 1666.

113. De Ponte FS, Brunelli A, Marchetti E, et al: Sublingual epidermoid cyst. *J Cranio Surg* 13:308, 2002.

114. Braun RP, Rabinovitz H, Oliviero M, et al: Dermoscopic diagnosis of seborrheic keratosis. *Clin Dermatol* 20:270, 2002.

115. Fu W, Cockerell CJ: The actinic (solar) keratosis. *Arch Dermatol* 139:66, 2003.

116. Lober BA, Lober CW: Actinic keratosis is squamous cell carcinoma. *South Med J* 93:650, 2000.

117. Robins P, Gupta AK: The use of topical fluorouracil to treat actinic keratosis. *Cutis* 70:4, 2002.

118. Castilla EE, DaGraca-Dutra M, Orioli-Parreiras IM: Epidemiology of congenital pigmented nevi: I. Incidence rates and relative frequencies. *Br J Dermatol* 104:307, 1981.

119. Rhodes AR, Melsk JW: Small congenital nevocellular nevi and the risk of cutaneous melanoma. *J Pediatr* 100:219, 1982.

120. Fishman SJ, Mulliken JB: Hemangiomas and vascular malformations of infancy and childhood. *Pediatr Clin North Am* 40:1177, 1993.

121. Lister W: The natural history of strawberry naevi. *Lancet* 1:1429, 1938.

122. Sadan N, Wolach B: Treatment of hemangiomas of infants with high doses of prednisone. *J Pediatr* 128:141, 1996.

123. Leikensohn J, Epstein L, Vasconez LO: Superselective embolization and surgery of noninvoluting hemangiomas and AV malformations. *Plast Reconstr Surg* 68:143, 1981.

124. Fleming ID, Amonette R, Monaghan T, et al: Principles of management of basal and squamous cell carcinoma of the skin. *Cancer* 75(Suppl 2):699, 1995.

125. Epstein JH: Photocarcinogenesis, skin cancer, and aging. *J Am Acad Dermatol* 9:487, 1983.

126. Gallagher RP, Hill GB, Bajdik CD, et al: Sunlight exposure, pigmentation factors, and risk of nonmelanocytic skin cancer: II. Squamous cell carcinoma. *Arch Dermatol* 131:164, 1995.

127. Luande J, Henschke CI, Mohammed N: The Tanzanian human albino skin: Natural history. *Cancer* 55:1823, 1985.

128. Marks R, Kopf AW: Cancer of the skin in the next century. *Int J Dermatol* 34:445, 1995.

129. Sober AJ, Burstein JM: Precursors to skin cancer. *Cancer* 75:645, 1995.

130. Novick M, Gard DA, Hardy SB, et al: Burn scar carcinoma: A review and analysis of 46 cases. *J Trauma* 17:809, 1977.

131. Luce EA: Oncologic considerations in nonmelanotic skin cancer. *Clin Plast Surg* 22:39, 1995.

132. Wang CY, Brodland DG, Su WP: Skin cancers associated with acquired immunodeficiency syndrome. *Mayo Clin Proc* 70:766, 1995.

133. Wade TR, Ackerman AB: The many faces of basal-cell carcinoma. *J Dermatol Surg Oncol* 4:23, 1978.

134. Nguyen AV, Whitaker DC, Frodel J: Differentiation of basal cell carcinoma. *Otolaryngol Clin North Am* 26:37, 1993.

135. Salasche SJ: Curettage and electrodesiccation in the treatment of midfacial basal cell epithelioma. *J Am Acad Dermatol* 8:496, 1983.

136. Wolf DJ, Zitelli JA: Surgical margins for basal cell carcinoma. *Arch Dermatol* 123:340, 1987.

137. Friedman HI, Cooper PH, Wanebo HJ: Prognostic and therapeutic use of microstaging of cutaneous squamous cell carcinomas of the trunk and extremities. *Cancer* 56:109, 1985.

138. Fleming MD, Hunt JL, Purdue GF, et al: Marjolin's ulcer: A review and reevaluation of a difficult problem. *J Burn Care Rehabil* 11:460, 1990.

139. Byers R, Kesler K, Redmon B, et al: Squamous carcinoma of the external ear. *Am J Surg* 146:447, 1983.

140. Mohs FE: *Chemosurgery, Microscopically Controlled Surgery for Skin Cancer.* Springfield: Charles C Thomas, 1978.

141. Dogan B, Harmanyeri Y, Baloglu H, et al: Intralesional alpha-2a interferon therapy for basal cell carcinoma. *Cancer Lett* 91:215, 1995.

142. Craven NM, Griffiths CE: Retinoids in the management of non-melanoma skin cancer and melanoma. *Cancer Surv* 26:267, 1996.

143. Ferlay J, Bray F, Pisani P, et al: *GLOBOCAN 2000: Cancer Incidence, Mortality and Prevalence Worldwide.* Version 1.0. IARC cancer base no. 5. Lyon: IARC Press, 2001.

144. Desmond RA, Soong S-J: Epidemiology of malignant melanoma. *Surg Clin North Am* 83:1, 2003.

145. Dennis LK: Analysis of the melanoma epidemic, both apparent and real. *Arch Dermatol* 135:275, 1999.

146. MacKie RM: Incidence, risk factors and prevention of melanoma. *Eur J Cancer* 34(Suppl 3):S3, 1998.

147. Tucker, MA, Halpern A, Holly EA, et al: Clinically recognized dysplastic nevi: A central risk factor for cutaneous melanoma. *JAMA* 277:1439, 1997.

148. Kopf AW, Hellman LJ, Rogers GS, et al: Familial malignant melanoma. *JAMA* 256:1915, 1986.

149. Langley RG, Fitzpatrick TB, Sober AJ: Clinical characteristics, in Balch CM, Houghton AN, Sober AJ, et al (eds): *Cutaneous Melanoma,* 3rd ed. St. Louis: Quality Medical Publishing, 1998, p 81.

150. Price NM, Rywlin AM, Ackerman AB: Histologic criteria for the diagnosis of superficial spreading melanoma. *Cancer* 38:2434, 1976.

151. Liu V, Mihm MC: Pathology of malignant melanoma. *Surg Clin North Am* 83:31, 2003.

152. Clark WH, Elder DE, Van Horn M: The biologic forms of malignant melanoma. *Hum Pathol* 5:443, 1986.

153. Koh HK: Cutaneous melanoma. *N Engl J Med* 325:1712, 1992.

154. Weinstock MA, Sober AJ: The risk of progression of lentigo maligna to lentigo maligna melanoma. *Br J Dermatol* 116:303, 1987.

155. Reintgen DS, McCarty KM Jr., Cox E, et al: Malignant melanoma in black American and white American populations. A comparison review. *JAMA* 248:1856, 1982.

156. Balch CM, Buzaid AC, Soong SJ, et al: Final version of the American Joint Committee on Cancer staging system for cutaneous melanoma. *J Clin Oncol* 19:3635, 2001.

157. Breslow A: Thickness, cross-sectional areas, and depth of invasion in the prognosis of cutaneous melanomas. *Ann Surg* 172:902, 1970.

158. Balch CM, Soong SJ, Gershenwald JE, et al: Prognostic factors analysis of 17,600 melanoma patients: Validation of the American Joint Committee on Cancer melanoma staging system. *J Clin Oncol* 19:3622, 2001.

159. Masback A, Olsson H, Westerdahl J, et al: Prognostic factors in invasive cutaneous malignant melanoma: A population-based study and review. *Melanoma Res* 11:435, 2001.

160. Balch CM, Soong SJ, Shaw HM, et al: An analysis of prognostic factors in 8500 patients with cutaneous melanoma, in Balch CM, Houghton AN, Milton GW, et al (eds): *Cutaneous Melanoma,* 2nd ed. Philadelphia: JB Lippincott, 1992, p 165.

161. Balch CM, Wilkerson JA, Murad TM, et al: The prognostic significance of ulceration on cutaneous melanoma. *Cancer* 45:3012, 1980.

162. Kashani-Sabet M, Sagebiel RW, Ferreira CM, et al: Tumor vascularity in the prognostic assessment of primary cutaneous melanoma. *J Clin Oncol* 20:1826, 2002.

163. Unger JM, Flaherty LE, Liu PY, et al: Gender and other survival predictors in patients with metastatic melanoma on Southwest Oncology Group trials. *Cancer* 91:1148, 2001.

164. Wells KE, Reintgen DS, Cruse CW: The current management and prognosis of acral lentiginous melanoma. *Am Plast Surg* 28:100, 1992.

165. Zettersten E, Shaikh L, Ramirez R, et al: Prognostic factors in primary cutaneous melanoma. *Surg Clin North Am* 83:61, 2003.

166. Essner R: Surgical treatment of malignant melanoma. *Surg Clin North Am* 83:109, 2003.

167. Heaton KM, Sussman JJ, Gershenwald JE, et al: Surgical margins and prognostic factors in patients with thick (>4 mm) primary melanoma. *Ann Surg Oncol* 5:322, 1998.

168. Roses DF, Provet JA, Harris MN, et al: Prognosis of patients with pathologic stage II cutaneous melanoma. *Ann Surg* 201:103, 1985.

169. Balch CM, Soong S, Ross MI, et al: Long-term results of a multi-institutional randomized trial comparing prognostic factors and surgical results for intermediate thickness melanomas (1.0 to 4.0 mm). *Ann Surg Oncol* 7:87, 2000.

170. Leong SPL: Selective lymphadenectomy for malignant melanoma. *Surg Clin North Am* 83:157, 2003.

171. Lee ML, Tomsu K, Von Eschen KB: Duration of survival for disseminated malignant melanoma: Results of a meta-analysis. *Melanoma Res* 10:81, 2000.

172. Karakousis CP, Velez A, Driscoll DL, et al: Metastasectomy in malignant melanoma. *Surgery* 115:295, 1994.

173. Kadison AS, Morton DL: Immunotherapy of malignant melanoma. *Surg Clin North Am* 83:343, 2003.

174. Sondak VK, Wolfe JA: Adjuvant therapy for melanoma. *Curr Opin Oncol* 9:184, 1997.

175. Creagan ET, Dalton RJ, Ahmann DL, et al: Randomized, surgical adjuvant clinical trial of recombinant interferon alfa-2a in selected patients with malignant melanoma. *J Clin Oncol* 13:2776, 1995.

176. Kirkwood JM, Strawderman MH, Ernstoff MS, et al: Interferon alfa-2b adjuvant therapy of high-risk resected cutaneous melanoma: The Eastern Cooperative Oncology Group trial EST 1684. *J Clin Oncol* 14:7, 1996.

177. Livingston PO, Wong GYC, Adluri S, et al: Improved survival in stage III melanoma patients with G$_{M2}$ antibodies: A randomized trial of adjuvant vaccination with G$_{M2}$ ganglioside. *J Clin Oncol* 12:1036, 1994.

178. Ang KK, Peters LJ, Weber RS, et al: Postoperative radiotherapy for cutaneous melanoma of the head and neck region. *Int J Radiat Oncol Biol Phys* 30:795, 1994.

179. Strom EA, Ross MI: Adjuvant radiation therapy after axillary lymphadenectomy for metastatic melanoma: Toxicity and local control. *Ann Surg Oncol* 2:445, 1995.

180. Ang KK, Geara FB, Byers RM, et al: Radiotherapy of melanoma, in Balch CM, Houghton AN, Sober AJ, et al (eds): *Cutaneous Melanoma,* 3rd ed. St. Louis: Quality Medical Publishing, 1998, p 389.

181. Eggermont AMM, van Geel AN, de Wilt JHW, et al: The role of isolated perfusion for melanoma confined to the extremities. *Surg Clin North Am* 83:371, 2003.

182. Cumberlin R, De Moss E, Lassus M, et al: Isolation perfusion for malignant melanoma of the extremity: A review. *J Clin Oncol* 3:1022, 1985.

183. Taber SW, Polk HC Jr.: Mortality, major amputation rates, and leukopenia after isolated limb perfusion with phenylalanine mustard for the treatment of melanoma. *J Surg Oncol* 4:440, 1997.

184. Lienard D, Ewalenko P, Delmotte J-J, et al: High-dose recombinant tumor necrosis factor alpha in combination with interferon gamma and melphalan in isolation perfusion of the limbs for melanoma and sarcoma. *J Clin Oncol* 10:52, 1992.

185. Fraker DL, Alexander HR, Andrich M, et al: Treatment of patients with melanoma of the extremity using Hyperthermic isolated limb perfusion with melphalan, tumor necrosis factor, and interferon gamma: Results of a tumor necrosis factor dose-escalation study. *J Clin Oncol* 14:479, 1996.

186. O'Connor WJ, Brodland DG: Merkel cell carcinoma. *Dermatol Surg* 22:262, 1996.

187. Chanda JJ: Extramammary Paget's disease: Prognosis and relationship to internal malignancy. *J Am Acad Dermatol* 13:1009, 1985.

188. Holden CA, Spittle MF, Jones EW: Angiosarcoma of the face and scalp: Prognosis and treatment. *Cancer* 5:1047, 1987.

189. Noel JC, Hermans P: Herpes virus–like DNA sequence and Kaposi's sarcoma: Relationship with epidemiology, clinical spectrum, and histologic features. *Cancer* 77:2132, 1996.

190. Beitler AJ, Ptaszynski K, Karpel JP: Upper airway obstruction in a woman with AIDS-related laryngeal Kaposi's sarcoma. *Chest* 109:836, 1996.

191. Barbagallo JS, Kolodzieh MS, Silverberg NB, et al: Neurocutaneous disorders. *Dermatol Clin* 20:547, 2002.

192. High AS, Robinson PA: Novel approaches to the diagnosis of basal cell nevous syndrome. *Expert Rev Mol Diagn* 2:321, 2002.

193. Goyal JL, Rao VA, Srinivasan R, et al: Oculocutaneous manifestations in xeroderma pigmentosa. *Br J Ophthalmol* 78:295, 1994.

194. Greene MH: The genetics of hereditary melanoma and nevi. 1998 update. *Cancer* 86:2464, 1999.

195. Hudson DA, Lazarus D, Silfen R: The use of serial tissue expansion in pediatric plastic surgery. *Ann Plast Surg* 45:589, 2000.

196. Takei T, Mills I, Arai K, et al: Molecular basis for tissue expansion: Clinical implications for the surgeon. *Plast Reconstr Surg* 102:247, 1998.

197. Gibstein LA, Abramson DL, Bartlett RA, et al: Tissue expansion in children: A retrospective study of complications. *Ann Plast Surg* 38:358, 1997.

198. Reinwald J, Green H: Serial cultivation strains of human epidermal keratinocytes: The formation of keratinizing colonies from a single cell. *Cell* 6:331, 1975.

199. Nunez-Gutierrez H, Castro-Munozledo F, Kuri-Harcuch W: Combined use of allograft and autograft epidermal cultures in therapy of burns. *Plast Reconstr Surg* 98:929, 1996.

200. Compton CC, Gill JM, Bradford DA, et al. Skin regenerated from cultured epithelial autografts on full-thickness burn wounds from 6 days to 5 years after grafting. A light, electron microscopic and immunohistochemical study. *Lab Invest* 60:600, 1989.

201. Klein MB, Chang J, Young DM: Update on skin replacements, in Habal M (ed): *Advances in Plastic and Reconstructive Surgery*. New York: Mosby, 1998, p 223.

202. Ryan CM, Schoenfeld DA, Malloy M, et al: Use of Integra artificial skin is associated with decreased length of stay for severely injured adult burn survivors. *J Burn Care Rehabil* 23:311, 2002.

203. Heimbach DM, Warden GD, Luterman A, et al: Multicenter postapproval clinical trial of Integra dermal regeneration template for burn treatment. *J Burn Care Rehabil* 24:42, 2003.

204. Haertsch P: Reconstructive surgery using an artificial dermis (Integra). *Br J Plast* Surg 55:362, 2002.

205. Terino EO: AlloDerm acellular dermal graft: Applications in aesthetic soft-tissue augmentation. *Clin Plast Surg* 28:83, 2001.

206. Pape SA, Byrne PO: Safety and efficacy of TransCyte for the treatment of partial-thickness burns. *J Burn Care Rehabil* 21:390, 2000.

207. Lukish JR, Eichelberger MR, Newman KD, et al: The use of a bioactive skin substitute decreases length of stay for pediatric burn patients. *J Pediatr Surg* 36:1118, 2001.

208. Jahoda CA, Reynolds AJ: Hair follicle dermal sheath cells: Unsung participants in wound healing. *Lancet* 358:1445, 2001.

209. Kuznetsov SA, Mankani MH, Gronthos S, et al: Circulating skeletal stem cells. *J Cell Biol* 153:1133, 2001.

210. Potten CS, Booth C: Keratinocyte stem cells: A commentary. *J Invest Dermatol* 119:888, 2002.

211. Bianco P, Robey PG: Stem cells in tissue engineering. *Nature* 414:118, 2001.

212. Griffith LG, Naughton G: Tissue engineering—Current challenges and expanding opportunities. *Science* 295:1009, 2002.

CHAPTER 16

The Breast

Kirby I. Bland, Samuel W. Beenken, and Edward M. Copeland III

Nonsurgical Breast Cancer Therapies

Radiation Therapy
Chemotherapy
    Adjuvant Chemotherapy
    Neoadjuvant Chemotherapy
    Chemotherapy for Distant Metastases
Antiestrogen Therapy
Ablative Endocrine Therapy
Anti-HER2/neu Antibody Therapy

Special Clinical Situations

Nipple Discharge
    Unilateral Nipple Discharge
    Bilateral Nipple Discharge
Axillary Lymph Node Metastases with Unknown Primary Cancer
Breast Cancer During Pregnancy
Male Breast Cancer
Phyllodes Tumors
Inflammatory Breast Carcinoma
Rare Breast Cancers
    Squamous Cell (Epidermoid) Carcinoma
    Adenoid Cystic Carcinoma
    Apocrine Carcinoma
    Sarcomas
    Lymphomas

A BRIEF HISTORY OF BREAST CANCER THERAPY[1-8]

Breast cancer, with its uncertain cause, has captured the attention of surgeons throughout the ages. Despite centuries of theoretical meandering and scientific inquiry, breast cancer remains one of the most dreaded of human diseases. The story of efforts to cope with breast cancer is complex, and there is no successful conclusion as in diseases for which cause and cure are known. However, progress has been made in lessening the horrors that formerly devastated the body and psyche. Currently, 50% of American women will consult their surgeon for breast disease, 25% will undergo breast biopsy, and 12% will develop some variant of breast cancer.

The Smith Surgical Papyrus (3000–2500 B.C.) is the earliest known document to refer to breast cancer. The cancer was in a man, but the description encompassed most of the common clinical features. In reference to this cancer, the author concluded, "There is no treatment." There were few other historical references to breast cancer until the first century. In *De Medicina*, Celsus commented on the value of operations for early breast cancer: "None of these may be removed but the cacoethes (early cancer), the rest are irritated by every method of cure. The more violent the operations are, the more angry they grow." In the second century, Galen inscribed his classical clinical observation: "We have often seen in the breast a tumor exactly resembling the animal the crab. Just as the crab has legs on both sides of his body, so in this disease the veins extending out from the unnatural growth take the shape of a crab's legs. We have often cured this disease in its early stages, but after it has reached a large size, no one has cured it. In all operations we attempt to excise the tumor in a circle where it borders on the healthy tissue."

The galenic system of medicine ascribed cancers to an excess of black bile and concluded that excision of a local bodily outbreak could not cure the systemic imbalance. Theories espoused by Galen dominated medicine until the Renaissance. The majority of respected surgeons considered operative intervention to be a futile

and ill-advised endeavor. However, beginning with Morgagni, surgical resections were more frequently undertaken, including some early attempts at mastectomy and axillary dissection. le Dran repudiated Galen's humoral theory in the eighteenth century and stated that breast cancer was a local disease that spread by way of lymph vessels to axillary lymph nodes. When operating on a woman with breast cancer, he routinely removed any enlarged axillary lymph nodes.

In the nineteenth century, Moore, of the Middlesex Hospital, London emphasized complete resection of the breast for cancer and stated that palpable axillary lymph nodes also should be removed. In a presentation before the British Medical Association in 1877, Banks supported Moore's concepts and advocated the resection of axillary lymph nodes even when palpable lymphadenopathy was not evident, recognizing that occult involvement of axillary lymph nodes was frequently present. In 1894, Halsted and Meyer reported their operations for treatment of breast cancer. By demonstrating superior locoregional control rates after radical resection, these surgeons established radical mastectomy as state-of-the-art treatment for that era. Both Halsted and Meyer advocated complete dissection of axillary lymph node levels I to III. Both routinely resected the long thoracic nerve and the thoracodorsal neurovascular bundle with the axillary contents.

In 1943, Haagensen and Stout described the grave signs of breast cancer, which included (1) edema of the skin of the breast, (2) skin ulceration, (3) chest wall fixation, (4) an axillary lymph node greater than 2.5 cm in diameter, and (5) fixed axillary lymph nodes. Women with two or more signs had a 42% local recurrence rate and only a 2% 5-year disease-free survival rate. Based on these findings, they declared that women with grave signs were beyond cure by radical surgery. Approximately 25% of women were excluded from surgery based on these criteria of inoperability. Today, with comprehensive mammography screening, only 10% of women are found to have such advanced breast cancers. In 1948, Patey and Dyson of the Middlesex Hospital, London, advocated a modified radical mastectomy for the management of advanced operable breast cancer, explaining, "Until an effective general agent for treatment of carcinoma of the breast is developed, a high proportion of these cases are doomed to die." Their technique included removal of the breast and axillary lymph nodes with preservation of the pectoralis major muscle. They showed that removal of the pectoralis minor muscle allowed access to and clearance of axillary lymph node levels I to III. Subsequently, Madden advocated a modified radical mastectomy that preserved both the pectoralis major and minor muscles even though this approach prevented complete dissection of the apical (level III) axillary lymph nodes.

In the 1970s, there was a transition from the Halsted radical mastectomy to the modified radical mastectomy as the surgical procedure most frequently used by American surgeons for breast cancer. This transition acknowledged that (1) extirpation of the pectoralis major muscle was not essential for locoregional control in stage I and stage II breast cancer, and (2) neither the modified radical mastectomy nor the Halsted radical mastectomy consistently achieved locoregional control of stage III breast cancer. The National Surgical Adjuvant Breast and Bowel Project B-04 (NSABP B-04) conducted by Fisher and colleagues compared local and regional treatments of breast cancer. Life table estimates were obtained for 1665 women enrolled and followed for a mean of 120 months (Fig. 16-1). This study randomized clinically node-negative women into three groups: (1) Halsted radical mastectomy (RM); (2) total mastectomy plus radiation therapy (TM+RT); and (3) total mastectomy alone (TM). Clinically node-positive women were treated with

PROBABILITY OF DISEASE-FREE SURVIVAL (%)

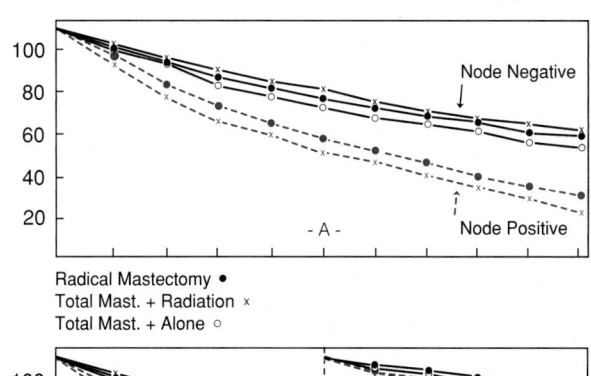

Radical Mastectomy •
Total Mast. + Radiation ×
Total Mast. + Alone ○

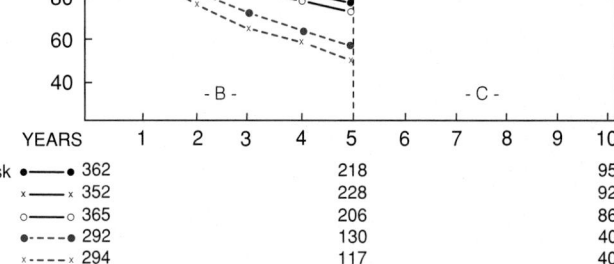

# At Risk				
•——•	362		218	95
×——×	352		228	92
○——○	365		206	86
•---•	292		130	40
×----×	294		117	40

Disease-Free Survival through 10 Years (*A*), during the First 5 Years (*B*), and during the Second 5 Years for Patients Free of Disease at the end of the 5th year (*C*).

FIG. 16-1. National Surgical Adjuvant Breast and Bowel Project B-04 (NSABP B-04) results. Disease-free survival for women treated by radical mastectomy *(solid circle)*, total mastectomy plus radiation *(x)*, or total mastectomy alone *(open circle)*. *(From Fisher B, et al: Ten-Year results of a randomized clinical trial comparing radical mastectomy and total mastectomy with or without radiation. N Engl J Med 312:674, 1985, with permission.)*

RM or TM+RT. There were no differences in survival between the three groups of node-negative women or between the two groups of node-positive women. (Fig. 16-1A). Correspondingly, there were no differences in survival during the first and second 5-year follow-up periods (Fig. 16-1B and C).

Other prospective clinical trials that compared the Halstead radical mastectomy to the modified radical mastectomy were the Manchester Trial, reported by Turner and colleagues, and the University of Alabama Trial, reported by Maddox and colleagues. In both studies, the type of surgical procedure did not influence recurrence rates for stage I and stage II breast cancer patients. The criterion for accrual to the Alabama Breast Cancer Project (1975–1978) was a T1-T3 breast cancer with no apparent distant metastases. Patients received a radical or a modified radical mastectomy. Node-positive patients received adjuvant cyclophosphamide, methotrexate, and 5-fluorouracil (CMF) chemotherapy or adjuvant melphalan. After a median follow-up period of 15 years, neither type of surgery nor type of chemotherapy was shown to affect locoregional disease-free or overall survival. Since the 1970s, considerable progress has been made in the integration of surgery, radiation therapy, and chemotherapy to control locoregional disease, enhance survival, and increase the possibility of breast conservation. Locoregional control is achieved for nearly 80% of women with advanced breast cancers.

EMBRYOLOGY AND FUNCTIONAL ANATOMY OF THE BREAST

Embryology[9]

At the fifth or sixth week of fetal development, two ventral bands of thickened ectoderm (mammary ridges, milk lines) are evident in the embryo. In most mammals, paired breasts develop along these ridges, which extend from the base of the forelimb (future axilla) to the region of the hind limb (inguinal area). These ridges are not prominent in the human embryo and disappear after a short time, except for small portions that may persist in the pectoral region. Accessory breasts (*polymastia*) or accessory nipples (*polythelia*) may occur along the milk line (Fig. 16-2) when normal regression

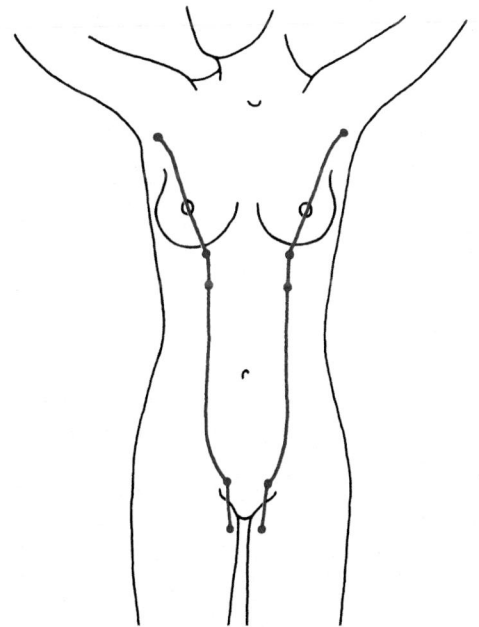

FIG. 16-2. The mammary milk line. *(From Bland et al,[9] p 214, with permission.)*

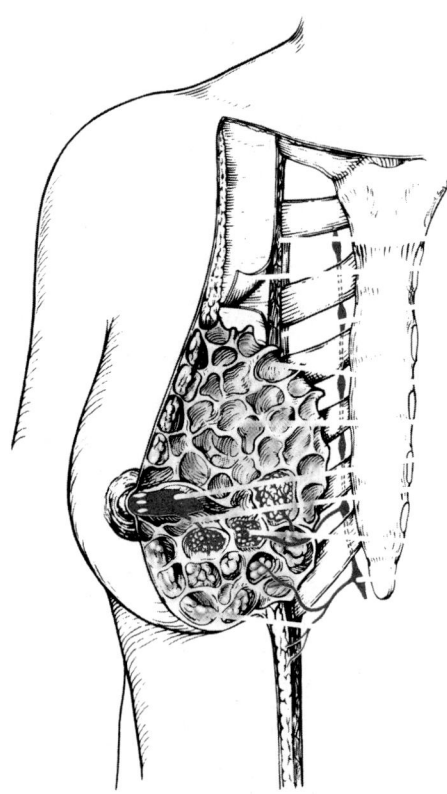

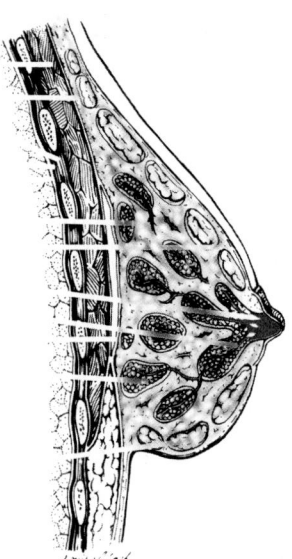

FIG. 16-3. Anatomy of the breast. Tangential and cross-sectional (sagittal) views of the breast and associated chest wall. *(From Romrell et al,[10] p 20, with permission.)*

fails. Each breast develops when an ingrowth of ectoderm forms a primary tissue bud in the mesenchyme. The primary bud, in turn, initiates the development of 15 to 20 secondary buds. Epithelial cords develop from the secondary buds and extend into the surrounding mesenchyme. Major (lactiferous) ducts develop, which open into a shallow mammary pit. During infancy, a proliferation of mesenchyme transforms the mammary pit into a nipple. If there is failure of a pit to elevate above skin level, an inverted nipple results. This congenital malformation occurs in 4% of infants. At birth, the breasts are identical in males and females, demonstrating only the presence of major ducts. Enlargement of the breast may be evident and a secretion, referred to as witch's milk, may be produced. These transitory events occur in response to maternal hormones that cross the placenta.

The breast remains undeveloped in the female until puberty, when it enlarges in response to ovarian estrogen and progesterone, which initiate proliferation of the epithelial and connective tissue elements. However, the breasts remain incompletely developed until pregnancy occurs. Absence of the breast (*amastia*) is rare and results from an arrest in mammary ridge development that occurs during the sixth fetal week. Poland's syndrome consists of hypoplasia or complete absence of the breast, costal cartilage and rib defects, hypoplasia of the subcutaneous tissues of the chest wall, and brachysyndactyly. Breast hypoplasia also may be iatrogenically induced prior to puberty by trauma, infection, or radiation therapy. *Symmastia* is a rare anomaly recognized as webbing between the breasts across the midline. Accessory nipples (polythelia) occur in less than 1% of infants and may be associated with abnormalities of the urinary tract (renal agenesis and cancer), abnormalities of the cardiovascular system (conduction disturbances, hypertension, congenital heart anomalies), and other conditions (pyloric stenosis, epilepsy, ear abnormalities, arthrogryposis). Supernumerary breasts may occur in any configuration along the mammary milk line, but

most frequently occur between the normal nipple location and the symphysis pubis. Turner's syndrome (ovarian agenesis and dysgenesis) and Fleischer's syndrome (displacement of the nipples and bilateral renal hypoplasia) may have polymastia as a component. Accessory axillary breast tissue is uncommon and usually is bilateral.

Functional Anatomy[10]

The breast is composed of 15 to 20 lobes (Fig. 16-3), which are each composed of several lobules. Fibrous bands of connective tissue travel through the breast (suspensory ligaments of Cooper), insert perpendicularly into the dermis, and provide structural support. The mature female breast extends from the level of the second or third rib to the inframammary fold at the sixth or seventh rib. It extends transversely from the lateral border of the sternum to the anterior axillary line. The deep or posterior surface of the breast rests on the fascia of the pectoralis major, serratus anterior, and external oblique abdominal muscles, and the upper extent of the rectus sheath. The retromammary bursa may be identified on the posterior aspect of the breast between the investing fascia of the breast and the fascia of the pectoralis major muscles. The axillary tail of Spence extends laterally across the anterior axillary fold. The upper outer quadrant of the breast contains a greater volume of tissue than do the other quadrants. The breast has a protuberant conical form. The base of the cone is roughly circular, measuring 10 to 12 cm in diameter. Considerable variations in the size, contour, and density of the breast are evident between individuals. The nulliparous breast has a hemispheric configuration with distinct flattening above the nipple. With the hormonal stimulation that accompanies pregnancy and lactation, the breast becomes larger and increases in volume and density, while with senescence, it assumes a flattened, flaccid, and more pendulous configuration with decreased volume.

Nipple–Areola Complex

The epidermis of the nipple–areola complex is pigmented and is variably corrugated. During puberty, the pigment becomes darker and the nipple assumes an elevated configuration. During pregnancy, the areola enlarges and pigmentation is further enhanced. The areola contains sebaceous glands, sweat glands, and accessory glands, which produce small elevations on the surface of the areola (Montgomery tubercles). Smooth-muscle bundle fibers, which lie circumferentially in the dense connective tissue and longitudinally along the major ducts, extend upward into the nipple where they are responsible for the nipple erection that occurs with various sensory stimuli. The dermal papilla at the tip of the nipple contains numerous sensory nerve endings and Meissner's corpuscles. This rich sensory innervation is of functional importance as the sucking infant initiates a chain of neurohumoral events that results in milk letdown.

Inactive and Active Breast

Each lobe of the breast terminates in a major (lactiferous) duct (2 to 4 mm in diameter), which opens through a constricted orifice (0.4 to 0.7 mm in diameter) into the ampulla of the nipple (see Fig. 16-3). Immediately below the nipple–areola complex, each major duct has a dilated portion (lactiferous sinus), which is lined with stratified squamous epithelium. Major ducts are lined with two layers of cuboidal cells, while minor ducts are lined with a single layer of columnar or cuboidal cells. Myoepithelial cells of ectodermal origin reside between the epithelial cells in the basal lamina and contain myofibrils. In the inactive breast, the epithelium is sparse and consists primarily of ductal epithelium (Fig. 16-4). In the early phase of the menstrual cycle, minor ducts are cord-like with small lumina. With estrogen stimulation at the time of ovulation, alveolar epithelium increase, in height, duct lumina become more prominent, and some secretions accumulate. When the hormonal stimulation decreases, the alveolar epithelium regresses.

With pregnancy, the breast undergoes proliferative and developmental maturation. As the breast enlarges in response to hormonal stimulation, lymphocytes, plasma cells, and eosinophils accumulate within the connective tissues. The minor ducts branch and alveoli develop. Development of the alveoli is asymmetric, and variations in the degree of development may occur within a single lobule

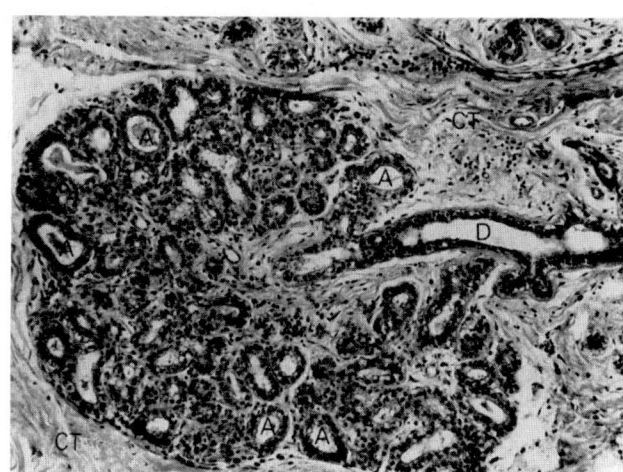

FIG. 16-5. Active human breast: pregnancy and lactation (x160). The alveolar epithelium becomes conspicuous during the early proliferative period. An alveolus (A) and a duct (D) are shown. The alveolus is surrounded by cellular connective tissue (CT). (From Romrell et al,[10] p 23, with permission.)

(Fig. 16-5). With parturition, enlargement of the breasts occurs via hypertrophy of alveolar epithelium and accumulation of secretory products in the lumina of the minor ducts. Alveolar epithelium contains abundant endoplasmic reticulum, large mitochondria, Golgi complexes, and dense lysosomes. Two distinct substances are produced by the alveolar epithelium: (1) the protein component of milk, which is synthesized in the endoplasmic reticulum (merocrine secretion), and (2) the lipid component of milk (apocrine secretion), which forms as free lipid droplets in the cytoplasm. Milk released in the first few days following parturition is called colostrum and has low lipid content but contains considerable quantities of antibodies. The lymphocytes and plasma cells that accumulate within the connective tissues of the breast are the source of the antibody component. With subsequent reduction in the number of these cells, the production of colostrum decreases and lipid-rich milk is released.

Blood Supply, Innervation, and Lymphatics

The breast receives its principal blood supply from (1) perforating branches of the internal mammary artery; (2) lateral branches of the posterior intercostal arteries; and (3) branches from the axillary artery, including the highest thoracic, lateral thoracic, and pectoral branches of the thoracoacromial artery (Fig. 16-6). The second, third, and fourth anterior intercostal perforators and branches of the internal mammary artery arborize in the breast as the medial mammary arteries. The lateral thoracic artery gives off branches to the serratus anterior, pectoralis major and minor, and subscapularis muscles. It also gives rise to lateral mammary branches. The veins of the breast and chest wall follow the course of the arteries with venous drainage being toward the axilla. The three principal groups of veins are (1) perforating branches of the internal thoracic vein; (2) perforating branches of the posterior intercostal veins; and (3) tributaries of the axillary vein. The vertebral venous plexus of Batson, which invests the vertebrae and extends from the base of the skull to the sacrum, may provide a route for breast cancer metastases to the vertebrae, skull, pelvic bones, and central nervous system. Lymph vessels generally parallel the course of blood vessels.

Lateral cutaneous branches of the third through sixth intercostal nerves provide sensory innervation of the breast (lateral mammary branches) and of the anterolateral chest wall. These branches exit the

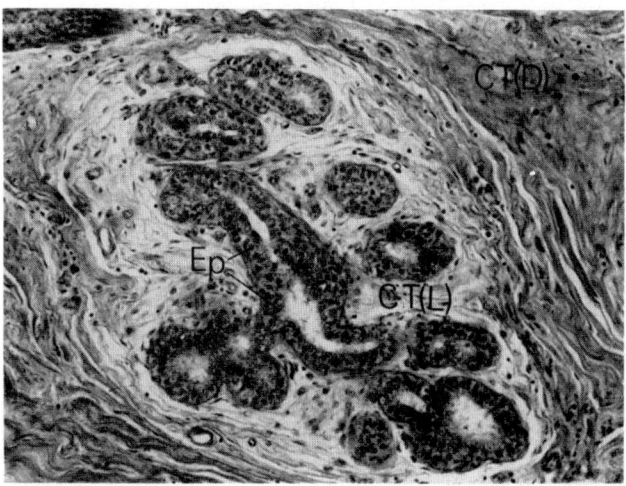

FIG. 16-4. Inactive human breast (x160). The epithelium (Ep), which is primarily ductal, is embedded in loose connective tissue (CT[L]). Dense connective tissue (CT[D]) surrounds the lobule. (From Romrell et al,[10] p 22, with permission.)

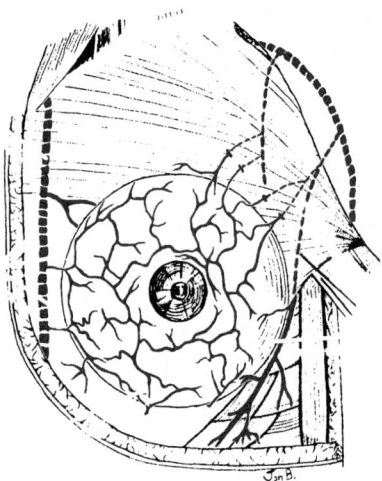

FIG. 16-6. Arterial supply to the breast, axilla, and chest wall. *(From Romrell et al,*[10] *p 28, with permission.)*

intercostal spaces between slips of the serratus anterior muscle. Cutaneous branches that arise from the cervical plexus, specifically the anterior branches of the supraclavicular nerve, supply a limited area of skin over the upper portion of the breast. The intercostobrachial nerve is the lateral cutaneous branch of the second intercostal nerve and may be visualized during surgical dissection of the axilla. Resection of the intercostobrachial nerve causes loss of sensation over the medial aspect of the upper arm.

The boundaries for lymph drainage of the axilla are not well demarcated, and there is considerable variation in the position of the axillary lymph nodes. The 6 axillary lymph node groups recognized by surgeons (Figs. 16-7 and 16-8) are (1) the axillary vein group (lateral) that consists of 4 to 6 lymph nodes, which lie medial or posterior to the vein and receive most of the lymph drainage from the upper extremity; (2) the external mammary group (anterior or pectoral group) that consists of 5 or 6 lymph nodes, which lie along

the lower border of the pectoralis minor muscle contiguous with the lateral thoracic vessels and receive most of the lymph drainage from the lateral aspect of the breast; (3) the scapular group (posterior or subscapular) that consists of 5 to 7 lymph nodes, which lie along the posterior wall of the axilla at the lateral border of the scapula contiguous with the subscapular vessels and receive lymph drainage principally from the lower posterior neck, the posterior trunk, and the posterior shoulder; (4) the central group that consists of 3 or 4 sets of lymph nodes, which are embedded in the fat of the axilla lying immediately posterior to the pectoralis minor muscle and receive lymph drainage both from the axillary vein, external mammary, and scapular groups of lymph nodes and directly from the breast; (5) the subclavicular group (apical) that consists of 6 to 12 sets of lymph nodes, which lie posterior and superior to the upper border of the pectoralis minor muscle and receive lymph drainage from all of the other groups of axillary lymph nodes; and (6) the interpectoral group (Rotter's) that consists of 1 to 4 lymph nodes, which are interposed between the pectoralis major and pectoralis minor muscles and receive lymph drainage directly from the breast. The lymph fluid that passes through the interpectoral group of lymph nodes passes directly into the central and subclavicular groups.

As indicated in Fig. 16-8, the lymph node groups are assigned levels according to their relationship to the pectoralis minor muscle. Lymph nodes located lateral to or below the lower border of the pectoralis minor muscle are referred to as level I lymph nodes, which include the axillary vein, external mammary, and scapular groups. Lymph nodes located superficial or deep to the pectoralis minor muscle are referred to as level II lymph nodes, which include the central and interpectoral groups. Lymph nodes located medial to or above the upper border of the pectoralis minor muscle are referred to as level III lymph nodes, which consist of the subclavicular group. The plexus of lymph vessels in the breast arises in the interlobular connective tissue and in the walls of the lactiferous ducts and communicates with the subareolar plexus of lymph vessels. Efferent lymph vessels from the breast pass around the lateral edge of the pectoralis major muscle and pierce the clavipectoral fascia ending in the external mammary (anterior, pectoral) group of lymph nodes. Some lymph vessels may travel directly to the subscapular (posterior, scapular) group of lymph nodes. From the upper part of the breast, a few lymph vessels pass directly to the subclavicular (apical) group of lymph nodes. The axillary lymph nodes usually receive more than 75% of the lymph drainage from the breast. The rest is derived primarily from the medial aspect of the breast, flows through the lymph vessels that accompany the perforating branches of the internal mammary artery, and enters the parasternal (internal mammary) group of lymph nodes.

PHYSIOLOGY OF THE BREAST

Breast Development and Function[11–13]

Breast development and function are initiated by a variety of hormonal stimuli, including estrogen, progesterone, prolactin, oxytocin, thyroid hormone, cortisol, and growth hormone. Estrogen, progesterone, and prolactin especially have profound trophic effects that are essential to normal breast development and function. Estrogen initiates ductal development, while progesterone is responsible for differentiation of epithelium and for lobular development. Prolactin is the primary hormonal stimulus for lactogenesis in late pregnancy and the postpartum period. It upregulates hormone receptors and stimulates epithelial development. Figure 16-9 depicts the secretion of neurotrophic hormones from the hypothalamus, which

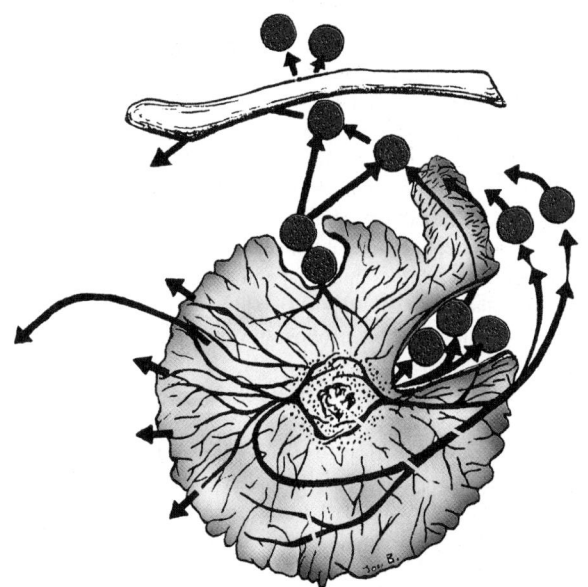

FIG. 16-7. Lymphatic pathways of the breast. Arrows indicate the direction of lymph flow. *(From Romrell et al,*[10] *p 30, with permission.)*

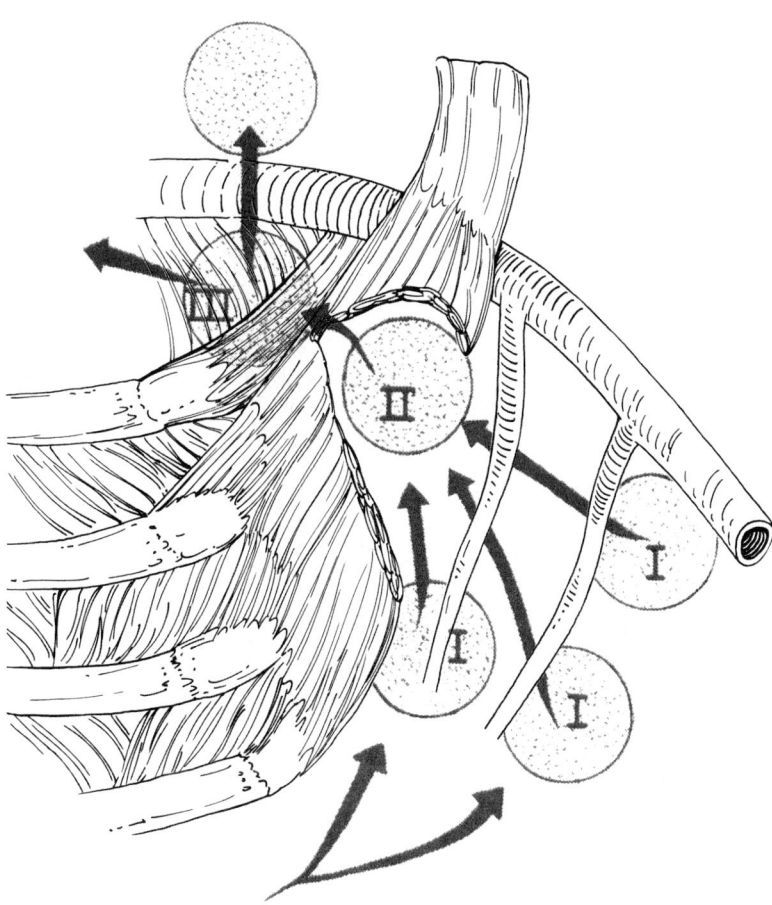

FIG. 16-8. *Axillary lymph node groups. Level I includes lymph nodes located lateral to the pectoralis minor muscle (PM); level II includes lymph nodes located deep to the PM; and level III includes lymph nodes located medial to the PM. Arrows indicate the direction of lymph flow. The axillary vein with its major tributaries and the supraclavicular lymph node group also are illustrated. (From Romrell et al,[10] p 32, with permission.)*

is responsible for regulation of the secretion of the hormones that affect the breast tissues. The gonadotropins luteinizing hormone (LH) and follicle-stimulating hormone (FSH) regulate the release of estrogen and progesterone from the ovaries. In turn, the release of LH and FSH from the basophilic cells of the anterior pituitary is regulated by the secretion of gonadotropin-releasing hormone (GnRH) from the hypothalamus. Positive and negative feedback effects of circulating estrogen and progesterone regulate the secretion of LH, FSH, and GnRH. These hormones are responsible for the development, function, and maintenance of breast tissues (Fig. 16-10). In the female neonate, circulating estrogen and progesterone levels decrease after birth and remain low throughout childhood because of the sensitivity of the hypothalamic pituitary axis to negative feedback by these hormones. With the onset of puberty, there is a decrease in the sensitivity of the hypothalamic pituitary axis to negative feedback and an increase in its sensitivity to positive feedback by estrogen. These physiologic events initiate an increase in GnRH, FSH, and LH secretion, and ultimately an increase in estrogen and progesterone secretion by the ovaries, leading to establishment of the menstrual cycle. At the beginning of the menstrual cycle, there is an increase in the size and density of the breasts, which is followed by engorgement of the breast tissues and epithelial proliferation. With the onset of menstruation, the breast engorgement subsides and epithelial proliferation decreases.

Pregnancy, Lactation, and Senescence[11–13]

A dramatic increase in circulating ovarian and placental estrogens and progestins is evident during pregnancy, which initiates striking alterations in the form and substance of the breast (see Fig. 16-10B).

The breast enlarges as the ductal and lobular epithelium proliferates, the areolar skin darkens, and the accessory areolar glands of Montgomery become prominent. In the first and second trimesters, the minor ducts branch and develop. During the third trimester, fat droplets accumulate in the alveolar epithelium and colostrum fills the alveolar and ductal spaces. In late pregnancy, prolactin stimulates the synthesis of milk fats and proteins.

Following delivery of the placenta, circulating progesterone and estrogen levels decrease, which permits full expression of the lactogenic action of prolactin. Milk production and release are controlled by neural reflex arcs that originate in nerve endings of the nipple–areola complex. Maintenance of lactation requires regular stimulation of these neural reflexes resulting in prolactin secretion and milk letdown. Oxytocin release results from the auditory, visual, and olfactory stimuli associated with nursing. Oxytocin initiates contraction of the myoepithelial cells resulting in compression of alveoli and expulsion of milk into the lactiferous sinuses. After weaning of the infant, prolactin and oxytocin release decrease. Dormant milk causes increased pressure within the ducts and alveoli resulting in atrophy of the epithelium (Fig. 16-10C). With menopause there is a decrease in the secretion of estrogen and progesterone by the ovaries and involution of the ducts and alveoli of the breast. The surrounding fibrous connective tissue increases in density, and breast tissues are replaced by adipose tissues (Fig. 16-10D).

Gynecomastia[14]

Gynecomastia refers to an enlarged breast in the male. Physiologic gynecomastia usually occurs during three phases of life: the neonatal period, adolescence, and senescence. Common to each of these

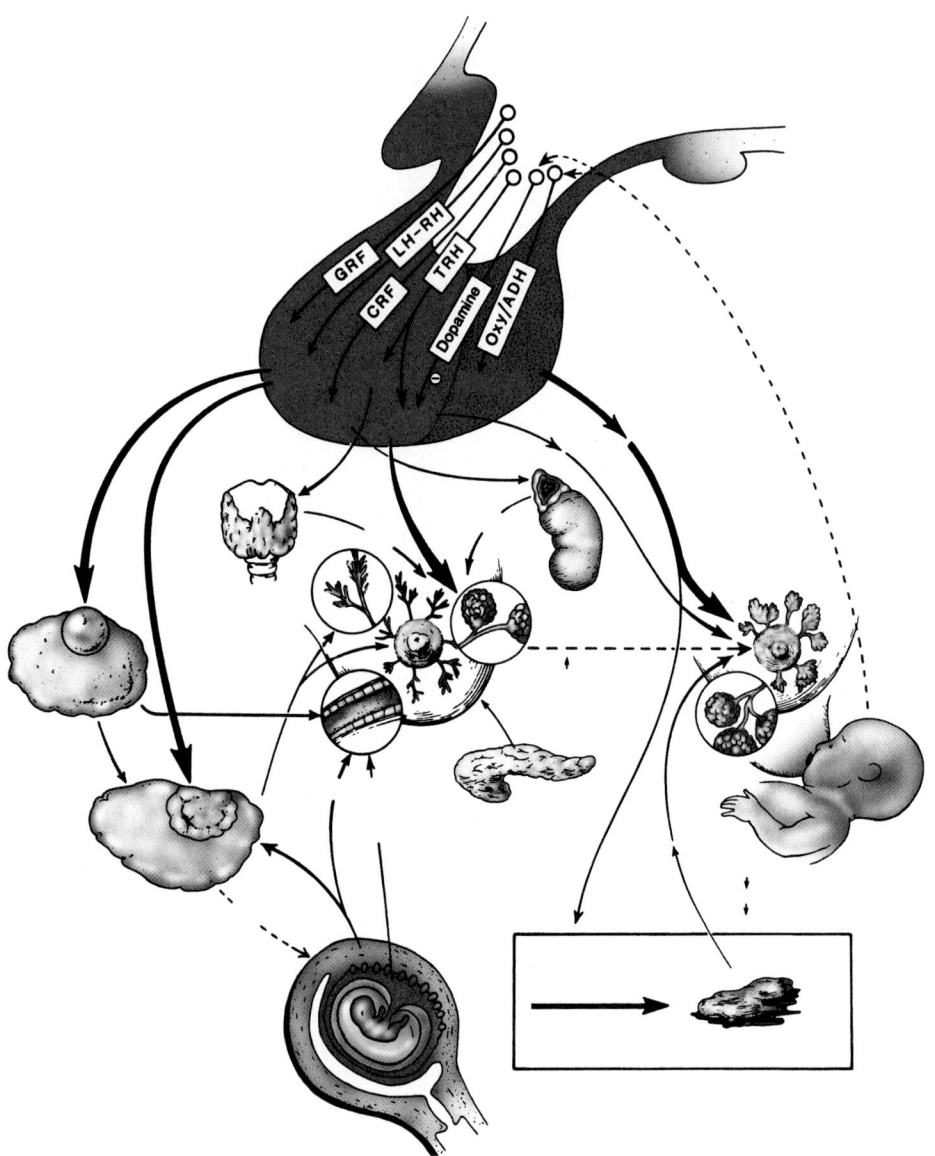

FIG. 16-9. Overview of the neuroendocrine control of breast development and function. [*Reproduced with permission from Keller-Wood M, et al: Breast physiology: Normal and abnormal development and function, in Bland KI, Copeland EM III (eds): The Breast: Comprehensive Management of Benign and Malignant Diseases. Philadelphia: WB Saunders, 1998, p 40.*]

phases is an excess of circulating estrogens in relation to circulating testosterone. Neonatal gynecomastia is caused by the action of placental estrogens on neonatal breast tissues, while in adolescence, there is an excess of estradiol relative to testosterone, and with senescence, the circulating testosterone level falls, resulting in relative hyperestrinism. In gynecomastia, the ductal structures of the male breast enlarge, elongate, and branch with a concomitant increase in epithelium. During puberty, the condition often is unilateral and typically occurs between ages 12 and 15 years. In contrast, senescent gynecomastia is usually bilateral. In the nonobese male, breast tissue measuring at least 2 cm in diameter must be present before a diagnosis of gynecomastia may be made. Mammography and ultrasonography are used to differentiate breast tissues. Dominant masses or areas of firmness, irregularity, and asymmetry suggest the possibility of a breast cancer, particularly in the older male. Gynecomastia generally does not predispose the male breast to cancer. However, the hypoandrogenic state of Klinefelter's syndrome (XXY), in which gynecomastia is usually evident, is associated with an increased risk of breast cancer. Table 16-1 presents a clinical classification of gynecomastia.

Table 16-2 identifies the pathophysiologic mechanisms that may initiate gynecomastia. Estrogen excess results from an increase in the secretion of estradiol from the testicles or from nontesticular tumors; nutritional alterations such as protein and fat deprivation; endocrine disorders (hyperthyroidism, hypothyroidism); and hepatic disease (nonalcoholic and alcoholic cirrhosis). Refeeding gynecomastia is related to the resumption of pituitary gonadotropin secretion after pituitary shutdown. Androgen deficiency may initiate gynecomastia. Concurrently occurring with decreased circulating testosterone levels is an elevated level of circulating testosterone-binding globulin, which results in a reduction of free testosterone. This senescent gynecomastia usually occurs in men age 50 to 70 years. Klinefelter's syndrome (XXY) is manifested by gynecomastia, hypergonadotropic hypogonadism, and azoospermia. Primary testicular failure also may be caused by adrenocorticotropic hormone (ACTH) deficiency, hereditary defects of androgen synthesis, and congenital anorchia (eunuchoidal males). Secondary testicular failure may result from trauma, orchitis, and cryptorchidism. Renal failure, regardless of cause, may also initiate gynecomastia. Drugs with estrogenic activity (digitalis, estrogens,

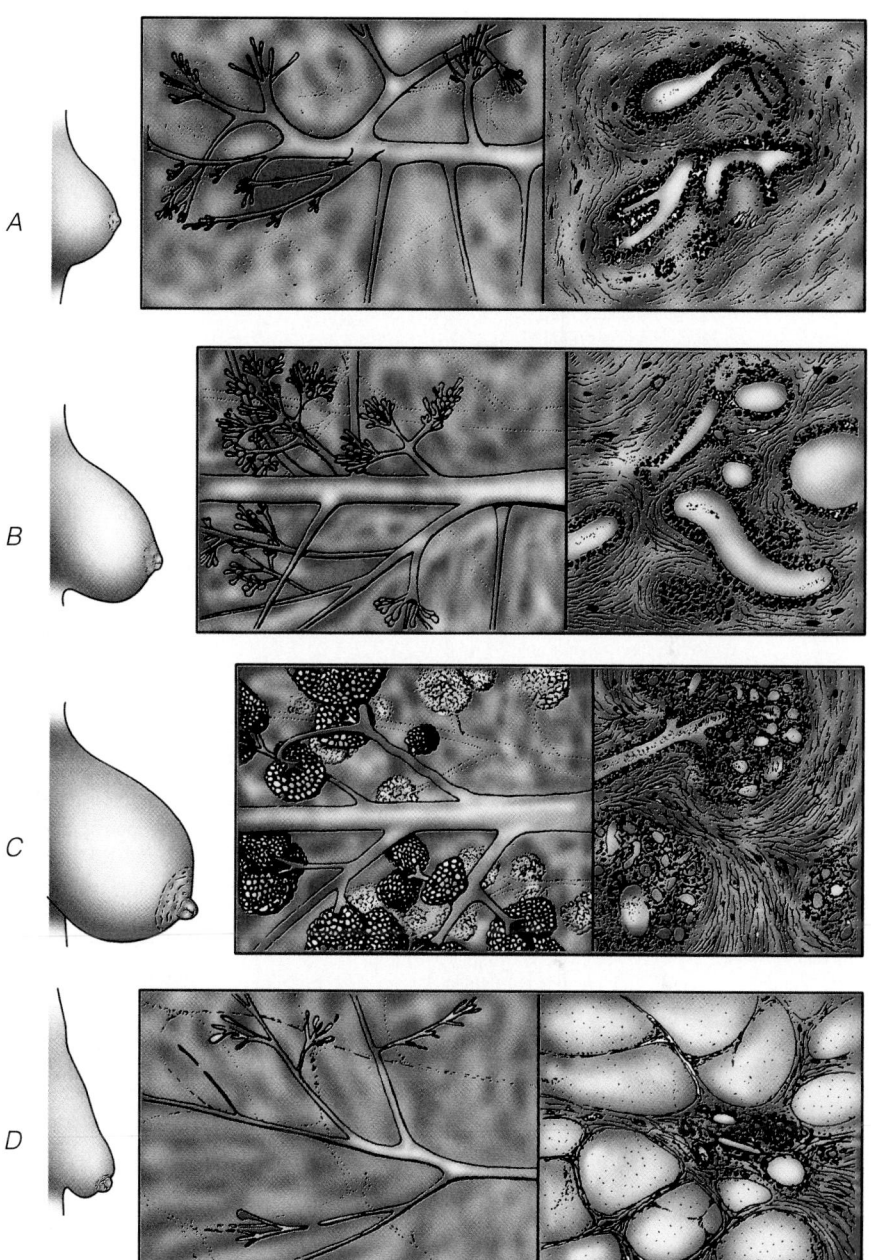

FIG. 16-10. The breast at different physiological stages. The central column contains three-dimensional depictions of microscopy structures. A. Adolescence. B. Pregnancy. C. Lactation. D. Senescence.

anabolic steroids, marijuana) or drugs that enhance estrogen synthesis (human chorionic gonadotropin) may cause gynecomastia. Drugs that inhibit the action or synthesis of testosterone (cimetidine, ketoconazole, phenytoin, spironolactone, antineoplastic agents, diazepam) also have been implicated. Drugs such as reserpine, theophylline, verapamil, tricyclic antidepressants, and furosemide

induce gynecomastia through idiopathic mechanisms. When gynecomastia is caused by (1) androgen deficiency, then testosterone administration may cause regression; (2) medications, then these are discontinued if possible; or (3) endocrine defects, then these receive specific therapy. When gynecomastia is progressive and does not respond to other therapies, surgical therapy is considered. Attempts to reverse gynecomastia with danazol have been successful, but the androgenic side effects of the drug are considerable.

INFECTIOUS AND INFLAMMATORY DISORDERS OF THE BREAST

Excluding the postpartum period, infections of the breast are rare and are classified as intrinsic (secondary to abnormalities in the breast) or extrinsic (secondary to an infection in an adjacent structure, e.g., skin, thoracic cavity).

Table 16-1
Clinical Classification of Gynecomastia

Grade I	Mild breast enlargement without skin redundancy
Grade IIa	Moderate breast enlargement without skin redundancy
Grade IIb	Moderate breast enlargement with skin redundancy
Grade III	Marked breast enlargement with skin redundancy and ptosis, which simulates a female breast

SOURCE: Modified with permission from Simon BE: Classification and surgical correction of gynecomastia. *Plas Reconstr Surg* 51:48, 1973.

Table 16-2
Pathophysiologic Mechanisms of Gynecomastia

I. Estrogen excess states
  A. Gonadal origin
    1. True hermaphroditism
    2. Gonadal stromal (nongerminal) neoplasms of the testis
      a. Leydig cell (interstitial)
      b. Sertoli cell
      c. Granulosa-theca
    3. Germ cell tumors
      a. Choriocarcinoma
      b. Seminoma, teratoma
      c. Embryonal carcinoma
  B. Nontesticular tumors
    1. Adrenal cortical neoplasms
    2. Lung carcinoma
    3. Hepatocellular carcinoma
  C. Endocrine disorders
  D. Diseases of the liver—nonalcoholic and alcoholic cirrhosis
  E. Nutrition alteration states
II. Androgen deficiency states
  A. Senescence
  B. Hypoandrogen states (hypogonadism)
    1. Primary testicular failure
      a. Klinefelter's syndrome (XXY)
      b. Reifenstein's syndrome
      c. Rosewater, Gwinup, Hamwi familial gynecomastia
      d. Kallmann's syndrome
      e. Kennedy's disease with associated gynecomastia
      f. Eunuchoidal males (congenital anorchia)
      g. Hereditary defects of androgen biosynthesis
      h. ACTH deficiency
    2. Secondary testicular failure
      a. Trauma
      b. Orchitis
      c. Cryptorchidism
      d. Irradiation
  C. Renal failure
III. Drug-related
IV. Systemic diseases with idiopathic mechanisms

Bacterial Infection[15]

Staphylococcus aureus and *Streptococcus* species are the organisms most frequently recovered from nipple discharge from an infected breast. Breast abscesses are typically seen in staphylococcal infections and present with point tenderness, erythema, and hyperthermia. These abscesses are related to lactation and occur within the first few weeks of breast-feeding. Figure 16-11 depicts progression of a staphylococcal infection, which may result in subcutaneous, subareolar, interlobular (periductal), and retromammary abscesses (unicentric or multicentric), necessitating operative drainage of fluctuant areas. Preoperative ultrasonography is effective in delineating the extent of the drainage procedure, which is best accomplished via circumareolar incisions or incisions paralleling Langer's lines. While staphylococcal infections tend to be more localized and may be located deep in the breast tissues, streptococcal infections usually present with diffuse superficial involvement. They are treated with local wound care, including warm compresses, and the administration of intravenous antibiotics (penicillins or cephalosporins). Breast infections may be chronic, possibly with recurrent abscess formation. In this situation, cultures are taken to identify acid-fast bacilli, anaerobic and aerobic bacteria, and fungi. Uncommon organisms may be encountered and long-term antibiotic therapy may be required.

Hospital-acquired puerperal infections of the breast are much less common now, but nursing women who present with milk stasis or noninfectious inflammation may still develop this problem.

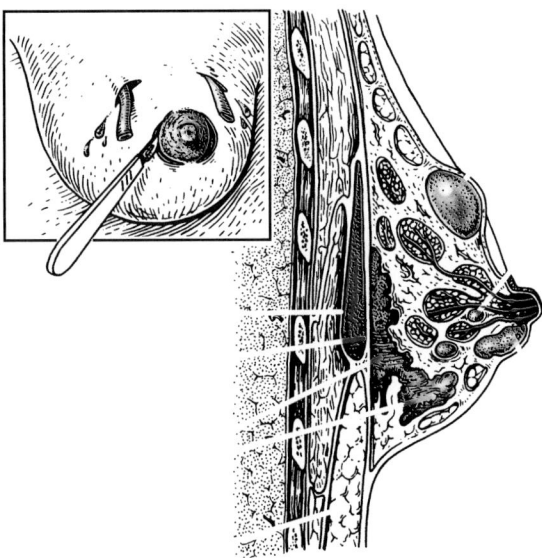

FIG. 16-11. *Breast abscesses. Sagittal view of the breast with sites of potential abscess formation. Deep abscesses may be multilocular and may communicate with subcutaneous or subareolar sites. Inset depicts drainage of a multilocular breast abscess through circumareolar incisions and other incisions that parallel Langer's lines.*

Epidemic puerperal mastitis is initiated by highly virulent strains of methicillin-resistant *S. aureus* that are transmitted via the suckling neonate and may result in substantial morbidity and occasional mortality. Pus frequently may be expressed from the nipple. In this circumstance, breast-feeding is stopped, antibiotics are started, and surgical therapy is initiated. Nonepidemic (sporadic) puerperal mastitis refers to involvement of the interlobular connective tissue of the breast by an infectious process. The patient develops nipple fissuring and milk stasis, which initiate a retrograde bacterial infection. Emptying of the breast by using breast suction pumps shortens the duration of symptoms and reduces the incidence of recurrences. The addition of antibiotics results in a satisfactory outcome in more than 95% of cases.

Mycotic Infections[15]

Fungal infestations of the breast are rare and usually involve blastomycosis or sporotrichosis. Intraoral fungi that are inoculated into the breast tissue by the suckling infant initiate these infections, which present as mammary abscesses in close proximity to the nipple–areola complex. Pus mixed with blood may be expressed from sinus tracts. Amphotericin B is the most effective antifungal agent for the treatment of systemic (noncutaneous) infections. This therapy generally eliminates the necessity of surgical intervention, but occasionally drainage of an abscess, or even partial mastectomy, may be necessary to eradicate a persistent fungal infection. *Candida albicans* affecting the skin of the breast presents as erythematous, scaly lesions of the inframammary or axillary folds. Scrapings from the lesions demonstrate fungal elements (filaments and binding cells). Therapy involves the removal of predisposing factors such as maceration and the topical application of nystatin.

Hidradenitis Suppurativa[15]

Hidradenitis suppurativa of the nipple–areola complex or axilla is a chronic inflammatory condition that originates within the accessory areolar glands of Montgomery or within the axillary sebaceous glands. Women with chronic acne are predisposed to developing hidradenitis. When located in and about the nipple–areola complex,

Table 16-3
ANDI Classification of Benign Breast Disorders

	Normal →	Disorder →	Disease
Early reproductive years (age 15–25)	Lobular development	Fibroadenoma	Giant fibroadenoma
	Stromal development	Adolescent hypertrophy	Gigantomastia
	Nipple eversion	Nipple inversion	Subareolar abscess
			Mammary duct fistula
Later reproductive years (age 25–40)	Cyclical changes of menstruation	Cyclical mastalgia	Incapacitating mastalgia
		Nodularity	
	Epithelial hyperplasia of pregnancy	Bloody nipple discharge	
Involution (age 35–55)	Lobular involution	Macrocysts	
		Sclerosing lesions	
	Duct involution		
	–Dilatation	Duct ectasia	Periductal mastitis
	–Sclerosis	Nipple retraction	
	Epithelial turnover	Epithelial hyperplasia	Epithelial hyperplasia with atypia

ANDI = Aberrations of normal development and involution.

SOURCE: Modified with permission from Hughes LE: in Hughes LE, Mansel RE, Webster DJT (eds): Aberrations of normal development and involution (ANDI): A concept of benign breast disorders based on pathogenesis. *Benign Disorders and Diseases of the Breast: Concepts and Clinical Management.* London: WB Saunders, 2000, p 23.

this disease may mimic other chronic inflammatory states, Paget's disease of the nipple, or invasive breast cancer. Involvement of the axillary skin is often multifocal and contiguous. Antibiotic therapy with incision and drainage of fluctuant areas is appropriate treatment. Excision of the involved areas may be required. Large areas of skin loss may necessitate coverage with advancement flaps or split-thickness skin grafts.

Mondor's Disease[16]

This variant of thrombophlebitis involves the superficial veins of the anterior chest wall and breast. In 1939, Mondor described the condition as "string phlebitis," a thrombosed vein presenting as a tender, cord-like structure. Frequently involved veins include the lateral thoracic vein, the thoracoepigastric vein, and, less frequently, the superficial epigastric vein. Typically, a woman presents with acute pain in the lateral aspect of the breast or the anterior chest wall. A tender, firm cord is found to follow the distribution of one of the major superficial veins. Rarely, the presentation is bilateral, and most women have no evidence of thrombophlebitis in other anatomic sites. This benign, self-limited disorder is not indicative of a cancer. When the diagnosis is uncertain, or when a mass is present near the tender cord, biopsy is indicated. Therapy for Mondor's disease includes the liberal use of anti-inflammatory medications and warm compresses that are applied along the symptomatic vein. Restriction of motion of the ipsilateral extremity and shoulder as well as brassiere support of the breast are important. The process usually resolves within 4 to 6 weeks. When symptoms persist or are refractory to therapy, excision of the involved vein segment is appropriate.

COMMON BENIGN DISORDERS AND DISEASES OF THE BREAST

Benign breast disorders and diseases encompass a wide range of clinical and pathologic entities. Surgeons require an in-depth understanding of benign breast disorders and diseases so that clear explanations may be given to affected women, appropriate treatment instituted, and unnecessary long-term follow-up avoided.

Aberrations of Normal Development and Involution[17]

The basic principles underlying the aberrations of normal development and involution (ANDI) classification of benign breast conditions are (1) benign breast disorders and diseases are related to the normal processes of reproductive life and to involution; (2) there is a spectrum of breast conditions that ranges from normal to disorder to disease; and (3) the ANDI classification encompasses all aspects of the breast condition, including pathogenesis and the degree of abnormality. The horizontal component of Table 16-3 defines ANDI along a spectrum from normal, to mild abnormality (disorder), to severe abnormality (disease). The vertical component defines the period during which the condition develops.

Early Reproductive Years[18]

Fibroadenomas are seen predominantly in younger women age 15 to 25 years (Fig. 16-12). Fibroadenomas usually grow to 1 or 2 cm in diameter and then are stable, but may grow to a larger size. Small fibroadenomas (1 cm in size or less) are considered normal,

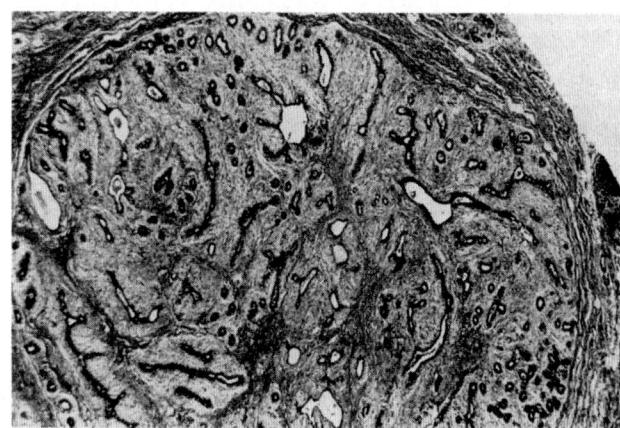

FIG. 16-12. Fibroadenoma (x10). *(Courtesy of Dr. R. L. Hackett.)*

while larger fibroadenomas (up to 3 cm) are disorders and giant fibroadenomas (larger than 3 cm) are disease. Similarly, multiple fibroadenomas (more than five lesions in one breast) are very uncommon and are considered disease. The precise etiology of adolescent breast hypertrophy is unknown. A spectrum of changes from limited to massive stromal hyperplasia (gigantomastia) is seen. Nipple inversion is a disorder of development of the major ducts, which prevents normal protrusion of the nipple. Mammary duct fistulas arise when nipple inversion predisposes to major duct obstruction, leading to recurrent subareolar abscess and mammary duct fistula.

Later Reproductive Years

Cyclical mastalgia and nodularity are usually associated with premenstrual enlargement of the breast and are regarded as normal. Cyclical pronounced mastalgia and severe painful nodularity are viewed differently than are physiologic discomfort and lumpiness. Painful nodularity that persists for more than 1 week of the menstrual cycle is considered a disorder. In epithelial hyperplasia of pregnancy, papillary projections sometimes give rise to bilateral bloody nipple discharge.

Involution

Involution of lobular epithelium is dependent on the specialized stroma around it. However, an integrated involution of breast stroma and epithelium is not always seen and disorders of the process are common. When the stroma involutes too quickly, alveoli remain and form microcysts, which are precursors of macrocysts. Macrocysts are common, are often subclinical in nature, and do not require specific treatment. Sclerosing adenosis is considered a disorder of both the proliferative and the involutional phases of the breast cycle. Duct ectasia (dilated ducts) and periductal mastitis are other important components of the ANDI classification. Periductal fibrosis is a sequela of periductal mastitis and may result in nipple retraction. Sixty percent of women age 70 years or older exhibit some degree of epithelial hyperplasia (Fig. 16-13). Atypical proliferative diseases include ductal and lobular hyperplasia, both of which display some features of carcinoma in situ. Women with atypical ductal or lobular hyperplasia have a fourfold increase in breast cancer risk (Table 16-4).

Pathology of Nonproliferative Disorders[19,20]

Of paramount importance for the optimal management of benign breast disorders and diseases is the histologic differentiation of benign, atypical, and malignant changes. Determining the clinical significance of these changes is a problem that is compounded by inconsistent nomenclature. The classification system developed by Page separates the various types of benign breast disorders and diseases into three clinically relevant groups: nonproliferative disorders, proliferative diseases without atypia, and proliferative disorders with atypia (Table 16-5). Nonproliferative disorders of the breast account for 70% of benign breast conditions and carry no increased risk for the development of breast cancer. This category includes cysts, duct ectasia, periductal mastitis, calcifications, fibroadenomas, and related disorders.

Breast macrocysts are an involutional disorder, have a high frequency of occurrence, and are often multiple. Duct ectasia is a clinical syndrome, which describes dilated subareolar ducts that are palpable and often associated with thick nipple discharge. Haagensen regarded duct ectasia as a primary event, which led to stagnation of secretions, epithelial ulceration, and leakage of duct secretions

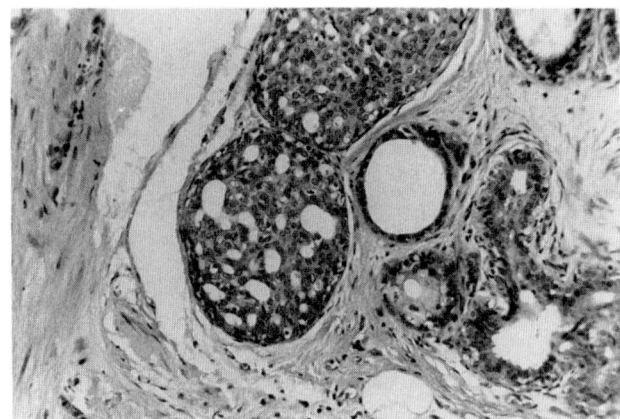

A

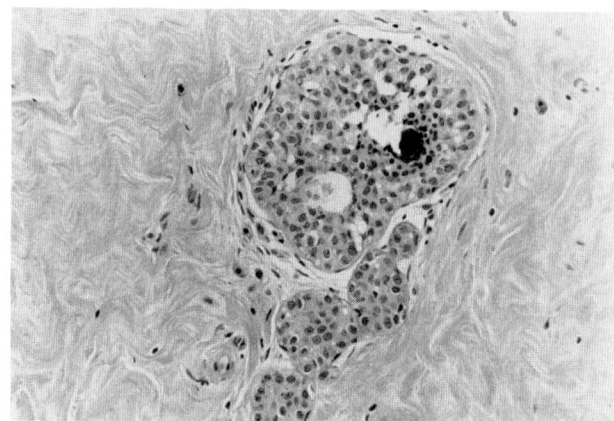

B

FIG. 16-13. *A. Ductal epithelial hyperplasia. The irregular intracellular spaces and variable cell nuclei distinguish this process from carcinoma in situ. B. Lobular hyperplasia. The presence of alveolar lumina and incomplete distention distinguish this process from carcinoma in situ. (Courtesy of Dr. R. L. Hackett.)*

(containing chemically irritant fatty acids) into periductal tissue. This sequence was thought to produce a local inflammatory process with periductal fibrosis and subsequent nipple retraction. An alternative theory considers periductal mastitis to be the primary process, which leads to weakening of the ducts and secondary dilatation. It

Table 16-4

Cancer Risk Associated with Benign Breast Disorders and In Situ Carcinoma of the Breast

Abnormality	Relative Risk
Nonproliferative lesions of the breast	No increased risk
Sclerosing adenosis	No increased risk
Intraductal papilloma	No increased risk
Florid hyperplasia	1.5 to 2-fold
Atypical lobular hyperplasia	4-fold
Atypical ductal hyperplasia	4-fold
Ductal involvement by cells of atypical ductal hyperplasia	7-fold
Lobular carcinoma in situ	10-fold
Ductal carcinoma in situ	10-fold

SOURCE: Modified with permission from Dupont WD, Page DL: Risk factors for breast cancer in women with proliferative breast disease *N Engl J Med* 312:146, 1985.

Table 16-5
Classification of Benign Breast Disorders

Nonproliferative disorders of the breast
Cysts and apocrine metaplasia
Duct ectasia
Calcifications
Fibroadenoma and related lesions
Proliferative breast disorders without atypia
Sclerosing adenosis
Radial and complex sclerosing lesions
Ductal epithelial hyperplasia
Intraductal papillomas
Atypical proliferative lesions
Atypical lobular hyperplasia (ALH)
Atypical ductal hyperplasia (ADH)

SOURCE: Modified with permission from Consensus Meeting: Is "fibrocystic disease" of the breast precancerous? *Arch Pathol Lab Med* 110:171, 1986.

is possible that both processes occur and together explain the wide spectrum of problems seen, which include nipple discharge, nipple retraction, inflammatory masses, and abscesses.

Calcium deposits are frequently encountered in the breast. Most are benign and are caused by cellular secretions and debris or by trauma and inflammation. Calcifications that are associated with cancer include microcalcifications, which vary in shape and density and are less than 0.5 mm in size, and fine, linear calcifications, which may show branching. Fibroadenomas have abundant stroma with histologically normal cellular elements. They show hormonal dependence similar to that of normal breast lobules in that they lactate during pregnancy and involute in the postmenopausal period. Adenomas of the breast are well circumscribed and are composed of benign epithelium with sparse stroma, which is the histologic feature that differentiates them from fibroadenomas. They may be divided into tubular adenomas and lactating adenomas. Tubular adenomas present in young nonpregnant women, while lactating adenomas present during pregnancy or during the postpartum period. Hamartomas are discrete breast tumors, which are usually 2 to 4 cm in diameter, firm, and sharply circumscribed. Adenolipomas consist of sharply circumscribed nodules of fatty tissue, which contain normal breast lobules and ducts.

Fibrocystic Disease

The term *fibrocystic disease* is nonspecific. Too frequently, it is used as a diagnostic term to describe symptoms, to rationalize the need for breast biopsy, and to explain biopsy results. Synonyms include fibrocystic changes, cystic mastopathy, chronic cystic disease, chronic cystic mastitis, Schimmelbusch's disease, mazoplasia, Cooper's disease, Reclus' disease, and fibroadenomatosis. Fibrocystic disease refers to a spectrum of histopathologic changes that are best diagnosed and treated specifically.

Pathology of Proliferative Disorders Without Atypia[19,20]

Proliferative breast disorders without atypia include sclerosing adenosis, radial scars, complex sclerosing lesions, ductal epithelial hyperplasia, and intraductal papillomas. Sclerosing adenosis is prevalent during the childbearing and perimenopausal years and has no malignant potential. Histologic changes are both proliferative (ductal proliferation) and involutional (stromal fibrosis, epithelial regression) in nature. Sclerosing adenosis is characterized by distorted breast lobules and usually occurs in the context of multiple microcysts, but occasionally presents as a palpable mass.

Benign calcifications are often associated with this disorder. Central sclerosis and varying degrees of epithelial proliferation, apocrine metaplasia, and papilloma formation characterize radial scars and complex sclerosing lesions of the breast. Lesions up to 1 cm in diameter are called radial scars, while larger lesions are called complex sclerosing lesions. Radial scars originate at sites of terminal duct branching where the characteristic histologic changes radiate from a central area of fibrosis. All of the histologic features of a radial scar are seen in the larger complex sclerosing lesions, but there is a greater disturbance of structure with papilloma formation, apocrine metaplasia, and, occasionally, sclerosing adenosis.

Mild ductal hyperplasia is characterized by the presence of three or four cell layers above the basement membrane. Moderate ductal hyperplasia is characterized by the presence of five or more cell layers above the basement membrane. Florid ductal epithelial hyperplasia occupies at least 70% of a minor duct lumen. It is found in more than 20% of breast tissue specimens, is either solid or papillary, and carries an increased cancer risk (see Table 16-4). Intraductal papillomas arise in the major ducts, usually in premenopausal women. They are generally less than 0.5 cm in diameter but may be as large as 5 cm. A common presenting symptom is nipple discharge, which may be serous or bloody. Grossly, intraductal papillomas are pinkish tan, friable, and are usually attached to the wall of the involved duct by a stalk. They rarely undergo malignant transformation, and their presence does not increase a woman's risk of developing breast cancer. However, multiple intraductal papillomas, which occur in younger women and are less frequently associated with nipple discharge, are susceptible to malignant transformation.

Pathology of Atypical Proliferative Diseases[21]

The atypical proliferative diseases have some of the features of carcinoma in situ (CIS) but either lack a major defining feature of CIS or have the features in less than fully developed form. In 1978, Haagensen and colleagues described lobular neoplasia, a spectrum of disorders ranging from atypical lobular hyperplasia to lobular carcinoma in situ.

Treatment of Selected Benign Breast Disorders and Diseases[22,23]

Cysts

Because needle biopsy of breast masses may produce artifacts that make mammography assessment more difficult, many radiologists prefer to image breast masses before needle biopsy. However, in practice, the first investigation of palpable breast masses is frequently needle biopsy, which allows for the early diagnosis of cysts. A 21-gauge needle attached to a 10-mL syringe is placed directly into the mass, which is fixed by fingers of the nondominant hand. The volume of a typical cyst is 5 to 10 mL, but it may be 75 mL or more. If the fluid that is aspirated is not bloodstained, then the cyst is aspirated to dryness, the needle is removed, and the fluid is discarded as cytologic examination of such fluid is not cost-effective. After aspiration, the breast is carefully palpated to exclude a residual mass. If one exists, ultrasound examination is performed to exclude a persistent cyst, which is reaspirated if present. If the mass is solid, a tissue specimen is obtained. When cystic fluid is bloodstained, 2 mL of fluid are taken for cytology. The mass is then imaged with ultrasound and any solid area on the cyst wall is biopsied by needle. The presence of blood is usually obvious, but in cysts with dark fluid, an occult blood test or microscopy examination will eliminate any doubt. The two cardinal rules of safe cyst aspiration are (1) the mass must disappear completely after aspiration, and (2) the fluid must not be bloodstained. If either of these conditions is not met, then ultrasound, needle biopsy, and perhaps excisional biopsy are recommended.

Fibroadenomas

Removal of all fibroadenomas has been advocated irrespective of patient age or other considerations, and solitary fibroadenomas in young women are frequently removed to alleviate patient concern. Yet most fibroadenomas are self-limiting and many go undiagnosed, so a more conservative approach is reasonable. Careful ultrasound examination with core-needle biopsy will provide for an accurate diagnosis. Subsequently, the patient is counseled concerning the biopsy results, and excision of the fibroadenoma may be avoided.

Sclerosing Disorders

The clinical significance of sclerosing adenosis lies in its mimicry of cancer. It may be confused with cancer on physical examination, by mammography, and at gross pathologic examination. Excisional biopsy and histologic examination are frequently necessary to exclude the diagnosis of cancer. The diagnostic work-up for radial scars and complex sclerosing lesions frequently involves stereoscopic biopsy. It is usually not possible to differentiate these lesions with certainty from cancer by mammography features, so biopsy is recommended.

Periductal Mastitis

Painful and tender masses behind the nipple–areola complex are aspirated with a 21-gauge needle attached to a 10-mL syringe. Any fluid obtained is submitted for cytology and for culture using a transport medium appropriate for the detection of anaerobic organisms. In the absence of pus, women are started on a combination of metronidazole and dicloxacillin while awaiting the results of culture. Antibiotics are then continued based on sensitivity tests. Many cases respond satisfactorily, but when there is considerable pus present, surgical treatment is recommended. Unlike puerperal abscesses, a subareolar abscess is usually unilocular and often is associated with a single duct system. Preoperative ultrasound will accurately delineate its extent. The surgeon may either undertake simple drainage with a view toward formal surgery, should the problem recur, or proceed with definitive surgery. In a woman of childbearing age, simple drainage is preferred, but if there is an anaerobic infection, recurrent infection frequently develops. Recurrent abscess with fistula is a difficult problem and may be treated by fistulectomy or by major duct excision, depending on the circumstances (Table 16-6).

When a localized periareolar abscess recur at the previous site and a fistula is present, the preferred operation is fistulectomy, which has minimal complications and a high degree of success. However, when subareolar sepsis is diffuse rather than localized to one segment or when more than one fistula is present, total duct excision is the preferred procedure. The first circumstance is seen in young women with squamous metaplasia of a single duct, while the latter circumstance is seen in older women with multiple ectatic ducts. However, age is not always a reliable guide, and fistula excision is the preferred initial procedure for localized sepsis irrespective of age. Antibiotic therapy is useful for recurrent infection after fistula excision, and a 2- to 4-week course is recommended prior to total duct excision.

Nipple Inversion

More women request correction of congenital nipple inversion than request correction for the nipple inversion that occurs secondary to duct ectasia. Although the results are usually satisfactory, women seeking correction for cosmetic reasons should always be made aware of the surgical complications of altered nipple sensation, nipple necrosis, and postoperative fibrosis with nipple retraction. Because nipple inversion is a result of shortening of the subareolar ducts, a complete division of these ducts is necessary for permanent correction of the disorder.

RISK FACTORS FOR BREAST CANCER

Hormonal and Nonhormonal Risk Factors[24-30]

Increased exposure to estrogen is associated with an increased risk for developing breast cancer, whereas reducing exposure is thought to be protective. Correspondingly, factors that increase the number of menstrual cycles, such as early menarche, nulliparity, and late menopause, are associated with increased risk. Moderate levels of exercise and a longer lactation period, factors that decrease the total number of menstrual cycles, are protective. The terminal differentiation of breast epithelium associated with a full-term pregnancy is also protective, so older age at first live birth is associated with an increased risk of breast cancer. Finally, there is an association between obesity and increased breast cancer risk. Because the major source of estrogen in postmenopausal women is the conversion of androstenedione to estrone by adipose tissue, obesity is associated with a long-term increase in estrogen exposure.

Nonhormonal risk factors include radiation exposure. Young women who receive mantle radiation therapy for Hodgkin's

Table 16-6
Treatment of Recurrent Subareolar Sepsis

Suitable for Fistulectomy	*Suitable for Total Duct Excision*
Small abscess localized to one segment	Large abscess affecting more than 50% of the areolar circumference
Recurrence involving the same segment	Recurrence involving a different segment
Mild or no nipple inversion	Marked nipple inversion
Patient unconcerned about nipple inversion	Patient requests correction of nipple inversion
Younger patient	Older patient
No discharge from other ducts	Purulent discharge from other ducts
No prior fistulectomy	Recurrence after fistulectomy

SOURCE: Modified with permission from Hughes LE: in Hughes LE, Mansel RE, Webster DJT (eds): *Benign Disorders and Diseases of the Breast: Concepts. The duct ectasia/periductal mastitis complex, Clinical Management.* London: WB Saunders, 2000, p 162.

Table 16-7
Relative Risk Estimates for the Gail Model

Variable	Relative Risk
Age at menarche (years)	
≥14	1.00
12–13	1.10
<12	1.21
Number of biopsies/history of benign breast disease, age <50 y	
0	1.00
1	1.70
≥2	2.88
Number of biopsies/history of benign breast disease, age ≥50 y	
0	1.02
1	1.27
≥2	1.62
Age at first live birth (years)	
<20 years	
Number of first-degree relatives with history of breast cancer	
0	1.00
1	2.61
≥2	6.80
20–24 years	
Number of first-degree relatives with history of breast cencer	
0	1.24
1	2.68
≥2	5.78
25–29 years	
Number of first-degree relatives with history of breast cancer	
0	1.55
1	2.76
≥2	4.91
= 30 years	
Number of first-degree relatives with history of breast cancer	
0	1.93
1	2.83
≥2	4.17

SOURCE: Modified with permission from Armstrong K, Eisen A, Weber B: Assessing the risk of breast cancer. *N Engl J Med* 342:564, 2000.

lymphoma have a breast cancer risk that is 75 times greater than that of age-matched control subjects. Survivors of the atomic bomb blasts in Japan during World War II have a very high incidence of breast cancer, likely because of somatic mutations induced by the radiation exposure. In both circumstances, radiation exposure during adolescence, a period of active breast development, magnifies the deleterious effect. Studies also suggest that the amount and duration of alcohol consumption are associated with an increased breast cancer risk. Alcohol consumption is known to increase serum levels of estradiol. Finally, evidence suggests that chronic consumption of foods with a high fat content contributes to an increased risk of breast cancer by increasing serum estrogen levels.

Risk-Assessment Models[31,32]

The average lifetime risk of breast cancer for newborn U.S. females is 12%. The longer a woman lives without cancer, the lower her risk of developing breast cancer. Thus, a woman age 50 years has an 11% lifetime risk of developing breast cancer, and a woman age 70 years has a 7% lifetime risk of developing breast cancer. As risk factors for breast cancer interact, evaluating the risk conferred by combinations of risk factors is difficult. Two risk-assessment models are currently used to predict the risk of breast cancer. From the Breast Cancer Detection Demonstration Project, a mammography screening program conducted in the 1970s, Gail and colleagues developed the most frequently used model, which incorporates age at menarche, the number of breast biopsies, age at first live birth, and

the number of first-degree relatives with breast cancer. It predicts the cumulative risk of breast cancer according to decade of life. To calculate breast cancer risk with the Gail model, a woman's risk factors are translated into an overall risk score by multiplying her relative risks from several categories (Table 16-7). This risk score is then compared to an adjusted population risk of breast cancer to determine a woman's individual risk. A software program incorporating the Gail model is available from the National Cancer Institute at http://bcra.nci.nih.gov/brc.

Claus and colleagues, using data from the Cancer and Steroid Hormone Study, a case-control study of breast cancer, developed the other frequently used risk-assessment model, which is based on assumptions about the prevalence of high-penetrance breast cancer susceptibility genes. Compared with the Gail model, the Claus model incorporates more information about family history, but excludes other risk factors. The Claus model provides individual estimates of breast cancer risk according to decade of life based on knowledge of first- and second-degree relatives with breast cancer and their age at diagnosis. Risk factors that are less-consistently associated with breast cancer (diet, use of oral contraceptives, lactation), or are rare in the general population (radiation exposure), are not included in either the Gail or Claus risk-assessment models.

Risk Management[33–41]

Several important medical decisions may be affected by a woman's underlying risk of breast cancer. These decisions include when to use postmenopausal hormone replacement therapy; at what age to begin mammography screening; when to use tamoxifen to prevent breast cancer; and when to perform prophylactic mastectomy to prevent breast cancer. Postmenopausal hormone replacement therapy reduces the risk of coronary artery disease and osteoporosis by 50%, but increases the risk of breast cancer by less than 30%. Because the average woman's risk of dying from coronary artery disease is much greater than her risk of dying from breast cancer, it may be argued that the benefits of hormone replacement therapy outweigh the risks. The balance between the risks and the benefits of hormone replacement therapy may shift for women who have a substantially increased risk of breast cancer. Hormone replacement therapy does not increase life expectancy for the small number of women with a breast cancer risk above 30% and an average risk of cardiac events. Finally, assessment of risk may also reassure the majority of women with a relatively low risk of breast cancer that the benefits of hormone replacement therapy outweigh its risks.

Routine use of screening mammography in women age 50 years and older reduces mortality from breast cancer by 33%. This reduction comes without substantial risks and at an acceptable economic cost. However, the use of screening mammography is more controversial in women younger than age 50 years for several reasons: (1) breast density is greater and screening mammography is less likely to detect early breast cancer; (2) screening mammography results in more false-positive tests, resulting in unnecessary biopsies; and (3) younger women are less likely to have breast cancer so fewer young women will benefit from screening. However, on a population basis, the benefits of screening mammography in women between the ages of 40 and 49 years still appear to outweigh the risks. Targeting mammography to women at higher risk of breast cancer may also improve the balance of risks and benefits. In one study of women ages 40 to 49 years, an abnormal mammography finding was three times as likely to be cancer in a woman with a family history of breast cancer.

Tamoxifen, a selective estrogen receptor modulator, was the first drug shown to reduce the incidence of breast cancer in healthy women. The Breast Cancer Prevention Trial (NSABP P-01) randomly assigned more than 13,000 women, with a 5-year Gail relative risk of breast cancer of 1.70 or greater, to tamoxifen or placebo. After a mean follow-up period of 4 years, tamoxifen had reduced the incidence of breast cancer by 49%. It is currently the only drug approved by the Food and Drug Administration for reducing the risk of breast cancer, but it is unclear whether the benefits of tamoxifen apply to women at lower risk. Tamoxifen currently is only recommended for women who have a Gail relative risk of 1.70 or greater. In addition, deep venous thrombosis occurs 1.6 times, pulmonary emboli 3.0 times, and endometrial cancer 2.5 times as often in women taking tamoxifen. The increased risk for endometrial cancer is restricted to early stage cancers in postmenopausal women. Cataract surgery is required almost twice as often among women taking tamoxifen. Although no formal risk-benefit analysis is currently available, the higher a woman's risk of breast cancer, the more likely it is that the reduction in the incidence of breast cancer conveyed by tamoxifen will outweigh the risk of serious side effects.

A retrospective study of women at high risk for breast cancer found that prophylactic mastectomy reduced their risk by more than 90%. However, the effects of prophylactic mastectomy on the long-term quality of life are poorly quantified. A study involving women who were carriers of a breast cancer susceptibility gene (BRCA) mutation found that the benefit of prophylactic mastectomy differed substantially according to the breast cancer risk conferred

by the mutations. For women with an estimated lifetime risk of 40%, prophylactic mastectomy added almost 3 years of life, whereas for women with an estimated lifetime risk of 85%, prophylactic mastectomy added more than 5 years of life.

BRCA Mutations

BRCA-1 [42–46]

Five to 10% of breast cancers are caused by inheritance of germline mutations such as BRCA-1 and BRCA-2, which are inherited in an autosomal dominant fashion with varying penetrance (Table 16-8). BRCA-1 is located on chromosome 17q, spans a genomic region of about 100 kb of DNA, and contains 22 coding exons. The full-length mRNA is 7.8 kb and encodes a protein of 1863 amino acids. Both BRCA-1 and BRCA-2 function as tumor-suppressor genes, and for each gene, loss of both alleles is required for the initiation of cancer. Data accumulated since the isolation of the BRCA-1 gene suggest a role in transcription, cell-cycle control, and DNA damage repair pathways. More than 500 sequence variations in BRCA-1 have been identified. It now is known that germline mutations in BRCA-1 represent a predisposing genetic factor in as many as 45% of hereditary breast cancers and in at least 80% of hereditary ovarian cancers. Female mutation carriers have up to a 90% lifetime risk for developing breast cancer and up to a 40% lifetime risk for developing ovarian cancer. Breast cancer in these families appears as an autosomal dominant trait with high penetrance. Approximately 50% of children of carriers inherit the trait. In general, BRCA-1–associated breast cancers are invasive ductal carcinomas, are poorly differentiated, and are hormone receptor–negative. BRCA-1 associated breast cancers have a number of distinguishing clinical features, such as an early age of onset when compared with sporadic cases; a higher prevalence of bilateral breast cancer; and the presence of associated cancers in some affected individuals, specifically ovarian cancer and possibly colon and prostate cancers.

Several founder mutations have been identified in BRCA-1. The two most common mutations are 185delAG and 5382insC, which account for 10% of all the mutations seen in BRCA-1. These two mutations occur at a tenfold higher frequency in the Ashkenazi Jewish population than in non-Jewish whites. The carrier frequency of the 185delAG mutation in the Ashkenazi Jewish population is 1% and, along with the 5382insC mutation, accounts for almost all BRCA-1 mutations in this population. Analysis of germline mutations in Jewish and non-Jewish women with early-onset breast cancer indicates

Table 16-8

Percent Incidence of Sporadic, Familial, and Hereditary Breast Cancer

Sporadic breast cancer	65–75%	
Familial breast cancer	20–30%	
Hereditary breast cancer	5–10%	↓
BRCA-1[a]		45%
BRCA-2		35%
p53 (*Li-Fraumeni syndrome*)		1%
STK11/LKB1 (*Peutz-Jeghers syndrome*)		<1%
PTEN (*Cowden disease*)		<1%
MSH2/MLH1 (*Muir-Torre syndrome*)		<1%
ATM (*Ataxia-telangiectasia*)		<1%
Unknown		20%

[a]Affected gene.

SOURCE: Adapted with permission from Martin AM et al.[47]

that 20% of Jewish women who develop breast cancer before age 40 years carry the 185delAG mutation.

BRCA-2[42,44–46,48]

BRCA-2 is located on chromosome 13q and spans a genomic region of about 70 kb of DNA. The 11.2-kb coding region contains 26 coding exons. It encodes a protein of 3418 amino acids. The BRCA-2 gene bears no homology to any previously described gene, and the protein contains no previously defined functional domains. The biologic function of BRCA-2 is not well defined, but like BRCA-1, it is postulated to play a role in DNA damage response pathways. BRCA-2 messenger RNA also is expressed at high levels in late G_1 and S phases of the cell cycle. The kinetics of BRCA-2 protein regulation in the cell cycle is similar to that of BRCA-1 protein, suggesting that these genes are coregulated. The mutational spectrum of BRCA-2 is not as well established as that of BRCA-1. To date, more than 250 mutations have been found. The breast cancer risk for BRCA-2 mutation carriers is close to 85% and the lifetime ovarian cancer risk, while lower than for BRCA-1, is still estimated to be close to 20%. Breast cancer in BRCA-2 families is an autosomal dominant trait and has a high penetrance. Approximately 50% of children of carriers inherit the trait. Unlike male carriers of BRCA-1 mutations, men with germline mutations in BRCA-2 have an estimated breast cancer risk of 6%, representing a 100-fold increase over the general male population risk. BRCA-2–associated breast cancers are invasive ductal carcinomas, which are more likely to be well differentiated and to express hormone receptors than BRCA-1–associated breast cancer. BRCA-2–associated breast cancer has a number of distinguishing clinical features, such as an early age of onset compared with sporadic cases; a higher prevalence of bilateral breast cancer; and the presence of associated cancers in some affected individuals, specifically ovarian, colon, prostate, pancreas, gallbladder, bile duct, and stomach cancers, as well as melanoma. A number of founder mutations have been identified in BRCA-2. The 6174delT mutation is found in Ashkenazi Jews with a prevalence of 1.2%. Another BRCA-2 founder mutation, 999del5, is observed in Icelandic and Finnish populations.

Identifying BRCA Mutation Carriers[49]

Identifying hereditary risk for breast cancer is a four-step process that includes: (1) obtaining a complete, multigenerational family history; (2) assessing the appropriateness of genetic testing for a particular patient; (3) counseling the patient; and (4) interpreting the results of testing. Genetic testing should not be offered in isolation, but only in conjunction with patient education and counseling, including referral to a genetic counselor. Initial determinations include whether the individual is an appropriate candidate for genetic testing and whether genetic testing will be informative for personal and clinical decision making. A thorough and accurate family history is essential to this process and the mother's and father's sides of the family are both assessed, because 50% of the women with a BRCA mutation have inherited the mutation from their fathers. To help surgeons advise women about testing, statistically based models that determine the probability that an individual carries a BRCA mutation have been developed. A hereditary risk of breast cancer is considered if a family includes two or more women who developed ovarian cancer or breast cancer before age 50 years. Any woman diagnosed with breast cancer before age 50 years or with ovarian cancer at any age is asked about first-, second-, and third-degree relatives on either side of the family with either of these

diagnoses. Breast and ovarian cancer in the same individual, and male breast cancer at any age, also suggest the possibility of hereditary breast and ovarian cancer. The threshold for genetic testing is lower in individuals who are members of ethnic groups in whom the mutation prevalence is increased. For instance, the possibility of hereditary cancer is considered for any Ashkenazi Jewish woman with early-onset breast cancer.

BRCA Mutation Testing[49,50]

Appropriate counseling for the individual being tested is strongly recommended, and documentation of informed consent is required. The test that is clinically available for analyzing BRCA mutation is gene sequence analysis. In a family with a history suggestive of hereditary breast cancer and no previously tested member, the most informative strategy is to first test an affected family member. This person undergoes complete sequence analysis of both the BRCA-1 and BRCA-2 genes. If a mutation is identified, relatives are usually only tested for that specific mutation. An individual of Ashkenazi Jewish ancestry is tested initially for the three specific mutations that account for hereditary breast and ovarian cancer in that population. If that test is negative, it may then be appropriate to fully analyze the BRCA-1 and BRCA-2 genes.

A positive test is one that discloses the presence of a BRCA mutation that interferes with translation or function of the BRCA protein. A woman who carries a deleterious mutation has a breast cancer risk of up to 85%, as well as a greatly increased risk of ovarian cancer. A negative test result is interpreted according to an individual's personal and family history, especially with regard to whether a mutation has been previously identified in the family, in which case the woman is generally tested only for that specific mutation. If the mutation is not present, the woman may be reassured that her risk of breast or ovarian cancer is no greater than that of the general population, regardless of family history, and no BRCA mutation can be passed on to the woman's children. In the absence of a previously identified mutation, a negative test result in an affected individual generally indicates that a BRCA mutation is not responsible for the familial cancer. However, the possibility remains of an unusual abnormality in one of these genes that cannot yet be identified through clinical testing. It also is possible that the familial cancer is indeed caused by an identifiable BRCA mutation, but that the individual tested had sporadic cancer, a situation known as "phenocopy." This is especially possible if the individual tested developed breast cancer close to the age of onset of the general population (age 60 years or older) rather than before age 50 years, as is characteristic of BRCA mutation carriers. Overall, the false-negative rate for BRCA mutation testing is less than 5%. Some test results, especially when a single base pair change (missense mutation) is identified, may be difficult to interpret. This is because single base pair changes do not always result in a nonfunctional protein. Thus, missense mutations not located within critical functional domains, or those that cause only minimal changes in protein structure, may not be disease-associated and are usually reported as indeterminate results. In communicating indeterminate results to women, care must be taken to relay the uncertain cancer risk associated with this type of mutation and to emphasize that ongoing research might clarify its meaning. In addition, testing other family members with breast cancer to determine if a genetic variant tracks with their breast cancer may provide clarification of its significance. Indeterminate genetic variance currently accounts for 12% of the test results.

Concern has been expressed that the identification of hereditary risk for breast cancer may interfere with access to affordable health insurance. This concern refers to discrimination directed against an individual or family based solely on an apparent or perceived genetic variation from the normal human genotype. The Health Insurance Portability and Accountability Act of 1996 (HIPAA) made it illegal in the United States for group health plans to consider genetic information a pre-existing condition or to use it to deny or limit coverage. Most states also have passed laws that prevent genetic discrimination in the provision of health insurance. In addition, individuals applying for health insurance are not required to report whether relatives have undergone genetic testing for cancer risk, only whether those relatives have actually been diagnosed with cancer. Currently there is little documented evidence of genetic discrimination resulting from available genetic tests.

Cancer Prevention for BRCA Mutation Carriers

Risk management strategies for BRCA-1 and BRCA-2 carriers include:

- Prophylactic mastectomy and reconstruction;
- Prophylactic oophorectomy and hormone replacement therapy;
- Intensive surveillance for breast and ovarian cancer; and
- Chemoprevention.

Although removal of breast tissue will reduce the likelihood of BRCA-1 and BRCA-2 carriers developing breast cancer, mastectomy does not remove all breast tissue and women continue to be at risk, because a germline mutation is present in any remaining breast tissue. For postmenopausal BRCA-1 and BRCA-2 carriers who have not had a mastectomy, it may be advisable to avoid hormone replacement therapy, because no data exist regarding the effect of the therapy on the penetrance of breast cancer susceptibility genes. Because breast cancers in BRCA mutation carriers have the same mammography appearance as breast cancers in noncarriers, a screening mammogram is likely to be effective in BRCA mutation carriers, provided it is performed and interpreted with a high level of suspicion by an experienced radiologist. Present screening recommendations for BRCA mutation carriers who do not undergo prophylactic mastectomy include clinical breast exam every 6 months and mammography every 12 months beginning at age 25 years, because the risk of breast cancer in BRCA mutation carriers increases after age 30 years. Despite a 49% reduction in the incidence of breast cancer in high-risk women taking tamoxifen, it is too early to recommend the use of tamoxifen uniformly for BRCA mutation carriers. Cancers arising in BRCA-1 carriers are usually high-grade and are hormone receptor–negative. Approximately 66% of BRCA-1–associated ductal carcinoma in situ (DCIS) is estrogen receptor–negative, suggesting early acquisition of the hormone-independent phenotype.

The risk of ovarian cancer in BRCA-1 and BRCA-2 carriers ranges from 20 to 40%, which is 10 times higher than that for the general population. Prophylactic oophorectomy is a reasonable prevention option in carriers. The American College of Obstetrics and Gynecology recommends that women with a documented BRCA-1 or BRCA-2 mutation consider prophylactic oophorectomy at the completion of childbearing or at the time of menopause. Hormone replacement therapy is discussed with the patient at the time of oophorectomy. The Cancer Genetics Studies Consortium recommended yearly transvaginal ultrasound timed to avoid ovulation and yearly serum CA 125 levels beginning at age 25 years as the best screening modalities for ovarian carcinoma in BRCA mutation carriers who have opted to defer prophylactic oophorectomy.

EPIDEMIOLOGY AND NATURAL HISTORY OF BREAST CANCER

Epidemiology[51,52]

Breast cancer is the most common site-specific cancer in women and is the leading cause of death from cancer for women age 40 to 44 years. It accounts for 33% of all female cancers and is responsible for 20% of the cancer-related deaths in women. It is predicted that approximately 211,300 invasive breast cancers will be diagnosed in women in the United States in 2003 and 39,800 of those diagnosed will die from that cancer. Breast cancer was the leading cause of cancer-related mortality in women until 1985, when it was surpassed by lung cancer (Fig. 16-14). In the 1970s, the probability of a woman in the United States developing breast cancer was estimated at 1 in 13, in 1980 it was 1 in 11, and in 2002 it was 1 in 8. Cancer registries in Connecticut and upper New York state document that the age-adjusted incidence of new breast cancer cases has steadily increased since the mid-1940s. This increase was about 1% per year from 1973 to 1980, and there was an additional increase in incidence to 4% between 1980 and 1987, which was characterized by frequent detection of small primary cancers. The increase in breast cancer incidence occurred primarily in women age 55 years or older and paralleled a marked increase in the percentage of older women who had mammograms. At the same time, incidence rates for regional metastatic disease dropped and breast cancer mortality declined. From 1960 to 1963, 5-year overall survival rates for breast cancer were 63 and 46% in white and African American women,

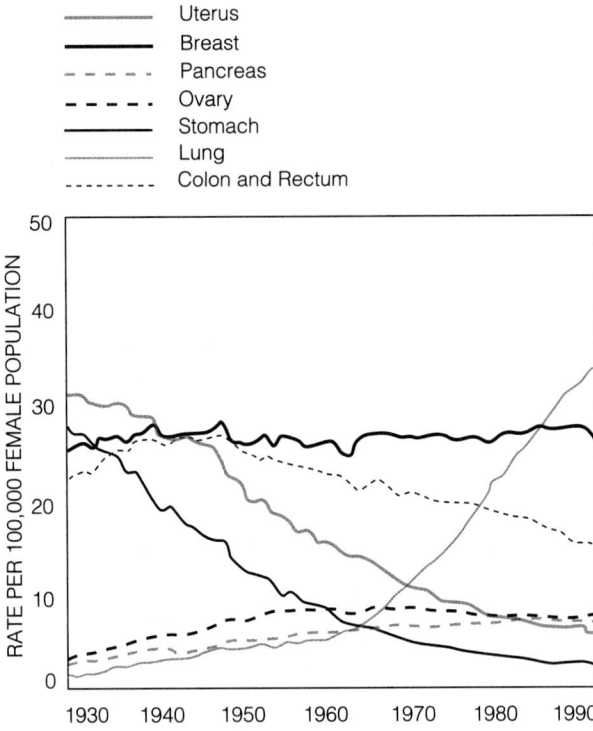

FIG. 16-14. Death rates for cancer at selected organ sites in U.S. women. These are age-adjusted rates per 100,000 population. The uterine cancer death rate is derived by combining the cervix and corpus death rates. Note the steep rise in the lung cancer death rate after 1960. (Reproduced with permission from Parker SL et al: Cancer statistics. CA Cancer J Clin 47:5, 1997.)

respectively, while the rates for 1981 to 1987 were 78 and 63%, respectively.

There is a tenfold variation in breast cancer incidence among different countries worldwide. England and Wales have the highest age-adjusted mortality for breast cancer (27.7 per 100,000 population), while South Korea has the lowest (2.6 cancers per 100,000 population). The United States has an age-adjusted mortality for breast cancer of 22.0 cases per 100,000 population. Women living in less-industrialized nations tend to have a lower incidence of breast cancer than women living in industrialized countries, although Japan is an exception. In the United States, Mormons, Seventh Day Adventists, American Indians, Eskimos, Mexican Americans, and Japanese and Filipino women living in Hawaii have a below average incidence of breast cancer, while nuns and Jewish women have an above average incidence.

Natural History[53]

Bloom and colleagues described the natural history of breast cancer based on the records of 250 women with untreated breast cancers who were cared for on charity wards in Middlesex Hospital, London, between 1805 and 1933. The median survival of this population was 2.7 years after initial diagnosis (Fig. 16-15). The 5- and 10-year survival rates for these women were 18.0 and 3.6%, respectively. Only 0.8% survived for 15 years or longer. Autopsy data confirmed that 95% of these women died of breast cancer, while the remaining 5% died of other causes. Almost 75% of the women developed ulceration of the breast during the course of the disease. The longest surviving patient died in the nineteenth year after diagnosis.

The Primary Breast Cancer

More than 80% of breast cancers show productive fibrosis that involves the epithelial and stromal tissues. With growth of the cancer and invasion of the surrounding breast tissues, the accompanying desmoplastic response entraps and shortens the suspensory ligaments of Cooper to produce a characteristic skin retraction.

Localized edema (peau d'orange) develops when drainage of lymph fluid from the skin is disrupted. With continued growth, cancer cells invade the skin and eventually ulceration occurs. As new areas of skin are invaded, small satellite nodules appear near the primary ulceration. The size of the primary breast cancer correlates with disease-free and overall survival, but there is a close association between cancer size and axillary lymph node involvement (Fig. 16-16B). In general, up to 20% of breast cancer recurrences

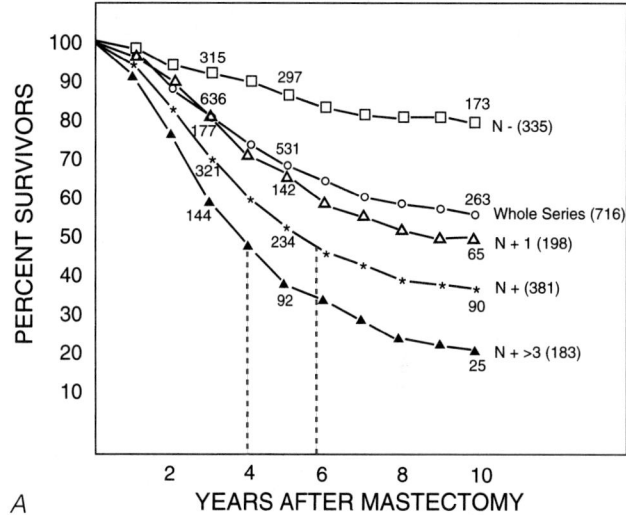

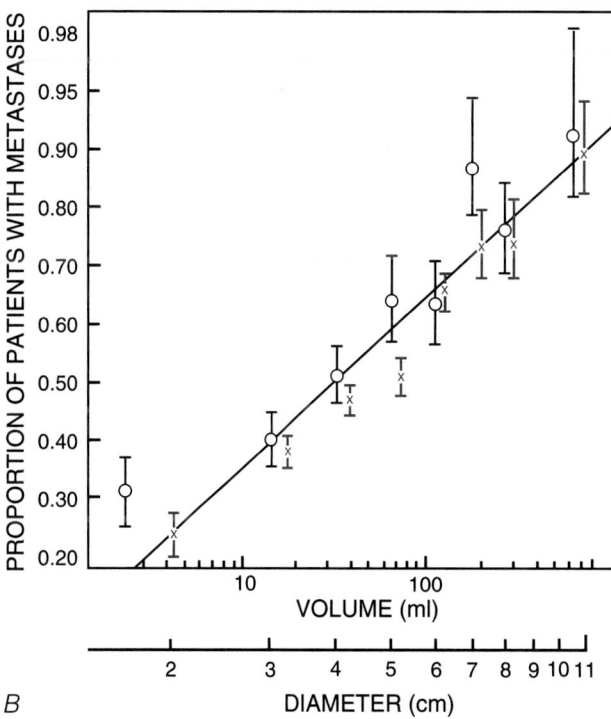

FIG. 16-16. *A. Overall survival for women with breast cancer according to axillary lymph node status. The time periods are years following radical mastectomy. (Reproduced with permission from Valagussa P et al: Patterns of relapse and survival following radical mastectomy. Cancer 41:1170, 1978.) B. Risk of metastases according to breast cancer volume and diameter (Reproduced with permission from Koscielny S et al: Breast cancer: Relationship between the size of the primary tumor and the probability of metastatic dissemination. Br J Cancer 49:709, 1984.)*

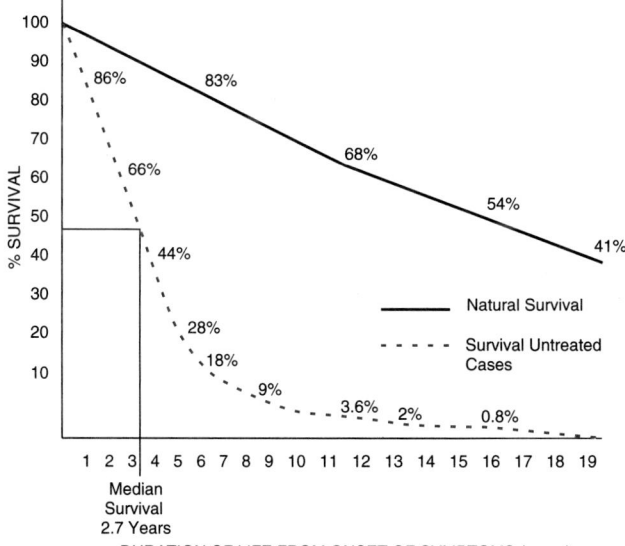

FIG. 16-15. *Survival of women with untreated breast cancer compared with natural survival. (Reproduced with permission from Bloom et al.[53])*

are locoregional, more than 60% are distant, and 20% are both locoregional and distant.

Axillary Lymph Node Metastases

As the size of the primary breast cancer increases, some cancer cells are shed into cellular spaces and transported via the lymphatic network of the breast to the regional lymph nodes, especially the axillary lymph nodes. Lymph nodes that contain metastatic cancer are at first ill-defined and soft, but become firm or hard with continued growth of the metastatic cancer. Eventually the lymph nodes adhere to each other and form a conglomerate mass. Cancer cells may grow through the lymph node capsule and fix to contiguous structures in the axilla including the chest wall. Typically, axillary lymph nodes are involved sequentially from the low (level I) to the central (level II) to the apical (level III) lymph node groups. While more than 95% of the women who die of breast cancer have distant metastases, the most important prognostic correlate for disease-free and overall survival is axillary lymph node status (see Fig. 16-16A). Node-negative women have less than a 30% risk of recurrence, compared to as much as a 75% risk for node-positive women.

Distant Metastases

At approximately the twentieth cell doubling, breast cancers acquire their own blood supply (neovascularization). Thereafter, cancer cells may be shed directly into the systemic venous blood to seed the pulmonary circulation via the axillary and intercostal veins or the vertebral column via Batson's plexus of veins, which courses the length of the vertebral column. These cells are scavenged by natural killer lymphocytes and macrophages. Successful implantation of metastatic foci from breast cancer predictably occurs after the primary cancer exceeds 0.5 cm in diameter, which corresponds to the twenty-seventh cell doubling. For 10 years following initial treatment, distant metastases are the most common cause of death in breast cancer patients. For this reason, conclusive results cannot be derived from breast cancer trials until at least 5 to 10 years have elapsed. While 60% of the women who develop distant metastases will do so within 24 months of treatment, metastases may become evident as late as 20 to 30 years after treatment of the primary cancer. Common sites of involvement, in order of frequency, are bone, lung, pleura, soft tissues, and liver.

HISTOPATHOLOGY OF BREAST CANCER

Carcinoma In Situ[54-57]

Cancer cells are in situ or invasive depending on whether or not they invade through the basement membrane. Broder's original description of in situ breast cancer stressed the absence of invasion of cells into the surrounding stroma and their confinement within natural ductal and alveolar boundaries. As areas of invasion may be minute, the accurate diagnosis of in situ cancer necessitates the analysis of multiple microscopy sections to exclude invasion. In 1941, Foote and Stewart published a landmark description of lobular carcinoma in situ (LCIS), which distinguished it from DCIS. In the late 1960s, Gallagher and Martin published their study of whole breast sections and described a stepwise progression from benign breast tissue to in situ cancer, and subsequently to invasive cancer. They coined the term *minimal breast cancer* (LCIS, DCIS, and invasive cancers smaller than 0.5 cm in size) and stressed the importance of early detection. It is now recognized that each type of minimal breast cancer has a distinct clinical and biologic behavior. Before the widespread use of mammography, diagnosis of breast cancer was by physical examination. At that time, in situ cancers constituted less than 6% of all breast cancers, and by a ratio of more than 2:1, LCIS was more frequently diagnosed than DCIS. However, when screening mammography became popular, a 14-fold increase in the incidence of in situ cancer (45%) was demonstrated, and by a ratio of more than 2:1, DCIS was more frequently diagnosed than LCIS. Table 16-9 lists the clinical and pathologic characteristics of DCIS and LCIS. Multicentricity refers to the occurrence of a second breast cancer outside the breast quadrant of the primary cancer, whereas multifocality refers to the occurrence of a second cancer within the same breast quadrant as the primary cancer. Multicentricity occurs in 60 to 90% of women with LCIS, while the rate of multicentricity for DCIS is 40 to 80%. LCIS occurs bilaterally in 50 to 70% of cases, while DCIS occurs bilaterally in 10 to 20% of cases.

Lobular Carcinoma In Situ

LCIS originates from the terminal duct lobular units and only develops in the female breast. It is characterized by distention and distortion of the terminal duct lobular units by cancer cells, which are large but maintain a normal nuclear:cytoplasmic ratio. Cytoplasmic

Table 16-9
Salient Characteristics of In Situ Ductal (DCIS) and Lobular (LCIS) Carcinoma of the Breast

	LCIS	*DCIS*
Age (years)	44–47	54–58
Incidence[a]	2–5%	5–10%
Clinical signs	None	Mass, pain, nipple discharge
Mammographic signs	None	Microcalcifications
Premenopausal	2/3	1/3
Incidence of synchronous invasive carcinoma	5%	2–46%
Multicentricity	60–90%	40–80%
Bilaterality	50–70%	10–20%
Axillary metastasis	1%	1–2%
Subsequent carcinomas:		
Incidence	25–35%	25–70%
Laterality	Bilateral	Ipsilateral
Interval to diagnosis	15–20 years	5–10 years
Histology	Ductal	Ductal

[a] Among biopsies of mammographically detected breast lesions.

SOURCE: Reproduced with permission from Frykberg ER, Bland KI: Current concepts on the biology and management of in situ (Tis, stage 0) breast carcinoma, in Bland KI, Copeland EM (eds): *The Breast.* Philadelphia: WB Saunders, 1998, p 1020.

mucoid globules are a distinctive cellular feature. LCIS may be observed in breast tissues that contain microcalcifications, but the calcifications associated with LCIS typically occur in adjacent tissues. This neighborhood calcification is a feature that is unique to LCIS and contributes to its diagnosis. The frequency of LCIS in the general population cannot be reliably determined because it usually presents as an incidental finding. The age at diagnosis is 44 to 47 years, which is approximately 15 to 25 years younger than the age at diagnosis for invasive breast cancer. LCIS has a distinct racial predilection, occurring 12 times more frequently in white women than in African American women. Invasive breast cancer develops in 25 to 35% of women with LCIS. Invasive lobular cancer may develop in either breast, regardless of which breast harbored the initial focus of LCIS, and is detected synchronously with LCIS in 5% of cases. In women with a history of LCIS, up to 65% of subsequent invasive cancers are ductal, not lobular in origin. For these reasons, LCIS is regarded as a marker of increased risk for invasive breast cancer rather than an anatomic precursor.

Ductal Carcinoma In Situ

While DCIS is predominantly seen in the female breast, it accounts for 5% of male breast cancers. Published series suggest a detection frequency of 7% in all biopsy tissue specimens. The term *intraductal carcinoma* is frequently applied to DCIS, which carries a high risk for progression to an invasive cancer. Histologically, DCIS is characterized by a proliferation of the epithelium that lines the minor ducts, resulting in papillary growths within the duct lumina. Early in their development, the cancer cells do not show pleomorphism, mitoses, or atypia, which leads to difficulty in distinguishing early DCIS from benign hyperplasia. The papillary growths (papillary growth pattern) eventually coalesce and fill the duct lumina so only scattered, rounded spaces remain between the clumps of atypical cancer cells, which show hyperchromasia and loss of polarity (cribriform growth pattern). Eventually pleomorphic cancer cells with frequent mitotic figures obliterate the lumina and distend the ducts (solid growth pattern). With continued growth, these cells outstrip their blood supply and become necrotic (comedo growth pattern). Calcium deposition occurs in the areas of necrosis and is a common mammography feature. DCIS is now frequently classified based on nuclear grade and the presence of necrosis (Table 16-10). The risk for invasive breast cancer is increased nearly fivefold in women with DCIS. The invasive cancers are observed in the ipsilateral breast, usually in the same quadrant as the DCIS that was originally detected, suggesting that DCIS is an anatomic precursor of invasive ductal carcinoma (Fig. 16-17).

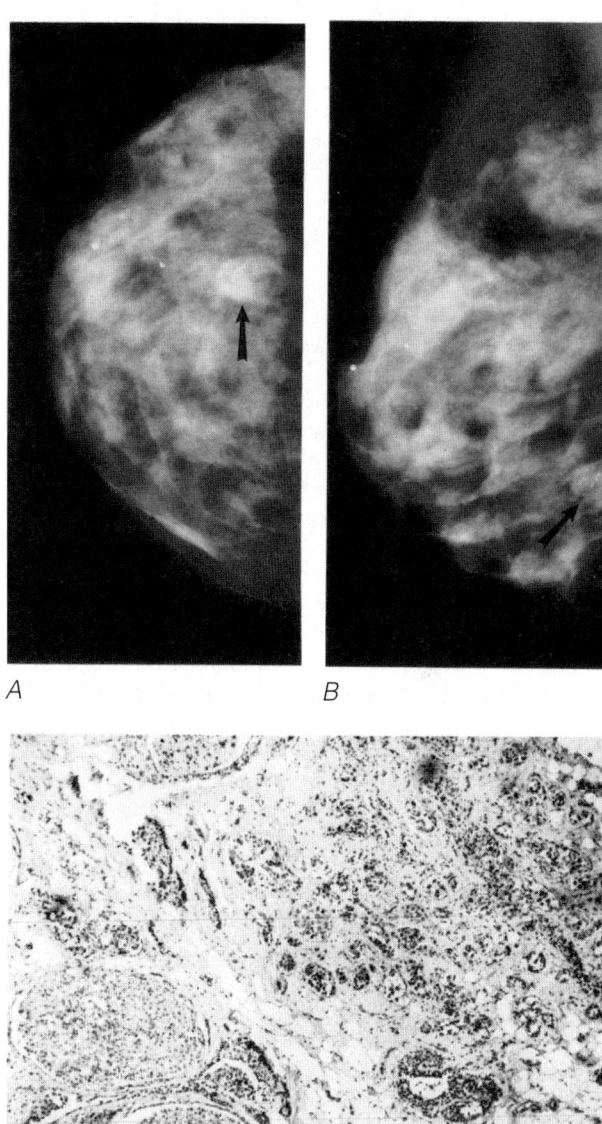

FIG. 16-17. Ductal carcinoma in situ (DCIS) *A.* Craniocaudal and (*B*) mediolateral oblique mammography views show a poorly defined 1.2-cm mass (arrow) containing microcalcifications. *C.* Histopathology of the surgical specimen confirms DCIS with areas of invasion (hematoxylin and eosin stain, x32).

Table 16-10
Classification of Breast Ductal Carcinoma In Situ (DCIS)

| Histology | Determining Characteristics | | DCIS Grade |
	Nuclear Grade	Necrosis	
Comedo	High	Extensive	High
Intermediate[a]	Intermediate	Focal or absent	Intermediate
Noncomedo[b]	Low	Absent	Low

[a] Often a mixture of noncomedo patterns.

[b] Solid, cribriform, papillary, or focal micropapillary.

SOURCE: Adapted with permission from Connolly JL, Nixon AJ: Ductal carcinoma in situ of the breast: Histologic subtyping and clinical signficance. *PPO Updates* 10 (10):1, 1996.

Invasive Breast Carcinoma[58-61]

Invasive breast cancers have been described as lobular or ductal in origin. Early classifications used the term *lobular* to describe invasive cancers that were associated with lobular carcinoma in situ, while all other invasive cancers were referred to as ductal. Current histologic classifications recognize special types of breast cancers (10% of total cases), which are defined by specific histologic features. To qualify as a special-type cancer, at least 90% of the cancer must contain the defining histologic features. Eighty percent of invasive breast cancers are described as invasive ductal carcinoma of no special type (NST). These cancers generally have a worse prognosis than special-type cancers. Foote and Stewart originally proposed the following classification for invasive breast cancer:

I. Paget's disease of the nipple
II. Invasive ductal carcinoma
    A. Adenocarcinoma with productive fibrosis (scirrhous, simplex, NST) 80%
    B. Medullary carcinoma 4%
    C. Mucinous (colloid) carcinoma 2%
    D. Papillary carcinoma 2%
    E. Tubular carcinoma (and ICC) 2%
III. Invasive lobular carcinoma 10%
IV. Rare cancers (adenoid cystic, squamous cell, apocrine)

Paget's disease of the nipple was described in 1874. It frequently presents as a chronic, eczematous eruption of the nipple, which may be subtle, but may progress to an ulcerated, weeping lesion. Paget's disease is usually associated with extensive DCIS and may be associated with an invasive cancer. A palpable mass may or may not be present. Biopsy of the nipple will show a population of cells that are identical to the underlying DCIS cells (pagetoid features or pagetoid change). Pathognomonic of this cancer is the presence of large, pale, vacuolated cells (Paget's cells) in the rete pegs of the epithelium. Paget's disease may be confused with superficial spreading melanoma. Differentiation from pagetoid intraepithelial melanoma is based on S-100 antigen immunostaining in melanoma and carcinoembryonic antigen (CEA) immunostaining in Paget's disease. Surgical therapy for Paget's disease may involve lumpectomy, mastectomy, or modified radical mastectomy, depending on the extent of involvement and the presence of invasive cancer.

Invasive ductal carcinoma of the breast with productive fibrosis (scirrhous, simplex, NST) accounts for 80% of breast cancers and presents with macroscopic or microscopic axillary lymph node metastases in 60% of cases. This cancer usually presents in perimenopausal or postmenopausal women in the fifth to sixth decades of life as a solitary, firm mass. It has poorly defined margins and its cut surfaces show a central stellate configuration with chalky white or yellow streaks extending into surrounding breast tissues. The cancer cells often are arranged in small clusters, and there is a broad spectrum of histologies with variable cellular and nuclear grades (Fig. 16-18).

Medullary carcinoma is a special-type breast cancer; it accounts for 4% of all invasive breast cancers and is a frequent phenotype of BRCA-1 hereditary breast cancer. Grossly, the cancer is soft and hemorrhagic. A rapid increase in size may occur secondary to necrosis and hemorrhage. On physical examination, it is bulky and often positioned deep within the breast. Bilaterality is reported in 20% of cases. Medullary carcinoma is characterized microscopically by (1) a dense lymphoreticular infiltrate composed predominantly of lymphocytes and plasma cells; (2) large pleomorphic nuclei that are poorly differentiated and show active mitosis; and (3) a sheet-like growth pattern with minimal or absent ductal or alveolar differentiation (Fig. 16-19). Approximately 50% of these cancers are associated with DCIS, which is characteristically present at the periphery of the cancer, and fewer than 10% demonstrate hormone receptors. In rare circumstances, mesenchymal metaplasia or anaplasia is noted. Because of the intense lymphocyte response associated with the cancer, benign or hyperplastic enlargement of the lymph nodes of the axilla may contribute to erroneous clinical staging. Women with this cancer have a better 5-year survival rate than those with NST or invasive lobular carcinoma.

Mucinous carcinoma (colloid carcinoma), another special-type breast cancer, accounts for 2% of all invasive breast cancers and

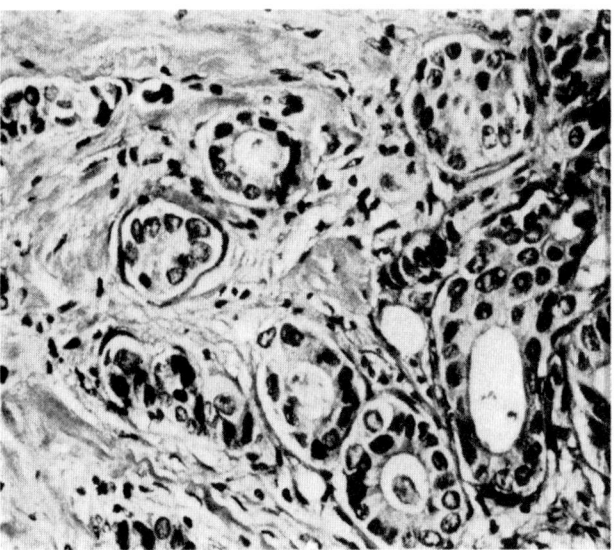

FIG. 16-18. Infiltrating ductal carcinoma with productive fibrosis (scirrhous, simplex, NST) (x62.5). *(Courtesy of Dr. R. L. Hackett.)*

typically presents in the elderly population as a bulky tumor. This cancer is defined by extracellular pools of mucin, which surround aggregates of low-grade cancer cells. The cut surface of this cancer is glistening and gelatinous in quality. Fibrosis is variable, and when abundant it imparts a firm consistency to the cancer. Approximately 66% of mucinous carcinomas display hormone receptors. Lymph node metastases occur in 33% of cases and 5- and 10-year survival rates are 73 and 59%, respectively. Because of the mucinous component, cancer cells may not be evident in all microscopy sections and analysis of multiple sections is essential to confirm the diagnosis of a mucinous carcinoma.

Papillary carcinoma is a special-type cancer of the breast that accounts for 2% of all invasive breast cancers. It generally presents in the seventh decade of life and occurs in a disproportionate number of nonwhite women. Typically, papillary carcinomas are small and rarely attain a size of 3 cm in diameter. These cancers are defined

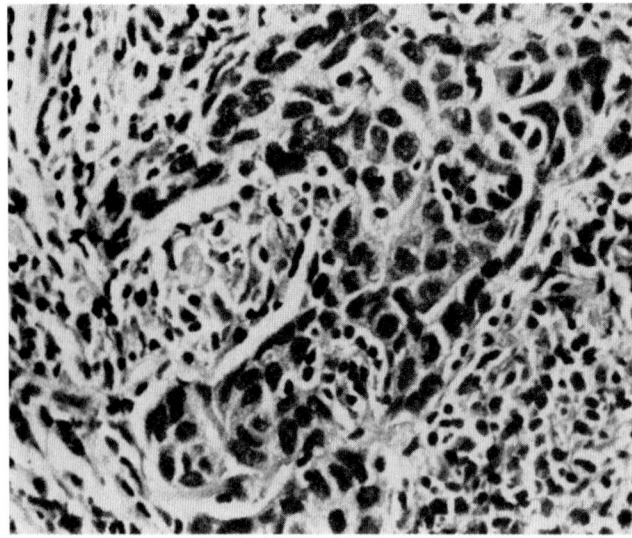

FIG. 16-19. Medullary breast carcinoma (x250). *(Reproduced with permission from Simpson JF et al,[60] p 285.)*

by papillae with fibrovascular stalks and multilayered epithelium. McDivitt and colleagues noted that it showed a low frequency of axillary lymph node metastases and had 5- and 10-year survival rates similar to those for mucinous and tubular carcinoma.

Tubular carcinoma is another special-type breast cancer and accounts for 2% of all invasive breast cancers. It is reported in as many as 20% of women whose cancers are diagnosed by mammography screening and is usually diagnosed in the perimenopausal or early menopausal periods. Under low-power magnification, a haphazard array of small, randomly arranged tubular elements is seen. Approximately 10% of women with tubular carcinoma or with invasive cribriform carcinoma, a special-type cancer closely related to tubular carcinoma, will develop axillary lymph node metastases, which are usually confined to the lowest axillary lymph nodes (level I). However, the presence of metastatic disease in one or two axillary lymph nodes does not adversely affect survival. Distant metastases are rare in tubular carcinoma and invasive cribriform carcinoma. Long-term survival approaches 100%.

Invasive lobular carcinoma accounts for 10% of breast cancers. The histopathologic features of this cancer include small cells with rounded nuclei, inconspicuous nucleoli, and scant cytoplasm (Fig. 16-20). Special stains may confirm the presence of intracytoplasmic mucin, which may displace the nucleus (signet-ring cell carcinoma). At presentation, invasive lobular carcinoma varies from clinically inapparent cancers to those that replace the entire breast with a poorly defined mass. It is frequently multifocal, multicentric, and bilateral. Because of its insidious growth pattern and subtle mammography features, invasive lobular carcinoma may be difficult to detect.

DIAGNOSING BREAST CANCER

In 33% of breast cancer cases, the woman discovers a lump in her breast. Other less frequent presenting signs and symptoms of breast cancer include (1) breast enlargement or asymmetry; (2) nipple changes, retraction, or discharge; (3) ulceration or erythema of the skin of the breast; (4) an axillary mass; and (5) musculoskeletal discomfort. However, up to 50% of women presenting with breast complaints have no physical signs of breast pathology. Breast pain usually is associated with benign disease.

Misdiagnosed breast cancer accounts for the greatest number of malpractice claims for errors in diagnosis and for the largest number of paid claims. Litigation often involves younger women whose physical examination and mammography may be misleading. If a young woman (age 45 years or less) presents with a palpable breast mass and equivocal mammography finding, ultrasound examination and biopsy are used to avoid a delay in diagnosis.

Examination[62,63]

Inspection

The surgeon inspects the woman's breast with her arms by her side (Fig. 16-21A), with her arms straight up in the air (Fig. 16-21B), and with her hands on her hips (with and without pectoral muscle contraction). Symmetry, size, and shape of the breast are recorded, as well as any evidence of edema (peau d'orange), nipple or skin retraction, and erythema. With the arms extended forward and in a sitting position, the woman leans forward to accentuate any skin retraction.

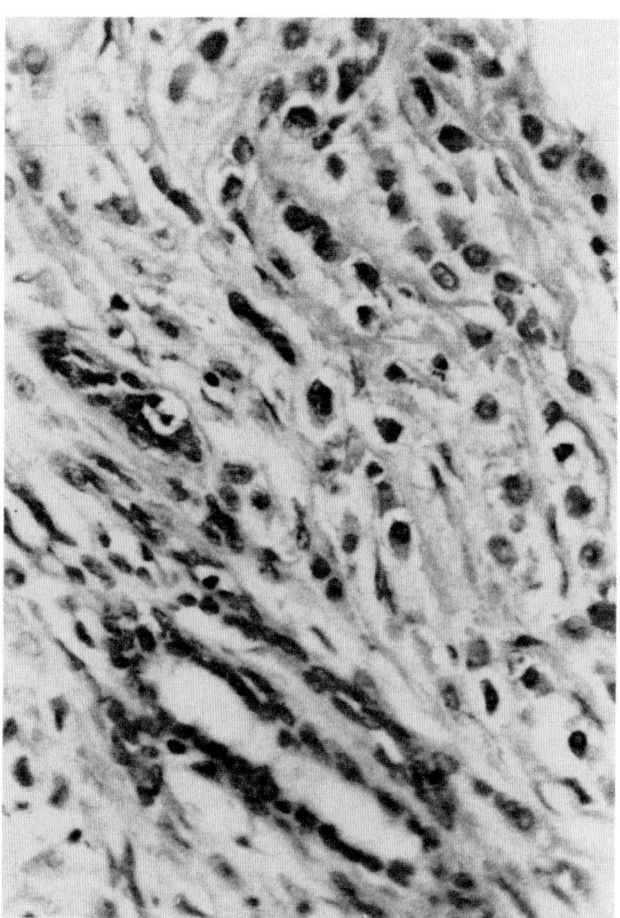

FIG. 16-20. Lobular carcinoma (x250). Uniform, relatively small lobular carcinoma cells are seen arranged in a single file orientation ("Indian file"). *(Reproduced with permission from Simpson JF et al,[60] p 285.)*

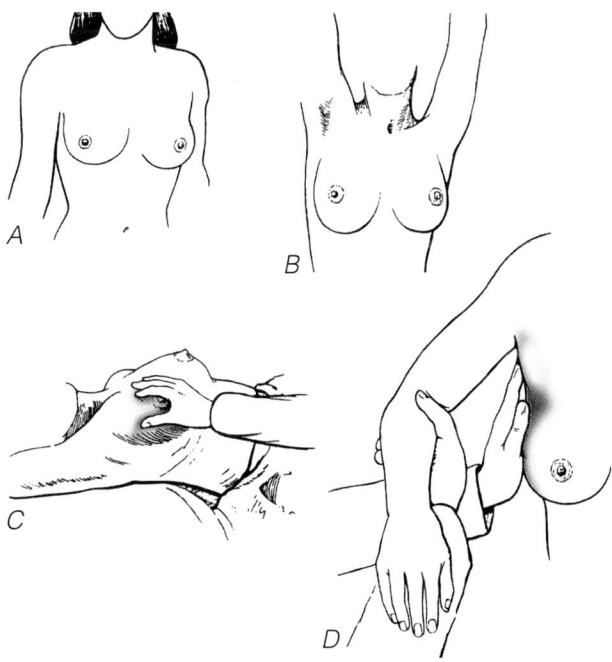

FIG. 16-21. Examination of the breast. *A.* Inspection of the breast with arms at sides. *B.* Inspection of the breast with arms raised. *C.* Palpation of the breast with the patient supine. *D.* Palpation of the axilla.

Palpation

As part of the physical examination, the breast is carefully palpated. Examination of the patient in the supine position (see Fig. 16-21C) is best performed with a pillow supporting the ipsilateral hemithorax. The surgeon gently palpates the breast from the ipsilateral side, making certain to examine all quadrants of the breast from the sternum laterally to the latissimus dorsi muscle, and from the clavicle inferiorly to the upper rectus sheath. The surgeon performs the examination with the palmar aspects of the fingers avoiding a grasping or pinching motion. The breast may be cupped or molded in the surgeon's hands to check for retraction. A systematic search for lymphadenopathy then is performed. Figure 16-21D shows the position of the patient for examination of the axilla. By supporting the upper arm and elbow, the shoulder girdle is stabilized. Using gentle palpation, all three levels of possible axillary lymphadenopathy are assessed. Careful palpation of supraclavicular and parasternal sites also is performed. A diagram of the chest and contiguous lymph node sites is useful for recording location, size, consistency, shape, mobility, fixation, and other characteristics of any palpable breast mass or lymphadenopathy (Fig. 16-22).

Imaging Techniques[64–67]

Mammography

Mammography has been used in North America since the 1960s and the techniques used continue to be modified and improved to enhance image quality (Fig. 16-23A and C). Conventional mammography delivers a radiation dose of 0.1 centigray (cGy) per study. By comparison, a chest x-ray delivers 25% of this dose. However, there is no increased breast cancer risk associated with the radiation dose delivered with screening mammography. Screening mammography is used to detect unexpected breast cancer in asymptomatic women.

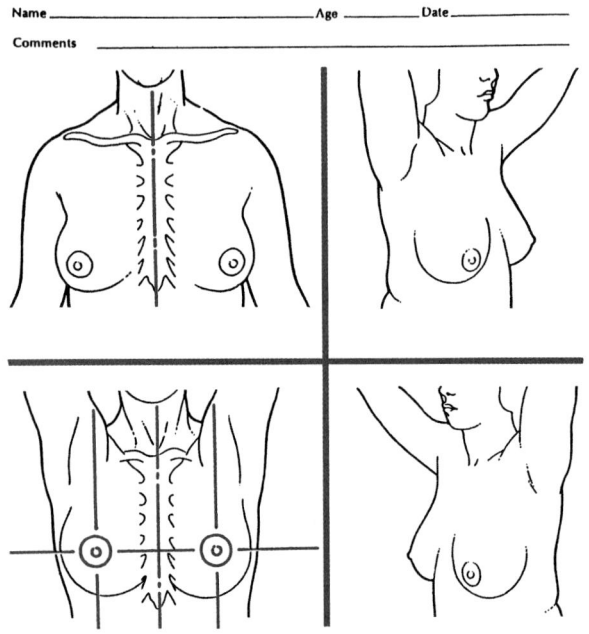

Breast Examination Record

Name _____ Age _____ Date _____

Comments _____

On this sheet, record the pertinent facts—positive and negative—of the patient's breast examination.
Attach the sheet to the patient's record.

FIG. 16-22. A breast examination record. (*Reproduced with permission from Cliggott Publishing Co: Darien, CT.*)

In this regard, it supplements history and physical examination. With screening mammography, two views of the breast are obtained, the craniocaudal (CC) view (Fig. 16-23D) and the mediolateral oblique (MLO) view (Fig. 16-23E). The MLO view images the greatest volume of breast tissue, including the upper outer quadrant and the axillary tail of Spence. Compared with the MLO view, the CC view provides better visualization of the medial aspect of the breast and permits greater breast compression. Diagnostic mammography is used to evaluate women with abnormal findings such as a breast mass or nipple discharge. In addition to the MLO and CC views, a diagnostic examination may use views that better define the nature of any abnormalities, such as the 90-degree lateral and spot compression views. The 90-degree lateral view is used along with the CC view to triangulate the exact location of an abnormality. Spot compression may be done in any projection by using a small compression device, which is placed directly over a mammography abnormality that is obscured by overlying tissues (Fig. 16-23F). The compression device minimizes motion artifact, improves definition, separates overlying tissues, and decreases the radiation dose needed to penetrate the breast. Magnification techniques ($\times 1.5$) often are combined with spot compression to better resolve calcifications and the margins of masses. Mammography also is used to guide interventional procedures, including needle localization and needle biopsy.

An experienced radiologist can detect breast cancer with a false-positive rate of 10% and a false-negative rate of 7%. Specific mammography features that suggest a diagnosis of a breast cancer include a solid mass with or without stellate features, asymmetric thickening of breast tissues, and clustered microcalcifications. The presence of fine, stippled calcium in and around a suspicious lesion is suggestive of breast cancer and occurs in as many as 50% of nonpalpable cancers. These microcalcifications are an especially important sign of cancer in younger women, in whom it may be the only mammography abnormality. The clinical impetus for screening mammography came from the Health Insurance Plan (HIP) study and the Breast Cancer Detection Demonstration Project (BCDDP), which demonstrated a 33% reduction in mortality for women after screening mammography. Mammography was more accurate than clinical examination for the detection of early breast cancers, providing a true positive rate of 90%. Only 20% of women with nonpalpable cancers had axillary lymph node metastases, as compared to 50% of women with palpable cancers. Current guidelines of the National Cancer Center Network (NCCN) suggest that normal-risk women age 20 years or older should have a breast exam at least every 3 years. At age 40 years, breast exams should be performed yearly along with a yearly mammogram. Prospective, randomized studies of mammography screening confirm a 40% reduction for stages II, III, and IV cancer in the screened population, with a 30% increase in overall survival.

Xeromammography techniques are identical to those of mammography with the exception that the image is recorded on a xerography plate, which provides a positive rather than a negative image (see Fig. 16-23B). Details of the entire breast and the soft tissues of the chest wall may be recorded with one exposure.

Ductography

The primary indication for ductography is nipple discharge, particularly when the fluid contains blood. Radiopaque contrast media is injected into one or more of the major ducts and mammography is performed. A duct is gently enlarged with a dilator and then a small, blunt cannula is inserted under sterile conditions into the nipple ampulla. With the patient in a supine position, 0.1 to 0.2 mL of dilute contrast media is injected and CC and MLO mammography views are obtained without compression. Intraductal papillomas are seen as small filling defects surrounded by contrast media (Fig. 16-24). Cancers may appear as irregular masses or as multiple intraluminal filling defects.

Ultrasonography

Second only to mammography in frequency of use for breast imaging, ultrasonography is an important method of resolving equivocal mammography findings, defining cystic masses, and demonstrating the echogenic qualities of specific solid abnormalities. On ultrasound examination, breast cysts are well circumscribed, with smooth margins and an echo-free center (Fig. 16-25). Benign breast masses usually show smooth contours, round or oval shapes, weak internal echoes, and well-defined anterior and posterior margins. Breast cancer characteristically has irregular walls (Fig. 16-26), but may have smooth margins with acoustic enhancement. Ultrasonography is used to guide fine-needle aspiration biopsy, core-needle biopsy, and needle localization of breast lesions. It is highly reproducible and has a high patient acceptance rate, but does not reliably detect lesions that are 1 cm or less in diameter.

Magnetic Resonance Imaging

In the process of evaluating MRI as a means of characterizing mammography abnormalities, additional breast lesions have been detected. However, in the circumstance of both a negative mammogram and a negative physical examination, the probability of a breast cancer being diagnosed by MRI is extremely low. There is current interest in using MRI to screen the breasts of high-risk women and of women with a newly diagnosed breast cancer. In the first case, women with a strong family history of breast cancer or who carry known genetic mutations require screening at an early age, but mammography evaluation is limited because of the increased breast density in younger women. In the second case, a study of MRI of the contralateral breast in women with a known breast cancer showed a contralateral breast cancer in 5.7% of these women.

Breast Biopsy

Nonpalpable Lesions[68]

Image-guided breast biopsies are frequently required to diagnose nonpalpable lesions. Ultrasound localization techniques are employed when a mass is present, while stereotactic techniques are used when no mass is present (microcalcifications only). The combination of diagnostic mammography, ultrasound or stereotactic localization, and fine-needle aspiration (FNA) biopsy is almost 100% accurate in the diagnosis of breast cancer. However, while FNA biopsy permits cytologic evaluation, core-needle or open biopsy also permits the analysis of breast tissue architecture and allows the pathologist to determine whether invasive cancer is present. This permits the surgeon and patient to discuss the specific management of a breast cancer before therapy begins. Core-needle biopsy is accepted as an alternative to open biopsy for nonpalpable breast lesions. The advantages of core-needle biopsy include a low complication rate, avoidance of scarring, and a lower cost.

Palpable Lesions[69]

FNA biopsy of a palpable breast mass is performed in an outpatient setting. A 1.5-inch, 22-gauge needle attached to a 10-mL

syringe is used. A syringe holder enables the surgeon performing the FNA biopsy to control the syringe and needle with one hand while positioning the breast mass with the opposite hand. After the needle is placed in the mass, suction is applied while the needle is moved back and forth within the mass. Once cellular material is seen at the hub of the needle, the suction is released and the needle is withdrawn. The cellular material is then expressed onto microscope slides. Both air-dried and 95% ethanol-fixed microscopy sections are prepared for analysis. When a breast mass is clinically and mammographically suspicious, the sensitivity and the specificity of FNA biopsy approaches 100%. Core-needle biopsy of palpable breast masses is performed using a 14-gauge needle, such as the Tru Cut needle. Automated devices also are available. Tissue specimens are placed in formalin and then processed to paraffin blocks. While the false-negative rate for core-needle biopsy is very low, a tissue specimen that does not show breast cancer cannot conclusively rule out that diagnosis because a sampling error may have occurred.

BREAST CANCER STAGING AND BIOMARKERS

Breast Cancer Staging[70]

The clinical stage of breast cancer is determined primarily through physical examination of the skin, breast tissue, and lymph nodes (axillary, supraclavicular, and cervical). However, clinical determination of axillary lymph node metastases has an accuracy of only 33%. Mammography, chest x-ray, and intraoperative findings (primary cancer size, chest wall invasion) also provide necessary staging information. Pathologic stage combines clinical stage data with findings from pathologic examination of the resected primary breast cancer and axillary lymph nodes. Fisher and colleagues found that accurate predictions regarding the occurrence of distant metastases were possible after resection and pathologic analysis of 10 or more level I and II axillary lymph nodes. A frequently used staging system is the TNM (tumor, nodes, and metastasis) system. The American Joint Committee on Cancer (AJCC) has modified the TNM system for breast cancer (Tables 16-11 and 16-12). Koscielny and colleagues demonstrated that tumor size correlates with the presence of axillary lymph node metastases (see Fig. 16-16B). Others have shown an association between tumor size, axillary lymph node metastases, and disease-free survival. The single most important predictor of 10- and 20-year survival rates in breast cancer is the number of axillary lymph nodes involved with metastatic disease. Routine biopsy of internal mammary lymph nodes is not recommended even though the frequency of internal mammary lymph node metastases increases in proportion to the size of central and medial quadrant cancers. Clinical or pathologic evidence of metastatic spread to supraclavicular lymph nodes is indicative of systemic (stage IV) disease, but routine scalene or supraclavicular lymph node biopsy is not indicated.

Biomarkers[71-75]

Breast cancer biomarkers are of several types. Risk-factor biomarkers are those associated with increased cancer risk. These include familial clustering and inherited germline abnormalities, proliferative breast disease with atypia, and mammography densities. Exposure biomarkers are a subset of risk factors that include measurement of carcinogen exposure such as DNA adducts. Surrogate endpoint biomarkers are biologic alterations in tissue that occur between initiation and cancer development. These biomarkers are used as endpoints in short-term chemoprevention trials and include histologic changes, indices of proliferation, and genetic alterations

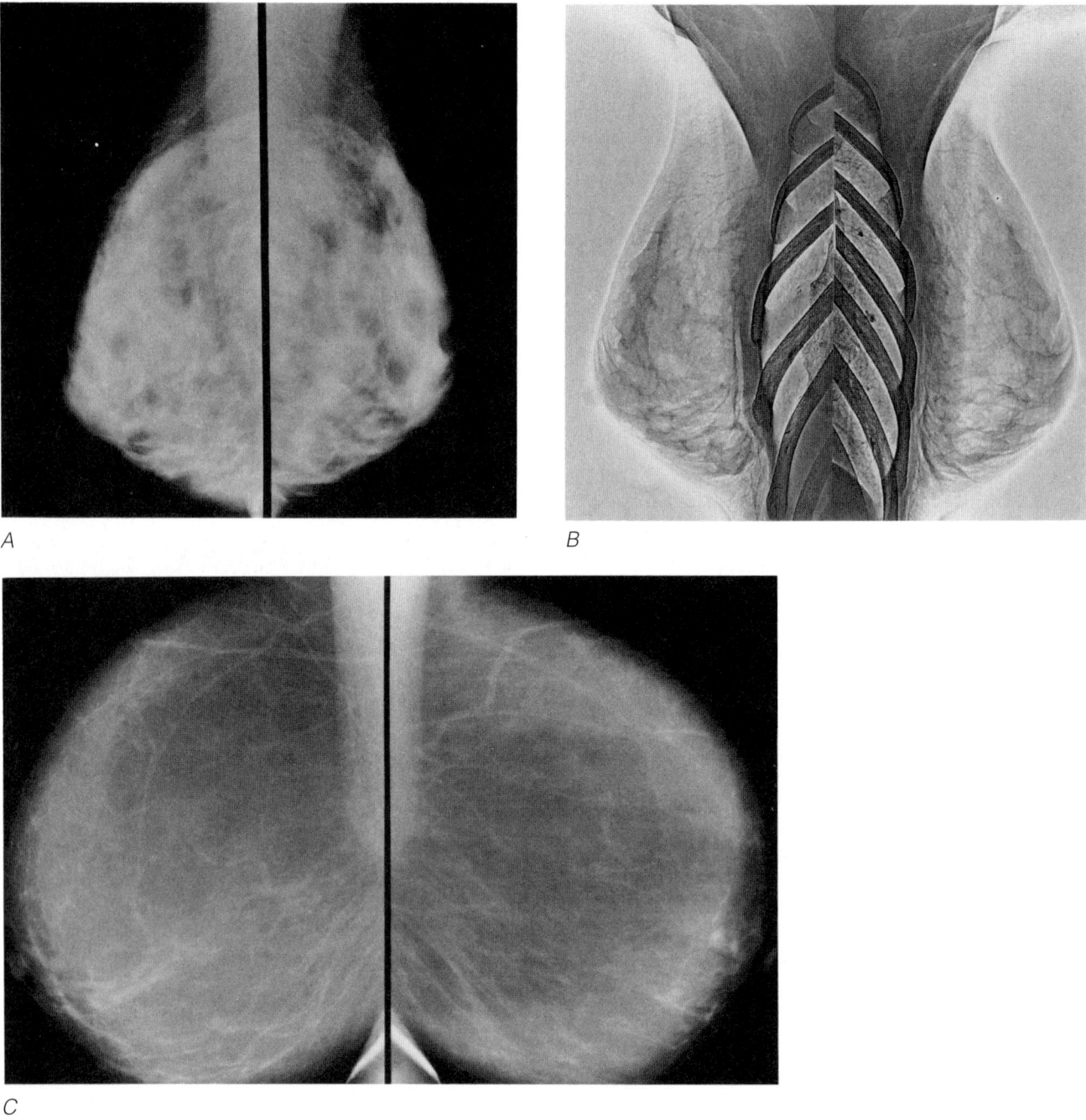

FIG. 16-23. Mammography and xeromammography. *A.* Mammogram of a premenopausal breast with a dense fibroglandular pattern. *B.* Xeromammogram of the breast shown in *A.* Xeromammography allows visualization from the nipple to the ribs, while mammography permits better visualization of the axillary tail of Spence. *C.* Mammogram of a postmenopausal breast with a sparse fibroglandular pattern. *(Continued)*

leading to cancer. Drug-effect biomarkers (serum glutathione reductase activity, ornithine decarboxylase activity), which may or may not be directly related to carcinogenesis, are used to monitor the biochemical effect of drugs. Prognostic biomarkers provide information regarding cancer outcome irrespective of therapy, while predictive biomarkers provide information regarding response to therapy. Candidate prognostic and predictive biomarkers for breast cancer include (1) indices of proliferation such as proliferating cell nuclear antigen (PCNA), BrUdR, and Ki-67; (2) indices of apoptosis

such as bcl-2 and the bax:bcl-2 ratio; (3) indices of angiogenesis such as vascular endothelial growth factor (VEGF) and the angiogenesis index; (4) growth factors and growth factor receptors such as human epidermal growth receptor (HER)-2/neu and epidermal growth factor receptor (EGFr); and (5) p53.

Indices of Proliferation[76–79]

PCNA is a nuclear protein associated with a DNA polymerase whose expression increases in G_1, reaches its maximum at the

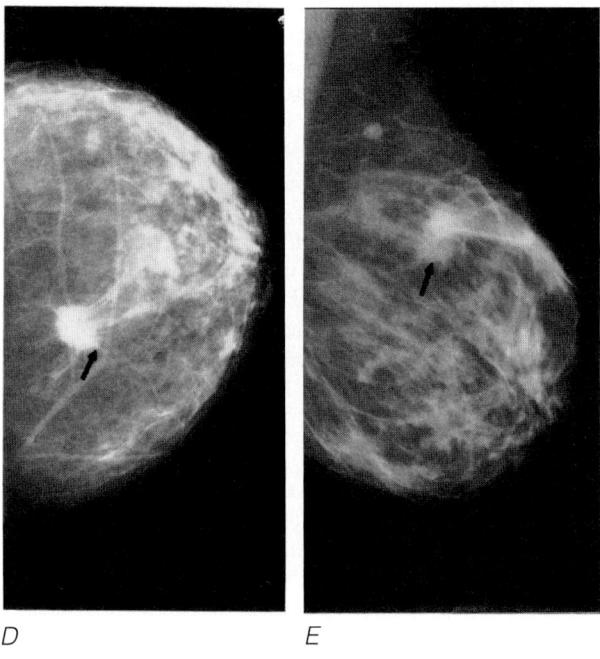

D E

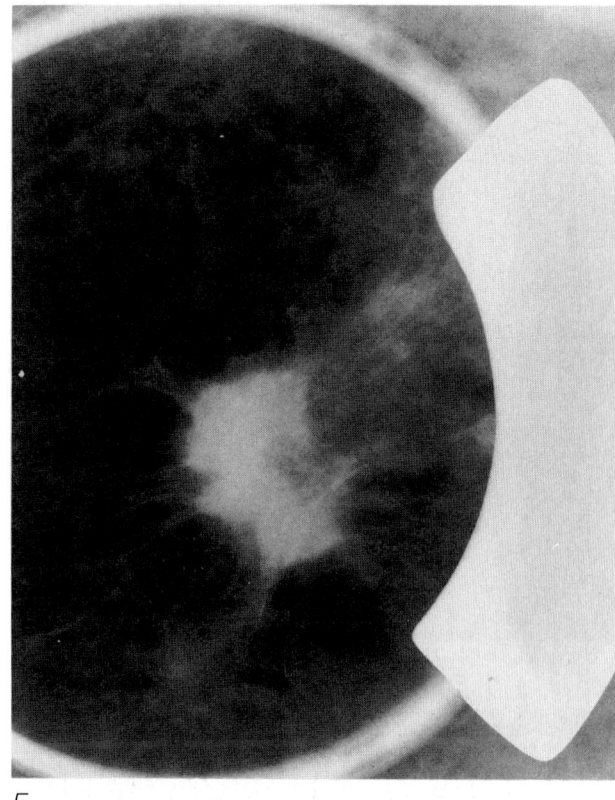

F

FIG. 16-23. *(continued) D.* Invasive breast cancer *(arrow)* shown in the craniocaudal mammography view. *E.* Invasive breast cancer *(arrow)* shown in the mediolateral oblique mammography view *F.* Cone-compression mammography view of the cancer seen in *D* and *E*. Note that the speculated margins of the cancer are accentuated by cone compression. *(Courtesy of Dr. B. Steinbach.)*

G_1/S interface, and then decreases through G_2. Immunohistochemical staining for PCNA outlines the proliferating compartments in breast tissue. Good correlation is seen between PCNA and (1) flow cytometrically determined cell cycle distributions based on DNA content, and (2) BrUdR and the proliferation-associated Ki-67 antigen. Individual proliferation markers are associated with slightly different phases of the cell cycle and are not equivalent. PCNA and Ki-67 expression are positively correlated with p53 overexpression, high S-phase fraction, aneuploidy, high mitotic index, and high histologic grade in human breast cancer specimens, and are negatively correlated with estrogen receptor content.

Indices of Apoptosis[80–82]

Alterations in programmed cell death (apoptosis), which may be triggered by p53-dependent or -independent factors, may be important prognostic and predictive biomarkers in breast cancer. Bcl-2–family proteins appear to regulate a step in the evolutionarily conserved pathway for apoptosis, with some members functioning as inhibitors of apoptosis and others as promoters of apoptosis. Bcl-2 is the only oncogene that acts by inhibiting apoptosis rather than by directly increasing cellular proliferation. The death-signal protein, bax, is induced by genotoxic stress and growth factor deprivation in the presence of wild-type (normal) p53 and/or APO-1/fos. The bax:bcl-2 ratio and the resulting formation of either bax–bax homodimers, which stimulate apoptosis, or bax–bcl-2 heterodimers, which

inhibit apoptosis, represent an intracellular regulatory mechanism with prognostic and predictive implications. In breast cancer, overexpression of bcl-2 and a decrease in the bax:bcl-2 ratio correlate with high histologic grade, the presence of axillary lymph node metastases, and reduced disease-free and overall survival rates. Similarly, decreased bax expression correlates with axillary lymph node metastases, a poor response to chemotherapy, and decreased overall survival.

Indices of Angiogenesis[83,84]

Angiogenesis is necessary for the growth and invasiveness of breast cancer and promotes cancer progression through several different mechanisms, including delivery of oxygen and nutrients and the secretion of growth-promoting cytokines by endothelial cells. Vascular endothelial growth factor (VEGF) induces its effect by binding to transmembrane tyrosine kinase receptors. Overexpression of VEGF in invasive breast cancer is correlated with increased microvessel density and recurrence in node-negative breast cancer. An angiogenesis index has been developed in which microvessel density (CD31 expression) is combined with thrombospondin expression (a negative modulator of angiogenesis) and p53 expression. Both VEGF expression and the angiogenesis index may have prognostic and predictive significance in breast cancer. Antiangiogenesis breast cancer therapy is now being studied in human trials.

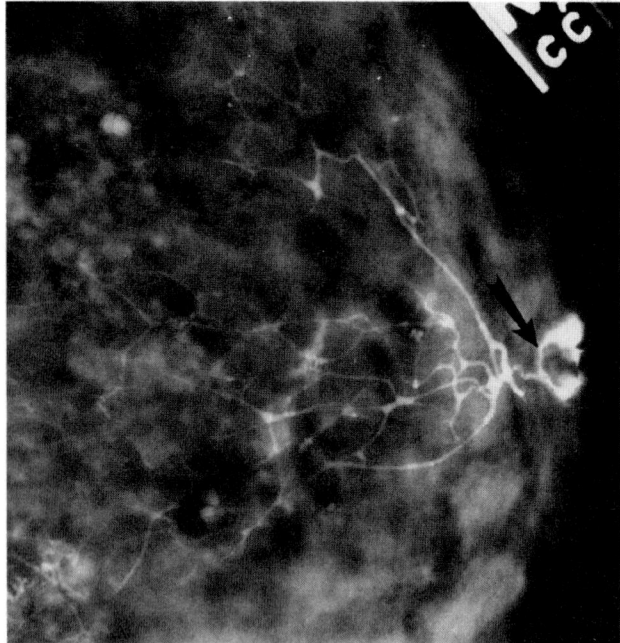

A

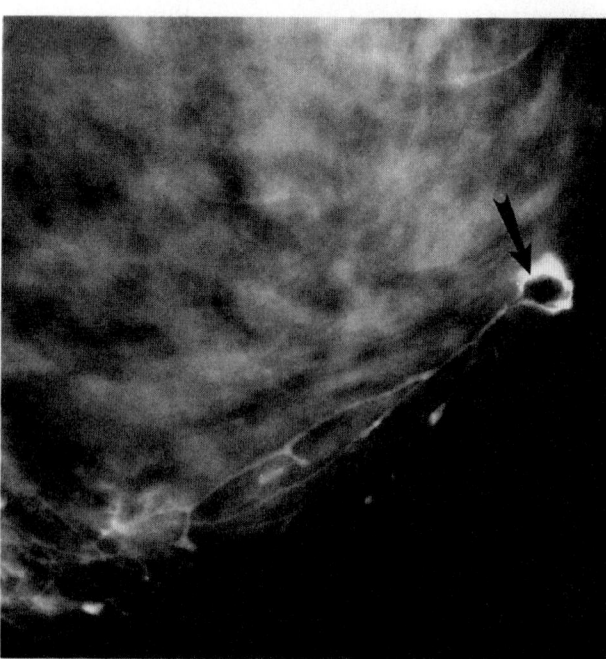

B

FIG. 16-24. Ductogram. *A.* Craniocaudal and *(B)* mediolateral oblique mammography views demonstrate a mass *(arrows)* posterior to the nipple and outlined by contrast, which also fills the proximal ductal structures. *(Courtesy of Dr. B. Steinbach.)*

Growth Factor Receptors and Growth Factors[85–87]

Overexpression of EGFr in breast cancer correlates with estrogen receptor–negative status and with p53 overexpression. Similarly, increased immunohistochemical membrane staining for the HER2/neu growth factor receptor in breast cancer is associated with p53 and Ki-67 overexpression and estrogen receptor–negative

status. HER2/neu is a member of the EGFr family of growth factor receptors in which ligand binding results in receptor homodimerization and tyrosine phosphorylation by tyrosine kinase domains within the receptor. Tyrosine phosphorylation is followed by signal transduction, resulting in changes in cell behavior. An important property of this family of receptors is that ligand binding to one receptor type may also result in heterodimerization between two different receptor types that are coexpressed, resulting in transphosphorylation and transactivation of both receptors in the complex (transmodulation). In this context, the lack of a specific ligand for the HER2/neu receptor suggests that HER2/neu may function solely as a coreceptor, modulating signaling by other EGFr family members. Anti–HER2/neu therapy is now an important breast cancer therapy.

p53

Wild-type (normal) p53 plays a central role in cell-cycle arrest, DNA repair, and programmed cell death. Mutation of the p53 gene causes conformational changes in the p53 protein, and results in increased protein half-life and overexpression in immunohistochemical assays. In breast cancer, p53 overexpression correlates with high nuclear grade, high proliferative fraction, aneuploidy, HER2/neu overexpression, and hormone receptor–negative status. Several retrospective studies of human breast cancer suggest a role for p53 in determining breast cancer prognosis and response to therapy.

Coexpression of Biomarkers

Selection of optimal therapy for breast cancer requires both an accurate assessment of prognosis and an accurate prediction of response to therapy. Unfortunately, current breast cancer biomarkers do not permit either of these. As a result, current therapy for breast cancer is empirical, based on the outcome of randomized clinical trials that examine average effects within populations. Clinicopathologic factors are used to separate breast cancer patients into broad prognostic groups, and treatment decisions are made on this basis (Table 16-13). With this approach, up to 70% of early breast cancer patients receive adjuvant chemotherapy that is either unnecessary or ineffective. As described above, a wide variety of biomarkers have been shown to individually predict prognosis and response to therapy, but they do not improve the accuracy of either the assessment of prognosis or the prediction of response to therapy.

As knowledge regarding cellular, biochemical, and molecular biomarkers for breast cancer increases, prognostic indices are being developed that combine the predictive power of several individual biomarkers with the relevant clinicopathologic factors. In laboratories at Brown University, molecular biomarkers (c-fos, c-myc, Ha-ras, p53) were studied in a series of patients with stages I, IIa, and IIb breast cancer. While single biomarker overexpression did not possess independent prognostic significance, the overexpression of three or more biomarkers was confirmed to endow breast cancers with an aggressive phenotype, accurately predicting worse disease-free and overall survival. At the University of Alabama at Birmingham, using archival breast tissues from women accrued prospectively to the Alabama Breast Cancer Project, an analysis of molecular biomarkers of breast cancer prognosis was undertaken. Following a 15-year follow-up period, the combination of HER2/neu and p53 overexpression more accurately predicted disease-free and overall survival than did clinicopathologic factors.

Exhaustive analysis of all relevant cellular, biochemical, and molecular abnormalities in breast cancer is a daunting task.

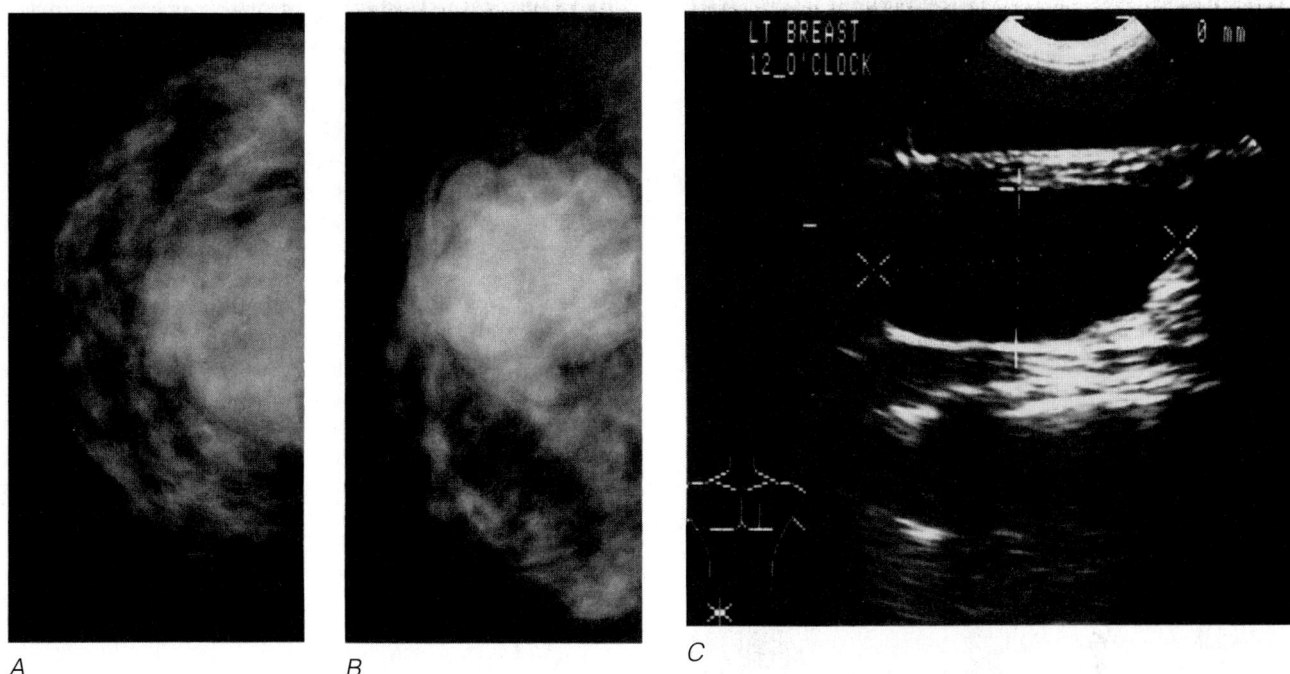

FIG. 16-25. Breast cyst. *A.* Craniocaudal and (*B*) mediolateral oblique mammography views show a large lobulated mass. *C.* Ultrasound image of the mass shows it to be anechoic with a well-defined back wall, characteristic of a cyst. (*Courtesy of Dr. B. Steinbach.*)

However, the technologies necessary for such a task have been developed. Microdissection techniques combined with high-density oligonucleotide arrays and other high-throughput analyses of gene expression now permit the simultaneous study of multiple alterations in breast cancer tissues. As bioinformatics provide the tools for categorizing and analyzing the immense amount of data being generated, these technologies will allow a detailed stratification of breast cancer patients for assessment of prognosis and for prediction of response to therapy.

OVERVIEW OF BREAST CANCER THERAPY

Before diagnostic biopsy, the surgeon must discuss with the patient the possibility that a suspicious mass or mammography finding may be a breast cancer that will require surgery and possibly radiation therapy and chemotherapy. Once a diagnosis of breast cancer is made, the type of therapy offered to a breast cancer patient is determined by the stage of the disease. Laboratory tests and imaging studies are performed based on the criteria presented in Table 16-14. Before therapy is initiated, the patient and the surgeon must share a clear perspective on the planned course of treatment.

In Situ Breast Cancer (Stage 0)[88–94]

Both LCIS and DCIS may be difficult to distinguish from atypical hyperplasia or from cancers with early invasion. Expert pathologic review is required in all cases. Bilateral mammography is performed to determine the extent of the in situ cancer and to exclude a second cancer. Because LCIS is considered a marker for increased risk rather than an inevitable precursor of invasive disease, the current treatment of LCIS is observation with or without tamoxifen. The goal of treatment is to prevent or detect at an early stage the invasive

cancer that subsequently develops in 25 to 35% of these women. There is no benefit to excising LCIS, as the disease diffusely involves both breasts and the risk of invasive cancer is equal for both breasts. The use of tamoxifen as a risk-reduction strategy should be considered in women with a diagnosis of LCIS.

Women with DCIS and evidence of widespread disease (two or more quadrants) require mastectomy. For women with limited disease, lumpectomy and radiation therapy are recommended. Low-grade DCIS of the solid, cribriform, or papillary subtype, which is less than 0.5 cm in diameter, may be managed by lumpectomy alone. For nonpalpable DCIS, needle localization techniques are used to guide the surgical resection. Specimen mammography is performed to ensure that all visible evidence of cancer is excised. Adjuvant tamoxifen therapy is considered for all DCIS patients. The gold standard against which breast conservation therapy for DCIS is evaluated is mastectomy. Women treated with mastectomy have local recurrence and mortality rates of less than 2%. Women treated with lumpectomy and adjuvant radiation therapy have a similar mortality rate, but the local recurrence rate increases to 9%. Forty-five percent of these recurrences will be invasive cancer. Both Lagios and Gump noted that recurrence of DCIS was greatest when the cancers were more than 2.5 cm in size, the criteria for histologic confirmation of clear margins were not rigorously applied, and the DCIS was of the comedo type. They noted that recurrences frequently occurred within the original surgery site, indicating that inadequate clearance of DCIS, rather than the biology of the cancer, was responsible.

Early Invasive Breast Cancer (Stage I, IIa, or IIb)[95–102]

NSABP B-06 compared total mastectomy to lumpectomy with or without radiation therapy in the treatment of stages I and II breast

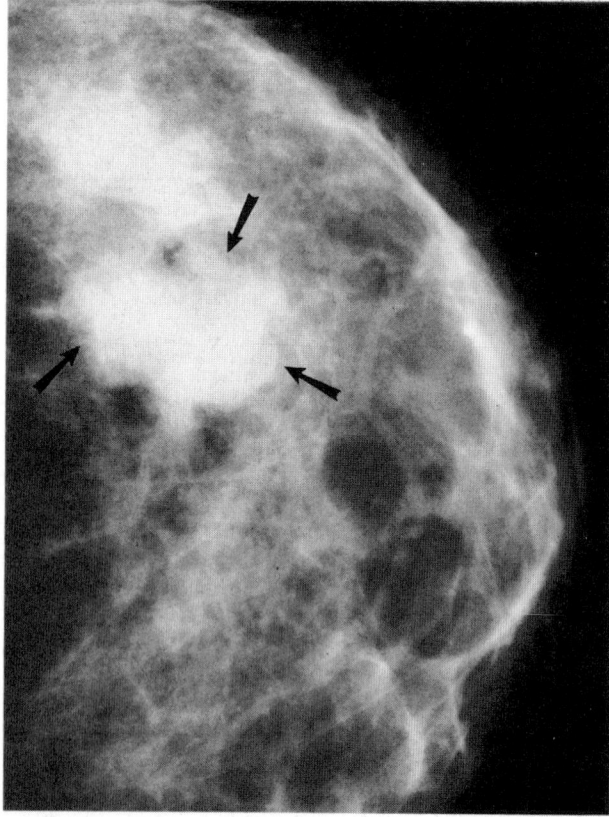

A

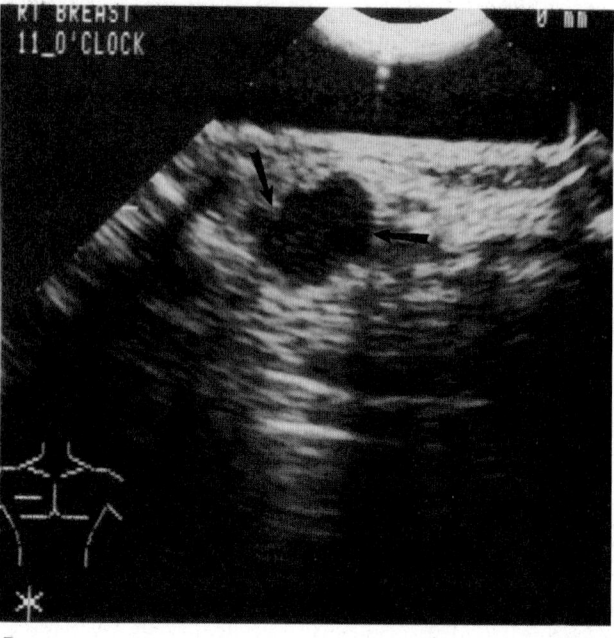

B

FIG. 16-26. *Breast cancer. A. Craniocaudal mammography view of a palpable mass (arrows). B. Ultrasound image demonstrates a solid mass with irregular borders (arrows) consistent with cancer.*

cancer. After 5- and 8-year follow-up periods, the disease-free, distant disease-free, and overall survival rates for lumpectomy with or without radiation therapy were similar to those observed after total mastectomy. However, the incidence of ipsilateral breast can-

cer recurrence (in-breast recurrence) was higher in the lumpectomy group not receiving radiation therapy. These findings supported the use of lumpectomy and radiation in the treatment of stages I and II breast cancer. Reanalysis of this study was undertaken after 12 years when it was found that one of the participating institutions had falsified information concerning the women enrolled. The reanalysis confirmed that there was no difference in disease-free survival rates after total mastectomy or after lumpectomy with or without adjuvant radiation therapy. The in-breast recurrence rate was higher in the lumpectomy alone group (35%) than in the lumpectomy plus adjuvant radiation therapy group (10%). These findings are detailed in Fig. 16-27.

Currently, mastectomy with assessment of axillary lymph node status and breast conservation (lumpectomy with assessment of axillary lymph node status and radiation therapy) are considered equivalent treatments for stages I and II breast cancer. Axillary lymphadenopathy or metastatic disease in a sentinel axillary lymph node (see below) necessitates an axillary lymph node dissection. Breast conservation is considered for all patients because of the important cosmetic advantages. Relative contraindications to breast conservation therapy include (1) prior radiation therapy to the breast or chest wall; (2) involved surgical margins or unknown margin status following re-excision; (3) multicentric disease; and (4) scleroderma or other connective-tissue disease.

Traditionally, dissection of axillary lymph node levels I and II has been performed in early invasive breast cancer. Sentinel lymph node biopsy is now being performed by many surgeons in the elective situation to assess axillary lymph nodes status. Candidates for this procedure have clinically uninvolved axillary lymph nodes, a T1 or T2 primary breast cancer, and have not had neoadjuvant chemotherapy. If the sentinel lymph node cannot be identified or is found to harbor metastatic disease, then an axillary lymph node dissection is performed. The performance of a sentinel lymph node biopsy is not warranted when the selection of adjuvant therapy will not be affected by the status of the axillary lymph nodes, such as in some elderly patients and in those with serious comorbid conditions.

Adjuvant chemotherapy for early invasive breast cancer is considered for all node-positive cancers, all cancers that are larger than 1 cm in size, and node-negative cancers larger than 0.5 cm in size when adverse prognostic features are present. Adverse prognostic factors include blood vessel or lymph vessel invasion, high nuclear grade, high histologic grade, HER2/neu overexpression, and negative hormone receptor status. Tamoxifen therapy is considered for hormone receptor–positive women with cancers that are larger than 1 cm in size. HER2/neu expression is determined for all newly diagnosed patients with breast cancer and may be used to provide prognostic information in patients with node-negative breast cancer, predict the relative efficacy of various chemotherapy regimens, and predict benefit from Herceptin in women with metastatic or recurrent breast cancer.

Advanced Locoregional Regional Breast Cancer (Stage IIIa or IIIb)[103,104]

Women with stages IIIa and IIIb breast cancer have advanced locoregional breast cancer but have no clinically detected distant metastases. In an effort to provide optimal locoregional disease-free survival, as well as distant disease-free survival for these women, surgery is integrated with radiation therapy and chemotherapy. Stage IIIa patients are divided into those who have operable disease and those who have inoperable disease (Fig. 16-28). Surgical therapy for

Table 16-11
TNM Staging System for Breast Cancer

Primary tumor (T) Definitions for classifying the primary tumor (T) are the same for clinical and for pathologic classification. If the measurement is made by physical examination, the examiner will use the major headings (T1, T2, or T3); if other measurements, such as mammographic or pathologic measurements, are used, the subsets of T1 can be used. Tumors should be measured to the nearest 0.1-cm increment

TX	Primary tumor cannot be assessed
T0	No evidence of primary tumor
Tis	Carcinoma in situ
Tis(DCIS)	Ductal carcinoma in situ
Tis(LCIS)	Lobular carcinoma in situ
Tis(Paget's)	Paget's disease of the nipple with no tumor (**Note:** Paget's disease associated with a tumor is classified according to the size of the tumor)
T1	Tumor 2 cm or less in greatest dimension
T1mic	Microinvasion 0.1 cm or less in greatest dimension
T1a	Tumor more than 0.1 cm but not more than 0.5 cm in greatest dimension
T1b	Tumor more than 0.5 cm but not more than 1 cm in greatest dimension
T1c	Tumor more than 1 cm but not more than 2 cm in greatest dimension
T2	Tumor more than 2 cm but not more than 5 cm in greatest dimension
T3	Tumor more than 5 cm in greatest dimension
T4	Tumor of any size with direct extension to (a) chest wall or (b) skin, only as described below
T4a	Extension to chest wall, not including pectoralis muscle
T4b	Edema (including peau d'orange), or ulceration of the skin of the breast, or satellite skin nodules confined to the same breast
T4c	Both T4a and T4b
T4d	Inflammatory carcinoma

Regional lymph nodes—Clinical (N)

NX	Regional lymph nodes cannot be assessed (e.g., previously removed)
N0	No regional lymph node metastasis
N1	Metastasis to movable ipsilateral axillary lymph node(s)
N2	Metastases in ipsilateral axillary lymph nodes fixed or matted, or in clinically apparent[a] ipsilateral internal mammary nodes in the absence of clinically evident axillary lymph node metastasis
N2a	Metastasis in ipsilateral axillary lymph nodes fixed to one another (matted) or to other structures
N2b	Metastasis only in clinically apparent[a] ipsilateral internal mammary nodes and in the absence of clinically evident axillary lymph node metastasis
N3	Metastasis in ipsilateral infraclavicular lymph node(s) with or without axillary lymph node involvement, or in clinically apparent[a] ipsilateral internal mammary lymph node(s) and in the presence of clinically evident axillary lymph node metastasis; or metastasis in ipsilateral supraclavicular lymph node(s) with or without axillary or internal mammary lymph node involvement
N3a	Metastasis in ipsilateral infraclavicular lymph node(s)
N3b	Metastasis in ipsilateral internal mammary lymph nodes(s) and axillary lymph node(s)
N3c	Metastasis in ipsilateral supraclavicular lymph node(s)

Regional lymph nodes—Pathologic (pN)

pNX	Regional lymph nodes cannot be assessed (e.g., previously removed, or not removed for pathologic study)
pN0[b]	No regional lymph node metastasis histologically, no additional examination for isolated tumor cells (**Note:** Isolated tumor cells (ITC) are defined as single tumor cells or small cell clusters not greater than 0.2 mm, usually detected only by immunohistochemical (IHC) or molecular methods but which may be verified on H&E stains; ITCs do not usually show evidence of malignant activity [e.g., proliferation or stromal reaction])
pN0(i−)	No regional lymph node metastasis histologically, negative IHC
pN0(i+)	No regional lymph node metastasis histologically, positive IHC, no IHC cluster greater than 0.2 mm
pN0(mol−)	No regional lymph node metastasis histologically, negative molecular findings (RT-PCR)
pN0(mol+)	No regional lymph node metastasis histologically, positive molecular findings (RT-PCR)
pN1	Metastasis in 1 to 3 axillary lymph nodes, and/or in internal mammary nodes with microscopic disease detected by sentinel lymph nodes dissection, not clinically apparent[c]
pN1mi	Micrometastasis (greater than 0.2 mm, none greater than 2.0 mm)
pN1a	Metastasis in 1 to 3 axillary lymph nodes
pN1b	Metastasis in internal mammary nodes with microscopic disease detected by sentinel lymph node dissection, not clinically apparent[c]
pN1c	Metastasis in 1 to 3 axillary lymph nodes and in internal mammary lymph nodes with microscopic disease detected by sentinel lymph node dissection but not clinically apparent[c] (if associated with greater than 3 positive axillary lymph nodes, the internal mammary nodes are classified as pN3b to reflect increased tumor burden)
pN2	Metastasis in 4 to 9 axillary lymph nodes, or in clinically apparent[a] internal mammary lymph nodes in the absence of axillary lymph node metastasis
pN2a	Metastasis in 4 to 9 axillary lymph nodes (at least one tumor deposit greater than 2.0 mm)
pN2b	Metastasis in clinically apparent[a] internal mammary lymph nodes in the absence of axillary lymph node metastasis
pN3	Metastasis in ≥10 axillary lymph nodes, or in infraclavicular lymph nodes, or in clinically apparent[a] ipsilateral internal mammary lymph nodes in the presence of 1 or more positive axillary lymph nodes; or in more than 3 axillary lymph nodes with clinically negative microscopic metastasis in internal mammary lymph nodes; or in ipsilateral supraclavicular lymph nodes
pN3a	Metastasis in 10 or more axillary lymph nodes (at lease one tumor deposit greater than 2.0 mm), or metastasis to the infraclavicular lymph nodes
pN3b	Metastasis in clinically apparent[a] ipsilateral internal mammary lymph nodes in the presence of 1 or more positive axillary lymph nodes; or in more than 3 axillary lymph nodes and in internal mammary lymph nodes with microscopic disease detected by sentinel lymph node dissection, not clinically apparent[c]
pN3c	Metastasis in ipsilateral supraclavicular lymph nodes

Distant metastasis (M)

MX	Distant metastasis cannot be assessed
M0	No distant metastasis
M1	Distant metastasis

[a] *Clinically apparent* is defined as detected by imaging studies (excluding lymphoscintigraphy) or by clinical examination or grossly visible pathologically.

[b] Classification is based on axillary lymph node dissection with or without sentinel lymph node dissection. Classification based solely on sentinel lymph node dissection without subsequent axillary lymph node dissection is designated (sn) for "sentinel node" e.g., pN-(l+) (sn).

[c] *Not clinically apparent* is defined as not detected by imaging studies (excluding lymphoscintigraphy) or by clinical examination.

RT-PCR = reverse transcriptase polymerase chain reaction.

SOURCE: Modified with permission from American Joint Committee on Cancer: *AJCC Cancer Staging Manual,* 6th ed. New York: Springer, 2002, pp 227–228.

Table 16-12
TNM Stage Groupings

Stage 0	Tis	N0	M0
Stage I	T1[a]	N0	M0
Stage IIA	T0	N1	M0
	T1[a]	N1	M0
	T2	N0	M0
Stage IIB	T2	N1	M0
	T3	N0	M0
Stage IIIA	T0	N2	M0
	T1[a]	N2	M0
	T2	N2	M0
	T3	N1	M0
	T3	N2	M0
Stage IIIB	T4	N0	M0
	T4	N1	M0
	T4	N2	M0
Stage IIIC	Any T	N3	M0
Stage IV	Any T	Any N	M1

[a]T1 includes T1 mic.

SOURCE: Modified with permission from American Joint Committee on Cancer: *AJCC Cancer Staging Manual,* 6th ed. New York: Springer, 2002, p 228.

women with operable stage IIIa disease is usually a modified radical mastectomy, followed by adjuvant chemotherapy, followed by adjuvant radiation therapy. Adjuvant chemotherapy is used to maximize distant disease-free survival, while radiation therapy is used to maximize locoregional disease-free survival. In selected stage IIIa patients, initial (neoadjuvant) chemotherapy is used to reduce the size of the primary cancer and permit conservation surgery. For inoperable stage IIIa and for stage IIIb breast cancer, neoadjuvant chemotherapy is used to decrease the locoregional cancer burden and may permit subsequent surgery to establish locoregional control. In this setting, surgery is followed by adjuvant chemotherapy and adjuvant radiation therapy.

Internal Mammary Lymph Nodes

Metastatic disease to internal mammary lymph nodes may be occult, evident on chest x-ray or CT scan, or may present as a painless parasternal mass with or without skin involvement. There is no consensus regarding the need for internal mammary lymph node radiation therapy in women who are at increased risk for occult involvement (cancers involving the medial aspect of the breast, axillary lymph node involvement), but who show no signs of internal mammary lymph node involvement. Systemic chemotherapy and

Table 16-13
Traditional Prognostic and Predictive Factors for Invasive Breast Cancer

Tumor Factors	Host Factors
Nodal status	Age
Tumor size	Menopausal status
Histologic/nuclear grade	Family history
Lymphatic/vascular invasion	Previous breast cancer
Pathologic status	Immunosuppression
Hormone receptor status	Nutrition
DNA content (ploidy, S-phase fraction)	Prior chemotherapy
Extensive intraductal component	Prior radiation therapy

SOURCE: Reproduced with permission from Beenken SW, Bland KI: Breast cancer genetics, in Ellis N (ed): *Inherited Cancer Syndromes.* New York: Springer-Verlag, 2003, p 112.

Table 16-14
Diagnostic Studies for Breast Cancer Patients

	Cancer Stage				
	0	I	II	III	IV
History & physical	X	X	X	X	X
CBC, platelets		X	X	X	X
Liver function tests		X	X	X	X
Chest x-ray		X	X	X	X
Bilateral mammograms	X	X	X	X	X
Hormone-receptor status		X	X	X	X
HER2/neu expression		X	X	X	X
Bone scan[a]			X	X	X
Abdominal CT scan or ultrasound or MRI				X	X

[a]Bone scan performed for stage II only if localized symptoms or elevated serum alkaline phosphatase.

SOURCE: Adapted with permission from Carlson RW et al: Breast cancer, in *National Comprehensive Cancer Network (NCCN) Practice Guidelines in Oncology* Vol. 2, 2002.

radiation therapy are used in the treatment of grossly involved internal mammary lymph nodes.

Distant Metastases (Stage IV)[105]

Treatment for stage IV breast cancer is not curative, but may prolong survival and enhance a woman's quality of life. Hormonal therapies that are associated with minimal toxicity are preferred to cytotoxic chemotherapy. Appropriate candidates for initial hormonal therapy include women with hormone receptor–positive cancers; women with bone or soft tissue metastases only; and women with limited and asymptomatic visceral metastases. Systemic chemotherapy is indicated for women with hormone receptor–negative cancers, symptomatic visceral metastases, and hormone refractory metastases. Women with stage IV breast cancer may develop anatomically localized problems that will benefit from individualized surgical treatment such as brain metastases; pleural effusion; pericardial effusion; biliary obstruction; ureteral obstruction; impending or existing pathologic fracture of a long bone; spinal cord compression; and painful bone or soft tissue metastases. Bisphosphonates, which may be given in addition to chemotherapy or hormone therapy, should be considered in women with bone metastases.

Locoregional Recurrence

Women with locoregional recurrence of breast cancer may be separated into two groups: those having had mastectomy and those having had lumpectomy. Women with a previous mastectomy undergo surgical resection of the locoregional recurrence and appropriate reconstruction. Chemotherapy and antiestrogen therapy are considered and adjuvant radiation therapy is given if the chest wall has not previously received radiation therapy. Women with previous breast conservation undergo a mastectomy and appropriate reconstruction. Chemotherapy and antiestrogen therapy are considered.

Breast Cancer Prognosis

Survival rates for women diagnosed with breast cancer between 1983 and 1987 have been calculated based on Surveillance, Epidemiology, and End Results (SEER) program data. The 5-year survival rate for stage I patients is 94%; for stage IIa patients, 85%; and for stage IIb patients, 70%, while for stage IIIa patients the 5-year survival rate is 52%; for stage IIIb patients, 48%; and for stage IV patients, 18%.

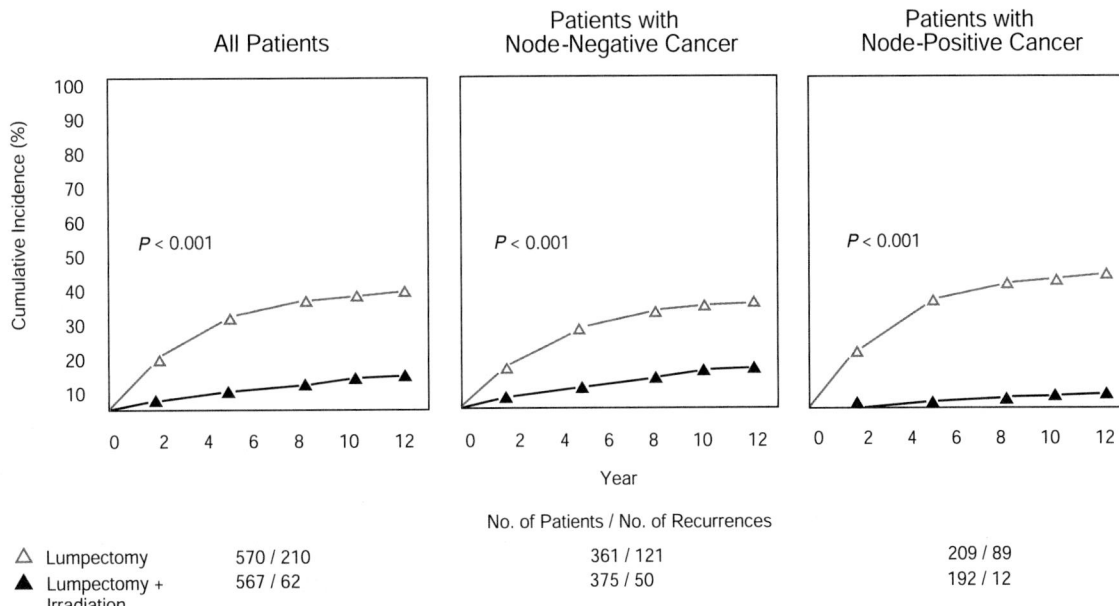

No. of Patients / No. of Recurrences

	All Patients	Node-Negative	Node-Positive
△ Lumpectomy	570 / 210	361 / 121	209 / 89
▲ Lumpectomy + Irradiation	567 / 62	375 / 50	192 / 12

FIG. 16-27. NSABP B-06 results. Life-table analysis showing the incidence of recurrent cancer in the ipsilateral breast after lumpectomy or lumpectomy with adjuvant radiation therapy in 1137 patients with clear surgical margins. *(Reproduced with permission from Fisher B et al.[98])*

SURGICAL TECHNIQUES IN BREAST CANCER THERAPY

Excisional Biopsy with Needle Localization[106]

Excisional biopsy implies complete removal of a breast lesion with a margin of normal-appearing breast tissue. Informed consent for the procedure may be written to allow the surgeon to proceed with definitive therapy (including mastectomy) if frozen section analysis of the biopsy tissue specimen confirms the presence of an invasive cancer. Figure 16-29 illustrates methods of obtaining a cosmetically acceptable breast scar. Excellent scars generally result from circum-areolar incisions through which subareolar and centrally located

FIG. 16-28. Treatment pathways for stage IIIa and stage IIIb breast cancer. *[Reproduced with permission from Beenken SW, Urist MM, Bland KI: Advanced breast carcinoma (stages IIIa and IIIb), in Bland KI (ed): The Practice of General Surgery. Philadelphia: WB Saunders, 2002, p 980.]*

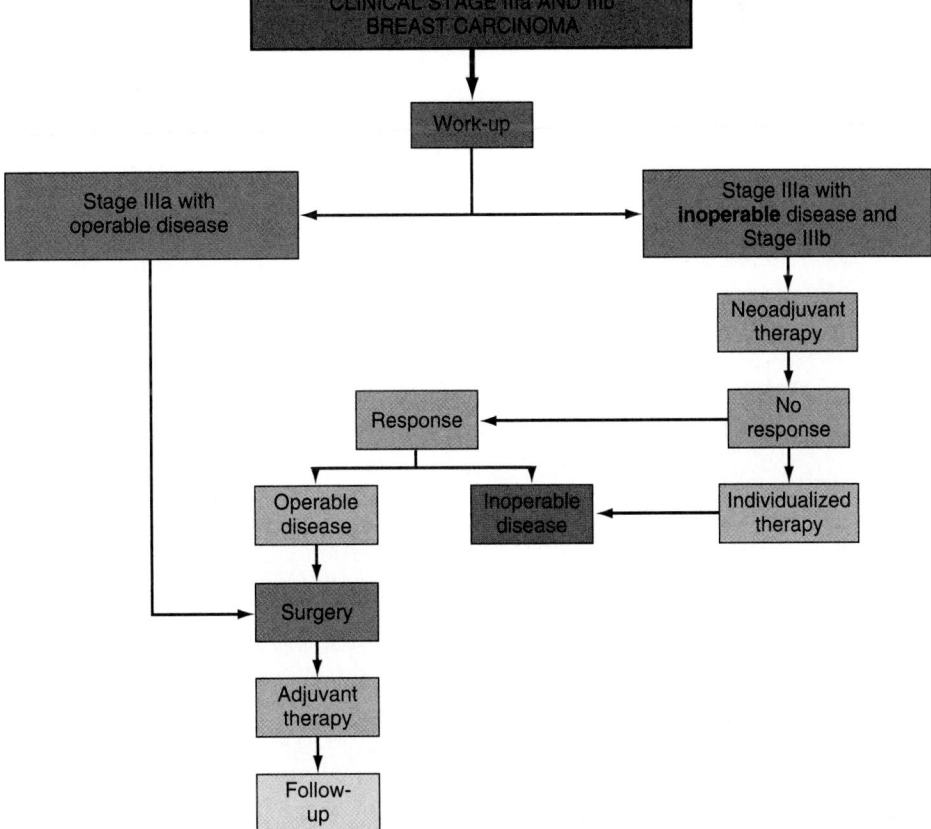

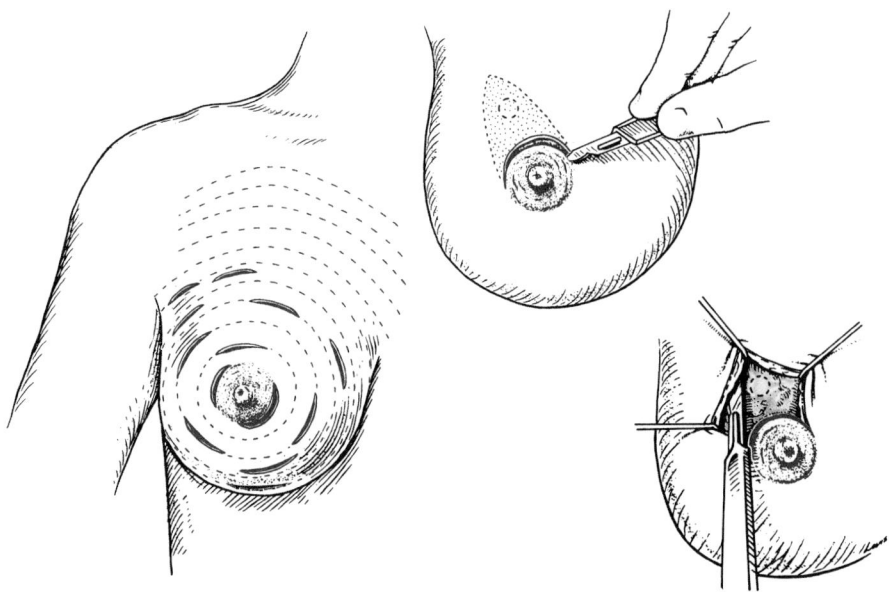

FIG. 16-29. Breast biopsy incisions. Circumareolar incisions or incisions that parallel Langer's lines are recommended. Thin skin flaps are avoided to ensure viable peri-areolar tissues and good cosmesis. (*Reproduced with permission from Souba WW et al.*[107])

breast lesions may be approached. Elsewhere, incisions that parallel Langer's lines, which are lines of tension in the skin that are generally concentric with the nipple–areola complex, result in acceptable scars. It is important to keep biopsy incisions within the boundaries of the skin excision that may be required as part of a subsequent mastectomy (Fig. 16-30). Radial incisions in the upper half of the breast are not recommended because of possible scar contracture resulting in displacement of the ipsilateral nipple–areola complex.

After excision of a suspicious breast lesion, the biopsy tissue specimen is orientated for the pathologist using sutures, clips, or dyes. Additional margins (superior, inferior, medial, lateral, superficial, and deep) may be taken from the surgical bed to confirm complete excision of the suspicious lesion. Electrocautery or absorbable ligatures are used to achieve wound hemostasis. Although approximation of the breast tissues in the excision bed is usually not necessary, cosmesis may occasionally be facilitated by approximation of the surgical defect using 3-0 absorbable sutures. A running subcuticular closure of the skin using 4-0 or 5-0 absorbable monofilament sutures is performed, followed by approximation of the skin edges with Steri-Strips. Wound drainage is avoided.

Excisional biopsy with needle localization requires a preoperative visit to the mammography suite for placement of a localization wire. The lesion to be excised is accurately localized by mammography, and the tip of a thin wire hook is positioned close to the

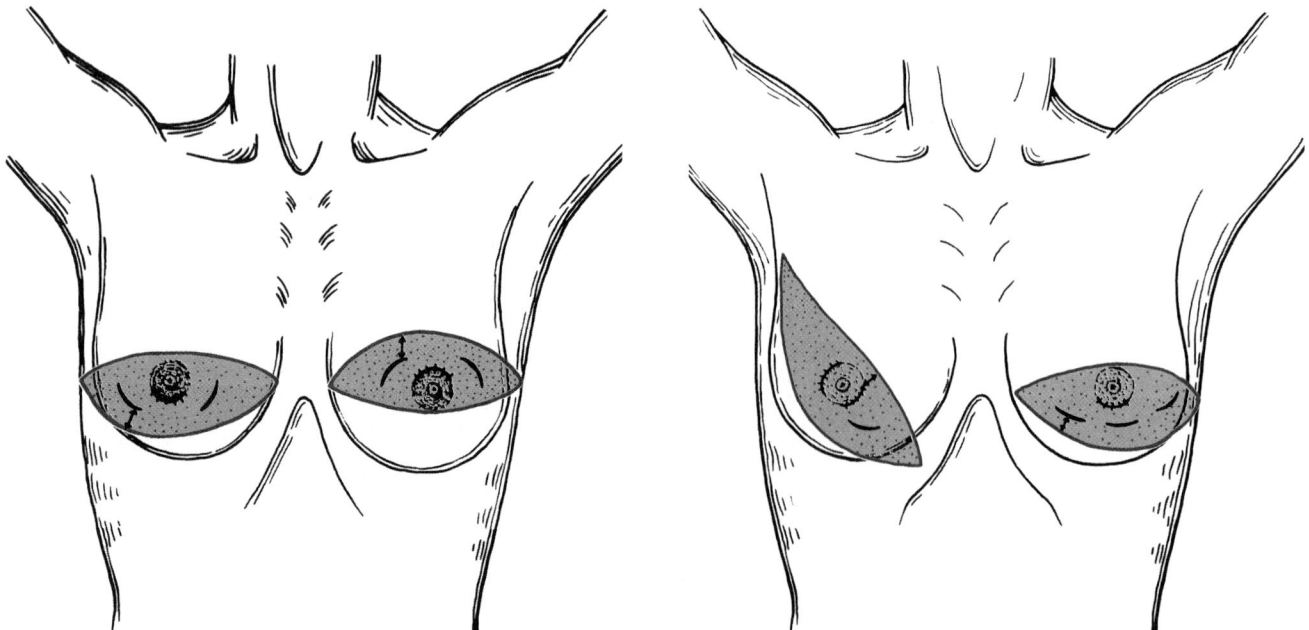

FIG. 16-30. Placement of breast biopsy incisions. Breast biopsy incisions are placed within the boundaries of subsequent mastectomy skin incisions, and their placement allows for 1-cm or larger margins (*arrows*) around the biopsy scar. (*Reproduced with permission from Souba WW et al.*[107])

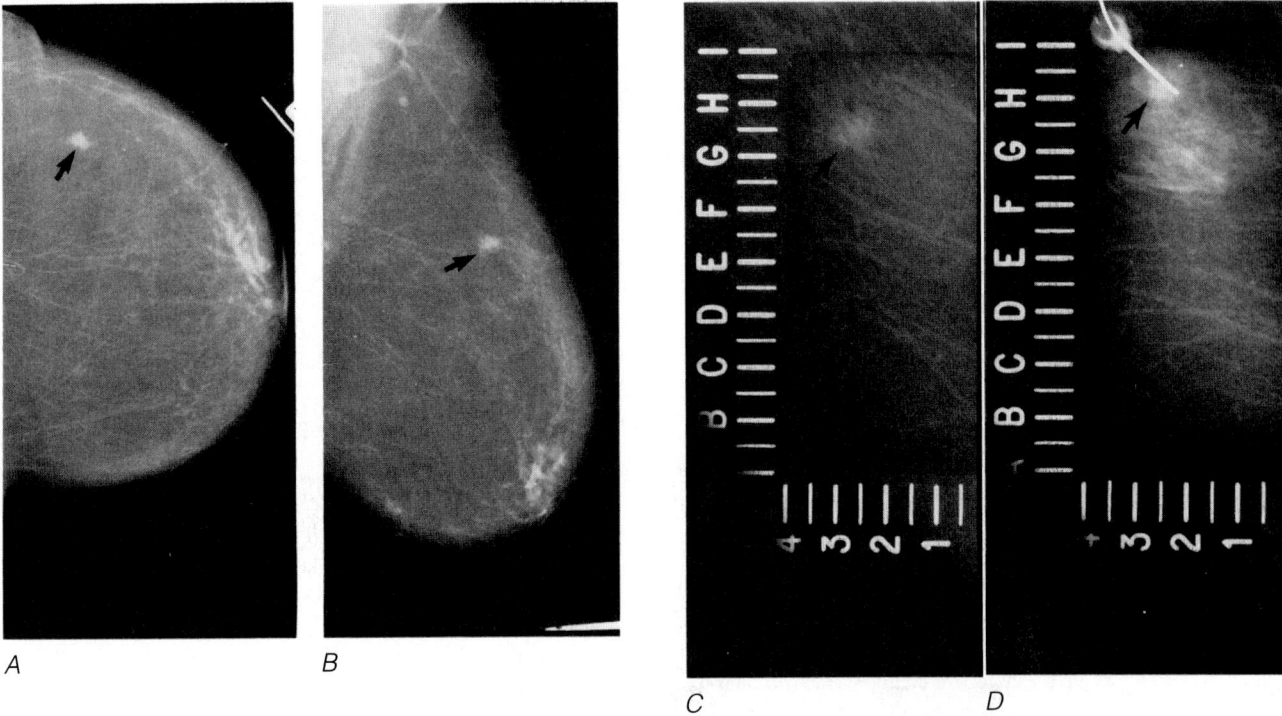

A   B

C   D

FIG. 16-31. Nonpalpable breast cancer. *A.* Craniocaudal and *(B)* mediolateral oblique mammography views of the breast demonstrate an 8-mm spiculated mass *(arrows)* subsequently shown to be a cancer. *C.* and *D.* Method of needle localization. The numbers and letters of the localization plate allow biplanar positioning of the guidewire *(arrows).* *(Courtesy of Dr. B. Steinbach.)*

lesion (Fig. 16-31). Using the wire hook as a guide, the surgeon subsequently excises the suspicious breast lesion while removing a margin of normal-appearing breast tissue. Before the patient leaves the operating room, specimen radiography is performed to confirm complete excision of the suspicious lesion (Fig. 16-32).

Sentinel Lymph Node Biopsy[107–116]

Sentinel lymph node biopsy is primarily used in women with early breast cancers (T1 and T2, N0). It also is accurate for T3 N0 cancers, but nearly 75% of these women will have nonpalpable axillary lymph node metastases. In women undergoing neoadjuvant chemotherapy to permit conservation surgery, sentinel lymph node biopsy may be used. Contraindications to the procedure include palpable lymphadenopathy, prior axillary surgery, chemotherapy or radiation therapy, and multifocal breast cancers.

Evidence from large prospective studies suggests that the combination of intraoperative gamma probe detection of radioactive colloid and intraoperative visualization of isosulfan blue dye (Lymphazurin) is more accurate than the use of either agent alone. Some surgeons employ preoperative lymphoscintigraphy, although it is not necessary. On the day prior to surgery, or on the morning of surgery, the radioactive colloid is injected. Using a tuberculin syringe and a 25-gauge needle, 0.5 mCi of 0.2-micron technetium-99 sulfur colloid in a volume of 0.2 to 0.5 mL is injected (three to four separate injections) at the cancer site or subdermally. Subdermal injections are given in proximity to the cancer site or subareolar. Subsequently, in the operating room, 4 mL of isosulfan blue dye (Lymphazurin) is injected in a similar fashion, but with an additional 1 mL injected between the cancer site and the overlying skin. For nonpalpable cancers, the injection is guided by either intraoperative ultrasound or by a localization wire that is placed preoperatively under ultrasound

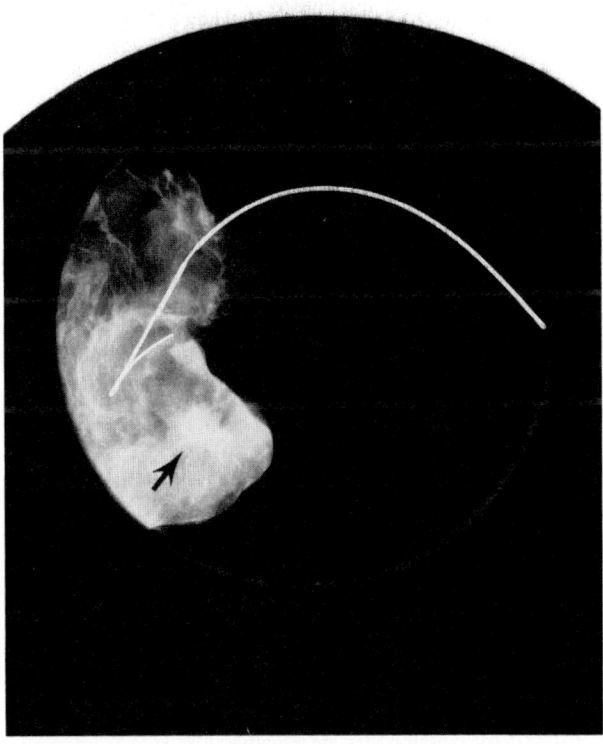

FIG. 16-32. Specimen mammography. The specimen mammogram contains the suspicious mass *(arrow)* seen on preoperative imaging. *(Courtesy of Dr. B. Steinbach.)*

or stereotactic guidance. It is helpful for the radiologist to mark the skin overlying the breast cancer at the time of needle localization using an indelible marker. In women who have undergone previous excisional biopsy, the injections are made around the biopsy cavity but not into it. Women are told preoperatively that the isosulfan blue dye injection will impart a change to the color of their urine and that there is a very small risk of allergic reaction to the dye (1 in 10,000). Anaphylactic reactions have been documented. The use of radioactive colloid is safe and radiation exposure is very low.

A hand-held gamma counter is then employed transcutaneously to identify the location of the sentinel lymph node. A 3- to 4-cm incision is made in line with that used for an axillary dissection, which is a curved transverse incision in the lower axilla just below the hairline. After dissecting through the subcutaneous tissue and identifying the lateral border of the pectoralis muscles, the clavipectoral fascia is divided to gain exposure to the axillary contents. The gamma counter is employed to pinpoint the location of the sentinel lymph node. As the dissection continues, the signal from the probe increases in intensity as the sentinel lymph node is approached. The sentinel lymph node also is identified by visualization of isosulfan blue dye in the afferent lymph vessel and in the lymph node itself. Before removing the sentinel lymph node, a 10-second in vivo radioactivity count is obtained. After removal of the sentinel lymph node, a 10-second ex vivo radioactive count is obtained, and the lymph node is then sent to pathology for either permanent or frozen section analysis. The lowest false-negative rates for sentinel lymph node biopsy have been obtained when all blue lymph nodes and all lymph nodes with radiation counts greater than 10% of the 10-second ex vivo count of the sentinel lymph node are harvested (10% rule). Based on this, the gamma counter is employed before closing the axillary wound to measure residual radioactivity in the surgical bed. When necessary, a search is made for a second sentinel lymph node. This procedure is repeated until residual radioactivity in the surgical bed is less that 10% of the 10-second ex vivo count of the most radioactive sentinel lymph node.

Breast Conservation[117,118]

Breast conservation involves resection of the primary breast cancer with a margin of normal-appearing breast tissue, adjuvant radiation therapy, and assessment of axillary lymph node status. Resection of the primary breast cancer is alternatively called segmental resection, lumpectomy, partial mastectomy, and tylectomy. Conservation surgery is currently the standard treatment for women with stage I or II invasive breast cancer. Women with DCIS require only resection of the primary cancer and adjuvant radiation therapy. When a lumpectomy is performed, a curvilinear incision lying concentric to the nipple–areola complex is made in the skin overlying the breast cancer. Skin encompassing any prior biopsy site is excised, but skin excision is not otherwise necessary. The breast cancer is removed with an envelope of normal-appearing breast tissue that is adequate to achieve at least a 2-mm cancer-free margin. Specimen orientation is performed and additional margins from the surgical bed are taken as described previously. Requests for hormone receptor status and HER2/neu expression are conveyed to the pathologist.

After closure of the breast wound, dissection of the ipsilateral axillary lymph nodes has traditionally been completed for cancer staging and for control of regional disease. Ten to 15 level I and level II axillary lymph nodes are usually considered adequate for staging purposes. Sentinel lymph node biopsy is now the preferred staging procedure in the clinically uninvolved axilla. When the sentinel lymph node does not contain metastatic disease, axillary lymph node dissection is avoided. It is the surgeon's responsibility to insure

complete removal of cancer in the breast. If viable cancer cells remain within the breast at the periphery of the resection site, they will be incorporated into the healing scar, become poorly oxygenated, and subsequently will be less susceptible to radiation therapy. Surgical margins that are free of breast cancer will minimize the chances of local recurrence and will enhance cure rates. Local recurrence of breast cancer after conservation surgery is determined primarily by the adequacy of surgical margins. Cancer size and the extent of skin excision are not significant factors in this regard. It is the practice of many North American and European surgeons to undertake re-excision when residual cancer within 2 mm of a surgical margin is determined by histopathologic examination. If clear margins are not obtainable with re-excision, mastectomy is required.

Mastectomy and Axillary Dissection[119,120]

A skin-sparing mastectomy removes all breast tissue, the nipple–areola complex, and only 1 cm of skin around excised scars. There is a recurrence rate of less than 2% when skin-sparing mastectomy is used for T1 to T3 cancers. A total (simple) mastectomy removes all breast tissue, the nipple–areola complex, and skin (see Fig. 16-30). An extended simple mastectomy removes all breast tissue, the nipple–areola complex, skin, and the level I axillary lymph nodes. A modified radical mastectomy removes all breast tissue, the nipple–areola complex, skin, and the level I and level II axillary lymph nodes. The Halstead radical mastectomy removes all breast tissue and skin, the nipple–areola complex, the pectoralis major and pectoralis minor muscles, and the level I, II, and III axillary lymph nodes. Chemotherapy, hormone therapy, and radiation therapy for breast cancer have nearly eliminated the need for the radical mastectomy.

For a variety of biologic, economic, and psychosocial reasons, some women desire mastectomy rather than breast conservation. Women who are less concerned about cosmesis may view mastectomy as the most expeditious and desirable therapeutic option because it avoids the cost and inconvenience of radiation therapy. Women whose primary breast cancers have an extensive intraductal component undergo mastectomy because of very high local failure rates in the ipsilateral breast after breast conservation. Women with large cancers that occupy the subareolar and central portions of the breast and women with multicentric primary cancers also undergo mastectomy.

Modified Radical Mastectomy[120]

A modified radical mastectomy preserves both the pectoralis major and pectoralis minor muscles, allowing removal of level I and level II axillary lymph nodes but not the level III (apical) axillary lymph nodes (Figs. 16-33 and 16-34). The Patey modification removes the pectoralis minor muscle and allows complete dissection of the level III axillary lymph nodes (Figs. 16-35 and 16-36). A modified radical mastectomy permits preservation of the medial (anterior thoracic) pectoral nerve, which courses in the lateral neurovascular bundle of the axilla and usually penetrates the pectoralis minor to supply the lateral border of the pectoralis major. Anatomic boundaries of the modified radical mastectomy are the anterior margin of the latissimus dorsi muscle laterally; the midline of the sternum medially; the subclavius muscle superiorly; and the caudal extension of the breast 2 to 3 cm inferior to the inframammary fold inferiorly (see Fig. 16-33 inset). Skin-flap thickness varies with body habitus, but ideally is 7 to 8 mm inclusive of skin and tela subcutanea. Once the skin flaps are fully developed, the fascia of the pectoralis major muscle and the overlying breast tissue are elevated off the

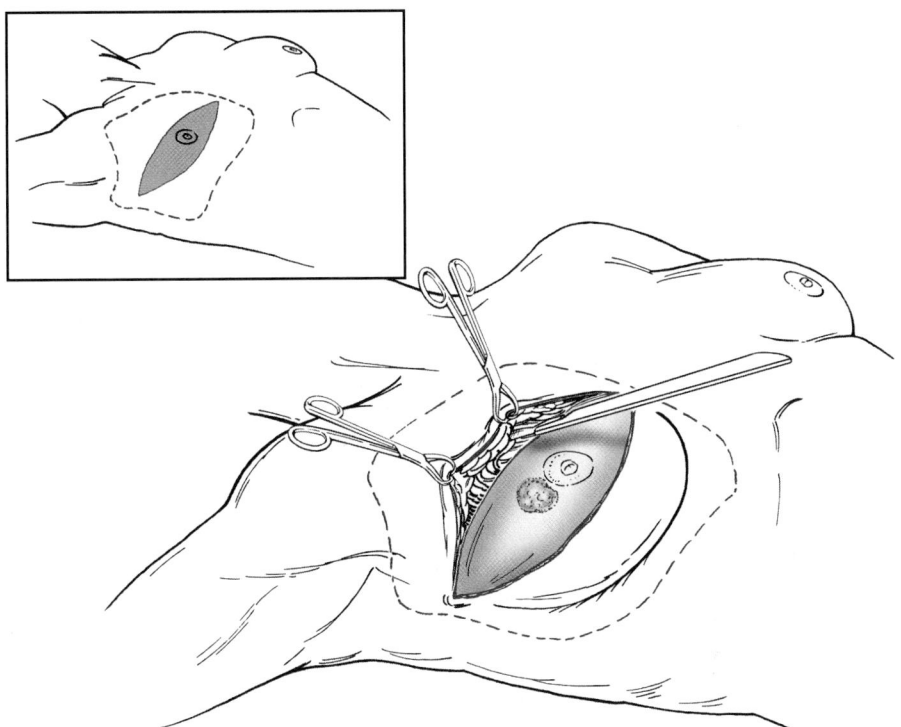

FIG. 16-33. Modified radical mastectomy: elevation of skin flaps. Skin flaps are 7 to 8 mm in thickness, inclusive of the skin and tela subcutanea. *Inset depicts the limits of the modified radical mastectomy.* [*Reproduced with permission from Bland KI et al: Modified radical mastectomy and total (simple) mastectomy, in Bland KI et al (eds): The Breast: Comprehensive Management of Benign and Malignant Diseases. Philadelphia, WB Saunders, 1998, p 905.*]

underlying musculature, allowing for the complete removal of the breast.

Subsequently, an axillary lymph node dissection is performed. The most lateral extent of the axillary vein is identified and the areolar tissue of the lateral axillary space is elevated as the vein is cleared on its anterior and inferior surfaces. The areolar tissues at the junction of the axillary vein with the anterior edge of the latissimus dorsi muscle, which include the lateral and subscapular lymph node groups (level I), are cleared in an inferomedial direction. Care is taken to preserve the thoracodorsal neurovascular bundle. The dissection then continues medially with clearance of the cen-

tral axillary lymph node group (level II). The long thoracic nerve of Bell is identified and preserved as it travels in the investing fascia of the serratus anterior muscle. Every effort is made to preserve this nerve because permanent disability with a winged scapula and shoulder weakness will follow denervation of the serratus anterior muscle. If there is palpable lymphadenopathy at the apex of the axilla, the tendinous portion of the pectoralis minor muscle is divided near its insertion onto the coracoid process (see Fig. 16-35 *inset*), which allows dissection of the axillary vein medially to the costoclavicular (Halsted's) ligament. Finally, the breast and axillary contents are removed from the surgical bed and are sent for pathologic

FIG. 16-34. Modified radical mastectomy: resection of breast tissue. The pectoralis major muscle is cleared of its fascia as the overlying breast is elevated. The latissimus dorsi muscle is the lateral boundary of the dissection. The cutaneous innervation of the skin of the lateral chest, axilla, and medial surface of the upper arm by lateral cutaneous branches of the intercostal nerves is illustrated. [*Reproduced with permission from Bland KI et al: Modified radical mastectomy and total (simple) mastectomy, in Bland KI et al (eds): The Breast: Comprehensive Management of Benign and Malignant Diseases. Philadelphia, WB Saunders, 1998, p 906.*]

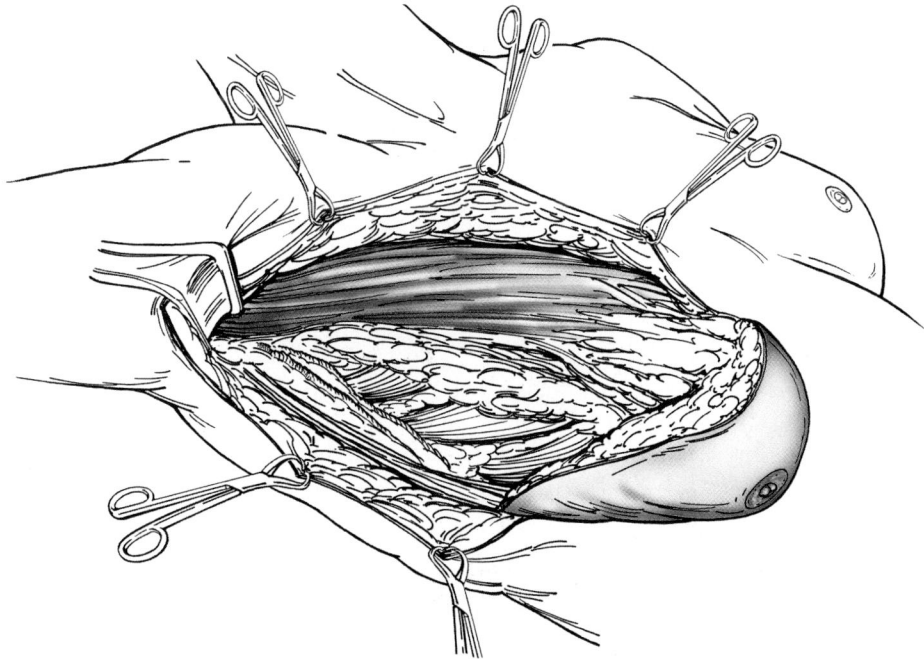

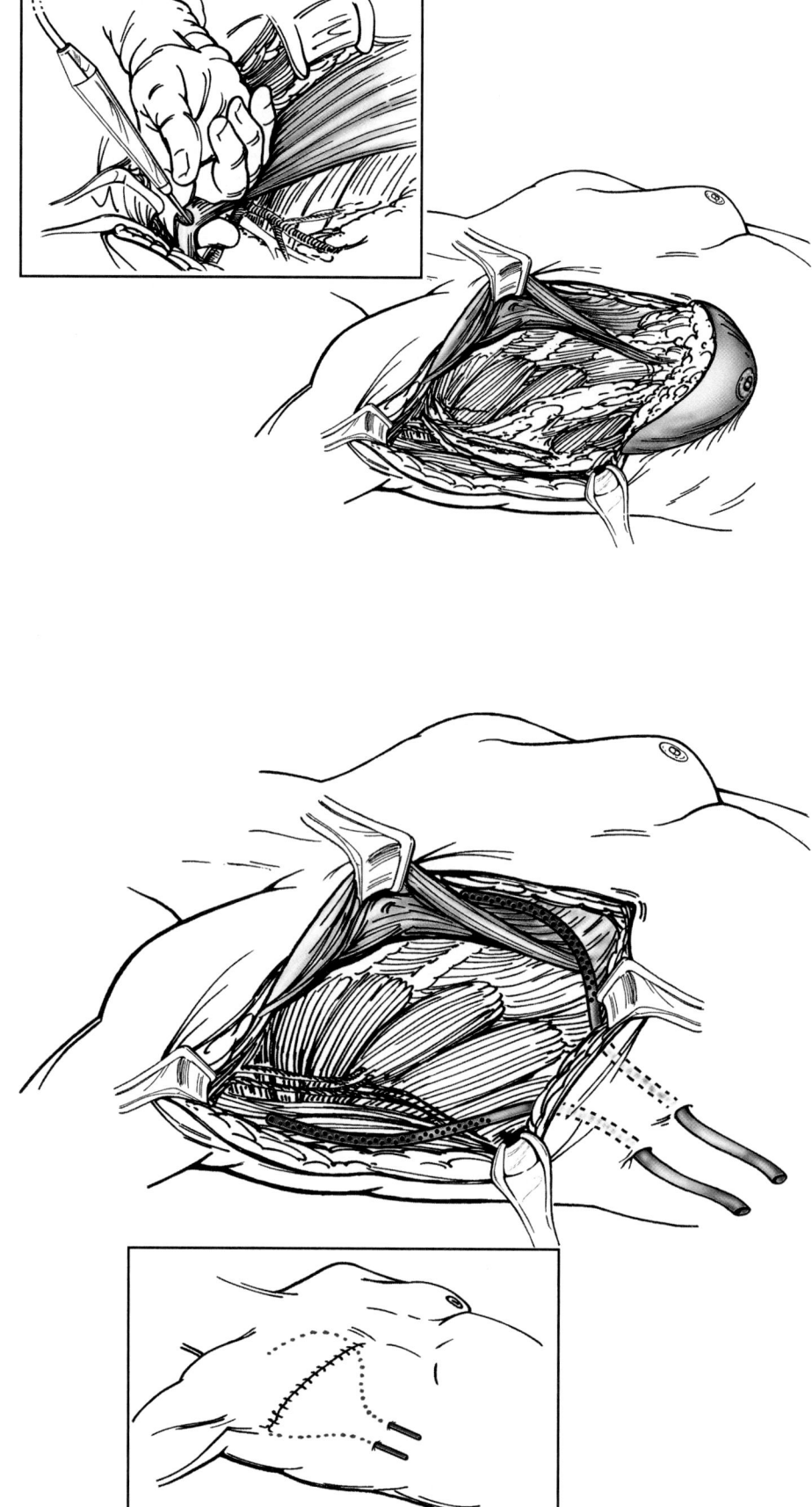

FIG. 16-35. Modified radical mastectomy (Patey modification): axillary lymph node dissection. The dissection proceeds from lateral to medial, with complete visualization of the anterior and inferior aspects of the axillary vein. Loose areolar tissue at the junction of the axillary vein and the anterior margin of the latissimus dorsi muscle is swept inferomedially inclusive of the lateral (axillary) lymph node group (level I). Care is taken to preserve the thoracodorsal artery, vein, and nerve in the deep axillary space. The lateral lymph node group is resected in continuity with the subscapular lymph node group (level I) and the external mammary lymph node group (level I). Dissection anterior to the axillary vein allows removal of the central lymph node group (level II) and the apical (subclavicular) lymph node group (level III). The superomedial limit of this dissection is the clavipectoral fascia (Halsted's ligament). *Inset* depicts division of the insertion of the pectoralis minor muscle at the coracoid process. The surgeon's finger shields the underlying brachial plexus. [*Reproduced with permission from Bland KI et al: Modified radical mastectomy and total (simple) mastectomy, in Bland KI et al (eds): The Breast: Comprehensive Management of Benign and Malignant Diseases. Philadelphia, WB Saunders, 1998, p 908.*]

FIG. 16-36. Modified radical mastectomy (Patey modification): completed dissection. The completed dissection includes the pectoralis minor muscle from its insertion to its origin from the second to fifth ribs. Rotter's lymph nodes (level I) are left attached to the pectoralis minor muscle as it is removed. Both medial and lateral pectoral nerves are preserved to ensure innervation of the lateral and medial heads (respectively) of the pectoralis major muscle. *Inset* depicts the positioning of closed-suction silastic catheters (10-F), which are brought out through the inferior flap. The lateral catheter is placed 2 cm inferior to the axillary vein. The medial catheter is positioned anterior to the pectoralis major muscle. [*Reproduced with permission from Bland KI et al: Modified radical mastectomy and total (simple) mastectomy, in Bland KI et al (eds): The Breast: Comprehensive Management of Benign and Malignant Diseases. Philadelphia, WB Saunders, 1998, p 909.*]

assessment. The Patey modification originally involved removal of the pectoralis muscle (see Fig. 16-36). However, some surgeons now only divide the tendon of the pectoralis minor muscle at its insertion onto the coracoid process while leaving the rest of the muscle intact.

Seromas beneath the skin flaps or in the axilla represent the most frequent complication of mastectomy and axillary lymph node dissection, reportedly occurring in as many as 30% of cases. The use of closed-system suction drainage reduces the incidence of this complication. Catheters are retained in the wound until drainage diminishes to less than 30 mL per day. Wound infections occur infrequently after a mastectomy and the majority occurs secondary to skin-flap necrosis. Culture of the infected wound for aerobic and anaerobic organisms, débridement, and antibiotics are effective management. Moderate or severe hemorrhage in the postoperative period is rare and is best managed with early wound exploration for control of hemorrhage and re-establishment of closed-system suction drainage. The incidence of functionally significant lymphedema after a modified radical mastectomy is 10%. Extensive axillary lymph node dissection, radiation therapy, the presence of pathologic lymph nodes, and obesity are predisposing factors. Individually fitted compressive sleeves and intermittent compression devices may be necessary.

Reconstruction of the Breast and Chest Wall[121]

The goals of reconstructive surgery following a mastectomy for breast cancer are wound closure and breast reconstruction, which is either immediate or delayed. For most women, wound closure after mastectomy is accomplished with simple approximation of the wound edges. However, if a more radical removal of skin and subcutaneous tissue is necessary, a skin graft provides functional coverage that will tolerate adjuvant radiation therapy. When soft-tissue defects are present that cannot be covered with a skin graft, myocutaneous flaps are employed. Breast reconstruction after prophylactic mastectomy or after mastectomy for early invasive breast cancer is performed immediately after surgery, while reconstruction following surgery for advanced breast cancer is delayed for 6 months after completion of adjuvant therapy to insure that locoregional control of disease is obtained. Many different types of myocutaneous flaps are employed for breast reconstruction, but the latissimus dorsi and the rectus abdominus myocutaneous flaps are most frequently used. The latissimus dorsi myocutaneous flap consists of a skin paddle based on the underlying latissimus dorsi muscle, which is supplied by the thoracodorsal artery with contributions from the posterior intercostal arteries. The transverse rectus abdominis myocutaneous (TRAM) flap consists of a skin paddle based on the underlying rectus abdominis muscle, which is supplied by vessels from the deep inferior epigastric artery. The free TRAM flap uses microvascular anastomoses to establish blood supply to the flap. When the bony chest wall is involved with cancer, resection of a portion of the bony chest wall is indicated. If only one or two ribs are resected and soft-tissue coverage is provided, reconstruction of the bony defect is usually not necessary as scar tissue will stabilize the chest wall. If more than two ribs are sacrificed, it is advisable to stabilize the chest wall with Marlex mesh, which is then covered with soft tissue by using a latissimus dorsi or TRAM flap.

NONSURGICAL BREAST CANCER THERAPIES

Radiation Therapy[122–128]

Radiation therapy is used for all stages of breast cancer. For women with limited DCIS (stage 0), in whom negative margins are achieved by lumpectomy or by re-excision, adjuvant radiation therapy is given to reduce the risk of local recurrence. Low-grade DCIS of the solid, cribriform, or papillary subtypes, which is less than 0.5 cm in diameter, is managed by excision alone. For women with stage I, IIa, or IIb breast cancer in which negative margins are achieved by lumpectomy or by re-excision, adjuvant radiation therapy is given to reduce the risk of local recurrence. Those women treated with mastectomy who have cancer at the surgical margins are at sufficiently high risk for local recurrence to warrant the use of adjuvant radiation therapy to the chest wall and supraclavicular lymph nodes. Women with metastatic disease involving four or more axillary lymph nodes and premenopausal women with metastatic disease involving one to three lymph nodes also are at increased risk for recurrence and are candidates for the use of chest wall and supraclavicular lymph node radiation therapy. In advanced locoregional breast cancer (stage IIIa or IIIb), women are at high risk for recurrent disease following surgical therapy and adjuvant radiation therapy is employed to reduce the recurrence rate (Fig. 16-37). Current recommendations for

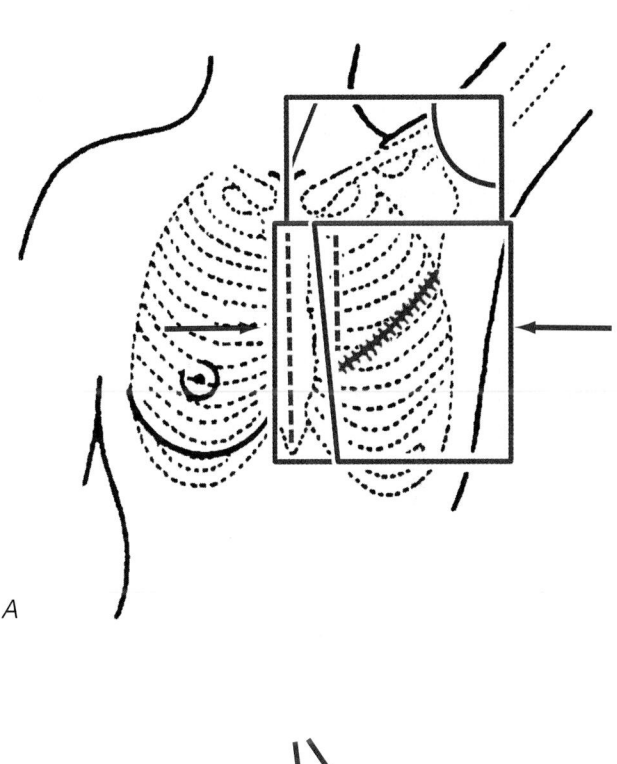

A

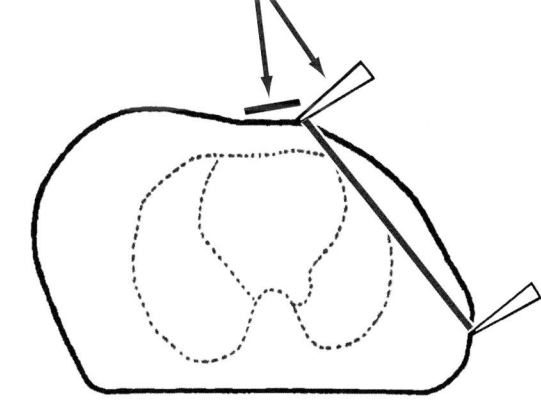

B

FIG. 16-37. Radiation therapy for stage IIIa and stage IIIb breast cancer. *A.* Comprehensive chest wall and regional lymph node radiation therapy. *B.* Cross-sectional view showing the tangential field. [*Reproduced with permission from Beenken SW et al: Advanced breast carcinoma (stages IIIa and IIIb), in Bland KI (ed): The Practice of General Surgery. Philadelphia: WB Saunders, 2002, p 983.*]

stages IIIa and IIIb breast cancer are (1) adjuvant radiation therapy to the breast and supraclavicular lymph nodes following neoadjuvant chemotherapy and lumpectomy with or without axillary lymph node dissection; (2) adjuvant radiation therapy to the chest wall and supraclavicular lymph nodes following neoadjuvant chemotherapy and mastectomy with or without axillary lymph node dissection; and (3) adjuvant radiation therapy to the chest wall and supraclavicular lymph nodes following lumpectomy or mastectomy with axillary lymph node dissection and adjuvant chemotherapy.

Chemotherapy

Adjuvant Chemotherapy[129–134]

The Early Breast Cancer Trialists' Collaborative Group overview analysis of adjuvant chemotherapy demonstrated reductions in the odds of recurrence and of death in women age 70 years or younger with stage I, IIa, or IIb breast cancer. For those age 70 years or older, the lack of definitive clinical trial data regarding adjuvant chemotherapy prevented definitive recommendations. Adjuvant chemotherapy is of minimal benefit to node-negative women with cancers 0.5 cm or less in size and is not recommended. Node-negative women with cancers 0.6 to 1.0 cm are divided into those with a low risk of recurrence and those with unfavorable prognostic features that portend a higher risk of recurrence and a need for adjuvant chemotherapy. Adverse prognostic factors include blood vessel or lymph vessel invasion, high nuclear grade, high histologic grade, HER2/neu overexpression, and negative hormone receptor status. Adjuvant chemotherapy is recommended for these women when unfavorable prognostic features are present. Table 16-15 lists the frequently used chemotherapy regimens for breast cancer.

For women with hormone receptor–negative cancers that are larger than 1 cm in size, adjuvant chemotherapy is appropriate. However, node-negative women with hormone receptor–positive cancers that are 1 to 3 cm in size are candidates for tamoxifen with or without chemotherapy. For special-type cancers (tubular, mucinous, medullary, etc), adjuvant chemotherapy or tamoxifen for cancers smaller than 3 cm in size is controversial. For node-positive women or women with a special-type cancer that is larger than 3 cm in size, the use of chemotherapy with or without tamoxifen is appropriate. Current treatment recommendations for operable stage IIIa breast cancer are a modified radical mastectomy followed by adjuvant chemotherapy with a doxorubicin-containing regimen followed by adjuvant radiation therapy. These recommendations are based in part on the results of NSABP B-15. In this study, node-positive women with tamoxifen-nonresponsive cancers who were age 59 years or younger were randomized to 2 months of therapy with Adriamycin and cyclophosphamide (AC) versus 6 months of cyclophosphamide, methotrexate, and CMF. There was no difference

Table 16-15
Chemotherapy Regimens for Breast Cancer

Node-Negative Women	Node-Positive Women
CMF	FAC or CEF
FAC	AC ± T
AC	A → CMF
	CMF
	EC

A = Adriamycin (doxorubicin); C = cyclophosphamide; E = epirubicin; F = 5-fluorouracil; M = methotrexate; T = Taxol (paclitaxel); → = "followed by."

SOURCE: Adapted with permission from Carlson RW et al: Breast cancer, in *National Comprehensive Cancer Network (NCCN) Practice Guidelines in Oncology* Vol. 2, 2002.

in relapse-free survival or overall survival rates and women preferred the shorter regimen.

Neoadjuvant Chemotherapy[135]

In the early 1970s, the National Cancer Institute in Milan, Italy, initiated two prospective, randomized, multimodality clinical trials for women with T3 or T4 breast cancer. The best results were achieved when surgery was interposed between chemotherapy courses, with 82% locoregional control and 25% 5-year disease-free survival. NSABP B-18 evaluated the role of neoadjuvant chemotherapy in women with operable stage III breast cancer. Women entered into this study were randomized to surgery followed by chemotherapy or neoadjuvant chemotherapy followed by surgery. There was no difference in the 5-year disease-free survival rate, but after neoadjuvant chemotherapy there was an increase in the number of lumpectomies performed. It was suggested that neoadjuvant chemotherapy be considered for the initial management of breast cancers judged too large for initial lumpectomy. Current recommendations for operable advanced locoregional breast cancer are neoadjuvant chemotherapy with an Adriamycin-containing regimen, followed by mastectomy or lumpectomy with axillary lymph node dissection if necessary, followed by adjuvant chemotherapy, followed by adjuvant radiation therapy. For inoperable stage IIIa and for stage IIIb breast cancer, neoadjuvant chemotherapy is used to decrease the locoregional cancer burden. This may then permit subsequent modified radical or radical mastectomy, which is followed by adjuvant chemotherapy and adjuvant radiation therapy.

Chemotherapy for Distant Metastases[136]

For women with stage IV breast cancer, an antiestrogen (usually tamoxifen) is the preferred therapy. However, women with hormone receptor–negative cancers with symptomatic visceral metastasis or with hormone refractory cancer may receive systemic chemotherapy. Pamidronate may be given to women with osteolytic bone metastases in addition to hormonal therapy or chemotherapy. Women with metastatic breast cancer may also be enrolled into clinical trials of high-dose chemotherapy with bone marrow or peripheral blood stem cell transplantation. No survival benefit for transplantation therapy has yet been shown.

Antiestrogen Therapy[129,137–141]

Within the cytosol of breast cancer cells are specific proteins (receptors) that bind and transfer steroid moieties into the cell nucleus to exert specific hormonal effects. The most widely studied hormone receptors are the estrogen receptor and progesterone receptor. Hormone receptors are detectable in more than 90% of well-differentiated ductal and lobular invasive cancers. Sequential studies of hormone receptor status reveal no differences between the primary cancer and metastatic disease in the same patient.

After binding to estrogen receptors in the cytosol, tamoxifen blocks the uptake of estrogen by breast tissue. Clinical responses to antiestrogen are evident in more than 60% of women with hormone receptor–positive breast cancers, but in less than 10% of women with hormone receptor–negative breast cancers. Diminished responsiveness at one-dose level may be overcome by escalation of the dose. An overview analysis by the Early Breast Cancer Trialists' Collaborative Group showed that adjuvant therapy with tamoxifen produced a 25% reduction in the annual risk of breast cancer recurrence and a 7% reduction in annual breast cancer mortality. The analysis also showed a 39% reduction in the risk of cancer in the contralateral breast. The major advantage of tamoxifen over chemotherapy is the absence of severe toxicity. Bone pain, hot flushes, nausea, vomiting, and fluid retention may occur. Thrombotic events occur in less than 3% of treated women. Cataract surgery is more frequently performed in patients receiving tamoxifen. A rare long-term risk of tamoxifen use is endometrial cancer. Tamoxifen therapy usually is discontinued after 5 years.

NSABP P-1 demonstrated a 49% reduction in the incidence of invasive breast cancer in high-risk women who were treated with tamoxifen. This reduction was demonstrated for all age groups treated, for all projected levels of risk, and for women with a prior history of either LCIS or atypical ductal hyperplasia. The reduction was demonstrable within the first year of follow-up and continued through a 6-year follow-up period. Women with a Gail relative risk assessment of 1.70 or greater are offered tamoxifen (20 mg/d) for up to 5 years to reduce the risk of breast cancer. Based on NSABP P-1, tamoxifen therapy is considered for all women with in situ cancer. The goals of such therapy are to decrease the risk of an ipsilateral recurrence after breast conservation for DCIS and to decrease the risk of a primary invasive breast cancer.

Node-negative women with hormone receptor–positive breast cancers that are 1 to 3 cm in size are candidates for adjuvant tamoxifen with or without chemotherapy. For node-positive women and for all women with a cancer that is more than 3 cm in size, the use of tamoxifen in addition to adjuvant chemotherapy is appropriate. Some oncologists recommend that tamoxifen be added to the neoadjuvant therapy regimen for women with advanced locoregional breast cancer, especially for women with hormone receptor–positive cancers. For women with stage IV breast cancer, an antiestrogen (usually tamoxifen), is the preferred initial therapy. For women with prior antiestrogen exposure, recommended second-line hormonal therapies include aromatase inhibitors in postmenopausal women and progestins, androgens, high-dose estrogen or oophorectomy (medical, surgical, or radioablative) in premenopausal women. Women who respond to hormonal therapy with either shrinkage of their breast cancer or with long-term stabilization of disease receive additional hormonal therapy at the time of progression. Women with hormone receptor–negative cancers, with symptomatic visceral metastasis, or with hormone refractory disease receive systemic chemotherapy rather than hormone therapy.

Ablative Endocrine Therapy[142]

In the past, oophorectomy, adrenalectomy, and/or hypophysectomy were the primary endocrine modalities used to treat metastatic breast cancer, but today, they are rarely employed. Oophorectomy was used for premenopausal breast cancer patients who presented with skin or bony metastases after a disease-free interval that exceeded 18 months. In contrast to this, pharmacologic doses of exogenous estrogens were given to similar postmenopausal women. For both groups, the response rates were nearly 30%. Adrenalectomy and hypophysectomy were effective in individuals who had previously responded to either oophorectomy or exogenous estrogen therapy, and the response to these additional procedures was nearly 30%. Visceral metastases (lung, liver) responded infrequently to any form of hormonal manipulation. Aminoglutethimide blocks enzymatic conversion of cholesterol to γ-5-pregnenolone and inhibits the conversion of androstenedione to estrogen in peripheral tissues. Dose-dependent and transient side effects include ataxia, dizziness, and lethargy. After treatment with this agent (medical adrenalectomy), adrenal suppression necessitates glucocorticoid therapy. Neither permanent adrenal insufficiency nor acute crises have been observed. Because the adrenal glands are the major site for production

of endogenous estrogens after menopause, aminoglutethimide has been compared prospectively with surgical adrenalectomy and hypophysectomy in postmenopausal women and is equally efficacious.

Anti-HER2/neu Antibody Therapy[143–145]

The determination of HER2/neu expression for all newly diagnosed patients with breast cancer is now recommended. It is used for prognostic purposes in node-negative patients; to assist in the selection of adjuvant chemotherapy because response rates appear to be better with Adriamycin-based adjuvant chemotherapy in patients with cancer that overexpress HER2/neu; and baseline information for when the patient develops recurrent disease that may benefit from anti-HER2/neu therapy (trastuzumab, Herceptin). Patients with cancers that overexpress HER2/neu may benefit if trastuzumab is added to paclitaxel chemotherapy. Considerable cardiotoxicity may develop if trastuzumab is added to Adriamycin-based chemotherapy.

SPECIAL CLINICAL SITUATIONS

Nipple Discharge

Unilateral Nipple Discharge

Nipple discharge is suggestive of cancer if it is spontaneous, unilateral, localized to a single duct, occurs in women age 40 years or more, is bloody, or is associated with a mass. A trigger point on the breast may be present where pressure induces discharge from a single duct. In this circumstance, mammography is indicated. A ductogram is also useful and consists of the cannulation of a single duct with a small nylon catheter or needle and the injection of 1.0 mL of water-soluble contrast solution. Nipple discharge associated with a cancer is clear, bloody, or serous. Testing for the presence of hemoglobin is helpful, but hemoglobin may also be detected when only an intraductal papilloma or duct ectasia is present. Definitive diagnosis depends on excisional biopsy of the offending duct and any mass lesion. A 3.0 lacrimal duct probe is used to identify the duct that requires excision. Needle localization biopsy is performed when the questionable mass lies more than 3.0 cm from the nipple.

Bilateral Nipple Discharge

Nipple discharge is suggestive of a benign condition if it is bilateral and multiductal in origin, occurs in women age 39 years or less, or is milky or blue green in color. Prolactin-secreting pituitary adenomas are responsible for bilateral nipple discharge in less than 2% of cases. If serum prolactin levels are repeatedly elevated, plain x-rays of the sella turcica are indicated and thin-section CT scan is required. Optical nerve compression, visual field loss, and infertility are associated with large pituitary adenomas.

Axillary Lymph Node Metastases with Unknown Primary Cancer[146]

A woman who presents with an axillary lymph node metastasis that is consistent with a breast cancer metastasis has a 90% probability of harboring an occult breast cancer. However, axillary lymphadenopathy is the initial presenting sign in only 1% of breast cancer patients. Fine-needle biopsy and/or open biopsy of an enlarged axillary lymph node is performed when metastatic disease cannot be excluded. When metastatic cancer is found, immunohistochemical analysis may classify the cancer as epithelial, melanocytic, or lymphoid in origin. The presence of hormone receptors suggests a breast cancer, but is not diagnostic. The search for a primary cancer includes careful examination of the thyroid, breast, and pelvis, including the rectum. Routine radiologic and laboratory studies include chest x-ray, liver function studies, and mammography. Chest, abdominal, and pelvic CT scans may be helpful. Suspicious mammography findings necessitate breast biopsy. When a breast cancer is found, treatment consists of an axillary lymph node dissection with a mastectomy or with whole-breast radiation therapy. Consideration is given to adjuvant chemotherapy and tamoxifen.

Breast Cancer During Pregnancy[147]

Breast cancer occurs in 1 of every 3000 pregnant women and axillary lymph node metastases are present in up to 75% of these women. The average age of the pregnant woman with breast cancer is 34 years. Less than 25% of the breast nodules developing during pregnancy and lactation will be cancerous. Ultrasonography and needle biopsy are used in the diagnosis of these nodules. Open biopsy may be required. Mammography is rarely indicated because of its decreased sensitivity during pregnancy and lactation and because of the risk of radiation injury to the fetus. Approximately 30% of the benign conditions encountered will be unique to pregnancy and lactation (galactoceles, lobular hyperplasia, lactating adenoma and mastitis or abscess). Once a breast cancer is diagnosed, CBC, chest x-ray (with shielding of the abdomen), and liver function studies are performed.

Because of the deleterious effects of radiation therapy on the fetus, a modified radical mastectomy is the surgical procedure of choice during the first and second trimesters of pregnancy, even though there is an increased risk of spontaneous abortion following first trimester anesthesia. During the third trimester, lumpectomy with axillary node dissection is considered if adjuvant radiation therapy is deferred until after delivery. Lactation is suppressed. Chemotherapy administered during the first trimester carries a risk of spontaneous abortion and a 12% risk of birth defects. There is no evidence of teratogenicity resulting from administration of chemotherapeutic agents in the second and third trimesters. Pregnant women with breast cancer present at a later stage of disease because breast tissue changes that occur in the hormone-rich environment of pregnancy obscure early cancers. However, pregnant women with breast cancer have a prognosis, stage by stage, that is similar to that of nonpregnant women with breast cancer.

Male Breast Cancer[148,149]

Less than 1% of all breast cancers occur in men. The incidence appears to be highest among North Americans and the British, in whom breast cancer constitutes as much as 1.5% of all male cancers. Jewish and African American males have the highest incidence. Male breast cancer is preceded by gynecomastia in 20% of men. It is associated with radiation exposure, estrogen therapy, testicular feminizing syndromes, and with Klinefelter's syndrome (XXY). Breast cancer is rarely seen in young males and has a peak incidence in the sixth decade of life. A firm, nontender mass in the male breast requires investigation. Skin or chest wall fixation is particularly worrisome.

DCIS makes up less than 15% of male breast cancer, while infiltrating NST makes up more than 85%. Special-type cancers, including infiltrating lobular carcinoma, have occasionally been reported. Male breast cancer is staged in an identical fashion to female breast cancer, and, stage by stage, men with breast cancer have the same survival rate as women. Overall, men do worse because of the advanced stage of their cancer (stage III or IV) at the time of diagnosis. The treatment of male breast cancer is surgical, with the most common procedure being a modified radical mastectomy. Adjuvant radiation therapy is appropriate in cases where there is a high risk for local recurrence. Eighty percent of male breast cancers

are hormone receptor–positive, and adjuvant tamoxifen is considered. Systemic chemotherapy is considered for men with hormone receptor–negative cancers and for men whose cancers relapse after tamoxifen therapy.

Phyllodes Tumors[150]

The nomenclature, presentation, and diagnosis of phyllodes tumors (including cystosarcoma phyllodes) have posed many problems for surgeons. These tumors are classified as benign, borderline, or malignant. Borderline tumors have a greater potential for local recurrence. Mammography evidence of calcifications and morphologic evidence of necrosis do not distinguish between benign, borderline, and malignant phyllodes tumors. Consequently, it is difficult to differentiate benign phyllodes tumors from the malignant variant and from fibroadenomas. Phyllodes tumors are usually sharply demarcated from the surrounding breast tissue, which is compressed and distorted. Connective tissue composes the bulk of these tumors, which have mixed gelatinous, solid, and cystic areas. Cystic areas represent sites of infarction and necrosis. These gross alterations give the gross cut tumor surface its classical leaf-like (phyllodes) appearance. The stroma of a phyllodes tumor generally has greater cellular activity than that of a fibroadenoma. Following microdissection to harvest clusters of stromal cells from fibroadenomas and from phyllodes tumors, molecular biology techniques have shown the stromal cells of fibroadenomas to be either polyclonal or monoclonal (derived from a single progenitor cell), while those of phyllodes tumors are always monoclonal in nature.

Most malignant phyllodes tumors (Fig. 16-38) contain liposarcomatous or rhabdomyosarcomatous elements rather than fibrosarcomatous elements. Evaluation of the number of mitoses and the presence or absence of invasive foci at the tumor margins may help to identify a malignant tumor. Small phyllodes tumors are excised with a 1-cm margin of normal-appearing breast tissue. When the diagnosis of a phyllodes tumor with suspicious malignant elements is made, re-excision of the biopsy site to insure complete excision of the tumor with a 1-cm margin of normal-appearing breast tissue is indicated. Large phyllodes tumors may require mastectomy. Axillary dissection is not recommended as axillary lymph node metastases rarely occur.

Inflammatory Breast Carcinoma[151]

Inflammatory breast carcinoma (stage IIIb) accounts for less than 3% of breast cancers. This cancer is characterized by the skin changes of brawny induration, erythema with a raised edge, and edema (peau d'orange). Permeation of the dermal lymph vessels by cancer cells is seen in skin biopsies. There may be an associated breast mass (Fig. 16-39). The clinical differentiation of inflammatory breast cancer may be extremely difficult, especially when a locally advanced scirrhous carcinoma invades dermal lymph vessels skin to produce peau d'orange and lymphangitis (Table 16-16). Inflammatory breast cancer may also be mistaken for a bacterial infection of the breast. More than 75% of women afflicted with inflammatory breast cancer present with palpable axillary lymphadenopathy and frequently also have distant metastases. A report of the SEER program found distant metastases at diagnosis in 25% of white women with inflammatory breast carcinoma.

Surgery alone and surgery with adjuvant radiation therapy have produced disappointing results in women with inflammatory breast cancer. However, neoadjuvant chemotherapy with an Adriamycin-containing regimen may effect dramatic regressions in up to 75% of cases. In this setting, mastectomy, modified radical mastectomy, or

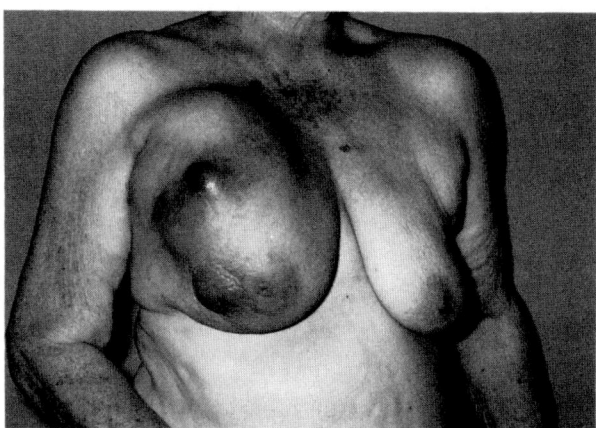

A

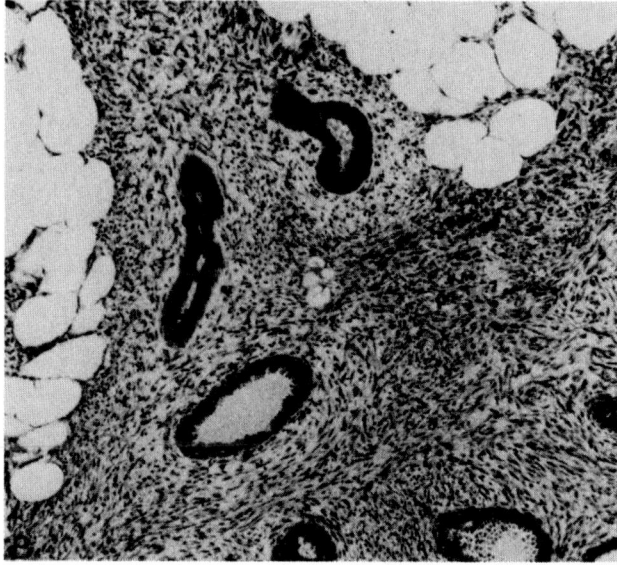

B

FIG. 16-38. *A. Malignant phyllodes tumor (cystosarcoma phyllodes). B. Histology of a malignant phyllodes tumor (hematoxylin and eosin stain, x100).*

radical mastectomy is performed to remove residual cancer from the chest wall and axilla. Adjuvant chemotherapy is then given. Finally, the chest wall and the supraclavicular, internal mammary, and axillary lymph node basins receive adjuvant radiation therapy. This multimodal approach results in 5-year survival rates that approach 30%.

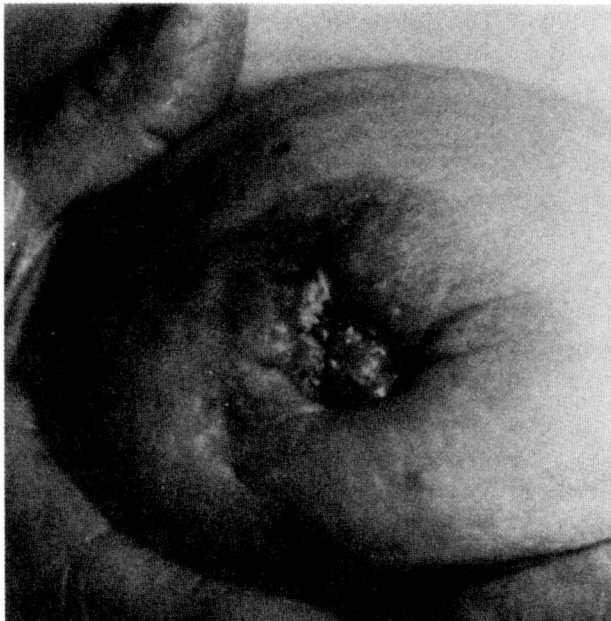

FIG. 16-39. *Inflammatory breast carcinoma. Stage IIIb cancer of the breast with erythema, skin edema (peau d'orange), nipple retraction, and satellite skin nodules.*

Rare Breast Cancers[152]

Squamous Cell (Epidermoid) Carcinoma

This rare cancer arises from metaplasia within the duct system and generally is devoid of distinctive clinical or radiographic characteristics. Regional metastases occur in 25% of patients, while distant metastases are rare.

Adenoid Cystic Carcinoma

This cancer is very rare, accounting for less than 0.1% of all breast cancers. It is typically indistinguishable from adenoid cystic carcinoma arising in salivary tissues. These cancers are generally 1 to 3 cm in diameter at presentation and are well circumscribed. Axillary lymph node metastases are rare, but deaths from pulmonary metastases from have been reported.

Apocrine Carcinoma

These well-differentiated cancers have rounded vesicular nuclei and prominent nucleoli. There is a very low mitotic rate and little variation in cellular features. However, apocrine carcinomas may display an aggressive growth pattern.

Table 16-16
Inflammatory vs. Noninflammatory Breast Cancer

Inflammatory	*Noninflammatory*
Dermal lymph vessel invasion is present with or without inflammatory changes.	Inflammatory changes are present without dermal lymph vessel invasion.
Cancer is not sharply delineated.	Cancer is better delineated.
Erythema and edema frequently involve more than 33% of the skin over the breast.	Erythema is usually confined to the lesion and edema is less extensive.
Lymph node involvement is present in more than 75% of cases.	Lymph nodes are involved in approximately 50% of the cases.
Distant metastases are present in 25% of cases.	Distant metastases are more common at initial presentation.
	Distant metastases are less common at presentation.

SOURCE: Modified from Chittoor SR, Swain SM: Locally advanced breast cancer: Role of medical oncology in Bland KI, Copeland EM (eds): *The Breast: Comprehensive Management of Benign and Malignant Diseases.* Philadelphia: WB Saunders, 1998, p 1281.

Sarcomas

Sarcomas of the breast are histologically similar to soft-tissue sarcomas at other anatomic sites. This diverse group includes fibrosarcoma, malignant fibrous histiocytoma, liposarcoma, leiomyosarcoma, malignant schwannoma, rhabdomyosarcoma, osteogenic sarcoma, and chondrosarcoma. The clinical presentation is typically that of a large, painless breast mass with rapid growth. Diagnosis is by core-needle biopsy or by open biopsy. Sarcomas are graded based on cellularity, degree of differentiation, nuclear atypia, and mitotic activity. Primary treatment is wide local excision, which may necessitate mastectomy. Axillary dissection is not indicated unless there is palpable lymphadenopathy. Angiosarcomas are classified as de novo, as postradiation, or as arising in postmastectomy lymphedema. In 1948, Stewart and Treves described lymphangiosarcoma of the upper extremity in women with ipsilateral lymphedema following radical mastectomy. Angiosarcoma is now the preferred name. The average interval between modified radical or radical mastectomy and the development of an angiosarcoma is 10.5 years. Sixty percent of women developing this cancer have a history of adjuvant radiation therapy. Forequarter amputation may be necessary to palliate the ulcerative complications and advanced lymphedema.

Lymphomas

Primary lymphomas of the breast are rare, and there are two distinct clinicopathologic variants. One type occurs in women age 39 years or less, is frequently bilateral, and has the histologic features of a Burkitt lymphoma. The second type is seen in women age 40 years or more and is usually of the B-cell type. Breast involvement by Hodgkin's lymphoma has been reported. An occult breast lymphoma may be diagnosed after detection of palpable axillary lymphadenopathy. Treatment depends on the stage of disease. Lumpectomy or mastectomy may be required. Axillary dissection for staging and for clearance of palpable disease is appropriate. Recurrent or progressive locoregional disease is best managed by chemotherapy and radiation therapy. The prognosis is favorable, with 5- and 10-year survival rates of 74 and 51%, respectively.

References

1. Breasted JH: *The Edwin Smith Surgical Papyrus. Classics of Med Lib.* Vol. III. Chicago: University of Chicago Press, 1930, p 405.
2. le Dran F: *Mémoire avec une précis de plusieurs observations sur le cancer. Mem Acad Roy Chir Paris* 3:1, 1757.
3. Moore C: On the influence of inadequate operations on the theory of cancer. *R Med Chir Soc Lond* 1:244, 1867.
4. Halsted WS: The results of operations for the cure of cancer of the breast performed at the Johns Hopkins Hospital from June 1889 to January 1894. *Johns Hopkins Hosp Rep* 4:297, 1894.
5. Meyer W: An improved method of the radical operation for carcinoma of the breast. *Med Rec* 46:746, 1894.
6. Patey DH, Dyson WH: The prognosis of carcinoma of the breast in relation to the type of operation performed. *Br J Cancer* 2:7, 1948.
7. Madden JL: Modified radical mastectomy. *Surg Gynecol Obstet* 121:1221, 1965.
8. Maddox MA, Carpenter JT, Laws HL, et al: A randomized prospective trial of radical (Halstead) mastectomy versus modified radical mastectomy in 311 breast cancer patients. *Ann Surg* 198:207, 1983.
9. Bland KI, Romrell LJ: Congenital and acquired disturbances of breast development and growth, in Bland KI, Copeland EM III (eds): *The Breast: Comprehensive Management of Benign Malignant Diseases.* Philadelphia: WB Saunders, 1998, p 214.
10. Romrell LJ, Bland KI: Anatomy of the breast, axilla, chest wall, and related metastatic sites in Bland KI, Copeland EM III (eds): *The Breast: Comprehensive Management of Benign Malignant Diseases.* Philadelphia: WB Saunders, 1998, p 19.
11. Rosenbloom AL: Breast physiology: Normal and abnormal development and function in Bland KI, Copeland EM III (eds): *The Breast: Comprehensive Management of Benign Malignant Diseases.* Philadelphia: WB Saunders, 1998, p 38.
12. Lonnerdal B: Nutritional and physiologic significance of human milk proteins. *Am J Clin Nutr* 77:1537S, 2003.
13. Van de Perre P: Transfer of antibody via mother's milk. *Vaccine* 21:3374, 2003.
14. Bland KI, Graves TA: Gynecomastia, in Bland KI, Copeland EM III (eds): *The Breast: Comprehensive Management of Benign Malignant Diseases.* Philadelphia: WB Saunders, 1998, p 153.
15. Bland KI: Inflammatory, infectious, and metabolic disorders of the breast in Bland KI, Copeland EM III (eds): *The Breast: Comprehensive Management of Benign Malignant Diseases.* Philadelphia: WB Saunders, 1998, p 75.
16. Camiel MR: Mondor's disease in the breast. *Am J Obstet Gynecol* 152:879, 1985.
17. Hughes LE, Mansel RE, Webster DJT: Aberrations of normal development and involution (ANDI): A concept of benign breast disorders based on pathogenesis, in Hughes LE, Mansel RE, Webster DJT (eds): *Benign Disorders and Diseases of the Breast Concepts and Clinical Management,* 2nd ed. Philadelphia: WB Saunders, 2000, p 21, 73.
18. Archer F, Omar N: The fine structure of fibroadenoma of the human breast. *J Pathol* 99:113, 1969.
19. Page DL, Anderson TJ: *Diagnostic Histopathology of the Breast.* Edinburgh: Churchill Livingstone, 1987.
20. Page DL, Simpson JF: Benign, high-risk, and premalignant lesions of the breast, in Bland KI, Copeland EM III (eds): *The Breast: Comprehensive Management of Benign Malignant Diseases.* Philadelphia: WB Saunders, 1998, p 191.
21. Haagensen CD: *Diseases of the Breast,* 3rd ed., Philadelphia: WB Saunders, 1986.
22. Gadd MA, Souba WW: Evaluation and treatment of benign breast disorders, in Bland KI, Copeland EM III (eds): *The Breast: Comprehensive Management of Benign Malignant Diseases.* Philadelphia: WB Saunders, 1998, p 233.
23. Marchant DJ: Benign breast disease. *Obstet Gynecol Clin North Am* 29:1, 2002.
24. Hulka BS: Epidemiologic analysis of breast and gynecologic cancers. *Prog Clin Biol Res* 396:17, 1997.
25. Bernstein L, Henderson BE, Hanisch R, et al: Physical exercise and reduced risk of breast cancer in young women. *J Natl Cancer Inst* 86:1403, 1994.
26. Pujol P, Galtier-Dereure F, Bringer J: Obesity and breast cancer risk, *Hum Reprod* 12(Suppl 1):116, 1997.
27. Goss PE, Sierra S: Current perspectives on radiation-induced breast cancer. *J Clin Oncol* 16:338, 1998.
28. Wynder EL, Cohen LA, Muscat JE, et al: Breast cancer: Weighing the evidence for a promoting role of dietary fat. *J Natl Cancer Inst* 89:766, 1997.
29. Singletary SE: Rating the risk factors for breast cancer. *Ann Surg* 237:474, 2003.
30. Blackburn GL, Copeland T, Khaodhiar L, Buckley RB: Diet and breast cancer. *J Womens Health (Larchmt)* 12:183, 2003.
31. Claus EB, Risch N, Thompson WD: Autosomal dominant inheritance of early-onset breast cancer: Implications for risk prediction. *Cancer* 73:643, 1994.
32. Domchek SM, Eisen A, Calzone K, et al: Application of breast cancer risk prediction models in clinical practice. *J Clin Oncol* 21:593, 2003.
33. Grodstein F, Stampfer MJ, Colditz GA, et al: Postmenopausal hormone therapy and mortality. *N Engl J Med* 336:1769, 1997.
34. Wu K, Brown P: Is low-dose tamoxifen useful for the treatment and prevention of breast cancer? *J Natl Cancer Inst* 95:766, 2003.

35. Kerlikowske K, Grady D, Rubin SM, et al: Efficacy of screening mammography: A meta-analysis. *JAMA* 273:149, 1995.

36. Rowe PM: ACS orders mammography for younger women. *Lancet* 349:928, 1997.

37. Fisher B, Costantino JP, Wickerham DL, et al: Tamoxifen for prevention of breast cancer: Report of the National Surgical Adjuvant Breast and Bowel Project P-1 Study. *J Natl Cancer Inst* 90:1371, 1998.

38. Hartmann LC, Schaid DJ, Woods JE, et al: Efficacy of bilateral prophylactic mastectomy in women with a family history of breast cancer. *N Engl J Med* 340:77, 1999.

39. Schrag D, Kuntz KM, Garber JE, et al: Decision analysis—Effects of prophylactic mastectomy and oophorectomy on life expectancy among women with *BRCA1* or *BRCA2* mutations. *N Engl J Med* 336:1465, 1997.

40. Sakorafas GH: The management of women at high risk for the development of breast cancer: Risk estimation and preventative strategies [review]. *Cancer Treat Rev* 29:79, 2003.

41. Vogel VG: Management of the high-risk patient [review]. *Surg Clin North Am* 83:733, 2003.

42. Wooster R, Weber BL: Breast and ovarian cancer. *N Engl J Med* 348:2339, 2003.

43. Gowen LC, Avrutskaya AV, Latour AM, et al: BRCA1 required for transcription-coupled repair of oxidative DNA damage. *Science* 281:1009, 1998.

44. Roa BB, Boyd AA, Bolcik K, et al: Ashkenazi Jewish population frequencies for common mutations in BRCA1 and BRCA2. *Nat Genet* 14:185, 1996.

45. Ford D, Easton DF, Stratton M, et al: Genetic heterogeneity and penetrance analysis of the BRCA1 and BRCA2 genes in breast cancer families. The Breast Cancer Linkage Consortium. *Am J Hum Genet* 62:676, 1998.

46. Rosen EM, Fan S, Pestell RG, Goldberg ID: BRCA1 gene in breast cancer. *J Cell Physiol* 196:19, 2003.

47. Martin AM, Weber BL: Genetic and hormonal risk factors in breast cancer. *J Natl Cancer Inst* 92:1126, 2000.

48. Oddoux C, Struewing JP, Clayton CM, et al: The carrier frequency of the BRCA2 6174delT mutation among Ashkenazi Jewish individuals is approximately 1%. *Nat Genet* 14:188, 1996.

49. Warner E, Foulkes W, Goodwin P, et al: Prevalence and penetrance of BRCA1 and BRCA2 gene mutations in unselected Ashkenazi Jewish women with breast cancer. *J Natl Cancer Inst* 91:1241, 1999.

50. Schneider KA: Genetic counseling for BRCA1/BRCA2 testing. *Genet Test* 1:91, 1997.

51. Guinee VF: Epidemiology of breast cancer, in Bland KI, Copeland EM III (eds): *The Breast: Comprehensive Management of Benign Malignant Diseases.* Philadelphia: WB Saunders, 1998, p 339.

52. Jemal A, Murray T, Samuels A, et al: Cancer statistics, 2003. *CA Cancer J Clin* 53:5, 2003.

53. Bloom HJG, Richardson WW, Harries EJ, et al: Natural history of untreated breast cancer (1805–1933): Comparison of untreated and treated cases according to histological grade of malignancy. *Br Med J* 5299:213, 1962.

54. Lagios MD, Page DL: In situ carcinomas of the breast: Ductal carcinoma in situ, Paget's disease, lobular carcinoma in situ, in Bland KI, Copeland EM III (eds): *The Breast: Comprehensive Management of Benign Malignant Diseases.* Philadelphia: WB Saunders, 1998, p 261.

55. Broders AC: Carcinoma in situ contrasted with benign penetrating epithelium. *JAMA* 99:1670, 1932.

56. Foote FW Jr., Stewart FW: Lobular carcinoma in situ: A rare form of mammary carcinoma. *Am J Pathol* 17:491, 1941.

57. Adamovich TL, Simmons RM: Ductal carcinoma in situ with microinvasion. *Am J Surg* 186:112, 2003.

58. Seth A, Kitching R, Landberg G, et al: Gene expression profiling of ductal carcinomas in situ and invasive breast tumors. *Anticancer Res* 23:2043, 2003.

59. Gallagher HS, Martin JE: The study of mammary carcinoma by mammography and whole organ sectioning. *Cancer* 23:855, 1969.

60. Simpson JF, Wilkinson EJ: Malignant neoplasia of the breast: Infiltrating carcinomas, in Bland KI, Copeland EM III (eds): *The Breast: Comprehensive Management of Benign Malignant Diseases.* Philadelphia: WB Saunders, 1998, p 285.

61. Devitt JE, Barr JR: The clinical recognition of cystic carcinoma of the breast. *Surg Gynecol Obstet* 159:130, 1984.

62. Jatoi I: Screening clinical breast examination. *Surg Clin North Am* 83:789, 2003.

63. Rosato FE, Rosato EL: Examination techniques: Roles of the physician and patient in evaluating breast diseases, in Bland KI, Copeland EM III (eds): *The Breast: Comprehensive Management of Benign Malignant Diseases.* Philadelphia: WB Saunders, 1998, p 615.

64. Bassett LW: Breast imaging, in Bland KI, Copeland EM III (eds): *The Breast: Comprehensive Management of Benign Malignant Diseases.* Philadelphia: WB Saunders, 1998, p 648.

65. Miller AB: Screening and detection, in Bland KI, Copeland EM III (eds): *The Breast: Comprehensive Management of Benign Malignant Diseases.* Philadelphia: WB Saunders, 1998, p 625.

66. Fletcher SW, Elmore JG: Clinical practice. Mammographic screening for breast cancer. *N Engl J Med* 348:1672, 2003.

67. Schnall MD: Breast MR imaging. *Radiol Clin North Am* 41:43, 2003.

68. Robinson DS, Sundaram M: Stereotactic imaging and breast biopsy, in Bland KI, Copeland EM III (eds): *The Breast: Comprehensive Management of Benign Malignant Diseases.* Philadelphia: WB Saunders, 1998, p 698.

69. Wilkinson EJ, Masood S: Cytologic needle samplings of the breast: Techniques and end results, in Bland KI, Copeland EM III (eds): *The Breast: Comprehensive Management of Benign Malignant Diseases.* Philadelphia: WB Saunders, 1998, p 705.

70. Yeatman TJ, Bland KI: Assessment and designation of breast cancer stage, in Bland KI, Copeland EM III (eds): *The Breast: Comprehensive Management of Benign Malignant Diseases.* Philadelphia: WB Saunders, 1998, p 400.

71. Haffty BG: Molecular and genetic markers in the local-regional management of breast cancer. *Semin Radiat Oncol* 12:329, 2002.

72. Esteva FJ, Sahin AA, Cristofanilli M, et al: Molecular prognostic factors for breast cancer metastasis and survival. *Semin Radiat Oncol* 12:319, 2002.

73. Dillon DA: Molecular markers in the diagnosis and staging of breast cancer. *Semin Radiat Oncol* 12:305, 2002.

74. Rogers CE, Loveday RL, Drew PJ, et al: Molecular prognostic indicators in breast cancer. *Eur J Surg Oncol* 28:467, 2002.

75. Morabito A, Magnani E, Gion M, et al: Prognostic and predictive indicators in operable breast cancer. *Clin Breast Cancer* 3:381, 2003.

76. Van Dierdendonck, Wijsman JH, Keijzer A, et al: Cell-cycle-related staining patterns of anti-proliferative cell nuclear antigen monoclonal antibodies. Comparison with BrdUrd labeling and Ki-67 staining. *Am J Pathol* 138:1165, 1991.

77. Monaghan P, Perusinghe NP, Nicholson RI, et al: Growth factor stimulation of proliferating cell nuclear antigen (PCNA) in human breast epithelium in organ culture. *Cell Biol Int Rep* 15:561, 1991.

78. Siitonen SM, Isola JJ, Rantala IS, et al: Intratumor variation in cell proliferation in breast carcinoma as determined by antiproliferating cell nuclear antigen monoclonal antibody automated image analysis. *Am J Clin Pathol* 99:226, 1993.

79. Tuccari G, Rizzo A, Muscara M, et al: PCNA/cyclin expression in breast carcinomas: Its relationships with Ki-67, ER, PgR immunostaining and clinico-pathologic aspects. *Pathologica* 85:47, 1993.

80. Allan DJ, Howell A, Roberts SA, et al: Reduction in apoptosis relative to mitosis in histologically normal epithelium accompanies fibrocystic change and carcinoma of the premenopausal human breast. *J Pathol* 167:25, 1992.

81. Binder C, Marx D, Binder L, et al: Expression of bax in relation to bcl-2 and other predictive parameters in breast cancer. *Ann Oncol* 7:129, 1996.

82. Bargou RC, Daniel PT, Mapara MY, et al: Expression of the bcl-2 gene family in normal and malignant breast tissue: Low bax-alpha

expression in tumor cells correlates with resistance towards apoptosis. *Int J Cancer* 60:854, 1995.

83. Brown LF, Berse B, Jackman RW, et al: Expression of vascular permeability factor (vascular endothelial growth factor) and its receptors in breast cancer. *Hum Pathol* 26:86, 1995.

84. Gasparini G, Toi M, Gion M, et al: Prognostic significance of vascular endothelial growth factor protein in node-negative breast carcinoma. *J Natl Cancer Inst* 89:139, 1997.

85. Tsutsumi Y, Naber SP, DeLellis RA, et al: Neu oncogene protein and epidermal growth factor receptor are independently expressed in benign and malignant breast tissues. *Hum Pathol* 21:750, 1990.

86. Van de Vijver MJ, Peterse JL, Mooi WJ, et al: Neu-protein overexpression in breast cancer: Association with comedo-type ductal carcinoma in situ and limited prognostic value in stage II breast cancer. *N Engl J Med* 319:1239, 1988.

87. Athanassiadou PP, Veneti SZ, Kyrkou KA, et al: Presence of epidermal growth factor receptor in breast smears of cyst fluids: Relationship to electrolyte ratios and pH concentration. *Cancer Detect Prev* 16:113, 1992.

88. Rosai J: Borderline epithelial lesions of the breast. *Am J Surg Pathol* 15:209, 1991.

89. Schnitt SJ, Connolly JL, Travassoli FA , et al: Interobserver reproducibility in the diagnosis of ductal proliferative breast lesions using standardized criteria. *Am J Surg Pathol* 16:1133, 1992.

90. Fisher B, Costantino JP, Wickerham DL, et al: Tamoxifen for the prevention of breast cancer: Report of the national surgical adjuvant breast and bowel project P-1 study *J Natl Cancer Inst* 90:1371, 1998.

91. Silverstein MJ, Lagios MD, Groshen S, et al: The influence of margin width on local control of ductal carcinoma in situ of the breast [see comments]. *N Engl J Med* 340:1455, 1999.

92. Lagios MD, Margolin FR, Groshen S, et al: Mammographically detected duct carcinoma in situ: Frequency of local recurrence following tylectomy and prognostic effect of nuclear grade on local recurrence. *Cancer* 63:618, 1989.

93. Julien JP, Bijker N, Fentiman IS, et al: Radiotherapy in breast-conserving treatment for ductal carcinoma in situ: First results of the EORTC randomized phase III trial 10853: EORTC Breast Cancer Cooperative Group and EORTC Radiotherapy group. *Lancet* 355:528, 2000.

94. Tan-Chiu E, Costantino J, Wang J, et al: The effect of tamoxifen on benign breast disease: Findings from the National Surgical Adjuvant Breast and Bowel Project (NSABP) breast cancer prevention trial (BCPT) [abstract 7]. *Breast Cancer Res Treat* 69:210, 2001.

95. Gump FE, Jicha DL, Ozello L, et al: Ductal carcinoma in situ (DCIS): A revised concept. *Surgery* 102:790, 1987.

96. Arriagada R, Le MG, Rochard F, et al: Conservative treatment versus mastectomy in early breast cancer: Patterns of failure with 15 years of follow-up data. Institut Gustave-Roussy Breast Cancer Group. *J Clin Oncol* 14:1558, 1996.

97. Early Breast Cancer Trialists' Collaborative Group: Effects of radiotherapy and surgery in early breast cancer: An overview of the randomized trials [erratum, *N Engl J Med* 1334:1003, 1996]. *N Engl J Med* 333:1444, 1995.

98. Fisher B, Anderson S, Redmond CK, et al: Reanalysis and results after 12 years of follow-up in a randomized clinical trial comparing total mastectomy with lumpectomy with or without irradiation in the treatment of breast cancer. *N Engl J Med* 333:1456, 1995.

99. Cooke T, Reeves J, Lanigan A, et al: HER2 as a prognostic and predictive marker for breast cancer. *Ann Oncol* 12(Suppl 1):S23, 2001.

100. Paik S, Bryant J, Tan-Chui E, et al: HER2 and choice of adjuvant chemotherapy for invasive breast cancer: National Surgical Adjuvant Breast and Bowel Project protocol B-15. *J Natl Cancer Inst* 92:1991, 2000.

101. Fisher B, Anderson S, Bryant J, et al: Twenty-year follow-up of a randomized trial comparing total mastectomy, lumpectomy, and lumpectomy plus irradiation for the treatment of invasive breast cancer. *N Engl J Med* 347:1233, 2002.

102. Veronesi U, Cascinelli N, Mariani L, et al: Twenty-year follow-up of a randomized study comparing breast-conserving surgery with radical mastectomy for early breast cancer. *N Engl J Med* 347:1227, 2002.

103. Slamon DJ, Leyland-Jones B, Shak S, et al: Use of chemotherapy plus a monoclonal antibody against HER2 for metastatic breast cancer that overexpresses HER2. *N Engl J Med* 334:783, 2001.

104. Hortobagy GN, Singletary SE, et al: Treatment of locally advanced and inflammatory breast cancer, in Harris JR (ed): *Diseases of the Breast.* Philadelphia: Lippincott, Williams and Wilkins, 2000, 645.

105. Favret AM, Carlson RW, Goffinet D, et al: Locally advanced breast cancer: Is surgery necessary? *Breast J* 7:131, 2001.

106. Brito RA, Valero V, Buzdar AU, et al: Long-term results of combined-modality therapy for locally advanced breast cancer with ipsilateral supraclavicular metastases: The University of Texas M. D. Anderson Cancer Center Experience. *J Clin Oncol* 19:628, 2001.

107. Souba WW, Bland KI: Indications and techniques for biopsy, in Bland KI, Copeland EM III (eds): *The Breast: Comprehensive Management of Benign Malignant Diseases.* Philadelphia: WB Saunders, 1998, p 802.

108. Bass SS, Lyman GH, McCann CR, et al: Lymphatic mapping and sentinel lymph node biopsy. *Breast J* 5:288, 1999.

109. Cox CE: Lymphatic mapping in breast cancer: Combination technique. *Ann Surg Oncol* 8:67S, 2001.

110. Cox CE, Nguyen K, Gray RJ, et al: Importance of lymphatic mapping in ductal carcinoma in situ (DCIS): Why map DCIS? *Am Surg* 67:513, discussion 519, 2001.

111. Krag D, Weaver D, Ashikaga T, et al: The sentinel node in breast cancer—A multicenter validation study. *N Engl J Med* 339:941, 1998.

112. McMasters KM, Giuliano AE, Ross MI, et al: Sentinel-lymph-node biopsy for breast cancer—Not yet the standard of care. *N Engl J Med* 339:990, 1998.

113. O'Hea BJ, Hill AD, El-Shirbiny AM, et al: Sentinel lymph node biopsy in breast cancer: Initial experience at Memorial Sloan-Kettering Cancer Center. *J Am Coll Surg* 186:423, 1998.

114. Veronesi U, Paganelli G, Galimberti V, et al: Sentinel-node biopsy to avoid axillary dissection in breast cancer with clinically negative lymph-nodes. *Lancet* 349:1864, 1997.

115. Wilke LG, Giuliano A: Sentinel lymph node biopsy in patients with early-stage breast cancer: Status of the National Clinical Trials. *Surg Clin North Am* 83:901, 2003.

116. Dupont E, Cox C, Shivers S, et al: Learning curves and breast cancer lymphatic mapping: Institutional volume index. *J Surg Res* 97:92, 2001.

117. Newman LA, Washington TA: New trend in breast conservation therapy. *Surg Clin North Am* 83:841, 2003.

118. Fisher B: Lumpectomy (segmental mastectomy and axillary dissection), in Bland KI, Copeland EM III (eds): *The Breast: Comprehensive Management of Benign Malignant Diseases.* Philadelphia: WB Saunders, 1998, p 917.

119. Simmons RM, Adamovich TL: Skin-sparing mastectomy. *Surg Clin North Am* 83:885, 2003.

120. Bland KI, Chang HR, et al: Modified radical mastectomy and total (simple) mastectomy, in Bland KI, Copeland EM III (eds): *The Breast: Comprehensive Management of Benign Malignant Diseases.* Philadelphia: WB Saunders, 1998, p 881.

121. McCraw JB, Papp C, et al: Breast reconstruction following mastectomy, in Bland KI, Copeland EM III (eds): *The Breast: Comprehensive Management of Benign Malignant Diseases.* Philadelphia: WB Saunders, 1998, p 962.

122. Hellman S: Stopping metastases at their source. *N Engl J Med* 337:996, 1997.

123. Overgaard M, Hansen PS, Overgaard J, et al: Postoperative radiotherapy in high-risk premenopausal women with breast cancer who receive adjuvant chemotherapy. Danish Breast Cancer Cooperative Group 82b Trial. *N Engl J Med* 337:949, 1997.

124. Overgaard M, Jensen MB, Overgaard J, et al: Postoperative radiotherapy in high-risk postmenopausal breast-cancer patients given adjuvant

tamoxifen: Danish Breast Cancer Cooperative Group DBCG 82c randomized trial. *Lancet* 353:1641, 1999.

125. Ragaz J, Jackson SM, Le N, et al: Adjuvant radiotherapy and chemotherapy in node-positive premenopausal women with breast cancer. *N Engl J Med* 337:956, 1997.

126. Recht A, Edge SB: Evidence-based indications for postmastectomy irradiation. *Surg Clin North Am* 83:995, 2003.

127. Fortin A, Dagnault A, Larochelle M, et al: Impact of locoregional radiotherapy in node-positive patients treated by breast-conservative treatment. *Int J Radiat Oncol Biol Phys* 56:1013, 2003.

128. Recht A, Edge SB, Solin LJ, et al: Postmastectomy radiotherapy: Clinical practice guidelines of the American Society of Clinical Oncology. *J Clin Oncol* 19:1539, 2001.

129. Loprinzi CL, Thome SD: Understanding the utility of adjuvant systemic therapy for primary breast cancer. *J Clin Oncol* 19:972, 2001.

130. Early Breast Cancer Trialists' Collaborative Group: Tamoxifen for early breast cancer: An overview of the randomized trials. *Lancet* 351:1451, 1998.

131. Early Breast Cancer Trialists' Collaborative Group: Polychemotherapy for early breast cancer: An overview of the randomized trials. *Lancet* 352:930, 1998.

132. Wood WC, Budman DR, Korzun AH, et al: Dose and dose intensity of adjuvant chemotherapy for stage II, node-positive breast carcinoma. *N Engl J Med* 330:1253, 1994.

133. Kelleher M, Miles D: The adjuvant treatment of breast cancer. *Int J Clin Pract* 57:195, 2003.

134. Fisher B, Brown AM, Dimitrov NV, et al: Two months of doxorubicin-cyclophosphamide with and without interval reinduction therapy compared with six months of cyclophosphamide methotrexate, and fluorouracil in positive-node breast cancer patients with tamoxifen-nonresponsive tumors: Results from NSABP B-15. *J Clin Oncol* 8:1483, 1990.

135. Fisher B, Bryant J, Wolkark N, et al: Effect of preoperative chemotherapy on the outcome of women with operable breast cancer. *J Clin Oncol* 16:2672, 1998.

136. Conte, PF, Latreille J, Mauriac L, et al: Delay in progression of bone metastases in breast cancer patients treated with intravenous pamidronate: Results from a multinational randomized controlled trial. The Aredia Multinational Cooperative Group. *J Clin Oncol* 145:2552, 1996.

137. Buzdar A, Douma J, Davidson N, et al: Phase III, multicenter, double-blind, randomized study of letrozole, an aromatase inhibitor, for advanced breast cancer versus megestrol acetate. *J Clin Oncol* 19:3357, 2001.

138. Buzdar AU, Jonat W, Howell A, et al: Anastrozole versus megestrol acetate in the treatment of postmenopausal women with advanced breast carcinoma: Results of a survival update based on a combined analysis of data from two mature phase III trials. Arimidex Study Group. *Cancer* 83:1142, 1998.

139. Bonneterre J, Thurlimann B, Buzdar A, et al: Anastrozole versus tamoxifen as first-line therapy for advanced breast cancer in 668 postmenopausal women: Results of the tamoxifen or Arimidex randomized group efficacy and tolerability study. *J Clin Oncol* 18:3748, 2000.

140. Baum M, Buzdar A: The current status of aromatase inhibitors in the management of breast cancer. *Surg Clin North Am* 83:973, 2003.

141. Campos SM, Winer EP: Hormonal therapy in postmenopausal women with breast cancer. *Oncology* 64:289, 2003.

142. Gradishar WJ, Jordan VC: Endocrine therapy of breast cancer, in Bland KI, Copeland EM III (eds): *The Breast: Comprehensive Management of Benign Malignant Diseases.* Philadelphia: WB Saunders, 1998, p 1350.

143. Paik S, Bryant J, Tan-Chiu E, et al: Real-world performance of HER2 testing: National Surgical Adjuvant Breast and Bowel Project experience. *J Natl Cancer Inst* 94:852, 2002.

144. Press MF, Slamon DJ, Flom KJ, et al: Evaluation of HER-2/neu gene amplification and overexpression: Comparison of frequently used assay methods in a molecularly characterized cohort of breast cancer specimens. *J Clin Oncol* 20:3095, 2002.

145. Volpi A, Nanni O, Depaola F, et al: HER-2 expression and cell proliferation: Prognostic markers in patients with node-negative breast cancer. *J Clin Oncol* 21:2708, 2003.

146. Tench DW, Page DL: The unknown primary presenting with axillary lymphadenopathy, in Bland KI, Copeland EM III (eds): *The Breast: Comprehensive Management of Benign Malignant Diseases.* Philadelphia: WB Saunders, 1998, p 1447.

147. Robinson DS, Sundaram M, et al: Carcinoma of the breast in pregnancy and lactation in Bland KI, Copeland EM III (eds): *The Breast: Comprehensive Management of Benign Malignant Diseases.* Philadelphia: WB Saunders, 1998, p 1433.

148. Giordana SH, Buzdar AU, Hortobagyi GN: Breast cancer in men. *Ann Intern Med* 137:163, 2002.

149. Wilhelm MC, Langenburg SE, et al: Cancer of the male breast, in Bland KI, Copeland EM III (eds): *The Breast: Comprehensive Management of Benign Malignant Diseases.* Philadelphia: WB Saunders, 1998, p 1416.

150. Khan SA, Badve S: Phyllodes tumors of the breast. *Curr Treat Options Oncol* 2:139, 2001.

151. Chittoor SR, Swain SM: Locally advanced breast cancer: Role of medical oncology, in Bland KI, Copeland EM III (eds): *The Breast: Comprehensive Management of Benign Malignant Diseases.* Philadelphia: WB Saunders, 1998, p 1403.

152. Mies C: Mammary sarcoma and lymphoma, in Bland KI, Copeland EM III (eds): *The Breast: Comprehensive Management of Benign Malignant Diseases.* Philadelphia: WB Saunders, 1998, p 307.

CHAPTER 17

Disorders of the Head and Neck

Richard O. Wein, Rakesh K. Chandra, and Randal S. Weber

The head and neck constitute a complex anatomic region where different pathologies may affect an individual's ability to see, smell, hear, speak, obtain nutrition and hydration, or breathe. The use of a multidisciplinary approach to many of the disorders in this region is essential in an attempt to achieve the best functional results with care. This chapter reviews many of the common diagnoses encountered in the field of otolaryngology—head and neck surgery—and aims to provide an overview that clinicians can use as a foundation for understanding head and neck diseases. As is the case with every field of surgery, care for patients with disorders of the head and neck is constantly changing as issues of quality of life and the economics of medicine continue to evolve.

BENIGN CONDITIONS OF THE HEAD AND NECK

Ear Infections

Infections may involve the external, middle, and/or internal ear. In each of these scenarios, the infection may follow an acute or chronic course and may be associated with both otologic and intracranial complications.

Otitis externa typically refers to infection of the skin of the external auditory canal.[1] Acute otitis externa is commonly known as "swimmer's ear," because moisture that persists within the canal after swimming often initiates the process and leads to skin maceration and itching. Typically, the patient subsequently traumatizes the canal skin by scratching (i.e., with a cotton swab or fingernail), thus eroding the normally protective skin/cerumen barrier. Because the environment within the external ear canal is already dark, warm, and humid, it then becomes susceptible to rapid microbial proliferation and tissue cellulitis. The most common organism responsible is *Pseudomonas aeruginosa*, although other bacteria and fungi may also be implicated. Table 17-1 summarizes the microbiology of common otolaryngologic conditions. Symptoms and signs of otitis externa include itching during the initial phases and pain with swelling of the canal soft tissues as the infection progresses. Infected, desquamated debris accumulates within the canal. In the chronic inflammatory stage of the infection, the pain subsides, but profound itching occurs for prolonged periods with gradual thickening of the external canal skin. Standard treatment requires removal of debris under otomicroscopy and application of appropriate topical antimicrobials such as neomycin/polymyxin or quinolone-containing eardrops. These preparations often include hydrocortisone to nonspecifically decrease pain and swelling. Nonantibiotic antimicrobial preparations, such as 2% acetic acid, may also have a role, particularly for mixed bacterial/fungal infections. The patient should also be instructed to keep the ear dry. Systemic antibiotics are reserved for those with severe infections, diabetics, and immunosuppressed patients.

Diabetic, elderly, and immunodeficient patients are susceptible to a condition called *malignant otitis externa,* a fulminant necrotizing infection of the otologic soft tissues combined with osteomyelitis of the temporal bone. In addition to the above findings, cranial neuropathies may be observed. The classic physical finding is granulation tissue along the floor of the external auditory canal. Symptoms include persistent otalgia for longer than 1 month and purulent otorrhea for several weeks. These patients require aggressive

Table 17-1
Microbiology of Common Otolaryngologic Infections

Condition	Microbiology
Otitis externa and malignant otitis externa	*Pseudomonas aeruginosa,* fungi (*Aspergillus* most common)
Acute otitis media	*Streptococcus pneumoniae, Haemophilus influenzae, Moraxella catarrhalis*
Chronic otitis media	Above bacteria, staphylococci, other streptococci; may be polymicrobial; exact role of bacteria unclear
Acute sinusitis	Viral URI, *S. pneumoniae, H. influenzae, M. catarrhalis*
Chronic sinusitis	Above bacteria, staphylococci, other streptococci; may be polymicrobial; exact role of bacteria unclear; may represent immune response to fungi
Pharyngitis	Viral, streptococci (usually pyogenes)

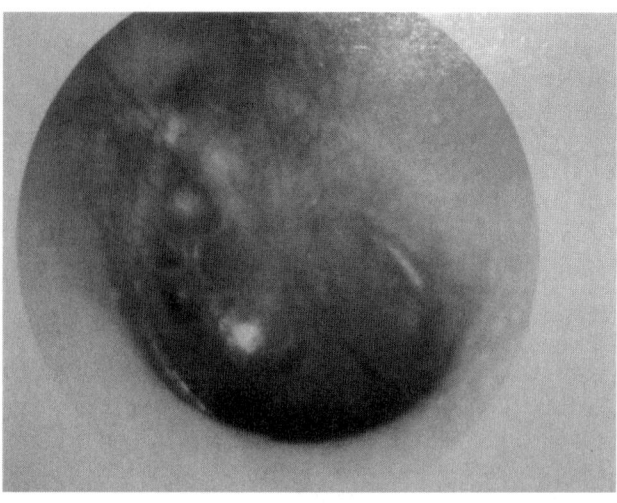

FIG. 17-2. Chronic serous otitis media.

medical therapy, including intravenous antibiotics covering *Pseudomonas.*[2] Other gram-negative bacteria and fungi are occasionally implicated, necessitating culture-directed therapy in those cases. Patients who do not respond to medical management require surgical débridement. This condition may progress to involvement of the adjacent skull base and soft tissues, meningitis, brain abscess, and death.

In its acute phase, otitis media typically implies a bacterial infection of the middle ear. This diagnosis accounts for 25% of all antibiotic prescriptions and is the most common bacterial infection of childhood. Most cases occur before 2 years of age and are secondary to immaturity of the eustachian tube. Contributing factors include upper respiratory viral infection and day-care attendance, as well as craniofacial conditions affecting eustachian tube function, such as cleft palate. Day-care attendance has been further correlated with antibiotic-resistant infecting organisms.[3]

Classification of the infection as acute is based upon the duration of the process being less than 3 weeks. In this phase, otalgia and fever are the most common symptoms and physical exam reveals a bulging, opaque tympanic membrane (Fig. 17-1). The most common organisms responsible are *Streptococcus pneumoniae, Haemophilus influenzae,* and *Moraxella catarrhalis.* If the process lasts 3 to 8 weeks, it is deemed subacute. Chronic otitis

media, lasting more than 8 weeks, usually results from an unresolved acute otitis media. Twenty percent of patients demonstrate a persistent middle ear effusion 8 weeks after resolution of the acute phase. Rather than a purely infectious process, however, it represents chronic inflammation and hypersecretion by the middle ear mucosa associated with eustachian tube dysfunction, viruses, allergy, ciliary dysfunction, and other factors. The bacteriology is variable, but often includes those found in acute otitis media and may be polymicrobial. The exact role of bacteria in the pathophysiology is controversial. The patient experiences otalgia, ear fullness, and conductive hearing loss. Physical exam reveals a retracted tympanic membrane that may exhibit an opaque character or an air-fluid level (Fig. 17-2). Bubbles may be seen behind the retracted membrane.

Treatment for uncomplicated otitis media is oral antibiotic therapy. However, penicillin resistance of the commonly implicated organisms is rising such that almost 100% of *Moraxella,* 50 to 70% of *Haemophilus,* and up to 40% of pneumococcal strains are resistant.[4] Beta-lactamase-resistant combinations, cephalosporins, and macrolides are often required, although amoxicillin and sulfas are still considered first-line drugs. Chronic otitis media is frequently treated with myringotomy and tube placement (Fig. 17-3). This is indicated for frequent acute episodes, chronic effusions persisting

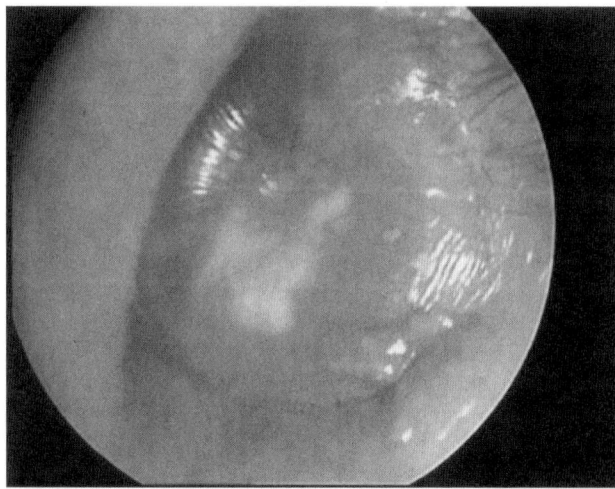

FIG. 17-1. Acute otitis media.

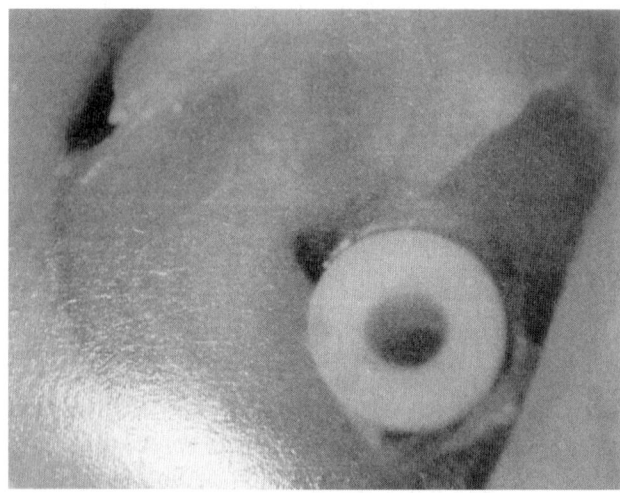

FIG. 17-3. Myringotomy and tube.

beyond 3 months, and those associated with significant conductive hearing loss. The purpose of this procedure is to remove the effusion and provide a route for middle ear ventilation.

Tympanic membrane perforation during acute otitis media frequently results in resolution of severe pain and provides for drainage of purulent fluid and middle ear ventilation. These perforations will heal spontaneously after the infection has resolved in the majority of cases. Chronic otitis media, however, may be associated with nonhealing tympanic membrane perforations. Patients may have persistent otorrhea, which is treated with topical drops. Preparations containing aminoglycoside are avoided, because this class of drugs is toxic to the inner ear. Solutions containing alcohol or acetic acid may be irritative or caustic to the middle ear, and are also avoided in the setting of a perforation. Nonhealing perforation requires surgical closure (tympanoplasty) after medical treatment of any residual acute infection. Chronic inflammation may also be associated with erosion of the ossicular chain, which can be reconstructed with various prostheses or autologous ossicular replacement techniques. Cholesteatoma is an epidermoid cyst of the middle ear and/or mastoid, which causes bone destruction secondary to its expansile nature and through enzymatic destruction. Cholesteatoma develops as a consequence of eustachian tube dysfunction and chronic otitis media secondary to retraction of squamous elements of the tympanic membrane into the middle ear space. Squamous epithelium may also migrate into the middle ear via a perforation. Chronic mastoiditis that fails medical management or is associated with cholesteatoma is treated by mastoidectomy.

Complications of otitis media may be grouped into two categories: intratemporal (otologic) and intracranial.[5,6] Fortunately, complications are rare in the antibiotic era, but mounting antibiotic resistance necessitates an increased awareness of these conditions. Intratemporal complications include acute coalescent mastoiditis, petrositis, facial nerve paralysis, and labyrinthitis. In acute coalescing mastoiditis, destruction of the bony lamellae by an acute purulent process results in severe pain, fever, and swelling behind the ear. The mastoid air cells coalesce into one common space filled with pus. Mastoid infection may also spread to the petrous apex, causing retro-orbital pain and sixth-nerve palsy. These diagnoses are confirmed by computed tomography (CT) scan (Fig. 17-4).[7]

Facial nerve paralysis may also occur secondary to an acute inflammatory process in the middle ear or mastoid. Intratemporal complications are managed by myringotomy tube placement in addition to appropriate intravenous (IV) antibiotics. In acute coalescent mastoiditis, and petrositis, mastoidectomy is also performed as necessary to drain purulent foci.

Labyrinthitis refers to inflammation of the inner ear. Most cases are idiopathic or are secondary to viral infections of the endolymphatic space. The patient experiences vertigo with sensorineural hearing loss and symptoms may smolder over several weeks. Labyrinthitis associated with middle ear infection may be serous or suppurative. In the former case, bacterial products and/or inflammatory mediators transudate into the inner ear via the round window membrane, establishing an inflammatory process therein. Total recovery is eventually possible after the middle ear is adequately treated. Suppurative labyrinthitis, however, is a much more toxic condition in which the acute purulent bacterial infection extends into the inner ear and causes marked destruction of the sensory hair cells and neurons of the eighth-nerve ganglion. This condition may hallmark impending meningitis and must be treated rapidly. The goal of management of inner ear infection which occurs

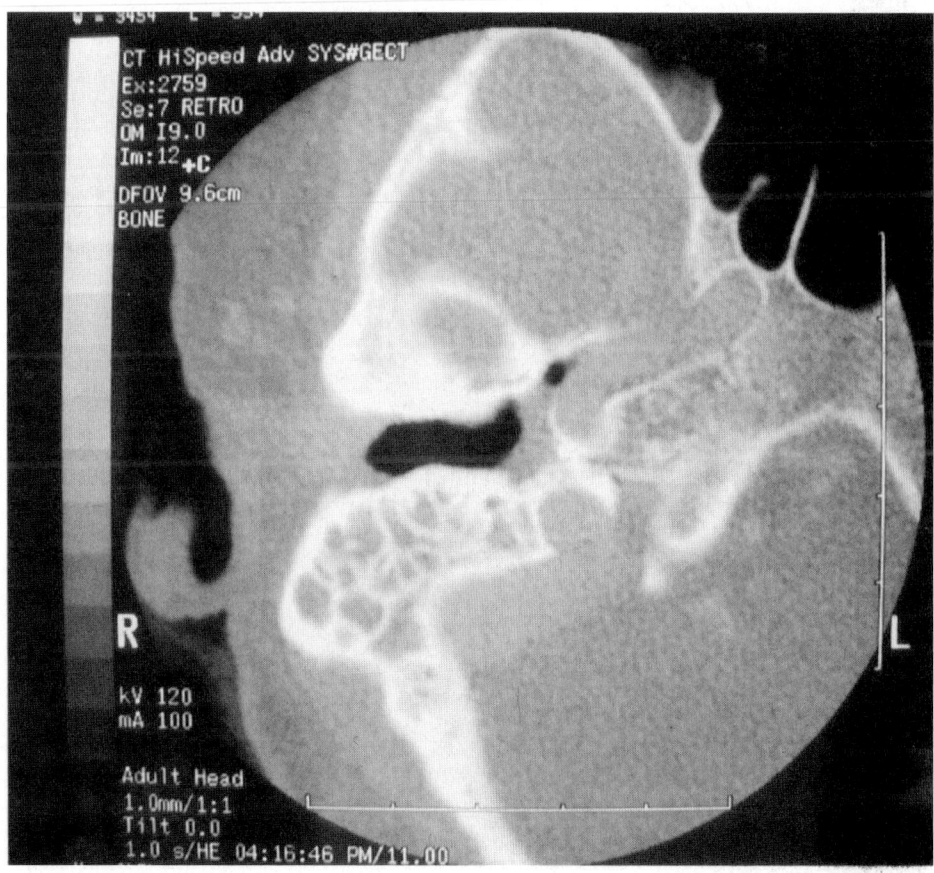

FIG. 17-4. Axial CT scan of mastoiditis revealing opacification of the mastoid air cells.

secondary to middle ear infection is to "sterilize" the middle ear space with antibiotics and the placement of a myringotomy tube.

Meningitis is the most common intracranial complication. Otologic meningitis in children is most commonly associated with a *H. influenzae* type B infection. Other intracranial complications include epidural abscess, subdural abscess, brain abscess, otitic hydrocephalus (pseudotumor), and sigmoid sinus thrombophlebitis. In these cases, the otogenic source must be urgently treated with antibiotics and myringotomy tube placement. Mastoidectomy and neurosurgical consultation may be necessary.

Bell's palsy, or idiopathic facial paralysis, may be considered within the spectrum of otologic disease given the facial nerve's course through the temporal bone. This entity is the most common etiology of facial nerve paralysis and is clinically distinct from that occurring as a complication of otitis media in that the otologic exam is normal. Historically, Bell's palsy was synonymous with "idiopathic" facial paralysis. It is now accepted, however, that the majority of these cases represent a viral neuropathy caused by herpes simplex. Treatment includes oral steroids plus antiviral therapy (i.e., acyclovir). Complete recovery is the norm, but does not occur universally, and selected cases may benefit from surgical decompression of the nerve within its bony canal. Electrophysiologic testing has been employed to identify those patients in whom surgery might be indicated.[8] The procedure involves decompression of the nerve via exposure in the middle cranial fossa. Varicella zoster virus may also cause facial nerve paralysis when the virus reactivates from dormancy in the nerve. This condition, known as Ramsey-Hunt syndrome, is characterized by severe otalgia followed by the eruption of vesicles of the external ear. Treatment is similar to Bell's palsy, but full recovery is only seen in approximately two thirds of cases.

Traumatic facial nerve injuries may occur secondary to accidental trauma or surgical injury. The former is detailed in the section below. Iatrogenic facial nerve trauma most often occurs during mastoidectomy.[9] When the facial nerve is injured intraoperatively, it is explored. Injuries to greater than 50% of the neural diameter are either reanastomosed primarily or with a nerve graft. Only partial recovery can be expected in these cases.

Sinus Inflammatory Disease

Sinusitis is a clinical diagnosis based on patient signs and symptoms.[10] The Task Force on Rhinosinusitis (sponsored by the American Academy of Otolaryngology–Head and Neck Surgery) has established criteria to define "a history consistent with sinusitis" (Table 17-2). To qualify for the diagnosis, the patient must exhibit at least two major factors or one major and two minor factors. The

Table 17-2
Factors Associated with a History of Rhinosinusitis[a]

Major Factors	Minor Factors
Facial congestion/fullness	Headache
Facial pain/pressure	Maxillary dental pain
Nasal drainage/discharge	Cough
Postnasal drip	Halitosis (bad breath)
Nasal obstruction/blockage	Fatigue
Hyposmia/anosmia (decreased or absent sense of smell)	Ear pain, pressure, or fullness
Fever (acute sinusitis only)	Fever
Purulence on nasal endoscopy (diagnostic by itself)	

[a]Either two major factors or one major and two minor factors are required. Purulence on nasal endoscopy is diagnostic. Fever is a major factor only in the acute stage.

classification of sinusitis as acute versus subacute or chronic is based on the time course over which those criteria have been met. If signs and symptoms are present for at least 7 to 10 days, but for less than 4 weeks, the process is designated acute sinusitis. Subacute sinusitis is present for 4 to 12 weeks and chronic sinusitis is diagnosed when the patient has had signs and symptoms for at least 12 weeks.

Acute sinusitis typically follows a viral upper respiratory infection whereby sinonasal mucosal inflammation results in closure of the sinus ostium. This results in stasis of secretions, tissue hypoxia, and ciliary dysfunction. These conditions promote bacterial proliferation and acute inflammation. The mainstay of treatment is oral antibiotics empirically directed toward the three most common organisms *S. pneumoniae, H. influenzae,* and *M. catarrhalis.*[11] As with otitis media, antibiotic resistance is a mounting concern. Nosocomial acute sinusitis frequently involves *Pseudomonas* or *S. aureus,* both of which may exhibit significant antibiotic resistance. Other treatments include topical and systemic decongestants, nasal saline spray, topical nasal steroids, and oral steroids in selected cases. In the acute setting, surgery is reserved for complications or pending complications, which may include extension to the eye (orbital cellulitis or abscess) or the intracranial space (meningitis, intracranial abscess). It should also be noted that, strictly speaking, a viral upper respiratory infection (common cold) is a form of acute sinusitis. The working definition outlined above, however, attempts to exclude these cases by requiring that symptoms be present for at least 7 to 10 days, by which time the common cold should be in a resolution phase. Use of this modified working definition avoids unnecessary antibiotic prescriptions and further promotion of resistance.

Chronic sinusitis represents a heterogeneous group of patients with multifactorial etiologies contributing to ostial obstruction, ciliary dysfunction, and inflammation. Components of genetic predisposition, allergy, anatomic obstruction, bacteria, fungi, and environmental factors play varying roles, depending on the individual patient. As of yet, no immunologic "final common pathway" has been defined, but the clinical picture is well described. Diagnosis is suspected according to the criteria described previously. Chronic sinusitis may also be associated with nasal polyps, which are manifestations of longstanding mucosal inflammatory disease. Polyps themselves may further block sinus outflow, resulting in further stasis of secretions and bacterial proliferation.

Nasal endoscopy is a critical element of the diagnosis of chronic sinusitis. Anatomic abnormalities, such as septal deviation, nasal polyps, and purulence may be observed (Figs. 17-5 and 17-6). The finding of purulence by nasal endoscopy is diagnostic of sinusitis, regardless of whether other criteria are met. In a setting in which symptoms persist for at least 12 weeks, purulence on nasal exam represents an acute exacerbation of chronic sinusitis. Pus found on endoscopic exam may be cultured, and subsequent antibiotic therapy can be directed accordingly. The spectrum of bacteria found in chronic sinusitis is highly variable and includes higher prevalences of polymicrobial infections and antibiotic-resistant organisms. Overall, *S. aureus,* coagulase-negative staphylococci, gram-negative bacilli, and streptococci are isolated, in addition to the typical pathogens of acute sinusitis.[11]

The diagnosis of chronic sinusitis can be confirmed by CT scan, which demonstrates mucosal thickening and/or sinus opacification (Fig. 17-7). It should be underscored, however, that CT scan is probably not the diagnostic gold standard because many asymptomatic patients will demonstrate findings on sinus CT scan. Also, patients with positive findings on nasal endoscopy may have normal CT scans. Overall, the decision to treat medically should be based upon patient history and nasal endoscopy, rather than results

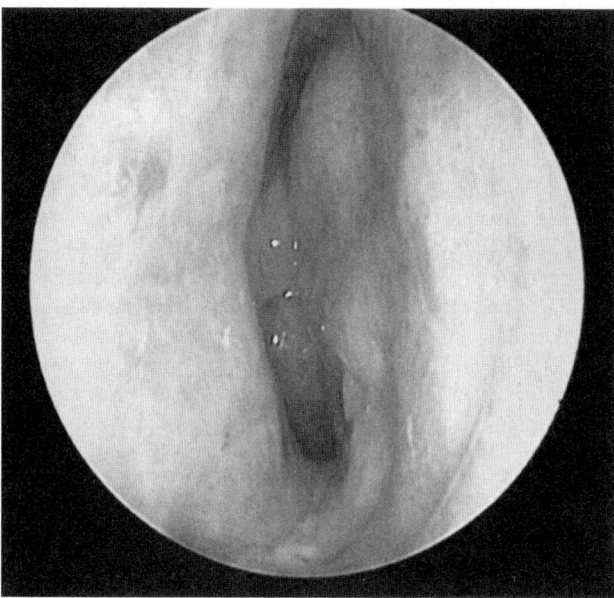

FIG. 17-5. Nasal polyps.

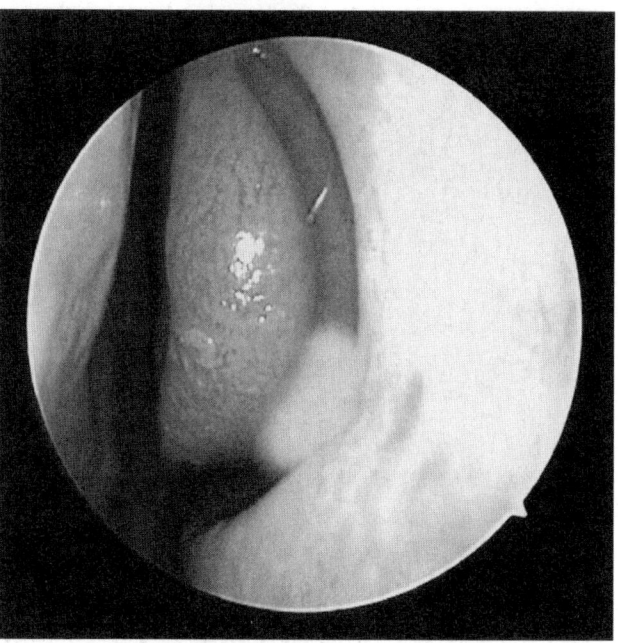

FIG. 17-6. Pus in the middle meatus seen in acute sinusitis.

of the CT scan. Furthermore, over 75% of patients with normal findings on nasal endoscopy will have normal CT scans, underscoring the importance of endoscopy in the decision-to-treat process. Although acute sinusitis is often treated empirically by the primary care practitioner, when clinical criteria for chronic sinusitis are met, this typically prompts otolaryngology referral for nasal endoscopy, aggressive medical therapy, and possibly surgery.

Medical management of chronic sinusitis includes a prolonged course of oral antibiotics for 3 to 6 weeks, oral steroids, and nasal irrigations with saline or antibiotic solutions.[12] Underlying allergic disease is managed with antihistamines and possible allergy immunotherapy. Those failing medical management are candidates

for elective surgery, where the goals are to enlarge the natural sinus ostia (Fig. 17-8) and to remove chronically infected bone to promote both ventilation and drainage of the sinus cavities. Eventual resolution of the chronic inflammatory process can be attained with a combination of surgery and aggressive medical therapy. Surgery is most often performed with endoscopic techniques.

The role of fungi in sinusitis is an area of active investigation.[13,14] Fungal sinusitis may take on both noninvasive and invasive forms. The noninvasive form includes the presence of a fungal ball and

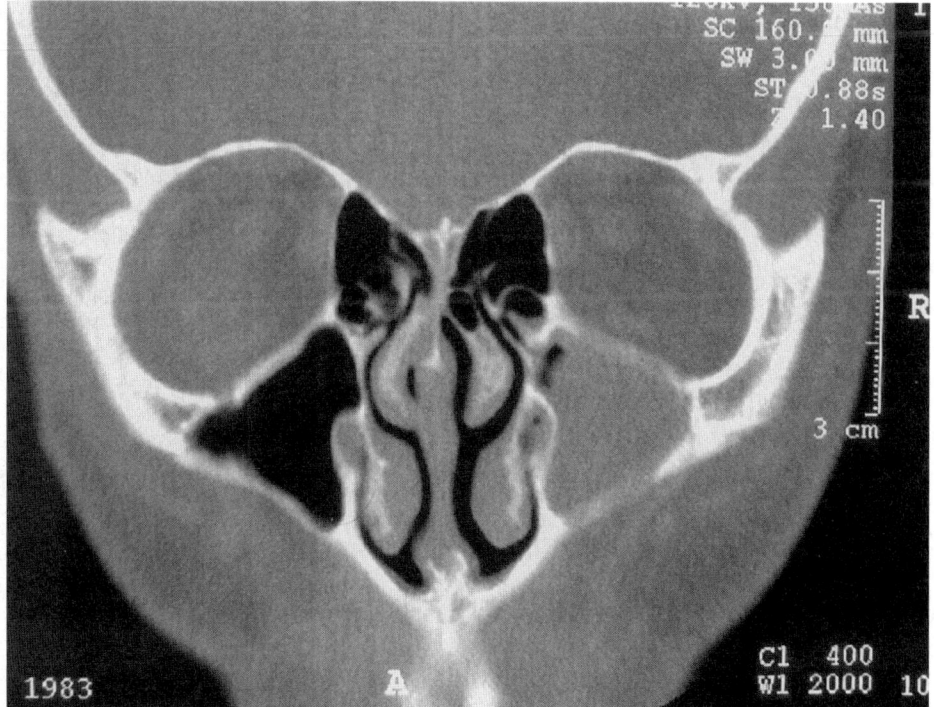

FIG. 17-7. Coronal CT scan of the sinus revealing near total opacification in the right maxillary sinus.

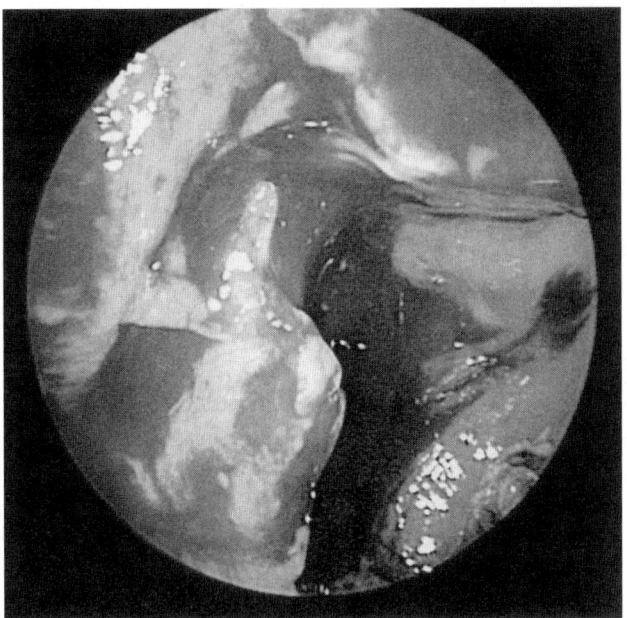

FIG. 17-8. Surgical enlargement of the maxillary sinus ostium and view into the sinus.

allergic fungal sinusitis, both of which occur in immunocompetent patients.

A fungal ball is typically seen in individuals with chronic (or recurrent acute) symptoms that are often subtle and limited to a single sinus. Patients may complain about the perception of a foul odor and occasionally report expelling fungal debris upon nose blowing. A fungal ball (Fig. 17-9) consisting of *Aspergillus fumigatus* is usually found in the maxillary sinus, with scant inflammatory cell infiltration. Surgery to remove the fungal ball and reestablish sinus ventilation is almost always curative. This can be accomplished endoscopically.

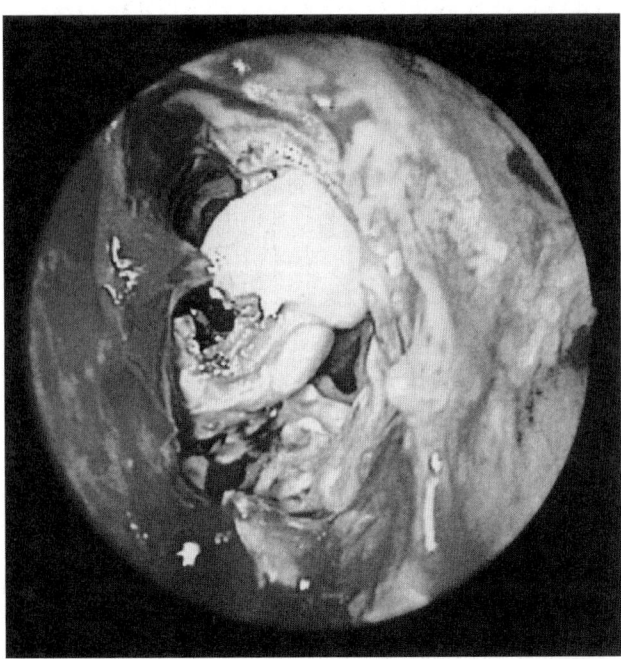

FIG. 17-9. Sinus fungal ball.

Allergic fungal sinusitis involves hypersensitivity (types I and III) reactions to fungal antigens within the nose and sinuses. Patients often present with chronic sinusitis that has been especially refractory to medical management. Endoscopic evaluation reveals florid polyposis and inspissated mucin containing fungal debris and products of eosinophil breakdown. The implicated organisms are usually those of the Dematiaceae family, but *Aspergillus* species are also seen. Treatment includes systemic steroids, surgery, and nasal irrigations. Oral antifungal therapy is sometimes indicated as well.

Immunocompetent patients may also develop an indolent form of invasive fungal sinusitis, but more commonly, invasive fungal sinusitis affects immunocompromised patients, diabetics, or the elderly.[15] Fungal invasion of the microvasculature causes ischemic necrosis and black, necrotic escharation of the sinonasal mucosa. *Aspergillus* and fungi of the Mucoraceae family are often implicated with the latter more common in diabetic patients. Treatment requires aggressive surgical débridement and IV antifungals, but the prognosis is dismal.

Pharyngeal and Adenotonsillar Disease

The pharyngeal mucosa contains significant concentrations of lymphoid tissue, predisposing this area to reactive inflammatory changes. Lymphoid tissue of various pharyngeal subsites forms the so-called Waldeyer's ring, consisting of the palatine tonsils ("the tonsils"), lingual tonsil (lymphoid tissue accumulation within the tongue base), and adenoid. The mucosa of the posterior and lateral pharyngeal walls is also rich with lymphoid cells. Infection, immune-mediated inflammatory disease, or local stressors, such as radiation or acid reflux, may initiate lymphoid reactivity and associated symptoms. Chronic or recurrent adenotonsillitis and adenotonsillar hypertrophy are the most common disorders affecting these structures.

In the vast majority of cases, infectious pharyngitis is viral rather than bacterial in origin. Most cases resolve without complication from supportive care and possibly antibiotics. Patients with tonsillitis present with sore throat, dysphagia, and fever. The mucosa is inflamed. Tonsillar exudates and cervical adenitis may be seen when the etiology is bacterial. If adenoiditis is present, the symptoms may be similar to those of sinusitis, but visual evaluation of the adenoid, at least in children, requires endoscopy and/or radiographic imaging (lateral neck soft-tissue x-ray). Tonsillitis and adenoiditis may follow acute, recurrent acute, and chronic temporal patterns.

It should be noted, however, that clinical diagnosis is often inaccurate for determining whether the process is bacterially induced. When the patient also has hoarseness, rhinorrhea, cough, and no evidence of exudates or adenitis, an upper respiratory viral infection can be presumed. When a bacterial cause is suspected,[16] antibiotics should be initiated to cover the usual organisms: group A beta-hemolytic streptococci (*Streptococcus pyogenes*), *S. pneumoniae,* and group C and G streptococci. *H. influenzae* and anaerobes also have been implicated. It is particularly important to identify group A beta-hemolytic streptococci in pediatric patients to initiate timely antibiotic therapy, given the risk of rheumatic fever, which may occur in up to 3% of cases if antibiotics are not used. Historically, if bacterial pharyngitis was suspected in a child, oropharyngeal swab with culture was performed to identify group A beta-hemolytic streptococci. Currently, rapid antigen assays are available with sensitivity and specificity of approximately 85 and 90%, respectively. Some authors advocate culture only when these are negative. Unnecessary antibiotic therapy for patients who are unlikely to have a bacterial etiology should be avoided, given the already mounting antibiotic resistance problem. When suspicion for a bacterial process is high, or with positive culture/antigen assay results, treatment may include penicillins, cephalosporins, or macrolides in penicillin-allergic patients.

Complications of *S. pyogenes* pharyngitis may be systemic, including rheumatic fever, poststreptococcal glomerulonephritis, and scarlet fever. The incidence of glomerulonephritis is not influenced by antibiotic therapy. Scarlet fever results from production of erythrogenic toxins by streptococci. This causes a punctate rash, first appearing on the trunk and then spreading distally, sparing palms and soles. The so-called strawberry tongue also is seen. Locoregional complications include peritonsillar abscess and, rarely, deep-neck space abscess. These conditions require surgical incision and drainage. Peritonsillar abscess may be drained transorally and some authors report that needle aspiration without incision is sufficient. Deep-neck space abscess, which more commonly is odontogenic in origin, usually requires operative incision and drainage.

Atypical cases of pharyngitis[17] may be caused by *Corynebacterium diphtheriae, Bordetella pertussis* (whooping cough), syphilis, *Neisseria gonorrhoeae,* and fungi. Diphtheria is a potentially fatal condition associated with toxin-mediated tissue necrosis and a gray membrane on the mucosal surface. Cardiorespiratory collapse may ensue from systemic circulation of the toxin. Treatment includes the use of antitoxin. Fortunately, diphtheria is rare in developed countries as a consequence of childhood vaccinations. Childhood vaccination also has almost eliminated whooping cough in developed nations. This entity follows a protracted, but usually self-limiting course. During the secondary phase of syphilis, ulcerations with raised red margins (resembling the chancre lesion) may be observed on the pharyngotonsillar mucosa. Identification of these less-typical organisms requires a high index of suspicion and application of appropriate culture techniques and/or serologic tests. *Candida albicans* is the most common fungal organism to cause pharyngitis. This organism is a normal component of the oral flora, but under conditions of immunosuppression, broad-spectrum antibacterial therapy, poor oral hygiene, or vitamin deficiency, it may become pathogenic. Whitish-cheesy or creamy mucosal patches are observed with underlying erythema, and diagnosis is easily established by Gram's stain of this material revealing budding yeast and pseudohyphae. Oral and topical antifungals are usually effective and immunosuppressed patients may require prophylactic therapy.

In addition to viral upper respiratory viruses, herpes simplex virus (HSV), Epstein-Barr virus (EBV), cytomegalovirus (CMV), and human immunodeficiency virus (HIV) are associated with pharyngitis. Systemic EBV infection represents clinical mononucleosis, although syphilis, CMV, and HIV are known to cause mononucleosis-like syndromes. These conditions, particularly EBV, may exhibit an exudative pharyngotonsillitis that may be confused with a bacterial etiology. Progression of the clinical picture reveals lymphadenopathy, splenomegaly, and hepatitis. Diagnosis is established based on the detection of heterophile antibodies or atypical lymphocytes in the peripheral blood. Occasionally, pharyngeal biopsy or cervical lymph node biopsy is required to establish the diagnosis.

Noninfectious causes of pharyngitis must also be considered. These include mucositis from chemoradiation therapy, which may be associated with fungal superinfection. Pharyngitis may also be seen in immune-mediated conditions such as erythema multiforme, bullous pemphigoid, and pemphigus vulgaris. In addition, reflux is being increasingly identified as a cause of both laryngitis and pharyngitis, particularly when the symptoms are chronic. A 24-hour pH probe is the gold standard diagnostic test.

Obstructive adenotonsillar hyperplasia may present with nasal obstruction, rhinorrhea, voice changes, dysphagia, and sleep-disordered breathing or obstructive sleep apnea, depending on the particular foci of lymphoid tissue involved.

Tonsillectomy and adenoidectomy are indicated for chronic or recurrent acute infection and for obstructive hypertrophy.[18] The *American Academy of Otolaryngology–Head and Neck Surgery Clinical Indicators Compendium (2000)* suggests tonsillectomy after three or more infections per year despite adequate medical therapy. Some feel that tonsillectomy is indicated in children who miss 2 or more weeks of school annually secondary to tonsil infections. Multiple techniques have been described, including electrocautery, sharp dissection, laser, and radiofrequency ablation. There is no consensus as to the best method. In cases of chronic or recurrent infection, surgery is considered only after failure of medical therapy. Patients with recurrent peritonsillar abscess should undergo tonsillectomy when the acute inflammatory changes have resolved. Selected cases, however, require tonsillectomy in the acute setting for the management of severe inflammation, systemic toxicity, or impending airway compromise. Adenoidectomy, in conjunction with myringotomy and tube placement, may be beneficial for children with chronic or recurrent otitis media.[19] This is because the adenoid appears to function as a bacterial reservoir that seeds the middle ear via the eustachian tube. Adenoidectomy is also the first-line of surgical management for children with chronic sinusitis. In addition to acting as a bacterial reservoir, an obstructive adenoid impairs mucociliary clearance from the sinonasal tract into the pharynx.

The primary complications of tonsillectomy[20] include bleeding, airway obstruction, death, and readmission for dehydration secondary to postoperative dysphagia. Complications of adenoidectomy also include hemorrhage, as well as nasopharyngeal stenosis and velopharyngeal insufficiency. In the latter condition, nasal regurgitation of liquids and hypernasal speech are experienced. Patients with significant airway obstruction secondary to adenotonsillar hypertrophy are also at risk for postobstructive pulmonary edema syndrome, once the obstruction is relieved by adenotonsillectomy. Overall, bleeding is the most significant risk and may require a return trip to the operating room for control. With the exception of bleeding, which is observed in 3 to 5% of patients, most of these complications are rare or self-limiting. It deserves special notation that adenotonsillectomy in a child with Down's syndrome requires attention to the cervical spine. Patients with this syndrome may exhibit atlantoaxial instability, resulting in cervical spine injury if the neck is extended for the procedure. Baseline radiographs, with appropriate orthopedic or neurosurgical consultation, are indicated preoperatively.

Surgery for adenotonsillar hypertrophy may be indicated when the patient exhibits sleep-disordered breathing. Sleep disorders represent a continuum from simple snoring to upper airway resistance syndrome (UARS) to obstructive sleep apnea (OSA).[21] UARS and OSA are associated with excessive daytime somnolence and frequent sleep arousals. In OSA, polysomnogram demonstrates at least 10 episodes of apnea or hypopnea per hour of sleep. The average number of apneas and hypopneas per hour can be used to calculate a respiratory disturbance index (RDI), which, along with oxygen saturation, can be used to grade the severity of OSA. These episodes occur as a result of collapse of the pharyngeal soft tissues during sleep. In adults, it should be noted that in addition to tonsil size, factors such as tongue size and body mass index are significant predictors of OSA. Other anatomic findings associated with OSA include obese neck, retrognathia, low hyoid bone, and enlarged soft palate. Surgery should be considered after failure of more conservative measures, such as weight loss, elimination of alcohol use, and continuous positive airway pressure, and should be tailored to the particular patient's pattern of obstruction. In children, surgical management typically involves tonsillectomy and/or adenoidectomy, because the disorder is usually caused by hypertrophy of these structures. In adults, uvulopalatoplasty is frequently performed to alleviate soft-palate collapse and is the most common operation performed for sleep-disordered breathing.[22] Multiple techniques have been described for this. Tongue base reduction, tongue advancement, hyoid suspension, and a variety of maxillomandibular advancement procedures also have been described with varying success. Adults with significant nasal obstruction may benefit from septoplasty or sinus surgery. Patients with severe OSA (RDI >40, lowest nocturnal oxygen saturation <70%) and unfavorable anatomy or comorbid pulmonary disease may require tracheotomy.

Benign Conditions of the Larynx

Disorders of voice may affect a wide array of patients with respect to age, gender, and socioeconomic status. The principle symptom of these disorders, at least when a mass lesion is present, is hoarseness. Other vocal manifestations include hypophonia or aphonia, breathiness, and pitch breaks. Benign laryngeal disorders may also be associated with airway obstruction, dysphagia, and reflux.[23] Smoking may also be a risk factor for benign disease, but this element of the history should raise the index of suspicion for malignancy.

Recurrent respiratory papillomatosis (RRP) reflects involvement of human papilloma virus (HPV) within the mucosal epithelium of the upper aerodigestive tract. The larynx is the most frequently involved site and subtypes 6 and 11 are the most often implicated. The disorder typically presents in the early childhood, secondary to viral acquisition during vaginal delivery. Many cases resolve after puberty, but the disorder may progress into adulthood. Adult-onset RRP typically occurs in the third or fourth decade of life, is usually less severe, and is more likely to involve extralaryngeal sites of the upper aerodigestive tract. With laryngeal involvement, RRP is most likely to present with hoarseness, although airway compromise may be observed. The diagnosis can be established with office endoscopy. Currently, there is no "cure" for RRP. Treatment involves operative microlaryngoscopy with excision or laser ablation, and the natural history is eventual recurrence. Therefore, surgery has an ongoing role for palliation of the disease. Multiple procedures are typically required over the patient's lifetime. Several medical therapies, including intralesional cidofovir injection and oral indole-3-carbinol, are currently being investigated to determine their abilities to retard recurrence.[24]

Laryngeal granulomas typically occur in the posterior larynx on the arytenoid mucosa (Fig. 17-10). These lesions develop secondary to multiple factors,[25] including reflux, voice abuse, chronic throat clearing, endotracheal intubation, and vocal fold paralysis. Effective management requires identification of the underlying cause(s). Patients report pain (often with swallowing) more commonly than vocal changes. In addition to fiberoptic laryngoscopy, work-up may include voice analysis, laryngeal electromyography (EMG), and pH probe testing.[26] Treatment is individualized, depending on the contributing factors identified. First-line modalities that may be employed include voice rest, voice retraining therapy, and antireflux therapy. The management of vocal cord paresis/paralysis is discussed later in this section. It is notable that the majority of cases demonstrate a component of reflux and when maximal medical therapy has failed, fundoplication may be indicated. Although some authors have described the use of botulism toxin for recalcitrant

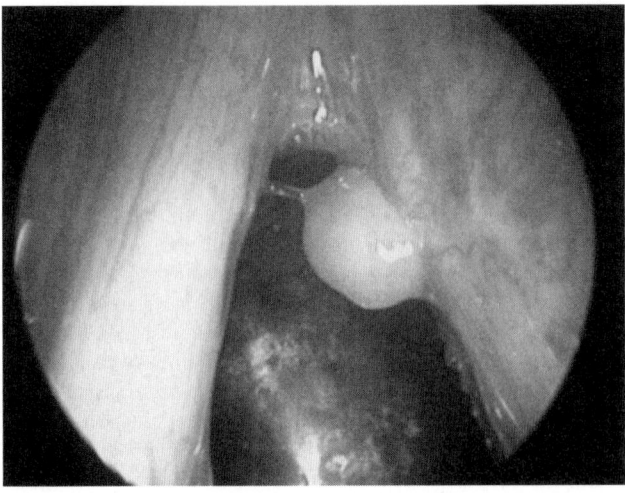

FIG. 17-10. *Laryngeal granulomas.*

granulomas to curtail chronic abusive vocal behaviors,[27] this is not appropriate for primary treatment. The role of surgical excision is also controversial, because it does not address the underlying etiology and is frequently associated with recurrence. Nonetheless, excision is indicated when carcinoma is suspected or when the patient has airway obstruction. Surgery may also be indicated in selected cases when a granuloma has matured into a fibroepithelial polyp, or when the patient (e.g., a performing artist) requires prompt removal for voice restoration. Surgical excision is optimally performed under jet ventilation so as to avoid endotracheal intubation. During surgery, it is important to preserve the arytenoid perichondrium to promote epithelialization postoperatively.

Edema in the superficial lamina propria of the vocal cord is known as polypoid corditis, polypoid laryngitis, polypoid degeneration of the vocal cord, or Reinke's edema. The superficial lamina propria just underlies the vibratory epithelial surface. Edema is thought to arise from injury to the capillaries that exist in this layer, with subsequent extravasation of fluid. Patients report progressive development of a rough, low-pitched voice. Females more commonly present for medical attention because the lowered vocal frequency is more evident, given the higher fundamental frequency of the female voice. The etiology is also multifactorial and may involve smoking, laryngopharyngeal reflux, hypothyroidism, and vocal hyperfunction. Most of these patients are heavy smokers. Findings are typically bilateral.

Focal, unilateral hemorrhagic vocal cord polyps (Fig. 17-11) are more common in men. These occur secondary to capillary rupture within the mucosa by shearing forces during voice abuse. Use of anticoagulant or antiplatelet drugs may be a risk factor. As with laryngeal granulomas, treatment of polypoid corditis and vocal cord polyps requires addressing the underlying factors. Conservative management includes absolute discontinuance of smoking, reflux management, and voice therapy. Notably, topical and systemic steroids are ineffective for these conditions. For polypoid corditis, elective surgery may be performed under microlaryngoscopy to evacuate the gelatinous matrix within the superficial lamina propria and trim excess mucosa. Focal polyps may be excised superficially under microlaryngoscopy. Surgery, particularly for polypoid corditis, will be less effective in patients who continue to smoke, although it should be noted that because of a heavy smoking history, surgery might be necessary to rule out occult malignancy. Surgery for polypoid corditis and hemorrhagic polyps may be accomplished either

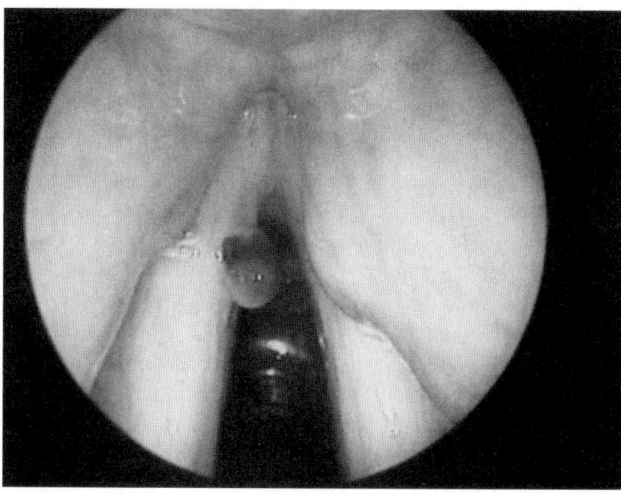

FIG. 17-11. Hemorrhagic vocal cord polyp.

with cold steel or by using the carbon dioxide laser. Postoperative voice therapy is usually indicated.

Cysts may occur under the laryngeal mucosa, particularly in regions containing mucous-secreting glands, such as the supraglottic larynx. Occasionally, they derive from minor salivary glands and congenital cysts may persist as remnants of the branchial arch. Cysts may present in a variety of ways depending on the size and site of origin (Fig. 17-12). Cysts of the vocal cord may be difficult to distinguish from vocal polyps and video stroboscopic laryngoscopy may be necessary to help establish the diagnosis. Cysts observed in children can be quite large, thus compromising the airway. Lesions of the true vocal cord usually present with hoarseness. Treatment again depends on the size and site of the cyst. Large cysts of the supraglottic larynx are treated by marsupialization with cold steel or a carbon dioxide laser. Those of the vocal cord itself require careful microsurgical technique for complete removal of the cyst while preserving the overlying mucosa.

Leukoplakia of the vocal fold represents a white patch (which cannot be wiped off) on the mucosal surface, usually on the superior surface of the true vocal cord. Rather than a diagnosis per se, the term leukoplakia describes a finding on laryngoscopic examination. The significance of this finding is that it may represent squamous

hyperplasia, dysplasia, and/or carcinoma. Lesions exhibiting hyperplasia have a 1 to 3% risk of progression to malignancy. In contrast, that risk is 10 to 30% for those demonstrating dysplasia. Furthermore, leukoplakia may be observed in association with inflammatory and reactive pathologies, including polyps, nodules, cysts, granulomas, and papillomas. The wide, differential diagnosis for leukoplakia necessitates sound clinical judgment when selecting lesions that require operative direct laryngoscopy with biopsy for histopathologic analysis. Features of ulceration and erythroplasia are particularly suggestive of possible malignancy. A history of smoking and alcohol abuse should also prompt a malignancy work-up. In the absence of suspected malignancy, conservative measures are employed for 1 month. These include reduction of caffeine and alcohol, which are dehydrating and promote laryngopharyngeal reflux, proper hydration, and elimination of vocal abuse behaviors. Antireflux therapy, including proton pump inhibitors, may be prescribed. Investigational therapies, including retinoids, also have been attempted. Any lesions that progress, persist, or recur should be considered for excisional biopsy.

Vocal cord paralysis is most commonly iatrogenic in origin, following surgery to the thyroid, parathyroid, carotid, or cardiothoracic structures. Vocal cord paralysis may also be secondary to malignant processes in the lungs, thoracic cavity, skull base, or neck.[28,29] In the pediatric population, up to one-fourth of cases may be neurologic in origin, with Arnold-Chiari malformation being the most common. Overall, the left vocal cord is more commonly involved secondary to the longer course of the recurrent laryngeal nerve (RLN) on that side, which extends into the thoracic cavity. When anterior approaches to the cervical spine are performed, however, the right RLN is at an increased risk, because it courses more laterally to the tracheoesophageal complex. Neurotoxic medications, trauma, intubation injury, and atypical infections are less-common causes of vocal cord paralysis. The cause remains idiopathic in up to 20% of adults and 35% of children. These cases should prompt an imaging work-up to examine the course of the vagal/RLN in question: from the skull base to the aortic arch on the left, and from skull base to the subclavian on the right. "Idiopathic" left true vocal cord paralysis may be a presenting sign of malignancy involving the lung, thyroid, or esophagus. Adults typically present with hoarseness and the voice may be breathy if the contralateral vocal cord has not compensated to close the glottic valve. If the proximal vagus nerve or the superior laryngeal nerve is involved, the patient may demonstrate aspiration secondary to diminished supraglottic sensation. Stridor, weak cry, and respiratory distress are seen in children, but adults typically do not exhibit signs of airway compromise unless paralysis is bilateral. Flexible fiberoptic laryngoscopy usually confirms the diagnosis, but laryngeal EMG may be necessary to distinguish vocal cord paralysis from mechanical fixation secondary to scar tissue or cricoarytenoid joint fixation. The position of the paralyzed fold depends on the residual innervation, pattern of reinnervation, and the degrees of atrophy and fibrosis of the laryngeal musculature. In bilateral vocal cord paralysis, the cords are often paralyzed in a paramedian position, creating airway compromise that necessitates tracheotomy. Once an airway is secure, vocal cord lateralization or arytenoidectomy may be performed electively to provide an adequate airway. Treatment of unilateral vocal cord paralysis includes speech therapy, which promotes glottic closure in order to optimize voice and prevent aspiration. Some patients do well with this modality alone.

Surgical treatment to augment or medialize the paralyzed vocal fold is performed to provide a surface against which the contralateral normal fold may make contact. Injection laryngoplasty may be performed under office or operative laryngoscopy with a variety of

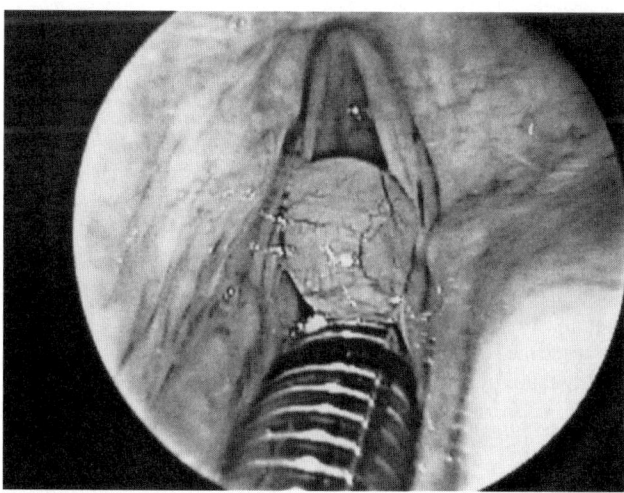

FIG. 17-12. Large cyst of vocal cord.

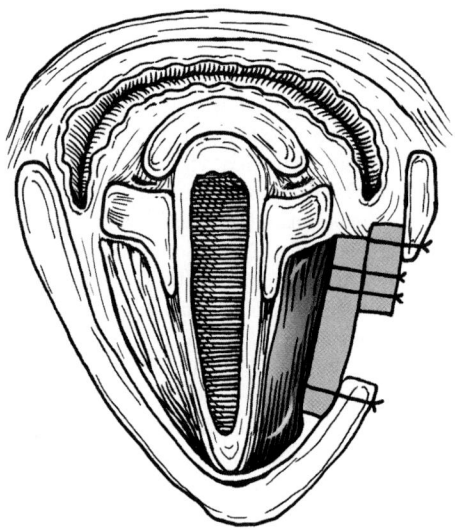

FIG. 17-13. Cross-section of the larynx demonstrating the principle of medialization laryngoplasty. An implant is used to push the paralyzed vocal cord toward the midline.

autologous (fat, collagen) or alloplastic (hydroxylapatite, silicone, Teflon) compounds. Autologous materials are preferred. Teflon injection is of historical significance only secondary to the incidence of severe foreign body inflammatory reactions. Injection of the vocal fold increases its bulk to optimize closure with the contralateral normal fold. This technique is also useful for vocal cord atrophy, which may occur with aging. Recent trends include the use of bovine collagen for this purpose, which has shown promising results. Laryngeal framework surgery involves the implantation of cartilage, hydroxylapatite, Gore-Tex, or silicone under the musculomembranous fold via an external approach through a window in the thyroid cartilage (Fig. 17-13).[30] This may be combined with procedures to adduct the vocal process of the arytenoids. Laryngeal reinnervation (with ansa cervicalis to recurrent laryngeal nerve transfer) and pacing have also been attempted with varying success.

Vascular Lesions

Vascular lesions can be broadly classified into two groups: hemangiomas and vascular malformations.[31] Hemangiomas (Fig. 17-14)

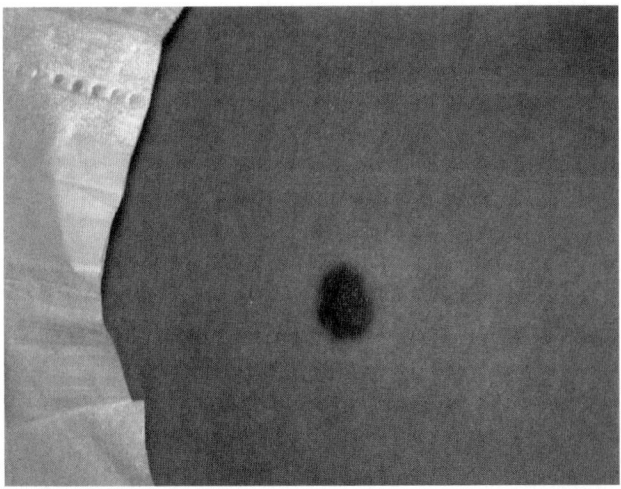

FIG. 17-14. Cutaneous hemangioma.

are the most common vascular lesions present in infancy and childhood. These lesions are present at birth in up to 30% of cases, but usually become apparent in the first few weeks of life. The lesions proliferate in size over the first year before beginning involution, which subsequently occurs over the next 2 to 12 years. Forty percent of cases will resolve completely, while the remainder require intervention. Once the proliferative phase has ended, the lesion should be observed every 3 months for involution, and surgery should be considered for those that have not significantly involuted by 3 to 4 years of age. Surgical treatment of proliferating hemangiomas is reserved for lesions associated with severe functional or cosmetic problems, such as those involving the nasal tip or periorbital region. Treatment is performed with either the flashlamp-pumped pulsed-dye laser (FPDL), the potassium titanyl phosphate (KTP) laser, or the neodymium yttrium-aluminum garnet (Nd:YAG) laser, repeated every 4 to 6 weeks until the lesion disappears. Systemic steroids may be employed to arrest rapidly proliferating lesions until the child reaches 12 to 18 months, after which growth should stabilize or involution begin. Subcutaneous interferon-α 2a may also be used for this purpose. This treatment, however, is associated with neurologic side effects and should be used with caution.[31–33]

Vascular malformations, in contrast, are almost always present at birth and slowly enlarge without proliferation.[34] These may arise from capillaries, venules, veins, arteriovenous channels, and/or lymphatics. Capillary malformations usually involve the midline neck or forehead, and may fade with age. Venular malformations are also known as port-wine stains. These lesions often follow facial dermatomes and usually thicken with age. Venous malformations are composed of ectatic veins within the lips, tongue, or buccal area. These may present as purple masses or subcutaneous/submucosal nodules. Arteriovenous malformations (AVMs) are rare malformations of arteriovenous channels that failed to regress during development. Lymphatic malformations (or lymphangiomas; Figs. 17-15 and 17-16) of the head and neck usually involve the cervical area, in which case they are more commonly macrocystic and well demarcated. Those arising above the hyoid bone tend to be microcystic and have an infiltrative quality. Lymphangiomas may become secondarily infected and may rapidly enlarge, causing airway compromise. These lesions may also be associated with feeding difficulties and failure to thrive.

Capillary hemangiomas and superficial port-wine stains are effectively treated by FPDL. The KTP laser or Nd:YAG laser is used for deeper port-wine stains. Venous malformations may be treated with laser, sclerotherapy, and/or surgical excision, depending on the depth, size, and location. Superficial lesions are treated with the Nd:YAG laser, which has deeper penetration than either the FPDL or KTP laser. Deeper venous malformations may benefit from Nd:YAG therapy of the superficial component followed by meticulous surgical excision of the deeper component.[31–33] Sclerotherapy should be undertaken with extreme caution in the head and neck, because the valveless quality of the veins in this region introduces significant risk of cavernous sinus thrombosis. AVMs require formal surgical resection with negative margins. Preoperative angiographic embolization is frequently employed to facilitate surgery. Microvascular reconstruction may be necessary, depending on the extent of the resection required. Surgical excision is also required for lymphatic malformations, although superficial lesions are sometimes treatable with the carbon dioxide laser. This is often difficult for microcystic cases given the infiltrative nature. Sclerotherapy with OK-432 is effective in macrocystic lymphangiomas and multiple other sclerosing agents have been explored.[35]

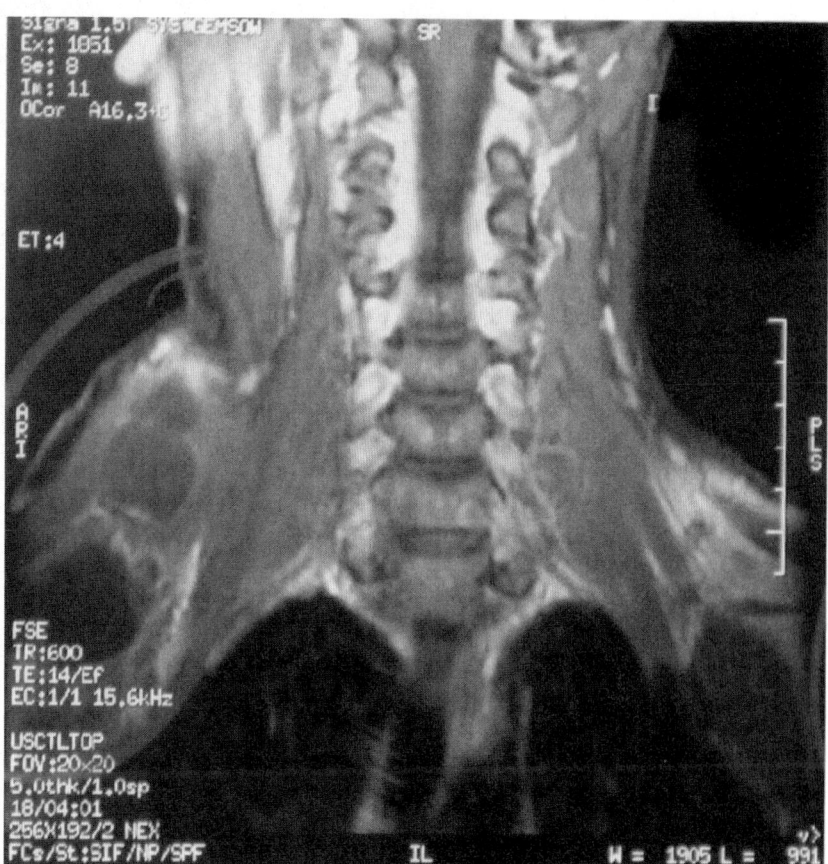

FIG. 17-15. Coronal MRI of cervical macrocystic lymphangioma (lymphatic vascular malformation).

TRAUMA OF THE HEAD AND NECK

Management of soft-tissue trauma in the head and neck has several salient features. Skin injuries may be classified as abrasions, contusions, or lacerations. Abrasions represent superficial epidermal injury and are treated with cleansing, saline irrigation, and removal of dirt or other foreign bodies. The latter step is important because retained materials may form a nidus for infection or foreign-body reaction and may cause tattooing of the skin after healing. Topical antibiotic dressing is applied until re-epithelialization is complete.

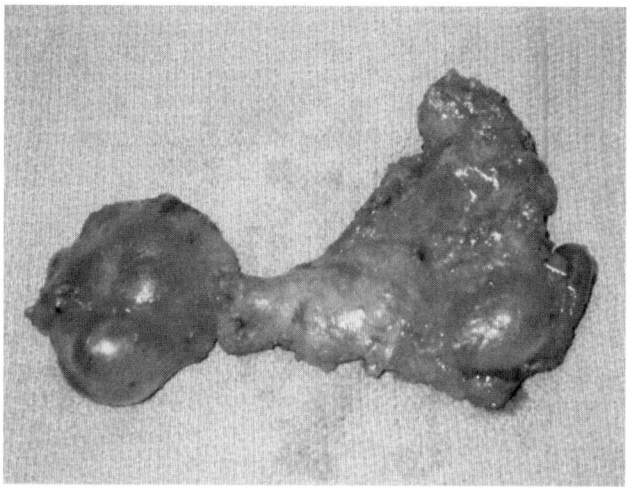

FIG. 17-16. Surgical specimen of case shown in Fig. 17-15.

The patient is instructed to avoid sunlight, because this can cause pigmentary abnormalities during the healing process, which matures over a 6- to 12-month period. Contusions may include ecchymosis and/or frank hematoma. Treatment includes head-of-bed elevation to decrease tissue edema, application of ice, and drainage of hematoma. Lacerations must also be cleansed and irrigated, with removal of any associated dirt or foreign bodies. Most lacerations without significant tissue loss can be closed primarily, and primary closure is preferred when possible. Closure of trapdoor lacerations requires conservative undermining of surrounding tissue and good approximation of subdermal levels prior to epidermal closure. A pressure dressing is also applied. These measures are employed to avoid a pincushion deformity (Fig. 17-17).

Typically, subdermal layers are approximated with an absorbable 3-0 or 4-0 suture such as Vicryl or polydioxanone, and the skin is closed using 5-0 or 6-0 monofilament nylon or Prolene. Sutures are removed after 4 to 5 days, but may be removed earlier in thin-skinned areas. The wound is treated with antibiotic ointments. Systemic antibiotics are indicated for through-and-through mucosal lacerations, contaminated wounds, bite injuries, and when delayed closure is performed (>72 hours). The chosen antibiotic should cover *S. aureus*. In many such wounds, healing by secondary intention may be preferable.

Wound closure must be understood in the context of the cosmetic and functional anatomic landmarks of the head and neck. Management of injuries to the eyelid requires identification of the orbicularis oculi, which is closed in a separate layer. The gray line (conjunctival margin; Fig. 17-18) must be carefully approximated to avoid lid notching or height mismatch. Management of lip injuries follows the same principle. The orbicularis oris must be closed, and

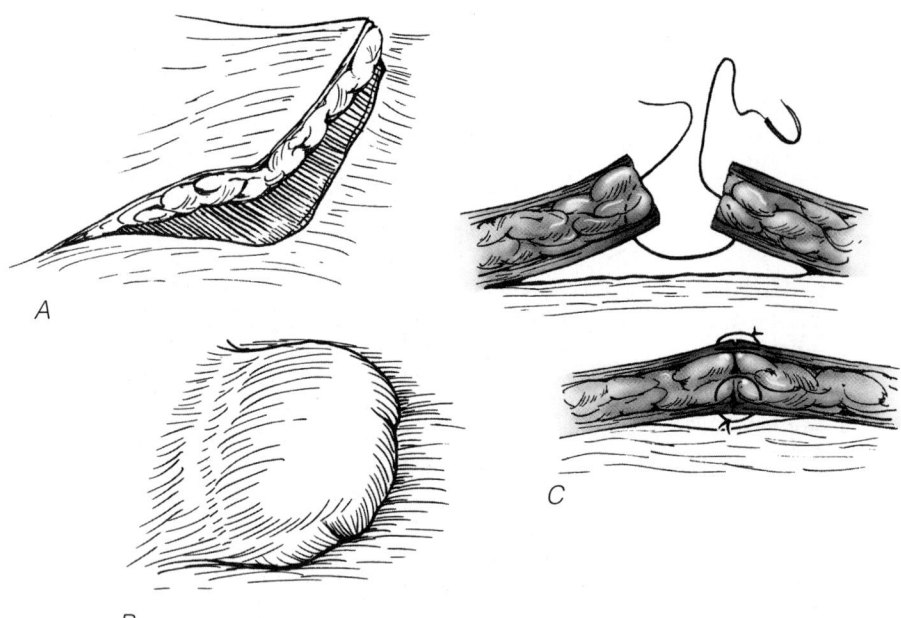

FIG. 17-17. Trapdoor laceration (A) healed with a "pin cushion" deformity (B). Soft-tissue layers must be meticulously approximated (C) to avoid this complication.

the vermilion border carefully approximated (Fig. 17-19). Injuries involving one-fourth the width of the eyelid or one-third the width of the lip may be closed primarily; otherwise, flap or grafting procedures may be required. With laceration of the auricle, key structures such as the helical rim and antihelix must be carefully aligned. These injuries must be repaired such that the cartilage is covered. The principles of auricular repair are predicated on the fact that the cartilage has no intrinsic blood supply and is thus susceptible to ischemic necrosis following trauma. The suture should be passed through the perichondrium, while placement though the cartilage itself should be avoided. Auricular hematomas should be drained promptly, with placement of a bolster as a pressure dressing. A pressure dressing is frequently advocated after closure of an ear laceration. It also deserves note that the surgeon must avoid the temptation to perform aggressive débridement after injuries to the eyelid or auricle. Given the rich vascular supply to the face and neck, many soft-tissue components that appear devitalized will indeed survive.

Most traumatic facial nerve injuries are secondary to temporal bone trauma, which is discussed below in this section. Soft-tissue injuries occurring in the midface may involve distal facial nerve branches. Those injured anterior to a vertical line dropped from the lateral canthus do not require repair secondary to collateral innervation in the anterior midface. Posterior to this line, the nerve should be repaired, primarily if possible, using 8-0 to 10-0 monofilament

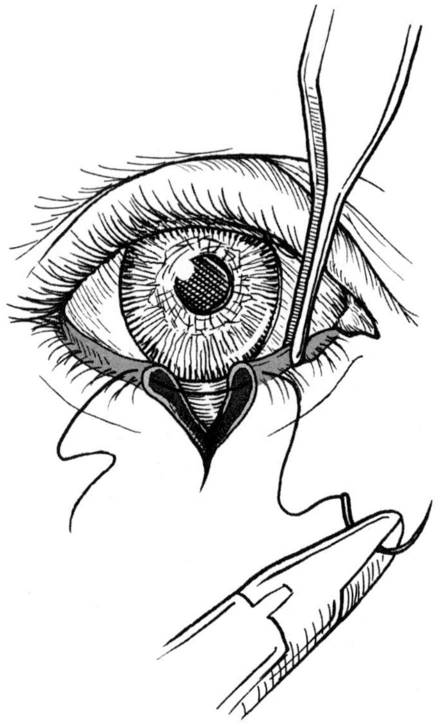

FIG. 17-18. Alignment of the gray line is the key step in the repair of eyelid lacerations.

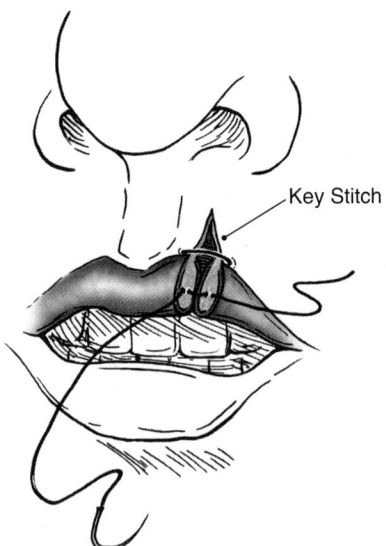

Key Stitch

FIG. 17-19. Approximation of the vermillion border is the key step in the repair of lip lacerations.

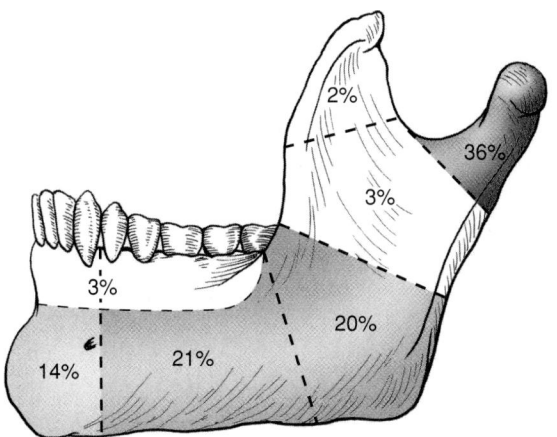

FIG. 17-20. Sites of common mandible fractures.

suture to approximate the epineurium under microscopic visualization. If neural segments are missing, cable grafting is performed using either the greater auricular (provides 7 to 8 cm) or sural nerve (up to 30 cm) as a donor. Injuries to the buccal branch should alert the examiner to a possible parotid duct injury. This structure lies along an imaginary line drawn from the tragus to the midline upper lip, running along with the buccal branch of the facial nerve. The duct should be repaired over a 22-gauge stent or marsupialized into the oral cavity.

The mandible is the most commonly fractured facial bone. Fractures most often involve the angle, body, or condyle, and in most cases, two or more sites are involved (Fig. 17-20). Fractures are described as either favorable or unfavorable, depending on whether or not the masticatory musculature tends to pull the fracture into reduction or distraction. Vertically favorable fractures are brought into reduction by the masseter, while horizontally favorable fractures are brought into reduction by the pterygoid musculature. The fracture is usually evaluated radiographically using a Panorex (Fig. 17-21), but specialized plain film views, and occasionally CT scan, are necessary in selected cases. Classical management of mandible fractures dictated closed reduction and a 6-week period of intermaxillary fixation (IMF) with arch bars applied via circumdental wiring (see Fig. 17-21). Comminuted, displaced, or unfavorable fractures

underwent open reduction and wire fixation in addition to IMF. Currently, arch bars and IMF are performed to establish occlusion. The fracture is then exposed and reduced, using transoral approaches where possible. Transcervical approaches are required to address fractures of the ramus or posterior body, with careful attention given to preserving the marginal mandibular branch of the facial nerve. Rigid fixation is then accomplished by the application of plates and screws. Selected fractures, such as those of the body, benefit from dynamic compression plating, which applies pressure toward the fracture line. With rigid fixation, IMF is required only to establish occlusion intraoperatively and not just for the 6-week period. This is preferable because IMF is associated with gingival and dental disease, as well as with significant weight loss and malnutrition, during the fixation period. In edentulous patients, determining the baseline occlusion is of less significance because dentures may be refashioned once healing is complete. If IMF is required to aid in immobilization of the fracture, interosseous wiring and/or the fabrication of custom-made splints is required.

Midface fractures are classically described in three patterns Le Fort I, II, and III. A full understanding of midface structure is first necessary (Fig. 17-22).[36] The midface is supported by three vertical buttresses: the nasofrontal-maxillary, the frontozygomaticomaxillary, and pterygomaxillary. The five weaker, horizontal buttresses include the frontal bone, nasal bones, upper alveolus, zygomatic arches, and the infraorbital region. Classical signs of midface fractures in general include subconjunctival hemorrhage; malocclusion; midface numbness or hypesthesia (maxillary division of the trigeminal nerve); facial ecchymoses/hematoma; ocular signs/symptoms; and mobility of the maxillary complex.

Le Fort I fractures occur transversely across the alveolus, above the level of the teeth apices. In a pure Le Fort I fracture, the palatal vault is mobile while the nasal pyramid and orbital rims are stable. The Le Fort II fracture extends through the nasofrontal buttress, medial wall of the orbit, across the infraorbital rim, and through the zygomaticomaxillary articulation. The nasal dorsum, palate, and medial part of the infraorbital rim are mobile. The Le Fort III fracture is

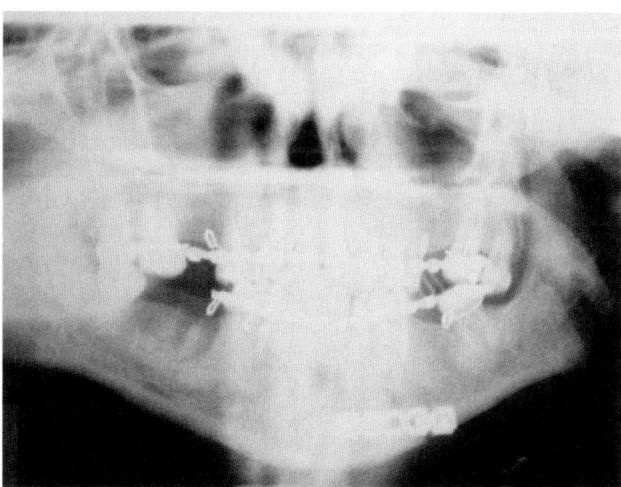

FIG. 17-21. Mandibular Panorex demonstrating intermaxillary fixation (maxillomandibular fixation) and plating of a parasymphysial fracture.

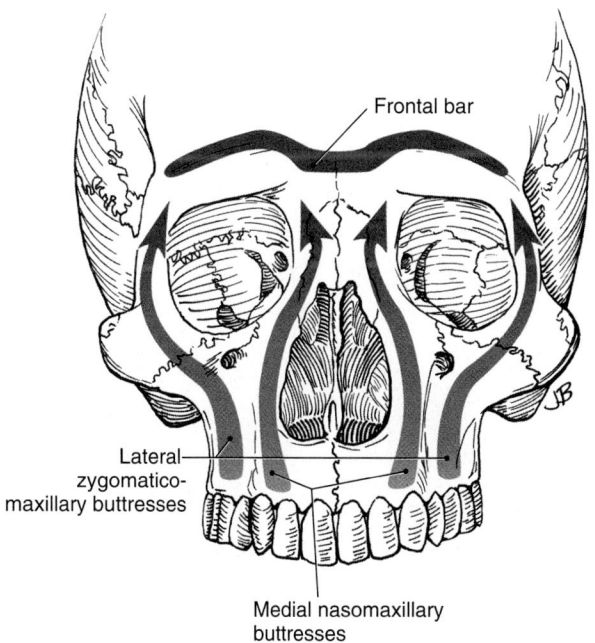

FIG. 17-22. Major buttresses of the midface.

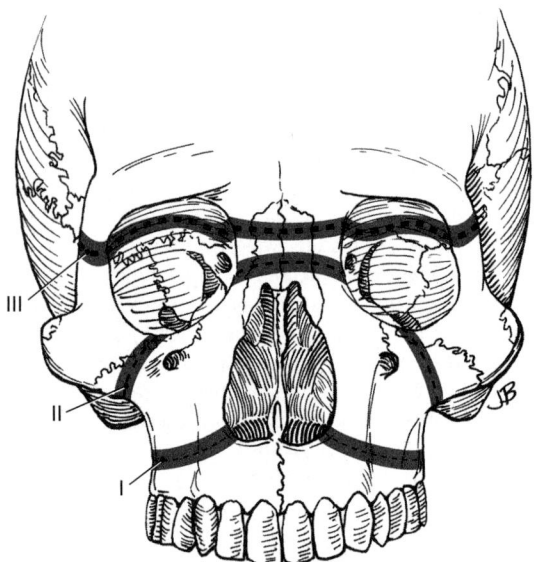

FIG. 17-23. Classic Le Fort fracture patterns.

also known as craniofacial disjunction. The frontozygomaticomaxillary, frontomaxillary, and frontonasal suture lines are disrupted. The entire face is mobile from the cranium. It is convenient to conceptualize complex midface fractures according to these patterns (Fig. 17-23); however, in reality, fractures reflect a combination of these three types. Also, the fracture pattern may vary between the left and right sides of the midface. Lateral blows to the cheek may be associated with isolated zygoma fractures. The zygoma is typically displaced inferiorly and medially with disruption of the suture lines between the temporal, frontal, and maxillary bones and the zygoma. Disruption of the latter articulation may be associated with depression into the maxillary sinus and blood in the sinus cavity. Fractures of the midface and/or zygoma may be associated with an orbital blow-out, whereas the orbital floor is disrupted and orbital soft tissues subsequently herniate into the maxillary sinus (Fig. 17-24). The mechanism of orbital blow-out may involve propagation of adjacent fracture lines or may be the result of a sudden increase in intraorbital pressure during the injury. This may be

associated with enophthalmos or entrapment of the inferior oblique muscle. The latter results in diplopia upon upward gaze. Entrapment is confirmed by forced duction testing, where, under topical or general anesthesia, the muscular attachment of the inferior oblique is grasped with forceps and manipulated to determine passive ocular mobility. Fractures of the midface, zygoma, and orbital floor are best evaluated using CT scan, and repair requires a combination of transoral and external approaches to achieve at least two points of fixation for each fractured segment.[37] Blow-out fractures demonstrating significant entrapment or enophthalmos are treated by orbital exploration and reinforcement of the floor with mesh or bone grafting.

Temporal bone fractures occur in approximately one-fifth of skull fractures. As with fractures of the mandible and midface, blunt trauma (from motor vehicle accident or assault) is usually implicated. Unfortunately, the incidence of temporal bone fracture from gunshot wounds to the head is rising. Fractures are divided into two patterns (Fig. 17-25), longitudinal and transverse, based on the clinical picture and CT imaging. In practice, most fractures are oblique. By classical descriptions, longitudinal fractures comprise 80% and are associated with lateral skull trauma. Signs and symptoms include conductive hearing loss, ossicular injury, bloody otorrhea, and labyrinthine concussion. The facial nerve is injured in approximately 20% of cases. In contrast, the transverse pattern comprises only 20% of temporal bone fractures and occurs secondary to fronto-occipital trauma. The facial nerve is injured in 50% of cases. These injuries frequently involve the otic capsule to cause sensorineural hearing loss and loss of vestibular function. Hemotympanum may be observed. A cerebrospinal fluid (CSF) leak must be suspected in temporal bone trauma. This resolves with conservative measures in most cases. The most significant consideration in the management of temporal bone injuries is the status of the facial nerve. Delayed or partial paralysis will almost always resolve

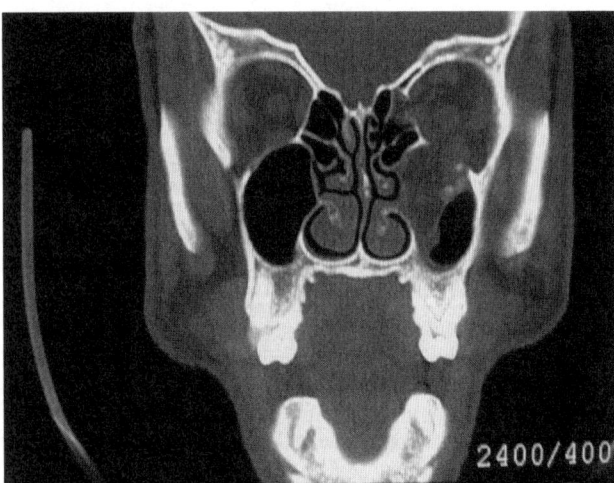

FIG. 17-24. Coronal CT demonstrating an orbital blow-out fracture with herniation of orbital contents into the maxillary sinus.

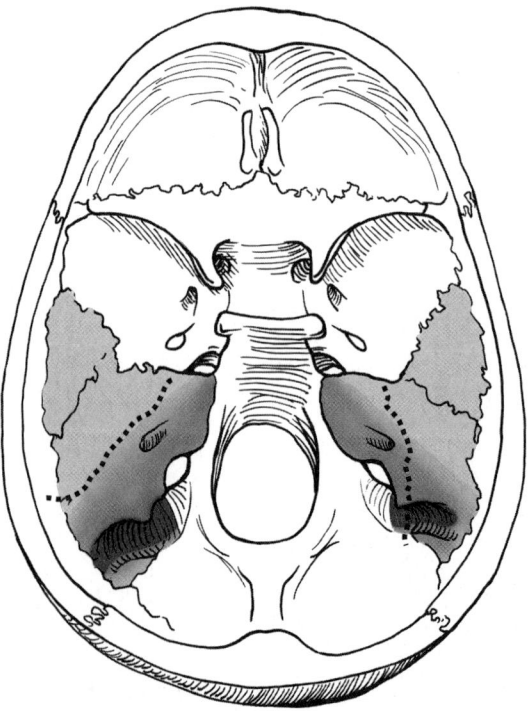

FIG. 17-25. View of cranial surface of skull base. Longitudinal (*left*) and transverse (*right*) temporal bone fractures.

with conservative management. However, immediate paralysis that does not recover within 1 week should be considered for nerve decompression. Electroneurography and EMG have been employed to help determine which patients with delayed onset complete paralysis will benefit from surgical decompression. The finding of greater than 90% degeneration more than 72 hours after the onset of complete paralysis is considered an indication for surgery.[38] Multiple approaches have been described for facial nerve decompression, some of which sacrifice hearing. These patients may have severe intracranial or vascular injuries such that the decision to operate must also be made in the context of the patient's overall medical stability. It is of paramount importance to protect the eye in patients with facial nerve paralysis of any etiology, because absence of an intact blink reflex will predispose to corneal drying and abrasion. This requires the placement of artificial tears throughout the day with lubricant ointment, eye taping, and/or a humidity chamber at night.[39,40]

TUMORS OF THE HEAD AND NECK

When a discussion of neoplasms of the head and neck is initiated, the conversation frequently focuses on squamous cell carcinoma. This is because the majority of malignancies of this region are represented by this pathology. The diagnosis and treatment of lesions spanning from the lips and oral cavity to the larynx requires a similar methodic approach. The evaluation of local, regional, and distant spread of tumor and the selection of treatment protocols vary for each site within the head and neck. Therapies aimed at organ preservation and the development of functional reconstructive options are some of the advances made within the field during the last decade. It appears that the future of head and neck cancer lies within the field of molecular biology as more is understood about the genetics of the pathology and additional treatment options developed with the goal of improving quality of life.

Etiology and Epidemiology

It should come as no surprise that abuse of tobacco and alcohol are the most common preventable risk factors associated with the development of head and neck cancers. This relationship is a synergistic rather than an additive one. Smoking confers a 1.9-fold increased risk to males and a threefold increased risk to females for developing a head and neck carcinoma, when compared to nonsmokers. The risk increases as the number of years smoking and number of cigarettes smoked per day increases. Alcohol alone confers a 1.7-fold increased risk to males drinking 1 to 2 drinks per day, when compared to nondrinkers. This increased risk rises to greater than threefold for heavy drinkers. Individuals who both smoke (two packs per day) and drink (four units of alcohol per day) had an odds ratio of 35 for the development of a carcinoma, when compared to controls.[41] Users of smokeless tobacco have a four times increased risk of oral cavity carcinoma, when compared nonusers.

Tobacco is the leading preventable cause of death in the United States and is responsible for 1 of every 5 deaths.[42] As of 1999, 23.5% of U.S. adults smoked tobacco products, with 25.7% of males and 21.5% of females comprising this population.[43] Recent trends have demonstrated an increase in the use of tobacco products by women, and the long-term affects have yet to be realized. The evidence supporting the need for head and neck cancer patients to pursue smoking cessation after treatment is compelling. In a study by Moore,[44] 40% of patients who continued to smoke after definitive treatment for an oral cavity malignancy went on to recur or develop a second

head and neck malignancy. For patients who stopped smoking after treatment, only 6% went on to develop a recurrence. Induction of specific p53 mutations within upper aerodigestive tract tumors has been noted in patients with histories of tobacco and alcohol use.[45,46]

When smokers who develop head and neck squamous cell carcinomas are compared to nonsmokers, differences between the two populations emerge. Koch and associates[47] noted that nonsmokers were represented by a disproportionate number of women and were more frequently at the extremes of age (<30 or >85 years of age). Tumors from nonsmokers presented more frequently in the oral cavity, specifically within the oral tongue, buccal mucosa, and alveolar ridge. Smokers presented more frequently with tumors of the larynx, hypopharynx, and floor of mouth. Former smokers, defined as those individuals who had quit greater than 10 years prior, demonstrated a profile more consistent with nonsmokers.

In India and Southeast Asia, the product of the Areca catechu tree, known as a betel nut, is chewed in a habitual manner and acts as a mild stimulant similar to that of coffee. The nut is chewed in combination with lime and cured tobacco as a mixture known as a quid. The long-term use of the betel nut quid can be destructive to oral mucosa and dentition and is highly carcinogenic.[48] Another habit associated with oral malignancy is that of reverse smoking, where the lighted portion of the tobacco product is within the mouth during inhalation. The risk of hard palate carcinoma is 47 times greater in reverse smokers, when compared to nonsmokers.

HPV is an epitheliotropic virus that has been detected to varying degrees within samples of oral cavity squamous cell carcinoma. Infection alone is not considered sufficient for malignant conversion; however, results of multiple studies suggest a role of HPV in a subset of head and neck squamous cell carcinoma. Approximately 40% of tonsillar carcinomas demonstrate evidence of HPV types 16 and 18.

Environmental ultraviolet light exposure has been associated with the development of lip cancer. The projection of the lower lip, as it relates to this solar exposure, has been used to explain why the majority of squamous cell carcinomas arise along the vermilion border of the lower lip. In addition, pipe smoking also has been associated with the development of lip carcinoma. Factors such as mechanical irritation, thermal injury, and chemical exposure have been described as etiologies associated with the practice of pipe smoking as an explanation for this finding.

Other entities associated with oral malignancy include Plummer-Vinson syndrome (achlorhydria, iron-deficiency anemia, mucosal atrophy of mouth, pharynx, and esophagus), chronic infection with syphilis, and immunocompromised status (30-fold increase with renal transplant).

Although evidence linking HIV infection to squamous cell carcinoma of the head and neck is lacking, several acquired immunodeficiency syndrome (AIDS)-defining malignancies, including Kaposi's sarcoma, non-Hodgkin's lymphoma, and Hodgkin's disease, may require the care of an otolaryngologist.

Anatomy and Histopathology

A brief overview of the anatomy of the head and neck can be accomplished by examining the upper aerodigestive tract and its related structures. The upper aerodigestive tract is divided into several distinct sites which include the oral cavity, pharynx, larynx, and nasal cavity/paranasal sinuses. Within these sites are individual subsites with specific anatomic relationships that affect diagnosis, spread, and treatment of tumors. The contiguous spread of tumors from one site to another is determined by the course of the nerves, blood vessels, lymphatic pathways, and by the fascial planes. These fascial

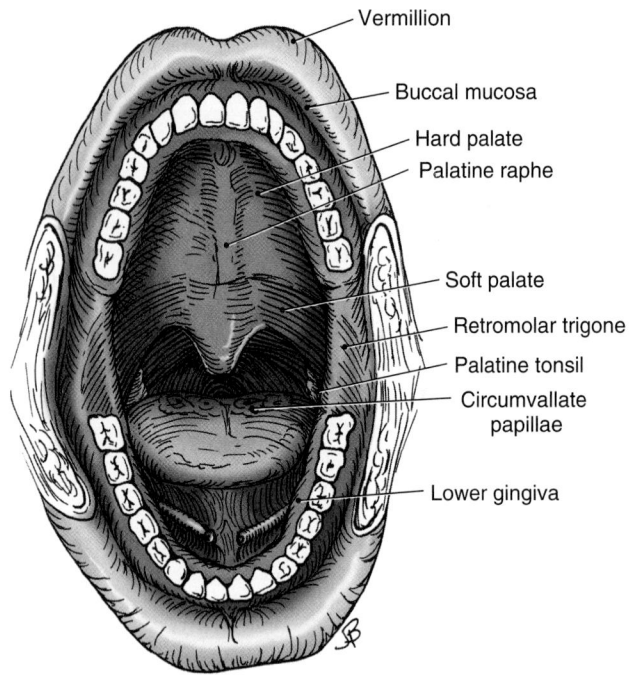

Vermillion
Buccal mucosa
Hard palate
Palatine raphe
Soft palate
Retromolar trigone
Palatine tonsil
Circumvallate papillae
Lower gingiva

FIG. 17-26. *Oral cavity landmarks.*

planes serve as barriers to the direct invasion of tumor and contribute to the pattern of spread to regional lymph nodes.

The oral cavity extends from the vermilion border of the lip to the hard-palate/soft-palate junction superiorly, to circumvallate papillae inferiorly, and to the anterior tonsillar pillars laterally (Fig. 17-26). It is divided into seven subsites: lips, alveolar ridges, oral tongue, retromolar trigone, floor of mouth, buccal mucosa, and hard palate. Advanced oral cavity lesions may present with mandible and/or maxillary involvement requiring consideration at the time of resection and reconstruction. Regional metastatic spread of lesions of the oral cavity spread to the lymphatics of the submandibular and the upper jugular region.

The pharynx is divided into three regions: nasopharynx, oropharynx, and hypopharynx. The nasopharynx extends from the posterior nasal septum and choana to the skull base and includes the fossa of Rosenmüller and torus of the eustachian tubes laterally. The inferior margin of the nasopharynx is the superior surface of the soft palate. The adenoids, typically involuted in adults, are located with the posterior aspect of this site. Given the midline location of the nasopharynx, bilateral regional metastatic spread is not uncommon for these lesions. Lymphadenopathy of the posterior triangle of the neck should provoke consideration for a nasopharyngeal primary.

The oropharynx extends from the hard-palate/soft-palate junction superiorly, the tonsillar pillars and linea terminalis anteriorly, the base of tongue to the vallecula inferiorly, and the palatoglossal and palatopharyngeal arches laterally. The major sites within the oropharynx are the tonsillar region, base of tongue, soft palate, and posterolateral pharyngeal walls. Regional lymphatic drainage for oropharyngeal lesions frequently occurs to the upper and lower cervical node chains. However, it should also be remembered that retropharyngeal metastatic lymphatic spread may occur with oropharyngeal lesions.

The hypopharynx extends from the vallecula to the lower border of the cricoid posterior and lateral to the larynx. The subsites of this region include the pyriform fossae, the postcricoid space, and posterior pharyngeal wall. Regional lymphatic spread is frequently bilateral and to the mid- and lower cervical nodes.

The larynx is divided into three distinct portions: the supraglottis, glottis, and subglottis. The supraglottic larynx includes the epiglottis, false vocal cords, medial surface of the aryepiglottic folds, and the roof of the laryngeal ventricles. The glottis includes the true vocal cords, anterior and posterior commissure, and the floor of the laryngeal ventricle. The subglottis extends from below the true vocal cords to the cephalic border of the cricoid within the airway. The supraglottis has a rich lymphatic network, which accounts for the high rate of bilateral spread of metastatic disease that is not typically seen with the glottis. Glottic and subglottic lesions, in addition to potential spread to the cervical chain lymph nodes, may also spread to the paralaryngeal and paratracheal lymphatics and require attention to prevent peristomal recurrence.

Carcinogenesis

Development of a tumor represents the loss of cellular signaling mechanisms involved in the regulation of growth. Following malignant transformation, the processes of replication (mitosis), programmed cell death (apoptosis), and the interaction of a cell with its surrounding environment are altered. Advances in molecular biology have allowed for the identification of many of the mutations associated with this transformation.

Overexpression of mutant p53 is associated with carcinogenesis at multiple sites within the body. Point mutations in p53 have been reported in up to 45% of head and neck carcinomas. Koch and associates[47] noted that p53 mutation is a key event in the malignant transformation of greater than 50% of head and neck squamous cell carcinomas in smokers.

Carcinogenesis has long been explained as a two-hit process, involving DNA damage and the progression of mutated cells through the cell cycle. These two events also are known as initiation and promotion. It has been proposed that up to 6 to 10 independent genetic mutations are required for the development of a malignancy. Overexpression of mitogenic receptors, loss of tumor-suppressor proteins, expression of oncogene-derived proteins that inhibit apoptosis, and overexpression of proteins that drive the cell cycle can allow for unregulated cell growth.

Genetic mutations may occur as a result of environmental exposure (e.g., radiation or carcinogen exposure), viral infection, or spontaneous mutation (deletions, translocations, frame shifts). Common genetic alterations, such as loss of heterozygosity at 3p, 4q, and 11q13, and the overall number of chromosomal microsatellite losses are found more frequently in the tumors of smokers than in the tumors of nonsmokers.[47]

The theory of field cancerization, introduced by Slaughter and associates[49] in the 1950s, attempted to explain why some patients presented with multiple primary tumors. It was hypothesized that repeated carcinogenic exposure of mucosal surfaces of the upper aerodigestive tract resulted in similar mutations at multiple sites and the development of multiple carcinomas. A separate theory developed later suggests that synchronous tumors in the head and neck represent separate and distinct clonal populations of tumor cells at each site. However, some evidence now exists that demonstrates that separate primary tumors may not represent distinct genetic mutational events. Rather, cells of the same clonal origin migrate to separate sites where they develop as geographically separate, but genetically identical tumors.[50]

Second Primary Tumors in the Head and Neck

Patients diagnosed with a head and neck cancer are predisposed to the development of a second tumor within the aerodigestive tract. The overall rate of second primary tumors is approximately 14%. A second primary tumor detected within 6 months of the diagnosis of the initial primary lesion is defined as a synchronous neoplasm. The prevalence of synchronous tumors is approximately 3 to 4%. The detection of a second primary lesion more than 6 months after the initial diagnosis is referred to as metachronous tumor. Eighty percent of second primaries are metachronous, and at least half of these lesions develop within 2 years of the diagnosis of the original primary. The incidence and site of the second primary tumor vary and depend on the site and the inciting factors associated with the initial primary tumor. The importance of advocating smoking cessation and addressing alcoholism in these patients cannot be underemphasized.

Patients with a primary malignancy of the oral cavity or pharynx are most likely to develop a second lesion within the cervical esophagus. A bimodal pattern of presentation is seen with second primary tumors in the esophagus. An early group presents within 2 years of treatment of the index tumor, and a later group presents 5 years after primary treatment. For patients with a carcinoma of the larynx, the second lesion usually arises in the lung. Hence, the presentation of a new-onset dysphagia in a patient with a history of oral cavity cancer or chronic cough, or for a patient with a history of laryngeal carcinoma, must be viewed with a reasonable degree of concern as representing a second primary tumor.

A staging examination is recommended at the initial evaluation of all patients with primary cancers of the upper aerodigestive tract. This may involve a direct laryngoscopy, rigid/flexible esophagoscopy, and rigid/flexible bronchoscopy known as panendoscopy. Some surgeons argue against the use of bronchoscopy because of the low yield of the examination in asymptomatic patients with a normal chest x-ray. Additionally, some surgeons prefer to use a barium swallow instead of esophagoscopy as a preoperative evaluation. Despite the different practices concerning pretreatment evaluation of asymptomatic patients, it should be noted that patients with symptoms potentially representing those of metastatic spread of disease require a work-up greater than a screening evaluation.

Staging

Staging for upper aerodigestive tract malignancies is defined by the American Joint Committee on Cancer (AJCC)[51] and follows the TNM (primary tumor, regional nodal metastases, distant metastasis) staging format. The T staging criteria for each site varies depending upon the relevant anatomy (e.g., vocal cord immobility is typical of T3 lesions). Table 17-3 demonstrates TNM staging for oral cavity

Table 17-3
TNM Staging for Oral Cavity Carcinoma

Primary tumor			
TX	Unable to assess primary tumor		
T0	No evidence of primary tumor		
Tis	Carcinoma in situ		
T1	Tumor is <2 cm in greatest dimension		
T2	Tumor >2 cm and <4 cm in greatest dimension		
T3	Tumor >4 cm in greatest dimension		
T4 (lip)	Primary tumor invading cortical bone, inferior alveolar nerve, floor of mouth, or skin of face (e.g., nose or chin)		
T4a (oral)	Tumor invades adjacent structures (e.g., cortical bone, into deep tongue musculature, maxillary sinus) or skin of face		
T4b (oral)	Tumor invades masticator space, pterygoid plates, or skull base and/or encases the internal carotid artery		
Regional lymphadenopathy			
NX	Unable to assess regional lymph nodes		
N0	No evidence of regional metastasis		
N1	Metastasis in a single ipsilateral lymph node, 3 cm or less in greatest dimension		
N2a	Metastasis in single ipsilateral lymph node, >3 cm and <6 cm		
N2b	Metastasis in multiple ipsilateral lymph nodes, all nodes <6 cm		
N2c	Metastasis in bilateral or contralateral lymph nodes, all nodes <6 cm		
N3	Metastasis in a lymph node >6 cm in greatest dimension		
Distant metastases			
MX	Unable to assess for distant metastases		
M0	No distant metastases		
M1	Distant metastases		
TMN staging			
Stage 0	Tis	N0	M0
Stage I	T1	N0	M0
Stage II	T2	N0	M0
Stage III	T3	N0	M0
	T1-3	N1	M0
Stage IVa	T4a	N0	M0
	T4a	N1	M0
	T1-4a	N2	M0
Stage IVb	Any T	N3	M0
	T4b	Any N	M0
Stage IVc	Any T	Any N	M1

SOURCE: *American Joint Committee on Cancer Staging Manual*, 6th ed.[51]

lesions. The N classification system is uniform for all head and neck sites except for the nasopharynx.

Upper Aerodigestive Tract

Lip

The lips represent a transition from external skin to internal mucous membrane that occurs at the vermilion border. The underlying musculature of the orbicularis oris, innervated by the facial nerve, creates a circumferential ring that allows the mouth to have a sphincter-like function. Cancer of the lip is most commonly seen in white men from the ages of 50 to 70 years, but can be seen in younger patients, particularly those with fair complexions. Risk factors include prolonged exposure to sunlight, fair complexion, immunosuppression, and tobacco use.

The majority of lip malignancies present on the lower lip (88 to 98%), followed by the upper lip (2 to 7%) and oral commissure (1%). The histology of lip cancers is predominantly squamous cell carcinoma; however, other tumors, such as keratoacanthoma, verrucous carcinoma, basal cell carcinoma, malignant melanoma, minor salivary gland malignancies, and tumors of mesenchymal origin (e.g., malignant fibrous histiocytoma, leiomyosarcoma, and rhabdomyosarcoma), may also present in this location. Basal cell carcinoma does disproportionately present more frequently on the upper lip than lower.

Clinical findings in lip cancer include an ulcerated lesion on the vermilion or cutaneous surface, or, less commonly, on the mucosal surface (Fig. 17-27). A nodular or sclerotic lesion may be palpable within the deeper tissues and careful palpation is important in determining the actual size of these lesions. The presence of paresthesias or dysesthesias in the area adjacent to the lesion may indicate mental nerve involvement.

Characteristics of lip primaries that negatively affect prognosis include perineural invasion, involvement of the underlying maxilla/mandible, cancer arising on the upper lip or commissure, regional lymphatic metastasis, and age younger than 40 years at onset. Lip cancer results in fewer than 200 patient deaths annually and is stage dependent. Early diagnosis coupled with adequate treatment results in high cure rates.

The treatment for lip cancer is determined by the overall health of the patient, size of the primary lesion, and the presence of regional metastases.[52] Small primary lesions may be treated with surgery or radiation with equal success and acceptable cosmetic results.

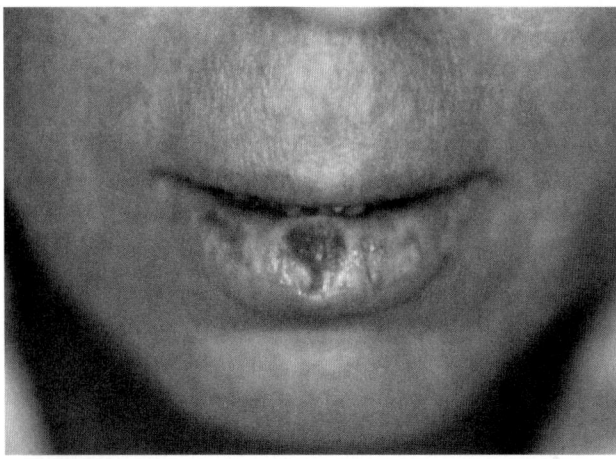

FIG. 17-27. Lower lip ulcerative lesion.

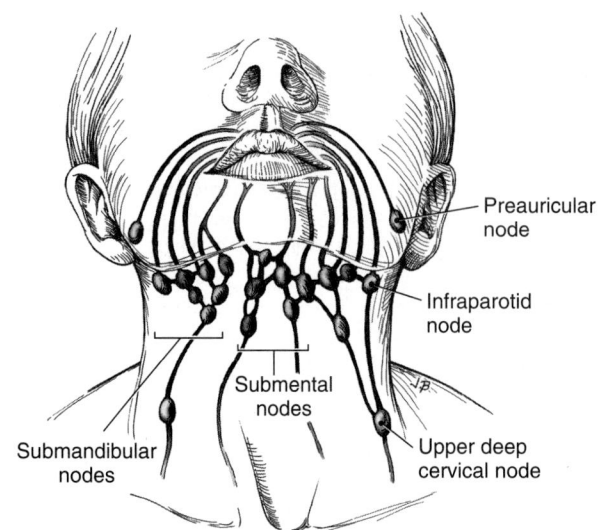

FIG. 17-28. Lymphatics of the lip.

However, surgical excision with histologic confirmation of tumor-free margins is the preferred modality. Lymph node metastasis occurs in fewer than 10% of patients with lip cancer (Fig. 17-28). The primary echelon of nodes at risk is in the submandibular and submental regions. In the presence of clinically evident neck metastasis, neck dissection is indicated. The overall 5-year cure rate of lip cancer approximates 90% and drops to 50% in the presence of neck metastases.[53] Postoperative radiation is administered to the primary site and neck for patients with close or positive margins, lymph node metastases, or perineural invasion.

The reconstruction of lip defects after tumor excision requires innovative techniques to provide oral competence, maintenance of dynamic function, and acceptable cosmesis. The typical lip length is 6 to 7 cm. This simple fact is important because the reconstructive algorithms available to the head and neck surgeon are based on the proportion of lip resected. Realignment of the vermilion border during the reconstruction and preservation of the oral commissure (when possible) are important principles in attempting to attain an acceptable cosmetic result. Resection with primary closure is possible with a defect of up to one-third of the lip (Fig. 17-29). When the resection includes one-third to one-half of the lip, rectangular excisions can be closed using Burow's triangles in combination with advancement flaps and releasing incisions in the mental crease.[52,54] Other medium-size defects can be repaired by borrowing tissue from the upper lip. For larger defects of up to 75%, the Karapandzic flap uses a sensate, neuromuscular flap that includes the remaining orbicularis oris muscle, conserving its blood supply from branches of the labial artery (Fig. 17-30). The lip-switch (Abbe-Estlander) flap or a stair-step advancement technique can be used to repair defects of either the upper or lower lip (Fig. 17-31). Microstoma is a potential complication with these types of lip reconstruction. For very large defects, Webster or Bernard types of repair using lateral nasolabial flaps with buccal advancement also have been described.[55] Details regarding specific techniques of reconstruction are not discussed in this chapter.

Oral Cavity

As previously mentioned, the oral cavity is composed of several sites with different anatomic relationships and associated risks with the presentation of a malignancy. The majority of tumors in

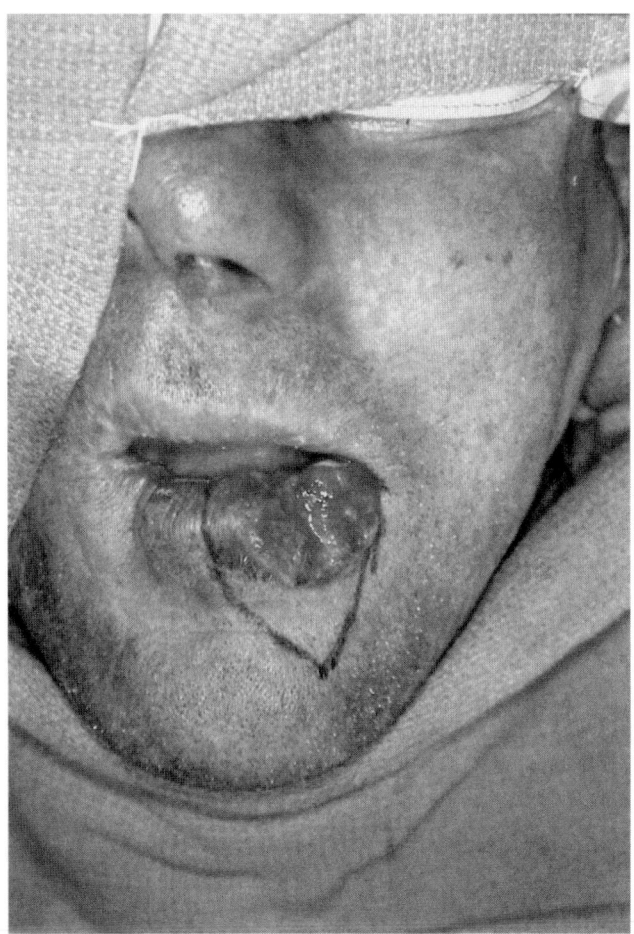

FIG. 17-29. Wedge resection of lower-lip squamous cell carcinoma.

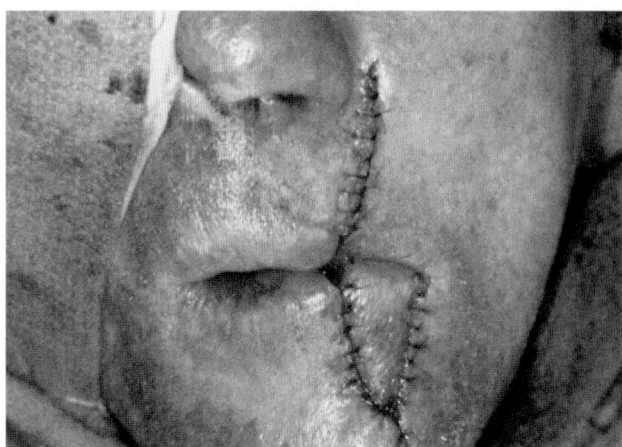

FIG. 17-31. Abbe-Estlander flap reconstruction of lip carcinoma resection.

the oral cavity are squamous cell carcinomas (>90%). Each site is briefly reviewed with emphasis placed on anatomy, diagnosis, and treatment options.

Oral Tongue. The oral tongue is a muscular structure with overlying nonkeratinizing squamous epithelium. The posterior limit of the oral tongue is the circumvallate papillae, whereas its ventral portion is contiguous with the anterior floor of mouth subsites including the lateral tongue, the tip the ventral tongue, and the posterior tongue. The tongue is composed of four intrinsic and four extrinsic muscles separated at the midline by the median fibrous lingual septum. Tumors of the tongue begin in the stratified epithelium of the surface and eventually invade into the deeper muscular structures. The presentation is commonly an ulcerated or exophytic mass (Fig. 17-32).[56] The regional lymphatics of the

oral cavity are to the submandibular space and the upper cervical lymph nodes (Fig. 17-33). The lingual nerve and the hypoglossal nerve may be invaded directly by tumors (Fig. 17-34). Their involvement produces the clinical findings of loss of sensation of the dorsal tongue surface and deviation on tongue protrusion, fasciculations, and atrophy. Tumors on the tongue may occur on any surface, but are most commonly seen on the lateral tongue and the ventral surfaces.[57] Primary tumors of the tongue musculature or mesenchymal components include leiomyomas, leiomyosarcoma, rhabdomyosarcoma, and neurofibromas.

Surgical treatment of small (T1-T2) primary tumors is wide local excision with either primary closure or healing by secondary intention (Fig. 17-35). The carbon dioxide laser may be used for excision of early tongue cancers or for ablation of premalignant lesions. A partial glossectomy, which removes a significant portion of the lateral oral tongue, permits reasonably effective postoperative function. Resection of larger tumors of the tongue that invade deeply can result in significant functional impairment. Removal of a significant portion of the tongue results in hypomobility and hypesthesia that impairs speech and swallowing function. Lingual contact with the palate, lip, and teeth is decreased and results in impaired articulation. The use of soft, pliable fasciocutaneous free flaps can provide intraoral bulk and preservation of tongue mobility. A palatal augmentation prothesis can allow for contact between the remaining tongue tissue and the palate, improving a patient's ability to speak and swallow. Treatment of the regional lymphatics is typically performed with the modality used to address the primary site, which most frequently is via modified radical or selective neck dissection. Depth of invasion of the primary tumor can direct the need for elective lymph node dissection with early stage lesions.[58]

FIG. 17-30. Karapandzic labioplasty for lower-lip carcinoma.

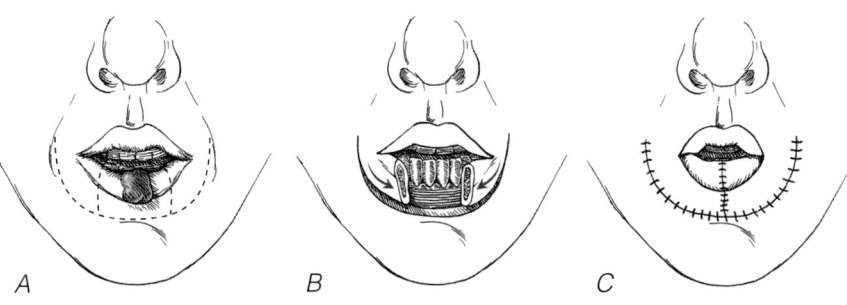

A   *B*   *C*

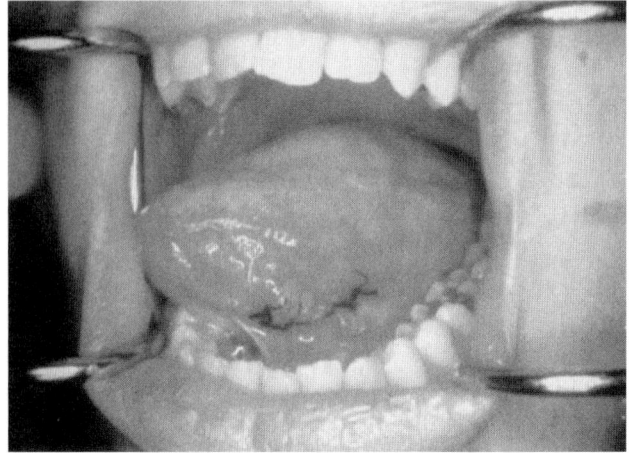

FIG. 17-32. *Oral tongue squamous cell carcinoma.*

Floor of Mouth. The floor of mouth is the mucosally covered semilunar area that extends from the anterior tonsillar pillar posteriorly to the frenulum anteriorly, and from the inner surface of the mandible to the ventral surface of the oral tongue. The ostia of the submaxillary and sublingual glands are contained in the anterior floor of mouth. The muscular floor of mouth is composed of the sling-like genioglossus, mylohyoid, and hyoglossus muscles, which serve as a barrier to spread of disease. Invasion into these muscles can lead to tongue hypomobility and poor articulation. Another pathway for spread of tumor is along the salivary ducts, which can result in direct extension into the sublingual space.

Anterior or lateral extension to the mandibular periosteum is of primary importance in preoperative treatment planning for these lesions. Imaging studies of the mandible, including CT scan, MRI, and Panorex radiography, are helpful for ascertaining bone invasion. These studies are useful in conjunction with a careful clinical evaluation, which includes bimanual palpation to assess adherence or fixation to adjacent bone (Fig. 17-36). The absence of fixation of the lesion to the inner mandibular cortex indicates that a mandible-sparing procedure is feasible.[59] Deep invasion into the

intrinsic musculature of the tongue causes fixation and mandates a partial glossectomy in conjunction with resection of the floor of mouth. Lesions in the anterior floor of mouth may directly invade the sublingual gland or submandibular duct and require resection of either of these glands in continuity with the primary lesion. Direct extension of tumors into or through the sublingual space and into the submaxillary space indicates the need for removal of the tumor and neck dissection specimen in continuity. Interruption of lymphatic channels when there is direct extension decreases the ability to obtain local control of disease.

The resection of large tumors of the floor of mouth may require a lip-splitting incision (Figs. 17-37 and 17-38) and usually require immediate reconstruction. The goals are to obtain watertight closure to avoid a salivary fistula and to avoid tongue tethering in order to maximize mobility. For small mucosal lesions, wide local excision can be followed by placement of a split-thickness skin graft over the muscular bed. Larger defects that require marginal or segmental mandibulectomy require complex reconstruction with a fasciocutaneous or a vascularized bone flap.

Alveolus/Gingiva. The alveolar mucosa overlies the bone of the mandible and maxilla. It extends from the gingivobuccal sulcus to the mucosa of the floor of mouth and hard palate. The posterior limits are the pterygopalatine arch and the ascending portion of the ramus of the mandible. Because of the tight attachment of the alveolar mucosa to the mandibular and maxillary periosteum, treatment of lesions of the alveolar mucosa frequently require resection of the underlying bone.

Marginal resection of the mandible can be performed for tumors of the alveolar surface that are associated with minimal bone invasion. Although access for such a procedure can be performed by using an anterior mandibulotomy (Fig. 17-39), use of transoral and pull-through procedures is preferred if a coronal or sagittal marginal mandibulotomy is performed. For more extensive tumors that invade into the medullary cavity, segmental mandibulectomy is necessary (Fig. 17-40). Preoperative radiographic evaluation of the mandible plays an important role in determining the type of bone resection required. For radiographic evaluation of the mandible, Panorex views demonstrate gross cortical invasion. MRI is the best modality for demonstrating invasion of the medullary cavity of the mandible. Sectional CT scanning with bone settings is the optimum modality for imaging subtle cortical invasion. Invasion of bone by radiographic or histologic evidence, involvement of the mandibular symphysis, advanced T stage, and presence of a high-grade lesion negatively impact locoregional control.[60]

Retromolar Trigone. The retromolar trigone is represented by tissue posterior to the posterior inferior alveolar ridge and ascends over the inner surface of the ramus of the mandible. Similar to alveolar lesions, early involvement of the mandible is common because of the lack of intervening soft tissue in the region. Presentation of trismus may indicate muscle of mastication involvement and potential spread to the skull base. Tumors of the region may extend posteriorly into the oropharyngeal anatomy or laterally to invade the mandible. As a result, resection of retromolar trigone tumors usually requires a marginal or segmental mandibulectomy with a soft-tissue and/or osseous reconstruction in order to maximize a patient's postoperative ability for functional speech and swallowing. Ipsilateral elective and therapeutic neck dissection is performed because of the risk of metastasis to the regional lymphatics. Huang and associates demonstrated a 5-year, disease-free survival rate for

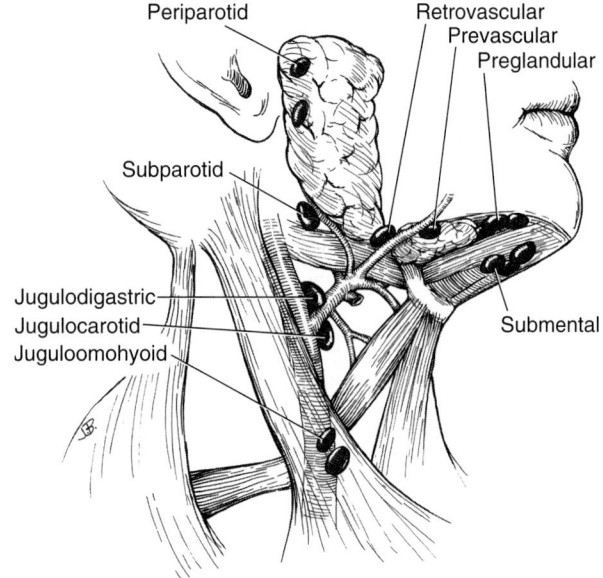

FIG. 17-33. *Primary lymphatics for oral cavity lesions.*

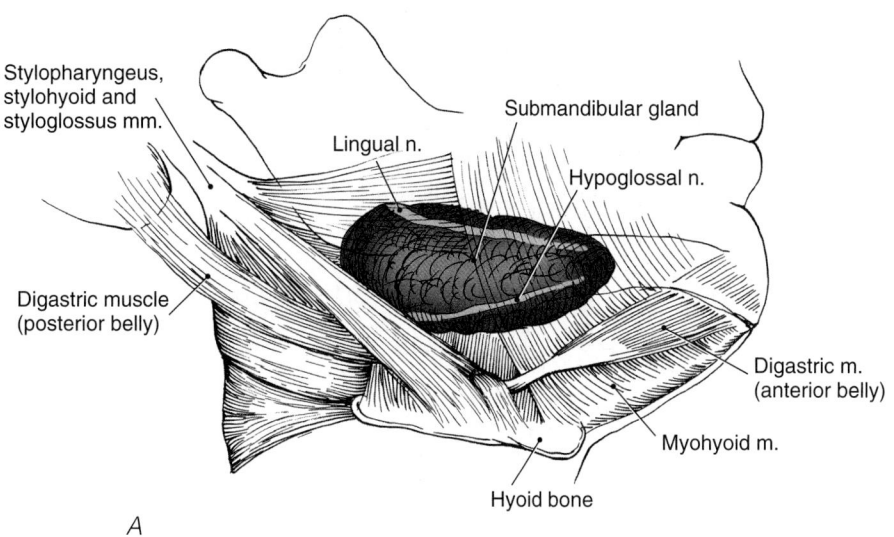

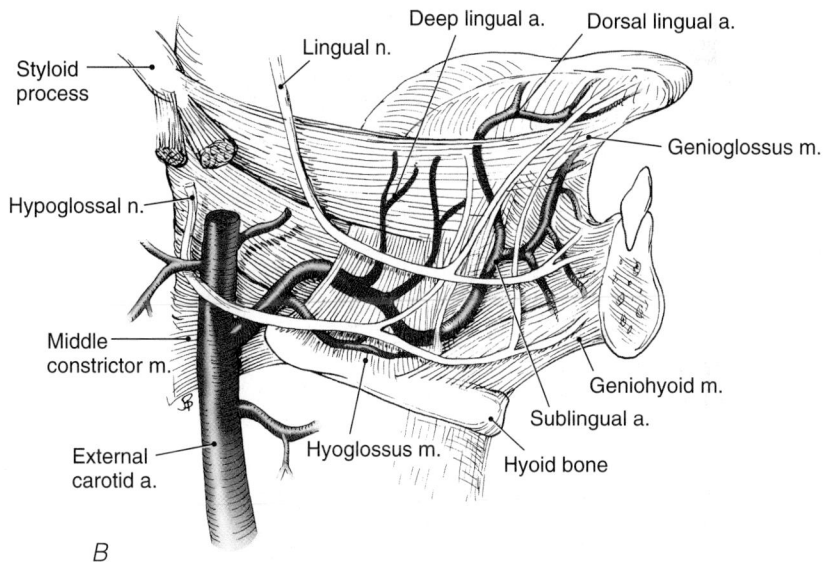

FIG. 17-34. *A* and *B*. Anatomy of the floor of mouth and submandibular space.

A

B

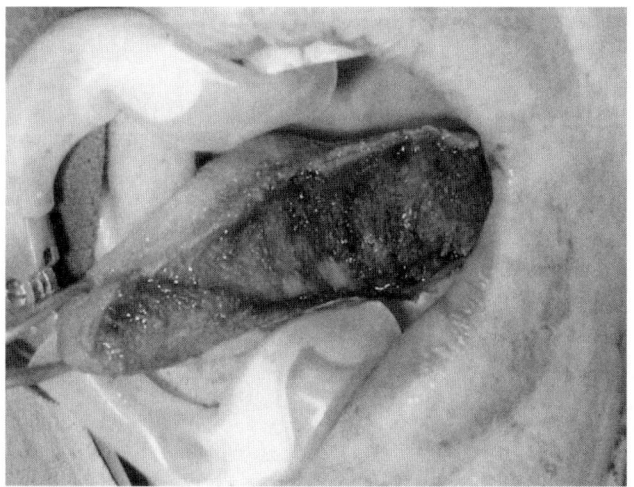

FIG. 17-35. Posttransoral resection of oral tongue squamous cell carcinoma.

T1 lesions of 76%, which declined to 54% for T4 disease. Patients with N0 disease had a 5-year survival rate of 69%.[61]

Buccal Mucosa. The buccal mucosa includes all of the mucosal lining from the inner surface of the lips to the line of attachment of mucosa of the alveolar ridges and pterygomandibular raphe. The etiologies of malignancies in the buccal area include lichen planus, chronic dental trauma, and the use of tobacco and alcohol. Tumors in this area have a propensity to spread locally and to metastasize to regional lymphatics (Fig. 17-41). Local intraoral spread may necessitate resection of the alveolar ridge of the mandible or maxilla. Lymphatic drainage is to the facial and the submandibular nodes (level I). Small lesions can be excised surgically, but more advanced tumors require combined surgery and postoperative radiation.[62] Deep invasion into the cheek may require through-and-through resection. Ideal reconstruction to provide both internal and external lining is best accomplished with a folded fasciocutaneous free flap.

Palate. The hard palate is defined as the semilunar area between the upper alveolar ridge and the mucous membrane covering the palatine process of the maxillary palatine bones. It extends from

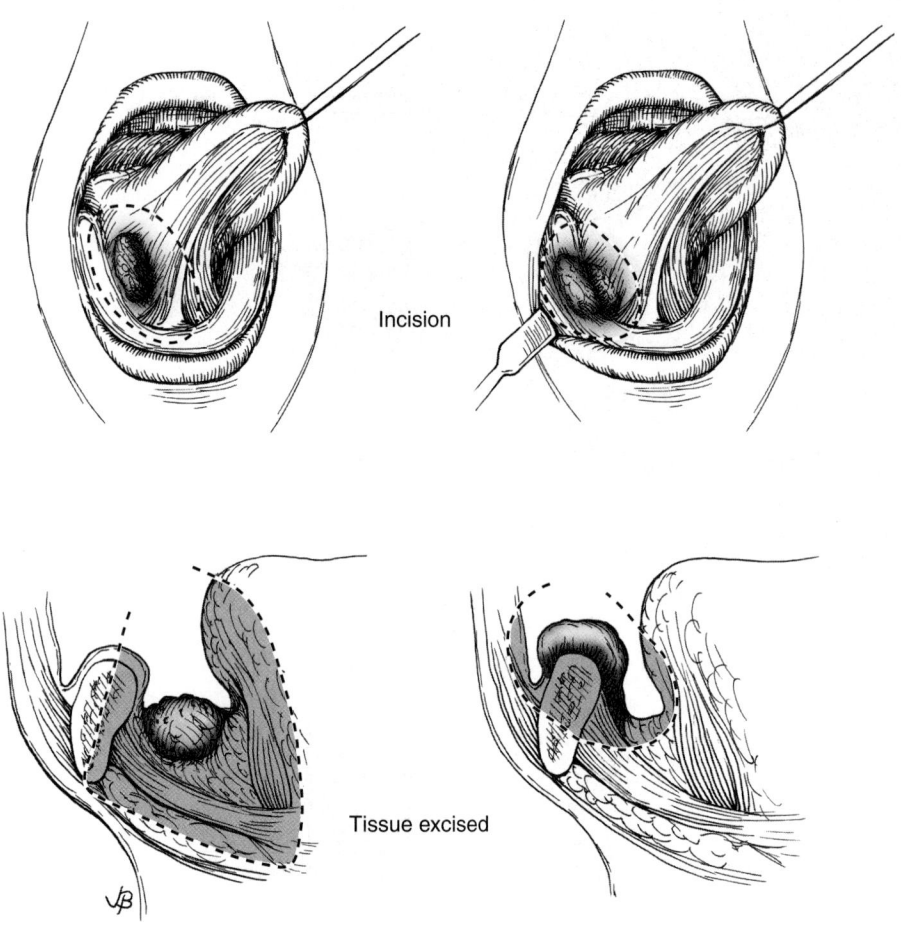

FIG. 17-36. *A* and *B*. Differences in the transoral resection of a floor of mouth and alveolar ridge lesion.

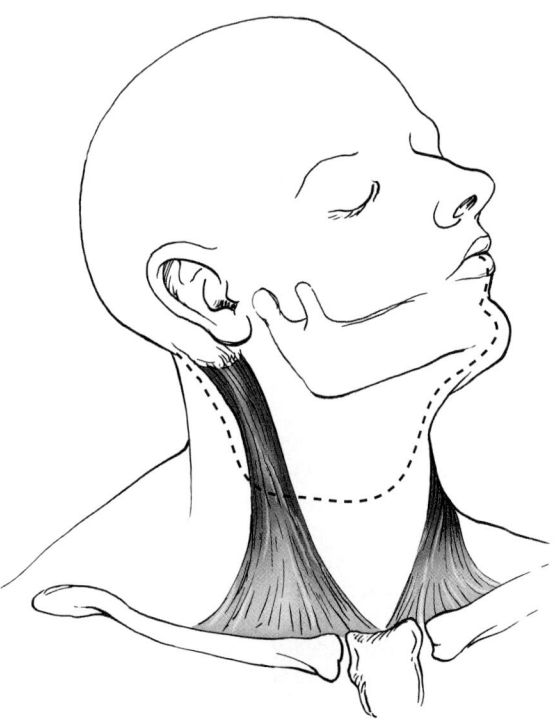

FIG. 17-37. Example of a lip-splitting incision used with mandibulotomy for access of oral cavity and oropharyngeal tumors.

the inner surface of the superior alveolar ridge to the posterior edge of the palatine bone. Most squamous cell carcinomas of the hard palate are caused by tobacco and alcohol use (Fig. 17-42). Chronic irritation from ill-fitting dentures also may play a causal role. Inflammatory lesions arising on the palate may mimic malignancy and can be differentiated by biopsy. Necrotizing sialometaplasia appears on the palate as a butterfly shaped ulcer and mimics carcinoma.

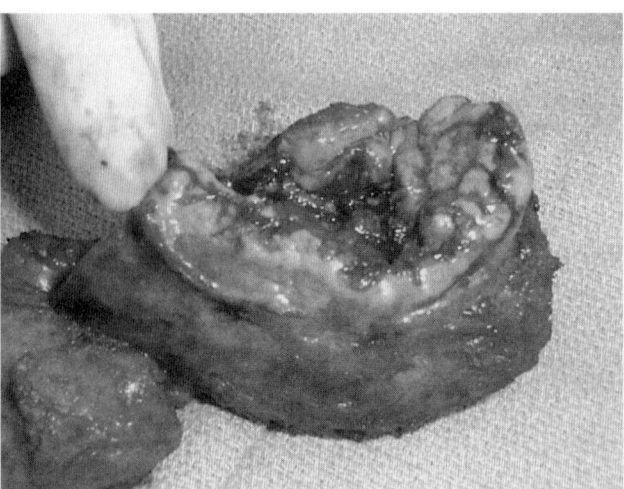

FIG. 17-38. Composite resection specimen of a T4 floor of mouth squamous cell carcinoma.

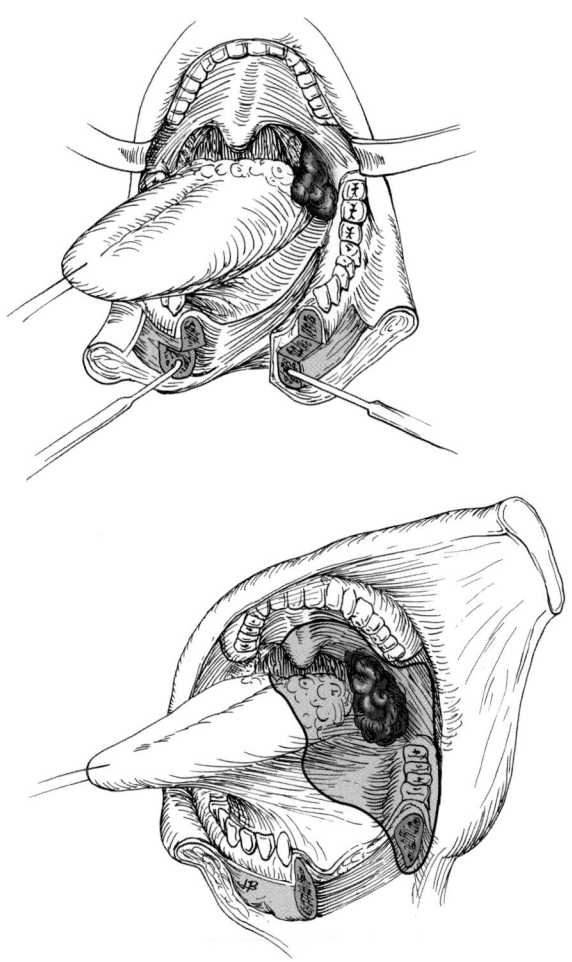

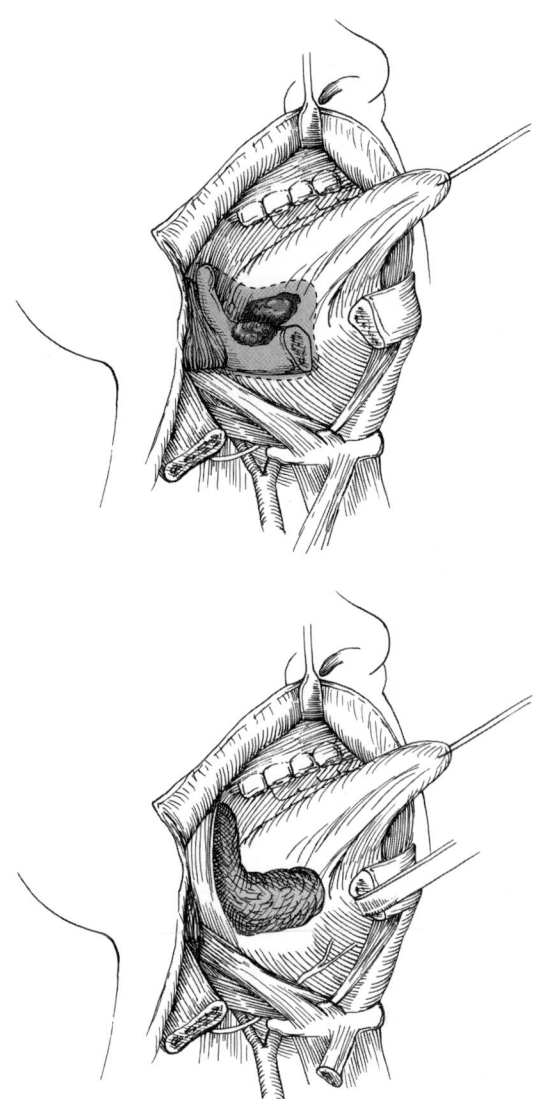

FIG. 17-39. Anterior mandibulotomy with mandibular swing to approach a posterior lesion.

FIG. 17-40. Composite resection with segmental resection of the mandible with a lateral oral cavity T4 lesion.

Treatment is symptomatic and biopsy confirms its benign nature. Torus palatini are exostoses or bony outgrowths of the midline palate and maxillary bone and do not specifically require surgical treatment unless symptomatic.

Squamous cell carcinoma and minor salivary gland tumors are the most common malignancies of the palate.[63,64] The latter include adenoid cystic carcinoma, mucoepidermoid carcinoma, adenocarcinoma, and polymorphous low-grade adenocarcinoma. Mucosal melanoma may occur on the palate and presents as a nonulcerated, pigmented plaque. Kaposi's sarcoma of the palate is the most common intraoral site for this tumor. Tumors may present as either an ulcer or an exophytic or submucosal mass. Minor salivary gland tumors tend to arise at the junction of the hard and soft palate. Direct infiltration of bone leads to extension into the floor of the nose or the maxillary antrum. Squamous cell carcinoma of the hard palate is treated surgically. Adjuvant radiation is indicated for advanced staged tumors. Because the periosteum of the palate bones acts as a barrier to spread, mucosal excision may be adequate for very superficial lesions. Involvement of the periosteum requires removal of a portion of the bony palate. Partial or subtotal maxillectomy is required for larger lesions or those involving the maxillary antrum. Malignancies may extend along the greater palatine nerve making biopsy of this nerve important for identifying neurotropic spread. Through-and-through defects of the palate require a dental prosthesis for rehabilitation of swallowing and speech.

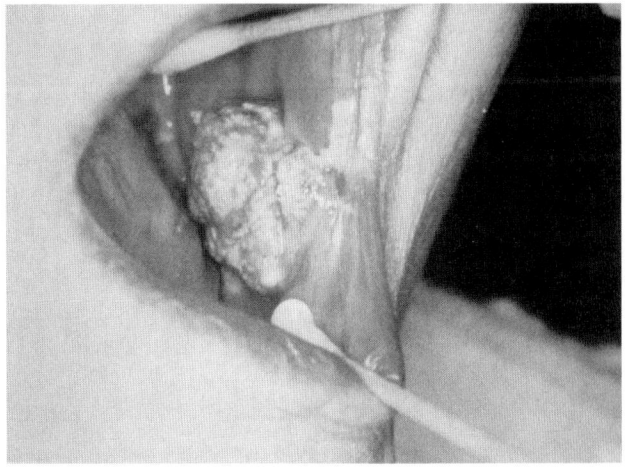

FIG. 17-41. Buccal mucosa squamous carcinoma.

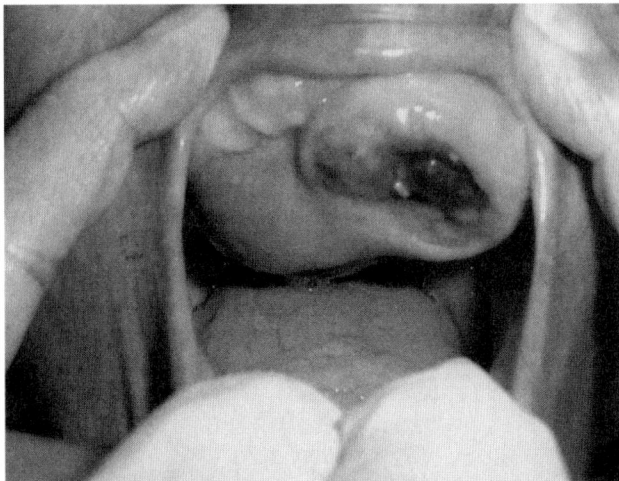

FIG. 17-42. *Hard-palate squamous carcinoma.*

Oropharynx

The oropharynx extends from the soft palate to the superior surface of the hyoid bone (or floor of the vallecula) and includes the base of tongue, the inferior surface of the soft palate and uvula, the anterior and posterior tonsillar pillars, the glossotonsillar sulci, the pharyngeal tonsils, and the lateral and posterior pharyngeal walls (Fig. 17-43). Laterally, the borders of this region are the pharyngeal constrictors and the medial aspect of the mandible. Direct extension of tumors from the oropharynx into these lateral tissues may involve spread through the pharyngeal constrictors into the parapharyngeal space. The ascending ramus of the mandible can be involved when tumors invade the medial pterygoid muscle.

As was true of the oral cavity, the histology of the majority of tumors in this region is squamous cell carcinoma. Although less

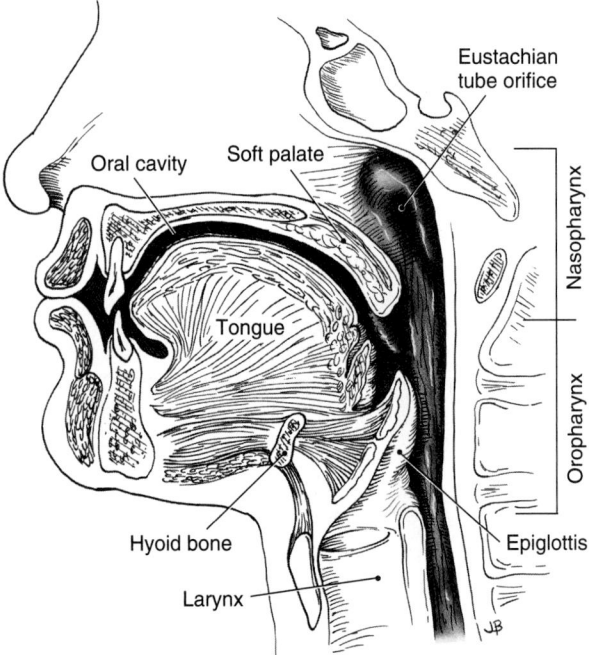

FIG. 17-43. *Sagittal view of the relationship of the oral cavity, nasopharynx, and oropharynx.*

common, minor salivary gland tumors may present as submucosal masses in the tongue base and palate. The palatine and lingual tonsils of Waldeyer's ring may be the presenting site of a lymphoma noted as an asymmetrically enlarged tonsil or tongue base mass.

Oropharyngeal cancer usually presents as an ulcerated, exophytic mass. Tumor fetor from tumor necrosis is common. A muffled or "hot potato" voice is seen with large tongue base tumors. Dysphagia and weight loss are common symptoms. Referred otalgia, mediated by the tympanic branches of CN IX and CN X, is a common complaint. Trismus may indicate advanced disease and usually results from involvement of the pterygoid musculature. The incidence of regional metastases from cancers of the tongue base and other oropharyngeal sites is high. Consequently, a neck metastasis is frequently a presenting sign.

Imaging studies are important for adequate staging and should assess for extension to the larynx, the constrictor muscles, parapharyngeal space, mandible, pterygoid muscles, and nasopharynx.

Lymph node metastasis from oropharyngeal cancer most commonly occurs in the subdigastric area of level II. Metastases also are found in levels III, IV, and V, in addition to the retropharyngeal and parapharyngeal lymph nodes. Forty to 50% of patients have metastases at the time of presentation. Bilateral metastases are common from tumors arising in the tongue base and soft palate.[65]

The treatment goals for patients with oropharyngeal cancer include maximizing survival and preserving function. Management of squamous cell cancers of this region includes surgery alone, primary radiation alone, surgery with postoperative radiation, and combined chemotherapy with radiation therapy. Many tumors of the oropharynx are poorly differentiated squamous cell carcinomas and tend to be radiosensitive.[66–68] Therefore, T1 and T2 lesions may be eradicated with radiation alone. Selected patients with T3 tumors without mandibular involvement and treated by radiation may have equal survival rates to those undergoing surgical resection. Additionally, adequate treatment of the neck is important with oropharyngeal squamous cancer because of the high risk of regional metastasis. More recently chemotherapy combined with radiotherapy has been used in patients with advanced stage oropharyngeal primary tumors. This approach has been effectively demonstrated to preserve function and is associated with survivorship comparable to surgery and radiation.

Tumors of the soft palate and tonsil extending to the tongue base are associated with poor survival. Extensive oropharyngeal cancers that are infiltrative usually are managed with surgical resection and postoperative radiotherapy.[69] Lesions that involve the mandible or its periosteum require composite resections, such as the classic jaw-neck resection or "commando" procedure. Tongue base involvement requires at least partial glossectomy, with the possibility of total glossectomy for lesions crossing the midline. With extensive resection of the tongue base, the possible need for laryngectomy to extirpate the tumor must be presented to the patient. Preservation of the larynx after total glossectomy is associated with the risk of postoperative aspiration and dysphagia.[70] Techniques to suspend the larynx to the mandible are used to minimize the risk of postoperative aspiration.

Swallowing rehabilitation in patients with oropharyngeal carcinoma is an important aspect of posttreatment care. For soft palate defects, palatal obturators provide a seal between the nasopharynx and the posterior pharyngeal wall.[71] Nasal regurgitation of air and liquids can be decreased or eliminated by their use. Close cooperation between the head and neck surgeon and the maxillofacial prosthodontist is essential in order to provide patients with the optimum prosthetic rehabilitation. Preoperative planning can result in the creation of a defect that better tolerates obturation. Additionally, skin grafting the defect can decrease contracture and provides a better contact surface for the obturator. For patients with major glossectomy defects, palatal augmentation prostheses can provide bulk extending inferiorly from the palate. The prosthesis decreases the volume of the oral cavity and allows the remaining tongue or soft tissue to articulate with the palate. It also facilitates posterior projection of the food bolus during the oral and pharyngeal phases of swallowing.

Hypopharynx and Cervical Esophagus

The hypopharynx extends from the vallecula to the lower border of the cricoid cartilage and includes the pyriform sinuses, the lateral and posterior pharyngeal walls, and the postcricoid region (Fig. 17-44). Squamous cancers of the hypopharynx frequently present at an advanced stage. Clinical findings are similar to those of lower oropharyngeal lesions and include a neck mass, muffled or hoarse voice, referred otalgia, dysphagia, and weight loss. A common symptom is dysphagia, starting with solids and progressing to liquids, leaving patients malnourished and catabolic at the time of presentation. Invasion of the larynx by direct extension can result in vocal cord paresis or paralysis and potential airway compromise.[72]

Routine office examination should include flexible fiberoptic laryngoscopy to properly assess the extent of tumor. During examination, the patient should be instructed to perform a Valsalva maneuver, which will result in passive opening of the pyriform sinuses and postcricoid regions, providing improved visualization. Manually displacing the larynx from side to side over the anterior cervical spine normally produces crepitus. Loss of crepitus can indicate the presence of a postcricoid tumor. Decreased laryngeal mobility or fixation indicates potential invasion of the prevertebral fascia and

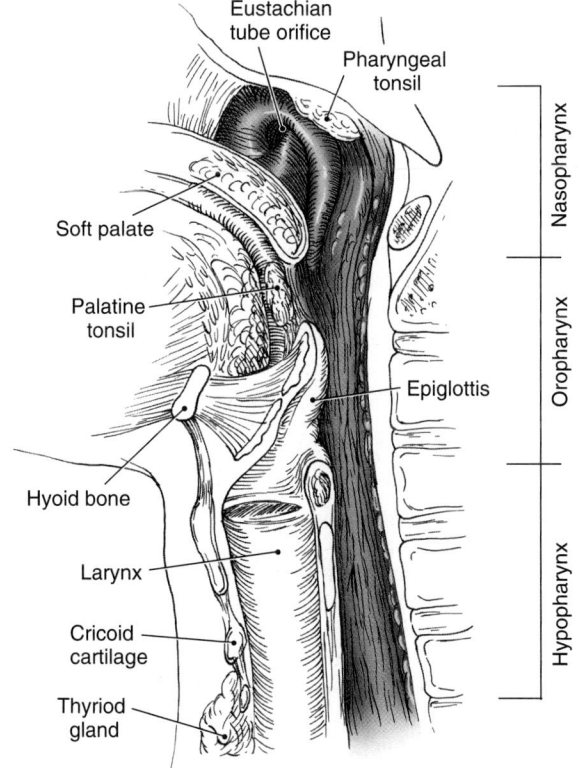

FIG. 17-44. Relationship of nasopharynx, oropharynx, and hypopharynx.

unresectability. Barium swallow can provide information regarding postcricoid and upper esophageal extension, potential multifocality within the esophagus, and document the presence of aspiration (Fig. 17-45). CT or MRI imaging should be obtained through the neck and upper chest to assess for invasion of the laryngeal framework and to identify for regional metastases, with special attention given to the paratracheal and upper mediastinal nodes (Fig. 17-46). Bilateral metastatic adenopathy in the paratracheal chain is common and approximately three-fourths of patients present with nodal disease at the time of diagnosis.

Tumors of the hypopharynx and cervical esophagus are associated with poorer survival rates than are other sites in the head and neck because of advanced primary stage and lymph node metastasis at presentation. Definitive radiation therapy is effective for smaller T1-T2 tumors. Surgery with postoperative radiation therapy improves locoregional control compared to single-modality therapy in the treatment of advanced stage tumors.[73] Surgical salvage after radiation failure has a success rate of less than 50% and can be associated with significant wound-healing complications.

Larynx-preserving surgical procedures for tumors of the hypopharynx are possible for only a limited number of lesions. Tumors of the medial pyriform wall or pharyngoepiglottic fold may be resected with partial laryngopharyngectomy. In this circumstance, the tumor must not involve the apex of the pyriform sinus, vocal cord mobility must be unimpaired, and the patient must have adequate pulmonary reserve. Available procedures that have the capacity to encompass the tumor include supraglottic laryngectomy or supracricoid hemilaryngopharyngectomy. Because of an increased risk for postoperative aspiration associated with these procedures, a history significant for pulmonary disease is a contraindication for performing the procedures. Because the majority of patients with tumors of the hypopharynx present with large lesions and significant submucosal spread, total laryngectomy is often required to achieve adequate margins. Resection of the primary tumor and surrounding pharyngeal tissue is performed en bloc by laryngopharyngectomy. Bilateral neck dissections are frequently indicated given the elevated risk of nodal metastases found with these lesions.

When laryngopharyngectomy is performed for hypopharyngeal tumors the surgical defect is preferentially repaired by primary closure when possible. Generally, 4 cm or more of pharyngeal mucosa is necessary for primary closure to provide an adequate lumen for swallowing and to minimize the risk of stricture formation. Larger surgical defects require closure with the aid of pedicled myocutaneous flaps or microvascular reconstruction with radial forearm or jejunal free flap. When total laryngopharyngoesophagectomy is necessary, gastric pull-up reconstruction is performed.

Organ preservation for hypopharyngeal cancer, using a platinum-based chemotherapy with radiation, has resulted in a laryngeal preservation rate of 30%. Diminished locoregional control rates have been observed when compared to surgery and postoperative radiation. No decrease was noted in the rate of distant metastases.[74]

Generally, cervical esophageal cancer is managed surgically. Preservation of the larynx has been described if the cricopharyngeus muscle is not involved. Unfortunately, this is not often the case and many patients with cervical esophageal cancer require a laryngectomy. Total esophagectomy is performed because of the tendency for multiple primary tumors and skip lesions seen with esophageal cancers. Recently, chemotherapy and external beam radiotherapy with and without surgery have been advocated.

Despite aggressive treatment strategies, the 5-year survival rate for cervical esophageal cancer is less than 20%. Because of the presence of paratracheal lymphatic disease, surgical treatment for

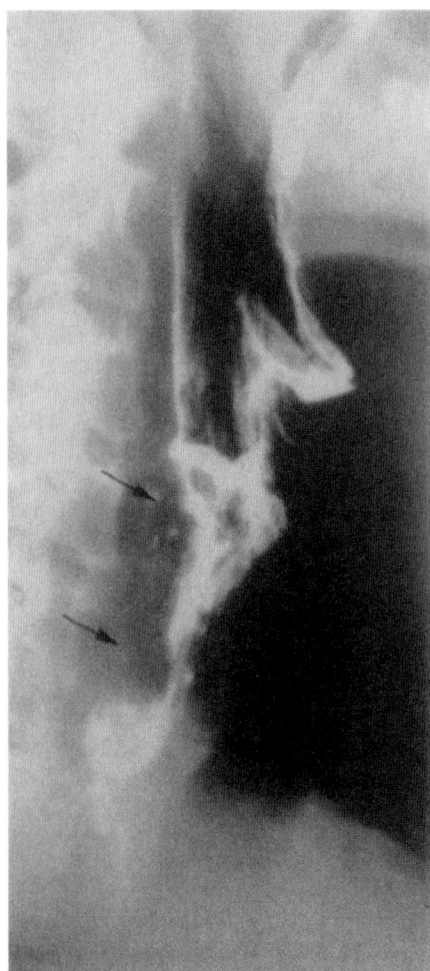
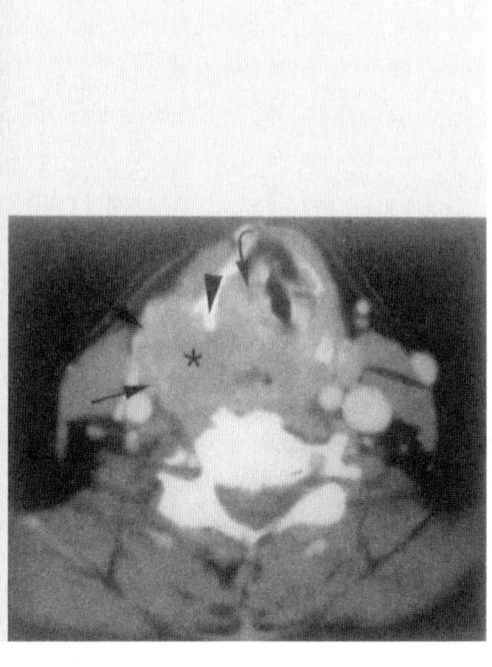

FIG. 17-45. Hypopharyngeal carcinoma: barium swallow and CT scan findings.

tumors of this area must include paratracheal lymph node dissection, in addition to treatment of the lateral cervical lymphatics.

Larynx

Laryngeal carcinoma is a diagnosis typically entertained in individuals with prominent smoking histories and the complaint of a prolonged hoarse voice (Fig. 17-47). The borders of the larynx span from the epiglottis superiorly to the cricoid cartilage inferiorly, and from the posterior commissure posteriorly to the lingual surface of the epiglottis, the thyrohyoid membrane, thyroid cartilage, and the anterior arch of the cricoid anteriorly. The lateral limits of the larynx are the aryepiglottic folds. The larynx is composed of three regions: the supraglottis, the glottis, and the subglottis (Fig. 17-48).

The supraglottis includes the epiglottis, aryepiglottic folds, arytenoids, and ventricular bands (false vocal folds). The inferior boundary of the supraglottis is a horizontal plane passing through the lateral margin of the ventricle. The glottis is composed of the true vocal cords (superior and inferior surfaces) and includes the anterior and posterior commissures. The subglottis extends from the inferior surface of the glottis to the lower margin of the cricoid cartilage. The soft-tissue compartments of the larynx are separated by fibroelastic membranes, which can act as barriers to the spread of cancer. These membranes thicken medially to form the false vocal fold and the vocal ligament (the true vocal cord).

The supraglottic larynx contains pseudostratified, ciliated respiratory epithelium that covers the false vocal cords. The epiglottis

and the vocal cords are lined by stratified, nonkeratinizing squamous epithelium. The subglottic mucosa is pseudostratified, ciliated respiratory epithelium. Minor salivary glands are also found in the supraglottis and subglottis. Tumor types that arise in the larynx are primarily squamous cell carcinoma but also include tumors of neuroendocrine origin, squamous papillomas, granular cell tumors, and tumors of salivary origin. Several histologic variants of squamous cell carcinoma exist and include verrucous carcinoma, basaloid squamous cell carcinoma, adenosquamous carcinoma, and spindle cell carcinoma. Tumors of the laryngeal framework include synovial sarcoma, chondroma, and chondrosarcoma.

The normal functions of the larynx are airway patency, protection of the tracheobronchial tree during swallowing, and phonation. Patients with tumors of the supraglottic larynx may present with symptoms of chronic sore throat, dysphonia ("hot potato" voice), dysphagia, or a neck mass secondary to regional metastasis. Supraglottic tumors may cause vocal cord fixation by inferior extension in the paraglottic space or direct invasion of the cricoarytenoid joint. Anterior extension of tumors arising on the laryngeal surface of the epiglottis into the pre-epiglottic space produces a muffled quality to the voice. Referred otalgia or odynophagia is encountered with advanced supraglottic cancers. Large bulky tumors of the supraglottis may result in airway compromise. In contrast to most supraglottic lesions, hoarseness is an early symptom in patients with tumors of the glottis.[75] Airway obstruction from a glottic tumor is usually a late symptom and is the result of tumor bulk or impaired vocal cord

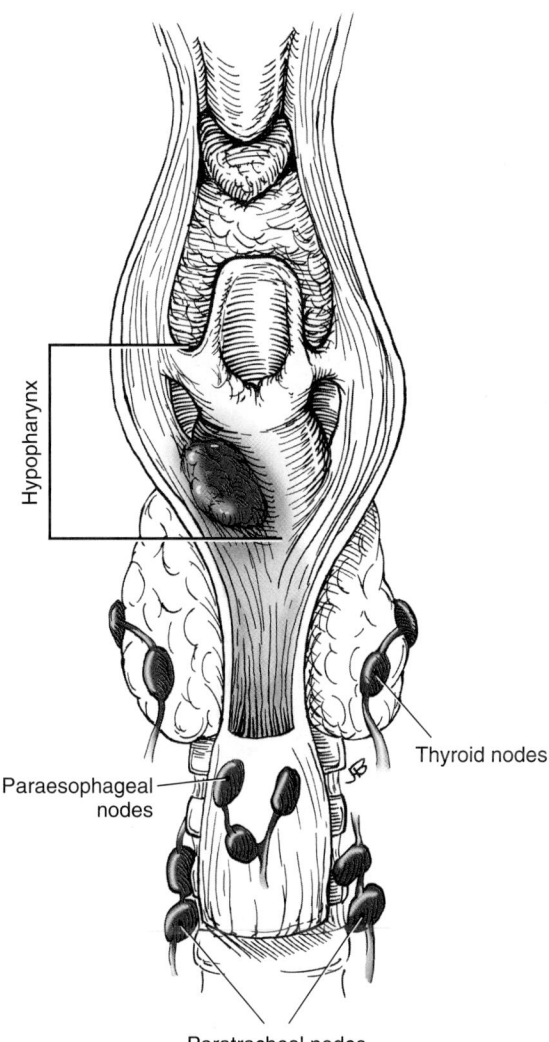

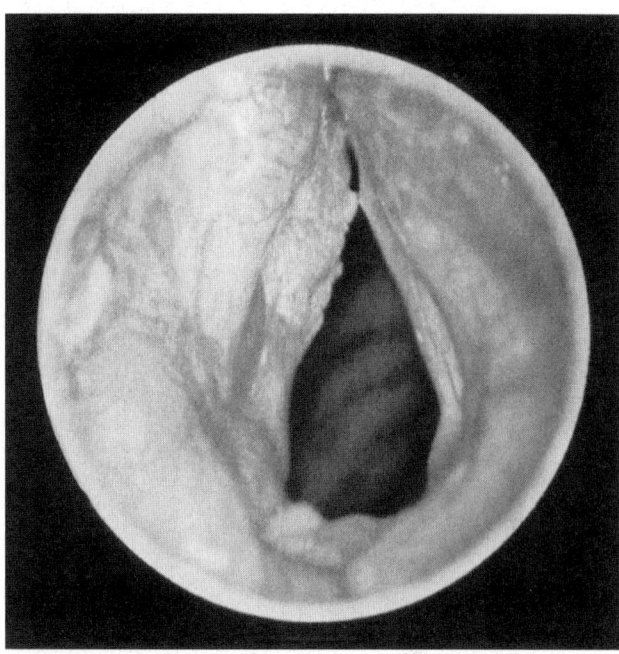

FIG. 17-47. Endoscopic view of a laryngeal squamous carcinoma.

erosion or invasion and extension into the pre-epiglottic and paraglottic spaces. High quality, thin-section images through the larynx should be obtained in patients with laryngeal tumors, and used along with clinical assessment to arrive at a final disease stage. Lymph node metastasis may be defined more readily with the use of imaging studies.

Lymphatic drainage of the larynx is distinct for each subsite and is determined by the presence of the fibroelastic membranes as well as the organ's embryogenesis. Two major groups of laryngeal lymphatic channels exist: those that drain areas superior to the fundus

FIG. 17-46. View of the hypopharynx demonstrating the potential pathways of spread of tumor and pertinent anatomy.

mobility. Decreased vocal cord mobility may be caused by direct laryngeal muscle invasion or involvement of the recurrent laryngeal nerve. Fixation of the vocal cord indicates invasion into the vocalis muscle, paraglottic space, or cricoarytenoid joint. Superficial tumors that are bulky may appear to cause cord fixation through mass effect. Subglottic cancers are relatively uncommon and typically present with laryngeal paralysis (usually unilateral), stridor, and/or pain.

The staging classification for squamous cell cancers of the larynx includes assessment of vocal cord mobility as well as the sites of tumor extension. Accurate clinical staging of laryngeal tumors requires fiberoptic endoscopy in the office and direct laryngoscopy of the larynx under general anesthesia. Direct laryngoscopy, used to assess the extent of local spread, may be combined with esophagoscopy or bronchoscopy to adequately stage the primary tumor and to exclude the presence of a synchronous lesion. Key areas to note for tumor extension in supraglottic tumors are the vallecula, base of tongue, ventricle, arytenoid, and anterior commissure. For glottic cancers, it is important to determine extension to the false cords, anterior commissure, arytenoid, and subglottis.

Radiographic imaging by CT or MRI (Fig. 17-49) provides important staging information and is crucial for identifying cartilage

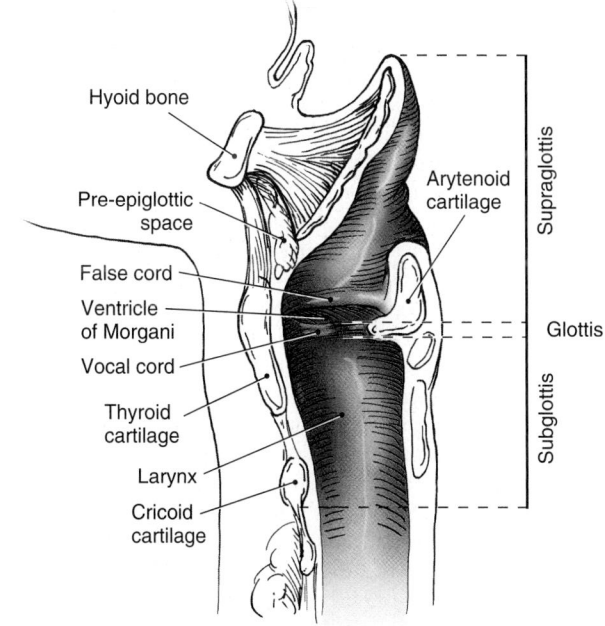

FIG. 17-48. Sagittal view of the larynx with the divisions of the supraglottis, glottis, and subglottis demonstrated.

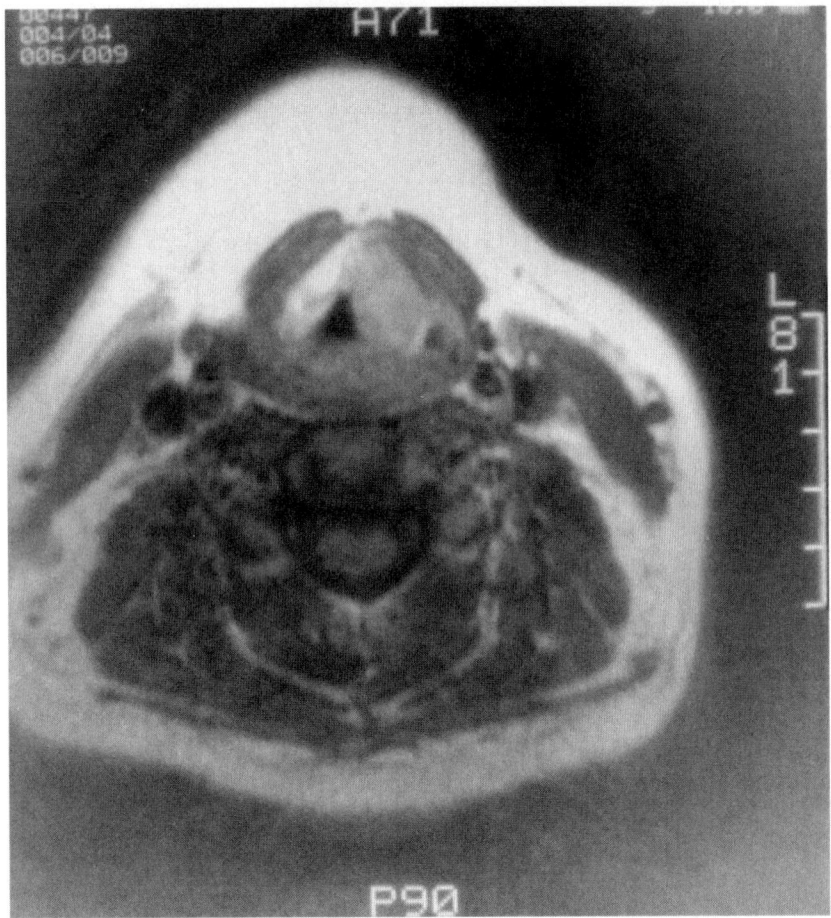

FIG. 17-49. MRI view of an invasive left true vocal cord squamous carcinoma.

of the ventricle, and those that drain areas inferior to it. Supraglottic drainage routes pierce the thyrohyoid membrane with the superior laryngeal artery, vein, and nerve, and drain mainly to the subdigastric and superior jugular nodes.[75] Those from the glottic and subglottic areas exit via the cricothyroid ligament and end in the prelaryngeal node (the Delphian node), the paratracheal nodes, and the deep cervical nodes along the inferior thyroid artery. Small glottic cancers rarely produce cervical metastases (1 to 4%). However, there is a high incidence of lymphatic spread from supraglottic (30 to 50%) and subglottic cancers (40%).

When considering treatment for laryngeal tumors, it is useful to categorize them as a continuum from early tumors (those with a small area of involvement or causing minimal or no functional impairment) to advanced tumors (those with significant airway compromise and local extension). For example, severe dysplasia and carcinoma in situ often can be treated successfully with laser ablation or conservative surgical procedures. In contrast, more advanced tumors may require substantial partial laryngeal resection[76] (Fig. 17-50) or even total laryngectomy (Fig. 17-51). Further complicating the treatment paradigm is the role of radiotherapy with or without chemotherapy for laryngeal preservation.[77]

Prognostic factors for patients with cancer of the larynx are tumor size, nodal metastasis, perineural invasion, and extracapsular spread of disease in cervical lymph nodes. Prognosis and patient comorbidity are two important considerations when arriving at a treatment plan for patients with laryngeal cancer.

For severe dysplasia or carcinoma in situ of the vocal cord, stripping of the surface mucosa is an effective treatment. Patients without

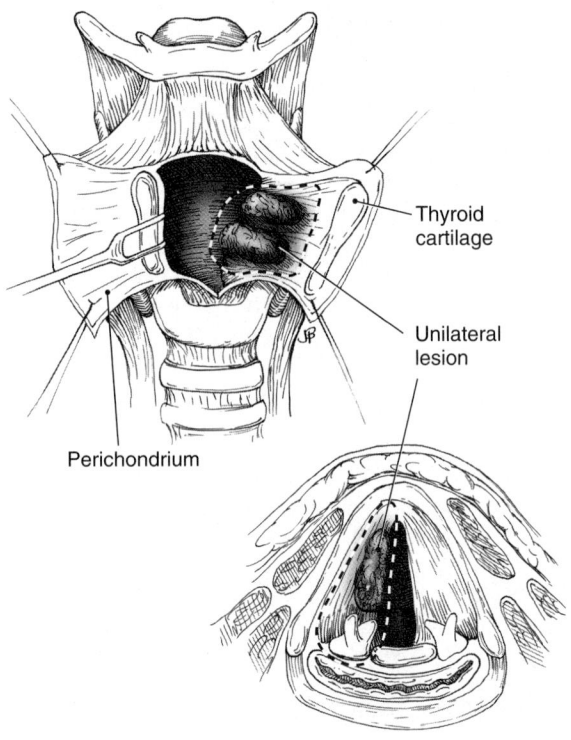

Thyroid cartilage

Unilateral lesion

Perichondrium

FIG. 17-50. Example of the resection of a vertical partial laryngectomy for an early stage glottic carcinoma.

(chronic obstructive pulmonary disease, cardiovascular, and renal disease), and tumor stage. Voice preservation and maintenance of quality of life are key issues and significantly impact therapeutic decisions. The use of radiation therapy for early stage disease of the glottis and supraglottis provides excellent disease control with reasonable, if not excellent, preservation of vocal quality. Partial laryngectomy for small glottic cancers provides excellent tumor control, but with some degree of voice impairment. For supraglottic cancers without arytenoid or vocal cord extension, standard supraglottic laryngectomy results in excellent disease control with good voice function. The goals of partial laryngeal surgery are to achieve local control of disease, reserving radiation therapy as an option for recurrent disease or a second primary tumor. For advanced tumors with extension beyond the endolarynx or with cartilage destruction, total laryngectomy followed by postoperative radiation is still considered the standard of care.[78] In this setting, pharyngeal reconstruction by means of a pectoralis major flap (Fig. 17-52) or free flap reconstruction is occasionally required.

Subglottic tumors are rare, constituting only 1% of laryngeal tumors and are best treated by total laryngectomy. Because these tumors present with adenopathy in 40% of patients, special attention must be given to the treatment of paratracheal lymph nodes and removal of one or both lobes of the thyroid.[79]

Laryngeal Preservation Techniques. Superficial cancers confined to the true vocal cord can be treated with a variety of surgical options. These include endoscopic vocal cord stripping, microflap dissection, partial cordectomy, and CO_2 ablation (Fig. 17-53). Although using a CO_2 laser can provide excellent hemostasis and minimize damage to the adjacent uninvolved tissue, scarring associated with its use is considered more significant than with conventional "cold" techniques. Microflap dissection, using a subepithelial infusion of a saline-epinephrine solution into Reinke's space, allows for assessment of depth of invasion and the potential to completely resect the lesion as one unit. Microscope visualization aids the precision of such dissections. Open laryngofissure and cordectomy may be reserved for more invasive tumors.

For larger tumors of the glottis with impaired vocal cord mobility, a variety of partial resections exist that permit preservation of reasonable vocal quality. For lesions involving the anterior commissure with limited subglottic extension, an anterofrontal partial laryngectomy is indicated. For T2 or T3 glottic tumors without cartilage destruction, a vertical partial laryngectomy is feasible. In this circumstance, reconstruction is accomplished by means of a false

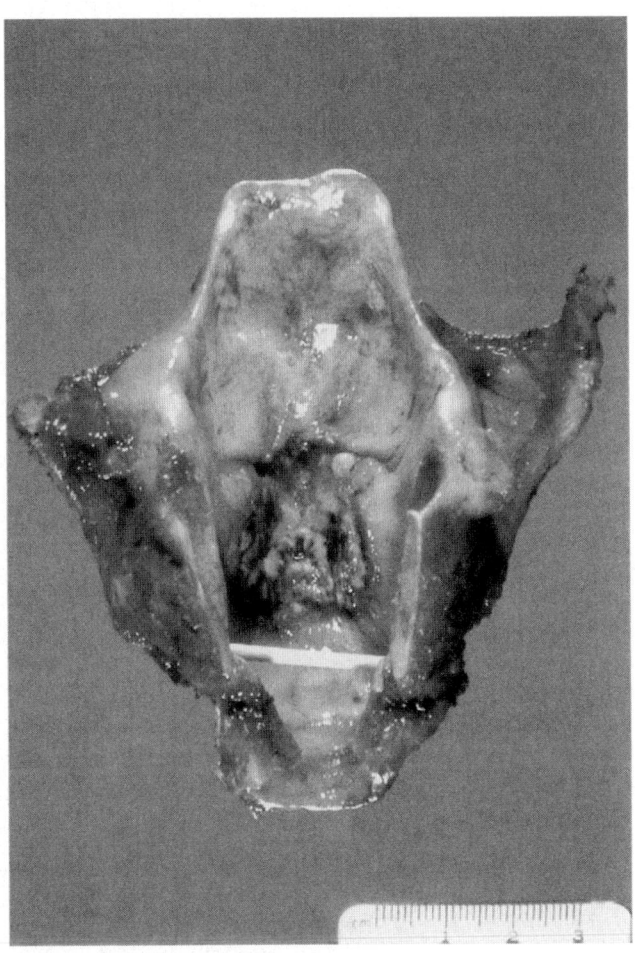

FIG. 17-51. Total laryngectomy specimen featuring a glottic squamous carcinoma.

extension to the arytenoid or anterior commissure are the best candidates for this approach. Multiple procedures may be necessary to control the disease and to prevent progression to an invasive cancer. Close follow-up examinations and smoking cessation are mandatory adjuncts of therapy. For early tumors of the glottis and the supraglottis, radiation therapy is equally as effective as surgery in controlling disease.

Critical factors in determining the appropriate treatment modality are the patient's wish to preserve voice, comorbid conditions

FIG. 17-52. Pectoralis flap reconstruction of a laryngectomy patient requires soft-tissue augmentation for pharynx closure.

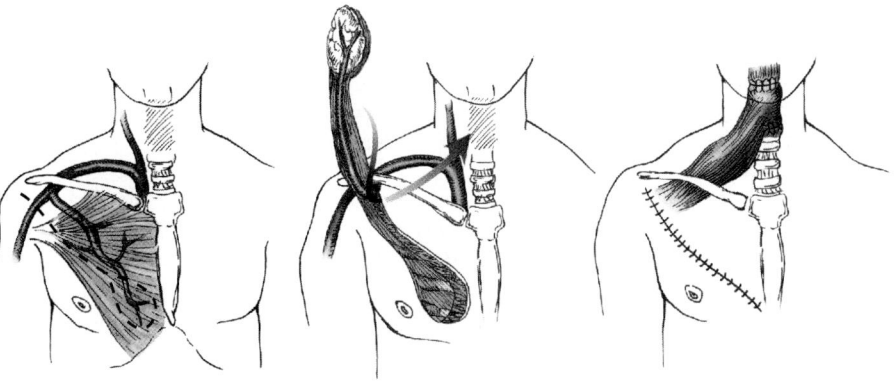

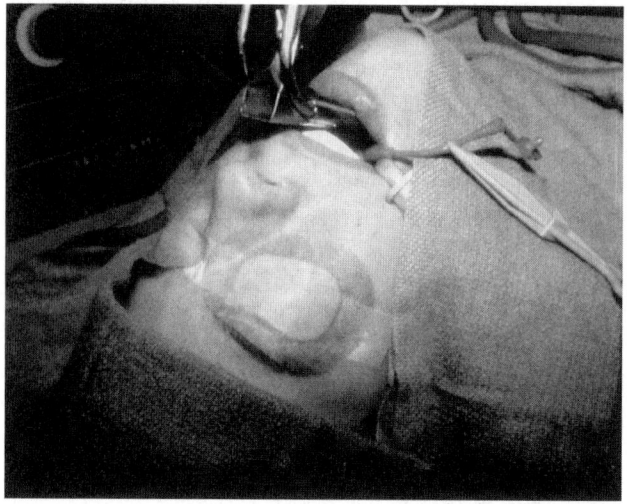

FIG. 17-53. Suspension laryngoscopy set-up for CO_2 laser resection of a glottic lesion.

vocal cord imbrication or pedicled muscle flap to create a pseudocord on the side of the resection.

For T3 glottic lesions not involving the pre-epiglottic space or cricoarytenoid joint, a supracricoid laryngectomy with cricohyoidopexy (CHP) or cricohyoidoepiglottopexy (CHEP) are options.[76] The supracricoid laryngectomy technique uses the remaining arytenoids as the phonatory structures, which come into apposition with epiglottic remnant in the CHEP, or with the tongue base in the CHP. Oncologic advantages of this procedure include the complete removal of the paraglottic spaces and thyroid cartilage. The supracricoid laryngectomy with CHEP is associated with excellent disease control and a high rate of tracheostomy decannulation. Favorable deglutition rates and a serviceable breathy voice are seen postoperatively with this procedure. For lesions with involvement of the cricoarytenoid joint and/or extension to the level of the cricoid, total laryngectomy is required. The near-total laryngectomy may also be used in this situation. However, widespread application of this technique has not been adopted and postprocedure the patient requires a permanent tracheostomy for maintenance of the airway.

Because of disturbances in swallowing function, the risk for aspiration is high following certain partial laryngectomies. Patient selection is vital to successful application of these techniques. Pulmonary function tests, such as spirometry and arterial blood gas measurements, are useful screening evaluations. One measurement of pulmonary functional reserve is to have the patient climb two flights of stairs. Those able to do so without stopping are candidates for the procedure. For patients who for functional or oncologic reasons are not candidates for partial laryngectomy, total laryngectomy is the best surgical option for locoregional control. Total laryngectomy may also be the preferred treatment for those patients who are noncompliant, given the importance of postoperative follow-up and monitoring for recurrence.

The approach to the treatment for patients with advanced tumors of the larynx and hypopharynx has evolved over time. Sequential and concomitant chemotherapy and radiation trials have demonstrated the feasibility of these approaches for organ preservation. The recently completed Radiation Therapy Oncology Group (RTOG) 91-11 trial for laryngeal preservation demonstrated a higher laryngeal preservation rate among patients receiving concomitant chemotherapy and radiotherapy than in those patients receiving radiation alone or sequential chemotherapy followed by radiation therapy.[80] A randomized laryngeal preservation trial of neoadjuvant induction chemotherapy followed by radiation therapy has yielded survival rates similar to those of laryngectomy, with the benefit of preservation of the larynx in 65% of patients.[77] Surgical salvage is available in cases of treatment failure or recurrent disease. The results of this study indicate that although overall survival rates are similar, patients who underwent total laryngectomy had better locoregional control, whereas patients treated with chemotherapy and radiation therapy had lower rates of distant metastases.

Speech and Swallowing Rehabilitation. Involvement of a speech and swallowing therapist in the preoperative counseling and postoperative rehabilitation of patients with laryngeal cancer is critical. Speech rehabilitation options after total laryngectomy include esophageal speech, tracheoesophageal puncture, and use of an electrolarynx. Esophageal speech is produced by actively swallowing and releasing air from the esophagus resulting in vibrations of the esophageal walls and pharynx. The sounds produced can be articulated into words. The ability to create esophageal speech depends on the motivation of the patient and their ability to control the upper esophageal sphincter, allowing injection and expulsion of air in a controlled fashion. Unfortunately, less than 20% of postlaryngectomy patients develop fluent esophageal speech.

In laryngectomized patients, a fistula created between the trachea and esophagus permits placement of a one-way valve that allows air from the trachea to enter the upper esophagus. The valve prevents retrograde passage of food or saliva into the trachea. Patients who are candidates for a speaking valve, also known as a tracheoesophageal puncture valve (TEP), have better than an 80% success rate in achieving fluent speech.

For patients unable to develop esophageal speech, the electrolarynx creates vibratory sound waves when held against the neck or cheek. The vibrations create sound waves that the patient articulates into words. A disadvantage of the electrolarynx is the mechanical quality of the sound produced. This device is most useful in the postoperative period prior to training for esophageal speech.

Postoperative swallowing rehabilitation is another important task performed by the speech and swallowing team. The ability to swallow, especially after partial laryngectomy, is impaired because of the loss of laryngeal sphincter function and loss of mucosal sensation. Patient instruction in various swallowing techniques and evaluation for the appropriate diet consistency allow a patient to initiate oral intake of nutrition while minimizing the risk of aspirating. Flexible fiberoptic laryngoscopy can be performed transnasally and provides valuable information to assist in the assessment of dysphagia. The oral intake of various consistencies of liquids and solids can be observed with endoscopic assessment and allow for the visualization of laryngeal penetrance. A similar assessment may be performed with modified barium swallow, with analysis of the various phases of swallowing.

Unknown Primary Tumors

When patients present with cervical nodal metastases without clinical or radiologic evidence of an upper aerodigestive tract primary tumor, they are referred to as having an unknown or occult primary tumor. Given the difficulty in examining regions such as the base of tongue, crevices within the tonsillar fossa, and the nasopharynx, examination under anesthesia with directed tissue biopsies has been advocated. Ipsilateral tonsillectomy, direct laryngoscopy with base of tongue and piriform biopsies, examination of the nasopharynx, and bimanual examination can allow for identification of a primary site in a portion of patients. In those individuals in whom a primary site cannot be ascertained, empiric treatment of the mucosal sources of the upper aerodigestive tract at risk and the cervical lymphatics with radiation therapy is performed. For patients with advanced neck disease (N2a or greater) or with persistent lymphadenopathy after radiation, a postradiation neck dissection is required. For patients with an identified primary lesion, standard protocols for that region are followed.

Nose and Paranasal Sinuses

As discussed previously, the nose and paranasal sinuses are the site of a great deal of infectious and inflammatory pathology. The diagnosis of tumors within this region is frequently made after a patient has been unsuccessfully treated for recurrent sinusitis and undergoes diagnostic imaging. Symptoms associated with sinonasal tumors are subtle and insidious. They include chronic nasal obstruction, facial pain, headache, epistaxis, and facial numbness. As such, tumors of the paranasal sinuses frequently present at an advanced stage. Orbital invasion can result in proptosis, diplopia, epiphora, and visual loss. Paresthesia within the distribution of CN V_2 is suggestive of pterygopalatine fossa or skull base invasion and is generally a poor prognostic factor. Maxillary sinus tumors can present with loose dentition indicating erosion of the alveolar and palatal bones. Tumors found to arise posterior to Ohngren's line are associated with a worse prognosis than are more anteriorly based lesions (Fig. 17-54).[81]

A variety of benign tumors arise in the nasal cavity and paranasal sinuses and include inverted papillomas, hemangiomas, hemangiopericytoma, angiofibroma, minor salivary tumors, and benign fibrous histiocytoma. Fibro-osseous and osseous lesions, such as fibrous dysplasia, ossifying fibroma, osteoma, and myxomas, can also arise in this region. Additionally, intranasal extension of intracranial tissues may result from erosion the skull base and present on clinical exam as a sinonasal mass.

Malignant tumors of the sinuses are predominantly squamous cell carcinomas.[82] Sinonasal undifferentiated carcinoma,[83] adenocarcinoma, mucosal melanoma, lymphoma, olfactory neuroblastoma,[84] rhabdomyosarcoma, and angiosarcoma are some of the malignancies that have been described. Metastases from the kidney, breast, lung, and thyroid may also present as an intranasal mass. Regional metastasis is uncommon with tumors of the paranasal sinuses (14 to 16%) and occurs in the parapharyngeal, retropharyngeal, and subdigastric nodes of the jugular chain.

The diagnosis of intranasal tumors is made with the assistance of a headlight and nasal speculum or nasal endoscope. The site of origin, involved bony structures, and the presence of pulsations or hypervascularity should be assessed. For paranasal sinus tumors, MRI and CT scanning are often complementary studies in determining orbital and intracranial invasion.[85] Benign processes frequently present as slow-growing expansile tumors with limited erosion of surrounding bone, as compared to the lytic destruction typically associated with malignancies. Neural foramina should be evaluated for expansion that may be suggestive of perineural invasion. Examination for cavernous sinus extension, cribriform plate erosion, and dural enhancement is necessary in order to assess for available treatment options. A meningocele or encephalocele will present as a unilateral pulsatile mass. Biopsy of a unilateral nasal mass should be deferred until imaging studies are obtained. Untimely biopsy might produce a cerebrospinal leak and/or meningitis. If hypervascularity is suspected, biopsy should be performed under controlled conditions in the operating room.

The standard treatment for malignant tumors of the paranasal sinuses is surgical resection and, in most cases, postoperative adjuvant radiation therapy. The extent of surgery is determined by the preoperative evaluation of disease spread. Tumors arising along the medial wall of the maxillary sinus may be treated by means of a medial maxillectomy (Fig. 17-55). The treatment of advanced tumors of the paranasal sinuses frequently involves a multispecialty approach. Members of this team include the head and neck surgeon, neurosurgeon, prosthodontist, ophthalmologist, and reconstructive surgeon. Each team member is necessary to facilitate the goal of safe and complete tumor removal. For vascular tumors,

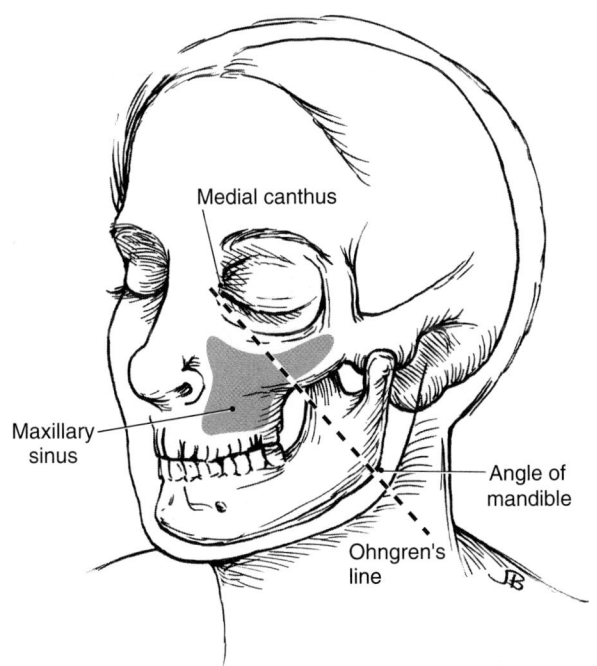

FIG. 17-54. *Example of the Ohngren's line and the relationship to the maxilla.*

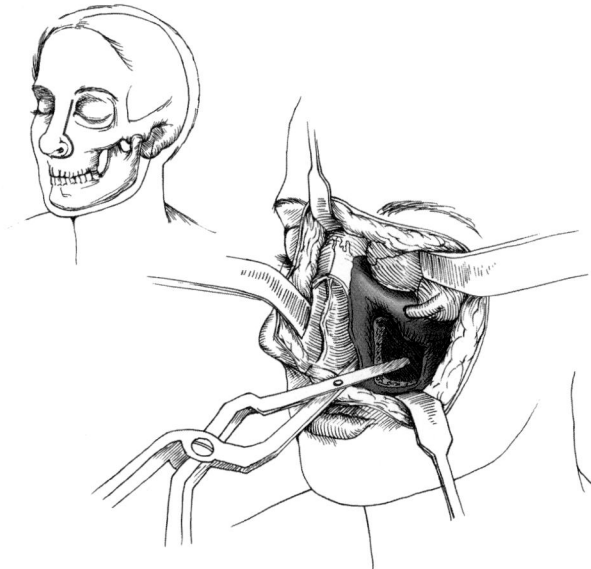

FIG. 17-55. *Example of the incision and bone cuts for medial maxillectomy.*

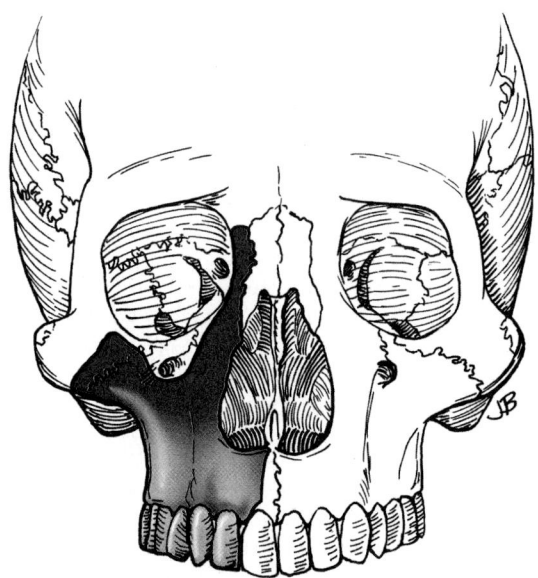

FIG. 17-56. Demonstration of the bone cuts made with an infrastructure maxillectomy.

preoperative embolization is frequently necessary to reduce intraoperative hemorrhage. The embolization is ideally performed within 24 hours of the planned surgical resection. When craniofacial resection is necessary for intracranial spread, cerebrospinal fluid decompression is performed through a lumbar drain.[86]

The prognosis for these patients depends on tumor location and extension to the adjacent sinuses, orbit, and intracranial cavity.[87] Infrastructure maxillectomy, which includes removal of the hard palate and the lower maxillary sinus, is necessary for inferiorly based tumors of the maxillary sinus (Fig. 17-56). For tumors in the upper portion of the maxillary sinus, complete maxillectomy (including removal of the orbital floor) is performed. If there is invasion of the orbital fat, exenteration of the orbital contents is required. Removal of the bony floor of the orbit and preservation of the globe are possible where there is absence of invasion through the orbital periosteum. However, reconstruction of the orbital floor to re-create a stable support for the orbital contents is essential. Removal of anterior cheek skin is rarely indicated, but is required when there is tumor extension into the subcutaneous fat and dermis.

For tumors involving the ethmoid sinuses, the integrity of the cribriform plate is of great importance in preoperative planning. Complete sphenoethmoidectomy or medial maxillectomy may suffice if the tumor is localized to the lateral nasal wall. Endoscopic resection with the assistance of image-guidance technology is gaining increasing acceptance for low-grade resectable lesions such as inverted papilloma. Additionally, endoscopic sinus techniques are being applied to assist in procedures such as craniofacial resection and optic nerve decompression.

If erosion of the cribriform has occurred, an anterior craniofacial resection is the standard approach. The head and neck surgeon and neurosurgeon work in concert to resect these neoplasms. The neurosurgeon performs a frontal craniotomy for exposure of the anterior cranial fossa floor, whereas the head and neck surgeon proceeds through a transfacial approach to resect the inferior bony attachments. Paranasal sinus malignancies that are deemed unresectable are those with bilateral optic nerve involvement, massive brain invasion, or carotid encasement.[88] Postoperative speech and cosmetic rehabilitation after orbital exenteration is accomplished by soft

tissue reconstruction and placement of a maxillofacial prosthesis. The goals of rehabilitation are to provide facial contour and separation of the oral cavity–oropharynx from the nasopharynx, which facilitates speech and swallowing.

Combined treatment with surgery and postoperative radiotherapy for squamous cell carcinoma of the sinuses consistently has been shown to provide survival superior to either radiation or surgery alone. Currently, systemic chemotherapy has a limited application and is administered for some sarcomas and sinonasal undifferentiated carcinoma. Rhabdomyosarcoma is treated with chemotherapy followed by radiation therapy and surgery is reserved for persistent disease after chemoradiation. Sinonasal undifferentiated carcinoma is highly aggressive and is not frequently controlled with standard therapy. Chemotherapy may help to reduce the tumor bulk and allow for orbital preservation. Trials with chemotherapy in addition to standard treatment with surgery and postoperative radiation have met with mixed success in the treatment of squamous cell carcinoma of the paranasal sinuses.[89]

Nasopharynx and Median Skull Base

The nasopharynx extends in a plane superior to the hard palate from the choana, to the posterior nasal cavity, to the posterior pharyngeal wall. It includes the fossa of Rosenmüller, the eustachian tube orifices (torus tubarius) and the site of the adenoid pad. Tumors arising in the nasopharynx are usually of squamous cell origin and range from lymphoepithelioma to well-differentiated carcinoma. However, the differential diagnosis for nasopharyngeal tumors is broad and also includes lymphoma, chordoma, chondroma, nasopharyngeal cysts (Tornwaldt's cyst), angiofibroma, minor salivary gland tumors, paraganglioma, teratoma, rhabdomyosarcoma, papilloma, extramedullary plasmacytoma, sarcomas, and neuroblastoma.[82]

Risk factors for nasopharyngeal carcinoma include area of habitation, ethnicity, environment, and tobacco use. There is a high incidence of nasopharyngeal cancer in southern China, Africa, Alaska, and in Greenland Eskimos. A strong correlation exists between nasopharyngeal cancer and the presence of EBV infection, such that EBV titers may be used as a means to follow a patient's response to treatment.

The symptoms associated with presentation of nasopharyngeal tumors include nasal obstruction, posterior (level V) neck mass, epistaxis, headache, serous otitis media with hearing loss, and otalgia. Cranial nerve involvement is indicative of skull base extension and advanced disease. Parapharyngeal involvement occurs from posterolateral infiltration of tumor beyond the pharyngobasilar fascia. Extension into the infratemporal fossa may produce trismus and occurs via spread anterior to the pterygoid musculature or lateral extension beyond the pterygomaxillary fissure. Lymphatic spread occurs to the posterior cervical, upper jugular, and retropharyngeal nodes, and is frequently bilateral. Distant metastasis is present in 5% of patients at presentation.

Examination of the nasopharynx is facilitated by the use of the flexible or rigid fiberoptic endoscope. Evaluation with imaging studies is important for staging and treatment planning. CT with contrast is best for determining bone destruction, and MRI is important for determining intracranial and soft-tissue extension. Erosion or enlargement of neural foramina (on CT imaging) or enhancement of cranial nerves (on MRI) is indicative of perineural spread of disease and portends a worse prognosis. The status of the cavernous sinus and optic chiasm should also be evaluated when reviewing imaging to determine the potential for treatment related morbidities.

For squamous cell carcinoma and undifferentiated nasopharyngeal carcinoma, the standard treatment is a combination of chemotherapy and radiation therapy. Combination therapy produces superior survival rates for nasopharyngeal carcinoma in comparison to radiation alone. A survival rate (3-year) of 76% has been reported for patients treated with concomitant cisplatin and 5-fluorouracil and radiotherapy. Intracavitary radiation boost with implants to the tumor may be included as an adjunct to external beam radiotherapy to improve local control of advanced tumors. Surgical treatment for nasopharyngeal carcinoma is rarely feasible, but may occasionally be considered as salvage therapy for patients with localized recurrences.[82]

For minor salivary gland and low-grade tumors of the nasopharynx, resection can be performed via a variety of approaches. Selection of the appropriate approach, whether it be transpalatal or with maxillotomy, requires that the approach provide adequate exposure with the least cosmetic and functional deformity. Awareness of the vasculature and associated cranial nerves in the region are essential to achieve an acceptably low morbidity. An example of a lesion that fits this scenario is juvenile nasopharyngeal angiofibroma, a vascular tumor of young males that is treated surgically. It requires preoperative angioembolization because of the extensive vascularity seen with this tumor. Lateral rhinotomy or midface degloving approaches can provide good access for removal of these tumors and excellent cosmetic results. Radiotherapy is reserved for patients with unresectable angiofibromas. Radiating benign tumors in children is associated with postradiation-induced tumors after a latency of 15 to 30 years. Malignant tumors arising in an irradiated field include sarcomas and epithelial carcinomas.

A variety of surgical approaches to tumors in the region of the nasopharynx, sphenoid, and clivus are described. Although many tumors are limited to the median skull base, extensive disease requires combined approaches. Transpalatal approaches are used with minimal functional impairment for the treatment of recurrent nasopharyngeal carcinoma, but may require combination with transmaxillary and transcervical routes to attain adequate control of the carotid artery. For tumors of the clivus, sphenoid sinus, and nasopharynx regions, approaches include the lateral rhinotomy, transfacial approach with bilateral medial maxillectomies, transpalatal approach, Le Fort I approach, or palatal split with extended maxillotomy.[87]

Anterior fossa approaches are also described for tumors high in the nasopharynx or sphenoid region and include the extended frontal, fronto-orbital, transfrontal nasal, and transfrontal nasal-orbital approaches. For access to both the lateral and central skull base compartments, an anterior median labiomandibulotomy with transection of the eustachian tube is described. With extensive disease that involves the lateral skull base and the infratemporal fossa, transmastoid-transcervical, translabyrinthine, transcochlear, and infratemporal fossa approaches may be required, alone or in combination with anterior approaches for resection. Cranial deficits after surgery may require rehabilitation of speech and swallowing secondary to palatal dysfunction and velopharyngeal incompetence.

Ear and Temporal Bone

Tumors of the ear and temporal bone are uncommon and account for less than 1% of all head and neck malignancies. Primary sites can include the external ear (pinna), external auditory canal (EAC), middle ear, mastoid, or petrous portion of the temporal bone. The most common site is the EAC and the most common histology is squamous cell carcinoma. Minor salivary gland tumors, including adenoid cystic carcinoma and adenocarcinoma, may also present in this region. The pinna, because of its exposure to ultraviolet light, is a site for basal cell and squamous cell carcinoma to arise. In the middle ear, squamous cell carcinoma related to the presence of chronic otitis media is a typical feature. Direct extension of tumors from

the parotid gland and periauricular skin can also occur. Metastases from distant sites occur primarily to the petrous bone and arise in the breast, kidney, lung, and prostate. In the pediatric population, tumors of the temporal bone are most commonly soft-tissue sarcomas. For advanced stage tumors with extensive temporal bone extension, the complex anatomy of the temporal bone makes removal of tumors with functional preservation challenging.[90]

The diagnosis of tumors of the ear and temporal bone is frequently delayed because the initial presentation of these patients appears consistent with benign infectious disease. When patients fail to improve with conservative care and symptoms evolve to include a facial nerve paralysis or worsening hearing loss, the need for imaging and biopsy are considered. Granulation tissue in the external auditory canal or middle ear should always be biopsied in patients with atypical presentations or histories consistent with chronic otologic disease.[91]

The complexity of the temporal bone anatomy makes the use of imaging studies of paramount importance in the diagnosis, staging, and treatment of tumors of the temporal bone. The temporal bone contains not only the middle ear but also the cochlea, the internal auditory canal and its contents, the vestibular system, the facial nerve, the jugular bulb, and the internal carotid artery. The posterior portion of the temporal bone is surrounded by the venous structures of the sigmoid and superior/inferior petrosal sinuses.

Temporal bone CT scans (thin cuts with axial and coronal planes), MRI imaging, and angiography can enable assessment of tumor extension of the skull base and involvement of the carotid.

Small skin cancers on the helix of the ear can be readily treated with simple excision and primary closure. Mohs microsurgery with frozen section margin control also can be used for cancer of the external ear. In lesions that are recurrent or that invade the underlying perichondrium and cartilage, rapid spread through tissue planes can occur. Tumors may extend from the cartilaginous external canal to the bony canal and invade the parotid, temporomandibular joint, and the skull base. For extensive pinna-based lesions, more radical procedures, such as auriculectomy, may be required, in combination with additional procedures. Radiation therapy is combined with surgery for advanced skin cancer or in the context of positive margins or perineural spread.

Tumors involving the external auditory canal and middle ear present with otorrhea, otalgia, external auditory canal or periauricular mass, hearing loss, facial palsy, vertigo, or tinnitus. The patient resembles the presentation of an external otitis unresponsive to standard medical therapy. Tumors involving the petrous apex or intracranial structures may present with headache and palsies of cranial nerves V and VI. The poor prognosis associated with these lesions is related to advanced stage of the disease at the time of diagnosis.

The optimal treatment for tumors of the middle ear and bony external canal is en bloc resection followed by radiation therapy. Management of the regional lymphatics is determined by the site and stage of the tumor at presentation. The involvement of the anterior external auditory canal requires removal of the parotid gland because of potential spread of disease anteriorly through the ear canal. The goals of surgery are to remove the tumor en bloc and to leave vital structures when possible. Sleeve resections are reserved for small superficial tumors involving the cartilaginous external canal. Temporal bone resections are classified as lateral or subtotal (Fig. 17-57). The lateral temporal bone resection removes the bony and cartilaginous canal, tympanic membrane, and ossicles. The subtotal temporal bone resection includes the removal of the ear canal, middle ear, inner ear, and facial nerve. It is indicated for malignant tumors extending into the middle ear.

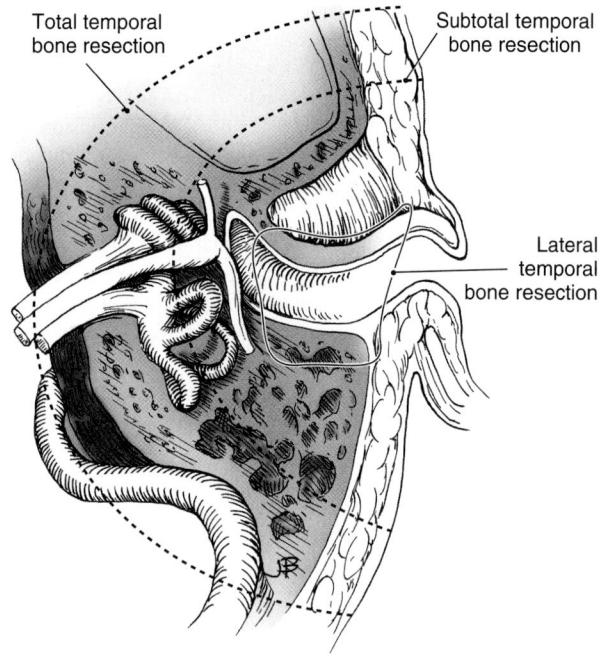

FIG. 17-57. *Examples of resection specimens for lateral temporal bone resection, subtotal temporal bone resection, and total temporal bone resection.*

Postoperative radiation therapy in the treatment of malignancies of the temporal bone is usually indicated and improves local control over surgery alone. Five-year survival rates are approximately 50% for patients with tumors confined to the external canal and decrease for more medial tumor extension. Prognosis is poor when tumor involves the petrous apex.[92]

The purpose of reconstruction after temporal bone resection is to provide vascularized tissue and bulk to the site of resection. Prevention of cerebrospinal fluid leak by watertight dural closure and prevention of meningitis is an important goal of repair. Additionally, the reconstruction enables protection of vascular structures and the surrounding bone in order to prepare the patient for postoperative radiation therapy. Commonly employed reconstruction methods are regional pedicle myocutaneous flaps (pectoralis major, latissimus dorsi myocutaneous trapezius flaps) and free flaps (rectus abdominis, parascapular, radial forearm, or latissimus dorsi). The loss of the pinna produces significant external deformity; however, a prosthetic ear may produce acceptable rehabilitation. When the facial nerve is sacrificed, rehabilitation is necessary and includes the use of interposition cable grafts, hypoglossal to facial anastomosis, and static and dynamic slings. Protection of the eye, by way of hydrating measures, in patients with facial paralysis is vital. In patients with poor eye closure, taping of the eyelids and the liberal use of eye lubrication prevent exposure keratitis. Additionally, tarsorrhaphy, lid-shortening procedures, and the use of gold weight implants can provide passive upper eyelid closure and protect the cornea.

Neck

The diagnostic evaluation of a neck mass requires a planned approach that does not compromise the effectiveness of future treatment options. A neck mass in a 50-year-old smoker/drinker with a synchronous oral ulcer is different from cystic neck mass in an 18-year-old that enlarges with an upper respiratory infection. As with all diagnoses, a complete history with full head and neck exam, including flexible laryngoscopy, are the core to this work-up.

The differential diagnosis of a neck mass is dependent on its location and the patient's age. In children, most neck masses are inflammatory or congenital. However, in the adult population, a neck mass greater than 2 cm in diameter has a greater than 80% probability of being malignant. Once the physician has developed a differential diagnosis, interventions to confirm or dispute diagnoses are initiated. Fine-needle aspiration, with or without the assistance of ultrasound or CT guidance, can provide a valuable tool for early treatment planning that provides less oncologic disruption to a tissue mass than an open biopsy. The use of CT scanning and/or MRI imaging is dictated by the patient's presentation. Imaging enables the physician to evaluate the anatomic relationships of the mass to the surrounding neck and sharpen the differential. A cystic lesion may represent benign pathology such as a branchial cleft cyst; however, it may also represent a regional metastasis of a tonsil/base of tongue squamous cell carcinoma or a papillary thyroid carcinoma. In this circumstance, evaluation of these potential primary sites, in addition to the characteristics of the neck mass, can alter the planned operative intervention such that a "lumpectomy" can be spared with the need for definitive surgery in a previously operated field.

If a variety of diagnoses are still being entertained after these evaluations, an open biopsy should be considered. For patients with the potential diagnosis of lymphoma, a radical biopsy sacrificing normal structures is not necessary. Ensuring appropriate processing of biopsied materials, sent in saline or in formalin, and sparing undue trauma to tissues can decrease the need for rebiopsy. Appropriate placement of the incision for an open biopsy should be considered if the need for neck dissection or composite resection is later required.

Patterns of Lymph Node Metastasis

The regional lymphatic drainage of the neck is divided into seven levels. These levels allow for a standardized format for radiologists, surgeons, pathologists, and radiation oncologists to communicate concerning specific sites within the neck and does not represent regions isolated by fascial planes (Fig. 17-58). The levels are defined as the following:

- Level I—the submental and submandibular nodes
- Level Ia—the submental nodes; medial to the anterior belly of the digastric muscle bilaterally, symphysis of mandible superiorly, and hyoid inferiorly

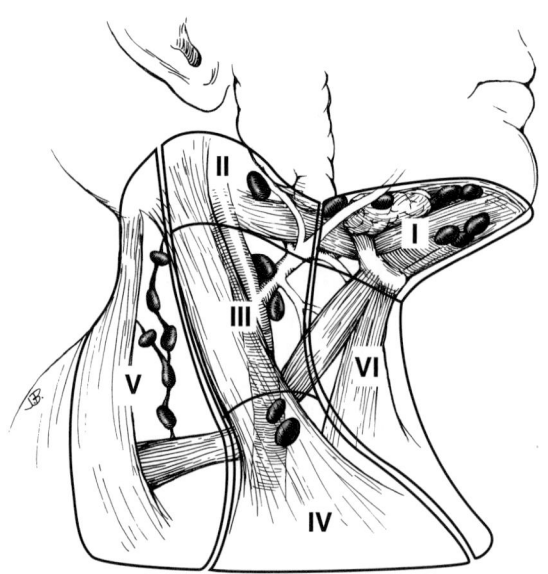

FIG. 17-58. *Levels of the neck denoting lymph node bearing regions.*

- Level Ib—the submandibular nodes and gland; posterior to the anterior belly of digastric, anterior to the posterior belly of digastric and inferior to the body of the mandible
- Level II—upper jugular chain nodes
- Level IIa—jugulodigastric nodes; deep to sternocleidomastoid (SCM) muscle, anterior to the posterior border of the muscle, posterior to the posterior aspect of the posterior belly of digastric, superior to the level of the hyoid, inferior to spinal accessory nerve (CN XI)
- Level IIb—submuscular recess; superior to spinal accessory nerve to the level of the skull base
- Level III—middle jugular chain nodes; inferior to the hyoid, superior to the level of the hyoid, deep to SCM from posterior border of the muscle to the strap muscles medially
- Level IV—lower jugular chain nodes; inferior to the level of the cricoid, superior to the clavicle, deep to SCM from posterior border of the muscle to the strap muscles medially
- Level V—posterior triangle nodes
- Level Va—lateral to the posterior aspect of the SCM, inferior and medial to splenius capitis and trapezius, superior to the spinal accessory nerve
- Level Vb—lateral to the posterior aspect of SCM, medial to trapezius, inferior to the spinal accessory nerve, superior to the clavicle
- Level VI—anterior compartment nodes; inferior to the hyoid, superior to suprasternal notch, medial to the lateral extent of the strap muscles bilaterally
- Level VII—paratracheal nodes; inferior to the suprasternal notch in the upper mediastinum

Patterns of spread from primary tumor sites in the head and neck to cervical lymphatics are well described.[93] The location and incidence of metastasis vary according to the primary site. Primary tumors within the oral cavity and lip metastasize to the nodes in levels I, II, and III. The occurrence of skip metastases with oral tongue lesions makes possible the involvement of nodes in level III or IV without involvement of higher-echelon nodes. Tumors arising in the oropharynx, hypopharynx, and larynx most commonly spread to the lymph nodes in levels II, III, and IV. Isolated level V nodes are uncommon with oral cavity, pharyngeal, and laryngeal primaries; however, level V adenopathy may be seen with concomitant involvement of higher echelon nodes. Malignancies of the nasopharynx and thyroid commonly spread to posterior lymph nodes in addition to the jugular chain nodes. Retropharyngeal nodes are sites for metastasis from tumors of the nasopharynx, soft palate, and lateral and posterior walls of the oropharynx and hypopharynx. Tumors of the hypopharynx, cervical esophagus, and thyroid frequently involve the paratracheal nodal compartment, and may extend to the lymphatics in the upper mediastinum (level VII). The Delphian node, a pretracheal lymph node, may become involved by advanced tumors of the glottis with subglottic spread.

The philosophy for the treatment of the cervical lymphatics in head and neck cancer patients has evolved significantly since the mid-1970s. The presence of cervical metastasis decreases the 5-year survival rate in patients with upper aerodigestive malignancies by approximately 50%. As such, adequate treatment of the N0 and N+ neck in these patients has always been viewed as a priority in an effort to increase disease-free survival rates. Traditionally, the gold standard for control of cervical metastasis has been the radical neck dissection (RND) first described by Crile. The classic RND removes levels I to V of the cervical lymphatics in addition the SCM muscle, internal jugular vein, and cranial nerve XI. Any modification of the RND that preserves nonlymphatic structures (i.e., cranial nerve XI, SCM, or internal jugular vein) is defined as a modified radical neck dissection (MRND). A neck dissection that preserves lymphatic compartments normally removed as part of a classic RND is termed a selective neck dissection (SND). Bocca[94] and colleagues demonstrated that the MRND, or "functional neck dissection," was equally effective in controlling regional metastasis as the RND, and found that the functional results were superior. With outcome data supporting the use of SND and MRND, these procedures have become the preferred alternative for the treatment cervical metastases.[95,96]

SND options have become increasingly popular given the benefits of improved shoulder function and cosmetic impact on neck contour when compared to MRND. The principle behind preservation of certain nodal groups is that specific primary sites preferentially drain their lymphatics in a predictable pattern, as mentioned previously. Types of SNDs include the supraomohyoid neck dissection, the lateral neck dissection, and the posterolateral neck dissection.[97] The supraomohyoid dissection, typically used with oral cavity primaries, removes lymph nodes in levels I to III (Fig. 17-59). The lateral neck dissection, frequently used for laryngeal malignancies, removes those nodes in levels II to IV (Fig. 17-60). The posterolateral neck dissection, used with thyroid cancer, removes the lymphatics in levels II to V (Fig. 17-61). In the clinically negative neck (N0), if the risk for occult metastasis is greater than 20%, an elective treatment of the nodes at risk is advocated. This may be in the form of elective neck irradiation or elective neck dissection, typically using a SND option. The treatment option selected for the primary lesion is frequently a factor for determining which treatment modality will be selected for elective treatment of the neck. An additional role of SND is as a staging tool to determine the need for postoperative adjuvant radiotherapy. Regional control after selective dissection has been shown to be as effective for controlling regional disease as the MRND in the N0 patient. Awareness of the potential for "skip metastases," in particular with lateral oral tongue lesions, may require extension of a standard SND to include additional levels for selected lesions.[98]

For clinically N+ necks, frequently the surgical treatment of choice is the MRND or RND. SND options have been advocated by some authors for treatment of limited N1 disease, however, do not have a role in the treatment of advanced N stage disease. When negative prognostic factors such as extracapsular spread, perineural

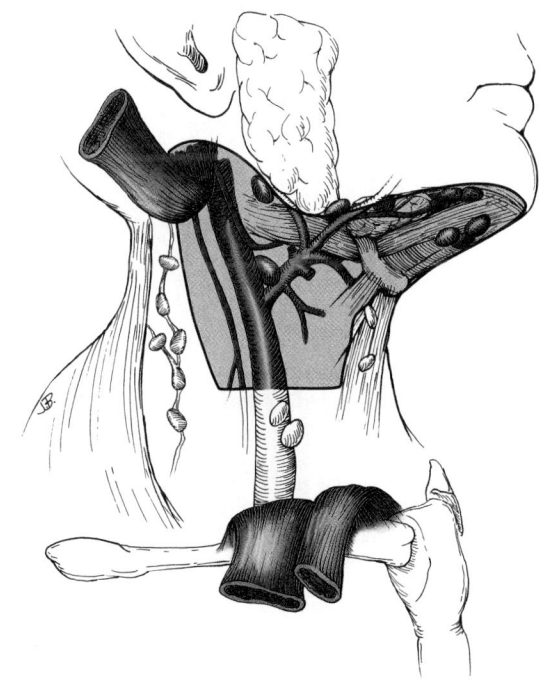

FIG. 17-59. Appearance of a supraomohyoid neck dissection.

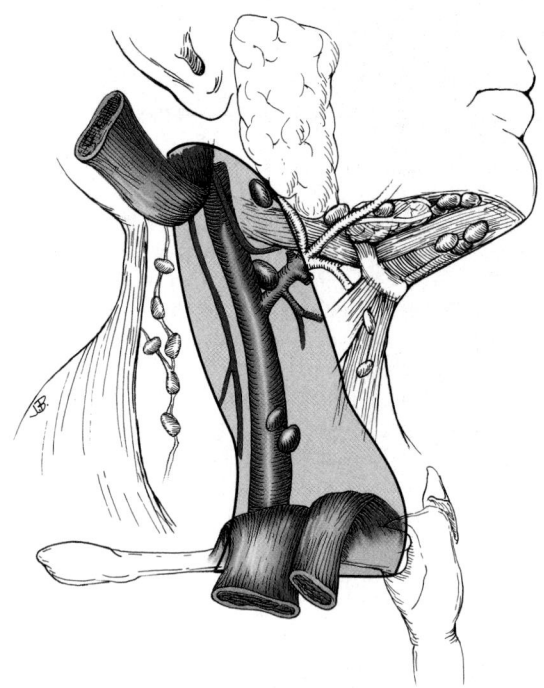

FIG. 17-60. *Appearance of a lateral neck dissection.*

invasion, vascular invasion, and the presence of multiple positive nodes, surgical management of the neck alone is not adequate.[99] Adjuvant radiation therapy is indicated in these cases.

A planned posttherapy neck dissection for patients undergoing radiation as a primary therapy is another indication for the use of neck dissection. In patients with existing advanced N stage disease (N2a or greater) or in patients with a partial response in the neck to therapy, neck dissection is performed 6 to 8 weeks after completion of treatment.

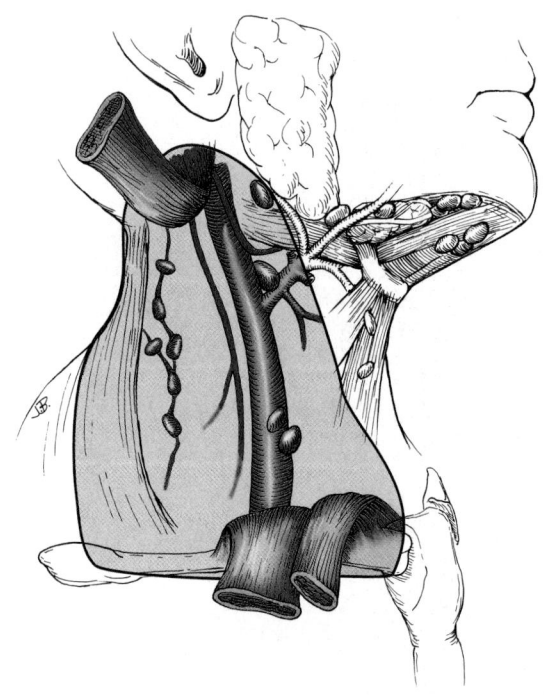

FIG. 17-61. *Appearance of a posterolateral neck dissection.*

Aggressive treatment for neck disease that encases the carotid artery or with fixation of nodes to surrounding structures (e.g., prevertebral muscles even with postoperative radiation) results in 5-year survival rates in the range of 15 to 22%. The associated morbidity is high with procedures involving carotid resection (cerebrovascular accident and death) and must be weighed carefully when deciding if surgery is to be pursued. Surgically debulking metastatic disease does not improve survival and is not advocated. Surgical salvage for recurrent neck disease after comprehensive neck dissection or radiation is associated with very poor survival.

Parapharyngeal Space Masses

The parapharyngeal space is a potential space, shaped like an inverted pyramid spanning the skull base to the hyoid. The boundaries of the space are separated by the styloid process and its associated fascial attachments into the "prestyloid" and "poststyloid" compartments.[100] The contents of the prestyloid space are the parotid, fat, and lymph nodes. The poststyloid compartment is composed of cranial nerves IX to XII, the carotid space contents, cervical sympathetic chain, fat and lymph nodes. Knowledge of these contents is pertinent because the pathology of the respective spaces is composed of tumors arising from these contents. Tumors in this space can produce displacement of the lateral pharyngeal wall medially into the oropharynx (Fig. 17-62), dysphagia, cranial nerve dysfunction, Horner's syndrome, or vascular compression.

Of the masses found in the parapharyngeal space, 40 to 50% of the tumors are of salivary gland origin. Tumors of neurogenic origin such as paragangliomas (glomus vagale, carotid body tumor) schwannomas, and neurofibromas are responsible for 20 to 25% of parapharyngeal masses. Lymph node metastases and primary lymphoma represent 15% of lesions. With this in mind, when reviewing preoperative imaging, one can assume that tumors arising anterior to the styloid process are most likely of salivary gland origin, whereas those of the retrostyloid compartment are vascular or neurogenic. This is helpful in that angiography is not as necessary for prestyloid lesions as it is for vascular poststyloid tumors. If a paraganglioma is suspected, a 24-hour urinary catecholamine collection should be obtained to allow for optimal premedication for patients with functional tumors. Embolization may be considered for vascular tumors prior to surgery in an attempt to decrease intraoperative blood loss; however, some believe that the inflammation that is provoked makes the resection more difficult.

Surgical access to these tumors may require mandibulotomy via a transoral approach, lateral cervical approach, or a combination of the two. It is inadvisable to approach parapharyngeal space tumors solely through the mouth without the necessary exposure and control of the associated vasculature that is afforded by the more appropriate transcervical or transmandibular approach. Tumors of the parapharyngeal space (e.g., the dumbbell tumors of deep parotid origin) may be amenable to removal by a transparotid and transcervical approach, dissecting the facial nerve, and removing the entire parotid gland.

Benign Neck Masses

A number of benign masses of the neck occur that require surgical management. Many of these masses are seen in the pediatric population. The differential diagnosis includes thyroglossal duct cyst, branchial cleft cyst, lymphangioma (cystic hygroma), hemangioma, and dermoid cyst.

Thyroglossal duct cysts represent the vestigial remainder of the tract of the descending thyroid gland from the foramen cecum, at

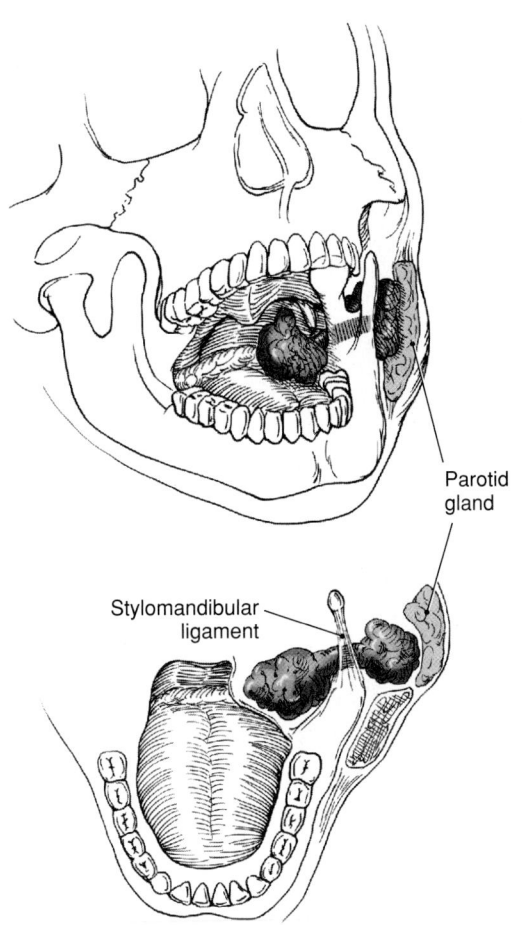

FIG. 17-62. *Parapharyngeal mass, prestyloid with prominent oropharyngeal presentation typical of a dumbbell tumor.*

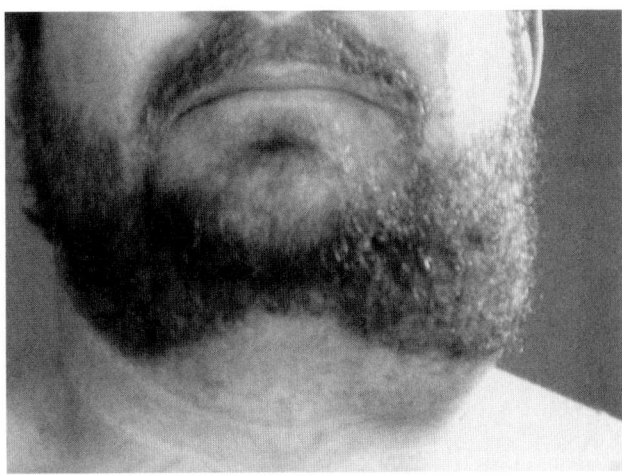

FIG. 17-63. *External appearance of a left-sided neck mass.*

the tongue base, into the lower anterior neck during fetal development. They present as a midline or paramedian cystic mass adjacent to the hyoid bone. After an upper respiratory infection, the cyst may enlarge or even suppurate. Surgical management of a thyroglossal duct cyst requires removal of the cyst, the tract, and the central portion of the hyoid bone (Sistrunk procedure), as well as a portion of the tongue base up to the foramen cecum. Prior to excision of a thyroglossal duct cyst, an imaging study is performed to identify functioning thyroid gland in the lower neck. This ensures that the cyst does not contain the only functioning thyroid tissue in the patient.

Congenital branchial cleft remnants are derived from the branchial cleft apparatus that persists after fetal development. There are several types, numbered according to their corresponding embryologic branchial cleft. First branchial cleft cysts and sinuses are associated intimately with the external auditory canal and the parotid gland. Second and third branchial cleft cysts are found along the anterior border of the sternocleidomastoid muscle and can produce drainage via a sinus tract to the neck skin (Figs. 17-63 and 17-64). Secondary infections can occur, producing enlargement, cellulitis, and neck abscess that requires operative drainage. The removal of branchial cleft cysts and fistula requires removal of the fistula tract to the point of origin in order to decrease the risk of recurrence. The second branchial cleft remnant tract courses between the internal and external carotid arteries and proceeds into the tonsillar fossa.

The third branchial cleft remnant courses posterior to the common carotid artery, ending in the pyriform sinus region. Surgical excision is preferred to establish the definitive diagnosis of a branchial cleft cyst and to avoid nontreatment of a masquerading head and neck regional metastasis. Cystic metastasis from squamous cell carcinoma of the tonsil or tongue base to a cervical lymph node can be confused for a branchial cleft cyst in an otherwise asymptomatic patient. Dermoid cysts tend to present as midline masses and represent trapped epithelium originating from the timing embryonic closure of the midline (Fig. 17-65).

Lymphatic malformations such as lymphangiomas and cystic hygromas can be difficult management problems. They typically present as mobile, fluid-filled masses with either a firm or doughy consistency. Because of their predisposition to track extensively into the surrounding soft tissues, complete removal to these lesions is often difficult. Recurrence and regrowth occur with incomplete removal and cosmetic deformity or nerve damage can result when extensive surgical dissection is performed for large lesions. In newborns and infants, there is higher associated morbidity when cystic hygromas and lymphangiomas become massive, require tracheostomy, and involve the deep neck and mediastinum.

Deep-Neck Fascial Planes

The fascial planes of the neck provide boundaries that are clinically applicable because they may determine the pathway of spread of an infection. The deep cervical fascia is composed of three layers. These are the investing (superficial deep), pretracheal, and the prevertebral fascias (Fig. 17-66). The superficial layer of the deep cervical fascia forms a cone around the neck and spans from skull base and mandible to the clavicle and manubrium. This layer surrounds the SCMs and covers the anterior and posterior triangles of the neck. The pretracheal fascia is found within the anterior compartment, deep to the strap muscles and surrounds the thyroid gland, trachea, and esophagus. This fascia blends laterally to the carotid sheath. Infections in this region may track along the trachea or esophagus into the mediastinum. The prevertebral fascia extends from the skull base to the thoracic vertebra and covers the prevertebral musculature and cervical spine. If an infection were to communicate anteriorly through the prevertebral fascia, it would enter the retropharyngeal space. Infectious extension into this space is complicated by the fact that this region, located posterior to the buccopharyngeal fascia, extends from the skull base to the mediastinum.

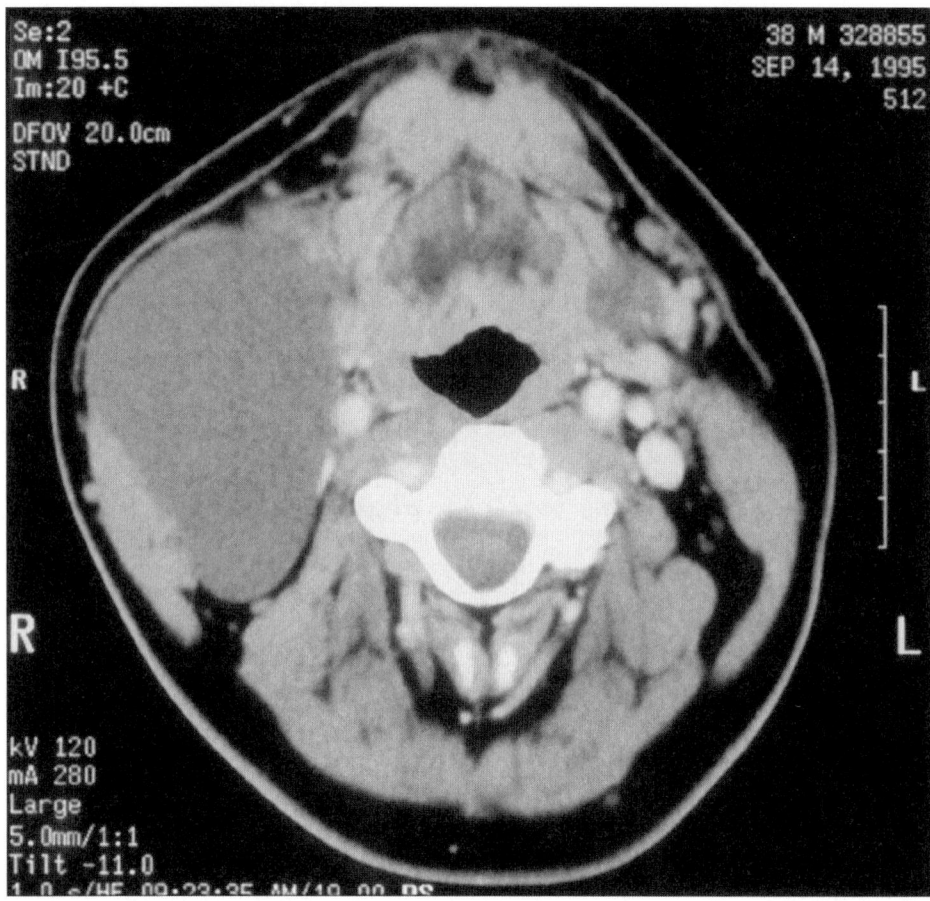

FIG. 17-64. CT scan demonstrating a branchial cleft cyst.

Salivary Gland Tumors

Tumors of the salivary gland are relatively uncommon and represent less than 2% of all head and neck neoplasms. The major salivary glands are the parotid, submandibular, and sublingual glands. Minor salivary glands are found throughout the submucosa of the upper aerodigestive tract with the highest density found within the palate.

Eighty-five percent of salivary gland neoplasms arise in the parotid gland (Fig. 17-67). The majority of these neoplasms are benign, with the most common histology being pleomorphic adenoma (benign mixed tumor). In contrast, approximately 50% of tumors arising in the submandibular and sublingual glands are malignant. Tumors arising from minor salivary gland tissue carry an even higher risk for malignancy (75%).[101]

Salivary gland tumors are usually slow growing and well circumscribed. Patients with a mass and findings of rapid growth, pain, paresthesias, and facial weakness are at increased risk of harboring

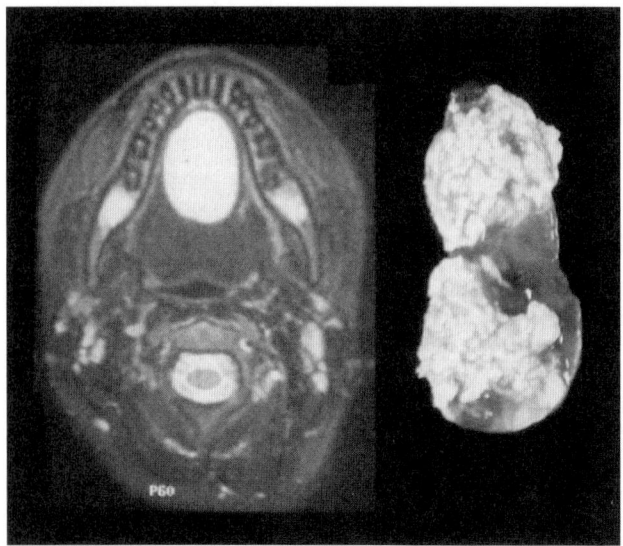

FIG. 17-65. CT scan revealing a dermoid cyst with operative specimen.

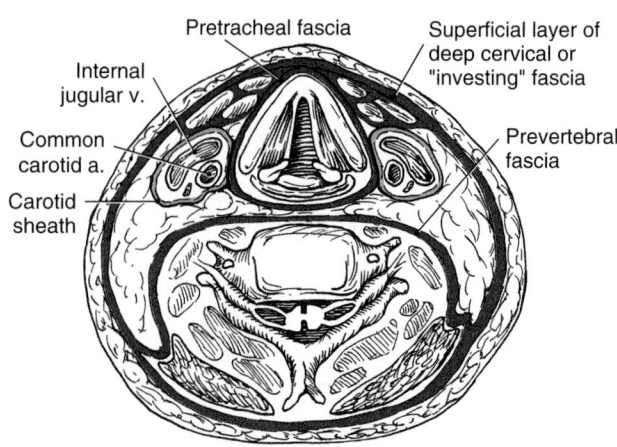

FIG. 17-66. Axial image of the neck demonstrating the fascial layers of the neck.

Pretracheal fascia

Internal jugular v.

Common carotid a.

Carotid sheath

Superficial layer of deep cervical or "investing" fascia

Prevertebral fascia

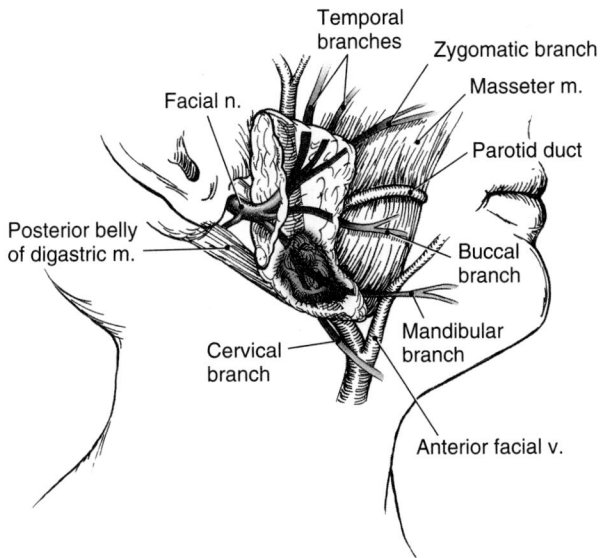

Temporal branches

Zygomatic branch

Masseter m.

Facial n.

Parotid duct

Posterior belly of digastric m.

Buccal branch

Cervical branch

Mandibular branch

Anterior facial v.

FIG. 17-67. *Example of a tumor in the parotid with the pattern of the facial nerve and associated anatomy.*

a malignancy. The facial nerve, which separates the superficial and deep lobes of the parotid, may be directly involved by tumors in 10 to 15% of patients. Additional findings ominous for malignancy include skin invasion and fixation to the mastoid tip. Trismus suggests invasion of the masseter or pterygoid muscles.[102]

Submandibular and sublingual gland tumors present as a neck mass or floor of mouth swelling, respectively. Malignant tumors of the sublingual or submandibular gland may invade the lingual or hypoglossal nerves, causing paresthesias or paralysis.[103] Bimanual examination is important for determining the size of the tumor and possible fixation to the mandible or involvement of the tongue.

Minor salivary gland tumors present as painless submucosal masses and are most frequently seen at the junction of the hard and soft palate (Fig. 17-68), but can occur throughout the upper aerodigestive tract. Minor salivary gland tumors arising in the prestyloid parapharyngeal space may produce medial displacement of the lateral oropharyngeal wall and tonsil.

The incidence of metastatic spread to cervical lymphatics is variable and depends on the histology, primary site, and stage of the

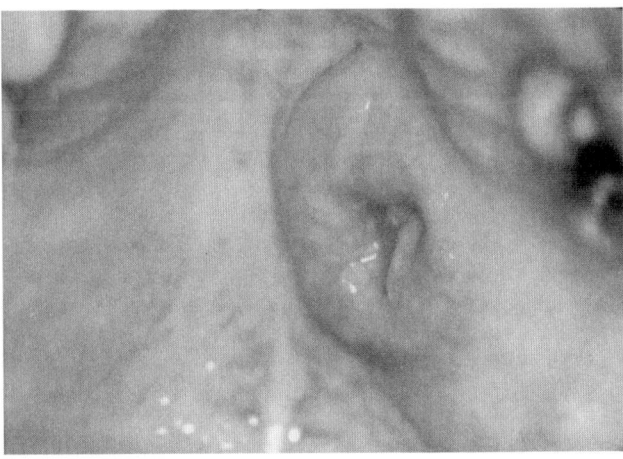

FIG. 17-68. *Palatal lesion typical of a minor salivary gland tumor at the junction of the hard palate and soft palate.*

tumor. Parotid gland malignancies can metastasize to the intra- and periglandular nodes. The next echelon of lymphatics for the parotid is the upper jugular nodal chain. Although the risk of lymphatic metastasis is low for most salivary gland malignancies, lesions that are considered high grade or that demonstrate perineural invasion and/or extraglandular spread have a higher propensity for regional spread. Tumors arising in patients of advanced age also tend to have more aggressive behavior. Initial nodal drainage for the submandibular gland is the prevascular facial lymph nodes and submental nodes followed by the upper and mid-jugular nodes. Extraglandular extension of tumor and lymph node metastases are adverse prognostic factors for submandibular gland tumors.

Imaging studies can be integral to the diagnostic evaluation of salivary gland tumors. MRI is the most sensitive study to determine soft tissue extension and involvement of adjacent structures. Unfortunately, imaging studies lack the specificity for differentiating benign and malignant neoplasms. Diagnosis of salivary gland tumors is frequently aided by the use of fine-needle aspiration. In the hands of an experienced cytologist familiar with salivary gland pathology, fine-needle aspiration can provide an accurate preoperative diagnosis in 70 to 80% of cases. This can help the operative surgeon with treatment planning and patient counseling, but should be viewed in the context that a more extensive procedure may be ultimately required. The final histopathologic diagnosis is confirmed by surgical excision.

Benign and malignant tumors of the salivary glands are divided into epithelial, nonepithelial, and metastatic neoplasms. Benign epithelial tumors include pleomorphic adenoma (80%), monomorphic adenoma, Warthin's tumor, oncocytoma, or sebaceous neoplasms. Nonepithelial benign lesions include hemangioma, neural sheath tumors, and lipoma. Treatment of benign neoplasms is surgical excision of the affected gland or, in the case of the parotid, excision of the superficial lobe with facial nerve dissection and preservation. The minimal surgical procedure for neoplasms of the parotid is superficial parotidectomy with preservation of the facial nerve. "Shelling out" of the tumor mass is not recommended because of the risk of incomplete excision and tumor spillage. Tumor spillage of a pleomorphic adenoma during removal can lead to recurrences and should be avoided.

Malignant epithelial tumors range in aggressiveness from low grade to high grade. Their behavior depends on tumor histology, degree of invasiveness, and the presence of regional metastasis. The most common malignant epithelial neoplasm of salivary glands is mucoepidermoid carcinoma. The low-grade mucoepidermoid carcinoma is composed of largely mucin-secreting cells, whereas in high-grade tumors, the epidermoid cells predominate. High-grade mucoepidermoid carcinomas resemble nonkeratinizing squamous cell carcinoma in their histologic features and clinical behavior. Adenoid cystic carcinoma, which has a propensity for neural invasion, is the second most common malignancy in adults. Skip lesions along nerves are common and can lead to treatment failures because of the difficulty in treating the full extent of invasion. Adenoid cystic carcinomas have a high incidence of distant metastasis, but display indolent growth. It is not uncommon for patients to experience lengthy survival despite the presence of disseminated disease. The most common malignancy in the pediatric population is mucoepidermoid carcinoma followed by acinic cell carcinoma. For minor salivary glands, the most common malignancies are adenoid cystic carcinoma, mucoepidermoid carcinoma, and low-grade polymorphous adenocarcinoma. Carcinoma ex pleomorphic adenoma is an aggressive malignancy that arises from a preexisting benign mixed tumor and is dominated by either an epithelial or mesenchymal component. In contrast, the malignant mixed tumor displays both neoplastic cell types and is considered a high-grade lesion. Additional uncommon tumor types that are encountered in salivary tissues are undifferentiated carcinoma and squamous cell carcinoma.

The primary treatment of salivary malignancies is surgical excision. In this setting, basic surgical principles include the en bloc removal of the involved gland with preservation of all nerves unless invaded directly by tumor. For parotid tumors that arise in the lateral lobe, superficial parotidectomy with preservation of CN VII is indicated. If the tumor extends into the deep lobe of the parotid, a total parotidectomy with nerve preservation is performed. Although malignant tumors may abut the facial nerve, if a plane of dissection can be developed without leaving gross tumor, it is preferable to preserve the nerve. If the nerve is encased by tumor and preservation would mean leaving gross residual disease, the nerve is sacrificed. Sacrifice of the facial nerve and temporal bone resection is a component of the surgical removal of advanced tumors with direct extension into the facial nerve or temporal bone. Radiation therapy is used as adjuvant treatment in the postoperative setting for specific indications.

The removal of submandibular malignancies includes en bloc resection of the gland and submental and submandibular lymph nodes. Radical resection is indicated with tumors that invade the mandible, tongue, or floor of mouth. Therapeutic removal of the regional lymphatics is indicated for clinical adenopathy or when the risk of regional metastasis exceeds 20% based on tumor characteristics. High-grade mucoepidermoid carcinomas, for example, have a high risk of regional disease and require neck dissection. Because the pattern of metastasis does not always follow an orderly progression, comprehensive neck dissection of nerves I through V is performed. When gross nerve invasion is found (lingual or hypoglossal), sacrifice of the nerve is indicated with retrograde frozen section biopsies to determine the extent of involvement. If the nerve is invaded at the level of the skull base foramina, a surgical clip is left in place to mark the area for inclusion in postoperative radiation fields. The presence of skip metastases in the nerve with adenoid cystic carcinoma makes recurrence common because of incomplete removal.

Postoperative radiation treatment plays an important role in the treatment of salivary malignancies. The presence of extraglandular disease, perineural invasion, direct invasion of regional structures, regional metastasis, and high-grade histology are all indications for radiation treatment.

RECONSTRUCTION IN HEAD AND NECK SURGERY

Defects of soft tissue and bony anatomy of the head and neck can occur after oncologic resection. Tumor surgery frequently necessitates removal of structures related to speech and swallowing. Loss of sensation and motor function can produce dysphagia through impairment of food bolus formation, manipulation, and propulsion. Removal of laryngeal, tongue base, and hypopharyngeal tumors can lead to impairment in airway protective reflexes and predisposes to aspiration. Cosmetic deformities that result from surgery also can significantly impact the quality of life of cancer survivors. Current surgical management of head and neck tumors requires restoration of form and function through application of contemporary reconstruction techniques.

Basic principles of reconstruction include attempting to replace resected tissue components (bone, skin, soft tissue) with like tissue. However, restoring functional ability, specifically speech and swallowing, does not always require strict observation of this rule. The head and neck reconstructive surgeon must consider a patient's preoperative comorbidities and anatomy when constructing a care plan. An example of this is the elderly edentulous patient with coronary artery disease who has prohibitive comorbidity for an extensive reconstructive procedure. Replacing the resected bone with like tissue will require a free flap reconstruction that will lengthen operative time and expose the patient to increased surgical morbidity. Nonbony reconstruction of the defect with a soft-tissue flap restores contour and allows oral intake and normal speech capacity.

A stepladder analogy has been used to describe the escalation in complexity of reconstructive options in the repair of head and neck defects. It is important to remember that the most complex procedure is not always the most appropriate. Progression for closure by secondary intention, primary closure, skin grafts, local flaps, regional flaps, and free-tissue transfer flaps (free flaps) run the gamut of options available. The most appropriate reconstructive technique used is based on the medical condition of the patient, the location and size of the defect to be repaired, and the functional impairment associated with the defect.

Small defects of the skin of the medial canthus, scalp, and nose may be allowed to heal by secondary intention with excellent cosmetic and functional results. When considering primary closure, the excision should be placed in the lines of relaxed skin tension and should not distort the hairline, nasal area, eyelid, or lips.

Skin Grafts

Split- and full-thickness skin grafts are used in the head and neck for a variety of defects. Following oral cavity resections, split-thickness grafts can provide adequate reconstruction of the mucosal surface if an adequate soft-tissue bed is available to support the blood supply needed for survival. These grafts incorporate into the recipient site in around 5 days and do not provide replacement of absent soft tissue; however, they are expeditious for covering mucosal defects and provide for ease of monitoring for recurrences of the primary tumor. Full-thickness grafts are used on the face when local rotational flaps are not available. These grafts have far less contracture than split-thickness grafts and also can provide a good color match for the defect area. Grafts can be harvested from the postauricular or supraclavicular areas to maximize the match of skin characteristics. Dermal grafts have been used to provide coverage for exposed vessels in the neck, reconstruct mucosal defects, and assist in providing soft-tissue bulk.

Local Flaps

Local flaps encompass a large number of mainly random-pattern flaps used to reconstruct defects in adjacent areas. It is beyond the scope of this chapter to enumerate all of these flaps, but they should be designed according to the relaxed skin tension lines of the face and neck skin. These lines are tension lines inherent in the facial regions and caused in part by the insertions of muscles of facial animation. Incisions paralleling the relaxed skin tension lines that respect the aesthetic subunits of the face heal with the least amount of tension and camouflage into a more appealing result. Poorly designed incisions or flaps result in widened scars and distortion of important aesthetic units. Flaps have many different configurations and sizes with the most common being the rotation and transposition flaps.

Regional Flaps

Regional flaps are those that are available as pedicled transfer of soft tissue or bone from areas adjacent to the defect. These flaps have an axial blood supply that traverses the flap longitudinally from proximal to distal between the fascia and subcutaneous tissue. Single-stage reconstruction is possible and harvest can occur simultaneously with the resection of primary disease, thus decreasing operative time.

The deltopectoral fasciocutaneous flap is a medially based flap from the anterior chest wall reliant on the perforators of the internal mammary artery. The flap provides a fair color match for surface defects. Its pliability permits folding, making it useful for reconstruction of pharyngoesophageal defects. Use of the flap requires a second stage for insetting approximately 2 weeks after the original procedure.

Several myocutaneous flaps exist for head and neck reconstruction. The cutaneous portions of these flaps are nourished by muscular perforating vessels which require care when harvesting to prevent undue torsion on the vessels. The vascular pedicle of these flaps permits a wide arc of rotation, making them ideal for a variety of different reconstructive needs. The trapezius muscle provides a number of soft-tissue flaps that can be rotated to reconstruct a number of defects in the head and neck. The superior trapezius flap is based on paraspinous perforators and is ideal for lateral neck defects. The lateral island trapezius flap, based on the transverse cervical and dorsal scapular vessels, allows for harvest of soft tissue below the inferior border of the scapula. This flap is ideal for reconstruction of scalp and lateral skull base defects.

The pectoralis myocutaneous flap is based on the pectoral branch of the thoracoacromial artery (medial) and the lateral thoracic artery (lateral). The latter vessel may be sacrificed to increase the arc of rotation. This flap includes the pectoralis major muscle, either alone or with overlying anterior chest skin. The pectoralis myocutaneous flap has enjoyed tremendous popularity because of its ease of harvest, the ability to tailor its thickness to the defect, and minimal donor site morbidity. It can be used for many reconstructive needs in the oropharynx, oral cavity, and the hypopharynx and can be tubed in some cases to replace cervical esophageal defects. Bulk associated with this flap may make certain applications less practical, and this problem is exacerbated in obese patients. The arc of rotation limits the superior extent of this flap to the zygomatic arch externally and the superior pole of the tonsil internally. It should be remembered that the least-reliable portion of this flap is the skin because it is the portion farthest from the blood supply. When portions of the flap are extended into regions beyond the underlying muscle, relying on random blood supply, healing at the primary site may be adversely affected. For patients that require expeditious recovery to initiate postoperative radiation therapy this can be a significant problem. This flap is still frequently used but has been replaced in many instances by free-tissue transfer for oral cavity and oropharyngeal defects because of its greater reliability and pliability.

The latissimus dorsi flap provides a large source of soft tissue, as well as a wide arc of rotation. The flap reaches farther cephalad than the pectoralis myocutaneous flap, such as to the superior skull base and scalp. Based on the thoracodorsal vessels, this flap can be used as a regional rotational flap or as a free flap. Lateral decubitus positioning is required for harvesting this flap, making it less attractive for simultaneous cancer ablation and reconstruction.

Free-Tissue Transfer

Free-tissue transfer with microvascular anastomosis (free flaps) affords the reconstructive surgeon unparalleled ability to replace tissue loss with tissues of similar characteristics. There are a number of donor sites available for various types of flaps, including

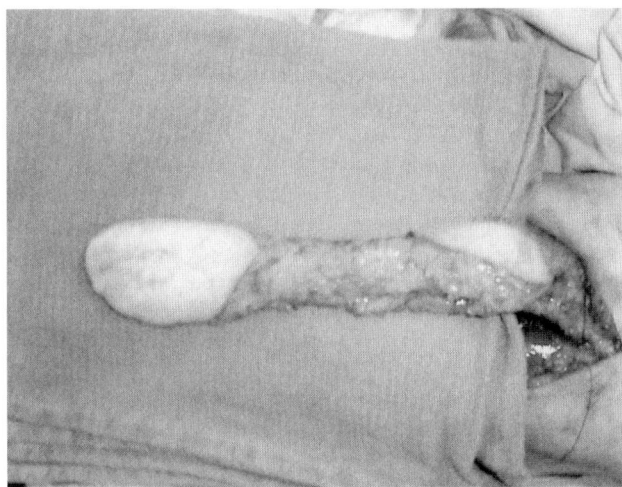

FIG. 17-69. *Radial forearm free flap with proximal monitoring paddle.*

osteomyocutaneous, myocutaneous, fasciocutaneous, fascial, and myoosseous flaps. The so-called sensate flaps include a superficial cutaneous nerve available for reanastomosis to the recipient site sensory nerve endings. The flaps most popular in head and neck reconstructive armamentarium are those with ease of harvesting from a standpoint of patient positioning and those that allow for a two-teamed approach for simultaneous flap harvesting and oncologic resection.[104]

The radial forearm fasciocutaneous flap (Fig. 17-69) is a hardy flap with constant vascular anatomy and a potentially long vascular pedicle, allowing for ease of insetting and choice in anastomotic vascular recipient sites. It is pliable and can be reinnervated as a sensate flap, making it ideal for repair of oral cavity and oropharyngeal defects. It can be tubed to repair hypopharyngeal and upper esophageal defects.[105,106]

The lateral thigh flap, based on perforators of the profunda femoris artery, provides relatively pliable tissue that can be tubed and is used to reconstruct similar defects as that of the radial forearm flap, as well as pharyngoesophageal defects extending from the thoracic inlet to the nasopharynx.

The lateral arm flap, based on the radial collateral artery, is another pliable, sensate fasciocutaneous flap that can be used in similar defects with minimal donor site morbidity.

The fibular osteocutaneous or osteomyocutaneous flap allows for one-stage reconstruction of resected mandible. In the adult, 25 cm of bone can be harvested and a cuff of soleus and flexor hallucis longus muscles can be included for additional soft-tissue bulk. The pedicle length can be extended by harvesting a long segment of bone, and the donor site defect is well tolerated as long as approximately 6 cm of bone are retained proximally and distally for knee and ankle stability.[107]

Iliac crest osteocutaneous flaps are frequently used for mandible defects involving the angle. The natural shape of this donor site bone is similar to the mandibular angle and eliminates the need for shaping of the bone flap prior to insetting into the defect. However, for long, mandibular defects, the fibular flap usually is chosen. For shorter mandible defects not involving the angle, other osteocutaneous flaps include scapular and radial forearm flaps. The scapular flap can provide 10 to 14 cm of lateral scapula bone and is based on the circumflex scapular artery. This flap can be combined with additional fasciocutaneous and myocutaneous components including separate parascapular and scapular skin islands and a portion of latissimus dorsi and serratus anterior. The radial forearm osteo-cutaneous flap can provide a limited quantity of bone with the soft tissue component of the flap but is associated with an increased risk of donor site fracture long-term.

Large soft-tissue defects can result from trauma, excision of skull base tumors, and tumors involving large segments of skin. Furthermore, after extensive skull base resections in the anterior and lateral skull base, the need for separation of the oropharyngeal and sinonasal tracts from the dura requires soft-tissue interposition between the dura and the contaminated upper aerodigestive tract. The rectus abdominis myocutaneous flap provides a large amount of soft tissue and is ideal for closure of wounds of the lateral skull base and dura.

For reconstruction of defects of the hypopharynx and cervical esophagus, both free flaps and regional pedicled flaps are available. The free transfer of a jejunal segment can be performed based on branches of the superior mesenteric artery. Other free flaps used in this area include fasciocutaneous flaps, such as tubed radial forearm, lateral thigh, and lateral arm flap. The gastric pull-up is a regional flap that is also in use for reconstruction of cervical esophageal defects. The stomach is mobilized and pedicled on the right gastric and gastroepiploic vessels into the defect via tunneling through the anterior mediastinum.[106]

TRACHEOSTOMY

Tracheostomy is indicated in the management of patients who require prolonged intubation, assisted ventilation, and pulmonary toilet, and in those patients with neurologic deficits that impair protective airway reflexes. Its use in head and neck surgery is often for the temporary management of the airway in the perioperative period. After surgical resection of oral cavity and oropharyngeal cancers, bleeding into the sublingual and submaxillary soft-tissue spaces may result in airway compromise, and elective tracheostomy is indicated to prevent loss of the airway.

The avoidance of prolonged orotracheal and nasotracheal intubation decreases the risk of laryngeal damage and subglottic stenosis, facilitates oral and pulmonary toilet, and decreases patient discomfort. When the tracheostomy is no longer needed, the tube is removed and prompt closure of the opening usually occurs. Complications of tracheostomy include pneumothorax or pneumomediastinum, recurrent laryngeal nerve injury, formation of granulation tissue, tracheal stenosis, wound infection with large-vessel erosion, and failure to close after decannulation. The use of cricothyroidotomy as an alternative to tracheostomy for patients who require prolonged intubation is associated with a higher incidence of vocal cord dysfunction and subglottic stenosis.[108] When cricothyroidotomy is used in the setting of establishing an emergency airway, conversion to a standard tracheostomy should be considered if decannulation is not anticipated within 5 to 7 days.

Placement of a tracheostomy does not obligate a patient to loss of speech. When a large cuffed tracheostomy tube is in place, expecting a patient to be capable of normal speech is impractical. However, after a patient is downsized to an uncuffed tracheostomy tube, intermittent finger occlusion or Passy-Muir valve placement will allow a patient to communicate while still using the tracheostomy to bypass the upper airway for inhalation. When a patient no longer has the original indication for the tracheostomy (secretion management, need for ventilatory support, upper airway edema) and can tolerate capping of the tracheal tube for greater than 24 hours, decannulation is considered safe. If an upper airway mass or tissue reconstruction

was the indication for the tracheostomy, pre-decannulation flexible laryngoscopic examination of the airway is recommended.[109]

LONG–TERM MANAGEMENT AND REHABILITATION

Palliative Care

For patients with unresectable disease or distant metastases, palliative care options exist. Palliative treatment is aimed at improving a patient's symptoms and may include radiation, chemotherapy, or consultation with a pain specialist. The head and neck surgeon has the options of tracheostomy and gastrostomy tube placement for patients progressing with worsening airway compromise and dysphagia, respectively. Hospice is also an option for patients with a limited short-term outlook; hospice allows a patient to retain dignity at the time of greatest adversity.

Follow-Up Care

Patients diagnosed and treated for a head and neck tumor require follow-up care aimed at monitoring for recurrence and the side effects of therapy. For malignancies of the upper aerodigestive tract, a proposed formula for follow-up appointments is as follows:[110]

Years posttreatment	Follow-up
1st year	1–3 months
2nd year	2–4 months
3rd year	3–6 months
4th year	4–6 months
After 5 years	Every 12 months

In addition to a formal head and neck examination, patients should be questioned about any emerging symptoms related to their primary tumor. New-onset pain, otalgia, hoarseness, and dysphagia are some of the problems that may indicate the need to evaluate further for recurrence. Worsening dysphagia may also be a presenting symptom for a patient developing a pharyngeal stricture. Such a patient may require dilatation and/or placement of a gastrostomy tube for nutrition. Additionally, a number of patients who undergo head and neck radiation will develop hypothyroidism months to years after treatment. Patients with shoulder dysfunction after neck dissection, or who underwent free-flap harvest, who have donor-site morbidity require physical therapy to minimize the long-term effects of their surgical care. Patients with chronic pain-related issues can benefit from consultation with a pain specialist in constructing a regimen to provide adequate control of long-term discomfort. Postoperative follow-up appointments can help a patient manage these problems as they present, in addition to allowing for surveillance for recurrence. Yearly chest radiographs are advised for patients to monitor for pulmonary metastases. Long-term follow-up for postradiation patients with a dentist experienced in caring for these patients is vital if prevention of osteoradionecrosis is to be achieved.

References

1. Senturia BA, Marcus MD, Lucente FE: *Diseases of the External Ear,* 2nd ed. New York: Grune and Stratton, 1980.
2. Kimmelman CP, Lucente FE: Use of ceftazidime for malignant external otitis. *Ann Otol Rhinol Laryngol* 98:721, 1989.
3. Teele DW, Klein JO, Rosner BA: Epidemiology of otitis media in children. *Ann Otol Rhinol Laryngol Suppl* 89:5, 1980.
4. Sutton D, Derkay CS, Darrow DH, et al: Resistant bacteria in the middle ear fluid at the time of tympanostomy tube surgery. *Ann Otol Rhinol Laryngol* 109:24, 2000.

5. Nissen AJ, Bui H: Complications of chronic otitis media. *Ear Nose Throat J* 75:284, 1996.

6. Arts HA, Neely JG: Intratemporal and intracranial complications of otitis media, in Calhoun KH, Healy GB, Jackler RK, et al (eds): *Byron J. Bailey Head and Neck Surgery—Otolaryngology,* 3rd ed. Philadelphia: Lippincott Williams and Wilkins, 2001, p 1759.

7. Antonelli PJ, Garside JA, Mancuso AA, et al: Computed tomography and the diagnosis of coalescent mastoiditis. *Otolaryngol Head Neck Surg* 120:350, 1999.

8. Gantz BJ, Rubinstein JT, Gidley P, et al: Surgical management of Bell's palsy. *Laryngoscope* 109:1177, 1999.

9. Green JD, Shelton C, Brackman DE: Surgical management of iatrogenic facial nerve injuries. *Otolaryngol Head Neck Surg* 111:606, 1994.

10. Lanza DC, Kennedy DW: Adult rhinosinusitis defined. *Otolaryngol Head Neck Surg* 117:S1, 1997.

11. Brook I: Microbiology and management of sinusitis. *J Otolaryngol* 25:249, 1996.

12. Benninger MS, Anon J, Mabry RL: The medical management of rhinosinusitis. *Otolaryngol Head Neck Surg* 117:S41, 1997.

13. Manning SC, Holman M: Further evidence for allergic pathophysiology in allergic fungal sinusitis. *Laryngoscope* 108:1485, 1998.

14. Cody DT, Neel HB, Ferrerio JA, et al: Allergic fungal sinusitis: The Mayo Clinic experience. *Laryngoscope* 104:1074, 1994.

15. deShazo RD, O'Brien M, Chapin K, et al: A new classification and diagnostic criteria for invasive fungal sinusitis. *Arch Otolaryngol Head Neck Surg* 123:1181, 1997.

16. Bisno AL, Gerber MA, Gwaltney JM, et al: Diagnosis and management of group A streptococcal pharyngitis: A practice guideline. *Clin Infect Dis* 25:574, 1997.

17. Thompson LDR, Wenig BM, Kornblut BM: Pharyngitis, in Calhoun KH, Healy GB, Jackler RK, et al (eds): *Byron J. Bailey Head and Neck Surgery—Otolaryngology,* 3rd ed. Philadelphia: Lippincott Williams and Wilkins, 2001, p 543.

18. Paradise J, Bluestone C, Bachman R, et al: Efficacy of tonsillectomy in recurrent throat infections in severely affected children. *N Engl J Med* 310:674, 1984.

19. Gates G, Cooper J, Avery C, et al: Chronic secretory otitis media: Effects of surgical management. *Ann Otol Rhinol Laryngol Suppl* 98:2, 1989.

20. Gerber ME, O'Connor DM, Adler E, et al: Selected risk factors in pediatric adenotonsillectomy. *Arch Otolaryngol Head Neck Surg* 122:811, 1996.

21. Friedman M, Tanyeri H, La Rossa M, et al: Clinical predictors of obstructive sleep apnea. *Laryngoscope* 109:1901, 1999.

22. Standards of Practice Committee of the American Sleep Disorders Association: Practice parameters for the use of laser assisted uvuloplasty. *Sleep* 17:744, 1994.

23. Zeitels SM, Casiano RR, Gardner GM, et al: Management of common voice problems: Committee report. *Otolaryngol Head Neck Surg* 126:333, 2002.

24. Rosen CA, Woodson GE, Thompson JW, et al: Preliminary results of the use of indole 3-carbinol for recurrent respiratory papillomatosis. *Otolaryngol Head Neck Surg* 118:810, 1998.

25. Gray S, Hammond E, Hanson DF: Benign pathologic responses of the larynx. *Ann Otol Rhinol Laryngol* 104:13, 1995.

26. Koufman JA: The otolaryngologic manifestations of gastroesophageal reflux disease (GERD). *Laryngoscope* 53(Suppl):1, 1991.

27. Nasri S, Sercarz JA, McAlpin T, et al: Treatment of vocal fold granuloma using botulism toxin type A. *Laryngoscope* 105:585, 1995.

28. Benninger MS, Crumley RL, Ford CN, et al: Evaluation and treatment of the unilateral paralyzed vocal fold. *Otolaryngol Head Neck Surg* 111:497, 1994.

29. Gentile RD, Miller RH, Woodson GE: Vocal cord paralysis in children 1 year of age and younger. *Ann Otol Rhinol Laryngol* 95:622, 1986.

30. Ishiki N: Vocal mechanics and the basis for phonosurgery. *Laryngoscope* 108:1761, 1998.

31. Hochman M, Vural E, Suen J, et al: Contemporary management of vascular lesions of the head and neck. *Curr Opin Otolaryngol Head Neck Surg* 7:161, 1999.

32. Waner M: The treatment of vascular lesions. *Facial Plast Surg Clin North Am* 4:275, 1996.

33. Waner M, Suen JY, Dinehart S: Treatment of hemangiomas of the head and neck. *Laryngoscope* 102:1123, 1992.

34. Kohut MP, Hansen M, Pribaz JJ, et al: Arteriovenous malformations of the head and neck: Natural history and management. *Plast Reconstr Surg* 102:643, 1998.

35. Giguere CM, Bauman NM, Smith RJH: New treatment options for lymphangioma in infants and children. *Ann Otol Rhinol Laryngol* 111:1066, 2002.

36. Gruss JS, Macinnon SE: Complex midface fractures: Role of buttress reconstruction and immediate bone grafts. *Plast Reconstr Surg* 78:9, 1988.

37. Shumrick K, Kersten R, Kulwin D, et al: Extended access/internal approaches for the management of facial trauma. *Arch Otolaryngol Head Neck Surg* 118:1105, 1992.

38. Coker NJ: Facial electroneurography: Analysis of techniques and correlation with degenerating motor neurons. *Laryngoscope* 102:747, 1992.

39. Brodie HA, Thompson TC: Management of complications from 820 temporal bone fractures. *Am J Otol* 18:188, 1997.

40. Darrouzet V, Duclos J, Liguoro D: Management of facial paralysis resulting from temporal bone fractures: Our experience in 115 cases. *Otolaryngol Head Neck Surg* 125:787, 2001.

41. Blot WJ, McLaughlin JK, Winn DM, et al: Smoking and drinking in relation to oral and pharyngeal cancer. *Cancer Res* 48:3282, 1988.

42. Rigotti NA: Treatment of tobacco use and dependence. *N Engl J Med* 346:506, 2002

43. Centers for Disease Control: Cigarette smoking among adults—United States, 1999. *Morb Mortal Wkly Rep* 50:869, 2001.

44. Moore C: Cigarette smoking and cancer of the mouth, pharynx and larynx. *JAMA* 218:553, 1971.

45. Brennan JA, Boyle JO, Koch WM, et al: Association between cigarette smoking and mutation of the p53 gene in squamous cell carcinoma of the head and neck. *N Engl J Med* 332:712, 1995.

46. Boyle JO, Koch W, Hrubin PA, et al: The incidence of P53 mutations increase with progression of head and neck cancer. *Cancer Res* 53:4477, 1993.

47. Koch WM, Lango M, Sewell D, et al: Head and neck cancer in nonsmokers: A distinct clinical and molecular entity. *Laryngoscope* 109:1544, 1999.

48. Jusawalla DJ, Despandi VA: Evaluation of cancer risk in tobacco chewers and smokers. An epidemiologic assessment. *Cancer* 28:244, 1971.

49. Slaughter DP, Southwick HW, Smejkal W: Field cancerization in oral stratified squamous epithelium: Clinical implications of multicentric origin. *Cancer* 6:963, 1953.

50. Scholes AGM, Woolgar JA, Boyle MA, et al: Synchronous oral carcinomas: Independent or common clonal origin? *Cancer Res* 58:2003, 1998.

51. Joint Committee on Cancer: *American Joint Committee on Cancer Staging Manual,* 6th ed. Chicago: American, 2002.

52. Baker SR: Current management of cancer of the lip. *Oncology* 4:107, 1990.

53. Zitsch RP, Park CW, Renner FJ, et al: Outcome analysis for lip carcinoma. *Otolaryngol Head Neck Surg* 113:589, 1995.

54. Calhoun K: Reconstruction of small- and medium-sized defects of the lower lip. *Am J Otolaryngol* 13:16, 1992.

55. Conley JJ, Donovan DT: A new technique for total reconstruction of the lower lip in a patient with malignant melanoma. *Otolaryngol Head Neck Surg* 94:393, 1986.

56. Franceschi D, Gupta R, Spiro RH, et al: Improved survival in the treatment of squamous carcinoma of the oral tongue. *Am J Surg* 166:360, 1993.

57. Lydiatt DD, Robbins KT, Byers RM, et al: Treatment of stage I and II oral cancer. *Head Neck* 15:308, 1993.

58. Spiro RH, Huvos AG, Wong GY, et al: Predictive value of tumor thickness in squamous carcinoma confined to the tongue and floor of mouth. *Am J Surg* 152:345, 1986.

59. Rodgers LW Jr., Stringer SP, Mendenhall WM, et al: Management of squamous cell carcinoma of the floor of mouth. *Head Neck* 15:16, 1993.

60. Overholt SM, Eicher SA, Wolf P, et al: Prognostic factors affecting outcome in lower gingival carcinoma. *Laryngoscope* 106:1335, 1996.

61. Huang CJ, Chao KSC, Tsai J, et al: Cancer of retromolar trigone: Long-term radiation therapy outcome. *Head Neck* 23:758, 2001.

62. Bloom ND, Spiro RH. Carcinoma of the cheek mucosa: A retrospective analysis. *Am J Surg* 154:411, 1987.

63. Evans JF, Shah JP. Epidermoid carcinoma of the palate. *Am J Surg* 142:451, 1981.

64. Beckhardt RN, Weber RS, Zane R, et al: Minor salivary gland tumors of the palate: Clinical and pathologic correlates of outcome. *Laryngoscope* 11:1155, 1995.

65. Bradford CR, Futran N, Peters G. Management of tonsil cancer. *Head Neck* 21:657, 1999.

66. Lee, HJ, Zelefsky MJ, Kraus DH, et al: Long-term regional control after radiation therapy and neck dissection for base of tongue carcinoma. *Int J Rad Oncology Biol Phys* 38:995, 1997.

67. Peters LJ, Weber RS, Morrison WH, et al: Neck surgery in patients with primary oropharyngeal cancer treated by radiotherapy. *Head Neck* 18:552, 1996.

68. Ang KK, Peters LJ, Weber RS, et al: Concomitant boost radiotherapy schedules in the treatment of carcinoma of the oropharynx and nasopharynx. *Int J Radiat Oncol Biol Phys* 19:1339, 1990.

69. Weber RS, Gidley P, Morrison WH, et al: Treatment selection for carcinoma of the base of tongue. *Am J Surg* 160:415, 1990.

70. Weber RS, Ohlms L, Bowman J, et al: Functional results after total or near total glossectomy with laryngeal preservation. *Arch Otolaryngol Head Neck Surg* 117:512, 1991.

71. Weber RS, Peters LJ, Wolf P, et al: Squamous cell carcinoma of the soft palate, uvula, and anterior faucial pillar. *Otolaryngol Head Neck Surg* 99:16, 1988.

72. Clayman G, Weber RS: Cancer of the hypopharynx and cervical esophagus, in Myers E, Suen JY (eds): *Cancer of the Head and Neck,* 3rd ed. Philadelphia: WB Saunders, 1996, p 423.

73. Frank J, Garb J, Kay S, et al: Postoperative radiotherapy improves survival in squamous cell carcinoma of the hypopharynx. *Am J Surg* 168:476, 1994.

74. Lefebve JL, Chevalier D, Luboinski B, et al: Larynx preservation in piriform sinus cancer: Preliminary results of a European organization for research and treatment of cancer phase III trial. *J Natl Cancer Inst* 88:890, 1996.

75. Hartig G, Truelson J, Weinstein GS. Supraglottic cancer. *Head Neck* 22:426, 2000.

76. Laccourreye H, Laccourreye O, Weinstein GS, et al: Supracricoid laryngectomy with cricohyoidoepiglottopexy: A partial laryngeal procedure for selected glottic carcinomas. *Ann Otol Rhinol Laryngol* 99:421, 1990.

77. Wolf GT, Hong WK, Fischer SG, et al: Induction chemotherapy plus radiation compared with surgery plus radiation in patients with advanced laryngeal cancer. *N Engl J Med* 324:1685, 1991.

78. Medina JE, Khafif A: Early oral feeding following total laryngectomy. *Laryngoscope* 111:368, 2001.

79. Weber RS, Marvel J, Smith P, et al: Paratracheal lymph node dissection for carcinoma of the larynx, hypopharynx, and cervical esophagus. *Otolaryngol Head Neck Surg* 108:11, 1993.

80. Weber RS, Berket BA, Forastiere A, et al: Outcome of salvage total laryngectomy following organ preservation therapy: The Radiation Therapy Oncology Group trial 91-11. *Arch Otolaryngol Head Neck Surg* 129:44, 2003.

81. Osguthorpe JD: Sinus neoplasia. *Arch Otolaryngol Head Neck Surg* 120:19, 1994.

82. Neel HB: A prospective evaluation of patients with nasopharyngeal carcinoma: An overview. *J Otolaryngol* 15:137, 1986.

83. Levine PA, Frierson HF, Mills SE, et al: Sinonasal undifferentiated carcinoma: A distinctive and highly aggressive neoplasm. *Laryngoscope* 97:905, 1987.

84. Levine PA, Gallager R, Cantrell RW: Esthesioneuroblastoma: Reflections of a 21-year experience. *Laryngoscope* 109:1539, 1999.

85. Senior BA, Lanza DC, Kennedy DW, et al: Computer-assisted resection of benign sinonasal tumors with skull base and orbital extension. *Arch Otolaryngol Head Neck Surg* 123:706, 1997.

86. Bales C, Kotapka M, Loevner LA, et al: Craniofacial resection of advanced juvenile nasopharyngeal angiofibroma. *Arch Otolaryngol Head Neck Surg* 128:1071, 2002.

87. Kennedy JD, Haines SJ: Review of skull base surgery approaches with special reference to pediatric patients. *J Neurooncol* 20:291, 1994.

88. Isaacs RS, Donald PJ: Sphenoid and sellar tumors. *Otolaryngol Clin North Am* 28:1191, 1995.

89. Al-Sarraf M, LeBlanc M, Giri PG, et al: Chemoradiotherapy versus radiotherapy in patients with advanced nasopharyngeal cancer: Phase III randomized intergroup 0099. *J Clin Oncol* 16:1310, 1998.

90. Arena S, Keen M: Carcinoma of the middle ear and temporal bone. *Am J Otol* 9:351, 1988.

91. Kuhel W, Hume CR, Selesnick SH: Cancer of the external auditory canal and temporal bone. *Otolaryngol Clin North Am* 29:827, 1996.

92. Prasad S, Janecka IP: Efficacy of surgical treatments for squamous cell carcinoma of the temporal bone: A literature review. *Otolaryngol Head Neck Surg* 110:270, 1994.

93. Shah JP: Patterns of cervical lymph node metastasis from squamous carcinomas of the upper aerodigestive tract. *Am J Surg* 160:405, 1990.

94. Bocca E, Pignataro O, Oldino C: Functional neck dissection: An evaluation and review of 843 cases. *Laryngoscope* 94:942, 1984.

95. Medina JE, Byers RM: Supraomohyoid neck dissection: Rationale, indications and surgical technique. *Head Neck* 11:111, 1989.

96. Eicher SA, Weber RS: Surgical management of cervical lymph node metastases. *Curr Opin Oncol* 8:215, 1996.

97. Robbins KT, Atkinson JLD, Byers RM, et al: The use and misuse of neck dissection for head and neck cancer. *J Am Coll Surg* 193:91, 2001.

98. Byers RM, Weber RS, Andrews T, et al: Frequency and therapeutic implications of "skip metastases" in the neck from squamous carcinoma of the oral tongue. *Head Neck* 19:14, 1997.

99. Myers EN, Fagan JJ: Treatment of the N+ neck in squamous cell carcinoma of the upper aerodigestive tract. *Otolaryngol Clin North Am* 31:671, 1998.

100. Eisele DE, Netterville J, Hoffman H, et al: Parapharyngeal space masses. *Head Neck* 21:154, 1999.

101. Chalian A, Weber RS: Salivary gland tumors, in Winchester DP, Jones RS, Murphy GP (eds): *Cancer Surgery for the General Surgeon.* Philadelphia: Lippincott Williams and Wilkins, 1999.

102. Frankenthaler RA, Luna MA, Lee S, et al: Prognostic variables in parotid gland cancer. *Arch Otol Head Neck Surg* 117:1251, 1991.

103. Weber RS, Byers RM, Petit B, et al: Submandibular gland tumors: Adverse histologic factors and therapeutic implications. *Arch Otolaryngol Head Neck Surg* 116:1055, 1990.

104. Blackwell KE, Buchbinder D, Biller HF: Reconstruction of massive defects in the head and neck: The role of simultaneous distant and regional flaps. *Head Neck* 19:620, 1997.

105. Anthony JP, Neligan PC, Rotstein LE, et al: Reconstruction of partial laryngopharyngectomy defects. *Head Neck* 19:541, 1997.

106. Schusterman M, Shestak K, de Vries EL, et al: Reconstruction of the cervical esophagus: Free jejunal transfer versus gastric pull-up. *Plast Reconstr Surg* 85:16, 1990.

107. Urken ML, Buchbinder D, Costantino PD, et al: Oromandibular reconstruction using microvascular composite flaps: Report of 210 cases. *Arch Otolaryngol Head Neck Surg* 124:46, 1998.

108. Kuriloff DB, Setzen M, Portnoy W, et al: Laryngotracheal injury following cricothyroidotomy. *Laryngoscope* 99:125, 1989.

109. Wenig BL, Applebaum EL: Indications for and technique for tracheostomy. *Clin Chest Med* 1293:545, 1991.

110. The American Society for Head and Neck Surgery and the Society of Head and Neck Surgeons. *Clinical Practice Guidelines for the Diagnosis and Management of Cancer of the Head and Neck.* 1996.

CHAPTER 18

Chest Wall, Lung, Mediastinum, and Pleura

Michael A. Maddaus and James D. Luketich

TRACHEA

Anatomy

An understanding of the relevant anatomy of the trachea is essential for surgeons of all specialties (Fig. 18-1). The cricoid cartilage is the first complete cartilage ring of the airway. It consists of an anterior arch and a posterior broad-based plate. The arytenoid cartilages articulate with the posterior cricoid plate. The vocal cords originate from these cartilages and then attach to the thyroid cartilage. The subglottic space begins at the inferior surface of the vocal cords and extends to the first tracheal ring. It is the narrowest part of the trachea, with an internal diameter of about 2.0 cm. The remainder of the distal trachea is 10.0 to 13.0 cm long, consists of 18 to 22 rings, and has an internal diameter of 2.3 cm.

The tracheal blood supply enters the airway near the junction of the membranous and cartilaginous portions of the airway (Fig. 18-2). It is segmental in nature, meaning that each entering small branch supplies a segment of 1.0 to 2.0 cm, thereby limiting circumferential mobilization to that same distance. The arteries supplying the trachea include the inferior thyroid and the bronchial arteries.

Tracheal Injury

Injury secondary to endotracheal intubation is most commonly the result of overinflation of the cuff. Although high volume–low pressure cuffs are now ubiquitous, they can easily be overinflated, and pressures can be generated that are high enough to cause ischemia of the contiguous airway wall. In some patients, periods of ischemia as short as 4 hours may be all that is required to induce an ischemic event significant enough to lead to scarring and stricture. With prolonged overinflation and consequent full-thickness destruction of the airway, fistula development between the innominate artery or esophagus may ensue. For these reasons, it is good practice in all intubations, no matter how brief, to only inflate the cuff to the level necessary to prevent air leakage around the cuff. In circumstances of prolonged ventilatory support and high airway pressures, cuff pressure monitoring (to maintain pressures below 20 mm Hg) is advisable.

Tracheal stenosis is nearly always iatrogenic. It is secondary to either endotracheal intubation or tracheostomy. Collectively, such tracheal injuries are referred to as postintubation injuries. If a

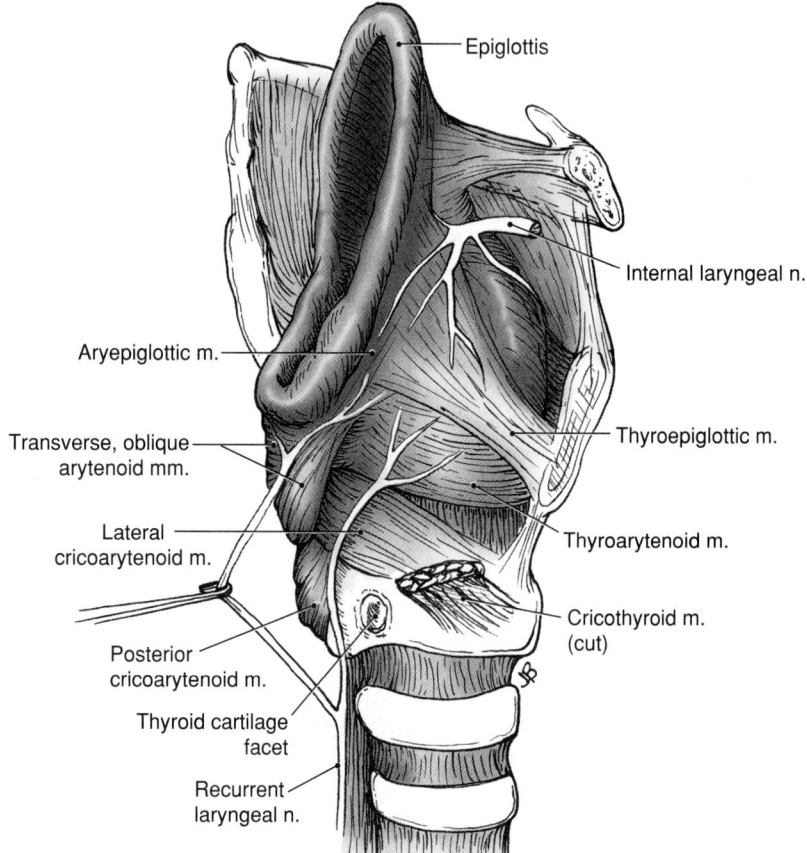

FIG. 18-1. Anatomy of the larynx and upper trachea.

Epiglottis

Internal laryngeal n.

Aryepiglottic m.

Thyroepiglottic m.

Transverse, oblique arytenoid mm.

Lateral cricoarytenoid m.

Thyroarytenoid m.

Cricothyroid m. (cut)

Posterior cricoarytenoid m.

Thyroid cartilage facet

Recurrent laryngeal n.

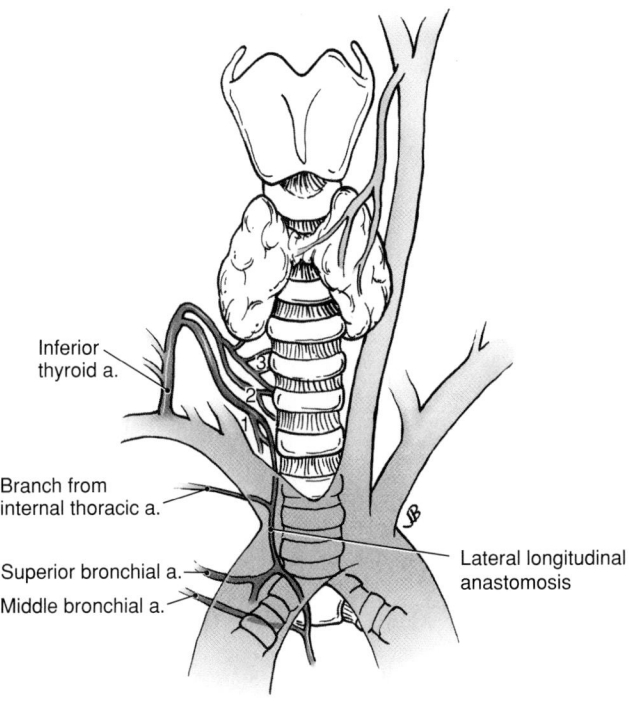

Inferior thyroid a.

Branch from internal thoracic a.

Superior bronchial a.

Middle bronchial a.

Lateral longitudinal anastomosis

FIG. 18-2. Arterial blood supply to the larynx and upper trachea.

tracheostomy is placed inappropriately high, through the first tracheal ring or the cricothyroid membrane where the airway is narrowest, tube-induced injury can lead to scarring and fibrosis. Even a properly placed tracheostomy can lead to tracheal stenosis secondary to scarring and local injury. Mild ulceration and stenosis are frequently seen after tracheostomy removal; however, clinically significant stenoses occur in 3 to 12% of tracheostomies. The larger the tracheostomy tube, the higher the rate of subsequent stenosis. The rate of stomal stenosis can be minimized by using a vertical tracheal incision without removing cartilage, and by using the smallest tracheostomy tube possible.

Clinically, stridor and dyspnea on exertion are the primary symptoms of tracheal stenosis. The length of time to onset of symptoms after extubation or after tracheostomy decannulation varies, usually ranging from 2 to 12 weeks; however, symptoms can appear immediately or as long as 1 to 2 years later. Frequently, patients are misdiagnosed as having asthma or bronchitis, and treatment for such illnesses can persist for some time before the correct diagnosis is discovered. Generally, the intensity of symptoms experienced is related to the degree of stenosis and to the patient's underlying pulmonary disease.

Acute Management

The treatment of tracheal stenosis is resection and primary anastomosis. In nearly all postintubation injuries the injury is transmural, and significant portions of the cartilaginous structural support are destroyed (Fig. 18-3). Measures such as laser ablation are temporizing. In the early phase of evaluating patients, dilatation using a rigid bronchoscope is useful to gain immediate dyspnea relief and to fully assess the lesion as well as its length, position, and relation to the vocal cords. Rarely if ever is a tracheostomy necessary. For patients unable to tolerate general anesthesia because of comorbidities, internal stents, typically silicone T tubes, are useful. Wire mesh stents should not be used, given their known propensity to erode through the wall of the airway.

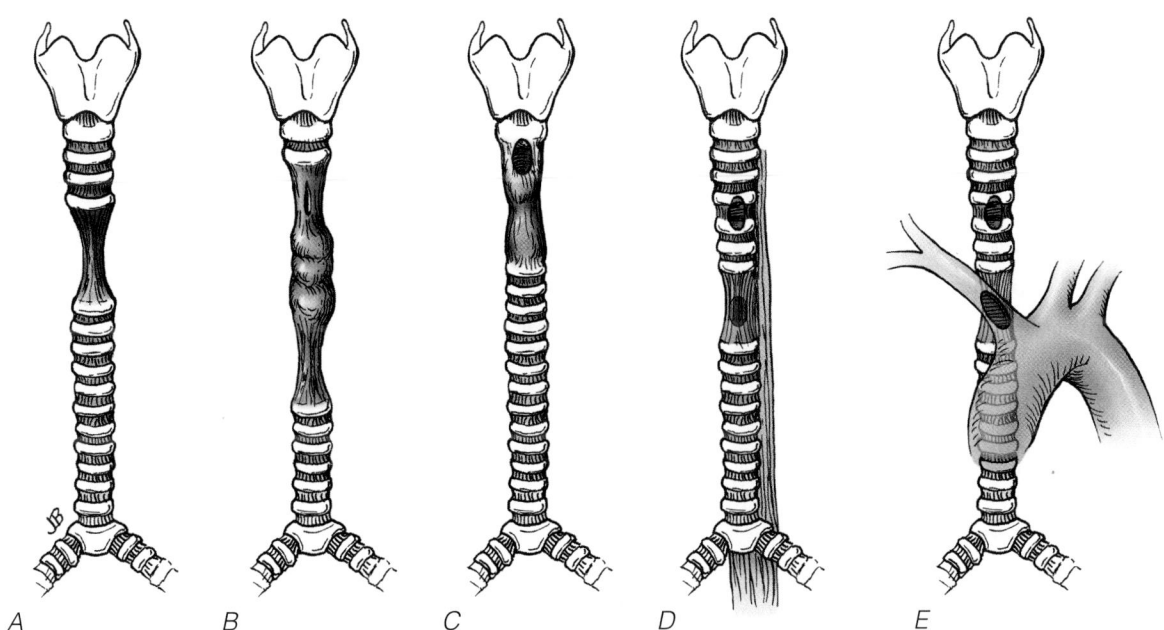

FIG. 18-3. Diagram of the principal postintubation lesions. *A.* A circumferential lesion at the cuff site after the use of an endotracheal tube. *B.* Potential lesions after the use of tracheostomy tubes. Anterolateral stenosis can be seen at the stomal level. Circumferential stenosis can be seen at the cuff level (lower than with an endotracheal tube). The segment in between is often inflamed and malacotic. *C.* Damage to the subglottic larynx. *D.* Tracheoesophageal fistula occurring at the level of the tracheostomy cuff; circumferential damage is usual at this level. *E.* Tracheoinnominate artery fistula. *(Adapted with permission from Grillo H: Surgical treatment of postintubation tracheal injuries. J Thorac Cardiovasc Surg 78:860, 1979.)*

A   B   C   D   E

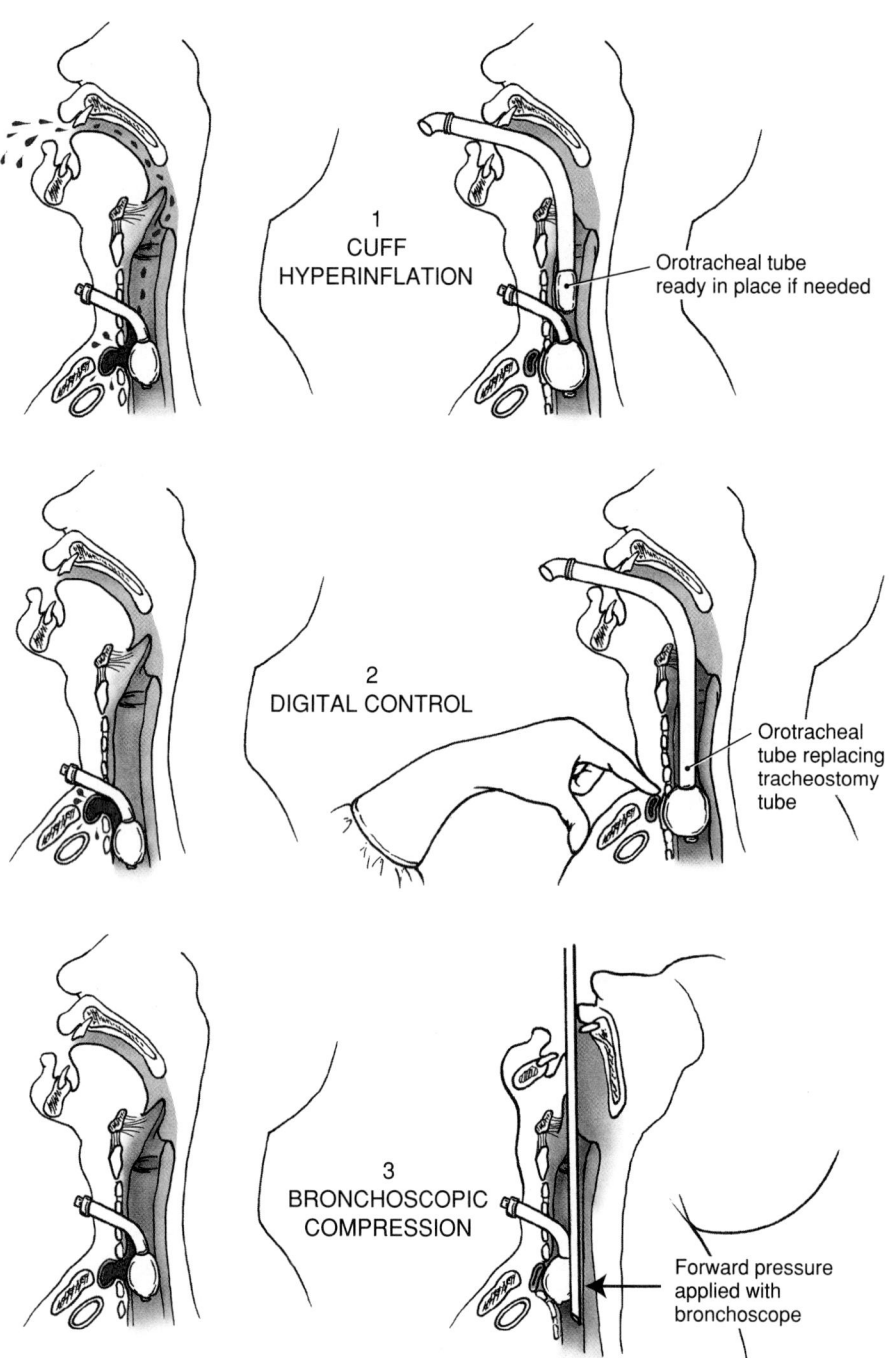

FIG. 18-4. Steps in the emergency management of a tracheoinnominate artery fistula.

Most intubation injuries are located in the upper third of the trachea, so tracheal resection is usually done through a collar incision. Remarkably, even if up to one half of the trachea needs to be resected, a primary anastomosis can still be performed without undue tension, although with benign stenosis removal of only 2 to 4 cm is usually required. In the case of postintubation injury, all inflamed and scarred tissue must be resected; postoperatively no tracheostomy or stent is required and the patient is extubated, often in the operating room.

Tracheal Fistulas

Tracheoinnominate Artery Fistula

Tracheoinnominate artery fistula has two causes. The first is from placing a tracheostomy too low. Tracheostomies should be placed

through the second to fourth tracheal rings without reference to the location of the sternal notch. With too low a placement, the inner curve of the tracheostomy cannula can come to rest and exert pressure on the upper surface of the innominate artery, leading to arterial erosion. The second cause is tracheal cuff injury of the airway, with erosion into the artery and fistula development. Most such fistulas develop within 2 weeks after tracheostomy creation.

Clinically, tracheoinnominate artery fistulas present with bleeding. A premonitory hemorrhage often occurs, and although it is usually not massive, it must not be ignored or simply attributed to general airway irritation or wound bleeding. With significant bleeding, the tracheostomy cuff can be hyperinflated in an effort to occlude the arterial injury. If such an effort is unsuccessful, the tracheostomy incision should be opened widely, and a finger inserted to compress the artery against the manubrium (Fig. 18-4). The patient is then

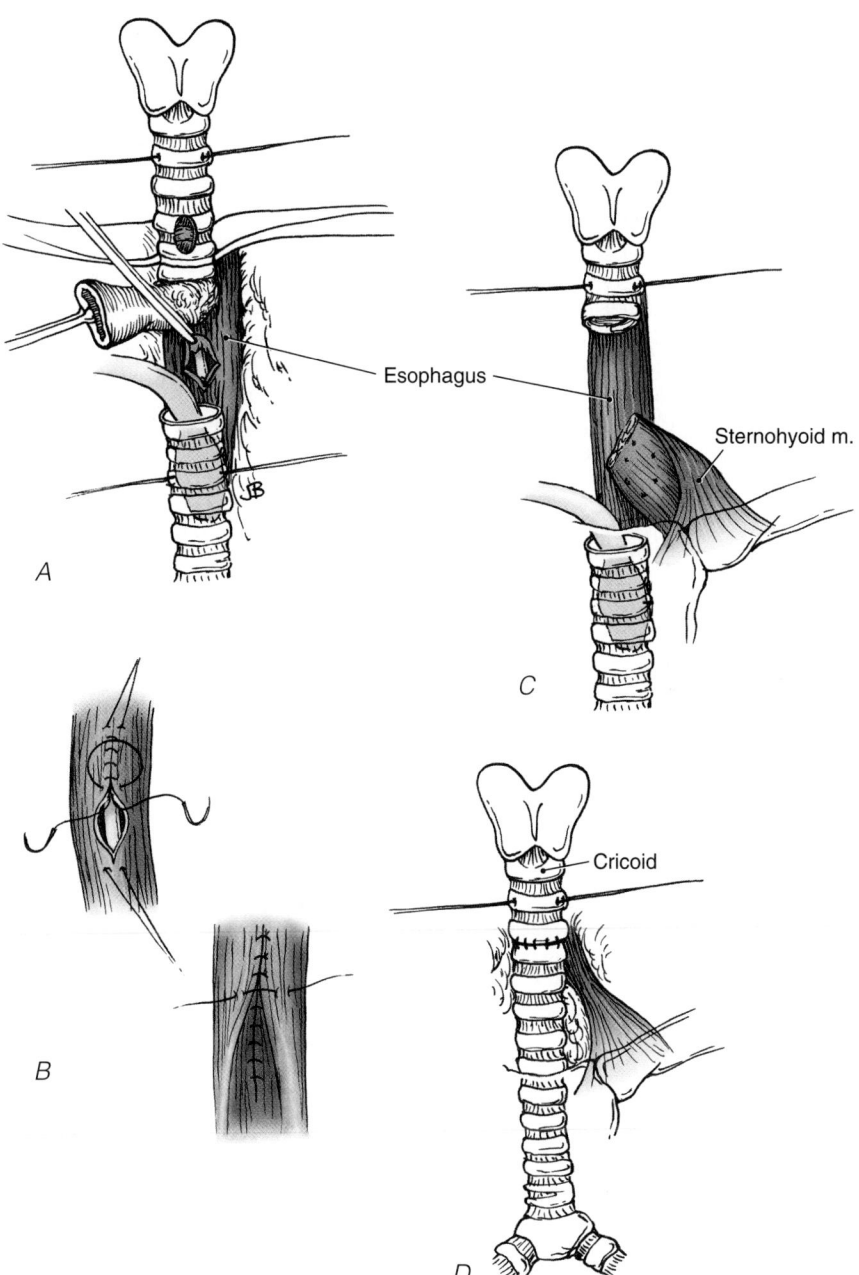

FIG. 18-5. *Single-stage operation for closure of a tracheoesophageal fistula and tracheal resection. A. The fistula is divided and the trachea is transected below the level of damage. B. The fistula is closed on the tracheal side in a single layer and the esophageal side in a double layer. The damaged trachea segment is resected. C. View of completed tracheal anastomosis.*

orally intubated, and suction is instituted. Next, surgical resection of the involved segment of artery is performed, usually without reconstruction.

Tracheoesophageal Fistula

Tracheoesophageal fistulas (TEFs) occur primarily in patients receiving prolonged mechanical ventilatory support concomitant with an indwelling nasogastric tube. Cuff compression of the membranous trachea against the nasogastric tube leads to airway and esophageal injury and fistula development. Clinically, saliva, gastric contents, or tube feeding contents are noted in the material suctioned from the airway. Distention of the stomach secondary to positive pressure ventilation can occur. Diagnosis of a suspected TEF is by bronchoscopy. By withdrawing the endotracheal tube with the bronchoscope inserted, the fistula at the cuff site can be seen. Alternatively, esophagoscopy will enable visualization of the cuff of the endotracheal tube in the esophagus.

First and foremost, treatment of a TEF requires weaning the patient from the ventilator and then extubating as soon as possible. During the weaning period, the nasogastric tube should be removed, ensuring that the cuff of the endotracheal tube is placed below the fistula and that it is not overinflated. Then a gastrostomy should be placed for aspiration (to prevent reflux) and a jejunostomy for feeding. If aspiration is relentless and not managed by the above steps, esophageal diversion with esophagostomy can be performed. Once the patient is weaned from the ventilator, a single-stage operation should be done, consisting of tracheal resection and primary anastomosis, repair of the esophageal defect, and interposition of a muscle flap between the trachea and esophagus (Fig. 18-5).

Tracheal Neoplasms

Primary tracheal tumors are unusual but frequent occurrences. The most common primary tracheal neoplasms are squamous cell carcinomas (related to smoking) and adenoid cystic carcinomas.

Clinically, tracheal tumors present with stridor, hemoptysis, dyspnea, or symptoms of invasion of contiguous structures (such as the recurrent laryngeal nerve or the esophagus). With tumors other than squamous cell carcinomas, symptoms may persist for months because of slow tumor growth rates.

Squamous cell carcinomas often present with regional lymph node metastases and are frequently not resectable at the time of presentation. Their biologic behavior is similar to that of squamous cell carcinomas of the lung. Adenoid cystic carcinomas, which are a type of salivary gland tumor, are generally slow-growing; they spread submucosally and tend to infiltrate along nerve sheaths and along the tracheal wall. Spread to regional lymph nodes can occur. Despite their somewhat indolent nature, adenoid cystic carcinomas are malignant and can spread to the lungs and bones. Other unusual tumors—small cell carcinomas, mucoepidermoid carcinomas, adenocarcinomas, lymphomas, and others—are rare occurrences.

Therapy

Evaluation and treatment of patients with such tumors should include neck and chest computed tomography (CT) and rigid bronchoscopy. Rigid bronchoscopy permits general assessment of the airway and tumor; it also allows débridement or laser ablation of the tumor to provide relief of dyspnea. If the tumor is judged to be completely resectable, primary resection and anastomosis is the treatment of choice for these tumors.

The length limit of tracheal resection is roughly 50% of the trachea. To prevent tension on the anastomosis postoperatively, specialized maneuvers are necessary such as anterolateral tracheal mobilization, suturing of the chin to the sternum with the head flexed forward for 7 days, laryngeal release, and right hilar release. In most tracheal resections (which involve much less than 50% of the airway), anterolateral tracheal mobilization and suturing of the chin to the sternum for 7 days are done routinely. Use of laryngeal and hilar release is determined at the time of surgery, based on the surgeon's judgment of the degree of tension present.

Due to their radiosensitivity, radiotherapy is frequently given postoperatively after resection of both adenoid cystic carcinomas and squamous cell carcinomas. A dose of 50 Gy or greater is usual. For patients with unresectable tumors, radiation may be given as the primary therapy, with an expectation of temporary local control, but is rarely curative. For recurrent airway compromise, stenting or laser therapy also are options.

LUNG

Anatomy

Segmental Anatomy

The segmental anatomy of the lungs and bronchial tree is illustrated in Fig. 18-6. Note the continuity of the pulmonary parenchyma between adjacent segments of each lobe. In contrast, separation of the bronchial and vascular stalks allows subsegmental and segmental resections, if the clinical situation requires it or if lung tissue can be preserved.

Lymphatic Drainage

Many lymphatic vessels are located beneath the visceral pleura of each lung, in the interlobular septa, in the submucosa of the bronchi, and in the perivascular and peribronchial connective tissue. Lymph nodes that drain the lungs are divided into two groups according to the tumor-node-metastasis (TNM) staging system for lung cancer:

RIGHT LUNG AND BRONCHI

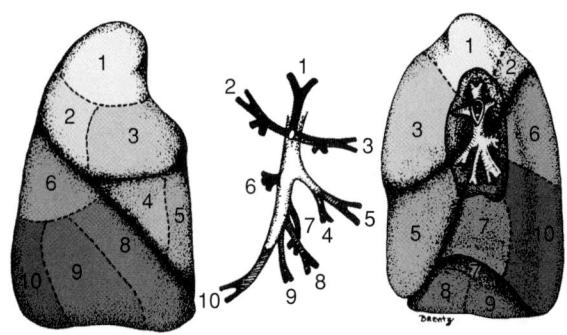

A

SEGMENTS	
1. Apical	6. Superior
2. Posterior	7. Medial Basal *
3. Anterior	8. Anterior Basal
4. Lateral	9. Lateral Basal
5. Medial	10. Posterior Basal

* Medial Basal (7) Not Present in Left Lung

LEFT LUNG AND BRONCHI

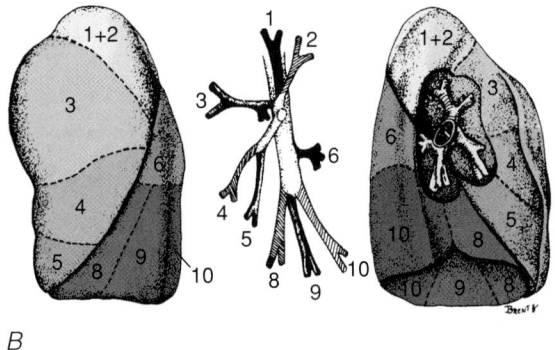

B

FIG. 18-6. The segmental anatomy of the lungs and bronchi.

the pulmonary lymph nodes, N1, and the mediastinal nodes, N2 (Fig. 18-7).

The N1 lymph nodes constitute the following: (1) intrapulmonary or segmental nodes that lie at points of division of segmental bronchi or in the bifurcations of the pulmonary artery, (2) lobar nodes that lie along the upper-, middle-, and lower-lobe bronchi, (3) interlobar nodes that are located in the angles formed by the bifurcation of the main bronchi into the lobar bronchi, and (4) hilar nodes that are located along the main bronchi. The interlobar lymph nodes lie in the depths of the interlobar fissure on each side and constitute a lymphatic sump for each lung, referred to as the *lymphatic sump of Borrie*; all of the pulmonary lobes of the corresponding lung drain into this group of nodes (Fig. 18-8). On the right side, the nodes of the lymphatic sump lie around the bronchus intermedius (bounded above by the right upper lobe bronchus and below by the middle lobe and superior segmental bronchi). On the left side, the lymphatic sump is confined to the interlobar fissure, with the lymph

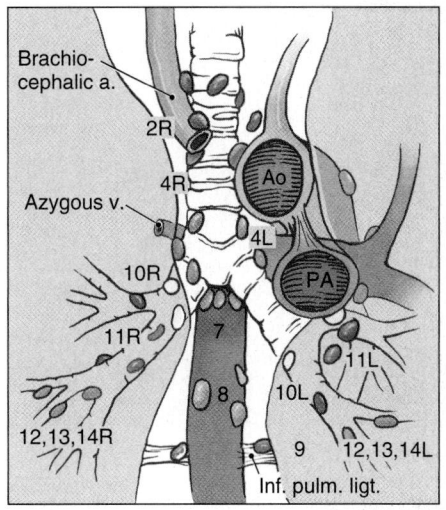
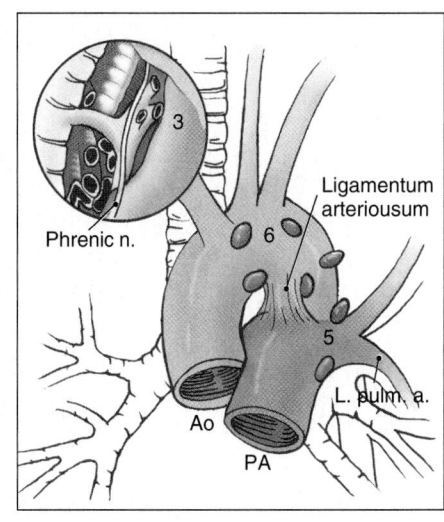

FIG. 18-7. The location of regional lymph node stations for lung cancer staging. *(Reproduced with permission from Mountain CF, Dresler CM: Regional lymph node classification for lung cancer staging. Chest 111:1718, 1997.)*

A   *B*

nodes lying in the angle between the lingular and lower lobe bronchi and in apposition to the pulmonary artery branches.

The N2 lymph nodes consist of four main groups: (1) anterior mediastinal, (2) posterior mediastinal, (3) tracheobronchial, and (4) paratracheal. The anterior mediastinal nodes are located in association with the upper surface of the pericardium, the phrenic nerves, the ligamentum arteriosum, and the left innominate vein. Within the inferior pulmonary ligament on each side are the paraesophageal lymph nodes, which are part of the posterior mediastinal group. Additional paraesophageal nodes can be located more superiorly, between the esophagus and trachea near the arch of the azygos vein. The tracheobronchial lymph nodes are made up of three subgroups that are located near the bifurcation of the trachea: the subcarinal nodes; the lymph nodes that lie in the obtuse angle between the trachea and each main stem bronchus; and nodes that lie anterior to the lower end of the trachea. The paratracheal lymph nodes are located in proximity to the trachea in the superior mediastinum. Those on the right side form a chain with the tracheobronchial nodes inferiorly, and with some of the deep cervical nodes above (scalene lymph nodes). Lymphatic drainage of the right lung is ipsilateral, except for occasional bilateral drainage to the superior mediastinum. Ipsilateral and contralateral drainage from the left lung to the superior mediastinum occur with the same frequency.

Computed Tomography

Spiral (helical) CT allows continuous scanning as the patient is moved through a scanning gantry so that an x-ray beam can trace a helical curve in relation to the patient's position. The entire thorax can be imaged during a solitary breath hold, so motion artifacts are eliminated, resulting in superior image quality (as compared with conventional CT) scanning, particularly in the detection of pulmonary nodules and central airway abnormalities. The shorter acquisition time of spiral CT allows for consistent contrast filling of the great vessels, resulting in markedly improved visualization of pathologic states and anatomic variation contiguous to vascular structures. In addition, three-dimensional spiral CT images can be reconstructed for enhanced visualization of spatial anatomic relationships.

In general, slice thickness is proportional to image resolution. As slice thickness increases, so does the amount of volume averaging, resulting in less resolution. Slice thickness is determined by the structure being imaged as well as by the indication for the study. Thin sections (1 to 2 mm collimation) at 1-cm intervals should be used to evaluate pulmonary parenchyma and peripheral bronchi. If the goal is to find any pulmonary metastases, thin sections at intervals of 5 to 7 mm collimation are recommended. For assessing the trachea and central bronchi, collimation of 3 to 5 mm is recommended. Virtually all institutions have protocols for spiral CT scanning. Providing accurate clinical history and data is of paramount importance to obtaining appropriate imaging. In addition, the astute clinician must be well versed in normal thoracic anatomy to appreciate pathologic changes and management strategies (Fig. 18-9).

Thoracic Surgical Approaches

Thoracic surgical approaches have changed over recent years with advancements in minimally-invasive approaches. A surgeon trained in advanced minimally-invasive techniques can now perform lobectomies and esophagectomies through multiple thoracoscopic/laparoscopic ports without the need for a substantial incision.

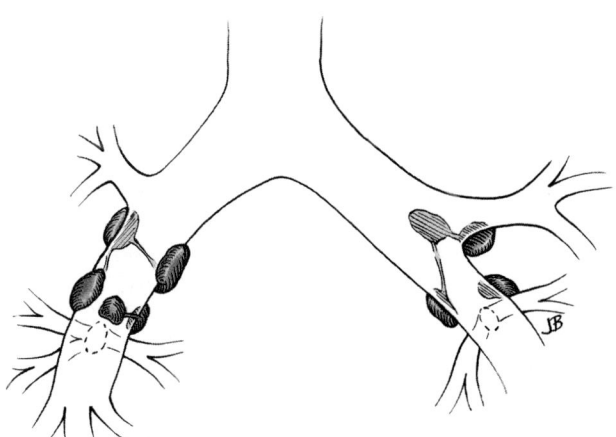

FIG. 18-8. The lymphatic sump of Borrie includes the groups of lymph nodes that receive lymphatic drainage from all pulmonary lobes of the corresponding lung.

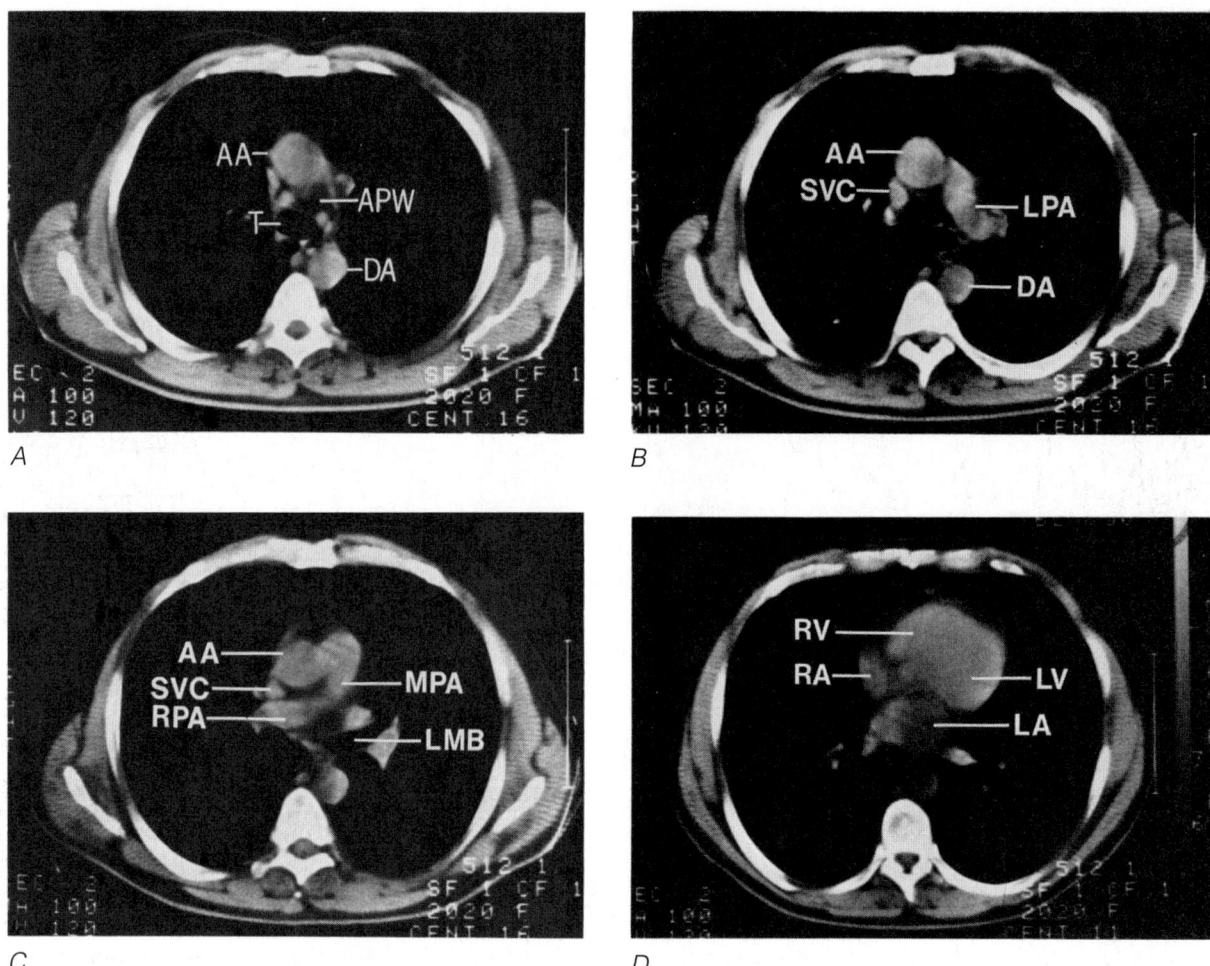

FIG. 18-9. Spiral CT scan showing normal transverse chest anatomy at four levels. *A.* At the level of the tracheal bifurcation, the aorticopulmonary window can be seen. *B.* The origin of the left pulmonary artery can be seen at a level 1 cm inferior to A. *C.* The origin and course of the right pulmonary artery can be seen at this next most cephalad level. The left upper lobe bronchus can be seen at its origin from the left main bronchus. *D.* Cardiac chambers and pulmonary veins are seen in the lower thorax. AA = ascending aorta; APW = aorticopulmonary window; DA = descending aorta; LA = left ventricle; LMB = left main bronchus; LPA = left pulmonary artery; MPA = main pulmonary artery; RA = right atrium; RPA = right pulmonary artery; RV = right ventricle; SVC = superior vena cava; T = trachea.

There has not been a documented change in mortality using these approaches; however, overall patients feel better and resume their activities of daily living sooner.

Mediastinoscopy is generally used for diagnostic assessment of mediastinal lymphadenopathy and staging of lung cancer. Mediastinoscopy is performed via a transverse 2- to 3-cm incision approximately 1 cm above the suprasternal notch. The incision is carried through the platysma. The midline of the strap muscles is identified and dissected laterally. Care is taken to avoid any venous structures that may overlie these muscles, which are highly variable in size and position. The pretracheal fascia is incised. Blunt dissection along the anterior trachea is performed to the level of the carina with careful note of the position of the innominate artery. The innominate artery can be located close to the suprasternal notch, particularly in women; therefore blind use of electrocautery is to be avoided. The mediastinoscope is inserted, and anatomic definition of the trachea, carina, and lateral aspect of both proximal bronchi is achieved with blunt dissection using a long suction catheter. Long biopsy forceps

can be inserted through the scope for sampling. The standard staging procedure for lung cancer includes biopsies of the paratracheal (stations 4R and 4L) and subcarinal lymph nodes (station 7).

A modified Chamberlain procedure can be used for evaluation of aortopulmonary window lymph nodes. A 4- to 5-cm incision is made over the left second costal cartilage, which on occasion is excised. The internal mammary vessels can be ligated or preserved. The dissection proceeds into the mediastinum along the aortic arch. Biopsy of the aortopulmonary window lymph nodes can then be performed. This approach also is used frequently to biopsy anterior mediastinal lymphomas, which are usually located just beneath the second and third costal cartilages. This procedure is less frequently performed with improved techniques of CT-guided biopsy and positron emission tomography (PET) scanning.

The most frequently used incision for an open procedure in thoracic surgery is the posterolateral thoracotomy. The posterolateral thoracotomy incision can be used for most pulmonary resections, esophageal operations, and for the approach to the posterior

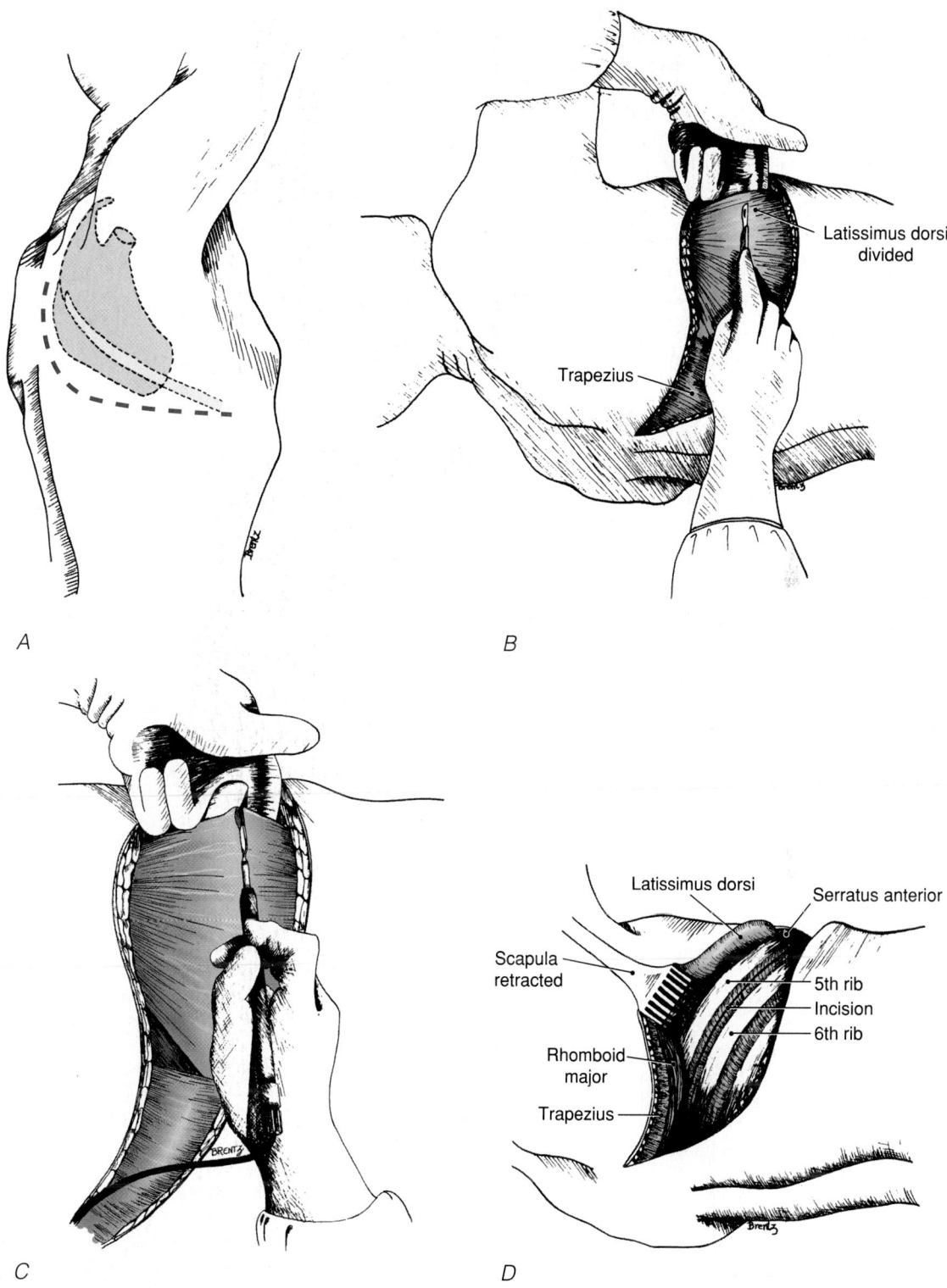

A

B

C

D

Latissimus dorsi
divided

Trapezius

Latissimus dorsi

Serratus anterior

Scapula
retracted

5th rib
Incision
6th rib

Rhomboid
major

Trapezius

FIG. 18-10. The posterolateral thoracotomy incision. *A.* Skin incision from the anterior axillary line to the lower extent of the scapula tip. *B* and *C.* Division of the latissimus dorsi and shoulder-girdle musculature. *D.* The pleural cavity is entered after dividing the intercostal muscles along the lower margin of the interspace, taking care not to injure the neurovascular bundle lying below each rib.

mediastinum and vertebral column (Fig. 18-10). The skin incision typically starts at the anterior axillary line just below the nipple level and extends posteriorly below the tip of the scapula. The incision then proceeds in a cranial direction halfway between the vertebral border of the scapula and the spinous processes of the vertebrae. The latissimus dorsi is divided and the serratus anterior is retracted. Typically at the fifth interspace the intercostal muscles are divided using electrocautery above the sixth rib, and the pleural space is entered after confirming that the anesthesiologist has excluded ventilation to the operative lung by clamping the proper lumen of a double-lumen endotracheal tube. A rib spreader is placed into the thoracic cavity and minimally opened. Cautery can then be used to perform an internal thoracotomy by continuing the division of the intercostal muscles more anteriorly (up to the level of the internal mammary artery) and posteriorly (up to the level of the paraspinous tendons). The internal thoracotomy will prevent rib fracture during subsequent spreading of the retractor. Injury to a rib can lead to increased postoperative pain and prolong restricted motion of the rib cage. It is recommended to resect any broken edges of a rib fracture should it occur.

The anterolateral thoracotomy has traditionally been used in trauma victims. This approach allows quick entry into the chest with the patient supine. In the face of hemodynamic instability, this approach is better than the lateral decubitus position, and gives the anesthesiologist control over the patient's cardiopulmonary system and resuscitation efforts. The incision is submammary, beginning at the sternal border overlying the fourth intercostal space and extending to the midaxillary line. The pectoralis major muscle and some of the pectoralis minor are divided, and the incision is carried through the serratus anterior. The intercostal muscles are divided with cautery over the top of the subjacent rib. Should more exposure be necessary, the sternum can be transected and the incision carried to the contralateral thoracic cavity ("clamshell" thoracotomy). A bilateral anterior thoracotomy incision with transection of the sternum ("clamshell" thoracotomy) is a standard operative approach to the heart and mediastinum in certain elective circumstances. It is the preferred incision for double-lung transplantation. A median sternotomy also can be added to an anterior thoracotomy ("trap-door" thoracotomy) for access to mediastinal structures. A hypesthetic nipple is a frequent complication of this approach.

A pitfall of thoracic incisions in a lateral decubitus position is potential for injury to the brachial plexus and axillary vascular structures secondary to displacement of the shoulder. Therefore careful attention must be paid to positioning the patient on the operating table after anesthesia has been induced.

The median sternotomy incision allows exposure of anterior mediastinal structures and is principally used for cardiac operations. Either pleural cavity may be entered, or incision into the pleural cavity may be avoided if it is unnecessary. Disadvantages of the incision include an increased risk of infection if a tracheostomy is needed concomitantly or before the sternotomy is completely healed. The skin incision extends from the suprasternal notch to the xiphoid process (Fig. 18-11). A saw is used to split the sternum. A sternotomy is associated with less pain and less compromise of pulmonary function than a lateral thoracotomy.

Video-Assisted Thoracoscopic Surgery

Video-assisted thoracoscopic surgery (VATS) has become an accepted approach to diagnosis and treatment of pleural effusions, recurrent pneumothoraces, lung biopsies, lobectomy, resection of bronchogenic and mediastinal cysts, esophageal myotomy, and intrathoracic esophageal mobilization for esophagectomy. VATS is performed via two to four incisions measuring 0.5 to 1.2 cm in length to allow insertion of the thoracoscope and instruments. The incision location varies according to the procedure. With respect to VATS lobectomy, port placement varies according to the lobe being resected and is highly variable among surgeons. The basic principle is to position the ports high enough on the thoracic cage to have

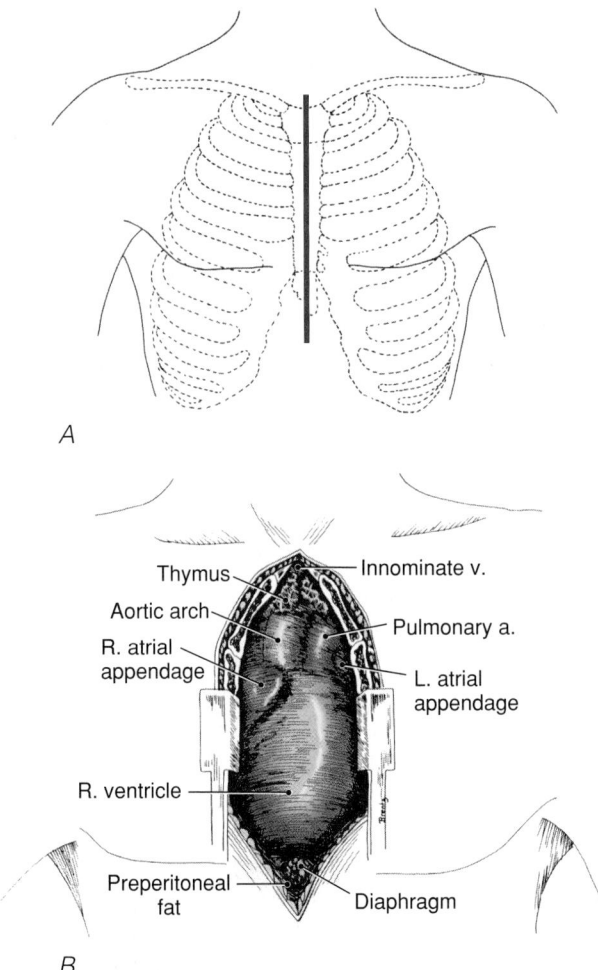

A

B

FIG. 18-11. *The median sternotomy incision. A. Skin incision from the suprasternal notch to the xiphoid process. B. Exposure of the pleural space.*

access to the hilar structures. Endoscopic staplers are used to divide the major vascular structures and bronchus.

At the conclusion of a thoracic operation, the pleural cavity typically is drained with a chest tube(s). Each chest tube is brought out through a separate stab incision in the chest wall below the level of the thoracotomy, or through a VATS port site. If the pleura has not been violated and no drainage is expected (i.e., after VATS sympathectomies), no chest tube is necessary. The lung is then ventilated and placed under positive pressure ventilation to assist with reexpansion of atelectatic segments. Thoracic incisions should be closed in layers: the costal space with three to four interrupted sutures, two running sutured musculofascial layers, and a running subcuticular suture for the skin (though staples also are utilized by some).

Postoperative Care

Chest Tube Management

At the conclusion of all operations involving resection or manipulation of lung tissue, chest tubes are routinely placed into the pleural space. Pleural tubes are left for two reasons: to drain fluid, thereby preventing pleural fluid accumulation, and to evacuate air if an air leak is present. The tube is removed when the volume of drainage decreases and when no air leak is present.

The ideal volume of drainage over a 24-hour period that predicts safe chest tube removal is unknown. The ability of the pleural lymphatics to absorb fluid is substantial. It can be as high as 0.40 mL/kg per hour in a healthy individual, possibly resulting in the absorption of up to 500 mL of fluid over a 24-hour period. The capacity of the pleural space to manage and absorb fluid is high if the pleural lining and lymphatics are healthy.

A drainage volume of 150 mL or less over 24 hours has been thought necessary in order to safely remove a chest tube. Recently, it has been shown that pleural tubes can be removed after VATS lobectomy with 24-hour drainage volumes as high as 400 mL, without subsequent development of pleural effusions. Currently, it is the practice of these authors to remove chest tubes with 24-hour outputs of 400 mL or less after lobectomy or lesser pulmonary resections.

If the pleural space is altered (e.g., malignant pleural effusion, pleural space infections or inflammation, and pleurodesis), strict adherence to a volume requirement before tube removal is appropriate (typically 100 to 150 mL over 24 hours). Such circumstances alter normal pleural fluid dynamics.

The use of suction and the management of air leaks vary. Suction levels of 20 cm H_2O have been routinely used after pulmonary surgery in an effort to eradicate residual air spaces and to control postoperative parenchymal air leaks. Recently it has been shown that the routine use of a water seal (with the patient off suction) actually promotes more rapid healing of parenchymal air leaks. The main guidelines for the use of a water seal are the degree of air leakage and the degree of expansion of the remaining lung. If the leak is significant enough to induce atelectasis or collapse during use of a water seal (off suction), suction should be used to achieve lung reexpansion.

It is important to remember the process of assessing an air leak. The chest tube and its attached tubing should be examined and the lack of kinks or external mechanical obstruction (e.g., patient lying on the tube) verified. The patient is asked to voluntarily cough. During the cough, the water seal chamber is observed. If bubbles pass through the water seal chamber, an air leak is presumed. Occasionally, if the chest tube is not secured snugly at the skin surface, air can entrain around the tube into the patient with respiration; thus an air leak will be present, although not emanating from the lung itself. During the voluntary cough, the fluid level in the water seal chamber should move up and down with the cough and with deep respiration, reflecting the pleural pressure changes occurring with these maneuvers. A stationary fluid level implies a mechanical blockage, either due to external tube compression or to a clot or debris within the tube.

Pain Control

Good pain control after posterolateral thoracotomy is critical. It permits the patient to actively participate in breathing maneuvers designed to clear and manage secretions, and promotes ambulation and a feeling of well being. The two most common techniques of pain management are epidural and intravenous. To maximize efficacy, epidural catheters should be inserted at about the T6 level, roughly at the level of the scapular tip. Lower placement risks inadequate pain control, and higher placement may provoke hand and arm numbness. Typically, combinations of fentanyl at 0.3 μg/mL, combined with either bupivacaine (0.125%) or ropivacaine (0.1%) are used. Ropivacaine has less cardiotoxicity than bupivacaine; thus in the case of inadvertent intravenous injection, the potential for refractory complete heart block that is seen with bupivacaine is significantly less.

When properly placed, a well-managed epidural can provide outstanding pain control without significant systemic sedation. Urinary retention is a frequent side effect, particularly in males who require an indwelling urinary catheter. In addition, the use of local anesthetics may cause sympathetic outflow blockade, leading to vasodilation and hypotension often requiring intravenous vasoconstrictors (an alpha agonist such as phenylephrine) and/or fluid administration. In such circumstances, fluid administration for hypotension may be undesirable in pulmonary surgery patients, particularly after pneumonectomy.

Alternatively, intravenous narcotics via patient-controlled analgesia can be used, often in conjunction with ketorolac. Titration of basal and intermittent dosing is often necessary to balance the degree of pain relief with the degree of sedation. Oversedated, narcotized patients are as ominous as patients without adequate pain control, because of the significant risk of secretion retention and development of atelectasis or pneumonia. Proper pain control with intravenous narcotics is a balance of pain relief and sedation. An alternative to epidural is the intercostal nerve catheter. A recent randomized trial demonstrated that a catheter placed along the intercostal nerves yielded equivalent pain control to epidural catheter in a postthoracotomy study.

Whether on epidural or intravenous pain control, the patient is typically transitioned to oral pain medication on the third or fourth postoperative day. During both the parenteral and oral phase of pain management, a standardized regimen of stool softeners and laxatives is advisable in order to prevent severe constipation.

Respiratory Care

Good respiratory care is the result of a commitment by the surgeon and by all other health care professionals involved. The team should be educated about the techniques of good respiratory care. The best respiratory care is achieved when the patient is able to deliver an effective cough to clear secretions. The process ideally begins preoperatively, with clear instructions on using pillows (or other support techniques) over the wound and then applying pressure. Postoperatively, proper pain control (as outlined above) is essential, without oversedation. Multiple studies have shown that a variety of adjunctive respiratory care techniques (e.g., intermittent positive pressure breathing and incentive spirometry) may not be of benefit. Those findings are consistent with the impression of these authors that routine respiratory care is best accomplished by a dedicated team and educated patients.

In patients whose pulmonary function preoperatively is significantly impaired, generating an effective cough postoperatively may be nearly impossible. In this setting, routine nasotracheal suctioning can be employed, but is uncomfortable for the patient. A better alternative is placement at the time of surgery of a percutaneous transtracheal suction catheter. This catheter is comfortable for the patient and allows regular and convenient suctioning.

Postoperative Complications

Postpneumonectomy pulmonary edema occurs in 1 to 5% of patients undergoing pneumonectomy, with a higher incidence after right pneumonectomy. Clinically, symptoms of respiratory distress manifest hours to days after surgery. Radiographically, diffuse interstitial infiltration or frank alveolar edema is seen. The pathophysiologic causes remain poorly understood, but are related to factors that increase permeability and filtration pressure, and that decrease lymphatic drainage from the affected lung. The syndrome reportedly has a nearly 100% mortality rate despite aggressive therapy. Treatment consists of ventilatory support, fluid restriction, and diuretics.

Postoperative air leak and bronchopleural fistula are two different problems, but distinguishing the two may be difficult. Postoperative air leaks are common after pulmonary resection. They occur more often and last longer in patients with emphysematous changes because the fibrotic changes and destroyed blood supply impairs healing of surface injuries. Prolonged air leaks—those lasting over 7 days—may be treated by diminishing or discontinuing suction (if used), by continuing chest drainage, or by instilling a pleurodesis agent, usually talcum powder.

If the leak is moderate to large and if a bronchopleural fistula from the resected bronchial stump is possible, flexible bronchoscopy is performed. Management options include continued prolonged chest tube drainage; reoperation and reclosure (with stump reinforcement with intercostals or a serratus muscle pedicle flap); or, for fistulas less than 4 mm, bronchoscopic fibrin glue application. Patients often have concomitant empyemas and open drainage may be necessary.

Solitary Pulmonary Nodule

A solitary pulmonary nodule or "coin lesion" is typically recognized as a single, well-circumscribed, spherical lesion. It is less than 3 cm in diameter and is completely surrounded by normal lung parenchyma. In large screening studies, a solitary pulmonary nodule was identified on 0.09 to 0.2% of all chest radiographs. About 150,000 solitary nodules are found incidentally each year. The clinical significance of such a lesion depends on whether or not it represents a malignancy.

Differential Diagnosis

Ideally, diagnostic approaches to a pulmonary nodule would allow for definitive surgical resection when it is malignant and avoid resection when it is not. In nonselected patient populations, a new solitary pulmonary nodule observed on a chest radiograph has a 20 to 40% likelihood of being malignant, with the risk approximating 50% or higher for smokers. The remaining causes of pulmonary nodules are numerous benign conditions. Infectious granulomas arising from a variety of organisms account for 70 to 80% of this type of solitary nodule; hamartomas are the next most common single cause, accounting for about 10%. The differential diagnosis of a solitary pulmonary nodule should include a broad variety of congenital, neoplastic, inflammatory, vascular, and traumatic disorders. No evidence-based guidelines are available that completely address the ideal approach to patients presenting with a solitary pulmonary nodule. The initial assessment of a pulmonary nodule should proceed from a clinical history and physical examination. Risk factors for malignancy include a history of smoking, prior neoplastic disease, hemoptysis, and age over 35 years.

Imaging

Chest thin-section CT scan is critical in characterizing nodule location, size, margin morphology, calcification pattern, and growth rate. The increased sensitivity of CT (as compared with radiography) for small nodules often reveals more than a single pulmonary nodule; up to 50% of patients thought to have a single lesion per chest x-ray were proven to harbor multiple nodules by CT. Beyond a certain number, multiple nodules more likely represent metastases or granulomatous disease, thereby altering work-up. Lesions larger than 3 cm are regarded as masses and are more likely malignant. Irregular, lobulated, or spiculated edges strongly suggest malignancy.

The corona radiata sign (consisting of fine linear strands extending 4 to 5 mm outward and appearing spiculated on radiographs) is highly cancer-specific (Fig. 18-12).

Calcification within a nodule suggests a benign lesion. Four patterns of benign calcification are common: diffuse, solid, central, and laminated or "popcorn." Granulomatous infections such as tuberculosis can demonstrate the first three patterns, whereas the popcorn pattern is most common in hamartomas.

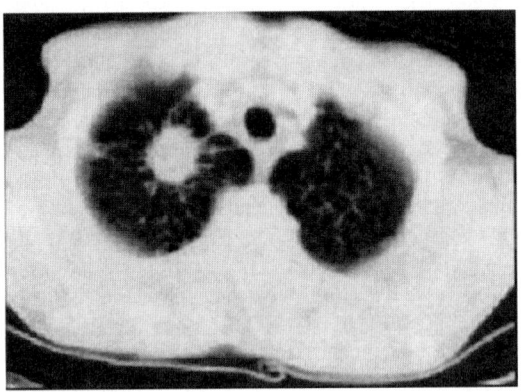

A

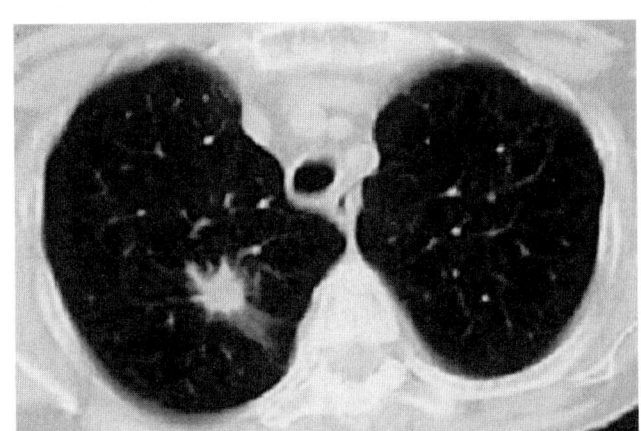

B

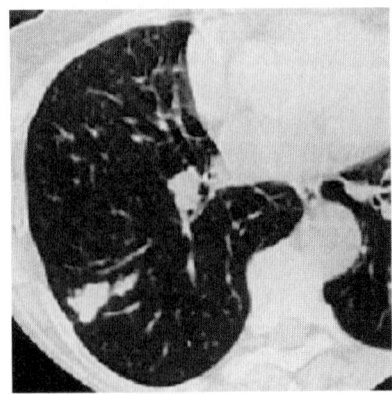

C

FIG. 18-12. CT scan images of solitary pulmonary nodules. *A.* The corona radiata sign demonstrated by a solitary nodule. Multiple fine striations extend perpendicularly from the surface of the nodule like the spokes of a wheel. *B.* A biopsy-proven adenocarcinoma demonstrating spiculation. *C.* A lesion with a scalloped border, an indeterminate finding suggesting an intermediate probability for malignancy.

Calcification that is stippled, amorphous, or eccentric is usually associated with cancer. Characteristically neoplasms grow, and several studies have confirmed that lung cancers have volume-doubling times from 20 to 400 days. Lesions with shorter doubling times are likely due to infection, as longer doubling times suggest benign tumors. Traditionally, 2-year size stability per chest radiography has been considered a sign of a benign tumor. This long-held notion has been challenged by recent investigations, which demonstrated only a 65% positive predictive value for chest radiographs. Thus size stability of a pulmonary mass on chest films is a relatively unreliable benign indicator that must be interpreted with caution.

PET scanning takes advantage of another biologic property of neoplasms: increased glucose uptake commensurate with increased metabolic activity. ^{18}F-fluorodeoxyglucose (FDG) is used to measure glucose metabolism in cells imaged by PET. Most lung tumors have increased signatures of glucose uptake, as compared with healthy tissues. PET is becoming widely used to help differentiate benign from malignant nodules. One meta-analysis estimated its sensitivity for identifying neoplasms as 97% and its specificity as 78%. False-negative results can occur (especially in patients who have bronchoalveolar carcinomas, carcinoids, and tumors less than 1 cm in diameter), as well as false-positive results (because of confusion with other infectious or inflammatory processes).

Biopsy versus Resection

Only a biopsy can definitively diagnose a pulmonary nodule. Bronchoscopy has a 20 to 80% sensitivity for detecting a neoplastic process within a solitary pulmonary nodule, depending on the nodule size, its proximity to the bronchial tree, and the prevalence of cancer in the population being sampled. Transthoracic fine-needle aspiration (FNA) biopsy can accurately identify the status of peripheral pulmonary lesions in up to 95% of patients; the false-negative rate ranges from 3 to 29%. Complications may occur at a relatively high rate (e.g., a 30% rate of pneumothorax). VATS is often used for excising and diagnosing indeterminate pulmonary nodules. Lesions most suitable for VATS are those that are located in the outer one-third of the lung and those that are less than 3 cm in diameter. Certain principles must be followed when excising potentially malignant lesions via VATS. The nodule must not be directly manipulated with instruments, the visceral pleura overlying the nodule must not be violated, and the excised nodule must be extracted from the chest within a bag to prevent seeding of the chest wall. Some groups advocate proceeding directly to VATS in the work-up of a solitary pulmonary nodule in appropriate clinical circumstances, citing superior diagnostic accuracy and low surgical risks.

Lung Neoplasms

Lung cancer is the leading cancer killer in the United States. Every year, it accounts for 30% of all cancer deaths—more than cancers of the breast, prostate, and ovary combined. It is the third most frequently diagnosed cancer in the United States, behind prostate cancer in men and breast cancer in women (Fig. 18-13).

Most patients are diagnosed at an advanced stage of disease, so therapy is rarely curative. The overall 5-year survival for all patients with lung cancer is 15%, making lung cancer the most lethal of the leading four cancers (Fig. 18-14). Survival of lung cancer varies according to several demographic and social factors. Positive survival factors are female sex (5-year survival of 18.3% for women versus 13.8% for men), younger age (5-year survival of 22.8% for those less than 45 years versus 13.7% for those over 65 years), and white race (5-year survival of 16.1% for whites versus 12.2% for blacks). The racial difference may be partially explained by less access to advanced medical care and later diagnosis.

Epidemiology

Cigarette smoking is the primary cause of lung cancer. Two lung cancer cell types, squamous cell carcinoma and small cell

2003 ESTIMATED U.S. CANCER DEATHS *

MEN
285,900

WOMEN
270,600

Lung & bronchus	31%	25%	Lung & bronchus
Prostate	10%	15%	Breast
Colon & rectum	10%	11%	Colon & rectum
Pancreas	5%	6%	Pancreas
Non-Hodgkin's lymphoma	4%	5%	Ovary
Leukemia	4%	4%	Non-Hodgkin's lymphoma
Esophagus	4%	4%	Leukemia
Liver/intrahepatic bile duct	3%	3%	Uterine corpus
Urinary bladder	3%	2%	Brain/other nervous system
Kidney	3%	2%	Multiple myeloma
All other sites	22%	23%	All other sites

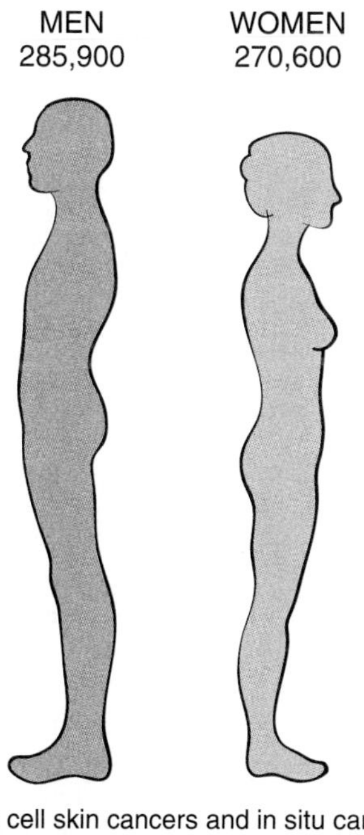

* Excludes basal and squamous cell skin cancers and in situ carcinomas except urinary bladder.
Source: American Cancer Society, 2003.

FIG. 18-13. Recent cancer statistics for the United States.

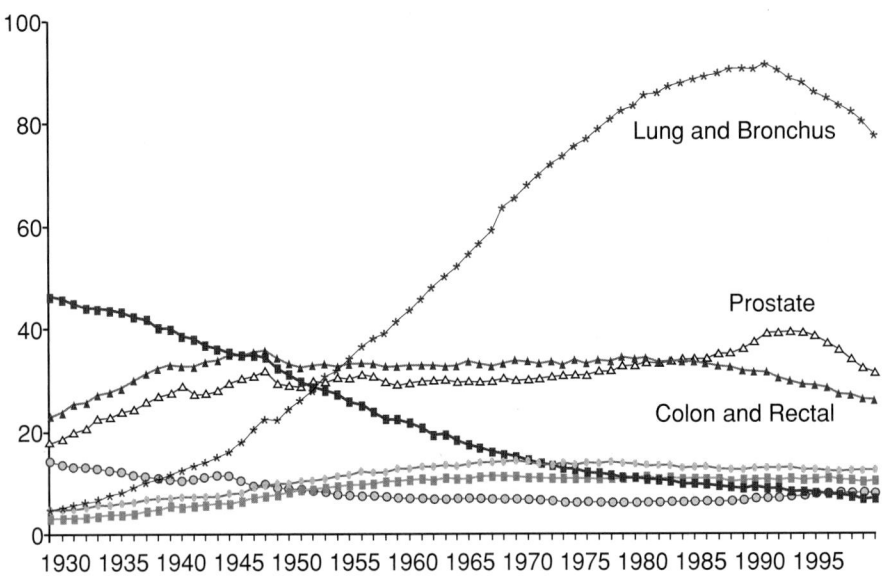

FIG. 18-14. Age-adjusted cancer-related mortality rates in men. (*Adapted with permission from U.S. Mortality Public Use Data Tapes, 1960 to 1999; U.S. Mortality Volumes 1930 to 1959; National Center for Health Statistics; and Centers for Disease Control and Prevention.*)

carcinoma, are extraordinarily rare in the absence of cigarette smoking. The risk of developing lung cancer escalates with the number of cigarettes smoked, the number of years smoked, and the use of unfiltered cigarettes. Conversely, the risk of lung cancer declines with smoking cessation (Table 18-1). However, even after smoking cessation, the risk never drops to that of people who never smoked, regardless of the length of abstinence. Only 15% of lung cancers are not related to smoking, and the majority of these are adenocarcinomas.

Secondhand (or passive) smoke exposure has been shown to confer an excess risk of 24% of developing lung cancer when a nonsmoker lives with a smoker. Preexisting lung disease confers an increased risk of lung cancer—up to 13%—for individuals who have never smoked. This increase is thought to be related to poor clearance of inhaled carcinogens and/or to the effects of chronic inflammation.

Other causes of lung cancer include exposure to a number of industrial compounds, including asbestos, arsenic, and chromium compounds. Of particular note is the ominous combination of asbestos exposure and cigarette smoking, which together have a multiplicative effect on risk, as opposed to an additive effect. Patients with chronic obstructive pulmonary disease (COPD) are at higher risk for lung cancer than would be predicted based on smoking risk alone. A previous history of tuberculosis with

secondary scar formation also leads to a higher risk of primary lung carcinoma.

Over 3000 chemicals have been identified in tobacco smoke, but the main chemical carcinogens are polycyclic aromatic hydrocarbons. Once inhaled and absorbed, these compounds become mutagenic through their activation by specific enzymes, binding to macromolecules such as deoxyribonucleic acid (DNA), and then induction of mutations.

In treating any patient with a previous smoking history, it is important to remember that field cancerization of the entire aerodigestive tract has likely occurred. The patient's risk is increased for cancers of the oral cavity, pharynx, larynx, tracheobronchial tree and lung, and esophagus. In examining such patients, a detailed history and physical examination of these organ systems must be performed.

Normal Lung Histology

The lung can be conveniently viewed as two linked components: the tracheobronchial tree (or conducting airways component) and the alveolar spaces (or gas exchange component). The tracheobronchial tree consists of approximately 23 airway divisions to the level of the alveoli. It includes the main bronchi, lobar bronchi, segmental bronchi (to designated bronchopulmonary segments), and terminal bronchioles (i.e., the smallest airway vessels that lack alveoli and are lined by bronchial epithelium). The tracheobronchial tree is normally lined by pseudostratified ciliated columnar cells and mucous (or goblet) cells, which both derive from basal cells (Fig. 18-15). Ciliated cells predominate. Goblet cells, which release mucus, can significantly increase in number in acute bronchial injury, such as exposure to cigarette smoke. The normal bronchial epithelium also contains bronchial submucosal glands, which are mixed salivary-type glands containing mucous cells, serous cells, and Kulchitsky cells. Kulchitsky cells are neuroendocrine cells; they are also found within the surface epithelium (see Fig. 18-15). The bronchial submucosal glands can give rise to salivary gland–type tumors (previously referred to as "bronchial gland tumors"), including mucoepidermoid carcinomas and adenoid cystic carcinomas.

Table 18-1
Relative Risk of Lung Cancer in Smokers

Smoking Category	Relative Risk
Never smokers	1.0
Current smokers	15.8–16.3
Former smokers	
Years of abstinence:	
1–9	5.9–19.5
10–19	2.0–6.1
>20	1.9–3.7

SOURCE: Adapted from Samet JM: Health benefits of smoking cessation. *Clin Chest Med* 12:673, 1991.

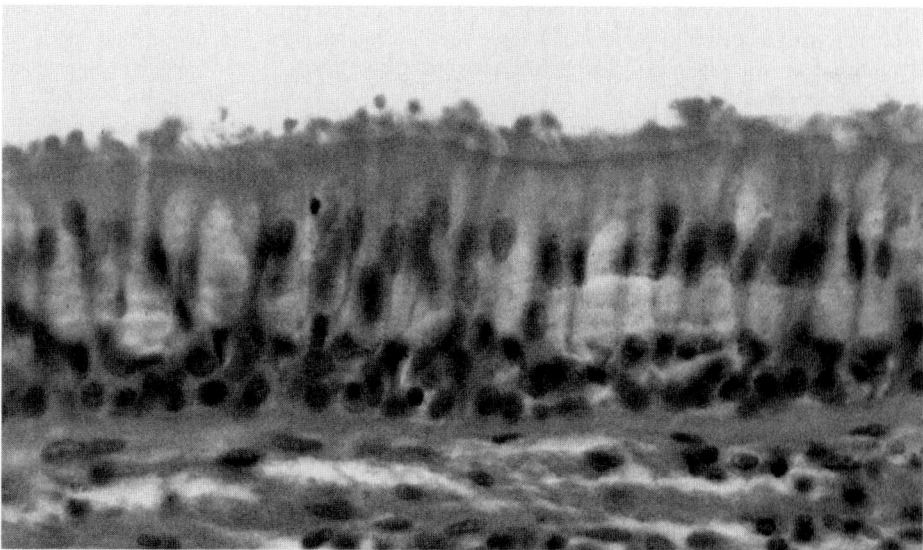

A

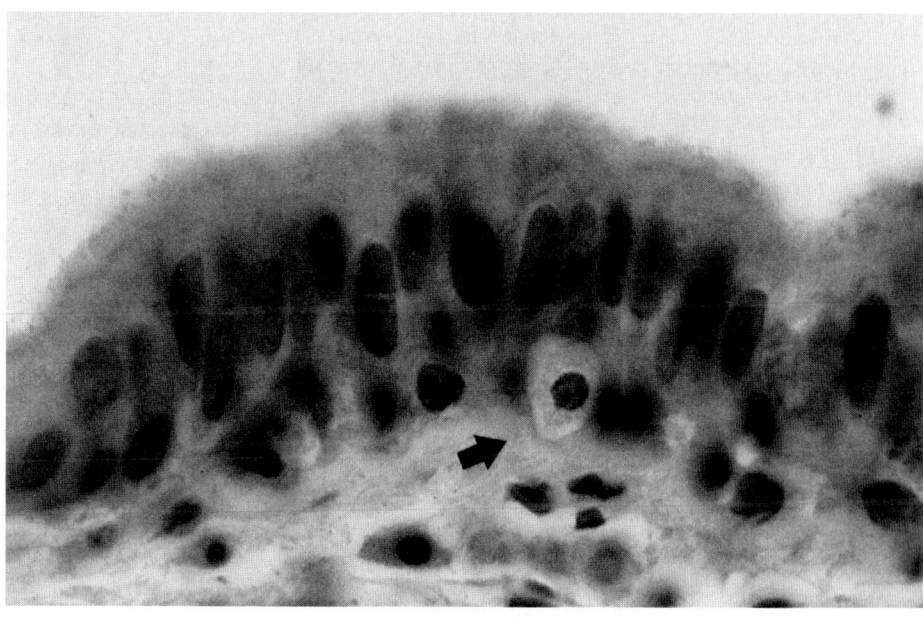

B

FIG. 18-15. Normal lung histology. *A*. Pseudostratified ciliated columnar cells and mucous cells normally line the tracheobronchial tree. *B*. A Kulchitsky cell is depicted (*arrow*).

The alveolar spaces or alveoli have two primary cell types, referred to as type I and II pneumocytes. Type I pneumocytes cover 95% of the surface area of the alveolar wall, but comprise only 40% of the total number of alveolar epithelial cells. These cells are not capable of regeneration because they have no mitotic potential. Type II pneumocytes cover only 3% of the alveolar surface, but comprise 60% of the alveolar epithelial cells. In addition, clusters of neuroendocrine cells are seen in the alveolar spaces.

Preinvasive Lesions

As with epithelial tumors of other organs, precancerous changes can be seen in the respiratory tract. Three precancerous lesions are currently recognized: squamous dysplasia and carcinoma in situ, atypical adenomatous hyperplasia (AAH), and diffuse idiopathic pulmonary neuroendocrine cell hyperplasia (DIPNECH). The term "precancerous" does not mean that an inevitable progression to invasive carcinoma will occur, but such lesions do constitute a clear marker of the potential for later development of invasive cancer.

Squamous Dysplasia and Carcinoma In Situ. Cigarette smoke can induce a metaplastic change of the tracheobronchial pseudostratified epithelium to squamous mucosa, which is a normal response to injury. With the development of cellular abnormalities in the metaplastic squamous mucosa, squamous dysplasia evolves. It involves increased cell size, an increased number of cell layers, an increased nuclear:cytoplasmic ratio, increased mitoses, and changes in cellular polarity. Gradations are considered mild, moderate, or severe. Carcinoma in situ represents carcinoma still confined by the basement membrane. Once the in situ tumor invades beyond the basement membrane, invasive squamous cell carcinoma is present.

Atypical Adenomatous Hyperplasia. AAH is defined as a lesion smaller than 5.0 mm, comprising epithelial cells lining the alveoli that are similar to type II pneumocytes. Histologically, AAH is similar to bronchoalveolar carcinoma. It represents the beginning stage of a stepwise evolution to bronchoalveolar carcinoma and then to adenocarcinoma.

Diffuse Idiopathic Pulmonary Neuroendocrine Cell Hyperplasia. This rare lesion represents a diffuse proliferation of neuroendocrine cells, but without invasion of the basement membrane. It can exist as a diffuse increase in the number of single neuroendocrine cells, or as small lesions less than 5.0 mm in diameter. Lesions that breach the basement membrane or that are over 5.0 mm in size are carcinoid tumors.

Invasive or Malignant Lesions

The term *bronchial carcinoma* is synonymous with lung cancer in general. Both terms refer to any epithelial carcinoma occurring in the bronchopulmonary tree. Currently, the pathologic diagnosis of the various types of lung cancer is based on light microscopic criteria. Immunohistochemical staining and electron microscopy are also used as adjuncts in diagnosis, particularly in the assessment of potential neuroendocrine tumors. Lung cancer is broadly divided into two main groups based primarily on light microscopic observations: *non-small-cell lung carcinoma* and neuroendocrine tumors (typical carcinoid, atypical carcinoid, large-cell neuroendocrine carcinoma, and small-cell carcinoma).

Non-Small-Cell Lung Carcinoma. The term *non-small-cell lung carcinoma (NSCLC)* is used to distinguish a group of tumors from small-cell carcinoma. Tumors in the NSCLC group include squamous cell carcinoma, adenocarcinoma (including bronchoalveolar carcinoma), and large-cell carcinoma. Although they differ in appearance histologically, their clinical behavior and treatment is similar. As such, they are usefully thought of as a uniform group. However, each type has unique features that affect their clinical presentation and findings.

Squamous Cell Carcinoma. Squamous cell carcinoma accounts for 30 to 40% of lung cancers. It is the cancer most frequently found in men and is highly correlated with cigarette smoking. Histologically, cells develop a pattern of clusters with intracellular bridges and keratin pearls. Importantly, squamous cell carcinoma is primarily located centrally and arises in the major bronchi, often causing the typical symptoms of centrally-located tumors, such as hemoptysis, bronchial obstruction with atelectasis, dyspnea, and pneumonia. Occasionally a more peripherally-based squamous cell carcinoma will develop in a tuberculosis scar or in the wall of a bronchiectatic cavity. Central necrosis is frequent and may lead to the radiographic findings of a cavity (possibly with an air-fluid level). Such cavities may become infected, with resultant abscess formation.

Adenocarcinoma. The incidence of adenocarcinoma has increased over the last several decades, and it now accounts for 25 to 40% of all lung cancers. It occurs with equal frequency in males and females. In contradistinction to squamous cell carcinoma, adenocarcinoma is most often a peripherally-based tumor, thus it is frequently discovered incidentally on routine chest radiographs. Symptoms of chest wall invasion or malignant pleural effusions dominate. Histologically, adenocarcinoma is composed of glands with or without mucin production, combined with destruction of contiguous lung architecture.

Bronchoalveolar Carcinoma. Bronchoalveolar carcinoma (BAC) is a relatively unusual (5% of all lung cancers) subtype of adenocarcinoma that has a unique growth pattern that differs from adenocarcinoma. Rather than invading and destroying contiguous

lung parenchyma, tumor cells multiply and fill the alveolar spaces. To be classified as a pure BAC, no evidence of destruction of surrounding lung parenchyma should be seen. When destruction is seen with areas of classic BAC, the tumor is instead classified as an adenocarcinoma with BAC features.

Because of their growth within alveoli, BAC tumor cells from one site can aerogenously seed other parts of the same lobe or lung, or the contralateral lung. This growth pattern and tendency to seed can produce three radiographic presentations: a single nodule, multiple nodules (in single or multiple lobes), or a diffuse form with an appearance mimicking that of a lobar pneumonia. Because tumor cells fill the alveolar spaces and envelop small airways rather than destroying them, air bronchograms can be seen, unlike with other carcinomas.

Large-Cell Carcinoma. Large-cell carcinoma accounts for 10 to 20% of lung cancers and may be located centrally or peripherally. As implied by the name, the cells are large, with diameters of 30 to 50 μm. They are often admixed with other cell types such as squamous cells or adenocarcinoma. Large-cell carcinoma can be confused with a large-cell variant of neuroendocrine carcinoma, with immunohistochemical staining usually allowing diagnostic distinction between the two.

Neuroendocrine Neoplasms. Neuroendocrine tumors of the lung have been plagued by a confusing array of differing classifications. Over the last decade, progress in understanding and classifying these tumors has been made based on detailed immunohistochemical and electron microscopic studies. In particular, immunohistochemical staining for neuroendocrine markers (including chromogranins, synaptophysin, CD57, and neuron-specific enolase) is essential to accurately diagnose most tumors.

Recently, neuroendocrine lung tumors have been reclassified into neuroendocrine hyperplasia and three separate grades of neuroendocrine carcinoma (NEC). Listed below is the grading system now applied to NEC (left column), with the previously used common name (right column):

Grade I NEC	Classic or typical carcinoid
Grade II NEC	Atypical carcinoid
Grade III NEC	Large-cell type
	Small-cell type

Grade I NEC (classic or typical carcinoid) is a low-grade NEC. An epithelial tumor, it arises primarily in the central airways, although 20% of the time it occurs peripherally. It occurs primarily in younger patients. Because of the central location, it classically presents with hemoptysis, with or without airway obstruction and pneumonia. Histologically, tumor cells are arranged in cords and clusters with a rich vascular stroma. This vascularity can lead to life-threatening hemorrhage with even simple bronchoscopic biopsy maneuvers. Regional lymph node metastases are seen in 15% of patients, but rarely spread systemically or cause death.

Grade II NEC (atypical carcinoid) describes a group of tumors with a degree of aggressive clinical behavior. Unlike Grade I NEC, these tumors are etiologically linked to cigarette smoking and are more likely to be peripherally located. Histologic findings may include areas of necrosis, nuclear pleomorphism, and higher mitotic rates. These tumors have a much higher malignant potential. Lymph node metastases are found in 30 to 50 percent of patients. At the time of their diagnosis, 25 percent of patients already have remote metastases.

Grade III NEC large-cell type tumors occur primarily in heavy smokers. These tumors tend to occur in the middle to peripheral lung fields. They are often large with central necrosis and a high mitotic rate. Their neuroendocrine nature is revealed by positive immunohistochemical staining for at least one neuroendocrine marker.

Grade III NEC small-cell type (small-cell lung carcinoma [SCLC]) is the most malignant NEC, and accounts for 25% of all lung cancers. These tumors are centrally located and consist of smaller cells with a diameter of 10 to 20 μm that have little cytoplasm and very dark nuclei. They also have a high mitotic rate and areas of extensive necrosis. Multiple mitoses are easily seen. Importantly, very small bronchoscopic biopsies can distinguish NSCLC from SCLC, but crush artifact may make NSCLC appear similar to SCLC. If uncertainty exists, special immunohistochemical stains or rebiopsy (or both) will be necessary. These tumors are the leading producer of paraneoplastic syndromes.

Salivary Gland–Type Neoplasms. The tracheobronchial tree has salivary-type submucosal bronchial glands interspersed throughout. These glands can give rise to tumors that are histologically identical to those seen in the salivary glands. The two most common are adenoid cystic carcinoma and mucoepidermoid carcinoma. Both tumors occur centrally due to their site of origin. Adenoid cystic carcinoma is a slow-growing tumor that is locally and systemically invasive. It tends to grow submucosally and infiltrate along perineural sheaths. Mucoepidermoid carcinoma consists of squamous and mucous cells and is graded as low or high grade, depending on the mitotic rate and degree of necrosis.

Clinical Presentation

Lung cancer displays one of the most diverse presentation patterns of all human maladies (Table 18-2). The wide variety of symptoms and signs is related to (1) histologic features, which often help determine the anatomic site of origin in the lung; (2) the specific tumor location in the lung and its relationship to surrounding structures; (3) biologic features, and the production of a variety of paraneoplastic syndromes; and (4) the presence or absence of metastatic disease.

Tumor Histology

Squamous cell and small-cell carcinomas frequently arise in main, lobar, or first segmental bronchi, which are collectively referred to as the central airways. Symptoms of airway irritation or obstruction are common, and include cough, hemoptysis,

wheezing (due to high-grade airway obstruction), dyspnea (due to bronchial obstruction with or without postobstructive atelectasis), and pneumonia (caused by airway obstruction with secretion retention and atelectasis).

In contrast, adenocarcinomas are often located peripherally. For this reason, they are often discovered incidentally as an asymptomatic peripheral lesion on chest x-ray. When symptoms occur, they are due to pleural or chest wall invasion (pleuritic or chest wall pain) or pleural seeding with malignant pleural effusion.

Bronchoalveolar carcinoma (a variant of adenocarcinoma) may present as a solitary nodule, as multifocal nodules, or as a diffuse infiltrate mimicking an infectious pneumonia (pneumonic form). In the pneumonic form, severe dyspnea and hypoxia may occur, sometimes with expectoration of large volumes (over 1 L/d) of light-tan colored fluid, with resultant dehydration and electrolyte imbalance. Because bronchoalveolar carcinoma tends to fill the alveolar spaces as it grows (as opposed to the typical invasion, destruction, and compression of lung architecture seen with other cell types), air bronchograms may be seen radiographically within the tumor.

Tumor Location

Symptoms related to the local intrathoracic effect of the primary tumor can be conveniently divided into two groups: pulmonary and nonpulmonary thoracic.

Pulmonary Symptoms. Pulmonary symptoms result from the direct effect of the tumor on the bronchus or lung tissue. Symptoms (in order of frequency) include cough (secondary to irritation or compression of a bronchus), dyspnea (usually due to central airway obstruction or compression, with or without atelectasis), wheezing (with narrowing of a central airway of greater than 50%), hemoptysis (typically, blood streaking of mucus that rarely is massive, and indicates a central airway location), pneumonia (usually due to airway obstruction by the tumor), and lung abscess (due to necrosis and cavitation, with subsequent infection).

Nonpulmonary Thoracic Symptoms. Nonpulmonary thoracic symptoms result from invasion of the primary tumor directly into a contiguous structure (e.g., chest wall, diaphragm, pericardium, phrenic nerve, recurrent laryngeal nerve, superior vena cava, and esophagus), or from mechanical compression of a structure (e.g., esophagus or superior vena cava) by enlarged tumor-bearing lymph nodes.

Table 18-2
Clinical Presentation of Lung Cancer

Category	Symptom	Cause
Pulmonary symptoms	Cough	Bronchus irritation/compression
	Dyspnea	Airway obstruction/compression
	Wheezing	>50% Airway obstruction
	Hemoptysis	Tumor erosion/irritation
	Pneumonia	Airway obstruction
Nonpulmonary thoracic symptoms	Pleuritic pain	Parietal pleural irritation/invasion
	Local chest wall pain	Rib and/or muscle involvement
	Radicular chest pain	Intercostal nerve involvement
	Pancoast syndrome	Stellate ganglion, chest wall, brachial plexus involvement
	Hoarseness	Recurrent laryngeal nerve involvement
	Swelling of head and arms	Bulky involved mediastinal lymph nodes Medial-based right upper lobe tumor

Peripherally-located tumors (often adenocarcinomas) extending through the visceral pleura lead to irritation or growth into the parietal pleura, and potentially to continued growth into the chest wall structures. Three types of symptoms, depending on the extent of chest wall involvement, are possible: (1) pleuritic pain, from noninvasive contact of the parietal pleura with inflammatory irritation and from direct parietal pleural invasion, (2) localized chest wall pain, with deeper invasion and involvement of the rib and/or intercostal muscles, and (3) radicular pain, from involvement of the intercostal nerve(s). Radicular pain may be mistaken for renal colic in the case of lower lobe tumors invading the posterior chest wall.

Tumors (usually adenocarcinomas) originating in the posterior apex of the chest, referred to as superior sulcus tumors, may produce the Pancoast syndrome. Depending on the exact tumor location, symptoms can include apical chest wall and/or shoulder pain (from involvement of the first rib and chest wall), Horner's syndrome (unilateral enophthalmos, ptosis, miosis, and facial anhidrosis from invasion of the stellate sympathetic ganglion), and radicular arm pain (from invasion of T1, and occasionally C8, brachial plexus nerve roots).

Invasion of the primary tumor into the mediastinum may lead to involvement of the phrenic or recurrent laryngeal nerves. The phrenic nerve traverses the thoracic cavity along the superior vena cava and anterior to the pulmonary hilum. Direct invasion of the nerve occurs with tumors of the medial surface of the lung, or with anterior hilar tumors. Symptoms may include shoulder pain (referred), hiccups, and dyspnea with exertion because of diaphragm paralysis. Radiographically, the diagnosis is suggested by unilateral diaphragm elevation on chest x-ray, and can be confirmed by fluoroscopic examination of the diaphragm with breathing and sniffing (the "sniff" test).

Recurrent laryngeal nerve (RLN) involvement most commonly occurs on the left side, given the hilar location of the left RLN as it passes under the aortic arch. Paralysis may occur from invasion of the vagus nerve above the aortic arch by a medially-based left upper lobe (LUL) tumor, from invasion of the RLN directly by a hilar tumor, or from invasion by hilar or aortopulmonary lymph nodes involved with metastatic tumor. Symptoms include voice change, often referred to as hoarseness, but more typically a loss of tone associated with a breathy quality, and coughing, particularly when drinking liquids.

Superior vena cava (SVC) syndrome most frequently occurs with small-cell carcinoma, with bulky enlargement of involved mediastinal lymph nodes and compression of the SVC. Occasionally, a medially-based right upper lobe (RUL) tumor can produce the syndrome with direct invasion. Symptoms include variable degrees of swelling of the head, neck, and arms; headache; and conjunctival edema. Pericardial invasion may lead to pericardial effusions (benign or malignant), associated with increasing levels of dyspnea and/or arrhythmias, and with the potential to develop pericardial tamponade. Diagnosis requires a high index of suspicion in the setting of a medially-based tumor with symptoms of dyspnea, and is confirmed by CT scan or echocardiography.

Direct invasion of a vertebral body produces symptoms of back pain, which is often localized and severe. If the neural foramina are involved, radicular pain may also be present. Involvement of the esophagus is usually secondary to external compression by enlarged lymph nodes involved with metastatic disease, usually with lower lobe tumors. Finally, invasion of the diaphragm by a tumor at the base of a lower lobe may produce dyspnea, pleural effusion, or referred shoulder pain.

Table 18-3
Paraneoplastic Syndromes in Patients with Lung Cancer

Endocrine
Hypercalcemia (ectopic parathyroid hormone)
Cushing's syndrome
Syndrome of inappropriate secretion of antidiuretic hormone
Carcinoid syndrome
Gynecomastia
Hypercalcitoninemia
Elevated growth hormone
Elevated prolactin, follicle-stimulating hormone, lutenizing hormone
Hypoglycemia
Hyperthyroidism

Neurologic
Encephalopathy
Subacute cerebellar degeneration
Progressive multifocal leukoencephalopathy
Peripheral neuropathy
Polymyositis
Autonomic neuropathy
Eaton-Lambert syndrome
Optic neuritis

Skeletal
Clubbing
Pulmonary hypertrophic osteoarthropathy

Hematologic
Anemia
Leukemoid reactions
Thrombocytosis
Thrombocytopenia
Eosinophilia
Pure red cell aplasia
Leukoerythroblastosis
Disseminated intravascular coagulation

Cutaneous
Hyperkeratosis
Dermatomyositis
Acanthosis nigricans
Hyperpigmentation
Erythema gyratum repens
Hypertrichosis lanuginosa acquista

Other
Nephrotic syndrome
Hypouricemia
Secretion of vasoactive intestinal peptide with diarrhea
Hyperamylasemia
Anorexia or cachexia

Tumor Biology

Lung cancers, both non-small-cell and small-cell, are capable of producing a variety of paraneoplastic syndromes, most often from tumor production and release of biologically active materials systemically (Table 18-3). The majority of such syndromes are caused by small-cell carcinomas, including many endocrinopathies. Paraneoplastic syndromes may produce symptoms even before symptoms are produced by the primary tumor, thereby leading to early diagnosis. Their presence does not influence resectability or the potential to successfully treat the tumor. Symptoms of the syndrome often will abate with successful treatment, and recurrence may be heralded by recurrent paraneoplastic symptoms. Many of the symptoms induced by these syndromes mimic those of the generalized debility caused by metastatic disease.

One of the more common paraneoplastic syndromes in patients with SCLC is hypertrophic pulmonary osteoarthropathy (HPO). Clinically, the syndrome is characterized by tenderness and swelling of the ankles, feet, forearms, and hands. It is due to periostitis of the

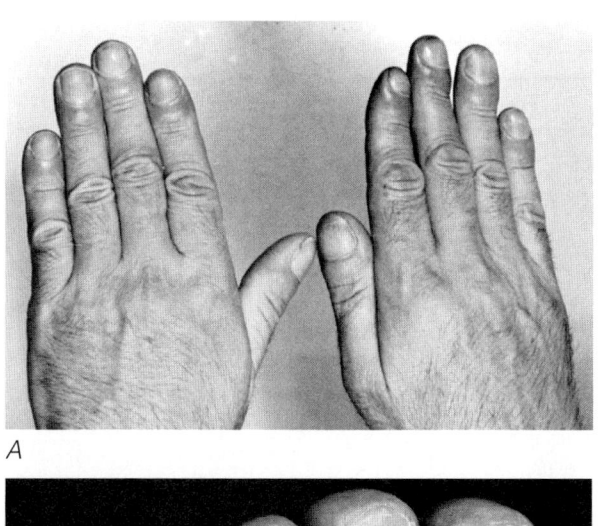

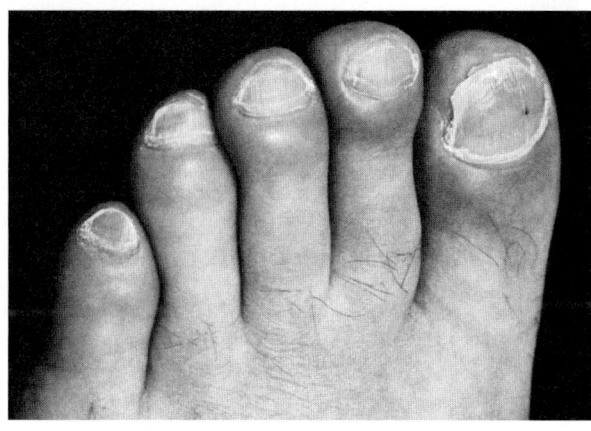

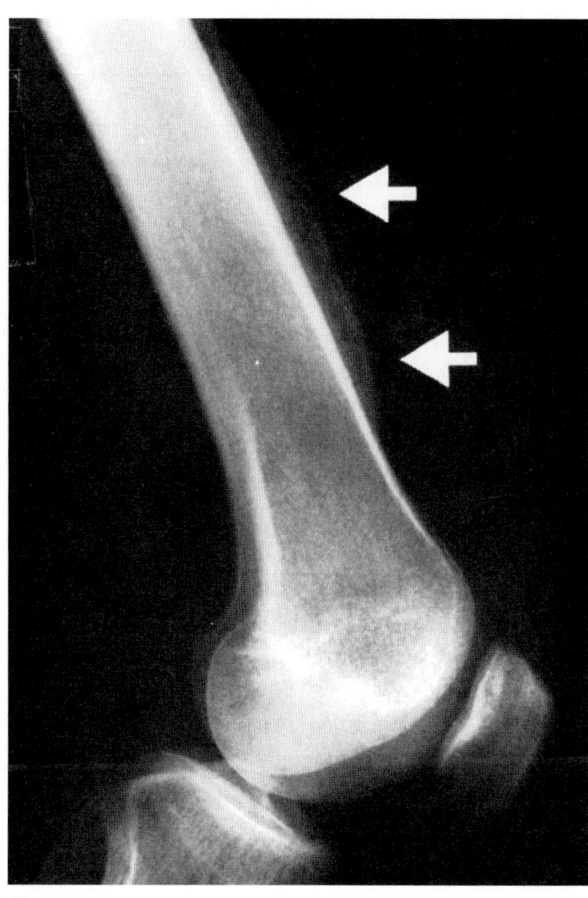

A

B

C

FIG. 18-16. Pulmonary hypertrophic osteoarthropathy associated with small-cell carcinoma. *A.* Painful clubbing of the fingers. *B.* Painful clubbing of the toes (close-up). *C.* The *arrows* point to new bone formation on the femur.

fibula, tibia, radius, metacarpals, and metatarsals. Symptoms may be severe and debilitating. Clubbing of the digits may occur with or be independent of HPO in up to 30% of patients with SCLC (Fig. 18-16). Symptoms of HPO may antedate the diagnosis of cancer by months. Radiographically, plain films of the affected areas show periosteal inflammation and elevation. A bone scan demonstrates intense but symmetric uptake in the long bones. Relief is afforded by aspirin or nonsteroidal anti-inflammatory agents and by successful surgical or medical eradication of the tumor.

Hypercalcemia occurs in up to 10% of patients with lung cancer and is most often due to metastatic disease. However, 15% of cases are due to secretion of ectopic parathyroid hormone–related peptide, most often with squamous cell carcinoma. A diagnosis of ectopic parathyroid hormone secretion can be made by measuring elevated serum levels of parathyroid hormone; however, the clinician must also rule out concurrent metastatic bone disease by a bone scan. Symptoms of hypercalcemia include lethargy, depressed level of consciousness, nausea, vomiting, and dehydration. Most patients have resectable tumors, and following complete resection the calcium level will normalize. Unfortunately, tumor recurrence is extremely common and may manifest as recurrent hypercalcemia.

Endocrinopathies are caused by the release of hormones or hormone analogues into the systemic circulation. Most occur with SCLCs. The syndrome of inappropriate secretion of antidiuretic hormone (SIADH) occurs in 10 to 45% of patients with SCLC. Characterized by confusion, lethargy, and possible seizures, it is diagnosed by the presence of hyponatremia, low serum osmolality, and high urinary sodium and osmolality. Another cause of hyponatremia can be the ectopic secretion of atrial natriuretic peptide (ANP).

Cushing's syndrome is due to production of an adrenocorticotropic hormone (ACTH)-like molecule and occurs principally in patients with SCLC. ACTH production is autonomous and not suppressible by dexamethasone. Immunoreactive ACTH is present in nearly all extracts of SCLC. A high percentage of patients with SCLC have elevated ACTH levels by radioimmunoassay, yet fewer than 5% have symptoms of Cushing's syndrome. Because the serum elevation of ACTH is rapid, the physical signs of Cushing's syndrome (e.g., truncal obesity, buffalo hump, striae) are unusual. Symptoms are primarily related to the metabolic consequences of severe hypokalemia, metabolic alkalosis, and hyperglycemia. Diagnosis is made by demonstrating hypokalemia (<3.0 mmol/L); nonsuppressible elevated plasma cortisol levels that lack the normal diurnal variation; elevated blood ACTH levels; or elevated urinary 17-hydroxycorticosteroids, all of which are not suppressible by administration of exogenous dexamethasone.

Peripheral and central neuropathies are among the most common in lung cancer, particularly in SCLC and squamous cell carcinoma. Unlike other paraneoplastic syndromes that are usually due to ectopic secretion of an active substance, these syndromes are felt to be immune mediated. Antigens normally expressed only by the nervous system are believed to be aberrantly expressed by the cancer

Table 18-4
Evaluation of Patients with Lung Cancer

	Primary Tumor	*Metastatic Disease*	*Functional Assessment*
History	Pulmonary Nonpulmonary thoracic Paraneoplastic	Weight loss Malaise New bone pain Neurologic Skin lesions	Two flights of stairs Flat surface
Physical exam	Voice	Supraclavicular node palpation Skin examination Neurologic examination	Accessory muscle usage Airflow by auscultation Force of cough
Radiographic	Chest CT	Chest CT PET	Chest CT: Tumor anatomy, atelectasis
Tissue analysis	Bronchoscopy Transthoracic needle aspiration and biopsy	Bone scan, head MRI, abdominal CT Bronchoscopic lymph node FNA Endoscopic ultrasound Mediastinoscopy Biopsy of suspected metastases	Quantitative perfusion scan
Other	Thoracoscopy		Pulmonary functions (FEV$_1$, D$_{LCO}$, O$_2$ consumption)

CT = computed tomography; FNA = fine-needle aspiration; MRI = magnetic resonance imaging; PET = positron emission tomography.

cells, generating antibodies leading either to interference with neurologic function or to immune neurologic destruction. Up to 16% of patients with lung cancer have evidence of neuromuscular disability, and of these patients, half have small-cell carcinomas and 25% have squamous cell carcinomas. In patients with neurologic or muscular symptoms, central nervous system (CNS) metastases must be ruled out with CT or magnetic resonance imaging (MRI) of the head. Other metastatic disease leading to disability must also be excluded.

Lambert-Eaton syndrome is a myasthenia-like syndrome usually seen in patients with SCLC. It is caused by a neuromuscular conduction defect. Gait abnormalities are due to proximal muscle weakness and fatigability, and particularly affect the thighs. Symptoms can occur before symptoms of the primary tumor and may actually precede radiographic evidence of the tumor. The syndrome is produced by immunoglobulin G (IgG) antibodies targeting voltage-gated calcium channels, which function in the release of acetylcholine from presynaptic sites at the motor end plate. Therapy is directed at the primary tumor with resection, radiation, and/or chemotherapy. Many patients have dramatic improvement after resection or successful medical therapy. For patients with refractory symptoms, treatment consists of guanidine hydrochloride, immunosuppressive agents such as prednisone and azathioprine, and occasionally plasma exchange. Unlike with myasthenia gravis patients, neostigmine is usually ineffective.

Metastatic Symptoms

Metastases occur most commonly in the CNS, vertebral bodies, bones, liver, adrenal glands, lungs, and skin and soft tissues. At diagnosis, 10% of patients with lung cancer have CNS metastases; another 10 to 15% will develop CNS metastases. Symptoms are often focal and include headache, nausea and vomiting, seizures, hemiplegia, and speech difficulty.

Bone metastases are seen in 25% of all patients with lung cancer. They are primarily lytic, producing localized pain; thus any new and localized skeletal symptoms should be evaluated radiographically. Lung cancer is the most common cause of spinal cord compression, which may occur from direct extension of a vertebral metastasis or by invasion of an intervertebral foramen from a primary tumor contiguous with the spine.

Liver metastases are most often an incidental finding on CT scan. Adrenal metastases are also typically asymptomatic and are usually discovered by routine CT scan. They lead to adrenal hypofunction. Skin and soft tissue metastases occur in 8% of patients dying of lung cancer, and generally present as painless subcutaneous or intramuscular masses. Occasionally, the tumor erodes through the overlying skin, with necrosis and creation of a chronic wound; excision may then be necessary for both mental and physical palliation.

Nonspecific Symptoms

Lung cancer often produces a variety of nonspecific symptoms such as anorexia, weight loss, fatigue, and malaise. The cause of these symptoms is often unclear, but should raise concern about possible metastatic disease.

Diagnosis, Evaluation, and Staging

In a patient with either a histologically-confirmed lung cancer or a pulmonary lesion suspected to be a lung cancer, assessment encompasses three areas: the primary tumor, presence of metastatic disease, and functional status (the patient's ability to tolerate a pulmonary resection). A discrete approach to these three areas allows the surgeon to systematically evaluate a patient, permits clinical stage assignment, and enables assessment of the patient's functional suitability for pulmonary resection (Table 18-4).

Assessment of the Primary Tumor. Assessment of the primary tumor begins with the history and directed questions regarding the presence or absence of pulmonary, nonpulmonary, thoracic, and paraneoplastic symptoms. Patients often have already undergone a chest x-ray or CT scan before their initial visit with the surgeon; the location of the tumor can then help direct the history.

Obtaining a chest CT scan is the next stage in evaluating a new patient. A routine chest CT scan should include intravenous contrast material to enable delineation of mediastinal lymph nodes relative to normal mediastinal structures. Chest CT allows assessment of the primary tumor and its relationship to surrounding and contiguous structures. It also indicates whether invasion of contiguous structures has occurred.

The determination of invasion often is made by the patient's history and the location of the primary tumor. For example, a tumor abutting the chest wall with underlying rib destruction is clear evidence of local invasion. It is common to see the primary tumor abutting the chest wall without evidence of rib destruction. In this circumstance, the history is an accurate guide to the presence or absence of parietal pleural, rib, or intercostal nerve involvement. Similar observations apply to tumors abutting the recurrent laryngeal nerve, phrenic nerve, diaphragm, vertebral bodies, and chest apex. Thoracotomy should not be denied because of presumptive evidence of invasion of the chest wall, vertebral body, or mediastinal structures; proof of invasion may require thoracoscopy or even thoracotomy.

MRI of pulmonary lesions and mediastinal nodes has been disappointing, offering no real improvement over CT scanning. However, due to its excellent imaging of vascular structures, MRI may be of value to define a tumor's relationship to a major vessel, especially if the use of contrast material is contraindicated. Thus routine use of MRI in lung cancer patients is reserved for those with contrast material allergies or with suspected mediastinal, vascular, or vertebral body invasion.

Tissue diagnosis of the primary tumor can be obtained through bronchoscopy or needle biopsy. Bronchoscopy provides additional useful information regarding tumor location within the airway and may guide operative planning. It is particularly useful for centrally-located tumors with a higher probability of being visualized and biopsied. In addition, it enables the entire tracheobronchial tree to be seen, allowing the surgeon to rule out the presence of additional unsuspected endobronchial lesions.

Diagnostic tissue from bronchoscopy can be obtained by one of four methods: (1) brushings and washings for cytology, (2) direct forceps biopsy of a visualized lesion, (3) fine-needle aspiration (FNA) with a Wang needle of an externally compressing lesion without visualized endobronchial tumor, and (4) transbronchial biopsy with the use of forceps guided to the lesion by fluoroscopy. For peripheral lesions (roughly the outer half of the lung), transbronchial fluoroscopic biopsy is often performed first, followed by brushings and washings. The intent is to improve the yield of the biopsy by picking up additional cells after disruption of the lesion by the biopsy forceps. For central lesions, direct forceps biopsy by bronchoscopic visualization is often possible, and again is followed by brushings and washings. For central lesions with external airway compression but no visible endobronchial lesions, Wang needle FNA through the bronchoscope is performed.

Transthoracic needle aspiration is ideally suited for peripheral lesions not easily accessible by bronchoscopy. Using image guidance (fluoroscopy or CT), either an FNA or core-needle biopsy is performed. The primary complication is pneumothorax (in up to 50% of patients), which is usually minor and requires no treatment. Three biopsy results are possible: malignant, a specific benign process, or indeterminate. The overall false-negative rate is 20 to 30%, therefore unless a specific benign diagnosis (such as granulomatous inflammation or hamartoma) is made, malignancy is not ruled out and further efforts at diagnosis are warranted.

Thoracoscopy is potentially a valuable staging tool for assessing the primary tumor's relationship to contiguous structures, since it is frequently difficult to discern whether the primary tumor has invaded a contiguous structure (such as the chest wall or mediastinal structures). Thoracoscopy can be useful for determining any invasion of such structures.

A thoracotomy occasionally is necessary to diagnose and stage a primary tumor. Although this occurs in fewer than 5% of patients, two circumstances may require such an approach: (1) a deep-seated lesion that yielded an indeterminate needle biopsy result or that could not be biopsied for technical reasons, or (2) inability to determine invasion of a mediastinal structure by any method short of palpation. In the circumstance of a deep-seated lesion without a diagnosis, FNA, a Tru-Cut biopsy, or preferably an excisional biopsy, can be performed with frozen-section analysis. If the biopsy result is indeterminate, a lobectomy may instead be necessary. When a pneumonectomy is required, a tissue diagnosis of cancer must be made before excision.

Assessment of Metastatic Disease. Distant metastases are found in about 40% of patients with newly diagnosed lung cancer. The presence of lymph node or systemic metastases may imply inoperability. A patient's risk of harboring metastatic disease must be carefully considered by the surgeon.

As with the primary tumor, assessment for the presence of metastatic disease should begin with the history and physical examination, focusing on the presence or absence of new bone pain, neurologic symptoms, and new skin lesions. In addition, constitutional symptoms (e.g., anorexia, malaise, and unintentional weight loss of greater than 5% of body weight) suggest either a large tumor burden or the presence of metastases. Physical examination should focus on the patient's overall appearance, noting any evidence of weight loss with muscle wasting. The appearance of cervical and supraclavicular lymph nodes as well as that of the oropharynx should also be examined for tobacco-associated tumors. The skin should be thoroughly examined. Routine laboratory studies should include checking the levels of hepatic enzymes (e.g., serum glutamic oxaloacetic transaminase and alkaline phosphatase), as well as those of serum calcium (to detect bone metastases or the ectopic parathyroid syndrome). Elevation of either hepatic enzymes or serum calcium levels typically occurs with extensive metastases.

Mediastinal Lymph Nodes. Chest CT scanning permits assessment of possible metastatic spread to the mediastinal lymph nodes. It continues to be the most effective noninvasive method available to assess the mediastinal and hilar nodes for enlargement. However, a positive CT result (i.e., nodal diameter more than 1.0 cm) predicts actual metastatic involvement in only about 70% of lung cancer patients. Thus even with enlarged mediastinal lymph nodes on a CT scan, up to 30% of such nodes are enlarged from noncancerous reactive causes such as inflammation due to atelectasis or pneumonia secondary to the tumor. Therefore, no patient should be denied an attempt at curative resection just because of a positive CT result for mediastinal lymph node enlargement. Any CT finding of metastatic nodal involvement must be confirmed histologically.

A negative CT result (lymph nodes less than 1.0 cm) generally is more accurate. With normal-size lymph nodes and a T1 tumor, the false-negative rate is less than 10%, leading many surgeons to omit mediastinoscopy. However, the false-negative rate increases to nearly 30% with centrally-located and T3 tumors. In this situation, mediastinoscopy is routinely recommended, as it has been demonstrated that T1 adenocarcinomas or large-cell carcinomas have a higher rate of early micrometastasis. Therefore all such patients should undergo mediastinoscopy.

PET scanning for metastatic disease is based on the detection of positrons emitted by FDG, a D-glucose analogue labeled with positron-emitting fluorine. After cellular uptake and phosphorylation, FDG is not metabolized further, leading to intracellular accumulation. This accumulation, combined with a cancer's intrinsically higher rate of glucose metabolism, leads to accumulation and potential visualization. A significant advantage of PET scanning is the ability to image the whole body after a single FDG injection, allowing simultaneous evaluation of the primary lung lesion, mediastinal lymph nodes, and distant organs.

Mediastinal lymph node staging by PET scanning appears to have greater accuracy than CT scanning. PET staging of mediastinal lymph nodes has been evaluated in two meta-analyses. The overall sensitivity of PET for detection of mediastinal lymph node metastases was 0.79 (95% CI 0.76 to 0.82), with a specificity of 0.91 (95% CI 0.89 to 0.93), and an accuracy of 0.92 (95% CI 0.90 to 0.94).

In comparing PET with CT scans in patients who also underwent lymph node biopsies, PET had a sensitivity of 88% and a specificity of 91%, while CT scanning had a sensitivity of 63% and a specificity of 76%. Combining CT and PET scanning may lead to even greater accuracy. In one study of CT, PET, and mediastinoscopy in 68 patients with potentially operable, non-small-cell lung carcinoma (NSCLC), CT correctly identified the nodal stage in 40 patients (59%). It understaged the tumor in 12 patients and overstaged it in 16. PET correctly identified the nodal stage in 59 patients (87%). It understaged the tumor in five patients and overstaged it in four. For detecting N2 and N3 disease, the combination of PET and CT scanning yielded a sensitivity, specificity, and accuracy of 93%, 95%, and 94%, respectively. CT scan alone yielded 75%, 63%, and 68%, respectively. With the recent development of combined PET-CT scanners, continued improvement in accuracy may be anticipated. However, with mediastinal lymph nodes, mediastinoscopy is recommended for histologic verification of nodes determined to be cancerous by PET.

Endoesophageal ultrasound (EUS) has recently emerged as a method of staging in NSCLC. EUS can accurately visualize mediastinal paratracheal lymph nodes (stations 4R, 7, and 4L) and other lymph node stations (stations 8 and 9). It is able to visualize primary lung lesions contiguous with or near the esophagus (see Fig. 18-7). Using FNA techniques, samples of lymph nodes or primary lesions can be obtained. However, EUS fails to visualize the anterior (pretracheal) mediastinum and thus does not provide as complete an assessment as mediastinoscopy.

Bronchoscopic FNA of paratracheal lymph nodes (primarily stations 4R, 7, and 4L) also can be performed. A significant disadvantage is the relatively blind nature of the aspiration. Station 7 can be reliably accessed, but other paratracheal lymph node locations must be estimated and aspiration attempted, therefore bronchoscopic FNA has limited usefulness. Both EUS and bronchoscopic FNA lack the complete staging afforded by mediastinoscopy, which enables sampling of all upper mediastinal nodal stations and determination of the degree of lymph node involvement (from microscopic to complete nodal replacement). Mediastinoscopy thus remains the standard method of tissue staging of the mediastinum.

Cervical mediastinoscopy has several advantages over other techniques of mediastinal lymph node staging (Fig. 18-17). It can provide a tissue diagnosis, allows sampling of all paratracheal and subcarinal lymph nodes, and permits visual determination of the presence of extracapsular extension of nodal metastasis. With complex hilar or right paratracheal primary tumors, it allows direct biopsies and assessment of invasion into the mediastinum.

An absolute indication for mediastinoscopy is mediastinal lymph node enlargement greater than 1.0 cm by CT scan. When the size of mediastinal lymph nodes is normal, mediastinoscopy is generally recommended for centrally located tumors, for T2 and T3 primary tumors, and occasionally for T1 adenocarcinomas or large-cell carcinomas (due to their higher rate of metastatic spread). Some surgeons perform mediastinoscopy in all lung cancer patients because of the poor survival associated with surgical resection of N2 disease.

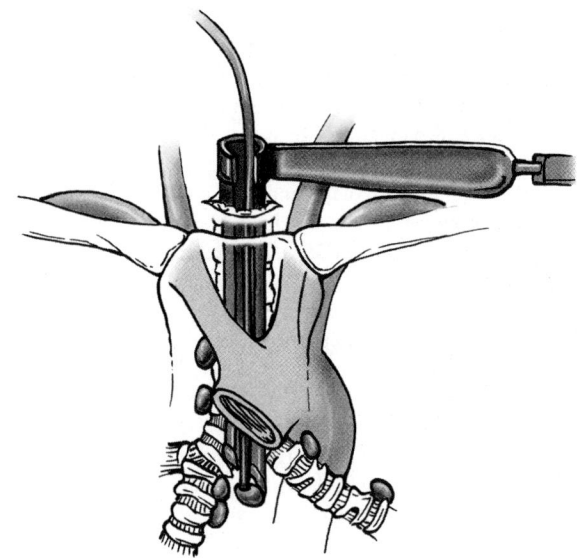

FIG. 18-17. Cervical mediastinoscopy. Paratracheal and subcarinal lymph node tissues (within the pretracheal space) can be sampled using a mediastinoscope introduced through a suprasternal skin incision.

Patients with LUL tumors may have localized regional spread to station 5 and 6 lymph nodes, without mediastinal paratracheal involvement (see Fig. 18-7). Traditionally, they undergo left anterior mediastinotomy (Chamberlain procedure). A left parasternal transverse incision is made with reflection of the mediastinal pleura laterally. The anterior mediastinal tissue is entered, allowing biopsy of station 5 and 6 lymph nodes and of primary tumors of the left hilum. Cervical mediastinoscopy should precede mediastinotomy, even if patients have normal paratracheal lymph nodes. Currently, the more common approach to station 5 and 6 lymph nodes is left thoracoscopy.

The current indications for prethoracotomy biopsy of station 5 and 6 lymph nodes are (1) required confirmation of N2 disease for entry into a preoperative adjuvant therapy protocol; (2) CT evidence of bulky nodal metastases or extracapsular spread, which could prevent complete resection; and (3) the need for tissue diagnosis of a hilar mass or of lymph nodes causing recurrent laryngeal nerve paralysis. However, if cervical mediastinoscopy results are negative and station 5 and 6 lymph nodes appear resectable, left thoracotomy and resection of the primary tumor and lymph nodes can be performed directly; the 5-year survival rate is 20 to 25%.

Pleural Effusion. The presence of pleural effusion on a CT scan (or chest x-ray) is not synonymous with a malignant effusion. Malignant pleural effusion can only be diagnosed by finding malignant cells in a sample of pleural fluid examined microscopically. Pleural effusion is often secondary to the atelectasis or consolidation seen with central tumors, or it can be reactive or secondary to cardiac dysfunction. However, pleural effusion associated with a peripherally-based tumor, particularly one that abuts the visceral or parietal pleural surface, does have a higher probability of being malignant. Regardless, no pleural effusion should be assumed to be malignant. Cytologic proof of the presence of malignant cells is required. Thoracoscopy may be indicated to rule out pleural metastases in select patients. It can be performed as part of a separate staging procedure, often with mediastinoscopy, or immediately before a planned thoracotomy.

Distant Metastases. Until recently, detection of distant metastases outside the thorax was performed with a combination of chest CT scan and multiorgan scanning (e.g., brain CT or MRI, abdominal CT, and bone scan). Chest CT scans always include the upper abdomen and allow visualization of the liver and adrenal glands. Liver abnormalities that are not clearly simple cysts or hemangiomas need to be further evaluated, typically by MRI scanning. Adrenal enlargement, nodules, or masses should also be further evaluated by MRI, and occasionally by needle biopsy. It must be remembered that adrenal adenomas, which are found in 2% of the general population and in up to 8% of patients with hypertension, may be mistakenly assumed to represent metastases. Adrenal adenomas have a high lipid content (secondary to steroid production), but metastases and most primary adrenal malignancies contain little if any lipid, thus MRI is usually able to distinguish the two.

In the absence of neurologic symptoms or signs, the probability of having a negative head CT scan is 95%. Bone scans are notorious for their high sensitivity but low specificity, with a known overall false-positive rate of 40%. False-positive findings with any organ often lead to further noninvasive and invasive evaluation, and may even lead to denial of surgical resection. For these reasons, routine preoperative multiorgan scanning is not recommended for patients with a negative clinical evaluation and clinical stage I disease. However, it is recommended for patients with regionally advanced (clinical stage II, IIIA, and IIIB) disease. Any patient—regardless of clinical stage—who has a positive clinical evaluation, whether organ-specific or not, should also undergo radiographic evaluation for metastatic disease.

PET scanning has supplanted multiorgan scanning in the search for distant metastases to the liver, adrenal glands, and bones. Currently, chest CT and PET are routine in the evaluation of patients with lung cancer. Brain MRI should be performed when the suspicion or risk of brain metastases is increased. Several reports show that PET scanning appears to detect an additional 10 to 15% of distant metastases not detected by routine chest or abdominal CT and bone scans. The finding of PET FDG uptake at a distant site must be proven not to be a metastasis. This is often accomplished with MRI and/or biopsies.

Integrated PET-CT scanners recently have become available. Early reports have demonstrated an improved accuracy of detection and localization of lymph node and distant metastases, as compared with independently performed PET and CT scans (Fig. 18-18). This technology appears to overcome the imprecise information on the exact location of focal abnormalities seen on PET and will likely become the standard imaging modality for lung cancer.

With any radiologic assessment for cancer, a common problem faced by surgeons is whether the results are true-positive or false-positive. Because a false-positive result can have a dramatic impact on a patient's therapeutic course, the accuracy of a given scan must be ensured. The patient must be given the benefit of any doubt about the accuracy of a scan; the result must be proven, most often by a biopsy, to be true-positive.

Assessment of Functional Status. For patients with a potentially resectable primary tumor, their functional status and ability to tolerate either lobectomy or pneumonectomy needs to be carefully assessed. The surgeon should first estimate the likelihood of pneumonectomy, lobectomy, or possibly sleeve resection, given the CT scan results (see section on surgical resection). A sequential process of evaluation then unfolds.

A patient's history is the most important tool for gauging risk. It must be emphasized that numbers alone (e.g., forced expiratory

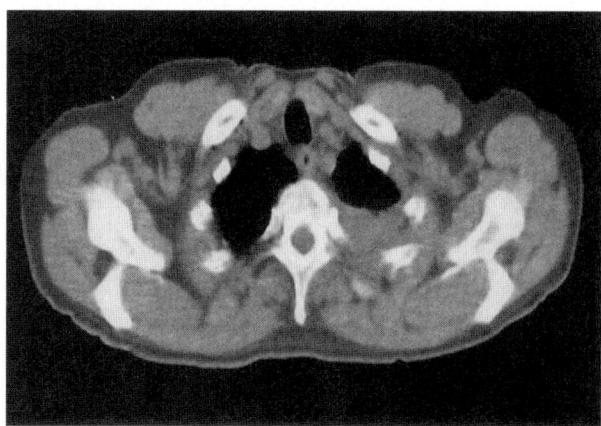

A

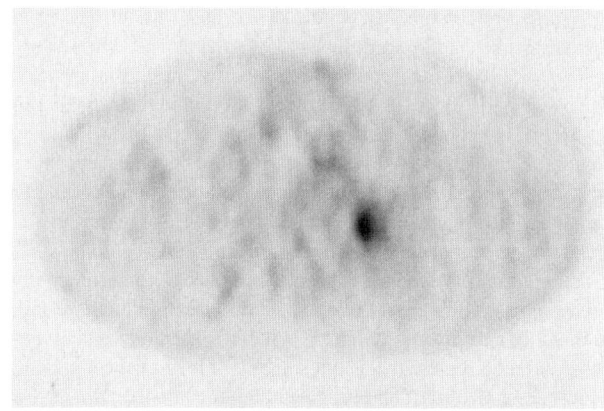

B

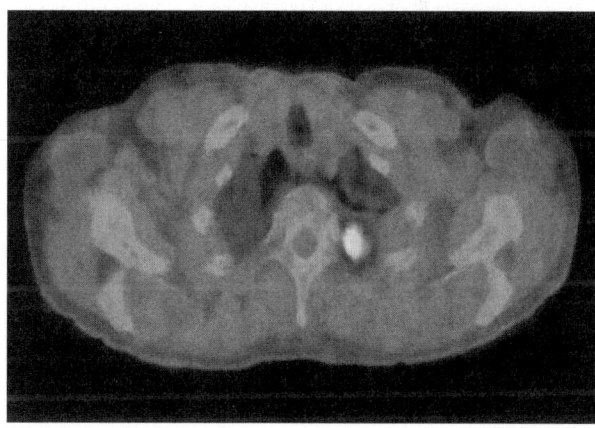

C

FIG. 18-18. Imaging of non-small-cell lung cancer by integrated PET-CT scan. *A.* CT of the chest showing a tumor in the left upper lobe. *B.* PET scan of the chest at the identical cross-sectional level. *C.* Coregistered PET-CT scan clearly showing tumor invasion (confirmed intraoperatively). (*Adapted with permission from Lardinois D, et al: Staging of non-small-cell lung cancer with integrated positron-emission tomography and computed tomography. N Engl J Med 348:2504.*)

volume in 1 second [FEV_1] and carbon monoxide diffusion capacity [D_{LCO}]) do not supplant the clinician's assessment. The clinical assessment entails the observation of the patient's general vigor and attitude. The late Dr. Robert Ginsberg best summarized the impact of a patient's vigor and attitude:

Other factors that may predict a poor outcome from surgical intervention are difficult to classify. It has been my distinct impression that the patient's attitude toward the disease, the desire to have a favorable outcome, and confidence in the doctor is predictive of success. A prospective analysis of quality of life following lung cancer treatment, performed by the Lung Cancer Study Group, confirmed that the patient's attitude toward the disease was the best indicator of long-term survival. Except in life-threatening situations, patients should never be cajoled or forced into accepting surgery. In most cases, this led to disastrous results. At times, it is best to defer surgical intervention to the patient with a significant negative outlook, especially if other curative options (e.g., radiotherapy for cancer) are available.

When obtaining the patient's history, specific questions should be routinely asked that help determine the amount of lung that the patient will likely tolerate having resected. Can the patient walk on a flat surface indefinitely, without oxygen and without having to stop and rest secondary to dyspnea? If so, the patient will be very likely to tolerate thoracotomy and lobectomy. Can the patient walk up two flights of stairs (up two standard levels), without having to stop and rest secondary to dyspnea? If so, the patient will likely tolerate pneumonectomy. Finally, nearly all patients, except those with CO_2 retention on arterial blood gas analysis, will be able to tolerate periods of single-lung ventilation and wedge resection.

Other pertinent elements of the history are current smoking status and sputum production. Current smokers have a significantly increased risk of postoperative complications. To diminish the risk significantly requires cessation of smoking at least 8 weeks preoperatively, a requirement that is often not feasible in a cancer patient. Nevertheless, efforts to abstain should be encouraged, ideally for 2 weeks before surgery. Smoking cessation on the day of surgery leads to increased sputum production and potential secretion retention postoperatively. Patients with chronic daily sputum production will have more problems postoperatively with retention and atelectasis; they are also at higher risk for pneumonia. Sputum culture, antibiotic administration, and bronchodilators may be warranted preoperatively.

The physical examination should focus on the following signs of COPD or airflow limitation: use of accessory muscles for breathing, fullness of breath sounds on auscultation, and the strength and "wetness" of a voluntarily-induced cough. The combination of the patient's answers to the above questions and the cough test allow the experienced thoracic surgeon to gauge operative risk remarkably well.

Pulmonary function studies are routinely performed when any resection greater than a wedge resection will be performed. Of all the measurements available, the two most valuable are FEV_1 and DLCO. General guidelines for the use of FEV_1 in assessing the patient's ability to tolerate pulmonary resection are as follows: greater than 2.0 L can tolerate pneumonectomy, and greater than 1.0 L can tolerate lobectomy. It must be emphasized that these are guidelines only. It is also important to note that the raw value is often imprecise because normal values are reported as "percent predicted" based on corrections made for age, height, and gender. For example, a raw FEV_1 value of 1.3 L in a 62-year-old, 6' 3" male has a percent predicted value of 30% (because the normal expected value is 4.31 L); in a 62-year-old, 5' 2" female, the predicted value is 59% (normal expected value 2.21 L). The male patient is at high risk for lobectomy, while the female could potentially tolerate pneumonectomy.

The percent predicted value of both FEV_1 and DLCO correlates with the risk of development of complications postoperatively, par-

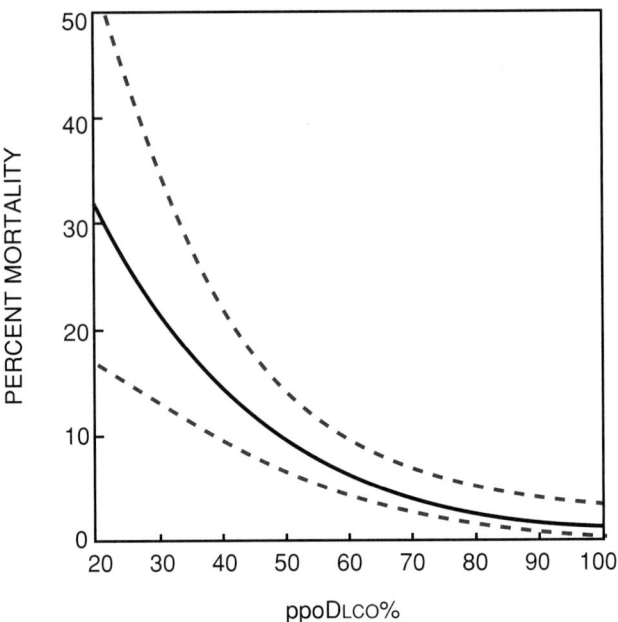

FIG. 18-19. Operative mortality after major pulmonary resection for non-small-cell lung cancer (334 patients) as a function of the predicted postoperative CO diffusing capacity expressed as percentage of predicted DLCO (ppoDLCO%). Solid line = logistic regression model; dashed lines = 95% confidence limits. *(Adapted with permission from Wang J, et al: Diffusing capacity predicts operative mortality but not long-term survival after resection for lung cancer. J Thorac Cardiovasc Surg 117:582, 1999.)*

ticularly pulmonary complications. Patients with predicted values of less than 50% show a significant increase in complication rates, with the risk of complications increasing in a stepwise fashion for each 10% decline. Figure 18-19 shows the relationship between predicted postoperative DLCO (ppoDLCO%) and estimated operative mortality. To calculate the predicted postoperative value for FEV_1 or DLCO, the percent predicted value of FEV_1 or DLCO is multiplied by the fraction of remaining lung after the proposed surgery. For example, with a planned right upper lobectomy, a total of three segments will be removed. Therefore, three of a total 20 segments will leave the patient with $(20 - 3/20) \times 100 = 85\%$ of their original lung capacity. In the two patients mentioned above, the man will have a ppoFEV₁ of $30\% \times 0.85 = 25\%$, while the woman will have a ppoFEV₁ of 50%.

The effect of the primary tumor on lung function must also be considered. Figure 18-20 shows a tumor with significant right main stem airway obstruction with associated atelectasis and volume loss of the right lung. At presentation, the patient was dyspneic with ambulation and the FEV_1 was 1.38 L. The referring physician told the patient that surgery was not feasible because he would require pneumonectomy, which he would not be able to tolerate. This case history illustrates a common pitfall made by clinicians: failure to determine a patient's functional status before the development of the tumor. Six months prior, this patient could walk up two flights of stairs without dyspnea. Similarly, if a patient with limited pulmonary function develops complete collapse of a lobe (e.g., right upper lobe [RUL]) and has only a mild decline in functional status, the surgeon can anticipate that the patient will tolerate lobectomy because the lobe is already not functioning, and in fact may be contributing to a shunt.

Quantitative perfusion scanning is used in select circumstances to help estimate the functional contribution of a lobe or whole lung.

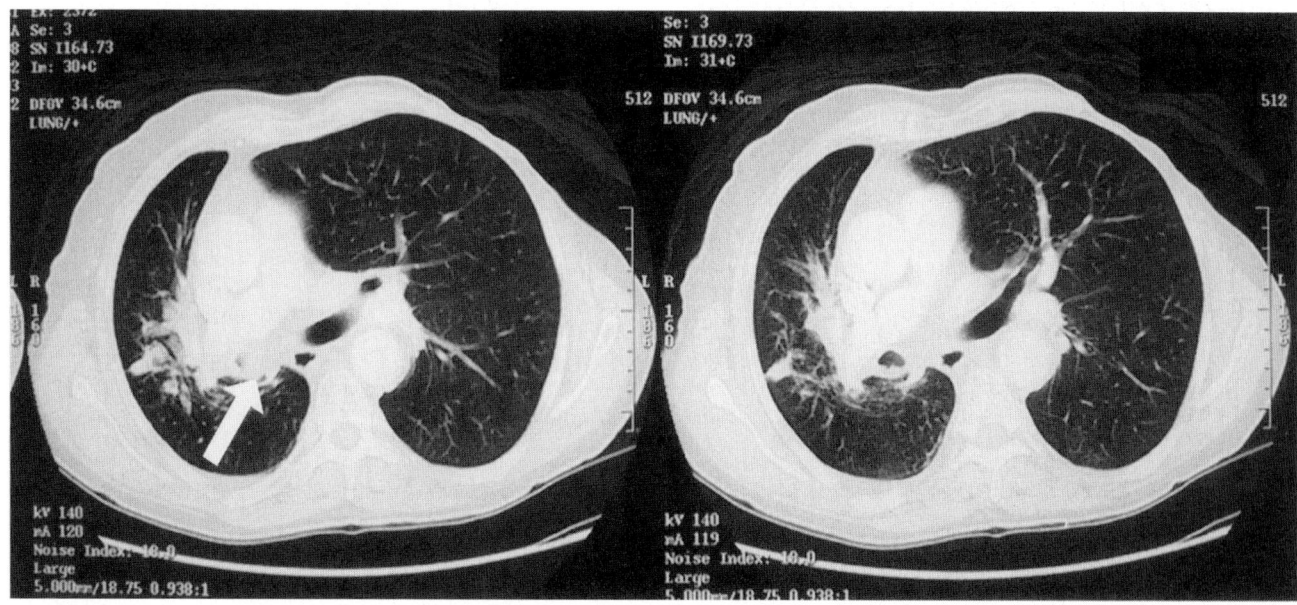

FIG. 18-20. *Chest CT scan of an obstructing right main stem lung tumor. Arrow indicates location of right main bronchus. The right lung volume is much less than the left lung volume.*

Such perfusion scanning is most useful when the impact of a tumor on pulmonary physiology is difficult to discern. With complete collapse of a lobe or whole lung, the impact is apparent, and perfusion scanning is usually unnecessary. However, with centrally-located tumors associated with partial obstruction of a lobar or main bronchus or of the pulmonary artery, perfusion scanning may be valuable in predicting the postoperative result of resection. For example, if the quantitative perfusion to the right lung is measured to be 21% (normal is 55%) and the patient's percent predicted FEV_1 is 60%, the predicted postoperative FEV_1 after a right pneumonectomy would be 60% x 0.79 = 47%, indicating the ability to tolerate pneumonectomy. If the perfusion value is 55%, the predicted postoperative value would be 27%, and pneumonectomy would pose a significantly higher risk.

Exercise testing that yields maximal oxygen consumption ($\dot{V}o_2$max) has emerged as a valuable decision-making technique to help patients with abnormal FEV_1 and $D\textsc{lco}$. It is not uncommon to encounter patients with significant reductions in their percent predicted FEV_1 and $D\textsc{lco}$ whose history shows a functional status that is inconsistent with the pulmonary function tests. In these circumstances, and in other situations in which decision making is difficult, the $\dot{V}o_2$max should be measured. Values of less than 10 mL/kg per minute generally prohibit any major pulmonary resection, while those greater than 15 mL/kg per minute generally indicate the patient's ability to tolerate pneumonectomy.

The risk assessment of a patient is an amalgam of clinical judgment and data. Commonly, there are gray areas in which data such as that described above can provide more accurate assessment of the risk. This risk must be integrated with the experienced clinician's sense of the patient, and with the patient's attitude toward the disease and toward life.

Lung Cancer Staging

The staging of any tumor is an attempt to measure or estimate the extent of disease present and in turn use that information to help determine the patient's prognosis. The staging of solid epithelial tumors is based on the TNM staging system. The "T" status provides information about the primary tumor itself, such as its size and relationship to surrounding structures; the "N" status provides information about regional lymph nodes; and the "M" status provides information about the presence or absence of metastatic disease. Table 18-5 lists the TNM descriptors that have been developed for use in NSCLC.

The designation of lymph nodes as N1, N2, or N3 requires familiarity with the lymph node map devised by Naruke and colleagues in 1978, which was subsequently modified by the American Thoracic Society and by Mountain and Dresler in 1997 (see Fig. 18-7). This map of lymph node stations is based on clearly delineated anatomic boundaries. It permits accurate designation of the exact location of thoracic lymph nodes, allowing detailed staging of the tumors of individual patients, and facilitating consistent assessment and reporting of patient outcomes.

A tumor in a given patient is typically classified into a clinical stage and a pathologic stage. The clinical stage (cTNM) is derived from an assessment of all data short of surgical resection of the primary tumor and lymph nodes. Thus clinical staging information would include the history and physical examination, radiographic test results, and diagnostic biopsy information. A therapeutic plan is then generated based on the clinical stage. After surgical resection of the tumor and lymph nodes, a postoperative pathologic stage (pTNM) is determined, providing further prognostic information.

In 1986, an international staging system for lung cancer was developed by Mountain and applied to a database of more than 3000 patients from the M. D. Anderson Hospital in Houston, Texas, and the Lung Cancer Study Group. In 1997, Mountain reviewed the survival data from an additional 1524 patients beyond the original database. Taking into account the combined total of 5319 patients, he revised the staging system. These changes were subsequently adopted by the American Joint Committee on Cancer. The 1997 version of the international staging system, which is still in use, is shown in Table 18-5.

It is important to recognize that significant variation in survival exists within stages (Table 18-6). For example, tumors 1.0 cm or less

Table 18-5

American Joint Committee on Cancer Staging System for Lung Cancer

Stage	TNM
IA	T1N0M0
IB	T2N0M0
IIA	T1N1M0
IIB	T2N1M0
	T3N0M0
IIIA	T3N1M0
	T1–3N2M0
IIIB	T4 Any N M0
	Any T N3 M0
IV	Any T Any N M1

TNM Definitions

T	**TX**	Positive malignant cell, but primary tumor not visualized by imaging or bronchoscopy
	T0	No evidence of primary tumor
	Tis	Carcinoma in situ
	T1	Tumor ≤3 cm, surrounded by lung or visceral pleura, without bronchoscopic evidence of invasion more proximal than the lobar bronchus
	T2	Tumor with any of the following features of size or extent:
		• >3 cm in greatest dimension
		• >Involves main bronchus, ≥2 cm distal to the carina
		• >Invades the visceral pleura
		• >Associated with atelectasis or obstructive pneumonitis that extends to the hilar region but does not involve the entire lung
	T3	Tumor of any size that directly invades any of the following: chest wall (including superior sulcus tumors), diaphragm, mediastinal pleura, parietal pericardium; or tumor in the main bronchus <2 cm distal to the carina, but without involvement of the carina; or associated atelectasis or obstructive pneumonitis of the entire lung
	T4	Tumor of any size that invades any of the following: mediastinum, heart, great vessels, trachea, esophagus, vertebral body, carina; or tumor with a malignant pleural or pericardial effusion, or with satellite tumor nodule(s) within the ipsilateral primary-tumor lobe of the lung
N	**NX**	Regional lymph nodes cannot be assessed
	N0	No regional lymph node metastasis
	N1	Metastasis to ipsilateral peribronchial and/or ipsilateral hilar lymph nodes, and intrapulmonary nodes involved by direct extension of the primary tumor
	N2	Matastasis to ipsilateral mediastinal and/or subcarinal lymph node(s)
	N3	Metastasis to contralateral mediastinal, contralateral hilar, ipsilateral or contralateral scalene, or supraclavicular lymph node(s)
M	**MX**	Presence of distant metastasis cannot be assessed
	M0	No distant metastasis
	M1	Distant metastasis present (including metastatic tumor nodule[s] in the ipsilateral nonprimary tumor lobe[s] of the lung)

Summary of Staging Definitions

Occult stage	Microscopically identified cancer cells in lung secretions on multiple occasions (or multiple daily collections); no discernible primary cancer in the lung
Stage 0	Carcinoma in situ
Stage IA	Tumor surrounded by lung or visceral pleura ≤3 cm arising more than 2 cm distal to the carina (T1 N0)
Stage IB	Tumor surrounded by lung >3 cm, or tumor of any size with visceral pleura involved arising more than 2 cm distal to the carina (T2 N0)
Stage IIA	Tumor ≤3 cm not extended to adjacent organs, with ipsilateral peribronchial and hilar lymph node involvement (T1 N1)
Stage IIB	Tumor >3 cm not extended to adjacent organs, with ipsilateral peribronchial and hilar lymph node involvement (T2 N1)
	Tumor invading chest wall, pleura, or pericardium but not involving carina, nodes negative (T3 N0)
Stage IIIA	Tumor invading chest wall, pleura, or pericardium and nodes in hilum or ipsilateral mediastinum (T3, N1–2) or tumor of any size invading ipsilateral mediastinal or subcarinal nodes (T1–3, N2)
Stage IIIB	Direct extension to adjacent organs (esophagus, aorta, heart, cava, diaphragm, or spine); satellite nodule same lobe, or any tumor associated with contralateral mediastinal or supraclavicular lymph-node involvement (T4 or N3)
Stage IV	Separate nodule in different lobes or any tumor with distant metastases (M1)

Table 18-6

Cumulative Percentage of Survival by Stage After Treatment for Lung Cancer

	Time After Treatment	
Pathologic Stage	**24 Months**	**60 Months**
pT1N0M0 ($n = 511$)	86%	67%
pT2N0M0 ($n = 549$)	76%	57%
pT1N1M0 ($n = 76$)	70%	55%
pT2N1M0 ($n = 288$)	56%	39%
pT3N0M0 ($n = 87$)	55%	38%

in diameter have a significantly better prognosis than tumors 2.0 to 3.0 cm in diameter. The wide range of postoperative 5-year survival rates (5 to 25%) after surgical resection with N2 nodal involvement demonstrates the effect of the number and location of involved nodal stations, and of the presence of extracapsular nodal extension. Such variations within stages should help the surgeon tailor preoperative decision making to individual patients. Tumors confined to one lobe without hilar invasion are nearly always resectable by lobectomy.

Treatment

Early-Stage Disease. Early-stage disease is typically defined as stages I and II. In this group are T1 and T2 tumors (with or without local N1 nodal involvement), and T3 tumors (without N1 nodal involvement). This group represents a small proportion of the total number of patients diagnosed with lung cancer each year (about 15% of 150,000 patients).

The current standard of treatment is surgical resection, accomplished by lobectomy or pneumonectomy, depending on the tumor location. Despite the term "early-stage," surgery as a single treatment modality remains disappointing. After surgical resection of postoperative pathologic stage IA disease, 5-year survival is only 67% as reported by Mountain in 1997. The figures decline with higher stages. The overall 5-year survival rate for stage I disease as a group is about 65%; for stage II disease it is about 41%.

Appropriate surgical procedures for patients with early-stage disease include lobectomy, sleeve lobectomy, and occasionally pneumonectomy with mediastinal lymph node dissection or sampling. Sleeve resection is performed for tumors located at airway bifurcations when an acceptable length bronchial margin cannot be obtained by standard lobectomy. Pneumonectomy is rarely performed; it is indicated primarily for larger central tumors involving the distal main stem bronchus when a bronchial sleeve resection is not possible, and when resection of involved N1 lymph nodes cannot be achieved short of pneumonectomy. The latter circumstance occurs with bulky adenopathy or with extracapsular nodal spread.

Pancoast tumor (apical tumor) resection should always be preceded by mediastinoscopy. In general, the treatment of these tumors has evolved to a multimodal approach in which radiation plays a constant role. Typically, an induction radiation dose of 30 to 35 Gy is administered to enhance the probability of complete resection, followed by surgery 4 to 5 weeks later. With this approach, 5-year survival rates of 35% have been achieved. Surgical excision usually includes a portion of the lower trunk of the brachial plexus, the stellate ganglion, and the chest wall, along with lobectomy.

With chest wall involvement, en bloc chest wall resection, along with lobectomy, is performed, with or without chest wall reconstruction. For small rib resections or those posterior to the scapula, chest wall reconstruction is usually unnecessary. Larger defects (two rib segments or more) are usually reconstructed with Gore-Tex to provide chest wall contour and stability. T3 tumors with direct invasion of the diaphragm or pericardium are also resected en bloc with the involved structure. If a large portion of the right-sided pericardium is removed, reconstruction with thin Gore-Tex membrane will be required to prevent cardiac herniation and venous obstruction.

If a patient is deemed medically unfit for major pulmonary resection due to inadequate pulmonary reserve or other medical conditions, then options include limited surgical resection or radiotherapy. Limited resection, defined as segmentectomy or wedge resection, can only be applied to more peripheral T1 or T2 tumors. Moreover, limited resection is associated with an increased rate of local recurrence and a decreased long-term survival rate, probably due to incomplete resection of occult intrapulmonary lymphatic tumor spread. Alternatively, definitive radiotherapy consisting of a total dose of 60 to 65 Gy has resulted in a 5-year survival rate of about 30% for patients with stage I disease.

The role of chemotherapy in early-stage NSCLC is evolving. Postoperative adjuvant chemotherapy previously was of no benefit in multiple prospective randomized trials; however, newer, more effective agents have been of benefit, though the final results of current trials are pending. Similarly, prospective phase II studies have shown a potential benefit for preoperative (or induction) chemotherapy.

Locoregional Advanced Disease. Surgical resection as sole therapy has a limited role in stage III disease. T3N1 tumors can be treated with surgery alone and have a 5-year survival rate of approximately 25%. Patients with N2 disease are a heterogeneous group. Patients with clinically evident N2 disease (i.e., bulky adenopathy present on CT scan or mediastinoscopy, with lymph nodes often replaced by tumor) have a 5-year survival rate of 5 to 10% with surgery alone. In contrast, patients with microscopic N2 disease discovered incidentally in one lymph node station after surgical resection have a 5-year survival rate that may be as high as 30%. Surgery generally does not play a role in the care of patients with N3 disease (IIIB); however, it is occasionally appropriate in select patients with a T4 primary tumor (superior vena caval, carinal, or vertebral body involvement) and no N2 or N3 disease. Survival rates remain low for these patients.

Definitive radiotherapy as a single modality can cure patients with N2 or N3 disease, albeit in less than 10%. Recent improvement has been seen with three-dimensional conformal radiotherapy and altered fractionation. Such poor results are reflective of the facts that radiotherapy is a locoregional treatment, and that most stage III patients die of systemic disease.

Therefore, definitive treatment of stage III disease (when surgery is not felt to be feasible at any time) is usually a combination of chemotherapy and radiation. Two strategies for delivery are available. "Sequential" chemoradiation involves full-dose systemic chemotherapy (i.e., cisplatin combined with a second agent) followed by standard radiotherapy (approximately 60 Gy). The combination of chemotherapy followed by radiation has been shown to improve the 5-year survival rate to 17%, as compared with 6% with radiotherapy alone.

An alternative approach, referred to as "concurrent chemoradiation," is to administer chemotherapy and radiation at the same time. When certain chemotherapeutic agents are given at the same time as radiation, tumor cells become sensitized to the radiation, thus enhancing the radiation effect. The advantages of this approach are improved local control of the primary tumor and associated lymph nodes and a lack of delay in administering radiotherapy. A disadvantage, however, is the necessary reduction in chemotherapy dosage in order to diminish overlapping toxicities, which thereby can potentially lead to undertreatment of systemic micrometastases. Randomized trials have shown a modest 5-year survival benefit as compared with chemotherapy.

Preoperative (Induction) Chemotherapy for NSCLC. The use of chemotherapy before possible surgical resection has a number of potential advantages:

1. The tumor's blood supply is still intact, allowing better chemotherapy delivery and avoiding tumor cell hypoxia (in any residual microscopic tumor remaining postoperatively), which would increase radioresistance.
2. The primary tumor may be downstaged with enhanced resectability.
3. Patients are better able to tolerate chemotherapy before surgery.
4. It functions as an in vivo test of the primary tumor's sensitivity to chemotherapy.
5. Responders are identified, thereby allowing tailoring of additional therapy.
6. Systemic micrometastases are treated.

Potential disadvantages include:

1. A possible increase in the perioperative complication rate.
2. Definitive surgical therapy may be delayed if the tumor is resistant.

In stage IIIA N2 disease, the response rates to such chemotherapy are high—in the range of 70%. The treatment is generally safe, as it does not cause a significant increase in perioperative morbidity. Two randomized trials have now compared surgery alone for

Table 18-7
Results of Randomized Trials of Surgery vs. Neoadjuvant Chemotherapy Plus Surgery for Advanced-Stage Non-Small-Cell Lung Cancer

Trial	Patients	Resection Rate (%)	Median Survival (Months)	3-Year Survival Rate (%)
Rosell et al, 1994				
Surgery (+ XRT)	30	90	8	0
Chemo + Surgery (+ XRT)	29	85	26	29
Roth et al, 1998				
Surgery	32	66	11	15
Chemo + Surgery	28	61	64	56

Chemo = chemotherapy; XRT = radiation therapy.

SOURCE: Roth JA, Atkinson EN, Fossella F, et al: Long-term follow-up of patients enrolled in a randomized trial comparing perioperative chemotherapy and surgery with surgery alone in resectable stage IIIA non-small-cell lung cancer. *Lung Cancer* 21(1):1, 1998.

patients with N2 disease to preoperative chemotherapy followed by surgery. Both trials were stopped before complete accrual because of a significant increase in survival for the chemotherapy arm. The initially observed survival differences have been maintained up to 3 years and beyond (5-year data not shown) (Table 18-7). Given these results, induction chemotherapy with cisplatin-based regimens (two to three cycles) has become standard for patients with N2 disease. The role of surgery remains to be determined.

The use of induction chemotherapy in stage I and II disease is undergoing investigation. Preliminary results from phase II studies have suggested an improvement in survival with preoperative chemotherapy. The question is currently being investigated in a large intergroup, cooperative randomized trial.

Surgery in Stage IV Disease. The treatment of patients with stage IV disease is chemotherapy. However, on occasion, patients with a single site of metastasis are encountered, particularly with adenocarcinomas presenting with a solitary brain metastasis. In this highly select group, 5-year survival rates of 10 to 15% can be achieved with surgical excision of the brain metastasis and the primary tumor, assuming it is early-stage.

Small-Cell Lung Carcinoma. Small-cell lung carcinoma (SCLC) accounts for about 20% of primary lung cancers and is not generally treated surgically. These aggressive neoplasms have early widespread metastases. Histologically, they can be difficult to distinguish from lymphoproliferative lesions and atypical carcinoid tumors. Therefore a definitive diagnosis must be established with adequate tissue samples. Three groups of SCLC are recognized: pure small-cell carcinoma (sometimes referred to as oat cell carcinoma), small-cell carcinoma with a large-cell component, and combined (mixed) tumors.

Unlike NSCLC, clinical staging of SCLC is broadly defined by the presence of local or distant disease. Patients present without evidence of distant metastatic disease, but often have bulky locoregional disease, termed "limited" SCLC. Most often, the primary tumor is large and associated with bulky mediastinal adenopathy, which may lead to obstruction of the superior vena cava. The other clinical stage, disseminated, usually presents with widely disseminated metastatic disease. Patients in either stage are treated primarily with chemotherapy and radiation. Surgery is appropriate for the rare patient with an incidentally discovered peripheral nodule that is found to be SCLC. If a stage I SCLC is identified after resection, postoperative chemotherapy is usually given.

Metastatic Lesions to the Lung. The cause of a new pulmonary nodule(s) in a patient with a previous malignancy can be difficult to discern. Features suggestive of metastatic disease are multiplicity; smooth, round borders on CT scan; and temporal proximity to the original primary lesion. One must always entertain the possibility that a single new lesion is a primary lung cancer. The probability of a new primary cancer versus metastasis in patients presenting with solitary lesions depends on the type of initial neoplasm. The highest likelihood of a new primary lung cancer is in patients with a history of uterine (74%), bladder (89%), lung (92%), and head and neck (94%) carcinomas.

Surgical resection of pulmonary metastases has a role in properly selected patients. General principles of selection include the following: (1) the primary tumor must already be controlled; (2) the patient must be able to tolerate general anesthesia, potential single-lung ventilation, and the planned pulmonary resection; (3) the metastases must be completely resectable according to CT imaging; (4) there must be no evidence of extrapulmonary tumor burden; and (5) alternative superior therapy must be unavailable. The technical aim of pulmonary metastasis resections is complete resection of all macroscopic tumor. In addition, any adjacent structure involved should be resected en bloc (i.e., chest wall, diaphragm, and pericardium). Multiple lesions and/or hilar lesions may require lobectomy. Pneumonectomy is rarely justified or employed.

Pulmonary metastasis resection can be approached through a thoracotomy or via VATS techniques. McCormack and colleagues reported their experience at Memorial Sloan-Kettering in a prospective study of 18 patients who presented with no more than two pulmonary metastatic lesions and underwent VATS resection. A thoracotomy was performed during the same operation; if palpation identified any additional lesions, they were resected. The study concluded that the probability that a metastatic lesion will be missed by VATS excision is 56%. The patients in that study were evaluated by standard chest CT scan before the advent of spiral CT scanning. It remains a controversial topic whether metastasis resection should be performed via thoracotomy or VATS. Proponents of an open approach refer to the above referenced study. Proponents of VATS techniques argue that the resolution of spiral CT scanning is so far superior that any data using the old standard CT scan are no longer applicable; they also point to the significantly less pain and faster recovery using VATS. To date, no subsequent prospective study using spiral CT scan has been performed to resolve this clinical dilemma.

The best data regarding outcomes of resection of pulmonary metastases come from the International Registry of Lung Metastases (IRLM). The registry was established in 1991 by 18 thoracic surgery departments in Europe, the United States, and Canada, and included data on 5206 patients. About 88% of patients underwent complete resection. Survival analysis at 5, 10 and 15 years (grouping

Table 18-8
Actuarial Survival Data from the International Registry
of Lung Metastases

Survival	Complete Resection	Incomplete Resection
5-Year	36%	13%
10-Year	26%	7%
15-Year	22%	

all primary tumor types) was performed (Table 18-8). Multivariate analysis showed a better prognosis for patients with germ-cell tumors, osteosarcomas, a disease-free interval over 36 months, and a single metastasis.

Pulmonary Infections

Lung Abscess

A *lung abscess* is a localized area of pulmonary parenchymal necrosis caused by an infectious organism; tissue destruction results in a solitary or dominant cavity measuring at least 2 cm in diameter. Less often, there may be multiple, smaller cavities (<2 cm). In that case, the infection is typically referred to as a necrotizing pneumonia. An abscess that is present for more than 6 weeks is considered chronic.

Based on the (Table 18-9), lung abscesses are further classified as primary or secondary. A primary lung abscess occurs, for example, in immunocompromised patients (as a result of malignancy, chemotherapy, or an organ transplant, etc.), in patients as a result of highly virulent organisms inciting a necrotizing pulmonary infection, or in patients who have a predisposition to aspirate

Table 18-9
Causes of Lung Abscess

I. Primary
   A. Necrotizing pneumonia
      1. *S. aureus, Klebsiella, Pseudomonas, Mycobacterium*
      2. *Bacteroides, Fusobacterium, Actinomyces*
      3. *Entamoeba, Echinococcus*
   B. Aspiration pneumonia
      1. Anesthesia
      2. Stroke
      3. Drugs or alcohol
   C. Esophageal disease
      1. Achalasia, Zenker's diverticulum, gastroesophageal reflux
   D. Immunodeficiency
      1. Cancer (and chemotherapy)
      2. Diabetes
      3. Organ transplantation
      4. Steroid therapy
      5. Malnutrition
II. Secondary
   A. Bronchial obstruction
      1. Neoplasm
      2. Foreign body
   B. Systemic sepsis
      1. Septic pulmonary emboli
      2. Seeding of pulmonary infarct
   C. Complication of pulmonary trauma
      1. Infection of hematoma or contusion
      2. Contaminated foreign body or penetrating injury
   D. Direct extension from extraparenchymal infection
      1. Pleural empyema
      2. Mediastinal, hepatic, subphrenic abscess

SOURCE: Adapted from Schwartz SI, et al: Chest wall, pleura, and mediastinum, in *Principles of Surgery*, 7th ed. New York: McGraw Hill,1999, p.735.

oropharyngeal or gastrointestinal secretions. A secondary lung abscess occurs in patients with an underlying condition such as a partial bronchial obstruction, a lung infarct, or adjacent suppurative infections (subphrenic or hepatic abscesses).

The incidence of bacterial lung abscess in the United States has declined significantly over the past 50 years, with a concomitant decrease in the mortality rate from between 30 and 40% to between 5 and 10%. This decrease has been attributed to the development of bactericidal antibiotics. Factors associated with a worse outcome include advanced patient age, prolonged symptoms, comorbid disease, nosocomial infection, and perhaps larger cavity size. More recently, a greater proportion of lung abscesses have been associated with pulmonary malignancies or immunosuppression, resulting in an increase in lung abscesses due to unusual or opportunistic organisms.

Pathogenesis. Lung abscess is the result of a lower respiratory tract infection only by organisms that cause necrosis. Microorganisms gain access to the respiratory tract via inhalation of aerosolized particles, aspiration of oropharyngeal secretions, or hematogenous spread from distant sites. Direct extension from a contiguous site is less frequent. Most primary lung abscesses are suppurative bacterial infections secondary to aspiration. Risk factors for increased aspiration include conditions of impaired consciousness, suppressed cough reflex, dysfunctional esophageal motility, and centrally acting neurologic diseases (e.g., stroke). At the time of aspiration, the composition of the oropharyngeal flora determines the etiologic organisms; those organisms that are most numerous or virulent proliferate and emerge as single or predominant pathogens. Secondary lung abscesses occur most often distal to an obstructing bronchial carcinoma. Infected cysts or bullae are not considered true abscesses.

The characteristic pathologic features of aspiration pneumonia include alveolar edema and infiltration with inflammatory cells. Because of the effect of gravity, foci of infection tend to develop in the subpleural regions of the superior segments of the lower lobes and in the posterior segments of the upper lobes. The right lung is involved more frequently, presumably because of the less acute angle of the right main bronchus. Thus, the right upper and lower lobes are most commonly affected, followed by the left lower lobe and right middle lobe.

Microbiology. In community-acquired pneumonia, the causative bacteria are predominantly gram-positive; in hospital-acquired pneumonia, 60 to 70% of the organisms are gram-negative. Gram-negative bacteria associated with nosocomial pneumonia include *Klebsiella pneumoniae, Haemophilus influenzae, Proteus* species, *Pseudomonas aeruginosa, Escherichia coli, Enterobacter cloacae,* and *Eikenella corrodens.* Immunosuppressed patients may develop abscesses because of the usual pathogens as well as less virulent and opportunistic organisms such as *Salmonella* species, *Legionella* species, *Pneumocystis carinii,* atypical mycobacteria, and fungi.

Normal oropharyngeal secretions contain many more *Streptococcus* species and more anaerobes (about 10^8 organisms/mL) than aerobes (about 10^7 organisms/mL). Pneumonia that follows from aspiration, with or without abscess development, is typically polymicrobial. An average of two to four isolates present in large numbers have been cultured from lung abscesses sampled percutaneously. Overall, at least 50% of these infections are caused by purely anaerobic bacteria, 25% are caused by mixed aerobes and anaerobes, and 25% or fewer are caused by aerobes only.

Clinical Features and Diagnosis. The typical presentation may include productive cough, fever (>38.9°C), chills, leukocytosis (>15,000 cells/ mm³), weight loss, fatigue, malaise, pleuritic chest pain, and dyspnea. Lung abscesses may also present in a more indolent fashion, with weeks to months of cough, malaise, weight loss, low-grade fever, night sweats, leukocytosis, and anemia. After aspiration pneumonia, 1 to 2 weeks typically elapse before cavitation occurs; 40 to 75% of such patients produce a putrid,

foul-smelling sputum. Severe complications such as massive hemoptysis, endobronchial spread to other portions of the lungs, rupture into the pleural space and development of pyopneumothorax, or septic shock and respiratory failure are rare in the modern antibiotic era. The mortality rate is about 5 to 10%, except in the presence of immunosuppression, where rates range from 9 to 28%.

The chest radiograph is the primary tool for diagnosing a lung abscess (Fig. 18-21). Its distinguishing characteristic is a density

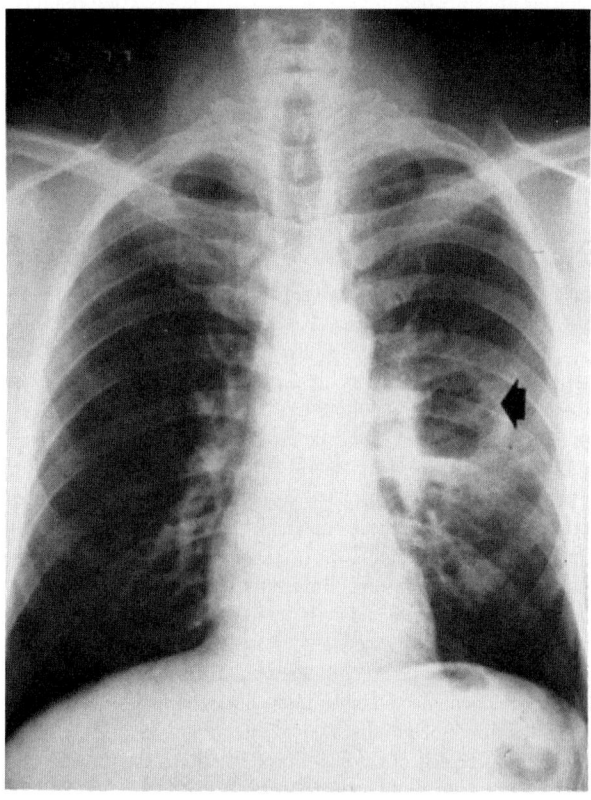

A

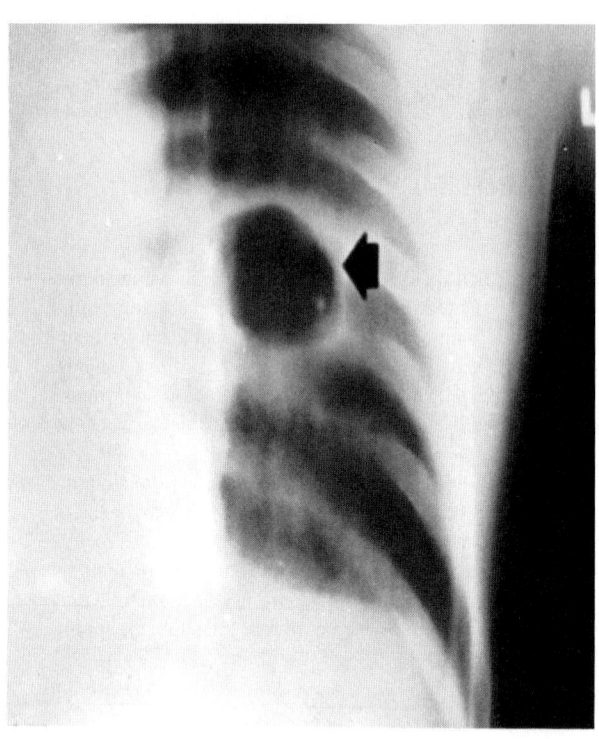

B

C

FIG. 18-21. Lung abscess resulting from emesis and aspiration after an alcoholic binge. *A.* Chest x-ray showing an abscess cavity in the left upper lobe. *B.* A coronal tomogram highlights the thin wall of the abscess. *C.* Healing of the abscess cavity after 4 weeks of antibiotic therapy and postural drainage.

or mass with a relatively thin-walled cavity. Frequently, an air-fluid level is observed within the abscess, indicating a communication with the tracheobronchial tree. A CT scan is useful to clarify the diagnosis when the radiograph is equivocal, to help rule out endobronchial obstruction, and to look for an associated mass or other pathologic anomalies. A cavitating lung carcinoma is frequently mistaken for a lung abscess. Other possible differential diagnoses include loculated or interlobar empyema, infected lung cysts or bullae, tuberculosis, bronchiectasis, fungal infections, and noninfectious inflammatory conditions (e.g., Wegener's granulomatosis).

The specific etiologic organism must be identified, ideally before antibiotic administration. Routine sputum cultures may be of limited usefulness because of contamination with upper respiratory tract flora. Bronchoscopy is essential to rule out endobronchial obstruction, which is usually due to a tumor, but occasionally is due to a foreign body. During bronchoscopy, uncontaminated cultures may be obtained by means of bronchoalveolar lavage. Culture samples can also be obtained by percutaneous, transthoracic FNA under ultrasound or CT guidance.

Management. Systemic antibiotics directed against the causative organism represent the mainstay of therapy. For community-acquired infections secondary to aspiration, likely pathogens are oropharyngeal streptococci and anaerobes. Penicillin G, ampicillin, or amoxicillin are the main therapeutic agents, but a beta-lactamase inhibitor or metronidazole should be added to cover the increasing prevalence of gram-negative anaerobes that produce beta-lactamase. Clindamycin is also a primary therapeutic agent. For hospital-acquired infections, *Staphylococcus aureus* and aerobic gram-negative bacilli are common organisms of the oropharyngeal flora. Piperacillin or ticarcillin with a beta-lactamase inhibitor (or equivalent alternatives) provide better coverage of likely pathogens. The duration of antimicrobial therapy is variable: 1 to 2 weeks for simple aspiration pneumonia and 3 to 12 weeks for necrotizing pneumonia and lung abscess. It is likely best to treat until the cavity is resolved or until serial radiographs show significant improvement. Parenteral therapy is generally used until the patient is afebrile and able to demonstrate consistent enteral intake. Oral therapy may then be needed.

Surgical drainage of lung abscesses is uncommon since drainage usually occurs spontaneously via the tracheobronchial tree. Indications for intervention include failure of medical therapy; an abscess under tension; an abscess increasing in size during appropriate treatment; contralateral lung contamination; an abscess larger than 4 to 6 cm in diameter; necrotizing infection with multiple abscesses, hemoptysis, abscess rupture, or pyopneumothorax; and inability to exclude a cavitating carcinoma. External drainage may be accomplished with tube thoracostomy, percutaneous drainage, or surgical cavernostomy. The choice between thoracostomy and radiologically-placed catheter drainage depends on the treating physician's preference and the availability of interventional radiology. Surgical resection is required in fewer than 10% of lung abscess patients. Lobectomy is the preferred intervention for bleeding from a lung abscess or pyopneumothorax. An important intraoperative consideration is to protect the contralateral lung with a double-lumen tube, bronchial blocker, or contralateral main stem intubation. Surgical treatment has a 90% success rate, with an associated mortality of 1 to 13%.

Bronchiectasis

Bronchiectasis is defined as a pathologic and permanent dilation of bronchi. This condition may be localized to certain bronchial segments or it may be diffuse throughout the bronchial tree, typically affecting the medium-sized airways. Overall, this is a rare clinical entity in the United States with a prevalence of less than 1 in 10,000.

Pathogenesis. Development of bronchiectasis can be attributed to either congenital or acquired causes. The principal congenital diseases that lead to bronchiectasis include cystic fibrosis, primary ciliary dyskinesia, and immunoglobulin deficiencies (e.g., selective IgA deficiency). Congenital causes tend to produce a diffuse pattern of bronchial involvement.

Acquired causes are categorized broadly as infectious and inflammatory. Adenoviruses and influenza viruses are the predominant childhood viral infections associated with the development of bronchiectasis. Chronic infection with tuberculosis remains an important worldwide cause of bronchiectasis. More significant in the United States is the occurrence of nontuberculous mycobacterial infections causing bronchiectasis, particularly *Mycobacterium avium* complex. Noninfectious causes of bronchiectasis include inhalation of toxic gases such as ammonia, which results in severe and destructive airway inflammatory responses. Allergic bronchopulmonary aspergillosis, Sjögren's syndrome, and alpha$_1$-antitrypsin deficiency are some additional examples of presumed immunologic disorders that may be accompanied by bronchiectasis.

The common pathway shared by all of these causes of bronchiectasis is impairment of airway defenses or deficits in immunologic mechanisms that permit bacterial colonization and establishment of chronic infection. Both the bacterial organisms and the inflammatory cells recruited to thwart the bacteria elaborate proteolytic and oxidative molecules, which progressively destroy the muscular and elastic components of the airway walls; those components are then replaced by fibrous tissue. Thus chronic airway inflammation is the essential pathologic feature of bronchiectasis. The dilated airways are usually filled with thick purulent material; more distal airways are often occluded by secretions or obliterated by fibrous tissue. The vascularity of affected bronchial walls increases, bronchial arteries become hypertrophied, and abnormal anastomoses form between the bronchial and pulmonary arterial circulation.

There are three principal types of bronchiectasis, based on pathologic morphology: cylindrical—uniformly dilated bronchi, varicose—an irregular or beaded pattern of dilated bronchi, and saccular (cystic)—peripheral balloon-type bronchial dilation. The saccular type is the most common after bronchial obstruction or infection (Fig. 18-22).

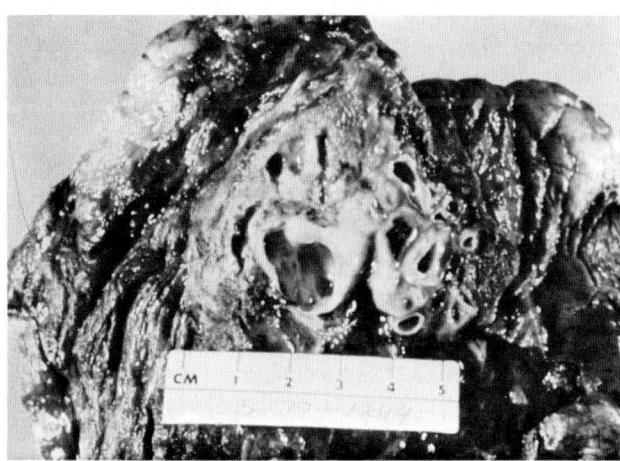

FIG. 18-22. Multiple cystic-type bronchiectatic cavities can be seen on a cut section of right lower lobe lung.

Clinical Manifestations and Diagnosis. A daily persistent cough and purulent sputum production are the typical symptoms of bronchiectasis. The quantity of daily sputum production (10 mL to >150 mL) tends to correlate with disease extent and severity. Often, patients with bronchiectasis may appear asymptomatic or have a dry nonproductive cough ("dry bronchiectasis"). These patients are prone to have involvement of the upper lobes. The clinical course is characterized by progressive symptoms and respiratory impairment. Increasing resting and exertional dyspnea are the result of progressive airway obstruction. Acute exacerbations may be triggered by viral or bacterial pathogens. Hemoptysis may become more frequent as the disease progresses, and bleeding is attributable to chronically inflamed, friable airway mucosa. In more advanced stages, massive bleeding may result from erosions of the hypertrophied bronchial arteries.

The current gold standard of diagnosis is chest CT scanning, which affords a highly-detailed, cross-sectional view of bronchial architecture. Both mild and severe forms of bronchiectasis are readily demonstrated with this imaging modality. A chest radiograph, although less sensitive, may reveal characteristic signs of bronchiectasis such as lung hyperinflation, bronchiectatic cysts, and dilated, thick-walled bronchi forming tram track–like patterns radiating from the lung hila. Sputum culture may identify characteristic pathogens including *H. influenzae, S. pneumoniae,* and *P. aeruginosa.* Sputum acid-fast bacillus smears and cultures should be performed to evaluate for the presence of nontuberculous mycobacteria, which may be common in this setting. The severity of airway obstruction should be determined with spirometry, which can also evaluate the course of disease.

Management. Standard therapy includes optimization of secretion clearance from the tracheobronchial tree, use of bronchodilators to reverse any airflow limitation, and correction of reversible underlying causes whenever possible. Chest physiotherapy based on vibration, percussion, and postural drainage is widely accepted as the basis for therapy. Acute exacerbations should be treated with courses of broad-spectrum antibiotics tailored to culture and sensitivity profiles. Usually, a 2- to 3-week course of intravenous antibiotics, followed by an oral regimen, will result in a longer-lasting remission. Surgical resection of a localized bronchiectatic segment or lobe may benefit patients with refractory symptoms while on maximal medical therapy. Multifocal disease must be excluded before any attempt at surgery; any uncorrectable predisposing factor (e.g., ciliary dyskinesia) also must be excluded. An important surgical tenet is to conserve as much normal parenchyma as possible. Patients with end-stage lung disease from bronchiectasis may be potential candidates for a bilateral lung transplant. Surgical resection is also indicated in patients with large hemoptysis secondary to hypertrophied bronchial arteries. Because resection may not always be clinically practical, bronchial artery embolization is an alternative.

Mycobacterial Infections

Epidemiology. Approximately 8 million new cases of tuberculosis are reported annually worldwide, which result in approximately 3 million deaths—more than for any other single infectious disease. In the United States, infection by mycobacteria is also a significant health problem, with an estimated 3 to 4% of infected individuals developing active disease within the first year, and 5 to 15% of all patients thereafter. During the 1980s the incidence of tuberculosis resurged, primarily related to the emergence of the acquired immunodeficiency syndrome (AIDS). More than 20,000 new cases of tuberculosis currently are reported annually in the United States.

More often, the elderly, minorities, and recent immigrants have clinical manifestations of infection, yet no age group, sex, or race is exempt from infection. In most large urban centers, reported cases of tuberculosis are more numerous among the homeless, prisoners, and drug-addicted populations. Immunocompromised patients additionally contribute to an increased incidence of tuberculosis infection, often developing unusual systemic as well as pulmonary manifestations. As compared with past decades, presently surgical intervention is required more frequently in patients with multiple-drug resistant tuberculosis organisms (MDRTB) who do not respond to medical treatment, and in selected patients with nontuberculous mycobacterial infections (NTM).

Microbiology. Mycobacterial species are obligate aerobes. They are primarily intracellular parasites with slow rates of growth. Their defining characteristic is the property of acid-fastness, which is the ability to withstand decolorization by an acid-alcohol mixture after being stained. *Mycobacterium tuberculosis* is the highly virulent bacillus of this species that produces invasive infection among humans, principally pulmonary tuberculosis. Because of improper application of antimycobacterial drugs and multifactorial interactions, MDRTB organisms have emerged that are defined by their resistance to two or more first-line antimycobacterial drugs. Approximately 10% of new tuberculosis cases, and as many as 40% of recurrent cases, are attributed to MDRTB organisms. The more important NTM organisms include *M. kansasii, M. avium* and *M. intracellulare* complex (MAC), and *M. fortuitum.* The highest incidence of *M. kansasii* infection is in midwestern U.S. cities among middle-aged males from good socioeconomic surroundings. MAC organisms are important infections in elderly and immunocompromised patient groups. *M. fortuitum* infections are common complications of underlying severe debilitating disease. None of these organisms are as contagious as *M. tuberculosis.*

Pathogenesis and Pathology. The main route of transmission is via airborne inhalation of viable mycobacteria. Three stages of primary infection have been described. In the first stage, alveolar macrophages ingest the bacilli. Infected macrophages release chemoattractants to recruit additional macrophages. In the second stage, from days 7 to 21, the bacteria continue to multiply in macrophages. The patient is often asymptomatic. The third stage is characterized by the onset of cell-mediated immunity (CD4$^+$ helper T cells) and delayed-type hypersensitivity. Activated macrophages acquire an increased capacity for bacterial killing. Macrophage death increases, resulting in the formation of a granuloma, the characteristic lesion found on pathologic examination.

Tuberculous granulomas are composed of blood-derived macrophages, degenerating macrophages or epithelioid cells, and multinucleated giant cells (which are fused macrophages with nuclei around the periphery), also called Langhans cells. T lymphocytes are found at the periphery of granulomas. Macrophage death results in central caseation. The low oxygen content of this environment inhibits macrophage function and bacillary growth. A Ghon complex is a single, small lung lesion that is often the only remaining trace of a primary infection. The primary infection is usually located in the peripheral portion of the middle zone of the lungs. Reactivation of tuberculosis infection may occur after hydrolytic enzymes liquify the caseum. Typically, the apical and posterior segments of the upper lobes and the superior segments of the lower lobes are involved. Edema, hemorrhage, and mononuclear cell infiltration are also present. The tuberculous cavity may become secondarily infected with other bacteria, fungi, or yeasts, all of which may contribute to enhanced tissue destruction.

The pathologic changes caused by NTM organisms are similar to those produced by *M. tuberculosis*. MAC infections not only commonly occur in immunocompromised patients, but also tend to develop in previously damaged lungs. Caseous necrosis is uncommon and is characterized by clusters of tissue macrophages filled with mycobacteria. It has a poor granulomatous response and confinement of immune cell infiltration to the interstitium and alveolar walls. Cavitary disease is infrequent, though nodules may be noted.

Clinical Presentation and Diagnosis. The clinical course of infection and the presentation of symptoms are influenced by many factors, including the site of primary infection, the stage of disease, and the degree of cell-mediated immunity. About 80 to 90% of tuberculosis patients present with clinical disease in the lungs. In 85 to 90% of these patients, involution and healing occur, leading to a dormant phase that may last a lifetime. The only evidence of tuberculosis infection may be a positive skin reaction to tuberculin challenge or a Ghon complex observed on chest radiograph. Within the first 2 years of primary infection, reactivation may occur in up to 10 to 15% of infected patients. In 80%, reactivation occurs in the lungs; other reactivation sites include the lymph nodes, pleura, and the musculoskeletal system.

After primary infection, pulmonary tuberculosis is frequently asymptomatic. Systemic symptoms of low-grade fever, malaise, and weight loss are subtle and may go unnoticed. A productive cough may develop, usually after tubercle cavitation. Many radiographic patterns can be identified at this stage, including local exudative lesions, local fibrotic lesions, cavitation, bronchial wall involvement, acute tuberculous pneumonia, bronchiectasis, bronchostenosis, and tuberculous granulomas. Hemoptysis often develops from complications of disease such as bronchiectasis or erosion into vascular malformations associated with cavitation. Extrapulmonary involvement is due to hematogenous or lymphatic spread from pulmonary lesions. Virtually any organ can become infected, giving rise to the protean manifestations of tuberculosis. Of note to the thoracic surgeon, the pleura, chest wall, and mediastinal organs may all be involved. More than one-third of immunocompromised patients have disseminated disease, with hepatomegaly, diarrhea, splenomegaly, and abdominal pain.

The definitive diagnosis of tuberculosis requires identification of the mycobacterium in a patient's bodily fluids or involved tissues. Skin testing using purified protein derivative is important for epidemiologic purposes, and can help exclude infection in uncomplicated cases. For pulmonary tuberculosis, sputum examination is inexpensive and has a high diagnostic yield. Bronchoscopy with alveolar lavage may also be a useful diagnostic adjunct and has high diagnostic accuracy. Chest CT scan can delineate the extent of parenchymal disease.

Management. Medical therapy is the primary treatment of pulmonary tuberculosis and is often initiated before a mycobacterial pathogen is definitively identified. Combinations of two or more drugs are routinely used in order to minimize resistance, which inevitably develops with only single-agent therapy. First-line drugs include isonicotinic acid hydrazine (isoniazid; INH), ethambutol, rifampin, and pyrazinamide. Second-line drugs include cycloserine, ethionamide, kanamycin, ciprofloxacin, and amikacin, among others. The initial therapy for patients with active pulmonary tuberculosis consists of various drug regimens lasting from 6 to 9 months. Bacterial sensitivity profiles help to tailor drug therapy. In the case of

MDRTB organisms, four or more antimycobacterial drugs are often used, generally for 18 to 24 months. Rifampin and INH augmented with one or more second-line drugs are most commonly used to treat NTM infections. Generally, therapy lasts about 18 months. The overall response rate is unsatisfactory in 20 to 30% of patients with *M. kansasii* infection, though most such patients do not require surgical intervention. In contrast, pulmonary MAC infections respond poorly, even to combinations of four or more drugs, thus most such patients become surgical candidates. Overall, sputum conversion is achieved in only 50 to 80% of NTM infections, and relapses occur in up to 20% of patients.

In the United States, surgical intervention is most often required in order to treat patients with MDRTB organisms whose lungs have been destroyed and who have persistent thick-walled cavitation. The indications for surgery related to mycobacterial pulmonary infections are as follows: (1) complications resulting from previous thoracic surgery to treat tuberculosis; (2) failure of optimized medical therapy (e.g., progressive disease, lung gangrene, or intracavitary aspergillosis superinfection); (3) tissue acquisition for a definitive diagnosis; (4) complications of pulmonary scarring (e.g., massive hemoptysis, cavernomas, bronchiectasis, or bronchostenosis); (5) extrapulmonary thoracic involvement; (6) pleural tuberculosis; and (7) NTM infections. The governing principle of mycobacterial surgery is to remove all gross disease while preserving any uninvolved lung tissue. Scattered nodular disease may be left intact, given its low mycobacterial burden. Antimycobacterial medications should be given preoperatively (for about 3 months) and continued postoperatively for 12 to 24 months. Overall, more than 90% of patients who were deemed good surgical candidates are cured when appropriate medical and surgical therapy is used.

Actinomycetic Infections

Actinomycosis. Members of the families Actinomycetaceae and Nocardiaceae were once considered fungi, but now are classified as bacteria. Actinomycosis is a chronic disease usually caused by *Actinomyces israelii*. It is characterized by chronic suppuration, sinus formation, and discharge of purulent material containing yellow-brown sulfur granules. About 15% of infections involve the thorax; organisms enter the lungs via the oral cavity (where they normally reside) of humans. The diagnosis is challenging because the disease is uncommon and thus not often suspected and appropriately cultured under anaerobic conditions. Lung involvement can present with progressive pulmonary fibrosis in the periphery. Pleural and chest wall involvement (periostitis of the ribs) is an associated finding. Prolonged, high-dose penicillin is effective. Because of an intense fibrotic reaction surrounding affected parenchyma, surgery is seldom possible.

Nocardiosis. *Nocardia asteroides* is an aerobic, acid-fast, gram-positive organism that usually causes nocardiosis, a disease similar to actinomycosis with additional CNS involvement. Additionally, hematogenous dissemination from a pulmonary focus may lead to generalized systemic infection. The disease process ranges from benign, self-limited suppuration of skin and subcutaneous tissues, to pulmonary (extensive parenchymal necrosis and abscesses) and systemic (e.g., CNS) manifestations. In immunosuppressed patients, pulmonary cavitation or hematogenous dissemination may be accelerated. Prolonged treatment (2 to 3 months) with sulfadiazine, minocycline, or trimethoprim-sulfamethoxazole is typically required. Surgery to drain abscesses and empyema is indicated.

Pulmonary Mycoses

An important differential diagnosis to consider in thoracic pathology in general is a mycotic lung infection that can mimic a bronchial carcinoma or tuberculosis. Most fungi are secondary or opportunistic pathogens that cause pulmonary and systemic infections in humans only when natural host resistance is impaired. Clinically significant examples include species of *Aspergillus, Cryptococcus, Candida,* and *Mucor.* However, some fungi are primary or true pathogens, able to cause infections in otherwise healthy patients. Some endemic examples in the United States include species of *Histoplasma, Coccidioides,* and *Blastomyces.*

The incidence of fungal infections has increased significantly, with many new opportunistic fungi emerging. This increase is attributed to the growing population of immunocompromised patients (i.e., organ transplant recipients, cancer patients undergoing chemotherapy, human immunodeficiency virus [HIV] patients, and young and elderly patients) who are more likely to become infected with fungi. Other at-risk patient populations include those who are malnourished, severely debilitated, diabetic, or who have hematologic disorders. Patients receiving high-dose, intensive antibiotic therapy are also susceptible. Fungal infections are definitively diagnosed by directly identifying the organism in body exudates or tissues, preferably grown in culture. Serologic testing to identify mycotic-specific antibodies may also be a useful diagnostic tool. Several new classes of antifungal agents are now available that are effective against many life-threatening fungi and are less toxic than older agents. Thoracic surgery may be a useful therapeutic adjunct for patients with pulmonary mycoses.

Aspergillosis. The genus *Aspergillus* comprises over 350 species, three of which are most commonly responsible for clinical disease: *A. fumigatus, A. flavus,* and *A. niger. Aspergillus* is a saprophytic, filamentous fungus with septate hyphae. Spores (2.5 to 3 μm in diameter) are released and easily inhaled by susceptible patients; the spores then are able to reach the distal bronchi and alveoli. Aspergillosis can manifest as one of three clinical syndromes: *Aspergillus* hypersensitivity lung disease, aspergilloma, or invasive pulmonary aspergillosis. Overlap occurs between these syndromes, depending on the patient's immune status. Hypersensitivity results in productive cough, fever, wheezing, lung infiltrates, eosinophilia, and elevation of IgE antibodies to *Aspergillus.*

Aspergilloma (fungal ball) tends to colonize preexisting cavities and is a matted sphere of hyphae, fibrin, and inflammatory cells, that grossly appears as a round or oval, friable, gray (or red, brown, or even yellow), necrotic-looking mass (Fig. 18-23). This form is the most common presentation of (noninvasive) pulmonary aspergillosis. The clinical features vary, with some patients remaining asymptomatic. Hemoptysis is most commonly associated with aspergilloma, followed by chronic and productive cough, clubbing, malaise, or weight loss. Sometimes the diagnosis is suggested by a routine chest radiograph, on which a crescentic radiolucency above a rounded radiopaque lesion (Monad sign) is observed. Therapy should be individualized; asymptomatic aspergilloma does not require treatment. For mild, non-life-threatening hemoptysis, initial treatment can be medical management. Amphotericin B is the drug of choice. Indications for surgical intervention include recurrent or massive hemoptysis, chronic cough with systemic symptoms, progressive infiltrate around the mycetoma, and a pulmonary mass of unknown cause. The goal of surgery is to encompass all diseased tissue with a limited pulmonary resection. The postresectional residual space in the thorax should be obliterated. Techniques to do so include pleural tent, pneumoperitoneum, decortication, muscle flap, omental transposition, and thoracoplasty. Long-term follow-up is necessary, given that the recurrence rate after surgery is about 7%.

Invasive pulmonary aspergillosis typically affects immunocompromised patients who have dysfunctional cellular immunity, namely defective polymorphonuclear leukocytes. Invasion of pulmonary parenchyma and blood vessels by a necrotizing bronchopneumonia may be complicated by thrombosis, hemorrhage, and then dissemination. Patients present with fever that is nonresponsive to antibiotic therapy in the setting of neutropenia. They may also have pleuritic chest pain, cough, dyspnea, or hemoptysis. A chest CT scan, in addition to routine radiography, may reveal finer details of the infective process and characteristic signs (e.g., halo sign and cavitary lesions). Empiric antifungal therapy (using amphotericin B) should be started in these high-risk patients. The mortality rate is high, ranging from 93 to 100% in bone marrow transplant recipients, to approximately 38% in kidney transplant recipients. To minimize the neutropenic period (which contributes to uncontrolled disease), hematopoietic growth factors may be considered. Surgical removal of the infectious nidus is advocated by some groups because medical treatment has such poor outcomes.

Cryptococcosis. Cryptococcosis is a subacute or chronic infection caused by *Cryptococcus neoformans,* a round, budding yeast (5 to 20 μm in diameter) that is sometimes surrounded by a characteristic wide gelatinous capsule. Cryptococci are typically present in soil and dust contaminated by pigeon droppings. When inhaled, such droppings can cause a nonfatal disease primarily affecting the pulmonary and central nervous systems. At present, cryptococcosis is the fourth most common opportunistic infection in patients with HIV infection, affecting 6 to 10% of that population. Four basic pathologic patterns are seen in the lungs of infected patients: granulomas; granulomatous pneumonia; diffuse alveolar or interstitial involvement; and proliferation of fungi in alveoli and lung vasculature. Symptoms are nonspecific, as are the radiographic findings. *Cryptococcus* may be isolated from sputum, bronchial washings, percutaneous needle aspiration of the lung, or cerebrospinal fluid. Multiple antifungal agents are effective against *C. neoformans,* including amphotericin B and the azoles.

Candidiasis. *Candida* organisms are oval, budding cells (with or without mycelial elements) that colonize the oropharynx of many healthy individuals. The fungi of this genus are common hospital and laboratory contaminants. Usually, *Candida albicans* causes disease in the oral or bronchial mucosa, among other anatomic sites. Other potentially pathogenic *Candida* species include *C. tropicalis, C. glabrata,* and *C. krusei.* An acute or chronic granulomatous reaction may result. Less common is the development of systemic or disseminated infections; these fungi can invade blood vessel walls and multiple tissues. The incidence of *Candida* infections has increased and they no longer are confined to immunocompromised patients, but now affect patients who are critically ill for prolonged duration, are taking multiple antibiotics long-term, have indwelling vascular catheters (or urinary catheters), sustain recurrent gastrointestinal perforations, or have burn wounds. With respect to the thorax, such patients commonly have candidal pneumonia, pulmonary abscess, esophagitis, and mediastinitis. Amphotericin B, often in combination with 5-fluorocytosine, is a proven therapeutic treatment for *Candida* tissue infections. In randomized trials, fluconazole has been found to be equally effective with less toxicity. For patients with *Candida* mediastinitis (which has a mortality rate over 50%),

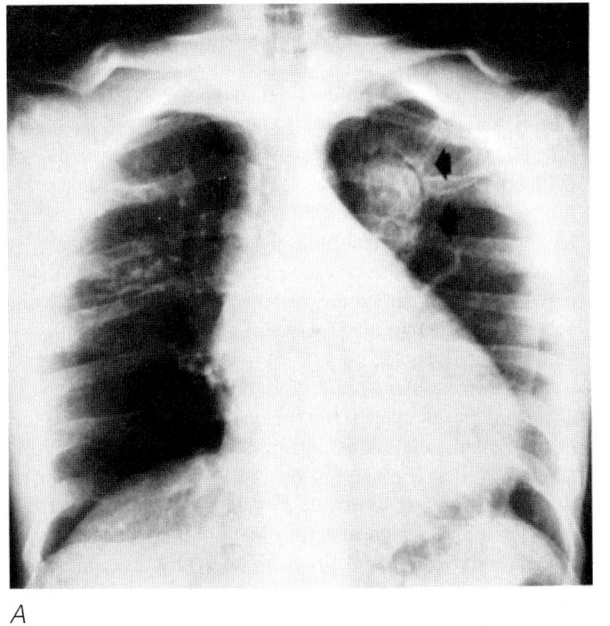

A

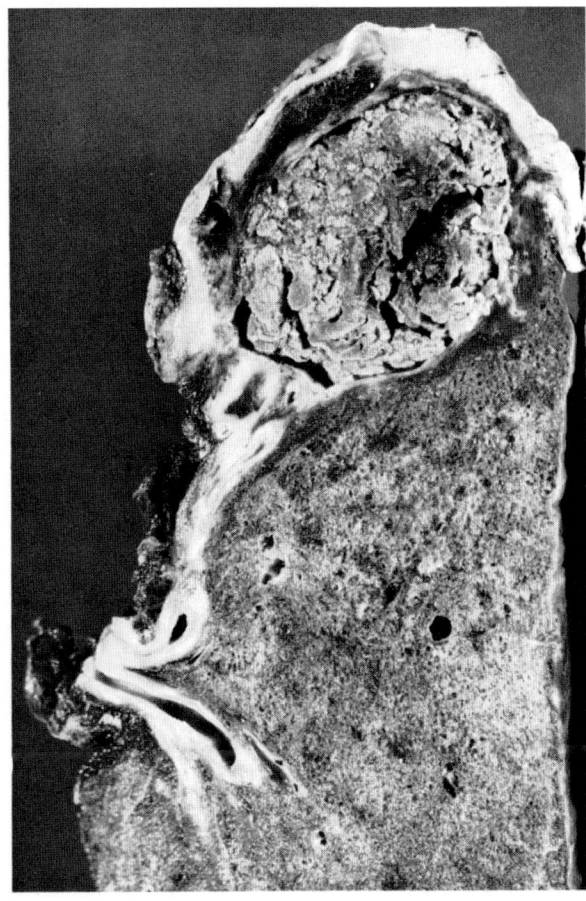

B

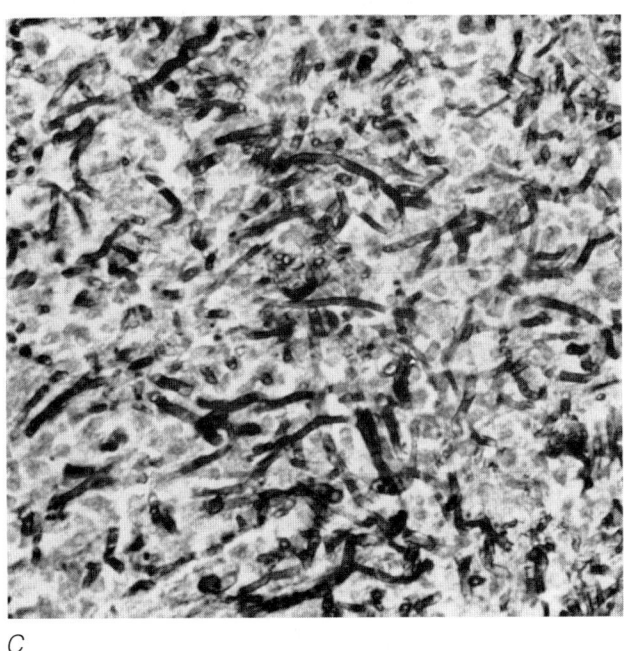

C

FIG. 18-23. *Pulmonary aspergilloma. A. The chest x-ray shows a solid mass within a cavity surrounded by a rim of air between the mass and cavity wall (Monad sign, arrows). B. A cut section shows the "fungus ball" occupying an old, fibrotic cavity. C. Histologic stain reveals characteristic Aspergillus hyphae invading the wall of the cavity.*

surgical intervention to débride all infected tissues is required, in addition to prolonged administration of antifungal drugs.

Mucormycosis. The *Mucor* species, rare members of the class Zygomycetes, are responsible for rapidly fatal disease in immunocompromised patients. Other disease-causing species of the class Zygomycetes include *Absidia, Rhizopus,* and *Mortierella.* Characteristic of these fungi are nonseptate, branching hyphae that are difficult to culture. Infection occurs via inhalation of spores. Neutropenia, acidosis, diabetes, and hematologic malignancy all predispose patients to clinical susceptibility. In the lungs, disease consists of blood vessel invasion, thrombosis, and infarction of infected organs. Tissue destruction is significant, along with cavitation and abscess formation. Initial treatment is to correct underlying risk factors and administer amphotericin B, although the optimal

duration and optimal total dose are unknown. Surgical resection of any localized disease should be performed after initial medical treatment attempts fail.

Primary Fungal Pathogens. *Histoplasma capsulatum* is a dimorphic fungus existing in mycelial form in soil contaminated by fowl or bat excreta, and in yeast form in human hosts. Histoplasmosis primarily affects the respiratory system after spores are inhaled. It is the most common of all fungal pulmonary infections. In the United States, this disease is endemic in the Midwest and Mississippi River Valley, where about 500,000 new cases arise each year. Active, symptomatic disease is uncommon. Acute forms of the disease present as primary or disseminated pulmonary histoplasmosis; chronic forms present as pulmonary granulomas (histoplasmomas), chronic cavitary histoplasmosis, mediastinal granulomas, fibrosing mediastinitis, or broncholithiasis. In immunocompromised patients, the infection becomes systemic and more virulent; because cell-mediated immunity is impaired, uninhibited fungal proliferation occurs within pulmonary macrophages and then spreads. Histoplasmosis is definitively diagnosed by fungal smear, culture, direct biopsy of infected tissues, or serologic testing.

The clinical presentation depends on the inoculum size and on host factors. Patients with acute pulmonary histoplasmosis commonly present with fever, chills, headache, chest pain, musculoskeletal pain, and nonproductive cough. Chest radiographs may be normal or may show mediastinal lymphadenopathy and patchy parenchymal infiltrates. Most patients improve in a few weeks and do not require antifungal therapy. Amphotericin B is the treatment of choice if moderate symptoms persist for 2 to 4 weeks; if the illness is extensive, including dyspnea and hypoxia; and if patients are immunosuppressed.

As the pulmonary infiltrates from acute histoplasmosis heal, consolidation into a solitary nodule or histoplasmoma may occur. This condition is asymptomatic and is usually seen incidentally on radiographs as a coin-shaped lesion. Central calcification may occur; if so, no further treatment is required. Noncalcification of the lesion requires further diagnostic work-up including chest CT scan, needle biopsy, or surgical excision to rule out a malignancy.

When lymph nodes and pulmonary granulomas calcify over time, pressure atrophy on the bronchial wall may result in erosion and migration of the granulomatous mass into the bronchus, causing broncholithiasis. Typical symptoms include cough, hemoptysis, and dyspnea. Life-threatening complications include massive hemoptysis or bronchoesophageal fistula. In addition to radiography, bronchoscopy should be performed to aid in diagnosis. Definitive treatment is surgical; the bronchial mass should be removed and any associated complications repaired.

Chronic cavitary histoplasmosis occurs in about 10% of patients who become symptomatic after infection. Most such patients have preexisting lung pathology such as COPD or emphysema. Colonization of diseased lung spaces occurs as the ongoing pneumonitis and necrosis that are characteristic of this disease lead to cavity enlargement, new cavity formation, and eventually spread to other areas of lung. Nonspecific symptoms are common, such as cough, sputum production, fever, weight loss, weakness, and hemoptysis. Cavitation, scarring, and partial resolution may be observed on radiographs. Itraconazole or ketoconazole can effectively treat this condition, although more severe infection may require amphotericin B. Surgical excision of localized thick-walled cavities unresponsive to courses of antifungal therapy should be considered if pulmonary reserve is adequate. Disseminated histoplasmosis presents as a spectrum of illness, ranging from nonspecific signs of fever, weight loss, and malaise, to shock, respiratory distress, and multiorgan failure. Use of amphotericin B has decreased the mortality rate to less than 25% in this type of serious infection.

Coccidioides immitis is an endemic fungus found in soil and dust of the southwestern United States. Infection results from inhalation of spores (arthroconidia), which individually swell into spherules that later subdivide into endospores. Positive culture results from sputum, other body fluid, or tissue are necessary for a definitive diagnosis. Acute pulmonary coccidioidomycosis occurs in about 40% of people who inhale spores. Symptoms consist of fever, sweating, anorexia, weakness, arthralgia, cough, sputum, and chest pain. When symptoms and radiographic findings persist for more than 6 to 8 weeks, the disease is considered to be persistent coccidioidal pneumonia. Caseous nodules, effusions, pneumonic areas, cavities, and calcified, fibrotic, or ossified lesions may be observed on chest radiographs. In a small minority of infected patients (0.5%) extrapulmonary disease may develop, with involvement of meninges, bones, joints, skin, or soft tissues. Immunocompromised patients are especially susceptible to disseminated coccidioidomycosis, which carries a mortality rate over 40%. Itraconazole and fluconazole are effective treatments for patients with mild to moderate disease with evidence of pulmonary cavitation or progressive chronic pulmonary lesions. Amphotericin B is warranted for patients with severe pulmonary or disseminated disease and for immunocompromised patients. Surgical resection by lobectomy may be considered if cavities persist for more than 2 years, are larger than 2 cm in diameter, rapidly enlarge, rupture, are thick-walled, or are associated with severe or recurrent hemoptysis.

Blastomyces dermatitidis is a round, single-budding yeast with a characteristic thick, refractile cell wall. It primarily infects the lungs of people who inhale contaminated soil that has been disturbed. Cutaneous and disseminated forms of blastomycosis also occur. *B. dermatitidis* has a worldwide distribution; in the United States it is endemic in the central states. The organism induces a granulomatous and pyogenic reaction with microabscesses and giant cells; caseation, cavitation, and fibrosis may also occur. Symptoms are nonspecific and include cough, mucoid sputum production, chest pain, fever, malaise, weight loss, and hemoptysis. In acute disease, consolidation is usually noted on radiographs; in chronic disease, fibronodular lesions (with or without cavitation) that are similar to tuberculosis are noted. Oral itraconazole for 6 months is the treatment of choice for most patients. Amphotericin B is warranted for patients with cavitary blastomycosis, disseminated disease, or extensive lung involvement and immunocompromised patients. After adequate drug therapy, surgical resection of known cavitary lesions should be considered because viable organisms are known to persist in such lesions.

Antifungals. Limitations in the treatment of fungal pneumonias still exist. Several antifungal agents are available and others are under study. Amphotericin B, a by-product of the actinomycete *Streptomyces nodosus,* has served as the mainstay for deep, systemic fungal infections. A complex lipophilic organic compound or polyene, amphotericin B binds to ergosterol in the cell membranes of fungi, causing disruption and ion leakage. However, nephrotoxicity limits its usefulness and applicability. Three lipid-based formulations of amphotericin B have now shown decreased nephrotoxicity and higher drug-dose delivery. Higher costs and limited data concerning better efficacy have tempered widespread adoption of these three drugs as first-line antifungal therapy. Susceptible fungi convert 5-fluorocytosine (flucytosine) to 5-fluorouracil, which inhibits DNA and RNA synthesis. Flucytosine is commonly used in combination with amphotericin B in patients with cryptococcal or candidal infections, in order to decrease the amount of amphotericin B necessary. The azole compounds include miconazole, ketoconazole, fluconazole, and itraconazole. This class of drugs inhibits the enzyme cytochrome P450, thereby interfering with fungal cell membrane synthesis; lanosterol is not converted to ergosterol, a necessary fungal component.

Echinocandins are a new class of antifungals that inhibit cell wall synthesis by interfering with glucan synthesis. Caspofungin is the first echinocandin to be approved by the U.S. Food and Drug Administration (FDA) for the treatment of invasive pulmonary aspergillosis that is refractory to first-line agents. The most common associated side effects include fever, nausea, vomiting, and infusion-related venous effects. In vitro, it has activity against *Candida* species, but human clinical trial results have not been published. It is likely that this class of antifungals will become an integral part of the management of candidiasis. Newer triazole antifungal agents with improved activity against *Aspergillus, Candida,* and *Histoplasma* species have been introduced. Voriconazole is the first such drug to be introduced into the clinical setting. Randomized trials need to be completed to establish its precise clinical applicability. Side effects include hepatotoxicity and visual disturbances.

Massive Hemoptysis

Massive hemoptysis is generally defined as expectoration of over 600 mL of blood within a 24-hour period. It is a medical emergency associated with a mortality rate of 30 to 50%. Most clinicians would agree that losing over a liter of blood via the airway within 1 day is significant, yet use of an absolute volume criterion presents difficulties. First, it is difficult for the patient or caregivers to quantify the volume of blood being lost. Second, and most relevant, the rate of bleeding necessary to incite respiratory compromise is highly dependent on the individual's prior respiratory status. For example, the loss of 100 mL of blood over 24 hours in a 40-year-old male with normal pulmonary function would be of little immediate consequence, because his normal cough would ensure his ability to clear the blood and secretions. In contrast, the same amount of bleeding in a 69-year-old male with severe COPD, chronic bronchitis, and an FEV_1 of 1.1 L may be life-threatening.

Anatomy

The lungs have two sources of blood supply: the pulmonary and bronchial arterial systems. The pulmonary system is a high-compliance, low-pressure system, and the walls of the pulmonary arteries are very thin and delicate. The bronchial arteries, part of the systemic circulation, have systemic pressures and thick walls; most branches originate from the proximal thoracic aorta. Most cases of massive hemoptysis involve bleeding from the bronchial artery circulation or from the pulmonary circulation pathologically exposed to the high pressures of the bronchial circulation. In many cases of hemoptysis, particularly those due to inflammatory disorders, the bronchial arterial tree becomes hyperplastic and tortuous. The systemic pressures within these arteries, combined with a disease process within the airway and erosion, lead to bleeding.

Causes

Significant hemoptysis has many causes, the most common of which are shown in Fig. 18-24. Most are secondary to inflammatory processes. An acute necrotizing pneumonic infection can lead to destruction and erosion of vascular structures and bleeding. Chronic inflammatory disorders (i.e., bronchiectasis, cystic fibrosis, tuberculosis, and others) lead to localized bronchial arterial proliferation, and with erosion, bleeding of these hypervascular areas occurs.

Tuberculosis also can cause hemoptysis by erosion of a broncholith (a calcified tuberculous lymph node) into a vessel, or when a tuberculous cavity is present, by erosion of a blood vessel within the cavity. Within such cavities, aneurysms of the pulmonary artery (referred to as Rasmussen's aneurysm) can develop that are accompanied by subsequent erosion and massive bleeding.

Hemoptysis due to lung cancer is usually mild, resulting in blood-streaked sputum. Massive hemoptysis in patients with lung cancer is typically caused by malignant invasion of pulmonary artery vessels by large central tumors; although rare, it is often a terminal event.

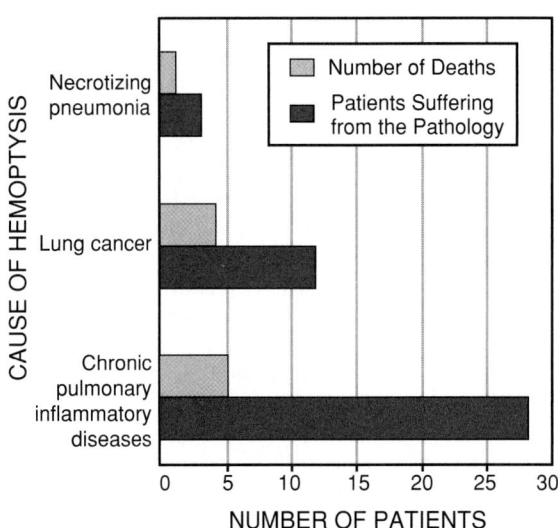

FIG. 18-24. *Cause of massive hemoptysis and in-hospital mortality. (Adapted with permission from Jougon J, Ballester M, Delcambre F, et al: Massive hemoptysis: What place for medical and surgical treatment. Eur J Cardiothorac Surg 22:345, 2002.)*

Management

The treatment of patients with life-threatening hemoptysis is best managed by a multidisciplinary team of intensive care physicians, interventional radiologists, and thoracic surgeons. Treatment priorities are as follows: (1) achieve respiratory stabilization and prevent asphyxiation, (2) localize the bleeding site, (3) stop the hemorrhage, (4) determine the cause, and (5) definitively prevent recurrence. The clinically pragmatic definition of massive hemoptysis is a degree of bleeding that threatens respiratory stability. Therefore clinical judgment of the risk of respiratory compromise is the first step in evaluating a patient. Two scenarios are possible: (1) bleeding is significant and persistent, but its rate allows a rapid but sequential diagnostic and therapeutic approach, and (2) bleeding is so rapid that emergency airway control and therapy are necessary.

Scenario 1: Significant, Persistent, But Nonmassive Bleeding. Although bleeding is brisk in scenario 1, the patient may be able to maintain clearance of the blood and secretions with his or her own respiratory reflexes. Immediate measures are admission to an intensive care unit, strict bedrest, Trendelenburg positioning with the affected side down (if known), administration of humidified oxygen, monitoring of oxygen saturation and arterial blood gases, and insertion of large-bore intravenous catheters. Strict bedrest with sedation may lead to slowing or cessation of bleeding, and the judicious use of intravenous narcotics or other relaxants to mildly sedate the patient and diminish some of the reflexive airway activity is often necessary. Also recommended are administration of aerosolized adrenaline, intravenous antibiotic therapy if needed, and correction of abnormal blood coagulation study results. Finally, unless contraindicated, intravenous vasopressin (20 U over 15 minutes, followed by an infusion of 0.2 U/min) can be given.

A chest x-ray is the first test, and often proves to be the most revealing. Localized lesions may be seen, but the effects of blood soiling of other areas of the lungs may predominate, obscuring the area of pathology. Chest CT scan provides more detail and is nearly always performed if the patient is stable. Pathologic areas may be obscured by blood soiling.

Flexible bronchoscopy is the next step in evaluating the patient's condition. Some clinicians argue that rigid bronchoscopy should always be performed. However, if the patient is clinically stable and the ongoing bleeding is not imminently threatening, flexible bronchoscopy is appropriate. It allows diagnosis of airway abnormalities and will usually permit localization of the bleeding site to either a lobe or even a segment. The person performing the bronchoscopy must be prepared with excellent suction and must be able to perform saline lavage with a dilute solution of epinephrine.

Most cases of massive hemoptysis arise from the bronchial arterial tree; therefore the next therapeutic option frequently is selective bronchial arteriography and embolization. Prearteriogram bronchoscopy is extremely useful to direct the angiographer. However, if bronchoscopy fails to localize the bleeding site, then bilateral bronchial arteriograms can be performed. Typically, the abnormal vascularity is visualized, rather than extravasation of the contrast dye. Embolization will acutely arrest the bleeding in 80 to 90% of patients. However, 30 to 60% of patients will have recurrences. Therefore, embolization should be viewed as an immediate but likely temporizing measure to acutely control bleeding. Subsequently, definitive treatment of the underlying pathologic process is appropriate. If bleeding persists after embolization, a pulmonary artery source should be suspected and a pulmonary angiogram performed.

If respiratory compromise is impending, orotracheal intubation should be performed. After intubation, flexible bronchoscopy should be performed to clear blood and secretions and to attempt localization of the bleeding site. Depending on the possible causes of the bleeding, bronchial artery embolization or (if appropriate) surgery can be considered.

Scenario 2: Significant, Persistent, and Massive Bleeding. Life-threatening bleeding requires emergency airway control and preparation for potential surgery. Such patients are best cared for in an operating room equipped with rigid bronchoscopy. Immediate orotracheal intubation may be necessary to gain control of ventilation and suctioning. However, rapid transport to the operating room with rigid bronchoscopy should be facilitated. Rigid bronchoscopy allows adequate suctioning of bleeding with visualization of the bleeding site; the nonbleeding side can be cannulated with the rigid scope and the patient ventilated. After stabilization, ice-saline lavage of the bleeding site can then be performed (up to 1 L in 50-mL aliquots); bleeding stops in up to 90% of patients.

Alternatively, blockade of the main stem bronchus of the affected side can be accomplished with a double-lumen endotracheal tube, with a bronchial blocker, or by intubation of the nonaffected side by an uncut standard endotracheal tube. Placement of a double-lumen endotracheal tube is challenging in these circumstances, given the bleeding and secretions. Proper placement and suctioning may be difficult, and attempts could compromise the patient's ventilation. The best option is to place a bronchial blocker in the affected bronchus with inflation. The blocker is left in place for 24 hours and the area is reexamined bronchoscopically. After this 24-hour period, bronchial artery embolization can be performed.

Surgical Intervention. In most patients, bleeding can be stopped, recovery can occur, and plans to definitively treat the underlying cause can be made. In scenario 1 (significant, persistent, but nonmassive bleeding), the patient may undergo further evaluation as an inpatient or outpatient. A chest CT scan and pulmonary function studies should be obtained preoperatively. In scenario 2 (patients with significant, persistent, and massive bleeding), surgery, if

appropriate, will usually be performed during the same hospitalization as the rigid bronchoscopy or main stem bronchus blockade. In less than 10% of patients, emergency surgery will be necessary, delayed only by efforts to localize the bleeding site by rigid bronchoscopy.

Surgical treatment is individualized according to the source of bleeding and the patient's medical condition, prognosis, and pulmonary reserve. General indications for urgent surgery include (1) presence of a fungus ball, (2) a lung abscess, (3) significant cavitary disease, or (4) failure to control the bleeding. In patients with significant cavitary disease or with fungus balls, the walls of the cavities are eroded and necrotic; rebleeding will likely ensue. In addition, bleeding from cavitary lesions may be due to pulmonary artery erosion, which requires surgery for control.

End-Stage Lung Disease

Lung Volume Reduction Surgery

Lung volume reduction surgery (LVRS) was originally described by Brantigan in the late 1950s, and the procedure was resurrected and refined by Cooper and associates in 1993. As described by Cooper, the ideal patient for LVRS has heterogeneous emphysema with apical predominance, meaning the worst emphysematous changes are in the apex (seen on chest CT scan) of both lungs. The physiologic lack of function of these areas is demonstrated by quantitative perfusion scan, which shows minimal or no perfusion. By surgically excising these nonfunctional areas, the volume of the lung is reduced, theoretically restoring respiratory mechanics. Diaphragm position and function are improved, and there may be an improvement in the dynamic small airway collapse in the remaining lung. After favorable outcomes were reported from the Barnes experience and other various smaller trials, application of LVRS rapidly escalated.

In the mid-1990s, analysis of Medicare claims for LVRS revealed an operative mortality of 16.9% and a 1-year mortality of 23%. In 1997 the National Emphysema Treatment Trial (NETT) conducted a randomized trial of 1218 patients in a noncrossover design to medical versus surgical management after a 10-week pretreatment pulmonary rehabilitation program. Subgroup analysis demonstrated that in patients with the anatomic changes delineated by Cooper and colleagues, LVRS significantly improved exercise capacity, lung function, quality of life, and dyspnea compared to medical therapy. After 2 years, functional improvements began to decline toward baseline. Similar parameters in medically treated patients steadily decline below baseline. LVRS was associated with increased short-term morbidity and mortality and did not confer a survival benefit over medical therapy.

Lung Transplantation

Cooper and associates at the University of Toronto performed the first successful single-lung transplant (SLT) in 1983. Pasque and colleagues introduced the modern technique of a bilateral sequential lung (BSL) transplant in 1990.

Today, the most common indications for referral for a lung transplant are COPD and idiopathic pulmonary fibrosis (IPF). Most patients with IPF and older patients with COPD are offered an SLT. Younger COPD patients and patients with alpha$_1$-antitrypsin deficiency and severe hyperinflation of the native lungs are offered a BSL. Most patients with primary pulmonary hypertension and almost all patients with cystic fibrosis are treated with a BSL. A heart-lung transplant is reserved for patients with irreversible ventricular failure or uncorrectable congenital cardiac disease.

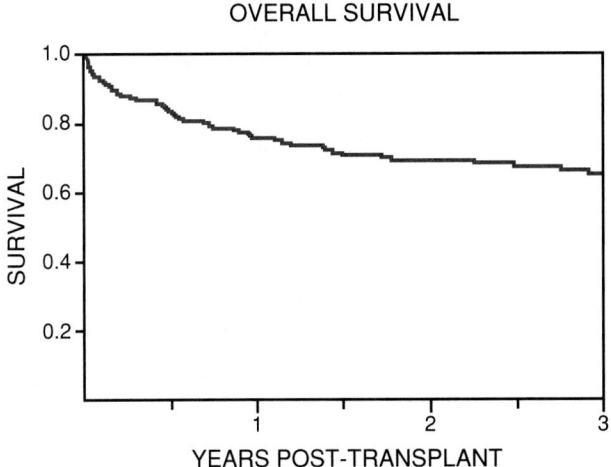

FIG. 18-25. The overall survival rate after lung transplantation at the University of Minnesota.

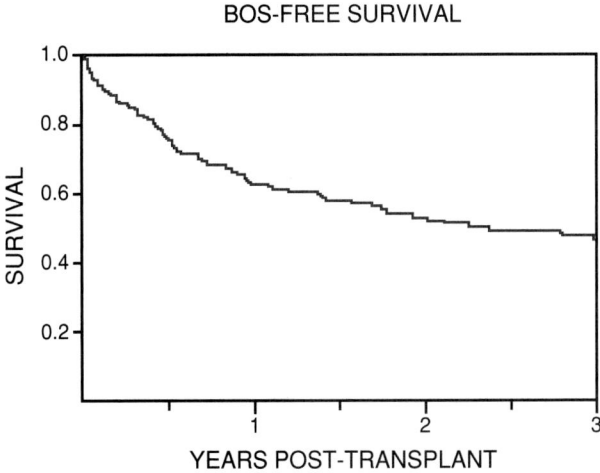

FIG. 18-26. The survival rate after lung transplantation in the absence of bronchiolitis obliterans syndrome (BOS) at the University of Minnesota.

Patients with COPD are considered for placement on the transplant waiting list when their forced expiratory volume in 1 second (FEV_1) has fallen to below 25% of its predicted value. Patients with significant pulmonary hypertension should be listed earlier. IPF patients should be referred when their forced vital capacity has fallen to less than 60%, or their carbon monoxide diffusion capacity (D_{LCO}) to less than 50% of their predicted values.

In the past, patients with primary pulmonary hypertension (PPH) and New York Heart Association (NYHA) class III or IV symptoms were listed for a lung transplant. However, treatment of such patients with intravenous prostacyclin and other pulmonary vasodilators has now markedly altered that old strategy. Virtually all patients with PPH are now treated with intravenous epoprostenol. Several of these patients have experienced a marked improvement in their symptoms associated with a decrease in their pulmonary arterial pressures and an increase in exercise capacity. Listing of these patients is deferred until they develop NYHA class III or IV symptoms or until their mean pulmonary artery pressure rises above 75 mm Hg. Medium-term and bronchiolitis obliterans syndrome (BOS)–free survival rates of patients who underwent a lung transplant during a recent 5-year period at the University of Minnesota are shown in Figs. 18-25 and 18-26. The mortality of patients while waiting for transplants is about 10%. In an effort to expand the number of lung donors, many transplant groups have liberalized their criteria for donor selection. Still, the partial pressure of arterial oxygen (Pao_2) should be greater than 300 mm Hg on a fraction of inspired oxygen (Fio_2) of 100%. In special circumstances, lungs may be used from donors with a smoking history; from donors older than 50 years of age; and from donors with positive Gram's stains or infiltrates on chest x-ray. The use of two living donors, each donating a single lower lobe, is another strategy for increasing the donor pool. Recipient outcomes are similar to those with cadaver donors in carefully selected patients.

Most of the early mortality after lung transplant is related to primary graft failure resulting from a severe ischemia-reperfusion injury to the lung(s) (Fig. 18-27). Reperfusion injury is characterized radiographically by interstitial and alveolar edema, and clinically by hypoxia and ventilation-perfusion mismatch. Donor neutrophils and recipient lymphocytes probably play an important role in the pathogenesis of reperfusion injury. The most important impediment to longer-term survival after a lung transplant is the development of

bronchiolitis obliterans syndrome (BOS), a manifestation of chronic rejection. Episodes of acute rejection are the major risk factors for developing BOS. Other injuries to the lung (including early reperfusion injury and chronic gastroesophageal reflux disease) may also adversely affect long-term outcomes of patients.

Spontaneous Pneumothorax

Spontaneous pneumothorax is secondary to intrinsic abnormalities of the lung, and the most common cause is rupture of an apical subpleural bleb. The cause of these blebs is unknown, but they occur more frequently in smokers and males, and they tend to predominate in young postadolescent males with a tall thin body habitus. Treatment is generally chest tube insertion with water seal. If a leak is present and it persists for greater than 3 days, thoracoscopic management (i.e., bleb resection with pleurodesis by talc or pleural abrasion) is performed. Recurrences or complete lung collapse with the first episode are generally indications for thoracoscopic intervention.

Other causes are emphysema (rupture of a bleb or bulla), cystic fibrosis, AIDS, metastatic cancer (especially sarcoma), asthma, lung

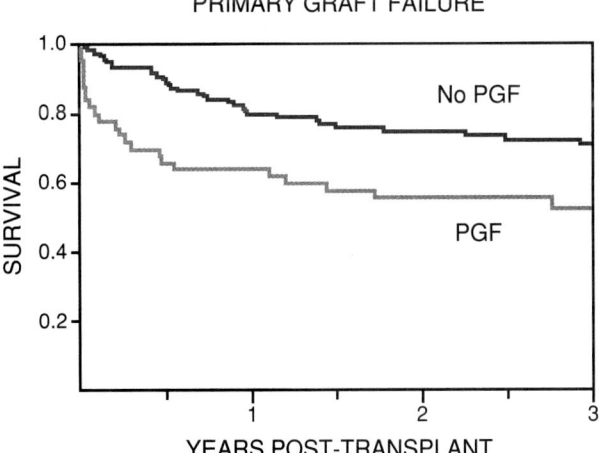

FIG. 18-27. The survival rate after lung transplantation at the University of Minnesota as a function of primary graft failure (PGF).

abscess, and occasionally lung cancer. Management of pneumothorax in these circumstances is often tied to therapy of the specific disease process and may involve tumor resection, thoracoscopic pleurectomy, or talc pleurodesis.

CHEST WALL

Chest Wall Mass

Clinical Approach

The overarching goal of any surgeon involved in caring for a patient with a chest wall mass is to *not compromise the patient's survival* should the lesion ultimately prove to be malignant. Both general and thoracic surgeons are asked to participate in the evaluation and subsequent managment of chest wall masses. Therefore the participating surgeons must be well versed in the principles of diagnosing and treating chest wall malignancies. If a less experienced surgeon participates as the technical provider of only a biopsy, it is highly likely that the ultimate surgical resection and reconstruction, and worse, the patient's survival, will be compromised. All chest wall tumors should be considered malignant until proven otherwise. A general approach is outlined in Figs. 18-28 and 18-29 and is discussed in further detail in the following text.

Patients with either a benign or malignant chest wall tumor typically present with complaints of a slowly enlarging palpable mass (50 to 70%), chest wall pain (25 to 50%), or both. When a patient notices a mass, it is often several months before medical consultation can be arranged. Masses may also be discovered after a local traumatic event.

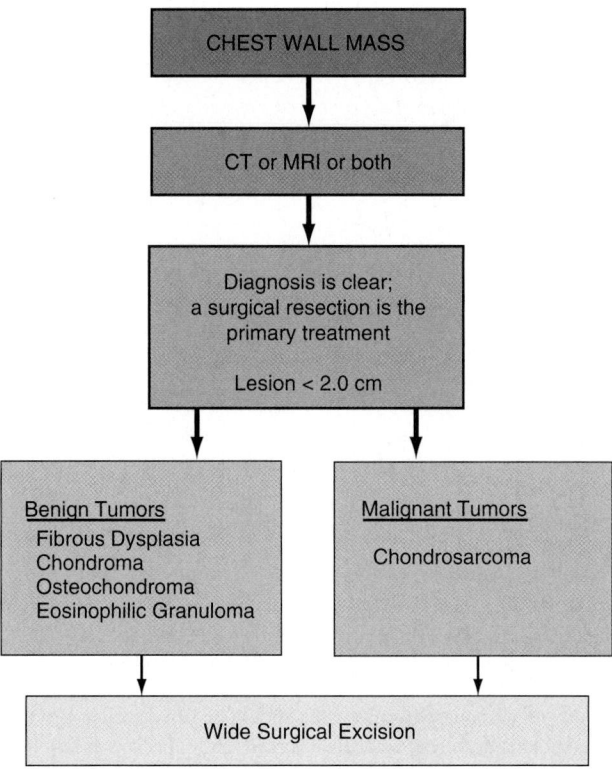

FIG. 18-28. Systematic approach for evaluating a chest wall mass. The clinical scenario is uncomplicated and initial imaging studies suggest a clear diagnosis.

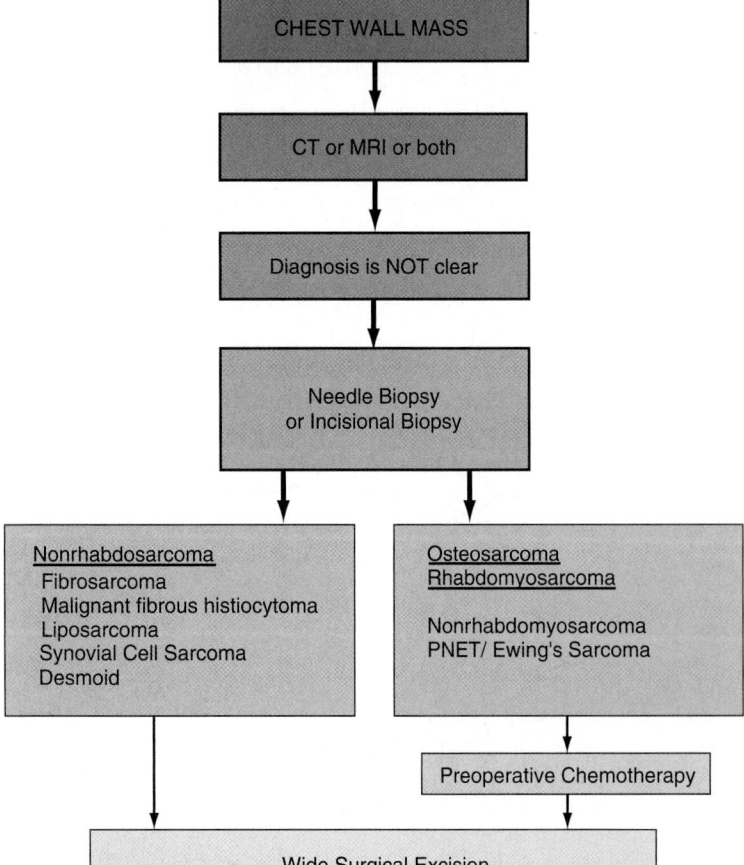

FIG. 18-29. Systematic approach for evaluating a chest wall mass in which the diagnosis is not unequivocal. A tissue diagnosis is critical in effective management of chest wall masses.

Pain from a chest wall mass is typically localized to the area of the tumor. Pain is more often present (and more intense) with malignant tumors, but it can also be present in up to one-third of patients with benign tumors. With Ewing's sarcoma, fever and malaise may also be present. Age can provide guidance as to the possibility of malignancy. Patients with benign chest wall tumors are on average 26 years old; the average age for patients with malignant tumors is 40 years old. Overall, the probability of a chest wall tumor being malignant is 50 to 80%.

Evaluation and Management

Laboratory evaluations are usually of little help in assessing chest wall masses. In plasmacytoma, there may be monoclonality of one of the immunoglobulins with normal levels of other immunoglobulins. Another exception is osteosarcoma, in which alkaline phosphatase levels may be elevated. Still another exception is Ewing's sarcoma, in which the erythrocyte sedimentation rate may be elevated.

Radiography. Radiographic evaluation begins with a chest x-ray, which may reveal evidence of rib destruction, calcification within the lesion, and if old films are available, a clue to growth rate. CT scanning should be done in all patients to evaluate the nature of the primary lesion, to determine its relationship to contiguous structures (e.g., mediastinum, lung, soft tissues, and other skeletal elements), and to search for possible pulmonary metastases. Importantly, contiguous involvement of underlying lung or other soft tissues or the presence of pulmonary metastases does not preclude successful surgery. CT is also valuable in assessing for the presence of extraosseous bone formation and bone destruction, both typically seen with osteosarcoma.

MRI has a number of advantages in the radiographic evaluation of chest wall masses, particularly those that may be malignant. Multiple planes of imaging (coronal, sagittal, and oblique) are possible. MRI may also better define the relationship between tumor and muscle. For tumors contiguous to or near neurovascular structures or the spine, MRI and magnetic resonance angiography (MRA) with multiple planes of imaging provides invaluable information about the tumor. Thus it greatly facilitates preoperative planning and may further delineate tissue abnormalities, potentially enhancing the ability to distinguish benign from malignant sarcomas.

Biopsy. The first step in the management of all chest wall tumors is to obtain a tissue diagnosis. Inappropriate or misguided attempts at tissue diagnosis through casual open biopsy techniques have the potential (if the lesion is a sarcoma) to seed surrounding tissues and contiguous body cavities (e.g., the pleural space) with tumor cells, potentially compromising local tumor control and patient survival. Accurately typing chest wall sarcomas has a profound impact on their management.

Tissue diagnosis can be made by one of three methods: a needle biopsy (typically CT-guided, FNA or a core biopsy), an incisional biopsy, or an excisional biopsy. Until recently, the thoracic surgery literature has been dogmatic in advocating only an excisional biopsy. Reasons for this dogmatic approach were that (1) the entire mass is removed, allowing 100% accurate sampling and diagnosis; (2) compared to incisional biopsy, the potential problem of seeding the surrounding soft tissues with tumor cells does not exist; and (3) adjuvant chemotherapy can be administered.

However, management of extremity sarcomas has changed dramatically in the last decade. Neoadjuvant therapy is now the standard of care for certain sarcomas. Since sarcomas of the thorax are the same as sarcomas of the extremities, management principles for both should be parallel, whenever technically and medically possible.

An excisional biopsy should still be done when the initial diagnosis (based on radiographic evaluation) indicates that it is a benign lesion, or when the lesion has the classic appearance of a chondrosarcoma (in which case definitive surgical resection can be undertaken). Any lesion less than 2.0 cm can be excised as long as the resulting wound is small enough to close primarily.

When the diagnosis cannot be made by radiographic evaluation, a needle biopsy (FNA or core) should be done. Pathologists experienced with sarcomas can accurately diagnose approximately 90% of patients using FNA techniques. A needle biopsy (FNA or core) has the advantage of avoiding wound and body cavity contamination (a potential complication with an incisional biopsy).

If a needle biopsy is nondiagnostic, an incisional biopsy may be performed, with caveats. When performing an incisional biopsy, the skin incision must be placed directly over the mass and oriented to allow subsequent excision of the scar. Development of skin flaps must be avoided, and in general no drains are used. A drain may be placed if a hematoma is likely to develop, as this can potentially limit soft tissue contamination by tumor cells. Subsequently, if definitive surgical resection is undertaken, the entire area of the biopsy (including skin) must be excised en bloc with the tumor.

Chest Wall Neoplasms

Benign

Chondroma. Chondromas are one of the more common benign tumors of the chest wall. They are primarily seen in children and young adults. Chondromas usually occur at the costochondral junction anteriorly. Given their typical location and the young age of most patients, chondromas may be confused with costochondritis. Clinically, a mass (usually without pain) is present in the case of chondromas. Radiographically, the lesion is lobulated and radiodense; it may have diffuse or focal calcifications, and may displace the bony cortex without penetration. Chondromas may grow to huge sizes if left untreated. Treatment is surgical resection with a 2-cm margin. One must be certain, however, that the lesion is not a well-differentiated chondrosarcoma. In this case, a wider 4-cm margin is required to prevent local recurrence. Therefore, large chondromas should be treated surgically as low-grade chondrosarcomas.

Fibrous Dysplasia. The ribs are a frequent site of origin of fibrous dysplasia. As with chondromas, fibrous dysplasia most frequently occurs in young adults. However, pain is infrequent, and the location is more often in the posterolateral aspect of the rib cage. Fibrous dysplasia may be associated with trauma. Radiographically, an expansile mass is present, with cortical thinning and no calcification. Local excision with a 2-cm margin is curative.

Osteochondroma. Osteochondromas are overall the most common benign bone tumor. Many are detected as incidental radiographic findings. Most are solitary; however, patients with multiple osteochondromas have a higher incidence of malignancy.

Osteochondromas occur in the first 2 decades of life and they arise at or near the growth plate of bones. The lesions are benign during youth or adolescence. Osteochondromas that enlarge after completion of skeletal growth have the potential to develop into chondrosarcomas.

When seen in the thorax they usually arise from the rib cortex and are often part of the autosomal dominant syndrome hereditary multiple exostoses. Key features in this circumstance are the known potential to degenerate into chondrosarcomas, which may be heralded by new onset of pain or gradual enlargement of the mass over time. Patients with multiple osteochondromatosis may have benign osteochondromas scattered throughout their rib cage. Thus, the presence of new or increasing localized pain would warrant excisional biopsy of the offending osteochondroma. Local excision of a benign osteochondroma is sufficient. If malignancy is determined, wide excision is performed with a 4-cm margin.

Eosinophilic Granuloma. Eosinophilic granulomas are benign osteolytic lesions. They were originally thought to be destructive lesions with large numbers of eosinophilic cells. Yet eosinophilic granulomas of the ribs can also occur as solitary lesions or as part of a more generalized disease process of the lymphoreticular system termed Langerhans cell histiocytosis (LCH). In LCH, the involved tissue is infiltrated with large numbers of histiocytes (similar to Langerhans cells seen in skin and other epithelia), which are often organized as granulomas. The cause is unknown. Of all LCH bone lesions, 79% are solitary eosinophilic granulomas, 7% involve multiple eosinophilic granulomas, and 14% belong to other forms of more systemic LCH.

Isolated single eosinophilic granulomas can occur in the ribs or skull, pelvis, mandible, humerus, and other sites. They are diagnosed primarily in children between the ages of 5 and 15 years. Because of the associated pain and tenderness, they may be confused with Ewing's sarcoma or with an inflammatory process such as osteomyelitis. Healing may occur spontaneously, but the typical treatment is limited surgical resection with a 2-cm margin.

Desmoid Tumors. Desmoid tumors are unusual soft tissue neoplasms that arise from fascial or musculoaponeurotic structures. Histologically, they consist of proliferations of benign-appearing fibroblastic cells, abundant collagen, and few mitoses. Accordingly, some authorities consider desmoid tumors to be a form of fibrosarcoma.

Although the cause is unknown, multiple associations with other diseases and conditions are well documented, such as familial polyposis (Gardner syndrome), states of increased estrogen (pregnancy), and trauma. Surgical incisions (abdominal and thorax) have been the site of desmoid development, either in or near the scar.

Clinically, patients are usually in the third to fourth decade of life, and have pain, a chest wall mass, or both. The tumor is usually fixed to the chest wall, but not to the overlying skin. No radiographic findings are typical, but MRI may delineate muscle or soft tissue infiltration. Histologic diagnosis may not be possible by a needle biopsy because of low cellularity. An open incisional biopsy for lesions over 3 to 4 cm is often necessary, following the caveats listed above (see biopsy section).

Desmoid tumors do not metastasize, but they have a significant propensity to recur locally, with local recurrence rates as high as 5 to 50%, sometimes despite complete initial resection with histologically negative margins. Such locally aggressive behavior is secondary to microscopic tumor infiltration of muscle and surrounding soft tissues.

Surgery consists of wide local excision with a margin of 2 to 4 cm, and with intraoperative assessment of resection margins by frozen section. Typically, a rib is removed above and below the tumor with a 4- to 5-cm margin of rib. A margin of less than 1 cm results in much higher local recurrence rates. If a major neurovascular structure would have to be sacrificed, leading to high morbidity, then a margin of less than 1 cm would have to suffice. Survival after wide local excision with negative margins is 90% at 10 years.

Table 18-10
Classification of Sarcomas by Therapeutic Response

Tumor Type	Chemotherapy Sensitivity
Osteosarcoma	+
Rhabdomyosarcoma	+
PNET	+
Ewing's sarcoma	+
MFH	+/−
Fibrosarcoma	+/−
Liposarcoma	+/−
Synovial sarcoma	+/−

MFH = malignant fibrous histiocytoma; PNET = primitive neuroectodermal tumor.

Primary Malignant Chest Wall Tumors

A wide variety of sarcoma cell types exist. Even though the diagnosis of chest wall tumors is classified by cell type, it is not the primary feature affecting prognosis. Rather, prognosis of sarcomas is determined more by two factors: responsiveness to chemotherapy and histologic grade.

Sarcomas can be divided into two broad groups by potential chemotherapeutic responsiveness (Table 18-10). Preoperative (neoadjuvant) chemotherapy offers the ability to (1) assess tumor chemosensitivity by the degree of tumor size reduction and microscopic necrosis, (2) determine which chemotherapeutic agents the tumor is sensitive to, and (3) lessen the extent of surgical resection by reducing tumor size. Patients whose tumors are responsive to preoperative chemotherapy (as judged by the reduction in the size of the primary tumor and/or by the degree of necrosis seen histologically following resection) have a much better prognosis than those with a poor response.

Given the tumor's potential response to chemotherapy or the presence of metastatic disease, the initial treatment is either (1) preoperative chemotherapy (for patients with osteosarcoma, rhabdomyosarcoma, primitive neuroectodermal tumor [PNET], or Ewing's sarcoma) followed by surgery and postoperative chemotherapy, (2) primary surgical resection and reconstruction (for patients with nonmetastatic malignant fibrous histiocytoma, fibrosarcoma, liposarcoma, or synovial sarcoma), or (3) neoadjuvant chemotherapy followed by surgical resection if indicated in patients presenting with metastatic soft tissue sarcomas. Exceptions to these guidelines may apply at specific centers where the impact of neoadjuvant chemotherapy on soft tissue sarcomas is under investigation. Typically this exception can apply to pediatric patients and to adult patients that have deep, high-grade, nonmetastatic tumors greater than 10 cm in diameter.

Malignant Chest Wall Bone Tumors

Chondrosarcoma. Chondrosarcomas are the most common primary chest wall malignancy. As with chondromas, they usually arise anteriorly from the costochondral arches. These slowly-enlarging, often painful masses of the anterior chest wall can reach massive proportions. CT scan shows a radiolucent lesion often with stippled calcifications pathognomonic for chondrosarcomas (Fig. 18-30). The involved bony structures are also destroyed. Metastatic disease to the lungs or bones should be ruled out by CT and bone scan.

Most chondrosarcomas are slow growing, low-grade tumors. For this reason, any lesion in the anterior chest wall likely to be a chondroma or a low-grade chondrosarcoma should be treated with wide (4-cm) resection. Chondrosarcomas are not sensitive to

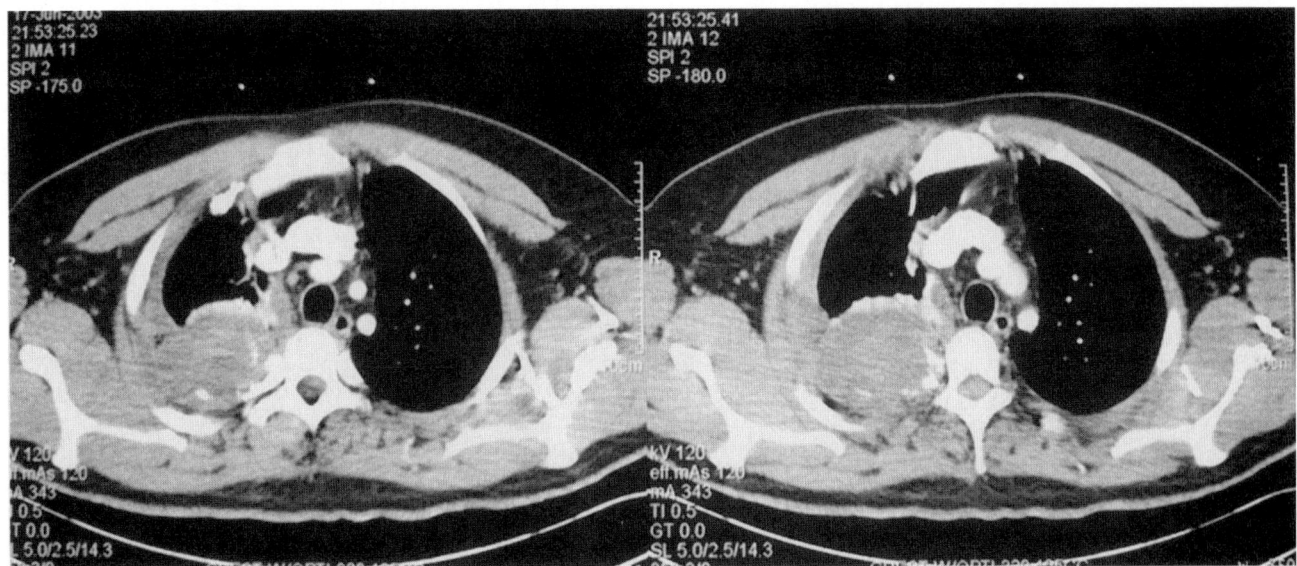

FIG. 18-30. Chest CT scan showing a right posterior lung tumor. In the appropriate clinical setting, stippled calcifications (white streaks in right lung mass) are highly indicative of chondrosarcomas.

chemotherapy or radiation therapy. Prognosis is determined by tumor grade and extent of resection. With a low-grade tumor and wide resection, patient survival at 5 to 10 years can be as high as 60 to 80%.

Osteosarcoma. Osteosarcomas are the most common bone malignancy, but they are an uncommon malignancy of the chest wall, representing only 10% of all malignant chest wall tumors. They present as rapidly-enlarging, painful masses. Although they primarily occur in young adults, osteosarcomas can occur in patients over the age of 40 years, sometimes in association with previous radiation, Paget's disease, or chemotherapy.

Radiographically, the typical appearance consists of spicules of new periosteal bone formation producing a sunburst appearance. As with chondrosarcomas, careful CT assessment of the pulmonary parenchyma for metastasis is necessary. Osteosarcomas have a propensity to spread to the lungs. Up to one-third of patients present with metastatic disease.

Osteosarcomas are potentially sensitive to chemotherapy. Currently, preoperative chemotherapy before surgical resection is common. After chemotherapy, complete resection is performed with wide (4-cm) margins, followed by reconstruction. In patients presenting with lung metastases that are potentially amenable to surgical resection, induction chemotherapy may be given, followed by surgical resection of the primary tumor and of the pulmonary metastases. Following surgical treatment of known disease, additional maintenance chemotherapy is usually recommended.

Other Tumors

Primitive Neuroectodermal Tumors. PNETs derive from primordial neural crest cells that migrate from the mantle layer of the developing spinal cord. This group of tumors includes neuroblastomas, ganglioneuroblastomas, and ganglioneuromas. Ewing's sarcomas and Askin's tumors are closely related to PNETs; together they are referred to as the Ewing's sarcoma/PNET family of tumors. Askin's tumors were originally described by Askin in 1979 as a "malignant, small-cell, round tumor of the thoracopulmonary region," and are now known to be members of the Ewing's sarcoma/PNET family. Ewing's sarcomas and PNETs have a common site: a genetic abnormality, a translocation between the long arms of chromosomes 11 and 22. They also share a consistent pattern of proto-oncogene

expression and have been found to express the product of the MIC2 gene. Histologically, they are small-round cell tumors.

Ewing's Sarcoma. Ewing's sarcomas occur in adolescents and young adults who present with progressive chest wall pain, but without the presence of a mass. Systemic symptoms of malaise and fever are often present. Laboratory studies reveal an elevated erythrocyte sedimentation rate and mild white blood cell elevation.

Radiographically, the characteristic onion peel appearance is produced by multiple layers of periosteum in the bone formation. Evidence of bony destruction is also common. The diagnosis can be made by a percutaneous needle biopsy or an incisional biopsy.

These tumors have a strong propensity to spread to the lungs and skeleton. Their aggressive behavior produces patient survival rates of only 50% or less at 3 years. Increasing tumor size is associated with decreasing survival. Treatment has improved significantly, now consisting of multiagent chemotherapy, radiation therapy, and surgery. Patients typically are treated preoperatively with chemotherapy; if residual disease is present, they can undergo surgical resection and reconstruction followed by maintenance chemotherapy.

Plasmacytoma. Solitary plasmacytomas of the chest wall are very rare, and only 25 to 30 cases are seen annually in the United States. Histologically, the lesion is identical to multiple myeloma, with sheets of plasma cells. It occurs at an average age of 55 years. The typical presentation is pain without a palpable mass. X-rays show an osteolytic lesion. Evaluation for systemic myeloma is performed with bone marrow aspiration, testing of calcium levels, and measurement of urinary Bence Jones proteins. If the results of these studies are negative, then a solitary plasmacytoma is diagnosed. Surgery is usually limited to a biopsy only, which may be excisional. Treatment consists of radiation with doses of 4000 to 5000 cGy. Up to 75% of patients go on to develop systemic multiple myeloma. Patient survival at 10 years is about 20%.

Malignant Chest Soft Tissue Sarcomas

Soft tissue sarcomas of the chest wall are uncommon (Fig. 18-31). They include fibrosarcomas, liposarcomas, malignant fibrous histiocytomas (MFHs), rhabdomyosarcomas, angiosarcomas, and other extremely rare lesions. With the exception of

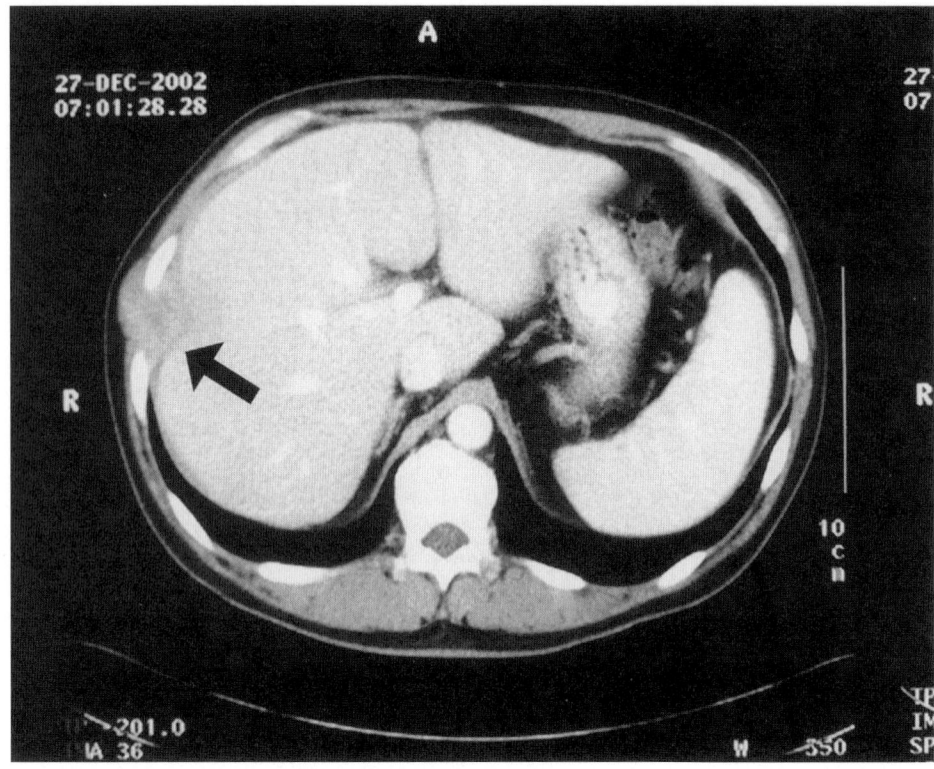

FIG. 18-31. Chest CT scan showing a right chest wall tumor (*arrow*). Tissue diagnosis revealed that this mass was a leiomyosarcoma.

rhabdomyosarcomas, the primary treatment of these lesions is wide surgical resection with 4-cm margins and reconstruction. Rhabdomyosarcomas are sensitive to chemotherapy and are often treated with preoperative chemotherapy. As with all sarcomas, soft tissue sarcomas of the chest wall have a propensity to spread to the lungs. The prognosis of such tumors, as noted above, heavily depends on their grade and stage.

Malignant Fibrous Histiocytoma. Malignant fibrous histiocytomas (MFHs) were originally thought to derive from histiocytes, because of the microscopic appearance of cultured tumor cells. Subsequently it was shown that their likely origin is the fibroblast. MFHs are generally the most common soft tissue sarcoma of late adult life, typically occurring between the age of 50 and 70 years, and they are rare under the age of 20. Presentation is pain, with or without a palpable mass. Radiographically, a mass is usually evident, with destruction of surrounding tissue and bone. Treatment is wide resection with a margin of 4 cm or more and reconstruction. Over two-thirds of patients suffer from distant metastasis or local recurrence.

Liposarcoma. Liposarcomas make up 15% of chest wall sarcomas. Most liposarcomas are low-grade tumors that have a propensity to recur locally, given their infiltrative nature. Clinically, they present most often as painless masses. Treatment is wide resection and reconstruction. Intraoperative margins should be evaluated (as with all sarcomas) and resection continued, if feasible, until margins are negative. Local recurrence can be treated with reexcision, with occasional use of radiotherapy.

Fibrosarcoma. Fibrosarcomas often present as large masses with pain. Radiographically, a mass is seen with surrounding tissue destruction. Treatment is wide local excision with intraoperative frozen-section analysis of margins, followed by reconstruction. Local and systemic recurrence is frequent. Patient survival at 5 years is about 50 to 60%.

Rhabdomyosarcoma. Rhabdomyosarcomas are rare tumors of the chest wall. Microscopically, they are a spindle cell tumor. The diagnosis often depends on immunohistochemical staining for muscle markers. Rhabdomyosarcomas are sensitive to chemotherapy. Treatment consists of preoperative chemotherapy with subsequent surgical resection.

Chest Wall Reconstruction

The principles of surgery for any malignant chest wall tumor are to strategically plan the anatomy of resection and to carefully assess what structures will need to be sacrificed to obtain a 4-cm margin. Prosthetic reconstruction is usually with 2-mm Gore-Tex, and with appropriate soft-tissue coverage to obtain good coverage of a potentially large defect and to achieve an acceptable cosmetic result.

The extent of resection depends on the tumor's location and on any involvement of contiguous structures. Laterally-based lesions often require simple wide excision, with resection of any contiguously involved lung, pleura, muscle, or skin. Anteriorly-based lesions contiguous with the sternum require partial sternectomy. Primary malignant tumors of the sternum may require complete sternectomy. Posterior lesions involving the rib heads over their articulations with the vertebral bodies may, depending on the extent of rib involvement, require partial en bloc vertebrectomy.

Reconstruction of the chest wall can always be accomplished with the use of 2-mm Gore-Tex, attached to the surrounding bony structures with stout sutures of Gore-Tex or polypropylene. Gore-Tex has become the standard material used in chest wall reconstruction at many institutions for several reasons. It is impervious to fluid, thus preventing pleural fluid from entering the chest wall; it is firm and provides excellent rigidity and stability when secured taut to the surrounding bony structures; and it provides a good platform for myocutaneous flap reconstruction.

Tissue coverage, except for smaller lesions, invariably involves the use of myocutaneous flaps using the latissimus dorsi, serratus anterior, rectus abdominis, or pectoralis major muscles. In all cases other than small excisions, an experienced plastic surgeon should be engaged with the thoracic surgeon in the preoperative planning and execution of the surgery, in order to ensure optimal physiologic and cosmetic results.

Because of the high rate of malignancy of chest wall neoplasms, any mass that likely represents a primary tumor must be aggressively managed. When malignancy is suspected, preliminary plans must be made for chest wall reconstruction that will allow resection of a generous margin of normal tissue around the neoplasm. The resection should include at least one normal adjacent rib above and below the tumor, with all intervening intercostal muscles and pleura. In addition, an en bloc resection of overlying chest wall muscles is often necessary, such as of the pectoralis minor or major, serratus anterior, or latissimus dorsi. When the periphery of the lung is involved with the neoplasm, it is appropriate to resect the adjacent part of the pulmonary lobe in continuity (Fig. 18-32). Involvement of the sternum by a malignant tumor requires total resection of the sternum with the adjacent cartilage. Techniques for postoperative respiratory support are now good enough that resection should not be compromised because of any concern about the patient's ability to be adequately ventilated in the early postoperative period.

Reconstruction of a large defect in the chest wall requires the use of some type of material to prevent lung herniation and to provide stability for the chest wall (see Fig. 18-32). Mild degrees of paradoxical motion are often well tolerated if the area of instability is relatively small. Several authors, notably Pairolero and Arnold from the Mayo Clinic, have reported extensive experience with chest wall reconstruction after removal of significant portions of the bony thorax. They emphasize that adequate resection and dependable reconstruction are essential ingredients to a successful operation. They strongly believe that both a thoracic surgeon and a

plastic surgeon must collaborate on these complicated problems. Historically, a wide variety of materials have been used to reestablish chest wall stability, including rib autografts, steel struts, acrylic plates, and numerous synthetic meshes. The current preference is either a 2-mm polytetrafluoroethylene (Gore-Tex) patch or a double-layer polypropylene (Marlex) mesh sandwiched with methyl methacrylate. If soft-tissue coverage is needed, myocutaneous flap reconstruction provides it.

MEDIASTINUM

General Concepts

Anatomy and Pathologic Entities

The mediastinum, the central part of the thoracic cavity, can be divided into compartments for classification of anatomic components and disease processes. There is much overlap, yet this compartmentalization facilitates understanding of general concepts of surgical interest. Several classification schemes exist, but for the purposes of this chapter, the three-compartment model is used (Fig. 18-33). This model includes the anterior compartment (often referred to as anterosuperior), the visceral compartment (middle), and the paravertebral sulci bilaterally (posterior compartment). The anterior compartment lies between the sternum and the anterior surface of the heart and great vessels. The visceral or middle compartment is located between the great vessels and the trachea. Posterior to these two compartments lies the paravertebral sulci, bilaterally, and the periesophageal area.

The normal content of the anterior compartment includes the thymus gland or its remnant, the internal mammary artery and vein, lymph nodes, and fat. During childhood, the size of the thymus gland is impressive, occupying the entire anterior mediastinum (Fig. 18-34). After adolescence, the thymus gland decreases in both thickness and length and it takes on a more fatty content, with only residual islands of thymic cellular components (Fig. 18-35). The middle mediastinal compartment contains the pericardium and its contents, the ascending and transverse aorta, the superior and inferior venae cavae, the brachiocephalic artery and vein, the

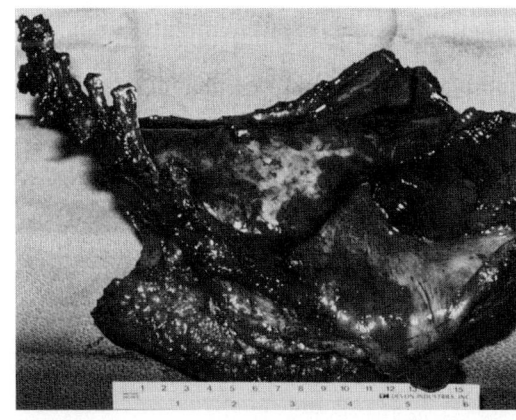 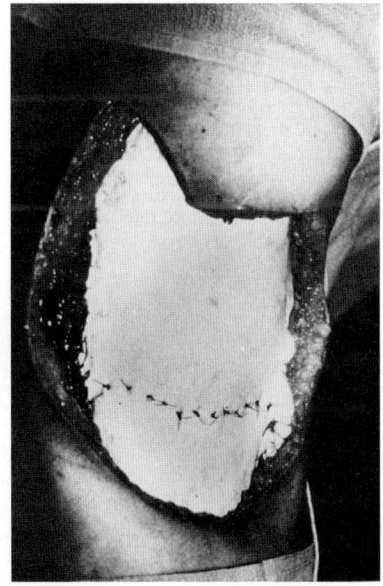

FIG. 18-32. Principles of reconstruction after resection of a chest wall tumor (osteogenic sarcoma) is shown. A. En bloc resection of the involved chest wall, including normal ribs above and below the tumor as well as pulmonary parenchyma, must be performed. The resected specimen is shown. B. A prosthesis has been sewn in place. In the lower third of the prosthesis, the line of diaphragm reattachment is seen. The skin defect was closed with a myocutaneous flap from the ipsilateral rectus muscle.   A   B

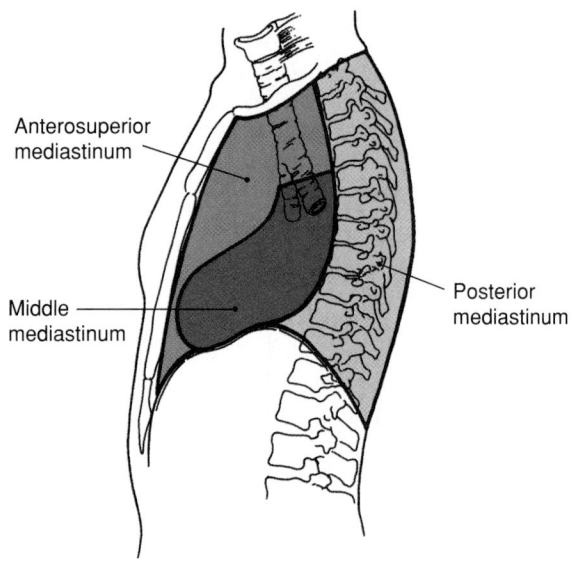

FIG. 18-33. *Anatomic division of the mediastinum.*

phrenic nerves, the upper vagus nerve trunks, the trachea, the main bronchi and their associated lymph nodes, and the central portions of the pulmonary arteries and veins. The posterior compartment contains the descending aorta, esophagus, thoracic duct, azygos and hemiazygos veins, and lymph nodes. Numerous pathologic variants may be present in the various compartments, with much overlap. Table 18-11 includes the most common pathologic entities listed by compartment.

History and Physical Examination

The type of mediastinal pathology encountered varies significantly by age of the patient. In adults, the most common tumors include neurogenic tumors of the posterior compartment, benign cysts occurring in any compartment, and thymomas of the anterior

mediastinum (Table 18-12). In children, neurogenic tumors of the posterior mediastinum are also common; lymphoma is the second most common mediastinal tumor, usually located in the anterior or middle compartment; and thymoma is rare (Table 18-13). In both age groups, about 25% of mediastinal tumors are malignant. Pediatric tumors will be discussed in Chap. 38.

In most recent series, up to two-thirds of mediastinal tumors in adults are discovered as asymptomatic abnormalities on radiologic studies ordered for other problems. Benign masses are even more likely to be asymptomatic. Characteristics such as size, location, rate of growth, and associated inflammation are important factors that correlate with symptoms. Large, bulky tumors, expanding cysts, and teratomas can cause compression of mediastinal structures, in particular the trachea, and lead to cough, dyspnea on exertion, or stridor. Chest pain or dyspnea may be reported secondary to associated pleural effusions, cardiac tamponade, or phrenic nerve involvement. Occasionally, a mediastinal mass near the aortopulmonary window may be identified in a work-up for hoarseness because of left recurrent laryngeal nerve involvement (Fig. 18-36). The patient in Fig. 18-36 presented with hoarseness and was found to have a primary lung cancer with metastases to the level 5 and 6 lymph nodes in the region of the aortopulmonary window, which led to compression of the left recurrent laryngeal nerve and hoarseness. In the era of screening CT examinations, a higher percentage of malignant tumors of the mediastinum are being discovered as asymptomatic, incidental masses.

The history and physical examination in conjunction with the imaging findings may suggest a specific diagnosis. The association of a mediastinal mass, enlarged lymph nodes, and a constitutional symptom such as night sweats or weight loss suggests a lymphoma. An anterior mediastinal mass in the setting of a history of fluctuating weakness and early fatigue or ptosis suggests a thymoma and myasthenia gravis. The neurologic examination may reveal ptosis, diplopia, or proximal muscle weakness, suggesting myasthenia gravis. The physical examination should include a careful search for extrathoracic adenopathy of the cervical, axillary, and inguinal locations. Adenopathy in these locations in association with

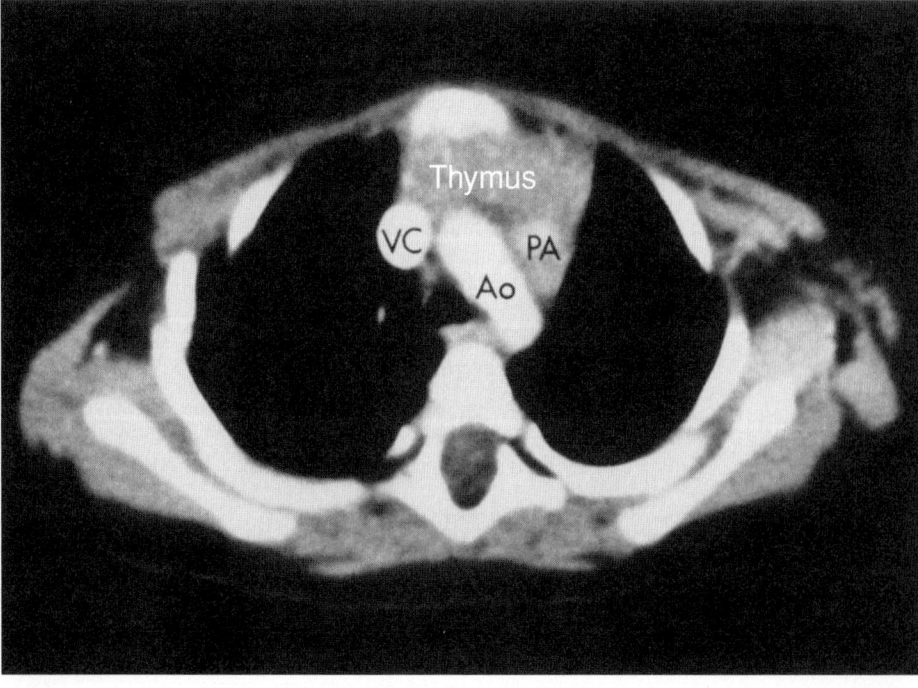

FIG. 18-34. *Normal appearance of the thymus gland in childhood. Ao = aorta; PA = pulmonary artery; VC = vena cava.*

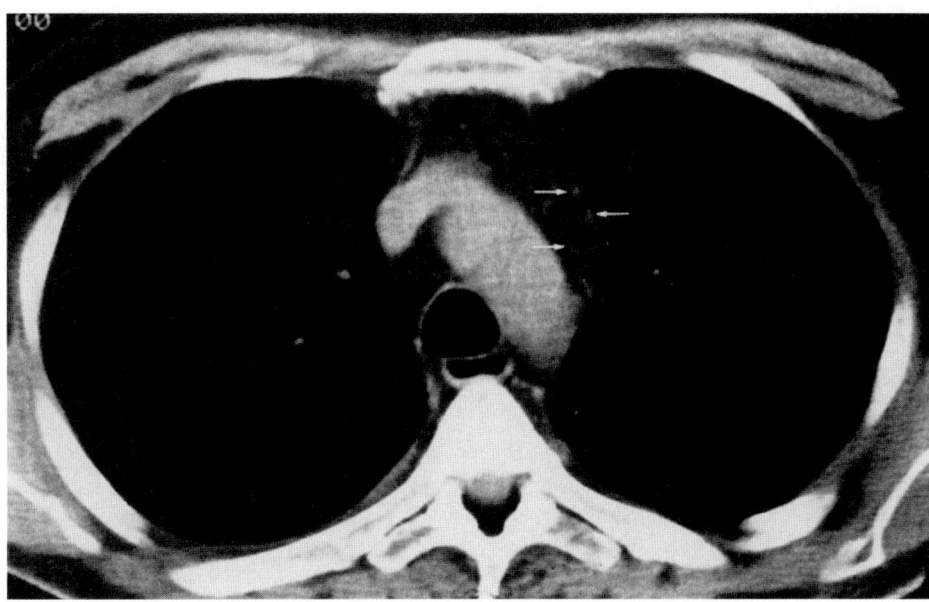

FIG. 18-35. CT scan of the normal appearance of an involuted thymus gland in an adult. Note the near-total fatty appearance of the gland with only tiny islands of soft tissue scattered within it (*small arrows*).

a mediastinal mass suggests a lymphoma. In young adult males, a mediastinal mass and a testicular mass suggest a germ cell tumor. In one recent series, systemic symptoms were present in 50% of patients with a mediastinal mass and a lymphoproliferative disorder, as compared with only 29% of patients with other masses (such as thymic or neurogenic). Laboratory signs of inflammation were also noted: the erythrocyte sedimentation rate (ESR) and C-reactive protein (CRP) levels were elevated and leukocytosis was present in 86% of patients with a lymphoproliferative disorder, as compared with only 58% of patients with other types of mediastinal masses.

Diagnostic Evaluation

Imaging and Serum Markers

A number of asymptomatic mediastinal masses are suggested by chest x-rays, but are generally poorly defined by this study. CT has become the most common imaging modality for evaluating mediastinal masses. Contrast-enhanced CT scans for clear delineation of anatomy is preferred. MRI may be indicated in the work-up of a mediastinal mass, particularly in patients contemplating surgical resection. Specifically, MRI is more accurate than CT scan in determining if there is invasion of vascular structures or spinal involvement.

Several other imaging modalities are available to evaluate mediastinal masses of suspected endocrine origin (Table 18-14). Single photon emission computed tomography (SPECT) technology may be used to improve image contrast and give information on three-dimensional localization of some tumors of endocrine origin. SPECT technology has largely replaced conventional two-dimensional nuclear imaging studies. If a thyroid origin is suspected, a thyroid scan using ^{131}I or ^{123}I can identify most intrathoracic goiters and identify the extent of functioning thyroid tissue. If indicated, the thyroid scan should precede other scans requiring iodine-containing contrast agents, because they would subsequently interfere with iodine tracer uptake by thyroid tissue and scanning. If a pheochromocytoma or neuroblastoma is suspected, the octreotide scan is helpful in diagnosis and localization. The sestamibi scan may be useful for diagnosing and localizing a mediastinal parathyroid gland.

PET scanning has improved the noninvasive staging of lung cancer and esophageal cancer. The utility of PET in staging the mediastinum for NSCLC is reviewed in the lung cancer section of this chapter. The utility of PET for staging other tumors of the mediastinum is not as clear. It is useful for distinguishing malignant from benign tumors. It may help detect distant metastases in some patients. For example, in patients with esophageal cancer, up to 10% of those with a negative metastatic survey by conventional imaging

Table 18-11
Usual Location of the Common Primary Tumors and Cysts of the Mediastinum

Anterior Compartment	*Visceral Compartment*	*Paravertebral Sulci*
Thymoma	Enterogenous cyst	Neurilemoma-schwannoma
Germ cell tumor	Lymphoma	Neurofibroma
Lymphoma	Pleuropericardial cyst	Malignant schwannoma
Lymphangioma	Mediastinal granuloma	Ganglioneuroma
Hemangioma	Lymphoid hamartoma	Ganglioneuroblastoma
Lipoma	Mesothelial cyst	Neuroblastoma
Fibroma	Neurenteric cyst	Paraganglioma
Fibrosarcoma	Paraganglioma	Pheochromocytoma
Thymic cyst	Pheochromocytoma	Fibrosarcoma
Parathyroid adenoma	Thoracic duct cyst	Lymphoma

SOURCE: Reproduced with permission from Shields TW: The mediastinum and its compartments, in *Mediastinal Surgery.* Philadelphia: Lea & Febiger, 1991, p 5.

Table 18-12
Mediastinal Tumors in Adults

Tumor Type	Incidence (%)	Location
Neurogenic tumors	21	Posterior
Cysts	20	All
Thymomas	19	Anterior
Lymphoma	13	Anterior/middle
Germ cell tumors	11	Anterior
Mesenchymal tumors	7	All
Endocrine tumors	6	Anterior/middle

SOURCE: Reproduced with permission from Shields TW: Primary lesions of the mediastinum and their investigation and treatment, in Shields TW (ed): *General Thoracic Surgery,* 4th ed. Baltimore: Williams & Wilkins, 1994, p 1731.

including CT scanning, will have a positive PET scan for distant metastases. The role of routine PET imaging for staging surgically resectable lesions of the mediastinum has not been established.

The use of serum markers to evaluate a mediastinal mass can be invaluable in some patients. For example, seminomatous and nonseminomatous germ cell tumors can frequently be diagnosed and often distinguished from one another by the levels of alpha-fetoprotein (AFP) and human chorionic gonadotropin (hCG). In over 90% of nonseminomatous germ cell tumors, either the AFP or the hCG level will be elevated. Results are close to 100% specific if the level of either AFP or hCG is greater than 500 ng/mL. Some centers institute chemotherapy based on this result alone, without a biopsy. In contrast, the AFP level is always normal in patients with mediastinal seminomas; only 10% will have an elevated hCG, which is usually less than 100 ng/mL. Other serum markers, such as intact parathyroid hormone level for ectopic parathyroid adenomas, may be useful for diagnosing and also for intraoperatively confirming complete resection. After successful resection of a parathyroid adenoma, this hormone level should rapidly normalize.

Diagnostic Nonsurgical Biopsies of the Mediastinum

The indications and decision-making steps for performing a diagnostic biopsy of a mediastinal mass remain somewhat controversial. In some patients, given noninvasive imaging results and the history, surgical removal may be the obvious choice; preoperative biopsy may be unnecessary and even hazardous. In other patients whose primary treatment is likely to be nonsurgical, a biopsy is essential. Even when a biopsy appears to be a reasonable goal, needle aspiration of the mediastinal mass may be considered hazardous or of low diagnostic yield.

Percutaneous biopsy may be technically difficult because of the overlying bony thoracic cavity and the proximity to lung tissue, the heart, and great vessels. FNA biopsy minimizes some of these

Table 18-13
Mediastinal Tumors in Children

Tumor Type	Incidence (%)	Location
Neurogenic tumors	40	Posterior
Lymphoma	18	Anterior/middle
Cysts	18	All
Germ cell tumors	11	Anterior
Mesenchymal tumors	9	All
Thymomas	Rare	Anterior

SOURCE: Reproduced with permission from Silverman NA, Sabiston DC Jr.: Mediastinal masses. *Surg Clin North Am* 60:760, 1980.

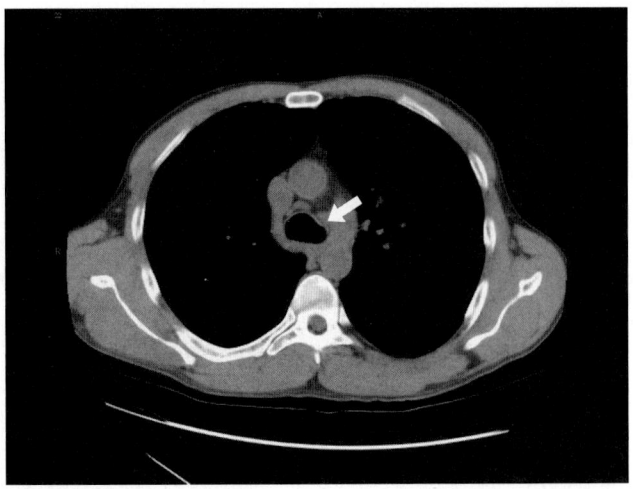

FIG. 18-36. A CT scan of a patient who presented with hoarseness due to compression of the left recurrent laryngeal nerve caused by mediastinal lymph node metastases to the aortopulmonary window area from a primary lung cancer.

potential hazards and may be effective in diagnosing mediastinal thyroid tissue, cancers, carcinomas, seminomas, inflammatory processes, and cysts. Other noncarcinomatous malignancies such as lymphoproliferative disorders, thymomas, and benign tumors may require larger pieces of tissue. Such biopsies may be obtained by a core-needle technique (which may not be safe depending on the location of the mass), or by surgery. In light of the issues cited, it is not surprising that the approach to biopsies of mediastinal masses may be different from center to center. Significant controversy exists in the literature regarding this topic. However, the treatment of up to 60% of patients with anterior mediastinal masses is ultimately nonsurgical, so it is essential to understand all options for obtaining adequate tissue for a definitive diagnosis using the least invasive approach. In one recent study, the authors used the medical history, physical examination, laboratory findings (ESR, CRP, and leukocytosis), and CT scan to assign patients to a possible lymphoproliferative diagnosis or a possible nonlymphoproliferative diagnosis. The authors concluded that, if features suggest the lymphoproliferative group of mediastinal masses, the patient should undergo a surgical biopsy, since larger pieces of tissues were required to make the diagnosis in their series. However, if a nonlymphoproliferative diagnosis was suggested, they recommended FNA before a potential surgical resection because the yield of accurate diagnoses by FNA was higher in that group.

In 1989, the American Thoracic Society published a position statement that declared that "cutting needles should not be used to biopsy diffuse infiltrative lung diseases or lesions in or adjacent to the mediastinum or hilar areas." However, since that time, institutions with significant interventional expertise have challenged that statement. In one series of 142 patients with mediastinal masses, CT-guided transthoracic core-needle biopsies were obtained with 14- to 22-gauge needles. The sensitivity was 98.9% with a specificity of 100%. Inadequate material was obtained in only 0.7% of patients, with no pneumothoraces or bleeding complications reported. The diagnostic yield is lower in series including a higher number of patients with lymphoproliferative disorders. Other series also reported a higher complication rate of pneumothorax, ranging from 8 to 23%, and of hemoptysis, up to 10%. In another series of anterior mediastinal masses, Herman reported that needle biopsies were greater

Table 18-14
Nuclear Imaging Relevant to the Mediastinum

Radiopharmaceutical, Radionuclide, or Radiochemical	Label	Disease of Interest
Iodine	^{131}I, ^{123}I	Retrosternal goiter, thyroid cancer
Monoclonal antibodies	^{111}In, ^{99m}Tc	Non-SCLC, colon and breast cancer, prostate cancer metastases
Octreotide	^{111}In	Amine precursor uptake decarboxylation tumors: carcinoid, gastrinoma, insulinoma, small-cell lung, pheochromocytoma, glucagonoma, medullary thyroid carcinoma, paraganglioma
Gallium	^{67}Ga	Lymphoma, non-SCLC, melanoma
Sestamibi	^{99m}Tc	Medullary thyroid carcinoma, nonfunctional papillary or follicular thyroid carcinoma, Hurthle cell thyroid carcinoma, parathyroid adenoma or carcinoma
Thallium	^{201}Tl	See sestamibi
MIBG	^{131}I, ^{123}I	Pheochromocytoma, neuroblastoma, see also octreotide
Fluorodeoxyglucose	^{18}F	General oncologic imaging, breast and colon cancer, melanoma

MIBG = metaiodobenzylguanidine; non-SCLC = non-small-cell lung cancer.
SOURCE: Reproduced with permission from McGinnis KM, Powers CN, Thomas FD, et al: Markers of the mediastinum, in Pearson FG, et al (eds): *Thoracic Surgery*, 2nd ed. New York: Churchill Livingstone, 2002, p 1675.

than 90% specific in diagnosing most carcinomatous tumors, but its accuracy for diagnosing lymphomas was less than 50%.

Similar controversy exists regarding the yield of needle biopsies for definitively diagnosing germ cell tumors and thymomas. Knapp described 56 patients with malignant germ cell tumors of the mediastinum. Various combinations of germ cell elements were present in 34% of tumors, so open biopsies with multiple tissue sections were seen as advisable. In another series of 79 patients with mediastinal masses suspected to be malignant, Larsen reported that endoscopic ultrasound-guided FNA had a sensitivity of 92% and a specificity of 100%.

CT-guided needle biopsy has proven most useful for investigating tumors that are clearly unresectable or for assessing suspected carcinomatous tumors, in these authors' experience. For mediastinal masses suggestive of a lymphoma, larger pieces of tissue obtained by mediastinoscopy for sampling paratracheal adenopathy are preferred. Thoracoscopic biopsies are preferred for other locations. If an anterior mediastinal mass appears localized and consistent with a thymoma, surgical resection is performed. Surgical resection without biopsies for most localized tumors of the posterior mediastinum suspected to be neurogenic in origin also is the preference of these authors.

Surgical Biopsies and Resection of Mediastinal Masses

For tumors of the mediastinum that are not amenable to a CT-guided needle biopsy or that do not yield sufficient tissue for diagnosis, a surgical biopsy is indicated. The definitive approach to a surgical biopsy of the anterior mediastinum is through a median sternotomy. At the time of sternotomy, if the lesion is easily resectable, it should be completely removed. Given the invasiveness of the procedure and the inability in some patients to obtain a definitive diagnosis by frozen section, less invasive procedures are preferable if the lesion is large or if the CT scan or history suggests that surgery is not the best definitive treatment. Masses in the paratracheal region are easily biopsied by mediastinoscopy. For tumors of the anterior or posterior mediastinum, a left or right VATS approach often allows safe and adequate surgical biopsies. In some patients, an anterior mediastinotomy (i.e., Chamberlain procedure) may be ideal for an anterior tumor or a tumor with significant parasternal extension. Before a surgical biopsy is pursued, a discussion should be held with the pathologist regarding routine histologic assessment, special stains and markers, and requirements for lymphoma work-up.

The gold standard for the resection of most mediastinal masses is through a median sternotomy or lateral thoracotomy. In some cases, a lateral thoracotomy with sternal extension (hemi-clamshell) provides excellent exposure for extensive mediastinal tumors that have a lateral component. This standard has been successfully challenged for some anterior mediastinal pathology. For example, good results have been reported using a cervical incision with a sternal retractor for thymus removal. The upward lift allows the surgeon reasonable access to the anterior mediastinum and has proven adequate in some centers for definitive resection of the thymus gland for myasthenia gravis. Similarly, several large series have now shown that a right or left VATS approach can be successful for removal of the thymus gland and for resection of small (1 to 2 cm) encapsulated thymomas. Most would agree that if a larger anterior mediastinal tumor is seen or malignancy is suspected, a median sternotomy with a more radical resection should be performed.

Neoplasms

Thymus

Thymic Enlargement
Thymic Hyperplasia. Diffuse thymic hyperplasia was first described in children after successful chemotherapy for lymphoma. It has now been described in adults and is referred to as "rebound thymic hyperplasia." It is most frequently reported after chemotherapy for lymphoma or germ cell tumors. Initially, atrophy of the thymic gland is seen; later, on follow-up scans, the patient is noted to have thymic gland enlargement, which can be dramatic. The usual time course for thymic hyperplasia to develop is about 9 months after cessation of chemotherapy, but it has been reported anywhere from 2 weeks to 12 months after chemotherapy. Benign hyperplasia must be clearly distinguished from recurrent lymphoma or germ cell tumors. Doing so may be difficult since thymic hyperplasia is dramatic in some patients, requiring careful follow-up, and at a minimum, serial CT scans. PET scanning may be helpful; a low standardized uptake value of tracer on PET scan suggests a benign tumor, but little has been published on this topic. Biopsies may be required if the clinical index of suspicion is high.

Thymic Tumors
Thymoma. Thymoma is the most frequently encountered neoplasm of the anterior mediastinum in adults (seen most frequently

between 40 and 60 years of age). They are rare in children. Most patients with thymomas are asymptomatic, but depending on the institutional referral patterns, between 10 and 50% have symptoms suggestive of myasthenia gravis or have circulating antibodies to acetylcholine receptor. However, less than 10% of patients with myasthenia gravis are found to have a thymoma on CT. Thymectomy leads to improvement or resolution of symptoms of myasthenia gravis in only about 25% of patients with thymomas. In contrast, in patients with myasthenia gravis and no thymoma, thymectomy results are superior: up to 50% of patients have a complete remission and 90% improve. In 5% of patients with thymomas, other paraneoplastic syndromes, including red cell aplasia, hypogamma-globulinemia, systemic lupus erythematosus, Cushing's syndrome, or SIADH may be present. Large thymic tumors may present with symptoms related to a mass effect, which may include cough, chest pain, dyspnea, or superior vena cava syndrome.

The diagnosis may be suspected based on CT scan and history, but imaging alone is not diagnostic. In most centers, the diagnosis is made after surgical resection because of the relative difficulty of obtaining a needle biopsy and the likelihood that removal will ultimately be recommended. However, CT-guided FNA biopsy has been reported to have a diagnostic sensitivity of 87% and a specificity of 95% in specialized centers. Cytokeratin is the marker that best distinguishes thymomas from lymphomas. In most patients, the distinction between lymphomas and thymomas can be made on CT scan, since most lymphomas have marked lymphadenopathy and thymomas most frequently appear as a solitary encapsulated mass.

The most commonly accepted staging system for thymomas is that of Masaoka. It is based on the presence or absence of gross or microscopic invasion of the capsule and of surrounding structures, as well as on the presence or absence of metastases (Table 18-15).

Histologically, thymomas are generally characterized by a mixture of epithelial cells and mature lymphocytes. Grossly, many thymomas remain well encapsulated. Even those with capsular invasion often lack histologic features of malignancy; they appear cytologically benign and identical to early-stage tumors. This lack of classic cellular features of malignancy is why most pathologists use the term "thymomas" or "invasive thymomas" rather than "malignant thymomas." Thymic tumors with malignant cytologic features are classified separately and referred to as "thymic carcinomas."

The definitive treatment for thymomas is complete surgical removal for all resectable tumors; local recurrence rates and survival vary according to stage (Fig. 18-37). Resection is generally accomplished by median sternotomy with extension to hemi-clamshell in more advanced cases. Even advanced tumors with local invasion of resectable structures such as the pericardium, superior vena cava, or innominate vessels should be considered for resection with reconstruction. VATS resection has been reported for small, encapsulated thymomas, but no large series or long-term results are available to support this approach.

The role of adjuvant or neoadjuvant therapies for advanced-stage tumors remains unclear. Traditionally, stage II thymomas have been

Table 18-15
Masaoka Classification of Thymoma Staging

Stage I: Encapsulated tumor with no gross or microscopic evidence of capsular invasion
Stage II: Gross capsular invasion or invasion into the mediastinal fat or pleura or microscopic capsular invasion
Stage III: Gross invasion into the pericardium, great vessels, or lung
Stage IV a: Pleural or pericardial dissemination
Stage IV b: Lymphogenous or hematogenous metastasis

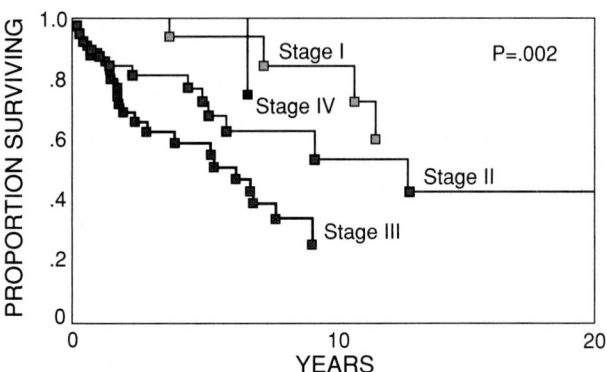

FIG. 18-37. *Stage-specific survival for thymomas.*

treated by complete surgical resection followed by mediastinal radiation, but due to the relatively small number of cases, randomized trials have not been done. A recent retrospective review of a single-institution series of stage II thymoma patients showed no difference in survival or local recurrence after complete surgical resection alone, as compared with surgical resection with radiotherapy. Advanced thymomas have been shown to respond to platinum-based chemotherapy and to corticosteroids. One summary of chemotherapy trials showed an overall response rate of about 70%. Combining radiotherapy and chemotherapy for local progression also has been successful in some small series the combination appears to prolong survival, although most advanced-stage, unresectable thymomas will recur. Therefore it is imperative that all patients with thymomas undergo a thorough evaluation for potential resection.

Thymic Carcinoma. Thymic carcinomas are unlike encapsulated or invasive thymomas in that they are unequivocally malignant at the microscopic level. Suster and Rosai classified thymic carcinomas into low-grade and high-grade tumors. Low-grade tumors are well differentiated with squamous cell, mucoepidermoid, or basaloid features. High-grade thymic carcinomas include those with lymphoepithelial, small-cell neuroendocrine, sarcomatoid, clear-cell, and undifferentiated or anaplastic features. Compared with thymomas, they are a more heterogeneous group of malignancies with a propensity for early local invasion and widespread metastases. Complete resection is occasionally curative, but most thymic carcinomas will recur and are refractory to chemotherapy. The prognosis of such patients remains poor.

Thymolipoma. Thymolipomas are rare benign tumors that may grow to a very large size before being diagnosed. On CT scan, their appearance can be dramatic, with a characteristic fat density dotted by islands of soft tissue density representing islands of thymic tissue (Fig. 18-38). Thymolipomas are generally well-encapsulated, soft, and pliable masses that do not invade surrounding structures. Resection is recommended for large masses.

Neurogenic Tumors

Most neurogenic tumors of the mediastinum arise from the cells of the nerve sheath, from ganglion cells, or from the paraganglionic system (Table 18-16). The incidence, cell types, and risk of malignancy strongly correlate with patient age. Tumors of nerve sheath origin predominate in adults. Most present as asymptomatic incidental findings and most are benign. In children and young adults, tumors of the autonomic ganglia predominate, with up to two-thirds being malignant.

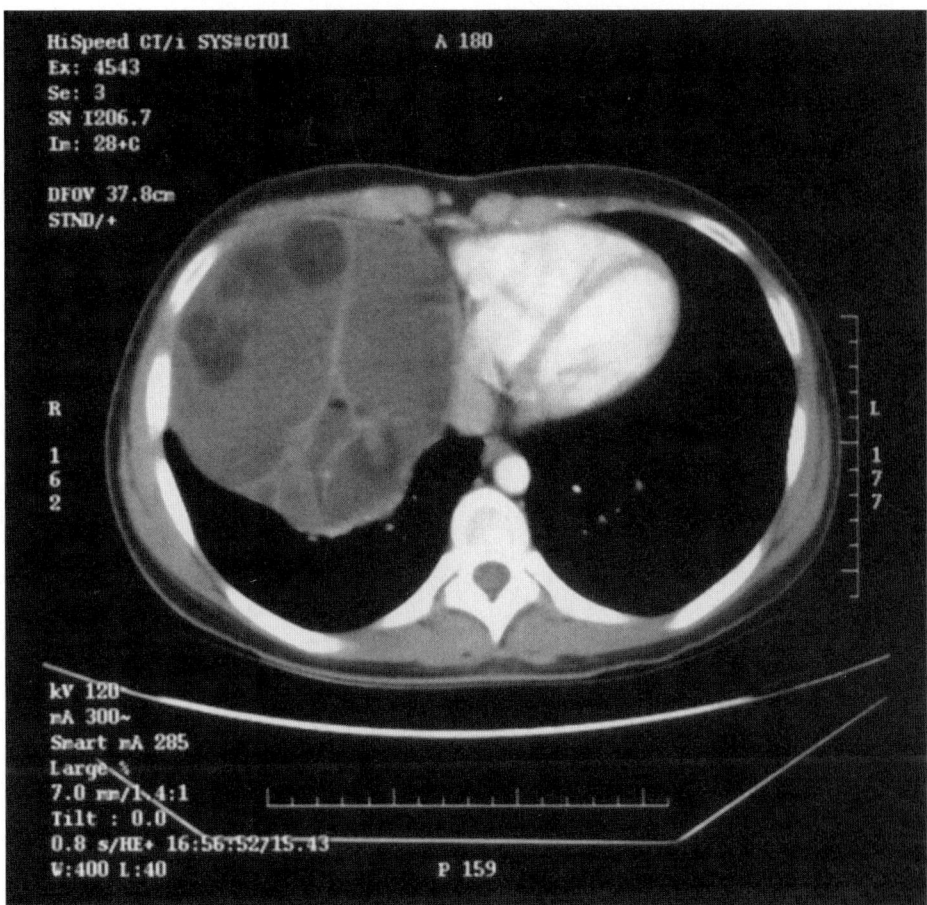

FIG. 18-38. Massive thymolipoma that was asymptomatic in an 18-year-old female.

Nerve Sheath Tumors. Nerve sheath tumors account for 20% of all mediastinal tumors. More than 95% of nerve sheath tumors are benign neurilemomas or neurofibromas. Malignant neurosarcomas are much less common.

Neurilemoma. Neurilemomas, also called schwannomas, arise from Schwann cells in intercostal nerves. They are firm, well-encapsulated, and generally benign. Two characteristic histologic components of benign neurilemomas exist and are referred to as Antoni type A and Antoni type B regions. Antoni type A regions contain compact spindle cells with twisted nuclei and nuclear palisading. Antoni type B regions contain loose and myxoid connective tissue with a haphazard cellular arrangement. These characteristics allow them to be distinguished from malignant, fibrosarcomatous tumors, which lack encapsulation and have no Antoni features. If routine CT scan suggests extension of a neurilemoma into the intervertebral foramen, MRI is suggested to evaluate the extent of this "dumbbell" configuration (Fig. 18-39). Such a configuration may lead to cord compression and paralysis, and requires a more complex surgical approach. It is recommended that most nerve sheath tumors be resected. Traditionally, this have been performed by open thoracotomy but more recently, a VATS approach has been established as safe and effective for simple operations. It is reasonable to follow small, asymptomatic paravertebral tumors in older patients or in patients at high risk for surgery. In children, ganglioneuroblastomas or neuroblastomas are more common; therefore all neurogenic tumors should be completely resected.

Neurofibroma. Neurofibromas have components of both nerve sheaths and nerve cells and account for up to 25% of nerve sheath

Table 18-16
Classification of Neurogenic Tumors of the Mediastinum

Tumor Origin	Benign	Malignant
Nerve sheath	Neurilemmoma, neurofibroma, melanotic schwannoma, granular cell tumor	Neurofibrosarcoma
Ganglion cell	Ganglioneuroma	Ganglioneuroblastoma, neuroblastoma
Paraganglionic	Chemodectoma, pheochromocytoma	Malignant chemodectoma, malignant pheochromocytoma

SOURCE: Reproduced with permission from Bousamra, M: Neurogenic tumors of the mediastinum, in Pearson FG et al (eds): *Thoracic Surgery,* 2nd ed. New York: Churchill Livingstone, 2002, p 1732.

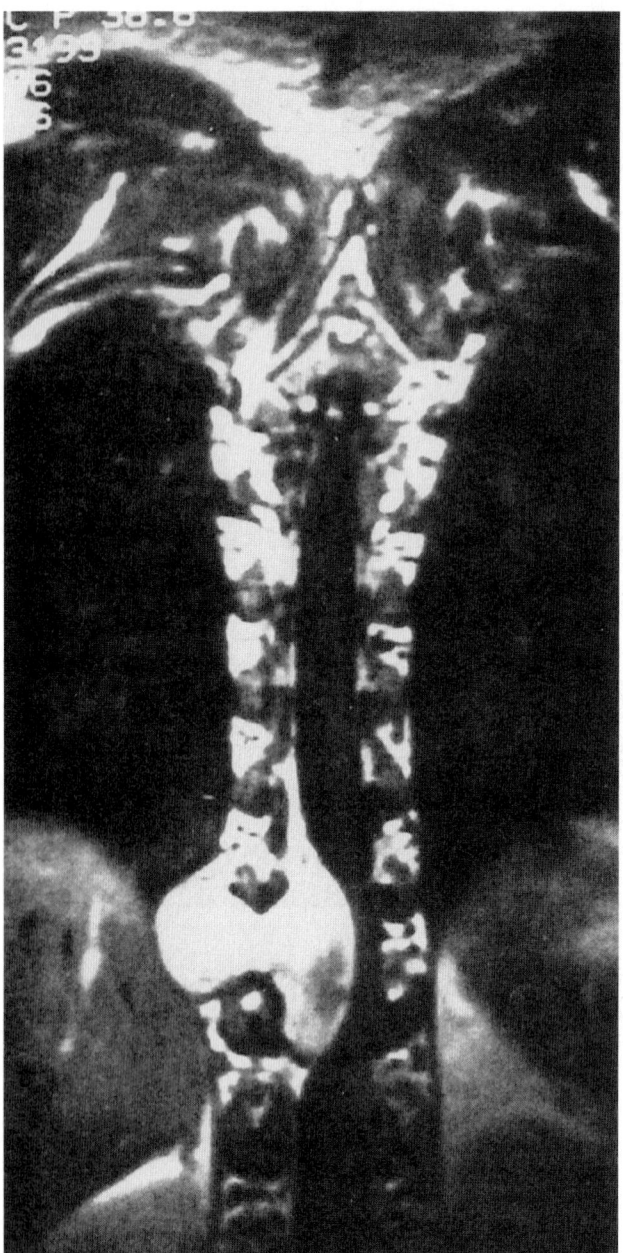

FIG. 18-39. MRI image of a neurogenic tumor with extension into the spinal canal via the foramen, giving a typical dumbbell appearance.

tumors. Up to 40% of patients with mediastinal fibromas have generalized neurofibromatosis (von Recklinghausen's disease). About 70% of neurofibromas are benign. Malignant degeneration to a neurofibrosarcoma may occur in 25 to 30% of patients. The risk of malignant degeneration increases with advancing age, with von Recklinghausen's disease, and with exposure to previous radiation. Neurofibrosarcomas carry a poor prognosis because of rapid growth and aggressive local invasion along nerve bundles. Complete surgical resection is the mainstay of treatment. Adjuvant radiotherapy or chemotherapy does not confer a significant benefit, but may be added if complete resection is not possible. The 5-year survival rate is 53%, but drops to 16% in patients with neurofibromatosis or with large tumors (>5 cm).

Ganglion Cell Tumors. Ganglion cell tumors arise from the sympathetic chain or from the adrenal medulla. Histologic cell types include ganglioneuromas, ganglioneuroblastomas, and neuroblastomas.

Ganglioneuroma. Ganglioneuromas are well-differentiated, benign tumors that are characterized histologically by well-differentiated ganglion cells with a background of Schwann cells. They tend to occur in asymptomatic young adults, although diarrhea related to secretion of a vasoactive intestinal peptide has been described. These tumors have a propensity for intraspinal canal extension, although they remain well-encapsulated; complete resection is curative, with a low risk of local recurrence.

Ganglioneuroblastoma. Ganglioneuroblastomas contain a mixture of benign ganglion cells and malignant neuroblasts. The distribution of these cells within the tumor is predictive of the clinical course. The nodular pattern is associated with a high incidence of metastatic disease; the diffuse pattern rarely metastasizes. On gross examination, these tumors often remain encapsulated; histologically, there are focal calcifications around regions of neuroblasts. Ganglioneuroblastomas arise most frequently in infants and children under 3 years old. The majority of tumors are resectable, with a 5-year survival rate of 80%.

Neuroblastoma. Neuroblastomas are highly malignant. They are the most common extracranial solid malignancy in pediatric patients and the most common intrathoracic malignancy of childhood. The adrenal gland is a common primary site, but 14% of all neuroblastomas arise in the thorax, where the tumors are commonly associated with extension into the spinal canal and osseous invasion. These thoracic tumors are not as recalcitrant to chemotherapy and surgical resection as other chest malignancies; they are more likely to be resectable, with less invasion of surrounding organs. More than half occur in children under 2 years old; 90% arise within the first decade of life and are therefore discussed in more detail in Chap. 38, Pediatric Surgery.

Paraganglionic Tumors. Paraganglionic tumors arising in the thoracic cavity include chemodectomas and pheochromocytomas. Only 10% of all pheochromocytomas are located in an extra-adrenal site. Intrathoracic pheochromocytomas are one of the most rare tumors. Approximately 10% of thoracic pheochromocytomas are malignant, a rate similar to that of adrenal tumors. The most common thoracic location is within the costovertebral sulcus, but paraganglionic tumors also arise within the visceral compartment of the mediastinum. These catecholamine-producing lesions can lead to life-threatening hemodynamic problems, so complete removal is important. Diagnosis is generally confirmed by measuring elevated levels of urinary catecholamines and their metabolites. Localization is by CT scan, aided by ^{131}I metaiodobenzylguanidine scintigraphy. Preoperative care includes alpha- and beta-adrenergic blockade to prevent intraoperative malignant hypertension and arrhythmias. These tumors tend to be highly vascular and should be approached with care. Chemodectomas are rare tumors that may be located around the aortic arch, vagus nerves, or aorticosympathetics. They rarely secrete catecholamines and are malignant in up to 30% of patients.

Lymphoma

Overall, lymphomas are the most common malignancy of the mediastinum. In about 50% of patients who have both Hodgkin's and non-Hodgkin's lymphoma, the mediastinum may be the primary site. The anterior compartment is most commonly involved, with occasional involvement of the middle compartment and hilar nodes.

The posterior compartment is rarely involved Chemotherapy and/or radiation results in a cure rate of up to 90% for patients with early-stage Hodgkin's disease, and up to 60% with more advanced stages.

Mediastinal Germ Cell Tumors

Germ cell tumors are uncommon neoplasms, with only about 7000 diagnosed each year. However, they are the most common malignancy in young men between age 15 and 35 years. Most germ cell tumors are gonadal in origin. Those with the mediastinum as the primary site are rare, constituting less than 5% of all germ cell tumors, and less than 1% of all mediastinal tumors (usually occurring in the anterior compartment). If a malignant mediastinal germ cell tumor is found, it is important to exclude a gonadal primary tumor. Primary mediastinal germ cell tumors (including teratomas, seminomas, and nonseminomatous malignant germ cell tumors) are a heterogeneous group of benign and malignant neoplasms thought to originate from primitive pluripotent germ cells "misplaced" in the mediastinum during embryonic development. Previously, most mediastinal germ cell tumors were thought to be metastatic. However, two lines of evidence suggest that many mediastinal germ cell tumors are primary, developing from pluripotent primordial germ cells in the mediastinum: (1) several autopsy series showed that patients with extragonadal sites of germ cell tumors, presumed previously to have originated from the gonads, had no evidence of an occult primary tumor or of any residual scar of the gonads, even after an exhaustive search; and (2) patients treated by surgery or radiation for their mediastinal germ cell tumors had long-term survival with no late testicular recurrences.

About one-third of all primary mediastinal germ cell tumors are seminomatous. Two-thirds are nonseminomatous tumors or teratomas. Treatment and prognosis vary considerably within these two groups. Mature teratomas are benign and can generally be diagnosed by the characteristic CT findings of multilocular cystic tumors, encapsulated with combinations of fluid, soft tissue, calcium, and/or fat attenuation in the anterior compartment. FNA biopsy alone may be diagnostic for seminomas, usually with normal serum markers, including hCG and AFP. In 10% of seminomas, hCG levels may be slightly elevated. FNA findings, along with high hCG and AFP levels, can accurately diagnose nonseminomatous tumors. If the diagnosis remains uncertain after assessment of FNA findings and serum marker levels, then core-needle biopsies or surgical biopsies may be required. An anterior mediastinotomy (Chamberlain procedure) or a thoracoscopy is the most frequent diagnostic surgical approach.

Teratoma. Teratomas are the most common type of mediastinal germ cell tumors, accounting for 60 to 70% of mediastinal germ cell tumors. They contain two or three embryonic layers that may include teeth, skin, hair (ectodermal), cartilage and bone (mesodermal), or bronchial, intestinal, or pancreatic tissue (endodermal). Therapy for mature, benign teratomas is surgical resection, which confers an excellent prognosis.

Rarely, teratomas may contain a focus of carcinoma; these malignant teratomas (or teratocarcinomas) are locally aggressive. Often diagnosed at an unresectable stage, they respond poorly to chemotherapy and in a limited manner to radiotherapy; the prognosis is uniformly poor.

Seminoma. Most patients with seminomas have advanced disease at the time of diagnosis and present with symptoms of local compression, including superior vena caval syndrome, dyspnea, or chest discomfort. With advanced disease, the preferred treatment is combination cisplatin-based chemotherapy regimens with bleomycin and either etoposide or vinblastine. Complete responses have been reported in over 75% of patients treated with these regimens. Surgical resection may be curative for small asymptomatic seminomas that are found incidentally with screening CT scans. Surgical resection of residual masses after chemotherapy may be indicated.

Nonseminomatous Germ Cell Tumors. Nonseminomatous germ cell tumors include embryonal cell carcinomas, choriocarcinomas, endodermal sinus tumors, and mixed types. They are often bulky, irregular tumors of the anterior mediastinum with areas of low attenuation on CT scan because of necrosis, hemorrhage, or cyst formation. Frequently, adjacent structures have been involved, with metastases to regional lymph nodes, pleura, and lungs. Lactate dehydrogenase (LDH), AFP, and hCG levels are frequently elevated. Chemotherapy is the preferred treatment and includes combination therapy with cisplatin, bleomycin, and etoposide. With this regimen, survival at 2 years is 67% and at 5 years is 60%. Surgical resection of residual masses is indicated, as it may guide further therapy. Up to 20% of residual masses contain additional tumors; in another 40%, mature teratomas; and the remaining 40%, fibrotic tissue.

Mediastinal Cysts

Primary Mediastinal Cyst

Benign cysts account for up to 25% of mediastinal masses. Most are located in the middle compartment. Benign cysts are the most frequent mass in the middle mediastinal compartment. A CT scan showing characteristic features of near water density in a typical location is virtually 100% diagnostic.

Pericardial Cyst

Pericardial cysts, the most common type of mediastinal cysts, are usually asymptomatic and detected incidentally. Typically they contain a clear fluid and appear in the right costophrenic angle. The cyst wall lining is a single layer of mesothelial cells. For most simple, asymptomatic pericardial cysts, observation alone is recommended. Surgical resection or aspiration may be indicated for complex cysts or large symptomatic cysts.

Bronchogenic Cyst

Bronchogenic cysts are developmental anomalies that occur during embryogenesis and occur as an abnormal budding of the foregut or tracheobronchial tree. Most frequently they arise in the mediastinum, but about 15% occur within the pulmonary parenchyma. The most frequent mediastinal location is just posterior to the carina or main stem bronchus. Thin-walled and lined with respiratory epithelium, they contain a protein-rich mucoid material and varying amounts of seromucous glands, smooth muscle, and cartilage. They may communicate with the tracheobronchial tree.

The management of bronchogenic cysts remains controversial. In children, most such cysts are symptomatic. Resection is generally recommended since serious complications may occur if the cyst becomes larger or infected. Complications include airway obstruction, infection, rupture, and rarely, malignant transformation.

In adults, over half of all bronchogenic cysts are found incidentally during work-up for an unrelated problem or during screening. The natural history of an incidentally diagnosed, asymptomatic bronchogenic cyst is unknown, but it is clear that many such cysts do not lead to clinical problems. In one study of young military personnel, 78% of all bronchogenic cysts found on routine chest x-rays were asymptomatic. However, in other reports with more comprehensive follow-up, up to 67% of adults with incidentally found bronchogenic cysts eventually became symptomatic. Symptoms include chest pain, cough, dyspnea, and fever. Serious complications are less common and include hemodynamic compromise, airway obstruction, pulmonary artery obstruction, hemoptysis, and malignant degeneration. Symptomatic bronchogenic cysts should be removed. Traditionally, removal has been via posterolateral thoracotomy. Resection of infected cysts may be quite difficult because of dense adhesions; elective removal is often recommended before infection has a chance to occur. Thoracoscopic exploration and resection are possible for small cysts with minimal adhesions. The goal of minimally-invasive or open surgery should be complete removal of the cyst wall.

Enteric Cyst

Most clinicians agree that in contrast to bronchogenic cysts, esophageal cysts should be removed, regardless of the presence or absence of symptoms. Esophageal cysts have a propensity for serious complications secondary to enlargement, leading to hemorrhage, infection, or perforation. Thus surgical resection is the treatment of choice in both adults and children.

Thymic Cyst

Thymic cysts are generally asymptomatic and are discovered incidentally during radiographic work-up for an unrelated problem. Simple cysts are of no consequence; however, the occasional cystic neoplasm must be ruled out. Cystic components occasionally are seen in patients with thymoma and Hodgkin's disease.

Ectopic Endocrine Glands

Up to 5% of all mediastinal masses are estimated to be of thyroid origin. However, most of these masses are simple extensions of thyroid masses. They are usually nontoxic and over 95% of such masses can be completely resected through a cervical approach. True ectopic thyroid tissue of the mediastinum is rare. About 10 to 20% of abnormal parathyroid glands are found in the mediastinum; most can be removed during exploration from a cervical incision. In cases of true mediastinal parathyroid glands, thoracoscopic or open resection may be indicated. Location can generally be pinpointed by a combination of CT scan and Sestamibi scans.

Mediastinitis

Acute Mediastinitis

Acute mediastinitis is a fulminant infectious process that spreads along the fascial planes of the mediastinum. Infections originate most commonly from esophageal perforations, sternal infections, and oropharyngeal or neck infections, but a number of less common etiologic factors can lead to this deadly process (Table 18-17). As infections from any of these sources enter the mediastinum, spread may be rapid along the continuous fascial planes connecting the cervical and mediastinal compartments. Clinical signs and symptoms include fever, chest pain, dysphagia, respiratory distress, and cervical and upper thoracic subcutaneous crepitus. In severe cases, the clinical course can rapidly deteriorate to florid sepsis, hemodynamic instability, and death. Thus, a high index of suspicion is required in the context of any infection with access to the mediastinal compartments.

A chest CT scan can be particularly helpful in determining the extent of spread and the best approach to surgical drainage. Acute

Table 18-17
Etiologic Factors in Acute Mediastinitis

Esophageal Perforation
Iatrogenic
    Balloon dilatation (for achalasia)
    Bougienage (for peptic stricture)
    Esophagoscopy
    Sclerotherapy (for variceal bleeding)
Spontaneous
    Postemetic (Boerhaave's syndrome)
    Straining during:
        Elimination
            Weight lifting
    Seizure
    Pregnancy
    Childbirth
Ingestion of Foreign Bodies
Trauma
    Blunt
    Penetrating
Postsurgical
    Infection
    Anastomotic leak
    Erosion by cancer
Deep sternotomy wound infection
Oropharynx and neck infections
Ludwig's angina
Quinsy
Retropharyngeal abscess
Cellulitis and suppurative lymphadenitis of neck
Infections of lung and pleura
Subphrenic abscess
Rib or vertebral osteomyelitis
Hematogenous or metastatic abscess

SOURCE: Reproduced with permission from Razzuk MA et al: Infections of the mediastinum, in Pearson FG et al (eds): *Thoracic Surgery,* 2nd ed. New York: Churchill Livingstone, 2002, p 1604.

mediastinitis is a true surgical emergency and treatment must be instituted immediately and must be aimed at correcting the primary problem, such as the esophageal perforation or oropharyngeal abscess. Another major concern is débridement and drainage of the spreading infectious process within the mediastinum, neck, pleura, and other tissue planes. Antibiotics, fluid resuscitation, and other supportive measures are important, but surgical correction of the problem at its source and open débridement of infected areas are critical measures. Surgical débridement may need to be repeated, and other planes and cavities explored depending on the patient's clinical status. Blood cell counts and serial CT scans may also be required. Persistent sepsis or collections on CT scan may require further radical surgical débridement.

Chronic Mediastinitis

Sclerosing or fibrosing mediastinitis is a result of chronic inflammation of the mediastinum, most frequently as a result of granulomatous infections such as histoplasmosis or tuberculosis. The process begins in lymph nodes and continues as a chronic, low-grade inflammation leading to fibrosis and scarring. In many patients, the clinical manifestations are silent. However, if the fibrosis is progressive and severe, it may lead to encasement of the mediastinal structures, causing entrapment and compression of the low-pressure veins (including the superior vena cava and innominate and azygos veins). This fibrotic process can compromise other structures such as the esophagus and pulmonary arteries. There is no definitive treatment. Surgery is indicated only for diagnosis or in specific patients to relieve airway or esophageal obstruction or to achieve vascular reconstruction. Reports of palliative success with less invasive procedures (such as dilation and stenting of airways, the esophagus, or the superior vena cava) are promising. In one series of 22 patients, ketoconazole was effective in controlling progression. In another series of 71 patients, 30% died during long-term follow-up. Chronic mediastinitis is similar to the fibrotic changes that occur in other sites including retroperitoneal fibrosis, sclerosing cholangitis, and Riedel's thyroiditis.

DISEASES OF THE PLEURA AND PLEURAL SPACE

Anatomy

The parietal pleura is a mesothelial lining of each hemithorax that invaginates at the hilum of each lung and continues on to cover each lung as the visceral pleura. Between these two surfaces is the potential pleural space, which is normally occupied only by a thin layer of lubricating pleural fluid. Two physiologic processes hold the visceral pleura of the lung in close apposition to the parietal pleura of the chest wall: those mechanisms that constantly remove pleural fluid and those that prevent an accumulation of free gas in the pleural space. A network of somatic, sympathetic, and parasympathetic fibers innervates the parietal pleura. Irritation of the parietal surface by inflammation, tumor invasion, trauma, and other processes can lead to a sensation of chest wall pain. The visceral pleura has no somatic innervation.

Pleural Effusion

Pleural effusion refers to any significant collection of fluid within the pleural space. Normally, there is an ongoing balance between the lubricating fluid flowing into the pleural space and its continuous absorption. Between 5 and 10 L of fluid normally enters the pleural space daily by filtration through microvessels supplying the parietal pleura (located mainly in the less dependent regions of the cavity). The net balance of pressures in these capillaries leads to fluid flow from the parietal pleural surface into the pleural space, and the net balance of forces in the pulmonary circulation leads to absorption through the visceral pleura. Normally, 15 to 20 mL of pleural fluid is present at any given time. Any disturbance in these forces can lead to imbalance and accumulation of pleural fluid. Common pathologic conditions in North America that lead to pleural effusion include congestive heart failure, bacterial pneumonia, malignancy, and pulmonary emboli (Table 18-18).

Diagnostic Work-Up

The initial diagnostic work-up for pleural effusion is guided in large part by the patient's history and physical examination. Bilateral pleural effusions are due to congestive heart failure in over 80% of patients. If the clinical history suggests this diagnosis, a trial of diuresis may be indicated (rather than thoracentesis). Up to 75% of effusions due to congestive heart failure resolve within 48 hours with diuresis alone.

A patient presenting with cough, fever, leukocytosis, and unilateral infiltrate and effusion is likely to have a parapneumonic process. If the effusion is small and the patient responds to antibiotics, a diagnostic thoracentesis may be unnecessary. However, a patient who has an obvious pneumonia and a large pleural effusion that is purulent and foul-smelling has an empyema. Aggressive drainage with chest tubes is required, possibly with surgical intervention. Outside of the setting of congestive heart failure or small effusions associated with an improving pneumonia, most patients with pleural effusions of unknown cause should undergo thoracentesis.

A general classification of pleural fluid collections into transudates and exudates is helpful in understanding the various causes (Table 18-19). Transudates are protein-poor ultrafiltrates of plasma that occur because of alterations in the systemic hydrostatic pressures or colloid osmotic pressures (for example, with congestive heart failure or cirrhosis). On gross visual inspection, a transudative effusion is generally clear or straw-colored. Exudates are protein-rich pleural fluid collections that generally occur because of inflammation or invasion of the pleura by tumors. Grossly, they are often turbid, bloody, or purulent. Grossly bloody effusions in the absence of trauma are frequently malignant, but may also occur in the setting of a pulmonary embolism or pneumonia. Several criteria have been traditionally used to differentiate transudates from exudates. An effusion is considered exudative if the pleural fluid to serum ratio of protein is greater than 0.5 and the LDH ratio is greater than 0.6 or the absolute pleural LDH level is greater than two-thirds of the normal upper limit for serum. If these criteria suggest a transudate, the patient should be carefully evaluated for congestive heart failure, cirrhosis, or conditions associated with transudates.

If an exudative effusion is suggested, further diagnostic studies may be helpful. If total and differential cell counts reveal a predominance of neutrophils (>50% of cells), the effusion is likely to be associated with an acute inflammatory process (such as a parapneumonic effusion or empyema, pulmonary embolus, or pancreatitis). A predominance of mononuclear cells suggests a more chronic inflammatory process (such as cancer or tuberculosis). Gram's stains and cultures should be obtained, if possible with inoculation into culture bottles at the bedside. Pleural fluid glucose levels are frequently decreased (<60 mg/dL) with complex parapneumonic effusions or malignant effusions. Cytologic testing should be done on exudative effusions to rule out an associated malignancy. Cytologic diagnosis is accurate in diagnosing over 70% of malignant effusions

Table 18-18

Leading Causes of Pleural Effusion in the United States, According to Analysis of Patients Subjected to Thoracentesis

Cause	Annual Incidence	Transudate	Exudate
Congestive heart failure	500,000	Yes	No
Pneumonia	300,000	No	Yes
Cancer	200,000	No	Yes
Pulmonary embolus	150,000	Sometimes	Sometimes
Viral disease	100,000	No	Yes
Coronary artery bypass surgery	60,000	No	Yes
Cirrhosis with ascites	50,000	Yes	No

SOURCE: Reproduced with permission from Light RW: Pleural effusion. *N Engl J Med* 346:1971, 2002.

Table 18-19
Differential Diagnosis of Pleural Effusions

I. Transudative pleural effusions
  A. Congestive heart failure
  B. Cirrhosis
  C. Nephrotic syndrome
  D. Superior vena caval obstruction
  E. Fontan procedure
  F. Urinothorax
  G. Peritoneal dialysis
  H. Glomerulonephritis
  I. Myxedema
  J. Cerebrospinal fluid leaks to pleura
  K. Hypoalbuminemia
  L. Pulmonary emboli
  M. Sarcoidosis

II. Exudative pleural effusions
  A. Neoplastic diseases
    1. Metastatic disease
    2. Mesothelioma
    3. Body cavity lymphoma
    4. Pyothorax-associated lymphoma
  B. Infectious diseases
    1. Bacterial infections
    2. Tuberculosis
    3. Fungal infections
    4. Parasitic infections
    5. Viral infections
  C. Pulmonary embolization
  D. Gastrointestinal disease
    1. Pancreatic disease
    2. Subphrenic abscess
    3. Intrahepatic abscess
    4. Intrasplenic abscess
    5. Esophageal perforation
    6. Postabdominal surgery
    7. Diaphragmatic hernia
    8. Endoscopic variceal sclerosis
    9. Post-liver transplant
  E. Heart diseases
    1. Post-coronary artery bypass graft surgery
    2. Post-cardiac injury (Dressler's) syndrome
    3. Pericardial disease
  F. Obstetric and gynecologic disease
    1. Ovarian hyperstimulation syndrome
    2. Fetal pleural effusion
    3. Postpartum pleural effusion
    4. Megis' syndrome
    5. Endometriosis
  G. Collagen-vascular disease
    1. Rheumatoid pleuritis
    2. Systemic lupus erythematosus
    3. Drug-induced lupus
    4. Immunoblastic lymphadenopathy
    5. Sjögren's syndrome
    6. Familial Mediterranean fever
    7. Churg-Strauss syndrome
    8. Wegener's granulomatosis
  H. Drug-induced pleural disease
    1. Nitrofurantoin
    2. Dantrolene
    3. Methysergide
    4. Ergot alkaloids
    5. Amiodarone
    6. Interleukin-2
    7. Procarbazine
    8. Methotrexate
    9. Clozapine

(Continued)

Table 18-19
Differential Diagnosis of Pleural Effusions (*continued*)

I. Miscellaneous diseases and conditions
  1. Asbestos exposure
  2. Post-lung transplant
  3. Post-bone marrow transplant
  4. Yellow nail syndrome
  5. Sarcoidosis
  6. Uremia
  7. Trapped lung
  8. Therapeutic radiation exposure
  9. Drowning
  10. Amyloidosis
  11. Milk of calcium pleural effusion
  12. Electrical burns
  13. Extramedullary hematopoiesis
  14. Rupture of mediastinal cyst
  15. Acute respiratory distress syndrome
  16. Whipple's disease
  17. Iatrogenic pleural effusions
J. Hemothorax
K. Chylothorax

SOURCE: Reproduced with permission from Light RW: Approach to the patient, in Light RW (ed): *Pleural Diseases.* Philadelphia: Lippincott, Williams & Wilkins, 2001, p 88.

associated with adenocarcinomas, but is less sensitive for mesotheliomas (<10%), squamous cell carcinomas (20%), or lymphomas (25 to 50%). If the diagnosis remains uncertain after drainage and fluid analysis, thoracoscopy and direct biopsies are indicated. Tuberculous effusions can now be diagnosed accurately by increased levels of pleural fluid adenosine deaminase (above 40 U per L). Pulmonary embolism should be suspected in a patient with a pleural effusion occurring in association with pleuritic chest pain, hemoptysis, or dyspnea out of proportion to the size of the effusion. These effusions may be transudative, but if an associated infarct near the pleural surface occurs, an exudate may be seen. If a pulmonary embolism is suspected in a postoperative patient, most clinicians would obtain a spiral CT scan. Alternatively, duplex ultrasonography of the lower extremities may yield a diagnosis of deep vein thrombosis, thereby indicating anticoagulant therapy and precluding the need for a specific diagnosis of pulmonary embolism. In some patients, a blood test for levels of D-dimer may be helpful; if a sensitive D-dimer blood test is negative, pulmonary embolism may be ruled out.

Malignant Pleural Effusion

Malignant pleural effusions may occur in association with a number of different malignancies, most commonly lung cancer, breast cancer, and lymphomas, depending on the patient's age and gender (Tables 18-20 and 18-21). Malignant effusions are exudative and often tinged with blood. An effusion in the setting of a malignancy means a more advanced stage; it generally indicates an unresectable tumor, with a mean survival of 3 to 11 months. Occasionally, benign pleural effusions may be associated with a bronchogenic NSCLC, and surgical resection may still be indicated if the cytology of the effusions is negative for malignancy. An important issue is the size of the effusion and the degree of dyspnea that results. Symptomatic, moderate to large effusions should be drained by chest tube, pigtail catheter, or VATS, followed by instillation of a sclerosing agent. Before sclerosing the pleural cavity, whether by chest tube or VATS, the lung should be nearly fully expanded. Poor expansion of the lung

Table 18-20
Primary Organ Site or Neoplasm Type in Male Patients with Malignant Pleural Effusions

Primary Site or Tumor Type	No. of Male Patients	Percentage of Male Patients
Lung	140	49.1
Lymphoma/leukemia	60	21.1
Gastrointestinal tract	20	7.0
Genitourinary tract	17	6.0
Melanoma	4	1.4
Miscellaneous less common tumors	10	3.5
Primary site unknown	31	10.9
Total	285	100

SOURCE: Reproduced with permission from Johnson WW: The malignant pleural effusion: A review of cytopathologic diagnoses of 584 specimens from 472 consecutive patients. *Cancer* 56:905, 1985.

(because of entrapment by tumor or adhesions) generally predicts a poor result. The choice of sclerosant includes talc, bleomycin, or doxycycline. Success rates of controlling the effusion range from 60 to 90%, depending on the exact scope of the clinical study, the degree of lung expansion after the pleural fluid is drained, and the care with which the outcomes were reported.

Empyema

Thoracic empyema is defined by a purulent pleural effusion. The most common causes are parapneumonic, but postsurgical or posttraumatic empyema is also common (Table 18-22). Grossly purulent, foul-smelling pleural fluid makes the diagnosis of empyema obvious on visual examination at the bedside. In the early stage, small to moderate turbid pleural effusions in the setting of a pneumonic process may require further pleural fluid analysis. Close clinical follow-up is also imperative to determine if progression to empyema is occurring. A deteriorating clinical course or a pleural pH of less than 7.20 and a glucose level of less than 40 mg/dL indicates the need to drain the fluid.

Patients of all ages can develop empyema, but the frequency is increased in older or debilitated patients. Common associated conditions include a pneumonic process in patients with pulmonary disorders and neoplasms, cardiac problems, diabetes mellitus, drug and alcohol abuse, neurologic impairments, postthoracotomy prob-

Table 18-21
Primary Organ Site or Neoplasm Type in Female Patients with Malignant Pleural Effusions

Primary Site or Tumor Type	No. of Female Patients	Percentage of Female Patients
Breast	70	37.4
Female genital tract	38	20.3
Lung	28	15.0
Lymphoma/leukemia	14	8.0
Gastrointestinal tract	8	4.3
Melanoma	6	3.2
Urinary tract	2	1.1
Miscellaneous less common tumors	3	1.6
Primary site unknown	17	9.1
Total	187	100.0

SOURCE: Reproduced with permission from Johnson WW: The malignant pleural effusion: A review of cytopathologic diagnoses of 584 specimens from 472 consecutive patients. *Cancer* 56:905, 1985.

Table 18-22
Pathogenesis of Empyema

Contamination from a source contiguous to the pleural space (50–60%)
Lung
Mediastinum
Deep cervical
Chest wall and spine
Subphrenic
Direct inoculation of the pleural space (30–40%)
Minor thoracic interventions
Postoperative infections
Penetrating chest injuries
Hematogenous infection of the pleural space from a distant site (<1%)

SOURCE: Reproduced with permission from Paris F, et al: Empyema and bronchopleural fistula, in Pearson FG et al (eds): *Thoracic Surgery,* 2nd ed. New York: Churchill Livingstone, 2002, p 1177.

lems, and immunologic impairments. The mortality of empyema frequently depends on the degree of severity of the comorbidity; it may range from as low as 1% to over 40% in immunocompromised patients.

Pathophysiology

The spectrum of organisms involved in pneumonic processes that progress to empyema is changing. Pneumococci and staphylococci continue to be the most common, but gram-negative aerobic bacteria and anaerobes are becoming more prevalent. Cases involving mycobacteria or fungi are rare. Multiple organisms may be found in up to 50% of patients, but cultures may be sterile if antibiotics were initiated before the culture or if the culture process was not efficient. Therefore, it is imperative that the choice of antibiotics be guided by the clinical scenario and not just the organisms found on culture. Broad spectrum coverage may be still required even when cultures have failed to grow out an organism or if a single organism is grown when the clinical picture is more consistent with a multiorganism process. Common gram-negative organisms include *Escherichia coli, Klebsiella, Pseudomonas,* and Enterobacteriaceae. Anaerobic organisms may be fastidious and difficult to document by culture and are associated with periodontal diseases, aspiration syndromes, alcoholism, general anesthesia, drug abuse, or other functional associations with gastroesophageal reflux.

The route of organism entry into the pleural cavity may be by contiguous spread from pneumonia, lung abscess, liver abscess, or another infectious process with contact with the pleural space. Organisms may also enter the pleural cavity by direct contamination from thoracentesis, thoracic surgical procedures, esophageal injuries, or trauma.

As organisms enter the pleural space, an influx of polymorphonuclear cells occurs, with a subsequent release of inflammatory mediators and toxic oxygen radicals. In an attempt to control the invading organisms, these mechanisms lead to variable degrees of endothelial injury and capillary instability. An influx of fluid into the pleural space then occurs, followed by a process that overwhelms the normal exit avenues of the pleural lymphatic network. This early effusion is watery and free-flowing in the pleural cavity. Thoracentesis at this stage yields fluid with a pH typically above 7.3, a glucose level greater than 60 mg/dL, and a low LDH level (<500 U/L). At this stage, the decision to use antibiotics alone or perform a repeat thoracentesis, chest tube drainage, thoracoscopy, or open thoracotomy depends on the amount of pleural fluid, its consistency, the clinical status of the patient, the degree of expansion of the lung after drainage, and the presence of loculated fluid in the pleural space (versus free-flowing purulent fluid). If relatively thin, purulent pleural fluid is diagnosed early in the setting of a pneumonic process, the fluid often can be completely drained with simple large-bore thoracentesis. If complete lung expansion is obtained and the pneumonic process is responding to antibiotics, no further drainage may be necessary. Pleural fluid with a pH lower than 7.2 and with a low glucose level means that a more aggressive approach to drainage should be pursued.

The pleural fluid may become thick and loculated over the course of hours to days, and may be associated with fibrinous adhesions (the fibrinopurulent stage). At this stage, chest tube insertion with closed-system drainage or drainage with thoracoscopy may be necessary to remove the fluid and adhesions and to allow complete lung expansion. Further progression of the inflammatory process leads to the formation of a pleural peel, which may be flimsy and easy to remove early on. However, as the process progresses, a thick pleural rind may develop, leaving a trapped lung; complete lung decortication by thoracotomy would then be necessary, or in some patients, thoracoscopy.

Management

If there is a residual space, persistent pleural infection is likely to occur. A persistent pleural space may be secondary to contracted, but intact, underlying lung; or it may be secondary to surgical lung resection. If the space is small and well-drained by a chest tube, a conservative approach may be possible. This requires leaving the chest tubes in place and attached to closed-system drainage until symphysis of the visceral and parietal surfaces takes place. At this point, the chest tubes can be removed from suction; if the residual pleural space remains stable, the tubes can be cut and advanced out of the chest over the course of several weeks. If the patient is stable, tube removal can frequently be done in the outpatient setting, guided by the degree of drainage and the size of the residual space visualized on serial CT scans. Larger spaces may require open thoracotomy and decortication in an attempt to reexpand the lung to fill this residual space. If reexpansion has failed or appears too high risk, then open drainage, rib resection, and prolonged packing may be required, with delayed closure with muscle flaps or thoracoplasty. Most chronic pleural space problems can be avoided by early specialized thoracic surgical consultation and complete drainage of empyemas, allowing space obliteration by the reinflated lung.

Chylothorax

Chylothorax develops most commonly after surgical trauma to the thoracic duct or a major branch, but may be associated with a number of other conditions (Table 18-23). It is generally unilateral; for example, it may occur on the right after esophagectomy where the duct is most frequently injured during dissection of the distal esophagus. The esophagus comes into close proximity to the thoracic duct as it enters the chest from its origin in the abdomen at the cisterna chyli (Fig. 18-40). If the mediastinal pleura is disrupted on both sides, bilateral chylothoraces may occur. Left-sided chylothoraces may develop after a left-sided neck dissection, especially in the region of the confluence of the subclavian and internal jugular veins. Chylothorax may also follow nonsurgical trauma, including penetrating or blunt injuries to the chest or neck area, central line placements, and other surgical misadventures. It is also seen in neonates, probably secondary to birth trauma. It may be seen in association with a variety of benign and malignant diseases that generally involve the lymphatic system of the mediastinum or neck. Given the significant variability of the course of the thoracic duct

Table 18-23
Etiology of Chylothorax

Congenital
Atresia of thoracic duct
Thoracic duct-pleural space fistula
Birth trauma
Traumatic and/or Iatrogenic
Blunt
Penetrating
Surgery
Cervical: excision of lymph nodes; radical neck dissection
Thoracic
Patent ductus arteriosus
Coarctation of the aorta
Vascular procedure reinvolving the origin of left subclavian artery
Esophagectomy
Sympathectomy
Resection of thoracic aneurysm
Resection of mediastinal tumors
Left pneumonectomy
Abdominal: sympathectomy; radical lymph node dissection
Diagnostic procedures
Translumbar arteriography
Subclavian vein catheterization
Left-sided heart catheterization
Neoplasms
Infections
Tuberculous lymphadenitis
Nonspecific mediastinitis
Ascending lymphangitis
Filariasis
Miscellaneous
Venous thrombosis
Left subclavian-jugular vein
Superior vena cava
Pulmonary lymphangiomatosis

SOURCE: Reproduced with permission from Cohen RG, et al: The pleura, in Sabiston DC, et al (eds): *Surgery of the Chest*, 6th ed. Elsevier, 1995.

within the chest, some injuries are inevitable. The direct relationship of chylothorax to a surgical procedure, traumatic event, or neoplastic process may not always be obvious. Understanding the anatomy and course of the thoracic duct and some of its more common variants is helpful.

Pathophysiology

Most commonly, the thoracic duct originates in the abdomen from the cisterna chyli, which is located in the midline, near the level of the second lumbar vertebra. From this origin, the thoracic duct ascends into the chest through the aortic hiatus at the level of T10 to T12, and courses just to the right of the aorta (see Fig. 18-40). As the thoracic duct courses cephalad above the diaphragm, it most commonly remains in the right chest, lying just behind the esophagus, between the aorta and azygos vein. The duct continues superiorly, lying just to the right of the vertebral column. Then, at about the level of the fifth or sixth thoracic vertebra, it crosses behind the aorta and the aortic arch into the left posterior mediastinum. From this location, it again courses superiorly, staying near the esophagus and mediastinal pleura as it exits the thoracic inlet. As it exits the thoracic inlet, it passes just to the left, just behind the carotid sheath and anterior to the inferior thyroid and vertebral bodies. Just medial to the anterior scalene muscle, it courses inferiorly and drains into the union of the internal jugular and subclavian veins. Given the extreme variability in the main duct and its branches, accumulation of chyle in the chest or flow from

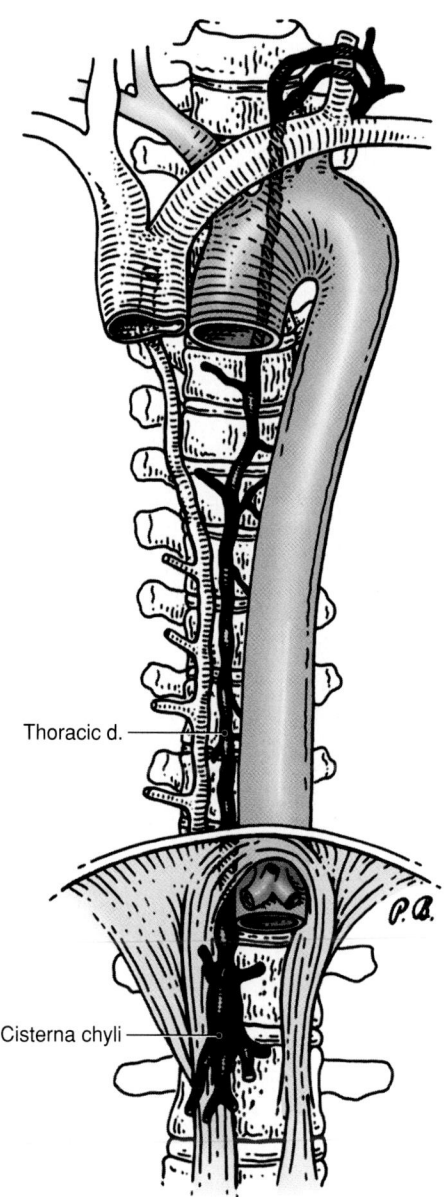

FIG. 18-40. Normal thoracic duct anatomy. The esophagus comes into close proximity with the thoracic duct as it enters the chest from its origin in the abdomen at the cisterna chyli.

Table 18-24
Composition of Chyle

Component	Amount (per 100 mL)
Total fat	0.4–5 g
Total cholesterol	65–220 mg
Total protein	2.21–5.9 g
Albumin	1.1–4.1 g
Globulin	1.1–3.1 g
Fibrinogen	16–24 g
Sugar	48–200 g
Electrolytes	Similar to plasma
Cellular elements	
Lymphocytes	400–6800/mm^3
Erythrocytes	50–600/mm^3
Antithrombin globulin	>25% plasma concentrate
Prothrombin	>25% plasma concentrate
Fibrinogen	>25% plasma concentrate

SOURCE: Reproduced with permission from Miller JI: Diagnosis and management of chylothorax. *Chest Surg Clin North Am* 6:139, 1996.

50 mg/mL, there is only a 5% chance of chylothorax. In many clinical situations, the accumulation of chyle may be slow, because of minimal digestive fat flowing through the gastrointestinal tract after major trauma or surgery, so the diagnosis may be more difficult to establish.

Management

The treatment plan for any chylothorax depends on its cause, the amount of drainage, and the clinical status of the patient (Fig. 18-41). In general, most patients are treated with a short period of chest tube drainage, NPO orders, total parenteral nutrition (TPN), and observation. Chest cavity drainage must be adequate to allow compete lung expansion. Somatostatin has been advocated by some authors, with variable results. If significant chyle drainage (>500 mL per day in an adult, >100 mL in an infant) continues despite TPN and good lung expansion, early surgical ligation of the duct is recommended. Ligation can be approached best by right thoracotomy, and in some experienced centers, by right VATS. Chylothoraces due to malignant conditions often respond to radiation and/or chemotherapy, so less commonly require surgical ligation. Untreated chylothoraces are associated with significant nutritional and immunologic depletion that leads to significant mortality. Before the introduction of surgical ligation of the thoracic duct, the mortality rate from chylothorax exceeded 50%. With the availability of TPN for nutritional supplementation and surgical ligation for persistent leaks, the mortality rate of chylothorax is less than 10%.

Access and Drainage of Pleural Fluid Collections

Approaches and Techniques

Once the decision is made to invasively access a pleural effusion, the next step is to determine if a sample of the fluid is required or if complete drainage of the pleural space is desired. This step is influenced by the clinical history, the type and amount of fluid present, the nature of the collection (such as free-flowing or loculated), the cause, and the likelihood of recurrence. For small, free-flowing effusions, an outpatient thoracentesis with a relatively small–bore needle or catheter (14- to 16-gauge) can be performed (Fig. 18-42). This approach can be used for sampling fluid or for completely

penetrating wounds may be seen after a variety of traumatic and medical conditions.

The main function of the duct is to transport fat absorbed from the digestive system. The composition of normal chyle is fat, with variable amounts of protein and lymphatic material (Table 18-24). Given the high volumes of chyle that flow through the thoracic duct, significant injuries can cause leaks in excess of 2 L per day; if left untreated, protein, volume, and lymphocyte depletion can lead to serious metabolic effects and death. The diagnosis generally requires thoracentesis, which may be grossly suggestive; often the pleural fluid is milky and nonpurulent. However, if the patient is nil per os (NPO, nothing by mouth), the pleural fluid may not be grossly abnormal. Laboratory analysis of the pleural fluid shows a high lymphocyte count and high triglyceride levels. If the triglyceride level is greater than 110 mg/100 mL, a chylothorax is almost certainly present (a 99% accuracy rate). If the triglyceride level is less than

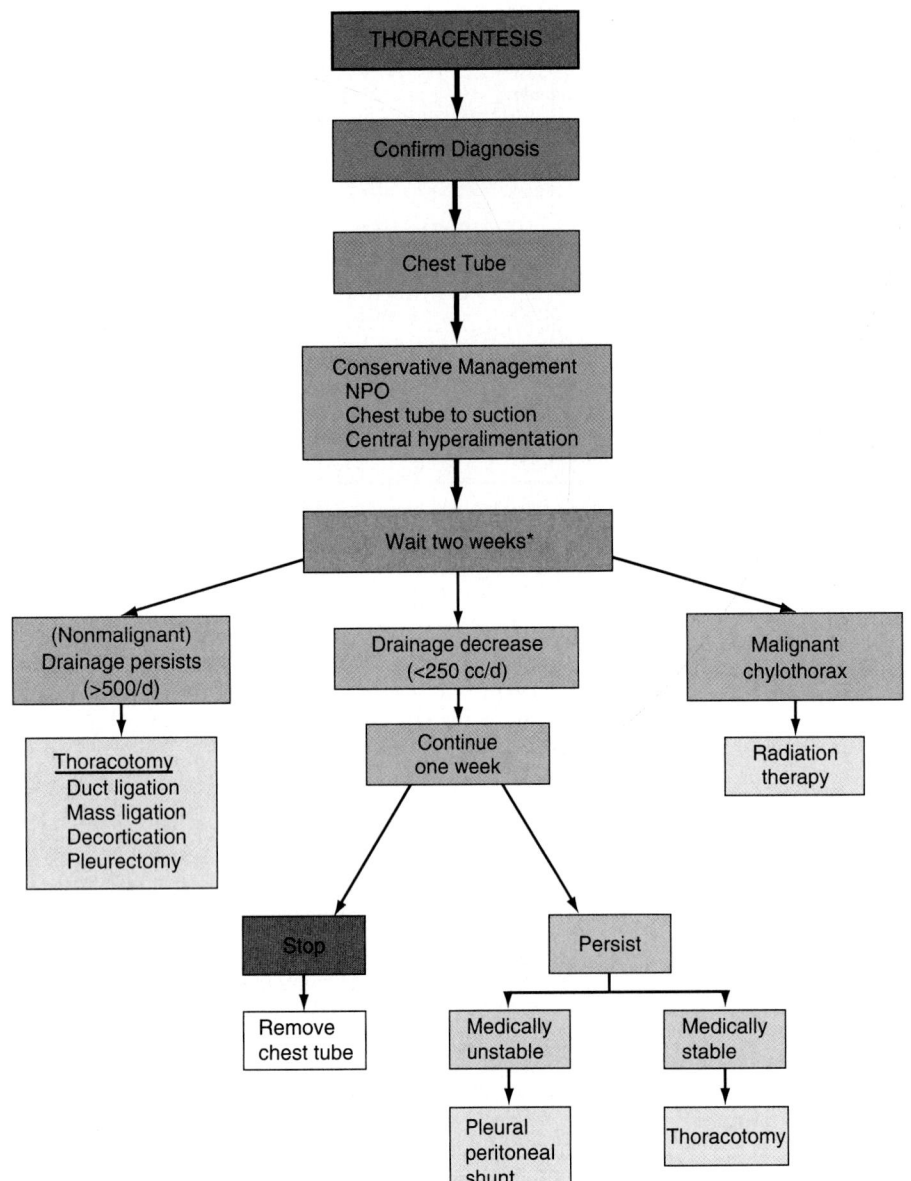

FIG. 18-41. Algorithm for the management of chylothorax. *If high output persists (>50 cc/d), early surgical ligation of the thoracic duct may be considered.

draining free-flowing pleural effusions. Fluid should be grossly examined as it is drained: clear straw-colored fluid is often transudative; turbid or bloody fluid is often exudative.

The site of entry for drainage of a pleural effusion or pneumothorax may be based on the chest x-ray alone if the effusion is demonstrated to be free-flowing. For large, free-flowing effusions, a low, posterolateral approach at the eighth or ninth intercostal space affords good access. If the effusion is more complex with loculations, a CT scan or ultrasound-guided approach may be indicated. If complete drainage is the goal and the fluid is nonbloody and nonviscous, a small-bore (14- to 16-gauge) pigtail catheter is inserted and connected to a Pleurovac or similar device for drainage. If the fluid is bloody or turbid, a larger-diameter drainage tube (such as a 28F chest tube) may be required. In general, the smallest-bore drainage catheter that will effectively drain the pleural space should be chosen. Smaller-diameter catheters significantly decrease the pain associated with the placement of chest tubes. For clinical situations requiring biopsy or for potential interventions such as adhesiolysis

or pleurodesis, minimally-invasive surgery may be indicated, using a VATS approach.

Complications of Pleural Drainage

The most common complication of invasive procedures to access the pleural space is inadvertent access to another cavity or organ. Examples include puncture of the underlying lung, with air leakage and pneumothorax; subdiaphragmatic entry, with damage to the liver, spleen, or other intra-abdominal viscera; bleeding secondary to intercostal vessel injury, or most commonly, larger vessel injury; and even cardiac puncture. Sometimes bleeding may be the result of an underlying coagulopathy or anticoagulant therapy. Other technical complications include loss of a catheter, guidewire, or fragment in the pleural space, and infections. Occasionally, rapid drainage of a large effusion can be followed by shortness of breath, clinical instability, and a phenomenon referred to as postexpansion pulmonary edema. For this reason, it is recommended to drain only up to 1 L

FIG. 18-42. *Techniques for aspiration and drainage of a pleural effusion. A. Needle aspiration. With careful appraisal of the x-ray findings, the best interspace is selected, and fluid is aspirated with a needle and syringe. Large volumes of fluid can be removed with a little patience and a large-bore needle. B. Chest tube insertion. After careful skin preparation, draping, and administration of local anesthesia, a short skin incision is made over the correct interspace. The incision is deepened into the intercostal muscles, and the pleura is penetrated (usually with a clamp). When any doubt exists about the status of the pleural space at the site of puncture, the wound is enlarged bluntly to admit a finger, which can be swept around the immediately adjacent pleural space to assess the situation and break down any adhesions. The tube is inserted, with the tip directed toward the optimal position suggested by the chest x-rays. In general, a high anterior tube is best for air (pneumothorax) and a low posterior tube is best for fluid. A 28 to 32F tube is adequate for most situations. A 36F tube is preferred for hemothorax or for a viscous empyema. Many surgeons prefer a very small tube (16 to 20F) for drainage of simple pneumothorax. C. The tube is connected to a water-seal drainage system. Suction is added, if necessary, to expand the lung; it usually will be required in a patient with a substantial air leak (bronchopleural fistula).*

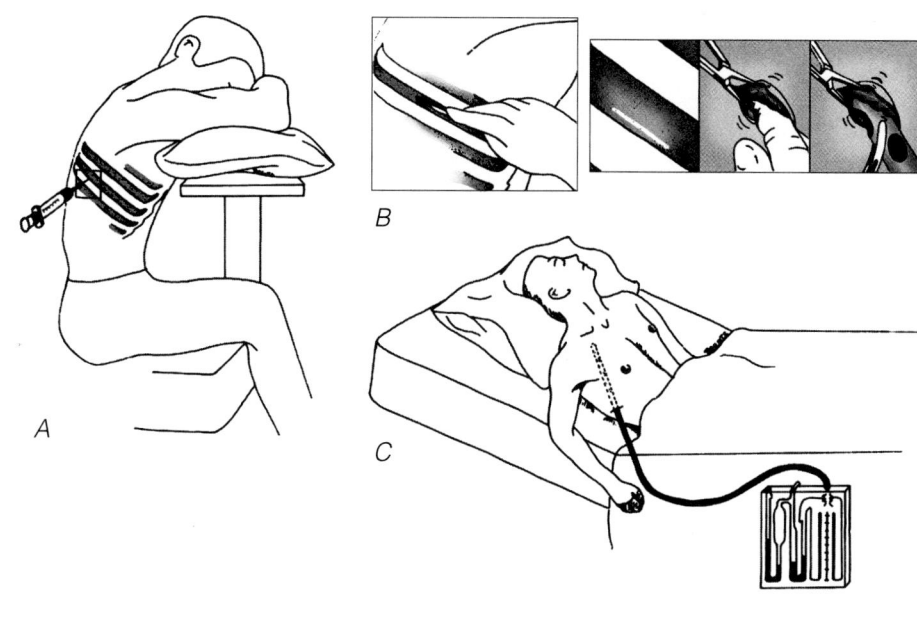

initially. Most complications can be avoided by consulting with a clinician experienced in pleural drainage techniques.

Tumors of the Pleura

Malignant Mesothelioma

Malignant mesothelioma is the most common type of tumor of the pleura. The annual incidence in the United States is about 3000 cases. Other tumors of the pleura are much less common and include benign and malignant fibrous tumors of the pleura, lipomas, and cysts. In 20% of malignant mesotheliomas, the tumor arises from the peritoneum. Exposure to asbestos is the only known risk factor; it can be established in over 50% of patients. Geographic areas of increased incidence are frequently associated with industries using asbestos in the manufacturing process, such as shipbuilding. The risk extends beyond the worker directly exposed to the asbestos; family members exposed to the dust of the clothing or the work environment are also at risk. Other risk factors have been identified, including exposure to fibers with similar physical properties to amphibole and exposure to radiation. Cigarette smoking does not appear to increase the risk of malignant mesothelioma, even though asbestos exposure and smoking synergistically increases the risk for lung cancer. Malignant mesotheliomas have a male predominance of 2:1, and are most common after the age of 40.

Pathophysiology. The exact etiologic role of asbestos fibers has not been elucidated; however, the physical characteristics of specific fibers (referred to as serpentine or amphibole) have been shown to be important. The serpentine fibers are large and curly and are generally not able to travel beyond larger airways. However, the narrow, straight amphibole fibers, in particular the crocidolite

fibers, may navigate distally into the pulmonary parenchyma and are most clearly associated with mesotheliomas. The latency period between asbestos exposure and the development of mesothelioma is at least 20 years. The tumor generally is multicentric, with multiple pleural-based nodules coalescing to form sheets of tumor. This process initially involves the parietal pleura, generally with early spread to the visceral surfaces and with a variable degree of invasion of surrounding structures. Autopsy studies have shown that most patients have distant metastases, but the natural history of the disease in untreated patients culminates in death due to local extension.

Clinical Presentation. Most patients present with dyspnea and chest pain. Over 90% have a pleural effusion. Thoracentesis is diagnostic in less than 10% of patients. Frequently, a thoracoscopy or open pleural biopsy with special stains is required to differentiate mesotheliomas from adenocarcinomas (Table 18-25). Once the diagnosis is confirmed, cell types can be distinguished (e.g., epithelial,

Table 18-25

Special Stains Required to Differentiate Mesothelioma from Adenocarcinoma

	Mesothelioma	Adenocarcinoma
CEA	Negative	Positive
Vimentin		
LMW cytokeratins	Positive	Negative
EM features	Long, sinuous villi	Short, straight villi, with fuzzy glycocalyx

CEA = carcinoembryonic antigen; EM = electron microscope; LMW = low molecular weight.

sarcomatous, and mixed). Epithelial types are associated with a more favorable prognosis, and in some patients long-term survival may be seen with no treatment. Sarcomatous and mixed tumors share a more aggressive course.

Management. The treatment of malignant mesotheliomas remains controversial. It has been the subject of a number of recent clinical trials, the vast majority with limited success. A new staging system has been devised that has clearly shown prognostic value (Table 18-26). However, while prognosis does depend on the stage of the disease, the problem is that many patients present with advanced local or distant disease beyond curative potential. Treatment options include supportive care only, surgical resection, and multimodality approaches (using a combination of surgery, chemotherapy, and radiation therapy).

Surgical options include palliative approaches such as pleurectomy or talc pleurodesis. Palliative approaches may lead to local control and a modest improvement in short-term survival. More radical surgical approaches (such as extrapleural pneumonectomy followed by adjuvant chemotherapy and radiation) have an increased morbidity rate; moreover, the mortality rate exceeds 10% in all but the most experienced centers. In one Japanese review, extrapleural pneumonectomy demonstrated no improvement in survival (as compared with debulking surgery), and showed no benefit over adjuvant therapy: the overall 5-year survival in all groups was less than 10%. However, several reports of trials of radical surgery combined with multimodality adjuvant therapy have shown reasonable improvements in survival for patients with early-stage tumors (as compared with historical controls). In one series of 183 patients undergoing extrapleural pneumonectomy and adjuvant chemotherapy and radiation, a subset of 31 patients had favorable prognostic features (i.e., epithelial cell type), negative resection margins, and negative extrapleural node status. This favorable subset had a 5-year survival rate of 46%, as compared with 15% for the entire group.

Table 18-26
International Mesothelioma Interest Group Staging System for Diffuse Malignant Pleural Mesothelioma

T Tumor

T1	T1a	Tumor limited to the ipsilateral parietal ± mediastinal ± diaphragmatic pleura
		No involvement of the visceral pleura
	T1b	Tumor involving the ipsilateral parietal ± mediastinal ± diaphragmatic pleura
		Tumor also involving the visceral pleura
T2		Tumor involving each of the ipsilateral pleural surfaces (parietal, mediastinal, diaphragmatic, and visceral pleurae) with at least one of the following features:
		Involvement of diaphragmatic muscle
		Extension of tumor from visceral pleura into the underlying pulmonary parenchyma
T3		Describes locally advanced but potentially resectable tumor
		Tumor involving all of the ipsilateral pleural surfaces (parietal, mediastinal, diaphragmatic, and visceral pleurae) with at least one of the following features:
		Involvement of the endothoracic fascia
		Extension into the mediastinal fat
		Solitary, completely resectable focus of tumor extending into the soft tissues of the chest wall
		Nontransmural involvement of the pericardium
T4		Describes locally advanced technically unresectable tumor
		Tumor involving all of the ipsilateral pleural surfaces (parietal, mediastinal, diaphragmatic, and visceral pleurae) wilh at least one of the following features:
		Diffuse extension or multifocal masses of tumor in the chest wall, with or without associated rib destruction
		Direct transdiaphragmatic extension of tumor to the peritoneum
		Direct extension of tumor to the contralateral pleura
		Direct extension of tumor to mediastinal organs
		Direct extension of tumor into the spine
		Tumor extending through to the internal surface of the pericardium with or without a pericardial effusion; or tumor involving the myocardium

N Lymph nodes

NX	Regional lymph nodes cannot be assessed
N0	No regional lymph node metastases
Nl	Metastases in the ipsilateral bronchopulmonary or hilar lymph nodes
N2	Metastases in the subcarinal or the ipsilateral mediastinal lymph nodes including the ipsilateral internal mammary nodes
N3	Metastases in the contralateral mediastinal, contralateral internal mammary, ipsilateral or contralateral supraclavicular lymph nodes

M Metastases

MX	Presence of distant metastases cannot be assessed
M0	No distant metastases
M1	Distant metastases present

Staging

Stage I			
Ia	T1a	N0	M0
Ib	T1b	N0	M0
Stage II	T2	N0	M0
Stage III	Any T3	Any N1	M0
		Any N2	
Stage IV	Any T4	Any N3	Any M1

SOURCE: Reproduced with permission from International Mesothelioma Interest Group: A proposed new international TNM staging system for malignant pleural mesothelioma. *Chest* 108:1122, 1995.

In another series, 88 patients with mesotheliomas were studied prospectively. Adjuvant radiation therapy was given to 54 patients after extrapleural pneumonectomy; the median survival was 17 months. However, in patients with stage I and II disease, the median survival was significantly better at 33.0 months.

The authors' current approach to malignant mesotheliomas is based on tumor stage and pulmonary performance status. For patients with early-stage mesotheliomas and good pulmonary function, extrapleural pneumonectomy is recommended, especially for epithelial mesotheliomas. Patients are referred for clinical trials of multimodality therapy, if available. For more advanced disease, or if patients have less-than-optimal pulmonary function or performance status, talc pleurodesis or supportive therapy is recommended.

Intrapleural therapy has been explored to improve the locoregional control of malignant mesotheliomas. In a phase II trial, 37 patients underwent pleurectomy with decortication, followed by intrapleural and systemic therapy with cisplatin and mitomycin C. Their median survival was 17 months, with a locoregional recurrence rate of 80%. According to another study, the addition of hyperthermic intrapleural perfusion seems to be pharmacokinetically advantageous; of seven patients, three underwent pleurectomy with decortication and received hyperthermic cisplatin. Systemic drug concentrations were greater after pleurectomy with decortication than after pleuropneumonectomy. The local tissue:perfusate ratio of platinum concentrations tended to be higher after hyperthermic perfusion rather than normothermic perfusion.

Another promising alternative to enhance the local efficacy of chemotherapy against malignant mesotheliomas is L-NDDP (cis-bis-neodecanoato-trans-R,R-1,2-diaminocyclohexane platinum), a new lipophilic cisplatinum analogue produced by the University of Texas M. D. Anderson Cancer Center in Houston, Texas. A phase II trial of L-NDDP enrolled 23 patients to receive a thoracoscopic biopsy and a cytologic examination before and after treatment. Of those 23 patients, 13 (56%) had a complete pathologic response; of the patients with positive cytologic results, 15 (83%) had a complete cytologic response. The findings of this phase II trial led to an ongoing phase II clinical trial at the University of Pittsburgh Cancer Institute to investigate intrapleural L-NDDP followed by surgical dissection and postoperative radiotherapy in patients with malignant mesotheliomas.

Fibrous Tumors of the Pleura

Fibrous tumors of the pleura are unrelated to asbestos exposure or malignant mesotheliomas. They generally occur as a single pedunculated mass arising from the visceral pleura. Frequently, they are discovered incidentally on routine chest x-rays, without an associated pleural effusion. Fibrous tumors of the pleura may be benign or malignant. Symptoms such as cough, chest pain, and dyspnea occur in 30 to 40% of patients. Less common are fever, hypertrophic pulmonary osteoarthropathy, hemoptysis, and hypoglycemia. Hypoglycemia occurs in only approximately 4% of patients and resolves with surgical resection, as do the other symptoms. Given the localized, pedunculated nature of both benign and malignant fibrous tumors of the pleura, most are cured by complete surgical resection. Incompletely resected malignant tumors may recur locally or metastasize; frequently, they are fatal within 2 to 5 years.

Acknowledgement

The authors wish to thank Chuong D. Hoang, MD, Denis R. Clohisy, MD, Mary Knatterud, PhD, Vita Sullivan, MD, and Jennifer Nichols for their invaluable help in compiling and editing this chapter. The authors also express appreciation to their spouses, Chris and Lee.

Bibliography

Trachea: Anatomy
Cusimano RJ, Pearson FG: Anatomy, physiology, and embryology of the upper airway, in Pearson FG, Cooper JD, Deslauriers J, et al (eds): *Thoracic Surgery,* 2nd ed. New York: Churchill Livingstone, 2002, p 215.

Tracheal Injury
Grillo HC: Surgical treatment of postintubation tracheal injuries. *J Thorac Cardiovasc Surg* 78:860, 1979.

Tracheal Fistulas
Couraaud L, Ballester MJ, Delaisement C: Acquired tracheoesophageal fistula and its management. *Semin Thorac Cardiovasc Surg* 8:392, 1996.
Mathisen DJ, Grillo HC, et al: Management of acquired nonmalignant tracheal esophageal fistula. *Ann Thorac Surg* 52:759, 1991.

Tracheal Neoplasms
Chow DC, Komaki R, et al: Treatment of primary neoplasms of the trachea. The role of radiation therapy. *Cancer* 71:2946, 1993.
Regnard JR, Fourquier P, et al: Results and prognostic factors in resections of primary tracheal tumors: A multicenter retrospective study. *J Thorac Cardiovasc Surg* 111:808, 1996.

Lung: Anatomy
Rice TW: Anatomy of the lung, in Pearson FG, Cooper JD, Deslauriers J, et al (eds): *Thoracic Surgery,* 2nd ed. New York: Churchill Livingstone, 2002, p 427.
Naidich DP: Helical computed tomography of the thorax. Clinical applications. *Radiol Clin North Am* 32:759, 1994.
Remy-Jardin M, Remy J, Giraud F, et al: Pulmonary nodules: Detection with thick-section spiral CT versus conventional CT. *Radiology* 187:513, 1993.

Thoracic Surgical Approaches
Dewey TM, Mack MJ: Lung cancer. Surgical approaches and incisions. *Chest Surg Clin North Am* 10:803, 2000.

Lung: Postoperative Care
Ayed AK: Suction versus water seal after thoracoscopy for primary spontaneous pneumothorax: Prospective randomized study. *Ann Thorac Surg* 75:1593, 2003.
Epstein SK, Faling JL, et al: Predicting complications after pulmonary resection: Preoperative exercise testing vs. a multi-factorial cardiopulmonary risk index. *Chest* 104:694, 1993.
Nagasaki F, Flehinger BJ, Martini N: Complications of surgery in the treatment of carcinoma of the lung. *Chest* 82:25, 1982.

Solitary Pulmonary Nodule
Marten K, Grabbe E: The challenge of the solitary pulmonary nodule: Diagnostic assessment with multislice spiral CT. *Clin Imaging* 27:156, 2003.
Ost D, Fein AM, Feinsilver SH: Clinical practice. The solitary pulmonary nodule. *N Engl J Med* 348:2535, 2003.

Lung Neoplasms
Cahan WG, Shah JP, Castro EB: Benign solitary lung lesions in patients with cancer. *Ann Surg* 187:241, 1978.
Cerilli LA, Ritter JH, Mills SE, et al: Neuroendocrine neoplasms of the lung. *Am J Clin Pathol* 116(Suppl):S65, 2001.
Davidson RS, Nwogu CE, Brentjens MJ, et al: The surgical management of pulmonary metastasis: Current concepts. *Surg Oncol* 10:35, 2001.
Dillman RO, Herndon J, Seagren SL, et al: Improved survival in stage III non-small-cell lung cancer: Seven-year follow-up of cancer and leukemia group b (calgb) 8433 trial. *J Natl Cancer Inst* 88:1210, 1996.

Feins RH: Multi-modality treatment of non-small-cell lung cancer. *Surg Clin North Am* 82:611, 2002.

Ginsberg RJ, Rubinstein LV: Randomized trial of lobectomy versus limited resection for T1 N0 non-small-cell lung cancer. Lung cancer study group. *Ann Thorac Surg* 60:615, 1995; discussion 622.

Goldberg M, Unger M: Lung cancer. Diagnostic tools. *Chest Surg Clin North Am* 10:763, vii, 2000.

Gould VE, Warren WH: Epithelial tumors of the lung. *Chest Surg Clin North Am* 10:709, 2000.

Hackshaw AK, Law MR, Wald NJ: The accumulated evidence on lung cancer and environmental tobacco smoke. *BMJ* 315:980, 1997.

Lau CL, Harpole DH Jr., Patz E: Staging techniques for lung cancer. *Chest Surg Clin North Am* 10:781, 2000.

McCormack PM, Bains MS, Begg CB, et al: Role of video-assisted thoracic surgery in the treatment of pulmonary metastases: Results of a prospective trial. *Ann Thorac Surg* 62:213, 1996; discussion 216.

Mountain CF: Revisions in the international system for staging lung cancer. *Chest* 111:1710, 1997.

Pastorino U, Buyse M, Friedel G, et al: Long-term results of lung metastasectomy: Prognostic analyses based on 5206 cases. *J Thorac Cardiovasc Surg* 113:27, 1997.

Pisters KM, Ginsberg RJ, Giroux DJ, et al: Induction chemotherapy before surgery for early-stage lung cancer: A novel approach. Bimodality lung oncology team. *J Thorac Cardiovasc Surg* 119:429, 2000.

Rosell R, Gomez-Codina J, Camps C, et al: A randomized trial comparing preoperative chemotherapy plus surgery with surgery alone in patients with non-small-cell lung cancer. *N Engl J Med* 330:153, 1994.

Roth JA, Atkinson EN, Fossella F, et al: Long-term follow-up of patients enrolled in a randomized trial comparing perioperative chemotherapy and surgery with surgery alone in resectable stage IIIa non-small-cell lung cancer. *Lung Cancer* 21:1, 1998.

Ruckdeschel JC, Piantadosi S: Quality of life in lung cancer surgical adjuvant trials. *Chest* 106:324S, 1994.

Samet JM: Health benefits of smoking cessation. *Clin Chest Med* 12:669, 1991.

Shon IH, O'Doherty MJ, Maisey MN: Positron emission tomography in lung cancer. *Semin Nucl Med* 32:240, 2002.

Stroobants S, Verschakelen J, Vansteenkiste J: Value of FDG-PET in the management of non-small cell lung cancer. *Eur J Radiol* 45:49, 2003.

Tockman MS, Mulshine JL: The early detection of occult lung cancer. *Chest Surg Clin North Am* 10:737, 2000.

Toloza EM, Harpole L, McCrory DC: Noninvasive staging of non-small cell lung cancer: A review of the current evidence. *Chest* 123:137S, 2003.

Walsh GL, Pisters KM, Stevens C: Treatment of stage I lung cancer. *Chest Surg Clin North Am* 11:17, vii, 2001.

Weigel TL, Martini N: Occult lung cancer treatment. *Chest Surg Clin North Am* 10:751, vii, 2000.

Pulmonary Infections

Barker AF: Bronchiectasis. *N Engl J Med* 346:1383, 2002.

Bradsher RW, Chapman SW, Pappas PG: Blastomycosis. *Infect Dis Clin North Am* 17:21, vii, 2003.

Conant EF, Wechsler RJ: Actinomycosis and nocardiosis of the lung. *J Thorac Imaging* 7:75, 1992.

Frieden TR, Sterling TR, Munsiff SS, et al: Tuberculosis. *Lancet* 362:887, 2003.

Gonzalez CE, Rinaldi MG, Sugar AM: Zygomycosis. *Infect Dis Clin North Am* 16:895, vi, 2002.

Haque AK: The pathology and pathophysiology of mycobacterial infections. *J Thorac Imaging* 5:8, 1990.

Iseman MD: Treatment of multidrug-resistant tuberculosis. *N Engl J Med* 329:784, 1993.

Kubak BM: Fungal infection in lung transplantation. *Transpl Infect Dis* 4(Suppl)3:24, 2002.

Mabeza GF, Macfarlane J: Pulmonary actinomycosis. *Eur Respir J* 21:545, 2003.

Mansharamani N, Balachandran D, Delaney D, et al: Lung abscess in adults: Clinical comparison of immunocompromised to non-immunocompromised patients. *Respir Med* 96:178, 2002.

Marr KA, Patterson T, Denning D: Aspergillosis. Pathogenesis, clinical manifestations, and therapy. *Infect Dis Clin North Am* 16:875, vi, 2002.

Mwandumba HC, Beeching NJ: Pyogenic lung infections. *Curr Opin Pulm Med* 5:151, 1999.

Ostrosky-Zeichner L, Rex JH, Bennett J, et al: Deeply invasive candidiasis. *Infect Dis Clin North Am* 16:821, 2002.

Pound MW, Drew RH, Perfect JR: Recent advances in the epidemiology, prevention, diagnosis, and treatment of fungal pneumonia. *Curr Opin Infect Dis* 15:183, 2002.

Wheat LJ, Goldman M, Sarosi G: State-of-the-art review of pulmonary fungal infections. *Semin Respir Infect* 17:158, 2002.

Wheat LJ, Kauffman CA: Histoplasmosis. *Infect Dis Clin North Am* 17:1, vii, 2003.

Massive Hemoptysis

Conlan AA, Hurwitz SS: Management of massive haemoptysis with the rigid bronchoscope and cold saline lavage. *Thorax* 35:901, 1980.

Conlan AA: Massive hemoptysis—diagnostic and therapeutic implications. *Surg Annu* 17:337, 1985.

End-Stage Lung Disease

Bhorade SM, Vigneswaran W, McCabe MA, et al: Liberalization of donor criteria may expand the donor pool without adverse consequence in lung transplantation. *J Heart Lung Transplant* 19:1199, 2000.

Dahlberg PS, Prekker ME, Hertz M, et al: Recent trends in lung transplantation: The University of Minnesota experience. *Clin Transpl* 243, 2002.

Kron IL, Tribble CG, Kern JA, et al: Successful transplantation of marginally acceptable thoracic organs. *Ann Surg* 217:518, 1993; discussion 522.

Palmer SM, Miralles AP, Howell DN, et al: Gastroesophageal reflux as a reversible cause of allograft dysfunction after lung transplantation. *Chest* 118:1214, 2000.

Pasque MK, Cooper JD, Kaiser LR, et al: Improved technique for bilateral lung transplantation: Rationale and initial clinical experience. *Ann Thorac Surg* 49:785, 1990.

Pierre AF, Sekine Y, Hutcheon MA, et al: Marginal donor lungs: A reassessment. *J Thorac Cardiovasc Surg* 123:421, 2002; discussion, 427.

Russi EW, Bloch KE, Weder W: Lung volume reduction surgery: What can we learn from the National Emphysema Treatment Trial? *Eur Respir J* 22:571, 2003.

Sundaresan S, Semenkovich J, Ochoa L, et al: Successful outcome of lung transplantation is not compromised by the use of marginal donor lungs. *J Thorac Cardiovasc Surg* 109:1075, 1995; discussion 1079.

Spontaneous Pneumothorax

Alfageme I, Moreno L, et al: Spontaneous pneumothorax: Long-term results with tetracycline pleurodesis. *Chest* 106:347, 1994.

Inderbitzi RGC, Leiser A, et al: Three years' experience in video-assisted thoracic surgery (VATS) for spontaneous pneumothorax. *J Thorac Cardiovasc Surg* 107:1410, 1994.

Chest Wall Mass

Cavanaugh DG, Cabellon S Jr., Peake JB: A logical approach to chest wall neoplasms. *Ann Thorac Surg* 41:436, 1986.

Chest Wall Neoplasms

Baliski CR, Temple WJ, Arthur K, et al: Desmoid tumors: A novel approach for local control. *J Surg Oncol* 80:96, 2002.

Deschamps C, Timaksiz BM, Darbandi R, et al: Early and long-term results of prosthetic chest wall reconstruction. *J Thorac Cardiovasc Surg* 117:588, 1999.

Graeber GM: Chest wall resection and reconstruction. *Semin Thorac Cardiovasc Surg* 11:251, 1999.

Liptay MJ, Fry WA: Malignant bone tumors of the chest wall. *Semin Thorac Cardiovasc Surg* 11:278, 1999.

Mansour KA, Thourani VH, Losken A, et al: Chest wall resections and reconstruction: A 25-year experience. *Ann Thorac Surg* 73:1720, 2002.

Somers J, Faber LP: Chondroma and chondrosarcoma. *Semin Thorac Cardiovasc Surg* 11:270, 1999.

Walsh GL, Davis BM, Swisher SG, et al: A single-institutional, multidisciplinary approach to primary sarcomas involving the chest wall requiring full-thickness resections. *J Thorac Cardiovasc Surg* 121:48, 2001.

Mediastinum: General Concepts

Kirschner PA: Anatomy and surgical access of the mediastinum, in Pearson FG, Cooper JD, Deslauriers J, et al (eds): *Thoracic Surgery,* 2nd ed. New York: Churchill Livingstone, 2002, p 1563.

Mediastinum: Diagnostic Evaluation

Baron RL, Levitt RG, et al: Computed tomography in the evaluation of mediastinal widening. *Radiology* 138:107, 1981.

Fraser RS, Pare PD, Bralow L, et al: *Diagnosis of Diseases of the Chest,* 4th ed, Vol. 1–4. Philadelphia: WB Saunders, 1999.

Mediastinum: Neoplasms

Blossom GB, Steiger Z, Stephenson LWL: Neoplasms of the mediastinum, in DeVita VT, Hellman S, Rosenberg SA (eds): *Cancer—Principles and Practice of Oncology,* 5th ed. Philadelphia: Lippincott-Raven, 1997, p 951.

Blumberg D, Port JL, Weksler B, et al: Thymoma: A multivariate analysis of factors predicting survival. *Ann Thorac Surg* 60:908, 1995.

Bousamra M: Neurogenic tumors of the mediastinum, in Pearson FG, Cooper JD, Deslauriers J, et al (eds): *Thoracic Surgery,* 2nd ed. New York: Churchill Livingstone, 2002, p 1732.

Bukowski RM, Wolf M, Kulander BG, et al: Alternating combination chemotherapy in patients with extragonadal germ cell tumors. *Cancer* 71:2631, 1993.

Chahanian A: Chemotherapy of thymomas and thymic carcinomas. *Chest Surg Clin North Am* 11:447, 2001.

Coleman BG, Arger PH, Dalinka MK: CT of sarcomatous degeneration in neurofibromatosis. *AJR* 140:383, 1983.

Davidson KG, Walbaum PR, McCormack RJ: Intrathoracic neural tumours. *Thorax* 33:359, 1978.

Deslauriers J, Letourneau L, Giubilei G: Diagnostic strategies in mediastinal tumors and masses, in Pearson FG, Cooper JD, Deslauriers J, et al (eds): *Thoracic Surgery,* 2nd ed. New York: Churchill Livingstone, 2002, p 1655.

Ducatman BS, Scheithauer BW, Peipgras DG: Malignant peripheral nerve sheath tumours: A clinicopathologic study of 120 cases. *Cancer* 57:2006, 1986.

Gale AW, Jelihovsky T, Grant AF: Neurogenic tumors of the mediastinum. *Ann Thorac Surg* 17:434, 1974.

Gunther RW: Percutaneous interventions in the thorax. Seventh Annual Charles Dotter Memorial Lecture. *J Vasc Intervent Radiol* 3:379, 1992.

Herman SJ, Holub RV, Weisbrod GL, et al: Anterior mediastinal masses: Utility of transthoracic needle biopsy. *Radiology* 180:167, 1991.

Hoerbelt R, Keunecke L, Grimm H, et al: The value of a noninvasive diagnostic approach to mediastinal masses. *Ann Thorac Surg* 75:1086, 2003.

Knapp RH, Hurt RD, Payne WS, et al: Malignant germ cell tumors of the mediastinum. *J Thorac Cardiovasc Surg* 89:82, 1985.

Larsen SS, Krasnik M, Vilmann P, et al: Endoscopic ultrasound-guided biopsy of mediastinal lesions has a major impact on patient management. *Thorax* 57:98, 2002.

Luketich JD, Ginsberg RJ: Current management of patients with mediastinal tumors. *Adv Surg* 30:311, 1996.

Luketich JD, Friedman DM, Weigel TL, et al: Evaluation of distant metastases in esophageal cancer: 100 consecutive positron emission tomography scans. *Ann Thorac Surg* 68:1133, 1999.

Masaoka A, Monden Y, Nakahara K, et al: Follow-up study of thymomas with special reference to their clinical stages. *Cancer* 48:2485, 1981.

Meyers BF, Cooper JD: Transcervical thymectomy for myasthenia gravis. *Chest Surg Clin North Am* 11:363, 2001.

Nichols CR, Saxman S, Williams SD, et al: Primary mediastinal nongerminomatous germ cell tumors: A modern single institute experience. *Cancer* 65:1641, 1989.

Oosterwijk WM, Swierenga J: Neurogenic tumours with an intrathoracic localization. *Thorax* 23:374, 1968.

Rosenstein BJ, Engelman K: Diarrhea in a child with catecholamine-secreting ganglioneuroma. *J Pediatr Surg* 63:217, 1963.

Small EJ, Venook AP, Damon LE: Gallium-avid thymic hyperplasia in an adult after chemotherapy for Hodgkin's disease. *Cancer* 72:905, 1998.

Strollo DC, Rosado-de-Christenson ML, Jett JR: Primary mediastinal tumors: part II. Tumors of the middle and posterior mediastinum. *Chest* 112:1344, 1997.

Suster S, Rosai J: Thymic carcinoma: A clinicopathological study of 60 cases. *Cancer* 67:1025, 1991.

Wick MR, Weiland LH, Scheithauer BW, et al: Primary thymic carcinomas. *Am J Surg Pathol* 6:616, 1982.

Yim APC, Kay LC, Izzat MB, et al: Video-assisted thoracoscopic thymectomy for myasthenia gravis. *Semin Thorac Cardiovasc Surg* 11:65, 1999.

Yim APC: Video-assisted thoracoscopic resection of anterior mediastinal masses. *Int Surg* 81:350, 1996.

Mediastinal Cysts

DiLorenzo M, Collin PP, Vaillancourt R, et al: Bronchogenic cysts. *J Pediatr Surg* 24:988, 1991.

Fontanelle LJ, Armstrong RG, Stanford W, et al: The asymptomatic mediastinal mass. *Arch Surg* 102:98, 1971.

Ribet ME, Copin MC, Gosselin B: Bronchogenic cysts of the mediastinum. *J Thorac Cardiovasc Surg* 109:1003, 1995.

Rice TW: Benign neoplasms and cysts of the mediastinum. *Semin Thorac Cardiovasc Surg* 4:25, 1992.

St. Georges R, Deslauriers J, Duranceau A, et al: Clinical spectrum of bronchogenic cysts of the mediastinum and lung in the adult. *Ann Thorac Surg* 52:6, 1991.

Mediastinitis

Razzuk MA, Razzuk LM, Hoover SJ, et al: Infections of the mediastinum, in Pearson FG, Cooper JD, Deslauriers J, et al (eds): *Thoracic Surgery,* 2nd ed. New York: Churchill Livingstone, 2002, p 1599.

Diseases of the Pleura and Pleural Space: Anatomy

Agostoni E: Mechanics of the pleural space, in: *American Physiological Society: Handbook of Physiology,* Vol. 3, Part 2. Bethesda, MD: American Physiological Society, 1986.

Lawrence GH: Considerations of the anatomy and physiology of the pleural space, in Lawrence GH (ed): *Problems of the Pleural Space.* Philadelphia: WB Saunders, 1983.

Pleural Effusion

Johnson WW: The malignant pleural effusion: A review of cytopathologic diagnosis of 584 specimens from 472 consecutive patients. *Cancer* 56:905, 1985.

Lee YCG, Rogers JT, Rodriguez RM, et al: Adenosine deaminase levels in nontuberculous and lymphocytic pleural effusions. *Chest* 120:356, 2001.

Light RW: Pleural effusion: Clinical practice. *N Engl J Med* 346:1971, 2002.

Ocana I, Martinez-Vazquez JM, Segura RM, et al: Adenosine deaminase in pleural fluids: Test for diagnosis of tuberculous pleural effusion. *Chest* 84:51, 1983.

Rusch VW: Pleural effusion: Benign and malignant, in Pearson FG, Cooper JD, Deslauriers J, et al (eds): *Thoracic Surgery,* 2nd ed. New York: Churchill Livingstone, 2002, p 1157.

Empyema

Light RW: Parapneumonic effusion and empyema. *Clin Chest Med* 6:55, 1985.

Miller JI Jr.: The history of surgery of empyema, thoracoplasty, eloesser flap, and muscle flap transposition. *Chest Surg Clin North Am* 10:45, viii, 2000.

Chylothorax

Malthaner RA, Inculet RI: The thoracic duct and chylothorax, in Pearson FG, Cooper JD, Deslauriers J, et al (eds): *Thoracic Surgery,* 2nd ed. New York: Churchill Livingstone, 2002, p 1228.

Miller JI Jr.: Diagnosis and management of chylothorax. *Chest Surg Clin North Am* 6:139, 1996.

Access and Drainage of Pleural Fluid Collections

Gammie JS, Banks MC, Fuhrman CR, et al: The pigtail catheter for pleural drainage: A less invasive alternative to tube thoracostomy. *JSLS* 3:57, 1999.

Luketich JD, Kiss M, Hershey J, et al: Chest tube insertion: A prospective evaluation of pain management. *Clin J Pain* 14:152, 1998.

Tumors of the Pleura

Cole FH Jr., Ellis RA, Goodman RC, et al: Benign fibrous pleural tumor with elevation of insulin-like growth factor and hypoglycemia. *South Med J* 83:690, 1990.

England DM, Hochholzer L, McCarthy MJ: Localized benign and malignant fibrous tumors of the pleura: A clinicopathologic review of 223 cases. *Am J Pathol* 13:647, 1989.

Khalil MY, Mapa M, Shin HJ, et al: Advances in the management of malignant mesothelioma. *Curr Oncol Rep* 5:334, 2003.

Ratto GB, Civalleri D, Esposito M, et al: Pleural space perfusion with cisplatin in the multimodality treatment of malignant mesothelioma: A feasibility and pharmacokinetic study. *J Thorac Cardiovasc Surg* 117:759, 1999.

Rusch V, Saltz L, Venkatraman E, et al: A phase II trial of pleurectomy/decortication followed by intrapleural and systemic chemotherapy for malignant pleural mesothelioma. *J Clin Oncol* 12:1156, 1994.

Rusch VW: The international mesothelioma interest group: A proposed new international staging system for malignant pleural mesothelioma. *Chest* 108:122, 1995.

Rusch VW, Rosenzweig K, Venkatraman E, et al: A phase II trial of surgical resection and adjuvant high-dose hemithoracic radiation for malignant pleural mesothelioma. *J Thorac Cardiovasc Surg* 122:788, 2001.

Sugarbaker DJ, Flores RM, Jaklitsch MT, et al: Resection margins, extrapleural nodal status, and cell type determine postoperative long-term survival in trimodality therapy of malignant pleural mesothelioma: Results in 183 patients. *J Thorac Cardiovasc Surg* 117:54, 1999.

Takagi K, Tsuchiya R, Watanabe Y: Surgical approach to pleural diffuse mesothelioma in Japan. *Lung Cancer* 31:57, 2001.

CHAPTER 19

Congenital Heart Disease

Tara B. Karamlou, Irving Shen, and Ross M. Ungerleider

Congenital heart surgery is a constantly evolving field. The last 20 years have brought about rapid developments in the technologic realm as well as a more thorough understanding of both the anatomy and pathophysiology of congenital heart disease, leading to the improved care of patients with this challenging disease.[1,2]

These new advancements created a paradigm shift in the field of pediatric heart surgery. The traditional strategy of initial palliation followed by definitive correction at a later age, which had pervaded the thinking of most surgeons, began to evolve to one emphasizing early repair, even in the tiniest patients.[2] Furthermore, some of the defects that were virtually uniformly fatal (such as hypoplastic left-heart syndrome) now can be successfully treated with aggressive forms of palliation using cardiopulmonary bypass, resulting in outstanding survival for many of these children.

Because the goal in most cases of congenital heart disease (CHD) is now early repair, as opposed to subdividing lesions into cyanotic or noncyanotic lesions, a more appropriate classification scheme divides particular defects into three categories based on the feasibility of achieving this goal: (1) defects that have no reasonable palliation and for which repair is the only option; (2) defects for which repair is not possible and for which palliation is the only option; and (3) defects that can either be repaired or palliated in infancy.[3] It bears mentioning that all defects in the second category are those in which the appropriate anatomic components either are not present, as in hypoplastic left-heart syndrome, or cannot be created from existing structures.

DEFECTS WHERE REPAIR IS THE ONLY OR BEST OPTION

Atrial Septal Defect

An atrial septal defect (ASD) is defined as an opening in the interatrial septum that enables the mixing of blood from the systemic venous and pulmonary venous circulations.

Embryology

The atrial and ventricular septa form between the third and sixth weeks of fetal development. After the paired heart tubes fuse into a single tube folded onto itself, the distal portion of the tube causes an indentation to form in the roof of the common atrium. Near this portion of the roof, the septum primum arises and extends into a crescentic formation toward the atrioventricular (AV) junction. The gap remaining between the septum primum and the developing tissues of the AV junction is called the ostium primum. Before the septum primum fuses completely with the endocardial cushions, a series of fenestrations appear in the septum primum that coalesce into the ostium secundum. During this coalescence, the septum secundum grows downward from the roof of the atrium, parallel to and to the right of the septum primum. The septum primum does not fuse, but creates an oblique pathway, called the foramen ovale, within the interatrial septum. After birth, the increase in left atrial pressure normally closes this pathway, obliterating the interatrial connection.[4]

Anatomy

ASDs can be classified into three different types: (1) sinus venosus defects, comprising approximately 5 to 10% of all ASDs; (2) ostium primum defects, which are more correctly described as partial atrioventricular canal defects; and (3) ostium secundum defects, which are the most prevalent subtype, comprising 80% of all ASDs (Fig. 19-1).[5]

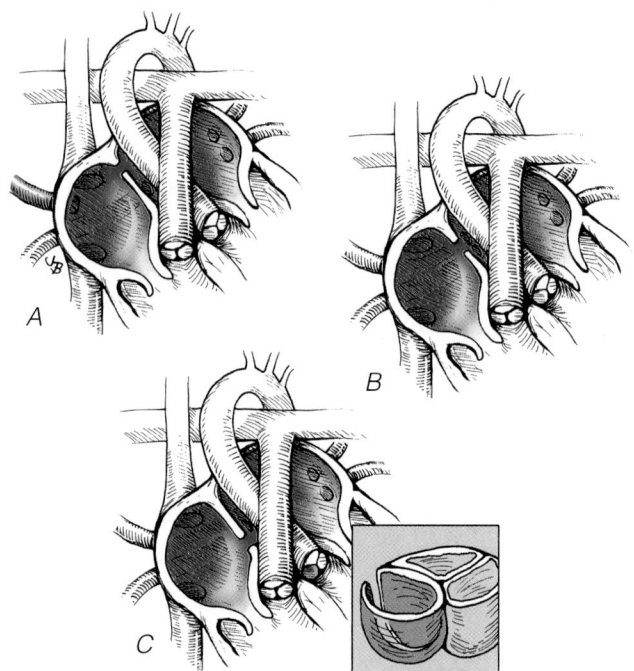

FIG. 19-1. The anatomy of atrial septal defects. In the sinus venosus type (A), the right upper and middle pulmonary veins frequently drain to the superior vena cava or right atrium. B. Secundum defects generally occur as isolated lesions. C. Primum defects are part of a more complex lesion and are best considered as incomplete atrioventricular septal defects. (Reproduced with permission from Mosca et al,[4] p 1444.)

Pathophysiology

ASDs result in an increase in pulmonary blood flow secondary to left-to-right shunting through the defect. The direction of the intracardiac shunt is predominantly determined by the compliance of the respective ventricles. In utero, the distensibility, or compliance, of the right and left ventricles is equal, but postnatally the left ventricle (LV) becomes less compliant than the right ventricle (RV). This shift occurs because the resistance of the downstream vascular beds changes after birth. The pulmonary vascular resistance falls with the infant's first breath, decreasing RV pressure, whereas the systemic vascular resistance rises dramatically, increasing LV pressure. The increased LV pressure creates a thicker muscle mass, which offers a greater resistance to diastolic filling than does the RV; thus, the majority of flow through the ASD occurs from left to right. The greater volume of blood returning to the right atrium causes volume overload in the RV, but because of its lower muscle mass and low-resistance output, it easily distends to accommodate this load.[5,6]

The long-term consequences of RV volume overload include hypertrophy with elevated RV end-diastolic pressure and a relative pulmonary stenosis across the pulmonary valve, because it cannot accommodate the increased RV flow. The resistance at the level of the pulmonary valve then contributes a further pressure load on the RV, which accelerates RV hypertrophy. Compliance gradually decreases as the right ventricular pressure approaches systemic pressure, and the size of the left-to-right shunt decreases. Patients at this stage have a balanced circulation and may deceptively appear less symptomatic.

A minority of patients with ASDs develop progressive pulmonary vascular changes as a result of chronic overcirculation. The increased pulmonary vascular resistance in these patients leads to an equalization of left and right ventricular pressures, and their ratio of pulmonary (Qp) to systemic flow (Qs), Qp:Qs, will approach 1.[5,7] This does not mean, however, that there is no intracardiac shunting, only that the ratio between the left-to-right component and the right-to-left component is equal.

The ability of the right ventricle to recover normal function is related to the duration of chronic overload, because those undergoing ASD closure before age 10 years have a better likelihood of achieving normal RV function in the postoperative period.[3]

The physiology of sinus venosus ASDs is similar to that discussed above except that these are frequently accompanied by anomalous pulmonary venous drainage. This often results in significant hemodynamic derangements that accelerate the clinical course of these infants.

The same increase in symptoms is true for those with ostium primum defects because the associated mitral insufficiency from the "cleft" mitral valve can lead to more atrial volume load and increased atrial level shunting.

Diagnosis

Patients with ASDs may present with few physical findings. Auscultation may reveal prominence of the first heart sound with fixed splitting of the second heart sound. This results from the relatively fixed left-to-right shunt throughout all phases of the cardiac cycle. A diastolic flow murmur indicating increased flow across the tricuspid valve may be discerned, and, frequently, an ejection flow murmur can be heard across the pulmonary valve. A right ventricular heave and increased intensity of the pulmonary component of the second heart sound indicates pulmonary hypertension and possible unrepairability.

Chest radiographs in the patient with an ASD may show evidence of increased pulmonary vascularity, with prominent hilar markings and cardiomegaly. The electrocardiogram shows right axis deviation with an incomplete bundle-branch block. When right bundle-branch block is associated with a leftward or superior axis, an AV canal defect should be strongly suspected.[8]

Diagnosis is clarified by two-dimensional echocardiography, and use of color-flow mapping facilitates an understanding of the physiologic derangements created by the defects.[9] Echocardiography also enables the clinician to estimate the amount of intracardiac shunting, can demonstrate the degree of mitral regurgitation in patients with ostium primum defects, and with the addition of microcavitation, can assist in the detection of sinus venosus defects.[5]

The advent of two-dimensional echocardiography with color-flow Doppler has largely obviated the need for cardiac catheterization because the exact nature of the ASD can be precisely defined by echo alone. However, in cases where the patient is older than age 40 years, catheterization can quantify the degree of pulmonary hypertension present, because those with a pulmonary vascular resistance (PVR) greater than 12 U/mL are considered inoperable.[10] Cardiac catheterization also can be useful in that it provides data that enable the calculation of Qp and Qs so that the magnitude of the intracardiac shunt can be determined. The ratio (Qp:Qs) can then be used to determine whether closure is indicated in equivocal cases, because a Qp:Qs greater than 1.5:1 is generally accepted as the threshold for surgical intervention. Finally, in patients older than age 40 years, cardiac catheterization can be important to disclose the presence of coronary artery disease.

In general, ASDs are closed when patients are between 4 and 5 years of age. Children of this size can usually be operated on without the use of blood transfusion and generally have excellent outcomes. Patients who are symptomatic may require repair earlier, even in infancy. Some surgeons, however, advocate routine repair in infants and children, as even smaller defects are associated with the risk of paradoxical embolism, particularly during pregnancy. In a recent review by Reddy and colleagues, 116 neonates weighing less than 2500 g who underwent repair of simple and complex cardiac defects with the use of cardiopulmonary bypass were found to have no intracerebral hemorrhages, no long-term neurologic sequelae, and a low operative-mortality rate (10%). These results correlated with the length of cardiopulmonary bypass and the complexity of repair.[11] These investigators also found an 80% actuarial survival at 1 year and, more importantly, that growth following complete repair was equivalent to weight-matched neonates free from cardiac defects.[11]

Treatment

ASDs can be repaired in a facile manner using standard cardiopulmonary bypass (CPB) techniques through a midline sternotomy approach.[7] The details of the repair itself are generally straightforward. An oblique atriotomy is made, the position of the coronary sinus and all systemic and pulmonary veins are determined, and the rim of the defect is completely visualized. Closure of ostium secundum defects is accomplished either by direct suture or by insertion of a patch. The decision of whether patch closure is necessary can be determined by the size and shape of the defect as well as by the quality of the edges.

Sinus venosus ASDs associated with partial anomalous pulmonary venous connection are repaired by inserting a patch, with redirection of the pulmonary veins behind the patch to the left atrium. Care must be taken with this approach to avoid obstruction of the pulmonary veins or the superior vena cava, although usually the superior vena cava is dilated and provides ample room for patch insertion.

These operative strategies have been well established, with a low complication rate and a mortality rate approaching zero. As such, attention has shifted to improving the cosmetic result and minimizing hospital stay and convalescence. Multiple new strategies have been described to achieve these aims, including the right submammary incision with anterior thoracotomy, limited bilateral submammary incision with partial sternal split, transxiphoid window, and limited midline incision with partial sternal split.[4,12-14] Some centers use video-assisted thoracic surgery (VATS) in the submammary and transxiphoid approaches to facilitate closure within a constricted operative field. The morbidity and mortality of all of these approaches are comparable to those of the traditional median sternotomy; however, each has technical drawbacks. The main concern is that operative precision be maintained with limited exposure. Luo and associates recently described a prospective randomized study comparing ministernotomy (division of the upper sternum for aortic and pulmonary lesions, and the lower sternum for septal lesions) to full sternotomy in 100 consecutive patients undergoing repair of septal lesions.[14] The patients in the ministernotomy group had longer procedure times (by 15 to 20 minutes), less bleeding, and shorter hospital stays. These results have been echoed by other investigators from Boston who maintain that ministernotomy provides a cosmetically acceptable scar without compromising aortic cannulation or limiting the exposure of crucial mediastinal structures.[12] This approach also can be easily extended to a full sternotomy should difficulty or unexpected anomalies be encountered.[13]

First performed in 1976, transcatheter closure of ASDs with the use of various occlusion devices is gaining widespread acceptance.[15] Certain types of ASDs, including patent foramen ovale, secundum defects, and some fenestrated secundum defects, are amenable to device closure. Complications reported to occur with transcatheter closure include air embolism (1 to 3%); thromboembolism from the device (1 to 2%); disturbed atrioventricular valve function (1 to 2%); systemic/pulmonary venous obstruction (1%); perforation of the atrium or aorta with hemopericardium (1 to 2%); atrial arrhythmias (1 to 3%); and malpositioning/embolization of the device requiring intervention (2 to 15%).[4,16] Thus, although percutaneous approaches are cosmetic and often translate into shorter periods of convalescence, their attendant risks are considerable, especially because their use may not result in complete closure of the septal defect.

Results

Surgical repair of ASDs should be associated with a mortality rate near zero.[4,5,7,8,11] Early repairs in neonates weighing less than 1000 g have been increasingly reported with excellent results.[11] Uncommonly, atrial arrhythmias or significant left atrial hypertension may occur soon after repair. The latter is caused by the noncompliant small, left atrial chamber and generally resolves rapidly.

Aortic Stenosis

Anatomy and Classification

The spectrum of aortic valve abnormality represents the most common form of CHD, with the great majority of patients being asymptomatic until midlife. Obstruction of the left ventricular outflow tract (LVOT) occurs at multiple levels: subvalvular, valvular, and supravalvular (Fig. 19-2). The critically stenotic aortic valve in the neonate or infant is commonly unicommissural or bicommissural, with thickened, dysmorphic, and myxomatous leaflet tissue and a reduced cross-sectional area at the valve level. Associated left-

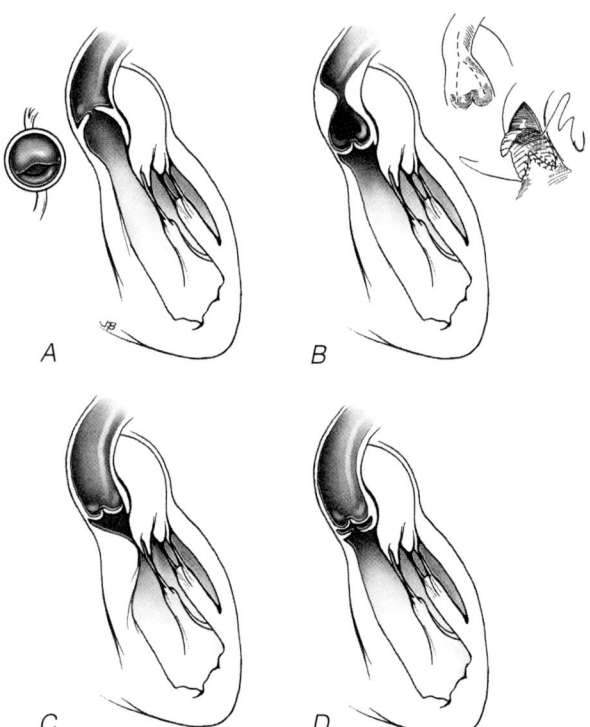

FIG. 19-2. *The anatomy of the types of congenital aortic stenosis. A. Valvular aortic stenosis. B. Supravalvular aortic stenosis and its repair (insert). C. Tunnel-type subvalvular aortic stenosis. D. Membranous subvalvular aortic stenosis. (Reproduced with permission from Mosca et al,[4] p 1247.)*

sided lesions are often present. In a review of 32 cases from the Children's Hospital in Boston, 59% had unicommissural valves and 40% had bicommissural valves.[17] Associated lesions were frequent, occurring in 88% of patients, most commonly patent ductus arteriosus, mitral regurgitation, and hypoplastic left ventricle. Endocardial fibroelastosis also is common among infants with critical aortic stenosis (AS).[18] In this condition, the LV is largely nonfunctional, and these patients are not candidates for simple valve replacement or repair, because the LV is incapable of supporting the systemic circulation. Often, the LV is markedly hypertrophic with a reduced cavity size, but on rare occasion, a dilated LV, reminiscent of overt heart failure, is encountered.[19]

Pathophysiology

The unique intracardiac and extracardiac shunts present in fetal life allow even neonates with critical AS to survive. In utero, left ventricular hypertrophy and ischemia cause left atrial hypertension, which reduces the right-to-left flow across the foramen ovale. In severe cases, a reversal of flow may occur, causing right ventricular volume loading. The RV then provides the entire systemic output via the patent ductus arteriosus. Although cardiac output is maintained, the LV suffers continued damage as the intracavitary pressure precludes adequate coronary perfusion, resulting in LV infarction and subendocardial fibroelastosis. The presentation of the neonate with critical AS is then determined by both the degree of left ventricular dysfunction and on the completeness of the transition from a parallel circulation to an in-series circulation (i.e., on closure of the foramen ovale and the ductus arteriosus). Those infants with mild-to-moderate AS in which LV function is preserved are asymptomatic at birth. The only abnormalities may be a systolic ejection murmur and electrocardiogram (ECG) evidence of left ventricular hypertrophy. However, those neonates with severe AS and compromised LV function are unable to provide adequate cardiac output at birth, and will present in circulatory collapse once the ductus closes, with dyspnea, tachypnea, irritability, narrowed pulse pressure, oliguria, and profound metabolic acidosis.[7,20] If ductal patency is maintained, systemic perfusion will be provided by the RV via ductal flow, and cyanosis may be the only finding.

Diagnosis

Neonates and infants with severe valvular AS may have a relatively nonspecific history of irritability and failure to thrive. Angina, if present, is usually manifested by episodic, inconsolable crying that coincides with feeding. As discussed previously, evidence of poor peripheral perfusion, such as extreme pallor, indicates severe LVOT obstruction. Differential cyanosis is an uncommon finding, but is present when enough antegrade flow occurs only to maintain normal upper body perfusion, while a large patent ductus arteriosus produces blue discoloration of the abdomen and legs.

Physical findings include a systolic ejection murmur, although a quiet murmur may paradoxically indicate a more severe condition with reduced cardiac output. A systolic click correlates with a valvular etiology of obstruction. As LV dysfunction progresses, evidence of congestive heart failure occurs.

The chest radiograph is variable, but may show dilatation of the aortic root, and the ECG often demonstrates LV hypertrophy. Echocardiography with Doppler flow is extremely useful in establishing the diagnosis, as well as quantifying the transvalvular gradient.[21] Furthermore, echocardiography can facilitate evaluation for the several associated defects that can be present in critical neonatal AS, including mitral stenosis, LV hypoplasia, LV endocardial fibroelastosis, subaortic stenosis, VSD, or coarctation. The presence of any or several of these defects has important implications related to treatment options for these patients. Although cardiac catheterization is not routinely performed for diagnostic purposes, it can be invaluable as part of the treatment algorithm if the lesion is amenable to balloon valvotomy.

Treatment

The infant with severe AS may require urgent intervention. Preoperative stabilization, however, has dramatically altered the clinical algorithm and outcomes for this patient population.[18,20] The preoperative strategy begins with endotracheal intubation and inotropic support. Prostaglandin infusion is initiated to maintain ductal patency, and confirmatory studies are performed prior to operative intervention.

Therapy is generally indicated in the presence of a transvalvular gradient of 50 mm Hg with associated symptoms including syncope, CHF, or angina, or if a gradient of 50 to 75 mm Hg exists with concomitant ECG evidence of LV strain or ischemia. In the critically ill neonate, there may be little gradient across the aortic valve because of poor LV function. These patients depend on patency of the ductus arteriosus to provide systemic perfusion from the RV, and all ductal-dependent patients with critical AS require treatment. However, the decision regarding treatment options must be based on a complete understanding of associated defects. For example, in the presence of a hypoplastic LV (left ventricular end-diastolic volume <20 mL/m^2), isolated aortic valvotomy should not be performed because studies have demonstrated high mortality in this population following isolated valvotomy.[22]

Relief of valvular AS in infants and children can be accomplished with standard techniques of CPB and direct exposure to the aortic valve. A transverse incision is made in the ascending aorta above the sinus of Valsalva, extending close to, but not into, the noncoronary sinus. Exposure is attained with placement of a retractor into the right coronary sinus. After inspection of the valve, the chosen commissure is incised to within 1 to 2 mm of the aortic wall (Fig. 19-3).

Balloon valvotomy performed in the cath lab has gained widespread acceptance as the procedure of choice for reduction of transvalvular gradients in symptomatic infants and children. This procedure is an ideal palliative option because mortality from surgical valvotomy can be high due to the critical nature of these patients' condition. Furthermore, balloon valvotomy provides relief of the valvular gradient by opening the valve leaflets without the trauma created by open surgery, and allows future surgical intervention to be performed on an unscarred chest. In general, most surgical groups have abandoned open surgical valvotomy and favor catheter-based balloon valvotomy. The decision regarding the most appropriate method to use depends on several crucial factors including the available medical expertise, the patient's overall status and hemodynamics, and the presence of associated cardiac defects requiring repair.[23] Although recent evidence is emerging to the contrary, simple valvotomy, whether performed percutaneously or open, is generally considered a palliative procedure. The goal is to relieve LVOT obstruction without producing clinically significant regurgitation, in order to allow sufficient annular growth for eventual aortic valve replacement. The majority of survivors of valvotomy performed during infancy will require further intervention on the aortic valve in 10 years.[24]

Valvotomy may result in aortic insufficiency. Eventually, the combination of aortic stenosis and/or insufficiency may result in the need for an aortic valve replacement. Neonates with severely

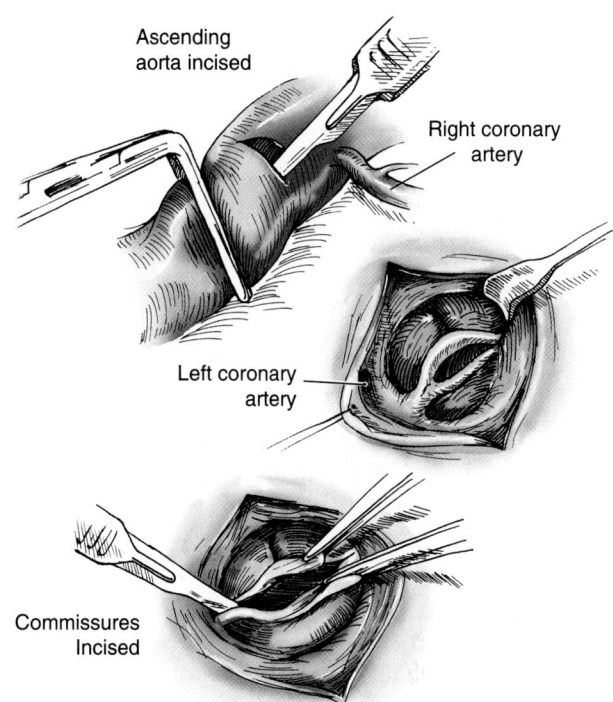

FIG. 19-3. *Aortic valvotomy with cardiopulmonary bypass. A transverse incision is made in the ascending aorta above the sinuses of Valsalva, extending close to, but not into, the noncoronary sinus. Exposure is accomplished with placement of a retractor into the right coronary sinus. After inspection of the valve, the chosen commissure is incised to within 1 to 2 mm of the aortic wall. (Reproduced with permission from Doty DB: Cardiac Surgery: A Looseleaf Workbook and Update Service. Chicago: Year Book, 1986.)*

hypoplastic LVs or significant LV endocardial fibroelastosis may not be candidates for two-ventricle repair and are treated the same as infants with the hypoplastic left-heart syndrome (HLHS), which is discussed later (see Hypoplastic Left-Heart Syndrome below).

Many surgeons previously avoided aortic valve replacement for aortic stenosis in early childhood because the more commonly used mechanical valves would be outgrown and require replacement later, and the obligatory anticoagulation for mechanical valves resulted in a substantial risk for complications. In addition, mechanical valves had an important incidence of bacterial endocarditis or perivalvular leak requiring re-intervention.

The use of allografts and the advent of the Ross procedure have largely obviated these issues and made early definitive correction of critical AS a viable option.[20,25,26] Donald Ross first described transposition of the pulmonary valve into the aortic position with allograft reconstruction of the pulmonary outflow tract in 1967,[25] in which a normal trileaflet semilunar valve made of a patient's native tissue was used to replace the damaged aortic valve (Fig. 19-4). Since then, the Ross procedure has become the optimal choice for aortic valve replacement in children, because it has improved durability and can be performed with acceptable morbidity and mortality rates. Lupinetti and Jones compared allograft aortic valve replacement with the Ross procedure and found a more significant transvalvular gradient reduction and regression of left ventricular hypertrophy in those patients who underwent the Ross procedure.[26] In some cases, the pulmonary valve may not be usable because of associated defects or congenital absence. These children are not candidates for the Ross procedure and are now most frequently treated with cryopreserved allografts (cadaveric human aortic valves). At times, there may be

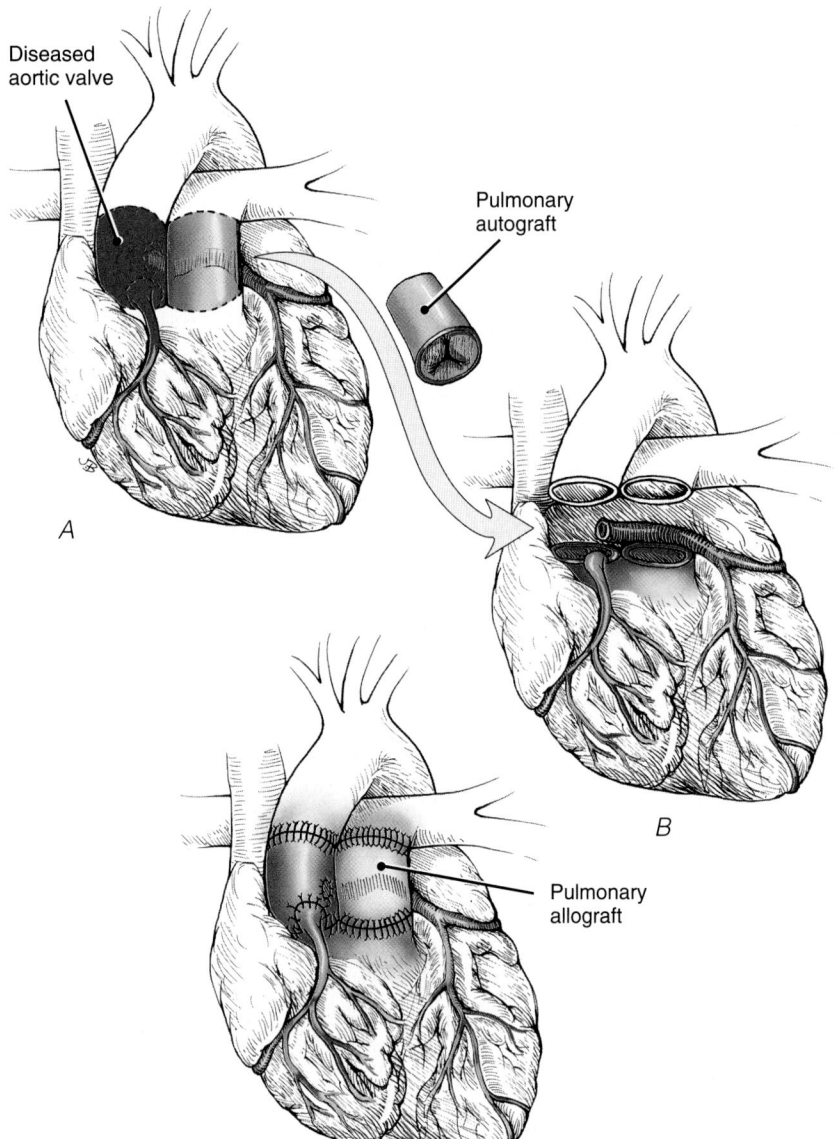

FIG. 19-4. *A to C.* The pulmonary autograft for aortic valve replacement. The aortic valve and adjacent aorta are excised, preserving buttons of aortic tissue around the coronary ostia. The pulmonary valve and main pulmonary artery are excised and transferred to the aortic position. The coronary buttons are then attached to the neoaortic root. A pulmonary allograft is inserted to reestablish the right ventricular outflow tract. *(Reproduced with permission from Kouchokos NT, Davila-Roman VG, Spray TL, et al: Replacement of the aortic root with a pulmonary autograft in children and young adults with aortic-valve disease. N Engl J Med 330:1, 1994.)*

a size discrepancy between the RVOT and the LVOT, especially in cases of severe critical AS in infancy. For these cases, the pulmonary autograft is placed in a manner that also provides enlargement of the aortic annulus (Ross/Konno) (Fig. 19-5).

Subvalvular AS occurs beneath the aortic valve and may be classified as discrete or tunnel-like (diffuse). A thin, fibromuscular diaphragm immediately proximal to the aortic valve characterizes discrete subaortic stenosis. This diaphragm typically extends for 180° degrees or more in a crescentic or circular fashion, often attaching to the mitral valve as well as the interventricular septum.[20] The aortic valve itself is usually normal in this condition, although the turbulence imparted by the subvalvular stenosis may affect leaflet morphology and valve competence.

Diffuse subvalvular AS results in a long, tunnel-like obstruction that may extend to the left ventricular apex. In some individuals, there may be difficulty in distinguishing between hypertrophic cardiomyopathy and diffuse subaortic stenosis. Operation for subvalvular AS is indicated with a gradient exceeding 30 mm Hg or when symptoms indicating LVOT obstruction are present. Some surgeons advocate repair in all cases of discrete AS, because it entails only simple membrane excision, to avoid aortic insufficiency,

which often occurs with this lesion.[27] Diffuse AS oftentimes requires aortoventriculoplasty as previously described. Results are generally excellent, with operative mortality less than 5%.[28]

Supravalvular AS occurs more rarely, and also can be classified into a discrete type, which produces an hourglass deformity of the aorta, and a diffuse form that can involve the entire arch and brachiocephalic arteries. The aortic valve leaflets are usually normal, but in some cases, the leaflets may adhere to the supravalvular stenosis, thereby narrowing the sinuses of Valsalva in diastole and restricting coronary artery perfusion. In addition, accelerated intimal hyperplastic changes in the coronary arteries can be demonstrated in these patients because the proximal position of the coronary arteries subjects them to abnormally high perfusion pressures.

The signs and symptoms of supravalvular AS are similar to other forms of LVOT obstruction. An asymptomatic murmur is the presenting manifestation in approximately half these patients. Syncope, poor exercise tolerance, and angina may all occur with nearly equal frequency. Occasionally, supravalvular AS is associated with Williams' syndrome, a constellation of elfin facies, mental retardation, and hypercalcemia.[29] Following routine evaluation, cardiac catheterization should be performed in order to delineate coronary

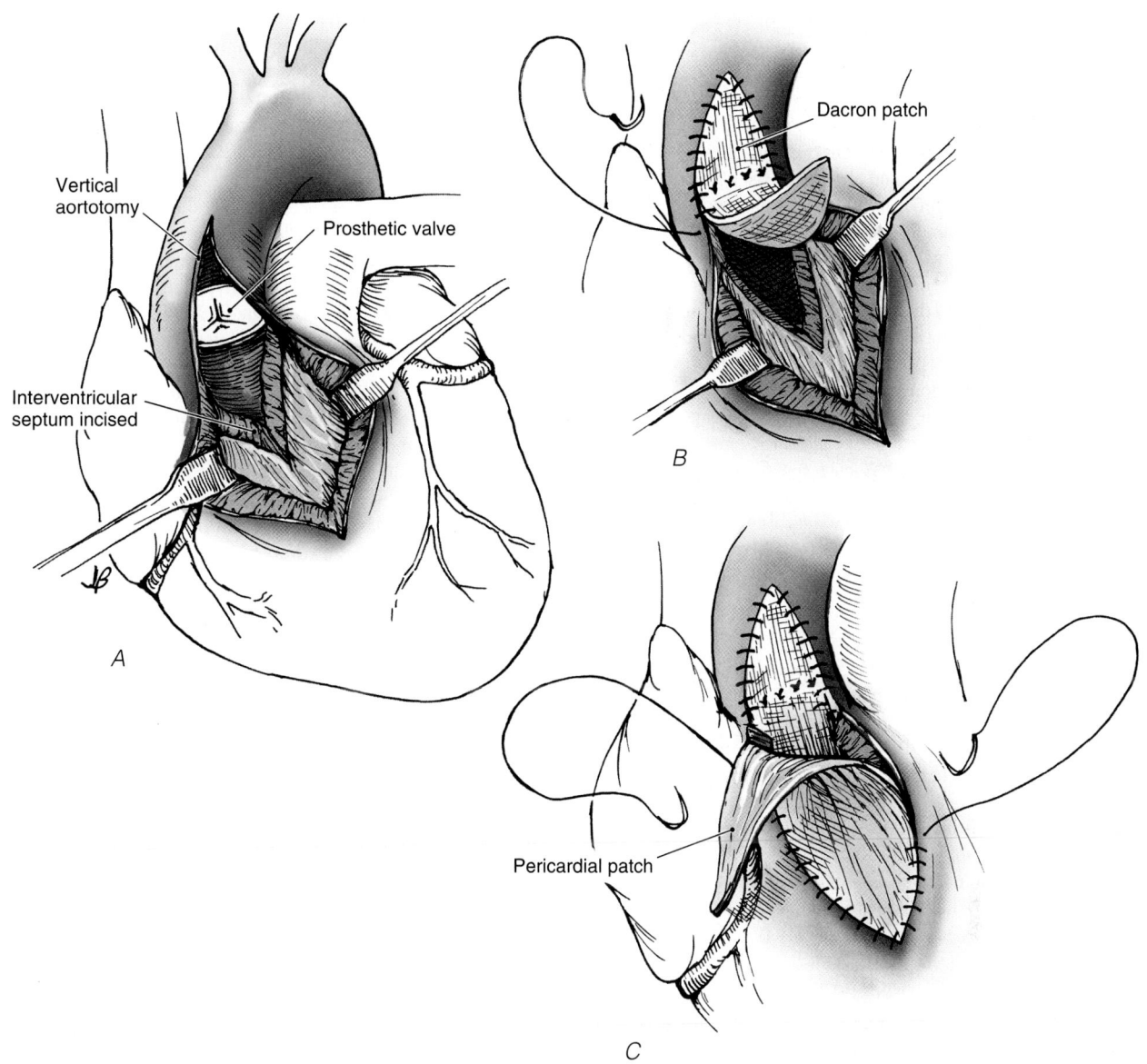

FIG. 19-5. The Konno-Rastan aortoventriculoplasty permits significant enlargement of the aortic annulus and subaortic region. *A.* A vertical aortotomy is made to the left of the right coronary artery and extended into the right ventricular outflow tract. After excising the aortic valve, the interventricular septum is incised and an aortic valve prosthesis is secured within the enlarged annulus. *B.* A Dacron patch that is attached to the sewing ring of the prosthesis closes the interventricular septum and the aortotomy. *C.* A separate pericardial patch closes the right ventriculotomy. *(Reproduced with permission from Misbach GA, Turley K, Ullyot DJ, et al: Left ventricular outflow enlargement by the Konno procedure. J Thorac Cardiovasc Surg 84:696, 1982.)*

anatomy, as well as to delineate the degree of obstruction. A gradient of 50 mm Hg or greater is an indication for operation. However, the clinician must be cognizant of any coexistent lesions, most commonly pulmonic stenosis, which may add complexity to the repair.

The localized form of supravalvular AS is treated by creating an inverted Y-shaped aortotomy across the area of stenosis, straddling the right coronary artery. The obstructing shelf is then excised and a pantaloon-shaped patch is used to close the incision.[20]

The diffuse form of supravalvular stenosis is more variable, and the particular operative approach must be tailored to each specific patient's anatomy. In general, either an aortic endarterectomy with patch augmentation can be performed, or if the narrowing extends past the aorta arch, a prosthetic graft can be placed between the ascending and descending aorta. Operative results for discrete

supravalvular AS are generally good, with a hospital mortality of less than 1% and an actuarial survival rate exceeding 90% at 20 years.[30] In contrast, however, the diffuse form is more hazardous to repair, and carried a mortality of 15% in a recent series.[30,31]

Patent Ductus Arteriosus

Anatomy

The ductus arteriosus is derived from the sixth aortic arch and normally extends from the main or left pulmonary artery to the upper descending thoracic aorta, distal to the left subclavian artery. In the normal fetal cardiovascular system, ductal flow is considerable (approximately 60% of the combined ventricular output), and is directed exclusively from the pulmonary artery (PA) to the aorta.[32]

In infancy, the length of the ductus may vary from 2 to 8 mm, with a diameter of 4 to 12 mm.

Locally produced and circulating prostaglandin E_2 (PGE_2) and prostaglandin I_2 (PGI_2) induce active relaxation of the ductal musculature, maintaining maximal patency during the fetal period.[33] At birth, increased pulmonary blood flow metabolizes these prostaglandin products, and absence of the placenta removes an important source of them, resulting in a marked decrease in these ductal-relaxing substances. In addition, release of histamines, catecholamines, bradykinin, and acetylcholine all promote ductal contraction. Despite all of these complex interactions, the rising oxygen tension in the fetal blood is the main stimulus causing smooth muscle contraction and ductal closure within 10 to 15 hours postnatally.[34] Anatomic closure by fibrosis produces the ligamentum arteriosum connecting the PA to the aorta.

Delayed closure of the ductus is termed prolonged patency, whereas failure of closure causes persistent patency, which may occur as an isolated lesion or in association with more complex congenital heart defects. In many of these infants with more complex congenital heart defects, either pulmonary or systemic perfusion may depend on ductal flow, and these infants may decompensate if exogenous PGE is not administered to maintain ductal patency.

Natural History

The incidence of patent ductus arteriosus (PDA) is approximately 1 in every 2000 births; however, it increases dramatically with increasing prematurity.[35] In some series, PDAs have been noted in 75% of infants of 28 to 30 weeks gestation. Persistent patency occurs more commonly in females, with a 2:1 ratio.[35]

PDA is not a benign entity, although prolonged survival has been reported. The estimated death rate for infants with isolated, untreated PDA is approximately 30%.[36] The leading cause of death is congestive heart failure, with respiratory infection as a secondary cause. Endocarditis is more likely to occur with a small ductus and is rarely fatal if aggressive antibiotic therapy is initiated early.

Clinical Manifestations and Diagnosis

After birth, in an otherwise normal cardiovascular system, a PDA results in a left-to-right shunt that depends on both the size of the ductal lumen and its total length. As the pulmonary vascular resistance falls 16 to 18 weeks postnatally, the shunt will increase, and its flow will ultimately be determined by the relative resistances of the pulmonary and systemic circulations.

The hemodynamic consequences of an unrestrictive ductal shunt are left ventricular volume overload with increased left atrial and pulmonary artery pressures, and right ventricular strain from the augmented afterload. These changes result in increased sympathetic discharge, tachycardia, tachypnea, and ventricular hypertrophy. The diastolic shunt results in lower aortic diastolic pressure and increases the potential for myocardial ischemia and underperfusion of other systemic organs, while the increased pulmonary flow leads to increased work of breathing and decreased gas exchange. Unrestrictive ductal flow may lead to pulmonary hypertension within the first year of life. These changes will be significantly attenuated if the size of the ductus is only moderate, and completely absent if the ductus is small.

Physical examination of the afflicted infant will reveal evidence of a hyperdynamic circulation with a widened pulse pressure and a hyperactive precordium. Auscultation demonstrates a systolic or continuous murmur, often termed a machinery murmur. Cyanosis is not present in uncomplicated isolated PDA.

The chest radiograph may reveal increased pulmonary vascularity or cardiomegaly, and the ECG may show LV strain, left atrial enlargement, and possibly RV hypertrophy. Echocardiogram with color mapping reliably demonstrates the patency of the ductus as well as estimates the shunt size. Cardiac catheterization is necessary only when pulmonary hypertension is suspected.

Therapy

The presence of a persistent PDA is sufficient indication for closure because of the increased mortality and risk of endocarditis.[2,4] In older patients with pulmonary hypertension, closure may not improve symptoms and is associated with much higher mortality.

In premature infants, aggressive intervention with indomethacin to achieve early closure of the PDA is beneficial.[37] Term infants, however, are generally unresponsive to pharmacologic therapy with indomethacin, so mechanical closure must be undertaken once the diagnosis is established. This can be accomplished either surgically or with catheter-based therapy.[12,38,39] Currently, transluminal placement of various occlusive devices, such as the Rashkind double-umbrella device or embolization with Gianturco coils, is in widespread use.[38] However, there are a number of complications inherent with the use of percutaneous devices, such as thromboembolism, endocarditis, incomplete occlusion, vascular injury, and hemorrhage secondary to perforation.[39] In addition, these techniques may not be applicable in very young infants, as the peripheral vessels do not provide adequate access for the delivery devices.

Video-assisted thoracoscopic occlusion, using metal clips, also has been described, although it offers few advantages over the standard surgical approach.[12] Preterm newborns and children, however, may do well with the thoracoscopic technique, while older patients (older than age 5 years) and those with smaller ducts (<3 mm) do well with coil occlusion. In fact, Moore and colleagues recently concluded from their series that coil occlusion is the procedure of choice for ducts smaller than 4 mm.[40] Complete closure rates using catheter-based techniques have steadily improved. Comparative studies of cost and outcome between open surgery and transcatheter duct closure, however, have shown no overwhelming choice between the two modalities.[12] Burke prospectively reviewed coil occlusion and VATS at Miami Children's Hospital, and found both options to be effective and less morbid than traditional thoracotomy.[12]

Standard surgical approach involves triple ligation of the ductus with permanent suture through either a left anterior or a posterior thoracotomy. Occasionally, a short, broad ductus, in which the dimension of its width approaches that of its length, will be encountered. In this case, division between vascular clamps with oversewing of both ends is advisable (Fig. 19-6). In extreme cases, the use of CPB to decompress the large ductus during ligation is an option.

Outcomes

In premature infants, the surgical mortality is very low, although the overall hospital death rate is significant as a consequence of other complications of prematurity. In older infants and children, mortality is less than 1%. Bleeding, chylothorax, vocal cord paralysis, and the need for reoperation occur infrequently. With the advent of muscle-sparing thoracotomy, the risk of subsequent arm dysfunction or breast abnormalities is virtually eliminated.[41]

Aortic Coarctation

Anatomy

Coarctation of the aorta (COA) is defined as a luminal narrowing in the aorta that causes an obstruction to blood flow. This narrowing

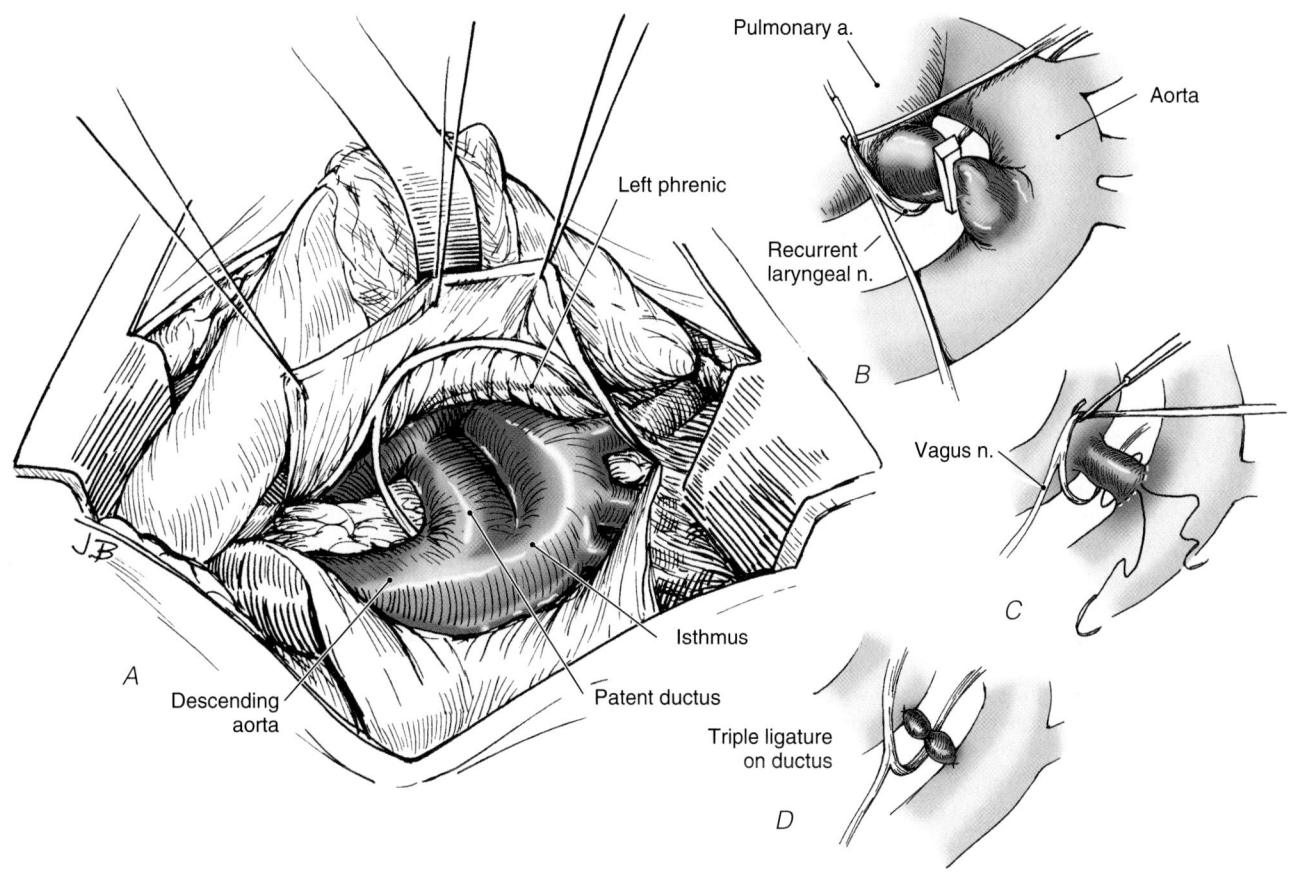

FIG. 19-6. *A. Surgeon's perspective of infant patent ductus arteriosus exposed via a left thoracotomy. B. The pleura over the aortic isthmus is incised and mobilized. C and D. Technique of triple ligation. (Reproduced with permission from Castaneda et al,[7] p 208.)*

is most commonly located distal to the left subclavian artery. The embryologic origin of COA is a subject of some controversy. One theory holds that the obstructing shelf, which is largely composed of tissue found within the ductus, forms as the ductus involutes.[42] The other theory holds that a diminished aortic isthmus develops secondary to decreased aortic flow in infants with enhanced ductal circulation.

Extensive collateral circulation develops, predominantly involving the intercostals and mammary arteries as a direct result of aortic flow obstruction. This translates into the well-known finding of "rib-notching" on chest radiograph, as well as a prominent pulsation underneath the ribs.

Other associated anomalies, such as ventricular septal defect, patent ductus arteriosus, and atrial septal defect, may be seen with COA, but the most common is that of a bicuspid aortic valve, which can be demonstrated in 25 to 42% of cases.[43]

Pathophysiology

Infants with COA develop symptoms consistent with left ventricular outflow obstruction, including pulmonary overcirculation and, later, biventricular failure. In addition, proximal systemic hypertension develops as a result of mechanical obstruction to ventricular ejection, as well as hypoperfusion-induced activation of the renin–angiotensin–aldosterone system. Interestingly, hypertension is often persistent after surgical correction despite complete amelioration of the mechanical obstruction and pressure gradient.[44] It has

been shown that early surgical correction may prevent the development of long-term hypertension, which undoubtedly contributes to many of the adverse sequelae of COA, including the development of circle of Willis aneurysms, aortic dissection and rupture, and an increased incidence of coronary arteriopathy with resulting myocardial infarction.[45]

Diagnosis

COA is likely to become symptomatic either in the newborn period if other anomalies are present or in the late adolescent period with the onset of left ventricular failure.

Physical examination will demonstrate a hyperdynamic precordium with a harsh murmur localized to the left chest and back. Femoral pulses will be dramatically decreased when compared to upper extremity pulses, and differential cyanosis may be apparent until ductal closure.

Echocardiography will reliably demonstrate the narrowed aortic segment, as well as define the pressure gradient across the stenotic segment. In addition, detailed information regarding other associated anomalies can be gleaned. Aortography is reserved for those cases in which the echocardiographic findings are equivocal.

Therapy

The routine management of hemodynamically significant COA in all age groups has traditionally been surgical. The most common technique in current use is resection with end-to-end anastomosis or extended end-to-end anastomosis, taking care to remove all residual ductal tissue.[46,47] The subclavian flap aortoplasty is another frequently used repair.[47] In this method, the left subclavian artery is transected and brought down over the coarcted segment as a vascularized patch. The main benefit of these techniques is that they do not involve the use of prosthetic materials.

However, end-to-end anastomosis may not be feasible when there is a long segment of coarctation, because sufficient mobilization of the aorta above and below the lesion may not be possible. In this instance, prosthetic materials, such as a patch aortoplasty, in which a prosthetic patch is used to enlarge the coarcted segment, or an interposition tube graft must be employed.

The most common complications after COA repair are late restenosis and aneurysm formation at the repair site.[48–50] Aneurysm formation is particularly common after patch aortoplasty when using Dacron material. In a large series of 891 patients, aneurysms occurred in 5.4% of the total, with 89% occurring in the group who received Dacron-patch aortoplasty, and only 8% in those who received resection with primary end-to-end anastomosis.[48] A further complication, although uncommon, is lower-body paralysis resulting from ischemic spinal cord injury during the repair. This dreaded outcome complicates 0.5% of all surgical repairs, but its incidence can be lessened with the use of some form of distal perfusion, preferably left-heart bypass with the use of femoral arterial or distal thoracic aorta for arterial inflow and the femoral vein or left atrium for venous return.[46]

Hypertension is also well-recognized following repair of COA. Bouchart and colleagues reported that in a cohort of 35 hypertensive adults (mean age 28 years) undergoing repair, despite a satisfactory anatomic outcome, only 23 patients were normotensive at a mean follow-up period of 165 months.[49] Likewise, Bhat and associates reported that in a series of 84 patients (mean age at repair was 29 years), 31% remained hypertensive at a mean follow-up of 5 years following surgery.[50]

Although operative repair is still the gold standard, treatment of COA by catheter-based intervention has become more widespread. Both balloon dilatation and primary stent implantation have been used successfully. The most extensive study of the results of balloon angioplasty reported on 970 procedures: 422 native and 548 recurrent COAs. Mean gradient reduction was 74 ± 24% for native and 70 ± 31% for recurrent COA.[51] This demonstrated that catheter-based therapy could produce equally effective results both in recurrent and in primary COA, a finding with far-reaching implications in the new paradigm of multidisciplinary treatment algorithms for CHD. In the valvuloplasty and angioplasty of congenital anomalies (VACA) report, higher preangioplasty gradient, earlier procedure date, older patient age, and the presence of recurrent COA were independent risk factors for suboptimal procedural outcome.[51]

The gradient after balloon dilatation in most series is generally acceptable. However, there is a significant minority (0 to 26%) for whom the procedural outcome is suboptimal, with a postprocedure gradient of 20 mm Hg or greater. These patients may be ideal candidates for primary stent placement. Restenosis is much less common in children, presumably reflecting the influence of vessel wall scarring and growth in the pediatric age group.

Deaths from the procedure also are infrequent (less than 1% of cases), and the main major complication is aneurysm formation, which occurs in 7% of patients.[46] With stent implantation, many authors have demonstrated improved resolution of stenosis compared with balloon dilatation alone, yet the long-term complications on vessel wall compliance remain largely unknown because only mid-term data are widely available.

In summary, children younger than age 6 months with native COA should be treated with surgical repair, while those requiring intervention at later ages may be ideal candidates for balloon dilatation or primary stent implantation.[46] Additionally, catheter-based therapy should be employed for those cases of restenosis following either surgical or primary endovascular management.

Truncus Arteriosus

Anatomy

Truncus arteriosus is a rare anomaly, comprising between 1 and 4% of all cases of congenital heart disease.[52] It is characterized by a single arterial conduit that arises from the heart, overrides the ventricular septum, and supplies the pulmonary, systemic, and coronary circulations.

The two major classification systems are those of Collett and Edwards, described in 1949, and Van Praagh and Van Praagh, described in 1965 (Fig. 19-7).[53,54] The Collett and Edwards classification focuses mainly on the origin of the pulmonary arteries from the common arterial trunk, whereas the Van Praagh system is based on the presence or absence of a VSD, the degree of formation of the aorticopulmonary septum, and the status of the aortic arch.

During embryonic life, the truncus arteriosus normally begins to separate and spiral into a distinguishable anterior pulmonary artery and posterior aorta. Persistent truncus, therefore, represents an arrest in embryologic development at this stage.[55] Other implicated events include twisting of the dividing truncus because of ventricular looping, subinfundibular atresia, and abnormal location of the semilunar valve anlages.[56]

The neural crest may also play a crucial role in the normal formation of the great vessels, as experimental studies in chick embryos have shown that ablation of the neural crest results in persistent truncus arteriosus.[57] The neural crest also develops into the pharyngeal pouches that give rise to the thymus and parathyroids, which likely explains the prevalent association of truncus arteriosus and DiGeorge's syndrome.[58]

The annulus of the truncal valve usually straddles the ventricular septum in a "balanced" fashion; however, it is not unusual for it to be positioned predominantly over the right ventricle, which increases the potential for left ventricular outflow tract (LVOT) obstruction following surgical repair. In the great majority of cases, the leaflets are thickened and deformed, which leads to valvular insufficiency. There are usually three leaflets (60%), but occasionally a bicuspid (50%), or even a quadricuspid valve (25%), is present.[59]

In truncus arteriosus, the pulmonary trunk bifurcates, with the left and right pulmonary arteries forming posteriorly and to the left in most cases. The caliber of the pulmonary arterial branches is usually normal, with stenosis or diffuse hypoplasia occurring in rare instances.

The coronary arteries may be normal; however, anomalies are not unusual and occur in 50% of cases.[59,60] Many of these are relatively minor, although two variations are of particular importance, because they have implications in the conduct of operative repair. The first is that the left coronary ostium may arise high in the sinus of Valsalva or even from the truncal tissue at the margin of the pulmonary artery tissue. This coronary artery can be injured during repair when the pulmonary arteries are removed from the trunk or when the resulting truncal defect is closed. The second is that the right coronary artery can give rise to an important accessory anterior descending artery, which often passes across the right ventricle in the exact location where the right ventriculotomy is commonly performed during repair.[59,60]

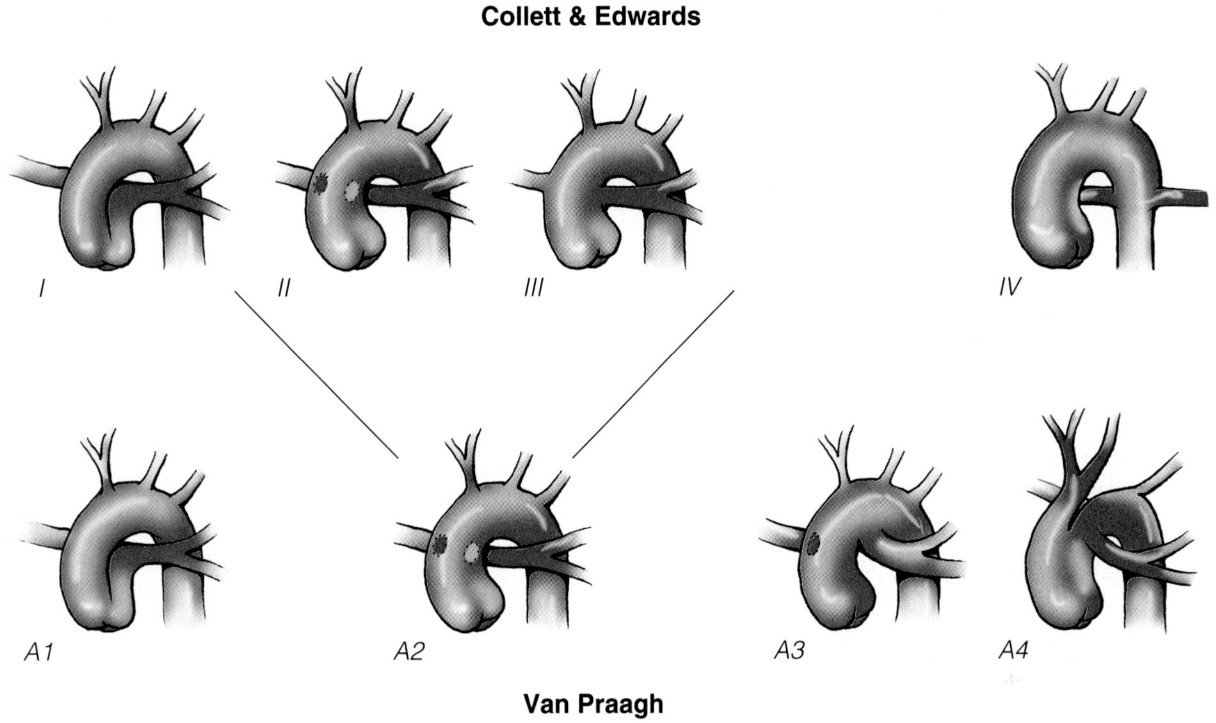

Collett & Edwards

Van Praagh

FIG. 19-7. There are similarities between the Collett and Edwards and the Van Praagh classifications of truncus arteriosus. Type I is the same as A1. Types II and III are grouped as a single type A2 because they are not significantly distinct embryologically or therapeutically. Type A3 denotes unilateral pulmonary artery with collateral supply to the contralateral lung (hemitruncus). Type A4 is truncus associated with interrupted aortic arch (13% of all cases of truncus arteriosus). [*Reproduced with permission from Fyler DC: Truncus arteriosus, in Fyler DC (ed): Nadas' Pediatric Cardiology. Philadelphia: Hanley and Belfus, 1992, p 676, as adapted from Hernanz-Schulman M, Fellows KE: Persistent truncus arteriosus: Pathologic, diagnostic and therapeutic considerations. Semin Roentgenol 20:121, 1985.*]

Physiology and Diagnosis

The main pathophysiologic consequences of truncus arteriosus are (1) the obligatory mixing of systemic and pulmonary venous blood at the level of the ventricular septal defect (VSD) and truncal valve, which leads to arterial saturations near 85%, and (2) the presence of a nonrestrictive left-to-right shunt, which occurs during both systole and diastole, the volume of which is determined by the relative resistances of the pulmonary and systemic circulations.[59] Additionally, truncal valve stenosis or regurgitation, the presence of important LVOT obstruction, and stenosis of pulmonary artery branches can further contribute to both pressure- and volume-loading of the ventricles. The presence of these lesions often results in severe heart failure and cardiovascular instability early in life. Pulmonary vascular resistance may develop as early as 6 months of age, leading to poor results with late surgical correction.

Patients with truncus arteriosus usually present in the neonatal period, with signs and symptoms of congestive heart failure and mild to moderate cyanosis. A pan-systolic murmur may be noted at the left sternal border, and occasionally a diastolic murmur may be heard in the presence of truncal regurgitation.

Chest radiography will be consistent with pulmonary overcirculation, and a right aortic arch can be appreciated 35% of the time. The ECG is usually nonspecific, demonstrating normal sinus rhythm with biventricular hypertrophy.

Echocardiography with Doppler color-flow or pulsed Doppler is diagnostic, and usually provides sufficient information to determine the type of truncus arteriosus, the origin of the coronary arteries, and

their proximity to the pulmonary trunk, the character of the truncal valves, and the extent of truncal insufficiency.[59] Cardiac catheterization can be helpful in cases where pulmonary hypertension is suspected, or to further delineate coronary artery anomalies prior to repair.

The presence of truncus is an indication for surgery. Repair should be undertaken in the neonatal period, or as soon as the diagnosis is established. Eisenmenger's physiology, which is found primarily in older children, is the only absolute contraindication to correction.

Repair

Truncus arteriosus was first managed with pulmonary artery banding as described by Armer and colleagues in 1961.[61] However, this technique led to only marginal improvements in 1-year survival rates because ventricular failure inevitably occurred. In 1967, however, complete repair was accomplished by McGoon and his associates based on the experimental work of Rastelli, who introduced the idea that an extracardiac valved conduit could be used to restore ventricular-to-pulmonary artery continuity.[62] Over the next 20 years, improved survival rates led to uniform adoption of complete repair even in the youngest and smallest infants.[52,59,63]

Generally, surgical correction entails the use of CPB. Repair is completed by separation of the pulmonary arteries from the aorta, closure of the aortic defect (occasionally with a patch) to minimize coronary flow complications, placement of a valved cryoreserved allograft to reconstruct the right ventricular outflow tract, and ventricular septal defect closure. Severe truncal valve insufficiency occasionally requires truncal valve replacement, which can be accomplished with a cryopreserved allograft.[64]

Results

The results of complete repair of truncus have steadily improved. Ebert reported a 91% survival rate in his series of 77 patients who were younger than 6 months of age; later reports by others confirmed these findings and demonstrated that excellent results could be achieved in even smaller infants with complex-associated defects.[11,63]

Newer extracardiac conduits also have been developed and used with success, which has widened the repertoire of the modern congenital heart surgeon and improved outcomes.[65] Severe truncal regurgitation, interrupted aortic arch, coexistent coronary anomalies, and age younger than 100 days are risk factors associated with perioperative death and poor outcome.

Total Anomalous Pulmonary Venous Connection

Total anomalous pulmonary venous connection (TAPVC) occurs in 1 to 2% of all cardiac malformations and is characterized by abnormal drainage of the pulmonary veins into the right heart, whether through connections into the right atrium or into its tributaries.[66] Accordingly, the only mechanism by which oxygenated blood can return to the left heart is through an ASD, which is almost uniformly present with TAPVC.

Unique to this lesion is the absence of a definitive form of palliation. Thus, TAPVC represents one of the only true surgical emergencies across the entire spectrum of congenital heart surgery.

Anatomy and Embryology

The lungs develop from an outpouching of the foregut, and their venous plexus arises as part of the splanchnic venous system. TAPVC arises when the pulmonary vein evagination from the posterior surface of the left atrium fails to fuse with the pulmonary venous plexus surrounding the lung buds. In place of the usual connection to the left atrium, at least one connection of the pulmonary plexus to the splanchnic plexus persists. Accordingly, the pulmonary veins drain to the heart through a systemic vein (Fig. 19-8).

Darling and colleagues classified TAPVC according to the site or level of connection of the pulmonary veins to the systemic venous system[67]: type I (45%), anomalous connection at the supracardiac level; type II (25%), anomalous connection at the cardiac level; type III (25%), anomalous connection at the infracardiac level; and type IV (5%), anomalous connection at multiple levels.[68] Within each category, further subdivisions can be implemented, depending on whether pulmonary venous obstruction exists. Obstruction to pulmonary venous drainage is a powerful predictor of adverse natural outcome and occurs most frequently with the infracardiac type, especially when the pattern of infracardiac connection prevents the ductus venosus from bypassing the liver.[69]

Pathophysiology and Diagnosis

Because both pulmonary and systemic venous blood return to the right atrium in all forms of TAPVC, a right-to-left intracardiac shunt must be present in order for the afflicted infant to survive. This invariably occurs via a nonrestrictive patent foramen ovale. Because of this obligatory mixing, cyanosis is usually present, and its degree depends on the ratio of pulmonary to systemic blood flow. Decreased pulmonary blood flow is a consequence of pulmonary venous obstruction, the presence of which is unlikely if the right ventricular pressure is less than 85% of systemic pressure.[70]

The child with TAPVC may present with severe cyanosis and respiratory distress necessitating urgent surgical intervention if a severe degree of pulmonary venous obstruction is present. However, in cases where there is no obstructive component, the clinical picture is usually one of pulmonary overcirculation, hepatomegaly, tachycardia, and tachypnea with feeding. In a child with serious obstruction, arterial blood gas analysis reveals severe hypoxemia (Po_2 less than 20 mm Hg), with metabolic acidosis.[71]

Chest radiography will show normal heart size with generalized pulmonary edema. Two-dimensional echocardiography is very useful in establishing the diagnosis, and also can assess ventricular septal position, which may be leftward secondary to small left ventricular volumes, as well as estimate the right ventricular pressure based on the height of the tricuspid regurgitant jet. Echocardiography can usually identify the pulmonary venous connections (types I–IV), and it is rarely necessary to perform other diagnostic tests.

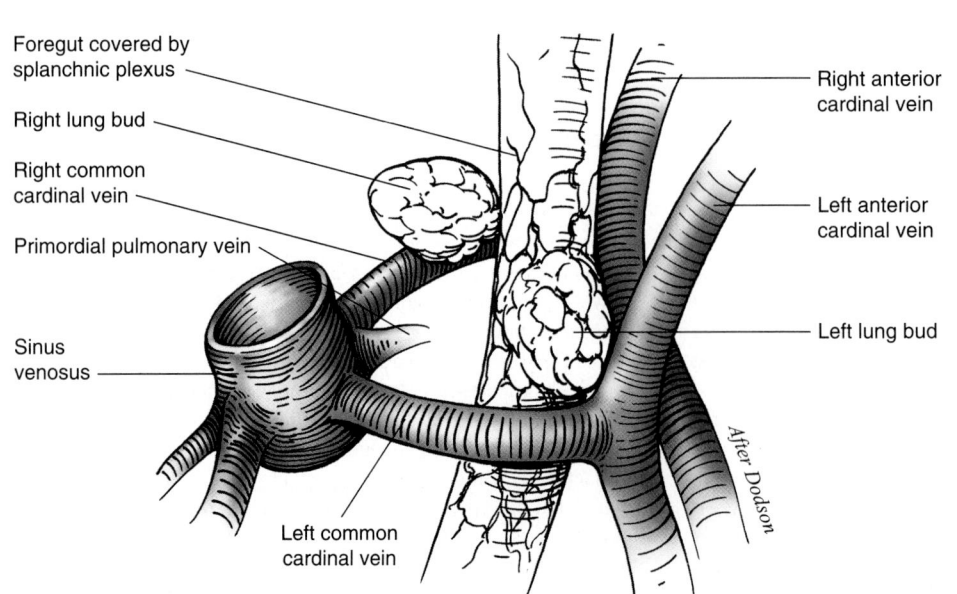

Foregut covered by splanchnic plexus

Right lung bud

Right common cardinal vein

Primordial pulmonary vein

Sinus venosus

Left common cardinal vein

Right anterior cardinal vein

Left anterior cardinal vein

Left lung bud

After Dodson

FIG. 19-8. Total anomalous pulmonary venous connection (TAPVC) results when the primordial pulmonary vein fails to unite with the plexus of veins that surround the lung buds and is derived from the splanchnic venous plexus, including the cardinal veins and umbilicovitelline veins. (*Reproduced with permission from Castaneda et al,[7] p 158.*)

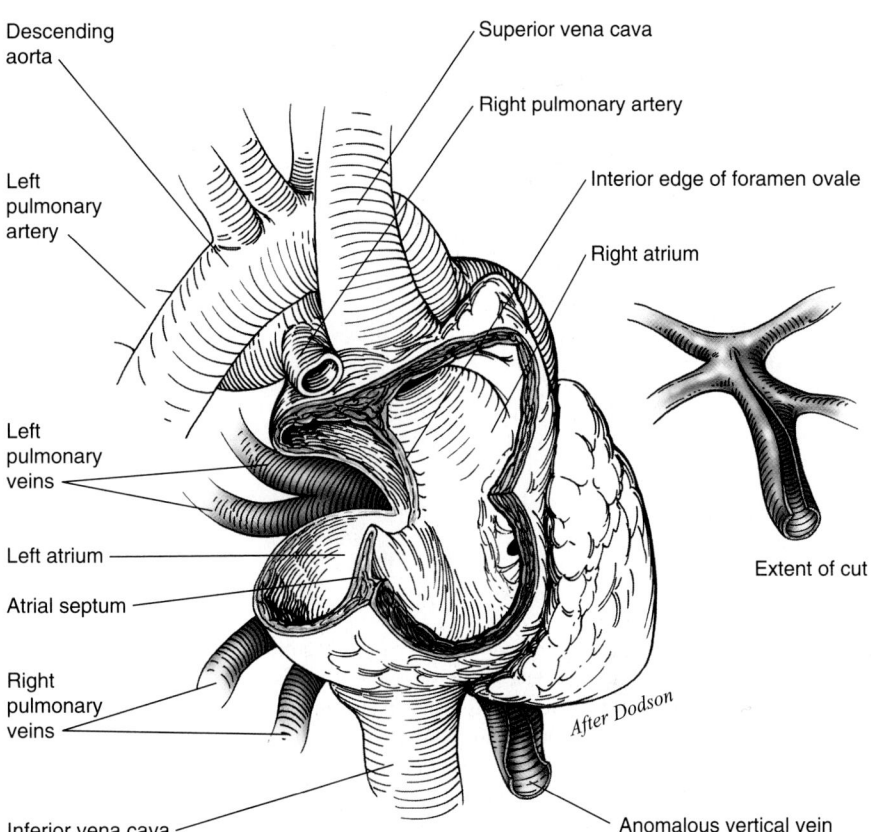

FIG. 19-9. Operative exposure obtained with infradiaphragmatic total anomalous pulmonary venous connection (TAPVC), using an approach from the right. *(Reproduced with permission from Castaneda et al,[7] p 161.)*

Cardiac catheterization is not recommended in these patients because the osmotic load from the intravenous contrast can exacerbate the degree of pulmonary edema.[72] When cardiac catheterization is performed, equalization of oxygen saturations in all four heart chambers is a hallmark finding in this disease since the mixed blood returned to the right atrium gets distributed throughout the heart.

Therapy

Operative correction of TAPVC requires anastomosis of the common pulmonary venous channel to the left atrium, obliteration of the anomalous venous connection, and closure of the atrial septal defect.[71,73]

All types of TAPVC are approached through a median sternotomy, and most surgeons use deep hypothermic circulatory arrest in order to achieve an accurate and widely patent anastomosis. The technique for supracardiac TAPVC includes early division of the vertical vein, retraction of the aorta and the superior vena cava laterally to expose the posterior aspect of the left atrium and the pulmonary venous confluence, and a side-to-side anastomosis between a long, horizontal biatrial incision and a longitudinal incision within the pulmonary venous confluence. The ASD can then be closed with an autologous pericardial patch.

In patients with TAPVC to the coronary sinus without obstruction, a simple unroofing of the coronary sinus can be performed through a single right atriotomy. If pulmonary venous obstruction is present, the repair should include generous resection of roof of the coronary sinus.[71]

Repair of infracardiac TAPVC entails ligation of the vertical vein at the diaphragm, followed by construction of a proximal, patulous longitudinal venotomy. This repair is usually performed by "rolling"

the heart toward the left, thus exposing the left atrium where it usually overlies the descending vertical vein (Fig. 19-9).

The perioperative care of these infants is crucial because episodes of pulmonary hypertension can occur within the first 48 hours, which contribute significantly to mortality following repair.[6,72,73] Muscle relaxants and narcotics should be administered during this period to maintain a constant state of anesthesia. Arterial PCO_2 should be maintained at 30 mm Hg with use of a volume ventilator and the FiO_2 should be increased to keep the pulmonary arterial pressure at less than two thirds of the systemic pressure.

Results

Results of TAPVC in infancy have markedly improved in recent years, with an operative mortality of 5% or less in some series.[71–74] This improvement is probably multifactorial, mainly as a consequence of early noninvasive diagnosis and aggressive perioperative management. The routine use of echocardiography; improvements in myocardial protection with specific attention to the right ventricle; creation of a large, tension-free anastomosis with maximal use of the venous confluence and atrial tissue; careful geometric alignment of the pulmonary venous sinus with the body of the left atrium avoiding tension and rotation of the pulmonary veins; and prevention of pulmonary hypertensive events have likely played a major role in reducing operative mortality. Risk factors such as venous obstruction at presentation, urgency of operative repair, and infradiaphragmatic anatomic type are no longer correlated with early mortality.[73,75]

The most significant postoperative complication of TAPVC repair is pulmonary venous obstruction, which occurs 9 to 11% of the time, regardless of the surgical technique employed. Mortality varies between 30 and 45% and alternative catheter interventions do not

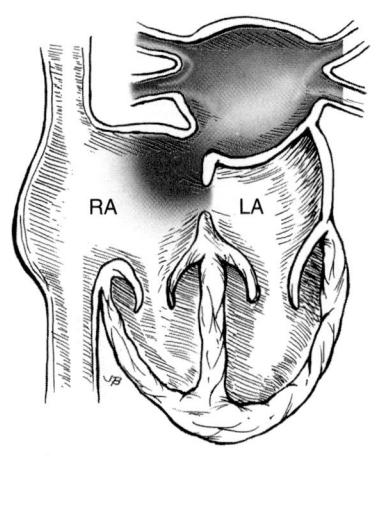

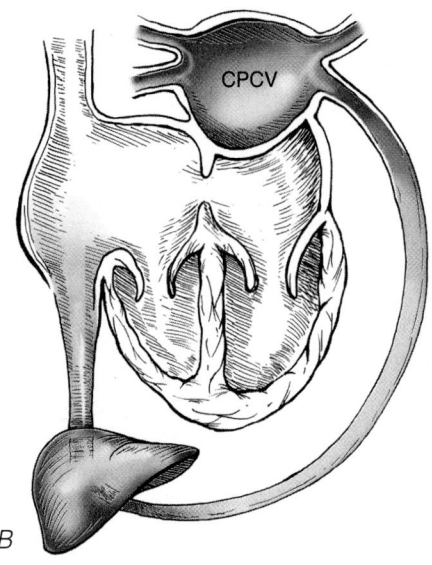

A   *B*

FIG. 19-10. Variants of cor triatriatum with imperforate membrane between common pulmonary venous chamber (*CPVC*) and left atrium (*LA*). A. Common chamber draining to right atrium directly. B. Common chamber draining into systemic venous circulation via anomalous vein. [*Adapted with permission from Lucas RV: Anomalous venous connections, pulmonary and systemic, in Adams FH, Emmanouilides GC (eds): Moss' Heart Disease in Infants, Children, and Adolescents, 3rd ed. Baltimore: Williams and Wilkins, 1983.*]

offer definitive solutions.[72] Recurrent pulmonary venous obstruction can be localized at the site of the pulmonary venous anastomosis (extrinsic), which can usually be cured with patch enlargement or balloon dilatation, or it may be secondary to endocardial thickening of the pulmonary venous ostia frequently resulting in diffuse pulmonary venous sclerosis (intrinsic), which carries a 66% mortality rate because few good solutions exist.[69] More commonly, postrepair left ventricular dysfunction can occur as the noncompliant left ventricle suddenly is required to handle an increased volume load from redirected pulmonary venous return. This can manifest as an increase in pulmonary artery pressure but is distinguishable from primary pulmonary hypertension (another possible postoperative complication following repair of TAPVC) from the elevated left atrial pressure found in LV dysfunction along with echocardiographic evidence of poor LV contractility. In pulmonary hypertension, the left atrial (LA) pressure may be low, the LV may appear "underfilled" (by echocardiography), and the RV may appear dilated. In *either* case, postoperative support for a few days with extracorporeal membrane oxygenation (ECMO) may be life-saving, and TAPVC should be repaired in centers that have this capacity.

Some investigators have speculated that preoperative pulmonary venous obstruction is associated with increased medial thickness within the pulmonary vasculature, which may predispose these infants to intrinsic pulmonary venous stenosis despite adequate pulmonary venous decompression.[74] Another complication following repair of TAPVC is the development of atrial arrhythmias secondary to altered atrial geometry and left atrial enlargement procedures. These arrhythmias may be asymptomatic, and certain surgeons therefore advocate routine long-term follow-up with 24-hour ECG monitoring to facilitate their detection and treatment.[75]

Cor Triatriatum

Anatomy

Cor triatriatum is a rare congenital heart disease characterized by the presence of a fibromuscular diaphragm that partitions the left atrium into two chambers: a superior chamber that receives drainage from the pulmonary veins, and an inferior chamber that communicates with the mitral valve and the left ventricle (Fig. 19-10). An ASD frequently exists between the superior chamber and the right atrium, or, more rarely, between the right atrium and the inferior chamber.

Pathophysiology and Diagnosis

Cor triatriatum results in obstruction of pulmonary venous return to the left atrium. The degree of obstruction is variable and depends on the size of fenestrations present in the left atrial membrane, the size of the atrial septal defect, and the existence of other associated anomalies. If the communication between the superior and inferior chambers is less than 3 mm, patients usually are symptomatic during the first year of life. The afflicted infant will present with the stigmata of low cardiac output and pulmonary venous hypertension, as well as congestive heart failure and poor feeding.

Physical examination may demonstrate a loud pulmonary S_2 sound and a right ventricular heave, as well as jugular venous distention and hepatomegaly. Chest radiography will show cardiomegaly and pulmonary vascular prominence, and the ECG will suggest right ventricular hypertrophy. Two-dimensional echocardiography provides a definitive diagnosis in most cases, with catheterization necessary only when echocardiographic evaluation is equivocal.

Therapy

Operative treatment for cor triatriatum is fairly simple. Cardiopulmonary bypass and cardioplegic arrest are used. A right atriotomy usually allows access to the left atrial membrane through the existing ASD, because it is dilated secondary to communication with the pulmonary venous chamber. The membrane is then excised, taking care not to injure the mitral valve or the interatrial septum, and the ASD is closed with a patch. Alternatively, if the right atrium is small, the membrane can be exposed through an incision directly into the superior left atrial chamber, just anterior to the right pulmonary veins.[76] Surgical results are uniformly excellent for this defect, with survival approaching 100%.

The utility of catheter-based intervention for this diagnosis remain controversial, although there have been two recent reports of successful balloon dilatation.[77]

Aortopulmonary Window

Embryology and Anatomy

Aortopulmonary window (APW) is a rare congenital lesion, occurring in about 0.2% of patients, characterized by incomplete development of the septum that normally divides the truncus into the aorta and the pulmonary artery.[78]

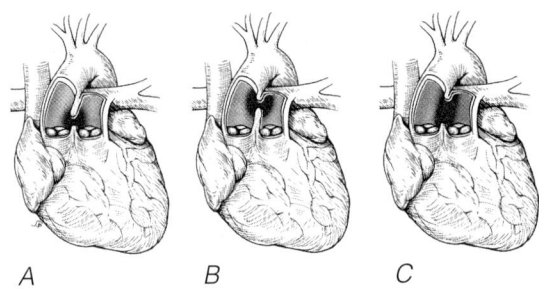

FIG. 19-11. *Classification of aortopulmonary window. A. Type I proximal defect; B. Type II distal defect; C. Type III total defect. (Reproduced with permission from Mori K, Ando M, Takao A: Distal type of aortopulmonary window: Report of 4 cases. Br Heart J 40:681, 1978.)*

In the vast majority of cases, APW occurs as a single defect of minimal length, which begins a few millimeters above the semilunar valves on the left lateral wall of the aorta (Fig. 19-11). Coronary artery anomalies, such as aberrant origin of the right or left coronary artery from the main pulmonary artery are occasionally present.

Pathophysiology and Diagnosis

The dominant pathophysiology of APW is that of a large left-to-right shunt with increased pulmonary flow and the early development of congestive heart failure. Like other lesions with left-to-right flow, the magnitude of the shunt is determined by both the size of the defect, as well as the pulmonary vascular resistance.

Infants with APW present with frequent respiratory tract infections, tachypnea with feeding, and failure to thrive. Cyanosis is usually absent because these infants deteriorate prior to the onset of significant pulmonary hypertension. The rapid decline with this defect occurs because shunt flow continues during both phases of the cardiac cycle, which limits systemic perfusion and increases ventricular work.[79]

The diagnosis of APW begins with the physical examination, which may demonstrate a systolic flow murmur, a hyperdynamic precordium, and bounding peripheral pulses. The chest radiograph will show pulmonary overcirculation and cardiomegaly, and the ECG will usually demonstrate either left ventricular hypertrophy or biventricular hypertrophy. Echocardiography can detect the defect and also provide information about associated anomalies. Retrograde aortography will confirm the diagnosis, but is rarely necessary.

Therapy

All infants with APW require surgical correction once the diagnosis is made. Repair is undertaken through a median sternotomy and the use of cardiopulmonary bypass. The pulmonary arteries are occluded once the distal aorta is cannulated, and a transaortic repair using a prosthetic patch for pulmonary artery closure is then carried out. The coronary ostia must be carefully visualized and included on the aortic side of the patch. Alternatively, a two-patch technique can be used, which may eliminate recurrent fistulas from suture line leaks that occasionally occur with the single-patch method (Fig. 19-12).[80]

Results

Results are generally excellent, with an operative mortality in most large series of less than 5%.[80]

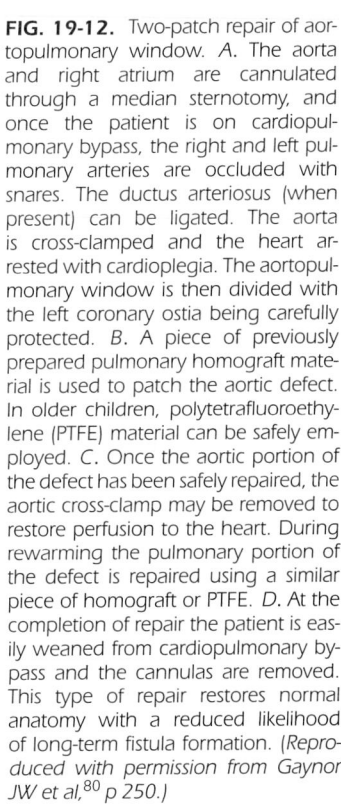

FIG. 19-12. *Two-patch repair of aortopulmonary window. A. The aorta and right atrium are cannulated through a median sternotomy, and once the patient is on cardiopulmonary bypass, the right and left pulmonary arteries are occluded with snares. The ductus arteriosus (when present) can be ligated. The aorta is cross-clamped and the heart arrested with cardioplegia. The aortopulmonary window is then divided with the left coronary ostia being carefully protected. B. A piece of previously prepared pulmonary homograft material is used to patch the aortic defect. In older children, polytetrafluoroethylene (PTFE) material can be safely employed. C. Once the aortic portion of the defect has been safely repaired, the aortic cross-clamp may be removed to restore perfusion to the heart. During rewarming the pulmonary portion of the defect is repaired using a similar piece of homograft or PTFE. D. At the completion of repair the patient is easily weaned from cardiopulmonary bypass and the cannulas are removed. This type of repair restores normal anatomy with a reduced likelihood of long-term fistula formation. (Reproduced with permission from Gaynor JW et al,[80] p 250.)*

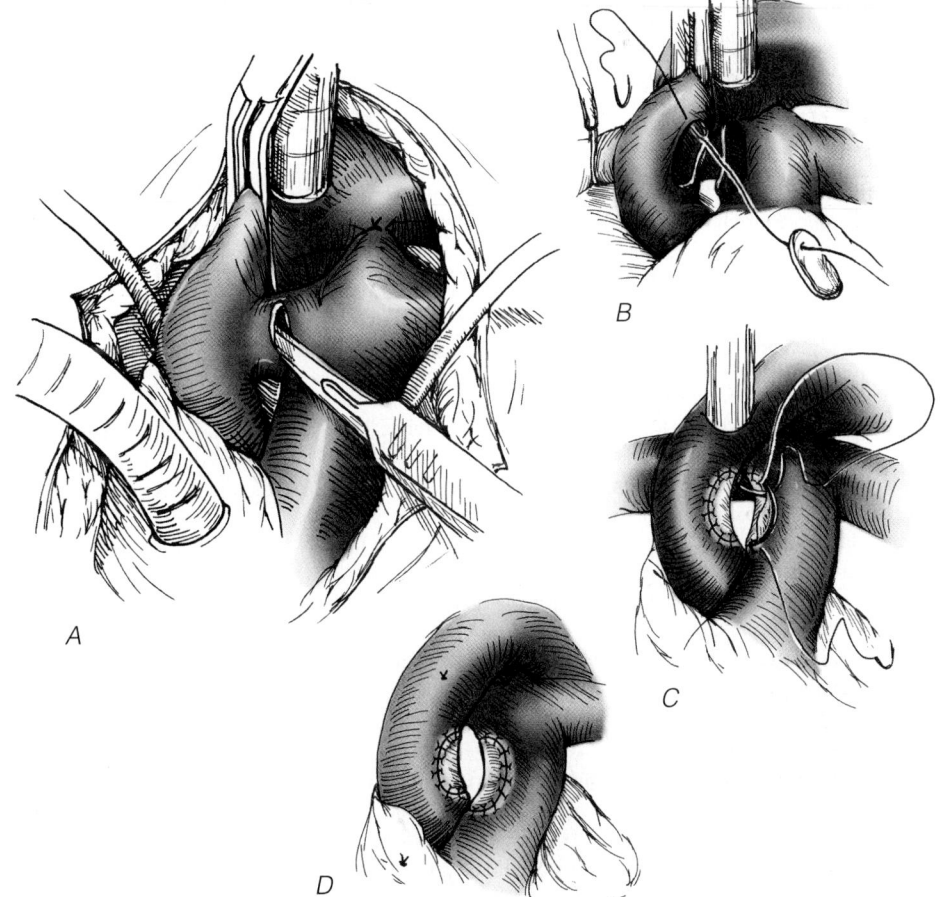

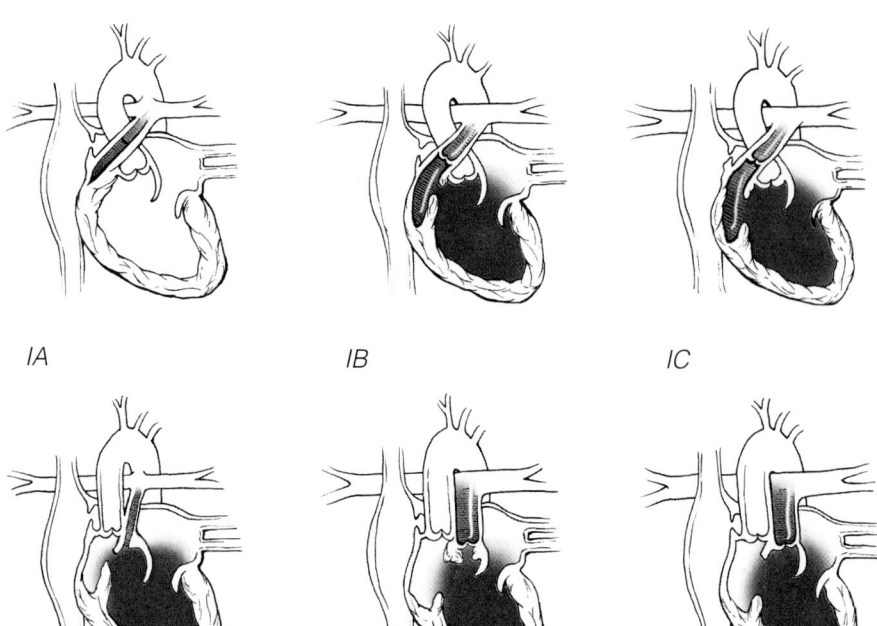

IA   IB   IC

IIA   IIB   IIC

FIG. 19-13. *Classification of tricuspid atresia. Type I, normally related great arteries with IA, pulmonary atresia with virtual absence of right ventricle; IB, pulmonary stenosis with small ventricular septal defect; IC, normal pulmonary valve, large VSD. Type II, transposed great arteries with IIA, pulmonary atresia; IIB, pulmonary or subpulmonary stenosis; IIC, normal or enlarged pulmonary valve and artery without subpulmonary stenosis. [Reproduced with permission from Backer CL, et al: Tricuspid atresia, in Mavroudis C, Backer CL (eds): Pediatric Cardiac Surgery, 2nd ed. St. Louis: Mosby, 1994, p 381.]*

DEFECTS REQUIRING PALLIATION

Tricuspid Atresia

Tricuspid atresia occurs in 2 to 3% of patients with congenital heart disease and is characterized by atresia of the tricuspid valve. This results in discontinuity between the right atrium and right ventricle. The right ventricle is generally hypoplastic, and left-heart filling is dependent on an atrial septal defect. Tricuspid atresia is the most common form of the single-ventricle complex, indicating that there is functionally only one ventricular chamber.

Anatomy

As mentioned, tricuspid atresia results in a lack of communication between the right atrium and the right ventricle, and in the majority of patients there is no identifiable valve tissue or remnant.[81] The right atrium is generally enlarged and muscular, with a fibrofatty floor. An unrestrictive ASD is usually present. The left ventricle is often enlarged as it receives both systemic and pulmonary blood flow, but the atrioventricular valve is usually normal.

The right ventricle, however, is usually severely hypoplastic, and there is sometimes a ventricular septal defect in its trabeculated or infundibular portion. In many cases, the interventricular communication is a site of obstruction to pulmonary blood flow, but obstruction may also occur at the level of the outlet valve or in the subvalvular infundibulum.[82] In most cases, pulmonary blood flow is dependent on the presence of a patent ductus arteriosus (PDA), and there may be no flow into the pulmonary circulation except for this PDA.

Tricuspid atresia is classified according to the relationship of the great vessels (Fig. 19-13).

Pathophysiology

The main pathophysiology in tricuspid atresia is that of a univentricular heart. That is, the left ventricle must receive systemic blood via the interatrial communication, and then distribute it to both the pulmonary circulation and the systemic circulation. Unless there is a VSD (as is found in some cases), pulmonary flow is dependent upon the presence of a PDA. As the ductus begins to close shortly after birth, infants become intensely cyaxotic. Re-establishing ductal patency (with PGE$_1$) restores pulmonary blood flow and stabilizes patients for surgical intervention. Pulmonary hypertension is unusual in tricuspid atresia. However, occasional patients have a large VSD between the left ventricle and the infundibular portion of the RV (just below the pulmonary valve). If there is no obstruction at the level of this VSD or at the valve, these infants may actually present with heart failure from excessive pulmonary blood flow. Regardless of whether these infants are "ductal-dependent" for pulmonary blood flow or have pulmonary blood flow provided across a VSD, they will be cyaxotic since the obligatory right-to-left shunt at the atrial level will provide complete mixing of systemic and pulmonary venous return so that the left ventricle ejects a hypoxemic mixture into the aorta.

Diagnosis

The signs and symptoms of tricuspid atresia are dependent on the underlying anatomic variant, but most infants are cyanotic and hypoxic as a result of decreased pulmonary blood flow and the complete mixing at the atrial level. When pulmonary blood flow is provided through a VSD, there may be a prominent systolic murmur. Tricuspid atresia with pulmonary blood flow from a PDA may present with the soft, continuous murmur of a PDA in conjunction with cyanosis.

In the minority of patients with tricuspid atresia, symptoms of congestive heart failure will predominate. This is often related to excessive flow across a VSD. The natural history of the muscular VSDs in these infants is that they will close and the congestive heart failure will dissipate and transform into cyanosis with reduced pulmonary blood flow. The predominant finding in all patients with tricuspid atresia is cyanosis. There is a subtype of tricuspid atresia that includes transposition of the great arteries. In these patient, the aorta arises from the dominative right ventricle and systemic

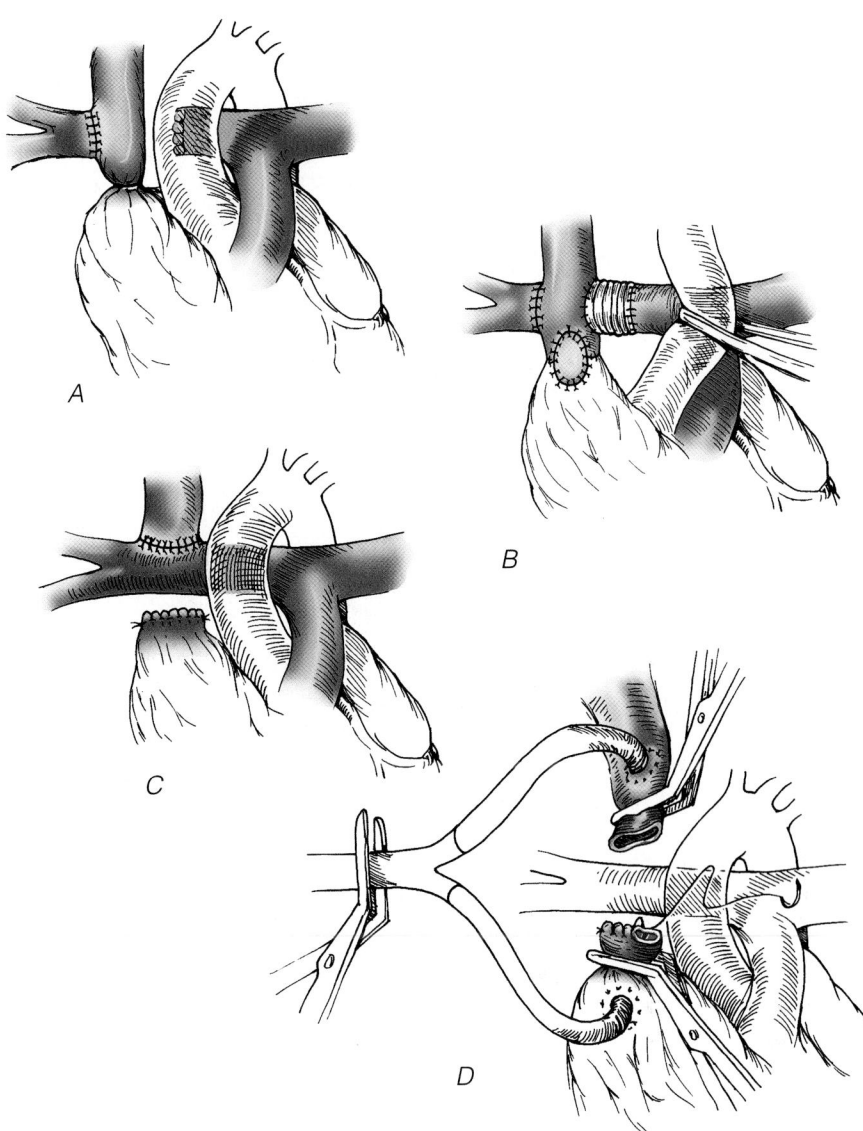

FIG. 19-14. Superior vena cava (SVC)–pulmonary artery shunts. *A.* Classical Glenn shunt. End-to-side right pulmonary artery-to-superior vena cava anastomosis with ligation of SVC–right atrial junction. *B.* Method of takedown of classic Glenn shunt and creation of total cavopulmonary anastomosis during Fontan operation. *C.* Bidirectional Glenn shunt (bidirectional SVC–pulmonary artery shunt), end-to-side SVC-to-RPA (right pulmonary artery) anastomosis. *D.* Method of construction of bidirectional Glenn shunt, one cannula in the high SVC or innominate vein, and another cannula in the right atrium connected to a Y-connector. *[Reproduced with permission from Backer CL, et al: Tricuspid atresia, in Mavroudis C, Backer CL (eds): Pediatric Cardiac Surgery, 2nd ed. St. Louis: Mosby, 1994, p 383.]*

blood flow requires a VSD or a PDA. These patient often have an associated aortic coarctation and usually require early intervention.

Chest radiography will show decreased pulmonary vascularity. The ECG is strongly suggestive, because uncharacteristic left axis deviation will be present, owing to underdevelopment of the right ventricle. Two-dimensional echocardiography readily confirms the diagnosis and the anatomic subtype.

Treatment

The treatment for tricuspid atresia in the earlier era of palliation was aimed at correcting the defect in the pulmonary circulation. That is, patients with too much pulmonary flow received a pulmonary band, and those with insufficient flow received a systemic-to-pulmonary artery shunt. Systemic-to-pulmonary artery shunts, or Blalock-Taussig (B-T) shunts, were first applied to patients with tricuspid atresia in the 1940s and 1950s.[83] Likewise pulmonary artery banding was applied to patients with tricuspid atresia and congestive failure in 1957. However, despite the initial relief of either cyanosis or congestive heart failure, long-term mortality was high, as the single ventricle was left unprotected from either volume or pressure overload.[84]

Recognizing the inadequacies of the initial repairs, Glenn described the first successful cavopulmonary anastomosis, an end-to-side right pulmonary artery (RPA)-to-superior vena cava (SVC) shunt in 1958, and later modified this to allow flow to both pulmonary arteries.[85] This end-to-side RPA-to-SVC anastomosis was known as the bidirectional Glenn, and is the first stage to final Fontan repair in widespread use today (Fig. 19-14). The Fontan repair was a major advancement in the treatment of congenital heart disease, as it essentially bypassed the right heart, and allowed separation of the pulmonary and systemic circulations. It was first performed by Fontan in 1971, and consisted of a classic Glenn anastomosis, ASD closure, and direct connection of the right atrium to the proximal end of the left pulmonary artery using an aortic homograft.[86] The main pulmonary artery was ligated, and a homograft valve was inserted into the orifice of the inferior vena cava.

Multiple modifications of this initial repair were performed over the next 20 years. One of the most important was the description by deLeval and colleagues of the creation of an interatrial lateral tunnel that allowed the inferior vena caval blood to be channeled exclusively to the superior vena cava.[87] A total cavopulmonary connection could then be accomplished by dividing the SVC and suturing the

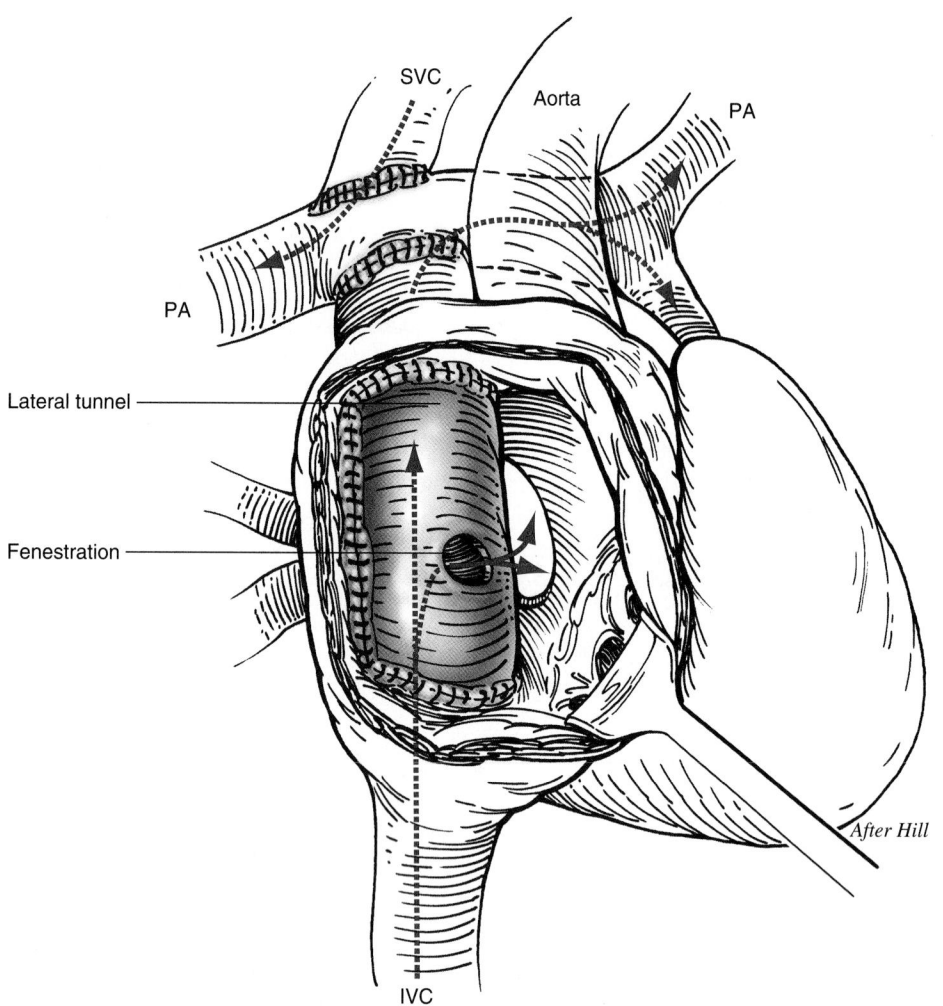

FIG. 19-15. The fenestrated Fontan procedure. Using a polytetrafluoro-ethylene patch, a tunnel is created in the lateral wall of the right atrium to direct inferior vena cava (IVC) flow to the superior vena cava (SVC) that is anastomosed to the pulmonary artery (PA). A 4- to 5-mm fenestration in the baffle diminishes systemic venous pressure and improves cardiac output at the expense of a small decrease in systemic arterial oxygen saturation. *(Reproduced with permission from Kopf GS, Kleinman CS, Hijazi ZM, et al: Fenestrated Fontan operation with delayed transcatheter closure of atrial septal defect: Improved results in high-risk patients. J Thorac Cardiovasc Surg 103:1039, 1992.)*

superior portion to the upper side of the right pulmonary artery and the inferior end to the augmented undersurface of the right pulmonary artery. Pulmonary flow then occurs passively, in a laminar fashion, driven by the central venous pressure. This repair became known as the modified Fontan operation.

Another important modification, the fenestrated Fontan repair, was introduced in the 1988s.[88] In this procedure, a residual 20 to 30% right-to-left shunt is either created or left unrepaired at the time of cavopulmonary connection to help sustain systemic output in the face of transient elevations in the pulmonary vascular resistance postoperatively (Fig. 19-15).[88]

The last notable variation on the original Fontan repair uses an extracardiac prosthetic tube graft, usually 20 mm in diameter, as the conduit directing inferior vena cava (IVC) blood to the pulmonary arteries.[89] This technique has the advantages of decreasing atrial geometric alterations by avoiding intra-atrial suture lines, and improving flow dynamics in the systemic venous pathway by maximizing laminar flow. Several investigators have shown a decrease in supraventricular arrhythmias, as well as an improvement in ventricular function, which may be secondary to decreased atrial tension and alleviation of chronic elevations in coronary sinus pressure.[89,90] The extracardiac Fontan operation can be completed without the use of cardiopulmonary bypass in selected cases, which may further improve outcomes.[91]

Despite these innovative approaches, the current strategy for operative management still relies on the idea of palliation. Patients are approached in a staged manner, to maximize their physiologic state so that they will survive to undergo a Fontan operation. The therapeutic strategy must begin in the neonatal period and should be directed toward reducing the patient's subsequent risk factors for a Fontan procedure. Accordingly, small systemic pulmonary shunts, which are usually performed through a median sternotomy, should be constructed for palliation of ductus-dependent univentricular physiology. This can easily be replaced with a bidirectional Glenn shunt at 6 months of life. In non-ductus-dependent univentricular physiology, the infant can be managed medically until primary construction of a bidirectional cavopulmonary anastomosis becomes feasible. This is possible in the majority of cases because the physiologically elevated pulmonary vascular resistance prevents pulmonary overcirculation during the neonatal period.

Occasionally, if a previous B-T shunt was performed, arterioplasty of the right pulmonary artery may be required to ensure adequate size and unobstructed bilateral flow.[2] The bidirectional Glenn shunt effectively avoids recirculation of both systemic and pulmonary venous return, thus preventing volume overload of the single ventricle and its attendant sequelae.[89] Pulmonary artery banding is necessary in 10 to 15% of patients with markedly increased pulmonary blood flow and florid congestive heart failure.

The Fontan is usually performed when the child is between 2 and 4 years of age, and it is generally successful if the infant was staged properly, with a protected single ventricle, and there is adequate PA growth. The pulmonary vascular resistance should be below

4 Woods Units, and the ejection fraction should be more than 45% to ensure success.[92] In patients with high pulmonary artery pressure, fenestration of the atrial baffle may be helpful because their PVR may preclude adequate flow postoperatively.[88,93]

Results

Recent reports of the Fontan procedure for tricuspid atresia have been encouraging, with an overall survival of 79% and an operative mortality of 2%.[94] The main complications are atrial arrhythmias, particularly atrial flutter; conduit obstruction requiring reoperation; protein-losing enteropathy; and decreased exercise tolerance.

Hypoplastic Left-Heart Syndrome

HLHS comprises a wide spectrum of cardiac malformations, including hypoplasia or atresia of the aortic and mitral valves and hypoplasia of the left ventricle and ascending aorta.[95] HLHS has a reported prevalence of 0.2 per 1000 live births and occurs twice as often in boys as in girls. Left untreated, HLHS is invariably fatal and is responsible for 25% of early cardiac deaths in neonates.[96] However, the recent evolution of palliative surgical procedures has dramatically improved the outlook for patients with HLHS, and an improved understanding of anatomic and physiologic alterations have spurred advances in parallel arenas such as intrauterine diagnosis and fetal intervention, echocardiographic imaging, and neonatal critical care.

Anatomy

As implied by its name, HLHS involves varying degrees of underdevelopment of left-sided structures, including the left ventricle and the aortic and mitral valves. Thus, HLHS can be classified into four anatomic subtypes based on the valvular morphology: (1) aortic and mitral stenosis; (2) aortic and mitral atresia; (3) aortic atresia and mitral stenosis; and (4) aortic stenosis and mitral atresia. Aortic atresia tends to be associated with more-severe degrees of hypoplasia of the ascending aorta than does aortic stenosis.

Even in cases without frank aortic atresia, however, the aortic arch is generally hypoplastic and, in severe cases, may even be interrupted. There is an associated coarctation shelf in 80% of patients with HLHS, and the ductus itself is usually quite large, as is the main pulmonary artery.[7] The segmental pulmonary arteries, however, are small, secondary to reduced intrauterine pulmonary blood flow, which is itself a consequence of the left-sided outflow obstruction. The left atrial cavity is generally smaller than normal, and is accentuated because of the leftward displacement of the septum primum. There is almost always an interatrial communication via the foramen ovale, which can be large, but more commonly restricts right-to-left flow. In rare cases, there is no atrial-level communication, which can be lethal for there infants since there is no way for pulmonary venous return to cross over to the right ventricle.

Associated defects can occur with HLHS, and many of them have importance with respect to operative repair. For example, if a ventricular septal defect is present, the left ventricle can retain its normal size during development even in the presence of mitral atresia. This is because a right-to-left shunt through the defect impels growth of the left ventricle.[97] This introduces the feasibility of biventricular repair for this subset of patients.

Although HLHS undoubtedly results from a complex interplay of developmental errors in the early stages of cardiogenesis, many investigators have hypothesized that the altered blood flow is responsible for the structural underdevelopment that characterizes HLHS. In other words, if the stimulus for normal development of the ascending aorta from the primordial aortic sac is high-pressure systemic blood flow from the left ventricle through the aortic valve, then an atretic or stenotic aortic valve, which impedes flow and leads to only low-pressure diastolic retrograde flow via the ductus, will change the developmental signals and result in hypoplasia of the downstream structures. Normal growth and development of the left ventricle and mitral valve can be secondarily affected, resulting in hypoplasia or atresia of these structures.[95]

Pathophysiology and Diagnosis

In HLHS, pulmonary venous blood enters the left atrium, but atrial systole cannot propel blood across the stenotic or atretic mitral valve into the left ventricle. Thus, the blood is shunted across the foramen ovale into the right atrium, where it contributes to volume loading of the right ventricle. The end result is pulmonary venous hypertension from outflow obstruction at the level of the left atrium, as well as pulmonary overcirculation and right ventricular failure. As the pulmonary vascular resistance falls postnatally, the condition is exacerbated because right ventricular output is preferentially directed away from the systemic circulation, resulting in profound underperfusion of the coronary arteries and the vital organs. Closure of the ductus is incompatible with life in these neonates.

Neonates with severe HLHS receive all pulmonary, systemic, and coronary blood flow from the right ventricle. Generally, a child with HLHS will present with respiratory distress within the first day of life, and mild cyanosis may be noted. These infants must be rapidly triaged to a tertiary center, and echocardiography should be performed to confirm the diagnosis. Prostaglandin E_1 must be administered to maintain ductal patency, and the ventilatory settings adjusted to avoid excessive oxygenation and increase carbon dioxide tension. These maneuvers will maintain pulmonary vascular resistance and promote improved systemic perfusion.[2,7,95] Cardiac catheterization should generally be avoided because it is not usually helpful and might result in injury to the ductus and compromised renal function secondary to the osmotic dye load.

Treatment

In 1983, Norwood and colleagues described a two-stage palliative surgical procedure for relief of HLHS[98] that was later modified to the currently used three-stage method of palliation.[99] Stage 1 palliation, also known as the modified Norwood procedure, bypasses the left ventricle by creating a single outflow vessel, the neoaorta, which arises from the right ventricle.

The current technique of arch reconstruction involves completion of a connection between the pulmonary root, the native ascending aorta, and a piece of pulmonary homograft used to augment the diminutive native aorta. There are several modifications of this anastomosis, most notably the Damus-Kaye-Stansel (DKS) anastomosis, which involves dividing both the aorta and the pulmonary artery at the sinotubular junction. The proximal aorta is anastomosed to the proximal pulmonary artery creating a "double-barreled" outlet from the heart. This outlet is anastomosed to the distal aorta, which can be augmented with homograft material if there is an associated coarctation. At the completion of arch reconstruction, a 3.5- or 4-mm shunt is placed from the innominate artery to the right pulmonary artery. The interatrial septum is then widely excised, thereby creating a large interatrial communication and preventing pulmonary venous hypertension (Fig. 19-16).

The DKS connection, as described above, might avoid postoperative distortion of the tripartite connection in the neoaorta, and thus decrease the risk of coronary insufficiency.[100] It can be used when

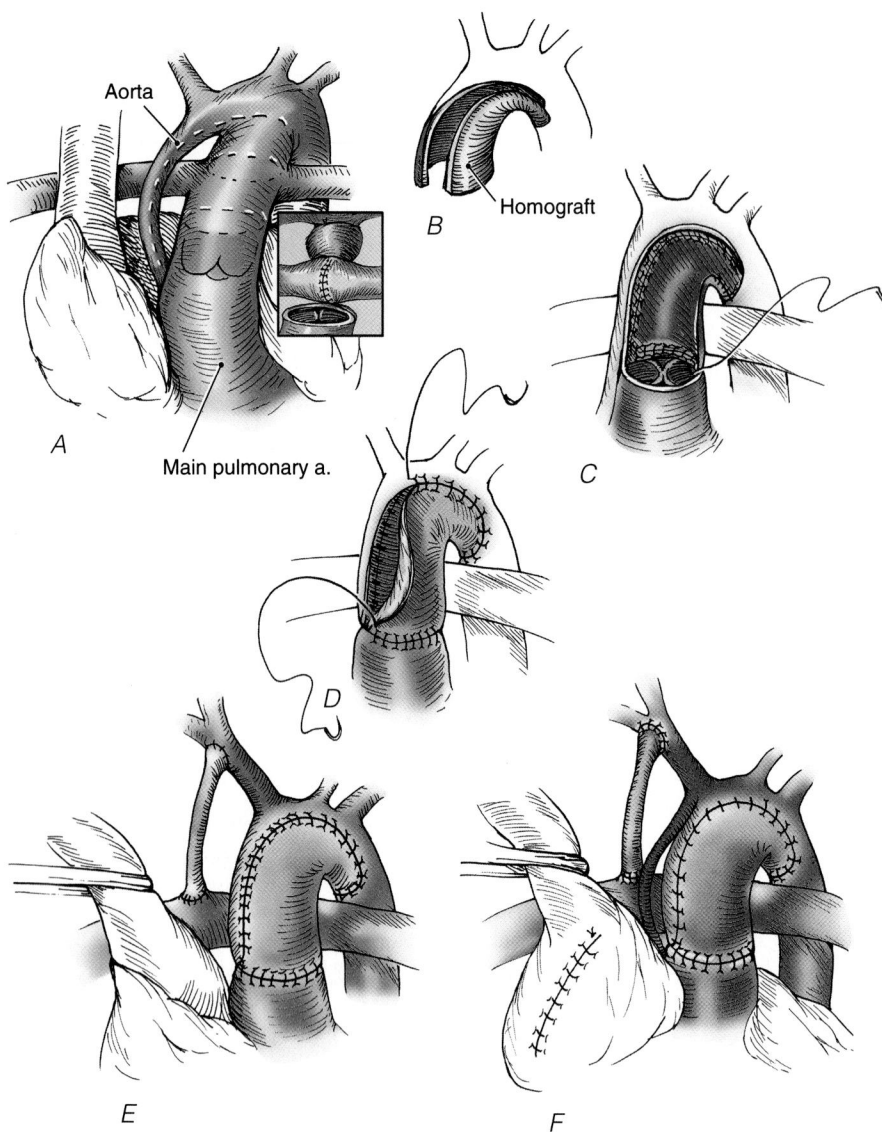

FIG. 19-16. Current techniques for first-stage palliation of the hypoplastic left-heart syndrome. *A*. Incisions used for the procedure, incorporating a cuff of arterial wall allograft. The distal divided main pulmonary artery may be closed by direct suture or with a patch. *B*. Dimensions of the cuff of the arterial wall allograft. *C*. The arterial wall allograft is used to supplement the anastomosis between the proximal divided main pulmonary artery and the ascending aorta, aortic arch, and proximal descending aorta. *D and E*. The procedure is completed by atrial septectomy and a 3- to 5-mm modified right Blalock shunt. *F*. When the ascending aorta is particularly small, an alternative procedure involves placement of a complete tube of arterial allograft. The tiny ascending aorta may be left in situ, as indicated, or implanted into the side of the neoaorta. (*Reproduced with permission from Castaneda et al,*[7] *p 371.*)

the aorta is 4 mm or larger. Unfortunately, in many infants with HLHS; especially if there is aortic atresia; the aorta is diminutive and often less than 2 mm in diameter.

The postoperative management of infants following stage 1 palliation is complex because favorable outcomes depend on establishing a delicate balance between pulmonary and systemic perfusion. Recent literature suggests that these infants require adequate postoperative cardiac output in order to supply *both* the pulmonary and the systemic circulations and that the use of oximetric catheters to monitor SvO_2 aids clinicians in both the selection of inotropic agents and in ventilatory management.[101] Recent introduction of a modification that includes arch reconstruction and placement of the shunt between the right ventricle and the pulmonary artery diminishes the diastolic flow created by the classical aortopulmonary shunt and may augment coronary perfusion, resulting in improved postoperative cardiac function.

Following stage 1 palliation, the second surgical procedure is the creation of a bidirectional cavopulmonary shunt, generally at 3 to 6 months of life when the pulmonary vascular resistance has decreased to normal levels. This is the first step in separating the pulmonary and systemic circulations, and it decreases the volume load on the

single ventricle. The existing innominate artery-to-pulmonary shunt (or RV-pulmonary shunt) is eliminated during the same operation (Fig. 19-17).

The third stage of surgical palliation, known as the modified Fontan procedure, completes the separation of the systemic and pulmonary circulations and is performed between 18 months and 3 years of age, or when the patient experiences increased cyanosis (i.e., has outgrown the capacity to perfuse the systemic circulation with adequately oxygenated blood). This has traditionally required a lateral tunnel within the right atrium to direct blood from the inferior vena cava to the pulmonary artery, allowing further relief of the volume load on the right ventricle, and providing increased pulmonary blood flow to alleviate cyanosis. More recently, many favor using an extracardiac conduit (e.g., 20-mm tube graft) to connect the inferior vena cava to the pulmonary artery.

Not all patients with HLHS require this three-stage palliative repair. Some infants afflicted with a milder form of HLHS, recently described as hypoplastic left-heart complex (HLHC), have aortic or mitral hypoplasia without intrinsic valve stenosis and antegrade flow in the ascending aorta. In this group, a two-ventricle repair can be achieved with reasonable outcome. Tchervenkov recently

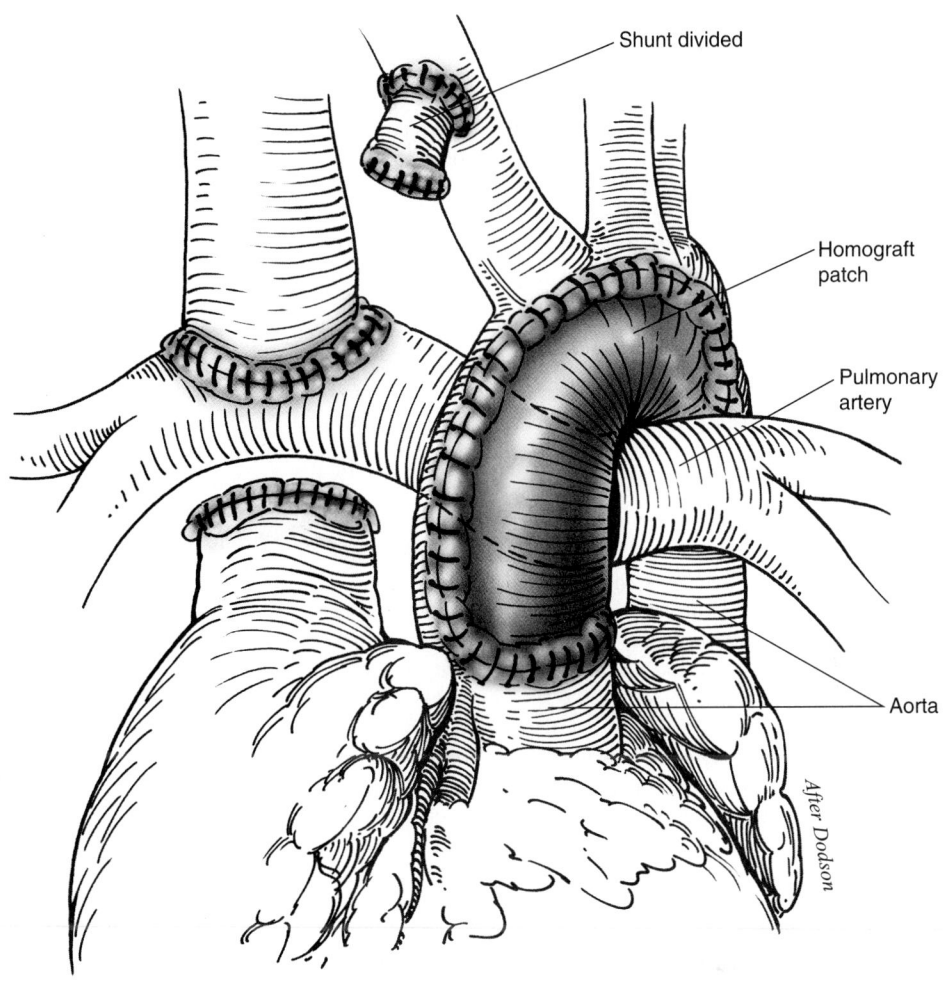

Shunt divided

Homograft
patch

Pulmonary
artery

Aorta

After Dodson

FIG. 19-17. Technique of a bidirectional Glenn shunt. The divided right superior vena cava has been anastomosed at the previous site of the distal anastomosis of the modified right Blalock shunt. The cardiac end of the divided superior vena cava may also be anastomosed to the right pulmonary artery, with the internal orifice being closed with a Gore-Tex patch. (*Reproduced with permission from Castaneda et al,[7] p 376.)*

published the results with 12 patients with HLHC who underwent biventricular repair at a mean age of 7 days.[102] The operative technique consisted of a pulmonary homograft patch aortoplasty of the aortic arch and ascending aorta and closure of the interatrial and interventricular communications.[102] The left heart was capable of sustaining systemic perfusion in 92% of patients, and early mortality was 15.4%. Four patients required reoperations to relieve left ventricular outflow tract obstruction, most commonly between 12 and 39 months following repair.

Transplantation can be used as a first-line therapy or when anatomic or physiologic considerations exist that preclude a favorable outcome with palliative repair. Significant tricuspid regurgitation, intractable pulmonary artery hypertension, or progressive right ventricular failure, are cases where cardiac replacement may be advantageous. The local probability of organ availability should be considered prior to electing transplantation, as 24% of infants died awaiting transplantation in the largest series to date.[103]

Results

Outcomes for HLHS are still significantly worse than those for other complex cardiac defects. However, with improvements in perioperative care and modifications in surgical technique, the survival following the Norwood procedure now exceeds 80% in experienced centers.[95,100,102,104] The outcome for low-birth-weight infants has improved, but low weight still remains a major predictor of adverse survival, especially when accompanied by additional cardiac

defects, such as systemic outflow obstruction, or extracardiac anomalies.[104]

DEFECTS THAT MAY BE PALLIATED OR REPAIRED

Ebstein's Anomaly

Anatomy

This is a rare defect, occurring in less than 1% of congenital heart disease patients. The predominant maldevelopment in this lesion is the inferior displacement of the tricuspid valve into the right ventricle. The anterior leaflet is usually attached in its normal position to the annulus, but the septal and posterior leaflets are displaced toward the ventricle. This effectively divides the RV into two parts: the inlet portion (atrialized RV) and the outlet portion (true RV). The atrialized RV is usually thin and dilated. Similarly, the tricuspid annulus and the right atrium are extremely dilated, and the tricuspid valve is usually regurgitant with a "sail-like" leaflet. There is commonly an ASD present, which results in a right-to-left shunt at the atrial level.

A Wolff-Parkinson-White syndrome type of accessory pathway with associated pre-excitation is present in 15% of patients.[105]

Pathophysiology

Right ventricular dysfunction occurs in patients with Ebstein's anomaly because of two basic mechanisms: the inflow obstruction at the level of the atrialized ventricle, which produces ineffective RV filling and contractile dysfunction. Inflow obstruction and tricuspid regurgitation, which is exacerbated by progressive annular dilatation, both produce ineffective RV filling. Contractile dysfunction of the right ventricle is a result of a decrease in the number of myocardial fibers, as well as the discordant contraction of the large atrialized portion.

The lack of forward flow at the right ventricular level leads to physiologic pulmonary atresia, and the infant is dependent on ductal patency for survival. All systemic venous return must be directed through an atrial septal defect to the left atrium, where it can be shunted through the ductus for gas exchange. However, the left ventricular function is usually compromised in infants with severe Ebstein's anomaly as well, because the enormous right ventricle and the to-and-fro flow within the atrialized RV prevent adequate intracardiac mixing.

Diagnosis

There is a spectrum of clinical presentation in the infants with Ebstein's anomaly that mirrors the anatomic spectrum of this anomaly. Some infants with less-severe forms may present with a mild degree of cyanosis, whereas the onset of clinical symptoms in patient's surviving childhood is gradual, with the average age of diagnosis in the mid-teens.

However, the infant with severe atrialization and pulmonary stenosis will be both cyanotic and acidotic at birth. The chest radiograph may demonstrate the classic appearance, which consists of a globular heart and a narrow waist, similar to that seen with pericardial effusion. The ECG may show right bundle-branch block and right axis deviation. Wolff-Parkinson-White (WPW) syndrome, as mentioned above, is a common finding in these patients. Echocardiography will confirm the diagnosis, as well as provide critical information including tricuspid valvular function, size of the atrialized portion of the RV, degree of pulmonary stenosis, and the atrial size.[6,105]

Electrophysiology study with radiofrequency ablation is indicated in patients with evidence of WPW syndrome, or in children with a history of supraventricular tachycardia, undefined wide-complex tachycardia, or syncope.

Treatment

Surgery is indicated for symptomatic infants and for older children with arrhythmias, progressive cyanosis, or NYHA class III or IV. However, the operative repair may be different, depending on the patient's age, because older children usually are candidates for a biventricular or one-and-a-half ventricle repair, whereas limited survival has been reported for neonates, except for some preliminary success with a procedure that converts the anatomy to a single ventricle physiology, as described by Starnes and coworkers.[106]

The surgical approach in widespread use today for patients surviving infancy was described by Danielson and colleagues in 1992.[6,105,107] This procedure entails excision of redundant right atrial tissue and patch closure of any associated ASD, plication of the atrialized portion of the ventricle with obliteration of the aneurysmal cavity, posterior tricuspid annuloplasty to narrow the tricuspid annulus, reconstruction of the tricuspid valve if the anterior leaflet is satisfactory, or replacement of the tricuspid valve if necessary.[107] If the tricuspid valve is not amenable to reconstruction, valve replacement should be considered. Care must be taken when performing the posterior annuloplasty, or during the conduct of tricuspid valve replacement, to avoid the conduction system, because

complete heart block can complicate this procedure. In addition, patients who demonstrated preoperative evidence of pre-excitation should undergo electrophysiologic mapping and ablation.

Neonatal Ebstein's anomaly is a separate entity. Results with surgical correction have been poor, and many neonates are not candidates for operative repair as previously described. Surgical options for the symptomatic neonate include palliative procedures, the one-and-a-half ventricle repair, or conversion to single ventricle physiology.[1,7,108] More recently there has been limited success in performing tricuspid valve repair in selected infants with Ebstein's anomaly.

The one-and-a-half ventricle repair was first described by Billingsly and coworkers as an attempt to achieve a more physiologic "pulsatile" pulmonary circulation in those patients with a hypoplastic or dysplastic right ventricle.[109] This is accomplished by diverting the superior vena caval blood directly into the pulmonary arterial system by a bidirectional cavopulmonary shunt while recruiting the right ventricle to propel the inferior vena caval blood directly to the pulmonary arteries via the right ventricular outflow tract. Thus the hemodynamics of the one-and-a-half ventricle repair are characterized by separate systemic and pulmonary circulations in series. The systemic circulation is fully supported by a systemic ventricle, and the pulmonary circulation is supported by both the bidirectional Glenn shunt and the hypoplastic (pulmonary) ventricle. Proponents of this approach report a decreased right atrial pressure and a decrease in IVC hypertension, which is theorized to be responsible for many of the dreaded complications of the Fontan circulation, including protein-losing encephalopathy, hepatic congestion, atrial arrhythmias, and systemic ventricular failure. In addition, the maintenance of pulsatile pulmonary blood flow, as opposed to continuous laminar flow as in the Fontan circulation, may be advantageous to the pulmonary microcirculation, although it has not been proven in any studies thus far.[109,110] Certain criteria, most notably an adequate tricuspid valve Z score, as well as the absence of severe pulmonary hypertension or concomitant defects requiring intricate intracardiac repair, should be satisfied prior to electing the one-and-a-half ventricle approach.[111] Patients who do not fulfill these criteria may be approached with a two-ventricle repair and atrial fenestration, or a Fontan repair.

In the infant with severe Ebstein's anomaly, initial stabilization with prostaglandin to maintain ductal patency, mechanical ventilation, and correction of cyanosis is mandatory. Many of these infants will improve over 1 to 2 weeks a pulmonary vascular resistance falls and they are able to improve antegrade flow into the pulmonary circulation through their abnormal right ventricle and tricuspid valve. When stabilization and medical palliation fails, surgical management remains an option, though its success depends on numerous anatomic factors (e.g., adequacy of the tricuspid valve, right ventricle and pulmonary outflow tract), and surgery for symptomatic neonates with Ebstein's anomaly carries a high risk. Recently, Knott-Craig and associates reported three cases where two-ventricle repair was undertaken by subtotal closure of the ASD, extensive resection of the right atrium, and vertical plication of the atrialized chamber.[112] Five-year follow-up revealed all patients to be asymptomatic and in sinus rhythm without medications.

Results

In the neonatal period, the most common postoperative problem, whether after a simple palliative procedure such as a Blalock-Taussig shunt or following a more extensive procedure such as attempted exclusion of the right ventricle, has been low cardiac output.

Supraventricular tachycardia also has been problematic postoperatively. Complete heart blockage necessitating pacemaker implantation should be uncommon if the techniques described to avoid suturing between the coronary sinus and the tricuspid annulus are used.

There are few published reports of outcomes, owing to the rarity of this defect. However, based on the natural history of this condition, which is remarkably benign for the majority of older patients, the outlook should be excellent for patients who have survived ASD closure, plication, and tricuspid annuloplasty.[7,105,107,112]

Transposition of the Great Arteries

Anatomy

Complete transposition is characterized by connection of the atria to their appropriate ventricles with inappropriate ventriculoarterial connections. Thus, the aorta arises anteriorly from the right ventricle, while the pulmonary artery arises posteriorly from the left ventricle. Van Praagh and coworkers introduced the term *D-transposition of the great arteries* (D-TGA) to describe this defect, while L-TGA describes a form of corrected transposition where there is concomitant atrioventricular discordance.[113,114]

D-TGA requires an obligatory intracardiac mixing of blood, which usually occurs at both the atrial and the ventricular levels or via a patent ductus. Significant coronary anomalies occur frequently in patients with D-TGA.[7] The most common pattern, occurring in 68% of cases, is characterized by the left main coronary artery arising from the leftward coronary sinus, giving rise to the left anterior descending and circumflex arteries. The most common varient is for the circumflex coronary artery to arise as a branch from the right coronary artery instead of from the left coronary artery.

Pathophysiology

D-TGA results in parallel pulmonary and systemic circulations, with patient survival dependent on intracardiac mixing of blood. After birth, both ventricles are relatively noncompliant, and thus, infants initially have higher pulmonary flow owing to the decreased downstream resistance. This causes left atrial enlargement and a left-to-right shunt via the patent foramen ovale.

Postnatally, the left ventricle does not hypertrophy because it is not subjected to systemic afterload. The lack of normal extrauterine left ventricular maturation has important implications for the timing of surgical repair because the LV must be converted to the systemic ventricle early enough to allow adaptation, usually within a few weeks after birth.

Clinical Manifestations and Diagnosis

Infants with D-TGA and an IVS are usually cyanotic at birth, with an arterial P_{O_2} between 25 and 40 mm Hg. If ductal patency is not maintained, deterioration will be rapid with ensuing metabolic acidosis and death. Conversely, those infants with a coexisting VSD may be only mildly hypoxemic and may come to medical attention after 2 to 3 weeks, when the falling PVR leads to symptoms of congestive heart failure.

The ECG will reveal right ventricular hypertrophy, and the chest radiograph will reveal the classic egg-shaped configuration. Definitive diagnosis is made by echocardiography, which reliably demonstrates ventriculoarterial discordance and any associated lesions. Cardiac catheterization is rarely necessary, except in those infants requiring surgery after the neonatal period to assess the suitability of the LV to support the systemic circulation. Limited catherization,

however, is useful for performance of atrial septostomy in those neonates with inadequate intracardiac mixing.

Surgical Repair

Blalock and Hanlon introduced the first operative intervention for D-TGA with the creation of an atrial septectomy to enhance intracardiac mixing.[115] This initial procedure was feasible in the precardiopulmonary bypass era, but carried a high mortality rate. Later, Rashkind and Causo developed a catheter-based balloon septostomy, which largely obviated the need for open septectomy.[38]

These early palliative maneuvers, however, met with limited success, and it was not until the late 1950s, when Senning and Mustard developed the first "atrial repair," that outcomes improved. The Senning operation consisted of rerouting venous flow at the atrial level by incising and realigning the atrial septum over the pulmonary veins and using the right atrial free wall to create a pulmonary venous baffle (Fig. 19-18).[116]

Although the Mustard repair was similar, it made use of either autologous pericardium or synthetic material to create the interatrial baffle.[117] These atrial switch procedures resulted in a physiologic correction, but not an anatomic one, as the systemic circulation is still based on the right ventricle. Still, survival rose to 95% in most centers by using an early balloon septostomy followed by an atrial switch procedure at 3 to 8 months of age.[116,117]

Despite the improved early survival rates, long-term problems, such as superior vena cava or pulmonary venous obstruction, baffle leak, arrhythmias, tricuspid valve regurgitation, and right ventricular failure, prompted the development of the arterial switch procedure

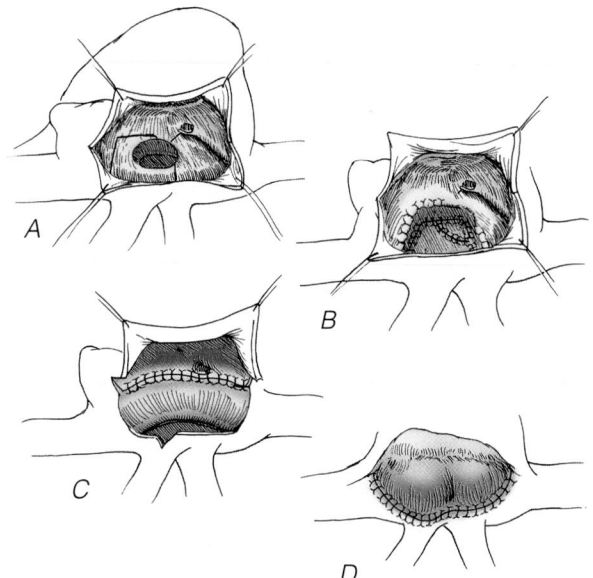

FIG. 19-18. *The Senning operation. A. The atrial septum is cut near the tricuspid valve, creating a flap attached posteriorly between the caval veins. B. The flap of atrial septum is sutured to the anterior lip of the orifices of the left pulmonary veins, effectively separating the pulmonary and systemic venous channels. C. The posterior edge of the right atrial incision is sutured to the remnant of the atrial septum, diverting the systemic venous channel to the mitral valve. D. The anterior edge of the right atrial incision (lengthened by short incisions at each corner) is sutured around the cava above and below to the lateral edge of the left atrial incision, completing the pulmonary channel and diversion of pulmonary venous blood to the tricuspid valve area. [Reproduced with permission from Backer CL, et al: D-Transposition of the great arteries, in Mavroudis C, Backer CL (eds): Pediatric Cardiac Surgery, 2nd ed. St. Louis: Mosby, 1994, p 345.]*

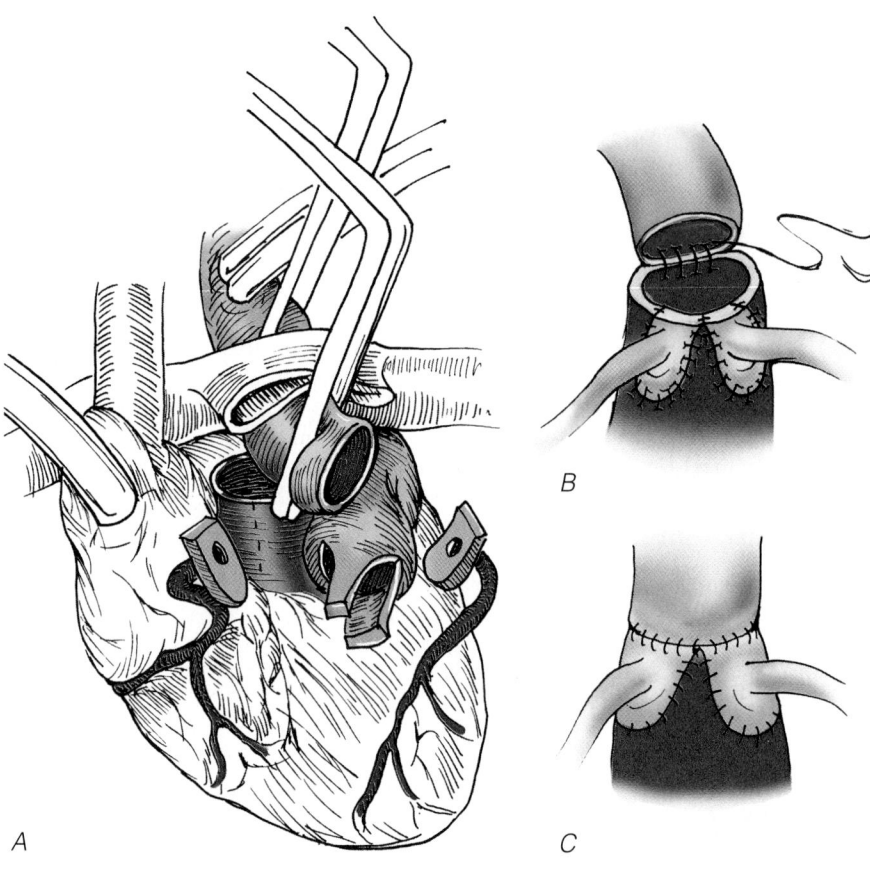

A

B

C

FIG. 19-19. *A.* The maneuver of LeCompte (positioning the pulmonary artery anterior to the aorta) is shown with aortic cross-clamp repositioning to retract the pulmonary artery during the neoaortic reconstruction. *B.* After the coronary patches are rotated for an optimal lie, they are sutured to the linearly incised sinuses of Valsalva at the old pulmonary artery (neoaorta). [Reproduced with permission from Backer CL, Idriss FS, Mavroudis C: Surgical techniques and intraoperative judgments to facilitate the arterial switch operation in transposition with intact ventricular septum, in Mavroudis C, Backer CL (eds): Arterial Switch. Cardiac Surgery: State of the Art Review. Philadelphia: Henley and Belfus, 1991, p 108.]

by Jatene in 1975.[118] The arterial switch procedure involves the division of the aorta and the pulmonary artery, posterior translocation of the aorta (LeCompte maneuver), mobilization of the coronary arteries, placement of a pantaloon-shaped pericardial patch, and proper alignment of the coronary arteries on the neoaorta (Fig. 19-19).

The most important consideration is the timing of surgical repair, because arterial switch should be performed within 2 weeks after birth, before the left ventricle loses its ability to pump against systemic afterload.[2,4,7] In patients presenting later than 2 weeks, the left ventricle can be retrained with preliminary pulmonary artery banding and aortopulmonary shunt followed by definitive repair. Alternatively, the unprepared left ventricle can be supported following arterial switch with a mechanical assist device for a few days while it recovers ability to manage systemic pressures. Echocardiography can be used to assess left ventricular performance and guide operative planning in these circumstances.

The subset of patients who present with D-TGA complicated by left ventricular outflow tract obstruction (LVOTO) and VSD may not be suitable for an arterial switch operation. The Rastelli operation, first performed in 1968, uses placement of an intracardiac baffle to direct left ventricular blood to the aorta and an extracardiac valved conduit to establish continuity between the right ventricle and the pulmonary artery, which has led to successful outcomes in these complex patients.[119]

Results

For patients with D-TGA, IVS, and VSD the arterial switch operation provides excellent long-term results with a mortality rate of less than 5%. Operative risk is increased when unfavorable coronary anatomic configurations are present, or when augmentation

of the aortic arch is required. The most common complication is supravalvular pulmonary stenosis, occurring 10% of the time, which may require reoperation.[4,7,120]

Results of the Rastelli operation have improved substantially, with an early mortality rate of 5% in a recent review.[121] Late mortality rate results were less favorable because conduit failure requiring reoperation, pacemaker insertion, or relief of left ventricular outflow obstruction were frequent.

Double-Outlet Right Ventricle

Anatomy

Double-outlet right ventricle (DORV) accounts for 5% of congenital heart disease and exists when both the aorta and pulmonary artery arise wholly, or in large part, from the right ventricle. DORV encompasses a spectrum of malformations, because the incomplete shift of the aorta toward the left ventricle is often associated with other abnormalities of cardiac development, such as ventricular looping and infundibular-truncal spiraling.[122] The vast majority of hearts exhibiting DORV have a concomitant VSD, which varies in its size and spatial association with the great vessels. The VSD is usually nonrestrictive and represents the only outflow for the left ventricle; its location relative to the great vessels dictates the dominant physiology of DORV, which can be analogous to that of a large isolated VSD, tetralogy of Fallot, or D-TGA. Thus, Lev and colleagues described a classification scheme for DORV based on the "commitment" of the VSD to either or both great arteries.[7,123] The VSD can be subaortic, doubly committed, noncommitted, or subpulmonic.

The subaortic type is the most common (50%) and occurs when the VSD is located directly beneath the aortic annulus. Doubly

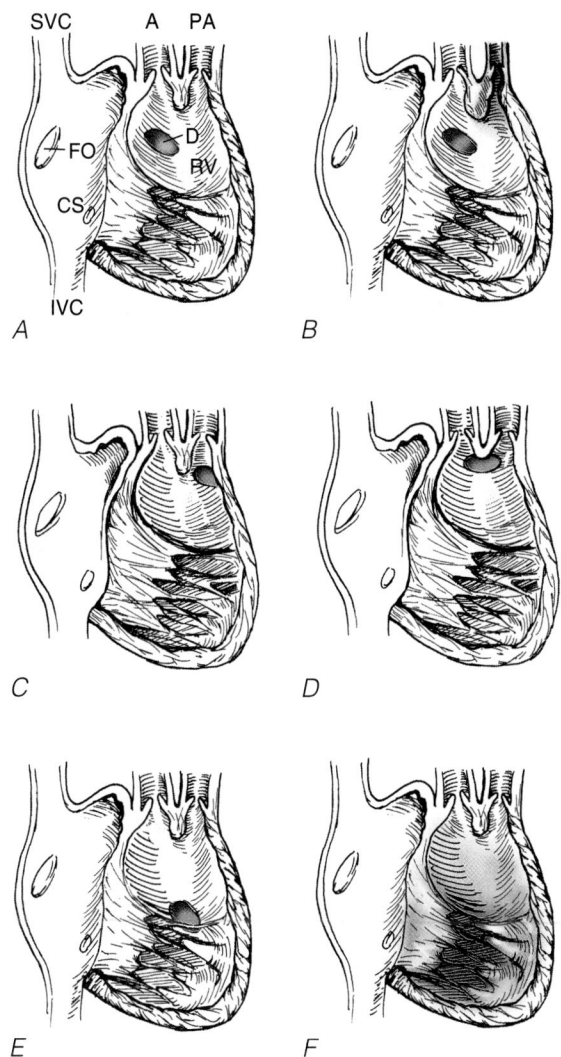

FIG. 19-20. The relationship of the ventricular septal defect (VSD) to the great arteries in double-outlet right ventricle (DORV). *A.* Subaortic VSD without pulmonary stenosis. *B.* Subaortic VSD with pulmonary stenosis. *C.* Subpulmonary VSD (Taussig-Bing malformation). *D.* Doubly committed VSD. *E.* Noncommitted (remote) VSD. *F.* Intact interventricular septum. A = aorta; CS = coronary sinus; D = ventricular septal defect; FO = foramen ovale; IVC = inferior vena cava; PA = pulmonary artery; RV = right ventricle; SVC = superior vena cava. (*Adapted with permission from Zamora R, Moller JH, Edwards JE: Double-outlet right ventricle. Chest 68:672, 1975.*)

committed VSD (10%) is present when the VSD lies beneath both the aorta and the pulmonary artery, which are usually side-by-side in this lesion. The noncommitted VSD (10 to 20%) exists when the VSD is remote from the great vessels. The subset of DORV hearts with the VSD located beneath the pulmonary valve also are classified as the Taussig-Bing syndrome.[124] This occurs in 30% of cases of DORV with VSD, and it occurs when the aorta rotates more anteriorly, with the pulmonary artery rotated more posteriorly (Fig. 19-20).

Clinical Manifestations and Diagnosis

Patients with DORV typically present with one of the following three scenarios: (1) those with doubly committed or subaortic VSD present with congestive heart failure and a high propensity for pulmonary hypertension, much like those infants with a large

single VSD; (2) those with a subaortic VSD and pulmonary stenosis present with cyanosis and hypoxia, much like those infants with tetralogy of Fallot; and (3) those with subpulmonic VSD present with cyanosis much like those with D-TGA, because streaming directs desaturated systemic venous blood to the aorta and oxygenated blood to the pulmonary artery.[122] Thus, the three critical factors influencing the clinical presentation and subsequent management of infants with DORV are the size of the VSD, the presence or absence of important right ventricular outflow tract obstruction, and the presence of other anomalies.

Echocardiography is the mainstay of diagnosis. Cardiac catheterization is rarely necessary, except to determine the degree of pulmonary hypertension and to determine the effects of previous palliative procedures on the pulmonary arterial anatomy.

Therapy

The goals of corrective surgery are to relieve pulmonary stenosis, to provide separate and unobstructed outflow pathways from each ventricle to the correct great vessel, and to achieve separation of the systemic and pulmonary circulations.

Double-Outlet Right Ventricle with Noncommitted VSD. The repair of hearts with DORV and noncommitted VSD can be accomplished by constructing an intraventricular tunnel connecting the VSD to the aorta, closing the pulmonary artery, and placing a valved extracardiac conduit from the right ventricle to the pulmonary artery. In those patients without pulmonary stenosis who have intractable congestive failure, a pulmonary artery band can be placed in the first 6 months to control PA overcirculation and prevent the development of pulmonary hypertension.

Those infants with pulmonary stenosis can be managed with a systemic-to-pulmonary shunt followed by biventricular repair as described by Belli and colleagues in 1999, or with a modified Fontan.[125] There is no consensus on the timing of repair, but recent literature suggests that repair within the first 6 months is associated with better outcome. However, in cases where an extracardiac valved conduit is necessary, it is better to delay definitive repair until the child is 2 to 3 years of age, because this allows placement of a larger conduit and possibly reduces the number of future obligatory conduit replacements.[7,122]

Double-Outlet Right Ventricle with Subaortic or Doubly Committed VSD without Pulmonary Stenosis. This group of patients can be treated by creating an intracardiac baffle that directs blood from the left ventricle into the aorta. Enlargement of the VSD may be necessary to allow ample room for the baffle; this should be done anterosuperiorly to avoid injury to the conduction system that normally lies inferoposteriorly along the border of the VSD. In addition, other important considerations in constructing the LV outflow tunnel include the prominence of the conal septum, the attachments of the tricuspid valve to the conal septum, and the distance between the tricuspid and pulmonary valves. In some instances, unfavorable anatomy may preclude placement of an adequate intracardiac baffle, necessitating single ventricle repair.

Double-Outlet Right Ventricle with Subaortic or Doubly Committed VSD with Pulmonary Stenosis. Repair of this defect is similar to the above except that concomitant RVOT reconstruction must be performed in addition to the intracardiac tunnel. The RVOT augmentation can be accomplished with the placement of a transannular patch or with placement of an extracardiac valved conduit when an anomalous left anterior descending artery precludes use of a patch.

Taussig-Bing Syndrome without Pulmonary Stenosis.
These infants are best treated with a balloon septostomy during the neonatal period to improve mixing, followed by VSD closure (creative transposition) and an arterial switch operation.

Taussig-Bing Syndrome with Pulmonary Stenosis.
This defect may be treated with a variety of techniques, depending on the specific anatomic details and the expertise of the treatment team. A Rastelli-type repair, which involves construction of an intraventricular tunnel through the existing VSD that connects the LV to both great vessels, followed by division of the pulmonary artery at its origin and insertion of a valved conduit from the RV to the distal PA, can be performed.[126]

Results

The results of DORV repairs are generally favorable, with operative mortality approaching zero in most centers. Older age at time of repair is the main risk factor for adverse outcome.

Tetralogy of Fallot

Anatomy

The four features of tetralogy of Fallot (TOF) are (1) malalignment ventricular septal defect, (2) dextroposition of the aorta, (3) right ventricular outflow tract obstruction, and (4) right ventricular hypertrophy. This combination of defects arises as a result of underdevelopment and anteroleftward malalignment of the infundibular septum.

Anomalous coronary artery patterns, related to either origin or distribution, have been described in TOF.[127] However, the most surgically important coronary anomaly occurs when the left anterior descending artery arises as a branch of the right coronary artery. This occurs in approximately 3% of cases of TOF and may preclude placement of a transannular patch, as the left anterior descending coronary artery crosses the RVOT at varying distances from the pulmonary valve annulus.[128]

Coexisting lesions are uncommon in TOF, but the most frequently associated lesions are atrial septal defect, patent ductus arteriosus, complete atrioventricular septal defect, and multiple VSDs.

Pathophysiology and Clinical Presentation

The initial presentation of a child afflicted with TOF depends on the degree of RVOT obstruction. Those children with cyanosis at birth usually have severe pulmonary annular hypoplasia with concomitant hypoplasia of the peripheral pulmonary arteries. Most children, however, present with mild cyanosis at birth, which then progresses as the right ventricular hypertrophy further compromises the RVOT. Cyanosis usually becomes significant within the first 6 to 12 months of life, and the child may develop characteristic "tet" spells, which are periods of extreme hypoxemia. These spells are characterized by decreased pulmonary blood flow and an increase in aortic flow. They can be triggered by any stimulus that decreases systemic vascular resistance, such as fever or vigorous physical activity. Cyanotic spells increase in severity and frequency as the child grows, and older patients with uncorrected TOF may often squat, which increases peripheral vascular resistance and relieves the cyanosis.

Physical examination in the older patient with TOF may demonstrate clubbing, polycythemia, or brain abscesses. Chest radiography will demonstrate a boot-shaped heart, and ECG will show the normal pattern of right ventricular hypertrophy. Echocardiography confirms the diagnosis because it demonstrates the position and nature

of the VSD, defines the character of the RVOT obstruction, and often visualizes the branch pulmonary arteries and the proximal coronary arteries. Cardiac catheterization is rarely necessary and is actually risky in TOF since it can create spasm of the RVOT muscle and result in a hypercyanotic episode (tet spell). Occasionally, aortography is necessary to delineate the coronary artery anatomy.

Treatment

The optimal age and surgical approach of repair of TOF have been debated for several decades. Currently, most centers favor primary elective repair in infancy, as contemporary perioperative techniques have improved outcomes substantially in this population.[4,7,129] In addition, definitive repair protects the heart and other organs from the pathophysiology inherent in the defect, as well as its palliated state.

However, systemic-to-pulmonary shunts, generally a B-T shunt, may still be preferred with an unstable neonate younger than 6 months of age, when an extracardiac conduit is required because of an anomalous left anterior descending coronary artery, or when pulmonary atresia, significant branch pulmonary artery hypoplasia, or severe noncardiac anomalies coexist with TOF.

Traditionally, TOF was repaired through a right ventriculotomy, providing excellent exposure for closure of the VSD and relief of the RVOT obstruction, but concerns that the resultant scar would significantly impair right ventricular function or lead to lethal arrhythmias led to the development of a transatrial approach. Transatrial repair, except in cases when the presence of diffuse RVOT hypoplasia requires insertion of a transannular patch, is now being increasingly advocated by many, although its superiority has not been conclusively demonstrated.[130]

The operative technique involves the use of cardiopulmonary bypass. All existing systemic-to-pulmonary arterial shunts, as well as the ductus arteriosus, are ligated. A right atriotomy is then made, and the anatomy of the VSD and the RVOT are assessed by retracting the tricuspid valve (Fig. 19-21). The outflow tract obstruction is relieved by resecting the offending portion of the infundibular septum as well as any muscle trabeculations. If necessary, a pulmonary valvotomy or, alternatively, a longitudinal incision in the main pulmonary artery can be performed to improve exposure. The diameter of the pulmonary valve annulus is assessed by inserting Hegar dilators across the outflow tract; if the PA/AA diameter is less than 0.5, or the estimated RV/LV pressure is greater than 0.7, a transannular patch is inserted.[21,130] Patch closure of the VSD is then accomplished, taking care when placing sutures along the posteroinferior portion to avoid the conduction system.

Results

Operative mortality for primary repair of TOF in infancy is less than 5% in most series.[4,7,129] Previously reported risk factors such as transannular patch insertion or younger age at time of repair have been eliminated secondary to improved intraoperative and postoperative care.

A major complication of repaired TOF is the development of pulmonary insufficiency, which subjects the RV to the adverse effects of acute and chronic volume overload. This is especially problematic if residual lesions such as a VSD or peripheral pulmonary stenosis exists. When significant deterioration of ventricular function occurs, insertion of a pulmonary valve may be required, although this is rarely necessary in infants.

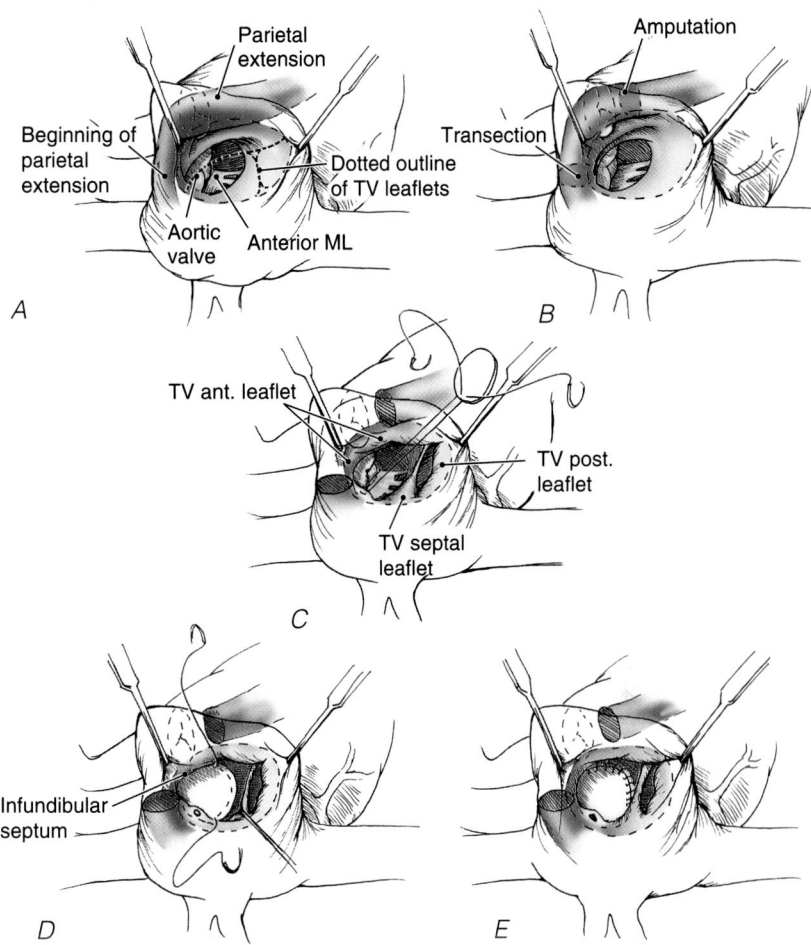

FIG. 19-21. The anatomy from the perspective of the RA approach, shown as if the right atrial free wall and tricuspid valve (TV) were translucent. The free edge of the tricuspid leaflets is shown by dashed lines. A. The difference from the RV perspective is in the apparent position of the parietal extension. From the RA perspective the surgeon looks beneath this, as the parietal extension arches over the right ventricular outflow tract. B. The same perspective without the outline of the tricuspid valve leaflets. The parietal extension is transected at its origin from the infundibular septum, dissected up toward the free wall, and amputated at the free wall. C. A pledgetted mattress suture is placed from the right atrial side through the base of the commissural tissue between septal and tricuspid leaflets and through the patch. D. The suturing is continued onto the parietal extension and infundibular septum, visualizing and staying close to the aortic valve leaflets to avoid leaving a hole between muscular bands. When working from the RA, it is particularly important to stay close to the aortic valve leaflets in the direction of the septum to avoid narrowing the RV outflow tract. E. The repair of the VSD is completed. Note that the suture line is away from the bundle of His and its branches, except where it crosses the right bundle branch anteroinferiorly. (Reproduced with permission from Kirklin JW, Barratt-Boyes BG: Cardiac Surgery, 2nd ed. New York: Churchill Livingstone, 1993, p 863.)

Ventricular Septal Defect

Anatomy

VSD refers to a hole between the left and right ventricles. These defects are common, comprising 20 to 30% of all cases of congenital heart disease, and may occur as an isolated lesion or as part of a more complex malformation.[132] VSDs vary in size from 3 to 4 mm to more than 3 cm, and are classified into four types based on their location in the ventricular septum: perimembranous, atrioventricular canal, outlet or supracristal, and muscular (Fig. 19-22).

Perimembranous VSDs are the most common type requiring surgical intervention, comprising approximately 80% of cases.[132] These defects involve the membranous septum and include the malalignment defects seen in tetralogy of Fallot. In rare instances, the anterior and septal leaflets of the tricuspid valve adhere to the edges of the perimembranous defect, forming a channel between the left ventricle and the right atrium. These defects result in a large left-to-right shunt owing to the large pressure differential between the two chambers.

Atrioventricular canal defects, also known as inlet defects, occur when part or all of the septum of the AV canal is absent. The VSD lies beneath the tricuspid valve and is limited upstream by the tricuspid annulus, without intervening muscle.

The supracristal or outlet VSD results from a defect within the conal septum. Characteristically, these defects are limited upstream by the pulmonary valve and are otherwise surrounded by the muscle of the infundibular septum.

Muscular VSDs are the most common type, and may lie in four locations: anterior, midventricular, posterior, or apical. These are surrounded by muscle, and can occur anywhere along the trabecular portion of the septum. The rare "Swiss-cheese" type of muscular VSD consists of multiple communications between the right and left ventricles, complicating operative repair.

Pathophysiology and Clinical Presentation

The size of the VSD determines the initial pathophysiology of the disease. Large VSDs are classified as nonrestrictive, and are at least equal in diameter to the aortic annulus. These defects allow free flow of blood from the left ventricle to the right ventricle, elevating right ventricular pressures to the same level as systemic pressure. Consequently, the pulmonary-to-systemic flow ratio (Qp:Qs) is inversely dependent on the ratio of pulmonary vascular resistance to systemic vascular resistance. Nonrestrictive VSDs produce a large increase in pulmonary blood flow, and the afflicted infant will present with symptoms of congestive heart failure. However, if untreated, these defects will cause pulmonary hypertension with a corresponding increase in pulmonary vascular resistance. This will lead to a reversal of flow (a right-to-left shunt), which is known as Eisenmenger's syndrome.

Small restrictive VSDs offer significant resistance to the passage of blood across the defect, and therefore right ventricular pressure is either normal or only minimally elevated and Qp:Qs rarely exceeds 1.5.[4,7] These defects are generally asymptomatic because there are few physiologic consequences. However, there is a

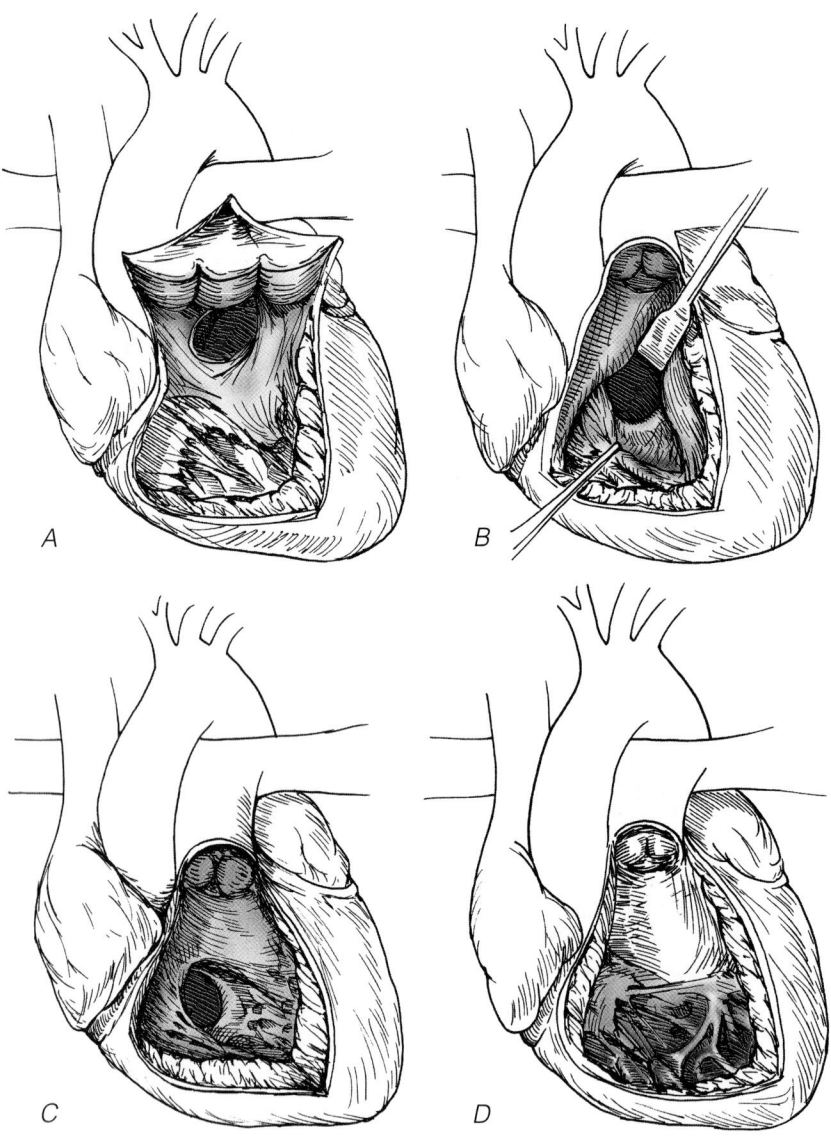

FIG. 19-22. Classic anatomic types of ventricular septal defect (VSD). A. Type I (conal, infundibular, supracristal, subarterial) VSD; (B) type II or perimembranous VSD; (C) type III VSD (AV canal type or inlet septum type); and (D) type IV VSD (single or multiple). [Reproduced with permission from Backer CL, et al: Ventricular septal defect, in Mavroudis C, Backer CL (eds): Pediatric Cardiac Surgery, 2nd ed. St. Louis: Mosby, 1994, p 70.]

long-term risk of endocarditis, because endocardial damage from the jet of blood through the defect may serve as a possible nidus for colonization.

Diagnosis

The child with a large VSD will present with severe congestive heart failure and frequent respiratory tract infections. Those children with Eisenmenger's syndrome may be deceptively asymptomatic until frank cyanosis develops.

The chest radiograph will show cardiomegaly and pulmonary overcirculation and the electrocardiogram will show signs of left ventricular or biventricular hypertrophy. Echocardiography provides definitive diagnosis, and can estimate the degree of shunting as well as pulmonary arterial pressures. Cardiac catheterization has largely been supplanted by echocardiography, except in older children where measurement of pulmonary resistance is necessary prior to recommending closure of the defect.

Treatment

VSDs may close or narrow spontaneously, and the probability of closure is inversely related to the age at which the defect is observed.

Thus, infants at 1 month of age have an 80% incidence of spontaneous closure, whereas a child at 12 months of age has only a 25% chance of closure.[133] This has an important impact on operative decision making, because a small or moderate-size VSD may be observed for a period of time in the absence of symptoms. Large defects and those in severely symptomatic neonates should be repaired during infancy to relieve symptoms and because irreversible changes in pulmonary vascular resistance may develop during the first year of life.

Repair of isolated VSDs requires the use of cardiopulmonary bypass with moderate hypothermia and cardioplegic arrest. The right atrial approach is preferable for most defects, except apical muscular defects, which often require a left ventriculotomy for adequate exposure. Supracristal defects may alternatively be exposed via a longitudinal incision in the pulmonary artery a transverse incision in the right ventricle below the pulmonary valve. Regardless of the type of defect present, a right atrial approach can be used initially to inspect the anatomy, as this may be abandoned should it offer inadequate exposure for repair. After careful inspection of the heart for any associated malformations, a patch repair is employed, taking care to avoid the conduction system (Fig. 19-23). Routine use

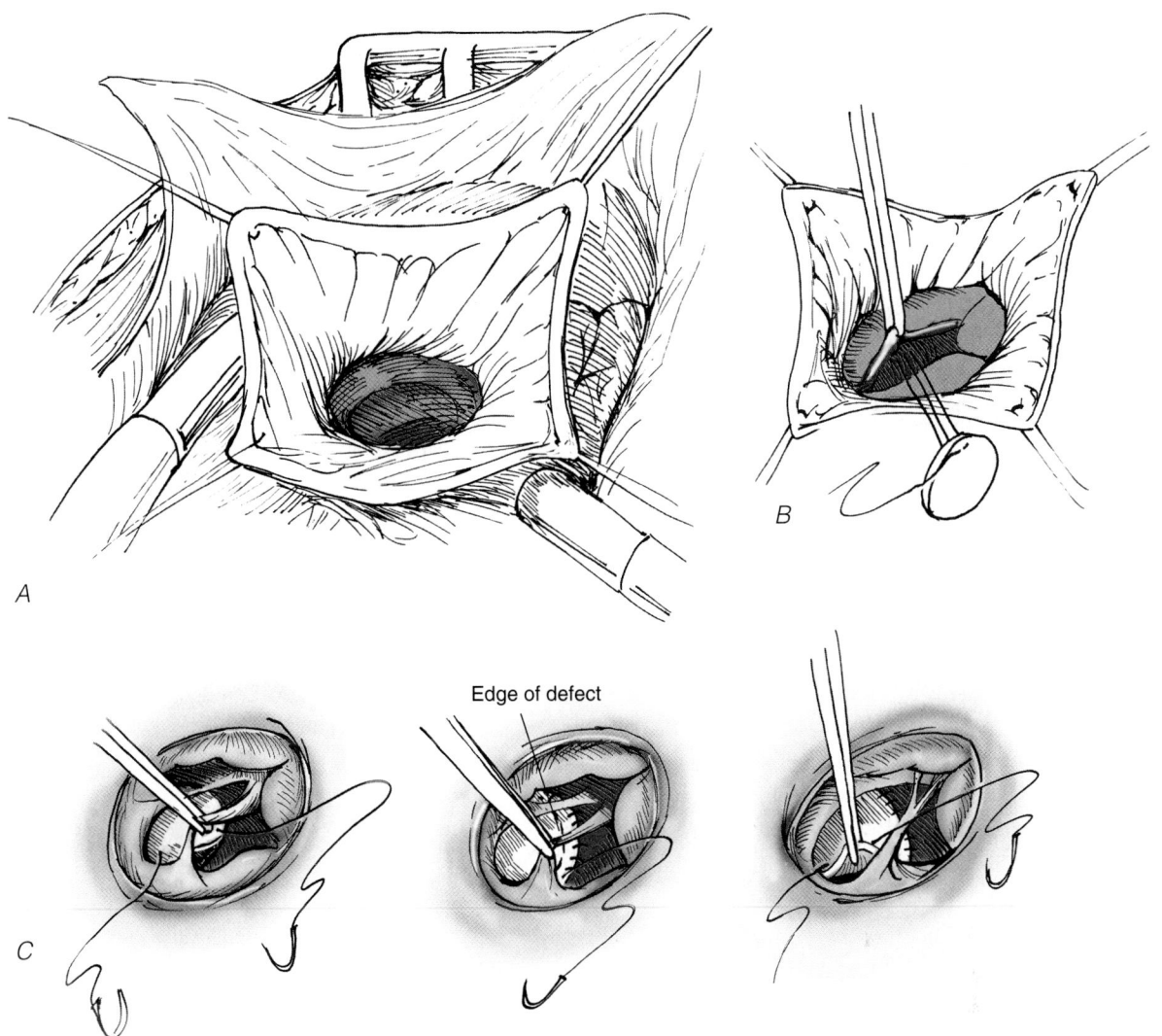

FIG. 19-23. *A.* Right atrial incision and exposure of perimembranous Ventricular sptal defect (VSD) in the region of the tricuspid anteroseptal commissure. Stay sutures have been placed to slightly evert the atrial wall. Note that initially the superior edge of this typical perimembranous defect is not visible. The atrioventricular (AV) node is in the muscular portion of the AV septum, just on the atrial side of the commissure between the tricuspid septal and anterior leaflets. The bundle of His thus penetrates at the posterior angle of the VSD, where it is vulnerable to injury. *B* and *C*. The repair of the perimembranous VSD is completed with use of a slightly oversized Dacron patch, taking care to place stitches 3 to 5 mm away from the edge of the defect itself to avoid injury to the conduction system. [*Reproduced with permission from Walters HL, Pacifico AD, Kirklin JK: Ventricular septal defects, in Sabiston DC, Lyerly HK (eds): Textbook of Surgery: The Biologic Basis of Modern Surgical Practice. Philadelphia: W.B. Saunders, 1997, p 2014.*]

of intraoperative transesophageal echocardiography should be used to assess for any residual defects.

Successful percutaneous device closure of VSDs using the Amplatzer muscular VSD was recently described.[134] The device has demonstrated a 100% closure rate in a small series of patients with isolated or residual VSDs, or as a collaborative treatment strategy for the VSD component in more complex congenital lesions. Proponents of device closure argue that their use can decrease the complexity of surgical repair, avoid reoperation for a small residual lesion, or avoid the need for a ventriculotomy.

Multiple or "Swiss-cheese" VSDs represent a special case, and many cannot be repaired during infancy. In those patients in whom definitive VSD closure cannot be accomplished, temporary placement of a pulmonary artery band can be employed to control

pulmonary flow. This allows time for spontaneous closure of many of the smaller defects, thus simplifying surgical repair.

Some centers, however, have advocated early definitive repair of the Swiss-cheese septum, by using oversize patches, fibrin glue, and combined intraoperative device closure, as well as techniques to complete the repair transatrially.[135] At the UCSF, 69% of patients with multiple VSDs underwent single-stage correction, and the repaired group had improved outcome as compared to the palliated group.[135]

Results

Even in very small infants, closure of VSDs can be safely performed with hospital mortality near 0%.[4,7,136] The main risk factor

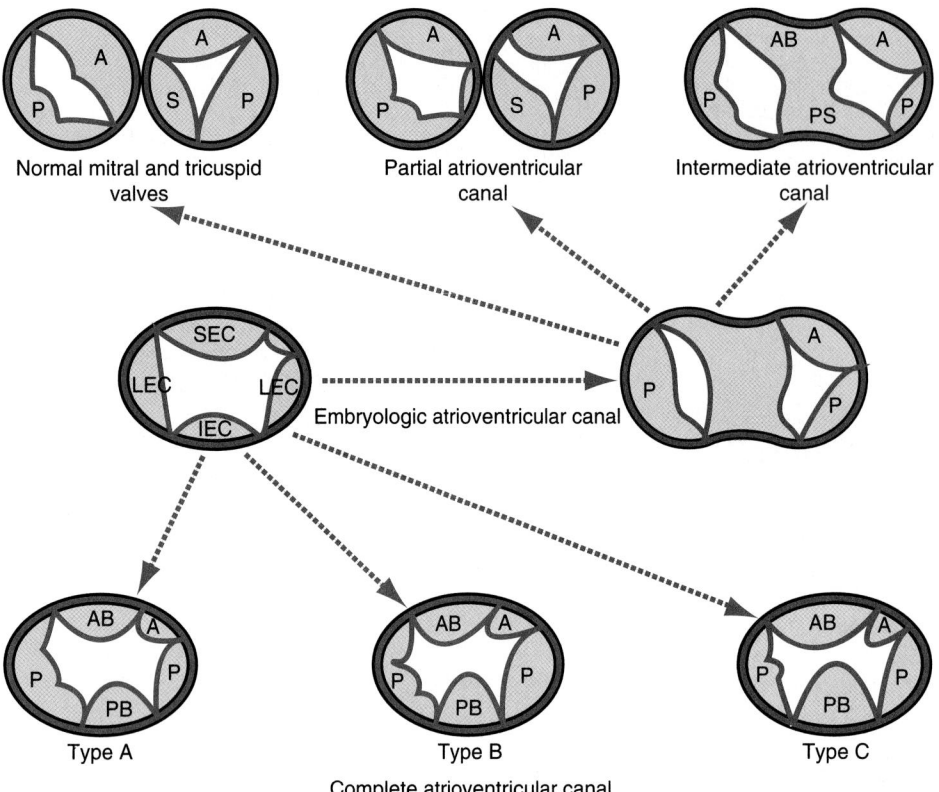

FIG. 19-24. Formation of mitral and tricuspid leaflets and probable embryogenesis of partial, intermediate, and complete forms of atrioventricular canal defects. A = anterior; AB = anterior bridging leaflet; DDCC = dorsodextral conus cushion; IEC = inferior endocardial cushion; LEC = lateral endocardial cushion; P = posterior; PB = posterior bridging leaflet; S = septal; SEC = superior endocardial cushion. [*Reproduced with permission from Feldt RH, Porter CJ, Edwards WD, et al: Defects of the atrial septum and the atrioventricular canal, in Adams FH, Emmanouilides GC (eds): Moss' Heart Disease in Infants, Children, and Adolescents, 4th ed. Baltimore: Williams and Wilkins, 1989*].

remains the presence of other associated lesions, especially when present in symptomatic neonates with large VSDs.

Atrioventricular Canal Defects

Anatomy

AV canal defects result from failure of fusion of the endocardial cushions in the central portion of the heart, causing a lesion that involves the atrial and the ventricular septum, as well as the anterior mitral and septal tricuspid valve leaflets. Defects involving primarily the atrial septum are known as partial AV canal defects and frequently occur in conjunction with a cleft anterior mitral leaflet. Complete AV canal defects have a combined deficiency of the atrial and ventricular septum associated with a common AV orifice rather than separate tricuspid and mitral valves. The common AV valve generally has five leaflets, three lateral (free wall) and two bridging (septal) leaflets. The defect in the ventricular septum can lie either between the two bridging leaflets, or beneath them. The relationship between the septal defect and the anterior bridging leaflet forms the basis of the Rastelli classification for complete AV canal defects (Fig. 19-24).[137]

Pathophysiology and Diagnosis

Partial AV canal defects, in the absence of AV valvular regurgitation, frequently resemble isolated atrial septal defects. Left-to-right shunting predominates as long as pulmonary vascular resistance remains low. However, 40% of patients with partial AV canal defects have moderate-to-severe valve incompetence, and progressive heart failure occurs early in this patient population.[138] Complete AV canal defects produce more severe pathophysiologic changes, because the large intracardiac communication and significant AV valve regurgitation contribute to ventricular volume loading and pulmonary

hypertension. Children with complete AV canal defects develop signs of congestive heart failure within the first few months of life.

Physical examination may reveal a right ventricular heave and a systolic murmur. Children may also present with endocarditis or paradoxical emboli as a result of the intracardiac communication. Chest radiography will be consistent with congestive heart failure, and the electrocardiogram demonstrates right ventricular hypertrophy with a prolonged PR interval.

Two-dimensional echocardiography with color-flow mapping is confirmatory, but cardiac catheterization can be employed to define the status of the pulmonary vasculature, with a pulmonary vascular resistance greater than 12 Woods Units indicating inoperability.[138]

Treatment

The management of patients with AV canal defects can be especially challenging. Timing of operation is individualized. Those patients with partial defects can be electively repaired between 2 and 5 years of age, whereas complete AV canal defects should be repaired within the first year of life to prevent irreversible changes in the pulmonary circulation. Complete repair in infancy should be accomplished, with palliative procedures such as pulmonary artery banding reserved for only those infants with other complex lesions, or who are too ill to tolerate cardiopulmonary bypass.

The operative technique requires the use of either continuous hypothermic cardiopulmonary bypass or, for small infants, deep hypothermic circulatory arrest. The heart is initially approached through an oblique right atriotomy, and the anatomy is carefully observed. In the case of a partial AV canal, the cleft in the mitral valve is repaired with interrupted sutures and the atrial septal defect is closed with a pericardial patch.[139] Complete AV canal defects are repaired by patch closure of the VSD, separating the common

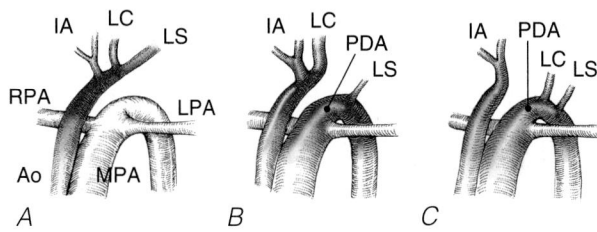

FIG. 19-25. Anatomic types of interrupted aortic arch. *Left,* Type A, interruption distal to the left subclavian artery. *Center,* Type B, interruption between the left subclavian and left carotid arteries. *Right,* Type C, interruption between the left carotid and innominate arteries. AO = aorta; IA = innominate artery; LC = left carotid artery; LPA = left pulmonary artery; LS = left subclavian artery; MPA = main pulmonary artery; PDA = patent ductus arteriosus; RPA = right pulmonary artery. [*Reproduced with permission from Jonas RA: Interrupted aortic arch, in Mavroudis C, Backer CL (eds): Pediatric Cardiac Surgery, 2nd ed. St. Louis, Mosby, 1994, p 184.*]

AV valve into tricuspid and mitral components and suspending the neovalves from the top of the VSD patch, and closing the ASD.

Results

Partial AV canal defects have an excellent outcome, with a mortality rate of 0 to 2% in most series.[138] Complete AV canal defects are associated with a poorer prognosis, with an operative mortality of 3 to 13%.

The most frequently encountered postoperative problems are complete heart block (1 to 2%), right bundle-branch block (22%), arrhythmias (11%), right ventricular outflow tract obstruction (11%), and severe mitral regurgitation (13 to 24%).[138] The increasing use of intraoperative transesophageal echocardiography may positively influence outcomes, as the adequacy of repair can be assessed and treated without need for subsequent reoperation.[138,140]

Interrupted Aortic Arch

Anatomy

Interrupted aortic arch (IAA) is a rare defect, comprising approximately 1% of all cases of congenital heart disease.[7,139] It is defined as an absence of luminal continuity between the ascending and descending aorta, and does not occur as an isolated defect in most cases, because a VSD or PDA is usually present. IAA is classified based on the location of the interruption (Fig. 19-25).

Clinical Manifestations and Diagnosis

Infants with IAA have ductal-dependent systemic blood flow and will develop profound metabolic acidosis and hemodynamic collapse upon ductal closure. In the rare instance of failed ductal closure, the diagnosis may be missed during infancy, and the child will present with symptoms of congestive heart failure from a persistent left-to-right shunt.

Once definitive diagnosis is made in infants, usually with echocardiography, preparations are made for operative intervention, and PGE_1 is infused to maintain ductal patency and correct acidosis. The infant's hemodynamic status should be optimized with mechanical ventilation and inotropic support. An effort should be made to increase pulmonary vascular resistance by decreasing the fractional inspired oxygen and avoiding hyperventilation, because this will preferentially direct blood into the systemic circulation.

Treatment

Initial strategies for the management of IAA involved palliation though a left thoracotomy by using one of the arch vessels as a conduit to restore aortic continuity. Pulmonary artery banding can be simultaneously performed to limit left-to-right shunting, because it is not feasible to repair the VSD or other intracardiac communications with this approach.

However, complete surgical repair in infants with IAA is now preferable. The operative technique involves use of a median sternotomy and cardiopulmonary bypass with short periods of circulatory arrest. Aortic arch reconstruction can be accomplished with either direct anastomosis or patch aortoplasty followed by closure of the VSD.[139]

In certain cases, the defect will involve hypoplasia of the left heart, precluding attempts at definitive repair. These infants should be managed with a Norwood procedure followed by a Fontan repair.

Results

Outcomes in infants with IAA have improved substantially over the last decades as a result of improved perioperative care. Operative mortality is now less than 10% in most series.[139] Some authors advocate the use of patch augmentation of the aorta to ensure adequate relief of LVOT obstruction and to diminish anastomotic tension, thus reducing the subsequent risk of restenosis and tracheobronchial compression.[7,139,141]

References

1. Ohye RG, Edward LB. Advances in congenital heart surgery. *Curr Opin Pediatr* 13:473, 2001.
2. Kouchoukos NT, Blackstone EH, Doty DB, et al: Atrial septal defect and partial anomalous pulmonary venous connection, in Kouchoukos NT, Blackstone EH, Doty DB, et al (eds): *Kirklin/Barrat-Boyes Cardiac Surgery,* 3rd ed. Philadelphia: Churchill Livingstone, 2003, p. 716.
3. Liberthson RR, Boucher CA, Strauss HW, et al: Right ventricular function in adult atrial septal defect. *Am J Cardiol* 47:56, 1981.
4. Mosca RS, Hirsch JC, Bove EL: Congenital heart disease and cardiac tumors, in Greenfield LJ, Mulholland MW, Oldham KT, et al (eds): *Surgery: Scientific Principles and Practice,* 3rd ed. Philadelphia: Lippincott Williams and Wilkins, 2001, p 1443.
5. Ungerleider RM: Atrial septal defects, ostium primum defects, and atrioventricular canals, in Sabiston DC, Lyerly HK (eds): *Surgery. The Biological Basis of Modern Surgical Practice,* 15th ed. Philadelphia: W.B. Saunders, 1997, p 1980.
6. Wenn S, Qayyum SR, Anderson RH, et al: Septation and separation within the outflow tract of the developing heart. *J Anat* 202(4):327, 2003.
7. Castaneda AR, Jonas RA, Mayer JE, et al: *Cardiac Surgery of the Neonate and Infant.* Philadelphia: W.B. Saunders, 1994.
8. Kirklin JW, Pacifico AD, Kirklin JK: The surgical treatment of atrioventricular canal defects, in Arciniegas E (ed): *Pediatric Cardiac Surgery.* Chicago: Yearbook Medical, 1985, 2398.
9. Peterson GE, Brickner ME, Reimold SC: Transesophageal echocardiography: Clinical indications and applications. *Circulation* 107:2398, 2003.
10. Kouchoukos NT, Blackstone EH, Doty DB, et al: Atrial septal defect and partial anomalous pulmonary venous connection, in Kouchoukos NT, Blackstone EH, Doty DB, et al (eds): *Kirklin/Barrat-Boyes Cardiac Surgery,* 3rd ed. Philadelphia: Churchill Livingstone, 2003, p 740.
11. Reddy VM: Cardiac surgery for premature and low birth weight neonates. *Semin Thorac Cardiovasc Surg Pediatr Card Surg Annu* 4:271, 2001.
12. Burke RP: Reducing the trauma of congenital heart surgery. *Semin Thorac Cardiovasc Surg Pediatr Card Surg Annu* 4:216, 2001.

13. Khan JH, McElhinney DB, Reddy M, et al: Repair of secundum atrial septal defect: Limiting the incision without sacrificing exposure. *Ann Thorac Surg* 66:1433, 1998.

14. Luo W, Chang C, Chen S: Ministernotomy versus full sternotomy in congenital heart defects: A prospective randomized study. *Ann Thorac Surg* 71:473, 2001.

15. King TD, Mills NL: Secundum atrial septal defects: Nonoperative closure during cardiac catheterization. *JAMA* 235:2506, 1976.

16. Rigby ML: The era of transcatheter closure of atrial septal defects [editorial]. *Heart* 81:227, 1999.

17. Zeevi B, Keane JF, Castaneda AR, et al: Neonatal critical valvular aortic stenosis. A comparison of surgical and balloon dilatation therapy. *Circulation* 80:831, 1989.

18. Brown JW, Stevens LS, Holly S, et al: Surgical spectrum of aortic stenosis in children: A thirty-year experience with 257 children. *Ann Thorac Surg* 45:393, 1988.

19. Kouchoukos NT, Blackstone EH, Doty DB, et al: Congenital aortic stenosis, in Kouchoukos NT, Blackstone EH, Doty DB, et al (eds): *Kirklin/Barrat-Boyes Cardiac Surgery,* 3rd ed. Philadelphia: Churchill Livingstone, 2003, p 1269.

20. Lupinetti FM, Bove EL: Left ventricular outflow tract obstruction, in Mavroudis C, Backer CL (eds): *Pediatric Cardiac Surgery,* 2nd ed. St. Louis: Mosby, 1994, p 435.

21. Gupta ML, Lantin-Hermoso MR, Rao PS: What's new in pediatric cardiology. *Indian J Pediatr* 70(1):41, 2003.

22. Hammon JW Jr., Lupinetti FM, Maples MD, et al: Predictors of operative mortality in critical aortic stenosis presenting in infancy. *Ann Thorac Surg* 45:537, 1988.

23. Mosca RS, Iannettoni MD, Schwartz SM, et al: Critical aortic stenosis in the neonate: A comparison of balloon valvuloplasty and transventricular dilatation. *J Thorac Cardiovasc Surg* 109:147, 1995.

24. Moore P, Egito E, Mowrey H, et al: Midterm results of balloon dilatation of congenital aortic stenosis: Predictors of success. *J Am Coll Cardiol* 27:1257, 1996.

25. Ross DN: Replacement of aortic and mitral valves with a pulmonary autograft. *Lancet* 57:956, 1967.

26. Jones TK, Lupinetti FM: Comparison of Ross procedures and aortic valve allografts in children. *Ann Thorac Surg* 66:S170, 1998.

27. Marasini M, Zannini L, Ussia GP, et al: Discrete subaortic stenosis: Incidence, morphology, and surgical impact of associated subaortic anomalies. *Ann Thorac Surg* 75:1763, 2003.

28. Somerville J, Stone S, Ross D: Fate of patients with fixed subaortic stenosis after surgical removal. *Br Heart J* 43:629, 1980.

29. Williams JCP, Barratt-Boyes BG, Lowe JB: Supravalvular aortic stenosis. *Circulation* 24:1311, 1961.

30. van Son JM, Danielson GK, Puga FJ, et al: Supravalvular aortic stenosis: Long-term results of surgical treatment. *J Thorac Cardiovasc Surg* 107:103, 1994.

31. Sharma BK, Fujiwara H, Hallman GL, et al: Supravalvular aortic stenosis: A 29-year review of surgical experience. *Ann Thorac Surg* 51:1031, 1991.

32. McElhinney DB, Petrossian E, Tworetzky W, et al: Issues and outcomes in the management of supravalvular aortic stenosis. *Ann Thorac Surg* 69:562, 2000.

33. Clyman RI, Mauray F, Roman C, et al: Circulating PGE$_2$ concentration and patent ductus arteriosus in fetal and neonatal lambs. *J Pediatr* 97:455, 1982.

34. McMurphy DM, Heymann MA, Rudolph AM, et al: Developmental change in constriction of the ductus arteriosus: Response to oxygen and vasoactive substances in the isolated ductus arteriosus of the fetal lamb. *Periatr Res* 6:231, 1972.

35. Mitchell SC, Korones SB, Berendes HW: Congenital heart disease in 56,109 births. Incidence and natural history. *Circulation* 43:323, 1971.

36. Campbell M: Natural history of persistent ductus arteriosus. *Br Heart J* 30:4, 1968.

37. Itabashi K, Ohno T, Nishida H: Indomethacin responsiveness of patent ductus arteriosus and renal abnormalities in preterm infants treated with indomethacin. *J Pediatr* 143:203, 2003.

38. Rashkind WJ, Cuaso CC: Transcatheter closure of patent ductus arteriosus. *Pediatr Cardiol* 1:3, 1979.

39. Moore JW, Schneider DJ, Dimeglio D: The duct-occlud device: Design, clinical results, and future directions. *J Interv Cardiol* 14:231, 2001.

40. Moore P, Egito E, Mowrey H, et al: Midterm results of balloon dilation of congenital aortic stenosis: Predictors of success. *J Am Coll Cardiol* 27:1257, 1996.

41. Mavroudis, C, Backer CL, Gevitz M: Forty-six years of patent ductus arteriosus division at Children's Memorial Hospital of Chicago. Standards for comparison. *Ann Thorac Surg* 220:402, 1994.

42. Elzenga NJ, Gittenberger-de Groot AC, Oppenheimer-Dekker A: Coarctation and other obstructive arch anomalies: Their relationship to the ductus arteriosus. *Int J Cardiol* 13:289, 1986.

43. Locher JP, Kron IL: Coarctation of the aorta, in Mavroudis C, Backer CL (eds): *Pediatric Cardiac Surgery.* St. Louis: Mosby, 1994, p 167.

44. Presbitero P, Demaie D, Villani M, et al: Long-term results (15–30 years) of surgical repair of coarctation. *Br Heart J* 57:462, 1987.

45. Cohen M, Fuster V, Steele PM, et al: Coarctation of the aorta: Long-term follow-up and prediction of outcome after surgical correction. *Circulation* 80:840, 1989.

46. Hornung TS, Benson LN, McLaughlin PR: Interventions for aortic coarctation. *Cardiol Rev* 10:139, 2002.

47. Waldhausen JA, Nahrwold DL: Repair of coarctation of the aorta with a subclavian flap. *J Thorac Cardiovasc Surg* 51:532, 1966.

48. Knyshov GV, Sitar LL, Glagola MD, et al: Aortic aneurysms at the site of the repair of coarctation of the aorta: A review of 48 patients. *Ann Thorac Surg* 61:935, 1996.

49. Bouchart F, Dubar A, Tabley A, et al: Coarctation of the aorta in adults: Surgical results and long-term follow-up. *Ann Thorac Surg* 70:1483, 2000.

50. Bhat MA, Neelakhandran KS, Unnikriahnan M, et al: Fate of hypertension after repair of coarctation of the aorta in adults. *Br J Surg* 88:536, 2001.

51. McCrindle BW, Jones TK, Morrow WR, et al: Acute results of balloon angioplasty of native coarctation versus recurrent aortic obstruction are equivalent. Valvuloplasty and Angioplasty of Congenital Anomalies (VACA) Registry Investigators. *J Am Coll Cardiol* 28:1810, 1996.

52. Hopkins RA, Wallace RB: Truncus arteriosus, in Sabiston DC, Lyerly HK (eds): *Textbook of Surgery: The Biologic Basis of Modern Surgical Practice,* 15th ed. Philadelphia: W.B. Saunders, 1997, p 2052.

53. Collett RW, Edwards JE: Persistent truncus arteriosus: A classification according to anatomic subtypes. *Surg Clin North Am* 29:1245, 1949.

54. Van Praagh R, Van Praagh S: The anatomy of common aorticopulmonary trunk (truncus arteriosus communis) and its embryologic implications: A study of 57 necroscopy cases. *Am J Cardiol* 16:406, 1965.

55. De la Cruz MV, Pio da Rocha J: An ontogenic theory for the explanation of congenital malformations involving the truncus and conus. *Am Heart J* 51:782, 1976.

56. Manner J: Cardiac looping in the chick embryo: A morphologic review with special reference to terminological and biomechanical aspects of the looping process. *Anat Rec* 259:242, 2000.

57. Hutson MR, Kirby ML: Neural crest and cardiovascular development: A 20-year perspective. *Birth Defects Res Part C Embryo Today* 69:2, 2003.

58. Kouchoukos NT, Blackstone EH, Doty DB, et al: Truncus arteriosus, in Kouchoukos NT, Blackstone EH, Doty DB, et al (eds): *Kirklin/Barrat-Boyes Cardiac Surgery,* 3rd ed. Philadelphia: Churchill Livingstone, 2003, p 1201.

59. Mavroudis C, Backer CL: Truncus arteriosus, in Mavroudis C, Backer CL (eds): *Pediatric Cardiac Surgery,* 2nd ed. St. Louis: Mosby, 1994, p 237.

60. Chiu IS, Wu SJ, Chen MR, et al: Anatomic relationship of the coronary orifice and truncal valve in truncus arteriosus and their surgical implication. *J Thorac Cardiovasc Surg* 123:350, 2002.

61. Armer RM, De Oliveira PF, Lurie PR: True truncus arteriosus. Review of 17 cases and report of surgery in 7 patients. *Circulation* 24:878, 1961.

62. McGoon DC, Rastelli GC, Ongley PA: An operation for the correction of truncus arteriosus. *JAMA* 205:69, 1968.

63. Ebert PA: Truncus arteriosus, in Glenn WWL, Baue AE, Geha AS (eds): *Thoracic and Cardiovascular Surgery,* 4th ed. Norwalk: Appleton-Century-Crofts, 1983, p 731.

64. Forbess JM, Shah AS, St Louis JD, et al: Cryopreserved homografts in the pulmonary position: Determinants of durability. *Ann Thorac Surg* 71:54, 2001.

65. Aupecle B, Serraf A, Belli E, et al: Intermediate follow-up of a composite stentless porcine valved conduit of bovine pericardium in the pulmonary circulation. *Ann Thorac Surg* 74:127, 2002.

66. Kouchoukos NT, Blackstone EH, Doty DB, et al: Total anomalous pulmonary venous connection, in Kouchoukos NT, Blackstone EH, Doty DB, et al (eds): *Kirklin/Barrat-Boyes Cardiac Surgery,* 3rd ed. Philadelphia: Churchill Livingstone, 2003, p 758.

67. Darling RC, Rothney WB, Craij JM: Total pulmonary venous drainage into the right side of the heart. *Lab Invest* 6:44, 1957.

68. Delisle G, Ando M, Calder AL, et al: Total anomalous pulmonary venous connection: Report of 93 autopsied cases with emphasis on diagnostic and surgical considerations. *Am Heart J* 91:99, 1976.

69. Michielon G, Di Donato RM, Pasquini L, et al: Total anomalous pulmonary venous connection: Long-term appraisal with evolving technical solutions. *Eur J Cardiothorac Surg* 22:184, 2002.

70. Jonas RA, Smolinsky A, Mayer JE, et al: Obstructed pulmonary venous drainage with total anomalous pulmonary venous connection to the coronary sinus. *Am J Cardiol* 59:431, 1987.

71. Austin EH: Disorders of pulmonary venous return, in Sabiston DC, Lyerly HK (eds): *Textbook of Surgery: The Biological Basis of Modern Surgical Practice,* 15th ed. Philadelphia: W.B. Saunders, 1997, p 2001.

72. Ricci M, Elliott M, Cohen GA, et al: Management of pulmonary venous obstruction after correction of TAPVC: Risk factors for adverse outcome. *Eur J Cardiothorac Surg* 24:28, 2003.

73. Serraf A, Bruniaux J, Lacour-Gayet F, et al: Obstructed total anomalous pulmonary venous return. Toward neutralization of a major risk factor. *J Thorac Cardiovasc Surg* 101:601, 1991.

74. Hyde JAJ, Stumper O, Barth MJ, et al: Total anomalous pulmonary venous connection: Outcome of surgical correction and management of recurrent venous obstruction. *Eur J Cardiothorac Surg* 15:735, 1999.

75. Korbmacher B, Buttgen S, Schulte HD, et al: Long-term results after repair of total anomalous pulmonary venous connection. *Thorac Cardiovasc Surg* 49:101, 2001.

76. Salomone G, Tiraboschi R, Bianchi T, et al: Cor triatriatum: Clinical presentation and operative results. *J Thorac Cardiovasc Surg* 101:1088, 1991.

77. Huang TC, Lee CL, Lin CC, et al: Use of an Inoue balloon dilatation method for treatment of cor triatriatum stenosis in a child. *Catheter Cardiovasc Interv* 57:252, 2002.

78. Cooley DA, McNamara DG, Latson JR: Aorticopulmonary septal defect: Diagnosis and surgical treatment. *Surgery* 42:101, 1957.

79. Ohtake S, Mault JR, Lilly MK, et al: Effect of a systemic-pulmonary artery shunt on myocardial function and perfusion in a piglet model. *Surg Forum* 42:200, 1991.

80. Gaynor JW, Ungerleider RM: Aortopulmonary window, in Mavroudis C, Backer CL (eds): *Pediatric Cardiac Surgery,* 2nd ed. St. Louis: Mosby, 1994, p 250.

81. Scalia D, Russo P, Anderson RH, et al: The surgical anatomy of hearts with no direct communication between the right atrium and the ventricular mass—So-called tricuspid atresia. *J Thorac Cardiovasc Surg* 87:743, 1984.

82. Cheung HC, Lincoln C, Anderson RH, et al: Options for surgical repair in hearts with univentricular atrioventricular connection and subaortic stenosis. *J Thorac Cardiovasc Surg* 100:672, 1990.

83. Trusler GA, Williams WG: Long-term results of shunt procedures for tricuspid atresia. *Ann Thorac Surg* 29:312, 1980.

84. Dick M, Gyler DC, Nadas AS: Tricuspid atresia: Clinical course in 101 patients. *Am J Cardiol* 36:327, 1975.

85. Glenn WWL, Patino JF: Circulatory by-pass of the right heart. Preliminary observations on the direct delivery of vena caval blood into the pulmonary arterial circulation. Azygous vein-pulmonary artery shunt. *Yale J Biol Med* 27:147, 1954.

86. Fontan F, Baudet E: Surgical repair of tricuspid atresia. *Thorax* 26:240, 1971.

87. deLeval MR, Kilner P, Gerwillig M, et al: Total cavopulmonary connection: A logical alternative to atriopulmonary connection for complex Fontan operations. *J Thorac Cardiovasc Surg* 96:682, 1988.

88. Laks H, Haas GS, Pearl JM, et al: The use of an adjustable interatrial communication in patients undergoing the Fontan and definitive heart procedures [abstract]. *Circulation* 78:357, 1988.

89. Haas GS, Hess H, Black M, et al: Extracardiac conduit Fontan procedure: Early and intermediate results. *Eur J Cardiothorac Surg* 17:648, 2000.

90. Tokunaga S, Kado H, Imoto Y, et al: Total cavopulmonary connection with an extracardiac conduit: Experience with 100 patients. *Ann Thorac Surg* 73:76, 2002.

91. Yetman AT, Drummond-Webb J, Fiser WP, et al: The extracardiac Fontan procedure without cardiopulmonary bypass: Technique and intermediate-term results. *Ann Thorac Surg* 74:S1416, 2002.

92. Mayer JE, Helgason H, Jonas RA, et al: Extending the limits for modified Fontan operation. *J Thorac Cardiovasc Surg* 92:1021, 1986.

93. Jacobs ML, Norwood WI: Fontan operation: Influence of modifications on morbidity and mortality. *Ann Thorac Surg* 58:945, 1994.

94. Mair DD, Puga FJ, Danielson GK: The Fontan procedure for tricuspid atresia: Early and late results of a 25-year experience with 216 patients. *J Am Coll Cardiol* 37:933, 2001.

95. Bardo DME, Frankel DG, Applegate KE, et al: Hypoplastic left heart syndrome. *Radiographics* 21:706, 2001.

96. Norwood WI: Hypoplastic left heart syndrome. *Ann Thorac Surg* 52:688, 1991.

97. Bronshtein M, Zimmer EZ: Early sonographic diagnosis of fetal small left heart ventricle with a normal proximal outlet tract: A medical dilemma. *Prenat Diagn* 249, 1997.

98. Norwood WI, Lang P, Hansen DD: Physiologic repair of aortic atresia-hypoplastic left heart syndrome. *N Engl J Med* 308:23, 1983.

99. Norwood WI: Hypoplastic left heart syndrome. *Ann Thorac Surg* 52:688, 1991.

100. Tweddell JS, Hoffman GM, Mussatto KA, et al: Improved survival of patients undergoing palliation of hypoplastic left heart syndrome: lessons learned from 115 consecutive patients. *Circulation* 106 (Suppl I):I-82, 2002.

101. Tweddell JS, Hoffan GM, Ghanayem NS, et al: Ventilatory control of pulmonary vascular resistance is not necessary to achieve a balanced circulation in the postoperative Norwood patient. *Circulation* 100 (18 Suppl):I-671, 1999.

102. Tchervenkov CI: Two-ventricle repair for hypoplastic left heart syndrome. *Semin Thorac Cardiovasc Surg Pediatr Card Surg Annu* 4:89, 2001.

103. Bailey LL, Gundry SR, Razzouk AJ, et al: Bless the babies: 115 late survivors of heart transplantation during the first year of life. The Loma Linda University Pediatric Heart Transplant Group. *J Thorac Cardiovas Surg* 105:805, 1993.

104. Gaynor JW, Mahle WT, Cohen MI, et al: Risk factors for mortality after the Norwood procedure. *Eur J Cardiothorac Surg* 22:88, 2002.

105. Matthew ST, Federico GF, Singh BK: Ebstein's anomaly presenting as Wolff-Parkinson-White syndrome in a postpartum patient. *Cardiol Rev* 11:208, 2003.

106. Starnes VA, Pitlick PT, Bernstein D, et al: Ebstein's anomaly appearing in the neonate. *J Thorac Cardiovasc Surg* 101:1082, 1991.

107. Danielson GK, Driscoll DJ, Mair DD, et al: Operative treatment of Ebstein's anomaly. *J Thorac Cardiovasc Surg* 104:1195, 1992.

108. Yetman AT, Freedom RM, McCrindle BW. Outcome in cyanotic neonates with Ebstein's anomaly. *Am J Cardiol* 81:749, 1998.

109. Billingsly AM, Laks H, Boyce SW, et al: Definitive repair in patients with pulmonary atresia and intact ventricular septum. *J Thorac Cardiovasc Surg* 97:746, 1989.

110. Stellin G, Vida VL, Milanesi O, et al: Surgical treatment of complex cardiac anomalies: The "one and one half ventricle repair." *Eur J Cardiothorac Surg* 22:435, 2002.

111. Chowdhury UK, Airan B, Sharma R, et al: One and a half ventricle repair with pulsatile Glenn: Results and guidelines for patient selection. *Ann Thorac Surg* 71:2000, 2001.

112. Knott-Craig CJ, Overholt ED, Ward KE, et al: Neonatal repair of Ebstein's anomaly: Indications, surgical technique, and medium-term follow-up. *Ann Thorac Surg* 69:1505, 2000.

113. Van Praagh R, Van Praagh S, Vlad P: Anatomic subtypes of congenital dextrocardia: Diagnostic and embryologic implications. *Am J Cardiol* 13:510, 1964.

114. Van Praagh R, Van Praagh S: Isolated ventricular inversion: A consideration of the morphogenesis, definition, and diagnosis of nontransposed and transposed great arteries. *Am J Cardiol* 17:395, 1966.

115. Blalock A, Hanlon CR: The surgical treatment of complete transposition of the aorta and the pulmonary artery. *Surg Gynecol Obstet* 90:1, 1950.

116. Senning A: Surgical correction of transposition of the great vessel. *Surgery* 45:966, 1959.

117. Mustard WT, Chute AL, Keith JD: A surgical approach to transposition of the great vessels with extracorporeal circuit. *Surgery* 36:39, 1954.

118. Jatene AD, Fontes VF, Paulista PP, et al: Successful anatomic correction of transposition of the great vessels: A preliminary report. *Arq Bras Cardiol* 28:461, 1975.

119. Rastelli GC: A new approach to the "anatomic" repair of transposition of the great arteries. *Mayo Clin Proc* 44:1, 1969.

120. Culbert EL, Ashburn DA, Cullen-Dean G, et al: Quality of life after repair of transposition of the great arteries. *Circulation* 108:857, 2003.

121. Dearani JA, Danielson GK, Puga FJ, et al: Late results of the Rastelli operation for transposition of the great arteries. *Semin Thorac Cardiovasc Surg Pediatr Card Surg Annu* 4:3, 2001.

122. Freedom RM, Yoo SJ: Double-outlet right ventricle: Pathology and angiocardiography. *Semin Thorac Cardiovasc Surg Pediatr Card Surg Annu* 3:3, 2000.

123. Lev M, Bharati S, Meng CCL, et al: A concept of double outlet right ventricle. *J Thorac Cardiovasc Surg* 64:271, 1972.

124. Taussig HB, Bing RJ: Complete transposition of the aorta and a levoposition of the pulmonary artery. *Am Heart J* 37:551, 1949.

125. Belli E, Serraf A, Lacour-Gayet F, et al: Double-outlet right ventricle with non-committed ventricular septal defect. *Eur J Cardiothorac Surg* 15:747, 1999.

126. Rastelli GC, McGoon DC, Wallace RB: Anatomic correction of transposition of the great arteries with ventricular septal defect and subpulmonic stenosis. *J Thorac Cardiovasc Surg* 58:545, 1969.

127. Brown JW, Ruzmetov M, Okada Y, et al: Surgical results in patients with double outlet right ventricle: A 20-year experience. *Ann Thorac Surg* 72:1630, 2001.

128. Need LR, Powell AJ, del Nido P, et al: Coronary echocardiography in tetralogy of Fallot: Diagnostic accuracy, resource utilization, and surgical implications over 13 years. *J Am Coll Cardiol* 36:1371, 2000.

129. Mahle WT, McBride MG, Paridon SM: Exercise performance in tetralogy of Fallot: The impact of primary complete repair in infancy. *Pediatr Cardiol* 23:224, 2002.

130. Alexiou C, Chen Q, Galogavrou M, et al: Repair of tetralogy of Fallot in infancy with a transventricular or a transatrial approach. *Eur J Cardiothorac Surg* 22:174, 2002.

131. Walsh EP, Rockenmacher S, Keane JF, et al: Late results in patients with tetralogy of Fallot repaired during infancy. *Circulation* 77:1062, 1988.

132. Kouchoukos NT, Blackstone EH, Doty DB, et al: Ventricular septal defect, in Kouchoukos NT, Blackstone EH, Doty DB, et al (eds): *Kirklin/Barrat-Boyes Cardiac Surgery,* 3rd ed. Philadelphia: Churchill Livingstone, 2003, p 851.

133. Turner SW, Hornung T, Hunter S: Closure of ventricular septal defects: A study of factors influencing spontaneous and surgical closure. *Cardiol Young* 12:357, 2002.

134. Waight DJ, Bacha EA, Khanana M, et al: Catheter therapy of swiss cheese ventricular septal defects using the Amplatzer muscular VSD occluder. *Catheter Cardiovasc Interv* 55:360, 2002.

135. Seddio F, Reddy VM, McElhinney DB, et al: Multiple ventricular septal defects: How and when should they be repaired? *J Thorac Cardiovasc Surg* 117:134, 1999.

136. Tsang VT, Hsia TY, Yates RW, et al: Surgical repair of supposedly multiple defects within the apical part of the muscular ventricular septum. *Ann Thorac Surg* 73:58, 2002.

137. Rastelli G, Kirklin JW, Titus JL: Anatomic observations on complete form of persistent common atrioventricular canal with special reference to atrioventricular valves. *Mayo Clin Proc* 41:296, 1966.

138. Ungerleider RM: Atrial septal defects, ostium primum defects, and atrioventricular canals, in Sabiston DC, Lyerly HK (eds): *Textbook of Surgery: The Biologic Basis of Modern Surgical Practice.* Philadelphia: W.B. Saunders, 1997, p 1993.

139. Kouchoukos NT, Blackstone EH, Doty DB, et al: Coarctation of the aorta and interrupted aortic arch, in Kouchoukos NT, Blackstone EH, Doty DB, et al (eds): *Kirklin/Barrat-Boyes Cardiac Surgery,* 3rd ed. Philadelphia: Churchill Livingstone, 2003, p 1353.

140. Ungerleider RM, Kisslo JA, Greeley WJ, et al: Intraoperative prebypass and postbypass epicardial color flow imaging in the repair of atrioventricular septal defects. *J Thorac Cardiovasc Surg* 98:1146, 1989.

141. Roussin R, Belli E, Lacour-Gayet F, et al: Aortic arch reconstruction with pulmonary autograft patch aortoplasty. *J Thorac Cardiovasc Surg* 123:443, 2002.

CHAPTER 20

Acquired Heart Disease

Aubrey C. Galloway, Ram Sharony, Charles F. Schwartz, Paul C. Saunders,
Eugene A. Grossi, and Stephen B. Colvin

INTRODUCTION

Clinical Evaluation

The importance of the history and physical examination when evaluating a patient with acquired heart disease for potential surgery cannot be overemphasized. It is imperative that the surgeon be well aware of the functional status of the patient and the clinical relevance of each symptom, since operative decisions depend upon the accurate assessment of the significance of a particular pathologic finding. Likewise, with the number of available diagnostic tests rapidly increasing, appropriate sequencing of the diagnostic work-up requires a clinical perspective that is obtained through the history and physical examination. Associated risk factors and coexisting conditions must be identified, as they significantly influence a patient's operative risk for cardiac or noncardiac surgery. Furthermore, the operative strategy is affected by specific physical findings and important history such as previous thoracic surgery, prior saphenous vein stripping, or peripheral vascular disease. The safe surgeon is one who can integrate clinical evidence and diagnostic information to establish a scientifically based operative plan.

Symptoms

The classic symptoms of heart disease are fatigue, angina, dyspnea, edema, cough or hemoptysis, palpitations, and syncope, as outlined by Braunwald. When a patient describes or complains of any of these symptoms, the clinical scenario leading to it must be explored in detail, including symptom intensity, duration, provocation, and conditions that lead to relief. The initial goal is to determine whether a symptom is cardiac or noncardiac in origin, as well as to determine the clinical significance of the complaint. An important feature of cardiac disease is that myocardial function or coronary blood supply that may be adequate at rest may become completely inadequate with exercise or exertion. Thus chest pain or dyspnea that occurs primarily during exertion is frequently cardiac in origin, while symptoms that occur at rest often are not.

In addition to evaluating the patient's primary symptoms, the history should include a family history, past medical history (prior surgery or myocardial infarction [MI], concomitant hypertension, diabetes, and other associated diseases), personal habits (smoking, alcohol or drug use), functional capacity, and a detailed review of systems. After a careful assessment of a patient's symptoms, appropriate diagnostic studies are ordered and interpreted. The classic symptoms are outlined below in detail.

Easy fatigability is a frequent but nonspecific symptom of cardiac disease that can arise from many causes. In some patients, easy fatigability reflects a generalized decrease in cardiac output or low-grade heart failure. The significance of subjective easy fatigability is vague and nonspecific.

Angina pectoris is the hallmark of myocardial ischemia secondary to coronary artery disease, although a variety of other conditions can produce chest pain, and it is up to the clinician to distinguish between chest pain of cardiac and noncardiac origin. Classic angina is precordial pain described as squeezing, heavy, or burning in nature, lasting from 2 to 10 minutes. The pain is usually substernal, often radiating into the left shoulder and arm, but occasionally occurring in the midepigastrium, jaw, right arm, or midscapular region. Angina is usually provoked by exercise, emotion, sexual activity, or eating, and is relieved by rest or nitroglycerin. Angina is present in its classic form in 75% of patients with coronary disease, while atypical symptoms occur in 25% of patients and more frequently in women. A small but significant number of patients have "silent" ischemia, most typically occurring in diabetics. Angina also is a classic symptom of aortic stenosis, occurring secondary to a combination of left ventricular hypertrophy, increased intracardiac pressure, increased ventricular wall tension (leading to higher oxygen requirements), and decreased cardiac output. This combination results in a myocardial oxygen supply-demand mismatch with resultant ischemia and angina.

Noncardiac causes of chest pain that may be confused with angina include gastroesophageal reflux disease or spasm, musculoskeletal pain, peptic ulcer disease, costochondritis (Tietze's syndrome), biliary tract disease, pleuritis, pulmonary embolus, pulmonary hypertension, pericarditis, and aortic dissection.

The physiologic change in most patients with heart failure is a rise in left ventricular end-diastolic pressure, followed by cardiac enlargement. While Starling's law describes the compensatory mechanism of the heart of increased work in response to increased diastolic fiber length, symptoms develop as this compensatory mechanism fails, resulting in a progressive rise in left ventricular end-diastolic pressure. Since this development is eventually damaging to the myocardial muscle and may ultimately result in a dilated cardiomyopathy, ample data suggest that surgery should be considered for many patients prior to the development of dyspnea or heart failure. Nevertheless, exertional dyspnea is often the first sign of left ventricular dysfunction, and when present the patient should be worked up thoroughly for underlying cardiac causes.

Dyspnea appears as an early sign in patients with mitral stenosis due to restriction of flow from the left atrium into the left ventricle. However, with other forms of heart disease dyspnea is a late sign, as it develops only after the left ventricle has failed and the end-diastolic pressure rises significantly. Dyspnea associated with mitral insufficiency, aortic valve disease, or coronary disease represents relatively advanced pathophysiology.

A number of other respiratory symptoms represent different degrees of pulmonary congestion. These include orthopnea, paroxysmal nocturnal dyspnea, cough, hemoptysis, and pulmonary edema. Occasionally dyspnea represents an "angina equivalent," occurring secondary to ischemia-related left ventricular dysfunction. This finding is more common in women and in diabetic patients.

Left-sided heart failure may result in fluid retention and pulmonary congestion, subsequently leading to pulmonary hypertension and progressive right-sided heart failure. A history of exertional dyspnea with associated edema is frequently due to heart failure.

Primary right heart failure may result from right ventricular injury and dysfunction or from primary tricuspid valve disease. Right atrial pressure, normally less than 5 to 8 mm Hg, may be elevated to 15 to 30 mm Hg or higher. Retention of more than 7 to 10 lb of fluid results in visible lower extremity edema, usually bilaterally symmetric. Additionally, jugulovenous distention and hepatomegaly develop with severe right heart failure. In chronic severe heart failure, generalized fluid retention may be quite severe, with marked deformities from accumulation of 20 or more pounds of fluid, accompanied by ascites and massive hepatomegaly.

Palpitations are secondary to rapid, forceful, ectopic, or irregular heartbeats. Palpitations frequently are innocuous, but they should not be ignored, as occasionally they represent significant or potentially life-threatening arrhythmias. The underlying cardiac arrhythmia may range from premature atrial or ventricular contractions to atrial fibrillation, atrial flutter, paroxysmal atrial or junctional tachycardia, or sustained ventricular tachycardia.

Atrial fibrillation is one of the most common causes of palpitations. It is a common arrhythmia in patients with mitral stenosis, and results from left atrial hypertrophy that evolves from sustained elevation in left atrial pressure. With other forms of heart disease, arrhythmias are less common, occurring sporadically. In general, arrhythmias are more frequent in older patients, resulting from intrinsic disease in the atrioventricular conduction mechanism resulting in "sick sinus syndrome" or intermittent heart block. Palpitations caused by a slow heart rate are frequently due to complete or intermittent atrioventricular nodal block.

Severe, life-threatening forms of ventricular tachycardia or ventricular fibrillation may occur in any patient with ischemic disease, either from ongoing ischemia or from prior infarction and myocardial scarring.

Syncope, or sudden loss of consciousness, is usually a result of sudden decreased perfusion of the brain. The differential diagnosis includes: (1) third-degree heart block with bradycardia or asystole, (2) malignant ventricular tachyarrhythmias or ventricular fibrillation, (3) aortic stenosis, (4) hypertrophic cardiomyopathy, (5) carotid artery disease, (6) seizure disorders, and (7) vasovagal reaction. Any episode of syncope must be worked up thoroughly, as many of these conditions can result in sudden death.

Functional Disability and Angina

An important part of the history is the assessment of the patient's overall cardiac functional disability, which is a good approximation of the severity of the patient's underlying disease. The New York Heart Association (NYHA) has developed a classification of patients with heart disease based on symptoms and functional disability (Table 20-1). The NYHA classification has been extremely useful in evaluating a patient's severity of disability, in comparing treatment regimens, and in predicting operative risk.

The NYHA functional classification system is widely used and adequate for the majority of patients. However, when a more precise functional analysis is necessary, the specific activity scale proposed by Goldman and based upon the estimated metabolic cost of various activities is utilized. A different grading system for patients with ischemic disease, developed by the Canadian Cardiovascular Society (CCS), is used to assess the severity of angina (Table 20-2).

Cardiac Risk Assessment in General Surgery Patients

Cardiac risk stratification for patients undergoing noncardiac surgery is an important part of the preoperative evaluation of the

Table 20-1
New York Heart Association Functional Classification

Class I: Patients with cardiac disease but without resulting limitation of physical activity. Ordinary physical activity does not cause undue fatigue, palpitation, dyspnea, or angina pain.

Class II: Patients with cardiac disease resulting in slight limitation of physical activity. They are comfortable at rest. Ordinary physical activity results in fatigue, palpitation, dyspnea, or angina pain.

Class III: Patients with cardiac disease resulting in marked limitation of physical activity. They are comfortable at rest. Less than ordinary physical activity causes fatigue, palpitation, dyspnea, or anginal pain.

Class IV: Patients with cardiac disease resulting in an inability to carry on any physical activity without discomfort. Symptoms of cardiac insufficiency or of the anginal syndrome may be present even at rest. If any physical activity is undertaken, discomfort is increased.

general surgery patient. The joint American College of Cardiology/American Heart Association (ACC/AHA) task force, chaired by Eagle, recently reported guidelines and recommendations, which are summarized here.[1] In general, the preoperative cardiovascular evaluation involves an assessment of clinical markers, the patient's underlying functional capacity, and various surgery-specific risk factors.

The *clinical markers* that predict an increased risk of a cardiac event during noncardiac surgery are divided into three grades. *Major* predictors include unstable coronary syndromes, including acute or recent MI and unstable angina (CCS class III or IV), decompensated heart failure (NYHA class IV), and significant arrhythmias and severe valvular disease. *Intermediate* predictors are mild angina (CCS class I or II), old MI, compensated heart failure (NYHA class II and III), diabetes, and renal insufficiency. *Mild* predictors are advanced age, uncontrolled systemic hypertension, nonsinus rhythm, prior stroke, abnormal electrocardiogram (ECG), and mild functional disability.

Specific *surgical risk factors or procedures* expose the patient to greater or lesser risk of a cardiovascular event. *High-risk* procedures include emergent, major procedures in the elderly; major vascular procedures (e.g., thoracic, abdominal aortic, or peripheral vascular); and long general surgical procedures with anticipated large fluid shifts and/or blood loss (e.g., pancreatectomy, hepatic resection, or abdominoperineal resection). *Intermediate-risk* procedures include any intraperitoneal or intrathoracic operation, carotid endarterectomy, and orthopedic, prostate, and head and neck procedures. *Low-risk* procedures include endoscopic, breast, cataract, and superficial operations.

Table 20-2
Canadian Cardiovascular Society

Class I: Ordinary physical activity, such as walking or climbing stairs, does not cause angina. Angina may occur with strenuous, rapid, or prolonged exertion at work or recreation.

Class II: There is slight limitation of ordinary activity. Angina may occur with walking or climbing stairs rapidly, walking uphill, walking or stair climbing after meals or in the cold, in the wind, or under emotional stress, or walking more than two blocks on the level, or climbing more than one flight of stairs under normal conditions at a normal pace.

Class III: There is marked limitation of ordinary physical activity. Angina may occur after walking one or more blocks on the level or climbing one flight of stairs under normal conditions at a normal pace.

Class IV: There is inability to carry on any physical activity without discomfort; angina may be present at rest.

Based upon the clinical markers, the functional class of the patient, and the proposed surgical procedure, the patient is assigned a high, intermediate, or low cardiac risk, and then managed appropriately. In some patients, further risk stratification is required, such as patients with intermediate cardiac risk factors who are undergoing a high-risk surgical procedure. These patients should undergo exercise stress testing or provocative testing (dipyridamole thallium or dobutamine stress echocardiography) prior to operation. In patients who are considered high cardiac risk due to clinical markers or by virtue of noninvasive testing, coronary angiography may be recommended prior to surgery. Coronary artery disease is then managed according to the classic indications. In patients who are thought to be low or moderate cardiac risk, medical management alone is sufficient.

Due to the common atherosclerotic etiology and the close association between clinically relevant coronary artery disease and peripheral vascular disease, patients undergoing major vascular surgery should be screened closely, either by history or provocative stress testing. Those patients with symptoms suggestive of ischemia, with a decreased ejection fraction due to prior MI, or with provocative stress testing suggestive of ischemia should undergo coronary angiography prior to vascular surgery. Any significant underlying coronary disease should be aggressively treated, either with intensive perioperative management or with coronary revascularization prior to surgery, using standard indications. This aggressive screening approach, followed by appropriate intervention in patients with significant coronary artery disease, has greatly lowered the operative risk of patients undergoing major vascular surgery.

Diagnostic Studies

Electrocardiogram and Chest X-Ray

ECG and the chest x-ray are the two classic diagnostic studies. The electrocardiogram is used to detect rhythm disturbances, heart block, atrial or ventricular hypertrophy, ventricular strain, myocardial ischemia, and MI. The chest x-ray is excellent for determining cardiac enlargement and pulmonary congestion, as well as for assessing associated pulmonary pathology.

Echocardiography

Echocardiography, which has become the most widely used cardiac diagnostic study, incorporates the use of ultrasound and reflected acoustic waves for cardiac imaging. Doppler flow velocity and frequency are assigned colors to help to visually evaluate direction and velocity of intracardiac blood flow. Intracardiac pressures, valvular insufficiency, and transvalvular gradients can be estimated from Doppler measurements. Color Doppler information is often superimposed onto the two-dimensional image, giving a graphic illustration of the directional intracardiac flow pattern and an assessment of valvular insufficiency.

Transthoracic echocardiography has become an excellent noninvasive screening test for evaluating cardiac size and wall motion and for assessing valvular pathology. Corrective operation for valvular disease is now frequently performed on younger patients based on these studies alone.

Transesophageal echocardiography (TEE), which is done by placement of the two-dimensional transducer in a flexible endoscope, improves the image quality by minimizing scatter from the chest wall and is particularly useful in evaluation of the left atrium, the mitral valve, and the aortic arch. TEE studies are used when more precise imaging is required or when the diagnosis is uncertain after the transthoracic study.

Dobutamine stress echocardiography has evolved as an important noninvasive provocative study. This study is used to assess cardiac wall motion in response to inotropic stimulation, as wall motion abnormalities reflect underlying ischemia. Several reports have documented the accuracy of dobutamine stress echocardiography in identifying patients with significant coronary artery disease. The predictive value of a positive test for MI or death after noncardiac surgery is approximately 10%, while 20 to 40% will have some cardiac event. A negative test is 93 to 100% predictive that no cardiac event will occur.

Radionuclide Studies

Currently the most widely used myocardial perfusion screening study is the thallium scan, which uses the nuclide thallium-201. Initial uptake of thallium-201 into myocardial cells is dependent on myocardial perfusion, while delayed uptake depends on myocardial viability. Thus, reversible defects occur in underperfused, ischemic, but viable zones, while fixed defects occur in areas of infarction. Fixed defects on the thallium scan suggest nonviable myocardium and may be of prognostic value.

The exercise thallium test is widely used to identify inducible areas of ischemia and is 95% sensitive in detecting multivessel coronary disease. This is the best overall test to detect myocardial ischemia, but it requires the patient to exercise on the treadmill. The study also gives excellent, specific information about the patient's cardiac functional status.

The dipyridamole thallium study is a provocative study using intravenous dipyridamole, which induces vasodilation and consequently unmasks myocardial ischemia in response to stress. This is the most widely used provocative study for risk stratification for patients who cannot exercise. In patients undergoing noncardiac surgery, the predictive value of a positive dipyridamole thallium study is 5 to 20% for MI or death, while a negative study is 99 to 100% predictive that a cardiac event will not occur. It is therefore a very effective screening study for moderate- to high-risk patients undergoing a general surgery procedure.

Global myocardial function is frequently evaluated by the gated blood pool scan (equilibrium radionuclide angiocardiography) using technetium-99m (^{99m}Tc). This study can detect areas of hypokinesis and measure left ventricular ejection fraction, end-systolic volume, and end-diastolic volume. An exercise-gated blood pool scan is an excellent method to assess a patient's global cardiac response to stress. Normally the ejection fraction will increase with exercise, but with significant coronary artery disease or valvular disease, the ejection fraction may remain unchanged or even decrease. The resting gated blood pool scan determines the degree of prior cardiac injury and assesses baseline cardiac function, whereas the exercise-gated blood pool scan assesses the functional response to stress.

Positron Emission Tomography Scan

The positron emission tomography (PET) scan is a special radionuclide imaging technique used to assess myocardial viability in underperfused areas of the heart. The technique may be more sensitive than the thallium scan for this purpose.[2] The PET scan is based on the myocardial metabolism of glucose or other compounds tagged with positron-emitting isotopes. PET allows the noninvasive functional assessment of perfusion, substrate metabolism, and cardiac innervation in vivo. The PET scan may be most useful in determining whether an area of apparently infarcted myocardium may in fact be hibernating and capable of responding to revascularization. These data can be used to determine whether patients with congestive heart failure might improve with operative revascularization.

Magnetic Resonance Imaging Viability Studies

Magnetic resonance imaging may be used to delineate the transmural extent of MI and to distinguish between reversible and irreversible myocardial ischemic injury.[3,4]

Cardiac Catheterization

The cardiac catheterization study remains an important part of cardiac diagnosis. While complete cardiac catheterization includes the measurement of intracardiac pressures and cardiac output, localization and quantification of intracardiac shunts, determination of internal cardiac anatomy and ventricular wall motion by cineradiography, and determination of coronary anatomy by coronary angiography (Fig. 20-1), most cardiac catheterizations today are more focused studies (e.g., coronary angiography alone), since echocardiography and other noninvasive studies can accurately evaluate valvular pathology and cardiac function.

During cardiac catheterization the cardiac output can be calculated using the Fick oxygen method, where cardiac index (1/min per square meter) = oxygen consumption (mL/min per square meter)/arteriovenous oxygen content difference (mL/min). For determining the arteriovenous oxygen difference, the oxygen content is calculated separately in the arterial and venous circulations by the formula: oxygen content (mL oxygen/L blood) = hemoglobin (g/100 mL) × percent hemoglobin saturation × 1.36 (mL oxygen/g hemoglobin) × 10. Calculation of systemic vascular resistance (SVR) is by the formula: SVR = (mean systemic arterial pressure − mean right atrial pressure) × 80/systemic blood flow (cardiac output). The normal SVR is 1200 dynes·sec·cm^{-5}. The pulmonary vascular resistance (PVR) is calculated by the formula: PVR = (mean pulmonary artery pressure − mean left atrial pressure) × 80/pulmonary blood flow (equal to the cardiac output when no shunt is present). The normal PVR is 70 to 80 dynes·sec·cm^{-5}.

The area of a cardiac valve can be determined from measured cardiac output and intracardiac pressures using Gorlin's formula. This formula relates the valve area to the flow across the valve divided by the square root of the transvalvular pressure gradient. The Gorlin formula indicates that a relatively small transvalvular pressure gradient may actually represent severe valvular stenosis when the patient's cardiac output is low, demonstrating the danger of basing a surgical decision on the transvalvular gradient alone. The significance of valvular stenosis should be based on the calculated valve area (the normal mitral valve area is 4 to 6 cm^2 and the normal aortic valve area is 2.5 to 3.5 cm^2 in adults).

Coronary angiography is currently the primary diagnostic procedure for determining the degree of coronary artery disease (see Fig. 20-1). The left coronary system supplies the major portion of the left ventricular myocardium, through the left main, left anterior descending, and circumflex coronary arteries. The right coronary artery supplies the right ventricle, and the posterior descending artery supplies the inferior wall of the left ventricle. The atrioventricular (AV) nodal artery arises from the right coronary artery in 80 to 85% of patients, termed *right dominant circulation*. In 15 to 20% of cases the circumflex branch of the left coronary system supplies the posterior descending branch and the AV nodal artery, termed *left dominant*, while 5% are codominant.

Computed Tomography Coronary Angiography

Technologic advances in computed tomography (CT) now allow less invasive imaging of the coronary anatomy. Newer rapid CT coronary angiography has been shown to be extremely sensitive in detecting coronary stenoses and comparable to traditional angiography in some recent studies.[3,4]

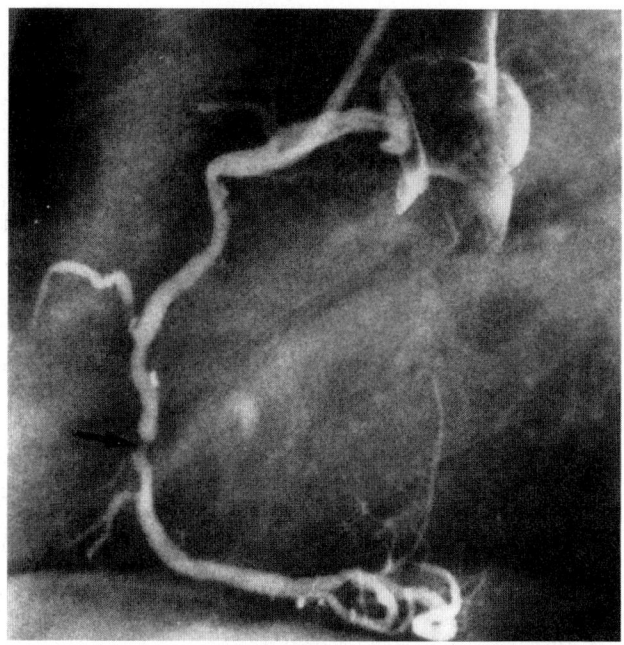

A

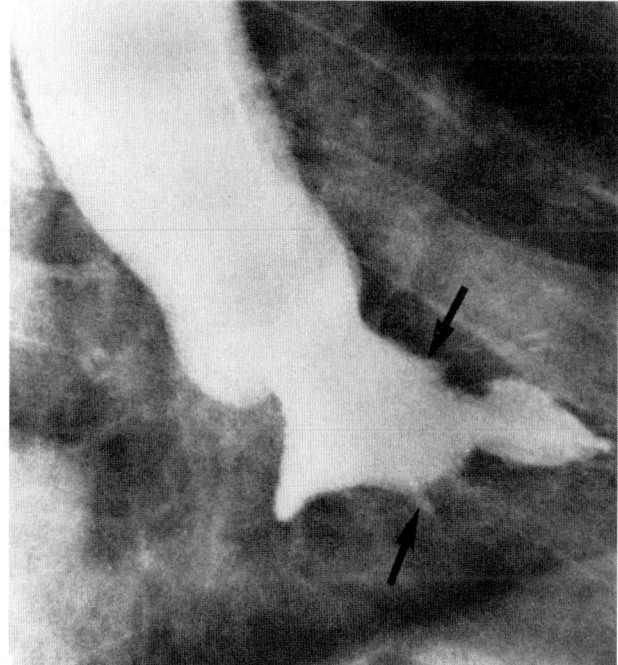

B

FIG. 20-1. *A.* Coronary angiogram demonstrating a severely stenotic atherosclerotic lesion in the right coronary artery. *B.* A systolic left ventriculogram of a patient with a normal ejection fraction.

Extracorporeal Perfusion

The pioneering imagination and efforts of Gibbon were largely responsible for the development of extracorporeal circulation (cardiopulmonary bypass [CPB] with pump-oxygenators). In 1932, Gibbon initiated laboratory investigations that continued for over 20 years, until he performed the first successful open heart operation in a human in 1953. Subsequently bubble oxygenators were developed, utilizing a blood-gas interface, while the membrane

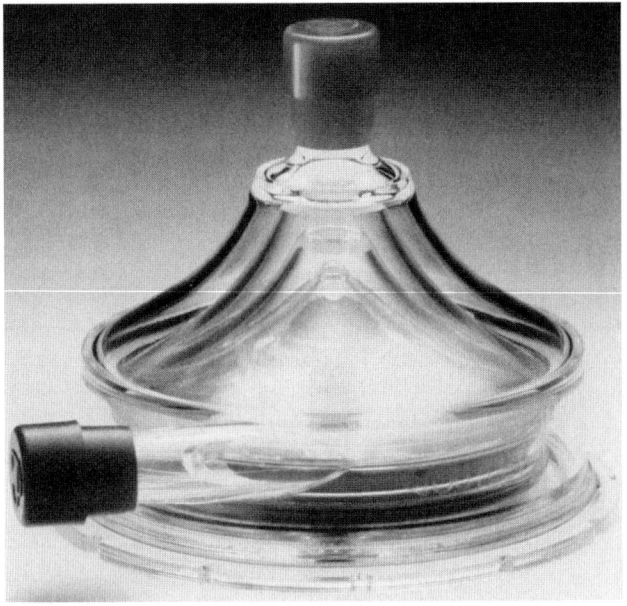

FIG. 20-2. Centrifugal pump (Medtronic Bio-Pump) designed to minimize trauma to the blood cells and platelets. (*Photo courtesy of Medtronic, Inc., Minneapolis, MN.*)

oxygenators that are now widely used utilize a blood-membrane-gas interface for oxygenation and gas exchange.

In addition to the oxygenator, the initial heart-lung machine used a simple roller pump, developed by DeBakey, for perfusion. A variety of other pumps have subsequently been used, such as the centrifugal pump (Fig. 20-2), which minimizes trauma to blood elements. In recent years the focus of perfusion technology has been on the development of perfusion systems that inflict less trauma on the patient's blood. One such advance was the introduction of biocompatible circuits to perfusion technology. This concept involves coating the plastic circuits with biocompatible materials that result in less activation of complement and other inflammatory cytokines during extracorporeal perfusion.

Technique

Sufficient heparin is given to elevate activated clotting time (ACT) above 500 seconds, starting with a heparin dose of 3 to 4 mg/kg. At New York University, a centrifugal pump is used for arterial perfusion, in combination with vacuum-assisted venous drainage and a membrane oxygenator. Venous blood was traditionally drained from the right atrium by gravity through large cannulas, but more recently vacuum-assisted venous drainage has been increasingly utilized, which allows use of smaller-diameter venous drainage cannulas. Systemic flow rates during extracorporeal perfusion depend on the body oxygen consumption requirements of the patient, which can vary based on the patient's body temperature. Normothermic perfusion is done at a flow rate of about 2.5 to 3.5 L/min per square meter, which is the normal cardiac index. Because hypothermia decreases the metabolic rate (approximately 50% for each 7°C), flow rates can be diminished as the patient is cooled. Safe bypass flow rates for 30°C are 1.8 to 2.3 L/min per square meter, for 25°C 1.5 to 1.8 L/min per square meter, and for 20°C 1.2 to 1.5 L/min per square meter. Oxygen flow through the oxygenator is adjusted to produce an arterial oxygen tension above 150 mm Hg. Systemic temperature is controlled with a heat exchanger in the circuit; the temperature is usually lowered to 25 to

32°C, although colder temperatures are occasionally necessary for some complicated procedures. Spilled intrapericardial or intracardiac blood is aspirated with a suction apparatus, filtered, and returned to the oxygenator. A cell-saving device is routinely used to aspirate spilled blood before and after bypass. Aspirated blood is washed and reinfused in order to avoid blood transfusion.

Arterial and venous blood gas parameters are continuously monitored with in-line trending devices, and periodically measured with point-of-care testing. Preferably, the arterial oxygen tension should be above 150 mm Hg, and the carbon dioxide tension 35 to 45 mm Hg. Venous blood returning to the heart-lung machine with the described flow rate will usually have an oxygen saturation greater than 60%. With flow rates and oxygen saturations in this range, metabolic acidosis of a significant degree does not occur. Patients are constantly monitored for signs of underoxygenation. Heparin is gradually metabolized by the body, and so additional heparin should be given as necessary to keep the ACT above 500 to 600 seconds, usually 1 mg/kg of body weight.

Once the operation is completed and the patient is systemically rewarmed to normothermic levels, perfusion is slowed and then stopped. Prior to discontinuing bypass, the surgeon should check several important variables: ECG (for rate, rhythm, and ST-segment changes), potassium level, hematocrit, contractility of the heart, and hemostasis of the suture lines. Both visual inspection and TEE are used to assess myocardial contractility. As the perfusion flow rate is slowed, the patient's blood is returned from the pump to the patient, restoring normal intracardiac pressures. As function is transferred from the perfusion pump back to the patient's native circulation, the patient's blood pressure and cardiac output are monitored closely. Careful observation for arrhythmias and adequate contractility is essential at this phase. Intraoperative TEE is useful in assessing myocardial wall motion and cardiac function. If a Swan-Ganz catheter is in place in the pulmonary artery, the cardiac output is measured and attempts are made to maintain the cardiac index at a normal level. The pulmonary capillary wedge pressure (PCWP) provides a guide to left atrial pressure or preload. The preload should be optimized with fluids. If, however, the cardiac output and blood pressure are inadequate despite an adequate preload, inotropic support is begun. Hypotension from a low peripheral vascular resistance and normal myocardial contractility is treated with vasoconstrictors.

After discontinuing bypass, heparin is neutralized with protamine, which is given to achieve the baseline ACT. If a coagulopathy is present, the ACT may not return to prebypass levels, indicating the need for coagulation products, such as fresh-frozen plasma or platelets. This occurs infrequently in routine cases, but is more common as the complexity of the procedure and the length of CPB increase.

Systemic Response

Significant changes in bodily functions occur during extracorporeal perfusion. These changes mainly involve platelet dysfunction and a generalized systemic inflammatory response syndrome (SIRS), which is apparently due to the activation of complement and other acute phase inflammatory components by extracorporeal circuits. The severity of the inflammatory response and the level of subsequent end-organ dysfunction are related to the length of the pump time, with complement and cytokine activation leading to an upregulation of white blood cell adhesion molecules and the ability of white blood cells to release superoxide. White blood cell upregulation or "priming" produced by extracorporeal circulation results in increased capillary permeability throughout the body, with the "primed" white blood cells placing the patient in a potentially vulnerable state for 24 to 48 hours, during which any secondary insult may result in various levels of multiorgan dysfunction. Other effects may include mental confusion, renal insufficiency, decreased oxygen exchange (pulmonary dysfunction), transient hepatic dysfunction, and hyperamylasemia. Platelet dysfunction may occur due to activation of platelets by artificial surfaces during bypass. Low levels of consumptive coagulopathy and hyperfibrinolysis from plasmin activation may also be present. Current research is focused on minimizing the body's systemic inflammatory response during extracorporeal circulation by coating circuits with biocompatible materials or by blockading specific cytokines. Aprotinin and steroids may attenuate the inflammatory response to bypass, while aprotinin and ε-aminocaproic acid diminish coagulopathy.

Zero-balance ultrafiltration (Z-BUF) is a method of ultrafiltration during CPB. This technique removes significant amounts of inflammatory mediators associated with CPB, and potentially attenuates the adverse effects of bypass while maintaining the patient's volume status. Recent studies have shown that Z-BUF reduces pulmonary edema and protects against lung injury.[5] Additionally, the use of Z-BUF has been shown to decrease the concentrations of interleukin-6 and interleukin-8 that are markers of systemic inflammation associated with CPB.

Myocardial Protection

The development of a myocardial protective solution (cardioplegia) to induce asystolic cardiac arrest and protect the heart muscle during cardiac surgery was a major advance. The primary theory is that when infused through the coronary circulation, cold high-potassium cardioplegic solution produces diastolic arrest, slowing the metabolic rate and protecting the heart from ischemia. The arrested heart allows the surgeon to work precisely on the heart in a bloodless field. With current cardioplegic techniques the heart can be stopped and protected for 2 to 3 hours quite safely, allowing time for complicated procedures to be performed with good recovery of cardiac function.

Both crystalloid and blood cardioplegic solutions are widely used, with the exact composition of the cardioplegic mixture varying among different institutions. With periods of cardiac arrest up to 90 minutes, there is little measurable difference in the two techniques, although blood cardioplegia may allow the heart to be safely arrested for longer periods.

CORONARY ARTERY DISEASE

History

Starting in the late 1930s, different investigators attempted to increase the blood supply to the ischemic heart by developing collateral circulation with vascular adhesions. Beck was the leading investigator, trying different methods for many years, but ultimately all failed. An ingenious concept arose in 1946, when Vineberg developed implantation of the internal mammary artery into a tunnel in the myocardium. This was applied clinically by Vineberg and Miller in 1951 and continued for many years. Interestingly, the artery remained patent in over 90% of patients, but the amount of flow through the artery was small and the procedure was subsequently abandoned. Coronary artery endarterectomy for coronary revascularization was attempted by Longmire in 1956 with short-term success. Late results were poor, however, due to progressive restenosis and occlusion. Shortly thereafter, CPB was utilized to facilitate

coronary revascularization, and Senning reported vein patch graft arterioplasty in 1961.

The development of the coronary artery bypass operation in the 1960s was a dramatic medical milestone. In the United States, the principal credit belongs to Favalaro and Effler from the Cleveland Clinic, who did the first series of coronary bypass grafts beginning in 1967, using CPB and saphenous vein grafts and launching the modern era of coronary bypass surgery. An additional breakthrough came in 1968 when Green and colleagues performed the first left internal mammary artery to left anterior descending artery bypass, using CPB and an operative microscope. Kolessov had independently performed internal mammary artery to left coronary artery bypass grafting on the beating heart in Russia in 1964, although his work was largely unknown for many years. Subsequently, coronary artery bypass surgery became one of the most widely applied surgical procedures in the United States and throughout the world.

Etiology and Pathogenesis

The etiology of coronary artery disease is atherosclerosis. The disease is multifactorial, with the primary risk factors being hyperlipidemia, smoking, diabetes, hypertension, obesity, sedentary lifestyle, and male gender. Newly identified risk factors include elevated levels of C-reactive protein, lipoprotein (a), and homocysteine. The atherosclerotic process results in the formation of obstructive lesions in the aorta, the peripheral vessels, and the coronary arteries. Atherosclerosis is the leading cause of death in the Western world, and acute MI alone accounts for 25% of the deaths in the United States each year. The most important factor in the long-term treatment of coronary disease is the modification of risk factors, including the immediate cessation of smoking, control of hypertension, weight loss, exercise, and reduction of serum cholesterol. If dietary control of cholesterol cannot be achieved in patients with coronary disease, evidence suggests that the use of medications (such as 3-hydroxy-3-methylglutaryl coenzyme A [HMG-CoA] reductase inhibitors) to lower cholesterol can significantly slow disease progression and lower the risk of subsequent cardiac events.

The basic lesion is a segmental plaque within the coronary artery. This segmental localization makes bypass grafts possible. Involvement of small distal vessels is usually less extensive, while arterioles and intramyocardial vessels are usually free of disease. Among the three major coronary arteries, the proximal anterior descending artery is frequently stenosed or occluded, with the distal half of the artery remaining patent. The right coronary artery is often stenotic or occluded throughout its course, but the posterior descending and left atrioventricular groove branches are almost always patent. The circumflex artery is often diseased proximally, but one or more distal marginal branches are usually patent. With progressive disease, platelet aggregation on the narrowed lumen or plaque hemorrhage or rupture may lead to unstable symptoms or to acute thrombosis and MI.

Clinical Manifestations

Myocardial ischemia from coronary artery disease may result in angina pectoris, MI, congestive heart failure, or cardiac arrhythmias and sudden death. Angina is the most frequent symptom, but MI may appear without prior warning. Congestive heart failure usually results as a sequela of MI, with significant muscular injury resulting in ischemic myopathy. Myocardial injury and scarring serve as a nidus for serious ventricular arrhythmias that may result in sudden death.

Angina pectoris, the most common manifestation, manifests by periodic chest discomfort, usually substernal, and typically appearing with exertion. Characteristically these symptoms subside within 3 to 5 minutes and are relieved by sublingual nitroglycerin. In 20 to 25% of patients the pain may be typical and radiate to the jaw, shoulder, or epigastrium. Some patients, especially women or diabetics, have no angina and experience primarily exertional dyspnea. Establishing a diagnosis of myocardial ischemia in these patients is difficult and perhaps impossible without provocative diagnostic studies. The differential diagnosis in patients with atypical symptoms includes aortic stenosis, hypertrophic cardiomyopathy, musculoskeletal disorders, pulmonary disease, gastritis or peptic ulcer disease, gastroesophageal reflux, diffuse esophageal spasm, and anxiety.

Myocardial infarction is the most common serious complication of coronary artery disease, with 900,000 occurring in the United States annually. Modern therapy, which involves early reperfusion with either thrombolytic therapy or emergent angioplasty, has lowered the mortality to less than 5%. MI may result in acute pump failure and cardiogenic shock, or in mechanical rupture of infarcted zones of the heart.

In a certain number of patients who have MI, congestive heart failure eventually develops, resulting from significant loss of left ventricular function. When areas of salvageable myocardium are still present, often manifest as angina associated with the heart failure, significant improvement can be obtained with coronary bypass grafting. In contrast, in patients with late-stage chronic congestive failure due to diffuse myocardial scarring, the outlook is ominous. Bypass grafting may not be beneficial in these patients unless viable myocardium is present with reversible ischemia. Cardiac transplantation or long-term support with a ventricular assist device may the only options in such patients.

Preoperative Evaluation

A complete history and physical examination should be performed in every patient with suspected coronary artery disease, along with a chest x-ray, ECG, and baseline echocardiogram. In patients with atypical symptoms, provocative stress tests, such as adenosine thallium or dobutamine echocardiography, may also be beneficial in deciding if cardiac catheterization is indicated. Cardiac catheterization remains the gold standard of evaluation, as it outlines the location and severity of the coronary disease and accurately assesses cardiac function. "Angiographically significant" coronary stenosis is considered to be present when the diameter is reduced by more than 50%, corresponding to a reduction in cross-sectional area greater than 75%. Furthermore, the number, location, and severity of the coronary stenoses are used to determine the appropriate method of revascularization.

Ventricular function is expressed as the left ventricular ejection fraction, with 0.55 to 0.70 considered as normal, 0.40 to 0.55 as mildly depressed, less than 0.40 as moderately depressed, and below 0.25 as severely depressed. An ejection fraction below 0.25 is usually associated with severe heart failure. The left ventricular ejection fraction is used to determine operative risk and the long-term prognosis. Regional wall motion may also be analyzed, either by cardiac catheterization or echocardiography.

Studies such as the PET scan, thallium scan, dobutamine echocardiogram, or magnetic resonance imaging (MRI) viability scan may be used to determine myocardial viability and the reversibility of ischemia in areas of the heart that might benefit from revascularization. A patient is not "inoperable" simply because the left

ventricular function is severely depressed, if a significant amount of myocardium has reversible ischemia and is thought to be viable but hibernating.

Coronary Artery Bypass Grafting

Indications

Coronary artery bypass grafting (CABG) may be indicated in patients with chronic angina, unstable angina, or postinfarction angina, and in asymptomatic patients or patients with atypical symptoms who have easily provoked ischemia during stress testing.

Chronic Angina. In some patients with chronic angina, CABG is associated with improved survival and improved complication-free survival when compared to medical management. In general, patients with more severe angina (CCS class III or IV symptoms) are most likely to benefit from bypass. For patients with less severe angina (CCS class I or II), other factors, such as the anatomic distribution of disease (left main disease or triple-vessel disease versus single-vessel disease) and the degree of left ventricular dysfunction, are used to determine which patients will most benefit from operative revascularization.

Three historic randomized trials attempted to determine which patients with mild degrees of chronic angina would have improved survival from coronary bypass surgery.

1. The Veterans Administration Cooperative Study. This study involved 668 males with mild to moderate angina, treated between 1972 and 1974, and demonstrated improved long-term survival in patients with left main disease treated with surgical therapy.[6] Largely based on this trial, surgery has been recommended for virtually all patients with significant left main arterial disease. Subsequent studies have shown that patients with left main arterial disease treated with surgery have a median survival of 13.3 years, versus 6.6 years in those treated medically.[7,8]
2. The European Coronary Surgery Study Group. This study, done between 1973 and 1976, randomized male patients with mild to moderate angina into medical or surgical therapy.[9] Surgery was found to be associated with improved survival in patients with triple-vessel disease and in patients with double-vessel disease with proximal left anterior descending and circumflex artery lesions.
3. Coronary Artery Surgery Study (CASS). This multicenter study performed between 1975 and 1979 randomized patients with mild angina (class I or II) into medical or surgical therapy. Late results demonstrated improved survival with surgery in patients with triple-vessel disease and depressed cardiac function.

Other nonrandomized trials and studies involving the overall CASS registry (of both randomized and nonrandomized patients) have suggested that surgical intervention might improve survival and event-free intervals in other patients with triple-vessel disease. A study by Jones and colleagues from Duke University evaluated the long-term benefits of bypass surgery and angioplasty versus medical therapy in 9263 patients with documented coronary artery disease treated between 1984 and 1990.[10] Treatment was nonrandomized, with 2449 patients receiving medical therapy, 3890 patients receiving bypass surgery, and 2924 patients receiving angioplasty. Both the surgery and angioplasty treatment groups had better long-term survival than medical therapy for all levels of disease severity, with surgery having the best survival benefit in patients with triple-vessel disease and in patients with double-vessel disease with proximal left anterior descending artery stenosis.

To summarize, while medical therapy may be appropriate for many patients with chronic stable angina, bypass surgery is indicated for most patients with multivessel disease and CCS class III or IV symptoms. In patients with milder (CCS class I or II) symptoms, surgery results in improved survival in those with left main stenosis and those with triple-vessel disease and depressed left ventricular function or diabetes. Certain other anatomic or physiologic subsets of patients, such as those with multivessel disease and tight proximal left anterior descending stenosis or easily provoked ischemia during stress testing, are also likely to have a survival benefit with surgery.

Unstable Angina. Unstable angina exists when angina is persistent or rapidly progressive despite optimal medical therapy. This occurs from severe ischemia and represents an unstable clinical situation, usually leading to myocardial infarction. It probably represents plaque rupture or hemorrhage, often with local thrombus and spasm, resulting in a sudden decrease in regional blood flow. Patients with unstable angina should be promptly hospitalized for intensive medical therapy and undergo prompt cardiac catheterization. Most patients with unstable angina will require urgent revascularization with either percutaneous coronary intervention (PCI) or coronary bypass grafting.

Acute Myocardial Infarction. CABG generally does not have a primary role in the treatment of uncomplicated acute MI, as PCI or thrombolysis is the preferred method of emergent revascularization in these patients. However, patients with subendocardial MI and underlying left main disease or postinfarction angina and multivessel involvement may require surgery.

The primary indication for surgery after acute transmural MI is in patients who develop late complications, such as postinfarction ventricular septal defect, papillary muscle rupture with mitral insufficiency, or left ventricular rupture. Postinfarction ventricular septal defect (VSD) typically occurs 4 to 5 days after MI, occurring in approximately 1% of patients. These patients usually present with congestive heart failure and pulmonary edema, and a new systolic murmur.[11] Once recognized, patients with postinfarction VSD should have an intra-aortic balloon pump placed and undergo emergent repair. The operative mortality ranges from 10 to 20%.[12] Another mechanical complication of acute MI is papillary muscle rupture with acute mitral insufficiency. These patients also typically present 4 to 5 days postinfarction with heart failure and a new murmur. Prompt valve repair or replacement offers the only meaningful chance for survival. Operative risk is 10 to 20%. The third mechanical complication of myocardial infarction is a left ventricular free wall rupture. These patients present with cardiogenic shock, often with acute tamponade. Emergent surgery has a success rate of approximately 50%.[13,14]

Percutaneous Coronary Intervention Versus Coronary Artery Bypass Grafting

PCI, or angioplasty, was developed by Gruentzig in 1977 and has significantly changed the treatment of patients with coronary artery disease.[15] Over 500,000 PCIs are now performed in the United States each year. The indications for PCI have continually expanded as the technology has advanced. Most recently, stents coated with pharmacologic agents (such as paclitaxel or sirolimus) aimed at reducing in-stent restenosis have been introduced.[16] A number of large, randomized studies have compared outcomes of patients with coronary disease treated with PCI and CABG.[17–28] These studies have attempted to identify the optimal therapy for patients with coronary disease, based on their anatomy and risk stratification. Two key representative studies are summarized here.

1. The BARI Trial (Bypass Angioplasty Revascularization Investigation). This trial, sponsored by the National Institutes of Health, randomized

1792 patients with multivessel coronary disease to either coronary bypass ($n = 914$) or PCI (n = 915).[17] In-hospital event rates for CABG and PCI were 1.3 and 1.1% for mortality, 4.6 and 2.1% for MI, and 0.8 and 0.2% for stroke. There was no significant difference in 5-year survival—89.3% for CABG and 86.3% for PCI. However, the PCI group required more repeat interventions, with 54% within 5 years versus only 8% for CABG. In diabetic patients with triple-vessel disease, CABG offered a clear survival advantage at 5 years, 80.6 versus 65.5% with PCI ($p = 0.003$).

2. Arterial Revascularization Therapies Study Group. This large trial compared outcomes in 1205 patients randomly assigned to CABG ($n = 605$) or PCI ($n = 600$).[20] Unlike the BARI trial, PCI patients in this trial received coronary stents. At 1 year, death, stroke, and MI rates were similar, although PCI patients had more recurrent symptoms, 16.8 versus 3.5% in CABG patients. The 1-year event-free survival rate was 73.8% with PCI compared with 87.8% with CABG.

Summary. When comparing CABG to PCI for the treatment of patients with coronary artery disease, results demonstrate that with appropriate patient selection both procedures are safe and effective, with little difference in mortality. PCI is associated with less short-term morbidity, decreased cost, and shorter hospital stay, but requires more late reinterventions. CABG provides more complete relief of angina, requires fewer reinterventions, and is more durable. CABG appears to offer a survival advantage in diabetic patients with multivessel disease.

Operative Techniques and Results

Conventional Coronary Artery Bypass Grafting. Conventional CABG is performed through a median sternotomy incision (Fig. 20-3), using cardiopulmonary bypass for extracorporeal

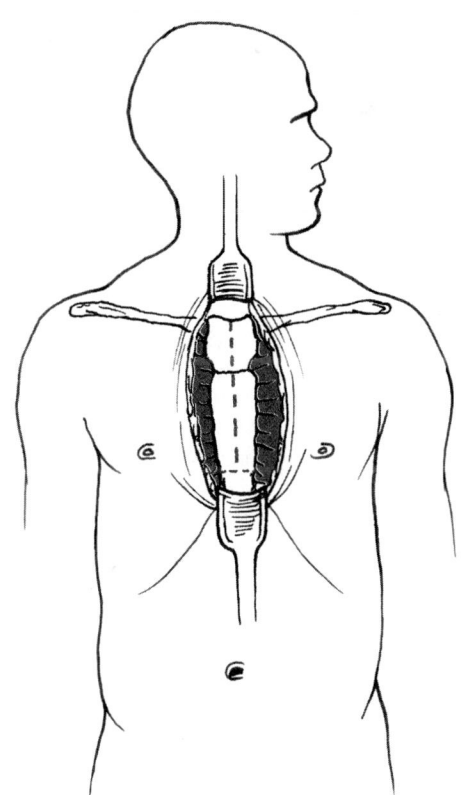

FIG. 20-3. *Median sternotomy incision. (Illustration courtesy of Heartport, Inc., Redwood City, CA.).*

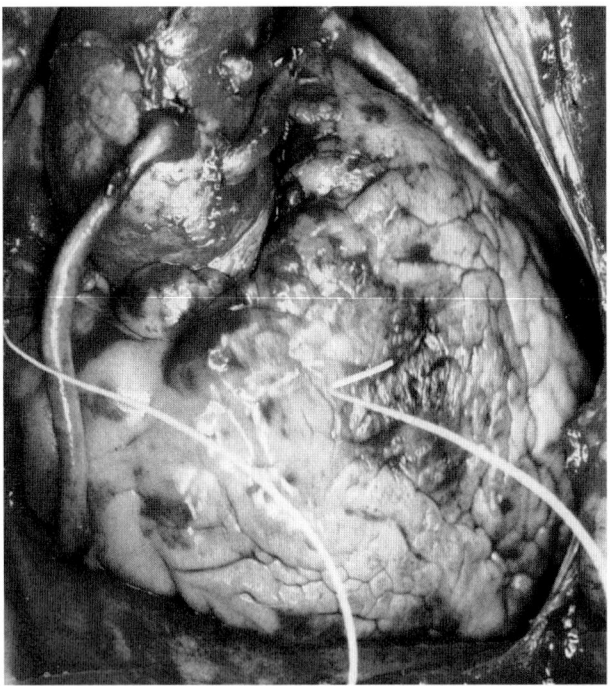

FIG. 20-4. Operative photograph of triple coronary artery bypass with reversed saphenous vein grafts.

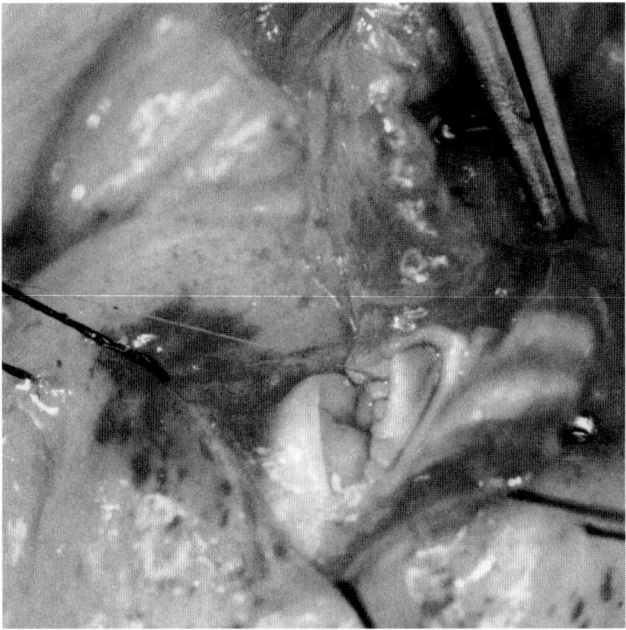

A

B

FIG. 20-5. *A.* Operative photograph of anastomosis between the left internal mammary artery and the left anterior descending artery. The anastomosis was completed using optical magnification, microvascular technique, and a continuous 8-0 suture. *B.* Fifteen-year follow-up of coronary angiogram demonstrating a widely patent left internal mammary artery–left anterior descending artery bypass graft. The arrow demonstrates the anastomotic site. The mammary artery is virtually free of graft atherosclerosis.

perfusion and cold cardioplegia for intraoperative myocardial protection of the heart (Fig. 20-4).

In the vast majority of patients the left internal mammary artery (IMA) is used as the primary conduit for bypassing the left anterior descending artery, which is the most important vessel in the heart (Fig. 20-5). The IMA is harvested from the chest wall and is usually used as an in situ graft, remaining connected proximally to the native subclavian artery. As such, the IMA remains metabolically active and enlarges over time in response to demand. The IMA is resistant to intrinsic atherosclerotic disease and its patency is rarely compromised by luminal stenosis. After cardiopulmonary bypass is initiated and the heart is arrested, the IMA to left anterior descending anastomosis is constructed end-to-side with fine sutures.

Loop reported a series of 2306 internal mammary grafts and 3625 vein grafts, demonstrating that use of an IMA graft significantly improved survival at 10 years. Patients who had IMA grafts also had fewer late complications with a decreased risk of MI and reoperation. The left IMA has a 10-year patency rate of approximately 95% when used as an in situ graft to the left anterior descending artery.

The excellent results obtained with in situ left IMA grafts prompted many other centers to use the right IMA in coronary revascularization. The right IMA can be used to provide a second arterial conduit as either an in situ or a free graft (Fig. 20-6). Dion reported 400 consecutive patients in whom both left and right IMAs were used, and found equivalent patency with the left and the right IMA.[29] Lytle and colleagues showed excellent late results and no increase in perioperative risk in over 500 cases in which both IMAs were used.[30] Even when the IMA is used as a "free" graft, patency rates are approximately 70 to 80% at 10 years.

Saphenous vein grafts, which were initially the primary conduits used for CABG, continue to be used widely, usually for grafting secondary targets on the side and back of the heart. Once CPB has been established and the heart arrested, a small arteriotomy is performed in the coronary artery, and the distal anastomosis is performed between the saphenous vein and the coronary artery. The proximal anastomosis then connects each vein graft to the ascending aorta. The 10-year patency of saphenous vein grafts is only approximately 65%, however, and patency is limited by the development of progressive intimal hyperplasia and late vein graft atherosclerosis.

In an attempt to achieve better long-term patency than that obtainable with saphenous vein grafts, and encouraged by the excellent late patency of internal mammary arterial grafts, surgeons have

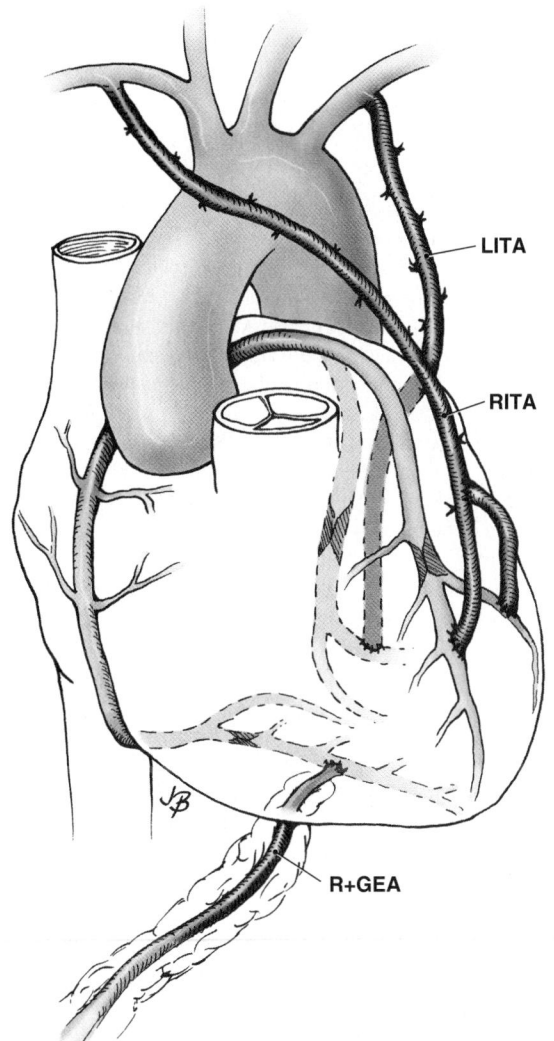

FIG. 20-6. Schematic of arterial conduits used in CABG, showing left internal mammary (or thoracic) artery (LITA), right internal mammary (or thoracic) artery (RITA), and composite graft using radial and gastroepiploic arteries (R+GEA). *(Reproduced with permission from Pevni D, Kramer A, Paz Y, et al: Composite arterial grafting with double skeletonized internal thoracic arteries. Eur J Cardiothorac Surg 20:299, 2001.)*

explored the use of other arterial conduits. The most widely used has been the radial artery graft. After an Allen test has been performed to assure adequate blood flow to the hand, the radial artery can be harvested and used as a free graft. Reports by Acar, Chen, and others have demonstrated excellent early and midterm patency rates with radial artery grafts.[31,32] Other alternative arterial grafts include the right gastroepiploic artery, which is usually used as an in situ pedicle graft, and the inferior epigastric artery, which is used as a free graft. Reports are mixed regarding late patency rates, however. While the expanded use of arterial grafts is appealing, improved patency of alternative arterial conduits compared to vein grafts has yet to be verified.

Results. The operative mortality for coronary artery bypass is 1 to 3%, depending on the number of risk factors present. Both the Society of Thoracic Surgeons (STS) and New York State have established large databases to establish risk factors and report outcomes. Variables that have been identified as influencing operative risk according to STS risk modeling include: female gender, age, race, body surface area, NYHA class IV status, low ejection fraction, hypertension, peripheral vascular disease, prior stroke, diabetes, renal failure, chronic obstructive pulmonary disease, immunosuppressive therapy, prior cardiac surgery, recent MI, urgent or emergent presentation, cardiogenic shock, left main disease, and concomitant valvular disease. Perioperative complications include MI, bleeding, stroke, arrhythmias, tamponade, wound infection, aortic dissection, pneumonia, respiratory failure, renal failure, gastrointestinal complications, and multiorgan failure.[33]

Late results demonstrate that relief of angina is striking after CABG. Angina is completely relieved or markedly decreased in over 98% of patients, and recurrent angina is rare in the first 5 to 7 years. Reintervention is required in less than 10% of patients within 5 years. Symptoms begin to recur more frequently between 8 and 15 years due to progression of disease or late graft occlusion. However, tight control of risk factors can minimize the risk of recurrence. Cessation of smoking and control of hypercholesterolemia are especially important, as late graft occlusion is five to seven times higher in patients who continue to smoke or have persistent hypercholesterolemia. If recurrent angina develops, angiography should be performed promptly, followed by repeat revascularization as indicated.

Exercise capacity generally improves significantly after CABG, with most patients demonstrating a markedly improved functional response to exercise secondary to improved blood flow. This functional improvement lasts up to 10 years, with longer improvement in patients receiving IMA grafts.

Late survival is similarly excellent after CABG, with a 5-year survival of over 90% and a 10-year survival of 75 to 90%, depending on the number of comorbidities present. Late survival is influenced by age, diabetes, left ventricular function, NYHA class, congestive heart failure, associated valvular insufficiency, completeness of revascularization, and nonuse of an IMA graft. Intense medical therapy for control of diabetes, hypercholesterolemia, and hypertension, and cessation of smoking significantly improves late survival.

Off-Pump Coronary Artery Bypass (OPCAB). One of the most significant developments in cardiac surgery in the last 15 to 20 years has been the introduction of off-pump coronary artery bypass (OPCAB). The main concept driving this approach is the elimination of the deleterious consequences of cardiopulmonary bypass. The initial experiences with beating heart techniques took place in Brazil under Benetti.

In order to perform coronary bypass on the beating heart, the surgeon has to address several issues: stabilization of the target vessel, maintenance of a bloodless field at the anastomotic site, avoidance of regional ischemia, and displacement of the beating heart in order to obtain exposure of posterior or inferior wall vessels and optimization of hemodynamics as the heart is displaced. During OPCAB surgery the coronary artery is temporarily snared or occluded to provide a relatively bloodless field for the creation of the anastomosis. Since this interval of regional ischemia may produce a critical reduction in cardiac function or arrhythmias, several methods, such as intracoronary shunts or preischemic conditioning, have been developed to minimize the risks of temporary coronary occlusion during construction of the anastomosis.

The manipulation and displacement of the heart often required during the OPCAB procedure, particularly while constructing posterior and inferior wall grafts, may lead to a reduction in cardiac output and subsequent hemodynamic instability. Several devices and intraoperative maneuvers have been proposed to minimize these

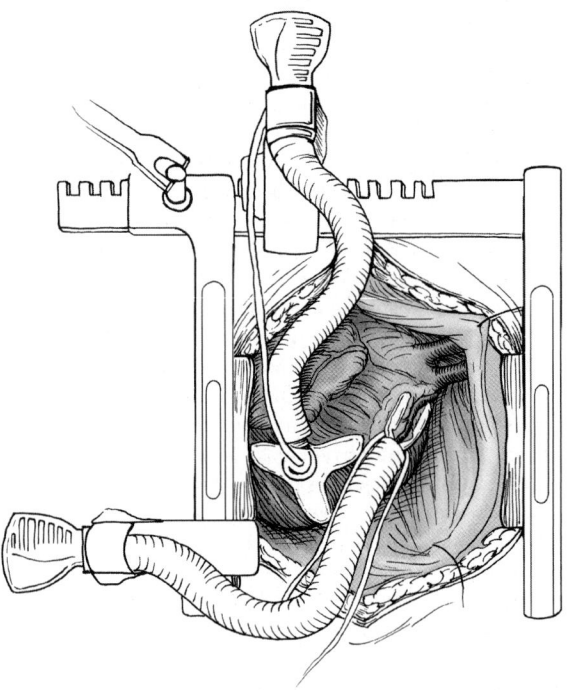

FIG. 20-7. Illustration demonstrating setup for off-pump coronary artery bypass (OPCAB). Shown are a retractor, a stabilizing device, and a displacement device. (Illustration courtesy of Medtronic, Inc., Minneapolis, MN.)

effects (Fig. 20-7). They include use of the right lateral decubitus and Trendelenburg ("head down") positions, administration of fluids, opening the right pleural cavity to minimize the compression of the right heart by the pericardium, use of pericardial sutures to aid in tilting the heart, and displacement devices that pull up the apex of the heart instead of compressing the left ventricle.[34] Temporary right heart support devices have also been used in select cases.

Results. The OPCAB technique has been extensively studied and results compared to conventional surgery. Initial attention was given to assessing the accuracy of graft placement with the OPCAB approach, which required grafting onto the beating heart. Puskas and associates assessed 421 grafts in 167 patients and found an overall early graft patency of 98.8%, with 100% patency of 163 internal mammary artery grafts.[35] These results were equivalent to those published for conventional CABG. Similarly, when evaluating patients receiving multiple arterial grafts, Kim and colleagues found no difference in the 1-year patency of arterial grafts performed with OPCAB compared with traditional methods.[36]

Sabik and coworkers compared overall results in 406 OPCAB patients with 406 conventional CABG patients.[37] The operative mortality and the risks of stroke, MI, and reoperation for bleeding were similar, while OPCAB patients had less risk of encephalopathy, sternal infection, blood transfusion, and renal failure. A prospective randomized comparison between OPCAB and conventional CABG, reported by Puskas,[38] demonstrated equivalent operative mortality and risk of stroke in each group, but less myocardial injury, fewer blood transfusions, earlier postoperative extubation, and earlier hospital discharge in OPCAB patients.

A study performed at New York University in high-risk patients with severe atheromatous aortic arch disease who required CABG compared outcomes in 245 OPCAB patients with outcomes in 245

conventional patients, using propensity case-matching methodology. In this high-risk patient population OPCAB was associated with a decreased risk of death (6.5 vs. 11.4%), stroke (1.6 vs. 5.7%), and all perioperative complications. Others have similarly shown significant reductions in both mortality and major neurologic events with the OPCAB technique.[39–42]

Minimally Invasive Direct Coronary Artery Bypass (MIDCAB). An even less invasive off-pump approach for CABG, termed minimally invasive direct coronary artery bypass, or MIDCAB, uses a small left anterior minithoracotomy incision to perform bypass grafting on the beating heart, without cardiopulmonary bypass. The technique utilizes a mechanical stabilizer to isolate the coronary artery and facilitate the anastomosis and an in situ left IMA graft. The technique is mainly useful in performing bypass to the anterior wall of the heart, primarily to the left anterior descending artery or to the diagonal branches.

Results. The operative mortality for MIDCAB has been less than 2%, and the patency rate of the IMA graft has been approximately 98%.[43] Since both the use of CPB and the need for sternotomy are eliminated, MIDCAB patients have less pain and blood loss, fewer perioperative complications, and a shorter recovery time than conventional CABG patients. Since the technique is generally only applicable to patients with single-vessel disease, outcomes after MIDCAB are probably best compared with PCI. Diegeler and associates reported a prospective, randomized trial that compared results of MIDCAB and PCI for treatment of isolated, proximal left anterior descending artery stenosis.[44] This study found that the combined perioperative risks of death and MI were equivalent, but the MIDCAB patients had better relief of angina and required fewer subsequent reinterventions. Similarly, a prospective, randomized study reported by Drenth and colleagues compared MIDCAB with PCI and stenting in patients with isolated high-grade left anterior descending artery stenosis. At 6 months, quantitative coronary angiography showed anastomotic stenosis in 4% after MIDCAB, but restenosis at the intervention site in 29% after PCI ($p < 0.001$).[45] Thus the late results with MIDCAB for revascularization of the left anterior descending artery appear to be significantly more durable than those achieved with PCI.

New Developments

Total Endoscopic Coronary Artery Bypass (TECAB). Minimal access coronary artery bypass performed using endoscopic instrumentation is facilitated with the latest generation of surgical robotic technology. Made possible by advancements in articulation of robotic instruments to more closely approximate the movement of human hands, total endoscopic coronary artery bypass (TECAB) has been reported on both the arrested and beating heart.[46,47] Robotic instrumentation also has been described to perform internal mammary artery harvests as part of the MIDCAB technique. While early results are promising, larger series with long-term data are necessary before TECAB moves out of the experimental phase.

Transmyocardial Laser Revascularization (TMR). TMR uses a high-powered carbon dioxide laser or holmium:yttrium-aluminum-garnet laser to drill multiple holes (1 cm^2) through the myocardium into the ventricular cavity. The procedure is performed on the beating heart with the laser pulses gated to the R wave on the ECG. The TMR procedure has been used primarily for patients with refractory angina who are unsuitable candidates for standard CABG due to poor distal coronary artery anatomy. The mechanism of benefit of TMR remains uncertain. It has been demonstrated that the transmyocardial laser channels are rapidly occluded and do not allow a direct flow from the ventricle to the myocardium. The most likely possibility is that TMR works by stimulating angiogenesis in the area of injury.[48]

Burkhoff and coworkers reported the results of a large, randomized, multicenter trial with TMR in 182 patients with CCS angina class III or IV, reversible ischemia, and incomplete response to other therapies. They found TMR to be associated with significant increases in exercise tolerance, reduction in angina score, and improvements in quality of life.[49] Despite subjective reports of improvement, however, the results of objective cardiac perfusion measurements after TMR have been inconclusive, and multiple randomized trials have failed to demonstrate any survival benefit with the procedure. Thus the exact role of TMR and its relationship to medical therapeutic angiogenesis remains to be determined.

Biomolecular Therapy and Tissue Engineering. Tissue engineering and biomolecular or gene therapy may be possible in the near future in order to replace the dysfunctional tissue or to improve organ function with an assembly that contains specific populations of living cells. Significant progress has been made in understanding the cellular and molecular mechanisms of cardiovascular disease, leading to new forms of molecular-genetic therapy. These innovations are currently being tried experimentally for genetically engineered or modified veins and arteries, engineered heart valves, stem cell or progenitor cell cardiomyocyte restoration therapy, and therapeutic angiogenesis. Much of this work has focused on vascular mitogens, on intracellular signaling pathways, and on the underlying genetic functions that control the cellular response.

In the field of coronary artery disease several gene therapy protocols are now under active investigation. These include: (1) genetic engineering of vein grafts that are resistant to atherosclerosis or restenosis; (2) gene therapy for coronary arteries to prevent restenosis after angioplasty or surgical endarterectomy; (3) genetic manipulation of the coronary and peripheral vascular system in an attempt to prevent lipid accumulation and progression of atherosclerosis; (4) the biomolecular delivery of growth factors or genetic material into the coronary system or myocardium to promote therapeutic angiogenesis; and (5) the total bioengineering of blood vessels using cell seeding techniques and a biodegradable scaffold. While these innovations are currently experimental, biomolecular adjuvant therapy offers great promise for the future.

Facilitated Anastomotic Devices. Significant technologic progress has led to the development of devices that mechanically construct proximal and distal vascular anastomoses, without the need for sutures or knot tying. The goals for these devices are to provide safe, rapid, and reproducible anastomoses; reduce operative time; limit anastomotic variability between surgeons; and improve graft patency. If perfected, such devices may facilitate newer minimally invasive endoscopic or robotic surgical techniques by eliminating the difficulties associated with suturing and knot tying in small spaces. Proximal anastomotic devices, some in early clinical trials, are designed to create aortosaphenous anastomoses without the need for aortic cross-clamping.[50] This may have particular significance in patients with severe atherosclerotic aortic disease in whom prevention of aortic manipulation is crucial in preventing embolic complications. Distal anastomotic devices are also in experimental use, and may facilitate off-pump or minimally invasive coronary artery bypass grafting.[51]

VENTRICULAR ANEURYSMS

Pathophysiology

Approximately 5 to 10% of transmural myocardial infarctions result in left ventricular aneurysms, which develop 4 to 8 weeks following transmural infarct as necrotic myocardium is replaced by fibrous tissue. Collateral circulation in the area of the infarct probably limits aneurysm formation in many other cases by maintaining partial myocardial viability.

The classic aneurysm is an avascular thin scar, 4 to 6 mm thick, which bulges outward when the remaining left ventricular muscle contracts in systole (Fig. 20-8A). This is termed *myocardial dyskinesis*, in contrast to hypokinesis (impaired contractility) or akinesis (absence of contractility). Mural thrombus is found attached to the ventricular surface of the aneurysm in over one half of patients, but arterial emboli are rare. The aneurysm usually enlarges to a moderate degree and is associated with a progressive deterioration of left ventricular function. Left ventricular aneurysms generally do not rupture, but manifest clinically as progressive heart failure, often with associated malignant ventricular arrhythmias.

Over 80% of aneurysms are in the anteroapical portion of the left ventricle, resulting from occlusion of the left anterior descending coronary artery. Patients with anteroapical aneurysms usually also have significant aneurysmal dilation of the upper part of the ventricular septum. Posterior ventricular aneurysms are less common (15 to 20%) and lateral wall aneurysms are rare. Posterior aneurysms can distort the mitral valve, resulting in concomitant mitral insufficiency.

Left ventricular aneurysms decrease ventricular function by dissipating the energy of ventricular contraction. The left ventricular end-diastolic and end-systolic volumes both increase, and the left ventricular end-diastolic pressure is usually markedly elevated. The combination of elevated intracavitary pressure and radius results in a significant elevation in wall tension according to Laplace's law (tension = pressure × radius), and therefore oxygen requirements are increased. The decrease in effective ventricular function results in congestive heart failure, and the increased wall tension and oxygen consumption may result in angina, which may be worsened by accompanying coronary disease in noninfarcted areas of the heart. Areas of scar tissue around the edge of the aneurysm frequently serve as foci for ventricular arrhythmias, which are prominent in 15 to 20% of patients with left ventricular aneurysms.

Diagnostic Evaluation

The diagnostic workup generally begins with echocardiography to assess wall motion in the various zones of the heart, to determine left ventricular end-systolic and end-diastolic size, and to assess for any associated mitral valve insufficiency. Cardiac MRI may also be useful in determining left ventricular size and shape and in assessing the amount of remaining functional myocardium. Dobutamine stress echocardiography may also be helpful in the latter regard. Cardiac catheterization is performed preoperatively to assess for the severity of coronary artery disease, and to determine the anatomic extent of the aneurysm and the areas of myocardium that still have good function. Workup of arrhythmias may include electrophysiologic studies.

Operative Treatment

Operative treatment requires excision or exclusion of the aneurysm and bypass grafting of diseased coronary arteries. The classic repair

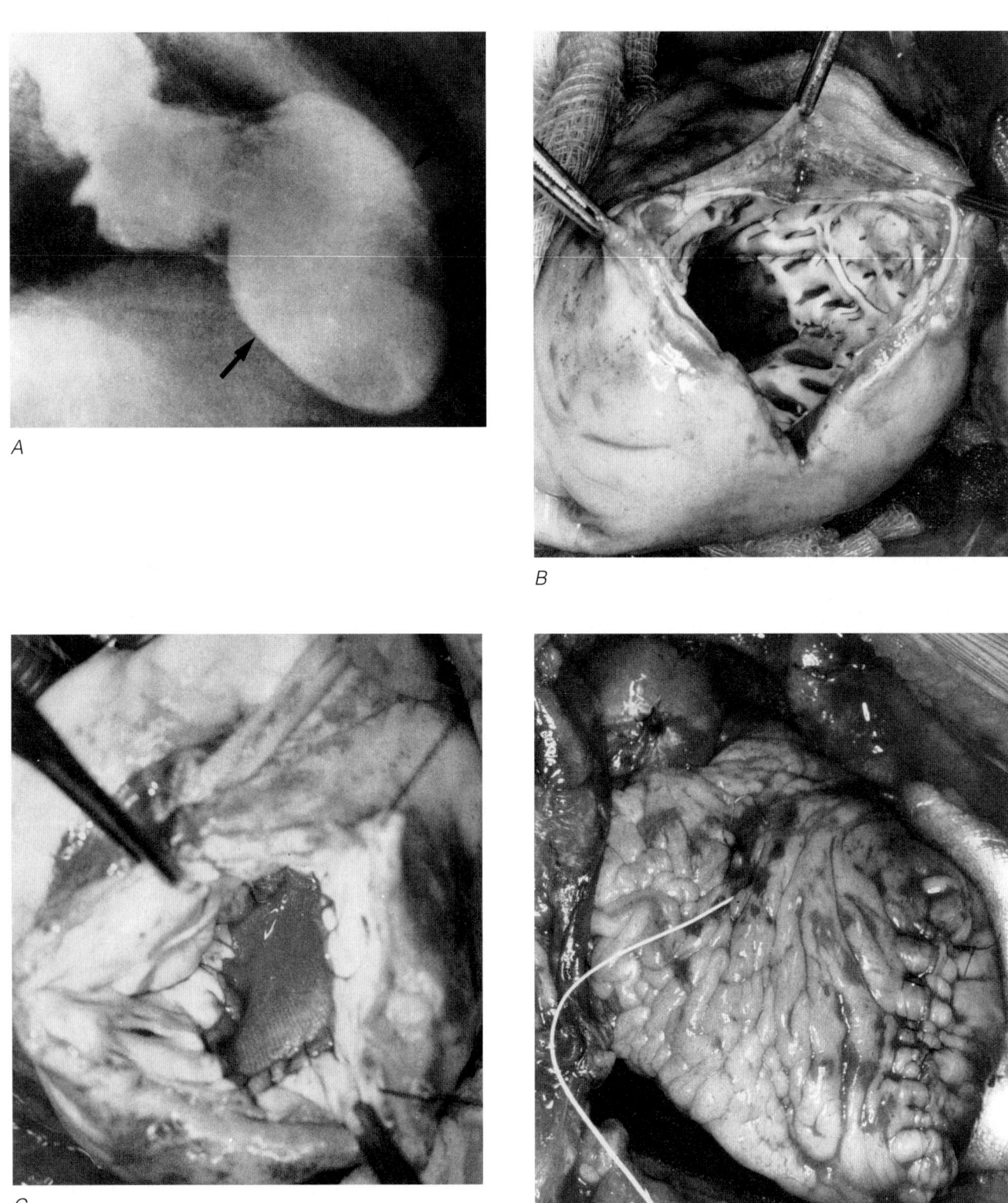

FIG. 20-8. *A.* A left ventriculogram demonstrating a large left ventricular aneurysm. Note the contrast to the normal left ventriculogram shown in Fig. 20-1B. *B.* Operative photograph of open left ventricular aneurysm. Aneurysmal involvement of the ventricular septum was present and significant subendocardial scar is seen. *C.* Aneurysm repair using a Dacron patch and the endoaneurysmorrhaphy technique, which excludes the aneurysm and the aneurysmal septum from the normal part of the left ventricular cavity. *D.* The wall of the aneurysm has been closed over the Dacron patch, completing the endoaneurysmorrhaphy.

was performed by excision of the aneurysm and linear closure of the ventricle. However, this technique had a geometrically deforming effect on the remaining left ventricle, and did not address aneurysmal deformity of the septum. Therefore, a more physiologic technique of intracavitary endoventricular patch reconstruction, or left ventricular restoration, was proposed by Jatene, Cooley, and Dor.[52-54]

Endoventricular patch reconstruction involves placement of a Dacron patch to obliterate the aneurysmal ventricle and septum, re-establishing a Dacron "roof" on the left ventricular cavity (see Fig. 20-8 B, C, and D). This repair remodels the ventricular cavity and obliterates the septal component of the aneurysm, which is not possible with linear aneurysm repair. The neck of the aneurysm is reduced with an encircling suture to ensure appropriate ventricular geometry, and the Dacron patch is sutured circumferentially to this zone at the junction of viable and nonviable myocardium. This technique may be combined with a subendocardial resection to obliterate conduction of arrhythmias. The endoventricular ventricular restoration technique results in lowering the diastolic volume without deforming the other walls of the heart, and it improves left ventricular systolic function.

Results

Following ventricular aneurysm repair, most patients experience considerable relief from heart failure and angina, with moderate improvement in left ventricular function. Dor and associates reported results in over 1000 cases, using an integrated approach of left ventricular reconstruction, CABG, and mitral repair as needed.[55] The hospital mortality rate was 7.3%. Postoperatively, the left ventricular ejection fraction had an average increase of 10 to 15%. Doss and colleagues compared the long-term results of linear closure and endoventricular patch reconstruction with 8 years follow-up.[56] The left ventricular ejection fraction increased significantly in patients who underwent endoventricular reconstruction, but decreased in those who underwent linear closure. The operative mortality was 1.9%, with an 8-year survival of 85.6%. In general, the published data suggest better results with the endoventricular patch reconstruction technique, although the classic linear repair remains useful in patients with smaller, anteroapical aneurysms, who do not have involvement of the ventricular septum.

ISCHEMIC CARDIOMYOPATHY

Patients with ischemic cardiomyopathy and heart failure are being evaluated and treated by surgeons with increasing frequency, as surgical options for the failing heart have expanded considerably over the last 10 to 20 years. This trend is expected to expand as the population continues to age and patients are able to survive longer with ischemic heart disease. Anatomically, ischemic cardiomyopathy results from multiple myocardial infarctions, which produce extensive myocardial scarring with decreased left ventricular systolic function. These patients may have a definable left ventricular aneurysm, but more commonly have diffuse myocardial scarring with large, nonfunctioning, akinetic zones of the heart. In addition to heart failure, the myocardial scarring serves as a nidus for ventricular arrhythmias and progressive cardiac dilation, along with injury to the papillary muscles, and may result in significant mitral valve insufficiency.

Ventricular Restoration Surgery

Left ventricular surgical restoration for ischemic cardiomyopathy is performed similarly to the endoventricular patch reconstruction

described above for repair of anteroapical left ventricular aneurysms. Dor extended the indications for endoventricular reconstruction to patients with dilated ischemic cardiomyopathy who had large areas of myocardial akinesis and scarring, but with no true dyskinetic aneurysm, and as such the technique has been referred to as the Dor procedure.[54] The goal of ventricular restoration is to restore the normal left ventricular size and shape, thus improving the efficiency of left ventricular ejection. To achieve this goal the surgeon must exclude the akinetic area of the anterior wall and septum. This produces a more normal left ventricular size and shape, resulting in reduced left ventricular wall tension and reduced end-diastolic fiber length. The left ventricular ejection fraction usually increases after repair, as the heart is allowed to work under more efficient loading conditions.

Most patients with ischemic myopathy who have documented reversible ischemia should undergo CABG, but it is currently unclear what degree of left ventricular dilation becomes an indication for concomitant ventricular restoration surgery. Certainly CABG alone may be inadequate when the heart is significantly dilated with increased left ventricular end-diastolic and end-systolic volumes, the left ventricular ejection is less than 20 to 25%, and regional wall motion abnormalities are associated with thinned ventricular walls.[57] Ventricular reconstruction is recommended in this group of patients and may be effective in decreasing the risk of progressive heart failure or avoiding possible cardiac transplantation.[58]

Results

A large international study (RESTORE) investigated outcomes after surgical anterior ventricular endocardial restoration (SAVER) in 439 patients with ischemic cardiomyopathy as a result of anterior infarction. They found an overall hospital mortality of 6.6%, with an increase in ejection fraction from 29.7 to 40% and a 3-year survival rate approaching 90%. These encouraging results suggest the benefit that patients with ischemic cardiomyopathy may gain from ventricular remodeling procedures.[57]

MECHANICAL CIRCULATORY SUPPORT AND MYOCARDIAL REGENERATION

Intra-Aortic Balloon Pump

The intra-aortic balloon pump (IABP) is the most common and effective technique for assisted circulation. Approximately 70,000 are inserted annually in the United States. The most frequent indications for use of IABP are to provide hemodynamic support during or after cardiac catheterization, cardiogenic shock, weaning from cardiopulmonary bypass, and for preoperative use in high-risk patients and refractory unstable angina. A balloon catheter is inserted through the femoral artery and advanced into the thoracic aorta. With electronic synchronization, the balloon is inflated during diastole and deflated during systole. Coronary blood flow is increased by improved diastolic perfusion, and afterload is reduced. The cardiac index typically improves after insertion, and the preload decreases. Total myocardial oxygen consumption is diminished by approximately 15%.

The use of a preoperative IABP in patients with severe left ventricular dysfunction or unstable angina with critical coronary anatomy has resulted in improved outcomes. Kang and associates reported that the risk-adjusted mortality was significantly lower in high-risk patients requiring CABG if a preoperative IABP was used, compared with emergent cases with intraoperative or postoperative IABP use.[59] The authors encourage the use of preoperative IABPs in selected high-risk patients undergoing heart surgery.

Generally, the IABP is used for a few days with minimal morbidity. Analysis of 911 patients undergoing coronary artery bypass grafting who received IABP revealed that the duration of IABP therapy ranged from 20 hours to 21 days (mean 3.8 days). Major complications occurred in 5.9% of the patients, and minor complications in 5.8%. Ischemia of the limb requiring thromboembolectomy developed in 2.7%.[60] Limb ischemia on the side of insertion is the most serious complication, and the extremity must be examined frequently for viability. A large multicenter registry including 203 hospitals collected 16,909 patient case records. Major IABP complications (limb ischemia, bleeding, balloon leakage, or death directly due to IABP insertion) occurred in 2.6% of cases. Female gender, advanced age, and peripheral vascular disease were independent predictors of the risk of complications.[61]

Ventricular Assist Devices

Mechanical circulatory support systems (ventricular assist devices; VADs) are designed for temporary assisted circulation ("bridge to recovery"), for long-term treatment ("bridge to transplantation"), or as a permanent substitute for the heart ("artificial heart" or "destination therapy"). Temporary assisted circulation is a valuable clinical modality in the treatment of transient cardiac injury. The most common indication for temporary assisted circulation is cardiac failure after cardiac surgery, manifested by a cardiac index of less than 1.5 L/min per square meter despite inotropic support. Often an IABP has been used in such situations without success. In these cases mechanical cardiac assistance for 24 to 48 hours or longer may permit recovery of cardiac function, probably by minimizing reperfusion injury and from resolution of myocardial edema. The most frequently used temporary left ventricular or biventricular circulatory assist systems are the BioMedicus centrifugal pump, the Thoratec ventricular assist system, and the Abiomed BVS 5000. Inflow for these devices is through either the left atrium or the apex of the left ventricle, and outflow is into the aorta. These devices can provide effective support for 5 to 7 days, and in rare cases, up to 2 weeks. External pulsatile assist devices deliver blood flow in synchrony with the native heart and are used for short-term support after cardiac surgery or as a long-term bridge to cardiac transplantation.

Long-term mechanical circulatory support has become more common in patients presenting with cardiogenic shock or those in end-stage heart failure who are waiting for heart transplantation. The three main types of devices available in the United States are the Thoratec ventricular assist system (VAS), the Novacor left ventricular assist system (LVAS), and the HeartMate LVAS. HeartMate is a rotating torque motor system that displaces blood from the left ventricle into the aorta. Blood is directed through the pump by inflow and outflow valves made of pig tissue. Prototypes of the continuous-flow VAD include the Jarvik 2000, Micro-Med DeBakey pump, and HeartMate II pumps, all now in clinical trials.[62] The unique characteristics and specific advantages and disadvantages of each system are beyond the scope of this chapter. With VADs, the right ventricle benefits from reduction of pulmonary arterial pressures, and in some cases the heart can recover. Mechanical circulatory support can be used in outpatients (mean support time of 454 days) without increased mortality and with an acceptable rate of readmissions (2.8/patient). This approach ensures the survival of the patient, enables recovery from multiorgan failure, and offers an acceptable quality of life.[63]

About 2000 patients receive heart transplants in the United States annually; however, about 50,000 patients who suffer from end-stage heart failure potentially could benefit from a transplant. A shortage of donors has created the need for an alternative. A definitive solution for heart failure may be a permanent artificial heart. In July 2001, surgeons from Louisville, Kentucky, removed a patient's heart and implanted a totally artificial heart in the patient, who survived for 151 days. Total cardiac replacement with an artificial heart, however, is still in the experimental arena. Long-term risks include thromboembolic complications, the risk of infection, and trauma to blood elements.

Myocardial Regeneration

Cell transplantation has been studied as a new alternative approach for repair or regeneration of the injured myocardium. Improved myocardial function after cell transplantation has been shown in animal studies. In humans, myoblast grafts can survive and show a switch to slow-twitch fiber, which might allow sustained improvement in cardiac function.[64] Recently, skeletal myoblasts have been evaluated in three patients who underwent coronary artery bypass grafting and implantation of autologous satellite cells isolated from muscle biopsies. At 3- to 4-month follow-up examination, increased left ventricular ejection fraction and decreased left ventricular diastolic diameter, as well as improved ventricular wall thickness and perfusion at the satellite cell implantation sites, were observed.[65] The feasibility and safety of autologous skeletal myoblast transplantation in patients with severe ischemic cardiomyopathy were assessed. The ejection fraction increased from 24 to 32% ($p < 0.02$). Echocardiographic analysis showed that 63% of the cell-implanted scars (14 of 22) demonstrated improved systolic thickening. However, four patients showed delayed episodes of sustained ventricular tachycardia. These preliminary data suggest good feasibility and safety of autologous skeletal myoblast transplantation in patients with severely ischemic cardiomyopathy, with the caveat of an arrhythmogenic potential.[66] The use of skeletal myoblasts for cardiomyoplasty has been initiated under clinical trials in Europe and the United States. Advances in stem cell biology may allow the further application of cellular myocardial regeneration therapy in the future.

VALVULAR HEART DISEASE

General Principles

According to the STS database, valve operations accounted for 14.0% of all classified procedures performed in 1996. By 2002, that percentage had increased by 45 to 20% of all classified procedures. Although CABG volume declined by 15.3% between 1996 and 1999, aortic valve replacements increased by 11.7% and mitral valve operations increased by 58% during the same period.[67]

Valvular heart disease can result in a *pressure load* (valvular stenosis), a *volume load* (valvular insufficiency), or both (mixed stenosis and insufficiency). Aortic stenosis increases the afterload of the left ventricle, resulting in left ventricular hypertrophy, while both aortic and mitral insufficiency result in a significant volume overload of the left ventricle, producing cardiac dilatation. Although the heart can effectively compensate for these hemodynamic changes for some time, progressive deterioration in cardiac function eventually develops, leading to valvular cardiomyopathy. The decision to proceed with surgical intervention is based on the patient's history, symptoms, physical findings, and the results of diagnostic studies, such as echocardiography, cardiac catheterization, and radionuclide studies. Demonstration of a decreased ejection fraction at rest (or a rise in the end-systolic volume by echocardiography) or a fall in the ejection fraction during exercise are probably the best signs that the systolic function of the heart is beginning to deteriorate and that surgery should be performed promptly. As surgeons have gained experience and as new technologies have been advanced, surgical risk has been reduced and long-term results have improved. Therefore surgical therapy is now recommended at a much earlier stage of the disease process in an attempt to maintain normal cardiac function long after valve surgery.

Survival after cardiac valve replacement is strongly influenced by the myocardial function at the time of operation. For example Chaliki and associates reported that the operative risk for aortic valve replacement for aortic insufficiency in patients with a low ejection fraction was 14%, compared to 3.7% in patients with preserved left ventricular function.[68] At 10 years, only 41 ± 9% of those patients with reduced ejection fraction had survived, compared with 70 ± 3% of those with normal ventricular function.

Postoperative cardiac function generally returns to normal if the operation is performed at an early phase of ventricular dysfunction. Even with impaired left ventricular function, NYHA class IV disability, and pulmonary hypertension, patients with valvular heart disease are rarely inoperable. After the hemodynamic burden on the ventricle has been removed with corrective surgery, the patient is treated with an aggressive medical heart failure regimen (digitalis, diuretics, afterload reduction, and beta blockers when indicated), usually with significant improvement. Except in the rare case of advanced cardiomyopathy combined with other systemic disease, surgery should not be denied to patients. The typical valve-related complications from valvular surgery include thromboembolic events, anticoagulant-related hemorrhage, prosthetic valve failure, endocarditis, prosthetic paravalvular leakage, and failure of valve repair.

Surgical Options

Two basic types of prosthetic valves are available: mechanical valves and tissue valves (xenografts). Valve replacement, in particular aortic valve replacement, also can be performed using human homografts or autografts. Finally, valve repair is increasingly an option, as opposed to valve replacement, especially for patients with mitral or tricuspid valve insufficiency. The recommendations for valve repair or replacement, type of prosthesis, and operative approach are based on multiple factors, such as the patient's age, lifestyle, associated medical conditions, access to follow-up health care, desire for future pregnancy, and experience of the surgeon. The risks, benefits, and options should be discussed in detail with the patient before arriving at a joint decision. General considerations regarding these choices are discussed in the following paragraphs.

Mechanical prostheses are highly durable but require permanent anticoagulation therapy to minimize the risk of valve thrombosis and thromboembolic complications. Such lifelong anticoagulation therapy carries the risk of hemorrhagic complications and may dictate lifestyle changes. For some patients, the typical mechanical valve closing sound adversely affects quality of life. Mechanical prostheses are usually preferable in patients with a long life expectancy who want to minimize the risk of reoperation and are suitable candidates for anticoagulation.

Tissue valves are more natural and less thrombogenic, and therefore generally do not require anticoagulation therapy. Consequently, tissue valves have lower risks of thromboembolic and anticoagulant-related complications, with the total yearly risk of all valve-related complications being considerably less than with mechanical valves. Unfortunately, tissue valves are more prone to structural failure due to late calcification of the xenograft tissue. However, because of improved methods of valve preservation and chemical impregnation to slow calcification of the tissue, the currently available tissue valves are becoming increasingly durable, and it is anticipated that it may take 15 to 20 years before structural failure will occur in these prostheses.

For aortic valve replacement, a mechanical prosthesis, a newer-generation tissue valve (either stented or nonstented), a homograft, or a pulmonary autograft (Ross procedure) may be recommended, depending on the patient's lifestyle and desire to avoid anticoagulation therapy. Some type of tissue valve is usually recommended for patients older than 65 years of age because anticoagulation therapy may be hazardous and valve durability is better in older patients. For patients over 65 years of age, Jamieson and colleagues demonstrated a risk of tissue valve structural deterioration of less than 10% at 15 years.[69]

While valve repair can be performed in the vast majority of patients with mitral insufficiency as discussed below, valve replacement may still be required in certain patients, and in the vast majority with rheumatic disease and valvular stenosis. When valve replacement is necessary, a tissue valve is an appropriate choice in women planning pregnancy or in patients over 60 to 65 years of age.[70] A mechanical prosthesis is recommended for younger patients, especially if the patient is in atrial fibrillation, since anticoagulation therapy is already required in this group.

Mechanical Valves

A common mechanical valve used in the United States is the St. Jude Medical bileaflet prosthesis (Fig. 20-9). Mechanical (disk) valves have excellent flow characteristics, an acceptably low risk of late valve-related complications, and an extremely low risk of mechanical valve failure. With proper anticoagulation and keeping the International Normalized Ratio (INR) at two to three times the normal for mechanical aortic valves and 2.5 to 3.5 times the

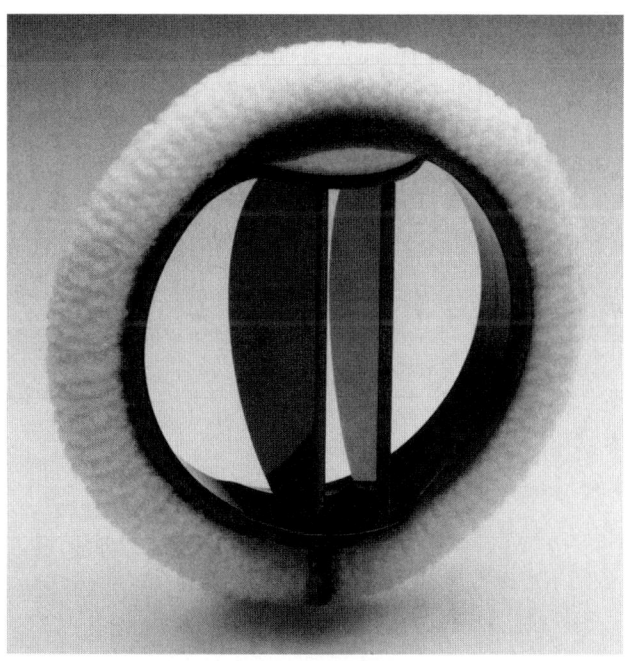

FIG. 20-9. Mechanical valve. St. Jude Medical bileaflet prosthesis. (Photo courtesy of St. Jude Medical, Inc., St. Paul, MN. All rights reserved.)

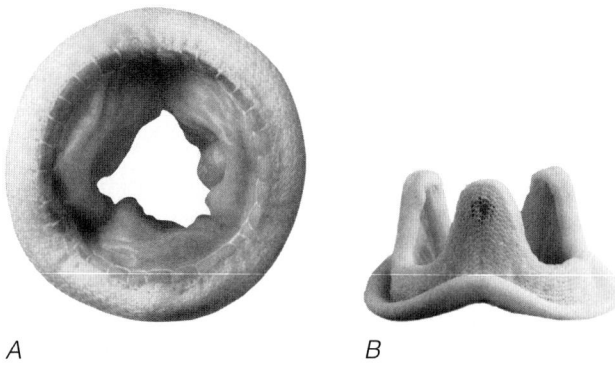

A   *B*

FIG. 20-10. Bioprosthetic valves. (*Photos courtesy of Medtronic, Inc., Minneapolis, MN.*)

normal for mechanical mitral valves, the incidence of thromboembolism is approximately 1 to 2% per patient per year, and the risk of anticoagulant-related hemorrhage is 0.5 to 2% per patient per year.[71–74] Careful monitoring of the INR reduces the risk of thromboembolic events, minimizes anticoagulation-related complications, and improves survival.[75]

Tissue Valves

Several types of xenograft tissue valves are available and widely used (Fig. 20-10). The stented valves are most common (either porcine or bovine pericardial), while stentless valves are being increasingly used by some groups. Again, the chief advantage of tissue valves is the low incidence of thromboembolism and the absence of the need for anticoagulation therapy. Stented tissue valves have the drawback of having higher gradients across the valve, particularly in smaller sizes (indexed prosthetic valve area <0.85 cm^2 valve area per square meter body surface area). Therefore, this group of patients may have less symptomatic improvement and a suboptimal hemodynamic response to exercise.[76] However, most patients experience excellent symptomatic improvement and have a normal response to exercise after stented tissue valve replacement.

Nevertheless, the limitations in flow characteristics observed in small sizes of stented tissue valves led to the development of stentless valves in an attempt to maximize the effective valve orifice area by eliminating the profile of the stent, and to take advantage of the natural dynamic nature of the aortic annulus. Since the first clinical report of a stentless porcine valve in 1990 by David and associates,[77] several stentless aortic bioprostheses have been introduced (Fig. 20-11). The technique of implantation varies (subcoronary or miniroot), but the results have been excellent in most series. Patients undergoing stentless valve replacement have been found to

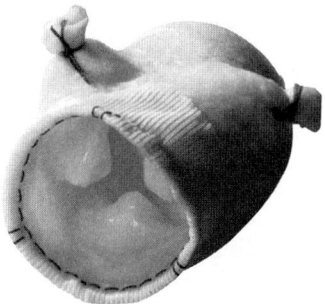

FIG. 20-11. Freestyle valve. (*Photo courtesy of Medtronic, Inc., Minneapolis, MN.*)

have a significant reduction in transvalvular gradient, both at rest and with exercise.[76,78,79] Although the long-term durability of stentless valves has not yet been established, these valves offer excellent hemodynamics, and durability is anticipated to be similar to that achieved with stented xenografts.[80]

Homografts

Surgical alternatives to prosthetic valve replacement have been developed in an attempt to utilize the body's natural tissue and lower the incidence of valve-related complications. In the 1960s, Ross in England and Barrett-Boyes in New Zealand described a procedure for aortic valve replacement using antibiotic-preserved aortic homograft (allograft) valves. Since this time, homografts have been used more frequently for aortic and pulmonary valve replacements. Similarly to patients receiving xenografts, the rate of thromboembolic complications is low, and long-term anticoagulation therapy is not required. In addition, homografts have much lower transvalvular pressure gradients than stented tissue valves. While homografts are attractive options in many instances, there are some limitations to their widespread use. During the first year of implantation, homograft valves rapidly lose their original cellular components and normal tissue architecture.[81] Newer methods of homograft preservation that result in significant retention of cellular viability are possible using cryopreservation techniques, widening the availability of homografts and potentially improving the long-term results. The main disadvantage of a homograft valve is its uncertain durability, especially in young patients, as structural degeneration of the valve tissue leads to graft dysfunction and valve failure. The 15-year durability is approximately that of a xenograft.

Autografts

Ross described a potentially durable but more complicated alternative for aortic valve replacement with natural autologous tissue, using the patient's native pulmonary valve as an autograft for aortic valve replacement and replacing the pulmonary valve with a homograft (Fig. 20-12). This operation, referred to as the Ross procedure, has the advantage of placing an autologous valve into the aortic position, which functions physiologically and does not require anticoagulation therapy. Results have shown minimal-to-absent transvalvular gradients, with improvement in left ventricular function both at rest and during exercise.[82] Ross reported late follow-up of 339 autograft patients with a rate of freedom from autograft replacement of 85% at 20 years, and a rate of freedom from all valve-related events of 70% at 20 years. Others have reported less durable results, with a combined failure rate of the autograft or pulmonary homograft of 30 to 40% at 12 to 15 years. The Ross procedure may be indicated for younger patients who require aortic valve replacement and want to avoid the need for anticoagulation.

Valve Repair

Valve repair has become the procedure of choice for most patients with mitral valve insufficiency, while repair of the aortic valve is feasible in certain situations. In the 1960s McGoon, Kay, and Reed each developed separate plication techniques for reconstruction of the mitral valve for mitral insufficiency. However, the primary advance in mitral valve repair resulted from work by Carpentier in the 1970s. Valve repair has subsequently proved to be highly reproducible for correction of mitral insufficiency, with excellent durability and freedom from late valve-related complications. The 15-year freedom from valve repair failure is over 90% in patients with degenerative mitral insufficiency. Valve repair offers significant

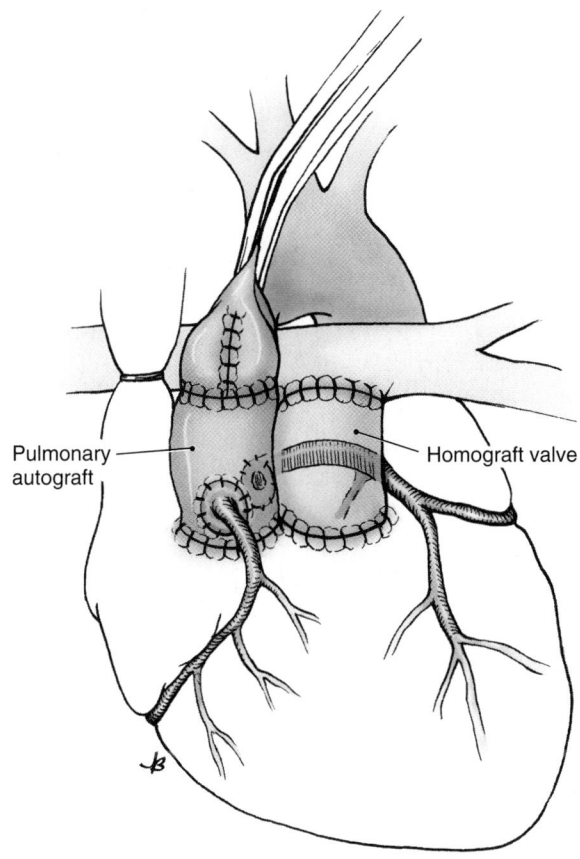

FIG. 20-12. Diagram of a completed Ross procedure. The aortic valve has been replaced with the patient's own pulmonary valve (pulmonary autograft), and the coronary arteries have been reimplanted. The pulmonary valve has been replaced with a homograft valve (aortic or pulmonary) obtained from a cadaver. (*Reproduced with permission from Oury JH: Clinical aspects of the Ross procedure: Indications and contraindications. Semin Thorac Cardiovasc Surg 8:328, 1996.*)

advantages over valve replacement, primarily lower risks of thromboembolic- and anticoagulant-related complications. Survival may also be improved in certain groups of patients after valve repair.

Mitral Valve Disease

Mitral Stenosis

Etiology. Mitral valve stenosis or mixed mitral stenosis and insufficiency almost always are caused by rheumatic heart disease, although a definite clinical history can be obtained in only 50% of patients. Congenital mitral stenosis is rarely seen in adults. Occasionally, intracardiac tumors such as left atrial myxoma may obstruct the mitral orifice and cause symptoms that mimic mitral stenosis.

Pathology. Although the rheumatic inflammatory process is associated with some degree of pancarditis involving endocardium, myocardium, and pericardium, permanent injury results predominantly from the endocarditis, with progressive fibrosis of the valves. Rheumatic valvulitis produces three distinct degrees of pathologic change: fusion of the commissures alone, commissural fusion plus subvalvular shortening of the chordae tendineae, and extensive fixation of the valve and subvalvular apparatus with calcification and scarring of both leaflets and chordae (Fig. 20-13). The degree of pathology present should be determined preoperatively, as this

predicts the suitability of balloon valvuloplasty, surgical commissurotomy, or valve replacement.

Pathophysiology. Mitral stenosis usually has a prolonged course after the initial rheumatic infection, and symptoms may not appear for 10 to 20 years. The progression to valvular fibrosis and calcification may be related to repeated episodes of rheumatic fever, or may result from scarring produced by inflammation and turbulent blood flow.

Mitral stenosis leads to a progressive decrease in the mitral valve area, which results in a transvalvular gradient across the stenotic valve during diastole. The normal cross-sectional area of the mitral valve is 4 to 6 cm^2. Symptoms may progressively develop with moderate stenosis, defined as a cross-sectional area 1.0 to 1.5 cm^2. Severe symptomatic stenosis occurs when the mitral valve area is less than 0.8 to 1.0 cm^2.

The pathophysiology associated with mitral stenosis results from an elevation in left atrial pressure, producing pulmonary venous congestion and pulmonary hypertension. As the left atrium dilates, atrial fibrillation may develop, exacerbating the patient's symptoms and resulting in an increased likelihood of clot formation and embolization. The left ventricular function usually remains normal since the ventricle is protected by the stenotic valve.

Clinical Manifestations. The main symptoms of mitral stenosis are exertional dyspnea and decreased exercise capacity. Dyspnea occurs when the left atrial pressure becomes elevated due to the stenotic valve, resulting in pulmonary congestion. Orthopnea and paroxysmal nocturnal dyspnea may also occur, or in advanced cases, hemoptysis. The most serious development is pulmonary edema. When the stenosis is chronic, with pulmonary hypertension, the patient may develop right-sided heart failure, manifest as jugular venous distention, hepatomegaly, ascites, or ankle edema.

Atrial fibrillation develops in a significant number of patients with chronic mitral stenosis, and in some patients arterial embolization is the initial presenting symptom. Atrial thrombi result from dilation and stasis of the left atrium, with the left atrial appendage being especially susceptible to clot formation. Angina is a rare symptom that may result from coronary embolization.

The characteristic auscultatory findings of mitral stenosis, called the auscultatory triad, are an increased first heart sound, an opening snap, and an apical diastolic rumble. A loud pansystolic murmur transmitted to the axilla usually indicates associated mitral insufficiency. A systolic murmur along the left lower sternal border, loudest near the xiphoid process, commonly occurs with associated tricuspid insufficiency.

Diagnostic Studies. The electrocardiogram may show atrial fibrillation, left atrial enlargement (P mitrale), and right-axis deviation, or it may be normal. On chest x-ray, enlargement of the left atrium is typically seen on the posteroanterior film as a double contour visible behind the right atrial shadow. The overall cardiac size may be normal, but enlargement of the left atrium and the pulmonary artery may obliterate the normal concavity between the aorta and the left ventricle, producing a "straight" left border of the heart. Calcifications of the mitral valve also may be seen. In the lung fields, the typical abnormalities consistent with pulmonary congestion may be present.

The Doppler echocardiogram is diagnostic. Transesophageal echocardiography is a particularly useful test because it provides enhanced resolution and unobstructed visualization of the mitral valve and the posterior cardiac structures, including the left atrium and the atrial appendage. Echocardiography gives a very accurate

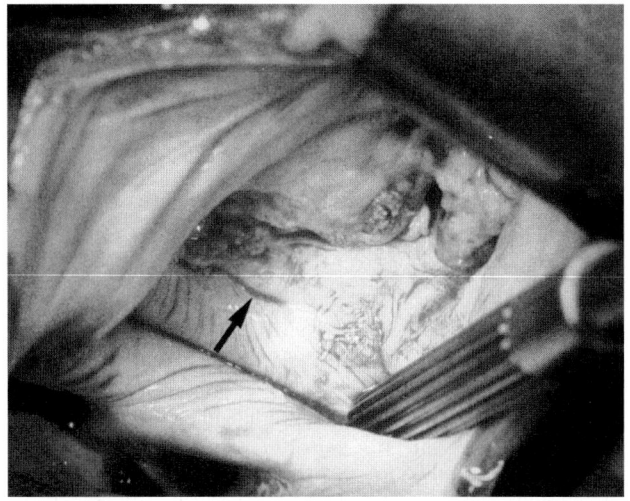

A

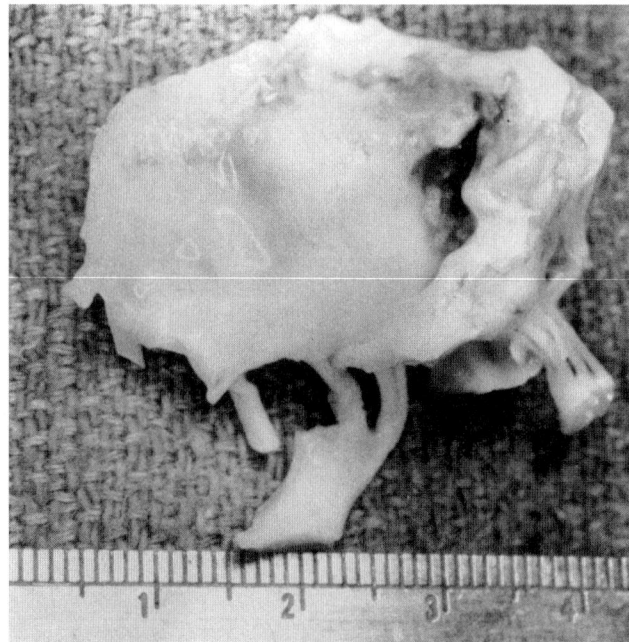

B

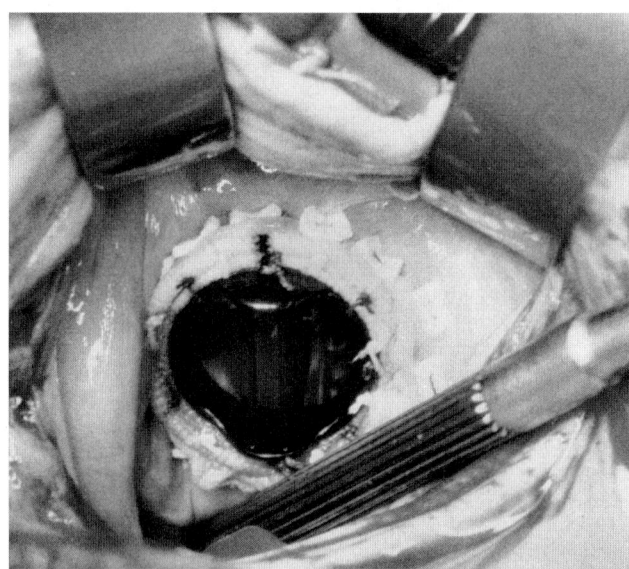

C

FIG. 20-13. *A.* Operative photograph of a rheumatic mitral valve with calcific mitral stenosis, viewed through a left atriotomy incision. *B.* Excised calcified mitral valve with fibrotic, shortened chordae tendineae. *C.* St. Jude mechanical mitral valve visualized through the open left atrium. Pledget-reinforced sutures were used to secure the valve in the native annulus.

measurement of the transvalvular gradient and the cross-sectional area of the mitral valve, and allows assessment of the degree of leaflet mobility, calcification, and subvalvular fusion, each of which may be important in predicting the feasibility of valve repair.

Cardiac angiography should be performed in patients in whom concomitant coronary artery disease is likely, based on the patient's history or risk factors, and in most patients older than 55 years of age. Right heart catheterization may be valuable in patients with pulmonary hypertension, although a reliable estimate of the pulmonary artery pressures can usually be determined from Doppler echocardiography.[71]

Indications for Valvuloplasty or Commissurotomy.
Although percutaneous balloon valvuloplasty has become an acceptable alternative for many patients with uncomplicated mitral

stenosis, open mitral commissurotomy remains an extremely reproducible and durable option. Commissurotomy has the advantage of allowing the surgeon to address nonpliable or calcified mitral valves, mobilize fused papillary muscles to correct subvalvular restrictive disease, effectively repair patients with mixed stenosis and insufficiency, and remove left atrial clot. Either balloon valvuloplasty or open surgical commissurotomy is indicated for symptomatic patients with moderate (mitral valve area <1.5 cm²) or severe (mitral valve area <1.0 cm²) mitral stenosis. Similarly, the development of pulmonary hypertension or embolic events in the presence of mitral stenosis is considered a relative indication for treatment. If the need for surgery is uncertain, exercise echocardiography may be useful, with a significant increase in the transvalvular gradient and a rise in pulmonary artery pressure being indications for intervention.

Mitral Insufficiency

Etiology. Degenerative disease is the most common cause of mitral insufficiency in the United States, accounting for 50 to 60% of the patients requiring surgery.[83] Other causes include rheumatic fever (15 to 20%), ischemic disease (15 to 20%), endocarditis, congenital abnormalities, and cardiomyopathy.

Pathology. The major structural components of the mitral valve are the annulus, the leaflets, the chordae tendinae, and the papillary muscles. A defect in any of these components may create mitral insufficiency. A functional classification for mitral insufficiency was proposed by Carpentier,[84] who characterized three basic types of functionally diseased valves. Type I insufficiency occurs from annular dilatation or leaflet perforation with normal leaflet motion. Type II occurs from leaflet prolapse or ruptured chordae tendinae with increased leaflet motion, typically occurring in patients with degenerative disease. Degenerative causes include myxomatous degeneration and fibroelastic deficiency. With myxomatous degeneration, thickened excessive leaflet tissue is present, with leaflet prolapse occurring from chordal elongation or chordal rupture. The valve usually has a billowing appearance (Barlow's syndrome). By contrast, patients with fibroelastic deficiency have thinned leaflets and chordae, with chordal elongation or rupture. In both types the mitral annulus is invariably dilated. Type III insufficiency occurs from restricted leaflet motion, with the leaflets not reaching the proper plane of closure during systole. Type III insufficiency typically occurs in rheumatic patients and in patients with chronic ischemic insufficiency.

In patients with rheumatic disease, the chordae tendinae are thickened and foreshortened, producing restrictive leaflet motion. Posterior dilatation of the mitral annulus is also usually present. With ischemic insufficiency, ventricular injury results in tethering of the mitral leaflets, producing restrictive leaflet motion, and central insufficiency, often with secondary annular dilation.

Pathophysiology. The basic physiologic abnormality in patients with mitral insufficiency is regurgitation of a portion of the left ventricular stroke volume into the left atrium. This results in decreased forward blood flow and an elevated left atrial pressure, producing pulmonary congestion and volume overload of the left ventricle.

As mitral insufficiency progresses there is a corresponding increase in the size of the left atrium, and eventually atrial fibrillation results. Concurrently, the left ventricle dilates. Initially the left ventricular stroke volume increases by Starling's law, but eventually this compensatory mechanism fails and the ejection fraction decreases. However, decreased systolic function of the heart is a relatively late finding, because the ventricle is "unloaded" as a result of the valvular insufficiency. Once left ventricular dysfunction and heart failure develop, the left ventricle usually has been significantly and often irreversibly injured.

Clinical Manifestations. In patients with acute mitral regurgitation, congestive heart failure develops suddenly, while in patients with chronic mitral insufficiency, the left atrium and ventricle become compliant, and symptoms do not develop until later in the course of the disease when the ventricle eventually fails, resulting in exertional dyspnea, decreased exercise capacity, and orthopnea. As left ventricular dysfunction progresses, symptoms of pulmonary congestion become more prominent, ultimately resulting in pulmonary hypertension and right-sided heart failure.

On physical examination the characteristic findings of mitral insufficiency are an apical holosystolic murmur and a forceful apical impulse. The apical murmur usually is harsh and transmitted to the axilla (in cases of anterior leaflet pathology), or to the left sternal border (typically in cases of posterior leaflet pathology), although this is variable. However, the severity of the insufficiency may not correlate with the intensity of the murmur.

Diagnostic Studies. The severity of mitral insufficiency can be determined accurately with echocardiography, along with the site of valvular prolapse or restriction, and the level of left ventricular function. An important measurement is the size of the cardiac chambers. The size of the left atrium reflects the chronicity and severity of the insufficiency. With severe, chronic mitral insufficiency, dilatation of the left atrium to 5 to 6 cm or greater is common. This is important because the propensity for atrial fibrillation is greatly increased when the left atrial size is more than 4.5 to 5 cm. The left ventricular diastolic dimensions become enlarged relatively early because of volume overload, but left ventricular systolic function is usually well maintained early in the course of the disease. Once the echocardiogram demonstrates a decrease in left ventricular systolic function, manifest as a rise in the end-systolic dimension of the heart and a drop in the ejection fraction, this is an indication that the left ventricle is beginning to decompensate. If there is uncertainty about the physiologic significance of mitral insufficiency, exercise stress-echocardiography may be used. Normally the ejection fraction rises with exercise, but a fall in ejection fraction with exercise is an early sign of left ventricular systolic dysfunction.

Indications for Operation. Delaying operation until the patient is severely symptomatic and the heart is markedly dilated often results in a certain degree of irreversible ventricular injury. According to ACC/AHA guidelines, mitral valve repair or replacement is recommended in any symptomatic patient with mitral insufficiency, even with normal left ventricular function (defined as ejection fraction greater than 60% and end-systolic dimension <45 mm).[71] Surgery also is currently recommended in asymptomatic patients with severe mitral insufficiency if there are signs of left ventricular systolic dysfunction (increased end-systolic dimension or decreased ejection fraction). Recent onset of atrial fibrillation, pulmonary hypertension, or an abnormal response to exercise testing are considered relative indications for surgery.

Mitral valve surgery should be strongly considered in most patients while they remain asymptomatic, prior to significant left ventricular dysfunction.[85] A retrospective study by David and associates compared 289 symptomatic with 199 asymptomatic patients undergoing mitral valve repair for degenerative disease.[86] Survival at 15 years was 76% for asymptomatic patients, identical to that for the general population matched for age and sex, compared to a survival of 53% for symptomatic patients.

Operative Techniques

The traditional approach for mitral valve surgery is through a median sternotomy incision with cardiopulmonary bypass and cardioplegic arrest. The mitral valve is exposed through a left atrial incision, made posterior and parallel to the intra-atrial groove. After the left atrial incision is made, self-retaining retractor blades are inserted to expose the mitral valve. In certain patients exposure through the posterior left atrial approach may not be optimal. This is particularly true in patients with a small left atrium, a deep chest, or an aortic prosthesis in place, and in reoperations in which the tissue is fixed and nonelastic. Alternative incisions for exposing the difficult mitral valve include a right atriotomy with transseptal incision, a superior approach through the dome of the atrium, and the biatrial transseptal approach.[87]

Commissurotomy.   Once cardiopulmonary bypass has been established and the heart has been arrested, the left atrium is opened and the mitral valve is visualized. Initially the atrial cavity is examined for thrombi, especially within the atrial appendage. The mitral valve is assessed by evaluating leaflet mobility, commissural fusion, and the degree of fibrosis in the subvalvular apparatus. A right-angle clamp often is placed beneath the commissures, gently applying horizontal tension to evaluate commissural fusion.

Once the commissure has been accurately identified and the chordae noted, a right-angle clamp is introduced beneath the fused commissure, stretching the adjacent chordae and leaflets, after which the commissure is carefully incised. The incision is made 2 to 3 mm at a time, serially confirming that the separated margins of the commissural leaflet remain attached to chordae tendineae. The usual commissurotomy curves slightly anteriorly and does not go directly laterally. The incision should stop 1 to 2 mm from the valve annulus where the leaflet tissue becomes thin, indicating the transition from the fused commissure to the normal commissural leaflet of the mitral valve. Once the commissurotomy is completed, any fused papillary muscle is incised as necessary to minimize restriction and improve mobility of the attached leaflet.

After separation of the commissure and mobilization of the underlying chordae tendineae and papillary muscle, leaflet mobility is assessed visually. The anterior leaflet is grasped with a forceps and moved throughout the entire range of motion, looking for subvalvular restriction or leaflet rigidity. In some patients, restricted motion may be further improved by dividing secondary chordae or by the selective débridement of calcium. Extremely thickened chordae can be mobilized by excision of a triangular portion of the fused cords. If extensive débridement and mobilization of the chordal structures are necessary, valve replacement usually is more appropriate. At least 30% of patients undergoing commissurotomy require more than simple incision of the commissure to produce an adequate mitral orifice and to restore mobility to the valve. Competence of the valve is assessed by injection of cold saline into the ventricle.

If the patient is in atrial fibrillation, the atrial appendage is closed with a continuous suture of 3-0 polypropylene to minimize the subsequent risk of emboli. Recently, intraoperative radiofrequency ablation procedures of the left atrium combined with mitral valve surgery have become widely used in an attempt to convert these patients to sinus rhythm.

Mitral Valve Replacement.   Mitral valve replacement is necessary when the extent of disease precludes commissurotomy or valve reconstruction. Valve replacement is most likely in patients with long-standing rheumatic disease. Once the valve is exposed and the need for valve replacement is determined, an incision is made in the anterior mitral leaflet, usually starting at the 12 o'clock position, and most of the anterior leaflet is resected. The posterior leaflet is preserved whenever possible, and the chordal attachments to both leaflets are preserved or reattached to the annulus, as this has been shown to improve left ventricular function and lower the risk of posterior left ventricular free wall rupture, a potentially lethal complication of valve replacement. However, chordal preservation is not always possible in patients with extensive rheumatic disease, because of extensive valvular thickening and calcification.

When the mitral valve is excised, an appropriate-sized replacement valve is selected. This valve usually is attached with 12 to 16 mattress sutures. A pledgeted mattress suture technique is recommended because it minimizes the risk of perivalvular leakage. The sutures may be inserted from the atrial to the ventricular side, everting the annulus and seating the valve intra-annularly, or from the ventricular side to the atrial side, resulting in supra-annular positioning of the prosthetic valve. Care is taken to insert the sutures precisely into the annular tissue because excessively deep insertion of sutures may injure critical structures, including the circumflex coronary artery posterolaterally (from the surgeon's perspective, at 7 to 8 o'clock), the atrioventricular node anteromedially (at 1 to 2 o'clock), or the aortic valve anterolaterally (at 10 to 12 o'clock). Once the sutures are placed through the mitral annulus, they are placed through the valve sewing ring. The valve is then lowered onto the annulus and the sutures are tied and cut. The atriotomy incision is closed, and after air is removed from the cardiac chambers, the aortic cross-clamp is removed and the heart is restarted.

Mitral Valve Reconstruction.   The basic techniques of mitral valve reconstruction include resection of the posterior leaflet, chordal shortening, chordal transposition, artificial chordal replacement, and triangular resection for repair of the anterior leaflet disease. An annuloplasty to correct associated annular dilation also is recommended in most cases.

The intraoperative assessment of the valvular pathology is an important step in valve reconstruction. A localized roughened area of atrial endocardium, termed a jet lesion, may be present from regurgitant blood striking the endocardium, providing a guide to the location of the insufficiency. Subsequently the commissures are examined, noting whether these are prolapsed, fused, or malformed. The closing plane of the leaflets in the area supported by commissural chordae is determined next, and the anterior and posterior leaflets are then examined, noting areas of prolapse or restriction. Such abnormalities as perforation, fibrosis, calcification, or leaflet clefts must also be recognized. Finally, the degree of annular enlargement is assessed.

Proper evaluation of the degree of leaflet prolapse is critical. The "billowing" mitral valve originally described by Barlow has excessive leaflet tissue, but may remain competent if the chordae are not elongated. In such cases, the rough free edge of the leaflet closes at the proper level, even though the midportion of the leaflet may contain excessive tissue. The anterolateral commissural chordae are seldom elongated, so elevating the commissural leaflet with a nerve hook provides a valuable reference point from which the degree of elongation of other chordae may be determined. Chordal rupture or total lack of structural support leads to prolapse and a completely flail leaflet.

Posterior Leaflet Procedures.   Quadrangular resection of the posterior leaflet has become the mainstay of mitral valve reconstruction (Figs. 20-14 and 20-15). A rectangular excision is performed, cutting directly down to, but not through, the mitral annulus. Diseased tissue in the posterior leaflet is excised with a quadrangular excision, usually removing 1 to 2 cm of tissue. Strong chordae of proper length are identified on each side of the excised leaflet and encircled with retraction sutures.

Once the quadrangular excision has been performed, the annulus of the excised segment of leaflet is corrected either by simple annular plication, folding plasty, or sliding plasty.[88] The simple annular plication is performed with several interrupted sutures placed about 5 mm apart. These are started centrally and extended to include a few millimeters of annulus adjacent to the remaining leaflets. When these annular sutures are tied, the leaflet margins are automatically

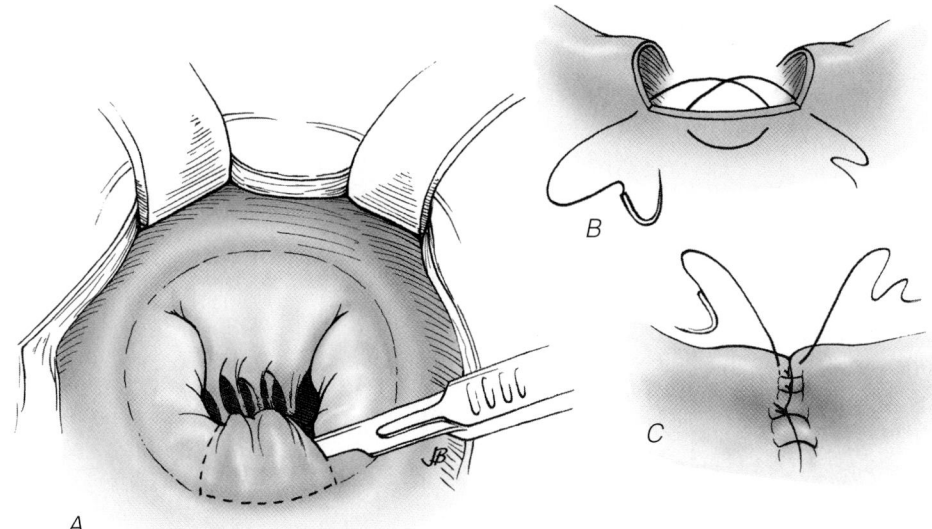

FIG. 20-14. Illustration of rectangular resection and repair for correction of posterior leaflet prolapse. (Reproduced with permission from Galloway AC, Colvin SB, Baumann SG, et al: Current concepts of mitral valve reconstruction for mitral insufficiency. Circulation 78:1087, 1988.)

brought into apposition without any tension. If there was tension on the leaflet tissues, there would be a serious possibility of dehiscence of the subsequent leaflet repair. Once the annular sutures have been tied, the leaflet margins are approximated with simple or figure-of-eight sutures, usually 4-0 or 5-0 polypropylene, depending on the thickness of the leaflets.

The folding plasty technique, described by the group from New York University (NYU), involves folding down the cut vertical edges of the posterior leaflet to the annulus and closing the ensuing cleft.[88] With this technique the central height of the posterior leaflet is reduced, the edge of leaflet coaptation is moved posteriorly, and annular plication is either eliminated or reduced. This elimination of annular plication avoids the serious complication of circumflex artery kinking, which may occur in the setting of left dominant coronary artery circulation and a large posterior leaflet resection. The sliding plasty technique reported by Carpentier and associates also is successful in reducing posterior leaflet height and moving the edge of leaflet coaptation posteriorly.[89]

Often the valve appears quite competent after the leaflet repair has been completed. Gently injecting saline into the ventricle with a bulb syringe and noting both the mobility of the leaflets and their apposition is an excellent visual guide for assessing competency. If localized insufficiency remains in other areas, additional procedures can be performed.

Anterior Leaflet Procedures. Four primary techniques are used for anterior leaflet reconstruction: chordal shortening, chordal transposition, artificial chordal replacement, and triangular resection of anterior leaflet tissue with primary repair. With chordal shortening, the elongated chord is imbricated either onto the free edge of the leaflet or onto the papillary muscle (Fig. 20-16). In contrast, the chordal transposition technique utilizes a segment of structurally intact posterior leaflet directly opposite the prolapsed anterior leaflet. A small quadrangular excision of the posterior leaflet with the attached chordae is performed, and the mobilized leaflet and chordae are then transposed onto the anterior leaflet to provide structural support. The defect created in the posterior leaflet is then repaired in the manner described above. Artificial chordae replacement has been used by some groups as an alternative for anterior leaflet repair, utilizing polytetrafluoroethylene sutures that are attached to both the papillary muscle and the free edge of the prolapsing leaflet

to re-establish structural support. Finally, triangular resection and primary repair has been increasingly used at NYU for treatment of anterior leaflet prolapse (Fig. 20-17). The adjacent intact chordae are identified, and triangular resection is performed to remove the prolapsing segment of the leaflet and any ruptured chordae. The technique is particularly helpful when a large amount of redundant anterior leaflet tissue is present, as in patients with myxomatous degeneration and Barlow's syndrome.

Repair of Leaflet Perforation. Leaflet perforations can be repaired by primary suture closure or by closure with a pericardial patch. Extensive leaflet destruction is best managed with mitral valve replacement.

Annuloplasty. Use of a mitral valve annuloplasty device (ring or partial band) to correct annular dilation during valve repair decreases the risk of late repair failure.[90,91] The primary purpose of an annuloplasty device is to correct the associated annular dilation that invariably occurs in patients with chronic mitral insufficiency, regardless of etiology, and results in worsening central insufficiency due to lack of leaflet coaptation. Various types of annuloplasty devices are available, including rigid or semirigid rings that geometrically remodel the annulus, flexible rings or bands that provide no geometric remodeling but restrict annular dilation while maintaining physiologic sphincter motion of the annulus, and semirigid bands that provide both annular remodeling and physiologic annular sphincter motion (Fig. 20-18). The relative advantages of the different types of devices remain under investigation, but it is widely accepted that use of an annuloplasty device to correct annular dilation improves long-term repair durability.

Results

Commissurotomy. The operative risk for open mitral commissurotomy is less than 1%, and long-term results have been excellent. Choudhary and associates reported a 10-year freedom from mitral valve failure after open commissurotomy of 87.0 ± 3.5%.[92] The incidence of thromboembolism was only 0.5% per patient-year. Antunes and colleagues reported favorable long-term results after open commissurotomy in 100 patients with a mean follow-up of 8.5 years.[93] The 9-year actuarial freedom from reoperation was 98%, and 93% were in NYHA functional class I or II. Open mitral

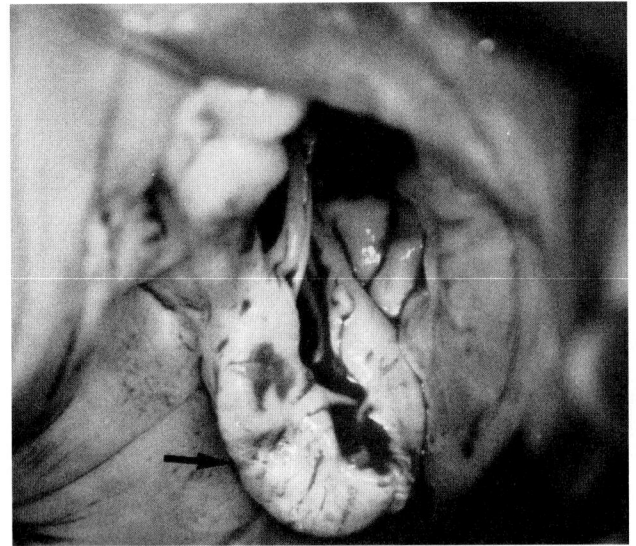

A

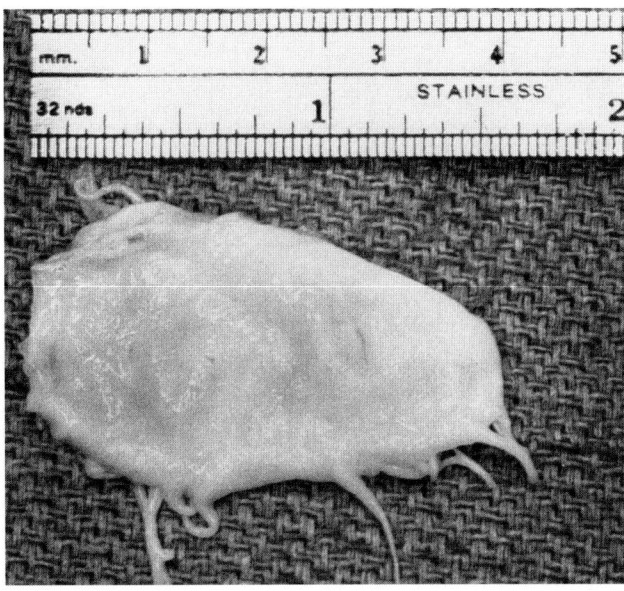

B

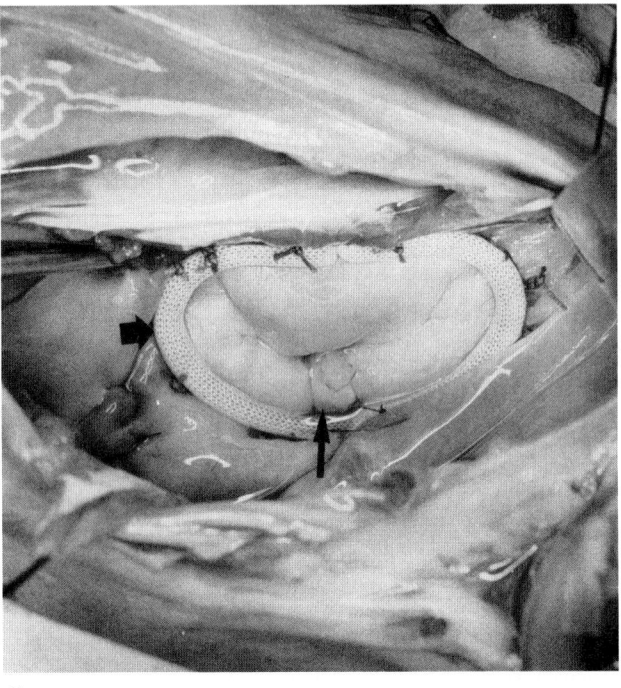

C

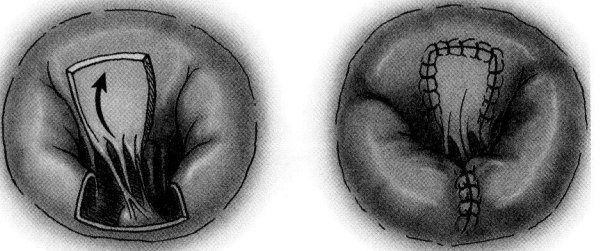

FIG. 20-16. Illustration of chordal transposition from the posterior leaflet to correct anterior leaflet prolapse. (*Reproduced with permission from Galloway AC, Colvin SB, Baumann SG, et al: Current concepts of mitral valve reconstruction for mitral insufficiency. Circulation 78:1087, 1988.*)

FIG. 20-15. *A.* Operative photograph demonstrating myxomatous mitral valve with massive prolapse and a flail posterior leaflet. *B.* Specimen of resected mitral valve posterior leaflet. *C.* Operative photograph of completed mitral valve reconstruction. The small arrow indicates the posterior leaflet repair, while the large arrow demonstrates the ring annuloplasty. Note the total correction of leaflet prolapse and annular dilatation.

commissurotomy is a well-established procedure, allowing effective correction of mitral stenosis.

Balloon Valvuloplasty. Percutaneous mitral balloon valvuloplasty has recently been developed as an alternative treatment for mitral stenosis. The choice between surgical commissurotomy and balloon valvuloplasty varies widely among centers. The main advantages of commissurotomy over balloon valvuloplasty are that during surgery the fused chordae can be surgically divided and mobility restored.

A prospective and randomized study has suggested that percutaneous balloon valvuloplasty and surgical commissurotomy result in comparable clinical improvement in selected patients with mitral stenosis.[94] Mitral valve areas were larger early after surgical

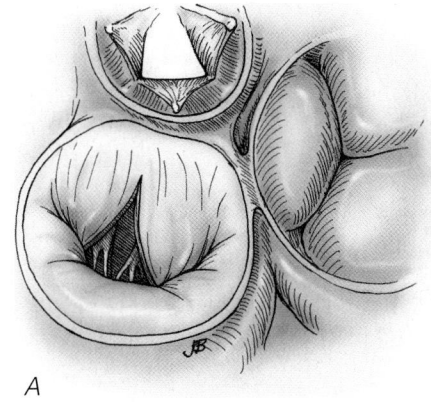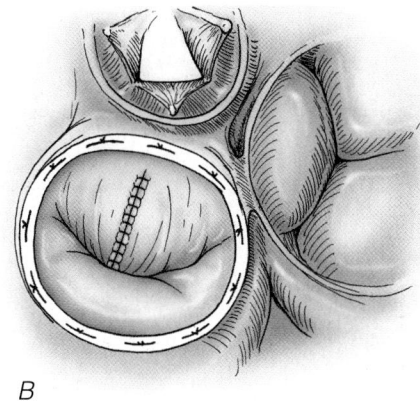

FIG. 20-17. *A. Illustration of triangular resection of the anterior mitral leaflet. B. Suture repair of the defect.*

A   *B*

commissurotomy, but were similar after 24 months. Patients receiving balloon valvuloplasty require more rigid selection criteria, as the procedure becomes less effective if the patient has significant calcification of the valve or fusion of the subvalvular apparatus.

Valve Replacement. The operative mortality rate for mitral valve replacement is 2 to 6%, depending on the number of comorbidities present. The major predictors of increased operative risk after mitral valve replacement are age, left ventricular function, emergency operation, NYHA functional status, previous cardiac surgery, associated coronary artery disease, and concomitant disease in another valve. Mohty and associates reported late survival rates after mitral valve replacement of $71 \pm 3\%$, $49 \pm 3\%$, and $29 \pm 4\%$ at 5, 10, and 15 years, respectively.[95] The major factors influencing long-term survival are age, urgency of operation, NYHA functional status, mitral insufficiency (versus stenosis), ischemic etiology, pulmonary hypertension, and the need for concomitant coronary bypass or procedures on another valve.

Improved engineering of mechanical prostheses has produced valves with lower intrinsic thrombogenicity and better durability, resulting in fewer late valve-related complications. Khan and coworkers compared late results in 513 patients receiving mechanical valves with 402 patients receiving tissue valves.[96] There was no difference

in survival or in thromboembolic or anticoagulation-related complications between the groups. However, freedom from reoperation at 15 years was 98% with mechanical valves and 79% with tissue valves. Thus while mechanical valves and tissue valves result in similar long-term survival, there is an increased risk of late reoperation in patients receiving tissue valves.

Valve Repair. The operative risk for mitral valve repair is less than 1 to 2%, and late results have demonstrated that compared to replacement, repair is associated with improved survival and better freedom from valve-related complications.[97,98] A recent report on 1195 patients undergoing valve repair and ring annuloplasty demonstrated that the actuarial freedoms from complications at 5 and 10 years, respectively, were as follows: thromboembolic, 92 and 88%; anticoagulant-related complications, 98 and 96%; endocarditis, 97 and 96%; and reoperation, 91 and 84%.[99] The need for anterior leaflet repair (as compared to posterior leaflet repair or annuloplasty alone) did not compromise the 5-year results in terms of patient survival, risk of reoperation, or freedom from valve-related complications. The freedom from reoperation, however, has been shown to be significantly better in nonrheumatic patients (93% at 5 years, 88% at 10 years) than in rheumatic patients (86% at 5 years, 73% at 10 years; $p < 0.005$).

Braunberger and associates reported long-term (20-year) results after mitral repair in 162 patients with nonrheumatic mitral valve insufficiency.[100] The 20-year Kaplan-Meier survival rate was 48%, which is similar to the normal age-matched population. Freedom from cardiac death was 92 and 81% at 10 and 20 years, respectively. The linearized risk of reoperation rate was 0.4% per patient-year, although the need for anterior leaflet repair did decrease late repair durability. Repair of posterior leaflet prolapse resulted in a 98.5% freedom from reoperation at 10 years, while anterior leaflet repair had an 86.2% percent freedom from reoperation at 10 years ($p < 0.03$).

Mohty and associates reported the results of 679 mitral valve repairs and 238 valve replacements performed at the Mayo Clinic between 1980 and 1995.[95] Survival after valve repair was better than after valve replacement (68 ± 2 vs. $49 \pm 3\%$ at 10 years and $37 \pm 5\%$ vs. $29 \pm 4\%$ at 15 years), with an adjusted odds ratio for death of 0.68 for repair versus replacement ($p < 0.002$). The overall late risk of reoperation after valve repair was only 16% at 15 years.

Minimally Invasive Mitral Valve Surgery. Newer techniques which allow mitral valve repair or replacement to be performed with a minimally invasive incision have been increasingly used over the last decade. Most techniques employ either

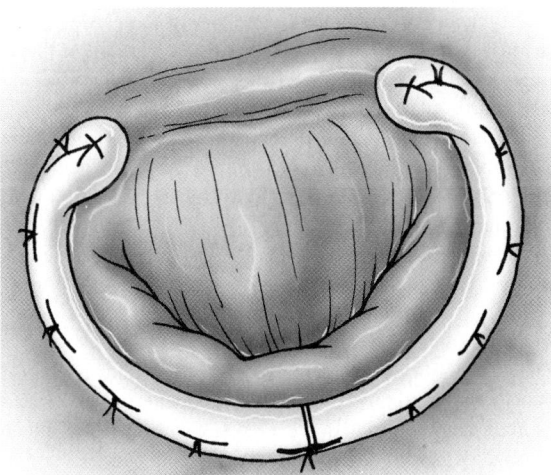

FIG. 20-18. *Illustration of Colvin-Galloway Future Band sewn into mitral valve annulus. This annuloplasty device corrects annular dilatation and restores appropriate geometric configuration to the annulus. (Illustration courtesy of Medtronic, Inc., Minneapolis, MN.)*

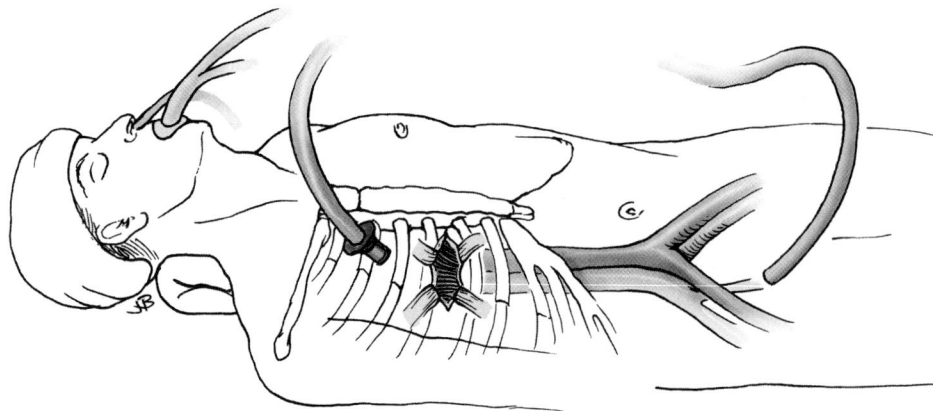

FIG. 20-19. Schematic diagram demonstrating operative approach for minimally invasive mitral valve surgery. A fourth interspace anterior minithoracotomy is shown, with direct aortic cannulation through the second interspace and percutaneous venous cannulation via the right femoral vein. (Reproduced with permission from Sharony R, Grossi EA, Saunders PC, et al: Operative techniques in thoracic and cardiovascular surgery. 8:4, 2004.)

minithoracotomy or a partial sternotomy incision. At NYU minimally invasive mitral valve surgery has been performed through a small right anterior thoracotomy incision, entering the chest through the third or fourth intercostal space (Fig. 20-19). Others have used partial upper sternotomy, partial lower sternotomy, or parasternal incisions. The ascending aorta may be directly cannulated for perfusion, or cannulation may be performed through the femoral artery, while venous drainage for cardiopulmonary bypass may be achieved either directly from the right atrium or from the femoral vein. Similar to traditional surgery, the operation is performed with moderate systemic hypothermia (28 to 30°C) and cardioplegia is used for myocardial protection. The aorta may be directly occluded with a flexible or special long cross-clamp or occluded internally with a balloon catheter. Long instruments are required but standard valve techniques are used.[101]

Grossi and associates analyzed the initial NYU minimally invasive mitral valve experience in 714 patients operated on between 1996 and 2001. Hospital mortality was 1.1% for isolated mitral valve repair and 5.8% for isolated valve replacement. The risk of complications was similar to that reported with conventional surgery, although minimally invasive patients needed less blood and had less pain, fewer infections, a shorter hospital stay, and a quicker overall recovery.[102,103] Galloway and colleagues reported late results after minimally invasive valve repair, demonstrating that repair durability, freedom from valve-related complications, and survival were equivalent to results achieved with the traditional sternotomy approach.[99] Thus the results after minimally invasive valve surgery are encouraging, and more widespread utilization of minimally invasive techniques is likely in the future.

New Developments

Edge-to-Edge Repair. In 1995, Alfieri described the "double-orifice" or "edge-to-edge" repair as an alternative technique for repair for mitral insufficiency.[104] With this technique the free edge of the anterior leaflet is sutured to the opposing free edge of the posterior leaflet, converting the valve into a double-orifice "bow tie." The edge-to-edge technique has been used for anterior leaflet pathology,[105] ischemic insufficiency,[106] endocarditis,[107] and dilated cardiomyopathy.[108] This method may be used as a primary repair technique or as an alternative after incomplete correction with other methods.[106] However, the late results after edge-to-edge repair are not well established, and some reports suggest that the edge-to-edge technique may negatively influence late repair durability.[107]

Robotic Mitral Valve Surgery. Recent technological achievements in optics and computerized telemanipulation have

enabled robotically assisted mitral valve operations. Chitwood and associates[109] and Mohr and associates[110] have reported encouraging results with robotically and videoscopically assisted mitral valve repair, with femoral perfusion and a transthoracic aortic cross-clamp. The da Vinci and Zeus robots are currently available for surgical use. Both are master-slave (console-effector) telemanipulation systems equipped with three-dimensional cameras. It has been reported that the articulated wrist-like instruments and three-dimensional visualization of the da Vinci surgical system enable precise tissue telemanipulation. These systems still have significant limitations, however, and may not be readily adaptable to performing the multiple complex tasks necessary for valve surgery.[111] While the use of robotics in valve surgery is exciting and may offer promise for the future, the current technique is limited by complexity and cost, with few cost-benefit outcome analyses yet available.

Aortic Valve Disease

Effective surgical treatment of aortic valve disease became possible in 1960 with the development of satisfactory prosthetic valves by Starr and Edwards and by Harken and associates.

Aortic Stenosis

Etiology. In the adult North American population the primary causes of aortic stenosis include acquired calcific disease, bicuspid aortic valve, and rheumatic disease.[112] Acquired calcific aortic stenosis typically occurs in the seventh or eighth decade of life, and is the most frequent etiology, accounting for over half of the cases. Acquired calcific stenosis, also termed degenerative aortic stenosis or senile aortic stenosis, appears to be related to the aging process, with progressive degeneration leading to valve damage and calcification, although a causative role of lipids has been demonstrated recently. Lipid-lowering drugs seem to slow the progression of acquired calcific stenosis.

Biscuspid aortic valve accounts for approximately one third of the cases of aortic stenosis in adults, typically presenting in the fourth or fifth decade of life, after years of turbulent flow through the bicuspid valve results in damage and calcification.

The third major cause of aortic stenosis, rheumatic heart disease, accounts for approximately 10 to 15% of patients in North America, but is more common in underdeveloped countries. With rheumatic disease the degree of stenosis progresses with time. Concomitant mitral valve disease almost always is present, although not always clinically significant.

Pathophysiology. Generally, the aortic valve must be reduced to one third its normal cross-sectional area before significant hemodynamic changes occur. A normal aortic valve has a cross-sectional area of 2.5 to 3.5 cm^2. Moderate aortic stenosis is defined as an aortic valve area between 0.8 and 1.2 cm^2, while severe stenosis is defined as a valve area less than 0.8 cm^2.[71] Patients with severe stenosis typically have a mean transvalvular pressure gradient greater than 50 mm Hg, although the gradient is dependent on both the valve area and the cardiac output, and therefore may not be severely elevated if the cardiac output is low. Once the valve area is less than 0.5 cm^2, with a transvalvular gradient of 100 mm Hg or greater, the degree of stenosis is considered critical.

Aortic stenosis results in increased myocardial work and progressive concentric left ventricular hypertrophy with little ventricular dilatation. This results in a thick, noncompliant ventricle, leading to early diastolic dysfunction. The significance of diastolic dysfunction has been intensively studied and has been implicated as a major cause of congestive heart failure in patients with aortic stenosis. The systolic function of the ventricle usually remains well preserved for many years, but eventually deteriorates due to long-standing increased afterload.

Myocardial ischemia develops in some patients with severe aortic stenosis, usually in response to exercise. The left ventricular mass and left ventricular systolic wall tension are increased, resulting in increased oxygen demand. Simultaneously, the cardiac output often is low and does not increase in response to exercise. The end-diastolic pressure of the ventricle becomes progressively elevated during exercise, resulting in increased demand, but with poor perfusion of the subendocardium.

Clinical Manifestations. The classic symptoms of aortic stenosis include exertional dyspnea, decreased exercise capacity, heart failure, angina, and syncope. Once the patient becomes symptomatic, prompt operation is indicated. If heart failure, angina, or syncope is present, the need for surgery is more urgent, as the risk of death exceeds 30 to 50% over the next 5 years. Sudden death, which accounts for a significant number of fatalities from aortic stenosis, possibly due to arrhythmias, becomes a more likely threat once the patient becomes severely symptomatic.

The most common symptoms are exertional dyspnea and decreased exercise capacity (NYHA class II or III), which are indicative of progressive left ventricular decompensation. The presence of NYHA class IV symptoms, manifest as congestive heart failure, orthopnea, pulmonary edema, and right-sided heart dysfunction, is a more ominous finding. Once congestive heart failure is present, the mortality approaches 40% over 2 to 3 years.

Angina pectoris, which may develop in patients with advanced disease, is a manifestation of increased left ventricular mass and increased myocardial strain, resulting in subendocardial ischemia. Subclinical ischemic episodes may be associated with silent myocardial necrosis, and patients with little history and few prior symptoms may present with markedly depressed left ventricular function, with large amounts of myocardium replaced by scar tissue.

Syncope may develop in patients with severe aortic stenosis secondary to the severe flow limitations imposed by the tightly stenotic valve and decreased cerebral blood flow. Syncope typically develops in response to exercise, but may occur when patients vasodilate from any cause after minimal effort and with little warning. In a small proportion of patients, syncope results from heart block. The average life expectancy once angina or syncope has appeared is 3 to 5 years.

With auscultation the principal finding is a harsh, diamond-shaped (crescendo-decrescendo) systolic murmur at the base of the heart (right second intercostal space) with radiation to the carotid arteries. The two components of the S_2 may become synchronous, or aortic valve closure may even follow pulmonic valve closure, causing paradoxical splitting of the S_2. An S_4 gallop at the apex reflects the presence of left ventricular hypertrophy or heart failure. The apical impulse has been described as a "prolonged heave," while the pulse pressure in the peripheral circulation is usually narrow and sustained (pulsus parvus et tardus).

Diagnostic Studies. On x-ray the heart size may be either normal or enlarged due to left ventricular hypertrophy. Calcification of the valve often is visible in older patients. The ECG may demonstrate left ventricular hypertrophy, but may also be normal. Conduction abnormalities are common, apparently from spicules of calcium projecting into the conduction bundle located at the base of the commissure between the right cusp and noncoronary cusp, and some patients may develop complete heart block. Atrial fibrillation generally indicates the presence of advanced disease with a prolonged elevation of intracardiac pressures.

The diagnosis of aortic stenosis is now most frequently made by echocardiography, which provides an accurate estimate of the peak and mean systolic transvalvular gradients, which allows calculation of the aortic valve area. Since the Doppler echocardiogram measures flow velocity, the peak instantaneous pressure gradient may overestimate the true peak gradient, and the mean gradient is usually more accurate. The echocardiogram also can demonstrate the amount of calcium in the leaflets, the degree of leaflet immobility, the left atrial size, the degree of left ventricular hypertrophy, the end-systolic and end-diastolic dimensions of the left ventricle, and the left ventricular function. Finally, the echocardiogram is important for identifying any occult subvalvular stenosis and for differentiating valvular stenosis from idiopathic hypertrophic subaortic stenosis (IHSS).

Cardiac catheterization readily confirms the diagnosis by measuring the aortic transvalvular gradient and permitting calculation of the cross-sectional area of the valve, but is often unnecessary for this purpose in the current era due to the accuracy of echocardiography. However, coronary angiography should be performed in patients over 55 years of age and in patients at high risk for coronary artery disease. The degree of pulmonary hypertension also should be measured in patients with severe congestive heart failure and NYHA class IV symptoms.

Operative Indications. Patients with aortic stenosis typically respond well to aortic valve replacement, which immediately relieves the increased afterload. A special subgroup of patients includes those with critical aortic stenosis and advanced left ventricular systolic dysfunction. These patients have an increased operative risk, but may still have significant improvement after valve replacement as long as the ventricle is not irreversibly damaged.[113] Echocardiographic signs of left ventricular dysfunction must be carefully assessed even in asymptomatic patients, since it is well documented that once ventricular systolic dysfunction occurs, symptoms progressively develop within 1 to 2 years, with congestive heart failure and ventricular damage progressing thereafter.

Aortic valve replacement is indicated for virtually all symptomatic patients with aortic stenosis. Even in patients with NYHA class IV symptoms and poor ventricular function, surgery has been found to improve both functional status and survival. In asymptomatic patients with moderate to severe stenosis, periodic echocardiographic studies are performed to assess the transvalvular gradient, valve area, left ventricular size, and left ventricular function. Surgery is indicated with the first sign of left ventricular systolic dysfunction, manifest on echocardiography as either a rise in the left ventricular end-systolic size or a drop in the left ventricular ejection fraction. Surgery may also be recommended for asymptomatic patients with aortic stenosis who have a progressive increase in the transvalvular gradient on serial echocardiographic studies, a rapid rise in diastolic dimensions, a valve area less than 0.80 cm^2, progressive pulmonary hypertension, or right ventricular dysfunction during exercise testing.[114]

Aortic Insufficiency

Etiology and Pathology. A variety of diseases can produce aortic valve insufficiency, including degenerative diseases, inflammatory or infectious diseases (endocarditis, rheumatic fever), congenital diseases, aortoannular ectasia or aneurysm of the aortic root, and aortic dissection. Mixed valvular stenosis and insufficiency can develop in any patient with aortic stenosis, regardless of etiology.

Degenerative valvular disease is a manifestation of fibroelastic deficiency or myxomatous degeneration that produces thin and elongated valvular tissue. The aortic valve leaflets sag into the ventricular lumen, often with no other tissue abnormality, producing central aortic insufficiency. The gross and histologic appearances suggest that this is a variant of the more common mitral valve prolapse.

Infectious and inflammatory etiologies of aortic insufficiency include bacterial endocarditis and rheumatic fever. Streptococci, staphylococci, or enterococci are the most common bacteria involved, in decreasing order of frequency. Syphilis is increasingly rare. Rheumatic fever often produces mixed stenosis and insufficiency, but may produce aortic insufficiency alone. Concomitant mitral valve disease is invariably present.

Patients who have a congenitally bicuspid aortic valve rarely become symptomatic during childhood, but prolonged turbulence may lead to aortic stenosis, mixed stenosis and insufficiency, or pure insufficiency later in life. Congenital causes of aortic insufficiency account for 10 to 15% of the patients operated on for aortic insufficiency as adults. Congenital aortic insufficiency may also occur secondary to subaortic ventricular septal defect, with valvular insufficiency developing from a Venturi effect that results in prolapse of the aortic valve leaflet into the septal defect.

Aneurysmal dilation of the aortic root is thought to be secondary to idiopathic or known connective tissue disorders, with the idiopathic variety seen with increasing frequency as the average age of the population increases. In the less severe forms of degenerative diseases of the aorta, such as idiopathic cystic medial necrosis, there may be a localized aneurysm in the ascending aorta or aortic root, with or without associated aortic valve insufficiency, depending on the degree of distortion of the sinotubular junction. Aortoannular ectasia with aneurysm of the aortic root occurs in its most extreme form in patients with Marfan's syndrome or Ehlers-Danlos syndrome. These connective tissue disorders involve defective genes coding for fibrillin cross-linkage or collagen synthesis, resulting in extensive weakness within the aortic wall with frequent involvement of the aortic root. A common presentation is aneurysmal dilation of the entire aortic root with concomitant aortic valve insufficiency. These patients also have an increased risk of aneurysmal disease elsewhere in the aorta, a high incidence of mitral valve prolapse, and a greatly increased risk of aortic dissection. Typically the aortic root gradually enlarges, starting in the sinuses of Valsalva and progressing until the entire root is involved. Valvular insufficiency results from dilatation of both the aortic sinotubular junction and the aortic valve annulus. The size and shape of the aneurysm is characteristic, resembling an inverted, truncated cone, with the narrow apex in the mid-to-distal ascending aorta and a large dilated aortic root.

Acute aortic dissection may produce aortic valve insufficiency by detachment of the commissures and prolapse of the valve cusps, usually involving the noncoronary cusp and the commissure between the left and right cusps. In patients with chronic dissection, the sinotubular junction is usually dilated and distorted, producing leaflet prolapse and valvular insufficiency. Both the aortic root and ascending aorta may be aneurysmal secondary to the chronic dissection.

Pathophysiology. With aortic valve insufficiency, blood regurgitates into the left ventricle during diastole, producing left ventricular volume overload (increased preload). The ventricle compensates by the Starling mechanism and increases the left ventricular stroke volume during systole. A widened pulse pressure and low diastolic pressure result in diminished coronary perfusion, while oxygen demand is increased secondary to the large stroke volume and increased cardiac work. Progressive valvular insufficiency results in ventricular dilation and eccentric left ventricular hypertrophy, with the heart initially compensating to maintain a normal ratio of wall thickness to cavity size. Since ventricular compliance is normal, the left ventricular diastolic pressure does not increase initially, and the patient usually remains asymptomatic for a long period of time despite significant diastolic volume overload. As the heart continues to dilate, however, the ventricular muscle can no longer compensate and the ratio of wall thickness to cavity size decreases. The systolic wall tension required for ejection eventually exceeds the ability of the ventricular muscle to contract, resulting in "afterload mismatch" and progressive systolic dysfunction. Further progression leads to left ventricular failure and pulmonary hypertension. In the advanced stages, fibrosis develops within the myocardium, which further contributes to systolic dysfunction, ultimately resulting in a dilated myopathic ventricle.

Clinical Manifestations. Symptoms develop at variable rates in patients with aortic insufficiency, depending on the acuity and severity of the insufficiency and the compliance and strength of the heart muscle. Frequently the patient who gradually develops moderate to severe insufficiency remains asymptomatic for many years, often 10 or more. Once symptoms appear, however, ventricular function usually is significantly depressed and rapid clinical deterioration occurs over the next 4 to 5 years. The terminal illness usually is progressive heart failure and arrhythmias.

The most common symptoms are dyspnea on exertion and decreased exercise capacity. These symptoms gradually increase in severity as the ventricle deteriorates. Palpitations are also common, apparently arising from forceful contraction of the dilated left ventricle. NYHA class IV symptoms, angina, and right heart failure occur with advanced disease or with severe incompetence in which the regurgitant flow exceeds 50% of forward flow.

Palpation reveals an enlarged heart and a prominent cardiac impulse described as a "forceful thrust," with the point of maximal impact displaced inferiorly and leftward. The hallmark of aortic insufficiency is a high-pitched decrescendo diastolic murmur heard best in the left third intercostal space with the patient erect and leaning forward. The length of the murmur may correspond with the severity of the insufficiency, but the intensity does not. If the murmur is loudest to the right of the sternum, aortoannular ectasia is likely. A light systolic ejection murmur due to increased flow across the aortic valve may also be present. An S_3 gallop, if present, is indicative of heart failure. A mid-diastolic rumble at the apex that simulates mitral stenosis has been described, the Austin Flint murmur. This murmur is produced by the aortic insufficiency impeding the opening of the mitral valve during diastole.

Examination of the peripheral arterial circulation may reveal several abnormalities. The pulse pressure is widened, partly from an increase in systolic pressure, but principally from a decrease in diastolic pressure, which may be in the range of 30 to 40 mm Hg. The true diastolic pressure, measured by direct arterial puncture, is never less than 30 to 35 mm Hg, even though on auscultation a diastolic pressure of zero may be obtained in some patients. Peripheral pulses usually are forceful, bounding, and quickly collapsing, termed Corrigan's or "water-hammer" pulses. "Pistol shot" sounds may be heard with the stethoscope over peripheral arteries. A wide variety of other auscultatory phenomena have been described, some over a century ago, all indicating vasodilatation and a hyperdynamic peripheral circulation.

Diagnostic Studies. The chest x-ray usually shows impressive cardiac enlargement, with the apex displaced downward and to the left and a markedly enlarged cardiac:thoracic ratio. The ECG is normal early in the disease, but with cardiac enlargement, signs of left ventricular hypertrophy become prominent. Sinus rhythm is usually present initially, although atrial fibrillation is common later in the course of the disease.

Echocardiography, which measures the degree of valvular insufficiency, the left ventricular end-diastolic and end-systolic dimensions, the left atrial size, and the left ventricular function, is the primary diagnostic tool. The echocardiogram also is used to assess the degree of mitral or tricuspid insufficiency and estimate the pulmonary artery pressure.

The classic finding on cardiac catheterization is the reflux of contrast material from the aortic root into the ventricle with aortic root angiography, graded from 1+ to 4+. However, due to the accuracy of current echocardiography, angiographic studies to diagnose aortic insufficiency are no longer necessary in most cases. Aortic root angiography or MRI studies may be performed if aneurysmal disease is suspected. If surgery is planned, coronary angiography should be performed to rule out coronary artery disease in patients with appropriate risk factors. In patients with heart failure the left ventricular end-diastolic pressure may be elevated to 15 to 20 mm Hg and sometimes higher, with an associated rise in the pulmonary artery pressure.

Operative Indications. The development of symptoms is an absolute indication for surgery in patients with aortic insufficiency. It has long been recognized, however, that postponing surgery until the patient becomes severely symptomatic is potentially dangerous, as many patients will have already developed substantial ventricular enlargement and cardiac dysfunction by that time. Therefore, echocardiographic studies are routinely used to determine the appropriate timing for surgical intervention, which should be performed prior to the development of symptoms and before the ventricular function severely deteriorates. Asymptomatic patients with severe aortic insufficiency should be referred for surgery at the first sign of deteriorating left ventricular systolic function on echocardiography, manifest as a rise in the end-systolic dimension of the ventricle or by a drop in the ejection fraction. Operative results indicate that cardiac function will return to normal and long-term survival will be improved significantly if an operation is done at this stage.

In the authors' experience valve replacement should be performed even in patients with low ejection fractions and advanced

NYHA class IV symptoms, especially if recruitable ventricular wall motion is present with inotropic stimuli. Most class IV patients will improve significantly after surgery, although the degree of improvement may be uncertain for 6 to 12 months. Intensive postoperative medical therapy with a heart failure regimen that includes afterload reduction, low-dose beta blockers, and diuretics is beneficial in this group of patients to help remodel the left ventricle. Since ventricular arrhythmias are a common cause of death in patients with markedly depressed left ventricular function, evidence supports routine electrophysiologic testing and implantation of an automatic internal cardiac defibrillator (AICD) if inducible arrhythmias are present.

Operative Techniques

Aortic Valve Replacement. Aortic valve replacement has traditionally been performed through a median sternotomy incision, and this approach remains the standard in most cardiac centers. Cardiopulmonary bypass with moderate systemic hypothermia is utilized, the aorta is cross-clamped, and the heart is protected by cardioplegia delivered antegrade into the aortic root, directly into the coronary ostia by hand-held cannulas, or retrograde through the coronary sinus. Typically a left ventricular vent is inserted through the right superior pulmonary vein to keep the field free of blood during the procedure and to aid in de-airing after blood flow is re-established to the heart.

After the heart has been arrested, an oblique or hockey-stick–shaped aortotomy incision is made, beginning approximately 1 cm above the right coronary artery and extending medially toward the pulmonary artery and inferiorly into the noncoronary sinus. The aortic valve is excised totally (Fig. 20-20), removing all leaflets and any fragments of calcium present in the annulus. A gauze pack is routinely placed in the ventricle before removal of the valve to minimize the risk of calcium spillage and embolization. Serial irrigations of the ventricle are performed after removal of the valve and débridement of calcium.

At NYU, pledgeted horizontal mattress sutures are routinely used, as this technique is thought to minimize the risk of paravalvular leakage. Other suturing techniques for placement of the valve include simple interrupted sutures, figure-of-eight sutures, and continuous sutures. Care is taken to avoid damage to the coronary ostia, to the conduction bundle adjacent to the membranous septum between the right and the noncoronary valve cusps, and to the mitral valve posteriorly. The valve may be seated on the annulus in either of two ways. For supra-annular placement (Fig. 20-21), the sutures are placed from below the annulus in an upward direction, through the annulus, and then through the valve sewing ring. For intra-annular placement the sutures are placed from above the annulus downward and then back up through the sewing ring, which results in the valve resting completely within the annulus.

Mechanical valves are widely used in younger patients. Two configurations are available, a single tilting disk and a bileaflet disk. The flow characteristics are extremely good with all current mechanical valves, and even better in newer designs that allow supra-annular valve placement and therefore increase the effective orifice size that can be implanted for a particular sized annulus. The flow characteristics of the valve become important when the aortic annulus is small, in order to minimize the postoperative gradient across the smaller prosthesis. Patients with mechanical valves routinely require lifelong anticoagulation with warfarin to minimize the risk of thromboembolic complications.

Tissue valves are most commonly used in older patients, although they now are increasingly used in younger patients who want to

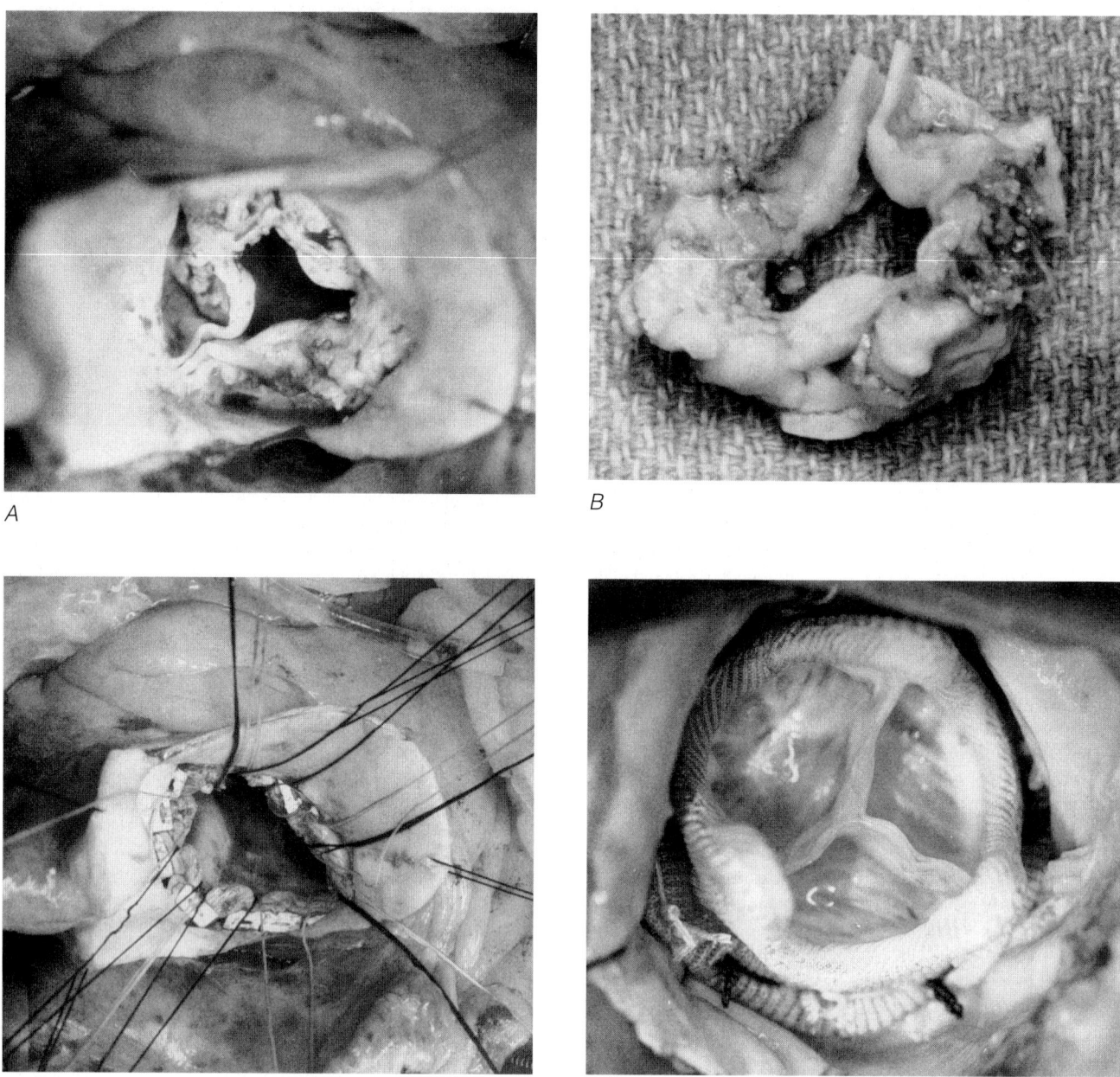

FIG. 20-20. *A.* Operative photograph of calcific aortic stenosis seen through an oblique aortotomy incision. *B.* Excised aortic valve. The valve leaflets were completely immobile and fixed in the midposition, producing a mixture of aortic stenosis and aortic insufficiency. *C.* After excising the valve, pledget-reinforced mattress sutures have been placed into the aortic valve annulus. The sutures will be subsequently placed through the sewing ring of the prosthetic valve. *D.* Porcine valve in the aortic position before closure of the aortotomy incision.

avoid the need for long-term anticoagulation therapy. Tissue valves may be either stented or stentless, with the traditional stented valves being easier to implant, and the stentless valves having better flow characteristics, particularly in smaller valve sizes. Current tissue valves have a projected durability of 15 years or longer and do not require long-term anticoagulation.

However, a small aortic root may be a particularly difficult problem when tissue valves are placed, as the stented tissue valves have relatively poor flow characteristics in smaller sizes. This can potentially result in patient-prosthesis mismatch, which may occur if the implanted prosthesis is equal to or less than 19 mm and the patient's body surface area is greater than 1.7 m^2, or when the

prosthetic valve area is less than 0.8 cm^2/m^2. Controversy exists regarding the impact of small prosthetic valves on late survival, although avoiding patient-prosthesis mismatch clearly results in better postoperative left ventricular mass regression. Surgical options to avoid patient-prosthesis mismatch include use of valves that have better flow characteristics in small sizes, such as supra-annular mechanical valves, stentless tissue valves, or homografts. Alternately, a larger size stented tissue valve can be placed using procedures to enlarge the aortic annulus.

Results. The operative risk for aortic valve replacement is 1 to 5% for most patients, but may be considerably higher in elderly

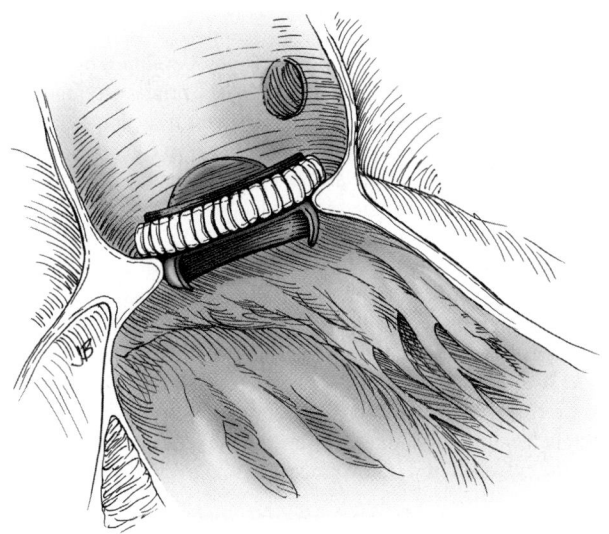

FIG. 20-21. *Supra-annular placement of a St. Jude HP valve in the aortic position. (Illustration courtesy of St. Jude Medical, Inc., St. Paul, MN. All rights reserved.)*

patients with multiple comorbidities and in patients with severely depressed left ventricular function. Chaliki and associates[68] reported that aortic valve replacement in patients with aortic insufficiency and poor left ventricular function (ejection fraction less than 35%) resulted in increased operative risk, 14% compared to 3.7% in patients with ejection fractions above 50%. Ten-year survival was 70% in patients with good ventricular function, but only 42% in patients with ejection fractions less than 35%.[68]

The Society of Thoracic Surgeons National Database lists the clinical variables affecting the operative risk associated with valve surgery.[33] The major risk factors are age, body surface area, diabetes, renal failure, hypertension, chronic lung disease, peripheral vascular disease, cerebrovascular accident, infectious endocarditis, prior cardiac operation, myocardial infarction, cardiogenic shock, NYHA functional status, and elevated pulmonary artery mean pressure. The overall incidence of perioperative stroke is 2.8 to 4.8%.[115]

The 10-year survival after aortic valve replacement in patients less than 65 years of age exceeds 80%, but may be significantly worse in patients with severely impaired ventricular function. The factors affecting late survival are age, NYHA functional status, ventricular function, concomitant coronary artery disease, concomitant disease in another valve and diabetes, previous myocardial infarction, congestive heart failure, and urgent or emergent surgery.[33]

Postoperative Care. Postoperative care is usually uneventful after aortic valve replacement in patients with normal left ventricular function. However, patients with significantly reduced left ventricular function may have a complicated postoperative course. Arrhythmias are relatively common, and continuous ECG monitoring is required for the first 48 hours. Anticoagulation therapy is started 1 day after mechanical valve replacement, targeting an INR (International Normalized Ratio) of 2.5 to 3 times normal. Antiplatelet therapy with aspirin is used in patients with tissue valves, homografts, or autografts. The postoperative hospital stay is usually approximately 5 days, depending on the patient's age and overall physical condition. Early cardiac rehabilitation is particularly helpful in elderly patients.

Except for patients with severe ventricular dysfunction, most patients become asymptomatic and regain a normal range of physical activity within 1 to 2 months after operation. Periodic medical

evaluations should be instituted for all patients because of the problems inherent with use of any prosthetic valve. The patient should have long-term monitoring for proper anticoagulation therapy (with the INR followed in patients on warfarin), and the valve function should be periodically assessed by echocardiography. Thromboembolism, anticoagulant-related hemorrhage, endocarditis, and prosthetic valve failure are the principal late complications. Both thromboembolism and anticoagulant-related hemorrhage occur with incidences of 1 to 2% per year after mechanical valve replacement, despite careful anticoagulation therapy and monitoring. Patients with tissue valves have a risk of thromboembolism of 0.5 to 1% per year, but anticoagulant-related hemorrhage is less common since warfarin is not required. Endocarditis remains an infrequent but serious late hazard after valve replacement, and routine antibiotic prophylaxis is recommended lifelong for any invasive procedure that might produce a transient bacteremia.

Aortic Valve Repair. Aortic valve repair rarely has been used as the primary treatment for aortic insufficiency because of the high risk of late repair failure. Recently, however, David, Yacoub, and Casselman independently described different techniques for valve repair in patients with aortic insufficiency, with encouraging results.[116-119]

David's approach is based on the principle that aortic insufficiency in patients with aortoannular ectasia is secondary to annular dilatation and distortion of the sinotubular junction. David's approach involved excising the aneurysmal portion of the aortic root and reimplanting the aortic valve inside a tubular Dacron graft, using a technique similar to homograft implantation, with reimplantation of the coronary arteries.[116] Late results were reported in 230 patients who underwent aortic valve-sparing operations for aortic insufficiency.[117] The 8-year survival was 83% and the 8-year freedom from reoperation was 99%.

Yacoub reported a similar valve-sparing technique for patients with annuloaortic ectasia.[118] With Yacoub's technique the aortic wall and sinuses of Valsalva are excised down to the anatomic annulus. The Dacron graft is sutured to the annulus, the valve is resuspended, and the coronary buttons are reimplanted.

The technique described by Casselman and associates for repair of aortic insufficiency in patients with bicuspid aortic valves involves triangular resection of the redundant segment of the involved valve cusp in an attempt to achieve cusp symmetry, followed by annular plication of one or both commissures.[119] Results were reported after repair in 94 patients. The freedom from reoperation was 95%, 87%, and 84% at 1, 5, and 7 years, respectively.

Ross Procedure. The Ross procedure involves replacement of the aortic valve with an autograft from the patient's native pulmonary valve. The resected pulmonary valve is then replaced with a pulmonary homograft. Variations of the technique of implantation of the autograft for the aortic valve replacement include free-hand replacement with resuspension of the valve commissures, and cylinder root replacement with reimplantation of the coronary artery ostia (see Fig. 20-12).

The cylinder root replacement technique is the most reproducible. With this method the native aorta is transected 5 mm above the sinotubular ridge. The aortic valve leaflets and the aortic tissue in the sinuses of Valsalva are totally removed, preserving the left main and right coronary arteries on buttons of aortic tissue. The main pulmonary artery is transected at the bifurcation, and a separate incision is made below the pulmonary valve in the right ventricular outflow tract. The pulmonary valve and artery are enucleated en bloc from the outflow tract bed, with care being taken to avoid injury to the first septal perforator as the valve is removed from the septum medially. The pulmonary autograft annulus is sutured to the aortic annulus with continuous or interrupted sutures, and the coronary arteries are reimplanted into the autograft. The pulmonary valve and right ventricular outflow are reconstructed in standard fashion with a homograft.

The Ross procedure has risks similar to those associated with standard aortic valve replacement, although the risk of bleeding may be slightly higher. The primary benefit is that patients do not require long-term anticoagulation and the risk of thromboembolism is negligible. Midterm durability of both the autograft and the pulmonary homograft has been good at 7 to 12 years postoperatively. Paparella and associates reported results in 155 patients, with an 86% 7-year period of freedom from severe recurrent insufficiency. However, progressive late aortic insufficiency has been described in a number of patients, along with calcification of the pulmonary homograft and pulmonary stenosis.[120,121] The risk of late reoperation ranges from 30 to 50% at 15 to 20 years.

Minimally Invasive Aortic Valve Surgery. Minimally invasive approaches for aortic valve surgery have recently become an acceptable alternative to conventional median sternotomy. Both ministernotomy and minithoracotomy approaches have been utilized with excellent success.[122–125] Although the proposed benefits of minimally invasive aortic valve replacement remain controversial, several centers have reported results that are at least comparable to standard surgery, but with less need for blood transfusions and shorter hospital stays.[124,126]

At NYU, minimally invasive aortic valve replacement is performed through a right anterior minithoracotomy incision, with central aortic cannulation and vacuum-assisted venous drainage. An external cross-clamp is applied directly to the aorta, and the heart is protected with traditional cardioplegic methods. This approach has now been used in over 1000 patients. A report by Grossi and colleagues demonstrated that patients treated with the minimally invasive approach had less need for blood transfusions, fewer infections, and a shorter hospital stay than matched patients receiving traditional surgery.[102] Sharony and coworkers reported results in elderly patients, demonstrating shorter hospital stay and rehabilitation time.[125] Thus, minimally invasive approaches for aortic valve replacement appear promising and deserve further investigation.

Idiopathic Hypertrophic Subaortic Stenosis

Patients with hypertrophic cardiomyopathy or IHSS have varying degrees of subaortic left ventricular outflow tract obstruction, usually associated with systolic anterior motion of the mitral valve. Systolic anterior motion of the valve has been explained by the presence of Venturi forces created by the high-velocity flow in the narrowed outflow tract, which pulls the adjacent anterior leaflet of the mitral valve into the outflow tract, worsening outflow obstruction.[127] The subaortic obstruction may have a dynamic component, and can usually be provoked with volume depletion, vasodilators, or inotropes. The intracavitary pressure of the left ventricle is usually markedly elevated, and the ventricle is hypercontractile with impaired diastolic relaxation. The degree of left ventricular outflow tract obstruction at rest is a strong predictor of progression to severe symptoms of heart failure and death.[128] However, most patients with hypertrophic cardiomyopathy and subaortic obstruction will respond to medical therapy, and only a minority will require surgical intervention.

Operative Techniques

Surgical septal myotomy and myectomy, developed by Morrow, has shown consistent results and remains the primary technique for treatment of IHSS.[129] This approach requires resection of a trough of muscle from the subaortic outflow tract. Typically the resection is 1 cm wide and 1 cm deep, and extends the length of the septum to below the lower edge of the anterior leaflet of the mitral valve. The resected trough should remain leftward of the right coronary ostium to avoid heart block, but should routinely produce a left bundle-branch block. A modification of the Morrow myectomy, termed extended myectomy, involves mobilization and partial excision of the papillary muscles. The extended approach has been suggested in order to resect the deeper portion of the septal bulge and redirect the flow medially and anteriorly away from the mitral valve, abolishing systolic anterior motion.[130] However, there are few data to suggest that the extended myectomy procedure improves late outcomes.

Tricuspid Stenosis and Insufficiency

Acquired tricuspid valve disease can be classified as organic or functional. Organic disease is almost always a result of either rheumatic fever or endocarditis. In patients with rheumatic disease, tricuspid stenosis or insufficiency virtually never occurs as an isolated lesion, but only in association with extensive disease of the mitral valve. With mitral disease the frequency of associated tricuspid disease is 10 to 15%, although an incidence as high as 30% has been reported. Rarely, blunt trauma produces rupture of a papillary muscle or chordae tendineae with resultant tricuspid insufficiency.

Functional tricuspid regurgitation is much more common than insufficiency from organic disease. Functional tricuspid regurgitation develops from dilatation of the tricuspid annulus and right ventricle as a result of pulmonary hypertension and right ventricular failure. These abnormalities usually result from mitral valve disease or from other conditions that result in left ventricular failure and pulmonary hypertension.

With tricuspid stenosis the pathologic changes are similar to those found with the more familiar mitral stenosis, with fusion of the commissures. Because right atrial pressure is normally only 4 to 5 mm Hg, significant tricuspid stenosis may be present with a valve orifice considerably larger than that seen with mitral stenosis. With rheumatic disease, mixed tricuspid stenosis and insufficiency or pure insufficiency may result from fibrosis and contraction of the valve leaflets, often in association with shortening and fusion of chordae tendineae. Calcification is rare.

Functional dilatation of the tricuspid annulus results in tricuspid insufficiency. The valve leaflets appear stretched, but otherwise are pliable and seemingly normal, even though serious regurgitation is present. The dilatation and deformity of the annulus are irreversible. Valves with severe functional insufficiency and a markedly dilated annulus usually do not regain competency, even after the mitral valve disease is corrected and pulmonary artery systolic pressure returns to normal.

Pathophysiology

With tricuspid stenosis or severe insufficiency, the mean right atrial pressure becomes elevated to 10 to 20 mm Hg or higher. The higher pressures are found with a tricuspid valve orifice smaller than 1.5 cm^2 and a mean diastolic gradient between the atrium and ventricle of 5 to 15 mm Hg or in patients with pulmonary hypertension and severe insufficiency. When the mean right atrial pressure remains above 15 mm Hg, hepatomegaly, ascites, and leg edema usually appear.

Clinical Manifestations

The symptoms and signs of tricuspid valve disease are similar to those of right heart failure resulting from mitral valve disease. They result from chronic elevation of right atrial pressure above the range of 15 to 20 mm Hg. Clinical manifestations include jugulovenous distention, hepatomegaly, pedal edema, and ascites. With longstanding severe tricuspid insufficiency, hepatic dysfunction and clotting abnormalities may develop.

The characteristic murmur of tricuspid stenosis is best heard as a diastolic murmur at the lower end of the sternum. It is a low-pitched murmur of medium intensity and can easily be overlooked because it is well localized at the lower end of the sternum. During inspiration the intensity of the murmur increases as the volume of blood returning to the heart is temporarily raised by an increase in intrathoracic negative pressure. Tricuspid insufficiency produces a prominent systolic murmur heard best at the left lower sternal border. The murmur often is found in association with an enlarged, pulsating liver and prominent and engorged jugular veins. A prominent jugular venous pulsation, especially when the cardiac rhythm is sinus, may be the best clue to unsuspected tricuspid disease. A hepatojugular reflex may also be noted.

Diagnostic Studies

The x-ray shows enlargement of the right atrium and right ventricle. Echocardiography confirms the diagnosis and differentiates stenosis from insufficiency. Cardiac catheterization is no longer necessary in most cases.

Indications for Surgery

Indications for surgery are based primarily on clinical findings, which are correlated with echocardiographic findings and hemodynamics. Severe insufficiency is indicated by echocardiography when the area of the regurgitant jet occupies a large part of the atrium, the effective regurgitant orifice is greater than 40 mm^2, or the width of the vena contracta (narrowest flow) is greater than 6.5 mm.[131,132] Severe tricuspid regurgitation should clearly be repaired since it has been widely demonstrated that annuloplasty provides excellent late results with little added morbidity.[133] Mild degrees of tricuspid insufficiency are usually left alone, especially in the absence of pulmonary hypertension, while repair of moderate insufficiency requires further consideration of the clinical findings and symptoms present. However, effective tricuspid valve repair minimizes the risk of late right-sided heart failure and reoperation.

Operative Techniques

In the small minority of patients whose tricuspid stenosis is secondary to pure commissural fusion, a commissurotomy may be performed, usually combined with an annuloplasty. More commonly, valve replacement is necessary when significant tricuspid stenosis is present, since the entire valve and subvalvular apparatus are damaged. When a prosthetic valve is inserted, care is required in suture placement along the septal leaflet where the conduction bundle is located, and sutures should be placed more superficially in this area.

In patients with functional tricuspid insufficiency the annulus is markedly dilated, while the leaflets appear entirely normal. Virtually all such patients can be treated by annuloplasty. The suture annuloplasty techniques proposed by Kay and Boyd and the De Vega annuloplasty technique have been highly reliable. Alternatively, a flexible or rigid annuloplasty device may be used.[134–137]

Results

Data on more than 300 patients from the authors' institution show that the suture annuloplasty repair for functional tricuspid insufficiency is reproducible in the absence of significant intrinsic leaflet disease. Valve repair using a posterior suture annuloplasty technique was 98% durable at 7 years. Similar results have been reported with the De Vega annuloplasty.[136] Other centers prefer the use of rigid or flexible annuloplasty devices for correction of tricuspid insufficiency, especially if the right heart pressures are expected to remain chronically elevated.

When tricuspid valve replacement is required, the options include use of either a tissue valve or a mechanical valve. Carrier and associates reported follow-up on 97 patients who underwent tricuspid valve replacement with either tissue valves ($n = 82$) or mechanical valves ($n = 15$).[138] The 5-year freedom from reoperation was 92% in patients with mechanical valves and 97% in patients with tissue valves ($p = 0.2$). Data suggest that the risk of valve thrombosis is increased in mechanical valves placed in the tricuspid position, as emphasized in a report by Kawano and colleagues that demonstrated a 30% risk of mechanical valve thrombosis in the tricuspid position over 15 years, with a linearized rate of 2.9% per patient-year.[139] Bioprostheses are therefore preferred for most patients requiring tricuspid valve replacement.

Multivalve Disease

Disease involving multiple valves is relatively common, particularly in patients with rheumatic disease. Prominent signs in one valve can readily mask disease in others. With aortic valve disease, functional mitral insufficiency can result from a progressive rise in the left ventricular end-diastolic pressure and volume. Similarly, mitral valve disease may result in pulmonary hypertension, right heart failure, and functional tricuspid insufficiency. Often these secondary functional changes resolve without treatment if the primary pathology is corrected in a timely fashion. Certainly multiple-valve surgery has a higher operative risk than single-valve procedures, in part because the condition often represents more advanced disease and is associated with significant cardiac dysfunction.

In a 1992 report by Galloway and colleagues, 513 patients with multiple-valve disease treated surgically between 1976 and 1985 were studied to assess factors influencing operative risk and long-term survival.[140] Three groups accounted for the majority of the cases: 58% had aortic and mitral valve disease (AV + MV), 29% had mitral and tricuspid valve disease (MV + TV), and 12% had triple-valve disease (AV + MV + TV). Preoperative congestive heart failure was present in 91%, 41% were NYHA class III, and 54% were NYHA class IV. The average pulmonary artery systolic pressure was 60 mm Hg. Despite chronic symptoms and severe disease, the overall operative mortality rate was 12.5% and the 5-year survival rate was 67%. The variables predicting decreased survival time were systolic pulmonary artery pressure, age, triple-valve procedures, concomitant coronary bypass grafting, previous heart surgery, and diabetes. After operation 80% of the patients improved to NYHA class I or II, demonstrating that most patients will have significant clinical improvement despite advanced symptoms preoperatively. The 5-year freedom from late cardiac-related death or complications was 82%.

Aortic and Mitral Valve Disease

Nine combinations of valvular pathology can produce aortic and mitral valve disease (AV + MV), because each valve can be stenotic, insufficient, or both. Stenosis in both valves may lead to underestimation of the degree of aortic stenosis, because return of blood to the left ventricle is limited as a result of mitral stenosis. Aortic insufficiency, which produces the Austin Flint murmur, might overshadow and mask true mitral stenosis. With functional mitral insufficiency resulting from severe aortic disease, aortic valve replacement can lead to resolution of insufficiency in some patients, but patients with more severe mitral insufficiency may require mitral repair or replacement. Patients presenting with AV + MV should be examined closely for these and other considerations.

Mitral and Tricuspid Valve Disease

Multiple combinations of valvular pathology are possible with mitral and tricuspid disease, but mitral disease with functional tricuspid insufficiency is the most common scenario, resulting from chronic pulmonary hypertension and right heart failure. The presence of associated tricuspid insufficiency increases the operative risk for patients undergoing mitral valve surgery. The risk for isolated mitral and tricuspid valve disease (MV + TV) is approximately 6%.

Triple-Valve Disease

Triple-valve surgery can be challenging because the clinical condition usually is a result of chronic aortic and mitral disease with severe pulmonary hypertension, biventricular failure, and functional tricuspid insufficiency. Occasionally rheumatic disease affects all three valves. The degree of pulmonary hypertension is the most significant predictor of survival in patients with triple-valve disease. The operative morality for 61 triple-valve procedures in the above-cited NYU report was only 5.6% when the pulmonary artery systolic pressure was less than 60 mm Hg, but over 25% when the pulmonary artery pressures were above 60 mm Hg and the patients were over 70 years of age.[140] This emphasizes the value of early operation, before the development of irreversible ventricular dysfunction and chronic pulmonary hypertension.

PERICARDIAL DISEASES

Acute Pericarditis

Pericarditis results from acute inflammation of the pericardial space, resulting in substernal chest pain, ECG changes, and a pericardial friction rub on physical examination. The pain often is inspiratory, worsened in the supine position, and relieved by leaning forward. Associated ECG changes frequently occur, most commonly sinus tachycardia with concave upward ST-segment elevation throughout the precordium. The ECG typically progresses to T-wave inversion, followed by the total resolution of all changes. The cause of acute pericarditis is variable, including infection, myocardial infarction, trauma, neoplasm, radiation, autoimmune diseases, drugs, nonspecific causes, and others. Untreated pericarditis may result in progressive development of a pericardial effusion with subsequent cardiac tamponade. Infectious causes may result in septic complications. Chronic constrictive pericarditis may develop after resolution of the acute process.

Diagnosis

The diagnostic workup should attempt to determine the underlying cause of the pericarditis. Blood tests should include erythrocyte sedimentation rate, hematocrit level, white blood cell count, bacterial cultures, viral titers, blood urea nitrogen, T_3, T_4, thyroid-stimulating hormone, antinuclear antibody, rheumatoid factor, and myocardial enzyme levels. The ECG may be typical or nonspecific. The chest x-ray may be normal or may demonstrate an enlarged

cardiac silhouette or a pleural effusion. An echocardiogram to evaluate the degree of pericardial effusion is essential. A pericardiocentesis or pericardial biopsy may be necessary when the diagnosis is uncertain.

Treatment

The preferred treatment depends on the underlying cause. Purulent pyogenic pericarditis requires drainage and prolonged intravenous antibiotic therapy. Postpericardiotomy syndrome, post–myocardial infarction syndrome, viral pericarditis, and idiopathic pericarditis often are self-limiting, but can require a short course of treatment with nonsteroidal anti-inflammatory agents. If a significant pericardial effusion is present, surgical drainage is indicated if tamponade is suspected or if resolution is not prompt with anti-inflammatory agents. A 5- to 7-day course of steroids is occasionally necessary. Follow-up studies should be done to document resolution of pericardial effusion or to assess for late constrictive pericarditis.

Chronic Constrictive Pericarditis

Etiology

In the majority of patients, the cause of chronic constrictive pericarditis is unknown and probably is the end stage of an undiagnosed viral pericarditis. Tuberculosis is a rarity. Intensive radiation is a significant cause in some series. Constrictive pericarditis may develop after an open-heart operation. Previous cardiac surgery was reported to be the cause in 39% of the patients treated surgically for constrictive pericarditis at the authors' institution.

Pathology and Pathophysiology

The pericardial cavity is obliterated by fusion of the parietal pericardium to the epicardium, forming dense scar tissue that encases and constricts the heart. In chronic cases, areas of calcification develop, adding an additional element of constriction.

The physiologic handicap is limitation of diastolic filling of the ventricles. This results in a decrease in cardiac output from a decrease in stroke volume. The right ventricular diastolic pressure is increased, with a corresponding increase in right atrial and central venous pressure ranging from 10 to 30 mm Hg. The venous hypertension produces hepatomegaly, ascites, peripheral edema, and a generalized increase in blood volume.

Clinical Manifestations

The disease is slowly progressive with increasing ascites and edema. Fatigability and dyspnea on exertion are common, but dyspnea at rest is unusual. The ascites often is severe, and the diagnosis is easily confused with cirrhosis.

Hepatomegaly and ascites often are the most prominent physical abnormalities. Peripheral edema is moderate in some patients, but severe in others. These findings are manifestations of advanced congestive failure from any form of heart disease. With constrictive pericarditis, however, the usual cardiac findings are a heart of normal size without murmurs or abnormal sounds. Atrial fibrillation is present in about one third of the patients, and a pleural effusion is common in more severe cases. A paradoxical pulse is found in a small proportion of patients.

Laboratory Findings

Venous pressure is elevated, often to 15 to 20 mm Hg or higher. The ECG, though not diagnostic, usually is abnormal with a low voltage and inverted T waves. The chest x-ray usually shows a heart of normal size, but pericardial calcification may be seen in a significant proportion of cases and often is the first clue to the diagnosis. Echocardiogram, MRI, or CT scan may demonstrate a thickened pericardium.

Findings on cardiac catheterization are highly characteristic. There is elevation of the right ventricular diastolic pressure with a change in contour, showing an early filling with a subsequent plateau, called the "square root" sign. There also is "equalization" of pressures in the different cardiac chambers, because right atrial pressure, right ventricular diastolic pressure, pulmonary artery diastolic pressure, pulmonary wedge pressure, and left atrial pressure are similar. The one condition that cannot be excluded without myocardial biopsy is a restrictive cardiomyopathy.

Treatment

When the diagnosis has been made, pericardiectomy should be done promptly, because the disease relentlessly progresses. Operation can be done through a sternotomy incision or a long left anterolateral thoracotomy. The constricting pericardium should be removed from all surfaces of the ventricle, mobilizing the heart so it can be held freely upward in the hand. Removal of the pericardium over the atria and the venae cavae is considered optional, although this usually is done as well. Cardiopulmonary bypass is not usually necessary, but may be needed in the event of significant hemorrhage. If this occurs, the patient can be heparinized and the blood aspirated and returned to the patient until the laceration is repaired. The pericardium is removed from the pulmonary veins on the right to the pulmonary veins on the left. Both phrenic nerves are mobilized and protected. Particular care is taken to remove pericardium over the pulmonary artery, where residual constriction can seriously impair the operative results.

As the constricting scar develops from organization of an exudate between the pericardium and the epicardium, the plane of dissection may be external to the epicardium, which will greatly decrease operative hemorrhage. If the epicardium is thickened, it must be removed from the underlying myocardium, though this is tedious and results in diffuse bleeding.

Intracardiac pressures should be measured by direct needle puncture before and after pericardiectomy. Often with a complete pericardiectomy the characteristic pressure abnormalities are eliminated or greatly improved. If significant abnormalities remain, the operative field should be carefully checked for any residual sites of constriction. In the past, slow recovery over many months probably was a result of inadequate pericardiectomy, not underlying ventricular atrophy.

Results

After a radical pericardiectomy that corrects the hemodynamic abnormalities, patients improve promptly with a massive diuresis. The risk of operation varies with the age of the patient and the severity of the disease; the mortality rate usually is less than 5%. A good result can be anticipated for more than 95% of the patients. Culliford and associates reported surgical treatment for chronic constrictive pericarditis with total pericardiectomy, with an operative mortality rate of 3%. After operation hemodynamic abnormalities were promptly corrected, ascites and peripheral edema resolved, and functional status improved dramatically.[141]

CARDIAC NEOPLASMS

Primary cardiac neoplasms are rare, reported to occur with incidences ranging from 0.001 to 0.3% in autopsy series. Benign tumors account for 75% of primary neoplasms and malignant tumors account for 25%. The most frequent primary cardiac neoplasm is myxoma, comprising 30 to 50%. Other benign neoplasms, in decreasing order of occurrence, include lipoma, papillary fibroelastoma, rhabdomyoma, fibroma, hemangioma, teratoma, lymphangioma, and others. Most primary malignant neoplasms are sarcomas (angiosarcoma, rhabdomyosarcoma, fibrosarcoma, leiomyosarcoma, and liposarcoma), with malignant lymphomas accounting for 1 to 2%.

Metastatic cardiac neoplasms are more common than primary neoplasms, occurring in 4 to 12% of patients dying of cancer. Symptoms include dyspnea, fever, malaise, weight loss, arthralgias, and dizziness. Clinical findings may include murmurs of mitral stenosis or insufficiency, heart failure, pulmonary hypertension, and systemic embolization.

Usually, the diagnosis is readily established by two-dimensional echocardiography. Transesophageal echocardiography may be useful when transthoracic findings are equivocal or confusing. MRI has been of value in diagnosis, providing excellent cardiac definition. Cardiac catheterization is not necessary in the majority of cases, but may be necessary when other cardiac disease is suspected or if other diagnostic studies are equivocal.

Excision is the treatment of choice for most benign tumors. Care is taken to avoid deformity or destruction of adjacent cardiac structures, and reconstruction of the involved cardiac chamber is sometimes necessary. Total excision of metastatic or primary malignant neoplasms is less frequently possible but should be attempted. Otherwise incisional diagnostic biopsy is performed. Multimodality therapy with excision, chemotherapy, and radiotherapy is indicated for most malignant cardiac neoplasms.

Myxomas

Sixty to 75% of cardiac myxomas develop in the left atrium, almost always from the atrial septum near the fossa ovalis. Most other myxomas develop in the right atrium. Fewer than 20 have been reported in the right or left ventricle. The curious predilection for a myxoma to develop from the rim of the fossa ovalis in the left atrium has been studied, but no satisfactory explanation has been found.

Myxomas are true neoplasms, although their similarity to an organized atrial thrombus has led to considerable debate. The occurrence of myxomas in the absence of other organic heart disease, histochemical studies of myxomas demonstrating mucopolysaccharide and glycoprotein, and a distinct histologic appearance indicate that myxomas are true neoplasms. While they can recur locally, they do not invade or metastasize and are considered benign.

Pathology

The tumors usually are polypoid, projecting into the atrial cavity from a 1- to 2-cm stalk attached to the atrial septum. The size ranges from 0.5 cm to larger than 10.0 cm. Only the superficial layer of the septum is involved; invasion of the septum does not occur. Some myxomas grow slowly; a few patients have symptoms for many years. There is no tendency to invade other areas of the heart and distant metastases are rarely reported. The friable consistency of a myxoma is of particular significance because fatal emboli have occurred after digital manipulation of the tumor at operation.

Histologically, a myxoma is covered with endothelium and composed of a myxomatous stroma with large stellate cells mixed with fusiform or multinucleated cells. Mitoses are infrequent. Lymphocytes and plasmacytes are regularly found. Hemosiderin, a result of hemorrhage into the tumor, is commonly present. Myxoma cells usually express interleukin-6, and some tumors have abnormal cellular DNA content.[142]

Sporadic myxomas usually present in the fifth or sixth decade of life, but have been described in younger and older patients. Autosomal dominant genetically transmitted familial myxomas can occur, usually presenting before 30 years of age. Familial myxoma syndrome includes myxomas, freckles, pigmented nevi, nodular adrenal cortical disease, and mammary myomatous fibroadenomas. Testicular tumors and pituitary adenomas with two or more components are required for diagnosis.

Pathophysiology

A myxoma may be completely asymptomatic until it grows large enough to obstruct the mitral or tricuspid valve or fragments to produce emboli. Embolization has been estimated to occur in 40 to 50% of patients. This is not surprising given the degree of motion that is seen on echocardiography and angiography, as the myxoma swings on a small pedicle with each cardiac contraction. Intermittent acute obstruction of the mitral orifice has been reported to produce syncope and even sudden death. In a series of 49 patients it has been reported that most myxomas originated from the left atrium (87.7%), but also much less frequently from the mitral valve (6.1%), from the right atrium (4.1%), and from the left and right atria (2.0%). The myxomas produced a prolapse into the left ventricle in 40.8% of the patients, mitral stenosis in 10.2%, and threatened left ventricular outflow tract obstruction in 2.0%.[143] Some myxomas produce generalized symptoms resembling an autoimmune disorder, including fever, weight loss, digital clubbing, myalgia, and arthralgia. These patients may have an immune reaction to the neoplasm, as elevated levels of interleukin-6 and elevated levels of antimyocardial antibodies have been described.

Clinical Manifestations

Symptoms may include those of mitral valve obstruction that resemble mitral stenosis; peripheral embolization; or generalized autoimmune symptoms. The diagnosis often is made after an embolic episode from histologic examination of the surgically removed embolus, or as a result of subsequent diagnostic studies to determine the reason for embolism. The precision and reliability of two-dimensional echocardiography has greatly simplified diagnosis. Angiography is optional unless additional disease is suspected. CT scan has been reported to be helpful with small tumors, but MRI is more definitive.

Treatment

Surgery should be performed as soon as possible after the diagnosis has been established, due to the inherent risk of a disabling or fatal cerebral embolus. Either a sternotomy or a minimally invasive approach can be used. Once extracorporeal circulation has been established, the aorta is clamped to avoid embolism. Palpation is avoided. The right atrium is opened and the fossa ovalis incised to expose the stalk of the myxoma. The left atrium is then opened in the interatrial groove. With the tumor visualized, the segment of atrial septum from which the tumor arises is excised, after which the tumor is removed through the left atrium (Fig. 20-22). The defect in the atrial septum is closed primarily or with a small patch. This technique is simple and allows exploration of atria and ventricles.

A few cases of recurrent myxoma have been reported, some of which have been re-excised successfully. While thought to result from inadequate excision of the site of origin, some have recurred at more remote sites in the atrium, indicating the multipotential source

of these unusual neoplasms. Periodic echocardiography should be routinely performed for several years after operation.

Keeling and associates described their experience with a series of 49 patients with cardiac myxomas over 20 years. Cardiac myxomas represented 86% of all surgically treated cardiac tumors. The early mortality rate was 2%, while the rate of reoperation was 2% after 24 years.[143]

Metastatic Neoplasms

Cardiac metastases have been found in 4 to 12% of autopsies performed for neoplastic disease. Although they have occurred from primary neoplasms developing in almost every known site of the body, the most common have been carcinoma of the lung or breast, melanoma, and lymphoma. Cardiac metastases involving only the heart are very unusual. Similarly, a solitary cardiac metastasis is rare; usually there are multiple areas of involvement. Cardiac involvement is common with leukemia or lymphoma, developing in 25 to 40% of patients. All areas of the heart are involved with equal frequency except the cardiac valves, perhaps because lymphatics are absent in valves.

The diagnosis of a primary cardiac malignant tumor may be suspected in a patient in whom an unexplained hemorrhagic pericardial effusion develops, especially in association with a bizarre cardiac shadow on the radiograph. Echocardiography should confirm the presence of an abnormal cardiac mass. Thoracotomy or sternotomy usually is required to establish the diagnosis. Combined chemotherapy and radiation is indicated, but only rarely is effective therapy possible.

Miscellaneous Tumors

A radical approach has been reported for cardiac sarcoma. Combined heart and lung resection followed by en bloc heart and bilateral lung transplantation was reported in four patients: two with inoperable pulmonary arterial sarcoma and two with left atrial sarcoma extending into the pulmonary vein. Median survival after transplantation was 31 months. All patients had tumor recurrence. Therefore, although combined heart and lung transplantation is a technically feasible treatment for highly selected patients with localized advanced primary cardiac sarcomas, the high incidence of metastatic disease limits its utility.[144]

Unusual benign lesions of the heart include fibromas, lipomas, angiomas, teratomas, and cysts. Fewer than 50 of each of these types of lesion have been reported. Fibromas have been found most frequently in the left ventricle, often as 2- to 5-cm nodules within the muscle. Sudden death, probably from a cardiac arrhythmia, has been reported with these tumors, and may be the reason that only 18% of tumors that have been reported have been found in adults.

Lipomas are rare asymptomatic tumors found projecting from the epicardial or endocardial surface of the heart in older patients. Angiomas are small, focal, vascular malformations of no clinical significance, although may be associated with heart block. Pericardial teratomas and bronchogenic cysts are rare lesions that can cause symptoms from compression of the right atrium and obstruction of venous return. Most of these occur in children. Some of the larger cysts, up to 10 cm in diameter, may produce grotesque deformities from extensive invagination of the right atrial wall. Myxomas are by far the most common benign tumor in adults; they are seldom found in children except as part of the familial syndrome described in the previous section.

Renal cell carcinoma, Wilms' tumor, uterine tumors, and adrenal tumors may have intracardiac extension. Excision of these

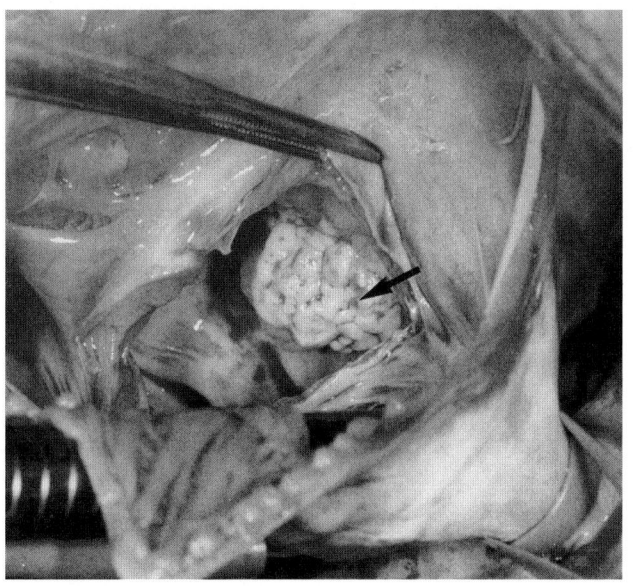

A

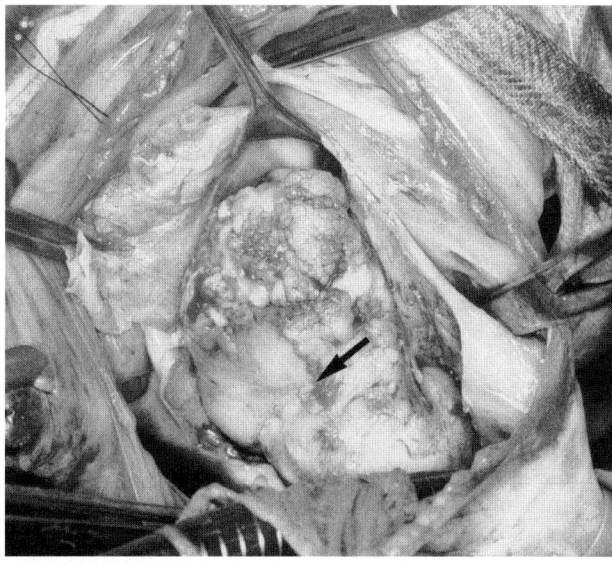

B

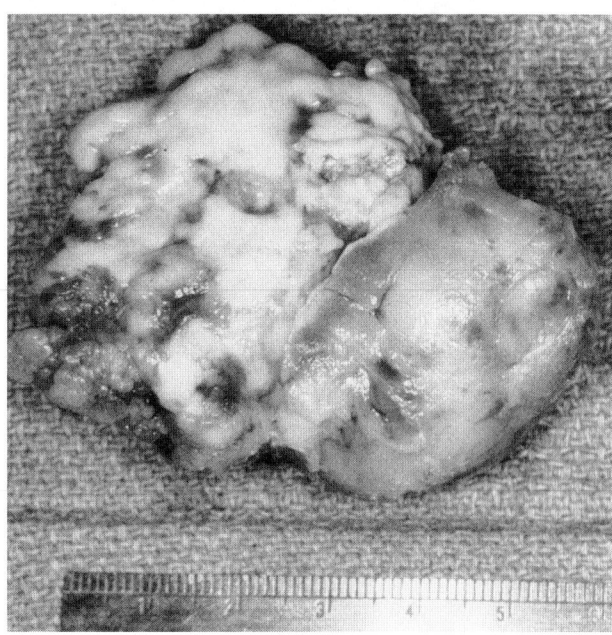

C

FIG. 20-22. *A.* Operative photograph of a patient who presented with nonspecific symptoms and a large left atrial mass, diagnosed preoperatively as a left atrial myxoma. The photograph demonstrates a large left atrial mass *(arrow)* attached to the atrial septum. *B.* The tumor completely fills the left atrial cavity. It was excised by removing a portion of the atrial septum. *C.* The specimen (>6 cm) has none of the classic features of an atrial myxoma. Pathologic examination revealed an extremely rare histiocytoid hemangioendothelioma. The resected portion of the atrial septum was closed with a pericardial patch, and the patient recovered uneventfully.

infradiaphragmatic tumors by radical surgery associated with cavoatrial thrombectomy has been suggested, and extracorporeal circulation and deep circulatory arrest provide an optimal technique for removing the tumor thrombus, even in the presence of metastatic disease, and have good early and long-term results.[145]

POSTOPERATIVE CARE AND COMPLICATIONS

General Considerations

Postoperative care of cardiac surgical patients involves prevention, recognition, and correction of the metabolic and hemodynamic derangements that are frequently seen after cardiac surgery. Important areas include myocardial and pulmonary support, fluid and electrolyte management, and control of bleeding and coagulopathy. All patients are observed in a specialized recovery room or intensive care unit after cardiac surgery, where hemodynamic data are continuously analyzed using both invasive and noninvasive monitoring. Additionally, important laboratory parameters, including arterial blood gases, enzymatic markers of cardiac injury, and mixed venous O_2 saturation, are measured serially. Data are evaluated and interpreted in context so the general trends may be identified.

Early postoperative complications include bleeding, cardiac tamponade, arrhythmias, myocardial infarction, graft occlusion, coronary spasm, low cardiac output syndrome, cardiac arrest, and stroke. Later complications include delayed bleeding, postpericardiotomy syndrome with pericardial effusion, renal dysfunction, ileus, mesenteric ischemia, gastrointestinal hemorrhage, pneumothorax, respiratory insufficiency, pneumonia, wound infection, and wound dehiscence. While the incidence of serious complications is relatively low (3 to 6%), each complication is potentially life-threatening and can be associated with significant morbidity.

Hemodynamics

Maintenance of cardiac function is critical in any patient following heart surgery. While adequate cardiac output may be reflected in the blood pressure and the urine output, exact determination may be obtained with invasive monitoring equipment. A Swan-Ganz catheter equipped with a thermistor allows measurement of the cardiac output and pulmonary capillary wedge pressure. Derived from the measured cardiac output, the cardiac index is a more accurate assessment of an individual patient's myocardial performance. A normal cardiac index is 2.5 to 3.0 L/min per square meter. A cardiac index less than 2 L/min per square meter is an ominous finding, and should prompt immediate investigation into possible causes of decreased cardiac performance. The classic clinical findings of low cardiac output with inadequate oxygen transport include hypotension, vasoconstriction, oliguria, and metabolic acidosis. Untreated low cardiac output is ultimately fatal from either progressive renal failure or arrhythmias.

When evaluating low cardiac output in the postoperative setting, the first consideration is to exclude cardiac tamponade or hypovolemia due to intrathoracic bleeding. Once these have been excluded, the physiologic causes of low output should be reviewed in terms of *preload, afterload,* and *intrinsic contractility* of the heart. If the patient is hypovolemic, therapy consists of volume resuscitation to raise the left atrial pressure or pulmonary capillary wedge pressure. As defined by the Starling principle, cardiac stroke volume rises with a rise in left atrial pressure. The cardiac output can be plotted against preload, assuming pulse and afterload are constant, to determine the optimal filling pressure of the heart.

Afterload reduction consists of reduction in peripheral vascular resistance with specific drugs that cause vasodilatation. If peripheral vascular resistance is elevated above the normal 1200 dynes/sec/cm^2, afterload reduction should be one of the initial forms of therapy. The most popular drugs for intravenous infusion are nitroprusside or nitroglycerin. Vasodilation, or decreased peripheral resistance, should be treated with vasoconstrictors such as phenylephrine to maintain an adequate perfusion pressure. In general, afterload should be controlled to keep the systolic blood pressure greater than 100 mm Hg but less than 150 mm Hg, and the mean arterial blood pressure greater than 70 mm Hg but less than 90 to 95 mm Hg, with a nearly normal vascular resistance.

Once bleeding and tamponade are excluded and preload and afterload have been optimized, inotropic agents may be used to augment myocardial contractility. First-line medications include milrinone and dobutamine, which may be augmented with norepinephrine or phenylephrine when the peripheral vascular resistance is low. Alpha-adrenergic agents may be administered directly into the left atrium to minimize pulmonary hypertension. Dopamine and epinephrine are useful second-line inotropic agents.

If the intrinsic cardiac rhythm is not sufficient to maintain optimal hemodynamics, cardiac pacing should be used to maintain both an adequate rate and rhythm. If a sinus mechanism is too slow or not present, atrial pacing or atrioventricular pacing is valuable for augmenting cardiac output. An optimal heart rate to maximize cardiac output without unduly increasing myocardial oxygen consumption generally is 80 to 90 beats per minute.

If low cardiac output persists despite optimizing preload, afterload, and inotropic support, an intra-aortic balloon pump (IABP) may be useful. An IABP: (1) decreases afterload, which improves cardiac output while decreasing wall tension and oxygen requirements; (2) decreases preload in a failing heart, again lowering wall tension and oxygen demand; and (3) provides diastolic counterpulsation to augment both systemic blood pressure and diastolic coronary perfusion. The balloon pump lowers oxygen consumption by approximately 20% while augmenting cardiac output by about 700 mL/min per square meter. The need for an IABP can be determined in the operating room by performing serial measurements of cardiac output following the cessation of CPB. If the cardiac index remains below 1.5 to 1.7 L/min per square meter despite inotropic support, an IABP is usually recommended.

An unexpected fall in cardiac output in the recovery room is frequently due to a correctable mechanical problem. A quick, thorough search for all causes of low output syndrome is essential. If correctable problems are not present and the low output syndrome does not respond to a combination of inotropes and a balloon pump, temporary placement of a left ventricular assist device may be necessary.

Electrocardiogram and Arrhythmias

The postoperative ECG is important for determining heart block, bundle-branch block, infarction (Q waves), ischemia (ST-segment elevation, T-wave inversion), and other signs of intraoperative injury. The ECG should be repeated periodically, and patients with signs of ischemia or injury should be monitored carefully. Acute ischemia or evolving infarction should be treated initially with nitrates and beta blockade. If ECG changes do not resolve promptly, acute graft occlusion should be considered, particularly if the patient is hemodynamically unstable.

In addition to serial 12-lead ECGs, continuous monitoring of the cardiac rhythm remains important in the postoperative setting. Life-threatening arrhythmias may develop unexpectedly despite the presence of a normal cardiac output and without any other signs of circulatory failure. Delayed detection of a significant arrhythmia is a major cause of unexpected sudden death following cardiac operations. Postoperative bradyarrhythmias and heart block are not uncommon, and for this reason temporary cardiac pacing wires are routinely placed in the right ventricle and right atrium at operation.

Other arrhythmias, including ventricular extrasystoles and ventricular tachycardia, may herald the development of ventricular fibrillation. Hypokalemia is an important cause of ventricular arrhythmias, as many patients undergoing cardiac surgery may have significant depletion of total body potassium stores from chronic diuretic therapy. Postoperatively serum potassium should be kept above 4.0 mEq/L. Continuous intravenous lidocaine, 1 to 4 mg/min, is a valuable form of therapy for temporary control of ventricular arrhythmias. Amiodarone has proven to be effective in controlling postoperative ventricular arrhythmias. Other agents useful in the treatment of serious ventricular arrhythmias include procainamide and bretylium.

Atrial fibrillation remains the most common postoperative arrhythmia. Beta blockers should be initiated early postoperatively unless contraindicated, as this has been found to lower the risk of developing postoperative atrial fibrillation. If atrial fibrillation does develop, initial treatment involves heart rate control with beta blockers and intravenous digitalis. If atrial fibrillation persists, anticoagulation with heparin is indicated, followed by an attempt at cardioversion, usually pharmacologically. Amiodarone has proven to be quite effective in converting postoperative patients to sinus rhythm and may be initiated intravenously, which aids in rate control, or may be given orally. If atrial fibrillation results in hemodynamic instability, the patient should be cardioverted with 50 to 100 J.

Patients who remain in atrial fibrillation should be anticoagulated, initially with heparin and subsequently with warfarin. A significant number of patients with persistent postoperative atrial fibrillation will spontaneously convert to normal sinus rhythm within 6 weeks; those who do not can be electrically cardioverted after assessing for clot in the left atrium with transesophageal echocardiography.

Cardiac Arrest and Resuscitation

Complete circulatory collapse in the postoperative cardiac surgical patient can occur without warning. Circulation must be restored within minutes or the brain and myocardium may suffer irreversible injury. Treatment should not be delayed, even if the exact cause is unknown. A high incidence of survival without any permanent disability is possible when cardiac arrest is promptly recognized, circulation is quickly restored, and the underlying cause is treated. Frequent causes of postoperative cardiac arrest include cardiac tamponade, arrhythmias, ischemia or graft occlusion, hypoxia, and drug toxicity.

Cardiac tamponade is a serious complication following cardiac surgery. It may occur early in the postoperative period from the accumulation of intrapericardial blood or later from a pericardial effusion. The classic findings of tamponade include: (1) elevation of central venous pressure; (2) equalization of central venous pressure, pulmonary artery diastolic pressure, and left atrial pressure; and (3) pulsus paradoxus of more than 10 mm Hg during inspiration. Clinical signs may include distended neck veins, muffled heart sounds, and hypotension. Extreme cases of tamponade may present with life-threatening hypotension or sudden circulatory collapse. The diagnosis must be considered in any patient with hypotension and a low cardiac output. A widening of the mediastinal shadow on chest x-ray or detection of significant pericardial effusion by echocardiography is suggestive of the diagnosis. No single test can exclude tamponade short of surgical exploration. Therefore any patient with suspected tamponade should be promptly returned to the operating room for definitive diagnosis and treatment. Moreover, any postoperative patient in extremis with suspected tamponade should undergo emergent re-exploration or subxiphoid drainage performed at the bedside in order to rule out tamponade. Surgical treatment includes clot and fluid removal along with rapid volume resuscitation.

Ongoing ischemia and myocardial injury secondary to poor intraoperative myocardial protection are probably the two most common causes of postoperative ventricular fibrillation. Ischemia and ventricular irritability may be due to graft occlusion, preoperative ischemia or injury, intraoperative injury, coronary spasm, or an area of myocardium that is not sufficiently revascularized.

Electrolyte imbalance, such as a deficiency of potassium or magnesium, also can cause serious arrhythmias leading to cardiac arrest or ventricular fibrillation. A serum potassium level below 3.0 mEq can produce severe cardiac irritability postoperatively, though the precise influence is determined by the coexisting concentration of calcium ions and the presence of acidosis or alkalosis. Hypothermia, when present, predisposes to arrhythmias.

Difficulties with ventilation and hypoxia may lead to cardiac arrhythmias from low arterial oxygen tension and progressive metabolic acidosis. Common causes include inadequate ventilation from pneumothorax, dislodgment of the endotracheal tube, and plugging of the airway with secretions.

Drugs may induce bradycardia, heart block, ventricular fibrillation, or cardiac arrest, either from toxicity or from an idiosyncratic reaction. Digitalis is a common example because of its widespread use. The sensitivity of the myocardium to digitalis varies with a number of factors, one of the most important of which is the concentration of potassium. Procainamide and quinidine are examples of drugs with known proarrhythmic effects.

Profound bradycardia (heart rate <60 beats per minute) from any cause may result in escape beats leading to ventricular fibrillation and cardiac arrest. Ventricular arrhythmias may progress to bigeminy, ventricular tachycardia, and ventricular fibrillation. This well-known sequence is the reason for constant monitoring of the electrocardiogram postoperatively.

Treatment

Advanced Cardiac Life Support (ACLS) guidelines include specific algorithms for the treatment of cardiac arrest and other causes of circulatory arrest. Although the treatment of cardiac arrest described in the remainder of this section relates mainly to postoperative cardiac surgery patients, the principles discussed follow ACLS guidelines and are applicable to noncardiac surgical patients as well.

Cerebral anoxia associated with circulatory arrest produces brain injury within 3 to 4 minutes, so the diagnosis must be made and treatment begun rapidly to avoid serious brain injury. Periods of anoxia of 6 to 8 minutes may produce extensive but reversible brain injury, whereas longer periods regularly cause irreversible injury. Closed-chest massage and ventilation should be started promptly. Thus the ABCs of cardiopulmonary resuscitation (CPR), airway, breathing, and circulation, apply.

The immediate first steps in CPR are to secure an adequate airway and provide prompt ventilation (breathing). Cardiac massage for more than a few seconds without securing the airway and providing adequate ventilation is futile. The mouth and throat are cleared of secretions, and ventilation is quickly accomplished by mask inflation with an oral airway. This can be begun immediately and continued until endotracheal intubation is achieved. With a laryngoscope, an endotracheal tube can easily be inserted by a physician or other trained personnel. In some patients, as in those with a short, thick neck, the anatomy is such that intubation is difficult, at times almost impossible, even for highly experienced staff. Unless intubation can be accomplished quickly and with certainty, oral insufflation should be continued until a cricothyroidotomy has been performed.

An infrequent but serious error can occur when the endotracheal tube is inadvertently placed in the esophagus. Because of this, immediate auscultation of the lungs for breath sounds is essential after attempted intubation. If any uncertainty exists after auscultation, the tube should be removed and intubation should be repeated. A tightly fitting face mask can provide a method of temporary ventilation. If endotracheal intubation is difficult, requiring repeated attempts, or simply cannot be performed, a cricothyroidotomy should be promptly performed. The patient cannot recover unless the airway is rapidly controlled and ventilation established.

The third step is to provide effective perfusion (circulation) with closed-chest massage or with inotropes or pressors as necessary. Effective CPR depends upon adequate intermittent compression of the heart between the sternum and the vertebral column. The patient must be placed on a firm surface, usually by placing a board behind the back. The heel of the hand should be applied over the lower third of the sternum with the other hand above it to depress the sternum intermittently for 3 to 4 cm. Massage should be at a rate of about 60/min. The sternal compression should be brisk, depressing the sternum sharply and then releasing it to permit cardiac filling. Mechanical ventilation must be synchronized with massage.

In the postoperative cardiac surgery patient with cardiac arrest, closed-chest massage may be initiated immediately as part of a resuscitative effort that may also include defibrillation and the administration of pharmacologic agents. If cardiac activity is not quickly restored or if the cardiac arrest is thought to be due to a mechanical cause such as tamponade or hemorrhage, the sternotomy incision is reopened immediately at the bedside and internal cardiac massage is instituted. Open cardiac massage is extremely effective if instituted promptly. For this reason, postoperative resuscitative efforts employing closed cardiac massage and external defibrillation are quickly aborted unless immediately successful. Rarely, open-chest massage may be effectively continued for more than an hour until the basic condition causing refractory arrhythmias or cardiac arrest is corrected. More commonly, the patient is returned to the operating room once the chest is opened, and CPB is initiated for support. After the patient is resuscitated the surgeon must determine if further therapy such as mechanical support or additional bypass grafting is indicated.

Drugs and Fluids

Epinephrine, sodium bicarbonate, and calcium are the most useful pharmacologic agents. Again, the protocols suggested by the ACLS program are followed. Epinephrine, 1 mg, may be given intravenously or alternately by direct intracardiac injection. Calcium, 3 to 4 mL of a 10% solution, is another powerful stimulant of myocardial contraction. Calcium administration in cardiac arrest may be valuable in some circumstances, but harmful in others and should not be used indiscriminately. Lidocaine is given primarily for ventricular arrhythmias, followed by amiodarone for refractory ventricular tachycardia. Medications are usually ineffective if severe myocardial anoxia or significant acidosis is present. Anoxia can be corrected only by the combination of effective cardiac massage and ventilation. Large amounts of sodium bicarbonate may be required to treat the acidosis. Excessive use of drugs before hypoxia and acidosis have been treated is probably futile.

Small amounts of fluid should be rapidly infused because vasodilatation is usually present. An intravenous infusion of a vasoconstrictor, norepinephrine or phenylephrine, is often helpful in order to maintain perfusion pressure. Blood transfusion may be required in the postoperative patient for volume resuscitation and improved oxygen-carrying capacity.

Defibrillation

Ventricular fibrillation can be differentiated from asystole only by the electrocardiogram or by direct inspection of the myocardium. Initial treatment of cardiac arrest should include a precordial thump, because it is often effective in converting ventricular tachycardia or ventricular fibrillation. Intravenous lidocaine is promptly administered. If this is not quickly effective and an electrocardiogram is not available, empiric defibrillation may be tried briefly because most resuscitations are effective when defibrillation is done promptly. Asystole is treated by pacing the heart with a transcutaneous pacemaker, a transvenous pacemaker if access is readily available, or a temporary pacing lead that can be placed directly on the myocardium if the chest is open.

Closed-chest defibrillation is usually done by applying electrodes over the base and apex of the heart. Defibrillation is best done with a direct current of 200 to 360 J. When open-chest defibrillation is used, the electrodes are applied directly to the heart and an impulse of 20 to 40 J is delivered. Vigorous cardiac massage should precede defibrillation to oxygenate the myocardium sufficiently. Perfusion pressure must be maintained to obtain successful defibrillation because ongoing subendocardial ischemia occurs when the perfusion

pressure is inadequate. Correction of acidosis with bicarbonate can be confirmed by blood gas determinations. Intramyocardial injection of epinephrine may stimulate myocardial tone and improve the chances of successful defibrillation. Unless a massive myocardial infarction has occurred, it should be possible to defibrillate the majority of fibrillating hearts, though the ensuing cardiac arrest may be refractory to therapy. The most significant factor influencing survival is the institution of defibrillation within 1 minute of onset of fibrillation or the ability to defibrillate with less than five shocks.

Following restoration of an adequate heart beat and blood pressure, the critical question is the extent of injury to the heart and to the central nervous system. A thorough search for reversible causes of the arrhythmia is undertaken immediately. If ischemia or graft occlusion is suspected, the patient is taken for cardiac catheterization or back to the operating room.

A detailed neurologic evaluation to elicit specific normal and abnormal reflexes should be done promptly. Permanent brain injury is common after more than 5 minutes of cardiac arrest, even though under experimental conditions cerebral neurons can tolerate nearly 20 minutes of normothermic ischemic anoxia. Intravenous steroid therapy is usually given for 24 to 48 hours to minimize cerebral edema, although the efficacy is difficult to measure. If serious cardiac or cerebral injury is not present following resuscitation, the prognosis is excellent. This fact is the basis for the enthusiastic advocacy of widespread training in cardiopulmonary resuscitation for all physicians, paramedical personnel, and lay people, because resuscitation is most effective when it is begun within 1 to 2 minutes after the onset of cardiac arrest.

Blood Loss

Blood conservation and minimization of bleeding associated with cardiac surgery begin preoperatively. Preoperative workup routinely includes a prothrombin time (PT), partial thromboplastin time (PTT), and platelet count. Patients with a history of abnormal bleeding or with chronic passive congestion of the liver receive full coagulation profiles and evaluation by a hematologist. Patients taking warfarin are instructed to discontinue the drug 3 to 4 days preoperatively so the PT can return to normal.

Since blood conservation is highly desirable, many patients operated on electively are able to donate autologous blood 1 to 3 weeks before surgery. Often erythropoietin is used after autologous donation to enhance the patient's red blood cell mass. Donor-directed blood units are solicited from family and friends. Intraoperatively, patients with a large blood volume and an adequate hematocrit may have one unit of fresh whole blood removed before bypass. The unit is saved and reinfused postbypass in order to take advantage of the fresh plasma and noninjured platelets. All blood in the operative field is collected during the procedure, either by suction into the CPB pump or into a cell-saver device. Similarly, mediastinal blood shed postoperatively through the chest tubes is collected sterilely and reinfused. By reinfusion of blood from the pump, cell-saver, and chest tubes, the need for blood transfusion associated with heart surgery has been diminished significantly, and many patients avoid transfusion altogether.

Postoperative Bleeding

For most open heart cases coagulopathy is nonexistent and the postoperative blood loss is low. On completion of CPB, heparinization is reversed with protamine and chest closure commences only when hemostasis is achieved. The normal total postoperative blood loss should range from 300 to 800 mL. *Blood loss in excess of*

300 to 500 mL/h or over 1 to 1.5 L total usually indicates active surgical bleeding, and is associated with a high incidence of hemodynamic compromise or cardiac tamponade. For this reason it is usually mandatory that patients with active bleeding or with a total blood loss greater than 1 to 1.5 L be returned to the operating room to control any active bleeding and avoid tamponade. If surgical bleeding is not found and a coagulopathy is present, appropriate treatment is initiated.

In some patients the effects of CPB can be quite damaging to the blood coagulation system, resulting in abnormal bleeding. The incidence of coagulopathy relates most strongly to the duration of CPB, but coagulopathy also is more frequent when hemodilution is excessive, after severe hypothermia, in patients having received aspirin or recent thrombolytic therapy, and in reoperations where ongoing blood loss from scar tissue results in progressive loss of coagulation factors.

The diagnosis of coagulopathy is made by the operating surgeon with the observation of abnormal bleeding from the operative field in the absence of a surgical source. Laboratory tests can confirm the diagnosis, but treatment should not be delayed until test results return, as this might further worsen the coagulation deficit, with fatal consequences. Nonsurgical causes of abnormal bleeding after heart surgery include (1) inadequate neutralization of heparin from insufficient protamine; (2) a functional platelet deficit, either from aspirin effect, or from the activation of platelets by the CPB circuit; (3) dilutional coagulopathy from the combination of crystalloid priming volume and transfusions; (4) a consumptive coagulopathy from a low-grade activation of the clotting factors by the bypass oxygenator and circuit; and (5) abnormal fibrinolysis.

Treatment of coagulopathy is urgent. Hypothermia should be corrected and extra protamine should be given until the activated clotting time returns to normal or until no further drop is seen in the activated clotting time. If abnormal bleeding persists, transfusion of platelets, fresh-frozen plasma, and cryoprecipitate is given until the clotting deficit is corrected. Antifibrinolytic agents such as ε-aminocaproic acid may be given to correct fibrinolysis. Recent advances used to minimize coagulopathy in high-risk cases include the use of heparin-bonded pump circuits and oxygenators. The pharmacologic prevention of coagulopathy is more effective if the protease inhibitor aprotonin is given preoperatively.

Ventilatory Support and Pulmonary Care

Nearly all cardiac surgical patients return to the recovery room intubated. While ventilating a patient after heart surgery, the physician should periodically assess the breath sounds, particularly in the posterior bases of the lungs, to determine the adequacy of ventilation. Tidal volumes on the respirator are usually set at 10 mL/kg, but occasionally up to 15 mL/kg is necessary in patients with chronic obstructive disease. For most cases, auscultation of the bases and determination of lung compliance (static lung compliance = tidal volume/end-inspiratory pressure) are the best ways to determine the optimal tidal volume, with the maximum lung compliance considered optimal for most cases. The adequacy of ventilation and oxygenation is then checked by periodic blood gas determinations. For difficult patients with marginal oxygenation, the optimal tidal volume and positive end-expiratory pressure (PEEP) may be better determined on the basis of oxygen delivery, with oxygen delivery equal to cardiac output times arterial oxygen content.

Weaning the patient is done via the intermittent mandatory ventilation (IMV) mode or via progressive continuous positive airway

pressure (CPAP) trials. Criteria for extubation include adequate blood gases on CPAP, with an inspired oxygen of less than 50%, a respiratory rate of less than 15 to 20 breaths per minute, a spontaneous tidal volume of 5 mL/kg, a forced vital capacity of 10 mL/kg, and a negative inspiratory pressure of 15 mL of water as determined by bedside pulmonary function tests. The patient should be awake enough to control the airway. Most patients are extubatable within 6 to 12 hours of surgery.

Postextubation pulmonary care involves use of the incentive spirometer, coughing, and deep breathing. Control of secretions is essential. Difficult cases might require the use of inhaled bronchodilators, such as the β_2-adrenergic agonist albuterol, or use of intravenous aminophylline. Rarely a short course of steroids is beneficial. Tracheobronchitis should be promptly treated with antibiotics. Observation of daily sputum specimens has been found by these authors to be important in infected patients, as clearing of the sputum and a drop in the white blood cell count indicate effective therapy. Clearing of secretions by coughing or suctioning is essential if the patient with tracheobronchitis is to recover. Flexible bronchoscopy has been effective in assessing the adequacy of suction and for evaluating the clearance of secretions in the refractory ventilator-dependent patient with tracheobronchitis.

Operation on the patient with a long smoking history and chronic obstructive pulmonary disease (COPD) poses a special problem. These patients should be strongly counseled on the need to stop smoking preoperatively, with the aid of transdermal nicotine patches if necessary. Evidence suggests that discontinuing smoking for even 1 week is markedly beneficial. However, poor pulmonary function usually does not prohibit cardiac surgery. For example, if a patient can function, albeit poorly, with substandard pulmonary reserve and critical aortic stenosis, the patient's overall cardiorespiratory function should significantly improve after correction of the valvular pathology. Fortunately, sternotomy has relatively little deleterious effect on pulmonary reserve.

With current preoperative preparation and intraoperative management, significant postoperative impairment of pulmonary function is uncommon, except in patients with pre-existing pulmonary disease or advanced cardiac failure. Most patients are now extubated within 8 to 12 hours, although mechanical ventilation for 24 to 72 hours is well tolerated by most patients. If periods of ventilation longer than 3 to 4 days are anticipated, a cricothyroidotomy or tracheostomy should be considered. In addition to providing patient comfort and safety and eliminating dead space, pulmonary toilet is more effective when done through a tracheostomy or cricothyroidotomy. Fortunately, ventilatory support for more than a short time is seldom necessary except in chronically ill or elderly patients in whom simple physical weakness may significantly impair the effectiveness of breathing and coughing. Such patients may require ventilatory support for days or even weeks.

General Care

Nutrition

The need for adequate postoperative nutrition cannot be overemphasized, particularly in elderly or chronically ill patients. The sick postoperative heart patient may require approximately 25 to 35 kcal/kg per day. Care should be taken to give adequate protein to patients with normal renal and hepatic function, while special formulas are available for patients with kidney or liver failure. Ill patients who remain intubated in the intensive care unit should have nutritional support started early, either as tube feeding or as intravenous hyperalimentation.

Wound Care

Early postoperative care of the surgical wound consists of the use of a sterile occlusive dressing for the first 24 hours. Wounds should be examined daily for redness, drainage, or sternal instability. Prophylactic antibiotics are started preoperatively and continued for 24 to 48 hours postoperatively, usually until indwelling catheters and chest tubes are removed. The prophylactic antibiotic used should be chosen based on the common organisms causing infection in the hospital.

Fever

All fever should be duly recorded and the patient examined for signs of infection. A moderate fever of 100 to 101°F is common in the first 1 to 2 days, usually resulting from the systemic inflammatory response induced by the extracorporeal circulation and the stress of major surgery or from atelectasis. A fever occurring from 3 to 7 days postoperatively with a normal white blood cell count is frequently due to postpericardiotomy syndrome. This syndrome is due to a combination of a generalized inflammatory response and localized irritation of the pericardium from surgical trauma. Postpericardiotomy syndrome may be associated with a friction rub and pericardial or pleural effusions. The syndrome can be treated with nonsteroidal anti-inflammatory agents or occasionally with a short course of steroids. Significant fevers should be evaluated with a chest x-ray and blood and urine cultures.

A serious sternal wound infection occurs in 1 to 2% of all open heart operations. Risk factors include diabetes, obesity, impaired nutrition, COPD, prolonged ventilatory support, harvest of bilateral internal mammary arteries, older age, low cardiac output, excessive mediastinal bleeding, re-exploration for bleeding, multiple transfusions, and prolonged CPB. The incidence is highest in diabetics receiving bilateral internal mammary artery grafts. Signs of infection include redness or pain in the wound, purulent drainage, sternal instability, fever, and an elevated white blood cell count. The diagnosis is easily made by sternal aspiration. Early diagnostic sternal aspiration is strongly recommended for any patient with persistent localized sternal pain or unexplained sepsis. *Staphylococcus aureus* and *Staphylococcus epidermidis* are the most common organisms isolated. Treatment requires prompt operation with either débridement and closure over antibiotic irrigation/drainage catheters or débridement followed by immediate or delayed closure with muscle flaps. The mortality rate from a sternal infection after cardiac surgery is 10 to 20%.

Renal Function

Close attention to renal function is necessary. The urine output for most adults should be 0.5 to 1 mL/kg per hour. The blood urea nitrogen (BUN) and creatinine levels are followed for several days postoperatively. Patients with a marginal urine output or with borderline renal function may benefit from low-dose (3 μg/kg per minute) dopamine. Some degree of salt and fluid retention is often present during postoperative days 3 to 5, even in patients with normal renal function, and diuretics may be necessary until the patients return to their preoperative weight. In patients with progressive renal dysfunction, early ultrafiltration or dialysis is indicated to control volume overload and to minimize the risk of arrhythmias and infection. Permitting the BUN level to rise above 90 to 100 mg/dL may result in serious cardiac arrhythmias and immunocompromise. The mortality rate is increased in patients with anuric renal failure after heart surgery, but newer techniques of aggressive management have dramatically improved results in these patients.

Rehabilitation

Most patients will benefit from early initiation of physical therapy and a cardiac rehabilitation program, but these treatments are especially important in elderly and debilitated patients. Physical therapy should begin early during the hospital stay and continue with a formalized rehabilitation program for an additional 1 to 2 weeks. Formal cardiac rehabilitation is usually available as either an inpatient or an outpatient program, depending on the patient's age and physical condition. After completing early cardiac rehabilitation, progressive exercise, such as walking up to 2 miles per day, is recommended for the first 4 to 6 weeks. More vigorous exercise may commence thereafter, but should be preceded by an exercise stress test.

References

1. Eagle KA, Berger PB, Calkins H, et al: ACC/AHA guideline update for perioperative cardiovascular evaluation for noncardiac surgery—executive summary report of the American College of Cardiology/American Heart Association Task Force on Practice Guidelines (Committee to Update the 1996 Guidelines on Perioperative Cardiovascular Evaluation for Noncardiac Surgery). *Circulation* 105:1257, 2002.
2. Gould KL, Nakagawa Y, Nakagawa K, et al: Frequency and clinical implications of fluid dynamically significant diffuse coronary artery disease manifest as graded, longitudinal, base-to-apex myocardial perfusion abnormalities by noninvasive positron emission tomography. *Circulation* 101:1931, 2000.
3. Nieman K, Oudkerk M, Rensing BJ, et al: Coronary angiography with multi-slice computed tomography. *Lancet* 357:599, 2001.
4. Treede H, Becker C, Reichenspurner H, et al: Multidetector computed tomography (MDCT) in coronary surgery: First experiences with a new tool for diagnosis of coronary artery disease. *Ann Thorac Surg* 74:S1398, 2002.
5. Darling E, Searles B, Nasrallah F, et al: High-volume, zero balanced ultrafiltration improves pulmonary function in a model of post-pump syndrome. *J Extra Corpor Technol* 34:254, 2002.
6. The Veterans Administration Coronary Artery Bypass Surgery Cooperative Study Group: Eleven-year survival in the Veterans Administration randomized trial of coronary bypass surgery for stable angina. *N Engl J Med* 311:1333, 1984.
7. Caracciolo EA, Davis KB, Sopko G, et al: Comparison of surgical and medical group survival in patients with left main coronary artery disease. Long-term CASS experience. *Circulation* 91:2325, 1995.
8. Chaitman BR, Fisher LD, Bourassa MG, et al: Effect of coronary bypass surgery on survival patterns in subsets of patients with left main coronary artery disease. Report of the Collaborative Study in Coronary Artery Surgery (CASS). *Am J Cardiol* 48:765, 1981.
9. Varnauskas E: Twelve-year follow-up of survival in the randomized European Coronary Surgery Study. *N Engl J Med* 319:332, 1988.
10. Jones RH, Kesler K, Phillips HR 3rd, et al: Long-term survival benefits of coronary artery bypass grafting and percutaneous transluminal angioplasty in patients with coronary artery disease. *J Thorac Cardiovasc Surg* 111:1013, 1996.
11. Chaux A, Blanche C, Matloff JM, et al: Postinfarction ventricular septal defect. *Semin Thorac Cardiovasc Surg* 10:93, 1998.
12. David TE: Operative management of postinfarction ventricular septal defect. *Semin Thorac Cardiovasc Surg* 7:208, 1995.
13. Pretre R, Benedikt P, Turina MI: Experience with postinfarction left ventricular free wall rupture. *Ann Thorac Surg* 69:1342, 2000.
14. Mantovani V, Vanoli D, Chelazzi P, et al: Post-infarction cardiac rupture: Surgical treatment. *Eur J Cardiothorac Surg* 22:777, 2002.
15. Gruentzig AR: Percutaneous transluminal coronary angioplasty. *Semin Roentgenol* 16:152, 1981.

16. Morice MC, Serruys PW, Sousa JE, et al: A randomized comparison of a sirolimus-eluting stent with a standard stent for coronary revascularization. *N Engl J Med* 346:1773, 2002.

17. The Bypass Angioplasty Revascularization Investigation (BARI) Investigators: Comparison of coronary bypass surgery with angioplasty in patients with multivessel disease. *N Engl J Med* 335:217, 1996.

18. Writing Group for the Bypass Angioplasty Revascularization Investigation (BARI) Investigators: Five-year clinical and functional outcome comparing bypass surgery and angioplasty in patients with multivessel coronary disease. A multicenter randomized trial. *JAMA* 277:715, 1997.

19. Coronary artery bypass surgery versus percutaneous coronary intervention with stent implantation in patients with multivessel coronary artery disease (the Stent or Surgery Trial): A randomised controlled trial. *Lancet* 360:965, 2002.

20. Abizaid A, Costa MA, Centemero M, et al: Clinical and economic impact of diabetes mellitus on percutaneous and surgical treatment of multivessel coronary disease patients: Insights from the Arterial Revascularization Therapy Study (ARTS) trial. *Circulation* 104:533, 2001.

21. de Feyter PJ, Serruys PW, Unger F, et al: Bypass surgery versus stenting for the treatment of multivessel disease in patients with unstable angina compared with stable angina. *Circulation* 105:2367, 2002.

22. Sedlis SP, Morrison DA, Lorin JD, et al: Percutaneous coronary intervention versus coronary bypass graft surgery for diabetic patients with unstable angina and risk factors for adverse outcomes with bypass: Outcome of diabetic patients in the AWESOME randomized trial and registry. *J Am Coll Cardiol* 40:1555, 2002.

23. Serruys PW, Unger F, Sousa JE, et al: Comparison of coronary-artery bypass surgery and stenting for the treatment of multivessel disease. *N Engl J Med* 344:1117, 2001.

24. Srinivas VS, Brooks MM, Detre KM, et al: Contemporary percutaneous coronary intervention versus balloon angioplasty for multivessel coronary artery disease: A comparison of the National Heart, Lung and Blood Institute Dynamic Registry and the Bypass Angioplasty Revascularization Investigation (BARI) study. *Circulation* 106:1627, 2002.

25. King SB 3rd, Lembo NJ, Weintraub WS, et al: A randomized trial comparing coronary angioplasty with coronary bypass surgery. Emory Angioplasty versus Surgery Trial (EAST). *N Engl J Med* 331:1044, 1994.

26. Coronary angioplasty versus coronary artery bypass surgery: The Randomized Intervention Treatment of Angina (RITA) trial. *Lancet* 341:573, 1993.

27. First-year results of CABRI (Coronary Angioplasty versus Bypass Revascularisation Investigation). CABRI Trial Participants. *Lancet* 346:1179, 1995.

28. Rodriguez A, Boullon F, Perez-Balino N, et al: Argentine randomized trial of percutaneous transluminal coronary angioplasty versus coronary artery bypass surgery in multivessel disease (ERACI): In-hospital results and 1-year follow-up. ERACI Group. *J Am Coll Cardiol* 22:1060, 1993.

29. Dion R, Etienne PY, Verhelst R, et al: Bilateral mammary grafting. Clinical, functional and angiographic assessment in 400 consecutive patients. *Eur J Cardiothorac Surg* 7:287, 1993; discussion 294.

30. Lytle BW, Cosgrove DM, Loop FD, et al: Perioperative risk of bilateral internal mammary artery grafting: Analysis of 500 cases from 1971 to 1984. *Circulation* 74:III37, 1986.

31. Chen AH, Nakao T, Brodman RF, et al: Early postoperative angiographic assessment of radial grafts used for coronary artery bypass grafting. *J Thorac Cardiovasc Surg* 111:1208, 1996.

32. Acar C, Ramsheyi A, Pagny JY, et al: The radial artery for coronary artery bypass grafting: Clinical and angiographic results at five years. *J Thorac Cardiovasc Surg* 116:981, 1998.

33. Society of Thoracic Surgeons National Adult Cardiac Surgery Database, 2003.

34. Grundeman PF: Vertical displacement of the beating heart by the Utrecht Octopus tissue stabilizer: Effects on haemodynamics and coronary flow. *Perfusion* 13:229, 1998.

35. Puskas JD, Thourani VH, Marshall JJ, et al: Clinical outcomes, angiographic patency, and resource utilization in 200 consecutive off-pump coronary bypass patients. *Ann Thorac Surg* 71:1477, 2001; discussion 1483.

36. Kim KB, Lim C, Lee C, et al: Off-pump coronary artery bypass may decrease the patency of saphenous vein grafts. *Ann Thorac Surg* 72:S1033, 2001.

37. Sabik JF, Gillinov AM, Blackstone EH, et al: Does off-pump coronary surgery reduce morbidity and mortality? *J Thorac Cardiovasc Surg* 124:698, 2002.

38. Puskas JD, Williams WH, Duke PG, et al: Off-pump coronary artery bypass grafting provides complete revascularization with reduced myocardial injury, transfusion requirements, and length of stay: A prospective randomized comparison of two hundred unselected patients undergoing off-pump versus conventional coronary artery bypass grafting. *J Thorac Cardiovasc Surg* 125:797, 2003.

39. Patel NC, Pullan DM, Fabri BM: Does off-pump total arterial revascularization without aortic manipulation influence neurological outcome? A study of 226 consecutive, unselected cases. *Heart Surg Forum* 5:28, 2002.

40. Novick RJ, Fox SA, Stitt LW, et al: Effect of off-pump coronary artery bypass grafting on risk-adjusted and cumulative sum failure outcomes after coronary artery surgery. *J Card Surg* 17:520, 2002.

41. Loop FD, Lytle BW, Cosgrove DM, et al: Influence of the internal mammary artery graft on 10-year survival and other cardiac events. *N Engl J Med* 314:1, 1986.

42. Calafiore AM, Di Mauro M, Canosa C, et al: Early and late outcome of myocardial revascularization with and without cardiopulmonary bypass in high-risk patients (EuroSCORE ≥ 6). *Eur J Cardiothorac Surg* 23:360, 2003.

43. Oliveira SA, Lisboa LA, Dallan LA, et al: Minimally-invasive single-vessel coronary artery bypass with the internal thoracic artery and early postoperative angiography: Midterm results of a prospective study in 120 consecutive patients. *Ann Thorac Surg* 73:505, 2002.

44. Diegeler A, Thiele H, Falk V, et al: Comparison of stenting with minimally-invasive bypass surgery for stenosis of the left anterior descending coronary artery. *N Engl J Med* 347:561, 2002.

45. Drenth DJ, Winter JB, Veeger NJ, et al: Minimally-invasive coronary artery bypass grafting versus percutaneous transluminal coronary angioplasty with stenting in isolated high-grade stenosis of the proximal left anterior descending coronary artery: Six months' angiographic and clinical follow-up of a prospective randomized study. *J Thorac Cardiovasc Surg* 124:130, 2002.

46. Detter C, Boehm DH, Reichenspurner H, et al: Robotically-assisted coronary artery surgery with and without cardiopulmonary bypass—from first clinical use to endoscopic operation. *Med Sci Monit* 8:MT118, 2002.

47. Falk V, Walther T, Autschbach R, et al: Robot-assisted minimally-invasive solo mitral valve operation. *J Thorac Cardiovasc Surg* 115:470, 1998.

48. Hughes GC, Kypson AP, Annex BH, et al: Induction of angiogenesis after TMR: A comparison of holmium:YAG, CO_2, and excimer lasers. *Ann Thorac Surg* 70:504, 2000.

49. Burkhoff D, Schmidt S, Schulman SP, et al: Transmyocardial laser revascularisation compared with continued medical therapy for treatment of refractory angina pectoris: A prospective randomised trial. ATLANTIC Investigators. Angina Treatments, Lasers and Normal Therapies in Comparison. *Lancet* 354:885, 1999.

50. Carrel TP, Eckstein FS, Englberger L, et al: Pitfalls and key lessons with the symmetry proximal anastomotic device in coronary artery bypass surgery. *Ann Thorac Surg* 75:1434, 2003.

51. Caskey MP, Kirshner MS, Alderman EL, et al: Six-month angiographic evaluation of beating-heart coronary arterial graft interrupted anastomoses using the coalescent U-CLIP anastomotic device: A prospective clinical study. *Heart Surg Forum* 5:319, 2002; discussion 327.

52. Jatene AD: Left ventricular aneurysmectomy. Resection or reconstruction. *J Thorac Cardiovasc Surg* 89:321, 1985.

53. Cooley DA: Ventricular endoaneurysmorrhaphy: A simplified repair for extensive postinfarction aneurysm. *J Card Surg* 4:200, 1989.

54. Dor V, Saab M, Coste P, et al: Left ventricular aneurysm: A new surgical approach. *Thorac Cardiovasc Surg* 37:11, 1989.

55. Dor V, Di Donato M, Sabatier M, et al: Left ventricular reconstruction by endoventricular circular patch plasty repair: A 17-year experience. *Semin Thorac Cardiovasc Surg* 13:435, 2001.

56. Doss M, Martens S, Sayour S, et al: Long term follow up of left ventricular function after repair of left ventricular aneurysm. A comparison of linear closure versus patch plasty. *Eur J Cardiothorac Surg* 20:783, 2001.

57. Athanasuleas CL, Stanley AW Jr., Buckberg GD, et al: Surgical anterior ventricular endocardial restoration (SAVER) in the dilated remodeled ventricle after anterior myocardial infarction. RESTORE group. Reconstructive Endoventricular Surgery, returning Torsion Original Radius Elliptical Shape to the LV. *J Am Coll Cardiol* 37:1199, 2001.

58. Mickleborough LL, Merchant N, Provost Y, et al: Ventricular reconstruction for ischemic cardiomyopathy. *Ann Thorac Surg* 75:S6, 2003.

59. Kang N, Edwards M, Larbalestier R: Preoperative intra-aortic balloon pumps in high-risk patients undergoing open heart surgery. *Ann Thorac Surg* 72:54, 2001.

60. Meharwal ZS, Trehan N: Vascular complications of intra-aortic balloon insertion in patients undergoing coronary reavscularization: Analysis of 911 cases. *Eur J Cardiothorac Surg* 21:741, 2001.

61. Ferguson JJ 3rd, Cohen M, Freedman RJ Jr., et al: The current practice of intra-aortic balloon counterpulsation: Results from the Benchmark Registry. *J Am Coll Cardiol* 38:1456, 2001.

62. McCarthy PM, Smith WA: Mechanical circulatory support—a long and winding road. *Science* 295:998, 2002.

63. Drews TN, Loebe M, Jurmann MJ, et al: Outpatients on mechanical circulatory support. *Ann Thorac Surg* 75:780, 2003; discussion 785.

64. Hagege AA, Carrion C, Menasche P, et al: Viability and differentiation of autologous skeletal myoblast grafts in ischaemic cardiomyopathy. *Lancet* 361:491, 2003.

65. Zhang F, Yang Z, Chen Y, et al: Clinical cellular cardiomyoplasty: Technical considerations. *J Card Surg* 18:268, 2003.

66. Menasche P, Hagege AA, Vilquin JT, et al: Autologous skeletal myoblast transplantation for severe postinfarction left ventricular dysfunction. *J Am Coll Cardiol* 41:1078, 2003.

67. Northrup WF 3rd, Kshettry VR, DuBois KA: Trends in mitral valve surgery in a large multi-surgeon, multi-hospital practice, 1979–1999. *J Heart Valve Dis* 12:14, 2003.

68. Chaliki HP, Mohty D, Avierinos JF, et al: Outcomes after aortic valve replacement in patients with severe aortic regurgitation and markedly reduced left ventricular function. *Circulation* 106:2687, 2002.

69. Jamieson WR, David TE, Feindel CM, et al: Performance of the Carpentier-Edwards SAV and Hancock-II porcine bioprostheses in aortic valve replacement. *J Heart Valve Dis* 11:424, 2002.

70. Marchand MA, Aupart MR, Norton R, et al: Fifteen-year experience with the mitral Carpentier-Edwards PERIMOUNT pericardial bioprosthesis. *Ann Thorac Surg* 71:S236, 2001.

71. Bonow RO, Carabello B, de Leon AC Jr., et al: Guidelines for the management of patients with valvular heart disease: Executive summary. A report of the American College of Cardiology/American Heart Association Task Force on Practice Guidelines (Committee on Management of Patients with Valvular Heart Disease). *Circulation* 98:1949, 1998.

72. Stein PD: Antithrombotic therapy in valvular heart disease. *Clin Geriatr Med* 17:163, 2001.

73. Emery RW, Van Nooten GJ, Tesar PJ: The initial experience with the ATS Medical mechanical cardiac valve prosthesis. *Ann Thorac Surg* 75:444, 2003.

74. Minakata K, Wu Y, Zerr KJ, et al: Clinical evaluation of the carbomedics prosthesis: Experience at providence health system in Portland. *J Heart Valve Dis* 11:844, 2002.

75. Butchart EG, Payne N, Li HH, et al: Better anticoagulation control improves survival after valve replacement. *J Thorac Cardiovasc Surg* 123:715, 2002.

76. Pibarot P, Dumesnil JG, Jobin J, et al: Hemodynamic and physical performance during maximal exercise in patients with an aortic bioprosthetic valve: Comparison of stentless versus stented bioprostheses. *J Am Coll Cardiol* 34:1609, 1999.

77. David TE, Pollick C, Bos J: Aortic valve replacement with stentless porcine aortic bioprosthesis. *J Thorac Cardiovasc Surg* 99:113, 1990.

78. Milano AD, Blanzola C, Mecozzi G, et al: Hemodynamic performance of stented and stentless aortic bioprostheses. *Ann Thorac Surg* 72:33, 2001.

79. Silberman S, Shaheen J, Merin O, et al: Exercise hemodynamics of aortic prostheses: Comparison between stentless bioprostheses and mechanical valves. *Ann Thorac Surg* 72:1217, 2001.

80. Dellgren G, Eriksson MJ, Brodin LA, et al: Eleven years' experience with the Biocor stentless aortic bioprosthesis: Clinical and hemodynamic follow-up with long-term relative survival rate. *Eur J Cardiothorac Surg* 22:912, 2002.

81. Koolbergen DR, Hazekamp MG, de Heer E, et al: Structural degeneration of pulmonary homografts used as aortic valve substitute underlines early graft failure. *Eur J Cardiothorac Surg* 22:802, 2002.

82. Legarra JJ, Concha M, Casares J, et al: Left ventricular remodeling after pulmonary autograft replacement of the aortic valve (Ross operation). *J Heart Valve Dis* 10:43, 2001.

83. Olson LJ, Subramanian R, Ackermann DM, et al: Surgical pathology of the mitral valve: A study of 712 cases spanning 21 years. *Mayo Clin Proc* 62:22, 1987.

84. Carpentier A: Cardiac valve surgery—the "French correction." *J Thorac Cardiovasc Surg* 86:323, 1983.

85. Enriquez-Sarano M: Timing of mitral valve surgery. *Heart* 87:79, 2002.

86. David TE, Ivanov J, Armstrong S, et al: Late outcomes of mitral valve repair for floppy valves: Implications for asymptomatic patients. *J Thorac Cardiovasc Surg* 125:1143, 2003.

87. Smith CR: Septal-superior exposure of the mitral valve. The transplant approach. *J Thorac Cardiovasc Surg* 103:623, 1992.

88. Grossi EA, Galloway AC, Kallenbach K, et al: Early results of posterior leaflet folding plasty for mitral valve reconstruction. *Ann Thorac Surg* 65:1057, 1998.

89. Carpentier A, Relland J, Deloche A, et al: Conservative management of the prolapsed mitral valve. *Ann Thorac Surg* 26:294, 1978.

90. Gillinov AM, Cosgrove DM, Blackstone EH, et al: Durability of mitral valve repair for degenerative disease. *J Thorac Cardiovasc Surg* 116:734, 1998.

91. Gillinov AM, Cosgrove DM: Mitral valve repair for degenerative disease. *J Heart Valve Dis* 11(Suppl 1):S15, 2002.

92. Choudhary SK, Dhareshwar J, Govil A, et al: Open mitral commissurotomy in the current era: Indications, technique, and results. *Ann Thorac Surg* 75:41, 2003.

93. Antunes MJ, Vieira H, Ferrao de Oliveira J: Open mitral commissurotomy: The "golden standard." *J Heart Valve Dis* 9:472, 2000.

94. Cardoso LF, Grinberg M, Rati MA, et al: Comparison between percutaneous balloon valvuloplasty and open commissurotomy for mitral stenosis. A prospective and randomized study. *Cardiology* 98:186, 2002.

95. Mohty D, Orszulak TA, Schaff HV, et al: Very long-term survival and durability of mitral valve repair for mitral valve prolapse. *Circulation* 104:I1, 2001.

96. Khan SS, Trento A, DeRobertis M, et al: Twenty-year comparison of tissue and mechanical valve replacement. *J Thorac Cardiovasc Surg* 122:257, 2001.

97. Galloway AC, Colvin SB, Baumann FG, et al: A comparison of mitral valve reconstruction with mitral valve replacement: Intermediate-term results. *Ann Thorac Surg* 47:655, 1989.

98. Yun KL, Miller DC: Mitral valve repair versus replacement. *Cardiol Clin* 9:315, 1991.

99. Galloway AC, Grossi EA, Bizekis CS, et al: Evolving techniques for mitral valve reconstruction. *Ann Surg* 236:288, 2002; discussion 293.

100. Braunberger E, Deloche A, Berrebi A, et al: Very long-term results (more than 20 years) of valve repair with Carpentier's techniques in nonrheumatic mitral valve insufficiency. *Circulation* 104:I8, 2001.

101. Spencer FC, Galloway AC, Grossi EA, et al: Recent developments and evolving techniques of mitral valve reconstruction. *Ann Thorac Surg* 65:307, 1998.

102. Grossi EA, Galloway AC, Ribakove GH, et al: Impact of minimally-invasive valvular heart surgery: A case-control study. *Ann Thorac Surg* 71:807, 2001.

103. Grossi EA, Zakow PK, Ribakove G, et al: Comparison of post-operative pain, stress response, and quality of life in port access vs. standard sternotomy coronary bypass patients. *Eur J Cardiothorac Surg* 16(Suppl 2):S39, 1999.

104. Fucci C, Sandrelli L, Pardini A, et al: Improved results with mitral valve repair using new surgical techniques. *Eur J Cardiothorac Surg* 9:621, 1995; discussion 626.

105. Totaro P, Tulumello E, Fellini P, et al: Mitral valve repair for isolated prolapse of the anterior leaflet: An 11-year follow-up. *Eur J Cardiothorac Surg* 15:119, 1999.

106. Umana JP, Salehizadeh B, DeRose JJ Jr., et al: "Bow-tie" mitral valve repair: An adjuvant technique for ischemic mitral regurgitation. *Ann Thorac Surg* 66:1640, 1998.

107. Lorusso R, Fucci C, Pentiricci S, et al: "Double-orifice" technique to repair extensive mitral valve excision following acute endocarditis. *J Card Surg* 13:24, 1998.

108. McCarthy PM, Starling RC, Wong J, et al: Early results with partial left ventriculectomy. *J Thorac Cardiovasc Surg* 114:755, 1997; discussion 763.

109. Chitwood WR Jr., Elbeery JR, Chapman WH, et al: Video-assisted minimally-invasive mitral valve surgery: The "micro-mitral" operation. *J Thorac Cardiovasc Surg* 113:413, 1997.

110. Mohr FW, Falk V, Diegeler A, et al: Minimally-invasive port-access mitral valve surgery. *J Thorac Cardiovasc Surg* 115:567, 1998; discussion 574.

111. Nifong LW, Chu VF, Bailey BM, et al: Robotic mitral valve repair: Experience with the da Vinci system. *Ann Thorac Surg* 75:438, 2003; discussion 443.

112. Dare AJ, Veinot JP, Edwards WD, et al: New observations on the etiology of aortic valve disease: A surgical pathologic study of 236 cases from 1990. *Hum Pathol* 24:1330, 1993.

113. Green GR, Miller DC: Continuing dilemmas concerning aortic valve replacement in patients with advanced left ventricular systolic dysfunction. *J Heart Valve Dis* 6:562, 1997.

114. Rosenhek R, Maurer G, Baumgartner H: Should early elective surgery be performed in patients with severe but asymptomatic aortic stenosis? *Eur Heart J* 23:1417, 2002.

115. Bucerius J, Gummert JF, Borger MA, et al: Stroke after cardiac surgery: A risk factor analysis of 16,184 consecutive adult patients. *Ann Thorac Surg* 75:472, 2003.

116. David TE, Feindel CM: An aortic valve-sparing operation for patients with aortic incompetence and aneurysm of the ascending aorta. *J Thorac Cardiovasc Surg* 103:617, 1992; discussion 622.

117. David TE, Ivanov J, Armstrong S, et al: Aortic valve-sparing operations in patients with aneurysms of the aortic root or ascending aorta. *Ann Thorac Surg* 74:S1758, 2002; discussion S1792.

118. Sarsam MA, Yacoub M: Remodeling of the aortic valve annulus. *J Thorac Cardiovasc Surg* 105:435, 1993.

119. Casselman FP, Gillinov AM, Akhrass R, et al: Intermediate-term durability of bicuspid aortic valve repair for prolapsing leaflet. *Eur J Cardiothorac Surg* 15:302, 1999.

120. Paparella D, David TE, Armstrong S, et al: Mid-term results of the Ross procedure. *J Card Surg* 16:338, 2001.

121. David TE, Omran A, Ivanov J, et al: Dilation of the pulmonary autograft after the Ross procedure. *J Thorac Cardiovasc Surg* 119:210, 2000.

122. Gundry SR, Shattuck OH, Razzouk AJ, et al: Facile minimally-invasive cardiac surgery via ministernotomy. *Ann Thorac Surg* 65:1100, 1998.

123. Byrne JG, Hsin MK, Adams DH, et al: Minimally-invasive direct access heart valve surgery. *J Card Surg* 15:21, 2000.

124. Cosgrove DM 3rd, Sabik JF, Navia JL: Minimally-invasive valve operations. *Ann Thorac Surg* 65:1535, 1998; discussion 1538.

125. Sharony R, Grossi EA, Saunders PC, et al: Minimally-invasive aortic valve surgery in the elderly: A case-control study. *Circulation* 108(Suppl 1):II43, 2003.

126. Byrne JG, Aranki SF, Couper GS, et al: Reoperative aortic valve replacement: Partial upper hemisternotomy versus conventional full sternotomy. *J Thorac Cardiovasc Surg* 118:991, 1999.

127. Sherrid MV, Chaudhry FA, Swistel DG: Obstructive hypertrophic cardiomyopathy: Echocardiography, pathophysiology, and the continuing evolution of surgery for obstruction. *Ann Thorac Surg* 75:620, 2003.

128. Maron MS, Olivotto I, Betocchi S, et al: Effect of left ventricular outflow tract obstruction on clinical outcome in hypertrophic cardiomyopathy. *N Engl J Med* 348:295, 2003.

129. Morrow AG, Fogarty TJ, Hannah H 3rd, et al: Operative treatment in idiopathic hypertrophic subaortic stenosis. Techniques and the results of preoperative and postoperative clinical and hemodynamic assessments. *Circulation* 37:589, 1968.

130. Nakatani S, Schwammenthal E, Lever HM, et al: New insights into the reduction of mitral valve systolic anterior motion after ventricular septal myectomy in hypertrophic obstructive cardiomyopathy. *Am Heart J* 131:294, 1996.

131. Tribouilloy CM, Enriquez-Sarano M, Capps MA, et al: Contrasting effect of similar effective regurgitant orifice area in mitral and tricuspid regurgitation: A quantitative Doppler echocardiographic study. *J Am Soc Echocardiogr* 15:958, 2002.

132. Tribouilloy CM, Enriquez-Sarano M, Bailey KR, et al: Quantification of tricuspid regurgitation by measuring the width of the vena contracta with Doppler color flow imaging: A clinical study. *J Am Coll Cardiol* 36:472, 2000.

133. Groves PH, Hall RJ: Late tricuspid regurgitation following mitral valve surgery. *J Heart Valve Dis* 1:80, 1992.

134. Kay J, Maselli-Campagna G, Tsuji H: Surgical treatment of tricuspid insufficiency. *Ann Surg* 162:53, 1965.

135. Boyd AD, Engelman RM, Isom OW, et al: Tricuspid annuloplasty. Five and one-half years' experience with 78 patients. *J Thorac Cardiovasc Surg* 68:344, 1974.

136. De Vega NG: Selective, adjustable and permanent annuloplasty. An original technic for the treatment of tricuspid insufficiency. *Rev Esp Cardiol* 25:555, 1972.

137. McCarthy JF, Cosgrove DM 3rd: Tricuspid valve repair with the Cosgrove-Edwards Annuloplasty System. *Ann Thorac Surg* 64:267, 1997.

138. Carrier M, Hebert Y, Pellerin M, et al: Tricuspid valve replacement: An analysis of 25 years of experience at a single center. *Ann Thorac Surg* 75:47, 2003.

139. Kawano H, Oda T, Fukunaga S, et al: Tricuspid valve replacement with the St. Jude medical valve: 19 years of experience. *Eur J Cardiothorac Surg* 18:565, 2000.

140. Galloway AC, Grossi EA, Baumann FG, et al: Multiple valve operation for advanced valvular heart disease: Results and risk factors in 513 patients. *J Am Coll Cardiol* 19:725, 1992.

141. Culliford AT, Lipton M, Spencer FC: Operation for chronic constrictive pericarditis: Do the surgical approach and degree of pericardial resection influence the outcome significantly? *Ann Thorac Surg* 29:146, 1980.

142. Acebo E, Val-Bernal JF, Gomez-Roman JJ, et al: Clinicopathologic study and DNA analysis of 37 cardiac myxomas: A 28-year experience. *Chest* 123:1379, 2003.

143. Keeling IM, Oberwalder P, Anelli-Monti M, et al: Cardiac myxomas: 24 years of experience in 49 patients. *Eur J Cardiothorac Surg* 22:971, 2002.

144. Talbot SM, Taub RN, Keohan ML, et al: Combined heart and lung transplantation for unresectable primary cardiac sarcoma. *J Thorac Cardiovasc Surg* 124:1145, 2002.

145. Chiappini B, Savini C, Marinelli G, et al: Cavoatrial tumor thrombus: Single-stage surgical approach with profound hypothermia and circulatory arrest, including a review of the literature. *J Thorac Cardiovasc Surg* 124:684, 2002.

CHAPTER 21

Thoracic Aortic Aneurysms and Aortic Dissection

Joseph S. Coselli and Scott A. LeMaire

The aorta consists of two major segments—the proximal aorta and the distal aorta—each of which has anatomic characteristics that impact clinical manifestations and treatment strategies (Fig. 21-1). The proximal aortic segment includes the ascending aorta and the transverse aortic arch. The ascending aorta begins at the aortic valve and ends at the origin of the innominate artery. The first portion of the ascending aorta is the aortic root, which includes the aortic valve annulus and the three sinuses of Valsalva; the coronary arteries originate from two of these sinuses. The aortic root joins the tubular portion of the ascending aorta at the sinotubular ridge. The transverse aortic arch is the segment from which the brachiocephalic branches arise. The distal aortic segment includes the descending thoracic aorta and the abdominal aorta. The descending thoracic aorta begins distal to the origin of the left subclavian artery and extends to the diaphragmatic hiatus, where it joins the abdominal aorta. The descending thoracic segment gives rise to multiple bronchial and esophageal branches as well as the segmental intercostal arteries, which provide circulation to the spinal cord.

The large volume of blood that flows through the thoracic aorta at high pressure is incomparable to that of any other vascular structure. For this reason, any condition that disrupts the integrity of the thoracic aorta, such as aortic dissection, aneurysm rupture, or traumatic injury, will have catastrophic consequences.

THORACIC AORTIC ANEURYSMS

Aortic aneurysm is defined as a permanent localized dilatation resulting in at least a 50% increase in diameter compared with the normal expected aortic diameter at the same anatomic level. The incidence of thoracic aortic aneurysms is estimated to be 5.9 per 100,000 persons annually. The clinical manifestations, methods of treatment, and treatment results in patients with aortic aneurysms vary according to the cause and aortic segment involved. Causes of thoracic aortic aneurysms include degenerative disease of the aortic wall, aortic dissection, aortitis, infection, and trauma. Aneurysms can be localized to a single aortic segment, or can involve multiple segments. Thoracoabdominal aortic aneurysms, for example, involve both the descending thoracic aorta and abdominal aorta. In the most extreme situation, the entire aorta is aneurysmal; this is often described as "mega-aorta."

Aneurysms of the thoracic aorta consistently increase in size and progress to serious complications including rupture, which is usually a fatal event. Therefore, aggressive treatment is indicated in all but the poorest surgical candidates. Small asymptomatic thoracic aortic aneurysms can be followed, especially in poor-risk patients, and later treated surgically if the patient develops symptoms or complications, or if progressive enlargement occurs. Meticulous control of hypertension is the primary medical treatment.

Elective resection with graft replacement is indicated in asymptomatic patients with an aortic diameter of at least twice the normal diameter for the involved segment (5 to 6 cm in most thoracic segments). Contraindications to elective repair are extreme operative

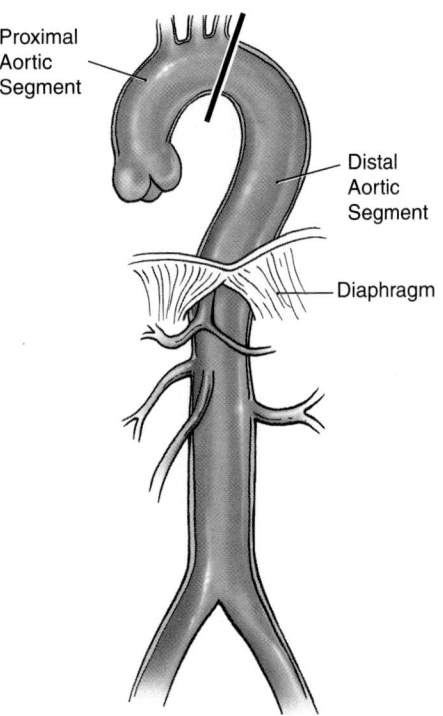

FIG. 21-1. *Drawing of the aorta, divided into the proximal segment and the distal segment.*

risk because of severe coexisting cardiac or pulmonary disease, or a limited life expectancy due to other conditions, such as malignancy. An emergency operation is required for any patient in whom a ruptured aneurysm is suspected.

Patients with thoracic aortic aneurysm often have coexisting aneurysms of other aortic segments. A common cause of death following repair of a thoracic aortic aneurysm is rupture of a different aortic aneurysm. Therefore staged repair of multiple aortic segments is often necessary. As with any major operative procedure, careful preoperative evaluation regarding coexisting disease and subsequent medical optimization are essential for successful surgical treatment.

Etiology and Pathogenesis

General Considerations

The normal aorta derives its elasticity and tensile strength from the medial layer, which contains approximately 45 to 55 lamellae of elastin, collagen, smooth muscle cells, and ground substance. Elastin content is highest within the ascending aorta, as would be expected with its compliant nature, and decreases distally into the descending and abdominal aorta. Maintenance of the aortic matrix involves complex interactions between smooth muscle cells, macrophages, proteases, and protease inhibitors. Any alteration within this delicate balance can lead to aortic pathology.

Causes of thoracic aortic aneurysms are listed in Table 21-1. Although these disparate pathologic processes differ in biochemical and microscopic terms, they share the final common pathway of progressive aortic expansion and eventual rupture. Hemodynamic factors clearly contribute to the process of aortic dilatation. The vicious cycle between increasing diameter and increasing wall tension, as characterized by Laplace's law (tension = pressure × radius), is well established. Turbulent blood flow is also recognized as a factor. Poststenotic aortic dilatation, for example, occurs in some patients with aortic valve stenosis or coarctation of the descending thoracic

Table 21-1
Causes of Thoracic Aortic Aneurysms

Nonspecific medial degeneration
Aortic dissection
Genetic disorders
Marfan syndrome
Ehlers-Danlos syndrome
Familial aortic aneurysms
Bicuspid aortic valves
Poststenotic dilatation
Infection
Aortitis
Takayasu's arteritis
Giant cell arteritis
Rheumatoid aortitis
Trauma

aorta. Hemodynamic derangements, however, are only one piece within a complex puzzle.

Atherosclerosis is commonly cited as a cause of thoracic aortic aneurysms. However, while atherosclerotic disease is often found in conjunction with aortic aneurysms, the notion that atherosclerosis is a distinct cause of aneurysm formation has been challenged. In thoracic aortic aneurysms, atherosclerosis appears to be a coexisting process rather than the underlying cause.

Recent research into the pathogenesis of abdominal aortic aneurysms has focused on the molecular mechanisms of aortic wall degeneration and dilatation. For example, imbalances between proteolytic enzymes (e.g., matrix metalloproteinases) and their inhibitors contribute to abdominal aortic aneurysm formation. Building on these advances, current investigations are exploring whether similar inflammatory and proteolytic mechanisms are involved in thoracic aortic disease, in hope of identifying potential molecular targets for pharmacologic therapy.

Nonspecific Medial Degeneration

Nonspecific medial degeneration is the most common cause of thoracic aortic disease. Histologic findings of mild medial degeneration, including fragmentation of elastic fibers and loss of smooth muscle cells, are expected in the aging aorta. However, an advanced, accelerated form of medial degeneration leads to progressive weakening of the aortic wall, aneurysm formation, and eventual rupture and/or dissection. The underlying causes of medial degenerative disease remain unknown.

Aortic Dissection

Aortic dissections usually begin as a tear in the inner aortic wall, which initiates a progressive separation of the medial layers, creating two channels within the aorta and a profoundly weakened outer wall. As the most common catastrophe involving the aorta, dissection represents a major, distinct cause of thoracic aortic aneurysms, and is discussed in detail in the second half of this chapter.

Genetic Disorders

Marfan Syndrome. Marfan syndrome is an autosomal dominant genetic disorder characterized by a specific connective tissue defect that leads to aneurysm formation. The phenotype of patients with Marfan syndrome typically includes a tall stature, high palate, joint hypermobility, lens disorders, mitral valve prolapse, and aortic aneurysms. The aortic wall is weakened by fragmentation of elastic fibers and deposition of extensive amounts of mucopolysaccharides (cystic medial degeneration). Patients with

Marfan syndrome have a mutation involving the fibrillin gene located on the long arm of the chromosome 15. Abnormal fibrillin in the extracellular matrix decreases connective tissue strength in the aortic wall and produces abnormal elastic properties that predispose the aorta to dilatation from wall tension resulting from left ventricular ejection impulses. Seventy-five to 85% of patients with Marfan syndrome exhibit dilation of the ascending aorta with annuloaortic ectasia (dilation of the aortic sinuses and annulus).

Ehlers-Danlos Syndrome. Ehlers-Danlos syndrome includes a spectrum of inherited connective tissue disorders of collagen synthesis; the subtypes represent differing defective steps of collagen production. Type IV Ehlers-Danlos syndrome is characterized by an autosomal dominant defect in type III collagen synthesis, and may produce life-threatening cardiovascular manifestations. Spontaneous arterial rupture, usually involving the mesenteric vessels, is the most common cause of death in these patients. Thoracic aortic aneurysms and dissections represent less common entities associated with Ehlers-Danlos syndrome, but nonetheless are reported and require challenging surgical management secondary to altered tissue integrity.

Familial Aortic Aneurysms. Guo and colleagues demonstrated a linkage to the 5q locus in nine of 15 families with strong family histories (i.e., autosomal dominant transmission) of ascending aortic aneurysms and dissections. Linkage to the fibrillin gene on chromosome 15 was not identified in any of the 15 families. Similar studies have found linkages to chromosomes 3 and 11. With the initiation of the International HapMap Project, which aims to establish a haplotype map of the human genome, aneurysms currently classified as idiopathic may eventually be described in terms of a specific genetic susceptibility that is exacerbated with certain environmental exposures, such as smoking.

Congenital Bicuspid Aortic Valve. Bicuspid aortic valve is the most common congenital malformation of the heart or great vessels, affecting nearly 1 to 2% of Americans. Compared to patients with normal trileaflet aortic valves, patients with bicuspid aortic valves have an increased incidence of ascending aortic aneurysm formation and exhibit a more rapid rate of aortic enlargement. Additionally, aortic dissection occurs 10 times more often in patients with bicuspid valves than in the general population. Recent investigations suggest that aneurysms associated with bicuspid aortic valves have a fundamentally different pathophysiology than those that occur in patients with trileaflet valves. The exact mechanism responsible for aneurysm formation in these patients remains controversial. The two main theories posit that the dilatation is caused by (1) a congenital defect involving the aortic wall matrix that results in progressive degeneration, or (2) ongoing hemodynamic stress caused by turbulent flow through the diseased valve. Ultimately, a combination of both hypotheses seems most likely; patients with bicuspid aortic valves may have a congenital connective tissue abnormality that predisposes them to aneurysm formation in the setting of chronic turbulent flow through a deformed valve.

Infection

Primary infection of the aortic wall resulting in aneurysm formation is rare. Although termed *mycotic aneurysms,* the responsible pathogens are usually bacteria rather than fungi. Bacterial invasion of the aortic wall may result from bacterial endocarditis, endothelial trauma caused by an aortic jet lesion, or extension from an infected laminar clot within a pre-existing aneurysm. The most common organisms include *Staphylococcus aureus, S. epidermidis,*

Salmonella, and *Streptococcus* spp. In contrast to most other causes of thoracic aortic aneurysms, which generally produce fusiform aneurysms, infection often produces saccular aneurysms localized in areas destroyed by the infectious process.

While once the most common cause of ascending aortic aneurysms, the advent of effective antibiotic therapy has made syphilitic aneurysms a rarity in developed nations. In other parts of the world, however, syphilitic aneurysms remain a major cause of morbidity and mortality. The spirochete *Treponema pallidum* causes an obliterative endarteritis of the vasa vasorum, resulting in medial ischemia and loss of the elastic and muscular elements of the aortic wall. The ascending aorta and arch are the most common areas of involvement. The emergence of the human immunodeficiency virus (HIV) in the 1980s has been associated with a substantial increase in the incidence of syphilis in both HIV-infected and non–HIV infected patients. Because syphilitic aortitis often presents 10 to 30 years after the primary infection, the incidence of associated aneurysms may increase in the near future.

Aortitis

Patients with pre-existing degenerative thoracic aortic aneurysms can develop localized transmural inflammation and subsequent fibrosis. The dense aortic infiltrate consists of lymphocytes, plasma cells, and giant cells. The cause of the intense inflammatory reaction is unknown. Although the severe inflammation is a superimposed problem rather than a primary cause, its onset within an aneurysm can further weaken the aortic wall and precipitate expansion.

Systemic autoimmune disorders also cause thoracic aortitis. While Takayasu's arteritis generally produces obstructive lesions related to severe intimal thickening, associated medial necrosis can lead to aneurysm formation. Patients with giant cell arteritis (temporal arteritis) may develop granulomatous inflammation involving the entire thickness of the aortic wall, causing intimal thickening and medial destruction. Rheumatoid aortitis is an uncommon systemic disease that is associated with rheumatoid arthritis and ankylosing spondylitis; the resulting medial inflammation and fibrosis can affect the aortic root, causing annular dilatation, aortic valve insufficiency, and ascending aortic aneurysm formation.

Pseudoaneurysms

Pseudoaneurysms, or false aneurysms, of the thoracic aorta usually represent chronic leaks that are contained by surrounding tissue and fibrosis. By definition, the wall of a pseudoaneurysm is not formed by intact aortic tissue; rather, the wall develops from organized thrombus and associated fibrosis. Pseudoaneurysms can arise from primary defects in the aortic wall (e.g., after trauma or contained aneurysm rupture) or anastomotic leaks after cardiovascular surgery. Anastomotic pseudoaneurysms can be caused by technical error or deterioration of the native aortic tissue, graft material, or suture. Tissue deterioration is usually related to either progressive degenerative disease or infection. Improvements in sutures, graft materials, and surgical techniques have decreased the incidence of thoracic aortic pseudoaneurysms.

Natural History

Decisions regarding treatment options in patients with thoracic aortic aneurysms are guided by our current understanding of the natural history. Classically, the natural history is characterized as progressive aortic dilatation and eventual rupture and/or dissection. Elefteriades' analysis of 1600 patients with thoracic aortic disease has helped quantify these well-recognized risks. Average expansion rates were 0.07 cm per year in ascending aortic aneurysms and 0.19 cm per year for descending thoracic aortic aneurysms. As expected, aortic diameter was a strong predictor of rupture, dissection, and mortality. For thoracic aortic aneurysms greater than 6 cm in diameter, annual rates of catastrophic complications were 3.6% for rupture, 3.7% for dissection, and 10.8% for death. Critical diameters, at which the incidence of natural complications significantly increased, were 6.0 cm for aneurysms of the ascending aorta and 7.0 cm for aneurysms of the descending thoracic aorta; the corresponding risks of rupture after reaching these diameters were 31 and 43%, respectively.

Certain patient subgroups have an increased propensity for expansion and rupture. Patients with Marfan syndrome, for example, have aneurysms that dilate at an accelerated rate and rupture or dissect at smaller diameters than non-Marfan aneurysms. Before the era of surgical treatment, this aggressive form of aortic disease resulted in an average life expectancy of 32 years for Marfan patients, with aortic root complications causing the majority of deaths. Saccular aneurysms, which are commonly associated with aortic infection, also grow more rapidly than degenerative fusiform aneurysms.

A common clinical scenario deserves special attention. A moderately dilated ascending aorta (i.e., 4 to 5 cm) is often encountered during aortic valve replacement or coronary artery bypass operations. The natural history of these ectatic ascending aortas has been defined by several studies. Michel and colleagues studied patients whose ascending aortic diameters exceeded 4 cm at the time of aortic valve replacement; 25% of these patients required reoperation for ascending aortic replacement. Prenger and colleagues reported that aortic dissection occurred in 27% of patients who had aortic diameters exceeding 5 cm at the time of aortic valve replacement.

Clinical Manifestations

In many patients with thoracic aortic aneurysms, the aneurysm is discovered incidentally when imaging studies are obtained for unrelated reasons. Therefore patients are often asymptomatic at the time of diagnosis. However, when thoracic aortic aneurysms go undetected, they ultimately create symptoms and signs that correspond with the segment of aorta that is involved. These aneurysms produce a wide variety of manifestations, including compression or erosion of adjacent structures, aortic valve insufficiency, distal embolism, and rupture.

Local Compression and Erosion

Initially, expansion and impingement on adjacent structures causes mild chronic pain. The most common symptom in patients with ascending aortic aneurysms is anterior chest discomfort; the pain is frequently precordial in location, but may radiate to the neck and jaw, mimicking angina. Aneurysms of the ascending aorta and transverse aortic arch can cause symptoms related to compression of the superior vena cava, the pulmonary artery, the airway, or the sternum. Although unusual, erosion can occur into the superior vena cava or right atrium, causing acute high-output failure. Expansion of the distal aortic arch can stretch the recurrent laryngeal nerve, resulting in left vocal cord paralysis and hoarseness. Descending thoracic and thoracoabdominal aneurysms frequently cause back pain localized between the scapulae. When the aneurysm is largest in the region of the aortic hiatus, middle back and epigastric pain may occur. Thoracic or lumbar vertebral body erosion typically causes severe, chronic back pain; extreme cases can present with spinal instability and neurologic deficits from spinal cord compression. Although

mycotic aneurysms have a peculiar propensity to destroy vertebral bodies, spinal erosion also occurs with degenerative aneurysms. Descending thoracic aortic aneurysms may cause varying degrees of airway obstruction, manifested as cough, wheezing, stridor, or pneumonitis. Pulmonary or airway erosion presents as hemoptysis. Compression or erosion of the esophagus creates dysphagia and hematemesis, respectively. Thoracoabdominal aortic aneurysms can cause duodenal obstruction, or upon bowel wall erosion, gastrointestinal bleeding. Jaundice due to compression of the liver or porta hepatis is uncommon. Erosion into the inferior vena cava or iliac vein will present with an abdominal bruit, widened pulse pressure, edema, and heart failure.

Aortic Valve Insufficiency

Ascending aortic aneurysms that involve the aortic root cause commissural displacement and annular dilatation, resulting in progressive aortic valve insufficiency. These patients may present with progressive heart failure, and will exhibit a widened pulse pressure and a diastolic murmur.

Distal Embolization

Thoracic aortic aneurysms—particularly those involving the descending and thoracoabdominal aorta—are commonly lined with friable, atheromatous plaque and mural thrombus. This debris may embolize distally, causing occlusion and thrombosis of the visceral, renal, or lower-extremity branches.

Rupture

Patients with ruptured thoracic aortic aneurysms often experience sudden, severe pain in the anterior chest (ascending aorta), upper back or left chest (descending thoracic aorta), or left flank or abdomen (thoracoabdominal aorta). When ascending aortic aneurysms rupture, they usually bleed into the pericardial space, producing acute cardiac tamponade and death. Descending thoracic aortic aneurysms rupture into the pleural cavity, producing a combination of severe hemorrhagic shock and respiratory compromise. External rupture is extremely rare; syphilitic aneurysms have been noted to rupture externally after eroding through the sternum.

Diagnostic Evaluation

Although certain constellations of symptoms and signs are highly suggestive of thoracic aortic aneurysm, the diagnosis and characterization of thoracic aortic aneurysm requires imaging studies. Besides their role in establishing the diagnosis, imaging studies provide critical information that guides the selection of treatment options. Optimal imaging techniques for the thoracic and thoracoabdominal aorta are somewhat institution-specific, based on the availability of imaging equipment and expertise.

Plain Radiographs

Plain radiographs of the chest, abdomen, or spine often provide enough information to support the initial diagnosis of thoracic aortic aneurysm. Ascending aortic aneurysms produce a convex shadow to the right of the cardiac silhouette. The anterior projection of an ascending aneurysm results in the loss of the retrosternal space in the lateral view. The presence of an aneurysm may be indistinguishable from elongation and tortuosity. It is important to recognize that chest radiographs are commonly normal in patients with thoracic aortic disease and cannot exclude the diagnosis of aortic aneurysm. Aortic root aneurysms, for example, are often hidden within the cardiac silhouette. Plain chest radiographs may demonstrate convexity

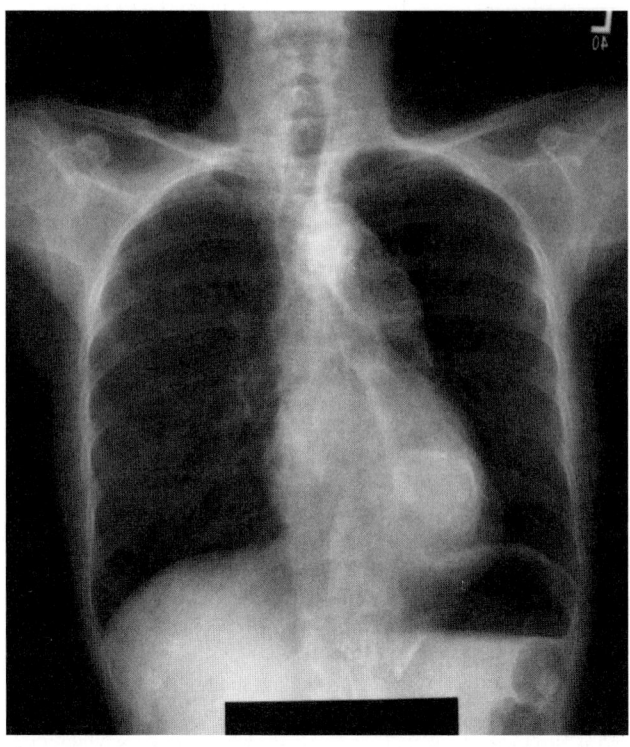

A

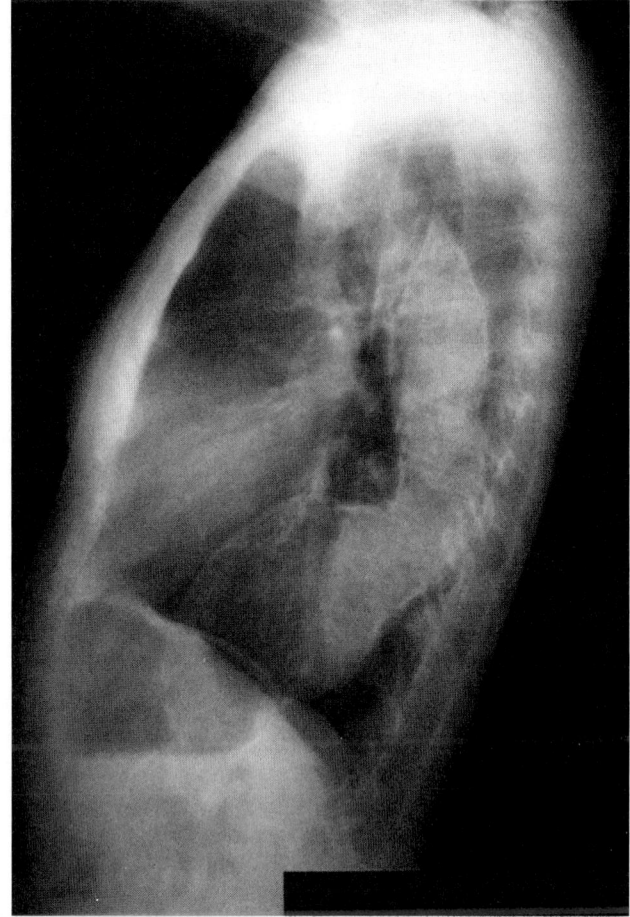

B

FIG. 21-2. *Chest roentgenogram. A. Anteroposterior view. B. Lateral view demonstrating calcified rim in the aortic wall of a thoracoabdominal aortic aneurysm.*

in the right superior mediastinum, loss of the retrosternal space, or widening of the descending thoracic aortic shadow, which may be highlighted by a rim of calcification outlining the dilated aneurysmal aortic wall. Aortic calcification may also be seen in the upper abdomen on a standard roentgenogram made in the anteroposterior or lateral projections (Fig. 21-2). Once a thoracic aortic aneurysm is detected on plain radiographs, additional studies are required to define the extent of aortic involvement.

Ultrasonography

Although useful in evaluating infrarenal abdominal aortic aneurysms, standard transabdominal ultrasonography does not allow visualization of the thoracic aorta. During ultrasound evaluation of a suspected infrarenal abdominal aortic aneurysm, if a definitive neck cannot be demonstrated at the level of the renal arteries, thoracoabdominal aortic involvement should be suspected and investigated with other imaging modalities.

Echocardiography

Ascending aortic aneurysms are commonly discovered during echocardiography in patients presenting with symptoms or signs of aortic valve insufficiency. Both transthoracic and transesophageal echocardiography provide excellent visualization of the ascending aorta, including the aortic root. The latter modality also allows visualization of the descending thoracic aorta, but has limitations in evaluating the transverse aortic arch, which is obscured by

air in the tracheobronchial tree, and the upper abdominal aorta. Effective echocardiography requires considerable technical skill both in obtaining adequate images and in interpretation.

Computed Tomography

Computed tomographic (CT) scanning is widely available and provides visualization of the entire thoracic and abdominal aorta. Consequently, it is the most common—and arguably the most useful—imaging modality for evaluating thoracic aortic aneurysms. Systems capable of constructing multiplanar images and three-dimensional aortic reconstructions are becoming increasingly available. In addition to establishing the diagnosis, CT provides information regarding location, extent, anatomic anomalies, and relationship to major branch vessels. Contrast-enhanced CT provides information regarding the aortic lumen, and can detect mural thrombus, aortic dissection, inflammatory periaortic fibrosis, and mediastinal or retroperitoneal hematoma due to contained aortic rupture. It is particularly useful in determining the absolute diameter of the aorta, especially in the presence of laminated clot.

Magnetic Resonance Angiography

Magnetic resonance angiography (MRA) is becoming widely available and has the capability of assessing the entire aorta. Compared to contrast-enhanced CT, MRA provides comparable aortic images, while offering the advantage of avoiding exposure to nephrotoxic contrast and ionizing radiation. MRA offers excellent visualization of branch vessel details, and it is useful when assessing the presence of branch vessel stenosis. Current limitations of MRA include high expense and the susceptibility to artifacts created by ferromagnetic materials. Furthermore, the MRA environment is not appropriate for many critically ill patients.

Aortography and Cardiac Catheterization

Although diagnostic aortography was until recently considered the gold standard for evaluating thoracic aortic disease, CT and MRA have largely replaced this modality. Technologic improvements in CT and MRA have enabled these modalities to provide excellent aortic imaging with less morbidity than catheter-based studies. Therefore the role of diagnostic angiography in these patients is currently limited. In selected cases, aortography is used to gain important information when other studies are contraindicated or have not provided satisfactory results. For example, information regarding obstructive lesions of the brachiocephalic, visceral, renal, or iliac arteries is useful when planning surgical treatment; if other imaging studies have not provided adequate detail, aortography can be obtained in patients with suspected branch vessel occlusive disease.

In contrast to standard aortography, cardiac catheterization continues to play a major role in diagnosis and preoperative planning, especially in patients with ascending aortic involvement. In addition to assessing the status of the coronary arteries and left ventricular function, proximal aortography evaluates the degree of aortic valve insufficiency, the extent of aortic root involvement, coronary ostial displacement, and the relationship of the aneurysm to the arch vessels.

The benefits of obtaining information from catheter-based diagnostic studies should be weighed against the established limitations and potential complications. A key limitation of aortography is that it only images the lumen, and may therefore underestimate the size of large aneurysms that contain laminated thrombus. Manipulation of intraluminal catheters can result in embolization of laminated thrombus or atheromatous debris. Proximal aortography carries a 0.6 to 1.2% risk of stroke. Other risks include allergic reaction to contrast, iatrogenic aortic dissection, and bleeding at the arterial access site. The volumes of contrast required to adequately fill large aneurysms can cause significant renal toxicity. To minimize the risk of contrast nephropathy, patients receive periprocedural intravenous fluids for hydration, mannitol for diuresis, and acetylcysteine. If possible, surgery is performed 1 or more days after angiography in order to observe renal function and to permit diuresis of the contrast agent. If renal insufficiency occurs or is worsened, elective surgical procedures are postponed until renal function returns to normal or stabilizes.

Management

Indications for Surgery

Thoracic aortic aneurysms are repaired in order to prevent fatal rupture. Therefore, based on the natural history studies discussed above, elective operation is recommended when the diameter exceeds 5 to 6 cm, or when the rate of dilatation exceeds 1 cm/y. In patients with connective tissue disorders, such as Marfan's and Ehlers-Danlos syndromes, the threshold for operation is lower for both absolute size and rate of growth. Smaller ascending aortic aneurysms (4 to 5 cm) are also considered for repair when they are associated with significant aortic valve insufficiency.

The acuity of presentation is a major factor when deciding the timing of surgical intervention. Many patients are asymptomatic at the time of presentation and can undergo thorough preoperative evaluation and optimization. In contrast, urgent operations should be considered in patients presenting with symptoms. Symptomatic patients are at increased risk of rupture and warrant expeditious evaluation. The onset of new pain in patients with known aneurysms is especially concerning, and may herald significant expansion, leakage, or impending rupture. Emergent intervention is reserved for patients presenting with rupture or superimposed acute dissection.

Preoperative Assessment and Preparation

Given the impact of comorbid conditions on perioperative complications, a careful preoperative assessment of physiologic reserve is critical in evaluating operative risk. Therefore most patients undergo a thorough evaluation—with emphasis placed on cardiac, pulmonary, and renal function—prior to undergoing elective surgery.

Cardiac Evaluation. Coronary artery disease is common in patients with thoracic aortic aneurysms and is responsible for a substantial proportion of early and late postoperative deaths. Similarly, valvular pathology and myocardial dysfunction have important implications when planning anesthetic management and surgical approaches for aortic repair. Transthoracic echocardiography is a satisfactory noninvasive method for evaluating both valvular and biventricular function. Dipyridamole-thallium myocardial scanning identifies regions of myocardium that have reversible ischemia, and is more practical than exercise testing in older patients with concomitant lower extremity peripheral vascular disease. Cardiac catheterization with coronary arteriography is obtained in patients with evidence of coronary disease—based on history or noninvasive studies—or an ejection fraction of 30% or less. If significant valvular or coronary artery disease is identified prior to proximal aortic operations, it can be addressed directly during the procedure. Patients who have asymptomatic distal aortic aneurysms and severe coronary artery occlusive disease undergo percutaneous transluminal angioplasty or surgical revascularization prior to aneurysm replacement.

Pulmonary Evaluation. Pulmonary function screening with arterial blood gases and spirometry are routinely obtained prior to thoracic aortic operations. Patients with a forced expiratory volume in 1 second (FEV_1) greater than 1.0 L and a partial pressure of carbon dioxide (Pco_2) less than 45 mm Hg are considered surgical candidates. In suitable patients, borderline pulmonary function can be improved by implementing a regimen that includes smoking cessation, weight loss, exercise, and treatment of bronchitis for a period of 1 to 3 months before surgery. While surgery is not withheld in patients with symptomatic aortic aneurysms and poor pulmonary function, adjustments in operative technique can be made to optimize the chance of recovery. In such patients, preservation of the left recurrent laryngeal nerve, phrenic nerves, and diaphragmatic function is particularly important.

Renal Evaluation. Renal function is assessed preoperatively via serum electrolytes, blood urea nitrogen, and creatinine measurements. Information regarding kidney size and perfusion can be obtained from the CT scan or aortogram obtained to evaluate the aorta. Accurate information regarding baseline renal function has important therapeutic and prognostic implications. For example, perfusion strategies and perioperative medications are adjusted based on renal function. Patients with severely impaired renal function frequently require at least temporary hemodialysis after surgery; these patients also have a significantly higher mortality rate. Patients with thoracoabdominal aortic aneurysms and poor renal function secondary to severe proximal renal occlusive disease undergo renal artery end-arterectomy, stenting, or bypass grafting during the aortic repair.

Operative Repair

Proximal Thoracic Aortic Aneurysms. Operations for proximal aortic aneurysms—which involve the ascending aorta and/or transverse aortic arch—are performed through a midsternal incision and require cardiopulmonary bypass. The technique of aortic replacement varies according to the extent of the aneurysm and the condition of the aortic valve. The spectrum of operations ranges from simple graft replacement of the tubular portion of the ascending aorta (Fig. 21-3) to graft replacement of the entire proximal aorta, including the aortic root, with reattachment of the coronary arteries and brachiocephalic branches. The options for managing aortic valve pathology, the aortic aneurysm, and perfusion each deserve detailed consideration (Table 21-2).

Many patients undergoing proximal aortic operations have aortic valve pathology that requires concomitant surgical correction. When aortic valvular disease is present and the sinus segment is normal, separate repair or replacement of the aortic valve and graft replacement of the tubular segment of the ascending aorta are carried out. Mild to moderate valve insufficiency with annular dilatation in this setting can be addressed by plicating the annulus with mattress sutures placed below each commissure. Valve replacement with a stented biologic or mechanical prosthesis is performed in patients with more severe valvular insufficiency or with valvular stenosis. Separate replacement of the aortic valve and ascending aorta are not performed in patients with Marfan syndrome, because progressive dilatation of the remaining sinus segment eventually leads to complications requiring reoperation. Therefore, patients with Marfan syndrome or annuloaortic ectasia require some form of aortic root replacement.

In most cases, aortic root replacement employs a mechanical or biologic graft that has both a valve and aortic conduit. There

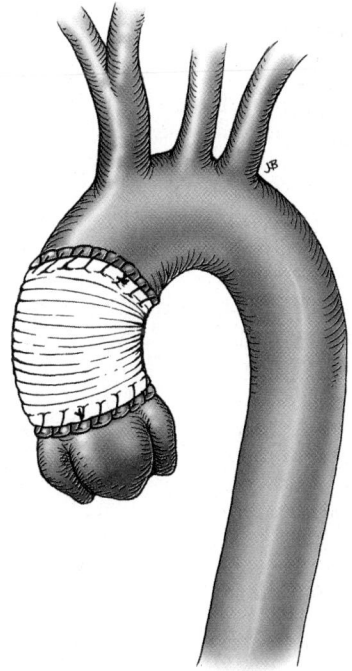

FIG. 21-3. *Illustration of graft replacement of the tubular portion of the ascending aorta.*

Table 21-2
Surgical Options During Proximal Aortic Surgery

Options for treating aortic valve pathology
  Aortic valve annuloplasty (annular plication)
  Aortic valve replacement with mechanical or biologic prosthesis
  Aortic root replacement
    Composite valve graft
    Aortic homograft
    Stentless porcine root
    Valve-sparing techniques
    Pulmonary autograft (Ross procedure)
Options for graft repair of the aortic aneurysm
  Patch aortoplasty
  Ascending replacement only
  Beveled hemiarch replacement
  Total arch replacement with reattachment of brachiocephalic
    branches
  Total arch replacement with separate grafts to each brachiocephalic
    branch
  Elephant trunk technique
Perfusion options
  Standard cardiopulmonary bypass
  Profound hypothermic circulatory arrest without adjuncts
  Profound hypothermic circulatory arrest with adjuncts
    Retrograde cerebral perfusion
    Selective antegrade cerebral perfusion
    Combined antegrade and retrograde cerebral perfusion

are currently three commercially available graft options: (1) composite valve grafts, which consist of a bileaflet mechanical valve attached to a polyester tube graft; (2) aortic root homografts, which are harvested from cadavers and cryopreserved; and (3) stentless porcine aortic root grafts. Another option for selected patients is the Ross procedure, in which the patient's pulmonary artery root is excised and placed in the aortic position. The right ventricular outflow tract is reconstructed using a cryopreserved pulmonary homograft. This option is rarely used in these patients, largely due to its technical demands and concerns regarding the potential for autograft dilatation in the setting of connective tissue disorders. A final option is valve-sparing aortic root replacement, which has evolved substantially during the past decade. The valve-sparing technique that is currently favored is called aortic root reimplantation, which involves excision of the aortic sinuses, attachment of a prosthetic graft to the patient's annulus, and resuspension of the native aortic valve inside the graft. The superior hemodynamics of the native valve and the avoidance of anticoagulation are major advantages to the valve-sparing approach. Long-term results in carefully selected patients have been excellent. The durability of this procedure in patients with Marfan syndrome has been controversial and is currently being investigated.

Regardless of the type of conduit used, aortic root replacement requires reattachment of the coronary arteries to openings in the graft. As originally described by Bentall and DeBono, this was accomplished by suturing the intact aortic wall surrounding each coronary artery to the openings in the graft. The aortic wall was then wrapped around the graft to create hemostasis. However, this technique frequently resulted in pseudoaneurysm formation originating from leaks at the coronary reattachment sites. Cabrol's modification—in which a separate, small tube graft is sutured to the coronary ostia and the main aortic graft—achieves tension-free coronary anastomoses and reduces the risk of pseudoaneurysm formation. Kochoucous' button modification of the Bentall procedure is currently the most widely used technique. The aneurysmal aorta is excised, leaving buttons of aortic wall surrounding both coronary

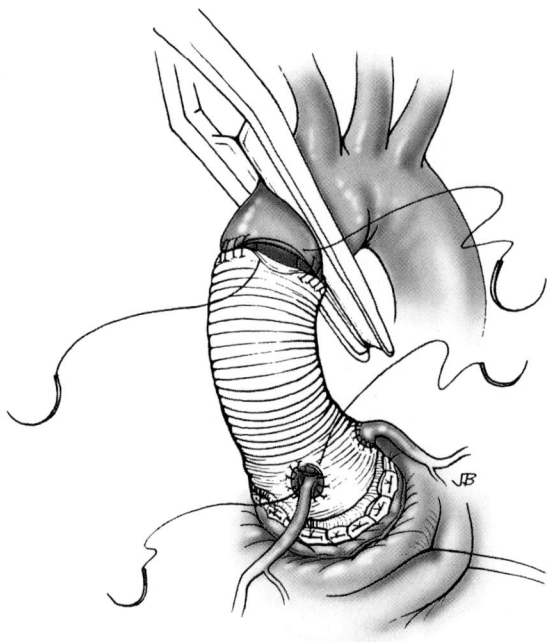

FIG. 21-4. Illustration of the modified Bentall procedure for aortic root replacement, during which buttons of aortic wall surrounding coronary arteries are mobilized and sutured to the aortic graft.

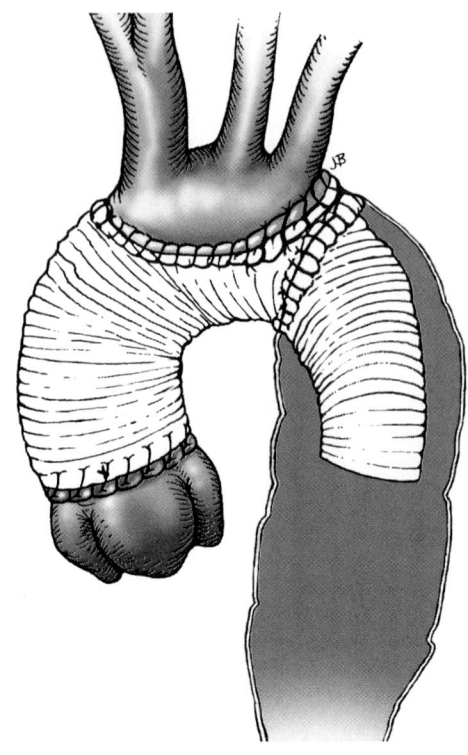

FIG. 21-5. Illustration demonstrating total aortic arch replacement using Borst's elephant trunk technique, in which the distal anastomosis is constructed so that a portion of the graft is left suspended within the proximal descending thoracic aorta. This is used to facilitate the subsequent operation to repair the descending thoracic aorta.

arteries, which are then mobilized and sutured to the aortic graft (Fig. 21-4). The coronary suture lines may be reinforced with polytetrafluoroethylene (PTFE) felt or pericardium to enhance hemostasis. When adequate mobilization of the coronary arteries is not feasible due to extremely large aneurysms or scarring from previous surgery, the Cabrol technique or bypass using interposition saphenous vein grafts can be used.

There are also several options for dealing with aneurysms that extend into the transverse aortic arch. The surgical approach depends on the extent of involvement and the need for cardiac and cerebral protection. Saccular aneurysms arising from the lesser curvature of the distal transverse arch that encompass less than 50% of the aortic circumference are treated by patch graft aortoplasty. For fusiform aneurysms, when the distal portion of the arch is a reasonable size, a single beveled replacement of the lower curvature (hemiarch) is performed. More extensive arch aneurysms require total replacement, with a distal anastomosis to the proximal descending thoracic aorta and separate reattachment of the brachiocephalic branches. The brachiocephalic vessels are reattached to one or more openings made in the graft, or are replaced with separate smaller grafts if they also are aneurysmal. In the most extreme cases, the aneurysm will involve the entire arch and extend into the descending thoracic aorta. This is approached using Borst's elephant trunk technique of total arch replacement (Fig. 21-5). The distal anastomosis is constructed so that a portion of the graft is left suspended within the proximal descending thoracic aorta. During a subsequent operation, this "trunk" is used to facilitate repair of the descending thoracic aorta.

Perfusion strategies during proximal aortic surgery also depend upon the extent requiring repair. Aneurysms that are isolated to the ascending segment can be replaced using standard cardiopulmonary bypass and distal ascending aortic clamping. This provides constant perfusion of the brain and other vital organs during the repair. Aneurysms involving the transverse aortic arch, however, cannot be clamped during the repair, and therefore require a period without cardiopulmonary bypass support; this is called circulatory arrest. In

order to protect the brain and other vital organs during the circulatory arrest period, the patient undergoes profound cooling prior to stopping pump flow. An electroencephalogram is monitored during cooling. Once electrocerebral silence is achieved—indicating cessation of brain activity and minimization of metabolic requirements—the pump flow is stopped and the arch is repaired. Electrocerebral silence usually occurs when the patient's nasopharyngeal temperature falls below 20°C. Although brief periods of circulatory arrest are generally well tolerated, this technique does have substantial limitations. The well-recognized risks of brain injury and death increase dramatically as the time of circulatory arrest increases.

Two perfusion strategies have been developed in order to reduce the risks of circulatory arrest: retrograde cerebral perfusion and selective antegrade cerebral perfusion (Fig. 21-6). Retrograde cerebral perfusion delivers cold, oxygenated blood from the pump into a cannula placed in the superior vena cava. The initial hope was that the retrograde delivery of blood would provide oxygen to the brain. Unfortunately, accumulating evidence suggests that this technique does not provide cerebral oxygenation as was once hoped. The apparent benefits of this technique are more likely due to maintenance of cerebral hypothermia and retrograde flushing of air and debris. Selective antegrade cerebral perfusion delivers blood directly into the brachiocephalic arteries while circulatory arrest is maintained in the rest of the body. This technique originally required cumbersome bypass grafts and cannulas, and consequently fell out of favor. However, recent improvements in technology and new strategies for delivery have resulted in a resurgence of interest in this adjunct. One common way of delivering antegrade cerebral perfusion employs small, flexible, balloon perfusion catheters that are inserted into one or more of the branch arteries. Another method,

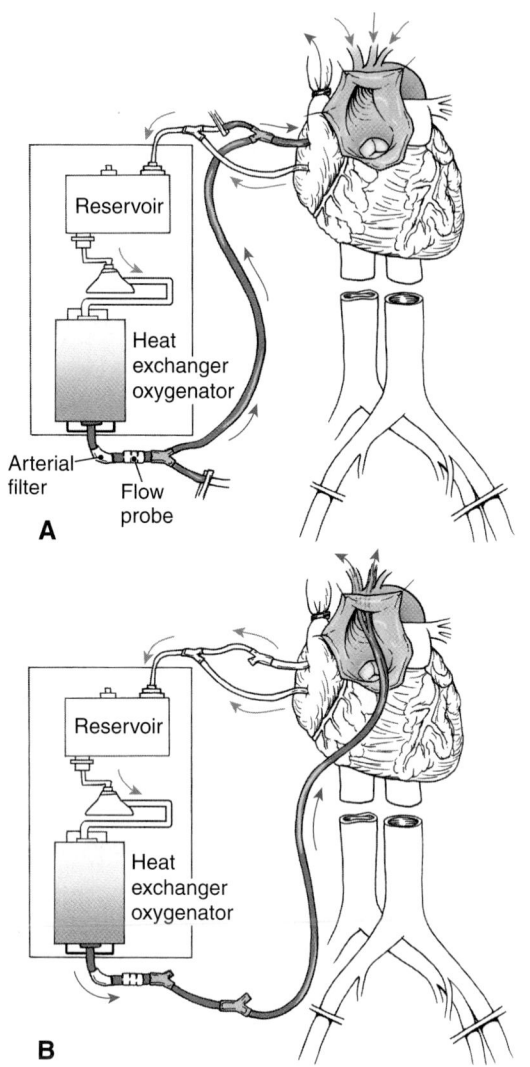

FIG. 21-6. *Diagrams of perfusion strategies during ascending and aortic arch aneurysm repair. A. Retrograde cerebral perfusion. B. Antegrade cerebral perfusion.*

which is rapidly gaining popularity due to its relative simplicity, involves cannulation of the right axillary artery. Upon initiating circulatory arrest and occluding the proximal innominate artery, the axillary artery cannula delivers blood flow into the cerebral circulation via the right common carotid artery. Because antegrade and retrograde cerebral perfusion have distinct mechanisms of providing cerebral protection, it is the preference of these authors often to combine them during aortic arch repairs. In the combined approach, antegrade perfusion is delivered during the arch reconstruction, and a brief period of retrograde perfusion is used to provide flushing immediately prior to resuming full cardiopulmonary bypass. The relative efficacy of these different perfusion strategies has never been established via an appropriately designed clinical trial.

Patients who require proximal aortic aneurysm repair after previous cardiac operations present special problems. If sternal re-entry appears unsafe, cardiopulmonary bypass and systemic cooling are initiated with the chest closed, using cannulas placed in the femoral artery and vein. Median sternotomy is performed after profound hypothermia has been achieved, allowing immediate conversion to circulatory arrest if bleeding occurs. When multiple previous median

sternotomies have been performed, or a large descending aneurysm precludes staged repair via the elephant trunk technique, total arch replacement can be accomplished through the left chest. In this setting, hypothermic circulatory arrest is usually achieved using a combination of femoral, aortic, and left atrial cannulas.

Many patients require staged operative procedures to achieve complete repair of extensive aneurysms involving the ascending aorta, transverse arch, and descending thoracic or thoracoabdominal aorta. When the descending segment is not disproportionately large (compared to the proximal aorta) and is not causing symptoms, the proximal aortic repair is carried out first. An important benefit of this approach is that it allows treatment of valvular and coronary artery occlusive disease at the first operation. The elephant trunk technique is used to perform the aortic arch repair in these patients. This technique permits access to the distal portion of the graft at the second operation, without the need to dissect around the distal transverse aortic arch, reducing the risk of injuring the left recurrent laryngeal nerve, esophagus, and pulmonary artery.

Distal Thoracic Aortic Aneurysms. In patients with descending thoracic or thoracoabdominal aortic aneurysms, several aspects of management—including preoperative risk assessment, anesthetic management, choice of incision, and use of protective adjuncts—are dictated by the overall extent of aortic involvement. By definition, descending thoracic aortic aneurysms involve the aorta in between the left subclavian artery and the diaphragm. Thoracoabdominal aneurysms can involve the entire thoracoabdominal aorta, from the origin of the left subclavian artery to the aortic bifurcation, and are categorized based on the Crawford classification (Fig. 21-7). Extent I thoracoabdominal aortic aneurysms involve most of the descending thoracic aorta, usually beginning near the left subclavian artery, and extend down to encompass the aorta at the origins of the celiac axis and superior mesenteric arteries; the renal arteries may also be involved. Extent II aneurysms also arise near the left subclavian artery, but extend distally into the infrarenal abdominal aorta and often reach the aortic bifurcation. Extent III aneurysms originate in the lower descending thoracic aorta (below the sixth rib) and extend into the abdomen. Extent IV aneurysms begin within the diaphragmatic hiatus and often involve the entire abdominal aorta.

Descending thoracic aortic aneurysms are repaired through a left thoracotomy. In patients with thoracoabdominal aortic aneurysms, the thoracotomy is extended across the costal margin and into the abdomen. A double-lumen endobronchial tube allows selective ventilation of the right lung and deflation of the left lung. Transperitoneal exposure of the thoracoabdominal aorta is achieved by performing medial visceral rotation and circumferential division of the diaphragm. During a period of aortic clamping, the diseased segment is replaced with a polyester tube graft. Important branch arteries—including intercostal, celiac, superior mesenteric, and renal arteries—are reattached to openings made in the side of the graft. Visceral and renal artery occlusive disease is commonly encountered during aneurysm repair; options for correcting branch vessel stenosis include endarterectomy, direct arterial stenting, and bypass grafting.

Clamping the descending thoracic aorta creates ischemia of the spinal cord and abdominal viscera. Clinically significant manifestations of hepatic, pancreatic, and bowel ischemia are relatively uncommon. However, spinal cord injury resulting in paraplegia or paraparesis and acute renal failure remain major causes of morbidity and mortality after these operations. Therefore several aspects of the operation are devoted to minimizing spinal and renal

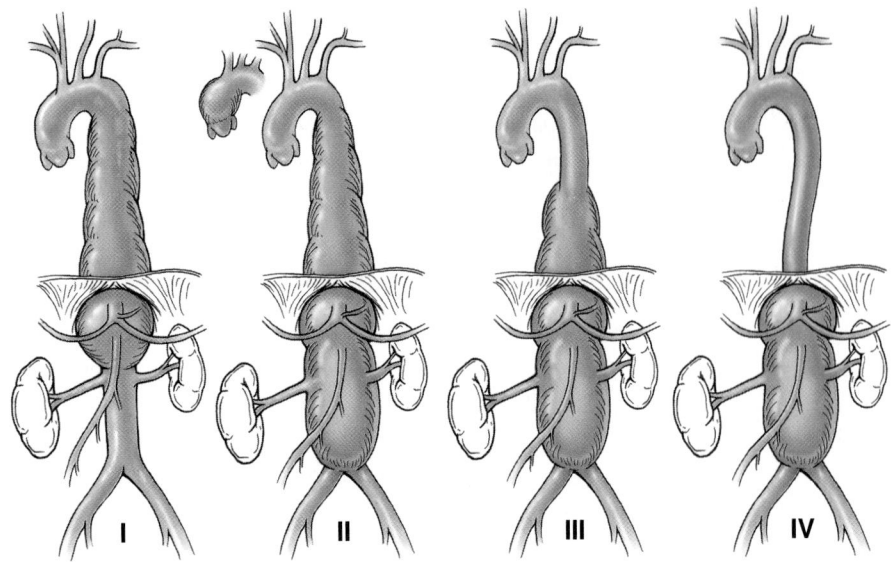

FIG. 21-7. The Crawford classification of thoracoabdominal aortic aneurysms based on the extent of aortic involvement.

ischemia (Table 21-3). The authors multimodality approach to spinal cord protection includes expeditious repair to minimize aortic clamping time, moderate systemic heparinization (1.0 mg/kg) to prevent small-vessel thrombosis, mild permissive hypothermia (32 to 34°C nasopharyngeal temperature), and reattachment of segmental intercostal and lumbar arteries. As the aorta is replaced from proximal to distal, the aortic clamp is moved sequentially to lower positions along the graft to restore perfusion to newly reattached branch vessels. During extensive thoracoabdominal aortic repairs (i.e., Crawford extents I and II), cerebrospinal fluid drainage is used. The benefits of this adjunct—which improves spinal perfusion by reducing cerebrospinal fluid pressure—have been confirmed by a prospective randomized trial performed by the authors' group. Left heart bypass—which provides perfusion of the distal aorta and its branches during the clamping period—is also used during extensive thoracoabdominal aortic repairs. Because it unloads the heart, left heart bypass also is useful in patients with poor cardiac reserve. Balloon perfusion cannulas connected to the left heart bypass circuit can be used to deliver blood directly to the celiac axis and superior mesenteric artery during their reattachment. The potential benefits of reducing hepatic and bowel ischemia include reduced risks of postoperative coagulopathy and bacterial translocation,

Table 21-3
Current Strategy for Spinal Cord, Visceral, and Renal Protection During Repair of Distal Thoracic Aortic Aneurysms

All extents
- Permissive mild hypothermia (32–34°C, nasopharyngeal)
- Moderate heparinization (1 mg/kg)
- Aggressive reattachment of segmental arteries, especially between T8 and L1
- Sequential aortic clamping when possible
- Perfusion of renal arteries with 4°C crystalloid solution when possible

Crawford extent I and II thoracoabdominal repairs
- Cerebrospinal fluid drainage
- Left heart bypass during proximal anastomosis
- Selective perfusion of celiac axis and superior mesenteric artery during intercostal and visceral/renal anastomoses

respectively. Whenever possible, renal protection is achieved by perfusing the kidneys with cold (4°C) crystalloid. In a recent randomized clinical trial conducted by these authors, reduced kidney temperature was associated with renal protection, and the use of cold crystalloid was an independent predictor of preserved renal function.

In selected cases, hypothermic circulatory arrest is required for descending thoracic or thoracoabdominal aortic repairs. The primary indication for this approach is the inability to clamp the aorta due to rupture, extremely large aneurysms, and extension of the aneurysm into the distal transverse aortic arch.

As discussed above, patients with extensive aneurysms involving the ascending, transverse arch, and descending thoracic aorta generally undergo staged operations to achieve complete repair. In this setting, when the descending or thoracoabdominal component is symptomatic (e.g., back pain or rupture) or disproportionately large (compared to the ascending aorta), the distal segment is treated during the initial operation, and repair of the ascending aorta and transverse aortic arch is performed as a second procedure. A reversed elephant trunk repair—in which a portion of the proximal end of the aortic graft is inverted down into the lumen—can be employed during the first operation; this facilitates the second-stage repair of the ascending aorta and transverse aortic arch (Fig. 21-8).

While spinal cord ischemia and renal failure receive the most attention, several other complications warrant consideration. The most common complication following these repairs is pulmonary dysfunction. In aneurysms located adjacent to the left subclavian artery, the vagus and left recurrent laryngeal nerves are often adherent to the aortic wall and susceptible to injury. Vocal cord paralysis should be suspected in patients who have postoperative hoarseness, and it is confirmed by endoscopic examination. Effective treatment of vocal cord paralysis can be provided by direct cord medialization (type 1 thyroplasty). Injury to the esophagus during the proximal anastomosis can have catastrophic consequences. Careful separation of the proximal descending thoracic aorta from the underlying esophagus prior to performing the proximal anastomosis minimizes the risk of a secondary aortoesophageal fistula. In patients who have undergone previous coronary artery bypass surgery using the left internal thoracic artery, clamping proximal to the left subclavian artery can precipitate severe myocardial ischemia and cardiac arrest. When clamping at this location is anticipated in these patients,

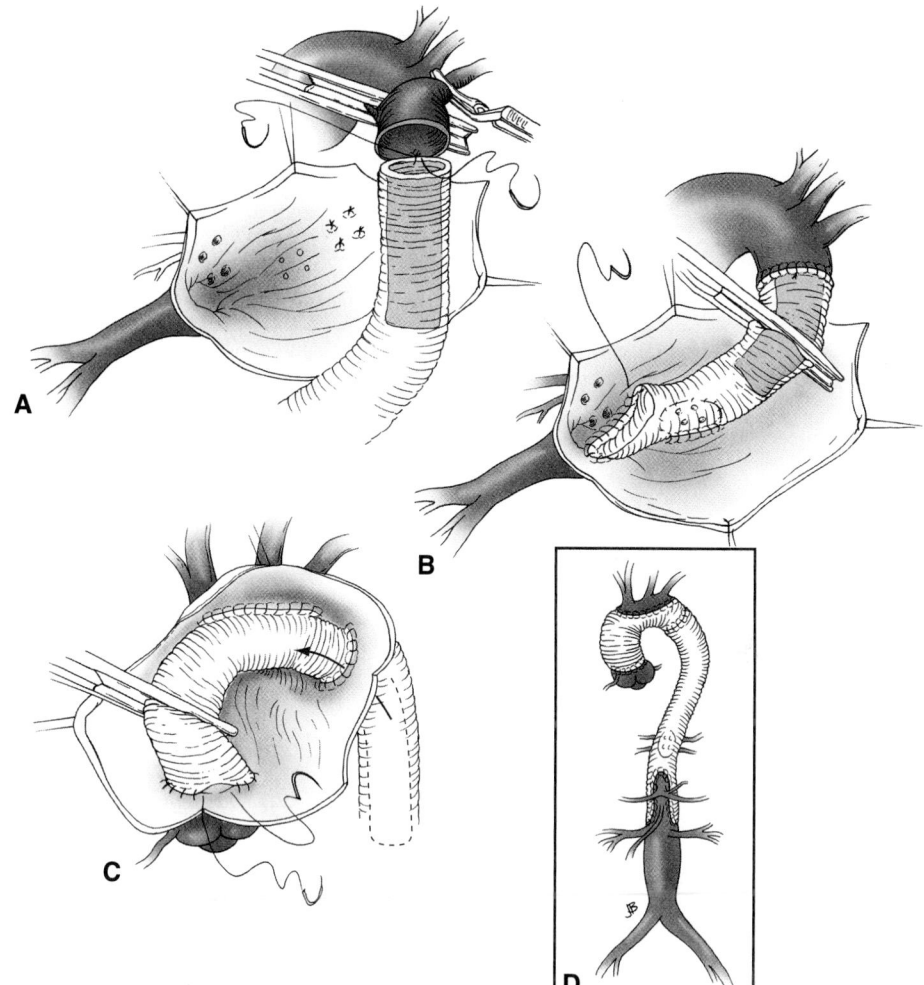

FIG. 21-8. *The reversed elephant trunk technique. A. During the first operation, the distal aortic segment is repaired through a left thoracoabdominal approach. The aneurysm is opened after clamping the distal aortic arch and left subclavian artery. Prior to performing the proximal anastomosis, the end of the graft is invaginated. B. After completing the proximal anastomosis, the clamps are repositioned to restore perfusion of the left subclavian artery. In this case, the repair is completed by reattaching intercostals arteries to a side-opening in the graft and performing a beveled distal anastomosis at the level of the visceral branches. C. During the second operation, performed through a median sternotomy, the aortic arch is opened during hypothermic circulatory arrest. The invaginated segment of graft is pulled out and used to replace the aortic arch and ascending aorta. This eliminates the need for a new distal anastomosis, thereby reducing the circulatory arrest time and the attendant risks. D. The completed two-stage repair of the entire thoracic aorta.*

a left common carotid to subclavian bypass is performed to avoid cardiac complications.

Recent Results

Improvements in anesthesia, surgical technique, and perioperative care have led to substantial improvements in outcome following thoracic aortic aneurysm repair. When performed in specialized centers, these operations achieve excellent survival with acceptable morbidity. Tables 21-4 and 21-5 display the authors' results with surgical repair of proximal and distal aortic aneurysms, respectively. Replacement of the entire thoracoabdominal aorta (extent II repairs) carries the highest risk of death, bleeding, renal failure, and paraplegia. As expected, stroke rates after distal aortic repairs are highest when the clamp site is near the left subclavian artery.

Postoperative Considerations

Aortic anastomoses are often extremely fragile during the early postoperative period. Even brief episodes of postoperative hypertension can disrupt suture lines and precipitate severe bleeding or pseudoaneurysm formation. Therefore, during the initial 24 to 48 hours, meticulous blood pressure control is maintained to protect the integrity of the anastomoses. Generally, the authors liberally use nitroprusside and intravenous beta antagonists to maintain the mean arterial blood pressure between 80 and 90 mm Hg. In patients with extremely friable aortic tissue, such as those with Marfan syndrome, we lower the target range to 70 to 80 mm Hg.

A second threat to anastomotic integrity is graft infection. In an attempt to prevent this complication, intravenous antibiotics are

Table 21-4
Results of Surgical Repair of Proximal Thoracic Aortic Aneurysms (Without Dissection)

No. of Patients	30-Day Mortality	Stroke	Bleeding[a]	Renal Failure[b]	Paraplegia or Paraparesis
784	49 (6.3%)	23 (2.9%)	18 (2.3%)	14 (1.8%)	6 (0.8%)

[a] Bleeding requiring reoperation.
[b] Acute renal failure requiring hemodialysis.

Table 21-5
Results of Surgical Repair of Distal Thoracic Aortic Aneurysms (Without Dissection)

Extent[a]	No. of Patients	30-Day Mortality	Stroke	Bleeding[b]	Renal Failure[c]	Paraplegia or Paraparesis
DTAA	282	12 (4.3%)	9 (3.2%)	6 (2.1%)	6 (2.1%)	6 (2.1%)
TAAA I	436	21 (4.8%)	7 (1.6%)	7 (1.6%)	7 (1.6%)	17 (3.9%)
TAAA II	411	36 (8.8%)	9 (2.2%)	19 (4.6%)	44 (10.7%)	33 (8.0%)
TAAA III	283	16 (5.7%)	2 (0.7%)	5 (1.8%)	20 (7.1%)	7 (2.5%)
TAAA IV	337	10 (3.0%)	1 (0.3%)	10 (3.0%)	25 (7.4%)	5 (1.5%)
Total	1749	95 (5.4%)	28 (1.6%)	47 (2.7%)	102 (5.8%)	68 (3.9%)

[a]Thoracoabdominal aortic aneurysm extents I–IV based on Crawford's classification.
[b]Bleeding requiring reoperation.
[c]Acute renal failure requiring hemodialysis.
DTAA = descending thoracic aortic aneurysm; TAAA = thoracoabdominal aortic aneurysm.

continued throughout the postoperative course until all drains, chest tubes, and central venous lines are removed.

AORTIC DISSECTION

Pathology and Classification

Aortic dissection—the most common catastrophic event involving the aorta—is the progressive separation of the aortic wall layers that usually occurs after a tear forms in the intima and inner media. Propagation of the separation within the layers of the media results in the formation of two or more channels (Fig. 21-9). The original lumen, which remains lined by the intima, is called the true lumen. The newly formed channel within the layers of the media is called the false lumen. The dissecting membrane separates the true and false lumens. Additional tears in the dissecting membrane allow communication between the two channels and are called re-entry sites. Although the progressive separation of layers primarily progresses distally along the length of aorta, it also can proceed in a proximal direction; this process is often referred to as proximal extension or retrograde dissection.

The relationship between dissection and aneurysmal disease requires clarification. Dissection and aneurysms are separate entities, despite the fact that they often coexist and serve as mutual risk factors. In most cases, dissection occurs in patients without aneurysms. The subsequent progressive dilatation of the weakened outer aortic wall results in an aneurysm. Alternatively, in patients with degenerative aneurysms, the ongoing deterioration of the aortic wall can lead to a superimposed dissection; the overused term "dissecting aneurysm" should be reserved for this specific situation.

The extensive disruption of the aortic wall has severe anatomic consequences (Fig. 21-10). First, the outer wall of the false lumen is extremely thin, inflamed, and fragile, making it prone to expansion or rupture in the face of ongoing hemodynamic stresses. Secondly, the expanding false lumen can compress the true lumen and interfere with blood flow in the aorta or any of the aortic branch vessels, including the coronary, carotid, intercostal, visceral, renal, and iliac arteries. Finally, when the separation of layers occurs within the aortic root, the aortic valve commissures can become unhinged, resulting in an acutely incompetent valve. The clinical consequences of each of these sequelae will be addressed in detail in the section on clinical manifestations, below.

Dissection of the aorta is classified based on several important variables, including which parts of the aorta are involved, when the

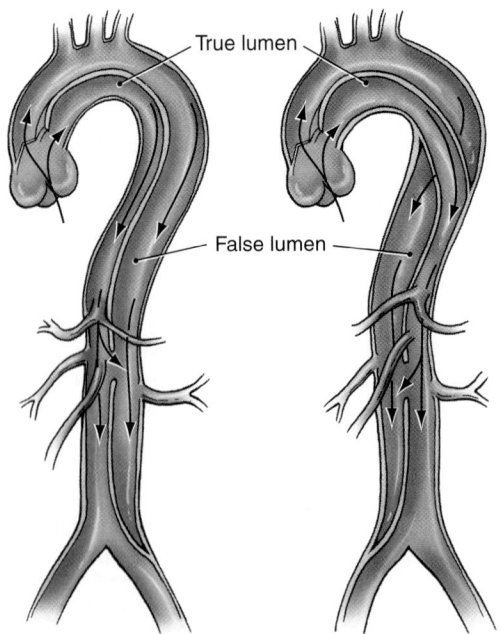

FIG. 21-9. Drawing of the aorta demonstrating aortic dissection, with the separation of the layers of the aortic wall that forms two or more channels.

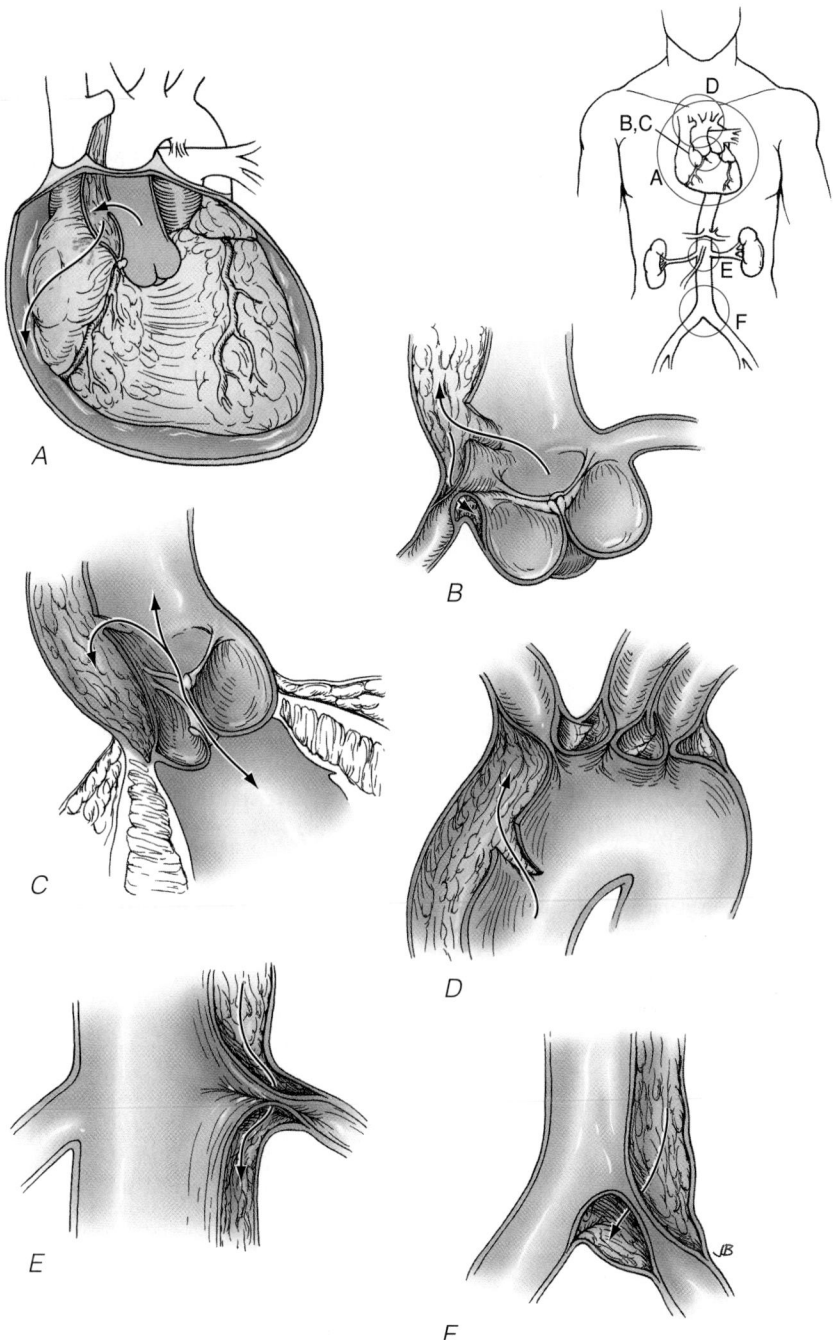

FIG. 21-10. Figure illustrating the anatomic consequences of aortic dissection. *A*. Cardiac tamponade. *B*. Disruption of coronary blood flow. *C*. Injury to the aortic valve. *D*, *E*, and *F*. Compromised blood flow to branch vessels due to dissection, causing ischemic complications.

dissection occurred, and the cause of the initial tear, among others. Dissections are categorized based on anatomic location and extent in order to guide treatment. There are two traditional classification schemes that remain in common use: the DeBakey classification and the Stanford classification (Fig. 21-11). In their current use, both of these methods describe the segments of aorta that are involved in the dissection, rather than the site of the initial intimal tear. The main drawback of the Stanford classification is that it does not distinguish between patients with isolated ascending aortic dissection and patients with dissection involving the entire aorta; both patients would be classified as type A, despite the fact that their treatment, follow-up, and prognosis are substantially different. Borst and associates advocated a more simplified, descriptive classification of aortic dissection instead of the traditional DeBakey and Stanford schemes. In this system, the proximal aortic segment (ascending and transverse arch) and distal aortic segment (descending thoracic and thoracoabdominal) are considered independently. This is useful because treatment strategies are based on which segments are involved. For example, patients with isolated proximal aortic dissections often undergo emergent operation. In contrast, when only the distal aorta is involved, the initial treatment is usually medical; surgery is reserved for patients who develop complications. Patients with dissections that involve both the proximal and distal segments often undergo surgical repair of the proximal segment, followed by aggressive medical treatment for the remaining distal dissection.

Aortic dissection also is categorized based on the time elapsed since the initial event. Dissection is considered acute within the first 14 days following the initial tear. After 14 days, the dissection is

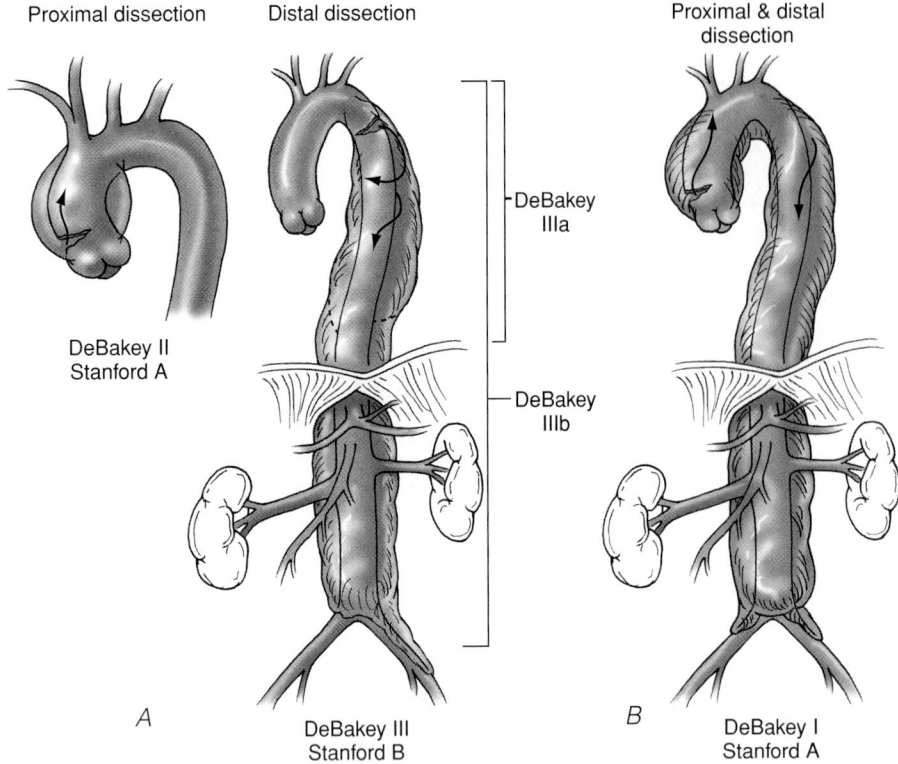

FIG. 21-11. The classification schemes of aortic dissection. A. Isolated dissection of the proximal (left) or distal (right) aorta. B. Diffuse dissection involving the proximal and distal aortic segments.

described as chronic. Although arbitrary, the distinction between acute and chronic dissections has important implications in perioperative management strategies, operative techniques, and surgical results. In light of the implications of acuity, Borst and associates have proposed a third phase—termed subacute—to describe the transition between the acute and chronic phases. The subacute period encompasses days 15 through 60 after the initial event. Although past the traditional 14-day acute phase, patients with subacute dissection continue to have extremely fragile aortic tissue that may complicate operative management and may increase the risk of surgery.

Two rare but important variants of aortic dissection are penetrating aortic ulcers and intramural hematomas. Penetrating aortic ulcers are essentially disrupted atherosclerotic plaques. Eventually the ulcer can penetrate through the aortic wall, leading to dissection or rupture. An intramural hematoma is a collection of blood within the aortic wall without an intimal tear; accumulation of the hematoma ultimately results in dissection. Although somewhat controversial, the current consensus is that in most cases, these variants of dissection should be treated identically to classic dissection.

Etiology and Natural History

Aortic dissection occurs in approximately 5 to 10 patients per million population per year and is highly lethal. Without treatment, nearly one half of patients with acute proximal aortic dissection die within 24 hours, and 60% of patients with acute distal aortic dissections die within 1 month.

Although several risk factors for aortic dissection have been identified, the specific causes remain unknown. Ultimately, any condition that weakens the aortic wall increases the risk of aortic dissection. Common general cardiovascular risk factors, such as smoking, hypertension, atherosclerosis, and hypercholesterolemia, are associated with aortic dissection. Patients with connective tissue disorders, aortitis, bicuspid aortic valve, or pre-existing medial degenerative disease are at risk for dissection, especially if they have already developed a thoracic aortic aneurysm. Aortic injury during cardiac catheterization or surgery is a common cause of iatrogenic dissection. Other situations that are associated with aortic dissection include pregnancy, cocaine abuse, and amphetamine abuse. Recent advances in the understanding of the molecular mechanisms behind abdominal aortic aneurysms have prompted similar investigations regarding thoracic aortic dissection.

Clinical Manifestations

The onset of dissection is often associated with severe chest or back pain—classically described as "tearing"—that migrates distally as the dissection progresses along the length of the aorta. The location of the pain often indicates which aortic segments are involved. Pain in the anterior chest suggests involvement of the proximal aorta, while pain in the back and abdomen generally indicates involvement of the distal segment. Additional clinical sequelae of acute aortic dissection are best considered in terms of the potential anatomic manifestations at each level of the aorta.

Proximal aortic dissection can directly injure the aortic valve. The severity of aortic valve insufficiency varies with the degree of commissural disruption, which may range from partial separation of only one commissure (producing mild valvular insufficiency) to full separation of all three commissures and complete prolapse of the valve into the left ventricle, producing severe acute heart failure. Patients with acute aortic valve regurgitation may complain of worsening dyspnea.

Proximal dissections also can extend into the coronary arteries or shear the coronary ostia off of the true lumen, creating acute coronary occlusion; when this occurs, it most often involves the right coronary artery. The sudden disruption of coronary blood flow can cause a myocardial infarction. By producing symptoms and

Table 21-6
Anatomic Complications of Aortic Dissection and Their Associated Symptoms and Signs

Anatomic Manifestation	Symptoms and Signs
Aortic valve insufficiency	Dyspnea
	Murmur
	Pulmonary rales
	Shock
Coronary malperfusion	Chest pain with characteristics of angina
	Nausea/vomiting
	Shock
	Ischemic changes on electrocardiogram
	Elevated cardiac enzymes
Pericardial tamponade	Dyspnea
	Jugular venous distention
	Pulsus paradoxus
	Muffled cardiac tones
	Shock
	Low-voltage electrocardiogram
Subclavian or iliofemoral artery malperfusion	Cold, painful extremity
	Extremity sensory and motor deficits
	Peripheral pulse deficit
Carotid artery malperfusion	Syncope
	Focal neurologic deficit (transient or persistent)
	Carotid pulse deficit
	Coma
Spinal malperfusion	Paraplegia
	Incontinence
Visceral malperfusion	Nausea/vomiting
	Abdominal pain
Renal malperfusion	Oliguria or anuria
	Hematuria

signs consistent with myocardial ischemia, this presentation can mask the presence of aortic dissection, resulting in delayed diagnosis and treatment.

The thin and inflamed outer wall of a dissected ascending aorta will often produce a serosanguineous pericardial effusion that can accumulate and cause tamponade. Suggestive signs include jugular venous distention, muffled heart tones, pulsus paradoxus, and low-voltage electrocardiogram (ECG) tracings. Free rupture into the pericardial space produces rapid tamponade and is generally fatal.

Any branch vessel from the aorta can become involved during progression of the dissection, resulting in compromised blood flow and ischemic complications. Therefore, depending on which arteries are involved, the dissection can produce acute stroke, paraplegia, hepatic failure, bowel infarction, renal failure, or a threatened ischemic limb.

Diagnostic Evaluation

Because of variations in severity and the wide variety of potential clinical manifestations, the diagnosis of acute aortic dissection can be challenging. Only three out of every 100,000 patients presenting to an emergency department with acute chest, back, or abdominal pain are eventually diagnosed with aortic dissection. Not surprisingly, diagnostic delays are common; delays beyond 24 hours after hospitalization occur in up to 39% of cases. Unfortunately, delays in diagnosis lead to delays in management, which can have disastrous consequences. The European Society of Cardiology Task Force on Aortic Dissection stated, "the main challenge in managing acute aortic dissection is to suspect and thus diagnose the disease as early as possible." A high index of suspicion is critical, particularly

in younger, atypical patients, who may have connective tissue disorders or other less common risk factors.

Most patients with acute aortic dissection (80 to 90%) experience severe pain in the chest, back, or abdomen. Classically, the pain occurs suddenly, has a "tearing" quality, and migrates distally as the dissection progresses along the aorta. For classification purposes (acute vs. subacute vs. chronic), the onset of pain is generally considered to represent the beginning of the dissection process. Most of the other common symptoms are either nonspecific or are caused by the secondary manifestations of dissection (Table 21-6).

A discrepancy in extremity pulse and/or blood pressure is the classic physical finding in patients with aortic dissection. This often occurs due to changes in flow in the true and false lumens, and does not necessarily indicate extension into an extremity branch vessel. Involvement of the proximal aorta often creates differences between the right and left arms, while distal aortic dissection often causes differences between the upper and lower extremities. Like symptoms, most of the physical signs after dissection are related to the secondary manifestations, and therefore vary considerably (see Table 21-6). For example, signs of stroke or a threatened ischemic limb may dominate the physical findings in patients with carotid or iliac malperfusion, respectively.

Unfortunately, laboratory studies are of little help in diagnosing acute aortic dissection. Tests that are commonly used to detect acute coronary events—including serum markers for myocardial injury and electrocardiograms—deserve special consideration and need to be interpreted carefully. Normal ECGs and serum markers in the setting of acute chest pain should raise suspicion regarding the presence of aortic dissection. It is important to remember that when ECG changes and elevated serum markers indicate a myocardial infarction, they do not exclude the diagnosis of aortic dissection, since

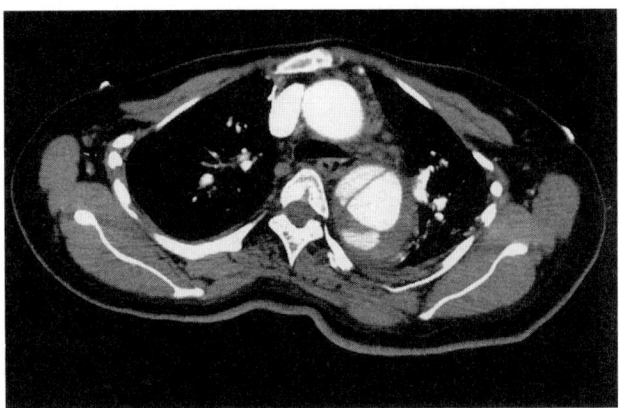

FIG. 21-12. Computed tomography (CT) scan demonstrating aortic dissection.

dissection can cause coronary malperfusion. Ultimately, although not well-studied, electrocardiograms seem to have little utility for detecting or ruling out dissection. Similarly, while chest radiographs may demonstrate a widened mediastinum or abnormal aortic contour, up to 16% of patients with dissection have a normal-appearing chest radiograph.

Once the diagnosis of dissection is considered, the thoracic aorta should be imaged with CT, MRA, or echocardiography. The accuracy of these noninvasive imaging tests has all but eliminated the need for diagnostic aortography in most patients with suspected aortic dissection. Currently, the diagnosis is usually established via contrast-enhanced CT. The classic diagnostic feature is a double-lumen aorta (Fig. 21-12). In addition, CT scans provide essential information regarding the segments of the aorta involved; the acuity of the dissection; aortic dilatation, including the presence of pre-existing degenerative aneurysms; and the development of threatening sequelae, including pericardial effusion, early aortic rupture, and branch vessel compromise. While MRA also provides excellent imaging, the MRI suite is not well-suited for critically ill patients. In patients who cannot undergo contrast-enhanced CT or MRA, transthoracic echocardiography can be used to establish the diagnosis. Transesophageal echocardiography is excellent for determining and distinguishing the presence of dissection, aneurysm, and intramural hematoma in the ascending aorta.

In patients with proximal aortic dissection, coronary angiography is obtained prior to surgery in selected patients (i.e., those who have evidence of pre-existing coronary artery disease). Specific relative indications in these patients include a history of angina or myocardial infarction, recent abnormal myocardial perfusion study, previous coronary artery bypass or angioplasty, and acute ischemic changes on an ECG. Contraindications include hemodynamic instability, aortic rupture, and pericardial effusion.

Management

Initial Assessment and Management

Regardless of the location of the dissection, the initial management is the same for all patients with suspected or confirmed acute aortic dissection. Furthermore, because of the potential for rupture before the diagnosis is confirmed, aggressive pharmacologic management is started once there is clinical suspicion of dissection, and is continued during the diagnostic evaluation. The goals of pharmacologic treatment are to stabilize the dissection and prevent rupture.

Patients are monitored closely in an intensive care unit. Indwelling radial arterial catheters are used to monitor blood pressure and optimize titration of antihypertensive agents. Measuring blood pressures in a malperfused limb will cause an underestimation of the central aortic pressure; therefore the arm with the best pulse is selected. Central venous catheters assure reliable intravenous access for delivery of vasoactive medications. Pulmonary artery catheters are reserved for patients with severe cardiopulmonary dysfunction.

In addition to confirming the diagnosis of dissection and defining its acuity and extent, the initial evaluation focuses on determining whether any of the various life-threatening complications are present. Particular attention is paid to changes in neurologic status, peripheral pulses, and urine output. Serial laboratory studies—including arterial blood gases, complete blood cell count, prothrombin and partial thromboplastin times, serum electrolytes, creatinine, blood urea nitrogen, and liver enzymes—are useful for determining the presence of organ ischemia and optimizing management.

The initial management strategy—commonly described as "antihypertensive therapy" or "blood pressure control"—focuses on reducing aortic wall stress, the force of left ventricular ejection, and the rate of change in blood pressure (dP/dT). Reductions in dP/dT are achieved by lowering both cardiac contractility and blood pressure. The drugs initially used to accomplish these goals include intravenous beta adrenergic blockers, direct vasodilators, calcium channel blockers, and angiotensin-converting enzyme inhibitors. These agents are used to achieve a heart rate between 60 and 80 beats/min, a systolic blood pressure between 100 and 110 mm Hg, and a mean arterial blood pressure between 60 and 75 mm Hg. These hemodynamic targets are maintained as long as urine output remains adequate and neurologic function is not impaired. Achieving adequate pain control with intravenous opiates such as morphine or fentanyl is an important step to maintaining acceptable blood pressure control.

Beta antagonists are administered to all patients with acute aortic dissections, unless there are strong contraindications such as severe heart failure, bradyarrhythmia, high-grade atrioventricular conduction block, or bronchospastic disease. Esmolol is an ultra-fast-acting agent with a short half-life; because it is cardioselective, it can be useful in patients with bronchospastic disease. Labetalol, which provides both nonselective beta blockade and postsynaptic alpha$_1$-blockade, reduces systemic vascular resistance without impairing cardiac output. The dose of beta antagonists is titrated to achieve a heart rate of 60 to 80 beats/min. In patients who cannot receive beta antagonists, calcium channel blockers such as diltiazem are an effective alternative. Nitroprusside, a direct vasodilator, can be administered once beta blockade is adequate. When used alone, however, nitroprusside can cause reflex increases in heart rate and contractility, elevated dP/dT, and progression of aortic dissection. Enalapril and other angiotensin-converting enzyme inhibitors are useful in patients with renal malperfusion; the decrease in rennin release may improve renal blood flow.

Management of Proximal Aortic Dissection

Acute Proximal Dissection. Proximal aortic repairs performed in the chronic phase uniformly have better outcomes than those performed in the acute phase. Unfortunately, the risk of a fatal complication such as aortic rupture during medical management outweighs the risk associated with early operation. Therefore, the presence of an acute proximal aortic dissection has traditionally been considered an absolute indication for emergency surgical repair. However, specific patient groups may benefit from nonoperative management or delayed operation. Situations that warrant consideration of delayed repair include: (1) patients presenting with acute stroke or mesenteric ischemia; (2) elderly patients with substantial comorbidity; (3) stable patients who may benefit from transfer to specialized centers; and (4) patients who have undergone a cardiac operation in the remote past. As a caveat to the last situation, it must be emphasized that dissections occurring during the initial 3 weeks after cardiac surgery are at high risk for rupture and tamponade; these patients should undergo early operation.

In the absence of the circumstances listed above, most patients with acute proximal aortic dissection undergo urgent graft replacement of the ascending aorta. The operation is conducted in a manner similar to that described for aneurysms of the transverse aortic arch in the previous section. Intraoperative transesophageal echocardiography is commonly performed before beginning the operation to further assess baseline myocardial and valvular function and, if necessary, to confirm the diagnosis. The operation is performed via a median sternotomy with cardiopulmonary bypass and hypothermic circulatory arrest (Fig. 21-13). In preparation for circulatory arrest, cannulas are placed in the right axillary artery (arterial inflow) and the superior and inferior vena cavae (venous drainage). After initiating cardiopulmonary bypass, the patient is cooled until electroencephalographic monitoring demonstrates electrocerebral silence. Cardiopulmonary bypass is then stopped and the ascending aorta is opened. The dissecting membrane that separates the true and false lumens is completely excised. After occluding the innominate artery with a clamp or balloon catheter, flow from the axillary artery cannula is used to provide selective antegrade cerebral perfusion. The transverse aortic arch is carefully inspected. Replacement of the entire arch is performed only if a primary tear is located in the arch or if the arch is aneurysmal; in most cases, a less extensive beveled "hemiarch" repair is adequate. This strategy of performing the distal anastomosis during circulatory arrest, often termed "open distal anastomosis," avoids placement of a clamp across the fragile aorta, which can produce further aortic damage. The distal aortic cuff is prepared by tacking the inner and outer walls together and using surgical adhesive to obliterate the false lumen and strengthen the tissue. A polyester tube graft is sutured to the distal aortic cuff. The anastomosis between the graft and the aorta is fashioned so that blood flow will be directed into the true lumen; this often alleviates any distal malperfusion problems that were present preoperatively. After reinforcing the distal anastomosis with additional adhesive, retrograde cerebral perfusion is briefly delivered via the superior vena caval cannula, the graft is deaired and clamped, full cardiopulmonary bypass is resumed, rewarming is initiated, and the proximal portion of the repair is started. In the absence of annuloaortic ectasia or Marfan syndrome—which generally require aortic root replacement—aortic valve insufficiency can be corrected by resuspending the commissures onto the outer aortic wall. The proximal aortic cuff is prepared with tacking sutures and surgical adhesive prior to performing the proximal aortic anastomosis.

In the majority of patients who undergo surgical repair of acute proximal dissection, the dissection persists distal to the site of the operative repair. Extensive dilatation of the distal aortic segment develops in 16% of the survivors, and rupture of the dilated distal aorta is the most common cause of late death. Therefore, following proximal aortic repair, most of these patients require aggressive management of the remaining acute distal aortic dissection, as described in detail below.

Chronic Proximal Dissection. Occasionally, patients with proximal aortic dissection will present for repair in the chronic phase. In most regards, the operation is conducted in a manner similar to acute dissection repair. The improved tissue strength in the chronic setting, making suturing safer, is a notable difference. Additionally, instead of obliterating the false lumen at the distal anastomosis, the dissecting membrane is fenestrated into the arch to assure perfusion of both lumens and prevent postoperative malperfusion complications.

Management of Distal Aortic Dissection

Nonoperative Management. Nonoperative management of acute distal aortic dissection results in lower morbidity and mortality rates than those achieved with surgical treatment. Therefore, these patients are primarily managed with pharmacologic treatment. However, the most common causes of death during nonoperative treatment are aortic rupture and end-organ malperfusion. Therefore, patients are continually reassessed for the development of complications. At least two serial CT scans—usually obtained on day 2 or 3 and on day 8 or 9—are compared to the initial scan to rule out significant aortic expansion.

Once the patient has been stabilized, pharmacologic management is gradually shifted from intravenous to oral medications. Oral therapy, usually including a beta antagonist, is initiated when systolic pressure is consistently 100 to 110 mm Hg and the neurologic, renal, and cardiovascular systems are stable. Many patients can be discharged after the blood pressure is well controlled on oral agents and serial CT scans confirm the absence of aortic expansion.

Long-term pharmacologic therapy is important for patients with chronic aortic dissection. Beta blockers remain the drugs of choice. In a 20-year follow-up study, DeBakey and colleagues reported that inadequate blood pressure control was associated with late aneurysm formation. Aneurysms developed in only 17% of patients with "good" blood pressure control, compared to 45% of patients with "poor" control.

Aggressive imaging follow-up is recommended for all patients with chronic aortic dissection. Both contrast-enhanced CT and MRA scans provide excellent aortic imaging and facilitate serial comparisons to detect progressive aortic expansion. The first surveillance scan is obtained approximately 6 weeks after the onset of dissection. Subsequent scans are obtained at least every 3 months for the first year, every 6 months for the second year, and annually thereafter. More frequent scans are obtained in high-risk patients, such as those with Marfan syndrome, or if significant aortic expansion is detected. Patients who have undergone graft repair also are evaluated with annual CT or MRA scans to detect false aneurysm formation or dilatation of unrepaired segments of aorta. Early detection of worrisome changes allows timely elective intervention before rupture or other complications develop. The importance of the careful follow-up was illustrated by Glower and associates, who reported long-term outcomes in patients with chronic aortic dissection; nearly 20% of late deaths were caused by aortic rupture and 25% of patients required surgical repair during the follow-up period.

Indications for Surgery. Surgery is reserved for patients who experience complications. In general terms, surgical intervention for acute distal aortic dissection is directed toward prevention or repair of rupture and relief of ischemic manifestations.

During the acute phase, the specific indications for operative intervention include (1) aortic rupture, (2) increasing periaortic or pleural fluid, (3) rapidly expanding aortic diameter, (4) uncontrolled hypertension, and (5) persistent pain despite adequate medical

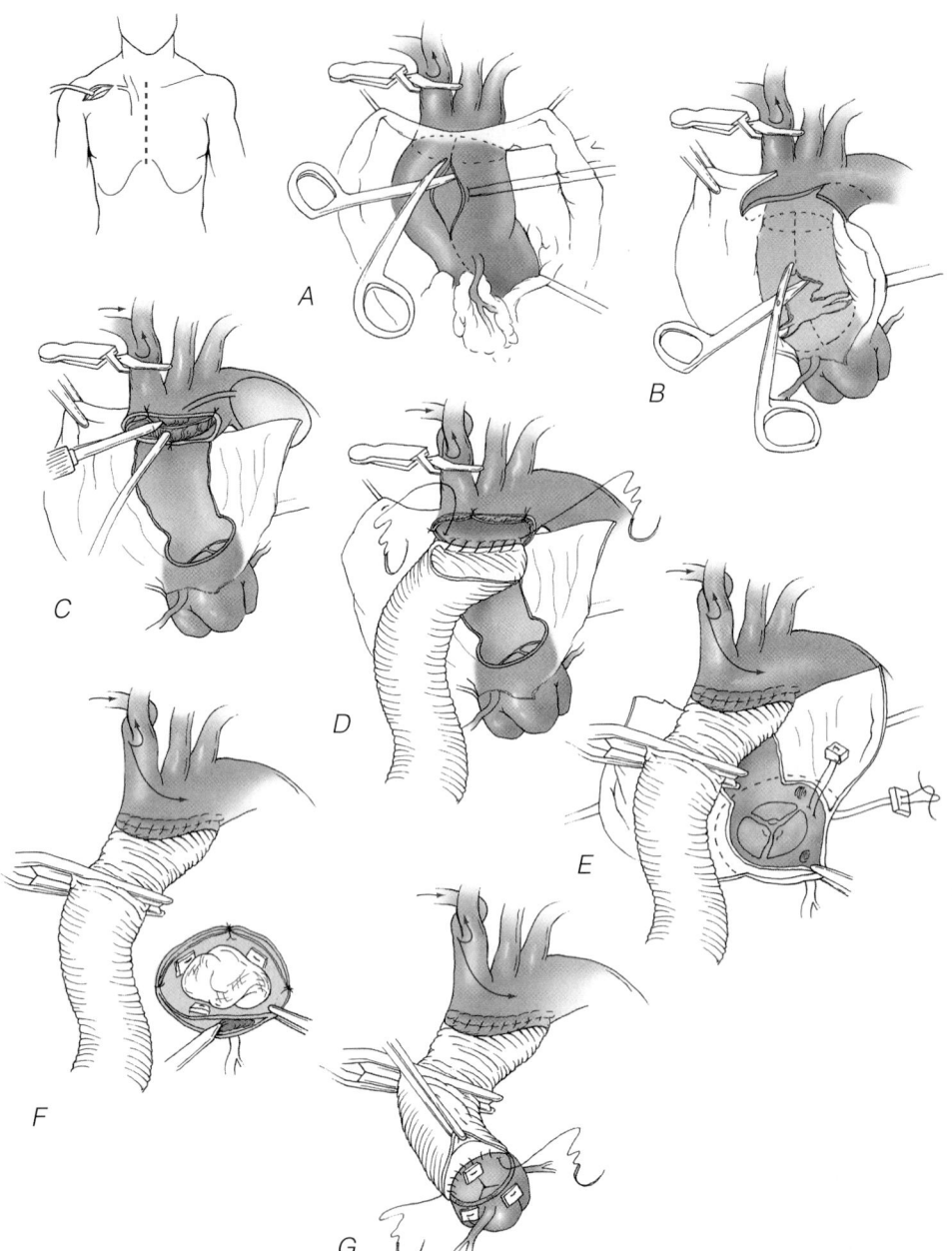

FIG. 21-13. *A.* Proximal aortic operations are performed through a median sternotomy and require cardiopulmonary bypass. Axillary artery can-nulation is used for cerebral protection. Under hypothermic circulatory arrest, the aorta is opened. *B.* The dissecting membrane is opened and the true lumen is entered. *C.* Surgical adhesive is used to obliterate the false lumen and prepare the aorta for the distal anastomosis. To help contain the adhesive, pockets within the false lumen are created by gently tacking the dissecting membrane to the outer wall using three to five interrupted 6-0 sutures. A moist gauze sponge is placed in the true lumen to prevent the adhesive from running into the brachiocephalic vessels. A balloon catheter is placed into the true lumen to compress the distal false lumen, which helps keep the adhesive within the proximal false lumen, optimizing the strength of the repair and preventing distal embolization of the adhesive through re-entry sites. *D.* An open distal anastomosis is always employed to avoid fracturing the distal intima with a clamp and to allow inspection of all of the transverse aortic arch internally. Provided the origin of the dissection (i.e., intimal tear or disruption) does not extensively involve the greater curvature of the transverse aortic arch, and there is no evidence of a pre-existing transverse arch aneurysm, the distal anastomosis is carried out in a beveled fashion, preserving most of the greater curvature of the arch. The aorta is transected beginning at the greater curvature immediately proximal to the origin of the innominate artery and extending distally toward the lesser curvature to the level of the left subclavian artery. Consequently, most of the transverse aortic arch, except for the dorsal segment containing the brachiocephalic arteries, is removed. An appropriately sized sealed (collagen or gelatin) Dacron tube graft is selected, and the beveled distal anastomosis is performed using continuous 4-0 or 5-0 monofilament suture. *E.* After resuming cardio pulmonary bypass, the aortic valve is assessed for incompetence and any disruption due to proximal extension of the dissection. The aorta is generally transected at the sinotubular junction. Aortic valve competence may be restored by resuspending the commissures with pledgeted mattress sutures. *F.* The aorta is generally transected at the sinotubular junction, and a saline-soaked 4 x 4 gauze sponge is placed within the true lumen to prevent the adhesive from injuring the aortic valve leaflets or entering the coronary artery ostia. As before, pockets within the false lumen can be created by gently tacking the dissecting membrane to the outer wall. After all clotted and fresh blood is thoroughly removed from the false lumen, the adhesive is used to obliterate the false lumen within the proximal aortic stump. *G.* After the adhesive has set for 2 to 3 minutes, the proximal anastomosis is carried out in the region between the sinotubular junction and the distal margin of the commissures.

therapy. Acute dissection superimposed on a pre-existing aneurysm is considered a life-threatening condition and also is an indication for operation. Finally, patients who have a history of noncompliance with medical therapy present a problematic situation; surgical treatment should be considered if these patients are otherwise reasonable operative candidates.

Acute malperfusion syndromes also warrant intervention. In the recent past, visceral and renal malperfusion were considered indications for operation. Advances in percutaneous interventions, however, have largely replaced open surgery for these complications. Therefore, patients who develop evidence of visceral or renal malperfusion undergo urgent aortography. Percutaneous fenestration of the dissecting membrane or placement of branch artery stents can restore organ perfusion. When this approach is unavailable or unsuccessful, surgical options—which include graft replacement of the aorta, open aortic fenestration, and visceral/renal artery bypass—can be employed. Lower extremity ischemia is usually addressed surgically via extra-anatomic revascularization, such as femoral-to-femoral crossover bypass.

In the chronic phase, the indications for operative intervention are similar to those for degenerative thoracic aortic aneurysms. Rapid expansion of the aneurysm and factors that increase the likelihood of rupture are indications for surgery. Elective operation is considered when the affected segment has reached 5 to 6 cm, or when an aneurysm has enlarged more than 1 cm during a 1-year period. A lower threshold is often used for patients with Marfan syndrome.

Operative Repair. Surgical repair of the descending thoracic or thoracoabdominal aorta in the setting of acute aortic dissection is associated with high morbidity and mortality. Therefore, the primary goals of surgery are to prevent fatal rupture and restore branch vessel perfusion. A limited graft repair of the symptomatic segment achieves these goals while minimizing risks. Since the most common site of rupture in distal aortic dissection is in the proximal third of the descending thoracic aorta, the upper half of the descending thoracic aorta is usually repaired. The distal half may also be replaced if it exceeds 4 cm in diameter. Graft replacement of the entire thoracoabdominal aorta is not attempted in this setting unless a large coexisting aneurysm mandates this radical approach. Similarly, the repair is not extended into the aortic arch unless it is aneurysmal, even if the primary tear is located there. Patients with chronic dissection who require emergency repair due to acute pain or rupture also undergo limited graft replacement of the symptomatic segment.

In patients with acute dissection, adjuncts that provide spinal cord protection are used liberally because of the increased risk of paraplegia. Therefore, cerebrospinal fluid drainage and left heart bypass often are employed, even if the repair is localized to the upper descending thoracic aorta. Proximal control is usually obtained between the left common carotid and left subclavian artery; any mediastinal hematoma near the proximal descending thoracic aorta is avoided until proximal control is established. After opening the aorta, the dissecting membrane is excised from the section undergoing graft replacement. The proximal and distal anastomoses utilize all layers of aortic wall, thereby excluding the false lumen in the suture lines and directing all blood flow into the true lumen. While the relative lack of mural thrombus assures the presence of multiple patent intercostal arteries, the extreme tissue fragility may preclude their reattachment.

A more aggressive replacement is usually performed during elective aortic repairs in patients with chronic dissection. In many regards, the operative approach in these patients is identical to that used for descending thoracic and thoracoabdominal aortic aneurysms, as described in the first half of this chapter (Fig. 21-14). One key difference is the need to excise as much dissecting membrane as possible in order to clearly identify the true and false lumens and locate all important branch vessels. When the dissection extends into the visceral or renal arteries, the membrane can be fenestrated or the false lumen can be obliterated using sutures or intraluminal stents. Asymmetric expansion of the false lumen can create wide separation of the renal arteries. This is addressed by reattaching the mobilized left renal artery to a separate opening in the graft or by performing a left renal artery bypass using a side graft. Wedges of dissecting membrane also are excised proximally and distally from within the aortic cuffs, allowing blood to flow through both true and false lumens. When a distal dissection has progressed retrograde into the transverse aortic arch and placement of the proximal clamp is not technically feasible, hypothermic circulatory arrest can be used to facilitate the proximal portion of the repair.

Recent Results

Proximal Aortic Dissection. Table 21-7 displays these authors results with proximal aortic dissection repair in 489 patients. Over 40% of repairs were performed in the acute setting. Compared to patients who underwent repairs in the chronic phase, those who had repairs of acute dissection had a stroke rate that was two times higher and a mortality rate that was nearly three times higher. Nonetheless, compared to the lethality of unrepaired acute proximal aortic dissection, contemporary results of surgical treatment are excellent.

Distal Aortic Dissection. Despite aggressive pharmacologic management, 10 to 20% of patients die during the initial treatment phase. The primary causes of death during nonoperative management include rupture, malperfusion, and cardiac failure. Risk factors associated with treatment failure—defined as death or need for surgery—include an enlarged aorta, persistent hypertension despite maximal treatment, oliguria, and peripheral ischemia.

Table 21-8 displays the results of these authors with distal aortic dissection repair in 714 patients. The majority of these repairs (80.3%) were performed in patients with chronic dissection. The overall results compare favorably to those obtained in patients without dissection.

ENDOVASCULAR TREATMENT OF THORACIC AORTIC DISEASE

While not yet considered standard therapy, endovascular stent-graft repairs are poised to play a major role in the armamentarium for treating thoracic aortic disease. As such, this therapeutic strategy deserves consideration. Recent technologic developments have made the endovascular repair of descending thoracic aortic disease a reality. In 1991, Parodi and associates reported using stent-grafts to achieve endovascular repair of abdominal aortic aneurysms. Only 3 years after this seminal report, Dake and colleagues reported endovascular descending thoracic aortic repair using "homemade" stent-grafts in 13 patients. Subsequent reports have applied this new, less-invasive option in patients with aortic dissection and traumatic, mycotic, and ruptured aneurysms of the descending thoracic aorta. In elderly patients with severe comorbidity or patients who have undergone previous complex thoracic aortic procedures, endovascular repair is a particularly attractive alternative to standard surgical procedures. Several prospective trials using differing commercially available stent-graft systems are underway. Data demonstrating long-term effectiveness are not currently available.

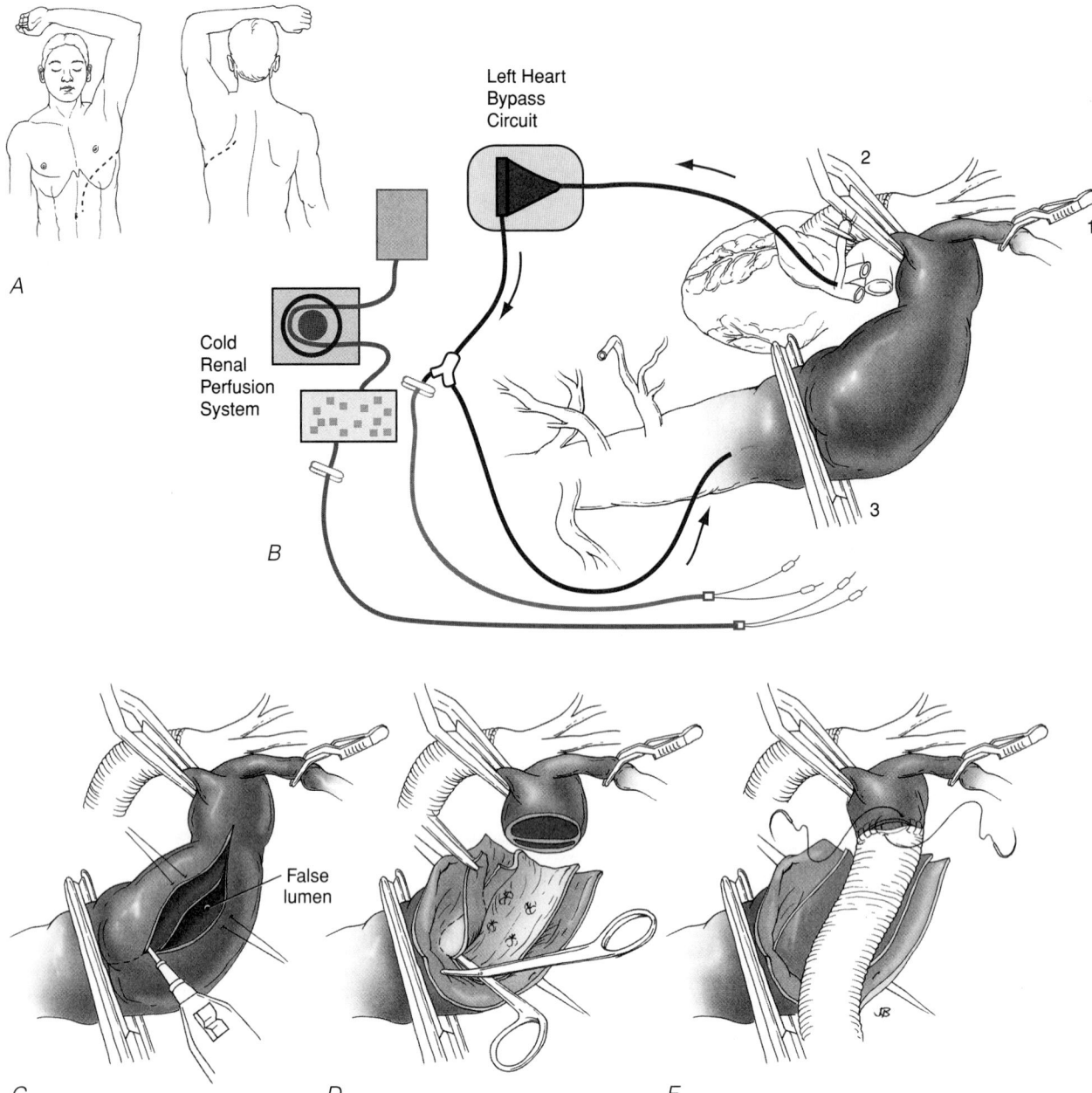

FIG. 21-14. *A.* Thoracoabdominal incision. *B.* Extent II thoracoabdominal aortic aneurysm resulting from chronic aortic dissection. The patient has undergone composite valve graft replacement of the aortic root in the past. After initiating left heart bypass, the proximal portion of the aneurysm is isolated by placing clamps (1) on the left subclavian artery, (2) between the left common carotid and left subclavian arteries, and (3) across the upper mid-descending thoracic aorta. *C.* The isolated segment of aorta is opened using electrocautery. *D.* The dissecting membrane is excised, and bleeding intercostal arteries are oversewn. The aorta is prepared for the proximal anastomosis by transecting it distal to the proximal clamp and separating this portion from the esophagus. *E.* The proximal anastomosis between the aorta and an appropriately sized Dacron graft is completed using continuous polypropylene suture. *F.* After stopping the left heart bypass and removing the distal aortic cannula, the proximal clamp is repositioned onto the graft and the remainder of the aneurysm is opened. *G.* The rest of the dissecting membrane is excised and the openings to the celiac, and superior mesenteric arteries are identified. *H.* Selective visceral perfusion with oxygenated blood from the bypass circuit is delivered through balloon perfusion catheters placed in the celiac, renal, and superior mesenteric arterial ostia. Cold crystalloid is delivered to the vena/arteries. The critical intercostal arteries are reattached to an opening cut in the graft. *I.* In order to minimize spinal cord ischemia, the proximal clamp is repositioned distal to the intercostal reattachment site. A second oval opening is fashioned in the graft adjacent to the visceral vessels. Selective perfusion of the visceral arteries continues during their reattachment to the graft. A separate anastomosis is often required to reattach the left renal artery. *J.* After completing the visceral anastomosis, the balloon perfusion catheters are removed and the clamp is again moved distally, restoring flow to the celiac, renal, and superior mesenteric arteries. The final anastomosis is created between the graft and the distal aorta. *(Continued)*

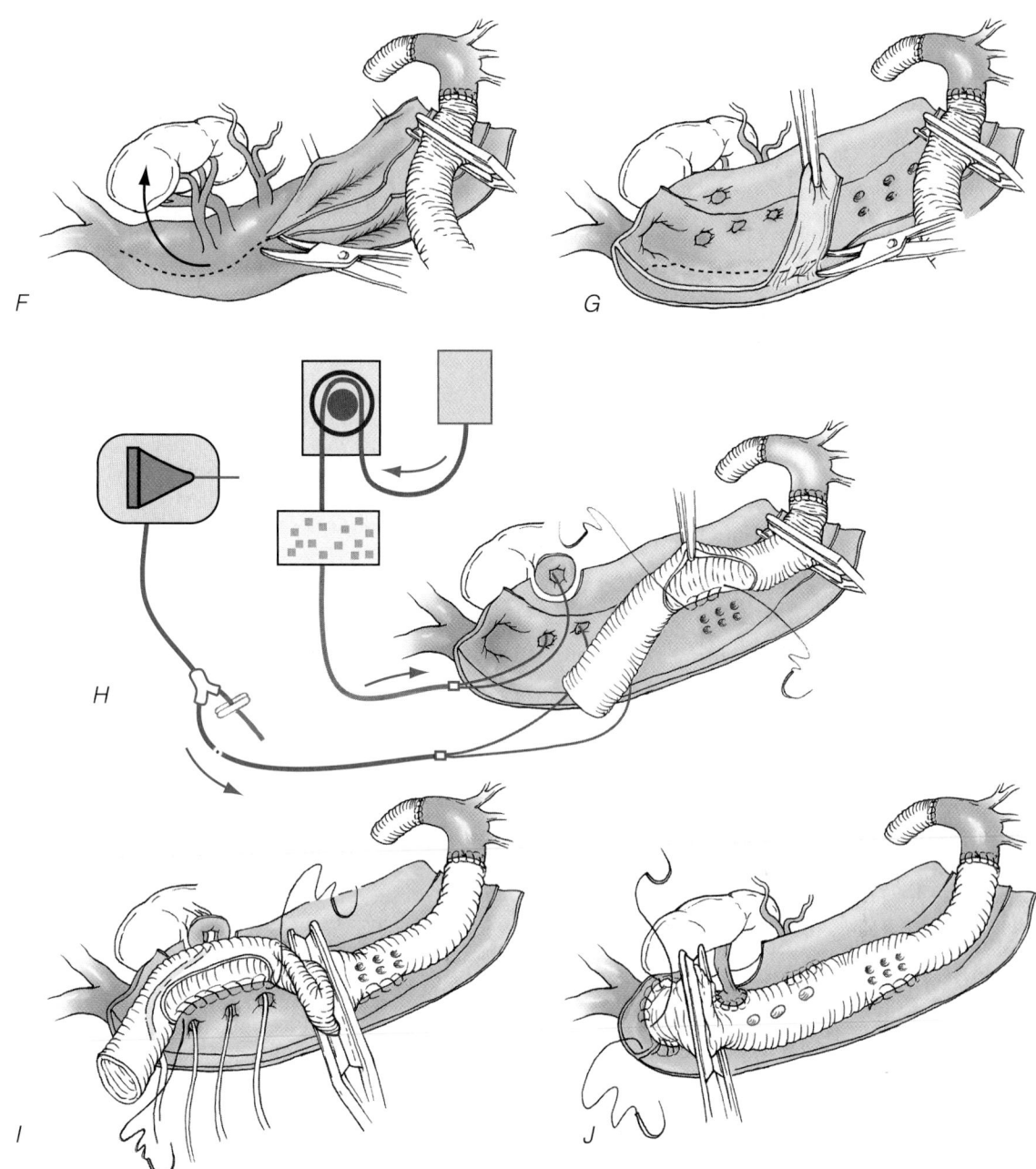

FIG. 21-14. *(Continued)*

Table 21-7

Results of Surgical Repair of Proximal Thoracic Aortic Dissection

Dissection	No. of Patients	30-Day Mortality	Stroke	Bleeding[a]	Renal Failure[b]	Paraplegia or Paraparesis
Acute	209	23 (11.0%)	13 (6.2%)	8 (3.8%)	4 (1.9%)	2 (1.0%)
Chronic	280	12 (4.3%)	9 (3.2%)	11 (3.9%)	2 (0.7%)	2 (0.7%)
Total	489	35 (7.2%)	22 (4.5%)	19 (3.9%)	6 (1.2%)	4 (0.8%)

[a] Bleeding requiring reoperation.
[b] Acute renal failure requiring hemodialysis.

Table 21-8
Results of Surgical Repair of Distal Thoracic Aortic Dissection

Extent[a]	No. of Patients	30-Day Mortality	Stroke	Bleeding[b]	Renal Failure[c]	Paraplegia or Paraparesis
DTAA	146	3 (2.1%)	1 (0.7%)	6 (4.1%)	3 (2.1%)	5 (3.4%)
TAAA I	218	13 (6.0%)	9 (4.1%)	2 (0.9%)	7 (3.2%)	6 (2.8%)
TAAA II	273	10 (3.7%)	6 (2.2%)	5 (1.8%)	13 (4.8%)	17 (6.2%)
TAAA III	44	3 (6.8%)	1 (2.3%)	1 (2.3%)	1 (2.3%)	1 (2.3%)
TAAA IV	33	2 (6.1%)	1 (3.0%)	0 (0.0%)	1 (3.0%)	1 (3.0%)
Total	714	31 (4.3%)	18 (2.5%)	14 (2.0%)	25 (3.5%)	30 (4.2%)

[a]Thoracoabdominal aortic aneurysm extents I–IV based on Crawford's classification.
[b]Bleeding requiring reoperation.
[c]Acute renal failure requiring hemodialysis.
DTAA = descending thoracic aortic aneurysm; TAAA = thoracoabdominal aortic aneurysm.

General mortality and morbidity following endovascular repair of descending thoracic aortic aneurysms is currently difficult to assess. Most of the reported series are small and contain a large proportion of high-risk patients with substantial comorbidity. For example, in the Stanford experience with "first generation" stent-grafts in 103 patients with descending thoracic aortic aneurysms, the operative mortality rate was 9%, stroke occurred in 7%, paraplegia/paraparesis occurred in 3%, and actuarial survival was only 73 ± 5% at 2 years. However, 62 (60%) patients were not considered candidates for thoracotomy and open surgical repair; as expected, this group experienced the majority of the morbidity and mortality. Future reports with larger series and healthier patients will help clarify risks and likely demonstrate relatively low overall morbidity and mortality.

As the experience with descending thoracic aortic stent-grafts continues to increase, reports regarding complications specifically related to device deployment are emerging in the literature. Many of these complications are directly related to manipulation of the delivery system within the iliac arteries and aorta. Patients with small, calcified, tortuous iliofemoral arteries are at particular risk for life-threatening iliac artery rupture. The potential for aortic injury precipitating immediate operation is well described in abdominal aortic stent-graft literature; thus far, reports of thoracic aortic rupture during stent-graft procedures are rare. A more common and equally deadly complication is acute iatrogenic aortic dissection into the aortic arch and ascending aorta. There are already several reports of this complication, most involving "new generation" devices and requiring emergency repair of the ascending aorta and aortic arch via sternotomy and cardiopulmonary bypass. Such a dissection converts a localized descending thoracic aortic disease into an acute problem involving the entire thoracic aorta. Although early reports have documented a 20 to 25% incidence of endoleak, this is expected to decline as stent-graft technology continues to advance. Early type I endoleaks—which result from an incomplete seal between the graft and aorta at attachment sites—can precipitate aortic rupture. Therefore, aggressive intervention is recommended, if feasible, when type I endoleaks develop within weeks after the initial procedure. Other device-related problems include stent-graft misdeployment, device migration, and endograft kinking. While not all complications related to stent-grafts are fatal, endovascular repairs should be performed by expert teams qualified to address the variety of unanticipated problems that may arise.

In contrast to endovascular repair of descending thoracic aortic aneurysms, experience with endovascular treatment of proximal aortic disease remains limited and purely experimental. The unique anatomy of the aortic arch and need for uninterrupted cerebral perfusion pose difficult challenges. In 1999, Inoue and colleagues reported placement of a triple-branched stent-graft in a patient with an aneurysm of the aortic arch. The three brachiocephalic branches were positioned using percutaneous wires placed in the right brachial, left carotid, and left brachial arteries. The patient required two subsequent procedures: surgical repair of a right brachial pseudoaneurysm, and placement of a distal stent-graft extension to control a major perigraft leak. Dorros and colleagues repaired an ascending aortic dissection with a short covered stent. Several authors have reported successful hybrid procedures in which extra-anatomic bypasses are performed to the brachiocephalic arteries prior to placing a stent-graft across the aortic arch.

Similarly, the experience with endovascular thoracoabdominal aortic aneurysm repair remains anecdotal and has had mixed results. Thoracoabdominal aortic aneurysms have been repaired using hybrid approaches, with stent-graft coverage of the entire aneurysm including branch vessel ostia, followed by open visceral bypass grafting to restore organ perfusion. Custom-made endografts with fenestrations or single side branches have been used to successfully exclude thoracoabdominal aneurysms while preserving perfusion of branch vessels. Chuter and colleagues used a stent-graft with four separate visceral branch-grafts to perform an extent III repair; this case was complicated by delayed paraplegia and kinking of the celiac and superior mesenteric stumps, which required revision with additional stents. Two groups have reported fatal ruptures due to distal type I endoleak following repair of extent I thoracoabdominal aortic aneurysms using straight stent-grafts. Until prospective studies demonstrate consistent and favorable results, endovascular thoracoabdominal aortic aneurysm repair must be considered purely investigational.

Acknowledgment

The authors gratefully acknowledge Autumn Jamison and Stacey Carter for their invaluable assistance while preparing this manuscript.

Bibliography

Thoracic Aortic Aneurysms

Etiology and Pathogenesis

Bonderman D, Gharehbaghi-Schnell E, Wollenek G, et al: Mechanisms underlying aortic dilatation in congenital aortic valve malformation. *Circulation* 99:2138, 1999.

Fedak PW, de Sa MP, Verma S, et al: Vascular matrix remodeling in patients with bicuspid aortic valve malformations: Implications for aortic dilatation. *J Thorac Cardiovasc Surg* 126:797, 2003.

Guo D, Hasham S, Kuang SQ, et al: Familial thoracic aortic aneurysms and dissections: Genetic heterogeneity with a major locus mapping to 5q13-14. *Circulation* 103:2461, 2001.

Keane MG, Wiegers SE, Plappert T, et al: Bicuspid aortic valves are associated with aortic dilatation out of proportion to coexistent valvular lesions. *Circulation* 102:III35, 2000.

LeMaire SA, Wang X, Wilks J, et al: Matrix metalloproteinases in ascending aortic aneurysms: Bicuspid vs. trileaflet aortic valves. *J Surg Res* 2004, in press.

Lesauskaite V, Tanganelli P, Sassi C, et al: Smooth muscle cells of the media in the dilatative pathology of ascending thoracic aorta: Morphology, immunoreactivity for osteopontin, matrix metalloproteinases, and their inhibitors. *Hum Pathol* 32:1003, 2001.

Marsalese DL, Moodie DS, Vacante M, et al: Marfan's syndrome: Natural history and long-term follow-up of cardiovascular involvement. *J Am Coll Cardiol* 14:422, 1989.

Nataatmadja M, West M, West J, et al: Abnormal extracellular matrix protein transport associated with increased apoptosis of vascular smooth muscle cells in Marfan syndrome and bicuspid aortic valve thoracic aortic aneurysm. *Circulation* 108(Suppl 1):II329, 2003.

Robicsek F: Aortic media in bicuspid valve disease. *Ann Thorac Surg* 76:337, 2003.

Schmid FX, Bielenberg K, Schneider A, et al: Ascending aortic aneurysm associated with bicuspid and tricuspid aortic valve: Involvement and clinical relevance of smooth muscle cell apoptosis and expression of cell death-initiating proteins. *Eur J Cardiothorac Surg* 23:537, 2003.

Segura AM, Luna RE, Horiba K, et al: Immunohistochemistry of matrix metalloproteinases and their inhibitors in thoracic aortic aneurysms and aortic valves of patients with Marfan's syndrome. *Circulation* 98(Suppl 1): II331, 1998.

Yasuda H, Nakatani S, Stugaard M, et al: Failure to prevent progressive dilation of ascending aorta by aortic valve replacement in patients with bicuspid aortic valve: Comparison with tricuspid aortic valve. *Circulation* 108(Suppl 1):II291, 2003.

Natural History

Bickerstaff LK, Pairolero PC, Hollier LH, et al: Thoracic aortic aneurysms: A population-based study. *Surgery* 92:1103, 1982.

Davies RR, Goldstein LJ, Coady MA, et al: Yearly rupture or dissection rates for thoracic aortic aneurysms: Simple prediction based on size. *Ann Thorac Surg* 73:17, 2002.

Elefteriades JA: Natural history of thoracic aortic aneurysms: Indications for surgery, and surgical versus nonsurgical risks. *Ann Thorac Surg* 74:S1877, 2002.

Faggioli GL, Stella A, Gargiulo M, et al: Morphology of small aneurysms: Definition and impact on risk of rupture. *Am J Surg* 168:131, 1994.

Juvonen T, Ergin MA, Galla JD, et al: Prospective study of the natural history of thoracic aortic aneurysms. *Ann Thorac Surg* 63:1533, 1997.

Michel PL, Acar J, Chomette G, et al: Degenerative aortic regurgitation. *Eur Heart J* 12:875, 1991.

Murdoch JL, Walker BA, Halpern BL, et al: Life expectancy and causes of death in the Marfan syndrome. *N Engl J Med* 286:804, 1972.

Prenger K, Pieters F, Cheriex E: Aortic dissection after aortic valve replacement: Incidence and consequences for strategy. *J Card Surg* 9:495, 1994.

Diagnostic Evaluation

Danias P, Eldeman R, Manning W: Magnetic resonance angiography of the great vessels and the coronary arteries, in Pohost G, O'Rourke R, Berman D, et al (eds): *Imaging in Cardiovascular Disease.* Philadelphia: Lippincott, Williams, & Wilkins, 2000, p 449.

Fillinger MF: Imaging of the thoracic and thoracoabdominal aorta. *Semin Vasc Surg* 13:247, 2000.

Goldstone J: Vascular imaging techniques, in Rutherford R (ed): *Vascular Surgery,* 3rd ed. Philadelphia: WB Saunders, 1989, p 119.

Schappert T, Sadony V, Schoen F, et al: Diagnosis and therapeutic consequences of intramural aortic hematoma. *J Card Surg* 9:508, 1994.

Wiet SP, Pearce WH, McCarthy WJ, et al: Utility of transesophageal echocardiography in the diagnosis of disease of the thoracic aorta. *J Vasc Surg* 20:613, 1994.

Management

Borst HG, Frank G, Schaps D: Treatment of extensive aortic aneurysms by a new multiple-stage approach *J Thorac Cardiovasc Surg* 95:11, 1988.

Cambria RP, Clouse WD, Davison JK, et al: Thoracoabdominal aneurysm repair: Results with 337 operations performed over a 15-year interval. *Ann Surg* 236:471, 2002.

Carrel TP, Berdat P, Englberger L, et al: Aortic root replacement with a new stentless aortic valve xenograft conduit: Preliminary hemodynamic and clinical results. *J Heart Valve Dis* 12:752, 2003.

Coady MA, Rizzo JA, Elefteriades JA: Developing surgical intervention criteria for thoracic aortic aneurysms. *Cardiol Clin* 17:827, 1999.

Coselli JS, Conklin LD, LeMaire SA: Thoracoabdominal aortic aneurysm repair: Review and update of current strategies. *Ann Thorac Surg* 74:S1881, 2002.

Coselli JS, LeMaire SA, Büket S: Marfan syndrome: The variability and outcome of operative management. *J Vasc Surg* 21:432, 1995.

Coselli JS, LeMaire SA, Conklin LD, et al: Left heart bypass during descending thoracic aortic aneurysm repair does not prevent paraplegia. *Ann Thorac Surg* 77:1298, 2004.

Coselli JS, LeMaire SA, Conklin LD, et al: Morbidity and mortality after extent II thoracoabdominal aortic aneurysm repair. *Ann Thorac Surg* 73:1107, 2002.

Coselli JS, LeMaire SA: Experience with retrograde cerebral perfusion during proximal aortic surgery in 290 patients. *J Card Surg* 12:322, 1997.

Coselli JS, LeMaire SA, Köksoy C, et al: Cerebrospinal fluid drainage reduces paraplegia after thoracoabdominal aortic aneurysm repair: Results of a randomized clinical trial. *J Vasc Surg* 35:635, 2002.

Coselli JS, LeMaire SA, Köksoy C: Thoracic aortic anastomoses. *Operative Tech Thorac Cardiovasc Surg* 5:259, 2000.

Coselli JS, LeMaire SA: Left heart bypass reduces paraplegia rates following thoracoabdominal aortic aneurysm repair. *Ann Thorac Surg* 67:1931, 1999.

Coselli JS, LeMaire SA, Miller CC III, et al: Mortality and paraplegia after thoracoabdominal aortic aneurysm repair: A risk factor analysis. *Ann Thorac Surg* 69:404, 2000.

Coselli JS, LeMaire SA: Surgical techniques: Thoracoabdominal aorta. *Cardiol Clin* 17:751, 1999.

Coselli JS, Oberwalder PJ: Successful repair of mega aorta using reversed elephant trunk procedure. *J Vasc Surg* 27:183, 1998.

David TE, Ivanov J, Armstrong S, et al: Aortic valve-sparing operations in patients with aneurysms of the aortic root or ascending aorta. *Ann Thorac Surg* 74:S1758, 2002.

Gott VL, Cameron DE, Alejo DE, et al: Aortic root replacement in 271 Marfan patients: A 24-year experience. *Ann Thorac Surg* 73:438, 2002.

Hagl C, Ergin MA, Galla JD, et al: Neurologic outcome after ascending aorta-aortic arch operations: Effect of brain protection technique in high-risk patients. *J Thorac Cardiovasc Surg* 121:107, 2001.

Köksoy C, LeMaire SA, Curling PE, et al: Renal perfusion during thoracoabdominal aortic operations: Cold crystalloid is superior to normothermic blood. *Ann Thorac Surg* 73:730, 2002.

Kouchoukos NT, Masetti P, Rokkas CK, et al: Hypothermic cardiopulmonary bypass and circulatory arrest for operations on the descending thoracic and thoracoabdominal aorta. *Ann Thorac Surg* 74:S1885, 2002.

LeMaire SA, Miller CC III, Conklin LD, et al: A new predictive model for adverse outcomes after elective thoracoabdominal aortic aneurysm repair. *Ann Thorac Surg* 71:1233, 2001.

LeMaire SA, Miller CC III, Conklin LD, et al: Estimating group mortality and paraplegia rates after thoracoabdominal aortic aneurysm repair. *Ann Thorac Surg* 75:508, 2003.

LeMaire SA, Rice DC, Schmittling ZC, et al: Emergency surgery for thoracoabdominal aortic aneurysms with acute presentation. *J Vasc Surg* 35:1171, 2002.

Mezrow CK, Sadeghi AM, Gandsas A, et al: Cerebral effects of low-flow cardiopulmonary bypass and hypothermic circulatory arrest. *Ann Thorac Surg* 57:532, 1994.

Safi HJ, Miller CC III, Huynh TT, et al: Distal aortic perfusion and cerebrospinal fluid drainage for thoracoabdominal and descending thoracic aortic repair: Ten years of organ protection. *Ann Surg* 238:372, 2003.

Schepens MA, Dossche KM, Morshuis WJ, et al: The elephant trunk technique: Operative results in 100 consecutive patients. *Eur J Cardiothorac Surg* 21:276, 2002.

Sinclair MC, Singer RL, Manley NJ, et al: Cannulation of the axillary artery for cardiopulmonary bypass: Safeguards and pitfalls. *Ann Thorac Surg* 75:931, 2003.

Strauch JT, Spielvogel D, Haldenwang PL, et al: Cerebral physiology and outcome after hypothermic circulatory arrest followed by selective cerebral perfusion. *Ann Thorac Surg* 76:1972, 2003.

van Dongen EP, Schepens MA, Morshuis WJ, et al: Thoracic and thoracoabdominal aortic aneurysm repair: Use of evoked potential monitoring in 118 patients. *J Vasc Surg* 34:1035, 2001.

Wong CH, Bonser RB: Retrograde cerebral perfusion: Clinical and experimental aspects. *Perfusion* 14:247, 1999.

Yacoub MH, Gehle P, Chandrasekaran V, et al: Late results of a valve-preserving operation in patients with aneurysms of the ascending aorta and root. *J Thorac Cardiovasc Surg* 115:1080, 1998.

Aortic Dissection

Pathology and Classification

Borst HG, Heinemann MK, Stone CD: *Surgical Treatment of Aortic Dissection.* New York: Churchill Livingstone, 1996, p 1.

Maraj R, Rerkpattanapipat P, Jacobs LE, et al: Meta-analysis of 143 reported cases of aortic intramural hematoma. *Am J Cardiol* 86:664, 2000.

O'Gara PT, DeSanctis RW: Acute aortic dissection and its variants: Toward a common diagnostic and therapeutic approach. *Circulation* 92:1376, 1995.

Sundt TM: Management of intramural hematoma of the ascending aorta: Still room for debate [editorial]. *J Thorac Cardiovasc Surg* 125:894, 2002.

Etiology and Natural History

Hagan PG, Nienaber CA, Isselbacher EM, et al: The International Registry of Acute Aortic Dissection (IRAD): New insights into an old disease. *JAMA* 283:897, 2000.

Ishii T, Asuwa N: Collagen and elastin degradation by matrix metalloproteinases and tissue inhibitors of matrix metalloproteinase in aortic dissection. *Hum Pathol* 31:640, 2000.

Juvonen T, Ergin MA, Galla JD, et al: Risk factors for rupture of chronic type B dissections. *J Thorac Cardiovasc Surg* 117:776, 1999.

Larson EW, Edwards WD: Risk factors for aortic dissection: A necropsy study of 161 cases. *Am J Cardiol* 53:849, 1984.

Schneiderman J, Bordin GM, Adar R, et al: Patterns of expression of fibrinolytic genes and matrix metalloproteinase-9 in dissecting aortic aneurysms. *Am J Pathol* 152:703, 1998.

Diagnostic Evaluation

Erbel R, Alfonso F, Boileau C, et al: Diagnosis and management of aortic dissection: Recommendations of the Task Force on Aortic Dissection, European Society of Cardiology. *Eur Heart J* 22:1642, 2001.

Klompas M: Does this patient have an acute thoracic aortic dissection? *JAMA* 87:2262, 2002.

Miller JS, LeMaire SA, Coselli JS: Evaluating aortic dissection: When is coronary angiography indicated? [editorial] *Heart* 83:615, 2000.

Panneton JM, Hollier LH: Dissecting descending thoracic and thoracoabdominal aortic aneurysms: Part II. *Ann Vasc Surg* 9:596, 1995.

Rizzo RJ, Aranki SF, Aklog L, et al: Rapid noninvasive diagnosis and surgical repair of acute ascending aortic dissection: Improved survival with less angiography. *J Thorac Cardiovasc Surg* 108:567, 1994.

Management

Bachet J, Goudot B, Dreyfus GD, et al: Surgery for acute type A aortic dissection: The Hospital Foch experience (1977–1998). *Ann Thorac Surg* 67:2006, 1999.

Bavaria JE, Pochettino A, Brinster DR, et al: New paradigms and improved results for the surgical treatment of acute type A dissection. *Ann Surg* 234:336, 2001.

Coselli JS, Crawford ES, Beall AC, et al: Determination of brain temperatures for safe circulatory arrest during cardiovascular operation. *Ann Thorac Surg* 45:638, 1988.

Coselli JS, LeMaire SA, Poli de Figueiredo L, et al: Paraplegia following thoracoabdominal aortic aneurysm repair: Is dissection a risk factor? *Ann Thorac Surg* 63:28, 1997.

Coselli JS, LeMaire SA, Walkes JC: Surgery for acute type A dissection. *Operative Tech Thorac Cardiovasc Surg* 4:13, 1999.

DeBakey ME, McCollum CH, Crawford ES, et al: Dissection and dissecting aneurysms of the aorta: Twenty year follow-up of five hundred twenty-seven patients treated surgically. *Surgery* 92:1118, 1982.

Elefteriades JA: What operation for acute type A dissection? [Editorial]. *J Thorac Cardiovasc Surg* 123:201, 2002.

Elefteriades JA, Hartlerroad J, Gusberg RJ, et al: Long-term experience with descending aortic dissection: The complication specific approach. *Ann Thorac Surg* 53:11, 1992.

Fann JI, Smith JA, Miller DC, et al: Surgical management of aortic dissection during a 30 year period. *Circulation* 92:113, 1995.

Genoni M, Paul M, Jenni R, et al: Chronic beta-blocker therapy improves outcome and reduces treatment costs in chronic type B aortic dissection. *Eur J Cardiothorac Surg* 19:606, 2001.

Gillinov AM, Lytle BW, Kaplon RJ, et al: Dissection of the ascending aorta after previous cardiac surgery: Differences in presentation and management. *J Thorc Cardiovasc Surg* 117:252, 1999.

Glower DD, Speier RF, White WD, et al: Management and long-term outcome of aortic dissection. *Ann Surg* 214:31, 1991.

Gysi J, Schaffner T, Mohacsi P, et al: Early and late outcome of operated and non-operated acute dissection of the descending aorta. *Eur J Cardiothorac Surg* 11:1163, 1997.

Israel DH, Sharma SK, Ambrose JA, et al: Cardiac catheterizaton and selective coronary angiography in ascending aortic aneurysm or dissection. *Cathet Cardiovasc Diagn* 32:232, 1994.

Kirsch M, Soustelle C, Houel R, et al: Risk factor analysis for proximal and distal reoperations after surgery for acute type A aortic dissection. *J Thorac Cardiovasc Surg* 123:318, 2002.

Pasic M, Schubel J, Bauer M, et al: Cannulation of the right axillary artery for surgery of acute type A aortic dissection. *Eur J Cardiothorac Surg* 24:231, 2003.

Safi HJ, Miller CC, Reardon MJ, et al: Operation for acute and chronic aortic dissection: Recent outcome with regard to neurologic deficit and early death. *Ann Thorac Surg* 66:402, 1998.

Scholl FG, Coady MA, Davies R, et al: Interval or permanent nonoperative management of acute type A aortic dissection. *Arch Surg* 134:402, 1999.

Schor JS, Yerlioglu ME, Galla JD, et al: Selective management of acute type B aortic dissection: Long-term follow-up. *Ann Thorac Surg* 61:1339, 1996.

Westaby S, Saito S, Katsumata T: Acute type A dissection: Conservative methods provide consistently low mortality. *Ann Thorac Surg* 73:707, 2002.

Yavuz S, Goncu MT, Turk T: Axillary artery cannulation for arterial inflow in patients with acute dissection of the ascending aorta. *Eur J Cardiothorac Surg* 22:313, 2002.

Endovascular Treatment of Thoracic Aortic Disease

Bethuyne N, Bove T, Van den Brande P, et al: Acute retrograde aortic dissection during endovascular repair of a thoracic aortic aneurysm. *Ann Thorac Surg* 75:1967, 2003.

Bleyn J, Schol F, Vanhandenhove I, et al: Side-branched modular endograft system for thoracoabdominal aortic aneurysm repair. *J Endovasc Ther* 9:838, 2002.

Bortone AS, Schena S, Mannatrizio G, et al: Endovascular stent-graft treatment for diseases of the descending thoracic aorta. *Eur J Cardiothorac Surg* 20:514, 2001.

Chuter TA, Gordon RL, Reilly LM, et al: An endovascular system for thoracoabdominal aortic aneurysm repair. *J Endovasc Ther* 8:25, 2001.

Chuter TA, Schneider DB, Reilly LM, et al: Modular branched stent graft for endovascular repair of aortic arch aneurysm and dissection. *J Vasc Surg* 38:859, 2003.

Criado FJ, Clark NS, Barnatan MF: Stent graft repair in the aortic arch and descending thoracic aorta: A 4-year experience. *J Vasc Surg* 36:1121, 2002.

Dake MD: Endovascular stent-graft management of thoracic aortic diseases. *Eur J Radiol* 39:42, 2001.

Dake MD, Miller DC, Semba CP, et al: Transluminal placement of endovascular stent-grafts for the treatment of descending thoracic aortic aneurysms. *N Engl J Med* 331:1729, 1994.

Dorros G, Dorros AM, Planton S, et al: Transseptal guidewire stabilization facilitates stent-graft deployment for persistent proximal ascending aortic dissection. *J Endovasc Ther* 7:506, 2000.

Fanelli F, Salvatori FM, Marcelli G, et al: Type A dissection developing during endovascular repair of an acute type B dissection. *J Endovasc Ther* 10:254, 2003.

Inoue K, Hosokawa H, Iwase T, et al: Aortic arch reconstruction by transluminally placed endovascular branched stent graft. *Circulation* 100(Suppl II):II-316, 1999.

Inoue K, Iwase T, Sato M, et al: Transluminal endovascular branched graft placement for a pseudoaneurysm: Reconstruction of the descending thoracic aorta including the celiac axis. *J Thorac Cardiovasc Surg* 114:859, 1997.

Kinney EV, Kaebnick HW, Mitchell RA, et al: Repair of mycotic paravisceral aneurysm with a fenestrated stent-graft. *J Endovasc Surg* 7:192, 2000.

Kotsis T, Scharrer-Palmer R, Kapfer X, et al: Treatment of thoracoabdominal aortic aneurysms with combined endovascular and surgical approach. *Int Angiol* 22:125, 2003.

Lawrence-Brown M, Sieunarine K, van Schie G, et al: Hybrid open-endoluminal technique for repair of thoracoabdominal aneurysm involving the celiac axis. *J Endovasc Ther* 7:513, 2000.

Misfeld M, Notzold A, Geist V, et al: Retrograde type A dissection after endovascular stent grafting of type B dissection. *Z Kardiol* 91:274, 2002.

Mitchell RS, Miller DC, Dake MD, et al: Thoracic aortic aneurysm repair with an endovascular stent graft: The "first generation." *Ann Thorac Surg* 67:1971, 1999.

Modine T, Lions C, Destrieux-Garnier L, et al: Iatrogenic iliac artery rupture and type A dissection after endovascular repair of type B aortic dissection. *Ann Thorac Surg* 77:317, 2004.

Ohata T, Fukuda S, Kigawa I, et al: Limitation of implantation of endovascular stent-graft: Case report of a patient with thoracoabdominal aneurysm. *J Thorac Cardiovasc Surg* 116:876, 1998.

Parodi JC, Palmaz JC, Barone HD: Transfemoral intraluminal graft implantation for abdominal aortic aneurysms. *Ann Vasc Surg* 5:491, 1991.

Pasic M, Bergs P, Knollmann F, et al: Delayed retrograde aortic dissection after endovascular stenting of the descending thoracic aorta. *J Vasc Surg* 36:184, 2002.

Rachel ES, Bergamini TM, Kinney EV, et al: Endovascular repair of thoracic aortic aneurysms: A paradigm shift in standard of care. *Vasc Endovascular Surg* 36:105, 2002.

Rousseau H, Soula P, Perreault P, et al: Delayed treatment of traumatic rupture of the thoracic aorta with endoluminal covered stent. *Circulation* 99:498, 1999.

Saccani S, Nicolini F, Beghi C, et al: Thoracic aortic stents: A combined solution for complex cases. *Eur J Vasc Endovasc Surg* 24:423, 2002.

Schneider DB, Curry TK, Reilly LM, et al: Branched endovascular repair of aortic arch aneurysm with a modular stent-graft system. *J Vasc Surg* 38:855, 2003.

Semba CP, Kato N, Kee ST, et al: Acute rupture of the descending thoracic aorta: Repair with use of endovascular stent-grafts. *J Vasc Interv Radiol* 8:337, 1997.

Semba CP, Sakai T, Slonim SM, et al: Mycotic aneurysm of the thoracic aorta: Repair with the use of endovascular stent-grafts. *J Vasc Interv Radiol* 9:33, 1998.

Stanley BM, Semmens JB, Lawrence-Brown MM, et al: Fenestration in endovascular grafts for aortic aneurysm repair: New horizons for preserving blood flow in branch vessels. *J Endovasc Ther* 8:16, 2001.

Thompson CS, Gaxotte VD, Rodriguez JA, et al: Endoluminal stent grafting of the thoracic aorta: Initial experience with the Gore Excluder. *J Vasc Surg* 35:1163, 2003.

Wantabe Y, Ishimaru S, Kawaguchi S, et al: Successful endografting with simultaneous visceral artery bypass grafting for severely calcified thoracoabdominal aortic aneurysm. *J Vasc Surg* 35:397, 2002.

CHAPTER 22

Arterial Disease

Alan B. Lumsden, Peter H. Lin, Ruth L. Bush, and Changyi Chen

HISTORY

In 1888 Rudolph Matas reported the successful treatment of a traumatic brachial artery pseudoaneurysm by endoaneurysmorrhaphy; however, joining of two blood vessels together using sutures was first accomplished in 1897, and represented the birth of modern day reconstructive vascular surgery.[1] Credit for this first human anastomosis goes to John Murphy of Chicago, Illinois, who repaired a traumatic femoral arteriovenous fistula with resection and anastomosis of the femoral artery.[2] Later, Carrel and Guthrie (1905–1906) developed many of the currently used techniques.[3] In 1915, Bernheim used the first vein graft in the United States for reconstruction of a syphilitic popliteal artery aneurysm.[4]

The first report of successful repair of an abdominal aortic aneurysm and its reconstruction using human homograft was in 1952, which stimulated intense interest in development of artificial aortic grafts. In the same year, Voorhees reported the use of the parachute cloth Vinyon-N as a vascular prosthesis. In 1953 DeBakey developed the Dacron velour graft, which is used to this day.[5] The development of the synthetic arterial bypass graft heralded what is regarded as contemporary vascular surgery. However, today vascular disease management is in the midst of a revolution in clinical practice, namely catheter-based intervention. Angioplasty led to the evolution of stents, which spawned stent grafts. Currently, the stent is no longer simply a passive mechanical scaffold, but is being evaluated as a drug delivery platform. It is likely that this will lead to the third revolution in treating vascular disease, where catheter-delivered devices will pharmacologically or genetically produce temporary and perhaps permanent changes in the biology of the vessel wall. Among the ranks of surgical luminaries such as Carrel, Murphy, Voorhees, and DeBakey, the names of new endovascular pioneers must be added. Those who will shape the future of vascular therapy include Charles Dotter (endoluminal recanalization), Andreas Gruntzig (balloon angioplasty), Julio Palmaz (endoluminal stent), and Juan Parodi (stent graft).

EPIDEMIOLOGY

It is estimated that peripheral arterial disease, a manifestation of systemic atherosclerosis, occurs in approximately 12% of the adult population, affecting about 8 to 10 million people in the United States (Fig. 22-1). The most common symptomatic manifestation of mild to moderate atherosclerotic peripheral arterial disease (PAD) is intermittent claudication, which occurs at an annual incidence of 2% in people over the age of 65. These patients are at a significantly higher risk of death compared with healthy controls of similar age. Not only are cardiovascular morbidity and mortality increased, but functional status is often severely impaired in patients with intermittent claudication. Peak exercise performance in the claudicating patient is about 50% that of age-matched controls, an impairment equivalent to moderate to severe heart failure using New York Heart Association criteria.

PATHOPHYSIOLOGY OF ATHEROSCLEROSIS

Atherosclerosis accounts for most peripheral arterial occlusive disease. Many of the risk factors for atherosclerotic coronary artery disease (CAD) such as hyperlipidemia have been identified as risk

PREVALANCE

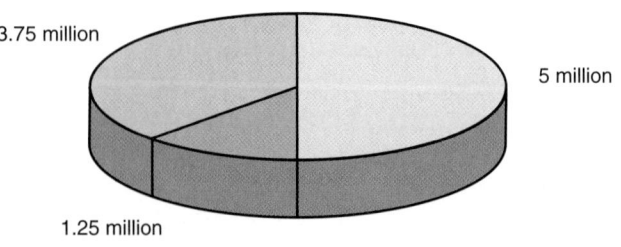

FIG. 22-1. Prevalence of arterial disease.

factors for peripheral arterial disease. The current concept is that a stable atherosclerotic plaque is well tolerated. Vessel remodeling can accommodate even large plaques on many occasions. However, plaque instability, which leads to rupture, exposure of the lipid core, and consequent activation of the coagulation system converts this previously stable situation into one which is limb- or life-threatening.

Atherosclerosis is clearly a complex disease in which numerous diverse etiologic factors play a role. Although there have been numerous hypotheses proposed, the concept that intimal injury incites a series of reactions, which ultimately culminate in development of fibrous plaques, remains the most appealing. This is the "response to injury" hypothesis.

Ross proposed that atherosclerosis reflected a continuing repair process occurring in the arterial wall secondary to persistent arterial injury.[6] The injurious factors could be multifactorial and include hyperlipidemia, shear stress, hypertension, and cigarette smoking. The common denominator is endothelial injury. This results in accumulation of blood-borne monocytes, which migrate into the subendothelial space. Such monocytic accumulation is one of the earliest detectable precursors in the genesis of atherosclerotic lesions. Within the subendothelial space the monocytes convert into cholesterol-laden foam cells. This accumulation distorts the endothelial covering, causing microseparation of endothelial cells and platelet deposition. Smooth muscle cells migrate into the intima from the media, also converting into foam cells (Fig. 22-2).

Relationship Between the Fatty Streak and the Fibrous Plaque

The fatty streak is the earliest identifiable lesion of atherosclerosis. It has been detected in children as young as 10 years of age and consists of lipid-laden macrophages overlying lipid-laden smooth muscle cells. They occur at the same anatomic sites as subsequent fibrous plaques. McGill demonstrated that increased surface involvement of fatty streaks precedes development of fibrous plaques, further supporting a precursor role for the fatty streak.[7]

Monocytes and Macrophages

In diet-induced hypercholesterolemic pigtail monkeys, Faggiotto and Ross demonstrated clustering of monocytes on arterial endothelium.[8] These cells appeared to be in motion and were often found in junctional areas between the endothelial cells from which they migrated and a subendothelial position, where they absorbed lipids and appeared to become foam cells. Monocytes preferentially adhere to injured or proliferating endothelium. Interleukin-1, a product of both macrophage and endothelial cells, will induce increased adherence of neutrophils and monocytes to arterial endothelium. The lesions produced by subendothelial accumulation of monocytes appear similar to fatty streaks. Such lesions enlarge by continued accumulation of monocytes and smooth muscle cell migration. Progressive lesion enlargement leads to disruption of endothelial continuity, exposing the underlying cells, and possibly inducing platelet deposition.

Monocytes have receptors for both native and modified low-density lipoproteins (LDLs). It is the capacity of these cells to remove de-esterified and re-esterified lipid, which may be important in their ability to transform into foam cells. The activated macrophage, derived from the blood monocyte, can release mitogens and chemoattractants, which may recruit more macrophage and smooth muscle cells to the developing plaque.

The Role of Platelet-Derived Growth Factor in Atherogenesis

Platelet-derived growth factor (PDGF) may be responsible for the intimal smooth muscle cell proliferation of atherosclerosis.[9] This concept originated from the observation that platelets contain a potent mitogen for smooth muscle cells, PDGF, and that platelets accumulate and degranulate at sites of endothelial disruption. Although PDGF remains of great interest, it is now apparent that many cells produce PDGF: macrophage, endothelial, and smooth muscle cells (at least in vitro). Therefore, although the platelet may be important in early PDGF release, it now seems likely that endogenous PDGF may be of greater long-term importance. In 1991, Ross demonstrated that antibodies to PDGF prevented the myointimal proliferation observed following balloon angioplasty, raising the question, "Could this have important implications for smooth muscle cells in atherosclerotic plaques?" These PDGF-producing cells also occur in human atherosclerotic plaque. PDGF gene expression has now been clearly demonstrated within human carotid plaque (probably smooth muscle). PDGF α-chain and β-chain messenger RNAs can

FIG. 22-2. *Time course of atherosclerosis.*

Atherosclerosis Time Course

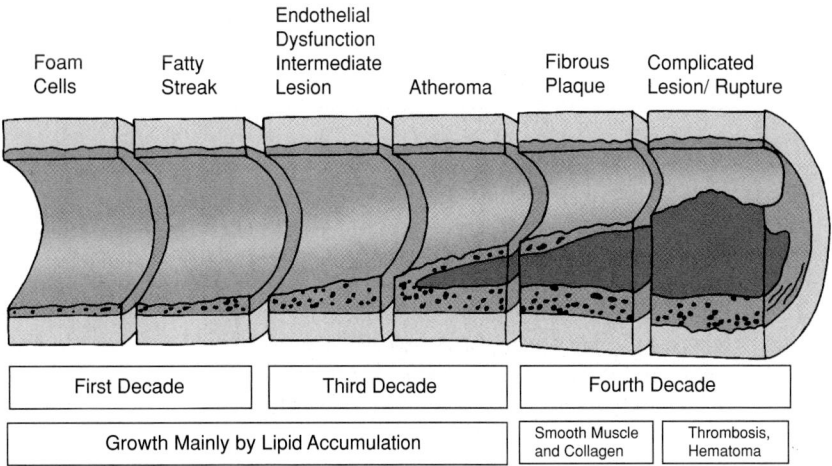

| Foam Cells | Fatty Streak | Endothelial Dysfunction Intermediate Lesion | Atheroma | Fibrous Plaque | Complicated Lesion/ Rupture |

be localized to mesenchymal-appearing intimal cells within the intima. PDGF receptor probes also localize to the intima. Smooth muscle cells (SMCs) in the media do not elaborate PDGF or receptor mRNA. Consequently, the PDGF hypothesis has been changed so that endogenous production of PDGF, locally produced within the plaque, may play an important role in smooth muscle cell proliferation.

Smooth Muscle and Endothelial Cells

Smooth muscle cells are found in variable amounts in fatty streaks, but are the main cell type in fibrous plaques. They contain receptors for PDGF and LDL. The phenotype of these intimal smooth muscle cells is altered from a contractile to a secretory type. Production of an extracellular matrix and further accumulation of lipid and foam cells enlarge these lesions until the core becomes ischemic and eventually necrotic. Following arterial injury, smooth muscle cell proliferation begins in the media. Cells then migrate into the intima where replication continues. The observation that smooth muscle cells may elaborate both PDGF and PDGF receptors heralds a new understanding in the complex, local hormonal environment in atherosclerotic plaque.[7–11] The fibrous plaque consists of multiple layers of smooth muscle cells, each of which lies in a panelled arrangement comprising alternating layers of basement membrane and proteoglycan. Deep to this cellular area is a region of cholesterol crystals, necrotic debris, and calcification. There is increasing interest in circulating stem cells as possible precursors of the transformed smooth muscle cells at sites of arterial injury.

Endothelial cells regulate which plasma constituents reach the subendothelial space. They bind LDLs through a specific receptor, transcytose, and modify it so it is recognized and ingested by cells such as macrophages. They further produce and release growth factors and inhibitors, which may have profound effects on smooth muscle cells and macrophages.[12–16]

Lipids and Atherosclerosis

Elevated plasma lipids have been reported in one third to one half of patients with peripheral vascular disease (PVD).[17] Low levels of high-density lipoprotein (HDL) cholesterol are associated with PVD. There are several apoprotein levels and apoprotein ratios which are predictive of PVD: A-I and A-II levels, and A-I:B and A-I:C-III ratios.

Lipoprotein (a) [Lp(a)], a cholesterol ester, is a low-density lipoprotein–like particle associated with an increased risk of cardiovascular disease. Elevated Lp(a) may represent the most prevalent inherited risk factor for atherosclerosis. Lp(a) levels are insensitive to dietary and drug manipulations.[18]

Elevated LDL and very low-density lipoprotein (VLDL) levels have long been associated with increased risk of atherosclerosis. Cells contain a specific receptor for LDL, and there is a correlation between LDL binding and control of 3-hydroxy-3-methylglutaryl coenzyme A (HMG CoA) reductase—the rate-limiting step for cholesterol synthesis. It is proposed that the number of receptors expressed by the cell varies, protecting the cell against excess cholesterol. However, as the number of expressed LDL receptors decreases, the rate of cholesterol clearance decreases and plasma levels rise. It is postulated that hypercholesterolemia may induce a subtle form of injury. Changes in the cholesterol:phospholipid cell membrane ratios may result in altered endothelial malleability.

Another possible mechanism of endothelial injury in hypercholesterolemia is via oxidization of LDLs. If LDLs are oxidized by macrophages, then toxic products may result in endothelial injury and explain the progression of fatty streaks to fibrous plaques.

Atherosclerosis and Hemodynamics

The effect of local hemodynamic factors on localization of plaque has been studied mainly in the carotid bifurcation, initially in glass models, but more recently it was validated with magnetic resonance angiographic (MRA) imaging and by computer modeling.[19,20] Intimal thickening develops largely in areas of low wall shear stress, in areas of flow separation, and areas with high particle residence time. The theory is that all of these factors facilitate particle (e.g., LDL) interaction with the arterial wall. Caro postulated that low wall shear stress results in slowed transport of circulating particles away from the wall, resulting in the increased intimal accumulation of lipids.

Oscillating shear stress, such as that which occurs in the carotid bulb with areas of transient flow reversal, has been implicated in early lesion formation.

The Modified Response to Injury Hypothesis of Atherosclerosis Development

The modified response to injury hypothesis, as it pertains to the development of atherosclerosis, proposes the following tenets: (1) endothelial injury results in growth factor secretion; (2) the local hemodynamic environment (low shear and oscillating shear) facilitates local injury and particle transfer; (3) circulating monocytes attach to the damaged endothelium; (4) subendothelial migration of monocytes may lead to fatty streak formation and further release of growth factors such as PDGF; (5) fatty streaks may then be converted to fibrous plaques via release of growth factors from macrophages, endothelial cells, or both; (6) macrophages may stimulate or injure the overlying endothelium, thus endothelial cell loss leads to platelet deposition; (7) platelet deposition leads to the release of growth factors and mitogenic factors for smooth muscle cells; and (8) some of the smooth muscle cells in the proliferative lesion itself may form and secrete growth factors.

Strategies for Atherosclerosis Modification

Lipid Modification

The most common cardiovascular risk factors for CAD and PVD include smoking, diabetes, hypertension, dyslipidemia, and abnormalities of homocysteine metabolism, as well as lower estrogen levels after menopause. Treatment of these risk factors may improve cardiovascular outcomes in persons with PVD.[21–24] Brown and Goldstein characterized the LDL receptor and showed how a number of genetic abnormalities are associated with reductions or abnormalities in the expression of this receptor, which in turn is responsible for an elevation of LDL cholesterol. However, reduction or abnormality of the LDL receptor mediated by mutation of a single gene appears to be responsible for only a minority of cases of hypercholesterolemia. Instead, like many other chronic conditions such as most forms of hypertension, diabetes, and asthma, most cases of hypercholesterolemia result from the interaction between multiple genes and environmental influences. The importance of genetic factors is underscored by the marked racial differences in the prevalence of coronary risk factors, as is reflected by the high incidence of diabetes mellitus in Pima Indians and South Pacific Islanders, as well as in the differing contributions that these risk factors make to the prevalence of coronary heart disease.

Several large clinical trials have determined the benefits of lowering cholesterol concentrations in patients with CAD. In patients with PAD, therapy with a statin not only lowers serum cholesterol concentrations, but also improves endothelial function as well as other markers of atherosclerotic risk, such as serum P-selectin concentrations.[25–27] A meta-analysis was performed of randomized trials of lipid-lowering therapy in 698 patients with PAD who were treated with a variety of therapies, including diet, cholestyramine, probucol, and nicotinic acid, for 4 months to 3 years.[24] The total mortality rate was 0.7% in the treated patients, as compared with 2.9% in the patients given placebo—an insignificant difference. This analysis also demonstrated that lipid-lowering therapy reduced disease progression, as measured by angiography, and the severity of claudication. In the Cholesterol Lowering Atherosclerosis Study, 188 men with evidence of both CAD and PVD were treated with diet and then randomly assigned to placebo or colestipol plus niacin. Lipid-lowering therapy was associated with stabilization or regression of femoral atherosclerosis.

Two studies evaluated the effects of lipid-lowering therapy on clinical endpoints in the leg. The Program on the Surgical Control of the Hyperlipidemias was a randomized trial of ileal-bypass surgery for the treatment of hyperlipidemia in 838 patients. After 5 years, the relative risk of an abnormal ankle-brachial index (ABI) value was 0.6 (95% confidence interval, 0.4 to 0.9; absolute risk reduction, 15 percentage points; $p < 0.01$), and the relative risk of claudication or limb-threatening ischemia was 0.7 (95% confidence interval, 0.2 to 0.9; absolute risk reduction, 7 percentage points; $p < 0.01$), as compared with the control group. In a subgroup of patients treated with simvastatin in the Scandinavian Simvastatin Survival Study, the relative risk of new claudication or worsening of pre-existing claudication was 0.6 (95% confidence interval, 0.4 to 0.9; absolute risk reduction, 1.3 percentage points), as compared with patients randomly assigned to placebo.

Therefore lipid-lowering therapy has benefits in patients with PAD, who often have coexisting coronary and cerebral arterial disease. In the recent recommendation, patients with PAD are to be treated in a similar manner as patients with CAD. Drug therapy should be initiated in patients with LDL-C greater than or equal to 130 mg/dL, with a target LDL-C of less than 100 mg/dL. Specific targets of therapy for HDL-C and triglycerides are not provided, but the definition of a low HDL-C is now less than or equal to 40 mg/dL, and optimal triglyceride levels are less than or equal to 150 mg/dL.[19,20]

Atherosclerosis and Inflammation

It is clear that atherosclerosis is associated with inflammation. The involvement of inflammatory cells such as macrophages and lymphocytes is critical to the progression of atherosclerosis. Increased concentrations of C-reactive protein (CRP), an acute phase reactant that reflects low-grade systemic inflammation, are known to be predictive of increased risk for CAD in apparently healthy men and women. Many current data suggest that lipoproteins or their derivatives (e.g., oxidized lipoproteins) contribute to nascent inflammation in atherosclerotic plaques. Other potential inciting stimuli may include infectious agents and autoantigens such as heat shock proteins, among other possible activators of T cells. The activated T cell secretes interferon-γ (IFN-γ), which may impair collagen synthesis. Macrophages and smooth muscle cells activated by inflammatory mediators such as the cytokines can elaborate enzymes that weaken the connective tissue framework of the plaque's fibrous cap. Reduction of inflammation should render atherosclerotic plaques more stable. Many studies have shown that statins have anti-inflammatory properties, including inhibition

of leukocyte-endothelium interactions and the reduction of inflammatory cell numbers within atherosclerotic plaques. Diomede and associates found that short-term lovastatin treatment was associated with a reduction in leukocyte recruitment due to an inhibition of interleukin-6 (IL-6), monocyte chemoattractant protein-1 (MCP-1), and the cytokine RANTES (meaning regulated upon activation, normal T-cell expressed and secreted). In addition, statins are able to reduce the expression of adhesion molecules, such as intercellular adhesion molecule-1 (ICAM-1), which are involved in the recruitment of circulating monocytes. Weitz-Schmidt and colleagues have shown that statins can inhibit the interaction between β_2-integrin leukocyte function antigen-1 (LFA-1) and ICAM-1. Reduced expression of the adhesion molecule P-selectin may also account for the inhibition of leukocyte-endothelial interactions by statins. Furthermore, several studies suggest that statins effectively lower plasma CRP levels in hyperlipidemic patients. It is therefore important to conduct further prospective clinical studies to fully elucidate the predictive value of inflammatory markers such as CRP.

Atherosclerosis and Thrombosis

The prothrombotic factors that have been evaluated include tissue factor expression, platelet aggregation, fibrinogen, plasma viscosity, and fibrinolytic factors. Tissue factor and corresponding messenger RNA have been localized in macrophages of human atherosclerotic plaque. Lipophilic statins (i.e., fluvastatin and simvastatin) suppress tissue factor expression by cultured human macrophages through inhibition of a geranylgeranylated protein involved in tissue factor biosynthesis.

Plaque Stabilization Strategies

Prevention of the rupture of atherosclerotic plaques is a critical step in the prevention of atherosclerotic complications (Fig. 22-3). Metalloproteinases are enzymes secreted by macrophages that are centrally involved in plaque rupture, and their inhibition could stabilize plaques and thereby prevent acute coronary events (Table 22-1). The prevention of thrombosis in disrupted plaques is another important objective. Although aspirin is a valuable antiplatelet agent, and heparin and warfarin are effective anticoagulants, they will be greatly improved upon. Platelet glycoprotein (Gp)IIb/IIIa–receptor blockers, tissue factor inhibitors, and antithrombins are all potentially more potent than the available drugs, and may also prove to be more effective in reducing the incidence of coronary events. Intravenously administered GpIIb/IIIa–receptor blockers reduce the incidence of acute coronary events in patients undergoing percutaneous catheter-based revascularization. The antithrombin bivalirudin has recently been shown to be as effective as GpIIb/IIIa inhibitors, with a reduced incidence of bleeding complications.

The presence of severe stenoses may merely serve as a marker for the presence of angiographically modest or even inapparent non–critically stenotic plaques that are actually more prone to precipitate acute myocardial infarction. The integrity of the fibrous cap overlying this lipid-rich core fundamentally determines the stability of an atherosclerotic plaque. Rupture-prone plaques tend to have thin, friable fibrous caps. Plaques not liable to precipitate events tend to have thicker fibrous caps that protect the blood compartment in the arterial lumen from potentially disastrous contact with the underlying thrombogenic lipid core (Fig. 22-4). Reductions in clinical events that have been observed without substantial change in the degree of luminal stenosis could reflect a stabilization of non-critically stenotic lesions. Stabilization might result from reducing the inflammatory stimuli provided by modified lipoproteins that

DETERMINANTS OF PLAQUE VULNERABILITY

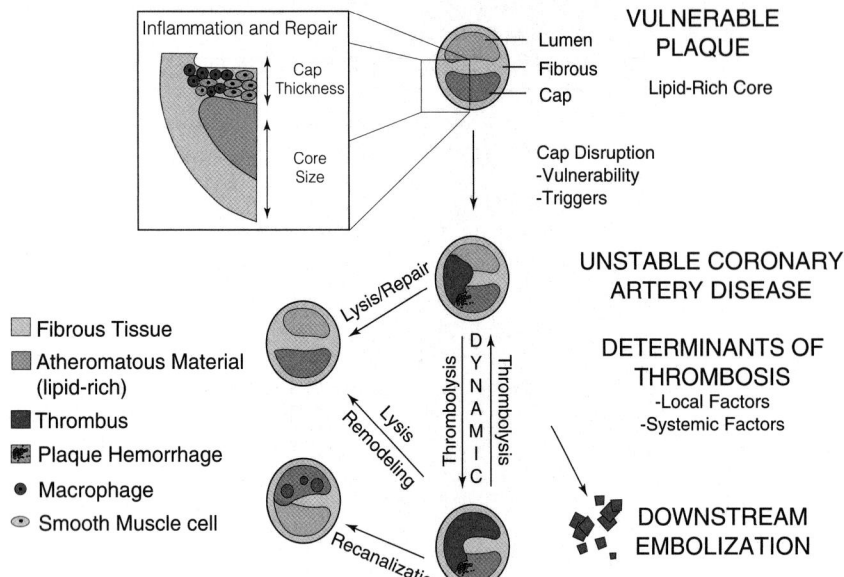

FIG. 22-3. Determinants of plaque vulnerability.

could contribute to activation of lesional foam cells and T lymphocytes. Consequently, strategies designed to stabilize plaque may be extremely important in reducing adverse clinical events in patients with PVD (Fig. 22-5).

CLINICAL MANIFESTATIONS OF VASCULAR DISEASE

Since the vascular system involves every organ system, the symptoms of vascular disease are as varied as those encountered in any medical specialty. Lack of adequate blood supply to target organs typically presents with pain; for example, calf pain with lower extremity claudication, postprandial abdominal pain from mesenteric ischemia, and arm pain with axillo-subclavian arterial occlusion. In contrast, stroke and transient ischemic attack (TIA) are the presenting symptoms from middle cerebral embolization as a consequence of a stenosed internal carotid artery. The pain syndrome of arterial disease is usually divided clinically into acute and chronic types, with all shades of severity between the two extremes. Sudden onset of pain can indicate complete occlusion of a critical vessel, leading

to more severe pain and critical ischemia in the target organ, resulting in lower limb gangrene or intestinal infarction. Chronic pain results from a slower, more progressive atherosclerotic occlusion, which can be totally or partially compensated by developing collateral vessels. Acute on chronic is another pain pattern in which a patient most likely has an underlying arterial stenosis that suddenly occludes; for example, the patient with a history of calf claudication who now presents with sudden, severe acute limb-threatening ischemia. The clinician should always try to understand and relate the clinical manifestations to the underlying pathologic process.

The Vascular History

Symptoms are elicited based on the presenting complaint (Table 22-2). The patient with lower extremity pain on ambulation has intermittent claudication that occurs in certain muscle groups; for example, calf pain upon exercise usually reflects superficial femoral artery disease, while pain in the buttocks reflects iliac disease. In most cases, the pain manifests in one muscle group below the level of the affected artery, occurs only with exercise, and is relieved with rest only to recur at the same location, hence the term

Table 22-1
Molecular Therapies for Vascular Disease

Pathologic Event	Therapeutic Target
Plaque rupture	Metalloproteinase inhibitors, leukoctye adhesion blockers
Thrombosis	GpIIa/IIIb–receptor blockers, tissue factor inhibitors, antithrombins
Endothelial dysfunction	Nitric oxide donors, antioxidants
Endothelial injury	VEGF, FGF
Dysregulated cell growth	Cell cycle inhibitors
Dysregulated apoptosis	Integrin antagonists
Matrix modification antagonists	Metalloproteinase inhibitors, plasmin

FGF = fibroblast growth factor, Gp = platelet glycoprotein, VEGF = vascular endothelial growth factor.

SOURCE: Reproduced with permission from Braunwald E: Shattuck lecture— cardiovascular medicine at the turn of the millennium: Triumphs, concerns, and opportunities. *N Engl J Med* 337:1360, 1997.

FACTORS CONTRIBUTING TO PLAQUE VULNERABILITY

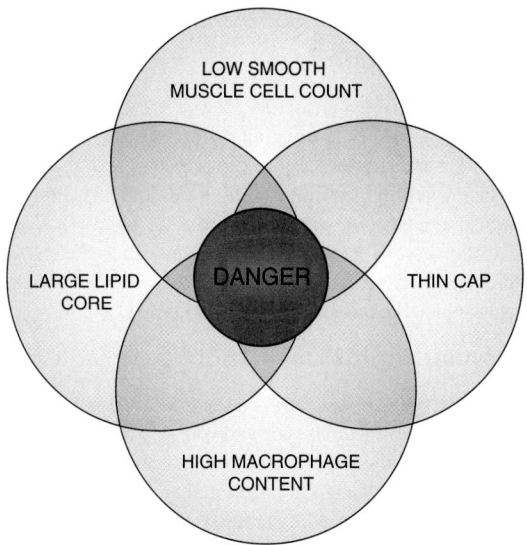

FIG. 22-4. *Factors contributing to plaque vulnerability.*

"window-gazers disease." Rest pain (a manifestation of severe underlying occlusive disease) is constant and occurs in the foot (not the muscle groups), typically at the metatarsophalangeal junction, and is relieved by dependency. Often the patient is prompted to sleep with their foot hanging off one side of the bed to increase the hydrostatic pressure.

The patient with carotid disease in most cases is totally asymptomatic, having been referred based on the finding of a cervical bruit or duplex finding of stenosis. Symptoms of carotid territory TIAs include transient monocular blindness (amaurosis), contralateral weakness or numbness, and dysphasia. Symptoms persisting longer than 24 hours constitute a stroke.

Chronic mesenteric ischemia presents with postprandial abdominal pain and weight loss. The patient fears eating because of the pain, avoids food, and loses weight. It is very unlikely that a patient with abdominal pain who has not lost weight has chronic mesenteric ischemia.

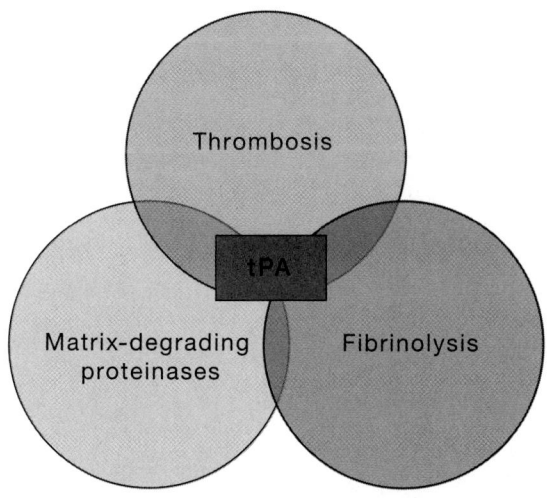

FIG. 22-5. *The fibrinolytic system and its inhibitors determine the stability of a thrombus formed at a site of plaque disruption.*

Table 22-2
Diagnosis and Patient History

Cardiovascular history
Relation between PVD, CAD, and cerebrovascular disease
TIAs, stroke
Angina, previous MI
Also determine history of:
Diabetes
Hypertension
Hyperlipidemia
Tobacco use

CAD = coronary artery disease; MI = myocardial infarction; PVD = peripheral vascular disease; TIA = transient ischemic attack.

Of particular importance in the previous medical history is noting prior vascular interventions (endovascular or open surgical), and all vascular patients should have inquiry made about their prior cardiac history and current cardiac symptoms. Approximately 30% of vascular patients will be diabetic. A smoking history should be elicited.

The Vascular Examination

Specific vascular examination includes pulse examination (femoral, popliteal, posterior tibial, and dorsalis pedis) of the lower extremity (Table 22-3). The femoral pulse is located at the midinguinal point (midway between the anterior superior iliac spine and the pubic tubercle). The popliteal artery is best palpated with the knee flexed to 45 degrees and the foot flat and supported on the examination table to relax the calf muscles. Palpation of the popliteal artery is a bimanual technique. Both thumbs are placed on the tibial tuberosity anteriorly and the fingers are placed into the popliteal fossa between the two heads of the gastrocnemius muscle. The popliteal artery is palpated by compressing it against the posterior aspect of the tibia just below the knee. The posterior tibial pulse is detected by palpation 2 cm posterior to the medial malleolus. The dorsalis pedis is detected 1 cm lateral to the hallucis longus extensor tendon (which dorsiflexes the great toe and is clearly visible) on the dorsum of the foot. Pulses are graded using a four-point scale: 2+ is normal; 1+ palpable, but reduced; 0 is absent to palpation (Doppler signals should be noted); and 3+ indicates aneurysmal enlargement. The foot should be carefully examined for pallor on elevation and rubor on dependency, as these findings are indicative of chronic ischemia. Ulceration and other findings specific to disease states are described in relevant sections below.

Upper extremity examination is necessary when an arteriovenous graft is to be inserted in patients who have symptoms of arm pain with exercise. Thoracic outlet syndrome (TOS) can result in occlusion or aneurysm formation of the subclavian artery. Distal embolization is a manifestation of TOS; consequently, the fingers should be examined for signs of ischemia and ulceration. The axillary artery enters the limb below the middle of the clavicle, where it can be palpated in thin patients. It is usually easily palpable in the axilla and medial upper arm. The brachial artery is most easily located at the antecubital fossa immediately medial to the biceps

Table 22-3
Lower Extremity Examination

Check pulses
Listen for bruits
Determine ankle-brachial index (ABI)
Evaluate color and skin nutrition
Compare lower extremities

tendon. The radial artery is palpable at the wrist anterior to the radius. The ulnar is palpable or present on Doppler examination on the medial side of the wrist. Doppler signals, particularly in the thumb, are usually detectable on either side of the digits. Digital Doppler signals also frequently can be detected in the fingers. The Allen test is a test of patency of the palmar arch. The radial and ulnar pulses are localized at the wrist, and the examiner occludes both by digital pressure. Then after the patient opens and closes the hand, pressure over one artery is released. Failure in hand reperfusion from one side indicates an incomplete palmar arch and indicates that occlusion of one artery (by catheter placement or by using it for an anastomosis) may be more likely to result in hand ischemia.

There is increasing interest in the use of the ankle-brachial index (ABI) to evaluate patients at risk for cardiovascular events. An ABI less than 0.9 correlates with increased risk of myocardial infarction and indicates significant, although perhaps asymptomatic, underlying peripheral vascular disease. The ankle-brachial index is determined in the following ways. Blood pressure is measured in both upper extremities using the highest systolic BP as the denominator for the ABI. The ankle pressure is determined by placing a blood pressure cuff above the ankle and measuring the return to flow of the posterior tibial and dorsalis pedis arteries using a pencil Doppler over each artery. The ratio of the systolic pressure in each vessel divided by the highest arm systolic pressure can be used to express the ABI in both the posterior tibial and dorsalis pedis arteries. Normal is more than 1. Claudicants are in the 0.6 to 0.9 range, with rest pain and gangrene occurring at less than 0.3. The test is less reliable in patients with heavily calcified vessels due to noncompressibility (i.e., diabetes and end-stage renal disease).

Aortic Examination

The abdomen should be palpated for an abdominal aortic aneurysm, detected as an expansile pulse above the level of the umbilicus. It should also be examined for the presence of bruits. Because the aorta typically divides at the level of the umbilicus, an aortic aneurysm is most frequently palpable in the epigastrium. In thin individuals a normal aortic pulsation is palpable, while in obese patients even large aortic aneurysms may not be detectable. Suspicion of a clinically enlarged aorta should lead to the performance of an ultrasound scan for a more accurate definition of aortic diameter.

Carotid Examination

The carotids should be auscultated for the presence of bruits, although there is a higher correlation with coronary artery disease than underlying carotid stenosis. A bruit at the angle of the mandible is a significant finding, leading to follow-up duplex scanning. The differential diagnosis is a transmitted murmur from a sclerotic or stenotic aortic valve. The carotid is palpable deep to the sternocleidomastoid muscle in the neck. Palpation, however, should be gentle and rarely yields clinically useful information.

The Vascular Graft Examination

After reconstructive vascular surgery, the graft may be available for examination, depending on its type and course. The in situ lower extremity graft runs in the subcutaneous fat and can be palpated along most of its length. A change in pulse quality, aneurysmal enlargement, or a new bruit should be carefully noted and may represent development of stenoses or aneurysmal enlargement. Axillofemoral grafts, femoral-to-femoral grafts, and arteriovenous access grafts can usually be easily palpated as well.

The Noninvasive Vascular Laboratory and Vascular Testing

The noninvasive vascular laboratory is under the supervision of vascular surgeons in most institutions, and appropriate use of noninvasive tests is important in the evaluation of the vascular patient.

Duplex Scanning

Duplex implies two forms of ultrasound: B-mode, which is typically used to create a gray-scale anatomic image, and Doppler ultrasound (Fig. 22-6). The latter allows moving structures to be imaged. Most physicians use the traditional pencil Doppler to detect nonpalpable blood vessels by sound. The more sophisticated duplex scanners display moving structures (in most cases red blood cells

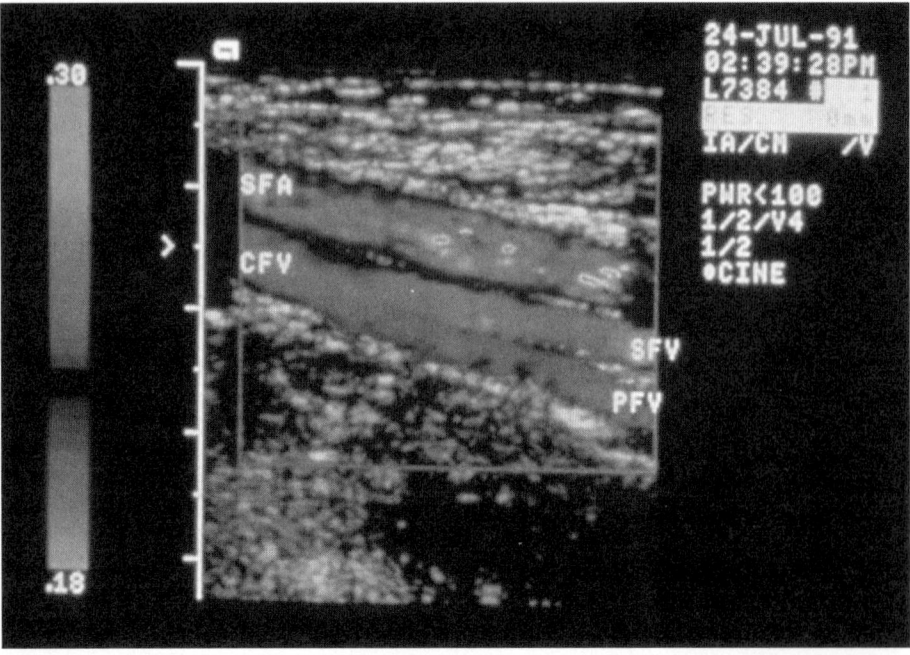

FIG. 22-6. Components of duplex ultrasound. It combines Doppler ultrasound and B-mode ultrasound. Color assignment to the Doppler shift permits real-time encoding of the Doppler flow signals as a color map, allowing direct visualization of flow within the vessels.

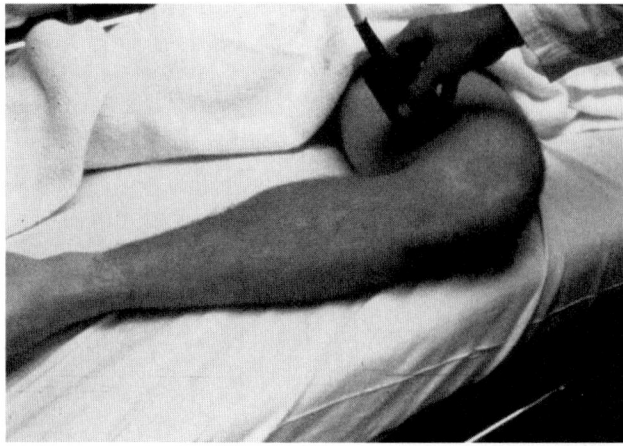

FIG. 22-7. Examining a femoral popliteal bypass graft.

moving within a vascular structure) as a color map proportional to the flow velocity and as an auditory signal. Furthermore, the scanner permits an accurate graphical depiction of the velocity of the moving red blood cells, and this permits measurement of peak systolic velocity and end-diastolic velocity. It is the measurement of the end-diastolic flow velocity that is used to determine the degree of narrowing of a carotid artery. The concept is somewhat like pinching a garden hose to accelerate the velocity of the water across the yard; the more it is pinched the greater the velocity. Velocity therefore is proportional to the degree of narrowing of the vessel under investigation.

Duplex scanning has become the first-line tool for imaging carotid arteries, lower extremity bypass grafts (Fig. 22-7), the abdominal aorta, and for diagnosis of deep venous thrombosis. A proper vascular laboratory is recognized by its Intersocietal Commission for Accreditation of Vascular Laboratories (ICAVL) accreditation and has technicians that are registered vascular technologist (RVT)-certified.

Although surgeons largely depend upon flow velocities in the arterial system, they rely even more on the anatomic appearance of the vessel when examining for thrombosis in the venous system. An occluded vein typically is larger than normal, not completely compressible, lacks respiratory variation, does not show flow augmentation with calf compression, and may have collateral flow.

Although duplex scanning has largely been performed in dedicated vascular laboratories, the advent of significantly less expensive portable scanners (Fig. 22-8) has led to the increased use of imaging in the vascular surgeon's office for diagnosis of pseudoaneurysms, mapping of veins for arteriovenous fistulas, and evaluation of patency of lower extremity bypass grafts. In the operating room, duplex scanning is helpful in image-guided venous access and completion ultrasound scanning. Competence in this type of imaging by the vascular surgeon will be increasingly necessary. Duplex arterial mapping of the lower extremity also is being used increasingly as an alternative to angiography.

Segmental Pressures

By placing serial blood pressure cuffs down the lower extremity and then measuring the pressure with a Doppler probe as flow returns to the artery below the cuff, it is possible to determine segmental pressures down the leg. This data can then be used to infer the level of the occlusion. The systolic pressure at each level is expressed as a ratio, with the highest systolic pressure in the upper extremities

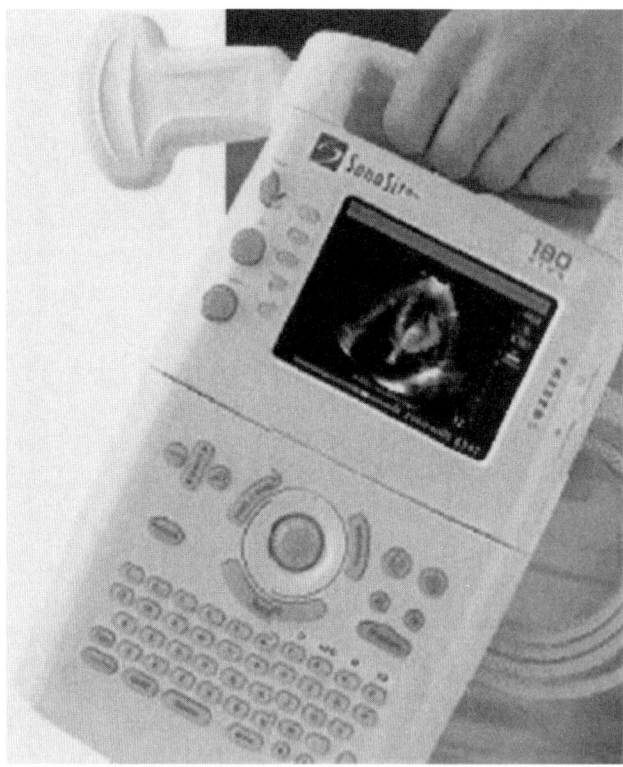

FIG. 22-8. Portable Duplex ultrasound will bring direct vascular imaging to the bedside.

as the denominator. A pressure gradient of 20 mm Hg between two subsequent levels is usually indicative of occlusive disease at that level. The most frequently used index is the ratio of the ankle pressure to the brachial pressure, the ABI. Normally the ABI is greater than 1.0, and a value less than 0.9 indicates some degree of arterial obstruction (Fig. 22-9) and has been shown to be correlated with an increased risk of coronary heart disease. Patients with claudication typically have an ABI in the 0.5 to 0.7 range, and those with rest pain are in the 0.3 to 0.5 range. Those with gangrene have an ABI less than 0.3. However, these ranges can vary depending on the degree of compressibility of the vessel. Patients with diabetes and end-stage renal disease have calcified vessels which are difficult to compress, rendering methods that depend on the detection of return to flow inaccurate, frequently showing falsely elevated pressure readings. This is usually noted on the report as a noncompressible vessel.

DIAGNOSIS - PHYSICAL EXAMINATION

ANKLE-BRACHIAL INDEX (ABI)
=
$$\frac{\text{Ankle Systolic Pressure}}{\text{Highest Brachial Systolic Pressure}}$$

≥ 1 = normal
> .5 to < 1 moderate disease
< .5 = severe disease

FIG. 22-9. Calculating the ankle-brachial index.

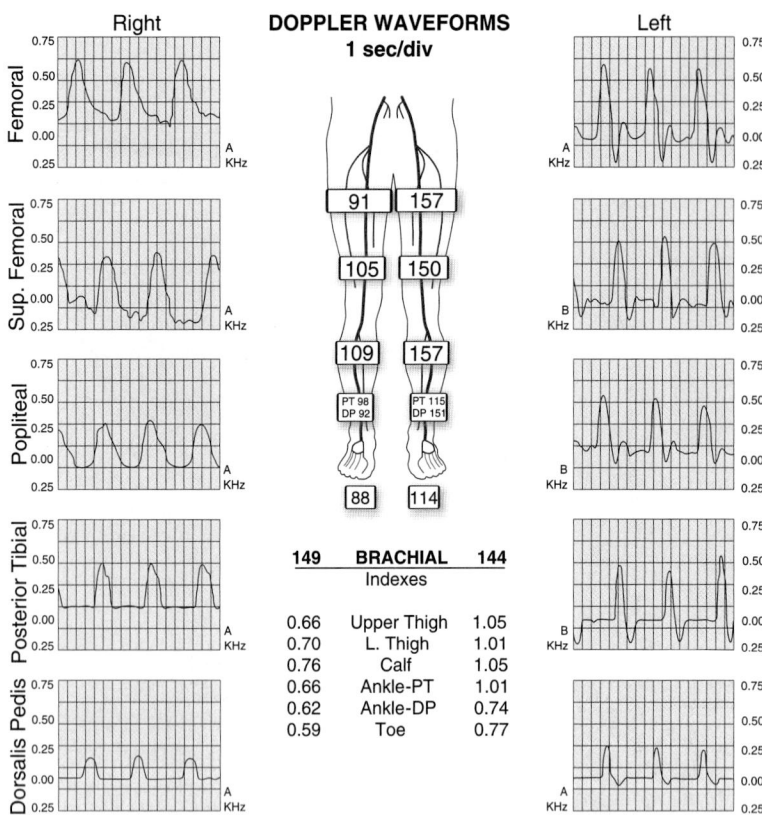

FIG. 22-10. Typical report of peripheral vascular resistance and segmental pressures.

Absolute pressures also can be measured, such as an ankle pressure of less than 50 mm Hg, which is indicative of critical limb ischemia.

In those patients with noncompressible vessels, segmental plethysmography can be useful. Cuffs placed at different levels on the leg detect changes in leg volume, which also can be used to localize levels of occlusion (Fig. 22-10).

Angiography

Diagnostic angiography has represented the gold standard in vascular imaging prior to an intervention. In many centers its use is rapidly decreasing due to the development of noninvasive imaging modalities such as duplex arterial mapping, computed tomographic angiography (CTA), and magnetic resonance angiography (MRA); nevertheless contrast angiography remains in widespread use today. The essential components to angiography are vascular access and catheter placement in the vascular bed to be imaged. The imaging system and the contrast agent are used to opacify the target vessel. Although in the past this function has largely been delegated to the interventional radiology service, an increasing number of surgeons are regaining this role and tying the imaging to immediate intervention.

The preangiography checklist includes serum creatinine; medications such as anticoagulants and oral hypoglycemics, specifically metformin (which can cause lactic acidosis when combined with contrast agents); history of dye allergy; and hydration status. Contrast angiography should be avoided if possible in all patients with a serum creatinine level greater than 3.0. It should be performed only if it is truly necessary, and other imaging modalities cannot provide equivalent information in patients with a serum creatinine level greater than 2.0. All patients with a serum creatinine level greater than 1.7 mg/dL are premedicated with acetylcysteine 600 mg by mouth twice daily on the day before and the day of angiography.

Many patients give a history of dye allergy, which may vary from trivial to life-threatening. In those with a history of anaphylaxis, contrast is best avoided. However, most patients can be safely given contrast after appropriate preparation. The usual prophylactic treatment is oral prednisone 40 mg 12 hours and 1 hour prior to the procedure, and oral diphenhydramine hydrochloride 50 mg 1 hour prior to the procedure.

For angiography, the right femoral artery is most commonly accessed. The puncture should be over the femoral head and its position should be determined fluoroscopically (not estimated using skin landmarks). The artery is entered with an 18-gauge Seldinger needle. Good pulsatile flow confirms arterial access. A Bentsen wire is then inserted up into the aorta under fluoroscopic guidance. After removing the needle, a catheter is inserted over the wire. The catheter and wire can be steered to the target vascular bed and dye injected to opacify the vessels. Contrast angiography provides a lumenogram, so thrombus-filled aneurysms can be easily missed. Digital subtraction angiography (where bony landmarks are electronically removed) provides the best delineation of vascular pathology. Once the procedure is complete, the catheter is removed from the femoral artery and pressure applied. This technique forms the basis for all interventional procedures.

There are numerous potential complications from angiography, some general and some specific to the vascular bed being studied. Access site complications are among the most common. Table 22-4 shows the acceptable rates of complications. Dye allergy (secondary to iodine content) is relatively common, but is extremely variable in its severity. Itching and skin rash are the more common manifestations; however, facial and laryngeal edema, bronchospasm, and cardiovascular collapse can occur. Nausea at the time of dye injection is relatively common and does not represent allergy. Patients at increased risk of dye allergy include those with multiple other

Table 22-4
Complications of Angiography[a]

Complication	Threshold (%)
Hematoma	3
Occlusion	0.5
Pseudoaneurysm	0.5
Arteriovenous fistula	0.1
Catheter-induced complications	
Arterial dissection	2
Subintimal injection	1
Cerebral arteriography	
All neurologic complications	4
Permanent neurologic complications	1
Contrast reactions	
All reactions	3
Major reactions	0.5
Contrast-induced renal failure	10

[a]Society of Cardiovascular & Interventional Radiology recommendations.

allergies, asthma, and those with known iodine allergy. With appropriate preintervention preparation (steroids and antihistamines), most patients with dye allergy can safely receive intravenous contrast. Exacerbation of chronic renal insufficiency, and on occasion precipitation of acute renal failure, can occur (contrast-mediated nephropathy). Those at increased risk are diabetics, dehydrated patients, and patients with renal insufficiency. Pretreatment with acetylcysteine or the dopa-1 agonist fenoldopam may be partially protective.

Modern contrast agents are low in osmolality (600 to 900 mOsm), compared with up to 2000 mOsm in the agents used in the past. The low-osmolar agents are associated with less pain during injection and may be associated with a reduced incidence of minor allergic reactions.

Other mechanical complications can occur from angiography, or more commonly with interventions such as angioplasty and stenting. The latter requires a larger-profile sheath in the femoral artery. Local complications include groin hematoma, pseudoaneurysm, and traumatic arteriovenous fistula. Catheters can enter the wall of an artery, producing dissection, rupture, or thrombosis. One of the most dangerous complications is retroperitoneal hematoma, in which blood leaking from the puncture site tracks superiorly into the retroperitoneum. Frequently the groin examination is totally normal, and the patient presents with hypotension. Diagnosis is established by CT scan, and the hole in the femoral or external iliac artery should be surgically repaired.

Brachial artery access is another option, but carries a significantly higher incidence of complications, mainly thrombosis and median nerve compression, and potential damage from extravasation.

Site-specific complications include stroke from arch angiography or selective carotid angiography. Distal embolization can occur from extensive catheter manipulation in a severely diseased vessel, particularly the aorta. This can result in renal failure, mesenteric infarction, and digit or limb loss.

Postcatheterization groin pseudoaneurysms present with local tenderness, swelling, and the presence of a tender pulsatile mass. The diagnosis is confirmed with ultrasound scanning. Treatment depends on the size of the pseudoaneurysm and whether the patient is anticoagulated. Spontaneous resolution is less likely if the patient is anticoagulated. Treatment has evolved from surgical repair of all pseudoaneurysms, through ultrasound-guided compression to the current standard therapy, which is ultrasound-guided thrombin injection. Surgical repair is reserved for those who fail injection or

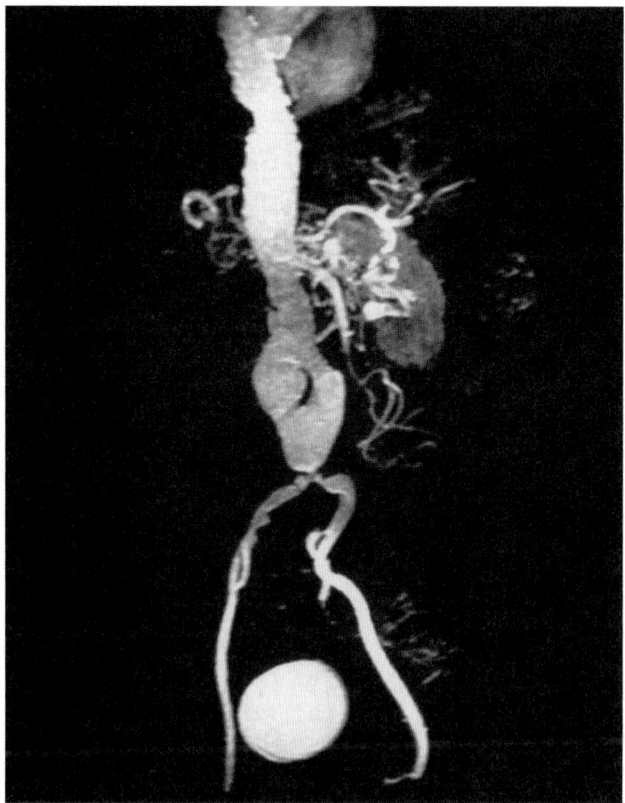

FIG. 22-11. Computed tomographic angiography (CTA) scan showing aortic aneurysm with dissection.

have a contraindication to thrombin injection such as wide neck, inability to compress the neck, or presence of an arteriovenous fistula.

Computed Tomographic Angiography

CTA is a noninvasive, contrast-dependent method for imaging the arterial system. It depends on intravenous infusion of iodine-based contrast agents. The patient is advanced through a rotating gantry, which images serial transverse slices. The contrast-filled vessels can be extracted from the slices and rendered in three-dimensional format (Fig. 22-11). The extracted image can be rotated and viewed from several different directions. This technology has been advanced as a consequence of aortic endografting. CTA provides images for postprocessing that can be used to display the aneurysm in a format that demonstrates thrombus, calcium, lumen, and the outer wall, and allows "fitting" of a proposed endograft into the aneurysm (Fig. 22-12). CTA is increasingly being used for imaging the carotid bifurcation, and as computing power increases, the speed of image acquisition and image resolution will continue to increase.

Magnetic Resonance Angiography

MRA has the advantage of not requiring iodinated contrast agents to provide vessel opacification (Fig. 22-13). Gadolinium is used as a contrast agent for MRA studies, and as it is generally not nephrotoxic, it can be used in patients with elevated creatinine. As with other MR tests, it is contraindicated in patients with pacemakers, severe claustrophobia, and most metallic foreign bodies. MRA tests are, however, relatively slow and very expensive. Like CTA, MRA is being increasingly used for imaging of the lower extremity vasculature, the carotid bifurcation, and the aorta and its branches.

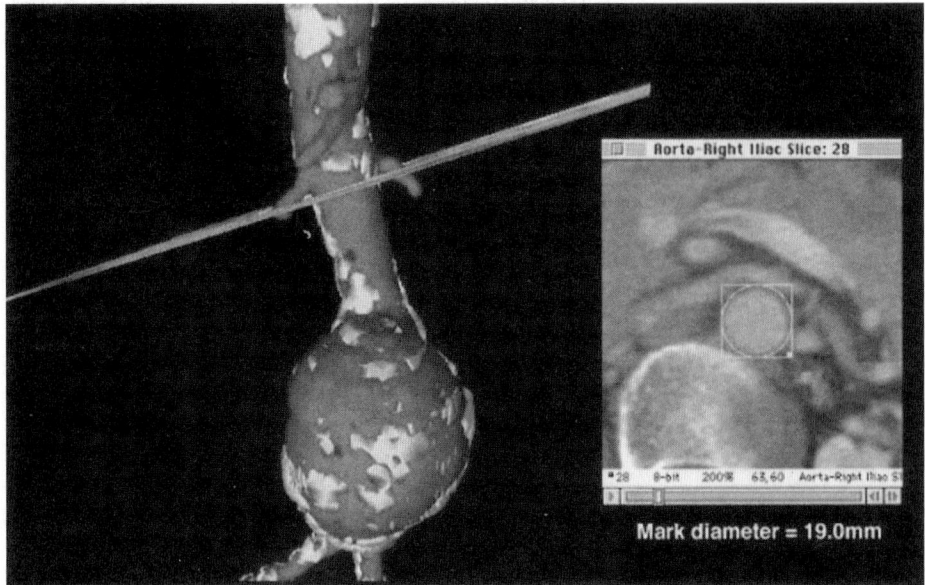

Mark diameter = 19.0mm

FIG. 22-12. Three-dimensional color reconstruction of computed tomographic angiography (CTA) scan.

Medical Management of the Vascular Patient

The presence of atherosclerotic peripheral arterial disease immediately places the patient in a very high-risk category for future major cardiovascular outcome events (MACE), and this has important implications for patients by reducing their life expectancy and increasing perioperative risk. The vascular specialist must understand how to appropriately manage risk factors for atherosclerosis and stratify risk in patients prior to planned intervention.

MEDICAL MANAGEMENT OF PERIPHERAL ARTERIAL DISEASE

Risk factors for peripheral arterial disease (PAD) are similar to those for coronary and cerebrovascular disease, but some factors appear to be even stronger for peripheral disease. Risk factors strongly linked to peripheral vascular disease include smoking, diabetes, elevated triglycerides, hyperhomocysteinemia, and low HDL cholesterol.[28] Although a positive family history has been definitely linked with coronary heart disease and stroke, it has not been confirmed as a significant risk factor for PAD.

The presence of PAD can most accurately be determined by measurement of the ankle-brachial index. An ABI of less than 0.9 is considered to be diagnostic of PAD and is associated with a 50% or greater risk for vessel stenosis. The majority of patients with peripheral arterial disease are asymptomatic. For every patient with intermittent claudication it is thought that there are three asymptomatic patients with significant disease. People at high risk for vascular disease should be screened with ABIs, because it is beneficial to intervene with medical management at an early stage. Those found to have a low ABI (less than 0.9) should be aggressively treated for atherosclerotic disease, even if they are asymptomatic. The goal of treatment is to prevent progression of peripheral vascular disease, reduce the risk of major atherosclerosis events elsewhere, and improve function in symptomatic patients. The risk of critical limb ischemia in patients with claudication is relatively low, about 1% per year, but the risk of death from coronary and cerebrovascular events is much higher, about 5 to 10% per year. The majority of patients can be treated medically, and even for those in whom surgical intervention is necessary, long-term outcome is significantly improved with maximal medical management. The cornerstone of medical management is reduction of vascular risk factors such as smoking cessation, control of blood pressure, reduction of blood lipid levels including statin therapy, correction of elevated homocysteine levels, and tight control of blood sugar in diabetics.

The relationship between smoking and PAD has been recognized since 1911, when it was reported that intermittent claudication was three times more common among smokers than nonsmokers. It has been suggested that the association between smoking and PAD may be even stronger than that between smoking and coronary artery disease. In the Framingham study, the risk at all ages for smokers was almost double for PAD compared with CAD. The severity of PAD tends to increase with the number of cigarettes smoked per day.

Smoking cessation is by far the most important factor in determining the outcome of patients with claudication. Nicotine replacement has been shown to double the success rate in the cigarette addict. Bupropion has similar efficacy when combined with supportive follow-up. Smoking cessation has been shown to result in a reduction of the 10-year mortality rate from 54 to 18%. In one clinical trial, at seven years 16% of smokers compared to 0% of quitters had progressed to rest pain. Alternative therapies such as hypnotherapy, acupuncture, or "aversive smoking" have not been proven to be beneficial.

It has been well established that the treatment of hypertension reduces the risk of stroke and coronary events. However, lowering of blood pressure may worsen intermittent claudication. Hypertension may delay the onset of symptoms of intermittent claudication in patients with PAD by elevating the central perfusion pressure; it is not uncommon for hypertensive patients to develop claudication when high blood pressure is discovered and treated. Hypertension is probably both a cause and an effect of atherosclerosis.

Although beta blockers have been thought to be particularly culpable as agents that aggravate claudication, there is no evidence to support that they are any worse than other agents. Angiotensin-converting enzyme (ACE) inhibitors have been shown to reduce cardiovascular morbidity and mortality in patients with PAD by 25%, regardless of the presence or absence of hypertension. Most patients with PAD would most likely benefit from therapy with an ACE inhibitor provided they do not have renal artery stenosis. Recent work

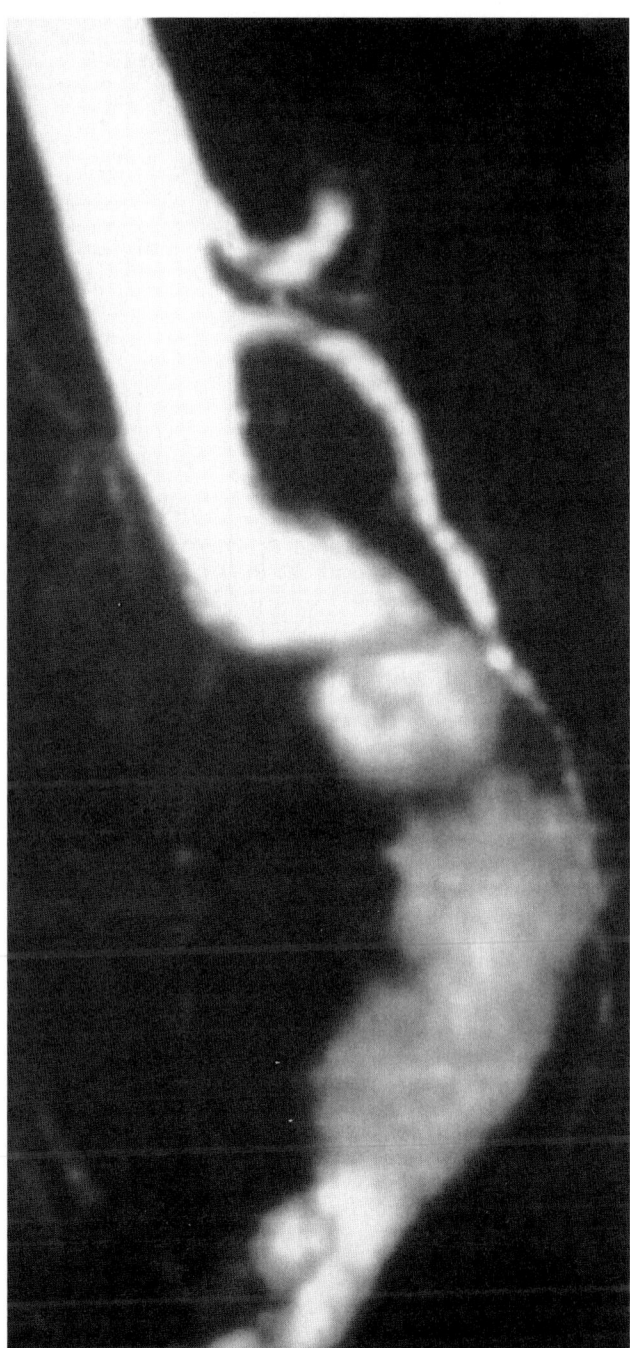

FIG. 22-13. *Magnetic resonance angiogram (MRA) of aorta. The advantage is the ability to examine the vessel in three dimensions, permitting in this case the origins of the celiac and superior mesenteric arteries to be viewed.*

showing an improvement in vessel wall function in patients on ACE inhibitors supports the idea that they could possibly improve symptoms of claudication.

Multiple studies have proven that lowering total cholesterol and LDL levels reduces mortality and morbidity in patients with PAD, regardless of their baseline cholesterol or LDL levels. There is good evidence that treatment of hyperlipidemia reduces both the progression of PAD and the incidence of intermittent claudication. Reduction of total cholesterol and LDL levels by 25% reduces mortality and morbidity by a corresponding 25%. This improvement is independent of age, sex, and baseline lipid levels. All patients with peripheral vascular disease should be on statin therapy, including those with normal baseline cholesterol levels. Patients with vascular disease should also be evaluated for other lipoprotein and metabolic abnormalities, such as elevated triglycerides, low HDL, high lipoprotein (a) [Lp(a)], and elevated homocysteine or complement levels that would indicate the need for additional medical therapy. An association between PAD and hypertriglyceridemia has been reported, but the strength of this association is unclear. Recently, it has been shown that Lp(a) is a significant independent risk factor for PAD.

Statin therapy is effective in the treatment of elevated LDL cholesterol, but has little effect on HDL, triglycerides, or Lp(a). Fibrates effectively lower triglycerides and raise HDL cholesterol. Niacin therapy has beneficial effects on all lipid parameters and is the only drug known to lower Lp(a). It is also the most effective agent for elevating HDL cholesterol. Slow-release niacin has increased tolerability and compliance and is emerging as an important therapy in patients with dyslipidemia.

Hyperhomocysteinemia

The incidence of hyperhomocysteinemia is as high as 60% in patients with vascular disease, compared with 1% in the general population. It has been reported that hyperhomocysteinemia was detected in 28 to 30% of patients with premature PAD. Hyperhomocysteinemia has been established as an independent risk factor for atherosclerosis by several studies. It may be a stronger risk factor for PAD than for CAD. A meta-analysis of studies concluded that the odds ratios for CAD were 1.6 and 1.8 in men and women, respectively, compared with 6.8 for patients with PAD. Elevated homocysteine levels can be treated with folic acid supplementation of 0.5 to 1.0 mg/d.

Diabetes Mellitus and Impaired Glucose Tolerance

Many studies have shown an association between diabetes mellitus and the development of vascular disease. Overall, intermittent claudication seems to be about twice as prevalent among patients with diabetes. PAD in diabetics is more aggressive, with early large vessel involvement coupled with microangiopathy. The risk of developing sudden ischemia and amputation is significantly higher in these patients. People with vascular disease should be screened carefully for diabetes. Accepting a fasting glucose of less than or equal to 126 mg/dL as normal will miss up to 20 to 30% of mild cases. Testing hemoglobin A_{1c} (Hgb A_{1c}) levels may help to prevent patients with mild glucose intolerance from being overlooked. Aggressive control of hyperglycemia in both type 1 and type 2 diabetics is associated with slowing the progression of atherosclerotic disease, and has been confirmed with studies on changes in the intima-media thickness of the carotid artery. Over the last decade, the importance and prevalence of the metabolic syndrome, which is characterized by obesity, non–insulin-dependent diabetes mellitus, hyperinsulinemia, hyperlipidemia, hypertension, hyperuricemia, and cardiovascular disease has become evident. Recognition of patients with metabolic syndrome is important so that they may be treated.

Exercise Programs

Exercise also is an important component of the treatment of peripheral vascular disease. Patients should exercise regularly, and those with symptoms should be enrolled in an exercise rehabilitation program. Exercise has been shown to improve function, reduce symptoms, and possibly prolong survival. It can produce an increase in walking distance of up to 150%—a clinically meaningful improvement—and has been associated with a 24% reduction in cardiovascular mortality. Exercise programs that consist of exercise for more than 30 minutes and more frequently than three times per week are most effective. More improvement is evident after 26 weeks, with walking the best form of exercise for intermittent claudication.

Specific Medical Therapy for Claudication

Other medical therapies directed specifically at peripheral disease rather than its risk factors include pentoxifylline and cilostazol.

Pentoxifylline improves symptoms of claudication by increasing red blood cell flexibility and thereby improving capillary blood flow. It has been shown to produce modest increases in treadmill walking time compared to placebo, rendering its overall clinical benefits questionable.

Cilostazol inhibits platelet aggregation, increases vasodilation, inhibits smooth muscle proliferation (via inhibition of phosphodiesterase type 3), and lowers HDL cholesterol and triglyceride levels.[29] This drug has been more effective than pentoxifylline in the treatment of claudication at doses of 100 mg twice daily (Fig. 22-14). Cilostazol has been shown to significantly increase walking distance in patients with claudication in several randomized trials and to result in improvement in physical functioning and quality of life. Improvement has ranged from 35 to 100%. A trial of the drug is indicated in symptomatic patients. It should be continued for at least 3 months before a decision is made about efficacy. The most common adverse effects are headache, transient diarrhea, palpitations, and dizziness. It is contraindicated in patients with congestive heart failure because of its effects on phosphodiesterase.

Antiplatelet medications have been used in the treatment of peripheral vascular disease, and aspirin has been found to reduce the vascular death rate in patients with any manifestation of atherosclerotic disease by about 25%. It has been shown to be equally effective in patients who present with coronary disease or PAD. Clopidogrel

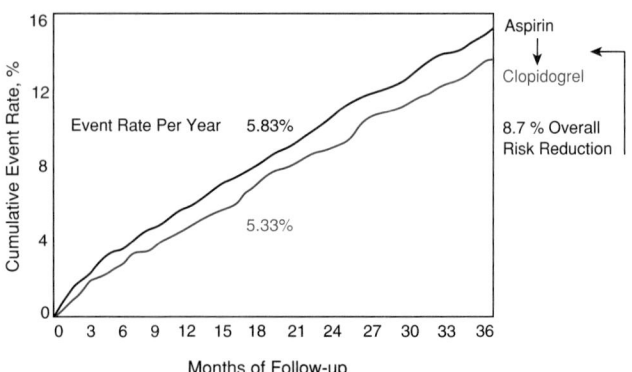

Efficacy of Clopidogrel Bisulfate in Primary Analysis of MI, Ischemic Stroke, or Vascular Death

FIG. 22-15. *CAPRIE Study. Efficacy of clopidogrel bisulfate in primary analysis of MI, ischemic stroke, or vascular death. Although the statistical significance favoring clopidogrel over aspirin was marginal ($p = 0.045$), and represents the result of a single trial that has not been replicated, the comparator drug, aspirin, is itself effective (vs. placebo) in reducing cardiovascular events in patients with recent MI or stroke. Thus, the difference between clopidogrel and placebo, although not measured directly, is substantial.*

is more effective than aspirin in reducing cardiovascular outcome events, especially in the patient with lower extremity occlusive disease, but is much more expensive and is usually reserved for patients who cannot tolerate aspirin (Fig. 22-15). There is no indication for clopidogrel and aspirin combination therapy.

Vasodilators have not been shown to be efficacious in the treatment of peripheral vascular disease and are not indicated. Anticoagulants also have not been shown to alter the course or symptoms of peripheral atherosclerosis.

Because of the systemic nature of atherosclerosis, all patients with PAD, whether they have a history of coronary disease or not, should benefit from medical prevention strategies. These include aggressive management of smoking, statin therapy with a goal of lowering LDL cholesterol to at least 100 mg/dL, treatment of blood pressure to attain 130/85 mm Hg, and management of diabetes mellitus to a glycohemoglobin level of 7%. Drugs shown to have particular benefit in these patients include the statins for LDL reduction, ACE inhibitors to treat blood pressure, and beta blockers for their cardioprotective effects. In addition, all patients should be given a trial of cilostazol, clopidogrel, or aspirin. Patients should also be investigated for other dyslipidemias and hyperhomocysteinemia and treated accordingly.

Risk Stratification for Intervention

Cardiac Evaluation in the Vascular Patient

Preoperative cardiac evaluation of vascular patients is imperative. Studies on the prevalence of CAD in patients with intermittent claudication have shown that history, clinical examination, and electrocardiography typically indicate the presence of CAD in 40 to 60% of these patients. However, in a study conducted at the Cleveland Clinic, in which all patients with intermittent claudication were studied with coronary angiography, only 10% had normal vessels and 28% had severe three-vessel disease, indicating an extremely high prevalence of coronary disease in patients with peripheral vascular

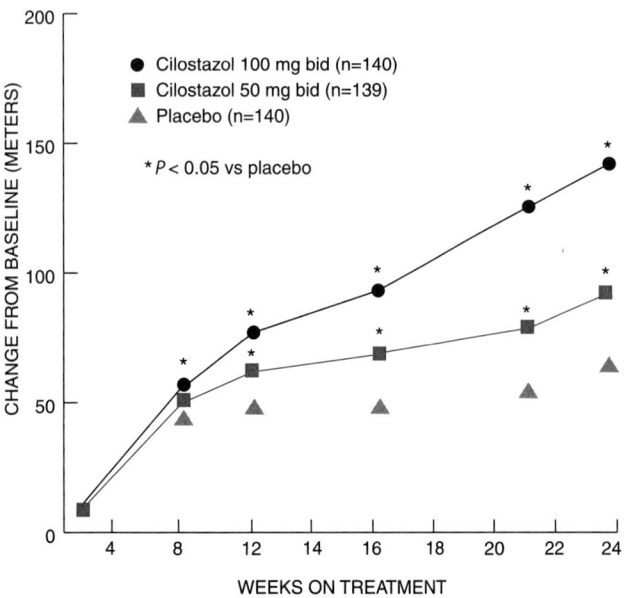

IMPROVEMENT IN MAXIMAL WALKING DISTANCE WITH CILOSTAZOL

- ● Cilostazol 100 mg bid (n=140)
- ■ Cilostazol 50 mg bid (n=139)
- ▲ Placebo (n=140)

* *P* < 0.05 vs placebo

FIG. 22-14. *Improvement in maximal walking distance with cilostazol. Improvements in both cilostazol-treated groups were significant at all time points compared with placebo.*

disease. Many of these patients may be asymptomatic, especially if exercise is severely limited by claudication.

Most perioperative cardiovascular complications occur in the early postoperative period, 1 to 4 days after surgery. The risk of intraoperative events is not much higher than during the preoperative period. Myocardial infarction (MI) is often asymptomatic in the immediate postoperative period. The pathogenesis of perioperative MI is unique. Unlike regular MI, perioperative MI is the result of an imbalance between coronary blood flow and myocardial oxygen demand in areas of coronary stenosis, and is therefore related to underlying coronary disease. The lack of cardiac reserve is exacerbated by adrenergic stimulation, rapid fluid shifts, hypotension, and other stresses of surgery. Perioperative MI is usually not secondary to plaque rupture and subsequent thrombosis, the most common etiology of MI outside of the perioperative period.

There have been multiple guidelines published for preoperative cardiac evaluation of surgical patients. One of the earliest set of guidelines, published in 1977, is commonly referred to as the Goldman criteria. The Goldman criteria are still frequently referenced in preoperative evaluations. Newer guidelines were published by the American College of Cardiology and the American Heart Association Task Force for noncardiac preoperative evaluation in 1996 and the American College of Physicians in 1997. The most recent guidelines were published by Lee and coworkers and are known as the Revised Cardiac Risk Index.[30] A recent Canadian study has shown the perioperative risk of cardiac complications to average 6.4% with application of the older guidelines and the Revised Cardiac Risk Index. However, the efficacy of the American College of Physicians and the American Heart Association Task Force guidelines has not been evaluated.

In the Guidelines for Preoperative Cardiac Evaluation published in 1996 by the American College of Cardiology and the American Heart Association (ACC/AHA) Task Force, noncardiac surgical procedures are stratified according to risk. Of the four high-risk procedures, two are vascular operations: aortic and other major vascular procedures, and peripheral vascular procedures. The other two are major emergency operations (especially in the elderly) and prolonged surgical procedures with large fluid shifts or blood loss.

According to these guidelines, evaluation of a patient for cardiac risk prior to surgery is accomplished by determining whether the patient is compromised by any of the major clinical predictors: unstable coronary syndromes, decompensated congestive heart failure, significant arrhythmias, or severe valvular disease. In the event that these problems are present, elective surgery should either be delayed until the problem can be treated and controlled or the patient should be thoroughly evaluated preoperatively, usually by coronary angiography. If none of the major clinical predictors are present, then evaluation for intermediate clinical predictors is sought including mild angina, prior MI, compensated or prior congestive heart failure, and diabetes.

In these patients the appropriate step is to determine their functional capacity. Functional capacity is measured in units called metabolic equivalents (METs) and can usually be determined by history. Strenuous sports such as swimming, skiing, and basketball are assigned a value of greater than 10 METs. Four METs is represented by activities such as golf, bowling, dancing, or climbing a flight of stairs. Activities of daily living such as grooming and preparing meals are considered to represent 1 to 4 METs. A patient is considered to have poor functional capacity if they are unable to perform activities requiring more than 4 METs. Poor functional capacity places the patient into a high-risk group, indicating the need for noninvasive testing for further evaluation such as a dobutamine

stress echo. Patients with a moderate or excellent functional capacity (greater than 4 METs) will need noninvasive testing only if undergoing a high-risk surgical procedure. All other patients with intermediate clinical predictors can proceed to surgery without further evaluation. Patients with planned low-risk procedures do not need further evaluation for intermediate clinical predictors, even if they have a low functional capacity.

Patients with a history of coronary disease and revascularization within the last 5 years who have remained asymptomatic can proceed to surgery without further evaluation. Patients with new symptoms or whose coronary surgery was done more than 5 years prior should have further evaluation based on their clinical predictors and the risk level of the planned procedure.

The most recent scheme of clinical assessment was written by Lee and colleagues and is known as the Revised Cardiac Risk Index.[30] Unlike the guidelines provided by the task force, it does not give advice on how to work up a patient preoperatively, it merely stratifies them into different risk groups and identifies six variables: high-risk surgical procedure, history of ischemic heart disease (excluding previous revascularization), history of heart failure, history of stroke or transient ischemic attack, preoperative insulin therapy, and preoperative serum creatinine level greater than 2 mg/dL. Patients are then stratified into risk levels based on the number of variables they have. After identifying these variables in over 2000 patients, they were applied in a different set of 1422 patients. This index has been studied and proven to have a significant predictive value (Table 22-5).[30]

Recently the paradigm of risk stratification has shifted from assessing risk by further testing to lowering risk with prophylactic medical therapy. Although much time and study has been put into refining methods to assess and stratify patient risk preoperatively, there is no good evidence that this practice has resulted in decreased morbidity and mortality. Recent studies have been unable to show that the pursuit of noninvasive cardiac imaging prior to surgery reduces the number of cardiac events or that further testing with cardiac catheterization improves outcomes. Regardless of the severity of the coronary disease, preoperative prophylactic coronary bypass or angioplasty does not decrease perioperative morbidity or mortality because of the inherent risk of bypass surgery or angioplasty and the delay and subsequent morbidity that results from postponing the originally planned procedure. Therefore, coronary bypass or angioplasty is not indicated as a prophylactic preoperative procedure unless it is indicated for clinical reasons independent of the planned noncardiac surgery. If bypass surgery is indicated by clinical symptoms, it should be done prior to the noncardiac surgery, not solely as preparation for that surgery.

Recent studies have produced compelling evidence that perioperative beta-blocker therapy reduces the risk of death and MI in association with noncardiac surgery. The perioperative use of beta blockers has been shown to reduce the incidence of ischemia and

Table 22-5
Major Cardiac Event Rates By the Revised Cardiac Risk Index

Class	Events/Patients	Event Rate	(95% CI, %)
I	(0 Risk factors)	0.4	(0.05–1.5)
II	(1 Risk factor)	0.9	(0.3–2.1)
III	(2 Risk factors)	6.6	(3.9–10.3)
IV	(3 Risk factors)	11.0	(5.8–18.4)

CI = confidence interval.

SOURCE: Adapted with permission from Lee et al.[30]

postoperative arrhythmia. Beta blockade reduces the incidence of perioperative cardiac complications in patients at low, intermediate, and high risk as defined by the Revised Cardiac Risk Index.[31] It is effective even in patients with inducible ischemia by dobutamine stress echo. Since recent studies have provided irrefutable evidence of the protective effects of beta blockade perioperatively, a strategy much simpler than that outlined by the ACC/AHA task force has been proposed based on the Revised Cardiac Risk Index. Patients with one to two risk variables should have beta blockade initiated perioperatively. If beta blockers are contraindicated, surgery can proceed without it since these patients are at relatively low risk. In patients with three or more risk variables, perioperative beta blockade is more strongly indicated. If beta blockade is contraindicated or the surgical risk seems excessive, canceling or deferring the surgery may be indicated. In those patients that are difficult to assess, dobutamine stress echo may be considered. If it is negative for ischemia, then the operative risk is low. A positive test confirms the importance of perioperative beta-adrenergic blocking agents and the fact that the patient is at higher risk. Unfortunately, patients with severe left ventricular systolic dysfunction were excluded from these studies, leaving no good data on how to handle these patients.

Other prophylactic medications such as intraoperative nitroglycerin have not been associated with an improved outcome. It is thought that intravenous nitroglycerin may result in excessive preload reduction when used in combination with anesthetic agents.

Preoperative Pulmonary Assessment

The risk of postoperative respiratory complications is increased by surgical procedures involving the thorax or upper abdomen, the presence of pre-existing pulmonary dysfunction, cigarette smoking, prolonged anesthesia, recent respiratory infection, chronic productive cough, and immunodeficiency syndrome. Preoperative interventions including smoking cessation, training in deep breathing techniques, control of infection, control of secretions, and weight loss have been shown to be beneficial. A preoperative FEV_1 (forced expiratory volume in 1 second) of less than 1 L is no longer a contraindication to surgery. Preoperative pulmonary function test results are useful only to direct pre- and postoperative care, not to determine surgical eligibility. However, preoperative pulmonary function testing has not been shown to improve perioperative management.

ANEURYSMAL DISEASE

An *aneurysm* is defined as a dilation of an artery greater than 1.5 times its normal diameter. They can occur in almost any artery in the body, but the most common locations are in the abdominal aorta, thoracic aorta, cerebral vessels, and iliac, popliteal, and femoral arteries. An aneurysmal artery can only contain the enclosed blood while the wall tension exceeds the distending pressure of the arterial blood. Rupture occurs when the tangential stress exceeds the tensile strength of the artery. The law of Laplace decrees that the tensile strength of the arterial wall is a function of the pressure multiplied by the radius. Consequently, larger aneurysms are more likely to rupture.

Classification of Aneurysms

Aneurysms are classified in a variety of ways based upon their shape, wall constituents, and etiology.

Shape

Fusiform, or spindle-shaped aneurysms, are the most commonly seen type in which the native vessel is diffusely dilated. However, *saccular aneurysms,* in which one wall is normal while the other is dilated, also occur.

Wall Constituents

True Aneurysms. In *true aneurysms,* the aneurysm wall is entirely composed of dilated arterial wall. This is in contrast to *pseudoaneurysms* or *false aneurysms* in which the aneurysm is composed partly of arterial wall and partly of adjacent structure such as the spine in eroding abdominal aortic aneurysms. Femoral anastomotic aneurysms are typical examples of pseudoaneurysms.

Etiology

Dissecting Aneurysm. Dissecting aneurysms occur when the vessel wall is split and the vessel enlarged. This most commonly affects the thoracic aorta. Initially the aorta may be of normal caliber, but the wall is weakened by the dissection and can undergo progressive enlargement.

Mycotic. The vessel wall is infected, and as a consequence of the ongoing inflammation undergoes progressive dilation. These aneurysms are rapidly progressive, surrounded by severe inflammation, and are challenging to reconstruct. Extra-anatomic bypass or reconstruction with autologous tissue covered by muscle flaps are frequently necessary.

Traumatic. Traumatic aneurysms can occur from any type of trauma. The most commonly encountered are from catheterization of the femoral artery, which fails to seal after the catheter is removed. This is a femoral pseudoaneurysm. Similar aneurysms can occur from blunt or penetrating trauma.

Abdominal Aortic Aneurysms

Natural History

Abdominal aortic aneurysms grow on average 0.4 cm/y. Risk of rupture is exponentially related to aneurysm diameter. Aneurysms 5.0 cm in diameter have an average yearly rupture rate of 3 to 5%[32–34] (Fig. 22-16). However, a 7-cm aneurysm carries a rupture rate of 19% per year. Szilagyi and colleagues demonstrated that repair of aneurysms greater than 6 cm prolonged patient survival, despite the fact that at that time a 14% operative mortality rate existed.[35]

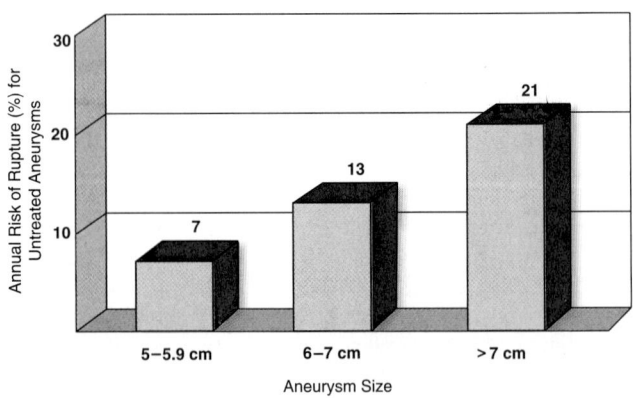

Rupture Risk of Untreated Aneurysms

FIG. 22-16. *Rupture risk of untreated aneurysms.*

Currently, with perioperative mortality rates of 3 to 5%, intervention is recommended for all aneurysms greater than 5 cm. Crawford reported a decline in the mortality rate from 19.2 to 1.9% over a 25-year period, despite increasingly complex repairs in higher-risk patients. Although an absolute measurement of aortic diameter was traditionally used to determine intervention, there is evidence from the UK Small Aneurysm Trial that women may rupture at smaller aneurysm diameters than men, suggesting that the ratio between native appropriate diameter and aneurysmal diameter may be more important.[36,37] Other factors that increase the risk of rupture are chronic obstructive pulmonary disease (COPD) and diastolic hypertension.

Epidemiology

Aneurysmal and occlusive disease of the abdominal aorta are significant problems for many older patients, and as the population of the United States ages, the prevalence of these diseases will likely increase (Fig. 22-17). Data from the U.S. Bureau of the Census indicate that 75 million people were born in the United States from 1946 to 1964. In 1990, 12.5% of the population, 31,079,000 people, were at least 65 years of age, including 10 million persons aged 75 to 84 years, and more than 3 million aged 85 years and older. Abdominal aortic aneurysms occur three times as frequently in males as in

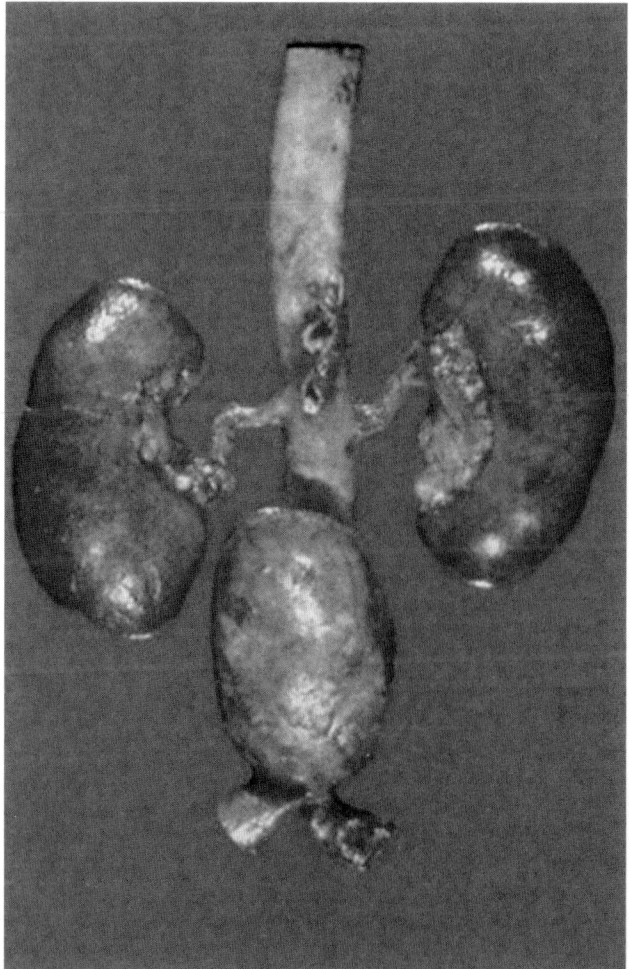

FIG. 22-17. Autopsy specimen of abdominal aortic aneurysm showing typical location below the renal arteries and extending to the aortic bifurcation. The presence of normal aorta below the renal arteries is a prerequisite for stent grafting.

females. On the basis of conservative estimates for birth, death, and immigration rates, by the year 2030, 20.1% of the U.S. population (70,175,000 people) will be aged at least 65 years, including more than 23 million people aged 75 to 84 years, and almost 9 million people aged 85 years and older. As the number of older individuals in the population continues to increase, physicians are faced with the need to acquire information to improve our ability to provide health care for geriatric patients.

History

The first successful excision of an abdominal aortic aneurysm was performed by Dubost in 1951, when he replaced the aneurysm with a human homograft. Shortly thereafter, DeBakey developed the Dacron graft, which arguably remains the gold standard to this date.[5] The most recent revolution in aortic surgery was initiated by Parodi when he developed the aortic endograft.[38] Currently the two competing approaches of open versus endograft repair are equally utilized.

Etiology and Pathology

Abdominal aortic aneurysms (AAA) are frequently referred to as atherosclerotic aneurysms, but it is clear that the etiology is more complex than simply being due to concurrent atherosclerosis. There is progressive loss of elastin in aortic aneurysms along with increased metalloprotease activity. Proteolysis and inflammation are the driving forces in AAA expansion. Normal aortic tissue contains 12% elastin, whereas aneurysmal tissue has only 1% elastin. There is a clear familial trend that is sex-linked and autosomally recessive. Presence of an aneurysm in a female usually is associated with aneurysms in family members. Estimated risk for first-degree relatives of affected family members is 11.6 times that of the rest of the population. Screening of siblings (over age 50) of patients with aneurysms revealed an aneurysm in 29% of brothers and 6% of sisters.

Smoking is a strong independent risk factor for AAA. Ninety percent of patients with AAA have reported a history of smoking, with risk directly correlated to quantity and duration of smoking.[54]

Clinical Manifestations

Symptoms. The vast majority of AAAs are completely asymptomatic, often being an incidental finding during evaluation of a concurrent condition. Occasionally, the calcified outer wall or a large soft tissue shadow is noted on a kidney, ureter, and bladder (KUB) radiograph (Fig. 22-18), or they are detected during performance of an ultrasound (Fig. 22-19) or CT scan (Figs. 22-20, 22-21, and 22-22) of the abdomen. Although rarely symptomatic, AAAs also present in myriad fashion. The most common symptoms are new-onset low-back pain and abdominal pain, which are occasionally due to compression/erosion of adjacent structures such as an aortocaval fistula, a ureteric obstruction, gastrointestinal (GI) bleeding from a primary aortoduodenal fistula, or rarely, they can be due to lower extremity embolization.

When aneurysms become symptomatic, they demand more expeditious evaluation and treatment. Pain arises from stretching of retroperitoneal tissues and is associated with increased risk of rupture.

Physical Examination. Inspection in a thin patient may show prominent epigastric/umbilical pulsatility. Careful palpation in all but obese patients usually reveals the expansile pulsatility of an AAA greater than 5 cm in diameter. In large patients it may be impossible to detect even large aneurysms. Most AAAs extend to

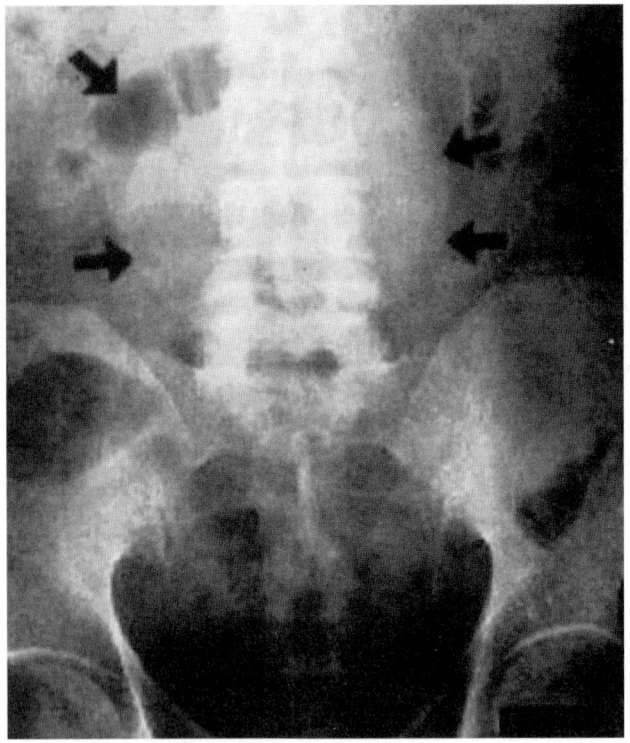

FIG. 22-18. Kidney, ureter, and bladder (KUB) radiograph showing a large soft tissue density, which is a large abdominal aortic aneurysm.

involve the common iliac arteries, which are occasionally of large diameter. This can lead to the finding of a pulsatile mass extending below the umbilicus. Part of the evaluation of AAAs includes careful evaluation of the femoral and distal pulses for several reasons:

(1) a concurrent femoral aneurysm may be evident and (2) a normal femoral pulse increases the likelihood for successful endografting. Distal pulses should be noted so that a change from baseline can be detected following AAA repair. Examination for carotid bruits should also be performed. Most surgeons will repair a high-grade carotid stenosis prior to an open AAA repair.

Testing. The extent of testing is dictated by aneurysm size. Risk of rupture, the driving force in treatment, is dictated by aneurysm diameter (see Fig. 22-16). As a general rule, aneurysms greater than 5 cm in diameter should be treated unless the patient has excessive comorbidities. However, the advent of aortic endografts has altered even this recommendation in that those with significant comorbidities can be safely treated if they are endograft candidates. For aneurysms in the 4.5- to 5-cm range, observation is reasonable, although recent expansion or high anxiety on the patient's part should lead to intervention. There are some recent data to suggest that smaller-diameter aneurysms in women should be treated.

Ultrasound scanning is the most cost-effective modality for following an aneurysm and typically should be performed on a yearly basis. As a preoperative scanning tool, CT scan is the gold standard. Thin-cut (3-mm) CT scanning with contrast has become the principal technique for evaluating patients preoperatively for endograft placement. CT permits measurement of the neck diameter; detection of neck thrombus; and measurement of neck length, aneurysm diameter, iliac diameter, and aneurysm length. It is particularly useful when combined with some of the newer techniques for CT reconstruction.

Angiography has largely been replaced by contrast CT scanning (Fig. 22-23). Nevertheless, it permits more accurate visualization of accessory renal arteries, and remains necessary in patients with coexistent horseshoe kidneys, mesenteric ischemia, and in those with lower extremity claudication. Table 22-6 summarizes the strengths and appropriate application of each imaging modality for AAAs.

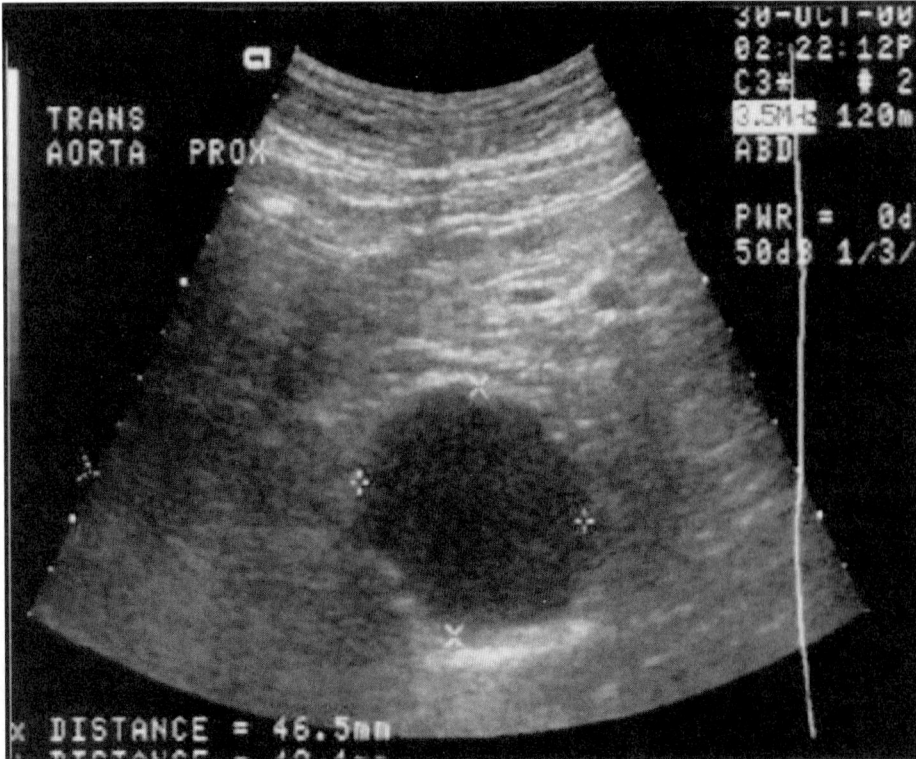

FIG. 22-19. Ultrasound is the least expensive technique for measuring the diameter of an abdominal aortic aneurysm.

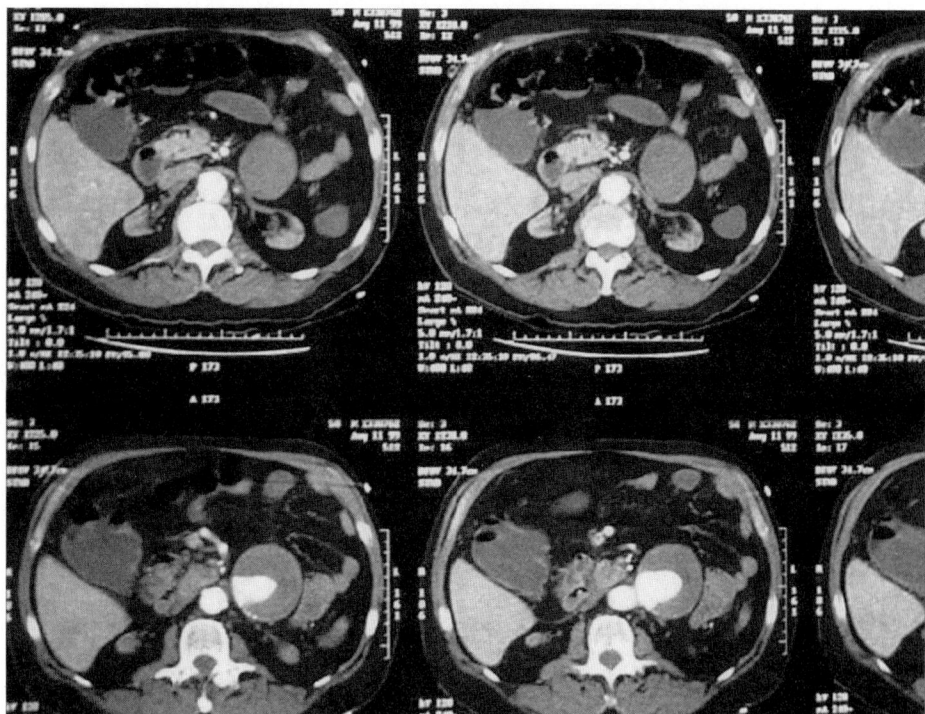

FIG. 22-20. Serial 3-mm slice computed tomography (CT) scans allow the aortic anatomy to be accurately defined. In this case CT shows acute angulation of the aortic neck into the aneurysm.

Guidelines for the treatment of AAAs, as reported by a subcommittee of the Joint Council of the American Association for Vascular Surgery and Society for Vascular Surgery, are as follows[39]:

1. The arbitrary setting of a single threshold diameter for elective AAA repair that is applicable to all patients is not appropriate, as the decision for repair must be individualized in each case.

2. Randomized trials have shown that the risk of rupture of small (<5 cm) AAAs is quite low and that a policy of careful surveillance up to a diameter of 5.5 cm is safe, unless rapid expansion (>1 cm/y) or symptoms develop. However, early surgery is comparable to surveillance with later surgery, so patient preference is important, especially for AAAs 4.5 to 5.5 cm in diameter.

3. Based upon the best available current evidence, a diameter of 5.5 cm appears to be an appropriate threshold for repair in an "average" patient. However, subsets of younger, low-risk patients with long projected life expectancy may prefer early repair. If the surgeon's personal documented operative mortality rate is low, repair may be indicated at smaller sizes (4.5 to 5.5 cm) if that is the patient's preference.

4. For women, or AAAs with greater-than-average rupture risk, 4.5 to 5.0 cm is an appropriate threshold for elective repair.

5. For high-risk patients, delay in repair until larger diameter is warranted, especially if endovascular aortic repair (EVAR) is not possible.

6. In view of its uncertain long-term durability and effectiveness, as well as the increased surveillance burden, EVAR is most appropriate for patients at increased risk for conventional open aneurysm repair.

7. EVAR may be the preferred treatment method if anatomy is appropriate for older, high-risk patients, those with "hostile" abdomens, or other clinical circumstances likely to increase the risk of conventional open repair.

8. Use of EVAR in patients with unsuitable anatomy markedly increases the risk of adverse outcomes, the need for conversion to open repair, or AAA rupture.

9. At present, there does not appear to be any justification that EVAR should change the accepted size thresholds for intervention in most patients.

10. In choosing between open repair and EVAR, patient preference is of great importance. It is essential that the patients be well informed to make such choices.

Options for Intervention

Patients should be informed of the two methods for aneurysm repair: traditional open repair and the newer aortic endografting. This section explains the advantages and disadvantages of each

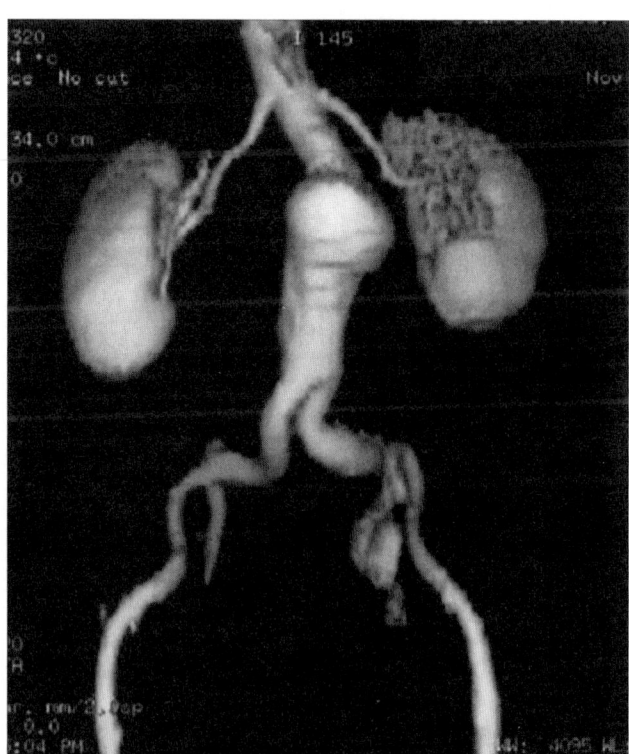

FIG. 22-21. Computed tomography (CT) three-dimensional reconstruction of abdominal aortic aneurysm.

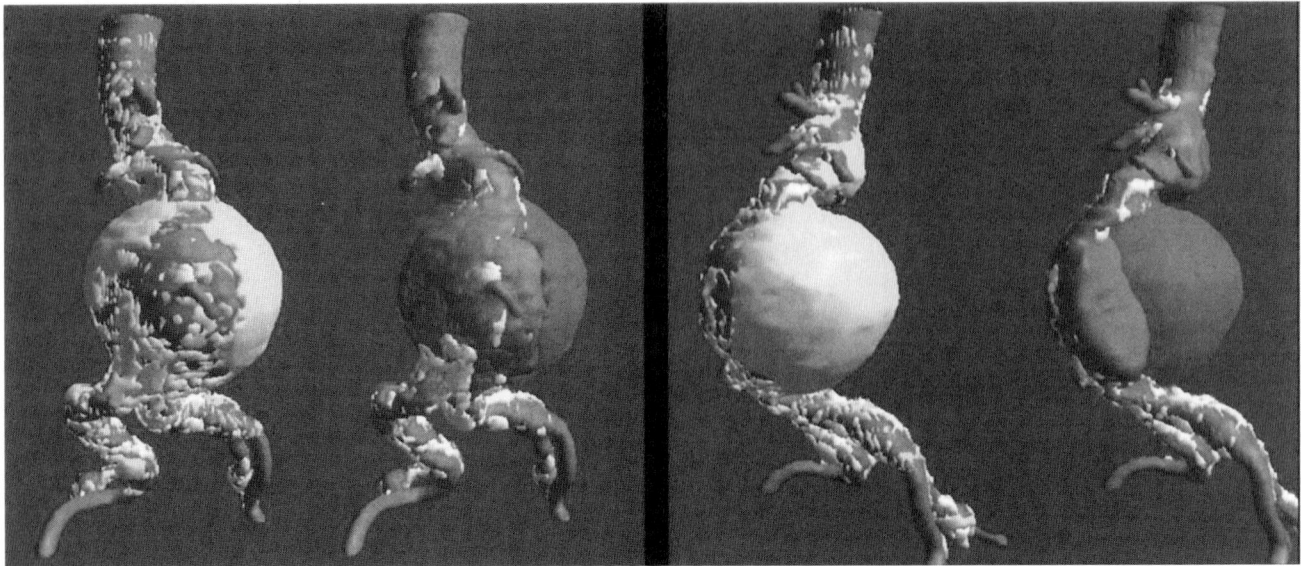

FIG. 22-22. Three-dimensional computed tomography (CT) scan depicting blood, calcification and thrombus. Such reconstructions greatly facilitate stent graft planning.

technique. Open repair requires a 1-day intensive care unit (ICU) stay, a 5- to 7-day hospitalization, and 2 months to return to baseline function. Thereafter follow-up is once per year and the incidence of long-term complications is 5 to 10%. Endografting is a smaller, up-front procedure that does not require an ICU stay, but does require a 2-day hospitalization, with return to baseline in 1 to 2 weeks. Ten percent of patients require an additional intervention within 2 years, and although the long-term efficacy remains unknown, data up to 5 years remain valid. There is no difference in the mortality rate in any of the clinical trials comparing open and endovascular

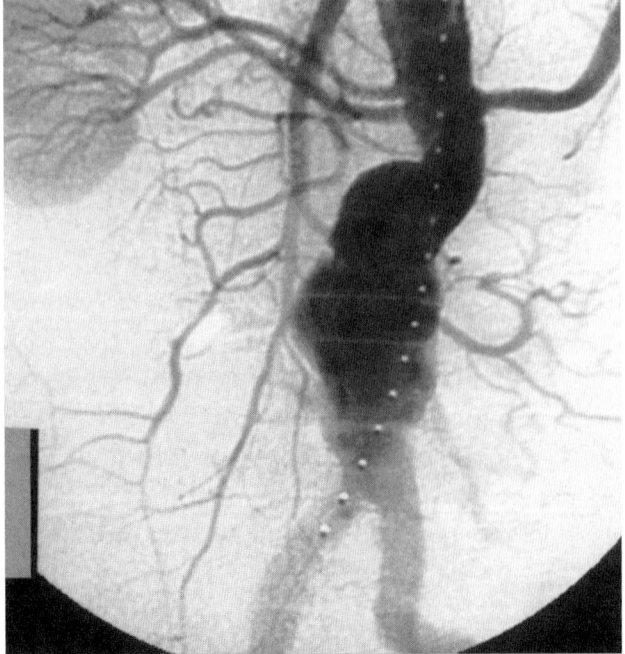

FIG. 22-23. Arteriogram of abdominal aortic aneurysm with marker catheter. Metal markers are spaced at 1-cm intervals, permitting accurate measurement.

repair. However, in high-risk patients who have anatomy suitable for endografting, there is benefit in avoiding a laparotomy.

Preoperative Preparation

Regardless of approach, all patients should have preoperative cardiac clearance. Risk factors for open aneurysm repair include myocardial infarction in the last 6 months without revascularization, congestive heart failure, and angina. An FEV_1 of less than 1 L and creatinine levels greater than 2.0 mg/dL are also risk factors. Preoperative pulmonary evaluation, with optimization of pulmonary function and renal protection with fenoldopam mesylate are used in patients with elevated creatinine levels.

Epidural anesthesia is a useful supplement for postoperative pain control and is essential in patients with compromised pulmonary function.

Surgery

AAAs can be addressed by either the open approach or via stent grafting. The open approach (Fig. 22-24) can be accomplished through either a midline transperitoneal abdominal incision or via a retroperitoneal approach (Fig. 22-25). The latter is particularly valuable in patients anticipated to have intra-abdominal adhesions and/or abdominal stoma, and may have value in patients with severe COPD. For some surgeons this is the preferred approach for most infrarenal aortic surgery. However, there are two limitations: the inability to reach the right renal artery, and difficulty may be encountered in exposing the right distal common iliac artery. Most surgeons still prefer the conventional midline incision, which extends from the xiphoid process to the pubic symphysis. After opening the peritoneum, exploratory laparotomy is performed to exclude concurrent intra-abdominal pathology. The transverse colon is then retracted superiorly and the small bowel is enclosed in a towel that is retracted to the patient's right. This exposes the base of the mesentery and the emerging fourth part of the duodenum. The peritoneum over the aorta is incised from the iliac bifurcation superiorly, around the duodenum, and up to the level of the left renal vein. The latter marks the upper limit of the dissection. Frequently, the inferior mesenteric

Table 22-6
Summary of Imaging Modalities for Abdominal Aortic Aneurysms (AAAs)

Studies	Overview	Pros	Cons
X-rays	Calcified aortic wall	Simple, inexpensive	Lower specificity; detects 60% of AAAs; calcified wall
B-mode ultrasound	Good screening tool	Accurate (80–90%), inexpensive	Bowel gas interference; operator-dependent
Computed tomography (CT)	Most accurate study for AAA diameter	Accurate; define anatomy and anomalies	Expensive; ionizing radiation
CT angiogram	New modality; combines CT and angiography	3-D images; avoids invasive angiogram	Expensive; same contrast load as angiogram; special protocol
Magnetic resonance angiography	New modality	3-D images; avoids radiation and invasive angiography	Expensive; limited resolution; patient contraindications
Angiogram	Popular due to endografting	Shows visceral and occlusive disease	Expensive; invasive; contrast load

vein is encountered crossing the aorta in the retroperitoneum. This can be safely divided and ligated. Once the peritoneum is incised, the duodenum can be further mobilized to the patient's right, exposing the underlying aorta. The distal extent of the dissection is determined by the extent of aneurysmal involvement of the iliac arteries (Fig. 22-26). If the iliac arteries are not involved, then they are dissected only to permit safe clamping. If the entire common iliac artery is aneurysmal, then dissection may be required down the bifurcation into the internal and external iliac arteries, which can be separately controlled. Almost invariably the aneurysmal disease stops at the common iliac bifurcation. Once the aneurysm is exposed, the patient is anticoagulated using 100 U/kg of heparin. Three minutes following heparin administration, the iliac arteries are clamped, fol-

lowed by the aorta. Clamps are placed anteroposteriorly, and it is unnecessary to circumferentially dissect the aorta or iliac arteries. The aneurysm is opened longitudinally. A large quantity of thrombus that lines the aneurysm is scooped out. Back-bleeding lumbar vessels are oversewn with 2-0 silk suture (Fig. 22-27). A tube (Fig. 22-28) or bifurcated graft (Fig. 22-29) is sewn end-to-end inside the aneurysm using 3-0 polypropylene suture for the aortic anastomoses. Prior to completion of the final anastomosis, the aorta is flushed, the iliac arteries allowed to back-bleed, and the graft flushed with heparinized saline. The anesthesiologist is informed prior to reperfusing the lower extremities to provide time for volume loading and to ensure that pressors are available if necessary. The surgeon, while continuously observing the patient's blood pressure, then performs slow and controlled reperfusion by releasing pressure on the graft.

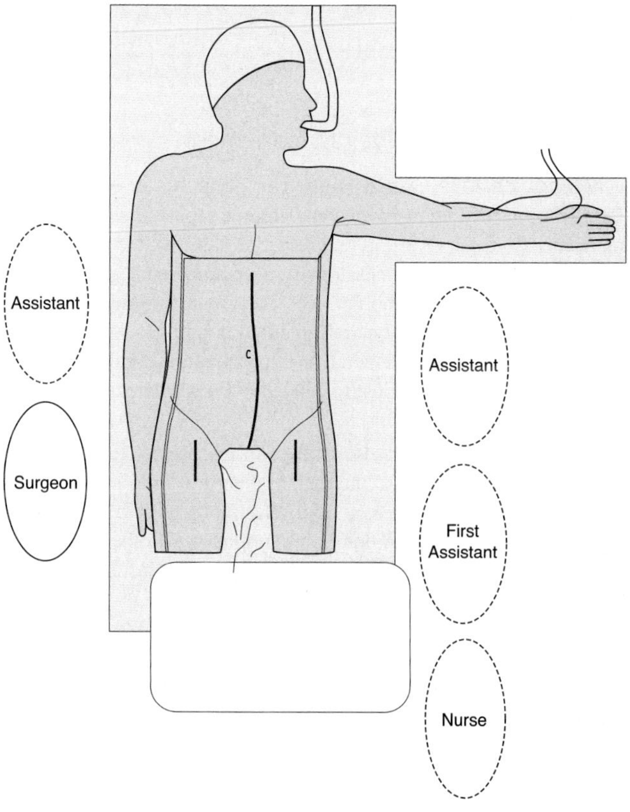

Femoral pulses are checked and the presence of a Doppler signal within the sigmoid mesocolon is noted. Absence of the latter would prompt exploration of the inferior mesenteric artery (IMA) and reimplantation into the aortic graft.

Anticoagulation is reversed using protamine sulfate. Once the operative field is hemostatic, the aneurysm sac is re-approximated over the graft using 2-0 polyglactic acid suture. The retroperitoneum is then also closed over the aneurysmal sac using running 2-0 polyglactic acid suture. Prior to leaving the operating room, the surgical team must ensure that there is adequate perfusion to the feet by checking Doppler signals or for the presence of palpable pulses. The distal IMA should also be studied to ensure that good Doppler signals are present in the sigmoid mesocolon. Absence of such signals would prompt reimplantation of the IMA into the aortic graft.

Postoperative Course

Patients are observed in the ICU overnight, with particular attention paid to hemodynamic stability and urine output, and aggressive pulmonary toilet is performed. Most patients are hospitalized for 4 to 5 days postprocedure; follow-up is at 1 month, 6 months, and then yearly. A CT scan is performed 3 years postprocedure, to look for evidence of pseudoaneurysm formation.

Morbidity and Mortality

The mortality rate in large institutions is 2 to 4% with a morbidity rate of 20%. There was no difference in mortality in the Ancure and Aneuryx endograft trials between open and endograft repair. Patients with endografts had fewer pulmonary complications.

FIG. 22-24. *Typical positioning of patient in the operating room for open abdominal aortic aneurysm (AAA) repair.*

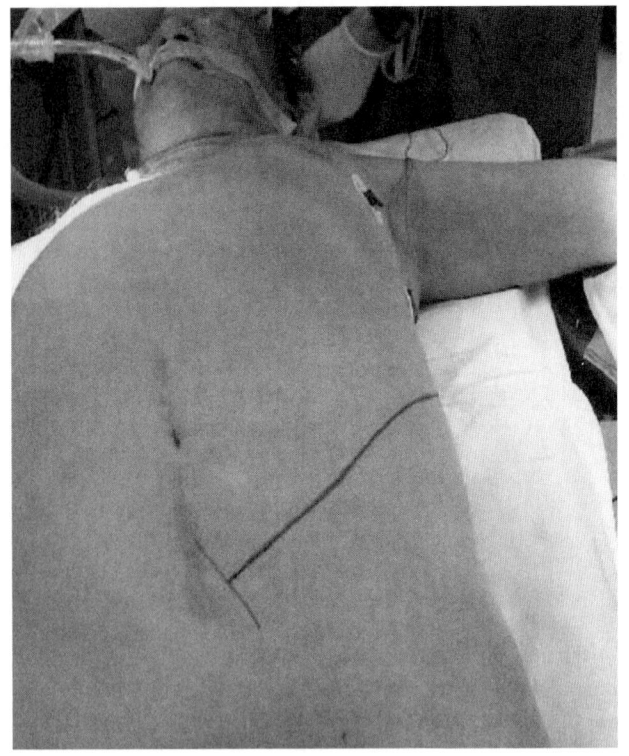

A

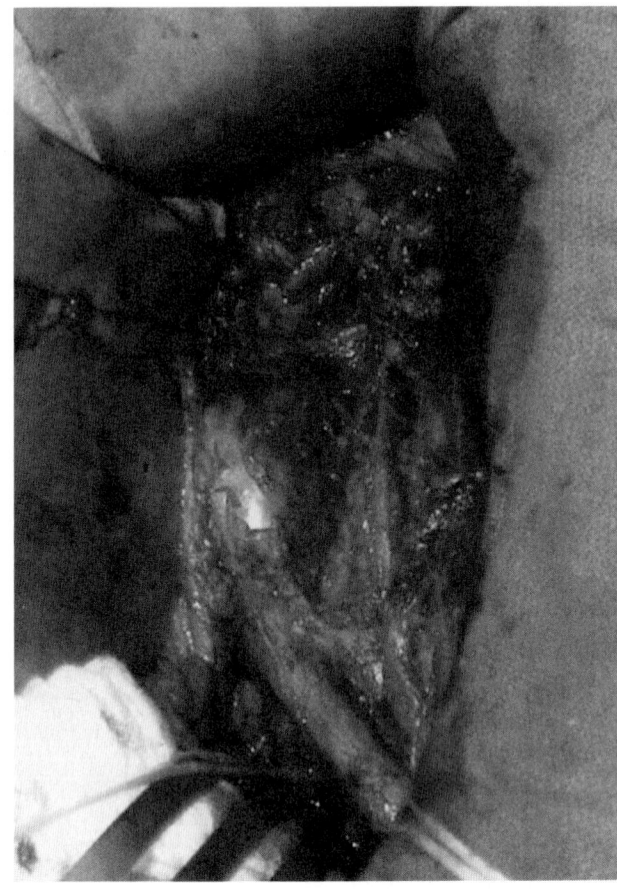

B

FIG. 22-25. *A.* Skin incision for a left retroperitoneal aortic aneurysm repair. *B.* Surgical exposure via a left retroperitoneal approach.

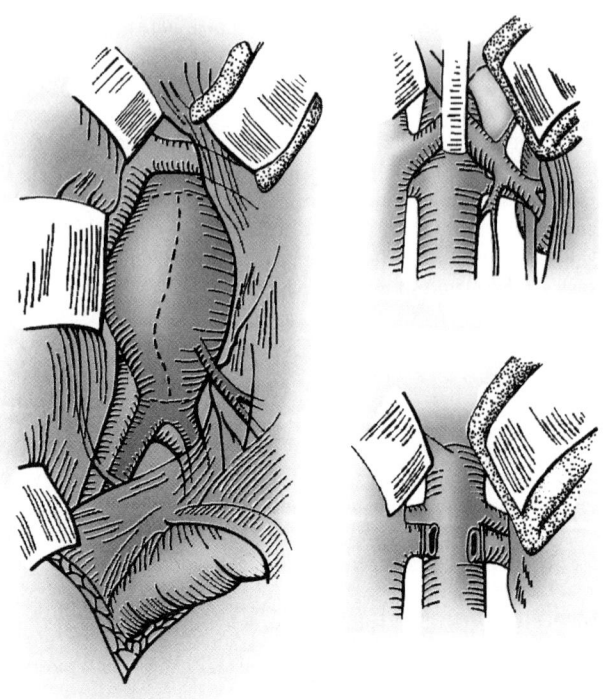

FIG. 22-26. Typical exposure of an abdominal aortic aneurysm (AAA) via a midline abdominal incision.

Complications and Their Management

Renal Failure. Renal failure can occur for several reasons, the most common being inadequate volume replacement. However, an aortic clamp close to the renal arteries can result in an embolic shower to the kidneys. Occasionally accessory renal arteries arise from the aneurysm. Although accessory renal arteries often can be sacrificed, they should be reimplanted in patients with compromised renal function. Preoperative impairment of renal function is the greatest predictor of postoperative renal insufficiency.

Lower Extremity Ischemia. The absence of a femoral pulse suggests acute occlusion of the limb of the graft. This is usually due to a technical error such as a poor anastomosis, graft kinking, or compression, or it can be due to a clamp injury to the iliac artery beyond the anastomosis. This usually requires immediate surgical correction.

If the femoral pulse is present, the limb is most likely ischemic due to either a distal embolus or acute thrombosis of the infrainguinal vessels resulting from pre-existing plaque or inadequate anticoagulation. Once again surgical exploration, thrombectomy, or bypass may be necessary.

Colonic Ischemia. Chronic ischemia is reported to occur at an incidence of 1 to 7%. However, with routine checking of the sigmoid perfusion at the completion of the case, the incidence has been significantly reduced. Other techniques include inserting a catheter

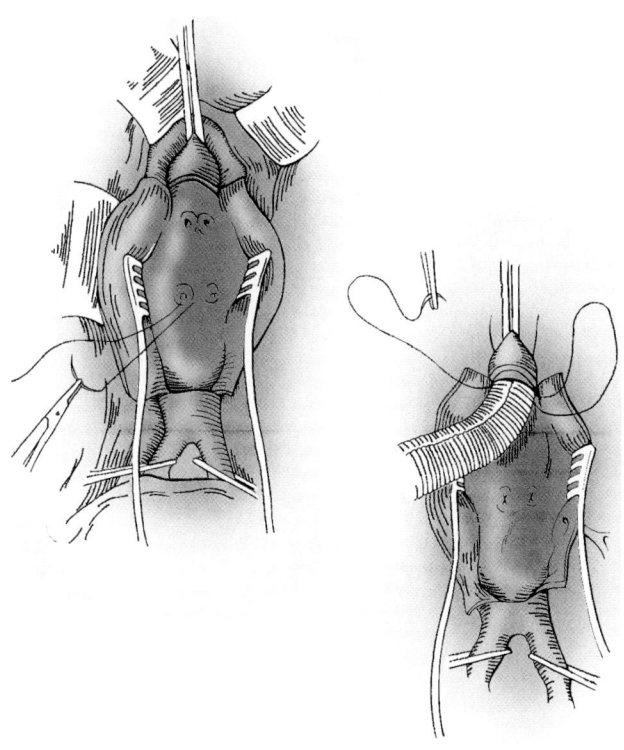

FIG. 22-27. After opening the aneurysm sac, back-bleeding lumbar arteries are oversewn.

FIG. 22-28. *A.* Schematic drawing of a prosthetic Dacron graft used to replace an abdominal aortic aneurysm. *B.* Intraoperative picture of a Dacron tube graft used to replace an abdominal aortic aneurysm.

into the inferior mesenteric arterial stump and measuring backpressure. Pressures greater than 40 mm Hg are indicative of adequate collateral flow and permit safe ligation of the IMA. Diagnosis of colon ischemia is often delayed because of sedation, analgesia, or misdiagnosis as an ileus. Difficulty in maintaining pelvic perfusion at the time of surgery should raise suspicion. Bloody diarrhea, elevated white blood cell count (WBC), or distention should prompt an aggressive search. The definitive diagnosis is established by colonoscopy. Early laparotomy and resection with colostomy is the only hope of survival in these critically ill patients.[40]

Spinal Cord Ischemia. Paraplegia is a rare (1:10,000) but devastating complication of abdominal aortic surgery. It is multifactorial in etiology, and is occasionally due to contributions from a sacrificed lumbar artery to the spinal cord. However, more commonly it is a manifestation of pelvic ischemia due to hypoperfusion (sacrifice of pelvic circulation) or due to embolization. Reimplantation of the inferior mesenteric artery or ensuring perfusion of an internal iliac artery will minimize the risk of this dreaded complication.

Complications of Prosthetic Repair of the Aorta

Prosthetic grafting of the abdominal aorta for aneurysmal or occlusive disease is a common vascular procedure. It has a high patency rate at 5 years and a low complication rate. Complications include anastomotic aneurysms, graft infection, graft thrombosis, and aortoenteric fistula (AEF). Anastomotic aneurysms involving the femoral or iliac arteries at the distal anastomosis are common.

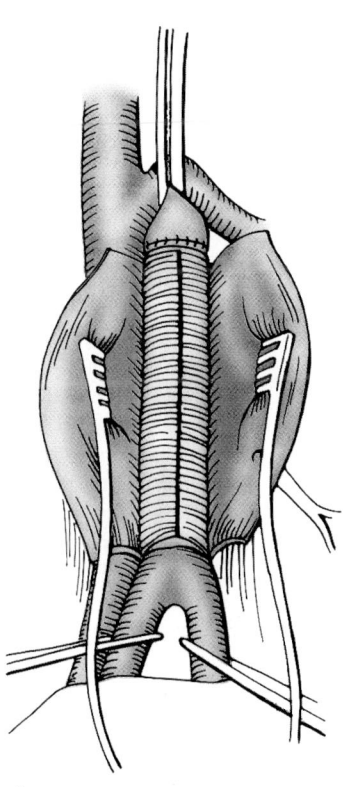

A

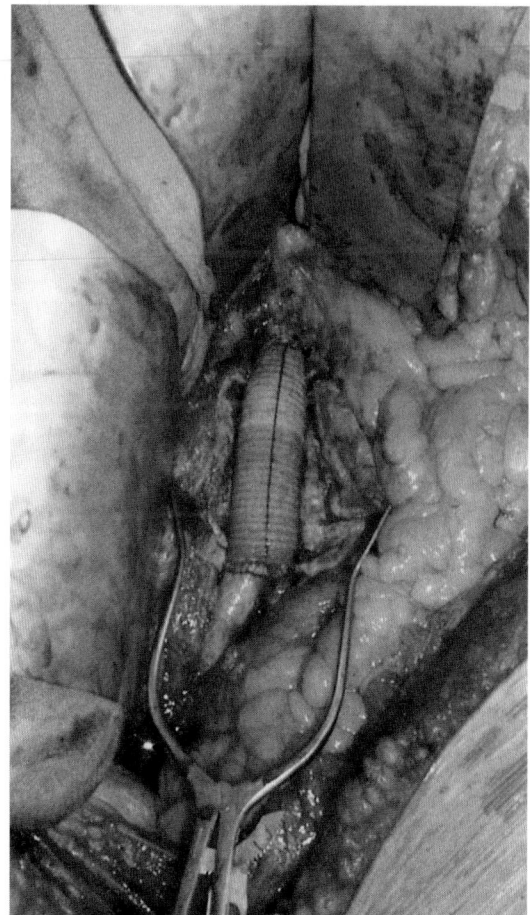

B

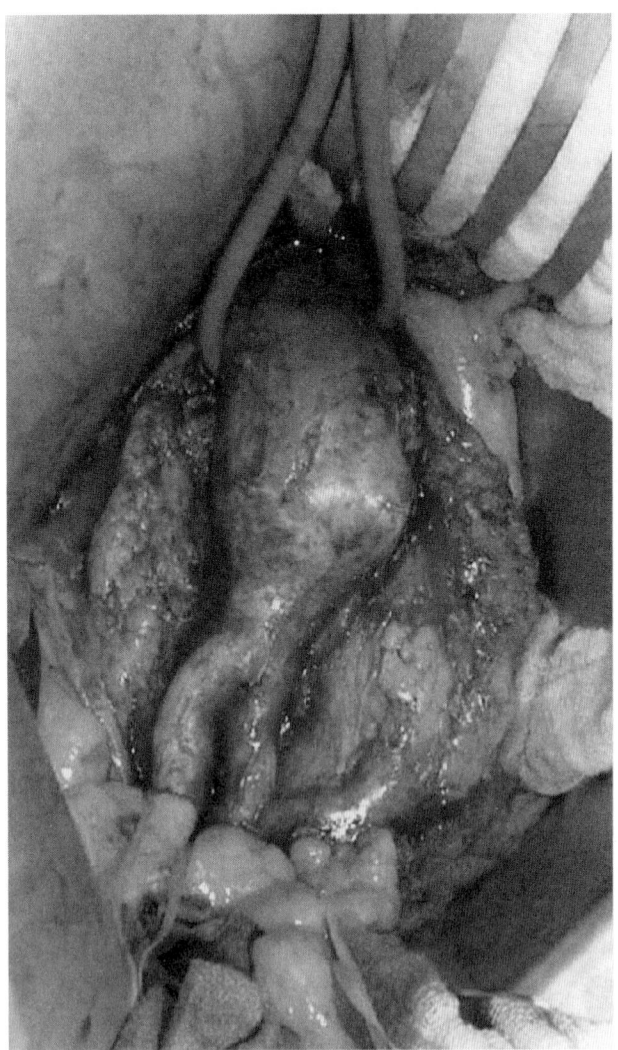

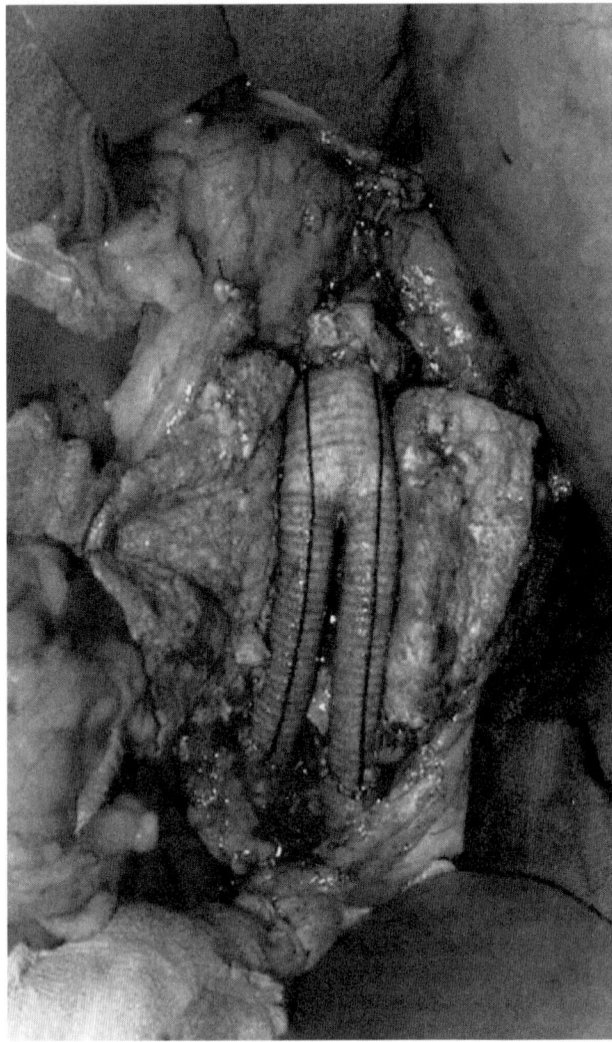

A

B

FIG. 22-29.   *A.* Intraoperative picture of an abdominal aortic aneurysms. *B.* A bifurcated graft has been used due to calcification at the aortic bifurcation, which precluded safe suturing.

Para-anastomotic aneurysms involving the abdominal aorta (PAAAs) also occur, but their incidence may be underestimated since routine screening after aortic grafting is presently not the standard of care.[41–43]

Aortoenteric Fistula. An aortoenteric fistula is an uncommon (<1%) occurrence, in which the proximal aortic graft erodes into the overlying duodenum (Figs. 22-30 and 22-31). The patient presents with GI bleeding that can be massive. Any patient with an upper GI bleed and a history of aortic surgery is presumed to have an aortoenteric fistula until proven otherwise. Positive diagnosis can be difficult, but upper GI endoscopy has the greatest yield. CT scanning and angiography may also be helpful. Treatment is by graft excision and closure of the duodenum. Vascular reconstruction can be performed using either extra-anatomic bypass (bilateral axillopopliteal grafts or axillobifemoral graft) or in situ replacement with antibiotic-impregnated Dacron grafts.

Aortic Endografting

Thirty to 50% of aneurysms are currently treated with endografts.[44–47] Endografts are inserted via a cutdown on each common femoral artery. The exposed artery is punctured with a Seldinger needle. Through the needle, a Bentsen guidewire is passed into the aortic artery using fluoroscopic guidance. Over the wire a marker pigtail is inserted and used to perform an angiogram (see Fig. 22-23). All preoperative measurements are then checked, and a stiff wire inserted up through the pigtail catheter, which is then removed. A second wire is advanced up through the contralateral groin and exchanged for a stiff wire. The patient is then fully anticoagulated and the ipsilateral femoral artery clamped. A transverse arteriotomy is made to permit insertion of the main body endograft. This is advanced up through the ipsilateral iliac system under fluoroscopic control (Fig. 22-32). The proximal markers are placed immediately below the lowest renal arteries and the device appropriately oriented (Fig. 22-33), then deployed (Figs. 22-34 and 22-35). The contralateral gate is then cannulated (Fig. 22-36) with a guidewire and its intragraft position confirmed by reconforming a pigtail catheter and ensuring that it spins freely within the lumen of the grafts. A stiff wire is reinserted though the pigtail catheter and the contralateral limb advanced into the gate and deployed (Figs. 22-37, 22-38, 22-39, and 22-40). Rapid changes in the type of endograft available and the options for the surgeon are

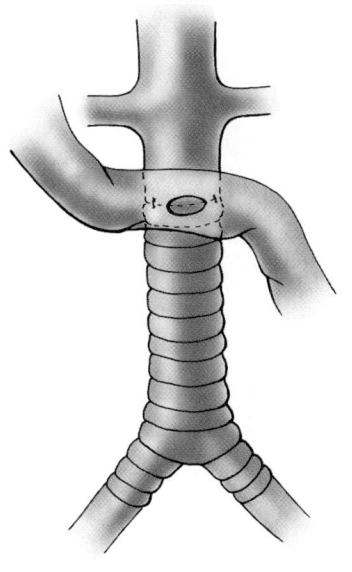
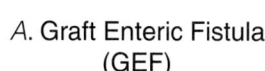

**A. Graft Enteric Fistula
(GEF)**

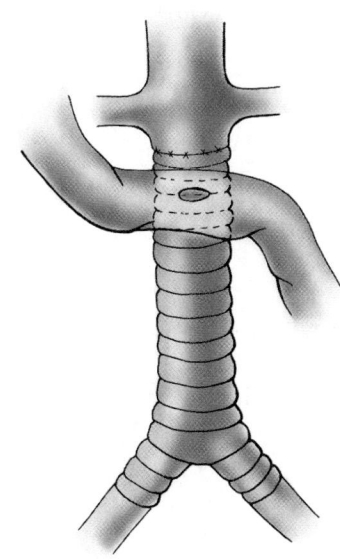

**B. Graft Enteric Erosion
(GEE)**

FIG. 22-30. *A.* Graft enteric fistula that is a communication between the bowel and arterial circulation at the level of an arterial prosthetic suture line. *B.* Graft enteric erosion that is a communication between the bowel and the interstices of an arterial prosthetic graft. The suture line is not involved.

presently occurring. Devices are now available for aortounilateral iliac aneurysms and for treatment of thoracic aortic aneurysms (Fig. 22-41). Iliac artery injuries can occur from insertion of the device, which may manifest as rupture, dissection, or limb occlusion postendografting. Renal dysfunction can occur form dye toxicity, embolization, and occasionally inadvertent coverage of the renal artery by the device.

The principal concern with endografting is the occurrence of endoleaks (Fig. 22-42). The most common is a type II leak, which occurs via the lumbar arteries or via the IMA. Management of type II leaks remains controversial and is based on whether the aneurysm is enlarging or stable. All type I endoleaks that are considered to be high-pressure leaks must be treated.[48,49]

Patients with endografts must be followed for life. Follow-up includes abdominal radiographs (e.g., anteroposterior [AP], lateral, and obliques), duplex ultrasound, and contrast-enhanced CT scanning. All patients are studied at 30 days, 6 months, and then yearly. Patients with an endoleak are examined more frequently.[50–53]

Juxtarenal Aneurysms

No specific definition exists of a juxtarenal aneurysm (Fig. 22-43). However, they are typically identified as those which extend to the renal arteries, thus requiring a suprarenal cross-clamp. Technical maneuvers that facilitate this are division of the left renal vein and a left retroperitoneal approach. Suprarenal clamping clearly increases the risk of renal dysfunction postprocedure. The graft can be sutured incorporating the inferior margin of the renal orifices.

Ruptured Abdominal Aortic Aneurysm

Fear of rupture is the driving force behind the elective repair of aneurysms. There has been almost no change in the mortality rate from ruptured AAAs in the last 20 years. Most patients die before reaching the hospital, and of those who do, the mortality remains close to 50%. This has led to some serious re-evaluation of the management of ruptured aneurysms, with increasing interest in the

use of permissive hypotension and the use of emergent stent graft placement. These developments, however, remain to be validated.

Most patients with a ruptured aneurysm are often unaware of the presence of an aneurysm.[54] Sudden-onset, severe abdominal pain and/or back pain are the principal presenting symptoms. Often there is a fainting episode that correlates with the initial aneurysm sac rupture, which is followed by a period of cardiovascular stability. Consequently the patient arrives in the emergency room with little to distinguish a ruptured AAA from other intra-abdominal catastrophes. Palpation of a pulsatile mass, the outline of a calcified AAA or soft tissue mass on abdominal x-rays (i.e., KUB) (Fig. 22-44), or a known history of AAA greatly facilitates the diagnosis. Where the diagnosis is clear-cut, the patient should go directly to the operating room for emergent repair. Often, however, the diagnosis is uncertain and established by CT scanning (Fig. 22-45). As in shock resuscitation for trauma, current thinking is to avoid aggressive resuscitation and infuse fluids or blood only to keep the patient stable and cerebrating, without creating hypertension that may accelerate additional bleeding. A systolic pressure of 70 mm Hg with a cerebrating patient is tolerable while preparations are made to go to the operating room.

In the operating room, the abdomen is prepped and draped with the patient awake. Decompensation can occur with the induction of anesthesia and loss of abdominal wall splinting. Once the patient is anesthetized, a long midline abdominal incision is created. Usually a large hematoma contained within the retroperitoneum is apparent (Fig. 22-46). The approach to control of the aorta depends on what preoperative data are available. If a preoperative CT scan is available, the surgeon can decide based on the extent and location of the hematoma whether to gain infrarenal control or supraceliac aortic control at the diaphragm. For the latter, the lesser omentum is incised between the lesser curve and the left lobe of the liver. The aorta is exposed by division of the median arcuate ligament of the diaphragm and the aorta clamped. In the unstable patient, an aortic compressor can be utilized. Exposure of the aorta at the diaphragm is not as easy or rapid as often portrayed. The inexperienced vascular surgeon should use an aortic compressor after opening the lesser sac.

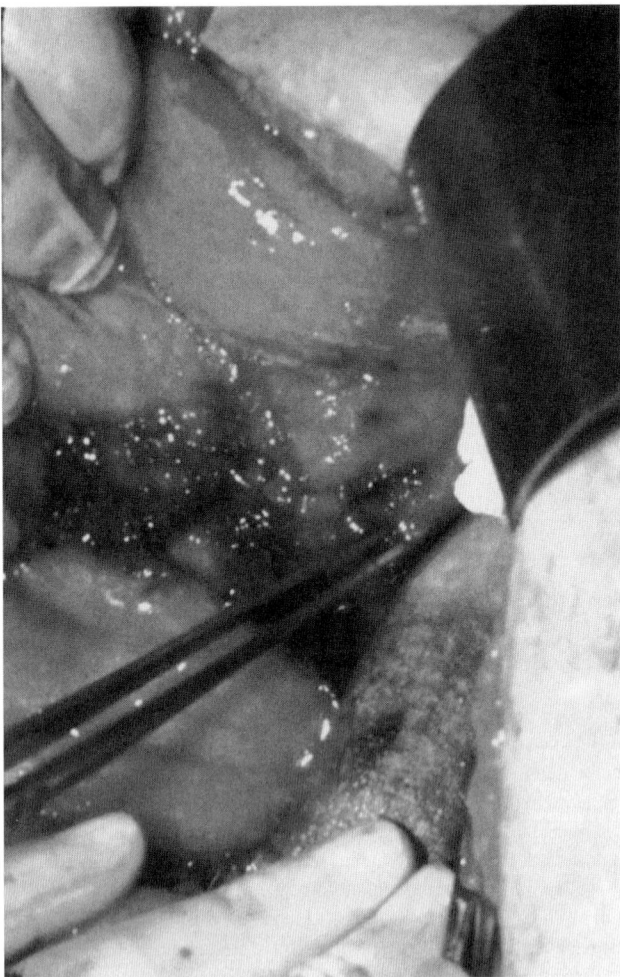

A

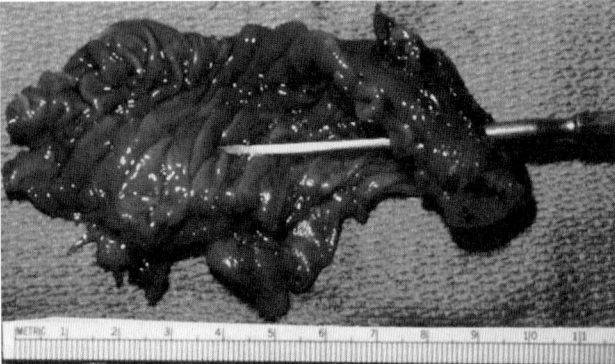

B

FIG. 22-31. *A.* Bile staining of the aortic graft. *B.* Defect in the duodenal wall.

This is entered bluntly with the fingers. Finger dissection is used to expose the peritoneum, which is divided superiorly, permitting the duodenum to be mobilized to the patient's right. The hand is used to dissect the aortic neck, a finger is inserted on either side of the neck of the aneurysm, and dissection is carried to the posterior spine. Care must be taken to avoid the left renal vein. Once the aneurysmal neck has been isolated, a coarctation clamp is placed and the supraceliac

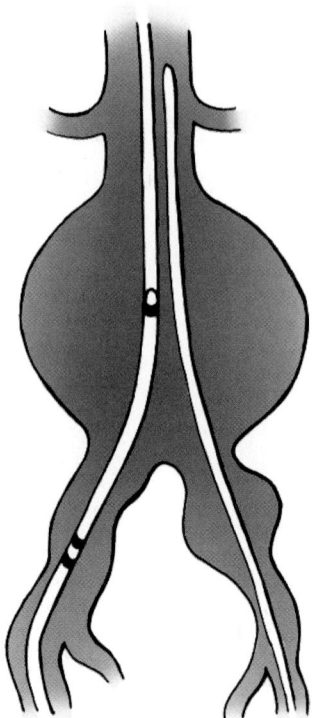

FIG. 22-32. Delivery catheter access for bifurcated segment.

control slowly released to ensure that inflow clamping is complete. With the fingers inside the aneurysm guiding the aortotomy, the aorta is opened inferiorly to the bifurcation. The iliac vessels can either be controlled endoluminally with Fogarty catheters, or externally by clamping, as judged by the surgeon. Aneurysm repair then proceeds as in elective cases. Declamping after rupture must be carefully controlled to prevent severe intractable hypotension. The surgeon must check colon perfusion with a pencil Doppler, blood flow to the feet, and ensure there is urine output.

Several technical complications occur more frequently in ruptured than elective aneurysm repair, including venous injury (i.e., renal, iliac or inferior vena cava [IVC]), ureteral injury, and injury to the duodenum. Multisystem organ failure is common in survivors who have suffered significant blood loss.

The emerging endovascular approach involves placement of a descending aortic occlusion balloon that is inflated only if the patient's blood pressure cannot be maintained in the range of the low 70s of systolic pressure. A CT scan is rapidly performed or intravascular ultrasound and angiography are done in the operating room to allow appropriate endoluminal graft selection. The device is then placed as expeditiously as possible.

Mycotic Aortic Aneurysm

Although mycotic aneurysms can occur in any artery, they are most frequently found in the aorta. The most common organisms cultured are staphylococci, followed by *Salmonella*. These aneurysms develop as a consequence of the infection, not as a result of infection in a pre-existing aneurysm. Mycotic aneurysms can occur as a result of infected emboli that lodge in the artery and spread in the wall. Most commonly they arise from infected aortic and mitral valves. Other mycotic aneurysms occur from direct extension of an area of infection into the adjacent arterial wall. Because patients who are immunosuppressed (i.e., acquired immunodeficiency

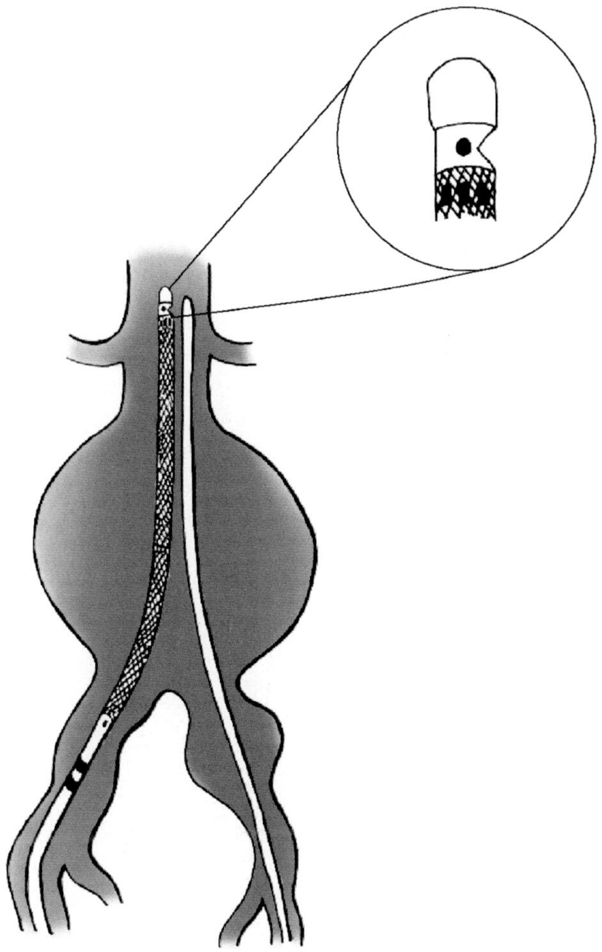

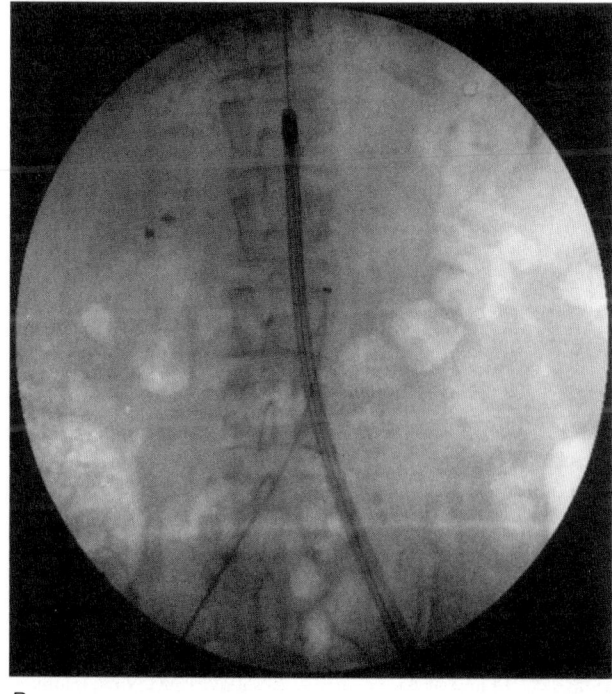

FIG. 22-33. *A.* Schematic drawing of an endovascular stent-graft positioned in the suprarenal aorta, with rotational orientation to ensure correct positioning. *B.* Intraoperative fluoroscopy demonstrates correct positioning of the endovascular stent-graft.

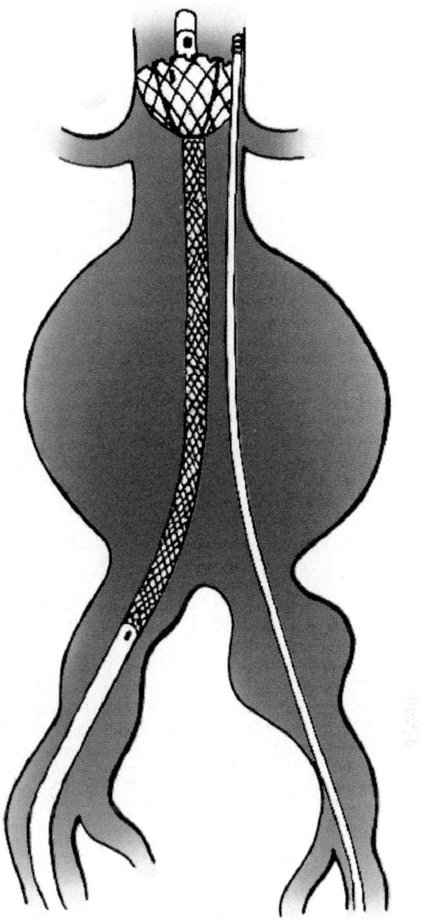

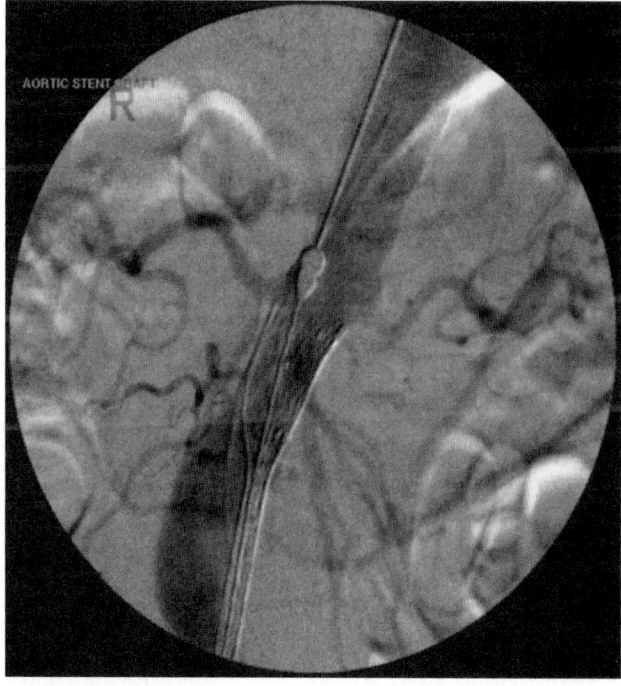

FIG. 22-34. *A.* Initial deployment of the stent-graft in the suprarenal aorta. *B.* Final positioning of the stent-graft in the aorta just below the renal arteries.

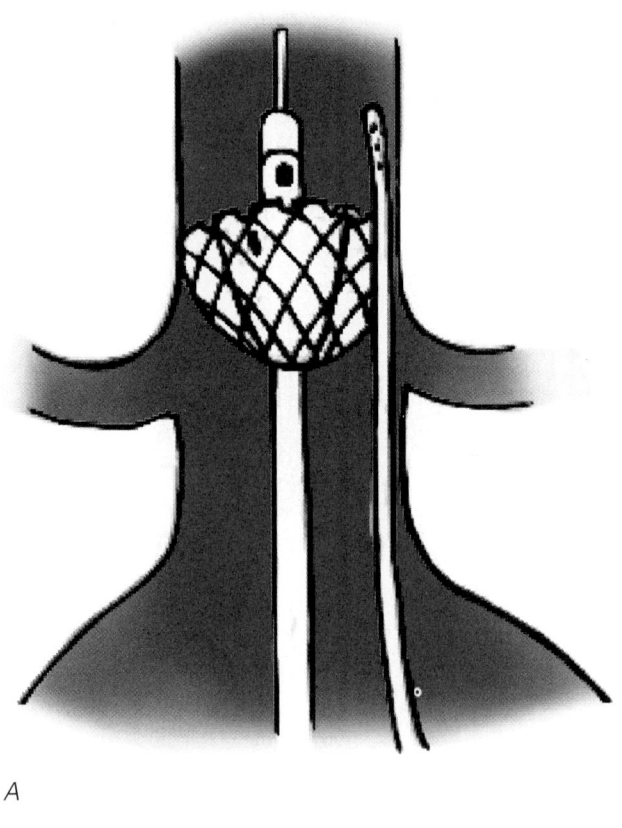

A

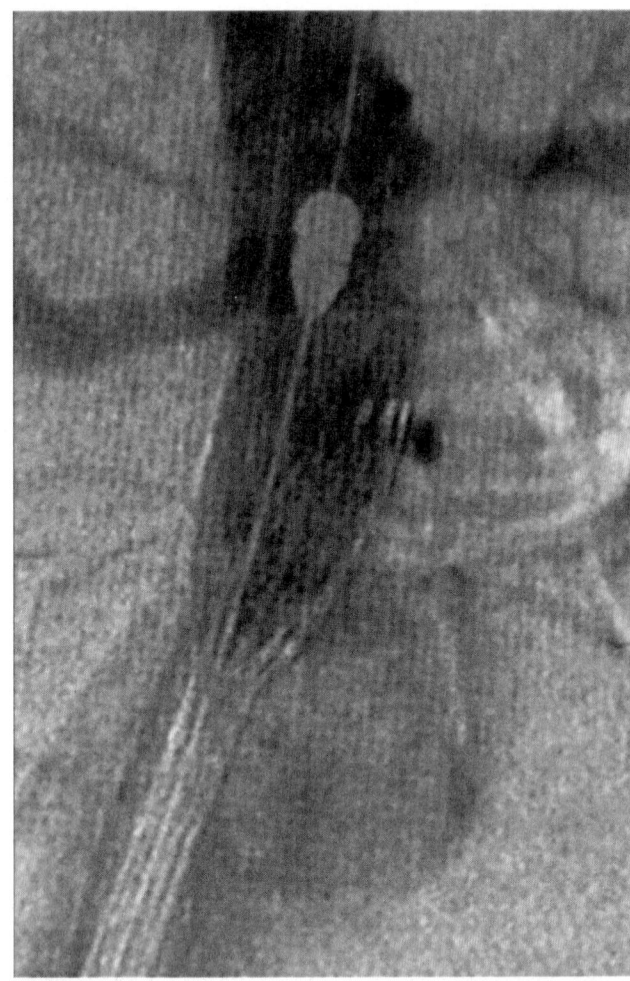

B

FIG. 22-35. *A. Schematic depiction of the initial endograft deployment in the aorta just above the renal arteries. B. Final position of the infrarenal aortic stent-graft.*

syndrome [AIDS] or organ transplant patients) are predisposed to infection, they are at an increased risk of developing mycotic aneurysms. Mycotic aneurysms often present with pain, are more rapidly progressive than degenerative aneurysms, and have a higher rupture rate. They also may erode into adjacent viscera. Mycotic aortic aneurysms are usually saccular, therefore the finding of a saccular aneurysm should raise concern of an infective etiology.

Treatment is determined by aneurysmal location. Those arising within the visceral aortic segment have to be treated by débridement and in situ reconstruction. Cryopreserved aorta has been widely used for this purpose. Expanded polytetrafluoroethylene (ePTFE) grafts may also be more infection resistant than Dacron grafts, although antibiotic-impregnated Dacron grafts are being increasingly utilized. Aneurysms that occur in the infrarenal aorta can be treated by several techniques. The traditional approach is to revascularize the lower extremities via an extra-anatomic approach (axillobifemoral bypass), followed by aortic excision and oversewing of the aortic stump. This is associated with an approximately 5% risk of aortic stump blow-out, which is usually fatal. This has led to a re-evaluation of in situ repair. Rifampin-soaked Dacron grafts have been placed into the aortic bed after excision, débridement, and irrigation. More recently, Clagett has popularized the use of bilateral superficial femoral vein to replace infected aortic grafts. This technique can also be useful for treatment of mycotic aneurysms. *Staphylococcus aureus* and *Pseudomonas* are particularly

aggressive organisms; hence extra-anatomic reconstruction should remain the procedure of choice.

Antibiotic therapy is used as directed by culture results, and long-term antibiotic therapy for 3 to 6 months is warranted. Careful follow-up with regular CT scanning should be utilized. Many different and unusual organisms have been associated with mycotic aneurysms, including *Mycobacterium tuberculosis, Pasteurella multocida,* and *Candida* spp.

Para-Anastomotic Aneurysms

Definition. Aneurysmal disease after bypass grafting of the abdominal aorta is defined radiographically as a focal dilatation juxtaposed to the aortic suture line or an adjacent aortic diameter that is greater than or equal to 4 cm (Fig. 22-47).

Incidence. A review of the recent literature reveals an apparent increase in the reported incidence (varying from 0.2 to 15%) of para-anastomotic aortic aneurysms (PAAAs) after bypass grafting for aneurysms of the abdominal aorta (AAA) or aortoiliac occlusive disease.[55–58] This increase in incidence seems paradoxical in light of advances in surgical technique and suture/graft material. However, patients with prostheses are living longer, and those with complicated vascular disease are receiving better medical care for their comorbid conditions. Edwards and colleagues have demonstrated, using life table analysis, an incidence of PAAA up to 27% at 15 years

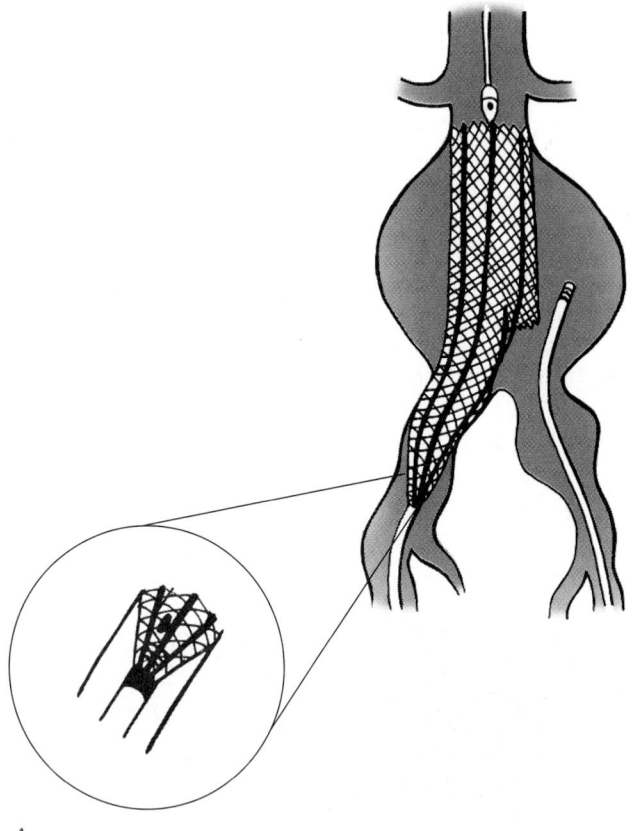

A

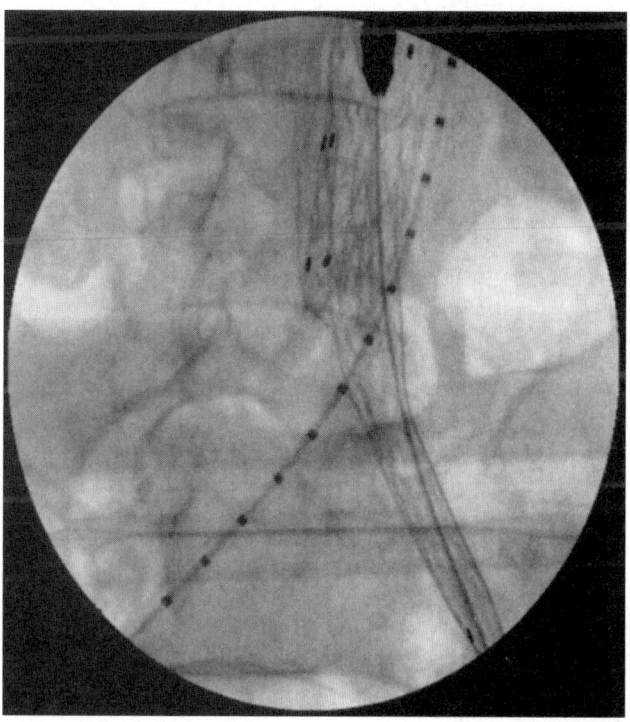

B

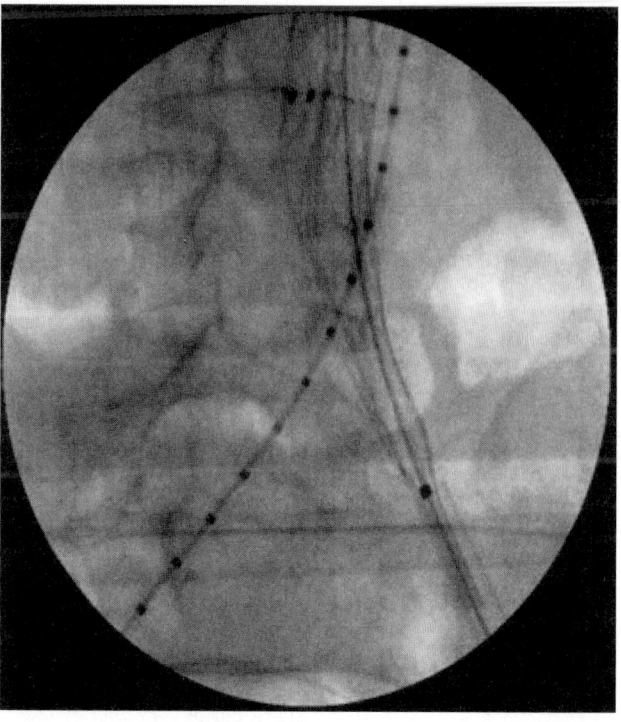

C

FIG. 22-36. *A.* Following the deployment of the main aortic endograft from the right femoral approach, a contralateral catheter is inserted from the left femoral artery to cannulate the main aortic endograft. *B* and *C.* Completed deployment of the main aortic bifurcated endograft.

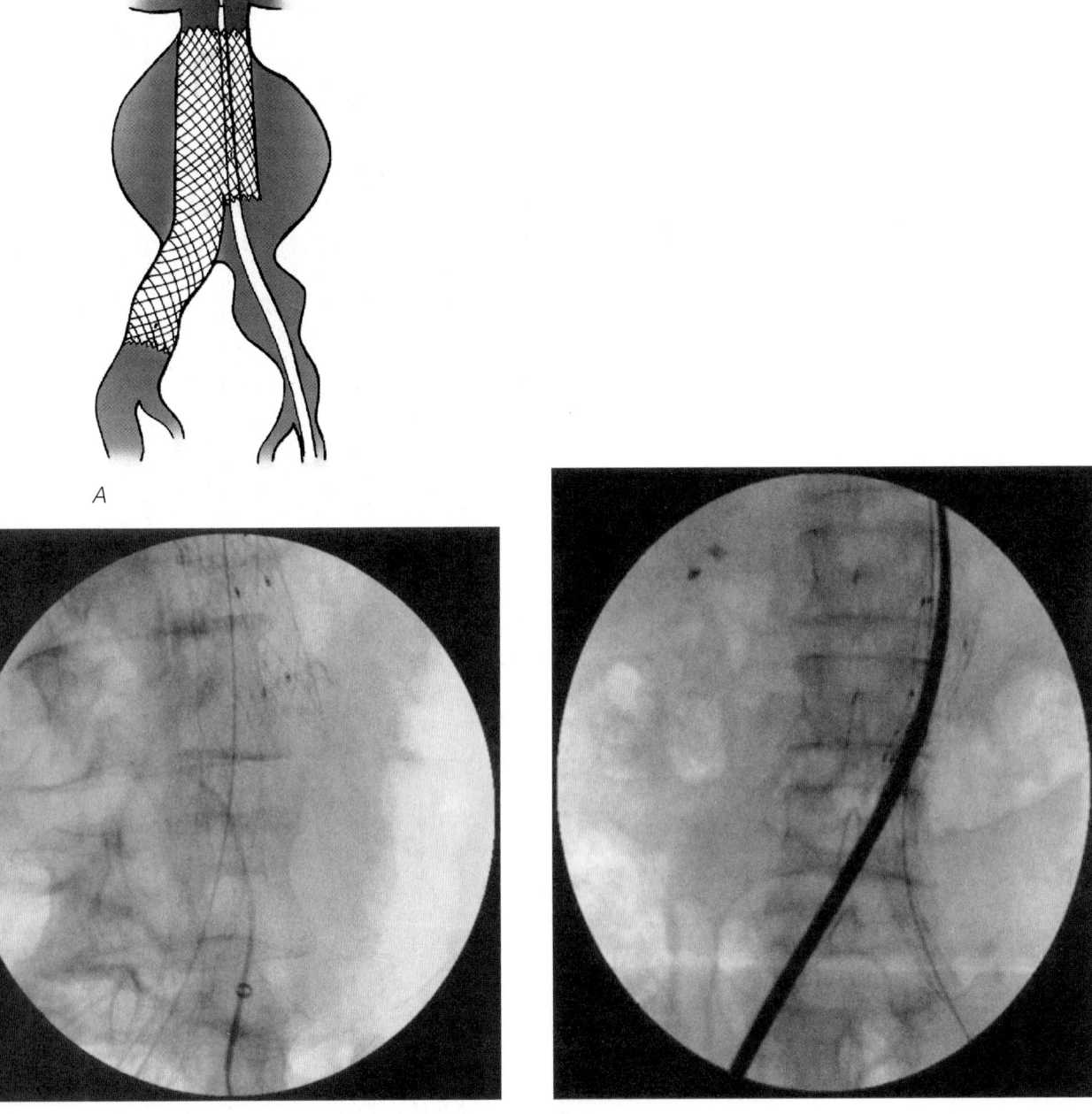

FIG. 22-37. *A.* Delivery catheter access via the contralateral femoral approach in cannulate the main aortic endograft. *B* and *C.* Deployment of the contralateral iliac endograft into the main aortic stent-graft.

after grafting.[55] This figure could be even higher since most patients receive no routine evaluation for development of a PAAA after bypass grafting.

Etiology. The etiology of PAAAs is speculative and is most likely multifactorial. It is important to distinguish true versus false aneurysms and to identify early versus late aneurysmal development. True aneurysms probably involve an intrinsic defect in the arterial wall, which may be due to an abnormality in collagen metabolism and may be inheritable. True PAAAs usually occur after bypass grafting for aneurysmal disease. Such aneurysms may

result from inadequate resection of the infrarenal aorta at the time of the initial operation. An alternate theory states that true aneurysms result from continued degeneration of an inherently abnormal vessel. False aneurysms may develop as a consequence of defects in the artery, suture, or graft. Factors implicated in their development include choice of suture material (e.g., silk or braided polyester), prosthesis dilatation (Dacron), type of anastomosis (end-to-side), severity/progression of atherosclerosis (multilevel disease), vessel versus graft compliance mismatch, and infection (periprosthetic) and AEF. Early PAAA formation has been associated with a complicated postoperative course following the primary aortic procedure.

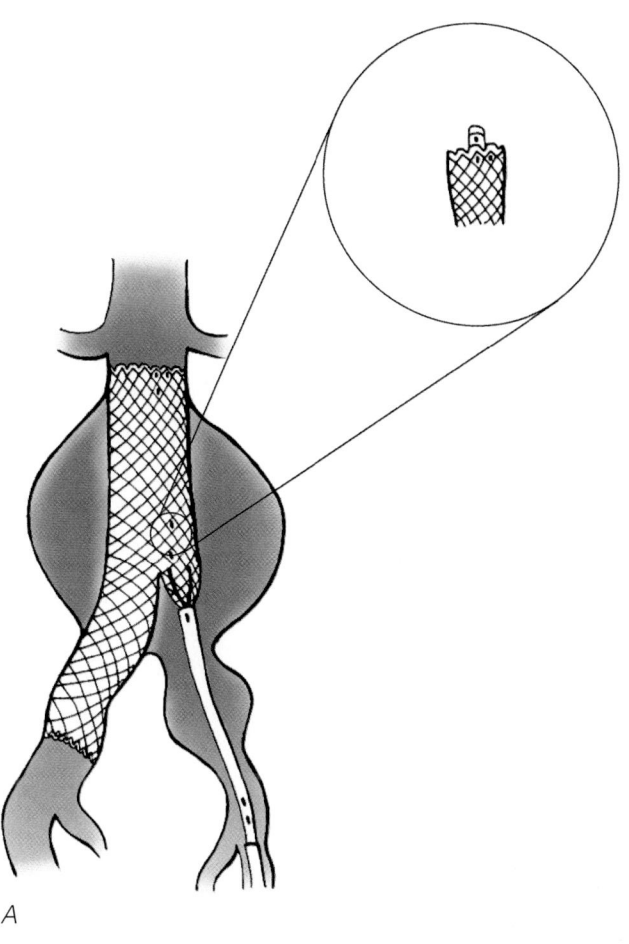

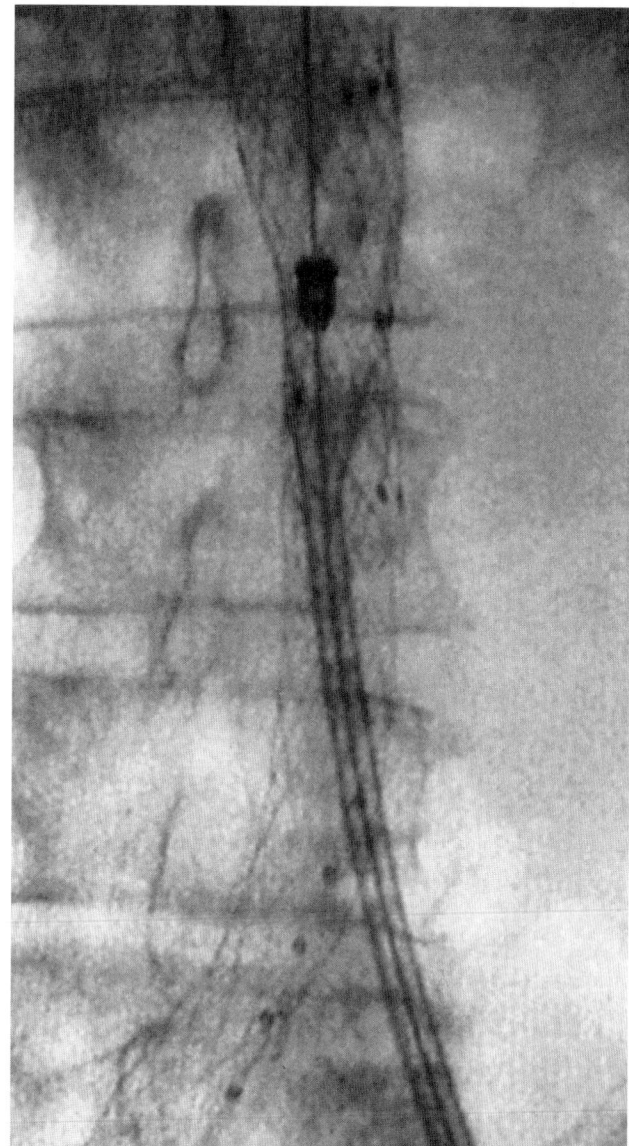

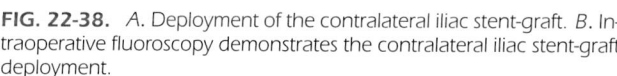

A

B

FIG. 22-38. *A. Deployment of the contralateral iliac stent-graft. B. Intraoperative fluoroscopy demonstrates the contralateral iliac stent-graft deployment.*

In these authors' experience it also has been linked to alpha$_1$-antitrypsin deficiency, recurrent PAAA, and graft infection.

Presentation. The clinical symptoms associated with a PAAA are varied and nonspecific. The patient can be totally asymptomatic, with the PAAA being detected by chance. For example, two patients in these authors' series were diagnosed serendipitously on abdominal CT and intravenous pyelogram examinations. Symptoms can include abdominal pain, back pain, and claudication. Physical examination may reveal a pulsatile mass in a patient who is otherwise asymptomatic. The majority of PAAAs are detected late, and therefore are large at the time of diagnosis, with an average size of approximately 7 cm in the series. The mean interval from the time of the primary aortic procedure to PAAA diagnosis is 8 to 10 years. Physical examination can be helpful if a mass is present, but frequently it is not diagnostic. A false aneurysm in the femoral artery is an associated finding in approximately 25% of patients with an aortic para-anastomotic aneurysm, and should be an indication to intensify surveillance. In contrast, approximately 15% of patients with a femoral pseudoaneurysm will have an associated PAAA. Rupture of a PAAA may present early or late during the postoperative

follow-up and is associated with a poor outcome. Two patients in these authors' study complaining of abdominal and back pain had a contained rupture of a false aneurysm early after bypass grafting. The characteristic presentation of AEF is a herald bleed and abdominal or back pain in a patient with a history of bypass grafting of the abdominal aorta. This classic triad was found in all three of the patients having a PAAA and associated AEF.

Diagnostic Studies. A high index of suspicion is required for diagnosis of PAAA in patients after abdominal aortic bypass grafting if routine screening is not employed. Ultrasonography (US) can be helpful diagnostically, and several academic centers have documented its high accuracy. However, this examination is operator-dependent, and results are variable between institutions. CT scanning also is effective in evaluating patients for complications after bypass grafting of the abdominal aorta. It demonstrates PAAA size and extent of involvement, as well as synchronous disease processes in the abdomen. Proper preoperative evaluation of PAAA patients prior to operative intervention is essential because of their frequently advanced age and multiple medical problems. Aortography, the gold standard for defining the aneurysm and associated anatomy,

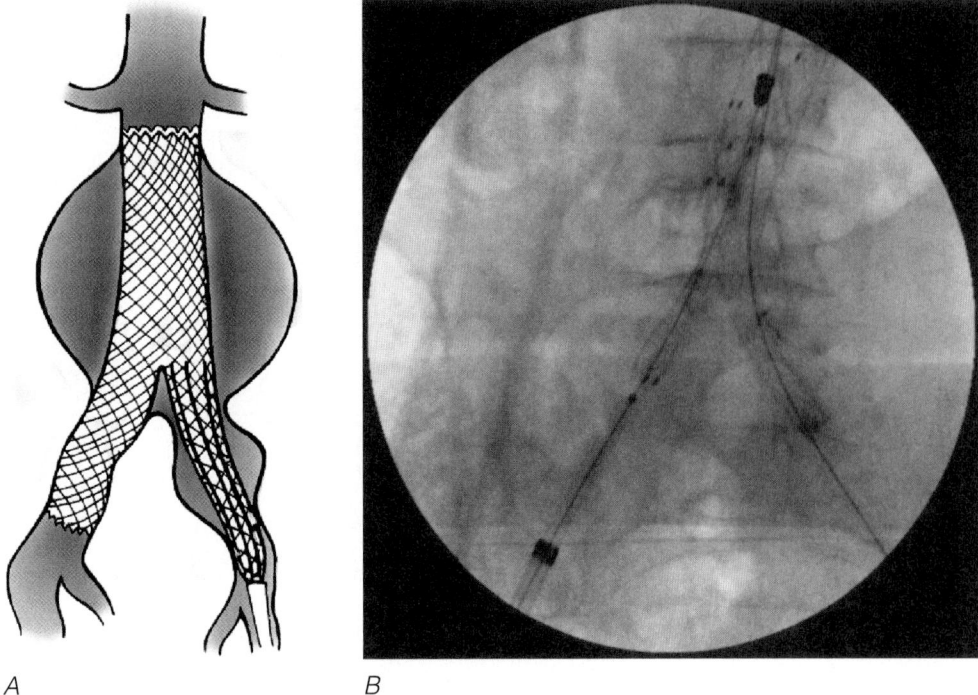

A   *B*

FIG. 22-39. *A. Completion deployment of the contralateral iliac stent-graft. B. Contralateral iliac stent-graft is fully docked in the aortic endograft.*

facilitates planning of the operative approach and selection of the appropriate surgical procedure. MRI will have an increasing role in the diagnosis of PAAA in the future and may supplant standard angiography.

Management. Elective surgical management of PAAA lesions is the treatment of choice since these lesions progressively increase in size and may rupture with time. Morbidity and mortality rates are acceptable in asymptomatic patients undergoing elective repair, as reported in these authors' series and by others. The operative repair most frequently involves excising the diseased segment of the artery and graft and placement of an interposition prosthesis. An end-to-side proximal anastomosis in patients with occlusive disease has been implicated as a causative factor of operative failure, but the importance of preserving the pelvic circulation must not be ignored. A bifurcated graft can be used if iliofemoral aneurysmal disease or generalized graft fatigue is present. Operative management of PAAA involving the renal and/or visceral vessels is more challenging, and a thoracoabdominal approach gives excellent proximal exposure and expedites repair. Operative complications are common and increase in the urgent setting or if other aortic graft complications are present (e.g., AEF or graft infection). Likewise, surgical mortality in these complicated reoperations is substantially higher than that associated with the initial aortic reconstruction (21% in the series of 29 patients). It is imperative to obtain operative cultures in every case, even if the index of suspicion for a graft infection is low. The clinical judgment of an experienced vascular surgeon is crucial in the management of these patients who are frequently elderly and frail. Observation with US surveillance should be considered as an option for patients with small asymptomatic PAAAs or for high-risk patients with an asymptomatic PAAA who are poor operative candidates.

More recently, use of endografts has become an increasingly popular method for treating anastomotic pseudoaneurysms. They are most easily utilized when the initial graft has been implanted well below the renal arteries such that a suitable landing and seal zone is available for positioning the device. In patients who are at high risk, stent grafting across the renal arteries with revascularization from the visceral or iliac vessels will avoid aortic cross-clamping.

Surveillance. Detection of aortic para-anastomotic aneurysms is usually a result of increasing size, symptom development, or serendipity. These aneurysms, when detected prior to development of complications, can be repaired with an acceptable risk. Accordingly, routine screening should be undertaken after aortic grafting. CT scanning is recommended on an annual basis beginning 4 years after graft implantation.

Other Anastomotic Aneurysms

The most common location for an aneurysm that develops at a suture line is at the femoral anastomosis of an aortobifemoral graft. In this location, either the Dacron degenerates, sutures deteriorate, or the sutures pull through the native artery, allowing a pseudoaneurysm to develop. Occasionally, degenerative changes in the host artery lead to graft-vessel separation. Other technical factors which may contribute to development of anastomotic pseudoaneurysms include excessive tension on the graft as a result of it being cut too short, or endarterectomy of recipient artery resulting in a thin vessel wall that cannot support the sutures. Infection of the graft extending to the suture line is another cause. Femoral anastomotic aneurysms are frequently bilateral.

They are detected by the presence of an enlarging pulsatile mass in the groin. Ultrasound confirms the diagnosis. Both groins should always be examined, and treatment is by surgical repair. The groin is entered via a vertical incision, and control of the inflow graft is necessary. Once this has been controlled, the patient is anticoagulated and the aneurysm opened. Fogarty catheters are used endoluminally

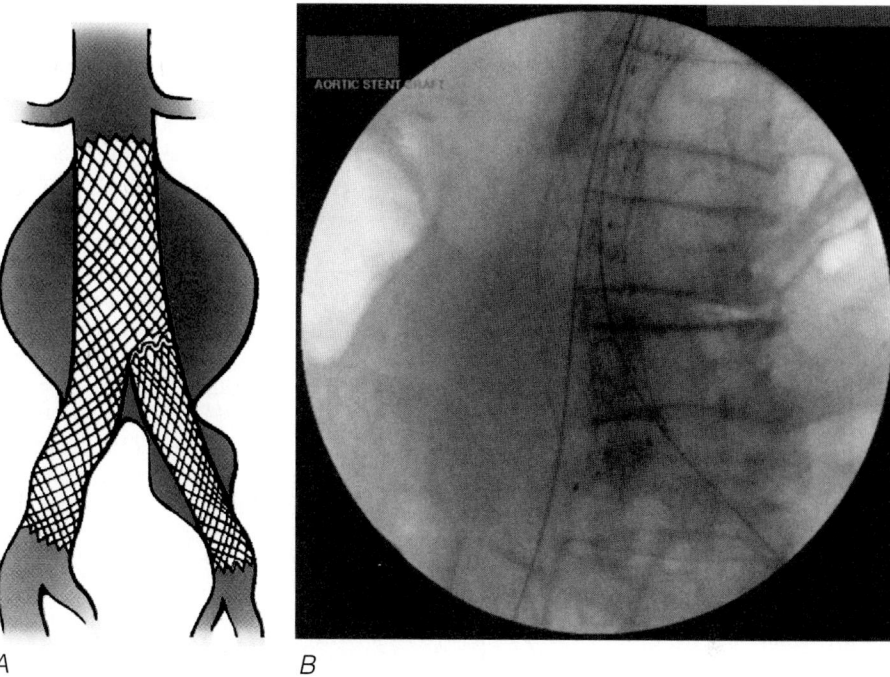

FIG. 22-40. *A.* Completion deployment of the bifurcated aortoiliac stent-graft. *B.* Intraoperative fluoroscopy demonstrates fully deployed bifurcated aortoiliac endograft.

A   *B*

to control the profunda femoris, the superficial femoral artery, and the native common femoral artery if it remains open. An interposition piece of Dacron or ePTFE is used to restore continuity. Proximally, it is sewn end-to-end to the previous graft. Distally, the graft usually has to be tailored around both the superficial femoral and profunda femoris arteries.

Iliac Artery Aneurysms

Most iliac aneurysms occur in conjunction with aortic aneurysms and as such are probably degenerative and atherosclerotic in etiology, therefore they are treated during the same operation.

Occasionally, however, isolated common iliac aneurysms are encountered. Internal iliac aneurysm may also be diagnosed, although isolated aneurysms of the external iliac artery are rare.

Common iliac aneurysms are often diagnosed incidentally, but can present with rupture or abdominal pain. Rare presentation includes the development of a fistula with the adjacent iliac vein or due to compression of the iliac vein. Iliac aneurysms greater than 3 cm should be treated. Treatment options include open surgical replacement with prosthetic graft or endovascular stent grafting. In patients with suitable anatomy, namely the presence of proximal and distal landing zones, stent grafting has become the treatment of choice.

FIG. 22-41. Alternate applications for endografts.

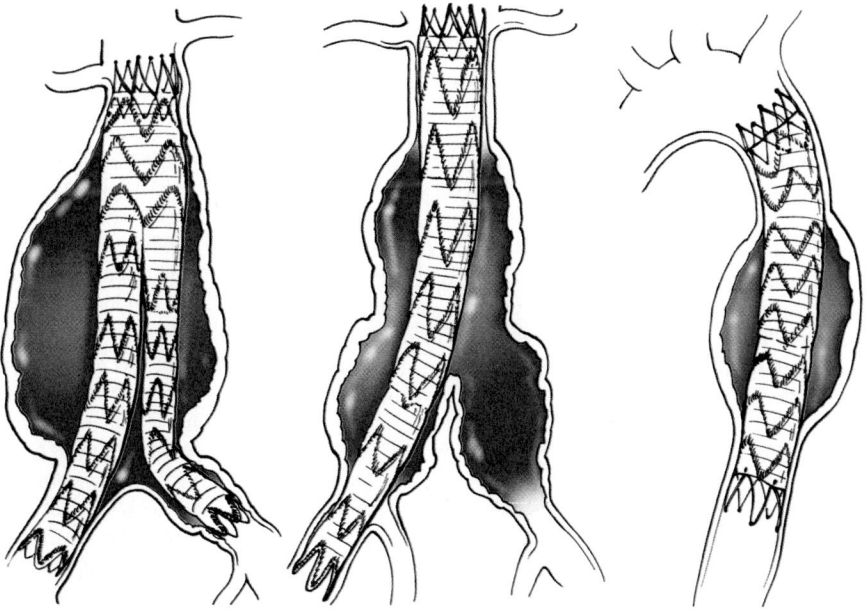

ENDOLEAK CLASSIFICATION

TYPE I   Attachment Site Leak
TYPE II   Lumbar or IMA Endoleak
TYPE III Junctional Leak (junctions
          of overlapping segments)
TYPE IV   Transgraft

A

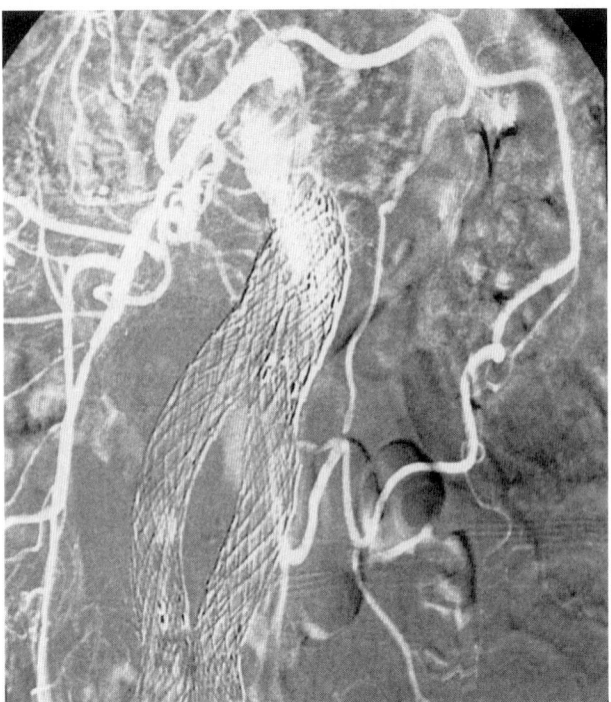

B

FIG. 22-42. *A. Endoleak classification. B. Type II endoleak via superior mesenteric artery–inferior mesenteric artery collateralization.*

Internal iliac artery aneurysms (Fig. 22-48) may be palpable on rectal examination. They are frequently bilateral and are treated by proximal ligation with opening of the aneurysm and oversewing of the distal branches. Because the distal end of the aneurysm may be located deep in the pelvis, an emerging approach is embolization and stent grafting across the orifice of the hypogastric. Although unilateral sacrifice of a hypogastric is well tolerated, bilateral ligation can result in pelvic ischemia. Consequently, an attempt should be made to revascularize one hypogastric. Follow-up by CT scanning is essential to ensure that the aneurysm is thrombosed and does not expand.

Popliteal Artery Aneurysms

Popliteal arterial aneurysms are the most common peripheral arterial aneurysms, accounting for 70%, and are commonly bilateral in 50 to 75%. Finding one popliteal aneurysm mandates evaluation of the contralateral popliteal artery, usually with ultrasound. They

are more common in males. These aneurysms present by a process of chronic distal embolization or sudden-onset acute occlusion of the popliteal artery. Consequently the clinical presentation is by development of claudication; chronic foot ischemia; or sudden-onset, limb-threatening, acute ischemia below the knee. Rupture is rare. Frequently a pattern of acute or chronic ischemia occurs, and the presence of chronic embolization of the infrapopliteal vessels can markedly complicate revascularization.[59–64]

Examination reveals a pulsatile mass, which can be massive in the popliteal fossa. Smaller aneurysms may not be palpable. Foot pulses may be diminished if embolization has been occurring. In patients with acute occlusion of the aneurysm or with embolization, many have all the clinical features of acute ischemia. A thrombosed aneurysm may be palpated as a hard mass, and pulsation is absent. Occasionally these aneurysms can be massive, filling the entire popliteal fossa. Large aneurysms compress the adjacent popliteal vein and occasionally present with acute deep venous thrombosis.

Ultrasound is performed when the patient presents electively, and aneurysms greater than 2 cm should be treated. Preoperative angiography (Fig. 22-49) is usually performed in both the acute and elective situation to facilitate treatment planning. MRA and duplex mapping are gaining in popularity. It is important to adequately demonstrate the run-off vessels because of the propensity of the aneurysms to chronically embolize and occlude the tibial and peroneal arteries. In the presence of limb-threatening ischemia, revascularization is undertaken emergently.

All aneurysms greater than 2 cm are repaired.[65,66] The approach is entirely dependent upon two factors: degree of ischemia and the ability to demonstrate distal target vessels for revascularization. Where no run-off is identifiable, the approach is to attempt thrombolysis via a catheter placed into, and ideally through, the aneurysm. Lytic agents are then infused in an attempt to open up the tibial vessels and permit a bypass graft to be created.[67–70] Alternately, surgical exploration is performed of the distal popliteal artery, and all three trifurcation vessels should be dissected and controlled. Fogarty embolectomy catheters (no. 3) are gently passed down each artery, inflated, and the thrombus removed. Once outflow is established, revascularization is performed as described for elective popliteal arterial aneurysms below. Completion angiography should be performed. Consideration should be given to fasciotomy in patients with severe ischemia.

In the elective situation in which target outflow vessels are evident, two approaches are open to the surgeon: medial and posterior. With a medial approach, incisions are made above and below the knee. Through the superior incision, the distal superficial femoral artery (SFA) is isolated (most popliteal aneurysms do not extend into the SFA), and the distal popliteal is controlled at its bifurcation. A reversed saphenous vein graft is tunneled from the superior to the inferior incision, and end-to-side anastomoses are created. The popliteal artery is then ligated distal and proximal to the bypass graft. One disadvantage of this incision is that up to 15% of aneurysms can continue to expand due to pressure from the geniculate arteries. However, risk of injury to the tibial and common peroneal nerves is minimal, and most surgeons are familiar with this approach.

The posterior approach (e.g., patient prone, foot supported on a pillow) is useful for smaller aneurysms limited to the midpopliteal artery or for exploring aneurysms which have continued to expand after ligation and bypass. A Z-type incision is made centered on the skin crease, with the superior arm extending medially toward the adductor hiatus. The common peroneal nerve courses along the superolateral margin of the popliteal fossa and must be carefully avoided. An endoaneurysmorrhaphy (Fig. 22-50) is easily

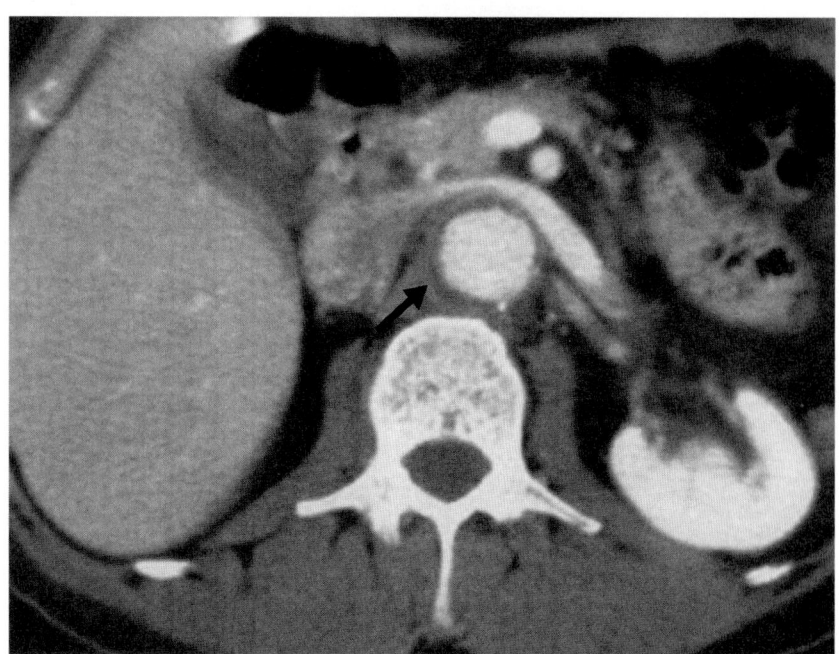

FIG. 22-43. Juxtarenal *(arrow)* aneurysm with thrombus in the neck. This precludes sealing of the endograft.

performed by opening the aneurysm, oversewing tributaries, and placing an interposition reversed saphenous vein graft.

Femoral Artery Aneurysms

Femoral arterial aneurysms (FAAs) are uncommon aneurysms that are usually diagnosed after noting a pulsatile mass in the groin. They occur in elderly men, often with other manifestations of atherosclerosis. One third are bilateral and nearly two thirds are associated with aneurysms elsewhere (e.g., popliteal and aortic). Ultrasound is used to confirm the diagnosis, and although most are considered atherosclerotic in etiology, mycotic femoral arterial aneurysms are encountered, particularly in intravenous drug abusers.[71]

Femoral aneurysms can reach a large size and via thrombosis can create symptoms such as limb-threatening ischemia, embolization, or skin erosion; however, rupture is rarely encountered. FAAs are often asymptomatic, but local pain, distal embolization, rupture, and venous compression may all be presenting features.

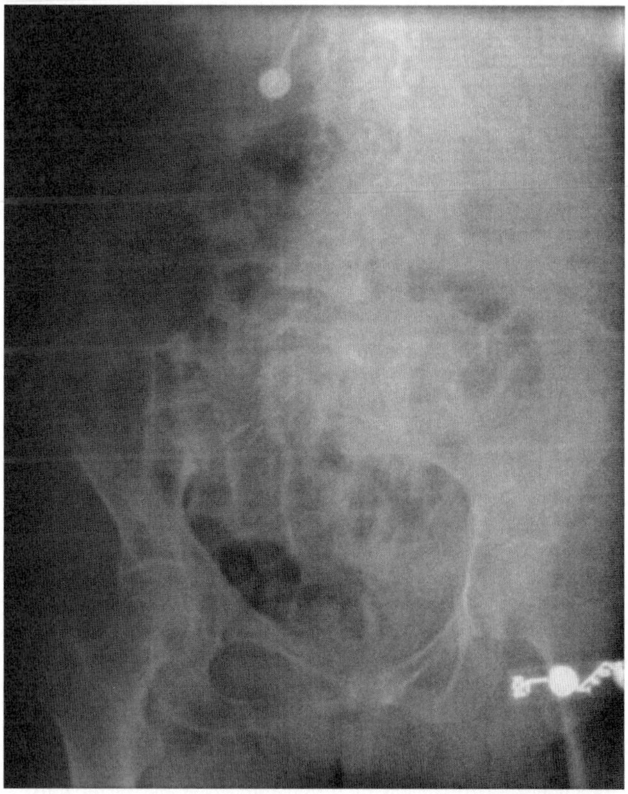

FIG. 22-44. Large, left-sided soft tissue shadow representing a contained retroperitoneal hematoma.

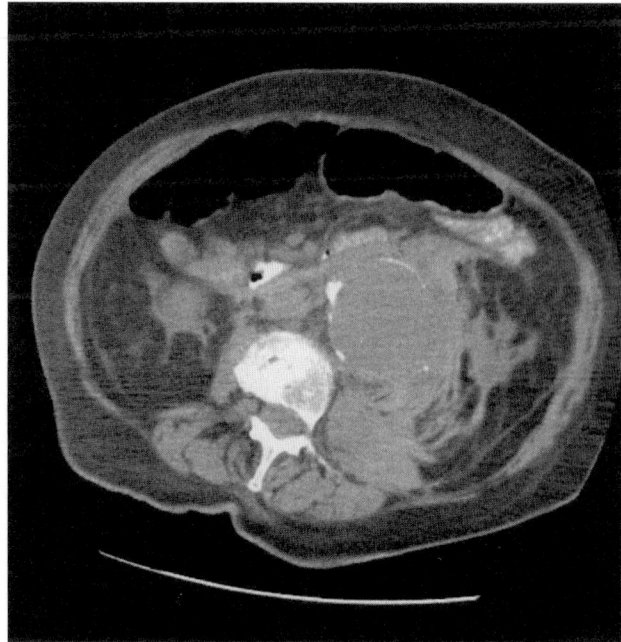

FIG. 22-45. CT scan showing an abdominal aortic aneurysm (AAA) with blood infiltrating the soft tissue in the retroperitoneum.

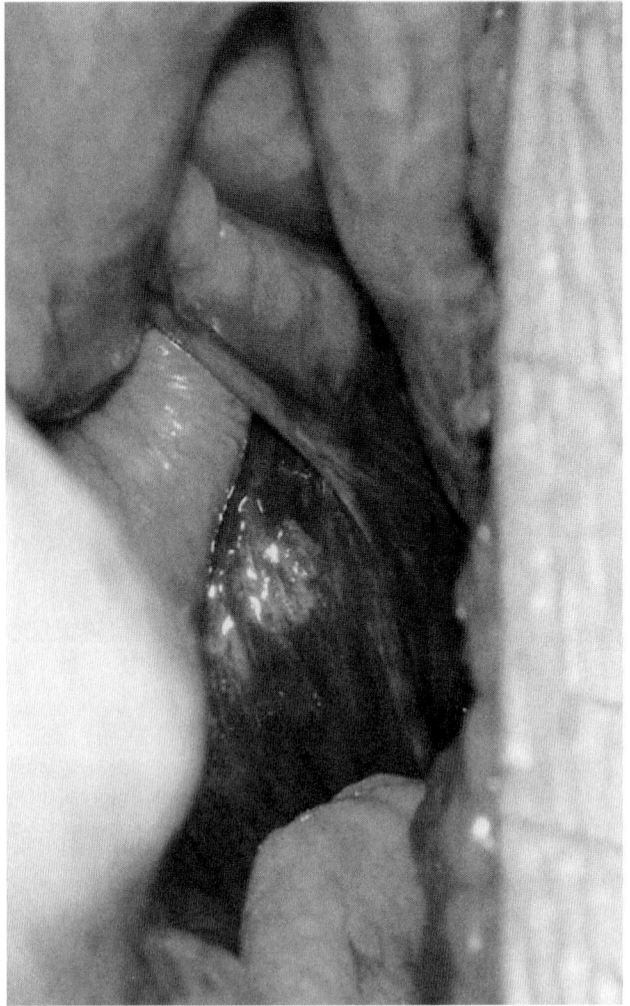

FIG. 22-46. *Large hematoma present in the retroperitoneal space.*

Treatment. All aneurysms greater than 2.5 cm should be treated with resection and interposition grafting. Prosthetic graft (8- to 10-mm Dacron or ePTFE) can be used in most cases, although reversed saphenous vein graft should be used for mycotic aneurysms. The aneurysm most often is confined to the common femoral artery, terminating at its bifurcation; however, it can extend to the superficial femoral artery, the profunda femoris, or both. When the profunda is involved, a side limb or reimplantation of the profunda into the graft is required for repair. In severe groin infections, obturator bypass should be considered to route the vein graft away from the area of sepsis, because vein blow-out can occur with ongoing infection.

Hepatic Artery Aneurysms

Hepatic arterial aneurysms (HAAs) compose 20% of splanchnic arterial aneurysms, which as a group are increasing in incidence. This is most likely as a result of a shift in etiologic factors and increased diagnostic opportunities.[72] Although not well-defined, the natural history of HAAs typically results in enlargement, rupture, and life-threatening hemorrhage. Hence, heightened clinical suspicion with conclusive diagnosis and effective treatment are imperative in the successful management of patients with these aneurysms.[73–75]

The true incidence of HAAs cannot be ascertained, but data from these authors' series indicate that HAAs are being encountered with increasing frequency.[76] This development may be due to a combination of several factors that include augmented referral patterns, enhanced clinical awareness, improved imaging techniques, and the result of a possible shift in etiology.[77,78] Traditionally, atherosclerosis has been the most common cause of HAAs, although there remain reservations about whether it is the primary process. Atherosclerotic aneurysms comprised the majority of early HAAs in the series, but an increased number of HAAs discovered in the later years were secondary to trauma or were of iatrogenic origin (50% of aneurysms in the last 6 years). Mycotic lesions were probably the single most common cause of HAAs at the start of the century, but gradually diminished in incidence and became rare by the late 1970s. Indeed, there was only one mycotic aneurysm in the series, but there is concern that these aneurysms, particularly in association with endocarditis, may reappear with increasing frequency due to the current rise in intravenous substance abuse and/or the prevalence of immunocompromised patients.

Controversy regarding the actual incidence of aneurysmal rupture is apparent, as values range from 20 to 80%. This wide variation is clearly influenced by the inability to detect asymptomatic aneurysms. It is likely that the risk of rupture has been overestimated, since reported data are weighted toward symptomatic and ruptured aneurysms. Hepatic aneurysms may come to attention due to erosion into the biliary tree, the portal vein with development of portal hypertension and its sequelae, or due to rupture into the retroperitoneum or peritoneal cavity.[2] Quincke's classic triad of jaundice, biliary colic, and gastrointestinal bleeding suggests hemobilia, and is reported to occur in one third of patients. In the series, hemobilia was present in six patients, while Quincke's triad was present in only two patients. Bleeding into the general abdominal cavity is a catastrophic event with a reported mortality rate of 82%. These authors have previously reported their experience in the management of hepatic arterioportal fistula. Interruption of the fistula by surgery or embolization leads, in most cases, to resolution of the portal hypertension.

Pseudoaneurysms typically affect younger male individuals and often reflect a traumatic etiology. However, the mean age of patients in this series with pseudoaneurysms was 53 years, which is probably explained by the fact that most of these lesions were the result of surgical trauma and not of societal violence. Also noted was the finding of a higher number of female patients, in contrast to the 2:1 male preponderance often cited in other reports. Again, this additional deviation from predicted values may be due to the increased proportion of pseudoaneurysms secondary to procedures for benign hepatobiliary disease in this series, which is more common in women.

As with other visceral aneurysms, HAAs are recognized for their ability to enlarge asymptomatically and suddenly rupture, causing life-threatening hemorrhage. When present, symptoms and signs are varied, and a high index of suspicion is required. The most common symptom is vague right-sided or epigastric abdominal pain, as demonstrated in 41% of patients. It is unclear, however, how pain correlates with the state of the aneurysm and whether it heralds impending rupture. Nevertheless, it serves the purpose of directing diagnostic efforts towards underlying abnormalities.

Plain abdominal x-rays or upper GI contrast studies may suggest an underlying HAA when a rim of calcification in the right hypochondrium or a smooth filling defect in the duodenum is demonstrated. Ultrasonography and contrast-enhanced CT scanning (Fig. 22-51) will provide the diagnosis in most cases. MRI has been

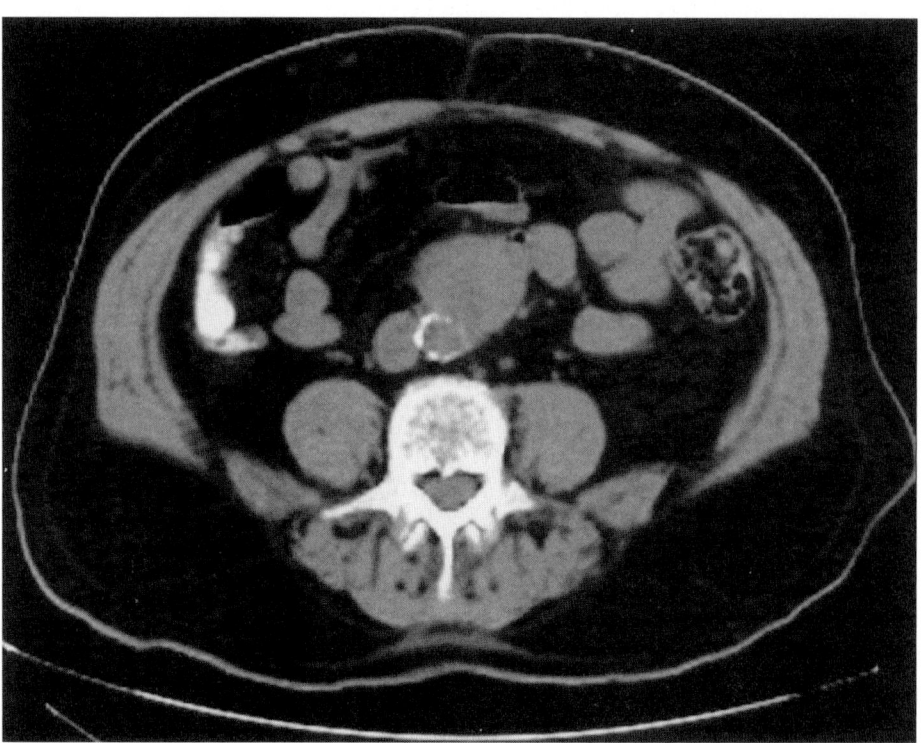

FIG. 22-47. Pseudoaneurysm at proximal anastomosis of aortic graft.

applied to good effect in the diagnosis of HAAs. Color-flow duplex ultrasonography is particularly effective in demonstrating intrahepatic lesions. It also has been used effectively to determine blood flow in some aneurysms, and will demonstrate arterialization of the portal system when a fistula is present. It is also useful to follow up intrahepatic aneurysms that have been embolized, to ensure their continued occlusion. However, the standard preoperative investigation in HAAs is selective angiography (Fig. 22-52). This modality defines the location of the lesion and its collateral pathways. If the

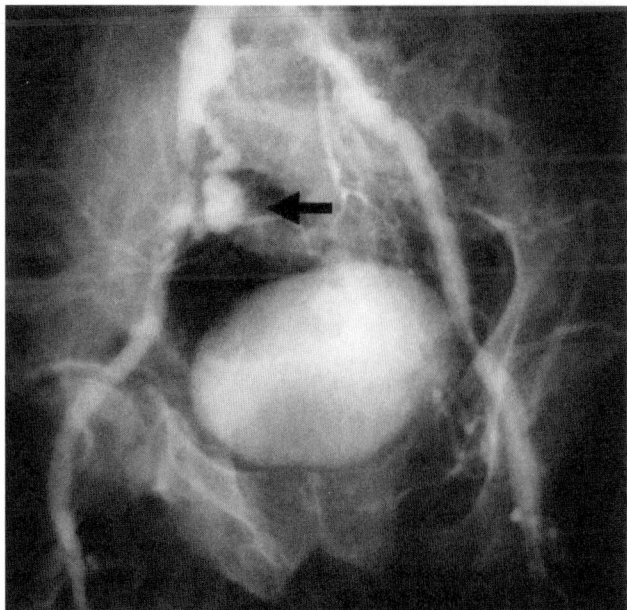

FIG. 22-48. Internal iliac artery aneurysm demonstrated by angiography.

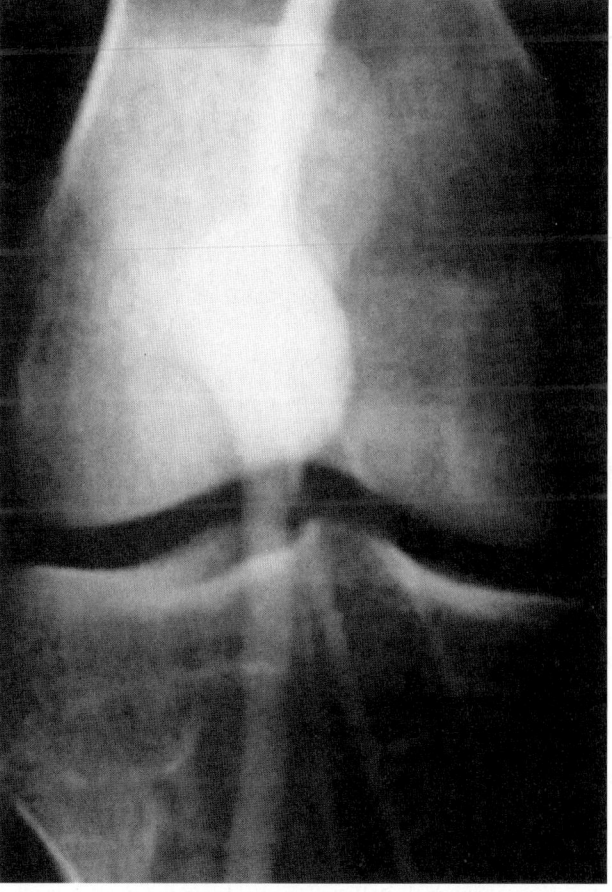

FIG. 22-49. Angiogram showing a popliteal artery aneurysm.

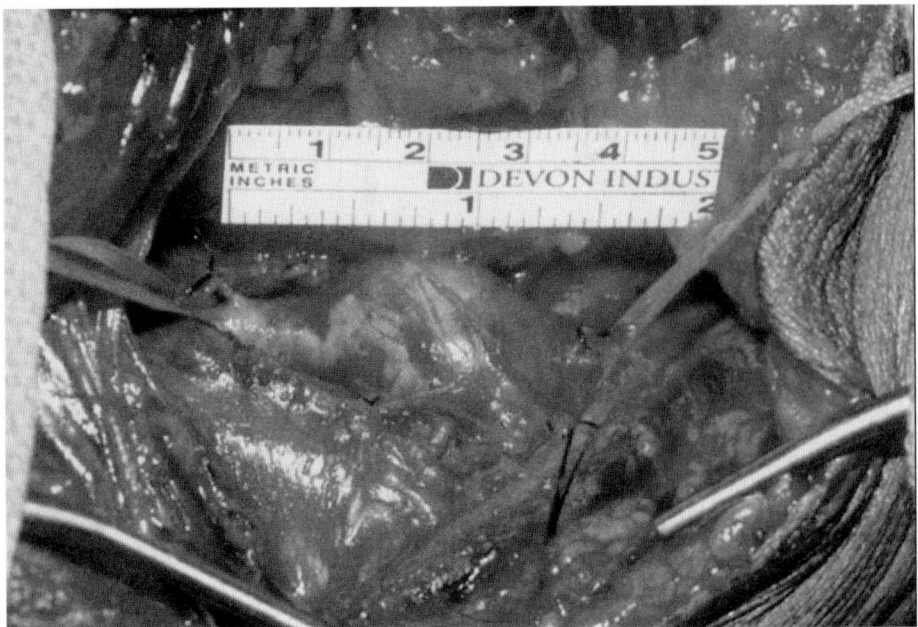

A

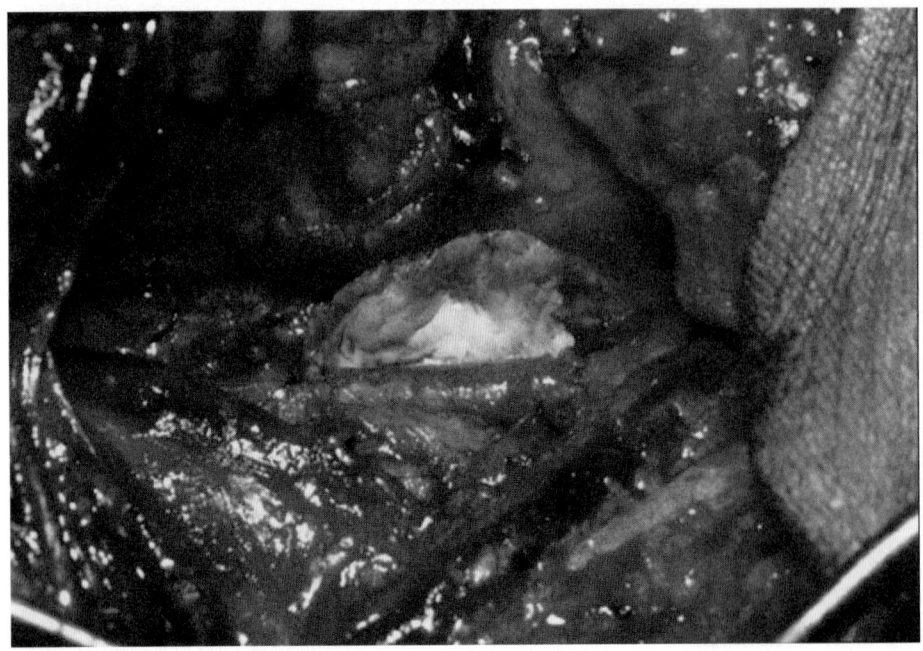

B

FIG. 22-50. *A*. Posterior exposure of popliteal artery aneurysm. *B*. The aneurysm has been opened and a reversed saphenous vein graft interposed.

gastroduodenal artery is not visualized, a superior mesenteric artery and/or left gastric artery injection should be performed. This procedure is valuable in the planning of surgical strategies for proximal aneurysms. It is likely, however, that spiral CT angiography or magnetic resonance angiography will become the studies of choice in the future.

Unless severe comorbidities disqualify the patient, all extrahepatic aneurysms greater than 2 cm in diameter should be treated. Usually these are atherosclerotic true aneurysms which are treated surgically. These patients have all the comorbidities associated with cardiovascular disease. Pseudoaneurysms, most of which are

intrahepatic and can be successfully embolized, are treated when greater than 1 cm.

In general, treatment options are largely determined by the anatomic location of the aneurysm. Extrahepatic aneurysms warrant surgical treatment, except in high-risk patients and in saccular aneurysms. Common HAAs (Fig. 22-53) (i.e., those proximal to a patent gastroduodenal artery) may be ligated and excised, as the liver will continue to receive arterial blood via collaterals such as the pancreaticoduodenal and gastroduodenal arteries (Fig. 22-54). However, the response of liver parenchyma to hepatic artery ligation is unpredictable. Countryman and associates suggest temporary

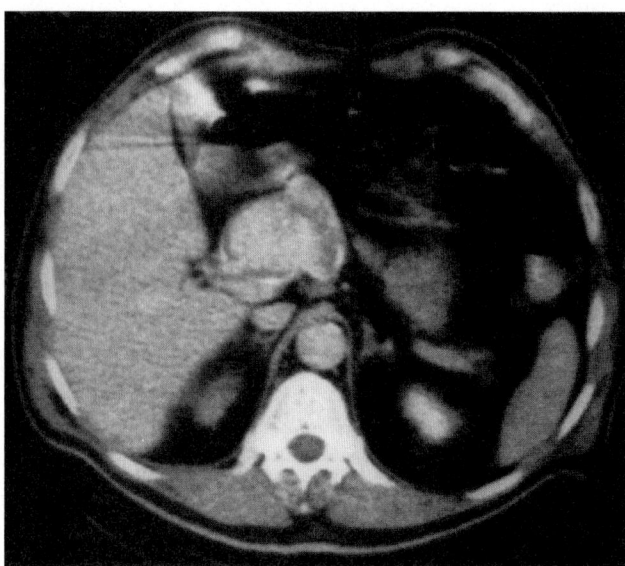

FIG. 22-51. CT scan showing a large hepatic artery aneurysm.

clamping of the hepatic artery with inspection of the liver for any change in color before definitive ligation.[73] Intraoperative Doppler ultrasonography performed pre- and postclamping is also used to help predict any subsequent compromise. In contrast, Dougherty and colleagues recommend vascular reconstruction at all times in low-risk patients.[74] Indeed, one patient in the series conducted by these authors unexpectedly sustained an area of central liver necrosis following ligation of a proximal aneurysm. If easily performed, it is recommended to reconstruct with reversed saphenous vein grafts.

As a rule, extrahepatic aneurysms involving the hepatic artery propria will need vascular reconstruction (Fig. 22-55). Simple ligation of the hepatic artery propria at sites beyond the gastroduodenal artery will probably result in significant liver ischemia. The

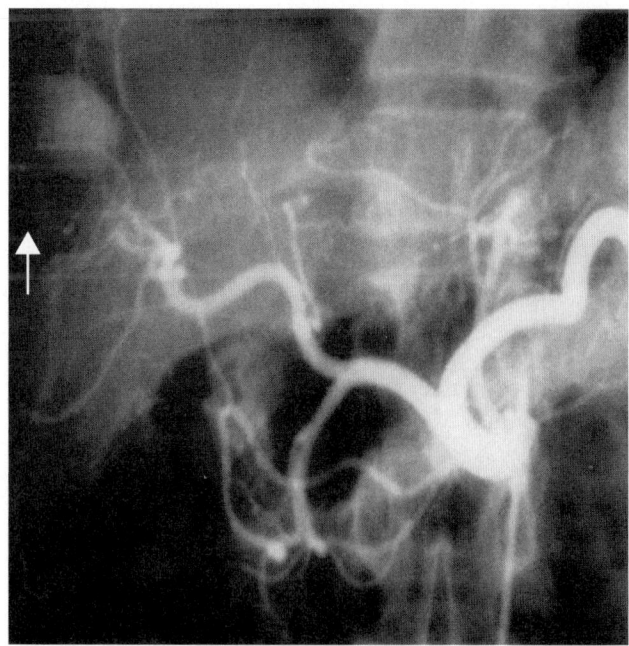

FIG. 22-52. Hepatic artery pseudoaneurysm (*arrow*).

COMMON HEPATIC ANEURYSMS

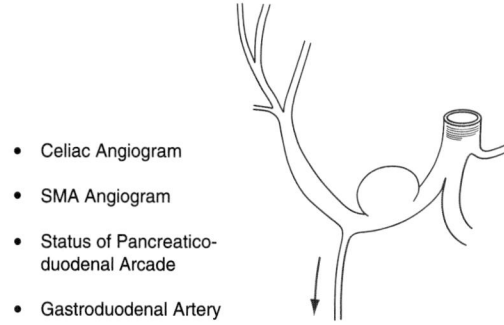

- Celiac Angiogram
- SMA Angiogram
- Status of Pancreatico-duodenal Arcade
- Gastroduodenal Artery

FIG. 22-53. Common hepatic artery aneurysms. It is important to demonstrate adequacy of the pancreaticoduodenal arcade by selective celiac and superior mesenteric artery (SMA) angiography.

preferred conduit in these procedures is the reversed autogenous saphenous vein graft.

Until the advent of transcatheter embolization, most intrahepatic HAAs inevitably warranted resection with relevant liver tissue. These hepatic resection procedures caused considerable morbidity, and in the authors' series, resulted in the formation of one postlobectomy abscess.[76] Successful percutaneous embolization was first reported in 1977, and several reports have been published that support the use of this technique.[79,80] An advantage of selective arterial embolization is its precision in limiting hepatic devascularization. It is of particular value in cases of posttraumatic pseudoaneurysms, and due to its lower morbidity, represents an attractive option in high-risk patients. A total of eight patients in the series underwent embolization. Percutaneous embolization has become the preferred method of treating intrahepatic aneurysms. The natural history of embolized aneurysms is unknown, but there is potential for recanalization and repeat aneurysmal formation. In the same series, three patients (42% of embolized patients) developed early recanalization, but were re-embolized without difficulty to achieve total aneurysmal occlusion. However, this serves to emphasize that follow-up imaging of the aneurysm is necessary following embolization. If the aneurysm has been effectively imaged by color-flow duplex, then this would be the follow-up modality of choice; otherwise repeat angiography is necessary. Table 22-7 summarizes recommended therapy for hepatic artery aneurysms.

COMMON HEPATIC ANEURYSMS

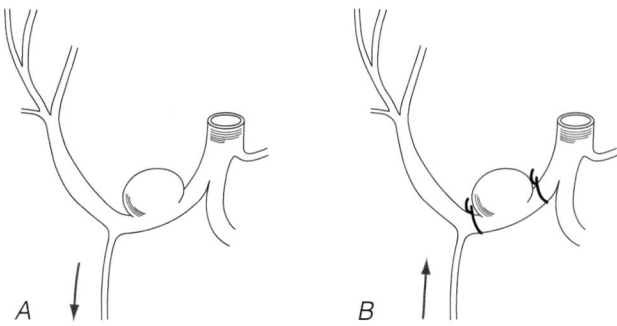

FIG. 22-54. *A.* Common hepatic artery aneurysms. *B.* Simple ligation will reverse flow in the pancreaticoduodenal arcade if it is patent, providing arterial supply to the liver.

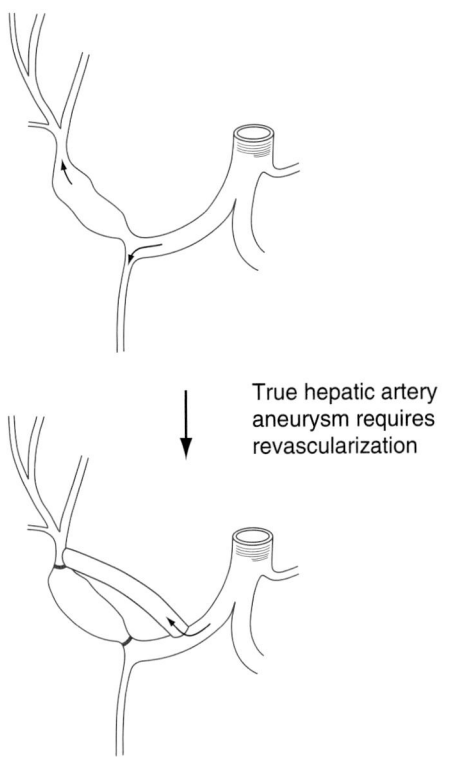

True hepatic artery aneurysm requires revascularization

FIG. 22-55. Extrahepatic aneurysm involving the hepatic artery requires revascularization.

Splenic Artery Aneurysms

The reported incidence of splenic arterial aneurysms (SAA) varies from 1.6% in an unselected autopsy population to 7.1% in autopsies performed on patients with cirrhotic portal hypertension. However, with increasing use of visceral angiography, Doppler ultrasound, and computed tomography, these lesions are being detected with greater frequency. Early reports documented a high risk (10%) of rupture, but more contemporary series suggest that this risk has been overestimated. They indicate that rupture rates are closer to 2%. Nevertheless, rupture does occur, and certain high-risk-groups can be identified. Although surgery has been the traditional method of treatment, percutaneous embolization has gained popularity.

The precise mechanism of aneurysmal dilatation of the splenic artery is unknown, but views have not changed markedly since the

Table 22-7
Recommended Therapy for Hepatic Artery Aneurysms

Site	Treatment
Intrahepatic	Embolization
Hepatic artery proper	Surgery
Good-risk candidate	Observation <2 cm diameter
Poor-risk candidate	Surgery >2 cm diameter
Saccular aneurysms	Embolization
Common hepatic artery	
Good-risk candidate	Aneurysmectomy
Poor-risk candidate	Embolization
Hepatic arterioportal fistula	
Intrahepatic	Embolization
Extrahepatic	Surgery, intra-aneurysmal oversewing of venous communicants

proposals published by Trimble and Hill in 1942. They identified two factors that were involved: preliminary weakness of the arterial wall, and a consecutive rise in blood pressure. Fibromuscular dysplasia is a recognized etiologic factor that is readily demonstrated by angiography. Stanley and Fry demonstrated internal elastic lamina disruption and diminution of elastic fibers in the SAAs of multiparous women. They suggested that pre-existing fibrodysplasia, in association with repeated pregnancies that cause increased intravascular volume and portal congestion, may promote aneurysmal dilatation. Furthermore, hormonal effects of pregnancy, particularly those of relaxin, may further weaken the arterial wall. This set of conditions also is present in patients with liver disease and portal hypertension with splenomegaly, in whom the incidence of SAA is reported to be as high as 20%.

The splenic artery is the visceral vessel that is most likely to develop pseudoaneurysms. These lesions occur either from disruption of the vessel wall as a result of the direct action of elastase and other digestive enzymes released by the inflamed pancreas, or due to penetrating or blunt trauma. In contrast to true aneurysms, pseudoaneurysms, particularly those secondary to pancreatitis, may be extremely fragile and are more likely to be a source of bleeding. These lesions, therefore, tend to be symptomatic and will have readily distinguishable etiologic factors. The finding of a "cyst within a cyst" on CT scan is suggestive of a pseudoaneurysm within a pseudocyst, but as in true SAAs, the most valuable investigative modality remains visceral angiography. In view of the expected difficulties with the operative approach, transcatheter embolization is the treatment of choice for pseudoaneurysms.

Symptoms and Signs. Symptoms and clinical findings are rare in SAAs. The overwhelming majority of patients in the series were asymptomatic. The aneurysms were discovered incidentally in the course of managing associated conditions, which were primarily the manifestations of portal hypertension. Chronic vague epigastric and left hypochondrial pain may be reported. The development of acute left upper quadrant pain indicates that rupture may have occurred, especially when signs of hypovolemia are present. Two patients in the series who were not previously diagnosed presented in this manner and received emergency treatment. Their aneurysms had ruptured. There are no reliable physical signs that indicate the presence of an SAA.[81–84]

Investigations. The presence of an SAA may be suspected with the appearance of calcification in a corresponding area on a KUB x-ray (Fig. 22-56). Most aneurysms reported in the literature were initially detected as calcified ring shadows on abdominal x-rays.

Contrast-enhanced CT scanning (Fig. 22-57) is valuable in demonstrating size and location of these aneurysms. Angiography confirms the diagnosis, delineates the location and number of these aneurysms, and assists in determining whether an endovascular or open surgical approach should be selected.

Treatment. Although there are no absolute determinants of impending rupture, several factors are important in the decision-making process for the interventional treatment of patients with SAAs. Sudden left upper quadrant pain usually indicates rupture has occurred, and clearly, any patient in this situation should undergo emergency surgery, particularly when signs of hypovolemia are present. About 25 to 30% of these patients may spontaneously stabilize, albeit temporarily. Sudden circulatory collapse and death usually ensues within 48 hours in untreated cases. These are the recognized features of the "double rupture" phenomenon in which

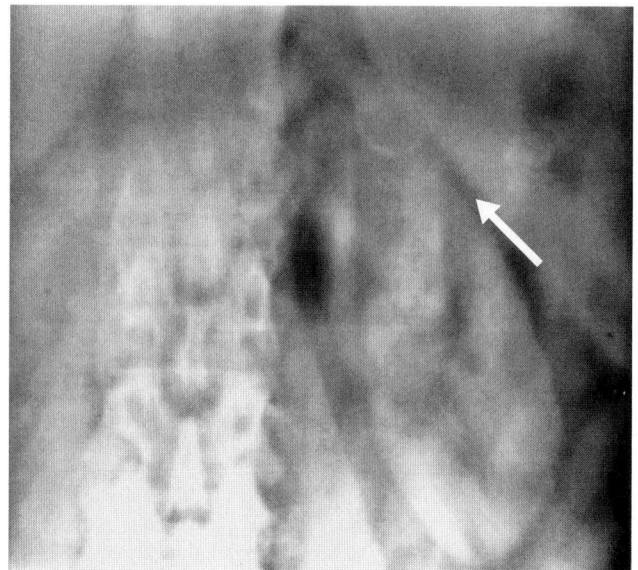

A

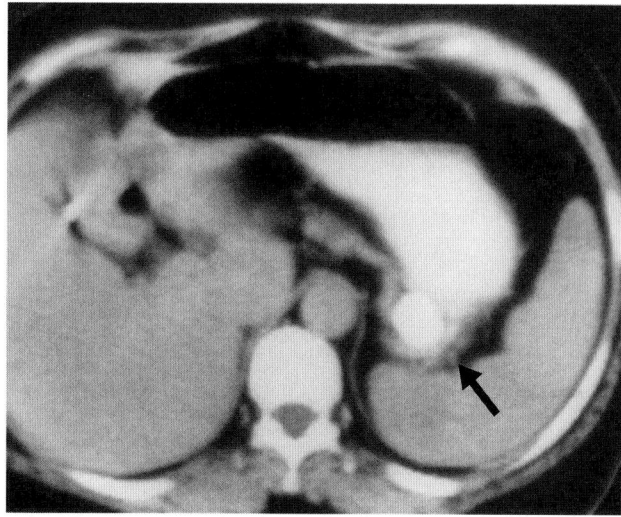

A

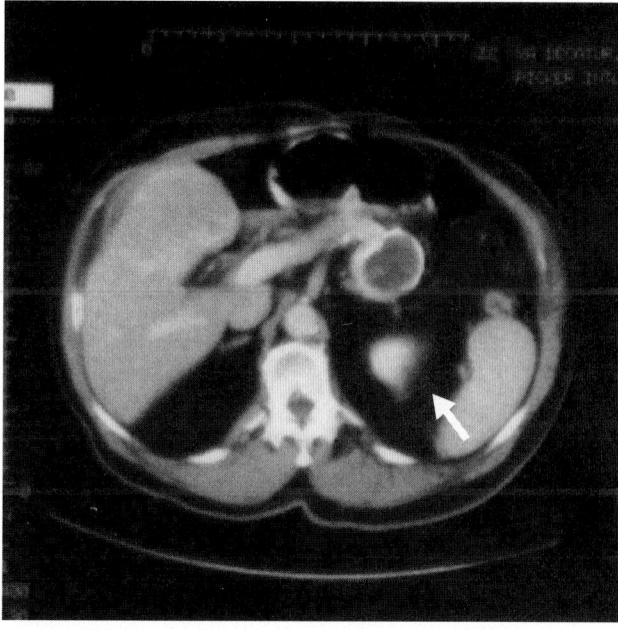

B

B

FIG. 22-56. *A.* Calcified ring shadow in left upper quadrant on renal tomogram *(arrow). B.* Calcified ring shadow seen in a barium swallow study.

FIG. 22-57. *A.* CT scan showing a proximal calcified splenic artery aneurysms *(arrow). B.* CT scan showing a distal calcified splenic artery aneurysm *(arrow).*

initial aneurysmal bleeding tamponades in the lesser sac, followed by inevitable flooding into the general peritoneal cavity.

There is a general consensus that women anticipating pregnancy should have surgical treatment, and patients with symptomatic aneurysms should be promptly treated. Although widely recommended, the indications for treating aneurysms that are larger than 2 cm are less definite.

The preservation of the spleen should be a consideration, although this may prove impossible in distal and intrasplenic aneurysms. Unfortunately, 70% of SAAs in patients with portal hypertension will be in this category, and one half of these aneurysms

will be of the multiple variety. The recommended procedure for more proximally situated aneurysms is exclusion of the lesion with proximal and distal ligation of the splenic artery. Occasionally, opening the aneurysm to oversew feeding vessels from within the lesion may be necessary. Distal ligation is mandatory to prevent back-filling of the aneurysm from the abundantly supplied spleen. Excision of the aneurysm is the operation of choice for middle-third lesions.

Successful endoscopic ligation has been reported. Percutaneous embolization with Gianturco coils and gelfoam sponges has been reported with favorable results[85–89] (Fig. 22-58).

Reports of ruptured SAAs following liver transplantation are appearing with increasing frequency. Ayalon recommends ligating the splenic artery in all patients undergoing orthotopic liver transplant who have documented SAAs.

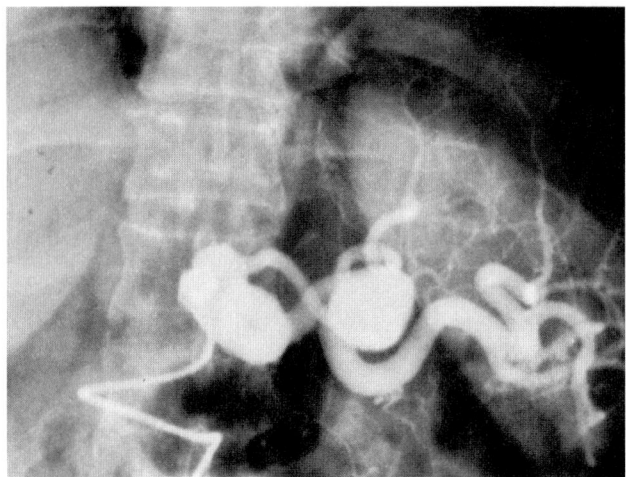

A

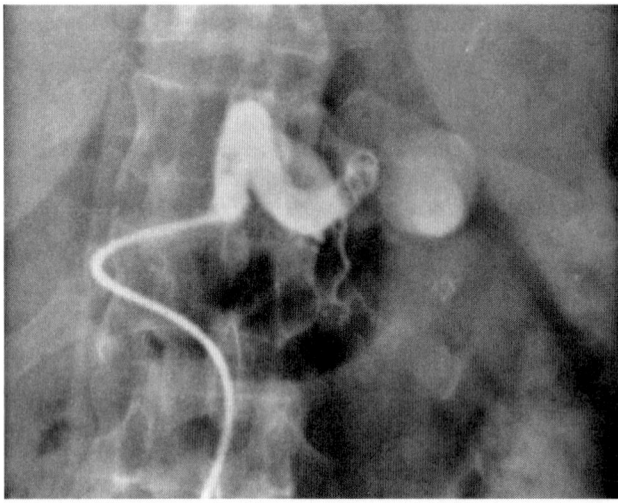

B

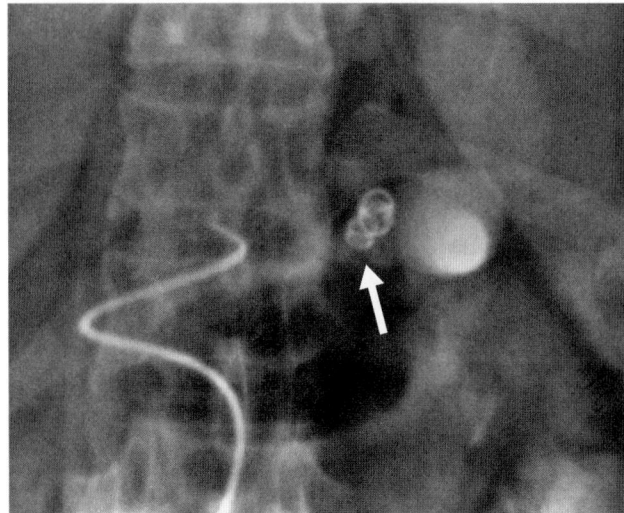

C

FIG. 22-58. *A, B,* and *C.* Embolization of two splenic artery aneurysms using coils (*arrow*).

Renal Artery Aneurysms

The incidence of renal arterial aneurysms (RAAs) is estimated to be between 0.09 and 0.7% of the population. The incidence rises to 2.5% among patients evaluated for hypertension, and is 9.2% among patients with fibromuscular disease (FMD) involving the renal artery. Complications are uncommon but can include renovascular hypertension; renal infarction from embolization, dissection, or thrombosis; and arteriovenous fistula formation.[90]

Etiologies are numerous, but FMD and congenital causes are the most common. Poststenotic dilation, false aneurysms, aneurysms secondary to renal artery dissections, inflammatory aneurysms, and arteritis-induced aneurysms also have been described.

Renal artery aneurysms are slightly more common in women than men and more frequently affect the right than the left renal artery, an observation reported previously and confirmed in this report. This sex and site predilection reflects the increased frequency of FMD in women and its occurrence in the right renal artery. Most renal arterial aneurysms are saccular, average 1.3 cm in diameter, and develop at the primary or secondary renal artery bifurcations (Fig. 22-59).

Hypertension may be both caused by and causative of renal artery aneurysms, as it is associated with up to 70 to 80% of cases. Preexisting hypertension in those patients with congenital defects of the internal elastic lamina and media may predispose to aneurysm formation. The mechanism of hypertension induction by renal artery aneurysms may be occult stenoses, arterial compression, parenchymal embolization, branch vessel compromise, or arteriovenous fistula. The detection of an aneurysm with significant hypertension is generally regarded as an indication for repair, even in the absence of demonstrable stenosis. However, without a lateralizing serum renin level, successful repair may occur in the absence of significant improvement in hypertension.

The true risk of rupture for renal arterial aneurysms has been overestimated. Early reports noted up to a 24% rupture rate, with occurrence most likely in those patients with aneurysms greater than 2 cm. More recent, larger series have refuted this finding, with one study in which 28 patients were followed for a mean of 36 months reporting no occurrence of ruptures.

A disproportionate number of ruptures have occurred in pregnancy, with more than 19 cases reported. Most occur in the third trimester, although not associated with labor, and have a 70% maternal mortality rate and near 100% fetal mortality rate. Most renal artery aneurysms occurring in pregnancy are situated within the left kidney, in contrast to aneurysms in the nonpregnant state, which are more common on the right. Due to the increased rupture risk and high morbidity and mortality, it is widely held that aneurysms detected in women planning pregnancy should be repaired prophylactically.

Management options include observation, transcatheter occlusion, or surgical intervention. Indications for intervention include aneurysm size greater than 2.5 cm, renovascular hypertension with lateralizing serum renin level, symptomatic aneurysms, documented expansion, renal embolization, and young women anticipating pregnancy (Table 22-8).

Embolization is particularly useful in patients with saccular aneurysms; small, bleeding aneurysms in patients with arteritis; and in high-risk patients. Transcatheter embolization is also the treatment of choice for intraparenchymal lesions.

Aneurysmectomy and arteriorrhaphy with or without patch angioplasty is the simplest method of aneurysm resection with reconstitution of the renal artery. It is most easily applied to saccular

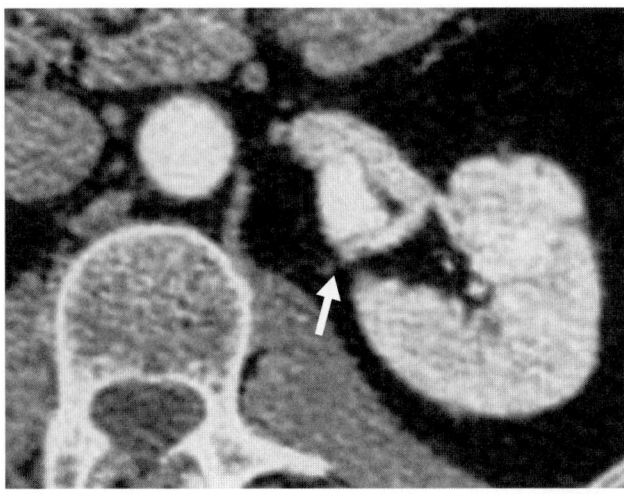

A

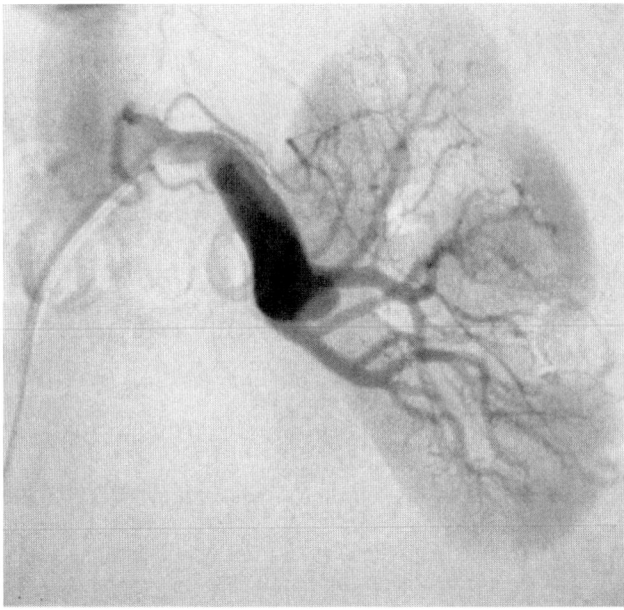

B

FIG. 22-59. A and B. Examples of renal artery aneurysms (arrow).

aneurysms with a narrow neck on the patent artery. Ligation and bypass are appropriately applied to fusiform aneurysms. Opening of the aneurysm with oversewing of feeding vessels from within the sac is optimal to preclude progressive enlargement of a ligated aneurysm. This technique may also be appropriately applied to closure of an arteriovenous fistula from within the aneurysm sac. When

Table 22-8
Indications for Repair of Renal Artery Aneurysms

Aneurysm >2.5 cm diameter
Renovascular hypertension with lateralizing renins
Symptomatic aneurysms
Aneurysms in women planning pregnancy
Aneurysm with distal embolization

there are multiple aneurysms, aneurysm associated with an abnormal renal artery (i.e., FMD or dissection), or there is intraparenchymal involvement, ex vivo repair with hypothermic perfusion is desirable.

If an observant approach is selected, then attentive, lifelong follow-up is necessary. Contrast-enhanced CT scanning is the imaging modality of choice. The patient should be instructed that flank pain or hematuria should prompt immediate evaluation. Blood pressure should be monitored, and development of hypertension will require arteriography.

ACUTE ARTERIAL OCCLUSION

One of the most common vascular emergencies is acute lower extremity ischemia; however, sudden-onset acute occlusion of any major vessel (e.g., mesenteric, renal, or upper extremity) presents with severe symptoms, which reflect ischemia in the organ supplied by those vessels. Arteries that undergo slow progressive occlusion permit the development of collaterals such that patients may be asymptomatic or lack the severe symptoms associated with acute ischemia. In the absence of collaterals, however, acute ischemia can result in nonreversible changes within the target organ within hours. Consequently, expeditious relief of the obstruction is mandatory, as well as revascularization of ischemic tissue, resulting in swelling and edema within the target tissues, and washout of lactic acid, myoglobin, and potassium. The vascular surgeon must know how to manage both the local and systemic effects of this postrevascularization syndrome.

Arterial Embolism

Cardiac Sources

The heart is the most common source of distal emboli (70%). Atrial fibrillation with dilated noncontractile atrial appendages is the most common source. Sudden cardioversion results in the appendage regaining contractile activity, which can dislodge the contained thrombus. Other cardiac sources include mural thrombus overlying a myocardial infarction, or thrombus forming within a dilated left ventricular aneurysm. Mural thrombi can also develop within a ventricle dilated by cardiomyopathy. Emboli which arise from a ventricular aneurysm or from a dilated cardiomyopathy can be very large and are the most common cause of a saddle embolus, an embolus that lodges at the aortic bifurcation and renders both legs ischemic.

Diseased valves are another source of distal embolization (Fig. 22-60). Historically, this was from rheumatic heart disease. Currently, subacute and acute bacterial endocarditis are the more common causes, as infected emboli can infect the recipient vessel wall, creating mycotic aneurysms.

Lower Extremity Acute Ischemia

Clinical Manifestations. Acute lower extremity ischemia manifests with the "five Ps": *p*ain, *p*allor (Fig. 22-61), *p*aresthesias, *p*aralysis, and *p*ulselessness, to which some add a sixth "P"— *p*oikilothermia or "*p*erishing cold." Pain, however, is what causes a patient to present to the emergency room. The most common location for an embolus to lodge in the leg is at the common femoral bifurcation. Typically a patient will complain of foot and calf pain. In addition to absent pulses, there is a variable diminution of sensation, which varies from a mild reduction in sensation compared to the contralateral side to being completely insensate. Inability to move

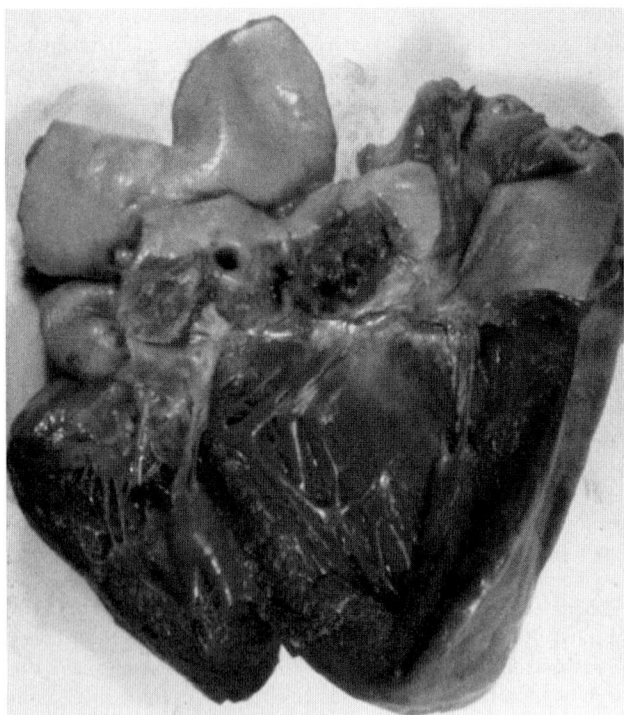

FIG. 22-60. Valvular vegetations occur from subacute bacterial endo-carditis.

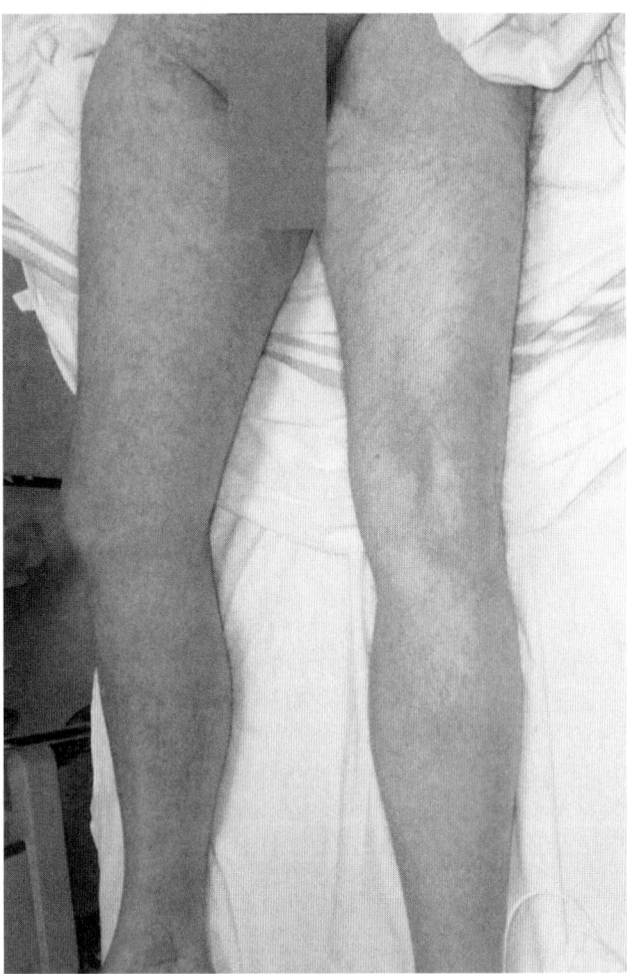

FIG. 22-61. Typical pallor in an acutely ischemic limb.

the affected muscle group is a sign of very severe ischemia and necessitates urgent revascularization. During evaluation of the affected extremity it is important to compare findings with the contralateral limb. Clinical evaluation is extremely important in determining the etiology and location of the obstruction. One of the most important pieces of information to obtain is whether the patient has had prior vascular procedures or if there is a history of lower extremity claudication. Either of these features suggests pre-existing vascular disease, renders revascularization more complicated, and usually mandates angiography to permit surgical planning. On the contrary, in a patient with no history suggestive of prior vascular disease, the etiology is most likely embolic and simple thrombectomy is more likely to be successful.

Absent bilateral femoral pulses in a patient with bilateral lower extremity ischemia is most likely due to saddle embolus to the aortic bifurcation. A palpable femoral pulse and absent popliteal and distal pulses may either be due to distal common femoral embolus (the pulse being palpable above the level of occlusion) or embolus to the superficial femoral or popliteal arteries. Typically, emboli lodge at bifurcations where there are sudden changes in arterial diameter. A popliteal trifurcation embolus will present with calf ischemia and absent pedal pulses, possibly with a popliteal pulse present. The finding of palpable contralateral pulses in the absence of ipsilateral pulses in the ischemic leg is suggestive of an embolus, even if Doppler signals are present. Arteriography is not necessary in the patient with no history suggestive of vascular disease; nevertheless, all patients should be positioned on the operating room table in such a way that fluoroscopic access to the entire inflow and outflow tract is achievable if necessary. In an era when most vascular surgeons have endovascular capability, it is unacceptable to be unable to easily switch to a catheter-based approach should it become necessary.

Medical Therapy. In the absence of any significant contraindication, the patient with an ischemic lower extremity should

be immediately anticoagulated. This will prevent propagation of the clot into unaffected vascular beds. Intravenous fluid should be started and a Foley catheter inserted to monitor urine output. Baseline labs should be obtained and creatinine levels noted.

Surgery. The abdomen, contralateral groin, and entire lower extremity are prepped in the field. The groin is opened through a vertical incision, exposing the common femoral artery and its bifurcation. Frequently, the location of the embolus at the femoral bifurcation is readily apparent by the presence of a palpable proximal femoral pulse, which disappears distally. The artery is clamped and opened transversely over the bifurcation. Thrombus is extracted by passing a Fogarty balloon embolectomy catheter (Fig. 22-62). Good back-bleeding and antegrade bleeding suggest that the entire clot has been removed (Fig. 22-63). Embolic material often forms a cast of the vessel and is sent for culture and histologic examination. Completion angiography is advisable. The artery is then closed and the patient fully anticoagulated.

When an embolus lodges in the popliteal artery, in most cases it can be extracted via a femoral incision using the techniques previously described. A femoral approach is preferred because the larger arterial size results in a lessened likelihood of arterial compromise when the artery is closed. The disadvantage is that the embolectomy catheter cannot be specifically directed into each of the infrapopliteal arteries. This can be achieved from the groin using fluoroscopic imaging and an over-the-wire thrombectomy catheter, which can be

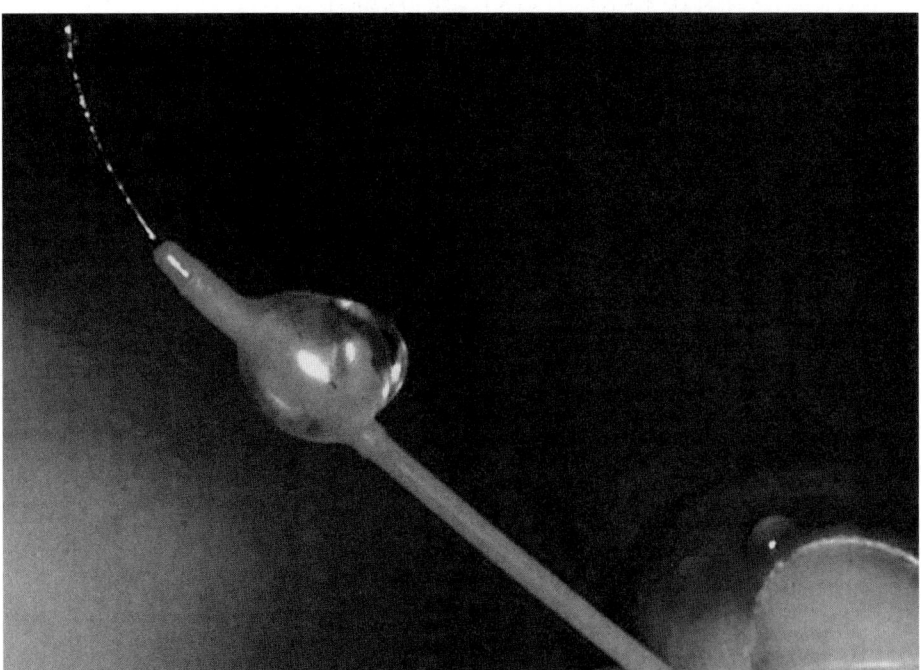

FIG. 22-62. Fogarty balloon embolectomy catheter.

specifically directed into each of the infrapopliteal vessels. Otherwise, a separate incision exposing the popliteal bifurcation may be necessary to ensure completeness of thrombectomy.

In the postoperative period it is important to seek the source of the embolus using echocardiography and CT scanning of the descending thoracic and abdominal aorta. A transthoracic or transesophageal echocardiogram should be performed looking for a cardiac source. An electrocardiogram (ECG) will diagnose atrial fibrillation. More unusual sources include mural thrombus from an aortic aneurysm;

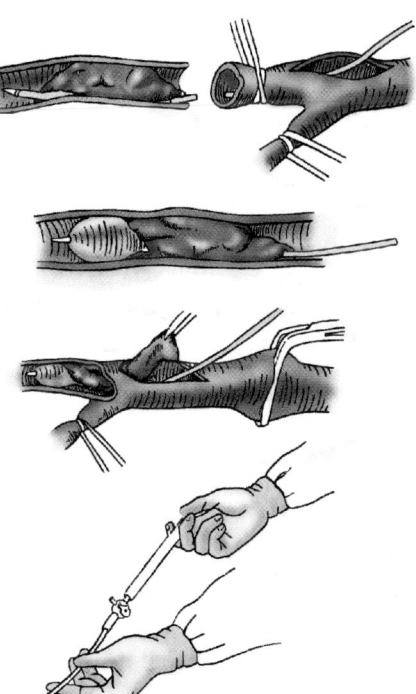

FIG. 22-63. Technique for removal of thrombus using balloon catheter.

occasionally idiopathic arterial-to-arterial thrombus occurs, usually from thrombus that has formed on a grossly normal descending thoracic aorta. The aortic arch may also be a source of embolus from severe atheroma. The presence of mobile plaque on transesophageal echocardiography (TEE) is suggestive of this source. Paradoxical embolus occurs when a patient has a patent foramen ovale and an embolus from a deep venous thrombosis (DVT) crosses through the atrial defect into the left side of the heart and passes into the peripheral circulation. This is diagnosed using a technique termed *bubble echocardiography,* in which air bubbles introduced into the venous circulation can be seen traversing the septal defect.

A more complex situation arises when a patient has pre-existing peripheral vascular disease and in situ thrombosis on top of pre-existing atheroma; frequently embolectomy catheters will not pass through these occlusions. Similarly, when a bypass graft fails, it is usually either due to progression of atheroma proximal or distal to the graft, or to intrinsic stenoses that develop within a vein graft. These are the more complex situations in which to revascularize the limb. There are essentially two options: surgical bypass or catheter-based lytic therapy. Angiography is necessary in both situations to determine the extent of the occlusion and to search for inflow and distal outflow vessels to which a bypass graft could be attached. Although the surgeon's preference tends to predominate in the approach to the ischemic limb, both approaches have been demonstrated to be fairly equivalent in terms of limb salvage. Criteria for selecting the appropriate approach are based on the presence or absence of good target vessels and availability of a suitable bypass conduit. If there are good distal vessels—usually inflow vessels are adequate or can be made adequate—and a good saphenous vein is available, surgical bypass is recommended, as it is fast and reliable. In the absence of a good distal target, absent saphenous vein, or in a patient at high risk for surgery, lysis is recommended.

Lysis. Prior to lysis, a wire traversal test is performed by puncturing the contralateral femoral artery and advancing a wire over the bifurcation and down the native vessels or occluded graft in the contralateral limb. The degree of ease with which the wire is passed

Table 22-9
Complications of Revascularization

Reperfusion syndrome
Hypotension
Hyperkalemia
Myoglobinuria
Renal failure
Compartment syndrome
Ischemic neuropathy
Muscle necrosis
Recurrent thrombosis

suggests fresh thrombus and is predictive of good results from lysis. A special catheter that allows a lytic agent to be sprayed into the clot along the length of the occlusion is inserted over the wire and lysis is begun. The agents most commonly used are urokinase and tissue plasminogen activator (t-PA). Lysis times are variable, ranging from 12 to 36 hours, and generally, the longer the lysis, the greater the risk of bleeding complications. Once the clot has been dissolved, underlying stenoses, which are predisposed to secondary thrombosis, are treated with balloon angioplasty, stenting, or bypass, as appropriate.

The principal risk of lysis is bleeding. Lytic agents are absolutely contraindicated in patients with intracranial surgery, intracranial hemorrhage within the last 3 months, or in the presence of any active bleeding. Most bleeding complications occur at the arterial puncture sites, but concealed retroperitoneal bleeding is possible. Rarely, patients can sustain intracerebral hemorrhage, which can be fatal or disabling.

Complications of Reperfusion of the Ischemic Limb. Reperfusion of the ischemic limb is variable in its physiologic effects, which directly relates to the severity and extent of the ischemia. Patients with a saddle embolus of the aortic bifurcation and severely ischemic limbs may sustain the full-blown "reperfusion syndrome." At the other end of the spectrum, patients with minimal muscle ischemia who are rapidly reperfused may have essentially no effects. However, many of these patients have severe underlying cardiac disease and poorly tolerate even short ischemic periods. Complications occurring after revascularization of the lower extremity and causes of recurrent thrombosis are listed in Tables 22-9 and 22-10. Therapy is directed toward forced alkaline diuresis by adding bicarbonate to the intravenous fluid. Alkalinization increases the solubility of myoglobin in the urine, preventing it from crystallizing in the tubules, which is what promotes acute renal failure.

Compartment Syndrome. Compartment syndrome occurs after prolonged ischemia followed by reperfusion. The capillaries leak fluid into the interstitial space in the muscles, which are enclosed within a nondistensible fascial envelope. When the pressure inside the compartment exceeds the capillary perfusion pressure, nutrient flow ceases and progressive ischemia occurs, even in the presence of peripheral pulses. Consequently, every patient who has

Table 22-10
Causes of Recurrent Thrombosis

Recurrent embolization
Inadequate thrombus removal
Arterial injury from thrombectomy catheter
Failure to treat critical lesion-causing thrombosis
Extensive muscle edema precluding distal flow
Underlying hypercoagulable state
Technical problem with bypass graft/arteriotomy closure

sustained an ischemic event and is reperfused is monitored for compartment syndrome, which is characterized by excessive pain in the compartment, pain on passive stretching of the compartment, and sensory loss due to nerve compression of the nerves coursing though the compartment. The most commonly affected compartment is the anterior compartment in the leg (Fig. 22-64). Numbness in the web space between the first and second toes is diagnostic due to compression of the deep peroneal nerve. When skin changes occur over the compartment, this indicates advanced ischemia. Compartment pressure is measured by inserting an arterial line into the compartment and recording the pressure. Although controversial, pressures greater than 30 mm Hg or below 30 mm Hg diastolic are frequently cited. Treatment is by fasciotomy. In the leg, medial and lateral incisions are utilized via the medial incision. Long openings are then made in the fascia of the superficial and deep posterior compartments. Through the lateral incision, the anterior and peroneal compartments are opened. Both skin and fascial incisions should be of adequate length to ensure full compartment decompression.[91]

Acute Aortic Occlusion

Acute aortic occlusion is a rare vascular catastrophe. It may result from an aortic saddle embolus (Fig. 22-65), in situ thrombosis of a previously atherosclerotic abdominal aorta, sudden thrombosis of small abdominal aortic aneurysms, distal aortic dissection (Fig. 22-66), or other etiologies that embolize to the aortic bifurcation. The diagnosis can easily go unrecognized and has a published mortality rate of 75% with conservative treatment. In addition, the condition often presents with leg paralysis that occasionally leads clinicians to perform an extensive neurologic workup, even if patients have absent femoral pulses, which can lead to delays in diagnosis and operative therapy.

In all patients, an acute onset of bilateral lower extremity ischemia or a sudden exacerbation of pre-existing chronic ischemia is the presenting syndrome. Extremity ischemia is characterized by rest pain, motor and sensory deficits, mottling, and tissue loss at initial presentation.

Etiologic Considerations. Significant coexisting medical conditions occur in these patients. A higher incidence of coronary atherosclerotic heart disease, recent myocardial infarction, and pre-existing peripheral vascular disease are found in the in situ thrombosis (IST) group, but the mortality rate was much higher in the embolic group. Thus, a higher operative risk exists for procedures in patients with saddle aortic embolization. If possible, co-existing conditions should be aggressively investigated and treated in both patient groups.[92–95]

Chronic aortic iliac occlusion as a consequence of atherosclerotic disease has a reported incidence of 1 to 8%. Although less common, *acute* aortic occlusion is associated with higher morbidity and mortality rates, up to 100% in some series. Acute aortic occlusion is a different entity than chronic obstruction, in which a well-developed collateral circulation (Fig. 22-67) may minimize symptoms. An exuberant collateral system may be responsible for the increased survival seen in the IST group in this series. When an embolus is large enough to occlude the aorta, the source is usually cardiac (i.e., mural thrombus over an infarct, a left ventricular aneurysm, or rheumatic heart disease). Large thrombi in the left atrial appendage may embolize following cardioversion. Mural thrombus from complicated myocardial infarction is now the more common source (17 to 66%). Thoracic or abdominal aortic aneurysms are occasionally the embolic source.[96–98]

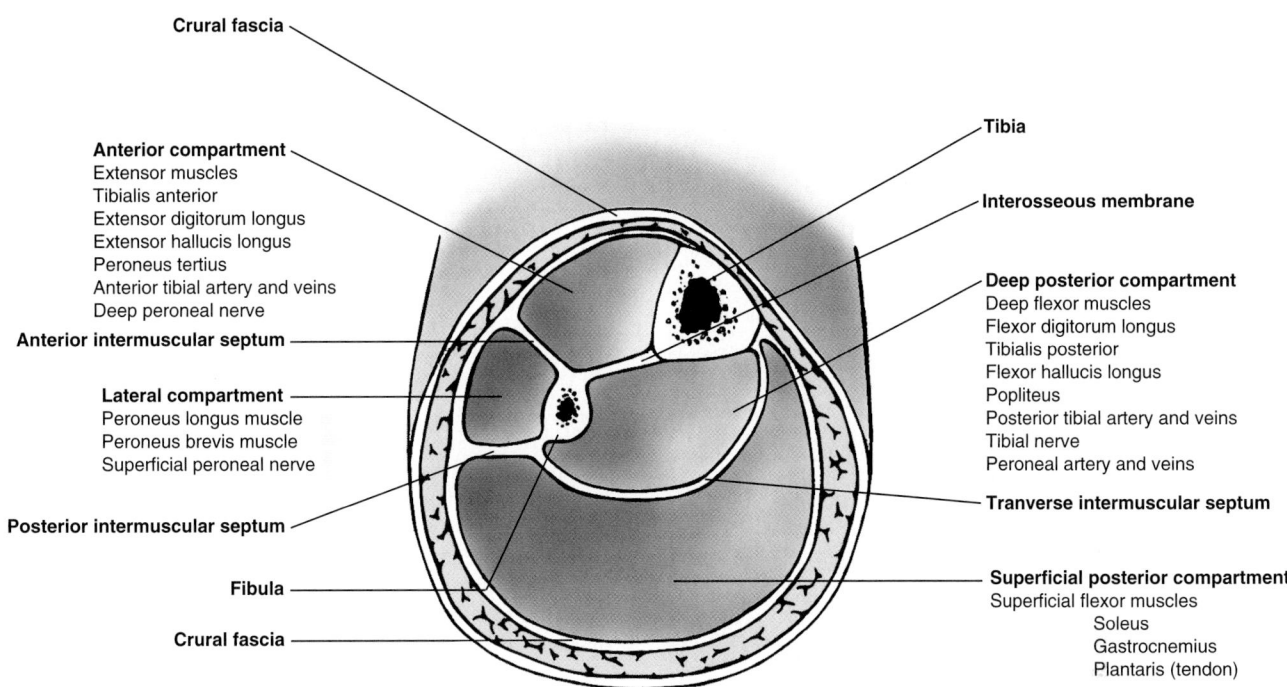

FIG. 22-64. *Fascial compartments of the lower leg.*

Presenting Symptoms. The degree and severity of symptoms in patients with pre-existing aortoiliac disease depends on the nature of collateral circulation. Symptoms in this group of patients include the sudden onset of bilateral limb pain, pallor, paralysis, paresthesia, and the absence of palpable pulses. Mottling of the lower extremities, often to the level of the umbilicus, may also be present. In the absence of collateral circulation, the patient usually experiences a sudden onset of low back, buttock, and lower extremity pain.

The diagnosis of acute aortic occlusion is difficult and can easily go unrecognized. Patients with a neurologic deficit often are referred to a neurologist or neurosurgeon, even with a physical finding of absent femoral pulses. The importance of early surgical intervention in this group of patients makes accurate diagnosis essential, and

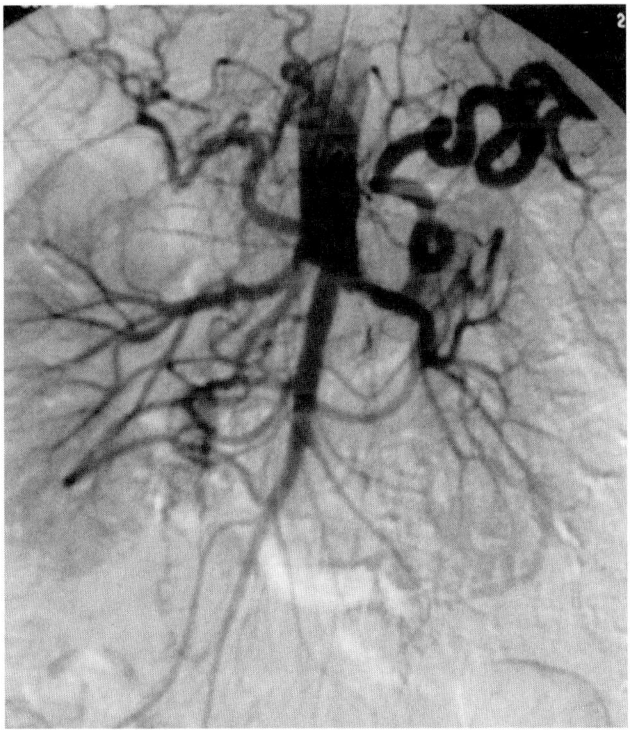

FIG. 22-65. Angiogram showing acute occlusion of the aorta below the renal arteries.

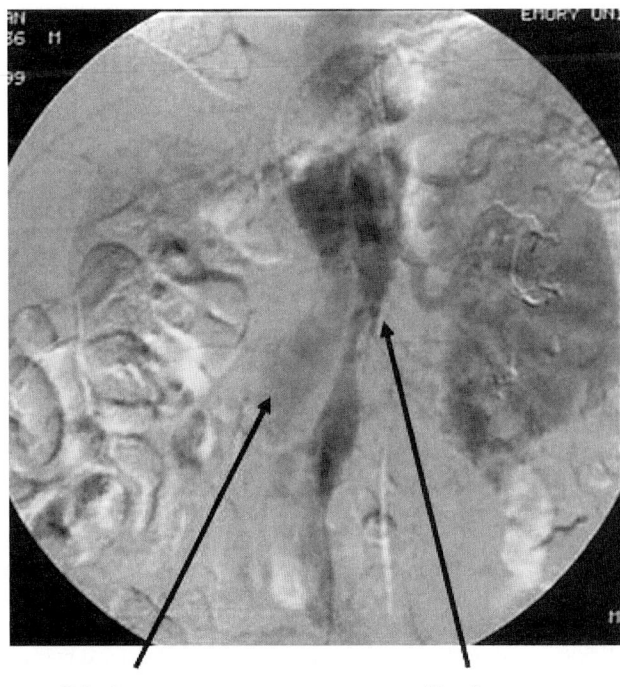

False lumen   True lumen

FIG. 22-66. *Dissection causing occlusion of the infrarenal aorta.*

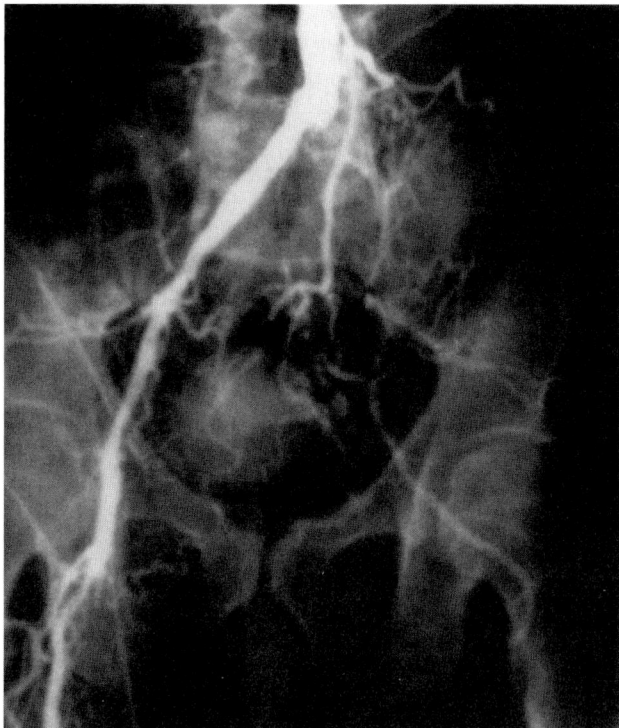

FIG. 22-67. Chronic occlusion of the left iliac system with well-developed collateral systems.

physicians in the emergency department or primary care centers need to perform a simple vascular examination on any patient with an apparent neurologic deficit in the lower extremities.

Physical Examination. If the physical examination shows the absence of both femoral pulses, the diagnosis of acute aortic occlusion is established. The cause of the occlusion will significantly alter patient management, and thus a detailed history is important. Severe coronary artery disease, known arrhythmias, or ventricular aneurysms suggest a saddle embolus, whereas known aortoiliac disease or a previously diagnosed aortic aneurysm suggests an in situ thrombosis.

Role of Angiography. Patients with suspected in situ abdominal aortic thrombosis with clinically unclear renal or mesenteric arterial involvement should have preoperative angiography. For all other patients, it is recommended that intraoperative angiography with a C-arm be used in the operating room, because it saves time and provides important information should it be needed.

Operative Considerations. Because patient prognosis is time-dependent, early recognition, institution of supportive care, and prompt diagnosis (if possible) are essential elements of management. The treatment of acute aortic occlusion is surgical. The cause of occlusion is important because transfemoral embolectomy is likely to restore perfusion in patients with saddle embolus, but is usually unhelpful in patients with in situ thrombosis. When the diagnosis is made, the patient should be heparinized immediately to prevent proximal and distal propagation of the thrombotic process. Bilateral transfemoral embolectomy is the first procedure of choice. If flow is re-established, the groin wounds are closed and postoperative anticoagulation is initiated. If flow cannot be re-established, more extensive surgery, such as aortoiliac bypass or axillobifemoral bypass, should be performed. The choice to perform axillobifemoral

bypass versus aortobifemoral bypass is guided by the clinical condition of the patient.

Postoperative Management. Postoperative management requires correction of any embolic diathesis. Transthoracic or transesophageal echocardiography should be obtained. A CT scan of the abdomen should be done if not performed preoperatively to rule out the presence of an abdominal aortic aneurysm. If an aneurysm is present and the patient is a reasonable candidate, the aneurysm may be ligated electively. If the patient is known to have an aneurysm that appears to have occluded, then replacement with a prosthetic graft is the procedure of choice. Long-term anticoagulation is necessary for all patients.

AORTOILIAC OCCLUSIVE DISEASE

The distal abdominal aorta and the iliac arteries are common sites of involvement with atherosclerosis. Aortoiliac occlusive disease occurs in a relatively younger group of patients (aged in their mid-50s), compared with patients with more femoropopliteal disease. It also differs from disease of the femoral-popliteal-tibial segment since it is rarely limb-threatening. Symptoms typically consist of bilateral thigh or buttock claudication and fatigue. Men report diminished penile tumescence, and there may later be complete failure of erectile function. These symptoms constitute Leriche's syndrome. Rest pain is unusual with isolated aortoiliac disease. Femoral pulses are usually diminished or absent. There are usually no stigmata of ischemia unless distal disease coexists.[99–102]

A small group of patients report a prolonged history of thigh and buttock claudication that has recently become more severe. It is likely that this group has underlying significant aortoiliac disease that has suddenly progressed to acute occlusion of the terminal aorta. Others may present with "trash foot," representing microembolization into the distal vascular bed (Fig. 22-68).

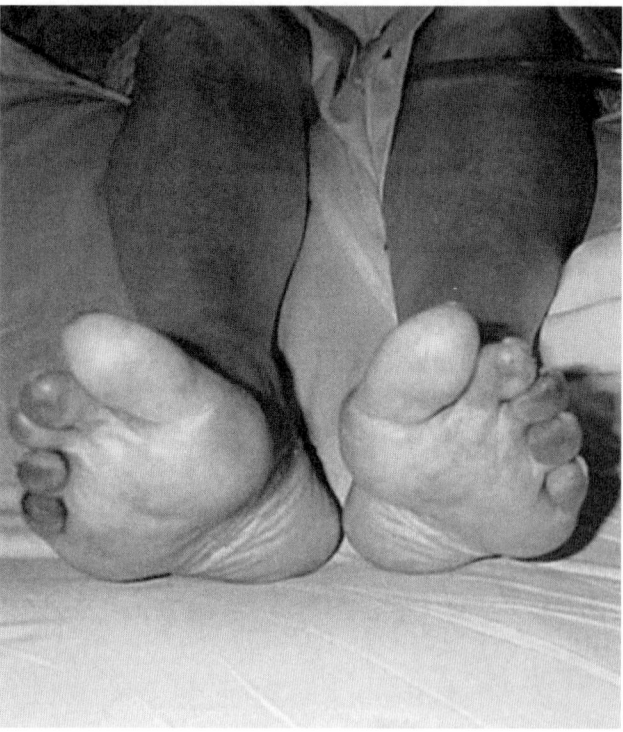

FIG. 22-68. Microembolization to the distal vessels from aortic atherosclerosis.

Noninvasive tests such as pulse volume recordings of the lower extremity with estimation or the thigh-brachial pressure index may be suggestive of aortoiliac disease. Definitive diagnosis, however, can only be established by arteriography. This further provides important information regarding distal arterial run-off (particularly the profunda femoris) and demonstrates pelvic collaterals that may be important in maintaining lower limb viability. It must be emphasized, however, that patients should be subjected to angiography only if their symptoms warrant surgical intervention.

Collateral Pathways in Chronic Aortic Occlusion

The principal collateral pathways in chronic aortic occlusion are: (1) the superior mesenteric artery to the distal inferior mesenteric artery via its superior hemorrhoidal branch to the middle and inferior hemorrhoidals to the internal iliac artery (39%); (2) the lumbar arteries to the superior gluteal artery to the internal iliac system (37%); (3) the lumbar arteries to the lateral and deep circumflex arteries to the common femoral artery (12%); and (4) Winslow's pathway from the subclavian to the superior epigastric artery to the inferior epigastric artery to the external iliac arteries at the groin.

Preferred Approach to Therapeutic Alternatives

Medical Treatment

There is no effective medical therapy for the management of aortoiliac disease. Patients should have hypertension, hyperlipidemia, and diabetes mellitus controlled. They should be advised to stop smoking. Despite these measures there is usually no improvement in exercise tolerance. A graduated exercise program may facilitate collateral development. Most patients are empirically placed on antiplatelet therapy.

Open Surgical Treatment or Endovascular Therapy

The decision to pursue an open rather than an endovascular approach is made based on the extent of the occlusive disease. The Trans-Atlantic Intersocietal Commission (TASC) has classified the distribution and extent of atherosclerosis and has suggested a therapeutic approach based on this classification (Fig. 22-69).[101] TASC type A lesions are best treated with a catheter-based approach. TASC type D lesions should have open bypass (Fig. 22-70). TASC types B and C remain controversial. However, this is a rapidly evolving field and it is likely that aortoiliac disease will be increasingly treated with a catheter-based approach.

Indications for Surgery. Indications for surgery include disabling claudication (severely limiting work or lifestyle), rest pain, limb-threatening ischemia, and microembolization of the toes in which no other source is identified.

Surgical Options. Surgical options consist of aortobifemoral bypass grafting, extra-anatomic bypass grafting, and aortoiliac endarterectomy. The procedure selected is determined by several factors, including anatomic distribution of the disease, clinical condition of the patient, and personal preference of the surgeon.

In most cases aortobifemoral bypass grafting is the procedure of choice of these authors. Bilateral bypass is virtually always performed since patients usually have disease in both iliac systems. Although one side may be more severely affected than the other, progression may occur, and bilateral bypass adds little to the procedure. Aortobifemoral bypass grafting is a satisfactory operation, it reliably relieves symptoms, has an excellent long-term patency of 60 to 75% at 10 years, and can be completed with a tolerable mortality of 2 to 3%.[103-108]

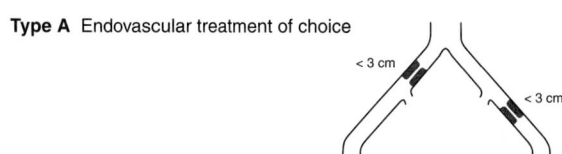

Type A Endovascular treatment of choice

< 3 cm   < 3 cm

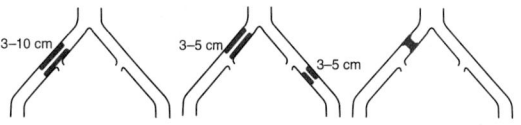

Type B Currently, endovascular treatment is more often used but insufficient evidence for recommendation.

3–10 cm   3–5 cm   3–5 cm

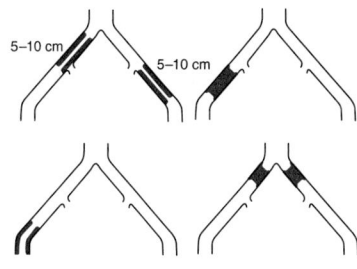

Type C Currently, surgical treatment is more often used but insufficient evidence for recommendation.

5–10 cm   5–10 cm

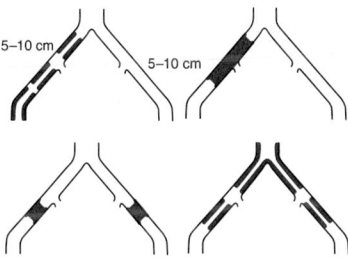

Type D Surgical treatment of choice

5–10 cm   5–10 cm

FIG. 22-69. TASC classification of aortoiliac occlusive disease.

Procedure. Both femoral arteries are initially exposed to ensure that they are adequate for the distal anastomoses. The abdomen is then opened at the midline, the intestine is retracted, and the posterior peritoneum overlying the aorta is incised.

A retroperitoneal approach may be an alternative in selected situations. This approach involves making a flank incision and displacing the peritoneum and its contents to the right. Such an approach is contraindicated if the right renal artery is acutely occluded, since visualization from the left flank is very poor. Tunneling of a graft to the right femoral artery is also more difficult from a retroperitoneal approach, but can be achieved. The retroperitoneal approach is generally regarded as being better tolerated than is a laparotomy in those with severe pulmonary disease.

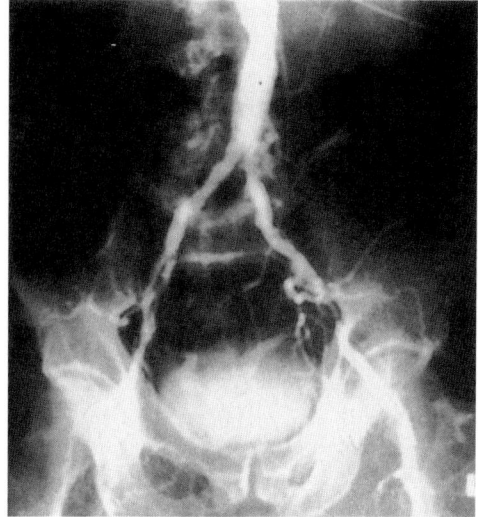

A

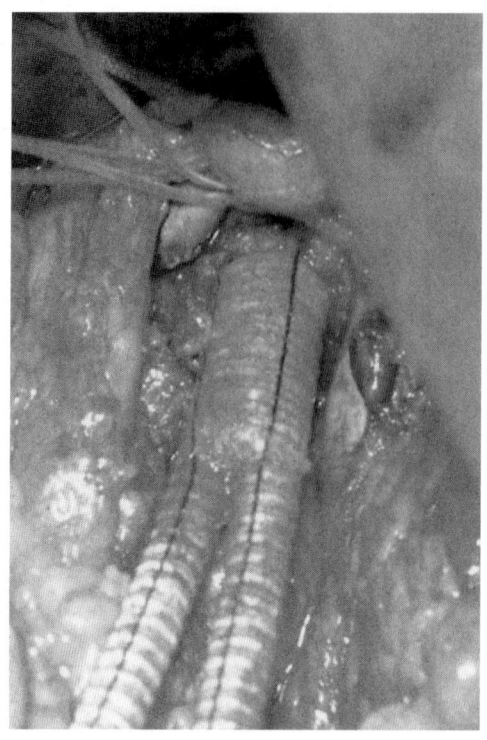

B

FIG. 22-70. *A. Angiogram shows severe aortoiliac occlusive disease (TASC type D), B. Surgical repair with aortoiliac bypass grafting.*

A collagen-impregnated, knitted Dacron graft is used prior to the proximal aortic anastomosis, which can then be made in either end-to-end or end-to-side fashion using 3-0 polypropylene suture.

An end-to-end anastomosis provides a better long-term hemodynamic result and is necessary in those patients with an aortic aneurysm. Relative indications for an end-to-side anastomosis include the presence of a large aberrant renal artery, an unusually large inferior mesenteric artery with poor back-bleeding suggesting inadequate collateralization, or a very small aorta. An end-to-side anastomosis may also be less deleterious to sexual function than end-to-end anastomoses. However, disadvantages of an end-to-side anastomosis do occur; for example, application of a partial occluding clamp may precipitate distal embolization. Furthermore, the distal aorta often proceeds to total occlusion after an end-to-side anastomosis. There also may be a higher incidence of aortoenteric fistula following end-to-side procedures because of the anterior projection of the graft.

The limbs of the graft are then tunneled through the retroperitoneum to the groin, where an end-to-side anastomosis is fashioned between the graft and the bifurcation of the common femoral artery using 5-0 polypropylene suture. Endarterectomy or patch angioplasty of the profunda femoris may be required concurrently. Once the anastomoses have been fashioned, the clamps are removed and the surgeon carefully controls the degree of aortic occlusion until full flow is re-established. During this period the patient must be carefully monitored for hypotension. Declamping shock is a complication of sudden restoration of aortic flow, particularly following prolonged occlusion. Once flow has been re-established, the peritoneum is carefully reapproximated over the prosthesis to prevent fistulization into the intestine.

Aortoiliac endarterectomy is rarely performed, as it is associated with greater blood loss, greater sexual dysfunction, and is more difficult to perform. However, long-term patency is comparable with aortobifemoral grafting, and it remains a reasonable option in cases in which the risk of infection of a graft is excessive, because it involves no prosthetic tissue. It also is useful if there is disease localized to either the aorta or common iliac arteries. However, this is a scenario in which balloon angioplasty and stenting is being more frequently used. Endarterectomy should not be performed if the aorta is at all aneurysmal.

Extra-anatomic (axillofemoral) bypass grafting from the axillary artery is an option for those patients with intercurrent medical problems that prohibit a laparotomy. It may be performed under local anesthesia, but because this procedure is confined to high-risk patients, it is used only for limb salvage. Before performing this operation, the surgeon should check pulses and blood pressure in both arms to ensure that there is no obvious disease affecting flow through the axillary system. Angiography is not necessary, but can be helpful if performed at the time of aortography. The axillary artery is exposed below the clavicle, and a 6- to 8-mm externally reinforced polytetrafluoroethylene graft is tunneled subcutaneously down the lateral chest wall and lateral abdomen to the groin. It is anastomosed to the ipsilateral distal common femoral artery over its bifurcation into the superficial femoral and profunda femoris arteries. A femoral-to-femoral crossover graft using a 6- to 8-mm externally reinforced polytetrafluoroethylene graft is then used to revascularize the opposite extremity if necessary. Reported patency rates over 5 years vary from 30 to 80%. Paradoxically, although it is a less complex procedure than aortofemoral grafting, the mortality rate is higher (10%), reflecting the risky nature of these patients.[104] Numerous complications may be encountered following

Table 22-11

Postoperative Complications of Aortobifemoral Bypass Grafting

Medical complications
    Perioperative myocardial infarction
    Respiratory failure
    Ischemia-induced renal failure
    Bleeding from intercurrent heparinization
    Stroke
Procedure-related complications
    Early
        Declamping shock
        Graft thrombosis
        Retroperitoneal bleeding
        Groin hematoma
        Bowel ischemia/infarction
        Peripheral embolization
        Loss of sexual function
        Lymphatic fistula
        Chylous ascites
        Paraplegia
    Late
        Graft infection
        Anastomotic pseudoaneurysm
        Aortoenteric fistula
        Aortourinary fistula
Reocclusion of graft

aortobifemoral bypass (Table 22-11). Patients with unilateral occlusion of the common iliac or external iliac arteries may be satisfactorily managed by femoral-to-femoral crossover grafting.

Postoperative Management. All patients who have undergone aortic replacement, endarterectomy, or extra-anatomic bypass require careful observation. All aortic patients are observed in the ICU overnight. Numerous complications, both medical and surgical, may arise in the postoperative period. It has been reported that the presence of significant left ventricular dysfunction is an important indicator of mortality. Careful hemodynamic support via optimizing volume status and judicious pressor therapy is necessary. Continuous intravenous nitroglycerin is used by the authors in all nonhypotensive patients. Perioperative myocardial infarction accounts for one half of all deaths. A 12-lead ECG is recommended on the first postoperative follow-up.

Distal pulses are monitored hourly. Loss of a pulse that had been present postoperatively is suggestive of graft occlusion and warrants angiography to assess for re-exploration if the graft has failed (Fig. 22-71).

The patient gets out of bed and into a chair on the second postoperative day and ambulates on the third day. Most patients may be discharged from the hospital 5 to 7 days postoperatively. Lifelong follow-up is necessary since delayed complications may occur.

Percutaneous Transluminal Dilatation

Angioplasty is most useful in the treatment of isolated iliac stenoses of less than 4 cm in length. When used for stenoses rather than occlusion, a 2-year patency of 86% can be achieved[109,110] (Fig. 22-72). The complication rate is approximately 2%, consisting of distal embolization, medial dissection, and acute thrombosis. Angioplasty is occasionally used in long segment stenoses, but with less favorable results. Angioplasty and stenting is recommended for TASC type A lesions, can be used in TASC type B (see Fig. 22-69) and type C lesions, but is best avoided for TASC type D (see Fig. 22-69) lesions. It is further useful as an adjunct to laser recanaliza-

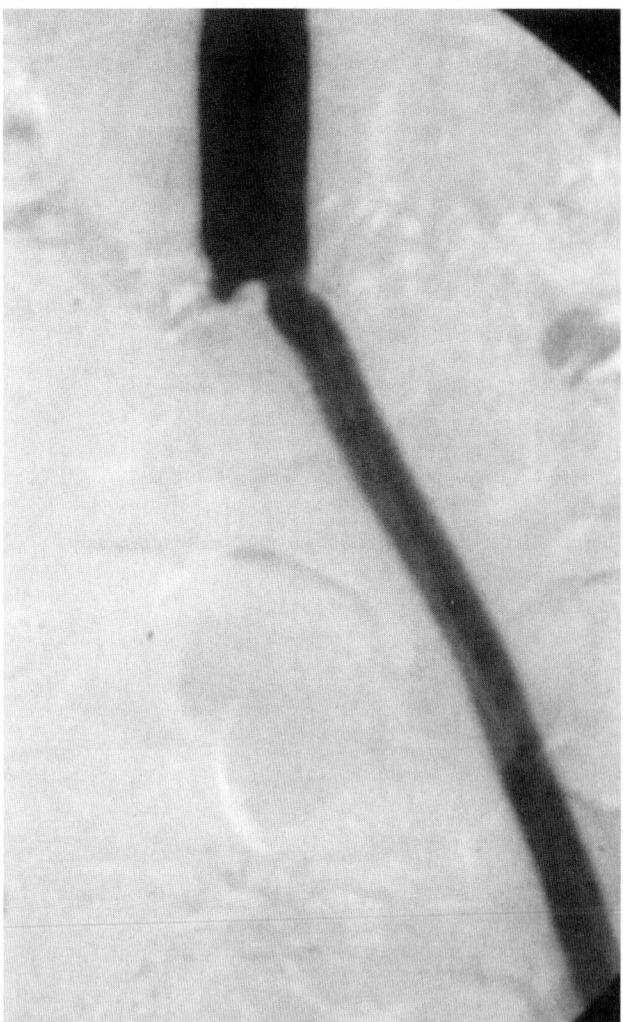

FIG. 22-71. Occluded right limb of an aortobifemoral graft.

tion of a completely occluded iliac vessel. This technique remains experimental, and further data are required before such an approach can be recommended.

Femoropopliteal Occlusive Disease

One of the most common sites for occlusive disease is in the distal superficial femoral artery (SFA) as it passes deep through the adductor canal. It may be that the entrapment by the adductor hiatus prevents the compensatory dilation that occurs in atherosclerotic vessels. Stenoses, which develop here, progress to occlusion of the distal third of the superficial femoral artery (Fig. 22-73). Although often originating in this location, the SFA is frequently the site of diffuse disease with posterior plaque, which spirals along the artery. When distal SFA occlusion develops slowly it may be totally asymptomatic, and collaterals from the proximal SFA or the profunda femoris artery (PFA) bypass the occlusion and reconstitute the popliteal artery. Symptom development is a function of the extent of occlusion, adequacy of collaterals, and also the activity level of the patients.

Clinical Manifestations

Presenting symptoms of femoropopliteal occlusive disease are broadly classified into two types: limb-threatening and

Kissing Stents at the Aortic Bifurcation

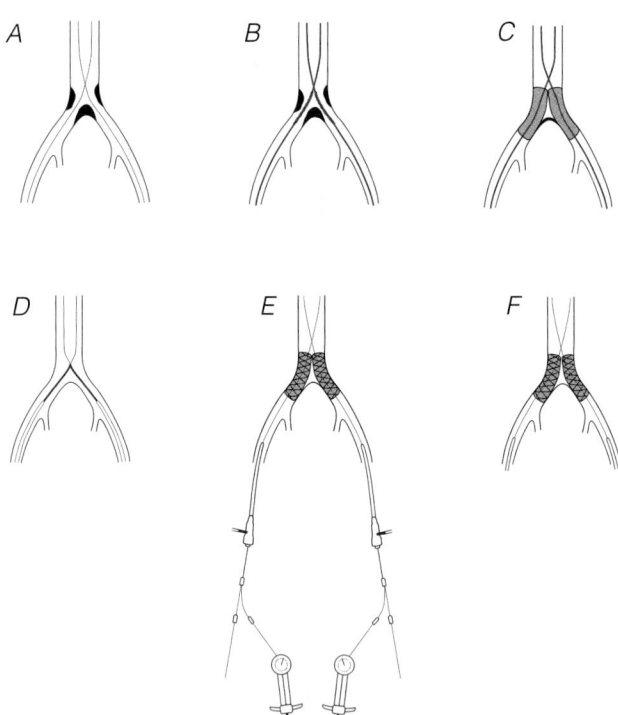

FIG. 22-72. *A.* Bilateral guidewire placement across the iliac artery stenoses. *B.* Bilateral angioplasty balloon catheter placement across the iliac artery stenoses. *C.* Balloon angioplasty of bilateral iliac artery stenoses. *D.* Removal of the bilateral balloon angioplasty catheters. *E.* Deployment of bilateral common iliac balloon-expandable stents. *F.* Completion of bilateral iliac kissing stent placement.

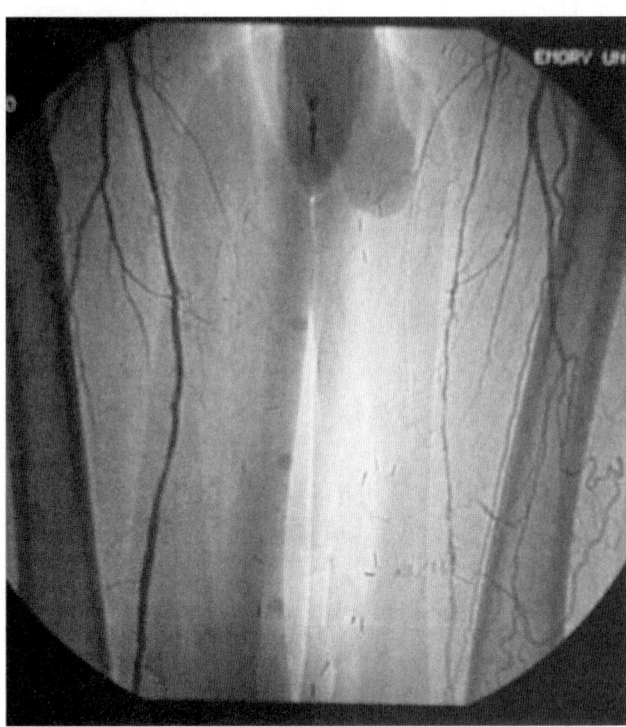

FIG. 22-73. Occluded left superficial femoral artery.

non–limb-threatening ischemia. Claudication is non–limb-threatening. Rest pain, ulceration, and gangrene are limb-threatening and demand intervention.

Occlusive disease of the femoral artery may be isolated or in conjunction with multilevel disease involving both the aortoiliac segment and the tibial vessels. Symptoms in patients with multilevel disease are always much more severe than those with single level disease. Pain from isolated SFA and popliteal occlusion is typically calf claudication. Cramping pain develops in the calf on ambulation, occurs at a reproducible distance, and is relieved by rest, hence the associated name "window gazer's disease." Because it recurs with further exercise, activities such as climbing stairs or going uphill exacerbate pain. Additionally, many patients report a worsening of symptoms during cold weather. It is important to evaluate whether the symptoms are progressive or static. In greater than 70% of patients the disease is stable, particularly with risk factor modification. It does not lead to progressive occlusion, and in most cases is not limb-threatening. This is extremely important for both the patient and physician to understand. Progression is more likely to occur in patients with diabetes and those who continue to smoke or fail to modify their atherosclerotic risk factors.

In contrast, rest pain is constant, usually occurring in the forefoot across the metatarsophalangeal joint. It is worse at night and requires foot dependency to improve symptoms. Patients may report that they either sleep in a chair or hang the foot off the side of the bed. The pain is severe and relentless, even with narcotics.

Ischemic ulceration most commonly involves the toes. Any toe can be affected. Occasionally ulcers develop on the dorsum of the foot. Ulceration can occur in atypical positions in an ischemic foot from trauma such as friction from new shoes. Injury to a foot with borderline ischemia can convert an otherwise stable situation into one which is limb-threatening. The initial development of gangrene also commonly involves the digits. As with all vascular patients, it is important to evaluate their risk factors, intercurrent cardiac diseases, and any prior vascular interventions.

Natural History

It is important to reassure patients that most do not need an intervention and that the majority of patients do not have progressive, aggressive occlusive disease leading to limb loss. With such reassurance, many patients can live with minor disability and can be treated medically. In contrast, young patients with short-distance claudication have significant lifestyle impairment, cannot work, and need improvement in walking distance. In this situation, it is recommended that the surgeon ensure that the patient understands the risks of intervention as well as the realistic benefits. True informed consent is mandatory in this situation. Of 1400 patients followed with claudication, Boyd noted that only 7% required amputation at 5 years, and the Framingham study showed that only 2% required amputation at 10 years follow-up. The risks for patients with claudication are in marked contrast to those of patients who present with limb-threatening ischemia, in whom over 50% will lose their limb if left untreated.

Differential Diagnosis

Night cramps often wake patients from sleep with painful calf muscle spasms and are not associated with arterial disease. However, foot ulceration, arterial ulcers that occur on the toes or lateral side of the foot, and venous ulcers, which are quite common and occur above the medial malleolus, usually in an area with the skin changes of lipodermatosclerosis, are associated with arterial disease.

Physical Examination

The physical examination focuses on the peripheral pulse. A normal femoral, but diminished popliteal, pulse indicates SFA occlusive disease. In contrast, a diminished popliteal pulse and diminished ankle pulses tells the examiner nothing about popliteal and tibial disease, although occasionally patients with an SFA occlusion have excellent collaterals that support palpable ankle pulses. Although the majority of patients who have SFA disease will have diminished ankle pulses, occasionally patients with symptoms that are suggestive of claudication will have palpable pedal pulses. Occasionally, patients with a high-grade stenosis will have palpable pulses. Nevertheless, the astute clinician should listen to and examine the patient with lower extremity pain, and feel for the pedal pulses (i.e., the finding of palpable pulses makes the diagnosis of significant lower extremity occlusive disease unlikely). A search for another causative factor should be undertaken.

Investigations

Segmental pressure measurement and pulse volume recordings (PVRs) will demonstrate the level at which the pressure fall occurs and assist in localizing the affected segment. A pressure drop of greater than 30 mm Hg between two adjacent segments is suggestive of significant occlusive disease at that level. Exercise testing with measurement of the ABI after exercise will help identify those patients who, despite significant occlusive disease, have palpable pedal pulses by showing an abrupt fall in ABI after exercise. In patients with calcified vessels that cannot be occluded with a cuff, the PVRs are valuable since they detect changes in limb volume at this level, and are not dependent on the ability to compress the underlying artery.

Angiography continues to be the best and most reliable test for imaging the entire lower extremity vasculature. An aortogram and bilateral run-off is performed. A pigtail catheter is placed in the aorta immediately above the renal arteries. Using 20 mL/s for a total of 30 mL of dye, the aorta and pelvic vessels are imaged using digital subtraction angiography (DSA). In large patients the catheter is then positioned above the aortic bifurcation, and the remainder of the pelvic vessels are imaged down to the level of the common femoral arteries. Using an injection rate of 12 mL/s for a total of 84 mL (7-second injection duration), and a step table that moves as the dye passes down the legs, the entire lower extremity vasculature can be imaged using DSA. This technique provides high-quality images from the renal arteries to the pedal arch.

Although MRA continues to improve, it has not yet replaced DSA for lower-extremity angiography as anticipated. Lower-extremity duplex arterial mapping is increasing in popularity, but there remain only a few select centers that routinely use this technique for preoperative planning. Treatment recommendations for lower extremity occlusive disease are based on the severity of presenting symptoms, understanding the natural history, the age and comorbidities of the patient, and the extent of disease.[111–113]

Age and Comorbidities. Choosing whether or not to perform a vascular procedure involves balancing the risks against the benefits of an intervention. Although this is true of all surgical procedures, it is particularly so in patients with atherosclerosis, where multisystem involvement is the norm and limited life expectancy is in the background. Studies suggest a 70% 5-year and a 50% 10-year survival rate in patients with lower extremity occlusive disease. A femoral-popliteal bypass in the 50-year-old patient who has to walk as part of their employment is warranted. In contrast, the same operation in an 80-year-old patient is usually not indicated. Likewise,

even the operation in the 50-year-old patient that has had two myocardial infarctions and is limited by chest pain and shortness of breath is not warranted.

Extent of Disease. Generally, localized disease (i.e., stenoses and short segment occlusions) is more amenable to a catheter-based approach. There is debate in vascular surgery circles as to whether ease of intervention should result in a lowering of the threshold for intervention. It is the opinion of these authors that this is inevitable and that appropriate catheter-based interventions carry less morbidity than does bypass grafting. Therefore, the extent of the disease and ease of performing catheter-based recanalization should play a part in the decision making. At the other end of the disease spectrum, where there is extensive involvement of the femoral popliteal and tibial vessels, perhaps with only a single vessel running to the foot, intervention for claudication is fraught with hazard. Loss of that vessel will convert a non–limb-threatening situation into a limb-threatening one.

Medical Therapy

Cilostazol has been demonstrated to be effective when compared with both placebo and pentoxifylline in improving walking distance. Likewise, for patients with non–limb-threatening ischemia, an exercise program should be initiated.

Open Surgical Procedures

Endarterectomy. Endarterectomy has a limited, albeit important role in lower extremity occlusive disease. It is most frequently used when there is disease of the common femoral artery or involving the profunda femoris artery. In this procedure, the surgeon opens the diseased segment longitudinally and develops a cleavage plane within the media that is developed proximally and distally. This permits the inner layer containing the atheroma to be excised. Great care must be taken at the distal end of the endarterectomy to ensure either a smooth transition or to tack down the distal endpoint to prevent the flow from elevating a potentially occlusive atheromatous flap. Currently, there is essentially no role for long open SFA endarterectomy or for its use in treating short segment stenoses or occlusions. The high incidence of restenosis occurring in the SFA is what limits utility of endarterectomy in this location. Short segment stenoses are more appropriately treated with balloon angioplasty. Endarterectomy using a catheter-based approach (e.g., Moll endarterectomy device) supplemented with stent grafting or stenting across the endpoint of the endarterectomy is currently being re-evaluated; however, no long-term data are available.

Bypass Grafting. Bypass grafting remains the primary intervention for lower-extremity occlusive disease. The type of bypass and the type of conduit are important variables. Those patients with occlusive disease limited to the SFA, with reconstitution of at least 4 cm (ideally 10 cm) of normal popliteal artery above the knee joint, and with at least one continuous vessel to the foot are treated with an above-knee femoral-to-popliteal bypass graft. In this location (i.e., not crossing the knee joint) the differential in patency between prosthetic (ePTFE) and vein graft is relatively small, although it is consistently better with the vein graft. However, use of the prosthetic graft in this location is acceptable, although the argument that saving the vein for future use for coronary artery bypass grafting or distal leg bypass grafting has been shown to be flawed. When the disease extends to involve the popliteal artery or the tibial vessels, the surgeon then must select an appropriate outflow vessel. These are usually defined as having a continuous channel beyond the anastomosis into the foot, and are listed in order of descending preference: above-knee popliteal, below-knee popliteal, posterior tibial, anterior tibial, and peroneal artery. In patients with diabetes, it is frequently the peroneal artery which is spared. Although it has no direct flow into the foot, the appropriate outflow vessel's terminal branches collateralize to the posterior tibial and anterior tibial arteries. The dorsalis pedis (i.e., the continuation of the anterior tibial in the foot) frequently also is spared. Patency is affected by the length of the bypass (longer bypasses have reduced patency), quality of the recipient artery, patent run-off to the foot, and quality of the saphenous vein graft.

Two techniques are used for distal bypass grafting: reversed saphenous vein grafting and in situ saphenous vein grafting. In the former, the vein is excised in its entirety from the leg using open or endoscopic vein harvest, reversed to render the valves nonfunctional, and tunneled from the common femoral artery inflow to the distal target vessels. End-to-side anastomoses are then created. The in situ technique was developed using the concept that minimizing trauma to the vein (i.e., minimal disruption of vasa vasorum), would lead to prolonged patency. Although improved patency has never been demonstrated, many favor this technique. The vein is exposed only at its proximal and distal extent. A valvulotome is passed in a retrograde fashion and used to disrupt the valves. The proximal anastomosis is created and flow established. Side branches are identified either by duplex scanning intraoperatively, Doppler examination, or angiography, and are exposed and ligated. Recently, an angioscopic method for coil embolization of the side branches was described. The principal advantage of the in situ technique is that the small distal vein is sewn to the smaller distal arteries, thereby providing a better size match.

Several adjunctive techniques have been used to try and improve the patency of vein grafts to tibial arteries. Creation of an arteriovenous fistula at the distal anastomosis is designed to increase flow through the graft. Another method is to create a large patch at the distal anastomosis in an attempt to streamline the flow and to reduce the likelihood of narrowing at the anastomosis from neointimal hyperplasia. As a result, experience gained from the vein patch techniques led to a modified ePTFE graft that is now available with a built-in distal hood, which has shown some encouraging early results.

Complications.   Fifteen percent of vein grafts will develop intrinsic stenoses within the first 18 months following implantation. Consequently all patients with a vein graft should enter a duplex surveillance protocol. Scanning should be performed in the postoperative period at 3, 6, 12, and 18 months. Stenoses greater than 50% should be repaired, usually with patch angioplasty. Grafts in which stenoses are identified and repaired prior to thrombus have assisted primary patency identical to primary patency. Those who thrombose have limited longevity resulting from ischemic injury to the vein wall. Limb swelling is common following revascularization and usually returns to baseline within 2 to 3 months. However, it tends to worsen with repeat revascularization (Table 22-12).

Table 22-12
Causes of Graft Thrombosis

Early postoperative failure is due either to a technical flaw or from vein injury or intrinsic vein abnormalities
Thrombosis from 30 days to 18 months is usually due to development of vein stenoses
Graft occlusions >18 months postprocedure are often due to progression of atherosclerosis in either inflow or, more commonly, the outflow vessels

Wound Infection.   Since the most common inflow vessel for distal bypass is the common femoral artery, groin infection occurs in 7% of cases. When an autogenous conduit such as saphenous vein is used, most infection can be managed with local wound care. However, when a prosthetic graft has been used, graft infection is a major concern. Infection of a lower extremity prosthetic bypass graft is associated with an amputation rate greater than 50%. Prosthetic graft infections cannot be eradicated with antibiotics and mandate graft excision and complex revascularization using a vein if it is available. In contrast, vein grafts do not get infected.

Alternate Bypass Techniques

In diabetic patients the SFA may be spared, and it is appropriate to shorten the bypass graft by performing popliteal-to-tibial grafts. In patients in whom both greater saphenous veins (GSVs) have been harvested, alternate vein sources include the short saphenous veins and upper extremity cephalic and basilic veins. Occasionally, sequential bypass such as ePTFE to above-the-knee popliteal artery with a second reversed saphenous vein graft from the popliteal to distal tibial vessels is warranted. A composite graft, in which a vein graft is sewn to an ePTFE graft for bypass, has patency similar to that of a prosthetic graft, and tends to develop neointimal hyperplasia at the graft-vein interface. Alternate conduit options include cryopreserved human saphenous vein graft, and umbilical vein graft. These are both used in limb salvage situations in which no alternate conduit is available.

Endovascular Procedures

Endovascular procedures are undergoing rapid change. Presently, endovascular procedures in the infrainguinal area have a limited role and are confined to short segment stenoses or occlusions. Longer lesions, although treatable, have limited durability due to neointimal hyperplasia. Most surgeons will primarily use angioplasty alone and employ stenting only for severe dissections. However, with the advent of drug-eluting stents, there exists the real possibility to control restenosis. Should these trials confirm restenosis control, a greatly expanded role for endovascular techniques in the infrainguinal vessels may then be realized.

Mesenteric Artery Occlusive Disease

Blood flow to the intestine is supplied by three vessels: the celiac artery (CA), the superior mesenteric artery (SMA) (Fig. 22-74), and the IMA. These are the arteries to the foregut (stomach to second part of duodenum), midgut (second part of duodenum to right two thirds of transverse colon), and hind gut (distal third of the transverse colon to the rectum), respectively. Anastomoses exist between the celiac and superior mesenteric arteries via the pancreaticoduodenal arcade, and between the SMA and IMA via the marginal artery of Drummond and the Riolan arc; however, these collateral pathways are inconsistent and cannot be relied on to suffice in either acute or chronic occlusion of the visceral arteries.

Occlusive disease of the mesenteric arteries usually occurs in individuals who are medically debilitated with generalized atherosclerosis. The disease process may evolve in a chronic fashion, as in the case of progressive luminal plaque narrowing due to atherosclerotic progression. On the other hand, mesenteric ischemia can occur suddenly, as in the case of thromboembolism. Despite recent progress in perioperative management and better understanding in pathophysiology, mesenteric ischemia is one of the most lethal vascular disorders, with mortality rates ranging from 50 to 75%. Delay in diagnosis and treatment are the main contributing factors to the high mortality

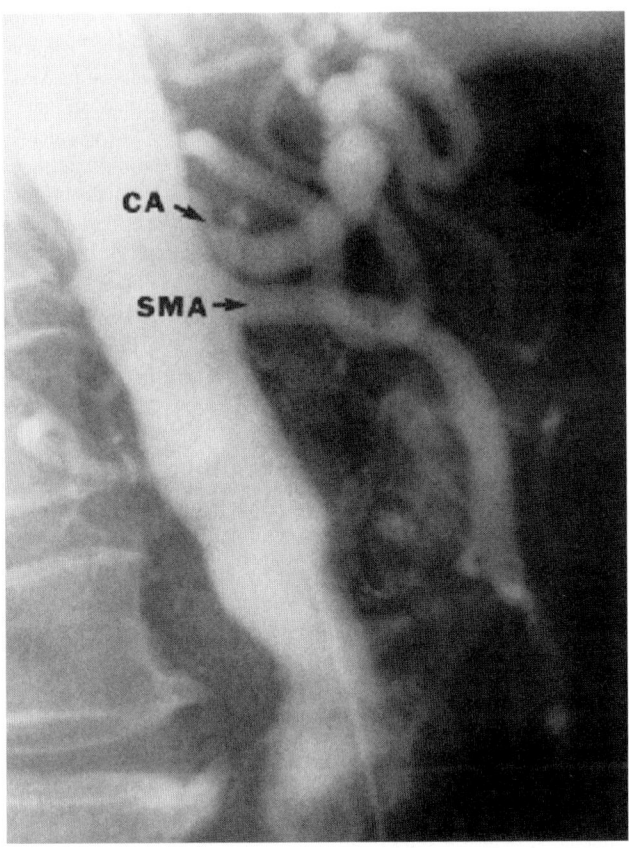

FIG. 22-74. *Lateral aortogram demonstrating normal origins of celiac and superior mesenteric arteries.*

rate. It is estimated that mesenteric ischemia accounts for one in every 1000 hospital admissions in this country. The prevalence is rising due in part to the increased awareness of this disease, the advanced age of the population, and the significant comorbidities

of these elderly patients. Early recognition and prompt treatment prior to the onset of irreversible intestinal ischemia are essential to improve the outcome.

Types of Mesenteric Artery Occlusive Disease

There are four major types of visceral ischemia involving the mesenteric arteries: (1) acute embolic mesenteric ischemia (Fig. 22-75), (2) acute thrombotic mesenteric ischemia, (3) chronic mesenteric ischemia, and (4) nonocclusive mesenteric ischemia.[114–117] Despite the variability of these syndromes, a common anatomic pathology is involved in these processes. The SMA is the most commonly involved vessel in acute mesenteric ischemia. Acute thrombotic mesenteric ischemia frequently occurs in patients with underlying mesenteric atherosclerosis, which usually involves the origin of the mesenteric arteries while sparing the collateral branches. The development of collateral vessels is more likely when the occlusive process is a gradual, rather than a sudden, ischemic event. In acute embolic mesenteric ischemia, the emboli typically originate from a cardiac source, and frequently occur in patients with atrial fibrillation or following myocardial infarction. Nonocclusive mesenteric ischemia is characterized by a low-flow state in otherwise normal mesenteric arteries. In contrast, chronic mesenteric ischemia is a functional consequence of a long-standing atherosclerotic process that typically involves at least two of the three main mesenteric vessels, the CA, the SMA, and the IMA.

Several less common syndromes of visceral ischemia involving the mesenteric arteries can also cause serious debilitation. Chronic mesenteric ischemic symptoms can occur due to extrinsic compression of the celiac artery by the diaphragm, which is termed the *median arcuate ligament syndrome*. Acute visceral ischemia may occur following an aortic operation, due to ligation of the IMA in the absence of adequate collateral vessels. Furthermore, acute visceral ischemia may develop in aortic dissection, which involves the mesenteric arteries. Finally, other unusual causes of ischemia include mesenteric arteritis, radiation arteritis, and cholesterol emboli.

FIG. 22-75. *A. and B. Superior mesenteric artery embolus appearing as a meniscus in the artery 5 cm from the origin.*

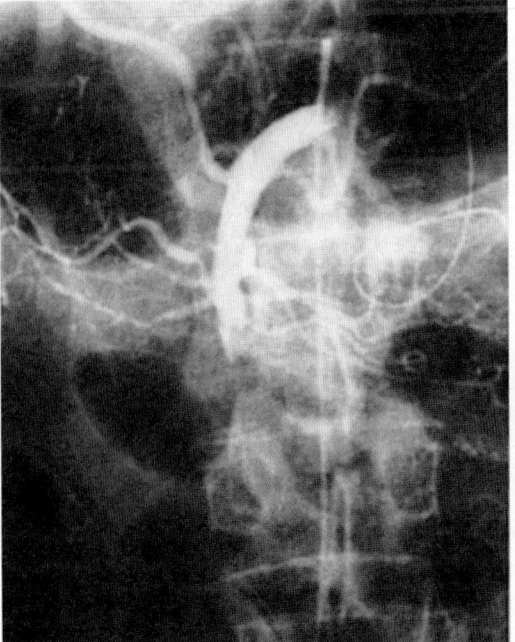

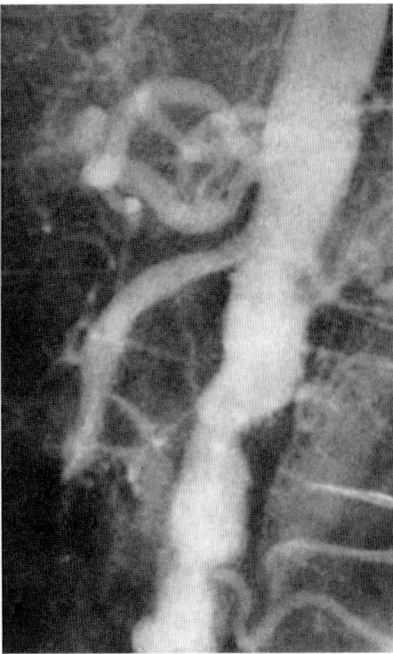

A　　　　*B*

Clinical Presentation

Abdominal pain out of proportion to physical findings is the classic presentation in patients with acute mesenteric ischemia, and occurs frequently following an embolic or thrombotic ischemic event involving the SMA. Clinical manifestations may include sudden onset of abdominal cramps in patients with underlying cardiac or atherosclerotic diseases. Pain out of proportion to the initial findings on abdominal examination is typical in the early stage. The abdominal pain is often associated with bloody diarrhea resulting from mucosal sloughing secondary to ischemia. Frequently, bowel emptying occurs with the onset of ischemia secondary to intestinal spasm as a consequence of the ischemia. Fever, diarrhea, nausea, vomiting, and abdominal distention are common but nonspecific manifestations. Diffuse abdominal tenderness, rebound, and rigidity are ominous signs and usually herald bowel infarction.[118,119]

Symptoms of thrombotic mesenteric ischemia may initially be more insidious than those of embolic mesenteric ischemia. Approximately 70% of patients with chronic mesenteric ischemia have a history of abdominal angina. In these patients, the chronicity of mesenteric atherosclerosis is important, as it permits collateral vessel formation. The precipitating factor leading to chronic mesenteric occlusion is often an unrelated illness that results in dehydration, such as diarrhea or vomiting, which may further confuse the actual diagnosis. If the diagnosis is not recognized promptly, symptoms may worsen that can lead to progressive abdominal distention, oliguria, increasing fluid requirements, and severe metabolic acidosis.

Abdominal pain is only present in approximately 70% of patients with nonocclusive mesenteric ischemia. When present, pain is usually severe, but may vary in location, character, and intensity. In the absence of abdominal pain, progressive abdominal distention with acidosis may be an early sign of ischemia and impending bowel infarction. The diagnosis of nonocclusive mesenteric ischemia should be considered in elderly patients with sudden abdominal pain who have any of the following risk factors: congestive heart failure, acute myocardial infarction with cardiogenic shock, hypovolemic or hemorrhagic shock, sepsis, pancreatitis, and administration of digitalis or vasoconstrictor agents such as epinephrine.

Diagnostic Studies

Laboratory evaluation is neither sensitive nor specific in the diagnosis of mesenteric ischemia. Complete blood count (CBC) may reveal hemoconcentration and leukocytosis. Metabolic acidosis develops as a result of anaerobic metabolism. Elevated serum amylase and lactate levels are nonspecific findings. Hyperkalemia and azotemia may occur in the late stages of ischemia. Plain abdominal radiographs may provide helpful information to exclude other abdominal pathologies such as bowel perforation, obstruction, or volvulus, which may exhibit symptoms mimicking intestinal ischemia. Radiographic appearance of an adynamic ileus with a gasless abdomen is the most common finding in patients with acute mesenteric ischemia. Embolic sources should be sought as described under acute ischemia.

The definitive diagnosis of mesenteric thrombosis is made by biplanar mesenteric arteriography, which should be performed promptly in any patient with suspected mesenteric occlusion. It typically shows occlusion or near-occlusion of the CA and SMA at or near their origins from the aorta. In most cases, the IMA has been previously occluded secondary to diffuse infrarenal aortic atherosclerosis. The differentiation of the four different types of mesenteric arterial occlusion may be suggested with a biplanar

mesenteric arteriogram. Mesenteric emboli typically lodge in the SMA at the origin of the middle colic artery, creating a "meniscus sign" with an abrupt cutoff (see Fig. 22-75) of a normal proximal SMA several centimeters from its origin on the aorta. Mesenteric thrombosis, in contrast, occurs at the most proximal SMA, which tapers off at 1 to 2 cm from its origin. In the case of chronic mesenteric occlusion, the appearance of collateral circulation is usually present. Nonocclusive mesenteric ischemia produces an arteriographic image of segmental mesenteric vasospasm with a relatively normal-appearing main SMA trunk.

Mesenteric arteriography also can play a therapeutic role. Once the diagnosis of nonocclusive mesenteric ischemia is made on the arteriogram, an infusion catheter can be placed at the SMA orifice, and vasodilating agents such as papaverine can be administered intra-arterially. The papaverine infusion may be continued postoperatively to treat persistent vasospasm, a common occurrence following mesenteric reperfusion. Transcatheter thrombolytic therapy has little role in the management of thrombotic mesenteric occlusion. Although thrombolytic agents may transiently recannulate the occluded vessels, the underlying occlusive lesions require definitive treatment. Furthermore, thrombolytic therapy typically requires a prolonged period of time to restore perfusion, and the intestinal viability may be difficult to assess.[120–125]

Treatment

Initial management of patients with acute mesenteric ischemia includes fluid resuscitation and systemic anticoagulation with heparin sulfate to prevent further thrombus propagation. Significant metabolic acidosis should be corrected with sodium bicarbonate if possible. A central venous catheter, peripheral arterial catheter, and a Foley catheter should be placed for fluid resuscitation and hemodynamic status monitoring. Appropriate antibiotics are given prior to surgical exploration. The operative management of acute mesenteric ischemia is dictated by the cause of the occlusion. It is helpful to obtain a preoperative mesenteric arteriogram to confirm the diagnosis and to plan appropriate treatment options. However, the diagnosis of mesenteric ischemia frequently cannot be established prior to surgical exploration, and therefore patients in a moribund condition with acute abdominal symptoms should undergo immediate surgical exploration, avoiding the delay required to perform an arteriogram.

Acute Embolic Mesenteric Ischemia. The primary goal of surgical treatment in embolic mesenteric ischemia is to restore arterial perfusion with removal of the embolus from the vessel. The abdomen is explored through a midline incision, which often reveals variable intestinal ischemia from the midjejunum to the ascending or transverse colon. The transverse colon is lifted superiorly, and the small intestine is reflected toward the right upper quadrant. The SMA is approached at the root of the small bowel mesentery (Fig. 22-76), usually as it emerges from beneath the pancreas to cross over the junction of the third and fourth portions of the duodenum. Alternatively, the SMA can be approached by incising the retroperitoneum lateral to the fourth portion of the duodenum, which is rotated medially to expose the SMA. Once the proximal SMA is identified and controlled with vascular clamps, a transverse arteriotomy is made to extract the embolus, using standard balloon embolectomy catheters (Fig. 22-77). In the event the embolus has lodged more distally, exposure of the distal SMA may be obtained in the root of the small bowel mesentery by isolating individual jejunal and ileal branches to allow a more comprehensive thromboembolectomy. Following the restoration of SMA flow, an assessment of intestinal viability must

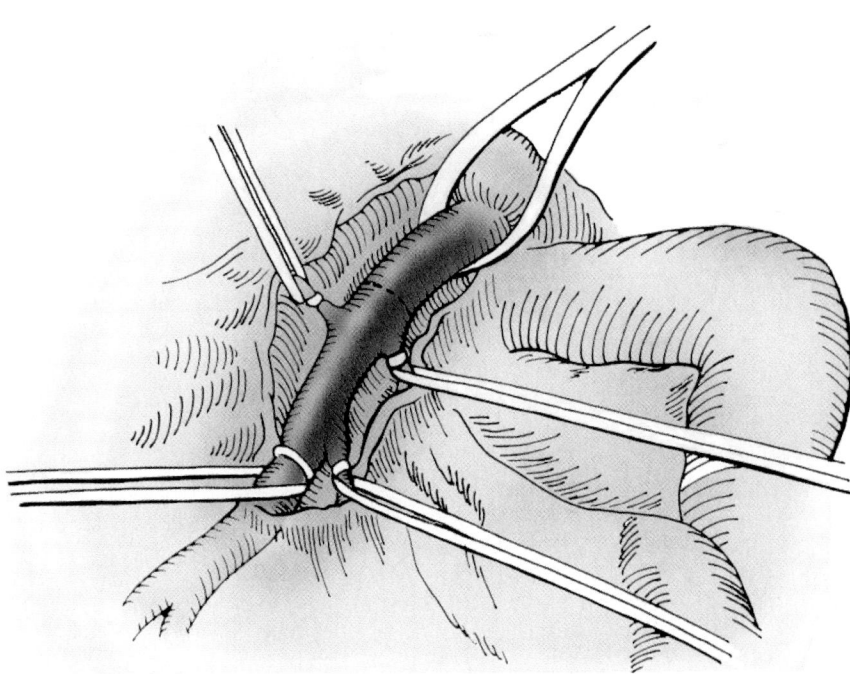

FIG. 22-76. The superior mesenteric artery is exposed as it emerges from below the pancreas.

be made, and nonviable bowel must be resected. Several methods have been described to evaluate the viability of the intestine, which include intraoperative intravenous fluorescein injection and inspection with a Wood's lamp, and Doppler assessment of antimesenteric intestinal arterial pulsations. A second-look procedure should be considered in many patients, and is performed 24 to 48 hours following embolectomy. The goal of the procedure is reassessment of the extent of bowel viability, which may not be obvious immediately following the initial embolectomy. If nonviable intestine is evident in the second-look procedure, additional bowel resections should be performed at that time.

Acute Thrombotic Mesenteric Ischemia. The treatment of thrombotic mesenteric ischemia differs from that of mesenteric embolism, due to the nature of the SMA. In embolic mesenteric ischemia, the SMA itself is otherwise normal, and

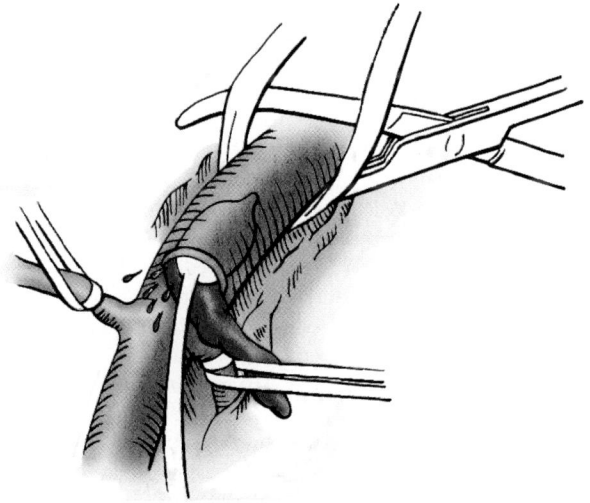

FIG. 22-77. After making a transverse arteriotomy, a balloon catheter is inserted proximally and distally in the SMA to remove all embolic material.

thromboembolectomy will usually suffice to restore mesenteric circulation. However, thrombotic mesenteric ischemia usually involves a severely atherosclerotic vessel, typically the proximal CA and SMA (Fig. 22-78). Therefore, these patients require a reconstructive procedure to the distal SMA to bypass the proximal occlusive lesion and restore adequate mesenteric flow. Exploration in patients with thrombotic mesenteric ischemia often reveals a much more extensive intestinal necrosis than in patients with embolic mesenteric ischemia, due to the extensive atherosclerotic process. The saphenous vein is the graft material of choice, and prosthetic materials should be avoided in patients with nonviable bowel, due to the risk of bacterial contamination if resection of necrotic intestine is performed. The bypass graft may originate from either the aorta or iliac artery. The supraceliac infradiaphragmatic aorta offers several advantages as the origin of the graft when compared to the infrarenal aorta. The supraceliac aorta is often devoid of atherosclerotic plaque, which minimizes the potential embolic complications associated with clamping of the frequently calcified infrarenal aorta. In addition, revascularization from the supraceliac aorta to the distal SMA permits an antegrade graft placement, which is less prone to kinking when the small intestine is returned to its normal location following the bypass procedure.

Chronic Mesenteric Ischemia. The therapeutic goal in patients with chronic mesenteric ischemia is to revascularize mesenteric circulation and prevent the development of bowel infarction. Mesenteric occlusive disease can be treated successfully by either transaortic endarterectomy or mesenteric artery bypass. Transaortic endarterectomy is indicated for ostial lesions of patent CA and SMA. This can be accomplished by a left medial visceral rotation to expose the aorta and its mesenteric branches. A lateral aortotomy is performed encompassing both the CA and SMA. The visceral arteries must be adequately mobilized so that the termination site of endarterectomy can be visualized. Otherwise, an intimal flap may develop, which can lead to early thrombosis or distal embolization.

For occlusive lesions located 1 to 2 cm distal to the mesenteric origin, mesenteric artery bypass should be performed.

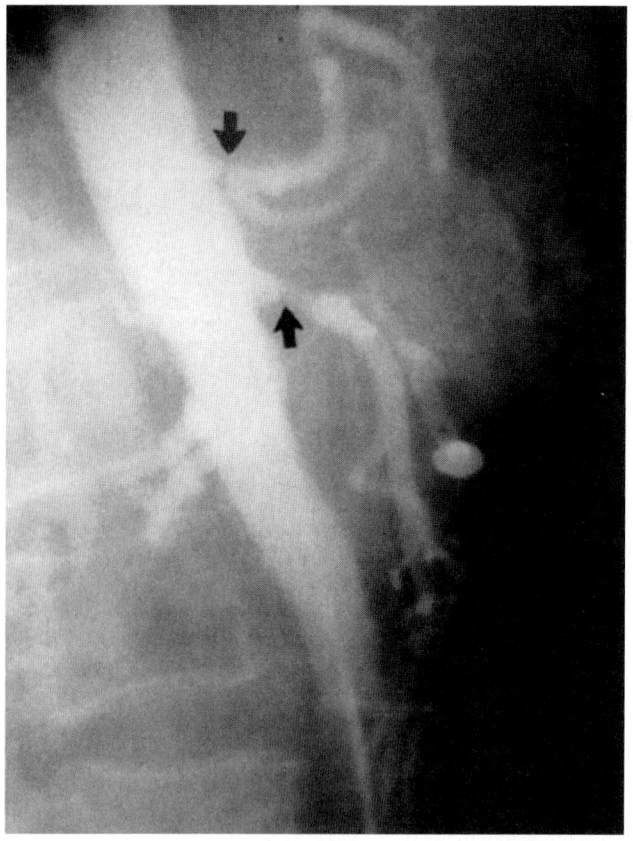

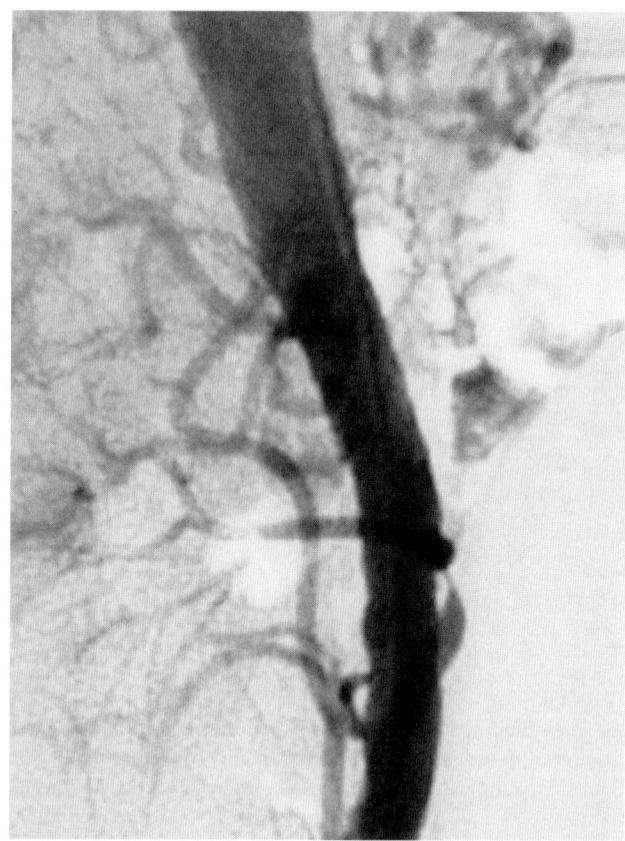

A

B

FIG. 22-78.   *A. and B. Chronic mesenteric ischemia. Stenoses are evident at the origin of both the celiac artery and the superior mesenteric artery.*

Multiple mesenteric arteries are typically involved in chronic mesenteric ischemia, and both the CA and SMA should be revascularized whenever possible; a collateral called the arc of Riolan may fill the distal SMA from the IMA (Fig. 22-79). In general, bypass grafting may be performed either antegrade from the supraceliac aorta or retrograde from either the infrarenal aorta or iliac artery. Both autogenous saphenous vein grafts and prosthetic grafts have been used with satisfactory and equivalent success (Fig. 22-80). An antegrade bypass also can be performed using a small-caliber bifurcated graft from the supraceliac aorta to both the CA and SMA, which yields an excellent long-term result.[126–129]

Nonocclusive Mesenteric Ischemia. The treatment of nonocclusive mesenteric ischemia is primarily pharmacologic, with selective mesenteric arterial catheterization followed by infusion of vasodilatory agents such as tolazoline or papaverine. Once the diagnosis is made via mesenteric arteriography, intra-arterial papaverine is given at a dose of 30 to 60 mg/h. This must be coupled with the cessation of other vasoconstricting agents. Concomitant intravenous heparin should be administered to prevent thrombosis in the cannulated vessels. The treatment strategy thereafter is dependent on the patient's clinical response to the vasodilator therapy. If abdominal symptoms improve, mesenteric arteriography should be repeated to document the resolution of vasospasm. The patient's hemodynamic status must be carefully monitored during papaverine infusion, as significant hypotension can develop in the event that the infusion catheter migrates into the aorta, which can lead to systemic circulation of papaverine. Surgical exploration is indicated if the

patient develops signs of continued bowel ischemia or infarction as evidenced by rebound tenderness or involuntary guarding. In these circumstances, papaverine infusion should be continued intraoperatively and postoperatively. The operating room should be kept as warm as possible and warm irrigation fluid and laparotomy pads should be used to prevent further intestinal vasoconstriction during exploration.

Celiac Artery Compression Syndrome

Abdominal pain due to narrowing of the origin of the celiac artery (CA) may occur as a result of extrinsic compression or impingement by the median arcuate ligament. This condition is known as celiac artery compression syndrome or median arcuate ligament syndrome. Celiac artery compression syndrome has been implicated in some variants of chronic mesenteric ischemia. However, significant compression of the celiac artery can be observed frequently on a lateral aortogram in the complete absence of symptoms. A decision to intervene is therefore based on both an appropriate symptom complex and the finding of celiac artery compression in the absence of other findings to explain the symptoms. The patient should be cautioned that relief of the celiac compression cannot be guaranteed to relieve the symptoms. Most patients are young females between 20 and 40 years of age. Abdominal symptoms are nonspecific, but the pain is localized in the upper abdomen and may be precipitated by meals. The treatment goal is to release the ligamentous structure that compresses the proximal CA and to correct any persistent stricture by bypass grafting.

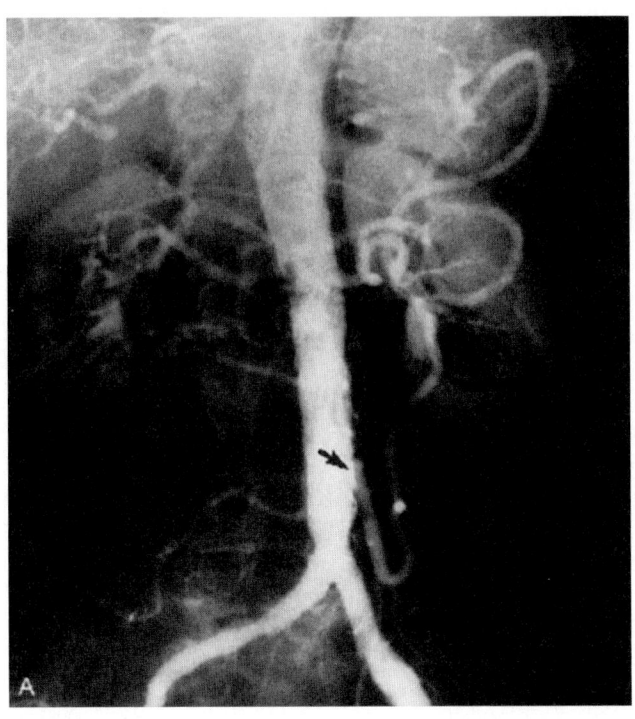

A

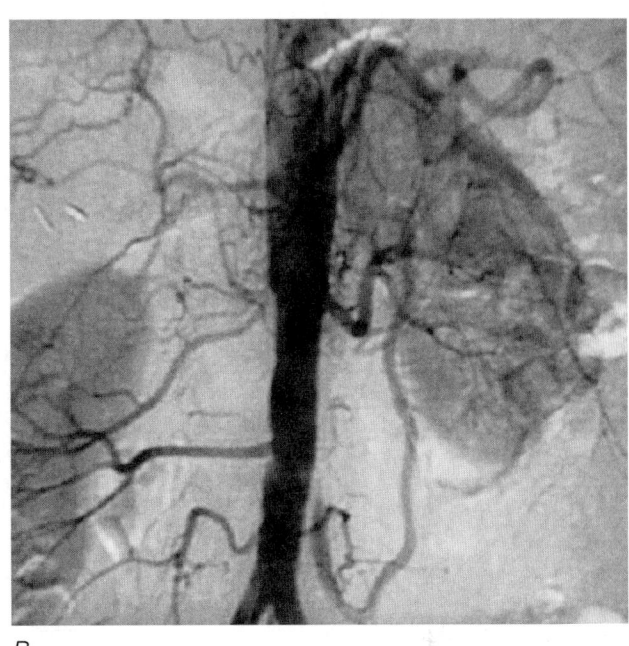

B

FIG. 22-79. The arc of Riolan, a collateral that connects the IMA to the SMA.

Other Causes of Mesenteric Ischemia

While atherosclerotic occlusion of the main mesenteric arteries accounts for the majority of cases of chronic intestinal ischemia, other conditions also exist that can compromise mesenteric circulation and should be considered in the differential diagnosis. They include radiation arteritis, polyarteritis nodosa, lupus erythematosus, Kawasaki's disease, and fibromuscular dysplasia. Patients who smoke heavily or young women who are taking oral contraceptives may be at risk of developing intimal hyperplasia of the visceral arteries, which also can lead to mesenteric ischemia.

Renal Artery Occlusive Disease

Obstructive lesions of the renal artery can produce hypertension, resulting in a condition known as renovascular hypertension, which is the most common form of hypertension amenable to therapeutic intervention. Renovascular hypertension is believed to affect 5 to 10% of all hypertensive patients in the United States. Patients with renovascular hypertension are at an increased risk for irreversible renal dysfunction if inappropriate pharmacologic therapies are used to control the blood pressure (e.g., angiotensin-converting enzyme [ACE] inhibitors). In the rare event that a critically ischemic kidney

FIG. 22-80. Infrarenal aorta-to-SMA bypass.

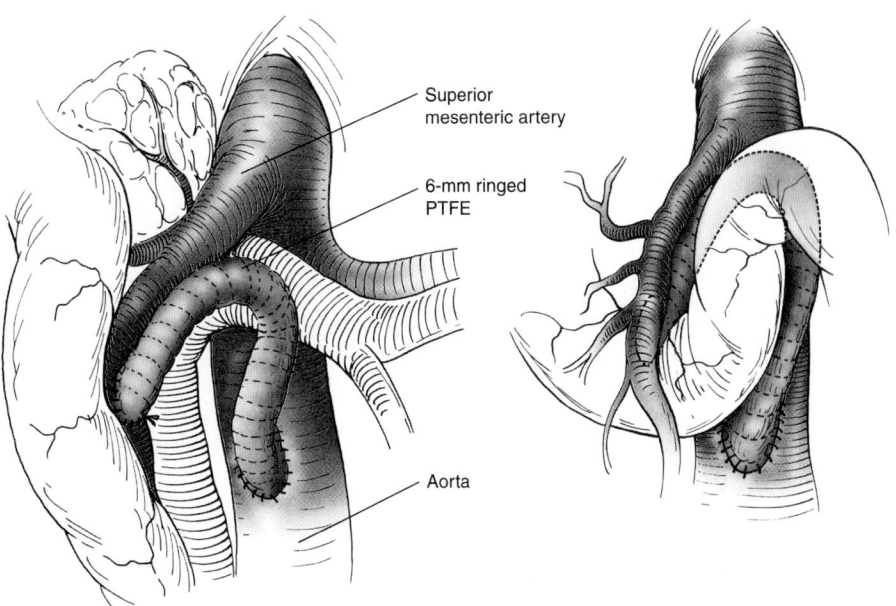

Superior mesenteric artery

6-mm ringed PTFE

Aorta

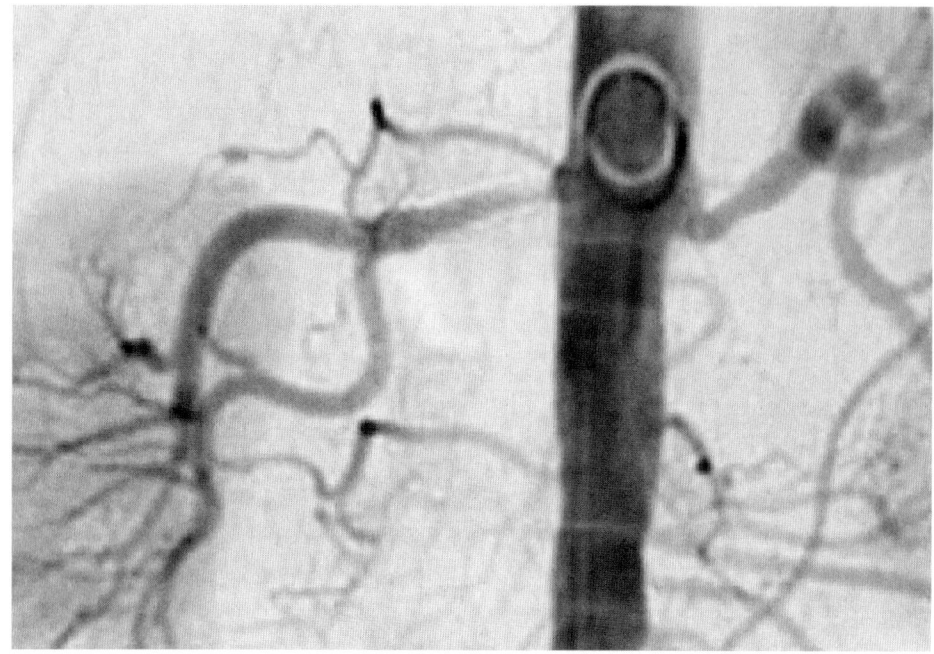

FIG. 22-81. In-stent restenosis in a stented right renal artery.

cannot be revascularized, nephrectomy may also be effective in improving hypertension and preserving contralateral renal function.

Causes of Renal Artery Stenosis

Nearly 70% of all renal artery occlusive lesions are caused by atherosclerosis, typically occur near the renal artery ostia, and are usually less than 1 cm in length.

Patients with this disease are usually elderly males that have other atherosclerotic disease such as ischemic heart disease and peripheral vascular disease; however, a growing number of patients develop restenosis of previously placed stents (Fig. 22-81).

The second most common cause of renal artery stenosis is fibromuscular dysplasia. Fibromuscular dysplasia of the renal artery represents a heterogeneous group of lesions that produce specific pathologic lesions in various regions of the vessel wall, including the intima, media, or adventitia. The most common variety consists of medial fibroplasia, in which thickened fibromuscular ridges alternate with attenuated media, producing the classic angiographic "string of beads" appearance. The cause of medial fibroplasia remains unclear, but it appears to be associated with modification of arterial smooth muscle cells in response to estrogenic stimuli during the reproductive years, unusual traction forces on affected vessels, and mural ischemia from impairment of vasa vasorum blood flow. Fibromuscular hyperplasia usually affects the distal two thirds of the main renal artery, and the right renal artery is affected more frequently than the left (Fig. 22-82). The entity occurs most commonly in young women, who are often multiparous.

Other less common causes of renal artery stenosis include renal artery aneurysm (compressing the adjacent normal renal artery), arteriovenous malformations, neurofibromatosis, renal artery dissections, renal artery trauma, Takayasu's disease (an arteritis causing stenosis of branch vessels arising from the aorta), and renal artery thrombosis.[130–136]

Pathophysiology of Renovascular Hypertension

A high-grade stenosis of the renal artery can induce a pressure gradient sufficient to cause increased renin release by the juxtaglomerular cells around renal afferent arterioles. Renin secretion is stimulated by decreased blood pressure and extracellular fluid volume. Once released into the systemic circulation, renin converts the glycoprotein angiotensinogen into angiotensin I in the liver. An angiotensin-converting enzyme subsequently splits angiotensin I into angiotensin II. The most important consequence of renal artery occlusive disease is the production of angiotensin II. Angiotensin II acts directly on arteriolar smooth muscle of nearly all vascular beds, with the splanchnic, renal, and cutaneous circulations being most sensitive to its effects. Angiotensin II exerts its pressor effect via the following four mechanisms: (1) it causes vasoconstriction by increasing systemic vascular resistance, thereby raising the

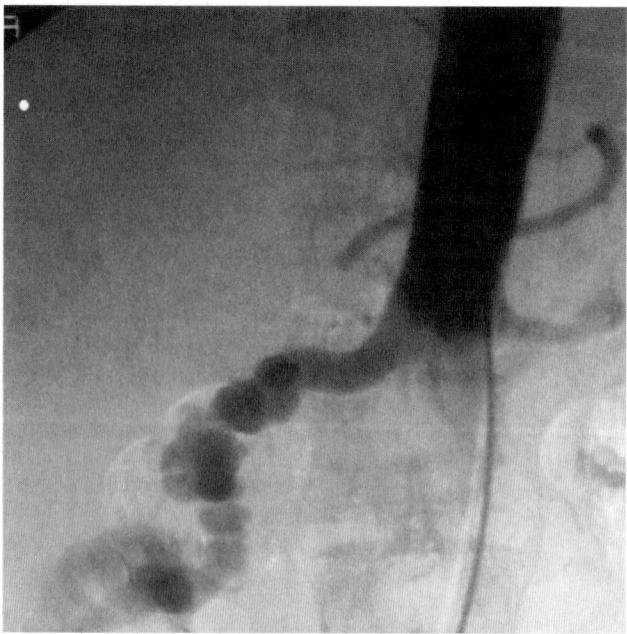

FIG. 22-82. Severe right renal artery fibromuscular disease.

arterial pressure; (2) it acts on the adrenal cortex to release aldosterone, which in turn acts on the kidneys to increase sodium and fluid retention; (3) it stimulates the release of vasopressin, an antidiuretic hormone, from the posterior pituitary, which causes the kidneys to increase fluid retention; and (4) it stimulates norepinephrine release from the sympathetic nerve endings and inhibits norepinephrine reuptake by nerve endings, thereby enhancing sympathetic adrenergic function.

In the case of renovascular hypertension caused by unilateral renal artery stenosis, a normal contralateral kidney can partially compensate for the elevated renin level by increasing natriuresis. Although renin levels remain elevated indefinitely, the administration of angiotensin II inhibitor is effective in lowering blood pressure in the setting of unilateral renal artery disease. By contrast, the compensatory response of increased natriuresis by the normal contralateral kidney does not occur in the presence of bilateral renovascular hypertension or unilateral renal artery disease in patients with a solitary kidney. In this setting, elevated renin secretion is transient because it is suppressed by volume expansion from sodium and water retention, and the hypertension is maintained by volume expansion rather than by renin-mediated vasoconstriction. As a result, the administration of angiotensin II inhibitor is generally ineffective in alleviating the hypertensive state caused by either bilateral renal artery stenosis or unilateral solitary renal artery stenosis.

Diagnostic Studies

Nearly all diagnostic studies for renovascular hypertension evaluate either the anatomic stenosis or renal parenchymal dysfunction attributed to the stenosis. The benefits and limitations of these tests are important in the proper selection of patients for renal artery intervention.

Renal duplex scanning is a noninvasive test assessing renal artery stenosis both by visualization of the vessel and by measurement of the effect of stenosis on blood flow velocity and waveforms. The presence of a severe renal artery stenosis correlates with peak systolic velocities of greater than 180 cm/s and a ratio of these velocities to those in the aorta of greater than 3.5. However, many renal artery ultrasounds are difficult to perform or interpret due to obesity or increased bowel gas pattern. In addition, renal ultrasonography does not differentiate among renal artery stenoses exceeding 60% cross-sectional stenosis. Because this test is highly dependent on the operator's expertise, its role as an effective screening test remains limited.[137]

Conventional renal artery angiography is critical to the evaluation of patients with possible renovascular hypertension. A flush aortogram is performed first so that any accessory renal arteries can be detected and the origins of all the renal arteries are adequately displayed. The presence of collateral vessels circumventing a renal artery stenosis strongly supports the hemodynamic importance of the stenosis. A pressure gradient of 10 mm Hg or greater is necessary for collateral vessel development, which is also associated with activation of the renin-angiotensin cascade.

Magnetic Resonance Angiography. Magnetic resonance angiography (MRA), particularly with gadolinium contrast enhancement, has become a useful diagnostic tool for renal artery occlusive disease, because of its ability to provide high-resolution images (Fig. 22-83). The minimally invasive nature of MRA plus the low risk of nephrotoxicity of gadolinium contrast makes it an appealing diagnostic modality. With continuous refinement in imaging

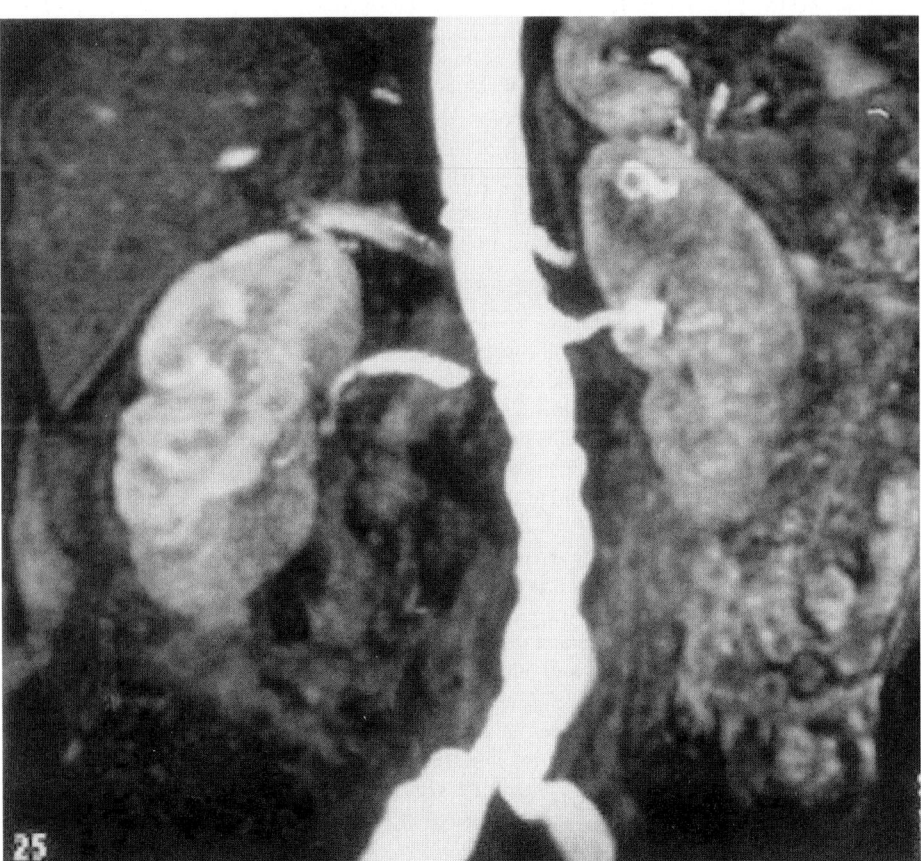

FIG. 22-83. Bilateral renal artery stenoses demonstrated by MRA.

software, it will likely become a widely accepted imaging modality in patients suspected of renovascular hypertension.[138-142]

Selective catheterization of the renal vein via a femoral vein approach for assessing renin activity is a more invasive test of detecting the functional status of renal artery disease. If unilateral disease is present, the affected kidney should secrete high levels of renin, while the contralateral kidney should have low renin production. A ratio between the two kidneys, or the renal vein renin ratio (RVRR), of greater than 1.5 is indicative of functionally significant renovascular hypertension, and it also predicts a favorable response to renovascular revascularization. Since this study assesses the RVRR between the two kidneys, it is not useful in patients with bilateral disease, since both kidneys may secrete abnormally elevated renin levels.

The renal systemic renin index (RSRI) is calculated by subtracting systemic renin activity from individual renal vein renin activity and dividing the remainder by systemic renin activity. This value represents the degree of renin that an individual kidney secretes. In normal individuals without renovascular hypertension, the renal vein renin activity from each kidney is typically 24% or 0.24 higher than the systemic level. As a result, the total of both kidneys' renin activity is usually 48% or 0.48 greater than the systemic activity. This value of 0.48 reflects a steady state of renal renin activity.

The RSRI of the affected kidney in patients with renovascular hypertension is greater than 0.24. In the case of unilateral renal artery stenosis with a normal contralateral kidney, the increase in ipsilateral renin release is normally balanced by suppression of the contralateral kidney renin production, which results in a drop in its RSRI to less than 0.24. Bilateral renal artery disease may negate the contralateral compensatory response, and the autonomous release of renin from both diseased kidneys may result in the sum of the individual RSRIs to be considerably greater than 0.48. The prognostic value of ischemic kidney renin hypersecretion (RSRI more than 0.48) and contralateral kidney renin suppression (RSRI between 0.0 and 0.24) as a means of discriminating between expected cured and favorable surgical response has been thoroughly studied. However, the prognostic accuracy of RSRI remains limited in that approximately 10% of patients with favorable surgical responses following renovascular revascularization do not exhibit contralateral renin suppression. The clinical usefulness of RSRI must be applied with caution in the management of patients with renovascular hypertension.

Treatment

Medical Therapy. The development of a new generation of antihypertensive medications including beta blockers, calcium channel blockers, and ACE inhibitors has greatly enhanced the ability to control high blood pressure in many patients with renovascular hypertension. Refractory hypertension, particularly that due to bilateral disease or unilateral renal artery stenosis with contralateral parenchymal disease, may respond to the addition of diuretic medications.

If the renal function remains stable and the blood pressure is satisfactorily controlled by medications, it is appropriate to maintain medical therapy for renovascular hypertension. However, a reduction in systemic pressure by drug therapy frequently reduces renal perfusion, which may lead to progressive renal failure. While ACE inhibitors have proved to be extremely effective in treating renovascular hypertension, these medications often have a deleterious effect on renal function by markedly reducing intrarenal blood pressure and altering intrarenal autoregulation. This harmful effect is particularly likely to occur when there is a critical stenosis in a solitary

kidney or bilateral disease. Since renal artery occlusive disease frequently progresses with concomitant loss of renal mass and function, a definitive therapy to restore normal renal blood flow may provide a greater long-term benefit than antihypertensive medical therapy.

Transluminal Balloon Angioplasty and Stenting. Percutaneous transluminal angioplasty of the renal artery is being performed with increasing frequency. A guidewire is inserted into the renal artery from a femoral artery approach and then passed across the stenosis. An angioplasty balloon catheter is next inserted over the guidewire and positioned across the renal artery stenosis. Inflation of the balloon creates a controlled disruption of the vessel wall, thereby eliminating the intraluminal stenosis.

Percutaneous balloon angioplasty has a high success and low recurrence rate as a treatment for fibromuscular dysplasia, particularly of the medial fibroplastic type. More than two thirds of patients with fibromuscular dysplasia are cured following balloon angioplasty and maintain diastolic pressure below 90 mm Hg without antihypertensive medication. Most of the remainder of patients have significant improvement in their renovascular hypertension, although they may require antihypertensive medication.

Patients with renal artery atherosclerotic lesions do less well with percutaneous balloon angioplasty alone. Renal artery atherosclerotic lesions are typically an extension of aortic disease and are limited to the renal artery ostium where it joins the aorta (Fig. 22-84). Balloon angioplasty in this setting is usually ineffective in achieving satisfactory dilatation because of recoil. Contraindications to balloon angioplasty include lesions involving renal artery bifurcations and bilateral renal artery stenoses.

Intravascular stents placed during balloon angioplasty are now widely used to support renal angioplasty as primary stenting has become common (Fig. 22-85). Current data suggest that stenting may prove useful in patients with ostial disease, those who develop restenosis after percutaneous balloon angioplasty, or those with complications resulting from percutaneous transluminal renal angioplasty (PTRA), such as dissection. Primary renal artery stenting in patients with atherosclerotic ostial renal artery stenosis has a high technical success rate, with restenosis rates ranging from 10 to 20% at 4 years.[143-146]

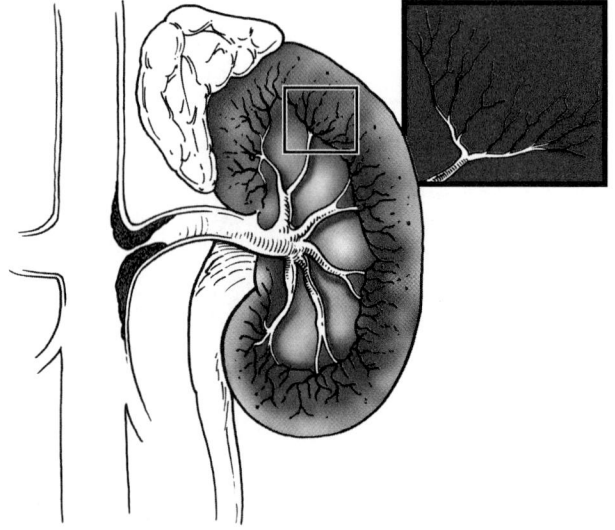

FIG. 22-84. Atherosclerotic disease of the renal artery often involves the ostium and distal arterial segments in the renal parenchyma.

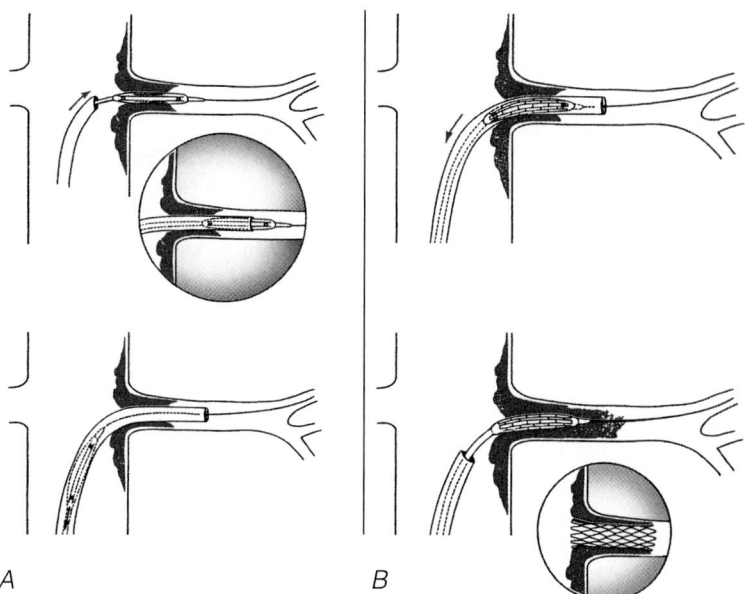

FIG. 22-85. *A. Renal artery stenting begins with the initial balloon angioplasty of the renal ostial lesion. B. A balloon-expandable renal stent is delivered to the renal artery lesion through a guiding sheath, which is followed by the deployment of the renal stent.*

A   B

Surgical Revascularization. A variety of surgical revascularization techniques can be utilized to correct stenosis or occlusion of the renal arteries. The proper selection of an operative approach relates to the extent of the renal artery occlusive disease, the degree of concomitant aortic atherosclerotic disease, and the preference of the surgeon performing the procedure.

Transaortic renal artery endarterectomy (Fig. 22-86) is appropriate for atherosclerotic lesions, but is not applicable in fibrodysplastic disease of the renal artery. The procedure may be accomplished through a transaortic exposure in which the aorta is clamped and opened at the level of the renal arteries via a transverse aortotomy.

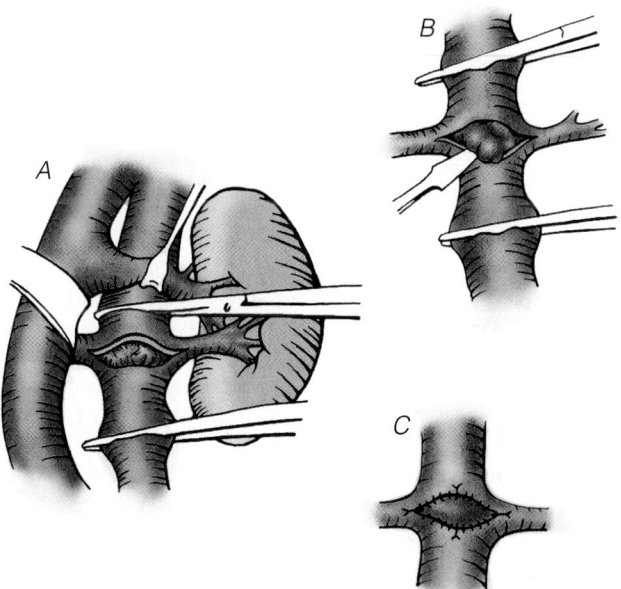

FIG. 22-86. *A. Transaortic endarterectomy begins with a proximal and distal aortic control followed by a transverse aortotomy. B. The aortic plaque is endarterectomized through the transverse aortotomy. C. The aortotomy is closed with an aortic patch angioplasty.*

A local endarterectomy of one or both vessels is performed. This procedure is useful in bilateral renal arterial ostial lesions. It should not be used if the disease is in the distal portion of the renal artery.

Renal artery bypass is another important operative approach to correct renal artery stenoses and occlusions. The choice of the type of renal reconstruction depends on the status of the abdominal aorta. An aortorenal bypass using autogenous saphenous vein is the procedure of choice when the aorta is relatively spared from atherosclerotic change and clamping will not produce injury or distal embolization. Prosthetic grafts with ePTFE or Dacron are acceptable alternatives to use of the saphenous vein. Use of the saphenous vein should be avoided in children, because it is prone to the development of aneurysmal change. The hypogastric artery is the best choice for aortorenal grafting in the pediatric patient.

In the event that the aorta is so heavily calcified that it poses a daunting technical challenge to perform an aortorenal grafting procedure, an alternative donor vessel source can be considered. Saphenous vein bypass from the hepatic artery to the right renal artery or splenic artery bypass to the left renal artery are the most appropriate alternatives. Both procedures avoid the embolic and hemodynamic consequences of aortic clamping. Splenorenal grafts are performed by transecting the splenic artery and constructing an anastomosis of one end of the splenic artery to one end or side of the left renal artery, and collateral flow from the short gastric vessels obviates the need for splenectomy. Alternatively, the gastroduodenal artery itself, which communicates between the celiac artery and superior mesenteric artery, can be divided distally and anastomosed to the right renal artery if it is long enough. Reconstructions based on the visceral arteries should only be performed if significant mesenteric artery occlusive disease has been excluded on angiography. Occasionally concurrent aortic disease mandates synchronous aortic reconstruction (Fig. 22-87).

Kidney autotransplantation may be a useful treatment modality when dealing with distal renal artery occlusive disease. Disease involving the distal renal artery or smaller renal artery branches may be difficult to expose and revascularize with the kidney left in situ. Correction of these lesions requires microvascular anastomosis using vein graft. In order for this to be performed, the kidney is

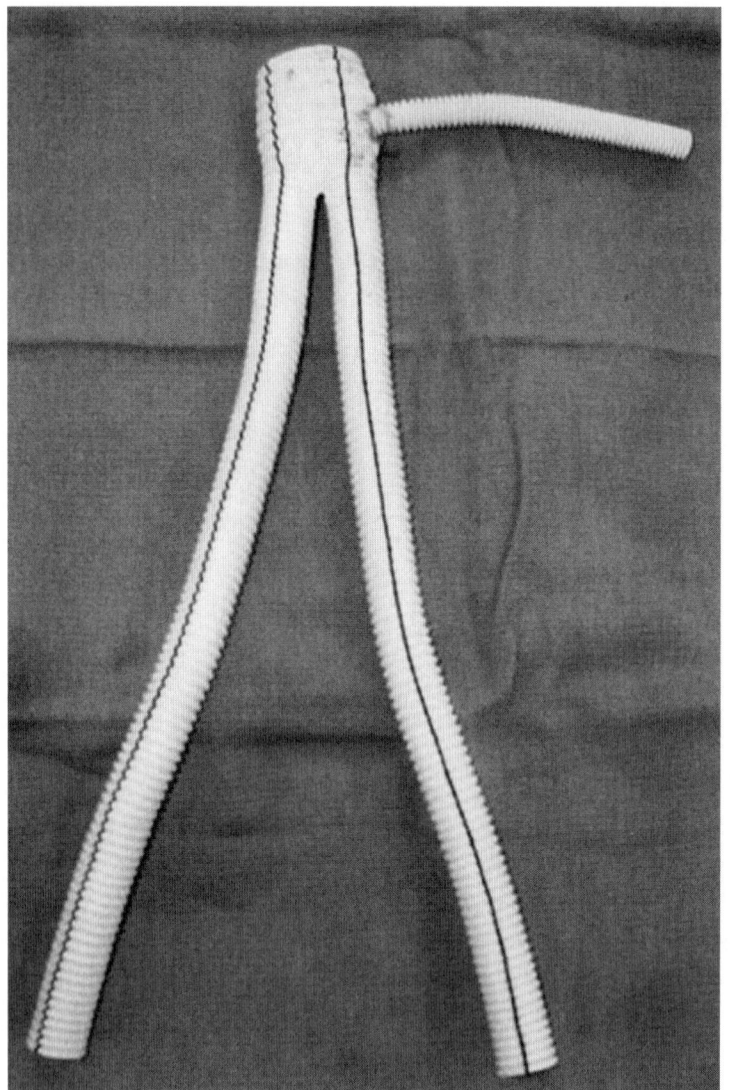

A

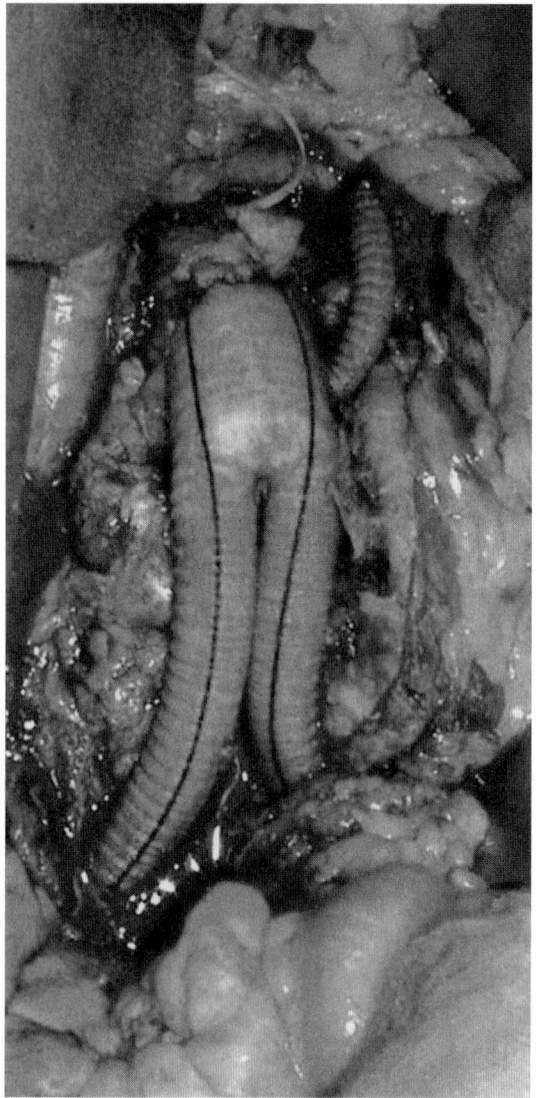

B

FIG. 22-87. *A. A prosthetic side limb is sewn to an aortic bifurcated graft for a concomitant aortic and renal bypass grafting. B. Completion image of an aortorenal bypass grafting.*

usually removed from the body and perfused with cold fluid to protect against ischemic damage. It is autotransplanted in the iliac fossa with the renal artery and vein anastomosing to the iliac vessels.

Nephrectomy is appropriate in patients with severe renovascular hypertension when the involved kidney is the source of renin production but is so severely damaged from chronic ischemia (<6 cm in length) that the prospects for retrieval of renal function are poor. In other patients it may prove impossible to safely bypass the renal artery while the contralateral kidney is functioning, either because of the extent of disease or the frailty of the patient. In these circumstances nephrectomy may provide a simple and safe treatment option for renovascular hypertension.[147–153]

Carotid Artery Occlusive Disease

An occlusive lesion at the origin of the internal carotid artery remains the most common cause of cerebrovascular accidents, which is the third most common cause of death and accounts for 160,000 deaths annually in the United States. Management of cerebrovascular accidents consumes $45 billion annually and is responsible for more than 1 million hospital admissions each year in the United States. The morbidity caused by a cerebrovascular accident is more disabling than that encountered with other arterial ischemic events, including myocardial infarction. Neurologic sequelae related to cerebrovascular accidents, including aphasia, paralysis, blindness, and weakness, can severely limit patients' ability to carry out routine daily activities and invariably create an enormous burden on the cost of health care. As a result, prevention of cerebrovascular accidents, particularly the treatment of extracranial carotid occlusive disease, will remain an important health care issue.

Nomenclature of Cerebrovascular Ischemia

Focal cerebral ischemic disease, or stroke, is defined as a loss of cerebral function lasting more than 24 hours that is due to ischemic vascular etiology. Stroke is responsible for 4.5 million deaths worldwide, with the majority occurring in nonindustrialized countries. The incidence of stroke is 0.2% per year in the general population, but rises significantly with concurrent risk factors such as age, sex, and ethnic background. Overall, the 20-year risk for a 45-year-old male is 3%, and this risk increases to 25% for a 40-year risk. The annual incidence of stroke doubles for each decade in patients greater than 55 years of age. The largest incidence of stroke is observed in patients more than 80 years of age, in whom the prevalence is 2%.

A *transient ischemic attack* (TIA) is defined in the same manner as is stroke, but lasts less than 24 hours. In fact most TIAs resolve within minutes rather than hours. In the United States, the prevalence of TIA in males aged between 65 and 69 years is 2.7%, which increases markedly to 3.6% for males aged between 75 and 79 years. When the frequency of TIAs is greater than two or three per day, it is referred to as *crescendo TIA*. When the ischemic focal neurologic symptoms last longer than 24 hours, but resolve within 3 weeks, the term *reversible ischemic neurologic deficit* (RIND) is applied. Neurologic deficits lasting longer than 3 weeks are considered completed strokes.

Pathogenesis of Stroke and Transient Ischemic Attacks

Approximately 80% of all strokes are caused by ischemic etiologies, while the remainder are caused by hemorrhage. Patients with ischemic neurologic deficit can be further classified into anterior or hemispheric symptoms and posterior or vertebrobasilar symptoms. Hemispheric symptoms are frequently caused by emboli from the carotid circulation. Vertebrobasilar symptoms originate from either flow-limiting or embolic lesions of the aortic arch vessels, the vertebral arteries, or the basilar artery. The predominant causes of stroke and TIA arise from the occlusive lesion of the extracranial carotid artery, and include internal carotid artery thrombosis, flow-related ischemic events, and cerebral embolization.

Carotid Artery Thrombosis. Thrombosis of the internal carotid artery represents the terminal event of the atherosclerotic progression of the carotid artery bifurcation. The clinical sequelae of carotid thrombosis depend on several factors, including the presence of cerebral collateral vessels provided by the circle of Willis, the chronicity of the thrombosis, and the extent of the thrombosis. Once the internal carotid artery becomes thrombosed, the column of thrombus usually propagates distally to the ophthalmic artery. However, the thrombus may occasionally extend beyond the ophthalmic artery and propagate into the circle of Willis. If the distal propagation of the thrombus stops at the ophthalmic artery and remains stable, the event of total occlusion may be silent if collateral flow is sufficient. If the thrombus progresses beyond the ophthalmic artery into the middle cerebral artery, a hemispheric event varying from a TIA to a profound stroke occurs.

Infrequently, carotid artery thrombosis may cause posterior or vertebrobasilar territory strokes. This occurs due in part to the embryologic development of the carotid circulation, in which the internal carotid artery provides the blood flow to the developing posterior cerebral hemispheres and brain stem via the posterior communicating and posterior cerebral arteries. If this anatomic circuitry persists into adult life, vertebrobasilar ischemic symptoms can occur as the result of carotid artery thrombosis.

Flow-Related Ischemic Events. Flow-related ischemic events (hypoperfusion) occur due to the development of hemodynamically significant stenosis involving multiple arteries, or secondary to a stenosis in an artery supplying a vascular territory for which there is a poor collateral network. This was once thought to be the most common cause of cerebral symptoms in conjunction with carotid artery disease. Although transient decreases in cerebral perfusion through a stenotic carotid artery can produce symptoms, this occurrence is rare and accounts for less than 15% of all cerebrovascular ischemic events. Patients who are susceptible to this type of stroke include those with critical internal carotid artery (ICA) stenoses, poor collateralization via the circle of Willis, and a secondary trigger such as hypotension following an acute cardiac event. Due in part to vast collateral pathways for cerebral perfusion through the circle of Willis, coupled with the rich contralateral carotid artery and transcranial external-to-internal carotid artery connections, cerebral perfusion is rarely diminished to a critical level despite the presence of a severe carotid artery stenosis.

Carotid Artery Embolization. Nearly one half of all ischemic carotid territory strokes are due to cholesterol or platelet-fibrin emboli that dislodged from atherosclerotic plaques within the ICA and subsequently occluded distal branches of the ICA, including territories supplied by either the middle cerebral artery and/or the anterior cerebral artery. This mechanism accounts for the occurrence of the Hollenhorst plaques, which are platelet-fibrin aggregates or cholesterol crystals obstructing branches of the retinal artery which are frequently observed during an ophthalmologic exam. TIA or stroke as a consequence of a carotid stenosis has been extensively studied, with clear benefit established in the NASCET trial for stenoses greater than 75%. The ACAS trial demonstrated benefit even in asymptomatic patients for stenoses greater than 60%.[154–162]

Cardiogenic Embolization. Cardiogenic embolization is responsible for less than 10% of all ischemic carotid territory strokes. The emboli materials consist of varying combinations of fibrin, cholesterol, calcified debris, and atheroma, depending on the underlying cardiac pathology. Sources include valvular heart disease, prosthetic valves, atrial myxoma, ventricular aneurysmal thrombus, cardiomyopathy, and infective endocarditis. The most common source for cardiogenic emboli is mural thrombus overlying a dyskinetic segment of myocardium following a myocardial infarction.

Hematologic Causes. Various hematologic pathologies predisposing to a hypercoagulable state are responsible for about 5% of ischemic strokes, and include polycythemia, sickle cell disease, leukemia, thrombocythemia, malignancies, lupus anticoagulant (antiphospholipid antibody syndrome), antithrombin III deficiency, and protein S or protein C deficiency.

Miscellaneous Causes. Miscellaneous causes account for less than 5% of ischemic carotid territory strokes, and include migraine, oral contraceptive use, trauma, dissection, giant cell arteritis, Takayasu's arteritis, systemic lupus erythematosus, polyarteritis nodosa, amyloid angiopathy, cocaine abuse, fibromuscular dysplasia, and radiation arteritis.

Pathology of Carotid Artery Disease

Atherosclerosis. Atherosclerosis is the most common pathology affecting the carotid artery bifurcation. The tendency for atherosclerotic plaque to occur at the carotid bifurcation is related to a number of factors, including geometry, velocity profile, and shear stress. It has been demonstrated that plaque formation in the carotid artery bifurcation is increased in areas of low flow velocity and low shear stress, and decreased in areas of high flow velocity and elevated shear stress (Figs. 22-88 and 22-89). Postmortem specimens showed that atherosclerosis was particularly pronounced along the outer (lateral) aspect of the proximal ICA and carotid bulb. This zone corresponds to areas of low velocity and low shear stress. Conversely, the medial or inner aspect of the cadaveric carotid bulb,

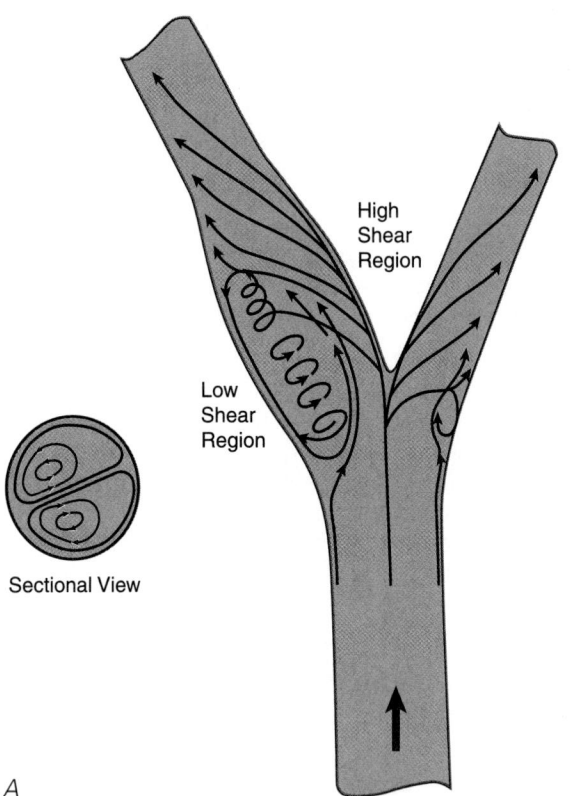

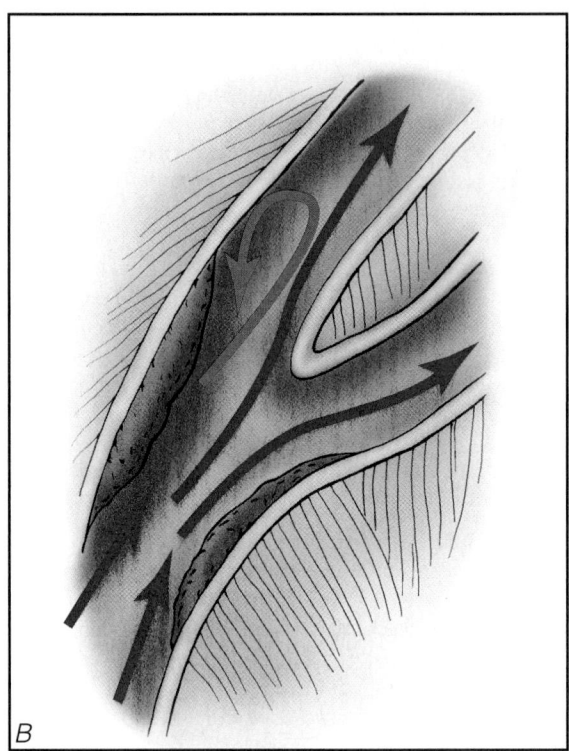

FIG. 22-88. *A. Relative low shear stress is present along the lateral portion of the carotid bifurcation, which predisposes to atherosclerotic plaque development. B. The low shear stress can also result in transient reversal of blood flow during cardiac cycle, which further predisposes carotid lesion formation.*

which was associated with high blood flow velocity and high shear stress in the flow model, were relatively free of plaque formation.

The majority of carotid plaques have a necrotic core consisting of loose cellular debris and cholesterol crystals. The necrotic core is separated from the carotid lumen by a fibrous cap, which is composed of a rim of variable thickness comprising cellular components and extracellular matrix. The structural integrity of the fibrous cap is crucial to the final stage of plaque disruption and its clinical and pathologic sequelae. It is now generally accepted that acute changes within the plaque, with exposure of the deeper lipid contents, predisposes toward thromboembolization.

Another feature characteristic of advanced atherosclerotic plaques is intraplaque hemorrhage that can occur in the absence of a disrupted fibrous cap. Symptomatic carotid disease is associated with increased neovascularization within the atherosclerotic plaque and fibrous cap. These vessels are larger and more irregular and may contribute to plaque instability and the onset of thromboembolic events.

Fibromuscular Dysplasia. Fibromuscular dysplasia (FMD) is the most common nonatherosclerotic disease affecting the ICA (Fig. 22-90). Approximately one quarter of patients with carotid FMD have associated intracranial aneurysms, and up to two thirds of these patients will have bilateral carotid FMD.

FMD can be divided into three distinct pathologic subtypes. Medial fibroplasia is the most common form (>85% of cases) and is usually found in long segment arteries with few side branches. It is characterized by stenoses alternating with intervening fusiform dilatations that resemble a string of beads, particularly in the upper ICA. Pathologically, smooth muscle cells in the outer media are replaced by compact fibrous connective tissue, while the inner me-

dia contains excess collagen and ground substance in disorganized smooth muscle cells. Because of its prevalence in females, a possible role for estrogen and progesterone has been postulated. Others have suggested that the absence of vasa vasorum in long nonbranching arteries such as the ICA or renal arteries may predispose to mural ischemia that leads to the development of FMD.

Intimal fibroplasia accounts for less than 10% of cases of FMD and affects men and women equally. It typically appears as a focal narrowing in older patients and long segmental stenoses in younger patients. The lesion is confined to the intimal layer, while the medial and adventitial structures are always normal. Its pathophysiology is due to irregularly aligned subendothelial mesenchymal cells within a loose matrix of connective tissue. Perimedial dysplasia is characterized by accumulation of elastic tissue between the media and the adventitia. This subtype predominantly affects the ICA and renal arteries, and may be associated with secondary aneurysm formation.

Coils and Kinks of the Extracranial Carotid Arteries. Redundancy of the extracranial carotid artery is thought to be due to abnormalities in development. Occasionally, the internal carotid artery may undergo a complete 360-degree rotation. The carotid artery is derived embryologically from the third aortic arch and the dorsal aortic root. In its early stages, a normally occurring redundancy is straightened as the heart and great vessels descend into the mediastinum. Incomplete descent of the heart and great vessels may result in the development of complex coils and kinks. These will be bilateral in approximately 50% of affected patients.

Elongation of the ICA, which can also result in kinking of the artery, may usually be due to degenerative changes associated with increasing age and atherosclerosis. The loss of elasticity of the

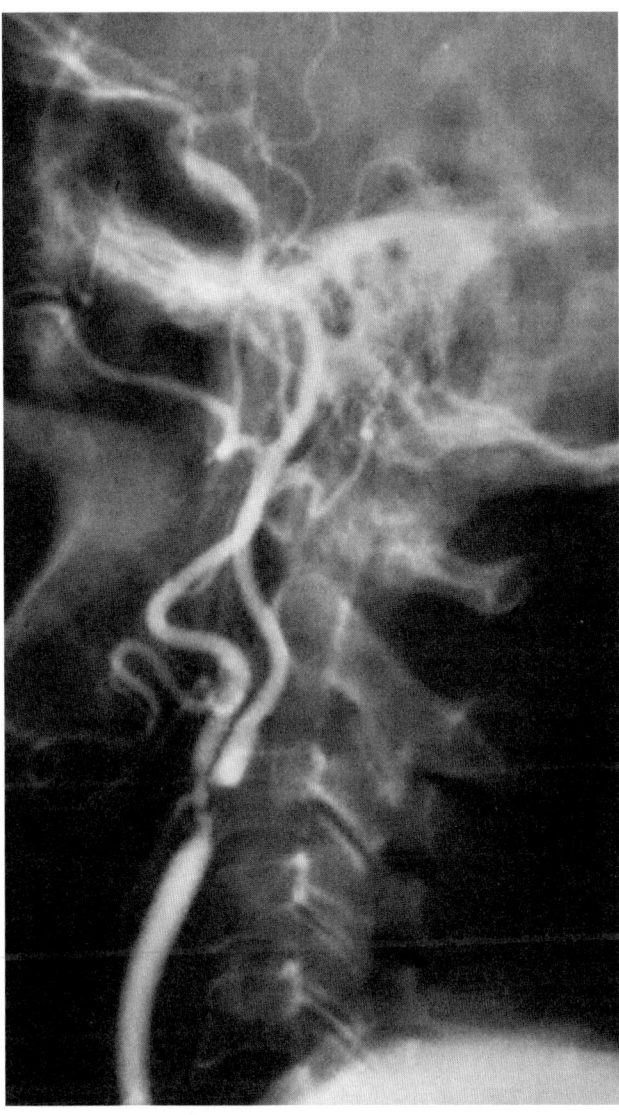

FIG. 22-89. Typical location of bifurcation disease.

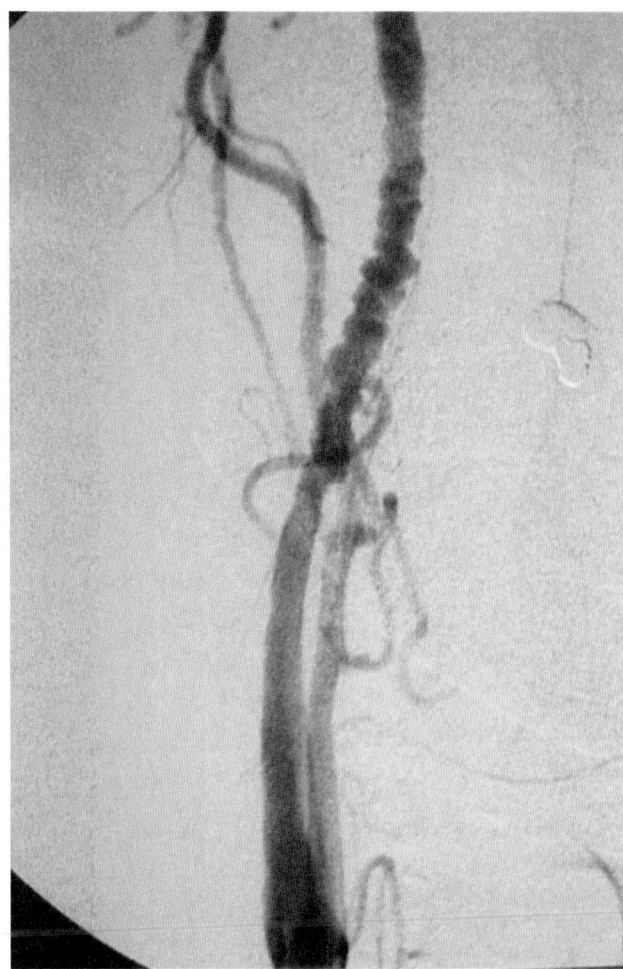

FIG. 22-90. Fibromuscular disease of the internal carotid artery.

arterial wall due to the aging process, coupled with hemodynamic shear stresses, predisposes toward kinks of the elongated carotid artery between the proximal and distal fixed points of the skull base and thoracic inlet.[163-165]

Carotid Artery Aneurysms. As with aneurysms anywhere else in the body, carotid aneurysms may be either true or false (Fig. 22-91). In the past, most true aneurysms have traditionally been classified as part of the atherosclerotic process. However, emerging evidence suggests that aneurysmal disease may be yet another manifestation of abnormalities of matrix metalloproteinase unless it is associated with other distinct pathologies (e.g., arteritis [giant cell or Takayasu's] or FMD). False aneurysms may arise as a consequence of iatrogenic injury, blunt trauma, or carotid patch infection due to prior carotid endarterectomy.

Carotid Dissection (Fig. 22-92). Acute carotid dissection can complicate atherosclerosis, FMD, cystic medial necrosis, and blunt trauma. Angiographic studies suggest that the most likely mechanism of acute carotid dissection is an intimal tear followed by an acute intimal dissection, which produces luminal occlusion due to secondary thrombosis. This appears as a flame-shaped occlusion 2 to 3 cm beyond the bifurcation. Autopsy studies typically reveal a

sharply demarcated transition between the normal carotid artery and the dissected carotid segment. The ICA is commonly affected, with the dissection plane typically occurring in the outer medial layer. Treatment is with anticoagulation, and in most cases this results in complete resolution within 1 to 2 months. Recently there has been increasing use of stenting in severely symptomatic patients.

Takayasu's Arteritis. Takayasu's arteritis is a nonspecific arteritis typically affecting the thoracic and abdominal aorta and their major branches. While this lesion is uncommon in Western countries, it is more prevalent in Asia and usually affects young females. Its pathogenesis relates to an inflammatory process involving all three layers of the arterial wall with proliferation of connective tissue and degeneration of the elastic fibers. Granulomatous lesions may also develop, and the condition may also be associated with fusiform or saccular aneurysms.

Radiation Arteritis. The principal effects of radiation on arteries include immediate arterial spasm and endothelial denudation, intimal disruption, subintimal edema, and collagen and smooth muscle cell degeneration. These acute changes predispose toward an increase in vessel wall permeability to circulating lipids, which produce a plaque characterized by fibrosis, fatty infiltration, and elastic tissue destruction. Hyperlipidemia and hypercholesterolemia appear to predispose patients who have received radiation therapy to

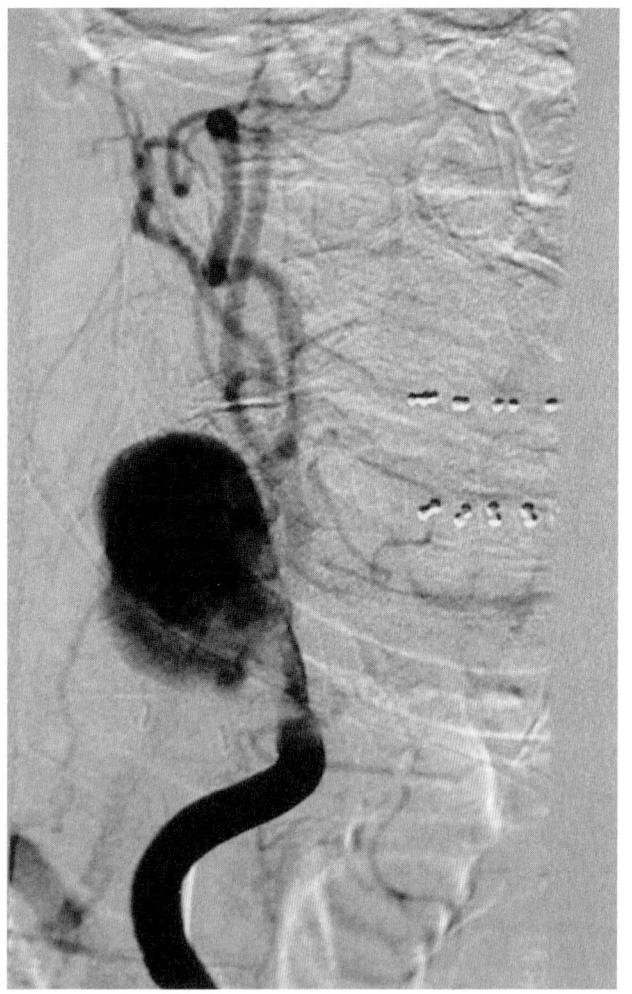

A

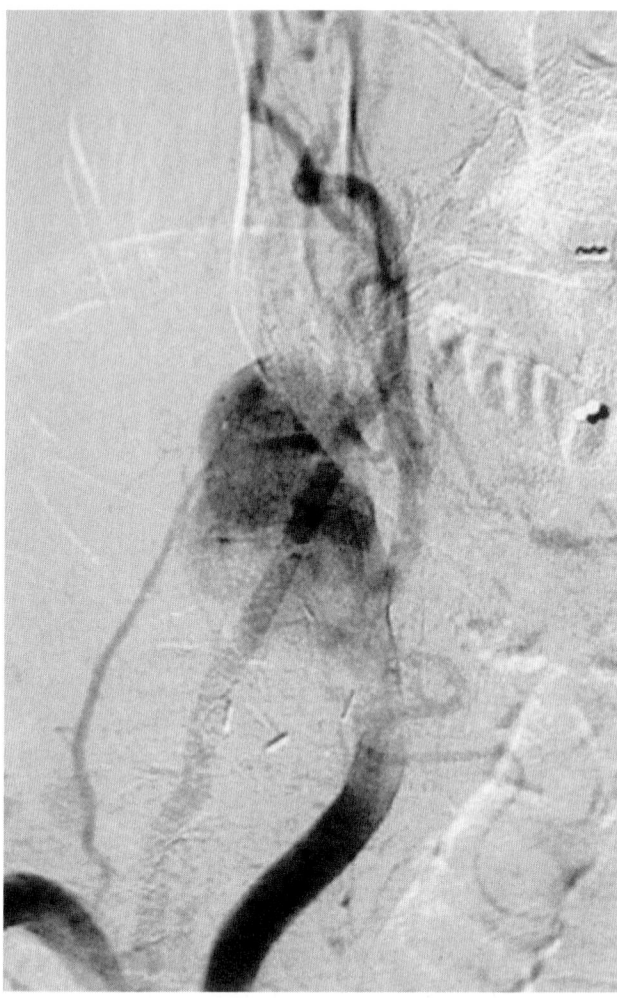

B

FIG. 22-91. *A and B. Selective carotid artery injection reveals a large carotid artery pseudoaneurysm.*

develop accelerated atherosclerotic lesions. The sensitivity of elastic tissue to radiation may account for the mechanism of structural weakening and eventual rupture in elastic arteries.

As a result of the increased use of external radiation to treat cervical malignancy, a rise in radiation-induced atherosclerotic disease in association with symptomatic carotid stenosis has been noted. Radiation-induced carotid lesions can present either in a segmental or diffuse manner. The affected carotid segments typically lie within the field of radiation treatment. One or both common carotid arteries may be involved, while the carotid bifurcation is often spared. The severity of carotid injury is related to radiation dose. Smaller doses cause less cellular damage, while larger doses may lead to arterial wall necrosis.

Carotid Body Tumor. Carotid body tumors originate from the chemoreceptor cells located at the carotid bifurcation (Fig. 22-93). Because the cells of the carotid body typically detect changes in partial oxygen pressure (Po_2), partial pressure of carbon dioxide (Pco_2), and pH levels, carotid body tumors have been reported to be more prevalent in individuals who live at high altitudes, suggesting that chronic hypoxia may be a causative factor in carotid body cell hyperplasia. A carotid body tumor typically presents as a palpable and painless mass over the carotid bifurcation region in the neck. Cranial nerve palsy may occur in up to 25% of patients,

particularly involving the vagus and hypoglossal nerves. The differential diagnosis includes cervical lymphadenopathy, carotid artery aneurysm, brachial cleft cyst, laryngeal carcinoma, and metastatic tumor.

The treatment of choice of carotid body tumors is surgical excision. Because these tumors are highly vascularized, preoperative tumor embolization may be an advantage to minimize operative blood loss when dealing with tumors greater than 3 cm in diameter. An important surgical principle in carotid body tumor resection is to maintain a dissecting plane along the subadventitial space, which will invariably allow complete tumor removal without interrupting the carotid artery integrity.

Carotid Trauma. Blunt trauma to the neck can cause carotid artery injury either by forceful compression or extension of the artery. Common scenarios include motor vehicle or motorcycle accidents, pedestrian injuries, hangings, or strangulations. Patients with carotid trauma may present with focal physical findings such as neck hematoma, pulsatile cervical mass, carotid bruit, or localized bleeding. More generalized physical findings include loss of consciousness and lateralizing neurologic deficits. Arteriography remains the diagnostic test of choice for carotid trauma, since it has the highest sensitivity and specificity compared to all other imaging modalities. Treatment of all blunt carotid artery injuries involves

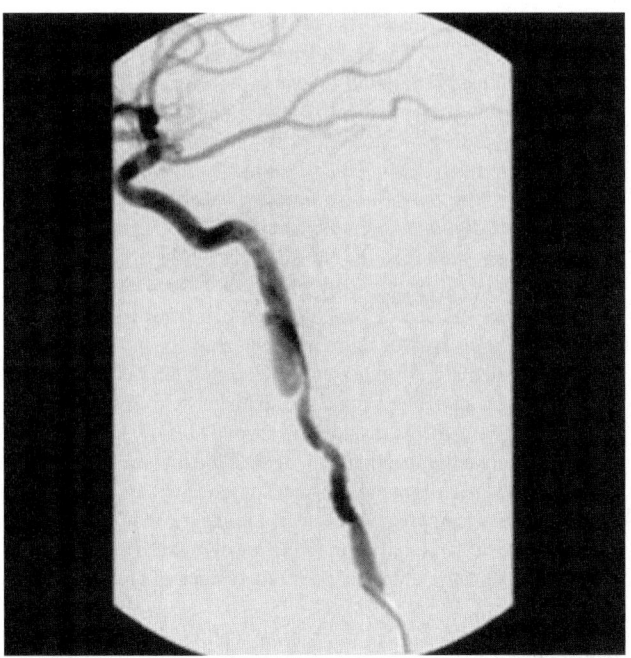

FIG. 22-92. Internal carotid artery (ICA) dissection extending close to the base of the skull.

anticoagulation. Antiplatelet therapy should be considered if systemic anticoagulation is contraindicated.

Diagnosis

The most important tool in the diagnosis of carotid artery disease is a careful history and complete neurologic examination, which should localize the area of cerebral ischemia responsible for the neurologic deficit. The neurologic examination of the patient should be complemented by a complete physical examination to determine the presence of vascular occlusive disease in either the coronary or peripheral arteries, as well as to define the other risk factors for stroke, such as acute arrhythmia. The diagnosis of carotid bifurcation disease is facilitated by the relatively superficial location of the carotid artery, rendering it accessible to auscultation and palpation. The cervical carotid pulse is usually normal in patients with carotid bifurcation disease, since the common carotid artery is the only palpable vessel in the neck and is rarely diseased. Carotid bifurcation bruits may be heard just anterior to the sternocleidomastoid muscle near the angle of the mandible. Bruits do not become audible until the stenosis is severe enough to reduce the luminal diameter by at least 50%. Bruits may be absent in extremely severe lesions because of the extreme reduction of flow across the stenosis.

The utility of noninvasive carotid imaging modalities has provided more accurate information regarding the nature and severity of the carotid artery lesion. Color-flow duplex scanning uses real-time, B-mode ultrasound and color-enhanced pulsed Doppler flow measurements to determine the extent of the carotid stenosis

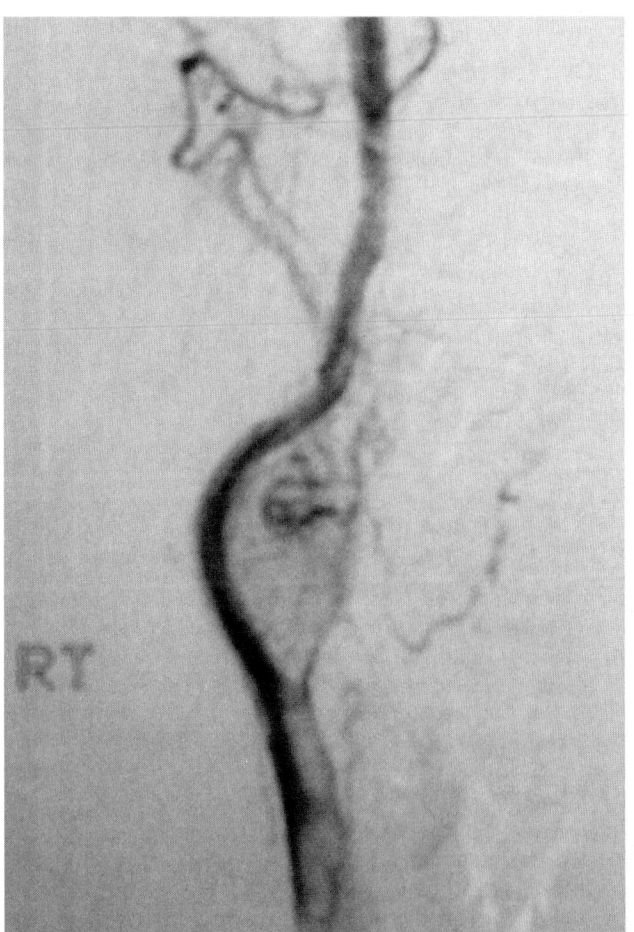

A

B

FIG. 22-93. Carotid body tumor. *A.* Splaying of the carotid bifurcation with a hypervascular tumor. *B.* Internal carotid artery stretched over the tumor.

with reliable sensitivity and specificity. Real-time, B-mode imaging permits localization of the disease and determination of the presence or absence of calcification within the plaque. Determination of the extent of stenosis is based largely on velocity criteria. As the stenosis increasingly obliterates the lumen of the vessel, the velocity of blood must increase in the area of the stenosis so that the total volume of flow remains constant within the vessel. Thus, the velocity is correlated with the extent of carotid artery stenosis. The ICA velocity profile is one of a low-resistance artery characterized by a significant period of carotid blood flow during diastole. In contrast, the external carotid artery reflects a signal typically found in a high-resistance artery, in which little blood flow occurs during diastole. Standard color-flow duplex scans cannot assess the cerebral arterial circulation beyond the first several centimeters of the ICA. A transcranial Doppler has been developed to evaluate the middle cerebral artery and other intracranial vessels, using a low-frequency Doppler signal to penetrate the thin bone of the temporal and occipital regions.

Magnetic resonance imaging (MRI) and MRA have been evaluated as a means of imaging the carotid arteries. These are highly sensitive imaging tools for the evaluation of patients with symptomatic cerebrovascular disease. MRI is more sensitive than computed tomography (CT) scanning for the detection of an acute stroke. MRI can detect a stroke immediately after the infarction occurs, whereas CT scanning cannot. MRA, which is evolving rapidly, permits evaluation of both the extracranial and intracranial cerebral circulations. The precision of MRA in determining the extent of stenosis, although improving rapidly, remains inferior to that achieved by conventional angiography. Nonetheless, MRA will likely play an increasingly important role in the diagnostic evaluation of patients with cerebrovascular disease.

Carotid angiography has been the traditional diagnostic tool for the evaluation of cerebrovascular disease. However, fewer hospitals now perform routine contrast angiography on all patients prior to surgery. This is partly because of the potential for angiography-related complications, as well as improved diagnostic accuracy of noninvasive imaging modalities. Angiography remains the only method that allows complete and detailed visualization of both the intracranial and extracranial arterial circulations. Complications associated with angiography include dye allergy; renal toxicity, particularly in patients with diabetes mellitus; chronic renal insufficiency; and neurologic complications such as stroke, which ranges from 1 to 3%.

Surgical Treatment

The first successful carotid artery operation for occlusive disease, or carotid endarterectomy, was performed by DeBakey and colleagues in 1953.[5] Since then, carotid endarterectomy has been subjected to intense, large-scale prospective randomized clinical trials. Presently, carotid endarterectomy is indicated for treatment of patients with hemispheric TIAs and stroke associated with carotid bifurcation occlusive disease. In addition, prophylactic carotid endarterectomy for asymptomatic patients with high-grade stenosis or complex ulcerated plaques is indicated. A brief overview of three important clinical trials, including the European Carotid Surgery Trial (ECST), the North American Symptomatic Carotid Endarterectomy Trial (NASCET), and the Asymptomatic Carotid Atherosclerosis Study (ACAS) is discussed below.[159–161]

Overview of the European Carotid Surgery Trial (ECST) and the North American Symptomatic Carotid Endarterectomy Trial (NASCET). The benefit of carotid endarterectomy for patients with symptomatic cerebrovascular

disease has recently been established by both the ECST and NASCET trials.[160,161] These studies randomized nearly 6000 patients in 200 hospitals around the world comparing "best medical therapy" against "best medical therapy" plus carotid endarterectomy. These studies documented a significant reduction in cerebrovascular events following the procedure compared with patients managed only medically. Both trials showed that carotid endarterectomy conferred significant benefit in symptomatic patients with a 70 to 99% stenosis. Although the NASCET trial observed a small but significant benefit in patients with 50 to 69% stenoses, the ECST trial found no evidence of benefit in patients with lesser degrees of disease. The reason for these apparent discrepancies lies in the method for calculating the degree of stenosis. ECST compared the residual luminal diameter against the diameter of the carotid artery at the level of the stenosis (usually the carotid bulb). NASCET compared the residual luminal diameter against the diameter of the ICA at least 1 cm above the stenosis. As a consequence, ECST tends to systematically overestimate stenoses (as compared with NASCET), particularly in those with mild to moderate disease. In reality, a 60% NASCET stenosis is approximately equivalent to an 80% ECST stenosis.[160,161]

The ECST and NASCET trials have identified predictive factors that are associated with a significantly higher risk of late stroke in medically treated patients. These factors include male sex, 90 to 94% stenosis, surface irregularity/ulceration, coexistent intracranial disease, no recruitment of intracranial collaterals, hemispheric symptoms, cerebral events within 2 months, multiple cerebral events, contralateral occlusion, multiple concurrent risk factors, and age of more than 75 years.[160,161]

Overview of the Asymptomatic Carotid Atherosclerosis Study (ACAS). The Asymptomatic Carotid Atherosclerosis Study (ACAS) trial was a prospective study that randomized 1600 patients with asymptomatic stenosis of 60% or greater to either carotid endarterectomy and aspirin or aspirin alone.[159] This study was interrupted because of a significant benefit identified in patients undergoing carotid endarterectomy. At the time of interruption of the study, a relative reduction in stroke rate by 50% was observed by patients undergoing carotid endarterectomy. The benefit was much greater in men than in women. This study used stroke as its primary endpoint. This group has since substantiated unequivocally the effectiveness of carotid endarterectomy in good-risk patients identified to have high-grade stenosis.[159]

These prospective trials firmly established the role of carotid endarterectomy in the prevention of strokes in patients with high-grade carotid artery stenosis, regardless whether the lesion is symptomatic or asymptomatic. All the patients in these clinical trials were carefully selected, and the carotid endarterectomy was performed by surgeons with proven successful outcomes and low complication rates. For patients with carotid occlusive disease to benefit from surgical intervention, the operation must be performed by experienced surgeons with proven low operative morbidity and mortality rates.

Technique of Carotid Endarterectomy (Figs. 22-94, 22-95, 22-96, and 22-97). The carotid bifurcation is usually approached via a longitudinal incision based on the anterior border of the sternocleidomastoid muscle, and any superficial veins are ligated and divided. Dissection continues medial to the sternocleidomastoid muscle to reveal the common facial vein. This large tributary of the internal jugular vein often overlies the carotid bifurcation and is a useful landmark. The common facial vein is divided.

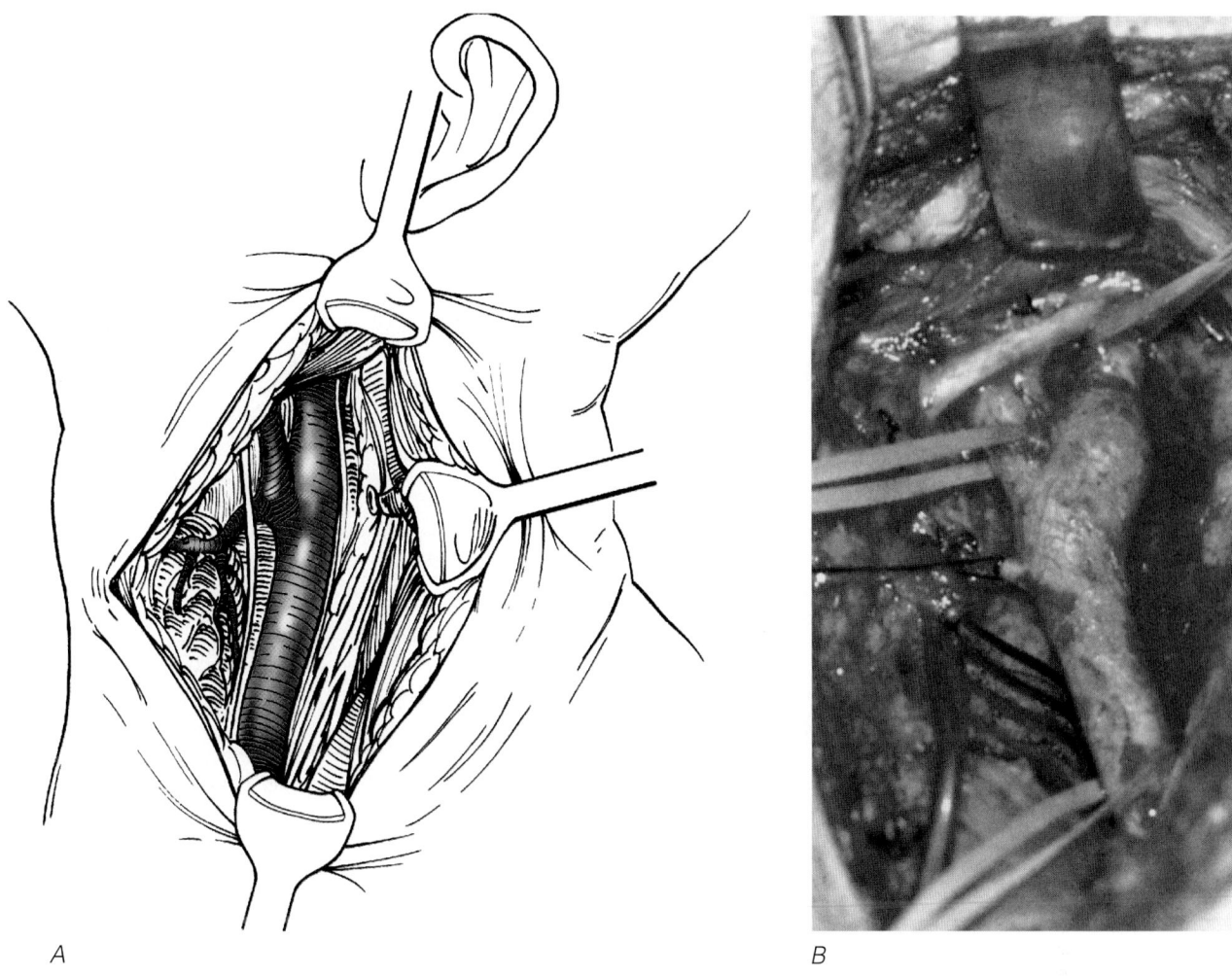

FIG. 22-94. *A.* Carotid endarterectomy is performed via an oblique incision in the anterior neck. *B.* Intraoperative exposure of the carotid bifurcation.

Dissection continues medial to the jugular vein, and the common carotid bifurcation is mobilized and exposed. The external carotid artery (ECA) can be identified by locating its first branch (the superior thyroid artery). Minimal manipulation of the carotid bulb is performed to prevent embolization from the atherosclerotic plaque.

The patient is systemically heparinized and the carotid arteries cross-clamped. If the surgeon chooses to shunt the patient, it is inserted at this time. The plaque is endarterectomized, tacking sutures are inserted if required, and the ECA origin is cleared of plaque using the eversion technique. The carotid arteriotomy is closed primarily using a running suture, and if the ICA is small, a patch angioplasty can be performed using either a vein or a prosthetic patch. First, flow is restored up the ECA, followed by the ICA. Once hemostasis is achieved, the wound is closed with absorbable suture to reconstitute the platysma muscle layer, followed by skin layer closure.

Although carotid endarterectomy has been performed for more than four decades, a wide variety of surgical and anesthetic approaches can be utilized. This operation can be performed under general endotracheal anesthesia, regional cervical block, or local anesthesia. The advantage of local anesthesia is that the surgeon is keenly aware of the patient's mental status at all times, especially when the carotid artery is clamped. Changes in level of consciousness or motor deficits at the time of interruption of blood flow signal the need for placement of an intraoperative shunt. In contrast,

general anesthesia confers the advantages of ventilatory support and increased cerebral blood flow with the use of halogenated agents, but alternative methods of assessing the adequacy of cerebral perfusion must be implemented. A variety of methods have been described to monitor cerebral perfusion during temporary carotid occlusion. The most common method includes the use of temporary shunts to maintain intracranial blood flow. Other methods include neurologic assessment of the awake patient being operated on under local or regional anesthesia, measurement of the ICA back-pressure in the anesthetized patient, or using continuous electronic encephalographic monitoring.[166–171]

Complications of Carotid Endarterectomy. The most serious complication of carotid endarterectomy is that of perioperative stroke. Stroke can occur during or after carotid endarterectomy secondary to a variety of mechanisms, including inadequate collateral blood flow to the brain during temporary ICA occlusion, embolization during dissection of the carotid artery, or embolism or thrombosis of the reconstruction during the early postoperative period. Embolization after carotid endarterectomy is usually secondary to platelet aggregates forming on the surface of the endarterectomized vessel. In contrast, thrombosis after carotid endarterectomy usually is a result of sudden intimal dissection due to a loose flap or inadequate distal endarterectomy endpoint.

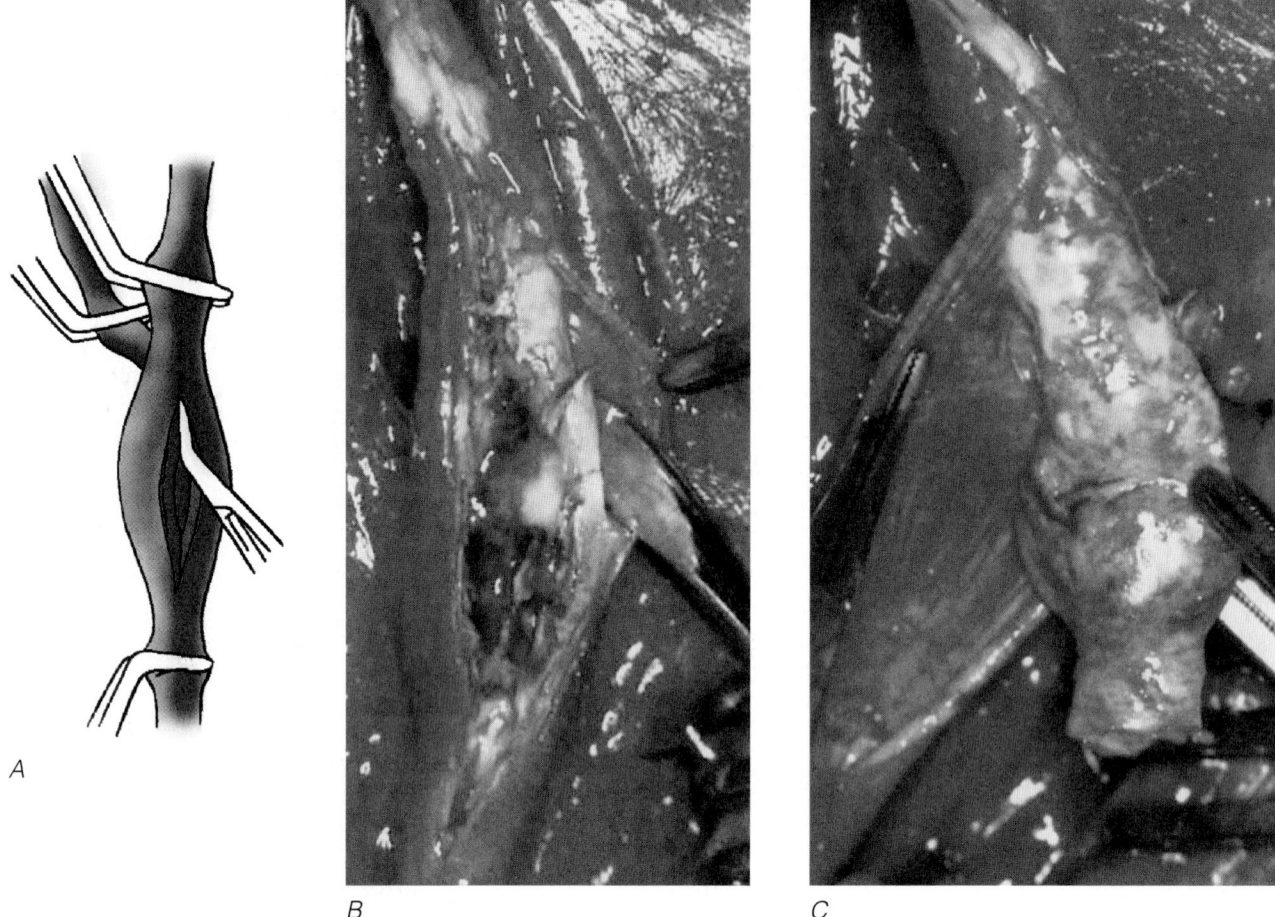

A

B   *C*

FIG. 22-95. *A. A vertical incision is made along the carotid bifurcation. B. The carotid plaque is carefully elevated from the carotid artery. C. The carotid plaque is next endarterectomized from the carotid artery.*

Postoperative cranial nerve dysfunction can occur in up to 35% of patients undergoing carotid endarterectomy, which can occur due to cranial nerve damage resulting from nerve division, excessive traction, or perineural dissection. Common cranial nerve injuries include dysfunction of the recurrent laryngeal nerve, causing hoarseness; dysfunction of the hypoglossal nerve, causing deviation of the tongue toward the side of the injury; and superior laryngeal nerve dysfunction, causing easy fatigability of the voice. Less common is injury of the marginal mandibular nerve, which results in drooping of the nasolabial fold ipsilateral to the injury.

Recurrent carotid stenosis is a relatively common but only rarely serious complication after carotid endarterectomy. Residual or recurrent carotid artery stenosis can be detected in up to 30% of patients undergoing careful postoperative surveillance with carotid duplex scanning. However, less than 3% of patients experience symptomatic recurrence. Two forms of recurrent disease have been described. Recurrent carotid stenosis that occurs within 6 months of the initial endarterectomy usually is secondary to intimal hyperplasia, characterized by both proliferation of vascular smooth muscle cells and increased matrix deposition. When the recurrent stenosis develops 2 years or longer after endarterectomy, recurrent atherosclerosis is usually found at the time of reoperation.

Carotid Balloon Angioplasty and Stenting (Fig. 22-98). Intra-arterial balloon angioplasty is an accepted component of standard vascular therapy in virtually every vascular system apart from the cerebral circulation. The reason for the discrepancy is the potential risk of procedural embolization and stroke. Balloon angioplasty alone of carotid artery occlusive disease has not resulted in high clinical success rates, due in part to several factors including vessel recoil, intimal dissection, plaque dislodgment, and particulate embolization. The rationale for carotid stenting is that it would avoid the above problems as well as reduce the rate of restenosis. Numerous cerebral protection devices have been developed in an effort to improve the clinical success of carotid stenting and reduce the likelihood of cerebral embolization.

To date, the results from carotid stent registries and individual institutional results worldwide have clearly demonstrated that carotid angioplasty and stenting is feasible and accepted by patients. With continual refinement and innovation, cerebral protection devices will likely continue to improve the results of carotid stenting. Ultimately, the answer will be determined by prospective randomized trials, and it is inevitable that carotid stenting will have a role in the management of selected patients with cerebral vascular disease. Until more clinical evidence becomes available from prospective trials, carotid stenting should be reserved for certain patient groups that include those with severe synchronous carotid and coronary artery disease, prior neck operation or irradiation, postendarterectomy restenosis, high distal lesions, and pre-existing cranial nerve palsy.[172–174]

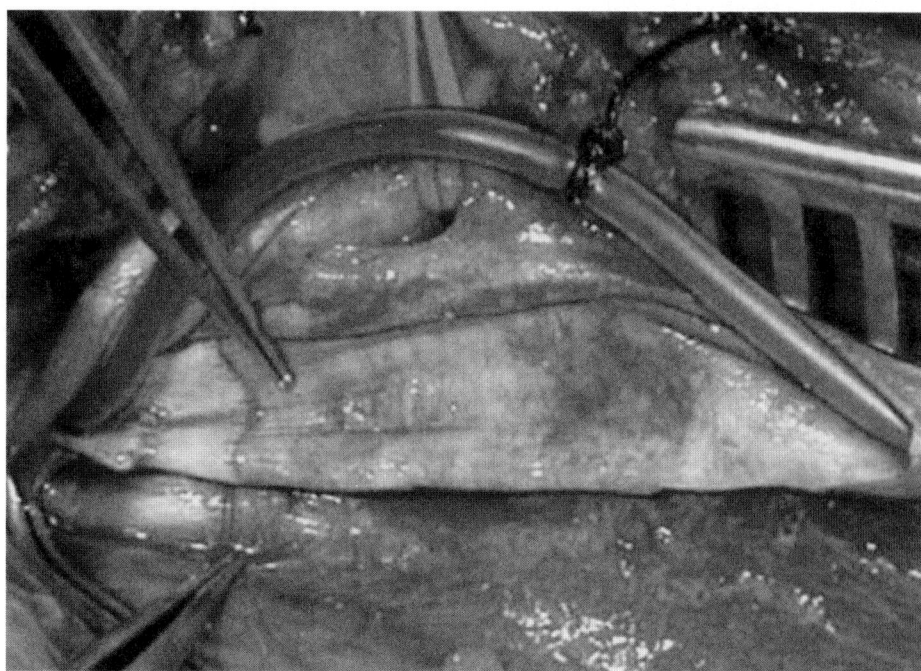

A

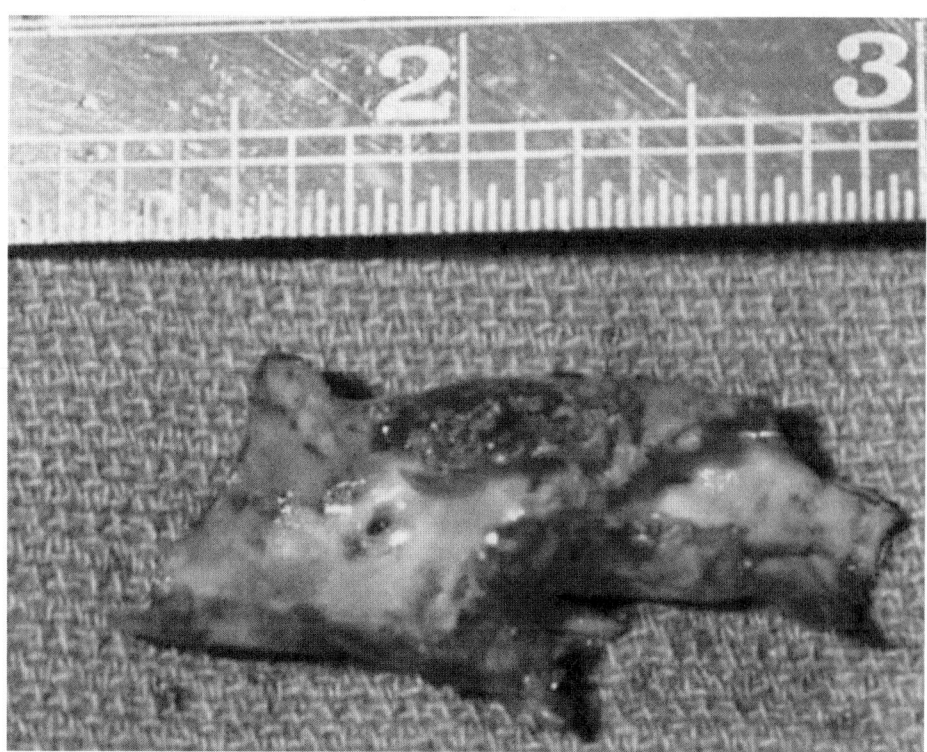

B

FIG. 22-96. *A.* A temporary carotid shunt is used to perfuse cerebral circulation during carotid endarterectomy. The distal internal artery media is tacked to the intima using 7-0 polypropylene suture to prevent distal dissection. *B.* Typical plaque removed during a carotid endarterectomy.

NONATHEROSCLEROTIC DISORDERS OF BLOOD VESSELS

The majority of cases of peripheral vascular disease that are seen by vascular surgeons are attributable to underlying atherosclerosis. Nonatherosclerotic disease states that result in arterial pathology are less commonly encountered, but are nonetheless important, as they are potentially treatable lesions that may mimic atherosclerotic lesions and result in vascular insufficiency. A thorough knowledge of these rare disease states is important for the practicing vascular surgeon in order to both make medical recommendations and provide appropriate surgical treatment. This chapter discusses the most commonly encountered nonatherosclerotic arterial pathologies and resulting vascular conditions.[175–185]

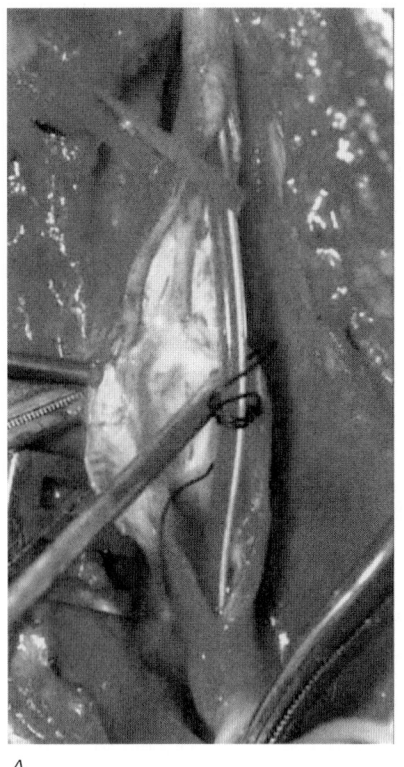

A

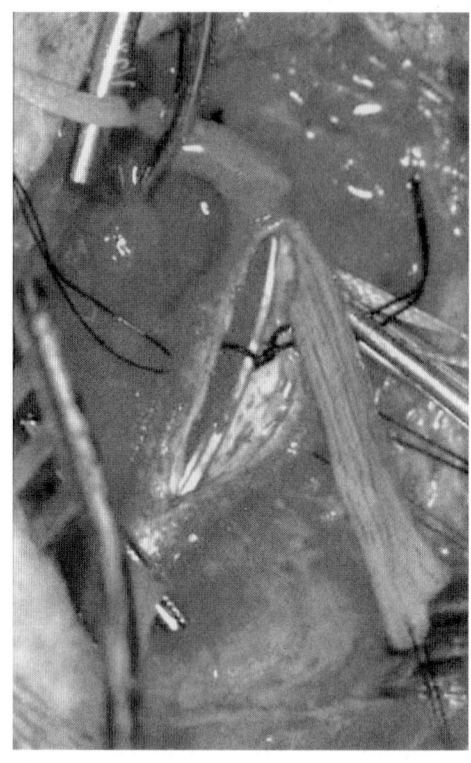

B

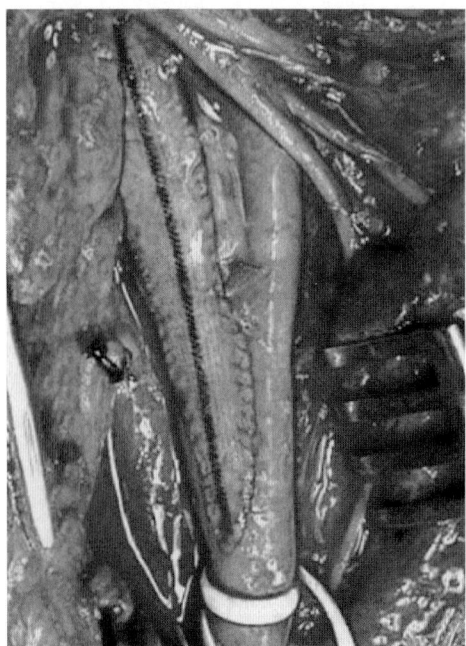

C

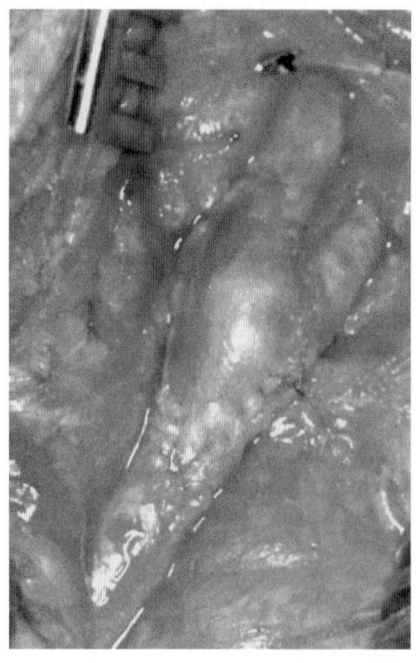

D

FIG. 22-97. Stages in carotid endarterectomy. *A.* A carotid shunt is used to allow temporary cerebral perfusion during endarterectomy. *B.* A carotid patch is used to close the carotid arteriotomy. *C.* Completion image of a carotid endarterectomy with a prosthetic patch closure. *D.* Completion image of a carotid endarterectomy with a saphenous vein patch closure.

Inheritable Disorders of Connective Tissue

Ehlers-Danlos Syndrome

Ehlers-Danlos syndrome is one of the more significant connective tissue disorders, along with Marfan's syndrome. This syndrome represents a heterogenous group of connective tissue disorders (types I through IV) that were first described in 1682 by van Meekeren. It is an autosomal dominant disorder affecting approximately 1 in 5000 persons that is characterized by skin elasticity, joint hypermobility, tissue fragility, multiple ecchymoses, and subcutaneous pseudotumors. Ehlers-Danlos syndrome is a disorder of fibrillar collagen metabolism with identifiable, specific defects that have been found in the collagen biosynthetic pathway that produce clinically distinct forms of this disease. Ten different phenotypes have been described, each with variable modes of inheritance and biochemical defects. Of the four basic types of collagen found

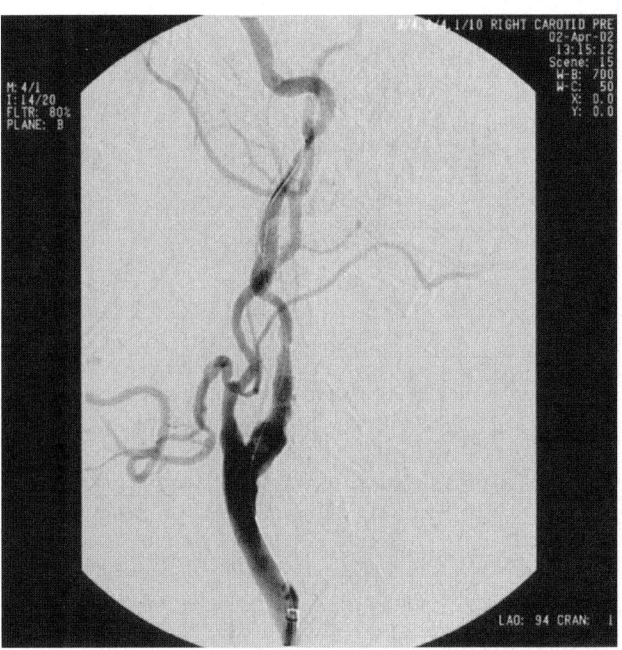

A

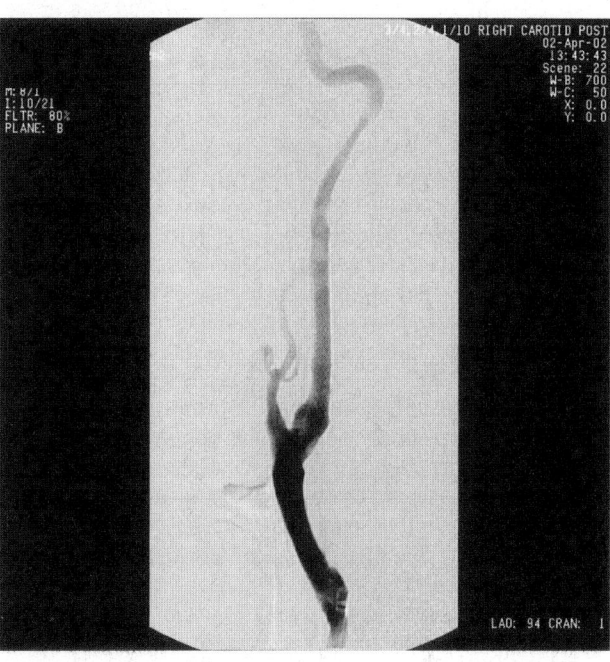

B

FIG. 22-98. *A. Carotid angiogram revealed multiple stenosis along a long segment of the internal carotid artery. B. Carotid stenting was performed which restored the carotid flow.*

in the body, the predominant type in blood vessels is type III. Within the vessel wall, type III collagen contributes to structural integrity and tensile strength, as well as playing a role in platelet aggregation and thrombus formation.

Of the three types of Ehlers-Danlos syndrome that have arterial complications, type IV represents 5% of cases and is the one most likely to be seen by a vascular surgeon. These patients synthesize abnormal type III collagen (mutation COL3A1), and represent 5% of all cases. Affected individuals do not show the typical skin and joint manifestations, and thus typically present for diagnosis when a major vascular catastrophe occurs.[175-177] In a review of 36 patients with this disorder, Cikrit and colleagues reported a 44% mortality rate from major hemorrhage prior to any surgical intervention.[178] In the 20 patients who underwent 29 vascular procedures, there was a 29% mortality rate. Arterial rupture, aneurysm formation, and acute aortic dissection may occur in any major artery, with the most frequent site of rupture being the abdominal cavity. Repair is problematic as the vessel wall is soft and sutures pull through the fragile tissue. Ligation may be the only option in many circumstances.[177,178]

Marfan's Syndrome

Another heterogeneous heritable disorder of connective tissue, Marfan's syndrome is characterized by abnormal musculoskeletal, ocular, and cardiovascular features first described by Antoine Marfan in 1896.[179] The inborn error of metabolism in this syndrome has been localized to the long arm of chromosome 15 (15q21.3). Defects occur in fibrillin, a basic protein in the microfibrillar apparatus that serves as a backbone for elastin, which is one of the main extracellular structural proteins in blood vessels. This is an autosomal dominant gene with high penetrance; however, approximately 15 to 20% of cases are secondary to new spontaneous mutations.[179-182]

Classic recognizable features of Marfan's syndrome include tall stature, long limbs (dolichostenomelia), long fingers (arachnodactyly), joint hyperextensibility, chest wall deformities, and sco-

liosis. Ocular manifestations are flattened corneas, lens subluxation, and myopia. Ninety-five percent of patients have cardiovascular involvement, which may include ascending aortic dilatation, mitral valve prolapse, valvular regurgitation, and aortic dissection. Skin, central nervous system, and pulmonary features may be present as well. Aortic root dilatation will generally occur in all patients.[178-181] This may not be evident on standard chest radiograph until dilatation has resulted in an ascending aortic aneurysm, aortic valve regurgitation, or dissection. Left untreated, the cardiovascular complications are devastating and reduce the life expectancy to about 40 years for men and slightly higher for women. Death is usually attributable to life-threatening complications of aortic regurgitation, dissection, and rupture after the ascending aorta has dilated to 6 cm or more.

Aggressive medical management with beta-adrenergic blocking agents and other blood pressure lowering regimens is crucial to treatment. Surgical intervention entails replacement of the aortic root with a composite valve graft (e.g., Bentall procedure).[8] Prophylactic operative repair is indicated for an aneurysm greater than 5.5 cm, with an acceptable perioperative mortality of less than 5%.

Pseudoxanthoma Elasticum

Pseudoxanthoma elasticum is a rare inherited disorder of connective tissue that is characterized by an unbalanced elastic fiber metabolism and synthesis, resulting in fragmentation and calcification of the fibers. Clinical manifestations occur in the skin, ocular, gastrointestinal, and cardiovascular systems.[182] Characteristic skin lesions are seen in the axilla, antecubital and popliteal fossae, and groin. The yellow, xanthoma-like papules occur in redundant folds of skin and are said to resemble plucked chicken skin. The inheritance pattern includes both autosomal dominant and recessive types and has a prevalence of 1 in 160,000 individuals.[183] The ATP-binding cassette subfamily C member 6 (ABCC6) gene has been demonstrated to be responsible, and 43 mutations have been identified, all of which lead to calcification of the internal elastic laminae of medium-sized vessel walls.[184,185]

Cardiovascular features are common and include premature coronary artery disease, cerebrovascular disease, renovascular hypertension, diminished peripheral pulses, and restrictive cardiomyopathy. Symptom onset typically occurs in the second decade of life, with onset at an average age of 13 years. Patients should be counseled to reduce potential contributing factors for atherosclerosis such as tobacco use and high cholesterol levels. Calcium intake should be restricted in adolescents, as a positive correlation has been found between disease severity and calcium intake.[184] Surgical management involves standard vascular techniques, with the exception that arterial conduits should not be employed in cardiac bypass.

Popliteal Artery Disease

There are three distinct nonatherosclerotic disease entities that may result in lower extremity claudication that predominantly occur in 40- to 50-year-old men. Adventitial cystic disease, popliteal artery entrapment syndrome, and Buerger's disease should be considered in any young patients presenting with intermittent claudication.

Adventitial Cystic Disease

The first successful operative repair of popliteal artery occlusion caused by a cyst arising from the adventitia was reported in 1954 by Ejrup and Hierton.[186] Adventitial cystic disease is a rare arterial condition occurring at an incidence of 0.1%, usually in the popliteal artery. This disease affects men in a ratio of approximately 5:1 and appears predominantly in the fourth and fifth decades. The incidence is approximately 1 in 1200 cases of claudication or 1 in 1000 peripheral arteriograms.[186] The predominance of reported cases is found in Japan and Europe. However, this disease may affect other vascular sites, such as the femoral, external iliac, radial, ulnar, and brachial arteries. Besides claudication as a symptom, this diagnosis should be considered in young patients who have a mass in a nonaxial vessel in proximity to a related joint. These synovial-like, mucin-filled cysts reside in the subadventitial layer of the vessel wall and have a similar macroscopic appearance to ganglion cysts. Despite this similarity and suggestion of a joint origin for these lesions, histochemical markers have failed to link the cystic lining to synovium.

Patients presenting at a young age with bilateral lower extremity claudication and minimal risk factors for atheroma formation should be evaluated for adventitial cystic disease, as well as the other two nonatherosclerotic vascular lesions described here. Because of luminal encroachment and compression, peripheral pulses may be present in the limb when extended, but then can disappear during knee joint flexion. Noninvasive studies may suggest arterial stenosis with elevated velocities. Color-flow duplex scanning followed by T2-weighted MRI now appears to be the best diagnostic choice.[187] Angiography will demonstrate a smooth, well-defined, crescent-shaped filling defect, the classic "scimitar" sign.[188] There may be associated calcification in the cyst wall and no other evidence of atherosclerotic occlusive disease.

Various therapeutic methods have been described for the treatment of adventitial cystic disease. The recommended treatments are excision of the cyst with the cystic wall, enucleation, or simple aspiration when the artery is stenotic. Retention of the cystic lining leads to continued secretion of the cystic fluid and recurrent lesions. In 30% of patients who have an occluded artery, resection of the affected artery, followed by an interposition graft using autogenous saphenous vein, is recommended.

Popliteal Artery Entrapment Syndrome

Love and colleagues first coined the term *popliteal artery entrapment* in 1965 to describe a syndrome combining muscular

Table 22-13
Types of Popliteal Entrapment

I. Popliteal artery is displaced medially around a normal medial head of the gastrocnemius
II. Medial head of gastrocnemius, which arises lateral to popliteal artery
III. Popliteal artery is compressed by an accessory slip of muscle from medial head of gastrocnemius
IV. Entrapment by a deeper popliteus muscle
V. Any of the above plus popliteal vein
VI. Functional

involvement with arterial ischemia occurring behind the knee, with the successful surgical repair having taken place 6 years earlier.[189,190] This is a rare disorder with an estimated prevalence of 0.16% that occurs with a male-to-female ratio of 15:1. Five types of anatomic entrapment have been defined, according to the position of the medial head of the gastrocnemius muscle, abnormal muscle slips or tendinous bands, or the course of the popliteal artery itself (Table 22-13). Concomitant popliteal vein impingement occurs in up to 30%. Twenty-five percent of cases are bilateral.

The typical patient presents with swelling and claudication of isolated calf muscle groups following vigorous physical activity. In a large series of 240 patients reported by Turnipseed, the median age for surgical treatment was 28.5 years.[191,192] Noninvasive studies with ankle-brachial indices should be performed with the knee extended and the foot in a neutral, forced plantar, and dorsiflexed position. A drop in pressure of 50% or greater or dampening of the plethysmographic waveforms in plantar or dorsiflexion is a classic finding. Contraction of the gastrocnemius should compress the entrapped popliteal artery. The sudden onset of signs and symptoms of acute ischemia with absent distal pulses is consistent with popliteal artery occlusion secondary to entrapment. Other conditions resulting from entrapment are thrombus formation with distal emboli or popliteal aneurysmal degeneration.[192] Although CT and MRI have been employed, angiography remains the most widely used test. Angiography performed with the foot in a neutral position may demonstrate classical medial deviation of the popliteal artery or normal anatomic positioning. Coexisting abnormalities may include stenosis, luminal irregularity, delayed flow, aneurysm, or complete occlusion. Diagnostic accuracy is increased with the use of ankle stress view-active plantar flexion and passive dorsiflexion.

The treatment of popliteal artery entrapment consists of surgical decompression of the impinged artery with possible arterial reconstruction.[193] Division of the anomalous musculotendinous insertion site with or without saphenous vein interposition grafting to bypass the damaged arterial segment has been described to be the procedure of choice.[194,195] The natural history of entrapment is progressive arterial degeneration leading to complete arterial thrombosis.[196] In such instances, thrombolytic therapy is needed with subsequent release of the functional arterial impairment. Lysis will improve distal runoff and may improve limb-salvage and bypass patency rates.

Buerger's Disease (Thromboangiitis Obliterans)

Buerger's disease, also known as thromboangiitis obliterans, is a progressive nonatherosclerotic segmental inflammatory disease that most often affects small and medium-sized arteries, veins, and nerves of the upper and lower extremities.[197] The clinical and pathologic findings of this disease entity were published in 1908 by Leo Buerger in a description of 11 amputated limbs.[198] The typical age range for occurrence is 20 to 50 years, and the disorder is more frequently found in males who smoke. The upper extremities may be involved, and a migratory superficial phlebitis may be present in up to 16% of patients, thus indicating a systemic inflammatory response.[199] In young adults presenting to the Mayo Clinic (1953–1981) with lower limb ischemia, Buerger's disease was diagnosed in 24%.[200] Conversely, the diagnosis was made in 9% of patients with ischemic finger ulcerations. The cause of thromboangiitis obliterans is unknown; however, use of or exposure to tobacco is essential to both the diagnosis and progression of the disease.

Pathologically, thrombosis occurs in small to medium size arteries and veins with associated dense polymorphonuclear leukocyte aggregation, microabscesses, and multinucleated giant cells. The chronic phase of the disease shows a decrease in the hypercellularity and frequent recanalization of the vessel lumen.[201] End-stage lesions demonstrate organized thrombus and blood vessel fibrosis. Although the disease is common in Asia, North American males do not appear to have any particular predisposition, as the diagnosis is made in less than 1% of patients with severe limb ischemia.

Buerger's disease typically presents in young male smokers, with symptoms beginning prior to age 40. Patients initially present with foot, leg, arm, or hand claudication, which may be mistaken for joint or neuromuscular problems. Progression of the disease leads to calf claudication and eventually ischemic rest pain and ulcerations on the toes, feet, or fingers. A complete history should exclude diabetes, hyperlipidemia, or autoimmune disease as possible etiologies for the occlusive lesions. Because it is likely that multiple limbs are involved, angiography should be performed of all four limbs. Even if symptoms are not yet present in a limb, angiographic findings may be demonstrated. Characteristic angiographic findings show disease confinement to the distal circulation, usually infrapopliteal and distal to the brachial artery. The occlusions are segmental and show "skip" lesions with extensive collateralization, the so-called "corkscrew collaterals."

The treatment of thromboangiitis obliterans revolves around strict smoking cessation. In patients who are able to abstain, disease remission is impressive and amputation avoidance is increased. In the experience reported from Oregon Health Sciences Center, no disease progression with associated tissue loss occurred after discontinuation of tobacco. The role of surgical intervention is minimal in Buerger's disease, as there is often no acceptable target vessel for bypass. Furthermore, autogenous vein conduits are limited secondary to coexisting migratory thrombophlebitis. Mills and associates reported their results of 31% limb loss in 26 patients over 15 years, thus authenticating the virulence of Buerger's disease involving the lower extremities.[202] In addition, others have described a significant discrepancy in limb loss in patients that continued to smoke versus those who discontinued tobacco use (35 versus 67%).[203]

Inflammatory Arteritis and Vasculitides

Chronic inflammatory arteritides and vasculitides (i.e., inflammatory changes within veins as well as arteries) include a spectrum of disease processes caused by immunologic mechanisms. These terms signify a necrotizing transmural inflammation of the vessel wall associated with antigen-antibody immune complex deposition within the endothelium. These conditions show pronounced cellular infiltration in the adventitia, thickened intimal fibrosis, and organized thrombus.[204] These disease processes may clinically mimic atherosclerosis, and most are treated by corticosteroid therapy or chemotherapeutic agents. Even so, it is important to recognize distinguishing characteristics of each disease in order to establish the

Table 22-14
Causes of Systemic Vasculitis

Large vessels	Takayasu's arteritis
	Giant cell arteritis
	Behçet's disease
Medium-sized vessels	Polyarteritis nodosa
	Kawasaki's disease
	Buerger's disease
Small vessels	Hypersensitivity angiitis

course of treatment and long-term prognosis. A classification system of systemic vasculitis by vessel size is shown in Table 22-14.[205]

Takayasu's Arteritis

First described in 1908 by a Japanese ophthalmologist, Takayasu's arteritis is an inflammatory disease of the large medial vessels, affecting primarily the aorta and its main branches and the pulmonary artery.[206] This rare autoimmune disease occurs predominantly in women between the ages of 10 and 40 years who are of Asian descent. Genetic studies have demonstrated a high frequency of human lymphocyte antigen (HLA) haplotypes in patients from Japan and Mexico, suggesting increased susceptibility to developing the disease in patients with certain alleles.[207] However, these associations have not been seen in North America. Vascular inflammation leads to arterial wall thickening, stenosis, and eventually, fibrosis and thrombus formation. The pathologic changes produce stenosis, dilation, aneurysm formation, and/or occlusion.

The clinical course of Takayasu's arteritis begins with a "prepulseless" phase in which the patient demonstrates constitutional symptoms. These include fever, anorexia, weight loss, general malaise, arthralgias, and malnutrition. As the inflammation progresses and stenoses develop, more characteristic features of the disease become evident. During the chronic phase, the disease is inactive or "burned out." It is during this latter stage that patients most frequently present with bruits and vascular insufficiency according to the arterial bed involved. Laboratory data may show elevations in erythrocyte sedimentation rate, C-reactive protein, white blood cell count, or conversely, anemia may predominate. Characteristic clinical features during the second phase vary according to the involved vascular bed, and include hypertension reflecting renal artery stenosis, retinopathy, aortic regurgitation, cerebrovascular symptoms, angina and congestive heart failure, abdominal pain or gastrointestinal bleeding, pulmonary hypertension, or extremity claudication.

The gold standard for diagnosis remains angiography showing narrowing or occlusion of the entire aorta or its primary branches, or focal or segmental changes in large arteries in the upper or lower extremities. Six types of Takayasu's arteritis exist and are graded in terms of severity: type I, affecting the aorta and arch vessels; type IIa, affecting the ascending aorta, aortic arch, and branches; type IIb, affecting the ascending aorta, aortic arch and branches, and thoracic descending aorta; type III, affecting the thoracic descending aorta, abdominal aorta, and/or renal arteries; type IV, affecting the abdominal aorta and/or renal arteries; and type V, with combined features of types IIb and IV.

Treatment consists of steroid therapy initially, with cytotoxic agents used in patients who do not achieve remission. Surgical treatment is performed only in advanced stages, and bypass needs to be delayed during active phases of inflammation. There is no role for endarterectomy, and synthetic or autogenous bypass grafts need to be placed onto disease-free segments of vessels. For focal lesions, there have been reports of success with angioplasty.[208–210]

Giant Cell Arteritis (Temporal Arteritis)

Giant cell arteritis is a systemic chronic inflammatory vascular disease with many characteristics similar to those of Takayasu's disease. The histologic and pathologic changes as well as laboratory findings are similar. Patients tend to be white women over the age of 50 years, with a high incidence in Scandinavia and women of Northern European descent.[211] Genetic factors may play a role in disease pathogenesis, with a HLA variant having been identified.[212] Differences exist between Takayasu's and giant cell arteritis in terms of presentation, disease location, and therapeutic efficacy. The inflammatory process typically involves the aorta and its extracranial branches, of which the superficial temporal artery is specifically affected.

The clinical syndrome begins with a prodromal phase of constitutional symptoms, including headache (most common), fever, malaise, and myalgias. The patients may be initially diagnosed with coexisting polymyalgia rheumatica; an HLA-related association may exist between the two diseases. As a result of vascular narrowing and end-organ ischemia, complications may occur such as visual alterations, including blindness and mural weakness, resulting in acute aortic dissection that may be devastating. Ischemic optic neuritis resulting in partial or complete blindness occurs in up to 40% of patients and is considered a medical emergency. Cerebral symptoms occur when the disease process extends to the carotid arteries. Jaw claudication and temporal artery tenderness may be experienced. Aortic lesions are usually asymptomatic until later stages and consist of thoracic aneurysms and aortic dissections.

The diagnostic gold standard is a temporal artery biopsy, which will show the classic histologic findings of multinucleated giant cells with a dense perivascular inflammatory infiltrate. Treatment regimens are centered on corticosteroids, and giant cell arteritis tends to rapidly respond. Remission rates are high, and treatment tends to have a beneficial and preventative effect on the development of subsequent vascular complications.

Behçet's Disease

Behçet's disease is a rare syndrome characterized by oral and genital ulcerations and ocular inflammation, affecting males in Japan and the Mediterranean. An HLA linkage has been found, indicating a genetic component to the etiology. Vascular involvement is seen in 7 to 38% of patients, and is localized to the abdominal aorta, femoral artery, and pulmonary artery.[213] Vascular lesions may also include venous complications such as deep venous thrombosis or superficial thrombophlebitis. Arterial aneurysmal degeneration can occur; however, this is an uncommon, albeit potentially devastating, complication. Multiple true aneurysms and pseudoaneurysms may develop, and rupture of an aortic aneurysm is the major cause of death in patients with Behçet's disease.[214]

Histologically, degeneration of the vasa vasorum with surrounding perivascular lymphocyte infiltration is seen, along with thickening of the elastic laminae around the tunica media.[215] Aneurysm formation is believed to be associated with a loss of the nutrient flow and elastic component of the vessels, leading to progressive dilatation. Multiple aneurysms are relatively common, with a reported occurrence of 36% in affected Japanese patients.[42] Furthermore, pseudoaneurysm formation after surgical bypass is common at anastomotic suture lines due to the vascular wall fragility and medial destruction. Systemic therapy with corticosteroids and

immunosuppressive agents may diminish symptoms related to the inflammatory process; however, they have no effect on the rate of disease progression and arterial degeneration.[216,217]

Polyarteritis Nodosa

Polyarteritis nodosa (PAN) is another systemic inflammatory disease process, which is characterized by a necrotizing inflammation of medium-sized or small arteries that spares the smallest blood vessels (i.e., arterioles and capillaries). This disease predominantly affects men over women by a 2:1 ratio. PAN develops subacutely, with constitutional symptoms that last for weeks to months. Intermittent, low-grade fevers, malaise, weight loss, and myalgias are common presenting symptoms. As medium-sized vessels lie within the deep dermis, cutaneous manifestations occur in the form of livedo reticularis, nodules, ulcerations, and digital ischemia.[218] Skin biopsies of these lesions may be sufficient for diagnosis. Inflammation may be seen histologically, with pleomorphic cellular infiltrates and segmental transmural necrosis leading to aneurysm formation.

Neuritis from nerve infarction occurs in 60% of patients, and gastrointestinal complications in up to 50%. Additionally, renal involvement is found in 40%, and manifests as microaneurysms within the kidney or segmental infarctions. Cardiac disease is a rare finding except at autopsy, where thickened, diseased coronary arteries may be seen, as well as patchy myocardial necrosis. Patients may succumb to renal failure, intestinal hemorrhage, or perforation. End-organ ischemia from vascular occlusion or aneurysm rupture can be disastrous complications with high mortality rates. The mainstay of treatment is steroid and cytotoxic agent therapy. Up to 50% of patients with active PAN will experience remission with high dosing.

Kawasaki's Disease

Kawasaki's disease was first described in 1967, as a mucocutaneous lymph node syndrome occurring in young children. In most studies, more than half the patients are younger than 2 years of age, with a higher prevalence in boys.[219] Although originally described in Japan, the disease is found worldwide. An infectious agent may be causative; however, no specific agent has been identified. Immune activation with the contribution of cytokines, elastases, growth factors, and metalloproteinases is believed to be a mechanism for inflammation and aneurysm formation. Coronary artery aneurysms, the hallmark of the disease, histologically demonstrate a panarteritis with fibrinoid necrosis. Coronary arteriography may show occlusions, recanalization, and localized stenosis, in addition to multiple aneurysms. A variety of constitutional symptoms and signs resulting from systemic vasculitis are present in the acute phase of the illness.[220]

Medical therapy for Kawasaki's disease clearly decreases the manifestations of coronary artery involvement. Intravenous gamma globulin and aspirin therapy are most successful if begun within the first 10 days of illness. Up to 20% of untreated patients will develop coronary arterial lesions. A long-term, low-dose aspirin therapy regimen is usually recommended.

Raynaud's Syndrome

First described in 1862 by Maurice Raynaud, the term *Raynaud's syndrome* applies to a heterogeneous symptom array associated with peripheral vasospasm, more commonly occurring in the upper extremities. The characteristically intermittent vasospasm classically follows exposure to various stimuli, including cold temperatures, tobacco, or emotional stress. Formerly, a distinction was made between Raynaud's "disease" and Raynaud's "phenomenon" for describing a benign disease occurring in isolation or a more severe disease secondary to another underlying disorder, respectively. However, many patients develop collagen vascular disorders at some point after the onset of vasospastic symptoms; progression to a connective tissue disorder ranges from 11 to 65% in reported series.[221–223] Therefore, the term Raynaud's syndrome is now used to encompass both the primary and secondary conditions.

Characteristic color changes occur in response to the arteriolar vasospasm, ranging from intense pallor to cyanosis to redness as the vasospasm occurs. The digital vessels then relax, eventually leading to reactive hyperemia. The majority of patients are young women less than 40 years of age. Up to 70 to 90% of reported patients are women, although many patients with only mild symptoms may never present for treatment. Geographic regions located in cooler, damp climates such as the Pacific Northwest and Scandinavian countries have a higher reported prevalence of the syndrome. Certain occupational groups, such as those that use vibrating tools, may be more predisposed to Raynaud's syndrome or digital ischemia. The exact pathophysiologic mechanism behind the development of such severe vasospasm remains elusive, and much attention has focused on increased levels of alpha$_2$-adrenergic receptors and their hypersensitivity in patients with Raynaud's syndrome, as well as abnormalities in the thermoregulatory response, which is governed by the sympathetic nervous system.[224–227]

The diagnosis of severe vasospasm may be made using noninvasive measurements in the vascular laboratory. Angiography is usually reserved for those who have digital ulceration and an embolic or obstructive cause is believed to be present and potentially surgically correctable. Different changes in digital blood pressure will occur in patients with Raynaud's syndrome. Normal individuals will show only a slight decrease in digital blood pressure in response to external cold stimuli, whereas those with Raynaud's syndrome will show a similar curve until a critical temperature is reached.[228] It is at this point that arterial closure acutely occurs.

There is no cure for Raynaud's syndrome, thus all treatments mainly palliate symptoms and decrease the severity and perhaps frequency of attacks. Conservative measures predominate, including the wearing of gloves, use of electric or chemically activated hand warmers, avoiding occupational exposure to vibratory tools, abstinence from tobacco, or relocating to a warmer, dryer climate. The majority (90%) of patients will respond to avoidance of cold and other stimuli. The remaining 10% of patients with more persistent or severe syndromes can be treated with a variety of vasodilatory drugs, albeit with only a 30 to 60% response rate. Calcium-channel blocking agents such as diltiazem and nifedipine are the drugs of choice. The selective serotonin reuptake inhibitor fluoxetine has been shown to reduce the frequency and duration of vasospastic episodes.[229] Intravenous infusions of prostaglandins have been reserved for nonresponders with severe symptoms.

Surgical therapy is limited to débridement of digital ulcerations and amputation of gangrenous digits, which are rare complications. Upper extremity sympathectomy may provide relief in 60 to 70% of patients; however, the results are short-lived with a gradual recurrence of symptoms in 60% within 10 years.[230–232]

OTHER NONATHEROSCLEROTIC VASCULAR PATHOLOGIES

Radiation-Induced Arteritis

Radiation-induced arteritis results from progressive stenosis due to endothelial damage that leads to cellular proliferation and fibrosis.

These are well-described complications of combined irradiation and chemotherapy, often for the treatment of malignancy. Arterial lesions are known complications of radiation and are similar to those found in atherosclerotic occlusive disease. Venous stenoses are becoming more recognizable complications. The angiographic findings of radiation arteritis include focal arterial irregularities in early lesions, diffuse arterial stenosis, and complete occlusion in chronic, older lesions.[233] Angiographically, radiation-induced vascular injuries are indistinguishable from atherosclerotic lesions. The former are simply limited to a prior radiation field.

Treatment of radiation injury to larger vessels includes standard techniques of endarterectomy or bypass grafts. In the carotid artery, percutaneous transluminal angioplasty with stent placement has been advocated recently for radiation-induced stenosis.[234–236] At this writing, several randomized trials comparing endarterectomy with carotid stenting are underway; however, guarded optimism is necessary until the most effective treatments, emboli protection devices and adjuvant pharmacotherapy, are fully scrutinized.

Arteriomegaly

In 1942, Rene Leriche described a syndrome of elongated and dilated arteries involving the aorta and iliofemoral vessels that was later designated *arteriomegaly*.[237] The expressions *arteria magna* and *arteria magna et dolicho* have been used to signify a diffuse ectasia of the arteries. This syndrome applies to patients with unusually large arteries (diameter greater than maximal normal vessel size) who have a high incidence of aneurysm formation. Studies have demonstrated an approximately 60% incidence of aneurysms in patients with arteriomegaly.[238,239] Familial patterns have been shown to exist, and there is a predominance among men. Aneurysms in these patients need to be differentiated from atherosclerotic aneurysms; this is usually done by the angiographic finding of ectatic arterial segments between aneurysms.

Arteriomegaly carries similar risks to those of other aneurysms: thrombosis, rupture, and peripheral embolism. For these reasons, aneurysms reaching 2 to 2.5 times the size of adjacent arterial segments should be repaired. Patients with diffuse aneurysmal disease may need to undergo staged reconstructions, depending on individual patient risk factors and urgency of the presentation of the patient.

Fibromuscular Dysplasia

Fibromuscular dysplasia (FMD) is a vasculopathy of uncertain etiology that is characterized by segmental arterial involvement. Histologically, fibrous tissue proliferation, smooth muscle cell hyperplasia, and elastic fiber destruction alternate with mural thinning.[240] The characteristic beaded appearance of FMD is due to areas of medial thinning alternating with areas of stenosis. The most commonly affected are medium-sized arteries, including the internal carotid, renal, vertebral, subclavian, mesenteric, and iliac arteries. The internal carotid artery is the second most common site of involvement after the renal arteries. FMD occurs most frequently in women (90%) and is recognized at approximately 55 years of age. Only 10% of patients with FMD will have complications attributable to the disease.[241,242] Pathologically, FMD is a heterogenous group of four distinct types of lesions which are subgrouped based on the predominant site of involvement within the vessel wall. Of the four types (medial fibroplasia, intimal fibroplasia, medial hyperplasia, and perimedial dysplasia), medial fibroplasia is the most common pathologic type, affecting the ICA and the renal artery, and occurring in 85% of reported cases.[243]

The two main clinical syndromes associated with FMD are transient ischemic attacks from disease in the ICA, and hypertension from renal artery involvement. Symptoms produced by FMD are generally secondary to associated arterial stenosis, and are clinically indistinguishable from those caused by atherosclerotic disease. Often, asymptomatic disease is found incidentally on conventional angiographic studies being performed for other reasons. Within the ICA, FMD lesions tend to be located higher in the extracranial segment than with atherosclerotic lesions, and may not be readily demonstrated by duplex scan.

Clinically, symptoms are due to encroachment on the vessel lumen and a reduction in flow. Additionally, thrombi may form in areas of mural dilatation from a stagnation of flow, leading to distal embolization. Surgical treatment has been favored for symptomatic patients with angiographically proven disease. Owing to the distal location of FMD lesions in the extracranial carotid artery, resection and repair is not usually feasible. Instead, graduated luminal dilatation under direct vision has been used successfully in patients, with antiplatelet therapy continued postoperatively. Percutaneous transluminal angioplasty has been used effectively in patients with FMD-induced hypertension. Several series have documented a high technical success rate, with recurrence rates of 8 to 23% at more than 1 year.[244,245] However, the therapeutic effect of blood pressure control may continue to be observed despite restenosis. Surgical reconstruction of the renal arteries for FMD has good long-term results and is recommended for recurrent lesions after angioplasty.[246] Open balloon angioplasty of the ICA has been described, which allows for precise fluoroscopic guidance, rather than blind dilatation with calibrated metal probes, and back-bleeding after dilatation to eliminate cerebral embolization.[247] Distal neuroprotective devices may allow this procedure to be performed completely percutaneously, by lessening the threat of cerebral emboli.

UPPER EXTREMITY ARTERIAL DISEASE

Upper extremity arterial disease is much less common than disease in the lower extremity. Indeed most arterial problems in the arms are related to the establishment of arteriovenous access grafts. Although atherosclerosis remains the most common cause of naturally occurring upper extremity vascular disease, there is a much higher incidence of nonatherosclerotic arterial disease in the upper extremity than in the leg. The details of these nonatherosclerotic vascular disorders are described in more detail in that section.

Symptoms

The most common location for atherosclerosis affecting the upper limb is at the origin of the subclavian artery, most commonly the left subclavian artery. Frequently there are no symptoms, due to rich collaterals and reversed flow in the ipsilateral vertebral artery. Symptoms when they do occur manifest as arm pain, described as aching and weakness in the extremity, made worse with exercise of the arm and relieved by rest. Subclavian steal syndrome occurs when posterior circulation symptoms (dizziness, drop attacks, and diplopia) occur during arm exercise in patients with proximal subclavian artery occlusion. This syndrome is relatively rare. Another unusual manifestation of subclavian artery occlusion is coronary-subclavian steal syndrome. This occurs in the setting of proximal (usually left) subclavian artery occlusion in a patient with a prior left internal mammary artery (LIMA) to left anterior descending artery (LAD) graft. Arm exercise may lead to reversed flow in the LIMA and lead to development of chest pain from myocardial ischemia.

Because of the collaterals, the limb is threatened only rarely; however, distal embolization can occur from atherosclerotic stenoses or from an axillosubclavian aneurysm, both of which can complicate thoracic outlet syndrome. Embolization usually manifests as small areas of digital gangrene.[248,249]

Examination

This begins with pulse examination: axillary, brachial, radial, and ulnar. Both the infraclavicular and supraclavicular fossae should be palpated and auscultated for aneurysms and bruits. The blood pressure should be recorded for both brachial arteries. A difference of greater than 20 mm Hg is likely to be significant and suggestive of proximal occlusive disease.

Investigations

The subclavian artery is inaccessible for examination and duplex scanning. However, the finding of a pressure difference between the arms and reversed flow in the ipsilateral vertebral artery by duplex scanning is highly suggestive of proximal subclavian stenosis. If this is not associated with symptoms, then further investigation may not be necessary. However, in a symptomatic patient or in a patient in whom an IMA to LAD bypass has been performed, further investigation is warranted. Spiral CT and MRA can be utilized, but the definitive procedure remains arch angiography. The angiographer should specifically look for reversed flow in the ipsilateral vertebral artery, which leads to late filling of the distal subclavian artery. This is an important observation to determine treatment options and select a distal site for bypass grafting.

Treatment

Intervention is indicated only for patients who are symptomatic. In patients with symptoms suggestive of subclavian steal syndrome and concurrent carotid stenoses, the carotid stenosis is usually treated first. If the carotid lesion is at the origin of the carotid required for carotid subclavian bypass, then synchronous retrograde stenting of the common carotid artery (CCA) origin prior to creating the bypass can be performed.

Both endovascular and open treatment options are available for subclavian disease. We prefer angioplasty and stenting for stenoses and reserve carotid subclavian bypass for total occlusion or for stenoses that have been actively embolizing or where there is intraluminal thrombus on angiography. The open procedure most commonly performed is carotid to subclavian bypass. This is performed through a supraclavicular incision, exposing the proximal CCA. The subclavian is exposed by dividing the scalenus anterior muscle. A short 8-mm Dacron graft is tunneled posterior to the jugular vein between the two arteries and should restore a palpable pulse to the extremity. Transposition of the subclavian artery into the common carotid is another option, made easier if the subclavian is high and tortuous. Although subclavian endarterectomy has been described, these authors believe this is fraught with hazard and should be abandoned. Other revascularization options employed when there is concurrent occlusive disease involving the other supraortic trunks include subclavian to subclavian bypass, axillosubclavian bypass, and in patients with disease involving all the supra-aortic vessels, direct revascularization from the aorta may be necessary.

When arm ischemia occurs due to more distal axillary or brachial artery disease, the physician must verify that the patient does not have atherosclerotic disease. In most cases bypass with reversed saphenous vein is the treatment of choice.

Subclavian stenting can be performed by either a transfemoral or retrograde brachial approach. Primary stenting is most commonly performed to minimize the risk of embolization down the limb or up the vertebral artery.

Subclavian Artery Aneurysms

Subclavian artery aneurysms are uncommon and difficult to treat. They are typically atherosclerotic in etiology and located at the origin of the subclavian artery. Clinical manifestations include pain from arm ischemia secondary to thrombosis or embolization. In addition, right-sided aneurysms can present with hoarseness due to stretching of the recurrent laryngeal nerve.

An aberrant right subclavian artery, arising from the aortic arch distal to the left subclavian artery, is particularly predisposed to undergoing aneurysmal degeneration, often referred to as a Kommerell diverticulum. Aneurysms of an aberrant right subclavian artery also can present with dysphagia due to compression of the esophagus.

The left subclavian artery and an aberrant right subclavian artery surgically are in very inaccessible locations. An aneurysm of the left subclavian artery is best approached through a left posterolateral thoracotomy. This permits both proximal subclavian or aortic control. The aneurysm is opened, and a 10-mm interposition Dacron graft can be inserted. Care is required when clamping the aorta due to the presence of the left recurrent laryngeal nerve hooking around the aorta medial to the left subclavian artery. On the right side, proximal control is gained via a median sternotomy. Depending on the extent of the aneurysm, distal control can be achieved via either a supraclavicular or infraclavicular incision.

Because of the difficulty in approaching these aneurysms, there has been increasing interest in the use of endovascular grafts to repair these aneurysms. Endografts can be delivered via either a femoral approach or via a retrograde brachial approach. Aneurysms with an adequate proximal and distal neck (>1 cm) are suitable for endografting. Ideally the vertebral artery should be spared; however, if the contralateral vertebral is normal, the ipsilateral vertebral can be sacrificed.

An alternate approach to a proximal subclavian artery aneurysm is ligation with embolization of the vertebral stump and carotid subclavian bypass to maintain antegrade perfusion to the arm and retrograde perfusion to the vertebral artery.

Minimally Invasive Vascular Procedures: Concepts and Techniques

The concept of a minimally invasive approach to the treatment of surgical diseases within the peritoneal cavity has become widely accepted by the surgical community since the initial reports of laparoscopic cholecystectomy in the mid-1980s. The benefits of this technique, including a shorter hospital stay and recovery time, have been well recognized. The technique of percutaneous access for both the diagnostic and therapeutic management of vascular disease has been the basis for entire subspecialties, including interventional radiology, invasive cardiology, and most recently, endovascular surgery.[250]

The development of catheter and endoscopic technology has laid the groundwork for advancement in related instrumentation. This has allowed the vascular surgeon to operate via an intra- or extraluminal route. However, catheter-based approaches to the treatment of vascular disease are rapidly expanding, while endoscopic applications such as endoscopic vein harvest and endoscopic subfascial perforator interruption have had a more limited adoption. Endovascular techniques are now able to treat the full spectrum of vascular

pathology, including stenoses and occlusions of arteriosclerotic and thrombotic etiologies, aneurysmal dilatation, and traumatic lesions. Many of these procedures only recently have been developed, and as such have not been investigated in a manner that would enable an accurate comparison with the more traditional methods of treatment. Additionally, long-term follow-up for these procedures is frequently lacking. Nevertheless, endovascular skills and techniques have matured sufficiently to be considered part of mainstream vascular surgery.

Endovascular Instrumentation and Technique

Needles. Needles are used for vascular access, primarily from a percutaneous location. The size of the needle will be dictated by the diameter of the guidewire used. Most often an 18-gauge needle is used, as it will accept a 0.035-in. guidewire. The most popular access needle is the Seldinger needle, which can be used for single- and double-wall puncture techniques. Femoral arterial puncture is the most common site for access. The artery, which is detected fluoroscopically, is punctured over the femoral head.

The single-wall puncture technique requires a sharp, beveled needle tip and no central stylet. The anterior wall of the vessel is punctured, with pulsatile back-bleeding indicating an intraluminal position. This method is most useful for graft punctures, patients with abnormal clotting profiles, or if thrombolytic therapy is anticipated.

Once the needle assumes an intraluminal position, verified by pulsatile back-bleeding, the guidewire may be advanced. This is always passed gently and under fluoroscopic guidance to avoid subintimal dissection or plaque disruption. A wide variety of guidewires exist that differ in the length and diameter of the wire, shape of the tip, the ability of the wire to cross tight stenoses, and the overall stiffness of the wire. The most commonly used guidewire is the Bentson wire. The straight, flexible tip and variety of sizes makes this the most versatile of the guidewires. The ability to cross tight stenoses is facilitated by a guidewire with a hydrophilic coating, angled at the tip to permit the ability to steer, and with a pliable tip to prevent subintimal dissection. Stiff wires are useful to maintain a position across a lesion and as a guide for catheter exchange.

Hemostatic Sheath. The hemostatic sheath is a device through which endovascular procedures are performed. The sheath acts to protect the vessel from injury as wires and catheters are introduced. A one-way valve prevents bleeding through the sheath, and a side-port allows contrast or heparin flushes during the procedure. Sheaths differ in diameter, with the most commonly used sheaths for percutaneous access having a 5- to 9-F inner diameter, and larger sizes for use when the vessel is exposed surgically. Sheaths also vary in length; however, the most commonly used are 10 cm long. Longer sheaths are available for interventions in remote locations.

Catheters. A wide variety of catheters exist that differ primarily in the configuration of the tip. The multiple shapes permit access to vessels of varying dimensions and angulations. Catheters are used to perform angiography, protect the passage of balloons and stents, and can be used to direct the guidewire through tight stenoses or tortuous vessels.

Angioplasty Balloons. Balloons differ primarily in their length and diameter, as well as the length of the catheter shaft. As balloon technology has advanced, lower profiles have been manufactured (i.e., the size that the balloon assumes upon deflation). Balloons are used to perform angioplasty on vascular stenoses, to deploy stents, and to assist with additional expansion in self-expanding stents. Lower-profile balloons are less likely to get caught during their withdrawal through stents and are easier to pull through sheaths.

Stents. Vascular stents are available in self-expanding or balloon-expandable varieties. The flexible nature of this stent allows for deployment through a small-diameter introducer; however, it also accounts for its considerable shortening upon expansion. Stents were initially used for suboptimal angioplasty, but primary stenting is being increasingly utilized. The stent exerts an outward hoop strength against the vessel wall.

Contrast Agents. Prior to choosing an endovascular treatment for a particular lesion, the patient must be carefully assessed in terms of the risk of administering intravenous contrast. A known allergy to contrast agents or iodine preparations should alert the clinician either to avoid the use of contrast dye or to pretreat the patient with corticosteroids and antihistamines. All necessary medications should be readily available in case of an unanticipated anaphylactic reaction. Patients receiving contrast while taking the oral hypoglycemic agent metformin occasionally have been reported to experience profound metabolic acidosis. It is currently recommended to withhold metformin for 48 hours prior to contrast administration.

Contrast agents are available in low or high osmolarity, as well as ionic and nonionic varieties. Low osmolarity agents are ten times more expensive than high osmolarity agents, but are less painful on injection, and have less associated renal toxicity and fewer allergic reactions. The incidence of severe adverse reactions to high and low osmolarity agents is equivalent at 0.01%. Nonionic contrast agents have a lower associated incidence of adverse reactions, both severe and overall, including a lower incidence of nephrotoxicity in patients with renal impairment.

Intravascular Imaging

Improvements in endovascular visualization largely have been born out of necessity. Approximately 70% of atherosclerotic plaque occurs in an eccentric location within the blood vessel. Because angiography is limited to a uniplanar "lumenogram," the images obtained can be misleading when attempting to evaluate a stenotic lesion. With increased experience in intravascular stent deployment, it has been discovered that assessment of stent apposition against the vessel wall and its location in relation to surrounding branches is poorly evaluated by angiography. Furthermore, angiography exposes the patient to the risks of both ionizing radiation and intravascular contrast. Nevertheless, contrast angiography remains the most common invasive method of vascular investigation for both diagnostic and therapeutic intervention.

Intravascular Ultrasound. Intravascular ultrasound (IVUS) is an imaging modality that enables the transmural visualization of blood vessels via use of an ultrasound transducer of 20 to 30 MHz. Luminal dimensions obtained using IVUS correlate well with both histologic and angiographic findings. IVUS accurately identifies intimal flaps and dissections, and better defines the degree of luminal stenosis. Perhaps the greatest role for IVUS is in assessment of endoluminal stents and guiding stent graft deployment. IVUS is free of the many limitations of angiography, including a lack of exposure to ionizing radiation or contrast. Furthermore, IVUS overcomes the problems inherent in visualization of a three-dimensional plaque in a unidimensional plane, by providing an intraluminal, circumferential view.

IVUS catheters range in diameter from 2.7 to 9 F, with transducers most commonly found in a range from 12.5 to 40 MHz.

Larger vessels such as the aorta, in which penetration of the vessel wall is necessary for adequate visualization, typically require lower-frequency transducers (12.5 to 20 MHz). IVUS provides an accurate evaluation of vessel wall anatomy, as well as plaque morphology, based upon acoustic echogenicity.

From a diagnostic standpoint, IVUS is quite helpful in clarifying equivocal angiographic findings, such as in patients in whom angiography does not correlate with symptomatology. Intravascular ultrasound assessment following stent deployment has become routine in many centers, due in large part to the inaccuracies associated with angiographic assessment. IVUS investigation following stent deployment initially guided by angiography has demonstrated that the majority of stents are not fully deployed, a factor contributing to early stent thrombosis. Endovascular stents and stent-grafts can be placed with IVUS as the only intraoperative imaging modality, although it is more commonly employed as an adjunct to angiographic assessment. Because of the many advantages over conventional contrast angiography, IVUS has secured a niche in the area of vascular imaging.

Angioscopy. Fiberoptic angioscopy has received renewed popularity in recent years. Angioscopy can be used to assess surface plaque anatomy, quantify the degree of ulceration, differentiate between thrombus and embolus, and can be used to verify the results of vascular reconstruction. Angioscopic examination of thrombectomized vessels not only identifies critical stenoses, but can also demonstrate residual thrombus missed by angiogram. Several investigators have found that angioscopy may reveal clinically important information not detected by extraluminal inspection, intraluminal probing, or angiography in as many as 20 to 30% of cases. With the increasing popularity of in situ saphenous vein bypass grafts, angioscopy has become the modality of choice to detect uncut valve leaflets, unligated side branches, or significant anastomotic stenoses that angiography is less able to diagnose. Whether the detection of these technical errors allows for their correction or will improve long-term results remains to be seen.

Angioscopy has permitted in situ saphenous vein bypass to be performed in a less invasive manner. Rosenthal and colleagues have devised two different methods to reach these goals. Following angioscopic valvulotomy, an extraluminal, endoscopic-assisted approach for ligation of venous tributaries may be performed, limiting the incision to the proximal and distal arterial anastomoses. A variation of this idea is to place platinum coils to occlude the venous side branches from within the lumen of the saphenous vein using an electronically steered nitinol catheter. The initial reports of both methods have demonstrated feasibility and decreasing rates of wound complications. Long-term patency, particularly with the likelihood of endothelial injury from excessive venous manipulation, remains unknown.

Endoscopic Venous Procedures

Endoscopic Saphenous Vein Harvest. There is no surgical procedure performed through a longer incision than saphenous vein harvesting for coronary or extremity bypass. This maximally invasive procedure is often performed in an extremity with pre-existing vascular disease, with predictable consequences. In the only prospective study to date, saphenous vein harvest site healing was complicated in 24% of patients undergoing coronary revascularization. While most problems consist of minor delays in wound healing, amputation has been necessary in a few patients suffering more catastrophic complications. Saphenectomy is a procedure that readily lends itself to a less-invasive approach.

Endoscopic techniques have been applied to saphenous vein harvest with promising results. Through several small (3- to 4-cm) incisions, retraction of overlying soft tissue, dissection of the greater saphenous vein, and clip application to venous side branches can be accomplished under direct visualization. While this should theoretically result in fewer wound complications related to the length of the incision, experience with this technique is limited. The primary difficulty in endoscopic vein harvest is working in a coaxial manner, which translates into a much longer time required for endoscopic saphenectomy (average 57.5 minutes) than for the open method (average 35.5 minutes). Only after the procedure becomes technically easier with shorter operative times will endoscopic saphenous vein harvest become a more widely accepted procedure.

Subfascial Endoscopic Perforator Vein Ligation. Endoscopic venous exposure has become a popular method for subfascial endoscopic perforator vein ligation in the treatment of chronic venous insufficiency with ulceration. This is a minimally invasive modification of the Linton procedure, in which a long, medial calf incision is used to expose and interrupt the veins communicating between the superficial and deep systems. This operation achieved successful results in healing of venous stasis ulcers, although wound complications and prolonged hospitalizations limited its acceptance.

Employing a 10-mm endoscope, the subfascial space of the leg is entered with a 10-mm port for the camera and a second port for dissection and clip application. After carbon dioxide insufflation to 30 mm Hg, perforating veins are identified and clipped. This endoscopic technique has allowed access to the perforating veins remote from the lipodermatosclerotic skin. Early reports demonstrate a 6% risk of wound infection, with 88% of ulcers healing at 5.4-month follow-up. While this appears to compare favorably with both the conventional Linton procedure and nonoperative therapy, long-term results are not yet available.

Thrombolysis. Thrombolysis has been a controversial treatment option for DVT. While anticoagulation is effective in preventing pulmonary embolus, many patients go on to suffer the consequences of the postphlebitic syndrome. It is well documented that lytic therapy leads to a more rapid and complete dissolution of clot compared with heparin treatment alone. Complete clot dissolution is observed in approximately 35% of those undergoing lysis, compared to less than 5% of those treated with heparin alone. Short-term follow-up (i.e., 3 to 6 months) has revealed preservation of valve function in 50% of the thrombolytic group compared with approximately 7% of the heparin-treated group. There appears to be no differences in mortality or in the incidence of pulmonary embolism, though bleeding complications are seen in 17% of the lytic group and 4% of the heparin-treated group. Long-term follow-up of an average of 6.5 years resulted in normal venograms for only 20 percent of the group—all of which belonged to the streptokinase group. By clinical assessment, three quarters of patients in the lytic group had normal examinations, compared with one third of the group treated with heparin. Others have prospectively followed patients with proximal DVT treated with either heparin or streptokinase. After a 2.5-year follow-up, no major hemodynamic benefit was seen as measured by foot volumetry. The optimal treatment for DVT is not completely clear. While the occlusive effects of DVT can quickly and effectively be treated with thrombolytic therapy, bleeding complications are significantly increased. Whether lytic therapy lessens the destructive effects of DVT on valve function and leads to significantly improved clinical outcome remains the crucial question to be answered.

Extraluminal Arterial Procedures

Laparoscopic Aortic Surgery. Laparoscopic exposure of the aorta for lymph node dissection in both Hodgkin's lymphoma and gynecologic malignancy is a well-recognized method for tissue biopsy. Laparoscopically assisted aortic vascular reconstruction was first reported in humans in 1993, and has since been detailed in sporadic case reports. Early reports utilized carbon dioxide peritoneal insufflation and a 10-cm minilaparotomy incision, through which vascular control and aneurysmorrhaphy were performed. Despite demonstrating feasibility, peritoneal insufflation resulting in gas embolism remains a concern. After creating a 1-cm incision in the vena cava of euvolemic dogs under pneumoperitoneum, 18% were found to have gas bubbles in the right heart by transesophageal echocardiography, suggesting a prohibitive risk to vascular procedures performed under pneumoperitoneum.

Because of the concern over gas embolus during laparoscopic vascular bypass, a gasless technique of laparoscopically assisted aortobifemoral bypass employing a mechanical abdominal wall lifter has been described. This gasless technique provides less exposure and requires a larger minilaparotomy incision. A single case of transperitoneal laparoscopic aortobifemoral bypass without minilaparotomy incision has been performed in a human. The procedure was not unexpectedly prolonged (total operative time was 12 hours and 10 minutes, with aortic cross-clamp time of 3 hours and 30 minutes), yet the patient had minimal analgesia requirements and was discharged on the third postoperative day.

The technical challenge associated with the transperitoneal approach is primarily due to difficulty in adequate small bowel retraction. In order to circumvent this problem, a gasless approach via the retroperitoneum has been described using the Laparolift for retraction. Laparoscopic-assisted repair of an abdominal aortic aneurysm with creation of a 10-cm minilaparotomy incision has been reported as well.

Some of the difficulties with the transperitoneal laparoscopic approach to the aorta have been improved upon with a retroperitoneal approach assisted by the endoscopic retractor, including problems with small bowel retraction and the potential for gas embolus. However, aortic anastomosis does not easily lend itself to performance under the spatial confines of a laparoscopic procedure. As advances in laparoscopic instrumentation continue, laparoscopic anastomosis might become less technically challenging. Until that time, laparoscopic or laparoscopic-assisted aortic surgery remains in an experimental stage, with only case reports presently appearing in the literature. With the expansion of aortic stent graft trials for treatment of abdominal aortic aneurysms, and the growing use of stents and stent grafts in the treatment of iliac occlusive disease, enthusiasm has shifted from laparoscopic-assisted aortic surgery to these other techniques.

Endoluminal Arterial Procedures

Arterial Occlusive Disease. Transluminal access to treat arterial occlusive disease is not a new concept, as Dotter and Judkins first described this technique over 33 years ago. What has evolved since that time has led to an explosion in catheter-based technology, enabling interventionalist access to treat occlusive disease in nearly any vascular bed. While the technique of balloon angioplasty has been applied to nearly all areas of the body, success of this modality is often site-specific and dependent upon several factors. Most importantly, lesion morphology is predictive of immediate and long-term success. Ideal angioplasty lesions are nonocclusive, short stenotic lesions. Patency improves when these lesions occur in larger vessels with greater flow velocity.

The best long-term follow-up data for the results of angioplasty exist for iliac artery angioplasty. The common iliac arteries are ideal for angioplasty due to their large diameter and high flow rates. Patency rates for iliac stenoses are 87 to 74% for 1- to 4-year follow-up, respectively. However, when the initial treatment failures are included in these figures, patency rates fall to 78%, 69%, and 32% for 1-, 3-, and 5-year patency, respectively. Totally occlusive lesions account for the majority of technical failures.

As vessel diameter and flow rates change, so do success rates of angioplasty. This is exemplified by the differences in long-term patency rates after angioplasty of the common iliac and external iliac arteries. Following angioplasty of the common iliac artery, patency rates at 1 to 6 years are 81 to 52%, respectively. Success after external iliac artery angioplasty at 1 to 4 years is 74 to 48%, respectively.

Iliac artery angioplasty is associated with a 2 to 4% major complication rate and 4 to 15% minor complication rate. Many of these minor complications are related to the arterial puncture site (i.e., hematoma, pseudoaneurysm, and others). Mortality rates from this procedure range from 0.3 to 0.8%.

Compared with conventional bypass, common iliac angioplasty has a 10 to 20% lower overall patency rate. Five-year patency of aortoiliac bypass is 65 to 95%, and at 10 years is 62 to 78%, based on a review of 19 previously published reports. Despite its lower long-term success, it is a useful procedure in patients with focal disease and mild symptoms in whom a major surgical revascularization is not justified. Angioplasty of the iliac vessels can be a useful adjunct to distal surgical bypass as well, increasing the success of distal revascularization and eliminating the risks associated with aortoiliac bypass. Thus, with long-term patency slightly less than, but comparable to, open surgical bypass, and with acceptable morbidity rates, iliac angioplasty has become a well-accepted modality of treatment for iliac occlusive disease.

Angioplasty of the infrainguinal vessels has not had the success that iliac angioplasty has enjoyed. Patency in this region is more dependent upon factors such as the patient's presenting symptoms (e.g., claudication versus limb-threatening ischemia) and the status of the distal run-off vessels, in addition to lesion morphology. Initial success in femoropopliteal angioplasty is 80 to 90%, while failure to cross a lesion occurs in 7% of stenoses and 18% of occlusive lesions. While the initial technical success is better for stenoses than occlusions, long-term patency rates for stenoses and short occlusions are equivalent. Patients with optimal angioplasty lesions (i.e., stenoses less than 2 cm in length) appear to have long-term results slightly lower than those obtained with surgical revascularization, and with less morbidity and at a lower cost.

In a review of 12 published studies, the initial 30-day success rate of femoropopliteal angioplasty for claudication was 89%, while for limb salvage it was 77%. However, at 6 months, patency rates fell to 81 and 60%, respectively. Carried out to 3 years, rates of 62 and 43% were observed. Overall, angioplasty of femoropopliteal lesions provides 5-year patency rates of 38 to 68%. More recent studies have found similarly disappointing results with superficial femoral and popliteal artery angioplasty (performed primarily for claudication), with a 24-month cumulative patency rate of 46%. Angioplasty success is also related to the status of the distal vessels. If at least two tibial arteries are open, the 5-year patency for femoropopliteal angioplasty is 77 to 53%, but with poor run-off, patency rates fall to 59 and 31%.

Most patients with infrapopliteal disease have extensive, multilevel disease that is not well suited for angioplasty. Angioplasty of infrapopliteal, short-segment stenoses is usually reserved for patients with rest pain or tissue necrosis, provides acceptable results, and may be a viable option in appropriately selected patients. In the largest review of infrapopliteal angioplasty, technical success was obtained in 77% of cases. Two-year success rates (improvement by at least one clinical stage) were 83% for a single stenosis, 67% for multiple stenoses, and 52% for occlusions, with an overall 2-year patency rate of 62%. The major complication rate was quite high in this series, occurring in 11.3%. Although percutaneous transluminal angioplasty (PTA) is an important part of an aggressive, multidisciplinary approach to limb salvage, 81% of patients with limb-threatening ischemia require operative treatment at some point, leaving only 19% who can be treated with PTA alone.

Proponents of angioplasty for short segment disease list cost efficacy among its benefits over surgical endarterectomy. A cost analysis has been performed comparing balloon angioplasty with endarterectomy for short segment occlusions of the femoropopliteal segment. Following the primary procedure, 3-year patency rates were 87% for the group undergoing endarterectomy compared to 44% for the balloon angioplasty group. When evaluating the cost of maintaining patency by either method over a period of 3 years (i.e., the cost-to-patency ratio), initial balloon angioplasty failures resulted in a significantly higher overall cost than endarterectomy. In appropriately selected patients with ideal lesions located in higher-flow vessels, angioplasty provides a viable alternative to bypass procedures from a cost standpoint.

Renovascular hypertension as a result of renal artery stenosis is a disease in which angioplasty has been widely applied. However, the precise role of angioplasty and stent placement in the renal vasculature has yet to be clearly defined, primarily because of the variation among renal artery lesions. These lesions vary in location (e.g., main renal artery, branch lesions, or ostial lesions) and etiology (e.g., atherosclerotic or fibromuscular dysplasia). These differences may well affect technical success and long-term patency. Patients with fibromuscular lesions tend to have better long-term success and fewer procedural complications than those with atherosclerotic renal arterial disease. Tegtmeyer's group reported on 66 patients with 85 renal artery lesions due to fibromuscular dysplasia.[144] After a mean follow-up of 39 months, 39% of the hypertensive patients were cured and 59% were improved. Angioplasty appears to be the best initial treatment for such lesions if confined to the main renal artery, while bypass is more appropriate if the dysplastic lesions extend to branch vessels.

In the treatment of atherosclerotic renal artery lesions, the location of the occlusive lesion along the renal artery has been shown to influence angioplasty success. Martin and colleagues from Emory University compared the results of angioplasty of 129 ostial with 31 nonostial lesions.[143] At a mean follow-up period of 38 months, 10% of patients with ostial lesions were cured of their hypertension, while 46% were improved. In those with nonostial lesions, 22% were cured, while 48% were improved. Primary clinical success rates for these patients with ostial lesions were 78% at 1 year, 63% at 2 years, and 54% at 3 years. Repeat angioplasty in 16 patients improved patency rates to 87, 75, and 66%, respectively.

The indications for intervention can also affect success rates. Weibull reported on 71 renal artery angioplasties, 57% of patients having hypertension and azotemia, and 43% having hypertension alone. The overall technical success rate was 86%. After a mean follow-up period of 54 months, 15% of hypertensive patients were cured and 75% were improved. For those with both hypertension and azotemia, 38% were improved, 47% were unchanged, and 15% were worse.

Angioplasty has taken a primary role in the treatment of atherosclerotic and fibromuscular lesions of the main renal artery. The optimal management of ostial atherosclerotic lesions or fibromuscular lesions extending to branch vessels is less clear, with surgical bypass having better long-term success in exchange for greater morbidity.

Lesions of the supra-aortic trunk are, in certain aspects, ideally suited for endovascular intervention. The mainstay of treatment for innominate and proximal subclavian atherosclerotic occlusive lesions has traditionally been bypass or endarterectomy via median sternotomy. The potential advantage of decreasing morbidity by avoiding a chest-splitting incision appears great. Innominate lesion morphology is well suited for angioplasty, as these often occur as short segment stenoses rather than occlusions. The prime concern focuses on the risk of embolization to the cerebral circulation during angioplasty.

The surgical treatment of innominate occlusive disease is associated with a morbidity rate of 7 to 67% and a mortality rate of 0 to 5.5%. With an average follow-up period of 43 months, Cherry and colleagues at the Mayo Clinic found a 13% restenosis rate, while the Texas Heart Institute reported an early graft occlusion rate of 7%, failed endarterectomy in 9%, and a 2% stroke rate. These are the results to which angioplasty must compare. The first reported angioplasty of the innominate artery appeared in the surgical literature in 1981. In an attempt to protect the cerebral circulation from embolic debris, the right common carotid artery was exposed and clamped during angioplasty. Since that time, angioplasty has been performed without carotid occlusion with a very low risk of neurologic sequelae. The difficulty with evaluation of innominate angioplasty is the small number of cases appearing in the literature, precluding accurate comparison with surgical alternatives. Innominate angioplasty appears safe and avoids the potential morbidity of a thoracic incision. However, the risk of cerebral embolism remains uncertain, and the precautions necessary to prevent neurologic deficit are undetermined.

Subclavian arterial occlusive disease is more common than innominate disease, but it is similar to the innominate with regard to morbidity of surgical treatment. Beebe reported a 23% complication rate for both intra- and extrathoracic subclavian revascularization. Bypass is a durable procedure, with 5-year patency rates of 83 to 94% reported using synthetic graft material. Re-establishing patency has proven to be difficult in completely occluded subclavian segments, with success rates of 0 to 56% reported. If initially successful, patency rates equivalent to those of surgical bypass have been demonstrated up to 3 years postprocedure. Thereafter, PTA patency rates fall more rapidly, to a 5-year actuarial patency of 54%. This has proven to be a safe procedure, with a major complication rate of 0.2% and minor complication rate of 4.1% reported for over 400 subclavian angioplasties. When treating subclavian steal syndrome, there is a delay of 20 seconds to 4 minutes in flow reversing from retrograde to antegrade in the vertebral artery. This acts to protect against embolization via the vertebral artery during subclavian PTA. While totally occlusive lesions of the subclavian artery have been resistant in the past to short- or long-term success, the adjunctive use of thrombolytic therapy and intraluminal stents may improve upon the current mediocre results.

The treatment of carotid arterial occlusive disease by percutaneous angioplasty is likely the most controversial topic in vascular surgery today. The first large series appeared in the literature in 1987. In this report, 48 patients with atherosclerotic stenoses or postsurgical restenosis were treated. The procedure was successful in 45 patients, with three complications including one case of monocular blindness and two acute occlusions with one stroke. In 1990, this same author reported on an additional 13 patients treated with carotid PTA using a triple-axial catheter system to protect against cerebral embolization. This technique was successful in preventing neurologic complications in this small patient sample.

In 1991, Kachel reported on 43 PTAs for carotid stenosis of unspecified etiology, including 35 internal carotid artery lesions. Complications included one TIA as the result of carotid spasm, and one case of platelet deposition treated with emergent endarterectomy. There were no lasting neurologic symptoms or residual stenoses in an undefined percentage of patients followed for 3 to 109 months.

Bergeron and colleagues treated 38 patients with carotid PTA, including 24 with internal carotid stenoses and 7 with common carotid lesions. The majority of these lesions were postoperative restenoses (19 patients) and atherosclerotic (10 patients). In the entire series, there was one death due to hyperperfusion syndrome, one reversible stroke from an internal carotid dissection, and one TIA due to thrombosis. Other complications included arterial spasm, acute occlusion necessitating redilation with stenting, and a silent cerebral infarct. All the complications occurred in the group treated solely with PTA, whereas lesions which were stented were all successful and symptom-free.

A comparison between angioplasty with stenting and endarterectomy was recently reported. There was no significant difference between the groups with regard to the frequency of symptomatic lesions being treated. There was no difference in the risk of "major stroke" after PTA/stent or carotid endarterectomy (CEA) (1.9 versus 1.8%, respectively); however, the risk of "minor stroke" was significantly higher in the PTA group (6.5 as compared with 0.6% for CEA).

The role of angioplasty and stent deployment in the carotid artery is controversial. Many in the surgical community argue that carotid PTA is an unproven treatment with unknown results and risks. Furthermore, it is being compared with perhaps the most intensively scrutinized operative procedure to date. In those patients at increased risk of operative complications (i.e., history of ipsilateral neck dissection or radiation), endovascular therapy may well have an acceptable role in the treatment of carotid disease. Further refinement of techniques and instrumentation may permit carotid angioplasty to eventually become an accepted treatment.

Endoluminal Stent-Grafts. The most exciting of all the new vascular technologies is the transluminally placed stented graft. This allows insertion via an access site remote from the vascular lesion of a new prosthetic vascular conduit, which is brought into position from within the blood vessel lumen. The prosthesis is then anchored in place with appropriate fixation devices. This represents a significantly less-invasive approach to treat a variety of vascular lesions, including aneurysmal disease, traumatic pseudoaneurysms, and occlusive lesions. This concept is based on the work of Juan Parodi, an Argentinean surgeon who performed the first endoluminal graft repair of an aortic aneurysm in 1990.[38]

Since Parodi's initial paper, numerous reports have attested to the technical feasibility and short-term patency of stent-grafts placed for arterial trauma, for occlusive aortoiliac lesions, and for isolated aortic, iliac, and combined aortoiliac aneurysmal disease. Summarizing their initial stent-graft experience, Marin had a technical success rate of 91% with both aneurysmal and occlusive lesions, and a 100% success rate with traumatic arterial lesions.[44] Although follow-up was brief, 18-month primary and secondary patency rates for aortoiliac occlusive lesions were 77 and 95%, respectively.[45]

Several different types of abdominal aortic endoluminal stent-grafts are currently being evaluated throughout Europe, and in the United States by Food and Drug Administration (FDA) trials. These stents differ in graft composition, location of metallic support (e.g., internal vs. external and fully supported vs. support at the ends only), and overall design (tube vs. bifurcated). Currently, the most common reasons precluding the use of these devices are unfavorable aortic anatomy (i.e., too short a proximal neck) or iliac anatomy (i.e., extreme tortuosity or severe occlusive disease). As stent-graft technology improves, a greater number of patients with infrarenal abdominal aortic aneurysms will become suitable candidates.

Conclusion

As biomedical technology continues to grow, it can be anticipated that many of the devices used today will be improved upon. This will likely result in a greater ability to open completely occluded lesions. However, whether this will translate into acceptable patency rates has yet to be determined. Technologic advancement will also provide lower-profile instrumentation, permitting percutaneous access for procedures now requiring arterial cutdown (i.e., abdominal aortic aneurysm stent grafting). This raises the possibility that diseases now treated by vascular surgeons may soon be in the treatment realm of anyone adept at catheter-based intervention; therefore it is plausible that all vascular, and perhaps perivascular, diseases eventually will be targeted with a catheter-based approach.

Vascular surgeons are becoming increasingly aware of the role that endovascular procedures will play in the care of the vascular patient. This fact, along with the biomedical industry's facilitation of product development and physician education has led to rapid growth in a short period of time. The treatment of hemodynamically significant atheromatous lesions has suddenly become much easier to perform for the surgeon and more tolerable for the patient. As surgeons become more involved in angiography, a host of lesions easily amenable to angioplasty will be identified. The natural history of appropriate treatment for these lesions from a surgical standpoint is familiar. The appropriate treatment of minimally symptomatic, though significantly stenotic, lesions becomes more problematic when one realizes how much more difficult these lesions are to treat once occlusion begins. This is one of the more difficult questions raised by this new modality: "In which lesions should surgeons intervene prophylactically?" As imaging becomes less invasive and less expensive, it will be increasingly used to create "vascular maps." Consequently surgeons will be faced with diagnosis of vascular lesions, which had been hitherto undiagnosed, and will be forced to reappraise the indications for the treatment of specific lesions by a minimally invasive approach that is associated with fewer and less severe complications than traditional open procedures. Until then, surgeons must adhere to the current principles of vascular surgery, and continue to carefully investigate the potential application of new technology.

The versatility of the endovascular surgeon allows for the treatment (i.e., traditional surgical or catheter-based) to be tailored to the specifics of the lesion type and patient characteristics. In this regard, the endovascularly trained vascular surgeon is ideally suited to care for the patient with peripheral vascular disease.

References

1. Matas R: An operation for the radical cure of aneurysm based upon arteriorrhaphy. *Ann Surg* 37:161, 1903.
2. Murphy JB: Resection of arteries and veins injured in continuity—end to end suture—experimental and clinical research. *Med Rec* 51:73, 1897.
3. Carrel A, Guthrie CC: Uniterminal and terminal venous transplantations. *Surg Gynaecol Obstet* 2:266, 1906.
4. Bernheim BM: The ideal operation for aneurysm of the extremity: Report of a case. *Bull Johns Hopkins Hosp* 27:93, 1916.
5. DeBakey ME, Colley DA: Successful resection of an aneurysm of the thoracic aorta and replacement by graft. *Surgery* 152:673, 1953.
6. Ross R: The pathogenesis of atherosclerosis. *N Engl J Med* 314:488, 1986.
7. McGill HC Jr.: Persistent problems in the pathogenesis of atherosclerosis. *Arteriosclerosis* 4:443, 1984.
8. Faggiotto A, Ross R: Studies of hypercholesterolemia in nonhuman primate: II. Fatty streak conversion to fibrous plaque. *Arteriosclerosis* 4:341, 1984.
9. Wilcox JN, Smith KM, Williams LT, et al: Platelet derived growth factor mRNA detection in human atherosclerotic plaque by in situ hybridization. *J Clin Invest* 82:1134, 1988.
10. Barrett TB, Benditt EP: Sis (PDGF-B) gene transcript levels are elevated in human atherosclerotic lesions compared to normal artery. *Proc Natl Acad Sci USA* 84:1099, 1987.
11. Libby P, Warner SJC, Salomon RN, et al: Production of a platelet derived growth factor like mitogen by smooth muscle cells from human atheromata. *N Engl J Med* 318:1493, 1988.
12. Golden MA, Au YPT, Kenagy RT, et al: Growth factor gene expression by intimal cells in healing PTFE grafts. *J Vasc Surg* 11:580, 1990.
13. Golden MA, Au YPT, Kirkman TR et al: Platelet derived growth factor and mRNA expression in healing vascular grafts in baboons. The association in vivo of PDGF mRNA protein and cellular proliferation. *J Clin Invest* 87:406, 1991.
14. Barrett TB, Gajdusek CM, Schwartz SM, et al: Expression of the sis gene by endothelial cells in culture and in vivo. *Proc Natl Acad Sci USA* 81:6772, 1984.
15. Clowes AW, Schwartz SM: Significance of quiescent smooth muscle cell migration in the injured rat carotid artery. *Circ Res* 56:139, 1985.
16. Schwartz SM, Reidy MR, Clowes A: Kinetics of atherosclerosis, a stem cell model. *Ann NY Acad Sci* 454:292, 1985.
17. Rapp JH: Basic data related to lipid abnormalities in peripheral vascular disease. *Ann Vasc Surg* 4:604, 1990.
18. Scanu AM: Lipoprotein (a) and atherosclerosis. *Ann Intern Med* 115:209, 1991.
19. Ku DN, Giddens DP, Phillips DJ, et al: Hemodynamics of the normal human carotid bifurcation: In vitro and in vivo studies. *Ultrasound Med Biol* 11:13, 1985.
20. Zarins CK, Giddens DP, Bharadvaj BK, et al: Carotid bifurcation. *Atherosclerosis Circ Res* 53:502, 1983.
21. LaRosa JC, He J, Vupputuri S: Effect of statins on risk of coronary disease: A meta-analysis of randomized controlled trials. *JAMA* 282:2340, 1999.
22. Khan F, Litchfield SJ, Belch JJ: Cutaneous microvascular responses are improved after cholesterol-lowering in patients with peripheral arterial disease and hypercholesterolaemia. *Adv Exp Med Biol* 428:49, 1997.
23. Kirk G, McLaren M, Muir AH, et al: Decrease in P-selectin levels in patients with hypercholesterolaemia and peripheral arterial occlusive disease after lipid-lowering treatment. *Vasc Med* 4:23, 1999.
24. Leng GC, Price JF, Jepson RG: Lipid-lowering for lower limb atherosclerosis (Cochrane review), in: *The Cochrane Library*. Oxford, England: Update Software, 2001.
25. Blankenhorn DH, Azen SP, Crawford DW, et al: Effects of colestipol-niacin therapy on human femoral atherosclerosis. *Circulation* 83:438, 1991.

26. Lewis B: Randomised controlled trial of the treatment of hyperlipidaemia on progression of atherosclerosis. *Acta Med Scand Suppl* 701:53, 1985.

27. van Heek M, France CF, Compton DS, et al: In vivo metabolism-based discovery of a potent cholesterol absorption inhibitor, SCH58235, in the rat and rhesus monkey through the identification of the active metabolites of SCH48461. *J Pharmacol Exp Ther* 283:157, 1997.

28. Mohler ER 3rd: Peripheral arterial disease: Identification and implications. *Arch Intern Med* 163:2306, 2003.

29. Money SR, Herd A, Isaacsohn JL, et al: Effect of cilostazol in patients with intermittent claudication caused by peripheral vascular disease. *J Vasc Surg* 27:267, 1998.

30. Lee TH, Marcantonio CM, Thomas EJ, et al: Derivation and prospective validation of a simple index for prediction of cardiac risk of major noncardiac surgery. *Circulation* 100:1043, 1999.

31. Torella F, de Cossart L, Dimitri SK, et al: Routine beta-blockade in vascular surgery. *Cardiovasc Surg* 11:459, 2003.

32. Brown LC, Powell JT: Risk factors for aneurysm rupture in patients kept under ultrasound surveillance. *Ann Surg* 230:289, 1999.

33. Scott RA, Ashton HA, Kay DN: Abdominal aortic aneurysm in 4237 screened patients: Prevalence, development and management over 6 years. *Br J Surg* 78:1122, 1991.

34. Scott RAP, Wilson NM, Ashton HA, et al: Influence of screening on the incidence of ruptured abdominal aortic aneurysm: 5-year results of a randomised controlled study. *Br J Surg* 82:1066, 1995.

35. Szilagyi DE, Smith RF, Macksood AJ, et al: Expanding and ruptured abdominal aortic aneurysms. Problems of diagnosis and treatment. *Arch Surg* 83:395, 1961.

36. The United Kingdom Small Aneurysm Trial Participants: Long-term outcomes of immediate repair compared with surveillance for small abdominal aortic aneurysms. *N Engl J Med* 346:1445, 2002.

37. Lederle FA, Wilson SE, Johnson GR, et al: Immediate repair compared with surveillance of small abdominal aortic aneurysms. *N Engl J Med* 346:1437, 2002.

38. Parodi JC, Palmaz JC, Barone HD: Transfemoral intraluminal graft implantation for abdominal aortic aneurysms. *Ann Vasc Surg* 5:491, 1991.

39. Brewster DC, Cronenwett JL, Hallett JW, et al: Joint Council of the American Association for Vascular Surgery and Society for Vascular Surgery. Guidelines for the treatment of abdominal aortic aneurysms. Report of a subcommittee of the Joint Council of the American Association for Vascular Surgery and Society for Vascular Surgery. *J Vasc Surg* 37:1106, 2003.

40. Welborn MB 3rd, Seeger JM: Prevention and management of sigmoid and pelvic ischemia associated with aortic surgery. *Semin Vasc Surg* 14:255, 2001.

41. Van den Akker PJ, Brand R, van Schlifgaarde R, et al: False aneurysms after prosthetic reconstructions for aortoiliac obstructive disease. *Ann Surg* 210:658, 1989.

42. Dennis JW, Littooy FN, Greisler HP, et al: Anastomotic pseudoaneurysms: A continuing late complication of vascular reconstructive procedures. *Arch Surg* 121:314, 1986.

43. Curl GR, Faggioli GL, Stella A, et al: Aneurysmal change at or above the proximal anastomosis after infrarenal grafting. *J Vasc Surg* 16:855, 1992.

44. Marin M, Veith FJ, Panetta TF, et al: Transluminally placed endovascular stented graft repair for arterial trauma. *J Vasc Surg* 20:466, 1994.

45. Marin M, Veith FJ, Lyon RT, et al: Transfemoral endovascular repair of iliac artery aneurysms. *Am J Surg* 170:179, 1995.

46. Scott RA, Chuter TA: Clinical endovascular placement of bifurcated graft in abdominal aortic aneurysm without laparotomy. *Lancet* 343:413, 1994.

47. Bush RL, Lumsden AB, Dodson TF, et al: Mid-term results after endograft repair of abdominal aortic aneurysm. *J Vasc Surg.* 33(Suppl 2):S70, 2001.

48. Maleux G, Rousseau H, Otal P, et al: Modular component separation and reperfusion of abdominal aortic aneurysm sac after endovascular repair of abdominal aortic aneurysm: A case report. *J Vasc Surg* 28:349, 1998.

49. Bohm T, Soldner J, Rott A, et al: Perigraft leak of an aortic stent graft due to material fatigue. *AJR Am J Roentgenol* 172:1355, 1999.

50. Zarins CK, White RA, Fogarty TJ: Aneurysm rupture after endovascular repair using the AneuRx stent graft. *J Vasc Surg* 31:960, 2000.

51. Najibi S, Steinberg J, Katzen BT, et al: Detection of isolated hook fractures 36 months after implantation of Ancure endograft: A cautionary note. *J Vasc Surg* 34:353, 2001.

52. Chaikof EL, Blankensteijn JD, Harris PL, et al: Ad Hoc Committee for Standardized Reporting Practices in Vascular Surgery of The Society for Vascular Surgery/American Association for Vascular Surgery. Reporting standards for endovascular aortic aneurysm repair. *J Vasc Surg* 35:1048, 2002.

53. Eskandari MK, Yao JS, Pearce WH, et al: Surveillance after endoluminal repair of abdominal aortic aneurysms. *Cardiovasc Surg* 9:469, 2001.

54. Brady AR, Thompson SG, Greenhalgh RM, et al: Cardiovascular risk factors and abdominal aortic aneurysm expansion: Only smoking counts. *Br J Surg* 90:492, 2003.

55. Edwards JM, Teeffey FA, Zierler RE, et al: Intraabdominal paraanastomotic aneurysms after aortic bypass grafting. *J Vasc Surg* 15:344, 1992.

56. Allen RC, Schneider J, Longenecker L, et al: Paraanastomotic aneurysms of the abdominal aorta. *J Vasc Surg* 18:424, 1993.

57. Briggs RM, Jarstfer BS, Collins GJ: Anastomotic aneurysms. *Am J Surg* 146:770, 1983.

58. Gaylis H, Dewar G: Anastomotic aneurysms: Facts and fancy. *Surg Annu* 22:317, 1990.

59. Ramesh S, Michaels JA, Galland RB: Popliteal aneurysm: Morphology and management. *Br J Surg* 80:1531, 1993.

60. Szilagyi DE, Schwartz RL, Reddy DJ: Popliteal artery aneurysms. Their natural history and management. *Arch Surg* 116:724, 1981.

61. Vermilion BD, Kimmins SA, Pace WG, et al: A review of one hundred forty-seven popliteal aneurysms with long-term follow up. *Surgery* 90:1009, 1981.

62. Varga ZA, Locke-Edmunds JC, Baird RN: A multicenter study of popliteal aneurysms. Joint Vascular Research Group. *J Vasc Surg* 20:171, 1994.

63. Dawson I, Sie RB, van Bockel JH: Atherosclerotic popliteal aneurysm. *Br J Surg* 84:293, 1997.

64. Duffy ST, Colgan MP, Sultan S, et al: Popliteal aneurysms: A 10-year experience. *Eur J Vasc Endovasc Surg* 16:218, 1998.

65. Bowyer RC, Cawthorn SJ, Walker WJ, et al: Conservative management of asymptomatic popliteal aneurysm. *Br J Surg* 77:1132, 1990.

66. Lowell RC, Glovickzki P, Hallett JW Jr., et al: Popliteal artery aneurysms: The risk of nonoperative management. *Ann Vasc Surg* 8:14, 1994.

67. Barr H, Lancashire MJR, Torrie EPH, et al: Intra-arterial thrombolytic therapy in the management of acute and chronic limb ischaemia. *Br J Surg* 78:284, 1991.

68. Galland RB, Earnshaw JJ, Baird RN, et al: Acute limb deterioration during intra-arterial thrombolysis. *Br J Surg* 80:1118, 1993.

69. Thompson JF, Beard J, Scott DJ, et al: Intraoperative thrombolysis in the management of thrombosed popliteal aneurysms. *Br J Surg* 80:858, 1993.

70. Gouny P, Bertrand P, Duedal V, et al: Limb salvage and popliteal aneurysms: Advantage of preventive surgery. *Eur J Vasc Endovasc Surg* 19:496, 2000

71. Levi N, Schroeder TV: Lower extremity occlusive disease. Arteriosclerotic femoral artery aneurysms. A short review. *J Cardiovasc Surg (Torino)* 38:335, 1997.

72. Guida PM, Moore SW: Aneurysms of the hepatic artery. Report of five cases with a brief review of the previously reported cases. *Surgery* 60:299, 1966.

73. Countryman D, Norwood S, Register D, et al: Hepatic artery aneurysm. Report of an unusual case and review of the literature. *Am Surg* 49:51, 1983.

74. Dougherty MJ, Gloviczi P, Cherry KJ, et al: Hepatic artery aneurysms: Evaluation and current management. *Int. Angiol* 12:178, 1993.

75. Stouffer JT, Weinman MD, Bynum TE: Hemobilia in a patient with multiple artery aneurysms: A case report and review of the literature. *Am J Gastroenterol* 84:59, 1989.

76. Lumsden AB, Allen RC, Sreeram S, et al: Hepatic arterioportal fistulae. *Am Surg* 5:722, 1993.

77. Kibbler CC, Cohen DL, Cruicshank P, et al: Use of CAT scanning in the diagnosis and management of hepatic artery aneurysm. *Gut* 26:752, 1985.

78. Zalcman M, Matos C, Gansbeke D, et al: Hepatic artery aneurysm: CT and MR features. *Gastrointest Radiol* 12:203, 1987.

79. Baker KS, Tisnado J, Cho S, et al: Splanchnic artery aneurysms and pseudoaneurysms: Transcatheter embolization. *Radiology* 163:135, 1987.

80. Salam TA, Lumsden AB, Martin LG, et al: Nonoperative management of visceral aneurysms and pseudoaneurysms. *Am J Surg* 164:215, 1992.

81. Busuttil RW, Brin BJ: The diagnosis and management of visceral artery aneurysms. *Surgery* 88:619, 1980.

82. Graham JM, McCollum CH, DeBakey ME: Aneurysms of the splanchnic arteries. *Am J Surg* 140:797, 1980.

83. Lumsden AB, Riley JD, Skandalakis JE: Splenic artery aneurysms. *Prob Gen Surg* 7:113, 1990.

84. Mandel SR, Jaques PF, Mauro MA, et al: Nonoperative management of peripancreatic arterial aneurysms: A 10-year experience. *Ann Surg* 205:126, 1987.

85. Uflacker R, Diehl JC: Successful embolization of a bleeding splenic artery pseudoaneurysm secondary to necrotizing pancreatitis. *Gastrointest Radiol* 7:379, 1982.

86. Spigos DG, Jonasson O, Mozes M, et al: Partial splenic embolization in the treatment of hypersplenism. *AJR Am J Roentegenol* 132:777, 1979.

87. Kuroda C, Kawamoto S, Hori S, et al: Pancreatic pseudocyst hemorrhage controlled by transcatheter embolization. *Cardiovasc Intervent Radiol* 6:167, 1983.

88. Mercer D, Ghent WR: Gastroduodenal artery aneurysm associated with chronic relapsing pancreatitis. *Can Med Assoc J* 126:1065, 1982.

89. Thakker RV, Gajjar B, Wilkins RA, et al: Embolization of gastroduodenal artery aneurysm caused by chronic pancreatitis. *Gut* 24:1094, 1983.

90. Lumsden AB, Salam TA, Walton KG: Renal artery aneurysm: A report of 28 cases. *Cardiovasc Surg* 4:185, 1996.

91. Scott JR, Daneker G, Lumsden AB: Prevention of compartment syndrome associated with dorsal lithotomy position. *Am Surg* 63:801, 1997.

92. Albright HL, Leonard FC: Embolectomy from the abdominal aorta. *N Engl J Med* 242:271, 1950.

93. Meagher AP, Lord RSA, Graham AR, et al: Acute aortic occlusion presenting with lower limb paralysis. *J Cardiovasc Surg* 32:643, 1991.

94. Taylor FW: Saddle embolus of the aorta. *Arch Surg* 62:38, 1951.

95. Bell JW: Acute thrombosis of the subrenal abdominal aorta. *Arch Surg* 95:681, 1967.

96. Littooy FN, Baker WH: Acute aortic occlusion—-a multifaceted catastrophe. *J Vasc Surg* 4:211, 1986.

97. Webb KH, Jacocks MA: Acute aortic occlusion. *Am J Surg* 155:405, 1988.

98. Babu SC, Shah PM, Sharma P, et al: Adequacy of central hemodynamics versus restoration of circulation in the survival of patients with acute aortic thrombosis. *Am J Surg* 154:206, 1987.

99. Crawford ES, Bomberger RA, Glaeser DH, et al: Aortoiliac occlusive disease: Factors influencing survival and function following reconstructive operation over a 25 year period. *Surgery* 90:1055, 1981.

100. Rutherford RB: Aortobifemoral bypass, the gold standard: Technical considerations. *Semin Vasc Surg* 7:11, 1994.

101. Dormandy JA, Rutherford RB: Management of peripheral arterial disease (PAD). TASC Working Group. TransAtlantic Inter-Society Consensus (TASC). *J Vasc Surg* 31(1 Pt 2):S1, 2000.

102. Rutherford RB: Options in the surgical management of aorto-iliac occlusive disease: A changing perspective. *Cardiovasc Surg* 7:5, 1999.

103. Eugene G, Goldstone J, Moore WS: Fifteen year experience with subcutaneous bypass grafts for lower extremity ischemia. *Ann Surg* 186:177, 1977.

104. Imparato AM: Aortoiliac occlusive disease, in Cameron JL (ed): *Current Surgical Therapy 3*. Toronto: Mosby, 1989, p 553.

105. Ketonen P, Harjola PT, Ala-Kulju IT, et al: Surgical treatment of occlusion of the infrarenal abdominal aorta. *Acta Chir Scand* 152:665, 1986.

106. LeRiche R, Motel A: Syndrome of thrombotic obliteration of the aortic bifurcation. *Ann Surg* 127:193, 1948.

107. Moore WS, Hall AD, Blaidsell FW: Late results of axillary-femoral bypass grafting. *Am J Surg* 122:148, 1971.

108. Reilly LM, Sauer L, Weinstein ES, et al: Infrarenal aortic occlusion. Does it threaten renal perfusion or function? *J Vasc Surg* 11:216, 1990.

109. Palmaz JC, Laborde JC, Rivera FJ, et al: Stenting of the iliac arteries with the Palmaz stent: Experience from a multicenter trial. *Cardiovasc Intervent Radiol* 19:312, 1992.

110. Waltman AC: Percutaneous transluminal angioplasty of the iliac and deep femoral arteries, in Athanusoulis CA, Pfister RC, Greene RE, Robertson GH (eds): *Interventional Radiology*. Philadelphia: WB Saunders, 1982, p 273.

111. Smith JK, Rawly KS, Joseph IE, et al: Endovascular treatment of superficial femoral and popliteal arterial occlusive disease. *J Invasive Cardiol* 12:382, 2000.

112. van der Heijden FH, Eikelboom BC, Banga JD, et al: Management of superficial femoral artery occlusive disease. *Br J Surg* 80:959, 1993.

113. Lumsden AB, Besman A, Jaffe M, et al: Infrainguinal revascularization in end-stage renal disease. *Ann Vasc Surg* 8:107, 1994.

114. Edwards MS, Cherr GS, Craven TE, et al: Acute occlusive mesenteric ischemia: Surgical management and outcomes. *Ann Vasc Surg* 17:72, 2003.

115. Trompeter M, Brazda T, Remy CT, et al: Non-occlusive mesenteric ischemia: Etiology, diagnosis, and interventional therapy. *Eur Radiol* 12:1179, 2002.

116. Moawad J, Gewertz BL: Chronic mesenteric ischemia: Clinical presentation and diagnosis. *Surg Clin North Am* 77:357, 1997.

117. Sakai L, Keltner R, Kaminski D: Spontaneous and shock-associated ischemic colitis. *Am J Surg* 140:755, 1980.

118. Greenwald DA, Brandt LJ, Reinus JF: Ischemic bowel disease in the elderly. *Gastroenterol Clin North Am* 30:445, 2001.

119. Smerud MJ, Johnson CD, Stephens DH: Diagnosis of bowel infarction: A comparison of plain films and CT scans in 23 cases. *Am J Roentgenol* 154:99, 1990.

120. Sheehan SR: Acute mesenteric ischemia: Recent advances in diagnosis and endovascular therapy. *Emergency Radiology* 7:231, 2000.

121. Ha HK, Rha SE, Kim AY, et al: CT and MR diagnoses of intestinal ischemia. *Semin Ultrasound CT MR* 21:40, 2000.

122. Meaney JF, Prince MR, Nostrant TT, et al: Gadolinium-enhanced MR angiography of visceral arteries in patients with suspected chronic mesenteric ischemia. *J Magn Reson Imaging* 7:171, 1997.

123. Fitzgerald SF, Kaminski DL: Ischemic colitis. *Semin Colon Rectal Surg* 4:222, 1993.

124. Endean ED, Barnes SL, Kwolek CJ, et al: Surgical management of thrombotic acute intestinal ischemia. *Ann Surg* 233:801, 2001.

125. Simo G, Echenagusia AJ, Camunez F, et al: Superior mesenteric arterial embolism: Local fibrinolytic treatment with urokinase. *Radiology* 20:775, 1997.

126. Kihara TK, Blebea J, Anderson KM, et al: Risk factors and outcomes following revascularization for chronic mesenteric ischemia. *Ann Vasc Surg* 13:37, 1999.

127. Moaward J, McKinsey JF, Wyble CW, et al: Current results of surgical therapy for chronic mesenteric ischemia. *Arch Surg* 132:613, 1997.

128. Loomer DC, Johnson SP, Diffin DC, DeMaioribus CA: Superior mesenteric artery stent placement in a patient with acute mesenteric ischemia. *J Vasc Intervent Radiol* 10:29, 1999.

129. Johnston KW, Lindsay T, Walker PM, Kalman PG: Mesenteric arterial bypass grafts: Early and late results and suggested surgical approach for chronic and acute mesenteric ischemia. *Surgery* 118:1, 1995.

130. Sang CN, Whelton PK, Hamper U, et al: Etiologic factors in renovascular fibromuscular dysplasia: A case-controlled study. *Hypertension* 14:472, 1989.

131. Sawicki PT, Kaiser S, Heinemann I, et al: Prevalence of renal artery stenosis in diabetes mellitus—an autopsy study. *Ann Intern Med* 229:489, 1991.

132. Dean RH, Kieffer RW, Smith BM, et al: Renovascular hypertension: Anatomic and renal function changes during therapy. *Arch Surg* 116:1408, 1981.

133. Tollefson DF, Ernst CB: Natural history of atherosclerotic renal artery stenosis associated with aortic disease. *J Vasc Surg* 14:327, 1991.

134. Crowley JJ, Santos RM, Peter RH, et al: Progression of renal artery stenosis in patients undergoing cardiac catheterization. *Am Heart J* 136:913, 1998.

135. Caps MT, Perissinotto C, Zierler RE, et al: Prospective study of atherosclerotic disease progression in the renal artery. *Circulation* 98:2866, 1998.

136. Caps MT, Zierler RE, Polissar NL, et al: Risk of atrophy in kidneys with atherosclerotic renal artery stenosis. *Kidney Int* 53:735, 1998.

137. Zierler RE, Bergelin RO, Isaacson JA, Strandness DE Jr.: Natural history of atherosclerotic renal artery stenosis: A prospective study with duplex ultrasonography. *J Vasc Surg* 19:250, 1994.

138. An epidemiological approach to describing risk associated with blood pressure levels: Final report of the Working Group on Risk and High Blood Pressure. *Hypertension* 7:641, 1985.

139. Simon N, Franklin SS, Bleifer KH, Maxwell MH: Clinical characteristics of renovascular hypertension. *JAMA* 220:1209, 1972.

140. Hansen KJ, Tribble RW, Reavis SW, et al: Renal duplex sonography: Evaluation of clinical utility. *J Vasc Surg* 12:227, 1990.

141. Gedroyc WMW, Neerhut P, Negus R, et al: Magnetic resonance angiography of renal artery stenosis. *Clin Radiol* 50:436, 1995.

142. Beregi JP, Elkohen M, Deklunder G, et al: Helical CT angiography compared with arteriography in the detection of renal artery stenosis. *Am J Roentgenol* 167:495, 1996.

143. Martin LG, Rees CR, O'Bryant T: Percutaneous angioplasty of the renal arteries, in Strandness DE Jr., van Breda A (eds): *Vascular Diseases: Surgical & Interventional Therapy,* 3rd ed. New York: Churchill Livingstone, 1994, p 721.

144. Tegtmeyer CJ, Elson J, Glass TA, et al: Percutaneous transluminal angioplasty: The treatment of choice for renovascular hypertension due to fibromuscular dysplasia. *Radiology* 143:631, 1982.

145. White CJ, Ramee SR, Collins TJ, et al: Renal artery stent placement: Utility in lesions difficult to treat with balloon angioplasty. *J Am Coll Cardiol* 30:1445, 1997.

146. Dorros G, Jaff M, Jain A, et al: Follow-up of primary Palmaz-Schatz stent placement for atherosclerotic renal artery stenosis. *Am J Cardiol* 75:1051, 1995.

147. Dean RH, Tribble RW, Hansen KJ, et al: Evolution of renal insufficiency in ischemic nephropathy. *Ann Surg* 213:446, 1991.

148. Bredenberg CD, Sampson LN, Ray FS, et al: Changing patterns in surgery for chronic renal artery occlusive diseases. *J Vasc Surg* 15:1018, 1992.

149. Hansen KJ, Starr SM, Sands RE, et al: Contemporary surgical management of renovascular disease. *J Vasc Surg* 16:319, 1991.

150. Clair DG, Belkin M, Whittemore AD, et al: Safety and efficacy of transaortic renal endarterectomy as an adjunct to aortic surgery. *J Vasc Surg* 21:926, 1995.

151. Chaikof EL, Smith RB III, Salam AA, et al: Ischemic nephropathy and concomitant aortic disease: A ten-year experience. *J Vasc Surg* 19:135, 1994.

152. Dean RH, Keyser JE III, Dupont WD, et al: Aortic and renal vascular disease: Factors affecting the value of combined procedures. *Ann Surg* 200:336, 1984.

153. Reilly JM, Rubin BG, Thompson RW, et al: Long-term effectiveness of extraanatomic renal artery revascularization. *Surgery* 116:784, 1994.

154. Chang YJ, Golby AJ, Albers GW: Detection of carotid stenosis. From NASCET results to clinical practice. *Stroke* 26:1325, 1995.

155. Moore WS, Barnett HJ, Beebe HG, , et al: Guidelines for carotid endarterectomy. A multidisciplinary consensus statement from the Ad Hoc Committee, American Heart Association. *Circulation* 91:566, 1995.

156. Barnett HJ, Warlow CP: Carotid endarterectomy and the measurement of stenosis. *Stroke* 24:1281, 1993.

157. Barnett HJ, Haines SJ: Carotid endarterectomy for asymptomatic carotid stenosis. *N Engl J Med* 328:276, 1993.

158. Barnett HJM, Taylor DW, Eliasziw M, et al: The benefit of carotid endarterectomy in patients with symptomatic moderate or severe stenosis. *N Engl J Med* 339:1415, 1998.

159. Executive Committee for the Asymptomatic Carotid Atherosclerosis Study (ACAS). Endarterectomy for asymptomatic carotid artery stenosis. *JAMA* 273:1421, 1995.

160. North American Symptomatic Carotid Endarterectomy Trial Collaborators. Beneficial effect of carotid endarterectomy in symptomatic patients with high-grade carotid stenosis. *N Engl J Med* 325:445, 1991.

161. Randomized trial of endarterectomy for recently symptomatic carotid stenosis: Final results of the MRC European Carotid Surgery Trial. *Lancet* 351:1379, 1998.

162. Hobson RW II, Weiss DG, Fields WS, et al, for the Veterans Affairs Asymptomatic Cooperative Study Group: Efficacy of carotid endarterectomy for asymptomatic carotid stenosis. *N Engl J Med* 328: 221, 1993.

163. Vannix RS, Joergenson EJ, Carter R: Kinking of the internal carotid artery: Clinical significance and surgical management. *Am J Surg* 134:82, 1977.

164. Stanton PE, McClusky DA, Lamis PA: Hemodynamic assessment and surgical correction of kinking of the internal carotid artery. *Surgery* 84:793, 1978.

165. Coyle KA, Smith RB 3rd, Chapman RL, et al: Carotid artery shortening: A safe adjunct to carotid endarterectomy. *J Vasc Surg* 22:257, 1995.

166. Hamann H: Carotid endarterectomy: Prevention of stroke in asymptomatic (Stage I) and symptomatic (Stage II) patients? *Thorac Cardiovasc Surg* 36:272, 1988.

167. Chino ES: A simple method for combined carotid endarterectomy and correction of internal carotid artery kinking. *J Vasc Surg* 6:197, 1987.

168. Nicholls SC, Phillips DI, Bergelin RO, et al: Carotid endarterectomy: Relation of outcome to early restenosis. *J Vasc Surg* 2:375, 1985.

169. Edwards WH, Edwards WH, Mulherin L, Martin RS: Recurrent carotid artery stenosis. *Ann Surg* 209:662, 1989.

170. Bernstein EF, Toren S, Dilley RB: Does carotid restenosis predict an increased risk of late symptoms, stroke, or death? *Ann Surg* 212:629, 1990.

171. Kieny R, Seiller C, Petit H: Evolution of carotid restenosis after endarterectomy. *Cardiovasc Surg* 2:555, 1994.

172. Hobson RW: CREST (Carotid Revascularization Endarterectomy versus Stent Trial): Background, design, and current status. *Semin Vasc Surg* 13:139, 2000.

173. Lin PH, Bush RL, Lumsden AB: Carotid artery stenting: Current status and future directions. *Vasc Endovascular Surg* 37:315, 2003.

174. Bush RL, Lin PH, Dodson TF, et al: Endoluminal stent placement and coil embolization for the management of carotid artery pseudoaneurysms. *J Endovasc Ther* 8:53, 2001.

175. Roseborough GS, Williams GM: Marfan and other connective tissue disorders: Conservative and surgical considerations. *Semin Vasc Surg* 13:272, 2000.

176. Hunter GC, Malone JM, Moore WS, et al: Vascular manifestations in patients with Ehlers-Danlos syndrome. *Arch Surg* 117:495, 1982.

177. Mao JR, Bristow J: The Ehlers-Danlos syndrome: On beyond collagens. *J Clin Invest* 107:1063, 2001.

178. Cikrit DF, Miles JH, Silver D: Spontaneous arterial perforation: The Ehlers-Danlos specter. *J Vasc Surg* 5:248, 1987.

179. Marfan A: Un case de deformation congenitale des quatre members, plus prononcee aux extremitites, caracterisee par l'allongement des os avec un certain degree d'amincissement. *Bul Sco Chir Paris* 13:220, 1896.

180. Dietz HC, Pyeritz RE, Hall BD, et al: The Marfan syndrome locus: Confirmation of assignment to chromosome 15 and identification of tightly linked markers at 15q15-q21.3. *Genomics* 9:355, 1991.

181. Pyeritz RE: The Marfan syndrome. *Am Fam Physician* 34:83, 1986.

182. Baumgartner WA, Cameron DE, Redmond JM, et al: Operative management of Marfan syndrome: The Johns Hopkins experience. *Ann Thorac Surg* 67:1859, 1999; discussion 1868.

183. Sherer DW, Sapadin AN, Lebwohl MG: Pseudoxanthoma elasticum: An update. *Dermatology* 199:3, 1999.

184. Ohtani T, Furukawa F: Pseudoxanthoma elasticum. *J Dermatol* 29:615, 2002.

185. Renie WA, Pyeritz RE, Combs J, Fine SL: Pseudoxanthoma elasticum: High calcium intake in early life correlates with severity. *Am J Med Genet* 19:235, 1984.

186. Ejrup B, Hiertonn T: Intermittent claudication. Three cases treated by a free vein graft. *Acta Chir Scandinav* 108:217, 1954.

187. Tsolakis IA, Walvatne CS, Caldwell MD: Cystic adventitial disease of the popliteal artery: Diagnosis and treatment. *Eur J Vasc Endovasc Surg* 15:188, 1998.

188. Levien LJ, Benn CA: Adventitial cystic disease: A unifying hypothesis. *J Vasc Surg* 28:193, 1998.

189. Tracy GD, Ludbrook J, Rundle FF: Cystic adventitial disease of the popliteal artery. *Vasc Surg* 3:10, 1969.

190. Love J: Popliteal artery entrapment syndrome. *Am J Surg* 109:620, 1965.

191. Hamming J: Intermittent claudication at an early age, due to an anomalous course of the popliteal artery. *Angiology* 10:369, 1959.

192. Turnipseed WD: Popliteal entrapment syndrome. *J Vasc Surg* 35:910, 2002.

193. Levien LJ, Veller MG: Popliteal artery entrapment syndrome: More common than previously recognized. *J Vasc Surg* 30:587, 1999.

194. Ohara N, Miyata T, Oshiro H, Shigematsu H: Surgical treatment for popliteal artery entrapment syndrome. *Cardiovasc Surg* 9:141, 2001.

195. di Marzo L, Cavallaro A, Sciacca V, et al: Surgical treatment of popliteal artery entrapment syndrome: A ten year experience. *Eur J Vasc Surg* 5:59, 1991.

196. di Marzo L, Cavallaro A, Sciacca V, et al: Natural history of entrapment of the popliteal artery. *J Am Coll Surg* 178:553, 1994.

197. Sasaki S, Sakuma M, Yasuda K: Current status of thromboangiitis obliterans (Buerger's disease) in Japan. *Int J Cardiol* 75(Suppl 1):S175, 2000.

198. Buerger L: Thrombo-angiitis obliterans: A study of the vascular lesions leading to presenile spontaneous gangrene. *Am J Med Sci* 136:567, 1908.

199. Mills JL, Friedman EI, Taylor LM, et al: Upper extremity ischemia caused by small artery disease. *Ann Surg* 206:521, 1987.

200. Pairolero PC, Joyce JW, Skinner CR, et al: Lower limb ischemia in young adults: Prognostic implications. *J Vasc Surg* 1:459, 1984.

201. Mills JL, Porter JM: Buerger's disease: A review and update. *Semin Vasc Surg* 6:14, 1993.

202. Mills JL, Taylor LM Jr., Porer JM: Buerger's disease in the modern era. *Am J Surg* 154:123, 1987.

203. Sasajima T, Kubo Y, Inaba M, et al: Role of infrainguinal bypass in Buerger's disease: An eighteen-year experience. *J Vasc Endovasc Surg* 13:186, 1997.

204. Watts RA, Scott DG: Epidemiology of the vasculitides. *Curr Opin Rheumatol* 15:11, 2003.

205. Numano F: Vasa vasoritis, vasculitis and atherosclerosis. *Int J Cardiol* 75(Suppl 1):S1, 2000; discussion S17.

206. Takayasu M: A case with peculiar changes of the retinal central vessels. *Acta Soc Ophtal Jpn* 2:554, 1908.

207. Arend WP, Michael BA, Block DA, et al: The American College of Rheumatology 1990 criteria for the classification of Takayasu arteritis. *Arthritis Rheum* 33:1129, 1990.

208. Gradden C, McWilliams R, Williams P, et al: Multiple stenting in Takayasu arteritis. *J Endovasc Ther* 9:936, 2002.

209. Johnston SL, Lock RJ, Gompels MM: Takayasu arteritis: A review. *J Clin Pathol* 55:481, 2002.

210. Rodriguez-Cuartero A, Perez-Blanco FJ, Canora-Lebrato J: Takayasu arteritis and renovascular hypertension. *Clin Nephrol* 55:176, 2001.

211. Nordborg E, Nordborg C: Giant cell arteritis: Epidemiological clues to its pathogenesis and an update on its treatment. *Rheumatology (Oxford)* 42:413, 2003.

212. Weyand CM, Goronzy JJ: Pathogenic mechanisms in giant cell arteritis. *Cleve Clin J Med* 69(Suppl 2):SII28, 2002.

213. Hirose H, Takagi M, Noguchi M, et al: Coronary revascularization and abdominal aortic aneurysm repair in a patient with Behcet's disease. *J Cardiovasc Surg (Torino)* 39:751, 1998.

214. Okita Y, Ando M, Minatoya K, et al: Multiple pseudoaneurysms of the aortic arch, right subclavian artery, and abdominal aorta in a patient with Behcet's disease. *J Vasc Surg* 28:723, 1998.

215. Kizilkilic O, Albayram S, Adaletli I, et al: Endovascular treatment of Behcet's disease-associated intracranial aneurysms: Report of two cases and review of the literature. *Neuroradiology* 45:328, 2003.

216. Koike S, Matsumoto K, Kokubo M, et al: A case of aorto-enteric fistula after reconstruction of an abdominal aortic aneurysm associated with Behcet's disease and special reference to 95 reported cases in Japan. *Nippon Geka Gakkai Zasshi* 89:945, 1988.

217. Sasaki S, Yasuda K, Takigami K, et al: Surgical experiences with peripheral arterial aneurysms due to vasculo-Behcet's disease. *J Cardiovasc Surg (Torino)* 39:147, 1998.

218. Stone JH: Polyarteritis nodosa. *JAMA* 288:1632, 2002.

219. Freeman AF, Shulman ST: Recent developments in Kawasaki disease. *Curr Opin Infect Dis* 14:357, 2001.

220. Kitamura S: The role of coronary bypass operation on children with Kawasaki disease. *Coron Artery Dis* 13:437, 2002.

221. Priollet P, Vayssairat M, Housset E: How to classify Raynaud's phenomenon. Long-term follow-up study of 73 cases. *Am J Med* 83:494, 1987.

222. Landry GJ, Edwards JM, Porter JM: Current management of Raynaud's syndrome. *Adv Surg* 30:33, 1996.

223. Luggen M, Belhorn L, Evans T, et al: The evolution of Raynaud's phenomenon: A long long-term prospective study. *J Rheumatol* 22:2226, 1995.

224. McLafferty RB, Edwards JM, Taylor LM, et al: Diagnosis and long-term clinical outcome in patients diagnosed with hand ischemia. *J Vasc Surg* 22:361, 1995; discussion 367.

225. McLafferty RB, Edwards JM, Ferris BL, et al: Raynaud's syndrome in workers who use vibrating pneumatic air knives. *J Vasc Surg* 30:1, 1999.

226. Landry GJ, Edwards JM, Porer JM: Raynaud's syndrome in women. *Semin Vasc Surg* 8:327, 1995.

227. Bowling JC, Dowd PM: Raynaud's disease. *Lancet* 361:2078, 2003.

228. Landry GJ, Edwards JM, McLafferty RB, et al: Long-term outcome of Raynaud's syndrome in a prospectively analyzed patient cohort. *J Vasc Surg* 23:76, 1996; discussion 85.

229. Coleiro B, Marshall SE, Denton CP, et al: Treatment of Raynaud's phenomenon with the selective serotonin reuptake inhibitor fluoxetine. *Rheumatology (Oxford)* 40:1038, 2001.

230. Wright HR, Drake DB, Gear AJ, et al: Refractory Raynaud's phenomenon in scleroderma: An indication for surgery. *Am J Emerg Med* 15:328, 1997.

231. Wigley FM: Clincial practice. Raynaud's phenomenon. *N Engl J Med* 347;1001, 2002.
232. Rajesh YS, Pratap CP, Woodyer AB: Thoracoscopic sympathectomy for palmar hyperhidrosis and Raynaud's phenomenon of the upper limb and excessive facial blushing: A five-year experience. *Postgrad Med J* 78:682, 2002.
233. Chuang VP: Radiation-induced arteritis. *Semin Roentgenol* 29:64, 1994.
234. Hobson RW 2nd, Lal BK, Chaktoura E, et al: Carotid artery stenting: Analysis of data for 105 patients at high risk. *J Vasc Surg* 37:1234, 2003.
235. Houdart E, Mounayer C, Chapot R, et al: Carotid stenting for radiation-induced stenoses: A report of 7 cases. *Stroke* 32:118, 2001.
236. Al-Mubarak N, Roubin GS, Iyer SS, et al: Carotid stenting for severe radiation-induced extracranial carotid artery occlusive disease. *J Endovasc Ther* 7:36, 2000.
237. Leriche R: Dolicho et mega-artere dolicho et mega-veine. *Presse Med* 51:554, 1943.
238. Lawrence PF, Wallis C, Dobrin PB, et al: Peripheral aneurysms and arteriomegaly: Is there a familial pattern? *J Vasc Surg* 28:599, 1998.
239. Hollier LH, Stanson AW, Gloviczki P, et al: Arteriomegaly: Classification and morbid implications of diffuse aneurysmal disease. *Surgery* 93:700, 1983.
240. Luscher TF, Lie JT, Stanson AW, et al: Arterial fibromuscular dysplasia. *Mayo Clinic Proc* 62:931, 1987.
241. Schievink WI, Bjornsson J: Fibromuscular dysplasia of the internal carotid artery: A clinicopathological study. *Clin Neuropathol* 15:2, 1996.
242. Stewart MT, Moritz MW, Smith RB, et al: The natural history of carotid fibromuscular dysplasia. *J Vasc Surg* 3:305, 1986.
243. Collins GJ Jr., Rich NM, Clagett GP, et al: Fibromuscular dysplasia of the internal carotid arteries. Clinical experience and follow-up. *Ann Surg* 194:89, 1981.
244. Tegtmeyer CJ, Selby JB, Hartwell GD, et al: Results and complications of angioplasty in fibromuscular disease. *Circulation* 83:1155, 1991.
245. Birrer M, Do DD, Mahler F, et al: Treatment of renal artery fibromuscular dysplasia with balloon angioplasty: A prospective follow-up study. *Eur J Vasc Endovasc Surg* 23:146, 2002.
246. Reiher L, Pfeiffer T, Sandmann W: Long-term results after surgical reconstruction for renal artery fibromuscular dysplasia. *Eur J Vasc Endovasc Surg* 20:556, 2000.
247. Smith LL, Smith DC, Killeen JD, Hasso AN: Operative balloon angioplasty in the treatment of internal carotid artery fibromuscular dysplasia. *J Vasc Surg* 6:482, 1987.
248. Salam TA, Lumsden AB, Smith RB 3rd: Subclavian artery revascularization: A decade of experience with extrathoracic bypass procedures. *J Surg Res* 56:387, 1994.
249. Lin PH, Bush RL, Weiss VJ, et al: Subclavian artery disruption resulting from endovascular intervention: Treatment options. *J Vasc Surg* 32:607, 2000.
250. Weiss VJ, Lumsden AB: Minimally invasive vascular surgery: Review of current modalities. *World J Surg* 23:406, 1999.

CHAPTER 23

Venous and Lymphatic Disease

Everett Y. Lam, Mary E. Giswold, and Gregory L. Moneta

VENOUS ANATOMY

Veins are part of a dynamic and complex system that returns venous blood to the heart against the force of gravity in an upright individual. Venous blood flow is dependent upon multiple factors such as gravity, venous valves, the cardiac and respiratory cycles, blood volume, and the calf muscle pump. Alterations in the intricate balance of these factors can result in venous pathology.

Structure of Veins

Veins are thin-walled, highly distensible, and collapsible structures. Their structure specifically supports their two primary functions of transporting blood toward the heart and as a reservoir for preventing intravascular volume overload. The venous intima is composed of a nonthrombogenic endothelium with an underlying basement membrane and an elastic lamina. The endothelium produces endothelium-derived relaxing factor and prostacyclin, which help maintain a nonthrombogenic surface through inhibition of platelet aggregation and by promoting platelet disaggregation.[1] Circumferential rings of elastic tissue and smooth muscle located in the media of the vein allow for changes in vein caliber with minimal changes in venous pressure. When an individual is upright and standing still, the veins are maximally distended and their diameters may be several times greater than if the individual was in a horizontal position.

Unidirectional blood flow is achieved with multiple venous valves. The number of valves is greatest below the knee and decreases in number in the more proximal veins. The inferior vena cava (IVC), the common iliac veins, the portal venous system, and the cranial sinuses are valveless. Each valve is made of two thin cusps consisting of a fine connective tissue skeleton covered by endothelium. Venous valves close in response to cephalad-to-caudal blood flow at a velocity of at least 30 cm/s.[2]

Lower Extremity Veins

Lower extremity veins are divided into superficial, deep, and perforating veins. The superficial venous system lies above the uppermost fascial layer of the leg and thigh and consists of the greater saphenous vein (GSV) and lesser saphenous vein (LSV) and their tributaries. The GSV originates from the dorsal pedal venous arch and courses cephalad anterior to the medial malleolus and enters the common femoral vein approximately 4 cm inferior and lateral to the pubic tubercle. The saphenous nerve accompanies the GSV medially and supplies cutaneous sensation to the medial leg and ankle. The LSV originates laterally from the dorsal pedal venous arch and courses cephalad in the posterior calf and penetrates the popliteal fossa, most often between the medial and lateral heads of the gastrocnemius, to join the popliteal vein. The termination of the LSV is somewhat variable. It may enter the deep venous system as high as the mid-posterior thigh. The sural nerve accompanies the LSV laterally along its course and supplies cutaneous sensation to the lateral malleolar region.

The deep veins follow the course of major arteries in the extremities. In the lower leg, paired veins parallel the course of the anterior and posterior tibial and peroneal arteries and join behind the knee to form the popliteal vein. Venous bridges connect the paired veins in the lower leg. The popliteal vein continues through the adductor hiatus to become the femoral vein. In the proximal thigh, the femoral vein joins with the deep femoral vein to form the common femoral vein. In the groin, the common femoral vein lies medial to the common femoral artery. The common femoral vein becomes the external iliac vein at the inguinal ligament.

Multiple perforator veins traverse the deep fascia to connect the superficial and deep venous systems. Clinically important perforator veins are the Cockett and Boyd perforators. The Cockett perforator veins drain the medial lower leg and are relatively constant. They connect the posterior arch vein (a tributary of the GSV) and the posterior tibial vein. They may become varicose or incompetent in venous insufficiency states. Boyd's perforator veins connect the greater saphenous vein to the deep veins approximately 10 cm below the knee and 1 to 2 cm medial to the tibia.

Venous sinuses are thin-walled, large veins located within the substance of the soleus and gastrocnemius muscles. These sinuses are valveless and are linked by valved, small venous channels that prevent reflux. A large amount of blood can be stored in the venous sinuses. With each contraction of the calf muscle bed, blood is pumped out through the venous channels into the main conduit veins to return to the heart.

Upper Extremity Veins

As in the lower extremity, there are deep and superficial veins in the upper extremity. Deep veins of the upper extremity are paired and follow the named arteries in the arm. Superficial veins of the upper extremity are the cephalic and basilic veins and their tributaries. The cephalic vein originates at the lateral wrist and courses over the ventral surface of the forearm. In the upper arm, the cephalic vein terminates in the infraclavicular fossa, piercing the clavipectoral fascia to empty into the axillary vein. The basilic vein runs medially along the forearm and penetrates the deep fascia as it courses past the elbow in the upper arm. It then joins with the deep brachial veins to become the axillary vein. The median cubital vein joins the cephalic and the basilic veins on the ventral surface of the elbow.

The axillary vein becomes the subclavian vein at the lateral border of the first rib. At the medial border of the scalenus anterior muscle, the subclavian vein joins with the internal jugular vein to become the brachiocephalic vein. The left and right brachiocephalic veins join to become the superior vena cava, which empties into the right atrium.

EVALUATION OF THE VENOUS SYSTEM

Clinical Evaluation

The evaluation of the venous system begins with a detailed history and physical examination. Risk factors for acute and chronic venous disease are identified. They include increased age, history of prior venous thromboembolism, malignancy, trauma, obesity, pregnancy, and hypercoagulable states, as well as the postoperative state. Venous pathology is often, but not always, associated with visible or palpable signs that can be identified during the physical examination. There is variation among individuals in the prominence of superficial veins when standing. The superficial veins of a lean athletic person, even when normal, will appear large and easily visualized, but they will be far less obvious in the obese individual. Possible signs of superficial venous abnormalities are listed in Table 23-1. The deep veins cannot be directly assessed clinically, and abnormalities within them can only be inferred indirectly from changes found on clinical examination.

Chronic venous insufficiency (CVI) may lead to characteristic changes in the skin and subcutaneous tissues in the affected limb. CVI results from incompetence of venous valves, venous obstruction, or both. Most CVI involves venous reflux, and severe CVI often reflects a combination of reflux and venous obstruction. It is important to remember that while CVI originates with abnormalities of the veins, the target organ of CVI is the skin. A typical leg affected by CVI will be edematous, with edema increasing over the course of the day (Fig. 23-1). The leg may also be indurated and pigmented with eczema and dermatitis. These changes are due to excessive proteinaceous capillary exudate and deposition of a pericapillary fibrin cuff that may limit nutritional exchange. In addition, an increase in white blood cell trapping within the skin microcirculation in CVI patients may lead to microvascular congestion and thrombosis. Subsequently, white blood cells may migrate into the interstitium and release necrotizing lysosomal enzymes, resulting in tissue destruction and eventual ulceration.

Fibrosis occurs from impaired nutrition, chronic inflammation, and fat necrosis (lipodermatosclerosis). Hemosiderin deposition due to the exudation of red cells and subsequent lysis in the skin causes the characteristic pigmentation of chronic venous disease (Fig. 23-2). Ulceration can develop with long-standing venous hypertension and is associated with alterations in microcirculatory and cutaneous lymphatic anatomy and function. The most common location of venous ulceration is approximately 3 cm proximal to the medial malleolus (Fig. 23-3).

The Trendelenburg test is a clinical test that can help determine whether incompetent valves are present, and in which of the three venous systems (superficial, deep, or perforator) the valves are abnormal. There are two components to this test. First, with the patient supine, the leg is elevated 45° to empty the veins, and the GSV is occluded with the examiner's hand or with a rubber tourniquet. With the GSV still occluded, the patient stands and the superficial veins are observed for blood filling. Then compression on the GSV is

Table 23-1
Possible Signs of Superficial Venous Abnormality

Tortuosity
Varicosity
Venous saccule
Distended subdermal venules (corona phlebectatica)
Distended intradermal venules (spider angiomata)
Warmth, erythema, tenderness (superficial thrombophlebitis)

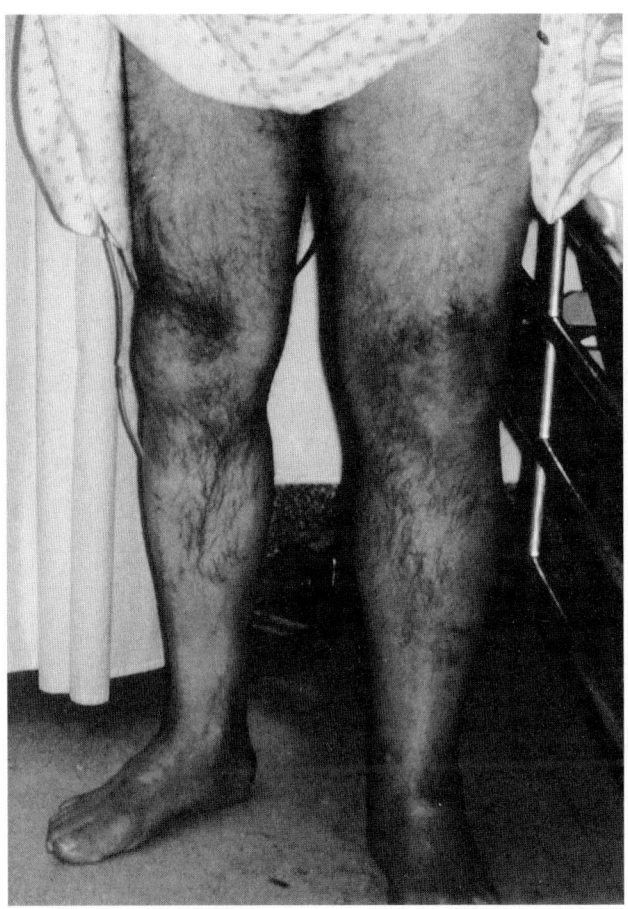

FIG. 23-1. Edematous left leg of patient with chronic venous insufficiency.

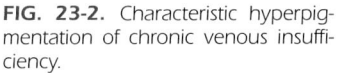

released and the superficial veins are observed for increased filling with blood. A negative result, indicating no clinically evident venous reflux, is the gradual filling of the veins from arterial inflow. A positive result is the sudden filling of veins with standing in the first

part of the test or with release of GSV compression in the second part of the test. The perforator veins are thought to be normal with competent valves if the first component of the test is negative. If this part of the test is positive, there are theoretically incompetent valves in both the deep and perforator veins. The GSV valves are competent if the second component of the test is negative, and the GSV valves are incompetent if the second component of the test is positive. Interpretation of the Trendelenburg test is obviously subjective. It has therefore been largely supplanted by the more objective noninvasive vascular laboratory tests to localize sites of venous reflux.

Noninvasive Evaluation

Prior to the development of vascular ultrasound, noninvasive techniques to evaluate the venous system were based on plethysmographic techniques. Although there are a variety of plethysmographic techniques used in the evaluation of both acute and chronic venous disease, they are all based on the detection of volume changes in the limb in response to blood flow.

Duplex ultrasonography (DUS) augmented by color flow imaging is now the most important noninvasive diagnostic method in the evaluation of the venous system. DUS has become standard for the detection of infrainguinal deep venous thrombosis (DVT), with near 100% sensitivity and specificity in symptomatic patients.[3] It is also the preferred method of evaluation for upper extremity venous thrombosis and is useful in the evaluation of CVI by documenting the presence of valvular reflux and venous obstruction.

Invasive Evaluation

With the improved accuracy of noninvasive techniques for diagnostic purposes, the use of invasive procedures has become more selective. Venography is now primarily used as an adjunct to percutaneous or operative therapy of venous disorders. Because the pelvic veins often cannot be visualized with DUS secondary to overlying bowel gas or body habitus, venography is often used to evaluate iliofemoral venous thrombosis in preparation for endovascular treatment or open surgical treatment.

Venography is performed by direct venipuncture with injection of contrast material. As with any invasive procedure, there are

FIG. 23-2. Characteristic hyperpigmentation of chronic venous insufficiency.

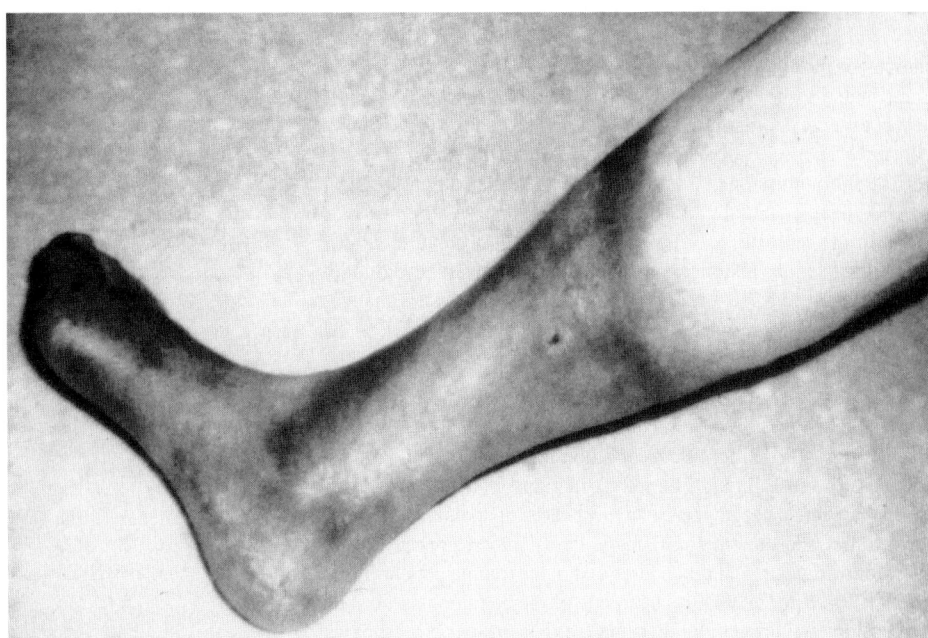

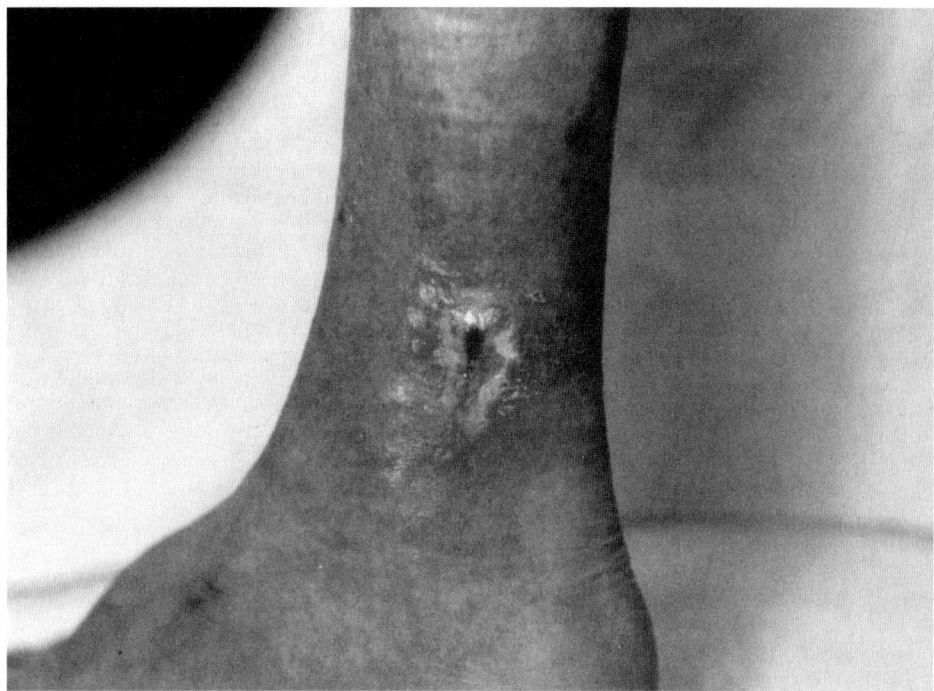

FIG. 23-3. Venous ulceration located proximal to the medial malleolus.

inherent risks associated with venography. Local effects include pain and local thrombosis at the puncture site and possible formation of a hematoma if larger veins are used for access. Pain developing from standard iodinated contrast injection is seen in up to 59% of patients undergoing venography for deep venous thrombosis.[4] Systemic effects of iodinated contrast include allergic reaction and risk of renal failure. Postvenography venous thrombosis occurs distal to the puncture site in 1 to 2% of patients undergoing venography and results from vein intimal damage from intravenous contrast.[5]

VENOUS THROMBOEMBOLISM

Epidemiology

Despite increased awareness and use of prophylactic modalities,[6] DVT and pulmonary embolism (PE) remain important preventable sources of morbidity and mortality. The annual incidence of DVT is estimated to be between 69 and 139 cases per 100,000 people in the general population. The prevalence of venous thromboembolism (VTE) in hospitalized patients is approximately 350 cases per 100,000 admissions,[7–9] and is a cause of death in approximately 250,000 people annually.[7] Not only does DVT pose an immediate threat to life with PE, it can also cause long-term impairment due to resultant venous insufficiency. The 20-year cumulative incidence rate is 26.8% and 3.7% for the development of venous stasis changes and venous ulcers, respectively, after an episode of DVT.[10]

Risk Factors

Three conditions, first described by Rudolf Virchow in 1862, contribute to VTE formation: stasis of blood flow, endothelial damage, and hypercoagulability. Of these risk factors, relative hypercoagulability appears most important in most cases of spontaneous DVT, while stasis and endothelial damage likely play a greater role in DVT following surgical procedures and in the trauma patient. Identified risk factors for VTE relate to one of the conditions described by Virchow, and often more than one factor is present. Specific risk

factors for VTE are listed in Table 23-2.[7,11–21] In one population-based study, over 90% of patients hospitalized for VTE had more than one risk factor.[12] The number of risk factors also increases with age.[22] The odds ratio for the development of symptomatic DVT in outpatients has been estimated at 1.26 for patients with one risk factor to 3.88 for patients with more than three risk factors.[23]

The risk for the development of VTE in surgical patients is multifactorial. Patients will have a period of activated coagulation, transient depression of fibrinolysis, and temporary immobilization. In addition, many patients may have a central venous catheter in place and have concomitant cardiac disease, malignancy, or intrinsic hypercoagulable states. In trauma patients, spinal cord injury (odds ratio 8.59) and fracture of the femur or tibia (odds ratio 4.82) are the strongest risk factors for VTE.[16] For otherwise healthy individuals, immobilization for a prolonged period of time in addition to pre-existing risk factors may be associated with VTE. Multiple reports have been published suggesting an association between prolonged periods with bent knees during travel and the development of VTE.[24,25] This has been referred to as the "economy-class syndrome."[26]

Table 23-2
Risk Factors for Venous Thromboembolism

History of venous thromboembolism
Age
Major surgery
Malignancy
Obesity
Trauma
Varicose veins/superficial thrombophlebitis
Cardiac disease
Hormones
Prolonged immobilization/paralysis
Pregnancy
Venous catheterization
Hypercoagulable states (most prevalent; resistance to activated protein C)

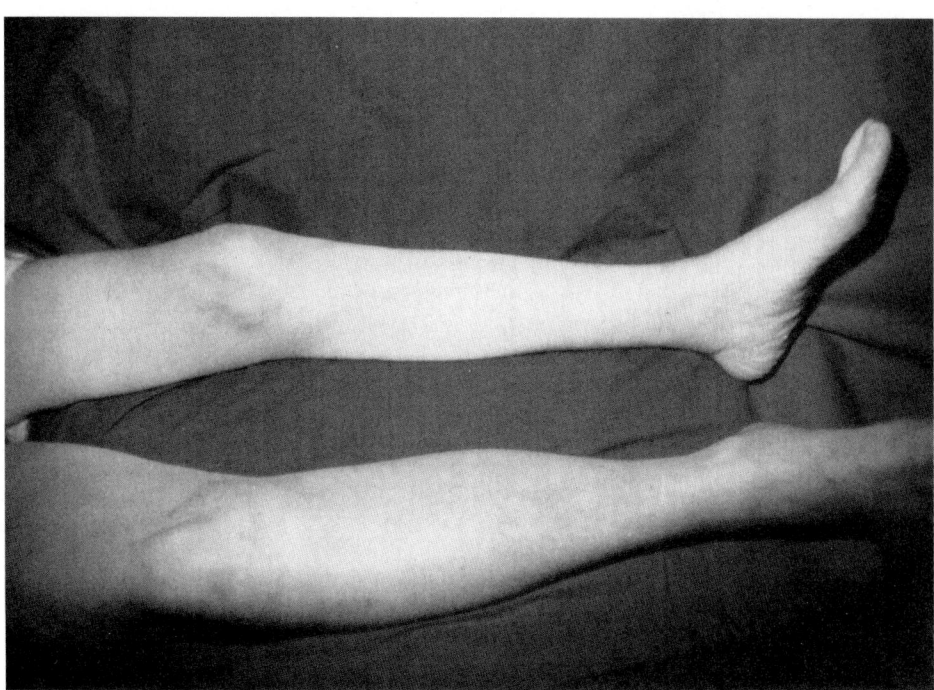

FIG. 23-4. Phlegmasia alba dolens of the right leg. Note the blanching and edema.

Diagnosis

Clinical Evaluation

Early in the course of DVT development, venous thrombosis is thought to begin in an area of relative stasis, such as a soleal sinus vein or immediately downstream to the cusps of a venous valve in the axial calf veins. Isolated proximal DVT without tibial vein thrombosis is unusual. Early in the course of a DVT, there may be no or few clinical findings such as pain or swelling. Even extensive DVT may sometimes be present without signs or symptoms. History and physical exam are therefore unreliable in the diagnosis of DVT. In addition, symptoms and signs generally associated with DVT, such as extremity pain and/or swelling, are nonspecific. In large studies, DVT has been found with venogram or DUS in 50% or less of patients where it was clinically suspected.[27,28] Objective studies are therefore required to confirm a diagnosis of DVT or to exclude the presence of DVT.

Clinical symptoms may worsen as DVT propagates and involves the major proximal deep veins. Massive DVT that obliterates the major deep venous channel of the extremity with relative sparing of collateral veins causes a condition called *phlegmasia alba dolens* (Fig. 23-4). This condition is characterized by pain, pitting edema, and blanching. There is no associated cyanosis. When the thrombosis extends to the collateral veins, massive fluid sequestration and more significant edema ensues, resulting in a condition known as *phlegmasia cerulea dolens*.[29] Phlegmasia cerulea dolens is preceded by phlegmasia alba dolens in 50 to 60% of patients. The affected extremity in phlegmasia cerulea dolens is extremely painful, edematous, and cyanotic, and may be associated with arterial insufficiency or compartment syndrome. If untreated, venous gangrene can ensue, leading to amputation.

Duplex Ultrasound. DUS is now the most commonly performed test for the detection of infrainguinal DVT, both above and below the knee, with sensitivity and specificity greater than 95% in symptomatic patients.[3] DUS combines real-time B-mode ultrasound with pulsed Doppler capability. Color flow imaging is useful in more technically difficult examinations such as in the evaluation of possible calf vein DVT. This combination offers the ability to noninvasively visualize the venous anatomy, detect occluded and partially occluded venous segments, and demonstrate physiologic flow characteristics using a mobile self-contained device.

In the supine patient, normal lower extremity venous flow is phasic (Fig. 23-5), decreasing with inspiration in response to increased intra-abdominal pressure with descent of the diaphragm with flow then increasing with expiration. When the patient is upright, the decrease in intra-abdominal pressure with expiration cannot overcome the hydrostatic column of pressure existing between the right atrium and the calf. Muscular contractions of the calf, along with the one-way venous valves, are then required to promote venous return to the heart. Flow also can be increased by leg elevation or compression and decreased by sudden elevation of intra-abdominal pressure (Valsalva maneuver). In a venous DUS examination performed with the patient supine, spontaneous flow, variation of flow with respiration, and response of flow to the Valsalva maneuver, are all assessed. However, the primary method of detecting DVT with ultrasound is demonstration of the lack of compressibility of the vein with probe pressure on B-mode imaging. Normally, in transverse section, the vein walls should coapt with pressure. Lack of coaptation indicates thrombus.

The examination begins at the ankle and continues proximally to the groin. Each vein is visualized and the flow signal is assessed with distal and proximal compression. Lower extremity DVT can be diagnosed by any of the following DUS findings: lack of spontaneous flow (Fig. 23-6), inability to compress the vein (Fig. 23-7), absence of color filling of the lumen by color flow DUS, loss of respiratory flow variation, and venous distention. Again, lack of venous compression on B-mode imaging is the primary diagnostic variable. Several studies comparing B-mode ultrasound to venography for the detection of femoropopliteal DVT in patients clinically suspected to have DVT report sensitivities greater than 91% and specificities greater than 97%.[30,31] The ability of DUS to assess isolated calf vein DVT varies greatly, with sensitivities ranging from 50 to 93% and specificities approaching 100%.[32,33]

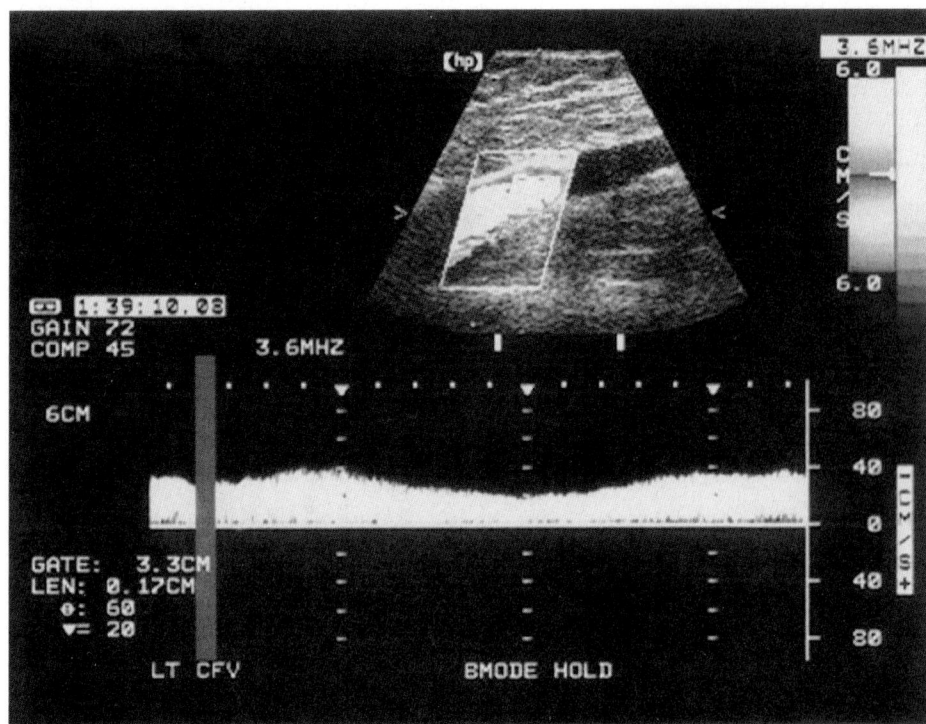

FIG. 23-5. Duplex ultrasound of a normal femoral vein with phasic flow signals.

Secondary Methods

Impedance Plethysmography (IPG). IPG was the primary non-invasive method of diagnosing DVT prior to the widespread use of DUS, but is infrequently used today. IPG is based on the principle that resistance to the flow of electricity between two electrodes, or electrical impedance, occurs as the volume of the extremity changes in response to blood flow. Two pairs of electrodes containing aluminum strips are placed circumferentially around the leg approximately 10 cm apart and a low-level current is delivered to the two outer electrodes. A pneumatic cuff is inflated over the thigh for venous outflow obstruction and then rapidly deflated. Changes in electrical resistance resulting from lower extremity blood volume changes are quantified. IPG is less accurate than DUS for detection of proximal DVT, with an 83% sensitivity in symptomatic patients. It is a poor detector of calf vein DVT.[34]

Iodine-125 Fibrinogen Uptake (FUT). FUT is a seldom used technique which involves intravenous administration of radioactive fibrinogen and monitoring for increased uptake in fibrin clots. An

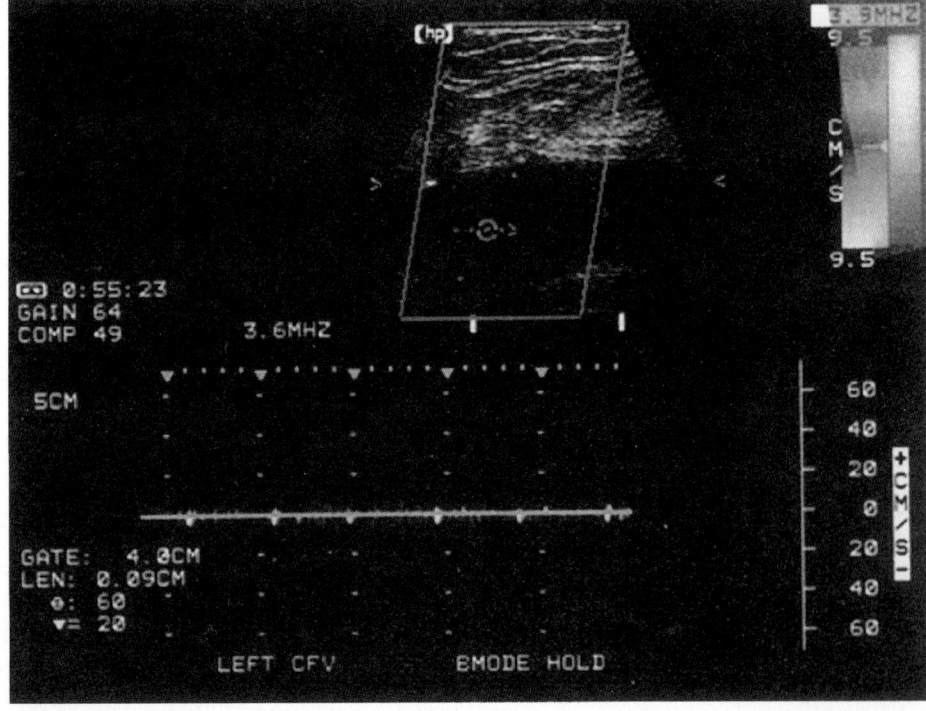

FIG. 23-6. Duplex ultrasound of a femoral vein containing thrombus, demonstrating no flow within the femoral vein.

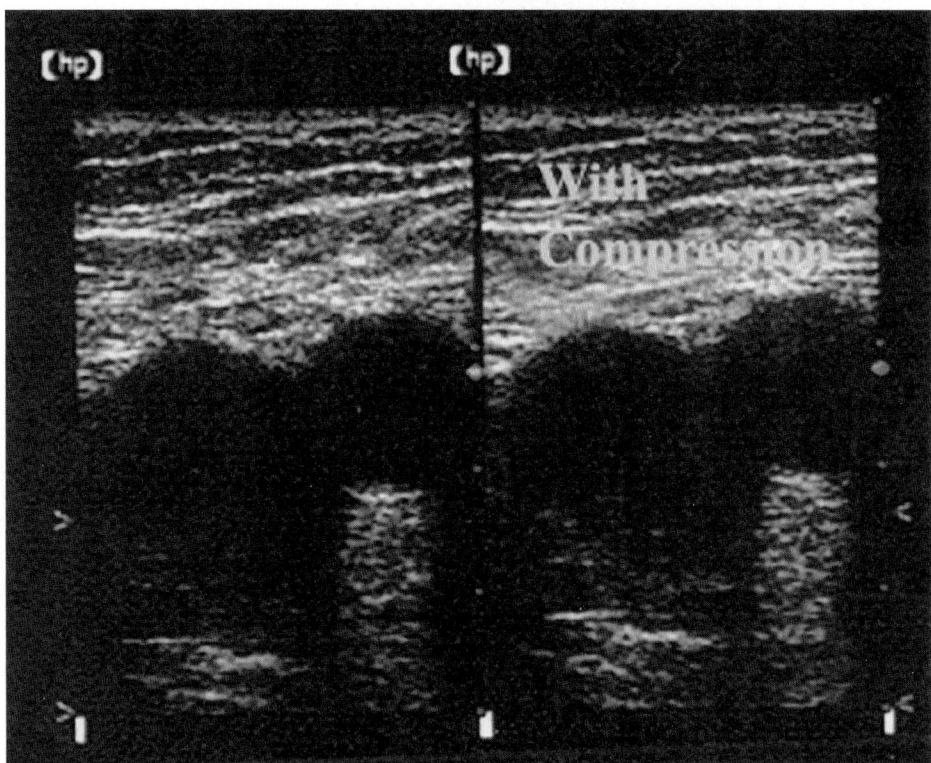

FIG. 23-7. B-mode ultrasound of the femoral vein in cross-section. The femoral vein does not collapse with external compression.

increase of 20% or more in one area of a limb indicates an area of thrombus.[35] FUT can detect DVT in the calf, but high background radiation from the pelvis and the urinary tract limits its ability to detect proximal DVT. It also cannot be used in an extremity that has been recently operated on or has active inflammation. In a prospective study, FUT had a sensitivity of 73% and specificity of 71% for DVT in a group of symptomatic and asymptomatic patients.[34] Currently, FUT is primarily a research tool of historic interest.

Venography. Venography is the most definitive test for the diagnosis of DVT in both symptomatic and asymptomatic patients. It is the gold standard to which other modalities are compared. This procedure involves placement of a small catheter in the dorsum of the foot and injection of radiopaque contrast. Radiographs are obtained in at least two projections. A positive study is failure to fill the deep systems with a passage of the contrast medium into the superficial system, or demonstration of discrete filling defects (Fig. 23-8). A normal study virtually excludes the presence of DVT. In a study of 160 patients with a normal venogram followed for 3 months, only two patients (1.3%) subsequently developed DVT and no patients suffered symptoms of pulmonary embolism.[5]

Venography is not routinely used for the evaluation of lower extremity DVT because of the associated complications previously discussed. Currently, venography is reserved for imaging prior to operative venous reconstruction and catheter-based therapy. It does, however, remain the procedure of choice in research studies evaluating methods of prophylaxis for DVT.

Prophylaxis

The goal of prophylaxis is to prevent the mortality and morbidity of VTE. The first manifestation of VTE may be a life-threatening PE (Fig. 23-9), and as indicated above, clinical evaluation to detect DVT prior to PE is unreliable. In surgical patients, the risk of VTE is dependent upon the type of operation and the presence of one or more risk factors.[36] Without prophylaxis, patients undergoing surgery for intra-abdominal malignancy have a 25% incidence of DVT, while orthopedic patients undergoing hip fracture surgery have a 40 to 50% incidence of DVT in the postoperative period. Patients at highest risk are elderly patients undergoing major surgery or those with previous VTE, malignancy, or paralysis.

Current recommendations for prophylaxis involve the use of one or more pharmacologic or mechanical modalities. The methods of VTE prophylaxis include low-dose heparin (LDH), low molecular weight heparin (LMWH), elastic stockings (ES), intermittent pneumatic compression (IPC), and warfarin. Aspirin therapy alone is not adequate for DVT prophylaxis. IPC devices aid in preventing VTE by decreasing venous stasis and stimulating fibrinolysis. Disadvantages of IPC devices include patient discomfort, noncompliance, and risk of skin erosion.

LMWH appears to be more effective than LDH, with a similar risk of major bleeding. In a large randomized, double-blind study comparing LDH (5000 U SC bid) and LMWH (enoxaparin 30 mg SC bid) in trauma patients without intracranial hemorrhage,[37] there was a 30% risk reduction ($p = 0.01$) of DVT in patients given LMWH. There was an overall major bleeding complication rate of 2% with no statistical difference between the two groups. Early use of LMWH for VTE prophylaxis is contraindicated in patients with intracranial bleeding, spinal hematoma, ongoing and uncontrolled hemorrhage, or uncorrected coagulopathy. Recommendations for VTE prophylaxis from the American College of Chest Physicians (ACCP) Consensus statement of 2001 are summarized in Table 23-3.[36]

Prophylactic insertion of IVC filters has been suggested for VTE prophylaxis in high-risk trauma patients and in some patients with malignancy who have contraindications for LMWH.[38] Trauma patients at a higher risk than the general trauma population include those with severe head injury, spinal cord injury, and severe fractures

Table 23-3
Recommendations for Venous Thromboembolism Prophylaxis

Indication	Prophylaxis Methods
Low-risk general surgery (minor surgery, age <40, no risk factors)	Early ambulation
Moderate-risk general surgery (minor surgery with risk factors; major surgery, age >40, no risk factors)	LDH, LMWH, ES, or IPC
High-risk general surgery (minor surgery with risk factors, age >60; major surgery, age >40 or additional risk factors)	LDH, LMWH, or IPC
Very high-risk general surgery (multiple risk factors present)	LDH or LMWH combined with ES or IPC
Elective hip replacement	LMWH (started 12 hours before surgery) or warfarin (started preoperatively or immediately after surgery with International Normalized Ratio [INR] target 2.5)
Elective knee replacement	LMWH or warfarin (INR = 2.5)
Hip fracture surgery	LMWH or warfarin (INR = 2.5)
Neurosurgery	IPC with or without ES and LMWH or LDH if feasible
Trauma	ES and/or IPC, LMWH if feasible
Acute spinal cord injury	LMWH with continuation of LMWH or conversion to warfarin (INR = 2.5) in the rehabilitation phase

ES = elastic compression stockings; IPC = intermittent pneumatic compression; LDH = low-dose heparin; LMWH = low molecular weight heparin.

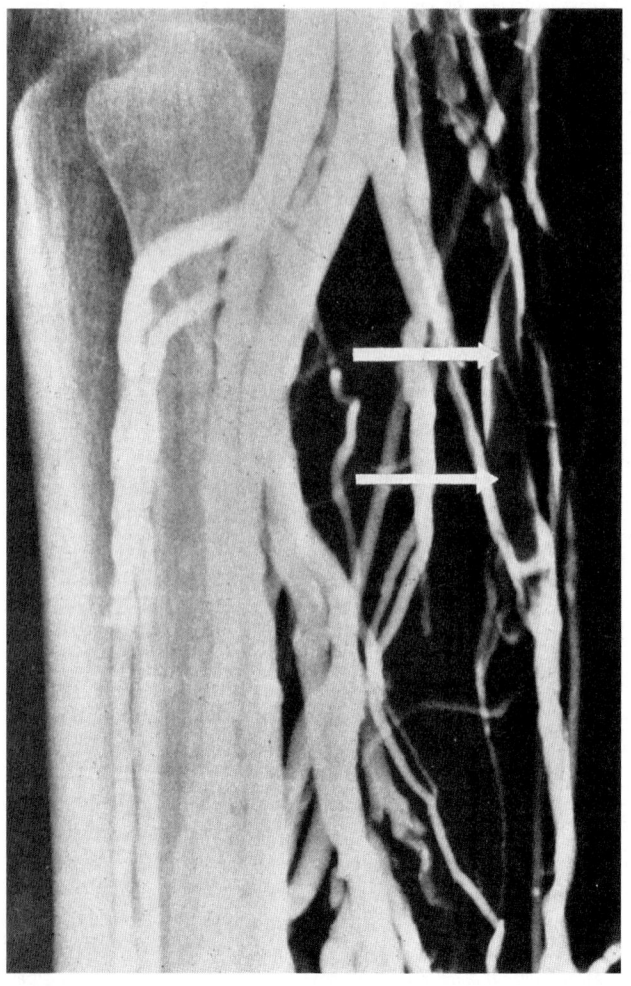

FIG. 23-8. *Venogram showing a filling defect in the popliteal vein (arrows).*

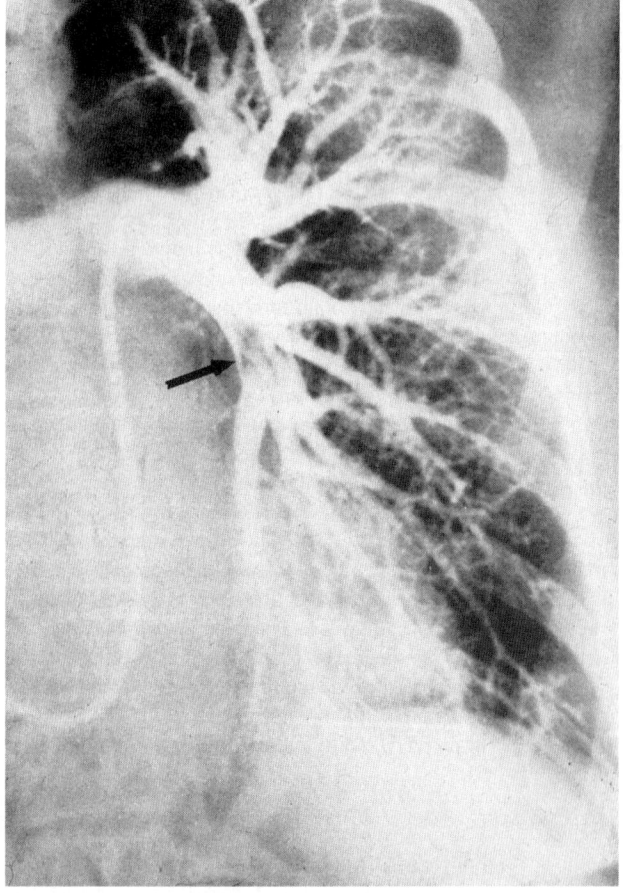

FIG. 23-9. *Pulmonary angiogram showing a pulmonary embolism (arrow).*

of the pelvis or long bones. A 5-year study of prophylactic IVC filter placement in 132 trauma patients at high risk of PE reported a 0% incidence of symptomatic PE in patients with a correctly positioned IVC filter.[39] Forty-seven patients with a malpositioned IVC filter (strut malposition or filter tilt) had a 6.3% incidence of symptomatic PE with three deaths. DVT occurred at the insertion site in 3.1% of the patients. IVC patency was 97.1% at 3 years by life table analysis.

Fatal and nonfatal PE can still occur in a patient with prophylactic vena cava interruption. Long-term complications associated with permanent IVC filters include IVC thrombosis and DVT. Currently, the ACCP recommends IVC filters be placed only if a proximal DVT is present and anticoagulation is contraindicated. Although widely practiced, IVC filter insertion is not recommended for primary prophylaxis.[36]

In an attempt to avoid long-term complications associated with permanent IVC filters, retrievable IVC filters have been developed for use in patients with a temporarily increased risk of PE (Fig. 23-10).[40] These devices may be removed up to 4 weeks postinsertion, even longer in some cases, assuming the period of increased PE risk has passed and no significant emboli are contained by the filter. Optimal patients for retrievable filter placement may include young trauma patients with transient immobility, patients undergoing surgical procedures associated with a high risk of PE, and patients with hypercoagulable states who cannot be anticoagulated for a short period of time. If the device traps a significant embolus, it may be left in place as a permanent filter.

Once the diagnosis of VTE has been made, treatment should be initiated. If clinical suspicion for VTE is high, it may be prudent to start treatment while an objective diagnosis is being obtained. The theoretic goals of VTE treatment are to prevent the mortality and morbidity associated with PE and to prevent the postphlebitic syndrome. However, the only proven benefit of anticoagulation treatment of DVT is to prevent death from pulmonary embolism. Treatment regimens may include thrombolytics, antithrombotics (heparin and warfarin), vena cava interruption, and operative thrombectomy.

Heparin

Unfractionated heparin (UFH) given intravenously has traditionally been the initial pharmacologic treatment for VTE since it was first determined to be useful in lowering mortality in patients with PE.[41] UFH acts as an anticoagulant by binding to antithrombin and potentiating antithrombin's inhibition of thrombin and activated factor X (Xa). In addition, UFH also catalyzes the inhibition of thrombin by heparin cofactor II independent of interaction with antithrombin.

Unfractionated heparin therapy should begin with a bolus intravenous injection followed by a continuous drip. The half-life of UFH is approximately 90 minutes. The level of anticoagulation should be monitored every 6 hours with activated partial thromboplastin time (aPTT) determinations until aPTT levels reach a steady state. Thereafter, aPTT can be obtained daily. aPTT levels must be kept at or above 1.5 times the control level for VTE treatment. Weight-based UFH dosages have been shown to be more effective than standard fixed boluses in rapidly achieving therapeutic levels.[42] Weight-based dosing of UFH is initiated with a bolus of 80 IU/kg IV, and a maintenance continuous infusion is started at 18 IU/kg per hour IV. Oral anticoagulation with warfarin is started after 1 day of UFH infusion. UFH and warfarin are then administered concurrently for approximately 4 to 5 days, and the daily dose of warfarin is adjusted to reach an International Normalized Ratio (INR) goal of 2 to 3. Because

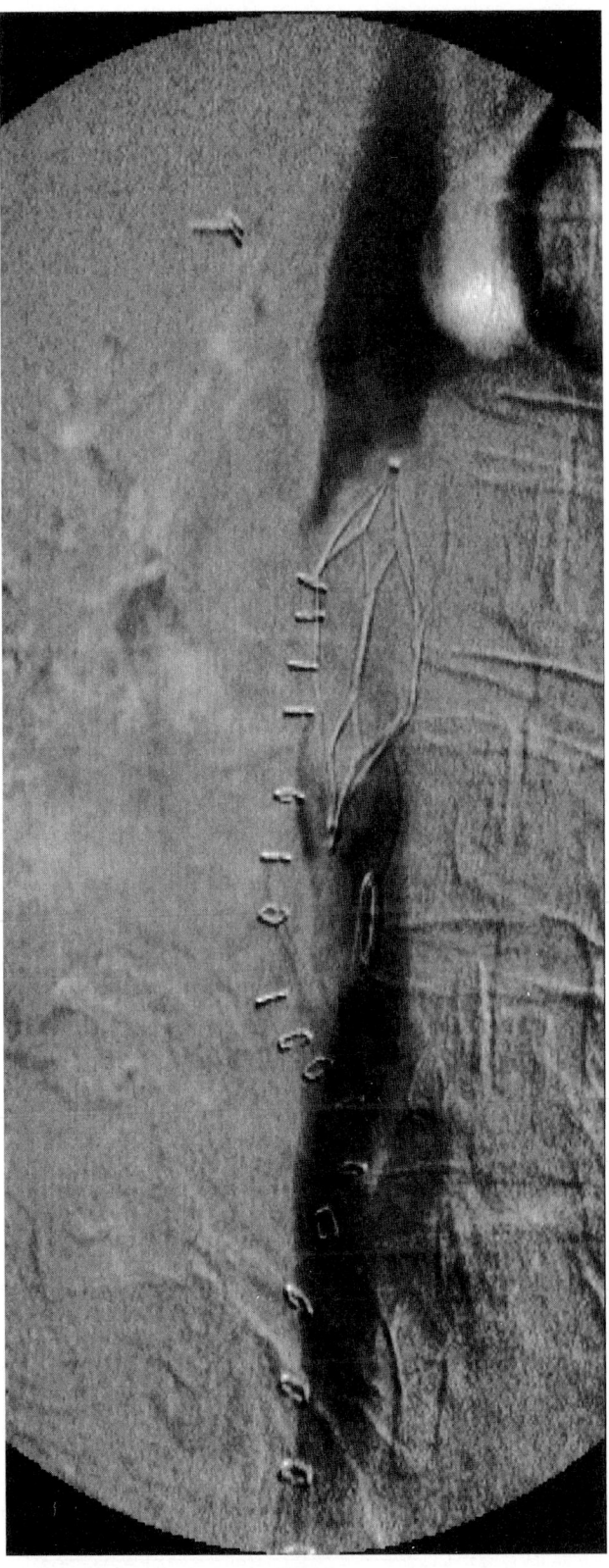

FIG. 23-10. Carbon dioxide venogram of emboli trapped within a retrievable inferior vena caval filter. The filter was not retrieved.

of the biochemistry of warfarin anticoagulation, UFH is stopped 2 days after the patient's INR reaches 2 to 3 on warfarin therapy.[43]

Hemorrhage is the primary complication of UFH therapy. The rate of major hemorrhage (fatal, intracranial, retroperitoneal, or requiring transfusion of greater than two units of packed red blood cells) is approximately 5% in hospitalized patients (1% in medical patients and 8% in surgical patients) undergoing UFH therapy.[44] For patients on UFH therapy who develop complications, cessation of UFH is required and anticoagulation can be reversed with protamine sulfate. Protamine sulfate binds to UFH and forms an inactive salt compound. Side effects of protamine sulfate include hypotension, pulmonary edema, and anaphylaxis. Typically, a dose of up to 50 mg IV is slowly administered and any development of side effects is monitored. The infusion is terminated if any side effects occur.

In addition to hemorrhage, heparin also has unique complications. Heparin-induced thrombocytopenia (HIT) results from antibodies directed against platelet factor 4 complexed with heparin.[45] It occurs in 1 to 5% of patients being treated with heparin.[46,47] HIT occurs most frequently in the second week of therapy and can lead to disastrous venous or arterial thrombotic complications. Because of HIT, platelet counts should be checked after 3 days of heparin therapy. Heparin should be stopped with a drop in platelet count to less than 100,000/μL. Another complication of prolonged high-dose heparin therapy is osteopenia, which results from impairment of bone formation and enhancement of bone resorption by heparin.

Warfarin

Warfarin is the only currently available oral anticoagulant, although other oral anticoagulants including oral heparins are currently under investigation. Warfarin acts in the liver by inhibiting the synthesis of vitamin K–dependent procoagulants (II, VII, IX, X) and anticoagulants (proteins C and S). Warfarin takes several days to achieve its full effect because residual normal coagulation factors have to be cleared. Therefore heparin should be continued along with warfarin for 2 days after achieving a therapeutic INR. The anticoagulation response to warfarin is variable and depends on liver function, diet, age, and concomitant medications. Warfarin has a long half-life of 40 hours and must be withheld 2 to 3 days prior to any invasive procedure that puts the patient at any significant bleeding risk. The level of anticoagulation is closely monitored with INR. The recommended INR for VTE therapy in most cases is between 2 and 3.

The major complication of warfarin is hemorrhage.[48] The risk of hemorrhage is related to the magnitude of INR prolongation. Bleeding complications can be treated with fresh-frozen plasma to replace depleted vitamin K–dependent factors or with intravenous vitamin K.

A unique complication associated with warfarin is the development of skin necrosis. This complication, which usually occurs in the first days of therapy, is associated with protein C or S deficiency and malignancy. When individuals with protein C or S deficiency are exposed to warfarin, the sudden decline in proteins C and S leads to thrombus formation in venules with extensive skin and subcutaneous fat necrosis.

Warfarin is not recommended for use in pregnant patients. In animal studies, it has been associated with spontaneous abortion and birth defects. Pregnant patients with VTE should be treated with heparin and monitored for the development of osteopenia. Heparin is discontinued 24 to 36 hours prior to labor induction.

Warfarin therapy following a period of initial heparin anticoagulation has been shown to reduce VTE recurrence after an acute event.[49,50] The duration of oral anticoagulation for VTE must be individualized and is dependent on the patient's risk factors for VTE. Patients with an initial VTE with identified reversible risk factors such as transient immobilization or estrogen use should be treated for at least 3 months, while those without identifiable risk factors who suffer a first episode of VTE should be treated for at least 6 months and perhaps longer, up to 2 to 3 years. Patients without identifiable risk factors are at a higher risk of recurrence. Patients with recurrent VTE or irreversible risk factors such as cancer or a hypercoagulable state should be treated for 12 months or longer.[43] A recent study[51] suggests that maintaining patients with idiopathic VTE who had been treated with 6 months of therapeutic full-dose anticoagulation on chronic low-intensity warfarin (target INR, 1.5 to 2.0) provides a risk reduction for late recurrent VTE of 64% (hazard ratio, 0.36; 95% confidence interval, 0.19 to 0.67). Current ACCP recommendations for duration of warfarin therapy are summarized in Table 23-4.

Low Molecular Weight Heparins (LMWHs)

LMWHs are derived from UFH using depolymerization techniques and differ from UFH in several ways.[52] LMWHs, like UFH, bind to antithrombin via a specific pentasaccharide sequence to expose an active site for the neutralization of factor Xa. However, unlike UFH, LMWHs lack the sufficient number of additional saccharide units (18 or more) to bind to and inactivate thrombin (factor IIa). In comparison to UFH, LMWHs have increased bioavailability, greater than 90% after a subcutaneous injection. Also in comparison to UFH, LMWHs also have a longer half-life and more predictable elimination rates.[53] Once- or twice-daily dosing with subcutaneous injections is therefore possible, a distinct advantage over the continuous IV infusions required for treatment of VTE with UFH.

The anticoagulant response of LMWHs is effective and predictable when given in a weight-based dose, thereby decreasing the need for routine laboratory monitoring. LMWHs are eliminated through the kidneys and must be used with caution in patients with creatinine clearance less than 30 mL/min.[43] In most patients, monitoring of LMWH's anticoagulant effect is generally not necessary. When required, monitoring of LMWHs is performed by assessing anti-Xa levels. Patients in whom high levels of LMWH may be anticipated and should be monitored include children less than 50 kg,

Table 23-4
Recommendations for Long-Term Anticoagulation

Indication	Duration
First VTE event with reversible risk factor (transient immobilization, estrogen use, surgery, trauma)	3–6 months
First idiopathic VTE event	≥6 months
Recurrent VTE or first VTE event in patient with irreversible risk factors (cancer or hypercoagulable state)	12 months to lifetime

VTE = Venous thromboembolism.

obese patients greater than 120 kg receiving weight-adjusted doses, pregnant patients, and patients with renal failure. There are several commercially available LMWHs. The various preparations of LMWHs differ in their anti-Xa and anti-IIa activities, and the treatment regimen recommended for one LMWH cannot be extrapolated for use with another one. LMWHs are only partially reversed with protamine sulfate.

Prospective, randomized trials of LMWHs versus UFH in the initial treatment of DVT have concluded that LMWHs are at least as effective as, and perhaps safer than, UFH.[54–56] HIT is seen in only 2 to 3% of patients receiving LMWHs.[54,57] A decrease in the incidence of heparin-associated osteoporosis has not been conclusively demonstrated in humans. Platelet counts should still be ascertained weekly in patients receiving LMWHs.

A major benefit of LMWHs is the ability to treat patients with VTE as outpatients.[54,57] In a randomized study comparing intravenous UFH and the LMWH nadroparin-Ca,[54] there was no significant difference in recurrent thromboembolism (8.6% for UFH versus 6.9% for LMWH) or major bleeding complications (2.0% for UFH versus 0.5% for LMWH). There was a 67% reduction in mean days in the hospital for the LMWH group.

A patient with VTE should meet several criteria prior to outpatient LMWH therapy.[43] First, the patient should not require hospitalization for any associated conditions that are risk factors for VTE. The patient should not have severe renal insufficiency, as LMWHs are eliminated renally. The patient should be hemodynamically stable with a low suspicion of PE and have a low bleeding risk. An established outpatient system to administer LMWH and warfarin, as well as to monitor recurrent VTE and bleeding complications, should be present. In addition, the patient's symptoms of pain and leg swelling should be controllable at home.

Pentasaccharide

Fondaparinux is the first chemically synthesized agent that contains the five-polysaccharide chain that binds and activates antithrombin, which then specifically inhibits factor Xa. It does not act against thrombin (factor IIa). Because it is chemically synthesized, fondaparinux does not contain any animal products. It is also specific to antithrombin and does not bind to platelets and therefore minimizes the risk of HIT. The results of a randomized double-blind trial comparing fondaparinux and the LMWH enoxaparin for the prevention of VTE after elective hip replacement surgery have recently been published.[58] There was no statistical difference between the two groups in the incidence of VTE. The incidence of VTE was 6% in the fondaparinux group and 8% in the enoxaparin group. There also was no difference in the incidence of major bleeding complications, with 20 events in the fondaparinux group and 11 events in the enoxaparin group. Fondaparinux is commercially available but has not been evaluated as prophylactic therapy for VTE in patients other than those undergoing surgery of the hip and knee.

Hirudin

Hirudin is a class of direct thrombin inhibitors that was first derived from the leech, *Hirudo medicinalis*. The commercially available hirudin, lepirudin, is manufactured by recombinant DNA technology. Hirudins form a tight complex with thrombin. They inhibit thrombin conversion of fibrinogen to fibrin as well as thrombin-induced platelet aggregation. These actions are independent of antithrombin. Unlike the larger heparin-antithrombin complex, the smaller hirudins can inhibit thrombin and fibrin deposition in the interstices of a developing thrombus. Hirudins do not bind to platelet

factor 4. They can be used in patients who develop HIT as a complication of heparin therapy.[59] Hirudin is administered intravenously with a loading dose of 0.4 mg/kg followed by a continuous infusion of 0.15 mg/kg per hour. The aPTT is used to monitor the effects of hirudins. The dose of hirudin must be adjusted in patients with renal failure because it is metabolized in the kidneys. There is no reversal agent currently available for hirudin. When necessary, plasma exchange may be useful to reverse the anticoagulant effect of hirudin.

Argatroban

Argatroban is a synthetic direct thrombin inhibitor that reversibly binds to thrombin. It is approved for use as an anticoagulant for prophylaxis or treatment of thrombosis in patients with heparin-induced thrombocytopenia. In addition, it is approved as an anticoagulant in patients with or at risk for heparin-induced thrombocytopenia who are undergoing percutaneous coronary intervention. As with hirudin, argatroban also does not require the presence of antithrombin to exert its anticoagulant effects. Argatroban has a short half-life of 39 to 51 minutes and reaches a steady state with intravenous infusion at 1 to 3 hours. The degree of anticoagulation achieved by argatroban can be monitored by the aPTT. There is no reversal agent for argatroban.

Oral Heparin

Ximelagatran is an investigational oral heparin that directly inhibits thrombin. Ximelagatran has several proposed advantages over UFH. It can be administered orally without food interactions and has predictable pharmacokinetics. There is also little variability in bioavailability among individual patients. Ximelagatran is rapidly absorbed and is converted into its active form, melagatran. An early phase II study comparing subcutaneous melagatran followed by ximelagatran with the LMWH dalteparin for prevention of VTE after total hip or knee replacement demonstrated that the rate of postoperative VTE in this population was dependent on the dose of the oral heparin. There was no difference in bleeding complications between the two groups.[60]

Treatment

Thrombolysis

Thrombolytic therapy can potentially reverse the hemodynamic consequences of PE and be lifesaving. However, in clinical practice, few patients with PE (<10%) are candidates for thrombolytic therapy[61] and its use must be highly individualized. A major complication of systemic thrombolytic therapy is bleeding. Thrombolytic therapy is absolutely contraindicated in patients with active internal bleeding, a recent (<2 months) cerebrovascular accident, and intracranial pathology. Relative major contraindications include major trauma, uncontrolled hypertension, active gastrointestinal pathology, recent (<10 days) major surgery, and ocular pathology.[62]

Three thrombolytic agents are currently available for clinical use: streptokinase, urokinase, and recombinant tissue plasminogen activator (rtPA). All three agents activate plasminogen to plasmin, leading to fibrin degradation and thrombolysis. Plasmin also limits thrombus formation by degrading coagulation factors V, VIII, XII, and prekallikrein.

First discovered in 1933, streptokinase is derived from beta-hemolytic streptococci. It is antigenic and can cause allergic reactions. It also can be inactivated by circulating antibodies. Streptokinase is not specific for fibrin-bound plasminogen and requires plasminogen as a cofactor. For PE, streptokinase is given as a 250,000-IU IV loading dose followed by 100,000 IU/h IV for

24 hours. Readministration of streptokinase is not recommended between 5 days and 1 to 2 years of initial use or after recent streptococcal infection because of the presence of neutralizing antibodies. These antibodies lead to reduced fibrinolytic activity or allergic reactions.[63]

Urokinase was isolated from urine in 1947.[64] It is currently produced by neonatal kidney cell culture and is also not specific for fibrin-bound plasminogen. It is not antigenic, but can still cause a febrile reaction. The systemic dosage for urokinase is 4400 IU/kg body weight loading dose followed by 2200 IU/kg per hour for 12 hours.

TPA is found in all human tissues and was first isolated in 1979.[65] A recombinant form, rtPA, is available for commercial use. It is more specific than streptokinase or urokinase for fibrin-bound plasminogen, but is not superior to the other agents for dissolution of thrombi or for reducing bleeding complications. rtPA to treat PE is given as a 100-mg infusion over 2 hours.

In patients with PE, urokinase has been shown to accelerate thrombolysis and decrease pulmonary resistance when compared to treatment with heparin alone. However, there were more bleeding complications with urokinase. No difference in mortality and recurrence rates were detected between those treated with urokinase versus those treated with heparin alone.[66,67] Subsequent studies with streptokinase and rtPA have found similar results.[67,68]

Thrombolytic therapy can be utilized in patients with massive iliofemoral DVT in an attempt to improve acute symptoms and to decrease the incidence of the postthrombotic syndrome. Currently, however, there is no clear benefit for thrombolytic therapy in a large majority of patients with DVT. Systemic administration of thrombolytic agents for DVT is largely ineffective as the majority of the thrombus is not exposed to the circulating agent. In studies comparing systemic streptokinase and heparin for the treatment of DVT, some degree of thrombolysis occurred 3.7 times more often with streptokinase than with heparin alone. However, there were 2.9 times more major bleeding complications in patients treated with streptokinase.[69] There appears to be no difference in the subsequent development of venous insufficiency in patients with DVT treated with systemic thrombolytic therapy versus those treated with heparin alone.[70]

In an effort to minimize bleeding complications and increase efficacy, catheter-directed thrombolytic techniques have been developed for the treatment of symptomatic DVT. In catheter-directed therapy, the lytic agent is administered into the thrombus. Venous access is usually achieved through the ipsilateral popliteal vein. A venogram is then performed to determine the extent and level of the thrombus. A guidewire is placed across the thrombus and a multihole infusion catheter is positioned. The thrombolytic agent is then directly infused into the thrombus.

The efficacy of catheter-directed urokinase for the treatment of symptomatic lower extremity DVT has been reported.[71] Groups of 221 patients with iliofemoral DVT and 79 patients with DVT were treated with catheter-directed infusions of urokinase for a mean of 53 hours. This was not a controlled study, but rather a registry seeking to document the experience of catheter-directed thrombolysis for DVT in a number of centers. The data derived from this study, while useful, cannot be considered definitive. A mean of 6.77 million IU of urokinase was used. Adjunctive treatment with metallic stent placement was necessary to treat residual stenoses and/or short residual occlusions that were resistant to lytic therapy in 103 limbs. Complete lysis was seen in 31% of the limbs, 50 to 99% lysis in 52% of the limbs, and less than 50% lysis in 17%. Overall, 1-year primary patency was 60%. Primary patency at 1 year was higher in patients

with iliofemoral DVT than in patients with femoral-popliteal DVT (64% versus 47%, $p < 0.01$). In addition, acute (≤ 10 days) symptoms at the onset of lytic therapy was predictive of an improved lytic outcome. Complete lysis was achieved in 34% of patients with acute symptoms (≤ 10 days) and in 19% of patients with chronic symptoms (> 10 days). The major bleeding complication rate was 11%. This study suggests that catheter-directed thrombolytic therapy in patients with acute (≤ 10 days) iliofemoral DVT has a reasonable chance of clearing the thrombosis. The long-term benefit in preventing the post-thrombotic syndrome is unknown.

Currently, the ACCP recommends that the use of thrombolytic agents be individualized and be considered in patients with hemodynamically unstable PE or massive iliofemoral thrombosis with low bleeding potential.[43]

Inferior Vena Cava Filters

Since the introduction of the Kimray-Greenfield filter in the United States in 1973, numerous filters have been developed to filter emboli in patients with DVT while allowing continuation of venous blood flow through the IVC. Early filters were placed surgically through the femoral vein. Currently, less invasive techniques now allow filter placement through a percutaneous venotomy in the femoral or internal jugular vein under fluoroscopic or ultrasound guidance. Complications associated with IVC filter placement include insertion site thrombosis, filter migration, erosion of the filter into the IVC wall, and IVC obstruction. The rate of fatal complications is less than 0.12%.[72]

The major, generally accepted indications for IVC filter placement in a patient with DVT or PE are contraindications to anticoagulation and a failure of anticoagulation in a patient who has had a PE or is at high risk of PE. Such patients may include those with DVT and hypercoagulable states who develop PE despite optimal anticoagulation and trauma patients with cerebral injuries who develop DVT or PE. In a prospective study of Greenfield filters in consecutive patients with or without DVT, the incidence of death from PE was 0.7%.[72] Another study comparing anticoagulated patients randomized to either IVC filter placement or no IVC filter[73] demonstrated that IVC filter placement did not prolong early or late survival in patients with proximal DVT, but did decrease the rate of PE (hazard ratio, 0.22; 95% confidence interval, 0.05 to 0.90). An increased rate of recurrent DVT was seen in patients with IVC filters (hazard ratio, 1.87; 95% confidence interval, 1.10 to 3.20).

Surgical Treatment

Iliofemoral DVT. In patients with acute iliofemoral DVT, surgical therapy is generally reserved for patients who worsen with anticoagulation therapy and those with phlegmasia cerulea dolens and impending venous gangrene. If the patient has phlegmasia cerulea dolens, a fasciotomy of the calf compartments is first performed. In iliofemoral DVT, a longitudinal venotomy is made in the common femoral vein (CFV) and a venous balloon embolectomy catheter is passed through the thrombus into the IVC and pulled back several times until no further thrombus can be extracted. The distal thrombus in the leg is removed by manual pressure beginning in the foot. This is accomplished by application of a tight rubber elastic wrap beginning from the foot and extending to the thigh. If the thrombus in the femoral vein is old and cannot be extracted, the vein is ligated. For a thrombus that extends into the IVC, the IVC is exposed transperitoneally and the IVC is controlled below the renal veins. The IVC is opened and the thrombus is removed by gentle massage. An intraoperative completion venogram is performed

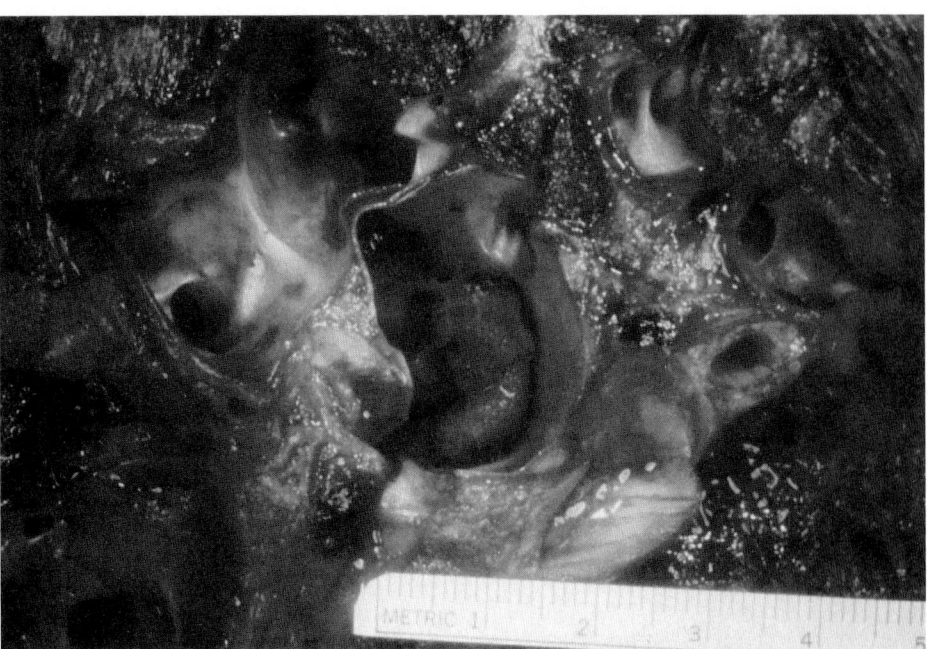

FIG. 23-11. Autopsy specimen showing a massive pulmonary embolism.

to determine if any residual thrombus or stenosis is present. If a residual iliac vein stenosis is present, intraoperative angioplasty and stenting can be performed. In most cases, an arteriovenous fistula is then created by anastomosing the GSV end-to-side with the superficial femoral artery in an effort to maintain patency of the thrombectomized iliofemoral venous segment. Heparin is administered postoperatively for several days. Warfarin anticoagulation is maintained for at least 6 months after thrombectomy. Complications of iliofemoral thrombectomy include PE in up to 20%[74] and death in less than 1%[75] of patients.

A recent study[76] followed 77 limbs for a mean of 8.5 years after thrombectomy for acute iliofemoral DVT. In limbs with successful thrombectomies, valvular competence in the thrombectomized venous segment was 80% at 5 years and 56% at 10 years. More than 90% of patients had minimal or no symptoms of post-thrombotic syndrome. There were 12 (16%) early thrombectomy failures. Patients were required to wear compression stockings for at least 1 year postthrombectomy.

Survival rates for surgical pulmonary embolectomy have improved over the past 20 years with the addition of cardiopulmonary bypass. Emergency pulmonary embolectomy for acute PE is rarely indicated. Patients with preterminal massive PE (Fig. 23-11) who have failed thrombolysis or have contraindications to thrombolytics may be candidates for this procedure. Open pulmonary artery embolectomy is performed through a posterolateral thoracotomy with direct visualization of the pulmonary arteries. Mortality rates range between 20 and 40%.[77–79]

Percutaneous catheter-based techniques for removal of PE involve mechanical thrombus fragmentation or embolectomy with suction devices. Mechanical clot fragmentation is followed by catheter-directed thrombolysis. Results of catheter-based fragmentation are based on small case series. In a study using a fragmentation device in 10 patients with acute massive PE, fragmentation was successful in seven patients with a mortality rate of 20%.[80] Transvenous catheter pulmonary suction embolectomy has also been performed for acute massive PE with a reported 76% successful extraction rate and a 30-day survival of 70%.[81]

OTHER FORMS OF VENOUS THROMBOSIS

Superficial Venous Thrombophlebitis

Superficial venous thrombophlebitis (SVT) most commonly occurs in varicose veins but can also occur in normal superficial veins. This condition also arises frequently in veins with indwelling catheters with or without associated extravasation of injected material. Upper extremity venous thrombosis has been reported to occur in 38% of patients with peripherally inserted central catheters, 57% of which developed in the cephalic vein (Fig. 23-12).[82] Suppurative SVT may occur in veins with indwelling catheters and may be associated with generalized sepsis. When SVT recurs at variable sites in normal superficial veins, it may signify a hidden visceral malignancy or a systemic disease such as a blood dyscrasia and/or a collagen vascular disease. This condition is known as *thrombophlebitis migrans.*

Clinical signs of SVT include redness, warmth, and tenderness along the distribution of the affected veins, often associated with a palpable cord. Patients with suppurative SVT may have fever and leukocytosis. DUS should be performed in patients with signs and symptoms of acute SVT to confirm the diagnosis by demonstrating thrombus within superficial veins, and also to determine if any associated DVT is present. Concomitant DVT is present in 5 to 40% of patients with SVT, most occurring in patients with SVT within 1 cm of the saphenofemoral junction.[75] A follow-up DUS should be performed in 5 to 7 days on patients without DVT on DUS who have SVT in the proximal GSV because these patients are at risk for the extension of thrombus into the deep venous system. Approximately 10 to 20% of patients with SVT involving the proximal GSV will develop progression to deep venous involvement within 1 week.[83,84]

Treatment of SVT is individualized and is dependent on the location of the thrombus and the severity of symptoms. In patients with SVT not within 1 cm of the saphenofemoral junction, treatment consists of compression and administration of anti-inflammatory medication such as indomethacin. In patients with suppurative SVT, removal of any existing indwelling catheters is mandatory and excision of the vein may be necessary. If the SVT extends proximally

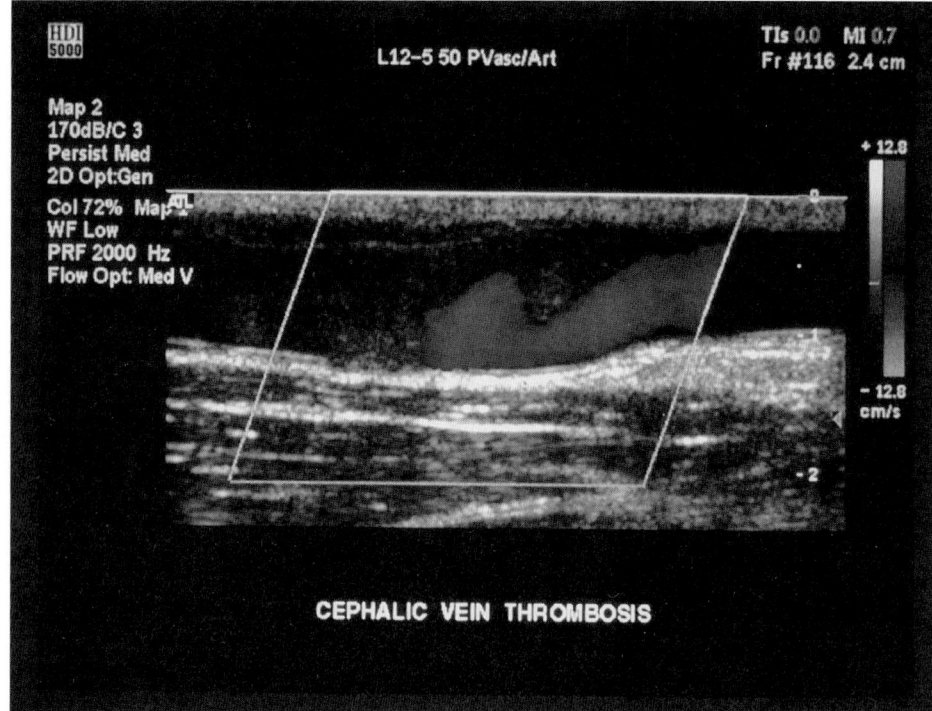

FIG. 23-12. Duplex ultrasound of a cephalic vein containing thrombus.

to within 1 cm of the saphenofemoral junction, extension into the common femoral vein is more likely to occur. In these patients, anticoagulation for 6 weeks or GSV ligation appear equally effective in preventing thrombus extension into the deep venous system.[85,86]

Axillary-Subclavian Vein Thrombosis

Axillary-subclavian vein thromboses (ASVTs) are classified into two forms. Primary ASVT comprises only a small minority of all patients with ASVT. In the primary form, no clear cause for the thrombosis is readily identifiable at initial evaluation. Patients with primary ASVT include patients who perform a prolonged, repetitive motion with their upper extremities in the raised position, resulting in damage to the subclavian vein, usually where it passes between the head of the clavicle and the first rib. This condition is known as venous thoracic outlet syndrome. Secondary ASVT is more common and is associated with an easily identified cause such as an indwelling catheter or a hypercoagulable state. Over 30% of patients with tunneled subclavian vein access devices develop ASVT.[87]

A patient with ASVT may be asymptomatic or may present with varying degrees of upper extremity swelling and tenderness. DUS can be performed initially to confirm the diagnosis. Anticoagulation should be initiated once ASVT is diagnosed to prevent PE and decrease symptoms.[88] Patients presenting with acute symptomatic primary ASVT may be candidates for thrombolytic therapy. A venogram is performed through a catheter placed via an ultrasound-guided percutaneous basilic vein approach to document the extent of the thrombus (Fig. 23-13). A guidewire is traversed through the thrombus and a catheter is placed within the thrombus. Typically, urokinase is infused with a loading dose of 250,000 IU followed by a continuous infusion of 10,000 IU/h. Heparin is administered concurrent with the urokinase infusion. After completion of thrombolytic therapy, a follow-up venogram is performed to identify any correctable anatomic abnormalities. Adjuvant procedures following thrombolytic therapy may include balloon angioplasty

for residual venous narrowing and cervical or first rib resection for thoracic outlet abnormalities.[89]

Mesenteric Venous Thrombosis

Five to fifteen percent of cases of acute mesenteric ischemia occur as a result of mesenteric venous thrombosis (MVT).[75] Mortality rates in patients with MVT are as high as 50%.[75] The major presenting symptom is nonspecific abdominal pain, followed by diarrhea and nausea and vomiting.[90] Peritoneal signs are present in less than

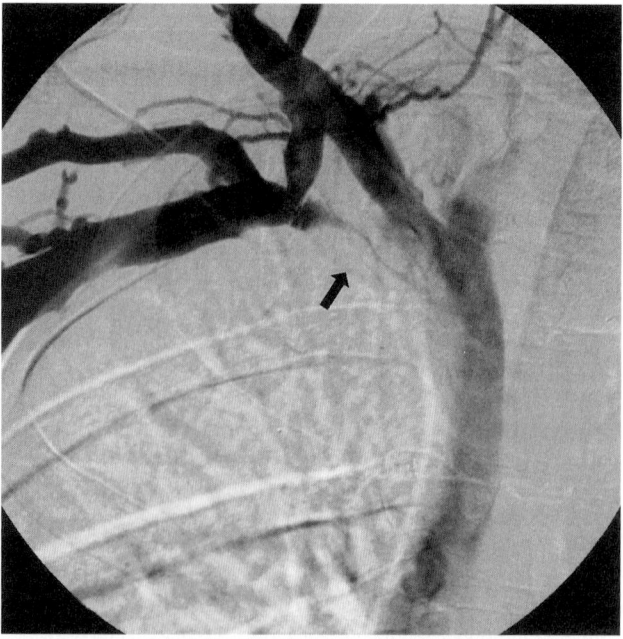

FIG. 23-13. Upper extremity venogram showing stenosis of the right subclavian vein.

half of MVT patients.[91] MVT is more common in patients with a hypercoagulable state and malignancy.[90]

Plain abdominal radiographs are usually obtained in patients with abdominal pain. Free air suggestive of a perforated viscus should be ruled out. In most patients with MVT, plain abdominal radiographs show a nonspecific bowel gas pattern and are generally nondiagnostic. Currently, contrast-enhanced abdominal CT scanning is the diagnostic study of choice in patients suspected of having MVT. In addition to MVT, CT scanning can accurately detect portal and ovarian vein thrombosis. In one series, contrast-enhanced abdominal CT scanning was diagnostic for MVT in 90% of patients.[90]

Patients with MVT should have adequate fluid resuscitation and be anticoagulated with heparin. Urgent laparotomy is undertaken in patients presenting with peritoneal findings. Perioperative broad-spectrum antibiotics are administered. Findings at laparotomy consist of edema and cyanotic discoloration of the mesentery and bowel wall with thrombus involving the distal mesenteric veins. Complete thrombosis of the superior mesenteric vein is rare, occurring in only 12% of patients undergoing laparotomy for suspected mesenteric vein thrombosis.[92] The arterial supply to the involved bowel is usually intact. Nonviable bowel is resected, and primary anastomoses can be performed. If the viability of the remaining bowel is in question, a second-look operation is performed within 24 to 48 hours.

In patients without peritoneal findings, anticoagulation with intravenous UFH is promptly initiated. Patients are maintained on bowel rest and are fluid resuscitated. Close clinical observation is warranted with serial abdominal examinations. Once the patient's clinical status improves, oral intake can be carefully started. The patient is transitioned to oral anticoagulation over 3 to 4 days and is usually maintained on lifelong oral anticoagulation.

VARICOSE VEINS

Varicose veins are a common medical condition present in at least 10% of the general population.[93] The findings of varicose veins may include dilated and tortuous veins, telangiectasias, and fine reticular varicosities. Risk factors for varicose veins include obesity, female sex, inactivity, and family history.[94] Varicose veins can be classified as primary or secondary. Primary varicose veins result from intrinsic abnormalities of the venous wall, while secondary varicose veins are associated with deep and/or superficial venous insufficiency.

In addition to an unsightly appearance, patients with varicose veins often complain of aching, heaviness, and early fatigue of the affected leg. These symptoms worsen with prolonged standing and sitting and are relieved by leg elevation above the level of the heart. A mild amount of edema is often present. More severe signs include thrombophlebitis, hyperpigmentation, lipodermatosclerosis, ulceration, and bleeding from attenuated vein clusters.

An important component of treatment for patients with varicose veins is the use of elastic compression stockings. Patients are prescribed 20- to 30-mm Hg elastic compression stockings to wear during the day. Stronger elastic stockings may be required for those who still complain of leg aching or fatigue. The majority of patients can be managed without additional therapy.

Additional interventions are warranted in patients whose symptoms worsen or are unrelieved despite compression therapy or who have signs of lipodermatosclerosis. Cosmetic concerns also can lead to intervention. Varicose veins may be managed by injection sclerotherapy or surgical therapy or a combination of both techniques. Injection sclerotherapy can be successful in varicose veins less than 3 mm in diameter and telangiectatic vessels. Sclerotherapy acts by destroying the venous endothelium. Sclerosing agents include hypertonic saline, sodium tetradecyl sulfate, and polidocanol. Concentrations of 11.7 to 23.4% hypertonic saline, 0.125 to 0.250% sodium tetradecyl sulfate, and 0.5% polidocanol are used for telangiectasias. Larger varicose veins require higher concentrations: 23.4% hypertonic saline, 0.50 to 0.75% sodium tetradecyl sulfate, and 0.75 to 1.0% polidocanol.[75] Elastic bandages are wrapped around the leg postinjection and worn continuously for 3 to 5 days to produce apposition of the inflamed vein walls and prevent thrombus formation. After bandage removal, elastic compression stockings should be worn for a minimum of 3 weeks. Complications from sclerotherapy include allergic reaction, pigmentation, thrombophlebitis, DVT, and possible skin necrosis.

In patients with symptomatic GSV reflux, the GSV should be removed. Small incisions are placed medially in the groin and just below the knee, and the GSV is stripped. Complications associated with GSV stripping include ecchymosis, lymphocele formation, infection, and transient numbness in the saphenous nerve distribution. GSV stripping has been documented in a randomized study to have a lower rate of recurrent varicose veins than GSV ligation alone (relative risk 0.28, 95% CI 0.13 to 0.59).[95] In another prospective study, patients with GSV stripping had significantly improved quality of life over a 2-year period when compared to patients who underwent saphenofemoral junction ligation alone.[96] Alternatively the greater saphenous vein can be left in situ and destroyed with catheter-based techniques using laser or radio frequency energy. Long-term follow-up and efficacy of such catheter-based techniques is currently not available, but studies are ongoing.

Larger varicose veins are best treated by surgical excision using the "stab avulsion" technique. Stab avulsions are performed by making 2-mm incisions directly over branch varicosities, and the varicosity is dissected from the surrounding subcutaneous tissue as far proximally and distally as possible through the small incisions (Fig. 23-14). In most cases the vein is simply avulsed with no attempt at ligation. Bleeding is easily controlled with leg elevation and manual pressure.

CHRONIC VENOUS INSUFFICIENCY

CVI is a major and costly medical problem affecting an estimated 600,000 patients in the United States.[97] Patients complain of leg fatigue, discomfort, and heaviness. Signs of CVI may include varicose veins, pigmentation, lipodermatosclerosis, and venous ulceration. Importantly, severe CVI can be present without varicose veins. In addition, chronic venous ulcers carry significant negative physical, financial, and psychologic implications. A quality-of-life study reported that 65% of chronic leg ulcer patients had severe pain, 81% had decreased mobility, and 100% experienced a negative impact of their disease upon their work capacity.[98] The socioeconomic impact of chronic venous leg ulcers is staggering, with an estimated 2 million workdays lost per year.[99] The annual health care cost in the United States to treat CVI is estimated at $1 billion.[100]

The signs and symptoms of CVI can be attributed to venous reflux, venous obstruction, calf muscle pump dysfunction, or a combination of these factors, as well as loss of venous wall elasticity.[101] The most important factor appears to be venous reflux in the majority of patients with CVI. Venous reflux results from abnormalities of the venous valve and can be classified as primary or secondary. Primary valvular reflux or incompetence is diagnosed when there is no known underlying etiology of valvular dysfunction. Secondary valvular reflux is diagnosed when an identifiable etiology is present.

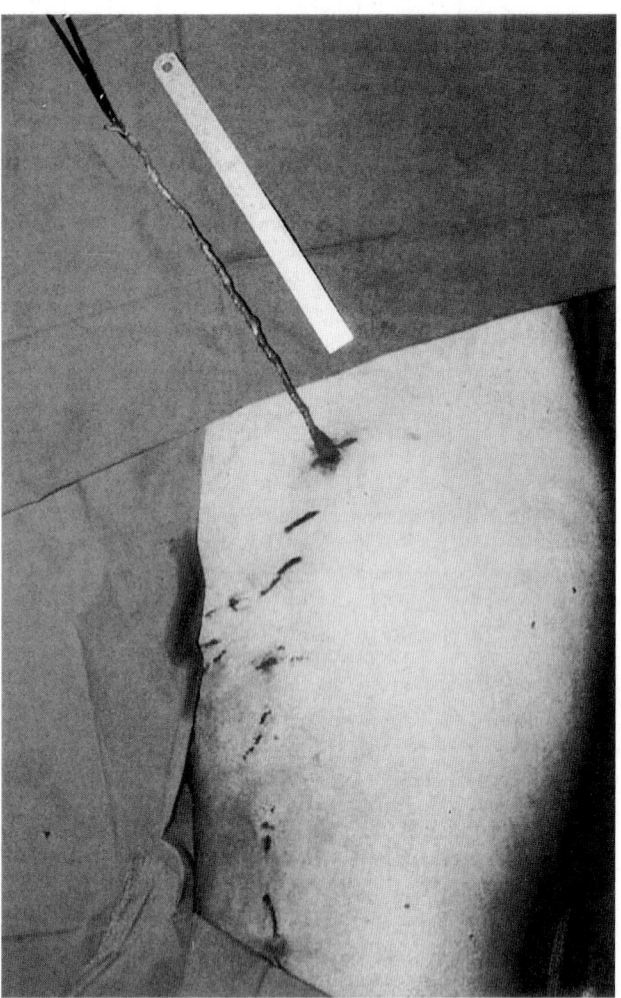

FIG. 23-14. *Removal of varicose veins via stab avulsions.*

The most frequent secondary etiology is DVT, which can lead to the dysfunction of venous valves. Signs of CVI include edema, hyperpigmentation, and ulceration.

Evaluation of Venous Insufficiency

Early diagnostic studies to evaluate CVI required invasive measurements of ambulatory venous pressure (AVP) and venous recovery times (VRT). To measure AVP and VRT, a needle is inserted into a dorsal foot vein and connected to a pressure transducer. Pressures measured in the dorsal veins of the foot are thought to reflect those in the deep veins of the calf. Once the needle is placed, the patient is asked to perform 10 tip-toe exercises. Initially there is often a slight upward deflection of pressure with the onset of exercise. With each subsequent tip-toe maneuver, the measured pressure should decrease. After approximately 10 tip-toes, the measured pressure stabilizes and reflects a balance of venous inflow and outflow. The pressure at this point is the AVP, which is measured in mm Hg. The patient is then asked to stop exercising to allow the vein to fill with return of the venous pressure to baseline. The time required for the venous pressure to return from the AVP level to 90% of baseline pressure is referred to as the VRT. Elevations of AVP indicate the presence of venous hypertension. The magnitude of AVP reflects the severity of CVI. There is an 80% incidence of venous ulceration in patients with AVP greater than 80 mm Hg.[102]

Plethysmography

Noninvasive plethysmography methods based on the measurement of volume changes in the leg have been used to evaluate CVI. Venous photoplethysmography (PPG) indirectly evaluates venous function through the use of infrared light. A light-emitting diode is placed just above the medial malleolus and the patient then performs a series of tip-toe maneuvers. PPG does not give accurate AVP measurements, but does provide adequate VRT determinations. In limbs with CVI, VRT is shortened compared to that of a normal limb. AVP and VRT are measures of overall function in the lower extremity venous system. They cannot localize the site of reflux or evaluate the function of the calf pump in patients with CVI.

Air plethysmography (APG) can be used to assess calf pump function as well as venous reflux and overall lower extremity venous function.[103] An air-filled plastic pressure bladder is placed on the calf to detect volume changes in the leg during a standard set of maneuvers. The patient is first supine and then the leg is elevated and the minimum volume of venous blood recorded. The patient is then asked to assume an upright position with the examined leg non–weight-bearing. The venous volume in the examined leg is determined when the volume curve flattens out. The venous filling index (VFI) is calculated by dividing the maximum venous volume by the time required to achieve maximum venous volume. The VFI is a measure of reflux. Next, the patient performs a single tip-toe maneuver and the ejection fraction (EF) is determined. The EF is the volume change between the recorded volume prior to and after the tip-toe maneuver, and is a measure of calf pump function. At this point, the veins of the leg are allowed to refill. The patient then performs 10 tip-toe maneuvers, and the residual volume fraction (RVF) is calculated by dividing the venous volume in the leg after 10 tip-toe exercises by the venous volume present before the exercises. The RVF is a reflection of overall venous function. Theoretically, patients with increased VFIs and normal EFs (indicating the presence of reflux with normal calf pump function) would benefit from antireflux surgery, while patients with normal VFIs and diminished EFs would not.

Venous Duplex Ultrasound

In addition to identifying patients with DVT, DUS can be used to evaluate reflux in individual venous segments of the leg. The examination is performed with the patient in the standing position and the examined leg in a non–weight-bearing position. Pneumatic pressure cuffs of appropriate size are placed around the thigh, calf, and around the forefoot. The ultrasound transducer is positioned over the venous segment to be examined, just proximal to the pneumatic cuff (Fig. 23-15). The cuff is then inflated to a standard pressure for 3 seconds and then rapidly deflated. Ninety-five percent of normal venous valves close within 0.5 second.[104] Reflux that is present for greater than 0.5 second is considered abnormal. Typically, the common femoral, femoral, popliteal, and posterior tibial, as well as the greater and lesser saphenous veins, are evaluated in a complete examination.

Nonoperative Treatment of Chronic Venous Insufficiency

Compression Therapy

Compression therapy is the mainstay of CVI management. Compression can be achieved using a variety of techniques, including elastic compression stockings, paste gauze boots (Unna's boot), multilayer elastic wraps/dressings (Fig. 23-16), or pneumatic

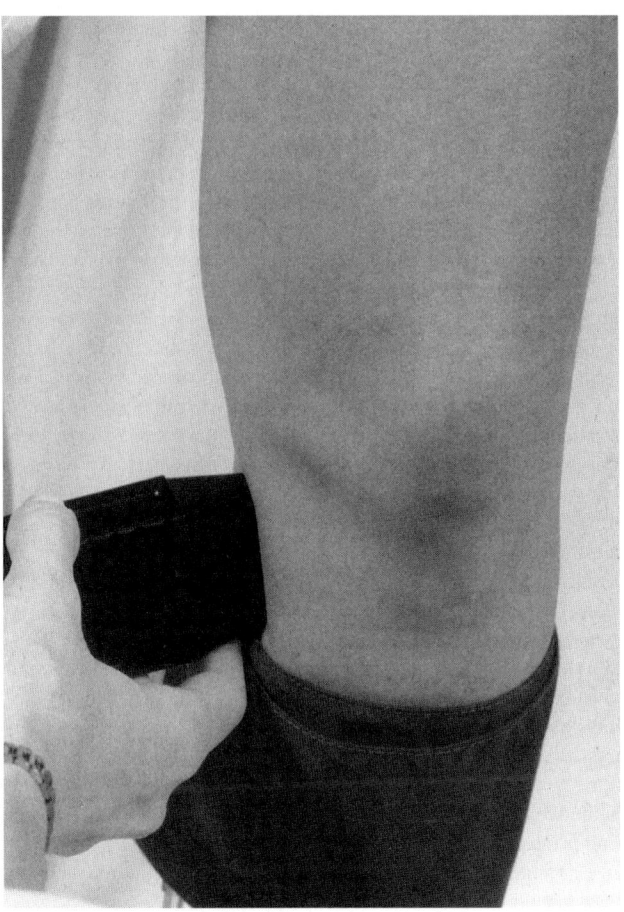

FIG. 23-15. Evaluation of a patient with chronic venous insufficiency with duplex ultrasonography.

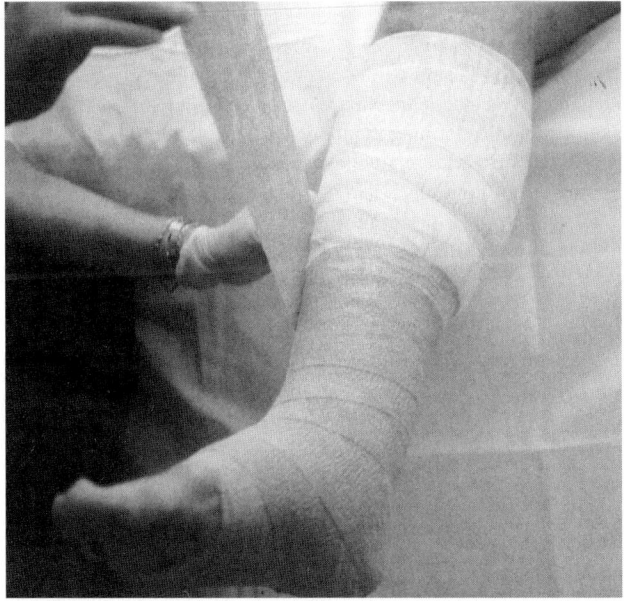

FIG. 23-16. Multilayered dressing for treatment of chronic venous insufficiency.

compression devices. The exact mechanism by which compression therapy can improve CVI remains uncertain. Improvement in skin and subcutaneous tissue microcirculatory hemodynamics as well as a direct effect on subcutaneous pressure have been hypothesized as the mechanism of compression therapy.[105] Clinically, routine use of elastic and nonelastic bandages reduces lower extremity edema in patients with CVI. In addition, supine perimalleolar subcutaneous pressure has been demonstrated to be increased with elastic compression.[106] With edema reduction, cutaneous metabolism may improve due to enhanced diffusion of oxygen and other nutrients to the cellular elements of skin and subcutaneous tissues. Increases in subcutaneous tissue pressure with elastic compression bandages may counteract transcapillary Starling forces, which favor leakage of fluid out of the capillary.

Prior to the initiation of therapy for CVI, patients must be educated about their chronic disease and the need to comply with their treatment plan in order to heal ulcers and prevent recurrence. A definitive diagnosis of venous ulceration must be made prior to undergoing treatment. A detailed history should be obtained from a patient presenting with lower extremity ulcerations, including medications and associated medical conditions that may promote lower extremity ulceration. Arterial insufficiency is assessed by physical examination or noninvasive studies. In addition, systemic conditions that affect wound healing and leg edema such as diabetes mellitus, immunosuppression, malnutrition, or congestive heart failure should be improved as much as possible.

Compression therapy is most commonly achieved with gradient elastic compression stockings. Gradient elastic compression stockings, initially developed by Conrad Jobst in the 1950s, were made to simulate the gradient hydrostatic forces exerted by water in a swimming pool. Elastic compression stockings are available in various compositions, strengths, and lengths, and can be customized for a particular patient.

The benefits of elastic compression stocking therapy for the treatment of CVI and healing of ulcerations have been well documented.[107–110] In a retrospective review of 113 venous ulcer patients,[108] the use of below-knee, 30- to 40-mm Hg elastic compression stockings, after first resolving edema and cellulitis if present, resulted in 93% healing. Complete ulcer healing occurred in 99 of 102 (97%) patients who were compliant with stocking use versus 6 of 11 patients (55%) who were noncompliant ($p < 0.0001$). The mean time to ulcer healing was 5 months. Ulcer recurrence was less in patients who were compliant with their compression therapy. By life table analysis, ulcer recurrence was 29% at 5 years for compliant patients and 100% at 3 years for noncompliant patients. In more recent studies, the reported rate of venous ulcer healing with compression therapy is approximately 40 to 50% at 6 months.[111,112]

In addition to promoting ulcer healing, elastic compression therapy can also improve quality of life in patients with CVI. In a recent prospective study,[113] 112 patients with CVI documented by DUS were administered a questionnaire to quantify the symptoms of swelling, pain, skin discoloration, cosmesis, activity tolerance, depression, and sleep alterations. Patients were treated with 30- to 40-mm Hg elastic compression stockings. There were overall improvements in symptom severity scores at 1 month after initiation of treatment. Further improvements were noted at 16 months posttreatment.

Patient compliance with compression therapy is crucial in treating venous leg ulcers. Many patients are often initially intolerant of compression in areas of hypersensitivity adjacent to an active ulcer or at sites of previously healed ulcers. They may also have difficulty applying elastic stockings. To improve compliance, patients

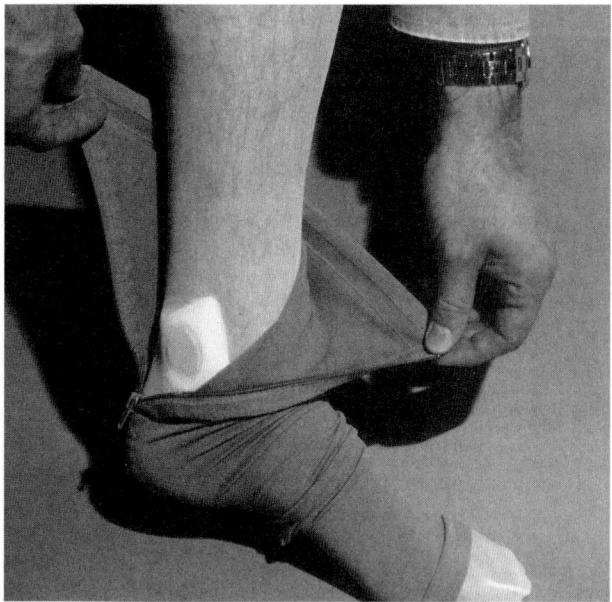

FIG. 23-17. Elastic compression stocking with zippered side for facilitating chronic venous insufficiency treatment.

should be instructed to initially wear their stockings only as long as it is easily tolerable and then gradually increase the amount of time stockings are worn. Alternatively, patients can be initially fitted with lower-strength stockings followed by higher-strength stockings over a period of several weeks. Many commercially available devices, such as silk inner toe liners, stockings with zippered sides (Fig. 23-17), and metal fitting aids (Fig. 23-18), are available to assist patients in applying elastic stockings.

Another method of compression was developed by the German dermatologist Paul Gerson Unna in 1896. Unna's boot has been used for many years to treat venous ulcers and is available in many versions. A typical Unna's boot consists of a three-layer dressing and requires application by trained personnel. A rolled gauze bandage impregnated with calamine, zinc oxide, glycerin, sorbitol, gelatin, and magnesium aluminum silicate is first applied with graded compression from the forefoot to just below the knee. The next layer consists of a 4-inch-wide continuous gauze dressing followed by an outer layer of elastic wrap, also applied with graded compression. The bandage becomes stiff after drying and the rigidity may aid in preventing edema formation. Unna's boot is changed weekly or

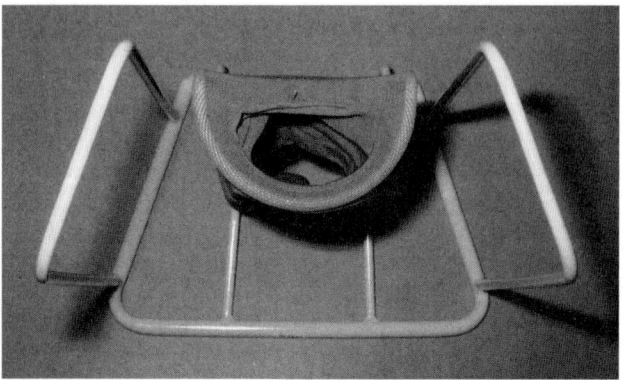

FIG. 23-18. Metal fitting aid to assist placement of elastic compression stockings.

sooner if the patient experiences significant drainage from the ulcer bed.

Once applied, Unna's boot requires minimal patient involvement and provides continuous compression and topical therapy. However, the Unna's boot has several disadvantages. It is uncomfortable to wear because of its bulkiness, which may affect patient compliance. In addition, the ulcer cannot be monitored after the boot is applied, the technique is labor intensive, and the degree of compression provided is operator-dependent. Occasionally, patients may develop contact dermatitis to the components of Unna's boot, which may require discontinuation of therapy.

The efficacy of Unna's dressing has been studied. In a retrospective 15-year review of 998 patients with one or more venous ulcers treated weekly with Unna's dressing,[114] 73% of ulcers healed in patients who returned for more than one treatment. The median time to healing for individual ulcers was 9 weeks. Unna's dressing has been compared to other forms of treatment. A randomized, prospective study[115] comparing Unna's boot to polyurethane foam dressing in 36 patients with venous ulcers demonstrated superior healing over 12 months in patients treated with Unna's boot (94.7% versus 41.2%).

Other forms of compression dressing, also available to treat CVI, include multilayered dressings and legging orthosis. The purported advantages of multilayered dressings include maintenance of compression for a longer period of time, more even distribution of compression, and better absorption of wound exudates. However, the efficacy of multilayered dressings is dependent on the wrapping technique of health care personnel. A commercially available legging orthosis consisting of multiple adjustable loop-and-hook closure compression bands provides compression similar to Unna's boot and can be applied daily by the patient.[116]

Skin Substitutes

Several types of skin substitutes are commercially available or under clinical study in the United States.[99] Bioengineered skin ranges in composition from acellular skin substitutes to partial-living skin substitutes. Their mechanism of action in healing venous ulcers is uncertain; however, they may serve as delivery vehicles for various growth factors and cytokines important in wound healing.

Apligraf is a commercially available bilayered living skin construct that closely approximates human skin for use in the treatment of venous ulcers. It contains a protective stratum corneum and a keratinocyte-containing epidermis overlying a dermis consisting of dermal fibroblasts in a collagen matrix.[117] Apligraf is between 0.5 mm and 1.0 mm thick and is supplied as a disk of living tissue on an agarose gel nutrient medium. It must be used within 5 days of release from the manufacturer[117] (Fig. 23-19). The disk is easily handled and applied, and easily conforms to irregularly contoured ulcer beds.

A prospective randomized study comparing multilayer compression therapy alone to treatment with Apligraf in addition to multilayered compression therapy has been performed to assess the efficacy of Apligraf in the treatment of venous ulcers.[111] More patients treated with Apligraf had ulcer healing at 6 months (63 vs. 49%, $p = 0.02$). The median time to complete ulcer closure was significantly shorter in patients treated with Apligraf (61 days vs. 181 days, $p = 0.003$). The ulcers that showed the greatest benefit with the living skin construct were ones that were large and deep (>1000 mm^2) or were long-standing (>6 months). No evidence of rejection or sensitization has been reported in response to Apligraf application.

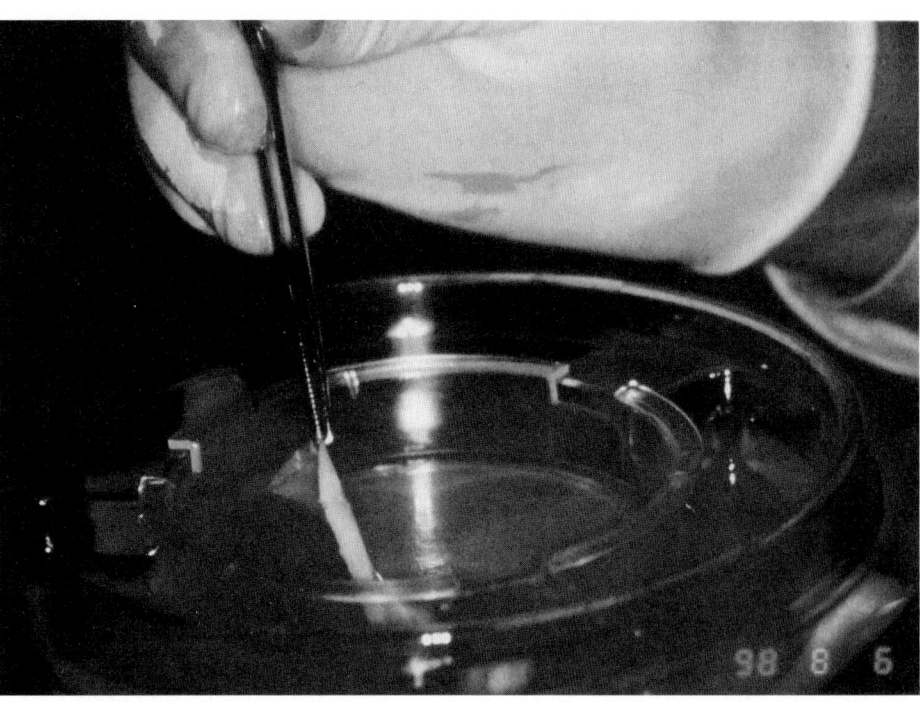

FIG. 23-19. *Apligraf supplied as a disk on an agarose gel nutrient medium.*

Surgical Therapy of Chronic Venous Insufficiency

Perforator Vein Ligation

Incompetence of the perforating veins connecting the superficial and deep venous systems of the lower extremities has been implicated in the development of venous ulcers. The classic open technique described by Linton in 1938 for perforator vein ligation has a high incidence of wound complications and has largely been abandoned.[118] A newer, minimally invasive technique termed *subfascial endoscopic perforator vein surgery* (SEPS) has evolved with the improvement in endoscopic equipment.

DUS is performed preoperatively in patients undergoing SEPS to document deep venous competence and to identify perforating veins in the posterior compartment. The patient is positioned on the operating table with the affected leg elevated at 45° to 60°. An Esmarque bandage and a thigh tourniquet are used to exsanguinate the limb. The knee is then flexed, and two small incisions are made in the proximal medial leg away from areas of maximal induration at the ankle. Laparoscopic trocars are then positioned, and the subfascial dissection is performed with a combination of blunt and sharp dissection. Carbon dioxide is then used to insufflate the subfascial space. The thigh tourniquet is inflated to prevent air embolism. The perforators are then identified and doubly clipped and divided. After completion of the procedure, the leg is wrapped in a compression bandage for 5 days postoperatively.

In a report from a large North American registry of 146 patients undergoing SEPS[119] (Fig. 23-20), healing was achieved in 88% of ulcers (75 of 85) at 1 year. Adjunctive procedures, primarily

FIG. 23-20. *Trocar placement for subfascial endoscopic perforator vein surgery (SEPS).*

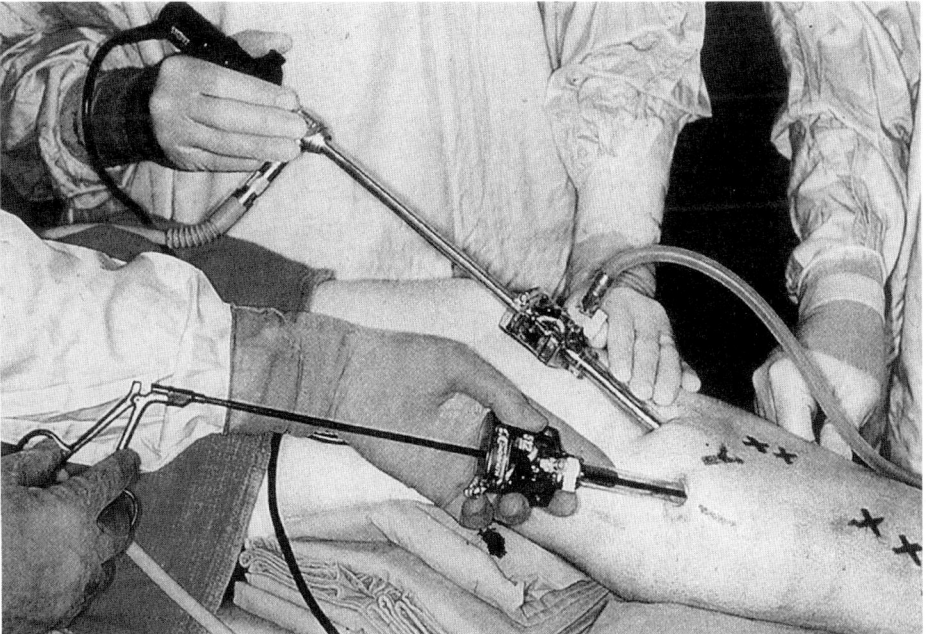

superficial vein stripping, were performed in 72% of patients. Ulcer recurrence was predicted to be 16% at 1 year and 28% at 2 years by life table analysis. The efficacy of the technique has not been confirmed in a randomized trial.

Venous Reconstruction

In the absence of significant deep venous valvular incompetence, saphenous vein stripping and perforator vein ligation can be effective in the treatment of CVI. However, in patients with a combination of superficial and deep venous valvular incompetence, the addition of deep venous valvular reconstruction theoretically may improve ulcer healing.[120] Numerous techniques of deep venous valve correction have been reported. These techniques consist of repair of existing valves, transplant of venous segments from the arm, and transposition of an incompetent vein onto an adjacent competent vein. Cryopreserved venous valve allografts placed below incompetent vein segments surgically or percutaneously are currently in the early phases of development, but do not seem effective.[121]

Successful long-term outcomes of 60 to 80% have been reported for venous valve reconstructions by internal suture repair.[120,122,123] However, in patients who initially had ulceration, 40 to 50% still had persistence or recurrence of ulcers in the long term.[122,123] Valve transplantation involves replacement of a segment of incompetent femoral vein or popliteal vein with a segment of axillary or brachial vein with competent valves. Early results are similar to those of venous valve reconstruction.[120,122,123] However, in the long term, the transplanted venous segments tend to develop incompetence, and long-term outcomes are poorer than those of venous valve reconstructions. The outcomes for venous transposition are similar to those of valve transplantation.

LYMPHEDEMA

Pathophysiology

Lymphedema is extremity swelling that results from a reduction in lymphatic transport, with resultant pooling of lymph within the inter-

stitial space. This is caused by anatomic problems such as lymphatic hypoplasia, functional insufficiency, or absence of lymphatic valves.

The original classification system, described by Allen, is based on the etiology of the lymphedema. Primary lymphedema is further subdivided into congenital, praecox, and tarda. *Congenital lymphedema* can involve a single lower extremity, multiple limbs, the genitalia, or the face. The edema is typically present at birth. *Lymphedema praecox* is the most common form of primary lymphedema, accounting for 94% of cases. Lymphedema praecox is far more common in women, with the gender ratio favoring women 10:1. The onset of swelling is during the childhood or teenage years and involves the foot and calf. *Lymphedema tarda* is uncommon, accounting for less than 10% of cases of primary lymphedema. The onset of edema is later in life than in lymphedema praecox.

Secondary lymphedema is far more common than primary lymphedema. Secondary lymphedema develops as a result of lymphatic obstruction or disruption. Lymphedema of the arm following axillary node dissection is the most common cause of secondary lymphedema in the United States. Other causes of secondary lymphedema include radiation therapy, trauma, or malignancy. Globally, filariasis, which causes elephantiasis, is the most common cause of secondary lymphedema.

Clinical Diagnosis

In most patients the diagnosis of lymphedema is made on the history and physical exam alone. Patients commonly complain of heaviness and fatigue in the affected extremity. The limb size increases throughout the day and decreases over the course of the night when the patient is in bed. The limb, however, never completely normalizes. The swelling involves the dorsum of the foot, and the toes have a squared-off appearance. In advanced cases, hyperkeratosis of the skin develops and fluid weeps from lymph-filled vesicles (Fig. 23-21).

Recurrent cellulitis is a common complication of lymphedema. Repeated infection results in further lymphatic damage, worsening existing disease. The clinical presentation of cellulitis ranges from

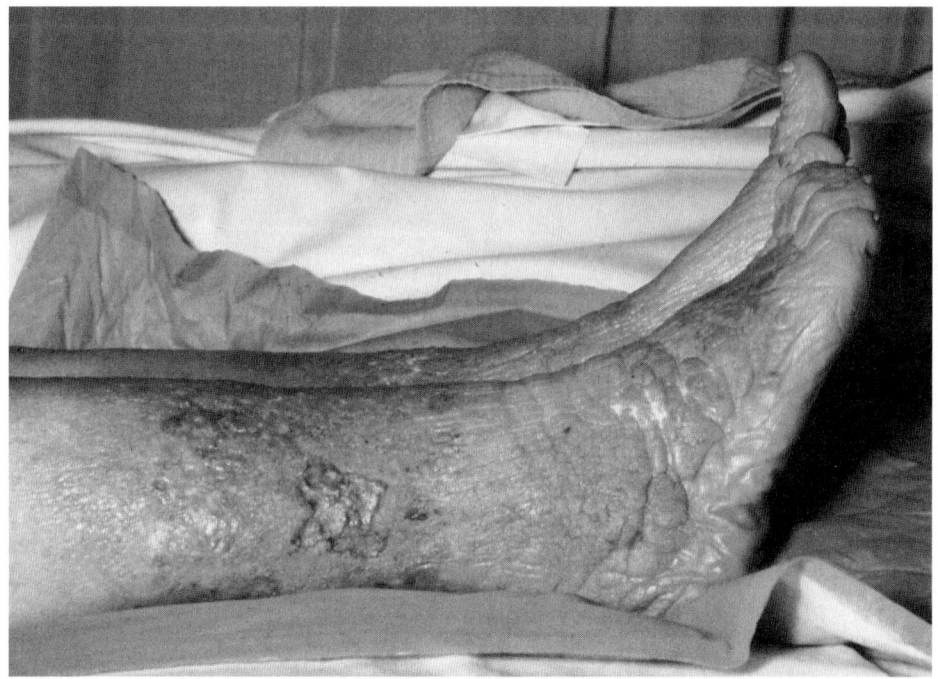

FIG. 23-21. Hyperkeratosis of the skin in a patient with long-standing lymphedema.

subtle erythema and worsening of edema to a rapidly progressive soft tissue infection with systemic toxicity.

Many medical conditions can cause edema. If the symptoms are mild, distinguishing lymphedema from other causes of leg swelling can be difficult. Venous insufficiency is often confused with lymphedema. However, patients with advanced venous insufficiency typically have lipodermatosclerosis in the gaiter region, skin ulceration, and/or varicose veins. Bilateral pitting edema is typically associated with congestive heart failure, renal failure, or a hypoproteinemic state.

Radiologic Diagnosis

Duplex Ultrasound

When evaluating a patient for edema, it is often difficult to distinguish the early stages of lymphedema from venous insufficiency. Duplex ultrasound of the venous system can determine if venous reflux is present and perhaps contributing to extremity edema. The diagnostic modalities discussed below have limited use in clinical practice. They are invasive, tedious, and rarely change the management of a patient with lymphedema. Most physicians rely on the patient's history and physical exam alone to make the diagnosis of lymphedema.

Lymphoscintigraphy

Isotope lymphoscintigraphy identifies lymphatic abnormalities. A radiolabeled sulfur colloid is injected into the subdermal, interdigital region of the affected limb. The lymphatic transport is monitored with a whole body gamma camera, and major lymphatics and nodes can be visualized (Fig. 23-22).

Radiologic Lymphology

Radiologic lymphology visualizes lymphatics with colored dye injected into the hand or foot. The visualized lymphatic is exposed through a small incision and cannulated. An oil-based dye is injected slowly into the lymphatics over several hours. The lymphatic channels and nodes are then visualized with traditional roentgenograms (Figs. 23-23 and 23-24).

Management

An important aspect in the management of lymphedema is patient understanding that there is no cure for lymphedema. The primary goals of treatment are to minimize swelling and to prevent recurrent infections. Controlling the chronic limb swelling can improve discomfort, heaviness, and tightness, and potentially reduce the progression of disease.[124]

Compression Garments

Graded compression stockings are widely used in the treatment of lymphedema. The stockings reduce the amount of swelling in the involved extremity by preventing the accumulation of edema while the extremity is dependent. When worn daily, compression stockings have been associated with long-term maintenance of reduced limb circumference.[125] They may also protect the tissues against chronically elevated intrinsic pressures, which lead to thickening of the skin and subcutaneous tissue.[126] Compression stockings also offer a degree of protection against external trauma.

The degree of compression required for controlling lymphedema ranges from 20 to 60 mm Hg and varies among patients. The stockings can be custom-made or prefabricated and are available in above- and below-knee lengths. The stockings should be worn

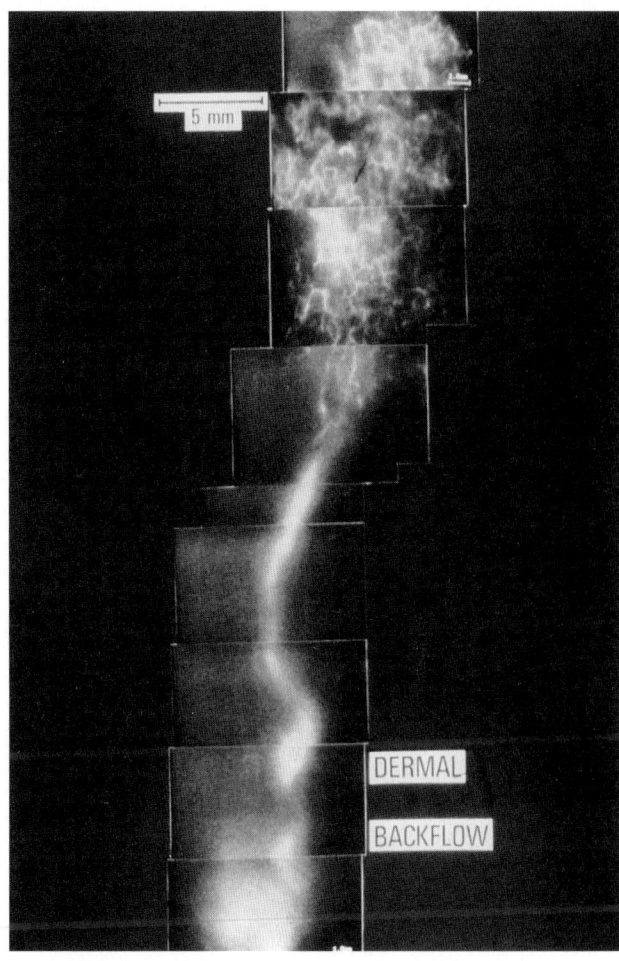

FIG. 23-22. Lymphoscintigraphy of the lower extremity.

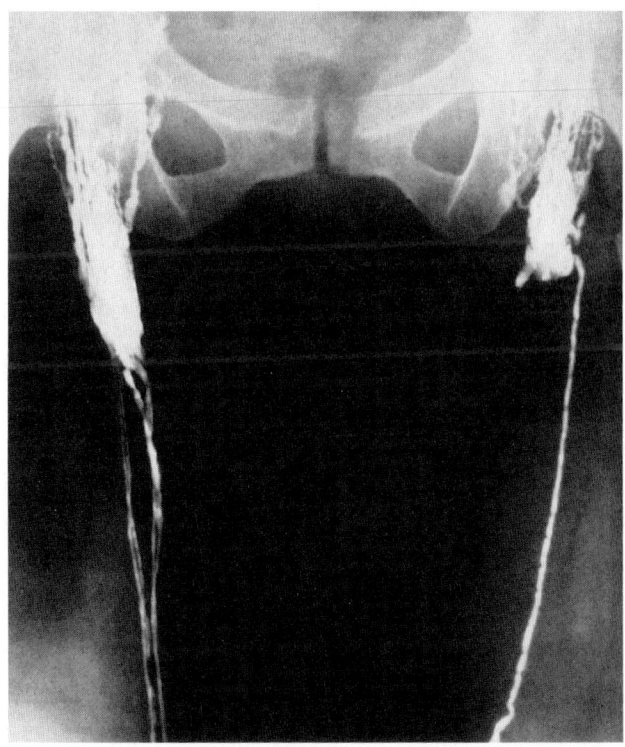

FIG. 23-23. Normal lymphangiogram of the pelvis.

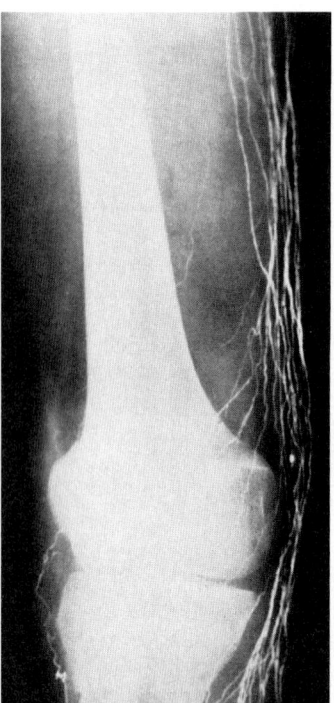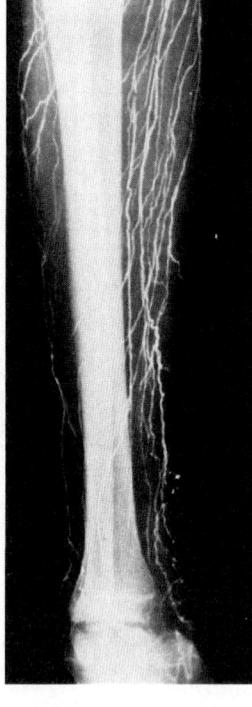

FIG. 23-24. *Normal lymphangiogram of the thigh and lower leg.*

during waking hours. The garments should be replaced approximately every 6 months when they lose elasticity.

Bed Rest and Leg Elevation

Elevation is an important aspect of controlling lower extremity swelling and is often the first recommended intervention. However, continuous elevation throughout the day can interfere with quality of life more than lymphedema itself. Elevation is an adjunct to lymphedema therapy, but is not the mainstay of treatment.

Sequential External Pneumatic Compression

The use of intermittent pneumatic compression with a single or multichamber pump temporarily reduces edema and provides an additional adjunct to compression stockings. These devices have been shown to be effective in reducing limb volume[127,128]; however, compression stockings are necessary to maintain the volume reduction when the patient is no longer supine. Typically, intermittent pneumatic compression is used for 4 to 6 hours per day at home when the patient is supine.

Lymphatic Massage

Manual lymphatic drainage is a form of massage developed by Vodder[129] that is directed at reducing edema. In combination with compression stockings, manual lymphatic drainage is associated with a long-term reduction in edema and fewer infections per patient per year.[130]

Antibiotic Therapy

Patients with lymphedema are at increased risk of developing cellulitis in the affected extremity. Recurrent infection can damage the lymphatics, aggravating the edema. *Staphylococcus* or beta-hemolytic *Streptococcus* are the most common organisms causing soft tissue infection. Aggressive antibiotic therapy is recommended at the earliest signs or symptoms of cellulitis. The drug of choice is penicillin, usually 500 mg orally 3 to 4 times per day. Patients with

a history of lymphedema and recurrent cellulitis should be given a prescription for antibiotics that can be kept at home and initiated at the first sign of infection.[75]

Surgery

There have been a variety of surgical procedures devised for the treatment of lymphedema. Surgical treatment involves either excision of extra tissue[131] or anastomoses of a lymphatic vessel to another lymphatic or vein.[132] With excisional procedures, part or all of the edematous tissue is removed. This does not improve lymphatic drainage, but debulks redundant tissue. The microsurgical procedures involve the creation of a lymphaticolymphatic or lymphaticovenous anastomosis, which theoretically improves lymphatic drainage. There are no long-term follow-up data available for these interventions, and therefore operative therapy for lymphedema is not well-accepted worldwide. Furthermore, operative intervention can further obliterate lymphatic channels, worsening the edema.[133]

Summary

Lymphedema is a chronic condition caused by ineffective lymphatic transport, which results in edema and skin damage. Lymphedema is not curable, but the symptoms can be controlled with a combination of elastic compression stockings, limb elevation, pneumatic compression, and massage. Controlling the edema protects the skin and potentially prevents cellulitis.

References

1. Moncada S, Radomski MW, Palmer RM: Endothelium-derived relaxing factor. Identification as nitric oxide and role in the control of vascular tone and platelet function. *Biochem Pharmacol* 37:2495, 1988.
2. van Bemmelen PS, Beach K, Bedford G, et al: The mechanism of venous valve closure. Its relationship to the velocity of reverse flow. *Arch Surg* 125:617, 1990.
3. Moneta GL, Strandness DE Jr.: Basic data concerning noninvasive vascular testing. *Ann Vasc Surg* 3:190, 1989.
4. Bettmann MA, Paulin S: Leg phlebography: the incidence, nature and modification of undesirable side effects. *Radiology* 122:101, 1977.
5. Hull R, Hirsh J, Sackett DL, et al: Clinical validity of a negative venogram in patients with clinically suspected venous thrombosis. *Circulation* 64:622, 1981.
6. Anonymous: Prevention of venous thrombosis and pulmonary embolism. NIH Consensus Development. *JAMA* 256:744, 1986.
7. Bick RL, Kaplan H: Syndromes of thrombosis and hypercoagulability. Congenital and acquired causes of thrombosis. *Med Clin North Am* 82:409, 1998.
8. Silverstein MD, Heit JA, Mohr DN, et al: Trends in the incidence of deep vein thrombosis and pulmonary embolism: a 25-year population-based study. *Arch Intern Med* 158:585, 1998.
9. Proctor MC, Greenfield LJ: Pulmonary embolism: diagnosis, incidence and implications. *Cardiovasc Surg* 5:77, 1997.
10. Mohr DN, Silverstein MD, Heit JA, et al: The venous stasis syndrome after deep venous thrombosis or pulmonary embolism: a population-based study. *Mayo Clin Proc* 75:1249, 2000.
11. Nordstrom M, Lindblad B, Bergqvist D, et al: A prospective study of the incidence of deep-vein thrombosis within a defined urban population. *J Intern Med* 232:155, 1992.
12. Anderson FA Jr., Wheeler HB, Goldberg RJ, et al: A population-based perspective of the hospital incidence and case-fatality rates of deep vein thrombosis and pulmonary embolism. The Worcester DVT Study. *Arch Intern Med* 151:933, 1991.
13. Clagett GP, Reisch JS: Prevention of venous thromboembolism in general surgical patients. Results of meta-analysis. *Ann Surg* 208:227, 1988.

14. Prandoni P, Lensing AW, Buller HR, et al: Deep-vein thrombosis and the incidence of subsequent symptomatic cancer. *N Engl J Med* 327:1128, 1992.

15. Venous thromboembolic disease and combined oral contraceptives: results of international multicentre case-control study. World Health Organization Collaborative Study of Cardiovascular Disease and Steroid Hormone Contraception. *Lancet* 346:1575, 1995.

16. Geerts WH, Code KI, Jay RM, et al: A prospective study of venous thromboembolism after major trauma. *N Engl J Med* 331:1601, 1994.

17. Jorgensen JO, Hanel KC, Morgan AM, et al: The incidence of deep venous thrombosis in patients with superficial thrombophlebitis of the lower limbs. *J Vasc Surg* 18:70, 1993.

18. Kotilainen M, Ristola P, Ikkala E, et al: Leg vein thrombosis diagnosed by 125I-fibrinogen test after acute myocardial infarction. *Ann Clin Res* 5:365, 1973.

19. Waring WP, Karunas RS: Acute spinal cord injuries and the incidence of clinically occurring thromboembolic disease. *Paraplegia* 29:8, 1991.

20. Ginsberg JS, Brill-Edwards P, Burrows RF, et al: Venous thrombosis during pregnancy: leg and trimester of presentation. *Thromb Haemost* 67:519, 1992.

21. Trottier SJ, Veremakis C, O'Brien J, et al: Femoral deep vein thrombosis associated with central venous catheterization: results from a prospective, randomized trial. *Crit Care Med* 23:52, 1995.

22. Anderson FA Jr., Wheeler HB, Goldberg RJ, et al: The prevalence of risk factors for venous thromboembolism among hospital patients. *Arch Intern Med* 152:1660, 1992.

23. Oger E, Leroyer C, Le Moigne E, et al: The value of a risk factor analysis in clinically suspected deep venous thrombosis. *Respiration* 64:326, 1997.

24. Iwama H, Furuta S, Ohmizo H: Graduated compression stocking manages to prevent economy class syndrome. *Am J Emerg Med* 20:378, 2002.

25. Hosoi Y, Geroulakos G, Belcaro G, et al: Characteristics of deep vein thrombosis associated with prolonged travel. *Eur J Vasc Endovasc Surg* 24:235, 2002.

26. Symington IS, Stack BH: Pulmonary thromboembolism after travel. *Br J Dis Chest* 71:138, 1977.

27. Markel A, Manzo RA, Bergelin RO, et al: Pattern and distribution of thrombi in acute venous thrombosis. *Arch Surg* 127:305, 1992.

28. Nicolaides AN, Kakkar VV, Field ES, et al: The origin of deep vein thrombosis: A venographic study. *Br J Radiol* 44:653, 1971.

29. Brockman SK, Vasko JS: The pathologic physiology of phlegmasia cerulea dolens. *Surgery* 59:997, 1966.

30. Lensing AW, Prandoni P, Brandjes D, et al: Detection of deep-vein thrombosis by real-time B-mode ultrasonography. *N Engl J Med* 320:342, 1989.

31. O'Leary DH, Kane RA, Chase BM: A prospective study of the efficacy of B-scan sonography in the detection of deep venous thrombosis in the lower extremities. *J Clin Ultrasound* 16:1, 1988.

32. Mussurakis S, Papaioannou S, Voros D, et al: Compression ultrasonography as a reliable imaging monitor in deep venous thrombosis. *Surg Gynecol Obstet* 171:233, 1990.

33. Habscheid W, Hohmann M, Wilhelm T, et al: Real-time ultrasound in the diagnosis of acute deep venous thrombosis of the lower extremity. *Angiology* 41:599, 1990.

34. Comerota AJ, Katz ML, Grossi RJ, et al: The comparative value of noninvasive testing for diagnosis and surveillance of deep vein thrombosis. *J Vasc Surg* 7:40, 1988.

35. Gomes AS, Webber MM, Buffkin D: Contrast venography vs. radionuclide venography: A study of discrepancies and their possible significance. *Radiology* 142:719, 1982.

36. Geerts WH, Heit JA, Clagett GP, et al: Prevention of venous thromboembolism. *Chest* 119:132S, 2001.

37. Geerts WH, Jay RM, Code KI, et al: A comparison of low-dose heparin with low-molecular-weight heparin as prophylaxis against venous thromboembolism after major trauma. *N Engl J Med* 335:701, 1996.

38. Rogers FB, Shackford SR, Ricci MA, et al: Routine prophylactic vena cava filter insertion in severely injured trauma patients decreases the incidence of pulmonary embolism. *J Am Coll Surg* 180:641, 1995.

39. Rogers FB, Strindberg G, Shackford SR, et al: Five-year follow-up of prophylactic vena cava filters in high-risk trauma patients. *Arch Surg* 133:406, 1998.

40. Millward SF, Oliva VL, Bell SD, et al: Gunther Tulip retrievable vena cava filter: Results from the Registry of the Canadian Interventional Radiology Association. *J Vasc Intervent Radiol* 12:1053, 2001.

41. Barritt DW, Jordan SC: Anticoagulant drugs in the treatment of pulmonary embolus: A controlled trial. *Lancet* 1:1309, 1960.

42. Raschke RA, Reilly BM, Guidry JR, et al: The weight-based heparin dosing nomogram compared with a standard care nomogram. A randomized controlled trial. *Ann Intern Med* 119:874, 1993.

43. Hyers TM, Agnelli G, Hull RD, et al: Antithrombotic therapy for venous thromboembolic disease. *Chest* 119:176S, 2001.

44. Hylek EM, Regan S, Henault LE, et al: Challenges to the effective use of unfractionated heparin in the hospitalized management of acute thrombosis. *Arch Intern Med* 163:621, 2003.

45. Amiral J, Bridey F, Dreyfus M, et al: Platelet factor 4 complexed to heparin is the target for antibodies generated in heparin-induced thrombocytopenia. *Thromb Haemost* 68:95, 1992.

46. Warkentin TE, Levine MN, Hirsh J, et al: Heparin-induced thrombocytopenia in patients treated with low-molecular-weight heparin or unfractionated heparin. *N Engl J Med* 332:1330, 1995.

47. Warkentin TE, Kelton JG: Heparin and platelets. *Hematol Oncol Clin North Am* 4:243, 1990.

48. Coon WW, Willis PW 3rd: Hemorrhagic complications of anticoagulant therapy. *Arch Intern Med* 133:386, 1974.

49. Coon WW, Willis PW 3rd, Symons MJ: Assessment of anticoagulant treatment of venous thromboembolism. *Ann Surg* 170:559, 1969.

50. Hull R, Delmore T, Genton E, et al: Warfarin sodium versus low-dose heparin in the long-term treatment of venous thrombosis. *N Engl J Med* 301:855, 1979.

51. Ridker P, Goldhaber S, Danielson E, et al: Long-term, low-intensity warfarin therapy for the prevention of recurrent venous thromboembolism. *N Engl J Med* 348:1425, 2003.

52. Fareed J, Walenga JM, Racanelli A, et al: Validity of the newly established low-molecular-weight heparin standard in cross-referencing low-molecular-weight heparins. *Haemostasis* 18:33, 1988.

53. Boneu B, Caranobe C, Cadroy Y, et al: Pharmacokinetic studies of standard unfractionated heparin and low-molecular-weight heparins. *Semin Thromb Hemostas* 14:18, 1988.

54. Koopman MM, Prandoni P, Piovella F, et al: Treatment of venous thrombosis with intravenous unfractionated heparin administered in the hospital as compared with subcutaneous low-molecular-weight heparin administered at home. The Tasman Study Group. *N Engl J Med* 334:682, 1996.

55. Prandoni P, Lensing AW, Buller HR, et al: Comparison of subcutaneous low-molecular-weight heparin with intravenous standard heparin in proximal deep-vein thrombosis. *Lancet* 339:441, 1992.

56. Merli G, Spiro TE, Olsson CG, et al: Subcutaneous enoxaparin once or twice daily compared with intravenous unfractionated heparin for treatment of venous thromboembolic disease. *Ann Intern Med* 134:191, 2001.

57. Levine M, Gent M, Hirsh J, et al: A comparison of low-molecular-weight heparin administered primarily at home with unfractionated heparin administered in the hospital for proximal deep-vein thrombosis. *N Engl J Med* 334:677, 1996.

58. Turpie AG, Bauer KA, Eriksson BI, et al: Postoperative fondaparinux versus postoperative enoxaparin for prevention of venous thromboembolism after elective hip-replacement surgery: A randomised double-blind trial. *Lancet* 359:1721, 2002.

59. Greinacher A, Volpel H, Janssens U, et al: Recombinant hirudin (lepirudin) provides safe and effective anticoagulation in patients with heparin-induced thrombocytopenia: A prospective study. *Circulation* 99:73, 1999.

60. Eriksson BI, Bergqvist D, Kalebo P, et al: Ximelagatran and melagatran compared with dalteparin for prevention of venous thromboembolism after total hip or knee replacement: The METHRO II randomised trial. *Lancet* 360:1441, 2002.

61. Markel A, Manzo RA, Strandness DE Jr.: The potential role of thrombolytic therapy in venous thrombosis. *Arch Intern Med* 152:1265, 1992.

62. Quinones-Baldrich W: Thrombolytic therapy for vascular disease, in Moore W (ed): *Vascular Surgery: A Comprehensive Review,* Vol. 1998. Philadelphia: WB Saunders, 1998, p 361.

63. Becker RC, Fintel DJ, Green D: *Antithrombotic Therapy.* Caddo, OK: Professional Communications, Inc, 2002, p 352.

64. MacFarlane R, Pilling J: Fibrinolytic activity of normal urine. *Nature* 159:779, 1947.

65. Rijken DC, Wijngaards G, Zaal-de Jong M, et al: Purification and partial characterization of plasminogen activator from human uterine tissue. *Biochim Biophys Acta* 580:140, 1979.

66. Anonymous: Urokinase pulmonary embolism trial. Phase 1 results: a cooperative study. *JAMA* 214:2163, 1970.

67. Anonymous: Urokinase-streptokinase embolism trial. Phase 2 results. A cooperative study. *JAMA* 229:1606, 1974.

68. Goldhaber SZ, Haire WD, Feldstein ML, et al: Alteplase versus heparin in acute pulmonary embolism: Randomised trial assessing right-ventricular function and pulmonary perfusion. *Lancet* 341:507, 1993.

69. Goldhaber SZ, Buring JE, Lipnick RJ, et al: Pooled analyses of randomized trials of streptokinase and heparin in phlebographically documented acute deep venous thrombosis. *Am J Med* 76:393, 1994.

70. Kakkar VV, Lawrence D: Hemodynamic and clinical assessment after therapy for acute deep vein thrombosis. A prospective study. *Am J Surg* 150:54, 1985.

71. Mewissen MW, Seabrook GR, Meissner MH, et al: Catheter-directed thrombolysis for lower extremity deep venous thrombosis: Report of a national multicenter registry. *Radiology* 211:39, 1999.

72. Becker DM, Philbrick JT, Selby JB: Inferior vena cava filters. Indications, safety, effectiveness. *Arch Intern Med* 152:1985, 1992.

73. Decousus H, Leizorovicz A, Parent F, et al: A clinical trial of vena caval filters in the prevention of pulmonary embolism in patients with proximal deep-vein thrombosis. Prevention du Risque d'Embolie Pulmonaire par Interruption Cave Study Group. *N Engl J Med* 338:409, 1998.

74. Plate G, Ohlin P, Eklof B: Pulmonary embolism in acute iliofemoral venous thrombosis. *Br J Surg* 72:912, 1985.

75. Gloviczki P, Yao JST (eds): *Handbook of Venous Disorders.* New York: Arnold, 2001, p 557.

76. Juhan CM, Alimi YS, Barthelemy PJ, et al: Late results of iliofemoral venous thrombectomy. *J Vasc Surg* 25:417, 1997.

77. Schmid C, Zietlow S, Wagner TO, et al: Fulminant pulmonary embolism: symptoms, diagnostics, operative technique, and results. *Ann Thorac Surg* 52:1102, 1991.

78. Kieny R, Charpentier A, Kieny MT: What is the place of pulmonary embolectomy today? *J Cardiovasc Surg* 32:549, 1991.

79. Gulba DC, Schmid C, Borst HG, et al: Medical compared with surgical treatment for massive pulmonary embolism. *Lancet* 343:576, 1994.

80. Schmitz-Rode T, Janssens U, Schild HH, et al: Fragmentation of massive pulmonary embolism using a pigtail rotation catheter. *Chest* 114:1427, 1998.

81. Greenfield LJ, Proctor MC, Williams DM, et al: Long-term experience with transvenous catheter pulmonary embolectomy. *J Vasc Surg* 18:450, 1993.

82. Allen AW, Megargell JL, Brown DB, et al: Venous thrombosis associated with the placement of peripherally inserted central catheters. *J Vasc Intervent Radiol* 11:1309, 2000.

83. Chengelis DL, Bendick PJ, Glover JL, et al: Progression of superficial venous thrombosis to deep vein thrombosis. *J Vasc Surg* 24:745, 1996.

84. Lutter KS, Kerr TM, Roedersheimer LR, et al: Superficial thrombophlebitis diagnosed by duplex scanning. *Surgery* 110:42, 1991.

85. Lohr JM, McDevitt DT, Lutter KS, et al: Operative management of greater saphenous thrombophlebitis involving the saphenofemoral junction. *Am J Surg* 164:269, 1992.

86. Ascer E, Lorensen E, Pollina RM, et al: Preliminary results of a nonoperative approach to saphenofemoral junction thrombophlebitis. *J Vasc Surg* 22:616, 1995.

87. Horne MK 3rd, May DJ, Alexander HR, et al: Venographic surveillance of tunneled venous access devices in adult oncology patients. *Ann Surg Oncol* 2:174, 1995.

88. Becker DM, Philbrick JT, Walker FB: Axillary and subclavian venous thrombosis. Prognosis and treatment. *Arch Intern Med* 151:1934, 1991.

89. Feugier P, Aleksic I, Salari R, et al: Long-term results of venous revascularization for Paget-Schroetter syndrome in athletes. *Ann Vasc Surg* 15:212, 2001.

90. Morasch MD, Ebaugh JL, Chiou AC, et al: Mesenteric venous thrombosis: A changing clinical entity. *J Vasc Surg* 34:680, 2001.

91. Abdu RA, Zakhour BJ, Dallis DJ: Mesenteric venous thrombosis—1911 to 1984. *Surgery* 101:383, 1987.

92. Rhee RY, Gloviczki P, Mendonca CT, et al: Mesenteric venous thrombosis: Still a lethal disease in the 1990s. *J Vasc Surg* 20:688, 1994.

93. Burkitt DP: Varicose veins, deep vein thrombosis, and haemorrhoids: Epidemiology and suggested aetiology. *Br Med J* 2:556, 1972.

94. Brand FN, Dannenberg AL, Abbott RD, et al: The epidemiology of varicose veins: The Framingham Study. *Am J Prev Med* 4:96, 1988.

95. Dwerryhouse S, Davies B, Harradine K, et al: Stripping the long saphenous vein reduces the rate of reoperation for recurrent varicose veins: Five-year results of a randomized trial. *J Vasc Surg* 29:589, 1999.

96. MacKenzie RK, Paisley A, Allan PL, et al: The effect of long saphenous vein stripping on quality of life. *J Vasc Surg* 35:1197, 2002.

97. Falanga V: Venous ulceration. *J Dermatol Surg Oncol* 19:764, 1993.

98. Phillips T, Stanton B, Provan A, et al: A study of the impact of leg ulcers on quality of life: Financial, social, and psychologic implications. *J Am Acad Dermatol* 31:49, 1994.

99. Skin Substitute Consensus Development Panel: Nonoperative management of venous ulcers: Evolving role of skin substitutes. *Vasc Surg* 33:197, 1999.

100. Abenhaim L, Kurz X: The VEINES study (VEnous Insufficiency Epidemiologic and Economic Study): An international cohort study on chronic venous disorders of the leg. VEINES Group. *Angiology* 48:59, 1997.

101. Clarke H, Smith SR, Vasdekis SN, et al: Role of venous elasticity in the development of varicose veins. *Br J Surg* 76:577, 1989.

102. Nicolaides AN, Hussein MK, Szendro G, et al: The relation of venous ulceration with ambulatory venous pressure measurements. *J Vasc Surg* 17:414, 1993.

103. Christopoulos DG, Nicolaides AN, Szendro G, et al: Air-plethysmography and the effect of elastic compression on venous hemodynamics of the leg. *J Vasc Surg* 5:148, 1987.

104. van Bemmelen PS, Bedford G, Beach K, et al: Quantitative segmental evaluation of venous valvular reflux with duplex ultrasound scanning. *J Vasc Surg* 10:425, 1989.

105. Nehler MR, Porter JM: The lower extremity venous system. Part II: The pathophysiology of chronic venous insufficiency. *Perspect Vasc Surg* 5:81, 1992.

106. Nehler MR, Moneta GL, Woodard DM, et al: Perimalleolar subcutaneous tissue pressure effects of elastic compression stockings. *J Vasc Surg* 18:783, 1993.

107. Dinn E: Treatment of venous ulceration by injection sclerotherapy and compression hosiery: A 5-year study. *Phlebology* 7:23, 1992.

108. Mayberry JC, Moneta GL, Taylor LM Jr., et al: Fifteen-year results of ambulatory compression therapy for chronic venous ulcers. *Surgery* 109:575, 1991.

109. Kitahama A, Elliott LF, Kerstein MD, et al: Leg ulcer. Conservative management or surgical treatment? *JAMA* 247:197, 1982.

110. Anning S: Leg ulcers: The results of treatment. *Angiology* 7:505, 1956.

111. Falanga V, Margolis D, Alvarez O, et al: Rapid healing of venous ulcers and lack of clinical rejection with an allogeneic cultured human skin equivalent. Human Skin Equivalent Investigators Group [see comments]. *Arch Dermatol* 134:293, 1998.

112. Phillips TJ: New skin for old: Developments in biological skin substitutes [editorial; comment]. *Arch Dermatol* 134:344, 1998.

113. Motykie GD, Caprini JA, Arcelus JI, et al: Evaluation of therapeutic compression stockings in the treatment of chronic venous insufficiency. *Dermatol Surg* 25:116, 1999.

114. Lippmann HI, Fishman LM, Farrar RH, et al: Edema control in the management of disabling chronic venous insufficiency. *Arch Phys Med Rehabil* 75:436, 1994.

115. Rubin JR, Alexander J, Plecha EJ, et al: Unna's boot vs. polyurethane foam dressings for the treatment of venous ulceration. A randomized prospective study. *Arch Surg* 125:489, 1990.

116. Vernick SH, Shapiro D, Shaw FD: Legging orthosis for venous and lymphatic insufficiency. *Arch Phys Med Rehabil* 68:459, 1987.

117. Sibbald RG: Apligraf living skin equivalent for healing venous and chronic wounds. *J Cutan Med Surg* 3(Suppl 1):S124, 1998.

118. Linton R: The communicating veins of the lower leg and the operative technique for their ligation. *Ann Surg* 107:582, 1938.

119. Gloviczki P, Bergan JJ, Rhodes JM, et al: Mid-term results of endoscopic perforator vein interruption for chronic venous insufficiency: Lessons learned from the North American subfascial endoscopic perforator surgery registry. The North American Study Group. *J Vasc Surg* 29:489, 1999.

120. Sottiurai VS: Surgical correction of recurrent venous ulcer. *J Cardiovasc Surg* 32:104, 1991.

121. Dalsing MC, Raju S, Wakefield TW, et al: A multicenter, phase I evaluation of cryopreserved venous valve allografts for the treatment of chronic deep venous insufficiency. *J Vasc Surg* 30:854, 1999.

122. Raju S, Fredericks R: Valve reconstruction procedures for nonobstructive venous insufficiency: Rationale, techniques, and results in 107 procedures with two- to eight-year follow-up. *J Vasc Surg* 7:301, 1988.

123. Masuda EM, Kistner RL: Long-term results of venous valve reconstruction: A four- to twenty-one-year follow-up. *J Vasc Surg* 19:391, 1994.

124. Rockson SG, Miller LT, Senie R, et al: American Cancer Society Lymphedema Workshop. Workgroup III: Diagnosis and management of lymphedema. *Cancer* 83:2882, 1998.

125. Yasuhara H, Shigematsu H, Muto T: A study of the advantages of elastic stockings for leg lymphedema. *Int Angiol* 15:272, 1996.

126. Grabois M: Breast cancer. Postmastectomy lymphedema. State of the art review. *Phys Med Rehabil Rev* 8:267, 1994.

127. Miranda F Jr., Perez MC, Castiglioni ML, et al: Effect of sequential intermittent pneumatic compression on both leg lymphedema volume and on lymph transport as semi-quantitatively evaluated by lymphoscintigraphy. *Lymphology* 34:135, 2001.

128. Richmand DM, O'Donnell TF Jr., Zelikovski A: Sequential pneumatic compression for lymphedema. A controlled trial. *Arch Surg* 120:1116, 1985.

129. Vodder E: *Le drainage lymphatique, une novelle methode therapeutique*. Paris: Sante pour tous, 1936.

130. Ko DS, Lerner R, Klose G, Cosimi AB: Effective treatment of lymphedema of the extremities. *Arch Surg* 133:452, 1998.

131. Miller TA, Wyatt LE, Rudkin GH: Staged skin and subcutaneous excision for lymphedema: A favorable report of long-term results. *Plast Reconstr Surg* 102:1486, 1998.

132. Baumeister RG, Siuda S: Treatment of lymphedemas by microsurgical lymphatic grafting: What is proved? *Plast Reconstr Surg* 85:64, 1990.

133. Bernas MJ, Witte CL, Witte MH: The diagnosis and treatment of peripheral lymphedema: draft revision of the 1995 Consensus Document of the International Society of Lymphology Executive Committee for discussion at the September 3–7, 2001, XVIII International Congress of Lymphology in Genoa, Italy. *Lymphology* 34:84, 2001.

CHAPTER 24

Esophagus and Diaphragmatic Hernia

Jeffrey H. Peters and Tom R. DeMeester

SURGICAL ANATOMY

The esophagus is a muscular tube that starts as the continuation of the pharynx and ends as the cardia of the stomach. When the head is in normal anatomic position, the transition from pharynx to esophagus occurs at the lower border of the sixth cervical vertebra. Topographically this corresponds to the cricoid cartilage anteriorly and the palpable transverse process of the sixth cervical vertebra laterally (Fig. 24-1). The esophagus is firmly attached at its upper end to the cricoid cartilage and at its lower end to the diaphragm; during swallowing, the proximal points of fixation move craniad the distance of one cervical vertebral body.

The esophagus lies in the midline, with a deviation to the left in the lower portion of the neck and upper portion of the thorax, and returns to the midline in the midportion of the thorax near the bifurcation of the trachea (Fig. 24-2). In the lower portion of the thorax, the esophagus again deviates to the left and anteriorly to pass through the diaphragmatic hiatus.

Three normal areas of esophageal narrowing are evident on the barium esophagogram or during esophagoscopy. The uppermost narrowing is located at the entrance into the esophagus and is caused by the cricopharyngeal muscle. Its luminal diameter is 1.5 cm, and it is the narrowest point of the esophagus. The middle narrowing is

due to an indentation of the anterior and left lateral esophageal wall caused by the crossing of the left main stem bronchus and aortic arch. The luminal diameter at this point is 1.6 cm. The lowermost narrowing is at the hiatus of the diaphragm and is caused by the gastroesophageal sphincter mechanism. The luminal diameter at this point varies somewhat, depending on the distention of the esophagus by the passage of food, but has been measured at 1.6 to 1.9 cm. These normal constrictions tend to hold up swallowed foreign objects, and the overlying mucosa is subject to injury by swallowed corrosive liquids due to their slow passage through these areas.

Figure 24-3 shows the average distance in centimeters measured during endoscopic examination between the incisor teeth and the cricopharyngeus, aortic arch, and cardia of the stomach. Manometrically, the length of the esophagus between the lower border of the cricopharyngeus and upper border of the lower sphincter varies according to the height of the individual.

The pharyngeal musculature consists of three broad, flat, overlapping fan-shaped constrictors (Fig. 24-4). The opening of the esophagus is collared by the cricopharyngeal muscle, which arises from both sides of the cricoid cartilage of the larynx and forms a continuous transverse muscle band without interruption by a median raphe. The fibers of this muscle blend inseparably with those of the inferior pharyngeal constrictor above and the inner circular muscle fibers of the esophagus below. Some investigators believe that the cricopharyngeus is part of the inferior constrictor; that is, that the inferior constrictor has two parts, an upper or retrothyroid portion having diagonal fibers, and a lower or retrocricoid portion having transverse fibers. Keith in 1910 showed that these two parts of the same muscle serve totally different functions. The retrocricoid portion serves as the upper sphincter of the esophagus and relaxes when the retrothyroid portion contracts, to force the swallowed bolus from the pharynx into the esophagus.

The cervical portion of the esophagus is approximately 5 cm long and descends between the trachea and the vertebral column, from the level of the sixth cervical vertebra to the level of the interspace between the first and second thoracic vertebrae posteriorly, or the level of the suprasternal notch anteriorly. The recurrent laryngeal nerves lie in the right and left grooves between the trachea and the esophagus. The left recurrent nerve lies somewhat closer to the esophagus than the right, owing to the slight deviation of the esophagus to the left, and the more lateral course of the right recurrent nerve around the right subclavian artery. Laterally, on the left and right sides of the cervical esophagus are the carotid sheaths and the lobes of the thyroid gland.

The thoracic portion of the esophagus is approximately 20 cm long. It starts at the thoracic inlet. In the upper portion of the thorax, it is in intimate relationship with the posterior wall of the trachea and the prevertebral fascia. Just above the tracheal bifurcation, the esophagus passes to the right of the aorta. This anatomic positioning can cause a notch indentation in its left lateral wall on a barium swallow radiogram. Immediately below this notch the esophagus crosses both the bifurcation of the trachea and the left main stem bronchus, owing to the slight deviation of the terminal portion of the trachea to the right by the aorta (Fig. 24-5). From there down, the esophagus passes over the posterior surface of the subcarinal lymph nodes, and then descends over the pericardium of the left atrium to reach the diaphragmatic hiatus (Fig. 24-6). From the bifurcation of the trachea downward, both the vagal nerves and the esophageal nerve plexus lie on the muscular wall of the esophagus.

Dorsally, the thoracic esophagus follows the curvature of the spine and remains in close contact with the vertebral bodies. From

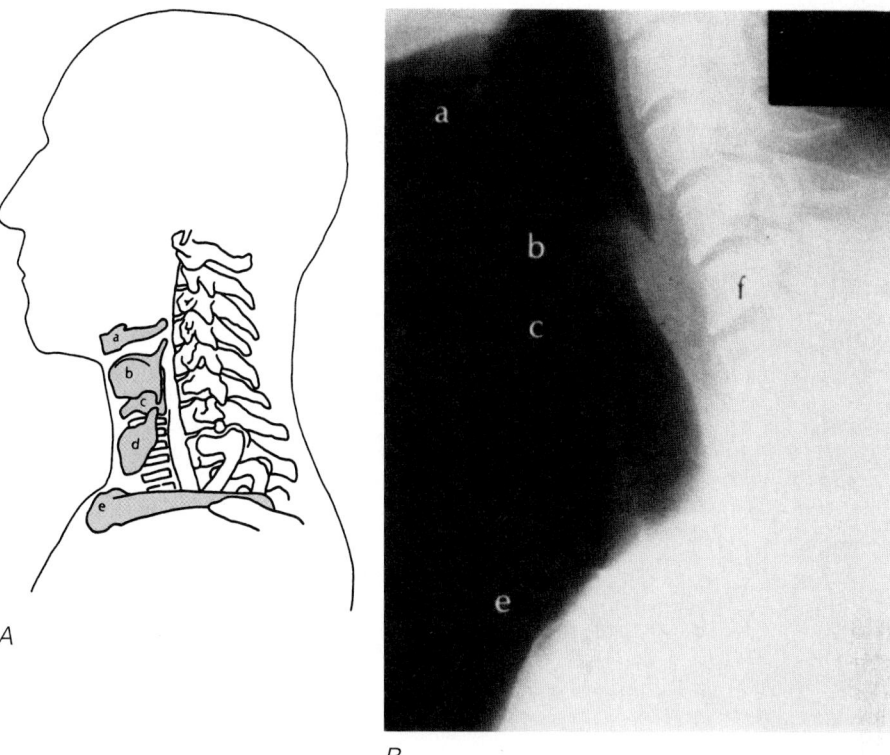

FIG. 24-1. A. Topographic relationships of the cervical esophagus: (a) hyoid bone, (b) thyroid cartilage, (c) cricoid cartilage, (d) thyroid gland, (e) sternoclavicular, and (f) C6 vertebra. B. Lateral radiographic appearance. [*Reproduced with permission from Rothberg M, DeMeester TR: Surgical anatomy of the esophagus, in Shields TW (ed): General Thoracic Surgery, 3rd ed. Philadelphia: Lea & Febiger, 1989, p 77.*]

A

B

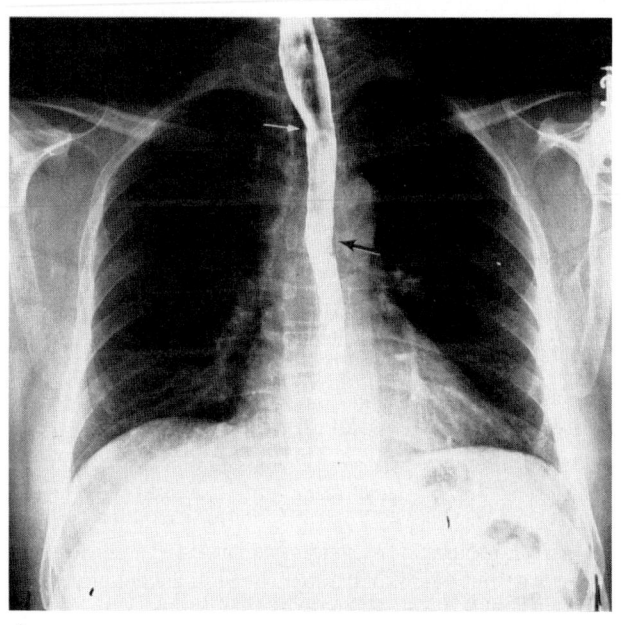

A

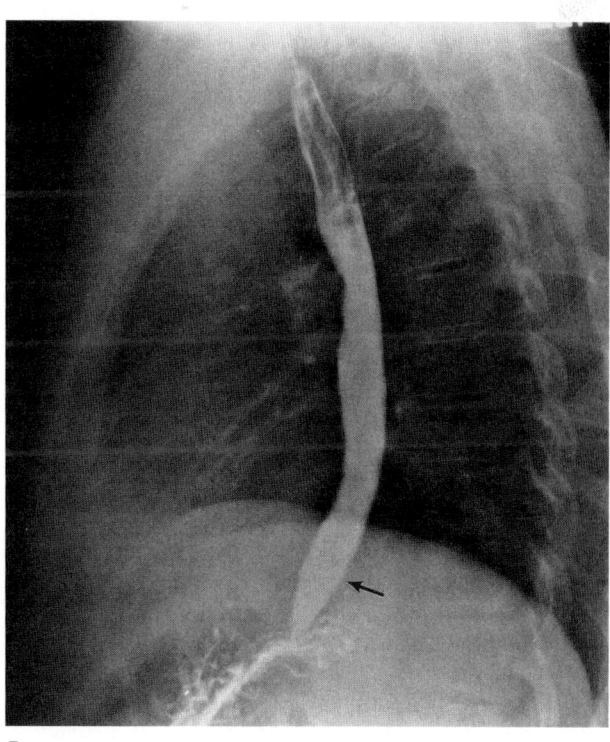

B

FIG. 24-2. Barium esophagogram. *A.* Posteroanterior view. *B.* Lateral view. White arrow shows deviation to the left. Black arrow shows return to midline. Black arrow on lateral view shows anterior deviation. [*Reproduced with permission from Rothberg M, DeMeester TR: Surgical anatomy of the esophagus, in Shields TW (ed): General Thoracic Surgery, 3rd ed. Philadelphia: Lea & Febiger, 1989, p 77.*]

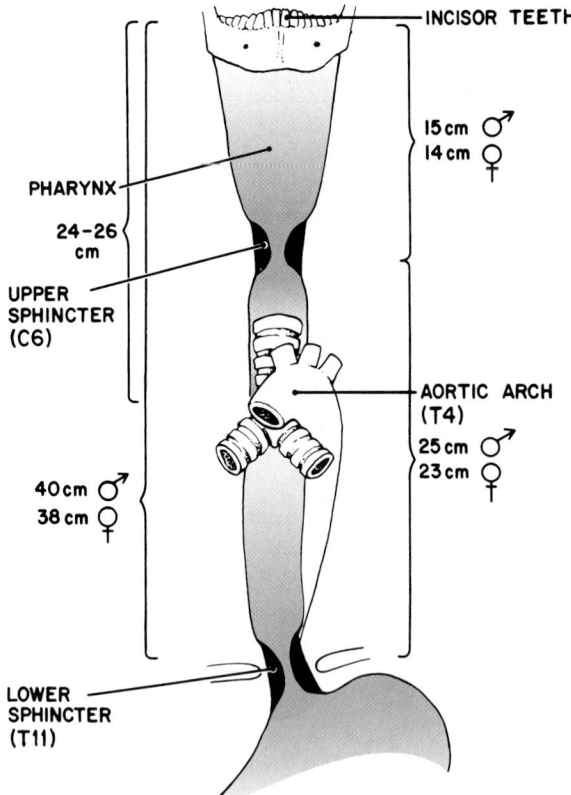

FIG. 24-3. Important clinical endoscopic measurements of the esophagus in adults. [*Reproduced with permission from Rothberg M, De-Meester TR: Surgical anatomy of the esophagus, in Shields TW (ed): General Thoracic Surgery, 3rd ed. Philadelphia: Lea & Febiger, 1989, p 78.*]

the eighth thoracic vertebra downward, the esophagus moves vertically away from the spine to pass through the hiatus of the diaphragm. The thoracic duct passes through the hiatus of the diaphragm on the anterior surface of the vertebral column behind the aorta and under the right crus. In the thorax, the thoracic duct lies dorsal to the esophagus between the azygos vein on the right and the descending thoracic aorta on the left.

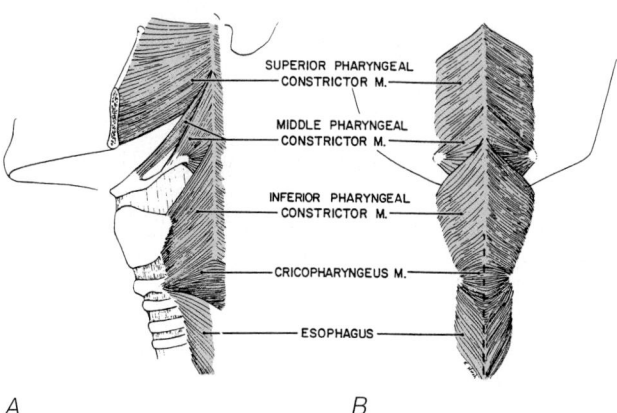

FIG. 24-4. External muscles of the pharynx. *A.* Posterolateral view. *B.* Posterior view. Dotted line represents usual site of myotomy. [*Reproduced with permission from Rothberg M, DeMeester TR: Surgical anatomy of the esophagus, in Shields TW (ed): General Thoracic Surgery, 3rd ed. Philadelphia: Lea & Febiger, 1989, p 78.*]

The abdominal portion of the esophagus is approximately 2 cm long and includes a portion of the lower esophageal sphincter (LES) (Fig. 24-7). It starts as the esophagus passes through the diaphragmatic hiatus and is surrounded by the phrenoesophageal membrane, a fibroelastic ligament arising from the subdiaphragmatic fascia as a continuation of the transversalis fascia lining the abdomen (Fig. 24-8). The upper leaf of the membrane attaches itself in a circumferential fashion around the esophagus, about 1 to 2 cm above the level of the hiatus. These fibers blend in with the elastic-containing adventitia of the abdominal esophagus and the cardia of the stomach. This portion of the esophagus is subjected to the positive-pressure environment of the abdomen.

The musculature of the esophagus can be divided into an outer longitudinal and an inner circular layer. The upper 2 to 6 cm of the esophagus contain only striated muscle fibers. From there on, smooth muscle fibers gradually become more abundant. Most clinically significant esophageal motility disorders involve only the smooth muscle in the lower two thirds of the esophagus. When a surgical esophageal myotomy is indicated, the incision needs to extend only this distance.

The longitudinal muscle fibers originate from a cricoesophageal tendon arising from the dorsal upper edge of the anteriorly located cricoid cartilage. The two bundles of muscle diverge and meet in the midline on the posterior wall of the esophagus about 3 cm below the cricoid (see Fig. 24-5). From this point on, the entire circumference of the esophagus is covered by a layer of longitudinal muscle fibers. This configuration of the longitudinal muscle fibers around the most proximal part of the esophagus leaves a V-shaped area in the posterior wall covered only with circular muscle fibers. Contraction of the longitudinal muscle fibers shortens the esophagus. The circular muscle layer of the esophagus is thicker than the outer longitudinal layer. In situ, the geometry of the circular muscle is helical and makes the peristalsis of the esophagus assume a worm-like drive, as opposed to segmental and sequential squeezing. As a consequence, severe motor abnormalities of the esophagus assume a corkscrew-like pattern on the barium swallow radiogram.

The cervical portion of the esophagus receives its main blood supply from the inferior thyroid artery. The thoracic portion receives its blood supply from the bronchial arteries, with 75% of individuals having one right-sided and two left-sided branches. Two esophageal branches arise directly from the aorta. The abdominal portion of the esophagus receives its blood supply from the ascending branch of the left gastric artery and from inferior phrenic arteries (Fig. 24-9). On entering the wall of the esophagus, the arteries assume a T-shaped division to form a longitudinal plexus giving rise to an intramural vascular network in the muscular and submucosal layers. As a consequence, the esophagus can be mobilized from the stomach to the level of the aortic arch without fear of devascularization and ischemic necrosis. Caution should be exercised as to the extent of esophageal mobilization in patients who have had a previous thyroidectomy with ligation of the inferior thyroid arteries proximal to the origin of the esophageal branches.

Blood from the capillaries of the esophagus flows into a submucosal venous plexus, and then into a periesophageal venous plexus from which the esophageal veins originate. In the cervical region, the esophageal veins empty into the inferior thyroid vein; in the thoracic region they empty into the bronchial, azygos, or hemiazygos veins; and in the abdominal region they empty into the coronary vein (Fig. 24-10). The submucosal venous networks of the esophagus and stomach are in continuity with each other, and in patients with portal venous obstruction, this communication functions as a

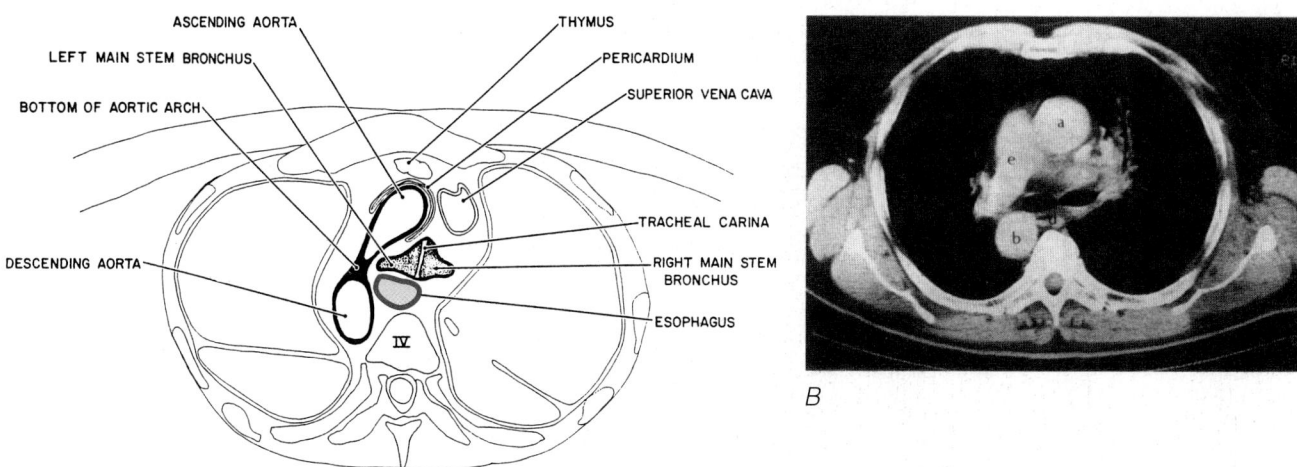

FIG. 24-5. *A.* Cross section of the thorax at the level of the tracheal bifurcation. *B.* Computed tomography (CT) scan at same level viewed from above: (*a*) ascending aorta, (*b*) descending aorta, (*c*) tracheal carina, (*d*) esophagus, and (*e*) pulmonary artery. [*Reproduced with permission from Rothberg M, DeMeester TR: Surgical anatomy of the esophagus, in Shields TW (ed): General Thoracic Surgery, 3rd ed. Philadelphia: Lea & Febiger, 1989, p 81.*]

collateral pathway for portal blood to enter the superior vena cava via the azygos vein.

The parasympathetic innervation of the pharynx and esophagus is provided mainly by the vagus nerves. The constrictor muscles of the pharynx receive branches from the pharyngeal plexus, which is on the posterior lateral surface of the middle constrictor muscle, and is formed by pharyngeal branches of the vagus nerves with a small contribution from cranial nerves IX and XI (Fig. 24-11). The cricopharyngeal sphincter and the cervical portion of the esophagus receive branches from both recurrent laryngeal nerves, which originate from the vagus nerves—the right recurrent nerve at the lower margin of the subclavian artery and the left at the lower

margin of the aortic arch. They are slung dorsally around these vessels and ascend in the groove between the esophagus and trachea, giving branches to each. Damage to these nerves interferes not only with the function of the vocal cords, but also with the function of the cricopharyngeal sphincter and the motility of the cervical esophagus, predisposing the individual to pulmonary aspiration on swallowing.

Afferent visceral sensory pain fibers from the esophagus end without synapse in the first four segments of the thoracic spinal cord, using a combination of sympathetic and vagal pathways. These pathways are also occupied by afferent visceral sensory fibers from the heart; hence, both organs have similar symptomatology.

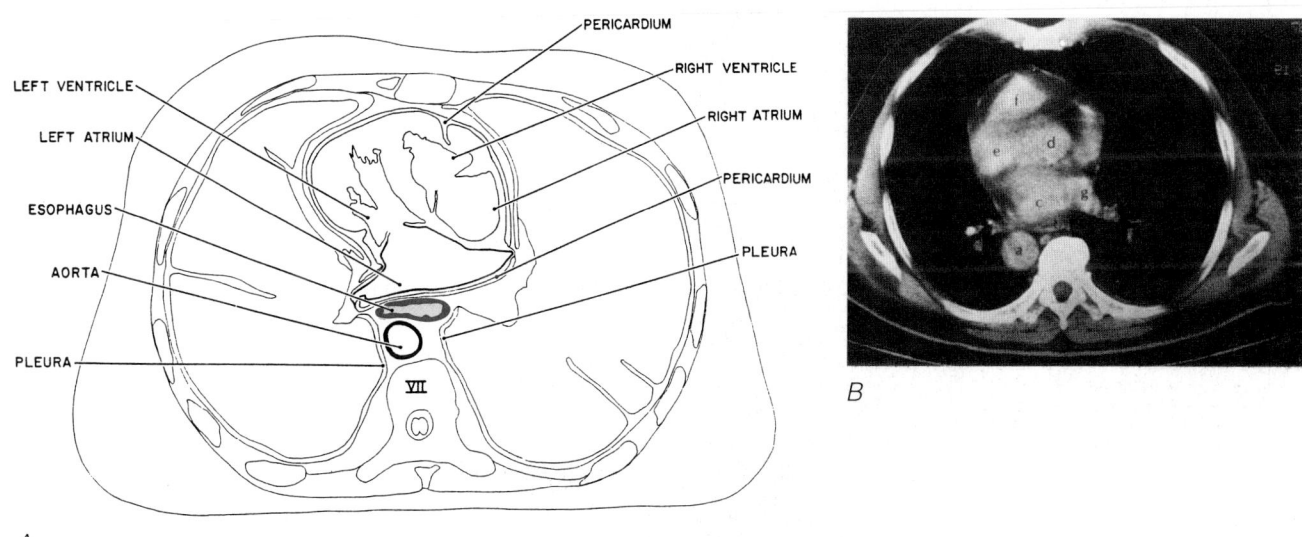

FIG. 24-6. *A.* Cross section of the thorax at the mid-left atrial level. *B.* CT scan at the same level viewed from above: (*a*) aorta, (*b*) esophagus, (*c*) left atrium, (*d*) right atrium, (*e*) left ventricle, (*f*) right ventricle, and (*g*) pulmonary vein. [*Reproduced with permission from Rothberg M, DeMeester TR: Surgical anatomy of the esophagus, in Shields TW (ed): General Thoracic Surgery, 3rd ed. Philadelphia: Lea & Febiger, 1989, p 82.*]

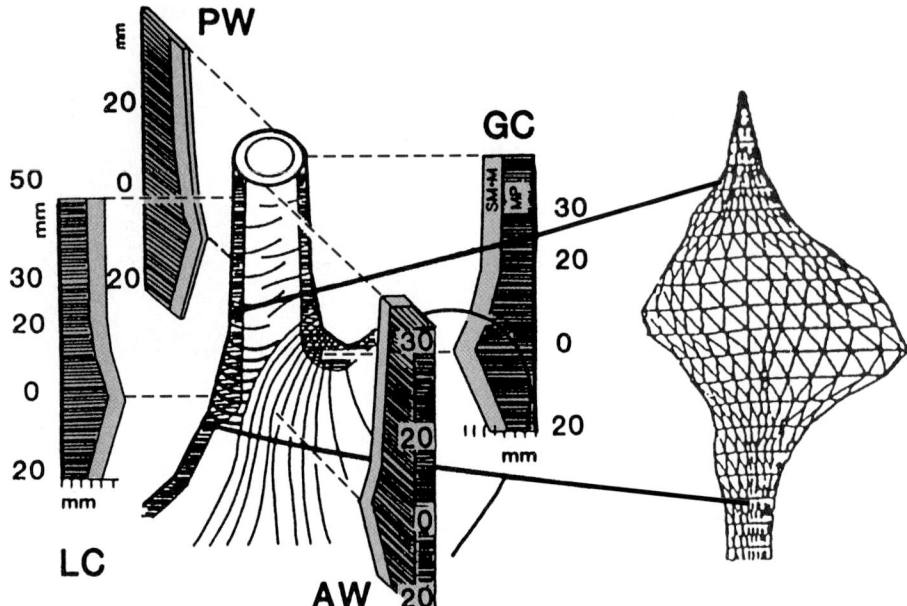

FIG. 24-7. Schematic drawing shows correlation between radial muscle thickness (*left*) and three-dimensional manometric pressure image (*right*) at the gastroesophageal junction. Muscle thickness across the gastroesophageal junction at the posterior gastric wall (PW), greater curvature (GC), anterior gastric wall (AW), and lesser curvature (LC) is shown in millimeters. Radial pressures at the gastroesophageal junction (in millimeters of mercury) are plotted around an axis representing atmospheric pressure. (*Reproduced with permission from Stein HJ, Liebermann-Meffert D, DeMeester TR, Siewert JR: Three-dimensional pressure image and muscular structure of the human LES. Surgery 117:692, 1995.*)

The lymphatics located in the submucosa of the esophagus are so dense and interconnected that they constitute a single plexus (Fig. 24-12). There are more lymph vessels than blood capillaries in the submucosa. Lymph flow in the submucosal plexus runs in a longitudinal direction, and on injection of a contrast medium, the longitudinal spread is seen to be about six times that of the transverse spread. In the upper two thirds of the esophagus the lymphatic flow is mostly cephalad, and in the lower third caudad. In the thoracic portion of the esophagus, the submucosal lymph plexus extends over a long distance in a longitudinal direction before penetrating the muscle layer to enter lymph vessels in the adventitia. As a consequence of this nonsegmental lymph drainage, a primary tumor can extend for a considerable length superiorly or inferiorly in the submucosal plexus. Consequently, free tumor cells can follow the submucosal lymphatic plexus in either direction for a long distance before they pass through the muscularis and on into the regional lymph nodes. The cervical esophagus has a more direct segmental lymph drainage into the regional nodes, and as a result, lesions in this portion of the esophagus have less submucosal extension and a more regionalized lymphatic spread.

The efferent lymphatics from the cervical esophagus drain into the paratracheal and deep cervical lymph nodes, and those from the upper thoracic esophagus empty mainly into the paratracheal lymph nodes. Efferent lymphatics from the lower thoracic esophagus drain into the subcarinal nodes and nodes in the inferior pulmonary

FIG. 24-8. Attachments and structure of the phrenoesophageal membrane. The transversalis fascia lies just above the parietal peritoneum. [*Reproduced with permission from Rothberg M, DeMeester TR: Surgical anatomy of the esophagus, in Shields TW (ed): General Thoracic Surgery, 3rd ed. Philadelphia: Lea & Febiger, 1989, p 83.*]

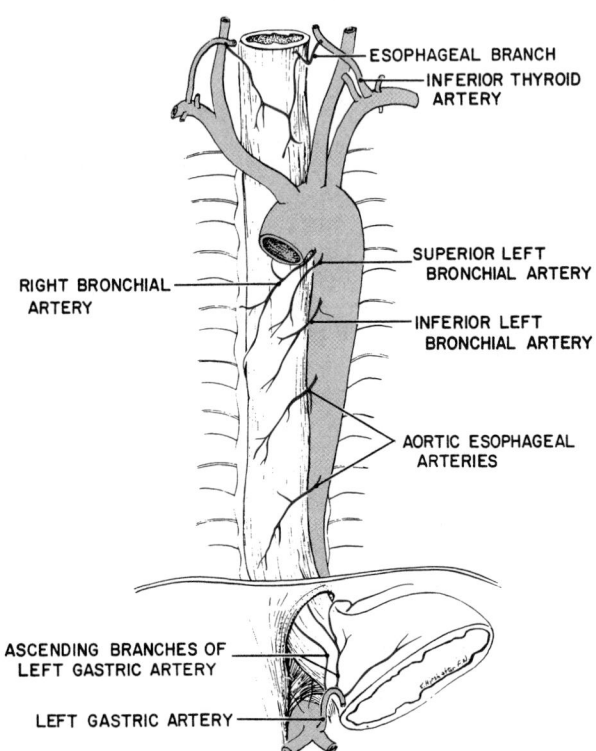

FIG. 24-9. Arterial blood supply of the esophagus. [*Reproduced with permission from Rothberg M, DeMeester TR: Surgical anatomy of the esophagus, in Shields TW (ed): General Thoracic Surgery, 3rd ed. Philadelphia: Lea & Febiger, 1989, p 84.*]

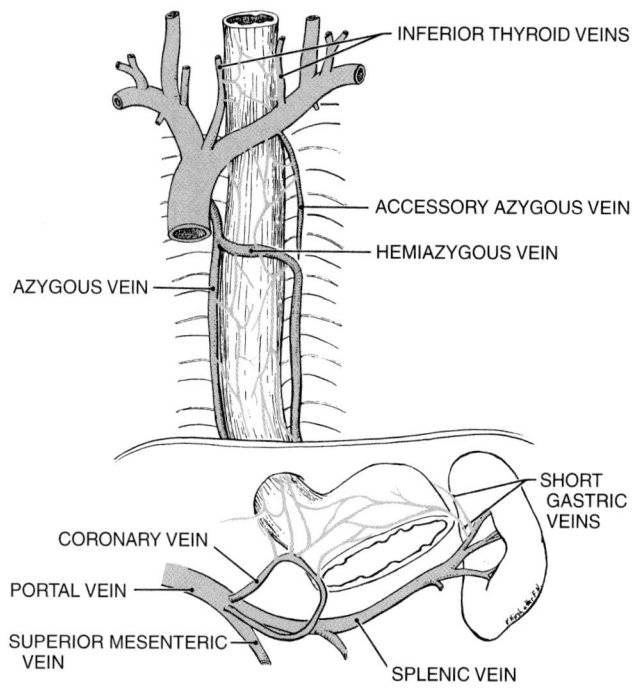

FIG. 24-10. Venous drainage of the esophagus. [*Reproduced with permission from Rothberg M, DeMeester TR: Surgical anatomy of the esophagus, in Shields TW (ed): General Thoracic Surgery, 3rd ed. Philadelphia: Lea & Febiger, 1989, p 85.*]

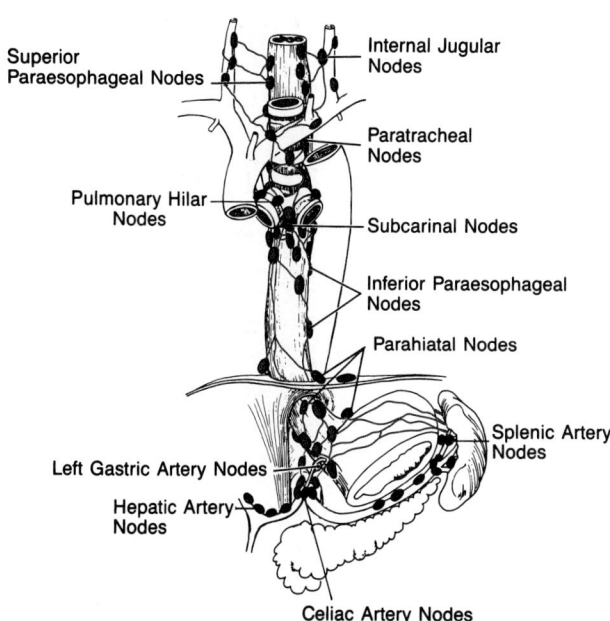

FIG. 24-12. Lymphatic drainage of the esophagus. (*Reproduced with permission from DeMeester TR, Barlow AP: Surgery and current management for cancer of the esophagus and cardia: Part I. Curr Probl Surg 25:498, 1988.*)

ligaments. The superior gastric nodes receive lymph not only from the abdominal portion of the esophagus, but also from the adjacent lower thoracic segment.

PHYSIOLOGY

Swallowing Mechanism

The act of alimentation requires the passage of food and drink from the mouth into the stomach. One third of this distance consists of the mouth and hypopharynx, and two thirds is made up by the esophagus. To comprehend the mechanics of alimentation, it is useful to visualize the gullet as a mechanical model in which the tongue and pharynx function as a piston pump with three valves, and the body of the esophagus and cardia function as a worm-drive pump with a single valve. The three valves in the pharyngeal cylinder are the soft palate, the epiglottis, and the cricopharyngeus. The valve of the esophageal pump is the LES. Failure of the valves or the pumps leads to abnormalities in swallowing—that is, difficulty in food propulsion from mouth to stomach—or regurgitation of gastric contents into the esophagus or pharynx.

Food is taken into the mouth in a variety of bite sizes, where it is broken up, mixed with saliva, and lubricated. Once initiated, swallowing is entirely a reflex act. When food is ready for swallowing, the tongue, acting like a piston, moves the bolus into the posterior oropharynx and forces it into the hypopharynx (Fig. 24-13). Concomitantly with the posterior movement of the tongue, the soft palate is elevated, thereby closing the passage between the oropharynx and nasopharynx. This partitioning prevents pressure generated in the oropharynx from being dissipated through the nose. When the soft palate is paralyzed, for example, after a cerebrovascular accident, food is commonly regurgitated into the nasopharynx. During swallowing, the hyoid bone moves upward and anteriorly, elevating the larynx and opening the retrolaryngeal space, bringing the epiglottis under the tongue (see Fig. 24-13). The backward tilt of the epiglottis

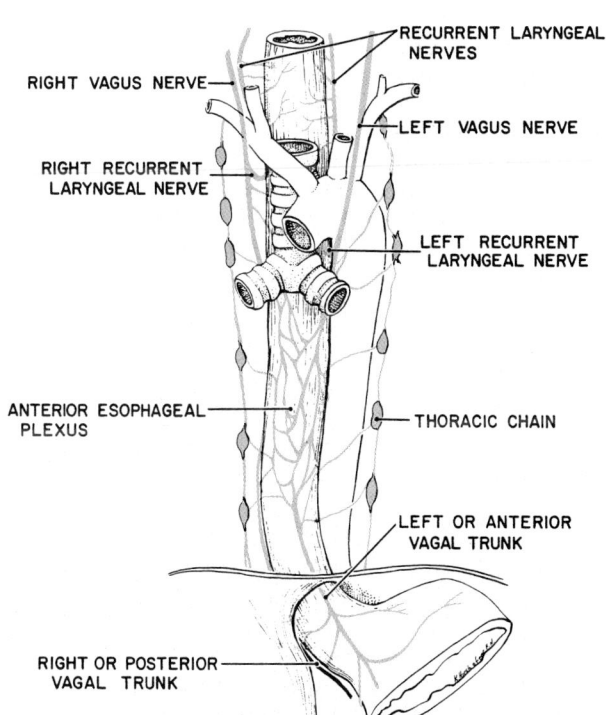

FIG. 24-11. Innervation of the esophagus. [*Reproduced with permission from Rothberg M, DeMeester TR: Surgical anatomy of the esophagus, in Shields TW (ed): General Thoracic Surgery, 3rd ed. Philadelphia: Lea & Febiger, 1989, p 85.*]

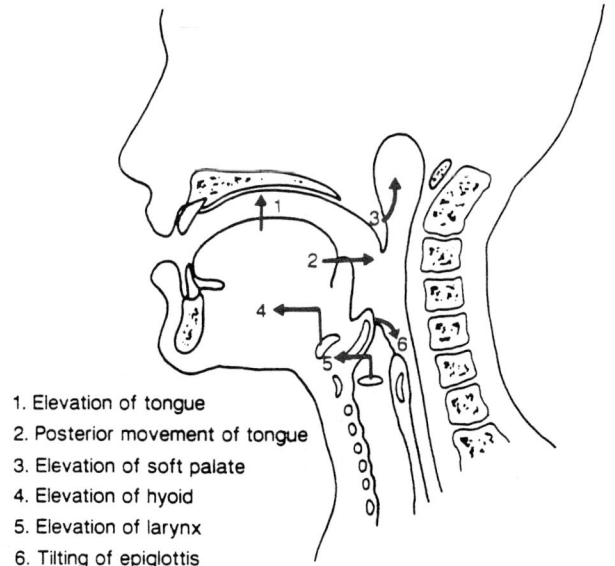

1. Elevation of tongue
2. Posterior movement of tongue
3. Elevation of soft palate
4. Elevation of hyoid
5. Elevation of larynx
6. Tilting of epiglottis

FIG. 24-13. Sequence of events during the oropharyngeal phase of swallowing. [Reproduced with permission from DeMeester TR, Stein HJ, Fuchs KH: Physiologic diagnostic studies, in Zuidema GD, Orringer MB (eds): Shackelford's Surgery of the Alimentary Tract, 3rd ed, Vol. I. Philadelphia: WB Saunders, 1991, p 95.]

covers the opening of the larynx to prevent aspiration. The entire pharyngeal part of swallowing occurs within 1.5 seconds.

During swallowing, the pressure in the hypopharynx rises abruptly, to at least 60 mm Hg, due to the backward movement of the tongue and contraction of the posterior pharyngeal constrictors. A sizable pressure difference develops between the hypopharyngeal pressure and the less-than-atmospheric midesophageal or intrathoracic pressure (Fig. 24-14). This pressure gradient speeds the movement of food from the hypopharynx into the esophagus when the

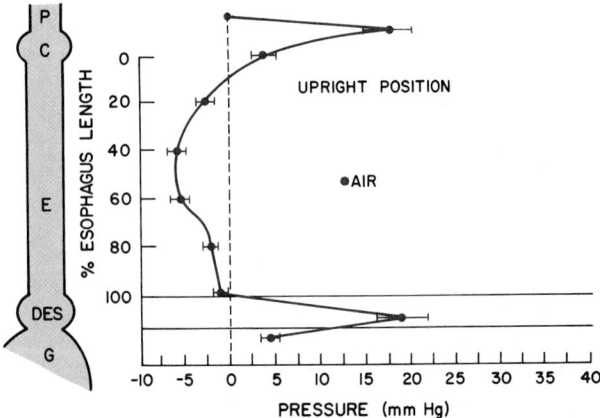

FIG. 24-14. Resting pressure profile of the foregut showing the pressure differential between the atmospheric pharyngeal pressure (P), the less-than-atmospheric midesophageal pressure (E), and the greater-than-atmospheric intragastric pressure (G), with the interposed high-pressure zones of the cricopharyngeus (C) and distal esophageal sphincter (DES). The necessity for relaxation of the cricopharyngeus and DES pressure in order to move a bolus into the stomach is apparent. Esophageal work occurs when a bolus is pushed from the midesophageal area (E), with a pressure less than atmospheric, into the stomach, which has a pressure greater than atmospheric (G). (Reproduced with permission from Waters PF, DeMeester TR: Foregut motor disorders and their surgical management. Med Clin North Am 65:1235, 1981.)

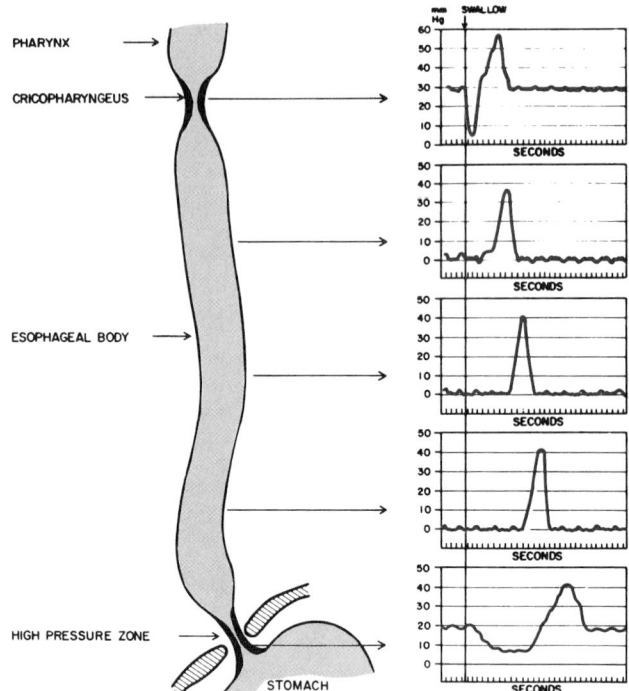

FIG. 24-15. Intraluminal esophageal pressures in response to swallowing. (Reproduced with permission from Waters PF, DeMeester TR: Foregut motor disorders and their surgical management. Med Clin North Am 65:1235, 1981.)

cricopharyngeus or upper esophageal sphincter relaxes. The bolus is both propelled by peristaltic contraction of the posterior pharyngeal constrictors and sucked into the thoracic esophagus. Critical to receiving the bolus is the compliance of the cervical esophagus; when compliance is lost due to muscle pathology, dysphagia can result. The upper esophageal sphincter closes within 0.5 second of the initiation of the swallow, with the immediate closing pressure reaching approximately twice the resting level of 30 mm Hg. The postrelaxation contraction continues down the esophagus as a peristaltic wave (Fig. 24-15). The high closing pressure and the initiation of the peristaltic wave prevents reflux of the bolus from the esophagus back into the pharynx. After the peristaltic wave has passed farther down the esophagus, the pressure in the upper esophageal sphincter returns to its resting level.

Swallowing can be started at will, or it can be reflexively elicited by the stimulation of areas in the mouth and pharynx, among them the anterior and posterior tonsillar pillars or the posterior lateral walls of the hypopharynx. The afferent sensory nerves of the pharynx are the glossopharyngeal nerves and the superior laryngeal branches of the vagus nerves. Once aroused by stimuli entering via these nerves, the swallowing center in the medulla coordinates the complete act of swallowing by discharging impulses through cranial nerves V, VII, X, XI, and XII, as well as the motor neurons of C1 to C3. Discharges through these nerves occur in a rather specific pattern and last for approximately 0.5 second. Little is known about the organization of the swallowing center, except that it can trigger swallowing after a variety of different inputs, but the response is always a rigidly ordered pattern of outflow. Following a cerebrovascular accident, this coordinated outflow may be altered, causing mild to severe abnormalities of swallowing. In more severe injury, swallowing can be grossly disrupted, leading to repetitive aspiration.

The striated muscles of the cricopharyngeus and the upper third of the esophagus are activated by efferent motor fibers distributed through the vagus nerve and its recurrent laryngeal branches. The integrity of innervation is required for the cricopharyngeus to relax in coordination with the pharyngeal contraction, and resume its resting tone once a bolus has entered the upper esophagus. Operative damage to the innervation can interfere with laryngeal, cricopharyngeal, and upper esophageal function, and predispose the patient to aspiration.

The pharyngeal activity in swallowing initiates the esophageal phase. The body of the esophagus functions as a worm-drive propulsive pump due to the helical arrangement of its circular muscles, and is responsible for transferring a bolus of food into the stomach. The esophageal phase of swallowing represents esophageal work done during alimentation, in that food is moved into the stomach from a negative-pressure environment of –6 mm Hg intrathoracic pressure, to a positive-pressure environment of 6 mm Hg intra-abdominal pressure, or over a gradient of 12 mm Hg (see Fig. 24-14). Effective and coordinated smooth muscle function in the lower third of the esophagus is therefore important in pumping the food across this gradient.

The peristaltic wave generates an occlusive pressure varying from 30 to 120 mm Hg (see Fig. 24-15). The wave rises to a peak in 1 second, lasts at the peak for about 0.5 seconds, and then subsides in about 1.5 seconds. The whole course of the rise and fall of occlusive pressure may occupy one point in the esophagus for 3 to 5 seconds. The peak of a primary peristaltic contraction initiated by a swallow (primary peristalsis) moves down the esophagus at 2 to 4 cm/s and reaches the distal esophagus about 9 seconds after swallowing starts (see Fig. 24-15). Consecutive swallows produce similar primary peristaltic waves, but when the act of swallowing is rapidly repeated, the esophagus remains relaxed and the peristaltic wave occurs only after the last movement of the pharynx. Progress of the wave in the esophagus is caused by sequential activation of its muscles, initiated by efferent vagal nerve fibers arising in the swallowing center.

Continuity of the esophageal muscle is not necessary for sequential activation if the nerves are intact. If the muscles, but not the nerves, are cut across, the pressure wave begins distally below the cut as it dies out at the proximal end above the cut. This allows a sleeve resection of the esophagus to be done without destroying its normal function. Afferent impulses from receptors within the esophageal wall are not essential for progress of the coordinated wave. Afferent nerves, however, do go to the swallowing center from the esophagus, because if the esophagus is distended at any point, a contractual wave begins with a forceful closure of the upper esophageal sphincter and sweeps down the esophagus. This secondary contraction occurs without any movements of the mouth or pharynx. Secondary peristalsis can occur as an independent local reflex to clear the esophagus of ingested material left behind after the passage of the primary wave. Current studies suggest that secondary peristalsis is not as common as once thought.

Despite the powerful occlusive pressure, the propulsive force of the esophagus is relatively feeble. If a subject attempts to swallow a bolus attached by a string to a counterweight, the maximum weight that can be overcome is 5 to 10 g. Orderly contractions of the muscular wall and anchoring of the esophagus at its inferior end are necessary for efficient aboral propulsion to occur. Loss of the inferior anchor, as occurs with a large hiatal hernia, can lead to inefficient propulsion.

The LES provides a pressure barrier between the esophagus and stomach and acts as the valve on the worm-drive pump of the

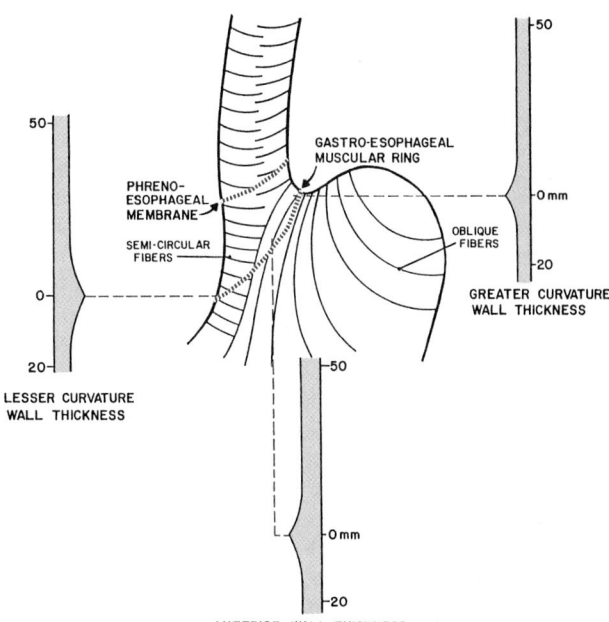

FIG. 24-16. Wall thickness and orientation of fibers on microdissection of the cardia. At the junction of the esophageal tube and gastric pouch, there is an oblique muscular ring composed of an increased muscle mass inside the inner muscular layer. On the lesser curve side of the cardia the muscle fibers of the inner layer are oriented transversely and form semicircular muscle clasps. On the greater curve side of the cardia, these muscle fibers form oblique loops that encircle the distal end of the cardia and gastric fundus. Both the semicircular muscle clasps and the oblique fibers of the fundus contract in a circular manner to close the cardia. [Reproduced with permission from DeMeester TR, Skinner DB: Evaluation of esophageal function and disease, in Glen WWL (ed): Thoracic and Cardiovascular Surgery, 4th ed. Norwalk, CT: Appleton & Lange, 1983, p 461.]

esophageal body. Although an anatomically distinct LES has been difficult to identify, microdissection studies show that in humans, the sphincter-like function is related to the architecture of the muscle fibers at the junction of the esophageal tube with the gastric pouch (Fig. 24-16). The sphincter actively remains closed to prevent reflux of gastric contents into the esophagus and opens by a relaxation that coincides with a pharyngeal swallow (see Fig. 24-15). The LES pressure returns to its resting level after the peristaltic wave has passed through the esophagus. Consequently, reflux of gastric juice that may occur through the open valve during a swallow is cleared back into the stomach.

If the pharyngeal swallow does not initiate a peristaltic contraction, then the coincident relaxation of the LES is unguarded and reflux of gastric juice can occur. This may be an explanation for the observation of spontaneous lower esophageal relaxation, thought by some to be a causative factor in gastroesophageal reflux disease. The power of the worm-drive pump of the esophageal body is insufficient to force open a valve that does not relax. In dogs, a bilateral cervical parasympathetic blockade abolishes the relaxation of the LES that occurs with pharyngeal swallowing or distention of the esophagus. Consequently, vagal function appears to be important in coordinating the relaxation of the LES with esophageal contraction.

The antireflux mechanism in human beings is composed of three components: a mechanically effective LES, efficient esophageal clearance, and an adequately functioning gastric reservoir. A defect of any one of these three components can lead to increased esophageal exposure to gastric juice and the development of mucosal injury.

Physiologic Reflux

On 24-hour esophageal pH monitoring, healthy individuals have occasional episodes of gastroesophageal reflux. This physiologic reflux is more common when awake and in the upright position than during sleep in the supine position. When reflux of gastric juice occurs, normal subjects rapidly clear the acid gastric juice from the esophagus regardless of their position.

There are several explanations for the observation that physiologic reflux in normal subjects is more common when they are awake and in the upright position than during sleep in the supine position. First, reflux episodes occur in healthy volunteers primarily during transient losses of the gastroesophageal barrier, which may be due to a relaxation of the LES or intragastric pressure overcoming sphincter pressure. Gastric juice can also reflux when a swallow-induced relaxation of the LES is not protected by an oncoming peristaltic wave. The average frequency of these "unguarded moments" or of transient losses of the gastroesophageal barrier is far less while asleep and in the supine position than while awake and in the upright position. Consequently, there are fewer opportunities for reflux to occur in the supine position. Second, in the upright position there is a 12-mm Hg pressure gradient between the resting, positive intra-abdominal pressure measured in the stomach and the most negative intrathoracic pressure measured in the esophagus at midthoracic level. This gradient favors the flow of gastric juice up into the thoracic esophagus when upright. The gradient diminishes in the supine position. Third, the LES pressure in normal subjects is significantly higher in the supine position than in the upright position. This is due to the apposition of the hydrostatic pressure of the abdomen to the abdominal portion of the sphincter when supine. In the upright position, the abdominal pressure surrounding the sphincter is negative compared with atmospheric pressure, and as expected, the abdominal pressure gradually increases the more caudally it is measured. This pressure gradient tends to move the gastric contents toward the cardia and encourages the occurrence of reflux into the esophagus when the individual is upright. By contrast, in the supine position the gastroesophageal pressure gradient diminishes, and the abdominal hydrostatic pressure under the diaphragm increases, causing an increase in sphincter pressure and a more competent cardia.

The LES has intrinsic myogenic tone, which is modulated by neural and hormonal mechanisms. Alpha-adrenergic neurotransmitters or beta blockers stimulate the LES, and alpha blockers and beta stimulants decrease its pressure. It is not clear to what extent cholinergic nerve activity controls LES pressure. The vagus nerve carries both excitatory and inhibitory fibers to the esophagus and sphincter. The hormones gastrin and motilin have been shown to increase LES pressure; and cholecystokinin, estrogen, glucagon, progesterone, somatostatin, and secretin decrease LES pressure. The peptides bombesin, l-enkephalin, and substance P increase LES pressure; and calcitonin gene-related peptide, gastric inhibitory peptide, neuropeptide Y, and vasoactive intestinal polypeptide decrease LES pressure. Some pharmacologic agents such as antacids, cholinergics, agonists, domperidone, metoclopramide, and prostaglandin F_2 are known to increase LES pressure; and anticholinergics, barbiturates, calcium channel blockers, caffeine, diazepam, dopamine, meperidine, prostaglandin E_1 and E_2, and theophylline decrease LES pressure. Peppermint, chocolate, coffee, ethanol, and fat are all associated with decreased LES pressure and may be responsible for esophageal symptoms after a sumptuous meal.

ASSESSMENT OF ESOPHAGEAL FUNCTION

A thorough understanding of the patient's underlying anatomic and functional deficits prior to making therapeutic decisions is fundamental to the successful treatment of esophageal disease. The diagnostic tests as presently employed may be divided into five broad groups: (1) tests to detect structural abnormalities of the esophagus; (2) tests to detect functional abnormalities of the esophagus; (3) tests to detect increased esophageal exposure to gastric juice; (4) tests to provoke esophageal symptoms; and (5) tests of duodenogastric function as they relate to esophageal disease.

Tests to Detect Structural Abnormalities

Radiographic Evaluation

The first diagnostic test in patients with suspected esophageal disease should be a barium swallow including a full assessment of the stomach and duodenum. Esophageal motility is optimally assessed by observing several individual swallows of barium traversing the entire length of the organ, with the patient in the horizontal position. Hiatal hernias are best demonstrated with the patient prone because the increased intra-abdominal pressure produced in this position promotes displacement of the esophagogastric junction above the diaphragm. To detect lower esophageal narrowing, such as rings and strictures, fully distended views of the esophagogastric region are crucial. The density of the barium used to study the esophagus can potentially affect the accuracy of the examination. Esophageal disorders shown clearly by a full-column technique include circumferential carcinomas, peptic strictures, large esophageal ulcers, and hiatal hernias. A small hiatal hernia is usually not associated with significant symptoms or illness, and its presence is an irrelevant finding unless the hiatal hernia is large (Fig. 24-17), the hiatal opening is narrow and interrupts the flow of barium into the stomach (Fig. 24-18), or the hernia is of the paraesophageal variety. Lesions extrinsic but adjacent to the esophagus can be reliably detected by the full-column technique if they contact the distended esophageal wall. Conversely, a number of important disorders may go undetected if this is the sole technique used to examine the esophagus. These include small esophageal neoplasms, mild esophagitis, and esophageal varices. Thus, the full-column technique should be supplemented with mucosal relief or double-contrast films to enhance detection of these smaller or more subtle lesions.

Motion-recording techniques greatly aid in evaluating functional disorders of the pharyngoesophageal and esophageal phases of swallowing. The technique and indications for cine- and videoradiography will be discussed later, as it is more useful to evaluate function and seldom used to detect structural abnormalities.

The radiographic assessment of the esophagus is not complete unless the entire stomach and duodenum have been examined. A gastric or duodenal ulcer, partially obstructing gastric neoplasm, or scarred duodenum and pylorus may contribute significantly to symptoms otherwise attributable to an esophageal abnormality.

When a patient's complaints include dysphagia and no obstructing lesion is seen on the barium swallow, it is useful to have the patient swallow a barium-impregnated marshmallow, a barium-soaked piece of bread, or a hamburger mixed with barium. This test may bring out a functional disturbance in esophageal transport that can be missed when liquid barium is used.

Endoscopic Evaluation

In any patient complaining of dysphagia, esophagoscopy is indicated, even in the face of a normal radiographic study. A barium

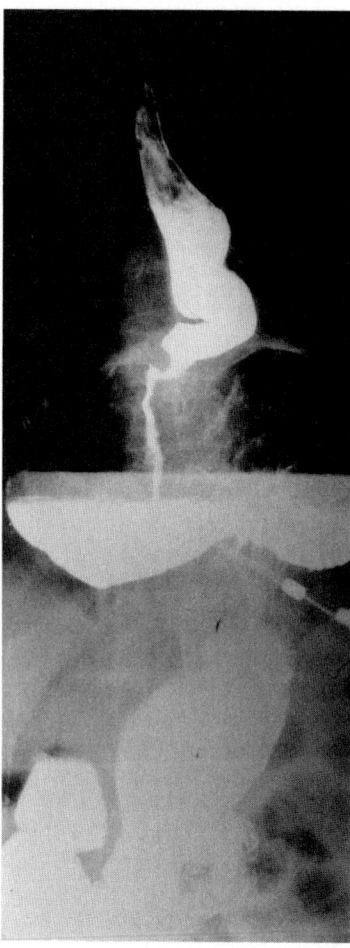

FIG. 24-17. Radiogram of an intrathoracic stomach. This is the end stage of a large hiatal hernia, regardless of its initial classification. *[Reproduced with permission from DeMeester TR, Stein HJ, Fuchs KH: Physiologic diagnostic studies, in Zuidema GD, Orringer MB (eds): Shackelford's Surgery of the Alimentary Tract, 3rd ed, Vol. I. Philadelphia: WB Saunders, 1991, p 111.]*

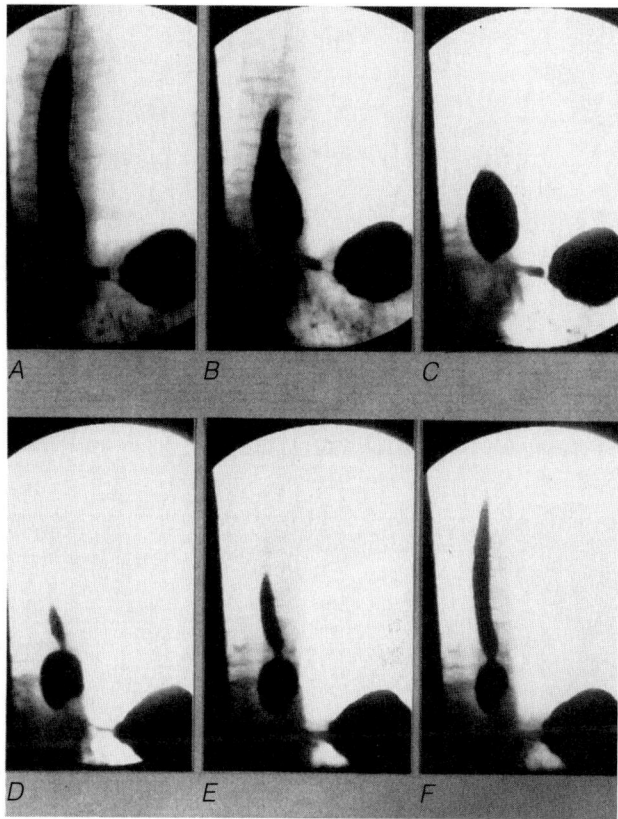

FIG. 24-18. Radiographic barium study showing a primary esophageal wave propelling liquid barium into the supradiaphragmatic portion of the stomach in a patient with a hiatal hernia (*A* and *B*). The diaphragmatic impingement on the stomach and the lack of contraction of the supradiaphragmatic stomach prevent passage of the bolus into the distal stomach (*C*). As a consequence, the contents in the supradiaphragmatic portion of the stomach are regurgitated into the thoracic esophagus (*D*, *E*, and *F*). The patient experiences dysphagia and regurgitation. On endoscopy, no anatomic abnormality other than a hiatal hernia was found, and on 24-hour pH monitoring, the patient had normal esophageal acid exposure. Symptoms of dysphagia and regurgitation were relieved by hiatal herniorrhaphy. *(Reproduced with permission from Kaul BJ, DeMeester TR, Oka M, et al: The cause of dysphagia in uncomplicated sliding hiatal hernia and its relief by hiatal herniorrhaphy. A roentgenographic, manometric, and clinical study. Ann Surg 211:409, 1990.)*

study obtained prior to esophagoscopy is helpful to the endoscopist by directing attention to locations of subtle change, and alerting the examiner to such potential danger spots as a cervical vertebral osteophyte, esophageal diverticulum, a deeply penetrating ulcer, or a carcinoma. Regardless of the radiologist's interpretation of an abnormal finding, each structural abnormality of the esophagus should be confirmed visually.

For the initial endoscopic assessment, the flexible fiberoptic esophagoscope is the instrument of choice because of its technical ease, patient acceptance, and the ability to simultaneously assess the stomach and duodenum. Rigid endoscopy may be required in specific instances and should be part of the armamentarium of the endoscopist. The rigid esophagoscope may be an essential instrument when deeper biopsies are required or the cricopharyngeus and cervical esophagus need closer assessment.

When gastroesophageal reflux disease is the suspected diagnosis, particular attention should be paid to detecting the presence of esophagitis and Barrett's columnar-lined esophagus. When endoscopic esophagitis is seen, severity and the length of esophagus involved are recorded. Grade I esophagitis is defined as small, circular, nonconfluent erosions. Grade II esophagitis is defined by the presence of linear erosions lined with granulation tissue that bleeds easily when touched. Grade III esophagitis represents a more

advanced stage, in which the linear or circular erosions coalesce into circumferential loss of the epithelium, or the appearance of islands of epithelium which on endoscopy appears as a "cobblestone" esophagus. Grade IV esophagitis is the presence of a stricture. Its severity can be assessed by the ease of passing a 36F endoscope. When a stricture is observed, the severity of the esophagitis above it should be recorded. The absence of esophagitis above a stricture suggests a chemical-induced injury or a neoplasm as a cause. The latter should always be considered and is ruled out only by evaluation of a tissue biopsy of adequate size.

Barrett's esophagus is a condition in which the tubular esophagus is lined with columnar epithelium, as opposed to the normal squamous epithelium. Histologically it appears as intestinal metaplasia. It is suspected at endoscopy when there is difficulty in visualizing the squamocolumnar junction at its normal location, and by the appearance of a redder, more luxuriant mucosa than is normally seen in the lower esophagus. Its presence is confirmed by biopsy. Multiple biopsies should be taken in a cephalad direction to determine the

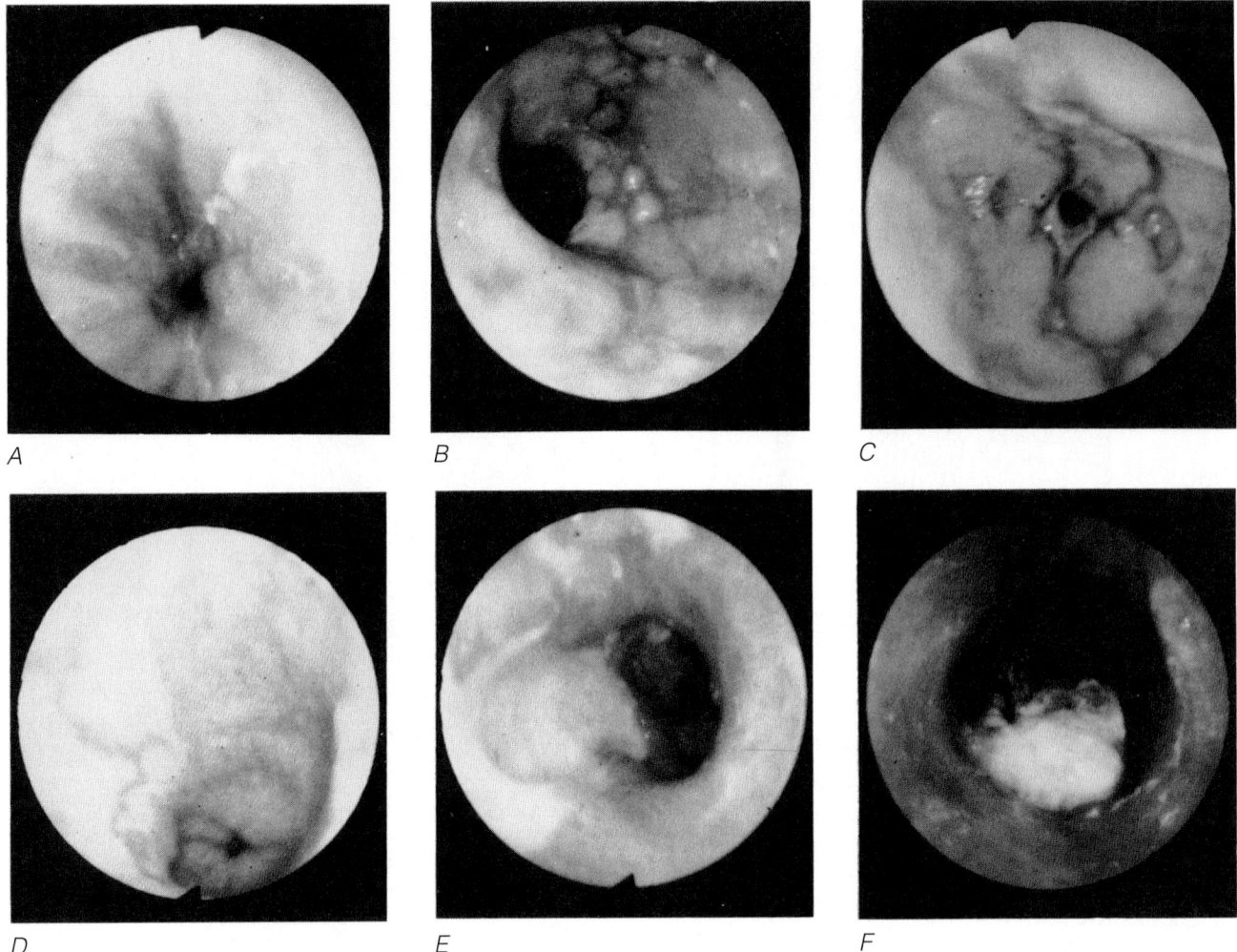

FIG. 24-19. Complications of reflux disease as seen on endoscopy. *A*. Linear erosion of grade II esophagitis. *B*. Cobblestone mucosa of grade III esophagitis. *C*. Stricture associated with grade III esophagitis. *D*. Uncomplicated Barrett's mucosa. *E*. Large ulcer in Barrett's mucosa. *F*. Adenocarcinoma arising in Barrett's mucosa.

level at which the junction of Barrett's epithelium with normal squamous mucosa occurs. Barrett's esophagus is susceptible to ulceration, bleeding, stricture formation, and most important, malignant degeneration. The earliest sign of the latter is severe dysplasia or intramucosal adenocarcinoma (Fig. 24-19). These dysplastic changes have a patchy distribution, so a minimum of four biopsy samples spaced 2 cm apart should be taken from the Barrett's-lined portion of the esophagus. Changes seen in one biopsy are significant. Nishimaki has determined that the tumors occur in an area of specialized columnar epithelium near the squamocolumnar junction in 85% of patients, and within 2 cm of the squamocolumnar junction in virtually all patients. Particular attention should be focused in this area in patients suspected of harboring a carcinoma.

Abnormalities of the gastroesophageal flap valve can be visualized by retroflexion of the endoscope. Hill has graded the appearance of the gastroesophageal valve from I to IV according to the degree of unfolding or deterioration of the normal valve architecture (Fig. 24-20). The appearance of the valve correlates with the presence of increased esophageal acid exposure, occurring predominantly in patients with grade III and IV valves.

A hiatal hernia is endoscopically confirmed by finding a pouch lined with gastric rugal folds lying 2 cm or more above the

margins of the diaphragmatic crura, identified by having the patient sniff. A prominent sliding hiatal hernia frequently is associated with increased esophageal exposure to gastric juice. When a paraesophageal hernia is observed, particular attention is taken to exclude a gastric ulcer or gastritis within the pouch. The intragastric retroflex or J maneuver is important in evaluating the full circumference of the mucosal lining of the herniated stomach.

When an esophageal diverticulum is seen, it should be carefully explored with the flexible endoscope to exclude ulceration or neoplasia. When a submucosal mass is identified, biopsies are usually not performed. Normally a submucosal leiomyoma or reduplication cyst can be easily dissected away from the intact mucosa, but if a biopsy sample is taken, the mucosa may become fixed to the underlying abnormality. This complicates the surgical dissection by increasing the risk of mucosal perforation.

Tests to Detect Functional Abnormalities

In many patients with symptoms of an esophageal disorder, standard radiographic and endoscopic evaluation fails to demonstrate a structural abnormality. In these situations, esophageal function tests are necessary to identify a functional disorder.

Stationary Manometry

Esophageal manometry is a widely used technique to examine the motor function of the esophagus and its sphincters. Manometry is indicated whenever a motor abnormality of the esophagus is suspected on the basis of complaints of dysphagia, odynophagia, or noncardiac chest pain, and the barium swallow or endoscopy does not show a clear structural abnormality. Esophageal manometry is particularly necessary to confirm the diagnosis of specific primary esophageal motility disorders (i.e., achalasia, diffuse esophageal

FIG. 24-20. *A.* Grade I flap valve appearance. Note the ridge of tissue which is closely approximated to the shaft of the retroflexed endoscope. It extends 3 to 4 cm along the lesser curve. *B.* Grade II flap valve appearance. The ridge is slightly less well defined than in grade I, and it opens rarely with respiration and closes promptly. *C.* Grade III flap valve appearance. The ridge is barely present, and there is often failure to close around the endoscope. It is nearly always accompanied by a hiatal hernia. *D.* Grade IV flap valve appearance. There is no muscular ridge at all. The gastroesophageal valve stays open all the time, and squamous epithelium can often be seen from the retroflexed position. A hiatal hernia is always present. (*Reproduced with permission from Hill LD, Kozarek RA, Kraemer SJ, et al: The gastroesophageal flap valve. In vitro and in vivo observations. Gastrointest Endosc 44:541, 1996.*) (*Continued*)

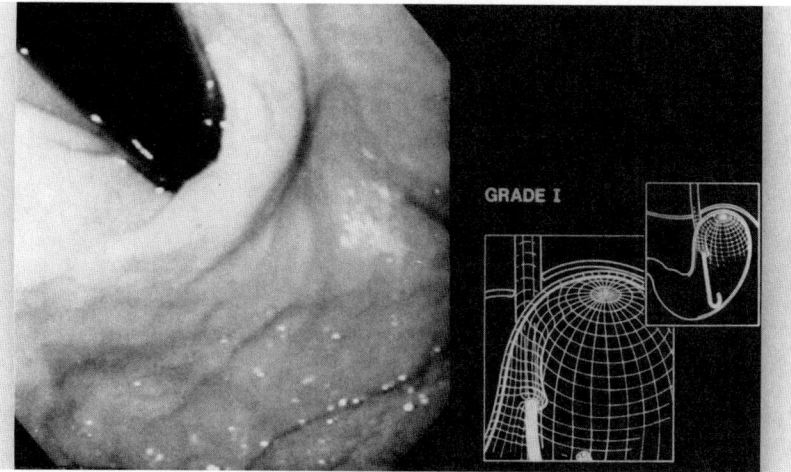

A

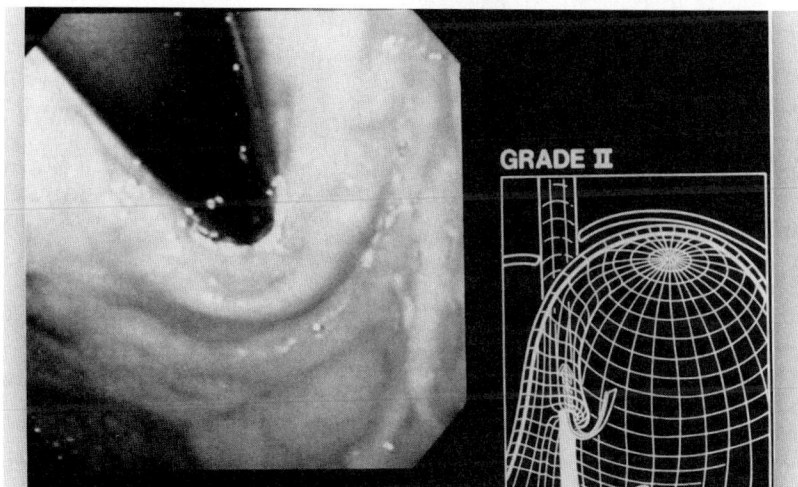

B

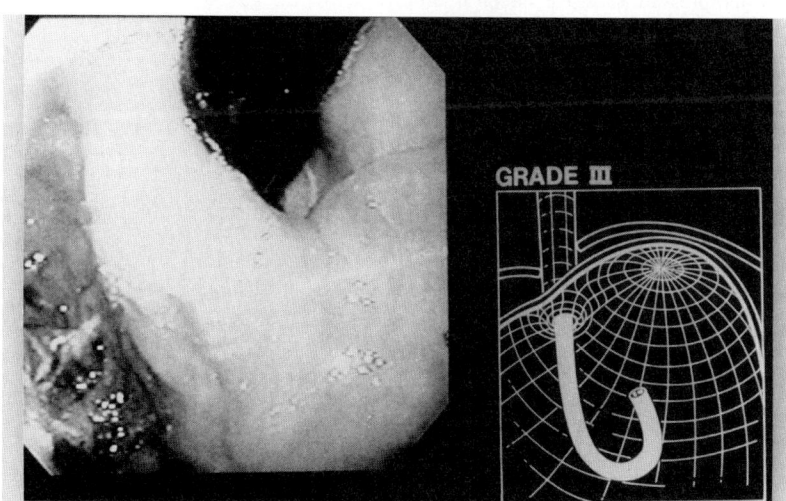

C

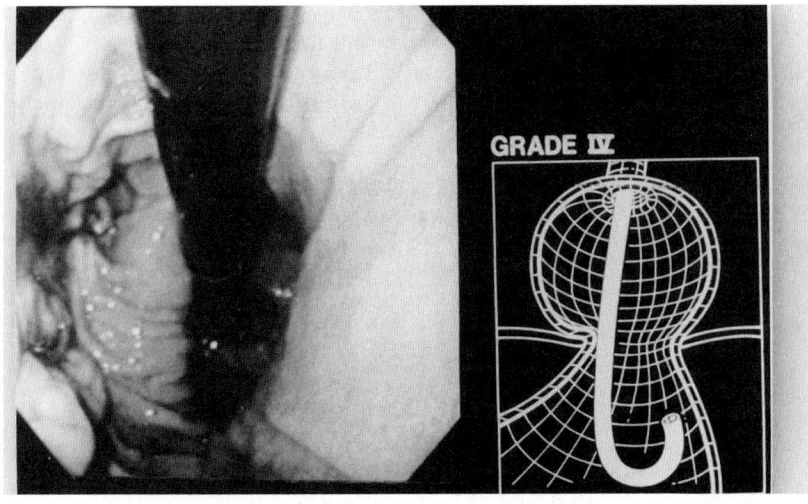

D

FIG. 24-20. (*continued*)

spasm, nutcracker esophagus, and hypertensive LES). It also identifies nonspecific esophageal motility abnormalities and motility disorders secondary to systemic disease such as scleroderma, dermatomyositis, polymyositis, or mixed connective tissue disease. In patients with symptomatic gastroesophageal reflux disease, manometry of the esophageal body can identify a mechanically defective LES, and evaluate the adequacy of esophageal peristalsis and contraction amplitude. Manometry has become an essential tool in the preoperative evaluation of patients prior to antireflux surgery, allowing selection of the appropriate procedure based upon the patient's underlying esophageal function.

Esophageal manometry is performed using electronic pressure-sensitive transducers located within the catheter, or water-perfused catheters with lateral side holes attached to transducers outside the body. The catheter usually consists of a train of five pressure transducers or five or more water-perfused tubes bound together. The transducers or lateral openings are placed at 5-cm intervals from the tip and oriented radially at 72° from each other around the circumference of the catheter. A special catheter assembly consisting of four lateral openings at the same level, oriented at 90° to each other, is of special use in measuring the three-dimensional vector volume of the LES. Other specially designed catheters can be used to assess the upper sphincter.

As the pressure-sensitive station is brought across the gastroesophageal junction, a rise in pressure above the gastric baseline signals the beginning of the LES. The respiratory inversion point is identified when the positive excursions that occur in the abdominal cavity with breathing change to negative deflections in the thorax. The respiratory inversion point serves as a reference point at which the amplitude of LES pressure and the length of the sphincter exposed to abdominal pressure are measured. As the pressure-sensitive station is withdrawn into the body of the esophagus, the upper border of the LES is identified by the drop in pressure to the esophageal baseline. From these measurements the pressure, abdominal length, and overall length of the sphincter are determined (Fig. 24-21). To account for the asymmetry of the sphincter (Fig. 24-22), the pressure profile is repeated with each of the five radially oriented transducers, and the average values for sphincter pressure above gastric baseline, overall sphincter length, and abdominal length of the sphincter are calculated.

Table 24-1 shows the values for these parameters in 50 normal volunteers without subjective or objective evidence of a foregut

disorder. The level at which a deficiency in the mechanics of the LES occurs was defined by comparing the frequency distribution of these values in the 50 healthy volunteers with a population of similarly studied patients with symptoms of gastroesophageal reflux disease. The presence of increased esophageal exposure to gastric juice was documented by 24-hour esophageal pH monitoring. Based on these studies, a mechanically defective sphincter is identified by having one or more of the following characteristics: an average LES pressure of less than 6 mm Hg, an average length exposed to the positive-pressure environment in the abdomen of 1 cm or less, and/or an average overall sphincter length of 2 cm or less. Compared with the normal volunteers, these values are below the 2.5 percentile for sphincter pressure and overall length and for abdominal length. It has been shown that the resistance of the sphincter to reflux of gastric juice is determined by the integrated effects of radial pressures extended over the entire length, resulting in three-dimensional computerized imaging of sphincter pressures. Calculating the volume of this image reflects the sphincter's resistance and is called the sphincter pressure vector volume (SPVV) (Fig. 24-23). A calculated SPVV less than the fifth percentile is an indication of a mechanically defective sphincter.

In a study of 50 normal volunteers and 150 patients with increased esophageal exposure to gastric juice and various degrees of esophageal mucosal injury, the calculation of the SPVV

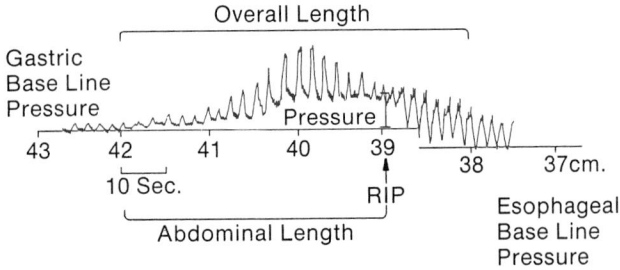

RIP = Respiratory Inversion Point

FIG. 24-21. Manometric pressure profile of the LES. The distances are measured from the nares. (*Reproduced with permission from Zaninotto G, DeMeester TR, Schwizer W, et al: The lower esophageal sphincter in health and disease. Am J Surg 155:104, 1988.*)

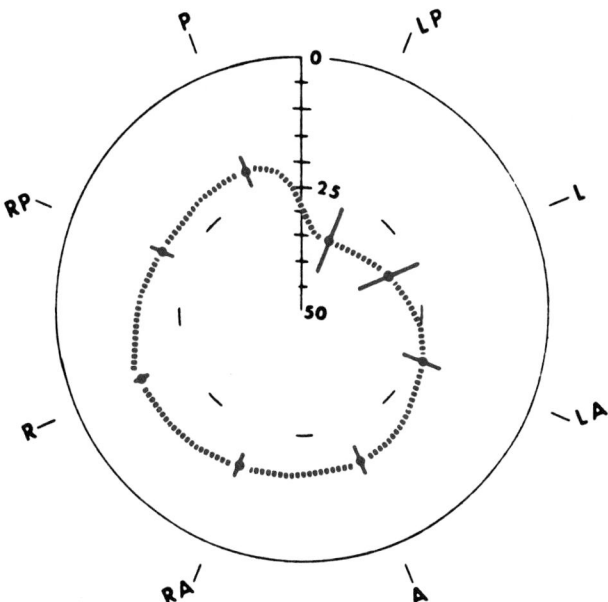

FIG. 24-22. Radial configuration of the LES. A = anterior; L = left; LA = left anterior; LP = left posterior; P = posterior; R = right; RA = right anterior; RP = right posterior. (*Reproduced with permission from Winans CS: Manometric asymmetry of the lower esophageal high pressure zone. Dig Dis Sci 22:348, 1977.*)

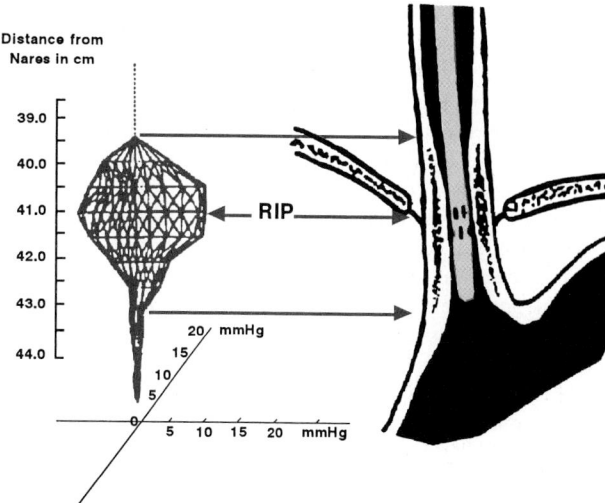

FIG. 24-23. Computerized three-dimensional imaging of the LES. A catheter with four to eight radial side holes is withdrawn through the gastroesophageal junction. For each level of the pullback, the radially measured pressures are plotted around an axis representing gastric baseline pressure. When a stepwise pullback technique is used, the respiratory inversion point (RIP) can be identified. (*Reproduced with permission from Stein HJ, DeMeester TR, Naspetti R, et al: Three-dimensional imaging of the lower esophageal sphincter in gastroesophageal reflux disease. Ann Surg 214:374, 1991.*)

increased the ability of manometry to identify a mechanically defective sphincter, compared with standard techniques (Fig. 24-24). This was particularly so in patients without mucosal injury and borderline sphincter abnormalities. Therefore, three-dimensional LES manometry and calculation of the vector volume should become the standard technique to assess the barrier function of the LES in patients with gastroesophageal reflux disease. Patients with gastroesophageal reflux disease and an SPVV below the fifth percentile of normal, or a deficiency of one, two, or all three mechanical components of an LES on standard manometry, have a mechanical defect of their antireflux barrier that a surgical antireflux procedure is designed to correct.

To assess the relaxation and postrelaxation contraction of the LES, a pressure transducer is positioned within the high-pressure zone, with the distal transducer located in the stomach and the proximal transducer within the esophageal body. Ten wet swallows (5 mL

water each) are performed. The normal pressure of the LES should drop to the level of gastric pressure during each wet swallow.

The function of the esophageal body is assessed with the five pressure transducers located in the esophagus. The standard procedure is to locate the most proximal pressure transducer 1 cm below the well-defined cricopharyngeal sphincter, allowing a pressure response throughout the whole esophagus to be obtained on one swallow. Ten wet swallows are recorded. Amplitude, duration, and morphology of contractions following each swallow are calculated at all recorded levels of the esophageal body. The delay between the onset or peak of esophageal contractions at the various levels of the esophagus is used to calculate the speed of wave propagation.

Table 24-1
Normal Manometric Values of the Distal Esophageal Sphincter, n = 50

		Percentile	
	Median	*2.5*	*97.5*
Pressure (mm Hg)	13	5.8	27.7
Overall length (cm)	3.6	2.1	5.6
Abdominal length (cm)	2	0.9	4.7
	Mean	*Mean −2 SD*	*Mean +2 SD*
Pressure (mm Hg)	13.8 ± 4.6	4.6	23.0
Overall length (cm)	3.7 ± 0.8	2.1	5.3
Abdominal length (cm)	2.2 ± 0.8	0.6	3.8

SOURCE: Reproduced with permission from DeMeester TR, Stein HJ: Gastroesophageal reflux disease, in Moody FG, Carey LC, et al (eds): *Surgical Treatment of Digestive Disease.* Chicago: Year Book Medical, 1990, p 89.

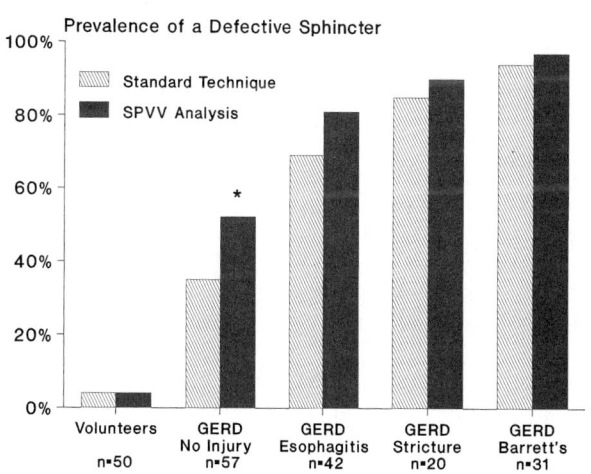

FIG. 24-24. Comparison of standard manometric techniques and SPVV analysis in the identification of a mechanically defective LES. * $p < 0.05$ vs. standard manometry. (*Reproduced with permission from Stein HJ, DeMeester TR, Naspetti R, et al: Three-dimensional imaging of the lower esophageal sphincter in gastroesophageal reflux disease. Ann Surg 214:374, 1991.*)

The relationship of the esophageal contractions following a swallow is classified as peristaltic or simultaneous. The data are used to identify motor disorders of the esophagus.

The position, length, and pressure of the cricopharyngeal sphincter are assessed with a stationary pull-through technique similar to that used for the LES. The manometric catheter is withdrawn in 0.5-cm intervals from the upper esophagus through the upper esophageal sphincter region into the pharynx. The relaxation of the upper esophageal sphincter is studied by straddling the eight pressure transducers across the sphincter so that some are in the pharynx and some are in the upper esophagus. High-speed graphic recordings (50 mm/s) are necessary to obtain an assessment of the coordination of cricopharyngeal relaxation with hypopharyngeal contraction. It has been difficult to consistently demonstrate a motility abnormality in patients with pharyngoesophageal disorders.

24-Hour Ambulatory Manometry

The development of miniaturized electronic pressure transducers and portable digital data recorders with large storage capacity has made ambulatory monitoring of esophageal motor function over an entire circadian cycle possible. The broad clinical application of this new technology in a large number of asymptomatic normal volunteers and patients with primary esophageal motor disorders or gastroesophageal reflux disease provides new insights into esophageal motor function in health and disease under a variety of physiologic conditions. In both normal volunteers and symptomatic patients, esophageal motor activity increases with the state of consciousness and focus on eating activity (i.e., from the supine, to the upright, to meal periods). In the normal situation, there is a higher prevalence of nonperistaltic contractions than appreciated on stationary manometry.

Compared with standard manometry, ambulatory esophageal manometry provides a more than 100 times larger database for the classification and quantification of abnormal esophageal motor function, and leads to a change in the diagnosis in a substantial portion of patients with symptoms suggestive of a primary esophageal motor disorder (Fig. 24-25). In patients with nonobstructive dysphagia, the circadian esophageal motor pattern is characterized by an inability to organize the motor activity into peristaltic contractions during a meal period (Fig. 24-26). This finding can be used to provide a new classification of motility disorders on the basis of when

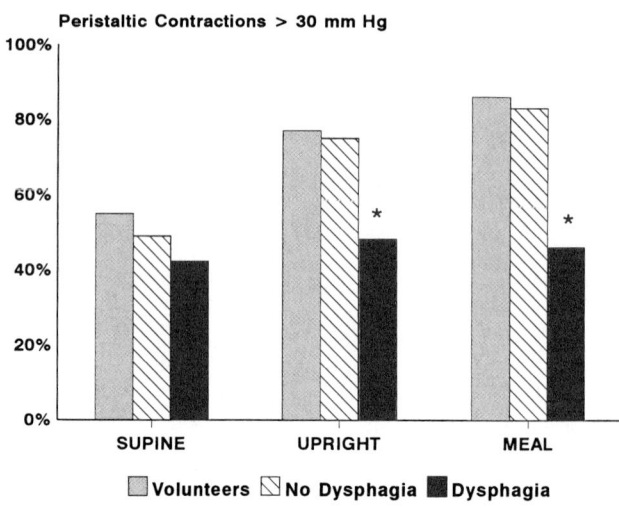

Peristaltic Contractions > 30 mm Hg

■ Volunteers ◫ No Dysphagia ■ Dysphagia

*: p < 0.01 vs "Volunteers" and "No Dysphagia"

FIG. 24-26. Frequency of peristaltic contractions with an amplitude <30 mm Hg during supine, upright, and meal periods, showing that patients with nonobstructive dysphagia are unable to organize their esophageal contractions with increasing states of awareness, from sleep (supine) to alertness (upright) to focus on eating (meals). *(Reproduced with permission from Stein HJ, DeMeester TR: Indications, technique, and clinical use of ambulatory 24-hour esophageal motility monitoring in a surgical practice. Ann Surg 217:128, 1993.)*

they may give rise to dysphagia (Fig. 24-27). In patients with noncardiac chest pain, ambulatory motility monitoring can document a direct correlation of abnormal esophageal motor activity with the symptom, and shows that the abnormal motor activity immediately preceding the pain episodes is characterized by an increased frequency of simultaneous double- and triple-peaked, high-amplitude long contractions. Ambulatory motility monitoring of patients with gastroesophageal reflux disease shows that the contractility of the esophageal body in these patients deteriorates with increasing severity of esophageal mucosal injury, compromising the clearance function of the esophageal body. Ambulatory esophageal

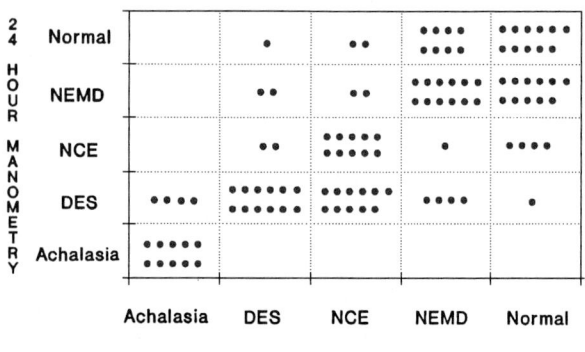

STANDARD MANOMETRY

FIG. 24-25. Classification of esophageal motility disorders on standard and ambulatory 24-hour manometry in 78 patients. DES = diffuse esophageal spasm; NCE = nutcracker esophagus; NEMD = nonspecific esophageal motility disorders. *[Reproduced with permission from DeMeester TR, Stein HJ: Surgery for esophageal motor disorders, in Castell DO (ed): The Esophagus. Boston: Little, Brown, 1992, p 412.]*

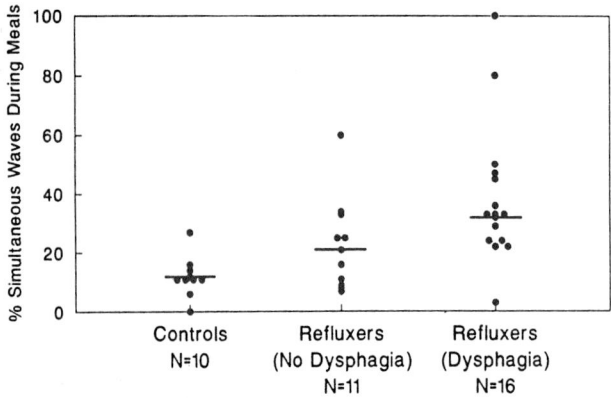

FIG. 24-27. Scattergram showing individual patient data for percentage of simultaneous waves during the meal periods in normal subjects and in patients. The bar denotes the median value for each group, with a significant difference between patients with reflux and dysphagia and the other groups. p < 0.05. *(Reproduced with permission from Singh S, Stein HJ, DeMeester TR, Hinder RA: Nonobstructive dysphagia in gastroesophageal reflux disease: A study with combined ambulatory pH and motility monitoring. Am J Gastroenterol 87:562, 1992.)*

manometry will replace standard manometry in the assessment of esophageal body function, and has the potential to improve the diagnosis and management of patients with esophageal motor abnormalities. The combination of ambulatory 24-hour esophageal manometry with esophageal and gastric pH monitoring is currently the most physiologic way to assess patients with foregut motility disorders.

Esophageal Impedance

New technology recently introduced into the clinical realm allows measurement of esophageal function and gastroesophageal reflux in a way that has heretofore not been possible. An intraluminal electrical impedance catheter has recently been developed for the measurement of gastrointestinal function. *Impedance* is the ratio of voltage to current, and is a measure of the electrical conductivity of a hollow organ and its contents. Intraluminal electrical impedance is inversely proportional to the electrical conductivity of the luminal contents and the cross-sectional area of the lumen. Air has a very low electrical conductivity and therefore high impedance. Saliva and food cause an impedance decrease because of their increased conductivity. Luminal dilatation results in a decrease in impedance, whereas luminal contraction yields an impedance increase. Investigators to date have established the impedance waveform characteristics that define esophageal bolus transport. This allows for the characterization of both esophageal function, via quantification of bolus transport, and gastroesophageal reflux. The probe measures impedance between adjacent electrodes, with measuring segments located at 2, 4, 6, 8, 14, and 16 cm from the distal tip. An extremely low electric current of 0.00025 microwatts is transmitted across the electrodes at a frequency of 1 to 2 kHz and is limited to 8 microamperes. This is below the stimulation threshold for nerves and muscles, and is three orders of magnitude below the threshold of cardiac stimulation. A standard pH electrode is located 5 cm from the distal tip.

Esophageal impedance has been validated as an appropriate method for the evaluation of gastrointestinal function. It has been compared to cineradiography showing that impedance waves correspond well with actual bolus transport illustrated by radiography. Bolus entry, transit, and exit can be clearly identified by impedance changes in the corresponding measuring segments. Preliminary studies comparing standard esophageal manometry with impedance measurements in healthy volunteers have been performed, and have validated the ability of esophageal impedance to correlate with peristaltic wave progression and bolus length. Clinical investigators are beginning to examine and validate impedance measurement in the evaluation of esophageal and small intestinal pathophysiology. Although the use of impedance technology in the assessment of esophageal function is still early in its development, it has the potential to add considerable understanding to both normal and abnormal esophageal physiology. For example, for the first time, all episodes of gastroesophageal reflux can be detected without regard for their chemical composition. Surprisingly, recent studies using this technology have shown that in normal subjects, proton pump inhibitor (PPI) therapy does not alter the number of reflux episodes; it simply converts them to neutral pH. This observation may have important implications in the treatment of gastroesophageal reflux disease.

Esophageal Transit Scintigraphy

The esophageal transit of a 10-mL water bolus containing technetium-99m (^{99m}Tc) sulfur colloid can be recorded with a gamma camera. Using this technique, delayed bolus transit has

been shown in patients with a variety of esophageal motor disorders, including achalasia, scleroderma, diffuse esophageal spasm, and nutcracker esophagus.

Video- and Cineradiography

High-speed cinematic or video recording of radiographic studies allows re-evaluation by reviewing the studies at various speeds. This technique is more useful than manometry in the evaluation of the pharyngeal phase of swallowing. Observations suggesting oropharyngeal or cricopharyngeal dysfunction include misdirection of barium into the trachea or nasopharynx, prominence of the cricopharyngeal muscle (Fig. 24-28), a Zenker's diverticulum, a narrow pharyngoesophageal segment, and stasis of the contrast medium in the valleculae or hypopharyngeal recesses (Fig. 24-29). These findings are usually not specific, but rather common manifestations of neuromuscular disorders affecting the pharyngoesophageal area. Studies using liquid barium, barium-impregnated solids, or radiopaque pills, aid the evaluation of normal and abnormal motility in the esophageal body. Loss of the normal stripping wave or segmentation of the barium column with the patient in the recumbent position correlates with abnormal motility of the esophageal body. In

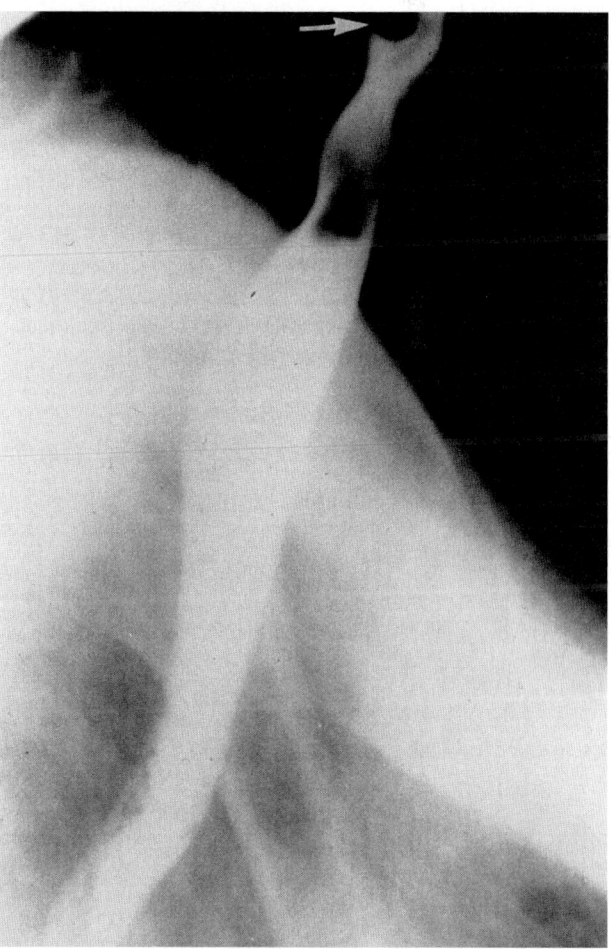

FIG. 24-28. Barium contrast radiogram of pharyngeal swallowing activity showing prominent cricopharyngeal indentation (*arrowhead*) in a patient who presented with dysphagia resulting from bulbar poliomyelitis. (*Reproduced with permission from Bonavina L, Khan NA, DeMeester TR: Pharyngoesophageal dysfunctions: The role of cricopharyngeal myotomy. Arch Surg 120:543, 1985.*)

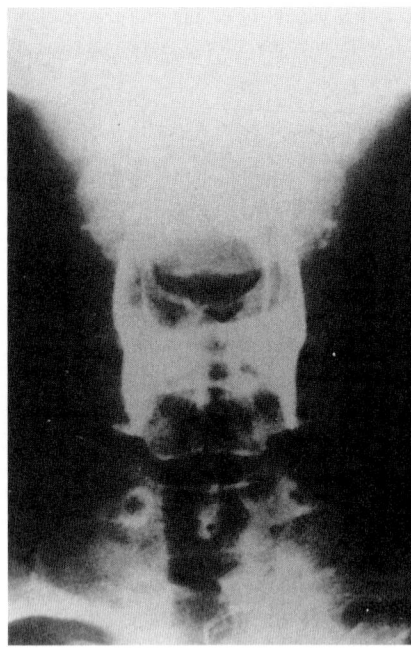
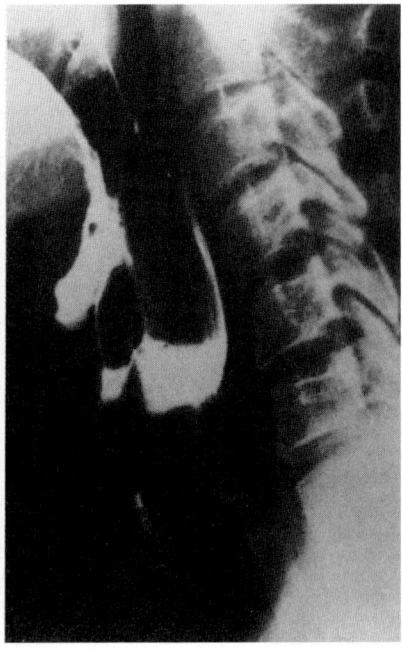

A   *B*

FIG. 24-29. *Esophagograms from a patient with cricopharyngeal achalasia. A. Anteroposterior film showing retention of the contrast medium at the level of the vallecula and piriform recesses, with no barium passing into the esophagus. B. Lateral film, taken opposite the C5–C6 vertebrae, showing posterior indentation of the cricopharyngeus, retention in the hypopharynx, and tracheal aspiration.* [Reproduced with permission from Lafontaine E: Pharyngeal dysphagia, in DeMeester TR, Matthews H (eds): International Trends in General Thoracic Surgery, Vol. 3, Benign Esophageal Disease. St. Louis: Mosby, 1987, p 345.]

addition, structural abnormalities such as small diverticula, webs, and minimal extrinsic impressions of the esophagus may be recognized only with motion-recording techniques. The simultaneous computerized capture of videofluoroscopic images and manonometric tracings is now available, and is referred to as manofluorography. Manofluorographic studies allow precise correlation of the anatomic events, such as opening of the upper esophageal sphincter, with manometric observations, such as sphincter relaxation. Manofluorography, while not widely available, is presently the best means available to evaluate complex functional abnormalities.

Tests to Detect Increased Exposure to Gastric Juice

24-Hour Ambulatory pH Monitoring

The most direct method of measuring increased esophageal exposure to gastric juice is by an indwelling pH electrode, or more recently via a radiotelemetric pH monitoring capsule that can be clipped to the esophageal mucosa. The latter consists of an antimony pH electrode fitted inside a small capsule-shaped device accompanied by a battery and electronics that allow 48-hour monitoring and transmission of the pH data via transcutaneous radio telemetry to a waist-mounted data logger. The device can be introduced either transorally or transnasally, and clipped to the esophageal mucosa utilizing endoscopic fastening techniques. It passes spontaneously within 1 to 2 weeks. Prolonged monitoring of esophageal pH is performed by placing the pH probe or telemetry capsule 5 cm above the manometrically measured upper border of the distal sphincter for 24 hours. It measures the actual time the esophageal mucosa is exposed to gastric juice, measures the ability of the esophagus to clear refluxed acid, and correlates esophageal acid exposure with the patient's symptoms. A 24- to 48-hour period is necessary so that measurements can be made over one or two complete circadian cycles. This allows measuring the effect of physiologic activity, such as eating or sleeping, on the reflux of gastric juice into the esophagus (Fig. 24-30).

The 24-hour esophageal pH monitoring should not be considered a test for reflux, but rather a measurement of the esophageal exposure to gastric juice. The measurement is expressed by the time the esophageal pH was below a given threshold during the 24-hour period. This single assessment, although concise, does not reflect how the exposure has occurred; that is, did it occur in a few long

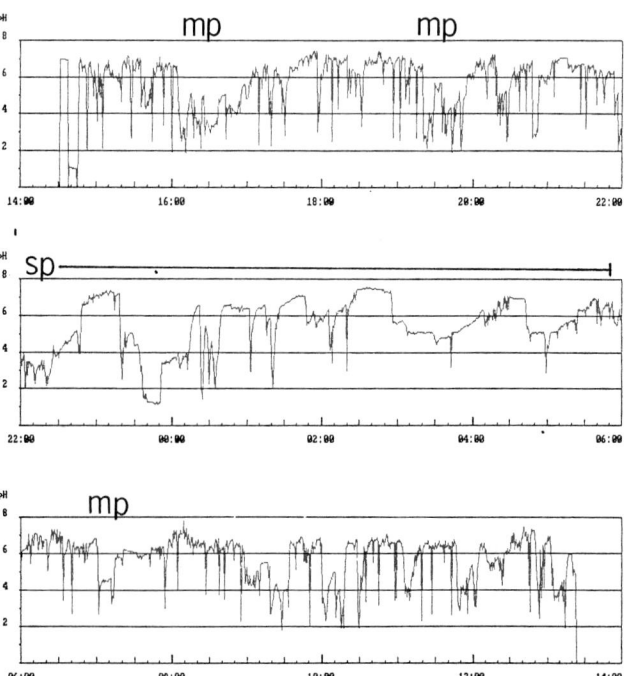

FIG. 24-30. *Strip chart display of a 24-hour esophageal pH monitoring study in a patient with increased esophageal acid exposure. mp = meal period; sp = supine period.* [Reproduced with permission from DeMeester TR, Stein HJ, Fuchs KH: Physiologic diagnostic studies, in Zuidema GD, Orringer MB (eds): Shackelford's Surgery of the Alimentary Tract, 3rd ed, Vol. I. Philadelphia: Saunders, 1991, p 119.]

Table 24-2
Normal Values for Esophageal Exposure to pH <4 (n = 50)

Component	Mean	SD	95%
Total time	1.51	1.36	4.45
Upright time	2.34	2.34	8.42
Supine time	0.63	1.0	3.45
No. of episodes	19.00	12.76	46.90
No. >5 min	0.84	1.18	3.45
Longest episode	6.74	7.85	19.80

SD = Standard deviation.

SOURCE: Reproduced with permission from DeMeester TR, Stein HJ: Gastroesophageal reflux disease, in Moody FG, Carey LC, et al (eds): *Surgical Treatment of Digestive Disease.* Chicago: Year Book Medical, 1990, p 68.

episodes or several short episodes? Consequently, two other assessments are necessary: the frequency of the reflux episodes and their duration.

The units used to express esophageal exposure to gastric juice are (1) cumulative time the esophageal pH is below a chosen threshold, expressed as the percentage of the total, upright, and supine monitored time; (2) frequency of reflux episodes below a chosen threshold, expressed as number of episodes per 24 hours; and (3) duration of the episodes, expressed as the number of episodes greater than 5 minutes per 24 hours, and the time in minutes of the longest episode recorded. Table 24-2 shows the normal values for these components of the 24-hour record at the whole-number pH threshold derived from 50 normal asymptomatic subjects. The upper limits of normal were established at the ninety-fifth percentile. Most centers use pH 4 as the threshold.

To combine the result of the six components into one expression of the overall esophageal acid exposure below a pH threshold, a pH score was calculated by using the standard deviation of the mean of each of the six components measured in the 50 normal subjects as a weighting factor. By accepting an abstract zero level 2 SD below the mean, the data measured in normal subjects could be treated as though they had a normal distribution. Thus, any measured patient value could be referenced to this zero point, and in turn be awarded points based on whether it was below or above the normal mean value for that component, according to this formula:

$$\text{Component score} = \frac{\text{Point value} - \text{mean}}{\text{SD}} + 1$$

The upper limits of normal for the composite score for each whole-number pH threshold are shown in Table 24-3.

Table 24-3
Normal Composite Score for Various pH Thresholds: Upper Level of Normal Value

pH Threshold	95th Percentile
<1	14.2
<2	17.37
<3	14.10
<4	14.72
<5	15.76
<6	12.76
>7	14.90
>8	8.50

SOURCE: Reproduced with permission from DeMeester TR, Stein HJ: Gastroesophageal reflux disease, in Moody FG, Carey LC, et al (eds): *Surgical Treatment of Digestive Disease.* Chicago: Year Book Medical, 1990, p 69.

The detection of increased esophageal exposure to acid gastric juice is more dependable than the detection of increased exposure to alkaline gastric juice. The latter is suggested by an increased alkaline exposure time above pH 7 or 8. Increased exposure in this pH range can be caused by abnormal calibration of the pH recorder; dental infection, which increases salivary pH; esophageal obstruction, which results in static pools of saliva with an increase in pH secondary to bacterial overgrowth; or regurgitation of alkaline gastric juice into the esophagus. Using a properly calibrated probe, in the absence of dental infections or esophageal obstruction, the percentage of time the pH is measured above 7 correlates with the concentration of bile acids continuously aspirated over a 24-hour period.

When done in a test population with an equal distribution of normal healthy subjects and patients with the classic reflux symptoms and a defective sphincter, 24-hour esophageal pH monitoring had a sensitivity and specificity of 96%. (*Sensitivity* is the ability to detect a disease when known to be present; *specificity* is the ability to exclude the disease when known to be absent.) This gave a predictive value of a positive and a negative test of 96%, and an overall accuracy of 96%. Based on these studies and extensive clinical experience, 24-hour esophageal pH monitoring has emerged as the gold standard for the diagnosis of gastroesophageal reflux disease.

24-Hour Ambulatory Bile Monitoring

The potentially injurious components that reflux into the esophagus include gastric secretions, such as acid and pepsin, as well as biliary and pancreatic secretions that regurgitate from the duodenum into the stomach. The presence of duodenal contents within the esophagus can now be determined via an indwelling spectrophotometric probe capable of detecting bilirubin (Fig. 24-31). Bilirubin serves as a marker for the presence of duodenal juice. Its absorbance is measured and recorded by a portable optoelectronic data logger capable of directly measuring bilirubin by spectrophotometry, based on its specific light absorption at a wavelength of 453 nm. Figure 24-32 shows the results of 24-hour ambulatory bilirubin monitoring in normal subjects compared to those with esophagitis and Barrett's esophagus. Ambulatory bilirubin monitoring can be used to identify patients who are at risk for esophageal mucosal injury, and are thus candidates for surgical antireflux treatment.

Radiographic Detection of Gastroesophageal Reflux

The definition of radiographic gastroesophageal reflux varies depending on whether reflux is spontaneous or induced by various maneuvers. In only about 40% of patients with classic symptoms of gastroesophageal reflux disease is spontaneous reflux (i.e., reflux of barium from the stomach into the esophagus with the patient in the upright position) observed by the radiologist. In most patients who show spontaneous reflux on radiography, the diagnosis of increased esophageal acid exposure is confirmed by 24-hour esophageal pH monitoring. Therefore, the radiographic demonstration of spontaneous regurgitation of barium into the esophagus in the upright position is a reliable indicator that reflux is present. Failure to see this does not indicate the absence of disease.

Tests of Duodenogastric Function

Esophageal disorders are frequently associated with abnormalities of duodenogastric function. Abnormalities of the gastric reservoir or increased gastric acid secretion can be responsible for increased esophageal exposure to gastric juice. Reflux of alkaline duodenal juice, including bile salts, pancreatic enzymes, and bicarbonate, is thought to have a role in the pathogenesis of esophagitis and

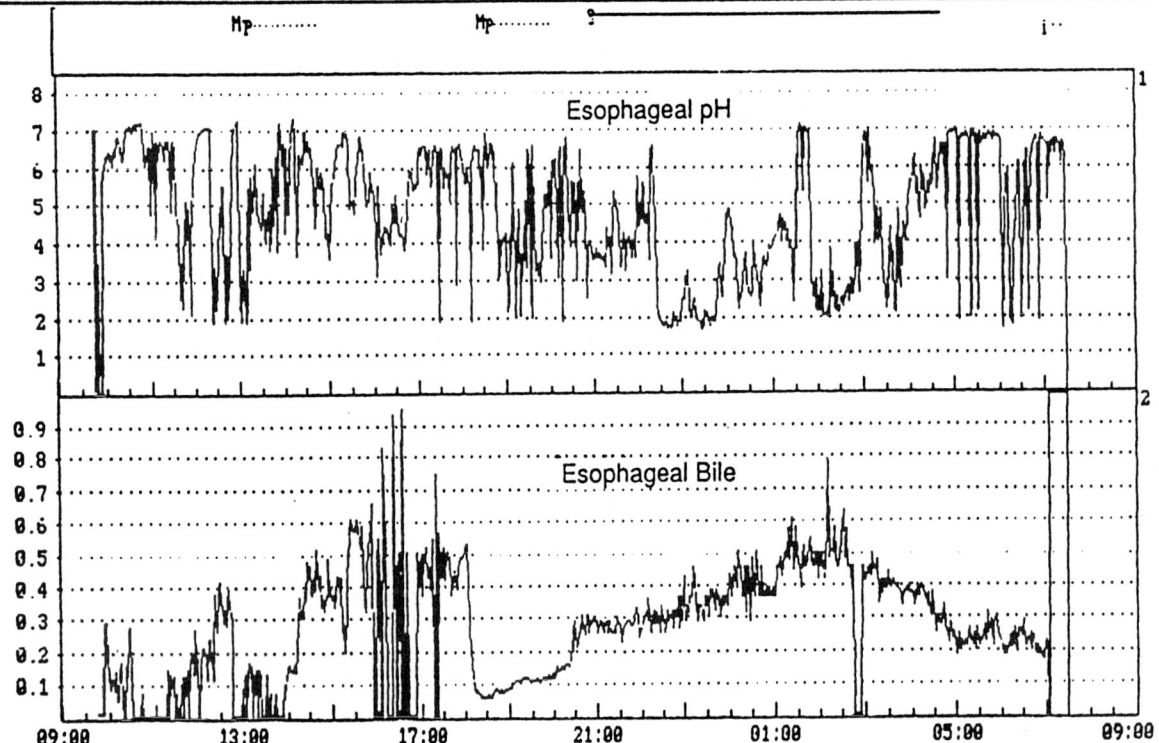

FIG. 24-31. Simultaneous 24-hour pH and bile monitoring in a young patient with gastroesophageal reflux.

complicated Barrett's esophagus. Furthermore, functional disorders of the esophagus are often not confined to the esophagus alone, but are associated with functional disorders of the rest of the foregut (i.e., stomach and duodenum). Tests of duodenogastric function that are helpful to investigate esophageal symptoms include gastric emptying studies, gastric acid analysis, and cholescintigraphy (for the diagnosis of pathologic duodenogastric reflux). The single test of

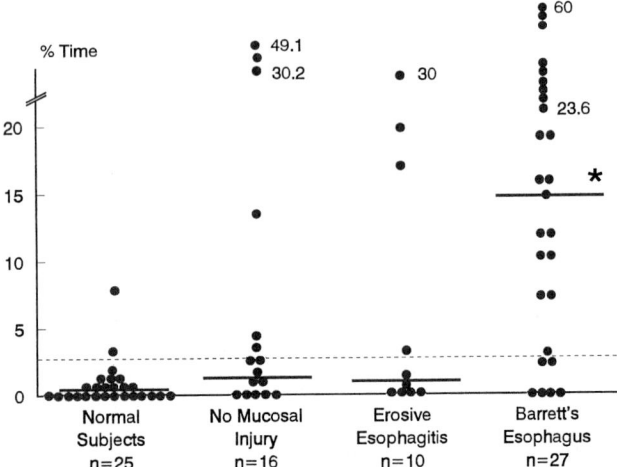

FIG. 24-32. Duration of esophageal bilirubin exposure in normal subjects and patients with gastroesophageal reflux disease with varied degrees of mucosal injury. (* $p < 0.05$ vs. all other groups). [Reproduced from Kauer WKH, Peters JH, DeMeester TR, et al: Mixed reflux of gastric and duodenal juice is more harmful to the esophagus than gastric juice alone. The need for surgical therapy re-emphasized. Ann Surg 222(4): 525–533, 1995.]

24-hour gastric pH monitoring can be used to identify gastric hypersecretion and imply the presence of duodenogastric reflux and delayed gastric emptying.

Gastric Emptying

Gastric emptying studies are performed with radionuclide-labeled meals. Emptying of solids and liquids can be assessed simultaneously when both phases are marked with different tracers. After ingestion of a labeled standard meal, gamma camera images of the stomach are obtained at 5- to 15-minute intervals for 1.5 to 2 hours. After correction for decay, the counts in the gastric area are plotted as the percentage of total counts at the start of the imaging. The resulting emptying curve can be compared with data obtained in normal volunteers. In general, normal subjects will empty 59% of a meal within 90 minutes.

Gastric Acid Analysis

The gastric secretory state is usually evaluated by determination of the titratable gastric acid in aspirated gastric juice. Interdigestive or basal gastric acid secretion is measured in the fasting state, and varies between 0 and 5 mmol/h in normal volunteers. The maximal acid secretory capacity of the stomach, which reflects the available parietal cell mass, is calculated following stimulation of gastric acid secretion with pentagastrin or histamine. Acid hypersecretors have a basal gastric acid secretory capacity of greater than 5 mmol/h and a maximal acid secretory capacity of over 30 mmol/h.

Cholescintigraphy

Scintigraphic hepatobiliary imaging is performed after intravenous injection of 5 μCi of technetium-99m iminodiacetic acid derivatives such as disofenin (^{99m}Tc-DISIDA). Gamma camera images of the upper abdomen including the gallbladder and stomach are obtained at 5-minute intervals for 60 minutes. Imaging is continued for an additional 30 minutes after stimulation of gallbladder contraction with 20 mg/kg of synthetic C-terminal octapeptide of cholecystokinin (CCK). Duodenogastric reflux is demonstrated as an increase of radioactivity in the stomach in the sequential images. The clinical value of this test is limited due to its short duration and a relatively high false-positive rate in normal volunteers.

24-Hour Gastric pH Monitoring

Monitoring is performed over a complete circadian cycle with a pH electrode placed 5 cm below the manometrically located LES. The patient is fully ambulatory during the test and is encouraged to perform normal daily activity. The gastric pH profile is assessed separately for the meal, postprandial period, and fasting period. The latter is divided into the time spent upright and supine.

The interpretation of continuous gastric pH recordings is more difficult than that of esophageal pH recordings. This is because the gastric pH environment is determined by a complex interplay of acid secretion; mucus secretion; ingested food; swallowed saliva; regurgitated duodenal, pancreatic, and biliary secretions; and the effectiveness of the mixing and evacuation of the chyme. Using 24-hour gastric pH monitoring to evaluate the gastric secretory state is based on studies that have shown that a good correlation exists between increased basal acid output on standard gastric acid analysis,

and a left shift on the frequency distribution graph of gastric pH recordings during the supine fasting period. The evaluation of gastric emptying by 24-hour gastric pH monitoring is based on studies demonstrating a good correlation between the emptying of a solid meal and the duration of the postprandial plateau and decline phase of the gastric pH record.

Using 24-hour gastric pH monitoring to evaluate duodenogastric reflux is based on the observation that reflux of alkaline duodenal juice into the stomach can alkalinize the gastric pH environment. The measurement is not straightforward because of the effect of meals, and reduction in acid secretion can result in changes in gastric pH that mimic alkaline reflux episodes. To overcome this problem, computerized measurements of the number and height of alkalinizing peaks, the baseline pH, the postprandial pH plateau, and the pattern of pH decline from the plateau can be used to identify the probability of duodenogastric reflux. The results are presented as an overall score that indicates the likelihood of pathologic duodenogastric reflux. Initial data indicate that this approach has a higher sensitivity and specificity for the diagnosis of pathologic duodenogastric reflux than scintigraphic methods do.

Combined 24-hour esophageal and gastric pH monitoring can identify excessive alkaline duodenogastric and alkaline gastroesophageal reflux in symptomatic patients. The combined tracings can often identify simultaneous gastric and esophageal alkalinization, suggesting a duodenal origin for the esophageal alkaline exposure (Fig. 24-33).

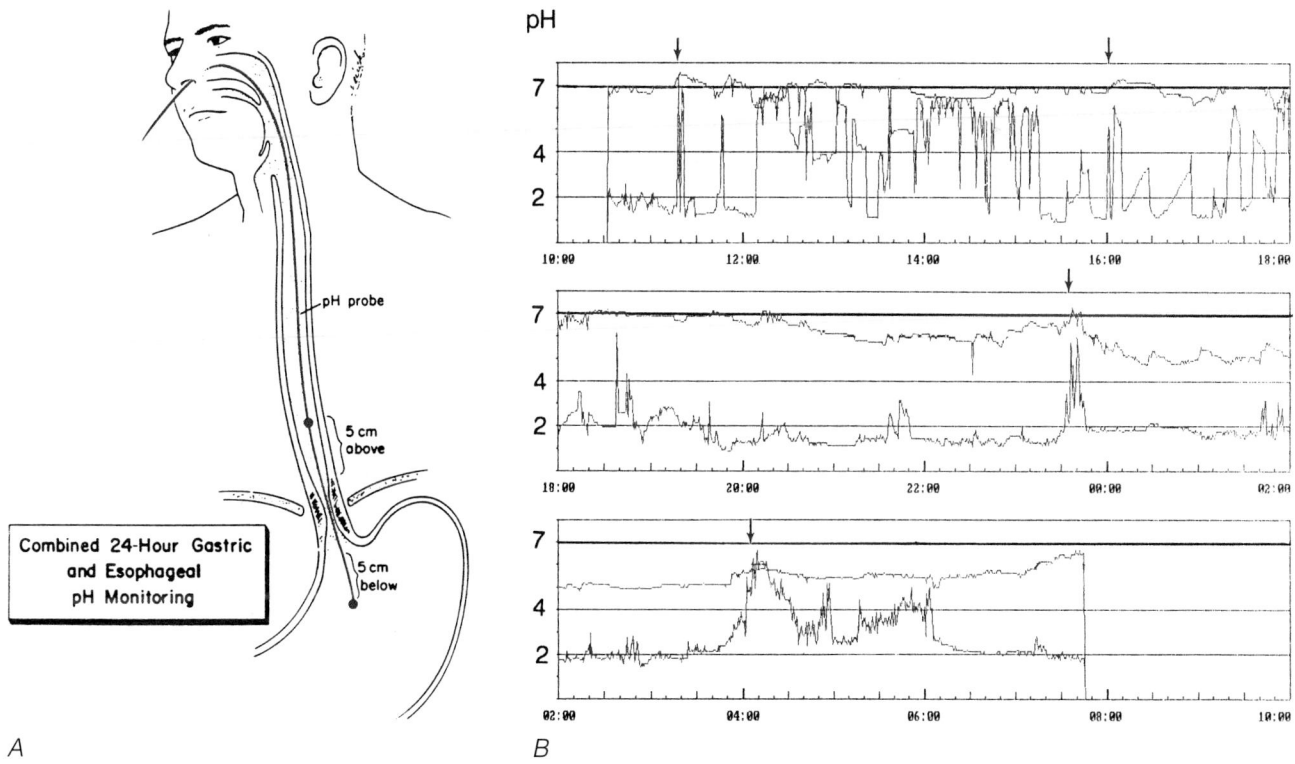

FIG. 24-33. *A.* Combined esophageal and gastric pH monitoring showing position of probes in relation to the LES. *B.* Combined ambulatory esophageal (*upper tracing*) and gastric (*lower tracing*) pH monitoring showing duodenogastric reflux (*arrows*) with propagation of the alkaline juice into the esophagus of a patient with complicated Barrett's esophagus. The gastric tracing is taken from a probe lying 5 cm below the upper esophageal sphincter. The esophageal tracing is taken from a probe lying 5 cm above the LES. Note that in only a small proportion of time does duodenogastric reflux move the pH of the esophagus above the threshold of 7, causing the iceberg effect. [*Reproduced with permission from DeMeester TR, Stein HJ, Fuchs KH: Physiologic diagnostic studies, in Zuidema GD, Orringer MB (eds): Shackelford's Surgery of the Alimentary Tract, 3rd ed, Vol. I. Philadelphia: WB Saunders, 1991, p 123.*]

24-Hour Gastric Bilirubin Monitoring

Ambulatory gastric bilirubin monitoring using the Bilitech 2000 spectrophotometic probe is now available for the detection of duodenogastric reflux, and the test may be superior to gastric pH monitoring, as it allows direct measurement of duodenal contents, rather than its inference via an alkaline pH. The probe is placed 5 cm below the LES and connected to a portable data logger, and a 24-hour ambulatory study is performed on an outpatient basis. The patient is allowed a solid diet consisting of food that does not interfere with the absorbance spectrum of bilirubin. Studies have suggested that duodenal juice is detected in the stomach of both normal subjects and patients most commonly during the supine period, and that duodenogastric reflux may be aggravated by previous cholecystectomy.

GASTROESOPHAGEAL REFLUX DISEASE

Gastroesophageal reflux disease (GERD) is a common disease that accounts for approximately 75% of esophageal pathology. Despite its high prevalence, it can be one of the most challenging diagnostic and therapeutic problems in benign esophageal disease. A contributing factor to this is the lack of a universally accepted definition of the disease.

The simplest approach is to define the disease by its symptoms. However, symptoms thought to be indicative of GERD, such as heartburn or acid regurgitation, are very common in the general population, and many individuals consider them to be normal and do not seek medical attention. Even when excessive, these symptoms are not specific for GERD, and can be caused by other diseases such as achalasia, diffuse spasm, esophageal carcinoma, pyloric stenosis, cholelithiasis, gastritis, gastric or duodenal ulcer, and coronary artery disease. In addition, patients with GERD can present with atypical symptoms, such as nausea, vomiting, postprandial fullness, chest pain, choking, chronic cough, wheezing, and hoarseness. Furthermore, bronchiolitis, recurrent pneumonia, idiopathic pulmonary fibrosis, and asthma can be primarily due to GERD. To confuse the issue more, GERD can coexist with cardiac and pulmonary disease. Thus using clinical symptoms to define GERD lacks sensitivity and specificity.

An alternative definition for GERD is the presence of endoscopic esophagitis. Using this criterion for diagnosis assumes that all patients who have esophagitis have excessive regurgitation of gastric juice into their esophagus. This is true in 90% of patients, but in 10% the esophagitis has other causes, the most common being unrecognized chemical injury from drug ingestion. In addition, the definition leaves undiagnosed those patients who have symptoms of gastroesophageal reflux but do not have endoscopic esophagitis.

A third approach to defining GERD is to measure the basic pathophysiologic abnormality of the disease; that is, increased exposure of the esophagus to gastric juice. In the past this was inferred by the presence of a hiatal hernia, later by endoscopic esophagitis, and more recently by a hypotensive LES pressure. The development of miniaturized pH electrodes and data recorders allowed measurement of esophageal exposure to gastric juice by calculating the percentage of time the pH was less than 4 over a 24-hour period. This provided an opportunity to objectively identify the presence of the disease, and stimulated a rational stepwise approach to determining the cause for the abnormal esophageal exposure to gastric juice.

The Human Antireflux Mechanism and the Pathophysiology of Gastroesophageal Reflux

The human antireflux mechanism consists of a pump, the esophageal body, and a valve, the LES. The common denominator for virtually all episodes of gastroesophageal reflux in both patients and normal subjects is the loss of the normal gastroesophageal barrier to reflux. This is usually secondary to low or reduced LES resistance. The loss of this resistance may be either permanent or transient. A structurally defective sphincter results in a permanent loss of LES resistance, and permits unhampered reflux of gastric contents into the esophagus throughout the circadian cycle. Transient loss of the gastroesophageal barrier may occur secondary to gastric abnormalities, including gastric distention with air or food, increased intragastric or intra-abdominal pressure, and delayed gastric emptying. These transient losses of sphincter resistance occur in the early stages of GERD, and are likely the mechanism for both physiologic and pathophysiologic postprandial reflux. Thus, GERD may begin in the stomach.

Data have shown that transient loss of sphincter resistance is due to gastric distention. This results in shortening of the LES, upright reflux, and inflammatory changes at the gastroesophageal junction secondary to prolapse of esophageal squamous mucosa into the gastric environment. Over time, persistent inflammation and the development of a hiatal hernia result in the permanent loss of LES function. Reflux in the supine position, erosive esophagitis, and Barrett's esophagus follow.

Several studies support the biomechanical effects of a distended stomach in the pathogenesis of GERD, and provide a mechanical explanation for why patients with a structurally normal LES may have increased esophageal acid exposure. In vivo baboon studies have shown that as gastric volume or distention increases, sphincter length decreases (Fig. 24-34). Furthermore, as the sphincter length decreases, its resting pressure, as measured by a perfused catheter, also decreases. The decrease usually occurs suddenly when an inefficient length of sphincter is reached usually between 1 and 2 cm. This phenomenon may explain how transient LES relaxations (TLESRs) are caused by gastric distention. If mechanical forces set in play by gastric distention are important in pulling open the sphincter and shortening its length, then the anatomic structure of the cardia (i.e., the presence of an acute angle of His or the dome architecture of a hiatal hernia) should influence the ease with which the sphincter was pulled open. Reflux episodes in this situation are more common after meals, when the stomach is distended.

The mechanism by which gastric distention contributes to shortening of sphincter length so that its resistance drops and reflux

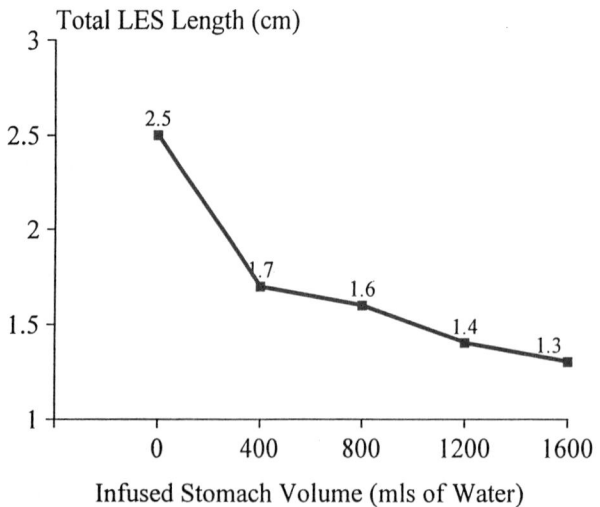

FIG. 24-34. Changes in LES length with increasing gastric volume. The data represent mean values from 10 baboons.

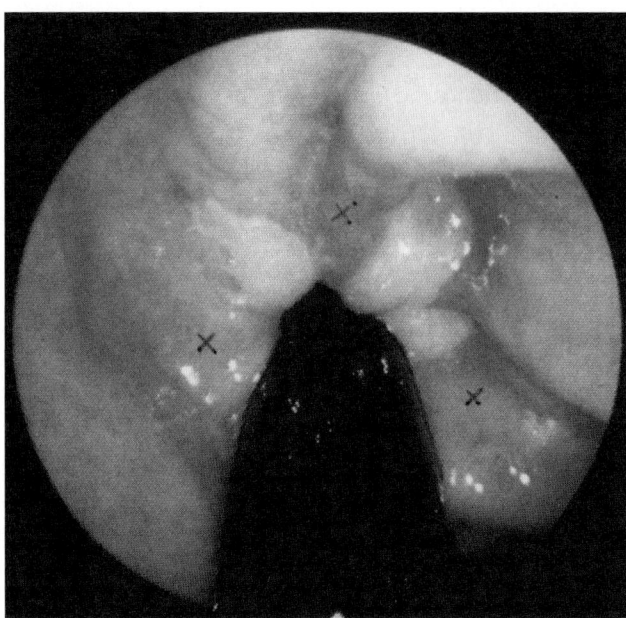

FIG. 24-35. *Endoscopic photograph illustrating prolapse of the squamous mucosa into the gastric lumen upon gastric distention. "X" marks areas of acquired cardiac epithelium following injury to squamous epithelium from gastric juice.*

occurs provides a mechanical explanation for "transient relaxations" of the LES without invoking a neuromuscular reflex. Rather than a "spontaneous" muscular relaxation, there is a mechanical shortening of the sphincter length as a consequence of gastric distention, to the point where it becomes incompetent. After gastric venting, sphincter length is restored and competence returns until distention again shortens the sphincter and encourages further venting and reflux. This sequence results in the common complaints of repetitive belching and bloating heard from patients with GERD. Gastric distention may initially occur due to overeating, stress aerophagia, or delayed gastric emptying, secondary to fatty diet or a systemic disorder. The distention is subsequently augmented by an increased swallowing frequency that occurs in patients as they repetitively swallow their saliva in an effort to neutralize the acid refluxed into their esophagus.

The consequence of fundic distention, with the LES being "taken up" into the stretched fundus, is that the squamous epithelium of the sphincter is exposed to gastric juice and mucosal injury. This initial step in the pathogenesis of GERD explains why mild esophagitis is usually limited to the very distal esophagus. Erosions in the terminal squamous epithelium caused by this mechanism may also explain the complaint of epigastric pain so often registered by patients with early disease. It may also be the stimulus to increase the swallowing of saliva to bathe the erosions in order to alleviate the discomfort induced by exposure to gastric acid. With increased swallowing come aerophagia, gastric distention, bloating, and repetitive belching. During this process there is repeated exposure of the squamous epithelium to gastric juice, due to the sphincter being "taken up" into the stretched fundus, which may cause erosion, ulceration, fibrosis (ring formation), and metaplasia of the terminal squamous mucosa (Figure 24-35).

This mechanism is supported by the finding that as the severity of GERD progresses, the length of columnar lining above the anatomic gastroesophageal junction is increased. This suggests that the presence and extent of columnar epithelium lining the distal esophageal sphincter result from a metaplastic process associated with a loss of sphincter function and increased esophageal acid exposure (Fig. 24-36). To interrupt the progression from early to late disease requires preventing gastric distention and the resultant unfolding of the sphincter. Currently, this can only be achieved with an antireflux operative procedure.

In summary, GERD starts in the stomach (Fig. 24-37). It is caused by gastric distention due to overeating or ingestion of fried foods, typical of the Western diet, which delays gastric emptying. Gastric distention causes unfolding of the sphincter as it is taken up by the distended fundus and exposure of the terminal squamous epithelium within the sphincter to noxious gastric juice. Signs of injury to the exposed squamous epithelium are erosions, ulceration, fibrosis, and columnar metaplasia, with an inflammatory infiltrate or foveolar hyperplasia. Intestinal metaplasia within the sphincter may result, as in Barrett's metaplasia of the esophageal body. This process results in the loss of muscle function, and the sphincter becomes mechanically defective, allowing free reflux with progressively higher degrees of mucosal injury.

Structural damage to the components of the LES, such as loss of pressure, inadequate overall length, or the loss of abdominal length—i.e., the portion exposed to the positive-pressure environment of the abdomen as measured by manometry—results in permanent failure of sphincter function. The probability of increased exposure to gastric juice is 73% if one component of the sphincter

FIG. 24-36. *Schematic illustration of the progression of gastroesophageal reflux disease. Increasing lengths of cardiac mucosa (brown area) are associated with deterioration of the LES, increasing esophageal acid exposure, and intestinal metaplasia.*

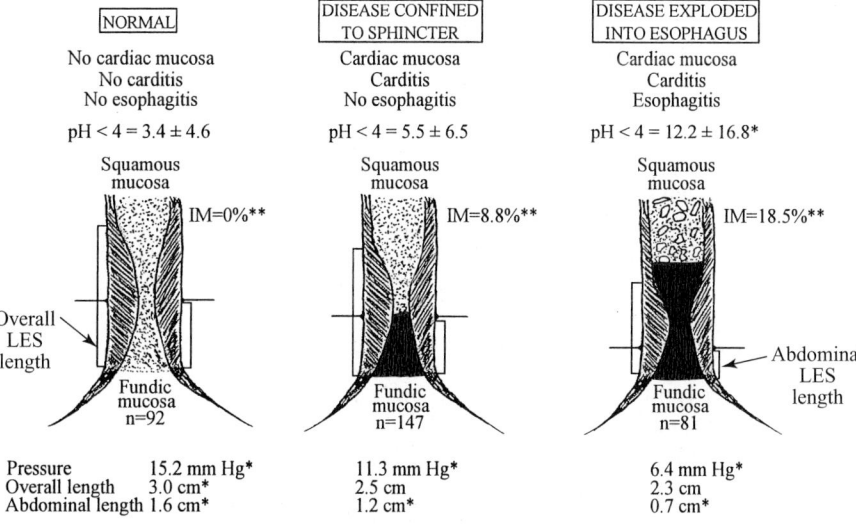

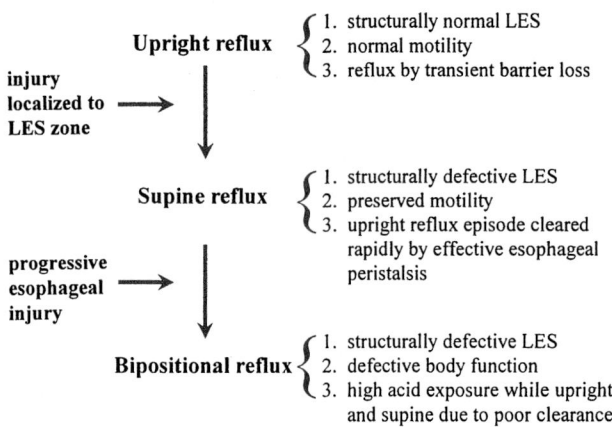

Upright reflux { 1. structurally normal LES
2. normal motility
3. reflux by transient barrier loss

injury localized to LES zone ⟶

Supine reflux { 1. structurally defective LES
2. preserved motility
3. upright reflux episode cleared rapidly by effective esophageal peristalsis

progressive esophageal injury ⟶

Bipositional reflux { 1. structurally defective LES
2. defective body function
3. high acid exposure while upright and supine due to poor clearance

FIG. 24-37. Proposed mechanisms of the progression of gastroesophageal reflux disease.

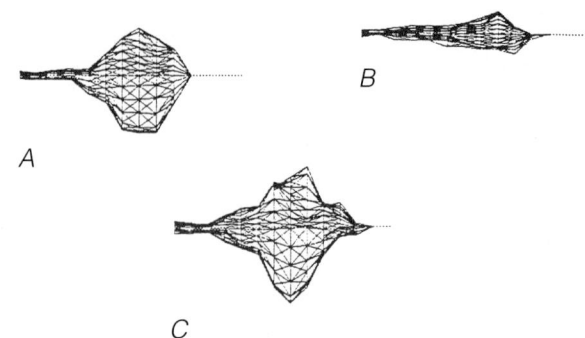

FIG. 24-38. Three-dimensional LES pressure profiles. *A.* A normal volunteer. *B.* A patient with a mechanically defective sphincter. *C.* The same patient 1 year after Nissen fundoplication. [*Reproduced with permission from DeMeester TR, Stein HJ: Surgical treatment of gastroesophageal reflux disease, in Castell DO (ed): The Esophagus. Boston: Little, Brown, 1992, p 619.*]

is abnormal, 74% if two components are abnormal, and 92% if all three are abnormal. This indicates that the failure of one or two of the components of the sphincter may be compensated for by the clearance of the esophageal body. Failure of all three sphincter components inevitably leads to increased esophageal exposure to gastric juice.

The most common cause of a structurally defective LES is inadequate sphincter pressure. The reduced pressure is most likely due to an abnormality of myogenic function. This is supported by two observations. First, the location of the LES, in either the abdomen or the chest, is not a major factor in the genesis of the sphincter pressure, since it can still be measured when the chest and abdomen are surgically opened and the distal esophagus is held free in the surgeon's hand. Second, Biancani and coworkers have shown that the distal esophageal sphincter's muscle response to stretch is reduced in patients with an incompetent cardia. This suggests that sphincter pressure depends on the length and tension properties of the sphincter's smooth muscle. Surgical fundoplication has been shown to restore the mechanical efficiency of the sphincter to normal by correcting the abnormal length-tension characteristics.

Although an inadequate pressure is the most common cause of a structurally defective sphincter, the efficiency of a sphincter with normal pressure can be nullified by an inadequate abdominal length or an abnormally short overall resting length. An adequate abdominal length is important in preventing reflux caused by increases in intra-abdominal pressure, and an adequate overall length is important in providing the resistance to reflux caused by gastric distention independent of intra-abdominal pressure. Therefore, patients with a low sphincter pressure or those with a normal pressure but a short abdominal length are unable to protect against reflux caused by fluctuations of intra-abdominal pressure that occur with daily activities or changes in body position. Patients with a low sphincter pressure or those with a normal pressure but short overall length are unable to protect against reflux related to gastric distention caused by outlet obstruction, aerophagia, gluttony, delayed gastric emptying associated with a fatty diet, or various gastropathies. Persons who have a short overall length on a resting motility study are at a disadvantage in protecting against excessive gastric distention secondary to eating, and suffer postprandial reflux. This is because with normal dilatation of the stomach, sphincter length becomes shorter, and if already shortened in the resting state, there is little tolerance for further shortening before incompetence occurs.

The combined effects of pressure, overall length, and abdominal length on the resistance of the sphincter to the reflux of gastric

juice can be determined by integrating the effects of radial pressures extended over the entire length of the sphincter. This can be quantified by three-dimensional computerized imaging of pressures throughout the sphincter length and calculating the volume of this image. This is referred to as the sphincter pressure vector volume. Figure 24-38 shows the three-dimensional sphincter representations for a normal volunteer and a patient with Barrett's esophagus before and after Nissen fundoplication. The marked improvement in the sphincter is apparent.

The second portion of the human antireflux mechanism is an effective esophageal pump that clears the esophagus after physiologic reflux episodes. Ineffective esophageal clearance can result in an abnormal esophageal exposure to gastric juice in individuals who have a normal LES and gastric function, but fail to clear physiologic reflux episodes. This situation is relatively rare, and ineffectual clearance is more apt to be seen in association with a structurally defective sphincter, which augments the esophageal exposure to gastric juice by prolonging the duration of each reflux episode.

Four factors important in esophageal clearance are gravity, esophageal motor activity, salivation, and anchoring of the distal esophagus in the abdomen. The loss of any one can augment esophageal exposure to gastric juice by contributing to ineffective clearance. This explains why in the absence of peristalsis, reflux episodes are prolonged in the supine position. The bulk of refluxed gastric juice is cleared from the esophagus by a primary peristaltic wave initiated by a pharyngeal swallow. Secondary peristaltic waves are initiated by either distention of the lower esophagus or a drop in the intraesophageal pH. Ambulatory motility studies indicate that secondary waves are less common and play less of a role in clearance than previously thought. The esophageal contractions initiated by a drop in esophageal pH rarely have a normal peristaltic pattern; they commonly have a broad-based, powerful synchronous pattern, which reduces the efficiency of esophageal clearance and encourages the regurgitation of refluxed material into the pharynx, predisposing the patient to aspiration.

Manometry of the esophageal body can detect failure of esophageal clearance by analysis of the pressure amplitude and speed of wave progression through the esophagus. The work of Kahrilas and Dodds has shown that the amplitude of an esophageal contraction required to clear the esophagus of liquid barium varies according to the level. Lower segments require a greater amplitude than upper segments. Inadequate amplitude results in ineffective clearance.

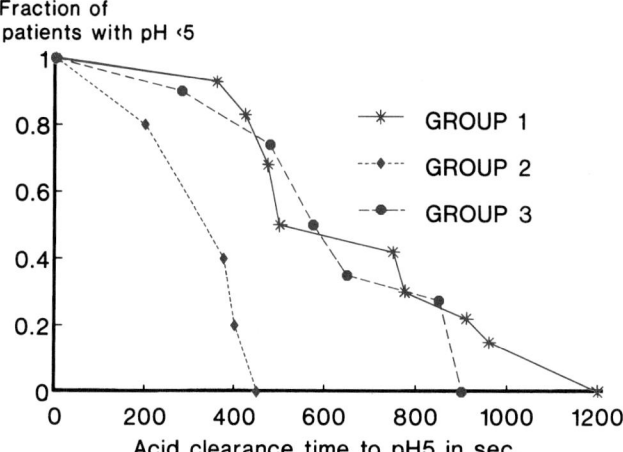

FIG. 24-39. *Acid clearance in subjects with hiatal hernia and symptoms of GERD (group 1), subjects with no hiatal hernia but symptoms of GERD (group 2), and subjects with hiatal hernia but no symptoms of GERD (group 3). The y axis shows the fraction of patients who persist with esophageal pH less than 5. The acid clearance time to pH 5 or greater is significantly faster in group 2 (symptomatic, no hiatal hernia) compared with group 1 (symptomatic, hiatal hernia) and group 3 (asymptomatic, hiatal hernia). Groups 1 and 3 have similar acid clearance times. (Reproduced with permission from Mittal RK, Lange RC, McCallum RW: Identification and mechanisms of delayed esophageal clearance in subjects with hiatus hernia. Gastroenterology 92:132, 1987.)*

Salivation contributes to esophageal clearance by neutralizing the minute amount of acid that is left following a peristaltic wave. Return of esophageal pH to normal takes significantly longer if salivary flow is reduced, such as after radiotherapy, and is shorter if saliva is stimulated by sucking lozenges. Saliva production may also be increased by the presence of acid in the lower esophagus. The patient experiences excessive mucus in the throat. Clinically, this is referred to as "water brash."

A hiatal hernia can also contribute to an esophageal propulsion defect due to loss of anchorage of the esophagus in the abdomen. This results in a reduction in the efficiency of acid clearance (Fig. 24-39). Kahrilas has shown that complete esophageal emptying without retrograde flow was achieved in 86% of test swallows in control subjects without a hiatal hernia, 66% in patients with a reducing hiatal hernia, and only 32% in patients with a nonreducing hiatal hernia. Impaired clearance in patients with nonreducing hiatal hernias suggests that the presence of a hiatal hernia contributes to the pathogenesis of GERD.

Gastric Reservoir

The third component of the human antireflux mechanism is the gastric reservoir. Abnormalities of the gastric reservoir that increase esophageal exposure to gastric juice include gastric dilatation, increased intragastric pressure, persistent gastric reservoir, and increased gastric acid secretion. The effects of gastric dilatation on reflux are discussed above. Increased intragastric pressure may be the result of outlet obstruction due to a scarred pylorus or duodenum, or the result of a vagotomy; it can also be found in the diabetic patient with gastroparesis. The latter two conditions are secondary to abnormalities of the normal adaptive relaxation of the stomach. The increase in intragastric pressure due to alteration in the pressure-volume relationship in these abnormalities can overcome the sphincter resistance and results in reflux.

A persistent gastric reservoir results from delayed gastric emptying and increases the exposure of the esophagus to gastric juice by accentuating physiologic reflux. It is caused by myogenic abnormalities such as gastric atony in advanced diabetes, diffuse neuromuscular disorders, anticholinergic medications, and postviral infections. Nonmyogenic causes are vagotomy, antropyloric dysfunction, and duodenal dysmotility. Delayed gastric emptying can result in increased exposure of the gastric mucosa to bile and pancreatic juice refluxed from the duodenum into the stomach, with the development of gastritis.

Gastric hypersecretion can increase esophageal exposure to gastric acid juice by the physiologic reflux of concentrated gastric acid. Barlow has shown that 28% of patients with increased esophageal exposure to gastric juice measured by 24-hour pH monitoring have gastric hypersecretion. A mechanically defective sphincter seems to be more important than gastric hypersecretion in the development of complications of reflux disease. In this respect, GERD differs from duodenal ulcer disease, as the latter is specifically related to gastric hypersecretion.

Complications of Gastroesophageal Reflux

The complications of gastroesophageal reflux result from the damage inflicted by gastric juice on the esophageal mucosa or respiratory epithelium, and changes caused by their subsequent repair and fibrosis. Complications due to repetitive reflux are esophagitis, stricture, and Barrett's esophagus; repetitive aspiration may lead to progressive pulmonary fibrosis. The severity of the complications is directly related to the prevalence of a structurally defective sphincter (Table 24-4). The observation that a structurally defective sphincter occurs in 42% of patients without complications (most of whom have one or two components failed) suggests that disease may be confined to the sphincter due to compensation by a vigorously contracting esophageal body. Eventually all three components of the sphincter fail, allowing unrestricted reflux of gastric juice into the esophagus and overwhelming its normal clearance mechanisms. This leads to esophageal mucosal injury with progressive deterioration of esophageal contractility, as is commonly seen in patients with strictures and Barrett's esophagus. The loss of esophageal clearance increases the potential for regurgitation into the pharynx with aspiration.

The potential injurious components that reflux into the esophagus include gastric secretions such as acid and pepsin, as well as biliary and pancreatic secretions that regurgitate from the duodenum

Table 24-4
Complications of Gastroesophageal Reflux Disease: 150 Consecutive Cases with Proven Gastroesophageal Reflux Disease (24-Hour Esophageal pH Monitoring Endoscopy, and Motility)

Complication	No.	Structurally Normal Sphincter	Structurally Defective Sphincter
None	59	58%	42%
Erosive esophagitis	47	23%	77%[a]
Stricture	19	11%	89%
Barrett's esophagus	25	0%	100%
Total	150		

[a]Grade more severe with defective cardia.

SOURCE: Reproduced with permission from DeMeester TR, Stein HJ: Gastroesophageal reflux disease, in Moody FG, Carey LC, et al (eds): *Surgical Treatment of Digestive Disease.* Chicago: Year Book Medical, 1990, p 81.

Table 24-5
Relation of the Type of Reflux to Injury

	No Injury	Esophagitis	Uncomplicated Barrett's	Complicated Barrett's
Gastric reflux	15 (54%)	13 (38%)	8 (32%)	1 (8%)
Gastroduodenal reflux	13 (38%)	21 (62%)	17 (68%)	12 (92%)

into the stomach. There is a considerable body of experimental evidence to indicate that maximal epithelial injury occurs during exposure to bile salts combined with acid and pepsin. These studies have shown that acid alone does minimal damage to the esophageal mucosa, but the combination of acid and pepsin is highly deleterious. Similarly, the reflux of duodenal juice alone does little damage to the mucosa, while the combination of duodenal juice and gastric acid is particularly noxious (Table 24-5).

Experimental animal studies have shown that the reflux of duodenal contents into the esophagus enhances inflammation, increases the prevalence of Barrett's esophagus, and results in the development of esophageal adenocarcinoma. The component of duodenal juice thought to be most damaging is bile acids. In order for bile acids to injure mucosal cells, it is necessary that they be both soluble and un-ionized, so that the un-ionized nonpolar form may enter mucosal cells. Before the entry of bile into the gastrointestinal tract, 98% of bile acids are conjugated with either taurine or glycine in a ratio of about 3:1. Conjugation increases the solubility and ionization of bile acids by lowering their pK_a. At the normal duodenal pH of approximately 7, over 90% of bile salts are in solution and completely ionized. At pH ranges from 2 to 7, there is a mixture of the ionized salt and the lipophilic, non-ionized acid. Acidification of bile to below pH 2 results in an irreversible bile acid precipitation. Consequently, under normal physiologic conditions, bile acids precipitate and are of minimal consequence when an acid gastric environment exists. On the other hand, in a more alkaline gastric environment, such as occurs with excessive duodenogastric reflux and after acid suppression therapy or vagotomy and partial or total

gastrectomy, bile salts remain in solution, are partially dissociated, and when refluxed into the esophagus can cause severe mucosal injury by crossing the cell membrane and damaging the mitochondria.

Complications of gastroesophageal reflux such as esophagitis, stricture, and Barrett's metaplasia occur in the presence of two predisposing factors: a mechanically defective LES and an increased esophageal exposure to fluid with a pH of less than 4 and greater than 7 (Fig. 24-40). The duodenal origin of esophageal contents in patients with an increased exposure to a pH greater than 7 has been confirmed by esophageal aspiration studies (Fig. 24-41). Studies have clarified and expanded these observations by measuring esophageal bilirubin exposure over a 24-hour period as a marker for the presence of duodenal juice. Direct measurement of esophageal bilirubin exposure as a marker for duodenal juice has shown that 58% of patients with GERD have increased esophageal exposure to duodenal juice, and that this exposure occurs most commonly when the esophageal pH is between 4 and 7 (Fig. 24-42). Furthermore, it is associated with more severe mucosal injury (Fig. 24-43).

The fact that the combination of refluxed gastric and duodenal juice is more noxious to the esophageal mucosa than gastric juice alone may explain the repeated observation that 25% of patients with reflux esophagitis develop recurrent and progressive mucosal damage, often despite medical therapy. A potential reason is that acid suppression therapy is unable to consistently maintain the pH of refluxed gastric and duodenal juice above the range of 6. Lapses into pH ranges from 2 to 6 encourage the formation of undissociated, nonpolarized, soluble bile acids, which are capable of penetrating the cell wall and injuring mucosal cells. To assure that bile acids remain completely ionized in their polarized form, and thus unable

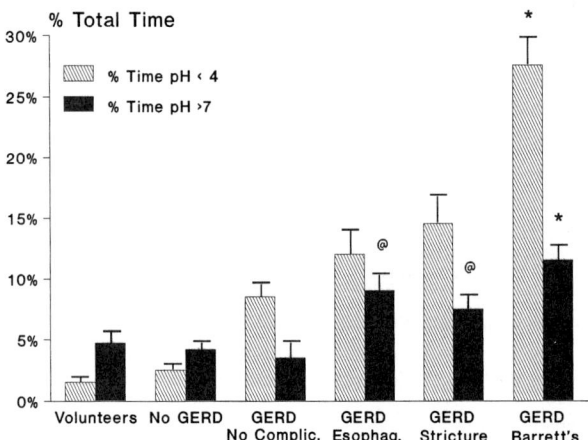

FIG. 24-40. Esophageal acid and alkaline exposure expressed as percentage of total time pH <4 and >7. * = p <0.01 vs. gastroesophageal reflux disease (GERD) patients with no complications. @ = p <0.05 vs. gastroesophageal reflux disease (GERD) patients with no complications. (Reproduced with permission from Stein HJ, Barlow AP, DeMeester TR, et al: Complications of gastroesophageal reflux disease: Role of the lower esophageal sphincter, esophageal acid and acid/alkaline exposure, and duodenogastric reflux. Ann Surg 216:35, 1992.)

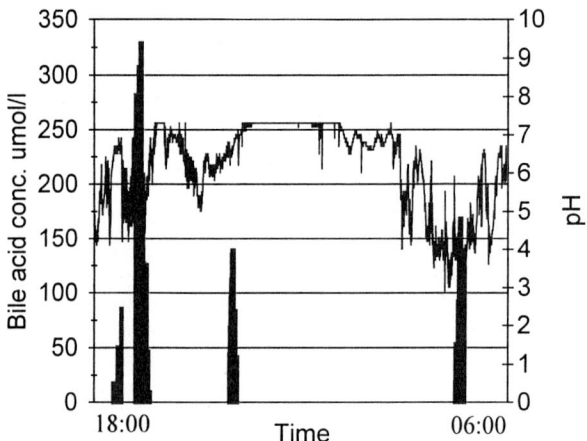

FIG. 24-41. Sample bile acid concentration and esophageal pH plotted against time to obtain detailed profiles, in this case showing both significant bile acid (vertical bars) and acid (linear plot) reflux. (Reproduced with permission from Nehra D, Watt P, Pye JK, Beynon J: Automated oesophageal reflux sampler—A new device used to monitor bile acid reflux in patients with gastro-oesophageal reflux disease. J Med Eng Technol 21:1, 1997.)

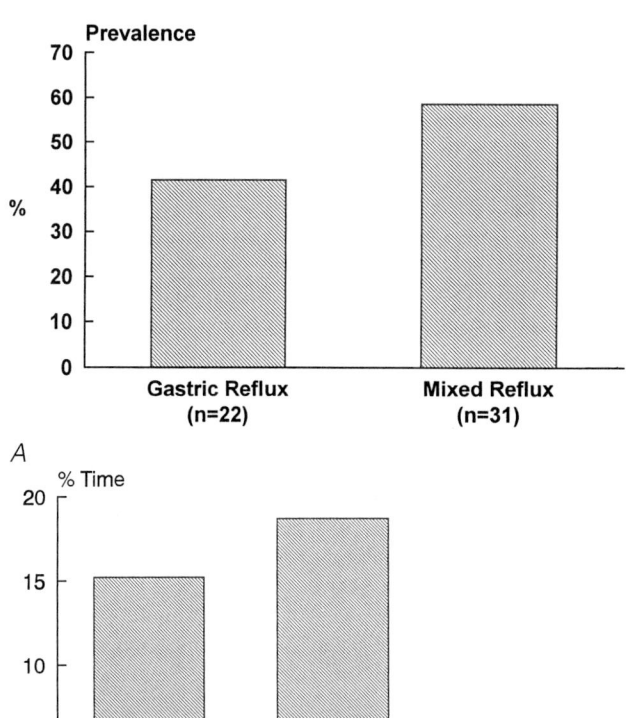

A

B

FIG. 24-42. *A. Prevalence of reflux types in 53 patients with GERD. B. Esophageal luminal pH during bilirubin exposure. (Reproduced with permission from Kauer WKH, Peters JH, DeMeester TR, et al: Mixed reflux of gastric and duodenal juices is more harmful to the esophagus than gastric juice alone. The need for surgical therapy re-emphasized. Ann Surg 222:525, 1995.)*

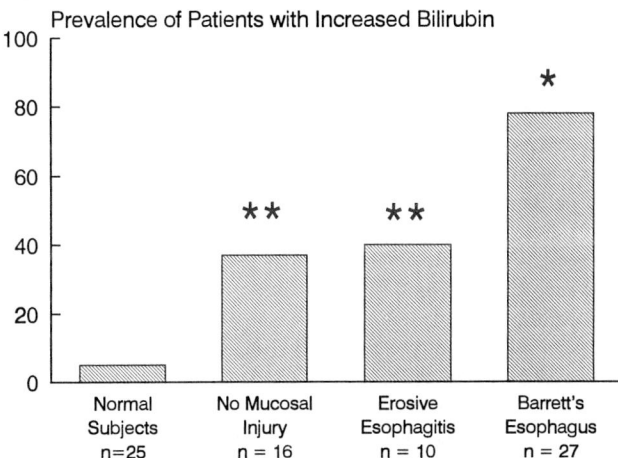

FIG. 24-43. *Prevalence of abnormal esophageal bilirubin exposure in healthy subjects and in patients with GERD with varied degrees of mucosal injury.* *p <0.03 vs. all other groups, **p <0.03 vs. healthy subjects. *(Reproduced with permission from Kauer WKH, Peters JH, De-Meester TR, et al: Mixed reflux of gastric and duodenal juices is more harmful to the esophagus than gastric juice alone. The need for surgical therapy re-emphasized. Ann Surg 222:525, 1995.)*

to penetrate the cell, requires that the pH of the refluxed material be maintained above 7, 24 hours a day, 7 days a week, for the patient's lifetime. In practice this would not only be impractical but likely impossible, unless very high doses of medications were used. The use of lesser doses would allow esophageal mucosal damage to occur while the patient was relatively asymptomatic. Antireflux operative procedures re-establish the barrier between stomach and esophagus, protecting the esophagus from damage in patients with mixed gastroesophageal reflux. If reflux of gastric juice is allowed to persist and sustained or repetitive esophageal injury occurs, two sequelae can result. First, a luminal stricture can develop from submucosal and eventually intramural fibrosis. Second, the tubular esophagus may become replaced with columnar epithelium. The columnar epithelium is resistant to acid and is associated with the alleviation of the complaint of heartburn. This columnar epithelium often becomes intestinalized, identified histologically by the presence of goblet cells. This specialized intestinal metaplasia is currently required for the diagnosis of Barrett's esophagus. Endoscopically, Barrett's esophagus can be quiescent or associated with complications of esophagitis, stricture, Barrett's ulceration, and dysplasia. The complications associated with Barrett's esophagus may be due to the continuous irritation from refluxed duodenogastric juice. This continued injury is pH dependent and may be modified by medical therapy. The incidence of metaplastic Barrett's epithelium becoming dysplastic and progressing to adenocarcinoma is approximately 1% per year.

An esophageal stricture can be associated with severe esophagitis or Barrett's esophagus. In the latter situation, it occurs at the site of maximal inflammatory injury (i.e., the columnar-squamous epithelial interface). As the columnar epithelium advances into the area of inflammation, the inflammation extends higher into the proximal esophagus, and the site of the stricture moves progressively up the esophagus. Patients who have a stricture in the absence of Barrett's esophagus should have the presence of gastroesophageal reflux documented before the presence of the stricture is ascribed to reflux esophagitis. In patients with normal acid exposure, the stricture may be due to cancer or a drug-induced chemical injury, the latter resulting from the lodgment of a capsule or tablet in the distal esophagus. In such patients, dilation usually corrects the problem of dysphagia. Heartburn, which may have occurred only because of the chemical injury, need not be treated. It is also possible for drug-induced injuries to occur in patients who have underlying esophagitis and a distal esophageal stricture secondary to gastroesophageal reflux. In this situation, a long string-like stricture progressively develops as a result of repetitive caustic injury from capsule or tablet lodgment on top of an initial reflux stricture. These strictures are often resistant to dilation.

When the refluxed gastric juice is of sufficient quantity, it can reach the pharynx, with the potential for pharyngeal tracheal aspiration, causing symptoms of repetitive cough, choking, hoarseness, and recurrent pneumonia. This is often an unrecognized complication of GERD, since either the pulmonary or the gastrointestinal symptoms may predominate in the clinical situation and focus the physician's attention on one to the exclusion of the other. Three factors are important in these patients. First, it may take up to 7 days for the loss of respiratory epithelium secondary to the aspiration of gastric contents to be recovered, and a chronic cough that is not related to a reflux episode may develop between episodes of aspiration. Second, the presence of an esophageal motility disorder is observed in 75% of patients with reflux-induced aspiration, and is believed to promote the aboral movement of the refluxate toward the pharynx. Third, if the pH in the cervical esophagus in patients with increased esophageal acid exposure is below 4 for less than 1% of the time, there is a high probability that the respiratory symptoms have been caused by aspiration. Increasingly, benign pulmonary pathology is recognized as being secondary to GERD, including asthma, idiopathic pulmonary fibrosis, and bronchiectases.

Symptomatic Assessment of Gastroesophageal Reflux Disease

Gastroesophageal reflux disease is a functional disorder often accompanied by non–reflux-related gastrointestinal and respiratory symptoms that will not improve or may be worsened by antireflux surgery. Symptoms consistent with irritable bowel syndrome, such as alternating diarrhea and constipation, bloating, and crampy abdominal pain, should be sought and detailed separately from GERD symptoms. Likewise, symptoms suggestive of gastric pathology including nausea, early satiety, epigastric abdominal pain, anorexia, and weight loss are important. It has become increasingly recognized that oral symptoms such as mouth and tongue burning and sore throat rarely improve with antireflux surgery.

The patient's perception of what each symptom means should be explored in an effort to avoid their misinterpretation. Of equal importance is the classification of symptoms as primary or secondary, for prioritization of therapy and to allow an estimate of the probability of relief of each of the particular symptoms. The response to acid-suppressing medications predicts success and symptom relief after surgery. In contrast to the widely held belief that failure of medical therapy is an indication for surgery, a good response to proton pump inhibitors is desirable, as it predicts that the symptoms are actually due to reflux of gastric contents.

GERD-related symptoms can be classified into "typical" symptoms of heartburn, regurgitation and dysphagia, and "atypical" symptoms of cough, hoarseness, asthma, aspiration, and chest pain. Because there are fewer mechanisms for their generation, typical symptoms are more likely to be secondary to increased esophageal acid exposure than are atypical symptoms. The relationship of atypical symptoms such as cough, hoarseness, wheezing, or sore throat to heartburn and/or regurgitation should be established. Other, more common factors that may contribute to respiratory symptoms also should be investigated. The patient must be made aware of the relatively diminished likelihood of success of surgery when atypical symptoms are the primary symptoms. Of note is the comparatively longer duration required for the respiratory symptoms to improve after surgery.

Medical Therapy

GERD is such a common condition that most patients with mild symptoms carry out self-medication. When first seen with symptoms of heartburn without obvious complications, patients can reasonably be placed on 8 to 12 weeks of simple antacids before extensive investigations are carried out. In many situations, this successfully terminates the attacks. Patients should be advised to elevate the head of the bed; avoid tight clothing; eat small, frequent meals; avoid eating their nighttime meal shortly before retiring; lose weight; and avoid alcohol, coffee, chocolate, and peppermint, which may aggravate the symptoms.

Used in combination with simple antacids, alginic acid may augment the relief of symptoms by creating a physical barrier to reflux, as well as by acid reduction. Alginic acid reacts with sodium bicarbonate in the presence of saliva to form a highly viscous solution that floats like a raft on the surface of the gastric contents. When reflux occurs, this protective layer is refluxed into the esophagus,

and acts as a protective barrier against the noxious gastric contents. Medications to promote gastric emptying such as metoclopramide, domperidone, or cisapride are beneficial in early disease, but of little value in more severe disease.

In patients with persistent symptoms, the mainstay of medical therapy is acid suppression. High-dosage regimens of hydrogen potassium proton pump inhibitors, such as omeprazole (up to 40 mg/d) can reduce gastric acidity by as much as 80 to 90%. This usually heals mild esophagitis. In severe esophagitis, healing may occur in only half of the patients. In patients who reflux a combination of gastric and duodenal juice, acid-suppression therapy may give relief of symptoms, while still allowing mixed reflux to occur. This can allow persistent mucosal damage in an asymptomatic patient. Unfortunately, within 6 months of discontinuation of any form of medical therapy for GERD, 80% of patients have a recurrence of symptoms.

Once initiated, most patients with GERD will require lifelong treatment with proton pump inhibitors, both to relieve symptoms and control any coexistent esophagitis or stricture. Although control of symptoms has historically served as the endpoint of therapy, the wisdom of this approach has recently been questioned, particularly in patients with Barrett's esophagus. Evidence suggesting that reflux control may prevent the development of adenocarcinoma and lead to regression of dysplastic and nondysplastic Barrett's segments has led many to consider control of reflux, and not symptom control, a better therapeutic endpoint. However, complete control of reflux can be difficult, as has been highlighted by studies of acid breakthrough while on PPI therapy, and of persistent reflux following antireflux surgery. Castell, Triadafilopoulos, and others have shown that 40 to 80% of patients with Barrett's esophagus continue to have abnormal esophageal acid exposure despite up to 20 mg twice daily of PPIs. Ablation trials have shown that mean doses of 56 mg of omeprazole were necessary to normalize 24-hour esophageal pH studies. It is likely that antireflux surgery results in more reproducible and reliable elimination of reflux of both acid and duodenal contents, although long-term outcome studies suggest that as many as 25% of post-Nissen patients will have persistent pathologic esophageal acid exposure confirmed by positive 24-hour pH studies.

Suggested Therapeutic Approach

The traditional stepwise approach to the therapy of GERD should be re-examined in view of a more complete understanding of the pathophysiology of gastroesophageal reflux, the rising incidence of Barrett's esophagus, and the increasing mortality rates associated with end-stage reflux disease. The approach should be to identify risk factors for persistent and progressive disease early in the course of the disease, and encourage surgical treatment when these factors are present. The following approach is suggested.

Patients presenting for the first time with symptoms suggestive of gastroesophageal reflux may be given initial therapy with H_2 blockers. In view of the availability of these as over-the-counter medications, many patients will have already self-medicated their symptoms. Failure of H_2 blockers to control the symptoms, or immediate return of symptoms after stopping treatment, suggests either that the diagnosis is incorrect or that the patient has relatively severe disease. Endoscopic examination at this stage of the patient's evaluation provides the opportunity for assessing the severity of mucosal damage and the presence of Barrett's esophagus. Both of these findings on initial endoscopy are associated with a high probability that medical treatment will fail. A measurement of the degree and pattern of esophageal exposure to gastric and duodenal juice, via 24-hour pH and bilirubin monitoring, should be obtained at this point. The status of the LES and the function of the esophageal body should also be measured. These studies identify features such as the following, which are predictive of a poor response to medical therapy, frequent relapses, and the development of complications: supine reflux, poor esophageal contractility, erosive esophagitis (or a columnar-lined esophagus at initial presentation), bile in the refluxate, and a structurally defective sphincter. Patients who have these risk factors should be given the option of surgery as a primary therapy, with the expectation of long-term control of symptoms and complications.

Selection of Patients for Surgery

Studies of the natural history of GERD indicate that most patients have a relatively benign form of the disease that is responsive to lifestyle changes and dietary and medical therapy, and do not need surgical treatment. Approximately 25 to 50% of the patients with GERD have persistent or progressive disease, and it is this patient population that is best suited to surgical therapy. These patients are identified by the same risk factors that predict a poor response to medical therapy. In the past, the presence of esophagitis and a structurally defective LES were the primary indications for surgical treatment, and many internists and surgeons were reluctant to recommend operative procedures in their absence. However, one should not be deterred from considering antireflux surgery in a symptomatic patient with or without esophagitis or a defective sphincter, provided the disease process has been objectively documented by 24-hour pH monitoring. This is particularly true in patients who have become dependent upon therapy with PPIs, or require increasing doses to control their symptoms. It is important to note that a good response to medical therapy in this group of patients predicts an excellent outcome following antireflux surgery.

A structurally defective LES is the most important factor predicting failure of medical therapy. While patients with normal sphincter pressures tend to remain well controlled with medical therapy, patients with a structurally defective LES do not respond well to medical therapy, usually developing recurrent symptoms within 1 to 2 years of beginning therapy, and these patients should be considered for an antireflux operation, regardless of the presence or absence of endoscopic esophagitis.

Young patients with documented reflux disease with or without a defective LES are also excellent candidates for antireflux surgery. They usually will require long-term medical therapy for control of their symptoms, and many will go on to develop complications of the disease. An analysis of the cost of therapy based on data from the Veterans Administration Cooperative trial indicates that surgery has a cost advantage over medical therapy in patients less than 49 years of age.

Severe endoscopic esophagitis in a symptomatic patient with a structurally defective LES is also an indication for early surgical therapy. These patients are prone to breakthrough of their symptoms while receiving medical therapy. Symptoms and mucosal injury can be controlled in such patients, but careful monitoring is required, and increasing dosages of PPIs are necessary. In everyday clinical practice, however, such treatment can be both difficult and impractical, and in such cases antireflux surgery should be considered early as a therapeutic option.

The development of a stricture in a patient represents a failure of medical therapy, and is also an indication for a surgical antireflux procedure. In addition, strictures are often associated with a structurally defective sphincter and loss of esophageal contrac-

tility. Before proceeding with surgical treatment, malignancy and a drug-related etiology of the stricture should be excluded, and the stricture progressively dilated up to a 60F bougie. When the stricture is fully dilated, the relief of dysphagia is evaluated and esophageal manometry is performed to determine the adequacy of peristalsis in the distal esophagus. If dysphagia is relieved and the amplitude of esophageal contractions is adequate, an antireflux procedure should be performed; if there is a global loss of esophageal contractility, caution should be exercised in performing an antireflux procedure with a complete fundoplication, and a partial fundoplication should be considered.

Barrett's columnar-lined esophagus is commonly associated with a severe structural defect of the LES and often poor contractility of the esophageal body. Patients with Barrett's esophagus are at risk of progression of the mucosal abnormality up the esophagus, formation of a stricture, hemorrhage from a Barrett's ulcer, and the development of an adenocarcinoma. An antireflux procedure may arrest the progression of the disease, heal ulceration, and resolve strictures. Evidence is accumulating that surgical treatment also reduces the risk of progression to cancer. If severe dysplasia or intramucosal carcinoma is found on mucosal biopsy specimens, an esophageal resection should be done.

The majority of patients requiring treatment have a relatively mild form of disease and will respond to antisecretory medications. Patients with more severe forms of disease, particularly those with risk factors predictive of medical failure and those who develop persistent or progressive disease, should be considered for early definitive therapy. Laparoscopic Nissen fundoplication will provide a long-term cure in the majority of these patients, with minimal discomfort and an early return to normal activity. If the disease has resulted in global failure of esophageal contractility, Barrett's metaplasia with high-grade dysplasia, or esophageal adenocarcinoma, an esophagectomy may be the best surgical treatment option.

Surgical Therapy

Preoperative Evaluation

Before proceeding with an antireflux operation, several factors should be evaluated. First, the propulsive force of the body of the esophagus should be evaluated by esophageal manometry to determine if it has sufficient power to propel a bolus of food through a newly reconstructed valve. Patients with normal peristaltic contractions do well with a 360 degree Nissen fundoplication. When peristalsis is absent or severely disordered, or the amplitude of the contraction is below 20 mm Hg throughout the lower esophagus, a two-thirds partial fundoplication may be the procedure of choice.

Second, anatomic shortening of the esophagus can compromise the ability to do an adequate repair without tension, and lead to an increased incidence of breakdown or thoracic displacement of the repair. Esophageal shortening is identified on a barium swallow roentgenogram by a sliding hiatal hernia that will not reduce in the upright position, or that measures larger than 5 cm between the diaphragmatic crura and gastroesophageal junction on endoscopy. When esophageal shortening is present, the motility of the esophageal body must be carefully evaluated, and if inadequate, a gastroplasty should be performed. In patients who have a global absence of contractility, more than 50% interrupted or dropped contractions, or a history of several failed previous antireflux procedures, esophageal resection should be considered as an alternative.

Third, the surgeon should specifically query the patient for complaints of nausea, vomiting, and loss of appetite. In the past, these symptoms were accepted as part of the reflux syndrome, but we now realize that they can be due to excessive duodenogastric reflux or gastric pathology. This problem is most pronounced in patients who have had previous upper gastrointestinal surgery, particularly cholecystectomy, although this is not always the case. In such patients, these symptoms may persist after an antireflux procedure, and patients should be given this information before the operation. In these patients, 24-hour bilirubin monitoring and gastric emptying studies can be performed to detect and quantify duodenogastric abnormalities. Antireflux surgery alone may influence these symptoms by improving the efficiency of gastric emptying.

Fourth, approximately 30% of patients with proven gastroesophageal reflux on 24-hour pH monitoring will have hypersecretion on gastric analysis, and 2 to 3% of patients who have an antireflux operation will develop a gastric or duodenal ulcer. The presence of *Helicobacter pylori* should be assessed in these patients and treated if present.

Principles of Surgical Therapy

The primary goal of antireflux surgery is to safely restore the structure of the sphincter or to prevent its shortening with gastric distention, while preserving the patient's ability to swallow normally, to belch to relieve gaseous distention, and to vomit when necessary. Regardless of the choice of the procedure, this goal can be achieved if attention is paid to five principles in reconstructing the cardia. First, the operation should restore the pressure of the distal esophageal sphincter to a level twice resting gastric pressure (i.e., 12 mm Hg for a gastric pressure of 6 mm Hg), and its length to at least 3 cm. This not only augments sphincter characteristics in patients in whom they are reduced prior to surgery, but prevents unfolding of a normal sphincter in response to gastric distention (Fig. 24-44). Preoperative and postoperative esophageal manometry measurements have shown that the resting sphincter pressure and the overall sphincter length can be surgically augmented over preoperative values, and that the change in the former is a function of the degree of gastric wrap around the esophagus (Fig. 24-45).

Second, the operation should place an adequate length of the distal esophageal sphincter in the positive-pressure environment of the abdomen by a method that ensures its response to changes in intra-abdominal pressure. The permanent restoration of 1.5 to 2 cm of abdominal esophagus in a patient whose sphincter pressure has been augmented to twice resting gastric pressure will maintain the competency of the cardia over various challenges of intra-abdominal pressure. All three of the popular antireflux procedures increase the length of the sphincter exposed to abdominal pressure by an average of 1 cm. When poorly performed, however, an operation may

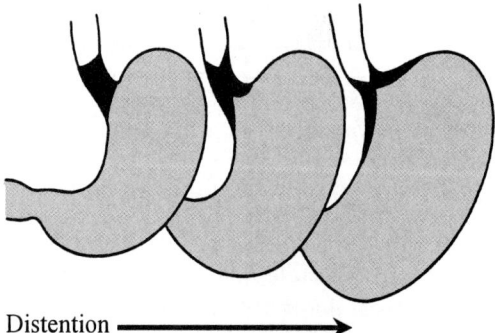

FIG. 24-44. A graphic illustration of the shortening of the LES that occurs as the sphincter is "taken up" by the cardia as the stomach distends.

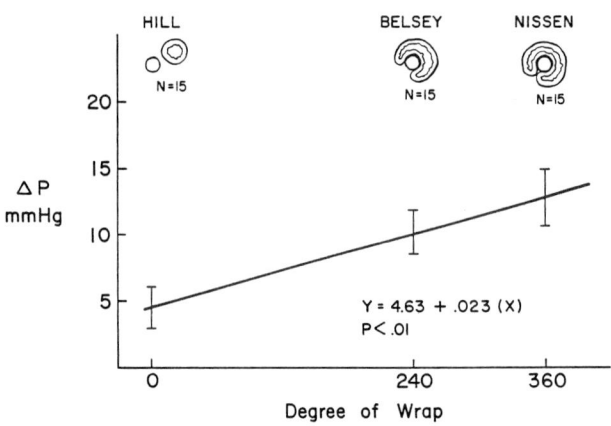

FIG. 24-45. The relationship between the augmentation of sphincter pressure over preoperative pressure (ΔP) and the degree of gastric fundic wrap in three popular antireflux procedures. (*Reproduced with permission from O'Sullivan GC, DeMeester TR, Joelsson BE, et al: Interaction of lower esophageal sphincter pressure and length of sphincter in the abdomen as determinants of gastroesophageal competence. Am J Surg 143:40, 1982.*)

result in a reduction of the length of abdominal sphincter. Increasing the length of sphincter exposed to abdominal pressure will improve competency only if it is acted on by challenges of intra-abdominal pressure. The creation of a conduit that will ensure the transmission of intra-abdominal pressure changes around the abdominal portion of the sphincter is a necessary aspect of surgical repair. The fundoplication in the Nissen and Belsey repairs serves this purpose.

Third, the operation should allow the reconstructed cardia to relax on deglutition. In normal swallowing, a vagally mediated relaxation of the distal esophageal sphincter and the gastric fundus occurs. The relaxation lasts for approximately 10 seconds and is followed by a rapid recovery to the former tonicity. To ensure relaxation of the sphincter, three factors are important: (1) only the fundus of the stomach should be used to buttress the sphincter, since it is known to relax in concert with the sphincter; (2) the gastric wrap should be properly placed around the sphincter and not incorporate a portion of the stomach or be placed around the stomach itself, since the body of the stomach does not relax with swallowing; and (3) damage to the vagal nerves during dissection of the thoracic esophagus should be avoided because it may result in failure of the sphincter to relax.

Fourth, the fundoplication should not increase the resistance of the relaxed sphincter to a level that exceeds the peristaltic power of the body of the esophagus. The resistance of the relaxed sphincter depends on the degree, length, and diameter of the gastric fundic wrap, and on the variation in intra-abdominal pressure. A 360 degree gastric wrap should be no longer than 2 cm and constructed over a 60F bougie. This will ensure that the relaxed sphincter will have an adequate diameter with minimal resistance. This is not necessary when constructing a partial wrap.

Fifth, the operation should ensure that the fundoplication can be placed in the abdomen without undue tension, and maintained there by approximating the crura of the diaphragm above the repair. Leaving the fundoplication in the thorax converts a sliding hernia into a paraesophageal hernia, with all the complications associated with that condition. Maintaining the repair in the abdomen under tension predisposes to an increased incidence of recurrence. This can occur in patients who have a stricture or Barrett's esophagus, and is due to shortening of the esophagus from the inflammatory process. This problem can be resolved by lengthening the esophagus by gastroplasty and constructing a partial fundoplication.

Procedure Selection

A laparoscopic approach is used in patients with normal esophageal contractility and length. Patients with questionable esophageal length may be best approached transthoracically, where full esophageal mobilization serves as a lengthening procedure. Those with a failed esophagus characterized by absent esophageal contractions and/or absent peristalsis such as those with scleroderma are best treated either medically or with a partial fundoplication in order to avoid the increased outflow resistance associated with a complete fundoplication. If the esophagus is short after it is mobilized from diaphragm to aortic arch, a Collis gastroplasty is done to provide additional length and avoid placing the repair under tension. In the majority of patients who have good esophageal contractility and normal esophageal length, the laparoscopic Nissen fundoplication is the procedure of choice for a primary antireflux repair. Experience and randomized studies have shown that the Nissen fundoplication is an effective and durable antireflux repair with minimal side effects, that provides long-lasting relief of reflux symptoms in over 90% of patients.

Primary Antireflux Repairs

Nissen Fundoplication

The most common antireflux procedure is the Nissen fundoplication. The procedure can be performed through an abdominal or a chest incision, as well as through a laparoscope. Rudolph Nissen described the procedure as a 360 degree fundoplication around the lower esophagus for a distance of 4 to 5 cm. Although this provided good control of reflux, it was associated with a number of side effects that have encouraged modifications of the procedure as originally described. These include using only the gastric fundus to envelop the esophagus in a fashion analogous to a Witzel jejunostomy, sizing the fundoplication with a 60F bougie, and limiting the length of the fundoplication to 1 to 2 cm. The essential elements necessary for the performance of a transabdominal fundoplication are common to both the laparoscopic and open procedures and include the following:

1. Crural dissection, identification, and preservation of both vagi, and the anterior hepatic branch
2. Circumferential dissection of the esophagus
3. Crural closure
4. Fundic mobilization by division of short gastric vessels
5. Creation of a short, loose fundoplication by placing the posterior fundic wall posterior, and the anterior fundus anterior, to the esophagus, meeting at the right lateral position

The Laparoscopic Approach. Laparoscopic fundoplication has become commonplace and has replaced the open abdominal Nissen fundoplication as the procedure of choice. Five 10-mm ports are utilized (Fig. 24-46). Dissection is begun by an incision of the portion of the gastrohepatic omentum above the hepatic branch of the anterior vagus nerve. The circumference of the diaphragmatic crura is dissected and the esophagus is mobilized by careful dissection of the anterior and posterior soft tissues within the hiatus. The esophagus is held anterior and to the left and the crura approximated with three to four interrupted 0 silk sutures, starting just above the aortic decussation and working anterior. Complete fundic mobilization allows construction of a tension-free fundoplication. Short gastric vessels along the upper third of the greater curvature

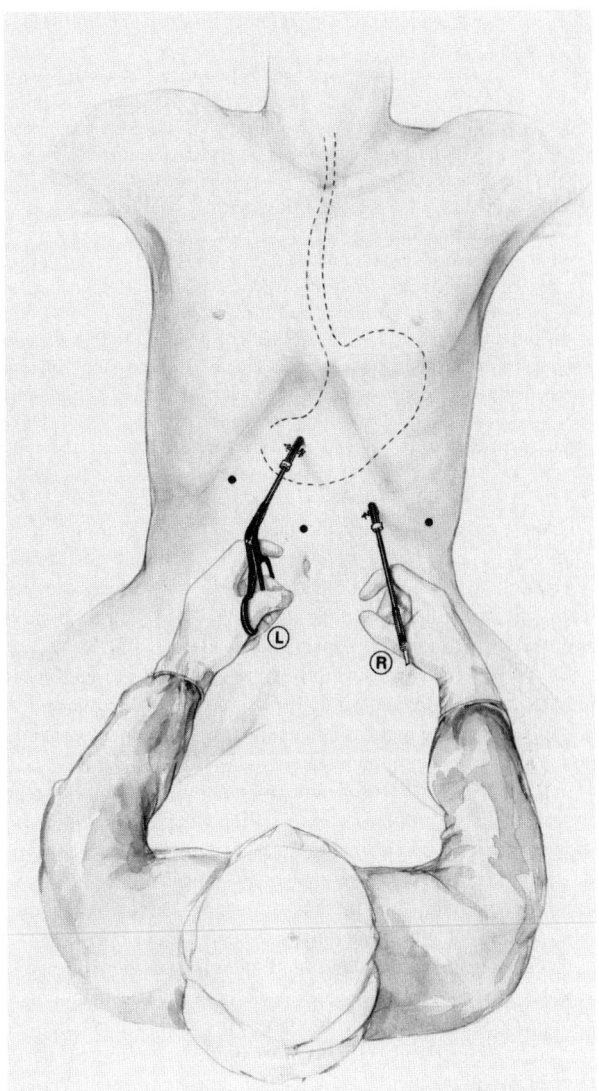

FIG. 24-46. *Patient positioning and trocar placement for laparoscopic antireflux surgery. The patient is placed with the head elevated 45 degree in the modified lithotomy position. The surgeon stands between the patient's legs and the procedure is completed using five abdominal access ports.*

are sequentially dissected and divided. Following complete mobilization, the posterior wall of the fundus is gently brought behind the esophagus to the right side. The anterior wall of the fundus is brought anterior to the esophagus, and the fundic lips are manipulated to allow the fundus to envelop the esophagus without twisting (Fig. 24-47). A 60F bougie is passed to properly size the fundoplication, and it is sutured utilizing a single U stitch of 2-0 polypropylene buttressed with felt pledgets.

Transthoracic Nissen Fundoplication. The indications for performing an antireflux procedure by a transthoracic approach are as follows:

1. A patient who has had a previous hiatal hernia repair. In this situation, a peripheral circumferential incision in the diaphragm is made to provide simultaneous exposure of the upper abdomen. This allows safe dissection of the previous repair from both the abdominal and thoracic sides of the diaphragm.

2. A patient who requires a concomitant esophageal myotomy for achalasia or diffuse spasm.
3. A patient who has a short esophagus. This is usually associated with a stricture or Barrett's esophagus. In this situation, the thoracic approach is preferred to allow maximum mobilization of the esophagus, and to perform a Collis gastroplasty in order to place the repair without tension below the diaphragm.
4. A patient with a sliding hiatal hernia that does not reduce below the diaphragm during a roentgenographic barium study in the upright position. This can indicate esophageal shortening, and again, a thoracic approach is preferred for maximum mobilization of the esophagus, and if necessary, the performance of a Collis gastroplasty.
5. A patient who has associated pulmonary pathology. In this situation, the nature of the pulmonary pathology can be evaluated and the proper pulmonary surgery, in addition to the antireflux repair, can be performed.
6. An obese patient. In this situation, the abdominal repair is difficult because of poor exposure, particularly in men, in whom the intra-abdominal fat is more abundant.

In the thoracic approach the hiatus is exposed through a left posterior lateral thoracotomy incision in the sixth intercostal space (i.e., over the upper border of the seventh rib). When necessary, the diaphragm is incised circumferentially 2 to 3 cm from the lateral chest wall for a distance of approximately 10 to 15 cm. The esophagus is mobilized from the level of the diaphragm to underneath the aortic arch. Mobilization up to the aortic arch is usually necessary to place the repair in a patient with a shortened esophagus into the abdomen without undue tension. Failure to do this is one of the major causes for subsequent breakdown of a repair and return of symptoms. The cardia is then freed from the diaphragm. When all the attachments between the cardia and diaphragmatic hiatus are divided, the fundus and part of the body of the stomach are drawn up through the hiatus into the chest. The vascular fat pad that lies at the gastroesophageal junction is excised. Crural sutures are then placed to close the hiatus, and the fundoplication constructed by enveloping the fundus around the distal esophagus in a manner similar to that described for the abdominal approach. When complete, the fundoplication is placed into the abdomen by compressing the fundic ball with the hand and manually maneuvering it through the hiatus.

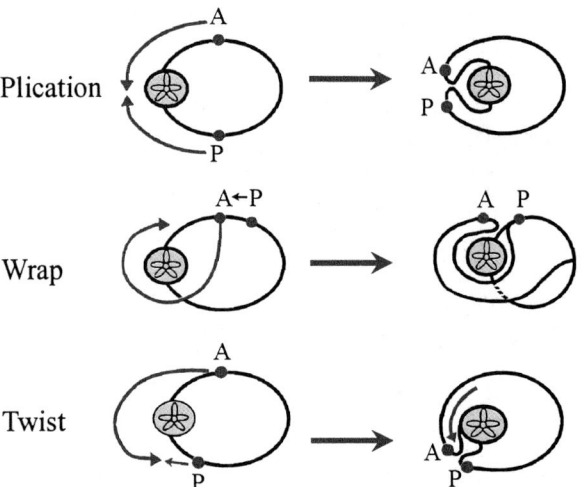

Plication

Wrap

Twist

FIG. 24-47. *Schematic representations of the various possibilities of orientation of a Nissen fundoplication. The top box represents the preferred approach; it can be seen that the approach shown in the bottom two boxes results in twisting of the fundoplication.*

Laparoscopic Toupet and Belsey Mark IV Partial Fundoplications

In the presence of severely altered esophageal motility, where the propulsive force of the esophagus is not sufficient to overcome the outflow obstruction of a complete fundoplication, a partial fundoplication is indicated. A partial fundoplication may be performed laparoscopically, a Toupet fundoplication, or transthoracically, a Belsey Mark IV repair. Both consist of a 270 degree gastric fundoplication around the distal 4 cm of esophagus, performed either laparoscopically or through a left chest incision (Fig. 24-48).

In patients with a short esophagus secondary to a stricture, Barrett's esophagus, or a large hiatal hernia, the esophagus is lengthened with a Collis gastroplasty (Fig. 24-49). The esophagus is lengthened by constructing a gastric tube along the lesser curvature. This allows a tension-free constriction of a Belsey Mark IV or Nissen fundoplication around the newly formed gastric tube, with placement of the repair in the abdomen. Because a short esophagus is commonly associated with a reduction in esophageal contraction amplitude and the gastric tube is inert, most surgeons prefer to combine the gastroplasty procedure with a 280 degree Belsey Mark IV fundoplication rather than a 360 degree Nissen fundoplication.

Outcome After Fundoplication

Nearly all published reports of laparoscopic fundoplication show that this procedure relieves the typical symptoms of gastroesophageal reflux—heartburn, regurgitation, and dysphagia—in greater than 90% of patients. Overall, there is a 4.2% conversion rate to open surgery, and a 0.5% rate of early reoperation. Persistent postoperative dysphagia occurred in approximately 9% of patients in the early series, a rate 2 to 3 times higher than what is accepted for open fundoplication. The incidence of dysphagia has decreased to the 3 to 5% range with increasing experience and attention to the technical details in constructing the fundoplication. Resting LES characteristics and esophageal acid exposure return to normal in nearly all patients (Fig. 24-50). Morbidity after laparoscopic fundoplication is similar to that after open fundoplication, averaging 10 to 15%. A pitfall unique to the laparoscopic approach is that 1 to 2% of patients develop a pneumothorax and surgical emphysema. This is related to excessive hiatal dissection, and has decreased as surgeons' experience has increased. Unrecognized perforation of the esophagus or stomach is the most life-threatening complication. Perforations occur most often during hiatal and circumferential dissection of the esophagus, and their incidence is also related to the surgeon's experience. Intraoperative recognition and repair are the keys to preventing a life-threatening complication.

It is recommended that the surgical approach to patients with GERD be selective (that is, that the specific antireflux procedure for any patient be based upon the patient's existing esophageal function). The benefit of a selective approach is shown in these authors' experience with 85 consecutive patients with different types of the disease (Table 24-6). In approximately 75 to 80% of the patients, a transabdominal Nissen fundoplication was the most suitable treatment. The remaining 20 to 25% were best treated by tailoring the antireflux procedure to their existing amplitude of esophageal contractility and esophageal length. Interestingly, patients selected for a Belsey partial fundoplication because of poor motility but normal esophageal length benefited the least. This suggests that in these patients the motility disorder may be a primary abnormality rather than secondary to reflux-induced injury.

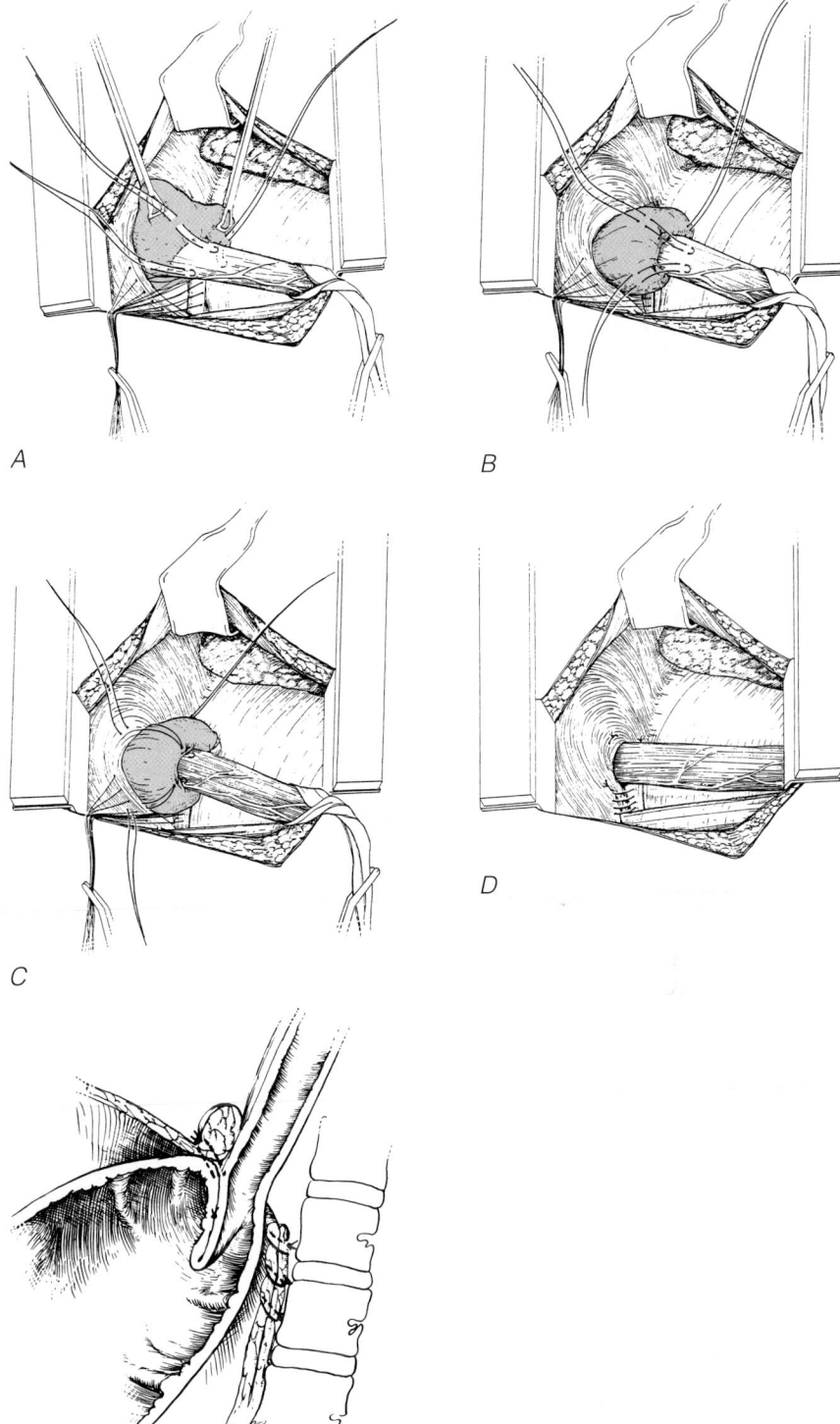

FIG. 24-48. *A.* Construction of a Belsey 240° gastric fundic wrap, showing placement of the first row of sutures 1.5 cm above the gastroesophageal junction. Particular attention must be given to placement of the right lateral suture. *B.* Continued construction of the Belsey 270 degree gastric fundic wrap, showing placement of the second row of sutures 1.5 to 2.0 cm above the previously tied sutures of the first row. *C.* Continued construction of the gastric fundic wrap, showing placement of the tails of the previously tied second row of sutures through the diaphragm, 0.5 cm apart and 1.0 to 1.5 cm from the edge of the hiatus. Note the placement of the sutures at the 4, 8, and 12 o'clock positions on an imaginary clockface oriented with the 6 o'clock position posterior in the hiatus between the right and left crura, just anterior to the aorta. *D.* The completed gastric fundic wrap showing the right and left crura approximated by tying the previously placed sutures. *E.* Sagittal section of the complete repair, showing posterior sutures in the crus and first and second row of sutures used to hold the partial fundoplication. Note the second row of sutures joins diaphragm, stomach, and esophagus. The position of the tied holding sutures is also shown. [*Reproduced with permission from DeMeester TR: Transthoracic antireflux procedures, in Nyhus LM, Baker RJ (eds): Mastery of Surgery. Boston: Little Brown & Company, 1984, p 388.*]

BARRETT'S ESOPHAGUS

The condition whereby the tubular esophagus is lined with columnar epithelium rather than squamous epithelium was first described by Norman Barrett in 1950. He incorrectly believed it to be congenital in origin. It is now realized that it is an acquired abnormality, occurs in 7 to 10% of patients with GERD, and represents the end stage of the natural history of this disease. It is also distinctly different from the congenital condition in which islands of gastric fundic epithelium are found in the upper half of the esophagus.

The definition of Barrett's esophagus (BE) has evolved considerably over the past decade. Traditionally, BE was identified by the presence of columnar mucosa extending at least 3 cm into the esophagus. It is now recognized that the specialized intestinal type

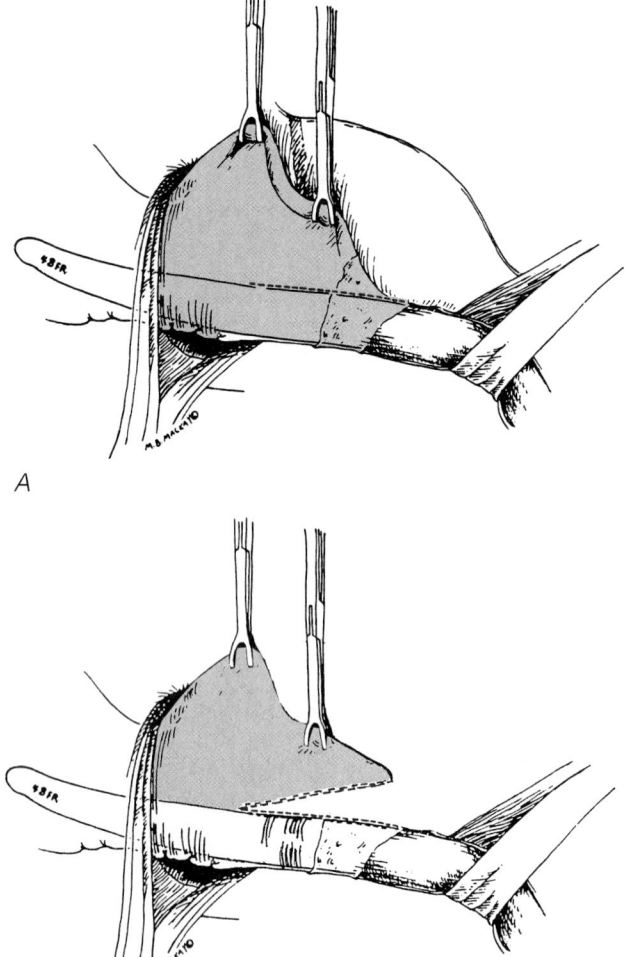

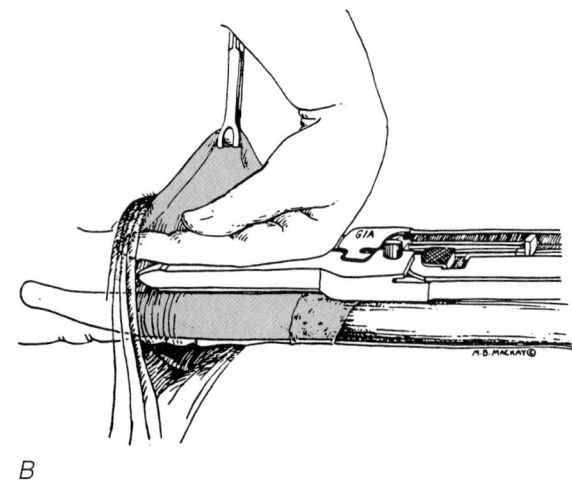

FIG. 24-49. *A.* Construction of a Collis gastroplasty. A 48F bougie is passed into the stomach. The dotted line indicates the site of division of the gastric wall for construction of the gastric tube in continuity with the esophagus. *B.* Continued construction of the Collis gastroplasty. The stomach is divided with a Endo-GIA stapler. Traction is exerted on the greater curvature side of the fundus before closing the jaws of the stapler. This ensures that the gastric tube closely approximates the diameter of the indwelling 48F bougie throughout its length. *C.* After stapling and division of the stomach, a 5-cm gastric tube is formed along the proximal portion of the lesser curvature. This effectively lengthens the esophagus and allows the construction of a Belsey partial fundoplication that can be placed below the diaphragm without tension. (*Reproduced with permission from Pearson FG, Cooper JD, et al: Gastroplasty and fundoplication for complex reflux problems. Ann Surg 206:473–81, 1987.*)

epithelium found in the Barrett's mucosa is the only tissue predisposed to malignant degeneration. Consequently, the diagnosis of BE is presently made given any length of endoscopically identifiable columnar mucosa that proves on biopsy to show intestinal metaplasia. While long segments of columnar mucosa without intestinal metaplasia do occur, they are uncommon and are probably congenital in origin.

The hallmark of intestinal metaplasia is the presence of intestinal goblet cells. There is a high prevalence of biopsy-demonstrated intestinal metaplasia at the cardia, on the gastric side of the squamocolumnar junction, in the absence of endoscopic evidence of a columnar-lined esophagus. Evidence is accumulating that these patches of what appears to be Barrett's in the cardia have a similar malignant potential as the longer segments, and are precursors for carcinoma of the cardia.

The long-term relief of symptoms remains the primary reason for performing antireflux surgery in patients with BE. Healing of esophageal mucosal injury and the prevention of disease progression are important secondary goals. In this regard, patients with BE are no different than the broader population of patients with gastroesophageal reflux. They should be considered for antireflux surgery when patient data suggest severe disease or predict the need for long-term medical management. Most patients with BE are symptomatic. Although it has been argued that some patients with BE may not

have symptoms, careful history taking will reveal the presence of symptoms in most, if not all, patients.

Patients with BE have a spectrum of disease ranging from visually identifiable but short segments, to long segments of classic BE. In general, however, they represent a relatively severe stage of gastroesophageal reflux, usually with markedly increased esophageal acid exposure, deficient LES characteristics, poor esophageal body function, and a high prevalence of duodenogastroesophageal reflux. Gastric hypersecretion occurs in 44% of patients. Most will require long-term proton pump inhibitor therapy for relief of symptoms and control of coexistent esophageal mucosal injury. Given such profound deficits in esophageal physiology, antireflux surgery is an excellent means of long-term control for most patients with BE. In years past, referral for antireflux surgery was reserved for patients with associated complications such as stricture, ulceration, or progression of the metaplastic segment. The advent of laparoscopic fundoplication and its successful control of gastroesophageal reflux in over 90% of patients has lowered the threshold for referral. Patients with quiescent, uncomplicated BE, particularly young patients, are now considered by many to be excellent candidates for antireflux surgery.

The typical complications in BE include ulceration in the columnar-lined segment, stricture formation, and a dysplasia-cancer sequence. Barrett's ulceration is unlike the erosive ulceration of

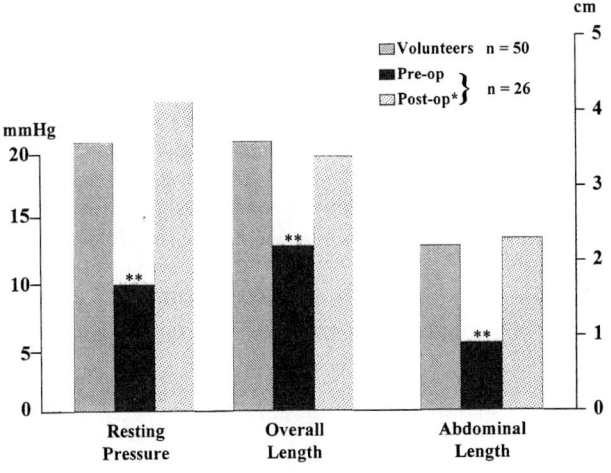

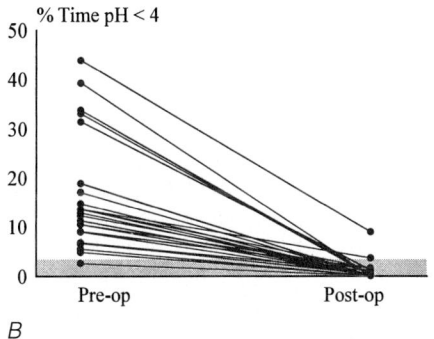

FIG. 24-50. *A.* Mean LES pressures before and after open and laparoscopic fundoplication. The line indicates the fifth percentile value for 50 normal volunteers (6 mm Hg). The average follow-up for these patients was 7.3 months for the laparoscopic and 54 months for the open group, respectively. * = p < 0.05 vs. preoperative values. *B.* Mean time of pH less than 4 on 24-hour esophageal pH monitoring before and after laparoscopic and open fundoplication. The line indicates the fifth percentile for 50 normal volunteers (4.3%). The average follow-up for these patients was 7.3 months for the laparoscopic and 54 months for the open group, respectively. * = p < 0.05 versus preoperative values.

reflux esophagitis in that it more closely resembles peptic ulceration in the stomach or duodenum, and has the same propensity to bleed, penetrate, or perforate. The strictures found in BE occur at the squamocolumnar junction, and are typically higher than peptic strictures in the absence of BE. Ulceration and stricture in association with BE were commonly reported prior to 1975, but with the advent of potent acid suppression medication they have become less common. In contrast, the complication of adenocarcinoma developing

in Barrett's mucosa has become more common. Adenocarcinoma developing in Barrett's mucosa was considered a rare tumor prior to 1975. Today it occurs in approximately one in every 100 patient-years of follow-up, which represents a risk 40 times that of the general population. Most if not all cases of adenocarcinoma of the esophagus arise in Barrett's epithelium (Fig. 24-51). About one third of all patients with BE present with malignancy.

The long-term risk of progression to dysplasia and adenocarcinoma, while not the driving force behind the decision to perform antireflux surgery, is a significant concern for both patient and physician. Although to date there have been no prospective randomized studies documenting that antireflux surgery has an effect on the risk of progression to dysplasia and carcinoma, complete control of reflux of gastric juice into the esophagus is clearly a desirable goal. As data accumulate regarding the relative impact of medical and surgical therapy on the natural history of Barrett's metaplasia, the risk of progression may play a larger role in therapeutic decisions.

Outcome of Antireflux Surgery in Patients with Barrett's Esophagus

Few studies have focused on the alleviation of symptoms after antireflux surgery in patients with BE (Table 24-7). Those that are available document excellent to good results in 72 to 95% of patients at 5 years following surgery.

Several studies have compared medical and surgical therapy. Attwood and associates, in a prospective but nonrandomized study, reported on 45 patients undergoing either medical (26) or surgical (19) treatment of BE. The groups were similar in age, length of Barrett's segment, the percentage of time during which pH was less than 4, and length of follow-up. Improvement of symptoms was dramatic after antireflux surgery. Symptoms of heartburn or dysphagia recurred in 88% of patients treated with medical therapy alone, and 21% after antireflux surgery. Complications, most commonly the development of an esophageal stricture, occurred in 38% of medically treated patients and 16 percent of surgically treated patients (p < 0.05) over the 3-year follow-up period. One patient in each group developed esophageal adenocarcinoma. It was concluded that antireflux surgery was superior to acid suppression for both the control of symptoms and the prevention of complications in patients with BE. Other nonrandomized comparisons of medical and surgical therapy have reported similar results.

Parrilla and colleagues recently reported an update of a study originally published in the *British Journal of Surgery* in 1996. One hundred one patients were enrolled over 18 years (1982 to 2000). Median follow-up was 6 years. Medical therapy consisted of 20 mg of omeprazole (PPI) twice daily since 1992 in all medically treated patients. Surgical therapy consisted of an open 1.5 to 3.0 cm Nissen, over a 48 to 50F bougie, with division of the short gastric arteries in 39% of patients, and crural closure in all. Symptomatic outcome

Table 24-6

Improvement of the Primary Symptom Responsible for Surgery After the Various Tailored Antireflux Procedures

	N	No. of Patients Cured	No. of Patients Failed	% Cured
Abdominal Nissen	49	44	5	90
Thoracic Nissen	20	19	1	95
Belsey	6	4	2	67
Collis-Belsey	10	8	2	80
Total	85	75	10	89

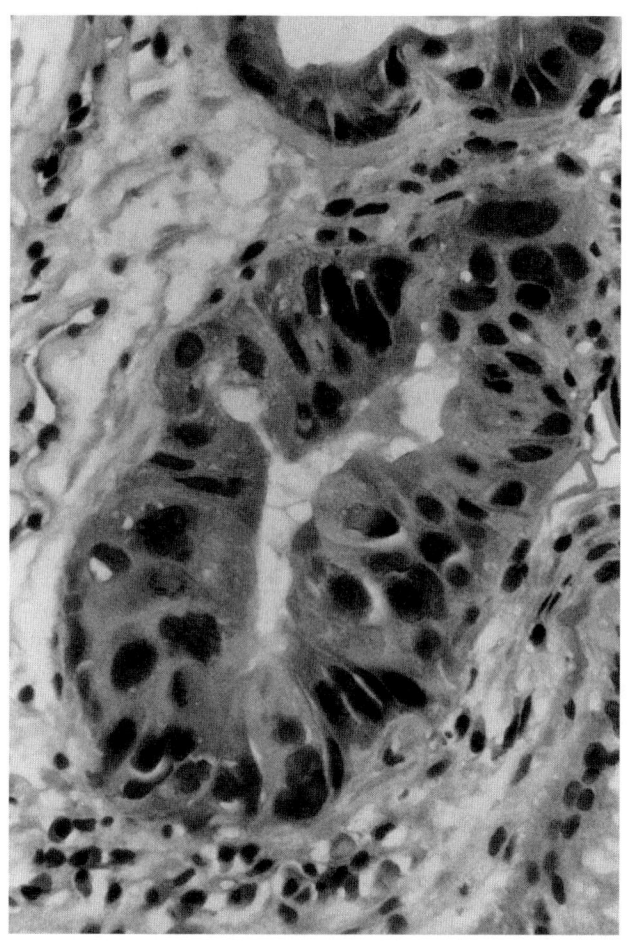

A

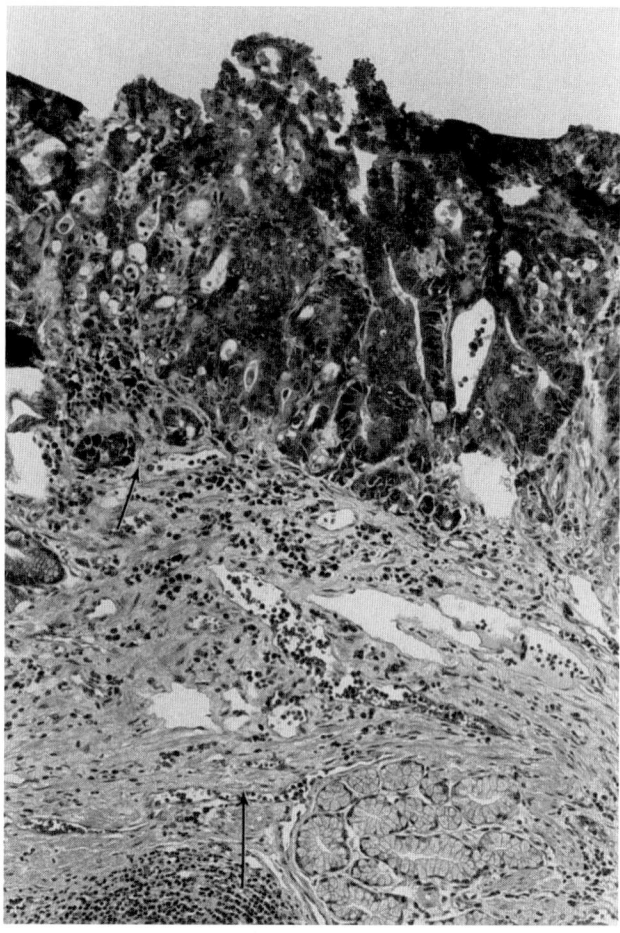

B

FIG. 24-51. Photomicrographs. *A*. Barrett's epithelium with severe dysplasia (×200). Note nuclear irregularity, stratification, and loss of polarity. *B*. Barrett's epithelium with intramucosal carcinoma (×66). Note malignant cells in the mucosa (*upper arrow*), but not invading the muscularis mucosae (*bottom arrow*). [Reproduced with permission from DeMeester TR, Stein HJ, Fuchs KH: Physiologic diagnostic studies, in Zuidema GD, Orringer MB (eds): Shackelford's Surgery of the Alimentary Tract, 3rd ed, Vol. I. Philadelphia: WB Saunders, 1991, p 113.]

in the two groups was nearly identical, although esophagitis and/or stricture persisted in 20% of the medically treated patients, compared to only 3 to 7% of patients following antireflux surgery. Fifteen percent of patients had abnormal acid exposure after surgery. Although pH data were not routinely collected in patients on PPI therapy, in the subgroup of 12 patients that did have 24-hour monitoring on treatment, three of 12 (25%) had persistently high esophageal acid exposure, and most (75%) had persistently high bilirubin exposure.

The outcome of laparoscopic Nissen fundoplication in patients with BE has been assessed at 1 to 3 years after surgery. Hofstetter and colleagues reported the experience at the University of Southern California (USC) with 85 patients with BE at a median of 5 years after surgery. Fifty-nine patients had long and 26 had short segment Barrett's; 50 had a laparoscopic approach. Reflux symptoms were absent in 67 of 85 patients (79%). Eighteen (20%) developed recurrent symptoms, while four patients were back on daily acid-suppressive medication. Seven patients underwent a secondary

Table 24-7
Symptomatic Outcome of Surgical Therapy for Barrett's Esophagus

Author	Year	No. of Patients	% Excellent to Good Response	Mean Follow-Up, Years
Starnes	1984	8	75	2
Williamson	1990	37	92	3
DeMeester	1990	35	77	3
McDonald	1996	113	82.2	6.5
Ortiz	1996	32	90.6	5

repair and were asymptomatic, raising the eventual successful outcome to 87%. Postoperative 24-hour pH was normal in 17 of 21 patents (81%). Ninety-nine percent of the patients considered themselves cured (77%) or improved (22%), and 97% were satisfied with the surgery.

Farrell and associates also reported symptomatic outcome of laparoscopic Nissen fundoplication in 50 patients with both long- and short-segment BE. Mean scores for heartburn, regurgitation, and dysphagia all improved dramatically post-Nissen. Importantly, there was no significant decrement in symptom scores when 1-year results were compared to those at 2 to 5 years postoperatively. They did find a higher prevalence of "anatomic" failures requiring re-operation in patients with BE when compared to non-Barrett's patients with GERD. Others have reported similar results. Taken together these studies document the ability of antireflux surgery to provide long-term symptomatic relief in patients with BE.

Long-Term Results

Three relevant questions arise concerning the fate, over time, of the metaplastic tissue found in Barrett's esophagus: (1) Does antireflux surgery cause regression of Barrett's epithelium? (2) Does it prevent progression? and (3) Can the development of Barrett's metaplasia be prevented by early antireflux surgery in patients with reflux disease?

The common belief that Barrett's epithelium cannot be reversed is likely false. DeMeester and associates reported that after antireflux surgery, loss of intestinal metaplasia (IM) in patients with visible BE was rare, but occurred in 73% of patients with inapparent IM of the cardia. This suggests that the metaplastic process may indeed be reversible if reflux is eliminated early in its process, that cardiac mucosa is dynamic, and that as opposed to IM extending several centimeters into the esophagus, IM of the cardia is more likely to regress following antireflux surgery. Gurski and colleagues recently reviewed pre- and posttreatment endoscopic biopsies from 77 Barrett's patients treated surgically and 14 treated with PPIs. Posttreatment histology was classified as having regressed if two consecutive biopsies taken more than 6 months apart, plus all subsequent biopsies, showed loss of IM or loss of dysplasia. Histopathologic regression occurred in 28 of 77 patients (36.4%) following antireflux surgery, and in one of 14 (7.1%) patients treated with PPIs alone ($p < 0.03$). After surgery, regression from low-grade dysplastic to nondysplastic BE occurred in 17 of 25 (68%) patients and from IM to no IM in 11 of 52 (21.2%) patients. Both types of regression were significantly more common in short- (<3 cm) compared to long-segment (>3 cm) Barrett's esophagus. Eight patients progressed; five from IM alone to low-grade dysplasia, and three from low- to high-grade dysplasia. All those who progressed had long-segment BE. On multivariate analysis, the presence of short-segment Barrett's, and the type of treatment, were significantly associated with regression; age, sex, surgical procedure, and preoperative LES and pH characteristics were not. The median time of biopsy-proven regression was 18.5 months after surgery, with 95% occurring within 5 years. Similar findings have been reported by the University of Washington group and Hunter and colleagues. Although these studies do not conclusively prove the ability of antireflux surgery to reverse the changes of early BE, they do provide encouragement that given early changes, the process may indeed be reversible.

Recent evidence suggests that the development of BE may even be preventable. Although a very difficult hypothesis to study, Oberg and coworkers followed a cohort of 69 patients with short-segment, nonintestinalized, columnar-lined esophagus (CLE) over a median of 5 years of surveillance endoscopy. Forty-nine of the patients were maintained on PPI therapy and 20 had antireflux surgery. Patients with antireflux surgery were 10 times less likely to develop IM in these CLE segments over a follow-up span of nearly 15 years than those on medical therapy. This rather remarkable observation supports the two-step hypothesis of the development of BE (cardiac metaplasia followed by intestinal metaplasia), and suggests that the second step can be prevented if reflux disease is recognized and treated early and aggressively.

Current data indicate that patients with BE should remain in an endoscopic surveillance program following antireflux surgery. Biopsy specimens should be reviewed by a pathologist with expertise in the field. If low-grade dysplasia is confirmed, biopsies should be repeated after 12 weeks of high-dose acid suppression therapy. If high-grade dysplasia is evident on more than one biopsy specimen, esophageal resection is advisable because of the more than 50% probability that an invasive cancer is already present. Early detection and resection have been shown to decrease the mortality rate from esophageal cancer in these patients.

Since BE results from chronic uncontrolled gastroesophageal reflux, and esophageal adenocarcinoma is virtually always associated with intestinal metaplasia, there are strong theoretical grounds for halting the progression toward malignancy by permanently and effectively stopping reflux of gastric contents. Thus prevention of progression, not regression, becomes the central issue. Although some cancers have developed after antireflux surgery, the absence of pre-existent dysplasia prior to surgery or the efficacy of the operative procedure in reducing 24-hour esophageal acid exposure to normal has not been documented. If the dysplasia is reported as lower grade or indeterminant, then inflammatory change often confused with dysplasia should be suppressed by a course of acid suppression therapy in high doses for 2 to 3 weeks, followed by rebiopsy of the Barrett's segment.

There is a growing body of evidence to attest to the ability of fundoplication to protect against dysplasia and invasive malignancy. Three studies suggest that an effective antireflux procedure can impact the natural history of BE in this regard. Two prospective randomized studies found less adenocarcinoma in the surgically treated groups. Parrilla and associates reported that although the development of dysplasia and adenocarcinoma was no different overall, the subgroup of surgical patients with normal postoperative pH studies developed significantly less dysplasia and had no adenocarcinoma. Spechler identified one adenocarcinoma 11 to 13 years after antireflux surgery, compared to four following medical treatment. Most of these authors concluded that there is a critical need for future trials exploring the role of antireflux surgery in protecting against the development of dysplasia in patients with BE.

Data from the Mayo Clinic strongly suggest that antireflux surgery impacts the development of adenocarcinoma in patients with BE. The authors reviewed the outcome of 118 patients with BE undergoing antireflux surgery between 1960 and 1990. Three cancers occurred over an 18.5-year follow-up period, all within the first 3 years after surgery. The fact that the development of adenocarcinoma was clustered in the early years after antireflux surgery, and not randomly dispersed throughout the follow-up period, suggests that antireflux surgery altered the natural history of the disease. Hammeetman has shown that once dysplasia has developed, carcinoma ensues in an average of 3 years. The occurrence of all observed cancers in the first few years suggests that the point of no return in the dysplasia-cancer sequence had already occurred prior to the time of antireflux surgery.

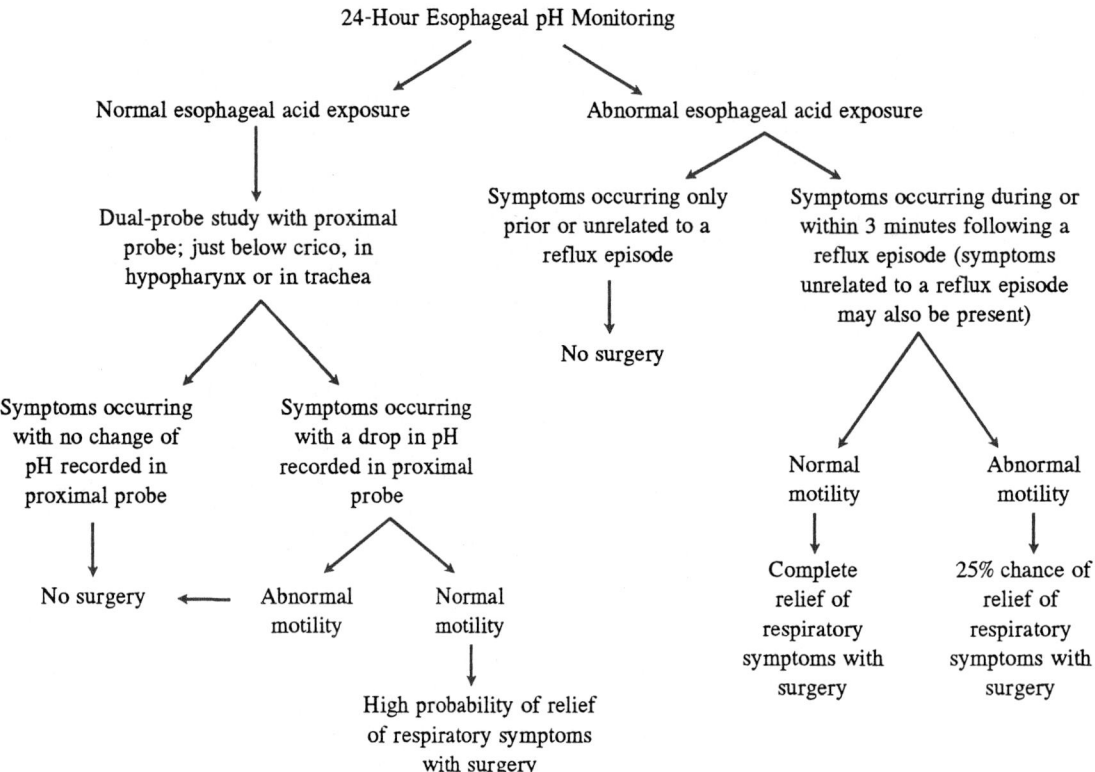

FIG. 24-52. Proposed management algorithm to select patients with unexplained recalcitrant respiratory symptoms for antireflux surgery.

Atypical Reflux Symptoms

Chronic respiratory symptoms, such as chronic cough, recurrent pneumonias, episodes of nocturnal choking, waking up with gastric contents in the mouth, or soilage of the bed pillow, may also indicate the need for surgical therapy (Fig. 24-52). The chest x-ray in patients suffering from repetitive pulmonary aspiration secondary to gastroesophageal reflux often shows signs of pleural thickening, bronchiectasis, and chronic interstitial pulmonary fibrosis. If 24-hour pH monitoring confirms the presence of increased esophageal acid exposure, and manometry shows normal esophageal body motility, an antireflux procedure can be done with an expected good result. However, these patients usually have a nonspecific motor abnormality of the esophageal body which tends to propel the refluxed material toward the pharynx. In some of these patients, the motor abnormality will disappear after a surgical antireflux procedure. In others, the motor disorder will persist and contribute to postoperative aspiration of swallowed saliva and food. Consequently, the results of an antireflux procedure in patients with a motor disorder of the esophageal body are variable.

Chest pain may be an atypical symptom of gastroesophageal reflux, and is often confused with coronary artery disease. Fifty percent of patients in whom a cardiac cause of the chest pain has been excluded will have increased esophageal acid exposure as a cause of the episode of pain. An antireflux procedure provides relief of the chest pain more consistently than medical therapy.

Dysphagia, regurgitation, or chest pain on eating in a patient with normal endoscopy and esophageal function studies can be an indication for an antireflux procedure. These symptoms are usually related to the presence of a large paraesophageal hernia, intrathoracic stomach, or a small hiatal hernia with a narrow diaphragmatic

hiatus. A Schatzki ring may be present with the latter. All these conditions are easily identified with an upper gastrointestinal radiographic barium examination done by a knowledgeable radiologist. These patients may have no heartburn, since the LES is usually normal and reflux of gastric acid into the esophagus does not occur. The surgical repair of the hernia usually includes an antireflux procedure because of the potential of destroying the competency of the cardia during the surgical dissection.

Reoperation for Failed Antireflux Repairs

Failure of an antireflux procedure occurs when after the repair the patient is unable to swallow normally, experiences upper abdominal discomfort during and after meals, or has recurrence or persistence of reflux symptoms. The assessment of these symptoms and the selection of patients who need further surgery are challenging problems. Functional assessment of patients who have recurrent, persistent, or emergent new symptoms following a primary antireflux repair is critical to identifying the cause of the failure. Analysis of patients requiring reoperation after a previous antireflux procedure shows that placement of the wrap around the stomach is the most frequent cause for failure after open procedures, while herniation of the repair into the chest is the most frequent cause of failure after a laparoscopic procedure. In both instances this is probably due to an unrecognized short esophagus. In the laparoscopic approach the elevated diaphragm allows the repair to be properly placed, but the tension from the short esophagus pulls the repair above the diaphragm when the crura are relaxed. Partial or complete breakdown of the fundoplication and construction of a too-tight or too-long wrap of a fundoplication occurs with both open and closed procedures. The fact that 10% of these patients had an undiagnosed underlying esophageal motor disorder underlines the critical role of preoperative esophageal function tests before the initial procedure.

The preferred surgical approach to a patient who has had a previously failed antireflux procedure is through a left thoracotomy with a peripheral circumferential incision in the diaphragm, to provide for simultaneous exposure of the upper abdomen and safe dissection of the previous repair from both abdominal and thoracic sides of the diaphragm. Patients who have recurrence of heartburn and regurgitation without dysphagia and have good esophageal motility are most amenable to reoperation, and can be expected to have an excellent outcome. When dysphagia is the cause of failure, the situation is more difficult to manage. If the dysphagia occurred immediately following the repair, it is usually due to a technical failure, most commonly a misplaced fundoplication around the upper stomach, and reoperation is usually satisfactory. When dysphagia is associated with poor motility and multiple previous repairs, serious consideration should be given to esophageal resection and replacement. With each reoperation the esophagus is damaged further, and the chances of preserving function become less. Also, blood supply is reduced, and ischemic necrosis of the esophagus can occur after several previous mobilizations.

MOTILITY DISORDERS OF THE PHARYNX AND ESOPHAGUS

Clinical Manifestations

Dysphagia (i.e., difficulty in swallowing) is the primary symptom of esophageal motor disorders. Its perception by the patient is a balance between the severity of the underlying abnormality causing the dysphagia, and the adjustment made by the patient in altering eating habits. Consequently, any complaint of dysphagia must include an assessment of the patient's dietary history. It must be known whether the patient experiences pain, chokes, or vomits with eating; whether the patient requires liquids with the meal, is the last to finish, or is forced to interrupt a social meal; and whether he or she has been admitted to the hospital for food impaction. These assessments, plus an evaluation of the patient's nutritional status, help to determine how severe the dysphagia is and evaluate the indications for surgical therapy.

A surgical myotomy is designed to improve the symptoms of dysphagia caused by a motility disorder. The results can profoundly improve the patient's ability to ingest food, but rarely return the function of the foregut to normal. The principle of the procedure is to destroy esophageal contractility in order to correct a defect in esophageal motility, resulting in improvement but never a return to normal function. To use a surgical myotomy to treat the problem of dysphagia, the surgeon needs to know the precise functional abnormality causing the symptom. This usually entails a complete esophageal motility evaluation. A clear understanding of the physiologic mechanism of swallowing, and determination of the motility abnormality giving rise to the dysphagia, are essential for determining if surgery is indicated and the extent of the myotomy to be performed. Endoscopy is necessary only to exclude the presence of tumor or inflammatory changes as the cause of dysphagia.

Motility Disorders of the Pharyngoesophageal Segment

Disorders of the pharyngoesophageal phase of swallowing result from a discoordination of the neuromuscular events involved in chewing, initiation of swallowing, and propulsion of the material from the oropharynx into the cervical esophagus. They can be categorized into one or a combination of the following abnormalities: (1) inadequate oropharyngeal bolus transport; (2) inability to pressurize the pharynx; (3) inability to elevate the larynx; (4) discoordination of pharyngeal contraction and cricopharyngeal relaxation; and (5) decreased compliance of the pharyngoesophageal segment secondary to muscle pathology. The latter results in incomplete anatomic relaxation of the cricopharyngeus and cervical esophagus.

Pharyngoesophageal swallowing disorders are usually congenital or due to acquired disease involving the central and peripheral nervous system. This includes cerebrovascular accidents, brain stem tumors, poliomyelitis, multiple sclerosis, Parkinson's disease, pseudobulbar palsy, peripheral neuropathy, and operative damage to the cranial nerves involved in swallowing. Muscular diseases such as radiation-induced myopathy, dermatomyositis, myotonic dystrophy, and myasthenia gravis are less common causes. Rarely, extrinsic compression by thyromegaly, cervical lymphadenopathy, or hyperostosis of the cervical spine can cause pharyngoesophageal dysphagia.

Diagnostic Assessment of the Cricopharyngeal Segment

Abnormalities of pharyngoesophageal swallowing are difficult to assess with standard manometric techniques because of the rapidity of the oropharyngeal phase of swallowing, the movement of the gullet, and the asymmetry of the cricopharyngeus. Video- or cineradiography is currently the most objective test to evaluate oropharyngeal bolus transport, pharyngeal compression, relaxation of the pharyngoesophageal segment, and the dynamics of airway protection during swallowing. It readily identifies a diverticulum (Fig. 24-53), stasis of the contrast medium in the valleculae, a cricopharyngeal bar, and/or narrowing of the pharyngoesophageal segment. These are anatomic manifestations of neuromuscular disease, and result from the loss of muscle compliance in portions of the pharynx and esophagus composed of skeletal muscle.

Careful analysis of video- or cineradiographic studies combined with manometry using specially designed catheters can identify the cause of a pharyngoesophageal dysfunction in most situations

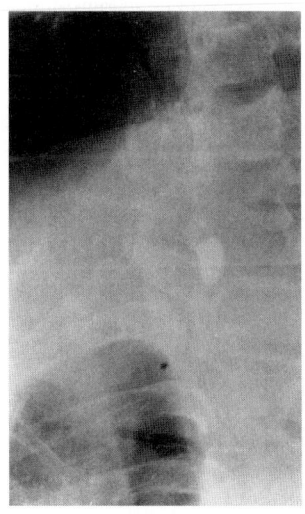 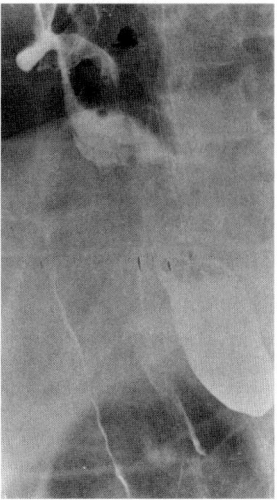

A   *B*

FIG. 24-53. *A.* Zenker's diverticulum, initially discovered 15 years ago and left untreated. *B.* Note its marked enlargement and evidence of laryngeal inlet aspiration on recent esophagogram. (*Reproduced with permission from Waters PF, DeMeester TR: Foregut motor disorders and their surgical management. Med Clin North Am 65:1235, 1981.*)

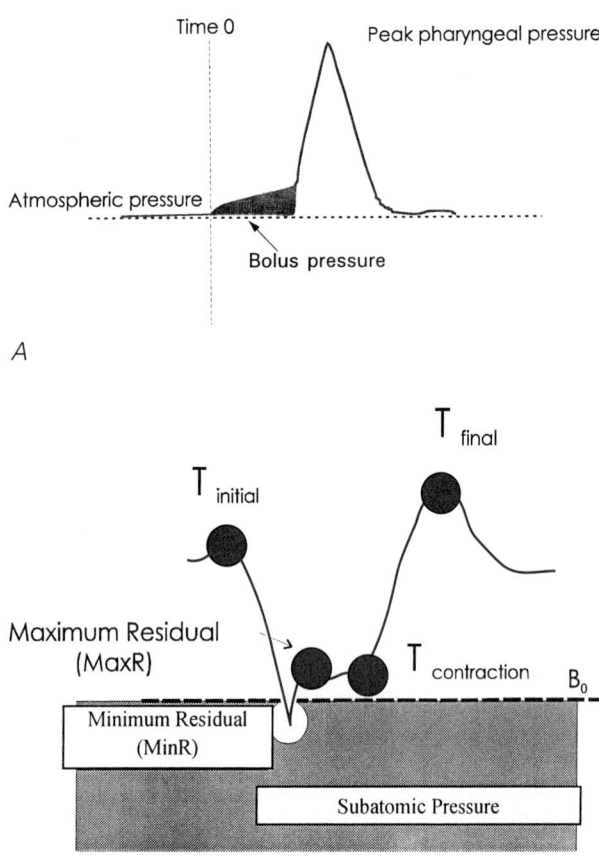

FIG. 24-54. *A.* Schematic drawing of a pharyngeal pressure wave indicating the presence of the bolus pressure. *B.* Schematic drawing of the manometric recording typically seen during cricopharyngeal sphincter relaxation.

(Fig. 24-54). Motility studies may demonstrate inadequate pharyngeal pressurization, insufficient or lack of cricopharyngeal relaxation, marked discoordination of pharyngeal pressurization, cricopharyngeal relaxation and cervical esophageal contraction, or a hypopharyngeal bolus pressure suggesting decreased compliance of the skeletal portion of the cervical esophagus (Fig. 24-55).

In many patients with cricopharyngeal dysfunction, including those with Zenker's diverticulum, it has been difficult to consistently demonstrate a motility abnormality or discoordination of pharyngoesophageal events. The abnormality most apt to be present is a loss of compliance in the pharyngoesophageal segment manifested by an increased bolus pressure. Cook and colleagues have demonstrated an increased resistance to the movement of a bolus through what appears on manometry to be a completely relaxed cricopharyngeal sphincter. Using simultaneous manometry and videofluoroscopy they showed that in these patients the cricopharyngeus is only partially relaxed; that is, the sphincter is relaxed enough to allow a drop of its pressure to esophageal baseline on manometry, but insufficiently relaxed to allow unimpaired passage of the bolus into the esophagus (Fig. 24-56). This incomplete relaxation is due to a loss of compliance of the muscle in the pharyngoesophageal segment, and may be associated with a cricopharyngeal bar or Zenker's diverticulum. This decreased compliance of the cricopharyngeal sphincter can be recognized on esophageal manometry by a "shoulder" on the pharyngeal pressure wave, the amplitude of which correlates directly with the degree of outflow obstruction (Fig. 24-57).

Increasing the diameter of this noncompliant segment reduces the resistance imposed on the passage of a bolus. Consequently, patients with low pharyngeal pressure (i.e., poor piston function of the pharynx), or patients with increased resistance of the pharyngocervical esophageal segment from loss of skeletal muscle compliance, are improved by a pharyngocricocervical esophageal myotomy. This enlarges the pharyngoesophageal segment and reduces outflow resistance. Esophageal muscle biopsy specimens from patients with Zenker's diverticulum have shown histologic evidence of the restrictive myopathy in the pharyngoesophageal segment. These findings correlate well with the observation of a decreased compliance of the upper esophagus demonstrated by videoradiography and the findings on detailed manometric studies of the pharynx and cervical esophagus. They suggest that the diverticulum develops as a consequence of the outflow resistance to bolus transport through the noncompliant muscle of the pharyngoesophageal segment.

The requirements for a successful pharyngoesophageal myotomy are (1) adequate oropharyngeal bolus transport; (2) the presence of an intact swallowing reflex; (3) reasonable coordination of pharyngeal pressurization with cricopharyngeal relaxation; and (4) a cricopharyngeal bar, Zenker's diverticulum, or a narrowed pharyngoesophageal segment on videoesophagogram and/or the presence of excessive pharyngoesophageal shoulder pressure on motility study.

Zenker's Diverticulum

In the past, the most common recognized sign of pharyngoesophageal dysfunction was the presence of a Zenker's diverticulum, originally described by Ludlow in 1769. The eponym resulted from Zenker's classic clinicopathologic descriptions of 34 cases published in 1878. Pharyngoesophageal diverticula have been reported to occur in 0.1% of 20,000 routine barium examinations, and classically occur in elderly, white males. Zenker's diverticula tend to enlarge progressively with time due to the decreased compliance of the skeletal portion of the cervical esophagus that occurs with aging.

Presenting symptoms include dysphagia associated with the spontaneous regurgitation of undigested, bland material, often interrupting eating or drinking. The symptom of dysphagia is due initially to the loss of muscle compliance in the pharyngoesophageal segment, later augmented by the presence of an enlarging diverticulum. On occasion, the dysphagia can be severe enough to cause debilitation and significant weight loss. Chronic aspiration and repetitive respiratory infection are common associated complaints. Once suspected, the diagnosis is established by a barium swallow. Endoscopy is usually difficult in the presence of a cricopharyngeal diverticulum, and potentially dangerous, owing to obstruction of the true esophageal lumen by the diverticulum and the attendant risk of diverticular perforation.

Pharyngocricoesophageal Myotomy

The low morbidity and mortality associated with cricopharyngeal and upper esophageal myotomy have encouraged a liberal approach toward its use for almost any problem in the oropharyngeal phase of swallowing. This attitude has resulted in an overall success rate in the relief of symptoms of only 64%. When patients are selected using radiographic or motility markers of disease as outlined above, it is unusual for patients not to see benefit.

The myotomy can be performed under local or general anesthesia through an incision along the anterior border of the left sternocleidomastoid muscle. The pharynx and cervical esophagus are exposed by retracting the sternocleidomastoid muscle and carotid sheath laterally, and the thyroid, trachea, and larynx medially (Fig. 24-58). When a pharyngoesophageal diverticulum is present, localization of the pharyngoesophageal segment is easy. The diverticulum is carefully freed from the overlying areolar tissue to expose its neck, just below the inferior pharyngeal constrictor and above the cricopharyngeus muscle. It can be difficult to identify the cricopharyngeus muscle in the absence of a diverticulum. A benefit of local anesthesia is that the patient can swallow and demonstrate an area of persistent narrowing at the pharyngoesophageal junction. Furthermore, before closing the incision, gelatin can be fed to the patient to ascertain whether the symptoms have been relieved, and to inspect the opening of the previously narrowed pharyngoesophageal segment. Under general anesthesia, and in the absence of a diverticulum, the placement of a nasogastric tube to the level of the manometrically determined cricopharyngeal sphincter helps in localization of the structures. The myotomy is extended cephalad by dividing 1 to 2 cm of inferior constrictor muscle of the pharynx,

and caudad by dividing the cricopharyngeal muscle and the cervical esophagus for a length of 4 to 5 cm. The cervical wound is closed only when all oozing of blood has ceased, since a hematoma after this procedure is common, and is often associated with temporary dysphagia while the hematoma absorbs. Oral alimentation is started the day after surgery. The patient is usually discharged on the first or second postoperative day.

If a diverticulum is present and is large enough to persist after a myotomy, it may be sutured in the inverted position to the prevertebral fascia using a permanent suture (i.e., diverticulopexy) (Fig. 24-59). If the diverticulum is excessively large so that it would be redundant if suspended, or if its walls are thickened, a diverticulectomy should be performed.

Endoscopic stapled diverticulotomy recently has been described. The procedure utilizes a Weerda diverticuloscope with two retractable valves passed into the hypopharynx. The lips of the diverticuloscope are positioned so that one lip lies in the esophageal

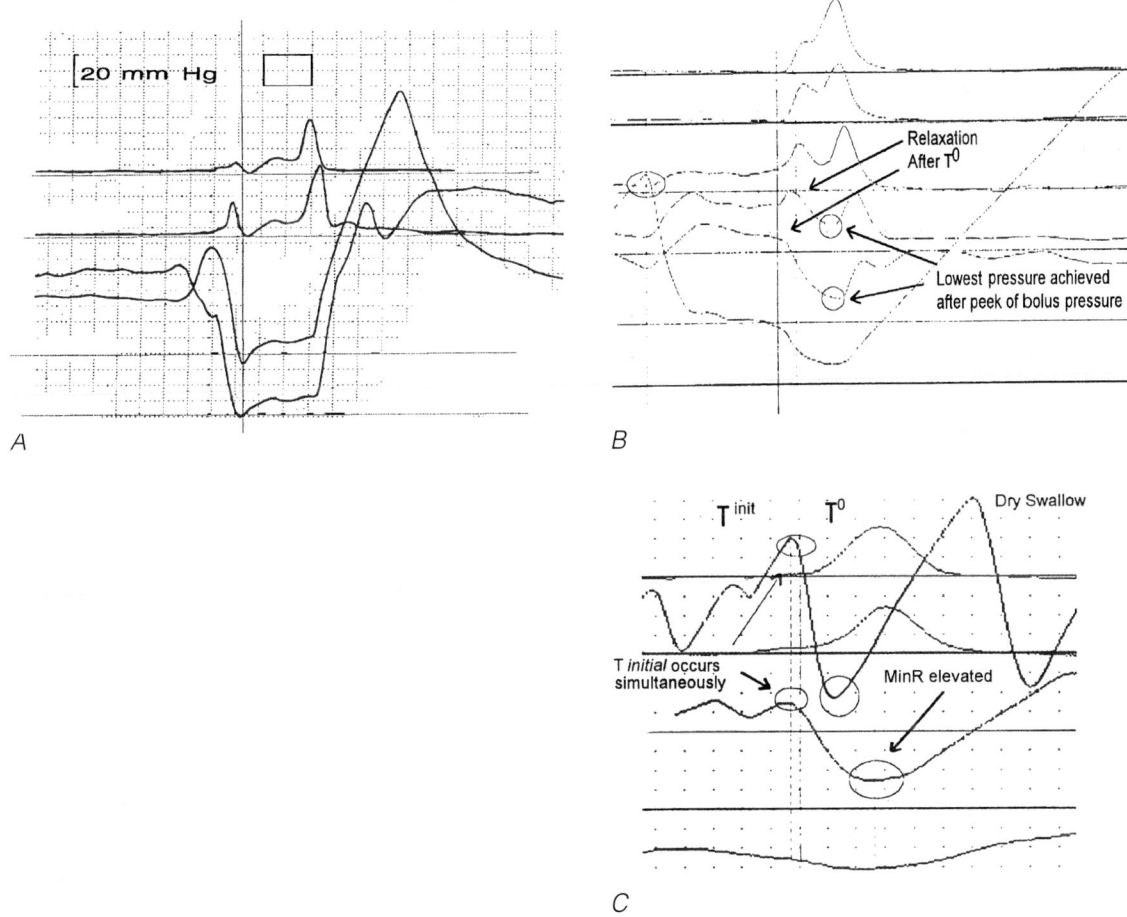

FIG. 24-55. *A.* Example of a detailed cricopharyngeal manometric study of a normal volunteer. The top two channels are in the pharynx and the bottom two in the cricopharyngeal sphincter. There is normal pharyngeal wave progression, no bolus pressure, and normal coordination (the minimum residual pressure of the cricopharyngeus occurs before the swallow). *B.* Detailed cricopharyngeal manometric tracing showing features consistent with a cricopharyngeal relaxation abnormality. Cricopharyngeal relaxation occurs after the initiation of the swallow, is simultaneous in both channels in the cricopharyngeal sphincter, and the minimal residual pressure is well above atmospheric pressure. *C.* Detailed cricopharyngeal manometric tracing showing features consistent with a defect in opening of the cricopharyngeal sphincter. The onset of the contraction (T-initial) occurs before the upstroke of the pharyngeal wave and is simultaneous in all channels recording the cricopharyngeal. *D. (Overleaf)* Detailed cricopharyngeal manometric tracing showing features consistent with increased outflow resistance and altered compliance of the cricopharyngeal muscle. The normal subatmospheric pressure drop seen in the cricopharyngeal sphincter is absent, the t-initial in the distal channels occurs before that of the proximal channels, and the pharyngeal bolus pressure and the bolus pressure within the sphincter increases with increasing volumes of water. *(Continued)*

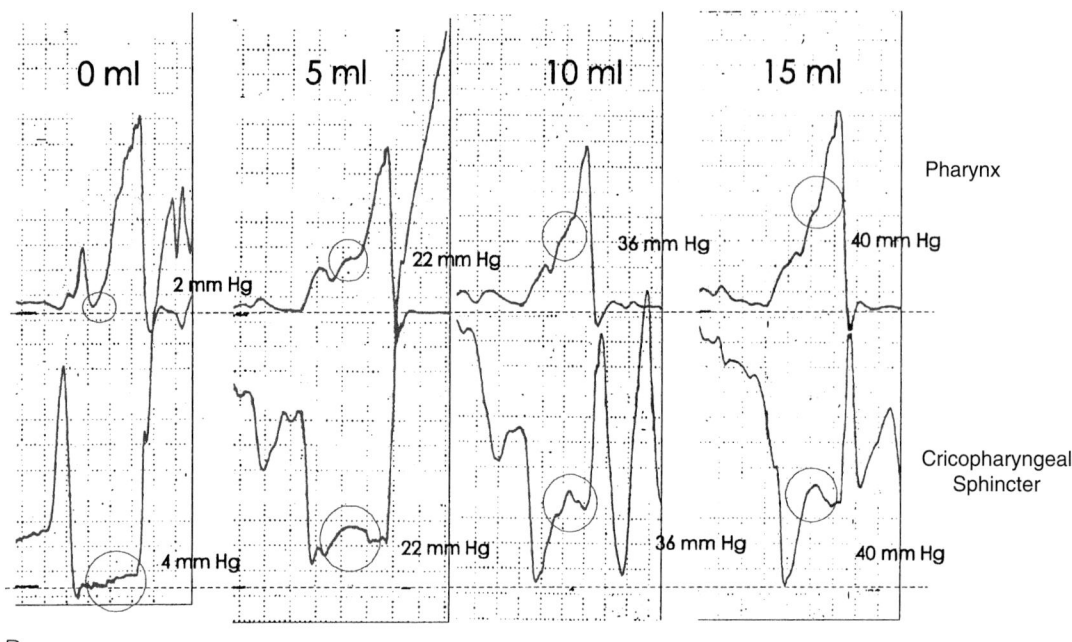

D

FIG. 24-55. (continued)

lumen and the other in the diverticular lumen. The valves of the diverticuloscope are retracted appropriately so as to visualize the septum interposed between the diverticulum and the esophagus. An endoscopic linear stapler is introduced into the diverticuloscope and positioned against the common septum with the anvil in the diverticulum and the cartridge in the esophageal lumen. Firing of the stapler divides the common septum between the posterior esophageal and the diverticular wall over a length of 30 mm, placing three rows of staples on each side. More than one stapler application may be needed, depending on the size of the diverticulum. The patient is allowed to resume liquid feeds either on the same day or the day after, and is usually discharged the day after surgery. Complications are rare and may include perforation at the apex of the diverticulum, and can be repaired with minimally invasive techniques.

Postoperative complications include fistula formation, abscess, hematoma, recurrent nerve paralysis, difficulties in phonation, and Horner's syndrome. The incidence of the first two can be reduced by performing a diverticulopexy. Recurrence of a Zenker's

diverticulum occurs late, and is more common after diverticulectomy without myotomy, presumably due to persistence of the underlying loss of compliance of the cervical esophagus when a myotomy is not performed.

Postoperative motility studies have shown that the peak pharyngeal pressure generated on swallowing is not affected, the resting cricopharyngeal pressure is reduced but not eliminated, and the cricopharyngeal sphincter length is shortened. Consequently, after myotomy there is protection against esophagopharyngeal regurgitation.

Motility Disorders of the Esophageal Body and Lower Esophageal Sphincter

Disorders of the esophageal phase of swallowing result from abnormalities in the propulsive pump action of the esophageal body or the relaxation of the LES. These disorders result from either primary esophageal abnormalities, or from generalized neural, muscular,

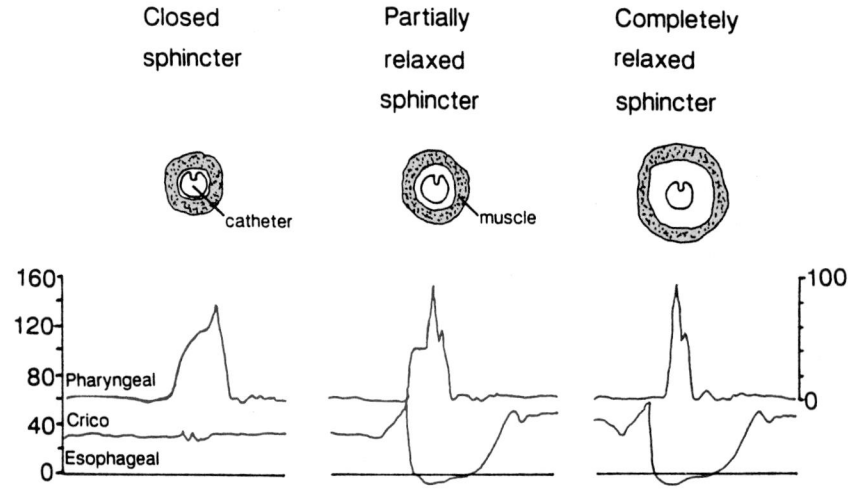

FIG. 24-56. Manometric record showing a hypopharyngeal pressure ramp and apparent normal relaxation of the upper esophageal sphincter. This finding indicates an increased intrabolus pressure during transsphincteric flow and is suggestive of decreased compliance of the upper esophageal sphincter.

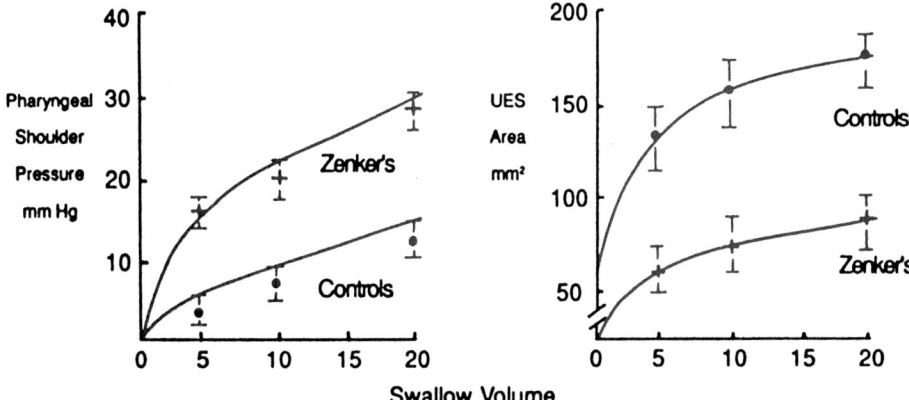

FIG. 24-57. Pharyngeal shoulder pressures and diameter of the pharyngo-esophageal segment in normals and patients with Zenker's diverticulum. UES = upper esophageal sphincter. [Data from Cook IJ, et al: Zenker's diverticulum: Evidence for a restrictive cricopharyngeal myopathy. Gastroenterology 96:A98, 1989.]

or collagen vascular disease (Table 24-8). The use of standard esophageal manometry techniques has allowed specific primary esophageal motility disorders to be identified out of a pool of nonspecific motility abnormalities. These include achalasia, diffuse esophageal spasm, the so-called nutcracker esophagus, and the hypertensive LES. The manometric characteristics of these disorders are shown in Table 24-9.

However, the boundaries between the primary esophageal motor disorders are vague, and intermediate types exist. This is because their diagnosis usually is based on the analysis of 10 wet swallows performed in a laboratory setting. The technique of ambulatory 24-hour monitoring of esophageal motor activity allows the classification of esophageal motor disorders to be performed on the basis of more than 1000 contractions recorded during different physiologic states (i.e., normal daily activities including eating and sleeping). There are significant differences in the classification of esophageal motor disorders based on standard manometry and classification based on ambulatory monitoring (see Fig. 24-25). The degree of reclassification that occurs when analysis of esophageal motor function is done on the basis of ambulatory manometry indicates that the classic categories of esophageal motor disorders are inappropriate. These findings indicate that esophageal motility disorders should be looked at as a spectrum of abnormalities that reflects various stages of destruction of esophageal motor function.

Achalasia

The best known and best understood primary motility disorder of the esophagus is achalasia, with an incidence of six per 100,000

population per year. Although complete absence of peristalsis in the esophageal body has been proposed as the major abnormality, present evidence indicates achalasia is a primary disorder of the LES. This is based on 24-hour outpatient esophageal motility monitoring, which shows that even in advanced disease up to 5% of contractions can be peristaltic. Simultaneous esophageal waves develop as a result of the increased resistance to esophageal emptying caused by the nonrelaxing LES. This is supported by experimental studies in which a Gore-Tex band placed loosely around the gastroesophageal junction in cats did not change sphincter pressures, but resulted in impaired relaxation of the LES and outflow resistance. This led to a markedly increased frequency of simultaneous waveforms and a decrease in contraction amplitude. The changes were associated with radiographic dilation of the esophagus and were reversible after removal of the band. Observations in patients with pseudoachalasia due to tumor infiltration, a tight stricture in the distal esophagus, or an antireflux procedure that is too tight, also provide evidence that dysfunction of the esophageal body can be caused by the increased outflow obstruction of a nonrelaxing LES. The observation that esophageal peristalsis can return in patients with classic achalasia following dilation or myotomy provides further support that achalasia is a primary disease of the LES.

The pathogenesis of achalasia is presumed to be a neurogenic degeneration, which is either idiopathic or due to infection. In experimental animals, the disease has been reproduced by destruction of the nucleus ambiguus and the dorsal motor nucleus of the vagus nerve. In patients with the disease, degenerative changes have been shown in the vagus nerve and in the ganglia in the Auerbach

FIG. 24-58. Cross section of the neck at the level of the thyroid isthmus, that shows the surgical approach to the hypopharynx and cervical esophagus. [Reproduced with permission from DeMeester TR, Stein HJ: Surgery for esophageal motor disorders, in Castell DO (ed): The Esophagus. Boston: Little, Brown, 1992, p 418.]

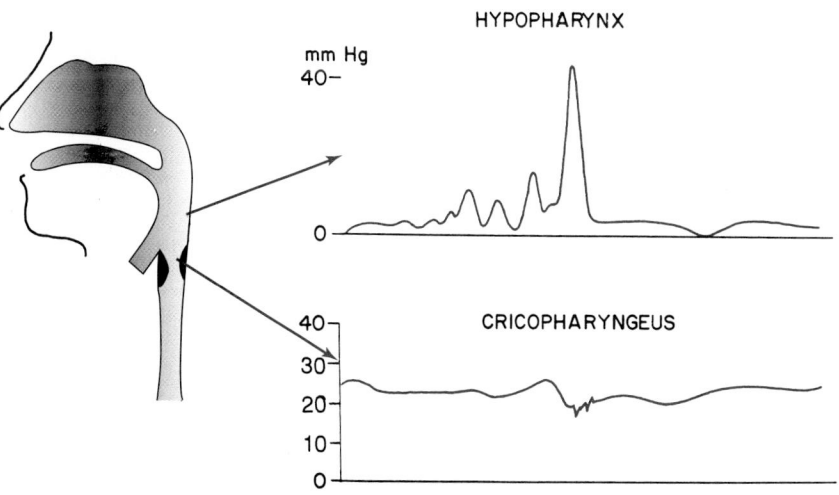

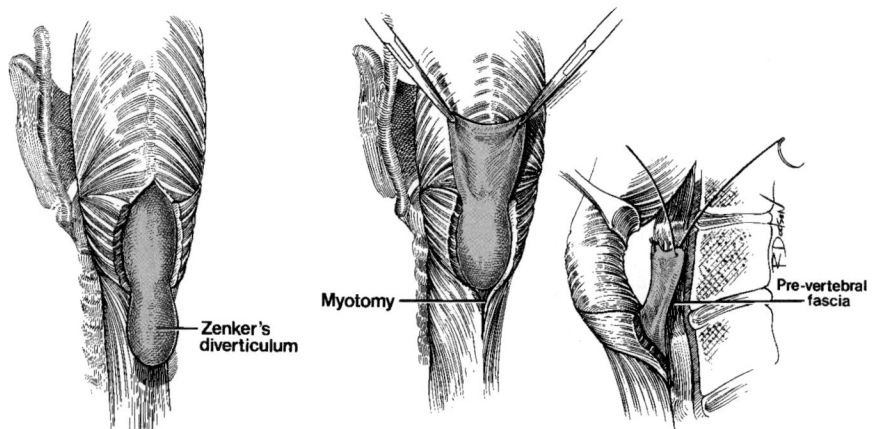

FIG. 24-59. *Posterior of the anatomy of the pharynx and cervical esophagus, showing pharyngoesophageal myotomy and pexis of the diverticulum to the prevertebral fascia.*

plexus of the esophagus itself. This degeneration results in hypertension of the LES, a failure of the sphincter to relax on deglutition, elevation of intraluminal esophageal pressure, esophageal dilatation, and a subsequent loss of progressive peristalsis in the body of the esophagus. The esophageal dilatation results from the combination of a nonrelaxing sphincter, which causes a functional retention of ingested material in the esophagus, and elevation of intraluminal pressure from repetitive pharyngeal air swallowing (Fig. 24-60). With time, the functional disorder results in anatomic alterations seen on radiographic studies, such as a dilated esophagus with a tapering, beak-like narrowing of the distal end (Fig. 24-61). There is usually an air-fluid level in the esophagus from the retained food and saliva, the height of which reflects the degree of resistance imposed by the nonrelaxing sphincter. As the disease progresses, the esophagus becomes massively dilated and tortuous.

A subgroup of patients with otherwise typical features of classic achalasia has simultaneous contractions of their esophageal body that can be of high amplitude. This manometric pattern has been termed "vigorous achalasia," and chest pain episodes are a common finding in these patients. Differentiation of vigorous achalasia from diffuse esophageal spasm can be difficult. In both diseases video-radiographic examination can show a corkscrew deformity of the esophagus and diverticulum formation.

Diffuse and Segmental Esophageal Spasm

Diffuse esophageal spasm is characterized by substernal chest pain and/or dysphagia. Diffuse esophageal spasm differs from classic achalasia in that it is primarily a disease of the esophageal body, produces a lesser degree of dysphagia, causes more chest pain, and has less effect on the patient's general condition. True symptomatic diffuse esophageal spasm is a rare condition, occurring about five times less frequently than achalasia.

The causation and neuromuscular pathophysiology of diffuse esophageal spasm are unclear. The basic motor abnormality is rapid wave progression down the esophagus secondary to an abnormality in the latency gradient. Hypertrophy of the muscular layer of

Table 24-8
Esophageal Motility Disorders

Primary Esophageal Motility Disorders

Achalasia, "vigorous" achalasia
Diffuse and segmental esophageal spasm
Nutcracker esophagus
Hypertensive lower esophageal sphincter
Nonspecific esophageal motility disorders

Secondary Esophageal Motility Disorders

Collagen vascular diseases: progressive systemic sclerosis, polymyositis
   and dermatomyositis, mixed connective tissue disease, systemic lupus
   erythematosus, et al
Chronic idiopathic intestinal pseudo-obstruction
Neuromuscular diseases
Endocrine and metastatic disorders

Table 24-9
Manometric Characteristics of the Primary Esophageal Motility Disorders

Achalasia

Incomplete lower esophageal sphincter (LES) relaxation
   (<75% relaxation)
Aperistalsis in the esophageal body
Elevated LES pressure ≤26 mm Hg
Increased intraesophageal baseline pressures relative to gastric baseline

Diffuse Esophageal Spasm (DES)

Simultaneous (nonperistaltic contractions) (>20% of wet swallows)
Repetitive and multi-peaked contractions
Spontaneous contractions
Intermittent normal peristalsis
Contractions may be of increased amplitude and duration

Nutcracker Esophagus

Mean peristaltic amplitude (10 wet swallows) in distal esophagus
   ≥180 mm Hg
Increased mean duration of contractions (>7.0 s)
Normal peristaltic sequence

Hypertensive Lower Esophageal Sphincter

Elevated LES pressure (≥26 mm Hg)
Normal LES relaxation
Normal peristalsis in the esophageal body

Ineffective Esophageal Motility Disorders

Decreased or absent amplitude of esophageal peristalsis (<30 mm Hg)
Increased number of nontransmitted contractions

SOURCE: Reproduced with permission from DeMeester TR, Stein HJ, Fuchs KH: Physiologic diagnostic studies, in Zuidema GD, Orringer MB (eds): *Shackelford's Surgery of the Alimentary Tract,* 3rd ed, Vol. I. Philadelphia: WB Saunders, 1991, p 115.

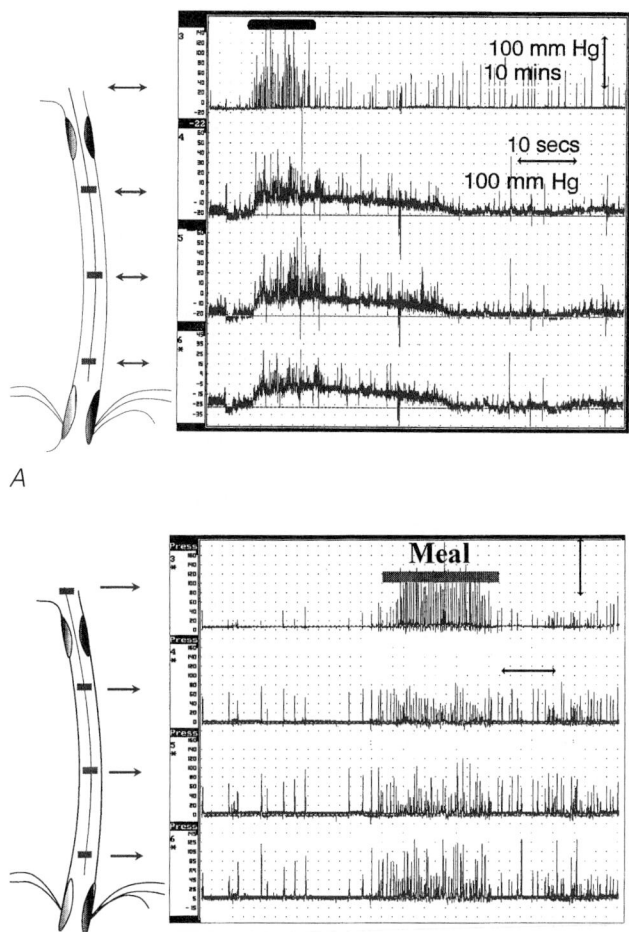

A

B

FIG. 24-60. *Pressurization of esophagus. Ambulatory motility tracing of a patient with achalasia. A. Before esophageal myotomy. B. After esophageal myotomy. The tracings have been compressed to exaggerate the motility spikes and baseline elevations. Note the rise in esophageal baseline pressure during a meal, represented by the rise off the baseline to the left of panel A. No such rise occurs postmyotomy (panel B).*

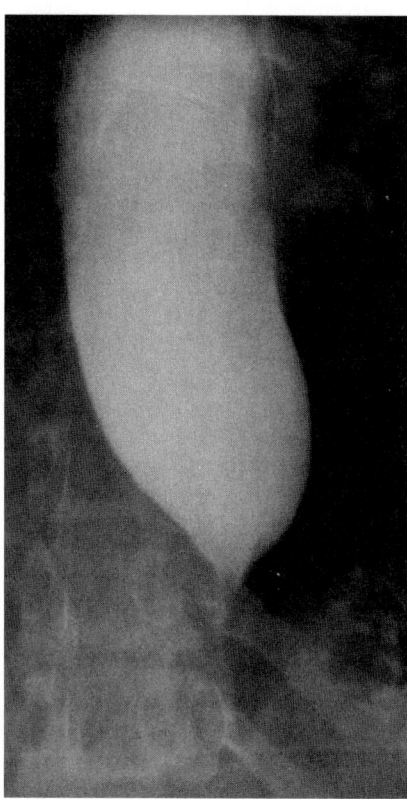

FIG. 24-61. Barium esophagogram showing a markedly dilated esophagus and characteristic "bird's beak" in achalasia. (*Reproduced with permission from Waters PF, DeMeester TR: Foregut motor disorders and their surgical management. Med Clin North Am 65:1235, 1981.*)

the esophageal wall and degeneration of the esophageal branches of the vagus nerve have been observed in this disease, although these are not constant findings. Manometric abnormalities in diffuse esophageal spasm may be present over the total length of the esophageal body, but usually are confined to the distal two thirds. In *segmental esophageal spasm,* the manometric abnormalities are confined to a short segment of the esophagus.

The classic manometric findings in these patients are characterized by the frequent occurrence of simultaneous waveforms and multipeaked esophageal contractions, which may be of abnormally high amplitude or long duration. Key to the diagnosis of diffuse esophageal spasm is that there remain some peristaltic waveforms in excess of those seen in achalasia. A criterion of 20% or more simultaneous waveforms out of 10 wet swallows has been used to diagnose diffuse esophageal spasm. However, this figure is arbitrary and often debated. Discriminate analysis has identified a series of abnormalities on the ambulatory motility record of patients with classic diffuse esophageal spasm. A composite score based on these parameters of the ambulatory motility record has allowed diagnosis of the disease with a sensitivity of 90% and a specificity of 100%. When applied prospectively, this scoring system identified severely

deteriorated esophageal motor function in symptomatic patients despite the absence of the classic motility abnormalities of diffuse spasm on standard manometry.

The LES in patients with diffuse esophageal spasm usually shows a normal resting pressure and relaxation on deglutition. A hypertensive sphincter with poor relaxation may also be present. In patients with advanced disease, the radiographic appearance of tertiary contractions appears helical, and has been termed *corkscrew esophagus* or *pseudodiverticulosis* (Fig. 24-62). Patients with segmental or diffuse esophageal spasm can compartmentalize the esophagus and develop an epiphrenic or midesophageal diverticulum (Fig. 24-63).

Nutcracker Esophagus

The disorder, termed "nutcracker" or "supersqueezer" esophagus, was recognized in the late 1970s. Other terms used to describe this entity are "hypertensive peristalsis" or "high-amplitude peristaltic contractions." It is the most common of the primary esophageal motility disorders. By definition the so-called nutcracker esophagus is a manometric abnormality in patients with chest pain characterized by peristaltic esophageal contractions with peak amplitudes greater than two standard deviations above the normal values in individual laboratories. Contraction amplitudes in these patients can easily be above 400 mm Hg. Ambulatory 24-hour monitoring of esophageal motor function in patients diagnosed as having nutcracker esophagus has identified a subgroup of patients with a motor pattern characteristic of diffuse esophageal spasm. These patients usually complain of dysphagia in addition to chest pain, and probably are misclassified on the basis of standard manometric findings. The identification of these patients is important, since

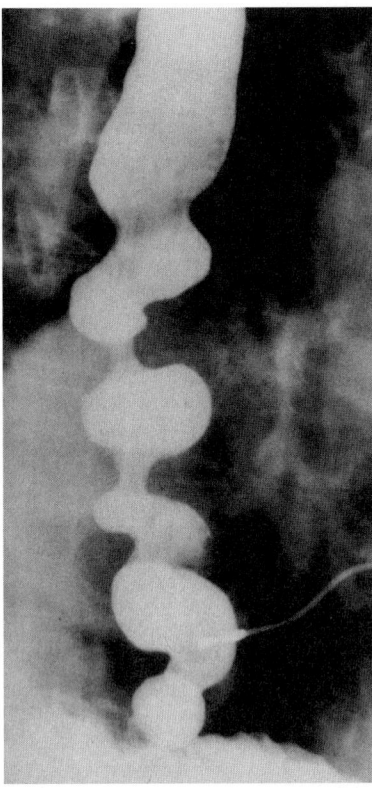

FIG. 24-62. Barium esophagogram of patient with diffuse spasm showing the corkscrew deformity.

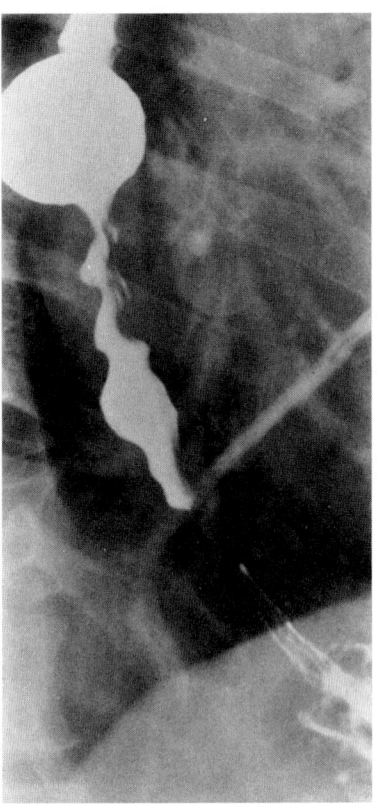

FIG. 24-63. Barium esophagogram showing a high epiphrenic diverticulum in a patient with diffuse esophageal spasm. [*Reproduced with permission from DeMeester TR, Stein HJ: Surgery for esophageal motor disorders, in Castell DO (ed): The Esophagus. Boston: Little, Brown, 1992, p 412.*]

esophageal myotomy is a therapeutic option for patients with dysphagia and diffuse esophageal spasm, but is of questionable value in patients with chest pain secondary to nutcracker esophagus.

Hypertensive Lower Esophageal Sphincter

Hypertensive LES in patients with chest pain or dysphagia was first described as a separate entity by Code and associates. This disorder is characterized by an elevated basal pressure of the LES with normal relaxation and normal propulsion in the esophageal body. About half of these patients, however, have associated motility disorders of the esophageal body, particularly hypertensive peristalsis and simultaneous waveforms. In the remainder, the disorder exists as an isolated abnormality. Dysphagia in these patients may be caused by a lack of compliance of the sphincter, even in its relaxed state. Myotomy of the LES may be indicated in patients not responding to medical therapy or dilation.

Nonspecific Esophageal Motor Disorders

Many patients complaining of dysphagia or chest pain of noncardiac origin demonstrate a variety of wave patterns and contraction amplitudes on esophageal manometry that are clearly out of the normal range, but do not meet the criteria of a primary esophageal motility disorder. Esophageal manometry in these patients frequently shows an increased number of multipeaked or repetitive contractions, contractions of prolonged duration, nontransmitted contractions, an interruption of a peristaltic wave at various levels of the esophagus, or contractions of low amplitude. These motility abnormalities have been termed nonspecific esophageal motility disorders. Their significance in the causation of chest pain or dysphagia is still unclear. Surgery plays no role in the treatment of these disorders unless there is an associated diverticulum.

A clear distinction between primary esophageal motility disorders and nonspecific esophageal motility disorders is often not possible. Patients diagnosed as having nonspecific esophageal motility abnormalities on repeated studies will occasionally show abnormalities consistent with nutcracker esophagus. Similarly, progression from a nonspecific esophageal motility disorder to classic diffuse esophageal spasm has been demonstrated. Therefore, the finding of a nonspecific esophageal motility disorder may represent only a manometric marker of an intermittent, more severe esophageal motor abnormality. Combined ambulatory 24-hour esophageal pH and motility monitoring has shown that an increased esophageal exposure to gastric juice is common in patients diagnosed as having a nonspecific esophageal motility disorder. In some situations, the motor abnormalities may be induced by the irritation of refluxed gastric juice; in other situations it may be a primary event unrelated to the presence of reflux.

Diverticula of the Esophageal Body

Radiographic abnormalities such as segmental spasm, corkscrewing, compartmentalization, and diverticulum are the anatomic results of disordered motility function. Of these, the most persistent and easiest to demonstrate is an esophageal diverticulum. Diverticula occur most commonly with nonspecific motility disorders, but can occur with all of the primary motility disorders. In the latter situation, the motility disorder is usually diagnosed before the development of the diverticulum. When present, a diverticulum may temporarily alleviate the symptom of dysphagia by becoming a receptacle for ingested food, and substitute the symptoms of postprandial pain and the regurgitation of undigested food. If a motility abnormality of the esophageal body or LES cannot be identified, a traction or congenital cause for the diverticulum should be considered. Because development in radiology preceded development in motility monitoring, diverticula of the esophagus were considered historically to be a primary abnormality, the cause, rather than the consequence, of motility disorders. Consequently, earlier texts focused on them as specific entities based upon their location.

Epiphrenic diverticula arise from the terminal third of the thoracic esophagus and are usually found adjacent to the diaphragm. They have been associated with distal esophageal muscular hypertrophy, esophageal motility abnormalities, and increased luminal pressure. They are "pulsion" diverticula, and have been associated with diffuse spasm, achalasia, or nonspecific motor abnormalities in the body of the esophagus.

Whether the diverticulum should be surgically resected or suspended depends on its size and proximity to the vertebral body. When diverticula are associated with esophageal motility disorders, esophageal myotomy from the distal extent of the diverticulum to the stomach is indicated; otherwise, one can expect a high incidence of suture line rupture due to the same intraluminal pressure that initially gave rise to the diverticulum. If the diverticulum is suspended to the prevertebral fascia of the thoracic vertebra, a myotomy is begun at the neck of the diverticulum and extended across the LES. If the diverticulum is excised by dividing the neck, the muscle is closed over the excision site and a myotomy is performed on the opposite esophageal wall, starting at the level of diverticulum. When a large diverticulum is associated with a hiatal hernia, the diverticulum is excised, a myotomy is performed if there is an associated esophageal motility abnormality, and the hernia is repaired because of the high incidence of postoperative reflux when it is omitted.

Midesophageal or traction diverticula were first described in the nineteenth century (Fig. 24-64). At that time they were frequently noted in patients who had mediastinal lymph node involvement with tuberculosis. It was theorized that adhesions form between the inflamed mediastinal nodes and the esophagus. By contraction, the adhesions exerted traction on the esophageal wall and led to a localized diverticulum (Fig. 24-65). This theory was based on the findings of early dissections, where adhesions between diverticula and lymph nodes were commonly found. It is now believed that some diverticula in the midesophagus may also be caused by motility abnormalities.

Most midesophageal diverticula are asymptomatic and incidentally discovered during investigation for nonesophageal complaints. In such patients, the radiologic abnormality may be ignored. Patients with symptoms of dysphagia, regurgitation, chest pain, or aspiration, in whom a diverticulum is discovered, should be thoroughly investigated for an esophageal motor abnormality and treated appropriately. Occasionally, a patient will present with a bronchoesophageal fistula manifested by a chronic cough on ingestion of meals. The diverticulum in such patients is most likely to have an inflammatory etiology.

The indication for surgical intervention is the degree of symptomatic disability. Usually midesophageal diverticula can be suspended due to their proximity to the spine. If motor abnormality is documented, a myotomy should be performed similarly to that described for an epiphrenic diverticulum.

Operations

Long Esophageal Myotomy for Motor Disorders of the Esophageal Body. A long esophageal myotomy is indicated for

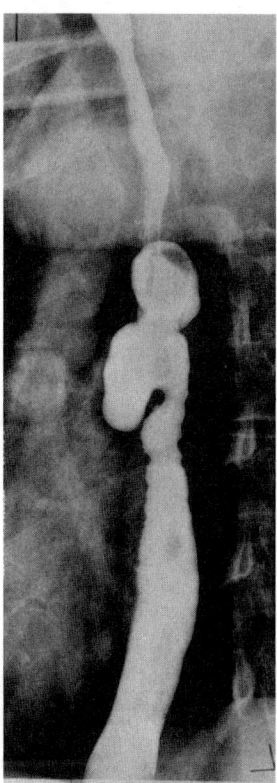

FIG. 24-64. Barium esophagogram showing a midesophageal diverticulum. Despite the anatomic distortion, the patient was asymptomatic. *(Reproduced with permission from Waters PF, DeMeester TR: Foregut motor disorders and their surgical management. Med Clin North Am 65:1235, 1981.)*

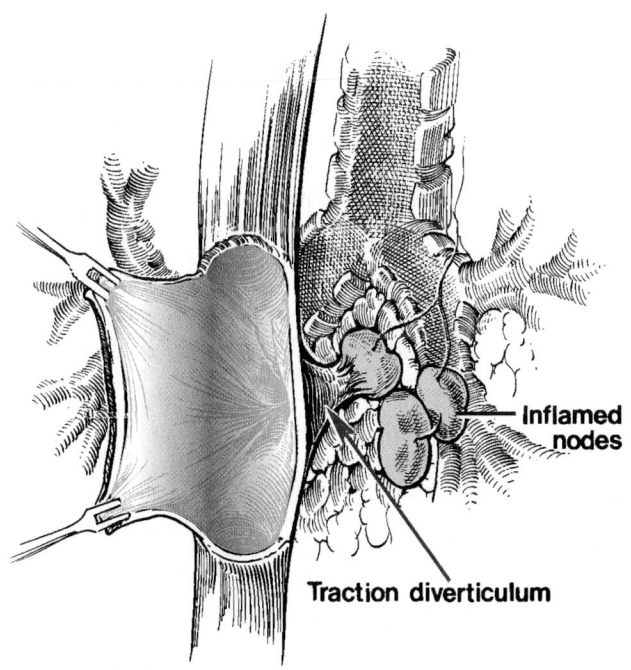

FIG. 24-65. Illustration of the pathophysiology of a midesophageal diverticulum, showing traction on the esophageal wall from adhesions to inflamed subcarinal lymph nodes.

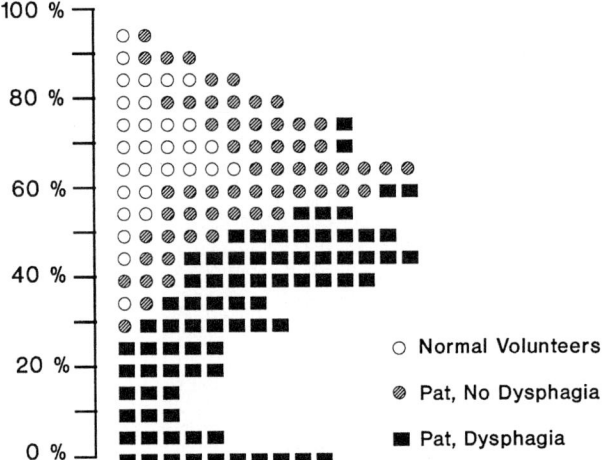

FIG. 24-66. Prevalence of effective contractions (i.e., peristaltic contractions with an amplitude >30 mm Hg) during meal periods in individual normal volunteers, patients without dysphagia, and patients with nonobstructive dysphagia.

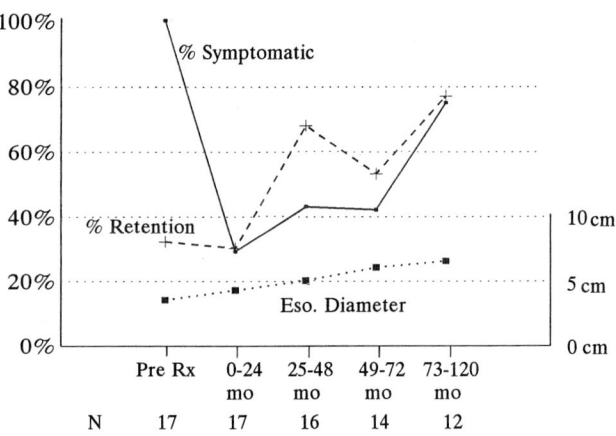

FIG. 24-67. Esophageal diameter, dysphagia, and esophageal retention in patients with achalasia treated with myotomy and Nissen fundoplication, 10 years after treatment. (*Based on Topart P, Deschamps C, Taillefer R, Duranceau A: Long-term effect of total fundoplication on the myotomized esophagus. Ann Thorac Surg 54:1046, 1992, with permission.*)

dysphagia caused by any motor disorder characterized by segmental or generalized simultaneous waveforms in a patient whose symptoms are not relieved by medical therapy. Such disorders include diffuse and segmental esophageal spasm, vigorous achalasia, and nonspecific motility disorders associated with a mid- or epiphrenic esophageal diverticulum. However, the decision to operate must be made by a balanced evaluation of the patient's symptoms, diet, lifestyle adjustments, and nutritional status, with the most important factor being the possibility of improving the patient's swallowing disability. The symptom of chest pain alone is not an indication for a surgical procedure.

Twenty-four-hour ambulatory motility monitoring has greatly aided in the identification of patients with symptoms of dysphagia and chest pain who might benefit from a surgical myotomy. Ambulatory motility studies have shown that when the prevalence of "effective contractions" (i.e., peristaltic waveforms consisting of contractions with an amplitude above 30 mm Hg) drops below 50% during meals, the patient is likely to experience dysphagia (Fig. 24-66). This would suggest that relief from the symptom can be expected with an improvement of esophageal contraction amplitude or amelioration of nonperistaltic waveforms. Prokinetic agents may increase esophageal contraction amplitude, but do not alter the prevalence of simultaneous waveforms. Patients in whom the efficacy of esophageal propulsion is severely compromised because of a high prevalence of simultaneous waveforms usually receive little benefit from medical therapy. In these patients, a surgical myotomy of the esophageal body can improve the patients' dysphagia, provided the loss of contraction amplitude in the remaining peristaltic waveforms, caused by the myotomy, has less effect on swallowing function than the presence of the excessive simultaneous contractions. This situation is reached when the prevalence of effective waveforms during meals drops below 30%, i.e., 70% of esophageal waveforms are ineffective.

In patients selected for surgery, preoperative manometry is essential to determine the proximal extent of the esophageal myotomy. Most surgeons extend the myotomy distally across the LES to reduce outflow resistance. Consequently, some form of antireflux protection is needed to avoid gastroesophageal reflux if there has been extensive dissection of the cardia. In this situation, most authors prefer a partial, rather than a full, fundoplication, in order not to

add back-resistance that will further interfere with the ability of the myotomized esophagus to empty (Fig. 24-67). If the symptoms of reflux are present preoperatively, 24-hour pH monitoring is required to confirm its presence.

The procedure may be performed either open or via thoracoscopy. The open technique is performed through a left thoracotomy in the sixth intercostal space (Fig. 24-68). An incision is made in the posterior mediastinal pleura over the esophagus, and the left lateral wall of the esophagus is exposed. The esophagus is not circumferentially dissected unless necessary. A 2-cm incision is made into the abdomen through the parietal peritoneum at the midportion of the left crus. A tongue of gastric fundus is pulled into the chest. This exposes the gastroesophageal junction and its associated fat pad. The latter is excised to give a clear view of the junction. A myotomy is performed through all muscle layers, extending distally over the stomach 1 to 2 cm below the gastroesophageal junction, and proximally on the esophagus over the distance of the manometric abnormality. The muscle layer is dissected from the mucosa laterally for a distance of 1 cm. Care is taken to divide all minute muscle bands, particularly in the area of the junction. The gastric fundic tongue is sutured to the margins of the myotomy over a distance of 3 to 4 cm and replaced into the abdomen. This maintains separation of the muscle and acts as a partial fundoplication to prevent reflux.

If an epiphrenic diverticulum is present, it is excised by dividing the neck and closing the muscle. The myotomy is then performed on the opposite esophageal wall. If a midesophageal diverticulum is present, the myotomy is made so that it includes the muscle around the neck, and the diverticulum is inverted and suspended by attaching it to the paravertebral fascia of the thoracic vertebra.

The results of myotomy for motor disorders of the esophageal body have improved in parallel with the improved preoperative diagnosis afforded by manometry. Previous published series report between 40 and 92% improvement of symptoms, but interpretation is difficult due to the small number of patients involved and the varying criteria for diagnosis of the primary motor abnormality. When myotomy is accurately done, 93% of the patients have effective palliation of dysphagia after a mean follow-up of 5 years, and 89% would have the procedure again if it was necessary. Most patients gain or maintain rather than lose weight after the operation. Postoperative motility studies show that the myotomy reduces the

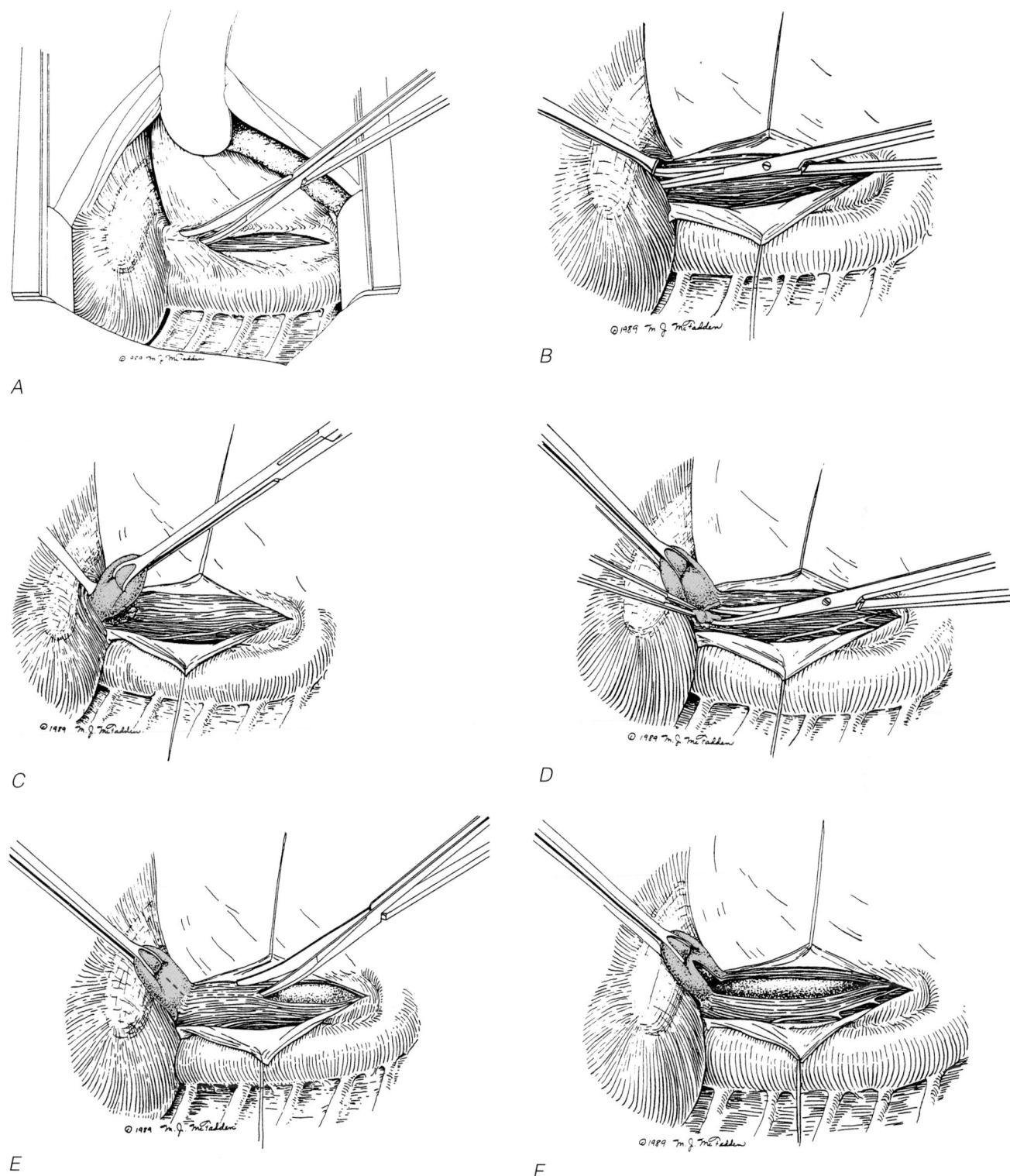

FIG. 24-68. Technique of long myotomy. *A.* Exposure of the lower esophagus through the left sixth intercostal space and incision of the mediastinal pleura in preparation for surgical myotomy. *B.* Location of a 2-cm incision made through the phrenoesophageal membrane into the abdomen along the midlateral border of the left crus. *C.* Retraction of tongue of gastric fundus into the chest through the previously made incision. *D.* Removal of the gastroesophageal fat pad to expose the gastroesophageal junction. *E.* A myotomy down to the mucosa is started on the esophageal body. *F.* Completed myotomy extending over the stomach for 1 cm. *G.* Reconstruction of the cardia after a myotomy, illustrating the position of the sutures used to stitch the gastric fundic flap to the margins of the myotomy. *H.* Reconstruction of the cardia after a myotomy, illustrating the intra-abdominal position of the gastric tongue covering the distal 4 cm of the myotomy. (*Continued*)

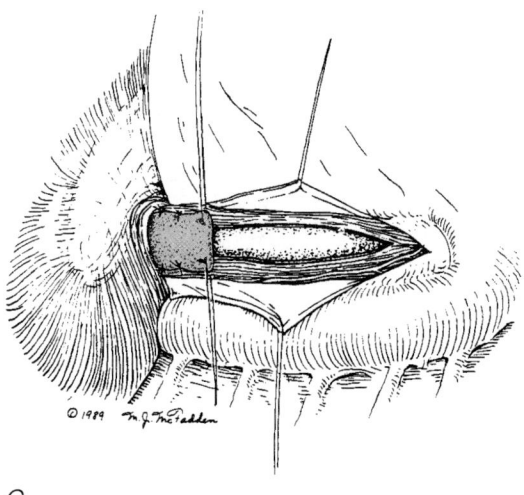

G

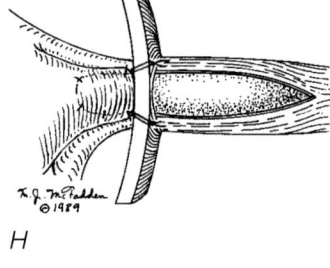

H

FIG. 24-68. *(continued)*

amplitude of esophageal contractions to near zero and eliminates simultaneous peristaltic waves. If the benefit of obliterating the simultaneous waves exceeds the adverse effect on bolus propulsion caused by the loss of peristaltic waveforms, the patient's dysphagia is likely to be improved by the procedure. If not, the patient is likely to continue to complain of dysphagia and to have little improvement as a result of the operation. Preoperative motility studies are thus crucial in deciding which patients are most likely to benefit from a long esophageal myotomy.

The thoracoscopic technique is complicated by the fact that it requires complete retraction of the lung anteriorly to expose the esophagus. Proper positioning of the patient is critical to achieving this exposure. A prone position is ideal, allowing the left lung to fall forward away from the esophagus. Because of the possibility of open thoracotomy, however, it is best to place the patient in the right lateral decubitus position with the left thorax up, and then to roll the patient anteriorly 45 degree toward prone. A beanbag secured to the table is used to hold the patient. The table can be rotated a further 30 to 40 degree so that the patient ends up nearly prone. Should thoracotomy become necessary, the table can be rotated back to the horizontal position and a thoracotomy performed without difficulty. Prone positioning is the key element in providing exposure for long myotomy. Four thoracoscopic ports in the left chest are utilized. With suitable lung retraction the myotomy is performed through all esophageal muscle layers, extending distally to the endoscopic gastroesophageal junction, and proximally over the distance of the manometric abnormality.

Few reports exist concerning the minimally invasive technique for performing long esophageal myotomy. Cuschieri has reported a preliminary experience with a thoracoscopically performed long esophageal myotomy for the treatment of nutcracker esophagus. Three patients with symptoms of chest pain and high-amplitude esophageal contractions and peristaltic waveforms were operated on. No major morbidity was encountered. Nasogastric tubes were removed the first postoperative day and oral feeding was started on the second postoperative day. Two patients were discharged on postoperative day 4 and one patient on day 5. All had symptomatic relief on short-term follow-up.

Myotomy of the Lower Esophageal Sphincter. Second only to reflux disease, achalasia is the most common functional disorder of the esophagus to require surgical intervention. The goal of treatment is to relieve the functional outflow obstruction secondary to the loss of relaxation and compliance of the LES. This requires disrupting the LES muscle. When performed adequately (i.e., reducing sphincter pressure to <10 mm Hg), and done early in the course of disease, LES myotomy results in symptomatic improvement with the occasional return of esophageal peristalsis. Reduction in LES resistance can be accomplished intraluminally by hydrostatic balloon dilation, which ruptures the sphincter muscle, or by a surgical myotomy that cuts the sphincter. The difference between these two methods appears to be the greater likelihood of reducing sphincter pressure to less than 10 mm Hg by surgical myotomy as compared with hydrostatic balloon dilation. However, patients whose sphincter pressure has been reduced by hydrostatic balloon dilation to less than 10 mm Hg have an outcome similar to those after surgical myotomy (Fig. 24-69). In performing a surgical myotomy of the LES, there are four important principles: (1) minimal dissection of the cardia, (2) adequate distal myotomy to reduce outflow resistance, (3) prevention of postoperative reflux, and (4) preventing rehealing of the myotomy site. In the past, the drawback of a surgical myotomy was the need for an open procedure. With the advent of limited-access technology, the myotomy can now be performed laparoscopically.

The therapeutic decisions regarding the treatment of patients with achalasia center around four issues. The first issue is the question of whether newly diagnosed patients should be treated with pneumatic dilation or a surgical myotomy. Long-term follow-up studies have shown that pneumatic dilation achieves adequate relief of dysphagia and pharyngeal regurgitation in 50 to 60% of patients (Fig. 24-70). Close follow-up is required, and if dilation fails, myotomy is indicated. For those patients who have a dilated and tortuous esophagus or an associated hiatal hernia, balloon dilation is dangerous and surgery is the better option. Whether it is better to treat a newly diagnosed esophageal achalasia patient by forceful dilation or by operative cardiomyotomy remains undecided. The outcome of the one controlled randomized study (38 patients) comparing the two modes of therapy suggests that surgical myotomy as a primary treatment gives better long-term results. There are several large retrospective series that report the outcome obtained with the two modes of treatment (Table 24-10). Despite objections regarding variations in surgical and dilation techniques and the number of

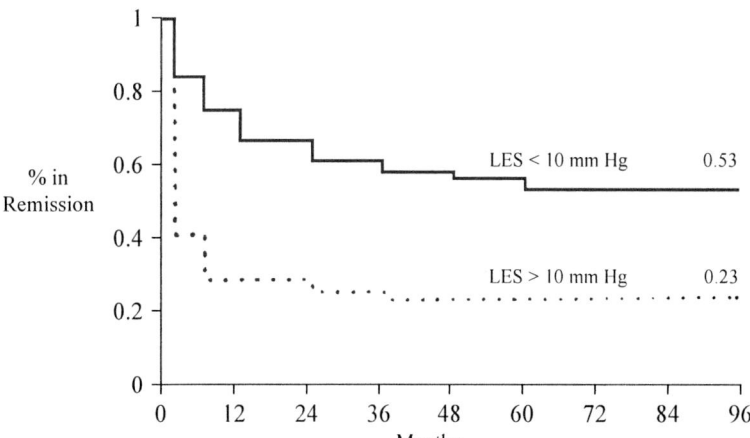

FIG. 24-69. Prevalence of clinical remission in 122 patients stratified according to postdilatation LES pressures greater than or less than 10 mm Hg. *(Reproduced with permission from Ponce, J, Garrigues V, Pertejo V, et al: Individual prediction of response to pneumatic dilation in patients with achalasia. Dig Dis Sci 41:2135, 1996.)*

physicians performing the procedures, these collective data would appear to support operative myotomy as the initial treatment of choice, when performed by a surgeon of average skill and experience. This view is confirmed by the large series of 899 patients reported by the Mayo Clinic spanning a 27-year period, and by the series of Csendes and colleagues on 100 patients followed for 5 to 7 years after surgery. Although it has been reported that a myotomy after previous balloon dilation is more difficult, this has not been the experience of these authors unless the cardia has been ruptured in a sawtooth manner. In this situation, operative intervention, either immediately or after healing has occurred, can be difficult.

The second issue is the question of whether a surgical myotomy should be performed through the abdomen or the chest.

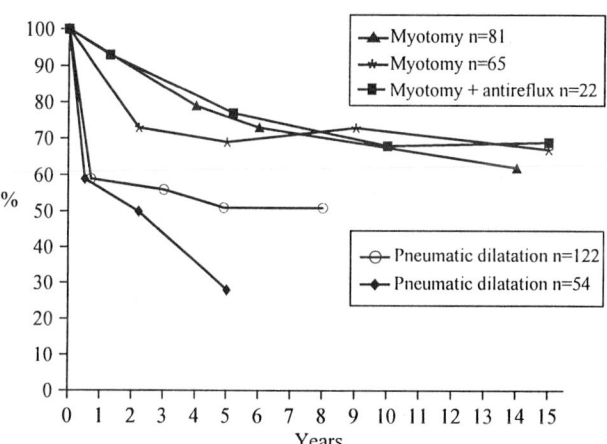

FIG. 24-70. Summary of long-term studies reporting the proportion of patients with complete relief or minimal dysphagia i.e., occasional episodes of short duration, stratified according to type of treatment.

▲ Ellis FH Jr: Oesophagomyotomy for achalasia: A 22-year experience. *Br J Surg* 80(7):882, 1993.
★ Goulbourne IA, Walbaum PR: Long-term results of Heller's operation for achalasia. *J Royal Coll Surg* 30:101, 1985.
■ Malthaner RA, Todd TR, Miller L, Pearson FG: Long-term results in surgically managed esophageal achalasia. *Ann Thorac Surg* 58:1343, 1994.
○ Ponce J, Garrigues V, Pertejo V, Sala T, et al: Individual prediction of response to pneumatic dilation in patients with achalasia. *Dig Dis Sci* 41(11):2135, 1996.
◆ Eckardt V, Aignherr C, Bernhard G: Predictors of outcome in patients with achalasia treated by pneumatic dilation. *Gastroenterol* 103:1732, 1992.

Myotomy of the LES can be accomplished via either an abdominal or thoracic approach. Recent data suggest that a transabdominal approach is preferable, particularly when done using minimally invasive techniques.

The third issue—and one that has been long debated—is the question of whether an antireflux procedure should be added to a surgical myotomy. Excellent results have been reported following meticulously performed myotomy without an antireflux component. Complicating the controversy is the virtual absence of studies including objective documentation of the presence or absence of pathologic reflux following myotomy. The results of published studies are mixed, although the majority support the need for antireflux protection, particularly if there is extensive dissection of the hiatus as occurs when a transabdominal myotomy is performed. Further support for an antireflux procedure is the fact that the development of a reflux-induced stricture after an esophageal myotomy is a serious problem, and usually necessitates esophagectomy for relief of symptoms. On the other hand, the complications of gastroesophageal reflux are paradoxically more common in patients who had a myotomy plus an antireflux procedure, than in those who only had a transthoracic myotomy. This indicates that the addition of an antireflux procedure does not protect against the complications of reflux. Consequently, there is little reason to accept the degree of dissection required for the performance of an antireflux procedure, if less dissection is beneficial in maintaining the competency of the cardia; similarly, there is little reason to accept the resistance an antireflux procedure imposes on esophageal emptying, when the elimination of this resistance is the purpose for performing a myotomy in the first place. If an antireflux procedure is used as an adjunct to esophageal myotomy, a complete 360 degree fundoplication should be avoided. Rather, a 270 degree Belsey fundoplication or a Dor hemifundoplication should be used to avoid the long-term esophageal dysfunction secondary to the outflow obstruction afforded by the fundoplication itself (see Fig. 24-67).

The fourth issue centers on whether or not a cure of this disease is achievable. Long-term follow-up studies after surgical myotomy have shown that late deterioration in results occurs after this procedure, regardless of whether an antireflux procedure is done, and also after balloon dilation, even when the sphincter pressure is reduced to below 10 mm Hg. It may be that even though a myotomy or balloon rupture of the LES muscle reduces the outflow obstruction at the cardia, the underlying motor disorder in the body of the esophagus persists and deteriorates further with the passage of time, leading to increased impairment of esophageal emptying. The earlier an effective reduction in outflow resistance can be accomplished, the better

Table 24-10
Series with >100 Patients Giving Follow-Up Results of Myotomy of Balloon Dilation for Achalasia

Author	Year	No. of Patients	Follow-Up Years	Good-to-Excellent Response
Surgical myotomy				
Black et al	1976	108	4	65%
Menzies Gow	1978	102	8	98%
Okike et al	1979	456	1–17	85%
Ellis et al	1984	113	3.5	91%
Csendes et al	1988	100	6.8	92%
Balloon dilation				
Sanderson et al	1970	408	...	81%
Vantrappen et al	1979	403	7.8	76%
Okike et al	1979	431	1–18	65%

SOURCE: Reproduced with permission from DeMeester TR, Stein HJ: Surgery for esophageal motor disorders, in Castell DO (ed): *The Esophagus.* Boston: Little, Brown, 1992, p 424.

the outcome will be, and the more likely some esophageal body function can be restored.

Open Esophageal Myotomy. Open techniques of distal esophageal myotomy are presently limited to the reoperative setting. Primary procedures can almost always be successfully completed via laparoscopy. A modified Heller myotomy can be performed through a left thoracotomy incision in the sixth intercostal space along the upper border of the seventh rib. The esophagus and a tongue of gastric fundus are exposed as described for a long myotomy. A myotomy through all muscle layers is performed, extending distally over the stomach to 1 to 2 cm below the junction, and proximally on the esophagus for 4 to 5 cm. The cardia is reconstructed by suturing the tongue of gastric fundus to the margins of the myotomy, to prevent rehealing of the myotomy site, and to provide reflux protection in the area of the divided sphincter. If an extensive dissection of the cardia has been done, a more formal Belsey repair is performed. The tongue of gastric fundus is allowed to retract into the abdomen. Postoperatively, nasogastric drainage is maintained for 6 days to prevent distention of the stomach during healing. An oral diet is resumed on the seventh day, after a barium swallow study shows unobstructed passage of the bolus into the stomach without extravasation.

In a randomized long-term follow-up by Csendes and colleagues of 81 patients treated for achalasia, either by forceful dilation or by surgical myotomy, myotomy was associated with a significant increase in the diameter at the gastroesophageal junction and a decrease in the diameter at the middle third of the esophagus on follow-up radiographic studies. There was a greater reduction in sphincter pressure and improvement in the amplitude of esophageal contractions after myotomy. Thirteen percent of patients regained some peristalsis after dilation, compared with 28% after surgery. These findings were shown to persist over a 5-year follow-up period, at which time 95% of those treated with surgical myotomy were doing well. Of those who were treated with dilation, only 54% were doing well, while 16% required redilation and 22% eventually required surgical myotomy to obtain relief.

If simultaneous esophageal contractions are associated with the sphincter abnormality, the so-called vigorous achalasia, then the myotomy should extend over the distance of the abnormal motility as mapped by the preoperative motility study. Failure to do this will result in continuing dysphagia and a dissatisfied patient. The best objective evaluation of improvement in the patient following either balloon dilation or myotomy is a scintigraphic measurement of esophageal emptying time. A good therapeutic response improves

esophageal emptying toward normal. However, some degree of dysphagia may persist despite improved esophageal emptying, due to disturbances in esophageal body function. When an antireflux procedure is added to the myotomy, it should be a partial fundoplication. A 360 degree fundoplication is associated with progressive retention of swallowed food, regurgitation, and aspiration to a degree that exceeds the patient's preoperative symptoms.

Laparoscopic Esophageal Myotomy. The laparoscopic approach is similar to the Nissen fundoplication in terms of the trocar placement and exposure and dissection of the esophageal hiatus. The procedure begins by division of the short gastric vessels in preparation for fundoplication. Exposure of the gastroesophageal junction (GEJ) via removal of the gastroesophageal fat pad follows. The anterior vagus nerve is swept right laterally along with the fat pad. Once completed, the GEJ and distal 4 to 5 cm of esophagus should be bared of any overlying tissue, and generally follows dissection of the GEJ. A distal esophageal myotomy is performed. It is generally easiest to begin the myotomy 1 to 2 cm above the GEJ, in an area above that of previous botulinum toxin injections or balloon dilation. Either scissors or a hook-type electrocautery can be used to initiate the incision in the longitudinal and circular muscle. Distally, the myotomy is carried across the GEJ and onto the proximal stomach for approximately 1.5 to 2 cm. After completion, the muscle edges are separated bluntly from the esophageal mucosa for approximately 50% of the esophageal circumference. An antireflux procedure follows completion of the myotomy. Either an anterior hemifundoplication augmenting the angle of His (Dor) or posterior partial fundoplication (Toupet) can be performed. The Dor type fundoplication is slightly easier to perform, and does not require disruption of the normal posterior gastroesophageal attachments (a theoretical advantage in preventing postoperative reflux).

Outcome Assessment of the Therapy for Achalasia.
Critical analysis of the results of therapy for motor disorders of the esophagus requires objective measurement. The use of symptoms alone as an endpoint to evaluate therapy for achalasia may be misleading. The propensity for patients to unconsciously modify their diet to avoid difficulty swallowing is underestimated, making an assessment of results based on symptoms unreliable. Insufficient reduction in outflow resistance may allow progressive esophageal digitation to develop slowly, giving the impression of improvement because the volume of food able to be ingested with comfort increases. A variety of objective measurements may be used to assess

success, including LES pressure, esophageal baseline pressure, and scintigraphic assessment of esophageal emptying time. Esophageal baseline pressure is usually negative when compared to gastric pressure. Given that the goal of therapy is to eliminate the outflow resistance of a nonrelaxing sphincter, measurement of improvements in esophageal baseline pressure and scintigraphic transit time may be better indicators of success, but are rarely reported.

Eckardt and associates investigated whether the outcome of pneumatic dilation in patients with achalasia could be predicted on the basis of objective measurements. Postdilation LES pressure was the most valuable measurement for predicting long-term clinical response. A postdilatation sphincter pressure less than 10 mm Hg predicted a good response. Fifty percent of the patients studied had postdilatation sphincter pressures between 10 and 20 mm Hg, with a 2-year remission rate of 71%. Importantly, 16 of 46 patients were left with a postdilatation sphincter pressure of greater than 20 mm Hg, and had an unacceptable outcome. Overall, only 30% of patients dilated remain in symptomatic remission at 5 years.

Bonavina and colleagues reported good to excellent results with transabdominal myotomy and Dor fundoplication in 94% of patients after a mean follow-up of 5.4 years. No operative mortality occurred in either of these series, attesting to the safety of the procedure. Malthaner and Pearson reported the long-term clinical results in 35 patients with achalasia, having a minimum follow-up of 10 years (Table 24-11). Twenty-two of these patients underwent primary esophageal myotomy and Belsey hemifundoplication at the Toronto General Hospital. Excellent to good results were noted in 95% of patients at 1 year, declining to 68, 69, and 67% at 10, 15, and 20 years, respectively. Two patients underwent early reoperation for an incomplete myotomy, and three underwent an esophagectomy for progressive disease. They concluded that there was a deterioration of the initially good results after surgical myotomy and hiatal repair for achalasia, which is due to late complications of gastroesophageal reflux.

Ellis reported his lifetime experience with transthoracic short esophageal myotomy without an antireflux procedure. One hundred seventy-nine patients were analyzed at a mean follow-up of 9 years, ranging from 6 months to 20 years. Overall 89% of patients were improved at the 9-year mark. He also observed that the level of improvement deteriorated with time, with excellent results (patients continuing to be symptom free) decreasing from 54% at 10 years to 32% at 20 years. He concluded that a short transthoracic myotomy without an antireflux procedure provides excellent long-term relief of dysphagia, and contrary to Malthaner and Pearson's experience, does not result in complications of gastroesophageal reflux. Both studies document nearly identical results 10 to 15 years following

the procedure, and both report deterioration over time, probably due to progression of the underlying disease. The addition of an antireflux procedure if the operation is performed transthoracically has no significant effect on the outcome.

The outcome of laparoscopic myotomy and hemifundoplication has been well documented. Two reports of over 100 patients have documented relief of dysphagia in 93% of patients. Richter and coworkers reviewed published reports to date, including 254 patients with an average success rate of 93% at 2.5 years. Conversion to an open procedure occurs in 0 to 5% of patients. Complications are uncommon, occurring in less than 5% of patients. Intraoperative complications consist largely of mucosal perforation, and have been more likely to occur after botulinum toxin injection. The incidence of objective reflux disease as evidenced by abnormal acid exposure is less than 10%.

Esophageal Resection for End-Stage Motor Disorders of the Esophagus. Patients with dysphagia and long-standing benign disease, whose esophageal function has been destroyed by the disease process or multiple previous surgical procedures, are best managed by esophagectomy. Fibrosis of the esophagus and cardia can result in weak contractions and failure of the distal esophageal sphincter to relax. The loss of esophageal contractions can result in the stasis of food, esophageal dilatation, regurgitation, and aspiration. The presence of these abnormalities signals end-stage motor disease. In these situations esophageal replacement is usually required to establish normal alimentation. Before proceeding with esophageal resection for patients with end-stage benign disease, the choice of the organ to substitute for the esophagus (i.e., stomach, jejunum, or colon) should be considered. The choice of replacement is affected by a number of factors, as described later in the section on techniques of esophageal reconstruction.

CARCINOMA OF THE ESOPHAGUS

Squamous carcinoma accounts for the majority of esophageal carcinomas worldwide. Its incidence is highly variable, ranging from approximately 20 per 100,000 in the United States and Britain, to 160 per 100,000 in certain parts of South Africa and the Honan Province of China, and even 540 per 100,000 in the Guriev district of Kazakhstan. The environmental factors responsible for these localized high-incidence areas have not been conclusively identified, though additives to local foodstuffs (nitroso compounds in pickled vegetables and smoked meats) and mineral deficiencies (zinc and molybdenum) have been suggested. In Western societies, smoking and alcohol consumption are strongly linked with squamous

Table 24-11
Reasons for Failure of Esophageal Myotomy

Reason	Ellis, Myotomy Only (n = 81)	Goulbourne, Myotomy Only (n = 65)	Malthaner, Myotomy + Antireflux (n = 22)
Reflux	4%	5%	18%
Inadequate myotomy	2%	...	9%
Megaesophagus	2%	...	...
Poor emptying	4%	3%	...
Persistent chest pain	1%	...	...

SOURCE: Reproduced with permission from Malthaner RA, Tood TR, Miller L, Pearson FG: Long-term results in surgically managed esophageal achalasia. *Ann Thorac Surg* 58:1343, 1994; Ellis FH Jr.: Oesophagomyotomy for achalasia: A 22-year experience. *Br J Surg* 80:882, 1993; and Goulbourne IA, Walbaum PR: Long-term results of Heller's operation for achalasia. *J Royal Coll Surg* 30, 1985.

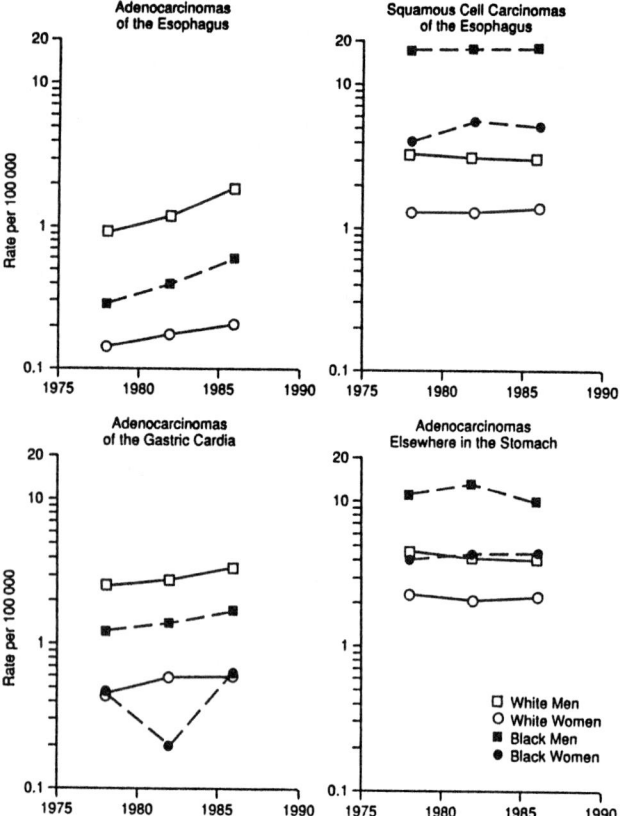

FIG. 24-71. Trends in age-adjusted incidence rates of esophageal and stomach cancers by histology and anatomic site, sex, and race, show a rise in the incidence of adenocarcinoma of both the esophagus and gastric cardia, suggesting that factors responsible for the development of these concerns may be similar. (*Reproduced with permission from Blot WJ, Devesa SS, Kneller RW, Fraumeni JF Jr.: Rising incidence of adenocarcinoma of the esophagus and gastric cardia. JAMA 265:1287, 1991.*)

carcinoma. Other definite associations link squamous carcinoma with long-standing achalasia, lye strictures, tylosis (an autosomal dominant disorder characterized by hyperkeratosis of the palms and soles), and human papillomavirus.

Adenocarcinoma of the esophagus, once an unusual malignancy, is diagnosed with increasing frequency (Fig. 24-71), and now accounts for over 50% of esophageal cancer in most Western countries. The shift in the epidemiology of esophageal cancer from predominantly squamous carcinoma seen in association with smoking and alcohol, to adenocarcinoma in the setting of Barrett's esophagus, is one of the most dramatic changes that have occurred in the history of human neoplasia. Although esophageal carcinoma is a relatively uncommon malignancy, its prevalence is exploding, largely secondary to the well-established association between gastroesophageal reflux, Barrett's esophagus, and esophageal adenocarcinoma. Once a nearly uniformly lethal disease, survival is improving with advances in the understanding of its molecular biology surveillance, improvements in staging surgical techniques, and neoadjuvant therapy are translated into clinically relevant improvements in the everyday care of patients.

Furthermore, the clinical picture of esophageal adenocarcinoma is changing. It now occurs not only considerably more frequently, but in younger patients, and is often detected at an earlier stage. These facts support rethinking the traditional approach of assuming palliation is appropriate in all patients. The historical focus on

palliation of dysphagia in an elderly patient with comorbidities should change when dealing with a young patient with dependent children and a productive life ahead. The potential for cure becomes of paramount importance.

The gross appearance resembles that of squamous cell carcinoma. Microscopically, adenocarcinoma almost always originates in metaplastic Barrett's mucosa, and resembles gastric cancer. Rarely it arises in the submucosal glands, and forms intramural growths that resemble the mucoepidermal and adenoid cystic carcinomas of the salivary glands.

The most important etiologic factor in the development of primary adenocarcinoma of the esophagus is a metaplastic columnar-lined or Barrett's esophagus, which occurs as a complication in approximately 10 to 15% of patients with GERD. When studied prospectively, the incidence of adenocarcinoma in a patient with Barrett's esophagus is one in 100 to 200 patient-years of follow-up (i.e., for every 100 patients with Barrett's esophagus followed for 1 year, one will develop adenocarcinoma). Although this risk appears to be small, it is at least 30 to 40 times that expected for a similar population without Barrett's esophagus. This risk is similar to the risk for developing lung cancer in a person with a 20-pack-per-year history of smoking. Endoscopic surveillance for patients with Barrett's esophagus is recommended for two reasons: (1) at present there is no reliable evidence that medical therapy removes the risk of neoplastic transformation, and (2) malignancy in Barrett's esophagus is curable if detected at an early stage.

Clinical Manifestations

Esophageal cancer generally presents with dysphagia, although increasing numbers of relatively asymptomatic patients are now identified on surveillance endoscopy, and/or present with nonspecific upper gastrointestinal symptoms and undergo upper endoscopy. Extension of the primary tumor into the tracheobronchial tree can cause stridor, and if a tracheoesophageal fistula develops, coughing, choking, and aspiration pneumonia result. Rarely, severe bleeding from erosion into the aorta or pulmonary vessels occurs. Either vocal cord may be invaded, causing paralysis, but most commonly, paralysis is caused by invasion of the left recurrent laryngeal nerve by the primary tumor or lymph node metastasis. Systemic organ metastases are usually manifested by jaundice or bone pain. The situation is different in high-incidence areas where screening is practiced. In these communities, the most prominent early symptom is pain on swallowing rough or dry food.

Dysphagia usually presents late in the natural history of the disease, because the lack of a serosal layer on the esophagus allows the smooth muscle to dilate with ease. As a result, the dysphagia becomes severe enough for the patient to seek medical advice only when more than 60% of the esophageal circumference is infiltrated with cancer. Consequently, the disease is usually advanced if symptoms herald its presence. Tracheoesophageal fistula may be present in some patients on their first visit to the hospital, and more than 40% will have evidence of distant metastases. With tumors of the cardia, anorexia and weight loss usually precede the onset of dysphagia. The physical signs of esophageal tumors are those associated with the presence of distant metastases.

Staging of Esophageal Carcinoma

At the initial encounter with a patient diagnosed as having carcinoma of the esophagus, a decision must be made as to whether he or she is a candidate for curative surgical therapy, palliative surgical therapy,

Table 24-12
Staging of Cancer of the Esophagus and Cardia (AJCC 1988)

Stage	Classification			No. of Patients	% 5-Year Survival	p Value
0	Tis	N_0	M_0	16	100	} NS
I	T_1	N_0	M_0	22	78.9	} 0.0021
IIA	T_2	N_0	M_0	80	37.9	
	T_3	N_0	M_0			
IIB	T_1	N_1	M_0	39	27.3	} NS
	T_2	N_1	M_0			
III	T_3	N_1	M_0	218	13.7	} NS
	T_4	Any N	M_0			
IV	Any T	Any N	M_1	$\dfrac{33}{408}$	0	} 0.0001

NS = not significant.

SOURCE: Reproduced with permission from Ellis FH, Heatly GJ, Krosna MJ, Williamson WA, Balogh K: Esophagogastrectomy for carcinoma of the esophagus and cardia: A comparison of findings and results after standard resection in three consecutive 8 year time intervals, using improved staging criteria. *J Thorac Cardiovasc Surg* 113:836, 1997.

or nonsurgical palliation. Making this decision is difficult, because evaluating the pretreatment disease stage of esophageal carcinoma is imprecise due to the difficulty of measuring the depth of tumor penetration of the esophageal wall and the inaccessibility of the organ's widespread lymphatic drainage.

The introduction of endoscopic ultrasound has made it possible to identify patients who are potentially curable prior to surgical therapy. Using an endoscope, the depth of the wall penetration by the tumor and the presence of five or more lymph node metastases can be determined with 80% accuracy. A curative resection should be encouraged if endoscopic ultrasound indicates that the tumor has not penetrated the esophageal wall, and/or fewer than five enlarged lymph nodes are imaged. Thoracoscopic and laparoscopic staging of esophageal cancer have been recommended; preliminary results indicate that using these techniques, correct staging of esophageal carcinomas approaches 90%. If these results are confirmed and the cost is not prohibitive, then thoracoscopic and laparoscopic staging are likely to become valuable tools to determine the extent of disease prior to therapy. At the present time, despite the modern techniques of computed tomography, magnetic resonance imaging, endoscopic ultrasound, and laparoscopic and thoracoscopic technology, pretreatment staging still remains imprecise. This underscores the need for an intraoperative assessment of the potential for cure in each individual patient.

Experience with esophageal resections in patients with early disease has identified characteristics of esophageal cancer that are associated with improved survival. A number of studies suggest that only metastasis to lymph nodes and tumor penetration of the esophageal wall have a significant and independent influence on prognosis. The beneficial effects of the absence of one factor persists, even when the other is present. Factors known to be important in the survival of patients with advanced disease, such as cell type, degree of cellular differentiation, or location of tumor in the esophagus, have no effect on survival of patients who have undergone resection for early disease. Studies also showed that patients having five or fewer lymph node metastases have a better outcome. Using these data, Skinner developed the wall penetration, lymph node, and distant organ metastases (WNM) system for staging.

The WNM system differed somewhat from the previous efforts to develop a satisfactory staging criteria for carcinoma of the esophagus. Most surgeons agreed that the 1983 TNM system left much to be desired. In the third edition of the manual for Staging of Cancer of the American Joint Committee on Cancer (1988), an effort was made to provide a finer discrimination between stages than had been contained in the previous edition in 1983. Table 24-12 shows the definitions for the primary tumor, regional lymph nodes, and distant metastasis, as listed in the 1988 manual. Recently, Ellis, in a study comparing different staging criteria, showed that the new staging criteria of the AJCC provide no better discrimination of stages as they relate to survival than the earlier version had. The 5-year survival of stage IIA patients was similar to that of stage IIB patients, and the survival of stage IIB patients was similar to that of stage III patients. Similarly, there was no difference between the 5-year survival of patients with T_1 and T_2 disease, nor was there a survival difference between those with T_3 and T_4 disease. He did confirm the observation that the depth of wall penetration and extent of lymph node involvement were reliable independent predictors of survival.

Ellis proposed adoption of Skinner's WNM staging system with some modifications (Table 24-13). In Ellis' proposal, tumors limited to above the muscularis mucosae would be equivalent to Skinner's W_0 designation, T_1 and T_2 tumors would equate with the W_1 classification, and T_3 and T_4 tumors to the W_2 classification. These classifications are illustrated in Fig. 24-72. He further reported a clear distinction between the 5-year survival of patients with negative nodes and those with fewer than five nodes involved, and a highly significant difference between the latter group and those with five or more nodes involved. Table 24-13 shows the definitions for the primary tumor, regional lymph nodes, and distant metastasis, for the Skinner WNM staging system as modified by Ellis.

Using an expanded base of 408 resected patients, Ellis compared the 1988 staging criteria with his modification of the Skinner WNM system and produced evidence that a modified WNM staging system was more useful from a prognostic standpoint (see Tables 24-12 and 24-13) than the 1988 criteria. Not only is the number of patients more evenly divided among the four stages in the modified Skinner system, but the comparison of the 5-year survival rates between stages is highly significant, with almost a 50% reduction in survival rates for each increasing stage. The major difference in the staging criteria of the proposed modification to the Skinner WNM system is the recognition that the number of nodes involved has a profound effect on prognosis. Ellis has been a proponent of a limited resection and lymph node dissection. The data used to validate the modified staging system represent what the outcome would be for simple tumor removal. Consequently, it serves as an excellent basis for

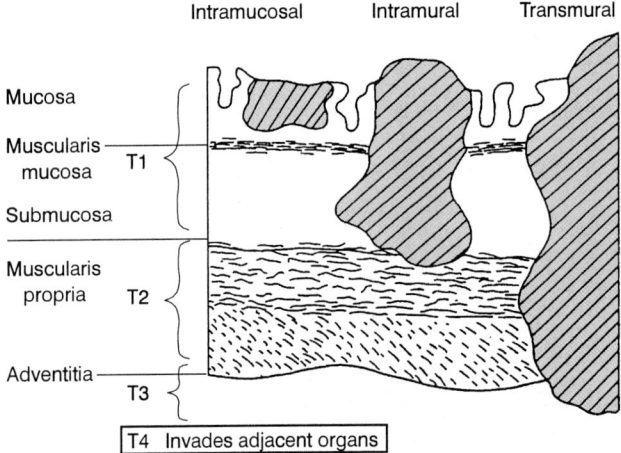

FIG. 24-72. *Staging of the primary tumor according to the depth of invasion, using standard anatomic landmarks: intramucosal carcinoma if tumor extent is through the basement membrane, but limited by the muscularis mucosae; intramural carcinoma if tumor extent is through the muscularis mucosae, but not the muscularis propria; and transmural if tumor invasion is through the muscularis propria. (Reproduced with permission from DeMeester TR, Attwood SEA, Smyrk TC, et al: Surgical therapy in Barrett's esophagus. Ann Surg 212:530, 1990.)*

comparison with the results for more extensive en bloc resections or preoperative chemotherapy programs.

Clinical Approach to Carcinoma of the Esophagus and Cardia

The selection of a curative versus a palliative operation for cancer of the esophagus is based on the location of the tumor, the patient's age and health, the extent of the disease, and intraoperative staging. Figure 24-73 shows an algorithm of the clinical decisions important in the selection of curative or palliative therapy.

Tumor Location

The selection of surgical therapy for patients with carcinoma of the esophagus depends not only on the anatomic stage of the disease and an assessment of the swallowing capacity of the patient, but also on the location of the primary tumor.

It is estimated that 8% of the primary malignant tumors of the esophagus occur in the cervical portion (Fig. 24-74). They are almost always squamous cell lesions, with a rare adenocarcinoma

arising from a congenital inlet patch of columnar lining. These tumors, particularly those in the postcricoid area, represent a separate pathologic entity for a number of reasons: (1) they are more common in females and appear to be a unique entity in this regard; and (2) the efferent lymphatics from the cervical esophagus drain completely differently from those of the thoracic esophagus. The latter drain directly into the paratracheal and deep cervical or internal jugular lymph nodes with minimal flow in a longitudinal direction. Except in advanced disease, it is unusual for intrathoracic lymph nodes to be involved.

Low cervical lesions that reach the level of the thoracic inlet are usually unresectable due to early invasion of the great vessels and trachea. The length of the esophagus below the cricopharyngeus is insufficient to allow intubation or construction of a proximal anastomosis for a bypass procedure. Consequently, palliation of these tumors is difficult, and patients afflicted with disease at this site have a poor prognosis. Upper airway obstruction or the development of tracheoesophageal fistulas in such tumors may require surgical intervention for palliation. If possible, these tumors should be resected after a preoperative course of chemotherapy has reduced their size.

Tumors that arise within the middle or upper third of the thoracic esophagus lie too close to the trachea and aorta to allow an en bloc resection without removal of these vital structures. Consequently, in this location only tumors that have not penetrated through the esophageal wall and have not metastasized to the regional lymph nodes are potentially curable. The resection for a tumor at this level is done similarly whether for palliation or cure, and long-term survival is a chance phenomenon. This does not mean that when resecting such tumors, efforts to remove the adjacent lymph nodes should be abandoned. To do so may inadvertently leave unrecognized metastatic disease behind and compromise the patient's overall survival, because of recurrent local disease and compression of the trachea. It is recommended that a course of preoperative chemoradiotherapy should be given before resection to shrink the size of the tumor. It is recommended that the radiotherapy be limited to 3.5 Gy to allow for tissue healing.

Tumors of the lower esophagus and cardia are usually adenocarcinomas. However, squamous cell carcinoma of the lower esophagus does occur. Both types of tumor are amenable to en bloc resection. Unless preoperative and intraoperative staging clearly demonstrate an incurable lesion, an en bloc resection in continuity with a lymph node dissection should be performed. Because of the propensity of gastrointestinal tumors to spread for long distances submucosally, long lengths of grossly normal gastrointestinal tract should be

Table 24-13
Staging of Cancer of the Esophagus and Cardia: Modified WNM Criteria

Stage	Classification			No. of Patients	% 5-Year Survival	p Value
0	W_0	N_0	M_0	38	88.2	} 0.0002
I	W_0	N_1	M_0	59	50.3	
	W_1	N_1	M_0			
II	W_1	N_1	M_0	95	22.5	} 0.0005
	W_2	N_0	M_0			
III	W_2	N_1	M_0	138	10.7	} 0.02
	W_1	N_2	M_0			
	W_0	N_2	M_0			
IV	Any W	Any N	M_1	$\frac{33}{408}$	0	} 0.0001

SOURCE: Reproduced with permission from Ellis FH, Heatley GJ, Krosna MJ, Williamson WA, Balogh K: Esophagogastrectomy for carcinoma of the esophagus and cardia: A comparison of findings and results after standard resection in three consecutive 8 year time intervals, using improved staging criteria. *J Thorac Cardiovasc Surg* 113:836, 1997.

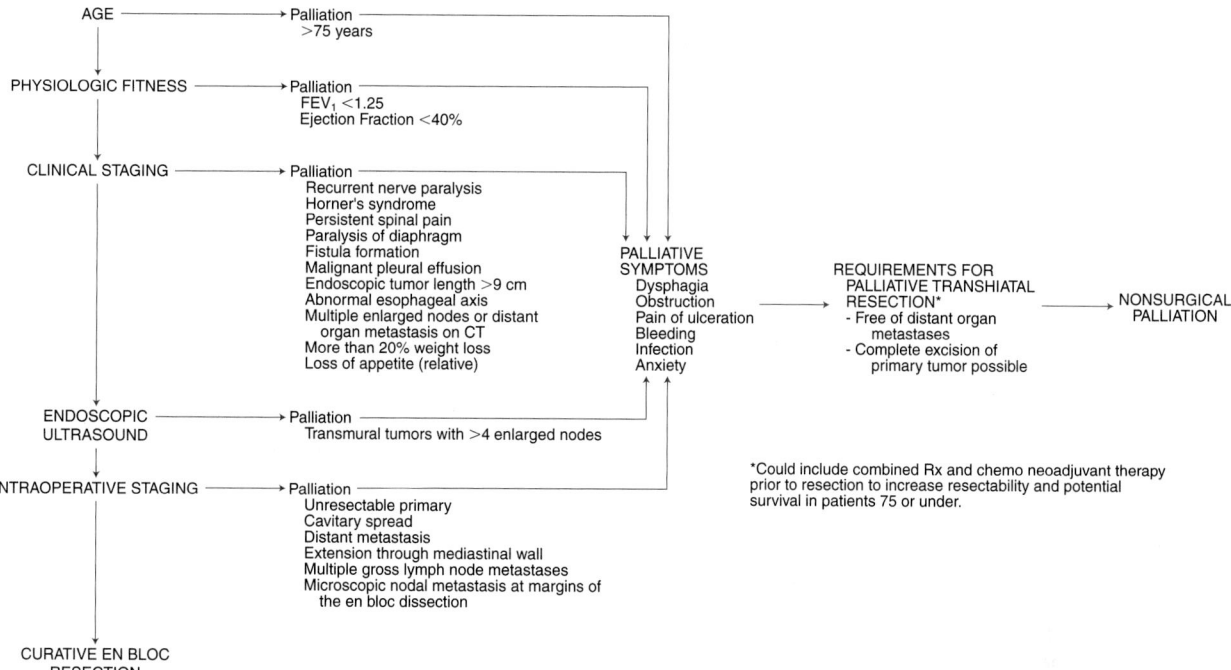

FIG. 24-73. Algorithm for the evaluation of esophageal cancer patients to select the proper therapy: curative en bloc resection, palliative transhiatal resection, or nonsurgical palliation. *(Reproduced with permission from DeMeester TR: Esophageal carcinoma: Current controversies. Semin Surg Oncol 13:217, 1997.)*

resected. The longitudinal lymph flow in the esophagus can result in skip areas, with small foci of tumor above the primary lesion, which underscores the importance of a wide resection of esophageal tumors. Wong has shown that local recurrence at the anastomosis can be prevented by obtaining a 10-cm margin of normal esophagus above the tumor. Anatomic studies have also shown that there is no

submucosal lymphatic barrier between the esophagus and the stomach at the cardia, and Wong has shown that 50% of the local recurrences in patients with esophageal cancer who are resected for cure occur in the intrathoracic stomach along the line of the gastric resection. Considering that the length of the esophagus ranges from 17 to 25 cm, and the length of the lesser curvature of the stomach is approximately 12 cm, a curative resection requires a cervical division of the esophagus and a greater than 50% proximal gastrectomy in most patients with carcinoma of the distal esophagus or cardia. This compromises the length of the stomach and esophagus remaining to re-establish gastrointestinal continuity, and necessitates a colon interposition.

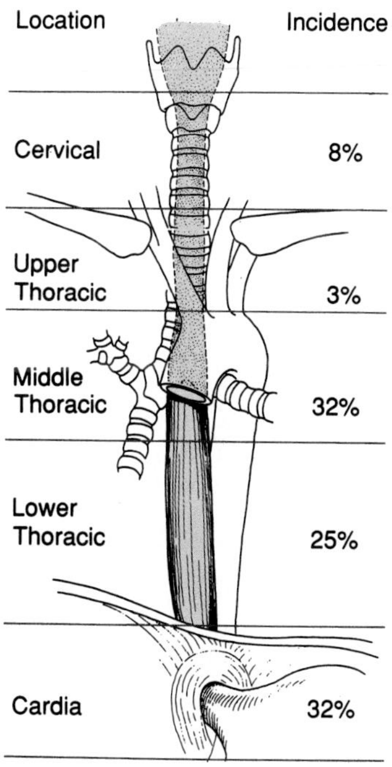

Age

An en bloc resection for cure of carcinoma of the esophagus in a patient older than 75 years is rarely indicated, because of the additional operative risk and the shorter life expectancy. Regardless of how favorable the staging criteria, a palliative resection is performed in these patients. This approach provides relief of symptoms with less extensive surgical procedures, and cure is still a chance possibility.

Cardiopulmonary Reserve

Patients undergoing esophageal resection should have sufficient cardiopulmonary reserve to tolerate the proposed procedure. The respiratory function is best assessed with the forced expiratory volume in 1 second (FEV_1), which ideally should be 2 L or more. Any patient with an FEV_1 of less than 1.25 L is a poor candidate for surgery, because he or she has a 40% risk of dying from respiratory insufficiency within 4 years. In such a patient, the chances of long-term survival, even if cured from the disease, do not justify an extensive en bloc resection. Clinical evaluation and electrocardiogram are not sufficient indicators of cardiac reserve. Echocardiography

Location	Incidence
Cervical	8%
Upper Thoracic	3%
Middle Thoracic	32%
Lower Thoracic	25%
Cardia	32%

FIG. 24-74. Incidence of carcinoma of the esophagus and cardia based on tumor location.

and dipyridamole thallium imaging provide accurate information on wall motion, ejection fraction, and myocardial blood flow. A defect on thallium imaging may require further evaluation with preoperative coronary angiography. A resting ejection fraction of less than 40%, particularly if there is no increase with exercise, is an ominous sign. The preference of these authors is to perform a palliative resection in such a patient, regardless of how favorable the other criteria are.

Clinical Stage

Clinical factors that indicate an advanced stage of carcinoma and exclude surgery with curative intent are recurrent nerve paralysis, Horner's syndrome, persistent spinal pain, paralysis of the diaphragm, fistula formation, and malignant pleural effusion. Factors that make surgical cure unlikely include a tumor greater than 8 cm in length, abnormal axis of the esophagus on a barium radiogram, enlarged lymph nodes on computed tomography (CT), a weight loss more than 20%, and loss of appetite. In patients in whom these findings are not present, staging depends primarily on the length of the tumor as measured with endoscopy, and the degree of wall penetration and lymph node metastasis seen with endoscopic ultrasound. Studies indicate that there are several favorable parameters associated with tumors less than 4 cm in length, there are fewer with tumors between 4 and 8 cm, and there are no favorable criteria for tumors greater than 8 cm in length. Consequently, the finding of a tumor over 8 cm in length should exclude curative resection, the finding of a smaller tumor should encourage an aggressive approach, and the smaller the tumor the more aggressive the approach should be. Endoscopic ultrasound imaging of esophageal tumors has recently become available, and provides further information regarding the size, wall penetration, and lymph node status of the lesion (Fig. 24-75).

Intraoperative Staging

Intraoperative staging allows selection of favorable candidates for a curative en bloc resection. It is based on the fact that there is a low survival rate for patients with a tumor that penetrates through the esophageal wall, or has multiple or distant lymph node metastasis, and requires an approach that allows switching from an en bloc curative dissection to a palliative resection if during the course of an operation one of the following features is revealed: an unresectable primary tumor, cavitary spread of the tumor, distant organ metastasis, extension of the tumor through the mediastinal pleura, multiple gross lymph node metastases, or microscopic evidence of lymph node involvement at the margins of an en bloc resection (i.e., low paratracheal, portal triad, subpancreatic, or periaortic lymph nodes). For cancers of the distal esophagus and cardia, patients with a favorable stage of disease can be identified by a combination of preoperative and intraoperative assessment with 86% accuracy. The overall 5-year survival of these selected patients after a curative en bloc resection is between 40 and 55%. If the tumor does not extend through the esophageal wall and there are less than five positive lymph nodes, the 5-year survival is 75%. These results support a clinical approach in which an en bloc resection of the esophagus and stomach is advocated only for patients most likely to benefit.

Management of Patients Excluded from Curative Resection

If the patient is considered incurable on preoperative or intraoperative evaluation, the severity of dysphagia or other incapacitating symptoms is assessed. Dysphagia of grade IV or higher (Table 24-14) is an indication for a palliative resection. If the patient is physiologically fit, simple esophageal resection and reconstruction with a cervical esophagogastrostomy offer the best palliation. This procedure allows the patient to eat without dysphagia and prevents the local complications of perforation, hemorrhage, fistula formation, and incapacitating pain. Occasionally a patient will be cured by a palliative resection, but this should not be used as justification for a palliative resection in the absence of dysphagia. Malignant pleural effusion, obvious mediastinal spread, or distant organ metastases are

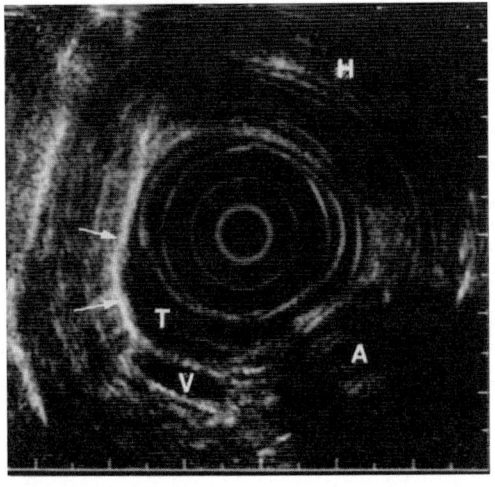

A

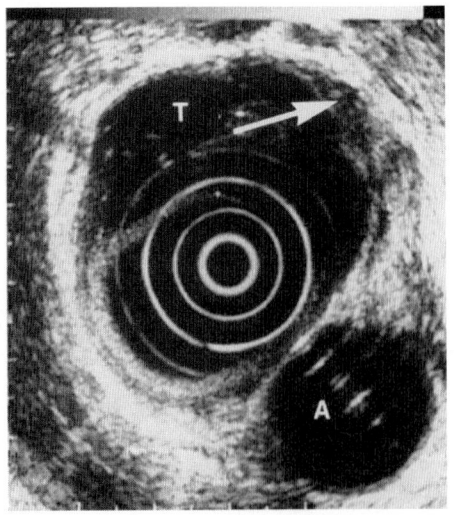

B

FIG. 24-75. *A.* Endoscopic ultrasound image of a tumor confined to the esophageal wall. T = tumor; V = azygos vein; H = heart; A = aorta; arrows = intact adventitia. *B.* Endoscopic ultrasound image of an advanced esophageal carcinoma with tumor penetrating through all layers of the esophagus. T = tumor; A = aorta; arrow shows tumor penetrating through the adventitia into periesophageal tissues. [*Reproduced with permission from Bremner RM, DeMeester TR: Surgical treatment of esophageal carcinoma, in Wong RKH (ed): Gastroenterology Clinics of North America, 20. Philadelphia: WB Saunders, 1991, p 13, 748.*]

Table 24-14
Functional Grades of Dysphagia

Grade	Definition	Incidence at Diagnosis (%)
I	Eating normally	11
II	Requires liquids with meals	21
III	Able to take semisolids but unable to take any solid food	30
IV	Able to take liquids only	40
V	Unable to take liquids, but able to swallow saliva	7
VI	Unable to swallow saliva	12

SOURCE: Modified with permission from Takita H, Vincent RG, et al: Squamous cell carcinoma of the esophagus: A study of 153 cases. *J Surg Oncol* 9:547, 1977.

usually contraindications for a palliative resection. In this setting, if dysphagia is not a problem, nothing more need be done.

If an obstructing tumor cannot be resected due to invasion of the trachea, aorta, or heart, or the patient's general condition precludes an operative procedure, relief of dysphagia by re-establishing the esophageal lumen is the focus of therapy. In this situation, the objective is to provide relief of dysphagia with the lowest mortality and the shortest hospital stay. A variety of techniques including bougienage, intubation, laser ablation, and electrical coagulation are available, and can be used alone or in combination. Most centers prefer intubation of the esophagus.

Figure 24-76 shows the correlation between grade of dysphagia and a patient's score on the Linear Analogue Self-Assessment test (LASA), which assesses the patient's physical and psychological well-being and symptom control, including dysphagia. There is a significant negative correlation between dysphagia grade and quality of life as measured by the LASA.

Surgical Treatment

A patient's nutritional status before surgery has a profound effect on the outcome of an esophageal resection. Low serum protein levels

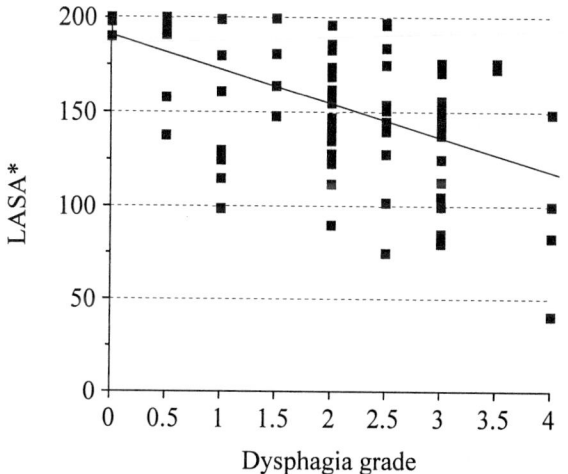

FIG. 24-76. Scatter diagram of relation between dysphagia grade and Linear Analogue Self-Assessment (LASA) in 38 patients with esophagogastric carcinoma. Eighty-six paired scores obtained at various times through the patients' survival have been plotted. The negative correlation shown is highly significant (p < 0.0001) with Spearman coefficients of −0.49 and −0.43, respectively. (*Reproduced with permission from Loizou LA, Grigg D, Atkinson M, Robertson C, Bown S: A prospective comparison of laser therapy and intubation in endoscopic palliation for malignant dysphagia. Gastroenterology 100:1303, 1991.*)

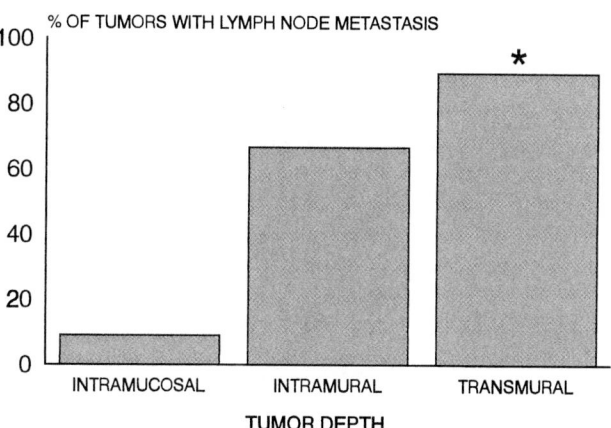

FIG. 24-77. Prevalence of nodal metastases according to the depth of the tumor in the pathology specimen. (* p < 0.01; X² = 9.3, 2df.) (*Reproduced with permission from Clark GW, Peters JH, Ireland AP, et al: Nodal metastasis and sites of recurrence after en-bloc esophagectomy for adenocarcinoma. Ann Thorac Surg 58:646, 1994.*)

have a deleterious effect on the cardiovascular system, and a poor nutritional status affects the host resistance to infection and the rate of anastomotic and wound healing. A serum albumin level of less than 3.4 g/dL on admission indicates poor caloric intake and an increased risk of surgical complications, including anastomotic breakdown. A feeding jejunostomy tube provides the most reliable and safest method for nutritional support in patients who cannot consume an oral diet and have a functionally normal small bowel. In severely malnourished patients, the jejunostomy is performed as a separate procedure to allow for preoperative nutritional support. In these patients the abdomen is entered through a small supraumbilical midline incision. Otherwise, the jejunostomy tube is placed at the time of esophageal resection, and feeding is begun on the third postoperative day.

In an analysis of patients undergoing curative en bloc resection for adenocarcinoma of the distal esophagus, lymph node metastases were present in 76%. Tumor depth was a good indicator of nodal involvement (Fig. 24-77). At the time of resection, 89% of transmural tumors, 60% of intramural tumors, and 6% of intramucosal lesions had lymph node metastasis. This finding has implications in the management of patients with high-grade dysplasia, where the prevalence of unexpected adenocarcinoma is up to 50%.

Adenocarcinomas of the lower esophagus and cardia spread widely to regional nodes, most commonly to nodes along the lesser curvature, celiac axis, and parahiatal regions (Table 24-15). Ten percent have subcarinal nodes and 18% had involved nodes of the splenic hilum, along the splenic artery, or along the greater curvature of the stomach; subcarinal and splenic nodes would remain following transhiatal resection. The involved nodes along the greater curvature of the stomach would by necessity be transposed into the chest if the stomach was used to re-establish gastrointestinal continuity. In addition, over 20% of patients had positive celiac axis nodes, an area not dissected by most surgeons during transhiatal esophagectomy.

Control of the local and regional disease forms the basis for the classic en bloc resection. In the experience of these authors, the site of nodal recurrence following en bloc resection in the field of the resection was only 1% (Fig. 24-78). All patients with thoracic nodal recurrence had disease in their upper mediastinum or aortopulmonary window, suggesting that these recurrences arose from nodes lying along the recurrent laryngeal nerve chains, which are not routinely

Table 24-15
Pattern of Lymph Node Spread in Resected Tumors of the Lower Esophagus and Cardia

Node Location	No. of Positive Patients (n = 43)	Percentage of Positive Patients	No. of Positive Nodes	Total No. of Nodes Resected	Percentage of Nodes Positive
Tracheobronchial	1	2.3%	1	42	2.4%
Subcarinal	4	9.3%	9	390	2.3%
Paraesophageal	12	27.9%	37	316	11.7%
Parahiatal	15	34.8%	35	247	14.2%
Splenic hilum	1	2.3%	3	39	7.7%
Splenic artery	2	4.7%	2	71	2.8%
Greater curvature	4	9.3%	10	89	11.2%
Lesser curvature	18	41.8%	64	261	24.5%
Left gastric	3	7%	8	94	8.5%
Celiac	9	20.9%	25	60	41.6%
Hepatic	1	2.3%	6	21	28.5%
Portal	1	2.3%	2	84	2.4%
Right gastric	1	23%	4	47	8.5%
Retropancreatic	0	0	0	23	0%

removed by the en bloc dissection. Performing a more extended mediastinal dissection combined with a radical neck dissection has been advocated by some authors in the treatment of esophageal squamous cell carcinoma. The increased morbidity and the possibility of permanent hoarseness associated with this approach have discouraged its widespread application. It has been reported that the finding of metastatic disease involving the celiac nodes precludes survival beyond 2 years. By contrast, these authors have reported prolonged survival in patients with celiac axis involvement.

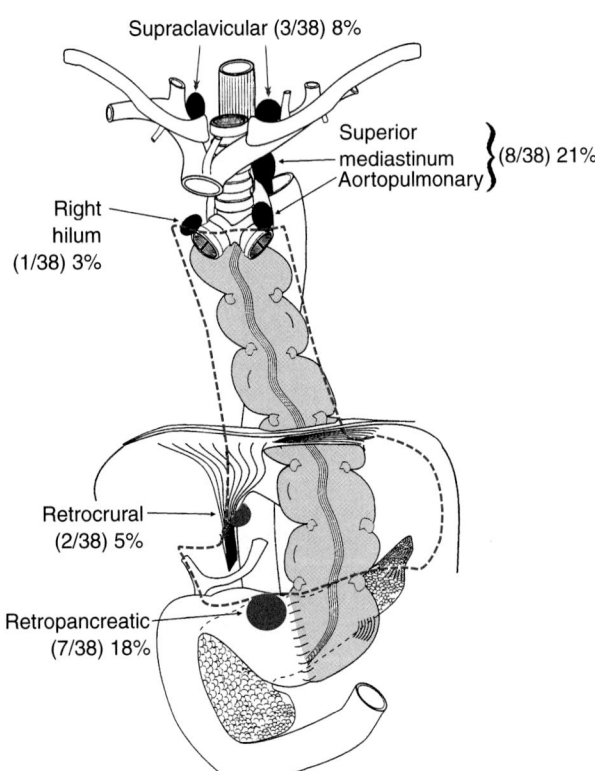

FIG. 24-78. Schematic drawing of the sites of lymph node recurrence after en bloc esophagectomy. Margins of the resection are indicated by the broken line. (*Reproduced with permission from Clark GW, Peters JH, Ireland AP, et al: Nodal metastasis and sites of recurrence after en-bloc esophagectomy for adenocarcinoma. Ann Thorac Surg 58:646, 1994.*)

Cervical and Upper Thoracic Esophageal Cancer

When considering resection, tumors of the esophagus are best divided into those above and those below the carina. Czerny reported the first successful resection of a carcinoma of the cervical esophagus in 1877. It was hoped that the prognosis for patients with this disease might be better than for those with carcinoma of the thoracic esophagus, but this has not proved to be the case. Early experience with resection of the cervical esophagus resulted in a high mortality rate, and reconstruction by neck flaps often required multiple operations. Because of these complexities and the generally disappointing results, radiotherapy frequently was elected. Immediate mortality decreased, but control of the tumor was not satisfactory.

The difference between the two forms of therapy is the manner in which the disease recurs. Tumors treated with radiation therapy initially tend to recur locally as well as systemically, and cause unmanageable local disease with eventual erosion into neck vessels and trachea, causing hemorrhage and dyspnea. Patients who undergo surgical therapy have few local recurrences of the tumor, provided total excision is possible, but they succumb to metastatic disease. Collin has reported a local failure rate of 80% after definitive radiation therapy, and 20% of these patients required palliative surgery in order to control the disease locally. Improvements in the techniques of immediate esophageal reconstruction have reduced the complications of the surgical treatment of this disease and encouraged a more aggressive surgical approach. The data reported by Collin suggest that an initial aggressive surgical resection yields longer survival than radiation therapy (Fig. 24-79). Positive surgical margins, tracheal invasion that cannot be removed, and vocal cord paralysis correlate with a significantly shorter survival following surgery. Palliation was better achieved in patients who underwent esophagectomy with immediate gastric pull-up than in those who underwent primary radiation therapy or chemotherapy.

Lesions that are not fixed to the spine, do not invade the vessels or trachea, and do not have fixed cervical lymph node metastases should be resected. If lymph node metastases are present or the tumor comes in close proximity to the cricopharyngeus muscle, a course of preoperative chemo- and radiotherapy should be given before surgical resection. This usually consists of two to three cycles of chemotherapy and no more than 3.5 Gy of radiation therapy. Neoadjuvant therapy is given in an attempt to salvage the larynx, since the larynx is often invaded by microscopic tumors, and in the past, a total laryngectomy in combination with esophagectomy was

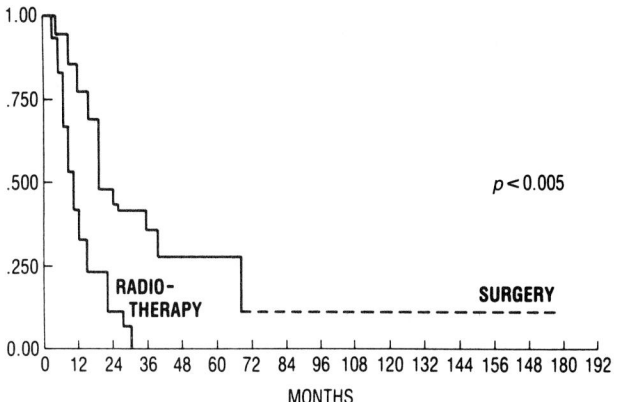

FIG. 24-79. Actuarial survival of patients with carcinoma of the cervical esophagus treated by surgery or 5000+ Gy of radiotherapy. (Reproduced with permission from Collin CF, Spiro RH: Carcinoma of the cervical esophagus: Changing therapeutic trends. Am J Surg 148:460, 1984, with permission.)

usually necessary. A simultaneous en bloc dissection of the superior mediastinum and cervical lymph nodes is done, sparing the jugular veins on both sides.

The thoracic esophagus is removed via a right posterolateral thoracotomy with a corresponding en bloc lymphadenectomy. The continuity of the gastrointestinal tract is re-established by pulling the stomach up through the esophageal bed. If removing the larynx is necessary, a permanent tracheostomy stoma is constructed in the lower flap of the cervical incision. The division of the trachea in some patients may preclude the possibility of a permanent cervical standard tracheostomy, since the remaining tracheal stump distal to the tumor will not reach the suprasternal notch. Removal of the medial head of the clavicles and the manubrium down to the sternal angle of Louis provides excellent exposure and allows the construction of a mediastinal tracheostomy. A bipedicle skin flap over the pectoralis muscle can be advanced upward, or a single-pedicle musculocutaneous flap including the pectoralis muscle and its overlying skin can be rotated to cover the defect. A circular incision in the flap can be used as a port through which the tracheal remnant is brought out to the skin.

Tumors of the Thoracic Esophagus and Cardia

For tumors that arise below the carina, the preference of these authors is either an en bloc resection for cure or a transhiatal removal for palliation. A curative procedure is performed according to the principles of an en bloc resection in continuity with the regional lymph nodes (Fig. 24-80). It is attempted in a patient whose preresection physical condition and tumor characteristics have the potential for long-term survival. The en bloc resection is done through three incisions in the following order: (1) right posterolateral thoracotomy, en bloc dissection of the distal esophagus, mobilization of the esophagus above the aortic arch, closure of the thoracotomy, repositioning of the patient in the recumbent position; (2) upper midline abdominal incision, en bloc dissection of the stomach and associated lymph nodes; and (3) left neck incision and proximal division of the esophagus. The specimen is removed transhiatally and the stomach is divided at the angulus, preserving the antrum. Gastrointestinal continuity is re-established with a left colon interposition. During the thoracic and abdominal dissection, intraoperative staging is done. If during the course of the operation an incurable situation is identified, the en bloc resection is abandoned

and a palliative resection is performed in a manner similar to that described for tumors of the middle and upper thoracic esophagus. The hospital mortality for patients undergoing a curative en bloc resection is similar to those undergoing a palliative transhiatal resection. If preoperative staging has shown that the patient is a candidate for palliative resection, a transhiatal esophagectomy is performed (Fig. 24-81). A standard left thoracotomy with intrathoracic anastomosis for lower lesions or an Ivor Lewis combined approach for higher lesions is not advocated because of (1) the proven need to resect long lengths of the esophagus to eradicate submucosal spread, (2) the higher morbidity associated with a thoracic anastomotic leak, and (3) the high incidence of esophagitis secondary to reflux following an intrathoracic anastomosis.

En Bloc Esophagogastrectomy Versus Transhiatal Resection for Carcinoma of the Lower Esophagus and Cardia

Many strategies for treatment of esophageal carcinoma limit the role of surgery to removing the primary tumor, with the hope that adjuvant therapy will increase cure rates by destroying systemic disease. This approach emphasizes the concept of biological determinism (i.e., that the outcome of treatment in esophageal cancer is determined at the time of diagnosis, and that surgical therapy aimed at removing more than the primary tumor is not helpful). Lymph node metastases are considered simply markers of systemic disease; the systematic removal of involved nodes is not considered beneficial. The belief that removal of the primary tumor by transhiatal esophagogastrectomy results in the same survival rates as a more extensive en bloc resection is based on the same kind of reasoning.

In the transhiatal procedure there is no specific attempt made to remove lymph node–bearing tissue in the posterior mediastinum. By contrast, the en bloc esophagectomy removes the tumor covered on all surfaces with a layer of normal tissue (see Fig. 24-80). A long length of foregut above and below the lesion is resected to incorporate submucosal spread of the tumor. Consistent with this is resection of the proximal two thirds of the stomach in patients with a tumor in the lower third of the thoracic esophagus or cardia. Appropriate cervical mediastinal and abdominal lymph node dissections are included using an en bloc technique to remove potentially involved regional nodes. Arguments to support the more extensive esophagectomy, gastrectomy, and lymph node dissection are listed in Table 24-16.

Hagen and colleagues recently reviewed 100 consecutive patients who underwent en bloc esophagectomy for esophageal adenocarcinoma. No patient received pre- or postoperative chemotherapy or radiation therapy. The aim of the study was to relate the extent of disease to prognostic features, timing and mode of recurrence, and survival following en bloc resection (Fig. 24-82). The median follow-up of surviving patients was 40 months, with 24 patients surviving 5 years or more. Overall actuarial survival at 5 years was 52%. Fifty-five of the tumors were transmural and 63 patients had lymph node involvement. Metastases to celiac (n = 16) or other distant node sites (n = 26) were not associated with decreased survival. Remarkably, local recurrence was seen in only one patient. Latent nodal recurrence outside the surgical field occurred in nine, and systemic metastases in 31. The authors concluded that long-term survival from adenocarcinoma of the esophagus can be achieved in over half of the patients who undergo en bloc resection. One third of patients with lymph node involvement survived 5 years, and the authors concluded that local control is excellent following en bloc resection.

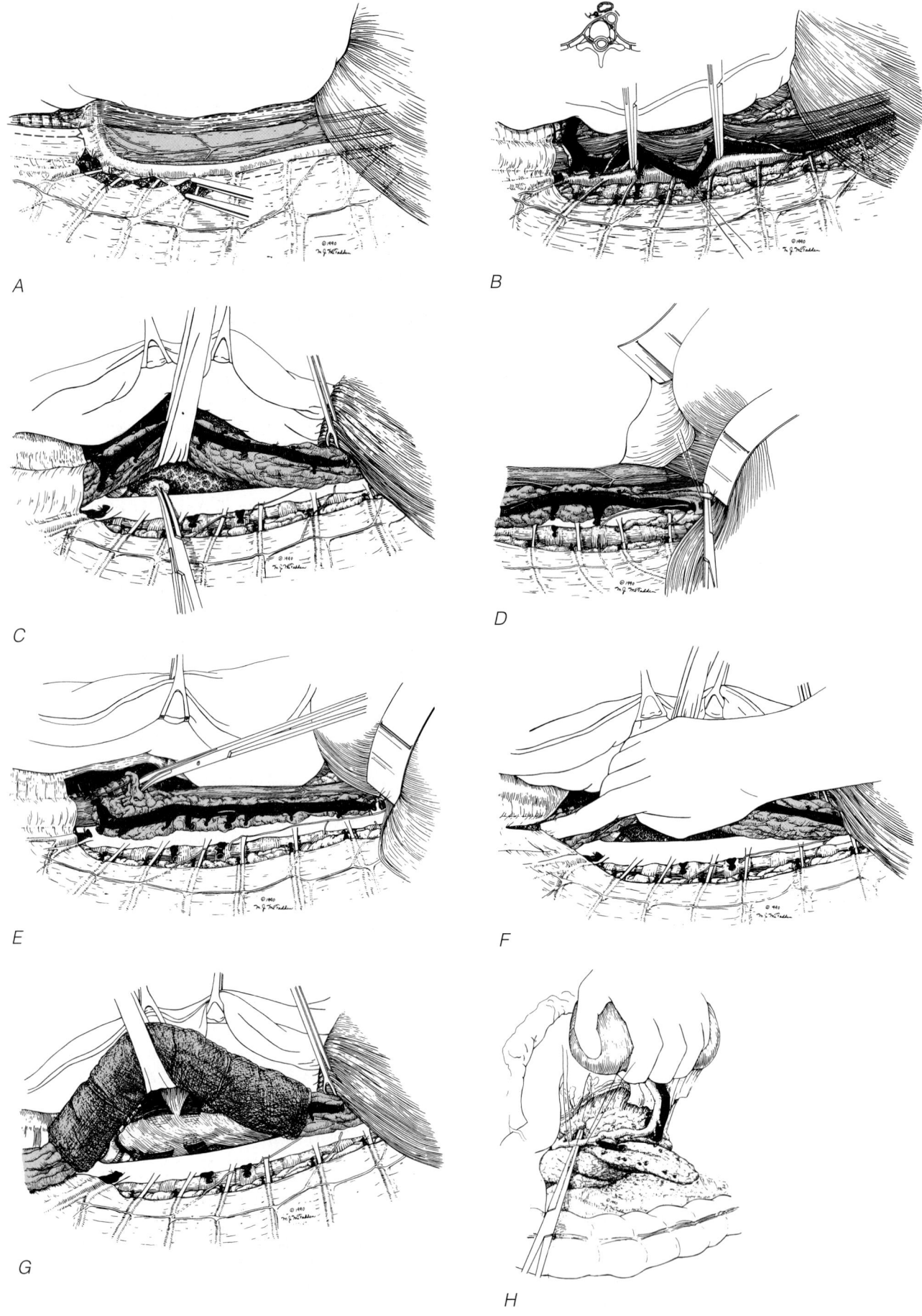

A

B

C

D

E

F

G

H

FIG. 24-80. *(Continued)*

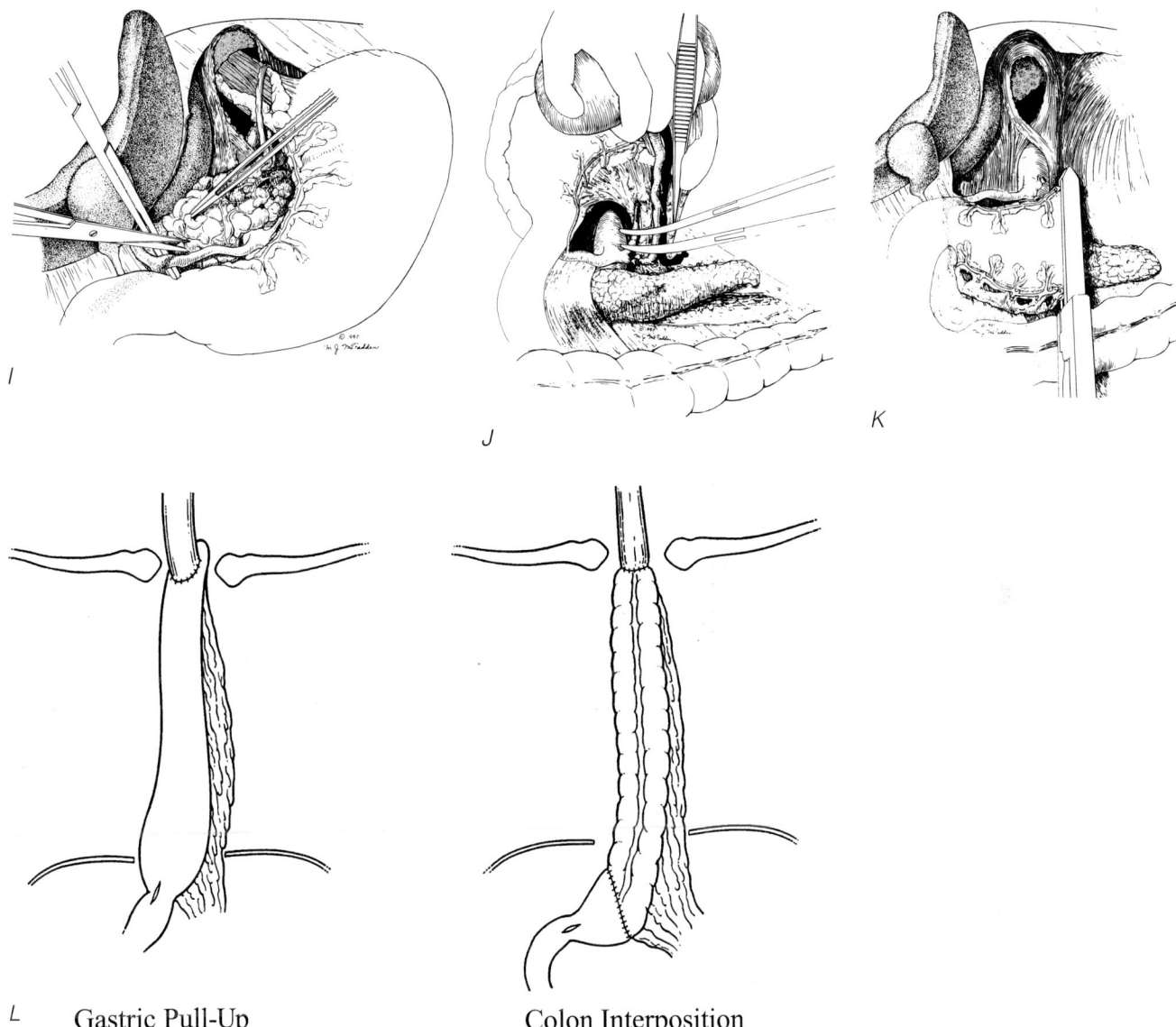

I

J

K

L   Gastric Pull-Up   Colon Interposition

FIG. 24-80. *(continued)* Technique of en bloc esophagogastrectomy. The procedure is performed through a right posterolateral thoracotomy followed by repositioning the patient and an upper abdominal laparotomy and left neck incision. The steps in the procedure are: *A.* Division of the intercostal veins over the course of the azygos vein. *B.* Division of the hemiazygos veins (insert shows plane of dissection). *C.* Dissection along the intercostal arteries and over the anterior surface of the aorta into the left chest. *D.* Ligation of the thoracic duct and terminal end of the azygos. *E.* Dissection of the subcarinal lymph nodes. *F.* Blunt finger dissection of the proximal esophagus. *G.* Specimen wrapped and left in the chest while the thoracotomy is closed and the patient is repositioned for the abdominal portion of the procedure. *H.* Dissection of the splenic artery in the beginning of the celiac and splenic lymphadenectomy. *I.* Opening of the gastrohepatic ligament and continuation of the lymphadenectomy along the common hepatic artery. *J.* Completion of the celiac and splenic lymphadenectomy with division of the left gastric artery. *K.* Transection of the stomach and removal of the specimen through the hiatus after division of the esophagus in the neck. *L.* Completed procedure with reconstruction of the gastrointestinal tract with left colon interposition. In patients with squamous cell tumor or small adenocarcinoma that do not extend down the lesser curve of the stomach a gastric tube is constructed along the greater curvature and used for reconstruction.

Controversy persists over the extent of resection necessary for cure of esophageal adenocarcinoma. Several retrospective studies have shown a benefit to the more extensive node dissection accomplished with a transthoracic en bloc esophagectomy as compared to the transhiatal esophagectomy. These studies have been criticized as suffering from selection bias and for inaccuracy in preoperative staging. Performance of a more complete node dissection also results in the potential for stage migration. Hulscher has reported a prospective randomized control trial that compared transthoracic en bloc to transhiatal esophagectomy. The results were inconclusive but showed a trend toward better survival with the en bloc resection. This trial eliminated many of the criticisms of the retrospective studies but included patients with various stages of disease. This may have obscured the benefits of systematic node dissection by the

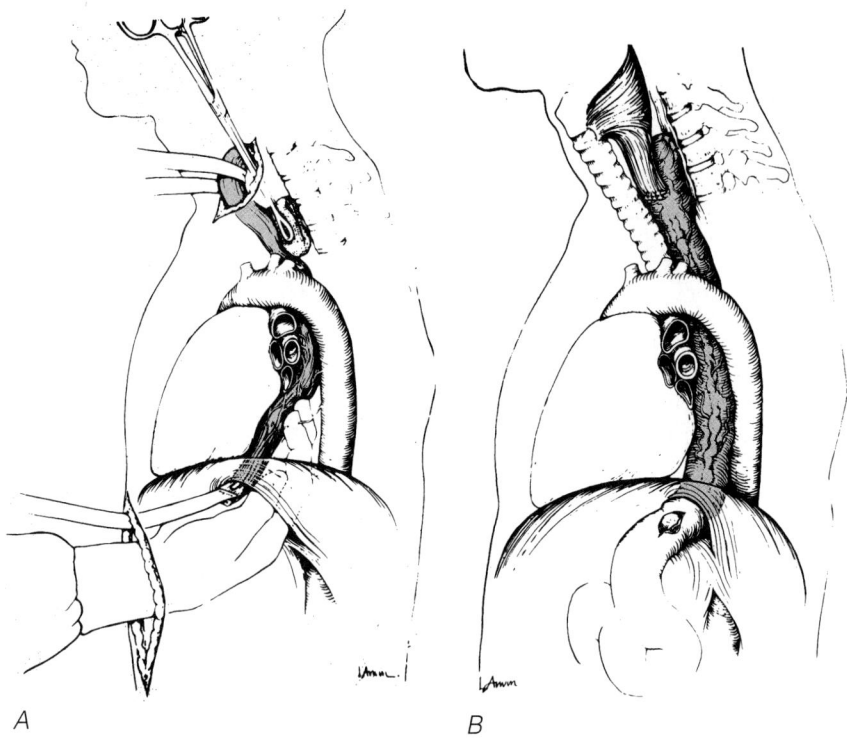

FIG. 24-81. Transhiatal esophagectomy. *A.* Illustration of blunt dissection of the thoracic esophagus through combined abdominal and neck incisions without thoracotomy. *B.* Reestablishment of gastrointestinal continuity using the stomach brought through the posterior mediastinum and cervical esophagogastrostomy.

unequal distribution of patients with early stage disease who did not need a formal lymphadenectomy, as well as those with advanced disease with extensive lymph node metastases who were not curable by surgery alone. An alternative approach to compare transthoracic en bloc to transhiatal resection has been done by Johansson using a retrospective case control study between nonrandomized patients having similar size transmural (T3) tumors with lymph node metastases (N1). The aim of the study was to determine whether patients with

locally advanced (T3N1) esophageal cancer benefit from the performance of a transthoracic en bloc resection. This approach removes the influence of inaccurate preoperative staging and minimizes the influence of postoperative stage migration on survival since all patients had N1 disease. Further, all patients had 20 or more lymph nodes in the surgical specimen which allowed confirmation that the extent of lymph node disease in both groups was comparable. These conditions focused the question as to which procedure was

Table 24-16
Arguments to Support Extensive Esophagectomy, Gastrectomy, and Lymph Node Dissection

Arguments to Support a More Extensive Esophagectomy

Injection of submucosal contrast medium shows that the length of longitudinal lymph flow is six times the transverse flow.
At least 10 cm of grossly normal esophagus proximal to the tumor must be resected to prevent local recurrence.
Special relation indicates that for an adequate proximal margin, a cervical anastomosis is almost always needed.

Arguments to Support a More Extensive Gastrectomy for Tumors of the Lower Third of the Esophagus or Cardia

No barrier to submucosal lymphatics between esophagus and stomach at the cardia.
Tumor cells in submucosal lymphatics can result in intragastric recurrence if too little of the stomach is resected.
Special relationships of the stomach don't allow for both adequate distal tumor margins and sufficient residual stomach to perform a cervical anastomosis.

Arguments for Lymph Node Dissection

Survival of lung cancer patients with metastases to the hilar lymph nodes (i.e., a cancer that also metastasizes to mediastinal lymph nodes) is dependent on removal of involved nodes.
Patients with esophageal carcinoma and lymph node metastases are cured by resections, whereas it is extremely rare for patients with lymph node metastases to be cured without their surgical removal.
Patients with esophageal and cardia cancer, like those with head and neck cancer, can die from lymph node metastasis alone.
Asian surgeons, who are incessant data keepers, accept unconditionally the benefit of lymph node dissection on survival in patients with carcinoma of the esophagus or stomach.
Forty-three percent of patients with esophageal carcinoma who have histologically node-negative disease have histochemical node-positive disease. Furthermore, after a median observation time of 12 months, patients with histochemical node-positive disease had a significantly shorter disease-free survival. On the basis of this finding, it is believed that when nodes are reported to be histologically free of tumor, more disease than is currently appreciated is removed if left behind, depending on the extent of resection.

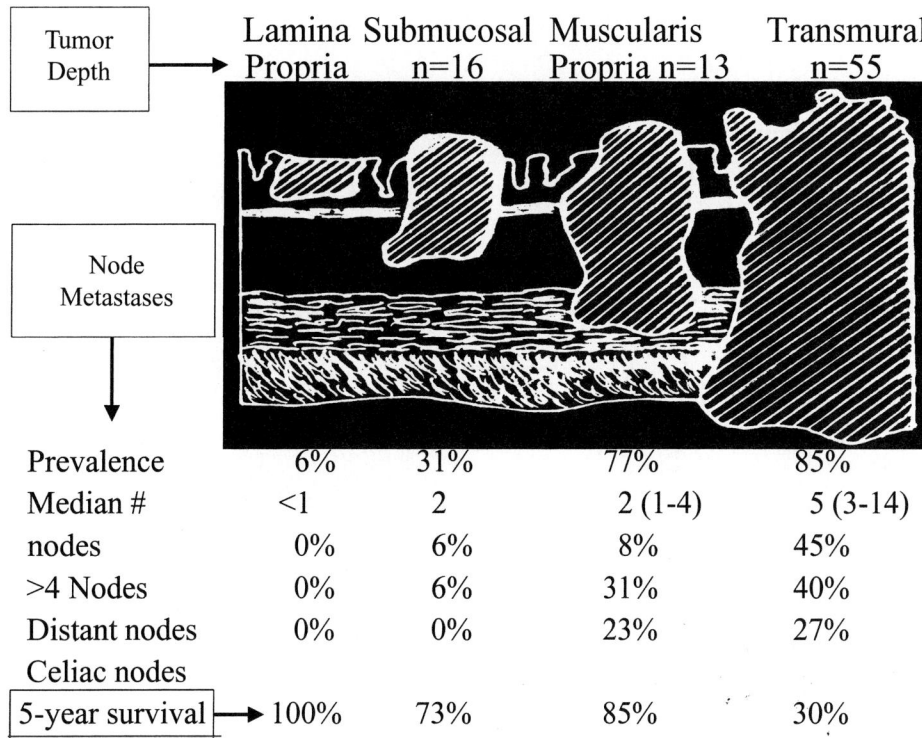

Tumor Depth	Lamina Propria	Submucosal n=16	Muscularis Propria n=13	Transmural n=55
Prevalence	6%	31%	77%	85%
Median # nodes	<1	2	2 (1-4)	5 (3-14)
>4 Nodes	0%	6%	8%	45%
Distant nodes	0%	6%	31%	40%
Celiac nodes	0%	0%	23%	27%
5-year survival	100%	73%	85%	30%

FIG. 24-82. The relationship of tumor depth to the prevalence, number, and location of metastatic nodes and patient survival obtained from the analysis of 100 consecutive en bloc esophagectomies for adenocarcinoma of the distal esophagus and the gastroesophageal junction.

associated with a better survival. The results, in Figures 24-83, 24-84, and 24-85, show that a transthoracic en bloc resection confers a survival benefit over a transhiatal resection in patients with transmural (T3) esophageal carcinomas when eight or fewer lymph nodes are involved (N1). The most likely explanation for the improved survival following transthoracic en bloc resection is a more complete removal of local-regional disease, which is unrecognized disease that is removed with an en bloc lymph node dissection but left behind with a tranhiatal lymph node dissection. Consequently, transthoracic en bloc resection results in better control of local-regional disease. Indeed, in clinical trials neoadjuvant radiochemotherapy has been added to transhiatal esophagectomy in an effort to control local-regional disease without great success. A more prudent approach would be to use a transthoracic en bloc dissection to control local-regional disease and focus postoperative adjuvant therapy on eliminating systemic disease.

FIG. 24-83. Cumulative survival rates in 49 patients with T3 N1 adenocarcinoma of the distal esophagus or gastroesophageal junction grouped by type of resection: transthoracic en bloc (n = 27) or trashiatal (n = 22), (p = 0.014). All deaths were due to cancer. All survivors were followed for a minimum of 5 years.

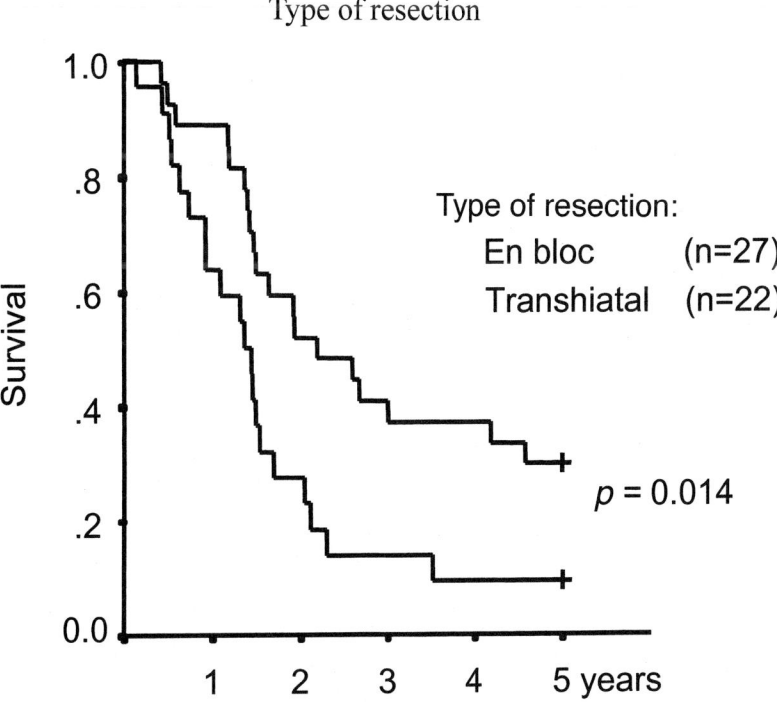

Type of resection

Type of resection:
En bloc (n=27)
Transhiatal (n=22)

$p = 0.014$

Patients with 1-8 metastatic nodes

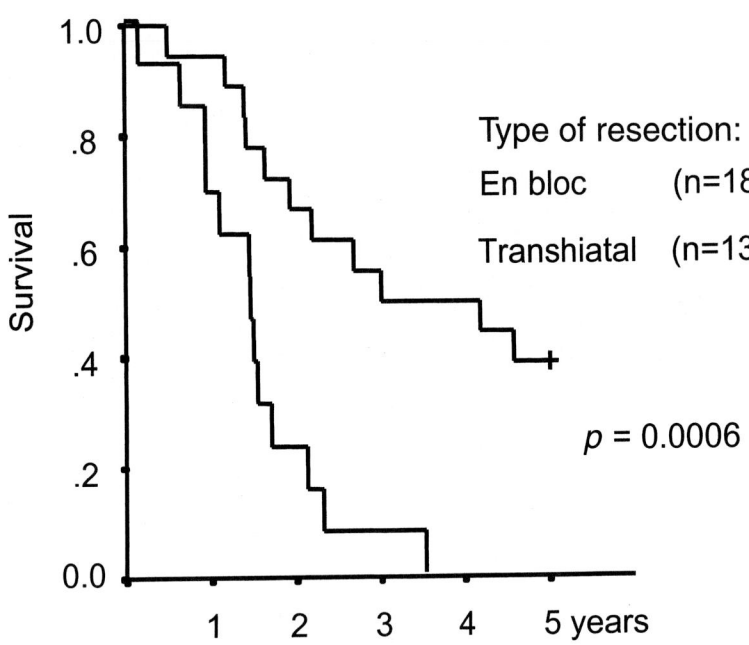

Type of resection:
En bloc   (n=18)
Transhiatal   (n=13)

p = 0.0006

FIG. 24-84. Survival of patients with 1-8 metastatic lymph nodes who had a transthoracic en bloc lymph node dissection (n = 18) and those who had a transhiatal lymph node dissection (n = 13). Log rank test statistic 10.25, df = 1, p = 0.0006. All deaths were due to cancer. All survivors were followed for a minimum of 5 years.

These studies showed that for early cancers of the lower esophagus and cardia, en bloc esophagogastrectomy results in significantly better survival rates than transhiatal esophagogastrectomy. This finding cannot be explained by a bias in the stage of disease resected, a difference in operative mortality, or death from nontumor causes. Rather, it appears to be due to the type of operation performed. Ideally, the question as to which procedure is the best should be resolved by a prospective randomized study of similiarly staged patients.

Extent of Resection to Cure Disease Confined to the Mucosa

The development of surveillance programs for the detection of early squamous cell carcinoma in endemic areas and for early

FIG. 24-85. Survival of patients with 9 or more metastatic lymph nodes who had a transthoracic en bloc lymph node dissection (n = 9) and those who had a transhiatal lymph node dissection (n = 9). Log rank test statistic 0.57, df = 1, p = 0.956. All deaths were due to cancer. All survivors were followed for a minimum of 5 years.

Patients with ≥ 9 metastatic nodes

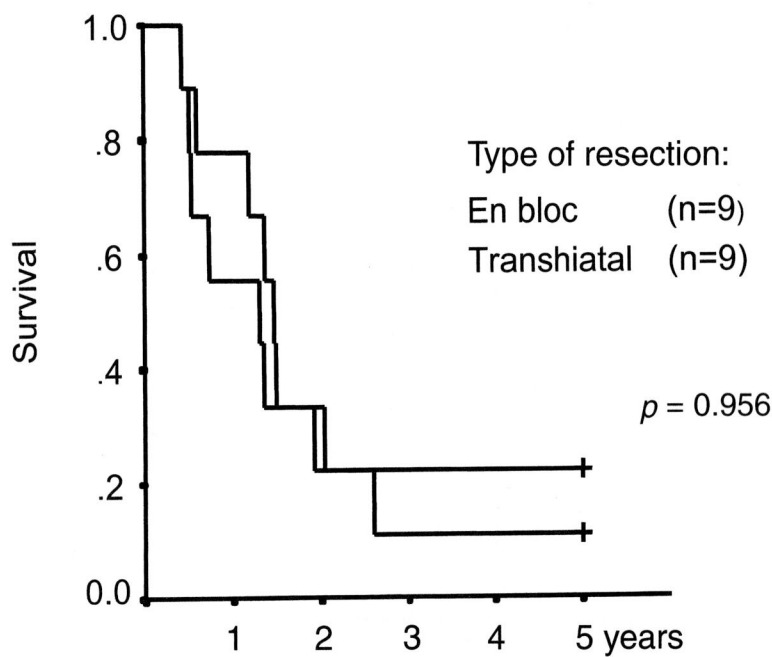

Type of resection:
En bloc   (n=9)
Transhiatal   (n=9)

p = 0.956

adenocarcinoma in patients with Barrett's esophagus has given rise to controversy over how to manage tumors confined to the mucosa. Some authors have endoscopically resected squamous carcinomas after using endoscopic ultrasound to determine that the depth of the tumor was limited to the mucosa. Surprisingly, large areas of squamous mucosa can be resected without perforation or bleeding, leaving the smooth surface of the muscularis mucosae intact. Re-epithelialization of the large artificially induced ulcer is usually complete in 3 weeks. In order not to miss a squamous cancer that has invaded deeper than expected, it is important to examine the deep margins of the resected specimen carefully, and to perform periodic endoscopic follow-up examinations with vital staining techniques. This technique is not appropriate for multiple and widespread or circumferential squamous lesions because of the risk of developing a stricture during the healing process. In this situation, those acquainted with endoscopic resection would advocate an esophagectomy.

Several studies have shown that intraepithelial carcinoma (i.e., carcinoma in situ or high-grade dysplasia), and intramucosal tumors (i.e., invasive cancer limited by the muscular mucosae), are quite different in their biologic behavior from submucosal tumors, regardless of their histologic characteristics, regardless of whether they are squamous cell carcinoma or adenocarcinoma arising in Barrett's mucosa. Vessel invasion and lymph node metastasis do not occur in severe dysplasia, are uncommon in the intramucosal tumors, but are the rule in submucosal tumors. Consequently, the 5-year survival for intramucosal tumors is significantly better than for submucosal tumors. These findings indicate that both severe dysplasia and intramucosal cancers represent early malignant lesions of the esophagus. A critical issue to be resolved is whether an intramucosal tumor can be correctly discriminated from a submucosal tumor before surgery. The results of using endoscopic ultrasound for determining the depth of tumors confined to the esophageal wall are of questionable accuracy. The resolution of present-day endoscopic ultrasonographic systems is not sufficient to predictably differentiate the fine detail of tumor infiltration when it is limited to the esophageal wall. Currently there is no dependable way, before surgery, of determining whether a tumor extends beyond the muscularis mucosae.

Another complicating factor is that up to 5% of patients with intramucosal tumors have lymph node metastases, although the number of involved nodes per patient is usually no more than one. Akiyama and others have reported that even though the number of involved nodes may be small, they can spread to distant nodal regions, including cervical and abdominal nodes.

These authors have recently utilized the presence or absence of an endoscopically visible lesion in patients with biopsy-proven high-grade dysplasia (HGD) or intramucosal carcinoma as a predictor of tumor depth and nodal metastases. The data indicate that a positive biopsy in the absence of an endoscopically visible lesion almost always corresponds to an intramucosal tumor without nodal metastases. Of patients with HGD, 43% proved to harbor occult adenocarcinoma at resection. Importantly, when there was no visible lesion on endoscopy, 88% of the tumors were intramucosal and 12% submucosal. Only one of 10 patients with no visible lesion had lymph node involvement, either histologically or immunohistochemically. In contrast, patients with endoscopically visible tumors had a high prevalence of tumors that penetrated beyond the mucosa (75%), and 56% had positive nodes.

Patients with HGD and intramucosal carcinoma are best treated by a total esophagectomy, removing all Barrett's tissue and any potential associated adenocarcinoma. Options include transhiatal

esophagectomy, or more recently, vagal-sparing esophagectomy. The vagal-sparing approach is suitable only given confidence of the absence of regional nodal disease. Reconstruction is accomplished with either the stomach (transhiatal) or colon (vagal sparing) with the anastomosis in the neck. The mortality associated with this procedure should be less than 5%, particularly in centers experienced in esophageal surgery. Functional recovery is excellent, particularly in the vagal-sparing group.

As the understanding of the pathology of esophageal cancer improves and experience with its resection increases, evidence is accumulating that the best chance for cure of patients with an intramural tumor in the distal esophagus or cardia is an en bloc esophagectomy and proximal gastrectomy, with gastrointestinal continuity re-established with a either gastric or colon interposition. For patients with a tumor in the upper or cervical esophagus, the best chance for cure is an en bloc esophagectomy and a cervical lymph node dissection with gastrointestinal continuity re-established with a gastric pull-up. Table 24-17 presents a summary of the extent of resection for tumors extending various depths into the esophageal wall.

Alternative Therapies

Radiation Therapy

Primary treatment with radiation therapy does not produce results comparable with those obtained with surgery. Currently, the use of radiotherapy is restricted to patients who are not candidates for surgery. Palliation of dysphagia is short term, generally lasting only 2 to 3 months. Furthermore, the length and course of treatment are difficult to justify in patients with a limited life expectancy. Consequently there is a reluctance to treat patients with advanced disease.

Adjuvant Chemotherapy

The proposal to use adjuvant chemotherapy in the treatment of esophageal cancer began when it became evident that most patients develop postoperative systemic metastasis without local recurrence. This observation led to the hypothesis that undetected systemic micrometastasis had been present at the time of diagnosis, and if effective systemic therapy was added to local regional therapy, survival should improve.

Recently this hypothesis has been supported by the observation of epithelial tumor cells in the bone marrow in 37% of patients with esophageal cancer who were resected for cure. These patients had a greater prevalence of relapse at 9 months after surgery compared to those patients without such cells. Such studies emphasize that hematogenous dissemination of viable malignant cells occurs early in the disease, and that systemic chemotherapy may be helpful if the cells are sensitive to the agent. On the other hand, systemic chemotherapy may be a hindrance, because of its immunosuppressive properties, if the cells are resistant. Unfortunately, current technology is not able to test tumor cell sensitivity to chemotherapeutic drugs. This requires that the choice of drugs be made solely on the basis of their clinical effectiveness against grossly similar tumors.

The decision to use preoperative rather than postoperative chemotherapy was based on the ineffectiveness of chemotherapeutic agents when used after surgery, and animal studies suggesting that agents given before surgery were more effective. The claim that patients who receive chemotherapy before resection are less likely to develop resistance to the drugs is unsupported by hard evidence. The claim that drug delivery is enhanced because blood flow is more robust before patients undergo surgical dissection is similarly flawed, due to the fact that if enough blood reaches the operative site

Table 24-17
Recommended Surgical Therapy for Esophageal Carcinoma

Lesion	Resection
1. Confined areas of high-grade dysplasia (intraepidermal cancer)	Endoscopic mucosal resection (at present only applicable to squamous carcinoma).
2. Widespread or circumferential area of high-grade dysplasia (intraepidermal cancer)	Transhiatal or vagal sparing esophagectomy.
3. Tumor invading through the basement membrane but not through the muscularis mucosae (intramucosal tumors)	Transhiatal or vagal sparing esophagectomy.
4. Tumor deeper than the muscularis mucosae but not through the esophageal wall (intramural tumors)	En bloc esophagectomy with appropriate systematic lymphadenectomy of the cervical, upper mediastinal (above the tracheal bifurcation), lower mediastinal (below the tracheal bifurcation) and abdominal nodes. (For upper and middle third cancers, mediastinal dissection must include the node along the left recurrent laryngeal nerve. For lower third esophageal and cardia cancers, omit cervical and upper mediastinal node dissection, but include the proximal stomach in the resection. For upper third esophageal cancers, omit abdominal lymph node dissection.) Reconstruction with gastric pull-up for middle and upper third tumors, and with colon interposition for lower third and cardia tumors that involve a segmental portion of the stomach.
5. Tumor extending through the muscularis propria (transmural tumors)	Same as for intramural tumors.

to heal the wound or anastomosis, then the flow should be sufficient to deliver chemotherapeutic drugs. There are, however, data supporting the claim that preoperative chemotherapy in patients with esophageal carcinoma can, if effective, facilitate surgical resection by reducing the size of the tumor. This is particularly beneficial in the case of squamous cell tumors above the level of the carina. Reducing the size of the tumor may provide a safer margin between the tumor and the trachea, and allow an anastomosis to a tumor-free cervical esophagus just below the cricopharyngeus. Involved margin at this level usually requires a laryngectomy to prevent subsequent local recurrence.

Preoperative Chemotherapy. Three randomized prospective studies with squamous cell carcinoma have shown no survival benefit with preoperative chemotherapy over surgery alone (Table 24-18). This includes a recent U.S. trial reported by Kelson. The possibility that preoperative neoadjuvant 5-fluorouracil (5-FU)/ platinum-based chemotherapy may indeed provide a small benefit was recently raised by a medical research council trial in the United Kingdom. This trial is one of the few to include enough patients (800) to detect small differences. Two thirds had adenocarcinoma and distal third tumors. The trial had a 10% absolute survival benefit at 2 years for the neoadjuvant chemotherapy group.

With the exception of the potential to improve resectability of tumors located above the carina, the benefits cited by those in favor of preoperative chemotherapy are questionable. Preoperative chemotherapy alone potentially can downstage the tumor, particularly squamous cell carcinoma. It can also potentially eliminate or delay the appearance of metastasis. There is little evidence, however, that it can prolong survival of patients with resectable carcinoma of the esophagus. Most failures are due to distant metastatic disease, underscoring the need for improved systemic therapy. Postoperative septic and respiratory complications may be more common in patients receiving chemotherapy.

Preoperative Combination Chemo- and Radiotherapy. Preoperative chemoradiotherapy using cisplatin and 5-FU in combination with radiotherapy has been reported by several investigators to be beneficial in both adenomatous and squamous cell carcinoma of the esophagus. There have been six randomized prospective studies: four with squamous cell carcinoma, one with both squamous and adenocarcinoma, and one with only adenocarcinoma (Table 24-19). Only one showed any survival benefit with preoperative chemoradiotherapy over surgery alone. Most authors report substantial morbidity and mortality to the treatment. However, many have been encouraged by the observation that some patients who had a complete response had remained free of recurrence at 3 years.

Caution must be exercised in trying to isolate the effects of chemotherapy, because the addition of preoperative radiation therapy to chemotherapy elevates the complete response rate and inflates the benefit of chemotherapy. With chemoradiation the complete response rates for adenocarcinoma range from 17 to 24%

Table 24-18
Esophageal Carcinoma: Randomized Preoperative Chemotherapy Versus Surgery Alone

Author	Year	No. Preop Chemotherapy/No. Surgery Alone	Cell Type	Regimen	Complete Response to Chemotherapy	Survival Chemotherapy vs. Surgery Alone
Roth	1988	19/20	Squamous	P, V, B	6%	NS
Nygaard	1992	50/41	Squamous	P, B	. . .	NS
Schlag	1992	21/24	Squamous	P, 5-FU	5%	NS
Low	1997	74/73	Squamous	P, 5-FU	. . .	NS
Kelson	1998	233/234	Squamous and adenomatous	P, 5-FU	2.5%	NS

B = bleomycin; 5-FU = 5-fluorouracil; NS = not significant; P=cisplatin; V = vindesine.

Table 24-19
Esophageal Carcinoma: Randomized Preoperative Chemo- or Radiotherapy Versus Surgery Alone

Author	Year	No. Preop Chemo-Radiotherapy/ No. Surgery Alone	Cell Type	Regimen	Survival Chemo-Radiotherapy vs. Surgery Alone
Nygaard	1992	47/41	Squamous	P, B, 35 Gy	NS
LePrise	1994	41/45	Squamous	P, 5-FU, 20 Gy	NS
Apinop	1994	35/34	Squamous	P, 5-FU, 40 Gy	NS
Urba	1995	50/50	Squamous and adenomatous	P, 5-FU, V, 45 Gy	NS
Walsh	1996	48/54	Adenomatous	P, 5-FU, 40 Gy	$p=0.01$
Bosset	1997	143/139	Squamous	P, 18.5 Gy	NS

B = bleomycin; 5-FU = 5-fluorouracil; NS = not significant; P = cisplatin; V = vindesine.

(Table 24-20). When radiation is removed, the complete response falls to 0 to 5%, which suggests that the effects of chemotherapy are negligible. If radiotherapy is the factor responsible for the improved response rate, surgery alone could do the job as well, since numerous studies in the past have shown that the combination of surgery and radiation does not provide any survival advantages.

The better question is whether a patient with carcinoma of the esophagus should go through three cycles of chemotherapy on the 5% chance that they may get a complete response in the primary tumor, and in the face of the paucity of evidence that such a response controls systemic disease. Studies have shown that the rates of infection, anastomotic breakdown, incidence of acute respiratory distress syndrome, and long-term use of a respirator were greater in patients receiving adjuvant therapy as compared with surgery alone.

Current data support giving chemoradiotherapy as a matter of routine in a limited number of clinical settings, including: (1) preoperatively to reduce tumor size in a young person with surgically incurable squamous cell carcinoma above the carina, and (2) chemotherapy as salvage therapy for patients who have not had previous chemotherapy and develop recurrent systemic disease after surgical resection (Fig. 24-86). Adjuvant therapy in patients not in those categories should be limited to the setting of a controlled clinical trial. At present, the strongest predictors of outcome of patients with esophageal cancer are the anatomic extent of the tumor at diagnosis and the completeness of tumor removal by surgical resection. After incomplete resection of an esophageal cancer, the 5-year survival rates are 0 to 5%. In contrast, after complete resection, independent of stage of disease, 5-year survival ranges from 15 to 40%, according to selection criteria and stage distribution. The importance of early recognition and adequate surgical resection cannot be overemphasized. Figure 24-86 is a global algorithm for the management of esophageal carcinoma.

SARCOMA OF THE ESOPHAGUS

Sarcomas and carcinosarcomas are rare neoplasms, accounting for approximately 0.1 to 1.5% of all esophageal tumors. They present with the symptom of dysphagia, which does not differ from the dysphagia associated with the more common epithelial carcinoma. Tumors located within the cervical or high thoracic esophagus can cause symptoms of pulmonary aspiration secondary to esophageal obstruction. Large tumors originating at the level of the tracheal bifurcation can produce symptoms of airway obstruction and syncope by direct compression of the tracheobronchial tree and heart (Fig. 24-87). The duration of dysphagia and age of the patients affected with these tumors are similar to those with carcinoma of the esophagus.

A barium swallow usually shows a large polypoid intraluminal esophageal mass, causing partial obstruction and dilatation of the esophagus proximal to the tumor (Fig. 24-88). The smooth polypoid nature of the lesion, although not diagnostic, is distinctive enough to suggest the presence of a sarcoma rather than the more common ulcerating, stenosing carcinoma.

Esophagoscopy commonly shows an intraluminal necrotic mass. When biopsy is attempted, it is important to remove the necrotic tissue until bleeding is seen on the tumor's surface. When this is not done, the biopsy specimen will show only tissue necrosis. Even when viable tumor is obtained on biopsy, it has been these authors' experience that it cannot be definitively identified as carcinoma, sarcoma, or carcinosarcoma on the basis of the histology of the portion biopsied. Biopsy results cannot be totally relied on to identify the presence of sarcoma, and it is often the polypoid nature of the lesion which arouses suspicion that it may be something other than carcinoma.

Polypoid sarcomas of the esophagus, in contrast to infiltrating carcinomas, remain superficial to the muscularis propria and are

Table 24-20
Results of Neoadjuvant Therapy in Adenocarcinoma of the Esophagus

Institution	Year	No. of Patients	Regimen	Complete Pathologic Response	Survival
M. D. Anderson	1990	35	P, E, 5-FU	3%	42% at 3 y
SLMC	1992	18	P, 5-FU, RT	17%	40% at 3 y
Vanderbilt	1993	39	P, E, 5-FU, RT	19%	47% at 4 y
Michigan	1993	21	P, VBL, 5-FU, RT	24%	34% at 5 y
MGH	1994	16	P, 5-FU	0%	42% at 4 y
MGH	1994	22	E, A, P	5%	58% at 2 y

A = doxorubicin; E = etoposide; 5-FU = 5-fluorouracil; MGH = Massachusetts General Hospital; P = cisplatin; RT = radiation therapy; SLMC = St. Louis University Medical Center; VBL = vinblastine.

SOURCE: Reproduced with permission from Wright CD, Mathisen DJ, Wain JC, et al: Evolution of treatment strategies for adenocarcinoma of the esophagus and gastroesophageal junction. *Ann Thorac Surg* 58:1574, 1994.

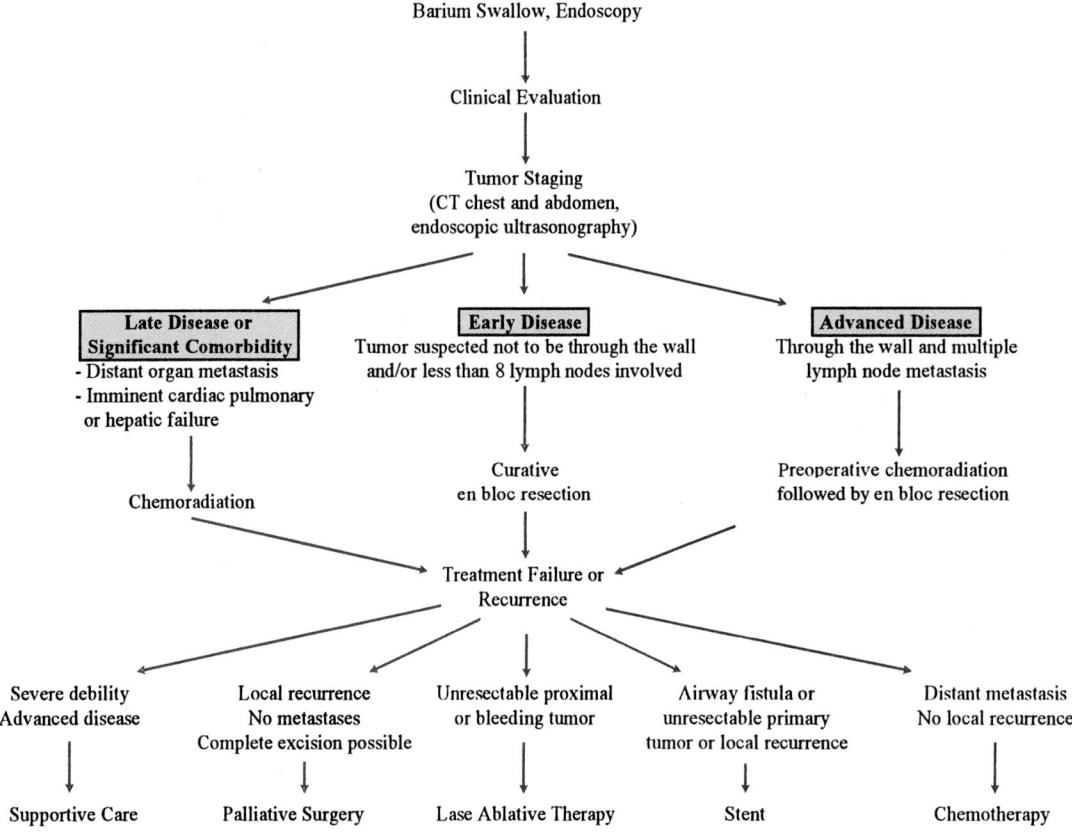

FIG. 24-86. *Suggested global algorithm for the management of carcinoma of the esophagus.*

less likely to metastasize to regional lymph nodes. In one series of 14 patients, local extension or tumor metastasis would have prevented a potentially curative resection in only five. Thus the presence of a large polypoid tumor should not deter the surgeon from resecting the lesion.

Sarcomatous lesions of the esophagus can be divided into epidermoid carcinomas with spindle cell features, such as carcinosarcoma, and true sarcomas that arise from mesenchymal tissue, such as leiomyosarcoma, fibrosarcoma, and rhabdomyosarcoma. Based on current histologic criteria for diagnosis, fibrosarcoma and rhabdomyosarcoma of the esophagus are extremely rare lesions and may not in fact exist.

Surgical resection of polypoid sarcoma of the esophagus is the treatment of choice, since radiation therapy has little success and the tumors remain superficial, with local invasion or distant metastases occurring late in the course of the disease. As with carcinoma, the absence of both wall penetration and lymph node metastases is necessary for curative treatment, and surgical resection is consequently responsible for the majority of the reported 5-year survivals. Resection also provides an excellent means of palliating the patient's symptoms. The surgical technique for resection and the subsequent restoration of the gastrointestinal continuity is similar to that described for carcinoma.

In these authors experience, four of the eight patients with carcinosarcoma survived for 5 years or longer. Even though this number is small, it suggests that resection produces better results in epithelial carcinoma with spindle cell features than in squamous cell carcinoma of the esophagus. Similarly, with leiomyosarcoma of the esophagus, the same scattered reports exist with little information on survival. Of seven patients with leimyosarcoma, two died from their

disease—one in 3 months and the other 4 years and 7 months after resection. The other five patients were reported to have survived more than 5 years.

It is difficult to evaluate the benefits of resection for leiomyoblastoma of the esophagus, due to the small number of reported patients with tumors in this location. Most leiomyoblastomas occur in the stomach, and 38% of these patients succumb to the cancer in 3 years. Fifty-five percent of patients with extragastric leiomyoblastoma also die from the disease, within an average of 3 years. Consequently, leiomyoblastoma should be considered a malignant lesion and apt to behave like a leiomyosarcoma. The presence of nuclear hyperchromatism, increased mitotic figures (more than one per high-power field), tumor size larger than 10 cm, and clinical symptoms of longer than 6 months' duration are associated with a poor prognosis.

BENIGN TUMORS AND CYSTS

Benign tumors and cysts of the esophagus are relatively uncommon. From the perspectives of both the clinician and the pathologist, benign tumors may be divided into those that are within the muscular wall and those that are within the lumen of the esophagus.

Intramural lesions are either solid tumors or cysts, and the vast majority are leiomyomas. They are made up of varying portions of smooth muscle and fibrous tissue. Fibromas, myomas, fibromyomas, and lipomyomas are closely related and occur rarely. Other histologic types of solid intramural tumors have been described, such as lipomas, neurofibromas, hemangiomas, osteochondromas, granular cell myoblastomas, and glomus tumors, but they are medical curiosities.

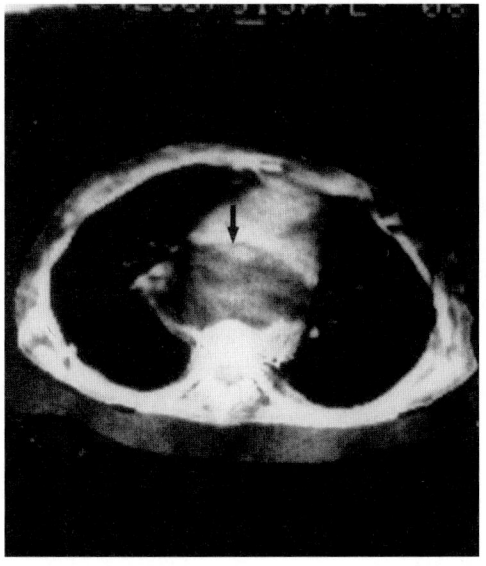

A

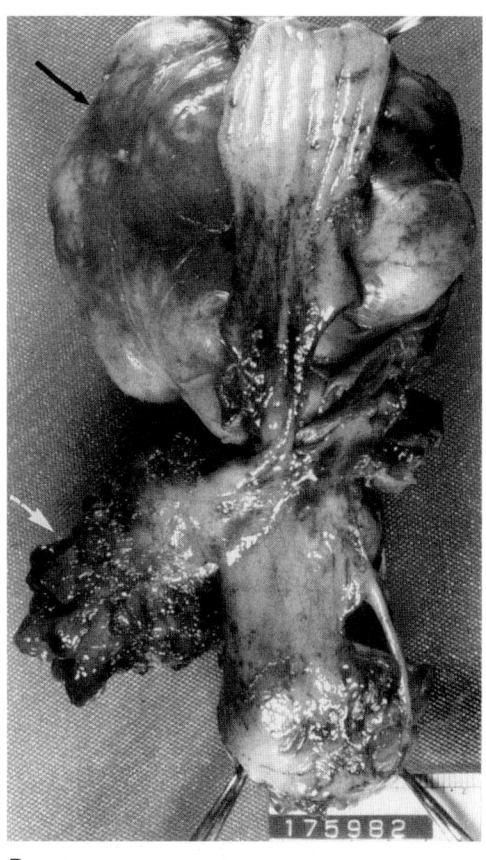

B

FIG. 24-87. *A.* CT scan of a leiomyosarcoma (*black arrow*) that caused compression of the heart and symptoms of syncope. *B.* Surgical specimen of the lesion in *A.*, with a pedunculated luminal lesion (*white arrow*) and a large extraesophageal component (*black arrow*). There was no evidence of lymph node metastasis at the time of surgery.

FIG. 24-88. *A.* Barium swallow showing a large polypoid intraluminal esophageal mass causing partial obstruction and dilation of the proximal esophagus. *B.* Operative specimen showing 9 cm polypoid leiomyoblastoma.

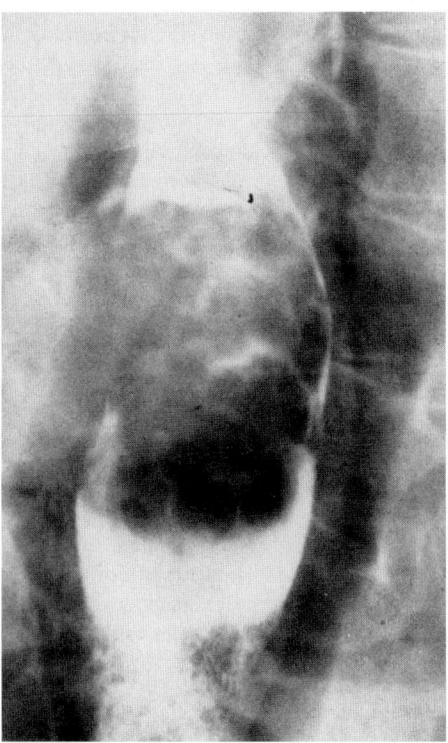

A

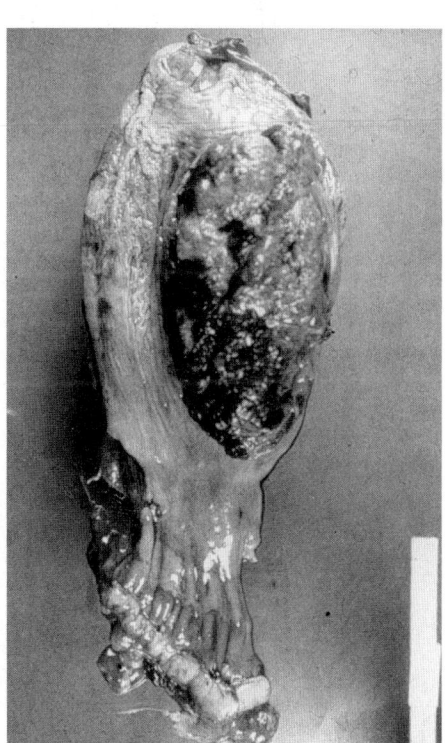

B

Intraluminal lesions are polypoid or pedunculated growths that usually originate in the submucosa, develop mainly into the lumen, and are covered with normal stratified squamous epithelium. The majority of these tumors are composed of fibrous tissue of varying degrees of compactness with a rich vascular supply. Some are loose and myxoid (e.g., myxoma and myxofibroma), some are more collagenous (e.g., fibroma), and some contain adipose tissue (e.g., fibrolipoma). These different types of tumor are frequently collectively designated as fibrovascular polyps, or simply as polyps. Pedunculated intraluminal tumors should be removed. If the lesion is not too large, endoscopic removal with a snare is feasible.

Leiomyoma

Leiomyomas constitute more than 50% of benign esophageal tumors. The average age at presentation is 38, which is in sharp contrast to that seen with esophageal carcinoma. Leiomyomas are twice as common in males. Because they originate in smooth muscle, 90% are located in the lower two thirds of the esophagus. They are usually solitary, but multiple tumors have been found on occasion. They vary greatly in size and shape. Tumors as small as 1 cm in diameter and as large as 10 lb have been removed.

Typically, leiomyomas are oval. During their growth, they remain intramural, having the bulk of their mass protruding toward the outer wall of the esophagus. The overlying mucosa is freely movable and normal in appearance. Neither their size nor location correlates with the degree of symptoms. Dysphagia and pain are the most common complaints, the two symptoms occurring more frequently together than separately. Bleeding directly related to the tumor is rare, and when hematemesis or melena occurs in a patient with an esophageal leiomyoma, other causes should be investigated.

A barium swallow is the most useful method to demonstrate a leiomyoma of the esophagus (Fig. 24-89). In profile the tumor appears as a smooth, semilunar, or crescent-shaped filling defect that moves with swallowing, is sharply demarcated, and is covered and surrounded by normal mucosa. Esophagoscopy should be performed to exclude the reported observation of a coexistence with carcinoma. The freely movable mass, which bulges into the lumen, should not

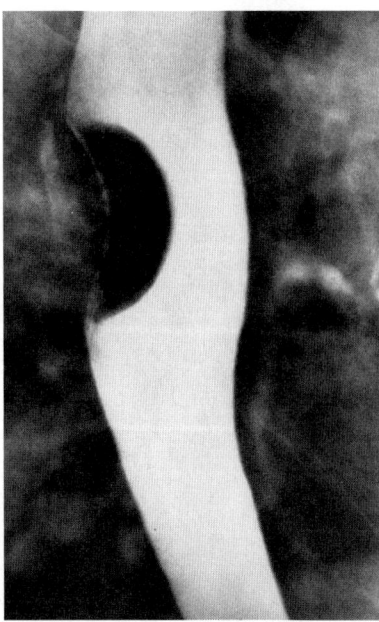

FIG. 24-89. *A. Barium esophagogram showing a classical smooch punched out defect of a leiomyoma.*

be biopsied because of an increased chance of mucosal perforation at the time of surgical enucleation.

Despite their slow growth and limited potential for malignant degeneration, leiomyomas should be removed unless there are specific contraindications. The majority can be removed by simple enucleation. If during removal the mucosa is inadvertently entered, the defect can be repaired primarily. After tumor removal, the outer esophageal wall should be reconstructed by closure of the muscle layer. The location of the lesion and the extent of surgery required will dictate the approach. Lesions of the proximal and middle esophagus require a right thoracotomy, whereas distal esophageal lesions require a left thoracotomy. Videothoracoscopic approaches have been reported. The mortality rate associated with enucleation is less than 2%, and success in relieving the dysphagia is near 100%. Large lesions or those involving the gastroesophageal junction may require esophageal resection.

Esophageal Cyst

Cysts may be congenital or acquired. Congenital cysts are lined wholly or partly by columnar ciliated epithelium of the respiratory type, by glandular epithelium of the gastric type, by squamous epithelium, or by transitional epithelium. In some, epithelial lining cells may be absent. Confusion over the embryologic origin of congenital cysts has led to a variety of names, such as enteric, bronchogenic, and mediastinal cysts. Acquired retention cysts also occur, probably as a result of obstruction of the excretory ducts of the esophageal glands.

Enteric and bronchogenic cysts are the most common, and arise as a result of developmental abnormalities during the formation and differentiation of the lower respiratory tract, esophagus, and stomach from the foregut. During its embryologic development, the esophagus is lined successively with simple columnar, pseudostratified ciliated columnar, and finally stratified squamous epithelium. This sequence probably accounts for the fact that the lining epithelium may be any or a combination of these; the presence of cilia does not necessarily indicate a respiratory origin.

Cysts vary in size from small to very large, and are usually located intramurally in the middle to lower third of the esophagus. Their symptoms are similar to those of a leiomyoma. The diagnosis similarly depends on radiographic and endoscopic findings. Surgical excision by enucleation is the preferred treatment. During removal, a fistulous tract connecting the cysts to the airways should be sought, particularly in patients who have had repetitive bronchopulmonary infections.

ESOPHAGEAL PERFORATION

Perforation of the esophagus constitutes a true emergency. It most commonly occurs following diagnostic or therapeutic procedures. Spontaneous perforation, referred to as Boerhaave's syndrome, accounts for only 15% of cases of esophageal perforation, foreign bodies for 14%, and trauma for 10%. Pain is a striking and consistent symptom and strongly suggests that an esophageal rupture has occurred, particularly if located in the cervical area following instrumentation of the esophagus, or substernally in a patient with a history of resisting vomiting. If subcutaneous emphysema is present, the diagnosis is almost certain.

Spontaneous rupture of the esophagus is associated with a high mortality rate because of the delay in recognition and treatment. Although there usually is a history of resisting vomiting, in a small number of patients the injury occurs silently, without any antecedent history. When the chest radiogram of a patient with an esophageal perforation shows air or an effusion in the pleural space, the condition is often misdiagnosed as a pneumothorax or pancreatitis. An elevated serum amylase caused by the extrusion of saliva through the perforation may fix the diagnosis of pancreatitis in the mind of an unwary physician. If the chest radiogram is normal, a mistaken diagnosis of myocardial infarction or dissecting aneurysm is often made.

Spontaneous rupture usually occurs into the left pleural cavity or just above the gastroesophageal junction. Fifty percent of patients have concomitant gastroesophageal reflux disease, suggesting that minimal resistance to the transmission of abdominal pressure into the thoracic esophagus is a factor in the pathophysiology of the lesion. During vomiting, high peaks of intragastric pressure can be recorded, frequently exceeding 200 mm Hg, but since extragastric pressure remains almost equal to intragastric pressure, stretching of the gastric wall is minimal. The amount of pressure transmitted to the esophagus varies considerably, depending on the position of the gastroesophageal junction. When it is in the abdomen and exposed to intra-abdominal pressure, the pressure transmitted to the esophagus is much less than when it is exposed to the negative thoracic pressure. In the latter situation, the pressure in the lower esophagus will frequently equal intragastric pressure if the glottis remains closed. Cadaver studies have shown that when this pressure exceeds 150 mm Hg, rupture of the esophagus is apt to occur. When a hiatal hernia is present and the sphincter remains exposed to abdominal pressure, the lesion produced is usually a Mallory-Weiss mucosal tear, and bleeding rather than perforation is the problem. This is due to the stretching of the supradiaphragmatic portion of the gastric wall. In this situation, the hernia sac represents an extension of the abdominal cavity, and the gastroesophageal junction remains exposed to abdominal pressure.

Diagnosis

Abnormalities on the chest radiogram can be variable and should not be depended upon to make the diagnosis. This is because the abnormalities are dependent on three factors: (1) the time interval between the perforation and the radiographic examination, (2) the site of perforation, and (3) the integrity of the mediastinal pleura. Mediastinal emphysema, a strong indicator of perforation, takes at least 1 hour to be demonstrated, and is present in only 40% of patients. Mediastinal widening secondary to edema may not occur for several hours. The site of perforation also can influence the radiographic findings. In cervical perforation, cervical emphysema is common and mediastinal emphysema rare; the converse is true for thoracic perforations. Frequently, air will be visible in the erector spinae muscles on a neck radiogram before it can be palpated or seen on a chest radiogram (Fig. 24-90). The integrity of the mediastinal pleura influences the radiographic abnormality in that rupture of the pleura results in a pneumothorax, a finding that is seen in 77% of patients. In two thirds of patients the perforation is on the left side, in one fifth it is on the right side, and in one tenth it is bilateral. If pleural integrity is maintained, mediastinal emphysema (rather than a pneumothorax) appears rapidly. A pleural effusion secondary to inflammation of the mediastinum occurs late. In 9% of patients the chest radiogram is normal.

The diagnosis is confirmed with a contrast esophagogram, which will demonstrate extravasation in 90% of patients. The use of a water-soluble medium such as Gastrografin is preferred. Of concern is that there is a 10% false-negative rate. This may be due to obtaining the radiographic study with the patient in the upright position. When the patient is upright, the passage of water-soluble contrast material

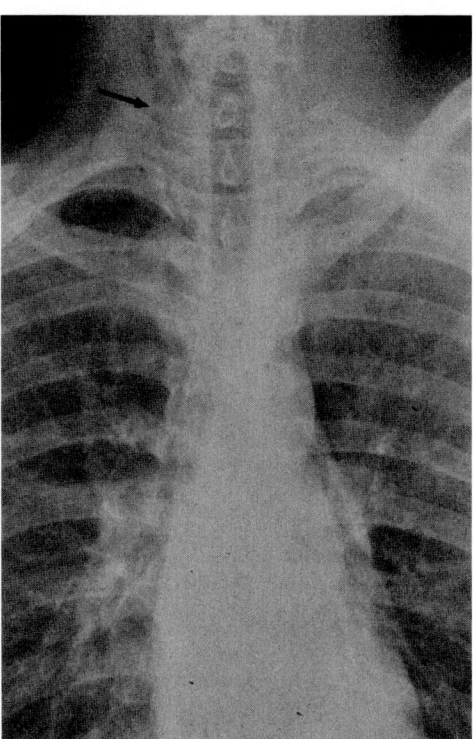

FIG. 24-90. Chest radiogram showing air in the deep muscles of the neck following perforation of the esophagus (arrow). This is often the earliest sign of perforation and can be present without evidence of air in the mediastinum.

can be too rapid to demonstrate a small perforation. The studies should be done with the patient in the right lateral decubitus position (Fig. 24-91). In this position the contrast material fills the entire length of the esophagus, allowing the actual site of perforation and its interconnecting cavities to be visualized in almost all patients.

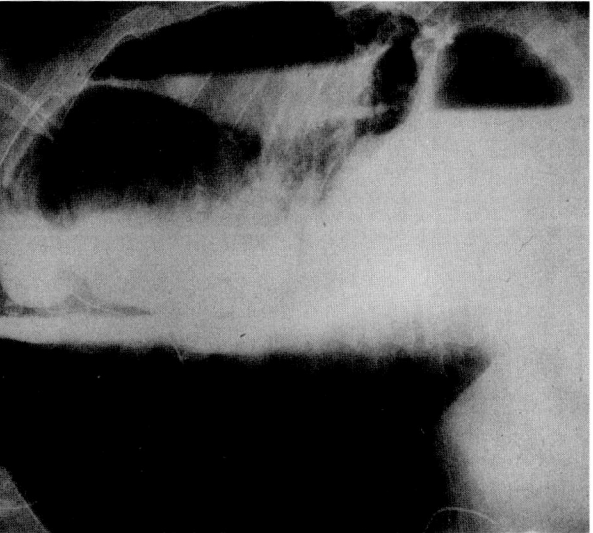

FIG. 24-91. Radiographic study of a patient with a perforation of the esophagus, using water-soluble contrast material. The patient is placed in the lateral decubitus position with the left side up to allow complete filling of the esophagus and demonstration of the defect.

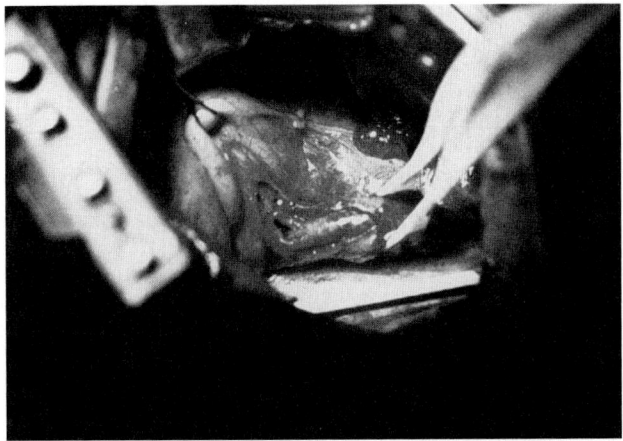

FIG. 24-92. Left thoracotomy in a patient with an esophageal rupture at the gastroesophageal junction following forceful dilation of the lower esophagus for achalasia (the surgical clamp is on the stomach, and the Penrose drain encircles the esophagus). The injury consists of a mucosal perforation and extensive splitting of the esophageal muscle from just below the Penrose drain to the stomach.

Management

The key to optimum management is early diagnosis. The most favorable outcome is obtained following primary closure of the perforation within 24 hours, resulting in 80 to 90% survival. Figure 24-92 is an operative photograph taken through a left thoracotomy of an esophageal rupture following a pneumatic dilation for achalasia. The most common location for the injury is the left lateral wall of the esophagus, just above the gastroesophageal junction. To get adequate exposure of the injury, a dissection similar to that described for esophageal myotomy is performed. A flap of stomach is pulled up and the soiled fat pad at the gastroesophageal junction is removed. The edges of the injury are trimmed and closed using a modified Gambee stitch (Fig. 24-93). The closure is reinforced by the use of a pleural patch or construction of a Nissen fundoplication.

Mortality associated with immediate closure varies between 8 and 20%. After 24 hours survival, decreases to less than 50%, and is not influenced by the type of operative therapy (i.e., drainage alone or drainage plus closure of the perforation). If the time delay prior to closing a perforation approaches 24 hours and the tissues are inflamed, division of the cardia and resection of the diseased portion of the esophagus are recommended. The remainder of the esophagus is mobilized, and as much normal esophagus as possible is saved and brought out as an end cervical esophagostomy. In some situations the retained esophagus may be so long that it loops down into the chest. The contaminated mediastinum is drained and a feeding jejunostomy tube is inserted. The recovery from sepsis is often immediate, dramatic, and reflected by a marked improvement in the patient's condition over a 24-hour period. On recovery from the sepsis, the patient is discharged and returns on a subsequent date for reconstruction with a substernal colon interposition. Failure to apply this aggressive therapy can result in a mortality rate in excess of 50% in patients in whom the diagnosis has been delayed.

Nonoperative management of esophageal perforation has been advocated in select situations. The choice of conservative therapy requires skillful judgment and necessitates careful radiographic examination of the esophagus. This course of management usually follows an injury occurring during dilation of esophageal strictures or pneumatic dilations of achalasia. Conservative management should not be used in patients who have free perforations into the

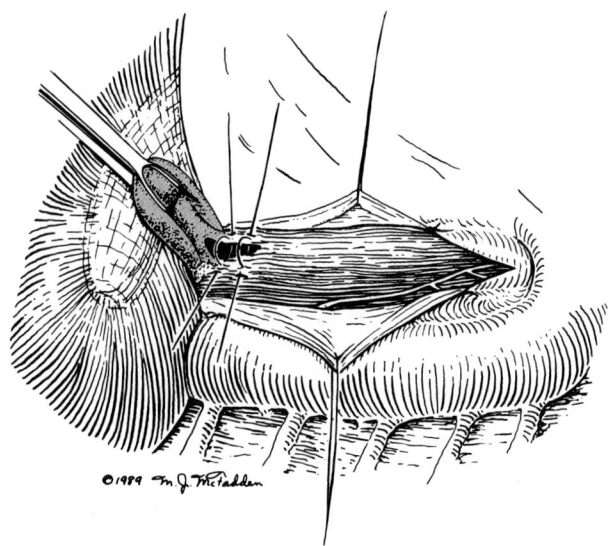

A

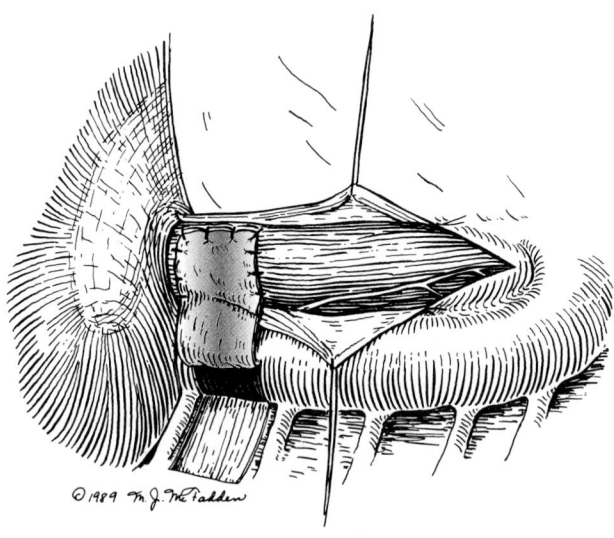

B

FIG. 24-93. The technique of closure of an esophageal perforation through a left thoracotomy. *A.* A tongue of stomach is pulled up through the esophageal hiatus and the gastroesophageal fat pad is removed. The edges of the mucosal injury are trimmed and closed using interrupted modified Gambee stitches. *B.* Reinforcement of the closure with a parietal pleural patch.

pleural space. Cameron proposed three criteria for the nonoperative management of esophageal perforation: (1) the barium swallow must show the perforation to be contained within the mediastinum and drain well back into the esophagus (Fig. 24-94), (2) symptoms should be mild, and (3) there should be minimal evidence of clinical sepsis. If these conditions are met, it is reasonable to treat the patient with hyperalimentation, antibiotics, and cimetidine to decrease acid secretion and diminish pepsin activity. Oral intake is resumed in 7 to 14 days, dependent on subsequent radiographic examinations.

CAUSTIC INJURY

Accidental caustic lesions occur mainly in children, and in general, rather small quantities of caustics are taken. In adults or teenagers, the swallowing of caustic liquids is usually deliberate, during suicide

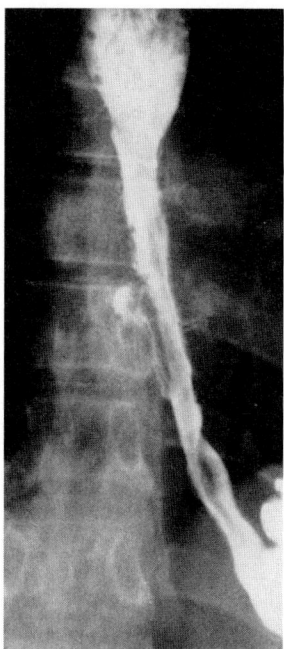

FIG. 24-94. *Barium esophagogram showing a stricture and a contained perforation following dilation. The injury meets Cameron criteria: it is contained within the mediastinum and drawn back into the esophagus; the patient had mild symptoms; and there was no evidence of clinical sepsis. Nonoperative management was successful.*

attempts, and greater quantities are swallowed. Alkalies are more frequently swallowed accidentally than acids, because strong acids cause an immediate burning pain in the mouth.

Pathology

The swallowing of caustic substances causes both an acute and a chronic injury. During the acute phase, care focuses on controlling the immediate tissue injury and the potential for perforation. During the chronic phase, the focus is on treatment of strictures and disturbances in pharyngeal swallowing. In the acute phase the degree and extent of the lesion are dependent on several factors: the nature of the caustic substance, its concentration, the quantity swallowed, and the time the substance is in contact with the tissues. Acids and alkalies affect tissue in different ways. Alkalies dissolve tissue, and therefore penetrate more deeply, while acids cause a coagulative necrosis that limits their penetration. Animal experiments have shown that there is a correlation between the depth of the lesion and the concentration of sodium hydroxide (NaOH) solution. When a solution of 3.8% comes into contact with the esophagus for 10 seconds, it causes necrosis of the mucosa and the submucosa, but spares the muscular layer. A concentration of 22.5% penetrates the whole esophageal wall and into the periesophageal tissues. Cleansing products can contain up to 90% NaOH. The strength of esophageal contractions varies according to the level of the esophagus, being weakest at the striated muscle–smooth muscle interface. Consequently, clearance from this area may be somewhat slower, allowing caustic substances to remain in contact with the mucosa longer. This explains why the esophagus is preferentially and more severely affected at this level than in the lower portions.

The lesions caused by lye injury occur in three phases. First is the acute necrotic phase, lasting 1 to 4 days after injury. During this period, coagulation of intracellular proteins results in cell necrosis, and the living tissue surrounding the area of necrosis develops an intense inflammatory reaction. Second is the ulceration and granulation phase, starting 3 to 5 days after injury. During this period the superficial necrotic tissue sloughs, leaving an ulcerated, acutely inflamed base, and granulation tissue fills the defect left by the sloughed mucosa. This phase lasts 10 to 12 days, and it is during this period that the esophagus is the weakest. Third is the phase of cicatrization and scarring, which begins the third week following injury. During this period the previously formed connective tissue begins to contract, resulting in narrowing of the esophagus. Adhesions between granulating areas occurs, resulting in pockets and bands. It is during this period that efforts must be made to reduce stricture formation.

Clinical Manifestations

The clinical picture of an esophageal burn is determined by the degree and extent of the lesion. In the initial phase, complaints consist of pain in the mouth and substernal region, hypersalivation, pain on swallowing, and dysphagia. The presence of fever is strongly correlated with the presence of an esophageal lesion. Bleeding can occur, and frequently the patient vomits. These initial complaints disappear during the quiescent period of ulceration and granulation. During the cicatrization and scarring phase, the complaint of dysphagia reappears and is due to fibrosis and retraction, resulting in narrowing of the esophagus. Of the patients who develop strictures, 60% do so within 1 month, and 80% within 2 months. If dysphagia does not develop within 8 months, it is unlikely that a stricture will occur. Serious systemic reactions such as hypovolemia and acidosis resulting in renal damage can occur in cases in which the burns have been caused by strong acids. Respiratory complications such as laryngospasm, laryngedema, and occasionally pulmonary edema can occur, especially when strong acids are aspirated.

Inspection of the oral cavity and pharynx can indicate that caustic substances were swallowed, but does not reveal that the esophagus has been burned. Conversely, esophageal burns can be present without apparent oral injuries. Because of this poor correlation, early esophagoscopy is advocated to establish the presence of an esophageal injury. To lessen the chance of perforation, the scope should not be introduced beyond the proximal esophageal lesion. The degree of injury can be graded according to the criteria listed in Table 24-21. Even if the esophagoscopy is normal, strictures may appear later. Radiographic examination is not a reliable means to identify the presence of early esophageal injury, but is important in later follow-up to identify strictures. The most common locations of caustic injuries are shown in Table 24-22.

Treatment

Treatment of a caustic lesion of the esophagus is directed toward management of both the immediate and late consequences of the injury. The immediate treatment consists of limiting the burn by administering neutralizing agents. To be effective, this must be done within the first hour. Lye or other alkali can be neutralized with

Table 24-21
Endoscopic Grading of Corrosive Esophageal and Gastric Burns

First degree: Mucosal hyperemia and edema
Second degree: Limited hemorrhage, exudate ulceration, and pseudomembrane formation
Third degree: Sloughing of mucosa, deep ulcers, massive hemorrhage, complete obstruction of lumen by edema, charring, and perforation

Table 24-22
Location of Caustic Injury (n = 62)

Pharynx	10%
Esophagus	70%
Upper	15%
Middle	65%
Lower	2%
Whole	18%
Stomach	20%
Antral	91%
Whole	9%
Both stomach and esophagus	14%

half-strength vinegar, lemon juice, or orange juice. Acid can be neutralized with milk, egg white, or antacids. Sodium bicarbonate is not used because it generates CO_2, which might increase the danger of perforation. Emetics are contraindicated, since vomiting renews the contact of the caustic substance with the esophagus and can contribute to perforation if too forceful. Hypovolemia is corrected and broad-spectrum antibiotics are administered to lessen the inflammatory reaction and prevent infectious complications. If necessary a feeding jejunostomy tube is inserted to provide nutrition. Oral feeding can be started when the dysphagia of the initial phase has regressed.

In the past, surgeons waited until the appearance of a stricture before starting treatment. Currently, dilations are started the first day after the injury, with the aim of preserving the esophageal lumen by removing the adhesions that occurred in the injured segments. However, this approach is controversial in that dilations can traumatize the esophagus, causing bleeding and perforation, and there are data indicating that excessive dilations cause increased fibrosis secondary to the added trauma. The use of steroids to limit fibrosis has been shown to be effective in animals, but their effectiveness in human beings is debatable.

Extensive necrosis of the esophagus frequently leads to perforation, and is best managed by resection. When there is extensive gastric involvement, the esophagus is nearly always necrotic or severely burned, and total gastrectomy and near-total esophagectomy are necessary. The presence of air in the esophageal wall is a sign of muscle necrosis and impending perforation and is a strong indication for esophagectomy.

Management of acute injury is summarized in the algorithm in Fig. 24-95. Some authors have advocated the use of an intraluminal esophageal stent (Fig. 24-96) in patients who are operated on and found to have no evidence of extensive esophagogastric necrosis. In these patients, a biopsy of the posterior gastric wall should be performed in order to exclude occult injury. If histologically there is a question of viability, a second-look operation should be done within 36 hours. If a stent is inserted it should be kept in position for 21 days, and removed after a satisfactory barium esophagogram. Esophagoscopy should be done and if strictures are present, dilations initiated.

Once the acute phase has passed, attention is turned to the prevention and management of strictures. Both antegrade dilation with a Hurst or Maloney bougie and retrograde dilation with a Tucker bougie have been satisfactory. Occasionally, particularly with severe strictures, the patient is instructed to swallow a string, over which metal Sippy dilators are passed until an adequate lumen can be obtained for passage of a mercury bougie. In a series of 1079 patients, early dilations started during the acute phase gave excellent results in 78%, good results in 13%, and poor results in 2%. Fifty-five patients died during the treatment. In contrast, of

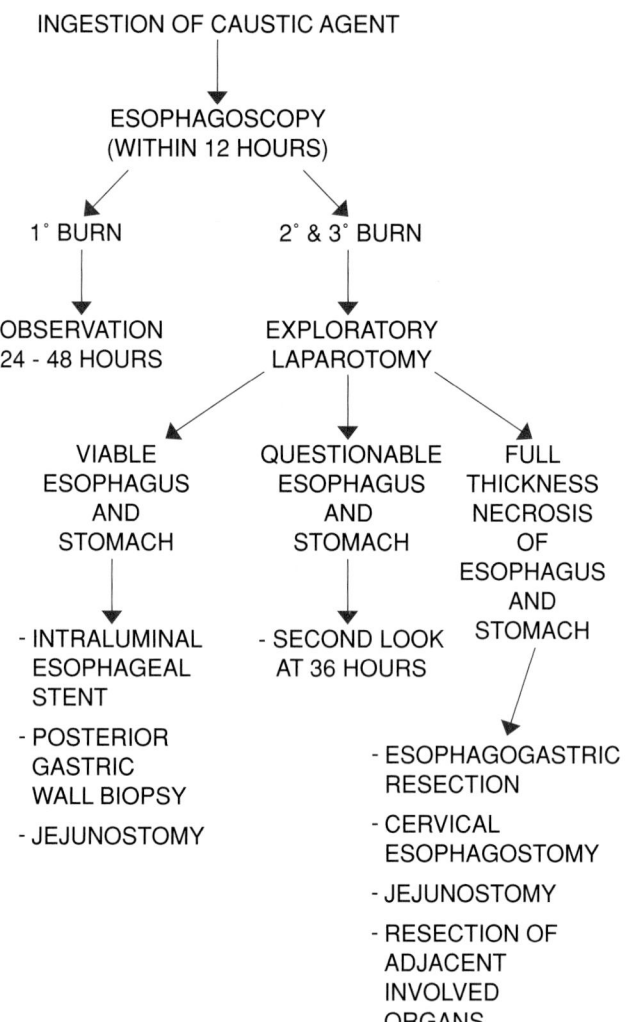

FIG. 24-95. Algorithm summarizing the management of acute caustic injury.

333 patients whose strictures were dilated when they became symptomatic, only 21% had excellent results, 46% good, and 6% poor, with three dying during the process. The length of time the surgeon should persist with dilation before consideration of esophageal resection is problematic. An adequate lumen should be re-established within 6 months to 1 year, with progressively longer intervals between dilations. If during the course of treatment an adequate lumen cannot be established or maintained (i.e., smaller bougies must be used), operative intervention should be considered. Surgical intervention is indicated when there is (1) complete stenosis in which all attempts from above and below have failed to establish a lumen, (2) marked irregularity and pocketing on barium swallow, (3) the development of a severe periesophageal reaction or mediastinitis with dilatation, (4) a fistula, (5) the inability to dilate or maintain the lumen above a 40F bougie, or (6) a patient who is unwilling or unable to undergo prolonged periods of dilation.

The variety of abnormalities seen requires that creativity be used when considering esophageal reconstruction. Skin tube esophagoplasties are now used much less frequently than they were in the past, and are mainly of historical interest. Currently the stomach, jejunum, and colon are the organs used to replace the esophagus, through either the posterior mediastinum or the retrosternal route. A

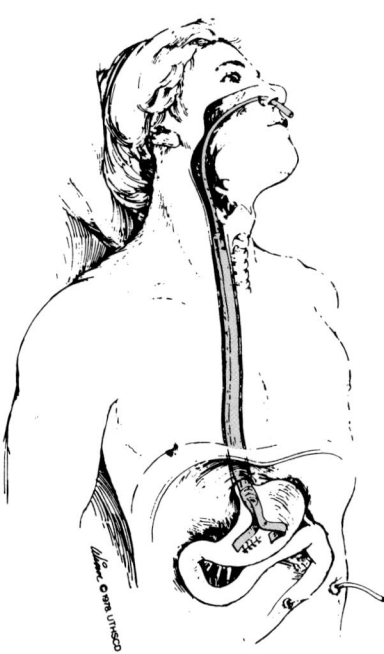

FIG. 24-96. *The use of an esophageal stent to prevent stricture. The stent is constructed from a chest tube and placed in the esophagus at the time of an exploratory laparotomy. A Penrose drain is placed over the distal end as a flap valve to prevent reflux. The stent is supported at its upper end by attaching it to a suction catheter which is secured to the nares. Continuous suction removes saliva and mucus trapped in the pharynx and upper esophagus.*

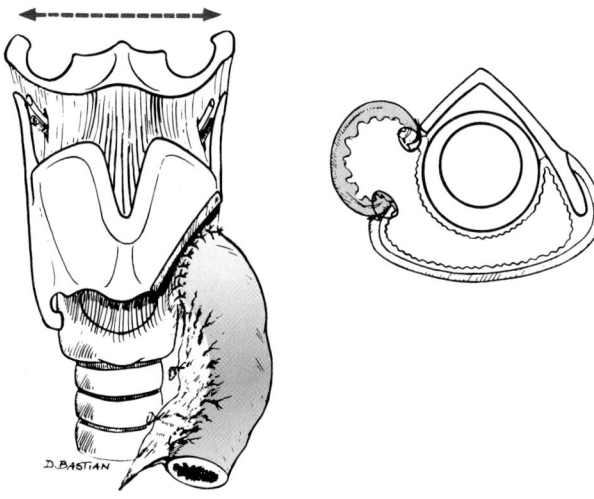

FIG. 24-97. *Anastomosis of the bowel to a preserved pyriform sinus. To identify the site, a finger is inserted into the free pyriform sinus through a suprahyoid incision (dotted line). This requires removing the lateral inferior portion of the thyroid cartilage as shown in cross section. (Reproduced with permission from Tran Ba Huy P, Celerier M: Management of severe caustic stenosis of the hypopharynx and esophagus by ileocolic transposition via suprahyoid or transepiglottic approach. Analysis of 18 cases. Ann Surg 207:439, 1988.)*

retrosternal route is chosen when there has been a previous esophagectomy or there is extensive fibrosis in the posterior mediastinum. When all factors are considered, the order of preference for an esophageal substitute is (1) colon, (2) stomach, and (3) jejunum. Free jejunal grafts based on the superior thyroid artery have provided excellent results. Whatever method is selected, it must be emphasized that these procedures cannot be taken lightly; minor errors of judgment or technique may lead to serious or even fatal complications.

Critical in the planning of the operation is the selection of cervical esophagus, pyriform sinus, or posterior pharynx as the site for proximal anastomosis. The site of the upper anastomosis depends on the extent of the pharyngeal and cervical esophageal damage encountered. When the cervical esophagus is destroyed and a pyriform sinus remains open the anastomosis can be made to the hypopharynx (Fig. 24-97). When the pyriform sinuses are completely stenosed, a transglottic approach is used to perform an anastomosis to the posterior oropharyngeal wall (Fig. 24-98). This allows excision of supraglottic strictures and elevation and anterior tilting of the larynx. In both of these situations, the patient must relearn to swallow. Recovery is long and difficult and may require several endoscopic dilations, and often reoperations. Sleeve resections of short strictures are not successful because the extent of damage to the wall of the esophagus can be greater than realized, and almost invariably the anastomosis is carried out in a diseased area.

The management of a bypassed damaged esophagus after injury is problematic. If the esophagus is left in place, ulceration from gastroesophageal reflux or the development of carcinoma must be considered. The extensive dissection necessary to remove the esophagus, particularly in the presence of marked periesophagitis, is associated with significant morbidity. Leaving the esophagus in place preserves the function of the vagus nerves, and in turn the function

of the stomach. On the other hand, leaving a damaged esophagus in place can result in multiple blind sacs and subsequent development of mediastinal abscesses years later. Most experienced surgeons recommend that the esophagus be removed unless the operative risk is unduly high.

DIAPHRAGMATIC HERNIAS

With the advent of clinical radiology, it became evident that a diaphragmatic hernia was a relatively common abnormality and was

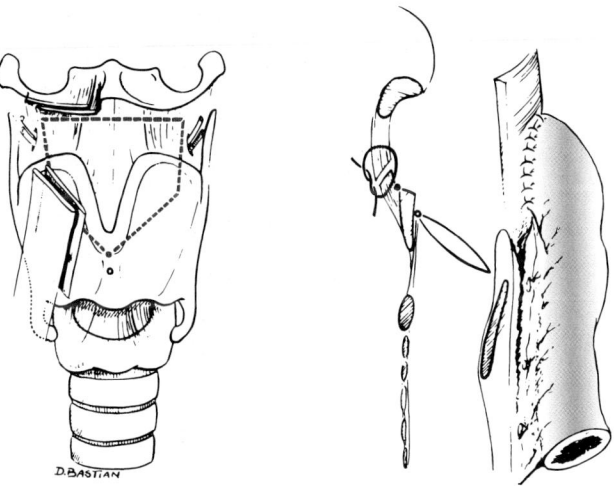

FIG. 24-98. *Anastomosis of the bowel to the posterior oropharynx. The anastomosis is done through an inverted trapezoid incision above the thyroid cartilage (dotted line). A triangle-shaped piece of the upper half of the cartilage is resected. Closure of the oropharynx is done so that the larynx is pulled up (sagittal section). (Reproduced with permission from Tran Ba Huy P, Celerier M: Management of severe caustic stenosis of the hypopharynx and esophagus by ileocolic transposition via suprahyoid or transepiglottic approach. Analysis of 18 cases. Ann Surg 207:439, 1988.)*

not always accompanied by symptoms. Three types of esophageal hiatal hernia were identified: (1) the sliding hernia, type I, characterized by an upward dislocation of the cardia in the posterior mediastinum (Fig. 24-99A); (2) the rolling or paraesophageal hernia, type II, characterized by an upward dislocation of the gastric fundus alongside a normally positioned cardia (Fig. 24-99B); and (3) the combined sliding-rolling or mixed hernia, type III, characterized by an upward dislocation of both the cardia and the gastric fundus (Fig. 24-99C). The end stage of type I and type II hernias occurs when the whole stomach migrates up into the chest by rotating 180 degree around its longitudinal axis, with the cardia and pylorus as fixed points. In this situation the abnormality is usually referred to as an intrathoracic stomach (Fig. 24-99D).

Incidence and Etiology

The true incidence of a hiatal hernia in the overall population is difficult to determine because of the absence of symptoms in a large number of patients who are subsequently shown to have a hernia. When radiographic examinations are done in response to gastrointestinal symptoms, the incidence of a sliding hiatal hernia is seven times higher than that of a paraesophageal hernia. The age distribution of patients with paraesophageal hernias is significantly different from that observed in sliding hiatal hernias. The median age of the former is 61; of the latter, 48. Paraesophageal hernias are more likely to occur in women by a ratio of 4:1.

Structural deterioration of the phrenoesophageal membrane over time may explain the higher incidence of hiatal hernias in the older age group. These changes involve thinning of the upper fascial layer of the phrenoesophageal membrane (i.e., the supradiaphragmatic continuation of the endothoracic fascia) and loss of elasticity in the lower fascial layer (i.e., the infradiaphragmatic continuation of the transversalis fascia). Consequently, the phrenoesophageal membrane yields to stretching in the cranial direction due to the persistent intra-abdominal pressure and the tug of esophageal shortening on swallowing. The upper fascial layer is formed only by loose connective tissue and is of little importance. The lower fascial layer is thick, stronger, and more important. It divides into an upper and lower leaf about 1 cm before attaching intimately with the esophageal adventitia. Due to stretching in the cranial direction, the attachment of the lower leaf protrudes upward and can frequently be identified in the thoracic cavity (Fig. 24-100).

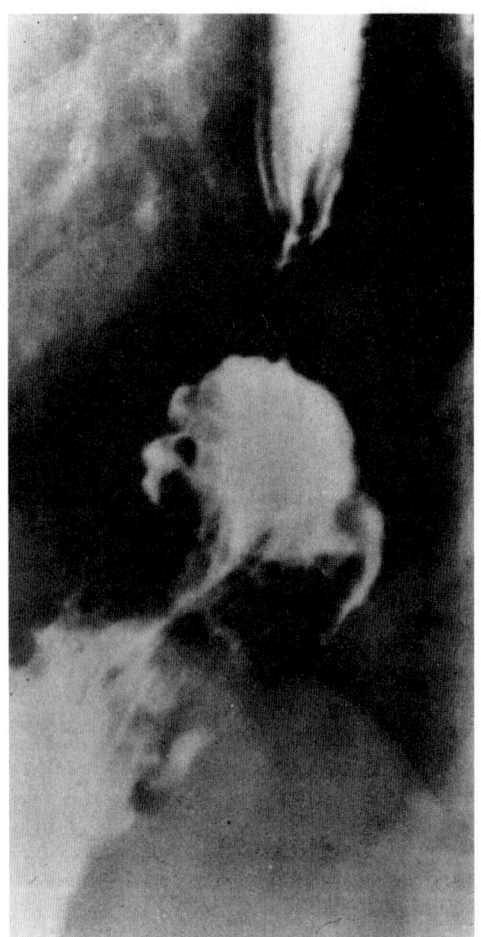

A

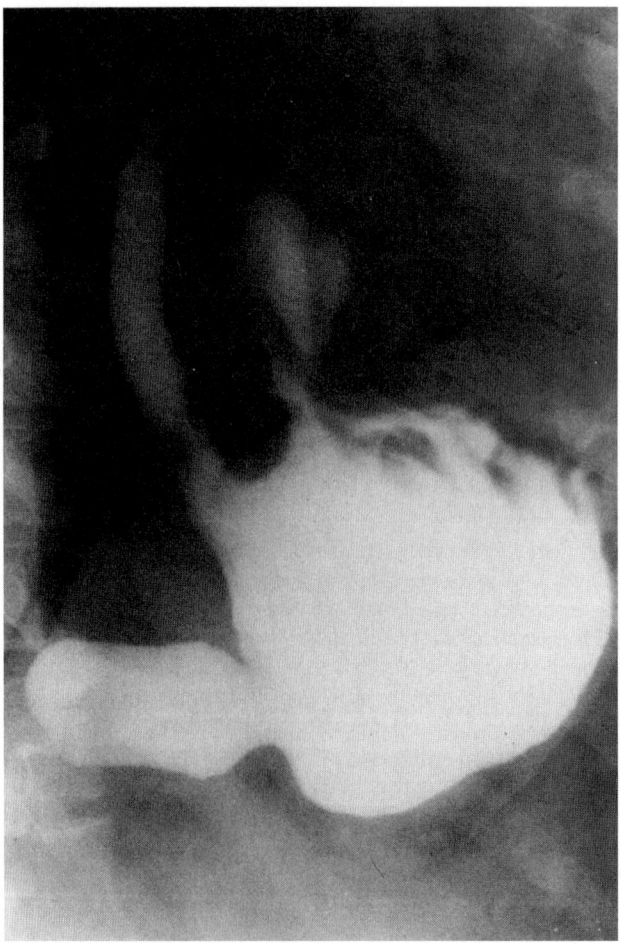

B

FIG. 24-99. *A.* Radiogram of a type I (sliding) hiatal hernia. *B.* Radiogram of a type II (rolling or paraesophageal) hernia. *C.* Radiogram of a type III (combined sliding-rolling or mixed) hernia. *D.* Radiogram of an intrathoracic stomach. This is the end stage of a large hiatal hernia, regardless of its initial classification. Note that the stomach has rotated 180 degree around its longitudinal axis, with the cardia and pylorus as fixed points. [*Reproduced with permission from DeMeester TR, Bonavina L: Paraesophageal hiatal hernia, in Nyhus LM, Condon RE (eds): Hernia, 3rd ed. Philadelphia: Lippincott, 1989, pp 684, 685, 686.*] (*Continued*)

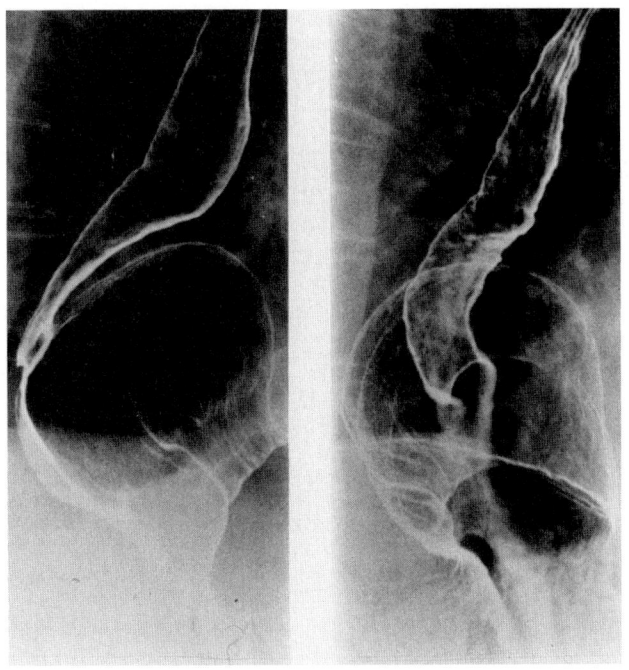

C

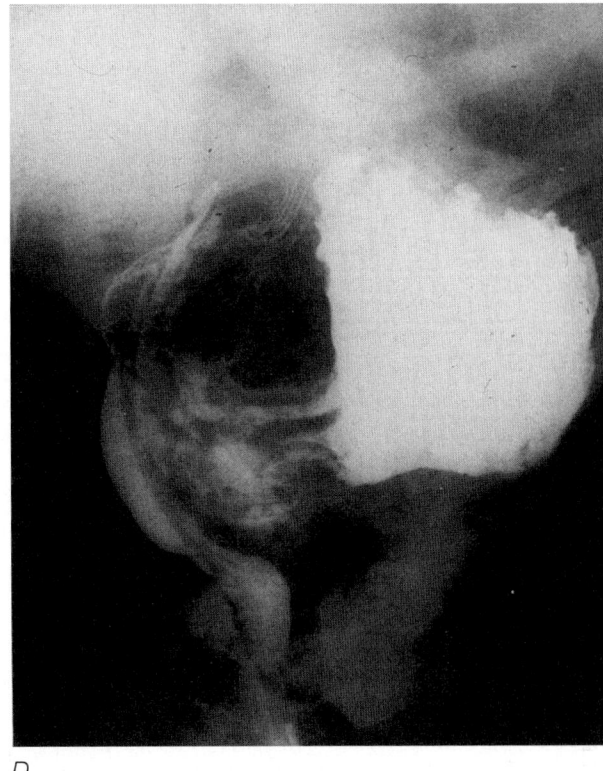

D

FIG. 24-99. *(continued)*

These observations point to the conclusion that the development of a hiatal hernia is an age-related phenomenon secondary to repetitive upward stretching of the phrenoesophageal membrane. A paraesophageal hernia rather than a sliding hernia develops when there is a defect, perhaps congenital, in the esophageal hiatus anterior to the esophagus. The persistent posterior fixation of the cardia to the preaortic fascia and the median arcuate ligament is the only essential difference between a sliding and a paraesophageal hernia. When an anterior defect in the hiatus occurs in association with a loss of fixation of the cardia, a mixed, or type III, hernia develops.

Clinical Manifestations

The clinical presentation of a paraesophageal hiatal hernia differs from that of a sliding hernia. There is usually a higher prevalence of symptoms of dysphagia and postprandial fullness with paraesophageal hernias, but the typical symptoms of heartburn and regurgitation present in sliding hiatal hernias can also occur. Both

FIG. 24-100. Changes in the anatomy of the phrenoesophageal membrane over time based on the dissection of 163 human cadavers from the fetal period to age 75. *A.* Fetus. *B.* Newborn and small infants and young adults 20 to 30 years of age. *C.* Adults 55 to 70 years of age. *D.* Adults 55 to 70 years of age in transition to a hiatal hernia. *E.* Adults 55 to 70 years of age with hiatal hernia. [*Reproduced with permission from DeMeester TR, Bonavina L: Paraesophageal hiatal hernia, in Nyhus LM, Condon RE (eds): Hernia, 3rd ed. Philadelphia: Lippincott, 1989, p 687.*]

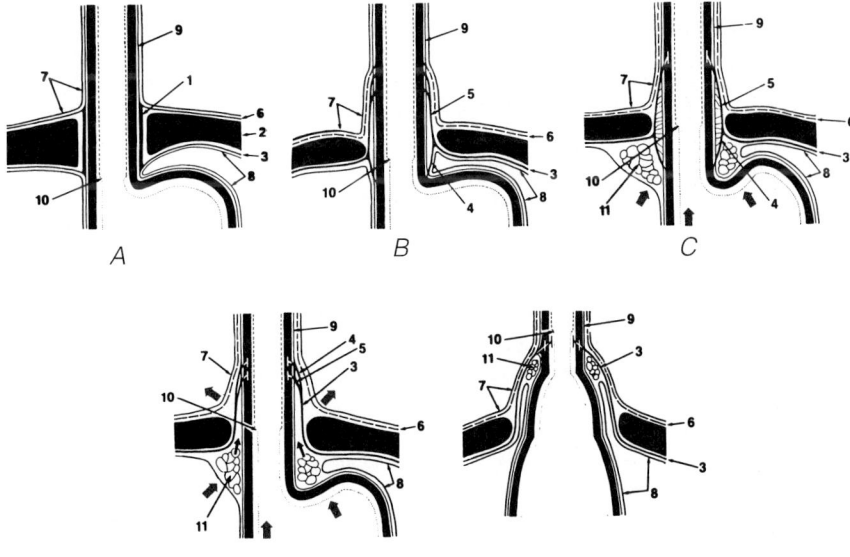

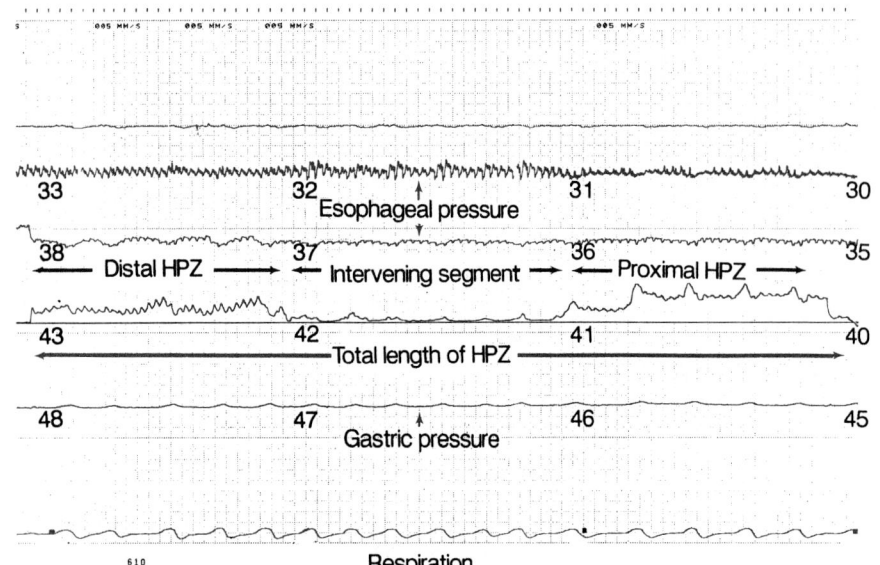

FIG. 24-101. The double-hump phenomenon seen on esophageal manometry, showing various divisions of the double-hump segment. HPZ = high pressure zone. *(Reproduced with permission from Kaul BK, DeMeester TR, Oka M, et al: The cause of dysphagia in uncomplicated sliding hiatal hernia and its relief by hiatal herniorrhaphy. A roentgenographic, manometric, and clinical study. Ann Surg 211:406, 1990.)*

are caused by gastroesophageal reflux secondary to an underlying mechanical deficiency of the cardia. The symptoms of dysphagia and postprandial fullness in patients with a paraesophageal hernia are explained by the compression of the adjacent esophagus by a distended cardia, or twisting of the gastroesophageal junction by the torsion of the stomach that occurs as it becomes progressively displaced in the chest.

Approximately one third of patients with a paraesophageal hernia are found to be anemic, which is due to recurrent bleeding from ulceration of the gastric mucosa in the herniated portion of the stomach. Respiratory complications are frequently associated with a paraesophageal hernia, and consist of dyspnea from mechanical compression and recurrent pneumonia from aspiration. With time the stomach migrates into the chest and can cause intermittent obstruction due to the rotation that has occurred. In contrast, many patients with paraesophageal hiatal hernia are asymptomatic or complain of minor symptoms. However, the presence of a paraesophageal hernia can be life-threatening in that the hernia can lead to sudden catastrophic events, such as excessive bleeding or volvulus with acute gastric obstruction or infarction. With mild dilatation of the stomach, the gastric blood supply can be markedly reduced, causing gastric ischemia, ulceration, perforation, and sepsis. The probability of incarceration is not well known, although recent analysis using mathematical modeling suggests the risk is small.

The symptoms of sliding hiatal hernias are usually due to functional abnormalities associated with gastroesophageal reflux and include heartburn, regurgitation, and dysphagia. These patients have a mechanically defective LES, giving rise to the reflux of gastric juice into the esophagus and the symptoms of heartburn and regurgitation. The symptom of dysphagia occurs from the presence of mucosal edema, Schatzki's ring, stricture, or the inability to organize peristaltic activity in the body of the esophagus as a consequence of the disease.

There is a group of patients with sliding hiatal hernias not associated with reflux disease who have dysphagia without any obvious endoscopic or manometric explanation. Video barium radiograms have shown that the cause of dysphagia in these patients is an obstruction of the swallowed bolus by diaphragmatic impingement on the herniated stomach. Manometrically, this is reflected by a double-humped high-pressure zone at the gastroesophageal junction (Fig. 24-101). The first pressure rise is due to diaphragmatic impingement on the herniated stomach, and the second to the true distal esophageal sphincter. These patients usually have a mechanically competent sphincter, but the impingement of the diaphragm on the stomach can result in propelling the contents of the supradiaphragmatic portion of the stomach up into the esophagus and pharynx, resulting in complaints of pharyngeal regurgitation and aspiration. Consequently this abnormality is often confused with typical gastroesophageal reflux disease. Surgical reduction of the hernia results in relief of the dysphagia in 91% of patients.

Diagnosis

A radiogram of the chest with the patient in the upright position can diagnose a hiatal hernia if it shows an air-fluid level behind the cardiac shadow (Fig. 24-102). This is usually caused by a paraesophageal hernia or an intrathoracic stomach. The accuracy of the upper gastrointestinal barium study in detecting a paraesophageal hiatal hernia is greater than for a sliding hernia, since the latter can often spontaneously reduce. The paraesophageal hiatal hernia is a permanent herniation of the stomach into the thoracic cavity, so a barium swallow provides the diagnosis in virtually every case. Attention should be focused on the position of the gastroesophageal junction, when seen, to differentiate it from a type II hernia (see Fig. 24-99B and C). Fiberoptic esophagoscopy is useful in the diagnosis and classification of a hiatal hernia because the scope can be retroflexed. In this position, a sliding hiatal hernia can be identified by noting a gastric pouch lined with rugal folds extending above the impression caused by the crura of the diaphragm (Fig. 24-103), or measuring at least 2 cm between the crura, identified by having the patient sniff, and the squamocolumnar junction on withdrawal of the scope (Fig. 24-104). A paraesophageal hernia is identified on retroversion of the scope by noting a separate orifice adjacent to the gastroesophageal junction into which gastric rugal folds ascend (Fig. 24-105). A sliding-rolling or mixed hernia can be identified by noting a gastric pouch lined with rugal folds above the diaphragm, with the gastroesophageal junction entering about midway up the side of the pouch (Fig. 24-106).

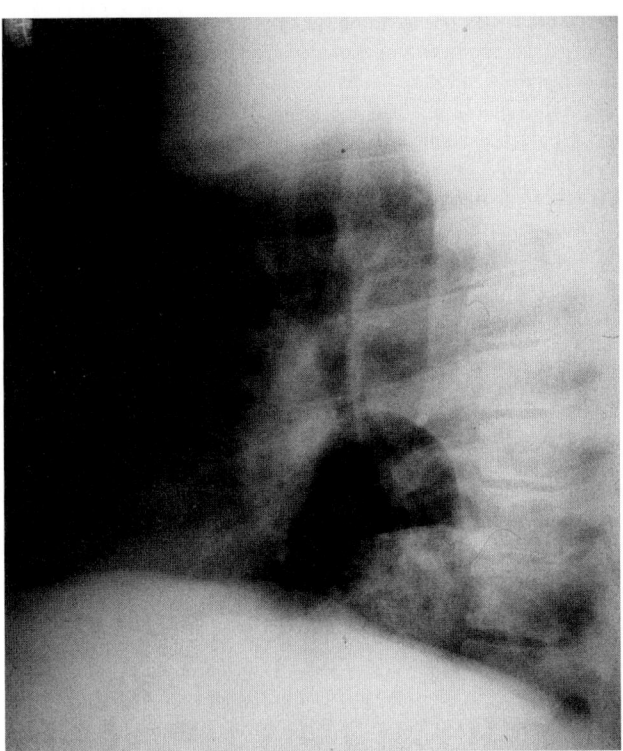

FIG. 24-102. Lateral chest radiogram showing a posterior mediastinal air-fluid level in a gas bubble, indicating the presence of a paraesophageal hernia. [*Reproduced with permission from DeMeester TR, Bonavina L: Paraesophageal hiatal hernia, in Nyhus LM, Condon RE (eds): Hernia, 3rd ed. Philadelphia: Lippincott, 1989, p 688.*]

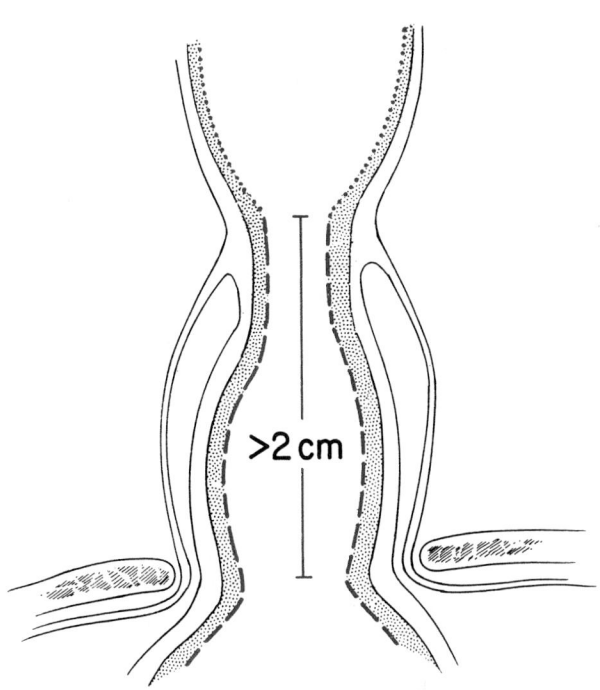

FIG. 24-104. Schematic diagram of the endoscopic criteria for diagnosing a sliding hiatal hernia. A gastric pouch above the crural impression measuring at least 2 cm between the crura, identified by having the patient sniff, and the squamocolumnar junction, with the patient resting in the left lateral position and breathing quietly. [*Reproduced with permission from DeMeester TR, Bonavina L: Paraesophageal hiatal hernia, in Nyhus LM, Condon RE (eds): Hernia, 3rd ed. Philadelphia: Lippincott, 1989, p 689.*]

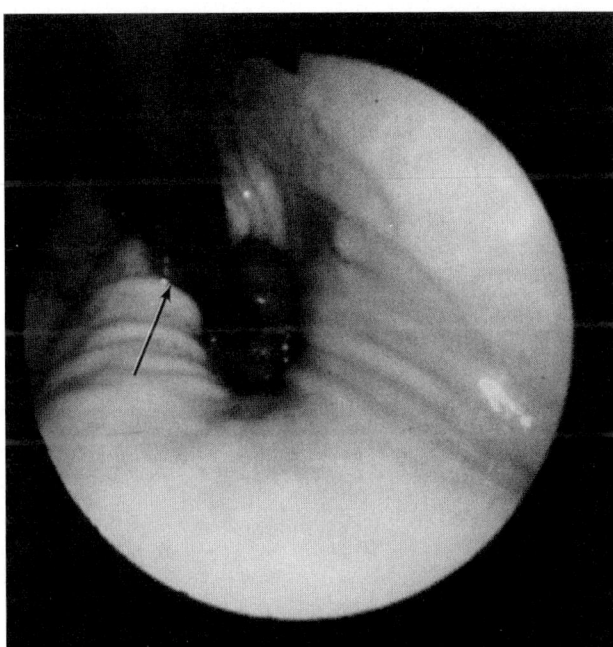

FIG. 24-103. Endoscopic view through a retroflexed fiberoptic gastroscope showing the shaft of the scope (arrow) coming down through a sliding hernia. Note the gastric rugal folds extending above the impression caused by the crura of the diaphragm. [*Reproduced with permission from DeMeester TR, Bonavina L: Paraesophageal hiatal hernia, in Nyhus LM, Condon RE (eds): Hernia, 3rd ed. Philadelphia: Lippincott, 1989, p 689.*]

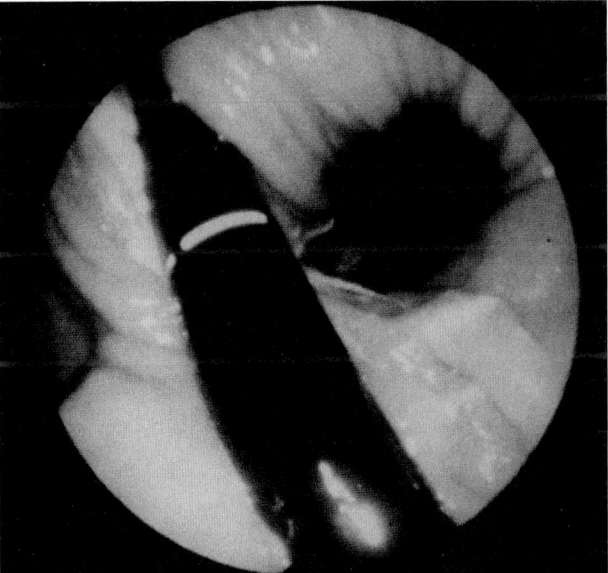

FIG. 24-105. Endoscopic view through a retroflexed fiberoptic gastroscope, showing the shaft of the scope coming down through the gastroesophageal junction adjacent to a separate orifice of the paraesophageal hernia into which the gastric rugal folds ascend. [*Reproduced with permission from DeMeester TR, Bonavina L: Paraesophageal hiatal hernia, in Nyhus LM, Condon RE (eds): Hernia, 3rd ed. Philadelphia: Lippincott, 1989, p 689.*]

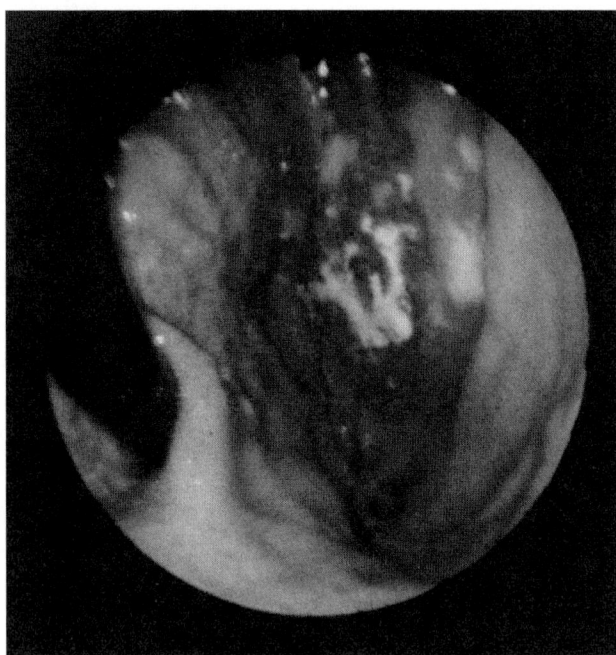

FIG. 24-106. Endoscopic view through a retroflexed fiberoptic gastro-scope, showing the shaft of the scope entering a hernia about midway up the side of a mixed hiatal hernial pouch that extends high into the thorax. [*Reproduced with permission from DeMeester TR, Bonavina L: Paraesophageal hiatal hernia, in Nyhus LM, Condon RE (eds): Hernia, 3rd ed. Philadelphia: Lippincott, 1989, p 689.*]

Pathophysiology

It has been assumed for a long time that a sliding hiatal hernia is associated with an incompetent distal esophageal sphincter, whereas a paraesophageal hiatal hernia constitutes a pure anatomic entity, and is not associated with an incompetent cardia. Accordingly, surgical therapy for patients with a sliding hernia has been directed toward restoration of the physiology of the cardia, but for patients with a paraesophageal hernia, treatment consisted of simply reducing the stomach into the abdominal cavity and closing the crura.

Physiologic testing with 24-hour esophageal pH monitoring has shown increased esophageal exposure to acid gastric juice in 60% of the patients with a paraesophageal hiatal hernia, compared with the observed 71% incidence in patients with a sliding hiatal hernia. It is now recognized that paraesophageal hiatal hernia can be associated with pathologic gastroesophageal reflux.

Physiologic studies have also shown that the competency of the cardia depends on an interrelationship between distal esophageal sphincter pressure, the length of the sphincter that is exposed to

the positive-pressure environment of the abdomen, and the overall length of the sphincter. A deficiency in any one of these manometric characteristics of the sphincter is associated with incompetency of the cardia regardless of whether a hernia is present. Patients with a paraesophageal hernia who have an incompetent cardia have been shown to have a distal esophageal sphincter with normal pressure, but a shortened overall length and displacement outside the positive-pressure environment of the abdomen (Fig. 24-107). In a sliding hernia, even though the sphincter appears to be within the chest on a radiographic barium study, it can still be exposed to abdominal pressure because of the surrounding hernial sac, which functions as an extension of the abdominal cavity. A high insertion of the phrenoesophageal membrane into the esophagus gives adequate length of the distal esophageal sphincter exposed to abdominal pressure. A low insertion gives inadequate length (Fig. 24-108). The importance of the anatomic length of esophagus within the hernial sac has been emphasized by Bombeck, Dillard, and Nyhus in their careful postmortem dissections of the hiatus in 55 patients. Of these patients, eight had a hiatal hernia. Five of the eight had no evidence of esophagitis, and therefore a competent cardia, and in these five patients, the phrenoesophageal membrane inserted 2 to 5 cm (with a mean of 3.6 cm) above the gastroesophageal junction. The other three patients had evidence of esophagitis and therefore an incompetent cardia, and in these patients the membrane inserted 1 cm or less (with a mean of 0.5 cm) above the gastroesophageal junction. This difference was significant and underscores the importance of an adequate length of intra-abdominal esophagus in maintaining competency of the cardia, even in the presence of a hiatal hernia.

In contrast to a paraesophageal hernia, in which the sphincter remains fixed in the abdomen, in a mixed (type III) hernia the sphincter moves extraperitoneally into the thorax through the widened hiatus along with a portion of the lesser curvature of the stomach and cardia, and forms part of the wall of the hernial sac. Consequently, the LES lies outside the abdominal cavity and is unaffected by its environmental pressures. The loss of normal esophageal fixation that occurs in a type I (sliding) hernia or a type III (mixed) hernia results in the body of the esophagus being less able to carry out its propulsive function. This contributes to a greater exposure of the distal esophagus to refluxed gastric juice when components of an incompetent cardia are present. The causes for mechanical incompetency of the cardia are similar regardless of the type of hernia, and are identical with those in patients who have an incompetent cardia and no hiatal hernia.

Treatment

The treatment of paraesophageal hiatal hernia is largely surgical. Controversial aspects include (1) indications for repair, (2) surgical approach, and (3) role of fundoplication.

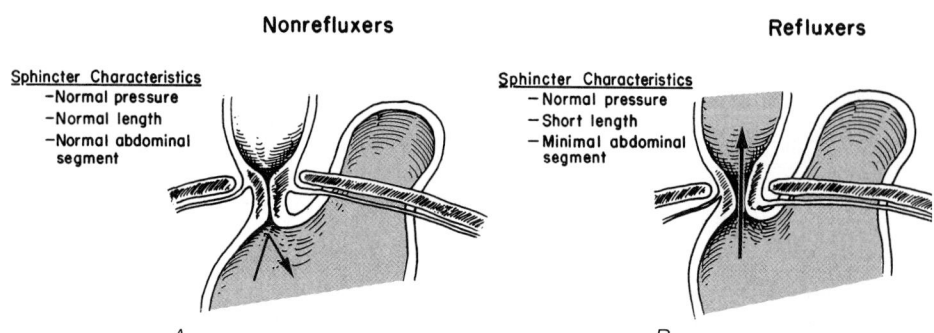

Nonrefluxers

Sphincter Characteristics
- Normal pressure
- Normal length
- Normal abdominal segment

Refluxers

Sphincter Characteristics
- Normal pressure
- Short length
- Minimal abdominal segment

A

B

FIG. 24-107. Schematic diagram of the anatomic and manometric difference between patients with a paraesophageal hiatal hernia with reflux and those without reflux, based on 24-hour esophageal pH monitoring. [*Reproduced with permission from DeMeester TR, Bonavina L: Paraesophageal hiatal hernia, in Nyhus LM, Condon RE (eds): Hernia, 3rd ed. Philadelphia: Lippincott, 1989, p 689.*]

Nonrefluxers   Refluxers

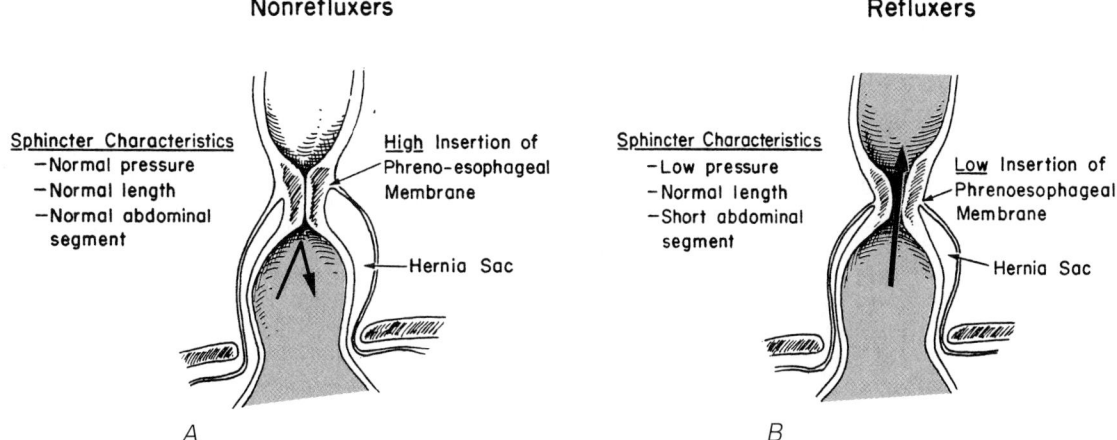

Sphincter Characteristics
  –Normal pressure
  –Normal length
  –Normal abdominal
   segment

High Insertion of
Phreno-esophageal
Membrane

Hernia Sac

Sphincter Characteristics
  –Low pressure
  –Normal length
  –Short abdominal
   segment

Low Insertion of
Phrenoesophageal
Membrane

Hernia Sac

A   B

FIG. 24-108. *Schematic diagram of the anatomic and manometric difference between patients with a sliding hiatal hernia with reflux and those without reflux, based on 24-hour esophageal pH monitoring. [Reproduced with permission from DeMeester TR, Bonavina L: Paraesophageal hiatal hernia, in Nyhus LM, Condon RE (eds): Hernia, 3rd ed. Philadelphia: Lippincott, 1989, p 689.]*

Indications

The presence of a paraesophageal hiatus hernia has traditionally been considered an indication for surgical repair. This recommendation is largely based upon two clinical observations. First, retrospective studies have shown a significant incidence of catastrophic, life-threatening complications of bleeding, infarction, and perforation in patients being followed with known paraesophageal herniation. Second, emergency repair carries a high mortality. In the classic report of Skinner and Belsey, six of 21 patients with a paraesophageal hernia, treated medically because of minimal symptoms, died from the complications of strangulation, perforation, exsanguinating hemorrhage, or acute dilatation of the herniated intrathoracic stomach. These catastrophes occurred for the most part without warning. Others have reported similar findings.

Recent studies suggest that catastrophic complications may be somewhat less common. Allen and colleagues followed 23 patients for a median of 78 months with only four patients progressively worsening. There was a single mortality secondary to aspiration that occurred during a barium swallow examination to investigate progressive symptoms. Although emergency repairs had a median hospital stay of 48 days compared to a stay of 9 days in those having elective repair, there were only three cases of gastric strangulation in 735 patient-years of follow-up.

If surgery is delayed and repair is done on an emergency basis, operative mortality is high, compared to less than 1% for an elective repair. With this in mind, patients with a paraesophageal hernia are generally counseled to have elective repair of their hernia, particularly if they are symptomatic. Watchful waiting of asymptomatic paraesophageal hernias may be an acceptable option.

Surgical Approach

The surgical approach to repair of a paraesophageal hiatal hernia may be either transabdominal (laparoscopic or open) or transthoracic. Each has its advantages and disadvantages. A transthoracic approach facilitates complete esophageal mobilization and removal of the hernia sac. Thoracotomy also allows for the occasional gastroplasty, which may be required for esophageal lengthening to achieve a tension-free repair.

The transabdominal approach facilitates reduction of the volvulus that is often associated with paraesophageal hernias. Although some degree of esophageal mobilization can be accomplished transhiatally, complete mobilization to the aortic arch is difficult or impossible without risk of injury to the vagal nerves.

Several authors have reported the successful repair of paraesophageal hernias using a laparoscopic approach. Laparoscopic repair of a pure type II, or mixed type III paraesophageal hernia is an order of magnitude more difficult than a standard laparoscopic Nissen fundoplication. Most would recommend that these procedures are best avoided until the surgeon has accumulated considerable experience with laparoscopic antireflux surgery. There are several reasons for this. First, the vertical and horizontal volvulus of the stomach often associated with paraesophageal hernias makes identification of the anatomy, in particular the location of the esophagus, difficult. Second, dissection of a large paraesophageal hernia sac usually results in significant bleeding, obscuring the operative field. Finally, redundant tissue present at the gastroesophageal junction following dissection of the sac frustrates the creation of a fundoplication, which these authors believe should accompany the repair of all paraesophageal hernias. Mindful of these difficulties, and given appropriate experience, patients with paraesophageal hernia may be approached laparoscopically, with expectation of success in the majority.

Role of Fundoplication

Controversy remains as to whether to perform an antireflux procedure at all, in selected cases only, or in all patients. The case against an antireflux procedure rests on the frequency of significant postoperative complications secondary to the fundoplication, as well as the slightly longer operative time and increased cost that additional surgery entails. Most advocate the routine addition of an antireflux procedure following repair of the hernia defect. There are several reasons for this. Physiologic testing with 24-hour esophageal pH monitoring has shown increased esophageal exposure to acid gastric juice in 60 to 70% of patients with a paraesophageal hiatal hernia, nearly identical to the observed 71% incidence in patients with a sliding hiatal hernia. Furthermore, there is no relation between the symptoms experienced by the patient with a paraesophageal hernia and the competency of the cardia. Finally, dissection of the gastroesophageal esophagus may lead to postoperative reflux despite a negative preoperative pH score.

Results

Most outcome studies report relief of symptoms following surgical repair of paraesophageal hernias in over 90% of patients. The current literature suggests that laparoscopic repair of a paraesophageal hiatal hernia can be successful. Most authors report symptomatic improvement in 80 to 90% of patients, and less than 10 to 15% prevalence of recurrent hernia. However, the problem of recurrent hernia following laparoscopic repair of *any* hiatal hernia is becoming increasingly appreciated. Recurrent hernia is now the most common cause of anatomic failure following laparoscopic Nissen fundoplication done for GERD. The problem of recurrent hernia following repair of large type III hiatal hernias has received less attention. Outcome following repair of these hernias is usually based on symptomatic assessment alone. Although recurrence rates of 6 to 13% have been reported, they have largely been based on the need for reoperation or investigations that are performed on a selective basis. Recent reports have shown some degree of anatomic recurrence in up to 45% of patients who underwent laparoscopic repair of their hernia.

The principles of laparoscopic repair of a large intrathoracic hernia are analogous to those for an open procedure, namely reduction of the hernia, excision of the peritoneal sac, crural repair, and fundoplication. However, there are several factors that make the laparoscopic repair of these large hernias complex. First, volvulus of the stomach often is associated with these hernias and makes identification of the anatomy, in particular the location of the esophagus, difficult. Second, type III hernias tend to be large, and the laparoscopic dissection of a large hernia sac frequently results in bleeding sufficient to obscure the field of view and impair the recognition of the anatomy. Third, the hiatal opening in a patient with a large hernia is wide, with the right and left muscular crura often separated by 4 cm or more. This can make closure problematic due to the tension required to bring the crura together. Fourth, the right crus may be devoid of stout tissue and sutures may pull through it easily. Finally, redundant tissue present at the gastroesophageal junction following dissection of the sac retards the creation of the fundoplication.

The use of prosthetic mesh as an adjunct to repair has been advocated for both open and laparoscopic repair of large hiatal hernias. Whether its use is beneficial or not remains controversial, but most prefer to avoid prosthetic material if possible. In contrast to groin hernias, the esophageal hiatus is a dynamic area with constant movement of the diaphragm, esophagus, stomach, and pericardium. Erosion of prosthetic material placed in this area into the gastrointestinal tract will occur, the only question is how often. The short-term follow-up of most studies is insufficient to provide insight into this problem.

MISCELLANEOUS LESIONS

Plummer-Vinson Syndrome

This uncommon clinical syndrome is characterized by dysphagia associated with atrophic oral mucosa, spoon-shaped fingers with brittle nails, and chronic anemia. It characteristically occurs in middle-aged edentulous women. Because iron-deficiency anemia is a common finding, another name for this condition is sideropenic dysphagia. The syndrome is more common in the Scandinavian countries than in the United States, and its presentation is variable. Not all patients exhibit the classic syndrome; some lack iron-deficiency anemia and others have the typical clinical stigmata, but lack dysphagia or the presence of an esophageal web.

Clinical observation suggests that the esophageal web once thought to be a component of the syndrome in some patients may actually be a drug-induced lesion, caused by ingestion of ferrous sulfate, a drug commonly prescribed in cases of iron-deficiency anemia. Ferrous sulfate is known to cause esophageal injury, and a number of patients may have had a drug-induced esophageal injury develop at the site where the web is commonly observed. Not knowing the cause of the esophageal abnormality, early observers reported the web as part of the syndrome. Malignant lesions of the oral mucosa, hypopharynx, and esophagus have been noted to occur in up to 100% of patients when followed long-term.

Videoradiographic study, as well as endoscopic findings, have demonstrated a fibrous web just below the cricopharyngeus muscle as the cause of dysphagia in these patients. Treatment consists of dilation of the web and iron therapy to correct the nutritional deficiency.

Schatzki's Ring

Schatzki's ring is a thin submucosal circumferential ring in the lower esophagus at the squamocolumnar junction, often associated with a hiatal hernia. Its significance and pathogenesis are unclear (Fig. 24-109). The ring was first noted by Templeton, but Schatzki and Gary defined it as a distinct entity in 1953. Its prevalence varies from 0.2 to 14% in the general population, depending on the technique of diagnosis and the criteria used. Stiennon believed the ring to be a pleat of mucosa formed by infolding of redundant esophageal mucosa due to shortening of the esophagus. Others believe the ring to be congenital, and still others suggest it is an early stricture resulting from inflammation of the esophageal mucosa caused by chronic reflux.

Schatzki's ring is a distinct clinical entity having different symptoms, upper gastrointestinal function studies, and response to

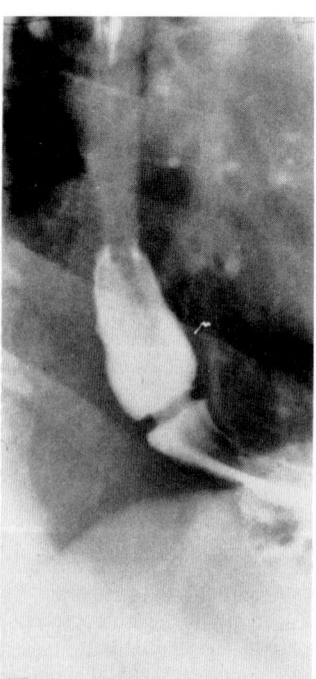

FIG. 24-109. Barium esophagogram showing Schatzki's ring, a thin circumferential ring in the distal esophagus at the squamocolumnar junction. Below the ring is a hiatal hernia.

treatment when compared with patients with a hiatal hernia, but without a ring. Twenty-four-hour esophageal pH monitoring has shown that patients with a Schatzki's ring have a lower incidence of reflux than hiatal hernia controls. They also have better LES function. This, together with the presence of a ring, could represent a protective mechanism to prevent gastroesophageal reflux.

Symptoms associated with Schatzki's ring are brief episodes of dysphagia during hurried ingestion of solid foods. Its treatment has varied from dilation alone to dilation with antireflux measures, antireflux procedure alone, incision, and even excision of the ring. Little is known about the natural progression of Schatzki's rings. Using radiologic techniques, Chen and colleagues showed progressive stenosis of rings in 59% of patients, whereas Schatzki found that the rings decreased in diameter in 29% of patients and remained unchanged in the rest.

Symptoms in patients with a ring are caused more by the presence of the ring than by gastroesophageal reflux. Most patients with a ring but without proven reflux respond to one dilation, while most patients with proven reflux require repeated dilations. In this regard, the majority of Schatzki's ring patients without proven reflux have a history of ingestion of drugs known to be damaging to the esophageal mucosa. Bonavina and associates have suggested drug-induced injury as the cause of stenosis in patients with a ring, but without a history of reflux. Since rings also occur in patients with proven reflux, it is likely that gastroesophageal reflux also plays a part. This is supported by the fact that there is less drug ingestion in the history of these patients. Schatzki's ring is probably an acquired lesion that can lead to stenosis from chemical-induced injury by pill lodgment in the distal esophagus, or from reflux-induced injury to the lower esophageal mucosa.

The best form of treatment of a symptomatic Schatzki's ring in patients who do not have reflux consists of esophageal dilation for relief of the obstructive symptoms. In patients with a ring who have proven reflux and a mechanically defective sphincter, an antireflux procedure is necessary to obtain relief and avoid repeated dilation.

Mallory-Weiss Syndrome

In 1929, Mallory and Weiss described four patients with acute upper gastrointestinal bleeding who were found at autopsy to have mucosal tears at the gastroesophageal junction. This syndrome, characterized by acute upper gastrointestinal bleeding following repeated vomiting, is considered to be the cause of up to 15% of all severe upper gastrointestinal bleeds. The mechanism is similar to spontaneous esophageal perforation: an acute increase in intra-abdominal pressure against a closed glottis in a patient with a hiatal hernia.

Mallory-Weiss tears are characterized by arterial bleeding, which may be massive. Vomiting is not an obligatory factor, as there may be other causes of an acute increase in intra-abdominal pressure, such as paroxysmal coughing, seizures, and retching. The diagnosis requires a high index of suspicion, particularly in the patient who develops upper gastrointestinal bleeding following prolonged vomiting or retching. Upper endoscopy confirms the suspicion by identifying one or more longitudinal fissures in the mucosa of the herniated stomach as the source of bleeding.

In the majority of patients the bleeding will stop spontaneously with nonoperative management. In addition to blood replacement, the stomach should be decompressed and antiemetics administered, as a distended stomach and continued vomiting aggravate further bleeding. A Sengstaken-Blakemore tube will not stop the bleeding, as the pressure in the balloon is not sufficient to overcome arterial pressure. Only occasionally will surgery be required to stop blood

loss. The procedure consists of laparotomy and high gastrotomy with oversewing of the linear tear. Mortality is uncommon and recurrence is rare.

Scleroderma

Scleroderma is a systemic disease accompanied by esophageal abnormalities in approximately 80% of patients. In most, the disease follows a prolonged course. Renal involvement occurs in a small percentage of patients and signals a poor prognosis. The onset of the disease is usually in the third or fourth decade of life, occurring twice as frequently in women as in men.

Small vessel inflammation appears to be an initiating event, with subsequent perivascular deposition of normal collagen, which may lead to vascular compromise. In the gastrointestinal tract, the predominant feature is smooth muscle atrophy. Whether the atrophy in the esophageal musculature is a primary effect or occurs secondary to a neurogenic disorder is unknown. The results of pharmacologic and hormonal manipulation, with agents that act either indirectly via neural mechanisms or directly on the muscle, suggest that scleroderma is a primary neurogenic disorder. Methacholine, which acts directly on smooth muscle receptors, causes a similar increase in LES pressure in normal controls and in patients with scleroderma. Edrophonium, a cholinesterase inhibitor that enhances the effect of acetylcholine when given to patients with scleroderma, causes an increase in LES pressure that is less marked in these patients than in normal controls, suggesting a neurogenic rather than myogenic etiology. Muscle ischemia due to perivascular compression has been suggested as a possible mechanism for the motility abnormality in scleroderma. Others have observed that in the early stage of the disease, the manometric abnormalities may be reversed by reserpine, an agent that depletes catecholamines from the adrenergic system. This suggests that in early scleroderma an adrenergic overactivity may be present that causes a parasympathetic inhibition, supporting a neurogenic mechanism for the disease. In advanced disease manifested by smooth muscle atrophy and collagen deposition, reserpine no longer produces this reversal. Consequently, from a clinical perspective, the patient can be described as having a poor esophageal pump and a poor valve.

The diagnosis of scleroderma can be made manometrically by the observation of normal peristalsis in the proximal striated esophagus, with absent peristalsis in the distal smooth muscle portion (Fig. 24-110). The LES pressure is progressively weakened as the disease advances. Because many of the systemic sequelae of the disease may be nondiagnostic, the motility pattern is frequently used as a specific diagnostic indicator. Gastroesophageal reflux commonly occurs in patients with scleroderma, since they have both hypotensive sphincters and poor esophageal clearance. This combined defect can lead to severe esophagitis and stricture formation. The typical barium swallow shows a dilated, barium-filled esophagus, stomach, and duodenum, or a hiatal hernia with distal esophageal stricture and proximal dilatation (Fig. 24-111).

Traditionally, esophageal symptoms have been treated with H_2 blockers, antacids, elevation of the head of the bed, and multiple dilations for strictures, with generally unsatisfactory results. The degree of esophagitis is usually severe and leads to marked esophageal shortening. Consequently a Collis gastroplasty in combination with a Belsey antireflux repair is the usual procedure for the surgical management of this problem. Surgery reduces esophageal acid exposure, but does not return it to normal because of the poor clearance function of the body of the esophagus. Only 50% of the patients have a good-to-excellent result. If the esophagitis is severe, or there has been a previous failed antireflux procedure and the disease is

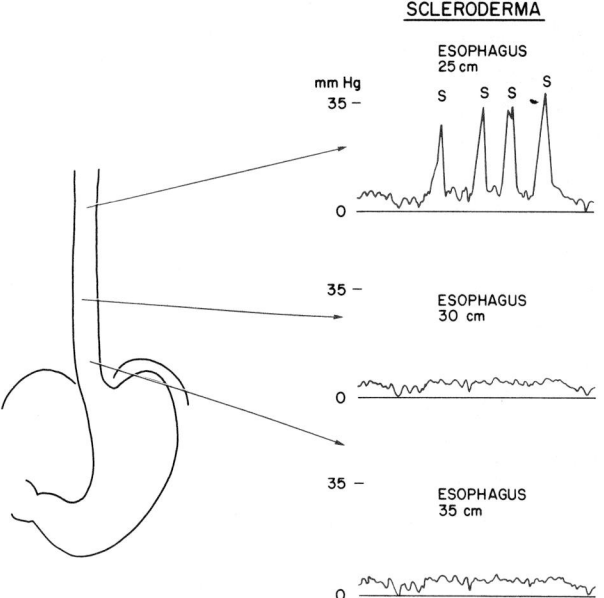

FIG. 24-110. Esophageal motility record in a patient with scleroderma, showing aperistalsis in the distal two thirds of the esophageal body with peristalsis in the proximal portion. *(Reproduced with permission from Waters PF, DeMeester TR: Foregut motor disorders and their surgical management. Med Clin North Am 65:1235, 1981.)*

associated with delayed gastric emptying, a gastric resection with Roux-en-Y esophagojejunostomy and a Hunt-Lawrence pouch has proved the best option.

Acquired Fistula

The esophagus lies in close contact with the membranous portion of the trachea and left bronchus, predisposing to the formation of fistula to these structures. Most acquired esophageal fistulas are to the tracheobronchial tree, and secondary to either esophageal or pulmonary malignancy. Traumatic fistulas and those associated with esophageal diverticula account for the remainder. Fistulas associated with traction diverticula are usually due to mediastinal inflammatory disease, and traumatic fistulas usually occur secondary to penetrating wounds, lye ingestion, or iatrogenic injury.

These fistulas are characterized by paroxysmal coughing following the ingestion of liquids, and by recurrent or chronic pulmonary infections. The onset of cough immediately after swallowing suggests aspiration, whereas a brief delay (30 to 60 seconds) suggests a fistula.

Spontaneous closure is rare, owing to the presence of malignancy or a recurrent infectious process. Surgical treatment of benign fistulas consists of division of the fistulous tract, resection of irreversibly damaged lung tissue, and closure of the esophageal defect. To prevent recurrence, a pleural flap should be interposed. Treatment of malignant fistulas is difficult, particularly in the presence of prior irradiation. Generally, only palliative treatment is indicated. This can best be done by using a specially designed esophageal endoprosthesis that bridges and occludes the fistula, allowing the patient to eat. Rarely, esophageal diversion, coupled with placement of a feeding jejunostomy, can be used as a last resort.

TECHNIQUES OF ESOPHAGEAL RECONSTRUCTION

Options for esophageal substitution include gastric advancement, colonic interposition, and either jejunal free transfer or advancement

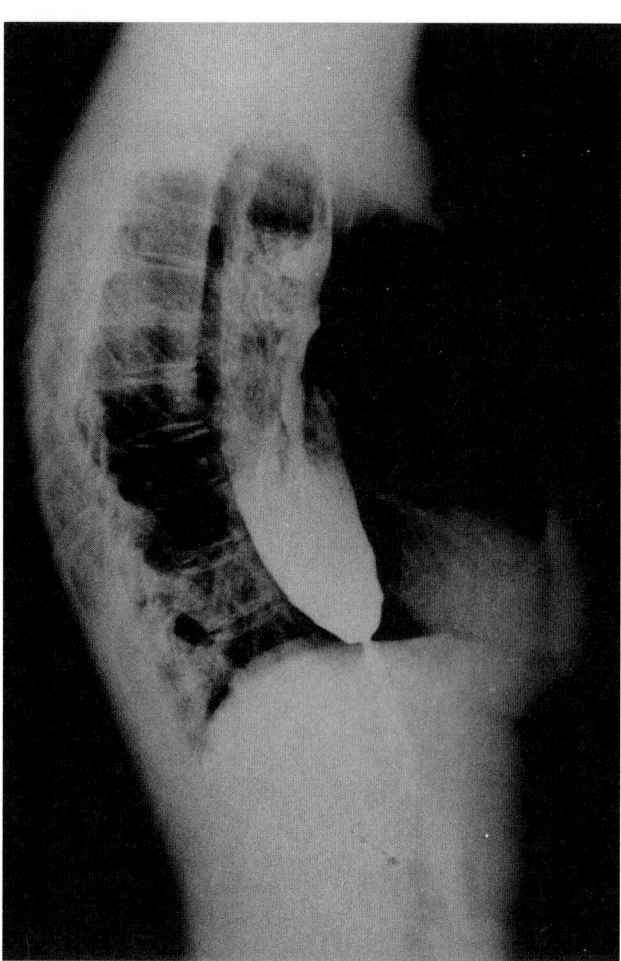

FIG. 24-111. Barium esophagogram of a patient with scleroderma and stricture. Note the markedly dilated esophagus and retained food material. *(Reproduced with permission from Waters PF, DeMeester TR: Foregut motor disorders and their surgical management. Med Clin North Am 65:1235, 1981.)*

into the chest. Rarely, combinations of these grafts will be the only possible option. The indications for esophageal resection and substitution include malignant and end-stage benign disease. The latter includes reflux- or drug-induced stricture formation that cannot be dilated without damage to the esophagus, a dilated and tortuous esophagus secondary to severe motility disorders, lye-induced strictures, and multiple previous antireflux procedures. The choice of esophageal substitution has significant impact upon the technical difficulty of the procedure, and influences the long-term outcome.

Partial Esophageal Resection

Low-lying benign lesions, with preserved proximal esophageal function, are best treated with the interposition of a segment of proximal jejunum into the chest and primary anastomosis. A jejunal interposition can reach to the inferior border of the pulmonary hilum with ease, but the architecture of its blood supply rarely allows the use of the jejunum above this point. Because the anastomosis is within the chest, a thoracotomy is necessary.

The jejunum is a dynamic graft and contributes to bolus transport, whereas the stomach and colon function more as a conduit. The stomach is a poor choice in this circumstance because of the propensity for the reflux of gastric contents into the upper esophagus following an intrathoracic esophagogastrostomy. It is now well

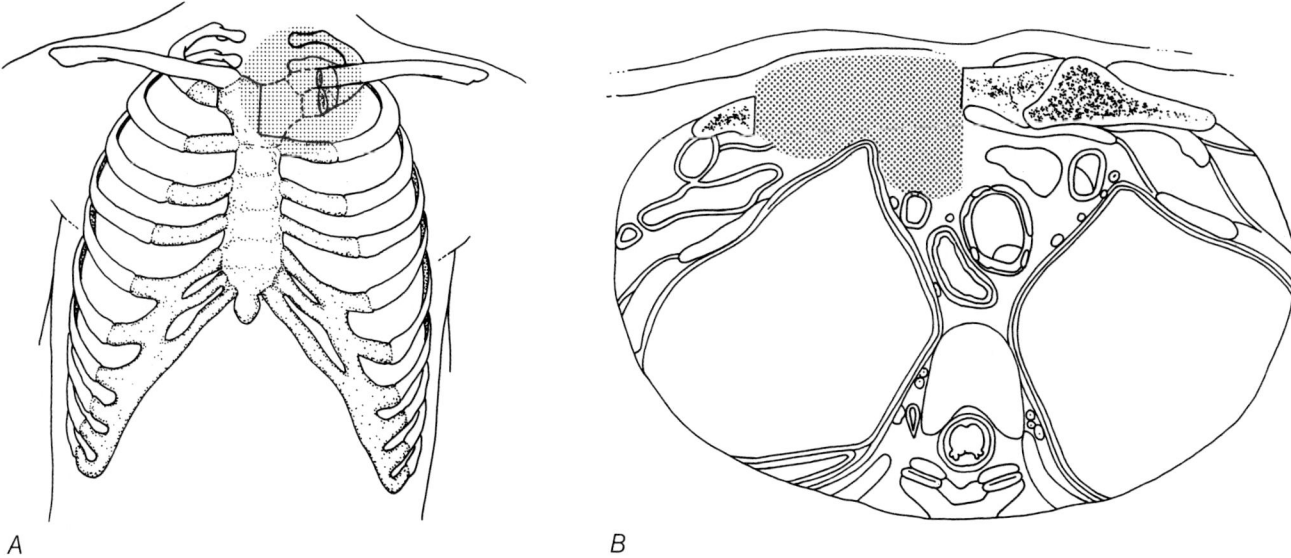

A   *B*

FIG. 24-112. *A.* The portion of the thoracic inlet to be resected in order to provide space for a free jejunal graft and access to the internal mammary artery. *B.* Cross section showing the space available after resection of the sternoclavicular joint and half of the manubrium. [*Reproduced with permission from Rothberg M, DeMeester TR: Exposure of the cervical esophagus, in Shields TW (ed): General Thoracic Surgery, 3rd ed. Philadelphia: Lea & Febiger, 1989, p 419.*]

recognized that this occurs, and can lead to incapacitating symptoms and esophageal destruction in some patients. Short segments of colon, on the other hand, lack significant motility and have a propensity for the development of esophagitis above the anastomosis.

Replacement of the cervical portion of the esophagus, while preserving the distal portion, is occasionally indicated in cervical esophageal or head and neck malignancy, and following the ingestion of lye. Free transfer of a portion of jejunum to the neck has become a viable option and is successful in the majority of cases. Revascularization is achieved via use of the internal mammary artery and the internal mammary or innominate vein. Removal of the sternoclavicular joint aids in performing the vascular and distal esophageal anastomosis (Fig. 24-112).

Reconstruction After Total Esophagectomy

Neither the intrathoracic stomach nor the intrathoracic colon functions as well as the native esophagus after an esophagogastrectomy. The choice between these organs will be influenced by several factors, such as the adequacy of their blood supply and the length of resected esophagus that they are capable of bridging. If the stomach shows evidence of disease, or has been contracted or reduced by previous gastric surgery, the length available for esophageal replacement may not be adequate. The presence of diverticular disease, unrecognized carcinoma, or colitis prohibits the use of the colon. The blood supply of the colon is more affected by vascular disease than the blood supply of the stomach, which may prevent its use. Of the two, the colon provides the longest graft. The stomach can usually reach to the neck if the amount of lesser curvature resected does not interfere with the blood supply to the fundus. Gastric interposition has the advantage that only one anastomosis is required. On the other hand, there is greater potential for aspiration of gastric juice or stricturing of the cervical anastomosis from chronic reflux when stomach is used for replacement.

Following an esophagogastrectomy, patients may have discomfort during or shortly after eating. The most common symptom is a postprandial pressure sensation or a feeling of being stuffed, which probably results from the loss of the gastric reservoir. This symptom is less common when the colon is used as an esophageal substitute, probably because the distal third of the stomach is retained in the abdomen and the interposed colon provides an additional reservoir function.

King and Hölscher have reported a 40 and 50% incidence of dysphagia after re-establishing gastrointestinal continuity with the stomach following esophagogastrectomy. This incidence is similar to Orringer's results after using the stomach to replace the esophagus in patients with benign disease. More than half of the patients experienced dysphagia postoperatively; two thirds of this group required postoperative dilation and one fourth had persistent dysphagia and required home dilation. By contrast, dysphagia is uncommon and the need for dilation is rare following a colonic interposition. Isolauri reported on 248 patients with colonic interpositions and noted a 24% incidence of dysphagia 12 months after the operation. When it occurred, the most common cause was recurrent mediastinal tumor. The high incidence of dysphagia with the use of the stomach is probably related to the esophagogastric anastomosis in the neck and the resulting difficulty of passing a swallowed bolus.

Another consequence of the transposition of the stomach into the chest is the development of postoperative duodenogastric reflux, probably due to pyloric denervation, and adding a pyloroplasty may worsen this problem. Following gastric advancement, the pylorus lies at the level of the esophageal hiatus, and a distinct pressure differential develops between the intrathoracic gastric and intra-abdominal duodenal lumina. Unless the pyloric valve is extremely efficient, the pressure differential will encourage reflux of duodenal contents into the stomach. Duodenogastric reflux is less likely to occur following colonic interposition, because there is sufficient intra-abdominal colon to be compressed by the abdominal pressure, and the pylorus and duodenum remain in their normal intra-abdominal position.

Although there is general acceptance of the concept that an esophagogastric anastomosis in the neck results in less postoperative esophagitis and stricture than one at a lower level, reflux esophagitis following a cervical anastomosis does occur, albeit at a slower rate than when the anastomosis is at a lower level. Most patients undergo cervical esophagogastrostomy for malignancy; thus the long-term sequelae of an esophagogastric anastomosis in the neck are not of concern. However, patients who have had a cervical esophagogastrostomy for benign disease may develop problems associated with the anastomosis in the fourth or fifth postoperative year that are severe enough to require anastomotic revision. This is less likely in patients who have had a colonic interposition for esophageal replacement. Consequently, in patients who have a benign process or a potentially curable carcinoma of the esophagus or cardia, a colonic interposition is used to obviate the late problems associated with a cervical esophagogastrostomy. Colonic interposition for esophageal substitution is a more complex procedure than gastric advancement, with the potential for greater perioperative morbidity, particularly in inexperienced hands.

Composite Reconstruction

Occasionally a combination of colon, jejunum, and stomach is the only reconstructive option available. This situation may arise when there has been previous gastric or colonic resection, when dysphagia has recurred after a previous esophageal resection, or following postoperative complications such as ischemia of an esophageal substitute. Although not ideal, combinations of colon, jejunum, and stomach used to restore gastrointestinal continuity function surprisingly well, and allow alimentary reconstruction in an otherwise impossible situation.

Vagal Sparing Esophagectomy

Traditional esophagectomy typically results in bilateral vagotomy and its attendant consequences. It is likely that symptoms such as dumping, diarrhea, early satiety, and weight loss seen in 15 to 20% of patients postesophagectomy are at least in part, if not completely, due to vagal interruption. The technique of vagal sparing esophagectomy has been described in an effort to avoid the morbidities associated with standard esophagectomy.

Through an upper midline abdominal incision the right and left vagal nerves are identified, circled with a tape, and retracted to the right. A limited, highly selective proximal gastric vagotomy is performed along the cephalad 4 cm of the lesser curvature. The stomach is divided with an Endo-GIA stapler just below the gastroesophageal junction. The colon is prepared to provide an interposed segment as previously described. A neck incision is made along the anterior border of the left sternocleidomastoid muscle and the strap muscles are exposed. The omohyoid muscle is divided at its pulley, and the sternohyoid and sternothyroid muscles are divided at their manubrial insertion. The left carotid sheath is retracted laterally and the thyroid and trachea medially. The left inferior thyroid artery is ligated laterally as it passes under the left common carotid artery. The left recurrent laryngeal nerve is identified and protected. The esophagus is dissected out circumferentially in an inferior direction, from the left neck to the apex of the right chest, to avoid injury to the right recurrent laryngeal nerve. The esophagus is divided at the level of the thoracic inlet, leaving about 3 to 4 cm of cervical esophagus. The proximal esophagus is retracted anteriorly and to the right with the use of two sutures to keep saliva and oral contents from contaminating the neck wound.

Returning to the abdomen, the proximal staple line of the gastric division is opened and the esophagus is flushed with povidone-iodine solution. A vein stripper is passed up the esophagus into the neck wound. The distal portion of the esophagus in the neck is

secured tightly around the stripping cable with "endoloops" and an umbilical tape for a trailer. The tip of the stripper is exchanged for a mushroom head, and the stripper is pulled back into the abdomen, inverting the esophagus as it transverses the posterior mediastinum. This maneuver strips the branches of the esophageal plexus off the longitudinal muscle of the esophagus, preserving the esophageal plexus along with the proximal vagal nerves and the distal vagal nerve trunks. In patients with end-stage achalasia, only the mucosa is secured around the stripping cable, so that it alone is stripped and the dilated muscular wall of the esophagus, with its enriched blood supply, remains. The resulting mediastinal tunnel, or in the case of achalasia the muscular tube, is dilated with a Foley catheter containing 90 mL of fluid in the balloon. The previously prepared interposed portion of the transverse colon is passed behind the stomach and up through the mediastinal tunnel into the neck. An end-to-end anastomosis is performed to the cervical esophagus using a single layer technique. The colon is pulled taut and secured to the left crus with four or five interrupted sutures. Five centimeters below the crura, an opening is made in the mesentery adjacent to the colon along its mesenteric border, through which an Endo-GIA stapler is passed and the colon is divided. The proximal end, which is the distal end of the interposed colon, is anastomosed high on the posterior fundic wall of the stomach, using a triangular stapling anastomotic technique. This is done by stapling longitudinally the stomach and colon together with a 75-mm Endo-GIA stapler, spreading the base of the incision apart, and closing it with a T-55 stapler. Colonic continuity is re-established by bringing the proximal right colon to the distal staple line in the left colon and performing an end-to-end anastomosis using a double layer technique.

Although conceptually appealing, preservation of vagal nerve integrity or the gastric reservoir function after vagal sparing esophagectomy only recently has been validated. Banki and associates compared patients undergoing vagal sparing esophagectomy to those with conventional esophagectomy and colon or gastric interposition. This study showed that vagal sparing esophagectomy preserved gastric secretion, gastric emptying, meal capacity, and body mass index, when compared to esophagogastrectomy with colon interposition or standard esophagectomy with gastric pull-up. Vagal sparing esophagectomy patients functioned, for the most part, similarly to normal subjects, allowing them to eat a normal meal, free of dumping or diarrhea. These results indicate that the vagal sparing esophagectomy procedure does indeed preserve the vagal nerves, and may be considered in the treatment of benign and early malignant lesions requiring esophagectomy.

Bibliography

General References

Balaji B, Peters JH: Minimally invasive surgery for esophageal motor disorders. *Surg Clin North Am* 82:763, 2002.

Bremner CG, DeMeester TR, Bremner RM: *Esophageal Motility Testing Made Easy*. St. Louis, MI: Quality Medical Publishing, 2001.

Castel DW, Richter J (eds): *The Esophagus*. Boston: Little, Brown & Co., 1999.

Demeester SR (ed): Barrett's esophagus. *Problems in General Surgery*, 18:2. Hagerstown, MD: Lippincott Williams & Wilkins, 2001.

DeMeester TR, Barlow AP: Surgery and current management for cancer of the esophagus and cardia: Part I. *Curr Probl Surg* 25:477, 1988.

DeMeester TR, Barlow AP: Surgery and current management for cancer of the esophagus and cardia: Part II. *Curr Probl Surg* 25:535, 1988.

DeMeester TR, Peters JH, Bremner CG, et al: Biology of gastroesophageal reflux disease; pathophysiology relating to medical and surgical treatment. *Annu Rev Med* 50:469, 1999.

DeMeester SR, Peters JH, DeMeester TR: Barrett's esophagus. *Curr Probl Surg* 38:549, 2001.

Hunter JG, Pellagrini CA: Surgery of the esophagus. *Surg Clin North Am* 77:959, 1997.

McFadyen BV, Arregui ME, Eubanks S, et al: *Laparoscopic Surgery of the Abdomen.* New York: Springer, 2003.

Stein HJ, DeMeester TR, Hinder RA: Outpatient physiologic testing and surgical management of functional foregut disorders. *Curr Probl Surg* 24:418, 1992.

Zuidema GD, Orringer MB (eds): *Shackelford's Surgery of the Alimentary Tract,* 3rd ed, Vol. I. Philadelphia: WB Saunders, 1991.

Surgical Anatomy

Daffner RH, Halber MD, Postlethwait RW, et al: CT of the esophagus. II. Carcinoma. *AJR* 133:1051, 1979.

Gray SW, Rowe JS Jr., Skandalakis JE: Surgical anatomy of the gastro-esophageal junction. *Am Surg* 45:575, 1979.

Liebermann-Meffert DMI, Meier R, Siewert JR: Vascular anatomy of the gastric tube used for esophageal reconstruction. *Ann Thorac Surg* 54:1110, 1992.

Liebermann-Meffert D, Siewert JR: Arterial anatomy of the esophagus; a review of the literature with brief comments on clinical aspects. *Gullet* 2:3, 1992.

Liebermann-Meffert D: The pharyngoesophageal segment; anatomy and innervation. *Dis Esophagus* 8:242, 1995.

Liebermann-Meffert DMI, Walbrun B, Hiebert CA, et al: Recurrent and superior laryngeal nerves; a new look with implications for the esophageal surgeon. *Ann Thorac Surg* 67:217, 1999.

Physiology

Barlow AP, DeMeester TR, et al: The significance of the gastric secretory state in gastroesophageal reflux disease. *Arch Surg* 124:937, 1989.

Biancani P, Zabinski MP, Behar J: Pressure, tension, and force of closure of the human LES and esophagus. *J Clin Invest* 56:476, 1975.

Bonavina L, Evander A, et al: Length of the distal esophageal sphincter and competency of the cardia. *Am J Surg* 151:25, 1986.

Davenport HW: *Physiology of the Digestive Tract,* 5th ed. Chicago: Year Book Medical, 1982, p 52.

DeMeester TR, Lafontaine E, et al: The relationship of a hiatal hernia to the function of the body of the esophagus and the gastroesophageal junction. *J Thorac Cardiovasc Surg* 82:547, 1981.

DeMeester TR, Stein HJ, Fuchs KH: Physiologic diagnostic studies, in Zuidema GD, Orringer MB (eds): *Shackelford's Surgery of the Alimentary Tract,* 3rd ed, Vol. I. Philadelphia: WB Saunders, 1991, p 94.

DeMeester TR: What is the role of intraoperative manometry? *Ann Thorac Surg* 30:1, 1980.

Helm JF, Dodds WJ, et al: Acid neutralizing capacity of human saliva. *Gastroenterology* 83:69, 1982.

Helm JF, Dodds WJ, et al: Effect of esophageal emptying and saliva on clearance of acid from the esophagus. *N Engl J Med* 310:284, 1984.

Helm JF, Dodds WJ, Hogan WJ: Salivary responses to esophageal acid in normal subjects and patients with reflux esophagitis. *Gastroenterology* 93:1393, 1982.

Helm JF, Riedel DR, et al: Determinants of esophageal acid clearance in normal subjects. *Gastroenterology* 85:607, 1983.

Joelsson BE, DeMeester TR, et al: The role of the esophageal body in the antireflux mechanism. *Surgery* 92:417, 1982.

Johnson LF, DeMeester TR: Evaluation of elevation of the head of the bed, bethanechol, and antacid foam tablets on gastroesophageal reflux. *Dig Dis Sci* 26:673, 1981.

Kahrilas PJ, Dodds WJ, Hogan WJ: Effect of peristaltic dysfunction on esophageal volume clearance. *Gastroenterology* 94:73, 1988.

Kaye MD, Showalter JP: Pyloric incompetence in patients with symptomatic gastroesophageal reflux. *J Lab Clin Med* 83:198, 1974.

Liebermann-Meffert D, Allgower M, et al: Muscular equivalent of the esophageal sphincter. *Gastroenterology* 76:31, 1979.

McCallum RW, Berkowitz DM, Lerner E: Gastric emptying in patients with gastroesophageal reflux. *Gastroenterology* 80:285, 1981.

Mittal RK, Lange RC, McCallum RW: Identification and mechanism of delayed esophageal acid clearance in subjects with hiatus hernia. *Gastroenterology* 92:130, 1987.

Price LM, El-Sharkawy TY, Mui HY, Diamant NE: Effects of bilateral cervical vagotomy on balloon-induced lower esophageal sphincter relaxation in the dog. *Gastroenterology* 77:324, 1979.

Rao SSC, Madipalli RS, Mujica VR, Patel RS, Zimmerman B: Effects of age and gender on esophageal biomechanical properties and sensation. *Am J Gastroenterol* 98:1688, 2003.

Zaninotto G, DeMeester TR, Schwizer W, et al: The lower esophageal sphincter in health and disease. *Am J Surg* 155:104, 1988.

Assessment of Esophageal Function

Adamek RJ, Wegener M, et al: Long-term esophageal manometry in healthy subjects: Evaluation of normal values and influence of age. *Dig Dis Sci* 39:2069, 1994.

Akberg O, Wahlgren L: Dysfunction of pharyngeal swallowing: A cineradiographic investigation in 854 dysphagial patients. *Acta Radiol Diagn* 26:389, 1985.

American Gastroenterological Association Patient Care Committee: Clinical esophageal pH recording: A technical review for practice guideline development. *Gastroenterology* 110, 1982.

Barish CF, Castell DO, Richter JE: Graded esophageal balloon distention: A new provocative test for non-cardiac chest pain. *Dig Dis Sci* 31:1292, 1986.

Battle WS, Nyhus LM, Bombeck CT: Gastroesophageal reflux: Diagnosis and treatment. *Ann Surg* 177:560, 1973.

Bechi P: Fiberoptic measurement of "alkaline" gastro-esophageal reflux: Technical aspects and clinical indications. *Dis Esophagus* 131, 1994.

Bechi P, Pucciani F, et al: Long-term ambulatory enterogastric reflux monitoring. Validation of a new fiberoptic technique. *Dig Dis Sci* 38:1297, 1991.

Behar J, Biancani P, Sheahan DG: Evaluation of esophageal tests in the diagnosis of reflux esophagitis. *Gastroenterology* 71:9, 1976.

Benjamin SM, Richter JE, et al: Prospective manometric evaluation with pharmacologic provocation of patients with suspected esophageal motility dysfunction. *Gastroenterology* 84:893, 1983.

Bennett JR, Atkinson M: Oesophageal acid-perfusion in the diagnosis of precordial pain. *Lancet* 2:1150, 1966.

Bernstein IM, Baker CA: A clinical test for esophagitis. *Gastroenterology* 34:760, 1958.

Castell DO, Richter JE, Dalton CB (eds): *Esophageal Motility Testing.* New York: Elsevier, 1987.

DeMeester TR, Johnson LF, et al: Patterns of gastroesophageal reflux in health and disease. *Ann Surg* 184:459, 1976.

DeMeester TR, Stein HJ, Fuchs KH: Physiologic diagnostic studies, in Zuidema GD, Orringer MB (eds): *Shackelford's Surgery of the Alimentary Tract,* 3rd ed, Vol. I. Philadelphia: Saunders, 1991, p 94.

DeMeester TR, Wang CI, et al: Technique, indications and clinical use of 24-hour esophageal pH monitoring. *J Thorac Cardiovasc Surg* 79:656, 1980.

DeMoraes-Filho JPP, Bettarello A: Lack of specificity of the acid perfusion test in duodenal ulcer patients. *Am J Dig Dis* 19:785, 1974.

Dent J: A new technique for continuous sphincter pressure measurement. *Gastroenterology* 71:263, 1976.

Dhiman RK, Saraswat VA, Naik SR: Ambulatory esophageal pH monitoring; technique interpretations and clinical indications. *Dig Dis Sci* 47:241, 2002.

Dodds WJ: Current concepts of esophageal motor function: Clinical implications for radiology. *AJR* 128:549, 1977.

Donner MW: Swallowing mechanism and neuromuscular disorders. *Semin Roentgenol* 9:273, 1974.

Emde C, Armstrong F, et al: Reproducibility of long-term ambulatory esophageal combined pH/manometry. *Gastroenterology* 100:1630, 1991.

Emde C, Garner A, Blum A: Technical aspects of intraluminal pH-metry in man: Current status and recommendations. *Gut* 23:1177, 1987.

Fein M, Fuchs K-H, et al: Fiberoptic technique for 24-hour bile reflux monitoring. Standards and normal values for gastric monitoring. *Dig Dis Sci* 41:216, 1996.

Fisher RS, Malmud LS, et al: Gastroesophageal (GE) scintiscanning to detect and quantitate GE reflux. *Gastroenterology* 70:301, 1976.

Fuchs KH, DeMeester TR, Albertucci M: Specificity and sensitivity of objective diagnosis of gastroesophageal reflux disease. *Surgery* 102:575, 1987.

Fuchs KH, DeMeester TR, et al: Concomitant duodenogastric and gastroesophageal reflux: The role of twenty-four-hour gastric pH monitoring, in Siewert JR, Holscher AH (eds): *Diseases of the Esophagus.* New York: Springer-Verlag, 1988, p 1073.

Glade MJ: Continuous ambulatory esophageal pH monitoring in the evaluation of patients with gastroesophageal reflux. *JAMA* 274:662, 1995.

Iascone C, DeMeester TR, et al: Barrett's esophagus: Functional assessment, proposed pathogenesis and surgical therapy. *Arch Surg* 118:543, 1983.

Johnson LF, DeMeester TR: Development of 24-hour intraesophageal pH monitoring composite scoring. *J Clin Gastroenterol* 8:52, 1986.

Johnson LF, DeMeester TR, Haggitt RC: Endoscopic signs for gastroesophageal reflux objectively evaluated. *Gastrointest Endosc* 22:151, 1976.

Johnson LF, DeMeester TR: Twenty-four-hour pH monitoring of the distal esophagus: A quantitative measure of gastroesophageal reflux. *Am J Gastroenterol* 62:325, 1974.

Kauer WKH, Burdiles P, Ireland A, et al: Does duodenal juice reflux into the esophagus in patients with complicated GERD? Evaluation of a fiberoptic sensor for bilirubin. *Am J Surg* 169:98, 1995.

Kramer P, Hollander W: Comparison of experimental esophageal pain with clinical pain of angina pectoris and esophageal disease. *Gastroenterology* 29:719, 1955.

Landon RL, Ouyang A, et al: Provocation of esophageal chest pain by ergonovine or edrophonium. *Gastroenterology* 81:10, 1981.

Mittal RK, Stewart WR, Schirmer BD: Effect of a catheter in the pharynx on the frequency of transient LES relaxations. *Gastroenterology* 103:1236, 1992.

Pandolfino JE, Richter JE, Ours T, et al: Ambulatory esophageal pH monitoring using a wireless system. *Am J Gastroenterol* 98:740, 2003.

Reid BJ, Weinstein WM, et al: Endoscopic biopsy can detect high-grade dysplasia or early adenocarcinoma in Barrett's esophagus without grossly recognizable neoplastic lesions. *Gastroenterology* 94:81, 1988.

Richter JE, Hackshaw BT, Wu WC: Edrophonium: A useful provocative test for esophageal chest pain. *Ann Intern Med* 103:14, 1985.

Russell COH, Hill LD, et al: Radionuclide transit: A sensitive screening test for esophageal dysfunction. *Gastroenterology* 80:887, 1981.

Schwesinger WH: Endoscopic diagnosis and treatment of mucosal lesions of the esophagus. *Surg Clin North Am* 69:1185, 1989.

Schwizer W, Hinder RA, DeMeester TR: Does delayed gastric emptying contribute to gastroesophageal reflux disease? *Am J Surg* 157:74, 1989.

Seaman WB: Roentgenology of pharyngeal disorders, in Margulis AR, Burhenne JH (eds): *Alimentary Tract Roentgenology,* 2nd ed, Vol. I. St Louis, MO: Mosby, 1973, p 305.

Shoenut JP, Yaffe CS: Ambulatory esophageal pH testing. Referral patterns, indications, and treatment in a Canadian teaching hospital. *Dig Dis Sci* 41:1102, 1996.

Smout AJPM: Ambulatory manometry of the oesophagus: The method and the message. *Gullet* 1:155, 1991.

Stein HJ, DeMeester TR, et al: Three-dimensional imaging of the LES in gastroesophageal reflux disease. *Ann Surg* 214:374, 1991.

Stein HJ, DeMeester TR, Peters JH, et al: Technique, indications, and clinical use of ambulatory 24-hour gastric pH monitoring in a surgical practice. *Surgery* 116:758, 1994.

Tolin RD, Malmud LS, et al: Esophageal scintigraphy to quantitate esophageal transit (quantitation of esophageal transit). *Gastroenterology* 76:1402, 1979.

Tutuian R, Vela MF, Balaji NS, et al: Esophageal function testing with combined multichannel intraluminal impedance and manometry; multicenter study in healthy volunteers. *Clin Gastroenterol Hepatol* 1:174, 2003.

Welch RW, Lickmann K, et al: Manometry of the normal upper esophageal sphincter and its alteration in laryngectomy. *J Clin Invest* 63:1036, 1979.

Wickremesinghe PC, Bayrit PQ, et al: Quantitative evaluation of bile diversion surgery utilizing 99mTc HIDA scintigraphy. *Gastroenterology* 84:354, 1983.

Winans CS: Manometric asymmetry of the lower esophageal high pressure zone. *Dig Dis Sci* 22:348, 1977.

Gastroesophageal Reflux Disease

Allison PR: Hiatus hernia: A 20 year retrospective survey. *Ann Surg* 178:273, 1973.

Allison PR: Peptic ulcer of the esophagus. *J Thorac Surg* 15:308, 1946.

Allison PR: Reflux esophagitis, sliding hiatus hernia and the anatomy of repair. *Surg Gynecol Obstet* 92:419, 1951.

Altorki NK, Sunagawa M, et al: High-grade dysplasia in the columnar-lined esophagus. *Am J Surg* 161:97, 1991.

Barlow AP, DeMeester TR, et al: The significance of the gastric secretory state in gastroesophageal reflux disease. *Arch Surg* 124:937, 1989.

Bonavina L, DeMeester TR, et al: Drug-induced esophageal strictures. *Ann Surg* 206:173, 1987.

Bremner RM, DeMeester TR, Crookes PF, et al: The effect of symptoms and non-specific motility abnormalities on surgical therapy for gastroesophageal reflux disease. *J Thorac Cardiovasc Surg* 107:1244, 1994.

Cadiot G, Bruhat A, et al: Multivariate analysis of pathophysiological factors in reflux oesophagitis. *Gut* 40:167, 1997.

Castell DO. Nocturnal acid breakthrough in perspective: Let's not throw out the baby with the bathwater. *Am J Gastroenterol* 98:517, 2003.

Chandrasoma P: Norman Barrett: So close, yet 50 years from the truth. *J Gastrointest Surg* 3:7, 1999.

Chen MF, Wang CS: A prospective study of the effect of cholecystectomy on duodenogastric reflux in humans using 24-hour gastric hydrogen monitoring. *Surg Gynecol Obstet* 175:52, 1992.

Clark GWB, Ireland AP, Peters JH, et al: Short segments of Barrett's esophagus: A prevalent complication of gastroesophageal reflux disease with malignant potential. *J Gastrointest Surg* 1:113, 1997.

DeMeester SR, Campos GMR, DeMeester TR, et al: The impact of an antireflux procedure on intestinal metaplasia of the cardia. *Ann Surg* 228:547; 1998.

DeMeester TR, Bonavina L, Albertucci M: Nissen fundoplication for gastroesophageal reflux disease: Evaluation of primary repair in 100 consecutive patients. *Ann Surg* 204:9, 1986.

DeMeester TR, Bonavina L, et al: Chronic respiratory symptoms and occult gastroesophageal reflux. *Ann Surg* 211:337, 1990.

DeMeester SR, DeMeester TR: Columnar mucosa and intestinal metaplasia of the esophagus: Fifty years of controversy. *Ann Surg* 231:303, 2000.

DeMeester TR: Management of benign esophageal strictures, in Stipa S, Belsey RHR, Moraldi A (eds): *Medical and Surgical Problems of the Esophagus.* New York: Academic Press, 1981, p 173.

DeMeester TR, Fuchs KH, et al: Experimental and clinical results with proximal end-to-end duodenojejunostomy for pathologic duodenogastric reflux. *Ann Surg* 206:414, 1987.

DeMeester TR, Johansson KE, et al: Indications, surgical technique, and long-term functional results of colon interposition or bypass. *Ann Surg* 208:460, 1988.

Desai KM, Klingensmith ME, Winslow ER, Frisella P, Soper NJ: Symptomatic outcomes of laparoscopic antireflux surgery in patients eligible for endoluminal therapies. *Surg Endosc* 16:1669, 2002.

Donahue PE, Samelson S, et al: The floppy Nissen fundoplication: Effective long-term control of pathologic reflux. *Arch Surg* 120:663, 1985.

Farrell TM, Smith CD, Metreveli RE, et al: Fundoplication provides effective and durable symptom relief in patients with Barrett's esophagus. *Am J Surg* 178:18, 1999.

Fass R: Epidemiology and pathophysiology of symptomatic gastroesophageal reflux disease. *Am J Gastroenterol* 98(Suppl):S2, 2003.

Fein M, Ireland AP, Ritter MP, et al: Duodenogastric reflux potentiates the injurious effects of gastroesophageal reflux. *J Gastrointest Surg* 1:27, 1997.

Fiorucci S, Santucci L, et al: Gastric acidity and gastroesophageal reflux patterns in patients with esophagitis. *Gastroenterology* 103:855, 1992.

Fletcher J, Wirz A, Young J, et al: Unbuffered highly acidic gastric juice exists at the gastroesophageal junction after a meal. *Gastroenterology* 121:775, 2001.

Freston JW: Long-term acid control and proton pump inhibitors: Interactions and safety issues in perspective. *Am J Gastroenterol* 92:51S, 1997.

Fuchs KH, DeMeester TR, et al: Computerized identification of pathologic duodenogastric reflux using 24-hour gastric pH monitoring. *Ann Surg* 213:13, 1991.

Gerson LB, Shetler K, Triadafilopoulos G: Prevalence of Barrett's esophagus in asymptomatic individuals. *Gastroenterology* 123:461, 2002.

Gillen P, Keeling P, et al: Implication of duodenogastric reflux in the pathogenesis of Barrett's oesophagus. *Br J Surg* 75:540, 1988.

Gotley DC, Ball DE, Owen RW, et al: Evaluation and surgical correction of esophagitis after partial gastrectomy. *Surgery* 111:29, 1992.

Graham DY: The changing epidemiology of GERD: Geography and *Helicobacter pylori*. *Am J Gastroenterol* 98:1462, 2003.

Gurski RR, Peters JH, Hagen JA, et al: Barrett's esophagus can and does regress following antireflux surgery: A study of prevalence and predictive features. *J Am Coll Surg* 196:706, 2003.

Henderson RD, Henderson RF, Marryatt GV: Surgical management of 100 consecutive esophageal strictures. *J Thorac Cardiovasc Surg* 99:1, 1990.

Hill LD, Kozarek RA, et al: The gastroesophageal flap valve. In vitro and in vivo observations. *Gastrointest Endosc* 44:541, 1996.

Hinder RA, et al: Relationship of a satisfactory outcome to normalization of delayed gastric emptying after Nissen fundoplication. *Ann Surg* 210:458, 1989.

Hinder RA, Filipi CJ: The technique of laparoscopic Nissen fundoplication. *Surg Laparosc Endosc* 2:265, 1992.

Hirota WK, Loughney TM, Lazas DJ, et al: Specialized intestinal metaplasia, dysplasia and cancer of the esophagus and esophagogastric junction: Prevalence and clinical data. *Gastroenterology* 116:277, 1999.

Hofstetter WA, Peters JH, DeMeester TR, et al: Long term outcome of antireflux surgery in patients with Barrett's esophagus. *Ann Surg* 234:532, 2001.

Ireland AP, Clark GWB, et al: Barrett's esophagus: The significance of p53 in clinical practice. *Ann Surg* 225:17, 1997.

Isolauri J, Luostarinen M, et al: Long-term comparison of antireflux surgery versus conservative therapy for reflux esophagitis. *Ann Surg* 225:295, 1997.

Iwakiri K, Kobayashi M, et al: Relationship between postprandial esophageal acid exposure and meal volume and fat content. *Dig Dis Sci* 41:926, 1996.

Jacob P, Kahrilas PJ, Herzon G: Proximal esophageal pH-metry in patients with "reflux laryngitis." *Gastroenterology* 100:305, 1991.

Jamieson JR, Hinder RA, et al: Analysis of 32 patients with Schatzki's ring. *Am J Surg* 158:563, 1989.

Johnson WE, Hagen JA, DeMeester TR, et al: Outcome of respiratory symptoms after antireflux surgery on patients with gastroesophageal reflux disease. *Arch Surg* 131:489, 1996.

Kahrilas PJ: Diagnosis of symptomatic gastroesophageal reflux disease. *Am J Gastroenterol* 98(Suppl):S15, 2003.

Kahrilas PJ, Dodds WP, Hogan WJ: Effect of peristaltic dysfunction on esophageal volume clearance. *Gastroenterology* 94:73, 1988.

Kahrilas PJ: Radiofrequency therapy of the lower esophageal sphincter for treatment of GERD. *Gastrointest Endosc* 57:723; 2003.

Kauer WKH, Peters JH, DeMeester TR, et al. Mixed reflux of gastric juice is more harmful to the esophagus than gastric juice alone. The need for surgical therapy reemphasized. *Ann Surg* 222:525, 1995.

Kaul BK, DeMeester TR, et al: The cause of dysphagia in uncomplicated sliding hiatal hernia and its relief by hiatal herniorrhaphy: A roentgenographic, manometric, and clinical study. *Ann Surg* 211:406, 1990.

Khaitan L, Ray WA, Holzman MD, et al: Health care utilization after medical and surgical therapy for gastroesophageal reflux disease. *Arch Surg* 138:1356, 2003.

Labenz J, Tillenburg B, et al. *Helicobacter pylori* augments the pH-increasing effect of omeprazole in patients with duodenal ulcer. *Gastroenterology* 110:725, 1996.

Liebermann-Meffert D: Rudolf Nissen: Reminiscences 100 years after his birth. *Dis Esophagus* 9:237, 1996.

Lin KM, Ueda RK, et al: Etiology and importance of alkaline esophageal reflux. *Am J Surg* 162:553, 1991.

Lind JF, et al: Motility of the gastric fundus. *Am J Physiol* 201:197, 1961.

Little AG, et al: Duodenogastric reflux and reflux esophagitis. *Surgery* 96:447, 1984.

Little AG, Ferguson MK, Skinner DB: Reoperation for failed antireflux operations. *J Thorac Cardiovasc Surg* 91:511, 1986.

Liu JY, Finlayson SRG, Laycock WS, Rothstein RI, et al: Determining the appropriate threshold for referral to surgery for gastroesophageal reflux disease. *Surgery* 133:5, 2003.

Lundell L, Miettinen P, Myrvold HE, et al: Long-term management of gastro-oesophageal reflux disease with omeprazole or open antireflux surgery: Results of a prospective randomized trial. *Eur J Gastroenterol Hepatol* 12:879, 2000.

Marshall RE, Anggiansah A, Owen WJ: Bile in the esophagus: Clinical relevance and ambulatory detection. *Br J Surg* 84:21, 1997.

Narayani RI, Burton MP, Young GS: Utility of esophageal biopsy in the diagnosis of non-erosive reflux disease. *Dis Esophagus* 16:187, 2003.

Nehra D, Watt P, Pye JK, et al: Automated oesophageal reflux sampler: A new device used to monitor bile acid reflux in patients with gastro-oesophageal reflux disease. *J Med Engr Tech* 21:1, 1997.

Nissen R: Eine einfache Operation zur Beeinflussung der Refluxoesophagitis. *Schweiz Med Wochenschr* 86:590, 1956.

Nissen R: Gastropexy and fundoplication in surgical treatment of hiatus hernia. *Am J Dig Dis* 6:954, 1961.

Notivol R, Coffin B, et al: Gastric tone determines the sensitivity of the stomach to distention. *Gastroenterology* 108:330, 1995.

Oberg S, Johansson H, Wenner J, et al: Endoscopic surveillance of columnar lined esophagus: Frequency of intestinal metaplasia detection and impact of antireflux surgery. *Ann Surg* 234:619, 2001.

Oleynikov D, Oelschlager B: New alternatives in the management of gastroesophageal reflux disease. *Am J Surg* 186:106, 2003.

Orlando RC: The pathogenesis of gastroesophageal reflux disease: The relationship between epithelial defense, dysmotility, and acid exposure. *Am J Gastroenterol* 92:3S, 1997.

Orringer MB, Skinner DB, Belsey RHR: Long-term results of the Mark IV operation for hiatal hernia and analyses of recurrences and their treatment. *J Thorac Cardiovasc Surg* 63:25, 1972.

O'Sullivan GC, DeMeester TR, et al: Twenty-four-hour pH monitoring of esophageal function: Its use in evaluation in symptomatic patients after truncal vagotomy and gastric resection or drainage. *Arch Surg* 116:581, 1981.

Ouatu-Lascar R, Triadafilopoulos G: Complete elimination of reflux symptoms does not guarantee normalization of intraesophageal acid reflux in patients with Barrett's esophagus. *Am J Gastroenterol* 93:711, 1998.

Parrilla P, Martinez de Haro LF, Ortiz A, et al: Long term results of a randomized prospective study comparing medical and surgical treatment in Barrett's esophagus. *Ann Surg* 237:291, 2003.

Patti MG, Debas HT, et al: Esophageal manometry and 24-hour pH monitoring in the diagnosis of pulmonary aspiration secondary to gastroesophageal reflux. *Am J Surg* 163:401, 1992.

Patti MG, Diener E, Tamburini A, et al: Role of esophageal function tests in diagnosis of gastroesophageal reflux disease. *Dig Dis Sci* 46:597, 2001.

Pearson FG, Cooper JD, et al: Gastroplasty and fundoplication for complex reflux problems. *Ann Surg* 206:473, 1987.

Pelligrini CA, DeMeester TR, et al: Gastroesophageal reflux and pulmonary aspiration: Incidence, functional abnormality, and results of surgical therapy. *Surgery* 86:110, 1979.

Peters JH, DeMeester TR: Indications, principles of procedure selection, and technique of laparoscopic Nissen fundoplication. *Semin Laparoscopy* 2:27, 1995.

Peters JH, Heimbucher J, Incarbone R, et al: Clinical and physiologic comparison of laparoscopic and open Nissen fundoplication. *J Am Coll Surg* 180:385, 1995.

Provenzale D, Kemp JA, et al: A guide for surveillance of patients with Barrett's esophagus. *Am J Gastroenterol* 89, 1994.

Richardson JD, Larson GM, Polk HC: Intrathoracic fundoplication for shortened esophagus: Treacherous solution to a challenging position. *Am J Surg* 143:29, 1982.

Richter JE: Long-term management of gastroesophageal reflux disease and its complications. *Am J Gastroenterol* 92:30S, 1997.

Romagnuolo J, Meier MA, Sadowski DC: Medical or surgical therapy for erosive reflux esophagitis: Cost utility analysis using a Markov model. *Ann Surg* 236:191, 2002.

Ropert A, Des Varannes SB, et al: Simultaneous assessment of liquid emptying and proximal gastric tone in humans. *Gastroenterology* 105:667, 1993.

Salama FD, Lamont G: Long-term results of the Belsey Mark IV antireflux operation in relation to the severity of esophagitis. *J Thorac Cardiovasc Surg* 100:17, 1990.

Schwizer W, Hinder RA, DeMeester TR: Does delayed gastric emptying contribute to gastroesophageal reflux disease? *Am J Surg* 157:74, 1989.

Shaker R, Castell DO, Schoenfeld PS, et al: Nighttime heartburn is an underappreciated clinical problem that impacts sleep and daytime function: The results of a Gallup survey conducted on behalf of the American Gastroenterologic Association. *Am J Gastroenterol* 98:1487, 2003.

Siewert JR, Isolauri J, Feussuer M: Reoperation following failed fundoplication. *World J Surg* 13:791, 1989.

Sontag SJ, O'Connell S, Khandelwal S, et al: Asthmatics with gastroesophageal reflux: Long term results of a randomized trial of medical and surgical antireflux therapies. *Am J Gastroenterol* 98:987, 2003.

Sontag SJ: The medical management of reflux esophagitis: Role of antacids and acid inhibition. *Gastroenterol Clin North Am* 19:683, 1990.

Spechler SJ, Department of Veterans Affairs Gastroesophageal Reflux Disease Study Group: Comparison of medical and surgical therapy for complicated gastroesophageal reflux disease in veterans. *N Engl J Med* 326:786, 1992.

Spechler SJ, Lee E, Ahmen D: Long term outcome of medical and surgical therapies for gastroesophageal reflux disease: Follow-up of a randomized controlled trial. *JAMA* 285:2331, 2001.

Stein HJ, Barlow AP, et al: Complications of gastroesophageal reflux disease: Role of the LES, esophageal acid and acid/alkaline exposure, and duodenogastric reflux. *Ann Surg* 216:35, 1992.

Stein HJ, Bremner RM, et al: Effect of Nissen fundoplication on esophageal motor function. *Arch Surg* 127:788, 1992.

Stein HJ, et al: Clinical use of 24-hour gastric pH monitoring vs. O-diisopropyl iminodiacetic acid (DISIDA) scanning in the diagnosis of pathologic duodenogastric reflux. *Arch Surg* 125:966, 1990.

Stein HJ, Smyrk TC, et al: Clinical value of endoscopy and histology in the diagnosis of duodenogastric reflux disease. *Surgery* 112:796, 1992.

Stirling MC, Orringer MB: Surgical treatment after the failed antireflux operation. *J Thorac Cardiovasc Surg* 92:667, 1986.

Vaezi MF, Hicks DM, Abelson TI, et al: Laryngeal signs and symptoms and gastroesophageal reflux disease (GERD): A critical assessment of cause and effect association. *Clin Gastroenterol Hepatol* 1:333, 2003.

Van Den Boom G, Go PMMYH, et al: Cost effectiveness of medical versus surgical treatment in patients with severe or refractory gastroesophageal reflux disease in the Netherlands. *Scand J Gastroenterol* 31:1, 1996.

Watson DI, Baigrie RJ, Jamieson GG: A learning curve for laparoscopic fundoplication. Definable, avoidable, or a waste of time? *Ann Surg* 224:198, 1996.

Wattchow DA, Jamieson GG, et al: Distribution of peptide-containing nerve fibers in the gastric musculature of patients undergoing surgery for gastroesophageal reflux. *Ann Surg* 290:153, 1992.

Welch NT, Yasui A, et al: Effect of duodenal switch procedure on gastric acid production, intragastric pH, gastric emptying, and gastrointestinal hormones. *Am J Surg* 163:37, 1992.

Weston AP, Krmpotich P, et al: Short segment Barrett's esophagus: Clinical and histological features, associated endoscopic findings, and association with gastric intestinal metaplasia. *Am J Gastroenterol* 91:981, 1996.

Wetscher GJ, Hinder RA, et al: Reflux esophagitis in humans is mediated by oxygen-derived free radicals. *Am J Surg* 170:552, 1995.

Williamson WA, Ellis FH Jr., et al: Effect of antireflux operation on Barrett's mucosa. *Ann Thorac Surg* 49:537, 1990.

Wright TA: High-grade dysplasia in Barrett's oesophagus. *Br J Surg* 84:760, 1997.

Zaninotto G, DeMeester TR, et al: Esophageal function in patients with reflux-induced strictures and its relevance to surgical treatment. *Ann Thorac Surg* 47:362, 1989.

Motility Disorders of the Pharynx and Esophagus

Achem SR, Crittenden J, et al: Long-term clinical and manometric follow-up of patients with nonspecific esophageal motor disorders. *Am J Gastroenterol* 87:825, 1992.

American Gastroenterologic Society: AGA technical review on treatment of patients with dysphagia caused by benign disorders of the distal esophagus. *Gastroenterology* 117:233, 1999.

Andreollo NA, Earlam RJ: Heller's myotomy for achalasia: Is an added antireflux procedure necessary? *Br J Surg* 74:765, 1987.

Anselmino M, Perdikis G, et al: Heller myotomy is superior to dilatation for the treatment of early achalasia. *Arch Surg* 132:233, 1997.

Bianco A, Cagossi M, et al: Appearance of esophageal peristalsis in treated idiopathic achalasia. *Dig Dis Sci* 90:978, 1986.

Bonavina L, Khan NA, DeMeester TR: Pharyngoesophageal dysfunctions: The role of cricopharyngeal myotomy. *Arch Surg* 120:541, 1985.

Bonavina L, Nosadinia A, et al: Primary treatment of esophageal achalasia: Long-term results of myotomy and Dor fundoplication. *Arch Surg* 127:222, 1992.

Browning TH, et al: Diagnosis of chest pain of esophageal origin. *Dig Dis Sci* 35:289, 1990.

Cassella RR, Brown AL Jr., et al: Achalasia of the esophagus: Pathologic and etiologic considerations. *Ann Surg* 160:474, 1964.

Chakkaphak S, Chakkaphak K, et al: Disorders of esophageal motility. *Surg Gynecol Obstet* 172:325, 1991.

Chen LQ, Chughtau T, Sideris L, et al: Long term effects of myotomy and partial fundoplication for esophageal achalasia. *Dis Esophagus* 15:171, 2002.

Code CF, Schlegel JF, et al: Hypertensive gastroesophageal sphincter. *Mayo Clin Proc* 35:391, 1960.

Cook IJ, Blumbergs P, et al: Structural abnormalities of the cricopharyngeus muscle in patients with pharyngeal (Zenker's) diverticulum. *J Gastroenterol Hepatol* 7:556, 1992.

Cook IJ, Gabb M, et al: Pharyngeal (Zenker's) diverticulum is a disorder of upper esophageal sphincter opening. *Gastroenterology* 103:1229, 1992.

Csendes A, Braghetto I, et al: Late results of a prospective randomized study comparing forceful dilatation and oesophagomyotomy in patients with achalasia. *Gut* 30:299, 1989.

Csendes A, Braghetto I, et al: Late subjective and objective evaluation of the results of esophagomyotomy in 100 patients with achalasia of the esophagus. *Surgery* 104:469, 1988.

Csendes A, Velasco N, et al: A prospective randomized study comparing forceful dilatation and esophagomyotomy in patients with achalasia of the esophagus. *Gastroenterology* 80:789, 1981.

Dalton CB, Castell DO, Richter JE: The changing faces of the nutcracker esophagus. *Am J Gastroenterol* 83:623, 1988.

DeMeester TR, Johansson KE, et al: Indications, surgical technique and long-term functional results of colon interposition or bypass. *Ann Surg* 208:460, 1988.

DeMeester TR, Lafontaine E, et al: The relationship of a hiatal hernia to the function of the body of the esophagus and the gastroesophageal junction. *J Thorac Cardiovasc Surg* 82:547, 1981.

DeMeester TR, Stein HJ: Surgery for esophageal motor disorders, in Castell DO (ed): *The Esophagus*. Boston: Little, Brown, 1992, p 401.

Donner MW: Swallowing mechanism and neuromuscular disorders. *Semin Roentgenol* 9:273, 1974.

Eckardt V, Aignherr C, Bernhard G: Predictors of outcome in patients with achalasia treated by pneumatic dilation. *Gastroenterol* 103:1732, 1992.

Eckardt VF, Köhne U, et al: Risk factors for diagnostic delay in achalasia. *Dig Dis Sci* 42:580, 1997.

Ekberg O, Wahlgren L: Dysfunction of pharyngeal swallowing: A cineradiographic investigation in 854 dysphagial patients. *Acta Radiol Diagn* 26:389, 1985.

Ellis FH Jr., Crozier RE: Cervical esophageal dysphagia: Indications for and results for cricopharyngeal myotomy. *Ann Surg* 194:279, 1981.

Ellis FH: Long esophagomyotomy for diffuse esophageal spasm and related disorders: An historical overview. *Dis Esophagus* 11:210; 1998.

Ellis Jr, FH: Oesophagomyotomy for achalasia: A 22-year experience. *Br J Surg* 80:882, 1993.

Evander A, Little AG, et al: Diverticula of the mid and lower esophagus. *World J Surg* 10:820, 1986.

Eypasch EP, Stein HJ, et al: A new technique to define and clarify esophageal motor disorders. *Am J Surg* 159:144, 1990.

Ferguson MK: Achalasia: Current evaluation and therapy. *Ann Thorac Surg* 52:336, 1991.

Ferguson MK, Skinner DB (eds): *Diseases of the Esophagus: Benign Diseases,* Vol. 2. Mount Kisco, NY: Futura Publishing, 1990.

Ferguson TB, Woodbury JD, Roper CL: Giant muscular hypertrophy of the esophagus. *Ann Thorac Surg* 8:209, 1969.

Foker JE, Ring WE, Varco RL: Technique of jejunal interposition for esophageal replacement. *J Thorac Cardiovasc Surg* 83:928, 1982.

Gillies M, Nicks R, Skyring A: Clinical, manometric, and pathologic studies in diffuse oesophageal spasm. *Br Med J* 2:527, 1967.

Goulbourne IA, Walbaum PR: Long-term results of Haller's operation for achalasia. *J Royal Coll Surg* 30:101, 1985.

Gutschow CA, Hamoir M, Rombaux P, et al: Management of pharyngo-esophageal (Zenker's) diverticulum: Which technique? *Ann Thorac Surg* 74:1677, 2002.

Hirano I, Tatum RP, Shi G, et al: Manometric heterogeneity in patients with idiopathic achalasia. *Gastroenterology* 120:789, 2001.

Kahrilas PJ, Logemann JA, et al: Pharyngeal clearance during swallowing: A combined manometric and videofluoroscopic study. *Gastroenterology* 103:128, 1992.

Lafontaine E: Pharyngeal dysphagia, in DeMeester TR, Matthews HR (eds): *Benign Esophageal Disease: International Trends in General Thoracic Surgery,* Vol. 3. St. Louis: CV Mosby, 1987.

Lam HGT, Dekker W, et al: Acute noncardiac chest pain in a coronary care unit. *Gastroenterology* 102:453, 1992.

Lang IM, Dantas RO, Cook IJ, et al: Videographic, manometric, and electromyographic analysis of canine upper esophageal sphincter. *Am J Physiol* 260:G911, 1991.

Lerut J, Elgariani A, et al: Zenker's diverticulum. Surgical experience in a series of 25 patients. *Acta Gastroenterol Belg* 46:189, 1983.

Lerut T, VanRaemdonck D, et al: Pharyngo-oesophageal diverticulum (Zenker's). Clinical, therapeutic and morphologic aspects. *Acta Gastroenterol Belg* 53:330, 1990.

Little AG, Correnti FS, et al: Effect of incomplete obstruction on feline esophageal function with a clinical correlation. *Surgery* 100:430, 1986.

Malthaner RA, Todd TR, Miller L, Pearson FG: Long-term results in surgically managed esophageal achalasia. *Ann Thorac Surg* 58:1343, 1994.

Mellow MH: Return of esophageal peristalsis in idiopathic achalasia. *Gastroenterology* 70:1148, 1976.

Meshkinpour H, Haghighat P, et al: Quality of life among patients treated for achalasia. *Dig Dis Sci* 41:352, 1996.

Migliore M, Payne H, et al: Pathophysiologic basis for operation on Zenker's diverticulum. *Ann Thorac Surg* 57:1616, 1994.

Moser G, Vacariu-Granser GV, et al: High incidence of esophageal motor disorders in consecutive patients with globus sensation. *Gastroenterology* 101:1512, 1991.

Moses PL, Ellis LM, Anees MR, et al: Antineural antibodies in idiopathic achalasia and gastro-oesophageal reflux disease. *Gut* 52:629, 2003.

Nehra D, Lord RV, DeMeester TR, et al: Physiologic basis for the treatment of epiphrenic diverticulum. *Ann Surg* 235:346, 2002.

Oelschlager BK, Chang L, Pellegrini CA: Improved outcome after extended gastric myotomy for achalasia. *Arch Surg* 138:490, 2003.

Patti MG, Fisichella PM, Peretta S, et al: Impact of minimally invasive surgery on the treatment of esophageal achalasia: A decade of change. *J Am Coll Surg* 196:698, 2003.

Pellegrini C, Wetter LA, et al: Thoracoscopic esophagomyotomy: Initial experience with a new approach for the treatment of achalasia. *Ann Surg* 216:291, 1992.

Peters JH: An antireflux procedure is critical to the long-term outcome of esophageal myotomy for achalasia. *J Gastrointest Surg* 5:17, 2001.

Peters JH, Kauer WKH, Ireland AP, Bremner CG, DeMeester TR: Esophageal resection with colon interposition for end-stage achalasia. *Arch Surg* 130:632, 1995.

Ponce J, Garrigues V, Pertejo V, Sala T, et al: Individual prediction of response to pneumatic dilation in patients with achalasia. *Dig Dis Sci* 41:2135, 1996.

Richter JE: Surgery or pneumatic dilation for achalasia: A head-to-head comparison. *Gastroenterology* 97:1340, 1989.

Shimi SM, Nathanson LK, Cuschieri A: Thoracoscopic long oesophageal myotomy for nutcracker oesophagus: Initial experience of a new surgical approach. *Br J Surg* 79:533, 1992.

Shoenut J, Duerksen D: A prospective assessment of gastroesophageal reflux before and after treatment of achalasia patients: Pneumatic dilation versus transthoracic limited myotomy. *Am J Gastroenterol* 92:1109, 1997.

Sivarao DV, Mashimo HL, Thatte HS, Goyal RK: Lower esophageal sphincter is achalasic in nNos(-/-) and hypotensive in W/W(v) mutant mice. *Gastroenterology* 121:34, 2001.

Spechler S, Castell DO: Classification of oesophageal motility abnormalities. *Gut* 49:145, 2001.

Stein HJ, DeMeester TR, Eypasch EP: Ambulatory 24-hour esophageal manometry in the evaluation of esophageal motor disorders and non-cardiac chest pain. *Surgery* 110:753, 1991.

Stein HJ, Eypasch EP, DeMeester TR: Circadian esophageal motility pattern in patients with classic diffuse esophageal spasm and nutcracker esophagus. *Gastroenterology* 96:491, 1989.

Streitz JM Jr., Glick ME, Ellis FH Jr.: Selective use of myotomy for treatment of epiphrenic diverticula: Manometric and clinical analysis. *Arch Surg* 127:585, 1992.

Vaezi MF, Baker ME, Achkar E, et al: Timed barium oesophogram: Better predictor of long term success after pneumatic dilation in achalasia than symptom assessment. *Gut* 50:765, 2002.

Vantrappen G, Janssens J: To dilate or to operate? That is the question. *Gut* 24:1013, 1983.

Verne G, Sallustio JE, et al: Anti-myenteric neuronal antibodies in patients with achalasia: A prospective study. *Dig Dis Sci* 42:307, 1997.

Waters PF, DeMeester TR: Foregut motor disorders and their surgical management. *Med Clin North Am* 54:1235, 1981.

Williams RB, Grehan MJ, Andre J, Cook IJ: Biomechanics, diagnosis, and treatment outcome in inflammatory myopathy presenting as oropharyngeal dysphagia. *Gut* 52:471, 2003.

Zhao X, Pasricha PJ: Botulinum toxin for spastic GI disorders: A systematic review. *Gastrointest Endosc* 57:219, 2003.

Carcinoma of the Esophagus

Akiyama H: Surgery for carcinoma of the esophagus. *Curr Probl Surg* 17:53, 1980.

Akiyama H, Tsurumaru M: Radical lymph node dissection for cancer of the thoracic esophagus. *Ann Surg* 220:364, 1994.

Akiyama H, Tsurumaru M, et al: Principles of surgical treatment for carcinoma of the esophagus: Analysis of lymph node involvement. *Ann Surg* 194:438, 1981.

Altorki N, Skinner D: Should en-bloc esophagectomy be the standard of care for esophageal carcinoma? *Ann Surg* 234:581, 2001.

Badwe RA, Sharma V, Bhansali MS, et al: The quality of swallowing for patients with operable esophageal carcinoma: A randomized trial comparing surgery with radiotherapy. *Cancer* 85:763, 1999.

Baker JW Jr., Schechter GL: Management of paraesophageal cancer by blunt resection without thoracotomy and reconstruction with stomach. *Ann Surg* 203:491, 1986.

Blazeby JM, Williams MH, et al: Quality of life measurement in patients with oesophageal cancer. *Gut* 37:505, 1995.

Bolton JS, Ochsner JL, et al: Surgical management of esophageal cancer. A decade of change. *Ann Surg* 219:475, 1994.

Borrie J: Sarcoma of esophagus: Surgical treatment. *J Thorac Surg* 37:413, 1959.

Cameron AJ, Ott BJ, Payne WS: The incidence of adenocarcinoma in columnar-lined (Barrett's) esophagus. *N Engl J Med* 313:857, 1985.

Clark GWB, Ireland AD, et al: Carcinoembryonic antigen measurements in the management of esophageal cancer. An indicator of subclinical recurrence. *Am J Surg* 170:597, 1995.

Clark GWB, Peters JH, Hagen JA, et al: Nodal metastases and recurrence patterns after en-bloc esophagectomy for adenocarcinoma. *Ann Thorac Surg* 58:646, 1994.

Clark GWB, Smyrk TC, et al: Is Barrett's metaplasia the source of adenocarcinomas of the cardia? *Arch Surg* 129:609, 1994.

Collin CF, Spiro RH: Carcinoma of the cervical esophagus: Changing therapeutic trends. *Am J Surg* 148:460, 1984.

Corley DA, Kerlikowske K, Verma R, et al: Protective association of aspirin/NSAIDs and esophageal cancer: A systematic review and meta-analysis. *Gastroenterology* 124:47, 2003.

Dallal HJ, Smith GD, Grieve DC, et al: A randomized trial of thermal ablative therapy versus expandable metal stents in the palliative treatment of patients with esophageal carcinoma. *Gastrointest Endosc* 54:549, 2001.

DeMeester TR, Attwood SEA, et al: Surgical therapy in Barrett's esophagus. *Ann Surg* 212:528, 1990.

DeMeester TR, Barlow AP: Surgery and current management for cancer of the esophagus and cardia: Part II. *Curr Probl Surg* 25:535, 1988.

DeMeester TR: Esophageal carcinoma: Current controversies. *Semin Surg Oncol* 13:217, 1997.

DeMeester TR, Skinner DB: Polypoid sarcomas of the esophagus. *Ann Thorac Surg* 20:405, 1975.

DeMeester TR, Zaninotto G, Johansson KE: Selective therapeutic approach to cancer of the lower esophagus and cardia. *J Thorac Cardiovasc Surg* 95:42, 1988.

Duhaylongsod FG, Wolfe WG: Barrett's esophagus and adenocarcinoma of the esophagus and gastroesophageal junction. *J Thorac Cardiovasc Surg* 102:36, 1991.

Ell C, May A, Gossner L, et al: Endoscopic mucosal resection of early cancer and high grade dysplasia in Barrett's esophagus. *Gastroenterology* 118:670, 2001.

Ellis FH, Heatley GJ, Krosna MJ, Williamson WA, Balogh K: Esophagogastrectomy for carcinoma of the esophagus and cardia: A comparison of findings and results after standard resection in three consecutive 8 year time intervals, using improved staging criteria. *J Thorac Cardiovasc Surg* 113:836, 1997.

Frenken M: Best palliation in esophageal cancer; surgery, stenting, radiation or what? *Dis Esophagus* 14:120, 2001.

Fujita H, Kakegawa T, et al: Mortality and morbidity rates, postoperative course, quality of life, and prognosis after extended radical lymphadenectomy for esophageal cancer. *Ann Surg* 222:654, 1995.

Gomes MN, Kroll S, Spear SL: Mediastinal tracheostomy. *Ann Thorac Surg* 43:539, 1987.

Goodner JT: Treatment and survival in cancer of the cervical esophagus. *Am J Surg* 20:405, 1975.

Guernsey JM, Knudsen DF: Abdominal exploration in the evaluation of patients with carcinoma of the thoracic esophagus. *J Thorac Cardiovasc Surg* 59:62, 1970.

Hagen JA, DeMeester TR, Peters JH, et al: Curative resection for esophageal adenocarcinoma analysis of 100 en bloc esophagectomies. *Ann Surg* 234:520, 2001.

Heatley RV, Lewis MH, Williams RHP: Preoperative intravenous feeding: A controlled trial. *Postgrad Med J* 55:541, 1979.

Heimlich HJ: Carcinoma of the cervical esophagus. *J Thorac Cardiovasc Surg* 59:309, 1970.

Heitmiller RF, Sharma RR: Comparison of prevalence and resection rates in patients with esophageal squamous cell carcinoma and adenocarcinoma. *J Thorac Cardiovasc Surg* 112:130, 1996.

Hofstetter W, Swisher SG, Correa AM: Treatment outcomes of resected esophageal cancer. *Ann Surg* 236:376, 2002.

Hulscher JBF, Van Sandick JW, DeBoer AGEM, et al: Extended transthoracic resection compared with limited transhiatal resection for adenocarcinoma of the esophagus. *N Engl J Med* 347:1662, 2002.

Iijima K, Henrey E, Moriya A, et al: Dietary nitrate generates potentially mutagenic concentrations of nitric oxide at the gastroesophageal junction. *Gastroenterology* 122:1248, 2002.

Ikeda M, Natsugoe S, Ueno S, et al: Significant host and tumor related factors for predicting prognosis in patients with esophageal carcinoma. *Ann Surg* 238:197, 2003.

Jankowski JA, Wight NA, Meltzer SJ, et al: Molecular evolution of the metaplasia-dysplasia-adenocarcinoma sequence in the esophagus. *Am J Pathol* 154:965, 1999.

Johansson J, DeMeester TR, Hoger JA, et al: En bloc is superior to transhiatal esophagectomy for T3 N1 adenocarcinoma of the distal esophagus and GE junction. *Arch Surg* 139:627, 2004.

Kaklamanos IG, Walker GR, Ferry K, et al: Neoadjuvant treatment for resectable cancer of the esophagus and the gastroesophageal junction: A meta-analysis of randomized clinical trials. *Ann Surg Oncol* 10:754, 2003.

Krasna MJ, Reed CE, Nedzwiecki D, et al: CALBG 9380: A prospective trial of the feasibility of thoracoscopy/laparoscopy in staging esophageal cancer. *Ann Thorac Surg* 71:1073, 2001.

Kirby JD: Quality of life after esophagectomy: The patients' perspective. *Dis Esophagus* 12:168, 1999.

Kron IL, Joob AW, et al: Blunt esophagectomy and gastric interposition for tumors of the cervical esophagus and hypopharynx. *Am Surg* 52:140, 1986.

Lagergren J, Bergstrom R, Lindgren A, et al: Symptomatic gastroesophageal reflux as a risk factor for esophageal adenocarcinoma. *N Engl J Med* 340:825, 1999.

Lavin P, Hajdu SI, Foote FW Jr.: Gastric and extragastric leiomyoblastomas. *Cancer* 29:305, 1972.

Law SYK, Fok M, Wong J: Pattern of recurrence after oesophageal resection for cancer: Clinical implications. *Br J Surg* 83:107, 1996.

Law SYK, Fok M, et al: A comparison of outcomes after resection for squamous cell carcinomas and adenocarcinomas of the esophagus and cardia. *Surg Gynecol Obstet* 175:107, 1992.

Law S, Kwong DLW, Kwok KF, et al: Improvement in treatment results and long term survival of patients with esophageal cancer: Impact of chemoradiation and change in treatment strategy. *Ann Surg* 238:339, 2003.

Lerut T, Coosemans W, et al: Surgical treatment of Barrett's carcinoma. Correlations between morphologic findings and prognosis. *J Thorac Cardiovasc Surg* 107:1059, 1994.

Lerut T, De Leyn P, et al: Surgical strategies in esophageal carcinoma with emphasis on radical lymphadenectomy. *Ann Surg* 216:583, 1992.

Leuketich JD, Alvelo-Rivera M, Buenaventura PO, et al: Minimally invasive esophagectomy: Outcomes in 222 patients. *Ann Surg* 238:486, 2003.

Levine DS, Reid BJ: Endoscopic diagnosis of esophageal neoplasms. *Gastrointest Clin North Am* 2:395, 1992.

Lewis I: The surgical treatment of carcinoma of the esophagus with special reference to a new operation for the growths of the middle third. *Br J Surg* 34:18, 1946.

Logan A: The surgical treatment of carcinoma of the esophagus and cardia. *J Thorac Cardiovasc Surg* 46:150, 1963.

Lund O, Hasenkam JM, et al: Time related changes in characteristics of prognostic significance of carcinomas of the esophagus and cardia. *Br J Surg* 76:1301, 1989.

Maerz LL, Deveney CW, et al: Role of computed tomographic scans in the staging of esophageal and proximal gastric malignancies. *Am J Surg* 165:558, 1993.

McCort JJ: Esophageal carcinosarcoma and pseudosarcoma. *Radiology* 102:519, 1972.

Medical Research Council Oesophageal Working Party: Surgical resection with or without preoperative chemotherapy in oesophageal cancer: A randomized controlled trial. *Lancet* 359:1727, 2002.

Moore TC, Battersby JS, et al: Carcinosarcoma of the esophagus. *J Thorac Cardiovasc Surg* 45:281, 1963.

Murray GF, Wilcox BR, Starek P: The assessment of operability of esophageal carcinoma. *Ann Thorac Surg* 23:393, 1977.

Naunheim KS, Petruska PJ, et al: Preoperative chemotherapy and radiotherapy for esophageal carcinoma. *J Thorac Cardiovasc Surg* 103:887, 1992.

Nicks R: Colonic replacement of the esophagus. *Br J Surg* 54:124, 1967.

Nigro JJ, Hagen JA, DeMeester TR, et al: Occult esophageal adenocarcinoma: Extent of disease and implications for effective therapy. *Ann Surg* 230:433, 1999.

Orringer MB, Marshall B, Iannettoni MD: Transhiatal esophagectomy: Clinical experience and refinements. *Ann Surg* 230:392, 1999.

Orringer MB: Transhiatal esophagectomy without thoracotomy for carcinoma of the thoracic esophagus. *Ann Surg* 200:282, 1984.

Orringer MB, Skinner DB: Unusual presentations of primary and secondary esophageal malignancies. *Ann Thorac Surg* 11:305, 1971.

Pacifico RJ, Wang KK, Wongkeesong LM, et al: Combined endoscopic mucosal resection and photodynamic therapy versus esophagectomy for management of early adenocarcinoma of the esophagus. *Clin Gastroenterol Hepatol* 1:252, 2003.

Pera M, Cameron AJ, et al: Increasing incidence of adenocarcinoma of the esophagus and esophagogastric junction. *Gastroenterology* 104:510, 1993.

Pera M, Trastek VF, et al: Barrett's esophagus with high-grade dysplasia: An indication for esophagectomy? *Ann Thorac Surg* 54:199, 1992.

Pera M, Trastek VF, et al: Influence of pancreatic and biliary reflux on the development of esophageal carcinoma. *Ann Thorac Surg* 55:1386, 1993.

Peters JH, Clark GWB, et al: Outcome of adenocarcinoma arising in Barrett's esophagus in endoscopically surveyed and non-surveyed patients. *J Thorac Cardiovasc Surg* 108:813, 1994.

Peters JH, Hoeft SF, et al: Selection of patients for curative or palliative resection of esophageal cancer based on preoperative endoscopic ultrasound. *Arch Surg* 129:534, 1994.

Peters JH: Surgical treatment of esophageal adenocarcinoma: Concepts in evolution. *J Gastrointest Surg* 6:518, 2002.

Piccone VA, Ahmed N, et al: Esophagogastrectomy for carcinoma of the middle third of the esophagus. *Ann Thorac Surg* 28:369, 1979.

Pouliquen X, Levard H, et al: 5-Fluorouracil and cisplatin therapy after palliative surgical resection of squamous cell carcinoma of the esophagus. *Ann Surg* 223:127, 1996.

Rasanen JV, Sihvo EIT, Knuuti J, et al: Prospective analysis of accuracy of proton emission tomography, computed tomography and endoscopic ultrasonography in staging of adenocarcinoma of the esophagus and esophagogastric junction. *Ann Surg Oncol* 10:954, 2003.

Ravitch M: *A Century of Surgery.* Philadelphia: Lippincott, 1981, p 56.

Reed CE: Comparison of different treatments for unresectable esophageal cancer. *World J Surg* 19:828, 1995.

Reid BJ, Weinstein WM, et al: Endoscopic biopsy can detect high-grade dysplasia or early adenocarcinoma in Barrett's esophagus without grossly recognizable neoplastic lesions. *Gastroenterology* 94:81, 1988.

Ribeiro U Jr., Posner MC, et al: Risk factors for squamous cell carcinoma of the oesophagus. *Br J Surg* 83:1174, 1996.

Rice TW, Boyce GA, et al: Esophageal ultrasound and the preoperative staging of carcinoma of the esophagus. *J Thorac Cardiovasc Surg* 101:536, 1991.

Robertson CS, Mayberry JF, Nicholson JA: Value of endoscopic surveillance in the detection of neoplastic changes in Barrett's esophagus. *Br J Surg* 75:760, 1988.

Rösch T, Lorenz R, et al: Endosonographic diagnosis of submucosal upper gastrointestinal tract tumors. *Scand J Gastroenterol* 27:1, 1992.

Rosenberg JC, Budev H, et al: Analysis of adenocarcinoma in Barrett's esophagus utilizing a staging system. *Cancer* 55:1353, 1985.

Rosenberg JC, Franklin R, Steiger Z: Squamous cell carcinoma of the thoracic esophagus: An interdisciplinary approach. *Curr Probl Cancer* 5:1, 1981.

Saidi F, Abbassi A, et al: Endothoracic endoesophageal pull-through operation: A new approach to cancers of the esophagus and proximal stomach. *J Thorac Cardiovasc Surg* 102:43, 1991.

Sarr MG, Hamilton SR, et al: Barrett's esophagus: Its prevalence and association with adenocarcinoma in patients with symptoms of gastroesophageal reflux. *Am J Surg* 149:187, 1985.

Schottenfeld D: Epidemiology of cancer of the esophagus. *Semin Oncol* 11:92, 1984.

Silver CE: Surgical management of neoplasms of the larynx, hypopharynx and cervical esophagus. *Curr Probl Surg* 14:2, 1977.

Skinner DB, Dowlatshahi KD, DeMeester TR: Potentially curable carcinoma of the esophagus. *Cancer* 50:2571, 1982.

Skinner DB, Ferguson MK, Little AG: Selection of operation for esophageal cancer based on staging. *Ann Surg* 204:391, 1986.

Smith R, Gowing WFC: Carcinoma of the esophagus with histological appearances simulating a carcinosarcoma. *Br J Surg* 40:487, 1953.

Sonnenberg A, Fennerty MB: Medical decision analysis of chemoprevention against esophageal adenocarcinoma. *Gastroenterology* 124:1758, 2003.

Spechler SJ: Endoscopic surveillance for patients with Barrett's esophagus: Does the cancer risk justify the practice? *Ann Intern Med* 106:902, 1987.

Stout AP, Humphreys GH, Rottenberg LA: A case of carcinosarcoma of the esophagus. *AJR Radium Ther Nucl Med* 61:461, 1949.

Streitz JM Jr., Ellis FH Jr., et al: Adenocarcinoma in Barrett's esophagus. *Ann Surg* 213:122, 1991.

Talbert JL, Cantrell JR: Clinical and pathologic characteristics of carcinosarcoma of the esophagus. *J Thorac Cardiovasc Surg* 45:1, 1963.

Thomas PA: Physiologic sufficiency of regenerated lung lymphatics. *Ann Surg* 192:162, 1980.

Turnbull AD, Rosen P, et al: Primary malignant tumors of the esophagus other than typical epidermoid carcinoma. *Ann Thorac Surg* 15:463, 1973.

Urschel JD, Ashiku S, Thurer R, et al: Salvage or planned esophagectomy after chemoradiation for locally advanced esophageal cancer: A review. *Dis Esophagus* 16:60, 2003.

Vigneswaran WT, Trastek VK, et al: Extended esophagectomy in the management of carcinoma of the upper thoracic esophagus. *J Thorac Cardiovasc Surg* 107:901, 1994.

Walsh TN, Noonan N, et al: A comparison of multimodal therapy and surgery for esophageal adenocarcinoma. *N Engl J Med* 335:462, 1996.

Watson WP, Pool L: Cancer of the cervical esophagus. *Surgery* 23:893, 1948.

Benign Tumors and Cysts

Bardini R, Segalin A, et al: Videothoracoscopic enucleation of esophageal leiomyoma. *Am Thorac Surg* 54:576, 1992.

Bonavina L, Segalin A, et al: Surgical therapy of esophageal leiomyoma. *J Am Coll Surg* 181:257, 1995.

Esophageal Perforation

Brewer LA III, Carter R, et al: Options in the management of perforations of the esophagus. *Am J Surg* 152:62, 1986.

Bufkin BL, Miller JI Jr., Mansour KA: Esophageal perforation. Emphasis on management. *Ann Thorac Surg* 61:1447, 1996.

Chang C-H, Lin PJ, et al: One-stage operation for treatment after delayed diagnosis of thoracic esophageal perforation. *Ann Thorac Surg* 53:617, 1992.

Engum SA, Grosfeld JL, et al: Improved survival in children with esophageal perforation. *Arch Surg* 131:604, 1996.

Gouge TH, Depan HJ, Spencer FC: Experience with the Grillo pleural wrap procedure in 18 patients with perforation of the thoracic esophagus. *Ann Surg* 209:612, 1989.

Jones WG II, Ginsberg RJ: Esophageal perforation: A continuing challenge. *Ann Thorac Surg* 53:534, 1992.

Pate JW, Walker WA, et al: Spontaneous rupture of the esophagus: A 30-year experience. *Ann Thorac Surg* 47:689, 1989.

Reeder LB, DeFilippi VJ, Ferguson MK: Current results of therapy for esophageal perforation. *Am J Surg* 169:615, 1995.

Salo JA, Isolauri JO, et al: Management of delayed esophageal perforation with mediastinal sepsis. Esophagectomy or primary repair? *J Thorac Cardiovasc Surg* 106:1088, 1993.

Sawyer R, Phillips C, Vakil N: Short- and long-term outcome of esophageal perforation. *Gastrointest Endosc* 41:130, 1995.

Segalin A, Bonavina L, et al: Endoscopic management of inveterate esophageal perforations and leaks. *Surg Endosc* 10:928, 1996.

Weiman DS, Walker WA, et al: Noniatrogenic esophageal trauma. *Ann Thorac Surg* 59:845, 1995.

Whyte RI, Iannettoni MD, Orringer MB: Intrathoracic esophageal perforation. The merit of primary repair. *J Thorac Cardiovasc Surg* 109:140, 1995.

Caustic Injury

Anderson KD, Rouse TM, Randolph JG: A controlled trial of corticosteroids in children with corrosive injury of the esophagus. *N Engl J Med* 323:637, 1990.

Ferguson MK, Migliore M, et al: Early evaluation and therapy for caustic esophageal injury. *Am J Surg* 157:116, 1989.

Jeng L-BB, Chen H-Y, et al: Upper gastrointestinal tract ablation for patients with extensive injury after ingestion of strong acid. *Arch Surg* 129:1086, 1994.

Lahoti D, Broor SL, et al: Corrosive esophageal strictures. Predictors of response to endoscopic dilation. *Gastrointest Endosc* 41:196, 1995.

Popovici Z: About reconstruction of the pharynx with colon in extensive corrosive strictures. *Kurume Med J* 36:41, 1989.

Sugawa C, Lucas CE: Caustic injury of the upper gastrointestinal tract in adults: A clinical and endoscopic study. *Surgery* 106:802, 1989.

Wu M-H, Lai W-W: Esophageal reconstruction for esophageal strictures or resection after corrosive injury. *Ann Thorac Surg* 53:798, 1992.

Wu M-H, Lai W-W: Surgical management of extensive corrosive injuries of the alimentary tract. *Surg Gynecol Obstet* 177:12, 1993.

Zargar SA, Kochhar R, et al: The role of fiberoptic endoscopy in the management of corrosive ingestion and modified endoscopic classification of burns. *Gastrointest Endosc* 37:165, 1991.

Diaphragmatic Hernias

Bombeck TC, Dillard DH, Nyhus LM: Muscular anatomy of the gastro-esophageal junction and role of the phrenoesophageal ligament. *Ann Surg* 164:643, 1966.

Bonavina L, Evander A, et al: Length of the distal esophageal sphincter and competency of the cardia. *Am J Surg* 151:25, 1986.

Casbella F, Sinanan M, et al: Systematic use of gastric fundoplication in laparoscopic repair of paraesophageal hernias. *Am J Surg* 171:485, 1996.

Dalgaard JB: Volvulus of the stomach. *Acta Chir Scand* 103:131, 1952.

DeMeester TR, Bonavina L: Paraesophageal hiatal hernia, in Nyhus LM, Condon RE (eds): *Hernia*, 3rd ed. Philadelphia: Lippincott, 1989, p 684.

DeMeester TR, Lafontaine E, et al: The relationship of a hiatal hernia to the function of the body of the esophagus and the gastroesophageal junction. *J Thorac Cardiovasc Surg* 82:547, 1981.

Eliska O: Phreno-oesophageal membrane and its role in the development of hiatal hernia. *Acta Anat* 86:137, 1973.

Fuller CB, Hagen JA, et al: The role of fundoplication in the treatment of type II paraesophageal hernia. *J Thorac Cardiovasc Surg* 111:655, 1996.

Hashemi M, Peters JH, DeMeester TR, et al: Laparoscopic repair of large type III hiatal hernia: Objective follow-up reveals high recurrence rate. *J Am Coll Surg* 190:539, 2000.

Kahrilas PJ, Wu S, et al: Attenuation of esophageal shortening during peristalsis with hiatus hernia. *Gastroenterology* 109:1818, 1995.

Kleitsch WP: Embryology of congenital diaphragmatic hernia. I. Esophageal hiatus hernia. *Arch Surg* 76:868, 1958.

Menguy R: Surgical management of large paraesophageal hernia with complete intrathoracic stomach. *World J Surg* 12:415, 1988.

Myers GA, Harms BA, et al: Management of paraesophageal hernia with a selective approach to antireflux surgery. *Am J Surg* 170:375, 1995.

Patti MG, Goldberg HI, et al: Hiatal hernia size affects LES function, esophageal acid exposure, and the degree of mucosal injury. *Am J Surg* 171:182, 1996.

Pierre AF, Luketich JD, Fernando HC, et al: Results of laparoscopic repair of giant paraesophageal hernias: 200 Consecutive patients. *Ann Thorac Surg* 74:1909, 2002.

Postlethwait RW: *Surgery of the Esophagus.* New York: Appleton-Century Crofts, 1979, p 195.

Skinner DB, Belsey RHR: Surgical management of esophageal reflux and hiatus hernia: Long-term results with 1030 patients. *J Thorac Cardiovasc Surg* 53:33, 1967.

Stylopoulos N, Gazelle GS, Ratner DW. Paraesophageal hernias: Operation or observation. *Ann Surg* 236:492. 2002.

Walther B, DeMeester TR, et al: The effect of paraesophageal hernia on sphincter function and its implication on surgical therapy. *Am J Surg* 147:111, 1984.

Miscellaneous Esophageal Lesions

Burdick JS, Venu RP, Hogan WJ: Cutting the defiant lower esophageal ring. *Gastrointest Endosc* 39:616, 1993.

Burt M, Diehl W, et al: Malignant esophagorespiratory fistula: Management options and survival. *Ann Thorac Surg* 52:1222, 1991.

Chen MYM, Ott DJ, Donati DL: Correlation of lower esophageal mucosal ring and LES pressure. *Dig Dis Sci* 39:766, 1994.

D'Haens G, Rutgeerts P, et al: The natural history of esophageal Crohn's disease. Three patterns of evolution. *Gastrointest Endosc* 40:296, 1994.

Eckhardt VF, Kanzler G, Willems D: Single dilation of symptomatic Schatzki rings. A prospective evaluation of its effectiveness. *Dig Dis Sci* 37:577, 1992.

Klein HA, Wald A, et al: Comparative studies of esophageal function in systemic sclerosis. *Gastroenterology* 102:1551, 1992.

Mathisen DJ, Grillo HC, et al: Management of acquired nonmalignant tracheoesophageal fistula. *Ann Thorac Surg* 52:759, 1991.

Poirier NC, Taillefer R, et al: Antireflux operations in patients with scleroderma. *Ann Thorac Surg* 58:66, 1994.

Soudah HC, Hasler WL, Owyang C: Effect of octreotide on intestinal motility and bacterial overgrowth in scleroderma. *N Engl J Med* 325:1461, 1991.

Stagias JG, Ciarolla D, Campo S, et al: Vascular compression of the esophagus. A manometric and radiologic study. *Dig Dis Sci* 39:782, 1994.

Toskes PP: Hope for the treatment of intestinal scleroderma (Letter to the Editor). *N Engl J Med* 325:1508, 1991.

Wilcox CM, Straub RF: Prospective endoscopic characterization of cytomegalovirus esophagitis in AIDS. *Gastrointest Endosc* 40:481, 1994.

Techniques of Esophageal Reconstruction

Akiyama H: Esophageal reconstruction. Entire stomach as esophageal substitute. *Dis Esophagus* 8:7, 1995.

Banki F, Mason RJ, DeMeester SR, et al: Vagal sparing esophagectomy: A more physiologic alternative. *Ann Surg* 236:324, 2002.

Bonavina L, Anselmino M, et al: Functional evaluation of the intrathoracic stomach as an oesophageal substitute. *Br J Surg* 79:529, 1992.

Burt M, Scott A, et al: Erythromycin stimulates gastric emptying after esophagectomy with gastric replacement. A randomized clinical trial. *J Thorac Cardiovasc Surg* 111:649, 1996.

Cheng W, Heitmiller RF, Jones BJ: Subacute ischemia of the colon esophageal interposition. *Ann Thorac Surg* 57:899, 1994.

Curet-Scott MJ, Ferguson MK, et al: Colon interposition for benign esophageal disease. *Surgery* 102:568, 1987.

DeMeester TR, Johansson K-E, et al: Indications, surgical technique, and long-term functional results of colon interposition or bypass. *Ann Surg* 208:460, 1988.

DeMeester TR, Kauer WKH: Esophageal reconstruction. The colon as an esophageal substitute. *Dis Esophagus* 8:20, 1995.

Dexter SPL, Martin IG, McMahon MJ: Radical thoracoscopic esophagectomy for cancer. *Surg Endosc* 10:147, 1996.

Ellis FH Jr., Gibb SP: Esophageal reconstruction for complex benign esophageal disease. *J Thorac Cardiovasc Surg* 99:192, 1990.

Finley RJ, Lamy A, et al: Gastrointestinal function following esophagectomy for malignancy. *Am J Surg* 169:471, 1995.

Fok M, Cheng SWK, Wong J: Pyloroplasty versus no drainage in gastric replacement of the esophagus. *Am J Surg* 162:447, 1991.

Gossot D, Cattan P, Fritsch S: Can the morbidity of esophagectomy be reduced by the thoracoscopic approach? *Surg Endosc* 9:1113, 1995.

Heitmiller RF, Jones B: Transient diminished airway protection after transhiatal esophagectomy. *Am J Surg* 162:442, 1991.

Honkoop P, Siersema PD, et al: Benign anastomotic strictures after transhiatal esophagectomy and cervical esophagogastrostomy. Risk factors and management. *J Thorac Cardiovasc Surg* 111:1141, 1996.

Liebermann-Meffert DMI, Meier R, Siewert JR: Vascular anatomy of the gastric tube used for esophageal reconstruction. *Ann Thorac Surg* 54:1110, 1992.

Maier G, Jehle EC, Becker HD: Functional outcome following oesophagectomy for oesophageal cancer. A prospective manometric study. *Dis Esophagus* 8:64, 1995.

Naunheim KS, Hanosh J, et al: Esophagectomy in the septuagenarian. *Ann Thorac Surg* 56:880, 1993.

Nishihra T, Oe H, et al: Esophageal reconstruction. Reconstruction of the thoracic esophagus with jejunal pedicled segments for cancer of the thoracic esophagus. *Dis Esophagus* 8:30, 1995.

Patil NG, Wong J: Surgery in the "new" Hong Kong. *Arch Surg* 136:1415, 2001.

Peters JH, Kronson J, Bremner CG, DeMeester TR: Arterial anatomic considerations in colon interposition for esophageal replacement. *Arch Surg* 130:858, 1995.

Stark SP, Romberg MS, et al: Transhiatal versus transthoracic esophagectomy for adenocarcinoma of the distal esophagus and cardia. *Am J Surg* 172:478, 1996.

Valverde A, Hay JM, Fingerhut A, Elhadad A: Manual versus mechanical esophagogastric anastomosis after resection for carcinoma. A controlled trial. French Associations for Surgical Research. *Surgery* 120:476, 1996.

Watson T, DeMeester TR, Kauer WKH, Peters JH, Hagen JA: Esophagectomy for end stage benign esophageal disease. *J Thorac Cardiovasc Surg* 115:1241, 1998.

Wu M-H, Lai W-W: Esophageal reconstruction for esophageal strictures or resection after corrosive injury. *Ann Thorac Surg* 53:798, 1992.

INTRODUCTION

The stomach is a remarkable organ with important digestive, nutritional, and endocrine functions. It stores and facilitates the digestion and absorption of ingested food and it helps regulate appetite. Treatable diseases of the stomach are common and the stomach is accessible and relatively forgiving; thus it is a favorite therapeutic target. In order to provide intelligent diagnosis and treatment, the physician and surgeon must understand gastric anatomy, physiology, and pathophysiology. This includes a sound understanding of the mechanical, secretory, and endocrine processes through which the stomach accomplishes its important functions. It also includes a familiarity with the common benign and malignant gastric disorders of clinical significance, especially peptic ulcer and gastric cancer.

HISTORY

The history of gastric surgery would fill a large portion of any objective historical account on the origins of abdominal operations. The existence of gastric ulceration was acknowledged by Diocles of Carystos (350 B.C.), Celsus, and Galen (131–201 A.D.). Marcellus Donatus of Mantua first described gastric ulcer at autopsy in 1586 and Muralto described duodenal ulcer at autopsy in 1688. In 1737, Morgagni described both gastric and duodenal ulcer at autopsy. In 1975, archeologists reported perforated prepyloric ulcer as the cause of death in a well-preserved Chinese corpse from 167 B.C.

Guy de Chauliac described the closure of a penetrating gastric wound in 1363. Throughout the 1600 and 1700s there were numerous reports of surgeons performing gastrotomy to remove foreign bodies, mostly knives. Many of these patients recovered. In 1833 William Beaumont reported his seminal studies in gastrointestinal physiology, which were made possible by his meticulous study and care of Alexis St. Martin, who developed a gastric fistula from a left upper quadrant musket wound. In 1875, the first successful gastrostomy for feeding was reported by Sidney Jones in London. However, it was Maury of Philadelphia who is said to have performed this operation successfully to palliate esophageal stricture in 1869, after consultation with Dr. Samuel Gross, the founder of the American Surgical Association. Thereafter, several different techniques of gastrostomy, many still used today, were described by Witzel (1891), Stamm (1894), and Janeway (1913).

Interestingly, gastric resection in humans was attempted before pyloroplasty or gastrojejunostomy. Paen performed the first (unsuccessful) distal gastrectomy and gastroduodenostomy for cancer in 1879. The patient died 5 days later. In 1880, Rydygier resected a distal gastric cancer and the patient died 12 hours later. Billroth was the first surgeon to successfully resect the distal stomach. The patient, Therese Heller, had distal gastric cancer, and continuity was reestablished with a gastroduodenostomy (Billroth I) using interrupted

silk suture. The patient recovered, but died 4 months later with abdominal carcinomatosis. Although initially Billroth anastomosed the duodenum to the lesser curvature side of the gastric remnant, eventually he came to prefer the greater curvature side for gastroduodenostomy. In 1881 one of Billroth's pupils, Anton Wolfler, at the suggestion of Nicoladonia, a visiting surgeon from Innsbruck, performed loop gastrojejunostomy to palliate an obstructing distal gastric cancer. In 1884 Rydygier reported an unsuccessful gastrojejunostomy for benign gastric outlet obstruction, and in 1885 Billroth performed a successful distal gastrectomy and gastrojejunostomy (Billroth II) for gastric cancer. The first successful gastrectomy in the U.S. was performed in Philadelphia by Rodman.

In 1886, Heineke performed the first pyloroplasty. One of Billroth's pupils, Johann von Mikulicz-Radecki, performed the same operation 2 years later. Their technique persists today as the Heineke-Mikulicz pyloroplasty. In 1892, Jaboulay described the gastroduodenostomy (pylorus remains intact), which today bears the moniker Jaboulay pyloroplasty. Shortly thereafter, Kocher described the mobilization of the duodenum which bears his name. In 1902, Finney from Baltimore described his pyloroplasty, a modification of the Jaboulay with the distal gastrotomy extended well into the duodenum, transecting the pylorus and closed with a gastroduodenostomy.

In the early decades of the 1900s, von Haberer and Finsterer touted subtotal gastrectomy as a better ulcer operation than gastrojejunostomy. By 1940 this was the operation of choice for peptic ulcer in the U.S. In 1943, Dragstedt and Owen described transthoracic truncal vagotomy to treat peptic ulcer disease. By the early 1950s it was well recognized that some patients developed gastric stasis after this procedure, and transabdominal truncal vagotomy and drainage (pyloroplasty or gastrojejunostomy) became a standard ulcer operation. In 1952, Farmer and Smithwick described good results with truncal vagotomy and hemigastrectomy for peptic ulcer. This evolved into truncal vagotomy and antrectomy, an operation which had a much lower recurrence rate than subtotal gastrectomy, and did not have the adverse nutritional consequences associated with the small gastric remnant after the latter operation. Vagotomy and antrectomy were described by Edwards and Herrington from Nashville in 1953. In 1957, Griffith and Harkins from Seattle described parietal cell vagotomy (highly selective vagotomy) for the elective treatment of peptic ulcer disease. Finally, between 1980 and 2000 there has been a growing worldwide awareness that a thorough and anatomic lymphadenectomy may improve survival in patients with gastric cancer.

ANATOMY

Embryology

During the fifth week of gestation the stomach arises as a dilatation in the tubular embryonic foregut (Fig. 25-1). It assumes its normal asymmetric shape and position by the end of the seventh week through descent, rotation, and progressive dilation, with disproportionate elongation of the greater curvature. It is likely that there is a congenital predisposition to some unusual benign gastric problems such as diverticulum or massive hiatal hernia with abnormal gastric rotation and fixation.

Gross Anatomy

Anatomic Relationships and Gross Morphology

The stomach is readily recognizable as the asymmetrical, pear-shaped, most proximal abdominal organ of the digestive tract

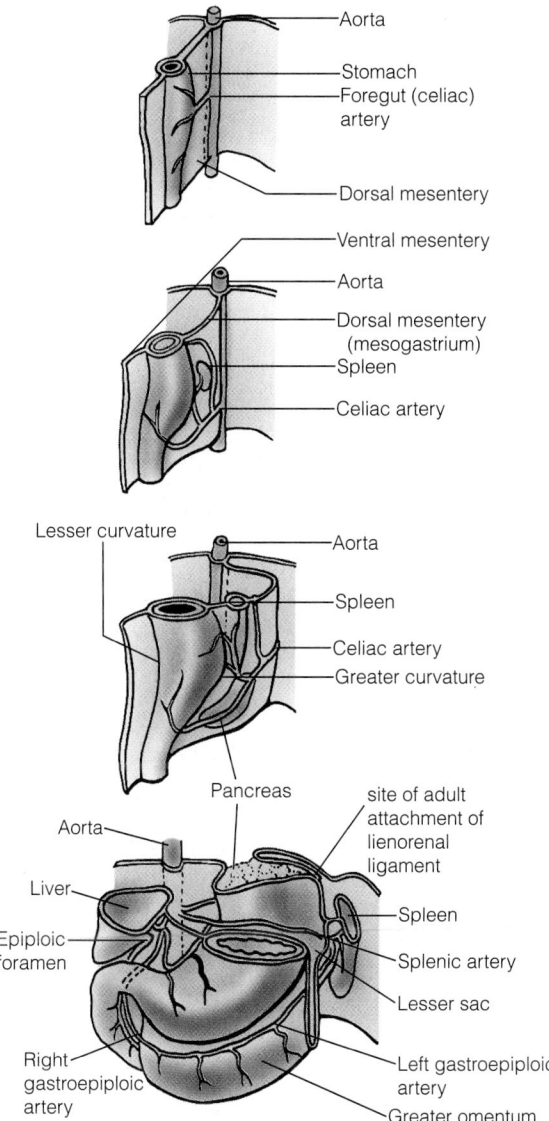

FIG. 25-1. Embryology of the stomach. (*Reproduced with permission from Moore KL: The Developing Human. Philadelphia: Saunders, 1974, p 175.*)

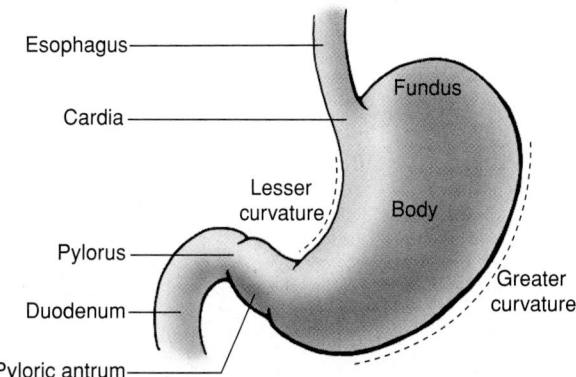

FIG. 25-2. Anatomic regions of the stomach [*Reproduced with permission from Mercer DW, Liu TH, Castaneda A: Anatomy and physiology of the stomach, in Zuidema GD, Yeo CJ (eds): Shackelford's Surgery of the Alimentary Tract, 5th ed., Vol. II. Philadelphia: Saunders, 2002, p 3.*]

beginning of the antrum, which comprises the distal 25 to 30% of the stomach.

The organs that commonly abut the stomach are the liver, colon, spleen, pancreas, and occasionally the kidney (Fig. 25-3). The left lateral segment of the liver usually covers a large part of the anterior stomach. Inferiorly, the stomach is attached to the transverse colon by the gastrocolic omentum. The lesser curvature is tethered to the liver by the hepatogastric ligament, also referred to as the lesser omentum. Posterior to the stomach is the lesser omental bursa and the pancreas.

Arterial and Venous Blood Supply

The stomach is the most richly vascularized portion of the alimentary canal. Both the quantity of blood delivered to the stomach and the richness of the intramural gastric vascular anastomotic network are impressive. The large majority of the gastric blood supply is from the celiac axis via four named arteries (Fig. 25-4). The left and right gastric arteries form an anastomotic arcade along the lesser curvature, and the right and left gastroepiploic arteries form an arcade along the greater gastric curvature. The consistently largest artery to the stomach is the left gastric artery, which usually arises directly from the celiac trunk and divides into an ascending and descending branch along the lesser gastric curvature. Approximately 15% of the time, the left gastric artery supplies an aberrant vessel which travels in the gastrohepatic ligament (lesser omentum) to the left side of the liver. Rarely, this is the only arterial blood supply to this part of the liver, and inadvertent ligation may lead to clinically significant hepatic ischemia. The second largest artery to the stomach is usually the right gastroepiploic artery, which arises fairly consistently from the gastroduodenal artery behind the first portion of the duodenum. The left gastroepiploic artery arises from the splenic artery, and together with the right gastroepiploic artery, forms the rich gastroepiploic arcade along the greater curvature. The right gastric artery usually arises from the hepatic artery near the pylorus and hepatoduodenal ligament, and runs proximally along the distal stomach. In the fundus along the proximal greater curvature, the short gastric arteries and veins arise from the splenic circulation. There also may be vascular branches to the proximal stomach from the phrenic circulation.

The veins draining the stomach generally parallel the arteries. The left gastric (coronary vein) and right gastric veins usually drain into the portal vein, though occasionally the coronary vein drains

(Fig. 25-2). The part of the stomach attached to the esophagus is called the cardia. Just proximal to the cardia at the gastroesophageal (GE) junction is the anatomically indistinct but physiologically demonstrable lower esophageal sphincter. At the distal end, the pyloric sphincter connects the stomach to the proximal duodenum. The stomach is relatively fixed at these points, but the large midportion is quite mobile.

The superior-most part of the stomach is the distensible floppy fundus, bounded superiorly by the diaphragm and laterally by the spleen. The angle of His is where the fundus meets the left side of the GE junction. Generally the inferior extent of the fundus is considered to be the horizontal plane of the GE junction, where the body (corpus) of the stomach begins. The body of the stomach contains most of the parietal (oxyntic) cells, some of which are also present in the cardia and fundus. The body is bounded on the right by the relatively straight lesser curvature and on the left by the more curved greater curvature. At the angularis incisura, the lesser curvature turns rather abruptly to the right, marking the anatomic

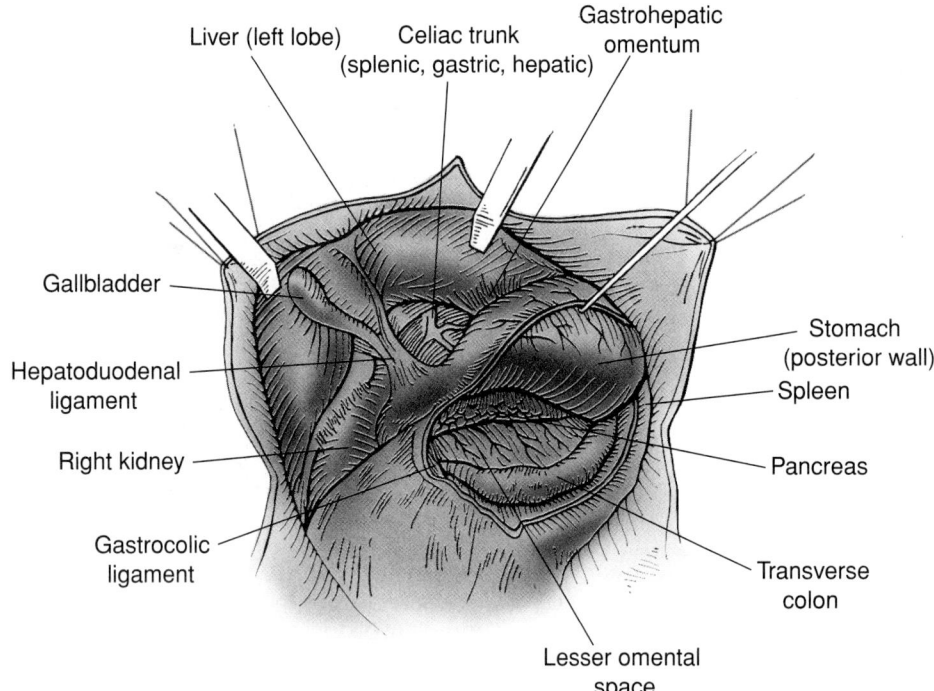

FIG. 25-3. Anatomic relationships of the stomach. [*Reproduced with permission from Mercer DW, Liu TH, Castaneda A: Anatomy and physiology of the stomach, in Zuidema GD, Yeo CJ (eds): Shackelford's Surgery of the Alimentary Tract, 5th ed., Vol. II. Philadelphia: Saunders, 2002, p 3.*]

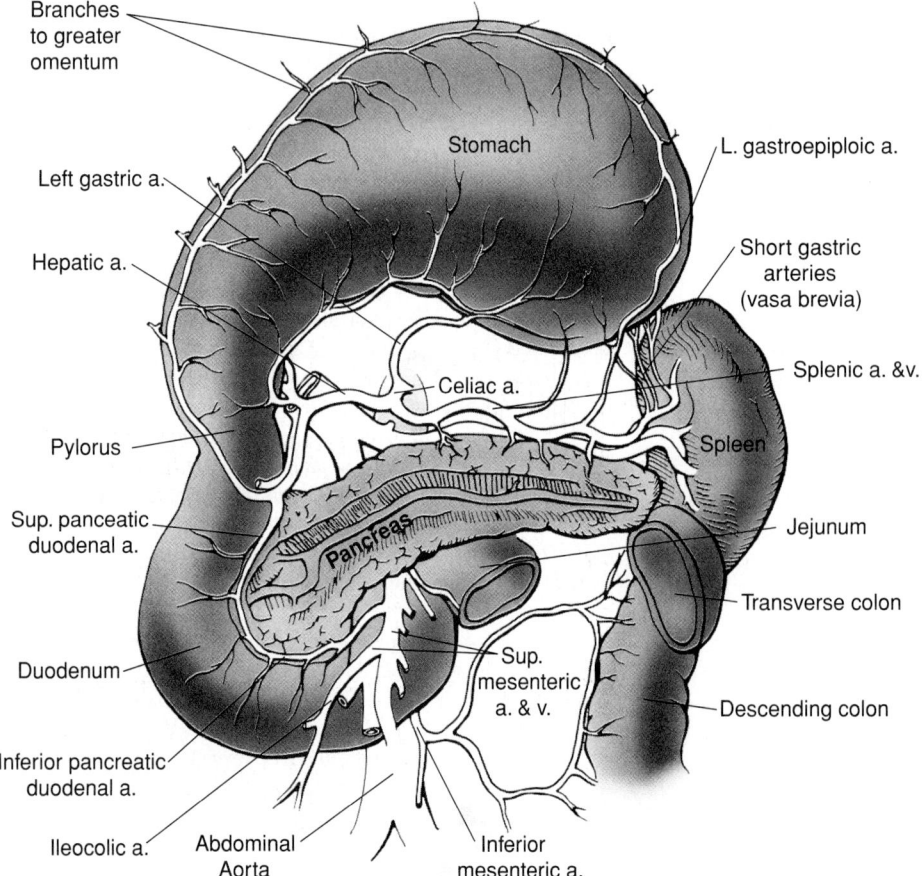

FIG. 25-4. Arterial blood supply to the stomach. [*Reproduced with permission from Mercer DW, Liu TH, Castaneda A: Anatomy and physiology of the stomach, in Zuidema GD, Yeo CJ (eds): Shackelford's Surgery of the Alimentary Tract, 5th ed., Vol. II. Philadelphia: Saunders, 2002, p 3.*]

into the splenic vein. The right gastroepiploic vein drains into the superior mesenteric vein near the inferior border of the pancreatic neck, and the left gastroepiploic vein drains into the splenic vein.

The richness of the gastric blood supply and the extensiveness of the anastomotic connections have some important clinical implications including: (1) erosion of a peptic ulcer or gastric cancer into a large perigastric vessel sometimes causes life-threatening hemorrhage; (2) because of the rich venous interconnections, a distal splenorenal shunt, which connects the distal end of the divided splenic vein to the side of the left renal vein, can effectively decompress esophagogastric varices in patients with portal hypertension; and (3) if necessary, at least two of the four named gastric arteries may be occluded or ligated with impunity. This is done routinely when the stomach is mobilized and pedicellated on the right gastric and right gastroepiploic vessels to reach into the neck as an esophageal replacement (see Chapter 24).

Lymphatic Drainage

Generally speaking, the gastric lymphatics parallel the blood vessels (Fig. 25-5). The cardia and medial half of the corpus commonly drain to nodes along the left gastric and celiac axis. The lesser curvature side of the antrum usually drains to the right gastric and pyloric nodes, while the greater curvature half of the distal stomach drains to the nodes along the right gastroepiploic chain. The proximal greater curvature side of the stomach usually drains into nodes along the left gastroepiploic or splenic hilum. The nodes along both the greater and lesser curvature commonly drain into the celiac nodal basin. There is a rich anastomotic network of lymphatics that drain the stomach, often in a somewhat unpredictable fashion. Thus a tumor arising in the distal stomach could give rise to positive lymph nodes in the splenic hilum. The rich intramural plexus of lymphatics and veins accounts for the fact that there may be microscopic evidence of malignant cells several centimeters from the resection margin of gross disease.

Extensive and meticulous lymphadenectomy is considered by many (particularly in Asia, but also in some centers in the U.S.) to be an important part of the operation for gastric cancer. Surgeons and pathologists have numbered the primary and secondary lymph node groups to which the stomach drains (Fig. 25-6).

Innervation

Both the extrinsic and intrinsic innervation of the stomach play an important role in gastric secretory and motor function. The vagus nerves provide the extrinsic parasympathetic innervation to the stomach, and acetylcholine is the most important neurotransmitter. From the vagal nucleus in the floor of the fourth cerebral ventricle, the vagus traverses the neck in the carotid sheath and enters the mediastinum, where it gives off the recurrent laryngeal nerve and divides into several branches around the esophagus. These branches come together again above the esophageal hiatus and form the *left* (*anterior*) and *right* (*posterior*) vagal trunks (mnemonic LARP). Near the gastroesophageal junction the anterior vagus sends a branch (or branches) to the liver in the gastrohepatic ligament, and continues along the lesser curvature as the anterior nerve of Latarjet (Fig. 25-7). Similarly, the posterior vagus sends branches to the celiac plexus and continues along the posterior lesser curvature. The nerves of Latarjet send segmental branches to the body of the stomach before they terminate near the angularis incisura as the "crow's foot," sending branches to the antropyloric region. There may be additional branches to the distal stomach and pylorus which travel near the right gastric and/or gastroepiploic arteries. In 50% of patients there are more than two vagal nerves at the esophageal hiatus. The branch that the posterior vagus sends to the posterior fundus is termed the criminal nerve of Grassi. This branch typically arises above the esophageal hiatus and is easily missed during truncal or highly selective vagotomy. Vagal fibers originating in the brain synapse with neurons in Auerbach's myenteric plexus and Meissner's submucosal plexus. Although clinicians are accustomed to thinking about the vagus nerves as important efferent nerves (i.e., carrying stimuli to the viscera), it is important to consider the fact that fully 75% of the axons contained in the vagal trunks are afferent (i.e., carrying stimuli from the viscera to the brain).

The extrinsic sympathetic nerve supply to the stomach originates at spinal levels T5 through T10 and travels in the splanchnic nerves to the celiac ganglion. Postganglionic sympathetic nerves then travel from the celiac ganglion to the stomach along the blood vessels.

Neurons in the myenteric and submucosal plexuses constitute the intrinsic nervous system of the stomach. There may be more

FIG. 25-5. Lymphatic drainage of the stomach. [*Reproduced with permission from Ritchie WP Jr.: Benign diseases of the stomach and duodenum, in Ritchie WP, Steele G, Dean RH (eds): General Surgery, Philadelphia: Lippincott, 1995, p 117.*]

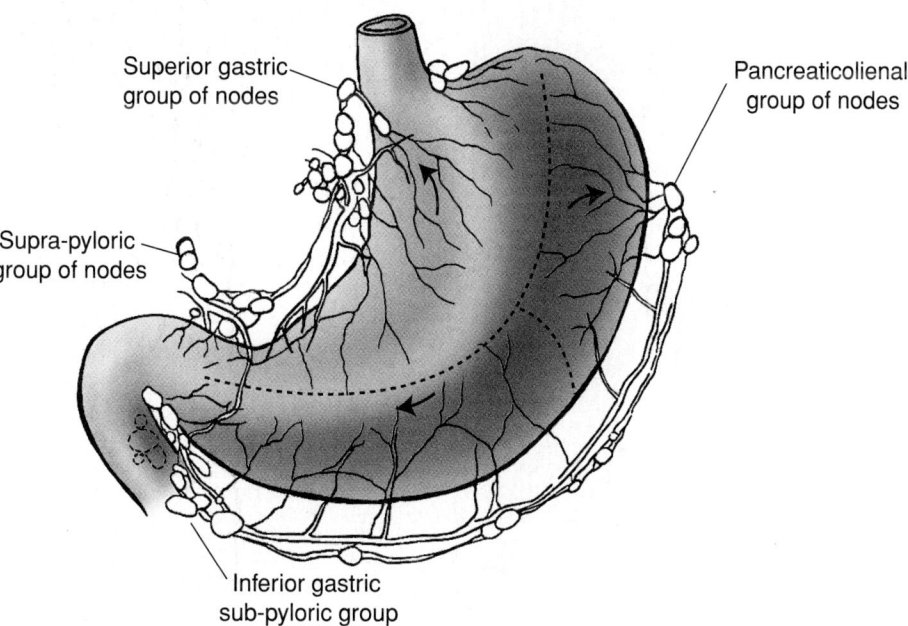

Superior gastric group of nodes

Pancreaticolienal group of nodes

Supra-pyloric group of nodes

Inferior gastric sub-pyloric group

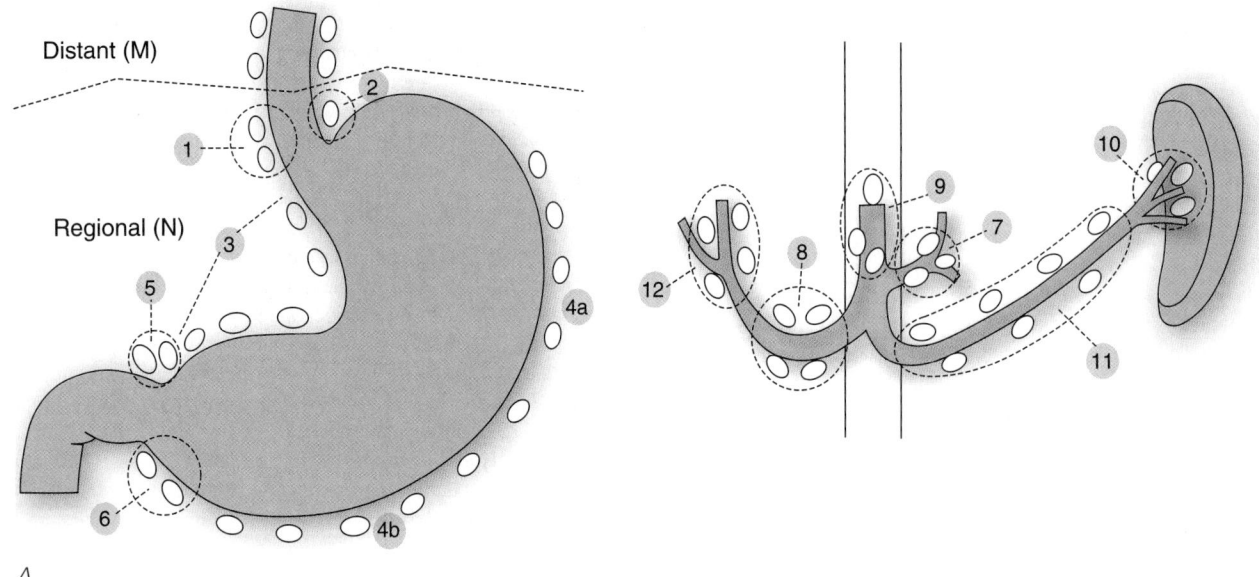

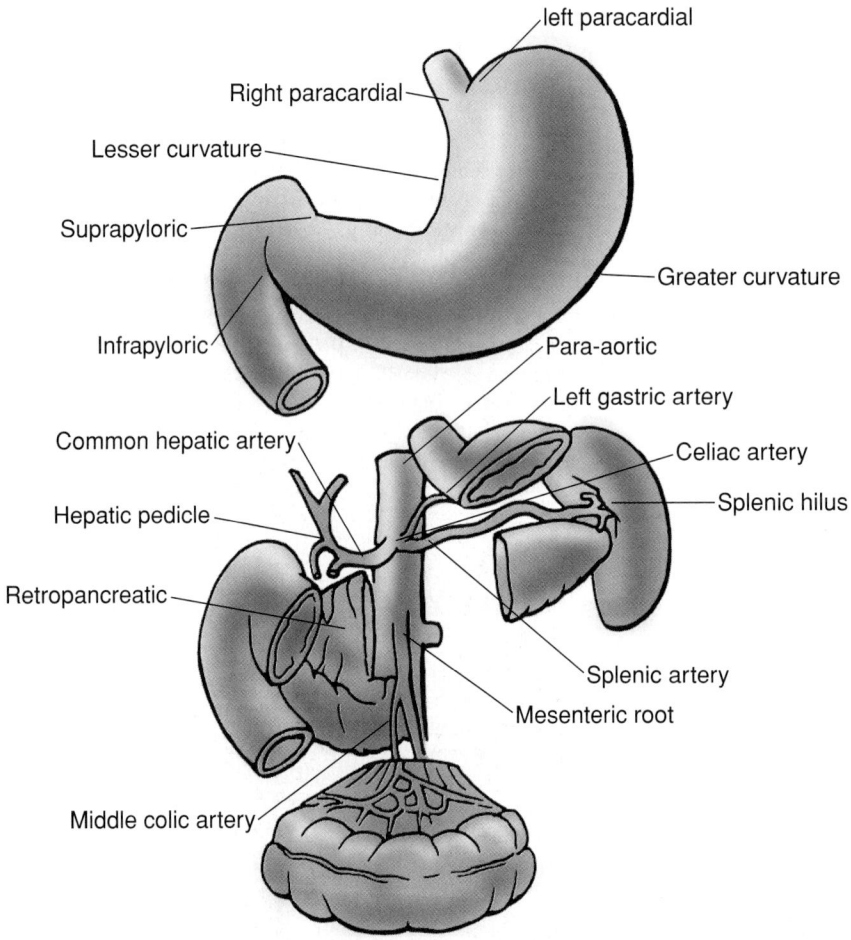

FIG. 25-6. Lymph node stations draining the stomach. *A.* Lymph node stations according to the Japanese Research Society for Gastric Cancer [*Reproduced with permission from Leung WK et al: Tumors of the stomach, in Yamada T, et al (eds): Textbook of Gastroenterology, 4th ed. Philadelphia: Lippincott, Williams & Wilkins, 2003, p 1416.*] *B.* Level 3 lymphadenectomy in stations shown in 25–6A, in addition to lymph nodes at mesenteric root, along middle colic artery, and in retropancreatic space.

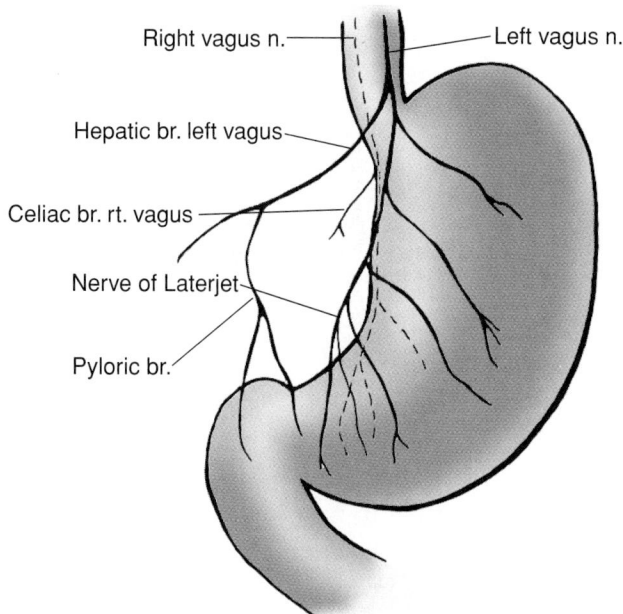

FIG. 25-7. Vagal innervation of the stomach. [Reproduced with permission from Mercer DW, Liu TH, Castaneda A: Anatomy and physiology of the stomach, in Zuidema GD, Yeo CJ (eds): Shackelford's Surgery of the Alimentary Tract, 5th ed., Vol. II. Philadelphia: Saunders, 2002, p 3.]

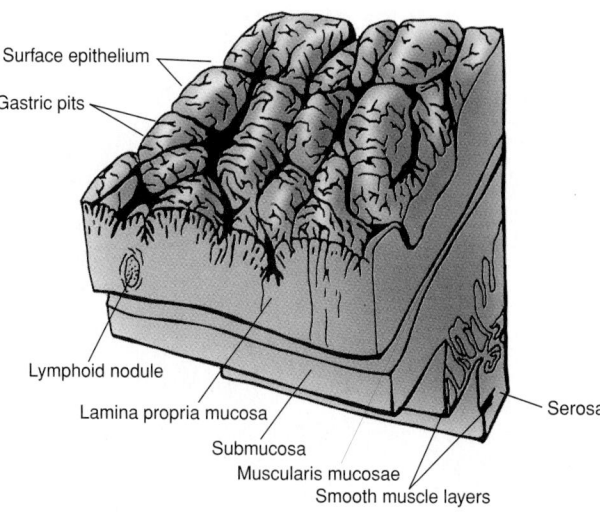

FIG. 25-8. Layers of the gastric wall. [Reproduced with permission from Mercer DW, Liu TH, Castaneda A: Anatomy and physiology of the stomach, in Zuidema GD, Yeo CJ (eds): Shackelford's Surgery of the Alimentary Tract, 5th ed., Vol. II. Philadelphia: Saunders, 2002, p 3.]

intrinsic gastric neurons than extrinsic neurons, but their function is poorly understood.

It is clearly a gross oversimplification (and most likely incorrect) to think of the vagus as the cholinergic system and the sympathetic system as the adrenergic system of innervation. Although acetylcholine is an important neurotransmitter mediating vagal function, and epinephrine is important in the sympathetic nerves, both systems (as well as the intrinsic neurons) have various and diverse

neurotransmitters including cholinergic, adrenergic, and peptidergic (e.g., substance P and somatostatin).

Histology

There are four distinct layers of the gastric wall: mucosa, submucosa, muscularis propria, and serosa (Fig. 25-8). The inner layer of the stomach is the mucosa, which is lined with columnar epithelial cells of various types. Beneath the basement membrane of the epithelial cells is the lamina propria, which contains connective tissue, blood vessels, nerve fibers, and inflammatory cells. Beneath the lamina propria is a thin muscle layer called the muscularis mucosa. The epithelium, lamina propria, and muscularis mucosa constitute

FIG. 25-9. Gastric mucosa. (Reproduced with permission from Bloom W, Fawcett DW: A Textbook of Histology. Philadelphia: Saunders, 1975, p 639.)

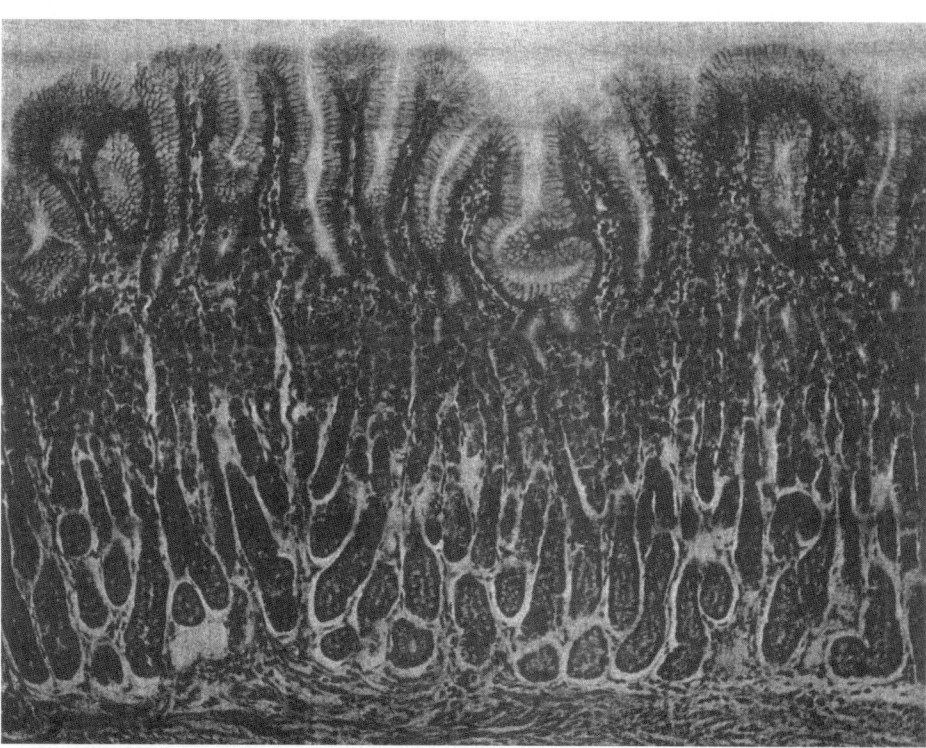

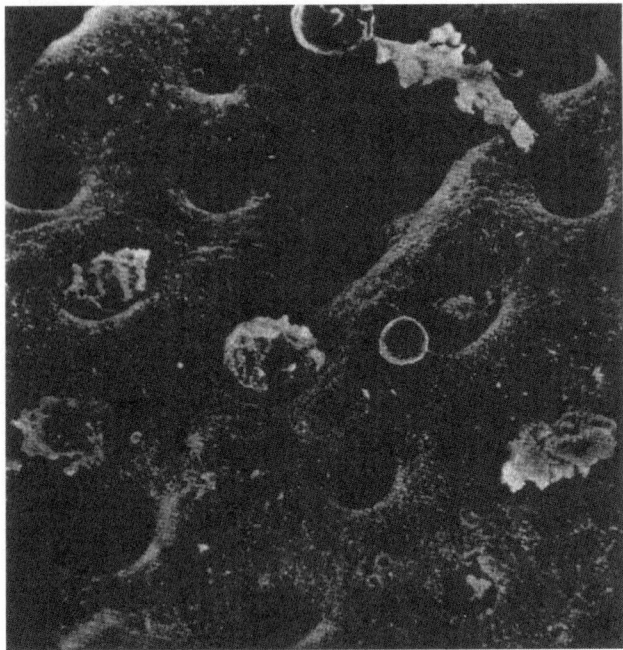

FIG. 25-10. *Scanning electron micrograph of the gastric surface (x400). [Reproduced with permission from Ashley SW, Evoy D, Daly JM: Stomach, in Schwartz SI (ed): Principles of Surgery, 7th ed. New York: McGraw-Hill, 1999, p 1181.]*

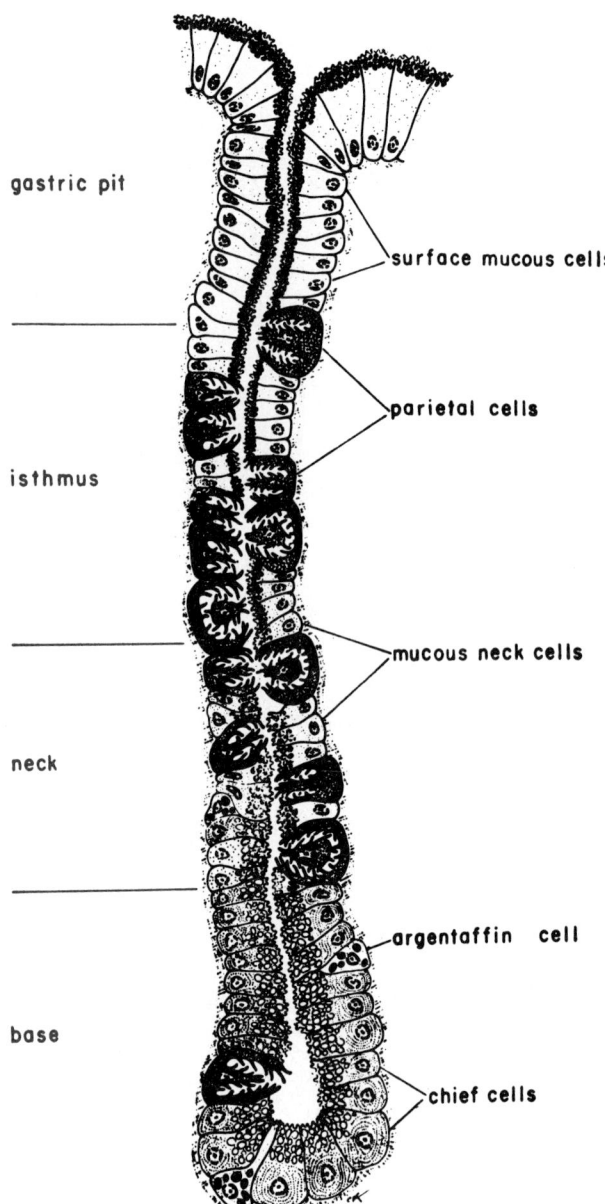

FIG. 25-11. *Gastric gland from the body of the stomach. [Reproduced with permission from Ashley SW, Evoy D, Daly JM: Stomach, in Schwartz SI (ed): Principles of Surgery, 7th ed. New York: McGraw-Hill, 1999, p 1181.]*

the mucosa (Fig. 25-9). The epithelium of the gastric mucosa is columnar glandular. A scanning electron micrograph shows a smooth mucosal carpet punctuated by the openings of the gastric glands (Fig. 25-10). The gastric glands are lined with different types of epithelial cells, depending upon their location in the stomach (Fig. 25-11; Table 25-1). There are also endocrine cells present in the gastric glands. Progenitor cells at the base of the glands differentiate and replenish sloughed cells on a regular basis. Throughout the stomach, the carpet consists primarily of mucus-secreting surface epithelial cells that extend down into the gland pits for variable distances. These cells also secrete bicarbonate and play an important role in protecting the stomach from injury due to acid, pepsin, and/or ingested irritants (see below). In fact, all epithelial cells of the stomach (except the endocrine cells) contain carbonic anhydrase and are capable of producing bicarbonate.

In the cardia, the gastric glands are branched and secrete primarily mucus and bicarbonate, but not much acid. In the fundus and body, the glands are more tubular and the pits are deep. Parietal and chief cells are common in these glands (see Fig. 25-11). Histamine-secreting enterochromaffin-like (ECL) cells and somatostatin-secreting D cells are also found. Parietal cells secrete acid and intrinsic factor into the gastric lumen, and bicarbonate into the intercellular space. They have a characteristic ultrastructural appearance with secretory canaliculi (deep invaginations of the surface membrane), and cytoplasmic tubulovesicles containing the acid-producing apparatus H^+/K^+-ATPase (proton pump) (Fig. 25-12). There are numerous mitochondria. When the parietal cell is stimulated, the cytoplasmic tubulovesicles fuse with the membrane of the secretory canaliculus; when acid production ceases the process is reversed. Arguably, the only truly essential substance produced by the stomach is produced by the parietal cell (i.e., intrinsic factor). Parietal cells tend to occupy the midportion of the gastric glands found in the corpus of the stomach.

Chief cells (also called zymogenic cells) secrete pepsinogen, which is activated at a pH below 2.5. They tend to be clustered toward the base of the gastric glands and have a low columnar shape. Ultrastructurally, chief cells have the characteristics of protein-synthesizing cells: basal granular endoplasmic reticulum, supranuclear Golgi apparatus, and apical zymogen granules (Fig. 25-13). When stimulated, the chief cells produce two immunologically distinct proenzyme forms of pepsinogen: pepsinogen I and II. These proenzymes are activated in an acidic luminal environment. Chief cells also produce lipase.

In the antrum, the gastric glands are again more branched and shallow, parietal cells are rare, and gastrin-secreting G cells and somatostatin-secreting D cells are present. A variety of hormone-secreting cells are present in various proportions throughout the gastric mucosa (Fig. 25-14). Histologic analysis suggests that in the normal stomach, 13% of the epithelial cells are oxyntic (parietal) cells, 44% are chief (zymogenic cells), 40% are mucous cells, and 3% are endocrine cells. In general terms, the antrum produces gastrin

Table 25-1
Epithelial Cells of the Stomach

Cell Type	Distinctive Ultrastructural Features	Major Functions
Surface-foveolar mucous cells	Apical stippled granules up to 1 μm in diameter	Production of neutral glycoprotein and bicarbonate to form a gel on the gastric luminal surface; neutralization of hydrochloric acid[a];
Mucous neck cell	Heterogeneous granules 1–2 μm in diameter dispersed throughout the cytoplasm	Progenitor cell for all other gastric epithelial cells; glycoprotein production; production of pepsinogens I and II
Oxyntic (parietal) cell	Surface membrane invaginations (canaliculi); tubulovesicle structures; numerous mitochondria;	Production of hydrochloric acid production of intrinsic factor production of bicarbonate
Chief cell	Moderately dense apical granules up to 2 μm in diameter; prominent supranuclear Golgi apparatus; extensive basolateral granular endoplasmic reticulum	Production of pepsinogens I and II, and of lipase
Cardiopyloric mucous cell	Mixture of granules like those in mucous neck and chief cells; extensive basolateral granular endoplasmic reticulum	Production of glycoprotein Production of pepsinogen II
Endocrine cells	See Figure 25-14	

[a]Bicarbonate is probably produced by other gastric epithelial cells in addition to surface-foveolar mucous cells.
SOURCE: Reproduced with permission from Antonioli DA, Madara JL, in Ming SC, Goldman H (eds): *Pathology of the Gastrointestinal Tract.* Baltimore: Williams & Wilkins, 1998, p 13.

but not acid, and the proximal stomach produces acid but not gastrin; however, it is important to recognize two facts: (1) the border between the corpus and antrum migrates proximally with age (especially on the lesser curvature side of the stomach), and (2) there are a few parietal cells in the antrum.

Deep to the mucosa is the submucosa, which is rich in branching blood vessels, lymphatics, collagen, various inflammatory cells, autonomic nerve fibers, and ganglion cells of Meissner's autonomic submucosal plexus. The collagen-rich submucosa gives strength to gastrointestinal anastomoses. The mucosa and submucosa are folded into the grossly visible gastric rugae, which tend to flatten out as the stomach becomes distended.

Below the submucosa is the thick muscularis propria (also referred to as the muscularis externa), which consists of an incomplete inner oblique layer, a complete middle circular layer (continuous with the esophageal circular muscle and the circular muscle of the pylorus), and a complete outer longitudinal layer (continuous with the longitudinal layer of the esophagus and duodenum). Within the muscularis propria is the rich network of autonomic ganglia and nerves that make up Auerbach's myenteric plexus.

The outer layer of the stomach is the serosa, also known as the visceral peritoneum. This layer provides significant tensile strength to gastric anastomoses. When tumors originating in the mucosa penetrate and breach the serosa, microscopic or gross peritoneal metastases are common, presumably from shedding of tumor cells which would not have occurred if the serosa had not been penetrated. In this way, the serosa may be thought of as a sort of outer envelope of the stomach.

PHYSIOLOGY

The stomach stores food and facilitates digestion through a variety of secretory and motor functions. Important secretory functions include the production of acid, pepsin, intrinsic factor, mucus, and a variety of gastrointestinal (GI) hormones. Important motor functions

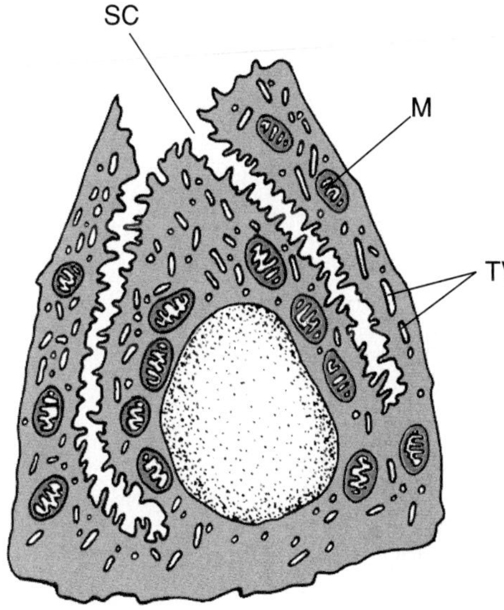

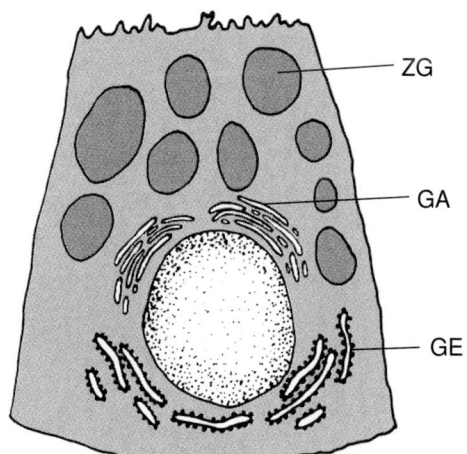

FIG. 25-12. Ultrastructural features of the parietal (oxyntic) cell. [Reproduced with permission from Antonioli DA, Madara JL: Functional anatomy of the gastrointestinal tract, in Ming S-C, Goldman H (eds): Pathology of the Gastrointestinal Tract, 2nd ed. Baltimore: Williams & Wilkins, 1998, p 13.] M = mitochondria; SC = secretory canaliculus; TV = tubulovesicle.

FIG. 25-13. Ultrastructural features of the chief (zymogenic) cell. [Reproduced with permission from Antonioli DA, Madara JL: Functional anatomy of the gastrointestinal tract, in Ming S-C, Goldman H (eds): Pathology of the Gastrointestinal Tract, 2nd ed. Baltimore: Williams & Wilkins, 1998, p 13.] GA = golgi apparatus; GE = granular endoplasmic reticulum; ZG = zymogen granule.

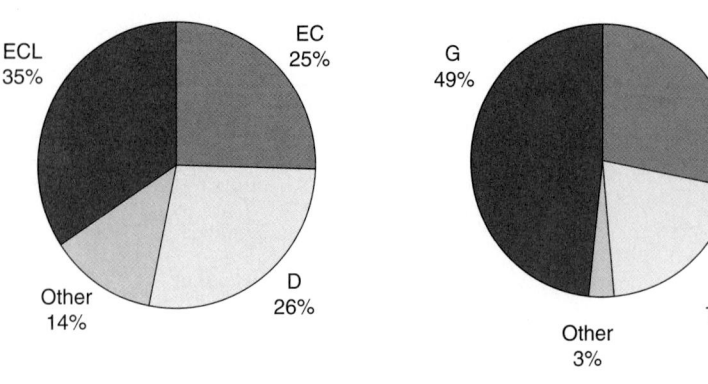

Oxyntic Mucosa   **Pyloric Mucosa**

FIG. 25-14. *Endocrine cells of the stomach. [Reproduced with permission from Feldman M: Gastric secretion, in Feldman M et al (eds): Sleisenger and Fordtran's Gastrointestinal and Liver Disease, 7th ed. Philadelphia: Saunders, 2002, p 715.]* ECL = enterochromaffin-like (histamine); EC = enterochromaffin serotonin; D = somatostatin; G = gastrin.

include food storage (receptive relaxation and accommodation), grinding and mixing, controlled emptying of ingested food, and periodic interprandial "housekeeping."

Acid Secretion

Hydrochloric acid in the stomach hastens both the physical and (with pepsin) the biochemical breakdown of ingested food. In an acidic environment, pepsin and acid facilitate proteolysis. Gastric acid also inhibits the proliferation of ingested bacteria, which probably protects against both infectious gastroenteritides and the nutritional side effects of intestinal bacterial overgrowth. When it enters the duodenum, gastric acid stimulates secretin release.

Parietal Cell

The parietal cell is stimulated to secrete acid (Fig. 25-15) when one or more of three membrane receptor types is stimulated by acetylcholine (from vagal nerve fibers), gastrin (from D cells), or

histamine (from ECL cells). The enzyme H^+/K^+-ATPase is the proton pump. It is stored within the intracellular tubulovesicles and is the final common pathway for gastric acid secretion. When the parietal cell is stimulated, there is a cytoskeletal rearrangement and fusion of the tubulovesicles with the apical membrane of the secretory canaliculus. The heterodimer assembly of the enzyme subunits into the microvilli of the secretory canaliculus results in acid secretion, with extracellular potassium being exchanged for cytosolic hydrogen. Although electro-neutral, this is an energy-requiring process since the hydrogen is secreted against a gradient of at least 1 millionfold, which explains why the parietal cell is the most mitochondria-dense mammalian cell (about one third by volume). During acid production, potassium and chloride are also secreted into the secretory canaliculus through separate channels, providing potassium for the H^+/K^+-ATPase, and chloride for the secreted hydrogen.

The normal human stomach contains approximately 1 billion parietal cells, and total gastric acid production is proportional to

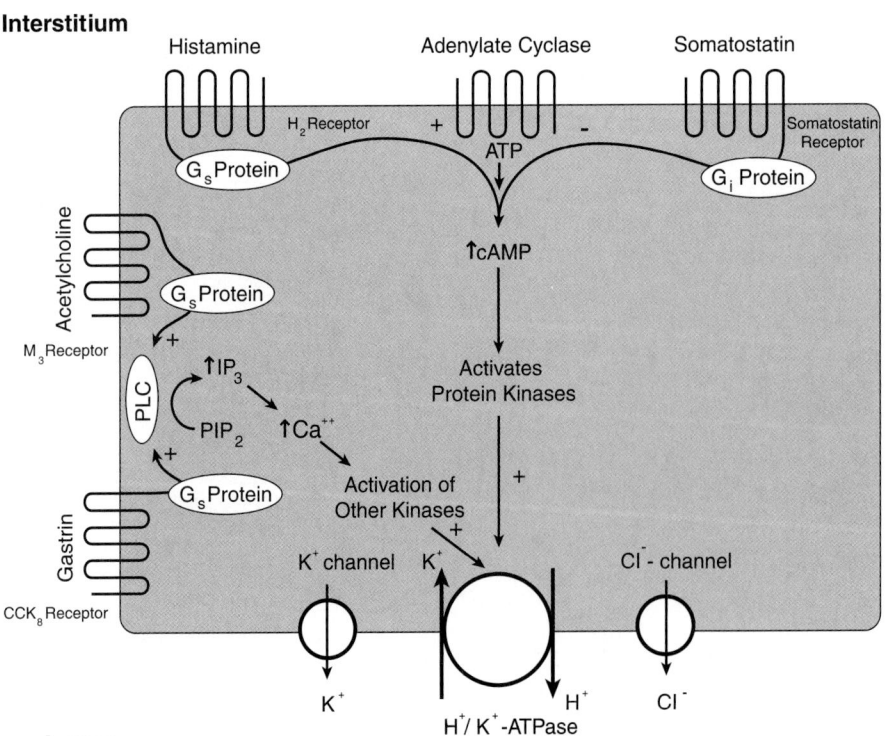

FIG. 25-15. *Control of acid secretion in the parietal cell. [Reproduced with permission from Mercer DW, Liu TH, Castaneda A: Anatomy and physiology of the stomach, in Zuidema GD, Yeo CJ (eds): Shackelford's Surgery of the Alimentary Tract, 5th ed., Vol. II. Philadelphia: Saunders, 2002, p 3.]*

parietal cell mass. The potent acid-suppressing proton pump inhibitor drugs irreversibly interfere with the function of the H^+/K^+-ATPase molecule. They must be incorporated into the activated enzyme to be effective, and thus work best when taken before or during a meal (when the parietal cell is stimulated). When proton pump inhibitor therapy is stopped, acid secretory capability returns as new H^+/K^+-ATPase is synthesized.

Gastrin, acetylcholine, and histamine stimulate the parietal cell to secrete hydrochloric acid (see Fig. 25-15). Gastrin binds to type B cholecystokinin (CCK) receptors, and acetylcholine binds to M_3 muscarinic receptors. Both stimulate phospholipase C via a G-protein linked mechanism leading to increased production of inositol trisphosphate (IP_3) from membrane bound phospholipids. IP_3 stimulates the release of calcium from intracellular stores, which leads to activation of protein kinases and activation of H^+/K^+-ATPase. Histamine binds to the histamine 2 (H_2) receptor, which stimulates adenylate cyclase, also via a G-protein–linked mechanism. Activation of adenylate cyclase results in an increase in intracellular cyclic adenosine monophosphate (AMP) which activates protein kinases, leading to increased levels of phosphoproteins and activation of the proton pump. Somatostatin from mucosal D cells binds to membrane receptors and inhibits the activation of adenylate cyclase through an inhibitory G protein.

Physiologic Acid Secretion

Food ingestion is the physiologic stimulus for acid secretion (Fig. 25-16). The acid secretory response that occurs after a meal is traditionally described in three phases: cephalic, gastric, and intestinal. The cephalic or vagal phase begins with the thought, sight, smell, and/or taste of food. These stimuli activate several cortical and hypothalamic sites (e.g., tractus solitarius, dorsal motor nucleus, and dorsal vagal complex), and signals are transmitted to the stomach by the vagal nerves. Acetylcholine is released, leading to stimulation of ECL cells and parietal cells. Although the acid secreted per unit of time in the cephalic phase is greater than in the other two phases, the cephalic phase is shorter. Thus the cephalic phase accounts for no more than 30% of total acid secretion in response to a meal. Sham feeding (chewing and spitting) stimulates gastric acid secretion only via the cephalic phase, and results in acid secretion which is about half of that seen in response to intravenous pentagastrin or histamine.

When food reaches the stomach, the gastric phase of acid secretion begins. This phase lasts until the stomach is empty, and accounts for about 60% of the total acid secretion in response to a meal. The gastric phase of acid secretion has several components. Amino acids and small peptides directly stimulate antral G cells to secrete gastrin, which is carried in the bloodstream to the parietal cells and stimulates acid secretion in an endocrine fashion. In addition, proximal gastric distention stimulates acid secretion via a vagovagal reflex arc, which is abolished by truncal or highly selective vagotomy. Antral distention also stimulates antral gastrin secretion. Acetylcholine stimulates gastrin release and gastrin stimulates histamine release from ECL cells.

The intestinal phase of gastric secretion is poorly understood. It is thought to be mediated by a hormone yet to be discovered that is released from the proximal small bowel mucosa in response to luminal chyme. This phase starts when gastric emptying of ingested food begins, and continues as long as nutrients remain in the proximal small intestine. It accounts for about 10% of meal-induced acid secretion.

Interprandial basal acid secretion is 2 to 5 mEq hydrochloric acid per hour, about 10% of maximal acid output, and it is greater at night. Basal acid secretion probably contributes to the relatively low bacterial counts found in the stomach. Basal acid secretion is reduced 75 to 90% by vagotomy or H_2-receptor blockade.

The pivotal role that ECL cells play in the regulation of gastric acid secretion is emphasized in Fig. 25-16. A large part of the acid-stimulatory effects of both acetylcholine and gastrin are mediated by histamine released from mucosal ECL cells. This explains why the H_2-receptor antagonists (H_2RAs) are such effective inhibitors of acid secretion, even though histamine is only one of three parietal cell stimulants. The mucosal D cell, which releases somatostatin, is also an important regulator of acid secretion. Somatostatin inhibits histamine release from ECL cells and gastrin release from D cells. The function of D cells is inhibited by *Helicobacter pylori* infection, and this leads to an exaggerated acid secretory response (see below).

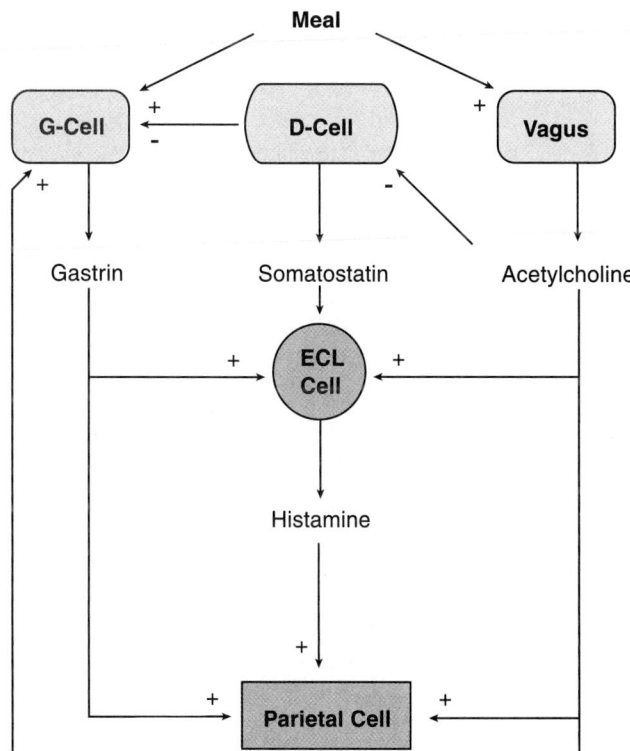

FIG. 25-16. *The physiologic control of acid secretion. [Reproduced with permission from Mercer DW, Liu TH, Castaneda A: Anatomy and physiology of the stomach, in Zuidema GD, Yeo CJ (eds): Shackelford's Surgery of the Alimentary Tract, 5th ed., Vol. II. Philadelphia: Saunders, 2002, p 3.]*

Pepsinogen Secretion

The most potent physiologic stimulus for pepsinogen secretion from chief cells is food ingestion; acetylcholine is the most important mediator. Somatostatin inhibits pepsinogen secretion. Pepsinogen I is produced by chief cells in acid-producing glands, whereas pepsinogen II is produced by chief cells in both acid-producing and gastrin-producing (i.e., antral) glands. Pepsinogen is cleaved to the active pepsin enzyme in an acidic environment and is maximally active at pH 2.5. The enzyme catalyzes the hydrolysis of proteins and is denatured at alkaline pH.

Intrinsic Factor

Activated parietal cells secrete intrinsic factor in addition to hydrochloric acid. Presumably the stimulants are similar, but acid secretion and intrinsic factor secretion may not be linked. Intrinsic factor binds to luminal vitamin B_{12}, and the complex is absorbed in the terminal ileum via mucosal receptors. Vitamin B_{12} deficiency can be life threatening, and patients with total gastrectomy or pernicious anemia require B_{12} supplementation by a nonenteric route. Some patients develop vitamin B_{12} deficiency following gastric bypass, presumably because there is insufficient intrinsic factor present in the small proximal gastric pouch. Under normal conditions, a significant excess of intrinsic factor is secreted, and acid-suppressive medication does not appear to inhibit intrinsic factor production and release.

Gastric Mucosal Barrier

The stomach's durable resistance to autodigestion by caustic hydrochloric acid and active pepsin is intriguing. Some of the important elements of gastric barrier function and cytoprotection are listed in Table 25-2. When these defenses break down, ulceration occurs. A variety of factors are important in maintaining an intact gastric mucosal layer. The mucus and bicarbonate secreted by surface epithelial cells forms an unstirred mucous gel with a favorable pH gradient. Cell membranes and tight junctions prevent hydrogen ions from gaining access to the interstitial space. Hydrogen ions that do break through are buffered by the alkaline tide created by basolateral bicarbonate secretion from stimulated parietal cells. Any sloughed or denuded surface epithelial cells are rapidly replaced by migration of adjacent cells, a process known as *restitution*. Mucosal blood flow plays a crucial role in maintaining a healthy mucosa, providing nutrients and oxygen for the cellular functions involved in cytoprotection. "Back-diffused" hydrogen is buffered and rapidly removed by the rich blood supply. When "barrier breakers" such as bile or aspirin lead to increased back-diffusion of hydrogen ions from the lumen into the lamina propria and submucosa, there is a protective increase in mucosal blood flow. If this protective response is blocked, gross ulceration can occur. Important mediators of these protective mechanisms include prostaglandins, nitric oxide, intrinsic nerves, and peptides (e.g., calcitonin gene-related peptide and gastrin). Misoprostol is a commercially available prostaglandin E analogue that has been shown to prevent gastric mucosal damage in chronic users of nonsteroidal anti-inflammatory drugs (NSAIDs). Some protective reflexes involve afferent sensory neurons, and can be blocked by the application of topical anesthetics to the gastric mucosa, or the experimental destruction of the afferent sensory nerves. In addition to these local defenses, there are important protective factors in swallowed saliva, duodenal secretions, and pancreatic or biliary secretions.

Gastric Hormones

Gastrin

Gastrin is produced by antral G cells and is the major hormonal stimulant of acid secretion during the gastric phase. A variety of molecular forms exist: big gastrin (34 amino acids; G_{34}), little gastrin (17 amino acids; G_{17}), and minigastrin (14 amino acids; G_{14}). The large majority of gastrin released by the human antrum is G_{17}. The biologically active pentapeptide sequence at the C-terminal end of gastrin is identical to that of CCK. Luminal peptides and amino acids are the most potent stimulants of gastrin release, and luminal acid is the most potent inhibitor of gastrin secretion. The latter effect is predominantly mediated in a paracrine fashion by somatostatin released from antral D cells. Gastrin-stimulated acid secretion is significantly blocked by H_2-antagonists, suggesting that the principal mediator of gastrin-stimulated acid production is histamine from mucosal ECL cells. In fact, chronic gastrin hypersecretion such as that seen with long-term use of potent acid suppressants or gastrinoma is associated with hyperplasia of gastric ECL cells, and rarely gastric carcinoid. Gastrin also is trophic to gastric parietal cells and to other GI mucosal cells. Important causes of hypergastrinemia include pernicious anemia, acid-suppressive medication, gastrinoma, retained antrum following distal gastrectomy and Billroth II surgery, and vagotomy.

Somatostatin

Somatostatin is produced by D cells located throughout the gastric mucosa. The predominant form in humans is somatostatin 14, though somatostatin 28 is present as well. The major stimulus for somatostatin release is antral acidification; acetylcholine from vagal nerve fibers inhibits its release. Somatostatin inhibits acid secretion from parietal cells and gastrin release from G cells. It also decreases histamine release from ECL cells. The proximity of the D cells to these target cells suggests that the primary effect of somatostatin is mediated in a paracrine fashion, but an endocrine (i.e., bloodstream) effect also is possible.

Gastrin-Releasing Peptide

Gastrin-releasing peptide (GRP) is the mammalian equivalent of bombesin, a hormone discovered over 2 decades ago in an extract of skin from a frog. In the antrum, GRP stimulates both gastrin and somatostatin release by binding to receptors on the G and D cells. There are nerve terminals ending near the mucosa in the gastric body and antrum, which are rich in GRP immunoreactivity. When GRP is given peripherally it stimulates acid secretion, but when it is given centrally into the cerebral ventricles of animals, it inhibits acid secretion, apparently via a pathway involving the sympathetic nervous system.

Ghrelin

Ghrelin is a small peptide described in 1999 that is produced primarily in the stomach. Ghrelin is a potent secretagogue of pituitary

Table 25-2
Important Components and Mediators of Mucosal Defenses in the Stomach

Components
Mucous barrier
Bicarbonate secretion
Epithelial barrier
Hydrophobic phospholipids
Tight junctions
Restitution
Microcirculation (reactive hyperemia)
Afferent sensory neurons
Mediators
Prostaglandins
Nitric oxide
Epidermal growth factor
Calcitonin gene-related peptide
Hepatocyte growth factor
Histamine

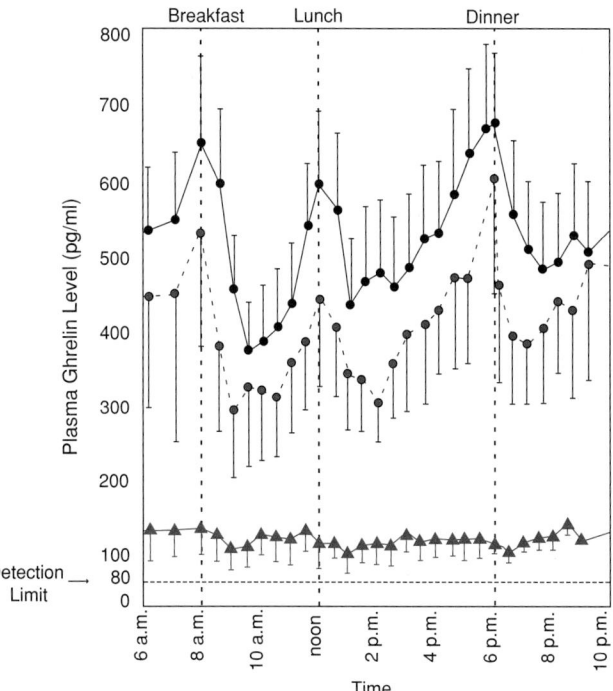

FIG. 25-17. *Ghrelin secretion after gastric bypass. (Reproduced with permission from Cummings DE, et al: N Engl J Med 346:1623, 2002.)*

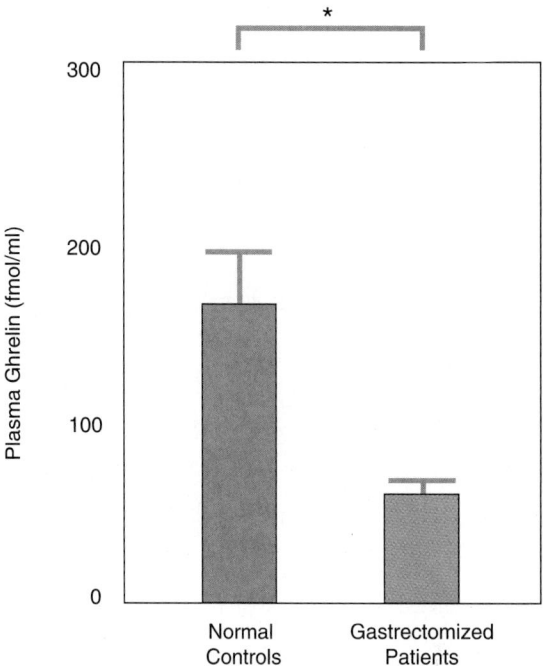

FIG. 25-18. *Ghrelin levels following gastrectomy (Reproduced with permission from Ariyasu H, Takaya K, Tagami T, et al: Stomach is a major source of circulating ghrelin, and feeding state determines plasma ghrelin-like immunoreactivity levels in humans. J Clin Endocrinol Metab 86:4753, 2001.)*

growth hormone (but not adrenocorticotropic hormone [ACTH], follicle-stimulating hormone [FSH], luteinizing hormone [LH], prolactin, or thyroid-stimulating hormone [TSH]). Ghrelin appears to be an orexigenic regulator of appetite (i.e., when ghrelin is elevated, appetite is stimulated, and when it is suppressed, appetite is suppressed). The gastric bypass operation, a very effective treatment for morbid obesity, is associated with suppression of plasma ghrelin levels (and appetite) in humans (Fig. 25-17). Resection of the primary source of this hormone (i.e., the stomach) may partly account for the anorexia and weight loss seen in some patients following gastrectomy (Fig. 25-18).

Gastric Motility and Emptying

Gastric motor function has several purposes. Interprandial motor activity clears the stomach of undigested debris, sloughed cells, and mucus. When feeding begins, the stomach relaxes to accommodate the meal. Regulated motor activity then breaks down the food into small particles, and controls the output into the duodenum. The stomach accomplishes these functions by coordinated smooth muscle relaxation and contraction of the various gastric segments (proximal, distal, and pyloric). Smooth muscle myoelectric potentials are translated into muscular activity, which is modulated by extrinsic and intrinsic innervation and hormones.

Intrinsic Gastric Innervation

The extrinsic parasympathetic and sympathetic gastric innervation was discussed above. The intrinsic innervation consists of ganglia and nerves that constitute the enteric nervous system (Fig. 25-19). There are a variety of neurotransmitters, which are generally grouped as excitatory (augment muscular activity) and inhibitory (decrease muscular activity). Important excitatory neurotransmitters include acetylcholine, the tachykinins, substance P and neurokinin A. Important inhibitory neurotransmitters include nitric oxide (NO) and vasoactive intestinal peptide (VIP). Serotonin

has been shown to modulate both contraction and relaxation. A variety of other molecules affect motility, including GRP, histamine, neuropeptide Y, norepinephrine, and endogenous opioids.

Specialized cells in the muscularis propria also are important modulators of gastrointestinal motility. These cells, called interstitial cells of Cajal, are distinguishable histologically from neurons and myocytes, and appear to amplify both cholinergic excitatory and nitrergic inhibitory input to the smooth muscle of the stomach and intestine.

Segmental Gastric Motility

In general the proximal stomach serves as short-term food storage function and helps regulate basal intragastric tone, and the distal stomach mixes and grinds the food. The pylorus helps the latter process when closed, facilitating retropulsion of the solid food bolus back into the body of the stomach for additional breakdown. The pylorus opens intermittently to allow metered emptying of liquids and small solid particles into the duodenum.

Most of the motor activity of the proximal stomach consists of slow tonic contractions and relaxations, lasting up to 5 minutes. This activity is the main determinant of basal intragastric pressure, an important determinant of liquid emptying. Rapid phasic contractions may be superimposed on the slower tonic motor activity. When food is ingested, intragastric pressure falls as the proximal stomach relaxes (Fig. 25-20). This proximal relaxation is mediated by two important vagovagal reflexes: receptive relaxation and gastric accommodation. Receptive relaxation refers to the reduction in proximal gastric tone associated with the act of swallowing. This occurs before the food reaches the stomach, and can be reproduced by mechanical stimulation of the pharynx or esophagus. Gastric accommodation refers to the proximal gastric relaxation associated with distention of the stomach. Accommodation is mediated through

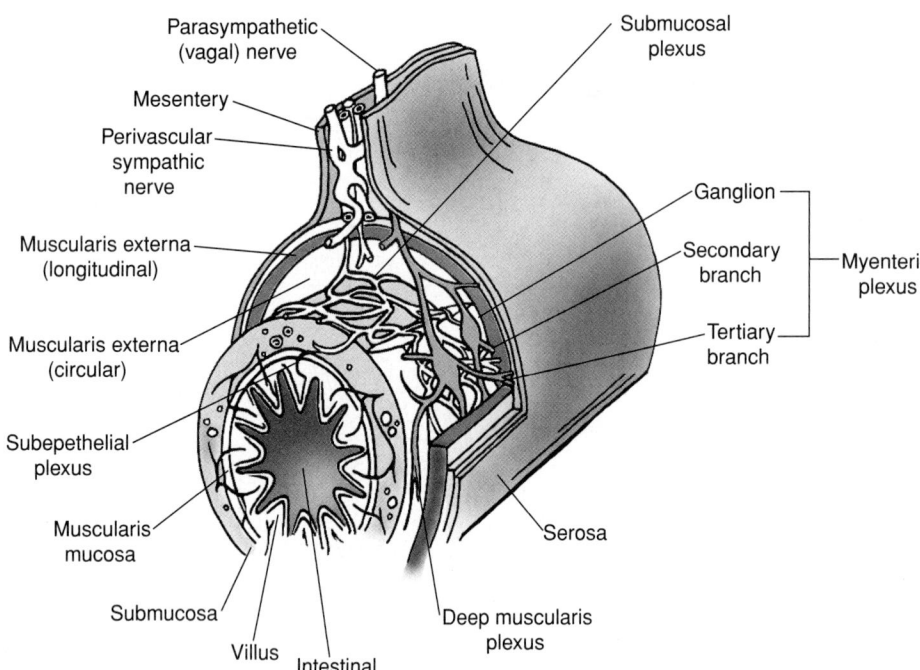

FIG. 25-19. *Enteric nervous system. [Reproduced with permission from Chial HJ, Camilleri M: Motility disorders of the stomach and small intestine, in Friedman SL, McQuaid KR, Grendell JH (eds): Current Diagnosis and Treatment in Gastroenterology, 2nd ed. New York: McGraw-Hill, 2003, p 355.]*

stretch receptors in the gastric wall and does not require esophageal or pharyngeal stimulation. Because both of these reflexes are mediated by afferent and efferent vagal fibers, they are significantly altered by truncal and highly selective vagotomy. Both these operations result in decreased gastric compliance and increased intragastric pressure after food ingestion due to interference with receptive relaxation and gastric accommodation. This tends to increase basal intragastric pressure and may increase the rate of liquid emptying.

NO and VIP are the principal mediators of proximal gastric relaxation. But a variety of other agents increase proximal gastric relaxation and compliance, including dopamine, gastrin, CCK, secretin, GRP, and glucagon. Proximal gastric tone also is decreased by duodenal distention, colonic distention, and ileal perfusion with glucose (ileal brake).

The distal stomach breaks up solid food and is the main determinant of gastric emptying of solids. Slow waves of myoelectric

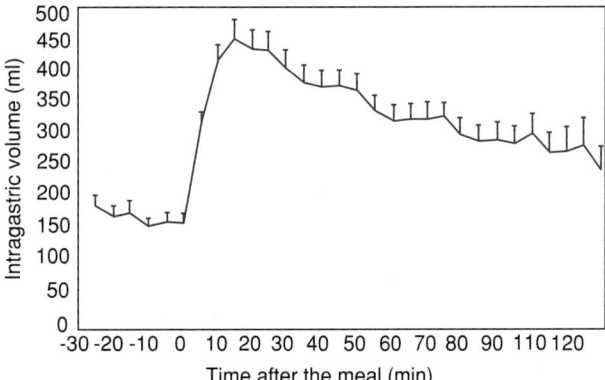

FIG. 25-20. *Gastric accommodation. Graph shows volume of intragastric balloon at constant pressure. As stomach relaxes with initiation of meal, balloon accomodates more volume without increase in pressure. (Reproduced with permission from Tack J, Piessevaux H, Coulie B, Caenepeel P, Janssens J: Role of impaired gastric accommodation to a meal in functional dyspepsia. Gastroenterology 115:1346, 1998.)*

depolarization sweep down the distal stomach at a rate of about three per minute. These waves originate from the proximal gastric pacemaker, high on the greater curvature (Fig. 25-21). The pacing cells may be the interstitial cells of Cajal, which have been shown to have a similar function in the small intestine and colon. Most of these myoelectric waves are below the threshold for smooth muscle contraction in the quiescent state, and thus are associated with negligible changes in pressure. Neural and/or hormonal input, which increases the plateau phase of the action potential, can trigger muscle contraction, resulting in a peristaltic wave associated with the electrical slow wave, and of the same frequency (three per minute) (Fig. 25-22).

During fasting, distal gastric motor activity is controlled by the migrating motor complex (MMC), the "gastrointestinal housekeeper" (Fig. 25-23). The function of the MMC is to sweep along any undigested food, debris, sloughed cells, and mucus after the fed phase of digestion is complete. The MMC lasts approximately 100 minutes (longer at night, shorter during daytime) and is divided into four phases. Phase I (about half the length of the entire cycle) is a period of relative motor inactivity. High-amplitude muscular contractions do not occur in phase I of the MMC. Phase II (about 25% of the entire MMC cycle) consists of some irregular high-amplitude generally nonpropulsive contractions. Phase III, a period of intense regular (about three per minute) propulsive contractions, only lasts about 5 to 10 minutes. Most phase III complexes of the gastrointestinal MMC begin in the stomach, and the frequency approximates that of the myoelectric gastric slow wave. Phase IV is a transition period.

Neurohormonal control of the MMC is poorly understood, but it appears that different phases are regulated by different mechanisms. For example, vagotomy abolishes phase II of the gastric MMC, but has little influence on phase III. In fact, phase III persists in the autotransplanted stomach, totally devoid of extrinsic neural input. This suggests that phase III is regulated by intrinsic nerves and/or hormones. Indeed, the initiation of phase III of the MMC in the distal stomach corresponds temporally to elevation in serum levels of motilin, a hormone produced in the duodenal mucosa. Resection

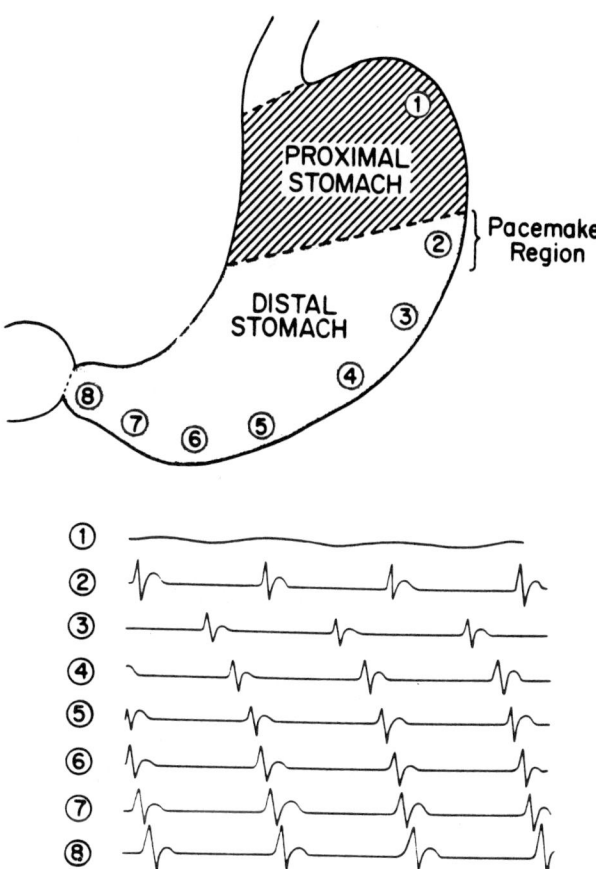

FIG. 25-21. *Regional myoelectric patterns in the stomach. [Reproduced with permission from Ashley SW, Evoy D, Daly JM: Stomach, in Schwartz SI (ed): Principles of Surgery, 7th ed. New York: McGraw-Hill, 1999, p 1181.]*

are retrograde, serving to mix and grind the solid components of the meal. The magnitude of gastric contractions and the duration of the pattern is influenced by the consistency and composition of the meal.

The pylorus functions as an effective regulator of gastric emptying, preventing large particles and large boluses of liquid from entering the duodenum, where they could overwhelm normal digestive and homeostatic mechanisms. It also is an effective barrier to duodenogastric reflux. Bypass, transection, or resection of the pylorus may lead to uncontrolled gastric emptying of food and the dumping syndrome (see below). Primary pyloric dysfunction and/or surgical interference with the pylorus also may result in uncontrolled entry of duodenal contents into the stomach, leading to bile reflux gastritis (see below). Perfusion of the duodenum with lipids, glucose, amino acids, hypertonic saline, or hydrochloric acid results in closure of the pylorus and decreased transpyloric flow. Ileal perfusion with fat has the same effect. A variety of neurohumoral pathways are involved with these physiologic responses, and there is evidence that different pathways may be involved for different stimuli.

The pylorus is readily apparent grossly as a thick ring of muscle and connective tissue. Histologically, it also is distinguishable from the distal stomach and proximal duodenum. The density of nerve tissue in the pyloric smooth muscle is severalfold higher than in the antrum, with increased numbers of neurons staining positive for substance P, neuropeptide Y, VIP, and galanin. Interstitial cells of Cajal are more closely associated with pyloric myocytes, and the myoelectric slow wave of the pylorus has the same frequency as that seen in the distal stomach. The motor activity of the pylorus is both tonic and phasic. During phase III of the MMC, the pylorus is open as gastric contents are swept into the duodenum. During the fed phase, the pylorus remains closed most of the time. It appears to relax intermittently, usually in synchronization with lower-amplitude minor antral contractions. The higher-amplitude, more major antral contractions are usually met with a closed pylorus, facilitating retropulsion and further grinding of food.

Modulation of pyloric motor activity is complex. There is evidence of both inhibitory and excitatory vagal pathways. Some contractile vagal effects are mediated by opioid pathways, since they are blocked by naloxone. Electrical stimulation of the duodenum causes the pylorus to contract, whereas electrical stimulation of the antrum causes pyloric relaxation. Generally, NO mediates pyloric relaxation; NO donors lead to pyloric relaxation and decreased resistance to flow in a variety of models, whereas NO synthetase inhibitors have the opposite effect. Other molecules that may play a physiologic role in controlling pyloric smooth muscle include serotonin, VIP, prostaglandin E_1, and galanin (pyloric relaxation); and histamine, CCK, and secretin (pyloric contraction).

Gastric Emptying

The control of gastric emptying is complex. In general, gastric emptying is slowed by increasing caloric content or osmolarity,

of the duodenum abolishes distal gastric phase III in dogs. There are clearly motilin receptors on antral smooth muscle and nerves. Other modulators of gastric MMC activity include NO, endogenous opioids, intrinsic cholinergic and adrenergic nerves, and duodenal pH (MMC phase III does not occur if the duodenal pH is below 7).

Feeding abolishes the MMC and leads to the fed motor pattern (Fig. 25-24). The neurohormonal initiator of this change is unknown, but CCK may play a role. Sham feeding transiently induces antral motor activity resembling the fed motor pattern, and this is blocked by the CCK receptor antagonist loxiglumide. The fed motor pattern of gastric activity starts within 10 minutes of food ingestion and persists until all the food has left the stomach. Gastric motility during the fed pattern resembles phase II of the MMC, with irregular but continuous phasic contractions of the distal stomach. During the fed state, about half of the myoelectric slow waves are associated with strong distal gastric contractions. Some are prograde and some

FIG. 25-22. The relationship between intracellular electrical activity and muscle cell contraction. *[Reproduced with permission from Hasler WL: Physiology of gastric motility and gastric emptying, in Yamada T et al (eds): Textbook of Gastroenterology, 4th ed. Philadelphia: Lippincott Williams & Wilkins, 2003, p 195.]*

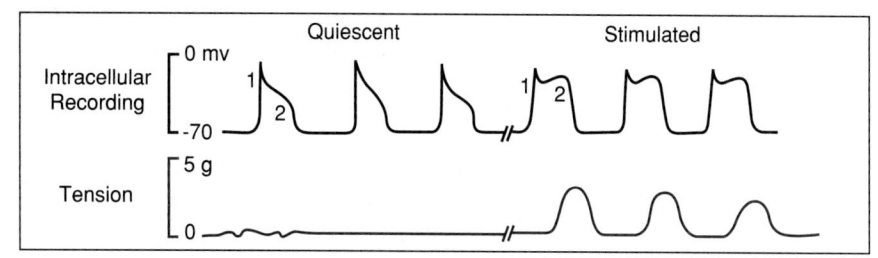

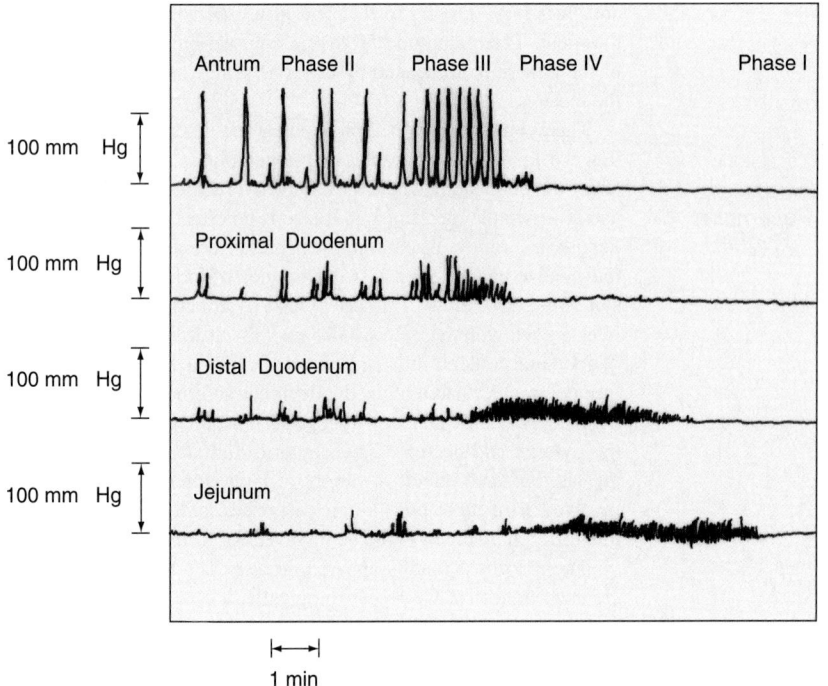

FIG. 25-23. Migrating motor complex. *[Reproduced with permission from Hasler WL: Physiology of gastric motility and gastric emptying, in Yamada T et al (eds): Textbook of Gastroenterology, 4th ed. Philadelphia: Lippincott Williams & Wilkins, 2003, p 195.]*

increased fat content, and increased particle size; liquid emptying is faster than solid emptying. Osmolarity, acidity, caloric content, and nutrient composition are important modulators. Duodenal osmoreceptors, glucoreceptors, and pH receptors clearly inhibit gastric emptying by a variety of neurohumoral mechanisms. Although many GI hormones can be shown to affect gastric emptying in the laboratory, only CCK has been consistently shown to inhibit gastric emptying at physiologic doses (Fig. 25-25). Recently it has been noted that the anorexic hormone leptin, secreted mostly by fat but also by gastric mucosa, inhibits gastric emptying, perhaps through the same pathway as CCK (which also has properties of a satiety hormone). The orexic hormone ghrelin has opposite effect.

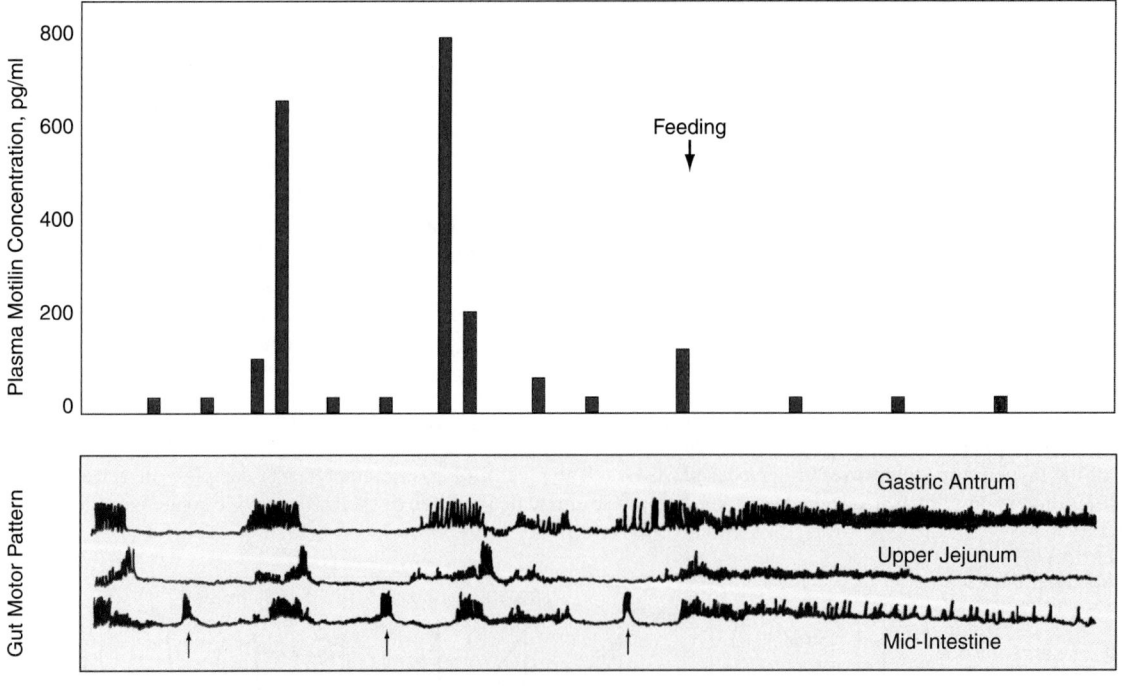

FIG. 25-24. Fasting pattern and fed pattern of GI motility, and motilin levels. *[Reproduced with permission from Hasler WL: Physiology of gastric motility and gastric emptying, in Yamada T et al (eds): Textbook of Gastroenterology, 4th ed. Philadelphia: Lippincott Williams & Wilkins, 2003, p 195.]*

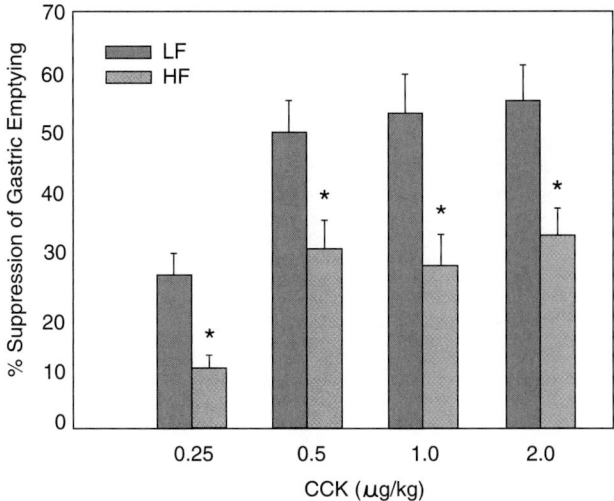

FIG. 25-25. Cholecystokinin inhibits gastric emptying in rats. LF = low fat diet, HF = high fat diet. *[Reproduced with permission from Hasler WL: Physiology of gastric motility and gastric emptying, in Yamada T et al (eds): Textbook of Gastroenterology, 4th ed. Philadelphia: Lippincott Williams & Wilkins, 2003, p 195.]*

Liquid Emptying

The gastric emptying of water or isotonic saline follows first-order kinetics, with a half emptying time around 12 minutes. Thus, if one drinks 200 mL of water, about 100 mL enters the duodenum by 12 minutes, whereas if one drinks 400 mL of water, about 200 mL enters the duodenum by 12 minutes. This emptying pattern of liquids is modified considerably as the caloric density, osmolarity, and nutrient composition of the liquid changes (Fig. 25-26). Up to an osmolarity of about 1 M, liquid emptying occurs at a rate of about 200 kcal per hour. Duodenal osmoreceptors and hormones (e.g.,

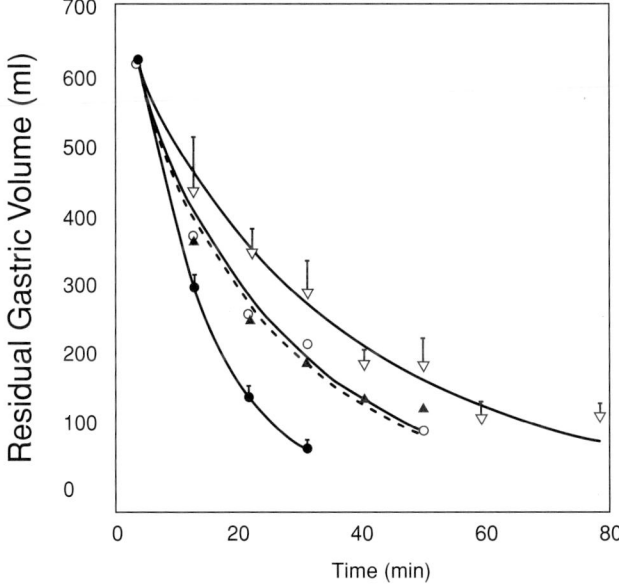

FIG. 25-26. Nutrient composition and caloric density affect liquid gastric emptying. Glucose = filled circles; milk protein = open triangles; two different peptide hydrolysates = open circles and closed triangles. *[Reproduced with permission from Hasler WL: Physiology of gastric motility and gastric emptying, in Yamada T et al (eds): Textbook of Gastroenterology, 4th ed. Philadelphia: Lippincott Williams & Wilkins, 2003, p 195.]*

secretin and VIP) are important modulators of liquid gastric emptying. Generally, liquid emptying is delayed in the supine position.

Traditionally, liquid emptying has been attributed to the activity of the proximal stomach, but it is probably more complicated than previously thought. Clearly, receptive relaxation and gastric accommodation play a role in gastric emptying of liquids. Patients with a denervated (e.g., vagotomy), resected, or plicated (e.g., fundoplication) proximal stomach have decreased gastric compliance and may show accelerated gastric emptying of liquids. A swallowed liquid meal induces receptive relaxation, but the same meal delivered via nasogastric tube bypasses this reflex and is associated with a higher intragastric pressure and accelerated emptying.

However, even if the proximal intragastric pressure is lower than duodenal pressure, normal gastric emptying of liquids occurs. Diabetic patients also may have normal proximal gastric motor function and profoundly delayed gastric emptying of liquids. These observations suggest an active role for the distal stomach in liquid emptying. Indeed, antral contractile activity does correlate with liquid gastric emptying, and this distal gastric activity appears to vary with the nutrient composition and caloric content of the liquid meal. Depending on the circumstances, distal gastric motor activity can promote or inhibit gastric emptying of liquids. Distal gastrectomy and pyloric stenting both accelerate the initial rapid phase of liquid gastric emptying.

Solid Emptying

Normally, the half-time of solid gastric emptying is about 2 hours. Unlike liquids, which display an initial rapid phase followed by a slower linear phase of emptying, solids have an initial lag phase during which little emptying of solids occurs (Fig. 25-27). It is during this phase that much of the grinding and mixing occurs. A linear emptying phase follows, during which the smaller particles are metered out to the duodenum. Solid gastric emptying is a function of meal particle size, caloric content, and composition (especially fat). When liquids and solids are ingested together, the liquids empty first. Solids are stored in the fundus and delivered to the distal stomach at constant rates for grinding. Liquids also are sequestered in the fundus, but they appear to be readily delivered to the distal stomach for early emptying. The larger the solid component of the meal, the slower the liquid emptying. Patients bothered by dumping syndrome are advised to limit the amount of liquid consumed with the solid meal, taking advantage of this effect.

Promotility Agents

A variety of prokinetic agents have been shown to be clinically useful in increasing gastric emptying. The commonly-used agents and mechanisms are shown in Table 25-3.

DIAGNOSIS OF GASTRIC DISEASE

Signs and Symptoms

The most common symptoms of gastric disease are pain, weight loss, early satiety, and anorexia. Nausea, vomiting, bloating, and anemia also are frequent complaints. Several of these symptoms (pain, bloating, nausea, and early satiety) are often described by physicians as dyspepsia, synonymous with the common lay term indigestion. Common causes of dyspepsia include gastroesophageal reflux disease (GERD) and disorders of the stomach, gallbladder, and pancreas. Although none of the above symptoms alone is specific for gastric disease, when elicited in the context of a careful

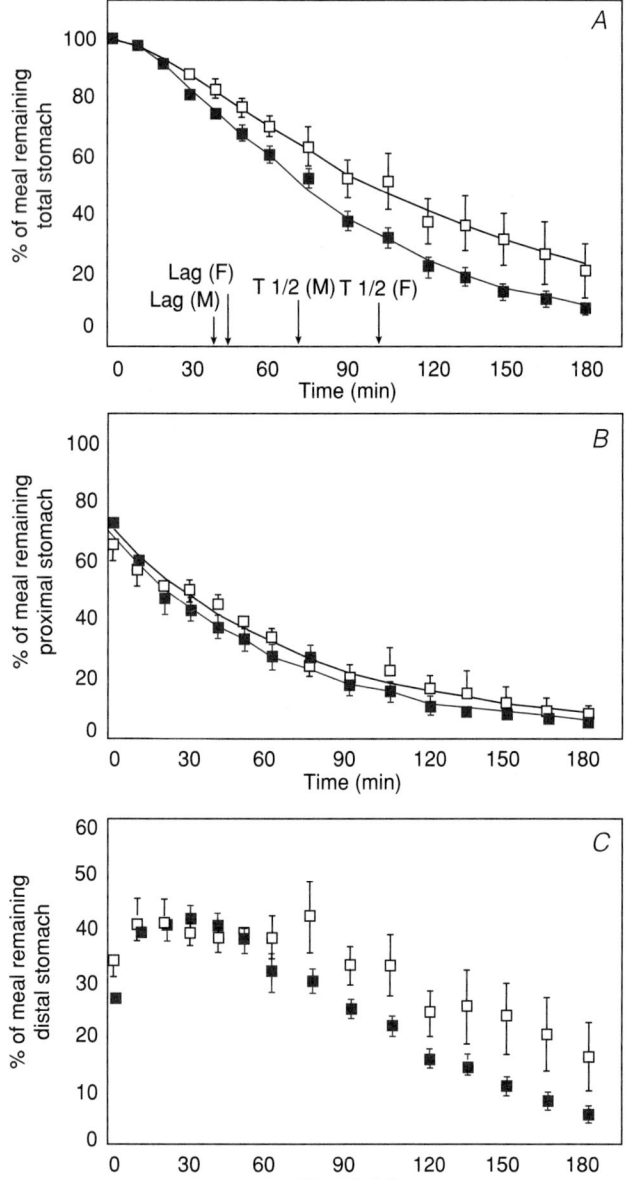

FIG. 25-27. Solid gastric emptying. Women = open squares, Men = filled squares. Note similarity between men and women in proximal (middle panel) but not distal (lower panel) emptying. *[Reproduced with permission from Hasler WL: Physiology of gastric motility and gastric emptying, in Yamada T et al (eds): Textbook of Gastroenterology, 4th ed. Philadelphia: Lippincott Williams & Wilkins, 2003, p 195.]*

history and physical examination they can clearly point to a probable differential diagnosis, which can then be refined with certain tests.

Epigastric pain that is exacerbated by eating may be indicative of benign gastric ulcer or a gastric tumor. Both may be associated with weight loss due to avoidance of food (sitophobia), but a more rapid rate of weight loss (e.g., 10% of body weight over several weeks) in a patient over 50 years of age suggests malignancy. Both gastric inflammation and tumor can decrease the compliance of the stomach, resulting in early satiety. Furthermore, in the presence of either benign or malignant gastric disease, appetite pathways may be affected, and the resulting anorexia and early satiety can result in significant weight loss. Vomiting could be due to diabetic or postsurgical gastroparesis, gastric ulcer, or distal gastric cancer.

Table 25-3
Promotility Agents That Accelerate Gastric Emptying

Drug	Mechanism
Metoclopramide	Dopamine antagonist
Domperidone	Dopamine antagonist
Erythromycin	Motilin agonist
Bethanecol	Cholinergic agonist
Neostigmine	Cholinergic agonist

The hypothesis of visceral hypersensitivity suggests that some patients perceive normal physiologic stimuli as painful. This is not uncommon in patients with irritable bowel syndrome, and may be an explanation for the occasional patient with pain suggestive of gastric disease, but with a negative (often extensive) work-up.

Diagnostic Tests

Esophagogastroduodenoscopy

Patients with one or more of the alarm symptoms listed in Table 25-4 should undergo expeditious upper endoscopy. Esophagogastroduodenoscopy (EGD) is a safe and accurate outpatient procedure performed under conscious sedation. Following an 8-hour fast, the flexible scope is advanced under direct vision into the esophagus, stomach, and duodenum. The fundus and GE junction are inspected by retroflexing the scope. To rule out cancer with a high degree of accuracy, all patients with gastric ulcer diagnosed on upper GI series or found at EGD should have multiple (six to eight) biopsies of the base and rim of the lesion. Brush cytology also should be considered. Gastritis should be biopsied both for histologic examination and for a tissue urease test to rule out the presence of *Helicobacter pylori*. The most serious complications of EGD are perforation (which is rare, but can occur anywhere from the cervical esophagus to the duodenum), aspiration, and respiratory depression from excessive sedation. Generally EGD is a more sensitive test than double contrast upper GI series, but these modalities should be considered complementary rather than mutually exclusive.

Radiologic Tests

Plain abdominal x-rays are helpful in the diagnosis of gastric perforations (from ulcer, tumor, or trauma), since free air is usually identified. Large gastric bezoars may be visible on plain abdominal x-ray, and a large air-filled or fluid-filled stomach suggests abnormal gastric emptying that may be due to tumor, ulcer, or motility disorder.

Compared to EGD, there may be some advantages to *double contrast upper GI series* performed by a skilled radiologist. Sedation is not required. Some anatomic abnormalities are more easily demonstrable or quantifiable on barium study than on EGD. These include diverticula, fistula, tortuosity or stricture location, and size of hiatal hernia. Although there are radiologic characteristics of ulcers which suggest the presence or absence of malignancy, it must be reiterated that gastric ulcers require adequate biopsy. Typically,

Table 25-4
Alarm Symptoms That Indicate the Need for Esophagogastroduodenoscopy

Weight loss
Recurrent vomiting
Dysphagia
Bleeding
Anemia

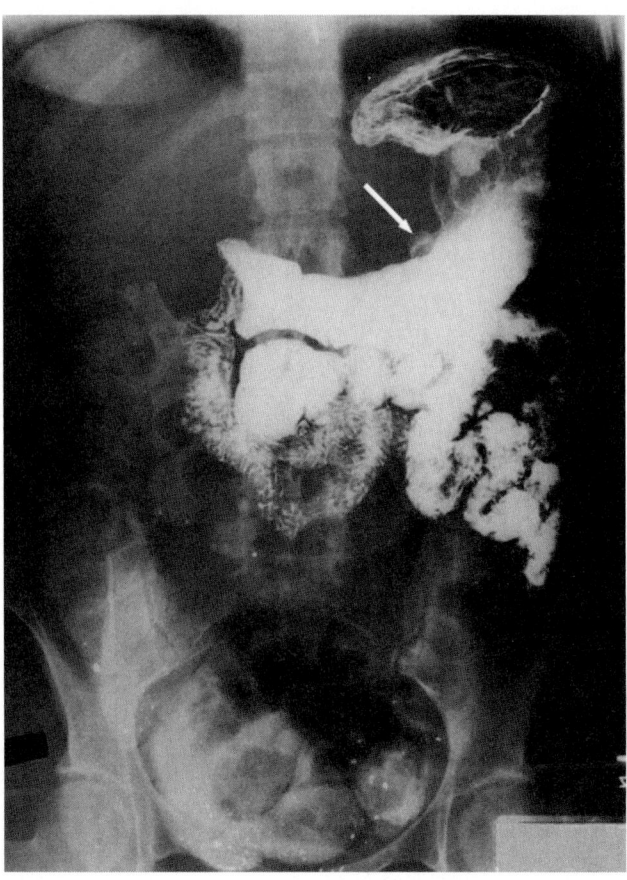

A

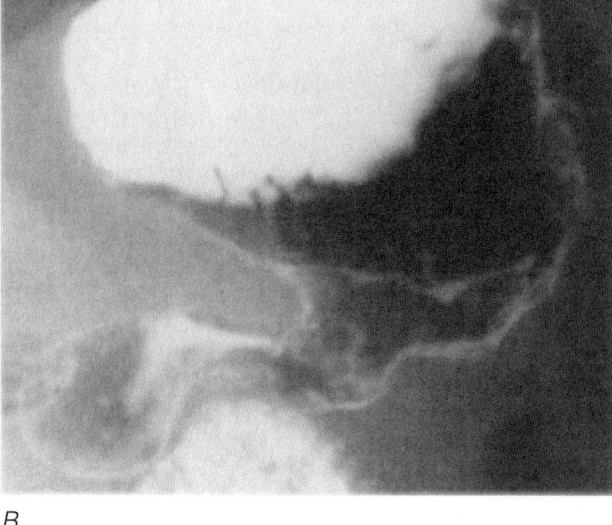

B

FIG. 25-28. Appearance of benign (*A*) and malignant (*B*) gastric ulcers on barium upper GI series.

benign ulcer craters extend beyond the luminal margin of the stomach and have radiating gastric folds, whereas malignant ulcers do not extend beyond the luminal margin and have parallel gastric folds (Fig. 25-28).

Computed Tomographic Scanning and Magnetic Resonance Imaging. Most cases of significant gastric disease can be diagnosed without these sophisticated imaging studies. However, one or the other should be part of the routine staging work-up for most patients with a malignant gastric tumor. Magnetic resonance imaging (MRI) may prove clinically useful as a quantitative test for gastric emptying, and may even hold some promise for the analysis of myoelectric derangements in patients with gastroparesis. Gastric thickening more than 1 cm may indicate malignancy and should be evaluated with endoscopy, but many patients will be found to have benign disease.

Advanced processing of high-resolution helical computed tomography (CT) data has made virtual endoscopy a reality. Currently a research tool, it may have potential as a screening tool for gastric disease since it is noninvasive and does not require a physician on site to perform. Digital transmission allows the images to be analyzed remotely. It is, however, doubtful that most of the curable gastric cancers (i.e., the early gastric cancers) could be detected with a nonendoscopic technique.

Arteriography rarely is necessary or useful in the diagnosis of gastric disease. It may be helpful in the occasional poor-risk patient with exsanguinating gastric hemorrhage, or in the patient with occult gastric bleeding that is difficult to diagnose. Extravasation of contrast indicates the location of the bleeding vessel, and embolization or selective infusion of vasopressin may be therapeutic. Occasionally empiric embolization of the suspected but unproven bleeding vessel helps. Arteriovenous malformations have a characteristic angiographic appearance.

Endoscopic Ultrasound. Endoscopic ultrasound (EUS) is useful in the evaluation of some gastric lesions. Local staging of gastric adenocarcinoma with EUS is quite accurate, and this modality can be used to plan therapy. At some centers, patients with biopsy-proven adenocarcinoma of the stomach that is transmural or associated with enlarged nodes are considered for preoperative chemoradiation therapy, and the need for this is best determined with EUS. Enlarged nodes can be sampled with EUS-guided endoscopic needle biopsy. Malignant tumors that are confined to the mucosa on EUS may be amenable to endoscopic resection. EUS also can be used to assess the response of gastric lymphoma to chemotherapy. Large submucosal masses should be resected because of the risk of malignancy, but small submucosal masses are common on endoscopy. EUS can provide reassurance, but cannot guarantee, that a small lesion under observation is likely to be benign because of characteristics associated with ultrasonography. Submucosal varices also can be assessed by EUS.

Gastric Secretory Analysis

Analysis of gastric acid output requires gastric intubation. This somewhat uncomfortable test may be useful in the evaluation of patients for Zollinger-Ellison syndrome, patients with refractory ulcer or GERD, and patients with recurrent ulcer after operation. Historically, gastric analysis was performed most commonly to test for the adequacy of vagotomy in postoperative patients with recurrent or persistent ulcer. However, this also can be done by assessing peripheral pancreatic polypeptide (PP) levels in response to sham feeding. A 50% increase in PP within 30 minutes of sham feeding suggests vagal integrity.

Gastric analysis is performed in the fasted state with the semi-recumbent patient in the left lateral position. After the position of the nasogastric tube is verified, the tube is hand aspirated every 5 minutes. Four successive 15-minute samples are created by pooling the 5-minute aliquots. An intravenous stimulant of acid secretion may then be administered (betazole or pentagastrin) or the patient is sham fed ("chew and spit"), and the process repeated. Samples are analyzed by titration. Normal basal acid output (BAO) is less than 5 mEq/h. Maximal acid output (MAO) is the average of the two final stimulated 15-minute periods and is usually 10 to 15 mEq/h. Peak acid output (PAO) is defined as the highest of the four stimulated periods. Patients with a gastrinoma commonly have a high BAO, often above 30 to 40 mEq/h. In these patients, the ratio of BAO to MAO exceeds 0.6. Normal acid output in the patient prescribed acid-suppressive medication usually means that the patient is noncompliant. To assess acid-secretory capacity in the absence of medication effect, H_2-blockers and proton pump inhibitors should be withheld for a week prior to gastric analysis.

Scintigraphy

Nuclear medicine tests can be helpful in the evaluation of gastric emptying and duodenogastric reflux. The standard scintigraphic evaluation of gastric emptying involves the ingestion of a test meal with one or two isotopes, and scanning the patient under a gamma camera. A curve for liquid and solid emptying is plotted and the half-time calculated. Normal standards exist for each facility. Duodenogastric reflux can be quantitated by the intravenous administration of hepatobiliary iminodiacetic acid (HIDA), which is concentrated and excreted by the liver into the duodenum. Software allows a semiquantitative assessment of how much of the isotope refluxes into the stomach.

Tests for *Helicobacter pylori*

Over the past two decades, *Helicobacter pylori* infection has emerged as a significant human pathogen. It is present in most patients with peptic ulcer disease, and has been associated with gastric lymphoma and adenocarcinoma. A variety of tests can help determine whether the patient has active *H. pylori* infection (Table 25-5). The predictive value (positive and negative) of any of these tests when used as a screening tool depends on the prevalence of *H. pylori* infection in the screened population. *A positive test is quite accurate in predicting H. pylori infection, but a negative test is characteristically unreliable.* Thus, in the appropriate clinical setting, treatment for *H. pylori* should be initiated on the basis of a positive test, but not necessarily withheld if the test is negative.

A positive serologic test is presumptive evidence of active infection if the patient has never been treated for *H. pylori*. Histologic examination of an antral mucosal biopsy using special stains is the gold standard test. Other sensitive tests include commercially available rapid urease tests, which assay for the presence of urease in mucosal biopsies (strong presumptive evidence of infection). Urease is an omnipresent enzyme in *H. pylori* strains that colonize the gastric mucosa. The labeled carbon urea breath test has recently

Table 25-5
Tests for *Helicobacter pylori*

Test	When to Use	Why	Why Not
Serologic test	Test of choice when endoscopy is not indicated and is not an option and when the patient has not received antimicrobial therapy for *H. pylori* infection	Noninvasive; sensitivity of >80%, specificity of about 90%	Does not confirm eradication, because serologic "scar" remains for indefinite period after microbiologic cure
Urea breath test	Preferred for confirming cure of *H. pylori* infection, but no sooner than 4 wk after completion of therapy	Simple; sensitivity and specificity of 90 to 99%	False-negatives possible if testing is done too soon after treatment with proton pump inhibitors, antimicrobials, or bismuth compounds; small radiation exposure with ^{14}C method; expensive
Histologic test	To directly ascertain presence of *H. pylori* when endoscopy is being used; also used when determination of neoplastic status of lesion is necessary	Sensitivity of 80 to 100%, specificity of >95%; hematoxylin-eosin and Diff-Quik stains are simplest; Genta stain has sensitivity of >95% and specificity of 99%	Requires laboratory facilities and experience; when hematoxylin-eosin stain is nondiagnostic, second staining method is required
Rapid urease test	Simplest method when endoscopy is necessary	Simple; rapid (once biopsy specimen has been obtained); sensitivity of 80 to 95%, specificity of 95 to 100%	Invasive; false-negatives possible if testing is done too soon after treatment with proton pump inhibitors, antimicrobials, or bismuth compounds
Culture	After repeated failure of appropriate combination antibiotic therapy; when antimicrobial resistance is suspected or high level of resistance exists in the population	Allows determination of antibiotic susceptibility	Time-consuming; expensive; usually not necessary unless resistance is suspected

SOURCE: Reproduced with permission from Graham DY, et al: *Postgraduate Medicine* 105:113, 1999.

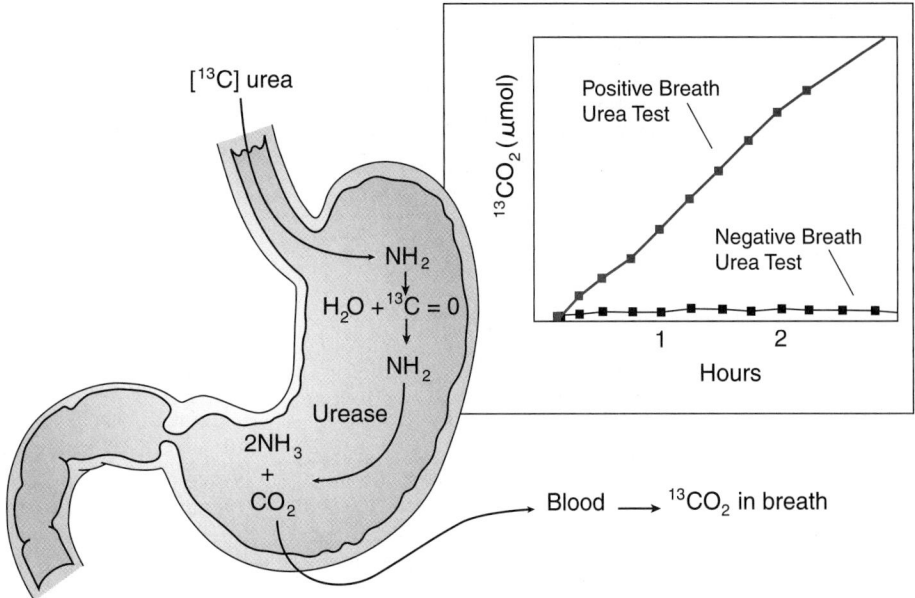

FIG. 25-29. Labeled urea breath test used to detect *H. pylori* infection. *(Reproduced with permission from Walsh JH, Peterson WL: N Engl J Med 333: 984,1995.)*

become available (Fig. 25-29). This has become the standard test to confirm eradication of *H. pylori* following appropriate treatment. In this test the patient ingests urea labeled with radioactive ^{14}C or nonradioactive ^{13}C. The labeled urea is acted upon by the urease present in the *H. pylori* and converted into ammonia and carbon dioxide. The radiolabeled carbon dioxide is excreted from the lungs and can be detected in the expired air. It also can be detected in a blood sample. The fecal antigen test also is quite sensitive and specific for active *H. pylori* infection and may prove useful in confirming a cure.

Antroduodenal Motility Testing and Electrogastrography

Antroduodenal motility testing and electrogastrography (EGG) are performed in specialized centers, and may be useful in the evaluation of the patient with anomalous epigastric symptoms. EGG consists of the transcutaneous recording of gastric myoelectric activity. Antroduodenal motility testing is done with a tube placed transnasally or transorally into the distal duodenum. There are pressure-recording sensors extending from the stomach to the distal duodenum. The combination of these two tests together with scintigraphy provides a thorough assessment of gastric motility.

PEPTIC ULCER DISEASE

Peptic ulcers are focal defects in the gastric or duodenal mucosa which extend into the submucosa or deeper (Fig. 25-30). They may be acute or chronic, and ultimately are caused by an imbalance between the action of peptic acid and mucosal defenses (Fig. 25-31). Peptic ulcer remains a common outpatient diagnosis, but the number of physician visits, hospital admissions, and elective operations for peptic ulcer disease have decreased steadily and dramatically over the past 3 decades (Fig. 25-32). These trends all predated the advent of fiberoptic endoscopy, highly selective vagotomy, and the use of H_2-blockers. However, the incidence of emergency surgery and the death rate associated with peptic ulcers are fairly stable (Fig. 25-33). These epidemiologic trends probably represent the net effect of several factors, including decreasing prevalence of *H. pylori* infection, better medical therapy, increases in outpatient management, and the use of NSAIDs and aspirin (with and without ulcer prophylaxis).

These epidemiologic facts notwithstanding, it is important to reiterate that peptic ulcer is a common disease in the U.S. In 2000, the total direct costs (hospital, physicians, and drugs) of peptic ulcer disease was about $3.3 billion, with indirect costs (lost work and productivity) of over $6 billion. The prevalence of peptic ulcer

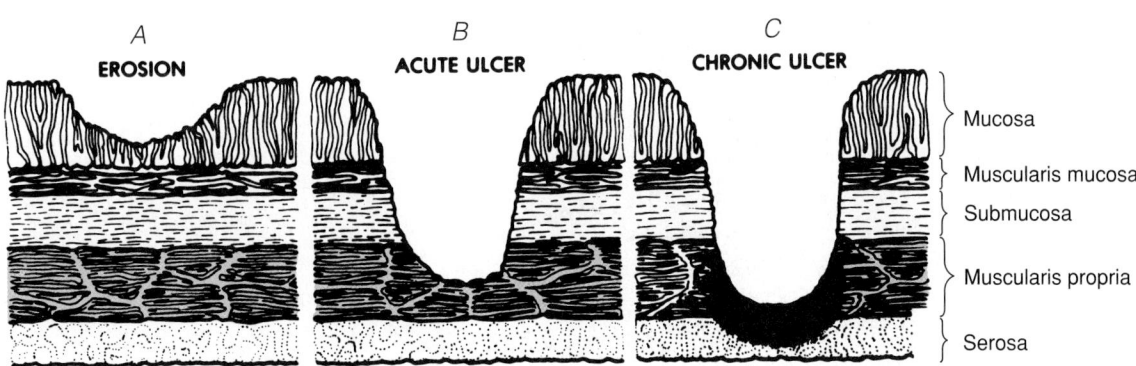

FIG. 25-30. Diagram of gastric erosions and ulcers. *[Reproduced with permission from Ashley SW, Evoy D, Daly JM: Stomach, in Schwartz SI (ed): Principles of Surgery, 7th ed. New York: McGraw-Hill, 1999, p 1181.]*

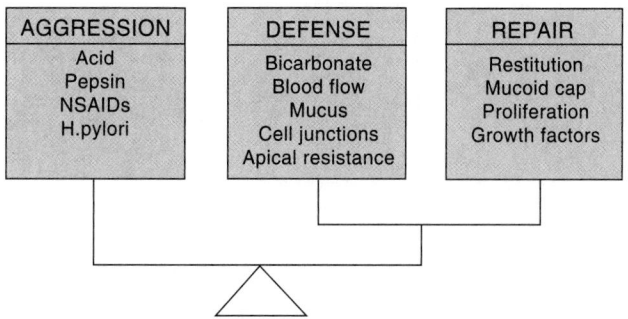

FIG. 25-31. *Balance of acid/peptic aggressive factors and mucosal defensive factors in the gastric mucosa. (Reproduced with permission from Mertz HR, Walsh JH: Peptic ulcer pathophysiology. Med Clin North Am 75:799, 1991.)*

in the U.S. is about 2%, and the lifetime risk is about 10%. In 1998, the crude mortality rate for peptic ulcer was 1.7 per 100,000 individuals. Gastric ulcer has a higher mortality than duodenal ulcer because of its increased prevalence in the elderly. Recent studies have shown an increase in the rates of hospitalization and mortality in elderly patients for the peptic ulcer complications of bleeding and perforation. Presumably this is due to the increasingly common use of NSAIDs and aspirin in this elderly cohort, many of whom have *H. pylori* infection.

Pathophysiology and Etiology

A variety of factors may contribute to the development of peptic ulcer disease. Although it is now recognized that the large majority of duodenal and gastric ulcers are caused by *H. pylori* infection and/or NSAID use (Fig. 25-34), the final common pathway to ulcer formation is peptic acid injury of the gastroduodenal mucosal barrier. Thus the adage "no acid, no ulcer" remains true even today. Acid suppression, either with medication or surgery, remains a mainstay in healing both duodenal and gastric ulcers and in preventing recurrence. It generally is thought that *H. pylori* predisposes to ulceration, both by acid hypersecretion, and by compromise of mucosal defense mechanisms. NSAID use is thought to lead to peptic ulcer disease predominantly by compromise of mucosal defenses. Duodenal ulcer has typically been thought of as a disease of increased peptic acid action on the duodenal mucosa, whereas gastric

ulcer has been viewed as a disease of weakened mucosal defenses in the face of relatively normal action of peptic acid. However, increased understanding of the pathophysiology of peptic ulcer has blurred this distinction. Clearly, weakened mucosal defenses play a role in many duodenal and most gastric ulcers (e.g., duodenal ulcer in an *H. pylori*–negative patient on NSAIDs or a patient with a typical type I gastric ulcer with acid hyposecretion), whereas increased aggressive activity of peptic acid may result in a duodenal or gastric ulcer in the setting of normal mucosal defenses (e.g., a duodenal ulcer in a patient with Zollinger-Ellison syndrome, or a gastric ulcer in a patient with gastric outlet obstruction, antral stasis, and acid hypersecretion).

Elimination of *H. pylori* infection or NSAID use is important for optimal ulcer healing, and perhaps is even more important in preventing ulcer recurrence and/or complications. A variety of other diseases are known to cause peptic ulcer, including Zollinger-Ellison syndrome (gastrinoma), antral G-cell hyperfunction and/or hyperplasia, systemic mastocytosis, trauma, burns, and major physiologic stress. Other causative agents include drugs (all NSAIDs, aspirin, and cocaine), smoking, alcohol, and psychologic stress. In the U.S., probably more than 90% of serious peptic ulcer complications can be attributed to *H. pylori* infection, NSAID use, or cigarette smoking.

Helicobacter pylori Infection

Helicobacter pylori is uniquely equipped for survival in the hostile environment of the stomach. It possesses the enzyme urease, which converts urea into ammonia and bicarbonate, thus creating an environment around the bacteria that buffers the acid secreted by the stomach. Mutant strains of *H. pylori* that do not produce urease are unable to colonize the stomach. The organism lives in the mucus layer atop the gastric surface epithelial cells, and some attach to these cells. There are a variety of possible mechanisms whereby *H. pylori* may produce mucosal injury (Table 25-6). One fundamental mechanism appears to be a disturbance in acid secretion. This is due at least in part to the inhibitory effect that *H. pylori* exerts on antral D cells that secrete somatostatin, a potent inhibitor of antral G-cell gastrin production. *H. pylori* infection is associated with decreased levels of somatostatin, decreased somatostatin messenger ribonucleic acid production, and fewer somatostatin-producing D cells. These effects are probably mediated by *H. pylori*–induced

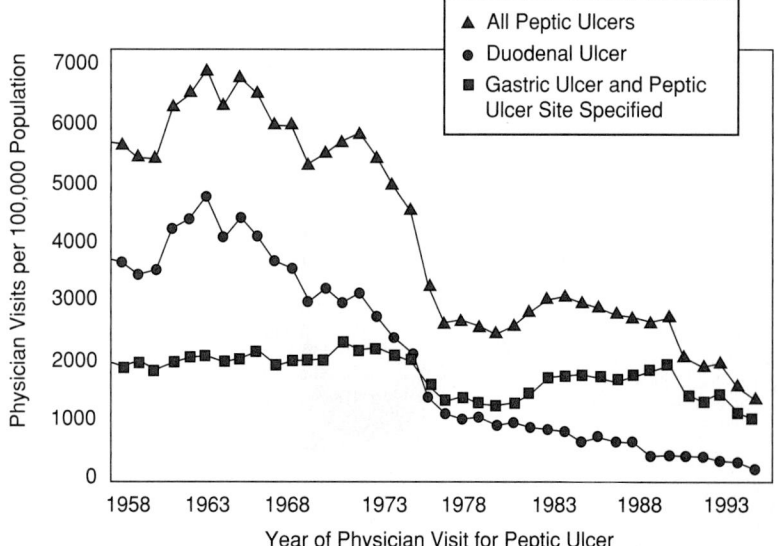

FIG. 25-32. *Physician visits for peptic ulcer. (Reproduced with permission from Munnangi S, Sonnenberg A: Time trends of physician visits and treatment patterns of peptic ulcer disease in the United States. Arch Intern Med 157:1489, 1997.)*

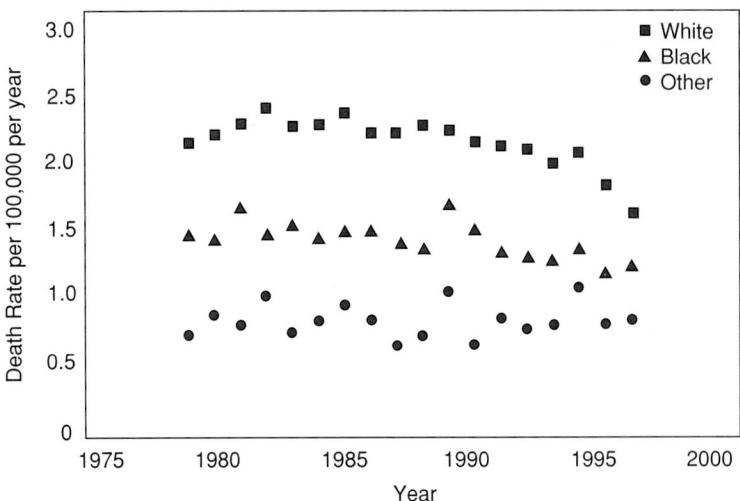

FIG. 25-33. Death rate for peptic ulcer. *(Reproduced with permission from Donahue PE: Arch Surg 134:1373, 1999.)*

local alkalinization of the antrum (antral acidification is the most potent antagonist to antral gastrin secretion), and *H. pylori*–mediated increases in other local mediators and cytokines, among other means. The end result is hypergastrinemia and acid hypersecretion (Fig. 25-35). This hypergastrinemia presumably leads to the parietal cell hyperplasia seen in many patients with duodenal ulcer. The acid hypersecretion and the antral gastritis are thought to lead to antral epithelial metaplasia in the postpyloric duodenum. This duodenal metaplasia allows *H. pylori* to colonize the duodenal mucosa, and in these patients the risk of developing a duodenal ulcer increases 50-fold. When *H. pylori* colonizes the duodenum, there is a significant decrease in acid-stimulated duodenal bicarbonate release. When *H. pylori* infection is successfully treated, acid secretory physiology tends to normalize (Fig. 25-36). Other mechanisms whereby *H. pylori* can induce gastroduodenal mucosal injury include the production of toxins (vacA and cagA), local elaboration of cytokines (particularly interleukin 8) by infected antral mucosa, recruitment of inflammatory cells and release of inflammatory mediators, and production of immunoglobulins. It is likely that *H. pylori* predisposes to gastric ulcer at least in part by weakening mucosal defenses.

The evidence supporting the central role of *H. pylori* in the pathophysiology of peptic ulcer disease is strong. Patients with *H. pylori* infection and antral gastritis are three and a half times more likely to develop peptic ulcer disease than patients without *H. pylori*

infection. Up to 90% of patients with duodenal ulcers, and 70 to 90% of patients with gastric ulcers, have *H. pylori* infection. It is clear from multiple randomized prospective studies that curing *H. pylori* infection dramatically alters the natural history of peptic ulcer disease, decreasing the recurrent ulcer rate from over 75% in patients treated with a course of acid-suppressive therapy alone (in whom *H. pylori* is not eradicated) to less than 20% in patients treated with a course of antibacterial therapy (Fig. 25-37).

Obviously, other factors are involved in the etiology of peptic ulcer disease, since everyone who has *H. pylori* (up to 50% of the adult population in some areas of the U.S.) does not get peptic ulcer disease. Only about 15 to 20% of patients colonized with *H. pylori* will develop peptic ulcer disease over their lifetime. Many patients on aspirin and NSAIDs develop peptic ulcer disease without *H. pylori* infection. These observations notwithstanding, it is clear from a variety of well-designed laboratory, clinical, and epidemiologic studies that *H. pylori* is indubitably an important factor in the development and recurrence of peptic ulcer disease. *H. pylori* also plays an etiologic role in gastric cancer and lymphoma (see below).

Acid Secretion and Peptic Ulcer

A variety of abnormalities related to mucosal acid exposure have been described in patients with duodenal ulcer (Fig. 25-38). As a

FIG. 25-34. *Causes of peptic ulcer disease. [Reproduced with permission from Spechler SJ: Peptic ulcer disease and its complications in Feldman M (ed): Sleisinger and Fordtran's Gastrointestinal and Liver Disease, 7th ed. Philadelphia: Saunders, 2002, p 747.]*

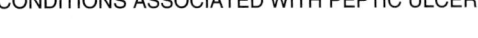

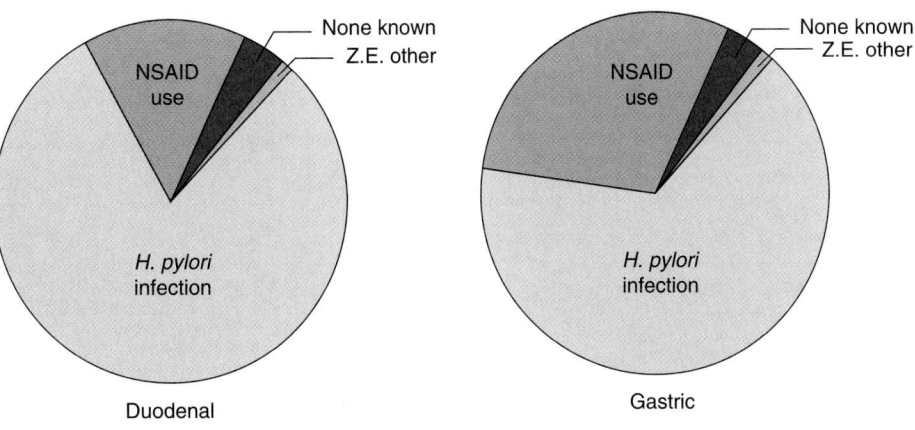

Table 25-6
Mechanisms by which *H. pylori* can Damage the Gastric Mucosa

Local effects
    Elaboration of toxins
        vacA
        cagA
Effect on immune response
    Elaboration of cytokines
    Elaboration of interleukin 8
    Recruitment of inflammatory cells
    Release of inflammatory mediators
    Production of immunoglobulins
Effect on acid secretion
    Initial hypochlorhydria
    Subsequent hyperchlorhydria
    Elevated serum gastric levels
    Reduced gastric antral somatostatin levels
    Increased levels of gastric fundic N-methylhistamine
    Hypergastrinemia may contribute to greater parietal cell mass
Effect on duodenal bicarbonate secretion
    Reduced secretion of duodenal bicarbonate in patients colonized
        with *H. pylori*

SOURCE: Kaufman GL: *Adv Surg* 34:121,2000.

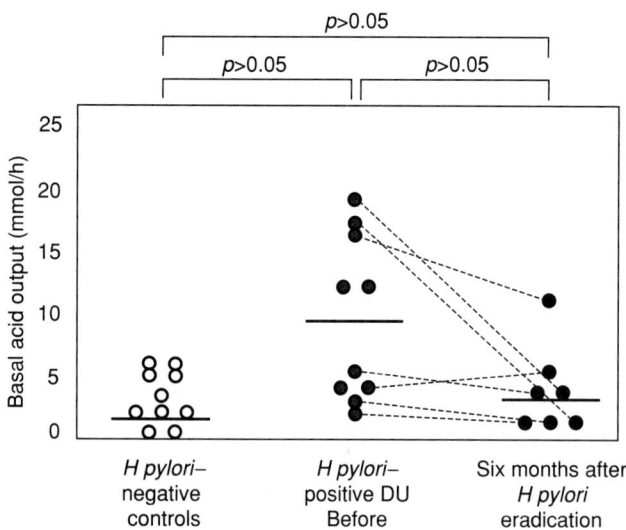

FIG. 25-36. *Basal acid output in normal controls and in patients with duodenal ulcer, before and after the eradication of H. pylori infection.*

rule, duodenal ulcer patients secrete more acid than patients with gastric ulcer. It has long been recognized that duodenal ulcer patients as a group have a higher mean BAO and also a higher mean MAO compared to normal controls (Fig. 25-39). Nocturnal acid secretion is more commonly elevated than daytime secretion. However, many duodenal ulcer patients have basal and peak acid outputs in the normal range, and there is no correlation between acid secretion and the severity of the ulcer disease. Duodenal ulcer patients produce more acid than normal controls in response to any known secretory stimulus for gastric acid output. Although duodenal ulcer patients usually have normal fasting gastrin concentrations, they often produce more gastric acid at any given dose of gastrin than controls. Considering that many duodenal ulcer patients do produce excessive gastric acid, it has been argued that a "normal" fasting

gastrin level in these patients is inappropriately high, and that there is an impaired feedback mechanism, especially in light of the apparently increased sensitivity of the parietal cell mass to gastrin. Many of these long-standing observations now seem reasonable in light of recently gained understanding of the perturbations in acid and gastrin secretion associated with *H. pylori* infection (described above). Some patients with duodenal ulcer also have increased rates of gastric emptying that delivers an increased acid load per unit of time to the duodenum. Finally, the buffering capacity of the duodenum in many patients with duodenal ulcer is compromised due to decreased duodenal bicarbonate secretion.

In patients with gastric ulcer, acid secretion is variable. Generally, four types of gastric ulcer are described. The most common, Johnson type I gastric ulcer, is typically located near the angularis incisura on the lesser curvature, close to the border between the antrum and the body of the stomach. These patients usually have

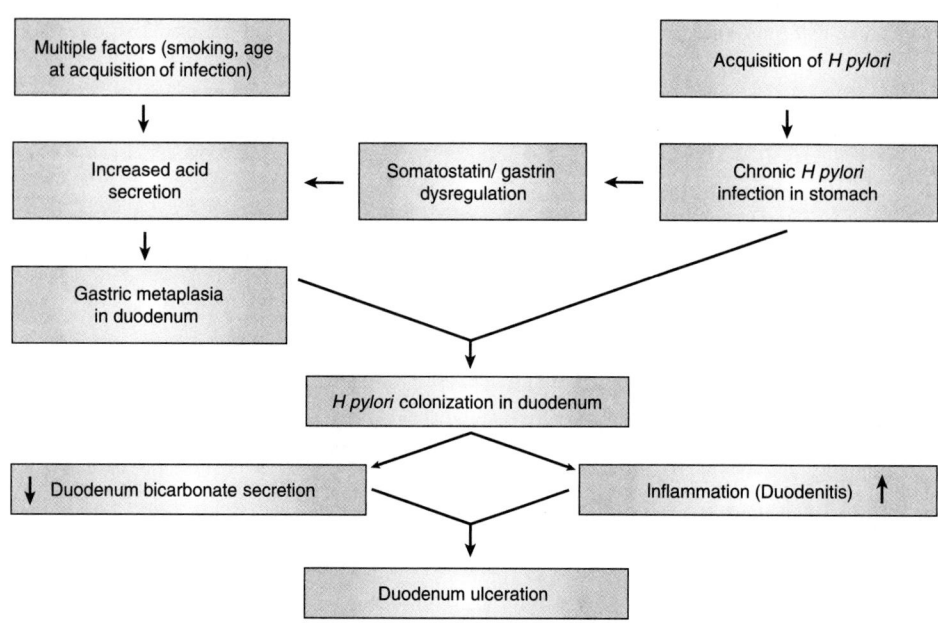

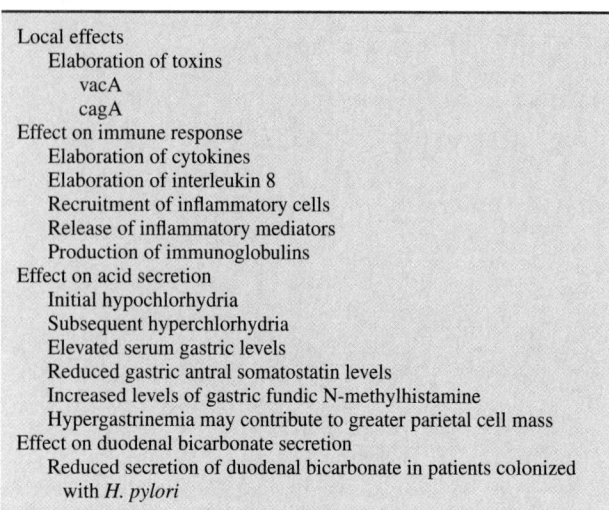

FIG. 25-35. Model of *H. pylori*–induced effects on duodenal ulcer pathogenesis. (*Reproduced with permission from Peek RM Jr., Blaser MJ: Pathophysiology of Helicobacter pylori-induced gastritis and peptic ulcer disease. Am J Med 102:200, 1997.*)

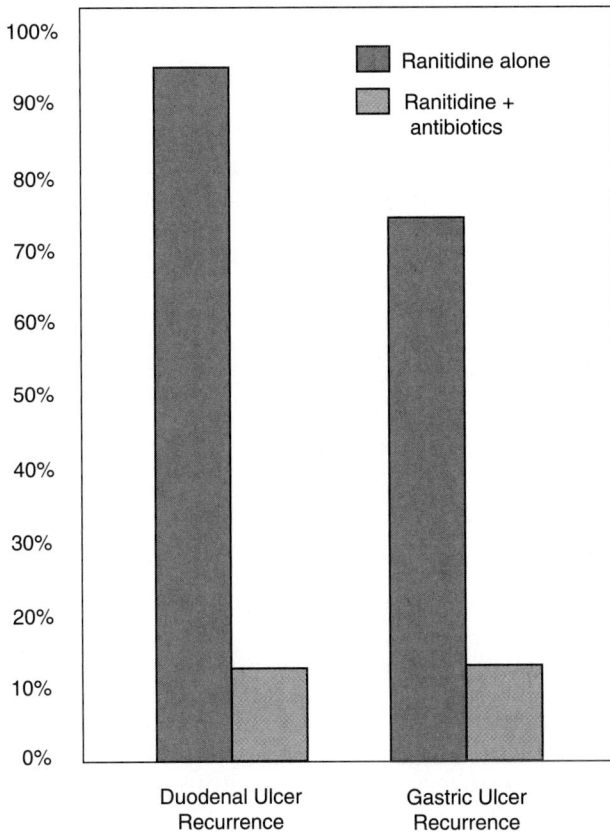

normal or decreased acid secretion. Type II gastric ulcer is associated with active or quiescent duodenal ulcer disease, and type III gastric ulcer is prepyloric. Both type II and type III gastric ulcers are associated with normal or increased gastric acid secretion. Type IV gastric ulcers occur near the gastroesophageal junction, and acid secretion is normal or below normal. Patients with type I or IV gastric ulcers may have weak mucosal defenses that permit an abnormal amount

of injurious acid back-diffusion into the mucosa. Duodenogastric reflux may play a role in weakening the gastric mucosal defenses in patients with gastric ulcer. A variety of components in duodenal juice, including bile, lysolecithin, and pancreatic juice, have been shown to cause injury and inflammation in the gastric mucosa. NSAIDs and aspirin have similar effects. Although chronic gastric ulcer is usually associated with surrounding gastritis, it is unproven that the latter leads to the former.

Nonsteroidal Anti-Inflammatory Drugs in Peptic Ulcer Disease

NSAIDs (including aspirin) are inextricably linked to peptic ulcer disease. Patients with rheumatoid arthritis and osteoarthritis who take NSAIDs have a 15 to 20% annual incidence of peptic ulcer, and the prevalence of peptic ulcer in chronic NSAID users is about 25% (15% gastric and 10% duodenal). Complications of peptic ulcer disease (specifically hemorrhage and perforation) are much more common in patients taking NSAIDs. More than half of patients who present with peptic ulcer hemorrhage or perforation report the recent use of NSAIDs, including aspirin. Many of these patients remain asymptomatic until they develop these life-threatening complications.

The overall risk of significant serious adverse GI events in patients taking NSAIDs is more than three times that of controls (Table 25-7). This risk increases to five times in patients over age 60. In elderly patients taking NSAIDs, the likelihood that they will require an operation related to a GI complication is 10 times that of the control group, and the risk that they will die from a GI cause is about four and a half times higher. This problem is put into prospective when one realizes that approximately 20 million patients in the United States take NSAIDs on a regular basis; perhaps as many regularly take aspirin. Persons who take NSAIDs also have a higher hospitalization rate for serious GI events than those who do not.

Factors that clearly put patients at increased risk for NSAID-induced GI complications include age over 60, prior GI event, high NSAID dose, concurrent steroid intake, and concurrent anticoagulant intake. *Any patient taking NSAIDs or aspirin who has one or more of these risk factors should receive concomitant acid suppressive medication or misoprostol at a therapeutic dose, or should be considered for alternative treatment with cyclooxygenase 2 (COX-2) inhibitors* (Table 25-8).

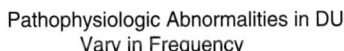

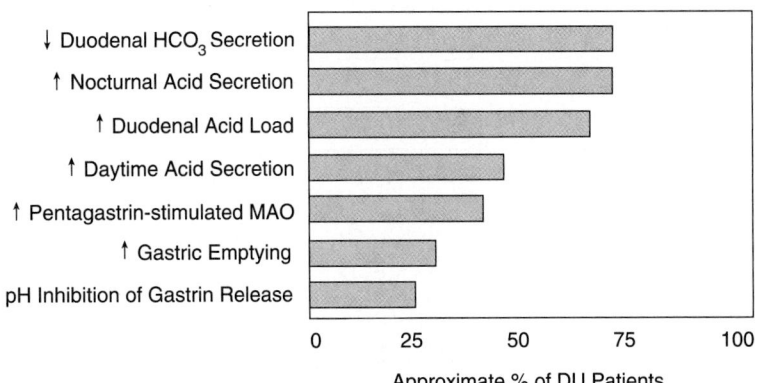

Pathophysiologic Abnormalities in DU
Vary in Frequency

Basal Acid Output
(mmol/h)

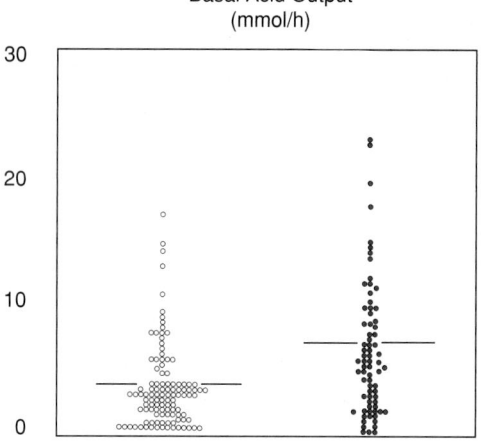

Peak Acid Output
(mmol/h)

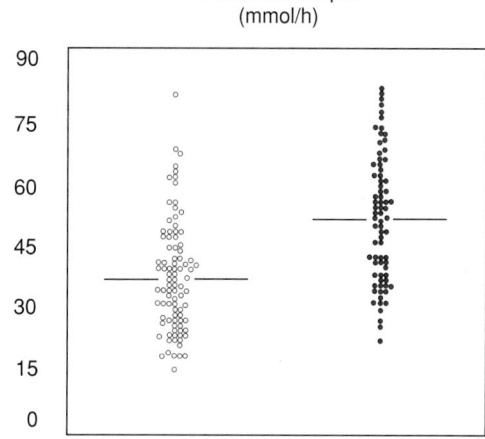

FIG. 25-39. Basal and peak acid output in normal (open circles) and duodenal ulcer (closed circles) patients. (*Reproduced with permission from Blair AJ, et al: JCI 79:582, 1987.*)

Smoking, Stress, and Other Factors

Epidemiologic studies suggest that smokers are about twice as likely to develop peptic ulcer disease as nonsmokers. Smoking increases gastric acid secretion and duodenogastric reflux. Smoking decreases both gastroduodenal prostaglandin production and pancreaticoduodenal bicarbonate production. These observations may be related, and any or all could explain the observed association between smoking and peptic ulcer disease.

Although difficult to measure, both physiologic and psychologic stress undoubtedly play a role in the development of peptic ulcer in some patients. In 1842, Curling described duodenal ulcer and/or duodenitis in burn patients. Decades later, Cushing described the appearance of acute peptic ulceration in patients with head trauma (Cushing ulcer). Even the ancients recognized the undeniable links between peptic ulcer disease and stress. Patients still present with ulcer complications (bleeding, perforation, and obstruction) that are seemingly exacerbated by stressful life events. Recently, the use of crack cocaine has been linked to juxtapyloric peptic ulcers with a propensity to perforate. Alcohol is commonly mentioned as a risk factor for peptic ulcer disease, but confirmatory data are lacking.

Clinical Manifestations

Over 90% of patients with peptic ulcer disease complain of abdominal pain. The pain is typically nonradiating, burning in quality, and located in the epigastrium. The mechanism of the pain is unclear. Patients with duodenal ulcer usually experience pain 2 to 3 hours after a meal and at night. Two thirds of patients with duodenal ulcers will complain of pain that awakens them from sleep. The pain of gastric ulcer more commonly occurs with eating and is less likely to awaken the patient at night. A history of peptic ulcer disease, use of NSAIDs, over-the-counter antacids, or antisecretory drugs, is suggestive of the diagnosis. Other signs and symptoms include nausea, bloating, weight loss, stool positive for occult blood, and anemia. Duodenal ulcer is about twice as common in men compared to women, but the incidence of gastric ulcer is similar in men and women. On average, gastric ulcer patients are 10 years older than duodenal ulcer patients, and the incidence is increasing in the elderly, probably because of increasing NSAID use in this cohort with a high incidence of *H. pylori* infection.

Diagnosis

In the young patient with dyspepsia and/or epigastric pain, it may be appropriate to initiate empiric therapy for peptic ulcer disease without confirmatory testing. All patients over 45 with the above symptoms should have an upper endoscopy, and all patients, regardless of age, should have this study if any alarm symptoms (see Table 25-4) are present. A double contrast upper GI x-ray study may be useful. All gastric ulcers should be adequately biopsied, and any sites of gastritis should be biopsied to rule out *H. pylori*, and for histologic evaluation. Additional testing for *H. pylori* may be indicated. Although somewhat controversial, it is not unreasonable to

Table 25-7

Hospitalization Rates for Gastrointestinal (GI) Events with and without Nonsteroidal Anti-inflammatory Drug (NSAID) Use in Selected Large Populations

Population Studied	Persons Observed		Annual GI Hospitalization Rate		
	NSAID Use	No NSAID Use	GI Event	NSAIDs	No NSAIDs
Tayside, Scotland >50 y	52,293	73,792	Any upper GI event	1.29%	0.53%
			Complicated event	0.74%	0.23%
Odense, Denmark	31,503	107,197	Ulcer/erosive bleeding	0.25%	0.05%
Tennessee Medicaid >65 y	27,067 person-years	134,560 person-years	Upper GI bleeding or ulcer	1.67%	0.42%
ARAMIS Arthritis data bank					
Osteoarthritis	2199 person-years	1035 person-years	Any GI event	0.73%	0.29%
Rheumatoid arthritis	8471 person-years	3753 person-years	Any GI event	1.46%	0.27%

SOURCE: Reproduced with permission from Laine L: *Gastroenterology* 120:76, 2001.

Table 25-8
Adverse Gastrointestinal Events in Patients Taking Nonsteroidal Anti-inflammatory Drugs (NSAIDs)

			Annualized Incidence[b]			
	Therapies Used		Clinical Upper GI Events[c]		Complicated Upper GI Events[d]	
Study[a]	NSAID Control	Study Drugs	Control	Study Drug	Control	Study Drug
MUCOSA	10 NSAIDs (N = 4439)	Misoprostol 200 µg qid + NSAID (N = 4404)	3.1%	1.6%	1.5%	0.7%
CLASS	Ibuprofen 800 mg tid, diclofenac 75 mg bid (N = 3987)	Celecoxib 400 mg bid (N = 3995)	3.5%	2.1%	1.5%	0.8%
			(No aspirin[e]: 2.9%	1.4%	1.3%	0.4%)
VIGOR	Naproxen 500 mg bid (N = 4047)	Rofecoxib 50 mg qd (N = 4029)	4.5%	2.1%	1.4%	0.6%

[a]MUCOSA and VIGOR trials included only rheumatoid arthritis patients; CLASS trial included osteoarthritis (73%) and rheumatoid arthritis (27%).

[b]Incidence for MUCOSA trial represents doubling of results provided at 6 months (although median follow-up was <6 months). Incidences for VIGOR and CLASS trials represent rates per 100 patient-years, although VIGOR median follow-up was 9 months and CLASS data include only the first 6 months of the study.

[c]Includes perforations, obstructions, bleeding, and uncomplicated ulcers discovered on clinically indicated work-up.

[d]Includes perforation, obstruction, bleeding (documented due to ulcer or erosions in MUCOSA and CLASS; major bleeding in VIGOR).

[e]21% of patients in CLASS study were taking low-dose aspirin.

NOTE: All differences between controls and study drugs were significant except clinical upper GI events in overall CLASS study ($p = 0.09$).

bid = twice a day; qd = once a day; qid = four times a day; tid = three times a day.

SOURCE: Reproduced with permission from Laine L: *Gastroenterology* 120:76, 2001.

test all peptic ulcer patients for *H. pylori*. A baseline serum gastrin level is appropriate to rule out gastrinoma.

Complications

The three most common complications of peptic ulcer disease, in decreasing order of frequency, are bleeding, perforation, and obstruction. Most peptic ulcer–related deaths in the U.S. are due to bleeding. Bleeding peptic ulcers account for about half of the clinically significant cases of upper GI bleeding at most medical centers (Table 25-9). Patients with a bleeding peptic ulcer typically present with melena and/or hematemesis. Nasogastric aspiration is usually confirmatory of the upper GI bleeding. Abdominal pain is quite uncommon. Shock may be present, necessitating aggressive resuscitation and blood transfusion. Early endoscopy is important to diagnose the cause of the bleeding and to assess the need for hemostatic therapy.

Three quarters of the patients who come to the hospital with bleeding peptic ulcer will stop bleeding if given acid suppression and kept NPO (non per os, meaning nothing by mouth). However,

Table 25-9
Causes of Upper Gastrointestinal Bleeding Requiring Hospitalization

Diagnosis	Number of Patients (%) (n = 948)
Peptic ulcer	524 (55)
Gastroesophageal varice	131 (14)
Angioma	54 (6)
Mallory-Weiss tear	45 (5)
Tumor	42 (4)
Erosion	41 (4)
Dieulafoy's lesion	6 (1)
Other	105 (11)

SOURCE: Data from the Center for Ulcer Research and Education (CURE) Hemostasis Research Group, UCLA School of Medicine and the West Los Angeles VA Medical Center, with permission.

one fourth will continue to bleed or will rebleed after an initial quiescent period, and virtually all the mortalities (and all the operations for bleeding) occur in this group. This group can be fairly well delineated based on clinical factors related to the magnitude of the hemorrhage and endoscopic findings (Table 25-10). Shock, hematemesis, transfusion requirement exceeding four units in 24 hours, and high-risk endoscopic stigmata (active bleeding or visible vessel) define this high-risk group. These patients benefit from endoscopic therapy to stop the bleeding. The most common endoscopic hemostatic modalities used are injection with epinephrine, and electrocautery. Persistent bleeding or rebleeding after endoscopic therapy is an indication for operation, although repeat endoscopic treatment has been successful in treating rebleeding. Elderly and high-risk patients do not tolerate repeated episodes of hemodynamically significant hemorrhage, and may benefit from early elective operation after initially successful endoscopic treatment, especially if they have one or more of the risk factors mentioned above or a high-risk ulcer. Planned surgery under controlled circumstances often yields better outcomes than emergent surgery performed in the middle of the night. Deep bleeding ulcers on the posterior duodenal bulb or lesser gastric curvature are high-risk lesions, because they often erode large arteries not amenable to nonoperative treatment, and early operation should be considered.

Perforated peptic ulcer usually presents as an acute abdomen. The patient can often give the exact time of onset of the excruciating abdominal pain. Initially, a chemical peritonitis develops from

Table 25-10
Factors that Predict the Need for Intervention to Stop the Hemorrhage in Patients with Bleeding Peptic Ulcer

Hypotension
Hematemesis
Transfusion
Visible vessel
Ongoing bleeding
Ulcer size and location

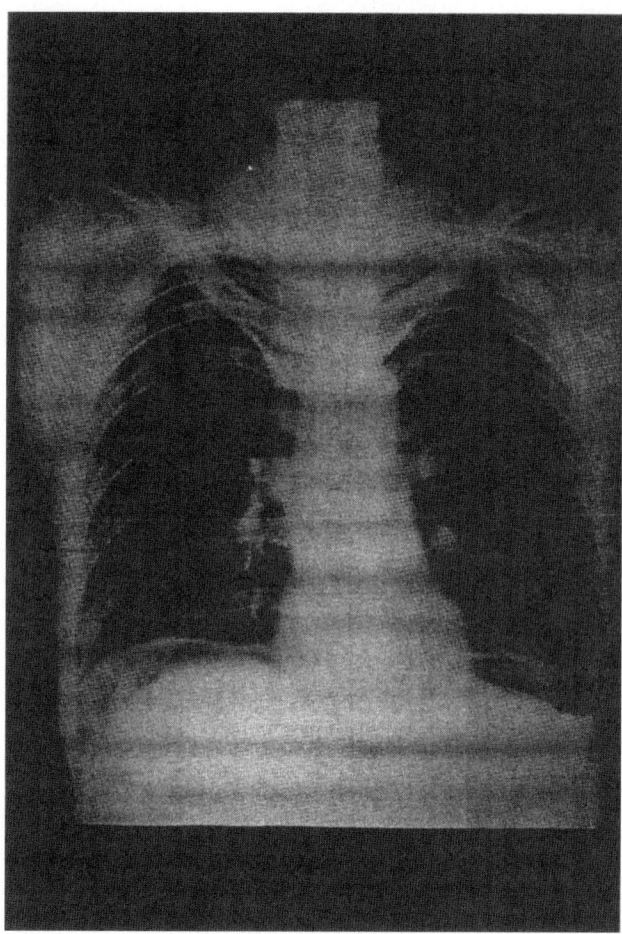

FIG. 25-40. *Pneumoperitoneum on upright chest x-ray in patient with perforated ulcer.*

Table 25-11
Treatment Regimens for *Helicobacter pylori* Infections

Bismuth triple therapy

Bismuth, 2 tablets four times daily
plus
Metronidazole, 250 mg three times daily
plus
Tetracycline, 500 mg four times daily

PPI triple therapy

PPI twice daily
plus
Amoxicillin, 1000 mg two times daily
plus
Clarithromycin, 500 mg two times daily
or
Metronidazole, 500 mg two times daily

Quadruple therapy

PPI twice daily
plus
Bismuth, 2 tablets four times daily
plus
Metronidazole, 250 mg three times daily
plus
Tetracycline, 500 mg four times daily

NOTE: Treatment for 10–14 days is recommended.

PPI = proton pump inhibitor.

obstructing ulcer disease require intervention, either balloon dilation or operation.

Medical Treatment

Patients with peptic ulcer disease should stop smoking and avoid alcohol and NSAIDs (including aspirin). If *H. pylori* infection is documented, it should be treated with one of several acceptable regimens (Table 25-11). Infectious disease consultation may be helpful in the compliant, symptomatic patient with persistent *H. pylori* infection following treatment; or another regimen could be tried (e.g., quadruple therapy). If initial *H. pylori* testing is negative, the ulcer patient may be treated with H$_2$-receptor blockers or proton pump inhibitors. Sucralfate or misoprostol may also be effective. If ulcer symptoms persist, an empiric trial of anti-*H. pylori* therapy is reasonable (false-negative *H. pylori* tests are common). Generally, antisecretory therapy can be stopped after 3 months if the ulcerogenic stimulus (usually *H. pylori*, NSAIDs, or aspirin) has been removed.

However, long-term maintenance therapy for peptic ulcer should be considered in all patients admitted to hospital with an ulcer complication, all high-risk patients on NSAIDs or aspirin (the elderly or debilitated), and all patients with a history of recurrent ulcer or bleeding. Consideration should be given to maintenance therapy in refractory smokers with a history of peptic ulcer. Misoprostol, sulcralfate, and acid suppression may be quite comparable in many of these groups, but misoprostol may cause diarrhea and cramps, and cannot be used in women of childbearing age because of its abortifacient properties.

Surgical Treatment

The indications for surgery in peptic ulcer disease are bleeding, perforation, obstruction, and intractability or nonhealing. Gastric cancer must always be considered in gastric ulcer, whereas malignancy is almost never an issue in duodenal ulcer. Fundamentally,

the gastric and/or duodenal secretions, but within hours a bacterial peritonitis supervenes. Fluid sequestration into the third space of the inflamed peritoneum can be impressive, and fluid resuscitation is mandatory. The patient is in obvious distress, and the abdominal exam shows peritoneal signs. Usually marked involuntary guarding and rebound tenderness is evoked by a gentle examination. Upright chest x-ray shows free air in about 80% of patients (Fig. 25-40). Once the diagnosis has been made, the patient is given analgesia and antibiotics, resuscitated with isotonic fluid, and taken to the operating room. Rarely, the perforation has sealed spontaneously by the time of presentation, and surgery can be avoided. Nonoperative management is appropriate only if there is objective evidence that the leak has sealed (i.e., radiologic contrast study), and in the absence of clinical peritonitis.

Gastric outlet obstruction occurs in no more than 5% of patients with peptic ulcer disease. It is usually due to duodenal or prepyloric ulcer disease, and may be acute (from inflammatory swelling and peristaltic dysfunction) or chronic (from cicatrix). Patients typically present with nonbilious vomiting and may have a profound hypokalemic hypochloremic metabolic alkalosis. Pain or discomfort is common. Weight loss may be prominent, depending on the duration of symptoms. Initial treatment is nasogastric suction, intravenous hydration and electrolyte repletion, and antisecretory medication. The diagnosis is confirmed by endoscopy. Cancer must be ruled out. Currently, most patients admitted to the hospital with

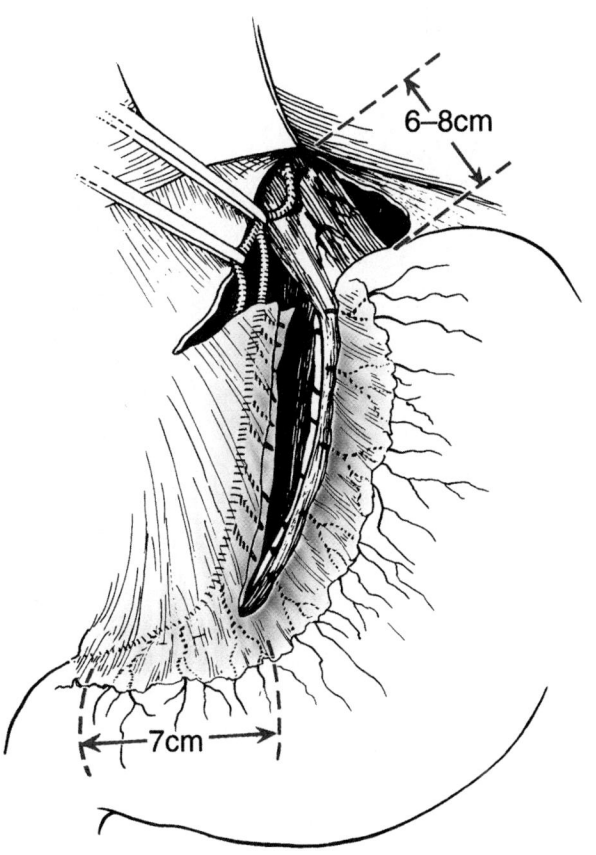

FIG. 25-41. *Highly selective vagotomy. [Reproduced with permission from Farrell TM, Hunter JG: Laparoscopic surgery of the stomach and duodenum, in Zuidema GD, Yeo CJ (eds): Shackelford's Surgery of the Alimentary Tract, 5th ed., Vol. II. Philadelphia: Saunders, 2002, p 202.]*

the vast majority of peptic ulcers are adequately treated by a variant of one of the three basic operations: highly selective vagotomy, vagotomy and drainage, and vagotomy and distal gastrectomy.

Highly Selective Vagotomy

Highly selective vagotomy (HSV), also called parietal cell vagotomy or proximal gastric vagotomy, is safe (mortality risk <0.5%) and causes minimal side effects. The operation severs the vagal nerve supply to the proximal two thirds of the stomach, where essentially all the parietal cells are located. It preserves the vagal innervation to the antrum and pylorus, and the remaining abdominal viscera (Fig. 25-41). Inadequate denervation of the proximal stomach due to technical error may lead to inadequate acid suppression and an unacceptably high incidence of ulcer recurrence. HSV decreases total gastric acid secretion by about 65 to 75%, which is quite comparable to the reduction seen with truncal vagotomy and acid-suppressive medication. Gastric emptying of solids is typically normal in patients after parietal cell vagotomy; liquid emptying may be normal or increased due to decreased compliance associated with loss of receptive relaxation and accommodation. When applied to uncomplicated duodenal ulcer, the recurrence rate is higher with HSV than with vagotomy and antrectomy. However, our increased understanding of the pathophysiologic role of *H. pylori* and NSAIDs in the development of recurrent ulcer may mitigate this concern. HSV has not performed particularly well as a treatment for type II (gastric and duodenal) and III (prepyloric) gastric ulcer, perhaps because of

hypergastrinemia caused by gastric outlet obstruction and persistent antral stasis.

HSV was accepted into the surgical armamentarium largely as a treatment for uncomplicated, intractable duodenal ulcer. Although the operation has been shown to be effective in treating selected patients with complicated peptic ulcer, its usefulness in this regard remains suspect for two reasons. First, many surgeons feel that complicated ulcer disease may call for a more radical operation than uncomplicated disease (a hypothesis that has not been proven). Second, HSV was conceived as an ulcer operation that preserves the pylorus and does not involve opening the GI tract. Most patients with complicated peptic ulcer disease need an ancillary procedure that invalidates these two technical advantages of HSV (e.g., pyloroduodenotomy to oversew a bleeding duodenal ulcer, or gastrojejunostomy to bypass an obstruction).

The Taylor procedure (anterior seromyotomy and posterior truncal vagotomy) is an attractive and simple alternative to HSV. This operation appears to have a similarly low incidence of side effects, and an acceptably low incidence of recurrent ulceration. Effective acid suppression is achieved and normal gastric emptying is maintained. Posterior truncal and anterior HSV are comparable. Although formal HSV is readily accomplished as a laparoscopic procedure, these shortcut operations are particularly attractive to the laparoscopic surgeon, and merit consideration.

Vagotomy and Drainage

Truncal vagotomy and pyloroplasty, and truncal vagotomy and gastrojejunostomy are the paradigmatic vagotomy and drainage (V+D) procedures. However, selective vagotomy and drainage, and HSV and gastrojejunostomy may be useful ulcer operations in selected patients. The advantage of V+D is that it can be performed safely and quickly by the experienced surgeon. The main disadvantages are the side effect profile (10% of patients have significant dumping and/or diarrhea), and a 10% recurrent ulcer rate. Whether the incidence of these postoperative problems (heretofore determined by studies predominantly involving patients with intractable uncomplicated duodenal ulcer) will be different in the current era, with our improved knowledge of complicated ulcer, *H. pylori*, and NSAIDs, is unknown. A serious attempt should be made to perform a complete truncal vagotomy (Fig. 25-42), keeping in mind that in many patients there are more than two vagal trunks at the esophageal hiatus. During truncal vagotomy, care must be taken not to perforate the esophagus, a potentially lethal complication. Intraoperative frozen section confirmation of at least two vagal trunks is prudent. Unlike HSV, V+D is widely accepted as a successful operation for complicated peptic ulcer disease. It has been described as a useful part of the operative treatment for bleeding duodenal and gastric ulcer, perforated duodenal and gastric ulcer, and obstructing duodenal and gastric (type II and III) ulcer. When applied to gastric ulcer, the ulcer should be excised or biopsied.

Truncal vagotomy denervates the antropyloric mechanism, and therefore some sort of procedure is necessary to ablate or bypass the pylorus; otherwise gastric stasis often results. Gastrojejunostomy is a good choice in patients with gastric outlet obstruction or a severely diseased proximal duodenum. The anastomosis is done between the proximal jejunum and the most dependent portion of the greater gastric curvature, in either an antecolic (Fig. 25-43) or retrocolic fashion (Fig. 25-44). On the other hand, pyloroplasty is useful in some patients who require a pyloroduodenotomy to deal with the ulcer complication (e.g., posterior bleeding duodenal ulcer), in those with limited or focal scarring in the pyloric region, or when

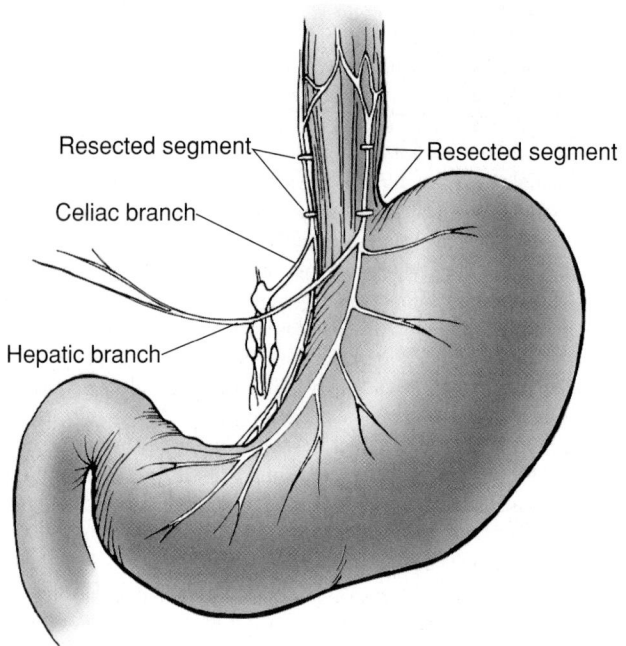

FIG. 25-42. Truncal vagotomy. [Reproduced with permission from Farrell TM, Hunter JG: Laparoscopic surgery of the stomach and duodenum, in Zuidema GD, Yeo CJ (eds): Shackelford's Surgery of the Alimentary Tract, 5th ed., Vol. II. Philadelphia: Saunders, 2002, p 202.]

gastrojejunostomy is technically difficult. The most commonly performed pyloroplasty is the Heineke-Mikulicz type, which closes a longitudinal transpyloric incision in a transverse fashion (Fig. 25-45). Other occasionally useful techniques include the Finney (Fig. 25-46) and the Jaboulay pyloroplasties (Fig. 25-47). These more extensive pyloroplasty techniques may make subsequent distal gastric resection more difficult and/or hazardous.

Vagotomy and Antrectomy

The advantages of vagotomy and antrectomy (V+A) are the extremely low ulcer recurrence rate and the applicability of the operation to many patients with complicated peptic ulcer disease (e.g., bleeding duodenal and gastric ulcer, obstructing peptic ulcer, nonhealing gastric ulcer, and recurrent ulcer). When applied to gastric ulcer disease, the resection is usually extended far enough

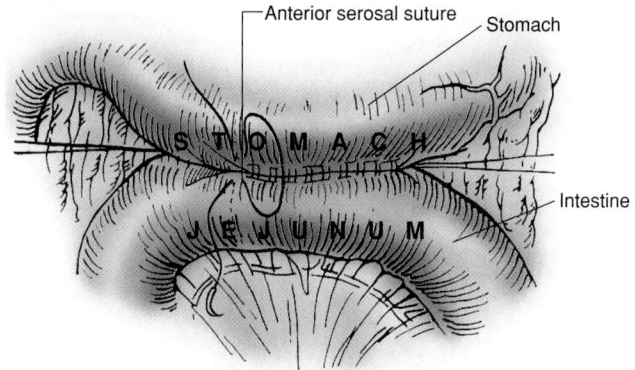

FIG. 25-43. Antecolic gastrojejunostomy. [Reproduced with permission from Farrell TM, Hunter JG: Laparoscopic surgery of the stomach and duodenum, in Zuidema GD, Yeo CJ (eds): Shackelford's Surgery of the Alimentary Tract, 5th ed., Vol. II. Philadelphia: Saunders, 2002, p 202.]

proximally to include the ulcer. The disadvantage of V+A is the somewhat higher operative mortality rate when compared with HSV or V+D. Following antrectomy, gastrointestinal continuity may be re-established, either via a Billroth I gastroduodenostomy (Fig. 25-48) or a Billroth II loop gastrojejunostomy (Fig. 25-49). Since antrectomy routinely leaves a 60 to 70% gastric remnant, reconstruction as a Roux-en-Y gastrojejunostomy should be avoided (Fig. 25-50). The Roux-en-Y operation is an excellent procedure for keeping duodenal contents out of the stomach and esophagus. However, in the presence of a large gastric remnant, this reconstruction will predispose to marginal ulceration and/or gastric stasis.

Although it is *not* clear that the long-term morbidity with vagotomy and antrectomy is greater than with truncal vagotomy and drainage, it *is* clear that the operative mortality rate is somewhat higher with the resectional procedure. Antrectomy should thus be avoided in hemodynamically unstable patients. It should also be avoided in patients with extensive inflammation and/or scarring of the proximal duodenum, since secure anastomosis (Billroth I) or duodenal closure (Billroth II) may be compromised.

Distal Gastrectomy

Distal gastrectomy without vagotomy (usually about a 50% gastrectomy to include the ulcer) has traditionally been the procedure of choice for type I gastric ulcer. Reconstruction may be done as a

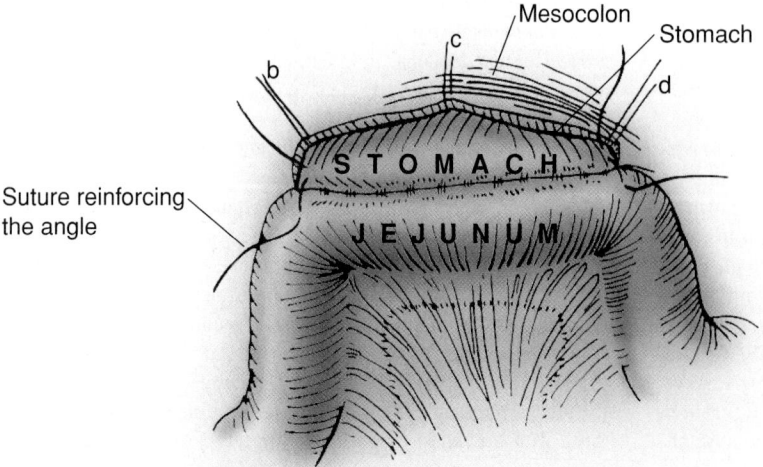

FIG. 25-44. Retrocolic gastrojejunostomy. [Reproduced with permission from Farrell TM, Hunter JG: Laparoscopic surgery of the stomach and duodenum, in Zuidema GD, Yeo CJ (eds): Shackelford's Surgery of the Alimentary Tract, 5th ed., Vol. II. Philadelphia: Saunders, 2002, p 202.]

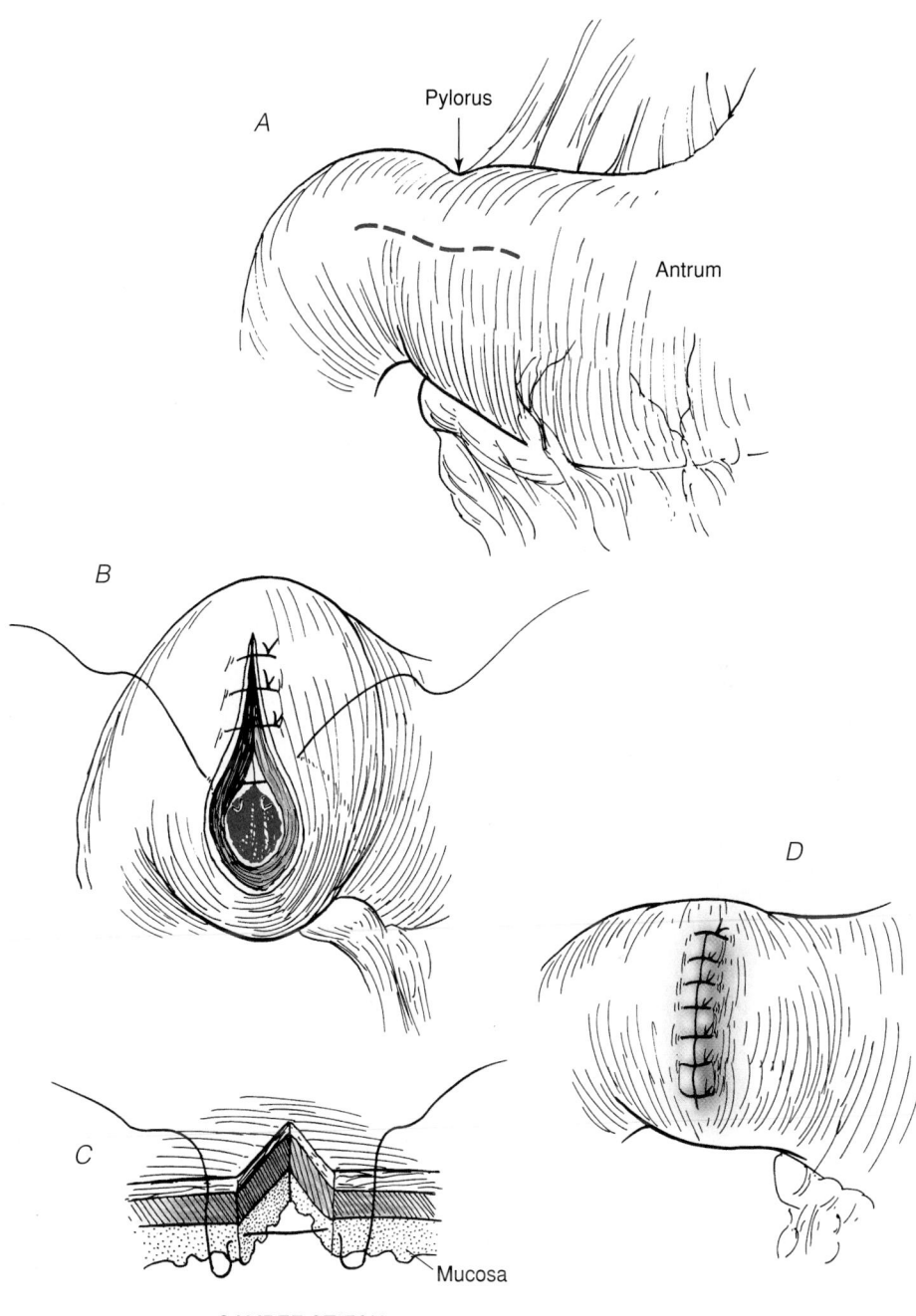

A

Pylorus

Antrum

B

D

C

Mucosa

GAMBEE STITCH

FIG. 25-45. Heineke-Mikulicz pyloro-plasty. *[Reproduced with permission from Farrell TM, Hunter JG: Laparoscopic surgery of the stomach and duodenum, in Zuidema GD, Yeo CJ (eds): Shackelford's Surgery of the Alimentary Tract, 5th ed., Vol. II. Philadelphia: Saunders, 2002, p 202.]*

Billroth I (preferable) or Billroth II. Truncal vagotomy is added for type II and III gastric ulcers, or if the patient is believed to be at increased risk for recurrent ulcer, and should be considered if Billroth II reconstruction is contemplated. Though not routinely used today in the surgical treatment of peptic ulcer, subtotal gastrectomy (75% distal gastrectomy) without vagotomy may be an appealing choice for an occasional ulcer patient. Periesophageal dissection is avoided (vagotomy is unnecessary if 75% gastrectomy is performed), and extensive periduodenal dissection is minimized (Billroth II is the reconstruction of choice). Finally, concomitant gastric ulcers (type II or III) are resected. However, subtotal gastrectomy is rarely the first operation of choice for any patient with duodenal ulcer, since it leaves an inadequate gastric reservoir, and since vagotomy and antrectomy has a lower recurrent ulcer rate, is at least as safe, and has a similar side effect profile.

Choice of Operation for Peptic Ulcer

The choice of operation for the individual patient with peptic ulcer disease depends on a variety of factors, including the type of ulcer (duodenal, gastric, recurrent, or marginal), the indication for operation, and the condition of the patient, among others. Other important considerations are intra-abdominal factors (duodenal scarring/inflammation, adhesions, or difficult exposure), the ulcer diathesis status of the patient, the surgeon's experience and personal preference, whether *H. pylori* infection is present, the need for NSAID therapy, previous treatment, and the likelihood of future compliance with treatment. Table 25-12 shows the surgical options for managing various aspects of peptic ulcer disease. In general, resective procedures have a lower ulcer recurrence rate, but a higher operative morbidity and mortality rate (Table 25-13) when compared

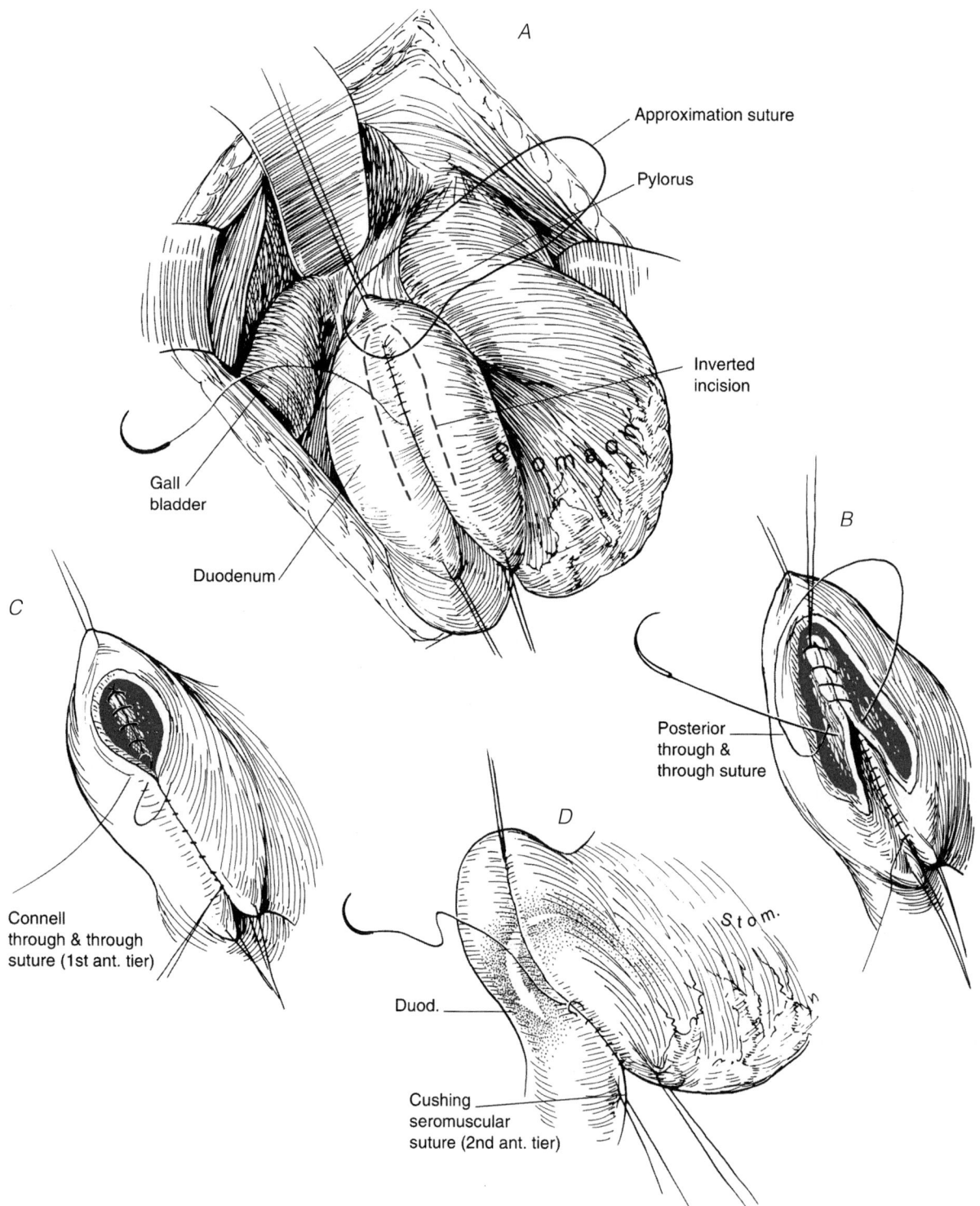

FIG. 25-46. Finney pyloroplasty. *[Reproduced with permission from Farrell TM, Hunter JG: Laparoscopic surgery of the stomach and duodenum, in Zuidema GD, Yeo CJ (eds): Shackelford's Surgery of the Alimentary Tract, 5th ed., Vol. II. Philadelphia: Saunders, 2002, p 202.]*

to nonresective ulcer operations. Because ulcer recurrence is often related to *H. pylori* and/or NSAIDs, it is usually managed adequately without reoperation. Thus, gastric resection to minimize recurrence in duodenal ulcer disease is often not justified today; resection for gastric ulcer remains the standard because of the risk of cancer.

Bleeding

Bleeding is the most common cause of ulcer-related death. Recently, the total number of operations for bleeding peptic ulcer in the U.S. appears to have increased, as has the ratio of operations for bleeding ulcer to total ulcer operations. It is not known if or how endoscopic

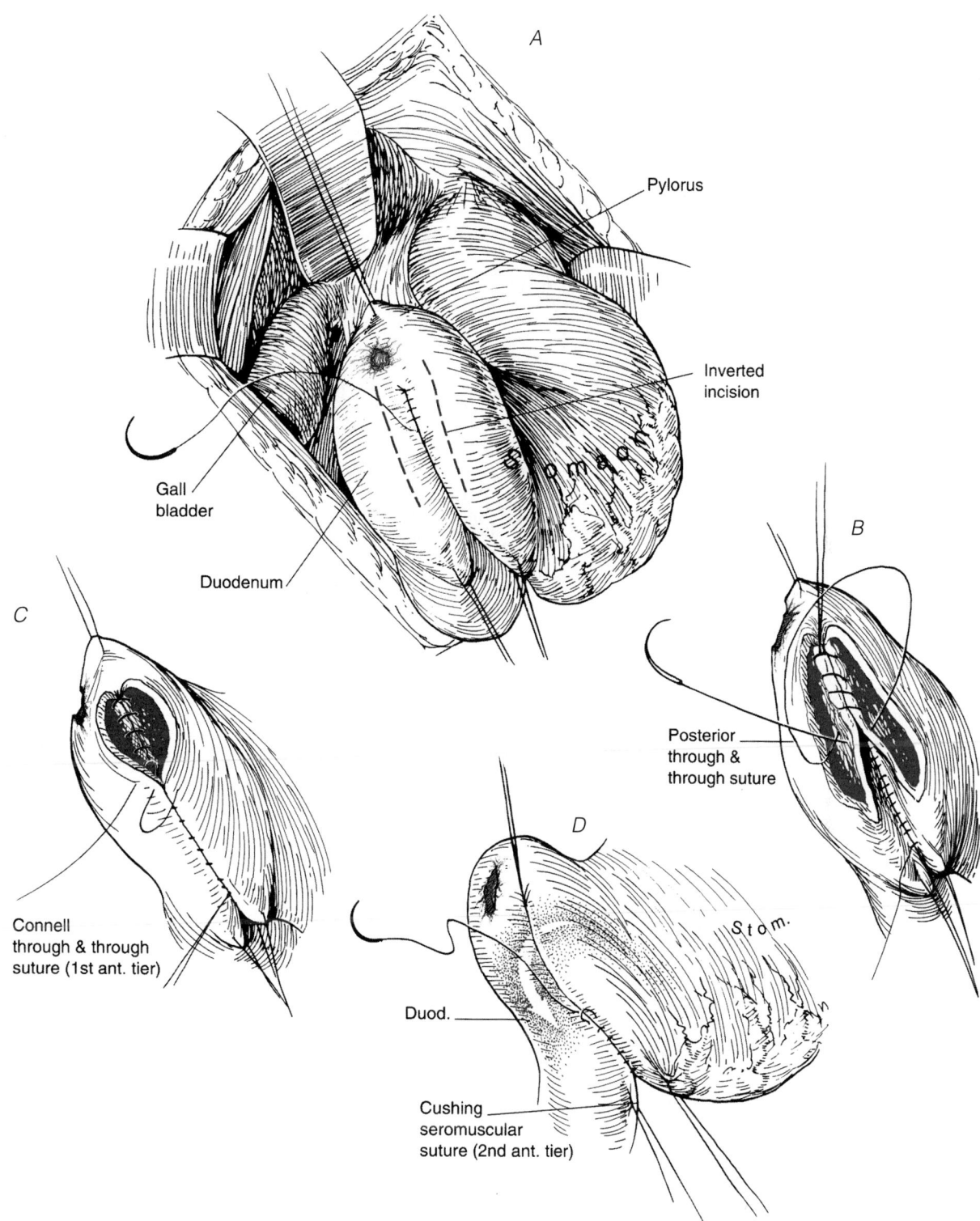

FIG. 25-47. Jaboulay pyloroplasty. *[Reproduced with permission from Farrell TM, Hunter JG: Laparo-scopic surgery of the stomach and duodenum, in Zuidema GD, Yeo CJ (eds): Shackelford's Surgery of the Alimentary Tract, 5th ed., Vol. II. Philadelphia: Saunders, 2002, p 202.]*

therapy, *H. pylori* treatment, and/or antisecretory drug use will affect this trend, which is no doubt due in part to the aging of the population and the epidemic of NSAID use. Although the surgeon treating patients with bleeding peptic ulcer disease needs to know when to operate and what operation to perform, the success of nonsurgical therapy in treating and preventing bleeding peptic ulcer disease has resulted in the selection of a subgroup of high-risk patients for to-day's surgeon. It is certainly likely that patients currently coming to operation for bleeding peptic ulcer disease are at higher risk, and thus more likely to have a poor surgical result than ever before.

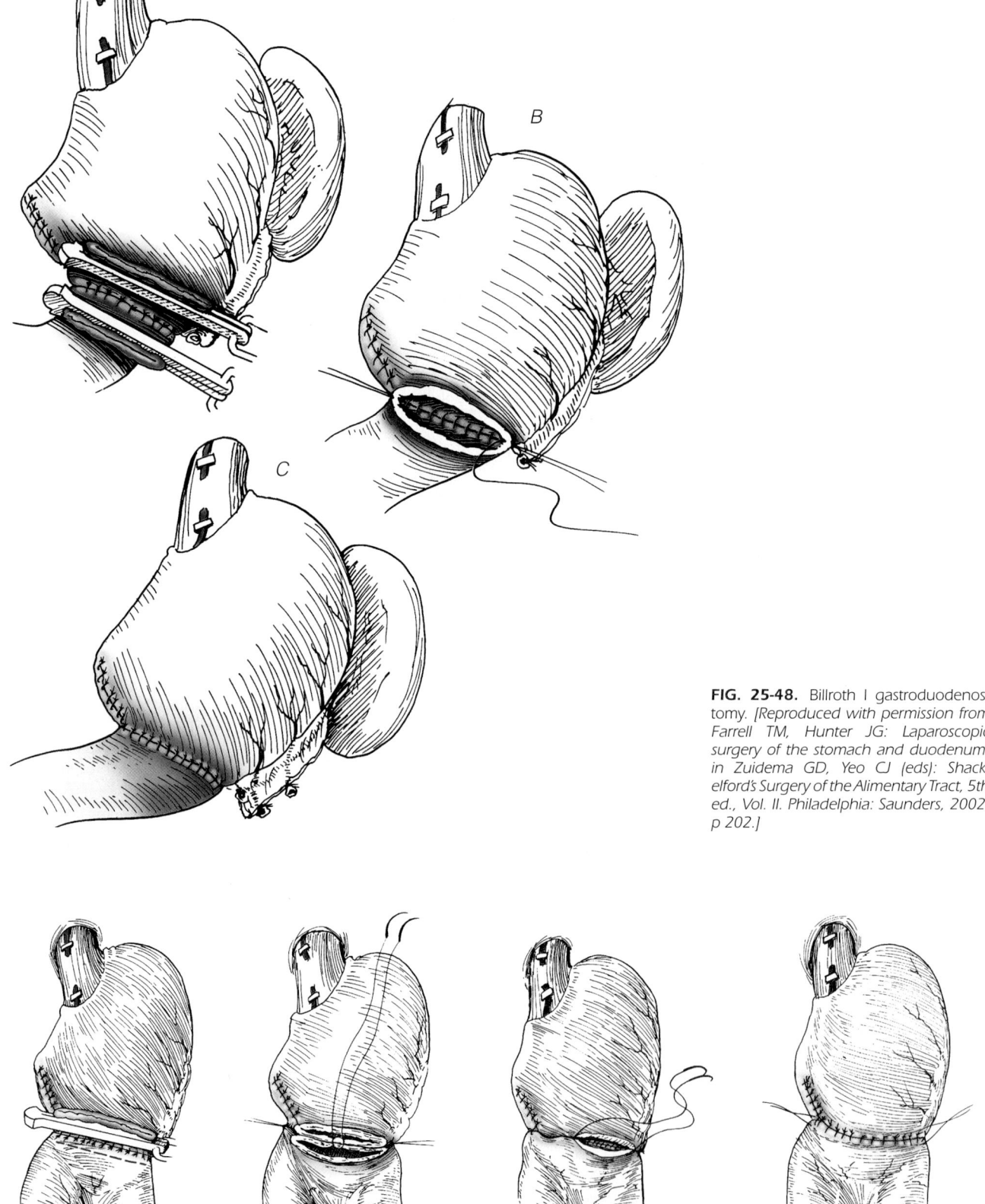

FIG. 25-48. Billroth I gastroduodenostomy. [Reproduced with permission from Farrell TM, Hunter JG: Laparoscopic surgery of the stomach and duodenum, in Zuidema GD, Yeo CJ (eds): Shackelford's Surgery of the Alimentary Tract, 5th ed., Vol. II. Philadelphia: Saunders, 2002, p 202.]

FIG. 25-49. Billroth II antecolic gastrojejunostomy. [Reproduced with permission from Farrell TM, Hunter JG: Laparoscopic surgery of the stomach and duodenum, in Zuidema GD, Yeo CJ (eds): Shackelford's Surgery of the Alimentary Tract, 5th ed., Vol. II. Philadelphia: Saunders, 2002, p 202.]

Table 25-13
Clinical Results of Surgery for Duodenal Ulcer

	Parietal Cell Vagotomy	Truncal Vagotomy and Pyloroplasty	Truncal Vagotomy and Antrectomy
Operative mortality rate (%)	0	<1	1
Ulcer recurrence rate (%)	5–15	5–15	<2
Dumping (%)			
Mild	<5	10	10–15
Severe	0	1	1–2
Diarrhea (%)			
Mild	<5	25	20
Severe	0	2	1–2

SOURCE: Modified with permission from Mulholland MW, Debas HT: Chronic duodenal and gastric ulcer. *Surg Clin North Am* 67:489, 1987.

The surgical options for treating bleeding peptic ulcer disease include suture ligation of the bleeder (and biopsy for gastric ulcer); suture ligation and definitive nonresective ulcer operation (HSV or V+D); and gastric resection (usually including vagotomy and ulcer excision).

Bleeding Duodenal Ulcer

Indications for operation for bleeding duodenal ulcers are massive hemorrhage that is unresponsive to endoscopic control, and transfusion requirement of more than 4 to 6 units of blood, despite attempts at endoscopic control. Lack of availability of a therapeutic endoscopist, recurrent hemorrhage after one or more attempts at endoscopic control, lack of availability of blood for transfusion, repeat hospitalization for bleeding duodenal ulcer, and concurrent indications for surgery such as perforation or obstruction, also are indications for surgery. The mortality rate for surgery for bleeding duodenal ulcer is 10 to 20%. Early operation should be considered in patients over 60 years of age, those presenting in shock, those requiring more than 4 units of blood in 24 hours or 8 units of blood in 48 hours, those with rebleeding, and those with ulcers greater than 2 cm in diameter or strategically located as described above.

The two operations most commonly used for bleeding duodenal ulcer are V+D combined with oversewing of the ulcer, or V+A. The trade-off appears to be an increased risk of rebleeding with V+D, compared to the increased operative mortality of V+A. When the mortality for reoperation for rebleeding is considered, the overall mortality is probably comparable for the two approaches. Patients who are in shock or medically unstable should not have gastric resection.

An initial pyloromyotomy incision allows access to the bleeding posterior duodenal ulcer, and an expeditious Kocher maneuver allows the surgeon to control the hemorrhage with the left hand if necessary. Heavy suture material on a stout needle is used to place figure-of-eight sutures or a U-stitch in order to secure the bleeding vessel at the base of the posterior duodenal ulcer. Multiple sutures are usually necessary. Once the surgeon is unequivocally convinced that hemostasis is secure, a pyloroplasty can be performed. A truncal vagotomy completes the operation. If V+A is selected, smaller ulcers are resected with the specimen, but larger bleeding duodenal ulcers must often be left behind in the duodenal stump. If this is the case, suture hemostasis must be attained and a secure duodenal closure accomplished. The anterior wall of the open duodenum

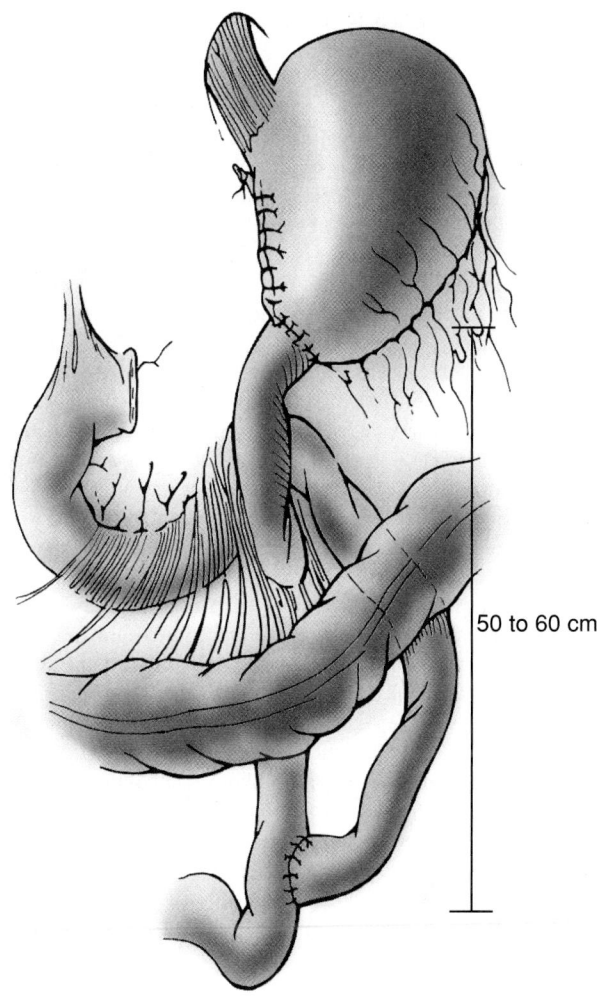

FIG. 25-50. Roux-en-Y gastrojejunostomy. *[Reproduced with permission from Farrell TM, Hunter JG: Laparoscopic surgery of the stomach and duodenum, in Zuidema GD, Yeo CJ (eds): Shackelford's Surgery of the Alimentary Tract, 5th ed., Vol. II. Philadelphia: Saunders, 2002, p 202.]*

50 to 60 cm

Table 25-12
Surgical Options in the Treatment of Duodenal and Gastric Ulcer Disease

Indication	Duodenal	Gastric
Bleeding	1. Oversew[a]	1. Oversew and biopsy[a]
	2. Oversew, V+D	2. Oversew, biopsy, V+D
	3. V+A	3. Distal gastrectomy[b]
Perforation	1. Patch[a]	1. Biopsy and patch[a]
	2. Patch, HSV[b]	2. Wedge excision, V+D
	3. Patch, V+D	3. Distal gastrectomy[b]
Obstruction	1. HSV + GJ	1. Biopsy; HSV + GJ
	2. V+A	2. Distal gastrectomy[b]
Intractability/ nonhealing	1. HSV[b]	1. HSV and wedge excision
	2. V+D	2. Distal gastrectomy
	3. V+A	

[a] Unless the patient is in shock or moribund, a definitive procedure should be considered.
[b] Operation of choice in low-risk patient.

GJ = gastrojejunostomy; HSV = highly-selective vagotomy; V+A = vagotomy and antrectomy; V+D = vagotomy and drainage.

can be sutured to either the proximal or distal lip of the posterior ulcer once the bleeding vessel has been sutured. The duodenal closure can be buttressed with omentum and the duodenum should be decompressed, either with a lateral duodenostomy or retrograde duodenostomy tube via the proximal jejunum. Use of a feeding jejunostomy is also considered. A Billroth II anastomosis is preferred because it avoids the extensive mobilization necessary for Billroth I, and because it keeps the ulcer out of the acid stream if it is left behind.

Bleeding Gastric Ulcer

Bleeding gastric ulcers tend to occur in older and/or medically complicated patients, and this fact tends to increase the operative risk. Although this has been used by some as an excuse not to operate early on these patients, experience shows that planned surgery in a resuscitated patient results in a better operative survival rate than emergent operation in a patient who has rebled and is in shock. Patients with gastric ulcer bleeding who are most likely to require surgery have bled more than 6 units and have presented in shock. Endoscopically, their ulcers tend to be on the lesser curvature with the usual stigmata of recent hemorrhage. Distal gastric resection to include the bleeding ulcer is the procedure of choice for bleeding gastric ulcer. Second best is V+D with oversewing and biopsy of the ulcer. Oversewing of the bleeder followed by long-term acid suppression is a reasonable alternative in extremely high-risk patients. The specter of cancer is ever present in the patient with gastric ulcer, whether it is bleeding or not.

Perforation

Perforation is the second most common complication of peptic ulcer. As with bleeding peptic ulcer disease, NSAID use has also been inextricably linked with perforated peptic ulcer disease, especially in the elderly population. Well over 20% of patients over the age of 60 presenting with a perforated ulcer are taking NSAIDs at the time of perforation. The mortality rate for perforated gastric ulcer is higher than that for duodenal ulcer, because the group with the former malady tend to be older and sicker. Surgery is almost always indicated, although occasionally nonsurgical treatment can be used in the stable patient without peritonitis, and in whom radiologic studies document a sealed perforation. Patients with acute perforation and GI blood loss (either chronic or acute) should be suspected of having a posterior "kissing" ulcer, and the appropriate definitive operation should then be performed.

The options for surgical treatment of perforated duodenal ulcer are simple patch closure, patch closure and HSV, or patch closure and V+D. Simple patch closure alone should be done in patients with hemodynamic instability and/or exudative peritonitis signifying a perforation over 24 hours old. In all other patients the addition of a definitive ulcer operation (HSV or V+D) should be considered. Numerous studies have reported a negligible mortality with this approach. Although in the U.S. and Western Europe there is clearly a trend away from definitive operation for perforated duodenal ulcer, it still seems prudent to add HSV to most stable patients with a perforated duodenal ulcer, especially in those with a chronic history, and in those who are unlikely to be compliant with *H. pylori* treatment or who require NSAIDs. In the pre-*H. pylori* era, it was shown that only 30% of patients with perforated duodenal ulcer treated by simple closure had good long-term results. Early data now suggest that simple closure of perforated duodenal ulcer may achieve satisfactory long-term results when *H. pylori* infection

(present in 50 to 75% of patients with perforated duodenal ulcer) is eliminated. However, it sometimes is difficult to determine the *H. pylori* status of the patient having emergent operation for perforated ulcer. Furthermore it is doubtful whether many of these patients will comply with the medication regimen required to eradicate *H. pylori*. Therefore, using possible *H. pylori* infection as an excuse not to do a definitive ulcer operation in any patient with perforated duodenal ulcer is irrational. While it must be acknowledged that laparoscopic patch repair for perforated ulcer is commonly done without definitive surgery, perhaps laparoscopic HSV or some variant thereof can be recommended for those patients who have persistent or recurrent ulcer symptoms.

Perforated gastric ulcer carriers a higher mortality rate than perforated duodenal ulcer (10 to 40%). This is generally thought to be due to the gastric ulcer patients' more advanced age, increased medical comorbidities, delay in seeking medical attention, and the larger size of gastric ulcers. Perforated gastric ulcers are associated with NSAID and tobacco use, and often present without prior symptoms. All perforated gastric ulcers are best treated by distal gastric resection with or without truncal vagotomy, depending upon ulcer type. Vagotomy is usually performed for type II and III gastric ulcers. Patch closure with biopsy; or local excision and closure; or biopsy, closure, truncal vagotomy, and drainage are alternative operations. All perforated gastric ulcers, even those in the prepyloric position, should be biopsied if they are not removed at surgery. HSV should generally not be used for perforated gastric ulcer. Simple patch closure has been shown to have a higher short-term complication rate (20 vs. 5%) and a higher ulcer recurrence rate (25 vs. 10%) than distal gastrectomy. The latter often eradicates *H. pylori,* which could partially explain this finding; other authors have cited lower ulcer recurrence rates following simple patch closure of perforated gastric ulcer with effective eradication of *H. pylori*. However, it should be recognized that many patients with perforated gastric ulcer are *H. pylori* negative.

Obstruction

Currently, gastric outlet obstruction is the least common indication for operation in peptic ulcer disease. Acute ulcers associated with obstruction due to edema and/or motor dysfunction may respond to intensive antisecretory therapy and nasogastric suction. But most patients with significant obstruction from chronic ulceration will require some sort of more substantial intervention. Endoscopic balloon dilation can often transiently improve obstructive symptoms, but many of these patients ultimately fail and come to operation. Even in patients who have a successful initial dilation, at least half will require subsequent surgery, usually for recurrent obstruction, although interval bleeding and perforation is also a possibility. Some investigators have speculated that effective treatment of *H. pylori* in patients with obstructing peptic ulcer disease will improve the results of balloon dilation and decrease the ulcer recurrence rate. But again, a significant percentage of patients with ulcer-related gastric outlet obstruction do not have demonstrable *H. pylori* infection.

The most common operations for obstructing peptic ulcer disease are V+A and V+D. HSV and drainage is comparable to vagotomy and antrectomy in this setting. HSV and gastrojejunostomy is an appealing operation for obstruction, both because it can be done as a laparoscopically assisted procedure, and because it does not complicate future resection should this be needed. All gastric ulcers associated with obstruction should be adequately biopsied if not resected.

Table 25-14

Differential Diagnosis of Intractability or Nonhealing Peptic Ulcer Disease

Cancer
    Gastric
    Pancreatic
    Duodenal
Persistent *H. pylori* infection
    Tests may be false-negative
    Consider empiric treatment
Noncompliant patient
    Failure to take prescribed medication
    Surreptitious use of nonsteroidal anti-inflammatory drugs
Motility disorder
Zollinger-Ellison syndrome

Intractability or Nonhealing

This should indeed be a rare indication for surgery performed today. Arguably, the patient referred for surgical evaluation because of intractable peptic ulcer disease should raise red flags for the surgeon. Acid secretion can be totally blocked and *H. pylori* eradicated with modern medication; therefore, the question remains: "Why does the patient have a persistent ulcer diathesis?" The surgeon should review the differential diagnosis of nonhealing ulcer prior to any consideration of operative treatment (Table 25-14).

Surgical treatment should be considered in patients with nonhealing or intractable peptic ulcer disease who have multiple recurrences, large ulcers (>2 cm), complications (obstruction, perforation, or hemorrhage), or suspected gastric cancer. Surgery should be approached most cautiously in the thin or marginally nourished individual.

It is important that the surgeon not fall into the trap of performing a large, irreversible operation on these patients, based on the unproven theory that if all other methods have failed, a larger operation is required. Today's patients are different than those of 3 or 4 decades ago. One might argue that modern medical care has healed the minor ulcer, and that patients presenting with true intractability or nonhealing will be more difficult to treat and are likely to have chronic problems after a major ulcer operation. If surgery is necessary, less is often better. It is the practice of this author never to perform a gastrectomy as the initial elective operation for intractable duodenal ulcer in the thin or asthenic patient. Instead, the preferred operation for this group of patients is HSV. In patients with nonhealing gastric ulcer, wedge resection with HSV should be considered in thin or frail patients. Otherwise distal gastrectomy (to include the ulcer) is recommended. It is unnecessary to add a vagotomy in patients with type I gastric ulcer. Juxtaesophageal gastric ulcers (type IV) are pathophysiologically akin to type I gastric ulcers (i.e., associated with gastric acid hyposecretion), but are often difficult to resect as part of a distal gastrectomy. A variety of techniques have been used to treat these ulcers surgically, including the Csendes operation, the Pauchet gastrectomy, and the Kelling-Madlener procedure (Fig. 25-51).

Zollinger-Ellison Syndrome

The Zollinger-Ellison syndrome (ZES) is caused by the uncontrolled secretion of abnormal amounts of gastrin by a pancreatic or duodenal neuroendocrine tumor (i.e., gastrinoma). Most cases (80%) are sporadic, but 20% are inherited. The inherited or familial form of gastrinoma is associated with multiple endocrine neoplasia type I (MEN I), which consists of parathyroid, pituitary, and pancreatic (or duodenal) tumors. Gastrinoma is the most common pancreatic tumor in patients with MEN I. Patients with MEN I usually have

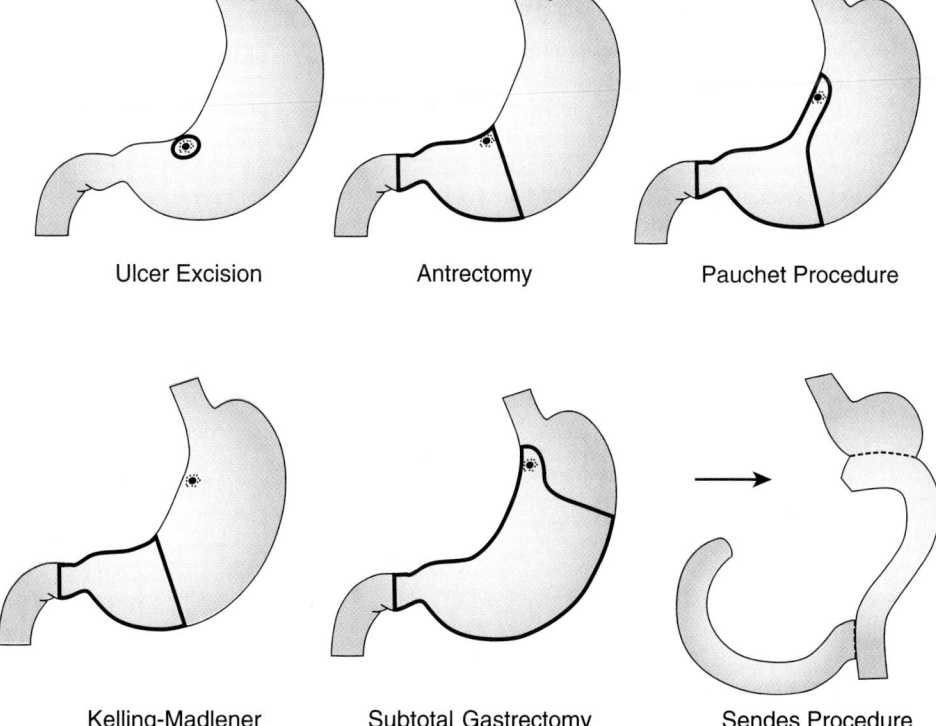

FIG. 25-51. Operations for gastric ulcer. *[Reproduced with permission from Farrell TM, Hunter JG: Laparoscopic surgery of the stomach and duodenum, in Zuidema GD, Yeo CJ (eds): Shackelford's Surgery of the Alimentary Tract, 5th ed., Vol. II. Philadelphia: Saunders, 2002, p 202.]*

Ulcer Excision

Antrectomy

Pauchet Procedure

Kelling-Madlener Procedure

Subtotal Gastrectomy Roux-en-Y Esophagogastrojejunostomy

Sendes Procedure

multiple gastrinoma tumors, and surgical cure is unusual. Sporadic gastrinomas are more often solitary and amenable to surgical cure. Currently, about 50% of gastrinomas are malignant, with lymph node, liver, or other distant metastases at presentation. Five-year survival in patients presenting with metastatic disease is approximately 40%.

The most common symptoms of ZES are epigastric pain, GERD, and diarrhea. The average age of presentation is 50 years, and over 90% of patients with gastrinoma have peptic ulcer. Most ulcers are in the typical location (proximal duodenum), but atypical ulcer location (distal duodenum, jejunum, or multiple ulcers) should prompt an evaluation for gastrinoma. Gastrinoma also should be considered in the differential diagnosis of recurrent or refractory peptic ulcer, secretory diarrhea, gastric rugal hypertrophy, esophagitis with stricture, bleeding or perforated ulcer, familial ulcer, and ulcer in the setting of hypercalcemia.

Hypergastrinemia in the presence of elevated BAO suggests gastrinoma. Despite this relatively simple guideline, most patients with ZES have been symptomatic for several years prior to diagnosis. In patients on antisecretory therapy, medication should be stopped for several days prior to checking the serum gastrin level, since acid suppression may falsely elevate gastrin levels. Causes of hypergastrinemia can be divided into those associated with hyperacidity and those associated with hypoacidity (Table 25-15). The diagnosis of ZES is confirmed by the secretin stimulation test. An intravenous bolus of secretin (2 U/kg) is given and gastrin levels are checked before and after injection. An increase in serum gastrin of 200 pg/mL or greater suggests the presence of gastrinoma. Other provocative tests such as calcium stimulation or standard meal are usually unnecessary. Patients with gastrinoma should have serum calcium and parathyroid hormone levels determined to rule out MEN I.

Eighty percent of primary tumors are found in the gastrinoma triangle (Fig. 25-52) and many tumors are small (<1 cm), making preoperative localization difficult. Transabdominal ultrasound is quite specific, but not very sensitive. CT will detect most lesions over 2 cm in size and magnetic resonance imaging (MRI) is comparable. Endoscopic ultrasound is more sensitive than these other noninvasive imaging tests, but it still misses many of the smaller lesions, and may confuse normal lymph nodes for gastrinomas. Currently, the imaging study of choice for gastrinoma is somatostatin receptor scintigraphy (SRS, the octreotide scan). When the pretest probability of gastrinoma is high, the sensitivity and specificity of this modality approach 100%. Gastrinoma cells contain type 2 somatostatin receptors which bind the indium-labeled somatostatin analogue (octreotide) with high affinity, making imaging with a gamma camera possible (Fig. 25-53). Currently, angiographic

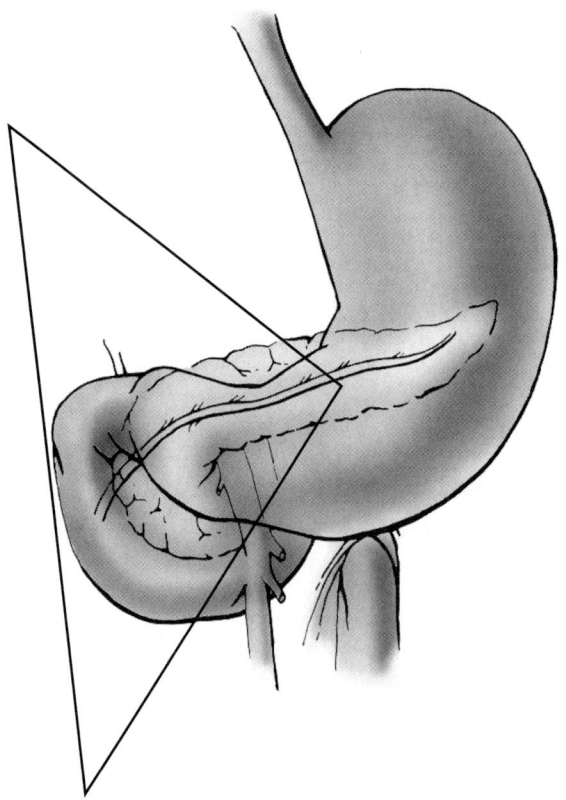

FIG. 25-52. Gastrinoma triangle. [Reproduced with permission from Ritchie WP Jr.: Benign diseases of the stomach and duodenum, in Ritchie WP, Steele G, Dean RH (eds): General Surgery. Philadelphia: Lippincott, 1995, p 117.]

localization studies are infrequently performed for gastrinoma. Both diagnostic angiography and transhepatic selective venous sampling of the portal system have been supplanted by selective secretin infusion, which helps to localize the tumor as inside or outside the gastrinoma triangle. In this test, an arterial catheter is selectively placed in a named vessel supplying the pancreas (e.g., gastroduodenal or splenic), and a venous catheter is placed in a hepatic vein. Secretin is injected into the visceral artery and gastrin is sampled in the hepatic vein. A significant elevation in hepatic venous gastrin indicates that the tumor is supplied by the injected artery. Probably the most important means of locating gastrinomas is intraoperative exploration.

All patients with sporadic (nonfamilial) gastrinoma should be considered for surgical resection and possible cure. The lesions should be located in 90% of patients, and 60% are cured by extirpation of the gastrinoma(s). A thorough intraoperative exploration of the gastrinoma triangle and pancreas is essential, but other sites (i.e., liver, stomach, small bowel, mesentery, and pelvis) should be evaluated as part of a thorough intra-abdominal evaluation to find the primary tumor, which is usually solitary. The duodenum and pancreas should be extensively mobilized and intraoperative ultrasound should be used. Intraoperative EGD with transillumination should be considered. If the tumor cannot be located, generous longitudinal duodenotomy with inspection and palpation should be considered. Lymph nodes from the portal, peripancreatic, and celiac drainage basins should be sampled. Ablation or resection of hepatic metastases should be considered. The management of gastrinoma in patients with MEN I is controversial because the patients are rarely cured by operation, and the tumors tend to be small and multiple.

Table 25-15
Differential Diagnosis of Hypergastrinemia

With excessive gastric acid formation (ulcerogenic)
    Zollinger-Ellison syndrome
    Gastric outlet obstruction
    Retained gastric antrum (after Billroth II reconstruction)
    G-cell hyperplasia
Without excessive gastric acid formation (nonulcerogenic)
    Pernicious anemia
    Atrophic gastritis
    Renal failure
    Postvagotomy
    Short gut syndrome (after significant intestinal resection)

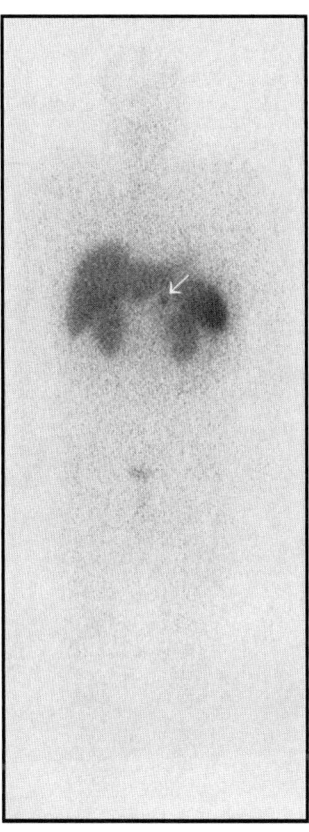

FIG. 25-53. *Positive octreotide scan in patient with gastrinoma (arrow).*

If tumor can be imaged preoperatively, operation by an experienced gastrinoma surgeon is reasonable.

Acid hypersecretion in patients with gastrinoma can always be managed with high-dose proton pump inhibitors. Highly selective vagotomy may make management easier in some patients and should be considered in those with surgically untreatable or unresectable gastrinoma.

GASTRITIS AND STRESS ULCER

Pathogenesis and Prevention

Gastritis is mucosal inflammation. The gross endoscopic diagnosis of gastritis correlates poorly with histologic findings, and is thus relatively useless as a diagnosis without confirmatory biopsy. Additionally, there is poor correlation between symptoms and histologic gastritis. The most common cause of gastritis is *H. pylori*. Other causes of gastritis include alcohol, NSAIDs, Crohn's disease, tuberculosis, and bile reflux (primary or secondary). These agents cause injury by a variety of different mechanisms. In general, the infectious and inflammatory causes result in immune cell infiltration and cytokine production which damage mucosal cells. The chemical agents (alcohol, aspirin, and bile) generally work to disrupt the mucosal barrier, allowing mucosal damage by back-diffusion of luminal hydrogen ions.

Stress gastritis is a peculiar entity that has all but disappeared from the clinical (if not endoscopic) lexicon, largely due to better critical care and acid suppression or cytoprotective agents (e.g., sucralfate) in the intensive care unit (ICU). Stress gastritis and stress ulcer are probably due to inadequate gastric mucosal blood flow

during periods of intense stress. Adequate mucosal blood flow is important to maintain the mucosal barrier, and to buffer any back-diffused hydrogen ions. When blood flow is inadequate, these processes fail and mucosal breakdown occurs. While it is still common to see small mucosal erosions when performing endoscopy in the ICU, it is rare for these lesions to coalesce into the larger bleeding erosions that plagued the ICU patient 30 years ago. In the extraordinarily rare patient requiring operation today for hemorrhagic stress gastritis, the surgical options include vagotomy and drainage with oversewing of the major bleeding lesions, or near total gastrectomy. Angiographic embolization and endoscopic hemostatic treatment should at least be considered as well.

MALIGNANT NEOPLASMS OF THE STOMACH

The three most common primary malignant gastric neoplasms are adenocarcinoma (95%), lymphoma (4%), and malignant gastrointestinal stromal tumor (GIST) (1%) (Table 25-16). Other rare primary malignancies include carcinoid, angiosarcoma, carcinosarcoma, and squamous cell carcinoma. Occasionally the stomach is the site of hematogenous metastasis from other sites (e.g., melanoma or breast). More commonly, malignant tumors from adjacent organs invade the stomach by direct extension (e.g., colon or pancreas) or by peritoneal seeding (e.g., ovary).

Adenocarcinoma

Epidemiology

In 1930 in the U.S., gastric cancer was the leading cause of cancer death among men and the third leading cause of death among women. Today it is not even included among the top 10 causes (Fig. 25-54). Over the past several decades there has been a dramatic decrease in the gastric cancer incidence and death rate in the U.S. (Fig. 25-55), as well as in most Western industrialized countries (Fig. 25-56). This decrease has been mostly in the so-called "intestinal form" rather than in the "diffuse form" of gastric cancer (see below). Worldwide, especially in Asia and Eastern Europe, gastric cancer remains the second most common cancer, and is the leading cause of cancer death. In 2003 in the U.S. there were approximately 22,400 new cases of stomach cancer (13,400 in men and 9000 in women), and 12,100 deaths from this disease (7000 men and 5100 women). The estimated 5-year survival rate is 22%, up from about 15% in 1975.

Table 25-16
Frequency of Gastric Tumors

Tumor Type	No. of Cases	Percent
Malignant tumors	4199	93.0
Carcinoma	3970	87.9
Lymphoma	136	3.0
Leiomyosarcoma	77	1.7
Carcinoid	11	0.3
Others	5	0.1
Benign tumors	315	7.0
Polyp	140	3.1
Leiomyoma	92	2.0
Inflammatory lesions	30	0.7
Heterotopic pancreas	20	0.4
Others	33	0.8

SOURCE: Modified with permission from Ming SC: Tumors of the esophagus and stomach, in *Atlas of Tumor Pathology,* Second Series, Fascicle 7. Washington: Armed Forces Institute of Pathology, 1973, p 82.

Leading Sites of New Cancer Cases and Deaths - 2003 Estimates

Estimated New Cases

Male	Female
Prostate	Breast
220,900 (33%)	211,300 (32%)
Lung & Bronchus	Lung & Bronchus
91,800 (14%)	81,100 (12%)
Colon & Rectum	Colon & Rectum
72,800 (11%)	74,700 (11%)
Urinary Bladder	Uterine Corpus
42,200 (6%)	40,100 (6%)
Melanoma of the Skin	Ovary
29,900 (4%)	25,400 (4%)
Non-Hodgkin's Lymphoma	Non-Hodgkin's Lymphoma
28,300 (4%)	24,300 (4%)
Kidney	Melanoma of the Skin
19,500 (3%)	24,300 (3%)
Oral Cavity	Thyroid
18,200 (3%)	18,200 (3%)
Leukemia	Pancreas
17,900 (3%)	15,800 (2%)
Pancreas	Urinary Bladder
14,900 (2%)	15,200 (2%)
All Sites	All Sites
675,300 (100%)	658,800 (100%)

Estimated Deaths

Male	Female
Lung & Bronchus	Lung & Bronchus
88,400 (31%)	68,800 (25%)
Prostate	Breast
28,900 (10%)	39,800 (15%)
Colon & Rectum	Colon & Rectum
28,300 (10%)	28,800 (11%)
Pancreas	Pancreas
14,700 (5%)	15,300 (6%)
Non-Hodgkin's Lymphoma	Ovary
12,200 (4%)	14,300 (5%)
Leukemia	Non-Hodgkin's Lymphoma
12,100 (4%)	11,200 (4%)
Esophagus	Leukemia
9,900 (4%)	9,800 (4%)
Liver	Uterine Corpus
9,200 (3%)	6,800 (3%)
Urinary Bladder	Brain
8,600 (3%)	5,800 (2%)
Kidney	Multiple Myeloma
7,400 (3%)	5,500 (2%)
All Sites	All Sites
285,900 (100%)	270,600 (100%)

Excludes basal and squamous cell skin cancers and in situ carcinoma except urinary bladder. Percentages may not total 100% due to rounding.

©2003, American Cancer Society, Inc., Surveilence Research.

FIG. 25-54. New cancer cases and estimated cancer deaths, 2003. *[Reproduced with permission from American Cancer Society: Cancer Facts and Figures 2003 (www.cancer.org).]*

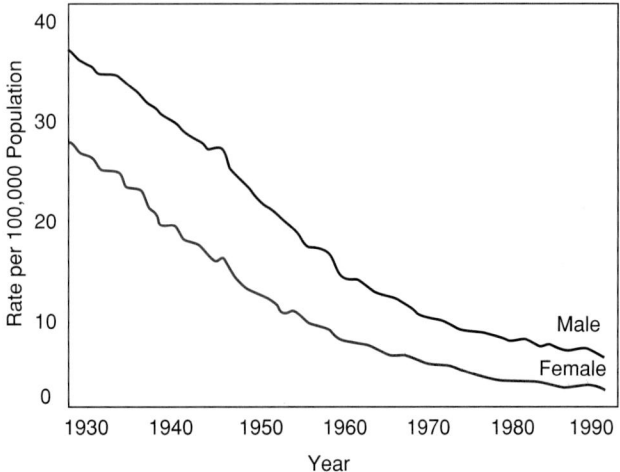

FIG. 25-55. Decline in deaths from gastric cancer in U.S. *[Reproduced with permission from Ming S-C, Hirota T: Malignant epithelial tumors of the stomach, in Ming C-J, Goldman H (eds): Pathology of the Gastrointestinal Tract, 2nd ed. Baltimore: Williams & Wilkins, 1998, p 607.]*

In general, gastric cancer is a disease of the elderly, and the male:female ratio is about 2:1. It is twice as common in blacks as in whites, with a similar sex ratio (2:1 male:female). Occasionally gastric cancer does occur in young adults (30 to 40 years of age). These tumors tend to be large and aggressive (large diffusely infiltrative tumors [linitis plastica] or signet ring histology), with a poor prognosis, seen predominantly in women (3:1). Gastric cancer has a higher incidence in groups of lower socioeconomic status.

Etiology

Gastric cancer is more common in patients with pernicious anemia, blood group A, or a family history of gastric cancer. When patients migrate from a high incidence region to a low incidence region, the risk of gastric cancer decreases in the subsequent generations born in the new region. This strongly suggests an environmental influence on the development of gastric cancer. Environmental factors appear to be more related etiologically to the intestinal form of gastric cancer than the more aggressive diffuse form. The commonly accepted risk factors for gastric cancer are listed in Table 25-17 and are discussed here.

Diet and Drugs. Typically, a starchy diet high in pickled, salted, or smoked food is found in many regions of high gastric

Age-Standardized Death Rates for Stomach Cancer per 100,00 Population

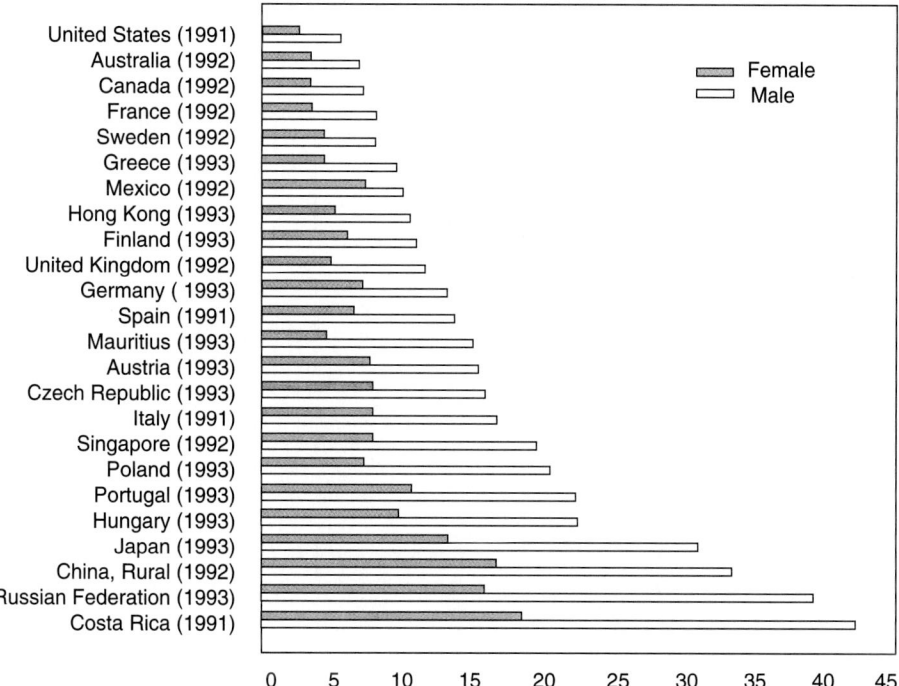

FIG. 25-56. Death rates for gastric cancer in different countries. [Reproduced with permission from Ming S-C, Hirota T: Malignant epithelial tumors of the stomach, in Ming C-J, Goldman H (eds): Pathology of the Gastrointestinal Tract, 2nd ed. Baltimore: Williams & Wilkins, 1998, p 607.]

cancer risk. Dietary nitrates have been impugned as a possible cause of gastric cancer. Gastric bacteria (more common in the achlorhydric stomach of patients with atrophic gastritis, a risk factor for gastric cancer) convert nitrate into nitrite, a proven carcinogen. A diet high in fresh fruits and vegetables and rich in vitamin C and E has been shown to decrease the population's risk of gastric cancer. The reduced consumption of nitrate-rich preserved foods seen with the growth of refrigeration has been suggested as a cause of the dramatic decrease in gastric cancer seen in North America and Western Europe. Tobacco use probably increases the risk of stomach cancer, and alcohol use probably has no effect. Regular aspirin use may be protective.

Helicobacter pylori. The risk of gastric cancer in patients with chronic *H. pylori* infection is increased about threefold. As discussed above, *H. pylori* is an important etiologic agent in the

Table 25-17
Factors Increasing and Decreasing the Risk for Gastric Cancer

Increase risk
  Family History
  Diet (high in nitrates, salt, fat)
  Familial polyposis
  Gastric adenomas
  Hereditary nonpolyposis colorectal cancer
  Helicobacter pylori infection
    Atrophic gastritis, intestinal metaplasia, dysplasia
  Previous gastrectomy or gastrojejunostomy (>10 years ago)
  Tobacco use
  Ménétrier's disease
Decrease risk
  Aspirin
  Diet (high fresh fruit and vegetable intake)
  Vitamin C

development of peptic ulcer disease. Interestingly, when compared to uninfected patients, patients with a history of gastric ulcer are more likely to eventually develop gastric cancer (incidence ratio 1.8, 95% confidence interval 1.6 to 2.0), and patients with a history of duodenal ulcer are at decreased risk for gastric cancer (incidence ratio 0.6, 95% confidence interval 0.4 to 0.7). As diagrammed in Fig. 25-57, this may be due to the fact that some patients develop antral-predominant disease (predisposing to duodenal ulcer and somehow protecting against gastric cancer), while other patients develop corpus-predominant gastritis, resulting in hypochlorhydria and somehow predisposing to gastric ulcer and gastric cancer. The theoretical sequence for development of gastric adenocarcinoma is diagrammed in Fig. 25-58. Interestingly, *H. pylori*–infected patients seem to be at decreased risk for the development of adenocarcinoma of the distal esophagus and cardia region. Perhaps the corporeal gastritis decreases acid secretion, creating a less damaging refluxate and thus reducing the risk for Barrett's esophagus, the precursor lesion for these tumors. Although *H. pylori* infection is clearly linked to the development of gastric cancer, it must be recognized that gastric adenocarcinoma is a multifactorial disease. Not all patients with gastric cancer have *H. pylori,* and there are some geographic areas with a high prevalence of chronic *H. pylori* infection and a low prevalence of gastric cancer (the "African enigma").

Epstein-Barr Virus. It appears that the Epstein-Barr virus (EBV) can infect the gastric epithelial cell. Some studies have demonstrated that the majority of gastric cancers show evidence of infection with EBV. These tumors tend to have more prominent lymphoid stroma.

Genetic Factors. A variety of genetic abnormalities have been described in gastric cancer (Table 25-18). Most gastric cancers are aneuploid. The most common genetic abnormalities in gastric

CHRONIC *H. PYLORI* INFECTION

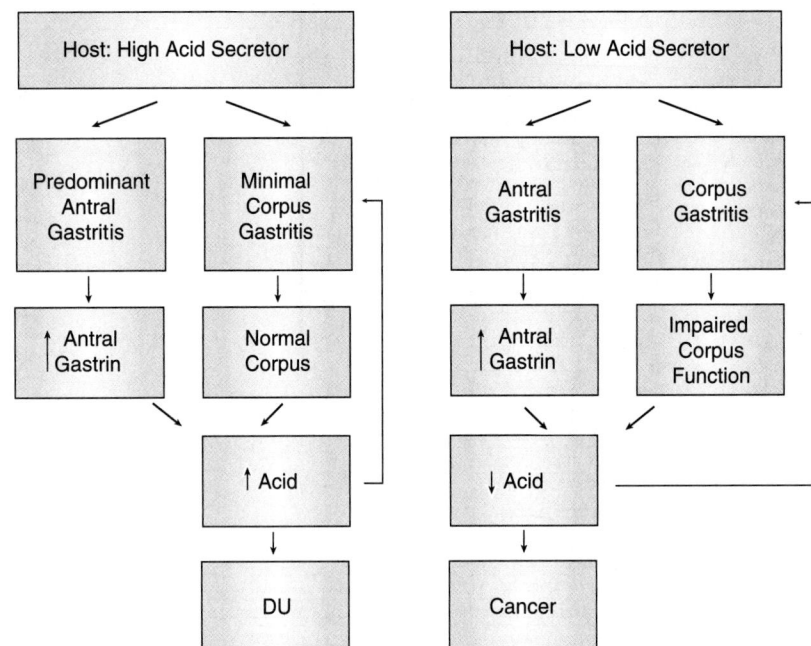

FIG. 25-57. *Helicobacter pylori and gastritis. [Reproduced with permission from Leung WK, Ng EKW, Sung JJY: Tumors of the stomach, in Yamada T et al (eds): Textbook of Gastroenterology, 4th ed. Philadelphia: Lippincott Williams & Wilkins, 2003, p 1416.]*

cancer affect the *p53* and *COX-2* genes. Over two thirds of gastric cancers have deletion or suppression of the important tumor suppressor gene *p53*. Additionally, approximately the same proportion have overexpression of *COX-2*. In the colon, tumors with upregulation of this gene have suppressed apoptosis, more angiogenesis, and higher metastatic potential. Gastric tumors that overexpress *COX-2* are more aggressive tumors.

Premalignant Conditions of the Stomach. Figure 25-59 shows the prevalence of some premalignant conditions associated with the development of early gastric cancer in a series of 1900 cases from Tokyo.

Polyps. There are five types of gastric epithelial polyps: inflammatory, hamartomatous, heterotopic, hyperplastic, and

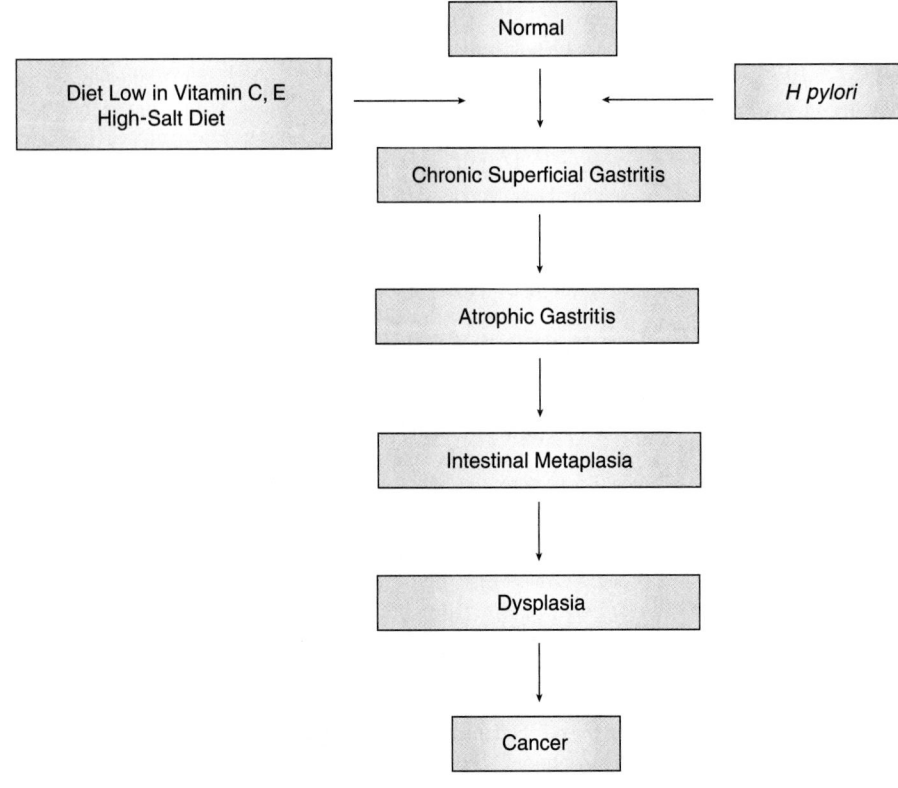

FIG. 25-58. *Gastric carcinogenesis. [Reproduced with permission from Leung WK, Ng EKW, Sung JJY: Tumors of the stomach, in Yamada T et al (eds): Textbook of Gastroenterology, 4th ed. Philadelphia: Lippincott Williams & Wilkins, 2003, p 1416.]*

Table 25-18
Genetic Abnormalities in Gastric Cancer

Abnormalities	Gene	Approximate Frequency (%)
Deletion/suppression	p53	60–70
	FHIT	60
	APC	50
	DCC	50
	E-cadherin	<5
Amplification/overexpression	COX-2	70
	HGF/SF	60
	VEGF	50
	c-met	45
	AIB-1	40
	β-catenin	25
	k-sam	20
	ras	10–15
	c-erb B-2	5–7
Microsatellite instability		25–40
DNA aneuploidy		60–75

SOURCE: Reproduced with permission from Koh TJ, Wang TC in *Sleisenger & Fordtran's Gastrointestinal and Liver Diseases*, 7th ed. Philadelphia: Saunders, 2002.

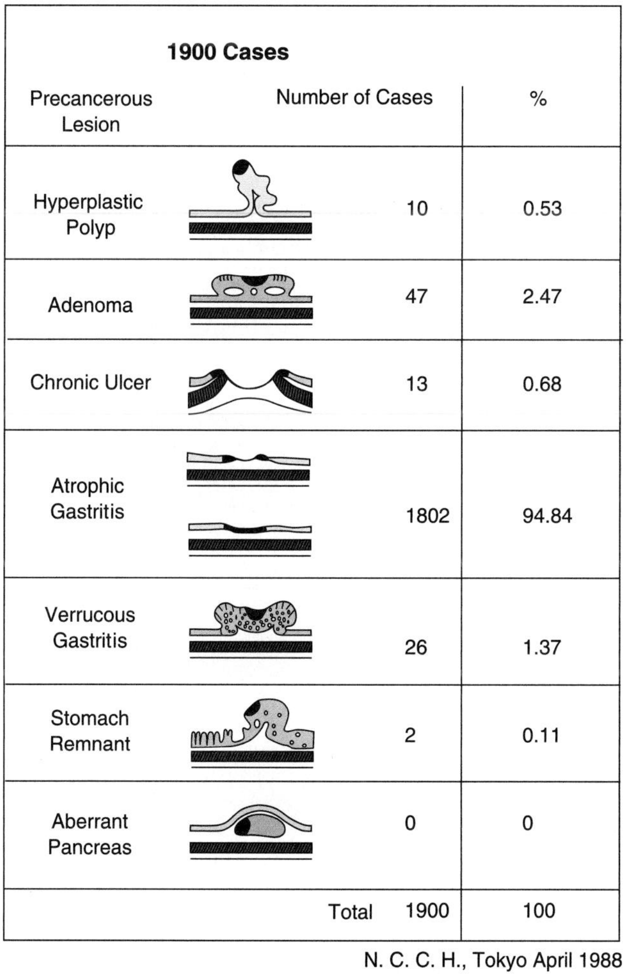

1900 Cases

Precancerous Lesion		Number of Cases	%
Hyperplastic Polyp		10	0.53
Adenoma		47	2.47
Chronic Ulcer		13	0.68
Atrophic Gastritis		1802	94.84
Verrucous Gastritis		26	1.37
Stomach Remnant		2	0.11
Aberrant Pancreas		0	0
	Total	1900	100

N. C. C. H., Tokyo April 1988

FIG. 25-59. Precancerous stomach lesions. [Reproduced with permission from Ming S-C, Hirota T: Malignant epithelial tumors of the stomach, in Ming C-J, Goldman H (eds): Pathology of the Gastrointestinal Tract, 2nd ed. Baltimore: Williams & Wilkins, 1998, p 607.]

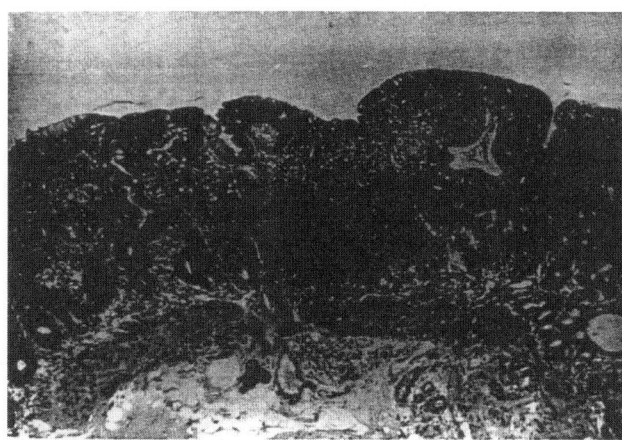

FIG. 25-60. Chronic atrophic gastritis. Compare to normal gastric mucosa seen in Fig. 25-9. [Reproduced with permission from Ming S-C, Hirota T: Malignant epithelial tumors of the stomach, in Ming C-J, Goldman H (eds): Pathology of the Gastrointestinal Tract, 2nd ed. Baltimore: Williams & Wilkins, 1998, p 607.]

adenoma. The first three types have negligible malignant potential. Adenomas can lead to carcinoma, just like in the colon, and should be removed when diagnosed. Occasionally, hyperplastic polyps can lead to carcinoma (<2%). Patients with familial adenomatous polyposis (FAP) have a high prevalence of gastric adenomatous polyps (about 50%), and are 10 times more likely to develop adenocarcinoma of the stomach than the general population.

Atrophic Gastritis. Chronic atrophic gastritis (Fig. 25-60) is the most common precursor for gastric cancer, particularly the intestinal subtype. In a Japanese study, 95% of patients with early gastric cancer had atrophic gastritis, and a Finnish study suggests that the risk of developing gastric carcinoma is close to 20% when there is severe gastritis involving the antrum, and 5% when the gastritis involves the body of the stomach. The prevalence of atrophic gastritis is higher in older age groups, but in areas with a high incidence of gastric cancer, the condition is common in younger people as well. In many patients, it is likely that *H. pylori* is involved in the pathogenesis of atrophic gastritis. Correa described three distinct patterns of chronic atrophic gastritis: autoimmune (involves the acid-secreting proximal stomach), hypersecretory (involving the distal stomach), and environmental (involving multiple random areas at the junction of the oxyntic and antral mucosa).

Intestinal Metaplasia. Gastric carcinoma often occurs in an area of intestinal metaplasia. Furthermore, an individual's risk of gastric cancer is proportional to the extent of intestinal metaplasia of the gastric mucosa. These observations strongly suggest that intestinal metaplasia is a precursor lesion to gastric cancer. There are different pathologic subtypes of intestinal metaplasia in the stomach, based upon the histologic and biochemical characteristics of the changed mucosal gland. In the complete type of intestinal metaplasia, the glands are completely lined with goblet cells and intestinal absorptive cells (Fig. 25-61). These cells are indistinguishable histologically and biochemically from their small bowel counterparts, and are not seen in the normal stomach. There is evidence that eradication of *H. pylori* infection leads to significant regression of intestinal metaplasia and improvement in atrophic gastritis. Therefore, treatment of *H. pylori* infection is a reasonable recommendation for patients with these pathologic diagnoses and *H. pylori* infection.

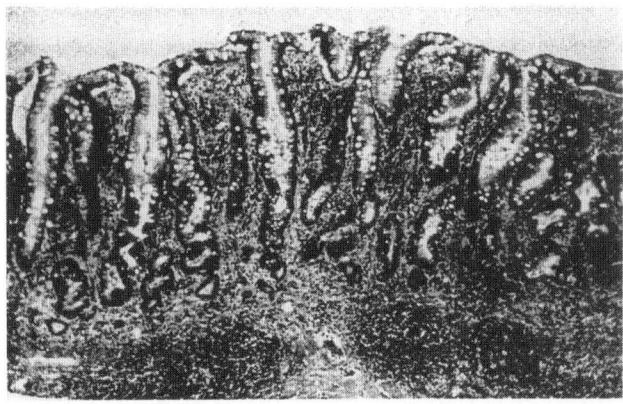

FIG. 25-61. *Complete intestinal metaplasia of the stomach. Note the intestinal-type crypts lined with goblet cells and intestinal absorptive cells. [Reproduced with permission from Ming S-C, Hirota T: Malignant epithelial tumors of the stomach, in Ming C-J, Goldman H (eds): Pathology of the Gastrointestinal Tract, 2nd ed. Baltimore: Williams & Wilkins, 1998, p 607.]*

Benign Gastric Ulcer. Although once considered a premalignant condition, it is likely that the older literature was confounded by mistakenly labeling inadequately biopsied ulcers and healing ulcers as "benign," when in fact they were malignant to begin with. It is now generally recognized that all gastric ulcers are cancer until proven otherwise with adequate biopsy and follow-up. Even today carcinomas are occasionally found when adequately biopsied "benign" ulcers are resected for nonhealing. It is more than likely that the factors discussed above are more significant etiologically in the development of gastric cancer than the history of a benign gastric ulcer.

Gastric Remnant Cancer. It has long been recognized that stomach cancer can develop in the gastric remnant, usually years following distal gastrectomy for peptic ulcer disease. The risk is controversial, but the phenomenon is real. Most tumors develop more than 10 years following the initial operation, and they usually arise in an area of chronic gastritis, metaplasia, and dysplasia. This is often near the stoma, but many of these tumors are quite large at presentation, and are equally divided between intestinal and diffuse subtypes. Most cases have been reported following Billroth II gastroenterostomy, but there also have been cases following Billroth I gastroduodenostomy. Whether simple loop gastrojejunostomy increases a patient's risk of gastric cancer, and whether a Roux-en-Y anastomosis following gastric resection lowers their risk of gastric cancer is unknown.

Other Premalignant States. It is not surprising that many of the above genetic and environmental factors will affect members of the same family. Up to 10% of gastric cancer cases appear to be familial, even without a clear-cut genetic diagnosis such as familial polyposis. First-degree relatives of patients with gastric cancer have a two- to threefold increased risk of developing the disease. Patients with hereditary nonpolyposis colorectal cancer have a 10% risk of developing gastric cancer, predominantly the intestinal subtype. The mucous cell hyperplasia of Ménétrier's disease is generally considered to carry a 5 to 10% risk of adenocarcinoma, but the glandular hyperplasia associated with gastrinoma is not premalignant.

Pathology

Dysplasia. It is generally accepted that gastric dysplasia is the universal precursor to gastric adenocarcinoma. There is significant controversy among pathologists as to what constitutes "dysplasia"

Table 25-19
Early Gastric Cancer

Type I	Exophytic lesion extending into the gastric lumen
Type II	Superficial variant
II A	Elevated lesions with a height no more than the thickness of the adjacent mucosa
IIB	Flat lesions
IIC	Depressed lesions with an eroded but not deeply ulcerated appearance
Type III	Excavated lesions that may extend into the muscularis propria without invasion of this layer by actual cancer cells

and what constitutes "early gastric cancer." Clearly, patients with severe dysplasia require some sort of ablative treatment, usually gastric resection. Patients with mild dysplasia should be followed carefully with endoscopic biopsy surveillance.

Early Gastric Cancer. Early gastric cancer is defined as adenocarcinoma limited to the mucosa and submucosa of the stomach, regardless of lymph node status. The entity is common in Japan, where gastric cancer is the number one cause of cancer death, and where aggressive surveillance programs have been established. Approximately 10% of patients with early gastric cancer will have lymph node metastases. There are several types and subtypes of early gastric cancer (Table 25-19 and Fig. 25-62). Approximately 70% of early gastric cancers are well differentiated, and 30% are poorly differentiated. The overall cure rate with adequate gastric resection and lymphadenectomy is 95%. In some Japanese centers, 50% of the gastric cancers treated are early gastric cancer. In the

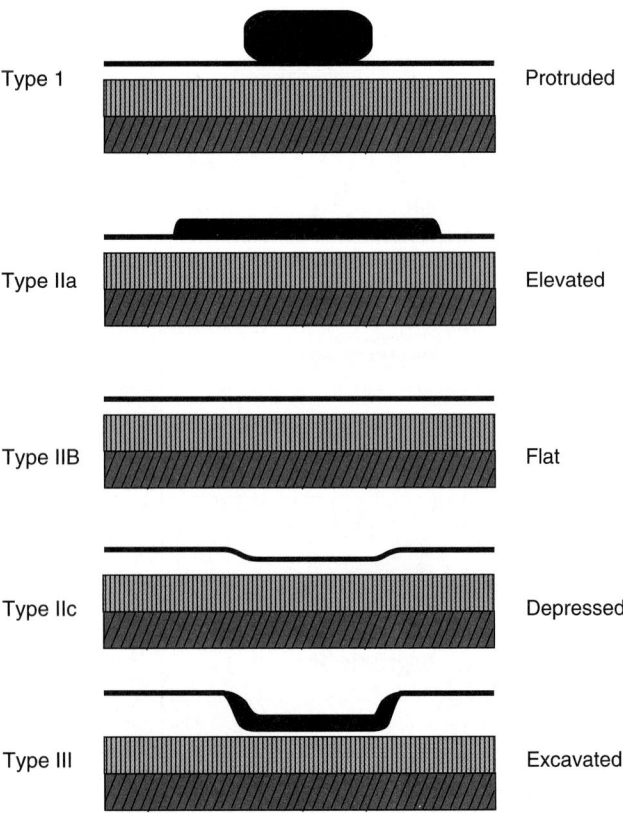

FIG. 25-62. *Pathologic types of early gastric cancer. [Reproduced with permission from Ashley SW, Evoy D, Daly JM: Stomach, in Schwartz SI (ed): Principles of Surgery, 7th ed. New York: McGraw-Hill, 1999, p 1181.]*

U.S., less than 20% of resected gastric adenocarcinomas are early gastric cancer.

Gross Morphology and Histologic Subtypes. There are four gross forms of gastric cancer: polypoid, fungating, ulcerative, and scirrhous. In the first two, the bulk of the tumor mass is intraluminal. Polypoid tumors are not ulcerated; fungating tumors are elevated intraluminally, but also ulcerated. In the latter two gross subtypes, the bulk of the tumor mass is in the wall of the stomach. Ulcerative tumors are self-descriptive; scirrhous tumors infiltrate the entire thickness of the stomach and cover a very large surface area. Scirrhous tumors (linitis plastica) have a particularly poor prognosis, and commonly involve the entire stomach. Although these latter lesions may be technically resectable with total gastrectomy, it is common for both the esophageal and duodenal margins of resection to show microscopic evidence of tumor infiltration. Death from recurrent disease within 6 months is the standard.

The location of the primary tumor in the stomach is important in planning the operation. Several decades ago, the large majority of gastric cancers were in the distal stomach. Recently, there has been a proximal migration of tumors, so that currently the distribution is closer to 40% distal, 30% middle, and 30% proximal.

Histology. The most important prognostic indicators in gastric cancer are both histologic: lymph node involvement and depth of tumor invasion. Tumor grade (degree of differentiation: well, moderately, or poorly) is also important prognostically.

There are several histologic classifications of gastric cancer. The World Health Organization (WHO) recognizes 10 histologic types (Table 25-20). The Japanese classification is similar but more detailed. The Lauren classification separates gastric cancers into intestinal type (53%), diffuse type (33%), and unclassified (14%). Clinically, this is an appealing classification because it relates to the above-noted risk factors. The intestinal subtype is associated with chronic atrophic gastritis, severe intestinal metaplasia, and dysplasia. The Ming classification also is useful and easy to remember, with only two types, expanding (67%) and infiltrative (33%).

Pathologic Staging. The most widespread system for staging of gastric cancer is the tumor-node-metastasis (TNM) staging system based on depth of tumor invasion, extent of lymph node metastases, and presence of distant metastases. This system was developed by the American Joint Committee on Cancer and the International Union Against Cancer, and has undergone several modifications since it was originally conceived (Table 25-21).

Clinical Manifestations

Most patients who are diagnosed with gastric cancer in the U.S. have advanced stage III or IV disease at the time of diagnosis. The

Table 25-20
World Health Organization Histologic Typing of Gastric Cancer

Adenocarcinoma
  Papillary adenocarcinoma
  Tubular adenocarcinoma
  Mucinous adenocarcinoma
  Signet-ring cell carcinoma
Adenosquamous carcinoma
Squamous cell carcinoma
Small cell carcinoma
Undifferentiated carcinoma
Others

SOURCE: Reproduced with permission from Ming SC, Hirota T: *Pathology of the Gastrointestinal Tract.*

Table 25-21
TNM Staging of Gastric Cancer by the International Union Against Cancer and American Joint Committee on Cancer

T: Primary tumor

Tis	Carcinoma in situ; Intraepithelial tumor without invasion of lamina propria
T1	Tumor invades lamina propria or submucosa
T2	Tumor invades muscularis propria or subserosa
T3	Tumor penetrates serosa (visceral peritoneum) without invasion of adjacent structures
T4	Tumor invades adjacent structures

N: Regional lymph node

N0	No regional lymph node metastasis
N1	Metastasis in 1 to 6 regional lymph nodes
N2	Metastasis in 7 to 15 lymph nodes
N3	Metastasis in more than 15 regional lymph nodes

M: Distant metastasis

M0	No distant metastasis
M1	Distant metastasis

Stage grouping

Stage	T	N	M
0	Tis	N0	M0
IA	T1	N0	M0
IB	T1	N1	M0
	T2	N0	M0
II	T1	N2	M0
	T2	N1	M0
	T3	N0	M0
IIIA	T2	N2	M0
	T3	N1	M0
	T4	N0	M0
IIIB	T3	N2	M0
IV	T4	N1–3	M0
	T1–3	N3	M0
	Any T	Any N	M1

SOURCE: Reproduced with permission from Koh TJ, Wang TC: Tumors of the stomach in *Sleisinger and Fordtran's Gastrointestinal and Liver Disease,* 7th ed. Philadelphia: Saunders, 2002.

most common symptoms are weight loss and decreased food intake due to anorexia and early satiety. Abdominal pain (usually not severe and often ignored) also is common. Other symptoms include nausea, vomiting, and bloating. Acute gastrointestinal bleeding is somewhat unusual (5%), but chronic occult blood loss is common and manifests as iron deficiency anemia and heme-positive stool. Dysphagia is common if the tumor involves the cardia of the stomach. Paraneoplastic syndromes such as Trousseau's syndrome (thrombophlebitis), acanthosis nigricans (hyperpigmentation of the axilla and groin), or peripheral neuropathy are rarely present.

Physical examination usually is normal. Other than signs of weight loss, specific physical findings usually indicate incurability. A focused exam in a patient in whom gastric cancer is a likely part of the differential diagnosis should include an exam of the neck, chest, abdomen, rectum, and pelvis. Cervical, supraclavicular (on the left referred to as Virchow's node), and axillary lymph nodes may be enlarged, and today can be sampled in the office with fine-needle aspiration cytology. There may be a metastatic pleural effusion, or aspiration pneumonitis in a patient with vomiting and/or obstruction. An abdominal mass could indicate a large (usually T4 incurable) primary tumor, liver metastases, or carcinomatosis (including Krukenberg tumor of the ovary). A palpable umbilical nodule (Sister Joseph's nodule) is pathognomonic of advanced disease, or there may be evidence on exam of malignant ascites. Rectal exam may reveal hard nodularity extraluminally and anteriorly, indicating so-called "drop metastases," or rectal shelf of Blumer in the pouch of Douglas.

Diagnostic Evaluation

Distinguishing between peptic ulcer and gastric cancer on clinical grounds alone is usually impossible. Patients over the age 45 who have new-onset dyspepsia, as well as all patients with dyspepsia and alarm symptoms (weight loss, recurrent vomiting, dysphagia, evidence of bleeding, or anemia) or family history should have *prompt upper endoscopy and biopsy* if a mucosal lesion is noted. Essentially all patients in whom gastric cancer is part of the differential diagnosis should have endoscopy and biopsy. If suspicion for cancer is high and the biopsy is negative, the patient should be re-endoscoped and more aggressively biopsied. In some patients with gastric tumors, upper GI series can be helpful in planning treatment. Although a good *double contrast barium upper GI examination* is sensitive for gastric tumors (up to 75% sensitive), in most centers endoscopy has become the gold standard for the diagnosis of gastric malignancy. The tests are often complementary in practice.

Preoperative staging of gastric cancer is best accomplished with abdominal/pelvic CT scanning with intravenous and oral contrast. MRI is probably comparable. The best way to stage the tumor locally is via endoscopic ultrasound, which gives accurate information about the depth of tumor penetration into the gastric wall, and can usually show enlarged (>5 mm) perigastric and celiac lymph nodes. In some centers, if the tumor is transmural (T3) or involves lymph nodes (enlarged nodes can usually be needled under ultrasound guidance), preoperative (neoadjuvant) therapy is given. However, there are limitations to tumor staging with EUS. It largely is operator dependent and tends to overestimate the T stage of the tumor, and may underestimate lymph node involvement since normal-sized nodes (<5 mm) can harbor metastases. EUS is most accurate in distinguishing early gastric cancer (T1) from more advanced tumors.

Positron Emission Tomography Scanning. Whole-body positron emission tomography (PET) scanning uses the principle that tumor cells preferentially accumulate positron-emitting 18^F fluorodeoxyglucose. This modality is most useful in the evaluation of distant metastasis in gastric cancer. It should be considered prior to major surgery in patients with particularly high-risk tumors or multiple medical comorbidities.

Staging Laparoscopy and Peritoneal Cytology. To some extent, the usefulness of these modalities depends on the individual patient's situation as well as the treatment philosophy of the cancer team. The fundamental question is "will it make a difference to this patient's management?" Peritoneal lavage can yield a positive cytology in up to 40% of patients with gastric cancer, and almost all of these patients go on to develop peritoneal metastases. Perhaps these patients should be treated with some sort of local therapy or protocol (e.g., intraperitoneal hyperthermic chemotherapy), but it is unclear that such treatment improves survival or quality of life, and most of these patients will have (and should have) gastric resection regardless of the cytology results. A quick laparoscopic examination can occasionally reveal small peritoneal implants or liver metastases that were not detected on preoperative imaging studies, and in some patients (e.g., high-risk for surgery or impressive carcinomatosis) this will change the operative plan. An extensive laparoscopic staging procedure, while quite accurate, has not been widely adopted.

Treatment

Surgery is the only curative treatment for gastric cancer. It also is the best palliation and provides the most accurate staging. Therefore

most patients with gastric adenocarcinoma should have gastric resection. Obvious exceptions include patients who cannot tolerate an abdominal operation, and patients with overwhelming metastatic disease. Occasional patients with relatively symptomatic primary tumors and systemic metastases challenge surgical judgment. Generally, palliation is poor with nonresective operations.

The goal of curative surgical treatment is resection of all tumor (i.e., R0 resection). Thus all margins (proximal, distal, and radial) should be negative and an adequate lymphadenectomy performed. Generally, the surgeon strives for a grossly negative margin of at least 5 cm, since some gastric tumors are quite infiltrative and tumor cells can extend well beyond the tumor mass. Therefore, frozen section confirmation of negative margins is important when performing operation for cure, but it is less important in obviously palliative operations. It should be strongly emphasized that many patients with positive lymph nodes are cured by adequate surgery. It should also be stressed that often lymph nodes that appear to be involved with tumor turn out to be benign or reactive on pathologic examination. Therefore therapeutic nihilism should be avoided, and in the low-risk patient an aggressive attempt to resect all tumor should be made.

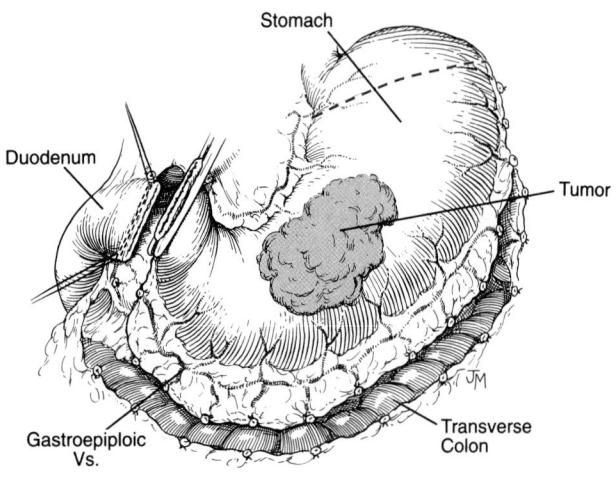

A

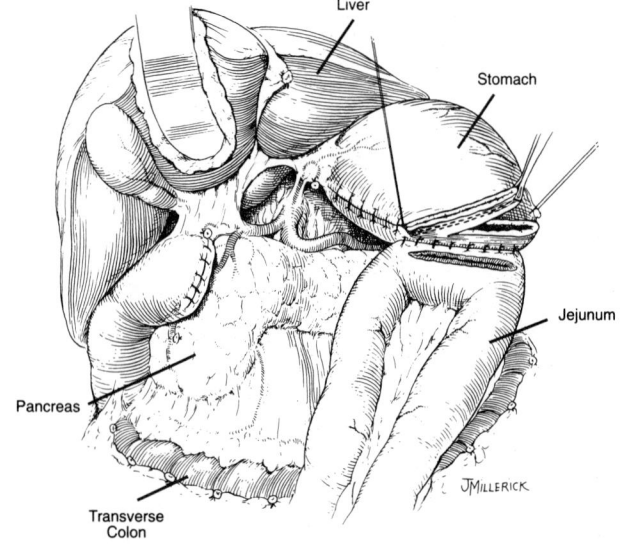

B

FIG. 25-63. Radical subtotal gastrectomy. [Reproduced with permission from Ashley SW, Evoy D, Daly JM: Stomach, in Schwartz SI (ed): *Principles of Surgery*, 7th ed. New York: McGraw-Hill, 1999, p 1181.]

The primary tumor may be resected en bloc with adjacent involved organs (e.g., distal pancreas, transverse colon, or spleen) during the course of curative gastrectomy.

Extent of Gastrectomy. The standard operation for gastric cancer is radical subtotal gastrectomy. This typically entails ligation of the left and right gastric and gastroepiploic arteries at the origin, as well as the en bloc removal of the distal 75% of the stomach, including the pylorus and 2 cm of duodenum, the greater and lesser omentum, and all associated lymphatic tissue (Fig. 25-63). Reconstruction is usually by Billroth II gastrojejunostomy, but if a small gastric remnant is left (<20%), a Roux-en-Y reconstruction is considered. The operative mortality is around 5%. Radical subtotal gastrectomy is generally deemed to be an adequate cancer operation in most Western countries, provided that the contingencies stated above obtain adequate margins and resection of all gross tumor. In the absence of involvement by direct extension, the spleen and pancreatic tail are not removed.

Total gastrectomy is not performed unless it is necessary to obtain an adequate margin (Fig. 25-64). There have been several large studies comparing subtotal gastrectomy to total gastrectomy for gastric cancer, and the survival results in the two groups have been the same. However, the complication rate in the total gastrectomy group is higher. Total gastrectomy with jejunal pouch/esophageal anastomosis may be the best operation for patients with proximal gastric adenocarcinoma. The alternative, proximal subtotal gastric resection, requires an esophagogastrostomy to a vagotomized distal gastric remnant. Pyloroplasty in this setting virtually guarantees bile esophagitis, and if the pylorus is left intact, gastric emptying may be problematic. An isoperistaltic jejunal interposition (Henley loop) between the esophagus and antrum could be considered.

Extent of Lymphadenectomy. The Japanese have labeled all the lymph node stations that potentially drain the stomach (see Fig. 25-6). Generally these are grouped into level N1 (i.e., stations 3 to 6), level N2 (i.e., stations 1, 2, 7, 8, and 11), and level N3

FIG. 25-64. Roux-en-Y esophagojejunostomy following total gastrectomy.

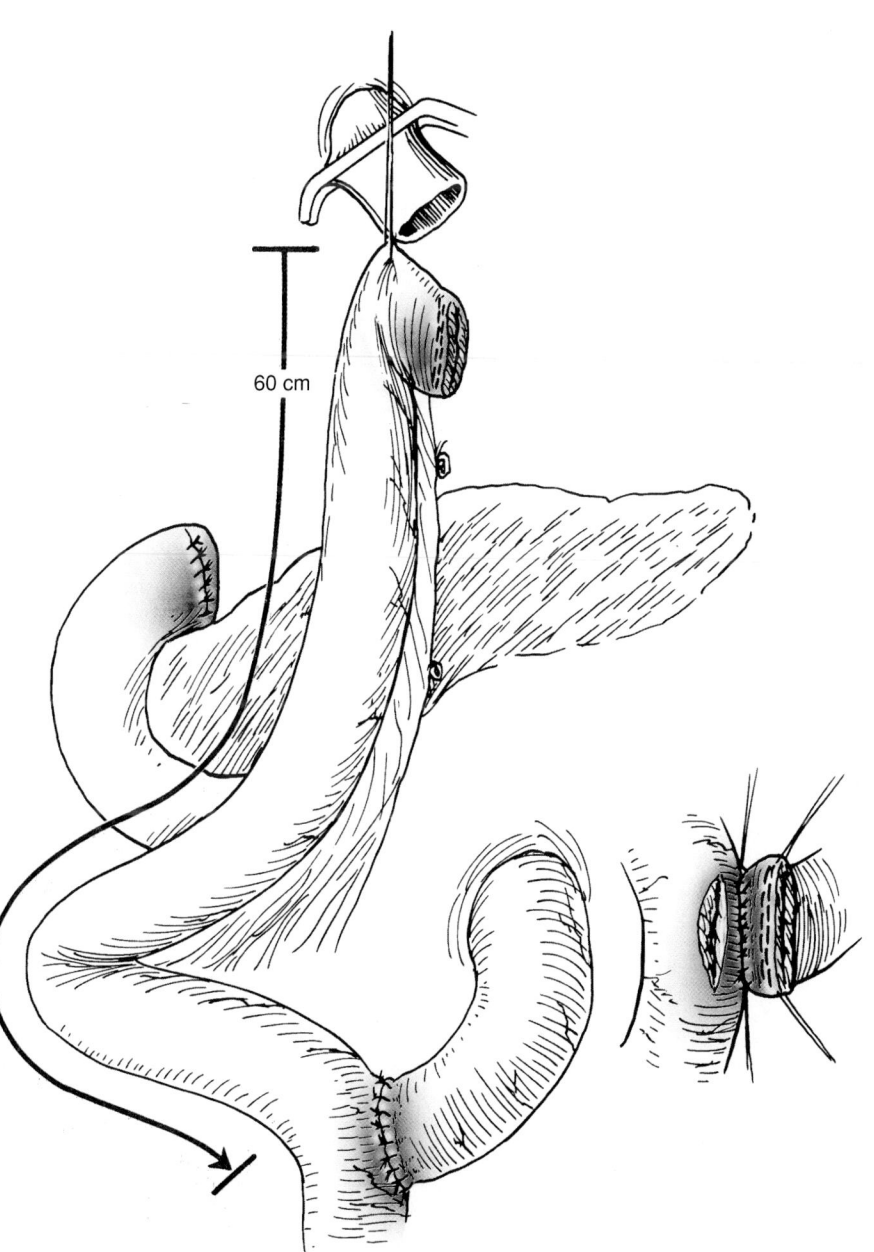

60 cm

Table 25-22
Gastric Cancer 5-Year Survival and Operative Mortality in the USA and Japan

	Maruyama (Japan), 1971–1985	*American College of Surgeons, 1982–1987*	*Memorial Sloan Kettering, 1985–1994*
No. Patients	3176	18365	675
Stage I	91%	50%	84%
Stage II	72%	29%	61%
Stage III	44%	13%	29%
Stage IV	9%	3%	25%
Operative mortality	1%	7%	3%

SOURCE: Reproduced with permission from Karpeh MS: in *Shackelford's Surgery of the Alimentary Tract,* 2002.

(i.e., stations 9, 10, and 12) nodes. The nodal stations defined as level N1, N2, and N3 vary depending on the location of the tumor. In general, N1 nodes are within 3 cm of the tumor, N2 nodes are along the hepatic and splenic arteries, and N3 nodes are the most distant. The operation described above (radical subtotal gastrectomy), which is by far the most commonly performed procedure in the U.S. for gastric cancer, is called a D1 resection since it removes the tumor and the N1 nodes. The standard operation for gastric cancer in Asia is the D2 gastrectomy, which involves a more extensive lymphadenectomy (removal of the N1 and N2 nodes). In addition to the tissue removed in a D1 resection, the standard D2 gastrectomy removes the peritoneal layer over the pancreas and anterior mesocolon, along with nodes along the hepatic and splenic arteries, and the crural nodes. Splenectomy and distal pancreatectomy are not routinely performed, since this clearly has been shown to increase the morbidity of the operation. The purported survival advantage of D2 gastrectomy in gastric cancer is shown in Table 25-22, which shows the 5-year survival rates for gastric cancer stratified by pathologic stage for the U.S. and Japan. Unfortunately, the randomized prospective trials that have been performed have not confirmed this survival advantage, but the morbidity and mortality in the D2 group was higher (Table 25-23). This was mostly attributable to the splenectomy and distal pancreatectomy, which are no longer routinely done as part of the D2 gastrectomy. Some experts have argued that the D2 operation is simply a better staging procedure, and that the apparent improved survival with this more extensive dissection is simply an epiphenomenon of improved pathologic staging. This stage shift suggests that many patients in U.S. series treated with D1 gastrectomy really had metastatic nodes at the D2 level that went unresected and undetected. Therefore, in the U.S. series, there were patients classified as stage I, who if they had undergone a D2 gastrectomy would be classified as stage II; and there were patients classified as stage II, who if they had undergone a D2 gastrectomy would be classified as stage III. The stage I survival in the U.S. would then actually be closer to the (more accurately staged) stage II survival in Japan, since this group includes some patients who

really *are* stage II, but the nodes were not found in the D1 resection. All experts would agree that in order to avoid understaging of gastric cancer, a minimum of 15 nodes should be resected with the gastrectomy specimen.

Chemotherapy and Radiation for Gastric Cancer. Adjuvant treatment with chemotherapy (5-fluorouracil and leucovorin) and radiation (4500 cGy) has demonstrated a survival benefit in resected patients with stage II and III adenocarcinoma of the stomach. There is no indication for the routine use of radiation alone in the adjuvant setting, but in certain patients it can be effective palliation for bleeding or pain. In patients with gross unresectable, metastatic, or recurrent disease, palliative chemotherapy has not been demonstrated to conclusively prolong survival, but occasionally a patient has a dramatic response. These patients should be considered for clinical trials. Agents that have shown activity against gastric cancer include 5-fluorouracil, cisplatin, doxorubicin, and methotrexate. Neoadjuvant treatment of gastric adenocarcinoma is being evaluated.

Endoscopic Resection. The Japanese have demonstrated that some patients with early gastric cancer can be adequately treated by an endoscopic mucosal resection. Small tumors (<3 cm) confined to the mucosa have an extremely low chance of lymph node metastasis (3%), which approaches the operative mortality rate for gastrectomy. If the resected specimen demonstrates no ulceration, no lymphatic invasion, and size less than 3 cm, the risk of lymph node metastases is less than 1%. Thus some patients with early gastric cancer might be better treated with the endoscopic technique. Currently, this should be limited to patients with tumors <2 cm in size that are node-negative and confined to the mucosa on EUS, in the absence of other gastric lesions.

Prognosis

The 5-year survival for gastric adenocarcinoma has increased from 15 to 22% in the U.S. over the past 25 years. Survival is

Table 25-23
Randomized Trials Comparing D1 and D2 Gastrectomy for Gastric Cancer

Authors	*Number of Patients*	*Type of Surgery*	*Postoperative Complications (%)*	*Postoperative Mortality (%)*	*5-Year Survival (%)*
Bonenkamp et al.	711	D1	25	4	45
		D2	43	10	47
Cuschieri et al.	400	D1	28	6.5	35
		D2	46	13	33

SOURCE: Data from Bonenkamp JJ, Hermans J, Sasako M, van de Velde CJH: Extended lymph node dissection for gastric cancer. *N Engl J Med* 340:908, 1999; and Cuschieri A, Fayers P, Fielding J, et al: Postoperative morbidity and mortality after D1 and D2 resections for gastric cancer: Preliminary results of the MRC randomized controlled surgical trial. *Lancet* 347:995, 1996.

dependent on pathologic stage (TNM stage) and degree of tumor differentiation.

Screening for Gastric Cancer

In Japan it clearly has been shown that patients participating in gastric cancer screening programs have a significantly decreased risk of dying from gastric cancer. Thus screening is effective in a high-risk population. Screening the general population in the U.S. (a low-risk country) does not make sense, but patients clearly at risk for gastric cancer probably should have periodic endoscopy and biopsy. This includes patients with familial adenomatous polyposis, hereditary nonpolyposis colorectal cancer, gastric adenomas, Ménétrier's disease, intestinal metaplasia or dysplasia, and remote gastrectomy or gastrojejunostomy.

Gastric Lymphoma

Gastric lymphomas generally account for about 4% of gastric malignancies. Over half of patients with non-Hodgkin's lymphoma have involvement of the GI tract. The stomach is the most common site of primary GI lymphoma, and over 95% are non-Hodgkin's type. Most are B-cell type, thought to arise in mucosa-associated lymphoid tissue (MALT). Interestingly, the normal stomach is relatively devoid of lymphoid tissue. However, in the setting of chronic gastritis, the stomach acquires MALT, which can undergo malignant degeneration. Again, *Helicobacter pylori* is thought to be the culprit. In populations with a high incidence of gastric lymphoma, there is a high incidence of *H. pylori* infection; patients with gastric lymphoma also usually have *H. pylori* infection.

Low-grade MALT lymphoma, essentially a monoclonal proliferation of B cells, presumably arises from a background of chronic gastritis associated with *H. pylori*. These relatively innocuous tumors then undergo degeneration to high-grade lymphoma, which is the usual variety seen by the surgeon. Remarkably, when the *H. pylori* is eradicated and the gastritis improves, the low-grade MALT lymphoma often disappears. Thus low-grade MALT lymphoma is not a surgical lesion. Careful follow-up is necessary.

High-grade gastric lymphoma is very different. These patients require aggressive oncologic treatment for cure, and present with many of the same symptoms as gastric cancer patients. However, systemic symptoms such as fever, weight loss, and night sweats occur in about 50% of patients with gastric lymphoma. The tumors may bleed and/or obstruct. Lymphadenopathy and/or organomegaly suggest systemic disease. Diagnosis is by endoscopy and biopsy. Much of the tumor may be submucosal, and an assiduous attempt at biopsy is necessary. Primary lymphoma is usually nodular with enlarged gastric folds. A diffusely infiltrative process akin to linitis plastica is more suggestive of secondary gastric involvement by lymphoma. A diligent search for extragastric disease is necessary before the diagnosis of localized primary gastric lymphoma is made. This includes EUS; CT scanning of the chest, abdomen, and pelvis; and bone marrow biopsy.

For gastric lymphoma limited to the stomach and regional nodes, radical subtotal gastrectomy may be performed, especially for bulky tumors with bleeding and/or obstruction. Palliative gastrectomy for tumor complications also has a role. Recently, patients have been treated with primary chemotherapy and radiation without operation, and the results have been quite good. Perforation and bleeding, especially from thick tumors, is a recognized complication of this approach. Certainly, a multidisciplinary team should be involved with the treatment plan for patients with primary gastric lymphoma.

Malignant Gastrointestinal Stromal Tumor

Gastrointestinal stromal tumors arise in mesenchymal tissue from an indistinct (probably multipotential) cell line of origin. There are varying patterns of differentiation, including smooth muscle type, formerly called leiomyosarcoma, and epithelioid type. Two thirds of all gut malignant GISTs occur in the stomach. Epithelial cell stromal GIST is the most common cell type arising in the stomach, and cellular spindle type is the next most common. The glomus tumor is seen only in the stomach.

GISTs are submucosal tumors that are slow growing. Smaller lesions are usually found incidentally, though they occasionally may ulcerate and cause impressive bleeding. Larger lesions generally produce symptoms of weight loss, abdominal pain, fullness, early satiety, and bleeding. An abdominal mass may be palpable. Spread is by the hematogenous route, often to liver and/or lung, though positive lymph nodes are occasionally seen in resected specimens. Diagnosis is by endoscopy and biopsy, though the interpretation of the latter may be problematic. Endoscopic ultrasound may be helpful, but symptomatic tumors and tumors over 2 cm in size should be removed. Metastatic workup entails CT of the chest, abdomen, and pelvis (chest x-ray may suffice in lieu of CT of the chest). Most gastric GISTs occur in the body of the stomach, but they also can occur in the fundus or antrum. They are almost always solitary. Wedge resection with clear margins is adequate treatment, and prognosis depends on tumor size and mitotic count. True invasion of adjacent structures is evidence of malignancy. If safe, en bloc resection of involved surrounding organs is appropriate to remove all tumor when the primary is large and invasive. Most patients with low-grade lesions are cured (80% 5-year survival), but most patients with high-grade lesions are not (30% 5-year survival).

GISTs are usually positive for the proto-oncogene, c-kit. Imatinib, a chemotherapeutic agent that blocks the activity of the tyrosine kinase product of c-kit, shows promising activity in patients with metastatic or unresectable GIST.

Gastric Carcinoid Tumors

Compared to midgut and hindgut locations, carcinoid tumors of the stomach are rather unusual. Gastric carcinoids comprise about 3% of gastrointestinal carcinoids (Table 25-24), and they clearly have malignant potential. Patients with pernicious anemia or atrophic gastritis are at risk for gastric carcinoid tumors, but thus far chronic pharmacologic suppression of acid has not been recognized as a risk factor. The tumors are submucosal and may be quite small. They are often confused with heterotopic pancreas or small leiomyomas. Biopsy may be difficult because of the submucosal location, and EUS can be helpful in defining the size and depth of the lesion. Gastric carcinoids should be resected. Small lesions confined to the mucosa may be removed endoscopically. Larger lesions should be removed by D1 gastrectomy. Survival is excellent for node-negative patients (>90% 5-year survival); node-positive patients have a 50% 5-year survival.

BENIGN GASTRIC NEOPLASMS
Polyps

Epithelial polyps are the most common benign tumor of the stomach (Table 25-25). There are essentially five types of benign epithelial polyps (Table 25-26): adenomatous, hyperplastic (regenerative), hamartomatous, inflammatory, and heterotopic (e.g., ectopic pancreas). The most common gastric polyp (about 75% in most series)

Table 25-24
Gastrointestinal Carcinoids

	Fraction of All Carcinoids	Average Age at Diagnosis[a]	Synchronous or Metachronous Noncarcinoid Tumors	Regional Spread[a,b]	Distant Metastases[a,b]	5-Year Survival[a] Rate
All carcinoids	—	—	13.0	25.7	19.6	50.35
Stomach	3.19	63.8	7.8	10.3	20.6	48.6
Small bowel	26.48	65.1	16.6	39.3	31.4	55.4
Appendix	18.9	42.2	14.6	26.8	8.5	85.9
Colon	9.95	65.6	13.1	33.4	37.8	41.6
Rectum	11.38	58.2	9.2	7.1	7.1	72.2

[a] Surveillance, Epidemiology, and End Results (SEER) data 1973–1991.

[b] At presentation.

Values other than age are given as percentages.

SOURCE: Data adapted with permission from Modlin IM, Sandor A: An analysis of 8305 cases of carcinoid tumors. *Cancer* 79:813, 1997.

is the hyperplastic or regenerative polyp, which frequently occurs in the setting of gastritis and has a low but real malignant potential. Adenomatous polyps may undergo malignant transformation, similarly to adenomas in the colon. They constitute about 10 to 15% of gastric polyps. Hamartomatous, inflammatory, and heterotopic polyps have negligible malignant potential. Polyps that are symptomatic, larger than 2 cm, or adenomatous should be removed, usually by endoscopic snare polypectomy. Consideration should also be given to removing hyperplastic polyps, especially if large. Repeat EGD for surveillance should be done following removal of adenomatous polyps, and perhaps after removal of hyperplastic polyps as well.

Leiomyoma

The term leiomyoma is decreasingly associated with lesions of the stomach. What was once called leiomyoma now is termed gastrointestinal stromal tumor. The typical leiomyoma is submucosal and firm. If ulcerated it has an umbilicated appearance and may bleed. Histologically, these lesions appear to be of smooth muscle origin. Lesions less than 2 cm are usually asymptomatic and benign. Larger lesions have greater malignant potential, and a greater likelihood to cause symptoms such as bleeding, obstruction, or pain. Asymptomatic lesions less than 2 cm may be observed; larger lesions and

symptomatic lesions should be removed by wedge resection (often possible laparoscopically). When these lesions are observed rather than resected, the patient should be made aware of their presence and the small possibility for malignancy.

Lipoma

Lipomas are benign submucosal fatty tumors which are usually asymptomatic, found incidentally on upper GI series or EGD. Endoscopically they have a characteristic appearance; there also is a characteristic appearance on endoscopic ultrasound. Excision is unnecessary unless the patient is symptomatic.

GASTRIC MOTILITY DISORDERS

Gastric motility disorders include delayed gastric emptying (gastroparesis), rapid gastric emptying, and motor and sensory

Table 25-26
Histology of Gastric Epithelial Polyps

I. Neoplastic polyp
  A. Benign: adenoma
    1. Flat (tubular) adenoma
    2. Papillary (villous) adenoma
  B. Malignant
    1. Primary polypoid carcinoma and carcinoid
    2. Secondary epithelial tumors
II. Nonneoplastic polyp
  A. Hyperplastic polyp
    1. Focal (polypoid) foveolar hyperplasia
    2. Hyperplastic (regenerative) polyp
    3. Hyperplastic polyp with dysplastic (adenomatous) lesion
  B. Hamartomatous polyp
    1. Peutz-Jeghers polyp
    2. Juvenile polyp
    3. Fundic gland polyp
  C. Inflammatory polyp
    1. Inflammatory pseudopolyp
    2. Inflammatory (retention) polyp
  D. Heterotopic polyp
    1. Ectopic pancreatic tissue
    2. Brunner gland hyperplasia
    3. Adenomyoma
  E. Nodular mucosal remnants

SOURCE: Reproduced with permission from Ming SC, Hirota T: *Pathology of the Gastrointestinal Tract.*

Table 25-25
Benign Polypoid Lesions of the Stomach

Type of Lesion	Total Number	Percent
Epithelial polyp	252	40.9
Leiomyoma	230	37.3
Inflammatory polyp	29	4.7
Heterotopic tissue	25	4.1
Lipoma	21	3.4
Neurogenic tumor	19	3.1
Vascular tumor	13	2.1
Eosinophilic granuloma	12	1.9
Fibroma	9	1.5
Miscellaneous lesions	6	1.0
Total	616	100.0

SOURCE: Modified with permission from Ming SC: Tumors of the esophagus and stomach, in *Atlas of Tumor Pathology,* Second Series, Fascicle 7. Washington: Armed Forces Institute of Pathology, 1973, p 101.

Table 25-27
Etiology of Gastroparesis

Idiopathic
Endocrine or metabolic
    Diabetes mellitus
    Thyroid disease
    Renal insufficiency
After gastric surgery
    After resection
    After vagotomy
Central nervous system disorders
    Brain stem lesions
    Parkinson's disease
Peripheral neuromuscular disorders
    Myotonia dystrophica
    Duchenne muscular dystrophy
Connective tissue disorders
    Scleroderma
    Polymyositis/dermatomyositis
Infiltrative disorders
    Lymphoma
    Amyloidosis
Diffuse gastrointestinal motility disorder
    Chronic intestinal pseudo-obstruction
Medication-induced
Electrolyte imbalance
    Potassium, calcium, magnesium
Miscellaneous conditions
    Infections (especially viral)
    Paraneoplastic syndrome
    Ischemic conditions
    Gastric ulcer

SOURCE: Reproduced with permission from Packman HP, Fisher RS: Disorders of gastric emptying in Yamada T (ed): *Textbook of Gastroenterology*, 2003.

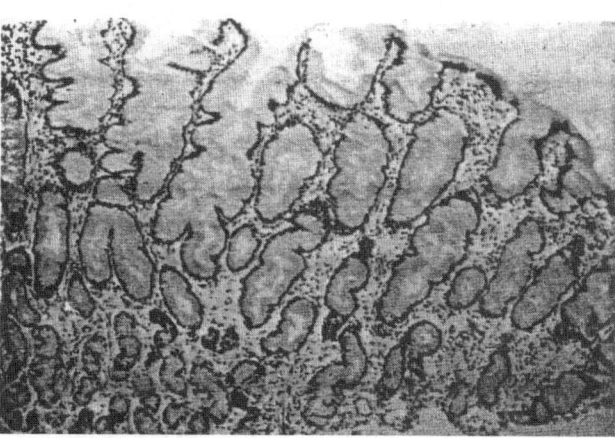

FIG. 25-65. Mucosal biopsy in Ménétrier's disease showing hyperplasia of surface cells. *[Reproduced with permission from Goldman H: Mucosal hypertrophy and hyperplasia of the stomach, in Ming C-J, Goldman H (eds): Pathology of the Gastrointestinal Tract, 2nd ed. Baltimore: Williams & Wilkins, 1998, p 577.]*

abnormalities (e.g., functional dyspepsia). Surgically relevant secondary disorders of gastric motility (e.g., dumping, gastric stasis, and Roux syndrome) are discussed below under postgastrectomy syndromes. Gastroparesis is the most surgically relevant primary disorder of gastric motility.

Most patients with primary gastroparesis present with nausea and vomiting. Bloating, early satiety, and abdominal pain are common. Eighty percent of these patients are women; some are diabetic. The gastroparesis and vomiting significantly complicate the management of the diabetes; frequently the patient takes parenteral insulin, eats, then vomits; they then become dangerously hypoglycemic. In patients with gastroparesis, it is important to rule out mechanical gastric outlet obstruction, and small bowel obstruction. Upper GI series may suggest slow gastric emptying and relative atony, or it may be normal. EGD may show bezoars, but is frequently normal. Gastric emptying scintigraphy shows delayed solid emptying, and often delayed liquid emptying. Gastroparesis can be a manifestation of a variety of problems (Table 25-27). Medical treatment includes promotility agents, antiemetics, and perhaps botulinum injection into the pylorus.

Surgeons need to understand the role of surgery in primary gastroparesis. If appropriate, the patient with severe diabetic gastroparesis should be evaluated for pancreas transplant prior to any invasive abdominal procedure, since some patients improve substantially after pancreas transplant. If the diabetic gastroparetic patient is not a candidate for pancreas transplant, both gastrostomy (for decompression) and jejunostomy tubes (for feeding and prevention of hypoglycemia) can be effective. Infection and wound problems are more common in diabetics with transabdominal tubes than in nondiabetics. Other surgical options include implantation of a gastric pacemaker, and gastric resection. Generally, gastric resection should be done infrequently, if at all, for primary gastroparesis.

MISCELLANEOUS LESIONS OF THE STOMACH

Hypertrophic Gastropathy (Ménétrier's Disease)

There are two clinical syndromes characterized by epithelial hyperplasia and giant gastric folds: Zollinger-Ellison syndrome (see above) and Ménétrier's disease. The latter is characteristically associated with protein-losing gastropathy and hypochlorhydria. There is a hyperplastic hypersecretory variant of Ménétrier's disease characterized by normal or increased acid secretion and no protein loss. There are large rugal folds in the proximal stomach, and the antrum is usually spared. Mucosal biopsy shows diffuse hyperplasia of the surface mucus-secreting cells (Fig. 25-65). The etiology is unclear, and there may be an increased risk of gastric cancer.

Most patients with Ménétrier's disease are middle-aged men who present with epigastric pain, weight loss, diarrhea, and hypoproteinemia. Sometimes the disease regresses spontaneously. Gastric resection may be indicated for bleeding, severe hypoproteinemia, or cancer in some patients with this rare problem. Present literature suggests that the risk of cancer in Ménétrier's disease may have been exaggerated.

Watermelon Stomach (Gastric Antral Vascular Ectasia)

The parallel red stripes atop the mucosal folds of the distal stomach give this rare entity its sobriquet. Histologically, gastric antral vascular ectasia is characterized by dilated mucosal blood vessels that often contain thrombi, in the lamina propria. Mucosal fibromuscular hyperplasia and hyalinization often are present (Fig. 25-66). The histologic appearance can resemble portal gastropathy, but the latter usually affects the proximal stomach, whereas watermelon stomach predominantly affects the distal stomach. Patients with gastric antral vascular ectasia are usually elderly women with chronic GI blood loss requiring transfusion. Most have an associated autoimmune connective tissue disorder, and at least 25% have chronic liver disease. Antrectomy may be required to control blood loss, but in patients with portal hypertension, transvenous intrahepatic portosystemic shunt should be considered first.

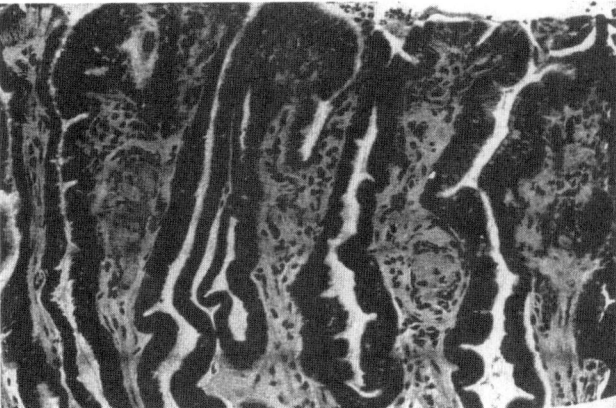

FIG. 25-66. Gastric antral vascular ectasia (watermelon stomach). *[Reproduced with permission from Goldman H: Mucosal hypertrophy and hyperplasia of the stomach, in Ming C-J, Goldman H (eds): Pathology of the Gastrointestinal Tract, 2nd ed. Baltimore: Williams & Wilkins, 1998, p 577.]*

Bezoars

Bezoars are concretions of undigestible matter that accumulate in the stomach. Trichobezoars, composed of hair, occur most commonly in young women who swallow their hair (Fig. 25-67). Phytobezoars are composed of vegetable matter and in the U.S. are usually seen in association with gastroparesis or gastric outlet obstruction. They also are associated with persimmon ingestion. Most commonly, bezoars produce obstructive symptoms, but they may cause ulceration and bleeding. Diagnosis is suggested by upper GI series and confirmed by endoscopy. Treatment options include enzyme therapy (papain, cellulase, or acetylcysteine), endoscopic disruption and removal, or surgical removal.

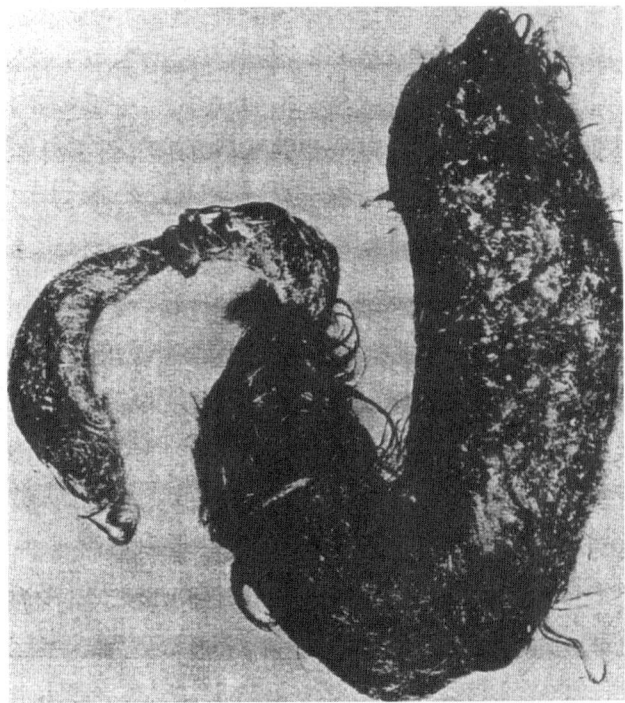

FIG. 25-67. Trichobezoar forming cast of stomach and duodenum removed from 15-year-old girl. *[Reproduced with permission from Ashley SW, Evoy D, Daly JM: Stomach, in Schwartz SI (ed): Principles of Surgery, 7th ed. New York: McGraw-Hill, 1999, p 1181.]*

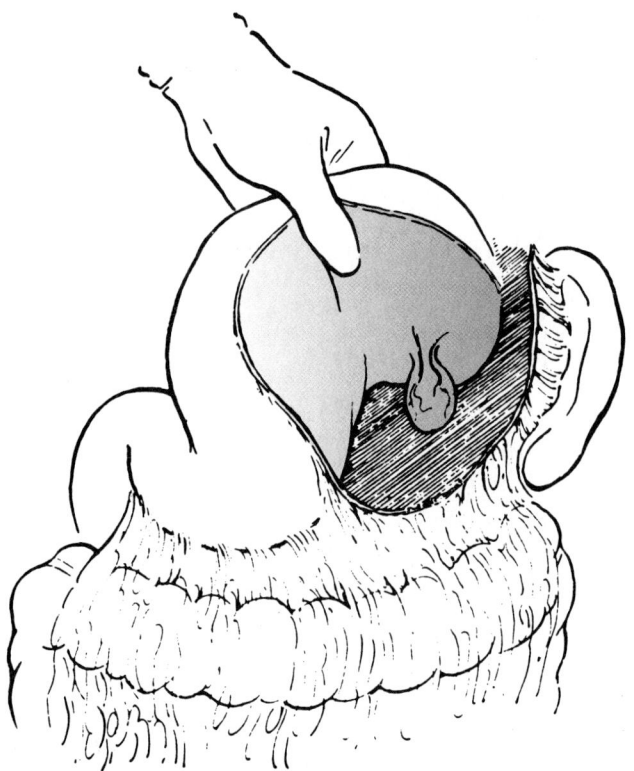

FIG. 25-68. Gastric diverticulum. *[Reproduced with permission from Ashley SW, Evoy D, Daly JM: Stomach, in Schwartz SI (ed): Principles of Surgery, 7th ed. New York: McGraw-Hill, 1999, p 1181.]*

Dieulafoy's Lesion

Dieulafoy's lesion is a congenital arteriovenous malformation characterized by an unusually large tortuous submucosal artery. If this artery is eroded, impressive bleeding may occur. To the operating surgeon, this appears as a stream of arterial blood emanating from what appears grossly to be a normal gastric mucosa. The lesion typically occurs in middle-aged or elderly men. Patients typically present with upper GI bleeding, which may be intermittent, and endoscopy can miss the lesion if it is not actively bleeding. Treatment options include endoscopic hemostatic therapy (usually injection), angiographic embolization, or operation. At surgery, the lesion may be oversewn or resected.

Diverticula

Gastric diverticula are usually solitary and may be congenital or acquired. Congenital diverticula are true diverticula and contain a full coat of muscularis propria, whereas acquired diverticula (perhaps caused by pulsion) usually have a negligible outer muscle layer. Most gastric diverticula occur in the posterior cardia or fundus (Fig. 25-68). Most of the time gastric diverticula are asymptomatic. However, they can become inflamed and may produce pain or bleeding. Perforation is rare. Asymptomatic diverticula do not require treatment, but symptomatic lesions should be removed. This can often be done laparoscopically.

Foreign Bodies

Ingested foreign bodies are usually asymptomatic. Removal of sharp or large objects should be considered. This can usually be done endoscopically, with an overtube technique. Recognized dangers include aspiration of the foreign body during removal, and rupture

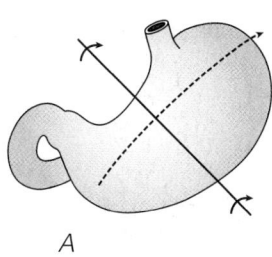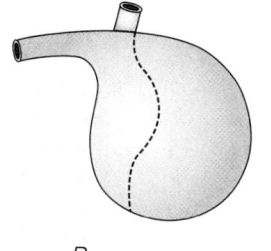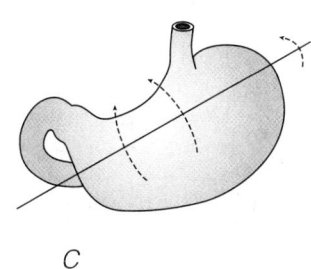

FIG. 25-69. Gastric volvulus (see text). *A, B* (mesenteroaxial rotation) and *C* (organoaxial rotation). [Reproduced with permission from Schirmer BD: Mechanical and motility disorders of the stomach and duodenum, in Zuidema GD, Yeo CJ (eds): Shackelford's Surgery of the Alimentary Tract, 5th ed., Vol. II. Philadelphia: Saunders, 2002, p 178.]

of drug-containing bags in "body packers." Both complications can be fatal. Surgical removal is recommended in body packers, and in patients with large jagged objects.

Mallory-Weiss Tear

The Mallory-Weiss lesion is a longitudinal tear in the mucosa of the gastroesophageal junction. It is presumably caused by forceful vomiting and/or retching, and is commonly seen in alcoholics. It commonly presents with impressive upper GI bleeding, often with hematemesis. Endoscopy confirms the diagnosis and may be useful in controlling the bleeding, but 90% of patients stop bleeding spontaneously. Other options to control the bleeding include balloon tamponade, angiographic embolization, or selective infusion of vasopressin, systemic vasopressin, and operation. Surgical treatment consists of oversewing the bleeding lesion through a long gastrotomy.

Volvulus

Gastric volvulus is a twist of the stomach that usually occurs in association with a large hiatal hernia. It also can occur in patients with an unusually mobile stomach without hiatal hernia. Typically, the stomach twists along its long axis (organoaxial volvulus), and the greater curvature flips up (Fig. 25-69C). If the stomach twists around the transverse axis, it is called mesenteroaxial rotation (Fig. 25-69A,B). Usually, volvulus is a chronic condition that can be surprisingly asymptomatic. In these instances, expectant nonoperative management is usually advised, especially in the elderly. The risk of strangulation and infarction has been overestimated in asymptomatic patients. Symptomatic patients should be considered for operation, especially if the symptoms are severe and/or progressive. Patients usually present with symptoms of pain and pressure related to the intermittently distending and poorly emptying twisted stomach. Pressure on the lung may produce dyspnea, pressure on the pericardium may produce palpitations, and pressure on the esophagus may produce dysphagia. Symptoms are often relieved with vomiting or passage of a nasogastric tube. Gastric infarction is a surgical emergency and the patient often presents moribund. Elective operation for gastric volvulus usually involves reduction of the stomach and repair of hiatal hernia, with or without gastropexy. Gastropexy alone may be considered for high-risk patients. A laparoscopic approach should be considered.

GASTROSTOMY

A gastrostomy is performed either for alimentation or for gastric drainage/decompression. Gastrostomy may be done percutaneously, laparoscopically, or via open technique. Currently, percutaneous endoscopic gastrostomy is the most common method used, usually with the Ponsky technique. In this procedure, the insufflated stomach is accessed percutaneously with a thin trocar needle under direct endoscopic vision. A long, braided wire is passed through the needle

into the stomach, snared endoscopically, and pulled out the mouth, where it is attached to the outside end of a special gastrostomy tube. The wire and attached tube are then pulled down the esophagus, into the stomach, and out the dilated trocar needle track and is secured.

The open techniques include the Stamm method (Fig. 25-70), the Witzel method (Fig. 25-71), and the Janeway method (Fig. 25-72). The latter is meant to create a permanent stoma that can be intubated as needed, but does not drain spontaneously. The Janeway gastrostomy is more complicated than the other open techniques, and is rarely necessary. By far the most common technique is the Stamm gastrostomy, which can be performed open or laparoscopically.

Complications of gastrostomy include infection, dislodgment, and aspiration pneumonia. Although gastrostomy tubes usually do prevent tense gastric dilatation, they may not adequately drain the stomach, especially when the patient is bedridden.

Postgastrectomy Problems

A variety of abnormalities affect some patients after a gastric operation that has usually been performed because of ulcer or tumor. Some of the more common disorders result from disturbance of the normal anatomic and physiologic mechanisms that control gastric motor function, and a discussion of these follows.

Dumping Syndrome

Dumping is a phenomenon caused by the destruction of the pyloric sphincter. However, other factors undoubtedly play a role since dumping can occur after operations that preserve the pylorus, such as parietal cell vagotomy. The appropriate stimulus can provoke dumping symptoms, even in some patients who have not undergone surgery. Clinically significant dumping occurs in 5 to 10% of patients after pyloroplasty, pyloromyotomy, or distal gastrectomy, and consists of a constellation of postprandial symptoms ranging in severity from annoying to disabling. The symptoms are thought to be the result of the abrupt delivery of a hyperosmolar load into the small bowel. This is usually due to ablation of the pylorus, but decreased gastric compliance with accelerated emptying of liquids (e.g., after highly selective vagotomy) is another accepted mechanism. Rapid fluid influx into the bowel lumen and wall results, along with an incompletely understood neuroendocrine response. There is peripheral and splanchnic vasodilatation. About 15 to 30 minutes after a meal, the patient becomes diaphoretic, weak, light-headed, and tachycardic. These symptoms may be ameliorated by recumbence or saline infusion. Diarrhea often follows. This is referred to as early dumping, and should be distinguished from postprandial (reactive) hypoglycemia, also called late dumping, which usually occurs later (2 to 3 hours following a meal), and is relieved by the administration of sugar. A variety of hormonal aberrations have been observed in early dumping, including increased vasoactive intestinal peptide, cholecystokinin, neurotensin, peripheral hormone

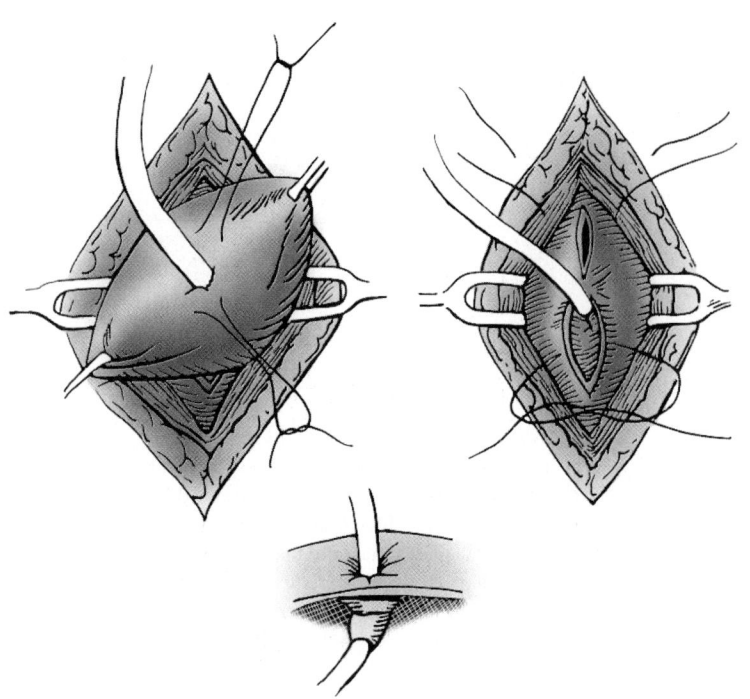

FIG. 25-70. Stamm gastrostomy. [Reproduced with permission from Tatum RP, Joehl RJ: Intubation of the stomach and small intestine, in Zuidema GD, Yeo CJ (eds): Shackelford's Surgery of the Alimentary Tract, 5th ed., Vol. II. Philadelphia: Saunders, 2002, p 46.]

FIG. 25-71. Witzel gastrostomy. [Reproduced with permission from Tatum RP, Joehl RJ: Intubation of the stomach and small intestine, in Zuidema GD, Yeo CJ (eds): Shackelford's Surgery of the Alimentary Tract, 5th ed., Vol. II. Philadelphia: Saunders, 2002, p 46.]

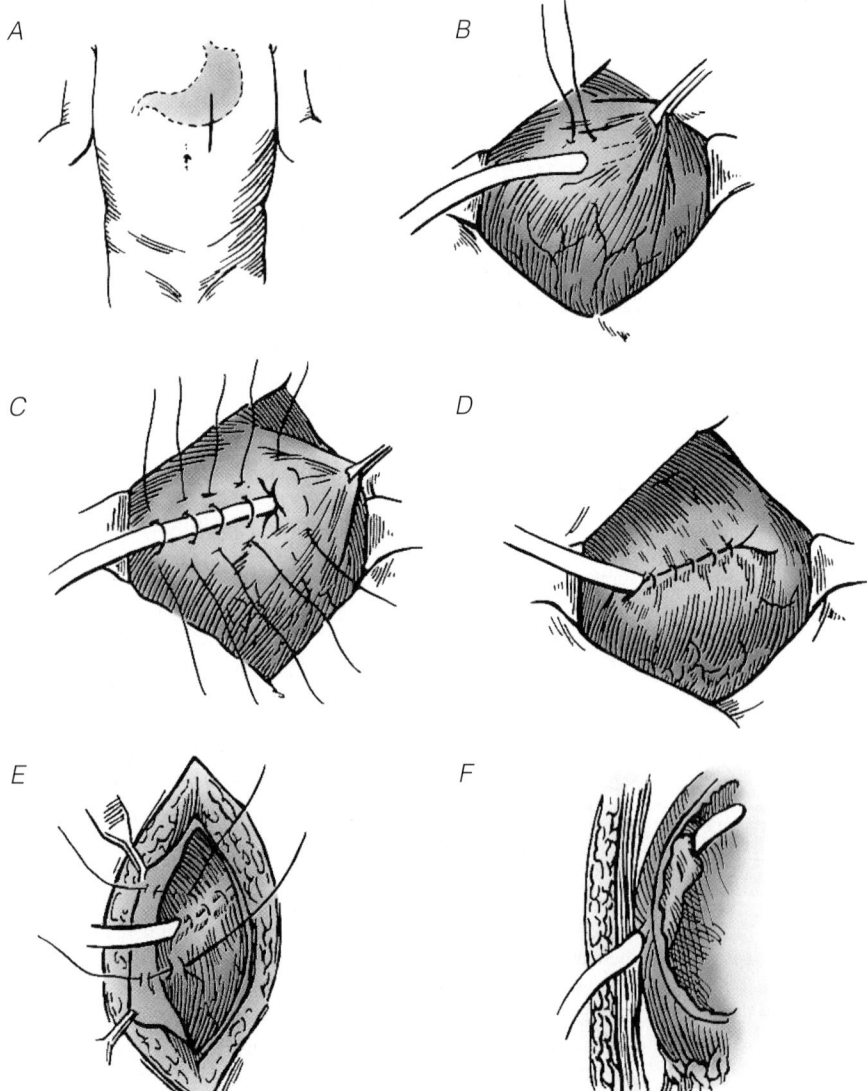

A

B

C

D

E

F

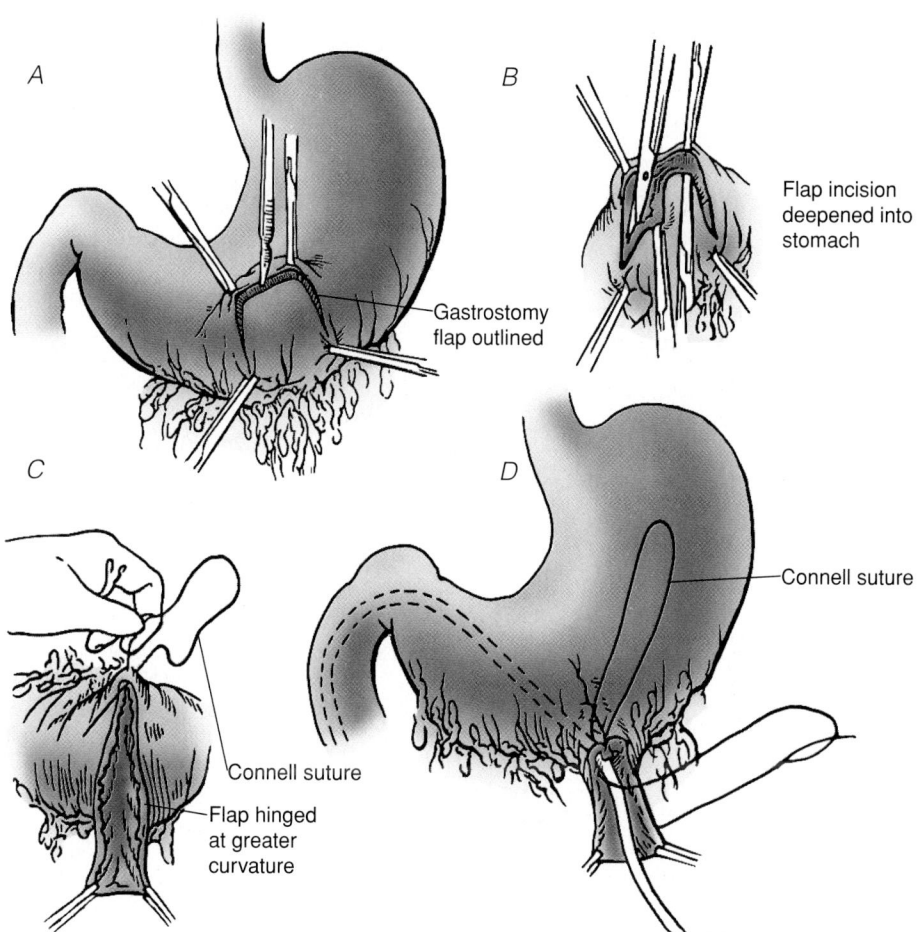

A

B

Flap incision
deepened into
stomach

Gastrostomy
flap outlined

C

D

Connell suture

Connell suture

Flap hinged
at greater
curvature

FIG. 25-72. Janeway gastrostomy. [Reproduced with permission from Tatum RP, Joehl RJ: Intubation of the stomach and small intestine, in Zuidema GD, Yeo CJ (eds): Shackelford's Surgery of the Alimentary Tract, 5th ed., Vol. II. Philadelphia: Saunders, 2002, p 46.]

peptide YY, renin-angiotensin-aldosterone, and decreased atrial natriuretic peptide. Late dumping is associated with hypoglycemia and hyperinsulinemia.

The medical therapy for the dumping syndrome consists of dietary management and somatostatin analogue (octreotide). Often symptoms improve if the patient avoids liquids during meals. Hyperosmolar liquids (e.g., milk shakes) may be particularly troublesome. There is some evidence that adding dietary fiber compounds at mealtime may improve the syndrome. If dietary manipulation fails, the patient is started on octreotide, 100 μg subcutaneously twice daily. This can be increased up to 500 μg twice daily if necessary. Octreotide ameliorates the abnormal hormonal pattern seen in patients with dumping symptoms. It also promotes restoration of a fasting motility pattern in the small intestine (i.e., restoration of the migrating motor complex). The alpha-glucosidase inhibitor acarbose may be particularly helpful in ameliorating the symptoms of late dumping.

Only a small percentage of patients with dumping symptoms ultimately require surgery. Most patients improve with time (months and even years), dietary management, and medication. Therefore the surgeon should by no means rush to reoperate on the patient with dumping symptoms. Multidisciplinary nonsurgical management must be optimized first. Prior to reoperation, a period of in-hospital observation is useful to define the severity of the patient's symptoms. Patient compliance with dietary and medical therapy also can be assessed.

The results of remedial operation for dumping are variable and unpredictable. There are a variety of surgical approaches, none of which work consistently well. Additionally, there is not a great deal of experience reported in the literature with any of these methods. Long-term follow-up is rare. Operations performed to treat disabling dumping syndrome include pyloric reconstruction, takedown of gastrojejunostomy, interposition of a 10-cm reversed intestinal segment between the stomach and duodenum, conversion of Billroth II to Billroth I anastomosis, and conversion to Roux-en-Y anastomosis.

Patients with disabling dumping after gastrojejunostomy can be considered for simple takedown of this anastomosis provided that (1) there is some vagal innervation to the antrum, and (2) the pyloric channel is open endoscopically. The reversed intestinal segment is rarely used today—and rightly so. This operation interposes a 10-cm reversed segment of intestine between the stomach and the intestine. This slows gastric emptying, but often leads to obstruction requiring reoperation. Isoperistaltic interposition (Henley loop) has not been successful in ameliorating severe dumping long term. The Roux-en-Y gastrojejunostomy is associated with delayed gastric emptying, probably on the basis of disordered motility in the Roux limb. Taking advantage of this disordered physiology, surgeons have used this operation successfully in the management of the dumping syndrome. Although this is probably the procedure of choice in the small group of patients requiring operation for severe dumping following gastric resection, gastric stasis may result, particularly if a large gastric remnant is left. In the presence of significant gastric acid secretion, marginal ulceration is common after both jejunal interposition and Roux-en-Y procedures; thus vagotomy and hemigastrectomy should be considered. The theoretical

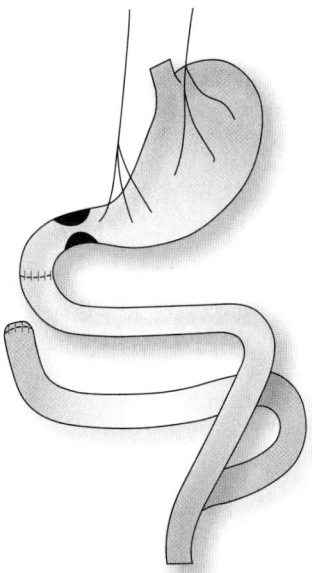

FIG. 25-73. Duodenal switch operation. Addition of highly selective vagotomy should be considered. *[Reproduced with permission from Schirmer BD: Mechanical and motility disorders of the stomach and duodenum, in Zuidema GD, Yeo CJ (eds): Shackelford's Surgery of the Alimentary Tract, 5th ed., Vol. II. Philadelphia: Saunders, 2002, p 178.]*

possibility of treating postpyloroplasty dumping with a Roux-en-Y to the proximal duodenum (the duodenal switch, a potentially reversible operation) has not been reported (Fig. 25-73). Since pyloric ablation seems to be the dominant factor in the etiology of dumping, it is not surprising that conversion of Billroth II to Billroth I anastomosis has not been successful in the treatment of dumping.

Diarrhea

Diarrhea following gastric surgery may be the result of truncal vagotomy, dumping, or malabsorption. Truncal vagotomy is associated with clinically significant diarrhea in 5 to 10% of patients. It occurs soon after surgery and usually is not associated with other symptoms, a fact that helps to distinguish it from dumping. The diarrhea may be a daily occurrence, or there may be significant periods of relatively normal bowel function. The symptoms tend to improve over the months and years after the index operation. The cause of postvagotomy diarrhea is unclear. Possible mechanisms include intestinal dysmotility and accelerated transit, bile acid malabsorption, rapid gastric emptying, and bacterial overgrowth. The latter problem is facilitated by decreased gastric acid secretion and (even small) blind loops. Although bacterial overgrowth can be confirmed with the hydrogen breath test, a simpler test is an empirical trial of oral antibiotics. Some patients with postvagotomy diarrhea respond to cholestyramine, while in others codeine or loperamide may be useful. Another theoretical cause of diarrhea following gastric surgery is fat malabsorption due to acid inactivation of pancreatic enzymes or poorly coordinated mixing of food and digestive juices. This can be confirmed with a qualitative test for fecal fat and treated with acid suppression. In the author's experience, postvagotomy diarrhea does not respond to treatment with pancreatic enzymes. In the rare patient who is debilitated by postvagotomy diarrhea that is unresponsive to medical management, the operation of choice is a 10-cm reversed jejunal interposition placed in continuity 100 cm distal to the ligament of Treitz. Another option is the onlay antiperistaltic distal

ileal graft. Both operations can cause obstructive symptoms and/or bacterial overgrowth.

Gastric Stasis

Gastric stasis following surgery on the stomach may be due to a problem with gastric motor function or be caused by an obstruction. The gastric motility abnormality may have been pre-existing and unrecognized by the operating surgeon. Alternatively, it may be secondary to deliberate or unintentional vagotomy or resection of the dominant gastric pacemaker. An obstruction may be mechanical (e.g., anastomotic stricture, efferent limb kink from adhesions or constricting mesocolon, or a proximal small bowel obstruction), or functional (e.g., retrograde peristalsis in a Roux limb). Gastric stasis presents with vomiting (often of undigested food), bloating, epigastric pain, and weight loss.

The evaluation of a patient with suspected postoperative gastric stasis includes esophagogastroduodenoscopy, upper GI series, gastric emptying scan, and gastric motor testing. Endoscopy shows gastritis and retained food or bezoar. The anastomosis and efferent limb should be evaluated for stricture or narrowing. Endoscopy may be facilitated by reviewing a recent upper GI series to help define the anatomy and to look for an area of obstruction. A dilated efferent limb suggests chronic stasis, either from a motor abnormality (e.g., Roux syndrome) or mechanical obstruction (e.g., chronic adhesion). Gastric emptying is best quantified clinically with scintigraphic techniques, which give a half-time for liquid and solid emptying. The former may be fairly normal, while the latter is profoundly delayed. If the problem is thought to be primarily a disorder of intrinsic motor function, newer techniques such as electrogastrography and gastrointestinal manometry should be considered. It should, however, be remembered that chronic mechanical obstruction may result in disordered motility in the proximal organ.

Once mechanical obstruction has been ruled out, medical treatment is successful in most cases of motor dysfunction following previous gastric surgery. This consists of dietary modification and promotility agents. Intermittent oral antibiotic therapy may be helpful in treating bacterial overgrowth, with its attendant symptoms of bloating, flatulence, and diarrhea.

Gastroparesis following vagotomy and drainage may be treated with subtotal (75%) gastrectomy. Billroth II anastomosis with Braun enteroenterostomy may be preferable to Roux-en-Y reconstruction. This latter option may be associated with persistent emptying problems that will subsequently require near-total or total gastrectomy, a nutritionally unattractive option. Delayed gastric emptying following ulcer surgery (vagotomy and drainage or vagotomy and antrectomy) may represent an anastomotic stricture (often due to recurrent ulcer), or proximal small bowel obstruction. The latter should be dealt with at reoperation. Recurrent ulcer usually responds to medical therapy. Endoscopic dilation is occasionally helpful. Gastroparesis following subtotal gastric resection is best treated with near-total (95%) or total gastric resection and Roux-en-Y reconstruction. If total gastrectomy is performed, a jejunal reservoir should be fashioned. Gastric pacing is promising, but it has not achieved widespread clinical usefulness in the treatment of postoperative gastric atony.

Bile Reflux Gastritis

Most patients who have undergone ablation or resection of the pylorus have bile in the stomach on endoscopic examination, along with some degree of gross or microscopic gastric inflammation. Therefore attributing postoperative symptoms to bile reflux is problematic, since most asymptomatic patients have bile reflux as well.

However, it is generally accepted that a small subset of patients have bile reflux gastritis, and present with nausea, bilious vomiting, and epigastric pain, and *quantitative evidence* of excess enterogastric reflux. Curiously, symptoms often develop months or years after the index operation. The differential diagnosis includes afferent or efferent loop obstruction, gastric stasis, and small bowel obstruction. Plain abdominal x-rays, upper endoscopy, upper GI series, abdominal CT scan, and gastric emptying scans are helpful in evaluating these possibilities.

Bile reflux may be quantified with gastric analysis, or more commonly with scintigraphy (bile reflux scan). Typically enterogastric reflux is greatest after Billroth II gastrectomy or gastrojejunostomy, and least after vagotomy and pyloroplasty, with Billroth I gastrectomy giving intermediate values. Patients who are well into the abnormal range may be considered for remedial surgery if symptoms are severe. Remedial surgery will eliminate the bile from the vomitus and may improve the epigastric pain, but it is quite unusual to render these patients completely asymptomatic, especially if they are narcotic dependent.

Bile reflux gastritis after distal gastric resection may be treated by one of the following options: Roux-en-Y gastrojejunostomy; interposition of a 40-cm isoperistaltic jejunal loop between the gastric remnant and the duodenum (Henley loop); or Billroth II gastrojejunostomy with Braun enteroenterostomy. To avoid bile reflux into the stomach, the Roux limb should be at least 45 cm long. The Braun enteroenterostomy should be placed a similar distance from the stomach. Excessively long limbs may be associated with obstruction or malabsorption. All operations can result in marginal ulceration on the jejunal side of the gastrojejunostomy, and thus are combined with a generous distal gastrectomy. If this has already been done at a previous operation, the Roux or Braun operations may be attractively simple. Whether truncal vagotomy is necessary is controversial in the current era of excellent acid-suppressing medications. The benefits of decreased acid secretion following vagotomy may be outweighed by problems with vagotomy-associated dysmotility in the gastric remnant. The Roux operation may be associated with an increased risk of emptying problems compared to the other two options, but controlled data are lacking. Patients with debilitating bile reflux after gastrojejunostomy can be considered for simple takedown of this anastomosis provided that (1) there is some vagal innervation to the antrum and (2) the pyloric channel is open.

Primary bile reflux gastritis (i.e., no previous operation) is rare, and may be treated with the duodenal switch operation, essentially an end-to-end Roux-en-Y to the proximal duodenum (see Fig. 25-73). The Achilles' heel of this operation is, not surprisingly, marginal ulceration. Thus it should be combined with highly selective vagotomy, and perhaps H_2-blockers.

Roux Syndrome

A subset of patients who have had distal gastrectomy and Roux-en-Y gastrojejunostomy will have great difficulty with gastric emptying in the absence of mechanical obstruction. These patients present with vomiting, epigastric pain, and weight loss. This clinical scenario has been labeled the Roux syndrome. Endoscopy may show bezoar formation, dilation of the gastric remnant, and/or dilation of the Roux limb. An upper GI series confirms these findings and may show delayed gastric emptying. This is better quantified by a gastric emptying scan, which always shows delayed solid emptying, and may show delayed liquid emptying as well.

Gastrointestinal motility testing shows abnormal motility in the Roux limb, with propulsive activity toward, rather than away from, the stomach. Gastric motility also may be abnormal. Presumably, the disordered motility in the Roux limb occurs in all patients with this operation. Why only a subset develops the Roux syndrome is unclear. Perhaps those patients with disordered gastric motility are at most risk. The disorder seems to be more common in patients with a generous gastric remnant. Truncal vagotomy also has been implicated.

Medical treatment consists of promotility agents. Surgical treatment consists of paring down the gastric remnant. If gastric motility is severely disordered, 95% gastrectomy should be done. The Roux limb should be resected if it is dilated and flaccid, and doing so does not put the patient at risk for short bowel problems. Gastrointestinal continuity may be re-established with another Roux, a Billroth II with Braun enteroenterostomy, or an isoperistaltic jejunal interposition between the stomach and the duodenum (Henley loop). Truncal vagotomy should probably not be done. Long-term acid suppression may be necessary.

Gallstones

Gallstone formation following gastric surgery generally is thought to be secondary to vagal denervation of the gallbladder with attendant gallbladder dysmotility. Presumably, vagotomy causes stasis of gallbladder bile with subsequent sludge and stone formation. Other possible but incompletely investigated possibilities include postoperative ampullary dysfunction and changes in bile composition. It is unclear whether simply dividing the hepatic branches of the anterior vagal trunk (as is frequently done during antireflux and bariatric operations, as well as subtotal gastric resection) increases gallstone formation. Although prophylactic cholecystectomy is not justified with most gastric surgery, it should be considered if the gallbladder appears abnormal, especially if subsequent cholecystectomy is likely to be difficult. If preoperative evaluation reveals sludge or gallstones, or if intraoperative evaluation reveals stones, cholecystectomy should be done if it appears straightforward and the gastric operation has gone well.

Weight Loss

Patients who have an operation on the stomach commonly lose weight. In the case of bariatric surgery, this is intentional and meant to be a permanent effect of the operation. In antireflux surgery, this is usually transient, and attributed to the temporary dietary modification required in the first few postoperative weeks as the patient compensates for mild dysphagia and early satiety. Severe (>10% ideal body weight) or permanent weight loss after antireflux surgery indicates a significant problem and should prompt a diagnostic work-up. Possible causes include a tight or slipped wrap, gastric stasis (due to vagal injury or a missed motor disorder), bacterial overgrowth and malabsorption, or an unrecognized preoperative problem (commonly a motor disorder).

Weight loss is common in patients who have had a vagotomy and/or gastric resection. The degree of weight loss tends to parallel the magnitude of the operation. It may be insignificant in the large person, or devastating in the asthenic female. The surgeon should always consider the possible consequences before performing a gastric resection for benign disease in a thin female. The causes of weight loss after gastric surgery generally fall into one of two categories: altered dietary intake or malabsorption. If a stool stain for fecal fat is negative, it is likely that decreased caloric intake is the cause. This is the most common cause of weight loss after gastric surgery, and may be due to small stomach syndrome, postoperative gastroparesis, or self-imposed dietary modification because of dumping and/or diarrhea. Specific problems may be treated as outlined above. Consultation with an experienced dietitian may prove invaluable.

Anemia

Iron absorption takes place primarily in the proximal gastrointestinal tract, and is facilitated by an acidic environment. Intrinsic factor, essential for the enteric absorption of vitamin B_{12}, is made by the parietal cells of the stomach. Vitamin B_{12} bioavailability also is facilitated by an acidic environment.

With this as background, it is easy to understand why patients who have had a gastric operation are at risk for anemia. Anemia is the most common metabolic side effect in patients who have had a gastric bypass for morbid obesity. It also occurs in up to one third of patients who have had a vagotomy and/or gastric resection. Iron deficiency is the most common cause, but vitamin B_{12} or folate deficiency also occurs, even in patients who have not had total gastrectomy. Of course, patients who have had a total gastrectomy will all develop B_{12} deficiency without parenteral vitamin B_{12}. Gastric bypass patients should be given oral iron supplements, and monitored for iron, B_{12}, and folate deficiency. Patients who have had a vagotomy and/or gastrectomy should be similarly monitored with periodic determination of hematocrit, red blood cell indices, iron and transferrin levels, B_{12}, and folate levels. Marginal nutrient status should be corrected with oral and/or parenteral supplementation.

Bone Disease

Gastric surgery sometimes disturbs calcium and vitamin D metabolism. Calcium absorption occurs primarily in the duodenum, which is bypassed with gastrojejunostomy. Fat malabsorption may occur because of blind loop syndrome and bacterial overgrowth, or because of inefficient mixing of food and digestive enzymes. This can significantly affect the absorption of vitamin D, a fat-soluble vitamin. Both abnormalities of calcium and vitamin D metabolism can contribute to metabolic bone disease in patients following gastric surgery. The problems usually manifest as pain and/or fractures years after the index operation. Musculoskeletal symptoms should prompt a study of bone density. Dietary supplementation of calcium and vitamin D may be useful in preventing these complications. Routine skeletal monitoring of patients at high-risk (e.g., elderly males and females and postmenopausal females) may prove useful in identifying skeletal deterioration that may be stopped with appropriate treatment.

LAPAROSCOPIC GASTRIC OPERATIONS

Perhaps the most common laparoscopic gastric operations performed today are for gastroesophageal reflux disease and obesity (see Chap. 26). However, all of the gastric operations described here can be performed with minimally invasive techniques. Some (e.g., partial or total gastric resection) are technically difficult or are of debatable merit (e.g., laparoscopic resection for cancer). The operations described in this chapter that lend themselves most readily to minimally invasive techniques are highly selective vagotomy, vagotomy and gastrojejunostomy, and gastrostomy. Laparoscopic wedge resection often is possible for GI stromal tumors, lipomas, or gastric diverticula. Combined endoscopic and laparoscopic techniques occasionally are useful. Diagnostic laparoscopy may prevent a futile laparotomy in some patients with gastric cancer.

Bibliography

Surgery of the Stomach
Ashley SW, Evoy D, Daly JM: Stomach, in Schwartz SI (ed): *Principles of Surgery*, 7th ed., New York: McGraw-Hill, 1999, p 1181.
Daly JM, Cady B, Low DW (eds): *Atlas of Surgical Oncology*. St. Louis: Mosby, 1993.
Dempsey DT: Concepts in surgery of the stomach and duodenum, in Scott-Conner CEH (ed): *Chassin's Operative Strategy in General Surgery*, 3rd ed. New York: Springer-Verlag, 2001.
Ritchie WP Jr.: Benign diseases of the stomach and duodenum, in Ritchie WP, Steele G, Dean RH (eds): *General Surgery.*, Philadelphia: Lippincott, 1995, p 117.
Sabiston DC Jr.: *Atlas of General Surgery*. Philadelphia: Saunders, 1994.
Scott HW Jr., Sawyers JL: *Surgery of the Stomach, Duodenum, and Small Intestine*, 2nd ed. Boston: Blackwell Scientific Publishers, 1992.
Soybel DI, Zinner MJ: Stomach and duodenum, in Zinner MJ, Schwartz SI, Ellis H (eds): *Maingot's Abdominal Operations*. Stamford, CT: Appleton & Lange, 1997.
Zollinger RM: *Atlas of Surgical Operations*. New York: Macmillan, 1975.

History
Beaumont W: Experiments and observations on the gastric juice and the physiology of digestion. Plattsburgh, NY: PP Allen, 1833.
Billroth T: Offenes screiben an Herrn Dr. L Wittelshofer. *Wien Med Woechenschr* 31:162, 1881.
Dragstedt LR: The pathogenesis of duodenal and gastric ulcers. *Am J Surg* 136:286, 1978.
Dragstedt LR: Vagotomy for the gastroduodenal ulcer. *Ann Surg* 122:973, 1945.
Herrington JL: Historical aspects of gastric surgery, in Scott HW Jr, Sawyers JL (eds): *Surgery of the Stomach, Duodenum, and Small Intestine*, 2nd ed. Blackwell, 1992.
Menguy R: *Surgery of Peptic Ulcer*. Philadelphia: Saunders, 1976.
Wangensteen OH, Wangensteen SD: Gastric surgery, in *The Rise of Surgery*. Minneapolis: University of Minnesota Press, 1978.
Zollinger RM, Ellison EH: Primary peptic ulcerations of the jejunum associated with islet cell tumors of the pancreas. *Ann Surg* 142:709, 1955.

Anatomy
Antonioli DA, Madara JL: Functional anatomy of the gastrointestinal tract, in Ming S-C, Goldman H (eds): *Pathology of the Gastrointestinal Tract*, 2nd ed. Baltimore: Williams & Wilkins, 1998, p 13.
Bloom W, Fawcett DW: *A Textbook of Histology*. Philadelphia: Saunders, 1975, p 639.
Gershon MD: The enteric nervous system. *Hosp Pract* 34:37, 1999.
Mercer DW, Liu TH, Castaneda A: Anatomy and physiology of the stomach, in Zuidema GD, Yeo CJ (eds): *Shackelford's Surgery of the Alimentary Tract*, 5th ed, Vol. II. Philadelphia: Saunders, 2002, p 3.
Moore KL: *The Developing Human*. Philadelphia: Saunders, 1974, p 175.
Raufman J-P: Stomach: Anatomy and structural anomalies, in Yamada T et al (eds): *Textbook of Gastroenterology*, 4th ed. Philadelphia: Lippincott Williams & Wilkins, 2003, p 1279.
Redel CA: Anatomy, histology, embryology, and developmental anomalies of the stomach and duodenum, in Feldman M (ed): *Sleisenger and Fordtran's Gastrointestinal and Liver Disease*, 7th ed. Philadelphia: Saunders, 2002, p 675.

Physiology
Allen A, Flemstrom G, et al: Gastroduodenal mucosal protection. *Physiol Rev* 73:823, 1993.
Ariyasu H, Takaya K, Tagami T, et al: Stomach is a major source of circulating ghrelin, and feeding state determines plasma ghrelin-like immunoreactivity levels in humans. *J Clin Endocrinol Metab* 86:4753, 2001.
Cullen JJ, Kelly KA: Gastric motor physiology and pathophysiology. *Surg Clin North Am* 73:1145, 1993.

Cummings DE, Weigle DS, Frayo RS, et al: Plasma ghrelin levels after diet-induced weight loss or gastric bypass surgery. *N Engl J Med* 346:1623, 2002.

Del Valle J, Todisco A: Gastric secretion, in Yamada T et al (eds): *Textbook of Gastroenterology*, 4th ed. Philadelphia: Lippincott Williams & Wilkins, 2003, p 266.

Feldman M: Gastric secretion, in Feldman M (ed): *Sleisenger and Fordtran's Gastrointestinal and Liver Disease*, 7th ed. Philadelphia: Saunders, 2002, p 715.

Hasler WL: Physiology of gastric motility and gastric emptying, in Yamada T et al (eds): *Textbook of Gastroenterology*, 4th ed., Philadelphia: Lippincott Williams & Wilkins, 2003, p 195.

Kim CH: Electrical activity of the stomach: Clinical applications. *Mayo Clin Proc* 61:205, 1986.

Lloyd KCK, Debas HT: Hormonal and neural regulation of gastric acid secretion, in Johnson LR (ed): *Physiology of the Gastrointestinal Tract*, 3rd ed. New York: Raven, 1993.

Murray CD, Kamm MA, Bloom SR, Emmanuel AV: Ghrelin for the gastroenterologist: History and potential. *Gastroenterology* 125:1492, 2003.

Quigley EMM: Gastric motor and sensory function, and motor disorders of the stomach, in Feldman M (ed): *Sleisenger and Fordtran's Gastrointestinal and Liver Disease*, 7th ed. Philadelphia: Saunders, 2002, p 691.

Rees WDW, Malagelada JR, Miller LJ, Go VLW: Human interdigestive and postprandial gastrointestinal hormone patterns. *Dig Dis Sci* 27:321, 1982.

Silen W, Ito S: Mechanisms for the rapid re-epithelization of the gastric mucosal surface. *Ann Rev Physiol* 47:217, 1985.

Wallace JL: Gastric resistance to acid: Is the "mucus-bicarbonate barrier" functionally redundant? *Am J Physiol* 256:31, 1989.

Wolfe MM, Soll AH: The physiology of gastric acid secretion. *N Engl J Med* 319:707, 1988.

Diagnosis of Gastric Disease

Allescher HD, Abraham-Fuchs K, Dunkel RE, Classen M: Biomagnetic 3-dimensional spatial and temporal characterization of electrical activity of human stomach. *Dig Dis Sci* 43:683, 1998.

Balaji NS, Crookes PF, Banki F, et al: A safe and noninvasive test for vagal integrity revisited. *Arch Surg* 137:954, 2002.

Caroline DF, Evers K: The stomach, in Grainger RG, Allison D, et al (eds): *Diagnostic Radiology, a Textbook of Medical Imaging*, 4th ed. London: Churchill Livingstone, 2001, p 1035.

Chieng DC, Jhala D, Jhala N, et al: Endoscopic ultrasound-guided fine-needle aspiration biopsy. A study of 103 cases. *Cancer* 96:232, 2002.

Dooley CP, Larson AW, Stace NH: Double-contrast barium meal and upper gastrointestinal endoscopy: A comparative study. *Ann Intern Med* 101:538, 1984.

Feinle C, Kunz P, Boesiger P, Fried M, Schwizer W: Scintigraphic validation of a magnetic resonance imaging method to study gastric emptying of a solid meal in humans. *Gut* 44:106, 1999.

Insko EK, Levine MS, Birnbaum BA, Jacobs JE: Benign and malignant lesions of the stomach: Evaluation of CT criteria for differentiation. *Radiology* 228:166, 2003.

Kawamoto K, Yamada Y, Utsunomiya T, et al: Gastrointestinal submucosal tumors: Evaluation with endoscopic US. *Radiology* 205:733, 1997.

Kelly S, Harris KM, Berry E, et al: A systematic review of the staging performance of endoscopic ultrasound in gastro-oesophageal carcinoma. *Gut* 49:534, 2001.

Ogata I, Komohara Y, Yamashita Y, et al: CT evaluation of gastric lesions with three-dimensional display and interactive virtual endoscopy: Comparison with conventional barium study and endoscopy. *Am J Roentgenol* 172:1263, 1999.

Ponsky JL, Dumot JA: Diagnostic evaluation of the stomach and duodenum, in Zuidema GD, Yeo CJ (eds): *Shackelford's Surgery of the Alimentary Tract*, 5th ed., Vol. II. Philadelphia: Saunders, 2002, p 34.

Puspok A, Raderer M, Chott A, et al: Endoscopic ultrasound in the follow up and response assessment of patients with primary gastric lymphoma. *Gut* 51:691, 2002.

Willmann JK, Weishaupt D, Bohm T, et al: Detection of submucosal gastric fundal varices with multi-detector row CT angiography. *Gut* 52:886, 2003.

Wood BJ, Razavi P: Virtual endoscopy: A promising new technology. *Am Fam Physician* 66:107, 2002.

Peptic Ulcer Disease

Pathophysiology

Blair AJ, Feldman M, Barnett C, et al: Detailed comparison of basal and food stimulated gastric acid secretion rates and serum gastrin concentrations in duodenal ulcer patients and normal subjects. *J Clin Invest* 79:582, 1987.

Cohen H: Peptic ulcer and *Helicobacter pylori*. *Gastroenterol Clin North Am* 29:775, 2000.

Cryer B, Feldman M: Peptic ulcer disease in the elderly. *Semin Gastrointest Dis* 5:166, 1994.

Donahue PE: Ulcer surgery and highly selective vagotomy—Y2K. *Arch Surg* 134:1373, 1999.

Fisher RS, Cohen S: Pyloric sphincter dysfunction in patients with gastric ulcer. *N Engl J Med* 288:273, 1976.

Harris AW, Gummett PA, Misiewicz JJ, Baron JH: Eradication of *Helicobacter pylori* in patients with duodenal ulcer lowers basal and peak acid outputs to gastrin releasing peptide and pentagastrin. *Gut* 38:663, 1996.

Isenberg JI: Impaired proximal duodenal mucosal bicarbonate secretion in patients with duodenal ulcer. *N Engl J Med* 316:374, 1987.

Laine L: Approaches to nonsteroidal anti-inflammatory drug use in the high-risk patient. *Gastroenterology* 120:594, 2001.

Mertz HR, Walsh JH: Peptic ulcer pathophysiology. *Med Clin North Am* 75:799, 1991.

Munnangi S, Sonnenberg A: Time trends of physician visits and treatment patterns of peptic ulcer disease in the United States. *Arch Intern Med* 157:1489, 1997.

NIH Consensus Development Panel: *Helicobacter pylori* in peptic ulcer disease. *JAMA* 272:65, 1994.

Peek RM Jr., Blaser MJ: Pathophysiology of *Helicobacter pylori*-induced gastritis and peptic ulcer disease. *Am J Med* 102:200, 1997.

Peterson WL, Graham DY: *Helicobacter pylori*, in Feldman M (ed): *Sleisenger and Fordtran's Gastrointestinal and Liver Disease*, 7th ed. Philadelphia: Saunders, 2002, p 732.

Diagnosis and Treatment

American Society for Gastrointestinal Endoscopy: An annotated algorithmic approach to upper gastrointestinal bleeding. *Gastrointest Endosc* 53:853, 2001.

Blatchford O, Murray WR: A risk score to predict need for treatment for upper gastrointestinal hemorrhage. *Lancet* 356:1318, 2000.

Boey J, Wong J: Perforated duodenal ulcers. *World J Surg* 11:319, 1987.

Chak A, Cooper GS, Lloyd LE, et al: Effectiveness of endoscopy in patients admitted to the intensive care unit with upper GI hemorrhage. *Gastrointest Endosc* 53:6, 2001.

Cook DJ, Guyatt GH, Salena BJ: Endoscopic therapy for acute nonvariceal upper gastrointestinal hemorrhage: A meta-analysis. *Gastroenterology* 102:139, 1992.

Cowles RA, Mulholland MW: Surgical management of peptic ulcer disease in the *Helicobacter* era—management of bleeding peptic ulcer. *Surg Laparosc Endosc Percutan Tech* 11:1, 2001.

Dayton MT: Vagotomy and drainage, in Zuidema GD, Yeo CJ (eds): *Shackelford's Surgery of the Alimentary Tract*, 5th ed., Vol. II. Philadelphia: Saunders, 2002, p 117.

Del Valle J, Chey WD, Scheiman JM: Acid peptic disorders, in Yamada T et al (eds): *Textbook of Gastroenterology*, 4th ed. Philadelphia: Lippincott Williams & Wilkins, 2003, p 1321.

Dempsey DT: Peptic ulcer disease: Obstruction, in Bland KI (ed): *The Practice of General Surgery*. Philadelphia: Saunders, 2001.

Donahue PE: Parietal cell vagotomy versus vagotomy-antrectomy: Ulcer surgery in the modern era. *World J Surg* 24:264, 2000.

Graham DY, Agrawal NM, Campbell DR, Haber MM, Collis C, et al: Ulcer prevention in long-term users of nonsteroidal anti-inflammatory drugs: Results of a double-blind, randomized, multicenter, active- and placebo-controlled study of misoprostol vs. lansoprazole. *Arch Intern Med* 162:169, 2002.

Graham DY, Lew GM, Klein PD, et al: Effect of treatment of *Helicobacter pylori* infection on the long-term recurrence of gastric or duodenal ulcer: A randomized controlled study. *Ann Intern Med* 116:705, 1992.

Graham DY, Rakel RE, Fendrick AM, et al: Recognizing peptic ulcer disease—keys to clinical and laboratory diagnosis. *Postgrad Med* 105:113, 1999.

Kate V, Ananthakrishnan N, Badrinath S: Effect of *Helicobacter pylori* eradication on the ulcer recurrence rate after simple closure of perforated duodenal ulcer: Retrospective and prospective randomized controlled studies. *Br J Surg* 88:1054, 2001.

Kauffman GL: Duodenal ulcer disease: Treatment by surgery, antibiotics, or both. *Adv Surg* 34:121, 2000.

Laine L, Peterson WL: Bleeding peptic ulcer. *N Engl J Med* 331:717, 1994.

Lau JYW, Sung JJY, Lam Y-H, et al: Endoscopic retreatment compared with surgery in patients with recurrent bleeding after initial endoscopic control of bleeding ulcers. *N Engl J Med* 340:751, 1999.

Lau JYW, Sung JJY, Lee KKC, et al: Effect of intravenous omeprazole on recurrent bleeding after endoscopic treatment of bleeding peptic ulcers. *N Engl J Med* 343:310, 2000.

Lin HJ, Lo WC, Lee FY, Perng CL, Tseng GY: A prospective randomized comparative trial showing that omeprazole prevents rebleeding in patients with bleeding peptic ulcer after successful endoscopic therapy. *Arch Intern Med* 158:54, 1998.

Liu CC, Lee CL, Chan CC, et al: Maintenance treatment is not necessary after *Helicobacter pylori* eradication and healing of bleeding peptic ulcer: A 5-year prospective, randomized, controlled study. *Arch Intern Med* 163:2020, 2003.

Millat B, Fingerhut A, Borie F: Surgical treatment of complicated duodenal ulcers: Controlled trials. *World J Surg* 24:299, 2000.

Moesinger RC, Yeo CJ: Duodenal ulcer, in Zuidema GD, Yeo CJ (eds): *Shackelford's Surgery of the Alimentary Tract*, 5th ed., Vol. II. Philadelphia: Saunders, 2002, p 57.

Murayama KM, Miller TA: Gastric ulcer, in Zuidema GD, Yeo CJ (eds): *Shackelford's Surgery of the Alimentary Tract*, 5th ed., Vol. II. Philadelphia: Saunders, 2002, p 74.

Rege RV, Jones DB: Current role of surgery in peptic ulcer disease, in Feldman M (ed): *Sleisenger and Fordtran's Gastrointestinal and Liver Disease*, 7th ed. Philadelphia: Saunders, 2002, p 797.

Schirmer B: Current status of proximal gastric vagotomy. *Ann Surg* 209:131, 1989.

Seymour NE, Andersen DK: Surgery for peptic ulcer disease and postgastrectomy syndromes, in Yamada T et al (eds): *Textbook of Gastroenterology*, 4th ed. Philadelphia: Lippincott Williams & Wilkins, 2003, p 1441.

Spechler SJ: Peptic ulcer disease and its complications, in Feldman M (ed): *Sleisenger and Fordtran's Gastrointestinal and Liver Disease*, 7th ed. Philadelphia: Saunders, 2002, p 747.

Talley NJ: Therapeutic options in nonulcer dyspepsia. *J Clin Gastroenterol* 32:286, 2001.

Thompson JC: The role of surgery in peptic ulcer. *N Engl J Med* 307:550, 1992.

Turner DJ, Mulholland MW: Gastric resection and reconstruction, in Zuidema GD, Yeo CJ (eds): *Shackelford's Surgery of the Alimentary Tract*, 5th ed., Vol. II. Philadelphia: Saunders, 2002, p 130.

Walsh JH, Peterson WL: The treatment of helicobacter pylori infection in the management of peptic ulcer disease. *N Engl J Med* 333:984, 1995.

Walsh RM, Anain P, Geisinger M, et al: Role of angiography and embolization for massive gastroduodenal hemorrhage. *J Gastrointest Surg* 3:61, 1999.

Wolfe MM, Sachs G: Acid suppression: Optimizing therapy for gastroduodenal ulcer healing, gastroesophageal reflux disease, and stress-related erosive syndrome. *Gastroenterology* 118:S9, 2000 (February supplement).

Zollinger-Ellison Syndrome

Del Valle J, Scheiman JM: Zollinger-Ellison syndrome, in Yamada T et al (eds): *Textbook of Gastroenterology*, 4th ed. Philadelphia: Lippincott Williams & Wilkins, 2003, p 1377.

Dolan JP, Norton JA: Zollinger-Ellison syndrome, in Zuidema GD, Yeo CJ (eds): *Shackelford's Surgery of the Alimentary Tract*, 5th ed., Vol. II. Philadelphia: Saunders, 2002, p 96.

Norton JA: Advances in the management of Zollinger-Ellison syndrome. *Adv Surg* 27:129, 1994.

Norton JA, Fraker DL, Alexander HR, et al: Surgery to cure the Zollinger-Ellison syndrome. *N Engl J Med* 341:635, 1999.

Pisegna JR: Zollinger-Ellison syndrome and other hypersecretory states, in Feldman M (ed): *Sleisenger and Fordtran's Gastrointestinal and Liver Disease*, 7th ed. Philadelphia: Saunders, 2002, p 782.

Wells SA Jr.: Surgery for the Zollinger-Ellison syndrome. *N Engl J Med* 341:689, 1999.

Gastritis and Stress Ulcer

Beejay U, Wolfe MM: Acute gastrointestinal bleeding in the intensive care unit. *Gastrointest Clin North Am* 29:309, 2000.

Cheung LY: Treatment of established stress ulcer disease. *World J Surg* 5:235, 1981.

Correa P: Chronic gastritis: A clinico-pathological classification. *Am J Gastroenterol* 83:504, 1988.

Genta RM: Gastritis and gastropathy, in Yamada T et al (eds): *Textbook of Gastroenterology*, 4th ed. Philadelphia: Lippincott Williams & Wilkins, 2003, p 1394.

Goldman H: Gastritis, in Ming C-J, Goldman H (eds): *Pathology of the Gastrointestinal Tract*, 2nd ed. Baltimore: Williams & Wilkins, 1998, p 525.

Goldman H: Stress ulcer and chronic peptic ulcer disease, in Ming C-J, Goldman H (eds): *Pathology of the Gastrointestinal Tract*, 2nd ed. Baltimore: Williams & Wilkins, 1998, p 559.

Hinder RA: Duodenal switch—a new form of pancreaticobiliary diversion. *Surg Clin North Am* 72:487, 1992.

Klingler PJ, Perdikis G, Wilson P, Hinder RA: Indications, technical modalities and results of the duodenal switch operation for pathologic duodenogastric reflux. *Hepatogastroenterology* 46:97, 1999.

Miller TA, Tornwall MS, Moody FG: Stress erosive gastritis. *Curr Probl Surg* 28:459, 1991.

Ritchie WP: Acute gastric mucosal damage produced by bile salts, acid, and ischemia. *Gastroenterology* 68:699, 1975.

Ritchie WP: Alkaline reflux gastritis: Late results of a controlled trial of diagnosis and treatment. *Ann Surg* 203:537, 1985.

Sung JJ, Lin SR, Ching JY, et al: Atrophy and intestinal metaplasia one year after cure of *H. pylori* infection: A prospective, randomized study. *Gastroenterology* 119:7, 2000.

Malignant Neoplasms of the Stomach

American Cancer Society: Cancer Facts and Figures 2003. (www.cancer.org)

Gunderson LL, Donohue JH, Burch PA: Stomach, in Abeloff M et al (eds): *Clinical Oncology*, 2nd ed. New York: Churchill Livingstone, 2000, p 1545.

Hermanek P, Huttler RVP, Sobin LH, et al (eds): *TNM Atlas*, 4th ed. Berlin: Springer, 1997.

Kalmar K, Cseke L, Zambo K, Horvath OP: Comparison of quality of life and nutritional parameters after total gastrectomy and a new type of pouch construction with simple Roux-en-Y reconstruction: Preliminary results of a prospective, randomized, controlled study. *Dig Dis Sci* 46:1791, 2001.

Karpeh MS Jr.: Tumors of the stomach, in Zuidema GD, Yeo CJ (eds): *Shackelford's Surgery of the Alimentary Tract*, 5th ed., Vol. II. Philadelphia: Saunders, 2002, p 86.

Koh TJ, Wang TC: Tumors of the stomach, in Feldman M (ed): *Sleisenger and Fordtran's Gastrointestinal and Liver Disease*, 7th ed. Philadelphia: Saunders, 2002, p 829.

Leung WK, Ng EKW, Sung JJY: Tumors of the stomach, in Yamada T et al (eds): *Textbook of Gastroenterology,* 4th ed. Philadelphia: Lippincott Williams & Wilkins, 2003, p 1416.

Parker SL, Tong T, Bolden S, et al: Cancer statistics 1997. *CA Cancer J Clin* 47:5, 1997.

Adenocarcinoma

Aarnio M, Salovaara R, Aaltonen L, et al: Features of gastric cancer in hereditary non-polyposis colorectal cancer syndrome. *Int J Cancer* 74:551, 1997.

Antonioli DA: Precursors of gastric carcinoma: A critical review with a brief description of early (curable) gastric cancer. *Hum Pathol* 25:994, 1994.

Bonenkamp JJ, Hermans J, Sasako M, van de Velde CJH: Extended lymph node dissection for gastric cancer. *N Engl J Med* 340:908, 1999.

Botterweck A, van den Brandt P, Goldbohm R: Vitamins, carotenoids, dietary fiber, and the risk of gastric carcinoma: Results from a prospective study after 6.3 years of follow-up. *Cancer* 88:737, 2000.

Bozzetti F, Marubini E, Bonfanti G, et al: Subtotal versus total gastrectomy for gastric cancer: Five-year survival rates in a multicenter randomized Italian trial. Italian Gastrointestinal Tumor Study Group. *Ann Surg* 230:170, 1999.

Csendes A, Burdiles P, Rojas J, et al: A prospective randomized study comparing D2 total gastrectomy versus D2 total gastrectomy plus splenectomy in 187 patients with gastric carcinoma. *Surgery* 131:401, 2002.

Cuschieri A, Fayers P, Fielding J, et al: Postoperative morbidity and mortality after D1 and D2 resections for gastric cancer: Preliminary results of the MRC randomized controlled surgical trial. *Lancet* 347:995, 1996.

Douglass HO Jr.: Gastric cancer, in Ritchie WP, Steele G, Dean RH (eds): *General Surgery.* Philadelphia: Lippincott, 1995, p 133.

Eslick G, Lim L, Byles J, et al: Association of *Helicobacter pylori* infection with gastric carcinoma: A meta-analysis. *Am J Gastroenterol* 94:2373, 1999.

EUROGAST Study Group: An international association between *Helicobacter pylori* infection and gastric cancer. *Lancet* 341:1359, 1993.

Fenoglio-Preiser CM, Noffsinger AE, Belli J, Stemmermann GN: Pathologic and phenotypic features of gastric cancer. *Semin Oncol* 23:292, 1996.

Hansson LE, Nyren O, et al: The risk of stomach cancer in patients with gastric or duodenal ulcer disease. *N Engl J Med* 335:242, 1996.

Harrison LE, Karpeh MS, Brennan MF: Proximal gastric cancers resected via a transabdominal only approach. Results and comparisons to distal adenocarcinoma of the stomach. *Ann Surg* 225:678, 1997.

Hartgrink HH, Bonenkamp HJ, van de Velde CJH: Influence of surgery on outcomes in gastric cancer. *Surg Oncol Clin North Am* 9:97, 2000.

Kitamura K, Nishida S, Ichikawa D, et al: No survival benefit from combined pancreaticosplenectomy and total gastrectomy for gastric cancer. *Br J Surg* 86:119, 1999.

Leung W, Kim J, Kim J, et al: Microsatellite instability in gastric intestinal metaplasia in patients with and without gastric cancer. *Am J Pathol* 156:537, 2000.

Lichtenstein P, Holm N, Verkasalo P, et al: Environmental and heritable factors in the causation of cancer: Analyses of cohorts of twins from Sweden, Denmark, and Finland. *N Engl J Med* 343:78, 2000.

Locke GR, Talley NJ, et al: Changes in the site- and histology-specific incidence of gastric cancer during a 50-year period. *Gastroenterology* 109:1750, 1995.

Macdonald JS, Schnall SF: Adjuvant treatment of gastric cancer. *World J Surg* 19:221, 1995.

Macdonald JS, Smalley SR, Benedetti J, et al: Chemoradiotherapy after surgery compared with surgery alone for adenocarcinoma of the stomach or gastroesophageal junction. *N Engl J Med* 345:725, 2001.

Maruyama K, Sasako M, et al: Surgical treatment for gastric cancer: The Japanese approach. *Semin Oncol* 23:360, 1996.

McColl KE, et al: *Helicobacter pylori* gastritis and gastric acid secretory function—an integrated approach, in Hunt RH, Tytgat GN (eds): *Basic Mechanisms to Clinical Cure.* Boston: Kluwer, 1996.

Meyer HJ, Jahne J: Lymph node dissection for gastric cancer. *Semin Surg Oncol* 17:117, 1999.

Ming S-C, Hirota T: Malignant epithelial tumors of the stomach, in Ming C-J, Goldman H (eds): *Pathology of the Gastrointestinal Tract,* 2nd ed. Baltimore: Williams & Wilkins, 1998, p 607.

Neugut AI, Hayek M, Howe G: Epidemiology of gastric cancer. *Semin Oncol* 23:281, 1996.

Noguchi M, Miyazaki I: Prognostic significance and surgical management of lymph node metastases in gastric cancer. *Br J Surg* 83:156, 1996.

Offerhaus GJ, Tersmette AC, Huibregtse K, et al: Mortality caused by stomach cancer after remote partial gastrectomy for benign conditions: 40 years of follow-up of an Amsterdam cohort of 2633 postgastrectomy patients. *Gut* 29:1588, 1988.

Ranaldi R, Santinelli A, et al: Long-term follow-up in early gastric cancer: Evaluation of prognostic factors. *J Pathol* 177:343, 1995.

Robertson CS, Chung SC, et al: A prospective randomized trial comparing R1 subtotal gastrectomy with R3 total gastrectomy for antral cancer. *Ann Surg* 220:176, 1994.

Rugge M, Cassaro M, et al: *Helicobacter pylori* in promotion of gastric carcinogenesis. *Dig Dis Sci* 41:950, 1996.

Schneider B, Gulley M, Eagan P, et al: Loss of p16/CDKN2A tumor suppressor protein in gastric adenocarcinoma is associated with Epstein-Barr virus and anatomic location in the body of the stomach. *Hum Pathol* 31:45, 2000.

Shimizu S, Tada M, Kawai K: Early gastric cancer: Its surveillance and natural course. *Endoscopy* 27:27, 1995.

Solcia E, Fiocca R, et al: Intestinal and diffuse gastric cancers arise in a different background of *Helicobacter pylori* gastritis through different gene involvement. *Am J Surg Pathol* 20:S8, 1996.

Stemmerman G, Heffelfinger SC, et al: The molecular biology of esophageal and gastric cancer and their precursors: Oncogenes, tumor suppressor genes, and growth factors. *Hum Pathol* 25:968, 1994.

World Health Organization. (www.who.int/cancer/en/)

Yamao T, Shirao K, et al: Risk factors for lymph node metastasis from intramucosal gastric carcinoma. *Cancer* 77:602, 1996.

Lymphoma

Fischbach W, Dragosics B, Kolve-Goebeler ME, Ohmann C, Greiner A, et al: Primary gastric B-cell lymphoma: Results of a prospective multicenter study. The German-Austrian Gastrointestinal Lymphoma Study Group. [erratum appears in *Gastroenterology* 119:1809, 2000.] *Gastroenterology* 119:1191, 2000.

Hsu C, Chen CL, Chen LT, et al: Comparison of MALT and non-MALT primary large cell lymphoma of the stomach: Does histologic evidence of MALT affect chemotherapy response? *Cancer* 91:49, 2001.

Isaacson PG: Lymphoproliferative disorders of the gastrointestinal tract, in Ming C-J, Goldman H (eds): *Pathology of the Gastrointestinal Tract,* 2nd ed. Baltimore: Williams & Wilkins, 1998, p 339.

Liu H, Ye H, Ruskone-Fourmestraux A, De Jong D, et al: T(11;18) is a marker for all stage gastric MALT lymphomas that will not respond to *H. pylori* eradication. *Gastroenterology* 122:1286, 2002.

Montalban C, Santon A, Boixeda D, Bellas C: Regression of gastric high grade mucosa associated lymphoid tissue (MALT) lymphoma after *Helicobacter pylori* eradication. *Gut* 49:584, 2001.

Ranaldi R, Goteri G, Baccarini MG, Mannello B, Bearzi I: A clinicopathological study of 152 surgically treated primary gastric lymphomas with survival analysis of 109 high grade tumours. *J Clin Pathol.* 55:346, 2002.

Stolte M, Bayerdorffer E, Morgner A, et al: *Helicobacter* and gastric MALT lymphoma. *Gut* 50(Suppl 3):III19, 2002.

Vaillant JC, Ruskone-Fourmestraux A, Aegerter P, et al: Management and long-term results of surgery for localized gastric lymphoma. *Am J Surg* 179:216, 2000.

Gastrointestinal Stromal Tumors

Appelman HD: Mesenchymal tumors of the gastrointestinal tract, in Ming C-J, Goldman H (eds): *Pathology of the Gastrointestinal Tract,* 2nd ed. Baltimore: Williams & Wilkins, 1998, p 361.

Burkill GJ, Badran M, Al-Muderis O, et al: Malignant gastrointestinal stromal tumor: Distribution, imaging features, and pattern of metastatic spread. *Radiology* 226:527, 2003.

Demetri GD: Targeting c-kit mutations in solid tumors: Scientific rationale and novel therapeutic options. *Semin Oncol* 28(5 Suppl 17):19, 2001.

Demetri GD, von Mehren M, Blanke CD, et al: Efficacy and safety of imatinib mesylate in advanced gastrointestinal stromal tumors. *N Engl J Med* 347:472, 2002.

Dempsey DT: Laparoscopic resection of gastric leiomyosarcoma. *J Laparoendoscopic Surg* 7:357, 1997.

Eisenberg BL, von Mehren M: Pharmacotherapy of gastrointestinal stromal tumours. *Expert Opin Pharmacother* 4:869, 2003.

Miettinen M, El-Rifai W, H L Sobin L, Lasota J: Evaluation of malignancy and prognosis of gastrointestinal stromal tumors: A review. *Hum Pathol* 33:478, 2002.

Toquet C, Le Neel JC, Guillou L, et al: Elevated (> or = 10%) MIB-1 proliferative index correlates with poor outcome in gastric stromal tumor patients: A study of 35 cases. *Dig Dis Sci* 47:2247, 2002.

Carcinoid

Granberg D, Wilander E, Stridsberg M, et al: Clinical symptoms, hormone profiles, treatment, and prognosis in patients with gastric carcinoids. *Gut* 43:223, 1998.

Kirshbom PM, Kherani AR, Onaitis MW, et al: Foregut carcinoids: A clinical and biochemical analysis. *Surgery* 126:1105, 1999.

Modlin IM, Lye KD, Kidd M: A 5-decade analysis of 13,715 carcinoid tumors. *Cancer* 97:934, 2003.

Solcia E, Capella C, Fiocca R, et al: Disorders of the endocrine system, in Ming C-J, Goldman H (eds): *Pathology of the Gastrointestinal Tract,* 2nd ed. Baltimore: Williams & Wilkins, 1998, p 295.

Tomassetti P, Migliori M, Caletti GC, et al: Treatment of type II gastric carcinoid tumors with somatostatin analogues. *N Engl J Med* 343:551, 2000.

Benign Gastric Neoplasms

Abraham SC, Nobukawa B, Giardiello FM, Hamilton SR, Wu TT: Fundic gland polyps in familial adenomatous polyposis: Neoplasms with frequent somatic adenomatous polyposis coli gene alterations. *Am J Pathol* 157:747, 2000.

Borch K, Skarsgard J, Franzen L, Mardh S, Rehfeld JF: Benign gastric polyps: Morphological and functional origin. *Dig Dis Sci* 48:1292, 2003.

Ming S-C: Benign epithelial polyps of the stomach, in Ming C-J, Goldman H (eds): *Pathology of the Gastrointestinal Tract,* 2nd ed. Baltimore: Williams & Wilkins, 1998, p 587.

Gastric Motility Disorders

Behrns KE, Sarr MG: Diagnosis and management of gastric emptying disorders. *Adv Surg* 27:233, 1994.

Chial HJ, Camilleri M: Motility disorders of the stomach and small intestine, in Friedman SL, McQuaid KR, Grendell JH (eds): *Current Diagnosis and Treatment in Gastroenterology,* 2nd ed. New York: McGraw-Hill, 2003, p 355.

Hornbuckle K, Barnett JL: The diagnosis and work-up of the patient with gastroparesis. *J Clin Gastroenterol* 30:117, 2001.

Parkman HP, Fisher RS: Disorders of gastric emptying, in Yamada T et al (ed): *Textbook of Gastroenterology,* 4th ed. Philadelphia: Lippincott Williams & Wilkins, 2003, p 1292.

Rabine JC, Barnett JL: Management of the patient with gastroparesis. *J Clin Gastroenterol* 32:11, 2001.

Schirmer BD: Mechanical and motility disorders of the stomach and duodenum, in Zuidema GD, Yeo CJ (eds): *Shackelford's Surgery of the Alimentary Tract,* 5th ed., Vol. II. Philadelphia: Saunders, 2002, p 178.

Tack J, Piessevaux H, Coulie B, Caenepeel P, Janssens J: Role of impaired gastric accommodation to a meal in functional dyspepsia. *Gastroenterology* 115:1346, 1998.

Miscellaneous Lesions of the Stomach

Burak KW, Lee SS, Beck PL: Portal hypertensive gastropathy and gastric antral vascular ectasia (GAVE) syndrome. *Gut* 49:866, 2001.

Chasse E, Buggenhout A, Zalcman M, et al: Gastric diverticulum simulating a left adrenal tumor. *Surgery* 133:447, 2003.

DeBakey M, Ochsner A: Bezoars and concretions: A comprehensive review of the literature with an analysis of 303 collected cases and a presentation of 8 additional cases. Part I. *Surgery* 4:934, 1938.

DeBakey M, Ochsner A: Bezoars and concretions: A comprehensive review of the literature with an analysis of 303 collected cases and a presentation of 8 additional cases. Part II. *Surgery* 5:132, 1939.

Goldman H: Mucosal hypertrophy and hyperplasia of the stomach, in Ming C-J, Goldman H (eds): *Pathology of the Gastrointestinal Tract,* 2nd ed. Baltimore: Williams & Wilkins, 1998, p 577.

Huang SP, Wang HP, Lee YC, et al: Endoscopic hemoclip placement and epinephrine injection for Mallory-Weiss syndrome with active bleeding. *Gastrointest Endosc* 55:842, 2002.

Lee EL, Feldman M: Gastritis and other gastropathies, in Feldman M (ed): *Sleisenger and Fordtran's Gastrointestinal and Liver Disease,* 7th ed. Philadelphia: Saunders, 2002, p 810.

Lee J: Bezoars and foreign bodies of the stomach. *Gastrointest Clin North Am* 6:605, 1996.

Park CH, Sohn YH, Lee WS, et al: The usefulness of endoscopic hemoclipping for bleeding Dieulafoy lesions. *Endoscopy* 35:388, 2003.

Rabine JC, Nostrant TT: Miscellaneous diseases of the stomach, in Yamada T et al (eds): *Textbook of Gastroenterology,* 4th ed. Philadelphia: Lippincott Williams & Wilkins, 2003, p 1455.

Schmulewitz N, Baillie J: Dieulafoy lesions: A review of 6 years of experience at a tertiary referral center. *Am J Gastroenterol* 96:1688, 2001.

Teague WJ, Ackroyd R, Watson DI, Devitt PG: Changing patterns in the management of gastric volvulus over 14 years. *Br J Surg* 87:358, 2000.

Gastrostomy

Duh Q-Y, Senokozlieff-Englehart AL, Choe YS, et al: Laparoscopic gastrostomy and jejunostomy—safety and cost with local vs. general anesthesia. *Arch Surg* 134:151, 1999.

Rosser JC, Rodas EB, Blancaflor J, et al: A simplified technique for laparoscopic jejunostomy and gastrostomy tube placement. *Am J Surg* 177:61, 1999.

Safadi BY, Marks JM, Ponsky JL: Percutaneous endoscopic gastrostomy. *Gastrointest Clin North Am* 8:551, 1998.

Tatum RP, Joehl RJ: Intubation of the stomach and small intestine, in Zuidema GD, Yeo CJ (eds): *Shackelford's Surgery of the Alimentary Tract,* 5th ed., Vol. II. Philadelphia: Saunders, 2002, p 46.

Postgastrectomy Syndromes

Aronow JS, Matthews JB, Garcia-Aguilar J, et al: Isoperistaltic jejunal interposition for intractable postgastrectomy alkaline reflux gastritis. *J Am Coll Surg* 180:648, 1995.

Carvajal SH, Mulvihill SJ: Postgastrectomy syndromes: Dumping and diarrhea. *Gastrointest Clin North Am* 23:261, 1994.

Delcore R, Cheung LY: Surgical options in postgastrectomy syndromes. *Surg Clin North Am* 71:57, 1991.

Dempsey DT: Reoperative gastric surgery and postgastrectomy syndromes, in Zuidema GD, Yeo CJ (eds): *Shackelford's Surgery of the Alimentary Tract,* 5th ed., Vol. II. Philadelphia: Saunders, 2002, p 161.

Eagon JC, Miedema BW, Kelly KA: Postgastrectomy syndromes. *Surg Clin North Am* 72:445, 1992.

Eckhauser FE, Conrad M, Knol JA, et al: Safety and long-term durability of completion gastrectomy in 81 patients with postsurgical gastroparesis syndrome. *Am Surg* 64:711, 1998.

Forster-Barthell AW, Murr MM, Nitecki S, et al: Near-total completion gastrectomy for severe postvagotomy gastric stasis: Analysis of early and long-term results in 62 patients. *J Gastrointest Surg* 3:15, 1999.

Hasler WL, Soudah HC, Owyang C: Mechanisms by which octreotide ameliorates symptoms in the dumping syndrome. *J Pharmacol Exp Ther* 277:1359, 1996.

Hocking MP, Vogel SB, Sninsky CA: Human gastric myoelectric activity and gastric emptying following gastric surgery and with pacing. *Gastroenterology* 103:1811, 1992.

Hopman WP, Wolberink RG, Lamers CB, Van Tongeren JH: Treatment of the dumping syndrome with the somatostatin analogue SMS 201-995. *Ann Surg* 207:155, 1988.

Lamers CB, Bijlstra AM, Harris AG: Octreotide, a long-acting somatostatin analog, in the management of postoperative dumping syndrome. An update. *Dig Dis Sci* 38:359, 1993.

Malagelada JR, Phillips SF, Shorter RG, et al: Postoperative reflux gastritis: Pathophysiology and long-term outcome after Roux-en-Y diversion. *Ann Int Med* 103:178, 1985.

Miedema BW, Kelly KA: The Roux operation for postgastrectomy syndromes. *Am J Surg* 161:256, 1991.

Miholic J, Reilmann L, Meyer HJ, et al: Extracellular space, blood volume, and the early dumping syndrome after total gastrectomy. *Gastroenterology* 99:923, 1990.

Nilas L, Christiansen C, Christiansen J: Regulation of vitamin D and calcium metabolism after gastrectomy. *Gut* 26:252, 1985.

Raimes SA, Smirniotis V, Wheldon EJ, et al: Postvagotomy diarrhea put into perspective. *Lancet* 2:851, 1986.

Richards WO, Geer R, O'Dorisio TM, et al: Octreotide acetate induces fasting small bowel motility in patients with dumping syndrome. *J Surg Res* 49:483, 1990.

Ritchie WP Jr.: Alkaline reflux gastritis. An objective assessment of its diagnosis and treatment. *Ann Surg* 192:288, 1980.

Tovey FI, Hall ML, Ell PJ, Hobsley M: A review of postgastrectomy bone disease. *J Gastroenterol Hepatol* 7:639, 1992.

Van der Milje HCJ, Kleibeuker JH, Limburg AJ, et al: Manometric and scintigraphic studies of the relation between motility disturbances in the Roux limb and the Roux-en-Y syndrome. *Am J Surg* 166:11, 1993.

Vecht J, Masclee AA, Lamers CB: The dumping syndrome. Current insights into pathophysiology, diagnosis and treatment. *Scand J Gastro* (Suppl) 223:21, 1997.

Vogel SB, Drane WE, Woodward ER: Clinical and radionuclide evaluation of bile diversion by Braun enteroenterostomy: Prevention and treatment of alkaline reflux gastritis. An alternative to Roux-en-Y diversion. *Ann Surg* 219:458, 1994.

Xynos E, Vassilakis JS, Fountos A, et al: Enterogastric reflux after various types of antiulcer gastric surgery: Quantitation by 99mTC-HIDA scintigraphy. *Gastroenterology* 101:991, 1991.

Laparoscopic Gastric Operations

Dubois F: New surgical strategy for gastroduodenal ulcer: Laparoscopic approach. *World J Surg* 24:270, 2000.

Farrell TM, Hunter JG: Laparoscopic surgery of the stomach and duodenum, in Zuidema GD, Yeo CJ (eds): *Shackelford's Surgery of the Alimentary Tract*, 5th ed., Vol. II. Philadelphia: Saunders, 2002, p 202.

Katkhouda N, Heimbucher J, Mouiel J: Laparoscopic posterior vagotomy and anterior seromyotomy. *Endosc Surg* 2:95, 1994.

CHAPTER 26

The Surgical Management of Obesity

Philip R. Schauer and Bruce D. Schirmer

THE DISEASE OF OBESITY

Obesity is a serious disease that carries substantial morbidity and mortality and has mixed genetic and environmental etiologies. Obesity is defined as the accumulation of excess body fat that leads to pathology. Severity is based on the degree of excess body fat, which is commonly assessed using the body mass index [BMI = weight (kg)/height (m)^2], which correlates body weight with height. Patients are classified as overweight, obese, or severely obese (sometimes referred to as morbidly obese) (Table 26-1). Obesity may also be defined as body weight that exceeds ideal body weight by 20%, with ideal body weight determined by population studies. Morbidly obese individuals generally exceed ideal body weight by 100 lb or more, or are 100% over ideal body weight. In 1991, the National Institutes of Health defined morbid obesity as a BMI of 35 kg/m^2 or greater with severe obesity-related comorbidity, or BMI of 40 kg/m^2 or greater without comorbidity.[1] *Superobesity* is a term sometimes used to define individuals who have a body weight exceeding ideal body weight by 225% or more, or a BMI of 50 kg/m^2 or greater.

Epidemiology and Risk Factors

Morbid obesity is reaching epidemic proportions in the United States. Since 1960, surveys of the prevalence of obesity have been conducted every decade by the National Center for Health Statistics. Twenty-five percent of adult Americans were overweight in 1980 compared to 34% in 1990. Over 58 million adult Americans (one third of the adult population) are overweight.[1] Approximately 4 million Americans have a BMI between 35 and 40 kg/m^2, and an additional 4 million have a BMI exceeding 40 kg/m^2. Despite the expenditure of over $30 billion annually on weight loss products, the prevalence of obesity is increasing. Obesity is most common in minorities, low-income groups, and women. Nearly half of African-American, Mexican-American, and Native American women are overweight.[2]

Genetics plays an important role in the development of obesity. While children of parents of normal weight have a 10% chance of becoming obese, the children of two obese parents have an 80 to 90% chance of developing obesity by adulthood. The weight of adopted children correlates strongly with the weight of their birth parents. Furthermore, concordance rates for obesity in monozygotic twins are doubled compared to those who are overweight to lesser degrees.[3]

Diet and culture are important factors as well; these environmental factors contribute significantly to the epidemic of obesity in the United States. The excess weight often limits physical activity in the morbidly obese, and the sedentary lifestyle and reduction in energy expenditure further hamper weight control.

Table 26-1
Assessing Disease Risk Using Body Mass Index and Waist Size

Category	BMI	Men (<40 in.) Women (<35 in.)	Men (>40 in.) Women (>35 in.)
Underweight	<18.5	−	−
Normal	18.5–24.9	−	−
Overweight	25.0–29.9	+	+
Obesity	^{3}30		
Class I	30.0–34.9	+	++
Class II	35.0–39.9	++	++
Class III (extreme obesity)	^{3}40	+++	

Etiology, Pathogenesis, and Natural History

An excess of caloric intake in relation to caloric expenditure results in deposition of fat or adipose tissue. However, this simplistic model does not adequately explain the etiology of morbid obesity; its causes are multiple and poorly understood. Obesity may be attributed to excessive caloric intake, inefficient utilization of calories, decreased energy expenditure from reduced physical or metabolic activity, a reduction in the thermogenic response to meals, an abnormally high set-point for body weight, or a decrease in the loss of heat energy. The Pima Indians have been described as having greater energy efficiency, and this may explain the tendency toward obesity in this group.[4]

Adipose tissue is deposited in subcutaneous tissues and the intra-abdominal compartment. Males have a greater tendency for abdominal fat distribution, while females typically have more gluteal or peripheral fat deposition. The size of adipose cells tends to parallel this gender pattern; larger fat cells are in the abdomen in males and in the gluteal area in females. Weight gain results from increase in both adipose cell size and number.[5]

Clinical Presentation

The morbidly obese patient often presents with chronic weight-related problems such as migraine headaches; back and lower extremity joint pain from degenerative joint disease; venous stasis ulcers; dyspnea on exertion; biliary colic; stress urinary incontinence; dysmenorrhea; infertility; gastroesophageal reflux; and inguinal, umbilical, and incisional hernias.[6] Those with central or android distribution of fat are more likely to develop complications related to obesity compared to those with peripheral or gynecoid fat distribution. There are a vast number of obesity-related comorbidities (see section on "Related Diagnoses").

The morbidly obese almost uniformly endure discrimination, prejudice, ridicule, and disrespectful treatment from the public. They are commonly viewed as lazy, ugly, and unmotivated, and are often considered to be to blame for their condition, which is unfairly attributed to gluttony and a lack of willpower. Consequently, the stigma of morbid obesity has a major impact on social function and emotional support.

Differential Diagnosis and Related Diagnoses

A few endocrine diseases are associated with obesity, including hypothyroidism, Cushing's disease, and adult-onset diabetes mellitus. However, patients who seek medical or surgical treatment for morbid obesity rarely have an endocrine etiology of their obesity. The combination of central obesity, glucose intolerance, dyslipidemia, and hypertension is known as syndrome X. Those with syndrome X have an elevated risk of developing coronary artery disease and

diabetes mellitus.[7] Once diagnosed with syndrome X, an individual should initiate dietary changes, exercise, and weight loss; medical intervention may be necessary as well.

Obesity has a profound effect on overall health and life expectancy. The morbidly obese are predisposed to developing serious weight-related comorbidities, including hypertension, coronary artery disease, adult-onset diabetes mellitus, sleep apnea and/or obesity hypoventilation syndrome (Pickwickian syndrome), deep venous thrombosis, pulmonary embolism, hypercoagulability, hyperlipidemia, and depression, among others. Mortality rates from cancers of the uterus, ovary, breast, colon, rectum, and prostate are increased in the morbidly obese.[8] Obesity is now considered to be the second leading cause of preventable death behind cigarette smoking.

Prognosis

The incidence of morbidity and mortality is directly related to the degree of obesity.[9] In a study with 12-year follow-up, mortality rates for those weighing 50% over average weight were doubled. Mortality and morbidity is largely attributable to the comorbidities of obesity. A study carried out by the Veterans Administration demonstrated a twelvefold increase in mortality among 200 morbidly obese men aged 25 to 34 years, and a sixfold increase among morbidly obese men aged 35 to 44 years. Average weight was 316 lb and mean follow-up was 7 years.[1,10]

MEDICAL AND SURGICAL MANAGEMENT

Goals and Initiation of Medical Treatment

The goal of treatment for morbid obesity is to reduce the excess body weight with maximum safety, minimum side effects or complications, control or prevention of obesity-related comorbidities, and long-term weight control.

Treatment of morbid obesity should begin with simple lifestyle changes, including moderation of diet and initiation of regular exercise such as walking. The treatment of associated comorbidities should be addressed expeditiously. However, because the only effective treatment for morbid obesity is bariatric surgery, these are the initial steps to be taken in preparation for the more definitive, albeit invasive, treatment (Fig. 26-1).

Lifestyle Changes

Lifestyle changes consisting of diet, exercise, and behavior modification constitute the first tier of therapy for obesity. The general objective that underlies the numerous obesity lifestyle change programs is the creation of a caloric deficit that results in loss of body fat over a period of time. Dietary restriction and exercise can each

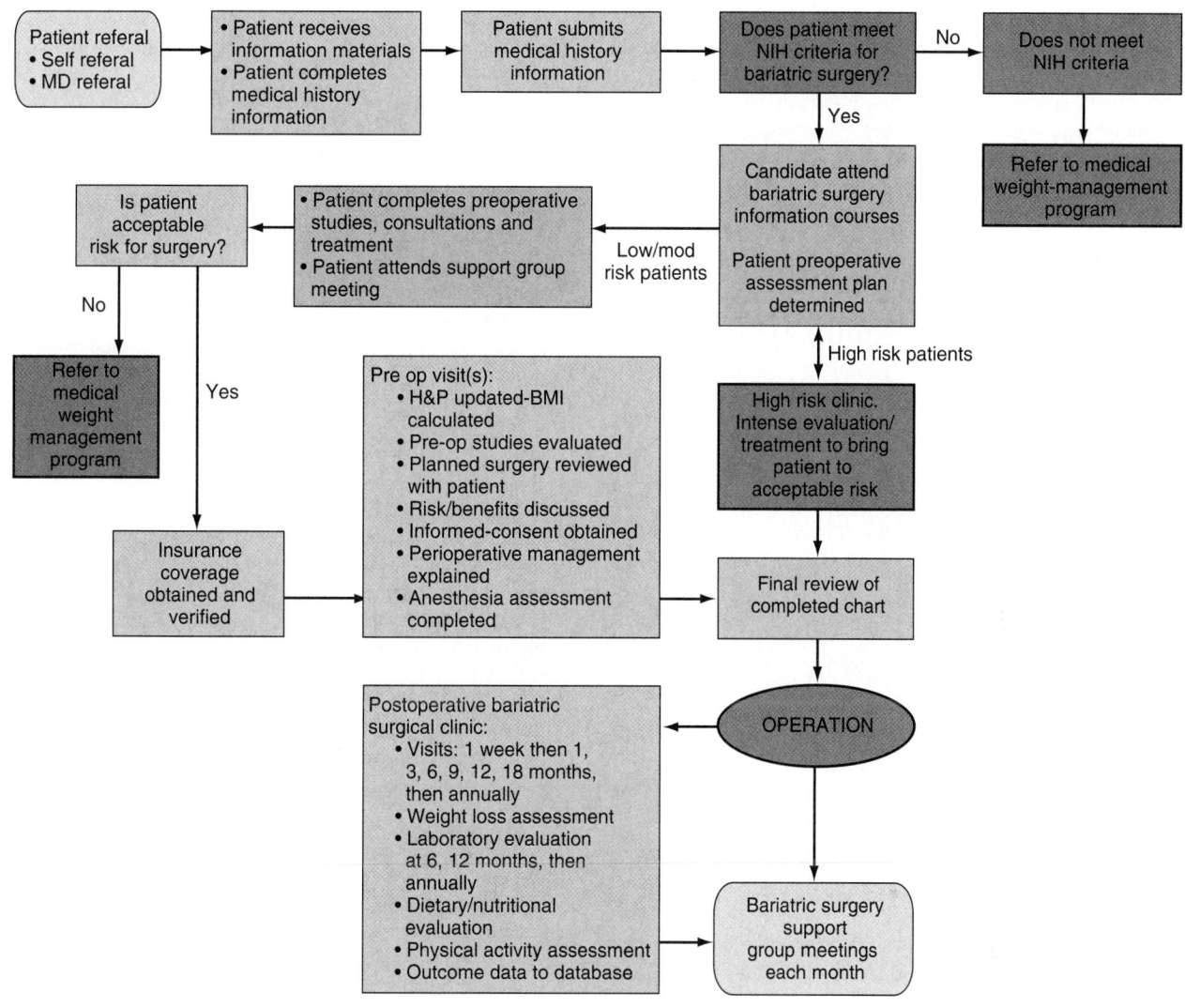

FIG. 26-1. Bariatric flow chart.

independently create an energy deficit. As a rule of thumb, a deficit of 500 kcal per day, resulting in a weekly deficit of 3500 kcal, translates to the loss of one pound of fat a week. Low-calorie diets (800 to 1500 kcal/d) are as effective as very low-calorie diets at 1 year, but carry a lower risk of nutritional deficiency.[11] They are able to achieve on average an 8% weight loss over a 6-month period. Physical activity (3 to 7 sessions a week, lasting 30 to 60 minutes each) can result in a 2 to 3% loss of body weight.[12] Behavior modification is intended to provide positive reinforcement for overcoming barriers to compliance with dietary therapy or increased physical activity. It consists of desirable and tangible nonculinary rewards for meeting short-term dietary or exercise targets. When combined with a dietary or exercise program, behavioral therapy achieved a 10% weight loss at 6 months that is sustained in 60% of patients at 40 weeks.[13] However, a meta-analysis of the long-term effect of this intervention showed that the weight loss maintained at 1 year was only 8.6% (SD 0.8).[14] Nevertheless, it is important to bear in mind that several comorbidities, especially diabetes mellitus, benefit from sustained weight loss as little as 2.3 to 3.7%,[15] and thus such therapies do have a role in the management of the obese patient. Lifestyle changes alone are appropriate for patients with a BMI less than 27,

but there are no published studies demonstrating any value of this approach in morbidly obese patients (BMI > 35).

Pharmacotherapy

Pharmacotherapy is a second tier therapy usually used in heavier patients (BMI > 27) or when lifestyle changes alone have failed. It is employed alone or in combination with lifestyle changes. The currently available agents are derived from the amphetamine class of central nervous system stimulants that exhibit a potent anorexigenic effect. Several agents, including phenylpropanolamine, phentermine, and fenfluramine also appeared, with varying efficacy and side-effect profiles. A randomized controlled study demonstrated the efficacy of combining phentermine and fenfluramine in patients with mild obesity in achieving 6% weight loss at 190 weeks, with 23% achieving a 10% or greater weight loss.[16] This combination (called Phen-Fen) allowed fewer side effects compared to using the individual agents, and was used in combination with a program of diet, exercise, and behavior modification. However, significant cardiac and pulmonary artery damage later led to the withdrawal of fenfluramine from the market. Phentermine alone has proved too ineffective to be widely used.

Sibutramine and orlistat are the only current Food and Drug Administration (FDA)–approved drugs for weight loss treatment. Orlistat is a potent and selective inhibitor of gastric and pancreatic lipases that reduces lipid intestinal absorption, while sibutramine is a noradrenaline and 5-hydroxytryptamine reuptake inhibitor that works as an appetite suppressant.[17] Despite their different mechanisms of action, they effectively produce weight loss of 6 to 10% of initial body weight at 1 year, but much of this weight is regained once the drug is stopped.[18]

The National Institutes of Health (NIH) consensus guidelines recommend that drugs should be used only as part of a comprehensive program that includes behavior therapy, diet, and physical activity.[19]

Overview of Bariatric Surgery

Goals and Mechanisms of Action

The goal of bariatric surgery is to improve health in morbidly obese patients by achieving long-term, durable weight loss. It involves reducing caloric intake and/or absorption of calories from food, and may modify eating behavior by promoting slow ingestion of small boluses of food.

Restrictive operations restrict the amount of food intake by reducing the quantity of food that can be consumed at one time, which results in a reduction in caloric intake. Malabsorptive procedures limit the absorption of nutrients and calories from ingested food by bypassing the duodenum and predetermined lengths of small intestine.

The operations currently in use for the management of morbid obesity involve gastric restriction with or without intestinal malabsorption. Gastric restrictive procedures include laparoscopic vertical banded gastroplasty (LVBG) and laparoscopic adjustable gastric banding (LAGB). Malabsorptive procedures include biliopancreatic diversion (BPD), and biliopancreatic diversion with duodenal switch (BPD-DS). Roux-en-Y gastric bypass has features of both restriction and malabsorption. The advent of laparoscopic techniques allowed surgeons to offer minimally-invasive approaches to these bariatric procedures.

Evolution of Bariatric Surgery

Surgery to treat morbid obesity was developed in 1950. Initially, intestinal bypass was performed in order to produce malabsorption, with the intent of producing weight loss through inability to absorb high-calorie foods. The initial jejunocolic bypasses caused electrolyte imbalance, intractable diarrhea, and liver failure unless reversed. This led to development of the jejunoileal bypass (JIB), in which a critical length of intestine was bypassed. However, the shortened intestine was associated with electrolyte imbalance. Liver failure also was not uncommon, especially in protein-deficient patients. Other problems such as oxalate renal stones and blind-loop syndrome also developed in these patients.[20]

In an attempt to restrict food intake, horizontal gastroplasty was developed. Its failure was due to proximal fundal pouch dilatation, outlet dilatation, and staple-line breakdown. In 1980, Mason began performing the vertical banded gastroplasty (VBG). It consists of a stapled vertical gastric channel along the lesser curvature, extending to the angle of His. Sufficient weight loss has been generally achieved; however, breakdown of the partition has produced concern.[21] Other complications of gastroplasty included Wernicke's encephalopathy and vitamin and iron deficiency.

In the late 1960s, a gastric bypass procedure was introduced by Mason and Itoh that achieved weight loss through the production of a small proximal gastric pouch that empties into a loop gastrojejunostomy.[21a] Later, the transverse pouch was changed to a vertical lesser curvature pouch. Gastric pouch problems such as marginal ulcers and staple-line disruption led to the development of a transected gastric pouch. Introducing Roux-loop modification prevented bile gastritis and decreased tension on the bowel loop. Vitamins (particularly vitamins A and B_{12} and folic acid), iron, calcium, and zinc must be replaced and levels monitored after gastric bypass surgery.[22]

In the late 1970s, Scopinaro developed the BPD. In this operation, small bowel is divided 250 cm proximal to the ileocecal valve. The proximal segment of the bowel is anastomosed to the gastric pouch. Protein malnutrition is a sequela of the procedure in some patients. The BPD produces the most effective and sustained loss of excess weight of any of bariatric procedure developed thus far.[23] Further modifications of the BPD included a duodenal switch, in which the pylorus is left intact. This prevents marginal ulceration and improves gastric emptying.

In the late 1970s, gastric banding was also introduced, which used various banding materials to create a small upper gastric pouch. This is the least invasive bariatric procedure, though complications like band migration and slippage occur. Indeed, although all bariatric operations are now being performed laparoscopically, gastric banding lends itself better to a laparoscopic approach than any other procedure. Inflatable bands can be adjusted according to actual outcome and side effects, and the procedure is easily reversible. Results from most European reports have been satisfactory; however, they have not yet been confirmed in American studies.

Indications

Patients that have a BMI of 35 kg/m^2 or more with comorbidity, or those with a BMI of 40 kg/m^2 or greater regardless of comorbidity, are eligible for bariatric surgery. Candidates must have attempted weight loss in the past by medically supervised diet regimens, exercise, or medications. Furthermore, they must be motivated to comply with postoperative dietary and exercise regimens and follow-up. Traditionally, surgeons have offered bariatric surgery to patients aged 18 to 60 years. However, bariatric surgery is now offered to some older adults at some institutions with no reported increase in morbidity or mortality. Adolescent patients with morbid obesity may be considered for bariatric surgery under select circumstances.

Contraindications

Patients who are unable to undergo general anesthesia because of cardiac, pulmonary, or hepatic disease, or those who are unwilling or unable to comply with postoperative lifestyle changes, diet, supplementation, or follow-up may not undergo these procedures. Patients with ongoing substance abuse, unstable psychiatric illness, or inadequate ability to understand the consequences of surgery are also considered to be poor surgical candidates.

Preparation for Surgery

Comorbidities are identified during the medical and surgical history taking and physical examination of the patient. Preoperative testing should be performed and additional studies should be considered, depending on the patient's comorbidities. The morbidly obese are at an increased risk of having hypertension, coronary artery disease, left ventricular hypertrophy, congestive heart failure, and pulmonary hypertension. A preoperative electrocardiogram should be obtained for all patients. Patients with cardiovascular disease should have preoperative evaluation by a cardiologist. Echocardiography, stress testing, and cardiac catheterization may be indicated for some patients.

Symptoms of loud snoring or daytime hypersomnolence in a morbidly obese patient should prompt a work-up for obstructive sleep apnea. The diagnosis is established by polysomnography at a sleep center. Patients with significant sleep apnea are treated with nasal continuous positive airway pressure. These patients are at risk for acute upper airway obstruction in the postoperative period and should be monitored closely. Obesity hypoventilation syndrome is characterized by hypoxemia (partial pressure of arterial oxygen [Pa_{O_2} < 55 mm Hg]) and hypercarbia (partial pressure of carbon dioxide [Pa_{CO_2} > 47 mm Hg]), with severe pulmonary hypertension and polycythemia. Patients diagnosed with obstructive sleep apnea, obesity hypoventilation syndrome, or severe asthma should have a preoperative evaluation by a pulmonologist. Patients with severe gastroesophageal reflux should undergo upper endoscopy with possible biopsy to rule out esophagitis or Barrett's esophagus. Due to the high incidence of gallstones in the obese population, many surgeons advocate routine preoperative sonography.

Nutritional evaluation and education is invaluable in the preoperative period. The dietitian may help determine whether the patient is able to understand the necessary changes in postoperative eating habits and food choices. The objective of psychologic screening for obesity surgery is to determine whether a patient has realistic expectations about the results of the procedure, as well as a fundamental understanding of the impact that it will have on his or her life. It may also help to identify patients suffering from depression or psychotic disorders that were previously unrecognized and that may require intervention.

Anesthesia for Bariatric Surgery

It is important for anesthesiologists to be familiar with the anatomic and physiologic implications and pharmacologic changes associated with obesity in order to offer optimal preoperative treatment. Hypertension, left ventricular hypertrophy, myocardial ischemia, and atherosclerosis are more common in morbidly obese patients. The greatest concern in these patients is development of myocardial infarction. Preoperative assessment of the cardiovascular system must be meticulous in all obese patients, and should be designed to carefully evaluate the cardiac risk. Laboratory testing should include hemoglobin and platelet count, glucose, blood urea nitrogen, and electrolyte levels. A 5-lead electrocardiogram (ECG) and chest x-ray must be performed, and in patients with a history of myocardial ischemia, an invasive assessment may be included, such as angiography and an estimation of ejection fraction.

One of the main concerns in anesthesia for morbidly obese patients is the difficulty that may be encountered in maintaining an airway. In pulmonary function tests, decreases in expiratory reserve volume, inspiratory capacity, vital capacity, and functional residual capacity are often seen. Drug pharmacokinetics differ in morbidly obese patients as well. Changes in volume of distribution include smaller-than-normal fraction of total body water, greater adipose tissue content, altered protein binding, and increased blood volume. Possible changes in renal and hepatic function have to be taken into consideration when administering drugs.

Pneumoperitoneum

In laparoscopic surgery, exposure is achieved by insufflation of the peritoneal cavity with CO_2 to create a pneumoperitoneum. CO_2 is the preferred gas for laparoscopy because it is inexpensive, readily available, and highly soluble, allowing relatively large quantities

to be safely absorbed and excreted by the lungs. It also is noncombustible, permitting the use of lasers and electrocautery. The flow of gas ceases automatically when a preset intra-abdominal pressure is reached. The intra-abdominal pressure is usually set at 15 mm Hg, and can be increased when required for better visualization. Use of two insulators is recommended for laparoscopic bariatric procedures to provide added compensation for gas leakage.[24]

Techniques Used in Bariatric Surgery

By minimizing the size of the access incisions, the laparoscopic surgeon can significantly reduce the recovery time and morbidity compared with laparotomy. Another factor favoring the laparoscopic approach for major abdominal operations is the reduction of the stress response to surgery. The gastrointestinal system also benefits from laparoscopy because postoperative ileus is less common and of shorter duration following some laparoscopic procedures. Laparoscopic access has dramatically reduced the incidence and magnitude of wound-related complications, including hematomas, seromas, infections, hernias, and dehiscence.[25]

The daunting technical hurdles involved in laparoscopic bariatric surgery have led to hand-assisted modifications to facilitate these operations. LVBG and Roux-en-Y gastric bypass (RYGB) have both been performed with hand-assisted techniques, although experience with these procedures is limited. Faster recovery after hand-assisted VBG compared to an open procedure has been confirmed.[26] DeMaria and colleagues recently reported that despite the increased cost, the hand-assisted approach could be valuable in bariatric surgery in the following five areas: (1) repair of an umbilical or ventral hernia, (2) to salvage a total laparoscopic case, (3) when a skilled assistant for a totally laparoscopic approach is not available, (4) in patients with a higher BMI, and (5) to aid in the learning curve of acquiring the skills to do a totally laparoscopic procedure.[27]

Assessment of Results

Weight loss has traditionally been used as the main outcome measure in bariatric surgery. Initially, the main criterion has been based on the concept of "ideal weight," and it was reasonable to attempt to achieve a postoperative weight closest to this desirable weight. It has become clear that weight loss is insufficient as a single outcome goal in bariatric treatment.

The NIH Conference recommended statistical reporting of surgical results, including quality of life, to provide a clearer assessment of outcomes. It underlines the fact weight loss should be considered the main postoperative outcome, but improvement of medical conditions associated with obesity is also desirable.[19] The Bariatric Analysis and Reporting Outcome System (BAROS) has been developed to standardize and compare outcomes of bariatric surgical series. This issue was further complicated by the many definitions of success that are used, and the usually poor long-term follow-up. The BAROS system defines five outcome groups (failure, fair, good, very good, and excellent), based on a scoring system that is used to evaluate three main areas: percentage of excess weight loss, changes in comorbid medical conditions, and quality of life (QOL). To assess changes in QOL after surgical treatment, a questionnaire has been developed that addresses self-esteem and four activities of daily living. Development of complications and the need for reoperation count against the final score. This system analyzes outcomes in a simple, objective, unbiased, and evidence-based fashion.[28]

Documentation

Documentation includes all necessary information about patients' current and past medical, surgical, and abdominal surgery history, including comorbidities. Meticulous medical, physical, psychologic, pulmonary, and dietary evaluation must be well documented.

The entire preoperative workup checklist should include body measurements and habitus, diagnostic tests (ECG, chest x-ray, sonogram, evaluation of the upper GI tract, endoscopy, motility, and pH studies), laboratory tests (complete blood count, platelets, prothrombin time, International Normalized Ratio, iron, electrolytes, blood urea nitrogen, creatinine, glucose, hemoglobin A_{1c}, liver function tests, albumin, calcium, phosphorus, magnesium, thyroid-stimulating hormone, lipids and cholesterol, urinalysis, and pregnancy test), consultations (nutritional, psychiatric, primary care provider, internal medicine, cardiac, pulmonary, high-risk evaluation, gynecologic/Pap smear, and hematology), cardiac testing (echocardiogram, stress test, and cardiac catheterization), and pulmonary testing (oxiflow screening, polysomnogram, and titration study). Imaging studies essential for bariatric patients include preoperative endoscopies, and in selected patients, postoperative computed tomography (CT) scanning and endoscopy.

A detailed operative report including impressions, step-by-step procedure, unexpected findings, problems, and intraoperative complications is essential. Use of a specific postoperative follow-up clinical evaluation form is strongly advised, and should include surgical procedure type and date, operating room (OR) height and weight, current height and weight, and weight at last clinic visit. Records of recovery must contain information regarding postoperative fever, pain, increased heart rate, bloating, breathing difficulty, and urinary problems. Wound and drain assessment (i.e., color, signs of infection, and healing) is important. Specific information about current patient diet should include any side effects when the diet is advanced, such as nausea or vomiting, and toleration of liquid and solid food. Various other problems such as dumping, diaphoresis, feeling faint, tremors, tachycardia, abdominal cramping, or loose stools should be noted. Bowel function difficulties (i.e., diarrhea, constipation, bloating, and increased flatulence) should be noted. Any postoperative upper GI x-rays, abdominal sonograms, upper endoscopy, and other imaging studies should be documented, if possible. Finally, the postsurgical treatment plan must be outlined, and should include impressions on weight loss, dietary counseling, drain and gastric tube status, exercise counseling, and planned lab work. All new complications occurring since the last visit or discharge must be described in detail.

Additional documentation includes correspondence, insurance issues, and patient requests. Electronically stored documents highly increase availability for follow-up and research. A systematically filled bariatric electronic database is very useful for further analyses.

Follow-Up

The American Society for Bariatric Surgery recommends visits during the immediate postoperative period, and then at variable intervals for life, with additional visits as needed, depending on the patient's condition.[29] The UPMC Center for Obesity Surgery recommends visits at 1 week, 1 month, 3 months, 6 months, 9 months, 1 year, 18 months, and yearly after surgery. During the first visit, a Jackson Pratt drain is usually removed and a more solid diet is introduced. At the 1-month visit, the diet is progressively advanced and exercises are recommended. Diet review usually is scheduled at 3 months after surgery. Laboratory studies are performed 6 months after surgery and then yearly. Malabsorptive procedures often require more frequent and extensive nutritional evaluation, due to the higher frequency of metabolic deficiencies.

Patients are encouraged to comply with lifelong follow-up, exercise, and vitamin supplementation after undergoing bariatric surgery. Follow-up includes assessment of weight loss trends, compliance with diet, and regular monitoring of metabolic and nutritional parameters.

Efficacy

Two randomized controlled trials have established the superiority of surgical weight loss procedures over nonsurgical approaches in achieving durable weight loss. Horizontal gastroplasty and a very low calorie diet produced equivalent weight loss at 12 months, but at 24 months, patients who had undergone the gastroplasty had lost significantly more weight 23 versus 2.8% excess body weight (EBW).[30] The vertical gastroplasty achieves superior weight loss compared to the horizontal gastroplasty,[31] with the difference apparent as early as 3 months postoperatively. The Dutch Obesity Project (DOP) trial showed that at 24 months, patients undergoing jejunoileostomy had lost significantly more weight than those treated medically.[9] Both surgical procedures tested in these randomized controlled trials now have been superseded or replaced by more effective procedures that have even fewer complications. The Swedish Obese Subjects (SOS) matched pair cohort study compared surgery (e.g., vertical banded gastroplasty, gastric banding, and gastric bypass) with nonsurgical treatment.[32] Weight loss at 2 years was 28 ± 15 kg among the operated patients and 0.5 ± 8.9 kg among the obese controls. At 8 years the weight loss was 20 ± 16 kg in the surgical group, with controls gaining weight (0.7 ± 12 kg). There was also a 32-fold reduction in the 2-year incidence of diabetes, rising to a fivefold reduction after 8 years. While the incidence of hypertension fell in the first 2 years, the incidence became equal in the two groups at 8 years. While 10-year data have yet to be gathered, there is no evidence at 8 years of a reduction in mortality in the surgically treated group. The SOS trial also provides evidence for improvement in quality-of-life measurements[33] of general health perception, mental well-being, mood disorders, social interaction (sickness impact profile), and obesity-related psychosocial problems and eating behavior. Peak values were obtained at 6 or 12 months, with a slight decrease at 24 months, and appear to closely mirror weight loss.

Randomized controlled trials also have compared gastric bypass with gastroplasty. Howard and colleagues showed that patients with a gastric bypass (n = 20) had a 78% excess weight loss (EWL), compared to 52% in patients undergoing vertical banded gastroplasty (n = 22) ($p < 0.05$) at 12 months, with the difference widening at 5 years to 70 and 37%, respectively.[34] This was previously confirmed by Sugerman,[35] with significantly more weight loss at 12 months (68 vs. 43%), 24 months (66 vs. 39%), and 36 months (62 vs. 37%) in the gastric bypass group.

Studies reporting gastric banding results collectively demonstrate a 40 to 60% mean EWL at 3 to 5 years. Mean hospital stay is less than 2 days, with a very low operative mortality (0.01%) rate.

Open RYGB results in a hospital stay ranging from 4 to 8 days with a perioperative complication rate of 3 to 20% and a mortality rate of about 1%. Long-term (5 to 14 years) EWL appears to be 49 to 62%. Pories and associates[36] showed a 65% excess body weight loss at 2 years, but with 15% weight regain over 14 years, after which it stabilizes. Laparoscopic and open approaches to RYGB appear to result in similar weight loss, at least in the medium term. The principal advantage of the laparoscopic approach has been in reducing perioperative morbidity, in particular the marked reduction in wound-related complications, including incisional hernias.[37–39]

Patients with malabsorption procedures had up to 78% EWL at 18 years, but with a major morbidity rate of 20 to 25%.[40]

Complications

Major complications after Roux-en-Y gastric bypass occur early (<30 days), and include pulmonary embolus (1 to 2%), gastrointestinal leak (1 to 5%), and anastomotic stricture (3 to 10%). Common late complications include hernia (5 to 24%), marginal ulcers (3 to 10%), and bowel obstructions (1 to 5%). Vitamin B_{12} deficiency and iron deficiency anemia are the most common nutritional sequelae after gastric bypass arising in approximately 15 and 30%, respectively. Both can be prevented with supplementation in most patients. Unlike malabsorptive procedures, significant protein-calorie malnutrition is rare in the absence of infection, obstruction, or other medical disorders.

The most common complications after malabsorptive procedures include hernia (10%), ulcer (8 to 12%), bowel obstruction (1%), wound infections (1%), wound dehiscence (1%), venous thrombosis (0.5%), and pulmonary embolus (0.5%). Late nutritional complications include anemia (5 to 40%) and protein malnutrition (7 to 12%).[23,40]

Bariatric Surgical Procedures

Vertical Banded Gastroplasty

The VBG is purely restrictive in nature, limiting the amount of solid food that can be consumed at one time, which leads to a calorie deficit. Of note, liquid intake is not limited by this procedure, and as such can be utilized to overcome the intended effect of the operation. A proximal gastric pouch empties through a calibrated stoma, which is reinforced by a strip of mesh or a Silastic ring.

Techniques Used in Vertical Banded Gastroplasty. Mason first described the vertical banded gastroplasty in 1982.[41] A 32F Ewald tube is passed through the mouth and into the stomach to facilitate isolation of the esophagus, and later facilitates pouch volume measurement and calibration of the stoma. The esophagus is encircled with a Penrose drain. The lesser omentum is opened and a 27F thoracostomy tube is passed from this opening behind the stomach and up to the angle of His through the gastrophrenic ligament.

An anvil for a circular stapler is held in the lesser sac against the posterior stomach wall. A trocar is pushed through both walls of the stomach at a point about 8 to 9 cm below the angle of His and into the anvil. A 2.5-cm window is created through the proximal stomach by firing a circular stapler with the Ewald tube pressed against the lesser curvature. A line of four rows of 90-mm staples leads from the circular opening to the angle of His to create a pouch 50 mL in size or smaller. Pouch volume is measured by instilling saline into the Ewald tube. Some surgeons use a linear cutting stapler to create the pouch. A strip of polypropylene mesh measuring 7 by 1.5 cm is placed around the lesser curvature channel and is sewn to itself to create a 5.0 to 5.5 cm collar circumference.

The laparoscopic technique follows the same principles. Using a five-trocar technique, the abdomen is entered and the left hepatic lobe is retracted anteriorly. The peritoneal reflection lateral to the angle of His is incised. The gastrohepatic omentum is incised and the lesser sac is entered. A 25-mm circular stapler is used to create a window through the stomach, 4 cm below the angle of His, near the lesser curvature of the stomach. A 60-mm linear stapler is inserted into this opening and is fired along a 9-mm esophageal bougie to create a divided staple line leading to the angle of His. A 5-cm band of polypropylene mesh is sutured around the gastric pouch.[42]

Another technique involves use of a linear cutting stapler to excise a wedge of fundus, thereby creating a 20-mL pouch without the use of a circular stapler. A polypropylene mesh or

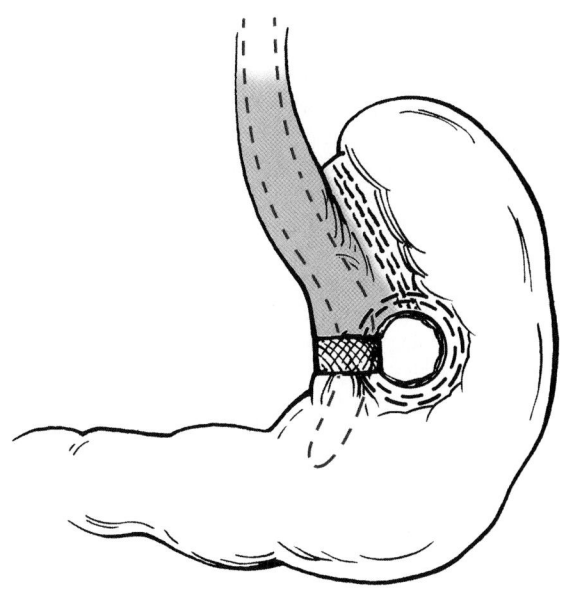

FIG. 26-2. Vertical banded gastroplasty.

polytetrafluoroethylene band is sutured around the distal end of the gastroplasty[43,44] (Fig. 26-2).

Efficacy of Vertical Banded Gastroplasty. Vertical banded gastroplasty achieves acceptable weight loss results. In a series of 305 patients followed for a minimum of 2 years, a mean excess weight loss of 61% was reported.[45] In a study of long-term results following VBG, 250 patients followed for 5 years had a mean excess weight loss of 60% for the morbidly obese and 52 percent for the superobese.[46] A study by van de Weijgert and associates demonstrated a mean excess weight loss of 63% after 7 years in 100 VBG patients.[47] All patients had lost at least 50% of excess weight preoperatively by dieting. Eckhout and colleagues reported on their experience with vertical Silastic ring gastroplasty in 1463 patients; the mean excess weight loss was 63.4%.[48]

A significant number of patients have required reoperation following vertical banded gastroplasty.[49] In a study from Spain, 100 patients followed for a minimum of 5 years after VBG had a mean excess weight loss of 54.3%. However, 25% of patients required reoperation for complications related to technique.[50] A prospective study of 71 patients who underwent VBG with a 99% 10-year follow-up reported that only 26% had maintained a loss of at least 50% of their excess weight, and 17% had a bariatric reoperation.[51] In a study of 60 patients followed for a median of 9.6 years, only 40% maintained the weight loss.[52] Sixty percent regained a significant amount of weight, and 31% returned to or exceeded their preoperative weight. These studies therefore cast doubt on the long-term success rate of vertical banded gastroplasty.

Complications. The overall morbidity rate with vertical banded gastroplasty is under 10%[53] and the mortality rate is 0 to 0.38%.[41] Early complications are infrequent and include splenectomy (0.3%) and peritonitis from leak (0.6%). Late complications include stomal stenosis[54] and staple line dehiscence, which occurs in up to 48%. In a series from MacLean and associates, 30% of all patients required reoperations for this problem.[55] Reflux esophagitis may occur in 16 to 38% of patients, and some patients may require conversion to Roux-en-Y gastric bypass for severe symptoms.[56] Intractable vomiting one or more times a week was seen in as many as 30 to 50% of patients in a series from the Mayo Clinic.[57]

Advantages and Disadvantages. With weight loss following vertical banded gastroplasty, there is significant improvement in comorbidities, including dyspnea, hypertension, diabetes mellitus, orthopedic problems, and quality of life.[58] VBG is associated with minimal long-term metabolic or nutritional deficiencies. Because it is technically easier to perform than Roux-en-Y gastric bypass, it requires less operative time. No anastomoses are required. It has a lower early morbidity rate than gastric bypass and a low mortality rate.

Long-term weight loss is less successful if patients eat sweets or drink high-calorie liquids, which are not restricted by this operation.[59] Patients who have difficulty digesting meat, bread, fruits, and vegetables may alter their eating behavior toward high-calorie soft foods. The vertical banded gastroplasty is less effective in terms of weight loss compared to the gastric bypass. Furthermore, the weight loss in superobese patients undergoing VBG is inferior to that seen with Roux-en-Y gastric bypass. Only 8% of superobese patients had "excellent" results, defined as a reduction of weight to within 25% of ideal body weight.[60]

Laparoscopic Adjustable Gastric Banding

Mechanism of Action. Adjustable gastric banding involves the minimally invasive (laparoscopic) or open-approach placement of a silicone band around the proximal stomach to restrict the amount of solid food that can be ingested at one time. Furthermore, the adjustable nature of the band allows the amount of restriction to be increased or decreased, depending upon the patient's weight loss. The Food and Drug Administration approved the laparoscopic adjustable gastric band for use in the United States in June 2001. Indications for laparoscopic adjustable gastric banding are the same as those for open gastric banding.

Technique. The patient is placed in the steep reverse Trendelenburg position. Six laparoscopic ports are placed. A 5-mm liver retractor is used to elevate the left hepatic lobe. A 15-mL gastric calibration balloon is used to identify the location for the initial dissection. A retrogastric tunnel is created starting at the base of the right diaphragmatic crus, using the parsflaccida technique. The silicone band is passed through the tunnel, toward the angle of His so that it encircles the cardia of the stomach about 1 cm below the gastroesophageal junction. The tail of the silicone band is passed through the buckle of the band and locked into place. A calibration tube is reinserted in order to determine the stoma diameter. Interrupted sutures are placed to secure the anterior stomach to the band. The end of the silicone tube is brought out through the left-sided 15-mm trocar, and is connected to the access port. The port, which will subsequently be used for injection or withdrawal of saline postoperatively for band volume adjustment, is secured to the anterior rectus sheath. It is preferable to place this port superficially so that it can be accessed without radiologic guidance.[61,62] (Fig. 26-3).

Postoperative Care. Patients are given clear liquids a few hours after the procedure. A Gastrografin swallow is obtained on the first postoperative day to confirm band position and patency. Patients can generally be discharged 1 to 2 days after surgery with a liquid diet for 4 weeks. At that time, a gradual transition to a regular diet is started.

Band adjustment may be performed with fluoroscopic guidance initially at 10 to 12 weeks. Patients are assessed monthly for weight loss and tolerance of oral intake. Band adjustments are made accordingly every 4 to 6 weeks during the first year following laparoscopic adjustable gastric banding.

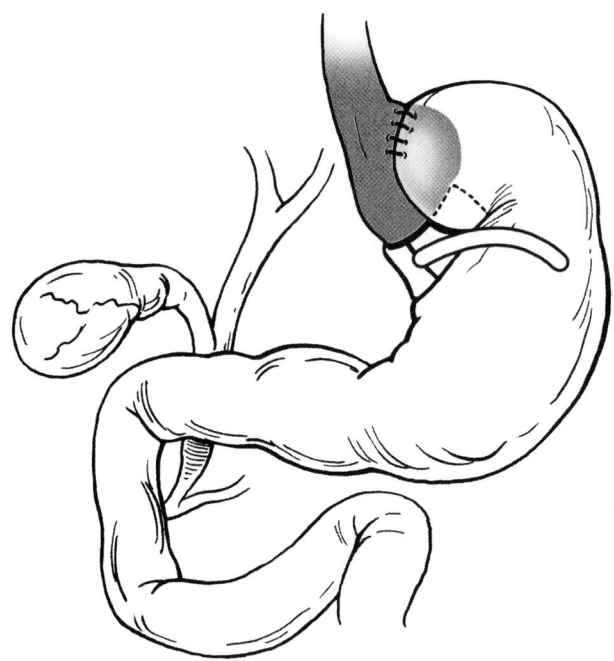

FIG. 26-3. Adjustable gastric band.

Efficacy. Suter and colleagues published their results with laparoscopic banding after 3 years of experience with this technique. One hundred fifty patients underwent laparoscopic adjustable gastric banding, with a mean body mass index of 44.6 kg/m^2 (range 35.1 to 64.1 kg/m^2), and mean initial excess body weight of 102.9% (range 58 to 191%). Mean follow-up was 17 months. Mean excess weight loss at 1 and 2 years was 55 and 56%, respectively.[63]

O'Brien and associates reported on a series of over 700 patients who underwent placement of a laparoscopic adjustable band. There have been no deaths perioperatively or during follow-up. Perioperative complications occurred in 1.2% of patients. Reoperation has been needed for prolapse (slippage) in 12.5%, erosion of the band into the stomach in 2.8%, and for tubing breaks in 3.6%. A steady progression of weight loss has occurred throughout the duration of the study, with 52 ± 19% EWL at 24 months (n = 333), 53 ± 22% EWL at 36 months (n = 264), 52 ± 24% EWL at 48 months (n = 108), 54 ± 24% EWL at 60 months (n = 30), and 57 ± 15% EWL at 72 months (n = 10). Major improvements have occurred in diabetes, asthma, gastroesophageal reflux, dyslipidemia, sleep apnea, and depression. Quality of life as measured by the RAND 36-Item Short Form Health Survey (SF-36) shows highly significant improvement.[64]

Data on 1893 patients who underwent laparoscopic adjustable gastric band placement in Italy (27 surgical centers) were collected and reported by the Italian Collaborative Study Group for the Lap-Band System. Weight loss was evaluated at 6, 12, 24, 36, 48, 60, and 72 months, with a BMI of 37.9, 33.7, 34.8, 34.1, 32.7, 34.8, and 32 kg/m^2, respectively. Postoperative mortality was 0.53%. Conversion to an open procedure occurred in 3.1%. Postoperative complications occurred in 10.2%, including tube port failure (40.9%), gastric pouch dilation (48.9%), and gastric erosion (10.8%). No deaths were recorded as a consequence of surgery.[65]

The impressive weight loss results following laparoscopic adjustable gastric banding reported in Australia and Europe have not been initially reproduced in the United States. In early U.S. experience, the weight loss result was lower compared to that in

Australia and Europe; intermediate results show a maximum weight loss of 34 to 42% in the United States. EWL from one of the original U.S. centers performing laparoscopic adjustable gastric banding was 18% (range 5 to 38%).[66] Recent American results, however, have showed success closer to that seen with this device outside America. In a group of 445 patients with a preoperative BMI of 49.6 kg/m^2, 99 patients have had a 1-year follow-up with an average loss of 44.3% excess body weight. One death was reported. Additional complications included band slippage in 3.1%, gastric obstruction without slippage in 2.7%, port migration in 0.4%, tubing disconnections in 0.7%, and port infection in 1.1%. Two bands (0.4%) were removed due to intra-abdominal abscess 2 months after placement.[67]

A prospective randomized trial from the Netherlands comparing open versus laparoscopic adjustable gastric band placement showed that both were of equal efficacy. Length of stay was significantly shorter for the laparoscopic group (5.9 vs. 7.2 days, $p < 0.05$). There also were fewer readmissions in the first postoperative year following laparoscopic adjustable gastric band placement (6 vs. 15, $p < 0.05$).[68]

Patients with diabetes mellitus, hyperinsulinemia, polycystic ovary syndrome, or a history of gestational diabetes have been shown to have a lower weight loss resulting from laparoscopic adjustable gastric banding.[69]

Complications. Intraoperative complications include splenic injury, esophageal or gastric injury (0 to 1%), conversion to an open procedure (1 to 2%), and bleeding (0 to 1%). Early postoperative complications include bleeding (0.5%), wound infection (0 to 1%), and food intolerance (0 to 11%). Late complications include slippage of the band (7.3 to 21%), band erosion (1.9 to 7.5%), tubing-related problems (4.2%), leakage of the reservoir, persistent vomiting (13%), pouch dilatation (5.2%) and gastroesophageal reflux.[70,71] Fixation of the band to the stomach has reduced the incidence of postoperative gastric prolapse.

In O'Brien's series of 700 patients, seven patients were converted to an open procedure, primarily because of hepatomegaly.[72] There were no mortalities. There were 10 significant adverse events (1.4%): seven port-site infections (1%), one deep venous thrombosis, one occurrence of hepatotoxicity, and one prolonged hospital stay because of failure of gastric emptying. Late complications requiring reoperation included gastric prolapse (15.1%), band erosions into the stomach (3.2%), and complications related to the tubing (4.7%). Among the patients requiring reoperation, 12 (1.7%) had the device removed.

In the FDA trial of laparoscopic adjustable gastric banding, which was initiated in the United States in 1995, the rate of reoperation for band slippage and removal of the band was significantly higher than that reported by investigators in Europe and Australia. DeMaria and colleagues removed 41% of bands from 37 patients, most commonly because of inadequate weight loss.[73] Seventy-two percent had dysphagia, vomiting, or reflux.

Pseudo-achalasia following laparoscopic adjustable gastric band placement has been reported in nine out of 120 patients from Switzerland, despite normal band position and stomal size. Patients with preoperative evidence of insufficiency of the lower esophageal sphincter appear to be at risk for this complication; preoperative manometry may help to identify these patients. Esophageal motility may be adversely affected by the band, and manifests as impairment of lower esophageal sphincter relaxation and abnormal esophageal peristalsis.[74]

Advantages. Laparoscopic adjustable gastric banding is a relatively simple procedure that takes less operative time than the more complex procedures such as laparoscopic RYGB or laparoscopic biliopancreatic diversion. The mortality rate is low (0.06%), as are conversion rates (0 to 4%). No staple lines or anastomoses are required. Recovery is rapid and hospital stay is short. The adjustable nature of the laparoscopic band allows the degree of restriction to be optimized for the patient's weight loss. Increasing band diameter may relieve postoperative vomiting.

Disadvantages. With this procedure, there is a potential for port site complications and the need for frequent postoperative visits for band adjustment. Some patients (5 to 10%) experience band slipping or gastric prolapse, which usually requires reoperation. Other potential problems include band erosion, port-related complications, gastroesophageal reflux, alterations in esophageal motility, and esophageal dilatation. Should inadequate weight loss occur, revision to Roux-en-Y gastric bypass is feasible, but may be technically difficult because of adhesions in the area surrounding the band.

Open Roux-en-Y Gastric Bypass

Mechanism of Action. RYGB is both a gastric restrictive procedure and a mildly malabsorptive procedure.[75] A small gastric pouch restricts food intake, while the Roux-en-Y configuration provides malabsorption of calories and nutrients. Mason described the optimal parameters for restriction necessary for adequate weight loss, including a gastrojejunostomy of 1.2 cm or less in diameter and a gastric pouch of 15 to 30 mL.[76]

Preparation. Patients must be counseled about the possibility of adverse nutritional sequelae following RYGB. For prevention of deep venous thrombosis, bilateral sequential compression devices are applied to the lower extremities, and perioperative subcutaneous unfractionated heparin or low-molecular-weight heparin is administered. Intravenous prophylactic antibiotics are used.

Technique. The abdomen is entered through a midline incision and is thoroughly explored. The gallbladder is inspected and palpated for gallstones. The distal esophagus is mobilized and encircled with a Penrose drain. The gastrohepatic omentum is bluntly entered over the caudate lobe. The phrenoesophageal ligament overlying the anterior and lateral distal esophagus is incised for subsequent esophageal mobilization. The mesentery between the first and second branches of the left gastric artery is divided with cautery. Blunt dissection is carried out between the opening in the gastrohepatic omentum and the angle of His. A 28F red rubber tube is placed from medial to lateral behind the stomach, and the open end of the tube is then brought through the opening in the mesentery.

All tubes and devices are removed from the stomach by the anesthesiologist. The red rubber tube is used to guide a 90-mm linear stapler with 4.8-mm staples across the stomach. Three superimposed staple lines are applied to the stomach so as to create a proximal pouch of 15 to 30 mL. Most surgeons advocate dividing the stomach rather than leaving it in continuity.

The ligament of Treitz is identified and a point 15 to 45 cm distally is identified. The jejunum is divided with a linear stapling device. The mesentery is divided between clamps and a side-to-side jejunojejunostomy is created with a linear stapler to create a 45- to 75-cm Roux limb for a standard gastric bypass, or a 150-cm limb for a long-limb modification in the superobese.[77] With a lengthened Roux limb, there is a greater degree of malabsorption for improvement of weight loss. The enterotomy is closed with a linear stapler and the mesenteric defect at the jejunojejunostomy is sutured closed.

The Roux limb is brought through the transverse mesocolon. A 1-cm gastrojejunal anastomosis is created between the gastric pouch and the jejunum, using a circular stapler or a hand-sewn, two-layer technique. The hand-sewn anastomosis is created over a 30F dilator. An 18F nasogastric tube is passed through the anastomosis into the jejunum with direct guidance by the surgeon after the anastomosis is completed. The integrity of the anastomosis is tested by injecting methylene blue into the nasogastric tube. The mesenteric defects are closed at this time, namely the transverse mesocolon opening and the space beneath the Roux limb, which would cause a Petersen hernia.

Postoperative Care. If a nasogastric tube is left in place at the time of surgery, it is removed within 24 hours. If deemed necessary, Gastrografin swallow is generally obtained on the second or third postoperative day and liquids are started thereafter. Patients are generally discharged 2 to 6 days after surgery.

Efficacy. Gastric bypass results in weight loss that is superior to that of purely restrictive operations. Five-year weight loss results have ranged from 48 to 74% excess weight loss.[1] One series of 608 patients followed over 14 years with less than 3% of patients lost to follow-up has demonstrated a 49% excess weight loss.[36]

RYGB has been demonstrated not only to prevent the progression of non–insulin-dependent diabetes mellitus, but also to reduce the mortality from diabetes mellitus, primarily due to a reduction in the number of deaths from cardiovascular disease.[78] Durable control of diabetes mellitus is achieved following gastric bypass, along with amelioration or resolution of other comorbidities such as hypertension, sleep apnea, and cardiopulmonary failure.

Other obesity-related medical illnesses that have shown improvement or resolution following RYGB include hyperlipidemia, hypertension, asthma, osteoarthritis, angina, venous stasis, and obesity-hypoventilation syndrome.

Complications. Early complications include anastomotic leak with peritonitis (1.2%), acute distal gastric dilatation, Roux limb obstruction, severe wound infection (4.4%), and minor wound infection or seroma (11.4%). Late complications include stomal stenosis (15%), marginal ulcer (13%), intestinal obstruction (2%), internal hernia (1%), staple line disruption (0 to 1%), incisional hernia (16.9%), cholecystitis (10%), and mortality (0.4%). Metabolic complications include deficiencies of calcium, thiamine, vitamin B_{12} (26 to 70%), folate (9 to 18%), iron (20 to 49%), and anemia (18 to 35%).

Advantages. The RYGB is more effective than vertical banded gastroplasty in terms of weight loss. A randomized, prospective trial with 95% follow-up demonstrated that patients addicted to sweets had lost significantly more weight 3 years after gastric bypass than after vertical banded gastroplasty (64 vs. 38% excess weight loss, respectively). The presence of dumping syndrome following gastric bypass may encourage patients to avoid sweets. In a more recent study in which sweet-eaters were assigned to gastric bypass and non–sweet-eaters were assigned to vertical banded gastroplasty, gastric bypass still had superior efficacy in terms of weight loss over vertical banded gastroplasty (69 vs. 50%).[79]

Disadvantages. Dumping syndrome occurs in a variable number of patients following gastric bypass. It is due to rapid emptying of hyperosmolar boluses into the small bowel. Patients may experience bloating, nausea, diarrhea, and abdominal pain after ingesting sweets or milk products. Vasomotor symptoms such as palpitations, diaphoresis, and lightheadedness also may occur. Dumping syndrome may provide a beneficial effect in promoting weight loss by causing patients to avoid sweets.

A few postoperative complications are specific to gastric bypass, including distal gastric distention and internal hernia. Distal gastric distention is often heralded by hiccups and left shoulder pain. If perforation is imminent, it may require percutaneous needle decompression or operative gastrostomy tube placement. Internal hernia may be difficult to diagnose. Patients may present with vague periumbilical pain, nausea, and vomiting. A radiographic upper gastrointestinal study is valuable in diagnosis. Operative repair is indicated, and involves reduction of the herniated bowel and suture closure of the mesenteric defect.[7]

Laparoscopic Roux-en-Y Gastric Bypass

Mechanism of Action. Like the open RYGB, the laparoscopic RYGB is both a gastric restrictive procedure and a mildly malabsorptive procedure. A small gastric pouch restricts food intake, while the Roux-en-Y configuration provides malabsorption of calories and nutrients.

Preparation. Patients must be informed about the possibility of conversion to an open procedure. Preoperative bowel preparation may be useful in reducing bingeing behavior prior to surgery. For prevention of deep venous thrombosis, bilateral sequential compression devices are applied to the lower extremities and perioperative subcutaneous unfractionated heparin or low-molecular-weight heparin is administered.

Technique. Laparoscopic RYGB was first described by Wittgrove, Clark, and Tremblay in 1994.[80] After pneumoperitoneum is established, five or six access ports are inserted. A vertically oriented proximal gastric pouch measuring 15 to 30 mL is created using sequential applications of a linear endoscopic stapler.

The ligament of Treitz is identified, and the jejunum is divided 10 to 12 cm distally with a linear stapler. A 75- to 150-cm Roux limb is constructed and a side-to-side jejunojejunostomy is created with linear endoscopic staplers. Some groups use an elongated Roux limb of 150–250 cm for superobesity.

The gastrojejunal anastomosis may be stapled or hand-sewn. Several stapling techniques have been described. For a circular stapled anastomosis with transoral passage of the anvil, upper endoscopy is then performed. A percutaneous intravenous cannula is placed by the surgeon and is used to introduce a loop of wire into the lumen of the gastric pouch, which is grasped by the endoscopist and attached to the anvil of a 21- or 25-mm circular stapler. The anvil is passed through the oropharynx, esophagus, and into the gastric pouch. Electrocautery is applied over the stem of the anvil to bring it through the gastric wall. A left-sided port site is enlarged for passage of a circular stapler. An incision is made in the Roux limb 8 to 10 cm from the stapled end to admit the circular stapler, which is mated with the anvil to create the stapled anastomosis. The enterotomy is closed with a linear stapler.[37]

To create a circular stapled anastomosis with transgastric anvil insertion, a gastrotomy is created on the anterior stomach and the anvil is introduced into the stomach. The tip is brought through the gastric wall; the pouch is then created using sequential firings of the linear stapler.[81,82]

For a combination hand-sewn and linear-stapled anastomosis, a posterior layer of continuous nonabsorbable sutures is placed to approximate the Roux limb to the pouch. A gastrotomy and an bleeding (0 to 3.3%), and pulmonary complications (0 to 5.8%). Stenosis of the gastrojejunostomy is observed in 1.6 to 6.3%. Other complications include internal hernia (2.5%), gallstones (1.4%), marginal ulcer (1.4%), and staple-line failure (1%). Conversion to an open procedure occurs in 3 to 9%. The mortality rate is 0 to 1.5%. Nguyen and Wolfe reported a case of hypopharyngeal perforation following transoral insertion of a circular stapler anvil.[81]

Advantages. With the laparoscopic gastric bypass, there is better cosmesis, less postoperative pain, and attenuation of the postoperative stress response. Patients recover rapidly and have a shorter hospital stay.[38] The laparoscopic approach to gastric bypass eliminates the midline laparotomy incision and therefore substantially reduces the morbidity from postoperative wound infections, dehiscence, and incisional hernias. Furthermore, there is a significant improvement in postoperative pulmonary function with the laparoscopic procedure compared to the open gastric bypass.[84]

Disadvantages. The laparoscopic gastric bypass, while safe and feasible, is a technically challenging, advanced laparoscopic procedure with a steep learning curve. This approach may be more difficult in superobese patients who have a preponderance of fat in the abdominal area, which may make exposure difficult. The presence of an enlarged fatty liver may also hinder the surgeon considerably.

Biliopancreatic Diversion

Mechanism of Action. The BPD is a procedure developed by Nicola Scopinaro of Italy. The procedure combines gastric restriction with an intestinal malabsorptive procedure. A 50- to 100-cm common absorptive alimentary channel is created proximal to the ileocecal valve; digestion and absorption are limited to this segment of bowel.

Indications. This procedure is primarily indicated for the superobese or for those who have failed restrictive bariatric procedures. Less commonly, some surgeons perform BPD as a primary operation in the non-superobese.

Contraindications. Patients with anemia, hypocalcemia, and osteoporosis, and those who are not motivated to comply with stringent postoperative supplementation regimens may not be appropriate for this procedure. The laparoscopic approach may be especially challenging in patients who have undergone multiple previous abdominal surgeries, previous weight loss surgery, patients with an enlarged fatty liver, and in those with a large amount of intra-abdominal fat.

Technique. A subtotal gastrectomy is performed, leaving a proximal 200-mL gastric pouch for the superobese patient, or 400-mL pouch for the others. A Roux-en-Y anastomosis is created 50 to 100 cm proximal to the ileocecal valve, and the distal 250 cm of small intestine is anastomosed to the gastric pouch with a 2- to 3-cm stoma. A concomitant cholecystectomy is performed because of the high incidence of postoperative cholelithiasis with this degree of malabsorption.

A modification of this technique with a duodenal switch involves a greater curvature sleeve gastrectomy, with maintenance of the continuity of the antrum, pylorus, and first portion of the duodenum. This allows for a lower marginal ulcer rate (0 to 1%) and a lower incidence of dumping syndrome.[85] For the laparoscopic approach, six to eight laparoscopic ports are inserted. A sleeve gastrectomy is performed to create a gastric reservoir of 150 to 200 mL.

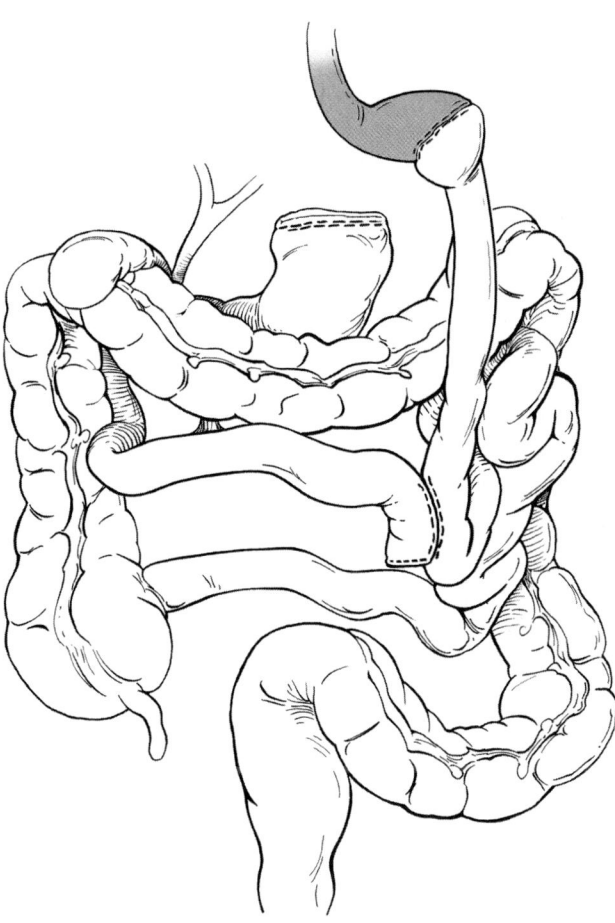

FIG. 26-4. Roux-en-Y gastric bypass.

enterotomy are made with ultrasonic dissection, and a 45-mm linear stapler is used to create the gastrojejunostomy. Upper endoscopy is performed and the flexible endoscope is passed through the anastomosis, which is completed with two layers of running nonabsorbable sutures. The gastrojejunal anastomosis may also be completely hand-sewn in two layers using absorbable suture.

Insufflation of the gastric pouch with air by endoscopy or via nasogastric tube is performed to test the integrity of the anastomosis, which is submerged in irrigation fluid. Alternately, methylene blue may be irrigated into a nasogastric tube. Port sites larger than 5 mm are closed at the fascial level (Fig. 26-4).

Postoperative Care. Some surgeons place a Jackson-Pratt or Blake drain at the anastomosis, which is left in place for a varying length of time, depending on surgeon preference. Nasogastric tubes are not used routinely. Early postoperative mobilization is emphasized.

Efficacy. Mean excess weight loss ranges from 69 to 82% with follow-up of 24 months or less. Wittgrove et al demonstrated a mean excess weight loss of 73% with follow-up of 60 months.[83] In the study by Schauer et al the mean excess weight loss was 83 and 77% at 24 and 30 months, respectively.[37] Most comorbidities were improved or eradicated, including diabetes mellitus, hypertension, sleep apnea, and reflux. Quality of life was improved significantly.

Complications. Postoperative complications include pulmonary embolism (0 to 1.5%), anastomotic leak (1.5 to 5.8%),

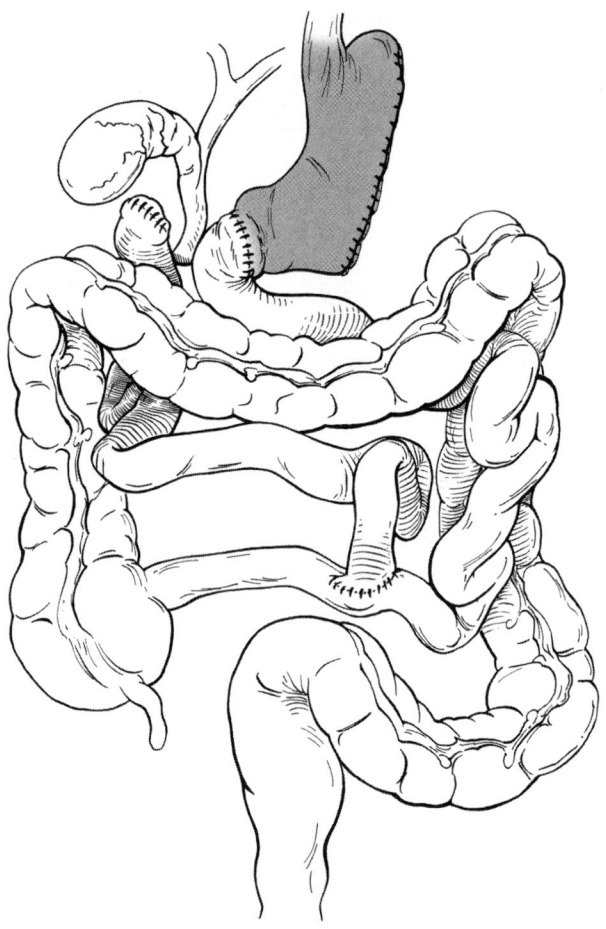

FIG. 26-5. *Biliopancreatic diversion with duodenal switch.*

To perform the biliopancreatic diversion with a duodenal switch, the continuity of the antrum, pylorus, and first portion of the duodenum is maintained. This allows for a lower marginal ulcer rate (0 to 1%), and a lower incidence of dumping syndrome because the pylorus is preserved.[85] The ileum is divided 250 cm proximal to the ileocecal valve and is anastomosed to the stomach. A Roux-en-Y anastomosis is created, leaving a common channel 100 cm long (Fig. 26-5).

Postoperative Care. The patient must be on lifelong vitamin, calcium, and iron supplementation, and must comply with lifelong follow-up because of the risk of malnutrition.

Efficacy. Weight loss results with BPD are excellent and durable. At 8 years, patients weighing up to 120% of ideal body weight, and those weighing more than 120% of ideal body weight maintained 72 and 77% mean excess weight loss, respectively. A group of 40 patients had a mean excess weight loss of 70% for a 15-year period.[40]

The results of laparoscopic BPD with duodenal switch in 40 patients with a mean follow-up of 12 months were reported.[85] Median BMI was 60 kg/m^2 (range 42 to 85 kg/m^2). There was one conversion to an open procedure (2.5%). Median operative time was 210 ± 9 minutes (range 110 to 360 minutes); this correlated significantly with BMI ($p = 0.04$). Median length of stay was 4 days (range 3 to 210 days). The mean excess weight loss at 6 and 9 months

was 46 ± 2% and 58 ± 3%, respectively, with a median follow-up of 6 months.

Complications. The incidence of postoperative complications is quite high following BPD. The most common morbidities include anemia (30%), protein-calorie malnutrition (20%), dumping syndrome, and marginal ulceration (10%). The duodenal switch modification is associated with a lower ulceration rate (1%) and a lower incidence of dumping syndrome. Other complications include vitamin B$_{12}$ deficiency, hypocalcemia, fat-soluble vitamin deficiencies, osteoporosis, night blindness, and prolongation of prothrombin time. The postoperative mortality rate ranges from 0.4 to 0.8%.

From Scopinaro's series, early surgical complications included wound infection and dehiscence (1.2%).[23] Late complications included incisional hernia (8.7%), intestinal obstruction (1.2%), protein malnutrition (7%), iron deficiency anemia (<5%), stomal ulcer (2.8%), and acute biliopancreatic limb obstruction. Bone demineralization was seen in 25% preoperatively; at 1 to 2 years, it was observed in 29%. At 3 to 5 years, it was present in 53%, and in 14% at 6 to 10 years.

In laparoscopic series from Ren and colleagues,[86] there was one death (2.5%). The major morbidity rate was 15%, including anastomotic leak (2.5%), venous thrombosis (2.5%), staple-line hemorrhage (10%), and subphrenic abscess (2.5%).

Advantages. Even if patients consume a great quantity of food, the malabsorptive component of the BPD allows for excellent results in terms of weight loss. This operation may be more effective than gastric bypass or restrictive surgery in patients with severe morbid obesity (e.g., BMI greater than 70 kg/m^2), or in those who have failed to maintain weight loss following gastric bypass or restrictive bariatric surgery.

The laparoscopic BPD with duodenal switch is an effective minimally invasive procedure for weight loss. It offers better weight loss than restrictive procedures because of the malabsorptive component of the operation. This operation may be valuable in patients with severe morbid obesity (e.g., BMI greater than 70 kg/m^2), or in those who have failed to maintain weight loss following gastric bypass surgery or restrictive procedures.

Disadvantages. The BPD is technically a more complex procedure than the restrictive procedures. Protein malnutrition with anemia, hypoalbuminemia, edema, and alopecia are among the serious adverse sequelae of this operation. Severe vitamin deficiencies may occur, leading to osteoporosis and night-blindness. Treatment requires prolonged hyperalimentation and supplementation. Patients have four to six foul-smelling stools per day, reflecting the fat malabsorption from this procedure. Patients may also experience bloating and heartburn following this procedure. Replacement of fat-soluble vitamins is needed for patients following BPD or BPD-DS.

The laparoscopic approach may be especially challenging in patients who have undergone multiple previous abdominal surgeries, previous weight loss surgery, in patients with an enlarged fatty liver, and in those with a large amount of intra-abdominal fat. The laparoscopic BPD is a technically demanding, lengthy laparoscopic procedure, with potential for nutritional sequelae similar to those of the open BPD. Patients may experience abdominal bloating, malodorous stools, heartburn, and abdominal pain. Protein malnutrition with anemia, hypoalbuminemia, edema, and alopecia are potential postoperative sequelae. Severe vitamin deficiencies may be observed. Treatment requires prolonged hyperalimentation and possibly reoperation to lengthen the common channel.

SPECIAL ISSUES RELATING TO THE BARIATRIC PATIENT

Bariatric Procedures in the Adolescent and the Elderly Patient

The prevalence of obesity (defined as a BMI $\geq$ 30 kg/m^2) in the United States has increased rapidly in recent years. A steady increase was observed across all age groups, but the greatest magnitude of increase was found in the 18- to 29-year-old group (7.1 to 14.1%) in a period from 1991 to 2001. In a group of elderly patients aged 60 to 69 years, the increase was 14.7 to 25.3%. Above 70 years of age, prevalence increased from 11.4 to 17.1%. The prevalence of obesity and diabetes among U.S. adults characteristically shows an increasing trend with age. Only 2.1% of obese young people (18 to 29 years old) have diabetes mellitus, whereas 15.5% of obese patients older than 70 years of age have this disease.[87]

Tracking the change in BMI that occurs from childhood to adulthood helps predict the probability of obesity in young adults in relation to the presence or absence of being overweight at various times during childhood. In children 10 to 15 years old, 10% of those with a BMI-for-age less than the eighty-fifth percentile were obese at age 25, whereas 75% of those with a BMI-for-age greater than or equal to the eighty-fifth percentile were obese as adults. Eighty percent of those with a BMI-for-age greater than or equal to the ninety-fifth percentile were obese at age 25. From this study, it is clear that an overweight child is more likely than a child of normal weight to be obese as an adult.[88]

Bariatric Surgery in Morbidly Obese Adolescents

Bariatric surgery in morbidly obese adolescents is controversial. It is generally believed that morbidly obese individuals should be of adult age before undergoing bariatric operations, despite the progressive and debilitating course of this increasingly common disease. An estimated 25% of children in the United States are obese, a number that has doubled over a 30-year period. Very little information has been published on the subject of obesity surgery in adolescents. However, review of the available literature shows that bariatric surgery in adolescents is safe and is associated with significant weight loss, correction of obesity comorbidity, and improved self-image and socialization.

Surgery may be indicated in this population because of the dismal failure of the conservative methods of weight control, the permanence of adult obesity following adolescent obesity, and the many disabling and deadly obesity-related comorbidities of adulthood. Bariatric surgery should be seriously considered after conservative methods have failed. All patients should meet NIH criteria for bariatric surgery.

Stanford and associates reported an average loss of 87% of excess body weight and nearly complete resolution of comorbidities (including hypertriglyceridemia, hypercholesterolemia, asthma, and gastroesophageal reflux disease) in a group of four adolescent patients during 20 months of follow-up. All patients who underwent laparoscopic Roux-en-Y gastric bypass were younger then 20 years of age, and all procedures were completed laparoscopically. There were no complications.[89]

Sugerman and associates described an experience with bariatric surgery in adolescents. Gastroplasty was the procedure of choice in the initial 3 years of the study, followed by gastric bypass. Thirty-three adolescents underwent the following bariatric operations: horizontal gastroplasty in one, vertical banded gastroplasty in two, and gastric bypass in 30. Mean BMI was 52 $\pm$ 11 kg/m^2. Early complications included pulmonary embolism in one patient, wound infection in five, stomal stenoses in three, and marginal ulcers in four. Late complications included small bowel obstruction in one and incisional hernias in six patients. There were two late sudden deaths (2 and 6 years postoperatively), but these were unlikely to have been caused by the bariatric surgical procedure. Significant weight loss was maintained in the majority of patients for up to 14 years after surgery. Most of comorbidities resolved at 1 year. Self-image was greatly enhanced, resulting in successful marriages and educational achievements.[90]

Capella and colleagues reported on 19 adolescent patients (aged 13 to 17) who underwent vertical banded gastroplasty Roux-en-Y gastric bypass. The average percentage of EWL at 3, 4, and 6 years was 80%. The initial average BMI was 49 kg/m^2. The postoperative BMI at the average follow-up time of 5.5 years was 28. One patient was a failure, with a reported EWL of only 35%. There were two revisions and no mortality or morbidity. All comorbidities disappeared and families and patients were satisfied with the surgery.[91]

Abu-Abeid reported on 11 adolescent patients (aged 11 to 17) with severe morbid obesity, who underwent laparoscopic adjustable gastric banding with a 4-year follow-up period. Some specific comorbidities such as amenorrhea and gallstones were noted in younger patients. Mean preoperative BMI was 46.4 kg/m^2. During the follow-up period, the mean BMI dropped from 46.6 to 32.1 kg/m^2, with marked improvement in medical conditions. No late complications developed. Authors noted difficulties involved in psychologically and cognitively preparing this population for surgery.[92]

Bariatric Surgery in Elderly Patients

In most studies, mean body weight increases with age up to about age 60, and then levels off; however, information about the association between body weight and mortality at higher ages is sparse. Some studies actually suggest a protective effect of being overweight in the oldest age groups. Indices of visceral obesity may be better indicators of risk than BMI in these age groups. Not only actual weight, but also weight development over the last decades of life may predict outcome. Most clinical trials exclude older patients, and little is known about the benefits of diets or drugs that induce weight loss in these age groups. More information is available suggesting multiple benefits of physical activity. Mechanical complications of obesity, such as osteoarthritis and static respiratory complications, seem to improve with weight loss, even at higher ages. For health-related and economic reasons it will become important to address treatment strategies in the elderly in the near future, since they will constitute a larger segment of the population. Recent studies suggest that bariatric surgery, previously considered contraindicated in obese patients above age 60, can be safely performed even in patients above age 70, with the same benefits as those seen in younger patients.[93]

Some surgeons have considered age 50 years or older as a relative contraindication to bariatric surgery. Gonzales and associates have reported interesting comparisons between laparoscopic technique and open technique for RYGB in older patients. They demonstrated safety and efficacy of RYGB in a group of patients of aged 50 years or older who underwent RYGB. The percentage of excess body weight lost was 66% at mean follow-up of 12 months. Blood samples drawn after a mean of 8 $\pm$ 2 months revealed no postoperative metabolic alterations. RYGB resulted in significant reduction of comorbidities such as hyperglycemia, hypertension, degenerative joint disease, gastroesophageal reflux disease, and continuous positive airway pressure–dependent sleep apnea. The laparoscopic approach resulted in fewer intensive care unit admissions and shorter length of stay when compared to open surgery. Authors concluded that RYGB is safe and well tolerated in patients 50 years or older, and resulted in no renal, hepatic, or electrolytic alterations. Weight loss and control of obesity-related comorbidities are satisfactory.[94]

In some previous reports other authors also indicated the effectiveness of bariatric surgery in elderly patients. Macgregor and Rand evaluated the long-term outcome of gastric restrictive surgery in morbidly obese patients aged 55 years and older. Seventy-seven patients had Roux-en-Y gastric bypass, four had vertical banded gastroplasty, and seven had silicone ring vertical gastroplasty. Patients had an average loss of 57% excess body weight and 20 to 48% reduction of comorbidities in a 6-year follow-up period. A BMI of less than 30 kg/m^2 was achieved and maintained by 42% of patients. The authors concluded that surgical treatment of obesity is appropriate for selected patients in the older age groups.[95]

Laparoscopic Gastric Banding in Older Patients

Older patients experience the same benefits from a laparoscopic gastric banding (LGB) operation as do younger patients. Nehoda and colleagues reported a series of 320 patients with an average preoperative BMI of 44.2 who underwent LGB. Patients were divided into two age groups: younger patients (18 to 49 years) and older patients (50 years or older). All patients received LGB with an adjustable gastric band. Clinical outcome, including weight loss, complications, length of hospital stay, and operative times, were reviewed. Sixty-eight older patients (21.5%) were identified. The excess weight loss after 12 months was 68%. Complications requiring reoperation occurred in 10.3% of patients. Ninety-seven percent of the patients reported an improvement in their comorbid conditions. The authors concluded that older patients receive the same benefits from laparoscopic gastric banding as do younger patients, with an acceptable postoperative complication rate. This has led to an increase in the upper age limit to 70 years in the authors' institution.[96]

The Female Patient: Pregnancy and Gynecologic Issues in the Bariatric Surgery Patient

Obesity-induced hormonal disorders could contribute to biologic imbalance, and thus favor the development of dysfunctional ovulation. Pregnancy in obese women should be managed as a high-risk pregnancy. The incidence of gestational diabetes and hypertension is increased. Macrosomia is common. There is a two- to threefold increase in the rate of cesarean sections, with more complications. Fetal morbidity does not appear to be changed when maternal weight gain is limited. With obesity, there is an increased risk for breast and endometrial cancer, due to elevated levels of circulating estrogens resulting from aromatization of male sex steroids in adipose tissue, and decreased levels of sex hormone–binding globulin.[97]

Women who suffer from morbid obesity are often infertile. If these women are able to become pregnant, they are considered high risk because of associated risk factors such as hypertension and diabetes. Following the pregnancy is difficult due to limitations of the physical examinations. More costly, more frequent ultrasound examinations are needed. Bariatric surgery reduces the woman's weight and the incidence of obesity-related comorbidities. Pregnancy in morbidly obese women soon after weight loss surgery may occur unexpectedly during a period of weight loss. Dixon and associates also suggest that morbidly obese women have higher obstetric risks and poorer neonatal outcomes.[98] However, weight loss reduces obstetric risk. They noticed decreased maternal weight gain during pregnancy for women who underwent laparoscopic gastric banding. No difference in birth weights was noted. Obstetric complications were minimal, and there were no premature or low birth weight infants. The ability to adjust gastric restriction allows optimal control of maternal weight change in pregnancy, and should help avoid the risks of excessive weight change.

Wittgrove and coworkers evaluated the rate of complications in patients identified as having been pregnant following gastric bypass for weight loss.[99] They found a lower risk of gestational diabetes, macrosomia, and cesarean section in surgical patients than in those who were obese and had not had the surgery. Because surgical patients have had an operation that restricts food intake, some dietary precautions should be taken in this patient population when they become pregnant. Early experience with pregnancy following gastric bypass in severely obese patients showed development of severe iron deficiency anemia resulting from malabsorption. This can complicate pregnancy following gastric bypass surgery. For women of childbearing age, this potential adverse effect must be considered.[100]

An interesting clinical study showed normalization of many gynecologic and obstetric changes after loss of massive amounts of body weight following bariatric surgery. Menstrual irregularities were present in 40.4% of premenopausal patients preoperatively; after massive weight loss, cycles were abnormal in 4.6%. Infertility problems were present preoperatively in 29.3%. During previous pregnancies, medical complications were frequent (hypertension 26.7%, pre-eclampsia 12.8%, diabetes 7.0%, and deep vein thrombosis 7.0%). After weight-loss stabilization, these obstetric complications did not occur. The incidence of urinary stress incontinence decreased from 61.2 to 11.6%.[101]

The polycystic ovary syndrome results from a systemic hormonal dysfunction. Women with polycystic ovaries are frequently obese and have a higher risk of infertility, anovulation, hyperandrogenism, dyslipidemia, insulin resistance, and abnormal menses.[102]

Obesity has a major impact on stress urinary incontinence. Women suffering from obesity manifest increased intra-abdominal pressures, which adversely stress the pelvic floor and may contribute to the development of urinary incontinence. In addition, obesity may affect the neuromuscular function of the genitourinary tract, thereby also contributing to incontinence. Accordingly, thorough evaluation of obese women must be performed prior to the institution of treatment. Weight loss may relieve urinary incontinence, but definitive therapy via operative procedures is effective, even in obese patients, and should be recommended with confidence.

Involuntary urinary leakage due to a rise in abdominal pressure is usually caused by stress (i.e., coughing, laughing, change in position, walking, running, or carrying heavy weights). The cure of an underlying condition, such as obesity, is sufficient in many cases. Subak and associates evaluated the effect of weight reduction on urinary incontinence in obese women. The study demonstrated an association between weight reduction and improved urinary incontinence.[103]

Dwyer and colleagues reported on results of a series of 368 incontinent women who underwent urodynamic assessment. Sixty-three percent were diagnosed as having genuine stress incontinence, and 27% as having detrusor instability. Obesity was significantly more common in women with genuine stress incontinence and detrusor instability than in the normal population. In those with detrusor instability, the BMI was found to increase with age and parity. In women with genuine stress incontinence, the BMI increased with age and the number of previous incontinence operations, and was higher in nulliparous than in parous women.[104] Kolbl and Riss confirmed similar findings. A markedly increased BMI was found to be correlated with a positive clinical stress test.[105]

Gallbladder Disease in the Bariatric Surgery Patient

Weight loss following laparoscopic Roux-en-Y gastric bypass (LRYGB) is accompanied by a rise in the incidence of gallstones, with 38 to 52.8% of patients who preoperatively did not have stones going on to develop stones in the first postoperative year.[106,107] Between 15 and 27% of all patients undergoing LRYGB will require urgent cholecystectomy within 3 years.[106,108]

Routine cholecystectomy concomitant with a LRYGB remains controversial.[109,110] The safety of combining laparoscopic cholecystectomy and LRYGB has been established, but performing both in one procedure may increase the length of hospital stay and adds an hour to the operative time.[111,112] An alternative is the prophylactic use of oral ursodiol for 6 months after LRYGB. This significantly reduces the incidence of gallstones,[113] but is hindered by poor patient compliance.[114] The decision to prophylactically remove the gallbladder is made by the surgeon based on the likelihood of the patient to take the postoperative ursodiol, compared to the risk of prolonging the procedure, especially in the superobese.

Choledocholithiasis becomes a difficult clinical problem because of a loss of endoscopic access to the duodenum. Anchoring the remnant stomach to the anterior abdominal wall, preferably with a radiologic marker, may provide a safe point for percutaneous access for endoscopic retrograde cholangiopancreatography.[115]

Gastroesophageal Reflux Disease in the Bariatric Surgery Patient

Symptomatic gastroesophageal reflux disease (GERD) is present in about 58% of morbidly obese individuals, and its presence is proven objectively in 21%.[37] The conventional approach of fundoplication and hiatal reconstruction as definitive treatment is associated with a poorer outcome in obese individuals.[142] Weight loss that results in a BMI less than 30 has been associated with more favorable results. The RYGB has been found to resolve GERD symptoms in the vast majority of patients.[143] In this study, there was a significant decrease in GERD-related symptoms, including heartburn (from 87 to 22%), water brash (from 18 to 7%), wheezing (from 40 to 5%), laryngitis (from 17 to 7%), and aspiration (from 14 to 2%). Furthermore, the postoperative use of medication decreased significantly, both for proton pump inhibitors (from 44 to 9%) and for H₂ blockers (from 60 to 10%).[143] The use of the adjustable gastric band is also associated with resolution of reflux esophagitis in 89%.[64]

After vertical banded gastroplasty, reflux esophagitis may occur in 16 to 38% of patients, who may require conversion to Roux-en-Y gastric bypass for severe symptoms.[56] Late complications after laparoscopic vertical banded gastroplasty that may require reoperation include new-onset gastroesophageal reflux (0.5 to 12%).

Diabetes in the Bariatric Surgery Patient

Paralleling the rise in incidence of morbid obesity is the incidence of type II diabetes, often as a component of the metabolic syndrome comprising central obesity, glucose intolerance, dyslipidemia, and hypertension.[7]

Several comorbidities, especially diabetes mellitus, benefit from sustained weight loss as little as 2.3 to 3.7%,[15] with lifestyle changes alone appropriate for patients with a BMI less than 27, but there are no published studies demonstrating any value of this approach

in morbidly obese patients (BMI > 35). However, several recently published outcome studies demonstrate the value of surgical procedures in improving diabetes in the morbidly obese. Laparoscopic adjustable gastric banding, reported in a series of 700 patients, showed complete resolution or definite improvement of diabetes in 97%.[62]

In a study by Schauer et al, 1160 patients undergoing laparoscopic LRYGB over a 5-year period were examined, with 240 (21%) demonstrating impaired fasting glucose or type II diabetes mellitus (T2DM). After surgery, fasting plasma glucose and glycosylated hemoglobin concentrations returned to normal levels (83%) or were markedly improved (17%) in all patients. A significant reduction in the use of oral antidiabetic agents (80%) and insulin (79%) was also observed following surgical treatment. Notably, patients with the shortest duration (<5 years), the mildest form of T2DM (diet-controlled), and the greatest weight loss after surgery, were most likely to achieve complete resolution of diabetes.[141]

Cardiovascular Disease and Hypertension in the Bariatric Surgery Patient

Both the cardiovascular and pulmonary systems appear to be abnormal in obese patients. The presence of pulmonary function abnormalities and correlation between the severity of lung function impairment and the degree of obesity have been well proven. Reduction in functional residual capacity and impairment of diffusion capacity were the most common abnormalities found in obese patients. Obstructive ventilatory impairment was found in some patients. Reduction in static lung volume correlated with the degree of obesity.[116] It also seems that the cardiopulmonary endurance to exercise in morbidly obese patients with upper body fat distribution is lower than in those with lower body fat distribution.[117]

During exercise, cardiopulmonary reserve is exhausted because of augmented requirements, leading to a significant intolerance. Exercise duration increases significantly 6 months following a weight loss surgical procedure. The mean O_2 consumption at peak exercise (peak VO_2) and at the anaerobic threshold (VO_{2AT}) was significantly higher after weight loss. Six months after vertical banded gastroplasty the left ventricle thickness decreased significantly. Diastolic indices, isovolumic relaxation time (IVRT), and early:late (E:A) velocity ratio significantly improved after weight loss. Peak VO_2 and VO_{2AT} were significantly correlated with IVRT and E:A velocity ratio. Weight loss resulting from bariatric surgery improves the cardiac diastolic function, and this is associated with an improvement in cardiopulmonary exercise performance. Left ventricular filling variables could be considered among the most important determinants of exercise intolerance in obese individuals.[118]

Obesity clearly correlates with the development of heart failure (HF). Obese and overweight patients have significantly higher rates of hypertension and diabetes, as well as higher levels of cholesterol, triglycerides, and low-density-lipoprotein cholesterol. However, in a large group of patients with advanced HF of multiple etiologies, obesity was not associated with increased mortality. Further studies are needed to delineate whether weight loss promotion in medically optimized patients with HF is a worthwhile therapeutic goal.[119] Reduced cardiac performance tolerance is linked with a reduced oxygen supply to the active muscles. Study results confirmed a relatively less efficient cardiac performance during progressive work rates in obese patients.[120] Increased left ventricular mass has been shown to be a significant independent predictor of cardiovascular risk. Hypertension and obesity each have significant independent associations with left ventricular mass and wall thickness. Obesity is particularly strongly associated with left ventricular internal diameter.[121]

Elevated arterial pressure in patients with obesity-related hypertension is associated with an increased cardiac output and total peripheral resistance. The elevated output is related to expanded intravascular volume that increases cardiopulmonary volume, venous return, and left ventricular preload; the elevated pressure and total peripheral resistance increase afterload. This dual ventricular overload promotes a dimorphic, concentric, and eccentric hypertrophy in response to the volume and pressure overload. Increased myocardial oxygen demand results from the elevated tension in the left ventricular wall, reflecting its increased diameter and pressure, and provides a physiologic rationale for the greater potential of coronary arterial insufficiency and cardiac failure. There are greater renal blood flow and lower renal vascular resistance in patients with obesity-related hypertension at any level of arterial pressure. This may be offset by an increased renal filtration fraction that may favor protein deposition and glomerulosclerosis, and predisposition of obese patients toward diabetes may aggravate this problem. With weight reduction, these hemodynamic derangements may be reversed: intravascular volume contracts, cardiac output decreases, and arterial pressure falls.[122] Reduction of weight in morbidly obese patients is significantly correlated with the fall in mean arterial pressure. Total circulating and cardiopulmonary blood volumes also are reduced, permitting a decreased venous return and cardiac output. Weight loss is also associated with reduced resting circulating levels of plasma norepinephrine, suggesting that diminished adrenergic function also may be related to weight reduction and its associated fall in arterial pressure.[123]

Sleep Apnea in the Bariatric Surgical Patient

Sleep apnea is defined by a respiratory disturbance index (number of apnea-hypopnea episodes per hour of sleep) of 5 or more in the presence of excessive daytime somnolence.[124] Patients with a BMI over 50, with hypersomnolence, hypertension, or with a history of loud snoring, should be assumed to have sleep apnea.[124] Preoperative administration of the Epworth sleepiness scale questionnaire[125] or a multivariable apnea prediction questionnaire[126] help in predicting a high probability of sleep apnea, and in identifying patients who need inpatient polysomnography.[127] Estimation of the positive airway pressure needed to keep the upper airway patent[128] also can be determined during this investigation.

Apneic arrest can complicate the postoperative course of patients whose sleep apnea has remained undiagnosed or mismanaged. Continuous positive airway pressure (CPAP) in the perioperative period has been shown to be effective in preventing apneic arrest without risk to the anastomosis.[129,130] The risk of apneic arrest is increased by narcotics,[128,131,132] requiring these patients to be in monitored beds and on CPAP when receiving postoperative opioid analgesia. A period of acclimatization to the face mask of at least 2 weeks prior to the surgery is valuable in improving postoperative compliance with CPAP.

A patient at high risk of apneic arrest may be deceptively comfortable with transient episodes of desaturation corrected by oxygen. However, it is the progressive hypercapnia that leads to CO_2 narcosis and respiratory acidosis, leading to cardiac arrest.

Plastic Surgery Following Weight Loss

Most massive weight loss patients are troubled by hanging skin and rolls of skin and fat. Though smaller in size, their clothes fit poorly. Skin macerates under abdominal pannus, hanging inner thighs, and ptotic breasts. Body aroma is unpleasant. Heavy flaps of skin burden the back and inhibit vigorous exercise. Intimate relations may be untenable. Plastic surgery can substantially improve or correct the skin changes resulting from weight loss. Since most insurance carriers maintain limited coverage for plastic surgery, many patients have limited access to its benefits.

Bariatric center staff members must anticipate these issues and encourage comprehensive body contouring surgery by a team of plastic surgeons. When patients are given time to describe their deformities and prioritize treatment, they are more likely to accept the risks, uncertainties, and obligations of body contouring surgery. Candidates with active psychiatric pathology and unrealistic expectations are excluded.

Body contouring surgery advanced considerably during the 1990s,[133–135] and these procedures have been modified for this new post–bariatric surgery population.[136–139]

The massive weight loss patient has a deflated shape that is related to genetically defined fat deposition patterns. The most susceptible regions are the anterior neck, upper arms, breasts, lower back, flanks, abdomen, mons pubis, and thighs. Problematic areas for women include the subcutaneous abdomen and hips and thighs; in men, they are the flanks, abdomen, and breasts. The deformity reflects the initial BMI and its change. Since the etiology of the skin laxity is not understood, there is no medical therapy. The widest possible areas of skin are excised and closed tightly.

Operative planning is based on the deformity and patient priorities. Most have excess tissue of the lower torso and thighs removed through a circumferential abdominoplasty and lower body lift.[136] Starting prone and then turning supine, the operation removes a wide swath of skin and fat along the bikini line. The lift of the buttocks and lateral thighs requires extensive undermining down the thighs followed by a very tight lateral subcutaneous fascial closure. This closure is aided by full abduction of the leg onto a utility table.[138] A panniculectomy that corrects the inflammatory sequelae of an overhanging pannus is included. As an isolated procedure, a panniculectomy is a long transverse excision of skin and fat between the umbilicus and pubis, without flap undermining or reconstruction of the umbilicus.

The circumferential abdominoplasty removes the redundant skin of the lower abdomen, flattens the abdomen, and incorporates the lower body lift. It requires central undermining to the xiphoid and minimal lateral undermining of the superior flap. Large, braided permanent sutures imbricate the central fascia from xiphoid to pubis. The operating table is flexed as the superior flap is approximated to the incision over the pubis and groins, with highest closure tension being lateral. That tension narrows the waist and advances the anterolateral thighs. Liposuction is performed as needed. A medial high transverse thighplasty usually accompanies the lower body lift in massive weight loss patients.

Unwanted skin redundancy distal to the mid-thighs requires long vertical medial excision of skin. Mid-back and epigastric rolls, along with sagging breasts, are corrected with an upper body lift. The upper body lift is a reverse abdominoplasty, removal of mid-torso excess skin, and reshaping of the breasts. For highly selected individuals, and with a well organized team, a single-stage total body lift, which includes a circumferential abdominoplasty, lower body lift, medial thighplasty, an upper body lift, and breast reshaping, can be performed safely in under 8 hours[139] (Figs. 26-6 and 26-7).

The opportunity that these large numbers of massive weight loss patients provide for plastic surgery innovation, treatment, and professional satisfaction is extraordinary, and is similar to the revolution

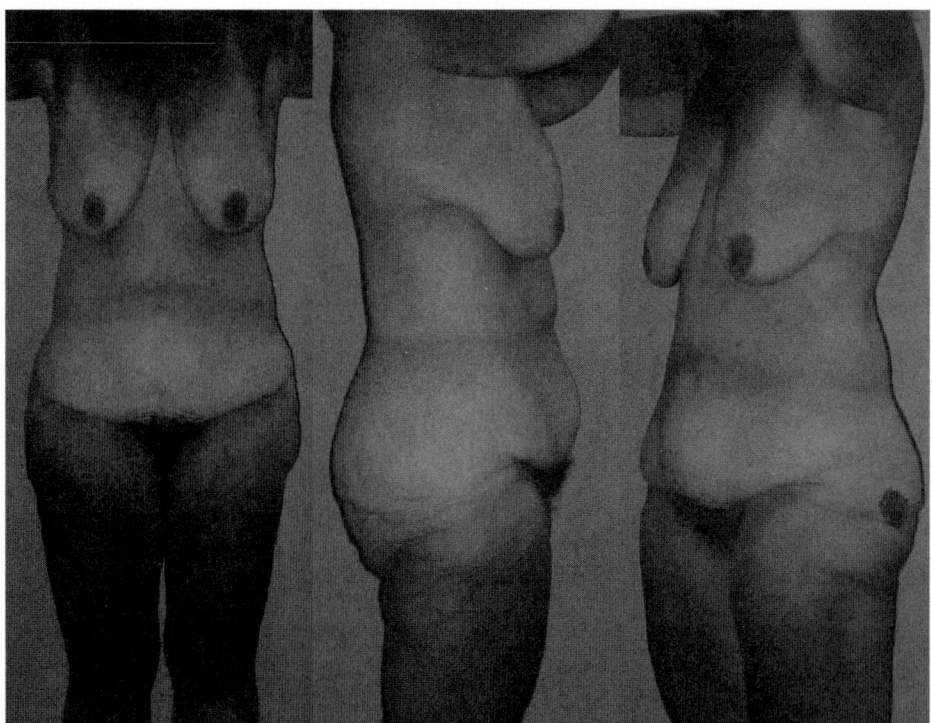

FIG. 26-6. These are the preoperative frontal, right lateral, and left anterior oblique views of a 36-year-old, 150-lb, 5'6" woman who lost 120 lb, 2 years after a laparoscopic Roux-en-Y gastric bypass procedure. She underwent a single-stage total body lift and bilateral brachioplasties. *(Courtesy of Dennis Hurwitz, M.D., Clinical Professor of Plastic Surgery, University of Pittsburgh.)*

of craniofacial surgery in the 1970s and breast reconstruction in the 1980s. Patients are uniformly pleased with their improvements, with the exception of pain and the minor complications noted above. Research in adipocyte physiology, skin biomechanics, and alternative surgical technique should lead to improved care.

ACKNOWLEDGEMENT

The authors would like to thank the following for their contributions to this chapter: Dennis Hurwitz, M. D., Clinical Professor of Plastic Surgery, University of Pittsburgh, Paul Thoidiyl, M. D., Fellow in Laparoscopic and Bariatric Surgery, University of Pittsburgh, and

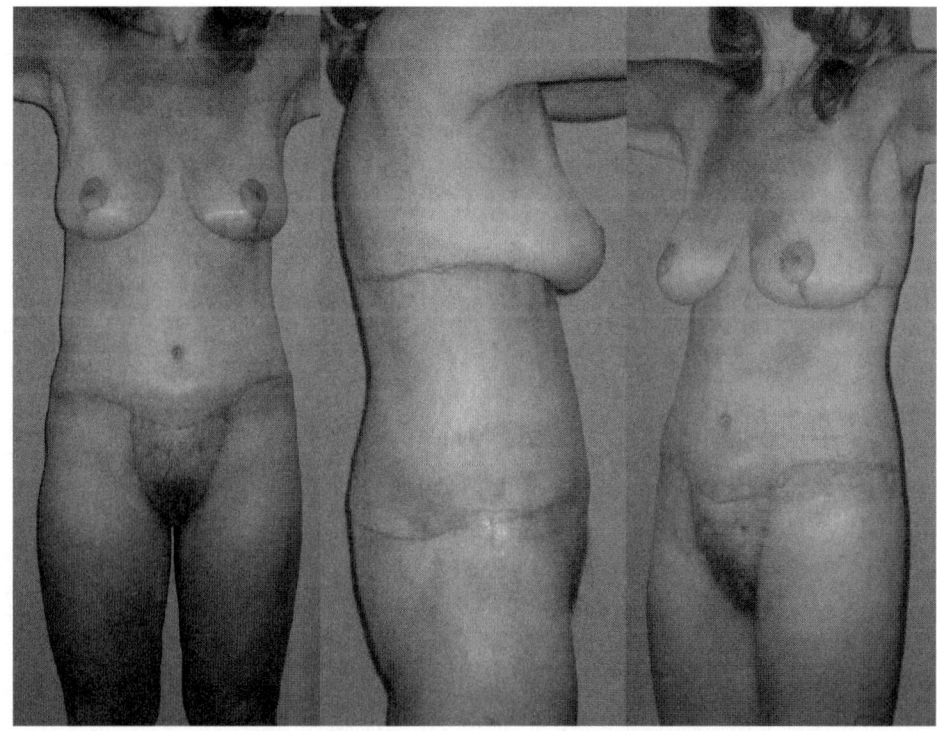

FIG. 26-7. These are the frontal, right lateral, and left anterior oblique views 6 weeks after surgery for the woman in Fig. 26-5. The scars indicate the circumferential abdominoplasty, lower body lift, upper body lift, breast reshaping, and autoaugmentation through a keyhole pattern and bilateral brachioplasties. All redundant skin has been removed, leaving well-positioned scars and feminine features. *(Courtesy of Dennis Hurwitz, M.D., Clinical Professor of Plastic Surgery, University of Pittsburgh.)*

Tomasz Rogula, M. D. Fellow in Laparoscopic and Bariatric Surgery
University of Pittsburgh.

References

1. Gastrointestinal surgery for severe obesity: National Institutes of Health Consensus Development Conference Statement. *Am J Clin Nutr* 55:615S, 1992.
2. Kuczmarski RJ, Flegal KM, Campbell SM, Johnson CL: Increasing prevalence of overweight among US adults. The National Health and Nutrition Examination Surveys, 1960 to 1991. *JAMA* 272:205, 1994.
3. Stunkard AJ, Foch TT, Hrubec Z: A twin study of human obesity. *JAMA* 256:51, 1986.
4. Ravussin E: Energy metabolism in obesity. Studies in the Pima Indians. *Diabetes Care* 16:232, 1993.
5. Brolin RE: Morbid obesity, in Levine BA, Copleland IEM, Howard RJ, Sugerman HJ, Warshaw AL (eds): *Current Practice of Gastrointestinal and Abdominal Surgery*. New York: Churchill Livingstone, 1994, p 1.
6. Sugerman HJ, DeMaria EJ, Kellum JM: Gastric surgery for morbid obesity, in Nyhus LM, Baker RJ, Fisher JE (eds): *Mastery of Surgery*. Boston: Little, Brown and Company, 1997, p 982.
7. Timar O, Sestier F, Levy E: Metabolic syndrome X: A review. *Can J Cardiol* 16:779, 2000.
8. Garfinkel L: Overweight and cancer. *Ann Intern Med* 103:1034, 1985.
9. Lew EA, Garfinkel L: Variations in mortality by weight among 750,000 men and women. *J Chronic Dis* 32:563, 1979.
10. Drenick EJ, Bale GS, Seltzer F, Johnson DG: Excessive mortality and causes of death in morbidly obese men. *JAMA* 243:443, 1980.
11. Wadden TA, Foster GD, Letizia KA: One-year behavioral treatment of obesity: Comparison of moderate and severe caloric restriction and the effects of weight maintenance therapy. *J Consult Clin Psychol* 62:165, 1994.
12. Wood PD, et al: Changes in plasma lipids and lipoproteins in overweight men during weight loss through dieting as compared with exercise. *N Engl J Med* 319:1173, 1988.
13. Wing RR: Behavioral strategies to improve long-term weight loss and maintenance. *Med Health RI* 82:123, 1999.
14. Miller WC, Koceja DM, Hamilton EJ: A meta-analysis of the past 25 years of weight loss research using diet, exercise or diet plus exercise intervention. *Int J Obes Relat Metab Disord* 21:941, 1997.
15. Eriksson KF, Lindgarde F: Prevention of type 2 (non-insulin-dependent) diabetes mellitus by diet and physical exercise. The 6-year Malmo feasibility study. *Diabetologia* 34:891, 1991.
16. Weintraub M: Long-term weight control study. IV (weeks 156 to 190). The second double-blind phase. *Clin Pharmacol Ther* 51:608, 1992.
17. Scheen AJ, Ernest P: New antiobesity agents in type 2 diabetes: Overview of clinical trials with sibutramine and orlistat. *Diabetes Metab* 28:437, 2002.
18. Bray GA: Drug treatment of obesity. *Rev Endocr Metab Disord* 2:403, 2001.
19. National Institutes of Health conference. Gastrointestinal surgery for severe obesity. Consensus Development Conference Panel. *Ann Intern Med* 115:956, 1991.
20. Deitel M: Jejunocolic and jejunoileal bypass: A historical perspective, in *Surgery for the Morbidly Obese Patients*. Philadelphia: Lea & Febiger, 1989, p 81.
21. Mason EE, Maher JW, Scott DH, et al: Ten years of vertical banded gastroplasty for severe obesity. *Probl Gen Surg* 9:280, 1992.
21a. Mason EE, Ito C: Gastric bypass. *Ann Surg* 170:329, 1969.
22. Miller DK, Goodman GN: Gastric bypass procedures, in Deitel M (ed): *Surgery for the Morbidly Obese Patients*. Philadelphia: Lea & Febiger, 1989, p 113.
23. Scopinaro N, Adami GF, Marinari GM, et al: Biliopancreatic diversion. *World J Surg* 22:936, 1998.
24. Ramanathan R, Gourash W, Ikramddin S, Schauer PR: Equipment and instrumentation for laparoscopic bariatric surgery, in Deitel M,

Cowan G (eds): *Update: Surgery for the Morbidly Obese Patients*. Toronto: FD-Communications, 2000, p 277.
25. Cottam DR, Mattar SG, Schauer PR: Laparoscopic era of operations for morbid obesity. *Arch Surg* 138:367, 2003.
26. Bleier JI, et al: Hand-assisted laparoscopic vertical banded gastroplasty: Early results. *Surg Endosc* 14:902, 2000.
27. DeMaria EJ, Schweitzer MA, Kellum JM, et al: Hand-assisted laparoscopic gastric bypass does not improve outcome and increases costs when compared with open gastric bypass for the surgical treatment of obesity. *Surg Endosc* 16:1452, 2002.
28. Oria HE, Moorehead MK: Bariatric analysis and reporting outcome system (BAROS). *Obes Surg* 8:487, 1998.
29. www.asbs.org
30. Andersen T, Backer OG, Stokholm KH, et al: Randomized trial of diet and gastroplasty compared with diet alone in morbid obesity. *N Engl J Med* 310:352, 1984.
31. Andersen T, Backer OG, Astrup A, et al: Horizontal or vertical banded gastroplasty after pretreatment with very-low-calorie formula diet: A randomized trial. *Int J Obes* 11:295, 1987.
32. Torgerson JS, Sjostrom L: The Swedish Obese Subjects (SOS) study—rationale and results. *Int J Obes Relat Metab Disord* 25(Suppl 1):S2, 2001.
33. Karlsson J, Sjostrom L, Sullivan M: Swedish obese subjects (SOS)—an intervention study of obesity. Two-year follow-up of health-related quality of life (HRQL) and eating behavior after gastric surgery for severe obesity. *Int J Obes Relat Metab Disord* 22:113, 1998.
34. Howard L, et al: Gastric bypass and vertical banded gastroplasty—a prospective randomized comparison and 5-year follow-up. *Obes Surg* 5:55, 1995.
35. Sugerman HJ, Starkey JV, Birkenhauer R: A randomized prospective trial of gastric bypass versus vertical banded gastroplasty for morbid obesity and their effects on sweets versus non-sweets eaters. *Ann Surg* 205:613, 1987.
36. Pories WJ, et al: Who would have thought it? An operation proves to be the most effective therapy for adult-onset diabetes mellitus. *Ann Surg* 222:339, 1995; discussion 350.
37. Schauer PR, Ikramuddin S, Gourash W, et al: Outcomes after laparoscopic Roux-en-Y gastric bypass for morbid obesity. *Ann Surg* 232:515, 2000.
38. Nguyen NT, et al: Laparoscopic versus open gastric bypass: A randomized study of outcomes, quality of life, and costs. *Ann Surg* 234:279, 2001; discussion 289.
39. Nguyen NT, Ho HS, Palmer LS, et al: A comparison study of laparoscopic versus open gastric bypass for morbid obesity. *J Am Coll Surg* 191:149, 2000; discussion 155.
40. Scopinaro N, et al: Biliopancreatic diversion for obesity at eighteen years. *Surgery* 119:261, 1996.
41. Mason EE: Vertical banded gastroplasty for obesity. *Arch Surg* 117:701, 1982.
42. Lonroth H, et al: Vertical banded gastroplasty by laparoscopic technique in the treatment of morbid obesity. *Surg Laparosc Endosc* 6:102, 1996.
43. Joffe J, Voitk A: A simple technique for laparoscopic vertical banded gastroplasty—the JOVO procedure. *Dig Surg* 18:90, 2001.
44. Cagigas JC, et al: "No punch" technique of laparoscopic vertical banded gastroplasty for morbid obesity. *Obes Surg* 9:407, 1999.
45. Willbanks OL: Long-term results of silicone elastomer ring vertical gastroplasty for the treatment of morbid obesity. *Surgery* 101:606, 1987.
46. Mason EE: Why the operation I prefer is vertical banded gastroplasty 5.0. *Obes Surg* 1:181, 1991.
47. van de Weijgert EJ, Ruseler CH, Elte JW: Long-term follow-up after gastric surgery for morbid obesity: Preoperative weight loss improves the long-term control of morbid obesity after vertical banded gastroplasty. *Obes Surg* 9:426, 1999.
48. Eckhout GV, Willbanks OL, Moore JT: Vertical ring gastroplasty for morbid obesity. Five year experience with 1463 patients. *Am J Surg* 152:713, 1986.

49. Sugerman HJ, Kellum JM, Jr., DeMaria EJ, et al: Conversion of failed or complicated vertical banded gastroplasty to gastric bypass in morbid obesity. *Am J Surg* 171:263, 1996.

50. Baltasar A, et al: Vertical banded gastroplasty at more than 5 years. *Obes Surg* 8:29, 1998.

51. Balsiger BM, Poggio JL, Mai J, et al: Ten and more years after vertical banded gastroplasty as primary operation for morbid obesity. *J Gastrointest Surg* 4:598, 2000.

52. Ramsey-Stewart G: Vertical banded gastroplasty for morbid obesity: Weight loss at short and long-term follow up. *Aust N Z J Surg* 65:4, 1995.

53. Capella JF, Capella RF: The weight reduction operation of choice: Vertical banded gastroplasty or gastric bypass? *Am J Surg* 171:74, 1996.

54. Greenway FL: Surgery for obesity. *Endocrinol Metab Clin North Am* 25:1005, 1996.

55. MacLean LD, Rhode BM, Forse RA: Late results of vertical banded gastroplasty for morbid and super obesity. *Surgery* 107:20, 1990.

56. Kim CH, Sarr MG: Severe reflux esophagitis after vertical banded gastroplasty for treatment of morbid obesity. *Mayo Clin Proc* 67:33, 1992.

57. Nightengale ML, et al: Prospective evaluation of vertical banded gastroplasty as the primary operation for morbid obesity. *Mayo Clin Proc* 66:773, 1991.

58. Bourdages H, Goldenberg F, Nguyen P, et al: Improvement in obesity-associated medical conditions following vertical banded gastroplasty and gastrointestinal bypass. *Obes Surg* 4:227, 1994.

59. Brolin RL, Robertson LB, Kenler HA, et al: Weight loss and dietary intake after vertical banded gastroplasty and Roux-en-Y gastric bypass. *Ann Surg* 220:782, 1994.

60. MacLean LD, Rhode BM, Forse RA: A gastroplasty that avoids stapling in continuity. *Surgery* 113:380, 1993.

61. Belachew M, et al: Laparoscopic placement of adjustable silicone gastric band in the treatment of morbid obesity: How to do it. *Obes Surg* 5:66, 1995.

62. O'Brien PE, Brown WA, Smith A, et al: Prospective study of a laparoscopically placed, adjustable gastric band in the treatment of morbid obesity. *Br J Surg* 86:113, 1999.

63. Suter M, Bettschart V, Giusti V, et al: A 3-year experience with laparoscopic gastric banding for obesity. *Surg Endosc* 14:532, 2000.

64. O'Brien PE, et al: The laparoscopic adjustable gastric band (Lap-Band): A prospective study of medium-term effects on weight, health and quality of life. *Obes Surg* 12:652, 2002.

65. Angrisani L, et al: Lap Band adjustable gastric banding system: The Italian experience with 1863 patients operated on 6 years. *Surg Endosc* 17:409, 2003.

66. Greenstein RJ, et al: The Lap-Band system as surgical therapy for morbid obesity: Intermediate results of the USA, multicenter, prospective study. *Surg Endosc* 13:S1, 1999.

67. Ren CJ, Weiner M, Allen JW: Favorable early results of gastric banding for morbid obesity: The American experience. *Surg Endosc* 17 (In press).

68. de Wit LT, et al: Open versus laparoscopic adjustable silicone gastric banding: A prospective randomized trial for treatment of morbid obesity. *Ann Surg* 230:800, 1999; discussion 805.

69. Dixon JB, Dixon ME, O'Brien PE: Pre-operative predictors of weight loss at 1-year after Lap-Band surgery. *Obes Surg* 11:200, 2001.

70. Silecchia G, et al: Laparoscopic adjustable silicone gastric banding: Prospective evaluation of intragastric migration of the lap-band. *Surg Laparosc Endosc Percutan Tech* 11:229, 2001.

71. Suter M: Laparoscopic band repositioning for pouch dilatation/slippage after gastric banding: Disappointing results. *Obes Surg* 11:507, 2001.

72. O'Brien P, Brown W, Dixon J: Revisional surgery for morbid obesity—conversion to the Lap-Band system. *Obes Surg* 10:557, 2000.

73. DeMaria EJ, et al: High failure rate after laparoscopic adjustable silicone gastric banding for treatment of morbid obesity. *Ann Surg* 233:809, 2001.

74. Weiss HG, et al: Treatment of morbid obesity with laparoscopic adjustable gastric banding affects esophageal motility. *Am J Surg* 180:479, 2000.

75. Mason EE, Ito C: Gastric bypass. *Ann Surg* 170:329, 1969.

76. Mason EE, Printen KJ, Hartford CE, Boyd WC: Optimizing results of gastric bypass. *Ann Surg* 182:405, 1975.

77. Brolin RE, Kenler HA, Gorman JH, Cody RP: Long-limb gastric bypass in the superobese. A prospective randomized study. *Ann Surg* 215:387, 1992.

78. MacDonald KG Jr., et al: The gastric bypass operation reduces the progression and mortality of non-insulin-dependent diabetes mellitus. *J Gastrointest Surg* 1:213, 1997.

79. Sugerman HJ, et al: Weight loss with vertical banded gastroplasty and Roux-Y gastric bypass for morbid obesity with selective versus random assignment. *Am J Surg* 157:93, 1989.

80. Wittgrove AC, Clark GW, Tremblay LJ: Laparoscopic gastric bypass, Roux-en-Y: Preliminary report of five cases. *Obes Surg* 4:353, 1994.

81. Nguyen NT, Wolfe BM: Hypopharyngeal perforation during laparoscopic Roux-en-Y gastric bypass. *Obes Surg* 10:64, 2000.

82. Scott DJ, Provost DA, Jones DB: Laparoscopic Roux-en-Y gastric bypass: Transoral or transgastric anvil placement? *Obes Surg* 10:361, 2000.

83. Wittgrove AC, Clark GW: Laparoscopic gastric bypass: A five-year prospective study of 500 patients followed from 3 to 60 months. *Obes Surg* 9:123, 1999.

84. Nguyen NT, et al: Comparison of pulmonary function and postoperative pain after laparoscopic versus open gastric bypass: A randomized trial. *J Am Coll Surg* 192:469, 2001; discussion 476.

85. Marceau P, et al: Biliopancreatic diversion with a new type of gastrectomy. *Obes Surg* 3:29, 1993.

86. Ren CJ, Patterson E, Gagner M: Early results of laparoscopic biliopancreatic diversion with duodenal switch: A case series of 40 consecutive patients. *Obes Surg* 10:514, 2000; discussion 524.

87. Mokdad AH, et al: Prevalence of obesity, diabetes, and obesity-related health risk factors, 2001. *JAMA* 289:76, 2003.

88. Whitaker RC, Wright JA, Pepe MS, et al: Predicting obesity in young adulthood from childhood and parental obesity. *N Engl J Med* 337:869, 1997.

89. Stanford A, et al: Laparoscopic Roux-en-Y gastric bypass in morbidly obese adolescents. *J Pediatr Surg* 38:430, 2003.

90. Sugerman HJ, et al: Bariatric surgery for severely obese adolescents. *J Gastrointest Surg* 7:102, 2003; discussion 107.

91. Capella JF, Capella RF: Bariatric surgery in adolescence. Is this the best age to operate? *Obes Surg* 13:826, 2003.

92. Abu-Abeid S, Gavert N, Klausner JM, et al: Bariatric surgery in adolescence. *J Pediatr Surg* 38:1379, 2003.

93. Rossner S: Obesity in the elderly—a future matter of concern? *Obes Rev* 2:183, 2001.

94. Gonzalez R, Lin E, Mattar SG, et al: Gastric bypass for morbid obesity in patients 50 years or older: Is laparoscopic technique safer? *Am Surg* 69:547, 2003; discussion 553.

95. Macgregor AM, Rand CS: Gastric surgery in morbid obesity. Outcome in patients aged 55 years and older. *Arch Surg* 128:1153, 1993.

96. Nehoda H, et al: Laparoscopic gastric banding in older patients. *Arch Surg* 136:1171, 2001.

97. Bongain A, Isnard V, Gillet JY: Obesity in obstetrics and gynaecology. *Eur J Obstet Gynecol Reprod Biol* 77:217, 1998.

98. Dixon JB, Dixon ME, O'Brien PE: Pregnancy after Lap-Band surgery: Management of the band to achieve healthy weight outcomes. *Obes Surg* 11:59, 2001.

99. Wittgrove AC, Jester L, Wittgrove P, et al: Pregnancy following gastric bypass for morbid obesity. *Obes Surg* 8:461, 1998; discussion 465.

100. Gurewitsch ED, Smith-Levitin M, Mack J: Pregnancy following gastric bypass surgery for morbid obesity. *Obstet Gynecol* 88:658, 1996.

101. Deitel M, Stone E, Kassam HA, et al: Gynecologic-obstetric changes after loss of massive excess weight following bariatric surgery. *J Am Coll Nutr* 7:147, 1988.

102. Gonzalez CA, Hernandez MI, Mendoza R, et al: [Polycystic ovarian disease: Clinical and biochemical expression.] *Ginecol Obstet Mex* 71:253, 2003.

103. Subak LL, et al: Does weight loss improve incontinence in moderately obese women? *Int Urogynecol J Pelvic Floor Dysfunct* 13:40, 2002.

104. Dwyer PL, Lee ET, Hay DM: Obesity and urinary incontinence in women. *Br J Obstet Gynaecol* 95:91, 1988.

105. Kolbl H, Riss P: Obesity and stress urinary incontinence: Significance of indices of relative weight. *Urol Int* 43:7, 1988.

106. Shiffman ML, Sugerman HJ, Kellum JM, et al: Changes in gallbladder bile composition following gallstone formation and weight reduction. *Gastroenterology* 103:214, 1992.

107. Iglezias Brandao de Oliveira C, Adami CE, Borges da Silva B: Impact of rapid weight reduction on risk of cholelithiasis after bariatric surgery. *Obes Surg* 13:625, 2003.

108. Amaral JF, Thompson WR: Gallbladder disease in the morbidly obese. *Am J Surg* 149:551, 1985.

109. Mason EE, Renquist KE: Gallbladder management in obesity surgery. *Obes Surg* 12:222, 2002.

110. Fobi M, et al: Prophylactic cholecystectomy with gastric bypass operation: Incidence of gallbladder disease. *Obes Surg* 12:350, 2002.

111. Hamad GG, Ikramuddin S, Gourash WF, Schauer PR: Elective cholecystectomy during laparoscopic Roux-en-Y gastric bypass: Is it worth the wait? *Obes Surg* 13:76, 2003.

112. Papavramidis S, et al: Laparoscopic cholecystectomy after bariatric surgery. *Surg Endosc* 2003.

113. Sugerman HJ, et al: A multicenter, placebo-controlled, randomized, double-blind, prospective trial of prophylactic ursodiol for the prevention of gallstone formation following gastric-bypass-induced rapid weight loss. *Am J Surg* 169:91, 1995; discussion 96.

114. Wudel LJ Jr., et al: Prevention of gallstone formation in morbidly obese patients undergoing rapid weight loss: Results of a randomized controlled pilot study. *J Surg Res* 102:50, 2002.

115. Fobi MA, Chicola K, Lee H: Access to the bypassed stomach after gastric bypass. *Obes Surg* 8:289, 1998.

116. Li AM, et al: The effects of obesity on pulmonary function. *Arch Dis Child* 88:361, 2003.

117. Li J, Li S, Feuers RJ, et al: Influence of body fat distribution on oxygen uptake and pulmonary performance in morbidly obese females during exercise. *Respirology* 6:9, 2001.

118. Kanoupakis E, et al: Left ventricular function and cardiopulmonary performance following surgical treatment of morbid obesity. *Obes Surg* 11:552, 2001.

119. Horwich TB, et al: The relationship between obesity and mortality in patients with heart failure. *J Am Coll Cardiol* 38:789, 2001.

120. Salvadori A, et al: Oxygen uptake and cardiac performance in obese and normal subjects during exercise. *Respiration* 66:25, 1999.

121. Lauer MS, Anderson KM, Levy D: Separate and joint influences of obesity and mild hypertension on left ventricular mass and geometry: The Framingham Heart Study. *J Am Coll Cardiol* 19:130, 1992.

122. Frohlich ED: Obesity and hypertension. Hemodynamic aspects. *Ann Epidemiol* 1:287, 1991.

123. Reisin E, et al: Cardiovascular changes after weight reduction in obesity hypertension. *Ann Intern Med* 98:315, 1983.

124. Flemons WW: Clinical practice. Obstructive sleep apnea. *N Engl J Med* 347:498, 2002.

125. Johns MW: A new method for measuring daytime sleepiness: The Epworth sleepiness scale. *Sleep* 14:540, 1991.

126. Maislin G, et al: A survey screen for prediction of apnea. *Sleep* 18:158, 1995.

127. Practice parameters for the indications for polysomnography and related procedures. Polysomnography Task Force, American Sleep Disorders Association Standards of Practice Committee. *Sleep* 20:406, 1997.

128. Rennotte MT, Baele P, Aubert G, Rodenstein DO: Nasal continuous positive airway pressure in the perioperative management of patients with obstructive sleep apnea submitted to surgery. *Chest* 107:367, 1995.

129. Ebeo CT, Benotti PN, Byrd RP Jr., et al: The effect of bi-level positive airway pressure on postoperative pulmonary function following gastric surgery for obesity. *Respir Med* 96:672, 2002.

130. Huerta S, et al: Safety and efficacy of postoperative continuous positive airway pressure to prevent pulmonary complications after Roux-en-Y gastric bypass. *J Gastrointest Surg* 6:354, 2002.

131. Benumof JL: Obstructive sleep apnea in the adult obese patient: Implications for airway management. *Anesthesiol Clin North Am* 20:789, 2002.

132. Cullen DJ: Obstructive sleep apnea and postoperative analgesia—a potentially dangerous combination. *J Clin Anesth* 13:83, 2001.

133. Lockwood T: Lower body lift with superficial fascial system suspension. *Plast Reconstr Surg* 92:1112, 1993; discussion 1123.

134. Van Geertruyden JP, et al: Circumferential torsoplasty. *Br J Plast Surg* 52:623, 1999.

135. Pascal JF, Le Louarn C: Remodeling bodylift with high lateral tension. *Aesthetic Plast Surg* 26:223, 2002.

136. Hurwitz DJ, Zewert T: Body contouring surgery in the bariatric surgical patient, in *Operative Techniques in Plastic Surgery and Reconstructive Surgery*. Philadelphia: Saunders, 2002, p 87.

137. Aly AS, et al: Belt lipectomy for circumferential truncal excess: The University of Iowa experience. *Plast Reconstr Surg* 111:398, 2003.

138. Hurwitz DJ, et al: Correction of saddlebag deformity in the massive weight loss patient with full thigh abduction. *Plast Reconst Surg* 2004 (In press).

139. Hurwitz DJ: Single stage total body lift after massive weight loss. *Ann Plast Surg* 52:435, 2004.

140. Zook EG: Abdominoplasty following gastrointestinal bypass surgery by savage RC. *Plast Reconstr Surg* 74:508, 1983.

141. Schauer PR, et al: Effect of laparoscopic Roux-en Y gastric bypass on type 2 diabetes mellitus. *Ann Surg* 238:467, 2003; discussion 84.

142. Perez AR, Moncure AC, Rattner DW: Obesity adversely affects the outcome of antireflux operations. *Surg Endosc* 15:986, 2001.

143. Frezza EE, et al: Symptomatic improvement in gastroesophageal reflux disease (GERD) following laparoscopic Roux-en-Y gastric bypass. *Surg Endosc* 16:1027, 2002.

CHAPTER 27

Small Intestine

Edward E. Whang, Stanley W. Ashley, and Michael J. Zinner

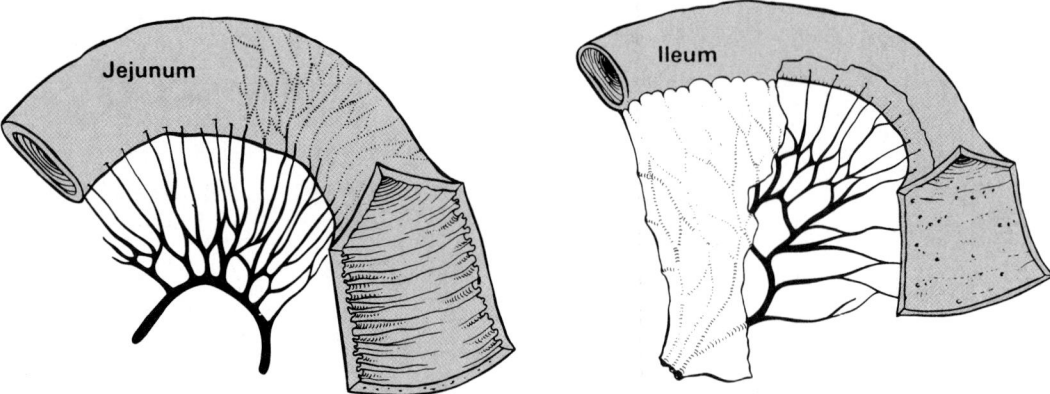

FIG. 27-1. *Gross features of jejunum contrasted with those of ileum. Relative to the ileum, the jejunum has a larger diameter, a thicker wall, more prominent plicae circulares, a less fatty mesentery, and longer vasa recta.*

The small intestine is the raison d'être of the gastrointestinal tract because it is the principal site of nutrient digestion and absorption.[1] The small intestine is also the body's largest reservoir of immunologically active and hormone-producing cells, and hence can be conceptualized as the largest organ of the immune and endocrine systems, respectively.

Recent scientific advances have led to new insights in intestinal physiology and pathophysiology. For example, the contributions of specific gene products to intestinal development, regeneration, and disease pathogenesis are being defined at an increasingly rapid rate. A peptide growth factor, glucagon-like peptide 2 (GLP-2), which has trophic activity specific for the intestinal epithelium, was previously characterized.[2] A signal transduction abnormality critical to the pathogenesis of gastrointestinal stromal tumors (GISTs) also was identified, facilitating the development of targeted therapy for this malignancy.[3,4]

Corresponding technologic advances include the increasingly prevalent application of minimally-invasive, and even robotic, surgical techniques in the therapy of intestinal disorders. Capsule enteroscopy—and with it the potential for the noninvasive visualization of the mucosa of the entire small intestine—also has been introduced.[5]

Despite these advances, the small intestine continues to pose formidable clinical and scientific challenges. For example, Crohn's disease is incurable and its etiology is unknown. Therapies for common conditions such as postoperative ileus are hardly more effective than those used at the dawn of the last century.[6] Mortality rates associated with acute mesenteric ischemia have not improved during the past 50 years.[7] Short bowel syndrome remains a devastating condition that continues to be approached with nihilism.

Furthermore, few high-quality, controlled data on the efficacy of surgical therapies for small-bowel diseases are available. In addition, for many of the diseases discussed in this chapter, currently available diagnostic tests lack sufficient predictive power to definitively guide clinical decision making for individual patients. Therefore, sound clinical judgment and a thorough understanding of anatomy, physiology, and pathophysiology remain essential to the care of patients with intestinal disorders.

GROSS ANATOMY

The small intestine is a tubular structure, with an estimated median length of 6 meters in adults, that consists of three segments lying in

series: the duodenum, the jejunum, and the ileum. The duodenum, the most proximal segment, lies in the retroperitoneum immediately adjacent to the head and inferior border of the body of the pancreas. The duodenum is demarcated from the stomach by the pylorus and from the jejunum by the ligament of Treitz. The jejunum and ileum lie within the peritoneal cavity and are tethered to the retroperitoneum by a broad-based mesentery. No distinct anatomic landmark demarcates the jejunum from the ileum; the proximal 40% of the jejunoileal segment is arbitrarily defined as the jejunum and the distal 60% as the ileum. The ileum is demarcated from the cecum by the ileocecal valve.

The small intestine contains mucosal folds known as *plicae circulares* or *valvulae conniventes* that are visible upon gross inspection. These folds are also visible radiographically and help to distinguish between small intestine and colon (which does not contain them) on abdominal radiographs. These folds are more prominent in the proximal intestine than in the distal small intestine. Other features evident on gross inspection that are more characteristic of the proximal than distal small intestine include larger circumference, thicker wall, less fatty mesentery, and longer vasa recta (Fig. 27-1). Gross examination of the small-intestinal mucosa also reveals aggregates of lymphoid follicles. Those follicles, located in the ileum, are the most prominent and are designated *Peyer's patches.*

Most of the duodenum derives its arterial blood from branches of both the celiac and the superior mesenteric arteries. The distal duodenum, the jejunum, and the ileum derive their arterial blood from the superior mesenteric artery. Their venous drainage occurs via the superior mesenteric vein. Lymph drainage occurs through lymphatic vessels coursing parallel to corresponding arteries. This lymph drains through mesenteric lymph nodes to the cisterna chyli, then through the thoracic duct, and ultimately into the left subclavian vein. The parasympathetic and sympathetic innervation of the small intestine is derived from the vagus and splanchnic nerves, respectively.

HISTOLOGY

The wall of the small intestine consists of four distinct layers: mucosa, submucosa, muscularis propria, and serosa (Figs. 27-2 and 27-3).

The mucosa is the innermost layer, which consists of three layers: epithelium, lamina propria, and muscularis mucosae. The epithelium is exposed to the intestinal lumen and is the surface through

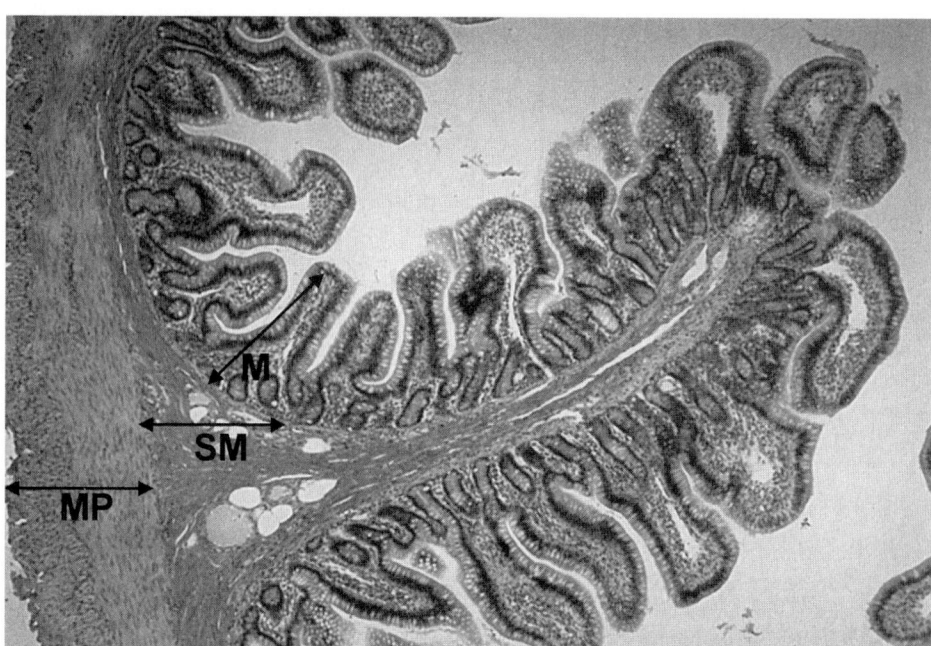

FIG. 27-2. Small intestine: histologic section. The muscularis propria (*MP*), submucosa (*SM*), and mucosa (*M*) are labeled. This section shows a fold of mucosa and underlying submucosa projecting to the upper right corner of the image. These folds, known as plicae circulares or valvulae conniventes, are grossly visible.

which absorption from and secretion into the lumen occurs. The lamina propria is located immediately external to the epithelium and consists of connective tissue and a heterogeneous population of cells. It is demarcated from the more external submucosa by the muscularis mucosae, a thin sheet of smooth-muscle cells.

The mucosa is organized into villi and crypts (crypts of Lieberkühn). *Villi* are finger-like projections of epithelium and underlying lamina propria that contain blood and lymphatic (lacteals) vessels that extend into the intestinal lumen. Intestinal, epithelial cellular proliferation is confined to the *crypts,* each of which carries an average census of 250 to 300 cells. All epithelial cells in each crypt

are derived from an unknown number of the yet uncharacterized multipotent stem cells located at or near the crypt's base. Their immediate descendants are amplified by undergoing several cycles of rapid division. These descendants then make a commitment to differentiate along one of four pathways that ultimately yield enterocytes and goblet, enteroendocrine, and Paneth cells. With the exception of Paneth cells, these lineages complete their terminal differentiation during an upward migration from each crypt to adjacent villi. The journey from the crypt to the villus tip is completed in 2 to 5 days and terminates with cells being removed by apoptosis and/or exfoliation. Thus, the small-intestinal epithelium undergoes continuous

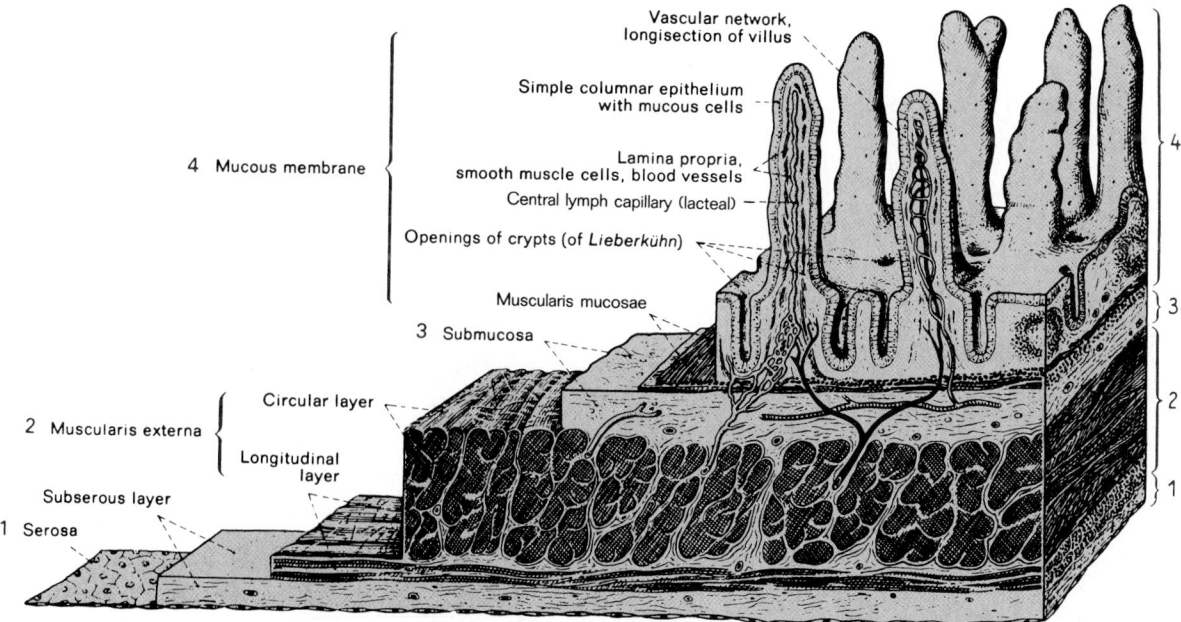

FIG. 27-3. Layers of wall of the small intestine. The individual layers and their prominent features are represented schematically.

renewal, making it one of the body's most dynamic tissues. The high cellular turnover rate contributes to mucosal resiliency, but also makes the intestine uniquely susceptible to certain forms of injury, such as that induced by radiation.

Enterocytes are the predominant absorptive cell of the intestinal epithelium. Their apical (lumen-facing) cell membrane contains specialized digestive enzymes, transporter mechanisms, and microvilli that are estimated to increase the absorptive surface area of the small intestine by up to 40-fold. *Goblet cells* produce mucin believed to play a role in mucosal defense against pathogens. *Enteroendocrine cells* are characterized by secretory granules containing regulatory agents and are discussed in greater detail later under "Endocrine Function." *Paneth cells* are located at the base of the crypt and contain secretory granules containing growth factors, digestive enzymes, and antimicrobial peptides. In addition, the intestinal epithelium contains M cells and intraepithelial lymphocytes. These two components of the immune system are discussed below.

The submucosa consists of dense connective tissue and a heterogeneous population of cells, including leukocytes and fibroblasts. The submucosa also contains an extensive network of vascular and lymphatic vessels, nerve fibers, and ganglion cells of the submucosal (Meissner's) plexus.

The muscularis propria consists of an outer, longitudinally oriented layer and an inner, circularly oriented layer of smooth-muscle fibers. Located at the interface between these two layers are ganglion cells of the myenteric (Auerbach's) plexus.

The serosa consists of a single layer of mesothelial cells and is a component of the visceral peritoneum.

DEVELOPMENT

The first recognizable precursor of the small intestine is the embryonic gut tube, formed from the endoderm during the fourth week of gestation. The gut tube initially communicates with the yolk sac; however, the communication between these two structures narrows by the sixth week to form the vitelline duct. The yolk sac and vitelline duct usually undergo obliteration by the end of gestation. Incomplete obliteration of the vitelline duct results in the spectrum of defects associated with Meckel's diverticula.

Also during the fourth week of gestation, the mesoderm of the embryo splits. The portion of mesoderm that adheres to the endoderm forms the visceral peritoneum, while the portion that adheres to the ectoderm forms the parietal peritoneum. This mesodermal division results in the formation of a coelomic cavity that is the precursor of the peritoneal cavity.

At approximately the fifth week of gestation, the bowel begins to lengthen to an extent greater than that which can be accommodated by the developing abdominal cavity, resulting in the extracoelomic herniation of the developing bowel. The bowel continues to lengthen during the subsequent weeks and is retracted back into the abdominal cavity during the tenth week of gestation. Subsequently, the duodenum becomes a retroperitoneal structure. Coincident with extrusion and retraction, the bowel undergoes a 270-degree counterclockwise rotation relative to the posterior abdominal wall. This rotation accounts for the usual locations of the cecum in the right lower quadrant and the duodenojejunal junction to the left of midline (Fig. 27-4).

The celiac and superior mesenteric arteries and veins are derived from the vitelline vascular system, which, in turn, is derived

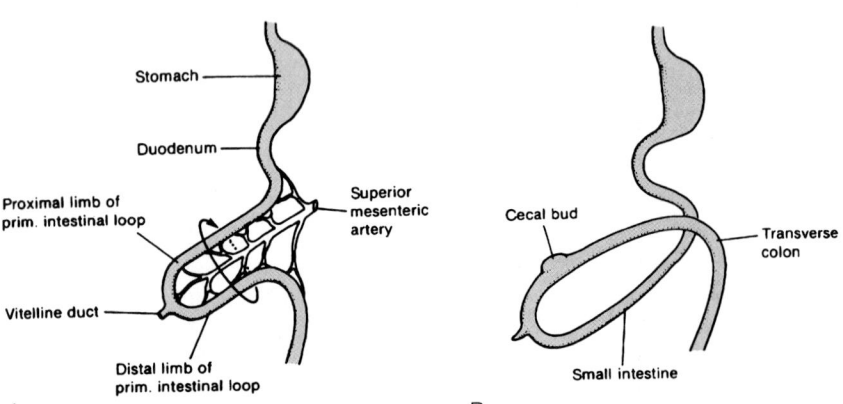

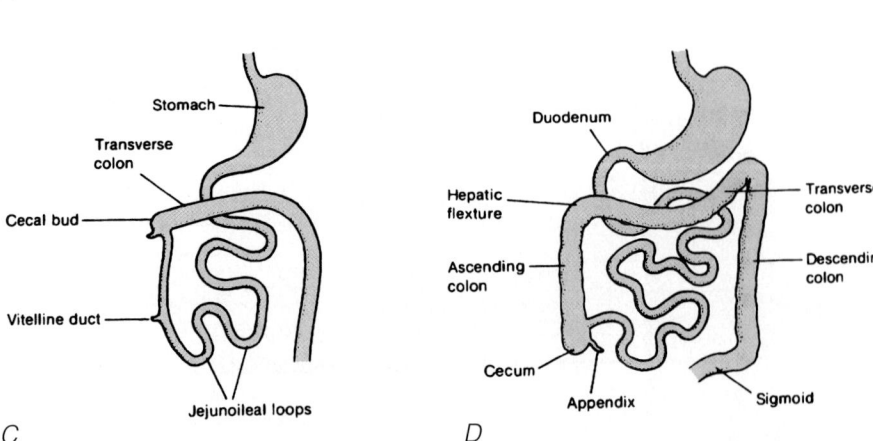

FIG. 27-4. Developmental rotation of the intestine. *A.* During the fifth week of gestation, the developing intestine herniates out of the coelomic cavity and begins to undergo a counterclockwise rotation about the axis of the superior mesenteric artery. *B* and *C.* Intestinal rotation continues, as the developing transverse colon passes anterior to the developing duodenum. *D.* Final positions of the small intestine and colon resulting from a 270-degree counterclockwise rotation of the developing intestine and its return into the abdominal cavity.

from blood vessels formed within the splanchnopleuric mesoderm during the third week of gestation. Neurons found in the small intestine are derived from neural crest cells that begin to migrate away from the neural tube during the third week of gestation. These neural crest cells enter the mesenchyme of the primitive foregut and subsequently migrate to the remainder of the bowel.

During the sixth week of gestation, the lumen of the developing bowel becomes obliterated as bowel epithelial proliferation accelerates. Vacuoles form within the bowel substance during the subsequent weeks and coalesce to form the intestinal lumen by the ninth week of gestation. Errors in this recanalization may account for defects such as intestinal webs and stenoses. Most intestinal atresias, however, are believed to be related to ischemic episodes occurring after organogenesis has been completed rather than to errors in recanalization.

During the ninth week of gestation, the intestinal epithelium develops intestine-specific features such as crypt-villus architecture. Organogenesis is complete by approximately the twelfth week of gestation.

Elucidation of the fundamental mechanisms regulating patterned intestinal development is an area of active investigation. For example, the roles played by products of specific genes, such as homeodomain-containing transcription factors encoded by *Hox* genes, in specific components of intestinal organogenesis are beginning to be defined.[8]

PHYSIOLOGY

Digestion and Absorption

The intestinal epithelium is the interface through which absorption and secretion occur. It has features characteristic of absorptive epithelia in general, including epithelial cells with cellular membranes possessing distinct apical (luminal) and basolateral (serosal) domains demarcated by intercellular tight junctions and an asymmetric distribution of transmembrane transporter mechanisms that promotes vectorial transport of solutes across the epithelium.

Solutes can traverse the epithelium by active or passive transport. Passive transport of solutes occurs through diffusion or convection and is driven by existing electrochemical gradients. *Active transport* is the energy-dependent net transfer of solutes in the absence of or against an electrochemical gradient.

Active transport occurs through transcellular pathways (through the cell), whereas passive transport can occur through either transcellular or paracellular pathways (between cells through the tight junctions). Transcellular transport requires solutes to traverse the cell membranes through specialized membrane proteins, such as channels, carriers, and pumps. The molecular characterization of transporter proteins is evolving rapidly. The Human Gene Nomenclature Database already includes over 35 different transporter families, each containing many individual genes encoding specific transporters.[9] Similarly, understanding of the paracellular pathway is evolving. In contrast to what was once believed, it is becoming apparent that paracellular permeability is substrate-specific, dynamic, and subject to regulation by specific tight junction proteins.[10]

Water and Electrolyte Absorption and Secretion

Eight to 9 L of fluid enter the small intestine daily. Most of this volume consists of salivary, gastric, biliary, pancreatic, and intestinal secretions. Under normal conditions, the small intestine absorbs more than 80% of this fluid, leaving approximately 1.5 L that enters the colon (Fig. 27-5). Small-intestinal absorption and secretion are

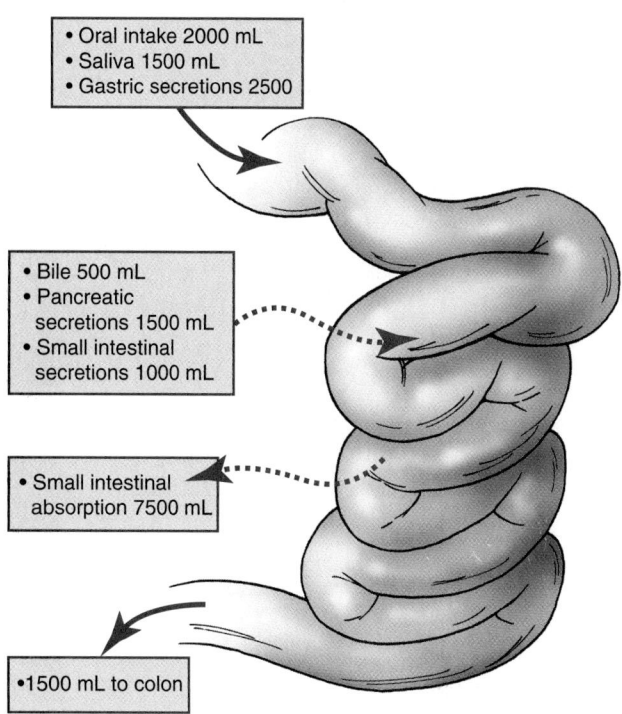

FIG. 27-5. Small-intestinal water transport. Typical quantities (in volume per day) of fluid entering and leaving the small intestinal lumen in a healthy adult are given.

tightly regulated; derangements in water and electrolyte homeostasis characteristic of many of the disorders discussed in this chapter play an important role in contributing to their associated clinical features.

Water absorption is believed to be driven by osmotic gradients created primarily by active transepithelial Na^+ absorption. Intestinal water secretion, in contrast, is believed to be driven by osmotic gradients created primarily by transepithelial Cl^- secretion. Most intestinal water transport is believed to occur through the transcellular pathway.[11] The specific transport mechanisms mediating water absorption are incompletely characterized. Aquaporins (water channels) are expressed in the intestinal epithelium; however, their contribution to overall intestinal water absorption appears to be relatively minor.[12]

Figure 27-6 shows the prevailing model for intestinal epithelial Na^+ absorption. Activity of the Na^+/K^+ ATPase enzyme, which is located in the basolateral membrane and exchanges three intracellular Na^+ for every two extracellular K^+ in an energy-dependent process, generates the electrochemical gradient that drives the transport of Na^+ from the intestinal lumen into the cytoplasm of enterocytes. Na^+ ions traverse the apical membrane through several distinct transporter mechanisms including nutrient-coupled sodium transport (e.g., sodium glucose cotransporter-1, SGLT1), sodium channels, and sodium-hydrogen exchangers (NHEs). Absorbed Na^+ ions are then extruded from enterocytes through the Na^+/K^+ ATPase located in the basolateral membrane. Similar mechanistic models that account for the transport of other common ions such as K^+ and HCO_3^- also exist.

Substantial heterogeneity, with respect to both crypt-villus and craniocaudal axes, exist for intestinal epithelial transport mechanisms. For example, nutrient-coupled Na^+ transporters are expressed in mature villus cells, but are absent in crypt cells. In contrast, the cystic fibrosis transmembrane regulator (CFTR, a chloride channel) is expressed to a greater extent in crypt cells. This spatial

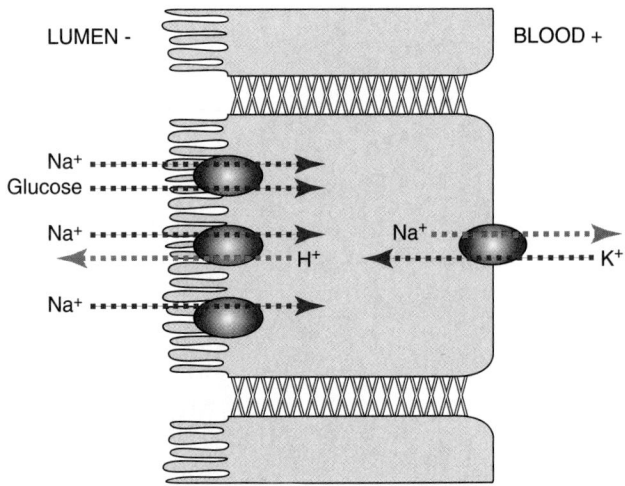

FIG. 27-6. *Model of transepithelial Na⁺ absorption. In the prevailing model, Na⁺ traverses the apical membrane of enterocytes through a variety of mechanisms, including nutrient-coupled Na⁺ transport, Na⁺/H⁺ exchange, and Na⁺ channels. Activity of the Na⁺/K⁺ ATPase located on the basolateral membrane generates the electrochemical gradient that provides the driving force for Na⁺ absorption.*

distribution of expression is consistent with a model in which absorptive function resides primarily in the villus and secretory function in the crypt.

Intestinal absorption and secretion are subject to modulation under physiologic and pathophysiologic conditions by a wide array of hormonal, neural, and immune regulatory mediators (Table 27-1).

Carbohydrate Digestion and Absorption

Approximately 45% of energy consumption in the average Western diet consists of carbohydrates, approximately half of which is in the form of starch (linear or branched polymers of glucose) derived from cereals and plants. Other major sources of dietary carbohydrates include sugars derived from milk (lactose), fruits, and

Table 27-1
Regulation of Intestinal Absorption and Secretion

Agents that stimulate absorption or inhibit secretion of water
  Aldosterone
  Glucocorticoids
  Angiotensin
  Norepinephrine
  Epinephrine
  Dopamine
  Somatostatin
  Neuropeptide Y
  Peptide YY
  Enkephalin
Agents that simulate secretion or inhibit absorption of water
  Secretin
  Bradykinin
  Prostaglandins
  Acetylcholine
  Atrial natriuretic factor
  Vasopressin
  Vasoactive intestinal peptide
  Bombesin
  Substance P
  Serotonin
  Neurotensin
  Histamine

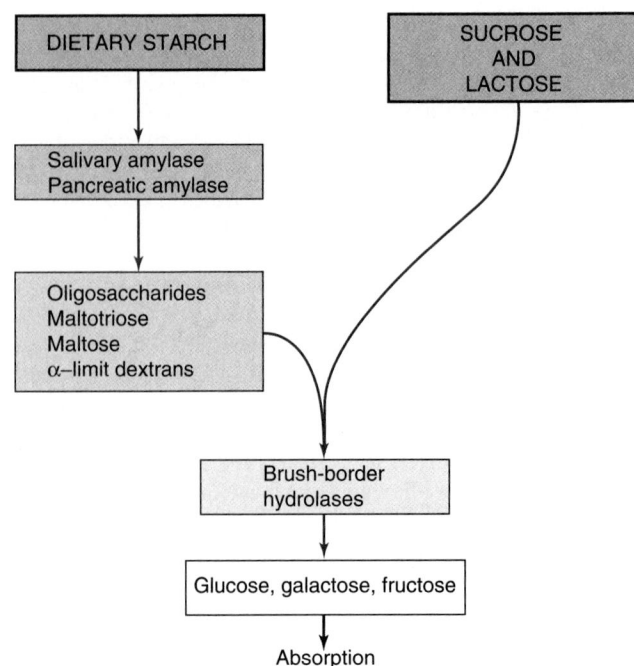

FIG. 27-7. *Carbohydrate digestion. Dietary carbohydrates, including starch and the disaccharides sucrose and lactose, must undergo hydrolysis into constituent monosaccharides glucose, galactose, and fructose before being absorbed by the intestinal epithelium. These hydrolytic reactions are catalyzed by salivary and pancreatic amylase and by enterocyte brush-border hydrolases.*

vegetables (fructose, glucose, and sucrose), or purified from sugar cane or beets (sucrose). Processed foods contain a variety of sugars, including fructose, oligosaccharides, and polysaccharides. Glycogen derived from meat contributes only a small fraction of dietary carbohydrate.

Pancreatic amylase is the major enzyme of starch digestion, although salivary amylase initiates the process. The terminal products of amylase-mediated starch digestion are oligosaccharides, maltotriose, maltose, and alpha-limit dextrins (Fig. 27-7). These products, as well as the major disaccharides in the diet (sucrose and lactose), are unable to undergo absorption in their intact forms. They must first undergo hydrolytic cleavage into their constituent monosaccharides; these hydrolytic reactions are catalyzed by specific brush-border membrane hydrolases that are expressed most abundantly in the villi of the duodenum and jejunum. The three major monosaccharides that represent the terminal products of carbohydrate digestion are glucose, galactose, and fructose.

Under physiologic conditions, most of these sugars are absorbed through the epithelium via the transcellular route. Glucose and galactose are transported through the enterocyte brush-border membrane via SGLT1 (Fig. 27-8). Fructose is transported through the brush-border membrane by facilitated diffusion via GLUT5 (a member of the facilitative glucose transporter family). All three monosaccharides are extruded through the basolateral membrane by facilitated diffusion. Extruded monosaccharides diffuse into venules and ultimately enter the portal venous system.

Protein Digestion and Absorption

Ten to 15% of energy consumption in the average Western diet consists of proteins. In addition to dietary proteins, approximately half of the protein load that enters the small intestine is derived from endogenous sources, including salivary and gastrointestinal

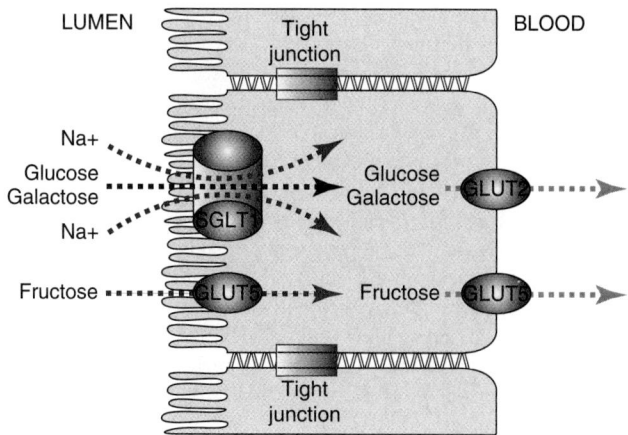

FIG. 27-8. *Glucose transporters. Glucose and galactose enter the enterocyte through secondary active transport via the sodium-glucose cotransporter (SGLT1) located on the apical (brush-border) membrane. Fructose enters through facilitated diffusion via glucose transporter 5 (GLUT5). Glucose and galactose are extruded basolaterally through facilitated diffusion via glucose transporter 2 (GLUT2). Fructose is extruded basolaterally via GLUT5.*

secretions and desquamated intestinal epithelial cells. Protein digestion begins in the stomach with the action of pepsins. Digestion continues in the duodenum with the actions of a variety of pancreatic peptidases. These enzymes are secreted as inactive proenzymes; this is in contrast to pancreatic amylase and lipase, which are secreted in their active forms. In response to the presence of bile acids, enterokinase is liberated from the intestinal brush border membrane to catalyze the conversion of trypsinogen to active trypsin; trypsin, in turn, activates itself and other proteases. The final products of intraluminal protein digestion consist of neutral and basic amino acids and peptides two to six amino acids in length (Fig. 27-9). Additional digestion occurs through the actions of peptidases that exist in the enterocyte brush border and cytoplasm. Epithelial absorption occurs for both single amino acids and di- or tripeptides via specific membrane-bound transporters. Absorbed amino acids and peptides then enter the portal venous circulation.

Of all amino acids, glutamine appears to be a unique, major source of energy for enterocytes. Active glutamine uptake into enterocytes occurs through both apical and basolateral transport mechanisms.

Fat Digestion and Absorption

Approximately 40% of the average Western diet consists of fat. More than 95% of dietary fat is in the form of long-chain triglycerides; the remainder includes phospholipids such as lecithin, fatty acids, cholesterol, and fat-soluble vitamins.

Ingested fat is converted into an emulsion by the mechanical actions of mastication and antral peristalsis. Although lipolysis of triglycerides to form fatty acids and monoglycerides is initiated in the stomach by gastric lipase, its principal site is the proximal intestine, where pancreatic lipase is the catalyst (Fig. 27-10).

Bile acids act as detergents by forming mixed micelles with the products of lipolysis to aid in their solubilization in water. These micelles are polymolecular aggregates, containing a hydrophobic core and a hydrophilic surface that act as shuttles, delivering the products of lipolysis to the enterocyte brush border membrane.

Dissociation of lipids from the micelles occurs in a thin layer of water (50 to 500 µm thick) with an acidic microenvironment immediately adjacent to the brush border called the *unstirred water layer.*

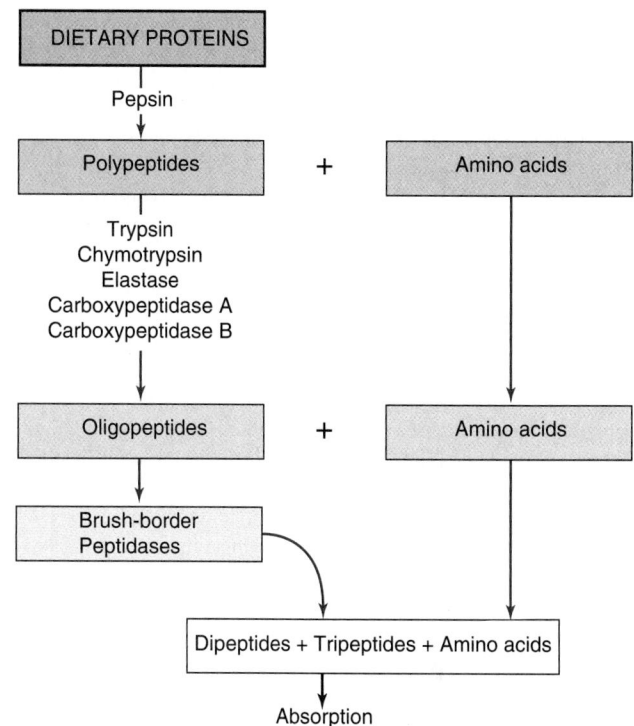

FIG. 27-9. *Protein digestion. Dietary proteins must undergo hydrolysis into constituent single amino acids and di- and tripeptides before being absorbed by the intestinal epithelium. These hydrolytic reactions are catalyzed by pancreatic peptidases (e.g., trypsin) and by enterocyte brush-border peptidases.*

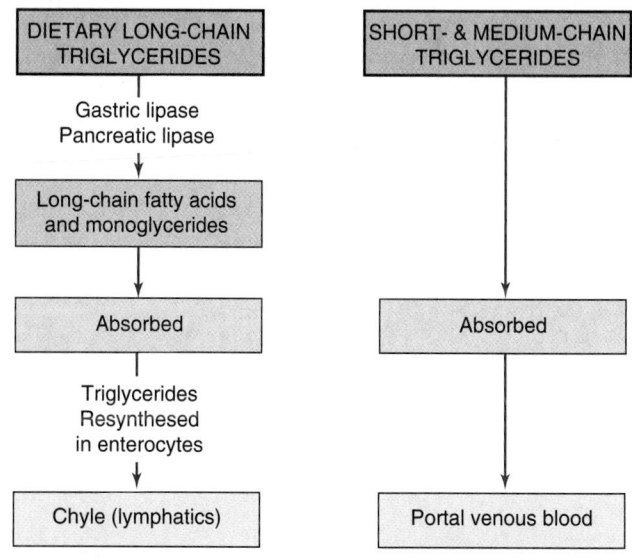

FIG. 27-10. *Fat digestion. Long-chain triglycerides, which constitute the majority of dietary fats, must undergo lipolysis into constituent long-chain fatty acids and monoglycerides before being absorbed by the intestinal epithelium. These reactions are catalyzed by gastric and pancreatic lipases. The products of lipolysis are transported in the form of mixed micelles to enterocytes, where they are resynthesized into triglycerides, which are then packaged in the form of chylomicrons that are secreted into the intestinal lymph (chyle). Triglycerides composed of short- and medium-chain fatty acids are absorbed by the intestinal epithelium directly, without undergoing lipolysis, and are secreted into the portal venous circulation.*

Most lipids are absorbed in the proximal jejunum, whereas bile salts are absorbed in the distal ileum through an active process. Fatty acid binding protein (FABP), a protein located in the brush-border membrane, facilitates diffusion of long-chain fatty acids across the brush-border membrane. Cholesterol crosses the brush-border membrane through an active process that is yet to be completely characterized. Within the enterocytes, triglycerides are resynthesized and incorporated into chylomicrons that are secreted into the intestinal lymphatics and ultimately enter the thoracic duct. In these chylomicrons, lipoproteins serve a detergent-like role similar to that served by bile salts in the mixed micelles.

The steps described above are required for the digestion and absorption of triglycerides containing long-chain fatty acids. However, triglycerides containing short- and medium-chain fatty acids are more hydrophilic and are absorbed without undergoing intraluminal hydrolysis, micellular solubilization, mucosal re-esterification, and chylomicron formation. Instead, they are directly absorbed and enter the portal venous circulation rather than the lymphatics. This information provides the rationale for administering nutritional supplements containing medium-chain triglycerides to patients with gastrointestinal diseases associated with impaired digestion and/or malabsorption of long-chain triglycerides.

Vitamin and Mineral Absorption

Vitamin B_{12} (cobalamin) malabsorption can result from a variety of surgical manipulations. The vitamin is initially bound by saliva-derived R protein. In the duodenum, R protein is hydrolyzed by pancreatic enzymes, allowing free cobalamin to bind to gastric parietal cell-derived intrinsic factor. The cobalamin-intrinsic factor complex is able to escape hydrolysis by pancreatic enzymes, allowing it to reach the terminal ileum, which expresses specific receptors for intrinsic factor. Subsequent events in cobalamin absorption are poorly characterized, but the intact complex probably enters enterocytes through translocation. Because each of these steps is necessary for cobalamin assimilation, gastric resection, gastric bypass, and ileal resection can each result in vitamin B_{12} insufficiency.

Other water-soluble vitamins for which specific carrier-mediated transport processes have been characterized include ascorbic acid, folate, thiamine, riboflavin, pantothenic acid, and biotin. Fat-soluble vitamins A, D, and E appear to be absorbed through passive diffusion. Vitamin K appears to be absorbed through both passive diffusion and carrier-mediated uptake.

Calcium is absorbed through both transcellular transport and paracellular diffusion. The duodenum is the major site for transcellular transport; paracellular transport occurs throughout the small intestine. A key step in transcellular calcium transport is mediated by calbindin, a calcium-binding protein located in the cytoplasm of enterocytes. Regulation of calbindin synthesis is the principal mechanism by which vitamin D regulates intestinal calcium absorption.

Iron and magnesium are each absorbed through both transcellular and paracellular routes. A divalent metal transporter capable of transporting Fe^{2+}, Zn^{2+}, Mn^{2+}, Co^{2+}, Cd^{2+}, Cu^{2+}, Ni^{2+}, and Pb^{2+} that was recently localized to the intestinal brush border may account for at least a portion of the transcellular absorption of these ions.[13]

Barrier and Immune Function

Although the intestinal epithelium allows for the efficient absorption of dietary nutrients, it must discriminate between pathogens and harmless antigens, such as food proteins and commensal bacteria, and it must resist invasion by pathogens. Factors contributing to epithelial defense include immunoglobulin A (IgA), mucins, and the relative impermeability of the brush border membrane and tight junctions to macromolecules and bacteria. Recently described factors likely to play important roles in intestinal mucosal defense include antimicrobial peptides such as the defensins.[14] The intestinal component of the immune system, known as the gut-associated lymphoid tissue (GALT), contains more than 70% of the body's immune cells.

The GALT is conceptually divided into inductive and effector sites.[15] Inductive sites include Peyer's patches, mesenteric lymph nodes, and smaller, isolated lymphoid follicles scattered throughout the small intestine (Fig. 27-11). Peyer's patches are macroscopic aggregates of B-cell follicles and intervening T-cell areas found in the lamina propria of the small intestine, primarily the distal ileum. Overlying Peyer's patches is a specialized epithelium containing microfold (M) cells. These cells possess an apical membrane with microfolds rather than microvilli, which is characteristic of most intestinal epithelial cells. Using transepithelial vesicular transport, M cells transfer microbes to underlying professional antigen-presenting cells (APCs), such as dendritic cells. Dendritic cells,

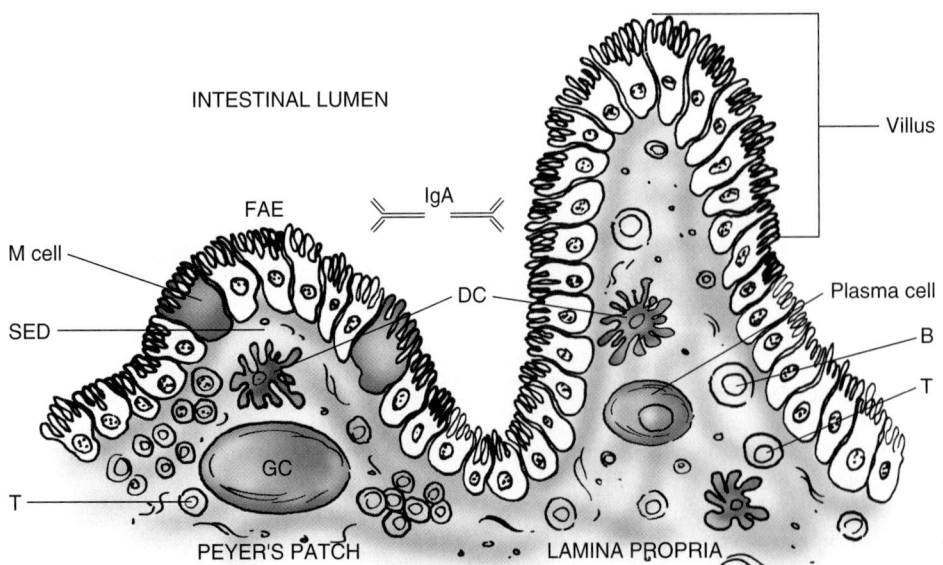

FIG. 27-11. Gut-associated lymphoid tissue (GALT). Select components of the GALT are schematically represented. Peyer's patches consist of a specialized follicle-associated epithelium (FAE) containing M cells, a subepithelial dome (SED) rich in dendritic cells, and B-cell follicle-containing germinal centers (GC). Plasma cells in the lamina propria produce IgA, which is transported to the intestinal lumen where it serves as the first line of defense against pathogens. Other components of the GALT include isolated lymphoid follicles, mesenteric lymph nodes, and regulatory and effector lymphocytes.

INTESTINAL LUMEN

FAE

IgA

M cell

SED

DC

GC

T

PEYER'S PATCH

LAMINA PROPRIA

Villus

Plasma cell

B

T

in addition, may sample luminal antigens directly through their dendrite-like processes that extend through epithelial tight junctions. APCs interact with and prime naïve lymphocytes, which then exit through the draining lymphatics to enter the mesenteric lymph nodes where they undergo differentiation. These lymphocytes then migrate into the systemic circulation via the thoracic duct, and ultimately accumulate in the intestinal mucosa at effector sites. Alternative induction mechanisms, such as antigen presentation within mesenteric lymph nodes, are also likely to exist.

Effector lymphocytes are distributed into distinct compartments. IgA-producing plasma cells are derived from B cells and are located in the lamina propria. CD4+ T cells also are located in the lamina propria. CD8+ T cells migrate preferentially to the epithelium, but also are found in the lamina propria. These T cells are central to immune regulation; in addition, the CD8+ T cells have potent cytotoxic activity. IgA is transported through the intestinal epithelial cells into the lumen, where it exists in the form of a dimer complexed with a secretory component. This configuration renders IgA resistant to proteolysis by digestive enzymes. IgA is believed to both help prevent the entry of microbes through the epithelium and to promote excretion of antigens or microbes that have already penetrated into the laminal propria.

Ineffective resistance to invasion by pathogens is hypothesized to play an etiologic role in sepsis by allowing translocation of bacteria and/or toxins into the systemic circulation. In contrast, overexuberant immune sensitivity or lack of tolerance to dietary antigens or commensal bacteria is believed to contribute to the pathogenesis of chronic inflammatory disorders such as celiac disease and Crohn's disease.[15]

Motility

Myocytes of the intestinal muscle layers are electrically and mechanically coordinated in the form of syncytia. Contractions of the muscularis propria are responsible for small-intestinal peristalsis. Contraction of the outer longitudinal muscle layer results in bowel shortening; contraction of the inner circular layer results in luminal narrowing. Contractions of the muscularis mucosae contribute to mucosal or villus motility, but not to peristalsis.

Several distinctive patterns of muscularis propria activity have been observed to occur in the small intestine. These patterns include *ascending excitation and descending inhibition* in which muscular contraction occurs proximal to a stimulus, such as the presence of a bolus of ingested food, and muscular relaxation occurs distal to the stimulus (Fig. 27-12). These two reflexes are present even in the absence of any extrinsic innervation to the small intestine and contribute to peristalsis when they are propagated in a coordinated fashion along the length of the intestine. The *fed* or *postprandial pattern* begins within 10 to 20 minutes of meal ingestion and abates 4 to 6 hours afterwards. *Rhythmic segmentations* or pressure waves traveling only short distances also are observed. This segmenting pattern is hypothesized to assist in mixing intraluminal contents and in facilitating their contact with the absorptive mucosal surface. The *fasting pattern* or *interdigestive motor cycle (IDMC)* consists of three phases: Phase I is characterized by motor quiescence; phase II by seemingly disorganized pressure waves occurring at submaximal rates; and phase III by sustained pressure waves occurring at maximal rates. This pattern is hypothesized to expel residual debris and bacteria from the small intestine. The median duration of the IDMC ranges from 90 to 120 minutes. At any given time, different portions of the small intestine can be in different phases of the IDMC.

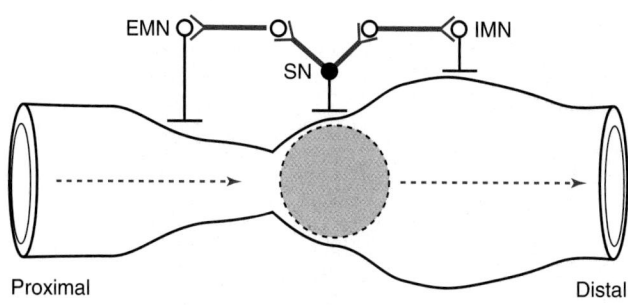

FIG. 27-12. *Ascending excitation and descending inhibition. The presence of a food bolus within the intestinal lumen is sensed by a sensory neuron (SN) that relays signals to (1) excitatory motor neurons (EMN) that have projections to intestinal muscle cells located proximal to the food bolus and (2) inhibitory motor neurons (IMN) that have projections to intestinal muscle cells located distal to the food bolus. This stereotypical motor reflex is controlled by the enteric nervous system and occurs in the absence of extra-intestinal innervation. It contributes to peristalsis.*

The regulatory mechanisms driving small-intestinal motility consist of both pacemakers intrinsic to the small intestine and external neurohumoral modulatory signals. The interstitial cells of Cajal are pleomorphic mesenchymal cells located within the muscularis propria of the intestine that generate the electrical slow wave (basic electrical rhythm or pacesetter potential) that plays a pacemaker role in setting the fundamental rhythmicity of small-intestinal contractions. The frequency of the slow wave varies along the longitudinal axis of the intestine: it ranges from 12 waves per minute in the duodenum to 7 waves per minute in the distal ileum. Smooth-muscle contraction occurs only when an electrical action potential (spike burst) is superimposed on the slow wave. Thus, the slow wave determines the maximum frequency of contractions; however, not every slow wave is associated with a contraction.

This intrinsic contractile mechanism is subject to neural and hormonal regulation. The enteric motor system provides both inhibitory and excitatory stimuli. The predominant excitatory transmitters are acetylcholine and substance P, and the inhibitory transmitters include nitric oxide, vasoactive intestinal peptide, and adenosine triphosphate. In general, the sympathetic motor supply is inhibitory to the enteric motor system; therefore, increased sympathetic input into the intestine leads to decreased intestinal smooth-muscle activity. The parasympathetic motor supply is more complex, with projections to both inhibitory and excitatory enteric motor system motor neurons. Correspondingly, the effects of parasympathetic inputs into intestinal motility are more difficult to predict.

Endocrine Function

Endocrinology as a discipline was born with the discovery of secretin, an intestinal regulatory peptide that was the first hormone to be identified. The small intestine is now recognized to be the largest hormone-producing organ in the body, both with respect to the number of hormone-producing cells and the number of individual hormones produced.[16] More than 30 peptide hormone genes have been identified as being expressed in the gastrointestinal tract. Because of differential posttranscriptional and posttranslational processing, more than 100 distinct regulatory peptides are produced. In addition, monoamines, such as histamine and dopamine, and eicosanoids with hormone-like activities are produced in the intestine.

"Gut hormones" were previously conceptualized as peptides produced by the enteroendocrine cells of the intestinal mucosa that are released into the systemic circulation to reach receptors in target

Table 27-2
Representative Regulatory Peptides Produced in the Small Intestine

Hormone	Source[a]	Actions
Somatostatin	D cell	Inhibits gastrointestinal secretion, motility, and splanchnic perfusion
Secretin	S cell	Stimulates exocrine pancreatic secretion; stimulates intestinal secretion
Cholecystokinin	I cell	Stimulates pancreatic exocrine secretion; simulates gallbladder emptying; inhibits sphincter of Oddi contraction
Motilin	M cell	Stimulates intestinal motility
Peptide YY	L cell	Inhibits intestinal motility and secretion
Glucagon-like peptide 2	L cell	Stimulates intestinal epithelial proliferation
Neurotensin	N cell	Stimulates pancreatic and biliary secretion; inhibits small bowel motility; stimulates intestinal mucosal growth

[a]This table indicates which enteroendocrine cell types located in the intestinal epithelium produce these peptides. These peptides are also widely expressed in nonintestinal tissues.

sites in the gastrointestinal tract. Now it is clear that "gut hormone" genes are widely expressed throughout the body, not only in endocrine cells, but also in central and peripheral neurons.[17] The products of these genes are general intercellular messengers that can act as endocrine, paracrine, autocrine, or neurocrine mediators. Thus, they may act as true blood-borne hormones, as well as through local effects.

There are notable homology patterns among individual regulatory peptides found in the gastrointestinal tract. Based on these homologies, approximately half of the known regulatory peptides can be classified into families.[17] For example, the secretin family includes secretin, glucagon, and glucagon-like peptides, gastric inhibitory peptide, vasoactive intestinal polypeptide, peptide histidine isoleucine, growth hormone-releasing hormone, and pituitary adenylyl cyclase-activating peptide. Other peptide families include those named for insulin, epidermal growth factor, gastrin, pancreatic polypeptide, tachykinin, and somatostatin.

Receptor subtype multiplicity and cell-specific expression patterns for these receptor subtypes that are characteristic of these regulatory mediators make definition of their actions complex. Detailed description of these actions is beyond the scope of this chapter; however, Table 27-2 summarizes examples of regulatory peptides produced by enteroendocrine cells of the small-intestinal epithelium and their most commonly ascribed functions. Some of these peptides, or their analogues, are used in routine clinical practice.[18] For example, therapeutic applications of octreotide, a long-acting analogue of somatostatin, include the amelioration of symptoms associated with neuroendocrine tumors (e.g., carcinoid syndrome), postgastrectomy dumping syndrome, enterocutaneous fistulas, and the initial treatment of acute hemorrhage caused by esophageal varices. The gastrin secretory response to secretin administration forms the basis for the standard test used to establish the diagnosis of Zollinger-Ellison syndrome. Cholecystokinin is used in evaluations of gallbladder ejection fraction, a parameter that may have utility in patients who have symptoms of biliary colic but are not found to have gallstones. Of the peptides listed in Table 27-2, GLP-2 is the most recently characterized (Fig. 27-13). This product of the proglucagon gene has potent trophic activity that is specific for the intestinal epithelium. GLP-2 both stimulates cellular proliferation and inhibits apoptosis in the intestinal epithelium. It has been demonstrated to induce intestinal regeneration and promote healing in numerous experimental models of intestinal disease. It is currently under clinical evaluation as an intestinotrophic agent in patients suffering from the short bowel syndrome, as discussed later under "Short-Bowel Syndrome."

Intestinal Adaptation

The small intestine has the capacity to adapt in response to varying demands imposed by physiologic and pathologic conditions. Of particular relevance to many of the diseases discussed in this chapter is the adaptation that occurs in the remnant intestine following surgical resection of a large portion of the small intestine (massive small-bowel resection). Postresection intestinal adaptation has been studied extensively using animal models. Within 24 to 48 hours after bowel resection, the remnant small intestine displays evidence of epithelial cellular hyperplasia; however, changes in enterocyte gene expression have been observed to occur even sooner.[19] With additional time, villi lengthen, intestinal absorptive surface area increases, and digestive and absorptive functions improve. Postresection intestinal adaptation in human patients, although less well-studied than in experimental models, appears to take place over the first 1 to 2 years following intestinal resection.[20]

The mechanisms responsible for inducing postresection intestinal adaptation are under active investigation. Several classes of effectors that stimulate intestinal growth include specific nutrients, peptide hormones and growth factors, pancreatic secretions, and some cytokines.[21] Nutritional components with intestinal growth-stimulating effects include fiber, fatty acids, triglycerides, glutamine, polyamines, and lectins. Peptide growth factors reported to induce growth include epidermal growth factor, transforming growth factor α, insulin-like growth factors I and II, keratinocyte growth factor, hepatocyte growth factor, gastrin, peptide YY,

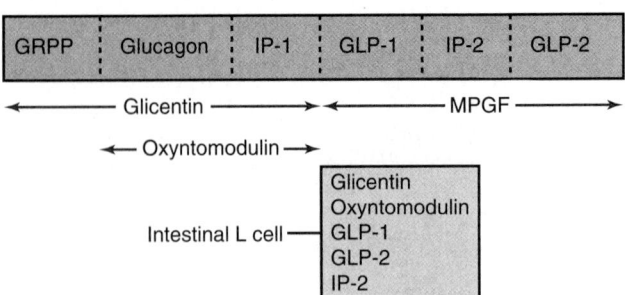

FIG. 27-13. Proglucagon cleavage products. Tissue-specific posttranslational processing of proglucagon in L cells of the intestinal mucosa yields the five peptide products shown. In the pancreas, posttranslation processing of this same gene product yields glucagon and the major proglucagon gene fragment (MPGF). GLP-1 = glucagon-like peptide 1; GLP-2 = glucagon-like peptide 2; GRPP = glicentin-related pancreatic polypeptide; IP-1 = intervening peptide-1; IP-2 = intervening peptide 2.

neurotensin, and bombesin. Cytokines that stimulate growth include interleukin (IL)-11, IL-3, and IL-15. The most recently characterized stimulator of enterocyte proliferation is GLP-2, which has potent trophic activity that is specific for the intestinal epithelium.[2] Because serum concentrations of GLP-2 rise following massive small-bowel resection and GLP-2 immunoneutralization inhibits postresection intestinal adaptation, GLP-2 is a promising candidate mediator of this response.

Postresection adaptation serves to compensate for the function of intestine that has been resected. However, the magnitude of this response is limited. If enough small intestine is resected, a devastating condition known as the short bowel syndrome results. This condition is discussed later under "Short-Bowel Syndrome."

SMALL-BOWEL OBSTRUCTION

Epidemiology

Mechanical small-bowel obstruction is the most frequently encountered surgical disorder of the small intestine. Although a wide range of etiologies for this condition exist, intra-abdominal adhesions related to prior abdominal surgery is the etiologic factor in up to 75% of cases of small-bowel obstruction. More than 300,000 patients are estimated to undergo surgery to treat adhesion-induced small-bowel obstruction in the United States annually.[22]

Less-prevalent etiologies for small-bowel obstruction include hernias (Fig. 27-14) and Crohn's disease. The frequency with which obstruction related to these conditions is encountered varies according to the patient population and practice setting. In contrast to colonic obstruction, small-bowel obstruction is uncommonly caused by neoplasms. Fewer than 3% of cases are caused by primary small-intestinal neoplasms.[23] Cancer-related small-bowel obstruction is more commonly caused by extrinsic compression or invasion by advanced malignancies arising in organs other than the small bowel (Fig. 27-15). Table 27-3 summarizes the most commonly encountered etiologies of small-bowel obstruction. Although congenital abnormalities capable of causing small-bowel obstruction usually become evident during childhood, they sometimes elude detection and are diagnosed for the first time in adult patients presenting with abdominal symptoms. For example, intestinal malrotation and mid-gut volvulus should not be forgotten when considering the differential diagnosis of adult patients with acute or chronic symptoms of small-bowel obstruction, especially those without a history of prior abdominal surgery. A rare etiology of obstruction is the superior mesenteric artery syndrome, characterized by compression of the third portion of the duodenum by the superior mesenteric artery as it crosses over this portion of the duodenum. This condition should be considered in young asthenic individuals who have chronic symptoms suggestive of proximal small-bowel obstruction.

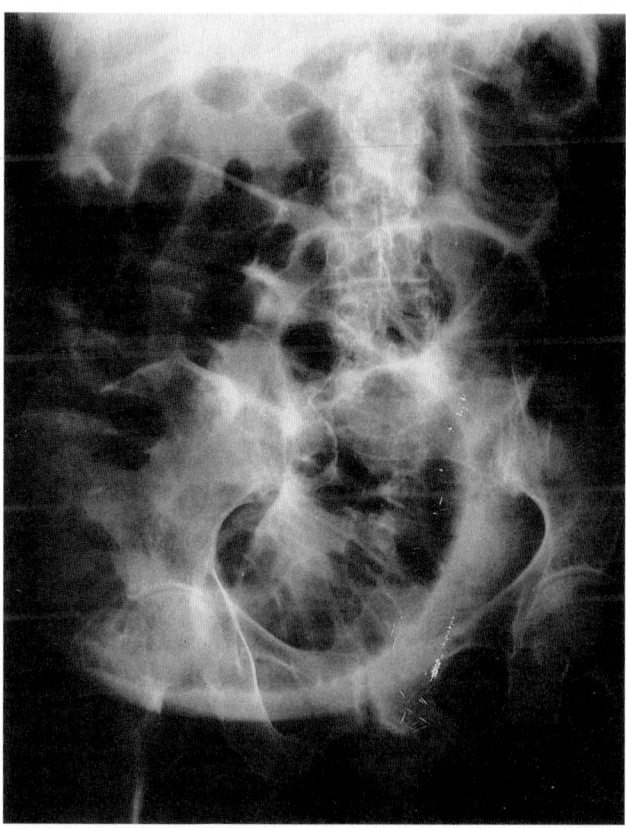

A

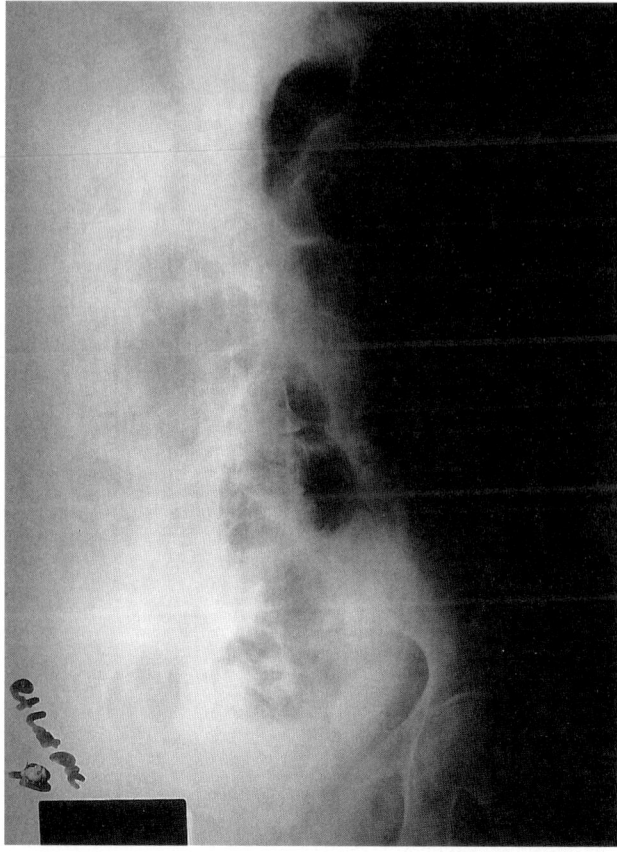

B

FIG. 27-14. *Small-bowel obstruction. Anteroposterior (A) and right lateral decubitus (B) radiographs demonstrate dilated loops of small bowel and a paucity of air in the colon. There is a collection of gas overlying the left obturator foramen. The etiology of this patient's small-bowel obstruction was found to be an incarcerated obturator hernia.*

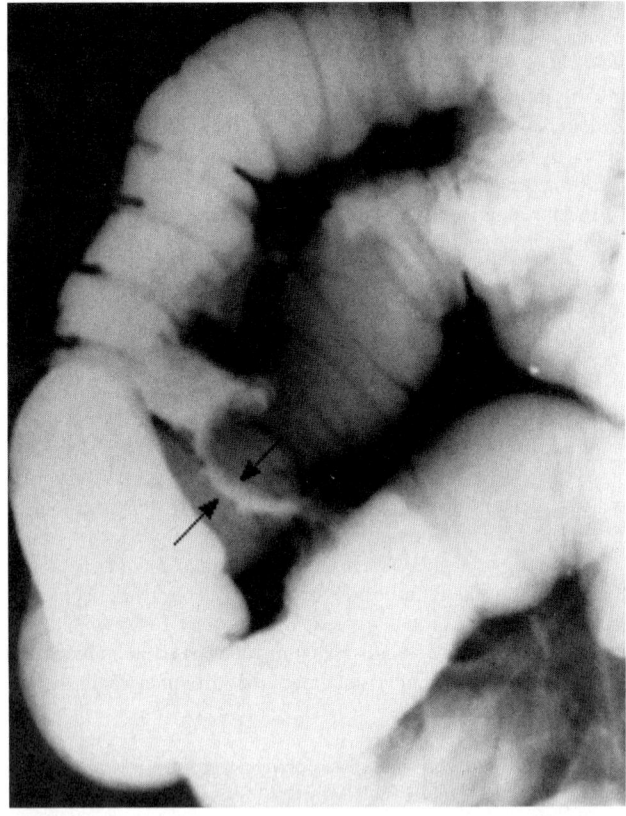

FIG. 27-15. Partial small-bowel obstruction. This small-bowel series demonstrates mildly dilated small-bowel loops and a stenotic lesion (arrows) caused by a colon-cancer derived metastasis.

Pathophysiology

The obstructing lesion can be conceptualized according to its anatomic relationship to the intestinal wall as (1) intraluminal (e.g., foreign bodies, gallstones, or meconium), (2) intramural (e.g., tumors, Crohn's disease-associated inflammatory strictures, or hematomas), or (3) extrinsic (e.g., adhesions, hernias, or carcinomatosis).

Table 27-3
Small-Bowel Obstruction: Common Etiologies

Adhesions
Neoplasms
Primary small-bowel neoplasms
Secondary small-bowel cancer (e.g., melanoma-derived metastasis)
Local invasion by intra-abdominal malignancy
Carcinomatosis
Hernias
External
Internal
Crohn's disease
Volvulus
Intussusception
Radiation-induced stricture
Postischemic stricture
Foreign body
Gallstone ileus
Diverticulitis
Meckel's diverticulum
Hematoma
Congenital abnormalities (e.g., webs, duplications, and malrotation)

With onset of obstruction, gas and fluid accumulate within the intestinal lumen proximal to the site of obstruction. Most of the gas that accumulates originates from swallowed air, although some is produced within the intestine. The fluid consists of swallowed liquids and gastrointestinal secretions (obstruction stimulates intestinal epithelial water secretion). With ongoing gas and fluid accumulation, the bowel distends and intraluminal and intramural pressures rise. If the intramural pressure becomes high enough, microvascular perfusion to the intestine is impaired, leading to intestinal ischemia, and, ultimately, necrosis. This condition is termed *strangulating bowel obstruction.*

With *partial small-bowel obstruction,* only a portion of the intestinal lumen is occluded, allowing passage of some gas and fluid. The progression of pathophysiologic events described above tends to occur more slowly than with *complete small-bowel obstruction,* and development of strangulation is less likely.

In contrast, progression to strangulation occurs especially rapidly with *closed loop obstruction* in which a segment of intestine is obstructed both proximally and distally (e.g., with volvulus). In such cases, the accumulating gas and fluid cannot escape either proximally or distally from the obstructed segment.

Clinical Presentation

The symptoms of small-bowel obstruction are colicky abdominal pain, nausea, vomiting, and obstipation. Continued passage of flatus and/or stool beyond 6 to 12 hours after onset of symptoms is characteristic of partial rather than complete obstruction. The signs of small-bowel obstruction include abdominal distention, which is most pronounced if the site of obstruction is in the distal ileum, or may be absent if the site of obstruction is in the proximal small intestine, and hyperactive bowel sounds. Laboratory findings reflect intravascular volume depletion and consist of hemoconcentration and electrolyte abnormalities. Mild leukocytosis is common.

Features of strangulated obstruction include tachycardia, localized abdominal tenderness, fever, marked leukocytosis, and acidosis. Serum levels of amylase, lipase, lactate dehydrogenase, phosphate, and potassium may be elevated. It is important to note that these parameters lack sufficient predictive value to allow for differentiation between simple and strangulated obstruction prior to the onset of irreversible intestinal ischemia. Indeed, 5 to 15% of patients who are demonstrated to have frank intestinal infarction have none of these features.[24] These features have an especially low prevalence in elderly patients. As a result, strangulated obstruction is particularly treacherous in this population.

Diagnosis

The diagnostic evaluation should focus on the following goals: distinguishing mechanical obstruction from ileus; determining the etiology of the obstruction; discriminating partial from complete obstruction; and discriminating simple from strangulating obstruction.

Important elements to obtain on history include prior abdominal operations (suggesting the presence of adhesions) and the presence of abdominal disorders (e.g., intra-abdominal cancer or inflammatory bowel disease) that may provide insights into the etiology of obstruction. Upon examination, a meticulous search for hernias (particularly in the inguinal and femoral regions) should be conducted. The stool should be checked for gross or occult blood, the presence of which is suggestive of intestinal strangulation.

The diagnosis of small-bowel obstruction is usually confirmed with radiographic examination. The *abdominal series* consists of a radiograph of the abdomen with the patient in a supine position, a radiograph of the abdomen with the patient in an upright position, and a radiograph of the chest with the patient in an upright position. The finding most specific for small-bowel obstruction is the triad of dilated small-bowel loops (>3 cm in diameter), air–fluid levels seen on upright films, and a paucity of air in the colon. The sensitivity of abdominal radiographs in the detection of small-bowel obstruction ranges from 70 to 80%.[25,26] Specificity is low, because ileus and colonic obstruction can be associated with findings that mimic those observed with small-bowel obstruction. False-negative findings on radiographs can result when the site of obstruction is located in the proximal small bowel and when the bowel lumen is filled with fluid but no gas, thereby preventing visualization of air–fluid levels or bowel distention. The latter situation is associated with closed-loop obstruction. Despite these limitations, abdominal radiographs remain an important study in patients with suspected small-bowel obstruction because of their widespread availability and low cost.

Computed tomographic (CT) scanning is 80 to 90% sensitive and 70 to 90% specific in the detection of small-bowel obstruction.[25,26] The findings of small-bowel obstruction include a discrete transition zone with dilation of bowel proximally, decompression of bowel distally, intraluminal contrast that does not pass beyond the transition zone, and a colon containing little gas or fluid. CT scanning may also provide evidence for the presence of closed-loop obstruction and strangulation (Fig. 27-16). Closed-loop obstruction is suggested by the presence of a U-shaped or C-shaped dilated bowel loop as-

sociated with a radial distribution of mesenteric vessels converging toward a torsion point. Strangulation is suggested by thickening of the bowel wall, pneumatosis intestinalis (air in the bowel wall), portal venous gas, mesenteric haziness, and poor uptake of intravenous contrast into the wall of the affected bowel. CT scanning also offers a global evaluation of the abdomen and may therefore reveal the etiology of obstruction. This feature also is important in the acute setting when intestinal obstruction represents only one of many diagnoses in patients presenting with acute abdominal conditions.

A limitation of CT scanning is its low sensitivity (<50%) in the detection of low-grade or partial small-bowel obstruction. A subtle transition zone may be difficult to identify in the axial images obtained during CT scanning. In such cases, contrast examinations of the small bowel, either *small-bowel series* (small-bowel follow-through) or *enteroclysis,* can be helpful. For standard small-bowel series, contrast is swallowed or instilled into the stomach through a nasogastric tube. Abdominal radiographs are then taken serially as the contrast travels distally in the intestine. Although barium can be used, water-soluble contrast agents, such as Gastrografin, should be used if the possibility of intestinal perforation exists. These examinations are more labor intensive and less-rapidly performed than CT scanning, but may offer greater sensitivity in the detection of luminal and mural etiologies of obstruction, such as primary intestinal tumors. For enteroclysis, 200 to 250 mL of barium followed by 1 to 2 L of a solution of methylcellulose in water is instilled into the proximal jejunum via a long nasoenteric catheter. Enteroclysis is rarely performed in the acute setting, but offers greater sensitivity than small-bowel series in the detection of lesions that may be causing partial small-bowel obstruction. The double-contrast technique

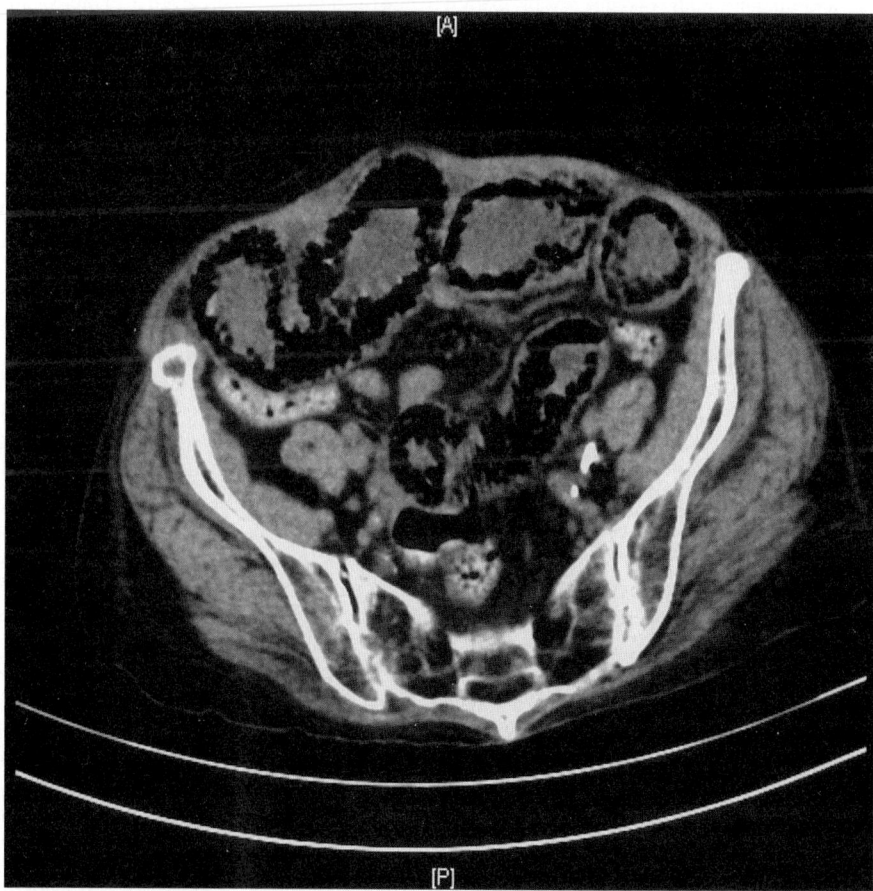

FIG. 27-16. *Small-bowel obstruction with strangulation. This CT scan of a patient with strangulating small-bowel obstruction shows dilated small-bowel loops with extensive pneumatosis intestinalis.*

used in enteroclysis permits assessment of mucosal surface detail and detection of relatively small lesions, even through overlapping small-bowel loops.

Therapy

Small-bowel obstruction is usually associated with a marked depletion of intravascular volume caused by decreased oral intake, vomiting, and sequestration of fluid in bowel lumen and wall. Therefore, fluid resuscitation is integral to treatment. Isotonic fluid should be given intravenously and an indwelling bladder catheter placed to monitor urine output. Central venous or pulmonary artery catheter monitoring may be necessary to assist with fluid management, particularly in patients with underlying cardiac disease. Broad-spectrum antibiotics are commonly administered because of concerns that bacterial translocation may occur in the setting of small-bowel obstruction; however, there are no controlled data to support or refute this approach.

The stomach should be continuously evacuated of air and fluid using a nasogastric (NG) tube. Effective gastric decompression decreases nausea, distention, and the risk of vomiting and aspiration. Longer nasoenteric tubes, with tips placed into the jejunum or ileum, were favored in the past, but are rarely used today. Although these long tubes are associated with higher complication rates than NG tubes, their greater efficacy in gastrointestinal decompression has not been demonstrated conclusively.

The standard therapy for small-bowel obstruction is expeditious surgery, with the exception of specific situations described below. The rationale for this approach is to minimize the risk for bowel strangulation, which is associated with an increased risk for morbidity and mortality. Clinical signs and currently available laboratory tests and imaging studies do not reliably permit the distinction between patients with simple obstruction and those with strangulated obstruction prior to the onset of irreversible ischemia. Therefore, the goal is to operate before the onset of irreversible ischemia.

The operative procedure performed varies according to the etiology of the obstruction. For example, adhesions are lysed, tumors are resected, and hernias are reduced and repaired. Regardless of the etiology, the affected intestine should be examined, and nonviable bowel resected. Criteria suggesting viability are normal color, peristalsis, and marginal arterial pulsations. Usually visual inspection alone is adequate in judging viability. In borderline cases, a Doppler probe may be used to check for pulsatile flow to the bowel, and arterial perfusion can be verified by visualizing intravenously administered fluorescein dye in the bowel wall under ultraviolet illumination. In general, if the patient is hemodynamically stable, short lengths of bowel of questionable viability should be resected and primary anastomosis of the remaining intestine performed. However, if the viability of a large proportion of the intestine is in question, a concerted effort to preserve intestinal tissue should be made. In such situations, the bowel of uncertain viability should be left intact and the patient reexplored in 24 to 48 hours in a "second-look" operation. At that time, definitive resection of nonviable bowel is completed.

Successful laparoscopic surgery for bowel obstruction is being reported with greater frequency. Reported data suggest that up to 60% of small-bowel obstruction cases caused by adhesions may be amenable to laparoscopic therapy.[27] However, the presence of bowel distention and multiple adhesions can cause these procedures to be difficult and potentially hazardous.

Exceptions to the recommendation for expeditious surgery for intestinal obstruction include partial small-bowel obstruction, obstruction occurring in the early postoperative period, intestinal obstruction as a consequence of Crohn's disease, and carcinomatosis.

Progression to strangulation is unlikely to occur with partial small-bowel obstruction, and an attempt at nonoperative resolution is warranted. Nonoperative management has been documented to be successful in 65 to 81% of patients with partial small-bowel obstruction. Of those successfully treated nonoperatively, only 5 to 15% have been reported to have symptoms that were not substantially improved within 48 hours after initiation of therapy.[28,29] Therefore, most patients with partial small obstruction whose symptoms do not improve within 48 hours after initiation of nonoperative therapy should undergo surgery. Patients undergoing nonoperative therapy should be closely monitored for signs suggestive of peritonitis, the development of which would mandate urgent surgery. The administration of hypertonic water-soluble contrast agents, such as Gastrografin used in upper GI and small-bowel follow-through examinations, causes a shift of fluid into the intestinal lumen, thereby increasing the pressure gradient across the site of obstruction. This effect may accelerate resolution of partial small-bowel obstruction; however, whether administration of water-soluble contrast agents increases the probability that an episode of bowel obstruction can be successfully managed nonoperatively remains controversial and requires further study.

Obstruction presenting in the early postoperative period has been reported to occur in 0.7% of patients undergoing laparotomy.[30] Patients undergoing pelvic surgery, especially colorectal procedures, have the greatest risk for developing early postoperative small-bowel obstruction. The presence of obstruction should be considered if symptoms of intestinal obstruction occur after the initial return of bowel function or if bowel function fails to return within the expected 3 to 5 days after abdominal surgery. Plain radiographs may demonstrate dilated loops of small intestine with air–fluid levels, but are interpreted as normal or nonspecific in up to a third of patients with early postoperative obstruction. CT scanning or small-bowel series is often required to make the diagnosis. Obstruction that occurs in the early postoperative period is usually partial and only rarely is associated with strangulation. Therefore, a period of extended nonoperative therapy consisting of bowel rest, hydration, and total parenteral nutrition (TPN) administration is usually warranted. However, if complete obstruction is demonstrated or if signs suggestive of peritonitis are detected, expeditious reoperation should be undertaken without delay.

Intestinal obstruction in patients with Crohn's disease often responds to medical therapy and is discussed in more detail later under "Crohn's Disease." Twenty-five to 33% of patients with a history of cancer who present with small-bowel obstruction have adhesions as the etiology of their obstruction and therefore should not be denied appropriate therapy.[31,32] Even in cases in which the obstruction is related to recurrent malignancy, palliative resection or bypass can be performed. Patients with obvious carcinomatosis pose a difficult challenge, given their limited prognosis. Management must be tailored to an individual patient's prognosis and desires.

Outcomes

Prognosis is related to the etiology of obstruction. Following laparotomy, there is a greater than 5% lifetime incidence of small-bowel obstruction caused by adhesions. Following surgery for small-bowel obstruction caused by adhesions, the probability of recurrent obstruction ranges from 20 to 30%. The perioperative mortality rate associated with surgery for nonstrangulating small-bowel obstruction is less than 5%, with most deaths occurring in elderly patients with significant comorbidities. Mortality rates associated with surgery for strangulating obstruction range from 8 to 25%.

ILEUS AND OTHER DISORDERS OF INTESTINAL MOTILITY

Epidemiology

Ileus and intestinal pseudo-obstruction designate clinical syndromes caused by impaired intestinal motility and are characterized by symptoms and signs of intestinal obstruction in the absence of a lesion-causing mechanical obstruction. Ileus is a major cause of morbidity in hospitalized patients. Postoperative ileus is the most frequently implicated cause of delayed discharge following abdominal operations; its economic impact has been estimated at between $750 million and $1 billion annually in the United States.[6]

Ileus is temporary and generally reversible if the inciting factor can be corrected. In contrast, chronic intestinal pseudo-obstruction comprises a spectrum of specific disorders associated with irreversible intestinal dysmotility.

Pathophysiology

Numerous factors capable of impairing intestinal motility, and thus inciting ileus, have been described (Table 27-4). The most frequently encountered factors are abdominal operations, infection and inflammation, electrolyte abnormalities, and drugs.

Following most abdominal operations or injuries, the motility of the gastrointestinal tract is transiently impaired. Among the proposed mechanisms responsible for this dysmotility are surgical stress-induced sympathetic reflexes, inflammatory response-mediator release, and anesthetic/analgesic effects; each of which can inhibit intestinal motility. The return of normal motility generally follows a characteristic temporal sequence, with small-intestinal motility returning to normal within the first 24 hours after laparotomy and gastric and colonic motility returning to normal by 48 hours and 3 to 5 days, respectively. Resolution of ileus may be delayed in the presence of other factors capable of inciting ileus

Table 27-4
Ileus: Common Etiologies

Abdominal surgery
Infection
  Sepsis
  Intra-abdominal abscess
  Peritonitis
  Pneumonia
Electrolyte abnormalities
  Hypokalemia
  Hypomagnesemia
  Hypermagnesemia
  Hyponatremia
Medications
  Anticholinergics
  Opiates
  Phenothiazines
  Calcium channel blockers
  Tricyclic antidepressants
Hypothyroidism
Ureteral colic
Retroperitoneal hemorrhage
Spinal cord injury
Myocardial infarction
Mesenteric ischemia

Table 27-5
Chronic Intestinal Pseudo-Obstruction: Etiologies

Primary causes
  Familial types
    Familial visceral myopathies (types I, II, and III)
    Familial visceral neuropathies (types I and II)
    Childhood visceral myopathies (types I and II)
  Sporadic types
    Visceral myopathies
    Visceral neuropathies
Secondary causes
  Smooth-muscle disorders
    Collagen vascular diseases (e.g., scleroderma)
    Muscular dystrophies (e.g., myotonic dystrophy)
    Amyloidosis
  Neurologic disorders
    Chagas disease, Parkinson's disease, spinal cord injury
  Endocrine disorders
    Diabetes, hypothyroidism, hypoparathyroidism
  Miscellaneous disorders
    Radiation enteritis
  Pharmacologic causes (e.g., phenothiazines and tricyclic antidepressants)
  Viral infections

such as the presence of intra-abdominal abscesses or electrolyte abnormalities.

Chronic intestinal pseudo-obstruction can be caused by a large number of specific abnormalities affecting intestinal smooth muscle, the myenteric plexus, or the extraintestinal nervous system (Table 27-5). Visceral myopathies constitute a group of diseases characterized by degeneration and fibrosis of the intestinal muscularis propria. Visceral neuropathies encompass a variety of degenerative disorders of the myenteric and submucosal plexuses. Both sporadic and familial forms of visceral myopathies and neuropathies exist. Systemic disorders involving the smooth muscle such as progressive systemic sclerosis and progressive muscular dystrophy, and neurologic diseases such as Parkinson's disease also can be complicated by chronic intestinal pseudo-obstruction. In addition, viral infections, such as those associated with Cytomegalovirus and Epstein-Barr virus can cause intestinal pseudo-obstruction.

Clinical Presentation

The clinical presentation of ileus resembles that of small-bowel obstruction. Inability to tolerate liquids and solids by mouth, nausea, and lack of flatus or bowel movements are the most common symptoms. Vomiting and abdominal distention may occur. Bowel sounds are characteristically diminished or absent, in contrast to the hyperactive bowel sounds that usually accompany mechanical small-bowel obstruction. The clinical manifestations of chronic intestinal pseudo-obstruction include variable degrees of nausea and vomiting and abdominal pain and distention.

Diagnosis

Routine postoperative ileus should be expected and requires no diagnostic evaluation. If ileus persists beyond 3 to 5 days postoperatively or occurs in the absence of abdominal surgery, diagnostic evaluation to detect specific underlying factors capable of inciting ileus and to rule out the presence of mechanical obstruction is warranted.

Patient medication lists should be reviewed for the presence of drugs, especially opiates, known to be associated with impaired intestinal motility. Measurement of serum electrolytes may demonstrate hypokalemia, hypocalcemia, hypomagnesemia, hypermagnesemia, or other electrolyte abnormalities commonly associated with ileus. Abdominal radiographs are often obtained, but the distinction between ileus and mechanical obstruction may be difficult based on this test alone. In the postoperative setting, CT scanning is the test of choice because it can demonstrate the presence of an intra-abdominal abscess or other evidence of peritoneal sepsis that may be causing ileus and can exclude the presence of complete mechanical obstruction.

The diagnosis of chronic pseudo-obstruction is suggested by clinical features and confirmed by radiographic and manometric studies. Diagnostic laparotomy or laparoscopy with full-thickness biopsy of the small intestine may be required to establish the specific underlying cause.

Therapy

The management of ileus consists of limiting oral intake and correcting the underlying inciting factor. If vomiting or abdominal distention are prominent, the stomach should be decompressed using a nasogastric tube. Fluid and electrolytes should be administered intravenously until ileus resolves. If the duration of ileus is prolonged, TPN may be required.

Given the frequency of postoperative ileus, a large number of investigations have been conducted to define strategies to reduce its duration. Although often used, the use of early ambulation, early postoperative feeding protocols, and routine nasogastric intubation have not been demonstrated to be associated with earlier resolution of postoperative ileus. The administration of nonsteroidal anti-inflammatory drugs such as ketorolac and concomitant reductions in opioid dosing have been shown to reduce the duration of ileus in most studies. Similarly, the use of perioperative thoracic epidural anesthesia/analgesia with regimens containing local anesthetics combined with limitation or elimination of systemically administered opioids has been shown to reduce duration of postoperative ileus.

Most other pharmacologic agents, including prokinetic agents, are associated with efficacy–toxicity profiles that are too unfavorable to warrant routine use. Recently, administration of a selective opioid receptor antagonist with limited oral absorption (ADL 8-2698) was demonstrated to reduce duration of postoperative ileus in a prospective, randomized, placebo-controlled trial.[33] Further studies will need to determine the clinical indications for this and other newer generations of pharmacologic agents designed to treat ileus.

The therapy of patients with chronic intestinal pseudo-obstruction focuses on palliation of symptoms as well as fluid, electrolyte, and nutritional management. Surgery should be avoided if at all possible. No standard therapies are curative or delay the natural history of any of the specific disorders causing intestinal pseudo-obstruction. Prokinetic agents, such as metoclopramide and erythromycin, are associated with poor efficacy. Cisapride has been associated with palliation of symptoms; however, because of cardiac toxicity and reported deaths, this agent is restricted to compassionate use.

Patients with refractory disease may require strict limitation of oral intake and long-term TPN administration. Despite these measures, some patients will continue to have severe abdominal pain or such copious intestinal secretions that vomiting and fluid and electrolyte losses remain substantial. These patients may require a decompressive gastrostomy or an extended small-bowel resection to remove abnormal intestine. Small-intestinal transplantation has been applied in these patients with increasing frequency; the ultimate role of this modality remains to be defined.

CROHN'S DISEASE

Epidemiology

Crohn's disease is a chronic, idiopathic inflammatory disease with a propensity to affect the distal ileum, although any part of the alimentary tract can be involved. Recent estimates of the incidence of Crohn's disease in the United States have ranged from 3.6 to 8.8 per 100,000.[34] A dramatic increase in incidence in the United States was observed to occur from the mid-1950s through the early 1970s. Incidence rates have been stable since the 1980s. Substantial regional variations in incidence have been observed, with the highest incidences reported to exist in northern latitudes. The incidence of Crohn's disease varies among ethnic groups within the same geographic region. For example, members of the East European Ashkenazi Jewish population are at two- to fourfold higher risk of developing Crohn's disease than are members of other populations living in the same location.

Most studies suggest that Crohn's disease is slightly more prevalent in females than in males. The median age at which patients are diagnosed with Crohn's disease is approximately 30 years; however, age of diagnosis can range from early childhood through the entire life span.

Both genetic and environmental factors appear to influence the risk for developing Crohn's disease. The relative risk among first-degree relatives of patients with Crohn's disease is 14 to 15 times higher than that of the general population. Approximately 1 of 5 patients with Crohn's disease will report having at least one affected relative. The concordance rate among monozygotic twins is as high as 67%; however, Crohn's disease is not associated with simple mendelian inheritance patterns. Although there is a tendency within families for either ulcerative colitis or Crohn's disease to be present exclusively, mixed kindreds also occur, suggesting the presence of some shared genetic traits as a basis for both diseases.

Higher socioeconomic status is associated with an increased risk of Crohn's disease. Most studies have found breast-feeding to be protective against the development of Crohn's disease. Crohn's disease is more prevalent among smokers. Furthermore, smoking is associated with the increased risk for both the need for surgery and the risk of relapse after surgery for Crohn's disease.

Pathophysiology

Crohn's disease is characterized by sustained inflammation. Whether this inflammation represents an appropriate response to a yet unrecognized pathogen or an inappropriate response to a normally innocuous stimulus is unknown. Various hypotheses on the roles of environmental and genetic factors in the pathogenesis of Crohn's disease have been proposed.

Many infectious agents have been suggested to be the causative organism of Crohn's disease. Candidate organisms have included *Chlamydia*, *Listeria monocytogenes*, *Pseudomonas* species, reovirus, *Mycobacterium paratuberculosis*, and many others. There is no conclusive evidence that any of these organisms is the causative agent.

Studies using animal models suggest that in a genetically susceptible host, nonpathogenic, commensal enteric flora are sufficient to induce a chronic inflammatory response resembling that associated with Crohn's disease. In these models, the sustained intestinal inflammation is the result of either abnormal epithelial barrier function or immune dysregulation. Poor barrier function is hypothesized to permit inappropriate exposure of lamina propria lymphocytes to antigenic stimuli derived from the intestinal lumen. In addition, a

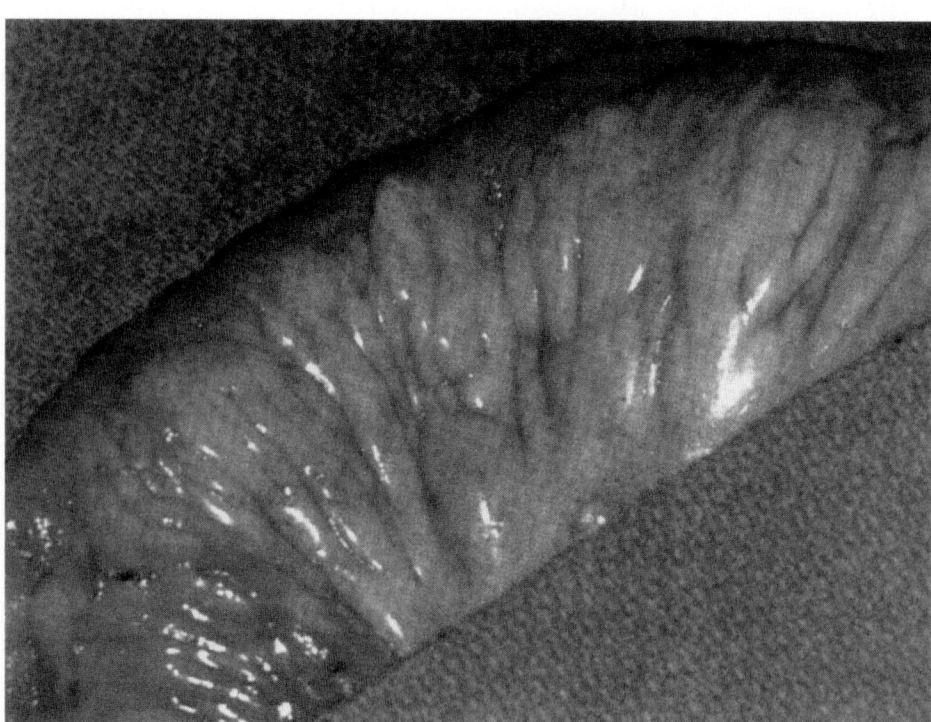

FIG. 27-17. Crohn's disease. This intraoperative photograph demonstrates encroachment of mesenteric fat onto the serosal surface of the intestine (fat wrapping) that is characteristic intestinal segments affected by active Crohn's disease.

variety of defects in immune regulatory mechanisms, e.g., overresponsiveness of mucosal T cells to enteric flora-derived antigens, can lead to defective immune tolerance and sustained inflammation.

Specific genetic defects associated with Crohn's disease in human patients are beginning to be defined. For example, the presence of a locus on chromosome 16 (the so-called IBD1 locus) has been linked to Crohn's disease. The IBD1 locus has been identified as the *NOD2* gene.[35,36] Persons with allelic variants on both chromosomes have a 40-fold relative risk of Crohn's disease when compared to those without variant *NOD2* genes. The relevance of this gene to the pathogenesis of Crohn's disease is biologically plausible, because the protein product of the *NOD2* gene mediates the innate immune response to microbial pathogens.

Pathology

Although the pathologic hallmark of Crohn's disease is focal, transmural inflammation of the intestine, a spectrum of pathologic lesions can be present. The earliest lesion characteristic of Crohn's disease is the aphthous ulcer. These superficial ulcers are up to 3 mm in diameter and are surrounded by a halo of erythema. In the small intestine, aphthous ulcers typically arise over lymphoid aggregates. Granulomas are highly characteristic of Crohn's disease and are reported to be present in up to 70% of intestinal specimens obtained during surgical resection. These granulomas are noncaseating and can be found in both areas of active disease and apparently normal intestine, in any layer of the bowel wall, and in mesenteric lymph nodes.

As disease progresses, aphthae coalesce into larger, stellate-shaped ulcers. Linear or serpiginous ulcers may form when multiple ulcers fuse in a direction parallel to the longitudinal axis of the intestine. With transverse coalescence of ulcers, a cobblestone appearance of the mucosa may arise.

With advanced disease, inflammation can be transmural. Serosal involvement results in adhesion of the inflamed bowel to other loops of bowel or other adjacent organs. Transmural inflammation also can result in fibrosis, with stricture formation, intra-abdominal

abscesses, fistulas, and, rarely, free perforation. Inflammation in Crohn's disease can affect discontinuous portions of intestine: so-called "skip lesions" that are separated by intervening normal-appearing intestine.

A feature of Crohn's disease that is grossly evident and helpful in identifying affected segments of intestine during surgery is the presence of *fat wrapping* (Fig. 27-17). This finding is virtually pathognomonic of Crohn's disease. It is the encroachment of mesenteric fat onto the serosal surface of the bowel. The presence of fat wrapping correlates well with the presence of underlying acute and chronic inflammation.

Features that allow for differentiation between Crohn's disease of the colon and ulcerative colitis include the layers of the bowel wall affected (inflammation in ulcerative colitis is limited to the mucosa and submucosa but may involve the full thickness of the bowel wall in Crohn's disease) and the longitudinal extent of inflammation (inflammation is continuous and characteristically affects the rectum in ulcerative colitis but may be discontinuous and spare the rectum in Crohn's disease). In the absence of full expression of features of advanced disease, Crohn's colitis can sometimes be difficult to distinguish from ulcerative colitis. It is also important to remember that although ulcerative colitis is a disease of the colon, it can be associated with inflammatory changes in the distal ileum (backwash ileitis).

Clinical Presentation

The most common symptoms of Crohn's disease are abdominal pain, diarrhea, and weight loss. However, the clinical features are highly variable among individual patients and depend on which segment(s) of the gastrointestinal tract is (are) predominantly affected, the intensity of inflammation, and the presence or absence of specific complications. Patients with Crohn's disease can be classified by their predominant clinical manifestation as having primarily fibrostenotic disease, fistulizing disease, or aggressive inflammatory disease. There is substantial overlap among these disease patterns

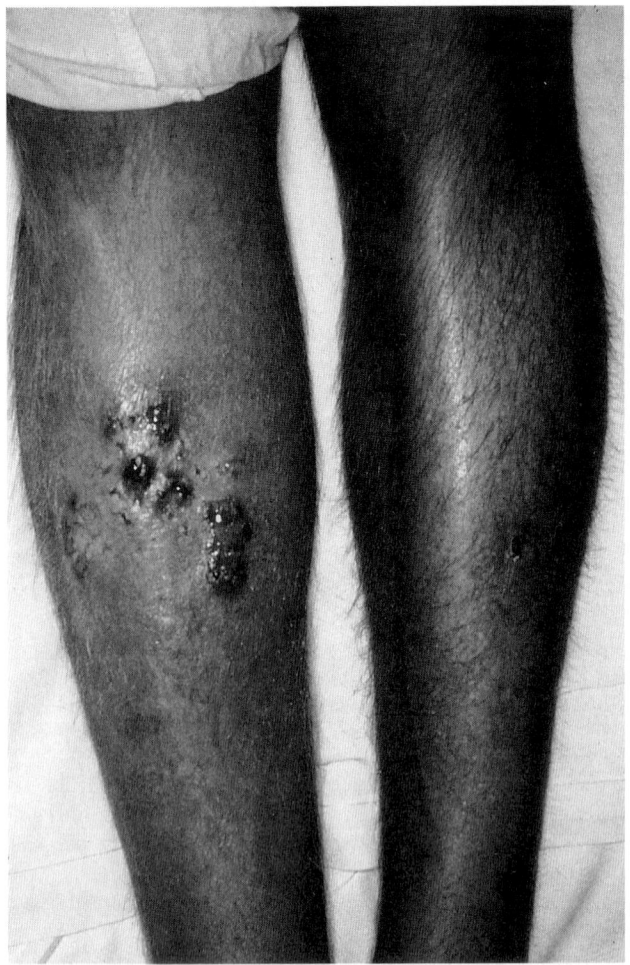

FIG. 27-18. *Pyoderma gangrenosum. This photograph depicts pretibial pyoderma gangrenosum in a patient with Crohn's disease. (Courtesy of Sonia Friedman, M.D., Department of Medicine, Brigham and Women's Hospital.)*

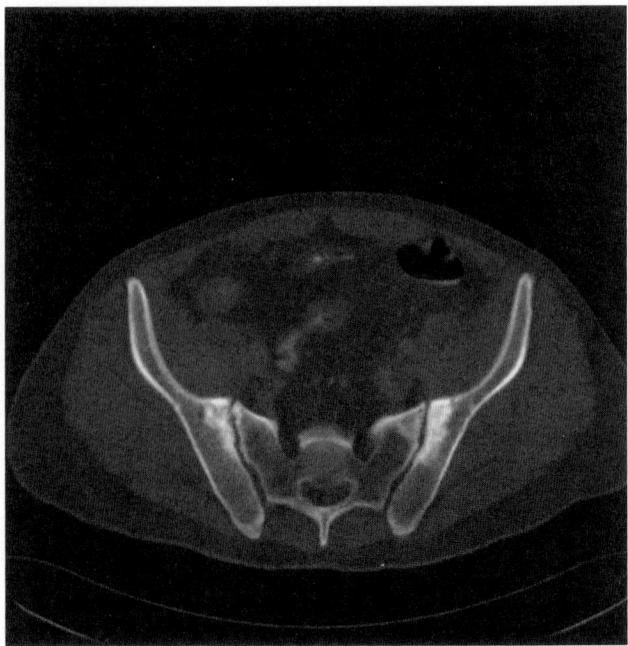

FIG. 27-19. Sacroiliitis. CT scan showing bilateral inflammation of the sacroiliac joints in a patient with Crohn's disease. *(Courtesy of John Braver, M.D., Department of Radiology, Brigham and Women's Hospital.)*

spondylitis, bear no apparent relationship to the severity of intestinal inflammation.

Diagnosis

Clinical situations in which the diagnosis of Crohn's disease should be considered include the presence of acute or chronic abdominal pain, especially when localized to the right lower quadrant, chronic

in individual patients, however. The onset of symptoms is insidious, and once present, their severity follows a waxing and waning course. Constitutional symptoms, particularly weight loss and fever, or growth retardation in children, may also be prominent and are occasionally the sole presenting features of Crohn's disease.

The distal ileum is the single most frequently affected site, being diseased at some time in 75% of patients with Crohn's disease. The small bowel alone is affected in 15 to 30% of patients, both the ileum and colon are affected in 40 to 60% of patients, and the colon alone is affected in 25 to 30% of patients. Isolated perineal and anorectal disease occurs in 5 to 10% of affected patients. Uncommon sites of involvement include the esophagus, stomach, and duodenum.

An estimated 25% of all patients with Crohn's disease will have an extraintestinal manifestation of their disease (Figs. 27-18 and 27-19). One-fourth of those affected will have more than one manifestation. Many of these complications are common to both Crohn's disease and ulcerative colitis, although as a whole, they are more prevalent among patients with Crohn's disease than those with ulcerative colitis. Table 27-6 lists the most common extraintestinal manifestations. The clinical severity of some of these manifestations, such as erythema nodosum and peripheral arthritis, are correlated with the severity of intestinal inflammation. The severity of other manifestations, such as pyoderma gangrenosum and ankylosing

Table 27-6
Extraintestinal Manifestations of Crohn's Disease

Dermatologic
    Erythema nodosum
    Pyoderma gangrenosum
Rheumatologic
    Peripheral arthritis
    Ankylosing spondylitis
    Sacroiliitis
Ocular
    Conjunctivitis
    Uveitis/iritis
    Episcleritis
Hepatobiliary
    Hepatic steatosis
    Cholelithiasis
    Primary sclerosing cholangitis
    Pericholangitis
Urologic
    Nephrolithiasis
    Ureteral obstruction
Miscellaneous
    Thromboembolic disease
    Vasculitis
    Osteoporosis
    Endocarditis, myocarditis, pleuropericarditis
    Interstitial lung disease
    Amyloidosis
    Pancreatitis

diarrhea, evidence of intestinal inflammation on radiography or endoscopy, the discovery of a bowel stricture or fistula arising from the bowel, and evidence of inflammation or granulomas on intestinal histology. Disorders associated with clinical presentations that resemble those of Crohn's disease include ulcerative colitis, functional bowel disorders such as irritable bowel syndrome, mesenteric ischemia, collagen vascular diseases, carcinoma and lymphoma, diverticular disease, and infectious enteritides. Infectious enteritides are most frequently diagnosed in immunocompromised patients but can also occur in patients with normal immune function. Acute ileitis caused by *Campylobacter* and *Yersinia* species can be difficult to distinguish from that caused by an acute presentation of Crohn's disease. Typhoid enteritis caused by *Salmonella typhosa* can lead to overt intestinal bleeding and perforation, most often affecting the terminal ileum. The distal ileum and cecum are the most common sites of intestinal involvement by infection caused by *Mycobacterium tuberculosis.* This condition can result in intestinal inflammation, strictures, and fistula formation, similar to those seen in Crohn's disease. Cytomegalovirus (CMV) can cause intestinal ulcers, bleeding, and perforation.

No single symptom, sign, or diagnostic test establishes the diagnosis of Crohn's disease. Instead, the diagnosis is based on a complete assessment of the clinical presentation with confirmatory findings derived from radiographic, endoscopic, and, in most cases, pathologic tests. Contrast examinations of the small bowel and colon may reveal strictures or networks of ulcers and fissures leading to the typical "cobblestone appearance" of the mucosa (Fig. 27-20).

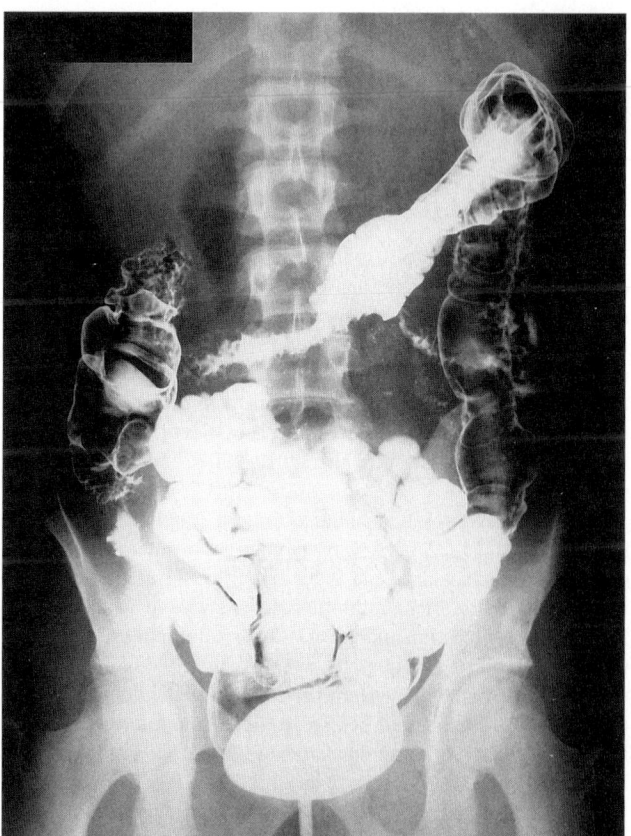

FIG. 27-20. *Crohn's disease. Contrast radiograph demonstrating that the lumen of the terminal ileum is narrowed and markedly separated from the surrounding small bowel by a thickened wall. There are skip lesions in the colon that have a cobblestone appearance.*

CT scanning may reveal intra-abdominal abscesses and is useful in acute presentations to rule out the presence of other intra-abdominal disorders. Colonoscopy is used to visualize and biopsy disease in the colon; occasionally the distal ileum can be reached as well. Esophagogastroduodenoscopy (EGD) is done for disease of the proximal alimentary tract.

Because of the insidious, and often nonspecific, presentation, the diagnosis of Crohn's disease is typically made only after symptoms have been present for several years. However, in acute presentations, the diagnosis is sometimes made intraoperatively or during surgical evaluation. The initial manifestation of Crohn's disease can consist of right lower quadrant abdominal mimicking the presentation of acute appendicitis. In patients with this presentation, Crohn's disease can be discovered for the first time during laparotomy or laparoscopy performed for presumed appendicitis. In some patients, the initial manifestation of Crohn's disease is an acute abdomen related to small-bowel obstruction, intra-abdominal abscess, or free intestinal perforation. In other patients, perianal abscesses and fistulas requiring surgical therapy may be the first manifestation of Crohn's disease.

Therapy

Because no curative therapies are available for Crohn's disease, the goal of treatment is to palliate symptoms rather than to achieve cure. Medical therapy is used to induce and maintain disease remission. Surgery is reserved for specific indications described below. In addition, nutritional support in the form of aggressive enteral regimens or, if necessary, parenteral nutrition, is used to manage the malnutrition that is common in patient's with Crohn's disease.

Medical Therapy

Pharmacologic agents used to treat Crohn's disease include antibiotics, aminosalicylates, corticosteroids, and immunomodulators. Antibiotics have an adjunctive role in the treatment of infectious complications associated with Crohn's disease. They are also used to treat patients with perianal disease, enterocutaneous fistulas, and active colonic disease.

Most studies have shown sulfasalazine, the parent compound of all aminosalicylates used to treat Crohn's disease, to be superior to placebo in inducing disease remission. Its efficacy in the maintenance of remission is less clear. Aminosalicylates are associated with minimal toxicity and are available in a variety of formulations that allow for their delivery to specific regions of the alimentary tract.

Orally administered glucocorticoids are used to treat patients with mildly to moderately severe disease that does not respond to aminosalicylates. Patients with severe active disease usually require intravenous administration of glucocorticoids. Although glucocorticoids are effective in inducing remission, they are ineffective in preventing relapse and their adverse side-effect profile makes long-term use hazardous. Therefore, they should be tapered once remission is achieved. Some patients are unable to undergo glucocorticoid tapering without suffering recurrence of symptoms. Such patients are said to have glucocorticoid dependence and are candidates for therapy with glucocorticoid-sparing immune modulators.

The thiopurine antimetabolites azathioprine and 6-mercaptopurine have demonstrated efficacy in inducing remission, in maintaining remission, and in allowing for glucocorticoid tapering in glucocorticoid-dependent patients. There is also some evidence that they decrease the risk of relapse after intestinal resection for Crohn's disease. These agents are relatively safe, but can induce bone marrow suppression and promote infectious complications. For patients who do not respond to the thiopurines, methotrexate is an alternative. There is little role for cyclosporine in Crohn's disease; its efficacy/toxicity profile in this disease is poor.

Infliximab is a chimeric monoclonal anti–tumor-necrosis-factor antibody that has efficacy in inducing remission and in promoting closure of enterocutaneous fistulas.[37] Infliximab is generally well tolerated but should not be used in patients with ongoing septic processes, such as undrained intra-abdominal abscesses.

Surgical Therapy

Seventy to 80% of patients with Crohn's disease will ultimately require surgical therapy for their disease.[38,39] Surgery is generally reserved for patients whose disease is unresponsive to aggressive medical therapy or who develop complications of their disease. Failure of medical management may be the indication for surgery if symptoms persist despite aggressive therapy for several months or if symptoms recur whenever aggressive therapy is tapered. Surgery should be considered if medication-induced complications arise, specifically corticosteroid-related complications, such as cushingoid features, cataracts, glaucoma, systemic hypertension, compression fractures, or aseptic necrosis of the femoral head.

One-third of patients with Crohn's disease will require surgery for intestinal obstruction. Abscesses and fistulas are frequently encountered during operations performed for intestinal obstruction in these patients, but are rarely the only indication for surgery. Most abscesses are amenable to percutaneous drainage, and fistulas unless associated with symptoms or metabolic derangements do not require surgical intervention. Growth retardation constitutes an indication for surgery in 30% of children with Crohn's disease. Less-common complications that require surgical intervention are acute gastrointestinal hemorrhage and cancer.

An uncommon, but not rare, scenario is the intraoperative discovery of inflammation limited to the terminal ileum during operations performed for presumed appendicitis. This scenario can result from an acute presentation of Crohn's disease or from acute ileitis caused by bacteria such as *Yersinia* or *Campylobacter*. Both conditions should be treated medically; ileal resection is not generally indicated. However, the appendix, even if normal appearing, should be removed (unless the cecum is inflamed, increasing the potential morbidity of this procedure) in order to eliminate appendicitis from the differential diagnosis of abdominal pain in these patients, particularly those with Crohn's disease who may be destined to have recurring symptoms.

If the diagnosis of Crohn's disease is known and surgery planned, extent of disease in the small and large intestine should be documented using a small-bowel contrast examination and either barium enema or colonoscopy, respectively. CT scanning should be performed in patients suspected of having intra-abdominal abscesses. Malnourished patients may benefit from preoperative nutritional support.

During surgery, thorough examination of the entire intestine should be performed. The presence of active disease is suggested by thickening of the bowel wall, narrowing of the lumen, serosal inflammation and coverage by creeping fat, and thickening of the mesentery. Skip lesions are present in approximately 20% of cases and should be sought. The length of uninvolved small intestine should be noted.

Segmental intestinal resection of grossly evident disease followed by primary anastomosis is the usual procedure of choice.

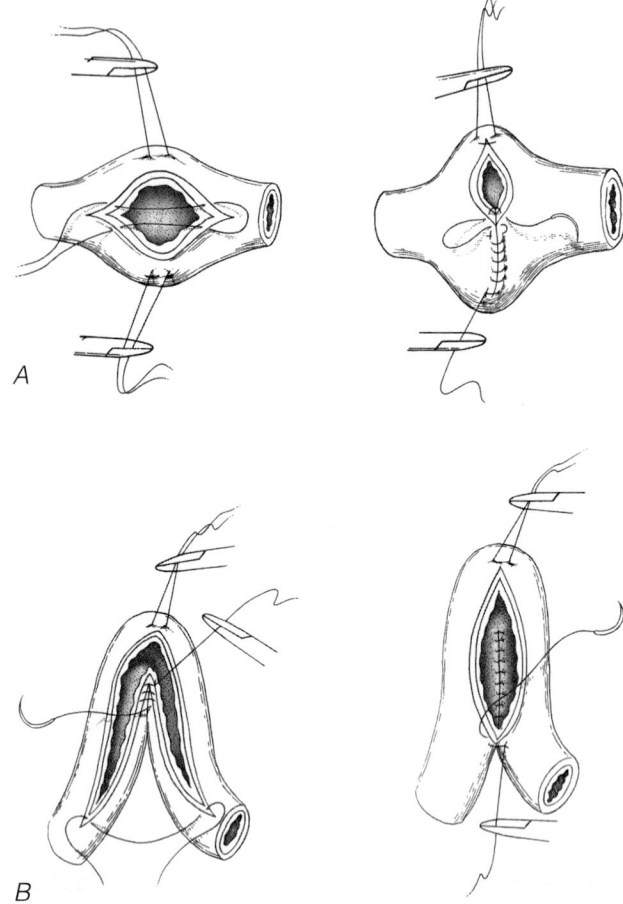

FIG. 27-21. *Stricturoplasty. The wall of the strictured bowel is incised longitudinally. Reconstruction is performed by closing the defect transversely in a manner similar to the Heinecke-Mikulicz pyloroplasty for short strictures (A) or the Finney pyloroplasty for longer strictures (B).*

Microscopic evidence of Crohn's disease at the resection margins does not compromise a safe anastomosis, and frozen-section analysis of resection margins is unnecessary. In a randomized prospective trial, the effects of achieving 2-cm resection margins beyond grossly evident disease were compared with achieving 12-cm resection margins.[40] There were no evident differences with respect to clinical recurrence rates or anastomotic recurrences. Recurrence rates were similar whether margins were histologically free of or involved with Crohn's disease.

An alternative to segmental resection for obstructing lesions is stricturoplasty (Fig. 27-21). This technique allows for preservation of intestinal surface area and is especially well-suited to patients with extensive disease and fibrotic strictures who may have undergone previous resection and are at risk for developing short-bowel syndrome. In this technique, the bowel is opened longitudinally to expose the lumen. Any intraluminal ulcerations should be biopsied to rule out the presence of neoplasia. Depending on the length of the stricture, the reconstruction can be fashioned in a manner similar to the Heinecke-Mikulicz pyloroplasty (for strictures less than 12 cm in length) or the Finney pyloroplasty (for longer strictures as much as 25 cm in length). Stricturoplasty sites should be marked with metallic clips to facilitate their identification on radiographs and during subsequent operations. Stricturoplasty is associated with recurrence rates that are no different from those associated with segmental resection.[41] Because the affected bowel is left in situ rather than resected, there is the potential for cancer developing at the stricturoplasty site. However, as data on this complication is limited to anecdotes, this risk remains a theoretic one. Stricturoplasty is contraindicated in patients with intra-abdominal abscesses or intestinal fistulas. The presence of a solitary stricture relatively close to a segment for which resection is planned is a relative contraindication.

Intestinal bypass procedures are sometimes required in the presence of intramesenteric abscesses or if the diseased bowel is coalesced in the form of a dense inflammatory mass, making its mobilization unsafe. Bypass procedures (gastrojejunostomy) are also used in the presence of duodenal strictures, for which stricturoplasty and segmental resection can be technically difficult.

Since the 1990s, laparoscopic surgical techniques have been applied to patients with Crohn's disease.[42] Theoretic advantages of laparoscopic surgery include less postoperative pain, earlier return of normal intestinal function that allows for shorter hospital stay, and superior cosmesis. In a prospective randomized trial comparing laparoscopic and open surgery for Crohn's disease conducted at a single institution, laparoscopic surgery was associated with faster recovery of pulmonary function, fewer complications, and shorter length of hospital stay. However, no differences in duration of ileus or analgesia usage were found between the two groups.[43]

Patient's undergoing initial surgery who present for elective ileocolectomy may be ideal candidates for laparoscopic surgery. It is important to remember that the inflammatory changes associated with Crohn's disease, such as thickened and foreshortened mesentery, obliterated tissue planes, and friable tissues with engorged vasculature, potentially make laparoscopic surgery difficult and dangerous. The risk of pancreatic, duodenal, and ureteral injury is substantial in patients in whom bowel is adherent to the retroperitoneum. Furthermore, the deficiency of tactile information characteristic of laparoscopic surgery may make detection of skip lesions difficult.

Outcomes

Overall complication rates following surgery for Crohn's disease range from 15 to 30%. Wound infections, postoperative intra-abdominal abscesses, and anastomotic leaks account for most of these complications.

Most patients whose disease is resected eventually develop recurrence. If recurrence is defined endoscopically, 70% recur within 1 year of a bowel resection and 85% by 3 years.[41] Clinical recurrence, defined as the return of symptoms confirmed as being caused by Crohn's disease, affects 60% of patients by 5 years and 94% by 15 years after intestinal resection. Reoperation becomes necessary in approximately one-third of patients by 5 years after the initial operation.

INTESTINAL FISTULAS

Epidemiology

A *fistula* is defined as an abnormal communication between two epithelialized surfaces. The communication occurs between two parts of the gastrointestinal tract or adjacent organs in an *internal fistula* (e.g., enterocolonic fistula or colovesicular fistula). An *external fistula* (e.g., enterocutaneous fistula or rectovaginal fistula) involves the skin or another external surface epithelium. Enterocutaneous fistulas that drain less than 200 mL of fluid per day are known as *low-output fistulas*, whereas those that drain more than 500 mL of fluid per day are known as *high-output fistulas*.

More than 80% of enterocutaneous fistulas represent iatrogenic complications that occur as the result of enterotomies or intestinal anastomotic dehiscences. Fistulas that arise spontaneously without antecedent iatrogenic injury are usually manifestations of progression of underlying Crohn's disease or cancer.

Pathophysiology

The manifestations of fistulas depend on which structures are involved. Low-resistance enteroenteric fistulas, which allow luminal contents to bypass a significant proportion of the small intestine, may result in clinically significant malabsorption. Enterovesicular fistulas often cause recurrent urinary tract infections. The drainage emanating from enterocutaneous fistulas are irritating to the skin and cause excoriation. The loss of enteric luminal contents, particularly from high-output fistulas originating from the proximal small intestine, results in dehydration, electrolyte abnormalities, and malnutrition.

Fistulas have the potential to close spontaneously. Factors inhibiting spontaneous closure, however, include malnutrition, sepsis, inflammatory bowel disease, cancer, radiation, obstruction of the intestine distal to the origin of the fistula, foreign bodies, high output, and epithelialization of the fistula tract.

Clinical Presentation

Iatrogenic enterocutaneous fistulas usually become clinically evident between the fifth and tenth postoperative days. Fever, leukocytosis, prolonged ileus, abdominal tenderness, and wound infection are the initial signs. The diagnosis becomes obvious when drainage of enteric material through the abdominal wound or through existing drains occurs. These fistulas are often associated with intra-abdominal abscesses.

Diagnosis

CT scanning following the administration of enteral contrast is the most useful initial test. Leakage of contrast material from the intestinal lumen can be observed. Intra-abdominal abscesses should be sought and drained percutaneously. If the anatomy of the fistula is not clear on CT scanning, a small-bowel series or enteroclysis examination can be obtained to demonstrate the fistula's site of origin in the bowel. This study is also useful to rule out the presence of intestinal obstruction distal to the site of origin. Occasionally, contrast administered into the intestine does not demonstrate the fistula tract. A *fistulogram,* in which contrast is injected under pressure through a catheter placed percutaneously into the fistula tract, may offer greater sensitivity in localizing the fistula origin (Fig. 27-22).

Therapy

The treatment of enterocutaneous fistulas should proceed through an orderly sequence of steps.[44] Step 1: *Stabilization.* Fluid and electrolyte resuscitation is begun. Nutrition is provided, usually through the parenteral route initially. Sepsis is controlled with antibiotics and drainage of abscesses. The skin is protected from the fistula effluent with ostomy appliances or fistula drains. Step 2: *Investigation.* The anatomy of the fistula is defined using the studies described above. Step 3: *Rehabilitation.* Probability of spontaneous closure is maximized. Nutrition and time are the key components of this phase. Most patients will require TPN; however, a trial of oral or enteral nutrition should be attempted in patients with low-output fistulas originating from the distal intestine. The somatostatin analogue octreotide is a useful adjunct, particularly in patients with high-output fistulas, because its administration reduces the volume of fistula output, thereby facilitating fluid and electrolyte management. Furthermore, octreotide may accelerate the rate at which fistulas close;

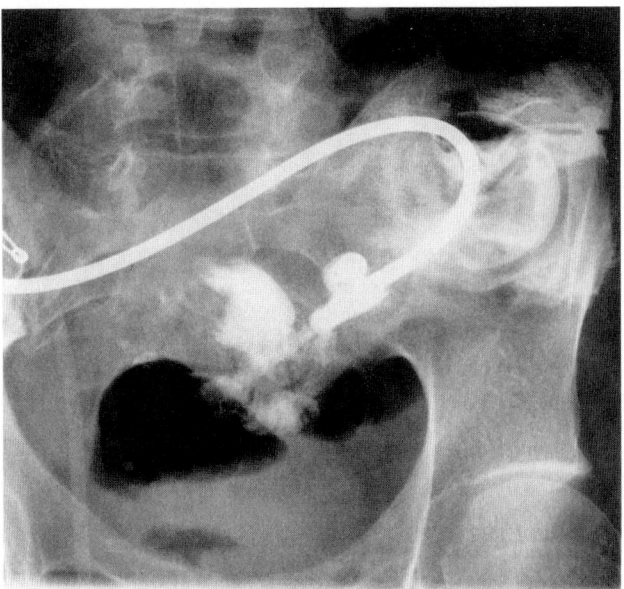

FIG. 27-22. Fistulogram. Contrast injected into a catheter placed into the fistula tract demonstrates communication with the small intestine in this patient with Crohn's disease. (*Courtesy of John Braver, M.D., Department of Radiology, Brigham and Women's Hospital.*)

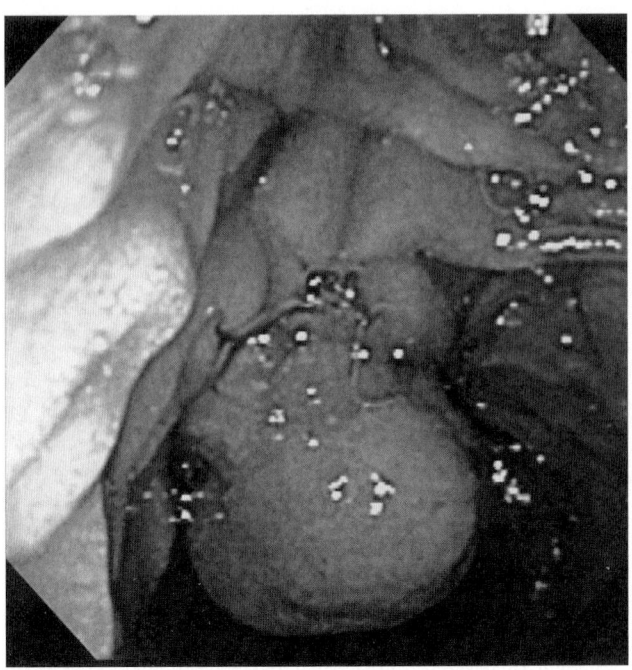

FIG. 27-23. Duodenal polyp. This polyp was incidentally encountered during EGD. It was biopsied and found to be an adenoma.

however, its administration has not clearly been demonstrated to increase the probability of spontaneous closure. Two to 3 months are allowed for spontaneous closure. Fistulas that do not close during this period are unlikely to do so.

If the fistula fails to resolve during this period, surgery may be required during which the fistula tract, together with the segment of intestine from which it originates, should be resected. Simple closure of the opening in the intestine from which the fistula originates is associated with high recurrence rates. Patients with intestinal fistulas typically have extensive and dense intra-abdominal adhesions. As a result, operations performed for nonhealing fistulas can present formidable challenges. Successful applications of alternative therapies to close intestinal fistulas such as the use of biologic sealants have been reported. The indications for their use remain to be defined.

Outcomes

Enterocutaneous fistulas are associated with a 10 to 15% mortality rate, mostly related to sepsis or underlying disease. Overall, 50% of intestinal fistulas close spontaneously. A useful mnemonic designates factors that inhibit spontaneous closure of intestinal fistulas: FRIEND (*f*oreign body within the fistula tract; *r*adiation enteritis; *i*nfection/inflammation at the fistula origin; *e*pithelialization of the fistula tract; *n*eoplasm at the fistula origin; *d*istal obstruction of the intestine). Surgery for fistulas is associated with a greater than 50% morbidity rate, including a 10% recurrence rate.

SMALL-BOWEL NEOPLASMS

Epidemiology

Adenomas are the most common benign neoplasm of the small intestine. Other benign tumors include fibromas, lipomas, hemangiomas, lymphangiomas, and neurofibromas. These lesions are most frequently encountered in the duodenum as incidental findings during EGD examinations (Fig. 27-23). Their reported prevalence rates,

as detected during EGD performed for other reasons, range from 0.3 to 4.6%.[45]

Primary small-bowel cancers are rare, with an estimated incidence of 5300 cases per year in the United States (Table 27-7).[46] Among small-bowel cancers, adenocarcinomas comprise 35 to 50% of all cases, carcinoid tumors comprise 20 to 40%, and lymphomas comprise approximately 10 to 15%. GISTs are the most common mesenchymal tumors arising in the small intestine and comprise up to 15% of small-bowel malignancies.[47–49] GISTs comprise the vast majority of tumors that were formerly classified as leiomyomas, leiomyosarcomas, and smooth muscle tumors of the intestine. The small intestine is frequently affected by metastases from or local invasion by cancers originating at other sites. Melanoma, in particular, is associated with a propensity for metastasis to the small intestine.

Most patients with small-intestinal cancers are in their fifth or sixth decade of life. Reported risk factors for developing small-intestinal adenocarcinoma include consumption of red meat, ingestion of smoked or cured foods, Crohn's disease, celiac sprue, hereditary nonpolyposis colorectal cancer (HNPCC), familial adenomatous polyposis (FAP), and Peutz-Jeghers syndrome. Patients with FAP have a nearly 100% cumulative lifetime risk of developing duodenal adenomas that have the potential to undergo malignant transformation. The risk of duodenal cancer in these patients is more than 100-fold than in the general population. Indeed, duodenal cancer is the leading cause of cancer-related death among patients with FAP who have undergone colectomy. Patients with Peutz-Jeghers syndrome develop hamartomatous polyps; however, these polyps can contain adenomatous foci that can undergo malignant transformation. Risk factors for developing other types of small-bowel cancers are not well delineated.

Pathophysiology

The small intestine contains more than 90% of the mucosal surface area of the gastrointestinal tract, but only 1.1 to 2.4% of all gastrointestinal malignancies. Proposed explanations for the low frequency

Table 27-7
Features of Small-Intestinal Malignancies

Tumor Type	Cell of Origin	Frequency[a]	Predominant Site
Adenocarcinoma	Epithelial cell	35–50%	Duodenum
Carcinoid	Enterochromaffin cell	20–40%	Ileum
Lymphoma	Lymphocyte	10–15%	Ileum
GIST	?Interstitial cell of Cajal	10–15%	—

[a]Frequencies given as percentages of small-intestinal malignancies comprised by each of the tumor types. Gastrointestinal stromal tumors display no regional variation in prevalence within the small intestine.

of small-intestinal neoplasms include (1) dilution of environmental carcinogens in the liquid chyme present in the small-intestinal lumen; (2) rapid transit of chyme, limiting the contact time between carcinogens and the intestinal mucosa; (3) a relatively low concentration of bacteria in small-intestinal chyme and, therefore, a relatively low concentration of carcinogenic products of bacterial metabolism; (4) mucosal protection by secretory IgA and hydrolases such as benzpyrene hydroxylase that may render carcinogens less active; and (5) efficient epithelial cellular apoptotic mechanisms that serve to eliminate clones harboring genetic mutations.[50]

Recent advances have begun to clarify the molecular pathogenesis of small-intestinal adenocarcinomas and GISTs; there has been less progress with respect to the pathogenesis of the other small-intestinal malignancies. Small-intestinal adenocarcinomas are believed to arise from preexisting adenomas through a sequential accumulation of genetic abnormalities in a model similar to that described for the pathogenesis of colorectal cancer.[51] Adenomas are histologically classified as tubular, villous, and tubulovillous. Tubular adenomas have the least-aggressive features. Villous adenomas have the most-aggressive features and tend to be large, sessile, and located in the second portion of the duodenum. Malignant degeneration has been reported to be present in up to 45% of villous adenomas by the time of diagnosis.[50]

A defining feature of GIST is its expression of the receptor tyrosine kinase KIT (CD117). Pathologic KIT signal transduction is believed to be a central event in GIST pathogenesis.[3,4] The majority of GISTs have activating mutations in the c-kit protooncogene, which cause KIT to become constitutively activated, presumably leading to persistence of cellular growth or survival signals. Because the interstitial cells of Cajal normally express KIT, these cells have been implicated as the cell of origin for GISTs.

Clinical Presentation

Most small-intestinal neoplasms are asymptomatic until they become large. Partial small-bowel obstruction, with associated symptoms of crampy abdominal pain and distention, nausea, and vomiting, is the most common mode of presentation. Obstruction can be the result of either luminal narrowing by the tumor itself or intussusception, with the tumor serving as the lead point. Hemorrhage, usually indolent, is the second most common mode of presentation.

Physical examination may be unrevealing. Up to 25% of patients with small-intestinal malignancies are reported to have a palpable abdominal mass. Findings of intestinal obstruction are reported to be present in 25% of patients. Fecal occult blood test may be positive. Jaundice secondary to biliary obstruction or hepatic metastasis may be present. Cachexia, hepatomegaly, and ascites may be present with advanced disease.

Although the clinical presentation is usually not specific for tumor type, some general comments are appropriate. Adenocarcino-

mas, as well as adenomas (from which most are believed to arise), are most commonly found in the duodenum, except in patients with Crohn's disease, in whom most are found in the ileum. Lesions in the periampullary location can cause obstructive jaundice or pancreatitis. Adenocarcinomas located in the duodenum tend to be diagnosed earlier in their progression than those located in the jejunum or ileum, which are rarely diagnosed prior to the onset of locally advanced or metastatic disease.

Carcinoid tumors of the small intestine are also usually diagnosed after the development of metastatic disease. These tumors are associated with a more aggressive behavior than the more common appendiceal carcinoid tumors. Approximately 25 to 50% of patients with carcinoid tumor-derived liver metastases will develop manifestations of the carcinoid syndrome. These manifestations include diarrhea, flushing, hypotension, tachycardia, and fibrosis of the endocardium and valves of the right heart. Candidate tumor-derived mediators of the carcinoid syndrome, such as serotonin, bradykinin, and substance P, undergo nearly complete metabolism during first passage through the liver. As a result, symptoms of carcinoid syndrome are rare in the absence of liver metastases.

Lymphoma may involve the small intestine primarily or as a manifestation of disseminated systemic disease. Primary small-intestinal lymphomas are most commonly located in the ileum, which contains the highest concentration of lymphoid tissue in the intestine. Although partial small-bowel obstruction is the most common mode of presentation, 10% of patients with small-intestinal lymphoma present with bowel perforation.

Sixty to 70% of GISTs are located in the stomach. The small intestine is the second most common site, containing 25 to 35% of GISTs. There appears to be no regional variation in the prevalence of GISTs within the small intestine. GISTs have a greater propensity to be associated with overt hemorrhage than the other small-intestinal malignancies (Fig. 27-24).

Metastatic tumors involving the small intestine can induce intestinal obstruction and bleeding.

Diagnosis

Because of the absent or nonspecific symptoms associated with most small-intestinal neoplasms, these lesions are rarely diagnosed preoperatively. Laboratory tests are nonspecific, with the exception of elevated serum 5-hydroxyindole acetic acid (5-HIAA) levels in patients with the carcinoid syndrome. Elevated carcinoembryonic antigen (CEA) levels are associated with small-intestinal adenocarcinomas, but only in the presence of liver metastases.

Contrast radiography of the small intestine may demonstrate benign and malignant lesions (Fig. 27-25). Enteroclysis is reported to have a sensitivity of greater than 90% in the detection of small-bowel tumors and is the test of choice, particularly for tumors located in the distal small bowel. Upper GI with small-bowel follow-through

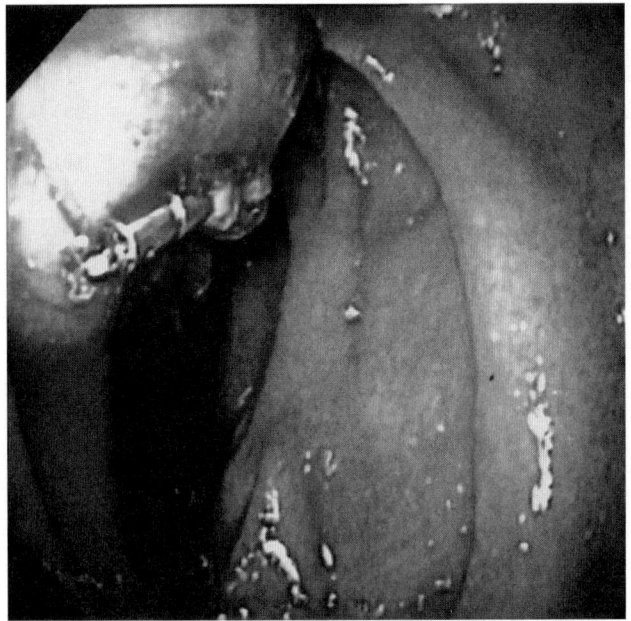

FIG. 27-24. *Gastrointestinal stromal tumor. This GIST located in the duodenum caused massive hemorrhage. Initial endoscopic control of the bleeding was achieved (endoscopically placed clips are shown). Recurrent bleeding prompted segmental duodenal resection.*

examinations have reported sensitivities ranging from only 30 to 44%.[50] CT scanning has low sensitivity for detecting mucosal or intramural lesions, but can demonstrate large tumors and is useful in the staging of intestinal malignancies (Fig. 27-26). Tumors associated with significant bleeding can be localized with angiography or radioisotope-tagged red blood cell (RBC) scans.

Tumors located in the duodenum can be visualized and biopsied on EGD. In addition, endoscopic ultrasonography (EUS) can offer additional information, such as the layers of the intestinal wall involved by the lesion (Fig. 27-27). Occasionally, the distal ileum can successfully be visualized during colonoscopy. Intraoperative enteroscopy can be used to directly visualize small-intestinal tumors beyond the reach of standard endoscopic techniques. Recently, swallowed radiotelemetry capsules that are capable of transmitting images of the bowel mucosa (capsule enteroscopy) were introduced. The accuracy of this technique for detecting small-intestinal neoplasms remains to be defined.

Therapy

Benign neoplasms of the small intestine that are symptomatic should be surgically resected or removed endoscopically, if feasible. Tumors located in the duodenum, including asymptomatic lesions incidentally found during EGD, can pose the greatest therapeutic challenges. These lesions should be biopsied; symptomatic tumors and adenomas, because of their malignant potential, should be removed. In general, duodenal tumors less than 1 cm in diameter are amenable to endoscopic polypectomy. Lesions greater than 2 cm in diameter are technically difficult to remove endoscopically and should therefore be removed surgically. Surgical options include transduodenal polypectomy and segmental duodenal resection. Tumors located in the second portion of the duodenum near the ampulla of Vater may require pancreaticoduodenectomy. EUS may offer utility for duodenal tumors ranging in size between 1 and 2 cm in diameter, with those limited to the mucosa being amenable to endoscopic polypectomy.[52] Adenomas can recur; therefore, surveillance endoscopy is required after these procedures.

Duodenal adenomas occurring in the setting of FAP require an especially aggressive approach to management. Patients with FAP should undergo screening EGD starting sometime during their

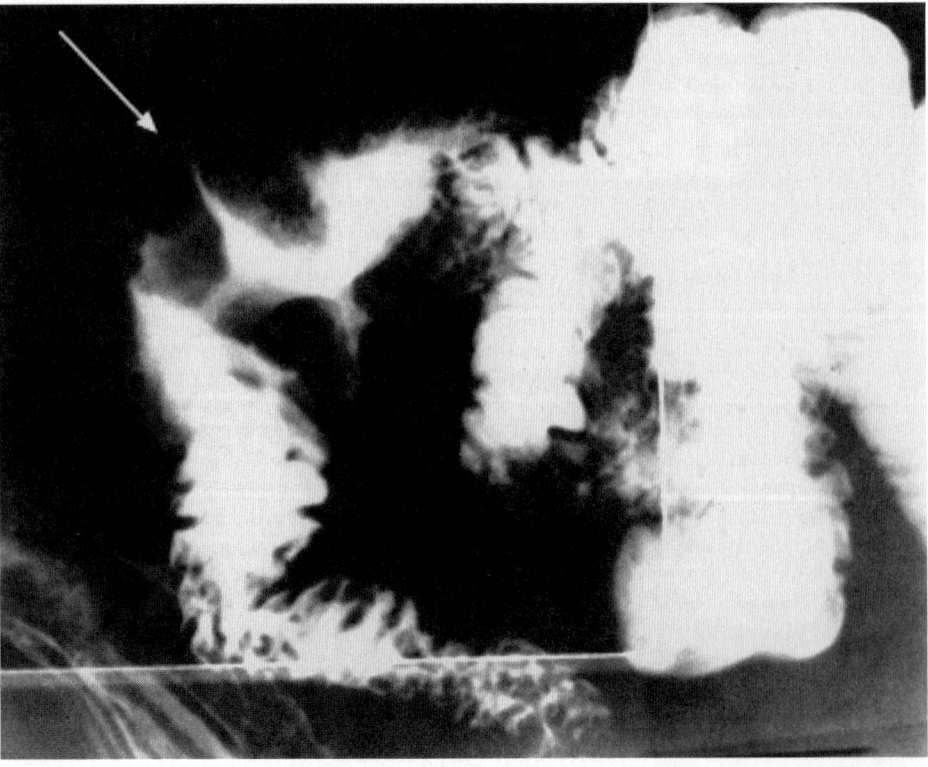

FIG. 27-25. *Jejunal adenocarcinoma. Contrast radiograph demonstrating a lesion in the proximal jejunum determined to be an adenocarcinoma of the small intestine at the time of surgery.*

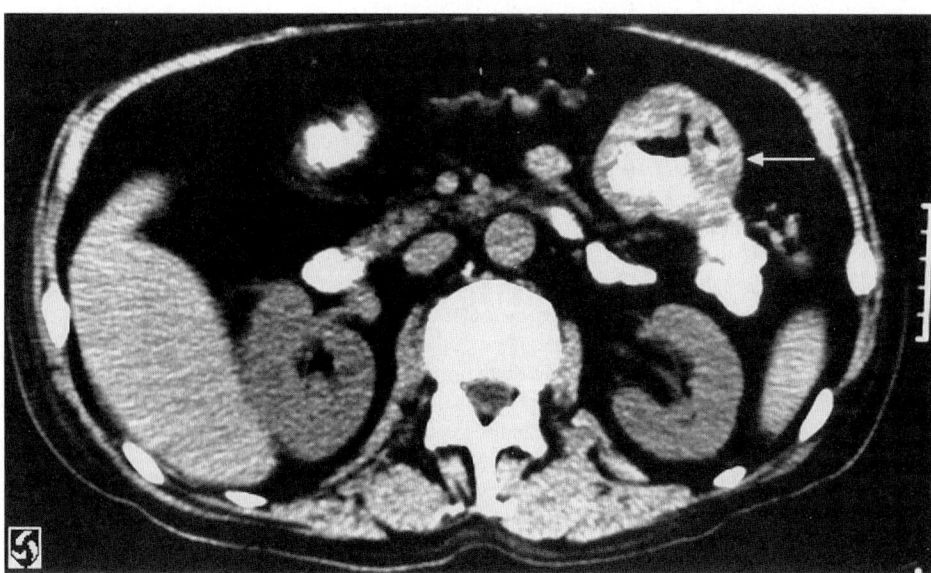

FIG. 27-26. Jejunal adenocarcinoma. CT scan demonstrating a small-bowel loop in the left upper quadrant with a irregularly thickened wall and areas of ulceration (*arrow*). This lesion proved to be a jejunal adenocarcinoma.

second or third decade of life. Adenomas detected should be removed endoscopically, if possible, followed by surveillance endoscopy in 6 months and yearly thereafter, in the absence of recurrence. If surgery is required, pancreaticoduodenectomy is generally necessary because adenomas in patients with FAP tend to be multiple and sessile, with a predilection for the periampullary region. Furthermore, localized resections are complicated by high recurrence rates. Given the potential for recurrences in the duodenal remnant following pylorus-preserving pancreaticoduodenectomy, there is rationale for recommending the application of standard pancreaticoduodenectomy in these patients. However, recurrences have been reported even following this procedure; therefore, continuing surveillance is necessary.

The surgical therapy of small-intestinal malignancies usually consists of wide–local resection of the intestine harboring the lesion. For adenocarcinomas, a wide excision of corresponding mesentery is done to achieve regional lymphadenectomy, as is done for adenocarcinomas of the colon. For most adenocarcinomas of the duodenum, except those in the distal duodenum, pancreaticoduodenectomy is required. In the presence of locally advanced or metastatic disease, palliative intestinal resection or bypass is performed. Chemotherapy has no proven efficacy in the adjuvant or palliative treatment of small-intestinal adenocarcinomas.

The goal of surgical therapy for carcinoids is resection of all visible disease. Localized small-intestinal carcinoid tumors should be treated with segmental intestinal resection and regional

FIG. 27-27. Duodenal adenoma. EUS revealed two mucosal lesions in the duodenum. The lesion at 11 o'clock proved to be an adenoma. (*Courtesy of Julia Liu, M.D., Department of Medicine, Brigham and Women's Hospital.*)

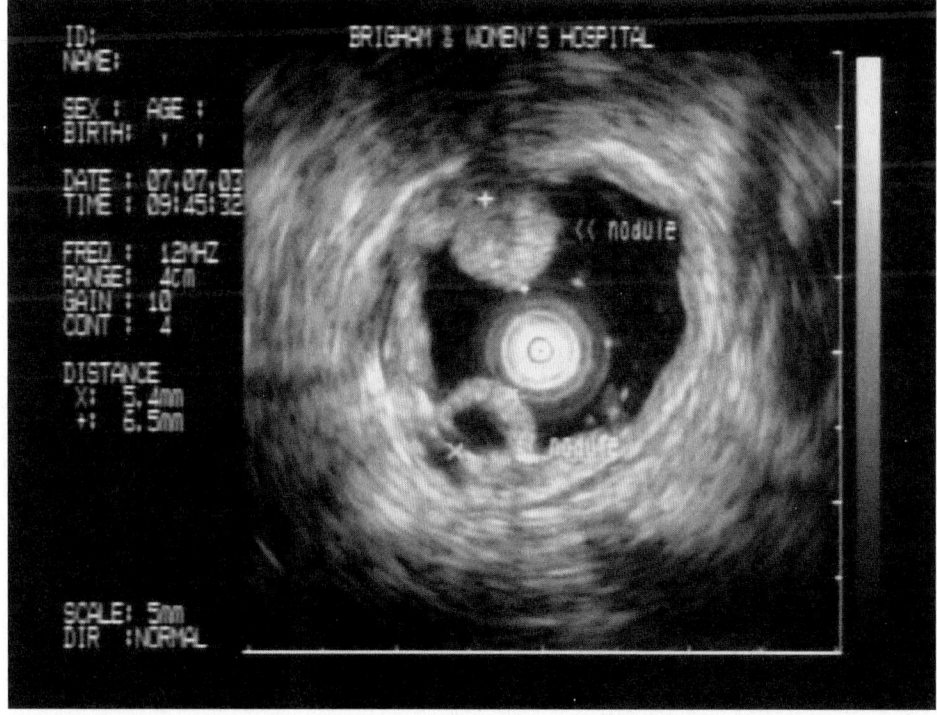

lymphadenectomy. Nodal metastases are rarely present with tumors less than 1 cm in diameter, but are present with 75 to 90% of tumors larger than 3 cm in diameter. In approximately 30% of cases, multiple small-intestinal carcinoid tumors are present. Therefore, the entire small intestine should be examined before planning the extent of resection. In the presence of metastatic disease, tumor debulking should be conducted because it can be associated with long-term survival and amelioration of symptoms of the carcinoid syndrome. Response rates of 30 to 50% have been reported to chemotherapy regimens based on agents such as doxorubicin, 5-fluorouracil, and streptozocin. However, none of these regimens is associated with a clearly demonstrable impact on the natural history of disease. Octreotide is the most effective pharmacologic agent for management of symptoms of carcinoid syndrome.

Localized small-intestinal lymphoma should be treated with segmental resection of the involved intestine and adjacent mesentery. If the small intestine is diffusely affected by lymphoma, chemotherapy, rather than surgical resection, should be the primary therapy. The value to adjuvant chemotherapy after resection of localized lymphoma is controversial.

Small-intestinal GISTs should be treated with segmental intestinal resection. If the diagnosis is known prior to resection, wide lymphadenectomy can be avoided because GISTs are rarely associated with lymph node metastases. GISTs are resistant to conventional chemotherapy agents. Imatinib (Gleevec, formerly known as ST1571) is a tyrosine kinase inhibitor with potent activity against tyrosine kinase KIT. Recent clinical trials show that 80% of patients with unresectable or metastatic GISTs derive clinical benefit from the administration of imatinib, with 50 to 60% having objective evidence of reduction in tumor volume.[53] The role of imatinib in the neoadjuvant and adjuvant therapy of GISTs is an active area of investigation.

Metastatic cancers affecting the small intestine that are symptomatic should be treated with palliative resection or bypass except in the most advanced cases. Systemic therapy may be offered if effective chemotherapy exists for the primary cancer.

Outcomes

Complete resection of duodenal adenocarcinomas is associated with postoperative 5-year survival rates ranging from 50 to 60%. Complete resection of adenocarcinomas located in the jejunum or ileum is associated with 5-year survival rates of only 5 to 30%. Five-year survival rates of 75 to 95% following resection of localized small-intestinal carcinoid tumors have been reported. In the presence of carcinoid tumor-derived liver metastases, 5-year survival rates of 19 to 54% have been reported. The overall 5-year survival rate for patients diagnosed with intestinal lymphoma ranges from 20 to 40%. For patients with localized lymphoma amenable to surgical resection, the 5-year survival rate is 60%.

The recurrence rate following resection of GISTs averages 35%. The 5-year survival rate following surgical resection has been reported to range from 35 to 60%. Both tumor size and mitotic index are independently correlated with prognosis. Low-grade tumors (mitotic index <10 per high-power field) less than 5 cm in diameter are associated with excellent prognosis.

RADIATION ENTERITIS

Epidemiology

Radiation therapy is a component of multimodality therapy for many intra-abdominal and pelvic cancers, such as those of the cervix,

endometrium, ovary, bladder, prostate, and rectum. An undesired side effect of radiation therapy is radiation-induced injury to the small intestine, which can present clinically as two distinct syndromes: acute and chronic radiation enteritis. Acute radiation enteritis is a transient condition that occurs in approximately 75% of patients undergoing radiation therapy for abdominal and pelvic cancers. Chronic radiation enteritis is inexorable and develops in approximately 5 to 15% of these patients.

Pathophysiology

Radiation induces cellular injury directly and through the generation of free radicals. The principal mechanism of radiation-induced cell death is believed to be apoptosis resulting from free radical-induced breaks in double-stranded DNA. Because radiation has its greatest impact on rapidly proliferating cells, the small-intestinal epithelium is acutely susceptible to radiation-induced injury. Pathologic correlates of this acute injury include villus blunting and a dense infiltrate of leukocytes and plasma cells within the crypts. With severe cases, mucosal sloughing, ulceration, and hemorrhage are observed. The intensity of injury is related to the dose of radiation administered, with most cases occurring in patients who have received at least 4500 cGy. Risk factors for acute radiation enteritis include conditions that may limit splanchnic perfusion such as hypertension, diabetes mellitus, coronary artery disease, and restricted motility of the small intestine caused by adhesions. Injury is potentiated by concomitant administration of chemotherapeutic agents that act as radiation-sensitizers such as doxorubicin, 5-fluorouracil, actinomycin D, and methotrexate. Because of the intestinal epithelium's capacity for regeneration, the mucosal injury that is characteristic of acute radiation enteritis resolves after the cessation of radiation therapy.

In contrast, chronic radiation enteritis is characterized by a progressive occlusive vasculitis that leads to chronic ischemia and fibrosis that affects all layers of the intestinal wall, rather than the mucosa alone. These changes can lead to strictures, abscesses, and fistulas, which are responsible for the clinical manifestations of chronic radiation enteritis.

Clinical Presentation

The most common manifestations of acute radiation enteritis are nausea, vomiting, diarrhea, and crampy abdominal pain. Symptoms are generally transient and subside after the discontinuation of radiation therapy. Because the diagnosis is usually obvious, given the clinical context, no specific diagnostic tests are required. However, if patients develop signs suggestive of peritonitis, CT scanning should be performed to rule out the presence of other conditions capable of causing acute abdominal syndromes.

The clinical manifestations of chronic radiation enteritis usually become evident within 2 years of radiation administration, although they can begin as early as several months or as late as decades afterwards. The most common clinical presentation is one of partial small-bowel obstruction with nausea, vomiting, intermittent abdominal distention, crampy abdominal pain, and weight loss being the most common symptoms. The terminal ileum is the most frequently affected segment. Other manifestations of chronic radiation enteritis include complete bowel obstruction, acute or chronic intestinal hemorrhage, and abscess or fistula formation.

Diagnosis

Evaluation of patients suspected of having chronic radiation enteritis should include review of the records of their radiation treatments

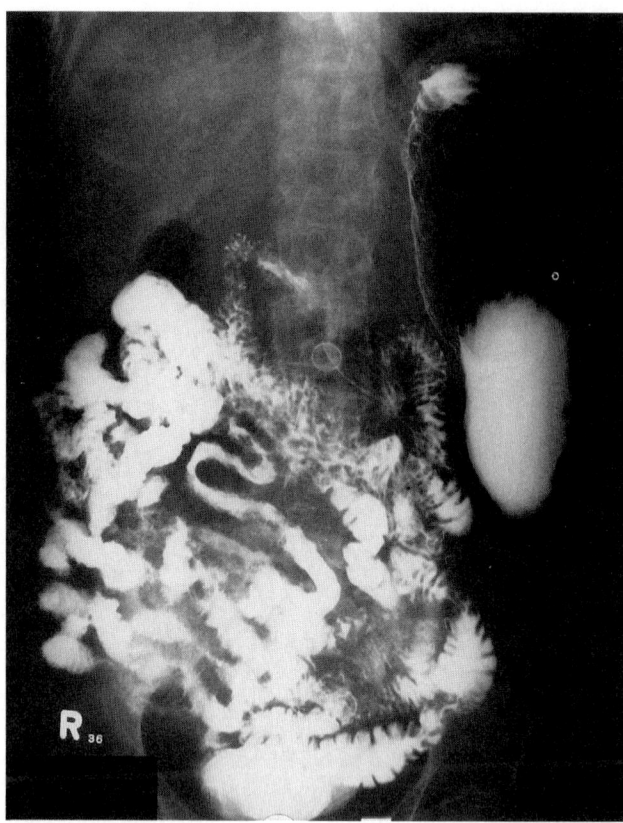

FIG. 27-28. Radiation enteritis. This contrast radiograph reveals widely separated loops of small bowel with luminal narrowing, loss of mucosal folds, and ulceration. This patient had received radiation therapy for a pelvic malignancy 8 years before this examination.

for information on total radiation dose administered, fractionation, and volume of treatment. Areas that received high doses should be noted, because lesions subsequently found in imaging studies usually localize to areas that had received high radiation doses. Enteroclysis is the most accurate imaging test for diagnosing chronic radiation enteritis, with reported sensitivities and specificities of greater than 90% (Fig. 27-28). CT scan findings are neither very sensitive nor specific for chronic radiation enteritis. However, CT scanning should be obtained to rule out the presence of recurrent cancer because its clinical manifestations may overlap with those of chronic radiation enteritis.

Therapy

Most cases of acute radiation enteritis are self-limited. Supportive therapy, including the administration of antiemetics, is usually sufficient. Patients with diarrhea-induced dehydration may require hospital admission and parenteral fluid administration. Rarely are symptoms severe enough to necessitate reduction in or cessation of radiation therapy.

In contrast, the treatment of chronic radiation enteritis represents a formidable challenge. Surgery for this condition is difficult, is associated with high morbidity rates, and should be avoided in the absence of specific indications such as high-grade obstruction, perforation, hemorrhage, intra-abdominal abscesses, and fistulas. The goal of surgery is limited resection of diseased intestine with primary anastomosis between healthy bowel segments. However, the characteristically diffuse nature of fibrosis and dense adhesions among bowel segments can make limited resection difficult to achieve.

Furthermore, it is difficult to distinguish between normal and irradiated intestine intraoperatively by either gross inspection or frozen-section analysis. This distinction is important because anastomoses between irradiated segments of intestine are associated with leak rates as high as 50%.[54] If limited resection is not achievable, an intestinal bypass procedure may be an option, except in cases for which hemorrhage is the surgical indication. There remain cases in which resections extensive enough to cause short-bowel syndrome are unavoidable. This condition is discussed in detail later under "Short-Bowel Syndrome."

Outcomes

Acute radiation injury to the intestine is self-limited; its severity is not correlated with the probability of chronic radiation enteritis developing. Surgery for chronic radiation enteritis is associated with high morbidity rates and reported mortality rates averaging 10%.

MECKEL'S DIVERTICULUM

Epidemiology

Meckel's diverticulum is the most prevalent congenital anomaly of the gastrointestinal tract, affecting approximately 2% of the general population.[55] A 3:2 male to female prevalence ratio has been reported. Meckel's diverticula are designated *true diverticula* because their walls contain all of the layers found in normal small intestine. Their location varies among individual patients, but they are usually found in the ileum within 100 cm of the ileocecal valve (Fig. 27-29). Approximately 60% of Meckel's diverticula contain heterotopic mucosa, of which more than 60% consist of gastric mucosa. Pancreatic acini are the next most common; others include Brunner's glands, pancreatic islets, colonic mucosa, endometriosis, and hepatobiliary tissues. A useful, although crude, mnemonic describing Meckel's diverticula is the "rule of twos": 2% prevalence, 2:1 female predominance, location 2 feet proximal to the ileocecal valve in adults, and half of those who are symptomatic are younger than 2 years of age.

Pathophysiology

During the eighth week of gestation, the omphalomesenteric (vitelline) duct normally undergoes obliteration. Failure or incomplete vitelline duct obliteration results in a spectrum of abnormalities, the most common of which is Meckel's diverticulum. Other abnormalities include omphalomesenteric fistula, enterocysts, and a fibrous band connecting the intestine to the umbilicus. A remnant of the left vitelline artery can persist to form a mesodiverticular band tethering a Meckel's diverticulum to the ileal mesentery.

Bleeding associated with Meckel's diverticulum is usually the result of ileal mucosal ulceration that occurs adjacent to acid-producing, heterotopic gastric mucosa located within the diverticulum. Intestinal obstruction associated with Meckel's diverticulum can result from several mechanisms: (1) volvulus of the intestine around the fibrous band attaching the diverticulum to the umbilicus; (2) entrapment of intestine by a mesodiverticular band (Fig. 27-30); (3) intussusception with the diverticulum acting as a lead point; or (4) stricture secondary to chronic diverticulitis. Meckel's diverticula can be found in inguinal or femoral hernia sacs (known as Littre's hernia). These hernias, when incarcerated, can cause intestinal obstruction.

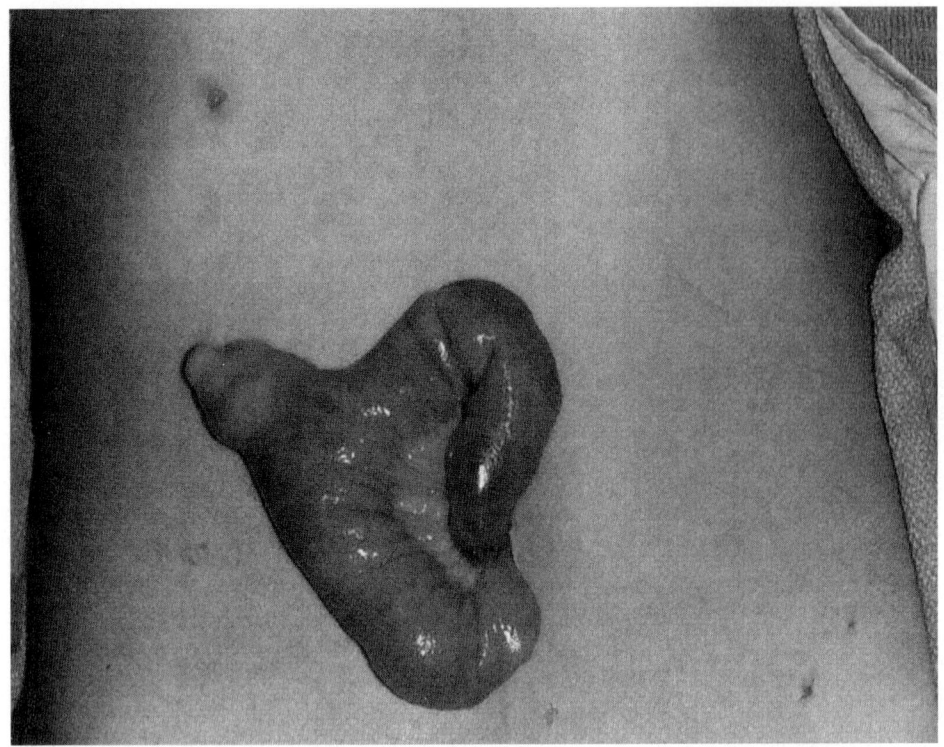

FIG. 27-29. Meckel's diverticulum. This intraoperative photograph shows Meckel's diverticulum in ileum that has been eviscerated.

Clinical Presentation

Meckel's diverticula are asymptomatic unless associated complications arise. The lifetime incidence rate of complications arising in patients with Meckel's diverticula has been estimated to be approximately 4%. More than 50% of patients who develop symptoms related to complications of Meckel's diverticula are younger than 10 years of age.

The most common presentations associated with symptomatic Meckel's diverticula are bleeding, intestinal obstruction, and diverticulitis. Bleeding is the most common presentation in children with Meckel's diverticula, representing more than 50% of Meckel's diverticulum-related complications among patients who are younger than 18 years of age. Bleeding associated with Meckel's diverticula is rare among patients who are older than 30 years of age.

Intestinal obstruction is the most common presentation in adults with Meckel's diverticula. Diverticulitis, present in 20% of patients with symptomatic Meckel's diverticula, is associated with a clinical syndrome that is indistinguishable from acute appendicitis. Neoplasms, most commonly carcinoid tumors, are present in 0.5 to 3.2% of symptomatic Meckel's diverticula that are resected.[56]

Diagnosis

Most Meckel's diverticula are discovered incidentally on radiographic imaging, during endoscopy, or at the time of surgery. In the absence of bleeding, Meckel's diverticula rarely are diagnosed prior to the time of surgical intervention. The sensitivity of CT scanning for the detection of Meckel's diverticula is too low to be clinically useful. Enteroclysis is associated with an accuracy of 75%,

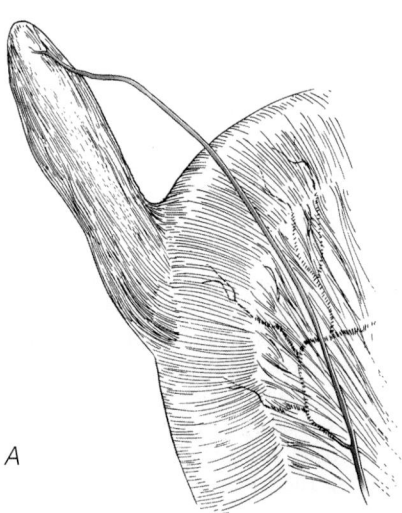
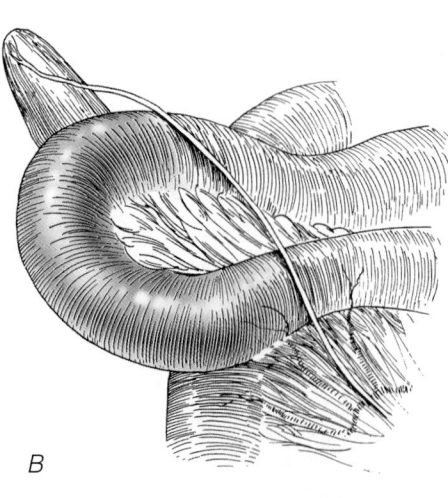

FIG. 27-30. *A.* Meckel's diverticulum with mesodiverticular band. *B.* One mechanism by which Meckel's diverticula can cause small-bowel obstruction is entrapment of the intestine by a mesodiverticular band.

A

B

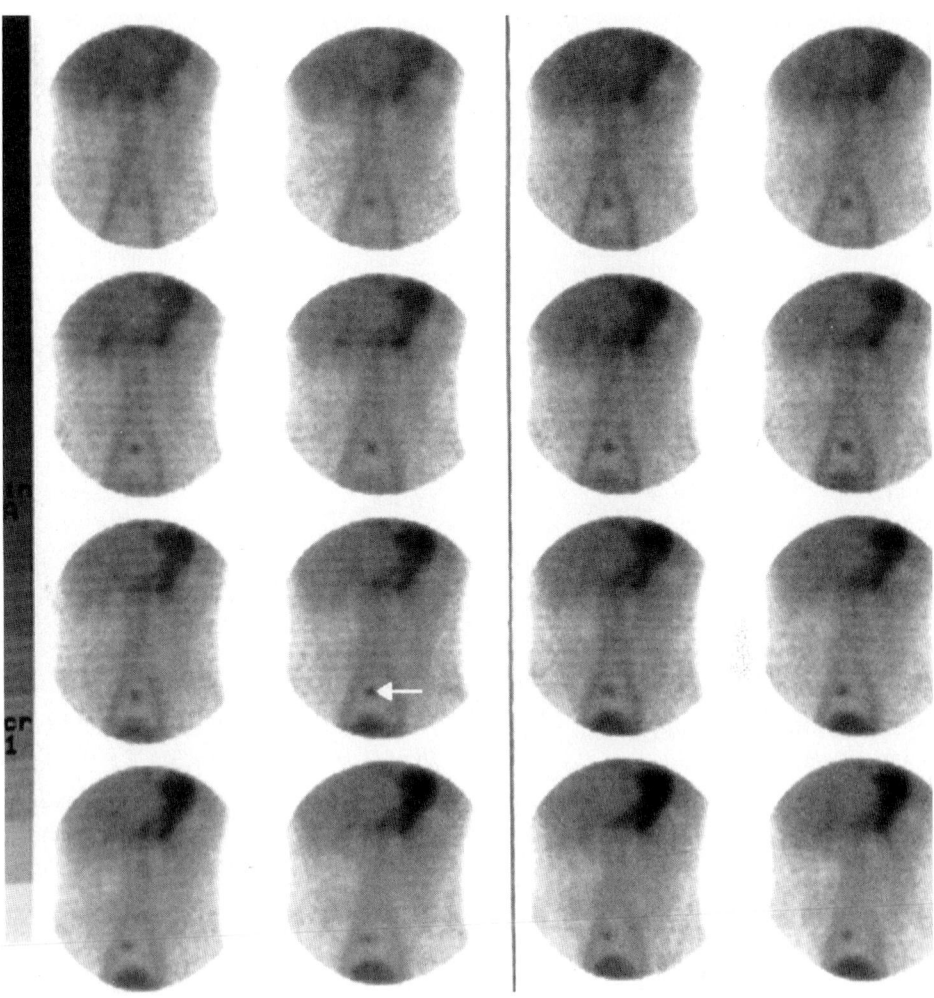

FIG. 27-31. Meckel's diverticulum with ectopic gastric tissue. The diagnosis was made in this patient with GI bleeding using ^{99m}Tc-pertechnetate scintigraphy. The study revealed an abnormal focus of radiotracer accumulation in the right lower quadrant (*arrow*).

but is usually not applicable during acute presentations of complications related to Meckel's diverticula. Radionuclide scans (^{99m}Tc-pertechnetate) suggest the diagnosis of Meckel's diverticulum when uptake occurs in associated ectopic gastric mucosa, or when extravasation occurs during active bleeding (Fig. 27-31). The accuracy of radionuclide scanning is reported to be 90% in pediatric patients, but less than 50% in adults. Angiography can localize the site of bleeding during acute hemorrhage related to Meckel's diverticula.

Therapy

The surgical treatment of symptomatic Meckel's diverticula should consist of diverticulectomy with removal of associated bands connecting the diverticulum to the abdominal wall or intestinal mesentery. If the indication for diverticulectomy is bleeding, segmental resection of ileum that includes both the diverticulum and the adjacent ileal peptic ulcer should be performed. Segmental ileal resection may also be necessary if the diverticulum contains a tumor, or if the base of the diverticulum is inflamed or perforated.

The management of incidentally found (asymptomatic) Meckel's diverticula is controversial. Until recently, most authors recommended against prophylactic removal of asymptomatic Meckel's diverticula, given the low lifetime incidence of complications. More recently, greater enthusiasm for prophylactic diverticulectomy has appeared in the literature.[55] Proponents of this approach cite the minimal morbidity associated with removing Meckel's diverticula and the possibility that previous estimates of the lifetime incidence

of complications related to Meckel's diverticula may be erroneously low. Other authors advocate a selective approach, with a recommendation to remove diverticula attached by bands and those with narrow bases, on the assumption that these diverticula are more likely to develop complications.[57] No controlled data supporting or refuting these recommendations exist.

ACQUIRED DIVERTICULA

Epidemiology

Acquired diverticula are designated *false diverticula* because their walls consist of mucosa and submucosa but lack a complete muscularis. Acquired diverticula in the duodenum tend to be located adjacent to the ampulla; such diverticula are known as *periampullary, juxtapapillary,* or *peri-Vaterian diverticula.* Approximately 75% of juxtapapillary diverticula arise on the medial wall of the duodenum. Acquired diverticula in the jejunum or ileum are known as *jejunoileal diverticula.* Eighty percent of jejunoileal diverticula are localized to the jejunum, 15% to the ileum, and 5% to both jejunum and ileum. Diverticula in the jejunum tend to be large and accompanied by multiple other diverticula, whereas those in the ileum tend to be small and solitary.

The prevalence of duodenal diverticula, as detected on upper GI examinations (Fig. 27-32), is reported to range from 0.16 to 6%.[56] Their prevalence, as detected during endoscopic retrograde

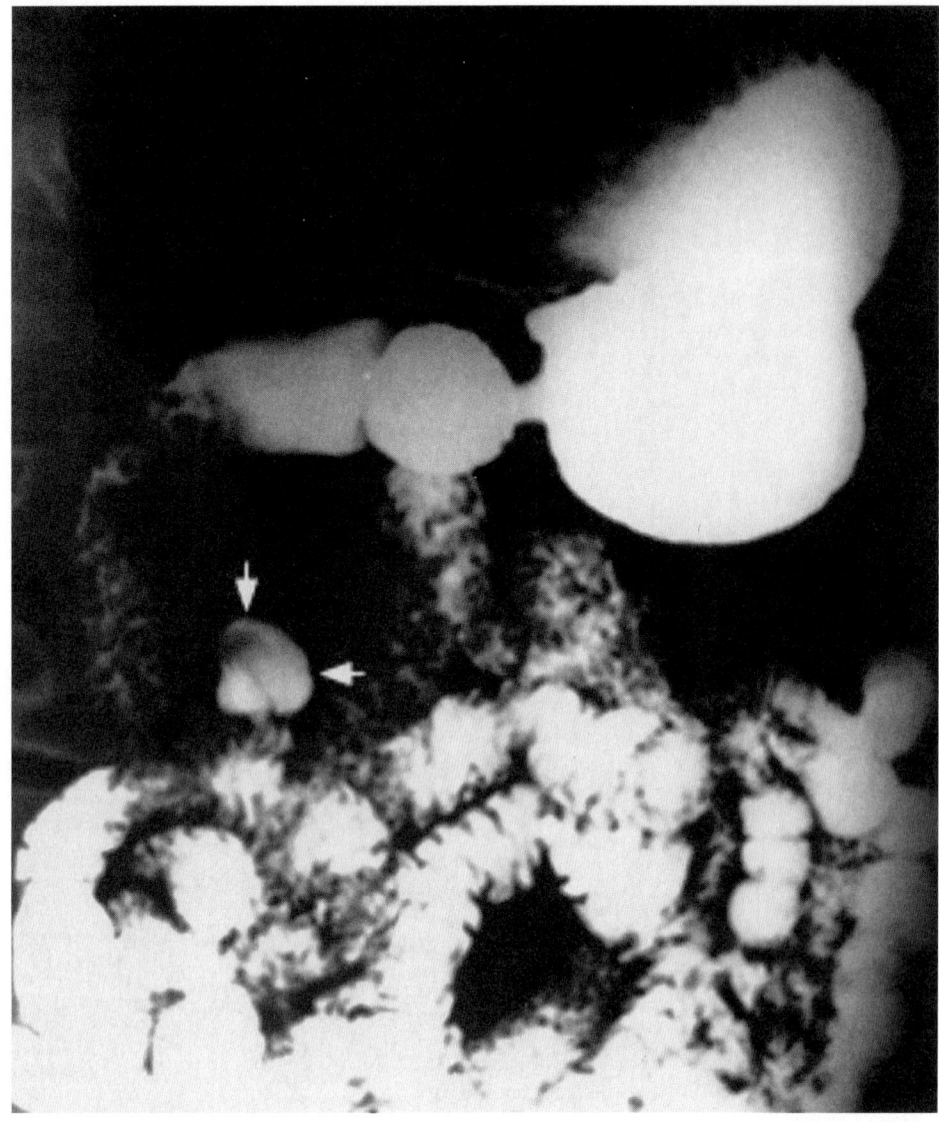

FIG. 27-32. Duodenal diverticulum. This contrast radiograph demonstrates a duodenal diverticulum (*arrows*) that extends medially into the substance of the head of the pancreas.

cholangiopancreatography (ERCP) examinations, is reported to range from 5 to 27%. A 23% prevalence rate was reported in an autopsy series. The prevalence of duodenal diverticula increases with age; they are rare in patients younger than age 40 years. The mean age of diagnosis ranges from 56 to 76 years.

The prevalence of jejunoileal diverticula (Fig. 27-33) has been estimated to range from 1 to 5%.[58] Their prevalence increases with age; most patients diagnosed with these diverticula are in the sixth and seventh decades of life.

Pathophysiology

The pathogenesis of acquired diverticula is hypothesized to be related to acquired abnormalities of intestinal smooth muscle or dysregulated motility, leading to herniation of mucosa and submucosa through weakened areas of muscularis.

Acquired diverticula can be associated with bacterial overgrowth, leading to vitamin B_{12} deficiency, megaloblastic anemia, malabsorption, and steatorrhea. Periampullary duodenal diverticula have been described to become distended with intraluminal debris and to compress the common bile duct or pancreatic duct, thus causing obstructive jaundice or pancreatitis, respectively.

Jejunoileal diverticula can also cause intestinal obstruction through intussusception or compression of adjacent bowel.

Clinical Presentation

Acquired diverticula are asymptomatic unless associated complications arise. Such complications are estimated to occur in 6 to 10% of patients with acquired diverticula and include intestinal obstruction, diverticulitis, hemorrhage, perforation, and malabsorption. Periampullary duodenal diverticula may be associated with choledocholithiasis, cholangitis, recurrent pancreatitis, and sphincter of Oddi dysfunction. However, a clear link between the presence of the diverticula and the development of these conditions has not been demonstrated. Symptoms such as intermittent abdominal pain, flatulence, diarrhea, and constipation are present in 10 to 30% of patients with jejunoileal diverticula. The relationship between these symptoms and the presence of the diverticula is similarly unclear.

Diagnosis

Most acquired diverticula are discovered incidentally on radiographic imaging, during endoscopy, or at the time of surgery. On ultrasound and CT scanning, duodenal diverticula may be mistaken

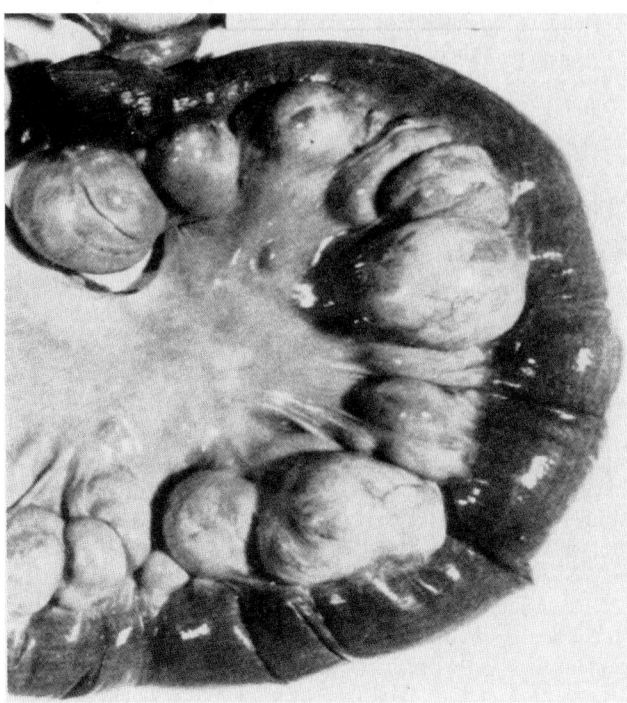

FIG. 27-33. Jejunoileal diverticula. This photograph demonstrates multiple diverticula located on the mesenteric aspect of the jejunum.

for pancreatic pseudocysts and fluid collections, biliary cysts, and periampullary neoplasms. These lesions can be missed on endoscopy, particularly with forward-viewing endoscopes, and are best diagnosed on upper gastrointestinal radiographs. Enteroclysis is the most sensitive test for detecting jejunoileal diverticula.

Therapy

Asymptomatic acquired diverticula should be left alone. Bacterial overgrowth associated with acquired diverticula is treated with antibiotics. Other complications, such as bleeding and diverticulitis, are treated with segmental intestinal resection for diverticula located in the jejunum or ileum. Bleeding and obstruction related to lateral duodenal diverticula are generally treated with diverticulectomy alone.

These procedures can be technically difficult for medial duodenal diverticula that penetrate into the substance of the pancreas. Complications related to these diverticula should be managed nonoperatively if possible. In emergent situations, bleeding related to medial duodenal diverticula can be controlled using a lateral duodenotomy and oversewing of the bleeding vessel. Similarly, perforation can be managed with wide drainage rather than complex surgery. Whether diverticulectomy should be done in patients with biliary or pancreatic symptoms is controversial and is not routinely recommended.[56]

MESENTERIC ISCHEMIA

Mesenteric ischemia can present as one of two distinct clinical syndromes: acute mesenteric ischemia and chronic mesenteric ischemia.

Pathophysiology

Four distinct pathophysiologic mechanisms can lead to acute mesenteric ischemia: arterial embolus, arterial thrombosis, vasospasm

(also known as nonocclusive mesenteric ischemia, or NOMI), and venous thrombosis. Embolus is the most common cause of acute mesenteric ischemia, and is responsible for more than 50% of cases. The embolic source is usually in the heart; most often the left atrial or ventricular thrombi or valvular lesions. Indeed, up to 95% of patients with acute mesenteric ischemia caused by emboli will have a documented history of cardiac disease. Embolism to the superior mesenteric artery accounts for 50% of cases; most of these emboli become wedged and cause occlusion at branch points in the mid to distal superior mesenteric artery, usually distal to the origin of the middle colic artery. In contrast, acute occlusions caused by thrombosis tend to occur in the proximal mesenteric arteries, near their origins. Acute thrombosis is usually superimposed on preexisting atherosclerotic lesions at these sites. NOMI is the result of vasospasm and is usually diagnosed in critically-ill patients who are receiving vasopressor agents.

Mesenteric venous thrombosis accounts for 5 to 15% of cases of acute mesenteric ischemia and involves the superior mesenteric vein in 95% of cases.[59] The inferior mesenteric vein is only rarely involved. Mesenteric venous thrombosis is classified as primary if no etiologic factor is identifiable, or as secondary if an etiologic factor, such as heritable or acquired coagulation disorders, is identified.

Regardless of the pathophysiologic mechanism, acute mesenteric ischemia can lead to intestinal mucosal sloughing within 3 hours of onset and full-thickness intestinal infarction by 6 hours.

In contrast, chronic mesenteric ischemia develops insidiously, allowing for development of collateral circulation, and, therefore, rarely leads to intestinal infarction. Chronic mesenteric arterial ischemia results from atherosclerotic lesions in the main splanchnic arteries (celiac, superior mesenteric, and inferior mesenteric arteries). In most patients with symptoms attributable to chronic mesenteric ischemia, at least two of these arteries are either occluded or severely stenosed. A chronic form of mesenteric venous thrombosis can involve the portal or splenic veins and may lead to portal hypertension, with resulting esophagogastric varices, splenomegaly, and hypersplenism.

Clinical Presentation

Abdominal pain for which the severity is out of proportion to the degree of tenderness on examination is the hallmark of acute mesenteric ischemia, regardless of the pathophysiologic mechanism. The pain is typically perceived to be colicky and most severe in the mid-abdomen. Associated symptoms can include nausea, vomiting, and diarrhea. Physical findings are characteristically absent early in the course of ischemia. With the onset of bowel infarction, abdominal distention, peritonitis, and passage of bloody stools occur.

Chronic mesenteric ischemia presents insidiously. Postprandial abdominal pain is the most prevalent symptom, producing a characteristic aversion to food ("food-fear") and weight loss. These patients are often thought to have a malignancy and suffer a prolonged period of symptoms before the correct diagnosis is made.

Most patients with chronic mesenteric venous thrombosis are asymptomatic because of the presence of extensive collateral venous drainage routes; this condition is usually discovered as an incidental finding on imaging studies. However, some patients with chronic mesenteric venous thrombosis present with bleeding from esophagogastric varices.

Diagnosis

It is important to consider and pursue the diagnosis of acute mesenteric ischemia in any patient who has the classic early finding of severe abdominal pain out of proportion to physical findings. Laboratory test abnormalities, such as leukocytosis, acidosis, and elevations in amylase and creatine kinase (BB isoenzyme), are late findings; no laboratory tests have clinically useful sensitivity for the detection of acute mesenteric ischemia prior to the onset of intestinal infarction.

Patients suspected of having acute mesenteric ischemia and who have physical findings suggestive of peritonitis should undergo emergent laparotomy. In the absence of such findings, diagnostic imaging should be performed.

Angiography is the most reliable method for diagnosing acute mesenteric arterial occlusion, with reported sensitivities ranging from 74 to 100% and specificities approaching 100%.[7] However, angiography is invasive, time-consuming, and costly. Hence, angiography should be performed only in select patients suspected of having acute mesenteric ischemia, as described below.

Most patients suspected of having acute mesenteric ischemia should undergo CT scanning as the initial imaging test. CT scans should be evaluated for (1) disorders other than acute mesenteric ischemia that might account for abdominal pain; (2) evidence of ischemia in the intestine and the mesentery; and (3) evidence of occlusion or stenosis of the mesenteric vasculature. The sensitivity of CT scanning for detecting acute arterial mesenteric ischemia is reported to range from 64 to 82%.[60] Because of this somewhat low sensitivity, a high clinical suspicion for the presence of mesenteric ischemia should prompt angiography if the CT scan reveals no

evidence of mesenteric ischemia or other conditions that could account for acute abdominal pain.

Because the CT findings of NOMI are nonspecific, patients at risk and suspected of having NOMI should undergo angiography without delay. The angiographic findings of NOMI include diffuse narrowing of mesenteric vessels in the absence of obstructing lesions and reduced opacification of bowel parenchyma.

CT scanning, with a sensitivity of 90%, is the test of choice for diagnosing acute mesenteric venous thrombosis. False-negative findings occur in patients with early thromboses of small mesenteric veins. Angiography, capable of demonstrating thromboses in these smaller veins, should therefore be reserved for patients with a history of thrombophilia in whom small-vessel mesenteric venous thrombosis is suspected.

Other imaging studies, such as plain radiographs and ultrasonography, are of little value in the evaluation of patients suspected of having acute mesenteric ischemia. There is only limited experience in the application of MRI in the evaluation of acute mesenteric ischemia.

The gold standard for the diagnosis of chronic arterial mesenteric ischemia is angiography, although CT angiography with three-dimensional reconstruction is noninvasive and offers good resolution (Fig. 27-34). CT findings suggestive of chronic mesenteric ischemia include the presence of atherosclerotic calcified plaques at or near the origins of proximal splanchnic arteries and obvious focal stenosis of proximal mesenteric vessels with prominent collateral

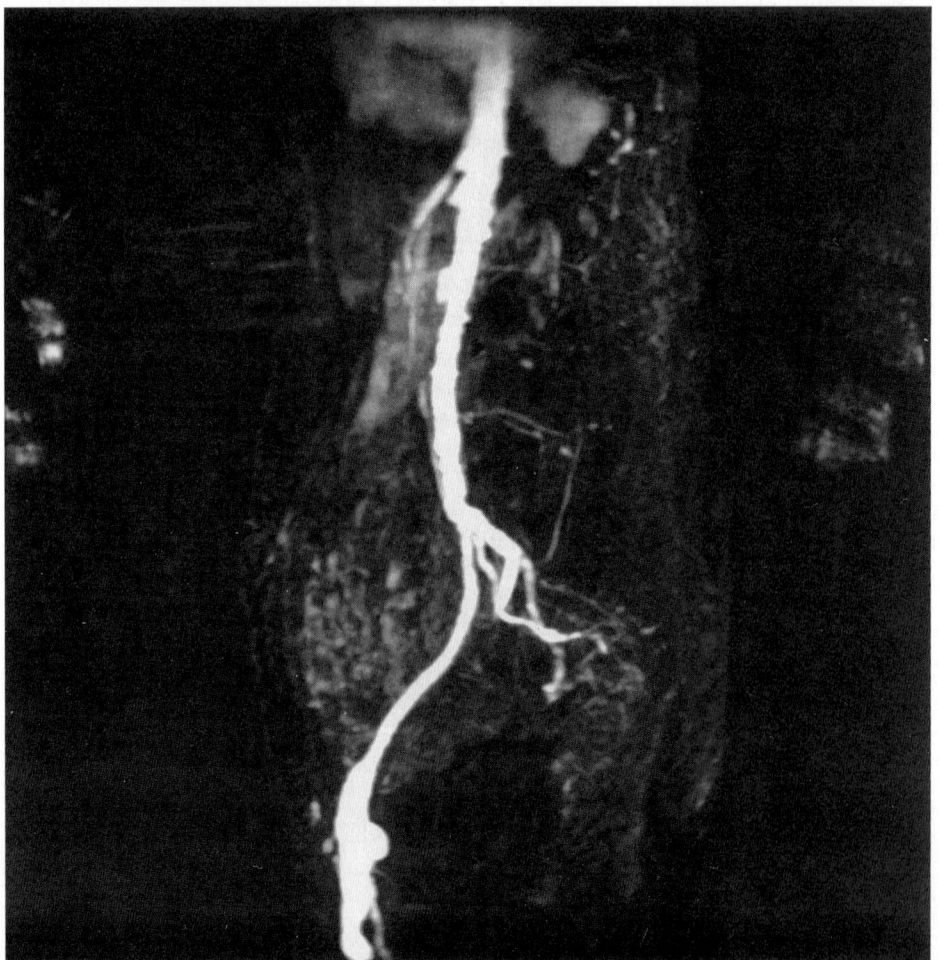

FIG. 27-34. Chronic mesenteric ischemia. This CT angiogram shows severe stenosis of the proximal celiac artery and occlusion of the superior mesenteric artery. (*Courtesy of Michael Conte, M.D., Department of Surgery, Brigham and Women's Hospital.*)

development. In patients suspected of having chronic mesenteric ischemia, duplex ultrasonography is often used as a screening test to detect stenoses at the origins of the superior mesenteric and celiac arteries.

Radiographic findings associated with chronic mesenteric venous thrombosis include the presence of luminal thrombus and extensive venous collaterals or the inability to visualize the superior mesenteric vein on duplex ultrasonography or CT scanning. Angiography can confirm the diagnosis but is rarely required.

Therapy

Important considerations in selecting among therapeutic options for acute mesenteric ischemia include the presence or absence of signs of peritonitis, the presence or absence of ischemic but viable intestine, the general condition of the patient, and the specific vascular lesion causing mesenteric ischemia.

If signs of peritonitis are detected at any time during the evaluation, laparotomy should be performed without delay. At the time of laparotomy, the intestine is assessed for viability, with the same criteria used for assessing viability in the context of small-bowel obstruction. Recommendations regarding intestinal resection and the application of second-look laparotomies are identical for acute mesenteric ischemia and for small-bowel obstruction with strangulation.

For embolus or thrombus-induced acute mesenteric ischemia, the standard treatment is surgical revascularization (embolectomy/thrombectomy/mesenteric bypass). These procedures are not indicated if most of the bowel supplied by the affected artery has already become infarcted, or if the patient is too unstable to undergo additional surgery beyond resection of infarcted intestine. For patients diagnosed with embolus or thrombus-induced acute mesenteric ischemia who do not have signs of peritonitis, thrombolysis, using agents such as streptokinase, urokinase, or recombinant tissue plasminogen activator, is an alternative therapeutic option. Thrombolytic therapy is most likely to be successful with smaller emboli lodged in the peripheral mesenteric circulation and with emboli that only partially obstruct, rather than completely occlude, the vessels in which they are lodged. Thrombolytic therapy is less likely to be successful when initiated 12 hours after onset of symptoms. Experience with thrombolytic therapy for acute mesenteric ischemia caused by superior mesenteric artery thrombosis is limited. It is important to remember that patients who develop signs of peritonitis during thrombolysis should undergo emergent laparotomy.

The standard treatment of NOMI is selective infusion of a vasodilator, most commonly papaverine hydrochloride, into the superior mesenteric artery. If signs of peritonitis develop, emergent laparotomy should be performed and infarcted intestine resected.

The standard treatment of acute mesenteric venous thrombosis is anticoagulation. Heparin administration is associated with reductions in mortality and recurrence rates, and should be initiated as soon as the diagnosis is made, even intraoperatively. As for mesenteric ischemia of arterial origin, signs of peritonitis mandate laparotomy, and infarcted bowel should be resected. Venous thrombectomy and thrombolysis can be attempted in the unusual circumstance in which the diagnosis is made soon after the onset of thrombosis; however, experience with these modalities is limited. Patients diagnosed with acute mesenteric venous thrombosis should be evaluated for the presence of hereditary and acquired thrombophilias. In the absence of an ongoing thrombotic disorder, patients should be maintained on warfarin to achieve chronic anticoagulation for 6 to 12 months.

The standard therapy for chronic arterial mesenteric ischemia is surgical revascularization using aortomesenteric bypass grafting and mesenteric endarterectomy procedures. An alternative therapy is percutaneous transluminal mesenteric angioplasty alone or with stent insertion. The durability of these procedures in inducing relief of symptoms appears to be less than that associated with surgical revascularization; as a result, they are generally applied in patients with substantial comorbidities for whom the risks of major surgery are deemed prohibitive.[7]

Patients with chronic venous mesenteric thrombosis who have an underlying thrombophilia identified should be treated with chronic anticoagulation. Additional therapy is indicated to control or prevent recurrent bleeding caused by esophagogastric varices. Pharmacologic agents such as propanol and endoscopic therapy are the first-line modalities. Surgical portosystemic shunts are indicated in patients whose bleeding cannot be controlled by conservative measures and who have a suitable vein for portosystemic venous anastomosis. When thrombosis is so extensive that no suitable vein is available, gastroesophageal devascularization or nonconventional shunts involving anastomosis of a large venous collateral vein with a systemic vein may be considered.

Outcomes

Recently reported mortality rates among patients with acute arterial mesenteric ischemia range from 59 to 93%.[7] Reported mortality rates among patients with acute mesenteric venous thrombosis range from 20 to 50%.[59] There is an approximately 30% recurrence rate in the absence of systemic anticoagulation, with most recurrences occurring within 30 days of presentation.

Reported perioperative mortality rates associated with surgery therapy for chronic mesenteric ischemia range from 0 to 16%, with lower mortality rates predominating in recent series. More than 90% of recently reported cases are associated with initial symptomatic relief; recurrence rates generally have been less than 10%. Recurrence rates associated with percutaneous angioplasty for chronic mesenteric ischemia appear to be higher in those with surgical revascularization, ranging from 10 to 67%.[7] The long-term efficacy of stenting for chronic mesenteric ischemia is currently unknown.

MISCELLANEOUS CONDITIONS

Obscure GI Bleeding

Obscure GI bleeding refers to gastrointestinal bleeding for which no source has been identified by routine endoscopic studies (EGD and colonoscopy). *Overt GI bleeding* refers to the presence of hematemesis, melena, or hematochezia. In contrast, *occult GI bleeding* occurs in the absence of overt bleeding and is identified on laboratory tests (e.g., iron-deficiency anemia) or examination of the stool (e.g., positive guaiac test). Obscure GI bleeding is occult in 20% of cases.

Up to 90% of lesions responsible for GI bleeding are within the reach of EGD and colonoscopy. Most of the small bowel, however, is beyond the reach of these examinations and, hence, contains most of the lesions responsible for obscure GI bleeding. Small-intestinal angiodysplasias account for approximately 75% of cases in adults; neoplasms account for approximately 10%. Meckel's diverticulum is the most common etiology of obscure GI bleeding in children. Other etiologies of obscure GI bleeding include Crohn's disease, infectious enteritides, nonsteroidal anti-inflammatory drug (NSAID)-induced ulcers and erosions, vasculitis, ischemia, varices, diverticula, and intussusception.

The diagnostic evaluation of patients with obscure GI bleeding should be tailored to the severity of bleeding and to the availability of technology and expertise. Enteroscopy is playing an increasingly important role in diagnosing obscure GI bleeding. Four endoscopic techniques for visualizing the small intestine are available: push enteroscopy, sonde enteroscopy, intraoperative enteroscopy, and wireless capsule enteroscopy.

Push enteroscopy entails advancing a long endoscope (such as a pediatric or adult colonoscope or a specialized instrument) beyond the ligament of Treitz into the proximal jejunum. This procedure can enable visualization of approximately 60 cm of the proximal jejunum. Reported diagnostic yield rates in patients with obscure GI bleeding range from 3 to 65%. In addition to diagnosis, push enteroscopy enables cauterization of bleeding sites.

In sonde enteroscopy, a long, thin fiberoptic instrument is propelled through the intestine by peristalsis following inflation of a balloon at the instrument's tip. Visualization is done during instrument withdrawal; approximately 50 to 75% of the small intestinal mucosa can be examined. However, this instrument lacks biopsy or therapeutic capability. Furthermore, it lacks tip deflection capability, limiting complete mucosal visualization. Reported diagnostic yield rates in patients with obscure GI bleeding range from 26 to 28%. Push and sonde enteroscopy can be complementary and are often used together in individual patients.

Intraoperative enteroscopy can be done during either laparotomy or laparoscopy. An endoscope (usually a colonoscope), is inserted into the small bowel through peroral intubation or through an enterotomy made in the small bowel or cecum. The endoscope is advanced by successively telescoping short segments of intestine onto the end to the instrument. In addition to the endoscopic image, the transilluminated bowel should be examined externally with the operating room lights dimmed, because this maneuver may facilitate the identification of angiodysplasias. Identified lesions should be marked with a suture placed on the serosal surface of the bowel; these lesions can be resected after completion of endoscopy. Examination should be performed during instrument insertion rather than withdrawal because instrument-induced mucosal trauma can be confused with angiodysplasias. Reported diagnostic yield rates when applied to patients with obscure GI bleeding range from 83 to 100%.

Wireless capsule enteroscopy relies on a radiotelemetry capsule enteroscope that is small enough to swallow and has no external wires, fiberoptic bundles, or cables. While the capsule is being propelled through the intestine by peristalsis, video images are transmitted using radiotelemetry to an array of detectors attached to the patient's body. These detectors capture the images and permit continuous triangulation of the capsule location in the abdomen, facilitating the localization of lesions detected. The entire system is portable, allowing the patient to be ambulatory during the entire examination. Initial comparative studies indicate that the diagnostic yield of wireless capsule enteroscopy in patients with obscure GI bleeding is as good or better than that of push enteroscopy. Further studies are needed to define the clinical impact of this new technology.

For patients in whom bleeding from an obscure GI source has apparently stopped, push and/or sonde enteroscopy or capsule enteroscopy (if available) is a reasonable initial study. If these examinations do not reveal a potential source of bleeding, then enteroclysis should be performed. Standard small-bowel follow-through examinations are associated with a low diagnostic yield in this setting, and should be avoided. If still no diagnosis has been made, a watch-and-wait approach is reasonable, although angiography should be considered if the prior episode of bleeding was overt. Angiography can reveal angiodysplasia and vascular tumors in the small intestine, even in the absence of ongoing bleeding.

For persistent mild bleeding from an obscure GI source, push and/or sonde enteroscopy should be used initially, if available. The role of capsule enteroscopy in this setting remains to be defined. If these examinations are nondiagnostic, then ^{99m}Tc-labeled RBC scanning should be performed and, if positive, followed by angiography to localize the source of bleeding. ^{99m}Tc-pertechnetate scintigraphy to diagnose Meckel's diverticulum should be considered, although its yield in patients older than 40 years of age is extremely low. Patients who remain undiagnosed but who continue to bleed, and those patients with recurrent episodic bleeding significant enough to require blood transfusions, should then undergo exploration with intraoperative enteroscopy.

Patients with persistent severe bleeding from an obscure source should undergo angiography. Push enteroscopy can be attempted, but sonde and capsule enteroscopy are too slow to be applicable in this setting. If these examinations fail to localize the source of bleeding, exploratory laparoscopy or laparotomy with intraoperative enteroscopy is indicated. If bleeding is massive enough to cause hemodynamic derangements, expeditious exploration avoiding the delays inherent with angiography may be necessary.

Small-Bowel Perforation

Prior to the 1980s, duodenal perforation as a consequence of peptic ulcer disease was the most common form of small-bowel perforation. Today, iatrogenic injury incurred during gastrointestinal endoscopy is the most common cause of small-bowel perforation. Other etiologies of small-bowel perforation include infections (especially tuberculosis, typhoid, and CMV), Crohn's disease, ischemia, drugs (e.g., potassium- and NSAID-induced ulcers), radiation-induced injury, Meckel's and acquired diverticula, neoplasms (especially lymphoma, adenocarcinoma, and melanoma), and foreign bodies.

Among iatrogenic injuries, duodenal perforation during ERCP with endoscopic sphincterotomy is the most common. This complication occurs in 0.3 to 2.1% of cases. Patients who have undergone Billroth II gastrectomy are at increased risk; duodenal perforation complicates 1.5 to 5% of the ERCPs in these patients. In addition jejunal perforation complicates 0.6 to 11% of ERCPs in patients who have undergone Billroth II gastrectomy.

Perforation of the jejunum and ileum occurs into the peritoneal cavity and usually causes overt symptoms and signs, such as abdominal pain, tenderness, and distention accompanied by fever and tachycardia. Perforations of the duodenum distal to its bulb, because of its retroperitoneal location, tend to be locally contained and can present insidiously. Manifestations of contained duodenal perforation following ERCP can resemble those of ERCP-induced pancreatitis, including hyperamylasemia.

Plain abdominal radiographs may reveal free intraperitoneal air if intraperitoneal perforation has occurred. If perforation is suspected but not clinically obvious, contrast radiography using a water-soluble contrast agent or CT scanning should be performed. CT scanning is the most sensitive test for diagnosing duodenal perforations; positive findings include pneumoperitoneum, retroperitoneal air, contrast extravasation, and paraduodenal fluid collections.

Iatrogenic small-bowel perforation incurred during endoscopy, if immediately recognized, can sometimes be repaired using endoscopic techniques. Ampullary injury incurred during ERCP can usually be managed by biliary stent placement. In addition, contained select cases of retroperitoneal perforations of the duodenum can be managed nonoperatively, in the absence of progression and sepsis. However, intraperitoneal duodenal perforations require surgical repair with pyloric exclusion and gastrojejunostomy or tube duodenostomy. Jejunal and ileal perforations require surgical repair or segmental resection. Hemodynamic instability or diffuse disease of the bowel may preclude primary anastomosis. If so, enterostomies should be created.

Chylous Ascites

Chylous ascites refers to the accumulation of triglyceride-rich peritoneal fluid with a milky or creamy appearance that is caused by the presence of intestinal lymph in the peritoneal cavity. Chylomicrons, produced by the intestine and secreted into lymph during the absorption of long-chain fatty acids, account for the characteristic appearance and triglyceride content of chyle.

The most common etiologies of chylous ascites in Western countries are abdominal malignancies and cirrhosis. In Eastern and developing countries, infectious etiologies, such as tuberculosis and filariasis, account for most cases. Chylous ascites can also develop as a complication of abdominal and thoracic operations and trauma. Operations particularly associated with this complication include abdominal aortic aneurysm repair, retroperitoneal lymph node dissection, inferior vena cava resection, and liver transplantation. Other etiologies of chylous ascites include congential lymphatic abnormalities (e.g., primary lymphatic hypoplasia), radiation, pancreatitis, and right-sided heart failure.

Three mechanisms have been postulated to cause chylous ascites: (1) exudation of chyle from dilated lymphatics on the wall of the bowel and in the mesentery caused by obstruction of lymphatic vessels at the base of the mesentery or the cisterna chili (e.g., by malignancies); (2) direct leakage of chyle through a lymphoperitoneal fistula (e.g., those which develop as a result of trauma or surgery); and (3) exudation of chyle through the wall of dilated retroperitoneal lymphatic vessels (e.g., in congenital lymphangiectasia or thoracic duct obstruction).

Patients with chylous ascites develop abdominal distention over a period of weeks to months. Postoperative chylous ascites can present acutely during the first postoperative week. Delayed presentations following surgery can occur if the mechanism of ascites formation is adhesion-induced lymphatic obstruction rather than lymphatic vessel disruption. Dyspnea may result if abdominal distention is severe enough.

Paracentesis is the most important diagnostic test. Chyle typically has a turbid appearance; however, it may be clear in fasting patients (such as those in the immediate postoperative period). Fluid triglyceride concentrations above 110 mg/dL are diagnostic. CT scanning may be useful in identifying pathologic intra-abdominal lymph nodes and masses and in identifying extent and localization of fluid. Lymphangiography and lymphoscintigraphy may help to localize lymph leaks and obstruction; this information is particularly useful for surgical planning.

Management of patients with chylous ascites should focus on evaluating and treating the underlying causes, especially for patients with infectious, inflammatory, or hemodynamic etiologies for this condition.

Most patients respond to administration of a high-protein and low-fat diet supplemented with medium-chain triglycerides. This regimen is designed to minimize chyle production and flow.

Medium-chain triglycerides are absorbed by the intestinal epithelium and are transported to the liver through the portal vein; they do not contribute to chylomicron formation.

Patients who do not respond to this approach should be fasted and placed on TPN. Octreotide can further decrease lymph flow. Paracentesis is indicated for respiratory difficulties related to abdominal distention. Overall, more than 60% of patients will respond to conservative therapy. However, approximately 30% of patients will require surgical therapy for chylous ascites. In general, postoperative and trauma-related cases that fail to respond to initial nonoperative therapy are best managed by surgical repair. Lymphatic leaks are localized and repaired with fine nonabsorbable sutures. If extravasation of chyle is localized to the periphery of the small-bowel mesentery, then a limited small-bowel resection can be performed instead. For patients who are poor surgical candidates and who do not respond to prolonged conservative therapy, peritoneovenous shunting may be an option. However, these shunts are associated with high rates of complications, including sepsis and disseminated intravascular coagulation. Because of the viscosity of chyle, these shunts are associated with a high occlusion rate.

SHORT-BOWEL SYNDROME

Epidemiology

Intestinal resection is performed for many of the diseases discussed in this chapter and generally is associated with minimal morbidity. However, when the extent of resection is great enough, a devastating condition known as the short-bowel syndrome can result. *Short-bowel syndrome* has been arbitrarily defined as the presence of less than 200 cm of residual small bowel in adult patients.[61] A functional definition, in which insufficient intestinal absorptive capacity results in the clinical manifestations of diarrhea, dehydration, and malnutrition, is more broadly applicable.

In adults, the most common etiologies of short-bowel syndrome are acute mesenteric ischemia, malignancy, and Crohn's disease. Seventy-five percent of cases result from resection of a large amount of small bowel at a single operation; 25% of cases result from the cumulative effects of multiple operations during which small intestine is resected. This latter pattern is typical of patients with Crohn's disease who develop short-bowel syndrome; the former is typical of patients with acute mesenteric ischemia who develop intestinal infarction. In pediatric patients, intestinal atresias, volvulus, and necrotizing enterocolitis are the most common etiologies of short-bowel syndrome.

The prevalence of short-bowel syndrome has been estimated to be as high as 2 million patients in the United States.[61] The most recent available data on chronic home TPN administration were obtained in 1992. At that time, approximately 40,000 patients were receiving TPN chronically at home.[62] The most prevalent indication for TPN among these patients was short-bowel syndrome; however, this estimate does not include patients with short-bowel syndrome who were not receiving TPN at home. It also fails to include those patients who had been weaned off of TPN.

Pathophysiology

Resection of less than 50% of the small intestine is generally well tolerated. However, clinically significant malabsorption occurs when greater than 50 to 80% of the small intestine has been resected.[63] Among adult patients who lack a functional colon, lifelong TPN dependence is likely to persist if there is less than 100 cm of residual small intestine. Among adult patients who have an intact and functional colon, lifelong TPN dependence is likely to persist if there is less than 60 cm of residual small intestine. Among infants with short-bowel syndrome, weaning from TPN-dependence has been achieved with as little as 10 cm of residual small intestine.

Residual bowel length is not the only factor predictive of achieving independence from TPN (enteral autonomy), however. There are several other determinants of the severity of malabsorption. First, is the presence or absence of an intact colon because the colon has the capacity to absorb large fluid and electrolyte loads. In addition, the colon can play an important, albeit small, role in nutrient assimilation by absorbing short-chain fatty acids. Second, an intact ileocecal valve is believed to be associated with decreased malabsorption. The ileocecal valve delays transit of chyme from the small intestine into the colon, thereby prolonging the contact time between nutrients and the small-intestinal absorptive mucosa. Third, a healthy, rather than diseased, residual small intestine is associated with decreased severity of malabsorption. Fourth, resection of jejunum is better tolerated than resection of ileum, because the capacity for bile salt and vitamin B_{12} absorption is specific to the ileum.

Malabsorption in patients who have undergone massive small-bowel resection is exacerbated by a characteristic hypergastrinemia-associated gastric acid hypersecretion that persists for 1 to 2 years postoperatively. The increased acid load delivered to the duodenum inhibits absorption by a variety of mechanisms, including the inhibition of digestive enzymes, most of which function optimally under alkaline conditions.

Also during the first 1 to 2 years following massive small-bowel resection, the remaining intestine undergoes compensatory adaptation, as discussed above. Clinically, the period of adaptation is associated with reductions in volume and frequency of bowel movements, increases in the capacity for enteral nutrient assimilation, and reductions in TPN requirements. Understanding the mechanisms mediating intestinal adaptation may suggest strategies for enhancing adaptation in patients with short-bowel syndrome who are unable to achieve independence from TPN. To date, the phenomenon of intestinal adaptation in human patients remains poorly understood.

Therapy

Medical Therapy

For patients having undergone massive small-bowel resection, the initial treatment priorities include management of the primary condition precipitating the intestinal resection and the repletion of fluid and electrolytes lost in the severe diarrhea that characteristically occurs. Most patients will require TPN, at least initially. Enteral nutrition should be gradually introduced, once ileus has resolved. High-dose histamine-2 receptor antagonists or proton pump inhibitors should be administered to reduce gastric acid secretion. Antimotility agents, such as loperamide hydrochloride or diphenoxylate, may be administered to delay small-intestinal transit. Octreotide can be administered to reduce the volume of gastrointestinal secretions, although its use is associated with an inhibition of intestinal adaptation in animal models.

During the period of adaptation, generally lasting 1 to 2 years postoperatively, TPN and enteral nutrition are titrated in an attempt to allow for independence from TPN. Patients who remain dependent on TPN face substantial TPN-associated morbidities, including catheter sepsis, venous thrombosis, liver and kidney failure, and osteoporosis. Costs associated with chronic TPN administration are estimated to be as high as $150,000 per patient annually.[20] Because

of these problems, alternative therapies for short-bowel syndrome are under investigation.

Nontransplant Surgical Therapy

Among patients with stomas, restoration of intestinal continuity should be performed, whenever possible, to capitalize on the absorptive capacity of all residual intestine. Other forms of nontransplant surgery designed to improve intestinal absorption are associated with unclear efficacy and/or substantial morbidities, and therefore should not be applied routinely.

The goal of these operations is to increase nutrient and fluid absorption by either slowing intestinal transit or increasing intestinal length. Operations designed to slow intestinal transit include segmental reversal of the small bowel, interposition of a segment of colon between segments of small bowel, construction of small-intestinal valves, and electrical pacing of the small intestine.[64] Reported experience with these procedures is limited to case reports or series of a few cases. Objective evidence of increased absorption is lacking; furthermore, these procedures are frequently associated with intestinal obstruction.

The intestinal lengthening operation for which there is the greatest experience is the longitudinal intestinal lengthening and tailoring (LILT) procedure, first described by Bianchi in 1980.[65] Approximately 100 of these procedures have been reported in the literature. The procedure entails separation of the dual vasculature of the small intestine, followed by longitudinal division of the bowel with subsequent isoperistaltic end-to-end anastomosis. This procedure has the potential to double the length of small intestine to which it is applied. This procedure has generally been used for pediatric patients with dilated residual small bowel. In a recently published uncontrolled series, 14 of 16 patients undergoing this procedure were subsequently weaned off of TPN.[66]

Recently, the serial transverse enteroplasty procedure (STEP) was described.[67] This procedure is designed to accomplish lengthening of dilated small intestine without the need for separating its dual vasculature (Fig. 27-35). Initial experimental and clinical experience with this procedure has been promising; however, its long-term efficacy needs to be determined.

Intestinal Transplantation

Approximately 100 intestinal transplants are performed in the United States annually, with most of these procedures applied to patients with short-bowel syndrome.[68] The currently accepted indication for intestinal transplantation is the presence of life-threatening complications attributable to intestinal failure and/or long-term TPN therapy. Specific complications for which intestinal transplantation is indicated include impending or overt liver failure, thrombosis of major central veins, frequent episodes of catheter-related sepsis, and frequent episodes of severe dehydration.

Currently, approximately 45% of transplants involving the small intestine are performed as isolated intestinal transplants, 40% are performed as combined intestine/liver transplants, and 15% are performed as multivisceral transplants.

Isolated intestinal transplantation is used for patients with intestinal failure who have no significant liver disease or failure of other organs. Combined intestine/liver transplantation is used for patients with both intestinal and liver failure. Multivisceral transplantation has been used for patients with giant desmoid tumors involving the vascular supply of the liver and pancreas, as well as that of the intestine, for diffuse gastrointestinal motility disturbances, and for diffuse splanchnic thrombosis.

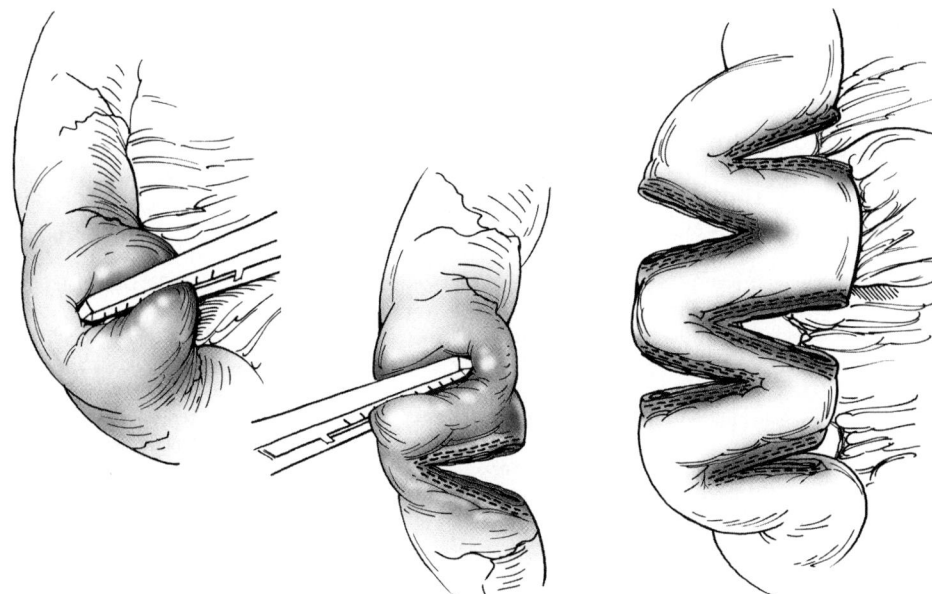

FIG. 27-35. STEP procedure. This illustration depicts the serial transverse enteroplasty procedure. Lengthening of dilated small intestine is accomplished by serial applications of an intestinal stapling device, with firings oriented perpendicular to the long axis of the intestine. (*Courtesy of Patrick Javid, M.D., and Tom Jaksic, M.D., Department of Surgery, Children's Hospital, Boston.*)

Nearly 80% of survivors have full intestinal graft function with no need for TPN. However, morbidities associated with intestinal transplantation are substantial and include acute and chronic rejection, CMV infection, and posttransplant lymphoproliferative disease.

Alternative Therapies

Pharmacologic and biologic therapies designed to expand intestinal mucosal surface area or to enhance the efficiency of intestinal absorption are beginning to undergo clinical evaluation. Promising regimens include GLP-2 and the combination of glutamine and growth hormone with a modified, high-carbohydrate diet.[20] Efficacy data with respect to these approaches are conflicting; multi-institutional prospective studies are currently underway. Prototype neointestinal constructs generated through a variety of tissue-engineering and stem cell isolation approaches have been reported; to date, their application has largely been limited to animal models.[69] For now, the short-bowel syndrome remains a formidable challenge for clinical surgeons and surgical scientists.

Outcomes

Approximately 50 to 70% of patients with short-bowel syndrome who initially require TPN are ultimately able to achieve independence from TPN.[61] Prognosis for achieving enteral autonomy is better among pediatric patients than among adults.

Information on survival among patients with short-bowel syndrome is limited. In a recently reported study of 124 adults with short-bowel syndrome caused by nonmalignant etiologies, the survival rates at 2 and 5 years of follow-up were 86 and 45%, respectively.[70] Patients with end-enterostomies, and patients having less than 50 cm of residual small intestine, had significantly worse survivals than did patients without these features.

No randomized trials comparing intestinal transplantation to chronic TPN administration among patients with short-bowel syndrome have been reported. In the most recent UNOS cohort evaluated, the 1-year patient and graft survival rates for isolated intestine recipients were 79 and 64%, respectively, and 50 and 49%, respectively, for intestine/liver recipients.[61] Five-year patient and graft survival rates for isolated intestine recipients were 50 and

38%, respectively, and for intestine/liver recipients, 37 and 36%, respectively.

References

1. Evers BM, Townsend CM, Thompson JC: Small intestine, in Schwartz S, Spencer F, Galloway A, et al (eds): *Principles of Surgery,* 7th ed. New York: McGraw-Hill, 1998, p. 1217.
2. Drucker DJ, Erlich P, Asa SL, et al: Induction of intestinal epithelial proliferation by glucagon-like peptide 2. *Proc Natl Acad Sci USA* 93:7911, 1996.
3. Hirota S, Isozaki K, Moriyama Y, et al: Gain-of-function mutations of *c-kit* in human gastrointestinal stromal tumors. *Science* 279:577, 1998.
4. Rubin BP, Fletcher JA, Fletcher CDM: Molecular insights into the histogenesis and pathogenesis of gastrointestinal stromal tumors. *Int J Surg Pathol* 8:5, 2000.
5. Appleyard M, Fireman Z, Glukhovsky A, et al: A randomized trial comparing wireless capsule endoscopy with push enteroscopy for the detection of small-bowel lesions. *Gastroenterol* 119:1431, 2000.
6. Luckey A, Livingston E, Tache Y: Mechanisms and treatment of postoperative ileus. *Arch Surg* 138:206, 2003.
7. Brandt LJ, Boley SJ: AGA technical review on intestinal ischemia. *Gastroenterol* 118:954, 2000.
8. Montgomery RK, Mulberg AE, Grand RJ: Development of the human gastrointestinal tract: Twenty years of progress. *Gastroenterol* 116:702, 1999.
9. http://www.gene.ucl.ac.uk/nomenclature
10. Thomson ABR, Keelan M, Thiesen A, et al: Small bowel review: Normal physiology part 2. *Dig Dis Sci* 46:2588, 2001.
11. Lane JS, Whang EE, Rigberg DA, et al: Paracellular glucose transport plays a minor role in the unanesthetized dog. *Am J Physiol* 276:G276, 1999.
12. Ma T, Verkman AS: Aquaporin water channels in gastrointestinal physiology. *J Physiol* 517 Pt 2:317, 1999.
13. Rolfs A, Hediger MA: Intestinal metal ion absorption: An update. *Curr Opin Gastroenterol* 17:177, 2001.
14. Nagler-Anderson C: Man the barrier! Strategic defenses in the intestinal mucosa. *Nat Rev Immunol* 1:59, 2001.
15. Mowat AM: Anatomical basis of tolerance and immunity to intestinal antigens. *Nat Rev Immunol* 3:331, 2003.
16. Ahlman H, Nilsson O: The gut as the largest endocrine organ in the body. *Ann Oncol* 12(Suppl 2):S63, 2001.

17. Rehfeld JF: The new biology of gastrointestinal hormones. *Physiol Rev* 78:1087, 1998.

18. Geoghegan J, Pappas TN: Clinical uses of gut peptides. *Ann Surg* 225:145, 1997.

19. Hines OJ, Bilchik AJ, McFadden DW, et al: Up-regulation of Na$^+$,K$^+$ adenosine triphosphatase after massive intestinal resection. *Surgery* 116:401, 1994.

20. Tavvakolizadeh A, Whang EE: Understanding and augmenting human intestinal adaptation: A call for more clinical research. *JPEN J* 26:251, 2002.

21. Drucker DJ: Epithelial cell growth and differentiation. I. Intestinal growth factors. *Am J Physiol* 273:G3, 1997.

22. Ray NF, Denton WG, Thamer M, et al: Abdominal adhesiolysis: Inpatient care and expenditures in the United States in 1994. *J Am Coll Surg* 186:1, 1998.

23. Mucha P Jr.: Small-intestinal obstruction. *Surg Clin North Am* 67:597, 1987.

24. Sarr MG, Bulkley GB, Zuidema GD: Preoperative recognition of intestinal strangulation obstruction: Prospective evaluation of diagnostic capability. *Am J Surg* 145:176, 1983.

25. Maglinte DD, Heitkamp DE, Howard TJ: Current concepts in imaging of small bowel obstruction. *Radiol Clin North Am* 41:263, 2003.

26. Suri S, Gupta S, Sudhakar PJ, et al: Comparative evaluation of plain films, ultrasound and CT in the diagnosis of intestinal obstruction. *Acta Radiol* 40:422, 1999.

27. Fischer CP, Doherty D: Laparoscopic approach to small bowel obstruction. *Semin Laparosc Surg* 9:40, 2002.

28. Brolin RE, Krasna MJ, Mast BA: Use of tubes and radiographs in the management of small bowel obstruction. *Ann Surg* 206:126, 1987.

29. Peetz DJ, Gamelli RL, Pilcher DB: Intestinal intubation in acute, mechanical small-bowel obstruction. *Arch Surg* 117:334, 1982.

30. Stewart RM, Page CP, Brender J, et al: The incidence and risk of early postoperative small bowel obstruction: A cohort study. *Am J Surg* 154:643, 1987.

31. Walsh HPJ, Schofield PF: Is laparotomy for small bowel obstruction justified in patients with previously treated malignancy? *Br J Surg* 71:933, 1984.

32. Krouse RS, McCahill LE, Easson A, et al: When the sun can set on an unoperated bowel obstruction: Management of malignant bowel obstruction. *J Am Coll Surg* 195:117, 2002.

33. Taguchi A, Sharma N, Saleem RM, et al: Selective postoperative inhibition of gastrointestinal opioid receptors. *N Engl J Med* 345:935, 2001.

34. Sands BE: Crohn's disease, in Feldman M, Tschumy WO, Friedman LS (eds): *Sleisenger and Fordtran's Gastrointestinal and Liver Disease,* 7th ed. Philadelphia: WB Saunders, 2002, p. 2005.

35. Hugot JP, Chamaillard M, Zouali H, et al: Association of NOD leucin-rich repeat variants with susceptibility to Crohn's disease. *Nature* 411:599, 2001.

36. Ogura Y, Bonen DK, Inohara N, et al: A frameshift mutation in NOD2 associated with susceptibility to Crohn's disease. *Nature* 411:603, 2001.

37. Present DH, Rutgeerts P, Targan S, et al: Infliximab for the treatment of fistulas in patients with Crohn's disease. *N Engl J Med* 340:1398, 1999.

38. Becker JM: Surgical therapy for ulcerative colitis and Crohn's disease. *Gastroenterol Clin North Am* 28:371, 1999.

39. Schraut WH: The surgical management of Crohn's disease. *Gastroenterol Clin North Am* 31:255, 2002.

40. Fazio VW, Marchetti F, Church JM, et al: Effect of resection margins on the recurrence of Crohn's disease of the small bowel. *Ann Surg* 224:563, 1996.

41. Delaney CP, Fazio VW: Crohn's disease of the small bowel. *Surg Clin North Am* 81:137, 2001.

42. Aleali M, Milsom JW: Laproscopic surgery in Crohn's disease. *Surg Clin North Am* 81:217, 2001.

43. Milsom JW, Hammerhofer KA, Bohm B, et al: Prospective, randomized trial comparing laparoscopic vs. conventional surgery for refractory ileocolic Crohn's disease. *Dis Colon Rectum* 44:1, 2001.

44. Moser AJ, Roslyn JJ: Enterocutaneous fistula, in Cameron JL (ed): *Current Surgical Therapy,* 6th ed. St. Louis: Mosby, 1998, p. 155.

45. Jepsen JM, Persson M, Jakobsen NO, et al: Prospective study of prevalence and endoscopic and histopathologic characteristics of duodenal polyps in patients submitted to upper endoscopy. *Scand J Gastroenterol* 29:483, 1994.

46. Jemal A, Murray T, Sammuels A, et al: Cancer statistics, 2003. *CA Cancer J Clin* 53:5, 2003.

47. Judson I: Gastrointestinal stromal tumors (GIST): Biology and treatment. *Ann Oncol* 13(Suppl 4):287, 2002.

48. Miettinen M, Majidi M, Lasota J: Pathology and diagnostic criteria of gastrointestinal stromal tumors (GISTs): A review. *Eur J Cancer* 38(Suppl 5):S39, 2002.

49. Roberts PJ, Eisenberg B: Clinical presentation of gastrointestinal stromal tumors and treatment. *Eur J Cancer* 38(Suppl 5):S37, 2002.

50. Coit DG: Cancer of the small intestine, in DeVita VT, Hellman S, Rosenberg SA (eds): *Cancer: Principles and Practice of Oncology,* 6th ed. Philadelphia: Lippincott Williams and Wilkins, 2001, p. 1204.

51. Rustgi AK: Small-intestinal neoplasms, in Feldman M, Tschumy WO, Friedman LS (eds): *Sleisenger and Fordtran's Gastrointestinal and Liver Disease,* 7th ed. Philadelphia: WB Saunders, 2002, p. 2169.

52. Perez A, Saltzman JR, Carr-Locke DL, et al: Benign nonampullary duodenal neoplasms. *J Gastrointest Surg* 7:536, 2003.

53. Demetri GD, Mehren M, Blanke C, et al: Efficacy and safety of imatinib mesylate in advanced gastrointestinal stromal tumors. *N Engl J Med* 347:472, 2002.

54. Girvent M, Carlson GL, Anderson I, et al: Intestinal failure after surgery for complicated radiation enteritis. *Ann R Coll Surg Engl* 82:198, 2000.

55. Yahchouchy EK, Marano AF, Etienne JC, et al: Meckel's diverticulum. *J Am Coll Surg* 192:654, 2001.

56. Lobo DN, Balfour TW, Iftikhar SY, et al: Periampullary diverticula and pancreaticobiliary disease. *Br J Surg* 86:588, 1999.

57. Williams RS: Management of Meckel's diverticulum. *Br J Surg* 68:477, 1981.

58. Chow DC, Babaian M, Taubin HL: Jejunoileal diverticula. *Gastroenterologist* 5:78, 1997.

59. Kumar S, Sarr MG, Kamath PS: Mesenteric venous thrombosis. *N Engl J Med* 345:1683, 2001.

60. Kim AY, Ha HK: Evaluation of suspected mesenteric ischemia: Efficacy of radiologic studies. *Radiol Clin North Am* 41:327, 2003.

61. Buchman AL, Solapio J, Fryer J: AGA technical review on short bowel syndrome and intestinal transplantation. *Gastroenterology* 124:1111, 2003.

62. Oley Foundation: *North American Home Parenteral and Enteral Nutrition Patient Registry Annual Report 1994.*

63. Vanderhoof JA, Langnas AN: Short-bowel syndrome in children and adults. *Gastroenterology* 113:1767, 1997.

64. Thompson JS, Langnas AN: Surgical approaches to improving intestinal function in the short-bowel syndrome. *Arch Surg* 134:706, 1999.

65. Bianchi A: Intestinal loop lengthening—A technique for increasing small-intestinal length. *J Pediatr Surg* 15:145, 1980.

66. Bianchi A: Longitudinal intestinal lengthening and tailoring: Results in 20 children. *J R Soc Med* 90:429, 1997.

67. Kim HB, Lee PW, Garza J, et al: Serial transverse enteroplasty for short bowel syndrome: A case report. *J Pediatr Surg* 38:881, 2003.

68. Fishbein TM, Gondolesi GE, Kaufman SS: Intestinal transplantation for gut failure. *Gastroenterology* 124:1615, 2003.

69. Tavakkolizadeh A, Ashley SW, Vacanti JP, et al: Tissue-engineered intestine: Progress toward a functional and physiological neomucosa. *Transplant Rev* 15:178, 2001.

70. Messing B, Crenn P, Beau P, et al: Long-term survival and parenteral nutrition dependence in adult patients with short bowel syndrome. *Gastroenterology* 117:1043, 1999.

CHAPTER 28

Colon, Rectum, and Anus

Kelli M. Bullard and David A. Rothenberger

The Immunocompromised Patient

Human Immunodeficiency Virus
Immunosuppression for Transplantation
The Neutropenic Patient

EMBRYOLOGY AND ANATOMY

Embryology

The embryonic gastrointestinal tract begins developing during the fourth week of gestation. The primitive gut is derived from the endoderm and divided into three segments: *foregut, midgut,* and *hindgut.* Both *midgut* and *hindgut* contribute to the colon, rectum, and anus.

The *midgut* develops into the small intestine, ascending colon, and proximal transverse colon, and receives blood supply from the superior mesenteric artery. During the sixth week of gestation, the midgut herniates out of the abdominal cavity, and then rotates 270 degrees counterclockwise around the superior mesenteric artery to return to its final position inside the abdominal cavity during the tenth week of gestation.

The *hindgut* develops into the distal transverse colon, descending colon, rectum, and proximal anus, all of which receive their blood supply from the inferior mesenteric artery. During the sixth week of gestation, the distal-most end of the hindgut, the *cloaca,* is divided by the urorectal septum into the urogenital sinus and the rectum.

The distal anal canal is derived from ectoderm and receives its blood supply from the internal pudendal artery. The dentate line divides the endodermal hindgut from the ectodermal distal anal canal.

Anatomy

The large intestine extends from the ileocecal valve to the anus. It is divided anatomically and functionally into the *colon, rectum,* and *anal canal.* The wall of the colon and rectum comprise five distinct layers: mucosa, submucosa, inner circular muscle, outer longitudinal muscle, and serosa. In the colon, the outer longitudinal muscle is separated into three *teniae coli,* which converge proximally at the appendix and distally at the rectum, where the outer longitudinal muscle layer is circumferential. In the distal rectum, the inner smooth-muscle layer coalesces to form the internal anal sphincter. The intraperitoneal colon and proximal one third of the rectum are covered by serosa; the mid and lower rectum lack serosa.

Colon Landmarks

The colon begins at the junction of the terminal ileum and cecum and extends 3 to 5 feet to the rectum. The rectosigmoid junction is found at approximately the level of the sacral promontory and is arbitrarily described as the point at which the three *teniae coli* coalesce to form the outer longitudinal smooth muscle layer of the rectum. The *cecum* is the widest diameter portion of the colon (normally 7.5 to 8.5 cm) and has the thinnest muscular wall. As a result, the cecum is most vulnerable to perforation and least vulnerable to obstruction. The ascending colon is usually fixed to the retroperitoneum. The hepatic flexure marks the transition to the transverse colon. The intraperitoneal transverse colon is relatively mobile, but is tethered by the gastrocolic ligament and colonic mesentery. The greater omentum is attached to the anterior/superior edge of the transverse colon. These attachments explain the characteristic triangular appearance of the transverse colon observed during colonoscopy. The splenic flexure marks the transition from the transverse colon to the descending colon. The attachments between the splenic flexure

and the spleen (the lienocolic ligament) can be short and dense, making mobilization of this flexure during colectomy challenging. The descending colon is relatively fixed to the retroperitoneum. The sigmoid colon is the narrowest part of the large intestine and is extremely mobile. Although the sigmoid colon is usually located in the left lower quadrant, redundancy and mobility can result in a portion of the sigmoid colon residing in the right lower quadrant. This mobility explains why volvulus is most common in the sigmoid colon and why diseases affecting the sigmoid colon, such as diverticulitis, may occasionally present as right-sided abdominal pain. The narrow caliber of the sigmoid colon makes this segment of the large intestine the most vulnerable to obstruction.

Colon Vascular Supply

The arterial supply to the colon is highly variable (Fig. 28-1). In general, the *superior mesenteric artery* branches into the *ileocolic artery* (absent in up to 20% of people), which supplies blood flow to the terminal ileum and proximal ascending colon, the *right colic artery,* which supplies the ascending colon, and the *middle colic artery,* which supplies the transverse colon. The *inferior mesenteric artery* branches into the *left colic artery,* which supplies the descending colon, several *sigmoidal branches,* which supply the sigmoid colon, and the *superior rectal artery,* which supplies the proximal rectum. The terminal branches of each artery form anastomoses with the terminal branches of the adjacent artery and communicate via the *marginal artery of Drummond.* This arcade is complete in only 15 to 20% of people.

Except for the *inferior mesenteric vein,* the veins of the colon parallel their corresponding arteries and bear the same terminology (Fig. 28-2). The inferior mesenteric vein ascends in the retroperitoneal plane over the psoas muscle and continues posterior to the pancreas to join the splenic vein. During a colectomy, this vein is often mobilized independently and ligated at the inferior edge of the pancreas.

Colon Lymphatic Drainage

The lymphatic drainage of the colon originates in a network of lymphatics in the muscularis mucosa. Lymphatic vessels and lymph nodes follow the regional arteries. Lymph nodes are found on the bowel wall (epicolic), along the inner margin of the bowel adjacent to the arterial arcades (paracolic), around the named mesenteric vessels (intermediate), and at the origin of the superior and inferior mesenteric arteries (main). The *sentinel lymph nodes* are the first one to four lymph nodes to drain a specific segment of the colon, and are thought to be the first site of metastasis in colon cancer. The utility of sentinel lymph node dissection and analysis in colon cancer remains controversial.

Colon Nerve Supply

The colon is innervated by both *sympathetic* (inhibitory) and *parasympathetic* (stimulatory) nerves, which parallel the course of the arteries. Sympathetic nerves arise from T6-T12 and L1-L3. The parasympathetic innervation to the right and transverse colon is from the vagus nerve; the parasympathetic nerves to the left colon arise from sacral nerves S2-S4 to form the nervi erigentes.

Anorectal Landmarks

The rectum is approximately 12 to 15 cm in length. Three distinct submucosal folds, the *valves of Houston,* extend into the rectal lumen. Posteriorly, the *presacral fascia* separates the rectum from the presacral venous plexus and the pelvic nerves. At S4, the

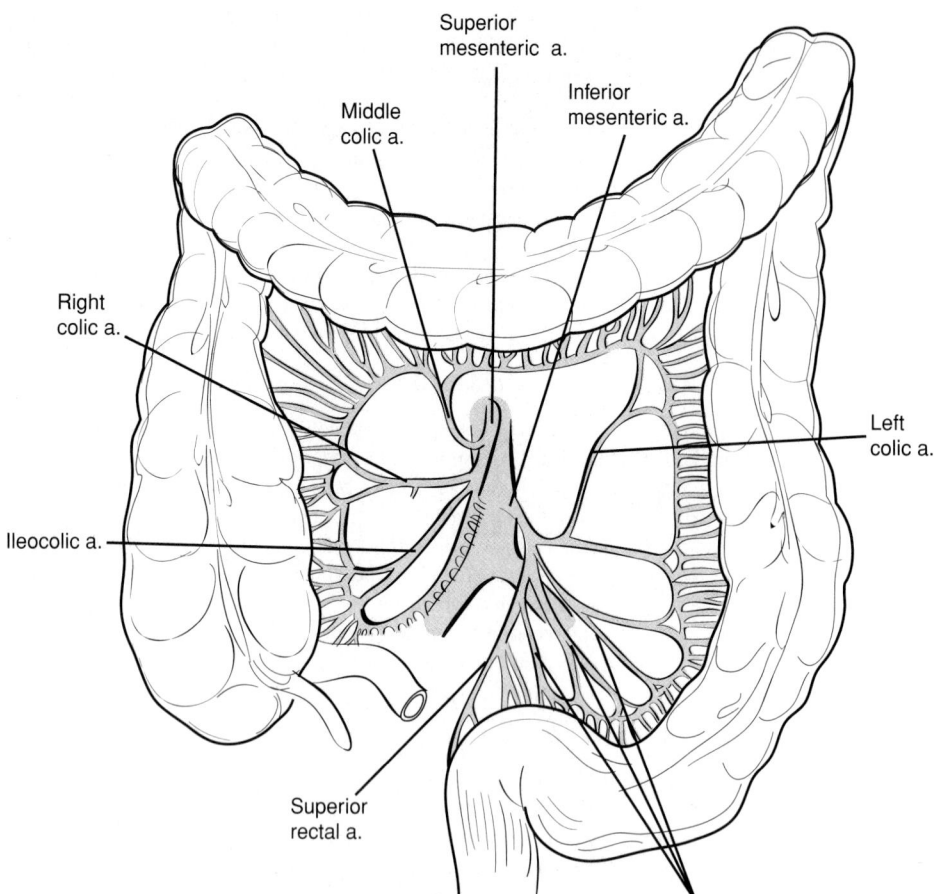

FIG. 28-1. Arterial blood supply to the colon. [*Reproduced with permission from Schwartz SI, Shires GT, Spencer FC (eds): Principles of Surgery. 5th ed. New York: McGraw-Hill, 1989, p 1226.*]

rectosacral fascia (*Waldeyer's fascia*) extends forward and downward and attaches to the fascia propria at the anorectal junction. Anteriorly, *Denonvilliers' fascia* separates the rectum from the prostate and seminal vesicles in men and from the vagina in women. The *lateral ligaments* support the lower rectum. The surgical anal canal measures 2 to 4 cm in length and is generally longer in men than in women. It begins at the anorectal junction and terminates at the anal verge. The *dentate* or *pectinate line* marks the transition point between columnar rectal mucosa and squamous anoderm. The 1 to 2 cm of mucosa just proximal to the dentate line shares histologic characteristics of columnar, cuboidal, and squamous epithelium and is referred to as the *anal transition zone*. The dentate line is surrounded by longitudinal mucosal folds, known as the *columns of Morgagni*, into which the anal crypts empty. These crypts are the source of cryptoglandular abscesses (Fig. 28-3).

In the distal rectum, the inner smooth muscle is thickened and comprises the *internal anal sphincter* that is surrounded by the *subcutaneous, superficial,* and *deep external sphincter*. The *deep external anal sphincter* is an extension of the *puborectalis muscle*. The *puborectalis, iliococcygeus,* and *pubococcygeus muscles* form the *levator ani muscle* of the pelvic floor (Fig. 28-4).

Anorectal Vascular Supply

The *superior rectal artery* arises from the terminal branch of the inferior mesenteric artery and supplies the upper rectum. The *middle rectal artery* arises from the internal iliac; the presence and size of these arteries are highly variable. The *inferior rectal artery* arises from the internal pudendal artery, which is a branch of the internal iliac artery. A rich network of collaterals connects the terminal arterioles of each of these arteries, thus making the rectum relatively resistant to ischemia (Fig. 28-5).

The venous drainage of the rectum parallels the arterial supply. The *superior rectal vein* drains into the portal system via the inferior mesenteric vein. The *middle rectal vein* drains into the internal iliac vein. The *inferior rectal vein* drains into the internal pudendal vein, and subsequently into the internal iliac vein. A submucosal plexus deep to the columns of Morgagni forms the *hemorrhoidal plexus* and drains into all three veins.

Anorectal Lymphatic Drainage

Lymphatic drainage of the rectum parallels the vascular supply. Lymphatic channels in the upper and middle rectum drain superiorly into the inferior mesenteric lymph nodes. Lymphatic channels in the lower rectum drain both superiorly into the inferior mesenteric lymph nodes and laterally into the internal iliac lymph nodes. The anal canal has a more complex pattern of lymphatic drainage. Proximal to the dentate line, lymph drains into both the inferior mesenteric lymph nodes and the internal iliac lymph nodes. Distal to the dentate line, lymph primarily drains into the inguinal lymph nodes, but can also drain into the inferior mesenteric lymph nodes and internal iliac lymph nodes.

Anorectal Nerve Supply

Both sympathetic and parasympathetic nerves innervate the anorectum. Sympathetic nerve fibers are derived from L1-L3 and join the preaortic plexus. The preaortic nerve fibers then extend

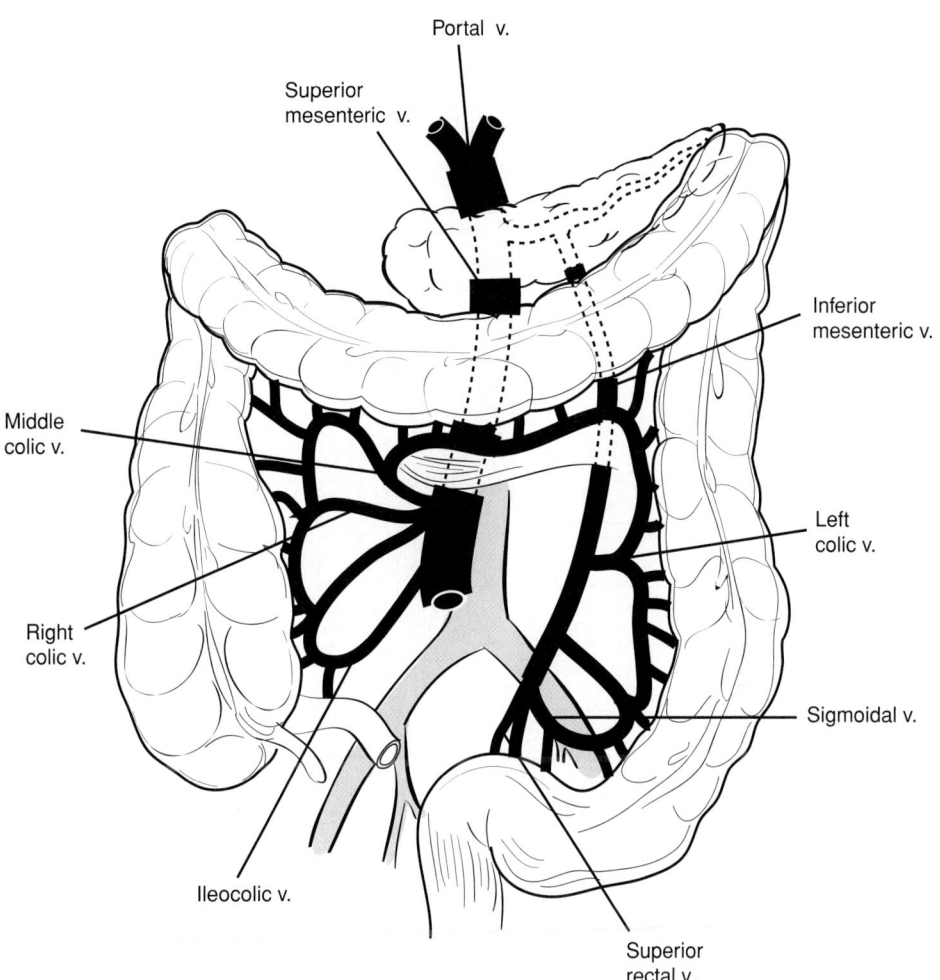

FIG. 28-2. Venous drainage of the colon. [*Reproduced with permission from Bell RH, Rikkers LF, Mulholland M (eds): Digestive Tract Surgery: A Text and Atlas. Philadelphia: Lippincott Williams & Wilkins, 1996, p 1459.*]

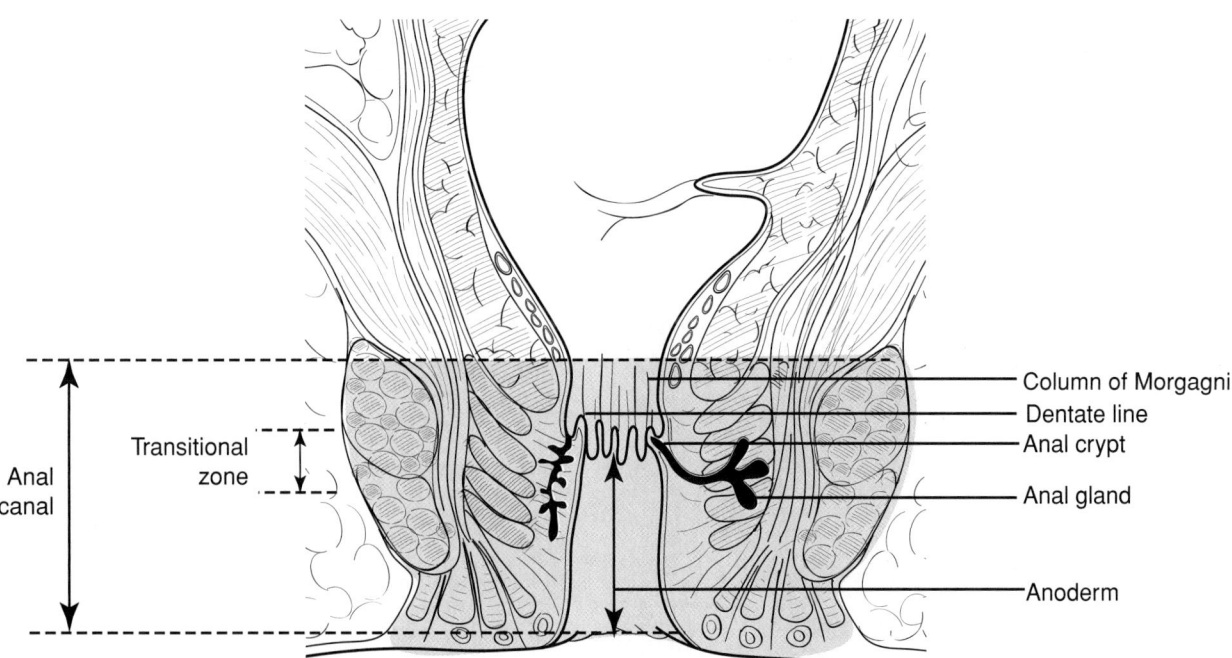

FIG. 28-3. The lining of the anal canal. [*From Goldberg SM, Gordon PH, Nivatvongs S (eds): Essentials of Anorectal Surgery. 1980, p 4. Reproduced with Permission from Stanley M. Goldberg, MD.*]

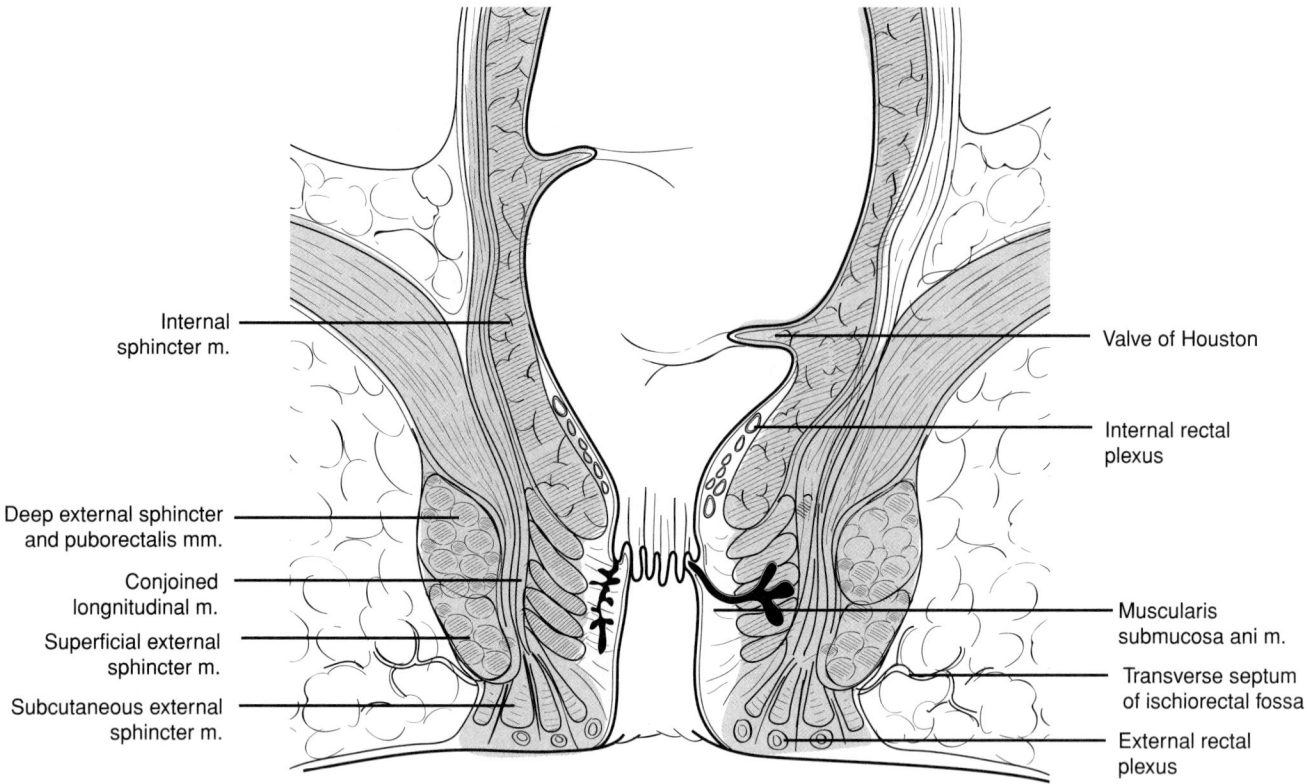

FIG. 28-4. The distal rectum and anal canal. [*Reproduced with permission from Schwartz SI, Shires GT, Spencer FC (eds): Principles of Surgery. 5th ed. New York: McGraw-Hill, 1989, p 1229.*]

Internal sphincter m.

Deep external sphincter and puborectalis mm.

Conjoined longnitudinal m.

Superficial external sphincter m.

Subcutaneous external sphincter m.

Valve of Houston

Internal rectal plexus

Muscularis submucosa ani m.

Transverse septum of ischiorectal fossa

External rectal plexus

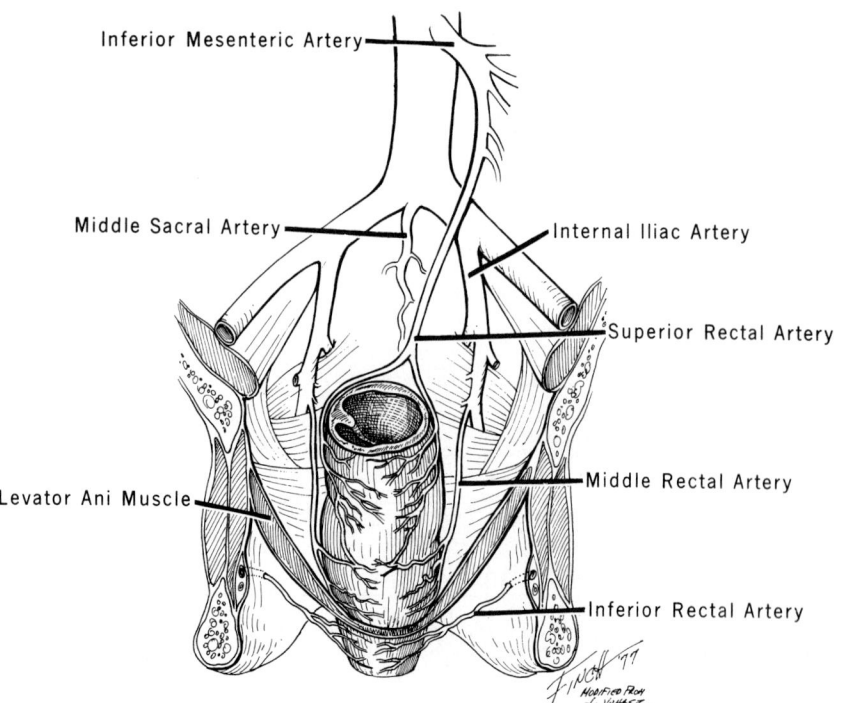

Inferior Mesenteric Artery

Middle Sacral Artery

Internal Iliac Artery

Superior Rectal Artery

Middle Rectal Artery

Levator Ani Muscle

Inferior Rectal Artery

FIG. 28-5. Arterial supply to the rectum and anal canal. [*Reproduced with permission from Schwartz SI, Shires GT, Spencer FC (eds): Principles of Surgery. 5th ed. New York: McGraw-Hill, 1989, p 1230.*]

below the aorta to form the *hypogastric plexus,* which subsequently joins the parasympathetic fibers to form the pelvic plexus. Parasympathetic nerve fibers are known as the *nervi erigentes* and originate from S2-S4. These fibers join the sympathetic fibers to form the pelvic plexus. Sympathetic and parasympathetic fibers then supply the anorectum and adjacent urogenital organs.

The internal anal sphincter is innervated by sympathetic and parasympathetic nerve fibers; both types of fibers inhibit sphincter contraction. The external anal sphincter and puborectalis muscles are innervated by the *inferior rectal branch* of the *internal pudendal nerve.* The levator ani receives innervation from both the *internal pudendal nerve* and direct branches of S3 to S5. Sensory innervation to the anal canal is provided by the *inferior rectal branch* of the *pudendal nerve.* While the rectum is relatively insensate, the anal canal below the dentate line is sensate.

Congenital Anomalies

Perturbation of the embryologic development of the midgut and hindgut may result in anatomic abnormalities of the colon, rectum, and anus. Failure of the midgut to rotate and return to the abdominal cavity during the tenth week of gestation results in varying degrees of intestinal malrotation and colonic nonfixation. Failure of canalization of the primitive gut can result in colonic duplication. Incomplete descent of the urogenital septum may result in imperforate anus and associated fistulas to the genitourinary tract. Many infants with congenital anomalies of the hindgut have associated abnormalities in the genitourinary tract.

NORMAL PHYSIOLOGY

Fluid and Electrolyte Exchanges

Water, Sodium, Potassium, Chloride, Bicarbonate, and Ammonia

The colon is a major site for water absorption and electrolyte exchange. Approximately 90% of the water contained in ileal fluid is absorbed in the colon (1000 to 2000 mL/d), and up to 5000 mL of fluid can be absorbed daily. Sodium is absorbed actively via a Na-K ATPase. The colon can absorb up to 400 mEq of sodium per day. Water accompanies the transported sodium and is absorbed passively along an osmotic gradient. Potassium is actively secreted into the colonic lumen and absorbed by passive diffusion. Chloride is absorbed actively via a chloride–bicarbonate exchange.

Bacterial degradation of protein and urea produces ammonia. Ammonia is subsequently absorbed and transported to the liver. Absorption of ammonia depends in part upon intraluminal pH. A decrease in colonic bacteria (e.g., broad spectrum antibiotic usage) and/or a decrease in intraluminal pH (e.g., lactulose administration) will decrease ammonia absorption.

Short-Chain Fatty Acids

Short-chain fatty acids (acetate, butyrate, and propionate) are produced by bacterial fermentation of dietary carbohydrates. Short-chain fatty acids are an important source of energy for the colonic mucosa, and metabolism by colonocytes provides energy for processes such as active transport of sodium. Lack of a dietary source for production of short-chain fatty acids, or diversion of the fecal stream by an ileostomy or colostomy, may result in mucosal atrophy and "diversion colitis."

Colonic Microflora and Intestinal Gas

Approximately 30% of fecal dry weight is composed of bacteria (10^{11} to 10^{12} bacteria/g of feces). Anaerobes are the predominant class of microorganism, and *Bacteroides* species are the most common (10^{11} to 10^{12} organisms/mL). *Escherichia coli* are the most numerous aerobes (10^8 to 10^{10} organisms/mL). Endogenous microflora are crucial for the breakdown of carbohydrates and proteins in the colon and participate in the metabolism of bilirubin, bile acids, estrogen, and cholesterol. Colonic bacteria also are necessary for production of vitamin K. Endogenous bacteria also are thought to suppress the emergence of pathogenic microorganisms, such as *Clostridium difficile.* However, the high bacterial load of the large intestine may contribute to sepsis in critically ill patients and may contribute to intra-abdominal sepsis, abscess, and wound infection following colectomy.

Intestinal gas arises from swallowed air, diffusion from the blood, and intraluminal production. Nitrogen, oxygen, carbon dioxide, hydrogen, and methane are the major components of intestinal gas. Nitrogen and oxygen are largely derived from swallowed air. Carbon dioxide is produced by the reaction of bicarbonate and hydrogen ions, and by the digestion of triglycerides to fatty acids. Hydrogen and methane are produced by colonic bacteria. The production of methane is highly variable. The gastrointestinal tract usually contains between 100 and 200 mL of gas and 400 to 1200 mL per day are released as flatus, depending upon the type of food ingested.

Motility, Defecation, and Continence

Motility

Unlike the small intestine, the large intestine does not demonstrate cyclic motor activity characteristic of the migratory motor complex. Instead, the colon displays intermittent contractions of either low or high amplitude. Low-amplitude, short-duration contractions occur in bursts and appear to move the colonic contents both antegrade and retrograde. It is thought that these bursts of motor activity delay colonic transit and thus increase the time available for absorption of water and exchange of electrolytes. High-amplitude contractions occur in a more coordinated fashion and create "mass movements." Bursts of "rectal motor complexes" also have been described. In general, cholinergic activation increases colonic motility.

Defecation

Defecation is a complex, coordinated mechanism involving colonic mass movement, increased intra-abdominal and rectal pressure, and relaxation of the pelvic floor. Distention of the rectum causes a reflex relaxation of the internal anal sphincter (the rectoanal inhibitory reflex) that allows the contents to make contact with the anal canal. This "sampling reflex" allows the sensory epithelium to distinguish solid stool from liquid stool and gas. If defecation does not occur, the rectum relaxes and the urge to defecate passes (the *accommodation response*). Defecation proceeds by coordination of increasing intra-abdominal pressure via the Valsalva maneuver, increased rectal contraction, relaxation of the puborectalis muscle, and opening of the anal canal.

Continence

The maintenance of fecal continence is at least as complex as the mechanism of defecation. Continence requires adequate rectal wall compliance to accommodate the fecal bolus, appropriate neurogenic control of the pelvic floor and sphincter mechanism, and functional internal and external sphincter muscles. At rest, the puborectalis muscle creates a "sling" around the distal rectum, forming a relatively acute angle that distributes intraabdominal forces onto the pelvic floor. With defecation, this angle straightens, allowing downward force to be applied along the axis of the rectum and anal canal. The internal and external sphincters are tonically active at rest. The internal sphincter is responsible for most of the resting, involuntary sphincter tone (resting pressure). The external sphincter is responsible for most of the voluntary sphincter tone (squeeze pressure). Branches of the pudendal nerve innervate both the internal and external sphincter. Finally, the hemorrhoidal cushions may contribute to continence by mechanically blocking the anal canal. Thus, impaired continence may result from poor rectal compliance, injury to the internal and/or external sphincter or puborectalis, or nerve damage or neuropathy.

CLINICAL EVALUATION

Clinical Assessment

A complete history and physical examination is the starting point for evaluating any patient with suspected disease of the colon and rectum. Special attention should be paid to the patient's past medical and surgical history to detect underlying conditions that might contribute to a gastrointestinal problem. If patients have had prior intestinal surgery, it is essential that one understand the resultant gastrointestinal anatomy. In addition, family history of colorectal disease, especially inflammatory bowel disease, polyps, and colorectal cancer, is crucial. Medication use must be detailed as many drugs cause gastrointestinal symptoms. Before recommending operative intervention, the adequacy of medical treatment must be ascertained. In addition to examining the abdomen, visual inspection of the anus and perineum and careful digital rectal exam are essential.

Endoscopy

Anoscopy

The anoscope is a useful instrument for examination of the anal canal. Anoscopes are made in a variety of sizes and measure approximately 8 cm in length. A larger anoscope provides better exposure for anal procedures such as rubber band ligation or sclerotherapy of hemorrhoids. The anoscope, with obturator in place, should be adequately lubricated and gently inserted into the anal canal. The obturator is withdrawn, inspection of the visualized anal canal is done, and the anoscope should then be withdrawn. It is rotated 90 degrees and reinserted to allow visualization of all four quadrants of the canal. If the patient complains of severe perianal pain and cannot tolerate a digital rectal examination, anoscopy should not be attempted without anesthesia.

Proctoscopy

The rigid proctoscope is useful for examination of the rectum and distal sigmoid colon and is occasionally used therapeutically. The standard proctoscope is 25 cm in length and available in various diameters. Most often, a 15- or 19-mm diameter proctoscope is used for diagnostic examinations. The large (25-mm diameter) proctoscope is useful for procedures such as polypectomy, electrocoagulation, or detorsion of a sigmoid volvulus. A smaller "pediatric" proctoscope (11-mm diameter) is better tolerated by patients with anal stricture. Suction is necessary for an adequate proctoscopic examination.

Flexible Sigmoidoscopy and Colonoscopy

Video or fiberoptic flexible sigmoidoscopy and colonoscopy provide excellent visualization of the colon and rectum. Sigmoidoscopes measure 60 cm in length. Full depth of insertion may allow visualization as high as the splenic flexure, although the mobility and redundancy of the sigmoid colon often limit the extent of the examination. Partial preparation with enemas is usually adequate for sigmoidoscopy and most patients can tolerate this procedure without sedation. Colonoscopes measure 100 to 160 cm in length and are capable of examining the entire colon and terminal ileum. A complete oral bowel preparation is usually necessary for colonoscopy and the duration and discomfort of the procedure usually require conscious sedation. Both sigmoidoscopy and colonoscopy can be used diagnostically and therapeutically. Electrocautery should generally not be used in the absence of a complete bowel preparation because of the risk of explosion of intestinal methane or hydrogen gases. Diagnostic colonoscopes possess a single channel through which instruments such as snares, biopsy forceps, or electrocautery can be passed; this channel also provides suction and irrigation capability. Therapeutic colonoscopes possess two channels to allow simultaneous suction/irrigation and the use of snares, biopsy forceps, or electrocautery.

Imaging

Plain X-Rays and Contrast Studies

Despite advanced radiologic techniques, plain x-rays and contrast studies continue to play an important role in the evaluation of patients with suspected colon and rectal diseases. Plain x-rays of the abdomen (supine, upright, and diaphragmatic views) are useful for detecting free intra-abdominal air, bowel gas patterns suggestive of small or large bowel obstruction, and volvulus. Contrast studies are useful for evaluating obstructive symptoms, delineating fistulous tracts, and diagnosing small perforations or anastomotic leaks. While Gastrografin cannot provide the mucosal detail provided by barium, this water-soluble contrast agent is recommended if perforation or leak is suspected. Double-contrast barium enema has been reported to be 70 to 90% sensitive for the detection of mass lesions greater than 1 cm in diameter.[1] Detection of small lesions can be extremely difficult, especially in a patient with extensive diverticulosis. For this reason, a colonoscopy is preferred for evaluating nonobstructing mass lesions in the colon. Double-contrast barium enema has been used as a back-up examination if colonoscopy is incomplete.

Computed Tomography

Computed tomography (CT) is commonly employed in the evaluation of patients with abdominal complaints. Its utility is primarily in the detection of extraluminal disease, such as intra-abdominal abscesses and pericolic inflammation, and in staging colorectal carcinoma, because of its sensitivity in detection of hepatic metastases.[2] Extravasation of oral or rectal contrast may also confirm the diagnosis of perforation or anastomotic leak. Nonspecific findings such as bowel wall thickening or mesenteric stranding may suggest inflammatory bowel disease, enteritis/colitis, or ischemia. A standard CT scan is relatively insensitive for the detection of intraluminal lesions.

Virtual Colonoscopy

Virtual colonoscopy is a new radiologic technique that is designed to overcome some of the limitations of traditional CT scanning. This technology uses helical CT and three-dimensional reconstruction to detect intraluminal colonic lesions. Oral bowel preparation, oral and rectal contrast, and colon insufflation are used to maximize sensitivity. Early evaluation of virtual colonoscopy suggests that accuracy may approach that of colonoscopy for detection of lesions 1 cm in diameter or greater.

Magnetic Resonance Imaging

The main use of magnetic resonance imaging (MRI) in colorectal disorders is in evaluation of pelvic lesions. MRI is more sensitive than CT for detecting bony involvement or pelvic sidewall extension of rectal tumors. MRI also can be helpful in the detection and delineation of complex fistulas in ano. The use of an endorectal coil may increase sensitivity.

Positron Emission Tomography

Positron emission tomography (PET) is used for imaging tissues with high levels of anaerobic glycolysis, such as malignant tumors. ^{18}F-fluorodeoxyglucose (FDG) is injected as a tracer; metabolism of this molecule then results in positron emission. PET has been used as an adjunct to CT in the staging of colorectal cancer and may prove useful in discriminating recurrent cancer from fibrosis. At present, the efficacy and utility of PET in the detection of recurrent and/or metastatic colorectal cancer remains unproven.

Angiography

Angiography is occasionally used for the detection of bleeding within the colon or small bowel. To visualize hemorrhage angiographically, bleeding must be relatively brisk (approximately 0.5 to 1.0 mL per minute). If extravasation of contrast is identified, infusion of vasopressin or angiographic embolization can be therapeutic.

Endorectal and Endoanal Ultrasound

Endorectal ultrasound is primarily used to evaluate the depth of invasion of neoplastic lesions in the rectum. The normal rectal wall appears as a five-layer structure (Fig. 28-6). Ultrasound can reliably differentiate most benign polyps from invasive tumors based upon the integrity of the submucosal layer. Ultrasound can also differentiate superficial T1-T2 from deeper T3-T4 tumors. Overall, the accuracy of ultrasound in detecting depth of mural invasion ranges between 81 and 94%.[3] This modality also can detect enlarged perirectal lymph nodes, which may suggest nodal metastases; accuracy of detection of pathologically positive lymph nodes is 58 to 83%. Ultrasound may also prove useful for early detection of local recurrence after surgery.

Endoanal ultrasound is used to evaluate the layers of the anal canal. Internal anal sphincter, external anal sphincter, and puborectalis muscle can be differentiated. Endoanal ultrasound is particularly useful for detecting sphincter defects and for outlining complex anal fistulas.

Physiologic and Pelvic Floor Investigations

Anorectal physiologic testing uses a variety of techniques to investigate the function of the pelvic floor. These techniques are useful in the evaluation of patients with incontinence, constipation, rectal prolapse, obstructed defecation, and other disorders of the pelvic floor.

Manometry

Anorectal manometry is performed by placing a pressure-sensitive catheter in the lower rectum. The catheter is then withdrawn

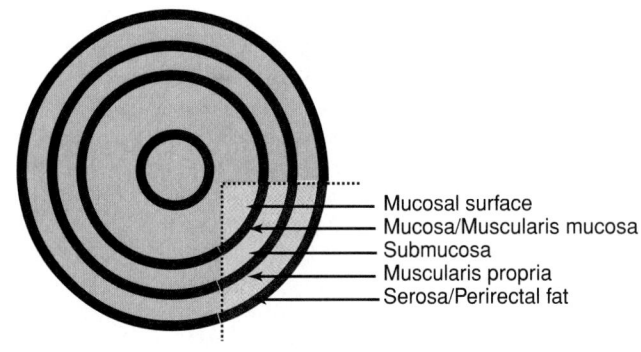

Mucosal surface
Mucosa/Muscularis mucosa
Submucosa
Muscularis propria
Serosa/Perirectal fat

A

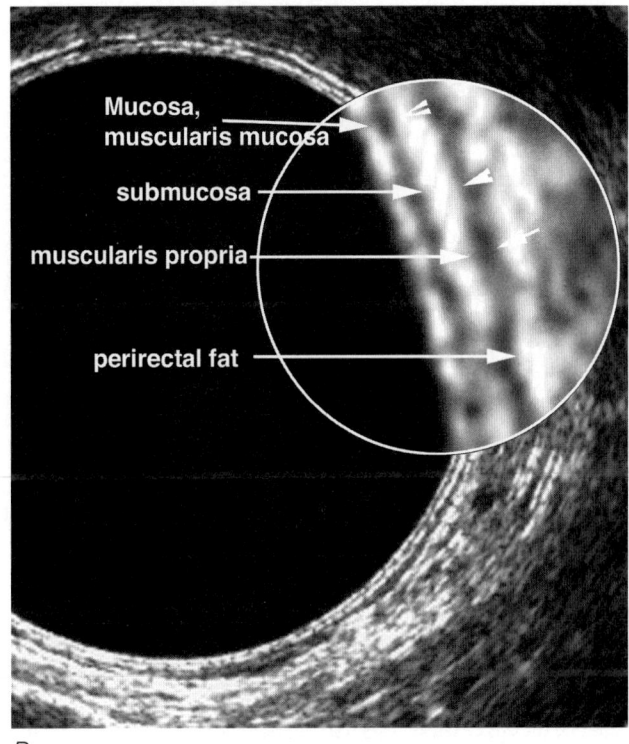

Mucosa, muscularis mucosa
submucosa
muscularis propria
perirectal fat

B

FIG. 28-6. *A. Schematic of the layers of the rectal wall observed on endorectal ultrasonography. (Courtesy of Charles O. Finne, III, MD, Minneapolis, MN.) B. Normal endorectal ultrasonography.*

through the anal canal and pressures recorded. A balloon attached to the tip of the catheter also can be used to test anorectal sensation. The *resting pressure* in the anal canal reflects the function of the internal anal sphincter (normal: 40 to 80 mm Hg), while the *squeeze pressure,* defined as the maximum voluntary contraction pressure minus the resting pressure, reflects function of the external anal sphincter (normal: 40 to 80 mm Hg above resting pressure). The *high-pressure zone* estimates the length of the anal canal (normal: 2.0 to 4.0 cm). The *rectoanal inhibitory reflex* can be detected by inflating a balloon in the distal rectum; absence of this reflex is characteristic of Hirschsprung's disease.

Neurophysiology

Neurophysiologic testing assesses function of the pudendal nerves and recruitment of puborectalis muscle fibers. Pudendal nerve terminal motor latency measures the speed of transmission of a nerve impulse through the distal pudendal nerve fibers (normal: 1.8 to 2.2 msec); prolonged latency suggests the presence of neuropathy. EMG recruitment assesses the contraction and relaxation of the puborectalis muscle during attempted defecation. Normally, recruitment increases when a patient is instructed to "squeeze," and decreases when a patient is instructed to "push." Inappropriate recruitment is an indication of paradoxical contraction (nonrelaxation of the puborectalis). Needle EMG has been used to map both the pudendal nerves and the anatomy of the internal and external sphincters. However, this examination is painful and poorly tolerated by most patients. Needle EMG has largely been replaced by pudendal nerve motor-latency testing to assess pudendal nerve function and endoanal ultrasound to map the sphincters.

Rectal Evacuation Studies

Rectal evacuation studies include the balloon expulsion test and video defecography. Balloon expulsion assesses a patient's ability to expel an intrarectal balloon. Video defecography provides a more detailed assessment of defecation. In this test, barium paste is placed in the rectum and defecation is then recorded fluoroscopically. Defecography is used to differentiate nonrelaxation of the puborectalis, obstructed defecation, increased perineal descent, rectal prolapse and intussusception, rectocele, and enterocele. The addition of vaginal contrast and intraperitoneal contrast is useful in delineating complex disorders of the pelvic floor.

Laboratory Studies

Fecal Occult Blood Testing

Fecal occult blood testing (FOBT) is used as a screening test for colonic neoplasms in asymptomatic, average-risk individuals. The efficacy of this test is based upon serial testing because the majority of colorectal malignancies will bleed intermittently. FOBT has been a nonspecific test for peroxidase contained in hemoglobin; consequently, occult bleeding from any gastrointestinal source will produce a positive result. Similarly, many foods (red meat, some fruits and vegetables, and vitamin C) will produce a false-positive result. Patients were counseled to eat a restricted diet for 2 to 3 days prior to the test. Increased specificity is now possible by using immunochemical FOBT. These tests rely on monoclonal or polyclonal antibodies to react with the intact globin portion of human hemoglobin. Because globin does not survive in the upper gastrointestinal tract, the immunochemical tests are more specific for identifying occult bleeding from the colon or rectum. Dietary restrictions are not necessary. Any positive FOBT mandates further investigation, usually by colonoscopy.

Stool Studies

Stool studies are often helpful in evaluating the etiology of diarrhea. Wet-mount examination reveals the presence of fecal leukocytes, which may suggest colonic inflammation or the presence of an invasive organism such as invasive *E. coli* or *Shigella*. Stool cultures can detect pathogenic bacteria, ova, and parasites. *C. difficile* colitis is diagnosed by detecting bacterial toxin in the stool.[4] Steatorrhea may be diagnosed by adding Sudan red stain to a stool sample.

Serum Tests

Specific laboratory tests that should be performed will be dictated by the clinical scenario. Preoperative studies generally include a complete blood count and electrolyte panel. The addition of coagulation studies, liver function tests, and blood typing/cross-matching depends upon the patient's medical condition and the proposed surgical procedure.

Tumor Markers

Carcinoembryonic antigen (CEA) may be elevated in 60 to 90% of patients with colorectal cancer. Despite this, CEA is not an effective screening tool for this malignancy. Many practitioners follow serial CEA levels after curative-intent surgery in order to detect early recurrence of colorectal cancer. However, this tumor marker is nonspecific, and no survival benefit has yet been proven. Other biochemical markers (ornithine decarboxylase, urokinase) have been proposed, but none has yet proven sensitive or specific for detection, staging, or predicting prognosis of colorectal carcinoma.[5]

Genetic Testing

Although familial colorectal cancer syndromes, such as familial adenomatous polyposis (FAP) and hereditary nonpolyposis colon cancer (HNPCC) are rare, information about the specific genetic abnormalities underlying these disorders has led to significant interest in the role of genetic testing for colorectal cancer.[6] Tests for mutations in the adenomatous polyposis coli (APC) gene responsible for FAP, and in mismatch repair genes responsible for HNPCC, are commercially available and extremely accurate in families with known mutations. Although many of these mutations are also present in sporadic colorectal cancer, the accuracy of genetic testing in average-risk individuals is considerably lower and these tests are not recommended for screening. Because of the potential psychosocial implications of genetic testing, it is strongly recommended that professional genetic counselors be involved in the care of any patient considering these tests.

Evaluation of Common Symptoms

Pain

Abdominal Pain. Abdominal pain is a nonspecific symptom with a myriad of causes. Abdominal pain related to the colon and rectum can result from obstruction (either inflammatory or neoplastic), inflammation, perforation, or ischemia. Plain x-rays and judicious use of contrast studies and/or a CT scan can often confirm the diagnosis. Gentle retrograde contrast studies (barium or Gastrografin enema) may be useful in delineating the degree of colonic obstruction. Sigmoidoscopy and/or colonoscopy performed by an experienced endoscopist can assist in the diagnosis of ischemic colitis, infectious colitis, and inflammatory bowel disease. However, if perforation is suspected, colonoscopy and/or sigmoidoscopy are generally contraindicated. Evaluation and treatment of abdominal pain from a colorectal source should follow the usual surgical principles of a thorough history and physical examination, appropriate diagnostic tests, resuscitation, and appropriately timed surgical intervention.

Pelvic Pain. Pelvic pain can originate from the distal colon and rectum or from adjacent urogenital structures. Tenesmus may result from proctitis or from a rectal or retrorectal mass. Cyclical pain associated with menses, especially when accompanied by rectal bleeding, suggests a diagnosis of endometriosis. Pelvic inflammatory disease also can produce significant abdominal and pelvic pain. The extension of a peridiverticular abscess or periappendiceal abscess into the pelvis may also cause pain. CT scan and/or MRI may be useful in differentiating these diseases. Proctoscopy (if tolerated) also can be helpful. Occasionally, laparoscopy will yield a diagnosis.

Anorectal Pain. Anorectal pain is most often secondary to an anal fissure or perirectal abscess and/or fistula. Physical examination can usually differentiate these conditions. Other, less common causes of anorectal pain include anal canal neoplasms, perianal skin infection, and dermatologic conditions. Proctalgia fugax results from levator spasm and may present without any other anorectal findings. Physical exam is critical in evaluating patients with anorectal pain. If a patient is too tender to examine in the office, an examination under anesthesia is necessary. MRI may be helpful in select cases where the etiology of pain is elusive.

Lower Gastrointestinal Bleeding

The first goal in evaluating and treating a patient with gastrointestinal hemorrhage is adequate resuscitation. The principles of ensuring a patent airway, supporting ventilation, and optimizing hemodynamic parameters apply and coagulopathy and/or thrombocytopenia should be corrected. The second goal is to identify the source of hemorrhage. Because the most common source of gastrointestinal hemorrhage is esophageal, gastric, or duodenal, nasogastric aspiration should always be performed; return of bile suggests that the source of bleeding is distal to the ligament of Treitz. If aspiration reveals blood or nonbile secretions, or if symptoms suggest an upper intestinal source, esophagogastroduodenoscopy is

performed. Anoscopy and/or limited proctoscopy can identify hemorrhoidal bleeding. A technetium-99 (^{99m}Tc)-tagged red blood cell (RBC) scan is extremely sensitive and is able to detect as little as 0.1 mL/h of bleeding; however, localization is imprecise. If the ^{99m}Tc-tagged RBC scan is positive, angiography can then be employed to localize bleeding. Infusion of vasopressin or angioembolization may be therapeutic. Alternatively, a catheter can be left in the bleeding vessel to allow localization at the time of laparotomy. If the patient is hemodynamically stable, a rapid bowel preparation (over 4 to 6 hours) can be performed to allow colonoscopy. Colonoscopy may identify the cause of the bleeding, and cautery or injection of epinephrine into the bleeding site may be used to control hemorrhage. Colectomy may be required if bleeding persists despite these interventions. Intraoperative colonoscopy and/or enteroscopy may assist in localizing bleeding. If colectomy is required, a segmental resection is preferred if the bleeding source can be localized. "Blind" subtotal colectomy may very rarely be required in a patient who is hemodynamically unstable with ongoing colonic hemorrhage of an unknown source. In this setting, it is crucial to irrigate the rectum and examine the mucosa by proctoscopy to ensure that the source of bleeding is not distal to the resection margin (Fig. 28-7).

Occult blood loss from the gastrointestinal tract may manifest as iron-deficiency anemia or may be detected with fecal occult blood

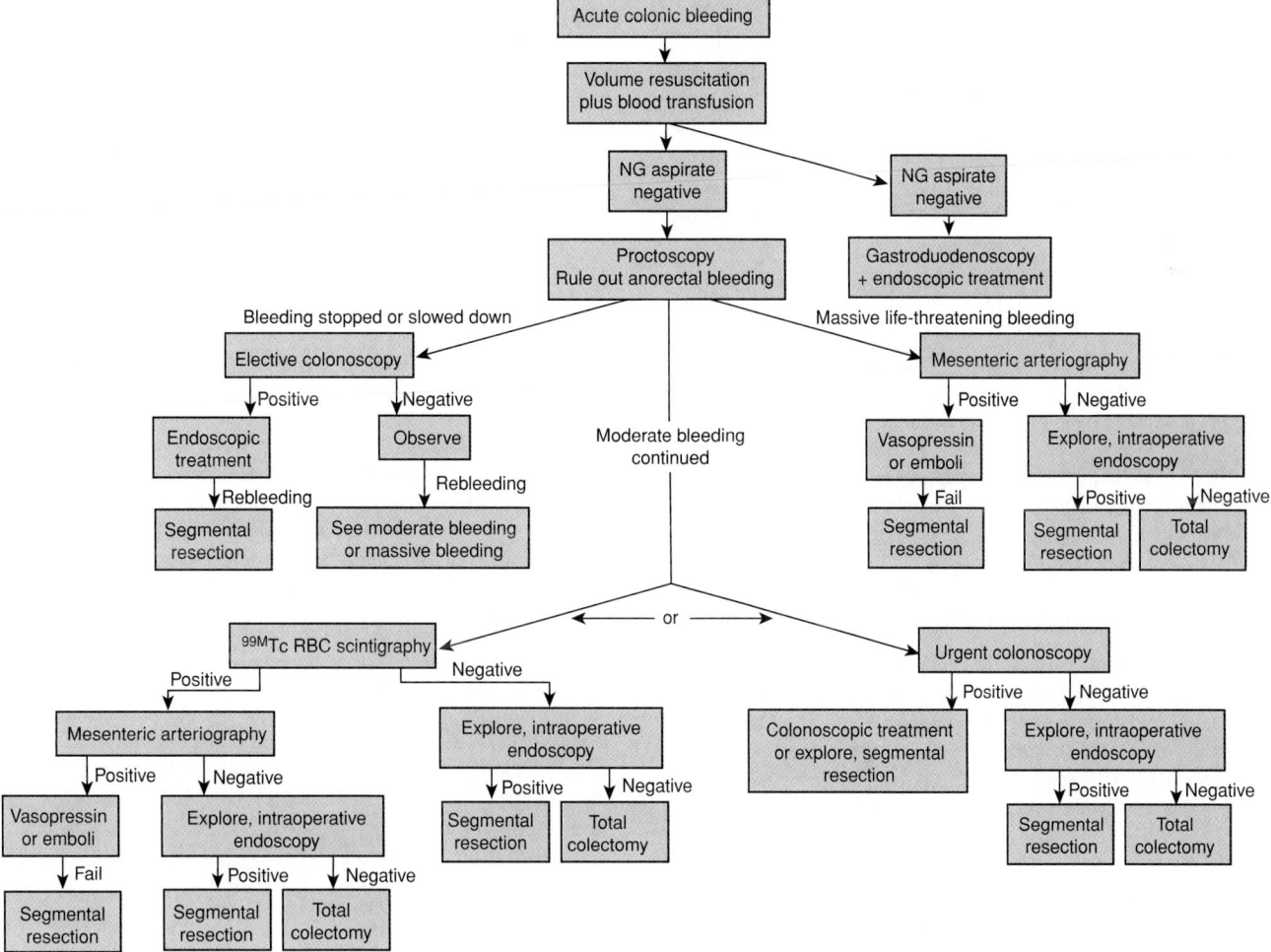

FIG. 28-7. Algorithm for treatment of colorectal hemorrhage. [*Reproduced with permission from Gordon PH, Nivatvongs S (eds): Principles and Practice of Surgery for the Colon, Rectum, and Anus, 2nd ed. New York: Marcel Dekker, Inc., 1999, p 1279.*]

testing. Because colon neoplasms bleed intermittently and rarely present with rapid hemorrhage, the presence of occult fecal blood should always prompt a colonoscopy. Unexplained iron-deficiency anemia is also an indication for colonoscopy.

Hematochezia is commonly caused by hemorrhoids or fissure. Sharp, knife-like pain and bright-red rectal bleeding with bowel movements suggest the diagnosis of fissure. Painless, bright-red rectal bleeding with bowel movements is often secondary to a friable internal hemorrhoid that is easily detected by anoscopy. In the absence of a painful, obvious fissure, any patient with rectal bleeding should undergo a careful digital rectal examination, anoscopy, and proctosigmoidoscopy. Failure to diagnose a source in the distal anorectum should prompt colonoscopy.

Constipation and Obstructed Defecation

Constipation is an extremely common complaint, affecting more than 4 million people in the United States. Despite the prevalence of this problem, there is lack of agreement about an appropriate definition of constipation. Patients may describe infrequent bowel movements, hard stools, or excessive straining. A careful history of these symptoms often clarifies the nature of the problem.

Constipation has a myriad of causes. Underlying metabolic, pharmacologic, endocrine, psychologic, and neurologic causes often contribute to the problem. A stricture or mass lesion should be excluded by colonoscopy or barium enema. After these causes have been excluded, evaluation focuses upon differentiating *slow-transit constipation* from *outlet obstruction*. Transit studies, in which radiopaque markers are swallowed and then followed radiographically, are useful for diagnosing slow-transit constipation. Anorectal manometry and electromyography can detect nonrelaxation of the puborectalis, which contributes to outlet obstruction. The absence of an anorectal inhibitory reflex suggests Hirschsprung's disease and may prompt a rectal mucosal biopsy. Defecography can identify rectal prolapse, intussusception, rectocele, or enterocele.

Medical management is the mainstay of therapy for constipation and includes fiber, increased fluid intake, and laxatives. Outlet obstruction from nonrelaxation of the puborectalis often responds to biofeedback.[7] Surgery to correct rectocele and rectal prolapse has a variable effect on symptoms of constipation, but can be successful in selected patients. Subtotal colectomy is considered only for patients with severe slow-transit constipation (colonic inertia) refractory to maximal medical interventions. While this operation almost always increases bowel movement frequency, complaints of diarrhea, incontinence, and abdominal pain are not infrequent, and patients should be carefully selected.[8]

Diarrhea and Irritable Bowel Syndrome

Diarrhea is also a common complaint and is usually a self-limited symptom of infectious gastroenteritis. If diarrhea is chronic or is accompanied by bleeding or abdominal pain, further investigation is warranted. Bloody diarrhea and pain are characteristic of colitis; etiology can be an infection (invasive *E. coli, Shigella, Salmonella, Campylobacter, Entamoeba histolytica,* or *C. difficile*), inflammatory bowel disease (ulcerative colitis or Crohn's colitis), or ischemia. Stool wet-mount and culture can often diagnose infection. Sigmoidoscopy or colonoscopy can be helpful in diagnosing inflammatory bowel disease or ischemia. However, if the patient has abdominal tenderness, particularly with peritoneal signs, or any other evidence of perforation, endoscopy is contraindicated.

Chronic diarrhea may present a more difficult diagnostic dilemma. Chronic ulcerative colitis, Crohn's colitis, infection, mal-

absorption, and short gut syndrome can cause chronic diarrhea. Rarely, carcinoid syndrome and islet cell tumors (vasoactive intestinal peptide-secreting tumor [VIPoma], somatostatinoma, gastrinoma) present with this symptom. Large villous lesions may cause secretory diarrhea. Collagenous colitis can cause diarrhea without any obvious mucosal abnormality. Along with stool cultures, tests for malabsorption, and metabolic investigations, colonoscopy can be invaluable in differentiating these causes. Biopsies should be taken even if the colonic mucosa appears grossly normal.

Irritable bowel syndrome is a particularly troubling constellation of symptoms consisting of crampy abdominal pain, bloating, constipation, and urgent diarrhea. Work-up reveals no underlying anatomic or physiologic abnormality. Once other disorders have been excluded, dietary restrictions and avoidance of caffeine, alcohol, and tobacco may help to alleviate symptoms. Antispasmodics and bulking agents may be helpful.

Incontinence

The incidence of fecal incontinence has been estimated to occur in 10 to 13 individuals per 1000 people older than age 65 years. Incontinence ranges in severity from occasional leakage of gas and liquid stool to daily loss of solid stool. The underlying cause of incontinence is often multifactorial and diarrhea is often contributory. In general, causes of incontinence can be classified as *neurogenic* or *anatomic*. Neurogenic causes include diseases of the central nervous system and spinal cord along with pudendal nerve injury. Anatomic causes include congenital abnormalities, procidentia, overflow incontinence secondary to impaction or neoplasm, and trauma. The most common traumatic cause of incontinence is injury to the anal sphincter during vaginal delivery. Other causes include anorectal surgery, impalement, and pelvic fracture.

After a thorough medical evaluation to detect underlying conditions that might contribute to incontinence, evaluation focuses on assessment of the anal sphincter and pudendal nerves. Pudendal nerve terminal motor latency testing may detect neuropathy. Anal manometry can detect low resting and squeeze pressures. Defecography can detect rectal prolapse. Endoanal ultrasound is invaluable in diagnosing sphincter defects (Fig. 28-8).

Therapy depends upon the underlying abnormality. Diarrhea should be treated medically. Even in the absence of frank diarrhea, the addition of dietary fiber may improve continence. Some patients may respond to biofeedback. Many patients with a sphincter defect are candidates for an overlapping sphincteroplasty.[9] Innovative technologies such as sacral nerve stimulation or artificial bowel sphincter are proving useful in patients who fail other interventions.[10,11]

GENERAL SURGICAL CONSIDERATIONS

Colorectal resections are performed for a wide variety of conditions, including neoplasms (benign and malignant), inflammatory bowel diseases, and other benign conditions. Although the indication and urgency for surgery will alter some of the technical details, the operative principles of colorectal resections, anastomoses, and use of ostomies are well established. These principles and general considerations for anesthesia and other operative preliminaries are outlined in this chapter.

Resections

The mesenteric clearance technique dictates the extent of colonic resection and is determined by the nature of the primary pathology (malignant or benign), the intent of the resection (curative or

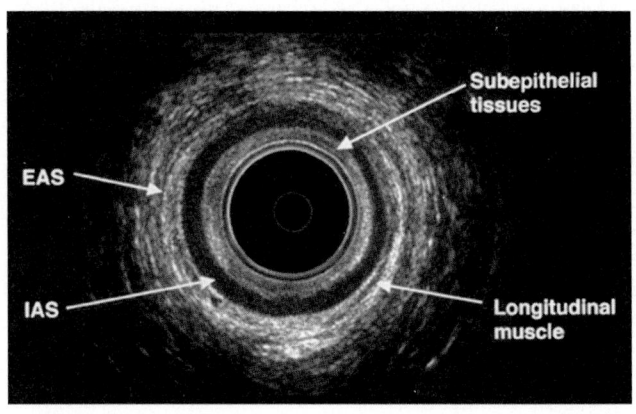

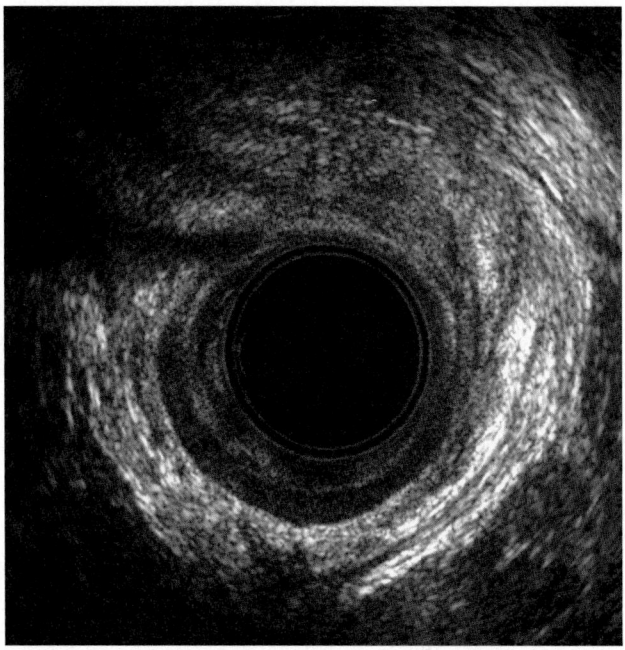

FIG. 28-8. *A. Endoanal ultrasonography showing the normal layers of the anal canal. B. Endoanal ultrasonography with anterior sphincter defect from birthing injury. (Both images courtesy of Charles O. Finne, III, MD, Minneapolis, MN.)*

B

palliative), the precise location(s) of the primary pathology, and the condition of the mesentery (thin and soft or thickened and indurated). In general, a proximal mesenteric ligation will eliminate the blood supply to a greater length of colon and require a more extensive "colectomy." Curative resection of a colorectal cancer is usually best accomplished by performing a proximal mesenteric vessel ligation and radical mesenteric clearance of the lymphatic drainage basin of the tumor site with concomitant resection of the overlying omentum (Fig. 28-9). Resection of a benign process does not require wide mesenteric resection and the omentum can be preserved if desired.

Emergency Resection

Emergency resection may be required because of obstruction, perforation, or hemorrhage. In this setting, the bowel is almost always unprepared and the patient may be unstable. The surgical principles described above apply and an attempt should be made to resect the involved segment along with its lymphovascular supply. If the resection involves the right colon or proximal transverse colon (right or extended right colectomy), a primary ileocolonic anastomosis can usually be performed safely as long as the remaining bowel appears healthy and the patient is stable. For left-sided tumors, the traditional approach has involved resection of the involved bowel and end colostomy, with or without a mucus fistula. However, there is an increasing body of data to suggest that a primary anastomosis with an on-table lavage, with or without a diverting ileostomy, may be equally safe in this setting. If the proximal colon looks unhealthy (vascular compromise, serosal tears, perforation), a subtotal colectomy can be performed with a small bowel to rectosigmoid anastomosis. Resection and diversion (ileostomy or colostomy) remains safe and appropriate if the bowel looks compromised or if the patient is unstable, malnourished, or immunosuppressed.

Laparoscopic Resection

With advances in minimally invasive technology, many procedures that previously have required laparotomy can now be performed *laparoscopically*.[12] Potential advantages of laparoscopy

include improved cosmetic result, decreased postoperative pain, and earlier return of bowel function. Moreover, some experimental data suggest that minimally invasive operations have less immunosuppressive impact on the patient and thus might improve postoperative outcome and even long-term survival. To date, most studies have demonstrated equivalence between laparoscopic and open resection in terms of extent of resection. However, laparoscopic colon resections are technically demanding and consistently require longer operative time than do open procedures. Return of bowel function and length of hospital stay are highly variable. Long-term outcome has yet to be determined.

Colectomy

A variety of terms are used to describe different types of colectomy (Fig. 28-10).

Ileocolic Resection. An ileocolic resection describes a limited resection of the terminal ileum, cecum, and appendix. It is used to remove disease involving these segments of the intestine (e.g., ileocecal Crohn's disease) and benign lesions or incurable cancers arising in the terminal ileum, cecum, and, occasionally, the appendix. If curable malignancy is suspected, more radical resections, such as a right hemicolectomy, are generally indicated. The ileocolic vessels are ligated and divided. A variable length of small intestine may be resected depending upon the disease process. A primary anastomosis is created between the distal small bowel and the ascending colon. It is technically difficult to perform an anastomosis at or just proximal to the ileocecal valve; therefore, if the most distal ileum needs to be resected, the cecum is generally also removed.

Right Colectomy. A right colectomy is used to remove lesions or disease in the right colon and is oncologically the most appropriate operation for curative intent resection of proximal colon carcinoma. The ileocolic vessels, right colic vessels, and right branches of the middle colic vessels are ligated and divided. Approximately 10 cm of terminal ileum are usually included in the resection. A primary ileal-transverse colon anastomosis is almost always possible.

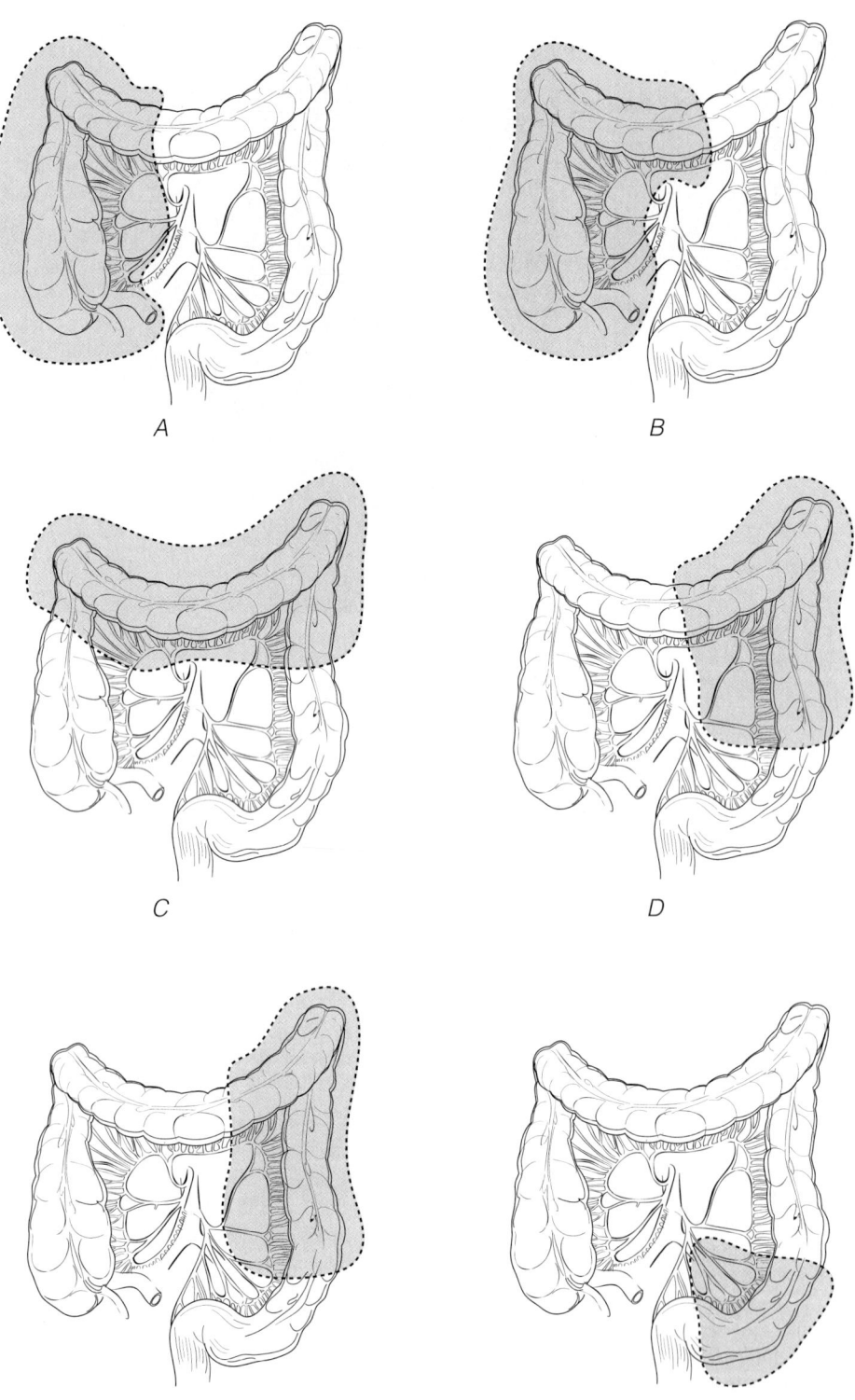

A

B

C

D

E

F

FIG. 28-9. Extent of resection for carcinoma of the colon. *A.* Cecal cancer. *B.* Hepatic flexure cancer. *C.* Transverse colon cancer. *D.* Splenic flexure cancer. *E.* Descending colon cancer. *F.* Sigmoid colon cancer. [*Reproduced with permission from Schwartz SI, Shires GT, Spencer FC (eds): Principles of Surgery. 5th ed. New York: McGraw-Hill, 1989, p 1279.*]

Extended Right Colectomy. An extended right colectomy may be used for curative intent resection of lesions located at the hepatic flexure or proximal transverse colon. A standard right colectomy is extended to include ligation of the middle colic vessels at their base. The right colon and proximal transverse colon are resected and a primary anastomosis is created between the ileum and distal transverse colon. Such an anastomosis relies on the marginal artery of Drummond. If the blood supply is questionable, the resec-

tion is extended to include the splenic flexure and the anastomosis of ileum is to the descending colon.

Transverse Colectomy. Lesions in the mid and distal transverse colon may be resected by ligating the middle colic vessels and resecting the transverse colon, followed by a colocolonic anastomosis. However, an extended right colectomy with an anastomosis between the terminal ileum and descending colon may be a safer anastomosis with an equivalent functional result.

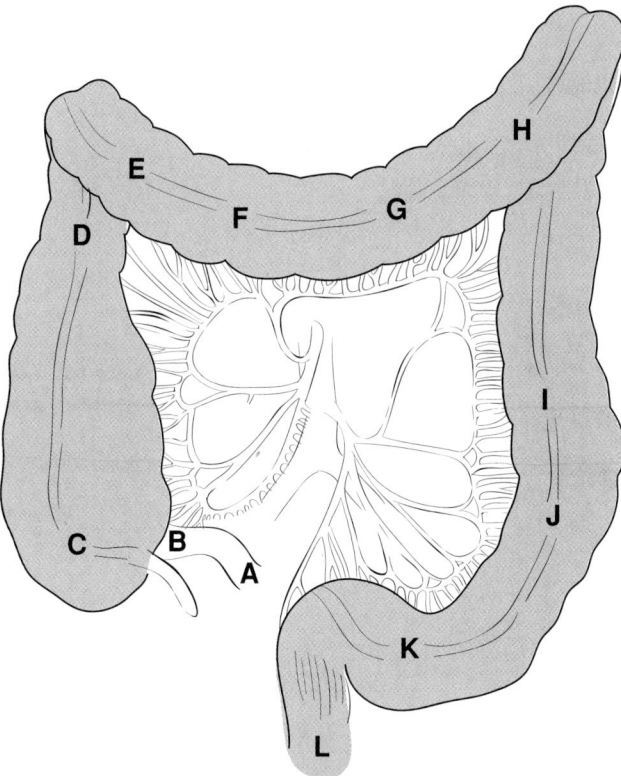

FIG. 28-10. Terminology of types of colorectal resections: A→C Ileocecectomy; + A + B→D Ascending colectomy; + A + B→F Right hemicolectomy; + A + B→G Extended right hemicolectomy; + E + F→G + H Transverse colectomy; G→I Left hemicolectomy; F→I Extended left hemicolectomy; J + K Sigmoid colectomy; + A + B→J Subtotal colectomy; + A + B→K Total colectomy; + A + B→L Total proctocolectomy. [Reproduced with permission from Fielding LP, Goldberg SM (eds): Rob & Smith's Operative: Surgery of the Colon, Rectum, and Anus. UK: Elsevier Science Ltd., 1993, p 349.]

Left Colectomy. For lesions or disease states confined to the distal transverse colon, splenic flexure, or descending colon, a left colectomy is performed. The left branches of the middle colic vessels, the left colic vessels, and the first branches of the sigmoid vessels are ligated. A colocolonic anastomosis can usually be performed.

Extended Left Colectomy. An extended left colectomy is an option for removing lesions in the distal transverse colon. In this operation, the left colectomy is extended proximally to include the right branches of the middle colic vessels.

Sigmoid Colectomy. Lesions in the sigmoid colon require ligation and division of the sigmoid branches of the inferior mesenteric artery. In general, the entire sigmoid colon should be resected to the level of the peritoneal reflection and an anastomosis created between the descending colon and upper rectum. Full mobilization of the splenic flexure is often required to create a tension-free anastomosis.

Total and Subtotal Colectomy. Total or subtotal colectomy is occasionally required for patients with fulminant colitis, attenuated familial adenomatous polyposis, or synchronous colon carcinomas. In this procedure, the ileocolic vessels, right colic vessels, middle colic vessels, and left colic vessels are ligated and divided. The superior rectal vessels are preserved. If it is desired to preserve the sigmoid, the distal sigmoid vessels are left intact and an

anastomosis is created between the ileum and distal sigmoid colon (subtotal colectomy with ileosigmoid anastomosis). If the sigmoid is to be resected, the sigmoidal vessels are ligated and divided, and the ileum is anastomosed to the upper rectum (total abdominal colectomy with ileorectal anastomosis). If an anastomosis is contraindicated, an end-ileostomy is created and the remaining sigmoid or rectum is managed either as a mucus fistula or a Hartmann pouch.

Proctocolectomy

Total Proctocolectomy. In this procedure, the entire colon, rectum, and anus are removed and the ileum is brought to the skin either as a Brooke ileostomy or a continent (Kock pouch) ileostomy.

Restorative Proctocolectomy (Ileal Pouch Anal Anastomosis). The entire colon and rectum are resected, but the anal sphincter muscles and a variable portion of the distal anal canal are preserved. Bowel continuity is restored by anastomosis of an ileal reservoir to the anal canal. The original technique included a transanal mucosectomy and handsewn ileoanal anastomosis. Proponents of this technique argue that mucosectomy guarantees removal of all of the diseased mucosa, including the anal transition zone, and therefore decreases the risk of ongoing disease, dysplasia, and carcinoma.[13] Opponents site the increased risk of incontinence after mucosectomy and argue that even meticulous technique invariably leaves behind mucosal "islands" that are subsequently hidden under the anastomosis. Moreover, the "double-staple" technique using the circular stapling devices is considerably simpler than mucosectomy and a handsewn anastomosis (Fig. 28-11).[14] Regardless of the anastomotic technique, many surgeons recommend that patients undergo annual surveillance of the anastomosis and/or anal transition zone by digital rectal exam and anoscopy or proctoscopy.

The neorectum is made by anastomosis of the terminal ileum aligned in a "J," "S," or "W" configuration. Because functional outcomes are similar and because the J-pouch is the simplest to construct, it has become the most used configuration. With increasing experience in laparoscopic colectomy, some centers have begun performing total proctocolectomy with ileal pouch anal reconstruction using minimally invasive surgical techniques.[15] Most surgeons perform a proximal ileostomy to divert succus from the newly created pouch in an attempt to minimize the consequences of leak and sepsis, especially in patients who are malnourished or immunosuppressed (Fig. 28-12). The ileostomy is then closed 6 to 12 weeks later, after a contrast study confirms the integrity of the pouch. In low-risk patients, however, there are reports of successful creation of an ileoanal pouch without diverting stoma.[16]

Anterior Resection

Anterior resection is the general term used to describe resection of the rectum from an abdominal approach to the pelvis with no need for a perineal, sacral, or other incision. Three types of anterior resection have been described.

High Anterior Resection. A *high anterior resection* is the term used to describe resection of the distal sigmoid colon and upper rectum and is the appropriate operation for benign lesions and disease at the rectosigmoid junction such as diverticulitis. The upper rectum is mobilized but the pelvic peritoneum is not divided and the rectum is not mobilized fully from the concavity of the sacrum. The inferior mesenteric artery is ligated at its base and the inferior mesenteric vein, which follows a different course than the artery, is ligated separately. A primary anastomosis (usually end-to-end)

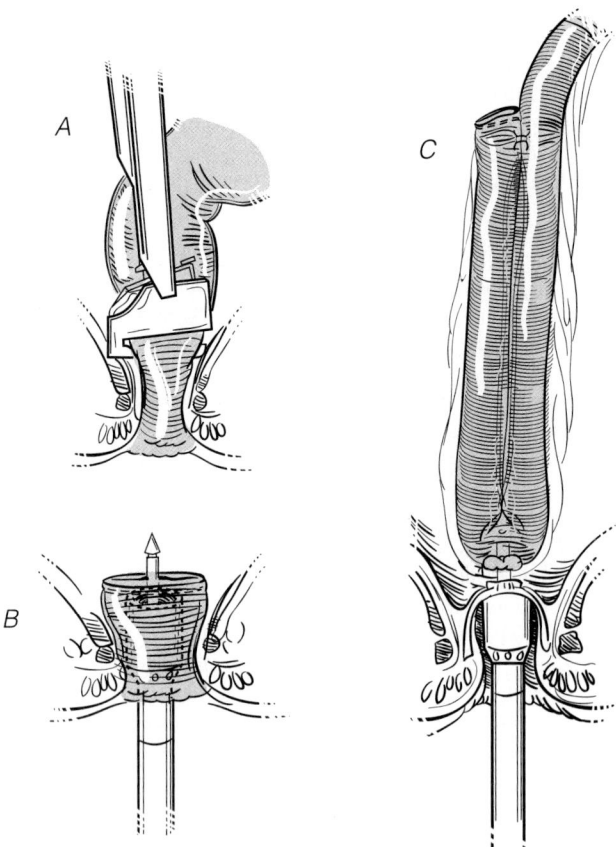

FIG. 28-11. After a total colectomy and resection of the rectum (A), the anal canal with a short cuff of transitional mucosa and sphincter muscles is preserved (B). An ileal J-pouch has been constructed and is anastomosed to the anal canal using a double-staple technique (C). *[Reproduced with permission from Bell RH, Rikkers LF, Mulholland M (eds): Digestive Tract Surgery: A Text and Atlas. Philadelphia: Lippincott Williams & Wilkins, 1996, p 1527.]*

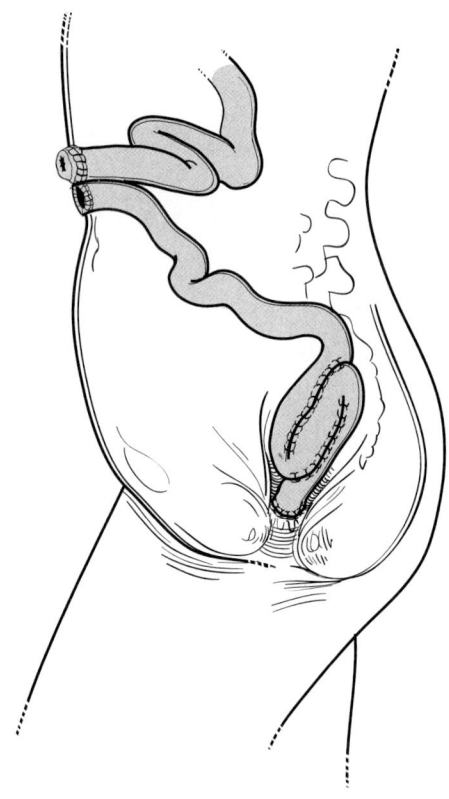

FIG. 28-12. Ileal S-pouch anal anastomosis with temporary loop ileostomy. *[Reproduced with permission from Bell RH, Rikkers LF, Mulholland M (eds): Digestive Tract Surgery: A Text and Atlas. Philadelphia: Lippincott Williams & Wilkins, 1996, p 1533.]*

between the colon and rectal stump with a short cuff of peritoneum surrounding its anterior two thirds can generally be performed.

Low Anterior Resection. A *low anterior resection* is used to remove lesions in the upper and mid rectum. The rectosigmoid is mobilized, the pelvic peritoneum is opened, and the inferior mesenteric artery is ligated and divided either at its origin from the aorta or just distal to the takeoff of the left colic artery. The rectum is mobilized from the sacrum by sharp dissection under direct view within the endopelvic fascial plane. The dissection may be performed distally to the anorectal ring, extending posteriorly through the rectosacral fascia to the coccyx and anteriorly through Denonvilliers' fascia to the vagina in women or the seminal vesicles and prostate in men. The rectum and accompanying mesorectum are divided at the appropriate level, depending upon the nature of the lesion. A low rectal anastomosis usually requires mobilization of the splenic flexure and ligation and division of the inferior mesenteric vein just inferior to the pancreas. Circular stapling devices have greatly facilitated the conduct and improved the safety of the colon to extraperitoneal rectal anastomosis.

Extended Low Anterior Resection. An *extended low anterior resection* is necessary to remove lesions located in the distal rectum, but several centimeters above the sphincter. The rectum is fully mobilized to the level of the levator ani muscle just as for a low

anterior resection, but the anterior dissection is extended along the rectovaginal septum in women and distal to the seminal vesicles and prostate in men. After resection at this level, a *coloanal anastomosis* can be created using one of a variety of techniques described below. Because the risk of an anastomotic leak and subsequent sepsis is higher when an anastomosis is created in the distal rectum or anal canal, creation of a temporary ileostomy should be considered in this setting.

Although an anastomosis may be technically feasible very low in the rectum or anal canal, it is important to note that postoperative function may be poor. Because the descending colon lacks the distensibility of the colon, the reservoir function may be compromised. Pelvic radiation, prior anorectal surgery, and obstetrical trauma may cause unsuspected sphincter damage. Finally, a very low anastomosis may involve and compromise the upper sphincter. Creation of a *colon J-pouch* or *coloplasty* may improve function.[17] A history of sphincter damage or any degree of incontinence is a relative contraindication for a coloanal anastomosis. In such patients, an end-colostomy may be a more satisfactory option.

Hartmann's Procedure and Mucus Fistula

Hartmann's procedure refers to a colon or rectal resection without an anastomosis in which a colostomy or ileostomy is created and the distal colon or rectum is left as a blind pouch. The term is typically used when the left or sigmoid colon is resected and the closed off rectum is left in the pelvis. If the distal colon is long enough to reach the abdominal wall, a *mucus fistula* can be created by opening the defunctioned bowel and suturing it to the skin.

Abdominoperineal Resection

An abdominoperineal resection involves removal of the entire rectum, anal canal, and anus with construction of a permanent colostomy from the descending or sigmoid colon. The abdominal–pelvic portion of this operation proceeds in the same fashion as described for an extended low anterior resection. The perineal dissection can be performed with the patient in lithotomy position (often by a second surgeon) or in the prone position after closure of the abdomen and creation of the colostomy. For cancer, the perineal dissection is designed to excise the anal canal with a wide circumferential margin. Primary wound closure is usually successful but the large perineal defect, especially if radiation has been used, may require flap closure in some patients. For benign disease, proctectomy may be performed using an *intersphincteric dissection* between the internal and external sphincters. This approach minimizes the perineal wound that is easier to close because the levator muscle remains intact.

Anastomoses

Anastomoses may be created between two segments of bowel in a multitude of ways. The geometry of the anastomosis may be *end-to-end, end-to-side, side-to-end,* or *side-to-side.* The anastomotic technique may be *handsewn (single* or *double layer)* or *stapled* (Fig. 28-13). The submucosal layer of the intestine provides the

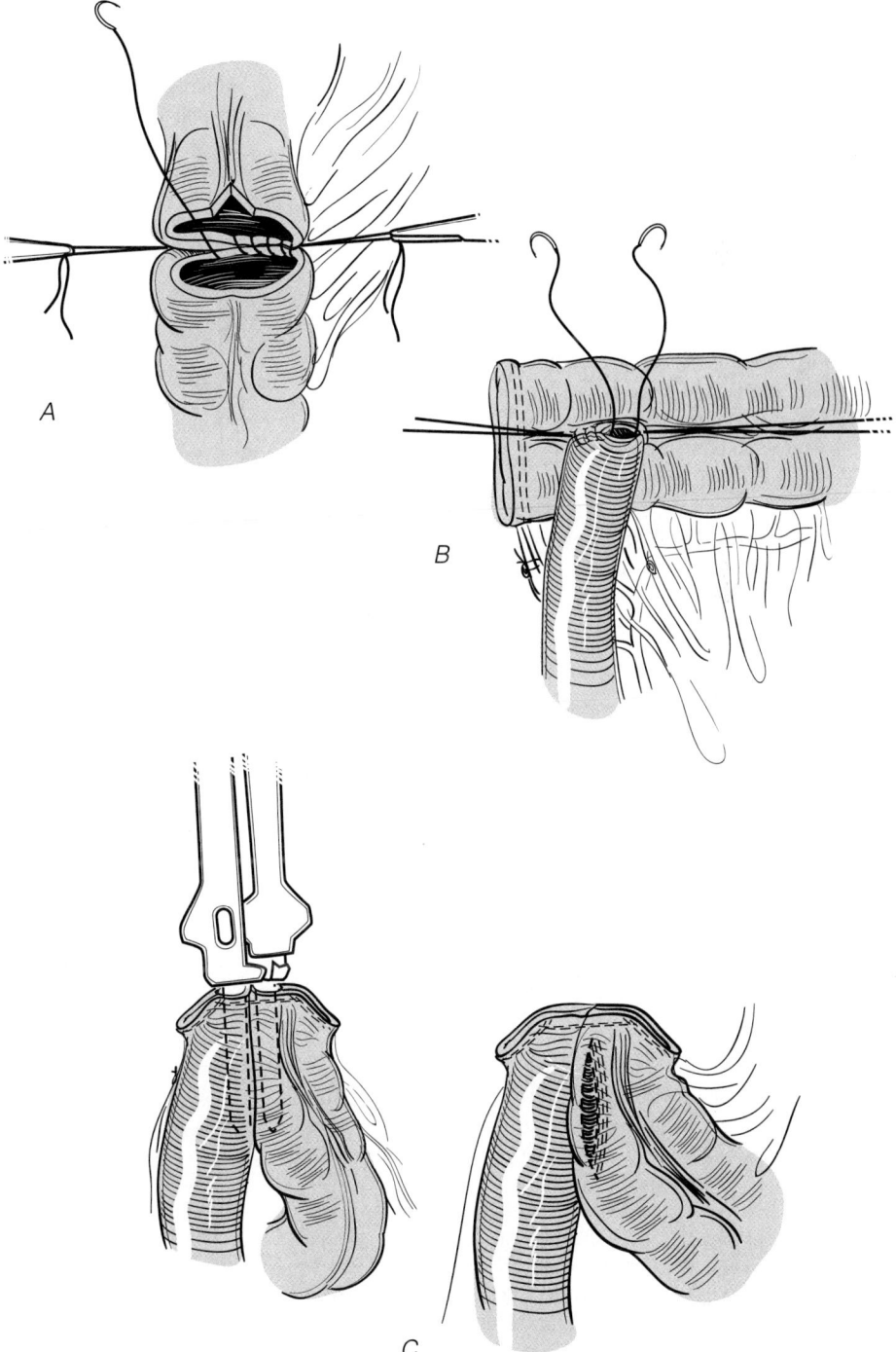

FIG. 28-13. *A.* Sutured end-to-end colocolic anastomosis. *B.* Sutured end-to-side ileocolic anastomosis. *C.* Stapled side-to-side, functional end-to-end ileocolic anastomosis. [*Reproduced with permission from Bell RH, Rikkers LF, Mulholland M (eds): Digestive Tract Surgery: A Text and Atlas. Philadelphia: Lippincott Williams & Wilkins, 1996, pp 1473, 1475, and 1479.*]

strength of the bowel wall and must be incorporated in the anastomosis to assure healing. The choice of anastomosis depends upon the operative anatomy and surgeon preference. Although many surgeons advocate one method over another, none has been proven to be superior. Accurate approximation of two well-vascularized, healthy limbs of bowel without tension in a normotensive, well-nourished patient almost always results in a good outcome. Anastomoses at highest risk of leak or stricture are those that are in the distal rectal or anal canal, involve irradiated or diseased intestine, or are performed in malnourished, ill patients.

Anastomotic Configuration

End-to-End. An end-to-end anastomosis can be performed when two segments of bowel are roughly the same caliber. This technique is most often employed in rectal resections, but may be used for colocolostomy or small bowel anastomoses.

End-to-Side. An end-to-side configuration is useful when one limb of bowel is larger than the other. This most commonly occurs in the setting of chronic obstruction.

Side-to-End. A side-to-end anastomosis is used when the proximal bowel is of smaller caliber than the distal bowel. Ileorectal anastomoses commonly make use of this configuration. A side-to-end anastomosis may have a less tenuous blood supply than an end-to-end anastomosis.

Side-to-Side. A side-to-side anastomosis allows a large, well-vascularized connection to be created on the antimesenteric side of two segments of intestine. This technique is commonly used in ileocolic and small bowel anastomoses.

Anastomotic Technique

Hand-Sutured Technique. Any of the configurations described above may be created using a hand-sutured or stapled technique. Hand-sutured anastomoses may be *single layer,* using either running or interrupted stitches, or *double layer.* A double-layer anastomosis usually consists of a continuous inner layer and an interrupted outer layer. Suture material may be either permanent or absorbable. After distal rectal or anal canal resection, a transanal, handsewn coloanal anastomosis may be necessary to restore bowel continuity. This can be done in conjunction with an anal canal mucosectomy to allow the anastomosis to be at the dentate line.

Stapled Techniques. Linear cutter stapling devices are used to divide the bowel and to create side-to-side anastomoses. The anastomosis may be reinforced with interrupted sutures if desired. Circular stapling devices can create end-to-end, end-to-side, or side-to-end anastomoses. These instruments are particularly useful for creating low rectal or anal canal anastomoses where the anatomy of the pelvis makes a handsewn anastomosis technically difficult or impossible.

Following resection of the colorectum, a stapled end-to-end colorectal, coloanal canal, or ileal pouch anal canal anastomosis may be created by one of two techniques. With the *open pursestring technique,* the distal rectal stump pursestring is placed by hand and the assembled circular stapler is inserted into the anus and guided up to the rectal pursestring. The stapler is opened and the distal pursestring is tied. A pursestring is placed in the distal end of the proximal colon; the proximal colon is placed over the anvil and the pursestring tightened. The stapler is closed and fired (Fig. 28-14). With the alternative *double-staple technique,* the distal rectum or anal canal is closed with a transverse staple line. The circular stapler is

inserted through the anus without its anvil until the cartridge effaces the transverse staple line. The stapler is opened, causing the trocar to perforate through the rectal stump adjacent to the transverse staple line. A pursestring is placed in the distal end of the proximal colon or the end of the ileal pouch. The stapler anvil is inserted into the proximal colon or ileal pouch and the pursestring is tightened around the anvil. The anvil is mated to the trocar and the stapler closed and fired (see Fig. 28-11). After firing and removing the stapler, the resulting anastomotic rings should be inspected to ensure that they are intact. A gap in an anastomotic ring suggests that the circular staple line is incomplete and the anastomosis should be reinforced with suture circumferentially, if technically feasible. A temporary proximal ileostomy may be indicated as well.

Ostomies

Depending upon the clinical situation, a stoma may be temporary or permanent. It may be end-on or a loop. However, regardless of the indication for a stoma, placement and construction are crucial for function. A stoma should be located within the rectus muscle to minimize the risk of a postoperative parastomal hernia. It should also be placed where the patient can see it and easily manipulate the appliance. The surrounding abdominal soft tissue should be as flat as possible to ensure a tight seal and prevent leakage. Preoperative evaluation by an enterostomal therapy nurse to identify the ideal stoma site and to counsel and educate the patient is invaluable (Fig. 28-15).

For all stomas, a circular skin incision is created and the subcutaneous tissue dissected to the level of the anterior rectus sheath. The anterior rectus sheath is incised in a cruciate fashion, the muscle fibers separated bluntly, and the posterior sheath identified and incised. The size of the defect depends upon the size of the bowel used to create the stoma, but should be as small as possible without compromising the intestinal blood supply (usually the width of two to three fingers). The bowel is then brought through the defect and secured. The abdominal incision is usually closed and dressed prior to maturing the stoma to avoid contaminating the wound. In order to make appliance use easier, a protruding nipple is fashioned by everting the bowel. Three or four interrupted absorbable sutures are placed through the edge of the bowel, then through the serosa, approximately 2 cm proximal to the edge, and then through the dermis (Brooke technique). After the stoma is everted, the mucocutaneous junction is sutured circumferentially with interrupted absorbable suture (Fig. 28-16).

Ileostomy

Temporary Ileostomy. A temporary ileostomy is often used to "protect" an anastomosis that is at risk for leakage (low in the rectum, in an irradiated field, in an immunocompromised or malnourished patient, and in some emergency operations). In this setting, the stoma is often constructed as a *loop ileostomy* (see Fig. 28-12). A segment of distal ileum is brought through the defect in the abdominal wall as a loop. An enterotomy is created and the stoma matured as described above. The loop may be secured with or without an underlying rod. A *divided loop* may also be created by firing a linear cutter stapler across the distal limb of the loop flush with the skin followed by maturation of the proximal limb of the loop. This technique prevents incomplete diversion that occasionally occurs with a loop ileostomy.

The advantage of a loop or divided loop ileostomy is that subsequent closure can often be accomplished without a formal laparotomy. An elliptical incision is created around the stoma and the

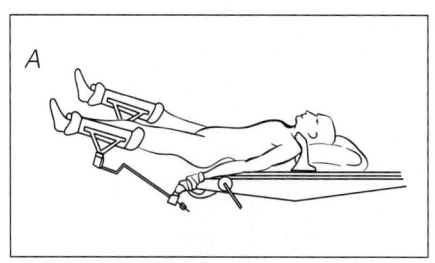

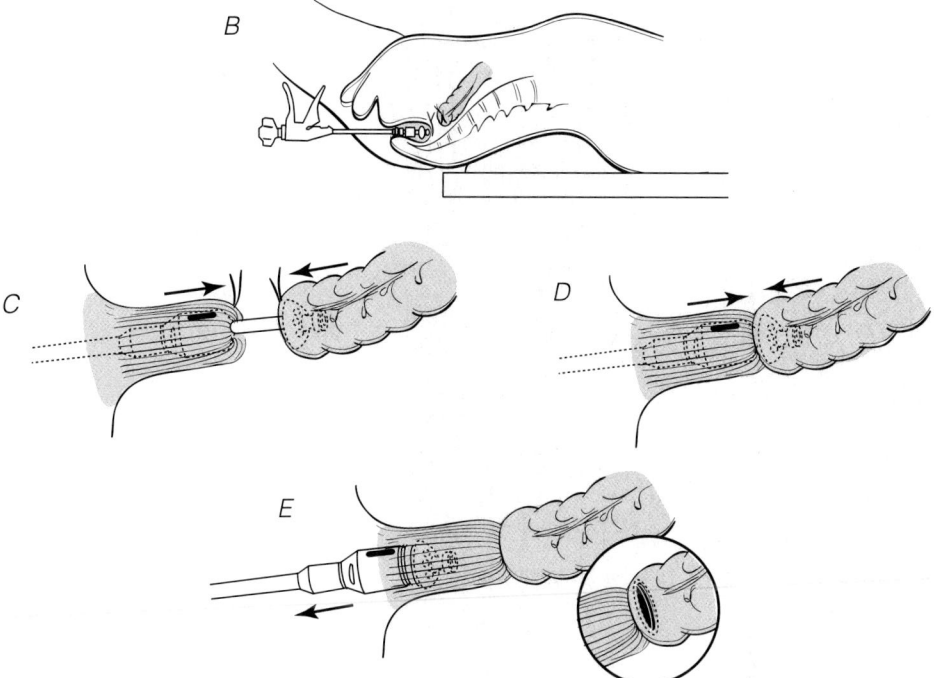

FIG. 28-14. Technique of end-to-end colorectal anastomosis using a circular stapler. *A.* The patient is in modified lithotomy position. *B.* After resection of the rectosigmoid and placement of pursestring sutures proximally and distally, the stapler is inserted into the anal canal and opened. *C.* Rectal pursestring suture is tied to secure the rectal stump to the rod of the stapler and the colonic pursestring is tied to secure the colon to the anvil of the stapler. *D.* The stapler is closed and fired. *E.* The stapler is removed leaving a circular stapled end-to-end anastomosis. [*Reproduced with permission from Schwartz SI, Shires GT, Spencer FC (eds): Principles of Surgery. 5th ed. New York: McGraw-Hill, 1989, p 1286.*]

bowel gently dissected free of the subcutaneous tissues and fascia. A handsewn or stapled anastomosis can then be created and the intestine returned to the peritoneal cavity. This avoids a long laparotomy incision and is generally well tolerated.

Permanent Ileostomy. A permanent ileostomy is sometimes required after total proctocolectomy or in patients with obstruction. An *end ileostomy* is the preferred configuration for a permanent ileostomy because a symmetric protruding nipple can be fashioned more easily than with a loop ileostomy (see Fig. 28-16). The end of the small intestine is brought through the abdominal wall defect and matured. Stitches are often used to secure the bowel to the posterior fascia. An alternative to the Brooke end ileostomy is the continent ileostomy described by Kock. An internal ileal reservoir stores effluent, and a nipple valve constructed of ileum maintains continence. The stoma is constructed flush with the skin in the lower abdomen and is intubated four to eight times per day to empty the reservoir.

Complications of Ileostomy. Stoma necrosis may occur in the early postoperative period and is usually caused by skeletonizing the distal small bowel and/or creating an overly tight fascial defect. Limited mucosal necrosis above the fascia may be treated expectantly, but necrosis below the level of the fascia requires surgical revision. Stoma retraction may occur early or late, and may

be exacerbated by obesity. Local revision may be necessary. The creation of an ileostomy bypasses the fluid-absorbing capability of the colon, and dehydration with fluid and electrolyte abnormalities is not uncommon. Ideally, ileostomy output should be maintained at less than 1500 mL/d to avoid this problem. Bulk agents and opioids (Lomotil, Imodium, tincture of opium) are useful. Skin irritation can also occur, especially if the stoma appliance fits poorly. Skin-protecting agents and custom pouches can help to solve this problem. Obstruction may occur intra-abdominally or at the site where the stoma exits the fascia. Parastomal hernia is less common after an ileostomy than after a colostomy, but can cause poor appliance fitting, pain, obstruction, or strangulation. In general, symptomatic parastomal hernias should be repaired. Repair usually requires resiting the stoma to the contralateral side of the abdomen. Prolapse is a rare, late complication and is often associated with a parastomal hernia. Valve slippage resulting in either leakage or obstruction is a common complication of a continent Kock pouch ileostomy.

Colostomy

Most colostomies are created as *end colostomies* rather than *loop colostomies* (Fig. 28-17). The bulkiness of the colon makes a loop colostomy awkward for an appliance, and prolapse is more likely with this configuration. Most colostomies are created on the left side of the colon. An abdominal wall defect is created and the end of the colon mobilized through it. Because a protruding stoma is

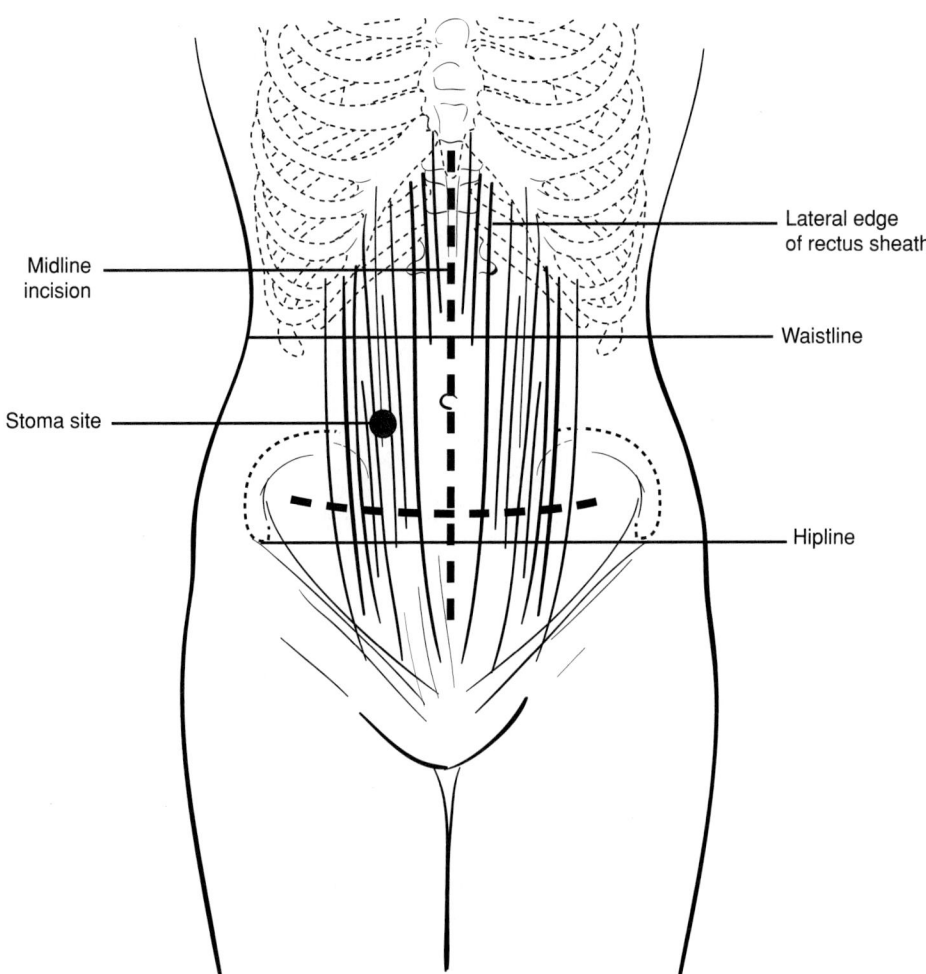

Midline incision

Lateral edge of rectus sheath

Waistline

Stoma site

Hipline

FIG. 28-15. Marking of an ideal site for ileostomy. [*Reproduced with permission from Bell RH, Rikkers LF, Mulholland M (eds): Digestive Tract Surgery: A Text and Atlas. Philadelphia: Lippincott Williams & Wilkins, 1996, p 1273.*]

considerably easier to pouch, colostomies should also be matured in a Brooke fashion. The distal bowel may be brought through the abdominal wall as a *mucus fistula* or left intra-abdominally as a *Hartmann's pouch*. Tacking the distal end of the colon to the abdominal wall or tagging it with permanent suture can make identification of the stump easier if the colostomy is closed at a later date. Closure of a colostomy usually requires laparotomy. The stoma is dissected free of the abdominal wall and the distal bowel identified. An end-to-end anastomosis is then created.

Complications of Colostomy. *Colostomy necrosis* may occur in the early postoperative period and results from an impaired vascular supply (skeletonization of the distal colon or a tight fascial defect). Like ileostomy necrosis, limited suprafascial necrosis may be followed expectantly, but necrosis below the fascia requires surgery. *Retraction* may also occur, but is less problematic with a colostomy than with an ileostomy because the stool is less irritating to the skin than *succus entericus*. *Obstruction* is unusual, but may also occur. *Parastomal hernia* is the most common late complication of a colostomy and requires repair if it is symptomatic. *Prolapse* occurs rarely. Dehydration is rare after colostomy and skin irritation is less common than with ileostomy.

Functional Results

Function following segmental colonic resection and primary anastomosis is generally excellent. A small percentage of patients

following subtotal or total colectomy and ileosigmoid or ileorectal anastomosis may experience diarrhea and bowel frequency. This is especially true if the patient is elderly, if significant length of small bowel has been resected, and if residual proctocolitis is poorly controlled. In general, the more distal the anastomosis, the more the risk of troublesome diarrhea and frequency.

Function following anterior resection is highly dependent on the level of anastomosis, the use of pre- or postoperative pelvic radiation, and underlying sphincter function. Following low anterior or extended low anterior resection, some surgeons prefer to do a coloplasty or construct a short (8 to 10 cm) colo-J-pouch to anastomose to the distal rectum or anal canal. The reservoir lessens urgency, frequency, and incontinence, but some patients have difficulty initiating defecation after construction of a colo-pouch.[17]

The physical and psychologic problems associated with a permanent Brooke ileostomy led to development of the continent Kock pouch ileostomy. Unfortunately, complications, especially complications related to valve slippage, are common. Despite variations of technique designed to improve the function of the continent ileostomy, most surgeons have abandoned this operation and instead perform restorative proctocolectomy with ileal pouch anal anastomosis.

Although ileal pouch anal reconstruction is anatomically appealing, functional outcome is far from perfect.[18,19] Patients should be counseled to expect eight to 10 bowel movements per day. Up to 50% have some degree of nocturnal incontinence. Pouchitis occurs in

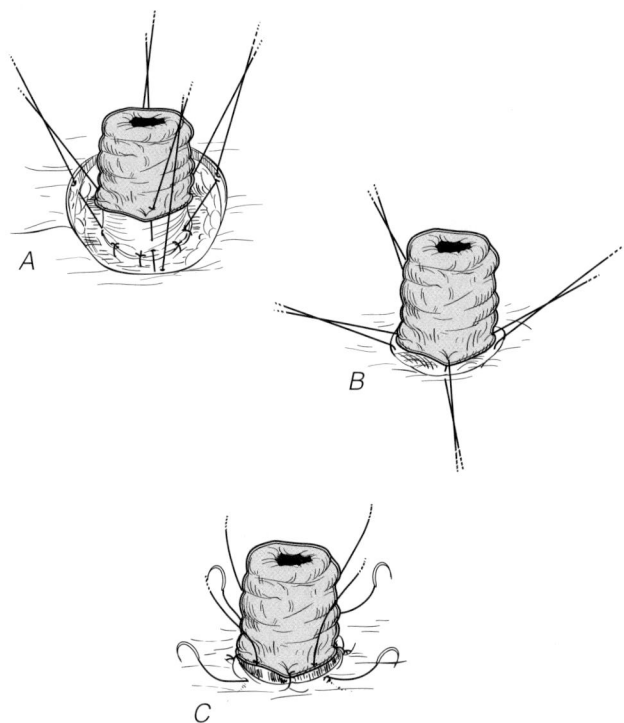

FIG. 28-16. Brooke ileostomy. *A.* Four sutures incorporating the cut end of the ileum, the seromuscular layer at the level of the anterior rectus fascia, and the subcuticular edge of the skin are placed at 90 degrees to each other. *B.* The sutures are tied to produce stomal eversion and (*C*) simple sutures from the cut edge of the bowel to the subcuticular tissue complete the maturation of the ileostomy. [*Reproduced with permission from Bell RH, Rikkers LF, Mulholland M (eds): Digestive Tract Surgery: A Text and Atlas. Philadelphia: Lippincott Williams & Wilkins, 1996, p 1278.*]

FIG. 28-17. Intraperitoneal end colostomy. [*Reproduced with permission from Schwartz SI, Shires GT, Spencer FC (eds): Principles of Surgery. 5th ed. New York: McGraw-Hill, 1989, p 1284.*]

nearly 50% of patients, and small-bowel obstruction is not uncommon. Other less common complications include difficulties with pouch evacuation, pouch–anal and/or pouch–vaginal fistula, and anal stricture. Pouch failure rate averages 5 to 10%. Patients who are subsequently diagnosed with Crohn's disease have a considerably higher pouch failure rate (approximately 50%), while patients with indeterminate colitis have an intermediate pouch failure rate (15 to 20%). Despite these drawbacks, the vast majority of patients are satisfied and prefer ileal pouch–anal reconstruction to permanent ileostomy.

Pouchitis is an inflammatory condition that affects both ileoanal pouches and continent ileostomy reservoirs. Incidence of pouchitis ranges from 30 to 55%. Symptoms include increased diarrhea, hematochezia, abdominal pain, fever, and malaise. Diagnosis is made endoscopically with biopsies. Differential diagnosis includes infection and undiagnosed Crohn's disease. The etiology of pouchitis is unknown. Some believe pouchitis results from fecal stasis within the pouch but emptying studies are not confirmatory. Antibiotics (metronidazole ± ciprofloxacin) are the mainstays of therapy and most patients will respond rapidly to either oral preparations or enemas.[20,21] Some patients develop chronic pouchitis that necessitates ongoing suppressive antibiotic therapy. Salicylate and corticosteroid enemas have also been used with some success. Reintroduction of normal flora by ingestion of *probiotics* has been suggested as a possible treatment in refractory cases. Occasionally, pouch excision is necessary to control the symptoms of chronic pouchitis.

Anesthesia Considerations

Local Anesthesia

Many anorectal procedures can be performed with local anesthetic alone. Intravenous sedation is often provided to calm the patient. Injection of 0.5% lidocaine (short acting) and 0.25% bupivacaine (long acting) into the perianal skin, sphincter, and area around the pudendal nerves usually provides an adequate block. The addition of dilute epinephrine decreases bleeding and prolongs the anesthetic effect.

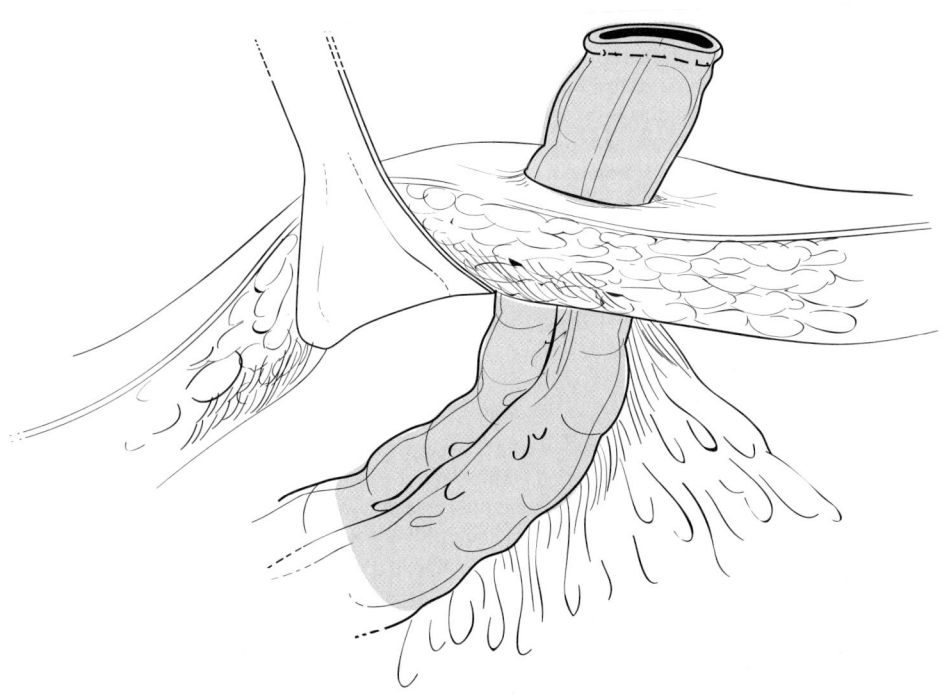

Regional Anesthesia

Epidural, spinal, and caudal anesthetics can be used for anorectal procedures and transanal resections. In patients with severe medical comorbidity, regional anesthesia may occasionally be used for laparotomy and colectomy. Postoperative epidural anesthesia provides excellent pain relief and improves pulmonary function.

General Anesthesia

General anesthesia is required for the vast majority of intra-abdominal procedures. Patients should undergo a thorough preoperative cardiovascular evaluation. In patients with significant comorbid disease, preadmission and an anesthesia consultation may be appropriate.

Positioning

Most abdominal colectomies can be performed in the supine position. Anterior and abdominoperineal resections require lithotomy positioning. Adequate padding should be provided for the patient's sacrum and care should be taken to avoid stirrup pressure on the peroneal nerves.

Anorectal procedures may be performed in lithotomy but the prone jackknife position is preferred for most procedures, especially if the anterior quadrant needs to be seen well. Distal posterior lesions can usually be accessed from either position, but more proximal posterior lesions are better accessed in prone position.

Operative Preliminaries

Bowel Preparation

The rationale for bowel preparation is that decreasing the bacterial load in the colon and rectum will decrease the incidence of postoperative infection. *Mechanical bowel preparation* uses cathartics to rid the colon of solid stool the night before surgery.[22,23] The most commonly used regimens include polyethylene glycol (PEG) solutions or sodium phosphate. PEG solutions require patients to drink a large volume and may cause bloating and nausea. Sodium phosphate solutions are generally better tolerated, but are more likely to cause fluid and electrolyte abnormalities. PEG and sodium phosphate are equally efficacious in bowel cleansing. *Antibiotic prophylaxis* also is recommended. The addition of oral antibiotics to the preoperative mechanical bowel preparation is thought to decrease postoperative infection by further decreasing the bacterial load of the colon. A combination of three doses of neomycin (1g) and erythromycin base (1g) is most commonly used. Some surgeons substitute metronidazole (500 mg) for erythromycin to avoid gastrointestinal upset. Ciprofloxacin has also been used in this setting. A broad-spectrum parenteral antibiotic(s) should be administered just prior to the skin incision. There is no proven benefit to using antibiotics postoperatively after an uncomplicated colectomy.

Stoma Planning

The preoperative preparation of a patient who is expected to require a stoma should include a consultation with an *enterostomal therapy (ET) nurse.* ET nurses are specially trained and credentialed by the Wound, Ostomy, and Continence Nurses Society. Preoperative planning includes counseling, education, and stoma siting. Postoperatively, the ET nurse assists with local skin care and pouching. Other considerations in stoma planning include evaluation of other medical conditions that may impact on a patient's ability to manage a stoma (e.g., eyesight, manual dexterity).

Preoperative stoma siting is crucial for a patient's postoperative function and quality of life. A poorly placed stoma can result in leakage and skin breakdown. Ideally, a stoma should be placed in a location that the patient can easily see and manipulate, within the rectus muscle, and below the belt line (see Fig. 28-15). Because the abdominal landmarks in a supine, anesthetized patient may be dramatically different from those in an awake, standing, or sitting patient, the stoma site should always be marked with a tattoo, skin scratch, or permanent marker preoperatively, if possible. In an emergency operation where the stoma site has not been marked, an attempt should be made to place a stoma within the rectus muscle and away from both the costal margin and iliac crest. In emergencies, placement high on the abdominal wall is preferred to a low-lying site.

Ureteral Stents

Ureteral stents may be useful for identifying the ureters intraoperatively and are placed via cystoscopy after the induction of general anesthesia and removed at the end of the operation. Stents can be invaluable in reoperative pelvic surgery or when there is significant retroperitoneal inflammation (such as complicated diverticulitis). Lighted stents may be helpful in laparoscopic resections. Patients often have transient hematuria postoperatively but major complications are rare.

Multidisciplinary Teams

Patients with complex colorectal disease often benefit from a multidisciplinary approach. Patients with pelvic floor disorders (especially incontinence) often require evaluation by both a colorectal surgeon and a urologist or urogynecologist. Preoperative evaluation of cancer patients by a medical oncologist and/or radiation oncologist is crucial for planning either neoadjuvant or adjuvant therapy. Intraoperatively, complex pelvic resections often require the involvement of not only a colorectal surgeon but also a urologist, gynecologic oncologist, neurosurgeon, and/or plastic surgeon. Radiation oncologists should be involved in the operation if brachytherapy catheters are to be placed for intracavitary radiation or if intraoperative radiation therapy is planned. Rarely, psychiatric disorders may manifest as colorectal problems (especially functional disorders and chronic pain) and involvement of a psychiatrist or psychologist may be beneficial.

INFLAMMATORY BOWEL DISEASE

General Considerations

Epidemiology

Inflammatory bowel disease includes *ulcerative colitis, Crohn's disease,* and *indeterminate colitis. Ulcerative colitis* occurs in 8 to 15 people per 100,000 in the United States and Northern Europe. The incidence is considerably lower in Asia, Africa, and South America, and among the nonwhite population in the United States. Ulcerative colitis incidence peaks during the third decade of life and again in the seventh decade of life. The incidence of Crohn's disease is slightly lower, 1 to 5 people per 100,000 population. Crohn's disease also affects Northern European and white populations disproportionately. Crohn's disease has a similar bimodal incidence, with most cases occurring between ages 15 to 30 years and ages 55 to 60 years. In 15% of patients with inflammatory bowel disease, differentiation between ulcerative colitis and Crohn's colitis is impossible; these patients are classified as having *indeterminate colitis.*

Etiology

Multiple etiologies for inflammatory bowel disease have been proposed, but none are proven. The consistent geographic differences in incidence suggest an environmental factor such as diet or infection. Smoking, alcohol, and oral contraceptive use have also been implicated. Family history may play a role because 10 to 30% of patients with inflammatory bowel disease report a family member with the same disease.[24] Other theories focus upon an autoimmune mechanism and/or a defect in the intestinal immune system.

Most mechanistic explanations for inflammatory bowel disease focus upon *infectious* or *immunologic* causes. Bacteria such as *Mycobacterium paratuberculosis* and *Listeria monocytogenes,* and viruses such as paramyxovirus and measles virus, have been suggested as etiologic agents in Crohn's disease. A defect in the gut mucosal barrier, which increases exposure to intraluminal bacteria, toxins, or proinflammatory substances, also has been suggested. Finally, an autoimmune mechanism has been postulated. Although there is no clear evidence linking an immunologic disorder to inflammatory bowel disease, the similarity of many of the extraintestinal manifestations to rheumatologic disorders has made this theory attractive. Regardless of the underlying cause of either ulcerative colitis or Crohn's disease, both disorders are characterized by intestinal inflammation and medical therapy is largely based upon reducing inflammation.

Pathology and Differential Diagnosis

Although ulcerative colitis and Crohn's colitis share many pathologic and clinical similarities, these conditions may be differentiated in 85% of patients. Ulcerative colitis is a mucosal process in which the colonic mucosa and submucosa are infiltrated with inflammatory cells. The mucosa may be atrophic and crypt abscesses are common. Endoscopically, the mucosa is frequently friable and may possess multiple inflammatory pseudopolyps. In long-standing ulcerative colitis, the colon may be foreshortened and the mucosa replaced by scar. In quiescent ulcerative colitis, the colonic mucosa may appear normal both endoscopically and microscopically. Ulcerative colitis may affect the rectum (proctitis), rectum and sigmoid colon (proctosigmoiditis), rectum and left colon (left-sided colitis), or the rectum and entire colon (pancolitis). Ulcerative colitis does not involve the small intestine, but the terminal ileum may demonstrate inflammatory changes ("backwash ileitis"). A key feature of ulcerative colitis is the continuous involvement of the rectum and colon; rectal sparing or skip lesions suggests a diagnosis of Crohn's disease. Symptoms are related to the degree of mucosal inflammation and the extent of colitis. Patients typically complain of bloody diarrhea and crampy abdominal pain. Proctitis may produce tenesmus. Severe abdominal pain and fever raises the concern of *fulminant colitis* or *toxic megacolon.* Physical findings are nonspecific and range from minimal abdominal tenderness and distention to frank peritonitis. In the nonemergent setting, the diagnosis is typically made by colonoscopy and mucosal biopsy.

In contrast to ulcerative colitis, Crohn's disease is a transmural inflammatory process that can affect any part of the gastrointestinal tract from mouth to anus. Mucosal ulcerations, an inflammatory cell infiltrate, and noncaseating granulomas are characteristic pathologic findings. Chronic inflammation may ultimately result in fibrosis, strictures, and fistulas in either the colon or small intestine. The endoscopic appearance of Crohn's colitis is characterized by deep serpiginous ulcers and a "cobblestone" appearance. Skip lesions and rectal sparing are common. Symptoms of Crohn's disease depend upon the severity of inflammation and/or fibrosis and the location

of inflammation in the gastrointestinal tract. Acute inflammation may produce diarrhea, crampy abdominal pain, and fever. Strictures may produce symptoms of obstruction. Weight loss is common, both because of obstruction and from protein loss. Perianal Crohn's disease may present with pain, swelling, and drainage from fistulas or abscesses. Physical findings are also related to the site and severity of disease.

In 15% of patients with colitis from inflammatory bowel disease, differentiation of ulcerative colitis from Crohn's colitis proves impossible either grossly or microscopically (indeterminate colitis). These patients typically present with symptoms similar to ulcerative colitis. Endoscopic and pathologic findings usually include features common to both diseases.

Further differential diagnoses include infectious colitides, especially *Campylobacter jejuni, Entamoeba histolytica, C. difficile, Neisseria gonococcus, Salmonella,* and *Shigella* species.

Extraintestinal Manifestations

The liver is a common site of extracolonic disease in inflammatory bowel disease. Fatty infiltration of the liver is present in 40 to 50% of patients and cirrhosis is found in 2 to 5%. Fatty infiltration may be reversed by medical or surgical treatment of colonic disease, but cirrhosis is irreversible. Primary sclerosing cholangitis is a progressive disease characterized by intra- and extrahepatic bile duct strictures. Forty to 60% of patients with primary sclerosing cholangitis have ulcerative colitis. Colectomy will not reverse this disease and the only effective therapy is liver transplantation.[25] Pericholangitis is also associated with inflammatory bowel disease and may be diagnosed with a liver biopsy. Bile duct carcinoma is a rare complication of long-standing inflammatory bowel disease. Patients who develop bile duct carcinoma in the presence of inflammatory bowel disease are, on average, 20 years younger than other patients with bile duct carcinoma.

Arthritis is also a common extracolonic manifestation of inflammatory bowel disease, and the incidence is 20 times greater than in the general population. Arthritis usually improves with treatment of the colonic disease. Sacroiliitis and ankylosing spondylitis are associated with inflammatory bowel disease, although the relationship is poorly understood. Medical and surgical treatment of the colonic disease does not impact symptoms.

Erythema nodosum is seen in 5 to 15% of patients with inflammatory bowel disease and usually coincides with clinical disease activity. Women are affected three to four times more frequently than men. The characteristic lesions are raised, red, and predominantly on the lower legs. Pyoderma gangrenosum is an uncommon but serious condition that occurs almost exclusively in patients with inflammatory bowel disease. The lesion begins as an erythematous plaque, papule, or bleb, usually located on the pretibial region of the leg and occasionally near a stoma. The lesions progress and ulcerate, leading to a painful, necrotic wound. Pyoderma gangrenosum may respond to resection of the affected bowel in some patients. In others, this disorder is unaffected by treatment of the underlying bowel disease.

Up to 10% of patients with inflammatory bowel disease will develop ocular lesions. These include uveitis, iritis, episcleritis, and conjunctivitis. They usually develop during an acute exacerbation of the inflammatory bowel disease. The etiology is unknown.

Principles of Nonoperative Management

Medical therapy for inflammatory bowel disease focuses upon decreasing inflammation and alleviating symptoms, and many of the agents used are the same for both ulcerative colitis and Crohn's disease. In general, mild to moderate flares may be treated in the outpatient setting. More severe signs and symptoms mandate hospitalization. Pancolitis generally requires more aggressive therapy than limited disease. Because ulcerative proctitis and proctosigmoiditis are limited to the distal large intestine, topical therapy with salicylate and/or corticosteroid suppositories and enemas can be extremely effective. Systemic therapy is rarely required in these patients.

Salicylates. Sulfasalazine (Azulfidine), 5-ASA, and related compounds are first-line agents in the medical treatment of mild to moderate inflammatory bowel disease. These compounds decrease inflammation by inhibition of cyclooxygenase and 5-lipoxygenase in the gut mucosa. They require direct contact with affected mucosa for efficacy. Multiple preparations are available for administration to different sites in the small intestine and colon (sulfasalazine, mesalamine [Pentasa], Asacol, Rowasa).

Antibiotics. Antibiotics are often used to decrease the intraluminal bacterial load in Crohn's disease. Metronidazole has been reported to improve Crohn's colitis and perianal disease, but the evidence is weak. Fluoroquinolones may also be effective in some cases. In the absence of fulminant colitis or toxic megacolon, antibiotics are not used to treat ulcerative colitis.

Corticosteroids. Corticosteroids (either oral or parenteral) are a key component of treatment for an acute exacerbation of either ulcerative colitis or Crohn's disease. Corticosteroids are nonspecific inhibitors of the immune system and 75 to 90% of patients will improve with the administration of these drugs. However, corticosteroids have a number of serious side effects and use of these agents should be limited to the shortest course possible. In addition, corticosteroids should be used judiciously in children because of the potential adverse affect on growth. Failure to wean corticosteroids is a relative indication for surgery.

Because of the systemic effects of corticosteroids, an effort has been made to develop drugs that act locally and have limited systemic absorption. Newer agents such as budesonide, beclomethasone dipropionate, and tixocortol pivalate undergo rapid hepatic degradation that significantly decreases systemic toxicity. Budesonide is available as an oral preparation. Corticosteroid enemas provide effective local therapy for proctitis and proctosigmoiditis and have fewer side effects than systemic corticosteroids.

Immunosuppressive Agents. Azathioprine and 6-mercatopurine (6-MP) are antimetabolite drugs that interfere with nucleic acid synthesis and thus decrease proliferation of inflammatory cells. These agents are useful for treating ulcerative colitis and Crohn's disease in patients who have failed salicylate therapy or who are dependent upon or refractory to corticosteroids. It is important to note, however, that the onset of action of these drugs takes 6 to 12 weeks, and concomitant use of corticosteroids is almost always required.[26]

Cyclosporine is an immunosuppressive agent that interferes with T-cell function. While cyclosporine is not routinely used to treat inflammatory bowel disease, up to 80% of patients with an acute flare of ulcerative colitis will improve with its use. However, the majority of these patients will ultimately require colectomy. Cyclosporine is also occasionally used to treat exacerbations of Crohn's disease and approximately two-thirds of patients will note some improvement. Improvement is generally apparent within 2 weeks of beginning cyclosporine therapy. Long-term use of cyclosporine is limited by its significant toxicity.

Methotrexate is a folate antagonist that also has been used to treat inflammatory bowel disease. Although the efficacy of this agent is unproven, there are reports that more than 50% of patients will improve with administration of this drug.[27]

Infliximab (Remicade) is a monoclonal antibody against tumor necrosis factor alpha (TNF-α). Intravenous infusion of this agent deceases inflammation systemically. More than 50% of patients with moderate to severe Crohn's disease will improve with infliximab therapy.[28,29] This agent also has been useful in treating patients with perianal Crohn's disease. Recurrence is common, however, and many patients require infusions on a bimonthly basis. Infliximab has not been used as extensively for treatment of ulcerative colitis; however, there are reports of efficacy in this setting.[30,31]

Nutrition. Patients with inflammatory bowel disease are often malnourished. Abdominal pain and obstructive symptoms may decrease oral intake. Diarrhea can cause significant protein loss. Ongoing inflammation produces a catabolic physiologic state. Parenteral nutrition should be strongly considered early in the course of therapy for either Crohn's disease or ulcerative colitis. The nutritional status of the patient should also be considered when planning operative intervention and nutritional parameters such as serum albumin, prealbumin, and transferrin should be assessed. In extremely malnourished patients, especially those who are also being treated with corticosteroids, creation of a stoma is often safer than a primary anastomosis.

Ulcerative Colitis

Ulcerative colitis is a dynamic disease characterized by remissions and exacerbations. The clinical spectrum ranges from an inactive or quiescent phase to low-grade active disease to fulminant disease. The onset of ulcerative colitis may be insidious, with minimal bloody stools, or the onset can be abrupt, with severe diarrhea and bleeding, tenesmus, abdominal pain, and fever. The severity of symptoms depends upon the degree and extent of inflammation. Although anemia is common, massive hemorrhage is rare. Physical findings are often nonspecific.

Diagnosis of ulcerative colitis is almost always made endoscopically. Because the rectum is invariably involved, proctoscopy may be adequate to establish the diagnosis. The earliest manifestation is mucosal edema, which results in a loss of the normal vascular pattern. In more advanced disease, characteristic findings include mucosal friability and ulceration. Pus and mucus may also be present. While mucosal biopsy is often diagnostic in the chronic phase of ulcerative colitis, biopsy in the acute phase will often reveal only nonspecific inflammation. A complete evaluation with colonoscopy or barium enema during an acute flare is contraindicated because of the risk of perforation.

Barium enema has been used to diagnose ulcerative colitis and to determine the extent of disease. However, this modality is less sensitive than colonoscopy and may not detect early disease. In long-standing ulcerative colitis, the colon is foreshortened and lacks haustral markings ("lead pipe" colon). Because the inflammation in ulcerative colitis is purely mucosal, strictures are highly uncommon. Any stricture diagnosed in a patient with ulcerative colitis must be presumed to be malignant until proven otherwise.

Indications for Surgery

Indications for surgery in ulcerative colitis may be emergent or elective. Emergency surgery is required for patients with massive life-threatening *hemorrhage, toxic megacolon,* or *fulminant colitis* who fail to respond rapidly to medical therapy. Patients with signs and symptoms of fulminant colitis should be treated aggressively with bowel rest, hydration, broad-spectrum antibiotics, and parenteral corticosteroids. Colonoscopy and barium enema are contraindicated and antidiarrheal agents should be avoided. Deterioration in clinical condition or failure to improve within 24 hours mandates surgery.

Indications for elective surgery include intractability despite maximal medical therapy and high-risk development of major complications of medical therapy such as aseptic necrosis of joints secondary to chronic steroid use. Elective surgery is also indicated in patients at significant risk of developing colorectal carcinoma. Risk of malignancy increases with pancolonic disease and the duration of symptoms is approximately 2% after 10 years, 8% after 20 years, and 18% after 30 years. Unlike sporadic colorectal cancers, carcinoma developing in the context of ulcerative colitis is more likely to arise from areas of *flat dysplasia* and may be difficult to diagnose at an early stage. For this reason, it is recommended that patients with long-standing ulcerative colitis undergo colonoscopic surveillance with multiple (40 to 50), random biopsies to identify dysplasia before invasive malignancy develops. Surveillance is recommended annually after 8 years in patients with pancolitis, and annually after 15 years in patients with left-sided colitis. Although low-grade dysplasia was long thought to represent minimal risk, more recent studies show that invasive cancer may be present in up to 20% of patients with low-grade dysplasia. For this reason, any patient with dysplasia should be advised to undergo proctocolectomy. Controversy exists over whether prophylactic proctocolectomy should be recommended for patients who have had chronic ulcerative colitis for greater than 10 years in the absence of dysplasia. Proponents of this approach note that surveillance colonoscopy with multiple biopsies samples only a small fraction of the colonic mucosa and dysplasia and carcinoma are often missed. Opponents cite the relatively low risk of progression to carcinoma if all biopsies have lacked dysplasia (approximately 2.4%). Neither approach has been definitively shown to decrease mortality from colorectal cancer.

Operative Management

Emergent Operation. In a patient with fulminant colitis or toxic megacolon, total abdominal colectomy with end ileostomy, rather than total proctocolectomy, is recommended. Although the rectum is invariably diseased, most patients improve dramatically after an abdominal colectomy, and this operation avoids a difficult and time-consuming pelvic dissection in a critically ill patient. Rarely, a loop ileostomy and decompressing colostomy may be necessary if the patient is too unstable to withstand colectomy. Definitive surgery may then be undertaken at a later date once the patient has recovered. Complex techniques, such as an ileal pouch anal reconstruction, are generally contraindicated in the emergent setting. However, massive hemorrhage that includes bleeding from the rectum may necessitate proctectomy and either a permanent ileostomy or ileal pouch anal anastomosis.

Elective Operation. In the past, *abdominal colectomy with ileorectal anastomosis* was often recommended for patients with relatively quiescent rectal disease. The risk of ongoing inflammation, the risk of malignancy, and the availability of restorative proctocolectomy have led most surgeons to now recommend elective operations that include resection of the rectum. Abdominal colectomy with ileorectal anastomosis is still an appropriate operation for a patient with indeterminate colitis and rectal sparing. *Total proctocolectomy with end ileostomy* has been the "gold standard" for patients with chronic ulcerative colitis. This operation removes the

entire affected intestine and avoids the functional disturbances associated with ileal pouch–anal reconstruction. Most patients function well physically and psychologically after this operation. *Total proctocolectomy with continent ileostomy (Kock's pouch)* was developed to improve function and quality of life after total proctocolectomy, but morbidity is significant and restorative proctocolectomy is generally preferred today. Since its reintroduction in 1980, *restorative proctocolectomy with ileal pouch–anal anastomosis* has become the procedure of choice for most patients who require total proctocolectomy but wish to avoid a permanent ileostomy (see Figs. 28-11 and 28-12).[18]

Crohn's Disease

Like ulcerative colitis, Crohn's disease is characterized by exacerbations and remissions. Crohn's disease, however, may affect any portion of the intestinal tract, from mouth to anus. Diagnosis may be made by colonoscopy or esophagogastroduodenoscopy, or by barium small bowel study or enema, depending upon which part of the intestine is most affected. Skip lesions are key in differentiating Crohn's colitis from ulcerative colitis, and rectal sparing occurs in approximately 40% of patients. The most common site of involvement in Crohn's disease is the terminal ileum and cecum (*ileocolic* Crohn's disease), followed by the small bowel, and then by the colon and rectum. Crohn's disease may also affect the distal rectum and anal canal and may present as complex perianal/perirectal fistulas and/or abscesses (*perianal Crohn's disease*).

Indications for Surgery

Because Crohn's disease can affect any part of the gastrointestinal tract, the therapeutic rationale is fundamentally different from that of ulcerative colitis. Ulcerative colitis may be cured by removal of the affected intestinal segment (the colon and rectum). In Crohn's disease, it is impossible to remove all of the at-risk intestine; therefore surgical therapy is reserved for complications of the disease.

Crohn's disease may present as an *acute inflammatory* process or as a *chronic fibrotic* process. During the acute inflammatory phase, patients may present with intestinal inflammation complicated by fistulas and/or intra-abdominal abscesses. Maximal medical therapy should be instituted, including anti-inflammatory medications, bowel rest, and antibiotics. Parenteral nutrition should be considered if the patient is malnourished. Most intra-abdominal abscesses can be drained percutaneously with the use of CT scan guidance. Although the majority of these patients will ultimately require surgery to remove the diseased segment of bowel, these interventions allow the patient's condition to stabilize, nutrition to be optimized, and inflammation to decrease prior to embarking upon a surgical resection.

Chronic fibrosis may result in strictures in any part of the gastrointestinal tract. Because the fibrotic process is gradual, free perforation proximal to the obstructing stricture is rare, and, instead, adjacent structures "wall off" the site of perforation. The result is often development of enteric and colonic internal fistulas to other segments of intestine and other viscera (bladder, uterus, vagina) and retroperitoneal sites. Chronic strictures almost never improve with medical therapy. Optimal timing for surgery should take into account the patient's underlying medical and nutritional status. Strictures may be treated with *resection* or *stricturoplasty*. Associated fistulas generally require resection of the segment of bowel with active Crohn's disease; the secondary sites of the fistula are often otherwise normal and do not generally require resection after division of the fistula. Simple closure of the secondary fistula site usually suffices.

Once an operation is undertaken for Crohn's disease, several principles should guide intraoperative decision making. In general, a laparotomy for Crohn's disease should be done through a *midline incision* because of the possible need for a stoma. *Laparoscopy* is also increasingly used in this setting. Because many patients with Crohn's disease will require multiple operations, *the length of bowel removed should be minimized.* Bowel should be resected to an area with *grossly normal margins; frozen sections are not necessary.* Finally, a primary anastomosis may be safely created if the patient is medically stable, nutritionally replete, and taking few immunosuppressive medications. *Creation of a stoma should be strongly considered* in any patient who is hemodynamically unstable, septic, malnourished, or receiving high-dose immunosuppressive therapy and in patients with extensive intra-abdominal contamination.

Ileocolic and Small-Bowel Crohn's Disease

The terminal ileum and cecum are involved in Crohn's disease in up to 41% of patients; the small intestine is involved in up to 35% of patients. The most common indications for surgery are *internal fistula or abscess* (30 to 38% of patients) and *obstruction* (35 to 37% of patients). *Psoas abscess* may result from ileocolic Crohn's disease. Sepsis should be controlled with percutaneous drainage of abscess(es) and antibiotics, if possible. Parenteral nutrition may be necessary in patients with chronic obstruction. The extent of resection depends upon the amount of involved intestine. Short segments of inflamed small intestine and right colon should be resected and a primary anastomosis created if the patient is stable, nutrition is adequate, and immunosuppression is minimal. Isolated chronic strictures should also be resected. In patients with multiple fibrotic strictures which would require extensive small-bowel resection, *stricturoplasty* is a safe and effective alternative to resection. Short strictures are amenable to a transverse stricturoplasty, while longer strictures may be treated with a side-to-side small-bowel anastomosis (Fig. 28-18).

Risk of recurrence after resection for ileocolic and small-bowel Crohn's disease is high. More than 50% of patients will experience a recurrence within 10 years and the majority of these will require a second operation.

Crohn's Colitis

Crohn's disease of the large intestine may present as *fulminant colitis* or *toxic megacolon.* In this setting, treatment is identical to treatment of fulminant colitis and toxic megacolon secondary to ulcerative colitis. Resuscitation and medical therapy with bowel rest, broad-spectrum antibiotics, and parenteral corticosteroids should be instituted. If the patient's condition worsens or fails to rapidly improve, total abdominal colectomy with end ileostomy is recommended. An elective proctectomy may be required if the patient has refractory Crohn's proctitis. Alternatively, if the rectum is spared, an ileorectal anastomosis may be appropriate once the patient has recovered.

Other indications for surgery in chronic Crohn's colitis are *intractability, complications of medical therapy,* and *risk of or development of malignancy.* Unlike ulcerative colitis, Crohn's colitis may be segmental and rectal sparing is often observed. A segmental colectomy may be appropriate if the remaining colon and/or rectum appear normal. An isolated colonic stricture may also be treated by segmental colectomy. Although it was long thought that Crohn's disease did not increase the risk of colorectal carcinoma, it is now recognized that Crohn's colitis (especially pancolitis) carries nearly the same risk for cancer as ulcerative colitis. Annual surveillance colonoscopy with multiple biopsies is recommended for patients

with long-standing Crohn's colitis (>7 years duration). As in ulcerative colitis, dysplasia is an indication for total proctocolectomy. Ileal pouch–anal reconstruction is not recommended in these patients because of the risk for development of Crohn's disease within the pouch and the high risk of complications—fistula, abscess, stricture, pouch dysfunction, and pouch failure.

Anal and Perianal Crohn's Disease

Anal and perianal manifestations of Crohn's disease are very common. Anal or perianal disease occurs in 35% of all patients with Crohn's disease. Isolated anal Crohn's disease is uncommon, affecting only 3 to 4% of patients. Detection of anal Crohn's disease, therefore, should prompt evaluation of the remainder of the gastrointestinal tract.

The most common perianal lesions in Crohn's disease are *skin tags* that are minimally symptomatic. *Fissures* are also common and tend to occur in unusual locations. A fissure that is particularly deep or broad and located in a lateral position (rather than anterior or posterior midline) should raise the suspicion of Crohn's disease. *Perianal abscess* and *fistulas* are common and can be particularly challenging. Fistulas tend to be complex and often have multiple tracts (Fig. 28-19). *Hemorrhoids* are not more common in patients with Crohn's disease than in the general population, although many patients tend to attribute any anal or perianal symptom to "hemorrhoids."

Treatment of anal and perianal Crohn's disease focuses on alleviation of symptoms. Perianal skin irritation from diarrhea often responds to medical therapy directed at small-bowel or colonic disease. In general, skin tags and hemorrhoids should *not* be excised unless they are extremely symptomatic because of the risk of creating chronic, nonhealing wounds. Fissures may respond to local or systemic therapy; sphincterotomy is relatively contraindicated because of the risk of creating a chronic, nonhealing wound, and because of the increased risk of incontinence in a patient with diarrhea from underlying colitis or small bowel disease. Examination under anesthesia is often necessary to exclude an underlying abscess or fistula and to assess the rectal mucosa in patients with severe anal pain. In the absence of active Crohn's proctitis, one can proceed cautiously with a partial internal sphincterotomy if the examination under anesthesia reveals a classic-appearing posterior or anterior fissure and anal stenosis.

Recurrent abscess(es) or complex anal fistulas should raise the possibility of Crohn's disease. Treatment focuses upon *control of sepsis, delineation of complex anatomy, treatment of underlying mucosal disease,* and *sphincter preservation.* Abscesses can often be drained locally, and mushroom catheters are useful for maintaining drainage. Endoanal ultrasound and pelvic MRI are useful for mapping complex fistulous tracts. Liberal use of setons can control many fistulas and avoid division of the sphincter. Many patients with anal Crohn's disease function well with multiple setons left in place for years. Endoanal advancement flaps may be considered for definitive therapy if the rectal mucosa is uninvolved. In 10 to 15% of cases, intractable perianal sepsis requires proctectomy.

Rectovaginal fistula can be a particularly difficult problem in these patients. A rectal or vaginal mucosal advancement flap may be used if the rectal mucosa appears healthy and scarring of the rectovaginal septum is minimal. Occasionally, proctectomy is the best option for women with highly symptomatic rectovaginal fistula. While proximal diversion is often employed to protect complex perianal reconstruction, there is no evidence that diversion alone increases healing of anal and perianal Crohn's disease.

Medical treatment of underlying proctitis with salicylate and/or corticosteroid enemas may be helpful; however, control of sepsis is

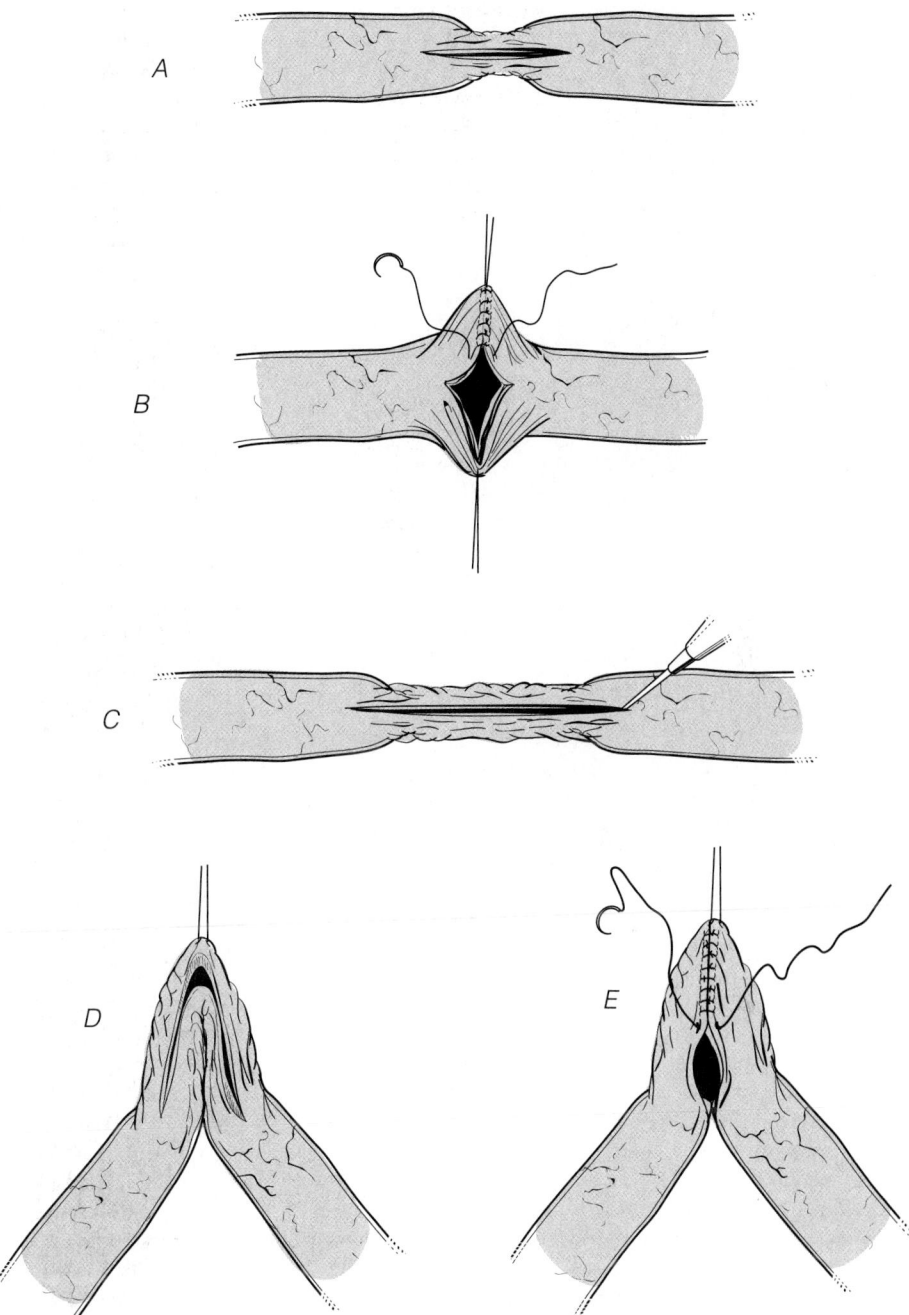

FIG. 28-18. Alternative stricture-plasty techniques. *A.* A short stricture is opened along the antimesenteric surface of the bowel wall. *B.* The enterotomy is closed transversely. *C.* A long stricture is opened along the antimesenteric surface of the bowel wall. *D.* The bowel is folded into an inverted "U." *E.* A side-to-side anastomosis is made. *(Reproduced with permission from Corman ML: Colon & Rectal Surgery, 2nd ed. Philadelphia: Lippincott Williams & Wilkins, 1989, p 832.)*

the primary goal of therapy. Metronidazole has also been used with some success in this setting. Infliximab has shown some efficacy in healing chronic fistulas secondary to Crohn's disease. However, it is of paramount importance to drain any and all abscesses before initiating immunosuppressive therapy such as corticosteroids or infliximab.

Indeterminate Colitis

Approximately 15% of patients with inflammatory bowel disease manifest clinical and pathologic characteristics of both ulcerative colitis and Crohn's disease. Endoscopy, barium enema, and biopsy may be unable to differentiate ulcerative colitis from Crohn's colitis in this setting. The indications for surgery are the same as those for ulcerative colitis: *intractability, complications of medical therapy,* and *risk of or development of malignancy.* In the setting of

indeterminate colitis in a patient who prefers a sphincter-sparing operation, a *total abdominal colectomy with end ileostomy* may be the best initial procedure. Pathologic examination of the entire colon may then allow a more accurate diagnosis. If the diagnosis suggests ulcerative colitis, an ileal pouch–anal anastomosis procedure can be performed. If the diagnosis remains in question, the safest surgical option is completion proctectomy with end ileostomy (similar to Crohn's colitis). Ileal pouch–anal reconstruction may also be considered with the understanding that the pouch failure rate is between 15 and 20%.

DIVERTICULAR DISEASE

Diverticular disease is a clinical term used to describe the presence of symptomatic diverticula. *Diverticulosis* refers to the presence

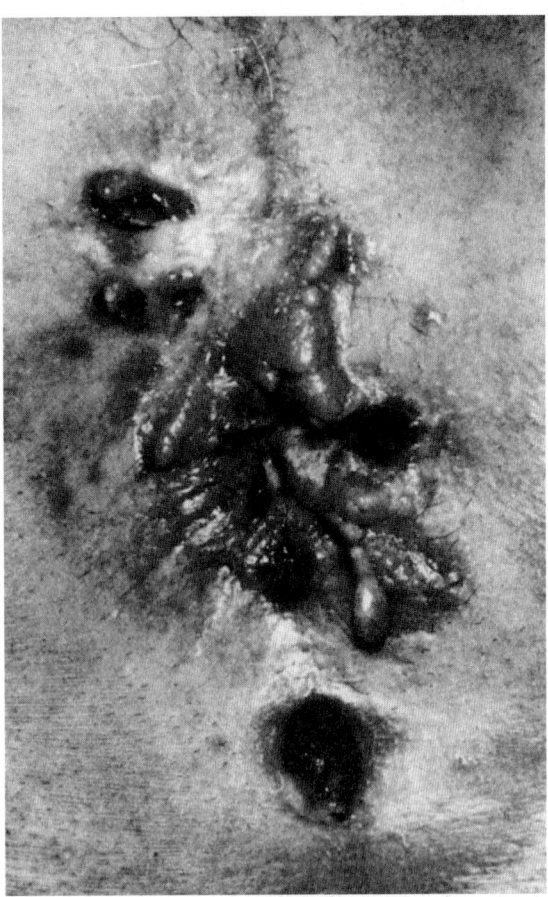

FIG. 28-19. Photograph of a patient with multiple perianal fistulas secondary to Crohn's disease. [*Reproduced with permission from Schwartz SI, Shires GT, Spencer FC (eds): Principles of Surgery. 5th ed. New York: McGraw-Hill, 1989, p 1248.*]

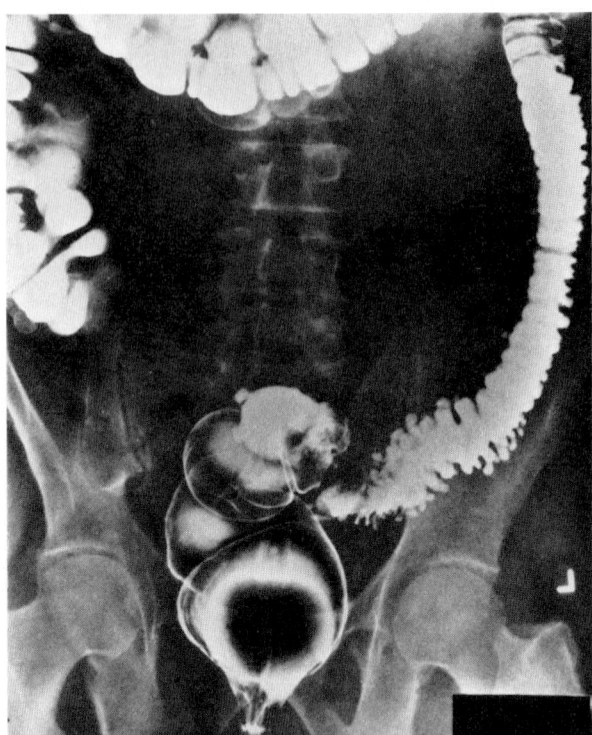

FIG. 28-20. Diverticulosis of sigmoid colon on barium enema. [*Reproduced with permission from Schwartz SI, Shires GT, Spencer FC (eds): Principles of Surgery. 5th ed. New York: McGraw-Hill, 1989, p 1256.*]

of diverticula without inflammation. *Diverticulitis* refers to inflammation and infection associated with diverticula. The majority of colonic diverticula are *false diverticula* in which the mucosa and muscularis mucosa have herniated through the colonic wall. These diverticula occur between the teniae coli, at points where the main blood vessels penetrate the colonic wall (presumably creating an area of relative weakness in the colonic muscle). They are thought to be *pulsion* diverticula resulting from high intraluminal pressure. *Diverticular bleeding* can be massive, but usually is self-limited. *True diverticula,* which comprise all layers of the bowel wall, are rare and are usually congenital in origin.

Diverticulosis is extremely common in the United States and Europe. It is estimated that half of the population older than age 50 years has colonic diverticula. The sigmoid colon is the most common site of diverticulosis (Fig. 28-20). Diverticulosis is thought to be an acquired disorder, but the etiology is poorly understood. The most accepted theory is that a lack of dietary fiber results in smaller stool volume, requiring high intraluminal pressure and high colonic wall tension for propulsion. Chronic contraction then results in muscular hypertrophy and pulsion diverticula. A loss of tensile strength and a decrease in elasticity of the bowel wall with age have also been proposed etiologies. While none of these theories has been proven, a high-fiber diet does appear to decrease the incidence of diverticulosis. Although diverticulosis is common, most cases are asymptomatic and complications occur in the minority of people with this condition.

Inflammatory Complications (Diverticulitis)

Diverticulitis refers to inflammation and infection associated with a diverticulum and is estimated to occur in 10 to 25% of people with diverticulosis. Peridiverticular and pericolic infection results from a perforation (either macroscopic or microscopic) of a diverticulum, which leads to contamination, inflammation, and infection. The spectrum of disease ranges from mild, uncomplicated diverticulitis that can be treated in the outpatient setting, to free perforation and diffuse peritonitis that requires emergency laparotomy. Most patients present with left-sided abdominal pain, with or without fever, and leukocytosis. A mass may be present. Plain radiographs are useful for detecting free intra-abdominal air. CT scan is extremely useful for defining pericolic inflammation, phlegmon, or abscess. Contrast enemas and/or endoscopy are relatively contraindicated because of the risk of perforation. The differential diagnosis includes malignancy, ischemic colitis, infectious colitis, and inflammatory bowel disease.

Uncomplicated Diverticulitis

Uncomplicated diverticulitis is characterized by left lower quadrant pain and tenderness. CT findings include pericolic soft-tissue stranding, colonic wall thickening, and/or phlegmon. Some patients with uncomplicated diverticulitis will respond to outpatient therapy with broad-spectrum oral antibiotics and a low-residue diet. Antibiotics should be continued for 7 to 10 days. Patients with more severe pain, tenderness, fever, and leukocytosis should be treated in the hospital with parenteral antibiotics and bowel rest. Most patients improve within 48 to 72 hours. Failure to improve may suggest abscess formation. CT can be extremely useful in this setting and many pericolic abscesses can be drained percutaneously (see below).

Deterioration in a patient's clinical condition and/or the development of peritonitis are indications for laparotomy.

Most patients with uncomplicated diverticulitis will recover without surgery and 50 to 70% will have no further episodes.[32] However, the risk of complications increases with recurrent disease. For this reason, elective sigmoid colectomy is often recommended after the second episode of diverticulitis, especially if the patient has required hospitalization. Resection may be indicated after the first episode in very young patients and in immunosuppressed patients, and is often recommended after the first episode of *complicated diverticulitis*. Medical comorbidity should be considered when evaluating a patient for elective resection, and the risks of recurrent disease weighed against the risks of the operation. Because colon carcinoma may have an identical clinical presentation to diverticulitis (either complicated or uncomplicated), all patients must be evaluated for malignancy after resolution of the acute episode. Sigmoidoscopy or colonoscopy is recommended 4 to 6 weeks after recovery. Inability to exclude malignancy is another indication for resection.

In the elective setting, a *sigmoid colectomy with a primary anastomosis* is the procedure of choice. The resection should always be extended to the rectum distally because the risk of recurrence is high if a segment of sigmoid colon is retained. The proximal extent of the resection should include all thickened or inflamed bowel; however, resection of all diverticula is unnecessary. Increasingly, laparoscopy is being used for elective sigmoid colectomy for diverticular disease.

Complicated Diverticulitis

Complicated diverticulitis includes diverticulitis with abscess, obstruction, diffuse peritonitis (free perforation), or fistulas between the colon and adjacent structures. Colovesical, colovaginal, and coloenteric fistulas are long-term sequelae of complicated diverticulitis. The *Hinchey staging system* is often used to describe the severity of complicated diverticulitis: Stage I includes colonic inflammation with an associated pericolic abscess; stage II includes colonic inflammation with a retroperitoneal or pelvic abscess; stage III is associated with purulent peritonitis; and stage IV is associated with fecal peritonitis. Treatment depends upon the patient's overall clinical condition and the degree of peritoneal contamination and infection. Small abscesses (<2 cm diameter) may be treated with parenteral antibiotics. Larger abscesses are best treated with CT-guided percutaneous drainage (Fig. 28-21).[2] The majority of these patients will ultimately require resection, but percutaneous drainage may allow a one-stage, elective procedure.

Urgent or emergent laparotomy may be required if an abscess is inaccessible to percutaneous drainage, if the patient's condition deteriorates or fails to improve, or if the patient presents with free intra-abdominal air or peritonitis. In almost all cases, an attempt should be made to resect the affected segment of bowel.[33,34] Patients with small, localized pericolic or pelvic abscesses (Hinchey stages I and II) may be candidates for a sigmoid colectomy with a primary anastomosis (a one-stage operation).[35] In patients with larger abscesses, peritoneal soiling, or peritonitis, sigmoid colectomy with end colostomy and Hartmann pouch is the most commonly used procedure.[36] Success also has been reported after sigmoid colectomy, primary anastomosis, ± on-table lavage, and proximal diversion (loop ileostomy). This option may be appropriate in stable patients and offers the great advantage that the subsequent operation to restore bowel continuity is simpler than is takedown of a Hartmann pouch. The presence of inflammation and phlegmon may increase the risk of ureteral damage during mobilization of the sigmoid colon, and preoperative placement of ureteral catheters can be invaluable. In extremely unstable patients, or in the presence of such severe inflammation that resection would harm adjacent organs, proximal diversion and local drainage have been employed. However, this approach is generally avoided because of high morbidity and mortality rates, along with the requirement for multiple operations.

Obstructive symptoms occur in approximately 67% of patients with acute diverticulitis, and complete obstruction occurs in 10%. Patients with incomplete obstruction often respond to fluid resuscitation, nasogastric suction, and gentle, low-volume water or Gastrografin enemas. Relief of obstruction allows full bowel preparation and elective resection. A high-volume oral bowel preparation is contraindicated in the presence of obstructive symptoms. Obstruction that does not rapidly respond to medical management mandates laparotomy. Sigmoid colectomy with end-colostomy is the safest procedure to perform in this setting. However, colectomy and primary

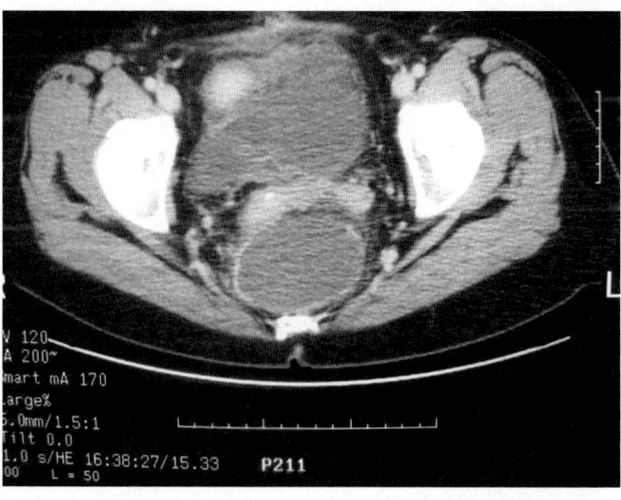

A

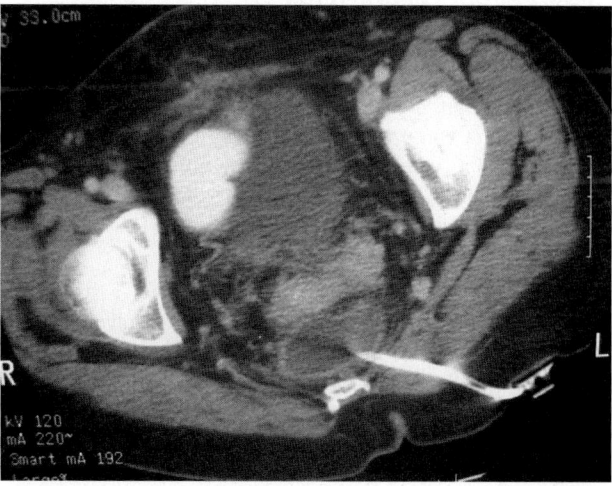

B

FIG. 28-21. *A.* CT scan demonstrating pelvic abscess from perforated diverticular disease. *B.* Posterolateral CT-guided drainage of abdominal abscess from perforated diverticular disease. (*Both images courtesy of Charles O. Finne, III, MD, Minneapolis, MN.*)

anastomosis, with or without on-table lavage (depending on extent of fecal load in the proximal colon), and proximal diversion may be appropriate if the patient is stable and the proximal and distal bowel appear healthy.

Approximately 5% of patients with complicated diverticulitis develop fistulas between the colon and an adjacent organ. *Colovesical* fistulas are most common, followed by *colovaginal* and *coloenteric* fistulas. *Colocutaneous* fistulas are a rare complication of diverticulitis. Two key points in the evaluation of fistulas are to *define the anatomy of the fistula* and *exclude other diagnoses*. Contrast enema and/or small bowel studies are extremely useful in defining the course of the fistula. CT scan can identify associated abscesses or masses. The differential diagnosis includes *malignancy, Crohn's disease,* and *radiation-induced fistulas.* While Crohn's disease and radiation injury may be suspected based upon the patient's medical history, colonoscopy or sigmoidoscopy is usually required to rule out malignancy. In addition, in a patient who has received radiation therapy, a fistula must be considered to be recurrent cancer until proven otherwise. Once the anatomy of the fistula has been defined and other diagnoses excluded, operative management should include resection of the affected segment of the colon involved with diverticulitis (usually with a primary anastomosis) and simple repair of the secondarily involved organ. Suspicion of carcinoma may mandate a wider, en bloc resection.

Hemorrhage

Bleeding from a diverticulum results from erosion of the peridiverticular arteriole and may result in massive hemorrhage. Most significant lower gastrointestinal hemorrhage occurs in elderly patients in whom both diverticulosis and angiodysplasia are common. Consequently, the exact bleeding source may be difficult to identify. Fortunately, in 80% of patients, bleeding stops spontaneously. Clinical management should focus upon resuscitation and localization of the bleeding site as described for lower gastrointestinal hemorrhage. Colonoscopy may occasionally identify a bleeding diverticulum that may then be treated with epinephrine injection or cautery. Angiography may be diagnostic and therapeutic in this setting. In the rare instance in which diverticular hemorrhage persists or recurs, laparotomy and segmental colectomy may be required.

Giant Colonic Diverticulum

Giant colonic diverticula are extremely rare. Most occur on the antimesenteric side of the sigmoid colon. Patients may be asymptomatic or may present with vague abdominal complaints such as pain, nausea, or constipation. Plain radiographs may suggest the diagnosis. Barium enema is usually diagnostic. Complications of a giant diverticulum include perforation, obstruction, and volvulus. Resection of the involved colon and diverticulum is recommended.

Right-Sided Diverticula

The cecum and ascending colon infrequently are involved in diverticulosis coli. Even more uncommon is a true solitary diverticulum, which contains all layers of the bowel wall and is thought to be congenital in origin. Right-sided diverticula occur more often in younger patients than do left-sided diverticula, and are more common in people of Asian descent than in other populations. Most patients with right-sided diverticula are asymptomatic. However, diverticulitis does occur occasionally. Because patients are young and present with right lower quadrant pain, they are often thought to suffer from acute appendicitis, and the diagnosis of right-sided diverticulitis is subsequently made in the operating room. If there is a single large diverticulum and minimal inflammation, a divertic-

ulectomy may be performed, but an ileocecal resection is usually the preferred operation in this setting. Hemorrhage rarely occurs and should be treated in the same fashion as hemorrhage from a left-sided diverticulum.

ADENOCARCINOMA AND POLYPS

Incidence

Colorectal carcinoma is the most common malignancy of the gastrointestinal tract. More than 145,000 new cases are diagnosed annually in the United States and more than 55,000 patients die of this disease each year, making colorectal cancer the second most lethal cancer in the United States. The incidence is similar in men and women and has remained fairly constant over the past 20 years. The widespread adoption of current national screening programs should dramatically decrease the incidence of this common and lethal disease. Early detection along with improvements in medical and surgical care are thought to be responsible for the decreasing mortality of colorectal cancer observed in recent years.

Epidemiology (Risk Factors)

Identification of risk factors for development of colorectal cancer is essential to establish screening and surveillance programs in appropriately targeted populations.

Aging

Aging is the dominant risk factor for colorectal cancer, with incidence rising steadily after age 50 years. More than 90% of cases diagnosed are in people older than age 50 years. This is the rationale for initiating screening tests of asymptomatic Americans at average risk of developing colorectal cancer at age 50 years. However, individuals of any age can develop colorectal cancer, so symptoms such as a significant change in bowel habits, rectal bleeding, melena, unexplained anemia, or weight loss require a thorough evaluation.

Hereditary Risk Factors

Approximately 80% of colorectal cancers occur sporadically, while 20% arise in patients with a known family history of colorectal cancer. Advances in the understanding of these familial disorders have led to interest in early diagnosis using genetic testing. Assays currently exist to detect the most common defects in the APC gene and in mismatch repair genes. Because of the medical, legal, and ethical considerations that are involved in this type of testing, all patients should be offered genetic counseling if a familial syndrome is suspected.

Environmental and Dietary Factors

The observation that colorectal carcinoma occurs more commonly in populations that consume diets high in animal fat and low in fiber has lead to the hypothesis that dietary factors contribute to carcinogenesis. A diet high in saturated or polyunsaturated fats increases risk of colorectal cancer, while a diet high in oleic acid (olive oil, coconut oil, fish oil) does not increase risk. Animal studies suggest that fats may be directly toxic to the colonic mucosa and thus may induce early malignant changes. In contrast, a diet high in *vegetable fiber* appears to be protective. A correlation between alcohol intake and incidence of colorectal carcinoma has also been suggested. Ingestion of calcium, selenium, vitamins A, C, and E, carotenoids, and plant phenols may decrease the risk of developing colorectal cancer. Obesity and sedentary lifestyle dramatically increase cancer-related mortality in a number of malignancies, including colorectal carcinoma. This knowledge is the basis for primary prevention strategies to eliminate colorectal cancer by altering diet and lifestyle.[37,38]

Inflammatory Bowel Disease

Patients with long-standing colitis from inflammatory bowel disease are at increased risk for the development of colorectal cancer.[39] It is hypothesized that chronic inflammation predisposes the mucosa to malignant changes. In general, the duration and extent of colitis correlate with risk. In ulcerative pancolitis, the risk of carcinoma is approximately 2% after 10 years, 8% after 20 years, and 18% after 30 years. Patients with Crohn's pancolitis have similar risk. Left-sided colitis carries somewhat less risk. For this reason, screening colonoscopy with multiple random mucosal biopsies has been recommended annually after 8 years of disease for patients with pancolitis and after 12 to 15 years of disease for patients with left-sided colitis. It is important to note, however, that intensive surveillance has not definitively been shown to improve survival, and some authors are questioning the efficacy of this approach.

Other Risk Factors

Cigarette smoking is associated with an increased risk of colonic adenomas, especially after more than 35 years of use. Patients with ureterosigmoidostomy are also at increased risk for both adenoma and carcinoma formation.[40] Acromegaly, which is associated with increased levels of circulating human growth hormone and insulin-like growth factor-1, increases risk as well.[41] Pelvic irradiation may increase the risk of developing rectal carcinoma, although it is unclear if this represents a direct effect of radiation damage or is instead a correlation between the development of rectal cancer and a history of another pelvic malignancy.

Pathogenesis of Colorectal Cancer

Genetic Defects

Over the past two decades, an intense research effort has focused on elucidating the genetic defects and molecular abnormalities associated with the development and progression of colorectal adenomas and carcinoma. Mutations may cause *activation of oncogenes* (K-ras) and/or *inactivation of tumor-suppressor genes* (APC, DCC [deleted in colorectal carcinoma], p53). Colorectal carcinoma is thought to develop from adenomatous polyps by accumulation of these mutations (Fig. 28-22).

Defects in the APC gene were first described in patients with *FAP*. By investigating these families, characteristic mutations in the APC gene were identified. They are now known to be present in 80% of sporadic colorectal cancers as well.

The APC gene is a *tumor-suppressor gene*. Mutations in both alleles are necessary to initiate polyp formation. The majority of mutations are premature stop codons, which result in a truncated

APC protein. In FAP, the site of mutation correlates with the clinical severity of the disease. For example, mutations in either the 3′ or 5′ end of the gene result in attenuated forms of FAP, while mutations in the center of the gene result in more virulent disease. Thus, knowledge of the specific mutation in a family may help guide clinical decision making.

APC inactivation alone does not result in a carcinoma. Instead, this mutation sets the stage for the accumulation of genetic damage that results in malignancy via mutations accumulated in the loss of heterozygosity (LOH) pathway. Additional mutations involved in this pathway include activation of the *K-ras* oncogene, and loss of the tumor-suppressor genes *DCC* and *p53*.

K-ras is classified as a *proto-oncogene* because mutation of only one allele will perturb the cell cycle. The K-ras gene product is a G-protein involved in intracellular signal transduction. When active, K-ras binds guanosine triphosphate (GTP); hydrolysis of GTP to guanosine diphosphate (GDP) then inactivates the G-protein. Mutation of K-ras results in an inability to hydrolyze GTP, thus leaving the G-protein permanently in the active form. It is thought that this then leads to uncontrolled cell division.

DCC is a tumor-suppressor gene and loss of both alleles is required for malignant degeneration. The role of the DCC gene product is poorly understood, but it might be involved in cellular differentiation. DCC mutations are present in more than 70% of colorectal carcinomas and may negatively impact prognosis.

The tumor-suppressor gene p53 has been well characterized in a number of malignancies. The p53 protein appears to be crucial for initiating apoptosis in cells with irreparable genetic damage. Mutations in p53 are present in 75% of colorectal cancers.

Genetic Pathways

Two major pathways for tumor initiation and progression have been described: the *LOH pathway* and the *replication error (RER) pathway*. The LOH pathway is characterized by chromosomal deletions and tumor aneuploidy. Eighty percent of colorectal carcinomas appear to arise from mutations in the LOH pathway. The remaining 20% of colorectal carcinomas are thought to arise from mutations in the RER pathway, which is characterized by errors in mismatch repair during DNA replication. A number of genes have been identified that appear to be crucial for recognizing and repairing DNA replication errors. These *mismatch repair genes* include hMSH2, hMLH1, hPMS1, hPMS2, and hMSH6/GTBP. A mutation in one of these genes predisposes a cell to mutations, which may occur in proto-oncogenes or tumor-suppressor genes. Accumulation of these errors then leads to genomic instability and ultimately to carcinogenesis.

The RER pathway is associated with *microsatellite instability*.[42] Microsatellites are regions of the genome in which short base-pair

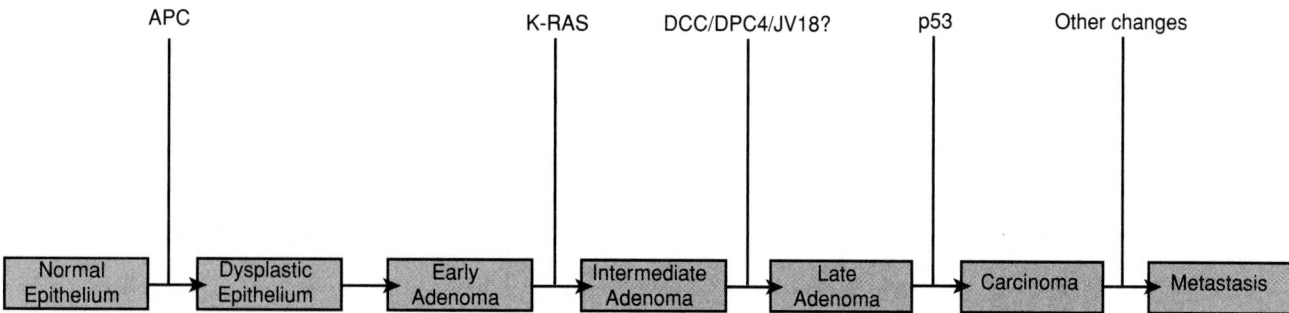

FIG. 28-22. Schematic showing progression from normal colonic epithelium to carcinoma of the colon.

segments are repeated several times. These areas are particularly prone to replication error. Consequently, a mutation in a mismatch repair gene produces variable lengths of these repetitive sequences, a finding that has been described as microsatellite instability.

Tumors associated with microsatellite instability (MSI) appear to have different biologic characteristics than do tumors that result from the LOH pathway. Tumors with MSI are more likely to be right sided, possess diploid DNA, and are associated with a better prognosis than tumors that arise from the LOH pathway that are microsatellite stable (MSS). Tumors arising from the LOH pathway tend to occur in the more distal colon, often have chromosomal aneuploidy, and are associated with a poorer prognosis.

Polyps

It is now well accepted that the majority of colorectal carcinomas evolve from adenomatous polyps; this sequence of events is the *adenoma–carcinoma sequence. Polyp* is a nonspecific clinical term that describes any projection from the surface of the intestinal mucosa regardless of its histologic nature. Colorectal polyps may be classified as *neoplastic (tubular adenoma, villous adenoma, tubulovillous adenomas), hamartomatous (juvenile, Peutz-Jeghers, Cronkite-Canada), inflammatory (pseudopolyp, benign lymphoid polyp),* or *hyperplastic.*

Neoplastic Polyps

Adenomatous polyps are common, occurring in up to 25% of the population older than 50 years of age in the United States. By definition, these lesions are dysplastic. The risk of malignant degeneration is related to both the size and type of polyp. Tubular adenomas are associated with malignancy in only 5% of cases, whereas villous adenomas may harbor cancer in up to 40%. Tubulovillous adenomas are at intermediate risk (22%). Invasive carcinomas are rare in polyps smaller than 1 cm; the incidence increases with size. The risk of carcinoma in a polyp larger than 2 cm is 35 to 50%. Although most neoplastic polyps do not evolve to cancer, most colorectal cancers originate as a polyp. It is this fact that forms the basis for secondary prevention strategies to eliminate colorectal cancer by targeting the neoplastic polyp for removal before malignancy develops.

Polyps may be *pedunculated* or *sessile.* Most pedunculated polyps are amenable to colonoscopic snare excision. Removal of sessile polyps is often more challenging. Special colonoscopic techniques, including saline lift and piecemeal snare excision, facilitate successful removal of many sessile polyps. For rectal sessile polyps, transanal operative excision is preferred because it produces an intact, single pathology specimen that can be used to determine the need for further therapy. Interpretation of the precise depth of invasion of a cancer arising in a sessile polyp after piecemeal excision is often impossible. The site of sessile polypectomies should be marked by injection of methylene blue or India ink to guide follow-up colonoscopy sessions to ensure that the polyp has been completely removed, and to facilitate identification of the involved bowel segment should operative resection be necessary. Colectomy is reserved for cases in which colonoscopic removal is impossible, such as large, flat lesions or if a focus of invasive cancer is confirmed in the specimen. These patients may be ideal candidates for laparoscopic colectomy.

Complications of polypectomy include *perforation* and *bleeding.* A small perforation (*microperforation*) in a fully prepared, stable patient may be managed with bowel rest, broad-spectrum antibiotics, and close observation. Signs of sepsis, peritonitis, or deterioration in clinical condition are indications for laparotomy. Bleeding may occur immediately after polypectomy or may be delayed. The bleeding will usually stop spontaneously, but colonoscopy may be required to re-snare a bleeding stalk or cauterize the lesion. Occasionally angiography and infusion of vasopressin may be necessary. Rarely, colectomy is required.

Hamartomatous Polyps (Juvenile Polyps)

In contrast to adenomatous polyps, hamartomatous polyps (juvenile polyps) are not usually premalignant. These lesions are the characteristic polyps of childhood but may occur at any age. Bleeding is a common symptom and intussusception and/or obstruction may occur. Because the gross appearance of these polyps is identical to adenomatous polyps, these lesions should also be treated by polypectomy.

Familial juvenile polyposis is an autosomal dominant disorder in which patients develop hundreds of polyps in the colon and rectum. Unlike solitary juvenile polyps, these lesions may degenerate into adenomas, and eventually carcinoma. Annual screening should begin between the ages of 10 and 12 years. Treatment is surgical and depends in part upon the degree of rectal involvement. If the rectum is relatively spared, a total abdominal colectomy with ileorectal anastomosis may be performed with subsequent close surveillance of the retained rectum. If the rectum is carpeted with polyps, total proctocolectomy is the more appropriate operation. These patients are candidates for ileal pouch–anal reconstruction to avoid a permanent stoma.

Peutz-Jeghers syndrome is characterized by polyposis of the small intestine, and to a lesser extent, polyposis of the colon and rectum. Characteristic melanin spots are often noted on the buccal mucosa and lips of these patients. The polyps of Peutz-Jeghers syndrome are generally considered to be hamartomas and are not thought to be at significant risk for malignant degeneration. However, carcinoma may occasionally develop. Because the entire length of the gastrointestinal tract may be affected, surgery is reserved for symptoms such as obstruction or bleeding or for patients in whom polyps develop adenomatous features. Screening consists of a baseline colonoscopy and upper endoscopy at age 20 years, followed by annual flexible sigmoidoscopy thereafter.

Cronkite-Canada syndrome is a disorder in which patients develop gastrointestinal polyposis in association with alopecia, cutaneous pigmentation, and atrophy of the fingernails and toenails. Diarrhea is a prominent symptom, and vomiting, malabsorption, and protein-losing enteropathy may occur. Most patients die of this disease despite maximal medical therapy, and surgery is reserved for complications of polyposis such as obstruction.

Cowden's syndrome is an autosomal dominant disorder with hamartomas of all three embryonal cell layers. Facial trichilemmomas, breast cancer, thyroid disease, and gastrointestinal polyps are typical of the syndrome. Patients should be screened for cancers. Treatment is otherwise based upon symptoms.

Inflammatory Polyps (Pseudopolyps)

Inflammatory polyps occur most commonly in the context of inflammatory bowel disease, but may also occur after amebic colitis, ischemic colitis, and schistosomal colitis. These lesions are not premalignant, but they cannot be distinguished from adenomatous polyps based upon gross appearance and therefore should be removed. Microscopic examination shows islands of normal, regenerating mucosa (the polyp) surrounded by areas of mucosal loss. Polyposis may be extensive, especially in patients with severe colitis, and may mimic familial adenomatous polyposis.

Hyperplastic Polyps

Hyperplastic polyps are extremely common in the colon. These polyps are usually small (<5 mm) and show histologic characteristics of hyperplasia without any dysplasia. They are not considered premalignant, but cannot be distinguished from adenomatous polyps colonoscopically and are therefore often removed. In contrast, large hyperplastic polyps (>2 cm) may have a slight risk of malignant degeneration. Moreover, large polyps may harbor foci of adenomatous tissue and dysplasia. *Hyperplastic polyposis* is a rare disorder in which multiple large hyperplastic polyps occur in young adults.

Inherited Colorectal Carcinoma

Many of the genetic defects originally described in hereditary cancers have subsequently been found in sporadic tumors. Although the majority of colorectal cancer is sporadic, several hereditary syndromes provide paradigms for the study of this disease. Insight gained from studying inherited colorectal cancer syndromes has led to better understanding of the genetics of colorectal carcinoma.

Familial Adenomatous Polyposis

This rare autosomal dominant condition accounts for only about 1% of all colorectal adenocarcinomas. Nevertheless, this syndrome has provided tremendous insight into the molecular mechanisms underlying colorectal carcinogenesis. The genetic abnormality in FAP is a mutation in the APC gene, located on chromosome 5q. Of patients with FAP, APC mutation testing is positive in 75% of cases. While most patients with FAP will have a known family history of the disease, up to 25% present without other affected family members. Clinically, patients develop hundreds to thousands of adenomatous polyps shortly after puberty. The lifetime risk of colorectal cancer in FAP patients approaches 100% by age 50 years.

Flexible sigmoidoscopy of first-degree relatives of FAP patients beginning at age 10 to 15 years has been the traditional mainstay of screening. Today, following genetic counseling, APC gene testing may be used to screen family members, providing an APC mutation has been identified in a family member. If APC testing is positive in a relative of a patient with a known APC mutation, annual flexible sigmoidoscopy beginning at age 10 to 15 years is done until polyps are identified. If APC testing is negative, the relative can be screened starting at age 50 years per average-risk guidelines. If APC testing is refused, annual flexible sigmoidoscopy beginning at age 10 to 15 years is performed until age 24 years. Screening flexible sigmoidoscopy is then done every 2 years until age 34 years, every 3 years until age 44 years, and then every 3 to 5 years. If an APC mutation is not found in the family, either APC testing can be done for at-risk family members or traditional screening by flexible sigmoidoscopy can be initiated.

FAP patients are also at risk for the development of adenomas anywhere in the gastrointestinal tract, particularly in the duodenum. Periampullary carcinoma is a particular concern. Upper endoscopy is therefore recommended for surveillance every 1 to 3 years beginning at age 25 to 30 years.

Once the diagnosis of FAP has been made and polyps are developing, treatment is surgical. Four factors affect the choice of operation: age of the patient; presence and severity of symptoms; extent of rectal polyposis; and presence and location of cancer or desmoid tumors. Three operative procedures can be considered: total proctocolectomy with either an end (Brooke's) ileostomy or continent (Kock's) ileostomy; total abdominal colectomy with ileorectal anastomosis; and restorative proctocolectomy with ileal pouch–anal anastomosis with or without a temporary ileostomy.[43,44] Most patients elect to have an ileal pouch–anal anastomosis in the absence of a distal rectal cancer, a mesenteric desmoid tumor that prevents the ileum from reaching the anus or poor sphincter function. Mucosectomy has been advocated in patients with FAP undergoing ileal pouch–anal anastomosis because of the risk of neoplasia in the anal transition zone, but the requirement for this procedure remains controversial. Although patient satisfaction with this procedure remains high, function may not be ideal and up to 50% of patients experience some degree of incontinence. Total proctocolectomy with continent ileostomy (Kock's pouch) has largely been abandoned because of the success of ileal pouch–anal reconstruction. Total abdominal colectomy with an ileorectal anastomosis is also an option in these patients, but requires vigilant surveillance of the retained rectum for development of rectal cancer.[45] There is increasing data suggesting that the administration of COX-2 inhibitors (celecoxib, sulindac) may slow or prevent the development of polyps.[46]

FAP may be associated with extraintestinal manifestations such as congenital hypertrophy of the retinal pigmented epithelium, desmoid tumors, epidermoid cysts, mandibular osteomas (Gardner's syndrome), and central nervous system tumors (Turcot's syndrome). Desmoid tumors in particular, can make surgical management difficult and are a source of major morbidity and mortality in these patients. Desmoid tumors are often hormone responsive and growth may be inhibited in some patients with tamoxifen. COX-2 inhibitors and nonsteroidal, anti-inflammatory drugs may also be beneficial in this setting.

Attenuated FAP

Attenuated FAP is a recently recognized variant of FAP associated with mutations at the 3′ or 5′ end of the APC gene. Patients present later in life with fewer polyps (usually 10 to 100) dominantly located in the right colon, when compared to classic FAP. Colorectal carcinoma develops in more than 50% of these patients, but occurs later (average age 50 years). Patients are also at risk for duodenal polyposis. APC mutation testing is positive in approximately 60% of patients. When positive, genetic counseling and testing may be used to screen at-risk family members. If the family mutation is unknown, screening colonoscopy is recommended beginning at age 13 to 15 years, then every 4 years to age 28 years, and then every 3 years. These patients are often candidates for a total abdominal colectomy with ileorectal anastomosis because the limited polyposis in the rectum can usually be treated by colonoscopic snare excision. Prophylaxis with COX-2 inhibitors may also be appropriate.

Hereditary Nonpolyposis Colon Cancer (Lynch's Syndrome)

Hereditary nonpolyposis colon cancer (HNPCC or Lynch's syndrome) is more common than FAP, but is still extremely rare (1 to 3%). The genetic defects associated with HNPCC arise from errors in *mismatch repair* and study of this syndrome has elucidated many of the details of the RER pathway. HNPCC is inherited in an autosomal dominant pattern and is characterized by the development of colorectal carcinoma at an early age (average age: 40 to 45 years).[47] Approximately 70% of affected individuals will develop colorectal cancer. Cancers appear in the proximal colon more often than in sporadic colorectal cancer and have a better prognosis regardless of stage. The risk of synchronous or metachronous colorectal carcinoma is 40%. HNPCC may also be associated with extracolonic malignancies, including endometrial, ovarian, pancreas, stomach, small bowel, biliary, and urinary tract carcinomas. The diagnosis of HNPCC is made based upon family history. The *Amsterdam*

Table 28-1
Advantages and Disadvantages of Screening Modalities for Asymptomatic Individuals

	Advantages	*Disadvantages*
Fecal occult blood testing	Ease of use and noninvasive Low cost Good sensitivity with repeat testing	May not detect most polyps Low specificity Colonoscopy required for positive result Poor compliance with serial testing
Sigmoidoscopy	Examines colon most at risk Very sensitive for polyp detection in left colon Does not require full bowel preparation (enemas only)	Invasive Uncomfortable Slight risk of perforation or bleeding May miss proximal lesions Colonoscopy required if polyp identified
Colonoscopy	Examines entire colon Highly sensitive and specific Therapeutic	Most invasive Uncomfortable and requires sedation Requires bowel preparation Risk of perforation or bleeding Costly
Double-contrast barium enema	Examines entire colon Good sensitivity for polyps >1 cm	Requires bowel preparation Less sensitivity for polyps <1 cm May miss lesions in the sigmoid colon Colonoscopy required for positive result
CT Colonography (virtual colonoscopy)	Examines entire colon Noninvasive Sensitivity may be as good as colonoscopy	Requires bowel preparation Insensitive for small polyps Minimal experience and data Colonoscopy required for positive result Costly

criteria for clinical diagnosis of HNPCC are three affected relatives with histologically verified adenocarcinoma of the large bowel (one must be a first-degree relative of one of the others) in two successive generations of a family with one patient diagnosed before age 50 years. The presence of other HNPCC-related carcinomas should raise the suspicion of this syndrome.

Screening colonoscopy is recommended annually for at-risk patients beginning at either age 20 to 25 years or 10 years younger than the youngest age at diagnosis in the family, whichever comes first.[48] Because of the high risk of endometrial carcinoma, transvaginal ultrasound or endometrial aspiration biopsy is also recommended annually after age 25 to 35 years. Because there is a 40% risk of developing a second colon cancer, total colectomy with ileorectal anastomosis is recommended once adenomas or a colon carcinoma is diagnosed, or if prophylactic colectomy is decided upon. Annual proctoscopy is necessary because the risk of developing rectal cancer remains high. Similarly, prophylactic hysterectomy and bilateral salpingo-oophorectomy should be considered in women who have completed childbearing.

Familial Colorectal Cancer

Nonsyndromic familial colorectal cancer accounts for 10 to 15% of patients with colorectal cancer. The lifetime risk of developing colorectal cancer increases with a family history of the disease. The lifetime risk of colorectal cancer in a patient with no family history of this disease (average-risk population) is approximately 6%, but rises to 12% if one first-degree relative is affected and to 35% if two first-degree relatives are affected. Age of onset also impacts risk and a diagnosis before the age of 50 years is associated with a higher incidence in family members. Screening colonoscopy is recommended every 5 years beginning at age 40 years or beginning 10 years before the age of the earliest diagnosed patient in the pedigree. While there are no specific genetic abnormalities that are associated with familial colorectal cancer, any of the defects found

in either the LOH pathway or RER pathway may be present in these patients.

Prevention: Screening and Surveillance

Because the majority of colorectal cancers are thought to arise from adenomatous polyps, preventive measures focus upon identification and removal of these premalignant lesions. In addition, many cancers are asymptomatic and screening may detect these tumors at an early and curable stage (Table 28-1). Although screening for colorectal cancer decreases the incidence of cancer and cancer-related mortality, the optimal method of screening remains controversial. Screening guidelines are meant for *asymptomatic* patients.[49–51] Any patient with a gastrointestinal complaint (bleeding, change in bowel habits, pain, etc) requires a complete evaluation, usually by colonoscopy.

Fecal Occult Blood Testing

The University of Minnesota Colon Cancer Control Study, a large, prospective, randomized trial, was the first of several large studies to conclude that FOBT screening reduces colorectal cancer mortality by 33% and metastatic cases by 50%. However, FOBT is relatively insensitive, missing up to 50% of cancers and the majority of adenomas. Its specificity is low because 90% of patients with positive tests do not have colorectal cancer. Compliance with annual testing is low and costs are significant if one includes the colonoscopy examinations done to evaluate patients with positive FOBT. Nonetheless, the direct evidence that FOBT screening is efficacious and decreases both the incidence and mortality of colorectal cancer is so strong that national guidelines recommend annual FOBT screening for asymptomatic, average-risk Americans older than 50 years of age as one of several accepted strategies. As noted earlier under "Clinical Evaluation," newer immunohistochemical methods for detecting human globin may prove to be more sensitive and specific.[51] A positive FOBT test should be followed by colonoscopy.

Rigid Proctoscopy

Case control studies show that the risk of dying of rectal cancer is decreased by prior screening via rigid proctoscopy while the risk of colon cancer death is not affected. A study from St. Mark's Hospital in London of more than 1500 patients who underwent rigid proctoscopy and treatment of rectal polyps showed that patients with a single, small tubular adenoma were at low risk of colorectal cancer. In contrast, those with larger tubular, tubulovillous, or villous adenomas were at increased risk for subsequent colon cancer, but at decreased risk for rectal cancer (if the rectal polyps were removed initially). Because of its limited range, proctoscopy has little place in modern screening programs.

Flexible Sigmoidoscopy

Screening by flexible sigmoidoscopy every 5 years may lead to a 60 to 70% reduction in mortality from colorectal cancer, chiefly by identifying high-risk individuals with adenomas. Presumed high cost has prohibited its use in mass screening in the past, but a randomized, multicenter, controlled trial of screening sigmoidoscopy was initiated by the National Cancer Institute in 1992, and results are expected in 2007. Studies show that trained nurse endoscopists may achieve similar results in polyp detection as their physician colleagues, which may reduce costs considerably. Patients found to have a polyp, cancer, or other lesion on flexible sigmoidoscopy will require colonoscopy.[52]

FOBT and Flexible Sigmoidoscopy

The FOBT trials from Mandel and associates (University of Minnesota), Hardcastle and associates (England), and Kronberg and associates (Denmark) all showed that FOBT screening was least effective at detecting rectosigmoid cancers. Two-thirds of interval cancers arose in the rectosigmoid in the English series. This is precisely the area screened by flexible sigmoidoscopy; thus, the combination of the two tests has been suggested as a reasonable screening strategy. Winawer, in a study of 12,479 subjects, showed that the combination of FOBT annually with flexible sigmoidoscopy every 5 years resulted in lower mortality from colorectal cancer and better survival in those patients with colorectal cancer. Such data led to the American Cancer Society recommendations that one of the acceptable screening regimens for average-risk Americans is the combination of FOBT annually and flexible sigmoidoscopy every 5 years; this combination was preferred over either test alone.

Colonoscopy

Colonoscopy is currently the most accurate and most complete method for examining the large bowel.[53] This procedure is highly sensitive for detecting even small polyps (<1 cm) and allows biopsy, polypectomy, control of hemorrhage, and dilation of strictures. However, colonoscopy does require mechanical bowel preparation and the discomfort associated with the procedure requires conscious sedation in most patients. Colonoscopy is also considerably more expensive than other screening modalities and requires a well-trained endoscopist. The risk of a major complication after colonoscopy (perforation and hemorrhage) is extremely low (0.2 to 0.3%). Nevertheless, deaths have been reported.

Air-Contrast Barium Enema

Air-contrast barium enema is also highly sensitive for detecting polyps greater than 1 cm in diameter (90% sensitivity). Unfortunately, there are no studies proving its efficacy for screening large populations. Accuracy is greatest in the proximal colon but may be compromised in the sigmoid colon if there is significant diverticulosis. For this reason, barium enema is often combined with flexible sigmoidoscopy for screening purposes. The major disadvantages of barium enema are the need for mechanical bowel preparation and the requirement for colonoscopy if a lesion is discovered.

CT Colonography (Virtual Colonoscopy)

Advances in imaging technology have created a number of less invasive, but highly accurate tools for screening. CT colonography makes use of helical CT technology and three-dimensional reconstruction to image the intraluminal colon. Patients require a mechanical bowel preparation. The colon is then insufflated with air, a spiral CT is performed, and both two-dimensional and three-dimensional images are generated. In the hands of a qualified radiologist, sensitivity appears to be as good as colonoscopy for colorectal cancers and polyps greater than 1 cm in size.[54] Colonoscopy is required if a lesion is identified. CT colonography may also prove useful for imaging the proximal colon in cases of obstruction. Limitations of this technique include false-positive results from retained stool, diverticular disease, haustral folds, motion artifacts, and an inability to detect flat adenomas.

Guidelines for Screening

Current American Cancer Society guidelines advocate screening for the average-risk population (asymptomatic, no family history of colorectal carcinoma, no personal history of polyps or colorectal carcinoma, no familial syndrome) beginning at age 50 years.[1] Recommended procedures include yearly FOBT, flexible sigmoidoscopy every 5 years, FOBT and flexible sigmoidoscopy in combination, air-contrast barium enema every 5 years, or colonoscopy every 10 years.[55] Patients with other risk factors should be screened earlier and more frequently (Table 28-2).

Routes of Spread and Natural History

Carcinoma of the colon and rectum arises in the mucosa. The tumor subsequently invades the bowel wall and eventually adjacent tissues and other viscera. Tumors may become bulky and circumferential, leading to colon obstruction. Local extension (especially in the rectum) may occasionally cause obstruction of other organs such as the ureter.

Regional lymph node involvement is the most common form of spread of colorectal carcinoma and usually precedes distant metastasis or the development of carcinomatosis. The likelihood of nodal metastasis increases with tumor size, poorly differentiated histology, lymphovascular invasion, and depth of invasion. The T stage (depth of invasion) is the single most significant predictor of lymph node spread. Carcinoma in situ (Tis) in which there is no penetration of the muscularis mucosa (basement membrane) has also been called *high-grade dysplasia* and should carry no risk of lymph node metastasis. Small lesions confined to the bowel wall (T1 and T2) are associated with lymph node metastasis in 5 to 20% of cases, while larger tumors that invade through the bowel wall or into adjacent organs (T3 and T4) are likely to have lymph node metastasis in more than 50% of cases. The number of lymph nodes with metastases correlates with the presence of distant disease and inversely with survival. Four or more involved lymph nodes predict a poor prognosis. In colon cancer, lymphatic spread usually follows the major venous outflow from the involved segment of the colon. Lymphatic spread from the rectum follows two routes. In the upper rectum, drainage ascends along the superior rectal vessels to the inferior mesenteric nodes. In the lower rectum, lymphatic drainage may course along the

Table 28-2
Screening Guidelines for Colorectal Cancer

Population	Initial Age	Recommended Screening Test
Average risk	50 years	Annual FOBT *or* Flexible sigmoidoscopy every 5 years *or* Annual FOBT and flexible sigmoidoscopy every 5 years *or* Air contrast barium enema every 5 years *or* Colonoscopy every 10 years
Adenomatous polyps	50 years	Colonoscopy at first detection; then colonoscopy in 3 years If no further polyps, colonoscopy every 5 yeaars If polyps, colonoscopy every 3 years Annual colonoscopy for >5 adenomas
Colorectal cancer	At diagnosis	Pretreatment colonoscopy; then at 12 months after curative resection; then colonoscopy after 3 years; then colonoscopy every 5 years, if no new lesions
Ulcerative colitis Crohn's colitis	At diagnosis; then after 8 years for pancolitis, after 15 years for left-sided colitis	Colonoscopy with multiple biopsies every 1–2 years
FAP	10–12 years	Annual flexible sigmoidoscopy Upper endoscopy every 1–3 years after polyps appear
Attenuated FAP	20 years	Annual flexible sigmoidoscopy Upper endoscopy every 1–3 years after polyps appear
HNPCC	20–25 years	Colonoscopy every 1–2 years Endometrial aspiration biopsy every 1–2 years
Familial colorectal cancer 1st degree relative	40 years or 10 years before the age of the youngest affected relative	Colonoscopy every 5 years Increase frequency if multiple family members are affected, especially before 50 years

SOURCES: Adopted from references 1, 49–51.

middle rectal vessels. Nodal spread along the inferior rectal vessels to the internal iliac nodes or groin is rare unless the tumor involves the anal canal or the proximal lymphatics are blocked with tumor (Fig. 28-23).

The most common site of distant metastasis from colorectal cancer is the liver. These metastases arise from hematogenous spread via the portal venous system. Like lymph node metastasis, the risk of hepatic metastasis increases with tumor size and tumor grade. However, even small tumors may produce distant metastasis. The lung is also a site of hematogenous spread for colorectal carcinoma. Pulmonary metastases rarely occur in isolation. Carcinomatosis (diffuse peritoneal metastases) occurs by peritoneal seeding and has a dismal prognosis.

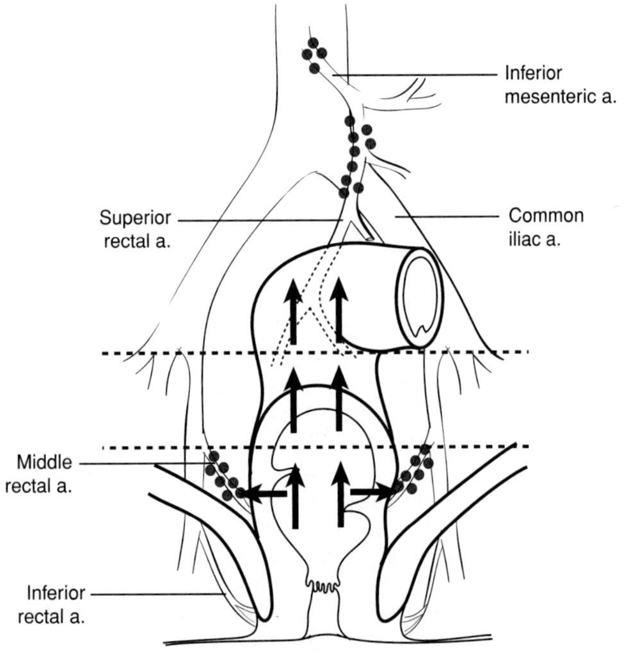

Staging and Preoperative Evaluation

Clinical Presentation

Symptoms of colon and rectal cancers are nonspecific and generally develop when the cancer is locally advanced. The classic first symptoms are a change in bowel habits and rectal bleeding. Abdominal pain, bloating, and other signs of obstruction typically occur with larger tumors and suggest more advanced disease. Because of the caliber of the bowel and the consistency of the stool, left-sided tumors are more likely to cause obstruction than are right-sided tumors. Rectal tumors may cause bleeding, tenesmus, and pain. Alternatively, patients may be asymptomatic and/or present with unexplained anemia, weight loss, or poor appetite.

Staging

Colorectal cancer staging is based upon tumor depth and the presence or absence of nodal or distant metastases. Older staging systems, such as the Dukes' Classification and its Astler-Coller modification, have been largely replaced by the TNM staging system (Table 28-3).[56] Stage I disease includes adenocarcinomas that are invasive through the muscularis mucosa but are confined to the submucosa (T1) or the muscularis propria (T2) in the absence of nodal metastases. Stage II disease consists of tumors that invade through the bowel wall into the subserosa or nonperitonealized pericolic or perirectal tissues (T3) or into other organs or tissues or through the

FIG. 28-23. Lymphatic drainage of the rectum. *[Reproduced with permission from Schwartz SI, Shires GT, Spencer FC (eds): Principles of Surgery. 5th ed. New York: McGraw-Hill, 1989, p 1232.]*

Table 28-3
TNM Staging of Colorectal Carcinoma

Tumor Stage (T)	Definition
Tx	Cannot be assessed
T0	No evidence of cancer
Tis	Carcinoma in situ
T1	Tumor invades submucosa
T2	Tumor invades muscularis propria
T3	Tumor invades through muscularis propria into subserosa or into nonperitonealized pericolic or perirectal tissues
T4	Tumor directly invades other organs or tissues or perforates the visceral peritoneum of specimen
Nodal Stage (N)	
NX	Regional lymph nodes cannot be assessed
N0	No lymph node metastasis
N1	Metastasis to one to three pericolic or perirectal lymph nodes
N2	Metastasis to four or more pericolic or perirectal lymph nodes
N3	Metastasis to any lymph node along a major named vascular trunk
Distant Metastasis (M)	
MX	Presence of distant metastasis cannot be assessed
M0	No distant metastasis
M1	Distant metastasis present

SOURCE: Adapted from Greene et al.[56]

visceral peritoneum (T4) without nodal metastases. Stage III disease includes any T stage with nodal metastases, and stage IV disease denotes distant metastases. The preoperative evaluation usually identifies stage IV disease. In colon cancer, differentiating stages I, II, and III depends upon examination of the resected specimen. In rectal cancer, endorectal ultrasound may predict the stage (ultrasound stage, uT_xN_x) preoperatively, but the final determination depends upon pathology examination of the resected tumor and adjacent lymph nodes (pathologic stage, pT_xN_x). Disease stage correlates with 5-year survival. Patients with stages I and II disease can expect excellent survival rates. The presence of nodal metastases (stage III) decreases survival to roughly 40% (Table 28-4). The 5-year survival rate with stage IV disease is less than 16%. While nodal involvement is the single most important prognostic factor in colorectal carcinoma, tumor characteristics, such as degree of differentiation, mucinous or signet-ring cell histology, vascular invasion, and DNA aneuploidy, also affect prognosis.

Preoperative Evaluation

Once a colon or rectal carcinoma has been diagnosed, a staging evaluation should be undertaken. The colon must be evaluated for synchronous tumors, usually by colonoscopy. Synchronous disease will be present in up to 5% of patients. For rectal cancers, digital rectal examination and rigid proctoscopy with biopsy should be done to assess tumor size, location, morphology, histology, and fixation. Endorectal ultrasound can be invaluable in staging rectal cancer

and is used to classify the ultrasound T and N stage of rectal cancers (Fig. 28-24). A chest x-ray and abdominal/pelvic CT scan should be obtained to evaluate for distant metastases. CT scan of the chest is only necessary if the chest x-ray is abnormal. Pelvic CT scan, and sometimes MRI, can be invaluable in large rectal tumors and in recurrent disease to determine the extent of local invasion. In patients with obstructive symptoms, a water-soluble contrast study (Gastrografin enema) may be useful for delineating the degree of obstruction. It is important to avoid mechanical bowel preparation (for either colonoscopy or surgery) in a patient who appears to be obstructed. PET scan may be useful in evaluating lesions seen on CT scan, and in patients in whom a risky or highly morbid operation is planned (pelvic exenteration, sacrectomy). Preoperative CEA is often obtained, and may be useful for postoperative follow-up.

Table 28-4
TNM Staging of Colorectal Carcinoma and 5-Year Survival

Stage	TNM	5-Year Survival
I	T1-2, N0, M0	70–95%
II	T3-4, N0, M0	54–65%
III	Tany, N1-3, M0	39–60%
IV	Tany, Nany, M1	0–16%

SOURCE: Adapted from Greene et al.[56]

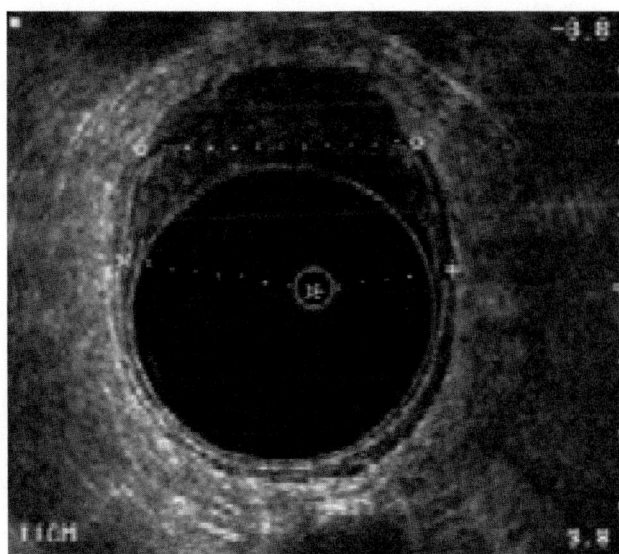

FIG. 28-24. Endorectal ultrasonography showing a T3 rectal carcinoma. The *dotted line* is being used to measure the diameter of the lesion. (*Courtesy of Charles O. Finne, III, M.D., Minneapolis, MN.*)

Therapy for Colonic Carcinoma

Principles of Resection

The objective in treatment of carcinoma of the colon is to remove the primary tumor along with its lymphovascular supply.[57] Because the lymphatics of the colon accompany the main arterial supply, the length of bowel resected depends upon which vessels are supplying the segment involved with the cancer. Any adjacent organ or tissue, such as the omentum that has been invaded, should be resected en bloc with the tumor. If all of the tumor cannot be removed, a palliative procedure should be considered.

The presence of synchronous cancers or adenomas or a strong family history of colorectal neoplasms suggests that the entire colon is at risk for carcinoma (often called a *field defect*) and a subtotal or total colectomy should be considered. Metachronous tumors (a *second primary colon cancer*) identified during follow-up studies should be treated similarly. However, the surgeon must be aware of which mesenteric vessels have been ligated at the initial colectomy because that may influence the choice of procedure.

If unexpected metastatic disease is encountered at the time of a laparotomy, the primary tumor should be resected, if technically feasible and safe. Consideration can be given to a primary anastomosis if the bowel appears healthy, is not involved in carcinomatosis, and the patient is stable. In the rare instance in which the primary tumor is not resectable, a palliative procedure can be performed and usually involves a proximal stoma or bypass. Hemorrhage in an unresectable tumor can sometimes be controlled with angiographic embolization.

Stage-Specific Therapy

Stage 0 (Tis, N0, M0). Polyps containing carcinoma in situ (high-grade dysplasia) carry no risk of lymph node metastasis. However, the presence of high-grade dysplasia increases the risk of finding an invasive carcinoma within the polyp. For this reason, these polyps should be excised completely and pathologic margins should be free of dysplasia. Most pedunculated polyps and many sessile polyps may be completely removed endoscopically. These patients should be followed with frequent colonoscopy to ensure that the polyp has not recurred and that an invasive carcinoma has not developed. In cases where the polyp cannot be removed entirely, a segmental resection is recommended.

Stage I: The Malignant Polyp (T1, N0, M0). Occasionally a polyp that was thought to be benign will be found to harbor invasive carcinoma after polypectomy. Treatment of a *malignant polyp* is based upon the risk of local recurrence and the risk of lymph node metastasis.[58] The risk of lymph node metastases depends primarily upon the depth of invasion. Invasive carcinoma in the head of a pedunculated polyp with no stalk involvement carries a low risk of metastasis (<1%) and may be completely resected endoscopically. However, lymphovascular invasion, poorly differentiated histology, or tumor within 1 mm of the resection margin greatly increases the risk of local recurrence and metastatic spread. Segmental colectomy is then indicated. Invasive carcinoma arising in a sessile polyp extends into the submucosa and is usually best treated with segmental colectomy (Fig. 28-25).

Stages I and II: Localized Colon Carcinoma (T1-3, N0, M0). The majority of patients with stages I and II colon cancer will be cured with surgical resection. Few patients with completely resected stage I disease will develop either local or distant recurrence, and adjuvant chemotherapy does not improve survival in these

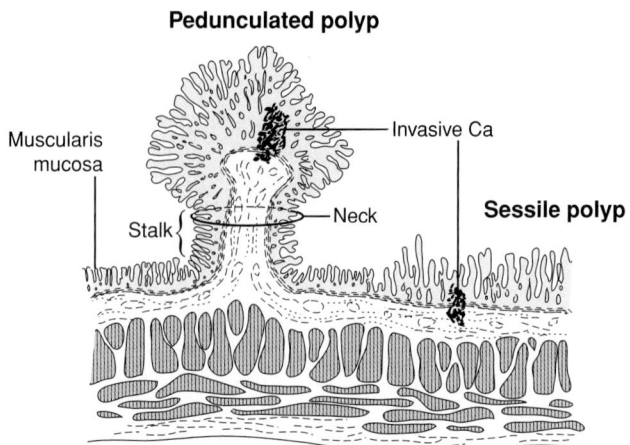

Pedunculated polyp

Muscularis mucosa — Invasive Ca — Neck — **Sessile polyp** — Stalk

FIG. 28-25. *Levels of invasive carcinoma in pedunculated and sessile polyps. [Reproduced with permission from Schwartz SI, Shires GT, Spencer FC (eds): Principles of Surgery. 5th ed. New York: McGraw-Hill, 1989, p 1266.]*

patients. However, up to 46% of patients with completely resected stage II disease will ultimately die from colon cancer. For this reason, adjuvant chemotherapy has been suggested for selected patients with stage II disease (young patients, tumors with "high-risk" histologic findings). Data is controversial as to whether chemotherapy improves survival rates in these patients. Improved staging to detect micrometastases and/or more sensitive prognostic tumor markers may improve patient selection for adjuvant therapy.

Stage III: Lymph Node Metastasis (Tany, N1, M0). Patients with lymph node involvement are at significant risk for both local and distant recurrence, and adjuvant chemotherapy has been recommended routinely in these patients. 5-Fluorouracil–based regimens (with levamisole or leucovorin) reduce recurrences and improve survival in this patient population.[59] Newer chemotherapeutic agents such as capecitabine, irinotecan, oxaliplatin, angiogenesis inhibitors, and immunotherapy also show promise.

Stage IV: Distant Metastasis (Tany, Nany, M1). Survival is extremely limited in stage IV colon carcinoma. Of patients with systemic disease, approximately 15% will have metastases limited to the liver. Of these, 20% are potentially resectable for cure. Survival is improved in these patients (20 to 40% 5-year survival) when compared to patients who do not undergo resection. Hepatic resection of synchronous metastases from colorectal carcinoma may be performed as a combined procedure or in two stages. All patients require adjuvant chemotherapy.

The remainder of patients with stage IV disease cannot be cured surgically and therefore the focus of treatment should be palliation. Many of these patients will require colon resection because of symptoms (primarily hemorrhage or obstruction). Methods such as colonic stenting for obstructing lesions of the left colon also provide good palliation. Some patients will respond to chemotherapy in this setting, but cure is rare.

Therapy for Rectal Carcinoma

Principles of Resection

The biology of rectal adenocarcinoma is identical to the biology of colonic adenocarcinoma, and the operative principles of complete resection of the primary tumor, its lymphatic bed, and any other involved organ apply to surgical resection of rectal carcinoma.

However, the anatomy of the pelvis and proximity of other structures (ureters, bladder, prostate, vagina, iliac vessels, and sacrum) make resection more challenging and often require a different approach than for colonic adenocarcinoma. Moreover, it is more difficult to achieve negative radial margins in rectal cancers that extend through the bowel wall because of the anatomic limitations of the pelvis.[60] Therefore, local recurrence is higher than with similar stage colon cancers. However, unlike the intraperitoneal colon, the relative paucity of small bowel and other radiation-sensitive structures in the pelvis makes it easier to treat rectal tumors with radiation. Therapeutic decisions, therefore, are based upon the location and depth of the tumor and its relationship to other structures in the pelvis.

Local Therapy

The distal 10 cm of the rectum are accessible transanally. For this reason, several local approaches have been proposed for treating rectal neoplasms. *Transanal excision* (full thickness or mucosal) is an excellent approach for noncircumferential, benign, villous adenomas of the rectum. Although this technique can be used for selected T1, and possibly some T2, carcinomas, local excision does not allow pathologic examination of the lymph nodes and might therefore understage patients. Local recurrence rates are high without the addition of adjuvant chemoradiation therapy.[61] *Transanal endoscopic microsurgery (TEM)* makes use of a specially designed proctoscope, magnifying system, and instruments similar to those used in laparoscopy to allow local excision of lesions higher in the rectum (up to 15 cm). Local excision of any rectal neoplasm should be considered an *excisional biopsy* because final pathologic examination of the specimen may reveal an invasive carcinoma that then mandates more radical therapy.

Ablative techniques, such as electrocautery or endocavitary radiation, have also been used. The disadvantage of these techniques is that no pathologic specimen is retrieved to confirm the tumor stage. Fulguration is generally reserved for extremely high-risk patients with a limited life span who cannot tolerate more radical surgery.

Radical Resection

Radical resection is preferred to local therapy for most rectal carcinomas. Radical resection involves removal of the involved segment of the rectum along with its lymphovascular supply. A 2-cm, distal mural margin is sought for curative resections.

Total mesorectal excision (TME) is a technique that uses sharp dissection along anatomic planes to ensure complete resection of the rectal mesentery during low and extended low anterior resections.[62] For upper rectal or rectosigmoid resections, a partial mesorectal excision of at least 5 cm distal to the tumor appears adequate. Total mesorectal excision both decreases local recurrence rates and improves long-term survival rates. Moreover, this technique is associated with less blood loss and less risk to the pelvic nerves and presacral plexus than is blunt dissection. The principles of total mesorectal excision should be applied to all radical resections for rectal cancer.

Recurrence of rectal cancer generally has a poor prognosis.[63,64] Extensive involvement of other pelvic organs (usually occurring in the setting of tumor recurrence) may require a *pelvic exenteration*. The rectal and perineal portions of this operation are similar to an abdominoperineal resection but en bloc resection of the ureters, bladder, and prostate or uterus and vagina are also performed. A permanent colostomy and an ileal conduit to drain the urinary tract may be necessary. The sacrum may also be resected if necessary

(sacrectomy) up to the level of the S2-S3 junction. These operations are best performed in tertiary centers with multidisciplinary teams consisting of a colon and rectal surgeon, urologist, neurosurgeon, and plastic surgeon.

Stage-Specific Therapy

Pretreatment staging of rectal carcinoma often relies on endorectal ultrasound to determine the T and N status of a rectal cancer.[65] Ultrasound is highly accurate at assessing tumor depth, but less accurate in diagnosing nodal involvement.[3] Ultrasound evaluation can guide choice of therapy in most patients.

Stage 0 (Tis, N0, M0). Villous adenomas harboring carcinoma in situ (high-grade dysplasia) are ideally treated with local excision. A 1-cm margin should be obtained. Rarely, radical resection will be necessary if transanal excision is not technically possible (large circumferential lesions).

Stage I: Localized Rectal Carcinoma (T1-2, N0, M0). Invasive carcinoma confined to the head of a pedunculated polyp carries a very low risk of metastasis (<1%). Polypectomy with clear margins is appropriate therapy. Although local excision has been used for small, favorable sessile uT1N0 and uT2N0 rectal cancers, local recurrence rates may be as high as 20 and 40%, respectively.[61] For this reason, radical resection is strongly recommended in all good-risk patients. Lesions with unfavorable histologic characteristics and those located in the distal third of the rectum, in particular, are prone to recurrence. In high-risk patients and in those patients who refuse radical surgery because of the risk of need for a permanent colostomy, local excision may be adequate, but strong consideration should be given to adjuvant chemoradiation to improve local control.

Stage II: Localized Rectal Carcinoma (T3-4, N0, M0). Larger rectal tumors are more likely to recur locally. There are two schools of thought, each differing in their approach to control local recurrences. Advocates of total mesorectal resection suggest that optimization of operative technique will obviate the need for any adjuvant chemoradiation to control local recurrence after resection of stages I, II, and III rectal cancers. The opposing school suggests that stages II and III rectal cancers will benefit from chemoradiation. They argue that such therapy reduces local recurrences and prolongs survival whether given preoperatively or postoperatively. The advantages of preoperative chemoradiation include tumor shrinkage, increased likelihood of resection and of a sphincter-sparing procedure, tumor downstaging by treating locally involved lymph nodes, and decreased risk to the small intestine. Disadvantages include possible overtreatment of early stage tumors, impaired wound healing, and pelvic fibrosis increasing the risk of operative complications. Postoperative radiation allows accurate pathologic staging of the resected tumor and lymph nodes, and avoids the wound healing problems associated with preoperative radiation. However, bulky tumors, tumors involving adjacent organs, and very low rectal tumors may be much more difficult to resect without preoperative radiation and may require a more extensive operation. Patients with T4 lesions probably benefit from neoadjuvant therapy followed by radical resection of the tumor and all other involved organs.

Stage III: Lymph Node Metastasis (T*any*, N1, M0). Many surgeons now recommend chemotherapy and radiation either pre- or postoperatively for node-positive rectal cancers. The advantages and disadvantages are similar to those listed for stage II disease, except that the likelihood of overtreating an early stage lesion is considerably less. For this reason, most patients currently receive neoadjuvant therapy followed by radical resection. Some surgeons believe that radical surgery with total mesorectal excision negates the need for chemoradiation to achieve local control.

Stage IV: Distant Metastasis (Tany, Nany, M1). Like stage IV colon carcinoma, survival is limited in patients with distant metastasis from rectal carcinoma. Isolated hepatic metastases are rare, but when present may be resected for cure in selected patients. Most patients will require palliative procedures. Radical resection may be required to control pain, bleeding, or tenesmus, but highly morbid procedures such as pelvic exenteration and sacrectomy should generally be avoided in this setting. Local therapy using cautery, endocavitary radiation, or laser ablation may be adequate to control bleeding or prevent obstruction. Intraluminal stents may be useful in the uppermost rectum, but often cause pain and tenesmus lower in the rectum. Occasionally, a proximal diverting colostomy will be required to alleviate obstruction. A mucus fistula should be created if possible to vent the distal colon.

Follow-Up and Surveillance

Patients who have been treated for one colorectal cancer are at risk for the development of recurrent disease (either locally or systemically) or metachronous disease (a second primary tumor). In theory, metachronous cancers should be preventable by using surveillance colonoscopy to detect and remove polyps before they progress to invasive cancer. For most patients, a colonoscopy should be performed within 12 months after the diagnosis of the original cancer (or sooner if the colon was not examined in its entirety prior to the original resection). If that study is normal, colonoscopy should be repeated every 3 to 5 years thereafter.

The optimal method of following patients for recurrent cancer remains controversial.[66,67] The goal of close follow-up observation is to *detect resectable recurrence* and to *improve survival*. Re-resection of local recurrence and resection of distant metastasis to liver, lung, or other sites is often technically challenging and highly morbid, with only a limited chance of achieving long-term survival. Thus, only selected patients who would tolerate such an approach should be followed intensively. Because most recurrences occur within 2 years of the original diagnosis, surveillance focuses on this time period. Patients who have undergone local resection of rectal tumors should probably also be followed with frequent endorectal ultrasound examinations (every 4 months for 3 years, then every 6 months for 2 years). The role of endorectal ultrasound after radical resection is less clear. CEA is often followed every 2 to 3 months for 2 years. CT scans are not routinely employed, but may be useful if CEA is elevated. More intensive surveillance is appropriate in high-risk patients such as those with possible HNPCC syndrome or T3 N+ cancers. Although intensive surveillance improves detection of resectable recurrences, it is important to note that a survival benefit has never been proven. Therefore, the risks and benefits of intensive surveillance must be weighed and treatment individualized.

Treatment of Recurrent Colorectal Carcinoma

Between 20 and 40% of patients who have undergone curative intent surgery for colorectal carcinoma will eventually develop recurrent disease. Most recurrences occur within the first 2 years after the initial diagnosis, but preoperative chemoradiation therapy may delay recurrence. While most of these patients will present with distant metastases, a small proportion will have isolated local recurrence and may be considered for *salvage surgery*. Recurrence after colon cancer resection usually occurs at the local site within the abdomen

or in the liver or lungs. Resection of other involved organs may be necessary. Recurrence of rectal cancer can be considerably more difficult to manage because of the proximity of other pelvic structures. If the patient has not received chemotherapy and radiation, then adjuvant therapy should be administered prior to salvage surgery. Radical resection may require extensive resection of pelvic organs (pelvic exenteration with or without sacrectomy). Pelvic MRI is useful for identifying tumor extension that would prevent successful resection (extension of tumor into the pelvic sidewall, involvement of the iliac vessels or bilateral sacral nerves, sacral invasion above the S2-S3 junction). Patients should also undergo a thorough preoperative evaluation to identify distant metastases (CT of chest, abdomen, and pelvis, and PET scan) before undergoing such an extensive procedure. Nevertheless, radical salvage surgery can prolong survival in selected patients.

Sentinel Lymph Node Biopsy for Colorectal Carcinoma

The technique of sentinel lymph node biopsy has been applied to a number of malignancies and is commonly employed in both breast cancer and melanoma. The goal of sentinel lymph node biopsy is to identify the first node(s) in the lymphatic basin, because this site should be most likely to harbor metastases. Unlike sentinel lymph node biopsy in breast cancer and melanoma, the goal of this technique in colorectal carcinoma is not to avoid radical lymphadenectomy, but instead to improve staging.[68] Intensive pathologic examination of the sentinel node(s) with multiple histologic sections, immunohistochemistry, and reverse-transcriptase polymerase chain reaction (RT-PCR) can detect micrometastases in a significant number of patients who were thought to be node-negative by conventional techniques. These patients may then be candidates for further adjuvant treatment. However, whether this increased sensitivity will translate into improved survival remains to be seen.

Laparoscopic Resection for Cancer

Laparoscopic technology has advanced rapidly over the past two decades and many centers are now performing laparoscopic or laparoscopically assisted colon resections. The applicability of this technology to colorectal cancer, however, remains controversial. Early experience with port-site recurrence has led to reluctance to adopt these techniques; however, greater experience shows that these recurrences are no more common than wound recurrences after open colectomy. There is also an increasing body of experimental data to suggest that minimally invasive operations have less immunosuppressive impact on the patient and thus might improve postoperative outcome. Although a few studies show equivalence in resection margins and node retrieval, few prospective studies exist and long-term follow up is not yet available.[69,70]

OTHER NEOPLASMS

Rare Colorectal Tumors

Carcinoid Tumors

Carcinoid tumors occur most commonly in the gastrointestinal tract and up to 25% of these tumors are found in the rectum. Most small rectal carcinoids are benign, and overall survival is greater than 80%. However, the risk of malignancy increases with size, and more than 60% of tumors greater than 2 cm in diameter are associated with distant metastases. Interestingly, rectal carcinoids appear to be less likely to secrete vasoactive substances than carcinoids in other locations, and carcinoid syndrome is uncommon in the absence of hepatic metastases. Small carcinoids can be locally resected, either transanally or using transanal endoscopic microsurgery. Larger tumors or tumors with obvious invasion into the muscularis require more radical surgery. Carcinoid tumors in the proximal colon are less common and are more likely to be malignant. Size also correlates with risk of malignancy, and tumors less than 2 cm in diameter rarely metastasize. However, the majority of carcinoid tumors in the proximal colon present as bulky lesions and up to two-thirds will have metastatic spread at the time of diagnosis. These tumors should usually be treated with radical resection. Because carcinoid tumors are typically slow growing, patients with distant metastases may expect reasonably long survival. Symptoms of carcinoid syndrome can often be alleviated with somatostatin analogues (octreotide) and/or interferon-α. Tumor debulking can offer effective palliation in selected patients.

Carcinoid Carcinomas

Composite carcinoid carcinomas (adenocarcinoids) have histologic features of both carcinoid tumors and adenocarcinomas. The natural history of these tumors more closely parallels that of adenocarcinomas than carcinoid tumors, and regional and systemic metastases are common. Carcinoid carcinoma of the colon and rectum should be treated according to the same oncologic principles as followed for management of adenocarcinoma.

Lipomas

Lipomas occur most commonly in the submucosa of the colon and rectum. They are benign lesions, but rarely may cause bleeding, obstruction, or intussusception, especially when greater than 2 cm in diameter. Small asymptomatic lesions do not require resection. Larger lipomas should be resected by colonoscopic techniques or by a colotomy and enucleation or limited colectomy.

Lymphoma

Lymphoma involving the colon and rectum is rare, but accounts for about 10% of all gastrointestinal lymphomas. The cecum is most often involved, probably as a result of spread from the terminal ileum. Symptoms include bleeding and obstruction, and these tumors may be clinically indistinguishable from adenocarcinomas. Bowel resection is the treatment of choice. Adjuvant therapy may be given based upon the stage of disease.

Leiomyoma and Leiomyosarcoma

Leiomyomas are benign tumors of the smooth muscle of the bowel wall and occur most commonly in the upper gastrointestinal tract. Most patients are asymptomatic, but large lesions can cause bleeding or obstruction. Because it is difficult to differentiate a benign leiomyoma from a malignant leiomyosarcoma, these lesions should be resected. Recurrence is common after local resection, but most small leiomyomas can be adequately treated with limited resection. Lesions larger than 5 cm should be treated with radical resection because the risk of malignancy is high.

Leiomyosarcoma is rare in the gastrointestinal tract. When this malignancy occurs in the large intestine, the rectum is the most common site. Symptoms include bleeding and obstruction. A radical resection is indicated for these tumors.

Retrorectal Tumors

Tumors occurring in the retrorectal space are rare. This region lies between the upper two-thirds of the rectum and the sacrum above the rectosacral fascia. It is bound by the rectum anteriorly, the presacral fascia posteriorly, and the endopelvic fascia laterally (lateral ligaments). The retrorectal space contains multiple embryologic remnants derived from a variety of tissues (neuroectoderm, notochord, and hindgut). Tumors that develop in this space are often heterogeneous.

Congenital lesions are most common, comprising almost two-thirds of retrorectal lesions. The remainder is classified as neurogenic, osseous, inflammatory, or miscellaneous lesions. Malignancy is more common in the pediatric population than in adults, and solid lesions are more likely to be malignant than are cystic lesions. Inflammatory lesions may be solid or cystic (abscess) and usually represent extensions of infection either in the perirectal space or in the abdomen.

Developmental cysts constitute the majority of congenital lesions and may arise from all three germ cell layers. Dermoid and epidermoid cysts are benign lesions that arise from the ectoderm. Enterogenous cysts arise from the primitive gut. Anterior meningocele and myelomeningocele arise from herniation of the dural sac through a defect in the anterior sacrum. A "scimitar sign" (sacrum with a rounded, concave border without any bony destruction) is the pathognomonic radiographic appearance of this condition.

Solid lesions include teratomas, chordomas, neurologic tumors, or osseus lesions. Teratomas are true neoplasms and contain tissue from each germ cell layer. They often contain both cystic and solid components. Teratomas are more common in children than in adults, but when found in adults, 30% are malignant. Chordomas arise from the notochord and are the most common malignant tumor in this region. These are slow-growing, invasive cancers that show characteristic bony destruction. Neurogenic tumors include neurofibromas and sarcomas, neurilemomas, ependymomas, and ganglioneuromas. Osseous lesions include osteomas and bone cysts, as well as neoplasms such as osteogenic sarcoma, Ewing's tumor, chondromyxosarcoma, and giant cell tumors.

Patients may present with pain (lower back, pelvic, or lower extremity), gastrointestinal symptoms, or urinary tract symptoms. Most lesions are palpable on digital rectal examination. While plain x-rays and CT scans are often used to evaluate these lesions, pelvic MRI is the most sensitive and specific imaging study. Myelogram is occasionally necessary if there is central nervous system involvement. Biopsy is not indicated, especially if the lesion appears to be resectable, because of the risk of infection and/or tumor seeding. Treatment is almost always surgical resection. The approach depends in part upon the nature of the lesion and its location. High lesions may be approached via a transabdominal route, whereas low lesions may be resected transsacrally. Intermediate lesions may require a combined abdominal and sacral operation.

Anal Canal and Perianal Tumors

Cancers of the anal canal are uncommon and account for approximately 2% of all colorectal malignancies. Neoplasms of the anal canal can be divided into those affecting the *anal margin* (distal to the dentate line) and those affecting the *anal canal* (proximal to the dentate line). Lymphatics from the anal canal proximal to the dentate line drain cephalad via the superior rectal lymphatics to the inferior mesenteric nodes and laterally along both the middle rectal vessels and inferior rectal vessels through the ischiorectal fossa to the internal iliac nodes. Lymph from the anal canal distal to the dentate line usually drains to the inguinal nodes. It can also drain to the superior rectal lymph nodes or along the inferior rectal lymphatics to the ischiorectal fossa if primary drainage routes are blocked with

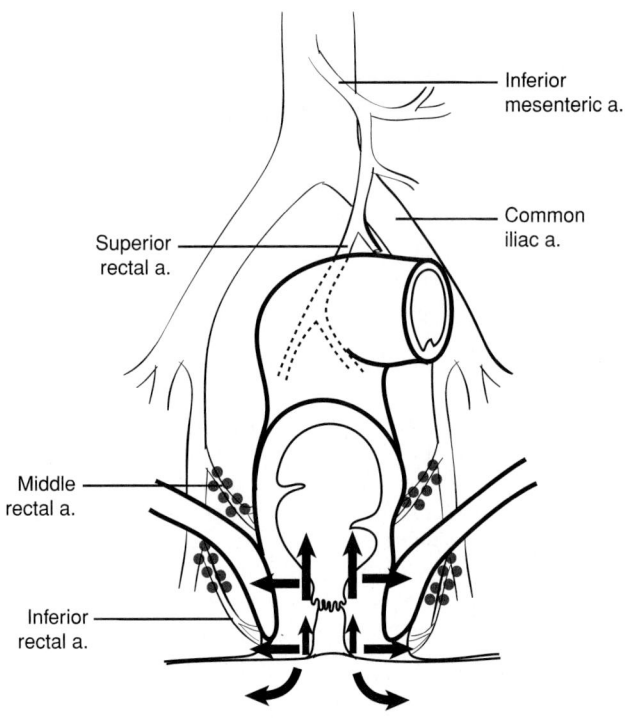

FIG. 28-26. Lymphatic drainage of the anal canal. *[Reproduced with permission from Schwartz SI, Shires GT, Spencer FC (eds): Principles of Surgery. 5th ed. New York: McGraw-Hill, 1989, p 1232.]*

tumor (Fig. 28-26). In many cases, therapy depends upon whether the tumor is located in the anal canal or at the anal margin.[71–73]

Anal Intraepithelial Neoplasia (Bowen's Disease)

Bowen's disease refers to squamous cell carcinoma in situ of the anus. Pathologically, carcinomas in situ and high-grade squamous intraepithelial dysplasia appear identical, and the term *anal intraepithelial neoplasia (AIN)* has recently been used to describe these lesions. Like cervical intraepithelial neoplasia (CIN), AIN is a precursor to an invasive squamous cell carcinoma (epidermoid carcinoma). AIN may appear as a plaque-like lesion, or may only be apparent with high-resolution anoscopy and application of acetic acid or Lugol's iodine solution. AIN is associated with infection with the human papilloma virus, especially HPV types 16 and 18. The incidence of both AIN and epidermoid carcinoma of the anus has increased dramatically among HIV-positive, homosexual men. This increase is thought to result from increased rates of HPV infection along with immunosuppression. Treatment of AIN is aimed at either *resection* or *ablation*. Extensive resection with flap closure may occasionally be required. Because of a high recurrence and/or reinfection rate, these patients require extremely close surveillance. High-risk patients should be followed with frequent anal Papanicolaou (Pap) smears every 3 to 6 months. An abnormal Pap smear should be followed by an examination under anesthesia and anal mapping using high-resolution anoscopy, biopsy, and ablation of dysplastic lesions.

Epidermoid Carcinoma

Epidermoid carcinoma of the anus includes squamous cell carcinoma, cloacogenic carcinoma, transitional carcinoma, and basaloid carcinoma.[74] The clinical behavior and natural history of these tumors is similar. Epidermoid carcinoma is a slow-growing tumor,

and usually presents as an anal or perianal mass. Pain and bleeding may be present. Epidermoid carcinoma of the anal margin may be treated in a similar fashion as squamous cell carcinoma of the skin in other locations because adequate surgical margins can usually be achieved without resecting the anal sphincter. Wide local excision is usually adequate treatment for these lesions. Epidermoid carcinoma occurring in the anal canal or invading the sphincter cannot be excised locally, and first-line therapy relies upon chemotherapy and radiation (the *Nigro protocol:* 5-fluorouracil, mitomycin C, and 3000 cGy external beam radiation). More than 80% of these tumors can be cured by using this regimen. Recurrence usually requires radical resection (abdominoperineal resection). Metastasis to inguinal lymph nodes is a poor prognostic sign.

Verrucous Carcinoma (Buschke-Lowenstein Tumor, Giant Condyloma Acuminata)

Verrucous carcinoma is a locally aggressive form of condyloma acuminata. Although these lesions do not metastasize, they can cause extensive local tissue destruction and may be grossly indistinguishable from epidermoid carcinoma. Wide local excision is the treatment of choice when possible, but radical resection may sometimes be required.

Basal Cell Carcinoma

Basal cell carcinoma of the anus is rare and resembles basal cell carcinoma elsewhere on the skin (raised, pearly edges with central ulceration). This is a slow-growing tumor that rarely metastasizes. Wide local excision is the treatment of choice, but recurrence occurs in up to 30% of patients. Radical resection and/or radiation therapy may be required for large lesions.

Adenocarcinoma

Adenocarcinoma of the anus is extremely rare, and usually represents downward spread of a low rectal adenocarcinoma. Adenocarcinoma may occasionally arise from the anal glands or may develop in a chronic fistula.[75] Radical resection with or without adjuvant chemoradiation is usually required.

Extramammary perianal *Paget's disease* is *adenocarcinoma in situ* arising from the apocrine glands of the perianal area. The lesion is typically plaque-like and may be indistinguishable from Bowen's disease. Characteristic *Paget's cells* are seen histologically. These tumors are often associated with a synchronous gastrointestinal adenocarcinoma, so a complete evaluation of the intestinal tract should be performed. Wide local excision is usually adequate treatment for perianal Paget's disease.

Melanoma

Anorectal melanoma is rare, comprising less than 1% of all anorectal malignancies and 1 to 2% of melanomas.[76,77] Despite many advances in the treatment of melanoma, prognosis for patients with anorectal disease remains poor. Overall 5-year survival is less than 10%, and many patients present with systemic metastasis and/or deeply invasive tumors at the time of diagnosis. A few patients with anorectal melanoma, however, present with isolated local or locoregional disease that is potentially resectable for cure, and both radical resection (abdominoperineal resection [APR]) and wide local excision have been advocated. Recurrence is common and usually occurs systemically regardless of the initial surgical procedure. Local resection with free margins does not increase the risk of local or regional recurrence and APR offers no survival advantage over local excision. Because of the morbidity associated with

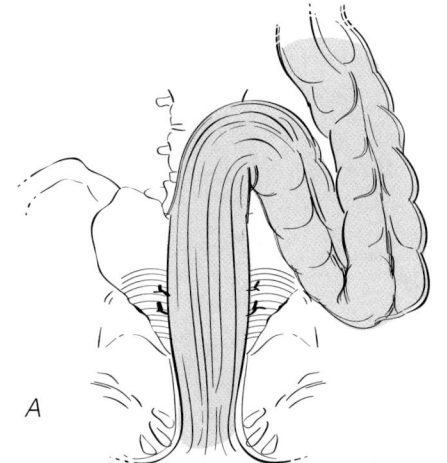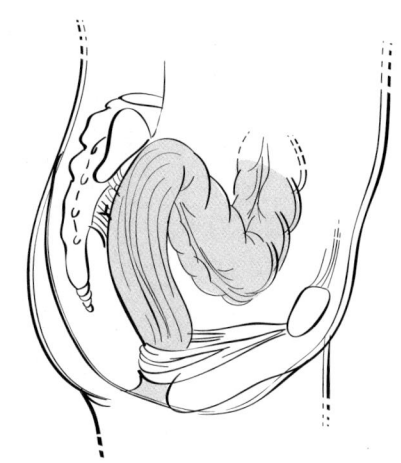

FIG. 28-27. Transabdominal proctopexy for rectal prolapse. The fully mobilized rectum is sutured to the presacral fascia. A. Anterior view. (B) Lateral view. If desired, a sigmoid colectomy can be performed concomitantly to resect the redundant colon. [Reproduced with permission from Schwartz SI, Shires GT, Spencer FC (eds): Principles of Surgery. 5th ed. New York: McGraw-Hill, 1989, p 1295.]

APR, wide local excision is recommended for initial treatment of localized anal melanoma. In some patients, wide local excision may not be technically feasible and APR may be required if the tumor involves a significant portion of the anal sphincter or is circumferential. The addition of adjuvant chemotherapy, biochemotherapy, vaccines, or radiotherapy may be of benefit in some patients, but efficacy remains unproven.

OTHER BENIGN COLORECTAL CONDITIONS

Rectal Prolapse and Solitary Rectal Ulcer Syndrome

Rectal Prolapse

Rectal prolapse refers to a circumferential, full-thickness protrusion of the rectum through the anus and has also been called "first-degree" prolapse, "complete" prolapse, or procidentia.[78] Internal prolapse occurs when the rectal wall intussuscepts but does not protrude, and is probably more accurately described as internal intussusception. Mucosal prolapse is a partial-thickness protrusion often associated with hemorrhoidal disease and is usually treated with banding or hemorrhoidectomy.

In adults, this condition is far more common among women, with a female:male ratio of 6:1. Prolapse becomes more prevalent with age in women and peaks in the seventh decade of life. In men, prevalence is unrelated to age. Symptoms include tenesmus, a sensation of tissue protruding from the anus that may or may not spontaneously reduce, and a sensation of incomplete evacuation. Mucus discharge and leakage may accompany the protrusion. Patients also present with a myriad of functional complaints, from incontinence and diarrhea to constipation and outlet obstruction.

A thorough preoperative evaluation, including colonic transit studies, anorectal manometry, tests of pudendal nerve terminal motor latency, electromyography, and cinedefecography, may be useful. The colon should be evaluated by colonoscopy or air-contrast barium enema to exclude neoplasms or diverticular disease. Cardiopulmonary condition should be thoroughly evaluated because comorbidities may influence the choice of surgical procedure.

The primary therapy for rectal prolapse is surgery and more than 100 different procedures have been described to treat this condition. Operations can be categorized as either *abdominal* or *perineal*. Abdominal operations have taken three major approaches: (a) reduction of the perineal hernia and closure of the cul-de-sac (*Moschowitz*

repair); (b) fixation of the rectum, either with a prosthetic sling (*Ripsten* and *Wells rectopexy*) or by *suture rectopexy;* or (c) resection of redundant sigmoid colon (Fig. 28-27). In some cases, resection is combined with rectal fixation (*resection rectopexy*). Abdominal rectopexy with or without resection is also increasingly performed laparoscopically. Perineal approaches have focused upon tightening the anus with a variety of prosthetic materials, reefing the rectal mucosa (*Delorme procedure*), or resecting the prolapsed bowel from the perineum (*perineal rectosigmoidectomy* or *Altemeier procedure*) (Fig. 28-28).

Because rectal prolapse occurs most commonly in elderly women, the choice of operation depends in part upon the patient's overall medical condition. Abdominal rectopexy (with or without sigmoid resection) offers the most durable repair, with recurrence occurring in fewer than 10% of patients. Perineal rectosigmoidectomy avoids an abdominal operation and may be preferable in high-risk patients, but is associated with a higher recurrence rate. Reefing the rectal mucosa is effective for patients with limited prolapse. Anal encirclement procedures have generally been abandoned.

Solitary Rectal Ulcer Syndrome

Solitary rectal ulcer syndrome and colitis cystica profunda are commonly associated with internal intussusception. Patients may complain of pain, bleeding, mucus discharge, or outlet obstruction. In solitary rectal ulcer syndrome, one or more ulcers are present in the distal rectum, usually on the anterior wall. In colitis cystica profunda, nodules or a mass may be found in a similar location. Evaluation should include anorectal manometry, defecography, and either colonoscopy or barium enema to exclude other diagnoses. Biopsy of an ulcer or mass is mandatory to exclude malignancy. Nonoperative therapy (high-fiber diet, defecation training to avoid straining, and laxatives or enemas) is effective in the majority of patients. Surgery (either abdominal or perineal repair of prolapse as described above) is reserved for highly symptomatic patients who have failed all medical interventions.

Volvulus

Volvulus occurs when an air-filled segment of the colon twists about its mesentery. The sigmoid colon is involved in up to 90% of cases, but volvulus can involve the cecum (<20%) or transverse colon. A volvulus may reduce spontaneously, but more commonly produces bowel obstruction, which can progress to strangulation, gangrene, and perforation. Chronic constipation may produce a large,

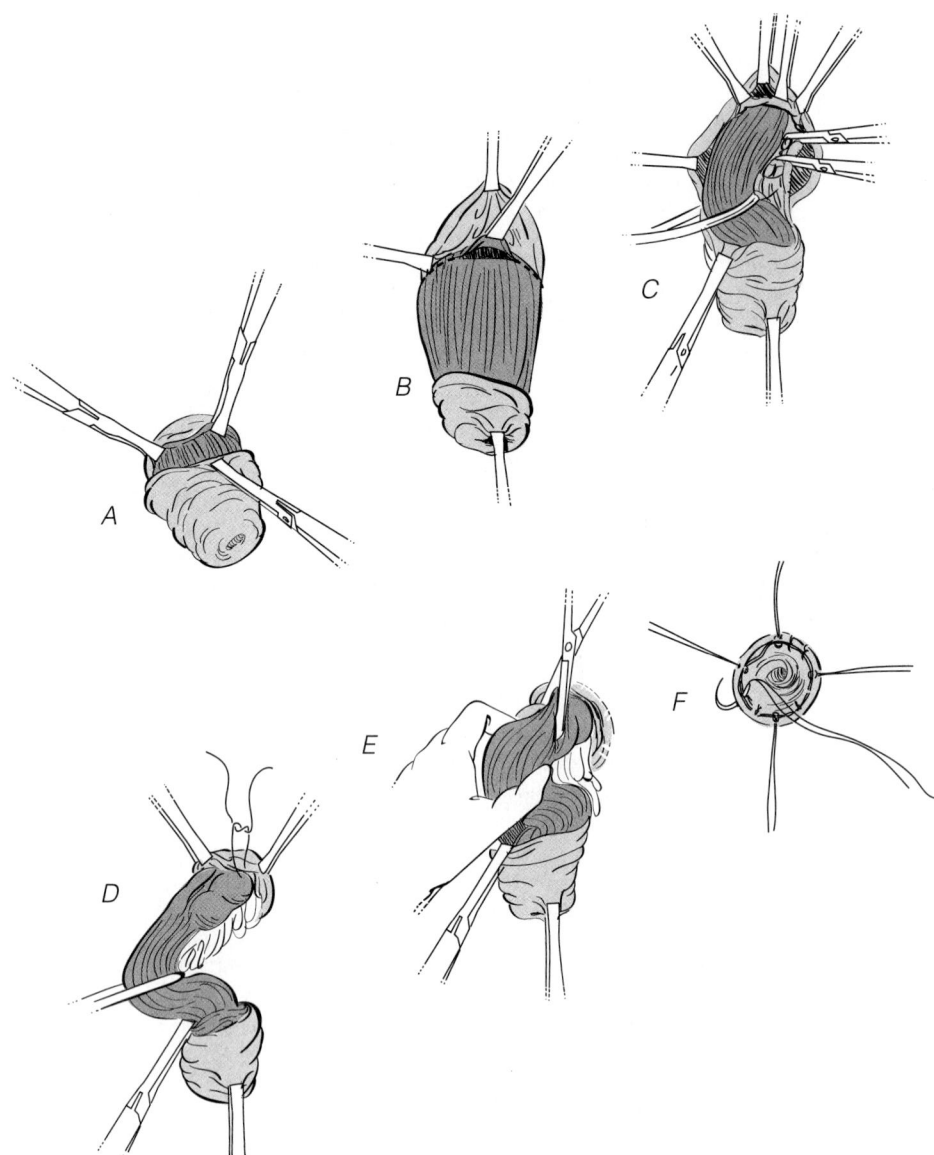

FIG. 28-28. Perineal rectosigmoidectomy shown in lithotomy position. *A.* A circular incision is made 2 cm proximal to the dentate line. *B.* The anterior peritoneal reflection is opened. *C.* The mesentery is divided and ligated. *D.* The peritoneum may be sutured to the bowel wall. *E.* The bowel is resected. *F.* A handsewn anastomosis is performed. [*Reproduced with permission from Schwartz SI, Shires GT, Spencer FC (eds): Principles of Surgery. 5th ed. New York: McGraw-Hill, 1989, p 1295.*]

redundant colon (*chronic megacolon*) that predisposes to volvulus, especially if the mesenteric base is narrow.

The symptoms of volvulus are those of acute bowel obstruction. Patients present with abdominal distention, nausea, and vomiting. Symptoms rapidly progress to generalized abdominal pain and tenderness. Fever and leukocytosis are heralds of gangrene and/or perforation. Occasionally, patients will report a long history of intermittent obstructive symptoms and distention, suggesting intermittent chronic volvulus.

Sigmoid Volvulus

Sigmoid volvulus can often be differentiated from cecal or transverse colon volvulus by the appearance of plain x-rays of the abdomen. Sigmoid volvulus produces a characteristic *bent inner tube* or *coffee bean* appearance, with the convexity of the loop lying in the right upper quadrant (opposite the site of obstruction). Gastrografin enema shows a narrowing at the site of the volvulus and a pathognomonic *bird's beak* (Fig. 28-29).

Unless there are obvious signs of gangrene or peritonitis, the initial management of sigmoid volvulus is resuscitation followed

by endoscopic detorsion. Detorsion is usually most easily accomplished by using a rigid proctoscope, but a flexible sigmoidoscope or colonoscope might also be effective. A rectal tube may be inserted to maintain decompression. Although these techniques are successful in reducing sigmoid volvulus in the majority of patients, the risk of recurrence is high (40%). For this reason, an elective sigmoid colectomy should be performed after the patient has been stabilized and undergone an adequate bowel preparation.

Clinical evidence of gangrene or perforation mandates immediate surgical exploration without an attempt at endoscopic decompression. Similarly, the presence of necrotic mucosa, ulceration, or dark blood noted on endoscopy examination suggests strangulation and is an indication for operation. If dead bowel is present at laparotomy, a sigmoid colectomy with end colostomy (Hartmann procedure) may be the safest operation to perform.

Cecal Volvulus

Cecal volvulus results from nonfixation of the right colon. Rotation occurs around the ileocolic blood vessels and vascular impairment occurs early. Plain x-rays of the abdomen show a characteristic

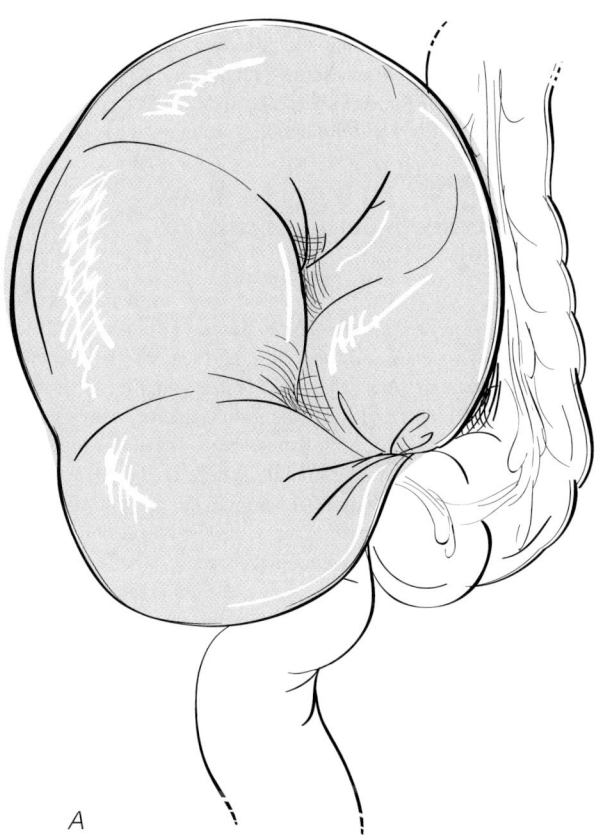 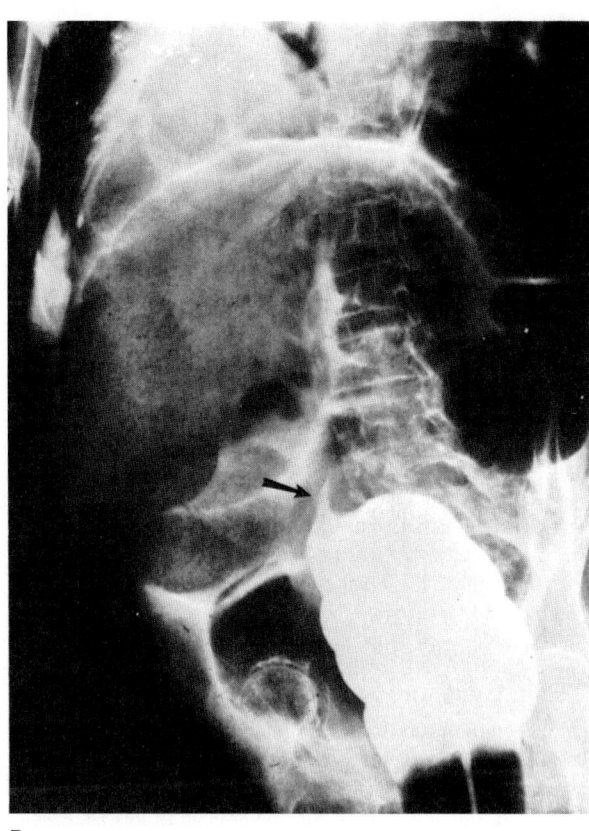

A   B

FIG. 28-29. Sigmoid volvulus: (A) Illustration and (B) Gastrografin enema showing "bird-beak" sign (arrow). [Reproduced with permission from Schwartz SI, Shires GT, Spencer FC (eds): Principles of Surgery. 5th ed. New York: McGraw-Hill, 1989, pp 1262 and 1263.]

kidney-shaped, air-filled structure in the left upper quadrant (opposite the site of obstruction), and a Gastrografin enema confirms obstruction at the level of the volvulus.

Unlike sigmoid volvulus, cecal volvulus can almost never be detorsed endoscopically. Moreover, because vascular compromise occurs early in the course of cecal volvulus, surgical exploration is necessary when the diagnosis is made. Right hemicolectomy with a primary ileocolic anastomosis can usually be performed safely and prevents recurrence. Simple detorsion or detorsion and cecopexy are associated with a high rate of recurrence.

Transverse Colon Volvulus

Transverse colon volvulus is extremely rare. Nonfixation of the colon and chronic constipation with megacolon may predispose to transverse colon volvulus. The radiographic appearance of transverse colon volvulus resembles sigmoid volvulus, but Gastrografin enema will reveal a more proximal obstruction. Although colonoscopic detorsion is occasionally successful in this setting, most patients require emergent exploration and resection.

Megacolon

Megacolon describes a chronically dilated, elongated, hypertrophied large bowel. Megacolon may be congenital or acquired and is usually related to chronic mechanical or functional obstruction. In general, the degree of megacolon is related to the duration of obstruction. Evaluation must always include examination of the colon and rectum

(either endoscopically or radiographically) to exclude a surgically correctable mechanical obstruction.

Congenital megacolon caused by Hirschsprung's disease results from the failure of migration of neural crest cells to the distal large intestine. The resulting absence of ganglion cells in the distal colon results in a failure of relaxation and causes a functional obstruction. The proximal, healthy bowel becomes progressively dilated. Surgical resection of the aganglionic segment is curative. Although Hirschsprung's disease is primarily a disease of infants and children, it occasionally presents later in adulthood, especially if an extremely short segment of the bowel is affected (*ultrashort-segment Hirschsprung's disease*).

Acquired megacolon may result from infection or chronic constipation. Infection with the protozoan *Trypanosoma cruzi (Chagas' disease)* destroys ganglion cells and produces both megacolon and megaesophagus. Chronic constipation from slow transit or secondary to medications (especially anticholinergic medications) or neurologic disorders (paraplegia, poliomyelitis, amyotrophic lateral sclerosis, multiple sclerosis) may produce progressive colonic dilatation. Diverting ileostomy or subtotal colectomy with an ileorectal anastomosis is occasionally necessary in these patients.

Colonic Pseudo-Obstruction (Ogilvie's Syndrome)

Colonic pseudo-obstruction (Ogilvie's syndrome) is a functional disorder in which the colon becomes massively dilated in the absence of mechanical obstruction. Pseudo-obstruction most commonly occurs in hospitalized patients and is associated with the use of narcotics, bedrest, and comorbid disease. Pseudo-obstruction is thought to result from autonomic dysfunction and severe adynamic ileus. The diagnosis is made based upon the presence of massive dilatation of the colon (usually predominantly the *right* and *transverse* colon) in the absence of a mechanical obstruction. Initial treatment consists of cessation of narcotics, anticholinergics, or other medications that may contribute to ileus. Strict bowel rest and intravenous hydration are crucial. Most patients will respond to these measures. In patients who fail to improve, colonoscopic decompression is often effective. However, this procedure is technically challenging and great care must be taken to avoid causing perforation. Recurrence occurs in up to 40% of patients. Intravenous neostigmine (an acetylcholinesterase inhibitor) is also extremely effective in decompressing the dilated colon and is associated with a low rate of recurrence (20%). However, neostigmine may produce transient but profound bradycardia and may be inappropriate in patients with cardiopulmonary disease. Because the colonic dilatation is typically greatest in the proximal colon, placement of a rectal tube is rarely effective. It is crucial to exclude mechanical obstruction (usually with a Gastrografin or barium enema) prior to medical or endoscopic treatment.

Ischemic Colitis

Intestinal ischemia occurs most commonly in the colon. Unlike small-bowel ischemia, colonic ischemia is rarely associated with major arterial or venous occlusion. Instead, most colonic ischemia appears to result from low flow and/or small-vessel occlusion. Risk factors include vascular disease, diabetes mellitus, vasculitis, and hypotension. In addition, ligation of the inferior mesenteric artery during aortic surgery predisposes to colonic ischemia. Occasionally, thrombosis or embolism may cause ischemia. Although the splenic flexure is the most common site of ischemic colitis, any segment of the colon may be affected. The rectum is relatively spared because of its rich collateral circulation.

Signs and symptoms of ischemic colitis reflect the extent of bowel ischemia. In mild cases, patients may have diarrhea (usually bloody) without abdominal pain. With more severe ischemia, intense abdominal pain (often out of proportion to the clinical examination), tenderness, fever, and leukocytosis are present. Peritonitis and/or systemic toxicity are signs of full-thickness necrosis and perforation.

The diagnosis of ischemic colitis is often based upon the clinical history and physical examination. Plain films may reveal *thumb printing,* which results from mucosal edema and submucosal hemorrhage. CT often shows nonspecific colonic wall thickening and pericolic fat stranding. Angiography is usually not helpful because major arterial occlusion is rare. While sigmoidoscopy may reveal characteristic dark, hemorrhagic mucosa, the risk of precipitating perforation is high. For this reason, *sigmoidoscopy is relatively contraindicated* in any patient with significant abdominal tenderness. Contrast studies (Gastrografin or barium enema) are similarly contraindicated during the acute phase of ischemic colitis.

Treatment of ischemic colitis depends upon clinical severity. Unlike ischemia of the small bowel, the majority of patients with ischemic colitis can be treated medically. Bowel rest and broad-spectrum antibiotics are the mainstay of therapy and 80% of patients will recover with this regimen. Hemodynamic parameters should be optimized, especially if hypotension and low flow appear to be the inciting cause. Long-term sequelae include stricture (10 to 15%) and chronic segmental ischemia (15 to 20%). Colonoscopy should be performed after recovery to evaluate strictures and to rule out other diagnoses such as inflammatory bowel disease or malignancy.

Failure to improve after 2 to 3 days of medical management, progression of symptoms, or deterioration in clinical condition is indication for surgical exploration. In this setting, all necrotic bowel should be resected. Primary anastomosis should be avoided. Occasionally, repeated exploration (a *second-look operation*) may be necessary.

Infectious Colitis

Pseudomembranous Colitis (*Clostridium difficile* Colitis)

Pseudomembranous colitis is caused by *C. difficile,* a gram-positive bacillus. *C. difficile colitis* is extremely common and is the leading cause of nosocomially acquired diarrhea.[4,79] The spectrum of disease ranges from watery diarrhea to fulminant, life-threatening colitis. *C. difficile* is carried in the large intestine of many healthy adults. Colitis is thought to result from overgrowth of this organism after depletion of the normal commensal flora of the gut with the use of antibiotics. Although clindamycin was the first antimicrobial agent associated with *C. difficile* colitis, almost any antibiotic may cause this disease. Moreover, although risk of *C. difficile* colitis increases with prolonged antibiotic usage, even a single dose of an antibiotic may cause the disease. Immunosuppression, medical comorbidities, prolonged hospitalization or nursing home residence, and bowel surgery increase the risk.

The pathogenic changes associated with *C. difficile* colitis result from production of two toxins: *toxin A* (an enterotoxin) and *toxin B* (a cytotoxin). Diagnosis of this disease was traditionally made by culturing the organism from the stool. Recently, detection of one or both toxins (either by cytotoxic assays or by immunoassays) has proven to be more rapid, sensitive, and specific. The diagnosis may also be made endoscopically by detection of characteristic ulcers, plaques, and pseudomembranes.

Management should include immediate cessation of the offending antimicrobial agent. Patients with mild disease (diarrhea but no fever or abdominal pain) may be treated as outpatients with a 10-day course of oral metronidazole. Oral vancomycin is a second-line agent used in patients allergic to metronidazole or in patients with recurrent disease. More severe diarrhea associated with dehydration and/or fever and abdominal pain is best treated with bowel rest, intravenous hydration, and oral metronidazole or vancomycin. Proctosigmoiditis may respond to vancomycin enemas. Recurrent colitis occurs in up to 20% of patients and may be treated by a longer course of oral metronidazole or vancomycin (up to 1 month). Reintroduction of normal flora by ingestion of *probiotics* has been suggested as a possible treatment for recurrent or refractory disease.[80] Fulminant colitis, characterized by septicemia and/or evidence of perforation, requires emergent laparotomy. A total abdominal colectomy with end ileostomy may be lifesaving.

Other Infectious Colitides

A variety of other infections with bacteria, parasites, fungi, or viruses may cause colonic inflammation. Common bacterial infections include enterotoxic *E. coli, Campylobacter jejuni, Yersinia enterocolitica, Salmonella typhi, Shigella,* and *Neisseria gonorrhoeae.* Less commonly, *Mycobacterium tuberculosis, Mycobacterium bovis, Actinomycosis israelii,* or *Treponema pallidum* (syphilis) may cause colitis or proctitis. Parasitic infections such as amebiasis, cryptosporidiosis, and giardiasis are also relatively common. Fungal infections (*Candida* species, histoplasmosis) are extremely rare in otherwise healthy individuals. The most common viral infections that produce colitic symptoms are the HIV, herpes simplex viruses, and cytomegalovirus.

Most symptoms are nonspecific and consist of diarrhea (with or without bleeding), crampy abdominal pain, and malaise. A thorough history may offer clues to the etiology (other medical conditions, especially immunosuppression; recent travel or exposures; and ingestions). Diagnosis is usually made by identification of a pathogen in the stool, either by microscopy or culture. Serum immunoassays may also be useful (amebiasis, HIV, CMV). Occasionally, endoscopy with biopsy may be required. Treatment is tailored to the infection.

ANORECTAL DISEASES

Any patient with anal/perianal symptoms requires a careful history and physical, including a digital rectal examination. Other studies such as defecography, manometry, CT scan, MRI, contrast enema, endoscopy, or exam under anesthesia may be required to arrive at an accurate diagnosis.

Hemorrhoids

Hemorrhoids are cushions of submucosal tissue containing venules, arterioles, and smooth-muscle fibers that are located in the anal canal (see Fig. 28-4). Three hemorrhoidal cushions are found in the left lateral, right anterior, and right posterior positions. Hemorrhoids are thought to function as part of the continence mechanism and aid in complete closure of the anal canal at rest. Because hemorrhoids are a normal part of anorectal anatomy, treatment is only indicated if they become symptomatic. Excessive straining, increased abdominal pressure, and hard stools increase venous engorgement of the hemorrhoidal plexus and cause prolapse of hemorrhoidal tissue. Outlet bleeding, thrombosis, and symptomatic hemorrhoidal prolapse may result.

External hemorrhoids are located distal to the dentate line and are covered with anoderm. Because the anoderm is richly innervated, thrombosis of an external hemorrhoid may cause significant pain. It is for this reason that external hemorrhoids should not be ligated or excised without adequate local anesthetic. A *skin tag* is redundant fibrotic skin at the anal verge, often persisting as the residual of a thrombosed external hemorrhoid. Skin tags are often confused with symptomatic hemorrhoids. External hemorrhoids and skin tags may cause itching and difficulty with hygiene if they are large. Treatment of external hemorrhoids and skin tags are only indicated for symptomatic relief.

Internal hemorrhoids are located proximal to the dentate line and covered by insensate anorectal mucosa. Internal hemorrhoids may prolapse or bleed, but rarely become painful unless they develop thrombosis and necrosis (usually related to severe prolapse, incarceration, and/or strangulation). Internal hemorrhoids are graded according to the extent of prolapse. *First-degree hemorrhoids* bulge into the anal canal and may prolapse beyond the dentate line on straining. *Second-degree hemorrhoids* prolapse through the anus but reduce spontaneously. *Third-degree hemorrhoids* prolapse through the anal canal and require manual reduction. *Fourth-degree hemorrhoids* prolapse but cannot be reduced and are at risk for strangulation.

Combined internal and external hemorrhoids straddle the dentate line and have characteristics of both internal and external hemorrhoids. Hemorrhoidectomy is often required for large, symptomatic, combined hemorrhoids. *Postpartum hemorrhoids* result from straining during labor, which results in edema, thrombosis, and/or strangulation. Hemorrhoidectomy is often the treatment of choice, especially if the patient has had chronic hemorrhoidal symptoms.

Portal hypertension was long thought to increase the risk of hemorrhoidal bleeding because of the anastomoses between the portal venous system (middle and upper hemorrhoidal plexuses) and the systemic venous system (inferior rectal plexuses). It is now understood that hemorrhoidal disease is no more common in patients with portal hypertension than in the normal population. *Rectal varices*, however, may occur and may cause hemorrhage in these patients. In general, rectal varices are best treated by lowering portal venous pressure. Rarely, suture ligation may be necessary if massive bleeding persists. Surgical hemorrhoidectomy should be avoided in these patients because of the risk of massive, difficult-to-control variceal bleeding.

Treatment

Medical Therapy. Bleeding from first- and second-degree hemorrhoids often improves with the addition of dietary fiber, stool softeners, increased fluid intake, and avoidance of straining. Associated pruritus may often improve with improved hygiene. Many over-the-counter topical medications are desiccants and are relatively ineffective for treating hemorrhoidal symptoms.

Rubber Band Ligation. Persistent bleeding from first-, second-, and selected third-degree hemorrhoids may be treated by rubber band ligation. Mucosa located 1 to 2 cm proximal to the dentate line is grasped and pulled into a rubber band applier. After firing the ligator, the rubber band strangulates the underlying tissue, causing scarring and preventing further bleeding or prolapse (Fig. 28-30). In general, only one or two quadrants are banded per visit. Severe pain will occur if the rubber band is placed at or distal to the dentate line where sensory nerves are located. Other complications of rubber band ligation include *urinary retention, infection,* and *bleeding.* Urinary retention occurs in approximately 1% of patients and is more likely if the ligation has inadvertently included a portion of the internal sphincter. *Necrotizing infection* is an uncommon, but life-threatening complication. Severe pain, fever, and urinary retention are early signs of infection and should prompt immediate evaluation of the patient usually with an exam under anesthesia. Treatment includes débridement of necrotic tissue, drainage of associated abscesses, and broad-spectrum antibiotics. *Bleeding* may occur approximately 7 to 10 days after rubber band ligation, at the time when the ligated pedicle necroses and sloughs. Bleeding is usually self-limited, but persistent hemorrhage may require exam under anesthesia and suture ligation of the pedicle.

Infrared Photocoagulation. Infrared photocoagulation is an effective office treatment for small first- and second-degree hemorrhoids. The instrument is applied to the apex of each hemorrhoid to coagulate the underlying plexus. All three quadrants may be treated during the same visit. Larger hemorrhoids and hemorrhoids with a significant amount of prolapse are not effectively treated with this technique.

Sclerotherapy. The injection of bleeding internal hemorrhoids with sclerosing agents is another effective office technique for treatment of first-, second-, and some third-degree hemorrhoids. One to 3 mL of a sclerosing solution (5-phenol in olive oil, sodium morrhuate, or quinine urea) are injected into the submucosa of each hemorrhoid. Few complications are associated with sclerotherapy, but infection and fibrosis have been reported.

Excision of Thrombosed External Hemorrhoids. Acutely thrombosed external hemorrhoids generally cause intense pain and a palpable perianal mass during the first 24 to 72 hours after thrombosis. The thrombosis can be effectively treated with an

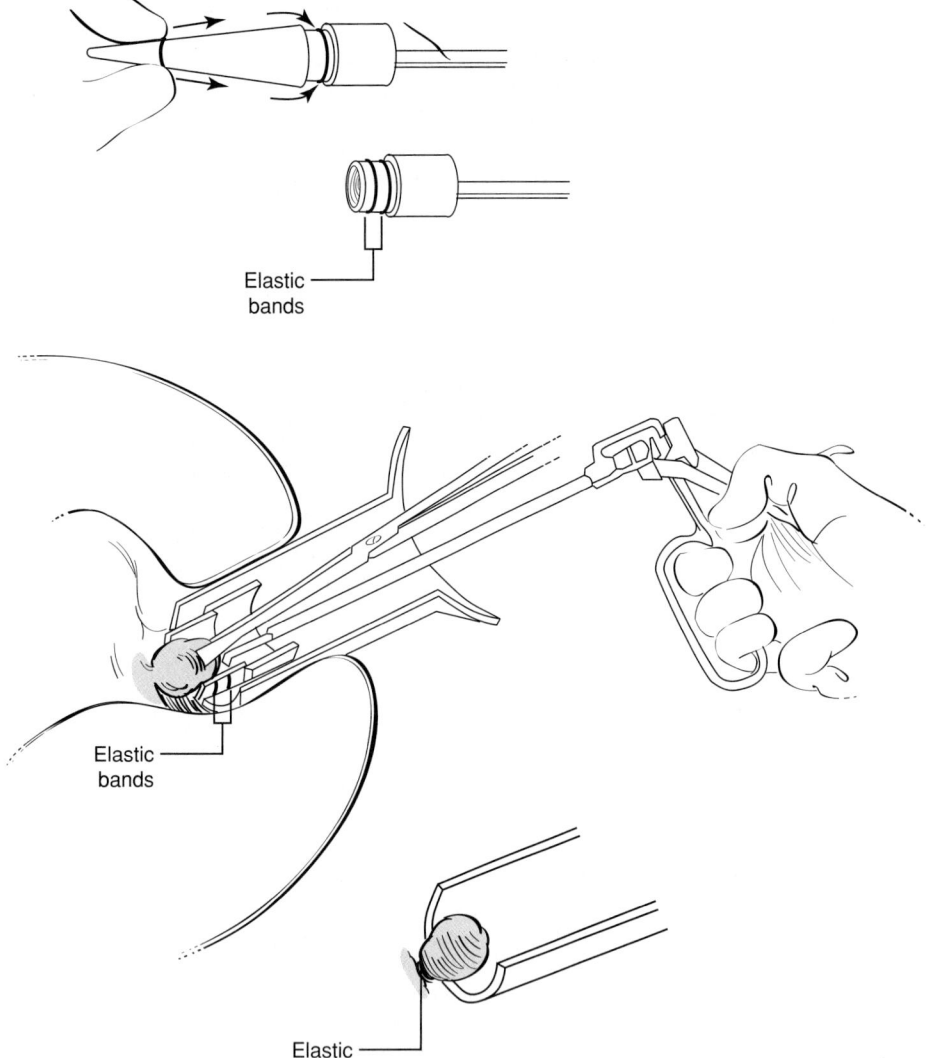

FIG. 28-30. Rubber band ligation of internal hemorrhoids. The mucosa just proximal to the internal hemorrhoids is banded. *[Reproduced with permission from Schwartz SI, Shires GT, Spencer FC (eds): Principles of Surgery. 5th ed. New York: McGraw-Hill, 1989, p 1303.]*

elliptical excision performed in the office under local anesthesia. Because the clot is usually loculated, simple incision and drainage is rarely effective. After 72 hours, the clot begins to resorb, and the pain resolves spontaneously. Excision is unnecessary, but sitz baths and analgesics are often helpful.

Operative Hemorrhoidectomy. A number of surgical procedures have been described for elective resection of symptomatic hemorrhoids. All are based on decreasing blood flow to the hemorrhoidal plexuses and excising redundant anoderm and mucosa.

Closed Submucosal Hemorrhoidectomy. The Parks or Ferguson hemorrhoidectomy involves resection of hemorrhoidal tissue and closure of the wounds with absorbable suture. The procedure may be performed in the prone or lithotomy position under local, regional, or general anesthesia. The anal canal is examined and an anal speculum inserted. The hemorrhoid cushions and associated redundant mucosa are identified and excised using an elliptical incision starting just distal to the anal verge and extending proximally to the anorectal ring. It is crucial to identify the fibers of the internal sphincter and carefully brush these away from the dissection in order to avoid injury to the sphincter. The apex of the hemorrhoidal plexus is then ligated and the hemorrhoid excised. The wound is then closed with a running absorbable suture. All three hemorrhoidal cushions

may be removed using this technique; however, care should be taken to avoid resecting a large area of perianal skin in order to avoid postoperative anal stenosis (Fig. 28-31).

Open Hemorrhoidectomy. This technique, often called the Milligan and Morgan hemorrhoidectomy, follows the same principles of excision described above, but the wounds are left open and allowed to heal by secondary intention.

Whitehead's Hemorrhoidectomy. Whitehead's hemorrhoidectomy involves circumferential excision of the hemorrhoidal cushions just proximal to the dentate line. After excision, the rectal mucosa is then advanced and sutured to the dentate line. While some surgeons still use the Whitehead hemorrhoidectomy technique, most have abandoned this approach because of the risk of ectropion (*Whitehead's deformity*).

Stapled Hemorrhoidectomy. Stapled hemorrhoidectomy has been proposed as an alternative surgical approach.[81–83] Unlike excisional hemorrhoidectomy, stapled hemorrhoidectomy does not aim to excise redundant hemorrhoidal tissue. Instead, stapled hemorrhoidectomy removes a short circumferential segment of rectal mucosa proximal to the dentate line using a circular stapler. This effectively ligates the venules feeding the hemorrhoidal plexus and fixes redundant mucosa higher in the anal canal. Critics suggest that this technique is only appropriate for patients with large, bleeding,

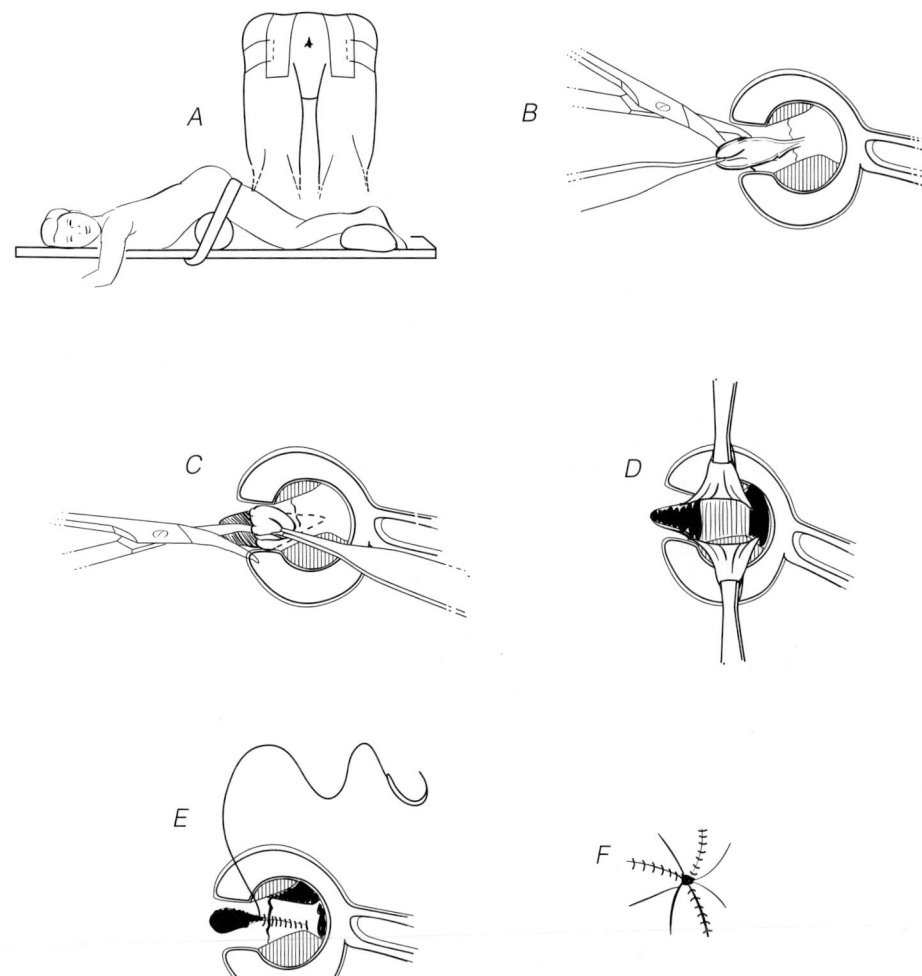

FIG. 28-31. Technique of closed submucosal hemorrhoidectomy. *A.* The patient is in prone jackknife position. *B.* A Fansler anoscope is used for exposure. *C.* A narrow ellipse of anoderm is excised. *D.* A submucosal dissection of the hemorrhoidal plexus from the underlying anal sphincter is performed. *E.* Redundant mucosa is anchored to the proximal anal canal and the wound is closed with a running absorbable suture. *F.* Additional quadrants are excised to complete the procedure. [*Reproduced with permission from Schwartz SI, Shires GT, Spencer FC (eds): Principles of Surgery. 5th ed. New York: McGraw-Hill, 1989, p 1304.*]

internal hemorrhoids, and is ineffective in management of external or combined hemorrhoids. Although stapled hemorrhoidectomy has not been widely accepted at this time, it remains a promising new technique.

Complications of Hemorrhoidectomy. Postoperative pain following excisional hemorrhoidectomy requires analgesia usually with oral narcotics. Nonsteroidal anti-inflammatory drugs, muscle relaxants, topical analgesics, and comfort measures, including sitz baths, are often useful as well. Several studies show that stapled hemorrhoidectomy is associated with a significant decrease in postoperative pain. Other complications are similar to those seen with excisional hemorrhoidectomy. Urinary retention is a common complication following hemorrhoidectomy and occurs in 10 to 50% of patients. The risk of urinary retention can be minimized by limiting intraoperative and perioperative intravenous fluids, and by providing adequate analgesia. Pain can also lead to *fecal impaction.* Risk of impaction may be decreased by preoperative enemas or a limited mechanical bowel preparation, liberal use of laxatives postoperatively, and adequate pain control. While a small amount of *bleeding,* especially with bowel movements, is to be expected, massive hemorrhage can occur after hemorrhoidectomy. Bleeding may occur in the immediate postoperative period (often in the recovery room) as a result of inadequate ligation of the vascular pedicle. This type of hemorrhage mandates an urgent return to the operating room where suture ligation of the bleeding vessel will often solve the problem. Bleeding may also occur 7 to 10 days after hemorrhoidectomy

when the necrotic mucosa overlying the vascular pedicle sloughs. While some of these patients may be safely observed, others will require an exam under anesthesia to ligate the bleeding vessel or to oversew the wounds if no specific site of bleeding is identified. *Infection* is uncommon after hemorrhoidectomy; however, necrotizing soft-tissue infection can occur with devastating consequences. Severe pain, fever, and urinary retention may be early signs of infection. If infection is suspected, an emergent examination under anesthesia, drainage of abscess, and/or débridement of all necrotic tissue are required.

Long-term sequelae of hemorrhoidectomy include *incontinence, anal stenosis,* and *ectropion (Whitehead's deformity).* Many patients experience transient incontinence to flatus, but these symptoms are usually short-lived and few patients have permanent fecal incontinence. Anal stenosis may result from scarring after extensive resection of perianal skin. Ectropion may occur after a Whitehead's hemorrhoidectomy. This complication is usually the result of suturing the rectal mucosa too far distally in the anal canal and can be avoided by ensuring that the mucosa is sutured at or just above the dentate line.

Anal Fissure

A fissure in ano is a tear in the anoderm distal to the dentate line. The pathophysiology of anal fissure is thought to be related to trauma from either the passage of hard stool or prolonged diarrhea. A tear in the anoderm causes spasm of the internal anal sphincter, which results in pain, increased tearing, and decreased blood supply to the anoderm. This cycle of pain, spasm, and ischemia contributes to development of a poorly healing wound that becomes a *chronic fissure*. The vast majority of anal fissures occur in the posterior midline. Ten to 15% occur in the anterior midline. Less than 1% of fissures occur off midline.

Symptoms and Findings

Anal fissure is extremely common.[84,85] Characteristic symptoms include tearing pain with defecation and hematochezia (usually described as blood on the toilet paper). Patients may also complain of a sensation of intense and painful anal spasm lasting for several hours after a bowel movement. On physical examination, the fissure can often be seen in the anoderm by gently separating the buttocks. Patients are often too tender to tolerate digital rectal examination, anoscopy, or proctoscopy. An *acute fissure* is a superficial tear of the distal anoderm and almost always heals with medical management. *Chronic fissures* develop ulceration and heaped-up edges with the white fibers of the internal anal sphincter visible at the base of the ulcer. There is often an associated external skin tag and/or a hypertrophied anal papilla internally. These fissures are more challenging to treat and may require surgery. A lateral location of a chronic anal fissure may be evidence of an underlying disease such as Crohn's disease, human immunodeficiency virus, syphilis, tuberculosis, or leukemia. If the diagnosis is in doubt or there is suspicion of another cause for the perianal pain such as abscess or fistula, an examination under anesthesia may be necessary.

Treatment

Therapy focuses on breaking the cycle of pain, spasm, and ischemia thought responsible for development of fissure in ano. First-line therapy to minimize anal trauma includes bulk agents, stool softeners, and warm sitz baths. The addition of 2% lidocaine jelly or other analgesic creams can provide additional symptomatic relief. Nitroglycerin ointment (0.2%) has been used locally to improve blood flow but often causes severe headaches.[86] Both oral and topical diltiazem have also been used to heal fissures and may have fewer side effects than topical nitrates.[87] Newer agents, such as arginine (a nitric oxide donor) and topical bethanechol (a muscarinic agonist), have also been used to treat fissures. Medical therapy is effective in most acute fissures, but will heal only approximately 50 to 60% of chronic fissures.

Botulinum toxin causes temporary muscle paralysis by preventing acetylcholine release from presynaptic nerve terminals. Injection of botulinum toxin has been proposed as an alternative to surgical sphincterotomy for chronic fissure. Although there is limited experience with this approach, results appear to be superior to other medical therapy, and complications such as incontinence are rare. However, healing is slower than after sphincterotomy and recurrence may be more common.[88]

Surgical therapy has traditionally been recommended for chronic fissures that have failed medical therapy, and lateral internal sphincterotomy is the procedure of choice for most surgeons.[89] The aim of this procedure is to decrease spasm of the internal sphincter by dividing a portion of the muscle. Approximately 30% of the internal sphincter fibers are divided laterally by using either an open (Fig. 28-32) or closed (Fig. 28-33) technique. Healing is achieved in more than 95% of patients by using this technique and most patients experience immediate pain relief. Recurrence occurs in less than 10% of patients and the risk of incontinence (usually to flatus) ranges from 5 to 15%.

Anorectal Sepsis and Cryptoglandular Abscess

Relevant Anatomy

The majority of anorectal suppurative disease results from infections of the anal glands (cryptoglandular infection) found in the intersphincteric plane. Their ducts traverse the internal sphincter and empty into the anal crypts at the level of the dentate line.

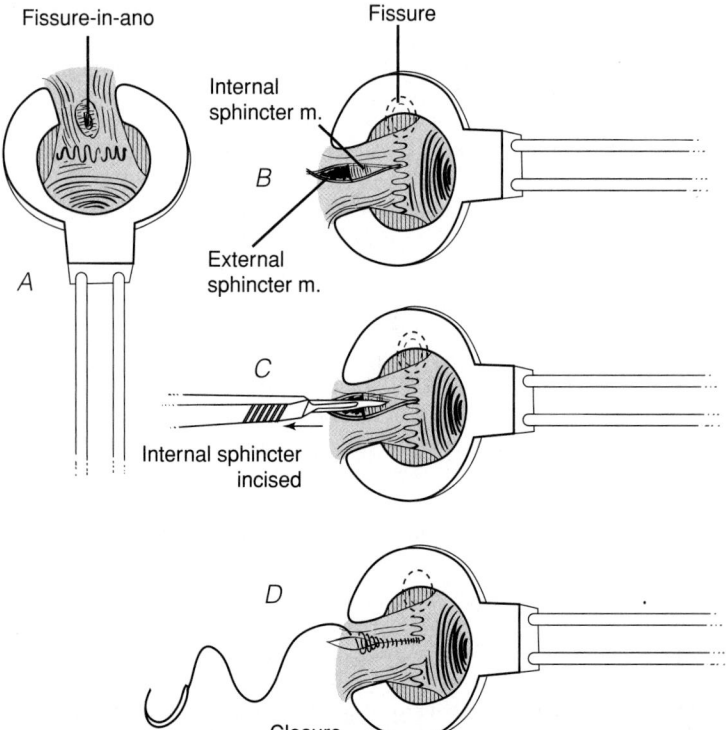

FIG. 28-32. Open lateral internal sphincterotomy for fissure in ano. [*Reproduced with permission from Schwartz SI, Shires GT, Spencer FC (eds): Principles of Surgery. 5th ed. New York: McGraw-Hill, 1989, p 1304.*]

Fissure-in-ano

Fissure

Internal sphincter m.

B

External sphincter m.

A

C

Internal sphincter incised

D

Closure

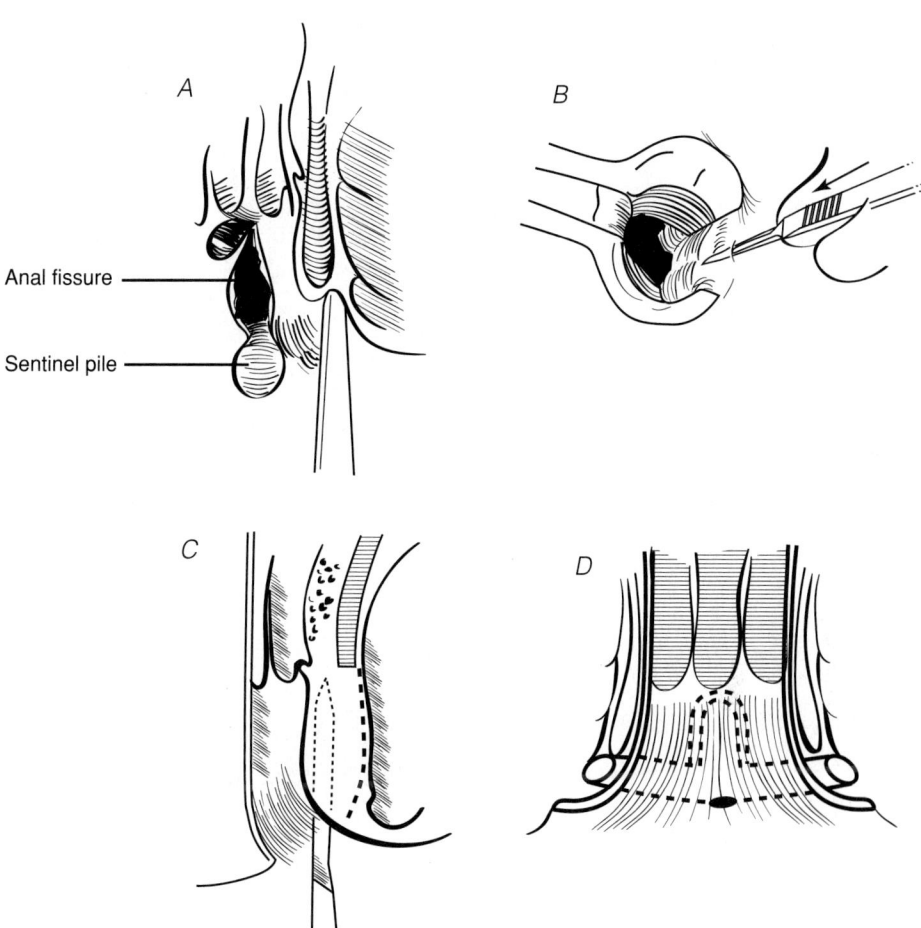

Anal fissure

Sentinel pile

FIG. 28-33. Closed lateral internal sphincterotomy for fissure in ano. [*Reproduced with permission from Schwartz SI, Shires GT, Spencer FC (eds): Principles of Surgery. 5th ed. New York: McGraw-Hill, 1989, p 1305.*]

Infection of an anal gland results in the formation of an abscess that enlarges and spreads along one of several planes in the perianal and perirectal spaces. The *perianal space* surrounds the anus and laterally becomes continuous with the fat of the buttocks. The *intersphincteric space* separates the internal and external anal sphincters. It is continuous with the perianal space distally and extends cephalad into the rectal wall. The *ischiorectal space (ischiorectal fossa)* is located lateral and posterior to the anus and is bounded medially by the external sphincter, laterally by the ischium, superiorly by the levator ani, and inferiorly by the transverse septum. The ischiorectal space contains the inferior rectal vessels and lymphatics. The two ischiorectal spaces connect posteriorly above the anococcygeal ligament but below the levator ani muscle, forming the *deep postanal space*. The *supralevator spaces* lie above the levator ani on either side of the rectum and communicate posteriorly. The anatomy of these spaces influences the location and spread of cryptoglandular infection (Fig. 28-34).

As an abscess enlarges, it spreads in one of several directions. A *perianal abscess* is the most common manifestation and appears as a painful swelling at the anal verge. Spread through the external sphincter below the level of the puborectalis produces an *ischiorectal abscess*. These abscesses may become extremely large and may not be visible in the perianal region. Digital rectal exam will reveal a painful swelling laterally in the ischiorectal fossa. *Intersphincteric abscesses* occur in the intersphincteric space and are notoriously difficult to diagnose, often requiring an examination under anesthesia. *Pelvic* and *supralevator abscesses* are uncommon and may result from extension of an intersphincteric or ischiorectal

abscess upward, or extension of an intraperitoneal abscess downward (Fig. 28-35).

Diagnosis

Severe anal pain is the most common presenting complaint. Walking, coughing, or straining can aggravate the pain. A palpable mass is often detected by inspection of the perianal area or by digital rectal examination. Occasionally, patients will present with fever, urinary retention, or life-threatening sepsis. The diagnosis of a perianal or ischiorectal abscess can usually be made with physical exam alone (either in the office or in the operating room). However, complex or atypical presentations may require imaging studies such as CT or MRI to fully delineate the anatomy of the abscess.

Treatment

Anorectal abscesses should be treated by drainage as soon as the diagnosis is established. If the diagnosis is in question, an examination under anesthesia is often the most expeditious way both to confirm the diagnosis and to treat the problem. Delayed or inadequate treatment may occasionally cause extensive and life-threatening suppuration with massive tissue necrosis and septicemia. Antibiotics are only indicated if there is extensive overlying cellulitis or if the patient is immunocompromised, has diabetes mellitus, or has valvular heart disease. Antibiotics alone are ineffective at treating perianal or perirectal infection.

Perianal Abscess. Most perianal abscesses can be drained under local anesthesia in the office, clinic, or emergency room.

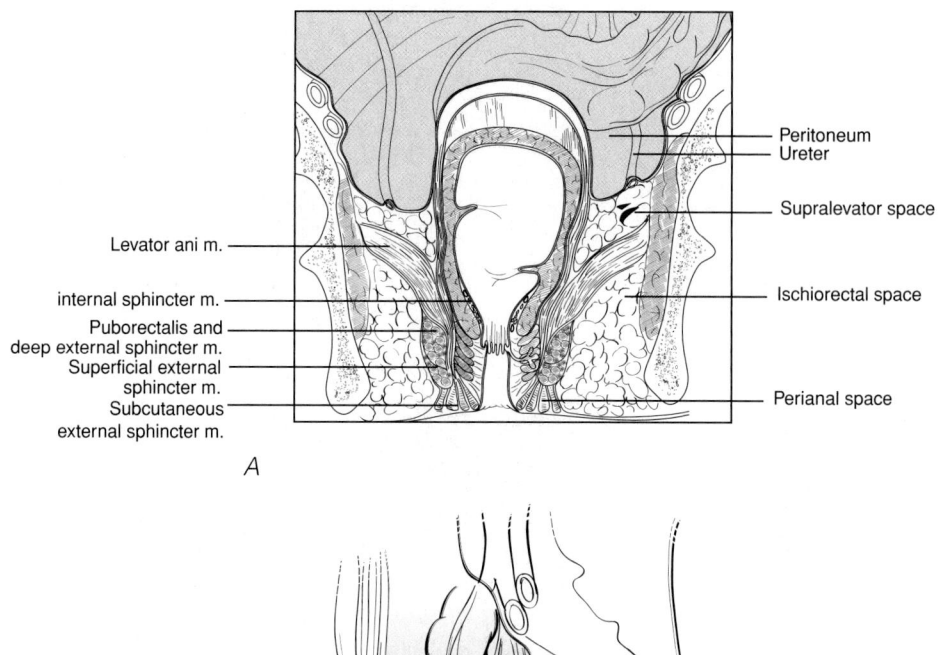

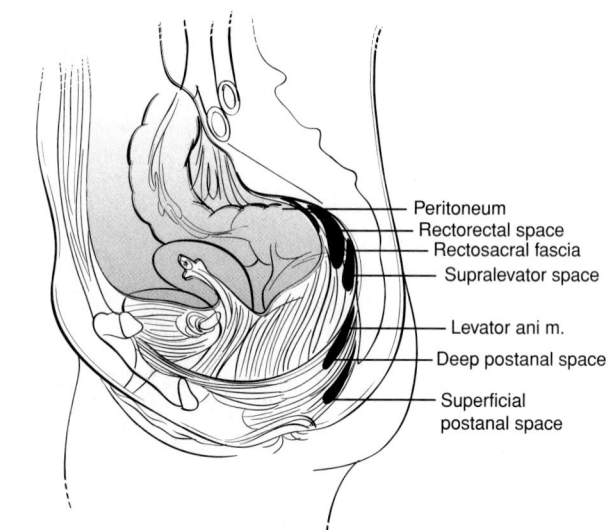

FIG. 28-34. Anatomy of perianorectal spaces. *A*. Anterior view and (*B*) lateral view. [*Reproduced with permission from Schwartz SI, Shires GT, Spencer FC (eds): Principles of Surgery. 5th ed. New York: McGraw-Hill, 1989, pp 1298 and 1299.*]

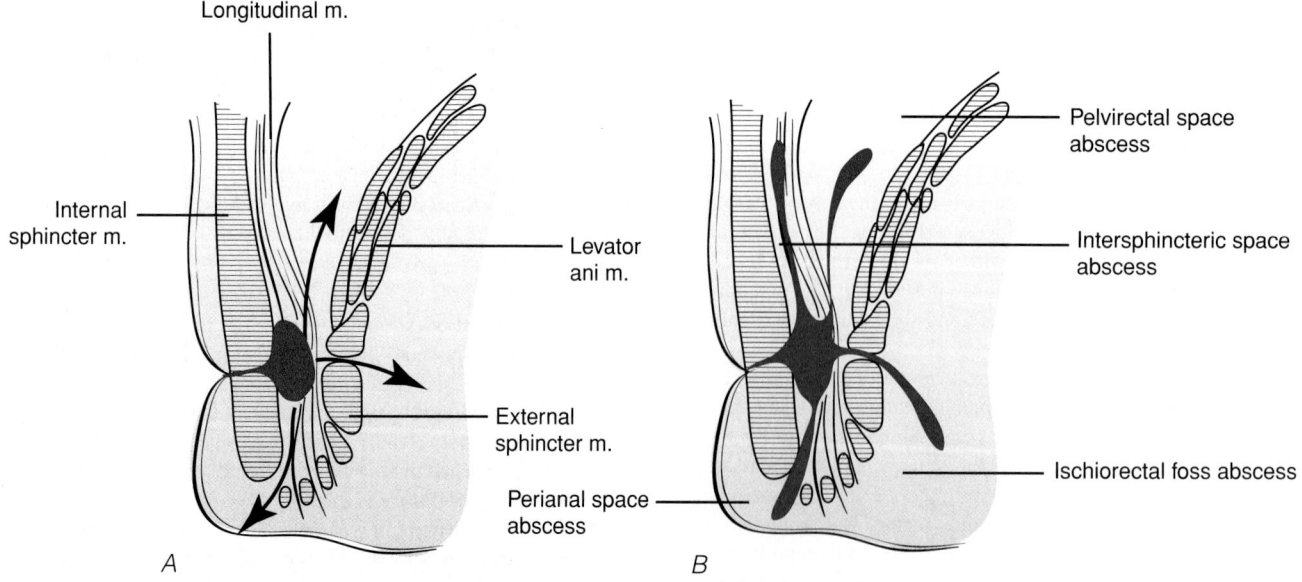

FIG. 28-35. Pathways of anorectal infection in perianal spaces. [*Reproduced with permission from Schwartz SI, Shires GT, Spencer FC (eds): Principles of Surgery. 5th ed. New York: McGraw-Hill, 1989, p 1299.*]

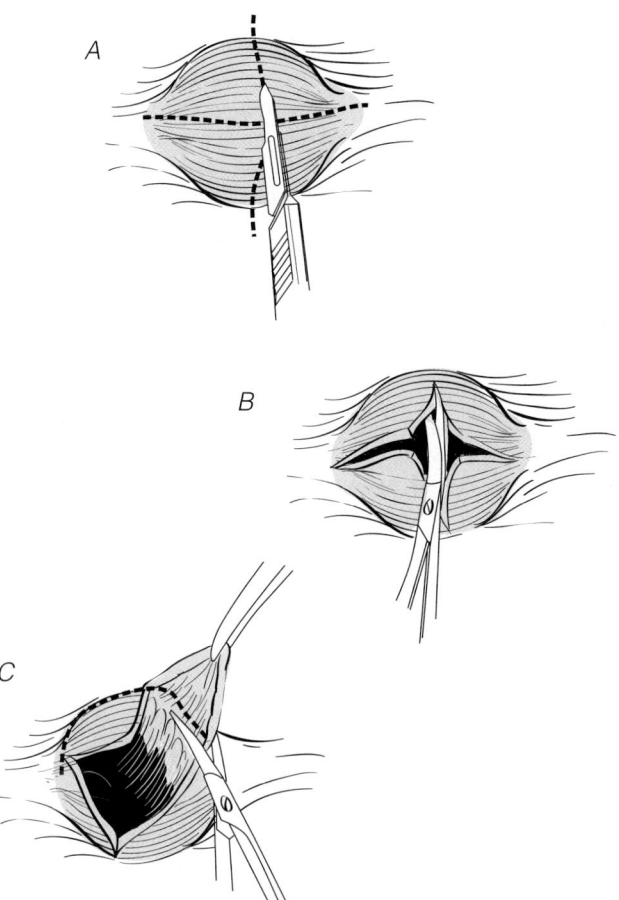

FIG. 28-36. Technique of drainage of perianal abscess. [Reproduced with permission from Schwartz SI, Shires GT, Spencer FC (eds): Principles of Surgery. 5th ed. New York: McGraw-Hill, 1989, p 1300.]

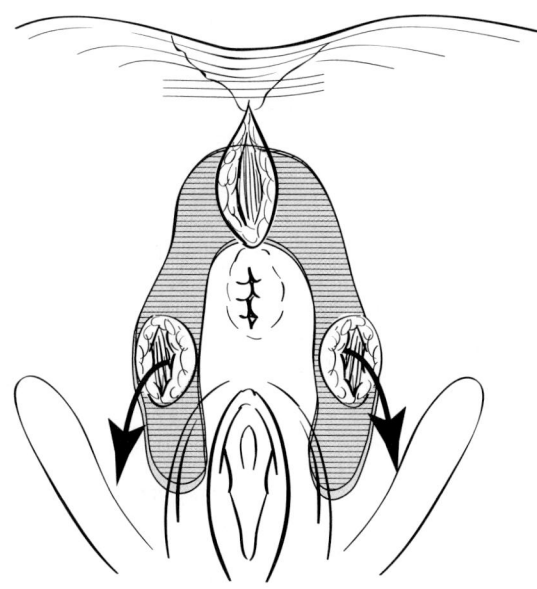

FIG. 28-37. Drainage of horseshoe abscess. The deep postanal space is entered, incising the anococcygeal ligament. Counter drainage incisions are made for each limb of the ischiorectal space. [Reproduced with permission from Schwartz SI, Shires GT, Spencer FC (eds): Principles of Surgery. 5th ed. New York: McGraw-Hill, 1989, p 1300.]

Larger, more complicated abscesses may require drainage in the operating room. A cruciate skin and subcutaneous incision is made over the most prominent part of the abscess and the "dog ears" are excised to prevent premature closure. No packing is necessary and sitz baths are started the next day (Fig. 28-36).

Ischiorectal Abscesses. An ischiorectal abscess causes diffuse swelling in the ischiorectal fossa that may involve one or both sides, forming a "horseshoe" abscess. Simple ischiorectal abscesses are drained through an incision in the overlying skin. Horseshoe abscesses require drainage of the deep postanal space and often require counterincisions over one or both ischiorectal spaces (Fig. 28-37).

Intersphincteric Abscess. Intersphincteric abscesses are notoriously difficult to diagnose because they produce little swelling and few perianal signs of infection. Pain is typically described as being deep and "up inside" the anal area, and is usually exacerbated by coughing or sneezing. The pain is so intense that it usually precludes a digital rectal examination. The diagnosis is made based upon a high index of suspicion and usually requires an examination under anesthesia. Once identified, an intersphincteric abscess can be drained through a limited, usually posterior, internal sphincterotomy.

Supralevator Abscess. This type of abscess is uncommon and can be difficult to diagnose. Because of its proximity to the peritoneal cavity, supralevator abscesses can mimic intra-abdominal

conditions. Digital rectal examination may reveal an indurated, bulging mass above the anorectal ring.

It is essential to identify the origin of a supralevator abscess prior to treatment. If the abscess is secondary to an upward extension of an intersphincteric abscess, it should be drained through the rectum. If it is drained through the ischiorectal fossa, a complicated, suprasphincteric fistula may result. If a supralevator abscess arises from the upward extension of an ischiorectal abscess, it should be drained through the ischiorectal fossa. Drainage of this type of abscess through the rectum may result in an extrasphincteric fistula. If the abscess is secondary to intra-abdominal disease, the primary process requires treatment and the abscess is drained via the most direct route (transabdominally, rectally, or through the ischiorectal fossa).

Perianal Sepsis in the Immunocompromised Patient. The immunocompromised patient with perianal pain presents a diagnostic dilemma. Because of leukopenia, these patients may develop serious perianal infection without any of the cardinal signs of inflammation. While broad-spectrum antibiotics may cure some of these patients, an exam under anesthesia should not be delayed because of neutropenia. An increase in pain or fever, and/or clinical deterioration mandates an exam under anesthesia. Any indurated area should be incised and drained, biopsied to exclude a leukemic infiltrate, and cultured to aid in the selection of antimicrobial agents.

Necrotizing Soft-Tissue Infection of the Perineum. Necrotizing soft-tissue infection of the perineum is a rare, but lethal, condition. Most of these infections are polymicrobial and synergistic. The source of sepsis is commonly an undrained or inadequately drained cryptoglandular abscess or a urogenital infection. Occasionally, these infections may be encountered postoperatively (e.g., after inguinal hernia repair). Immunocompromised patients and diabetic patients are at increased risk.

Physical examination may reveal necrotic skin, bullae, or crepitus. Patients often have signs of systemic toxicity and may be hemodynamically unstable. A high index of suspicion is necessary because perineal signs of severe infection may be minimal and prompt surgical intervention can be lifesaving.

Surgical débridement of all nonviable tissue is required to treat all necrotizing soft-tissue infections. Multiple operations may be necessary to ensure that all necrotic tissue has been resected. Broad-spectrum antibiotics are frequently employed, but adequate surgical débridement remains the mainstay of therapy. Colostomy may be required if extensive resection of the sphincter is required, or if stool contamination of the perineum makes wound management difficult. Despite early recognition and adequate surgical therapy, the mortality of necrotizing perineal soft-tissue infections remains approximately 50%.

Fistula in Ano

Drainage of an anorectal abscess results in cure for about 50% of patients. The remaining 50% develop a persistent *fistula in ano*. The fistula usually originates in the infected crypt (*internal opening*) and tracks to the *external opening*, usually the site of prior drainage. The course of the fistula can often be predicted by the anatomy of the previous abscess.

While the majority of fistulas are cryptoglandular in origin, trauma, Crohn's disease, malignancy, radiation, or unusual infections (tuberculosis, actinomycosis, and chlamydia) may also produce fistulas. A complex, recurrent, or nonhealing fistula should raise the suspicion of one of these diagnoses.

Diagnosis

Patients present with persistent drainage from the internal and/or external openings. An indurated tract is often palpable. While the external opening is often easily identifiable, identification of the internal opening may be more challenging. Goodsall's rule can be used as a guide in determining the location of the internal opening (Fig. 28-38). In general, fistulas with an external opening *anteriorly* connect to the internal opening by a *short, radial tract*. Fistulas with an external opening *posteriorly* track in a *curvilinear fashion to the posterior midline*. However, exceptions to this rule often occur if an anterior external opening is greater than 3 cm from the anal margin. Such fistulas usually track to the posterior midline. Fistulas are categorized based upon their relationship to the anal sphincter

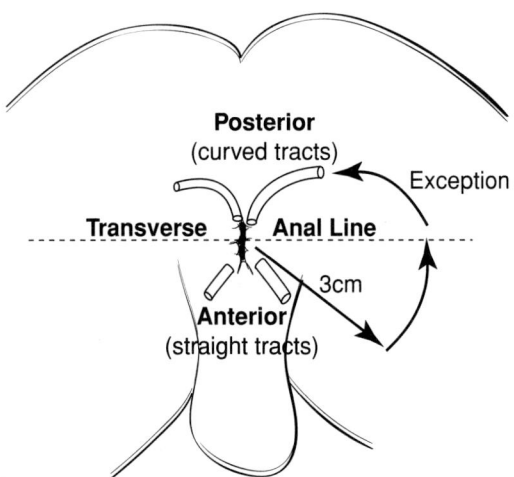

FIG. 28-38. Goodsall's rule to identify the internal opening of fistulas in ano. [*Reproduced with permission from Schwartz SI, Shires GT, Spencer FC (eds): Principles of Surgery. 5th ed. New York: McGraw-Hill, 1989, p 1305.*]

complex and treatment options are based upon these classifications. An *intersphincteric fistula* tracks through the distal internal sphincter and intersphincteric space to an external opening near the anal verge (Fig. 28-39A). A *transsphincteric fistula* often results from an ischiorectal abscess and extends through both the internal and external sphincters (Fig. 28-39B). A *suprasphincteric fistula* originates in the intersphincteric plane and tracks up and around the entire external sphincter (Fig. 28-39C). An *extrasphincteric fistula* originates in the rectal wall and tracks around both sphincters to exit laterally, usually in the ischiorectal fossa (Fig. 28-39D).

Treatment

The goal of treatment of fistula in ano is eradication of sepsis without sacrificing continence. Because fistulous tracks encircle variable amounts of the sphincter complex, surgical treatment is dictated by the location of the internal and external openings and the course of the fistula. The external opening is usually visible as a red elevation of granulation tissue with or without concurrent drainage. The internal opening may be more difficult to identify. Injection of hydrogen peroxide or dilute methylene blue may be helpful. Care must be taken to avoid creating an artificial internal opening (thus often converting a simple fistula into a complex fistula).

Simple intersphincteric fistulas can often be treated by *fistulotomy* (opening the fistulous tract), curettage, and healing by secondary intention (see Fig. 28-39A). *"Horseshoe"* fistulas usually have an internal opening in the posterior midline and extend anteriorly and laterally to one or both ischiorectal spaces by way of the deep postanal space. Treatment of a transsphincteric fistula depends upon its location in the sphincter complex. Fistulas that include less than 30% of the sphincter muscles can often be treated by sphincterotomy without significant risk of major incontinence (see Fig. 28-39B). High transsphincteric fistulas, which encircle a greater amount of muscle, are more safely treated by initial placement of a *seton* (see below). Similarly, suprasphincteric fistulas are usually treated with seton placement (see Fig. 28-39C). Extrasphincteric fistulas are rare, and treatment depends upon both the anatomy of the fistula and its etiology. In general, the portion of the fistula outside the sphincter should be opened and drained. A primary tract at the level of the dentate line may also be opened if present. Complex fistulas with multiple tracts may require numerous procedures to control sepsis and facilitate healing. Liberal use of drains and setons is helpful. Failure to heal may ultimately require fecal diversion (see Fig. 28-39D). Complex and/or nonhealing fistulas may result from Crohn's disease, malignancy, radiation proctitis, or unusual infection. Proctoscopy should be performed in all cases of complex and/or nonhealing fistulas to assess the health of the rectal mucosa. Biopsies of the fistula tract should be taken to rule out malignancy.

A *seton* is a drain placed through a fistula to maintain drainage and/or induce fibrosis. *Cutting setons* consist of a suture or a rubber band that is placed through the fistula and intermittently tightened in the office. Tightening the seton results in fibrosis and gradual division of the sphincter, thus eliminating the fistula while maintaining continuity of the sphincter. A *noncutting seton* is a soft plastic drain (often a vessel loop) placed in the fistula to maintain drainage. The fistula tract may subsequently be laid open with less risk of incontinence because scarring prevents retraction of the sphincter. Alternatively, the seton may be left in place for chronic drainage. Higher fistulas may be treated by an *endorectal advancement flap* (see below). *Fibrin glue* has also been used to treat persistent fistulas with variable results.

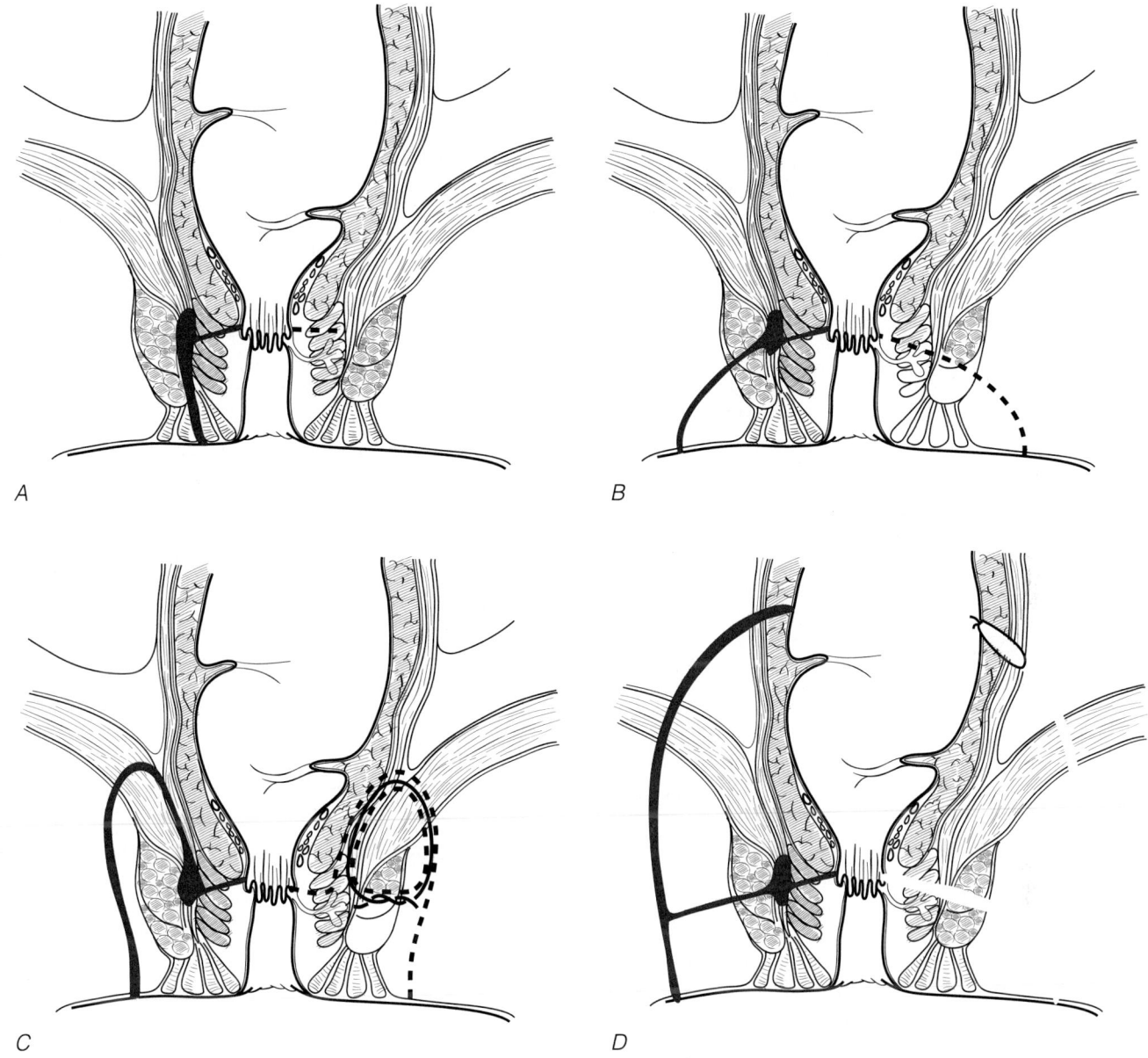

FIG. 28-39. The four major categories of fistula in ano (*left side of drawings*) and the usual operative procedure to correct the fistula (*right side of drawings*). A. Intersphincteric fistula with simple low tract. B. Uncomplicated transsphincteric fistula. C. Uncomplicated suprasphincteric fistula. D. Extrasphincteric fistula secondary to anal fistula. [*Reproduced with permission from Gordon PH, Nivatvongs S (eds): Principles and Practice of Surgery for the Colon, Rectum and Anus, 2nd ed. New York: Marcel Dekker, Inc., 1999, pp 256–260.*]

Rectovaginal Fistula

A rectovaginal fistula is a connection between the vagina and the rectum or anal canal proximal to the dentate line. Rectovaginal fistulas are classified as *low* (rectal opening close to the dentate line and vaginal opening in the fourchette), *middle* (vaginal opening between the fourchette and cervix), or *high* (vaginal opening near the cervix). Low rectovaginal fistulas are commonly caused by obstetric injuries or trauma from a foreign body. Mid-rectovaginal fistulas may result from more severe obstetric injury, but also occur after surgical resection of a mid-rectal neoplasm, radiation injury, or extension of an undrained abscess. High rectovaginal fistulas result from operative or radiation injury. Complicated diverticulitis may

cause a colovaginal fistula. Crohn's disease can cause rectovaginal fistulas at all levels, as well as colovaginal and enterovaginal fistulas.

Diagnosis

Patients describe symptoms varying from the sensation of passing flatus from the vagina to the passage of solid stool from the vagina. Most patients experience some degree of fecal incontinence. Contamination may result in *vaginitis*. Large fistulas may be obvious on anoscopic and/or vaginal speculum examination, but smaller fistulas may be difficult to locate. Occasionally, a barium enema or vaginogram may identify these fistulas. Endorectal ultrasound may also be useful. With the patient in the prone position, installation of

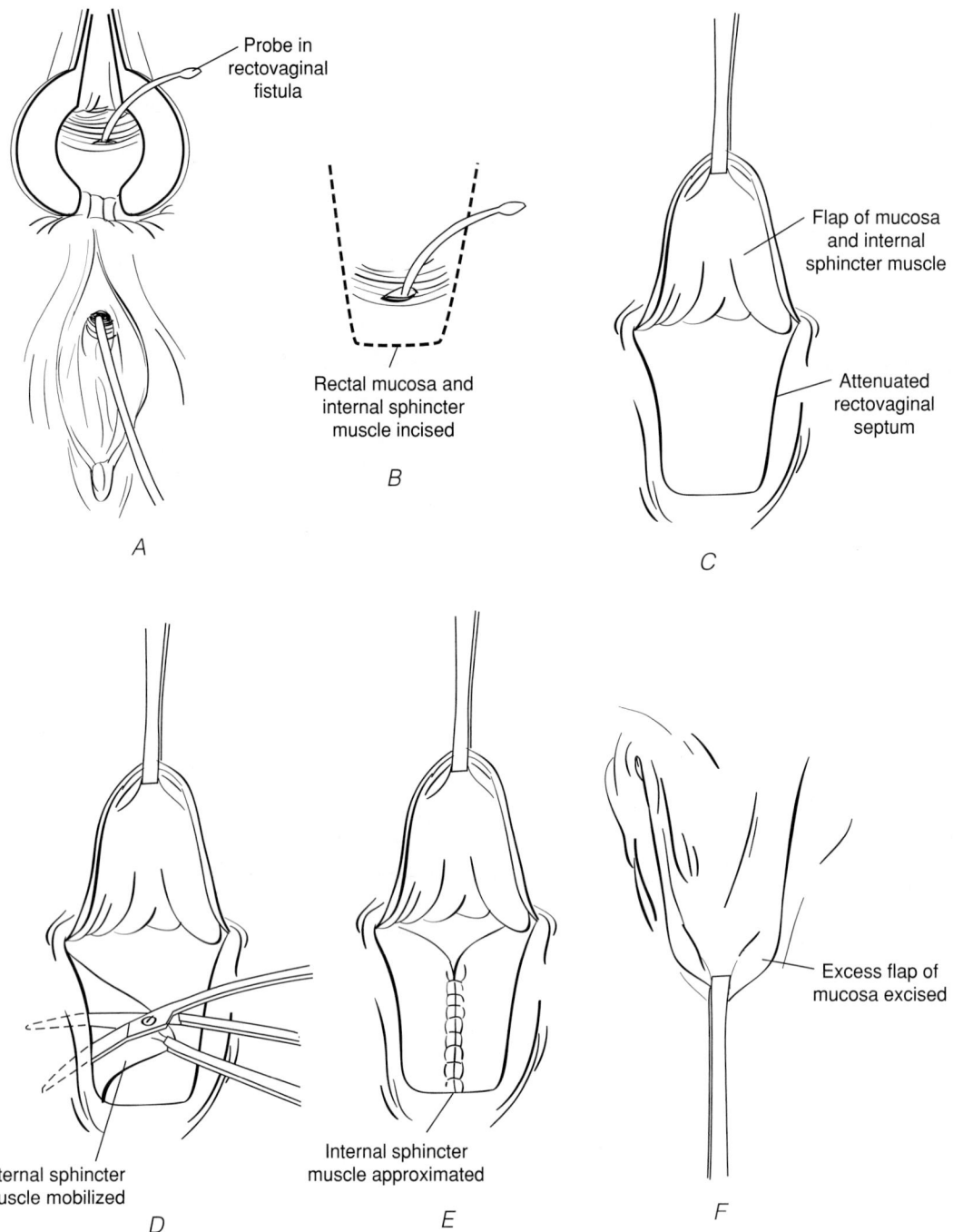

FIG. 28-40. Endorectal advancement flap for rectovaginal fistula. *[Reproduced with permission from Gordon PH, Nivatvongs S (eds): Principles and Practice of Surgery for the Colon, Rectum, and Anus, 2nd ed. New York: Marcel Dekker, Inc., 1999, p 412.]*

methylene blue into the rectum while a tampon is in the vagina may confirm the presence of a small fistula.

Treatment

The treatment of rectovaginal fistula depends upon the size, location, etiology, and condition of surrounding tissues. Because up to 50% of fistulas caused by obstetric injury heal spontaneously, it is prudent to wait 3 to 6 months before embarking upon surgical repair in these patients. If the fistula was caused by a cryptoglandular abscess, drainage of the abscess may allow spontaneous closure.

Low and mid-rectovaginal fistulas are usually best treated with an endorectal advancement flap. The principle of this procedure is based upon the advancement of healthy mucosa, submucosa, and circular muscle over the rectal opening (the high pressure side of the fistula) to promote healing (Fig. 28-40). If a sphincter injury is present, an overlapping sphincteroplasty should be performed concurrently. Fecal diversion is rarely required. High rectovaginal, colovaginal, and enterovaginal fistulas are usually best treated via a transabdominal approach. The diseased tissue, which caused the fistula (upper rectum, sigmoid colon, or small bowel), is resected and the hole in the vagina closed. Healthy tissue, such as omentum or muscle, is frequently interposed between the bowel anastomosis and the vagina to prevent recurrence.

Rectovaginal fistulas caused by Crohn's disease, radiation injury, or malignancy almost never heal spontaneously. In Crohn's disease, treatment is based on adequate drainage of perianal sepsis and nutritional support. An endorectal advancement flap may be performed if the rectum is spared from active Crohn's disease. Fistulas resulting from radiation damage are not amenable to local repair with an advancement flap because of damage to the surrounding rectal and vaginal tissues. Mid- and high rectovaginal fistulas are occasionally repaired successfully with a transabdominal approach in which healthy tissue (omentum, muscle, or nonradiated bowel) is interposed between the damaged rectum and vagina. Fistulas caused by malignancy should be treated with resection of the tumor. Because differentiating radiation damage from malignancy can be extremely difficult, all fistulas resulting from radiation should be biopsied to rule out cancer.

Perianal Dermatitis

Pruritus Ani

Pruritus ani (severe perianal itching) is a common problem with a multitude of etiologies. Surgically correctable (anatomic) causes include prolapsing hemorrhoids, ectropion, fissure, fistula, and neoplasms. Perianal infection may also present with pruritus ani. Infections may be caused by fungus (*Candida* species, *Monilia,* and *Epidermophyton* organisms), parasites (*Enterobius vermicularis* [pinworms], *Pediculus pubis* [a louse], and *Sarcoptes scabiei* [scabies]), bacteria (*Corynebacterium minutissimum* [erythrasma] and *Treponema pallidum* [syphilis]), or viruses (*human papilloma virus* [condyloma acuminata]). Antibiotic use may also cause itching, usually by precipitating fungal infection. Noninfectious dermatologic causes include seborrhea, psoriasis, and contact dermatitis. Contact dermatitis can be particularly troublesome because many over-the-counter topical agents used by patients to relieve itching may exacerbate the problem. Occasionally, systemic diseases such as jaundice and diabetes may present with pruritus ani.

Despite this myriad of causes, the majority of pruritus ani is idiopathic and probably related to local hygiene, neurogenic, or psychogenic causes. Treatment focuses upon removal of irritants, improving perianal hygiene, dietary adjustments, and avoiding scratching. Biopsy and/or culture may be required to rule out an infectious or dermatologic cause. Hydrocortisone ointment 0.5 to 1.0% can provide symptomatic relief but should not be used for prolonged periods of time because of dermal atrophy. Skin barriers such as Calmoseptine can also provide relief. Systemic antihistamines or tricyclic antidepressants have also been used with some success.

Nonpruritic Lesions

Several perianal skin conditions may present with perianal skin changes. Leprosy, amebiasis, actinomycosis, and lymphogranuloma venereum produce characteristic perianal lesions. Neoplasms such as Bowen's disease, Paget's disease, and invasive carcinomas may also appear first in the perianal skin. Biopsy can usually distinguish these diagnoses.

Sexually Transmitted Diseases[90,91]

Bacterial Infections

Proctitis is a common symptom of anorectal bacterial infection. *N. gonorrhoeae* is the most common bacterial cause of proctitis and causes pain, tenesmus, rectal bleeding, and mucus discharge.

C. trachomatis infection may be asymptomatic or may produce similar symptoms. *T. pallidum,* the microbe causing syphilis, causes a chancre at the site of inoculation, which may be asymptomatic or may present as an atypical fissure (primary syphilis). Condyloma lata are characteristic of secondary syphilis. Chancroid, caused by *Haemophilus ducreyi,* is a disease manifested by multiple painful, bleeding lesions. Inguinal lymphadenopathy and fluctuant, draining lymph nodes are characteristic. *Donovania granulomatis* infection produces shiny, red masses on the perineum (granuloma inguinale). Diarrheal illnesses caused by organisms such as *Campylobacter* or *Shigella* may also be sexually transmitted. Treatment consists of antimicrobial agents directed against the infecting organism.

Parasitic Infections

Entamoeba histolytica is an increasingly common sexually transmitted disease. Amebas produce ulcerations in the gastrointestinal mucosa and can infect any part of the gut. Symptoms include diarrhea, abdominal pain, and tenesmus. *Giardia lamblia* is also common and produces diarrhea, abdominal pain, and malaise.

Viral Infections

Herpes Simplex Virus. Herpes proctitis is extremely common. Proctitis is usually caused by type II herpes simplex virus and less commonly by type I herpes simplex virus. Patients complain of severe, intractable perianal pain and tenesmus. Pain often precedes the development of characteristic vesicles and these patients may require an examination under anesthesia to exclude another diagnosis such as an intersphincteric abscess. Diagnosis is confirmed by viral culture of tissue or vesicular fluid.

Human Papilloma Virus. HPV causes condyloma acuminata (anogenital warts) and is associated with anal intraepithelial neoplasia and squamous cell carcinoma (see "Anal Canal and Perianal Tumors" above). Condylomas occur in the perianal area or in the squamous epithelium of the anal canal. Occasionally, the mucosa of the lower rectum may be affected. There are approximately 30 serotypes of HPV. HPV types 16 and 18, in particular, appear to predispose to malignancy and often cause flat dysplasia in skin unaffected by warts. In contrast, HPV types 6 and 11 commonly cause warts, but do not appear to cause malignant degeneration.

Treatment of anal condyloma depends upon the location and extent of disease. Small warts on the perianal skin and distal anal canal may be treated in the office with topical application of bichloracetic acid or podophyllin. Although 60 to 80% of patients will respond to these agents, recurrence and reinfection are common. Imiquimod (Aldara) is an immunomodulator that was recently introduced for topical treatment of several viral infections, including anogenital condyloma.[92] Initial reports suggest that this agent is highly effective in treating condyloma located on the perianal skin and distal anal canal. Larger and/or more numerous warts require excision and/or fulguration in the operating room. Excised warts should be sent for pathologic examination to rule out dysplasia or malignancy. It is important to note that prior use of podophyllin may induce histologic changes that mimic dysplasia.

Human Immunodeficiency Virus. See "The Immunocompromised Patient" below.

Pilonidal Disease

Pilonidal disease (cyst, infection) consists of a hair-containing sinus or abscess occurring in the intergluteal cleft. Although the etiology is unknown, it is speculated that the cleft creates a suction that draws hair into the midline pits when a patients sits. These ingrown hairs may then become infected and present acutely as an abscess in the sacrococcygeal region. Once an acute episode has resolved, recurrence is common.

An acute abscess should be incised and drained as soon as the diagnosis is made. Because these abscesses are usually very superficial, this procedure can often be performed in the office, clinic, or emergency room under local anesthetic. Because midline wounds in the region heal poorly, some surgeons recommend using an incision *lateral* to the intergluteal cleft. A number of procedures have been proposed to treat a chronic pilonidal sinus. The simplest method involves unroofing the tract, curetting the base, and marsupializing the wound. The wound must then be kept clean and free of hair until healing is complete (often requiring weekly office visits for wound care). Alternatively, a small lateral incision can be created and the pit excised. This method is effective for most primary pilonidal sinuses. In general, extensive resection should be avoided. Complex and/or recurrent sinus tracts may require more extensive resection and closure with a Z-plasty, advancement flap, or rotational flap.

Hidradenitis Suppurativa

Hidradenitis suppurativa is an infection of the cutaneous apocrine sweat glands. Infected glands rupture and form subcutaneous sinus tracts. The infection may mimic complex anal fistula disease, but stops at the anal verge because there are no apocrine glands in the anal canal. Treatment involves incision and drainage of acute abscesses and unroofing of all chronically inflamed fistulas and debridement of granulation tissue. Radical excision and skin grafting is almost never necessary.

TRAUMA

Penetrating Colorectal Injury

Colorectal injury is common following penetrating trauma to the abdomen and has historically been associated with high mortality. In the first half of the twentieth century, the mortality rate from colorectal injury was as high as 90%. The introduction of exteriorization of colonic injuries and fecal diversion during World War II dramatically decreased mortality, and this principle has governed the management of large-bowel injury for over 50 years. Recently, however, this practice was challenged and trauma surgeons are increasingly performing primary repairs in selected patients.

Management of colonic injury depends upon the mechanism of injury, the delay between the injury and surgery, the overall condition and stability of the patient, the degree of peritoneal contamination, and the condition of the injured colon. A primary repair may be considered in hemodynamically stable patients with few additional injuries and minimal contamination if the colon appears otherwise healthy. Contraindications to primary repair include shock, injury to more than two other organs, mesenteric vascular damage, and extensive fecal contamination. A delay of greater than 6 hours between the injury and the operation is also associated with increased morbidity and mortality and is a relative contraindication to primary repair. Injuries caused by high-velocity gunshot wounds or blast injuries are often associated with multiple intra-abdominal injuries and tissue loss and therefore are usually treated by fecal diversion after debridement of all nonviable tissue. Patient factors, such as medical comorbidities, advanced age, and the presence of tumor or radiation injury, must also be considered (Table 28-5).

Like injuries to the intraperitoneal colon, penetrating trauma to the rectum traditionally has been associated with high morbidity

Table 28-5
Criteria for Use of an Ostomy

Injuring Agent Factors
High-velocity bullet wounds
Shotgun wounds
Explosive blast wounds
Crush injury

Patients Factors
Presence of tumor
Radiated tissue
Medical condition
Advanced age

Injury Factors
Inflamed tissue
Advanced infection
Distal obstruction
Local foreign body
Impaired blood supply
Mesenteric vascular damage
Shock with blood pressure <80/60 mm Hg
Hemorrhage >1000 mL
More than two organs (especially kidney) injured
Interval to operation >6 h (pancreatic, splenic, hepatic)
Extensive injury requiring resection
Major abdominal wall loss
Thoracoabdominal penetration

SOURCE: Reproduced with permission from Gordon PH, Nivatvongs F (eds). Principles and Practice of Surgery for the Colon, Rectum, and Anus, 2nd ed. New York: Marcel Dekker, Inc., 1999, p 1249.

and mortality. Primary repair of the rectum is more difficult than primary repair of the colon, however, and most rectal injuries are associated with significant contamination. For that reason, the majority of penetrating rectal injuries should be treated with proximal fecal diversion and copious irrigation of the rectum (distal rectal washout). If there is extensive fecal contamination, presacral drains may be useful. Small, clean rectal injuries may be closed primarily without fecal diversion in an otherwise stable patient. Intractable rectal bleeding may require angiographic embolization. Very rarely, hemorrhage or extensive tissue loss (especially if the anal sphincter is severely damaged) may require an emergent abdominoperineal resection. However, this operation should be avoided, if at all possible, because of the morbidity associated with an extensive pelvic dissection in a severely injured patient.

Blunt Colorectal Injury

Blunt injury to the colon and rectum is considerably less common than penetrating injury. Nevertheless, blunt trauma can cause colon perforation and shear injury to the mesentery can devascularize the intestine. Management of these injuries should follow the same principles outlined for management of penetrating injuries. Small perforations with little contamination in a stable patient may be closed primarily; more extensive injury requires fecal diversion. A serosal hematoma alone does not mandate resection, but the bowel should be carefully inspected to ensure that there is not an associated perforation or significant bowel ischemia.

Blunt injury to the rectum may result from significant trauma, such as a pelvic crush injury, or may result from local trauma caused by an enema or foreign body. Crush injuries, especially with an associated pelvic fracture, are often associated with significant rectal damage and contamination. These patients require débridement of all nonviable tissue, proximal fecal diversion, and a distal rectal washout, with or without drain placement. Blunt trauma from an enema or foreign body may produce a mucosal hematoma, which requires no surgical treatment if the mucosa is intact. Small mucosal tears may be closed primarily if the bowel is relatively clean and there is little contamination.

Iatrogenic Injury

Intraoperative Injury

The colon and rectum are at risk for inadvertent injury during other procedures, especially during pelvic operations. The key to managing these injuries is *early recognition.* The vast majority of iatrogenic colorectal injuries may be closed primarily if there is little contamination and if the patient is otherwise stable. Delayed recognition of colorectal injuries may result in significant peritonitis and life-threatening sepsis. In these cases, fecal diversion is almost always required and the patient may need repeated exploration for drainage of abscesses.

Injury from Barium Enema

Colorectal injury from a barium enema is an extremely rare complication associated with a high rate of morbidity and mortality. Perforation with spillage of barium, especially above the peritoneal reflection, may result in profound peritonitis, sepsis, and a systemic inflammatory response. If the perforation is recognized early, it may be closed primarily and the abdomen irrigated to remove stool and barium. However, if the patient has developed sepsis, fecal diversion (with or without bowel resection) is almost always required. Rarely, a small mucosal injury to the extraperitoneal rectum may be managed with bowel rest, broad-spectrum antibiotics, and close observation.

Colonoscopic Perforation

Perforation is the most common major complication after either diagnostic or therapeutic colonoscopy. Fortunately, this complication is rare and occurs in less than 1% of procedures. Perforation may result from trauma from the tip of the instrument, from shear forces related to the formation of a "loop" in the colonoscope, or from barotrauma from insufflation. Biopsy or fulguration can also cause perforation. Polypectomy using electrocautery may produce a full-thickness burn, resulting in *postpolypectomy syndrome* in which a patient develops abdominal pain, fever, and leukocytosis without evidence of diffuse peritonitis.

Management of colonoscopic perforation depends upon the *size of the perforation,* the *duration of time* since the injury, and the *overall condition of the patient.* A large perforation recognized during the procedure requires surgical exploration. Because the bowel has almost always been prepared prior to the colonoscopy, there is usually little contamination associated with these injuries and most can be repaired primarily. If there is significant contamination, if there has been a delay in diagnosis with resulting peritonitis, or if the patient is hemodynamically unstable, proximal diversion with or without resection is the safest approach. Occasionally, a patient will develop abdominal pain and localized signs of perforation after what was thought to be an uneventful colonoscopy. Many of these patients will have a "microperforation" which will resolve with bowel rest, broad-spectrum antibiotics, and close observation. Evidence of peritonitis or any deterioration in clinical condition mandates exploration. Similarly, free retroperitoneal or intraperitoneal air may be discovered incidentally after colonoscopy. In a completely asymptomatic patient, this finding is thought to result from barotrauma and dissection of air through tissue planes without a free perforation. Many of these patients can be successfully treated with bowel rest and broad-spectrum antibiotics. Surgical exploration is indicated for any clinical deterioration.

Anal Sphincter Injury and Incontinence

The most common cause of anal sphincter injury is obstetric trauma during vaginal delivery. The risk of sphincter injury is increased by a laceration that extends into the rectum (fourth-degree tear), infection of an episiotomy or laceration repair, prolonged labor, and possibly by use of a midline episiotomy. Sphincter damage may also result from hemorrhoidectomy, sphincterotomy, abscess drainage, or fistulotomy. Patients with incontinence and a suspected sphincter injury can be evaluated with anal manometry, electromyography (EMG), and endoanal ultrasound. Mild incontinence, even in the presence of a sphincter defect, may respond to dietary changes and/or biofeedback. More severe incontinence may require surgical repair.

The anal sphincter can also be injured by penetrating or blunt mechanisms (impalement, blast injury, crush injuries of the pelvis). Because damage to the anal sphincter is not life-threatening, definitive repair of the sphincter is often deferred until other injuries have been repaired and the patient's clinical condition is stable. Isolated sphincter injuries that do not involve the rectum may be repaired primarily. Rectal injury accompanied by sphincter injury should be treated with fecal diversion, distal rectal washout, and drain placement. Significant perineal tissue loss may require extensive débridement and a diverting colostomy.

Surgical Repairs

The most common method of repair of the anal sphincter is a *wrap-around sphincteroplasty* (Fig. 28-41).[9] The procedure involves mobilization of the divided sphincter muscle and reapproximation without tension. The internal and external sphincters may be overlapped together or separately. *Postanal intersphincteric levatorplasty* is less commonly used to repair sphincter defects but may be useful for incontinence caused by prolapse and/or loss of the anorectal angle (see "Continence" above). The approach is via the intersphincteric plane posteriorly. It may be performed concomitantly with a perineal repair of rectal prolapse. The levator ani muscle is approximated to restore the anorectal angle and the puborectalis and external sphincter muscle are tightened with sutures. These elective procedures do not usually require a diverting colostomy.

In cases where there has been significant loss of sphincter muscle, or in which prior repairs have failed, more complex techniques, such as *gracilis muscle transposition* with or without chronic, low-frequency electrostimulation, have been used with some success.[93] In this procedure, the gracilis muscle is mobilized from the thigh, detached from its insertion on the tibial tuberosity, tunneled through the perineum, and wrapped around the anal canal. Another alternative in patients who have failed other repairs is the *artificial anal sphincter.* This device consists of an inflatable silastic cuff, a pressure-regulating balloon, and a control pump. Patients deflate the cuff manually to open the anal canal; the cuff then reinflates spontaneously to maintain closure of the anal canal. *Sacral nerve stimulation* via an implanted pulse generator is a new technique used for neurogenic incontinence when the sphincter is intact.[10,11]

Foreign Body

Foreign-body entrapment in the rectum is not uncommon. Depending upon the level of entrapment, a foreign body may cause damage to the rectum, rectosigmoid, or descending colon. Generalized abdominal pain suggests intraperitoneal perforation. Evaluation of the

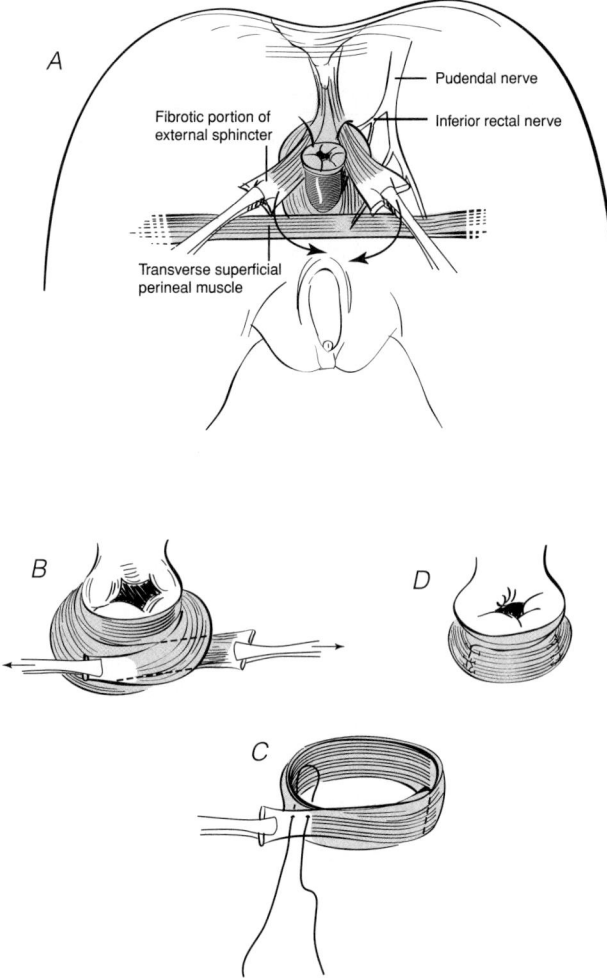

FIG. 28-41. Overlapping sphincteroplasty for incontinence from sphincter disruption. *A.* The external sphincter muscle with scar at site of injury is mobilized. *B.* The muscle edges are aligned in an overlapping fashion. *C.* Mattress sutures are used to approximate the muscle. *D.* The completed operation. [*Reproduced with permission from Schwartz SI, Shires GT, Spencer FC (eds): Principles of Surgery. 5th ed. New York: McGraw-Hill, 1989, p 1308.*]

patient includes inspection of the perineum and a careful abdominal examination to detect any evidence of perforation. Plain films of the abdomen are mandatory to detect free intra-abdominal air.

Foreign bodies lodged low in the rectum may often be removed under conscious sedation with or without a local anesthetic block. Objects impacted higher in the rectum may require regional or general anesthesia for removal. Only rarely will a laparotomy be required to remove the object. After removal of the foreign body, it is crucial to evaluate the rectum and sigmoid colon for injury. Proctoscopy and/or flexible sigmoidoscopy should be performed. A hematoma without evidence of perforation requires no surgical treatment. Perforation of the rectum or sigmoid colon should be managed as described in the preceding sections.

THE IMMUNOCOMPROMISED PATIENT

Human Immunodeficiency Virus

Patients infected with HIV may present with a myriad of gastrointestinal symptoms.[94] Diarrhea, in particular, is extremely common.

The severity of gastrointestinal disease depends in part upon the degree of immunosuppression; however, both ordinary and opportunistic pathogens may affect patients at any stage of the disease. Opportunistic infections with bacteria (*Salmonella, Shigella, Campylobacter, Chlamydia,* and *Mycobacterium* species), fungi (*Histoplasmosis, Coccidiosis, Cryptococcus*), protozoa *(Toxoplasmosis, Cryptosporidiosis, Isosporiasis),* and viruses (*Cytomegalovirus, herpes simplex virus*) can cause diarrhea, abdominal pain, and weight loss. *CMV* in particular may cause severe enterocolitis and is the most common infectious cause of emergency laparotomy in acquired immunodeficiency syndrome (AIDS) patients. *C. difficile colitis* is a major concern in these patients, especially because many patients are maintained on suppressive antibiotic therapy. The incidence of gastrointestinal malignancy is also increased in patients with HIV infection.[95] Kaposi's sarcoma is the most common malignancy in AIDS patients and can affect any part of the gastrointestinal tract. Patients may be asymptomatic or may develop bleeding or obstruction. Gastrointestinal lymphoma (usually non-Hodgkin's lymphoma) is also common. The incidence of colorectal carcinoma may also be increased in this population, although definitive data are lacking.

Perianal disease is extremely common in patients with HIV infection. Because HIV is sexually transmitted, it is common to find concomitant infection with other sexually transmitted diseases such as *Chlamydia, herpes simplex virus,* and *human papilloma virus (anal condyloma). Anal condyloma* in particular are very common and the incidence of dysplasia (anal intraepithelial neoplasia) is high in the HIV-infected population.[96–98] Abscesses and fistulas may be more difficult to diagnose in these patients and may be complex. Many patients require an examination under anesthesia with biopsy and cultures to determine the etiology of many of these perianal problems.

Immunosuppression for Transplantation

The gastrointestinal tract is a common site for posttransplantation complications that are responsible for significant morbidity and mortality. In these patients, infection and medication are the most common causes of diarrhea. Immunosuppressant medications, in particular, may cause diarrhea. CMV infection is common and may be severe. *C. difficile* colitis also occurs commonly. Diverticulitis appears to be more common in some populations of transplant patients and may be more likely to present with abscess or free perforation. Elective resection after recovery from one episode of confirmed diverticulitis may be indicated in the transplant population. Graft-versus-host disease is unique to transplant patients and often requires endoscopy and biopsy to diagnose gastrointestinal involvement. Patients are subject to the same opportunistic infections outlined above; however, sexually transmitted infections and Kaposi's sarcoma are somewhat less prevalent. Perianal disease is somewhat less common in the transplant population than in patients infected with HIV; however, similar infections may occur and immunosuppression often makes diagnosis challenging.

With increasing long-term survival among transplant recipients, the development of posttransplant malignancy has become a major concern. Posttransplant lymphoproliferative disease is increasingly common and may occur anywhere in the gastrointestinal tract. The risk of colorectal carcinoma is increased in patients with predisposing conditions such as ulcerative colitis. However, immunosuppression alone does not appear to increase the incidence of colorectal cancer, and current screening recommendations are similar to those for the average risk population. In contrast, the incidence of anal squamous cell carcinoma is dramatically increased in transplant patients and patients with known HPV infection should undergo more vigorous screening.

The Neutropenic Patient

Neutropenic enterocolitis (typhlitis) is a life-threatening problem with a mortality rate of greater than 50%. This syndrome is characterized by abdominal pain and distention, fever, diarrhea (often bloody), nausea, and vomiting in a patient with fewer than 1000 neutrophils from any cause (bone marrow transplantation, solid-organ transplantation, or chemotherapy). CT scan of the abdomen often shows a dilated cecum with pericolic stranding. However, a normal-appearing CT scan does not exclude the diagnosis. Some patients will respond to bowel rest, broad-spectrum antibiotics, parenteral nutrition, and granulocyte infusion or colony-stimulating factors. Evidence of perforation, generalized peritonitis, or deterioration in clinical condition are indications for operation.

Neutropenic patients often develop perianal pain, and diagnosis may be difficult because of a lack of inflammatory response to infection. While broad-spectrum antibiotics may cure some of these patients, an examination under anesthesia should not be delayed because of neutropenia. An increase in pain or fever, and/or clinical deterioration mandates an exam under anesthesia. Any indurated area should be incised and drained, biopsied to exclude a leukemic infiltrate, and cultured to aid in the selection of antimicrobial agents.

References

1. Smith RA, von Eschenbach AC, Wender R, et al: American Cancer Society guidelines for the early detection of cancer: Update of early detection guidelines for prostate, colorectal and endometrial cancers. *CA Cancer J Clin* 51:38, 2001.
2. Bernini A, Spencer MP, Wong WD, et al: Computed tomography-guided percutaneous abscess drainage in intestinal disease. Factors associated with outcome. *Dis Colon Rectum* 40:1009, 1997.
3. Garcia-Aguilar J, Pollack J, Lee SH, et al: Accuracy of endorectal ultrasonography in preoperative staging of rectal tumors. *Dis Colon Rectum* 45:10, 2002.
4. Turgeon D, Novicki T, Quick J, et al: Six rapid tests for direct detection of *Clostridium difficile* and its toxins in fecal samples compared with the fibroblast cytotoxic assay. *J Clin Microbiol* 41:667, 2003.
5. Qui H, Sirivongs P, Rothenberger M, et al: Molecular prognostic factors in rectal cancer treated by radiation and surgery. *Dis Colon Rectum* 43:451, 2000.
6. Offit K: Genetic prognostic markers for colorectal cancer. *N Engl J Med* 342:124, 2000.
7. Dailianas A, Skandalis N, Rimikis M, et al: Pelvic floor study in patients with obstructed defecation: Influence of biofeedback. *J Clin Gastroenterol* 30:176, 2000.
8. Fitzharris G, Garcia-Aguilar J, Parker S, et al: Quality of life after subtotal colectomy for slow transit constipation—Both quality and quantity count. *Dis Colon Rectum* 46:433, 2003.
9. Buie WD, Lowry AC, Rothenberger DA, et al: Clinical rather than laboratory predicts continence after anterior sphincteroplasty. *Dis Colon Rectum* 44:1255, 2001.
10. Ganio E, Ratto C, Masin A, et al: Neuromodulation for fecal incontinence: Outcome in 16 patients with definitive implant. *Dis Colon Rectum* 44:965, 2001.
11. Vaizey CF, Kamm MA, Roy AJ, et al: Double-blind crossover study of sacral nerve stimulation for fecal incontinence. *Dis Colon Rectum* 43:298, 2000.
12. Lezoche E, Feliciotti F, Paganini, et al: Laparoscopic colonic resections versus open surgery: A prospective non-randomized study on 310 unselected cases. *Hepatogastroenterology* 47:697, 2000.
13. Regimbeau J, Panis Y, Pocard M, et al: Handsewn ileal pouch–anal anastomosis on the dentate line after total proctocolectomy: Technique to avoid incomplete mucosectomy and the need for long-term follow-up of the anal transition zone. *Dis Colon Rectum* 44:43, 2001.
14. O'Riodan MG, Fazio VW, Lavery IC, et al: Incidence and natural history of dysplasia of the anal transitional zone after ileal pouch–anal anastomosis. *Dis Colon Rectum* 43:1660, 2000.
15. Ky A, Sonoda T, Milsom J, et al: One-stage laparoscopic restorative proctocolectomy: An alternative to the conventional approach? *Dis Colon Rectum* 45:207, 2002.
16. Heuschen U, Hinz U, Allemayer E, et al: One- or two-stage procedure for restorative proctocolectomy: Rationale for a surgical strategy in ulcerative colitis. *Ann Surg* 234:788, 2001.
17. Heah SM, Seow-Choen F, Eu KW, et al: Prospective randomized trial comparing sigmoid vs. descending colonic J-pouch after total rectal excision. *Dis Colon Rectum* 45:322, 2002.
18. Faroulk R, Pemberton JH, Wolff BG, et al: Functional outcomes after ileal pouch–anal anastomosis for chronic ulcerative colitis. *Ann Surg* 231:919, 2000.
19. Bullard K, Madoff R, Gemlo B: Is ileoanal pouch function stable over time? Results of a prospective audit. *Dis Colon Rectum* 45:299, 2002.
20. Sandborn W, McLeod R, Jewell D: Pharmacotherapy for inducing and maintaining remission in pouchitis. *Cochrane Database Syst Rev* 2:CD001176, 2000.
21. Stocchi L, Pemberton JH: Pouch and pouchitis. *Gastroenterol Clin North Am* 30:223, 2001.
22. Miettinen RPJ, Laitinen ST, Makela JT, et al: Bowel preparation with oral polyethylene glycol electrolyte solution vs. no preparation in elective open colorectal surgery. Prospective, randomized study. *Dis Colon Rectum* 43:669, 2000.
23. Zmora O, Pikarsky A, Wexner SD: Bowel preparation for colorectal surgery. *Dis Colon Rectum* 44:1537, 2001.
24. Bonen DK, Cho JH: The genetics of inflammatory bowel disease. *Gastroenterology* 124:521, 2003.
25. Dvorchik I, Subotin M, Demetris A, et al: Effect of liver transplantation on inflammatory bowel disease in patients with primary sclerosing cholangitis. *Hepatology* 35:380, 2002.
26. Mahadevan U, Loftus EV Jr., Tremaine WJ, et al: Azathioprine or 6-mercaptopurine before colectomy for ulcerative colitis is not associated with increased postoperative complications. *Inflamm Bowel Dis* 8:311, 2002.
27. Alfadhli A, McDonald J, Feagan B: Methotrexate for induction of remission in refractory Crohn's disease [Cochrane Review]. *Cochrane Database Syst Rev* 1:CD003459, 2003.
28. Present D, Rutgeerts P, Targan S, et al: Infliximab for the treatment of fistulas in patients with Crohn's disease. *N Engl J Med* 340:1398, 1999.
29. Hanauer S, Feagan B, Lichtenstein G: Maintenance infliximab for Crohn's disease: The ACCENT I randomised trial. *Lancet* 359:1541, 2002.
30. Actis G, Bruno M, Pinna-Pintor M: Infliximab for treatment of steroid-refractory ulcerative colitis. *Dig Liver Dis* 34:631, 2002.
31. Su C, Salzberg B, Lewis J, et al: Efficacy of anti-tumor necrosis factor therapy in patients with ulcerative colitis. *Am J Gastroenterol* 97:2577, 2002.
32. Chautems RC, Ambrosetti P, Ludwig A, et al: Long-term follow-up after first acute episode of sigmoid diverticulitis: Is surgery mandatory? A prospective study of 118 patients. *Dis Colon Rectum* 45:962, 2002.
33. Wong WD, Wexner SD, Lowry A, et al: The Standards Task Force. The American Society of Colon and Rectal Surgeons. Practice parameters for the treatment of sigmoid diverticulitis. *Dis Colon Rectum* 43:289, 2000.
34. Wong WD, Wexner SD, Lowry A, et al: The Standards Task Force. The American Society of Colon and Rectal Surgeons. Practice parameters for the treatment of sigmoid diverticulitis—Supporting documentation. *Dis Colon Rectum* 43:290, 2000.
35. Wolff BG, Devine RM: Surgical management of diverticulitis. *Am Surg* 66:153, 2000.

36. Schilling MK, Maurer CA, Kollmar O, et al: Primary vs. secondary anastomosis after sigmoid colon resection for perforated diverticulitis (Hinchey Stage II and IV): A prospective outcome and cost analysis. *Dis Colon Rectum* 44:699, 2001.

37. Janne PA, Mayer RD: Chemoprevention of colorectal cancer [review]. *N Engl J Med* 342:160, 2000.

38. Calle E, Rodriguez C, Walter-Thurmond K, et al: Overweight, obesity, and mortality from cancer in a prospective studied cohort of U.S. adults. *N Engl J Med* 348:1625, 2003.

39. Eaden J, Abrams K, Mayberry J: The risk of colorectal cancer in ulcerative colitis: A meta-analysis. *Gut* 48:526, 2001.

40. Woodhouse C: Guidelines for monitoring of patients with uretero sigmoidoscopy. *Gut* 51(Suppl V):v15, 2002.

41. Jenkins P, Fairclough PD: Screening guidelines for colorectal cancer and polyps in patients with acromegaly. *Gut* 51(Suppl V):v13, 2002.

42. Gryfe R, Kim H, Hsieth ET, et al: Tumor microsatellite instability and clinical outcome in young patients with colorectal cancer. *N Engl J Med* 342:69, 2000.

43. Van Duijvendijk P, Slors JF, Taat CW, et al: Quality of life after total colectomy with ileorectal anastomosis or proctocolectomy and ileal pouch–anal anastomosis for familial adenomatous polyposis. *Br J Surg* 87:590, 2000.

44. Vasen HF, van Duijvendijk P, Buskens E, et al: Decision analysis in the surgical treatment of patients with familial adenomatous polyposis: A Dutch-Scandinavian collaborative study including 659 patients. *Gut* 49:231, 2001.

45. Bulow C, Vasen H, Jarvinen H, et al: Ileorectal anastomosis is appropriate for a subset of patients with familial adenomatous polyposis. *Gastroenterology* 119:1454, 2000.

46. Steinbach G, Lynch PM, Phillips RK, et al: The effect of celecoxib, a cyclooxygenase-2 inhibitor, in familial adenomatous polyposis. *N Engl J Med* 342:1946, 2000.

47. Syngal S, Fox E, Li C: Interpretation of genetic test results for hereditary nonpolyposis colorectal cancer: Implications for clinical predisposition testing. *JAMA* 282:247, 1999.

48. Jarvinen HJ, Aarnio M, Mustonen H, et al: Controlled 15-year trial on screening for colorectal cancer in families with hereditary nonpolyposis colorectal cancer. *Gastroenterology* 118:829, 2000.

49. National Comprehensive Cancer Network: Colorectal cancer screening clinical practice guidelines in oncology. *J NCCN* 1:72, 2003.

50. Pignone M, Rich M, Teutsch SM, et al: Screening for colorectal cancer in adults at average risk: A summary of the evidence for the U.S. Preventive Services Task Force. *Ann Intern Med* 173:132, 2002.

51. Levin B, Brooks D, Smith R: Emerging technologies in screening for colorectal cancer: CT colography, immunochemical fecal occult blood tests, and stool screening using molecular markers. *CA Cancer J Clin* 53:44, 2003.

52. Imperiale TF, Wagner DR, Lin CY, et al: Risk of advanced proximal neoplasms in asymptomatic adults according to the distal colorectal findings. *N Engl J Med* 343:169, 2000.

53. Lieberman DA, Weiss DB, Bond JH, et al: Use of colonoscopy to screen asymptomatic adults for colorectal cancer. Veterans Affairs Cooperative Study Group 380. *N Engl J Med* 343:162, 2000.

54. Yee J, Akerkar GA, Hung RK, et al: Colorectal neoplasia: Performance characteristics of CT colonography for detection of 300 patients. *Radiology* 219:685, 2001.

55. Winawer SJ, Stewart ET, Zauber AG, et al: A comparison of colonoscopy and double-contrast barium enema for surveillance after polypectomy. National Polyp Study Work Group. *N Engl J Med* 342:1766, 2000.

56. Greene FL, Page DL, Fleming, et al: *AJCC Cancer Staging Manual,* 6th ed. New York: Springer-Verlag, 2002.

57. National Comprehensive Cancer Network: Colon cancer clinical practice guidelines in oncology. *J NCCN* 1:40, 2003.

58. Rothenberger DA, Garcia-Aguilar J: Management of cancer in a polyp, in Saltz L (ed): *Colorectal Cancer: Multimodality Management.* NJ: Humana Press, 2002, p. 325.

59. Marsoni S: International Multicenter Pooled Analysis of Colon Cancer Trial Investigators. Efficacy of adjuvant fluorouracil and leucovorin in stage B2 and C colon cancer. *Semin Oncol* 28(1 Suppl 1):14, 2001.

60. Hall NR, Finan PJ, Al-Jaberi T, et al: Circumferential margin involvement after mesorectal excision of rectal cancer with curative intent. *Dis Colon Rectum* 41:979, 1998.

61. Garcia-Aguilar J, Mellgren A, Sirivongs P, et al: Local excision of rectal cancer without adjuvant therapy: A word of caution. *Ann Surg* 231:345, 2002.

62. Heald R, Moran B, Ryall R, et al: Rectal cancer: The Basingstoke experience of total mesorectal excision, 1978–1997. *Arch Surg* 133:894, 1998.

63. Friel CM, Cromwell JW, Marra C, et al: Salvage radical surgery after failed local excision for early rectal cancer. *Dis Colon Rectum* 45:875, 2002.

64. Yiu R, Wong SK, Cromwell JW, et al: Pelvic wall involvement denotes a poor prognosis in T4 rectal cancer. *Dis Colon Rectum* 44:1676, 2001.

65. National Comprehensive Cancer Network: Rectal cancer clinical practice guidelines in oncology. *J NCCN* 1:54, 2003.

66. Beart RW Jr.: Follow-up: Does it work? Can we afford it? *Surg Oncol Clin North Am* 9:827, 2000.

67. Jeffrey GM, Hickey BE, Hider P: Follow-up strategies for patients treated for non-metastatic colorectal cancer [review]. *Cochrane Database Syst Rev* 2, 2002.

68. Saha S, Bilchik A, Wiese D, et al: Ultrastaging of colorectal cancer by sentinel lymph node mapping technique—A multicenter trial. *Ann Surg Oncol* 8:94, 2001.

69. Lacy A, Garcia-Valdecases J, Delgado S, et al: Laparoscopy-assisted colectomy versus open colectomy for treatment of non-metastatic colon cancer: A randomised trial. *Lancet* 359:2224, 2002.

70. Weeks J, Nelson H, Gelber, et al: Short-term quality-of-life outcomes following laparoscopic-assisted colectomy vs. open colectomy for colon cancer. *JAMA* 16:321, 2002.

71. National Comprehensive Cancer Network: Anal canal cancer clinical practice guidelines in oncology. *J NCCN* 1:64, 2003.

72. Beck D, Timmcke AE: Anal margin lesions. *Clin Colon Rectal Surg* 15:277, 2002.

73. Ryan D, Compton C, Mayer R: Medical progress: Carcinoma of the anal canal. *N Engl J Med* 342:792, 2000.

74. Nguyen W, Beck D: Epidermoid carcinoma of the anal canal. *Clin Colon Rectal Surg* 15:263, 2002.

75. Moore HG, Guillem JG: Adenocarcinoma of the anal canal. *Clin Colon Rectal Surg* 15:255, 2002.

76. Mutch MG, Roberts PL: Anal and peri-anal melanoma. *Clin Colon Rectal Surg* 15:271, 2002.

77. Bullard K, Tuttle T, Rothenberger D, et al: Surgical therapy for anorectal melanoma. *J Am Coll Surg* 196:206, 2003.

78. Bullard K, Madoff R: Rectal prolapse and intussusception, in Stollman N, Wexner S (eds): *The Colon.* New York: Marcel Dekker, 2003.

79. Joyce A, Burns D: Recurrent *Clostridium difficile* colitis. Tackling a tenacious nosocomial infection. *Postgrad Med* 112:53, 2002.

80. Cremonini F, DiCaro S, Santarelli L, et al: Probiotics in antibiotic-associated diarrhea. *Dig Liver Dis* 34(Suppl):S78, 2002.

81. Ganio E, Altomare DF, Gabrielli F, et al: Prospective randomized multicentre trial comparing stapled with open haemorrhoidectomy. *Br J Surg* 88:669, 2001.

82. Ho YH, Seow-Choen F, Tsang C, et al: Randomized trial assessing anal sphincter injuries after stapled hemorrhoidectomy. *Br J Surg* 88:1449, 2001.

83. Ho Y-H, Cheong W-K, Tsang C, et al: Stapled hemorrhoidectomy—Cost and effectiveness. Randomized, controlled trial including incontinence scoring, anorectal manometry, and endoanal ultrasound assessments at up to three months. *Dis Colon Rectum* 43:1666, 2000.

84. Madoff R, Fleshman J: AGA technical review on the diagnosis and care of patients with anal fissure. *Gastroenterology* 124:235, 2003.

85. Minguez M, Herreros B, Benages A: Chronic anal fissure. *Curr Treat Options Gastroenterol* 6:257, 2003.

86. Bailey H, Beck D, Billingham R, et al: A study to determine the nitroglycerin ointment dose and dosing interval that best promote the healing of chronic anal fissures. *Dis Colon Rectum* 45:1192, 2002.

87. Jonas M. Speake W, Scholefield J: Diltiazem heals glyceryl trinitrate-resistant chronic anal fissures: A prospective study. *Dis Colon Rectum* 45:1091, 2002.

88. Mentes B, Irkorucu, O, Akin M, et al: Comparison of botulinum toxin injection and lateral internal sphincterotomy for the treatment of chronic anal fissure. *Dis Colon Rectum* 46:232, 2003.

89. Richard CS, Gregoire R, Plewes EA, et al: Internal sphincterotomy is superior to topical nitroglycerin the treatment of chronic anal fissure. *Dis Colon Rectum* 43:1048, 2000.

90. Wexner SD: Sexually transmitted diseases of the colon, rectum, and anus. The challenge of the nineties. *Dis Colon Rectum* 33:1048, 1990.

91. Smith L: Sexually transmitted diseases, in Gordon P, Nivatvongs S (eds): *Principles and Practice of Surgery for the Colon, Rectum, and Anus.* St. Louis: Quality Medical Publishing, 1999, p 341.

92. Staley M: Imiquimod and the imidazoquinolones: Mechanism of action and therapeutic potential. *Clin Exp Dermatol* 27:571, 2002.

93. Baeten CGMI, Bailey HR, Bakka A, et al: Safety and efficacy of dynamic graciloplasty for fecal incontinence: Report of a prospective, multicenter trial. *Dis Colon Rectum* 43:743, 2000.

94. Orenstein J, Dieterich D: The histopathology of 103 consecutive colonoscopy biopsies from 82 symptomatic patients with acquired immunodeficiency syndrome: Original and look-back diagnosis. *Arch Pathol Lab Med* 125:1042, 2001.

95. Cooksley C, Hwang L, Wallder D, et al: HIV-related malignancies: community-based study using linkage of cancer registry and HIV registry data. *Int J STD AIDS* 10:795, 1999.

96. El-Attar SM, Evans DV: Anal warts, sexually transmitted diseases, and anorectal conditions associated with human immunodeficiency virus. *Prim Care* 26:81, 1999.

97. Palefsky J: Anal squamous intraepithelial lesions: Relation to HIV and human papilloma virus infection. *J Acquir Immune Defic Syndr* 21(Suppl 1):S42, 1999.

98. Chang G, Berry J, Jay N, et al: Surgical treatment of high-grade anal squamous intraepithelial lesions: A prospective study. *Dis Colon Rectum* 45:453, 2002.

99. Smith L: Traumatic injuries, in Gordon PH, Nivatvongs S (eds): *Principles and Practice of Surgery for the Colon, Rectum, and Anus,* 2nd ed. New York: Marcel Dekker, 1999, p 1249.

CHAPTER 29

The Appendix

Bernard M. Jaffe and David H. Berger

ANATOMY AND FUNCTION

The appendix first becomes visible in the eighth week of embryologic development as a protuberance off the terminal portion of the cecum. During both antenatal and postnatal development, the growth rate of the cecum exceeds that of the appendix, displacing the appendix medially toward the ileocecal valve. The relationship of the base of the appendix to the cecum remains constant, whereas the tip can be found in a retrocecal, pelvic, subcecal, preileal, or right pericolic position (Fig. 29-1). These anatomic considerations have significant clinical importance in the context of acute appendicitis. The three taenia coli converge at the junction of the cecum with the appendix and can be a useful landmark to identify the appendix. The appendix can vary in length from less than 1 cm to greater than 30 cm; most appendices are 6 to 9 cm in length. Appendiceal absence, duplication, and diverticula have all been described.[1–4]

For many years, the appendix was erroneously viewed as a vestigial organ with no known function. It is now well recognized that the appendix is an immunologic organ that actively participates in the secretion of immunoglobulins, particularly immunoglobulin A (IgA). Although the appendix is an integral component of the gut-associated lymphoid tissue (GALT) system, its function is not essential and appendectomy is not associated with any predisposition to sepsis or any other manifestation of immune compromise. Lymphoid tissue first appears in the appendix approximately 2 weeks after birth. The amount of lymphoid tissue increases throughout puberty, remains steady for the next decade, and then begins a steady decrease with age. After the age of 60 years, virtually no lymphoid tissue remains within the appendix, and complete obliteration of the appendiceal lumen is common.[1–4]

ACUTE APPENDICITIS

Historical Background

Although ancient texts have scattered descriptions of surgery being performed for ailments sounding like appendicitis, credit for performance of the first appendectomy goes to Claudius Amyand, a surgeon at St. George's Hospital in London and Sergeant Surgeon to Queen Ann, King George I, and King George II. In 1736, he operated on an 11-year-old boy with a scrotal hernia and a fecal fistula. Within the hernia sac, Amyand found the appendix perforated by a pin. He successfully removed the appendix and repaired the hernia.[5]

The appendix was not identified as an organ capable of causing disease until the nineteenth century. In 1824, Louyer-Villermay presented a paper before the Royal Academy of Medicine in Paris. He reported on two autopsy cases of appendicitis and emphasized the importance of the condition. In 1827, François Melier, a French physician, expounded on Louyer-Villermay's work. He reported six autopsy cases and was the first to suggest the antemortem recognition of appendicitis.[5] This work was discounted by many

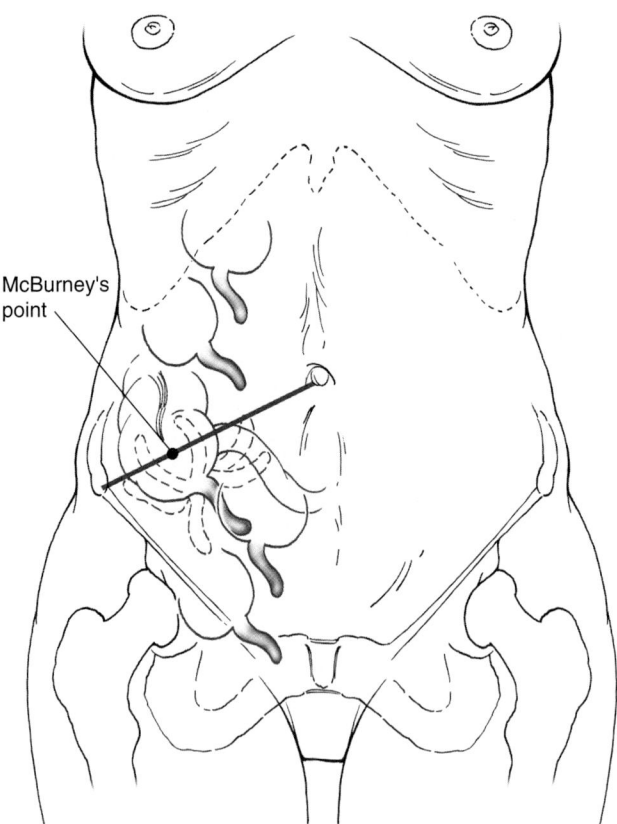

McBurney's point

FIG. 29-1. *Various anatomic positions of the vermiform appendix.*

physicians of the era, including Baron Guillaume Dupuytren. Dupuytren believed that inflammation of the cecum was the main cause of pathology of the right lower quadrant. The term "typhlitis" or "perityphlitis" was used to describe right lower quadrant inflammation. In 1839, a textbook authored by Bright and Addison titled *Elements of Practical Medicine* described the symptoms of appendicitis and identified the primary cause of inflammatory processes of the right lower quadrant.[6] Reginald Fitz, a professor of pathologic anatomy at Harvard, is credited for coining the term "appendicitis." His landmark paper definitively identified the appendix as the primary cause of right lower quadrant inflammation.[7]

Initial surgical therapy for appendicitis was primarily designed to drain right lower quadrant abscesses that occurred secondary to appendiceal perforation. It appears that the first surgical treatment for appendicitis or perityphlitis without abscess was made by Hancock in 1848. He incised the peritoneum and drained the right lower quadrant without removing the appendix. The first published account of appendectomy for appendicitis was by Krönlein in 1886. However, this patient died 2 days postoperatively. Fergus, in Canada, performed the first elective appendectomy in 1883.[5]

The greatest contributor to the advancement in the treatment of appendicitis is Charles McBurney. In 1889, he published his landmark paper in the *New York Medical Journal* describing the indications for early laparotomy for the treatment of appendicitis. It is in this paper that he described McBurney's point as the point of "maximum tenderness, when one examines with the fingertips is, in adults, one-half to two inches inside the right anterior spinous process of the ilium on a line drawn to the umbilicus."[8] McBurney subsequently published a paper describing the incision that bears his name in 1894. However, McBurney later credited McArthur with

first describing this incision.[9] Semm is widely credited with performing the first successful laparoscopic appendectomy in 1982.[10]

The surgical treatment of appendicitis is one of the great public health advancements of the last 150 years. Appendectomy for appendicitis is the most commonly performed emergency operation in the world. Additionally, appendicitis is a disease of the young, with 40% of the cases occurring in patients between the ages of 10 and 29 years.[11] In 1886, Fitz reported the associated mortality rate of appendicitis to be at least 67% without surgical therapy.[7] Currently, the mortality rate for acute appendicitis is reported to be less than 1%.[12] In the United States, more than 260,000 appendectomies are performed each year. If it is assumed that there is a 15% negative appendectomy rate and a median life expectancy of 80 years, the development of surgical therapy of appendicitis results in saving approximately 8 million lives per year in the United States alone.

Incidence

The lifetime rate of appendectomy is 12% for men and 25% for women, with approximately 7% of all people undergoing appendectomy for acute appendicitis. Over a 10-year period from 1987 to 1997, the overall appendectomy rate decreased parallel to a decrease in incidental appendectomy.[11,13] However, the rate of appendectomy for appendicitis has remained constant at 10 per 10,000 patients per year.[14] Appendicitis is most frequently seen in patients in their second through fourth decades of life, with a mean age of 31.3 years and a median age of 22 years. There is a slight male to female predominance (M:F 1.2 to 1.3:1).[11,13]

Despite an increased use of ultrasonography, computed tomography (CT) scanning, and laparoscopy between 1987 and 1997, the rate of misdiagnosis of appendicitis has remained constant (15.3%), as has the rate of appendiceal rupture. The percentage of misdiagnosis of appendicitis is significantly higher among women than men (22.2 vs. 9.3%). The negative appendectomy rate for women of reproductive age is 23.2%, with the highest rates identified in women age 40 to 49 years. The highest negative appendectomy rate is reported for women older than 80 years of age (Fig. 29-2).[13–15]

Etiology and Pathogenesis

Obstruction of the lumen is the dominant causal factor in acute appendicitis. Fecaliths are the usual cause of appendiceal obstruction. Less-common causes are hypertrophy of lymphoid tissue, inspissated barium from previous x-ray studies, tumors, vegetable and fruit seeds, and intestinal parasites. The frequency of obstruction rises with the severity of the inflammatory process. Fecaliths are found in 40% of cases of simple acute appendicitis, 65% of cases of gangrenous appendicitis without rupture, and nearly 90% of cases of gangrenous appendicitis with rupture.

There is a predictable sequence of events leading to eventual appendiceal rupture. The proximal obstruction of the appendiceal lumen produces a closed-loop obstruction, and continuing normal secretion by the appendiceal mucosa rapidly produces distention. The luminal capacity of the normal appendix is only 0.1 mL. Secretion of as little as 0.5 mL of fluid distal to an obstruction raises the intraluminal pressure to 60 cm H_2O. Distention of the appendix stimulates nerve endings of visceral afferent stretch fibers, producing vague, dull, diffuse pain in the mid-abdomen or lower epigastrium. Peristalsis is also stimulated by the rather sudden distention, so that some cramping may be superimposed on the visceral pain early in the course of appendicitis. Distention continues from continued mucosal secretion and from rapid multiplication of the resident bacteria

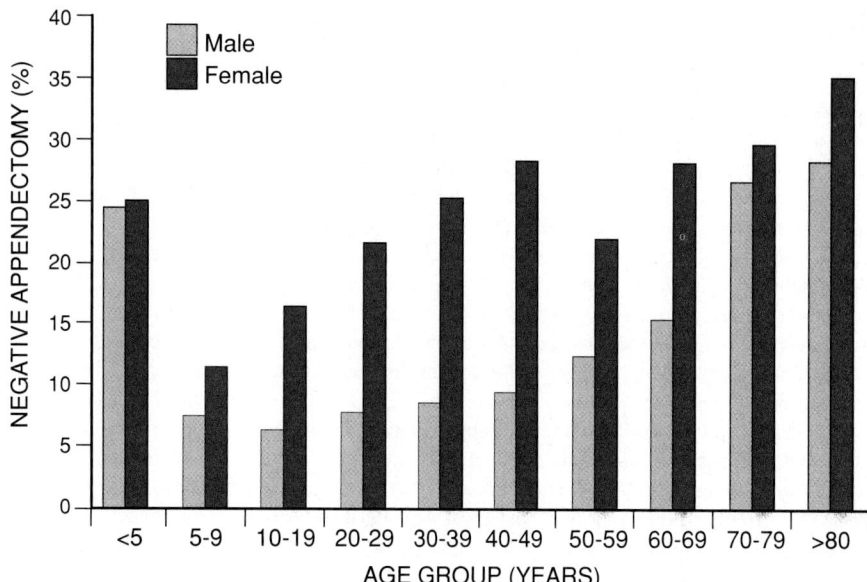

FIG. 29-2. The rate of negative appendectomy by age group. (*Adapted from Flum et al.*[14,15])

of the appendix. Distention of this magnitude usually causes reflex nausea and vomiting, and the diffuse visceral pain becomes more severe. As pressure in the organ increases, venous pressure is exceeded. Capillaries and venules are occluded, but arteriolar inflow continues, resulting in engorgement and vascular congestion. The inflammatory process soon involves the serosa of the appendix and in turn parietal peritoneum in the region, producing the characteristic shift in pain to the right lower quadrant.

The mucosa of the gastrointestinal tract, including the appendix, is susceptible to impairment of blood supply, thus its integrity is compromised early in the process, allowing bacterial invasion. As progressive distention encroaches upon first the venous return and subsequently the arteriolar inflow, the area with the poorest blood supply suffers most: ellipsoidal infarcts develop in the antimesenteric border. As distention, bacterial invasion, compromise of vascular supply, and infarction progress, perforation occurs, usually through one of the infarcted areas on the antimesenteric border. Perforation generally occurs just beyond the point of obstruction rather than at the tip because of the effect of diameter on intraluminal tension.

This sequence is not inevitable, however, and some episodes of acute appendicitis apparently subside spontaneously. Many patients who are found at operation to have acute appendicitis give a history of previous similar, but less severe, attacks of right lower quadrant pain. Pathologic examination of the appendices removed from these patients often reveals thickening and scarring, suggesting old, healed, acute inflammation.[16-18]

Bacteriology

The bacteriology of the normal appendix is similar to that of the normal colon. The appendiceal flora remains constant throughout life with the exception of *Porphyromonas gingivalis*. This bacterium is seen only in adults.[19] The bacteria cultured in cases of appendicitis are therefore similar to those seen in other colonic infections such as diverticulitis. The principal organisms seen in the normal appendix, in acute appendicitis, and in perforated appendicitis are *Escherichia coli* and *Bacteroides fragilis*.[19-22] However, a wide variety of both facultative and anaerobic bacteria and mycobacteria may be present (Table 29-1). Appendicitis is a polymicrobial infection, with some

series reporting up to 14 different organisms cultured in patients with perforation.[19]

The routine use of intraperitoneal cultures in patients with either perforated or nonperforated appendicitis is questionable. As discussed above, the flora is known and therefore broad-spectrum antibiotics are indicated. By the time culture results are available, the patient often has recovered from the illness. Additionally, the number of organisms cultured and the ability of a specific lab to culture anaerobic organisms vary greatly. Peritoneal culture should be reserved for patients who are immunosuppressed, as a result of either illness or medication, and for patients who develop an abscess after the treatment of appendicitis.[21-24] Antibiotic coverage is limited to 24 to 48 hours in cases of nonperforated appendicitis. For perforated appendicitis, 7 to 10 days is recommended. Intravenous antibiotics are usually given until the white blood cell count is normal and the patient is afebrile for 24 hours. The use of antibiotic irrigation of the peritoneal cavity and transperitoneal drainage through the wound are controversial.

Clinical Manifestations

Symptoms

Abdominal pain is the prime symptom of acute appendicitis. Classically, pain is initially diffusely centered in the lower epigastrium or umbilical area, is moderately severe, and is steady, sometimes with intermittent cramping superimposed. After a period varying from 1 to 12 hours, but usually within 4 to 6 hours,

Table 29-1

Common Organisms Seen in Patients with Acute Appendicitis

Aerobic and Facultative	Anaerobic
Gram-negative bacilli	Gram-negative bacilli
E. coli	*Bacteroides fragilis*
Pseudomonas aeruginosa	*Bacteroides* species
Klebsiella species	*Fusobacterium* species
Gram-positive cocci	Gram-positive cocci
Streptococcus anginosus	*Peptostreptococcus* species
Streptococcus species	Gram-positive bacilli
Enterococcus species	*Clostridium* species

the pain localizes to the right lower quadrant. This classic pain sequence, although usual, is not invariable. In some patients, the pain of appendicitis begins in the right lower quadrant and remains there. Variations in the anatomic location of the appendix account for many of the variations in the principal locus of the somatic phase of the pain. For example, a long appendix with the inflamed tip in the left lower quadrant causes pain in that area; a retrocecal appendix principally may cause flank or back pain; a pelvic appendix, principally suprapubic pain; and a retroileal appendix may cause testicular pain, presumably from irritation of the spermatic artery and ureter. Malrotation is also responsible for puzzling pain patterns. The visceral component is in the normal location, but the somatic component is felt in that part of the abdomen where the cecum has been arrested in rotation.

Anorexia nearly always accompanies appendicitis. It is so constant that the diagnosis should be questioned if the patient is not anorectic. Although vomiting occurs in nearly 75% of patients, it is neither prominent nor prolonged and most patients vomit only once or twice. Vomiting is caused both by neural stimulation and the presence of ileus.

Most patients give a history of obstipation beginning prior to the onset of abdominal pain, and many feel that defecation would relieve their abdominal pain. However, diarrhea occurs in some patients, particularly children, so that the pattern of bowel function is of little differential diagnostic value.

The sequence of symptom appearance has great differential diagnostic significance. In more than 95% of patients with acute appendicitis, anorexia is the first symptom, followed by abdominal pain, which is followed, in turn, by vomiting (if vomiting occurs). If vomiting precedes the onset of pain, the diagnosis of appendicitis should be questioned.[25]

Signs

Physical findings are determined principally by the anatomic position of the inflamed appendix, as well as by whether the organ has already ruptured when the patient is first examined.

Vital signs are minimally changed by uncomplicated appendicitis. Temperature elevation is rarely more than 1°C (1.8°F) and the pulse rate is normal or slightly elevated. Changes of greater magnitude usually indicate that a complication has occurred or that another diagnosis should be considered.[26]

Patients with appendicitis usually prefer to lie supine, with the thighs, particularly the right thigh, drawn up, because any motion increases pain. If asked to move, they do so slowly and with caution.

The classic right lower quadrant physical signs are present when the inflamed appendix lies in the anterior position. Tenderness is often maximal at or near McBurney's point.[8] Direct rebound tenderness is usually present. Additionally, referred or indirect rebound tenderness is present. This referred tenderness is felt maximally in the right lower quadrant, indicating localized peritoneal irritation.[26] Rovsing's sign—pain in the right lower quadrant when palpatory pressure is exerted in the left lower quadrant—also indicates the site of peritoneal irritation. Cutaneous hyperesthesia in the area supplied by the spinal nerves on the right at T10, T11, and T12 frequently accompanies acute appendicitis. In patients with obvious appendicitis, this sign is superfluous, but in some early cases, it may be the first positive sign. Hyperesthesia is elicited either by needle prick or by gently picking up the skin between the forefinger and thumb.

Muscular resistance to palpation of the abdominal wall roughly parallels the severity of the inflammatory process. Early in the disease, resistance, if present, consists mainly of voluntary guarding. As peritoneal irritation progresses, muscle spasm increases and becomes largely involuntary, i.e., true reflex rigidity due to contraction of muscles directly beneath the inflamed parietal peritoneum.

Anatomic variations in the position of the inflamed appendix lead to deviations in the usual physical findings. With a retrocecal appendix, the anterior abdominal findings are less striking and tenderness may be most marked in the flank. When the inflamed appendix hangs into the pelvis, abdominal findings may be entirely absent, and the diagnosis may be missed unless the rectum is examined. As the examining finger exerts pressure on the peritoneum of the cul-de-sac of Douglas, pain is felt in the suprapubic area, as well as locally within the rectum. Signs of localized muscle irritation may also be present. The psoas sign indicates an irritative focus in proximity to that muscle. The test is performed by having patients lay on their left side as the examiner slowly extends the right thigh, thus stretching the iliopsoas muscle. The test is positive if extension produces pain. Similarly, a positive obturator sign of hypogastric pain on stretching the obturator internus indicates irritation in the pelvis. The test is performed by passive internal rotation of the flexed right thigh with the patient supine.

Laboratory Findings

Mild leukocytosis, ranging from 10,000 to 18,000/mm^3, is usually present in patients with acute, uncomplicated appendicitis and is often accompanied by a moderate polymorphonuclear predominance. However, white blood cell counts are variable. It is unusual for the white blood cell count to be greater than 18,000/mm^3 in uncomplicated appendicitis. White blood cell counts above this level raise the possibility of a perforated appendix with or without an abscess. Urinalysis can be useful to rule out the urinary tract as the source of infection. Although several white or red blood cells can be present from ureteral or bladder irritation as a result of an inflamed appendix, bacteriuria in a catheterized urine specimen is not generally seen with acute appendicitis.[27]

Imaging Studies

Plain films of the abdomen, although frequently obtained as part of the general evaluation of a patient with an acute abdomen, are rarely helpful in diagnosing acute appendicitis. However, plain radiographs can be of significant benefit in ruling out other pathology. In patients with acute appendicitis, one often sees an abnormal bowel gas pattern, which is a nonspecific finding. The presence of a fecalith is rarely noted on plain films, but if present, is highly suggestive of the diagnosis. A chest x-ray is sometimes indicated to rule out referred pain from a right lower lobe pneumonic process.

Additional radiographic techniques include barium enema and radioactive-labeled leukocyte scans. If the appendix fills on barium enema, appendicitis is excluded. On the other hand, if the appendix does not fill, no determination can be made. To date, there has not been enough experience with radionuclide scans to assess their utility.[28]

Graded compression sonography has been suggested as an accurate way to establish the diagnosis of appendicitis. The technique is inexpensive, can be performed rapidly, does not require contrast, and can be used even in pregnant patients. Sonographically, the appendix is identified as a blind-ending, nonperistaltic bowel loop originating from the cecum. With maximal compression, the diameter of the appendix is measured in the anteroposterior dimension. A scan is considered positive if a noncompressible appendix 6 mm or greater in the anteroposterior direction is demonstrated

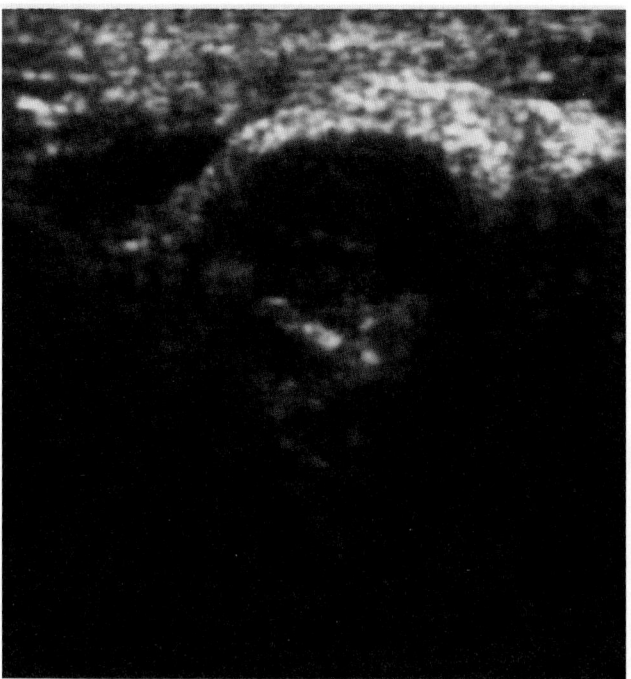

A

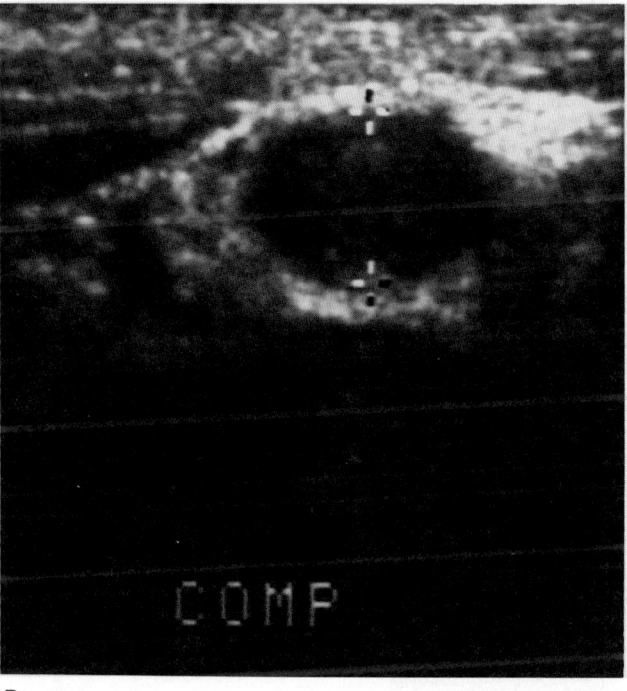

B

FIG. 29-3. *Sonogram of a 10-year-old female who presented with nausea, vomiting, and abdominal pain. The appendix measured 10.0 mm in maximal anteroposterior diameter in both the noncompression (A) and compression (B) views.*

(Fig. 29-3). The presence of an appendicolith establishes the diagnosis. The presence of thickening of the appendiceal wall and periappendiceal fluid is highly suggestive. Sonographic demonstration of a normal appendix, which is an easily compressible blind-ending tubular structure measuring 5 mm or less in diameter, excludes the diagnosis of acute appendicitis. The study is considered

inconclusive if the appendix is not visualized and there is no pericecal fluid or mass. When the diagnosis of acute appendicitis is excluded by sonography, a brief survey of the remainder of the abdominal cavity should be performed to establish an alternative diagnosis. In females of child-bearing age, the pelvic organs must be adequately visualized either by transabdominal or endovaginal ultrasonography in order to exclude gynecologic pathology as a cause of acute abdominal pain. The sonographic diagnosis of acute appendicitis has a reported sensitivity of 55 to 96% and a specificity of 85 to 98%.[29-31] Sonography is similarly effective in children and pregnant women, although its application is somewhat limited in late pregnancy.

Although sonography can easily identify abscesses in cases of perforation, the technique has limitations and results are user-dependent. A false-positive scan can occur in the presence of peri-appendicitis from surrounding inflammation, a dilated fallopian tube can be mistaken for an inflamed appendix, inspissated stool can mimic an appendicolith, and, in obese patients, the appendix may not be compressible because of overlying fat. False-negative sonograms can occur if appendicitis is confined to the appendiceal tip, the appendix is retrocecal in location, the appendix is markedly enlarged and mistaken for small bowel, or if the appendix is perforated and therefore compressible.[32]

Some studies have reported that graded compression sonography improved the diagnosis of appendicitis over clinical exam, specifically decreasing the percentage of negative explorations for appendectomies from 37 to 13%.[33] Sonography also decreases the time before operation. Sonography identified appendicitis in 10% of patients who were believed to have a low likelihood of the disease on physical examination.[34] The positive and negative predictive values of ultrasonography have impressively been reported as 91 or 92%, respectively. However, in a recent prospective multicenter study, routine ultrasonography did not improve the diagnostic accuracy or rates of negative appendectomy or perforation when compared to clinical assessment.

High-resolution, helical, computer tomography also has been used to diagnose appendicitis. On CT scan, the inflamed appendix appears dilated (greater than 5 cm) and the wall is thickened. There is usually evidence of inflammation, with "dirty fat," thickened mesoappendix, and even an obvious phlegmon (Fig. 29-4). Fecaliths can be easily visualized, but their presence is not necessarily pathognomonic of appendicitis. An important suggestive abnormality is the arrowhead sign. This is caused by thickening of the cecum, which funnels contrast toward the orifice of the inflamed appendix. CT scanning is also an excellent technique for identifying other inflammatory processes masquerading as appendicitis.

Several CT techniques have been used, including focused and nonfocused CT scans and enhanced and nonenhanced helical CT scanning. The nonenhanced helical CT scan is important because one of the disadvantages of using CT scanning in the evaluation of right lower quadrant pain is dye allergy. Surprisingly, all these techniques have yielded essentially identical rates of diagnostic accuracy, i.e., 92 to 97% sensitivity, 85 to 94% specificity, 90 to 98% accuracy, and 75 to 95% positive and 95 to 99% negative predictive values.[35-37] Similarly, the additional use of rectal contrast did not improve the results of CT scanning.

A number of studies have documented improvement in diagnostic accuracy with the liberal use of CT scanning in the workup of suspected appendicitis. Computed tomography lowered the rate of negative appendectomies from 19 to 12% in one study,[38] and the incidence of negative appendectomies in women from 24 to 5% in another.[39] The use of this imaging study altered the care of 24%

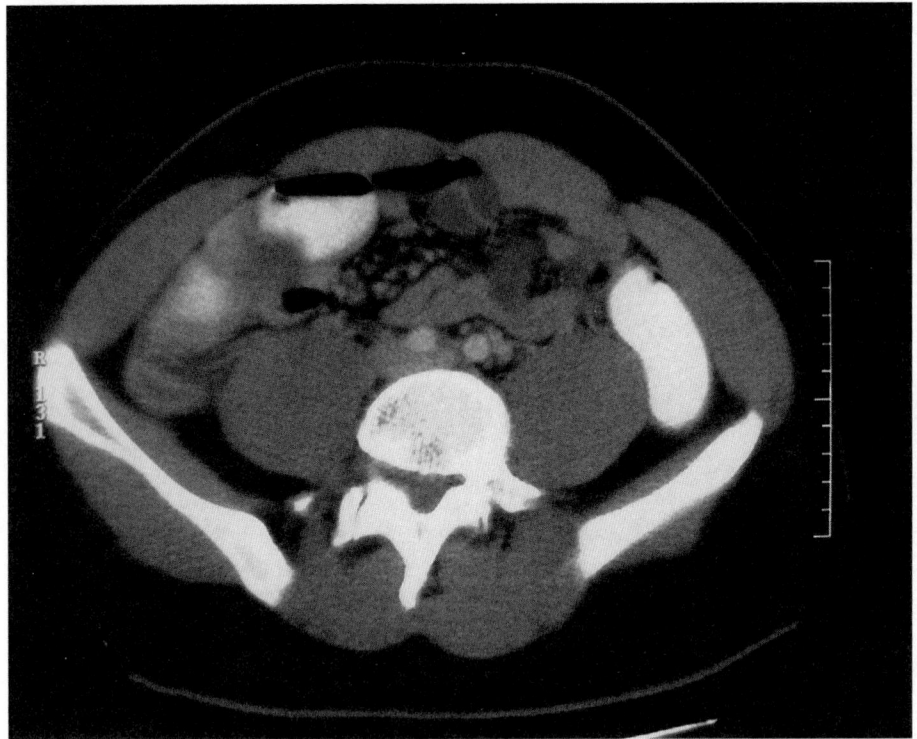

A

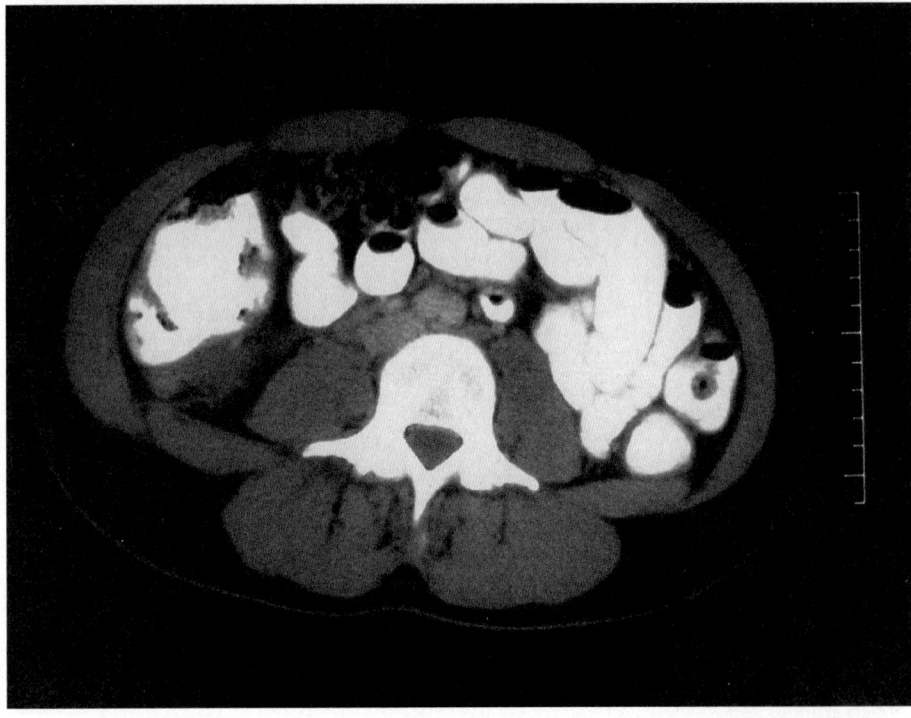

B

FIG. 29-4. CT scans positive for appendicitis. Note the thick-walled and dilated appendix (*A*) and mesenteric streaking and "dirty fat" (*B*).

of patients studied and provided alternative diagnoses in half of the patients with normal appendices on CT scan.[40]

Despite the potential usefulness of this technique, there are significant disadvantages. CT scanning is expensive, exposes the patients to significant radiation, and cannot be used during pregnancy. Allergy contraindicates the application of intravenous contrast in some patients, and others cannot tolerate the oral ingestion of luminal dye, particularly in the presence of nausea and vomiting. Finally, not all studies have documented the utility of CT scanning in all patients with right lower quadrant pain.[41]

A number of studies have compared the effectiveness of graded compression ultrasound and helical computed tomography in establishing the diagnosis of appendicitis. Although the differences are rather small, CT scanning has consistently proven superior. For example, in one study, 600 ultrasounds and 317 CT scans revealed sensitivities of 80 and 97%, specificities of 93 and 94%, diagnostic accuracies of 89 and 95%, positive predictive values of 91 and 92%, and negative predictive values of 88 and 98%, respectively.[31] In another study, ultrasound positively impacted the management of 19% of patients, as compared to 73% of patients for CT. Finally, in a third study, patients studied by ultrasonography had a 17% negative appendix rate compared to a 2% negative appendix rate in patients who underwent helical CT scanning.[42] One concern about ultrasonography is the high intraobserver variability.[43]

One issue that has not been resolved is which patients are candidates for imaging studies.[44] This question may be moot, because CT scanning is routinely ordered by emergency physicians before surgeons are even consulted. The concept that all patients with right lower quadrant pain should undergo CT scanning has been strongly supported by two reports by Rao and his colleagues at the Massachusetts General Hospital. In one, this group documented a fall in the negative appendectomy rate from 20 to 7%, and a decline in the perforation rate from 22 to 14%, as well as establishing an alternative diagnosis in 50% of patients.[45] In the second study, published in the *New England Journal of Medicine*, they documented that CT scanning prevented 13 unnecessary appendectomies, saved 50 inpatient hospital days, and lowered the per patient cost by $447.[46] In contrast, several studies failed to prove an advantage of routine CT scanning, documenting that surgeon accuracy approached that of the imaging study and expressing concern that the imaging studies could adversely delay appendectomy in affected patients.[47,48]

The rational approach is the selective use of CT scanning. This has been documented by several studies in which imaging was performed based on an algorithm or protocol.[49] The likelihood of appendicitis can be ascertained using the Alvarado scale (Table 29-2).[50] This scoring system was designed to improve the diagnosis of appendicitis and was devised by giving relative weight to specific clinical manifestation. Table 29-2 lists the eight specific indicators identified. Patients with scores of 9 to 10 are almost certain to have appendicitis; there is little advantage in further workup, and they should go to the operating room. Patients with scores of 7 to 8 have a high likelihood of appendicitis, while scores of 5 to 6 are compatible with, but not diagnostic of appendicitis. CT scanning is certainly appropriate for patients with Alvarado scores of 5 and 6, and a case can be built for imaging those with scores of 7 and 8. On the other hand, it is difficult to justify the expense, radiation exposure time, and possible complications of CT scanning in those patients whose scores of 0 to 4 make it extremely unlikely (but not impossible) that they have appendicitis.

Table 29-2
Alvarado Scale for the Diagnosis of Appendicitis

	Manifestations	*Value*
Symptoms	Migration of pain	1
	Anorexia	1
	Nausea/vomiting	1
Signs	RLQ tenderness	2
	Rebound	1
	Elevated temperature	1
Laboratory values	Leukocytosis	2
	Left shift	1
		Total Points 10

RLQ = right lower quadrant.
SOURCE: From Alvarado,[50] with permission.

Selective CT scanning based on the likelihood of appendicitis takes advantage of the clinical skill of the experienced surgeon and, when indicated, adds the expertise of the radiologist and his or her imaging study. Figure 29-5 proposes a treatment algorithm addressing the rationale use of diagnostic testing.[51]

Laparoscopy can serve as both a diagnostic and therapeutic maneuver for patients with acute abdominal pain and suspected acute appendicitis. Laparoscopy is probably most useful in the evaluation of females with lower abdominal complaints because appendectomy is performed on a normal appendix in as many as 30 to 40% of these patients. Differentiating acute gynecologic pathology from acute appendicitis can be effectively accomplished by using the laparoscope.

Appendiceal Rupture

Immediate appendectomy has long been the recommended treatment of acute appendicitis because of the known risk of progression to rupture. The overall rate of perforated appendicitis is 25.8%. Children younger than age 5 years and patients older than age 65 years have the highest rate of perforation (45 and 51%, respectively) (Fig. 29-6).[13–15] It has been suggested that delays in presentation are responsible for the majority of perforated appendices. There is no accurate way of determining when and if an appendix will rupture prior to resolution of the inflammatory process. Although it has been suggested that observation and antibiotic therapy alone may be an appropriate treatment for acute appendicitis, nonoperative treatment exposes the patient to the increased morbidity and mortality associated with a ruptured appendix.

Appendiceal rupture occurs most frequently distal to the point of luminal obstruction along the antimesenteric border of the appendix. Rupture should be suspected in the presence of fever greater than $39°C$ ($102°F$) and a white blood cell count greater than $18,000/mm^3$. In the majority of cases, rupture is contained and patients display localized rebound tenderness. Generalized peritonitis will be present if the walling-off process is ineffective in containing the rupture.

In 2 to 6% of cases, an ill-defined mass will be detected on physical examination. This could represent a phlegmon, which consists of matted loops of bowel adherent to the adjacent inflamed appendix, or a periappendiceal abscess. Patients who present with a mass have a longer duration of symptoms, usually at least 5 to 7 days. The ability to distinguish acute, uncomplicated appendicitis from acute appendicitis with perforation on the basis of clinical findings is often difficult, but it is important to make the distinction because their treatment differs. CT scan may be beneficial in guiding therapy. Phlegmons and small abscesses can be treated conservatively with intravenous antibiotics; well-localized abscesses can be managed with percutaneous drainage; complex abscesses should be considered for surgical drainage. If operative drainage is required, it should be performed by using an extraperitoneal approach, with appendectomy reserved for cases in which the appendix is easily accessible. Interval appendectomy performed at least 6 weeks following the acute event has classically been recommended for all patients treated either nonoperatively or with simple drainage of an abscess.[52–54]

Differential Diagnosis

The differential diagnosis of acute appendicitis is essentially the diagnosis of the "acute abdomen" (see Chap. 34). This is because clinical manifestations are not specific for a given disease, but are specific for disturbance of a physiologic function or functions. Thus, an essentially identical clinical picture can result from a wide variety

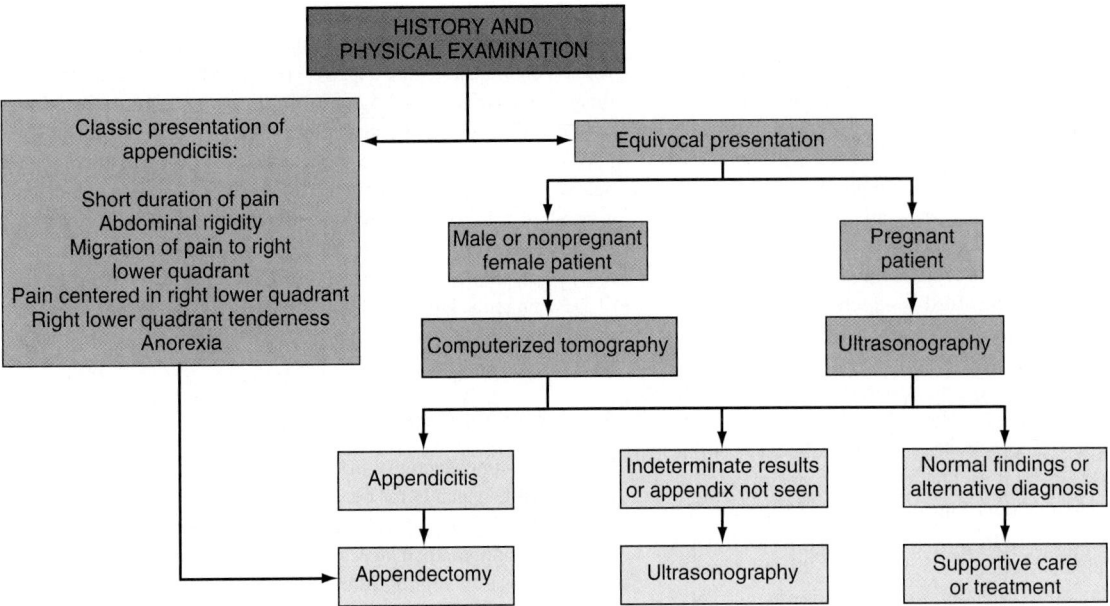

FIG. 29-5. Clinical algorithm for suspected cases of acute appendicitis. If gynecologic disease is suspected, a pelvic and endovaginal ultrasound examination is indicated. (*Reproduced with permission from Paulson EK, Kalady MF, Pappas TN: Suspected appendicitis. N Engl J Med 348:236, 2003.*)

of acute processes within or near the peritoneal cavity that produce the same alterations of function as acute appendicitis.

The accuracy of preoperative diagnosis should be approximately 85%. If it is consistently less, it is likely that some unnecessary operations are probably being performed, and a more rigorous preoperative differential diagnosis is in order. A diagnostic accuracy rate consistently greater than 90% should also cause concern, because this may mean that some patients with atypical, but bona fide cases of, acute appendicitis are being "observed" when they should have prompt surgical intervention. The Haller group has shown, however, that this is not invariably true.[55] Before the group's study, the perforation rate at the hospital where the study took place was 26.7%, and acute appendicitis was found in 80% of the operations.

By a policy of intensive in-hospital observation when the diagnosis of appendicitis was unclear, the group raised the rate of acute appendicitis found at operation to 94%, while the perforation rate remained unchanged at 27.5%.[55]

There are a few conditions in which operation is contraindicated. Other disease processes that are confused with appendicitis are also surgical problems, or, if not, are not made worse by surgical intervention. A common error is to make a preoperative diagnosis of acute appendicitis only to find some other condition (or nothing) at operation; much less frequently, acute appendicitis is found after a preoperative diagnosis of another condition. The most common erroneous preoperative diagnoses—accounting for more than 75%—in descending order of frequency are acute mesenteric lymphadenitis,

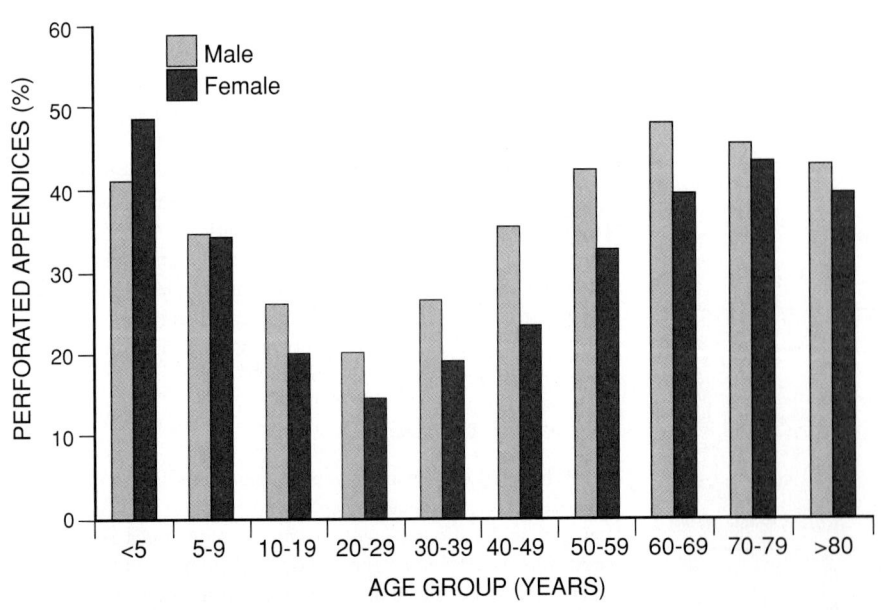

FIG. 29-6. The rate of appendiceal rupture by age group. (*Personal communication from David Flum, M.D.*)

no organic pathologic conditions, acute pelvic inflammatory disease, twisted ovarian cyst or ruptured graafian follicle, and acute gastroenteritis.

The differential diagnosis of acute appendicitis depends upon four major factors: the anatomic location of the inflamed appendix; the stage of the process (i.e., simple or ruptured); the patient's age; and the patient's sex.[56-60]

Acute Mesenteric Adenitis

Acute mesenteric adenitis is the disease most often confused with acute appendicitis in children. Almost invariably, an upper respiratory infection is present or has recently subsided. The pain is usually diffuse, and tenderness is not as sharply localized as in appendicitis. Voluntary guarding is sometimes present, but true rigidity is rare. Generalized lymphadenopathy may be noted. Laboratory procedures are of little help in arriving at the correct diagnosis, although a relative lymphocytosis, when present, suggests mesenteric adenitis. Observation for several hours is in order if the diagnosis of mesenteric adenitis seems likely, because mesenteric adenitis is a self-limited disease. However, if the differentiation remains in doubt, immediate exploration is the safest course of action.

Acute Gastroenteritis

Acute gastroenteritis is common in childhood but can usually be easily differentiated from appendicitis. Viral gastroenteritis, an acute self-limited infection of diverse causes, is characterized by profuse watery diarrhea, nausea, and vomiting. Hyperperistaltic abdominal cramps precede the watery stools. The abdomen is relaxed between cramps, and there are no localizing signs. Laboratory values are normal.

Salmonella gastroenteritis results from ingestion of contaminated food. Abdominal findings are usually similar to those in viral gastroenteritis, but in some cases, the abdominal pain is intense, localized, and associated with rebound tenderness. Chills and fever are common. The leukocyte count is usually normal. The causative organisms can be isolated from nearly 100% of patients. However, cultures may take too long to assist the clinician in making a timely differential diagnosis. Similar attacks in other persons eating the same food as the patient greatly strengthen the presumptive diagnosis of salmonella gastroenteritis.

Because typhoid fever is now a rare disease, its diagnosis is frequently missed. The onset is less acute than in appendicitis, with a prodrome of several days. Differentiation is usually possible because of prostration, maculopapular rash, inappropriate bradycardia, and leukopenia. Diagnosis is confirmed by culture of *Salmonella typhosa* from stool or blood. Intestinal perforation, usually in the lower ileum, develops in 1% of cases and requires immediate surgical therapy.

Diseases of the Male Urogenital System

Diseases of the male urogenital system must be considered in differential diagnosis of appendicitis, including torsion of the testis and acute epididymitis, because epigastric pain may overshadow local symptoms early in these diseases. Seminal vesiculitis may also mimic appendicitis, but can be diagnosed by palpating the enlarged, tender seminal vesicle on rectal examination.

Meckel's Diverticulitis

Meckel's diverticulitis causes a clinical picture similar to that of acute appendicitis. The Meckel's diverticulum is located within the distal 2 feet of the ileum. Meckel's diverticulitis is associated with the same complications as appendicitis and requires the same treatment—prompt surgical intervention. Resection of the segment of ileum bearing the diverticulum with end-to-end anastomosis can nearly always be done through a McBurney incision, extended if necessary, as well as laparoscopically.

Intussusception

In contrast to Meckel's diverticulitis, it is extremely important to differentiate intussusception from acute appendicitis as the treatment is different. Patient age is important: appendicitis is very uncommon in children younger than age 2 years, whereas nearly all idiopathic intussusceptions occur in children younger than age 2 years. Intussusception occurs typically in a well-nourished infant who is suddenly doubled up by apparent colicky pain. Between attacks of pain, the infant appears well. After several hours, the patient usually passes a bloody mucoid stool. A sausage-shaped mass may be palpable in the right lower quadrant. As the intussusception progresses distally, the right lower quadrant feels abnormally empty. The preferred treatment of intussusception, if seen before signs of peritonitis supervene, is reduction by barium enema, but treatment of acute appendicitis by barium enema may be catastrophic.

Crohn's Enteritis

The manifestations of acute regional enteritis—fever, right lower quadrant pain and tenderness, and leukocytosis—often simulate acute appendicitis. Diarrhea and the infrequency of anorexia, nausea, and vomiting favor a diagnosis of enteritis but are not sufficient to exclude acute appendicitis. In an appreciable percentage of patients with chronic regional enteritis, the diagnosis has been first made at the time of operation for presumed acute appendicitis. In the presence of an acutely inflamed distal ileum with no cecal involvement, and a normal appendix, appendectomy is indicated. Progression to chronic Crohn's ileitis is uncommon.

Perforated Peptic Ulcer

Perforated peptic ulcer closely simulates appendicitis if the spilled gastroduodenal contents gravitate down the right gutter to the cecal area and if the perforation spontaneously seals, minimizing upper abdominal findings.

Colonic Lesions

Diverticulitis or perforating carcinoma of the cecum, or of that portion of the sigmoid that lies on the right side, may be impossible to distinguish from appendicitis. These entities should be considered in older patients. CT scanning is often helpful in making a diagnosis in older patients with right lower quadrant pain and atypical clinical presentations.

Epiploic Appendagitis

Epiploic appendagitis probably results from infarction of the colonic appendage(s) secondary to torsion. Symptoms may be minimal, or there may be continuous abdominal pain in an area corresponding to the contour of the colon, lasting several days. Pain shift is unusual, and there is no diagnostic sequence of symptoms. The patient does not look ill, nausea and vomiting are unusual, and appetite is commonly unaffected. Localized tenderness over the site is usual and is often associated with marked rebound tenderness without rigidity. In 25% of reported cases, pain has persisted or recurred until the infarcted epiploic appendage was removed.

Urinary Tract Infection

Acute pyelonephritis, on the right side particularly, may mimic a retroileal acute appendicitis. Chills, right costovertebral angle tenderness, pyuria, and bacteriuria are usually sufficient to make the diagnosis.

Ureteral Stone

If the calculus is lodged near the appendix, it may simulate a retrocecal appendicitis. Pain referred to the labia, scrotum, or penis; hematuria; and/or absence of fever or leukocytosis suggest the presence of a ureteral stone. Pyelography and CT scanning without oral contrast usually confirm the diagnosis.

Primary Peritonitis

Primary peritonitis occurs most often in patients with nephrotic syndrome, cirrhosis, and endogenous or exogenous immunosuppression. It rarely mimics simple acute appendicitis, but presents a picture similar to diffuse peritonitis secondary to a ruptured appendix. The diagnosis is made by peritoneal aspiration. If only gram-positive cocci are seen on the Gram-stained smear, peritonitis is primary and treated with antibiotics; if the flora are mixed or gram-negative rods, secondary peritonitis should be suspected.

Henoch-Schönlein Purpura

This syndrome usually occurs 2 to 3 weeks after a streptococcal infection. Abdominal pain may be prominent, but joint pains, purpura, and nephritis are also frequently present.

Yersiniosis

Human infection with *Yersinia enterocolitica* or *Y. pseudotuberculosis* is transmitted through food contaminated by feces or urine. *Yersinia* infections cause a variety of clinical syndromes, including mesenteric adenitis, ileitis, colitis, and acute appendicitis. Many of the infections are mild and self-limited, but some lead to a systemic septic course with a high fatality rate if untreated. The organisms are usually sensitive to tetracyclines, streptomycin, ampicillin, and kanamycin. A preoperative suspicion of the diagnosis should not delay operative intervention because appendicitis caused by *Yersinia* cannot be clinically distinguished from appendicitis from other causes. Approximately 6% of cases of mesenteric adenitis and 5% of cases of acute appendicitis are caused by *Yersinia* infection.

Campylobacter jejuni causes diarrhea and pain that mimics that of appendicitis. The organism can be cultured from stool. *Salmonella typhimurium* infection causes mesenteric adenitis and paralytic ileus similar to the symptoms of appendicitis. The diagnosis can be established by serology.

Gynecologic Disorders

The rate of false-negative appendectomies is highest in young adult females. The finding of a normal appendix is seen in 32 to 45% of appendectomies performed in women 15 to 45 years of age.[15] Diseases of the female internal reproductive organs that may be erroneously diagnosed as appendicitis are, in approximate descending order of frequency, pelvic inflammatory disease, ruptured graafian follicle, twisted ovarian cyst or tumor, endometriosis, and ruptured ectopic pregnancy.

Pelvic Inflammatory Disease. The infection is usually bilateral, but if confined to the right tube, may mimic acute appendicitis. Nausea and vomiting often are present in patients with appendicitis, but only in approximately 50% of those with pelvic in-

flammatory disease. The greatest value of these symptoms for establishing a diagnosis of pelvic inflammatory disease is their absence. Pain and tenderness are usually lower, and motion of the cervix is exquisitely painful. Intracellular diplococci may be demonstrable on smear of the purulent vaginal discharge. The ratio of appendicitis to pelvic inflammatory disease is low in the early phase of the menstrual cycle and high during the luteal phase. The clinical use of all the above-mentioned distinctions has resulted in a reduction of the incidence of negative findings on laparotomy in young women to 15%.

Ruptured Graafian Follicle. Ovulation commonly results in the spillage of sufficient amounts of blood and follicular fluid to produce brief, mild, lower abdominal pain. If the amount of fluid is unusually copious and is from the right ovary, appendicitis may be simulated. Pain and tenderness are rather diffuse. Leukocytosis and fever are minimal or absent. Because this pain occurs at the midpoint of the menstrual cycle, it is often called mittelschmerz.

Ruptured Ectopic Pregnancy. Pregnancies may implant in the fallopian tube (usually the ampullary portion), ovary, and, rarely, the peritoneum. Rupture of right tubal or ovarian pregnancies can mimic appendicitis. Patients usually give a history of abnormal menses; either missing one or two periods or noting only slight vaginal bleeding. Unfortunately, patients do not always realize they are pregnant. The development of right lower quadrant or pelvic pain may be the first symptom. The diagnosis of ruptured ectopic pregnancy should be relatively easy. The presence of a pelvic mass and elevated levels of chorionic gonadotropin are characteristic. While the leukocyte count rises slightly (to approximately 14,000), the hematocrit level falls as a consequence of the intra-abdominal hemorrhage. Vaginal examination reveals cervical motion and adnexal tenderness, and a more definitive diagnosis can be established by culdocentesis. The presence of blood and particularly decidual tissue is pathognomonic. The treatment of ruptured ectopic pregnancy is emergency surgery.

Twisted Ovarian Cyst. Serous cysts of the ovary are common and generally remain asymptomatic. When right-sided cysts rupture or undergo torsion, the manifestations are similar to those of appendicitis. Patients develop right lower quadrant pain, tenderness, rebound, fever, and leukocytosis. If the mass is palpable on vaginal exam, the diagnosis can be made easily. Both transvaginal ultrasonography and CT scanning can be diagnostic if a mass is not palpable.

Torsion requires emergent operative treatment. If the torsion is complete or long-standing, the pedicle undergoes thrombosis, and the ovary and tube become gangrenous and require resection. However, leakage of ovarian cysts resolves spontaneously and is best treated nonoperatively.[25,56-61]

Other Diseases

Diseases not mentioned in the previous sections that occur in patients of all ages and both sexes and that must be considered in the differential diagnosis of appendicitis are foreign-body perforations of the bowel, closed-loop intestinal obstruction, mesenteric vascular occlusion, pleuritis of the right lower chest, acute cholecystitis, acute pancreatitis, and hematoma of the abdominal wall.

Acute Appendicitis in the Young

The establishment of a diagnosis of acute appendicitis in young children is more difficult than in the adult. The inability of young children to give an accurate history, diagnostic delays by both parents and physicians, and the frequency of gastrointestinal upset in children are all contributing factors. The more rapid progression to rupture and the inability of the underdeveloped greater omentum to contain a rupture lead to significant morbidity rates in children. Children younger than 5 years of age have a negative appendectomy rate of 25% and an appendiceal perforation rate of 45%. This is compared to a negative appendectomy rate of less than 10% and a perforated appendix rate of 20% for children 5 to 12 years of age.[14,15] The incidence of major complications after appendectomy in children is correlated with appendiceal rupture. The wound infection rate after the treatment of nonperforated appendicitis in children is 2.8% as compared to a rate of 11% after the treatment of perforated appendicitis. The incidence of intra-abdominal abscess is also higher after the treatment of perforated appendicitis as compared to nonperforated cases (6% vs. 3%).[24] The treatment regimen for perforated appendicitis generally includes immediate appendectomy and irrigation of the peritoneal cavity. Antibiotic coverage is limited to 24 to 48 hours in cases of nonperforated appendicitis. For perforated appendicitis, 7 to 10 days of antibiotics is recommended. Intravenous antibiotics are usually given until the white blood cell count is normal and the patient is afebrile for 24 hours. The use of antibiotic irrigation of the peritoneal cavity and transperitoneal drainage through the wound are controversial. Laparoscopic appendectomy has been shown to be safe and effective for the treatment of appendicitis in children.[62]

Acute Appendicitis in the Elderly

Although the incidence of appendicitis in the elderly is lower than in younger patients, the morbidity and mortality are significantly increased in this patient population. Delays in diagnosis, a more rapid progression to perforation, and comorbid disease are all contributing factors. The diagnosis of appendicitis may be subtler and less typical than in younger individuals, and a high index of suspicion should be maintained.[63] In patients older than age 80 years, perforation rates of 49% and mortality rates of 21% have been reported.[13–15,63]

Acute Appendicitis During Pregnancy

Appendicitis is the most frequently encountered extrauterine disease requiring surgical treatment during pregnancy. The incidence is approximately 1 in 2000 pregnancies. Acute appendicitis can occur at any time during pregnancy, but is more frequent during the first two trimesters. As fetal gestation progresses, the diagnosis of appendicitis becomes more difficult as the appendix is displaced laterally and superiorly (Fig. 29-7). Nausea and vomiting after the first trimester or new-onset nausea and vomiting should raise the consideration of appendicitis. Abdominal pain and tenderness will be present, although rebound and guarding are less frequent because of laxity of the abdominal wall. Elevation of the white blood cell count above the normal pregnancy levels of 15,000 to 20,000/μL, with a predominance of polymorphonuclear cells, is usually present. When the diagnosis is in doubt, abdominal ultrasound may be beneficial. Laparoscopy may be indicated in equivocal cases, especially early in pregnancy. The performance of any operation during pregnancy carries a risk of premature labor of 10 to 15%, and the risk is similar for both negative laparotomy and appendectomy for simple appendicitis. The most significant factor associated with both fetal and maternal death is appendiceal perforation. Fetal mortality increases from 3 to 5% in early appendicitis to 20% with perforation. The suspicion of appendicitis during pregnancy should prompt rapid diagnosis and surgical intervention.[64–66]

FIG. 29-7. Location of the appendix during pregnancy. ASIS = Anterior Superior Iliac Spine. [*Reproduced with permission from Metcalf A: The appendix, in Corson JD, Williamson RCN (eds): Surgery. London: Mosby, 2001.*]

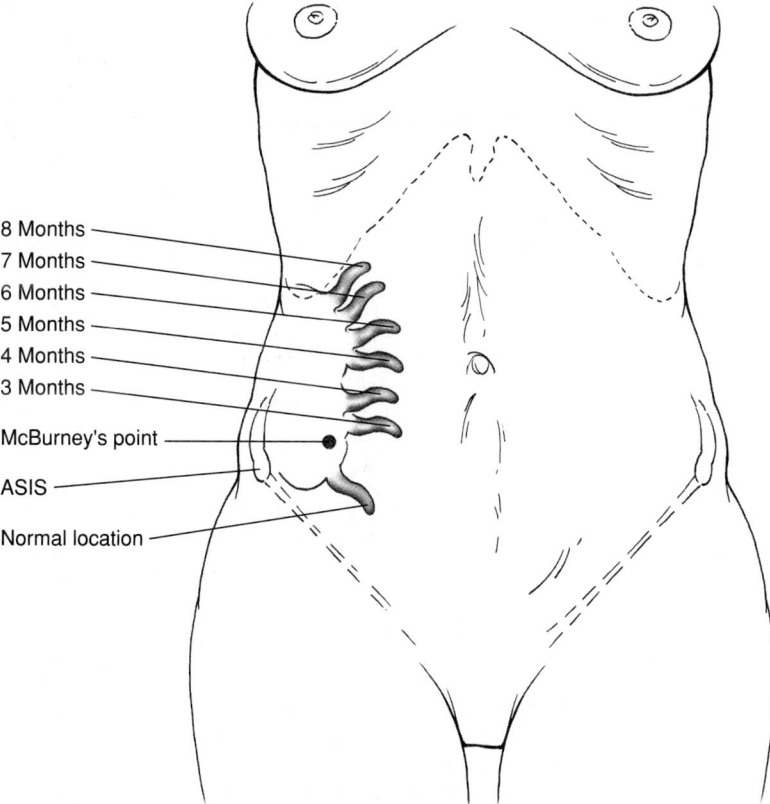

8 Months
7 Months
6 Months
5 Months
4 Months
3 Months
McBurney's point
ASIS
Normal location

Appendicitis in Patients with AIDS or HIV Infection

The incidence of acute appendicitis in HIV-infected patients is reported to be 0.5%.[67] This is higher than the 0.1 to 0.2% incidence reported for the general population.[68] The presentation of acute appendicitis in HIV-infected patients is similar to that of noninfected patients. The majority of HIV-infected patients with appendicitis will have fever, periumbilical pain radiating to the right lower quadrant (91%), right lower quadrant tenderness (91%), and rebound tenderness (74%). HIV-infected patients will not manifest an absolute leukocytosis; however, if a baseline leukocyte count is available, nearly all HIV-infected patients with appendicitis will demonstrate a relative leukocytosis.[68,69]

There appears to be an increased risk of appendiceal rupture in HIV-infected patients. In one large series of HIV-infected patients who underwent appendectomy for presumed appendicitis, 43% of patients were found to have perforated appendicitis at laparotomy.[70] The increased risk of appendiceal rupture may be related to the delay in presentation seen in this patient population.[68,70] The mean duration of symptoms prior to arrival in the emergency room has been reported to be increased in HIV-infected patients, with more than 60% of patients reporting the duration of symptoms to be longer than 24 hours.[68] In early series, significant hospital delay also may have contributed to high rates of rupture.[68] However, with increased understanding of abdominal pain in HIV-infected patients, hospital delay has become less prevalent.[68,70] A low CD4 count is also associated with an increase in appendiceal rupture. In one large series, patients with nonruptured appendices had CD4 counts of 158.75 ± 47 cells/mL^3 compared with 94.5 ± 32 cells/mL^3 in patients with appendiceal rupture.[68]

The differential diagnosis of right lower quadrant pain is expanded in HIV-infected patients when compared to the general population. In addition to the conditions discussed elsewhere in this chapter, opportunistic infections should be considered as a possible cause of right lower quadrant pain.[68–71] These opportunistic infections include cytomegalovirus (CMV), Kaposi's sarcoma, tuberculosis, lymphoma, and other causes of infectious colitis. CMV infection may be seen anywhere in the gastrointestinal tract. CMV causes a vasculitis of blood vessels in the submucosa of the gut, leading to thrombosis. Mucosal ischemia develops, leading to ulceration, gangrene of the bowel wall, and perforation. Spontaneous peritonitis may be caused by opportunistic pathogens including CMV, *Mycobacterium avian-intracellulare*, *M. tuberculosis*, *Cryptococcus neoformans*, and strongyloides. Kaposi's sarcoma and non-Hodgkin's lymphoma may present with pain and a right lower quadrant mass. Viral and bacterial colitis occur with a higher frequency in HIV-infected patients than in the general population. Colitis should always be considered in HIV-infected patients presenting with right lower quadrant pain. Neutropenic enterocolitis (typhlitis) should also be considered in the differential diagnosis of right lower quadrant pain in HIV-infected patients.[69,71]

It is important to obtain a thorough history and physical when evaluating any patient with right lower quadrant pain. In the HIV-infected patient with classic signs and symptoms of appendicitis, immediate appendectomy is indicated. In those patients with diarrhea as a prominent symptom, colonoscopy may be warranted. In patients with equivocal findings, CT scan is usually helpful. The majority of pathologic findings identified in HIV-infected patients who undergo appendectomy for presumed appendicitis are typical. The negative appendectomy rate is 5 to 10%. However, up to 25% of patients will have AIDS-related entities in the operative

specimens, including CMV, Kaposi's sarcoma, and *M. avium-intracellulare*.[68,70]

In an accumulated report of 77 HIV-infected patients from 1988 to 1995, the 30-day mortality rate for patients undergoing appendectomy was reported to be 9.1%.[68] More recent series report 0% mortality in this group of patients.[68,70] Morbidity rates for HIV-infected patients with nonperforated appendicitis are similar to those seen in the general population. Postoperative morbidity rates appear to be higher in HIV-infected patients with perforated appendicitis. Additionally, the length of hospital stay for HIV-infected patients undergoing appendectomy is twice that of the general population.[68,70] No series has been reported to date that addresses the role of laparoscopic appendectomy in the HIV-infected population.

Treatment

Despite the advent of more sophisticated diagnostic modalities, the importance of early operative intervention should not be minimized. Once the decision to operate for presumed acute appendicitis has been made, the patient should be prepared for the operating room. Adequate hydration should be ensured; electrolyte abnormalities corrected; and pre-existing cardiac, pulmonary, and renal conditions should be addressed. Many trials have demonstrated the efficacy of preoperative antibiotics in lowering the infectious complications in appendicitis. Most surgeons routinely administer antibiotics to all patients with suspected appendicitis. If simple acute appendicitis is encountered, there is no benefit in extending antibiotic coverage beyond 24 hours. If perforated or gangrenous appendicitis is found, antibiotics are continued until the patient is afebrile and has a normal white blood cell count. For intra-abdominal infections of gastrointestinal tract origin of mild to moderate severity, the Surgical Infection Society has recommended single-agent therapy with cefoxitin, cefotetan, or ticarcillin-clavulanic acid. For more severe infections, single-agent therapy with carbapenems or combination therapy with a third-generation cephalosporin, monobactam, or aminoglycoside plus anaerobic coverage with clindamycin or metronidazole is indicated.

Open Appendectomy

Most surgeons employ either a McBurney (oblique) or Rocky-Davis (transverse) right lower quadrant muscle-splitting incision in patients with suspected appendicitis. The incision should be centered over either the point of maximal tenderness or a palpable mass. If an abscess is suspected, a laterally placed incision is imperative to allow retroperitoneal drainage and to avoid generalized contamination of the peritoneal cavity. If the diagnosis is in doubt, a lower midline incision is recommended to allow a more extensive examination of the peritoneal cavity. This is especially relevant in older patients with possible malignancy or diverticulitis.

Several techniques can be used to locate the appendix. Because the cecum is usually visible within the incision, the convergence of the taeniae can be followed to the base of the appendix. A sweeping lateral to medial motion can aid in delivering the appendiceal tip into the operative field. Occasionally, limited mobilization of the cecum is needed to aid in adequate visualization. Once identified, the appendix is mobilized by dividing the mesoappendix, taking care to ligate the appendiceal artery securely.

The appendiceal stump can be managed by simple ligation or by ligation and inversion with either a purse-string or Z stitch. As long as the stump is clearly viable and the base of the cecum not involved with the inflammatory process, the stump can be safely ligated with a nonabsorbable suture. The mucosa is frequently obliterated to avoid the development of mucocele. The peritoneal cavity is irrigated and the wound closed in layers. If perforation or gangrene is found in adults, the skin and subcutaneous tissue should be left open and allowed to heal by secondary intent or closed in 4 to 5 days as a delayed primary closure. In children, who generally have little subcutaneous fat, primary wound closure has not led to an increased incidence of wound infection.

If appendicitis is not found, a methodical search for an alternative diagnosis must be performed. The cecum and mesentery should first be inspected. Next, the small bowel is examined in a retrograde fashion beginning at the ileocecal valve and extending at least 2 feet. In females, special attention should be paid to the pelvic organs. An attempt is also made to examine the upper abdominal contents. Peritoneal fluid should be sent for Gram's stain and culture. If purulent fluid is encountered, it is imperative that the source be identified. A medial extension of the incision (Fowler-Weir), with division of the anterior and posterior rectus sheath, is acceptable if further evaluation of the lower abdomen is indicated. If upper abdominal pathology is encountered, the right lower quadrant incision is closed and an appropriate upper midline incision performed.[9,25,72]

Laparoscopy

Semm first reported successful laparoscopic appendectomy in 1983, several years before the first laparoscopic cholecystectomy.[10] However, the widespread use of the laparoscopic approach to appendectomy did not occur until after the success of laparoscopic cholecystectomy. This may be due to the fact that appendectomy, by virtue of its small incision, is already a form of minimal-access surgery.[73]

Laparoscopic appendectomy is performed under general anesthesia. A nasogastric tube and a urinary catheter are placed prior to obtaining a pneumoperitoneum. Laparoscopic appendectomy usually requires the use of three ports. Four ports may occasionally be necessary to mobilize a retrocecal appendix. The surgeon usually stands to the patient's left. One assistant is required to operate the camera. One trocar is placed in the umbilicus (10 mm), with a second trocar placed in the suprapubic position. Some surgeons will place this second port in the left lower quadrant. The suprapubic trocar is either 10 or 12 mm, depending on whether a linear stapler will be used. The placement of the third trocar (5 mm) is variable and is usually either in the left lower quadrant, epigastrium, or right upper quadrant. Placement is based on location of the appendix and surgeon preference. Initially, the abdomen is thoroughly explored to exclude other pathology. The appendix is identified by following the anterior taeniae to its base. Dissection at the base of the appendix enables the surgeon to create a window between the mesentery and base of the appendix (Fig. 29-8A). The mesentery and base of the appendix are then secured and divided separately. When the mesoappendix is involved with the inflammatory process, it is often best to divide the appendix first with a linear stapler, and then to divide the mesoappendix immediately adjacent to the appendix with clips, electrocautery, Harmonic Scalpel, or staples (Fig. 29-8B and C). The base of the appendix is not inverted. The appendix is removed from the abdominal cavity through a trocar site or within a retrieval bag. The base of the appendix and the mesoappendix should be evaluated for hemostasis. The right lower quadrant should be irrigated. Trocars are removed under direct vision.[74,75]

The utility of laparoscopic appendectomy in the management of acute appendicitis remains controversial. Surgeons may be hesitant to implement a new technique because the conventional open approach has already proved to be simple and effective. There

are a number of articles in peer-reviewed journals that compare laparoscopic and open appendectomy, including more than 20 randomized, controlled trials and 6 meta-analyses.[62,73,76-80] The overall quality of these randomized, controlled trials has been limited by the failure to blind patients and providers as to the treatment modality used. Furthermore, there has been a failure to perform prestudy sample size analysis for the outcomes studied.[62] The largest meta-analysis comparing open to laparoscopic appendectomy included 47 studies, 39 of which were studies of adult patients. This analysis demonstrated that the duration of surgery and operation costs were higher for laparoscopic appendectomy than for open appendectomy. Wound infections were approximately half as likely after laparoscopic appendectomy than after open appendectomy. However, intra-abdominal abscess was three times greater after laparoscopic appendectomy than after open appendectomy.[62]

A principal proposed benefit of laparoscopic appendectomy has been decreased postoperative pain. Patient-reported pain on the first postoperative day is significantly less after laparoscopic appendectomy. However, the difference has been calculated to be only 8 on a 100-point visual analogue scale. This difference is under the level of pain that an average patient is able to perceive.[62] Hospital length of stay also is statistically significantly less after laparoscopic appendectomy. However, in most studies this difference is less than 1 day.[62,73] It appears that the more important determinant of length of stay after appendectomy is the pathology at operation, specifically whether a patient has perforated or nonperforated appendicitis. In nearly all studies, laparoscopic appendectomy is associated with a shorter period prior to return to normal activity, return to work, and return to sports.[62,73,76-80] However, treatment and subject bias may have a significant impact on the data. Although the majority of studies have been performed in adults, similar data has been obtained in children.[62]

There appears to be little benefit to laparoscopic appendectomy over open appendectomy in thin males between the ages of 15 and 45 years. In these patients, the diagnosis is usually straightforward. Open appendectomy has been associated with outstanding results for several decades. Laparoscopic appendectomy should be considered an option in these patients, based on surgeon and patient preference. Laparoscopic appendectomy may be beneficial in obese patients in whom it may be difficult to gain adequate access through a small right lower quadrant incision. Additionally, there may be a decreased risk of postoperative wound infection after laparoscopic appendectomy in obese patients.[81] Further study is warranted regarding the benefit of laparoscopic appendectomy in this patient subgroup.

Diagnostic laparoscopy has been advocated as a potential tool to decrease the number of negative appendectomies performed. However, the morbidity associated with laparoscopy and general anesthesia is acceptable only if pathology requiring surgical treatment is present and is amenable to laparoscopic techniques. The question of leaving a normal appendix in situ is a controversial one. Seventeen to 26% of normal-appearing appendices at exploration have a pathologic histologic finding.[76] The availability of diagnostic laparoscopy may actually lower the threshold for exploration, thus impacting the negative appendectomy rate adversely.[82] Fertile women with presumed appendicitis constitute the group of patients most likely to benefit from diagnostic laparoscopy. Up to one-third of these patients will not have appendicitis at exploration. Most of these patients without appendicitis will have gynecologic pathology identified.[83] A large meta-analysis demonstrated that in fertile women in whom appendectomy was deemed necessary, diagnostic laparoscopy reduced the number of unnecessary appendectomies.[62]

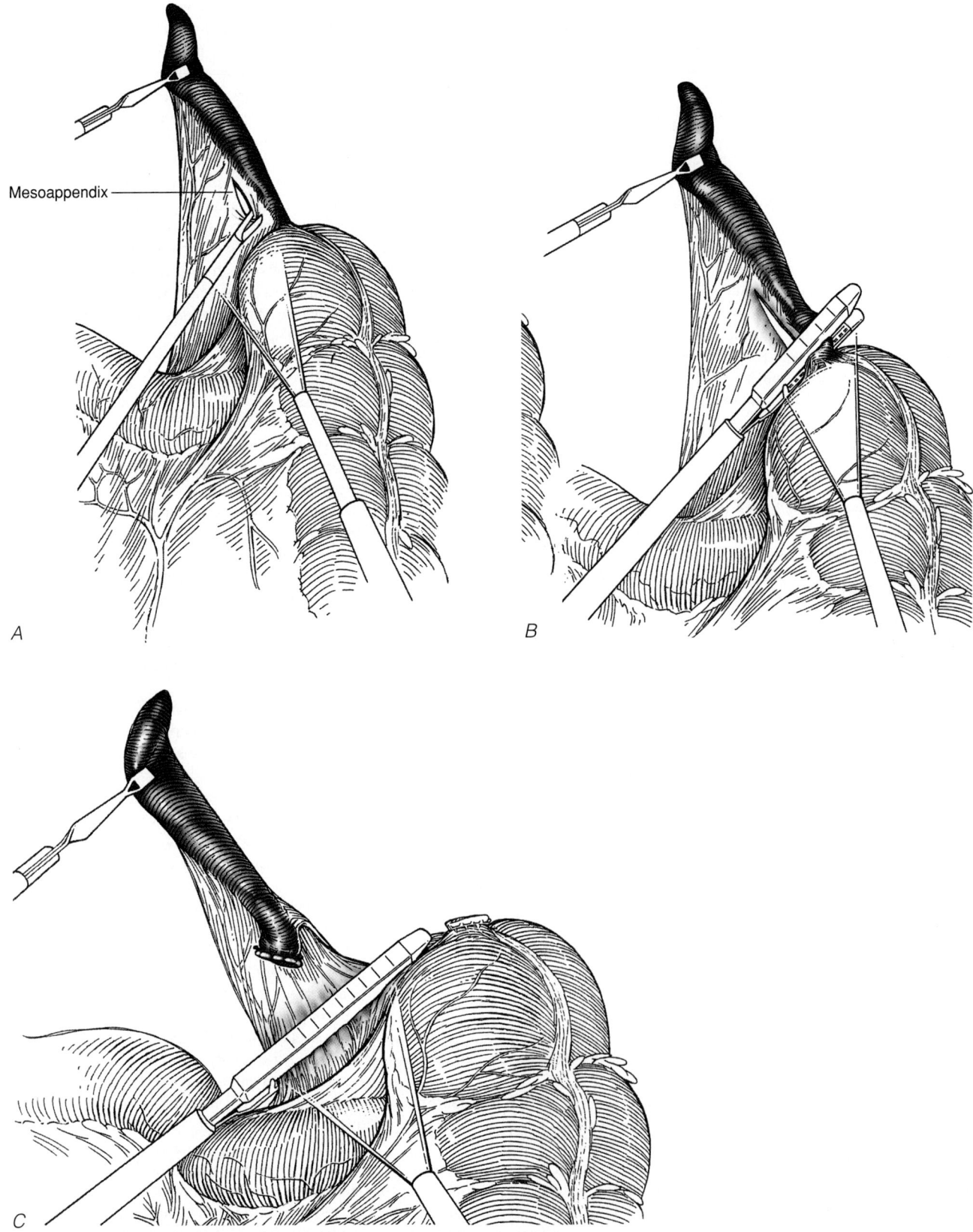

Mesoappendix

A

B

C

FIG. 29-8. Laparoscopic resection of the appendix. Occasionally, if the appendix and mesoappendix are extremely inflamed, it is easier to divide the appendix at its base prior to division of the mesoappendix. *A.* A window is created in the mesoappendix close to the base of the appendix. *B.* The linear stapler is then used to divide the appendix at its base. *C.* Finally the mesoappendix can be easily divided using the linear stapler. [*Reproduced with permission from Ortega JM, Ricardo AE: Surgery of the appendix and colon, in Moody FG (ed): Atlas of Ambulatory Surgery. Philadelphia: WB Saunders, 1999.*]

Additionally, the number of women without a final diagnosis was smaller. It appears that leaving a normal-appearing appendix in fertile women with identifiable gynecologic pathology is safe.[83]

In summary, it has not been resolved whether laparoscopic appendectomy is more effective at treating acute appendicitis than the time-proven method of open appendectomy. It does appear that laparoscopic appendectomy is effective in the management of acute appendicitis. Laparoscopic appendectomy should be considered part of the surgical armamentarium available to treat acute appendicitis. The decision regarding how to treat any single patient with appendicitis should be based on surgical skill, patient characteristics, clinical scenario, and patient preference. Additional well-controlled, prospective, blinded studies are needed to determine which subsets of patients may benefit from any approach to the treatment of appendicitis.

Interval Appendectomy

The accepted algorithm for the treatment of appendicitis associated with a palpable or radiographically documented mass (abscess or phlegmon) is conservative therapy with interval appendectomy 6 to 10 weeks later. This technique has been quite successful and provides much lower morbidity and mortality rates than immediate appendectomy. Unfortunately, this treatment is associated with added expense and longer hospitalization (8 to 13 vs. 3 to 5 days).[84]

The initial treatment consists of intravenous antibiotics and bowel rest. While generally effective, there is a 9 to 15% failure rate, with operative intervention required at 3 to 5 days after presentation. Percutaneous or operative drainage of abscesses is not considered a failure of conservative therapy.[85]

While the second stage of this treatment plan, interval appendectomy, has usually been performed, the need for subsequent operation has been questioned. The major argument against interval appendectomy is that approximately 50% of patients treated conservatively never develop manifestations of appendicitis, and those who do, can generally be treated nonoperatively. In addition, pathologic examination of the resected appendix is normal in 20 to 50% of cases.

On the other hand, the data clearly support the need for interval appendectomy. In a prospective series, 19 of 48 (40%) patients who were successfully treated conservatively needed appendectomy earlier (4.3 weeks) than the 10 weeks planned because of bouts of appendicitis.[84] Overall, the rate of late failure as a consequence of acute disease averages 20%. An additional 14% of patients either continue to have, or redevelop, right lower quadrant pain. While the appendix may occasionally be pathologically normal, persistent periappendiceal abscesses and adhesions are found in 80% of patients. In addition, almost 50% have histologic evidence of inflammation in the organ itself. Several neoplasms also have been detected in the resected appendix, even in those of children.[30]

The timing of interval appendectomy is somewhat controversial. Appendectomy may be required as early as 3 weeks following conservative therapy. Two thirds of the cases of recurrent appendicitis occur within 2 years, and this is the outside limit.

Interval appendectomy is associated with a morbidity rate of 3% or less and a hospitalization of 1 to 3 days in length. The laparoscopic approach has been used recently and has been successful in 68% of procedures.

Prognosis

The mortality from appendicitis in the United States has steadily decreased from a rate of 9.9 per 100,000 in 1939, to 0.2 per 100,000 as of 1986. Among the factors responsible are advances in anesthesia, antibiotics, intravenous fluids, and blood products. Principal factors in mortality are whether rupture occurs before surgical treatment and the age of the patient. The overall mortality rate for a general anesthetic is 0.06%. The overall mortality rate in ruptured acute appendicitis is about 3%—a 50-fold increase. The mortality rate of ruptured appendicitis in the elderly is approximately 15%—a fivefold increase from the overall rate.

Death is usually attributable to uncontrolled sepsis—peritonitis, intra-abdominal abscesses, or gram-negative septicemia. Pulmonary embolism continues to account for some deaths. Aspiration is a significant cause of death in the older patient group.

Morbidity rates parallel mortality rates, being significantly increased by rupture of the appendix and to a lesser extent by old age. In one report, complications occurred in 3% of patients with nonperforated appendicitis and in 47% of patients with perforations. Most of the serious early complications are septic and include abscess and wound infection. Wound infection is common, but is nearly always confined to the subcutaneous tissues and promptly responds to wound drainage, which is accomplished by reopening the skin incision. Wound infection predisposes the patient to wound dehiscence. The type of incision is relevant; complete dehiscence rarely occurs in a McBurney incision.

The incidence of intra-abdominal abscesses secondary to peritoneal contamination from gangrenous or perforated appendicitis has decreased markedly since the introduction of potent antibiotics. The sites of predilection for abscesses are the appendiceal fossa, pouch of Douglas, subhepatic space, and between loops of intestine. The latter are usually multiple. Transrectal drainage is preferred for an abscess that bulges into the rectum.

Fecal fistula is an annoying, but not particularly dangerous, complication of appendectomy that may be caused by sloughing of that portion of the cecum inside a constricting purse-string suture; by the ligature's slipping off a tied, but not inverted, appendiceal stump; or by necrosis from an abscess encroaching on the cecum.

Intestinal obstruction, initially paralytic but sometimes progressing to mechanical obstruction, may occur with slowly resolving peritonitis with loculated abscesses and exuberant adhesion formation. Late complications are quite uncommon. Adhesive band intestinal obstruction after appendectomy does occur, but much less frequently than after pelvic surgical therapy. The incidence of inguinal hernia is three times greater in patients who have had an appendectomy. Incisional hernia is like wound dehiscence in that infection predisposes to it, it rarely occurs in a McBurney incision, and it is not uncommon in a lower right paramedian incision.[25,86]

CHRONIC APPENDICITIS

The existence of chronic appendicitis as a true clinical entity has been questioned for many years. However, recent clinical data document the existence of this uncommon disease.[87,88] Histologic criteria have been established. Characteristically, the pain lasts longer and is less intense than that of acute appendicitis, but is in the same location. There is a much lower incidence of vomiting, but anorexia and occasionally nausea, pain with motion, and malaise are characteristic. Leukocyte counts are predictably normal and CT scans are generally nondiagnostic.

At operation, surgeons can establish the diagnosis with 94% specificity and 78% sensitivity. There is an excellent correlation between clinical symptomatology, intraoperative findings, and histologic abnormalities. Laparoscopy can be effectively used in the management of this clinical entity. Appendectomy is curative. Symptoms resolve postoperatively in 82 to 93% of patients. Many of those whose symptoms are not cured or recur are ultimately diagnosed with Crohn's disease.

APPENDICEAL PARASITES

A number of intestinal parasites cause appendicitis. While *Ascaris lumbricoides* is the most common, a wide spectrum of helminths have been implicated, including *Enterobius vermicularis*, *Strongyloides stercoralis*, and *Echinococcus granulosis*. The live parasites occlude the appendiceal lumen, causing obstruction. The presence of parasites in the appendix at operation makes ligation and stapling of the appendix technically difficult. Once appendectomy has been performed and the patient recovered, therapy with helminthicide is necessary to clear the remainder of the gastrointestinal tract.

Amebiasis can also cause appendicitis. Invasion of the mucosa by trophozoites of *Entamoeba histolytica* incites a marked inflammatory process. Appendiceal involvement is a component of more generalized intestinal amebiasis. Appendectomy must be followed by appropriate antibiotic therapy (metronidazole).

INCIDENTAL APPENDECTOMY

The decisions regarding the efficacy of incidental appendectomy should be based on the epidemiology of appendicitis. The best data were published by the Centers for Disease Control based on the period from 1979 to 1984.[11] During this period, there was an average of 250,000 cases of appendicitis in the United States. The highest annual incidence of appendicitis was in patients 9 to 19 years of age (23.3 per 10,000 population). Males were more likely to develop appendicitis than females. Accordingly, the incidence during teenage years was 27.6 in males and 20.5 in females per 10,000 population per year. Beyond age 19 years, the annual incidence fell. After 45 years of age, the annual incidence was 6 in 10,000 males and 4 in 10,000 females. Using the life table technique, the data identified a lifetime risk of appendicitis of 8.6% in men and 6.7% in women. While men were more likely to develop appendicitis, the preoperative diagnosis was correct in 91.2% of men and 78.6% of women. Similarly, perforation occurred more commonly in men (19.2 vs. 17.8% in women). In contrast to the cases of appendicitis, 310,000 incidental appendectomies were performed between 1979 and 1984, 62% of the total appendectomies in men and 17.7% in women. Based on these data, 36 incidental appendectomies had to be performed to prevent 1 patient from developing appendicitis.[89]

The financial aspects of the decision to perform incidental appendectomy were recently assessed.[90] Using open appendectomy, there was a financial disincentive to perform incidental appendectomy. On an annual basis, $20,000,000 had to be spent to save the $6,000,000 cost of appendicitis. With the laparoscopic approach, it was cost-effective to perform incidental appendectomy only in patients younger than age 25 years only if the reimbursement for surgeons was 10% of usual and customary changes. At a higher rate of reimbursement, it was not cost-effective in any age group.

While incidental appendectomy is generally neither clinically nor economically appropriate, there are some special circumstances during laparotomy or laparoscopy for other indications in which it should be performed. These include children about to undergo chemotherapy, the disabled who cannot describe symptoms or react normally to abdominal pain, Crohn's disease patients in whom the cecum is free of macroscopic disease, and individuals who are about to travel to remote places where there is no access to medical/surgical care.[91]

TUMORS

Appendiceal malignancies are extremely rare. Primary appendiceal cancer is diagnosed in 0.9 to 1.4% of appendectomy specimens.[92] These tumors are only rarely suspected preoperatively. Additionally, less than 50% of cases are diagnosed at operation.[93] Most series report that carcinoid is the most common appendiceal malignancy, representing more than 50% of the primary lesions of the appendix.[92,94,95] However, a recent review from The National Cancer Institute's Surveillance, Epidemiology, and End Results program found the age-adjusted incidence of appendiceal malignancies to be 0.12 cases per 1,000,000 people per year, and identified mucinous adenocarcinoma as the most frequent histologic diagnosis with 37% of total reported cases. Carcinoid was the second most frequent histologic diagnosis, comprising 33% of total cases.[93]

Carcinoid

The finding of a firm, yellow, bulbar mass in the appendix should raise the suspicion of an appendiceal carcinoid. The appendix is the most common site of gastrointestinal carcinoid, followed by the small bowel and then rectum. Carcinoid syndrome is rarely associated with appendiceal carcinoid unless widespread metastases are present, which occur in 2.9% of cases. Symptoms attributable directly to the carcinoid are rare, although the tumor can occasionally obstruct the appendiceal lumen much like a fecalith and result in acute appendicitis.[92,94,95]

The majority of carcinoids are located in the tip of the appendix. Malignant potential is related to size, with tumors less than 1 cm rarely resulting in extension outside of the appendix or adjacent to the mass. In one report, 78% of appendiceal carcinoids were less than 1 cm, 17% were 1 to 2 cm, and only 5% were greater than 2 cm.[94] Treatment rarely requires more than simple appendectomy. For tumors smaller than 1 cm with extension into the mesoappendix, and for all tumors larger than 1.5 cm, a right hemicolectomy should be performed.[92,94,95]

Adenocarcinoma

Primary adenocarcinoma of the appendix is a rare neoplasm of three major histologic subtypes: mucinous adenocarcinoma, colonic adenocarcinoma, and adenocarcinoid.[93] The most common mode of presentation for appendiceal carcinoma is that of acute appendicitis. Patients may also present with ascites or a palpable mass, or the neoplasm may be discovered during an operative procedure for an unrelated cause. The recommended treatment for all patients with adenocarcinoma of the appendix is a formal right hemicolectomy. Appendiceal adenocarcinomas have a propensity for early perforation, although they are not clearly associated with a worsened prognosis.[95] Overall 5-year survival is 55% and varies with stage and grade. Patients with appendiceal adenocarcinoma are at significant risk for both synchronous and metachronous neoplasms, approximately half of which will originate from the gastrointestinal tract.[93]

Mucocele

An appendiceal mucocele leads to progressive enlargement of the appendix from the intraluminal accumulation of a mucoid substance. Mucoceles are of four histologic types, and the type dictates the course of the disease and prognosis: retention cysts, mucosal hyperplasia, cystadenomas, and cystadenocarcinomas. A mucocele of benign etiology is adequately treated by a simple appendectomy.[95]

Pseudomyxoma Peritonei

Pseudomyxoma peritonei is a rare condition in which diffuse collections of gelatinous fluid are associated with mucinous implants on peritoneal surfaces and omentum. Pseudomyxoma is two to three times more common in females than males. There is controversy in the literature as to whether pseudomyxoma arises from the appendix or the ovary in female patients. Recent immunocytologic and molecular studies suggest that the appendix is the site of origin for most cases of pseudomyxoma. Pseudomyxoma is invariably caused by neoplastic mucous-secreting cells within the peritoneum. These cells may be difficult to classify as malignant because they may be sparse, widely scattered, and have a low-grade cytologic appearance. Patients with pseudomyxoma usually present with abdominal pain, distention, or a mass. Primary pseudomyxoma usually does not cause abdominal organ dysfunction. However, ureteral obstruction and obstruction of venous return can be seen.[96]

The use of imaging before surgery is advantageous in order to plan surgery. CT scanning is the preferred imaging modality. At surgery a variable volume of mucinous ascites is found together with tumor deposits involving the right hemidiaphragm, right retrohepatic space, left paracolic gutter, ligament of Treitz, and the ovaries in women. Peritoneal surfaces of the bowel are usually free of tumor. Thorough surgical debulking is the mainstay of treatment. All gross disease should be removed. Appendectomy is routinely performed. Hysterectomy with bilateral salpingo-oophorectomy is performed in women. Ultra-radical surgery has not been shown to be of significant benefit. Additionally, adjuvant intraperitoneal chemotherapy (with or without hyperthermia) or systemic postoperative chemotherapy have not been shown to be of benefit. Pseudomyxoma is a disease that progresses slowly and in which recurrences may take years to develop or become symptomatic.[96] In a series from the Mayo Clinic, 76% of patients developed recurrences within the abdomen.[97] Lymph node metastasis and distant metastasis are uncommon. Any recurrence should be investigated completely. Recurrences are usually treated by additional surgery. It is important to note that surgery for recurrent disease is usually difficult and associated with an increased incidence of unintentional enterotomies, anastomotic leaks, and fistulas. With adequate primary surgery and debulking of recurrences, the median survival of pseudomyxoma is 5.9 years, with 53% of patients surviving 5 years.[96,97]

Lymphoma

Lymphoma of the appendix is extremely uncommon. The gastrointestinal tract is the most frequently involved extranodal site for non-Hodgkin's lymphoma.[98] Other types of lymphoma, such as Burkitt's, as well as leukemia, have also been reported.[99] The frequency of primary lymphoma of the appendix ranges from 1 to 3% of gastrointestinal lymphomas. Appendiceal lymphoma usually presents as acute appendicitis and is rarely suspected preoperatively. Findings on CT scan of an appendiceal diameter greater than or equal to 2.5 cm or surrounding soft-tissue thickening should prompt suspicion of an appendiceal lymphoma. The management of appendiceal lymphoma confined to the appendix is appendectomy. Right hemicolectomy is indicated if there is extension of tumor beyond the appendix onto the cecum or mesentery. A postoperative staging workup is indicated prior to initiating adjuvant therapy. Adjuvant therapy is not indicated for lymphoma confined to the appendix.[99,100]

References

1. Buschard K, Kjaeldgaard A: Investigation and analysis of the position, fixation, length and embryology of the vermiform appendix. *Acta Chir Scand* 139:293, 1973.
2. Ajmani ML, Ajmani K: The position, length and arterial supply of vermiform appendix. *Anat Anz* 153:369, 1983.
3. Fitz RH: Persistent omphalo-mesenteric remains: Their importance in the causation of intestinal duplication, cyst formation, and obstruction. *Am J Med Sci* 88:30, 1884.
4. Skandalakis JE, Gray SW, Ricketts R: The colon and rectum, in Skandalakis JE, Gray SW (eds): *Embryology for Surgeons.* Baltimore: Williams and Wilkins, 1994, p 242.
5. Ellis H: Appendix, in Schwartz SI (ed): *Maingot's Abdominal Operations,* 8th ed. Vol. 2. Norwalk: Appleton-Century-Crofts, 1985, p 1255.
6. Lewis F: Appendix, in Davis JH (ed): *Clinical Surgery,* 1st ed. Vol. 1. St. Louis: Mosby, 1987, p 1581.
7. Fitz RH: Perforating inflammation of the vermiform appendix: With special reference to its early diagnosis and treatment. *Trans Assoc Am Physicians* 1:107, 1886.
8. McBurney C: Experience with early operative interference in cases of disease of the vermiform appendix. *NY State Med J* 50:676, 1889.
9. McBurney C: The incision made in the abdominal wall in cases of appendicitis. *Ann Surg* 20:38, 1894.
10. Semm K: Endoscopic appendectomy. *Endoscopy* 15:59, 1983.
11. Addiss DG, Shaffer N, Fowler BS, et al: The epidemiology of appendicitis and appendectomy in the United States. *Am J Epidemiol* 132:910, 1990.
12. Hale DA, Molloy M, Pearl RH, et al: Appendectomy: A contemporary appraisal. *Ann Surg* 225:252, 1997.
13. Korner H, Sondenaa K, Soreide JA, et al: Incidence of acute nonperforated and perforated appendicitis: Age-specific and sex-specific analysis. *World J Surg* 21:313, 1997.
14. Flum DR, Morris A, Koepsell T, et al: Has misdiagnosis of appendicitis decreased over time? A population-based analysis. *JAMA* 286:1748, 2001.
15. Flum DR, Koepsell T: The clinical and economic correlates of misdiagnosed appendicitis: Nationwide analysis. *Arch Surg* 137:799, 2002.
16. Burkitt DP: The aetiology of appendicitis. *Br J Surg* 58:695, 1971.
17. Butler C: Surgical pathology of acute appendicitis. *Hum Pathol* 12:870, 1981.
18. Miranda R, Johnston AD, O'Leary JP: Incidental appendectomy: Frequency of pathologic abnormalities. *Am Surg* 46:355, 1980.
19. Rautio M, Saxen H, Siitonen A, et al: Bacteriology of histopathologically defined appendicitis in children. *Pediatr Infect Dis J* 19:1078, 2000.
20. Allo MD, Bennion RS, Kathir K, et al: Ticarcillin/clavulanate versus imipenem/cilastatin for the treatment of infections associated with gangrenous and perforated appendicitis. *Am Surg* 65:99, 1999.
21. Soffer D, Zait S, Klausner J, et al: Peritoneal cultures and antibiotic treatment in patients with perforated appendicitis. *Eur J Surg* 167:214, 2001.
22. Kokoska ER, Silen ML, Tracy TF Jr., et al: The impact of intraoperative culture on treatment and outcome in children with perforated appendicitis. *J Pediatr Surg* 34:749, 1999.
23. Mosdell DM, Morris DM, Fry DE: Peritoneal cultures and antibiotic therapy in pediatric perforated appendicitis. *Am J Surg* 167:313, 1994.
24. Bilik R, Burnweit C, Shandling B: Is abdominal cavity culture of any value in appendicitis? *Am J Surg* 175:267, 1998.
25. Schwartz SI: Appendix, in Schwartz SI, Shires GT, Spencer FC (eds): *Principles of Surgery,* 5th ed. Vol. 2. New York: McGraw-Hill, 1989, p 1315.
26. Berry J, Malt RA: Appendicitis near its centenary. *Ann Surg* 200:567, 1984.
27. Bower RJ, Bell MJ, Ternberg JL: Diagnostic value of the white blood count and neutrophil percentage in the evaluation of abdominal pain in children. *Surg Gynecol Obstet* 152:424, 1981.

28. Smith DE, Kirchmer NA, Stewart DR. Use of the barium enema in the diagnosis of acute appendicitis and its complications. *Am J Surg* 138:829, 1979.

29. Douglas CD, Macpherson NE, Davidson PM, et al: Randomised controlled trial of ultrasonography in diagnosis of acute appendicitis, incorporating the Alvarado score. *Brit Med J* 321:1, 2000.

30. Franke C, Bohner H, Yang Q, et al: Ultrasonography for diagnosis of acute appendicitis: Results of a prospective multicenter trial. *World J Surg* 23:141, 1999.

31. Kaiser S, Frenckner B, Jorulf HK: Suspected appendicitis in children: US and CT—A prospective randomized study. *Radiology* 223:633, 2002.

32. Jeffrey RB, Jain KA, Nghiem HV: Sonographic diagnosis of acute appendicitis: Interpretive pitfalls. *Am J Roentgenol* 162:55, 1994.

33. Puig S, Hormann M, Rebhandl W, et al: US as a primary diagnostic tool in relation to negative appendectomy: Six years experience. *Radiology* 226:101, 2003.

34. Rettenbacher T, Hollerweger A, Gritzmann N, et al: Appendicitis: Should diagnostic imaging be performed if the clinical presentation is highly suggestive of the disease? *Gastroenterology* 123:992, 2002.

35. Funaki B, Grosskreutz SR, Funaki CN: Using unenhanced helical CT with enteric contrast material for suspected appendicitis in patients treated at a community hospital. *Am J Roentgenol* 171:997, 1998.

36. Raman SS, Lu DSK, Kadell BM, et al: Accuracy of nonfocused helical CT for the diagnosis of acute appendicitis: A 5-year review. *Am J Roentgenol* 178:1319, 2002.

37. Stroman DL, Bayouth CV, Kuhn JA, et al: The role of computed tomography in the diagnosis of acute appendicitis. *Am J Surg* 178:485, 1999.

38. Weyant MJ, Eachempati SR, Maluccio MA, et al: Interpretation of computed tomography does not correlate with laboratory or pathologic findings in surgically confirmed acute appendicitis. *Surgery* 128:145, 2000.

39. Fuchs JR, Schlamberg JS, Shortsleeve MJ, et al: Impact of abdominal CT imaging on the management of appendicitis: An update. *J Surg Res* 106:131, 2002.

40. Walker S, Haun W, Clark J, et al: The value of limited computed tomography with rectal contrast in the diagnosis of acute appendicitis. *Am J Surg* 180:450, 2000.

41. Ujiki MB, Murayama KM, Cribbins AJ, et al: CT scan in the management of acute appendicitis. *J Surg Res* 105:119, 2002.

42. Applegate KE, Sivit CJ, Salvator AE, et al: Effect of cross-sectional imaging on negative appendectomy and perforation rates in children. *Radiology* 220:103, 2001.

43. Wise SW, Labuski MR, Kasales CJ, et al: Comparative assessment of CT and sonographic techniques for appendiceal imaging. *Am J Roentgenol* 176:933, 2001.

44. Wilson EB, Cole JC, Nipper ML, et al: Computed tomography and ultrasonography in the diagnosis of appendicitis: When are they indicated? *Arch Surg* 136:670, 2001.

45. Rao PM, Rhea JT, Rattner DW, et al: Introduction of appendiceal CT: Impact on negative appendectomy and appendiceal perforation rates. *Ann Surg* 229:344, 1999.

46. Rao PM, Rhea JT, Novelline RA, et al: Effect of computed tomography of the appendix on treatment of patients and use of hospital resources. *N Engl J Med* 338:141, 1998.

47. Morris KT, Kavanagh M, Hansen P, et al: The rational use of computed tomography scans in the diagnosis of appendicitis. *Am J Surg* 183:547, 2002.

48. Lee SL, Walsh AJ, Ho HS: Computed tomography and ultrasonography do not improve and may delay the diagnosis and treatment of acute appendicitis. *Arch Surg* 136:556, 2001.

49. Garcia Pena BM, Taylor GA, Fishman SJ, et al: Effect of an imaging protocol on clinical outcomes among pediatric patients with appendicitis. *Pediatrics* 110:1088, 2002.

50. Alvarado A: A practical score for the early diagnosis of acute appendicitis. *Ann Emerg Med* 15:557, 1986.

51. Paulson EK, Kalady MF, Pappas TN: Clinical practice. Suspected appendicitis. *N Engl J Med* 348:236, 2003.

52. De U, Ghosh S: Acute appendicectomy for appendicular mass: A study of 87 patients. *Ceylon Med J* 47:117, 2002.

53. Tingstedt B, Bexe-Lindskog E, Ekelund M, et al: Management of appendiceal masses. *Eur J Surg* 168:579, 2002.

54. Willemsen PJ, Hoorntje LE, Eddes EH, et al: The need for interval appendectomy after resolution of an appendiceal mass questioned. *Dig Surg* 19:216, 2002.

55. Haller JA Jr., Shaker IJ, Donahoo JS, et al: Peritoneal drainage versus non-drainage for generalized peritonitis from ruptured appendicitis in children: A prospective study. *Ann Surg* 177:595, 1973.

56. Bongard F, Landers DV, Lewis F: Differential diagnosis of appendicitis and pelvic inflammatory disease. A prospective analysis. *Am J Surg* 150:90, 1985.

57. Jepsen OB, Korner B, Lauritsen KB, et al: *Yersinia enterocolitica* infection in patients with acute surgical abdominal disease. A prospective study. *Scand J Infect Dis* 8:189, 1976.

58. Knight PJ, Vassy LE: Specific diseases mimicking appendicitis in childhood. *Arch Surg* 116:744, 1981.

59. McDonald JC: Nonspecific mesenteric lymphadenitis: Collective review. *Surg Gynecol Obstet* 116:409, 1963.

60. Morrison JD: Yersinia and viruses in acute non-specific abdominal pain and appendicitis. *Br J Surg* 68:284, 1981.

61. Droegemueller W: Upper genital tract infections, in Herbst AL, Mishell DR, Stenchever MW, et al (eds): *Comprehensive Gynecology,* 2nd ed. St. Louis: Mosby Year Book, 1992, p 691.

62. Sauerland S, Lefering R, Neugebauer EA: Laparoscopic versus open surgery for suspected appendicitis. *Cochrane Database Syst Rev* (1):CD001546, 2002.

63. Hui TT, Major KM, Avital I, et al: Outcome of elderly patients with appendicitis: Effect of computed tomography and laparoscopy. *Arch Surg* 137:995, 2002.

64. Bailey LE, Finley RK Jr., Miller SF, et al: Acute appendicitis during pregnancy. *Am Surg* 52:218, 1986.

65. Masters K, Levine BA, Gaskill HV, et al: Diagnosing appendicitis during pregnancy. *Am J Surg* 148:768, 1984.

66. Musselman RC, Nunnelee JD, Ware DB: Appendicitis during pregnancy. *Clin Excell Nurse Pract* 2:338, 1998.

67. Wells SB, Beaton HL: Appendiceal disease in HIV-infected homosexual men. *AIDS Reader* Sept/Oct:173, 1991.

68. Flum DR, Steinberg SD, Sarkis AY, et al: Appendicitis in patients with acquired immunodeficiency syndrome. *J Am Coll Surg* 184:481, 1997.

69. Mueller GP, Williams RA: Surgical infections in AIDS patients. *Am J Surg* 169(5A Suppl):34S, 1995.

70. Bova R, Meagher A: Appendicitis in HIV-positive patients. *Aust NZ J Surg* 68:337, 1998.

71. Lowy AM, Barie PS: Laparotomy in patients infected with human immunodeficiency virus: Indications and outcome. *Br J Surg* 81:942, 1994.

72. Arnbjornsson E: Invagination of the appendiceal stump for the reduction of peritoneal bacterial contamination. *Curr Surg* 42:184, 1985.

73. Golub R, Siddiqui F, Pohl D: Laparoscopic versus open appendectomy: A meta-analysis. *J Am Coll Surg* 186:545, 1998.

74. Hunter JG: Advanced laparoscopic surgery. *Am J Surg* 173:14, 1997.

75. Scott-Conner CE: Laparoscopic gastrointestinal surgery. *Med Clin North Am* 86:1401, 2002.

76. Fingerhut A, Millat B, Borrie F: Laparoscopic versus open appendectomy: Time to decide. *World J Surg* 23:835, 1999.

77. Hunter JG: Clinical trials and the development of laparoscopic surgery. *Surg Endosc* 15:1, 2001.

78. McCall JL, Sharples K, Jadallah F: Systematic review of randomized controlled trials comparing laparoscopic with open appendicectomy. *Br J Surg* 84:1045, 1997.

79. Ortega AE, Hunter JG, Peters JH, et al: A prospective, randomized comparison of laparoscopic appendectomy with open appendectomy.

Laparoscopic Appendectomy Study Group. *Am J Surg* 169:208, 1995.

80. Pedersen AG, Petersen OB, Wara P, et al: Randomized clinical trial of laparoscopic versus open appendicectomy. *Br J Surg* 88:200, 2001.

81. Enochsson L, Hellberg A, Rudberg C, et al: Laparoscopic vs. open appendectomy in overweight patients. *Surg Endosc* 15:387, 2001.

82. McGreevy JM, Finlayson SR, Alvarado R, et al: Laparoscopy may be lowering the threshold to operate on patients with suspected appendicitis. *Surg Endosc* 16:1046, 2002.

83. Borgstein PJ, Gordijn RV, Eijsbouts QA, et al: Acute appendicitis—A clear-cut case in men, a guessing game in young women. A prospective study on the role of laparoscopy. *Surg Endosc* 11:923, 1997.

84. Samuel M, Hosie G, Holmes K: Prospective evaluation of nonsurgical versus surgical management of appendiceal mass. *J Pediatr Surg* 37:882, 2002.

85. Yamini D, Vargas H, Bongard F, et al: Perforated appendicitis: Is it truly a surgical urgency? *Am Surg* 64:970, 1998.

86. Cooperman M: Complications of appendectomy. *Surg Clin North Am* 63:1233, 1983.

87. Leardi S, Delmonaco S, Ventura T, et al: Recurrent abdominal pain and "chronic appendicitis." *Minerva Chir* 55:39, 2000.

88. Mussack T, Schmidbauer S, Nerlich A, et al: Chronic appendicitis as an independent clinical entity. *Chirurg* 73:710, 2002.

89. Wang HT, Sax HC: Incidental appendectomy in the era of managed care and laparoscopy. *J Am Coll Surg* 192:182, 2001.

90. Sugimoto T, Edwards D: Incidence and costs of incidental appendectomy as a preventive measure. *Am J Public Health* 77:471, 1987.

91. Fisher KS, Ross DS: Guidelines for therapeutic decision in incidental appendectomy. *Surg Gynecol Obstet* 171:95, 1990.

92. Connor SJ, Hanna GB, Frizelle FA: Appendiceal tumors: Retrospective clinicopathologic analysis of appendiceal tumors from 7970 appendectomies. *Dis Colon Rectum* 41:75, 1998.

93. McCusker ME, Cote TR, Clegg LX, et al: Primary malignant neoplasms of the appendix: A population-based study from the Surveillance, Epidemiology and End Results program, 1973–1998. *Cancer* 94:3307, 2002.

94. Roggo A, Wood WC, Ottinger LW: Carcinoid tumors of the appendix. *Ann Surg* 217:385, 1993.

95. Deans GT, Spence RA: Neoplastic lesions of the appendix. *Br J Surg* 82:299, 1995.

96. Hinson FL, Ambrose NS: Pseudomyxoma peritonei. *Br J Surg* 85:1332, 1998.

97. Gough DB, Donohue JH, Schutt AJ, et al: Pseudomyxoma peritonei. Long-term patient survival with an aggressive regional approach. *Ann Surg* 219:112, 1994.

98. Crump M, Gospodarowicz M, Shepherd FA: Lymphoma of the gastrointestinal tract. *Semin Oncol* 26:324, 1999.

99. Pickhardt PJ, Levy AD, Rohrmann CA Jr., et al: Non-Hodgkin's lymphoma of the appendix: Clinical and CT findings with pathologic correlation. *Am J Roentgenol* 178:1123, 2002.

100. Muller G, Dargent JL, Duwel V, et al: Leukaemia and lymphoma of the appendix presenting as acute appendicitis or acute abdomen. Four case reports with a review of the literature. *J Cancer Res Clin Oncol* 123:560, 1997.

CHAPTER 30

Liver

Timothy D. Sielaff and Steven A. Curley

ANATOMY

It is unclear if the ancient Greeks understood concepts like functional hepatic reserve and hepatic regeneration, but they may well have had some insight into the remarkable regenerative capacity of the liver based on the well-known myth of Prometheus. Zeus punished Prometheus for giving fire to humans. The eternal torment of Prometheus was to have his liver devoured daily by an apparently surgically adept eagle. His liver would regenerate completely over the next 24 hours, assuring a meal for the eagle the next day.

Around 2000 B.C. the Babylonians knew the liver had an impressive blood supply and capacity for hemorrhage, thus they considered it to be the seat of the soul. For many years, surgeons operated on

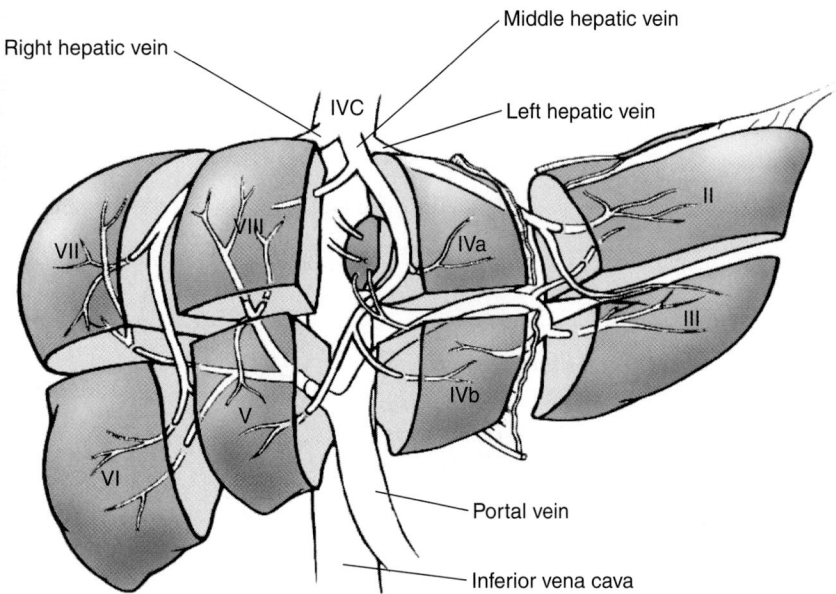

FIG. 30-1. *Segmental anatomy of the liver with the eight segments based on portal vein blood supply and hepatic venous outflow as designated by Couinaud. Segment I is also known as the caudate lobe; segments II and III comprise the lateral segment of the left lobe; segment IV is the medial segment of the left lobe; and segments V to VIII comprise the right lobe. (Adapted from www.ahpba.org, the website of The American Hepato-Pancreato-Biliary Association.)*

the liver only with trepidation, often being confronted with persistent or massive hemorrhage. However, recent advances in knowledge of hepatobiliary anatomy and advances in techniques for major liver resections have produced marked reductions in the high morbidity and mortality rates classically associated with hepatobiliary operations.

The liver is the largest solid organ in the body, weighing about 1.5 kg in the adult. It lies in the right upper quadrant of the abdomen and is completely protected by the thoracic rib cage. Its normal expanse is from the nipple line at the fourth intercostal space down to the costal margin in the midclavicular line. It is completely surrounded by a peritoneal membrane, known as Glisson's capsule. The cephalad aspect of the liver is in contact with the left and right hemidiaphragm, while the caudal surface is in contact with the stomach, duodenum, and colon. Glisson's capsule also envelops the portal triad structures as they enter the liver. The posterior aspect of the liver is in contact with the right kidney and adrenal gland. The gross anatomic landmarks include the falciform ligament and the ligamentum teres hepaticus (round ligament of the liver) separating the left lateral segment of the liver (segments II and III) from the remaining liver (Fig. 30-1). The round ligament is the vestigial remnant of the umbilical vein, and is an external marker for the location of the intrahepatic portion of the left portal vein. The ligamentum venosum is the vestigial remnant of the ductus venosus. It runs from the intrahepatic portal vein to the vena cava. It marks the border between the caudate lobe (segment I) and the left lateral sector. The gallbladder lies on the caudal surface of the liver. Two attachments, the left and right triangular ligaments (Fig. 30-2), secure the liver to the retroperitoneum. The gastrohepatic omentum, through which the hepatic branches of the vagus as well as an accessory or replaced left hepatic artery (if present) run, connects the caudal surface of the liver with the lesser curvature of the stomach.

Segments

One of the greatest advances in hepatic surgery is the understanding of the segmental anatomy of the liver. The Couinaud system for liver segmental nomenclature is widely accepted in practice.[1,2] The liver is divided into longitudinal planes drawn through each hepatic

vein to the vena cava, and a transverse plane at the level of the main portal bifurcation (see Fig. 30-2). The plane of the middle hepatic vein and the primary bifurcation of the portal vein divide the liver into a right and left lobe. This runs from the inferior vena cava to the tip of the gallbladder fossa (also known as Cantlie's line or the portal fissure). The secondary portal bifurcations on the right and left give rise to four sectors (or sections). On the right side this produces the anterior and posterior sectors, which are split by the plane of the right hepatic vein. The tertiary branches on the right supply four segments, two in each sector. On the left, the secondary bifurcation is less symmetrical (Fig. 30-3). The ascending branch of the left gives off recurrent branches to the medial sector of the left lobe.[3] However, the left lateral sector is supplied by separate branches that supply the two segments (segments II and III, Fig. 30-4). Segment I, the caudate lobe, receives blood supply from both the left and right portal pedicles; bile ducts from segment I also drain into the right and left hepatic ducts.

The translation of understanding surgical segmental anatomy to axial radiologic imaging is important in evaluating diagnostic computed tomographic (CT) or magnetic resonance imaging (MRI)

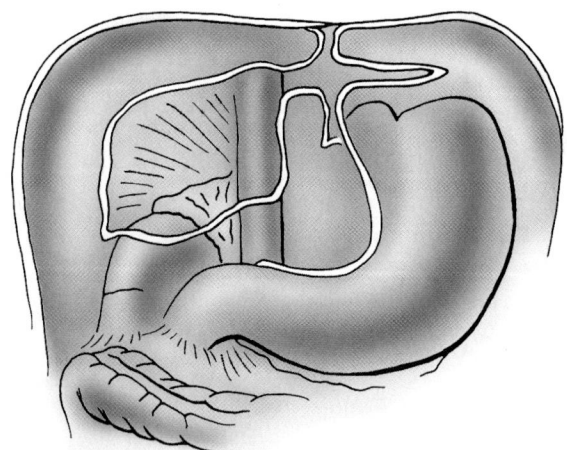

FIG. 30-2. The external and retroperitoneal attachments of the liver.

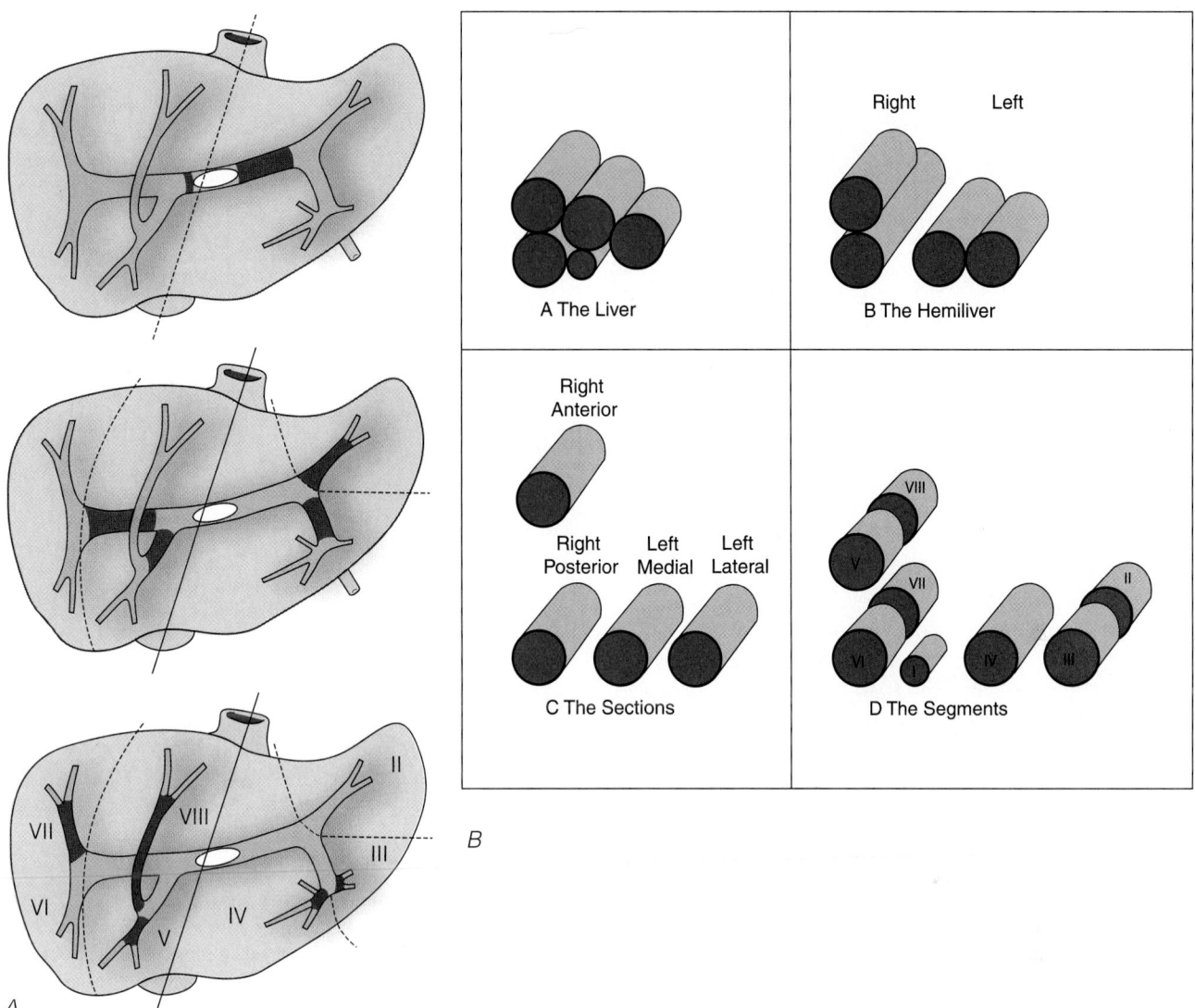

FIG. 30-3. *A.* Primary, secondary, and tertiary bifurcations of the portal pedicle as seen from the cephalad aspect of the liver. *B.* The liver lobes, sectors/sections, and segments are viewed as cylinders. The hemilivers are separated by the middle hepatic vein plane and are supplied by the primary branches of the main portal vein. The sections/sectors are divided by the right and left hepatic veins and are supplied by the secondary portal bifurcation within each lobe. The segments are supplied by the tertiary branches (bifurcation within a section/sector) and split along the coronal plane of the main portal bifurcation.

studies of the liver. Interpretation of axial studies should begin with the identification of the hepatic vein insertions into the vena cava and the plane of the portal bifurcation. Segments cephalad to the portal vein bifurcation are VII, VIII, IVA, or II. Those caudal to the portal vein bifurcation are VI, V, IVB, and III (Fig. 30-5). Post–liver resection, residual liver volumes can be calculated with CT volumetrics (Fig. 30-6). This information is important in planning extensive liver resections, particularly if preoperative portal vein embolization is considered, or in calculating the graft/recipient weight ratio in living donor or split cadaver donor liver transplantation.

Portal Vein

The portal vein is a valveless structure that is formed by the confluence of the superior mesenteric vein and the splenic vein. The portal vein provides approximately 75% of the total liver blood supply by volume. In the hepatoduodenal ligament, the portal vein is found most commonly posterior to the bile duct and hepatic artery. The normal pressure in the portal vein is between 3 and 5 mm Hg. Since the portal vein and its tributaries are without valves, increases in venous pressure are distributed throughout the splanchnic circulation. In the setting of portal venous hypertension, portosystemic collaterals develop secondary to the increased pressure (see portal hypertension below). The most clinically important portosystemic connections include those fed through the coronary (left gastric) and short gastric veins through the fundus of the stomach and distal esophagus to the azygos vein, resulting in gastroesophageal varices. Recanalization of the round ligament/umbilical vein leads to a caput medusa around the umbilicus. Portal hypertension through the inferior mesenteric veins and hemorrhoidal plexuses can lead to engorged external hemorrhoids.

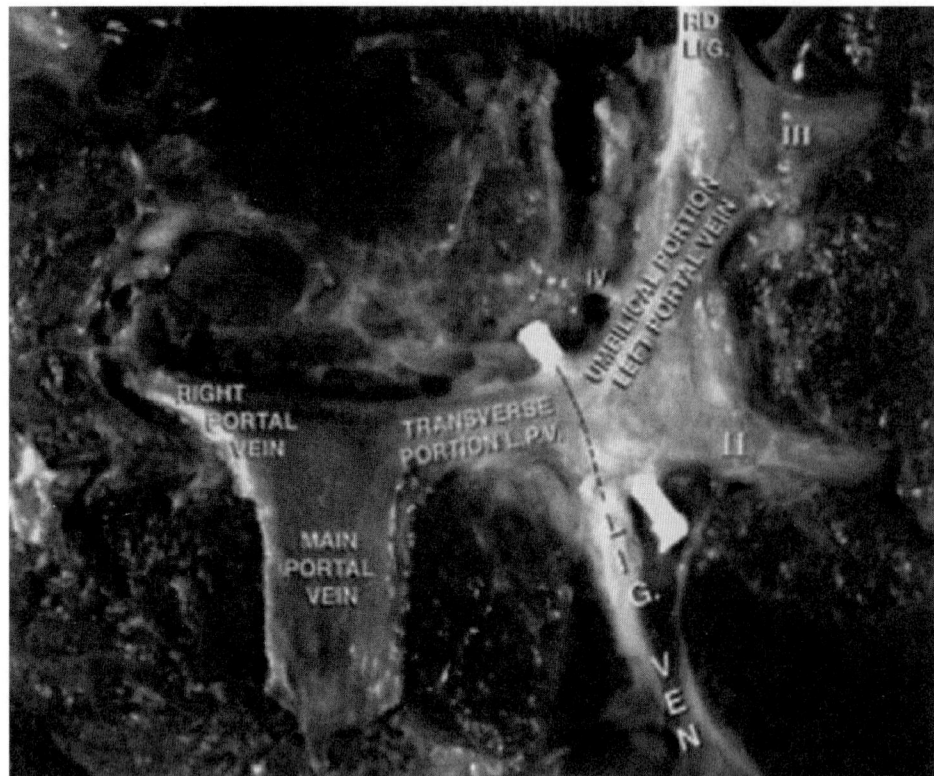

FIG. 30-4. *Branching of the portal structures in the left lobe of the liver. Lig ven = ligamentum venosum; L.P.V. = left portal vein; Rd lig = round ligament. (Reproduced with permission from Jones et al.[5])*

Hepatic Veins

The majority of the venous drainage of the liver occurs through three hepatic veins. The right hepatic vein drains segments V, VI, VII, and VIII, and enters directly into the vena cava. The middle hepatic vein drains segments IVA, IVB, V, and VIII, and enters into a common orifice with the left hepatic vein that drains segments II and III. A scissural branch of the left hepatic vein may run underneath the falciform ligament. A number of small short hepatic veins enter directly into the vena cava from the undersurface of the liver in segment I. Direct venous drainage into the vena cava is through small, short hepatic veins, although large segmental branches may also be present and are usually seen on high-quality preoperative imaging studies (Fig. 30-7). Major middle vein tributaries from segments V and VIII also can be detected by CT scan, and noting the location of such structures with intraoperative ultrasound can help avoid unnecessary blood loss during liver resection.

Hepatic Artery

From the level of the hepatic plate (the interface of the portal bifurcation with the liver capsule), the hepatic arterial anatomy is part of the portal triad and follows the segmental anatomy. The extrahepatic arterial anatomy can be highly variable[4,5] (Fig. 30-8). In roughly half of the population, the common hepatic artery arises from the celiac trunk, giving off the gastroduodenal artery followed by a right gastric artery. The proper hepatic artery gives rise to the right and left hepatic arteries. However, there is great variation in hepatic artery anatomy that is important to understand and detect in performing cholecystectomies, portal dissections, and liver resections. Replaced hepatic arteries are lobar vessels that arise from either the superior mesenteric artery (replaced right hepatic artery) or left gastric artery (replaced left hepatic artery). The replaced right hepatic artery travels posterior to the portal vein in close proximity to the posterior aspect of the pancreas and bile duct. A replaced right hepatic artery is felt behind both the bile duct and the portal vein when palpating the portal triad structures through the foramen of Winslow. The left hepatic artery, regardless of its origin, enters the liver at the base of the round ligament. A replaced or accessory left hepatic artery will run in the lesser omentum anterior to the caudate lobe and is typically very easily identified. In contrast to a replaced hepatic artery, an accessory hepatic artery is one that exists in addition to an anatomically typical originating vessel. Accessory right hepatic arteries often supply the posterior sector of the right lobe (segment VI and VII). An accessory left hepatic artery will typically supply the left lateral segment. The cystic artery most commonly arises from the right hepatic artery, but has a variety of common anomalies as well (see Chap. 31).

Biliary System

The bile duct arises at the cellular level from the hepatocyte membrane which coalesces with adjacent hepatocytes to form canaliculi. The canal of Hering results from the coalescence of canaliculi. Larger collections of canaliculi form small ducts. The bile ducts follow the segmental anatomy of the intrahepatic vasculature as previously described. The confluence of the right and left hepatic ducts may be intrahepatic. The right hepatic duct is found to be largely intrahepatic, while the left hepatic duct is extrahepatic and runs perpendicular to the common hepatic duct to the level of the round ligament, where it is formed by a confluence of ducts from segment IV and segments II/III. The confluence of the left and right hepatic ducts is cephalad and ventral to the portal vein bifurcation. On the right it is common to encounter multiple ducts at the level of the "bifurcation," especially when performing a right lobectomy for living donor liver transplantation.[6,7] In order to circumferentially

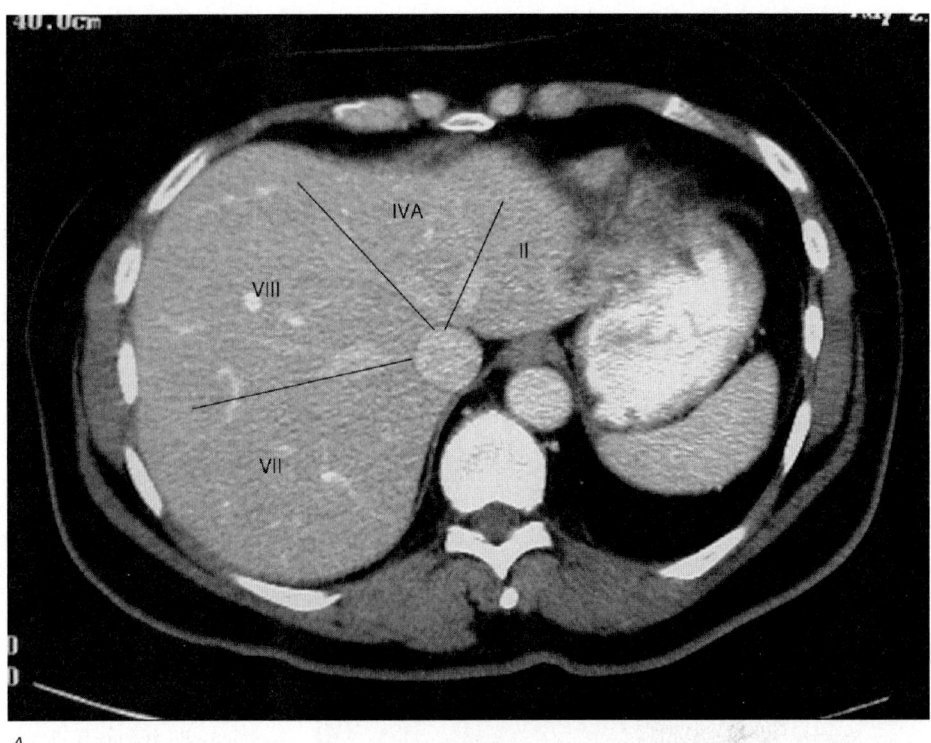

A

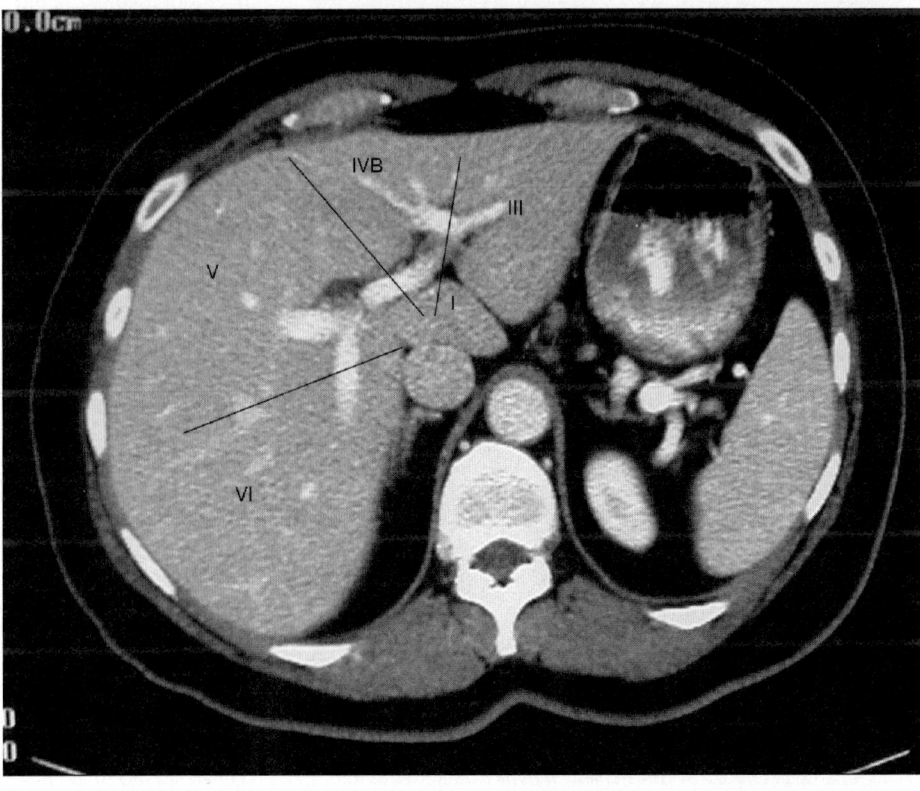

FIG. 30-5. Segmental anatomy of the liver by CT scan. *A.* The planes of the hepatic veins are demonstrated. These liver segments are cephalad to the portal vein bifurcation. *B.* The transverse plane of the portal bifurcation; the noted segments begin here and are caudal to the portal vein bifurcation.

B

isolate the right or left hepatic duct structures, one must fully encircle the Glissonian sheath from the level of the hilar plate posteriorly through the level of the caudate lobe.

The hepatic bile duct confluence gives rise to the common hepatic duct, the duct between the confluence and the cystic duct takeoff.

The common bile duct extends from the cystic duct to the ampulla of Vater. A normal common bile duct is less than 10 mm in diameter in the adult. The blood supply to the bile duct arises from the right hepatic artery superiorly and from the gastroduodenal artery inferiorly. A rich anastomosis between the right and left hepatic arteries

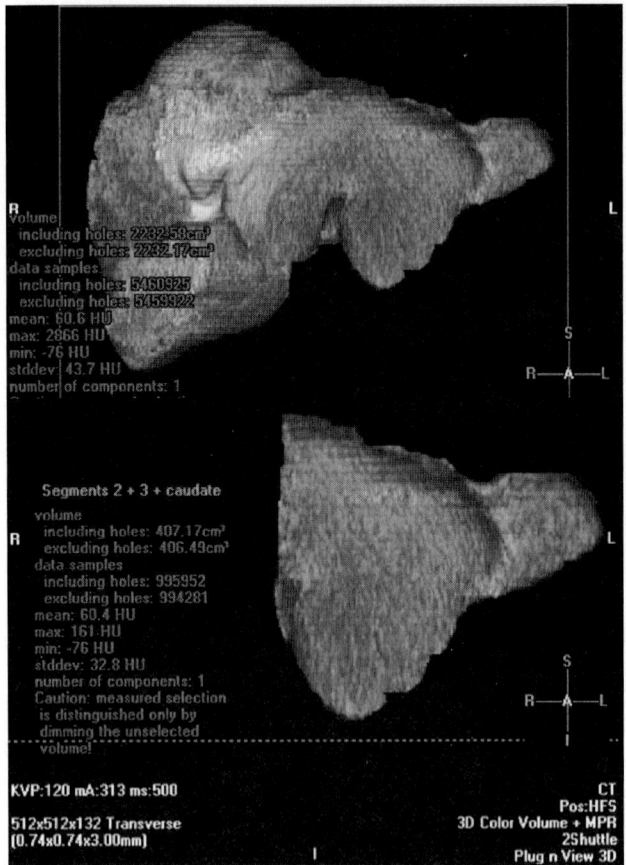

FIG. 30-6. A CT scan with three-dimensional reconstruction to calculate total liver volume and the predicted residual volume after a right trisectorectomy (leaving segments II and III).

has been demonstrated with corrosion cast analyses of the hilum, indicating that preservation of these intrahepatic anastomoses will preserve bile duct blood flow, even with extrahepatic ligation of one or the other arterial structures.

Lymphatics

The spaces of Disse and clefts of Mall produce lymph fluid at the cellular level that is collected through sub-Glissonian and periportal lymphatics that ultimately drain into larger lymphatics emptying through the porta hepatis into the cisterna chyli. The anatomy and physiology of lymphatic drainage is important in the development of ascites and in the process of tumor metastasis. Evaluation of portal lymph nodes must be included during surgical operations for hepatic malignancies to exclude the presence of extrahepatic nodal disease.

Neural Innervation

Parasympathetic fibers from the hepatic branches of the vagus nerve and both parasympathetic and sympathetic fibers derived from the celiac plexus innervate the liver and gallbladder, the latter traveling along the hepatic arteries. The functions of these nerves is not well understood,[8] but liver transplantation shows that the nerves are not essential for normal liver function. Irritation or stretching of the Glisson's capsule or gallbladder cause referred pain to the right shoulder through the third and forth cervical nerves.

Microscopic Liver Anatomy

The microscopic anatomy of the liver is best understood through the description of the acinar unit[9] (Fig. 30-9). This construct involves an afferent portal venule, hepatic arteriole, and a bile ductule flowing antegrade along plates of hepatocytes. Portal venous blood flows along sinusoids and comes in contact with hepatocytes through a perisinusoidal space of Disse. Blood in these sinusoids flows toward a hepatic venule. Concentration gradients of oxygen and solutes occur along the sinusoidal spaces; three zones have been described, with zone one being closest to the portal triad and zone three being closest to the terminal hepatic vein.

While hepatic venules feed the sinusoids most directly, the hepatic arterioles are more closely adherent to biliary ductule structures and may play an important role in bile homeostasis. Hepatic arterioles also ultimately feed into the sinusoids and contribute to the oxygen gradient across zones one, two, and three (Fig. 30-10).

The liver is also the largest repository of the reticuloendothelial system. Kupffer cells, which are tissue-based macrophages, line the sinusoidal spaces and are exposed to portal venous blood as a result.

The Hepatocyte

Hepatocytes are metabolically highly active, polarized cells found in plate-like orientations in the acinus. They are covered with microvilli and are in close approximation with each other, allowing their common membranes to generate vital canaliculi. They also are in close proximity through the perisinusoidal space to sinusoidal endothelial cells and blood. Sinusoidal endothelial cells are highly permeable, and there is generally free flow of both large- and small-molecular-weight substances to the hepatocyte.

SYNTHETIC FUNCTIONS

The liver is crucial to the production and release of a variety of circulating factors critical to the coagulation cascade (see Chap. 3). Indeed, the single most sensitive tests of liver function are measures of coagulation function—International Normalized Ratio (INR) and factor VII and factor V levels (Table 30-1). The liver also synthesizes a wide variety of plasma proteins, the most important of which is albumin, a serum protein that accounts for as much as one seventh of total liver protein synthesis. The liver also makes a variety of acute-phase proteins and cytokines that have important interactions with a variety of inflammatory, infectious, and regulatory processes.

Carbohydrate Metabolism

The liver is a critical storage site of glycogen and is essential to the maintenance of systemic glucose homeostasis through a complex process involving broad interactions with lipid metabolism.[10] The liver also metabolizes lactate, and the Cori cycle is important in maintaining peripheral glucose availability in the setting of anaerobic metabolism.

Lipid Metabolism

The liver is an important modulator of lipid metabolism, performing a critical role in the synthesis of lipoproteins, triglycerides, gluconeogenesis from fatty acids, and cholesterol metabolism. In humans, cholesterol is synthesized in the liver and is used most importantly for bile salt synthesis.

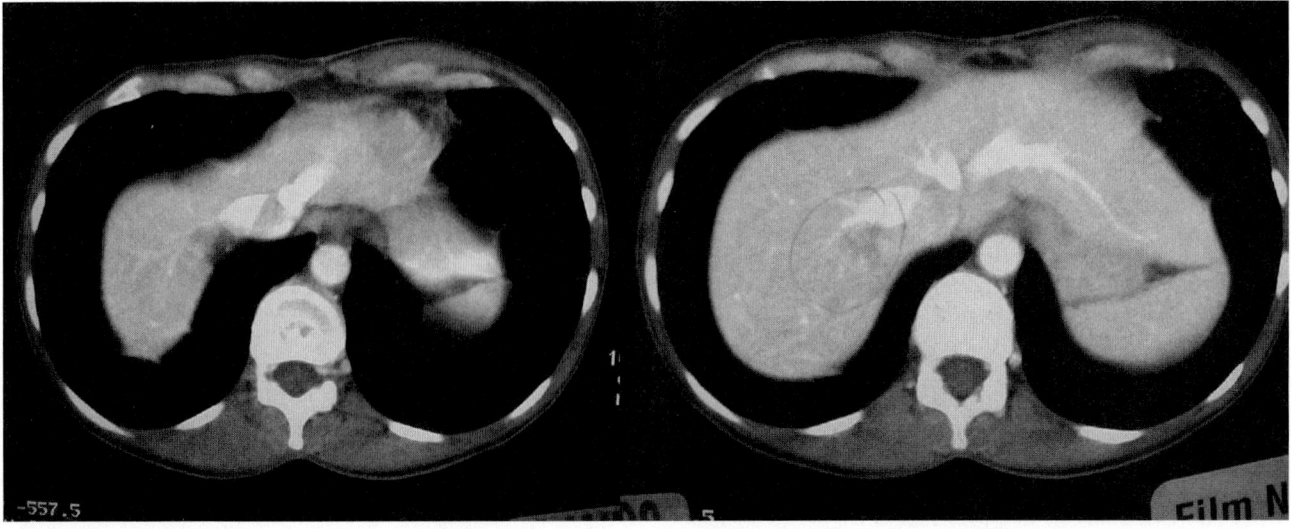

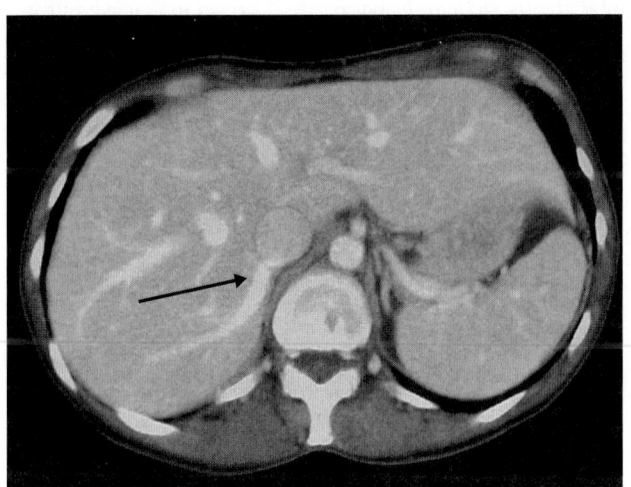

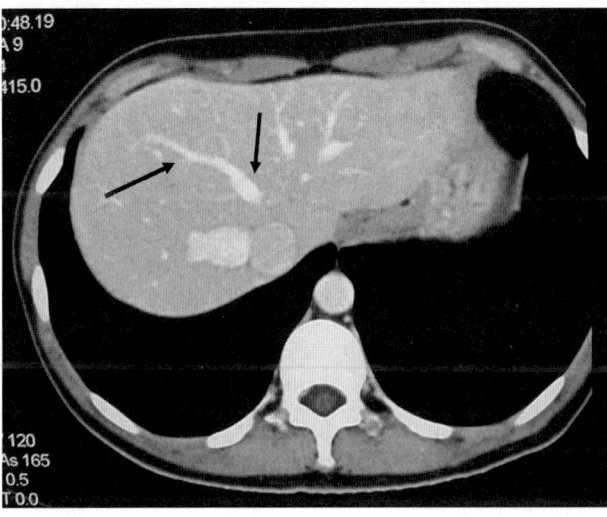

FIG. 30-7. Hepatic venous anatomy. *A.* The right hepatic vein and the middle/left confluence are demonstrated on these CT scans. The right hepatic vein can be isolated at its extrahepatic junction with the vena cava. Isolation of the left hepatic vein requires intrahepatic dissection and runs a risk of injury to the middle hepatic vein. *B.* A segment VI hepatic vein draining directly into the vena cava. *C.* A CT reconstruction demonstrating a large segment VIII vein (*left arrow*) draining into the middle hepatic vein (*right arrow*). Identifying these vessels preoperatively and marking them using intraoperative ultrasonography can help avoid needless blood loss during liver resection.

Bilirubin Metabolism

The excretion of bilirubin, a product of heme metabolism from erythrocytes, occurs in bile.[11] Bilirubin circulates bound to albumin in the blood. It is actively taken up by hepatocytes, where it is glucuronidated and actively secreted into bile. Benign disorders of bilirubin metabolism include Dubin-Johnson and Rotor's syndrome, which produce conjugated (direct) hyperbilirubinemia. Unconjugated hyperbilirubinemia is seen in Crigler-Najjar type II and Gilbert's syndromes.[12] Crigler-Najjar type I causes neonatal kernicterus and invariably is fatal. The liver has an immense capacity to metabolize bilirubin, such that correction of jaundice in hilar biliary obstruction requires drainage of only one liver sector. Even with complete lobar biliary obstruction, the serum bilirubin level may be normal (Fig. 30-11).

Bile and the Enterohepatic Circulation

Bile is a mixed micelle composed of bile acids and pigments, phospholipids and cholesterol, proteins, and electrolytes that is important for small intestinal absorption of fats and vitamins (Fig. 30-12). The production of bile by hepatocytes is an active process that occurs at the level of the canalicular membrane.[13,14] The bile ductules and ducts actively change the water content of bile, and the volume of bile secreted in an adult ranges from 500 to 1000 mL/24 h. An understanding of this volume may be important in understanding

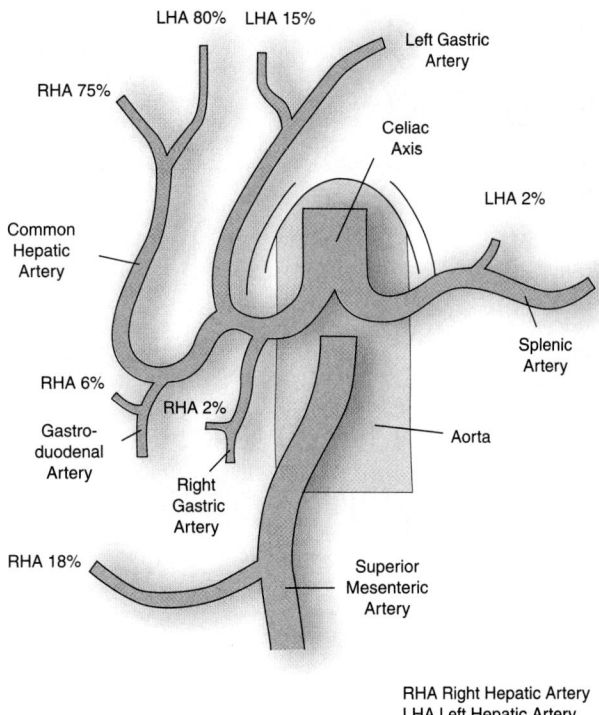

RHA Right Hepatic Artery
LHA Left Hepatic Artery

FIG. 30-8. Hepatic artery anatomy and common variants.

the severity of postoperative biliary fistulas. Since the electrolyte composition of bile is similar to plasma, intravenous volume replacement of a high-volume biliary fistula output can be made milliliter for milliliter with lactated Ringer's solution.

The important role of the distal ileum in the reabsorption of bile salts became clear when patients undergoing resection of the ileum for Crohn's ileitis developed malabsorption and steatorrhea. It was also noted that such patients had lower serum cholesterol levels, ultimately found to be a result of increased hepatic metabolism of cholesterol to bile acids to replace the bile acids not absorbed and recirculated.

Cholic acids and chenodeoxycholic acids are important primary bile acids. Secondary bile acids include deoxycholic and lithocholic acids, which are formed by intestinal bacteria. As a result of enterohepatic circulation, approximately 95% of bile acids are actively transported and returned back to the liver via the portal circulation. Bile acids are critical to the solubilization of intestinal lipids (fatty acids, monoglycerides, and the fat soluble vitamins A, D, E, and K). Bile acids form salt micelles that are critical for the absorption of intestinal lipids; likewise proteins within the intestinal mucosa combine with lipids to form lipoproteins. A complex series of molecular signals and enzymatic reactions occurs to regulate bile acid production. After ingestion of food, bile acid concentration in the portal blood decreases and inhibition of cholesterol 7-hydroxylase decreases, leading to increased bile acid synthesis. During fasting, high portal bile acid concentrations inhibit the activity of this enzyme, thereby downregulating bile acid synthesis.[13]

INTERPRETATION OF LIVER TESTS

Liver tests are broken down into tests of liver function, parenchymal injury, and biliary obstruction (see Table 30-1). The pattern of

FIG. 30-9. The hepatic acinus. BC = bile cannaliculus; BD = bile duct; CV = central vein; E = endothelial cell; HA = hepatic artery; H = hepatocyte; K = Kupffer cell; PV = portal vein.

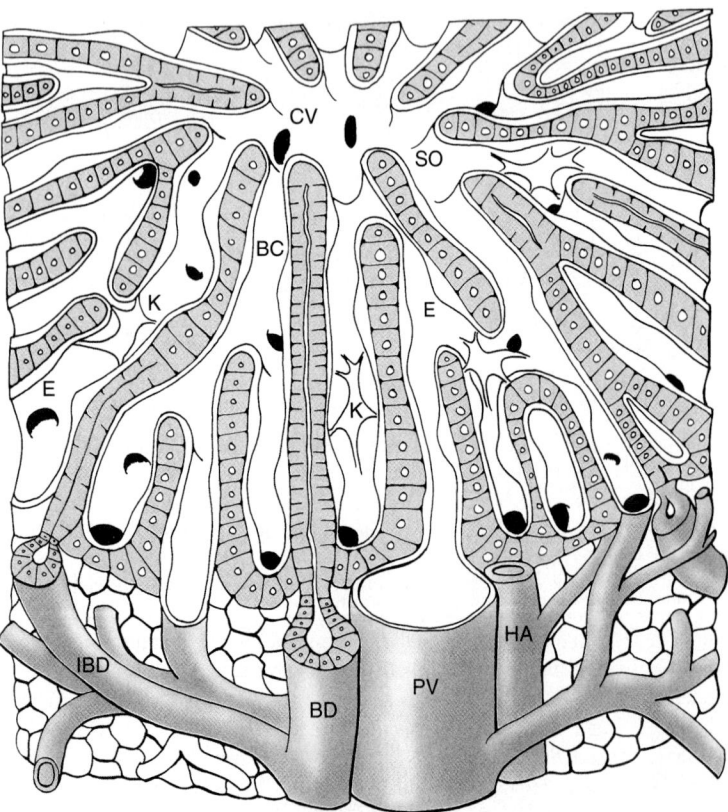

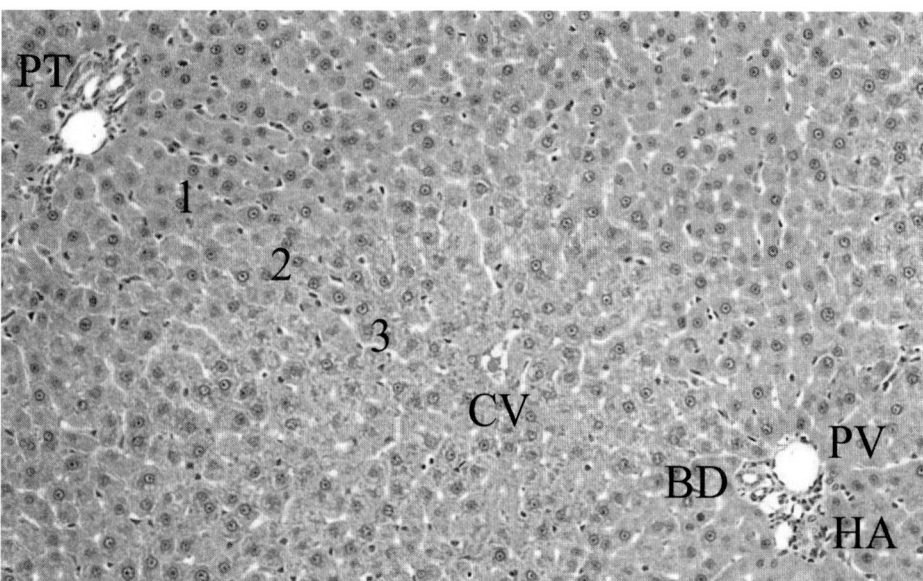

FIG. 30-10. *Light microscopy of the liver. The chords of hepatocytes are seen. The three zones of oxygen and nutrient gradients are noted. The portal triad (PT) is on the left, the central hepatic (CV) venule is on the right. BD = bile duct; PV = portal vein; HA = hepatic artery.*

liver test abnormalities is more important than any individual test result. Figure 30-13 shows the general time course for liver test abnormalities and recovery after a major liver resection. Deviation from this normal time course should prompt specific evaluation for potentially correctable vascular (portal vein thrombosis) or biliary (obstructive) pathology.

Radiologic Evaluation of the Liver

The liver is most commonly evaluated as part of right upper quadrant ultrasound studies for gallbladder disease. However, the indications for directed evaluation of the liver include screening or assessment of malignancy, the study of a newly diagnosed cirrhotic patient, or evaluation for living donor transplantation. A comprehensive understanding of the available tests is critical to patient management.[15]

Ultrasound

Transcutaneous ultrasound is frequently the first radiologic evaluation performed on the liver.[16] Ultrasound is an excellent test for identifying biliary tract stones and intrahepatic biliary ductal dilation. The echo-texture of the liver can suggest cirrhosis or fatty infiltration, and cystic and solid characteristics of tumors can be delineated (Fig. 30-14). Ultrasonography is rarely used as a screening or follow-up evaluation tool in patients with metastatic liver tumors, but because it is a readily available and relatively inexpensive technology, ultrasonography is commonly used in programs that screen high-risk populations for the development of hepatocellular carcinoma (HCC). In studies from the United States and Europe, ultrasonography has been shown to be superior to serum

alpha-fetoprotein (AFP) measurement to detect early HCC in patients who suffer from chronic viral hepatitis.[17,18]

The development of new ultrasound technologies including microbubble contrast agents and multidimensional imaging may increase the utility of ultrasound as a screening test for benign or malignant solid tumors, such as adenomas, focal nodular hyperplasia, metastases, and HCC and may allow differentiation among these entities. Many of these agents are taken up by cells of the reticuloendothelial system in the liver, and the microbubble contrast agents increase the visibility of metastases and HCC. Initial studies of these agents suggest that the sensitivity of ultrasound to detect metastatic disease can be improved as much as 20%, and the mean size of the smallest lesions detected is reduced to less than 1 cm.[19] Doppler ultrasound, even in the absence of contrast agents, is effective in determining the patency and flow direction of all major hepatic blood vessels. Tumor vascularity also can be evaluated.

Table 30-1
Serum Liver Tests

Parenchymal (hepatocytes)	AST, ALT
Canalicular (biliary)	ALP, 5'NT, GGT, bilirubin
Synthetic function and metabolism	INR, factors V and VII, bilirubin, albumin

ALP = alkaline phosphatase; ALT = alanine aminotransferase; AST = aspartate aminotransferase; 5'NT = 5' nucleotidase; GGT = gamma glutamyl transferase; INR = International Normalized Ratio.

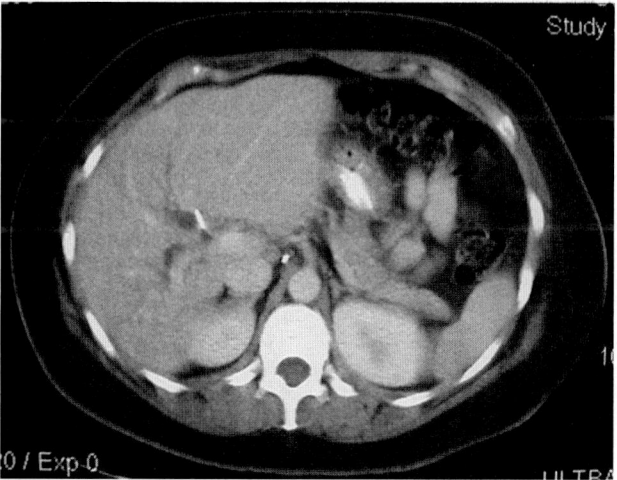

FIG. 30-11. *A CT scan from an asymptomatic patient 3 years after a complete ligation of the right hepatic duct during a laparoscopic cholecystectomy (note clip). The only liver test abnormality was an elevated alkaline phosphatase. There is atrophy of the right liver lobe, a dilated right biliary system, and hypertrophy of the left liver lobe.*

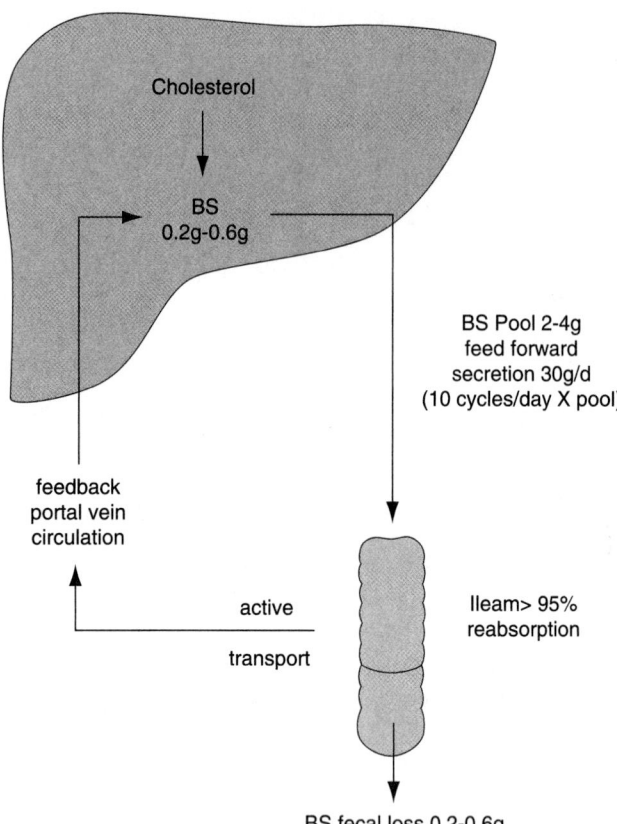

FIG. 30-12. Bile production by the liver and enterohepatic circulation. BS = bile salts.

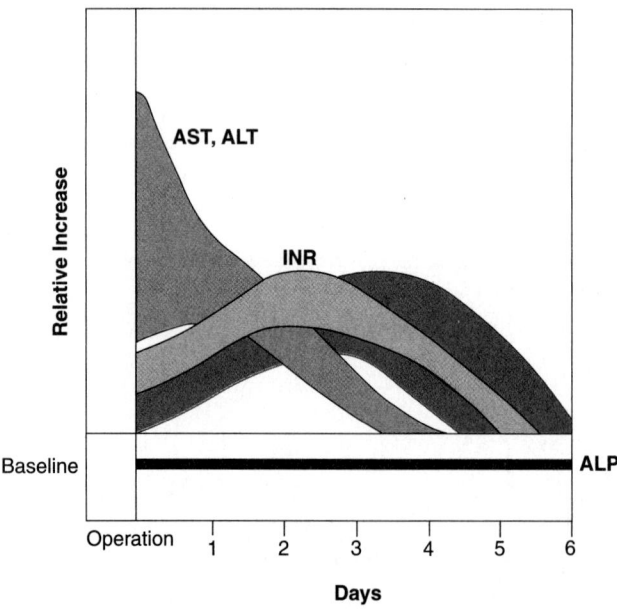

FIG. 30-13. The general time course of liver test changes after lobar liver resection. Progressive increases in serum aspartate aminotransferase/alanine aminotransferase (AST/ALT) and coagulation studies (INR) should prompt an evaluation of the patency of vascular inflow and outflow from the liver with duplex color flow ultrasonography or a contrast-enhanced CT scan. A rising serum alkaline phosphatase may indicate biliary obstruction. A progressive rise in bilirubin levels in the absence of a rising serum alkaline phosphatase level may signify a bile leak.

Intraoperative ultrasonography (IOUS) has become the gold standard against which all other diagnostic imaging modalities are compared to detect the number, extent, and association of tumors with intrahepatic blood vessels in both primary and metastatic liver tumors. IOUS can be performed laparoscopically or during laparotomy.[20] Placement of the probe directly on the surface of the liver enhances discrimination and sensitivity. Laparoscopy provides the additional advantage of a visual inspection to exclude the presence of extrahepatic disease on the peritoneal surfaces in the abdominal cavity. Laparoscopic evaluation and laparoscopic ultrasonography have reduced the rate of unwarranted exploratory laparotomies, and thereby increased the proportion of patients who undergo successful hepatic resection at the time of laparotomy.[21] Like IOUS, laparoscopic ultrasonography detects small metastatic or primary liver tumors not visualized on preoperative CT scans or MRI studies in up to 15% of patients.[21,22] Prior to proceeding with liver resection for malignancy, all patients should undergo IOUS as a way of excluding the presence of smaller lesions not detected by preoperative studies. IOUS also can be used to map the line of resection as it relates to relevant vascular structures, in order to avoid and anticipate possible sources of bleeding (Fig. 30-15). IOUS is necessary for intraoperative image-guided procedures such as biopsy and radiofrequency ablation (RFA).

Computed Tomography Scan

Modern CT scans are helical and are highly sensitive at spatial discrimination and quantitation of lesions in the liver.[23–25] Lesions can be characterized as solid or cystic and the enhancement characteristics can be evaluated during the arterial, portal, and delayed phases. The smallest detectable lesion size is approximately 1 cm. Rapid acquisition and multidetector technologies also allow for three-dimensional reconstructions (Fig. 30-16). These volume-rendered reconstructions are useful in preoperative planning, assessment of hepatic inflow and outflow blood vessels, and measurement of liver volume, which is useful in both resective surgery and living donor transplantation[26] (Fig. 30-17). Dual- and triple-phase bolus intravenous contrast helical CT scan is more accurate than standard CT or portal venous phase CT in detecting colorectal liver metastases. However, the overall detection rate compared to intraoperative and pathologic findings is still ~85% with a false-positive rate of up to 5%.[27,28] For HCC, the helical CT detection rate for small tumors is less than that for detecting hepatic metastases. The detection rate of small HCCs (<2 cm), 40 to 60%, is based on the difficulty of detecting small tumors in cirrhotic livers, particularly in reference to the problem of distinguishing HCC from macroregenerative nodules.[29,30] CT remains the preferred method for evaluating the remainder of the abdomen. Among patients with liver metastases, a CT scan is used to evaluate for the presence of peritoneal disease, portal lymphadenopathy, and other remote lesions.

Magnetic Resonance Imaging

MRI technology also is rapidly advancing.[29–31] MRI is somewhat less sensitive at spatial discrimination of lesions, but provides additional tumor characterization benefits that are not available with CT scanning.[23] MRI scans are slightly less accurate than helical CT in detecting the extent of colorectal liver metastases, but are more sensitive for detecting early HCC and in distinguishing HCC from macroregenerative nodules.[29,30] Contrast enhancement provides an evaluation of vascular enhancement similar to CT, but MRI allows

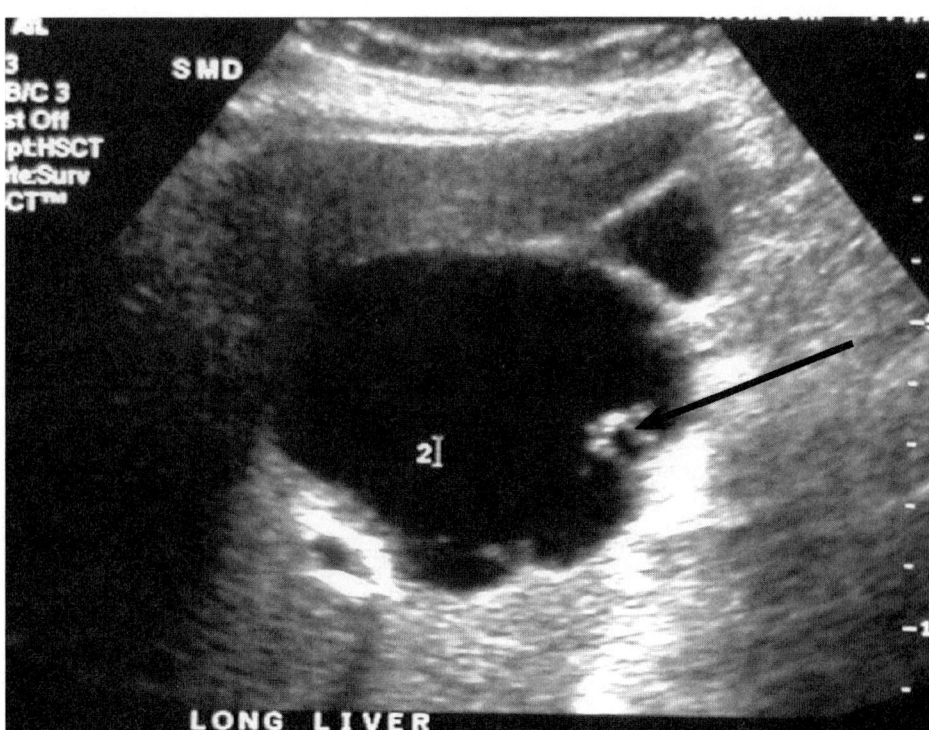

FIG. 30-14. Transcutaneous ultrasonography demonstrating a cystic lesion (arrow) of the right lobe of the liver (upper panel). Further characterization demonstrated papillary projections (arrows) and a septation consistent with a biliary cystadenoma (lower panel).

for better differentiation of cystic lesions and hemangiomas using T2-weighted images (Fig. 30-18). This technique also is useful in magnetic resonance cholangiography (MRC). MRC is an excellent study for the evaluation of the intrahepatic biliary tree, and is critical to the operative planning for hilar bile duct malignancies requiring liver resection. Magnetic resonance venography is a very sensitive technique for the noninvasive study of the extrahepatic portal

system, and is especially useful in confirming extrahepatic portal vein thrombosis.

Nuclear Medicine Studies

Positron Emission Tomography. Positron emission tomography (PET) is a whole-body, multiaxial technology that has

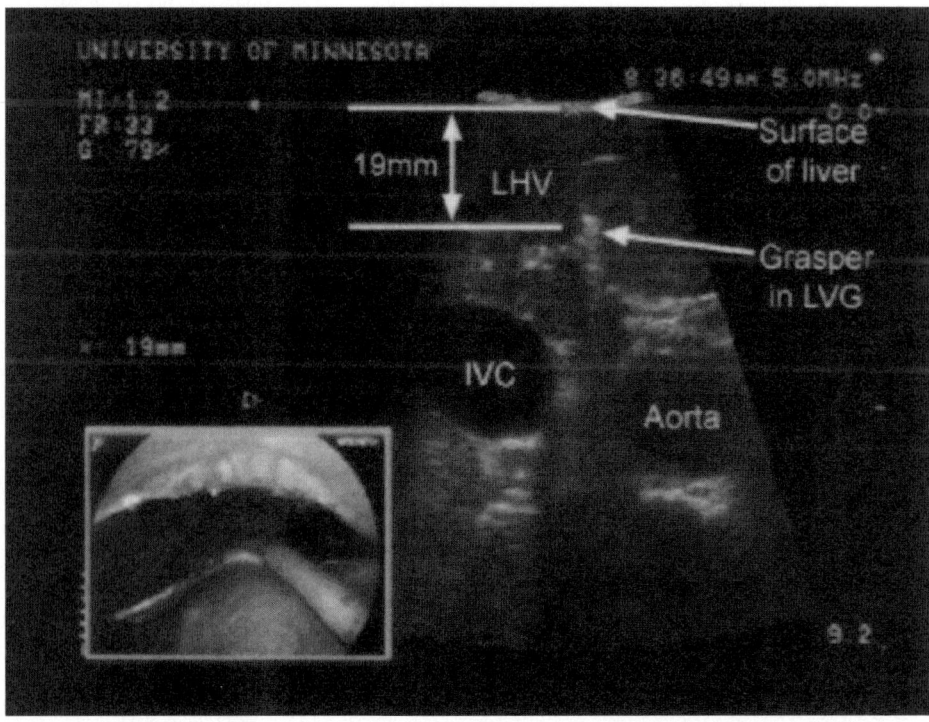

FIG. 30-15. The use of intraoperative ultrasonography in a laparoscopic left lateral sector liver resection. The ultrasound probe (inset photograph) is used to delineate the thickness of the liver and the location of the portal structures and left hepatic vein in the left lateral sector. Asterisk = inferior vena cava; white arrow = thickness of the liver at the ligamentum venosum groove.

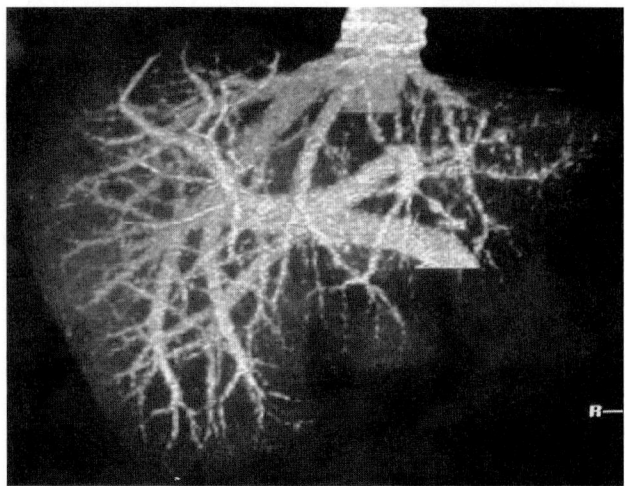

FIG. 30-16. A CT image with three-dimensional reconstruction demonstrating the relationship between the portal and hepatic veins in a liver donor study.

been used to detect a variety of cancers including melanoma, breast cancer, and colorectal cancer. ^{18}F-fluorodeoxyglucose (FDG) is injected systemically through an intravenous catheter, and axial tomography is performed of the entire body.[32] It has been called a metabolic imaging method since FDG is taken up by active tissues (e.g., the brain) and cancer. The FDG PET is especially useful in the evaluation of patients with hepatic metastases of colorectal cancer to rule out the presence of extrahepatic disease. Strasberg and colleagues have demonstrated significantly improved survival in patients undergoing PET scan screening prior to potentially curative liver resection.[33,34] PET may be used to exclude patients from surgical consideration because of the presence of extrahepatic disease that is imaged in up to 11% of patients who are considered for liver resection.[35,36] Similarly to other diagnostic studies, PET does have a false-negative rate of 7 to 10%, but the false-positive rate appears to be significantly lower than this value. In patients with a history of colorectal cancer, a rising serum carcinoembryonic antigen (CEA) level, and no recurrent or metastatic disease evident on CT or MRI images of the chest, abdomen, and pelvis, PET images demonstrating hypermetabolic areas may provide a clue as to the

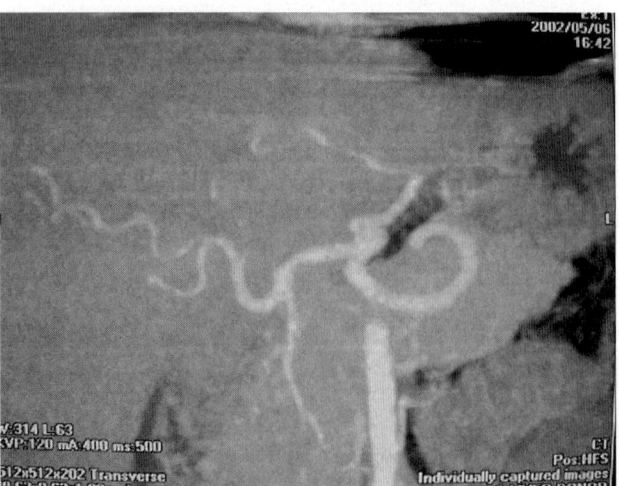

FIG. 30-17. The hepatic artery study in the same patient shown in Fig. 30-16 demonstrates a replaced left hepatic artery.

site of recurrent disease. PET has been less useful in the evaluation of patients with HCC, as many of these tumors do not have a significantly higher uptake of the radioisotope compared to the surrounding hepatic parenchyma.[37] Until further studies are undertaken, the use of PET scanning should be tied very closely to other forms of axial imaging studies. One method is fusion of PET scans with CT scanning (Fig. 30-19). If there is a failure to correlate a hypermetabolic focus on PET scan with a tumor mass on CT scan, then directed evaluation, including biopsy of the hypermetabolic focus, should be performed prior to proceeding with liver resection.

Other Nuclear Medicine Studies. Scans using radioactive octreotide, a somatostatin analogue, can be used in the evaluation and treatment of patients with neuroendocrine tumors.[38] These cells possess receptors to somatostatin, and the study can be used to document the extent of tumor burden. In the setting of carcinoid syndrome, liver-directed therapy, including resection or tumor ablation, is appropriate even in the presence of extrahepatic disease. However, an octreotide scan may document the bulk of systemic disease as a way of predicting the response to liver treatment. A radioactive technetium (^{99}Tc)-labeled albumin scan is occasionally useful in distinguishing complex focal nodular hyperplasia from an adenoma. This agent is taken up by Kupffer cells in focal nodular hyperplasia, while most adenomas are "cold" because they lack Kupffer cells. ^{99}Tc-labeled red blood cell scans are useful in identifying atypical hemangiomas; this study relies on the pooling of radiolabeled red blood cells within the vascular hemangioma.

Angiography

Angiography is becoming less important in the evaluation of liver tumors, as CT and MRI technology allows for the definition of vascular anatomy and characterization of tumors in the majority of circumstances. Rarely, angiography is diagnostic for confirming the presence of an atypical hemangioma, the presence of which cannot be established using other modalities. Angiography for hepatic arterial chemoembolization is a potential therapy for unresectable malignant tumors, including HCC and neuroendocrine liver metastases.

Percutaneous Biopsy

The role of image-guided percutaneous biopsy has become less important as the sensitivity and specificity of radiologic imaging studies had improved. In patients with a clinical picture and radiologic findings that point to a specific type of lesion, percutaneous biopsy is rarely indicated to initiate liver-directed therapy. In patients in whom the diagnosis is not evident based on clinical and radiographic grounds, a percutaneous biopsy can be done safely using either ultrasound or CT guidance. The target lesion should be accessed through a quantity of normal liver tissue sufficient to avoid free rupture of tumor into the peritoneum (Fig. 30-20). This is especially important with HCCs, which are friable and vascular lesions.

Diagnostic Laparoscopy

The last step in liver imaging to be considered is diagnostic laparoscopy.[39] The goal of the preoperative evaluation in hepatic neoplasms is to detect surgically treatable disease. In most malignancies, this includes identifying contraindications to resection or ablation such as extrahepatic disease, extensive intrahepatic disease, and portal hypertension. Although some controversy exists as to the utility of diagnostic laparoscopy, the ability to evaluate the entire abdomen, including the parietal and visceral peritoneal surfaces,

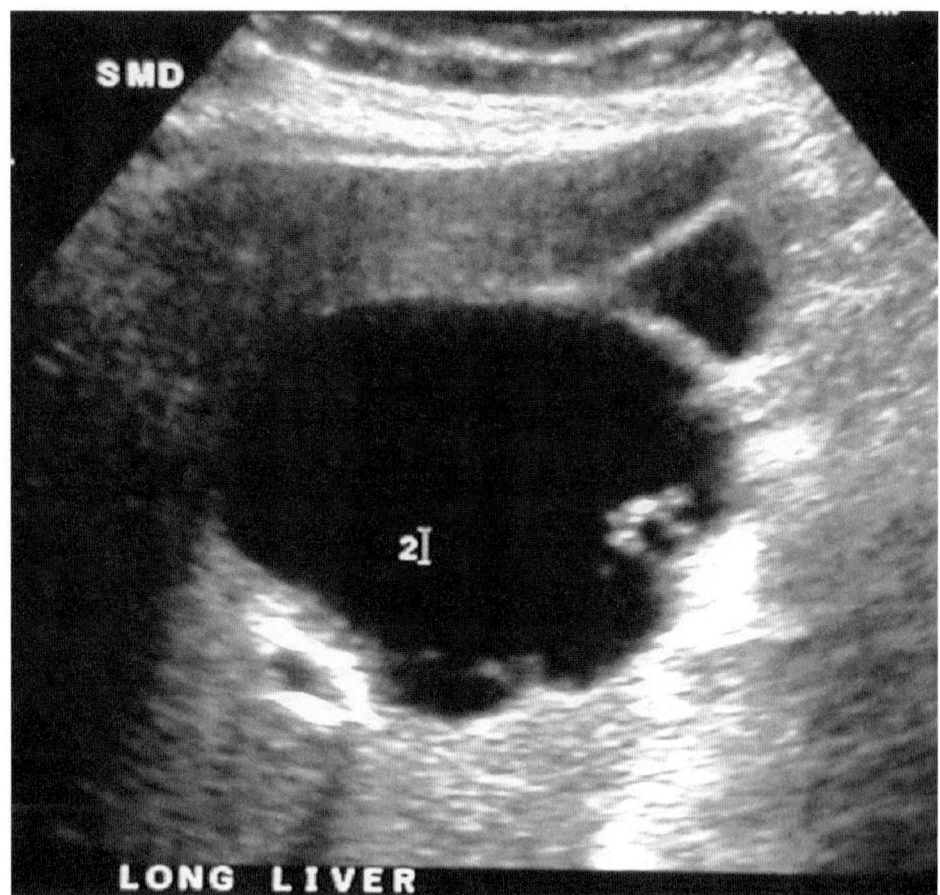

FIG. 30-18. A cavernous hemangioma of segment V on T2-weighted magnetic resonance imaging. Note that the cerebrospinal fluid in the spinal canal is bright as well.

FIG. 30-19. Fusion of positron emission tomography and computed tomography to demonstrate a large malignant tumor involving the right liver lobe.

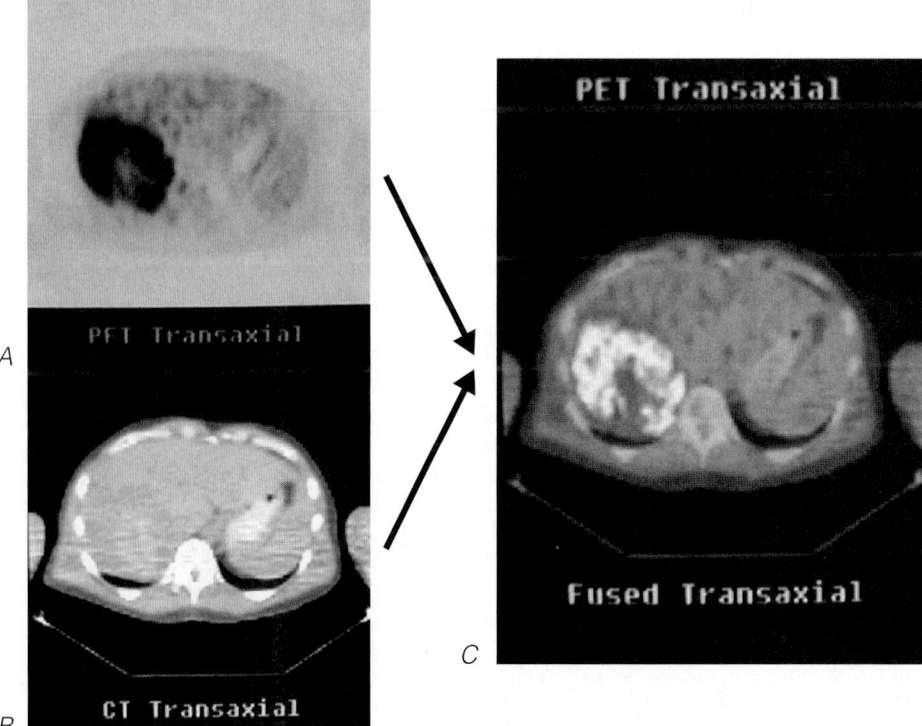

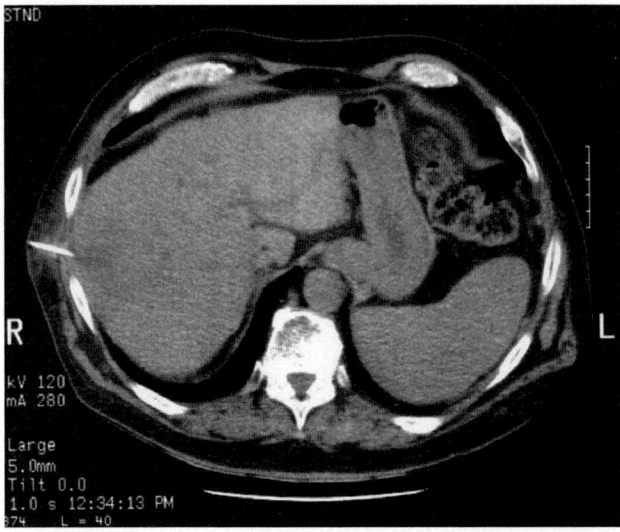

FIG. 30-20. Computed tomography (CT)-guided biopsy of a resectable hepatocellular cancer. The biopsy needle is directly in the tumor and resulted in intraperitoneal tumor cell spillage and eventual carcinomatosis.

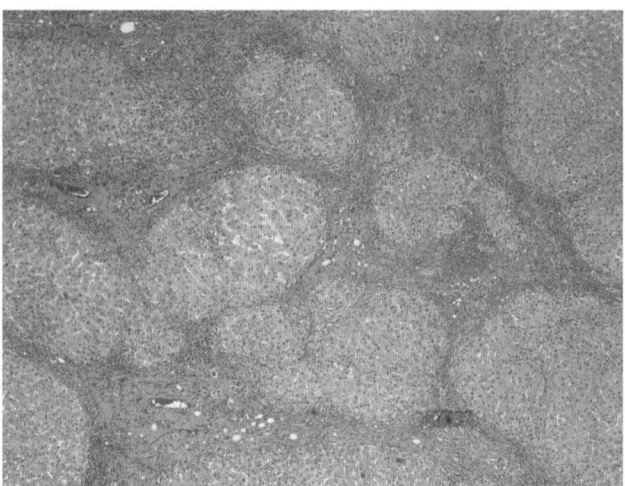

FIG. 30-21. Regenerative nodules and bridging fibrosis representative of cirrhosis seen on standard light microscopy. Hematoxylin and eosin stain, magnification x75.

perform intraoperative laparoscopic ultrasound, and evaluate the porta hepatis in a minimally invasive manner is compelling. A number of centers have published results indicating that up to 20% of patients undergoing exploration for liver malignancy will have evidence of unresectability.[40] Patients with metastatic colorectal cancer presenting with more than three lesions are at higher risk of having occult metastases identified compared with patients with solitary lesions. A complete diagnostic laparoscopy including laparoscopic ultrasound can be performed in less than 20 minutes. Strong consideration should be given for the use of diagnostic laparoscopy as the final step in patient staging for hepatic malignant disease. Avoiding morbidity and longer hospitalization in patients who are not candidates for a potentially curative resection is meritorious.

LIVER FAILURE

Liver failure can be divided into two general categories: *acute* and *chronic.* Acute liver failure is relatively uncommon, with approximately 5000 new cases reported annually in the United States. The pathophysiology is related to an acute, massive loss of hepatocyte functional mass. However, there are usually no long-term sequelae in survivors. In chronic liver failure (long-term liver injury)—whether derived from viral hepatitis, metabolic diseases, ethanol abuse, or toxins—ongoing and progressive hepatocyte necrosis produces a fibrotic response and liver cell regeneration that leads to cirrhosis. Twenty-five thousand people die each year from cirrhosis, making it the eighth leading cause of death from disease in the United States.

Cirrhosis is a histologic term that describes generalized hepatic fibrosis and nodular regeneration of the liver (Fig. 30-21). Despite the wide variety of etiologies of cirrhosis, the histologic end results are often indistinguishable. As described earlier, one of the unique physiologic capabilities of the liver is regeneration. The response of the liver to hepatocyte necrosis is collapse of portal tracks with fibrous replacement and nodular regeneration. Liver stellate cells (Ito cells) are the principal mediators of fibrosis in the liver,[41] and are stimulated by hepatocyte necrosis and cytokines (tumor necrosis factor-α, interleukin-1, interleukin-6), growth factors (epidermal growth factor, platelet-derived growth factor, transforming growth factor β_1) released by platelets, and Kupffer and endothelial

cells.[42,43] Type IV collagen, fibronectin, laminin, and heparin sulfate proteoglycans make up the principal connective tissue components of the normal liver. Hepatocyte inflammation and injury leads to a rapid proliferation of stellate cells and a marked increase in their production rates. In contrast, it decreases the degradation rate of these extracellular matrix components.[44,45] As stellate cells are activated they demonstrate characteristics of myofibroblasts, that additionally play a role in altering local blood flow and may exacerbate the formation of fibrous bands.[46] Sinusoidal blood also is shunted to the periphery of these nodules where sinusoids persist, thereby preventing this blood from being exposed to functional hepatocytes.

Grossly, cirrhosis can be described as micronodular, macronodular (Fig. 30-22), or mixed. The CT findings of cirrhosis can be subtle, but include right lobe atrophy, ascites, caudate lobe hypertrophy, recanalization of the umbilical vein, enlargement of the portal vein caliber and splenomegaly (Fig. 30-23). The physical examination findings of cirrhosis are shown in Table 30-2. Laboratory findings in the unsuspected and compensated cirrhotic patient may be absent or include mild elevations in serum transaminases, borderline thrombocytopenia, or elevations in INR. These findings should prompt consideration for further investigation, since cirrhosis and

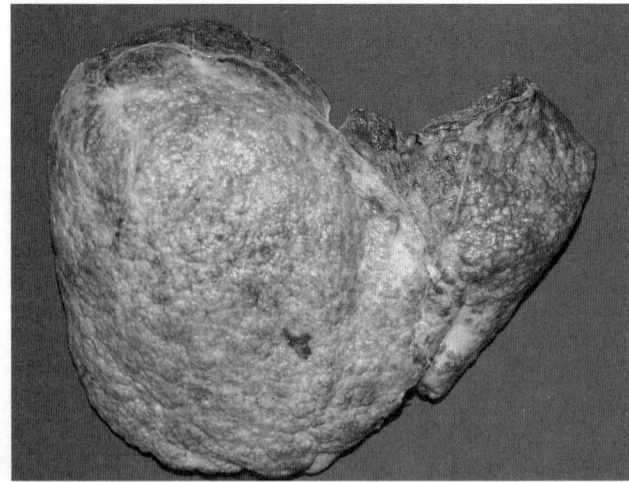

FIG. 30-22. A gross specimen photograph showing the appearance of macronodular cirrhosis.

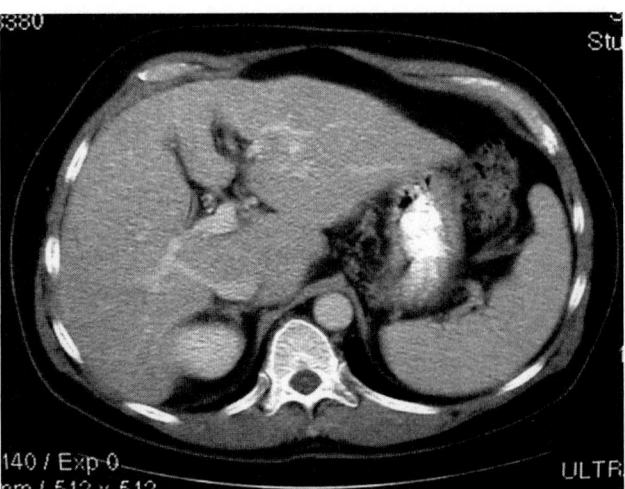

FIG. 30-23. A CT scan with subtle abnormalities of cirrhosis and portal hypertension. Caudate lobe hypertrophy, recanalization of the umbilical vein, left lobe hypertrophy, and mild splenomegaly are all evident. Note that the liver is not grossly nodular in this patient with micronodular cirrhosis.

portal hypertension will have a negative impact on the outcomes of nontransplant surgical procedures.

Risks of General Surgical Procedures in Portal Hypertension

The Child classification was originally developed to evaluate the risk of portocaval venous shunt surgery for portal hypertension, but it has also been shown to be useful in predicting the risks of other abdominal operations in cirrhotic patients and was subsequently modified by others (Table 30-3). General anesthesia and surgical stress lead to hepatic ischemia due to reduced hepatic and splanchnic blood flow, coupled with an increased hepatic catabolic response. Laparoscopic operations may be associated with a reduced rate of complications because of reduced catabolic stress on the liver.

A dysregulation of the compensatory blood flow response (e.g., increased hepatic arterial flow in response to decreased portal vein flow) is seen in cirrhosis. A variety of studies have shown that American Society of Anesthesiologists (ASA) score, renal insufficiency, and higher Child scores are adverse prognostic factors that predict an increased probability of complications and mortality after an operation. Laparoscopic cholecystectomy is safe in Child class A and B patients.[47] In elective procedures, attention to preoperative control of ascites, electrolyte abnormalities, and coagulopathy are critical to the success of elective surgery. Prevention of postoperative

Table 30-2
Physical Findings in Chronic Liver Disease

Jaundice
Caput medusa
Spider angiomata
Fetor hepaticus
Asterixis
Ascites
Hemorrhoids
Palmar erythema
Temporal wasting
Dupuytren's contracture
Gynecomastia
Testicular atrophy
Splenomegaly

ascites begins with restriction of sodium-containing intravenous fluids in the operating room. As ascites accumulates, continued fluid restriction, diuretic therapy, bedrest, and intermittent paracentesis may be needed. Chronic peritoneal catheter drainage should be avoided due to the risk of retrograde contamination of the peritoneal cavity. Ascites in this setting is highly morbid, especially if complicated by bacterial infection. Encephalopathy should also be anticipated. Administration of narcotic pain medicines and sedatives should be limited when possible, as the hepatic metabolism of most drugs is compromised.

Portal Hypertension

Portal hypertension may be classified as presinusoidal, sinusoidal, or postsinusoidal (Table 30-4).[48] Sinusoidal causes are the most common in the Western Hemisphere due to alcoholic cirrhosis that results from fibrous replacement in the space of Disse. Chronic liver insufficiency is common. Postsinusoidal portal hypertension often has a vascular etiology and also is associated with some degree of liver dysfunction. In contrast, patients with presinusoidal portal hypertension may have well-preserved hepatic function. Etiologies include schistosomiasis, extrahepatic portal vein thrombosis (Fig. 30-24), and congenital hepatic fibrosis (most commonly seen in children). The sequelae of portal hypertension are varied, and the long-term outcomes are related most strongly to the underlying degree of hepatic dysfunction. Upregulation of nitric oxide synthase has been shown to play an important role in augmented blood flow in portal hypertension.[48] Although excessive splanchnic blood flow is rarely a sole cause of portal hypertension, many cirrhotic patients have some increased splanchnic flow that may be attributed to nitric oxide.

The physical findings of portal hypertension should be sought in all patients with a presentation or history suggestive of liver disease. Figure 30-25 lists the variety of pathophysiologic portosystemic shunts that are both clinically evident and major causes of morbidity and mortality. When evaluating a patient with new-onset portal hypertension, the history and physical findings will be of great assistance in formulating a differential diagnosis. A variety of screening tests are also appropriate in the evaluation of patients (Table 30-5). The first imaging test should be a transcutaneous liver ultrasound with Doppler blood flow assessment. This study will provide information on the character of the liver parenchyma and the presence of altered blood flow, and is a useful screening test for the presence of hepatic tumors. If extrahepatic portal vein thrombosis is suspected, then a MRI venogram or contrast-enhanced helical CT scan can document the extent of the thrombus.

Budd-Chiari Syndrome

Budd-Chiari syndrome, which is a rare cause of postsinusoidal liver failure and cirrhosis, can occur as a spectrum of presentations that range from asymptomatic disease to fulminant liver failure. The pathophysiology is related to thrombosis of the three major hepatic veins at the level of the inferior vena cava. In patients from Asia, there may also be an associated web in the vena cava, but this is not commonly seen in patients from Western countries. The disease is more common in women and is associated with a variety of hypercoagulable states: protein C, S, or antithrombin III deficiency; polycythemia vera; lupus anticoagulant; estrogen exposure; myeloproliferative disorders; and Behçet's disease. Patients will often present with jaundice, ascites, and hepatomegaly. Transcutaneous Doppler-flow ultrasound will show thrombosed hepatic veins and may demonstrate large collaterals into the retrohepatic inferior vena cava. CT findings include striking caudate lobe hypertrophy

Table 30-3
Revised Child Classification of Clinical Severity of Cirrhosis

	Class		
	A	*B*	*C*
Nutritional status	Excellent	Good	Poor
Ascites	None	Minimal, controlled	Moderate to severe
Encephalopathy	None	Minimal, controlled	Moderate to severe
Serum bilirubin (mg/dL)	<2	2–3	>3
Serum albumin (g/dL)	>3.5	2.8–3.5	<2.8
Prothrombin time (% of control)	>70	40–70	<40

and inhomogeneous contrast enhancement (Fig. 30-26). Anticoagulation is the standard immediate therapy. Treatment of acute decompensated Budd-Chiari includes placement of a transjugular intrahepatic portosystemic shunt (TIPS) or a nonselective shunt.[49,50] The surgical shunt options include a side-to-side portocaval shunt or interposition mesocaval shunt. The latter procedure may be technically easier, as the side-to-side shunt may require resection of a portion of the hypertrophied caudate lobe. Liver transplantation is appropriate for patients with advanced liver disease, but is plagued by potential failure resulting from the underlying disorder.[51]

Acute Bleeding

Patients with portal hypertension may require surgical intervention after an episode of acute upper gastrointestinal (GI) bleeding. After intravenous fluid resuscitation and correction of coagulation abnormalities, the single most important diagnostic and potentially therapeutic procedure to be performed in the cirrhotic patient with an upper GI bleed is endoscopy. The differential diagnosis must include sources other than bleeding from esophageal varices, since as many as 20% of patients will have bleeding from gastritis or

Table 30-4
Classification of Site and Etiologies of Portal Hypertension

Presinusoidal
Sinistral/extrahepatic
  Splenic vein thrombosis
  Splenomegaly
  Splenic arteriovenous fistula
Intrahepatic
  Schistosomiasis
  Nodular regenerative hyperplasia
  Congenital hepatic fibrosis
  Idiopathic portal fibrosis
  Chronic active hepatitis
  Myeloproliferative disorders
  Sarcoid
  Graft-versus-host disease
Sinusoidal
Intrahepatic
  Cirrhosis
  Alcoholic hepatitis
Postsinusoidal
Intrahepatic
  Alcoholic terminal hyaline sclerosis
  Vascular occlusive disease
Posthepatic
  Budd-Chiari Syndrome
  Inferior vena caval web
  Chronic passive venous congestion

duodenal ulcer disease. However, these are usually associated with less severe bleeding.

Esophageal varices are the most common cause of massive bleeding in patients with cirrhosis, and result from shunting of blood through the coronary (left gastric) vein into the submucosal plexus of the esophagus.[52] When the pressure in these veins rises above 12 mm Hg, spontaneous rupture will occur in up to 30% of patients. In addition to increased pressure in the varix, mucosal ulceration can precipitate bleeding. Prevention of the first bleeding event with prophylactic beta-adrenergic blockade is more effective than placebo, and the addition of a systemic vasodilator agent is slightly more efficacious, but at the expense of increased peripheral edema.[53,54] Sclerotherapy, TIPS, or surgical shunts have not been associated with a reduction in first bleeding risk in Western, alcoholic-cirrhotic patients. Prophylaxis is important since variceal bleeding in cirrhotic patients is a grave prognostic event with 70% of patients dying within 1 year. Indeed, patients with Child class C cirrhosis and variceal bleeding have a 70% mortality rate at 6 weeks (most in the hospital setting).

Correction of circulating intravascular volume with packed red blood cells is necessary and replacement of clotting factors (with fresh frozen plasma, vitamin K, and platelets) must be employed aggressively. The most critical treatment for acute hemorrhage in cirrhotic patients is prompt endoscopic intervention and therapy. Acute esophageal variceal bleeding can be managed with endoscopic variceal banding in 85% of patients.[55] Sclerotherapy is being performed much less frequently. Administration of intravenous vasopressin or octreotide can decrease splanchnic blood flow, and are useful in reducing bleeding from esophageal varices in the acute phase of management. The systemic effects of vasopressin make it a less favorable drug in patients with concomitant cardiac problems. Paracentesis will reduce portal venous pressures in patients with tense ascites. Minnesota or Sengstaken-Blakemore tubes have inflatable reservoirs that serve to compress the lower esophagus, stomach, and gastroesophageal junction, and are reserved for control of rebleeding from documented esophageal varices. These tubes have a limited duration of safety and effectiveness, and should be considered as temporary methods to use while planning more definitive therapy. Patients should be endotracheally intubated when these tubes are used.

Hepatic encephalopathy from absorption of the intestinal blood load, as well as azotemia from large-volume blood replacement, should be anticipated. It may be necessary to use oral or nasogastric lactulose elixir to promote catharsis. Emergency TIPS is successful in treating acute bleeding and in preventing rebleeding in approximately 80% of patients. The procedure has supplanted the surgical shunt at most institutions for the treatment of refractory bleeding. It

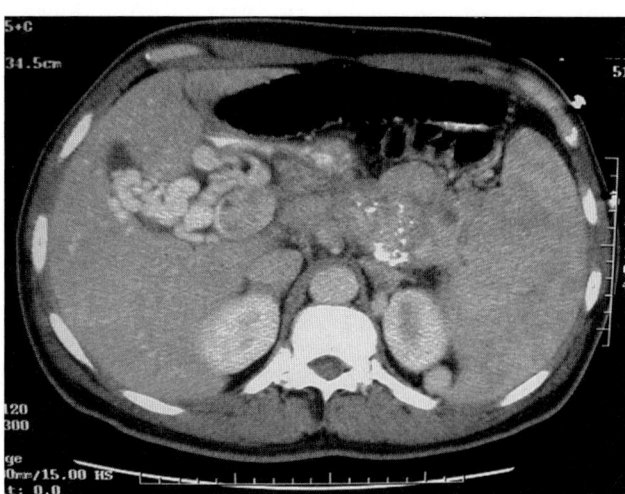

FIG. 30-24. Extrahepatic portal vein thrombosis with dilated periportal collaterals.

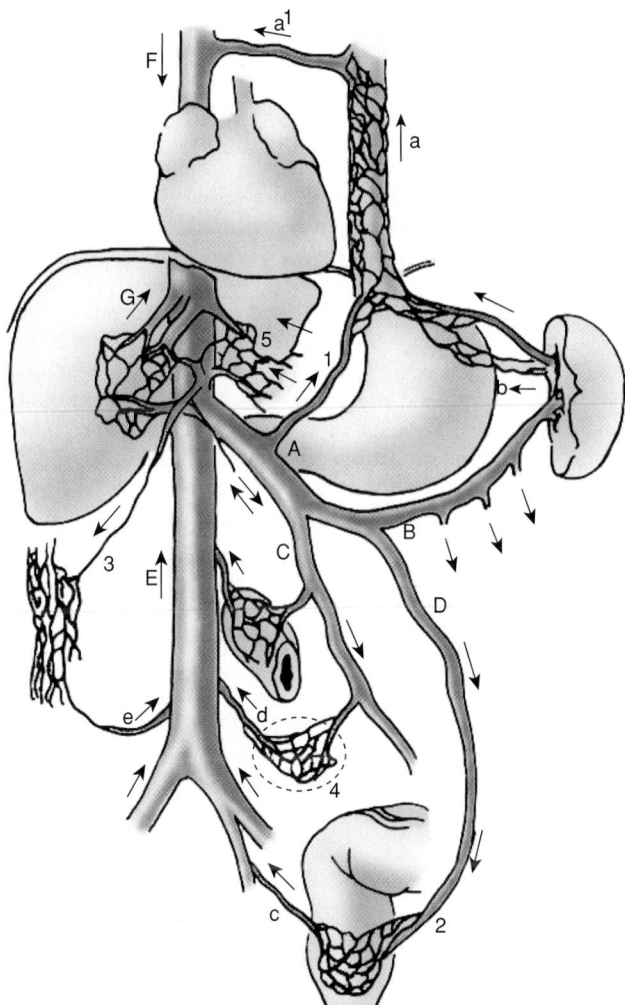

FIG. 30-25. Intra-abdominal venous flow pathways leading to engorged veins (varices) from portal hypertension. 1, coronary vein; 2, superior hemorrhoidal veins; 3, paraumbilical veins; 4, veins of Retzius; 5, veins of Sappey; A, portal vein; B, splenic vein; C, superior mesenteric vein; D, inferior mesenteric vein; E, inferior vena cava; F, superior vena cava; G, hepatic veins; a, esophageal veins; a¹, azygos system; b, vasa brevia; c, middle and inferior hemorrhoidal veins; d, intestinal; e, epigastric veins.

Table 30-5
Screening Tests for Portal Hypertension

Liver tests, albumin, platelet count
International Normalized Ratio
Serologies for viral hepatitis
Iron indices
Antinuclear antibody, antimitochondrial antibody, anti–smooth
 muscle antibody
Alpha$_1$-antitrypsin deficiency
Ceruloplasmin

should be noted, however, that surgical shunts are very effective at preventing rebleeding.

The selection of a surgical shunt in the emergency setting requires consideration of the surgeon's experience and the patient's future candidacy for liver transplantation. Surgical shunts are associated with long-term survival rates of more than 70% in Child class A and B patients. However, the number of surgeons experienced with these procedures is dwindling. A nonselective portocaval shunt will have the most immediate and durable effect in the acute setting. In patients who are potential liver transplant candidates, an interposition mesocaval shunt or central splenorenal shunt will avoid portal dissection and not complicate a subsequent liver transplant operation. If the patient has complete portal vein thrombosis, an end-to-side portocaval shunt will be effective and is technically straightforward.

Prevention of Rebleeding

After acute control of bleeding is achieved, a plan for the long-term prevention of rebleeding must be made. Repeated endoscopic therapy employing sclerotherapy or banding can eradicate varices and prevent rebleeding in up to 80% of patients in the first year.[55] Use of beta-adrenergic blockade or octreotide has been demonstrated to significantly reduce rebleeding rates in combination with endoscopic therapy.[56] In the cirrhotic patient with significant hepatic dysfunction, liver transplantation must be considered. The long-term outlook in patients with preserved hepatic function may be

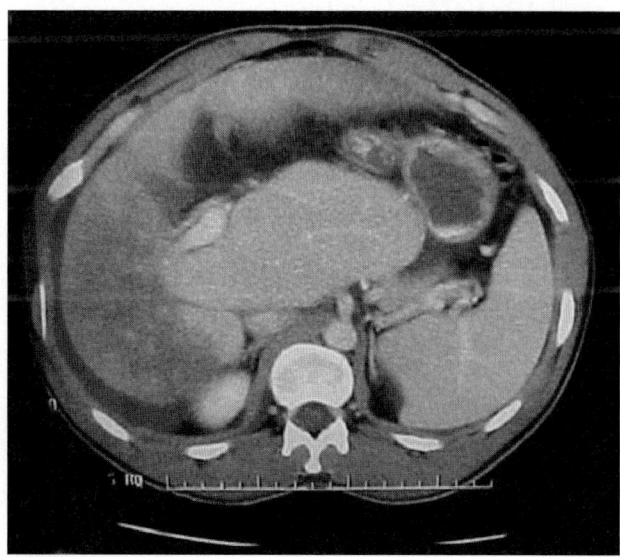

FIG. 30-26. Budd-Chiari syndrome. Note the ascites and caudate lobe hypertrophy. The contrast enhancement is primarily in the caudate lobe (segment I) with inhomogeneous contrast enhancement of the remaining liver.

significantly different, and these patients are candidates for surgical shunts.

Portosystemic Shunts

Transjugular Intrahepatic Portosystemic Shunt. The TIPS has revolutionized the management of the complications of portal hypertension. The procedure is minimally invasive and creates the equivalent of a nonselective surgical shunt. The indications for TIPS include bleeding refractory to endoscopic and medical management, refractory ascites, Budd-Chiari syndrome, and hepatopulmonary syndromes.[57,58] The procedure involves the placement of an expandable wire mesh stent between the middle hepatic vein and region of the portal bifurcation using ultrasound and radiographic direction. The stent is expanded to a diameter that reduces the portosystemic gradient to less then 12 mm Hg[58] (Fig. 30-27). TIPS is associated with postprocedure encephalopathy rates of approximately 25%, and patients with renal insufficiency are at risk for worsened renal function. The long-term problem with TIPS is stenosis of the shunt, which occurs in as many as two thirds of patients. Most centers advocate an aggressive Doppler ultrasound monitoring program with prompt balloon dilation for identified stenosis of the stent. The advent of new covered stents may improve the primary patency rates of this procedure.

Surgical Shunts. The advent of liver transplantation and TIPS has markedly reduced the need for surgical shunts in the management of portal hypertension and its complications of bleeding and ascites. Indeed, patients who are being considered for a surgical shunt should also be evaluated as potential liver transplant candidates. Surgical shunts are best used in patients with relatively well-preserved liver function (Child class A and B) who are not candidates for liver transplantation or who have limited access to the medical surveillance necessary for TIPS monitoring. Patients who

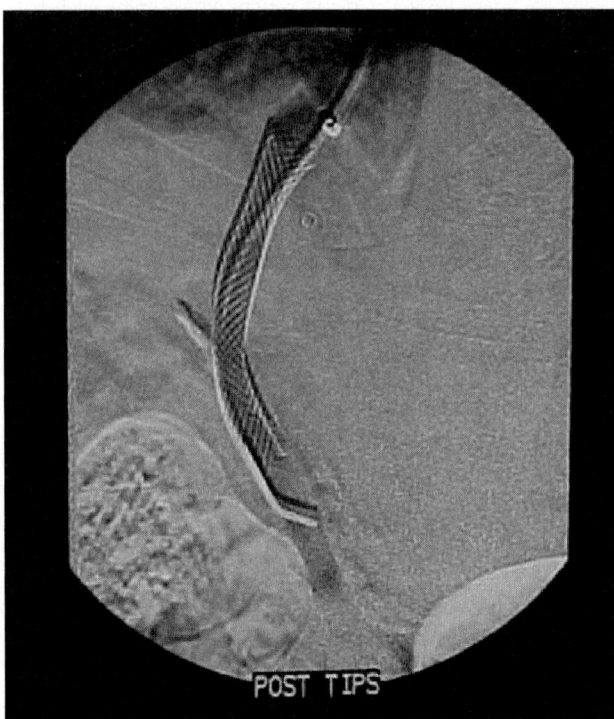

FIG. 30-27. Transjugular intrahepatic portosystemic shunt (TIPS) seen on an angiographic study.

Table 30-6
Surgical Shunts to Reduce Portal Venous Pressure

Nonselective
   End-to-side portacaval shunt
   Side-to-side portacaval shunt
   Large diameter interposition shunts (e.g., mesocaval)
   Central splenorenal shunt
Selective
   Distal splenorenal (Warren)
   Small-diameter portacaval H graft shunt

may require liver transplant in the future (>1 year) are also candidates for surgical shunts since surgical shunt patency is superior to that of TIPS.[59]

Surgical shunts can be divided into two general categories: selective and nonselective (Table 30-6). Nonselective shunts are associated with a high risk of encephalopathy, especially in patients with marginal liver function. Selective shunts are associated with a lower incidence of encephalopathy, as they maintain hepatopetal flow while lowering portal pressure. Currently, the most useful surgical shunts are the small-diameter portacaval H graft shunt[60] and distal splenorenal shunt (DSRS).[61,62] The small-diameter portacaval H graft shunt uses an 8-mm, ringed GoreTex graft anastomosed between the portal vein and the vena cava (Fig. 30-28). The portal vein and vena cava are approached from the right lateral side, where control of these vessels is easier and avoids dissection through omental and retroperitoneal varices. The success rate of the small-diameter portacaval H graft shunt at preventing rebleeding is 90% and the primary patency rate is near 80%. In patients who may require liver transplantation, the presence of this shunt increases the complexity of the transplant, but survival is not altered.

The DSRS is selective and has been shown to be most effective in nonalcoholic patients with preserved liver function who require a shunt for the elective treatment of refractory bleeding. This operation is more complex to perform, but the excellent outcomes coupled with the avoidance of portal dissection make it a preferred procedure in liver transplant candidates. The DSRS can exacerbate ascites and therefore should be avoided in patients already being treated for this problem. The interposition mesocaval shunt is a nonselective shunt that avoids portal dissection and also is useful in future liver transplant candidates. The shunt must be ligated at the time of hepatic transplantation.

In general, nonselective shunts are appropriate for the management of medically refractory bleeding in the patient with preserved liver function who is not a liver transplant candidate and who has intractable ascites. In patients with complete intrahepatic portal vein thrombosis, an end-to-side portacaval shunt is the easiest to perform and the most effective shunt.

Other Operations

Patients with extrahepatic portal vein thrombosis and refractory bleeding are candidates for esophagogastric devascularization (Sugiura procedure).[63] The results of this operation in Western countries have been limited compared to Asian data, possibly because of the higher rates of nonalcoholic etiologies in Asia. A retrograde minilaparotomy TIPS involves surgical mesenteric vein cannulation and a combined antegrade and retrograde TIPS by the interventional radiologist working with the surgeon, and has been successful in patients with very small, sclerotic livers. The surgical incision is very limited and a short limb of small bowel is delivered through the incision. A peripheral mesenteric vein is dilated and cannulated with a sheath,

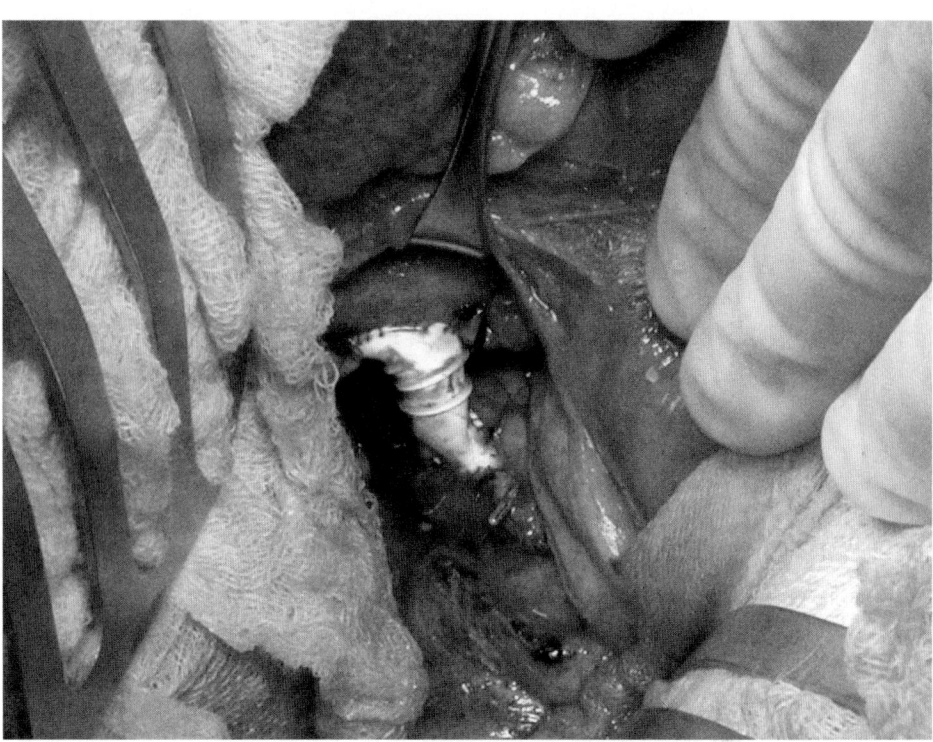

FIG. 30-28. Small-diameter porta-caval H graft shunt to treat portal hypertension.

after which the TIPS procedure is performed by the interventional radiologist. A watertight abdominal wall closure and careful restriction of use of intraoperative intravenous salt-containing electrolyte solutions will help avoid postoperative wound complications.

Ascites

Ascites is a common complication of portal hypertension and cirrhosis. Ascites forms as a result of a complicated interaction between portal hypertension, increased lymph production, and inadequate or inappropriate renal fluid and electrolyte responses. A variety of theories have been proposed to explain the etiology of ascites.[64] The "underfill" hypothesis suggests that pooling of blood in the splanchnic vasculature causes the kidneys to sense underfilling of the systemic circulation (decreased circulating volume), leading to increased activity of the renin-angiotensin-aldosterone system. Alternately, these alterations in splanchnic vascular flow may lead to peripheral arterial vasodilation and overactivity of the renin-angiotensin-aldosterone system. The "overfill" hypothesis contends that the vascular system is overfilled and there is intrinsic renal malfunction, which when combined with the portal hypertension, leads to ascites. However, the number of seemingly opposing hypotheses suggests that the process is indeed multifactorial. In disease processes such as Budd-Chiari syndrome there is clearly a relatively abrupt increase in lymph production, leading to ascites.

The medical management of ascites resulting from chronic liver failure is effective in 90% of patients with cirrhosis. Dietary sodium restriction to less than 100 mmol/day is recommended. The diuretics furosemide and spironolactone are the mainstays of medical therapy. Renal function and symptoms must be monitored closely in patients started on diuretics to avoid major electrolyte abnormalities. Bedrest is associated with spontaneous natriuresis because of decreased activation of the renin-angiotensin system. If symptomatic tense ascites is present, then large volume paracentesis may be necessary in the short term. Paracentesis of 4 to 6 L should be followed with IV replacement with 25% salt-poor albumin at a dose of 8 to 10 g per liter of ascites removed.

Medically refractory ascites is defined by the failure to correct ascites after 2 weeks of maximal diuretic therapy, especially when the urine sodium is less than 50 mmol/L. Treatment options include serial large-volume paracenteses with or without albumin replacement, TIPS, peritoneovenous shunting, or liver transplantation. In patients with advanced liver disease, no significant survival differences have been seen when comparing large-volume paracentesis and TIPS. However, patients with relatively well-preserved liver function can significantly benefit from TIPS. Peritoneovenous shunting has become less popular in the management of chronic, medically refractory ascites because of a high rate of perioperative complications including disseminated intravascular coagulation and shunt thrombosis.

Encephalopathy

Chronic encephalopathy in cirrhosis can be subtle and sometimes can manifest as sleep disturbances (day-night reversal) and forgetfulness.[65] Acute or chronic encephalopathy will frequently have a nonhepatic etiology that should be treated. The common precipitants are shown in Table 30-7. Treatment is directed at reducing the intestinal ammonia and bacterial load. Lactulose is an effective cathartic agent used to reduce intestinal ammonia and bacterial levels. The dose is titrated to the effect of two to three soft bowel movements per day. Use of the antimicrobial neomycin orally also is beneficial in the short term.

ACUTE LIVER FAILURE

Acute liver failure (ALF) denotes a spectrum of highly morbid conditions that result from a massive loss of hepatocyte function without pre-existing liver disease or portal hypertension. Fulminant hepatic failure (FHF) is defined as hepatic encephalopathy occurring within

Table 30-7

Common Precipitants of Hepatic Encephalopathy in Cirrhotic Patients

Increased nitrogen load
  Gastrointestinal bleeding
  Excess dietary protein
  Azotemia
  Constipation
Electrolyte imbalance
  Hyponatremia
  Hypokalemia
  Metabolic alkalosis/acidosis
  Hypoxia
  Hypovolemia
Drugs
  Narcotics, tranquilizers, sedatives
Miscellaneous
  Infection
  Surgery
  Superimposed acute liver disease
  Progressive liver disease
  Transjugular intrahepatic portosystemic shunt (TIPS)
  Surgical portosystemic shunts

Table 30-8

Criteria for Selection of Patients Most Likely to Benefit From Liver Transplantation

1. Acetaminophen toxicity
   a. pH <7.3 regardless of grade of encephalopathy
      or
   b. Prothrombin time >100 seconds (INR >6.5)
      and
      Creatinine >300 μmol/L (>3.4 mg/dL) in patients with grade 3 or 4 encephalopathy
2. Viral hepatitis/drug reaction (non-acetaminophen causes)
   a. Prothrombin time >100 seconds (INR >6.5 regardless of grade of encephalopathy)
      or
      Any 3 of the following (regardless of grade of encephalopathy)
   b. Age <11 and >40 years
   c. Duration of jaundice before the onset of encephalopathy >7 days
   d. Cause: non-A, non-B hepatitis, halothane hepatitis, idiosyncratic drug reactions
   e. Prothrombin time >50 seconds (INR >3.5)
   f. Serum bilirubin >300 μmol/L (>17.5 mg/dL)

INR = International Normalized Ratio.

8 weeks of the onset of acute liver injury. Subfulminant hepatic failure develops after 8 weeks, and the morbidity is more frequently associated with some degree of portal hypertension and renal insufficiency. Both diagnoses are associated with a high mortality rate, exceeding 80% when patients develop coma. The pathophysiology of FHF is directly related to hepatic insufficiency.[66] The balance between liver cell necrosis and regeneration will determine the outcome for each patient. Other than acetaminophen poisoning, identification of a treatable etiology is uncommon in the United States, although one should be explored. A transjugular liver biopsy is the safest method to obtain tissue in FHF patients. The liver biopsy may provide information regarding the etiology as well as the severity of hepatocyte necrosis. Viral hepatitis, acetaminophen overdose, and other drug toxicities are the most common causes of FHF in North America. The majority of cases of viral-induced FHF appear to be due to non-A, non-B, non-C, and non-E hepatitis. Despite advances in supportive medical therapy, there has been little impact on the prognosis of FHF. End-organ dysfunction (renal and cardiopulmonary failure), hypoglycemia, and infection must be anticipated. Systemic and oral antimicrobials administered as prophylaxis are of benefit in delaying infection. Approximately 20% of patients with FHF will survive and go on to have normal liver function and will not develop cirrhosis.[66] However, patients with FHF, progressive liver insufficiency, and encephalopathy should be cared for at a liver transplant program, as liver transplantation is the only potentially

curative therapy available today. Table 30-8 shows criteria for liver transplant candidacy in these patients.

Cerebral edema and intracranial hypertension are the complications of FHF most likely to result in adverse outcome and death.[67] Table 30-9 shows the clinical findings of progressive encephalopathy in FHF. As coma develops, the importance of monitoring intracranial hypertension dictates the liberal use of intracranial pressure (ICP) monitoring. This technology has been shown to be critical to the ongoing determination of a patient's candidacy for liver transplantation. Patients whose ICP rises above 20 mm Hg or whose cerebral perfusion pressure drops below 60 mm Hg will have a high risk of irreversible brain injury and are unlikely to benefit from transplantation.[68]

The pathogenesis of cerebral edema in FHF is controversial, but is likely related to a combination of impaired blood flow, metabolic derangements, and increased cerebral nervous system permeability. Insight into the pathogenesis is demonstrated by the efficacy of liver transplantation in the correction of the process.[69] Liver transplantation has become the therapy of choice and can improve mortality from 15% to a 1-year survival rate that exceeds 60%.[69] Although 4 to 6% of all liver transplants in the United States are now performed for FHF, one third of patients listed as candidates for liver transplantation die before a donor organ becomes available. These factors have intensified the interest in the development of liver-assist devices as a bridge to liver transplantation or full recovery.[70]

Table 30-9

Grading of Severity of Hepatic Encephalopathy in Fulminant Hepatic Failure

Grade	Level of Consciousness	Intellectual Function	Neurologic Findings	EEG
1	Lack of awareness; personality change; day/night reversal	Short attention	Incoordination; mild asterixis	Slowing (5–6 cps); triphasic
2	Lethargic; inappropriate behavior	Disoriented	Asterixis; abnormal reflexes	Slowing; triphasic
3	Asleep; arousable	Loss of meaningful communication	Asterixis; abnormal reflex	Slowing; triphasic
4	Unarousable	Absent	Decerebrate	Very slow (2–3 cps); delta waves present

CPS = cycles per second on EEG; EEG = electroencephalogram.

CYSTIC DISEASES OF THE LIVER

Noninfectious cystic lesions in the liver are common throughout all decades of life. The vast majority of hepatic cysts are asymptomatic and are found incidentally. Cysts can be categorized as congenital or neoplastic.

Congenital Cysts

Congenital cysts include simple hepatic cysts, which are the most common benign lesions found in the liver. Simple cysts result from excluded hyperplastic bile duct rests and they are commonly identified on imaging studies as unilocular, homogeneous fluid-filled structures with a thin wall without projections. The epithelium of the cyst secretes clear fluid that does not contain bile, and they rarely are symptomatic unless they are large, in which case patients may complain of pain, epigastric fullness or a mass, or early satiety related to gastric compression.[71] Often these cysts are aspirated prior to surgical referral, but the recurrence rate after simple percutaneous aspiration is extremely high. Simple aspiration is not recommended as an initial therapy; however, useful information about symptom resolution is often obtained. Percutaneous aspiration, instillation of absolute alcohol, and reaspiration (PAIR) has a success rate as high as 80%.[71,72] In patients with easily accessible lesions and appropriate interventional radiology support, PAIR is an excellent first line of therapy in the management of simple, congenital, hepatic cysts.

The surgical management of simple cysts centers on wide cyst fenestration.[73,74] These procedures are performed laparoscopically, if technically feasible. The recurrence rate after wide cyst fenestration is usually less than 5%. The excised cyst wall is sent for pathologic analysis, and the remaining cyst wall within the liver should be carefully examined for the presence of gross neoplastic changes. Cystic fluid analysis by cytology and tumor markers is not indicated unless there is concern for neoplasia. A symptomatic simple cyst rarely requires complete resection, either as an enucleation or as a formal liver resection.

Polycystic Liver Disease

Polycystic disease occurs as an autosomal dominant disease presenting in adulthood. An autosomal recessive process that is associated with hepatic fibrosis also occurs in rare instances in infancy. A wide spectrum of clinical and anatomic presentations is seen in polycystic liver disease (PCLD).[75] Symptoms of fullness, early satiety, dysphagia, and pain are often chronic and unrelenting, and as with any consideration for liver surgery of benign processes, other contributing factors should be ruled out. Three general anatomic presentations can be described, and often a specific distribution of the cystic disease can be ascribed to specific symptoms. Some patients will have a few dominant cysts that are clearly associated with a specific symptom, usually pain, even in the presence of widespread cystic disease. Other patients will have a limited anatomic distribution of their cysts (lobar or segmental) with compensatory hypertrophy in the unaffected liver. Finally, patients can present with significant hepatomegaly and a diffuse distribution of their disease.

In patients with dominant cysts and associated symptoms, PAIR should be used for the initial approach to manage symptoms. Obliteration of a treated cyst is normally seen in 80% of cases; however, careful patient selection is necessary to avoid recurrence. In patients who are not candidates for PAIR or who have failed PAIR, fenestration or resection of the cyst(s) should be undertaken based on anatomic considerations. Fenestration can be performed laparoscopically or as an open procedure, depending on the anatomic location.[74] Formal lobectomy along the border of the majority of the cystic disease may be required and is expected to be associated with a durable correction of symptoms in up to 90% of carefully selected patients. In patients with massive hepatomegaly but no dominant anatomic presentation, a transverse hepatectomy (resection of segments III, IVB, V, and VI at the level of the rib cage) has been reported to be associated with excellent improvement of symptoms[76] (Fig. 30-29).

FIG. 30-29. Transverse hepatectomy for symptomatic polycystic liver disease. The vascular loop is around the porta hepatis.

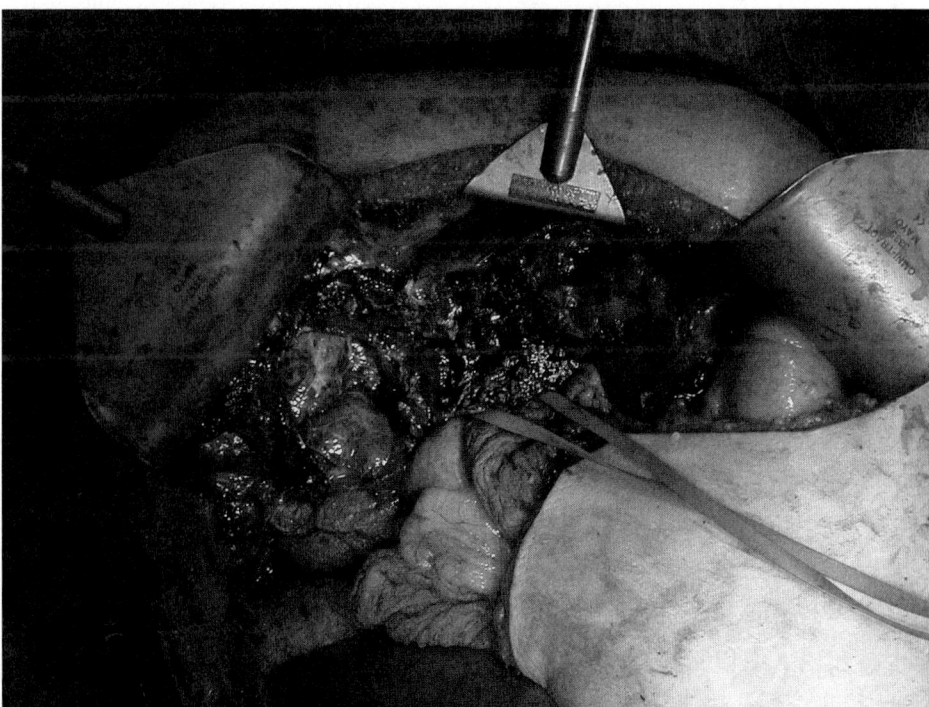

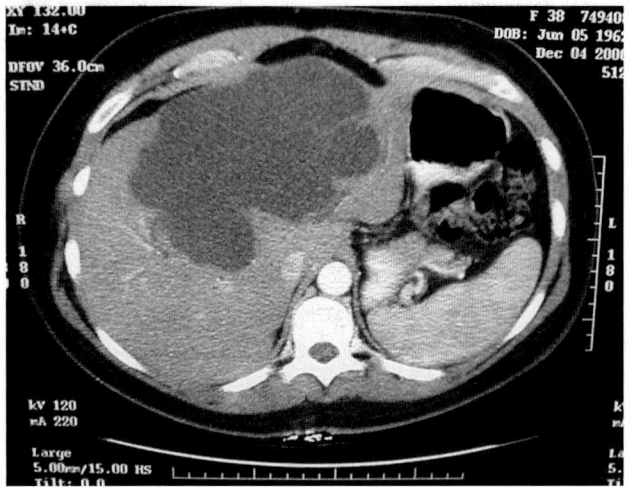

FIG. 30-30. CT scan of a large biliary cystadenoma causing pain and jaundice in a 37-year-old woman. The lesion was removed by a combination of medial enucleation of the cyst off the right portal structures and completion left hepatic lobectomy.

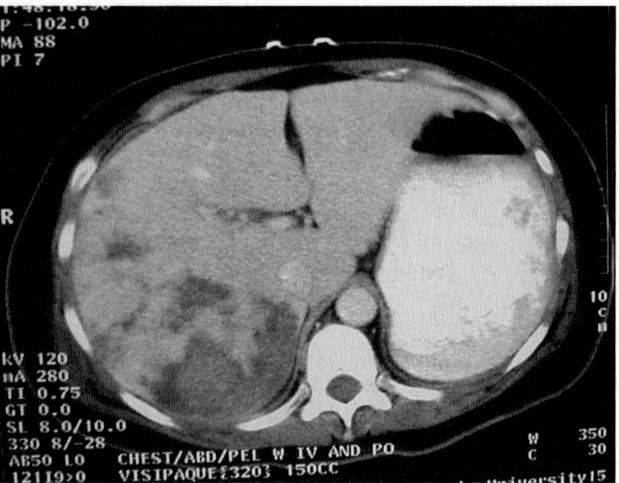

FIG. 30-31. A ruptured hepatic adenoma in segment VII.

The most common complication specific to surgery for PCLD is ascites, occurring in all patients undergoing resection for this disease; however, it is not always symptomatic. When patients develop symptomatic ascites, diuretic use and a low-salt diet will result in nearly uniform resolution of the process. An additional concern with resection in PCLD is bile leakage. Because these cysts compress intervening hepatic parenchyma, great care must be taken to ligate any open biliary radicals, and control of any bile leakage must be sought before completion of the surgical procedure. The application of fibrin sealants to the cut surface of the liver is promising, but has not clearly been shown to prevent bile leaks. Patients who develop progressive liver dysfunction from PCLD should be considered for orthotopic or living related donor liver transplantation.

Neoplastic Cysts

Neoplastic cysts are more common in women and in those individuals older than 40 years of age. These lesions are symptomatic and have a characteristic appearance on ultrasound and other axial imaging studies.[77] Neoplastic cysts tend to have papillary excrescences and may have multiple loculations within the cyst (Fig. 30-30). Percutaneous aspiration is rarely indicated, but if performed will typically yield mucinous fluid.

The surgical management of neoplastic cysts further relies on the initial differentiation between biliary cystadenoma and biliary cystadenocarcinoma.[78] Biliary cystadenocarcinoma is uncommon and is associated with marked thickening of the cyst wall and vascular enhancement on axial imaging studies. Biliary cystadenomas can be either enucleated or resected as dictated by the anatomy.[79] As with hemangiomas and PCLD, biliary cystadenomas compress the surrounding liver parenchyma and careful identification and control of the adjacent intrahepatic portal pedicles is necessary to avoid postoperative bile leakage. If any concern of biliary cystadenocarcinoma is present based on the axial imaging studies, a formal liver resection is indicated.

Other Cysts

Occasionally, cystic lesions can occur in patients who have suffered liver trauma. The general appearance is that of a simple hepatic cyst, and management should be conservative.

BENIGN SOLID LIVER TUMORS

Benign solid liver tumors are increasingly identified with the more common use of axial imaging studies. Differentiation of benign tumors from malignancies including metastatic lesions is achieved based on the clinical scenario and interpretation of radiologic images.[80,81] Therefore biopsy is rarely indicated.

Hepatic Adenoma

Hepatic adenomas (e.g., liver cell adenoma and hepatocellular adenoma) are the most significant benign liver tumors that surgeons encounter. These lesions occur in reproductive-aged women, and are an order of magnitude more common in women who use oral contraceptive pills (OCPs).[82,83] Histologically, these lesions are composed of sheets of hepatocytes with no nonparenchymal cells (Kupffer cells) or bile ducts present. Up to 75% of adenomas may be symptomatic at the time of presentation, with abdominal pain being the most common presenting symptom. Hepatocellular adenomas are significant in that they can rupture and as many as 25% of these lesions are identified after an acute episode of hemorrhage (Fig. 30-31).

Radiographically, it is difficult to distinguish hepatic adenomas from focal nodular hyperplasia (FNH).[84] Both lesions demonstrate rapid contrast enhancement followed by rapid washout of contrast within the tumor on CT scan and MRI. Adenomas may demonstrate increased fat signal on MRI when compared to FNH,[85] and do not have a central scar, which is frequently seen in FNH. If the diagnosis is unclear following contrast-enhanced CT scan or MRI, obtaining a ^{99}Tc-macroaggregated albumin (^{99}Tc-MAA) liver scan should be considered. Typically, adenomas will be "cold" and FNH "hot" owing to the presence of nonparenchymal cells in the latter. Unfortunately, the accuracy of this radioisotope liver scan is only approximately 80%.

The management of patients with hepatic adenomas is evolving. Cessation of OCPs in patients with lesions less than 4 cm in diameter is prudent. Regression of the lesion is commonly seen and such a regression may obviate or facilitate liver-directed intervention. Surgical intervention is recommended in patients with lesions larger than 4 cm in diameter, in patients whose lesions do not shrink after cessation of OCP use, those who medically cannot stop OCP use, or in patients who plan to become pregnant.[86,87] RFA is another potentially effective treatment option in managing hepatic adenomas, especially in patients with multiple adenomas.

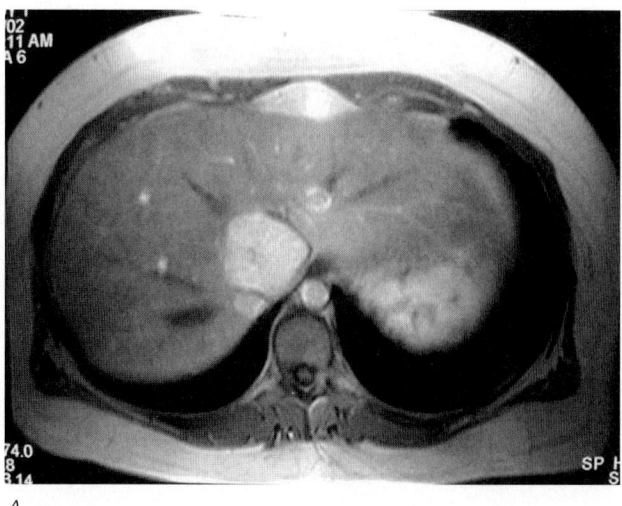

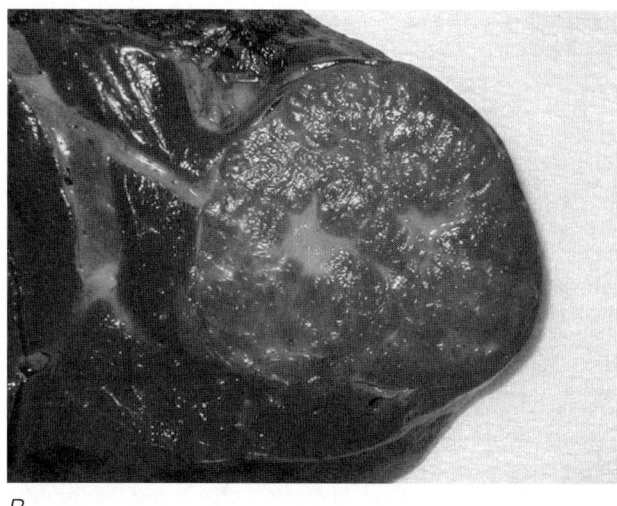

A   *B*

FIG. 30-32. *Focal nodular hyperplasia. A. Contrast-enhanced MRI reveals a hypervascular lesion with a central scar located in segments IVA and VIII. B. Resected specimen showing the characteristic central scar.*

However, until further follow-up data of this technology are available, resection remains the standard therapy. A number of patients with large adenomas undergoing resection have been found to have foci of well-differentiated hepatocellular carcinoma, although large longitudinal studies have not supported a strong association between OCP use and hepatocellular carcinoma.[88]

Focal Nodular Hyperplasia

In contrast to hepatic adenomas, focal nodular hyperplasia typically is not associated with symptoms and does not pose any risks of rupture or malignant degeneration.[84] These lesions intensely enhance on the arterial vascular phase of axial imaging studies (Fig. 30-32). Characteristically, up to two thirds of lesions will demonstrate a central scar. The lesions are often peripherally located and histologically composed of regenerative nodules with hyperplastic bile ducts and connective tissue septae. The etiology is thought to be a result of an early embryologic vascular injury and the histologic findings are a response to this event.

FNH is rarely symptomatic. Therefore other etiologies for symptoms should be explored. In patients with symptoms related to FNH, resection is indicated. Because the lesions are often peripheral, minimally invasive (laparoscopic) approaches to resection should be advocated for the experienced surgeon.[89] Resection of the lesion with a thin margin of normal liver parenchyma is curative, but formal segmental resection should be considered, as such procedures are associated with lower morbidity.

Hemangiomas

Hemangiomas, also known as cavernous hemangiomas, are common benign liver lesions generally discovered incidentally on axial imaging studies. Patients with hemangiomas may present with chronic low-intensity right upper quadrant abdominal pain, especially when the lesions are quite large.[90] Ultrasound can be helpful in identifying hemangiomas, but a CT scan or contrast-enhanced MRI are diagnostic. CT and MRI will demonstrate peripheral nodular contrast enhancement followed by gradual centripetal enhancement, and finally washout of contrast in the lesion on further delayed films (Fig. 30-33). On MRI, these lesions will be bright on T2-weighted evaluation. In rare instances, hemangiomas are difficult to differentiate on MRI and are termed

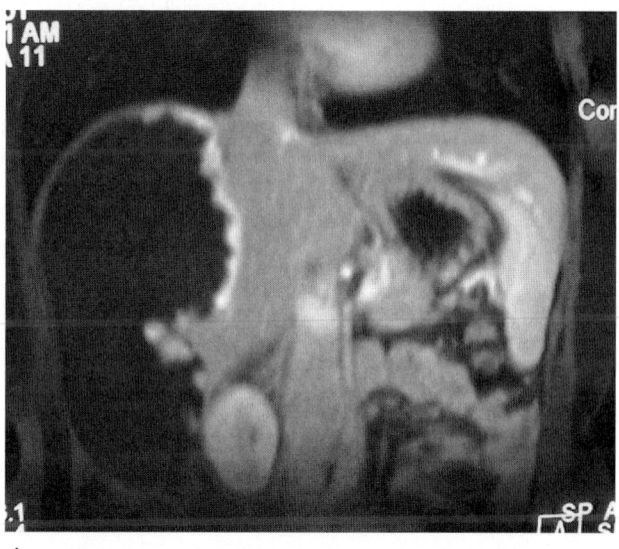

A

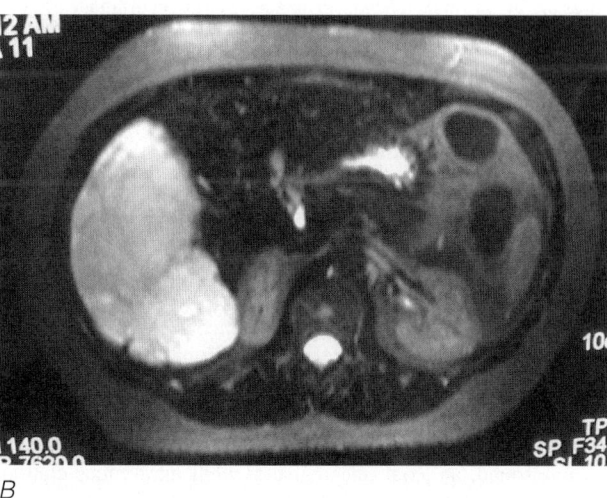

B

FIG. 30-33. *Hemangioma of the liver. A. Contrast-enhanced MRI demonstrating peripheral nodular enhancement. B. Bright signal characteristics of the same lesion on T2-weighted MRI.*

atypical hemangiomas. An atypical hemangioma can be further evaluated using ^{99}Tc-labeled red cell study. Angiography is rarely necessary.

As with other benign lesions, when symptoms are present other causes of abdominal pain should always be ruled out. Resection can be recommended if symptoms can be clearly ascribed to a large hemangioma. Hemangiomas can be resected by enucleation or more standard formal liver resection.[91,92] Enucleation of hemangiomas follows the line of compressed liver tissue, and great care must be taken to ensure control of any biliary radicals that are opened in the process.

Bile Duct Hamartomas

Bile duct hamartomas are the most common liver lesions seen at laparotomy. Hamartomas are peripheral in location, and are firm, smooth, and white in appearance. They are less than 1 cm in size and usually only 1 to 3 mm in diameter. The lesions can be difficult to differentiate from miliary metastatic lesions, especially those derived from colorectal cancer and bile duct cancers. Biopsy is indicated for grossly equivocal lesions.

LIVER INFECTIONS

The liver parenchyma is constantly exposed to a low level of enteric bacteria through the portal blood flow; however, liver infections are rare. The liver is the largest repository of the reticuloendothelial system and is therefore able to cope with this constant barrage. When the inoculum exceeds the capacity for control, infection and abscess occur. Liver abscess can be ascribed to two categories: pyogenic or parasitic.

Pyogenic Liver Abscesses

Pyogenic liver abscesses have been well known for over 100 years and were a common cause of morbidity and mortality in patients with untreated appendicitis and pylephlebitis. Currently, the most common etiologies of pyogenic liver abscesses include biliary tract manipulation, diverticular disease, inflammatory bowel disease, and systemic infections such as bacterial endocarditis.[93-95] Rarely, endoscopic retrograde cholangiography for ascending cholangitis or the management of biliary strictures may result in liver abscess.[96] Patients with contrast material injected proximal to undrained strictures are at high risk. The performance of targeted drainage after an initial noninvasive diagnostic magnetic resonance cholangiogram can aid in avoiding this complication.

The clinical presentation of patients with pyogenic liver abscesses is rarely subtle. Patients present with right upper quadrant abdominal pain, fever, and occasionally jaundice.[95] A careful history and physical examination are necessary to elicit findings of less obvious etiologies such as mild diverticular disease and poor dentition. In patients with chronic symptomatology, fever and weight loss with progressive fatigue may be seen. Significant liver test abnormalities are relatively uncommon and are typically mild. Interestingly, as many as one third of patients with pyogenic liver abscesses will not have an identifiable primary source of infection.

Ultrasound examination will demonstrate a cystic mass in the liver, often with multiple complex septations or inhomogeneous fluid characteristics. In patients who present with abnormalities on ultrasound, an axial imaging study with intravenous contrast should follow. CT findings will include a complex hypodense mass with peripheral enhancement (Fig. 30-34). In patients with a solitary dominant abscess, percutaneous aspiration with evaluation by

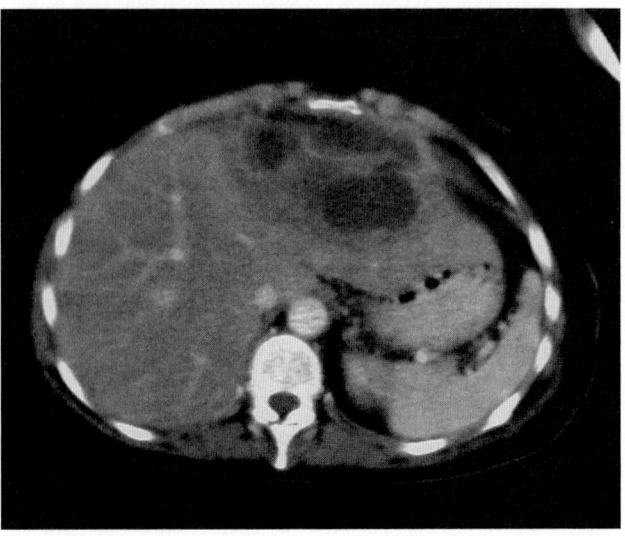

FIG. 30-34. *Left lobe hepatic abscess in a patient who underwent biliary tract instrumentation for common bile duct stones.*

Gram's stain and culture is essential to direct further antimicrobial and drainage therapy.[97] In patients with solitary abscesses, aspiration alone may be sufficient if the abscess can be significantly drained. The placement of a percutaneous drainage catheter at the time of aspiration is beneficial for patients with a complex abscess or an abscess containing particularly thick fluid. Occasionally patients presenting with multiple small abscesses are not amenable to percutaneous sampling. Under such circumstances, laparoscopic evaluation of the liver, including IOUS and a focused biopsy, can be beneficial.[98] In an immunosuppressed patient who has multiple abscesses, hepatosplenic candidiasis should be considered, as well as more conventional pyogenic etiologies (Fig. 30-35). The radiologic diagnosis of hepatosplenic candidiasis can be made based on serial MRI findings. Operative exploration should be reserved for indeterminate cases.

In patients with intra-abdominal sources leading to hepatic abscesses, Gram-negative aerobes, Gram-positive aerobes, and

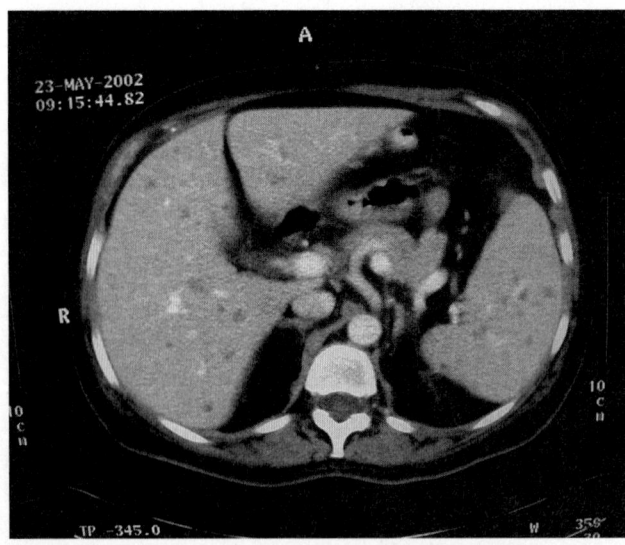

FIG. 30-35. *Multiple small abscesses consistent with hepatosplenic candidiasis in a bone marrow transplant recipient.*

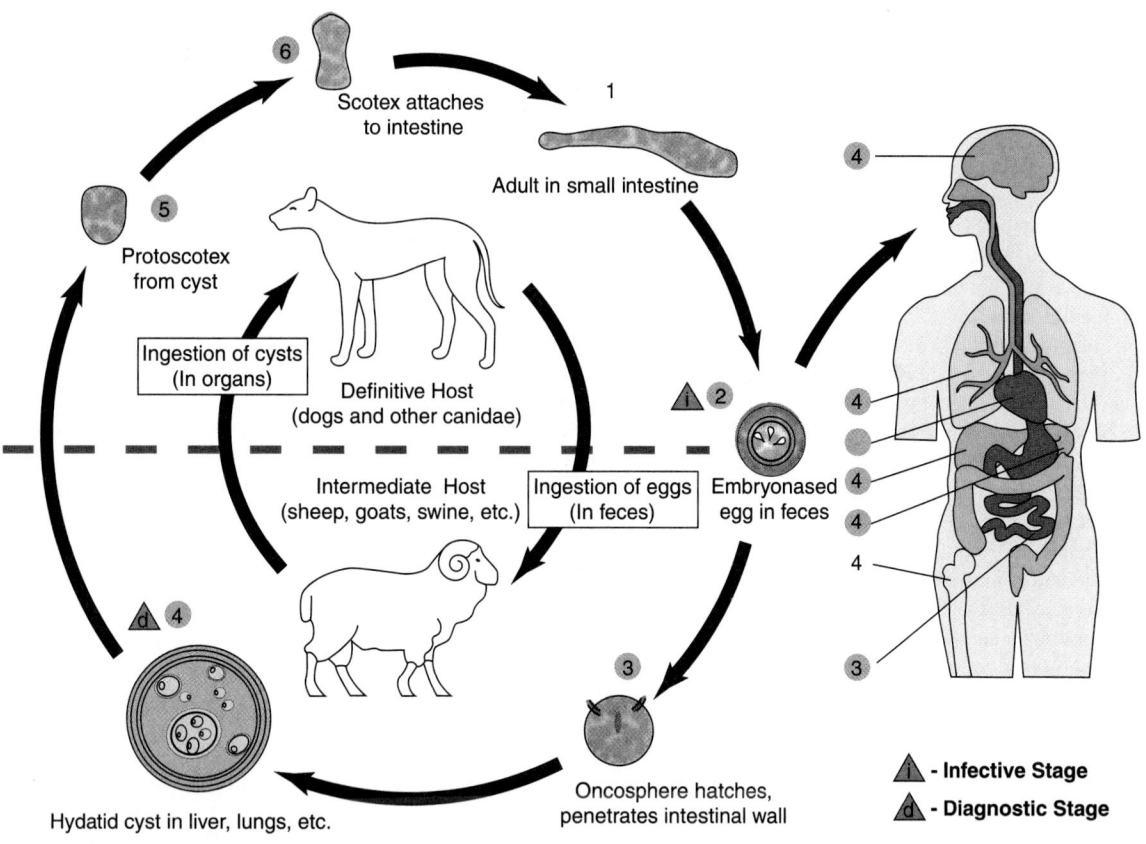

A

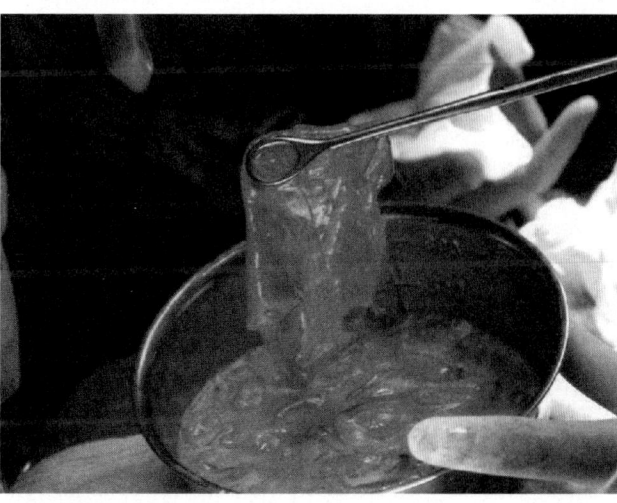

B

FIG. 30-36. Hydatid disease of the liver. *A.* Life cycle of *Echinococcus granulosus. B.* Hydatid cyst contents. (*Courtesy of Dr. William Gamble.*)

anaerobes are the predominant organisms found in liver abscesses. Commonly encountered organisms include *Escherichia coli, Klebsiella pneumoniae, Enterococcus faecalis* and *faecium,* and anaerobic or facultative anaerobic species such as *Bacteroides fragilis.* In patients with systemic infections from subacute bacterial endocarditis and indwelling catheter infections, *Staphylococcus* and *Streptococcus* species are more common. Monomicrobial abscesses are found in approximately 40% of patients, an additional 40% are polymicrobial, while the remaining cases are culture negative.

Antimicrobial therapy should be empiric, based on the etiology of the primary infection from the culture results following aspiration of the abscess. Since percutaneous aspiration is effective in 80 to 90% of patients, surgical intervention is typically unnecessary. However, when percutaneous drainage fails, laparoscopic or open surgical drainage may be necessary. Rarely, in patients with recalcitrant lesions, formal liver resection may be necessary.

Parasitic Liver Abscesses

Hydatid Disease

Cystic hydatid disease is caused by the larval/cyst stage of *Echinococcus granulosus,* in which humans are an intermediate host (Fig. 30-36A). Humans are infected by oral ingestion of excrement from animals (most commonly canines). This form of hydatid disease occurs throughout the world, predominantly in the Southern Hemisphere, Europe, Russia, and China.

Hydatid cysts can be uncomplicated and asymptomatic. However, these lesions may rupture, can become secondarily infected, or may infect other organs. The diagnosis is based on an enzyme-linked immunosorbent assay (ELISA) test for echinococcal antigens, which is positive in over 85% of infected patients.[99] Ultrasound and CT scanning will typically demonstrate either simple or complex cysts with a cyst wall of varying thickness. The treatment of hydatid disease involves the use of oral anthelmintics such as albendazole. Albendazole therapy is the mainstay of treatment in the majority of patients with hydatid disease. It is given alone and for prolonged periods of time in patients who are poor candidates for cyst-directed intervention. However, liver-directed treatment is preferred. In patients with anatomically appropriate lesions PAIR is the preferred initial treatment.[100] The efficacy of PAIR in managing hydatid cysts is greater than 75%. For patients whose disease is refractory to PAIR, laparoscopic or open complete cyst removal with instillation of a scolicidal agent generally is curative (see Fig. 30-36B).[101,102] If surgical cystectomy with removal of the germinal laminated layers is not technically feasible, then formal liver resection can be employed. During aspiration or surgical treatment of hydatid cysts, extreme caution must be taken to avoid rupture of the cyst with release of protoscolices into the peritoneal cavity.

Alveolar echinococcosis (*Echinococcus multilocularis*) occurs in the Northern Hemisphere, produces a more generalized granulomatous reaction, and can present in a manner similar to a malignancy. Resection is the treatment of choice.

Amebiasis

Entamoeba histolytica enters into humans in a cyst form but transforms into a trophozoite in the colon.[103] It enters into the colonic mucosa and invades the portal venous system, infecting the liver. Amebic abscesses result from local proteolytic destruction of the liver parenchyma with focal infarction. Amebiasis is a disease found in subtropical climates, especially in areas with poor sanitation. Although resulting from a colonic infection, a recent history of severe diarrhea is uncommon. Patients typically present with sweating and chills, usually of at least 1 week duration. Fevers can be high and patients typically have right upper quadrant abdominal pain and tenderness. The majority of patients have a positive fluorescent antibody test for *E. histolytica* as well as mild abnormalities in liver enzymes; hyperbilirubinemia is relatively uncommon.

In patients who live in or who have recently visited an endemic area and who present with right upper quadrant tenderness and hepatomegaly, an ultrasound showing an abscess should be considered diagnostic for the presence of amebiasis.[104] Patients diagnosed with amebic liver abscesses should be treated with metronidazole for at least 1 week. Most patients will respond rapidly with complete defervescence within 3 days. Aspiration of the abscess is rarely necessary and should be avoided, except in patients in whom secondary infection from pyogenic organisms is suspected.[105]

EVALUATION OF FUNCTIONAL HEPATIC RESERVE

Patients with normal hepatic parenchyma and serum liver tests can tolerate resection of as much as 80% of their liver volume. The remaining 20% of normal, perfused liver has the metabolic capacity to provide adequate hepatic function while liver regeneration occurs. However, patients with abnormal liver function related to extensive fatty infiltration or cirrhosis, most commonly caused by chronic ethanol ingestion or chronic hepatitis B or C viral infections, may not tolerate resection of a significant proportion of the liver and are at increased risk for postoperative liver insufficiency or liver failure and death. The size, number, and location of liver tumors will mandate the type of operation that must be performed to achieve a margin-negative resection. A significant amount of hepatic parenchyma is lost with major liver resections. The average amount of liver parenchyma resected during a right trisegmentectomy is 85%, a right lobectomy 65%, a left lobectomy 35%, and segmental or wedge resections involve a loss of 3 to 15%. In patients with abnormal liver function who are being considered for partial hepatic resection of malignant disease, assessing the functional hepatic reserve should be considered to determine the patient's risk for postoperative liver failure.

Patients with cirrhosis who develop HCC should undergo assessment of functional hepatic reserve. It may also be appropriate to evaluate functional hepatic reserve in patients with primary or metastatic liver tumors who have significant fatty infiltration of the liver, and in those undergoing resection of an extensive portion of the hepatic parenchyma, such as a right trisegmentectomy. Assessing the risk of postoperative liver failure based on a clinical classification system, such as the Child class (see Table 30-3) alone is inadequate; the postresection mortality rate from liver failure for Child class A or B patients ranges from 8 to 25%.[109] In cirrhotic patients being considered for resection of malignant liver disease, the addition of quantitative or functional hepatic studies can improve patient selection, determine the extent of hepatic parenchymal resection that will be tolerated, and reduce the postoperative mortality rate from liver failure to between 0 and 5%. Functional studies of the liver employ compounds that normally are rapidly acquired and metabolized or cleared by hepatocytes. Rates of metabolism and clearance are decreased in cirrhotic or diseased livers. Some of the compounds used in functional studies have a clearance rate that is determined principally by the route of delivery rather than metabolism. Hence these compounds reflect changes in hepatic microcirculation and reduction in hepatic blood flow associated with cirrhosis. Other compounds are less affected by blood flow rates, and their metabolism is a more accurate indicator of functional hepatocyte mass.

The most commonly used test to assess functional hepatic reserve is indocyanine green (ICG) clearance. ICG is an anionic dye bound by plasma lipoproteins which is rapidly cleared by the liver and excreted unconjugated in bile.[110] Hepatic clearance is limited by both the hepatic blood flow rate and uptake by hepatocytes. Following an intravenous bolus of ICG, the kinetics of its disappearance from plasma due to hepatic clearance can be used to estimate the functional hepatic reserve in patients with cirrhosis or extensive fatty infiltration, even in the presence of hyperbilirubinemia. ICG clearance determinations are widely used and readily available. The ICG clearance values can be used to predict risk of liver failure and mortality following major hepatic resection in the majority of cirrhotic patients. However, there are two principal disadvantages of ICG clearance. First, this test is not a true measure of hepatocyte function, as ICG delivery to the liver is limited in part by the reduced blood flow to the cirrhotic liver. Second, for patients whose values fall in the middle of the ICG clearance risk assessment range, the tests cannot accurately predict a given individual's risk for postoperative liver failure and death. This is particularly true if the patient will require more than a simple wedge or segmental resection to remove the malignant liver disease. There are several tests that assess functional hepatic reserve that are not dependent upon hepatic blood flow rate. These tests can provide a more accurate measure of hepatocyte uptake and metabolism. The aminopyrine and phenylalanine breath tests are noninvasive and reasonably simple to perform. The patient ingests an oral dose of radiolabeled [^{14}C] aminopyrine or L-[^{13}C] phenylalanine, then the individual breathes into an apparatus that collects expired CO_2 at intervals for up to 2 hours after the radiolabeled compound is ingested. The amount of exhaled $^{14}CO_2$ or $^{13}CO_2$ is then used to calculate the percentage of the original aminopyrine or phenylalanine dose undergoing hepatic demethylation or oxidation. Another test of hepatocyte microsomal capacity involves an intravenous injection of galactose followed by serial measurement of serum galactose levels to determine hepatic clearance of galactose. This test is not affected by altered hepatic blood flow rates that may occur with cirrhosis. Both of the radio label tracer studies and galactose eliminate rate have been shown to increase the predictive accuracy of postoperative liver failure in cirrhotic patients with borderline abnormal ICG clearance rates.[109–111]

Administering a known intravenous dose of lidocaine to determine the rate of hepatic microsomal metabolism of lidocaine to monoethylglycinexylidide (MEGX) is another method of evaluating liver function.[112] This test is less expensive, simpler, and provides an assessment of functional hepatic reserve more rapidly than other clearance studies. A measurement of the levels of MEGX in the serum 15 minutes after an intravenous injection of lidocaine (1 mg/kg) is useful in distinguishing patients with mild liver dysfunction from those with cirrhosis, but MEGX levels are not as accurate in predicting severity of cirrhosis when compared with the aminopyrine breath test or galactose elimination capacity. Unfortunately, measurements of metabolites like MEGX, galactose, aminopyrine, and phenylalanine, that are quantitative liver tests based on microsomal metabolism, may quantitate only particular enzymatic reactions. Thus these specific pathways may not be representative of the entire functional hepatic reserve. Nonetheless, using one or several of these tests in addition to ICG clearance can be useful in selecting patients to undergo partial hepatectomy who are at low risk of developing postoperative liver failure, despite the presence of a fatty or cirrhotic liver.

A recent prospective study of 61 cirrhotic patients being considered for resection of HCC used the hippurate ratio, a novel measurement of glycine conjugation of para-aminobenzoic acid to hippurated metabolites by the liver, as a preoperative study of functional hepatic reserve.[113] The hippurate ratio was compared to ICG clearance in the same patient population. ICG clearance rates did not predict the patients who developed postoperative liver failure, including three deaths; however, the hippurate ratio was an accurate predictor of liver failure. Although an interesting initial study, its results will need to be confirmed in a larger group of patients, as only 35 of the 61 cirrhotic patients actually underwent liver resection.

An additional application for nuclear medicine studies is the development of new compounds to assess functional hepatic reserve. Dynamic single photon emission computed tomography (SPECT) images have been used following intravenous injection of ^{99m}Tc-galactosyl-serum albumin (GSA) to assess functional hepatic reserve in patients with chronic liver disease before and after liver resection.[114] Initial results showed a good correlation between total hepatic ^{99m}Tc-GSA clearance and conventional hepatic studies including ICG clearance, cholinesterase levels, and hepaplastin tests. A total of 114 patients were studied, including 55 who underwent hepatic resection for malignant liver tumors. In the five patients who developed postoperative liver insufficiency, ^{99m}Tc-GSA clearance accurately predicted liver failure in each of the patients. PET using $H_2^{(15)}O$ has recently been shown to be a noninvasive method to measure portal venous and hepatic arterial blood flow.[115] There was excellent correlation between portal blood flow and severity of

cirrhosis. This technique will now be studied as a prognostic indicator in patients with cirrhosis who are undergoing liver resection for malignant disease.

MALIGNANT LIVER TUMORS

Surgical Treatment

The first recorded successful elective resection of a liver tumor in the United States was performed by Tiffany in 1890, followed in 1891 by Lucke in Europe.[106] If they were not already aware of the risk of massive hemorrhage from the liver, surgeons were reminded of it by Elliot in 1897 in his report of an attempted resection of a liver tumor, when he stated that the liver "is so friable, so full of gaping vessels and so evidently incapable of being sutured that it seemed impossible to successfully manage large wounds of its substance."[107] Most surgeons continued to choose judiciously which patients they would consider for an elective liver resection, if any, until a greater understanding of hepatobiliary anatomy was published by Couinaud in 1954.[108] Couinaud's description of the segmental liver anatomy based on portal venous inflow and hepatic venous outflow, and the identification of eight hepatic segments (numbered I through VIII) were key steps in the development of safe, anatomic hepatic resections (see Fig. 30-1; Fig. 30-37).

Building on the anatomic and surgical foundation laid down by investigators 50 to 100 years ago, modern surgeons are performing elective operations for liver tumors with increasing frequency. The persistent interest in improved and safer surgical treatments for malignant liver tumors is based on the fact that surgical extirpation or complete cytodestruction currently provides patients with the best chance for long-term disease-free and overall survival. This is true for disease confined to the liver, whether treating patients with primary or metastatic liver cancers.

Improved preoperative imaging studies, routine use of intraoperative ultrasonography, understanding of the vascular and segmental anatomy of the liver, application of new surgical instruments and technology, and improved perioperative anesthesia management have combined to increase the number of patients undergoing successful hepatic resections as treatment for primary or metastatic liver tumors. HCC is one of the most common solid human cancers, with an annual incidence estimated to be approximately 1 million new patients.[116,117] In addition to being a common site for the development of primary malignancy, the liver is second only to lymph nodes as a common site of metastasis from other solid cancers.[118] It is not uncommon, particularly in patients with colorectal adenocarcinoma, for the liver to be the only site of metastatic disease. Surgical resection of HCC, colorectal cancer hepatic metastases, and carefully selected patients with liver-only metastases from other types of primary tumors can result in significant long-term survival benefit in 20 to 45% of patients.[119,120]

Indications for Resection

The important role of liver resection as a treatment for colorectal cancer metastases was solidified by the report in 1988 from the Registry of Hepatic Metastases.[121] This retrospective chart review from 24 institutions identified 859 patients who underwent resection of colorectal liver metastases between 1948 and 1985. The 5-year actuarial survival rate in these patients was 33%, with a 5-year actuarial disease-free survival rate of 21%. Several indicators of poor prognosis also were established by a subset analysis, including a 0% 5-year survival rate when extrahepatic metastatic disease was present, a significantly reduced survival rate if the tumor-free

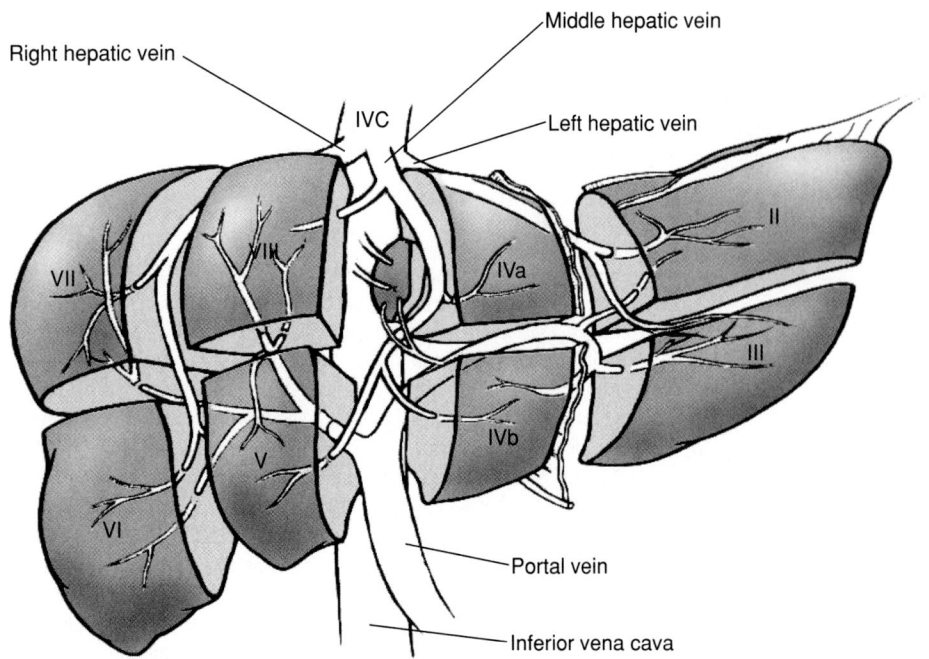

FIG. 30-37. Segmental liver anatomy and nomenclature for lobar, segmental, and extended liver resections. (*Adapted from www.ahpba.org, the Web site of The American Hepato-Pancreato-Biliary Association.*)

resection margin was less than 1 cm or if the primary tumor was stage III (node positive) versus stage II (node negative), and reduced 5-year overall and disease-free survival rates in patients who underwent resection of three or more metastases. The authors noted that patients with three metastases had a significantly poorer disease-free survival rate than those with a single metastasis or two metastases, and that patients with four or more metastases appeared to do at least as poorly. Based on those observations, the presence of four or more liver metastases from colorectal cancer became a contraindication to resection, even when technically feasible with an adequate remaining volume of perfused hepatic parenchyma.

The Registry of Hepatic Metastases report is a retrospective review of patients who underwent operation largely before the availability of adequate preoperative and intraoperative imaging modalities. Furthermore, careful pathologic analysis and an accurate count of the number of lesions were not available in all of the patients. Most of the patients were identified by the development of symptoms, abnormalities in serum liver tests, or an elevated serum tumor marker in the later period of the study. The study included 509 (59%) patients with a solitary liver metastasis, indicating that this was a highly selected group of patients. Of the 149 patients who had three or more metastases, a breakdown of survival by number of metastases was not provided, and the actuarial 5-year survival rate for this group was 18%.[121]

Recent re-evaluations of the number of metastases that should be considered for resection have demonstrated that there is a potential survival benefit in patients with four or more metastases. In contrast to the registry data, all patients in these modern series underwent thorough intraoperative ultrasonography to detect metastatic foci within the liver not identified by preoperative imaging studies, as well as to ensure that the resection be performed with a high probability of tumor-free margins. A study of 235 patients from Japan who underwent hepatic resection for metastatic colorectal cancer included 53 patients (22.6%) who had more than four metastases, including some patients with as many as 10 to 15 lesions.[122] The actuarial 10-year life expectancy of patients with four or more lesions was 29%, which was almost equivalent to the long-term survival of

patients who underwent resection of a solitary metastasis. Patients with two or three metastases actually had a slightly worse long-term survival than patients with more than four tumors. A study from the United States of 155 patients who underwent resection of more than four colorectal liver metastases revealed an overall 5-year survival rate of 23%.[123] As the number of resected metastases increased above nine, there was a significant reduction in long-term survival probability. On multivariate analysis, only positive resection margins and a large number of metastases were significant prognostic indicators for poor outcome.

The indications for resection of HCC also have been re-evaluated. Studies from the 1980s and early 1990s suggested that the presence of cirrhosis or multiple tumors were harbingers of poor outcome after resection of HCC.[109] However, these studies were performed during a time when operative mortality rates in cirrhotic HCC patients ranged from 6 to 15%, and the need for intraoperative and postoperative blood transfusion was common. Improved outcomes have been demonstrated in more recent studies in which modern hepatic resection techniques were employed.[124,125] Specifically, perioperative blood transfusion rates fell from 69 to 87% in the earlier time period to 23 to 39% in more recent series. The operative and hospital death rate was reduced from 13.2% to under 2%, and 5-year survival rates improved from 19 to 32% to 25 to 49%, despite all patients harboring pathologically proven cirrhosis.[124]

Stapling Devices in Liver Resection

Vascular staplers can be used in properly selected patients to reduce operative time and intraoperative blood loss.[126] Hepatic inflow and outflow control can be achieved with stapling devices. However, these techniques should be applied judiciously and should not be used if a tumor must be divided near the vasculature because of the significant negative prognostic impact of positive tumor margins. When a hepatic tumor is near the main right or left portal vein branches, the traditional technique of extrahepatic dissection in the porta hepatis with ligation of the portal vein, hepatic artery, and bile duct branch to the affected lobe should be performed.

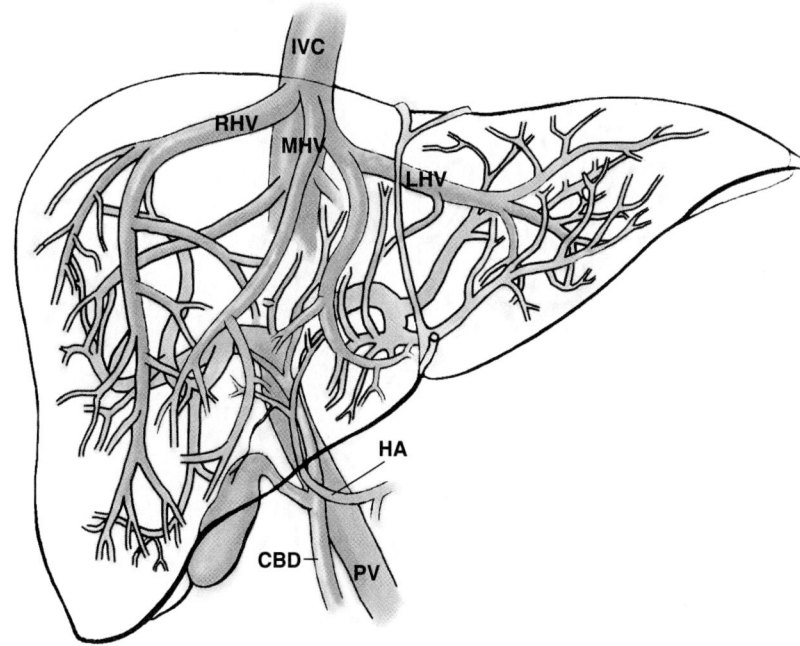

FIG. 30-38. Transparenchymal vascular stapling techniques in the liver can be performed safely using intraoperative ultrasonography to demonstrate the location and association of branches of the portal vein (*PV*), the right hepatic vein (*RHV*), the middle hepatic vein (*MHV*), and the left hepatic vein (*LHV*). Transparenchymal stapling of hepatic inflow vessels also controls hepatic arterial (*HA*) as well as bile duct (*BD*) branches.

A major advantage of stapling techniques is intrahepatic ligation and division of the vascular inflow to a lobe. A key point in the safe use of staplers for hepatic resection is that complete mobilization of the lobe to be resected is required. This is true whether achieving inflow control of the portal pedicles or outflow control of the major hepatic veins.[127] A vascular stapler can be used to divide the blood supply to the right hepatic lobe after performing cholecystectomy to establish the inferior liver surface landmarks

(Figs. 30-38 through 30-42). The stapler is introduced at the junction of segments IVB and V and exits posteriorly in segment VII; this maneuver is safe only if the right lobe of the liver has first been fully mobilized and the direct venous branches from the posterior aspect of the liver into the vena cava have been individually ligated and divided. The vascular Endo-GIA stapler can also be used to ligate and divide the inflow blood supply during left hepatic lobectomy (see Fig. 30-39; Figs. 30-43, 30-44, and 30-45), or

FIG. 30-39. An illustration demonstrating the anterior and inferior aspect of the liver following removal of the gallbladder. Transparenchymal stapling of the inflow blood supply and bile ducts to the right lobe of the liver is facilitated by using electrocautery to score the capsule of the liver along the medial aspect of the gallbladder fossa (*GBF*) as denoted by [*A*]. Transparenchymal stapling of the blood supply and bile ducts to the left lobe of the liver is facilitated by using electrocautery to score the liver capsule inferiorly at the hilar plate as denoted by [*B*].

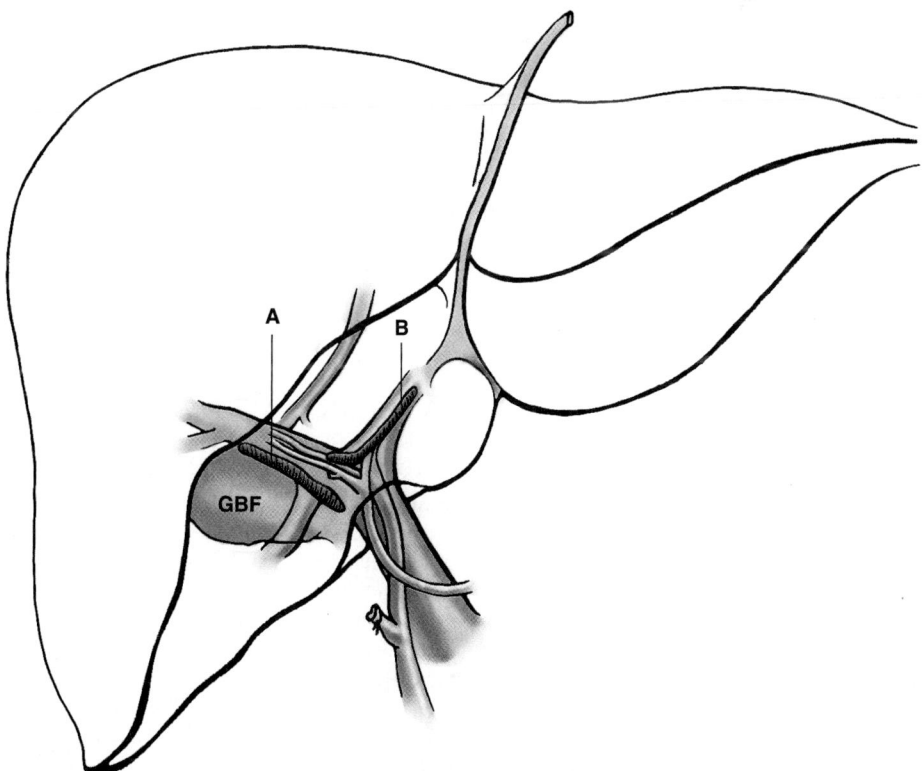

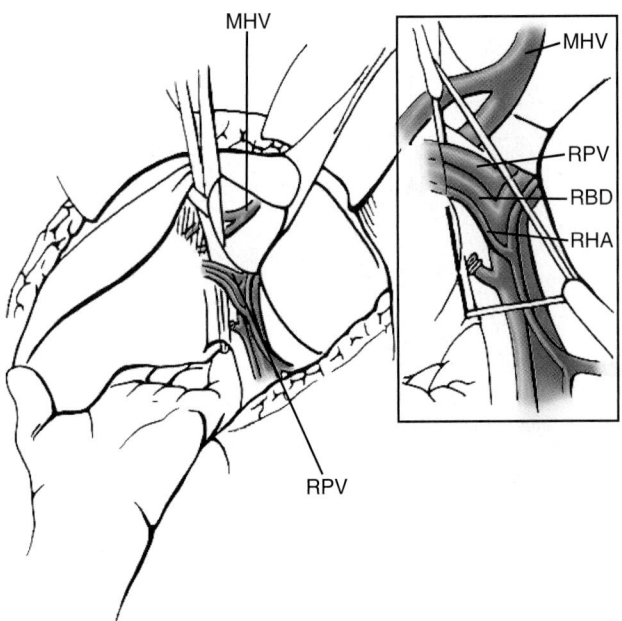

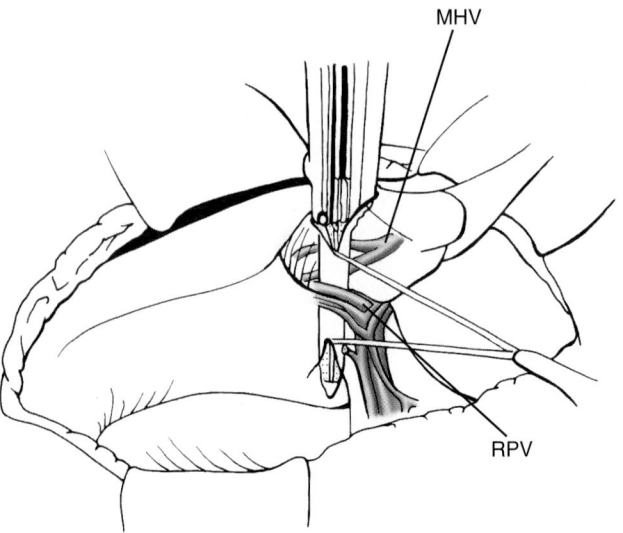

FIG. 30-40. *Illustration demonstrating the maneuvers used to perform transparenchymal stapling for a right hepatic lobectomy. The right lobe of the liver has been completely mobilized from its attachments to the retroperitoneum and the diaphragm, and all small direct perforating branches from the posterior aspect of the liver to the inferior vena cava have been ligated and divided. Through the score mark on the liver capsule along the medial aspect of the gallbladder fossa as denoted by [A] in Fig. 30-39, a long, fine dissecting clamp is used to gently push through the hepatic parenchyma superiorly for 3 to 5 cm, and then the clamp is directed posteriorly to exit in segment VII, just lateral to the inferior vena cava. This maneuver encircles the right portal vein (RPV), right bile duct (RBD), and right hepatic artery (RHA). It is imperative to use intraoperative ultrasonography to determine the length of superior dissection in the liver to encircle the inflow blood supply and bile duct to the right lobe of the liver, as well as to ensure that the clamp passes inferior and posterior to the middle hepatic vein branches (MHV) to avoid injury and hemorrhage from these branches.*

FIG. 30-41. *A suture is grasped and pulled back through the track by the clamp that was used for intraparenchymal dissection around the inflow blood vessels and bile duct to the right hepatic lobe. This suture encircles the vessels and bile duct and is used to guide placement of one piece of the vascular Endo-GIA stapler, as demonstrated in this illustration. Again, it is key to pass the stapler using the suture as a guide through the proper track to encircle the right portal vein (RPV) as well as the right hepatic artery and right bile duct, while also avoiding injury to middle hepatic vein (MHV) branches.*

when resecting segments II and III of the liver, a so-called left lateral segmentectomy.

The low profile, flexible neck, and long handle of a vascular Endo-GIA stapler makes it ideal for outflow control with ligation and division of the hepatic veins. This technique is used most commonly for the right hepatic vein (Fig. 30-46), but with proper hepatic mobilization and division of the parenchyma around the vessels, the middle and left hepatic veins also can be divided using this device.[127] Control of the inflow and outflow vessels of the lobe to be resected allows division of the hepatic parenchyma in a relatively bloodless field (Figs. 30-47, 30-48, and 30-49).

Laparoscopic Hepatic Resection

Laparoscopy has a definite role in the diagnosis and staging of patients with gastrointestinal malignancies. A therapeutic role for laparoscopic liver resection has yet to be established. The development of endoscopic vascular staplers and the harmonic scalpel have increased interest in laparoscopic approaches to benign and malignant liver tumors, although minimally invasive liver resection has not advanced as far as laparoscopic colon, adrenal, and spleen resection. Over the last several years, small series of patients treated with laparoscopic liver resection have been reported. The large majority of liver resection cases completed laparoscopically have been left lateral segmentectomies, segmental or partial segmental resections,

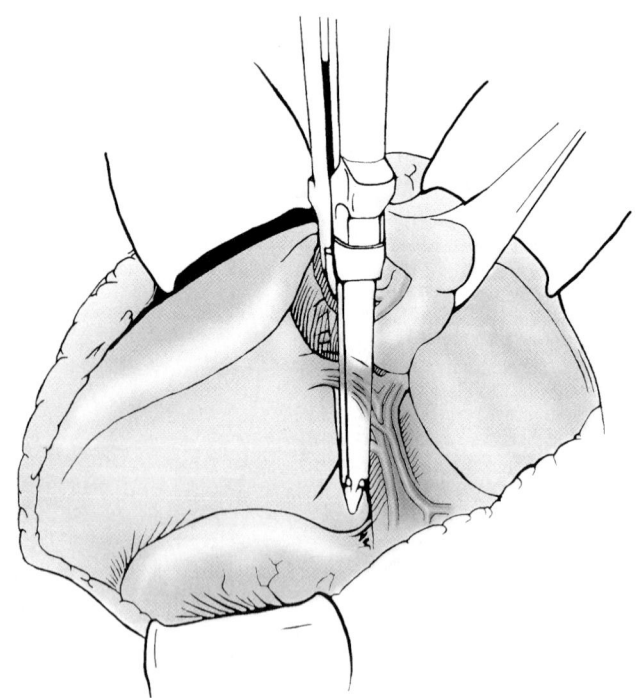

FIG. 30-42. *This illustration demonstrates that the second piece of a vascular Endo-GIA stapler has been joined to the end of the stapler that was passed transparenchymally to encircle the right portal vein, right hepatic artery, and right bile duct. The stapler is fired and released, ligating and dividing the inflow blood supply and bile ducts to the right lobe of the liver.*

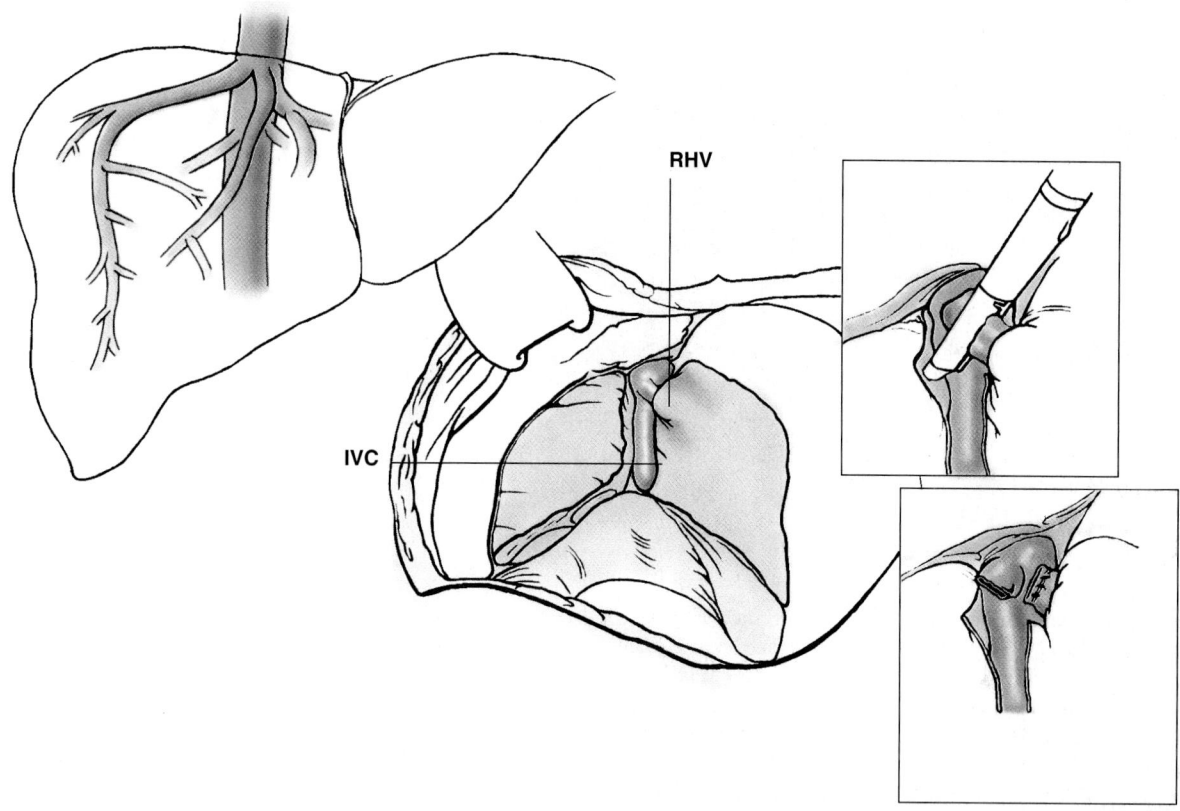

FIG. 30-43. After the inflow blood supply and bile duct to the right lobe of the liver has been ligated and divided as demonstrated in Fig. 30-42, this illustration demonstrates the previously completed dissection along the inferior vena cava (IVC) to expose the right hepatic vein (RHV). This dissection is done prior to dividing the inflow blood supply to the right lobe of the liver, both to ligate any small perforating branches from the liver to the inferior vena cava, and to dissect and encircle the right hepatic vein with a vessel loop. After the inflow blood supply to the right hepatic lobe has been divided, the RHV is divided with a single application of an Endo-GIA vascular stapler as denoted in the top right side panel. After the stapler is fired and released, the RHV is ligated and divided as seen in the lower right panel.

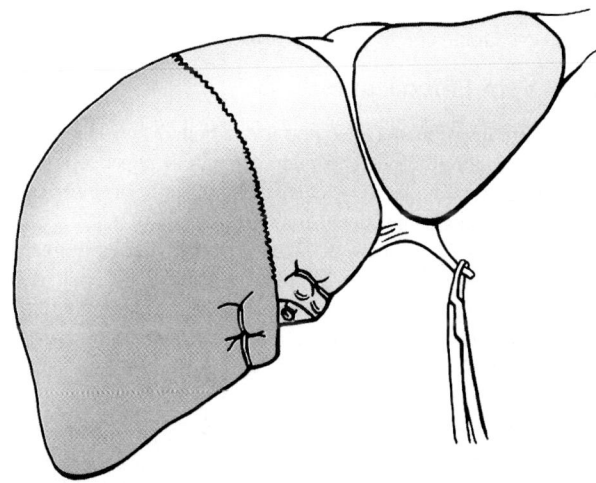

FIG. 30-44. This illustration demonstrates the devascularized right lobe of the liver which lies between segments IVA and IVB (medial segment of the left lobe of the liver) and segments V and VIII as seen in this anterior view. Transection of the hepatic parenchyma is initiated by placing two no. 1 chromic liver sutures on either side of the zone of demarcation between vascularized and devascularized liver. The parenchyma compressed by these sutures is then divided with electrocautery and the capsule of the liver is scored and divided with electrocautery to a depth of 2 to 3 mm along the line of vascular demarcation.

or wedge resections.[128,129] Laparoscopic ultrasonography is performed to localize tumors and to mark the surface of the liver with electrocautery to ensure an adequate margin-negative resection. The parenchyma can be transected using endovascular staplers, the harmonic scalpel, or with finger fracture through a hand port using a pneumosleeve. The reasons for converting a laparoscopic to an open liver resection include dense adhesions that preclude adequate laparoscopic visualization, inadequate tumor-free margins, or brisk hemorrhage during laparoscopic resection.

Repeat Hepatectomy for Recurrent Malignant Tumors

The long-term, disease-free survival rates for patients undergoing surgical resection of primary or metastatic liver tumors is usually below 40% in the most optimistic reports, and may be below 20% in others. Clearly, the majority of patients develop recurrent malignant disease after hepatic resection. In a subset of these patients, the only site of recurrence will be new tumor deposits in the liver. Yet a further subset of these patients may have undergone significant hepatic regeneration and have tumors in locations amenable to repeat liver resection.

The group of patients most frequently considered for repeat hepatectomy are those with recurrent colorectal metastases.[130,131] Only 10 to 15% of patients who develop recurrent disease after liver resection for colorectal metastases will be considered as candidates for a second or third resection. The incidence of extrahepatic disease

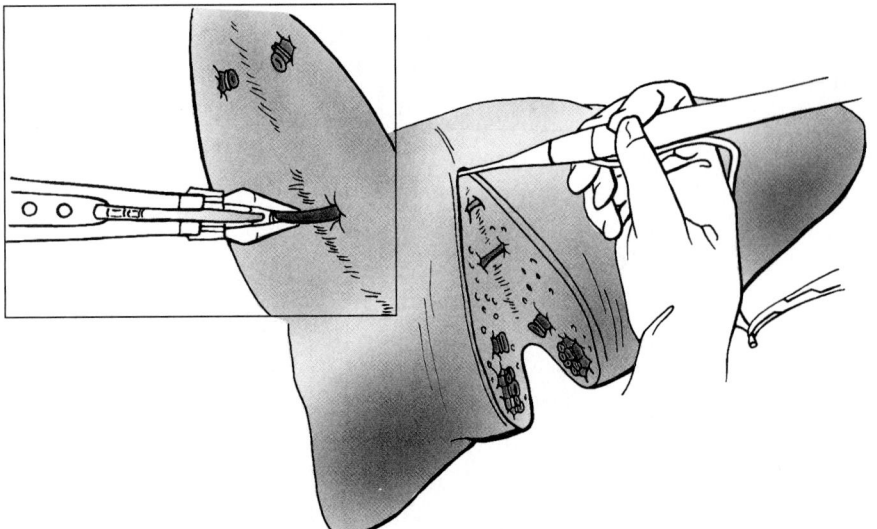

FIG. 30-45. Transection of the remaining hepatic parenchyma can be performed using a variety of techniques. This illustration demonstrates use of the CUSA (Cavitron Ultrasonic Aspirator) device. Vessels bridging between the left lobe and right lobe of the liver are exposed during this dissection and can be divided between hemoclips, as demonstrated in the inset illustration in the upper left, or can be tied or suture ligated.

in patients being considered for repeat hepatectomy may be as high as 30%; thus they should undergo thorough preoperative evaluation with state-of-the-art helical CT imaging and PET scans.[131] While technically challenging because of adhesions and altered vascular anatomy related to the previous hepatic resection, repeat hepatectomy can be performed with low morbidity and mortality rates. At the M.D. Anderson Cancer Center in Houston, Texas, these authors experienced 23 patients with colorectal cancer metastases who underwent a repeat resection with no perioperative deaths and a 22% complication rate.[130] The median survival in this small group of patients was 39 months, but the 5-year survival rate was only

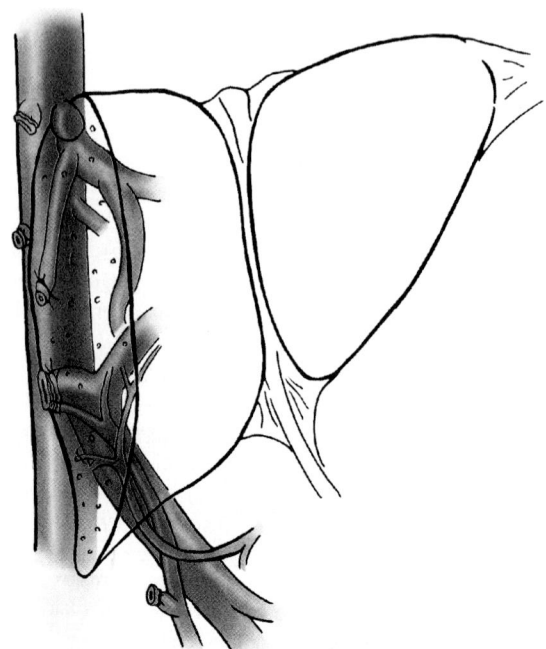

FIG. 30-46. Illustration demonstrating a completed right hepatic lobectomy, with the right portal vein, right hepatic artery, and right bile duct ligated and divided with vascular Endo-GIA staplers, and the right hepatic vein ligated and divided with an Endo-GIA vascular stapler. Middle hepatic vein branches can be controlled with additional firings of the vascular Endo-GIA stapler or with suture ligatures.

13%. In contrast, other authors report 5-year survival rates of up to 35%, attained with similar low operative morbidity and mortality rates.[131]

Repeat hepatic resection may also be applied in selected patients with HCC. Intrahepatic recurrence as the only site of disease is more common in HCC patients than those with metastatic liver tumors, but the number of patients who are candidates for repeated surgical treatment is less than 10% of those who develop recurrent disease. Patients who develop hepatic recurrence of HCC after hepatic resection of their primary tumor may not be candidates for repeat resection because of multifocality, vascular invasion by tumor, or the severity of underlying cirrhosis. In properly selected patients, repeat hepatic resection for HCC can be performed and result in long-term survival rates of up to 30%.[132,133] The incidence of postresection liver failure is no higher in patients who undergo a second hepatic resection, indicating the importance of carefully selecting individuals who will have adequate functional hepatic reserve following a second operation.

Portal Vein Embolization

Direct tumor invasion of a lobar portal vein branch may lead to ipsilateral hepatic lobe atrophy and contralateral lobe hypertrophy. The development of compensatory hypertrophy of a lobe or segments of the liver following tumor occlusion of contralateral portal venous branches led to the concept of planned portal vein embolization (PVE) to initiate hypertrophy in segments of the liver that would remain following a major liver resection. PVE was first reported as a potentially useful treatment to induce hepatic hypertrophy prior to liver resection in a small group of HCC patients in 1986.[134] These patients also were treated with hepatic arterial embolization of their primary liver tumor, but PVE was noted to induce hypertrophy rarely seen with hepatic arterial embolization alone.

Interest in preoperative PVE has increased because extended hepatectomy (resection of five or more hepatic segments) is now more commonly considered an appropriate and safe treatment option in patients with hepatobiliary malignancies. Surgical mortality from extended hepatic resections continues to be reduced as a result of improved patient selection and safer surgical and anesthetic techniques. However, complications related to postoperative hepatic insufficiency, including cholestasis, coagulopathy, bleeding, fluid retention, and impaired hepatic synthetic function, may cause a

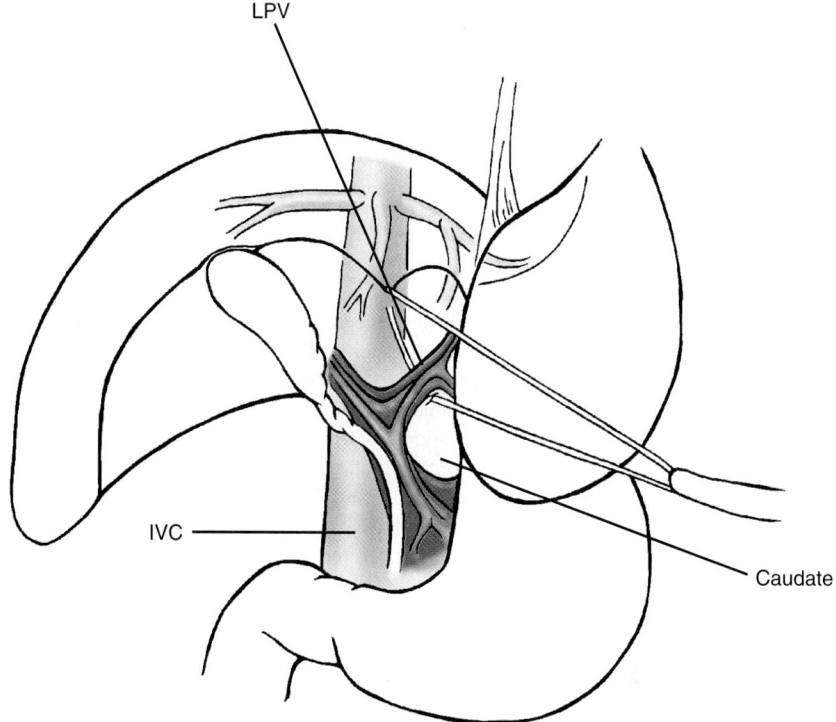

FIG. 30-47. Illustration demonstrating key anatomic points for performing a left hepatic lobectomy utilizing vascular staplers. The hilar plate of the liver is scored with electrocautery and opened along the line denoted [B] in Fig. 30-39. Similarly to the technique used for the right hepatic lobectomy, a long, slightly curved dissecting clamp is used to gently push through the hepatic parenchyma, exiting posteriorly in segments II and III just above the caudate lobe (segment I). A suture is pulled through this same track and is used as a guide to ensure that the stapler is placed around the left portal vein (LPV), left hepatic artery, and left bile duct, while avoiding injury to the inferior vena cava.

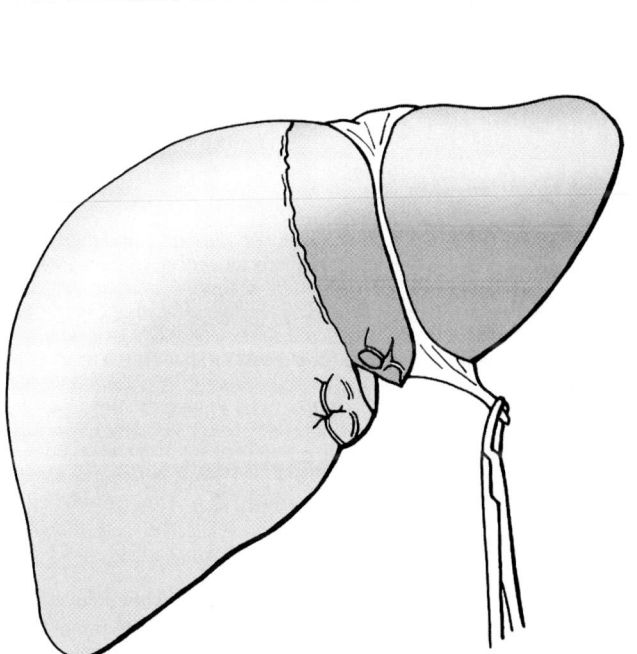

FIG. 30-48. After dividing the vascular inflow blood supply and the bile duct to the left lobe using an Endo-GIA vascular stapler, the left lobe demarcates and becomes darker than the still vascularized right lobe of the liver. Once again, the dissection is initiated by placing two no. 1 chromic liver sutures on either side of the zone of demarcation, tying these down, and then dividing the parenchyma between these sutures with electrocautery.

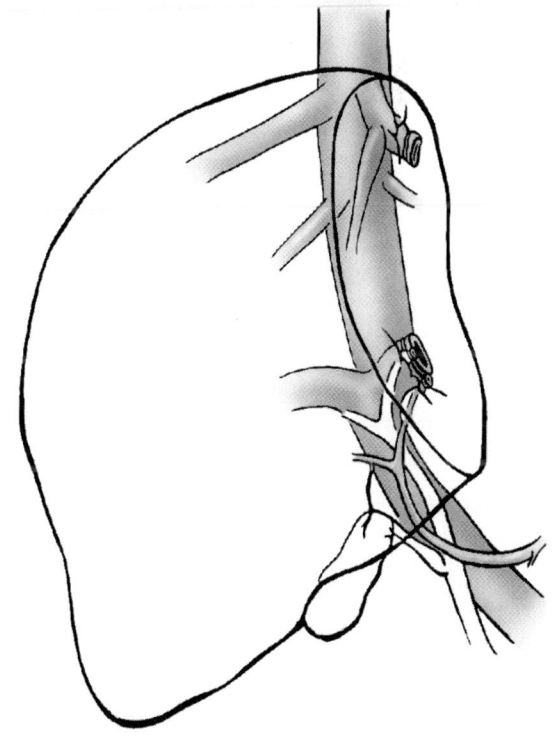

FIG. 30-49. A completed left hepatic lobectomy resecting segments II, III, and IV. Unlike right hepatic lobectomy, in which the right hepatic vein is dissected and divided in its extrahepatic portion, branches of the middle hepatic vein and left hepatic vein are divided intraparenchymally using additional firings of the vascular Endo-GIA stapler.

prolonged hospital stay and protracted recovery following extended hepatectomy.[135] Furthermore, during preoperative evaluation of patients for an extended hepatectomy, some patients will be excluded from the benefit of a potentially curative resection because the anticipated liver remnant will be too small.

Indications for Portal Vein Embolization

In patients with normal hepatic parenchyma, preservation of a perfused section of liver comprising 25% of the total hepatic volume is usually sufficient to prevent major postoperative complications and hepatic insufficiency. This 25% value has been determined somewhat empirically, and there is a paucity of data regarding the exact volume of liver that can be resected safely without postoperative liver failure when the remaining liver parenchyma is completely normal. In a recent series of 20 patients with normal liver parenchyma who underwent an extended right hepatic lobectomy, it was demonstrated that a future liver remnant of 25% or less of the total liver volume was associated with increases in severity of postoperative liver insufficiency, length of stay, and complications.[136] Another recent report described the results with extended liver resection in 55 patients with normal hepatic parenchyma.[137] Based on preoperative calculation of a future liver remnant that was 25% or less of the total liver volume, 18 of these patients underwent preoperative PVE. The median increase in the future liver remnant was 8%. As a result of the increase in the future liver remnant in the PVE group, there was no difference in the immediate preoperative volume of the future liver remnant between the PVE group (23% future liver remnant) and the group that did not receive preoperative PVE (25% future liver remnant). Importantly, there was no difference in the occurrence of major postoperative complications or length of stay between the two groups. Thus, preoperative PVE allowed a safe liver resection in 18 patients who otherwise would not have been candidates for an extended hepatic resection, and the median survival time following liver resection in the patients treated with PVE was not significantly different from those patients who did not require PVE.[137] The functional capacity of liver compromised by cholestasis, acute or chronic inflammation, steatosis, or cirrhosis is variable. A larger future liver remnant is required to avoid posthepatectomy hepatic insufficiency or failure in patients with diseased hepatic parenchyma. Two recent studies suggest that at least 40% of the total hepatic volume should remain in order to minimize postoperative complications in patients who have underlying chronic liver disease or who have received high-dose chemotherapy.[138,139] In addition to preoperative PVE, patients with underlying chronic liver disease also may require careful assessment of functional hepatic reserve before and after PVE to assess the risk of postoperative liver failure.

Preoperative Volumetric Determination of the Future Liver Remnant

Rapid-sequence, thin-section, helical CT is used to make direct measurements of total liver volume, volume of the liver to be resected, and volume of the future liver remnant (Fig. 30-50).[136] The total liver volume also can be estimated based on the described association between body surface area (BSA) and the total liver volume, where total liver volume = $706.2 \times BSA$ (in m^2) $+ 2.4$.[140] The future liver remnant volume, for example the volume of segments I, II, and III in a patient undergoing an extended right hepatectomy, can be directly measured on a helical CT, and then divided by the total estimated liver volume to calculate the percentage of the future liver remnant. If the future liver remnant is estimated to be too small

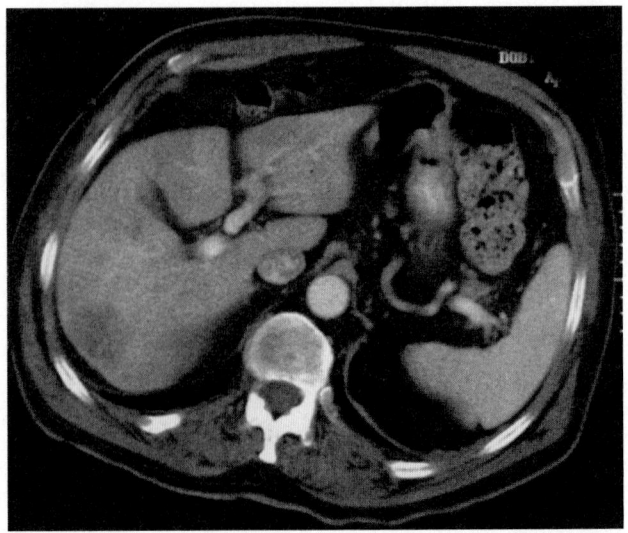

A

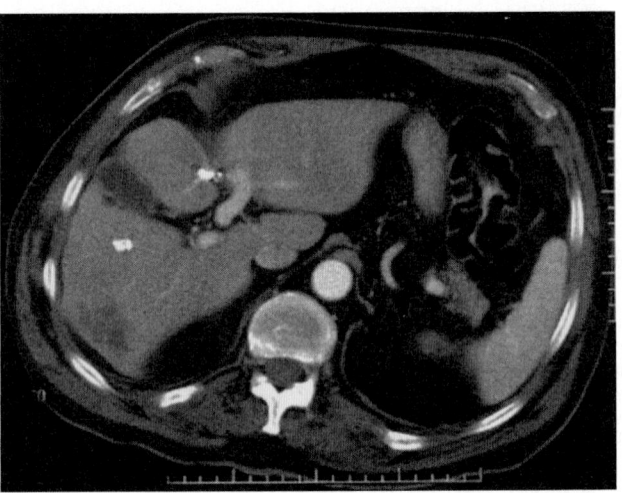

B

FIG. 30-50. *A.* CT image of a patient with right lobe and medial left lobe (segment IV) involvement by colorectal cancer liver metastases. An extended hepatic resection would be necessary to surgically excise all of the malignant disease; however, the lateral segment of the left lobe comprises less than 20% of the total hepatic volume, and the risk of postoperative liver failure would be excessive. *B.* CT scan from the same patient following portal vein embolization 4 weeks prior to this image being obtained. There has been significant compensatory hypertrophy of the left lateral segment, which on volumetric CT analysis now comprises between 25 and 30 percent of the total hepatic volume. The metallic coils used to embolize portal vein branches to the right lobe of the liver and the medial segment of the left lobe of the liver are clearly evident.

when also considering the presence or absence of chronic liver disease, PVE may be considered to increase the size of the future liver remnant.

Approach for Portal Vein Embolization

A percutaneous transhepatic approach has become the standard technique for PVE.[141] The principal advantage of this technique is that it allows direct access to the portal venous branches of the lobe and segments to be embolized via an ipsilateral approach. This technique minimizes the risk of thrombosis of the main trunk of the portal vein and vascular injury to the portal venous branches supplying the future liver remnant. The side effects are minor and transient and include pain from the transhepatic access site and low-grade fever.

It is important to embolize not only the main right portal vein, but also the portal venous branches to segment IV if an extended right hepatic lobectomy is planned.[141] Systematic embolization of segment IV branches is imperative for two reasons. First, all segments of the liver-bearing tumor are embolized to minimize the risk of accelerated tumor growth. Accelerated tumor growth has been reported when incomplete right trisectoral embolization has been performed.[142] Second, embolization of segment IV portal vein branches in addition to the main right portal vein may contribute to better hypertrophy of segments I, II, and III prior to the extended right hepatic lobectomy.

Results After Portal Vein Embolization

Preoperative PVE has been used to treat primary liver malignancies, including HCC and cholangiocarcinoma, and metastatic liver tumors, particularly colorectal cancer metastases. Studies that report outcome after PVE indicate that the predicted future liver remnant volume increased from 19 to 36% of total liver volume pre-embolization to 31 to 59% postembolization.[136,139,141–148] Complications are rare (0 to 10%) and there were no reported deaths after PVE (Table 30-10). Not all patients who undergo PVE undergo surgery, because some patients fail to develop adequate hypertrophy,

or more commonly will develop intrahepatic or extrahepatic progression of their disease in the interval between PVE and the planned resection (see Table 30-10).

Almost 250 reported extended liver resections have been performed following PVE[136,139,141–148] (see Table 30-10). Perioperative mortality rates range from 0 to 7%, with no significantly higher mortality rate in cirrhotic compared to noncirrhotic patients. The reported complication rate of more than 15% following extended hepatic resection in patients who first underwent PVE is equivalent or better than most reports describing complication rates following this type of procedure without preoperative PVE. Unfortunately, few of the studies report long-term outcome and survival data. In a small series of 13 HCC patients treated with PVE followed by extended hepatectomy, the 1- and 2-year survival rates were 69% and 40%, respectively.[147] In a study of 41 patients, most with colorectal cancer liver metastases, who underwent extended hepatic resection following PVE, the overall 5-year survival rate was 31%.[148] In another series of 19 patients with colorectal cancer liver metastases, the 5-year actuarial survival rate after extended hepatic resection following PVE was 40%, which compared favorably to the 38% 5-year actuarial survival rate following resection in a patient cohort with a similar extent of resection without PVE.[139] These promising early results suggest that PVE, when successful in increasing the volume of the future liver remnant, can increase the number of patients who can undergo a successful and safe extended hepatic resection with the goal of improving their long-term survival.[149]

Table 30-10

Changes in Future Liver Remnant (FLR) Volume and Complications of Embolization and Resection Following Portal Vein Embolization (PVE)

Year of Study	No. of Patients	Cancer Type	Mean % Increase in FLR Volume After PVE	Percentage of Embolized Patients Who Came to Resection	Major PVE Complications	Major Perioperative Complications (Other Than Death)	30-Day Operative Deaths
1991	54	31 HCC, 12 CAC, 8 metastatic, 3 other	14	85	0	3 abscess, 1 pneumonia	1 (cholangitis)
1993	10	CRC, HCC, CAC, 2 other	12	90	1 required re-embolization		
1993	20	GB, hilar CAC, HCC	10	NR	1 transient hemobilia		NR
1994	12	Hilar CAC	8	100	0	1 abscess, 1 pancreatic leak	0
1995	4	Hilar CAC	10	NR	0	1 transient liver insufficiency	0
1995	19	14 GB, 5 CAC	11	68	NR		NR
1996	31	22 CRC, 1 HCC, 1 CAC, 5 other	13	77	1 flushing(w/carcinoid)	1 ATN, 1 bile leak	2 PV thrombosis MOF and pneumonia
1997	7	HCC	27	100	0	1 bile leak, 1 abscess, 2 liver insufficiency	0
1997	13	HCC	11	100	0	5 prolonged jaundice	2 liver failure
1999	84	51 hilar CAC, 22 GB, 7 mets, 5 HCC, 1 benign	10	79	2 SBO, 1 reoperation (for SBO)		1 bleeding after liver failure
1999	49	27 CRC, 4 HCC, 10 other	12	84	0	2 bile leaks, 1 abscess, 2 GI anastomotic leaks	1 peritonitis
2000	12	6 CRC, 2 CAC, 1 GB, 3 HCC	10	58	0	1 ascites and wound breakdown	0
2000	30	30 CRC	11	63	1 (hepatic artery injury, septic liver necrosis)	1 technical; unrelated to PVE, 2 biliary fistulae	0 (1 death at 45 days)

ATN = acute tubular necrosis; CAC = cholangiocarcinoma; CRC = colorectal carcinoma liver metastases; GB = gallbladder carcinoma; GI = gastrointestinal; HCC = hepatocellular carcinoma; met = metastases; MOF = multiorgan failure; NR = not reported; PV = portal vein; SBO = small bowel obstruction.

SOURCE: Adapted and used with permission from Alvarez Perez et al.[95]

Radiofrequency Ablation

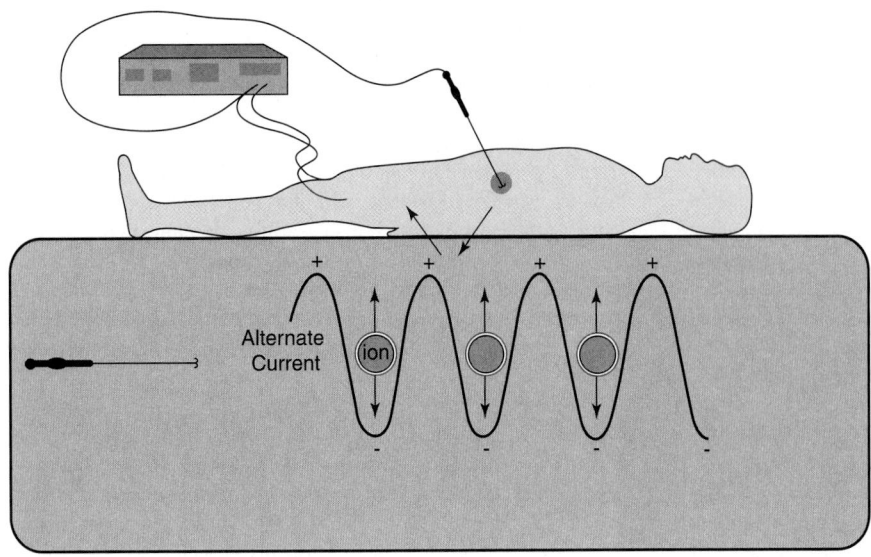

FIG. 30-51. A schematic diagram demonstrating a patient undergoing radiofrequency (RF) ablation of a malignant liver tumor (top half of illustration). The multiple array RF needle electrode is inserted into the liver tumor with the intent of producing complete coagulative necrosis of the tumor and a surrounding zone of nonmalignant hepatic parenchyma. The RF needle electrode and grounding pads from the patient are attached to a radiofrequency generator. The lower portion of the diagram shows the ionic agitation that occurs around the multiple array RF needle electrode when alternating current from the RF generator is applied. Ionic agitation produces frictional heating in the tissue, resulting in coagulative necrosis of tissue around the electrode.

Radiofrequency Ablation

Background and Basics of Radiofrequency Tissue Ablation

The use of radiofrequency (RF) energy to produce thermal tissue destruction has been the focus of increasing research and practice over the past several years. During the application of RF energy, a high-frequency alternating current moves from the tip of an electrode into the tissue surrounding that electrode. As the ions within the tissue attempt to follow the change in the direction of the alternating current, their movement results in frictional heating of the tissue (Fig. 30-51). As the temperature within the tissue becomes elevated beyond 60°C, cells begin to die, resulting in a region of necrosis surrounding the electrode.[150]

An RF needle electrode is advanced into the liver tumor to be treated via either a percutaneous, laparoscopic, or open (laparotomy) route. Using transcutaneous or intraoperative ultrasonography to guide placement, the needle electrode is advanced to the targeted area of the tumor, and then the individual wires or tines of the electrode are deployed into the tissues. Once the tines have been deployed, the needle electrode is attached to a RF generator and two dispersive electrodes (return or grounding pads) are placed on the patient, one on each thigh (see Fig. 30-51). The RF energy is then applied following an established treatment algorithm to create a sphere of cellular necrosis.[151] Tumors less than 2.5 cm in their greatest dimension can be ablated with the placement of a needle electrode with an array diameter of 3.5 to 4.0 cm when the electrode is positioned in the center of the tumor (Fig. 30-52). Tumors

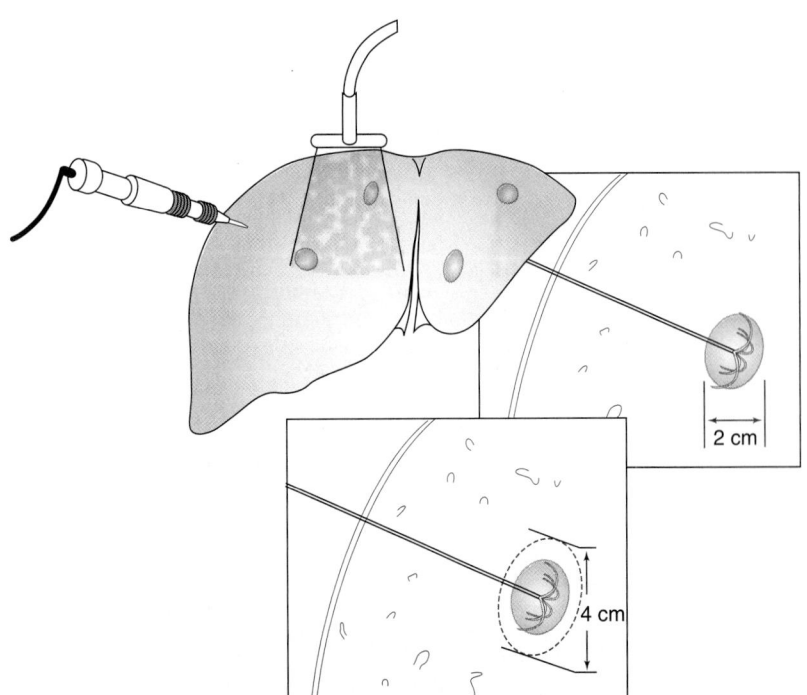

FIG. 30-52. The upper left illustration represents an intraoperative ultrasound probe placed on the surface of the liver to visualize small malignant tumors deep within the hepatic parenchyma. Intraoperative ultrasonography is used to guide placement of the RF needle electrode into the tumor. Once the needle is placed in the appropriate position within the tumor, the multiple array secondary electrodes are deployed from the needle tip (upper right inset illustration). When currently available RF generators and multiple array needle electrodes are used to treat a tumor nodule 2 cm in diameter or smaller, a single placement of the multiple array electrode is usually sufficient to produce a 4- to 5-cm diameter zone of coagulative necrosis to completely destroy the tumor and a surrounding zone of normal hepatic parenchyma (lower inset illustration).

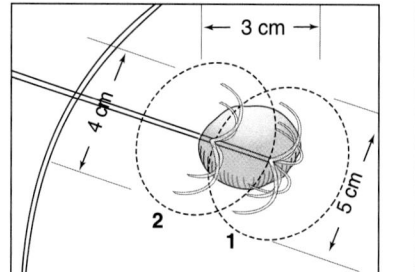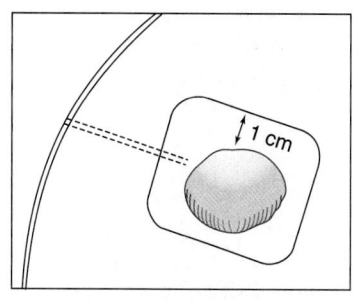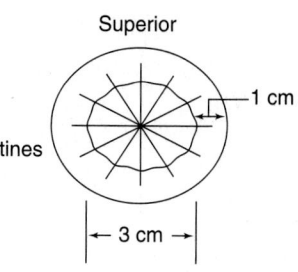

FIG. 30-53. Use of a multiple array RF needle electrode to treat a 3-cm diameter malignant liver tumor. The left side illustration demonstrates the use of a needle electrode with a multiple array diameter of 4 cm. The RF needle is first guided into the deepest portion of the tumor, and the multiple array is deployed at the interface of the posterior aspect of the tumor and normal hepatic parenchyma (area 1). This area is treated with RF energy until coagulative necrosis of the tumor and surrounding liver is complete. The multiple array is then retracted into the needle tip and the tip is withdrawn approximately 1.5 cm. The multiple array is again deployed to treat the more superficial interface of tumor and normal parenchyma (area 2). The central illustration shows that an ideal ablation destroys not only the tumor, but a 1-cm margin of surrounding hepatic parenchyma to ensure destruction of any microscopic extension of the tumor mass. The illustration on the right side of the figure shows an idealized superior view looking directly down on the tumor, again indicating the needle track placement centrally into the tumor with the multiple array tines radiating out through the tumor into the surrounding hepatic parenchyma to produce thermal ablation of the tumor and a 1-cm zone of surrounding hepatic parenchyma.

larger than 2.5 cm require more than one deployment of the needle electrode. For larger tumors, multiple placements and deployments of the electrode array may be necessary to completely destroy the tumor (Figs. 30-53 and 30-54). Treatment is planned such that the zones of coagulative necrosis overlap to ensure complete destruction of the tumor. Typically, the array is first placed at the most posterior interface between the tumor and nondiseased liver parenchyma, and then the needle is repositioned and the array is redeployed anteriorly at 2.0- to 2.5-cm intervals within the tissue. In order to mimic a surgical margin in these unresectable tumors, the needle electrode is used to produce a thermal lesion that incorporates not only the tumor, but also nonmalignant liver parenchyma in a zone 1 cm wide

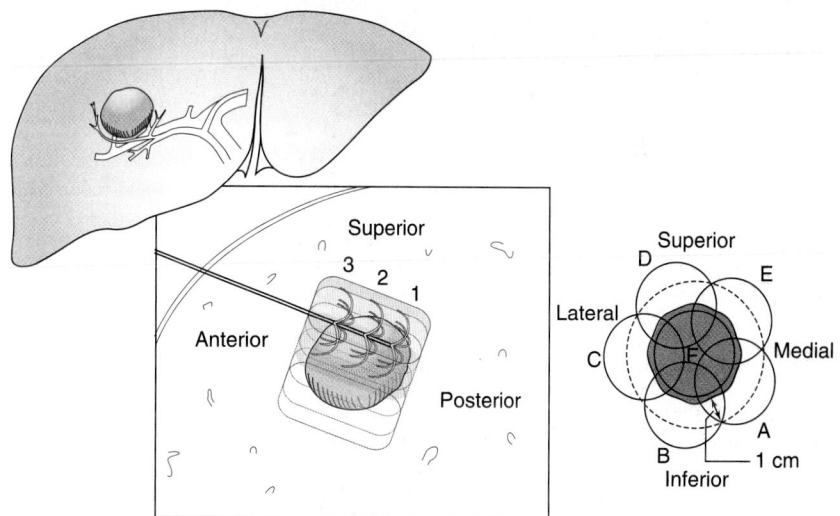

FIG. 30-54. A schematic illustration of a 5-cm diameter malignant tumor in the right lobe of the liver. The upper illustration shows the tumor in relation to the portal venous and hepatic arterial inflow blood supply to the tumor and the surrounding hepatic parenchyma. The inset illustration is a sagittal view showing the multiple overlapping cylinders of RF-induced thermal ablation that must be created to assure complete destruction of the tumor and a surrounding zone of normal hepatic parenchyma. The first areas treated are the more medial aspects of the tumor (A and B, far right illustration superior view) to destroy this region of the tumor and its inflow blood supply. The needle electrode is placed sequentially at the margin of the tumor in the normal parenchyma so that part of the secondary multiple array is opened within the tumor and part is in the surrounding hepatic parenchyma. As demonstrated in the central inset illustration, the needle is first placed at the posterior interface of tumor and normal parenchyma (area 1). After this area has been completely treated, the array is retracted and the needle is pulled back to area 2, and the array is deployed and treatment performed. Finally, the more anterior or superficial interface between tumor and parenchyma is treated (area 3) to produce a cylindrical zone of coagulative necrosis. The far right illustration shows an idealized view looking directly down on the tumor to emphasize the RF treatment planning. Overlapping cylinders of thermal ablation are created to destroy the entire tumor and a 1-cm zone of surrounding hepatic parenchyma. Included is the sequence of needle electrode placements (A through E) to first treat (A, B) the aspects of the tumor adjacent to its inflow blood supply.

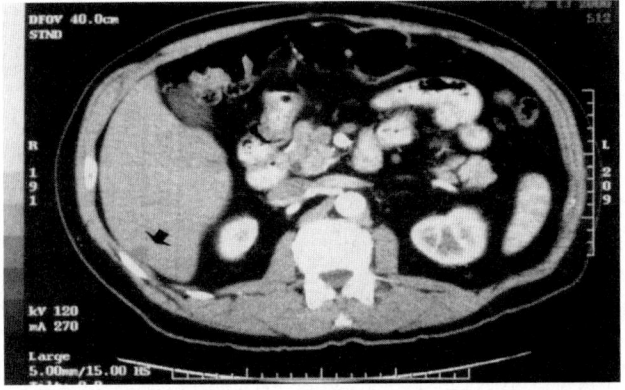

A

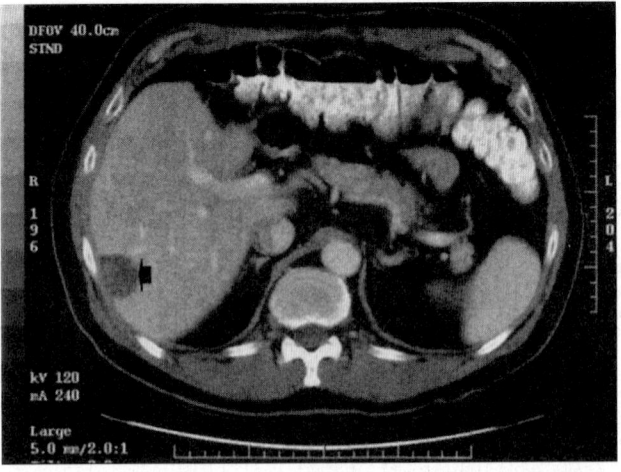

B

FIG. 30-55. *A. A CT scan of a patient demonstrating a metastatic liver tumor in the right lobe of the liver. This is one of six metastatic hepatic lesions identified. The patient underwent resection of tumors in the left lobe of the liver and RFA of tumors in the right lobe. B. CT scan performed 6 months after RFA of the tumor in the right lobe of the liver. The radiofrequency cavitary lesion is larger than the original treated tumor. Treatment is planned to destroy the entire tumor and a surrounding zone of normal parenchyma to reduce the probability of local recurrence.*

surrounding the tumor. Tumors in proximity to major blood vessels also may require additional probe deployment and duration of RFA, as these structures can act as heat sinks. CT scans performed after RFA of primary or metastatic liver tumors initially demonstrate a cystic-density lesion larger than the original tumor; the size of this cystic area decreases slightly over time (Fig. 30-55).

Indications for Radiofrequency Ablation of Liver Tumors

RF energy has been used to produce coagulative necrosis in hepatic malignancies in patients who did not meet the criteria for resectability of HCC and metastatic liver tumors, and yet were candidates for a liver-directed procedure based on the presence of disease confined to the liver.[151,152] The selection of patients to be treated with RFA is based on rational principles and goals. Any local therapy for malignant hepatic tumors, be it surgical resection, RFA, or some other tumor ablative technique, is generally performed with curative intent; however, a significant proportion of patients will

subsequently develop hepatic or extrahepatic recurrence from their coexistent micrometastatic disease. Occasionally, patients with tumor types usually associated with disseminated, systemic metastatic disease, such as breast or renal cancer, may be considered for RFA if they have been treated with at least 6 months of effective systemic chemotherapy, and have only liver metastasis. This latter group of patients is a small, highly selected subset from which a few patients will derive long-term survival benefit from aggressive liver-directed therapy.[153] Thus RFA should be performed only in patients with no preoperative or intraoperative evidence of extrahepatic disease, and only for tumor histologies with a reasonable probability of disease metastatic only to the liver. The notable exception to considering RFA in patients with low-volume extrahepatic disease and multiple liver metastases is the subgroup of patients with functional endocrine syndromes from neuroendocrine tumor liver metastases, as some patients can survive years with their disease. The goal of RFA in this group is to perform a safe, palliative, rather than curative, treatment.

RFA can be used to treat patients with a solitary hepatic tumor in a location that precludes a margin-negative hepatic resection, such as a tumor nestled between the inferior vena cava and the entry of the three hepatic veins into the liver (Fig. 30-56). The only area of the liver to avoid when treating a tumor with RFA is the hilar plate where the portal vein and hepatic arterial branches enter the liver. While these blood vessels can tolerate the heat associated with the RFA treatment, the large bile ducts coursing with them do not, and biliary fistulae or strictures are likely to occur. RFA-induced biliary injury can be minimized by excluding patients with tumors involving the perihilar region. Lastly, RFA is ideally suited to treat small HCCs in cirrhotic patients who may not be candidates for resection based on the severity of their liver dysfunction.[152]

With the exception of the previously noted group of patients with functional neuroendocrine tumor liver metastases, candidates for RFA should have primary or metastatic liver tumors with no clinically evident extrahepatic disease. Given the limitations of currently available RFA equipment, RF treatment for tumors greater than 5.0 cm in diameter must be applied judiciously, if at all. The local recurrence rate in larger tumors is much higher due to incomplete coagulative necrosis of malignant cells near the tumor periphery.[151,152]

When considering patients for a combined approach of liver resection of large tumors and RFA of smaller lesions in the opposite lobe, standard surgical considerations apply. Thus an adequate volume of perfused, functional hepatic parenchyma must remain to avoid postoperative liver failure. The volume of liver that must remain varies from patient to patient, depending on the presence of normal liver versus diseased liver related to chronic hepatitis viral infection, ethanol abuse, or some other cause of chronic hepatic inflammation leading to cirrhosis. RFA does not replace standard hepatic resection in patients with resectable disease. In contrast, RFA expands the population of patients who may be treated with aggressive liver-directed therapy in attempts to improve survival, quality of life, or palliation. Some patients heretofore not candidates for surgical therapy because of the presence of bilobar liver tumors now can be treated with a combination of liver resection and RFA.

Radiofrequency Ablation of Primary Liver Tumors

The use of RFA to treat primary liver tumors was recently reported.[152] The HCC tumor size treated with RFA in this patient population ranged from 1 to 7 cm in greatest dimension.[153] The patients who underwent RFA of HCC nodules less than 2 cm in diameter had either small satellite tumors treated near a larger tumor

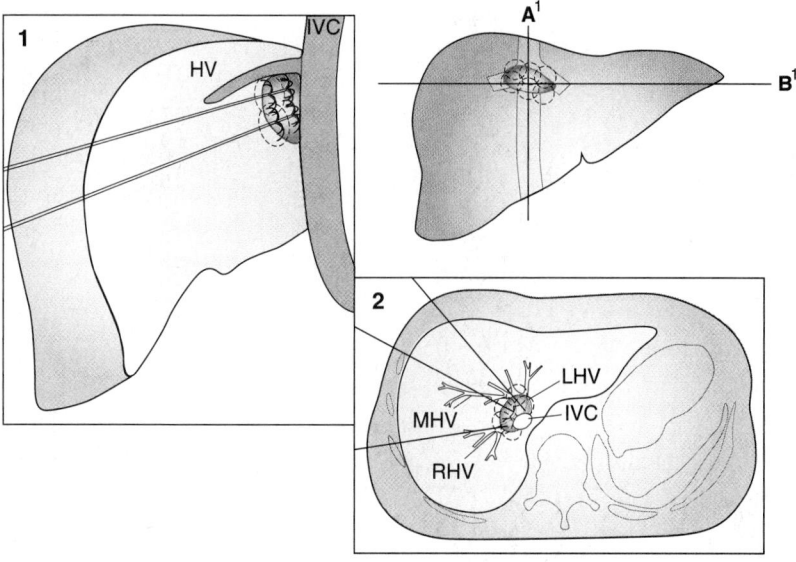

A

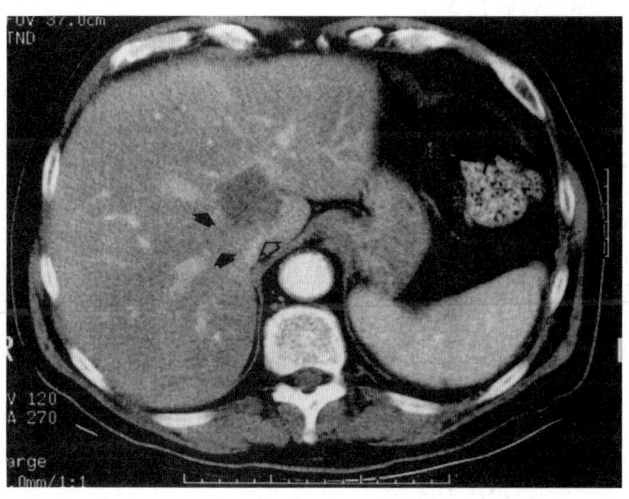

B

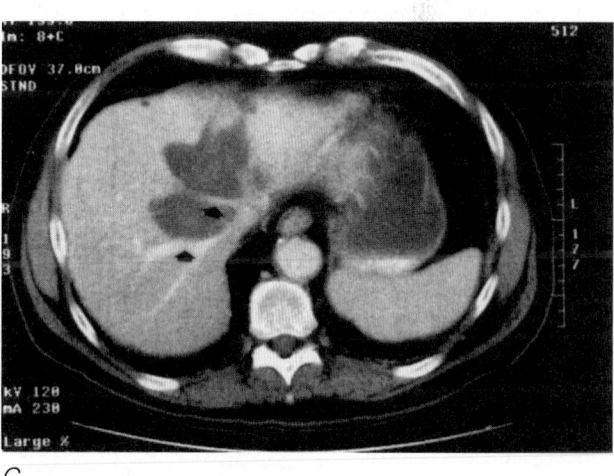

C

FIG. 30-56. *A.* Illustration of a malignant hepatic tumor abutting the inferior vena cava *(IVC)* and nestled under the right, middle, and left hepatic veins *(RHV, MHV,* and *LHV).* View (1) demonstrates the sagittal view of the tumor lying on the IVC and abutting a hepatic vein. Multiple insertions of the RF ablation needle electrode are required, with the secondary multiple array opened just outside the IVC first, and then sequentially withdrawn to treat the more anterior aspects of tumor. View (2) shows the axial view with lines indicating the multiple placements of the RF needle electrode needed to produce thermal ablation of the entire tumor and a surrounding zone of nondiseased hepatic parenchyma. Blood flow in the IVC and hepatic veins prevents thermal destruction or thrombosis of these major vessels. *B.* CT scan of a malignant liver tumor abutting the IVC and hepatic veins. *C.* CT scan 6 months after RFA shows no evidence of viable tumor and patent right and middle hepatic veins. The radiofrequency cavitary lesion is larger than the original tumor.

or multifocal small tumors involving more than one couinaud segment. As the size of the tumor increased, the number of deployments of the multiple array needle electrode and the total time of applying RF energy increased. Primary liver tumors tend to be highly vascular, therefore a vascular heat sink phenomenon may contribute to the extended ablation times.

All 110 HCC patients in this study were followed for a minimum of 12 months after RFA; the median follow-up period was 19 months.[152] Percutaneous or intraoperative RFA was performed in 76 (69%) and 34 patients (31%), respectively, and a total of 149 discrete HCC tumor nodules were treated with RFA. The median diameter of tumors treated percutaneously (2.8 cm) was smaller than lesions treated during laparotomy (4.6 cm). Local tumor recurrence at the RFA site developed in four patients (3.6%), all with tumors greater than 4.0 cm in diameter; all four subsequently developed recurrent HCC in other areas of the liver. New liver tumors or extrahepatic metastases developed in 50 patients (45.5%), but 56 patients (50.9%) had no evidence of recurrence. Clearly, a longer follow-up period is required to establish long-term, disease-free, and overall survival rates.

Procedure-related complications were minimal in patients with HCC. There were no treatment-related deaths, but complications developed in 12.7% of the HCC patients.[152] These complications included symptomatic pleural effusion, fever, pain, subcutaneous hematoma, subcapsular liver hematoma, and ventricular fibrillation. In addition, one patient with Child class B cirrhosis developed ascites, and another class B cirrhotic patient developed bleeding in the ablated tumor 4 days after RFA, requiring hepatic arterial embolization and transfusion of two units of packed red blood cells. All patient events resolved with appropriate clinical management within 1 week following the RFA procedure, with the exception of the development of ascites, which resolved with the use of diuretics within 3 weeks of the RFA treatment. Development of thermal injury to adjacent organs or structures, hepatic insufficiency, renal insufficiency, or coagulopathy following the application of RF energy to the target tumors was not reported for any of the patients. The overall complication rate following RFA of HCC was low, which is particularly notable because there were 50 Child class A, 31 class B, and 29 class C cirrhotic patients treated.

Radiofrequency Ablation of Metastatic Liver Tumors

In these authors' experience, the sizes of the metastatic liver tumors treated with RF energy ranged from 0.5 to 12 cm in greatest dimension.[151] As was expected, as the size of the tumor increased, the number of deployments of the needle electrode and the total elapsed time of applying RF energy increased.[152] For tumors in which the largest dimension was less than 1 cm, typically only one deployment was necessary, while those lesions greater than 1 cm in diameter were treated with two or more separate deployments of the needle electrode array. More than one deployment of the electrode array was used in metastatic tumors greater than 1 cm in diameter because over 70% of the metastatic tumors treated abutted a major intrahepatic blood vessel; additional RFA near the vessel was performed to ensure complete killing of tumor cells.

Procedure-related complications were infrequent in patients with metastatic liver tumors. A few of the sites (10%) of intraoperative RFA expressed bleeding when the needle was withdrawn from the needle electrode track, but in all cases this was minimal (less than 5 mL) and controlled easily with electrocauterization of the puncture site at the surface of the liver. Complications following RFA arose in less than 10% of the patients. The complications included a single intrahepatic abscess, fever, pain, two biliary fistulae, and perihepatic abscess in an area of liver resection in two patients. All events resolved with appropriate clinical management within 1 month following the procedure. Thermal injury to adjacent organs or tissues, hepatic insufficiency, renal insufficiency, or coagulopathy following RFA of the hepatic metastases was not reported in any of the patients.

Local recurrence or persistence of metastatic tumors at the site of the RFA occurred in approximately 7% of the patients, and over 80% of the local recurrences developed in tumors more than 5 cm in diameter. All regions of recurrence or persistence were at the periphery of the necrotic tissue of the ablated tumors (Fig. 30-57). No recurrence or persistence was noted within the center of the thermal lesions produced by RFA. New occurrences of additional hepatic or extrahepatic metastases were found in 46% of patients within 18 months post-RFA. The use of a combination of regional and systemic chemotherapy after RFA of colorectal cancer liver metastases to reduce recurrence and improve survival is currently under study by the authors.

In another recent report, the results of 109 patients with 172 metastatic hepatic lesions who underwent percutaneous RFA were described.[154] The median follow-up period was 3 years (range 5

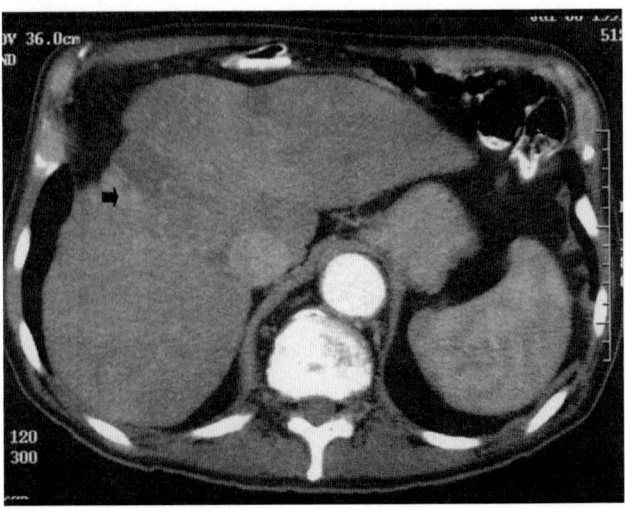

FIG. 30-57. A CT scan performed 6 months after RF ablation of a hepatocellular carcinoma. An area of contrast-enhancing ingrowth of tissue into the cavity represents incomplete thermal ablation and local recurrence.

to 52 months), and local control was achieved in 121 (70%) of the lesions, but local recurrence developed in 51 (30%). Of these 51 lesions, 24 had repeat RFA and 11 (45%) achieved local control. A significant difference in local recurrence rates was observed when comparing lesions less than 3 cm (16%) to those greater than 3 cm (56%) in diameter. Median time to local recurrence was 16 months. There were no deaths and only one major complication (colonic perforation) after 162 RFA sessions (0.6%), with seven minor complications (4%). New metastases developed in 50% of the patients at a median time to recurrence of 12 months after RFA. Overall 2- and 3-year survival rates were 67 and 33%, respectively, with a median survival of 30 months.[154] Thus percutaneous RFA was associated with a high incomplete treatment (local recurrence) rate due to less accurate resolution with transabdominal ultrasonography, making precise needle electrode placement to ablate the entire tumor and a surrounding rim of hepatic parenchyma more difficult.

Using a laparoscopic approach with a multiprobe array monopolar RFA electrode, the results from 43 patients with 181 lesions, of which 170 were metastatic tumors, were reported.[155] The size of the necrotic cavity produced by RFA was larger than the original tumor on posttreatment CT scans in all but three cases, two of which recurred locally. Local control was achieved in 88% of the lesions (72% of patients) with at least 3 months follow-up. Although the follow-up period is too short to establish long-term local and distant tumor recurrence rates, several predictors of local RFA treatment failure were identified. These included: (1) an ablation lesion size less than original tumor size (suggesting incomplete RFA) on posttreatment CT scans, (2) adenocarcinoma or sarcoma metastases (as compared to neuroendocrine metastases or HCC), (3) tumor size greater than 3 cm, and (4) laparoscopic ultrasound evidence of gross vascular invasion by tumor.[155]

In a larger series, 231 tumors in 84 patients were treated with 91 RFA procedures.[156] The majority of patients had metastatic lesions (213 lesions in 73 patients), and 51 of the 91 treatments were with RFA alone. The other 40 treatments included RFA combined with surgical resection, cryoablation, and/or hepatic artery infusion of chemotherapy. Of the 91 treatments, 39 patients underwent RFA at laparotomy, 27 during laparoscopy, and 25 were treated percutaneously. Tumors treated with RFA ranged in size from 0.3 to 9.0 cm. There were seven major complications (8%), resulting in three deaths (4%). At a median follow-up period of 9 months (range 1 to 27 months), 15 patients (18%) had developed a local recurrence. Of the remaining 69 patients, 34 were alive without disease, 14 were alive with new metastatic disease, and 21 had died from their disease; new hepatic tumors or extrahepatic disease had developed in 35 patients. Although this study is challenging to interpret due to the use of multiple therapies and the combination of primary and metastatic liver lesions in the analyses, a few points are worth highlighting. In agreement with other reports, recurrence rates were related to the original size of the tumor. The mean diameter of lesions that developed a local recurrence (4.1 cm) was significantly larger than the mean diameter of those that did not (2.8 cm). However, the likelihood of recurrence was not related to the numbers of lesions ablated, colorectal versus noncolorectal metastases, or RFA treatment approach (laparotomy, laparoscopy, or percutaneously). New hepatic tumors or extrahepatic disease developed in 42% of the patients, a number similar to other reports. The authors also noted that the use of intraoperative ultrasound (either open or laparoscopic) detected additional intrahepatic tumors that were subsequently ablated in 25 of 66 patients (38%) that were not evident on preoperative imaging, suggesting a major advantage for open or laparoscopic RFA combined with intraoperative ultrasound over the percutaneous approach.[156]

Neuroendocrine tumors metastatic to the liver often produce symptoms secondary to excessive hormone production and release. Although only a minority of patients with neuroendocrine liver metastases may be curable by surgical techniques, significant symptomatic relief can be obtained by debulking, which may include resection combined with RFA, or RFA alone. One group reported 18 patients with 115 neuroendocrine tumors (carcinoid, islet cell, or medullary thyroid cancers) treated with RFA.[157] The mean lesion size was 3.2 cm (range 1.3 to 10.0 cm), and the average number of lesions ablated per patient was six (range 1 to 14). There were two complications consisting of atrial fibrillation in one patient and upper GI bleeding in another. Fifteen patients (83%) with 100 lesions were followed for a mean of 12.1 months (range 3 to 35 months). Local recurrence in tumors treated with RFA was detected in six lesions (6%) in three of these 15 patients (20%); three patients died of progressive metastatic disease during follow-up. While the exact number was not indicated, the authors reported that most patients had significant improvement in hormone-related symptoms following RFA.[157]

Interstitial Laser Hyperthermic Ablation

Direct thermal destruction of hepatic tumors using laser energy is known by several acronyms: LTA (laser thermal ablation), ILT (interstitial laser thermotherapy), ILP (interstitial laser photocoagulation), and LITT (laser-induced interstitial thermotherapy). These acronyms and phrases all describe the same type of thermal treatment, and because LITT is the most common acronym that appears in the medical literature, it will be used throughout the remainder of this section.

Background and Principles of Laser-Induced Interstitial Thermotherapy

As described by the name of this thermal treatment modality, LITT requires placement of a laser fiber or fibers directly into the tumor or tissue to be treated. Thus LITT is a type of contact mode laser therapy. While the mechanism of action is different than that of RFA, LITT produces lethal thermal injury to tumor cells in an identical fashion. Prolonged heating of tumor cells to 45 to 55°C leads to cell death, while short exposure of cells to temperatures that exceed 60°C causes irreversible cell damage and death from protein denaturation, inhibition of protein synthesis, breaking of chemical bonds in DNA and RNA molecules, and loss of integrity in lipid bilayers. Application of LITT at low power produces a progressively enlarging zone of radiant and conductive tissue heating around the laser fiber or fibers. Irreversible cytotoxic effects develop in cells that are heated above 55 to 60°C.

LITT produces local tissue heating when photons from low-intensity laser energy interact with molecular chromophores that are inherent to all mammalian cells. Photochemical effects may be accentuated by the exogenous administration of photosensitizing agents like porfimer sodium, but the presence of natural cellular chromophores is sufficient to produce exothermic photochemical reactions. Naturally occurring chromophores that interact with laser light include hemoglobin, myoglobin, bilirubin, cytochrome pigments in mitochondria, melanin, xanthophyll, rhodopsin, and lipofuscin.[158]

Laser light in LITT is scattered, reflected, and absorbed to varying degrees, depending on the wavelength of light, the applied laser energy, and the specific photoabsorptive properties of the tissue. The photoabsorptive characteristics of tissues can vary markedly from area to area within a tumor or normal tissue depending on tissue composition, vascularity, fibrosis, and necrosis. Natural chromophores have a strong dependence on wavelengths in the near infrared range for photochemical reactions to occur. This is fortunate because penetration depth increases with increasing wavelength of light. Thus, LITT utilizes diode lasers (wavelength 800 to 980 nm), or more frequently, neodymium:yttrium aluminum garnet (Nd:YAG) lasers (wavelength 1064 nm).[158,159] Laser light at 1064 nm generated by Nd:YAG lasers has an tissue penetration depth of up to 10 to 12 mm.[158] In contrast to other medical laser applications, where high-energy laser light is applied briefly to achieve rapid photocoagulation, LITT uses low-energy (3 to 20 watts) laser energy in the continuous mode applied over 2 to 20 minutes. Slow heating of tissue must be achieved by LITT to avoid carbonization and vaporization of tissue near the light-emitting portion of the laser fiber. Rapid production of a tissue coagulum from carbonization reduces optical penetration into the tissue and severely limits expansion of the zone of heated tissue with temperatures sufficient to produce lethal injury to tumor cells. In general, penetration of tumor tissue is greater than in normal tissue by approximately 33% at the 1064-nm wavelength, but rapid coagulative necrosis reduces optical penetration by up to 25% in both normal and tumor tissues.[160]

Similarly to RFA, transient hepatic inflow occlusion during LITT can be used to double the volume of thermal injury using single-fiber systems, and can produce up to a fivefold increase in the volume of thermal coagulation by using a four-fiber system.[161] Portal venous occlusion has been shown to be more important than hepatic arterial occlusion in producing this increase in the volume of thermal necrosis, suggesting that pretreatment transarterial hepatic arterial embolization associated with percutaneous LITT is less useful than laparoscopic or open surgical occlusion of both portal venous and hepatic arterial flow with a Pringle maneuver.

Results of Laser-Induced Interstitial Thermotherapy for Malignant Hepatic Tumors

The majority of reports describing LITT for the treatment of liver malignancies describe a percutaneous approach for intratumoral placement of the laser fiber using ultrasonographic or MRI monitoring during therapy. There are recent reports of use of LITT via laparoscopy or open laparotomy, particularly using a multifiber beam splitting laser system, which also permits hepatic vascular

inflow occlusion during the treatment. The disadvantage of a laparoscopic or open surgical approach is the need for general anesthesia and a longer recovery time from a more invasive procedure.[158]
However, the benefits may outweigh these disadvantages in patients
who are undergoing treatment of multiple tumors, where the percutaneous treatment time in the MRI scanner is excessive, or if
tumors are located near key vascular or biliary structures where
intraoperative ultrasonographic guidance to place the laser fiber is
desirable. LITT suffers from the same problem inherent in the other
recently developed, thermal ablation techniques, namely a lack of
long-term follow-up data to establish disease-free and overall patient
survival rates.

A study of 55 patients with colorectal liver metastases treated
with LITT at a mean follow-up of only 10 months was reported.[162]
The mean number of percutaneous LITT sessions required to completely treat all detectable tumor was 2.2 sessions per patient.
The mean survival at 12 months was 86%. Another group studied
104 patients, 77 with HCC and 27 with hepatic metastases, treated
with ultrasound-guided percutaneous LITT with a mean follow-up
period of less than 5 months.[163] Complete destruction of tumor as assessed by triphasic contrast-enhanced CT scans was noted in 82%
of the HCC tumors and 77% of the hepatic metastases. Three of
the cirrhotic HCC patients developed liver failure after LITT, with
one of these patients dying 2 months after treatment. No data were
provided on any re-treatment sessions of the patients with incomplete destruction of the tumor after LITT, nor was there mention
of local recurrence rates in lesions thought to be completely destroyed based on the results of the initial posttreatment imaging
studies.

The largest reported experience with LITT consists of 705 patients with 1981 metastatic liver tumors.[164] A total of 1653 treatment
sessions consisting of 7148 laser applications were required to treat
the metastatic liver tumors in these patients. All treatments were
performed with percutaneous insertion of the laser fiber using real-
time MRI monitoring. The local tumor control rate was 98%, based
on MRI evaluation 6 months after completion of all LITT treatments in the individual patients. The mean survival time for patients
with unresectable colorectal liver metastases treated by LITT was
42 months, with a 3-year actuarial survival rate of 50%. In a smaller
subset of patients with breast cancer liver metastases, the mean survival was 4.3 years after LITT.[164] The overall complication rate
in this large series was 7.5%, but the authors report that most of
the complications were mild and were treated in the outpatient setting. The rate of more significant complications requiring hospitalization, interventional therapies, or prolonged treatment was 1.3%.
This is consistent with other reports of complication rates of less
than 2% in patients treated with LITT.[159] Reported complications
include pneumothorax, hemothorax, transient bile leaks, subcapsular hemorrhage or bleeding from the needle track, bradycardia,
tachycardia, right upper quadrant abdominal pain, and transient
hyperthermia.

The major limitation of single-fiber LITT is an inability to
achieve large volumes of tumor necrosis. Another disadvantage is
the need to perform multiple treatment sessions in most patients. It is
possible that LITT may become a more clinically useful and widely
applied treatment if improvements such as multiple fiber beam splitting systems, diffuser fiber tips, pharmacologic thermosensitization,
and radiologic or direct surgical occlusion of hepatic inflow are able
to overcome these problems. Presently, there are inadequate data on
local tumor recurrence rates and long-term survival rates after LITT
to perform a rigorous assessment of its future as a durable treatment
modality for hepatic malignancies.

Microwave Coagulation Therapy for Hepatic Tumors

Background and Principles of Microwave Coagulation Therapy

Microwave coagulation was initially developed in the early
1980s to achieve hemostasis along the plane of transection during hepatic resection.[165] Microwave coagulation of tissue surfaces
was slower than electrocautery units and produced deeper areas of
tissue necrosis. While microwave coagulation has not been useful
during hepatic resection, the extended area of tissue necrosis led
to investigation of use of microwave coagulation therapy (MCT) to
treat unresectable hepatic malignancies.

The microwave generators developed for MCT produce microwaves with a frequency of 2450 MHz and a wavelength of
12 cm.[166] Biologically, microwaves applied to living tissues produce dielectric heat by stimulation of water molecules within the
tissue and cells. The rapid agitation of water molecules within cells
and tissues with direct application of microwaves produces rapid
frictional heating and coagulative necrosis. The microwave generators available for clinical use have an output of 70 to 90 watts. The
microwave-emitting needle (14- to 22-gauge) is placed directly into
the hepatic tumor to be treated, usually using ultrasonographic guidance, then is attached to the microwave generator, the generator is
activated, and each area of the tumor is treated for 30 to 60 seconds
at 70 to 90 watts of power. The rapid generation of heat using MCT
produces 10- to 25-mm zones of coagulative necrosis after only
30 to 60 seconds. The lesions can range from spherical to elliptical in shape. The rapid development of coagulative necrosis within
the tissue around the MCT needle produces a tissue coagulum that
inhibits further dissipation of heat into the tissue.

The small areas of coagulation produced by MCT requires that
the needle be advanced at 5- to 10-mm intervals throughout the area
to be treated and surrounding parenchyma to create multiple overlapping zones of coagulative necrosis. For tumors larger than 2 cm in
diameter, multiple MCT needle placements are required to produce
overlapping zones of coagulative necrosis in the tumor and in a surrounding rim of hepatic parenchyma. Like RFA and LITT, MCT can
be performed percutaneously using ultrasound or CT guidance for
needle placement, or can be performed laparoscopically or during
an open surgical procedure using intraoperative ultrasound guidance
to place the MCT needle.

Results of Microwave Coagulation Therapy for Treatment of Malignant Hepatic Tumors

The overwhelming majority of reports describing MCT to treat
hepatic malignancies come from Japan, where this technique was
first used in 1988. There, MCT has been used principally to treat
cirrhotic HCC patients. Most of the patients treated with MCT, even
those with a solitary tumor less than 3 cm in size, were not candidates
for resection because of the severity of their cirrhosis. A study of
19 patients with unresectable HCC reported that MCT was performed during laparotomy in 12 patients, laparoscopically in five
patients, and using a thoracotomy approach in two patients with tumors at the dome of the liver.[167] A solitary HCC tumor was treated
in 13 patients, while the remaining six patients had between two and
five HCC tumors treated with MCT. MCT was performed to palliate
symptoms from a large tumor in six of the 19 patients who had additional intrahepatic or extrahepatic metastases. The mean size of the
tumors treated with MCT was 21 mm (range 5 to 90 mm), and the
mean duration of operation was 4.7 hours (range 1.8 to 7.0 hours).

The reproducible and reliable zone of complete coagulative necrosis around the MCT needle electrode is only 10 mm; thus the mean number of electrode insertions to treat the HCC tumors was 46 (range 10 to 135). The authors report that the follow-up period in these patients ranged from 4 to 64 months; there were two patients treated with curative intent who were alive 47 and 64 months, respectively, after MCT, with no evidence of recurrent or new metastatic HCC. In the entire group of 19 patients, six patients had died of recurrent HCC or progressive liver failure, 10 were alive without radiographic evidence of recurrent HCC, and three were alive with evidence of new HCC metastases.[167] The authors reported that there was no evidence of local recurrence in 28 of the 31 nodules (90%) treated with MCT. However, it is difficult to assess the true local recurrence rate, because most of the patients were treated with hepatic arterial chemoembolization after MCT.

A recent report evaluated the risk factors for distant recurrence of HCC after treatment with MCT or RFA.[168] A total of 92 patients with HCC tumors less than 3 cm in diameter were treated with MCT (68 patients) or RFA (16 patients). All patients were treated percutaneously or laparoscopically. This was a nonrandomized study, so MCT or RFA was selected as a treatment option based on the preference of the treating surgeon. Eighty-four patients were followed for 12 to 44 months after treatment (median follow-up period of 22 months); the remaining eight patients died before 12 months because of hepatic failure (five patients), HCC progression (two patients), or pneumonia (one patient). In the 84 evaluable patients, the 1-year survival rate was 99% and the 3-year survival rate was 78%. During the follow-up period, distant recurrence of HCC was observed in 22 patients (26%). There is no comment on local recurrence rates after MCT or RFA in any of these patients. The only variables found to be significant in predicting a higher risk for the development of distant metastatic HCC after MCT or RFA were the treatment of more than one HCC nodule, or the presence of chronic hepatitis C infection as the underlying etiology of chronic liver disease.[168]

There is a striking paucity of data on local recurrence rates and complications following MCT to treat HCC or other malignant liver tumors. Some authors mention that MCT should not be performed near the hepatic hilum, where major bile ducts and blood vessels are located, or near any major hepatic blood vessels, suggesting that there is experience with vascular and biliary complications related to treatment of tumors in these locations. It is unlikely that MCT will be widely applied to treat patients with unresectable malignant hepatic tumors unless modifications in equipment and treatment algorithms occur to produce larger zones of coagulative necrosis around the MCT needle.

Adjuvant Treatment of Liver Malignancies

There is no accepted or clinically superior single combination of agents used as postresection adjuvant therapy for colorectal metastases or HCC. A nonrandomized study of 57 patients with colorectal cancer liver metastases who underwent liver resection examined 31 patients who were treated with adjuvant hepatic arterial infusion consisting of 5-fluorouracil (5-FU), doxorubicin, and mitomycin C, while 26 patients were treated with resection alone.[169] The surgical complication rate was not mentioned, nor was there information provided on the incidence or types of toxicities associated with the adjuvant treatment. The 3- and 5-year survival rates in the 26 patients who did not receive adjuvant therapy were 35 and 12%, respectively, compared to 57 and 57%, respectively, for the 31 patients who received adjuvant regional chemotherapy.

Another nonrandomized, prospective study of 110 patients who underwent hepatic resection for colorectal liver metastases included 60 patients who received adjuvant hepatic arterial chemotherapy.[170] The surgical resection was not curative in 26% of patients. Individuals were treated with four different adjuvant chemotherapy regimens consisting of floxuridine (FUDR) alone, FUDR and folinic acid, or 5-FU and folinic acid. There was no difference in the postoperative morbidity or mortality rates comparing patients who did or did not undergo placement of a hepatic artery infusion pump at the time of liver resection. At least five cycles of adjuvant chemotherapy were administered in 48 of the 60 patients (80%). The remaining patients did not complete adjuvant therapy because of problems with occlusion, dislodgment, or leakage from the hepatic arterial catheter. The 3- and 5-year survival rates for patients treated with adjuvant hepatic arterial chemotherapy following curative surgery were 60% and 41%, respectively. These survival rates were significantly better compared to patients treated with curative surgery alone (3- and 5-year survival rates of 43 and 25%, respectively). The median survival time in patients treated with curative hepatic resection and adjuvant hepatic arterial chemotherapy was 54 months. The most common toxicity related to regional chemotherapy was stomatitis in patients who received 5-FU, while transient increases in serum hepatic enzyme levels was the most common occurrence noted after administration of FUDR. Of the 33 patients who received adjuvant hepatic arterial infusion with FUDR, two (6%) developed biliary sclerosis.

A retrospective, nonrandomized study of 174 patients who underwent resection of colorectal liver metastases compared the outcome of the 78 patients who received adjuvant hepatic arterial infusion chemotherapy to 30 who had adjuvant portal venous infusion chemotherapy and 66 who had no adjuvant treatment.[171] The adjuvant hepatic arterial infusion or portal venous infusion chemotherapy regimen consisted of 5-FU, aclarubicin suspended in an oily contrast medium, and mitomycin C. A total of six patients (3.4%), including one in the hepatic artery infusion group, one in the portal vein infusion group, and four in the resection alone group, died within 60 days of hepatic resection secondary to hepatic failure. The toxicity of adjuvant chemotherapy consisted of nausea, emesis, and diarrhea, which occurred in 59% of the patients receiving hepatic arterial infusion chemotherapy and in 77% of the patients receiving portal venous infusion chemotherapy. Most of the patients required dose reduction of their chemotherapy related to hematologic toxicity, but no patient developed biliary sclerosis or drug-induced hepatitis. The actuarial 5-year, disease-free survival rates for the hepatic arterial infusion, portal venous infusion, and resection-alone groups were 35%, 13%, and 9%, respectively. The corresponding overall 5-year survival rates were 40%, 17%, and 20%, respectively. The disease-free and overall survival rate was significantly better for the group of patients treated with hepatic arterial infusion chemotherapy compared to patients treated with portal venous infusion chemotherapy or surgery alone. Patients treated with hepatic arterial infusion chemotherapy had a significantly lower rate of recurrence of disease in the liver, while portal venous infusion chemotherapy did not reduce the incidence of hepatic recurrence compared to patients treated with surgery alone.

A randomized, prospective trial from the United States assigned 156 patients undergoing resection of colorectal cancer liver metastases to one of two adjuvant treatment arms.[172] Patients received either 6 monthly cycles of systemic 5-FU and folinic acid or hepatic arterial infusion chemotherapy with FUDR and dexamethasone plus systemic 5-FU, with or without folinic acid. The patients were assigned randomly at the time of liver resection to one of the two treatment arms, and were stratified according to previous systemic chemotherapy treatment and number of liver metastases. There was a significant improvement in actuarial overall 2-year survival and a lower rate of hepatic recurrence in the group treated with regional combined with systemic chemotherapy (86%, 2-year actuarial survival) compared to the group treated with adjuvant systemic chemotherapy alone (72%, 2-year actuarial survival). With a median follow-up period of 63 months, the median survival in the combined regional and systemic chemotherapy group was 72 months versus 59 months in the patients who received only adjuvant systemic therapy. Chemotherapy-related side effects occurred with equal frequency in the two treatment arms, but the rate of diarrhea and abnormalities in serum liver tests was higher in patients in the combined regional plus systemic chemotherapy arm. Many of the patients in the combined regional and systemic therapy arm were unable to complete the planned 6 months of adjuvant therapy because of chemotherapy-induced elevations in serum liver tests.

Adjuvant therapy after resection of HCC also has been studied. A randomized, prospective trial assigned patients to a single postoperative dose of ^{131}I-lipiodol or no further treatment.[173] Of the 43 patients recruited to the trial, 21 received a single hepatic arterial infusion of ^{131}I-lipiodol 6 weeks after liver resection and 22 received no adjuvant treatment. With a median follow-up period of 35 months, recurrent HCC developed in six of the 21 patients (29%) who received adjuvant ^{131}I-lipiodol, compared with 13 of the 22 (59%) control patients. There was a significant improvement in median disease-free survival in the treatment group (57.2 months) compared with the surgery alone group (13.6 months). Additionally, the 3-year overall survival was significantly improved in the treatment versus control group, 86.4% versus 46.3%, respectively. There was no significant toxicity related to the single postoperative intra-arterial infusion of ^{131}I-lipiodol.

Data regarding the effect of neoadjuvant therapy for unresectable colorectal cancer recently has been published. In 701 patients initially considered unresectable and then treated with systemic 5-FU, folinic acid, and oxaliplatin, 95 (13%) achieved significant reduction in tumor size and subsequently underwent a potentially curative hepatic resection.[174] The mean number of chemotherapy sessions required to achieve tumor reduction sufficient to allow resection was 10.6 over a 10-month period. There was no perioperative mortality and the postoperative complication rate was 23%. The overall 5-year survival rate in these 95 patients downstaged with neoadjuvant therapy was 34%. When 5-year survival was evaluated based on the initial reason the patients were felt to have unresectable disease, it was determined that 5-year survival was 60% in patients with large tumors, 49% for tumors located near major vascular structures preventing a margin-negative resection, 34% for patients with multinodular disease, and 18% for those with evidence of extrahepatic disease at the time of presentation.

Neoadjuvant and adjuvant therapy trials have indicated that an increased number of patients may be considered for resection with aggressive preoperative therapy, and the disease-free and overall survival rates of patients may be improved using adjuvant therapy after resection of colorectal cancer liver metastases and HCC. In a phase II trial at the University of Texas M.D. Anderson Cancer Center, these authors have found that adjuvant hepatic arterial infusion chemotherapy with either RFA alone or RFA combined with resection of colorectal cancer liver metastases reduced the incidence of hepatic recurrence of disease.[175] The follow-up period in this cohort of patients is not yet sufficient to allow analysis of long-term survival. Entry into clinical trials of neoadjuvant and

adjuvant therapy after resection or thermal ablation of malignant liver tumors should be considered in all patients undergoing surgical treatment.

Overall, the results from neoadjuvant therapy trials to downstage patients with primary or metastatic liver tumors in an attempt to convert unresectable to resectable disease indicates that only 10 to 20% of such patients will actually undergo a resection. Most patients will have disease that is too widespread or will fail to respond sufficiently to the preoperative treatment regimen to be considered for surgical treatment. Nonetheless, the survival rate in patients who do achieve significant tumor downstaging is similar to the long-term survival rates for patients who have resectable disease at the time of the initial diagnosis of their malignant liver tumors. Further investigation of multimodality neoadjuvant treatments is ongoing in an attempt to increase the proportion of patients who become resectable and to improve the overall outcome.

References

1. Couinaud C: *Le Foie. Etudes Anatomiques et chirugicales*. Paris: Masson & Cie, 1953, p 1.
2. Strasberg S, Belghiti J, Clavien P-A, et al: The Brisbane 2000 terminology of liver anatomy and resections. Terminology committee of the International Hepato-Pancreato-Biliary Association. *HPB Surg* 2:333, 2000.
3. Otero AC, Strasberg SM: Division of the left hemiliver in man—segments, sectors, or sections. *Liver Transp Surg* 4:226, 1998.
4. Gruttadauria S, Foglieni CS, Doria C, et al: The hepatic artery in liver transplantation and surgery: Vascular anomalies in 701 cases. *Clin Transplant* 15:359, 2001.
5. Jones RM, Hardy KJ: The hepatic artery: A reminder of surgical anatomy. *J R Coll Surg Edinb* 46:168, 2001.
6. Kawarada Y, Das BC, Taoka H: Anatomy of the hepatic hilar area: The plate system. *J Hepatobiliary Pancreat Surg* 7:580, 2000.
7. Launois B, Maddern G, Tay KH: The Glissonian approach of the hilum. *Swiss Surg* 5:143, 1999.
8. Jungermann K, Stumpel F: Role of hepatic, intrahepatic and hepatoenteral nerves in the regulation of carbohydrate metabolism and hemodynamics of the liver and intestine. *Hepatogastroenterology* 46:1414, 1999.
9. Crawford AR, Lin XZ, Crawford JM: The normal adult human liver biopsy: A quantitative reference standard. *Hepatology* 28:323, 1998.
10. Randle PJ: Regulatory interactions between lipids and carbohydrates: The glucose fatty acid cycle after 35 years. *Diabetes Metab Rev* 14:263, 1998.
11. Kamisako T, Kobayashi Y, Takeuchi K, et al: Recent advances in bilirubin metabolism research: The molecular mechanism of hepatocyte bilirubin transport and its clinical relevance. *J Gastroenterol* 35:659, 2000.
12. Okolicsanyi L, Cavestro GM, Guatti-Zuliani C: Hyperbilirubinemia: Does it matter? *Can J Gastroenterol* 13:663, 1999.
13. Redinger RN: The coming of age of our understanding of the enterohepatic circulation of bile salts. *Am J Surg* 185:168, 2003.
14. Trauner M, Boyer JL: Bile salt transporters: Molecular characterization, function, and regulation. *Physiol Rev* 83:633, 2003.
15. Ros PR, Mortele KJ: Hepatic imaging. An overview. *Clin Liver Dis* 6:1, 2002.
16. Abbitt PL: Ultrasonography of the liver. An update on new applications. *Clin Liver Dis* 6:17, 2002.
17. Tong MJ, Blatt LM, Kao VW: Surveillance for hepatocellular carcinoma in patients with chronic viral hepatitis in the United States of America. *J Gastroenterol Hepatol* 16:553, 2001.
18. Izzo F, Cremona F, Ruffolo F, et al: Outcome of 67 patients with

hepatocellular cancer detected during screening of 1125 patients with chronic hepatitis. *Ann Surg* 227:513, 1998.

19. Blomley MJ, Cooke JC, Unger EC, et al: Microbubble contrast agents: A new era in ultrasound. *BMJ* 322:1222, 2001.

20. John TG, Greig JD, Crosbie JL, et al: Superior staging of liver tumors with laparoscopy and laparoscopic ultrasound. *Ann Surg* 220:711, 1994.

21. Jarnagin WR, Bach AM, Winston CB, et al: What is the yield of intraoperative ultrasonography during partial hepatectomy for malignant disease? *J Am Coll Surg* 192:577, 2001.

22. Fuhrman GM, Curley SA, Hohn DC, et al: Improved survival after resection of colorectal liver metastases. *Ann Surg Oncol* 2:537, 1995.

23. Harisinghani MG, Hahn PF: Computed tomography and magnetic resonance imaging evaluation of liver cancer. *Gastroenterol Clin North Am* 31:759, 2002.

24. Fenchel S, Fleiter TR, Merkle EM: Multislice helical CT of the abdomen. *Eur Radiol* 12:S5, 2002.

25. Vauthey JN, Rousseau DL Jr.: Liver imaging. A surgeon's perspective. *Clin Liver Dis* 6:271, 2002.

26. Mortele KJ, McTavish J, Ros PR: Current techniques of computed tomography. Helical CT, multidetector CT, and 3D reconstruction. *Clin Liver Dis* 6:29, 2002.

27. Valls C, Andia E, Sanchez A, et al: Hepatic metastases from colorectal cancer: Preoperative detection and assessment of resectability with helical CT. *Radiology* 218:55, 2001.

28. Scott DJ, Guthrie JA, Arnold P, et al: Dual phase helical CT versus portal venous phase CT for the detection of colorectal liver metastases: Correlation with intra-operative sonography, surgical and pathological findings. *Clin Radiol* 56:235, 2001.

29. Rode A, Bancel B, Douek P, et al: Small nodule detection in cirrhotic livers: Evaluation with US, spiral CT, and MRI and correlation with pathologic examination of explanted liver. *J Comput Assist Tomogr* 25:327, 2001.

30. Peterson MS, Baron RL: Radiologic diagnosis of hepatocellular carcinoma. *Clin Liver Dis* 5:123, 2001.

31. Beavers KL, Semelka RC: MRI evaluation of the liver. *Semin Liver Dis* 21:161, 2001.

32. Akhurst T, Fong Y: Positron emission tomography in surgical oncology. *Adv Surg* 36:309, 2002.

33. Strasberg SM, Siegal BA: Survival of patients staged by FDG-PET before resection of hepatic metastases from colorectal cancer. *Ann Surg* 235:308, 2002.

34. Strasberg SM, Dehdashti F, Siegel BA, et al: Survival of patients evaluated by FDG-PET before hepatic resection for metastatic colorectal carcinoma: A prospective database study. *Ann Surg* 233:293, 2001.

35. Johnson K, Bakhsh A, Young D, et al: Correlating computed tomography and positron emission tomography scan with operative findings in metastatic colorectal cancer. *Dis Colon Rectum* 44:354, 2001.

36. Topal B, Flamen P, Aerts R, et al: Clinical value of whole-body emission tomography in potentially curable colorectal liver metastases. *Eur J Surg Oncol* 27:175, 2001.

37. Shiomi S, Nishiguchi S, Ishizu H, et al: Usefulness of positron emission tomography with fluorine-18-fluorodeoxyglucose for predicting outcome in patients with hepatocellular carcinoma. *Am J Gastroenterol* 96:1877, 2001.

38. Boushey RP, Dackiw AP: Carcinoid tumors. *Curr Treat Options Oncol* 3:319, 2002.

39. Giger U, Schafer M, Krahenbuhl L: Technique and value of staging laparoscopy. *Digestive Surg* 19:473, 2002.

40. D'Angelica M, Fong Y, Weber S, et al: The role of staging laparoscopy in hepatobiliary malignancy: Prospective analysis of 401 cases. *Ann Surg Oncol* 10:183, 2003.

41. Li D, Friedman SL: Liver fibrogenesis and the role of hepatic stellate cells: New insights and prospects for therapy. *J Gastroenterol Hepatol* 14:618, 1999.

42. Streetz KL, Wustefeld T, Klein C, et al: Mediators of inflammation and acute phase response in the liver. *Cell Mol Biol* 47:661, 2001.

43. Shi B, Wang X, Yang Z: Vascular endothelial growth factors and liver diseases. *Hepato-Gastroenterol* 48:1145, 2001.

44. Maher JJ: Interactions between hepatic stellate cells and the immune system. *Semin Liver Dis* 21:417, 2001.

45. Benyon RC, Arthur MJ: Extracellular matrix degradation and the role of hepatic stellate cells. *Semin Liver Dis* 21:373, 2001.

46. Reynaert H, Thompson MG, Thomas T, et al: Hepatic stellate cells: Role in microcirculation and pathophysiology of portal hypertension. *Gut* 50:571, 2002.

47. Fernandes NF, Schwesinger WH, Hilsenbeck SG, et al: Laparoscopic cholecystectomy and cirrhosis: A case-control study of outcomes. *Liver Transplant* 6:340, 2000.

48. Shah V: Cellular and molecular basis of portal hypertension. *Clin Liver Dis* 5:629, 2001.

49. Bass NM, Yao FY: The role of the interventional radiologist. Transjugular procedures. *Gastrointest Endosc Clin North Am* 11:131, 2001.

50. Slakey DP, Klein AS, Venbrux AC, et al: Budd-Chiari syndrome: Current management options. *Ann Surg* 233:522, 2001.

51. Gordon RD: Liver transplantation and venous disorders of the liver. *Liver Transplant Surg* 3:S41, 1997.

52. Harry R, Wendon J: Management of variceal bleeding. *Curr Opin Crit Care* 8:164, 2002.

53. Bosch J, Garcia-Pagan JC: Prevention of variceal rebleeding. *Lancet* 361:952, 2003.

54. Nagell W, Tonus C, Nier H, et al: Primary prophylactic therapy of esophageal varices—a literature review. *Hepato-Gastroenterol* 49:423, 2002.

55. Luketic VA: Management of portal hypertension after variceal hemorrhage. *Clin Liver Dis* 5:677, 2001.

56. Nader A, Grace ND: Pharmacological prevention of rebleeding. *Gastrointest Endosc Clin North Am* 9:301, 1999.

57. Schepke M, Sauerbruch T: Transjugular portosystemic stent shunt in treatment of liver diseases. *World J Gastroenterol* 7:170, 2001.

58. Rosch J, Keller FS: Transjugular intrahepatic portosystemic shunt: Present status, comparison with endoscopic therapy and shunt surgery, and future prospectives. *World J Surg* 25:337, 2001.

59. Helton WS, Maves R, Wicks K, et al: Transjugular intrahepatic portasystemic shunt vs. surgical shunt in good-risk cirrhotic patients: A case-control comparison. *Arch Surg* 136:17, 2001.

60. Hillebrand DJ, Kojouri K, Cao S, et al: Small-diameter portacaval H-graft shunt: A paradigm shift back to surgical shunting in the management of variceal bleeding in patients with preserved liver function. *Liver Transplant* 6:459, 2000.

61. Zacks SL, Sandler RS, Biddle AK, et al: Decision-analysis of transjugular intrahepatic portosystemic shunt versus distal splenorenal shunt for portal hypertension. *Hepatology* 29:1399, 1999.

62. Jenkins RL, Gedaly R, Pomposelli JJ, et al: Distal splenorenal shunt: Role, indications, and utility in the era of liver transplantation. *Arch Surg* 134:416, 1999.

63. Selzner M, Tuttle-Newhall JE, Dahm F, et al: Current indication of a modified Sugiura procedure in the management of variceal bleeding. *J Am Coll Surg* 193:166, 2001.

64. Wong F, Blendis L: The pathophysiologic basis for the treatment of cirrhotic ascites. *Clin Liver Dis* 5:819, 2001.

65. Ong JP, Mullen KD: Hepatic encephalopathy. *Eur J Gastroenterol Hepatol* 13:325, 2001.

66. Riordan SM, Williams R: Fulminant hepatic failure. *Clin Liver Dis* 4:25, 2000.

67. Blei AT: Pathophysiology of brain edema in fulminant hepatic failure, revisited. *Metab Brain Dis* 16:85, 2001.

68. Detry O, Arkadopoulos N, Ting P, et al: Intracranial pressure during liver transplantation for fulminant hepatic failure. *Transplantation* 67:767, 1999.

69. Farmer DG, Anselmo DM, Ghobrial RM, et al: Liver transplantation for fulminant hepatic failure: Experience with more than 200 patients over a 17-year period. Ann Surg 237:666, 2003.

70. Hui T, Rozga J, Demetriou AA: Bioartificial liver support. *J Hepato-Biliary-Pancreatic Surg* 8:1, 2001.

71. Regev A, Reddy KR, Berho M, et al: Large cystic lesions of the liver in adults: A 15-year experience in a tertiary center. *J Am Coll Surg* 193:36, 2001.

72. Ammori BJ, Jenkins BL, Lim PC, et al: Surgical strategy for cystic diseases of the liver in a western hepatobiliary center. *World J Surg* 26:462, 2002.

73. Katkhouda N, Hurwitz M, Gugenheim J, et al: Laparoscopic management of benign solid and cystic lesions of the liver. *Ann Surg* 229:460, 1999.

74. Gigot JF, Metairie S, Etienne J, et al: The surgical management of congenital liver cysts. *Surg Endosc* 15:357, 2001.

75. Geevarghese SK, Powers T, Marsh JW, et al: Screening for cerebral aneurysm in patients with polycystic liver disease. *South Med J* 92:1167, 1999.

76. Johnson LB, Kuo PC, Plotkin JS: Transverse hepatectomy for symptomatic polycystic liver disease. *Liver* 19:526, 1999.

77. Mortele KJ, Ros PR: Cystic focal liver lesions in the adult: Differential CT and MR imaging features. *Radiographics* 21:895, 2001.

78. Lauffer JM, Baer HU, Maurer CA, et al: Biliary cystadenocarcinoma of the liver: The need for complete resection. *Eur J Cancer* 34:1845, 1998.

79. Kim K, Choi J, Park Y, et al: Biliary cystadenoma of the liver. *J Hepato-Biliary-Pancreatic Surg* 5:348, 1998.

80. Semelka RC, Martin DR, Balci C, Lance T: Focal liver lesions: Comparison of dual-phase CT and multisequence multiplanar MR imaging including dynamic gadolinium enhancement. *J Magn Reson Imag* 13:397, 2001.

81. Horton KM, Bluemke DA, Hruban RH, et al: CT and MR imaging of benign hepatic and biliary tumors. *Radiographics* 19:431, 1999.

82. Trotter JF, Everson GT: Benign focal lesions of the liver. *Clin Liver Dis* 5:17, 2001.

83. Reddy KR, Kligerman S, Levi J, et al: Benign and solid tumors of the liver: Relationship to sex, age, size of tumors, and outcome. *Am Surg* 67:173, 2001.

84. De Carlis L, Pirotta V, Rondinara GF, et al: Hepatic adenoma and focal nodular hyperplasia: Diagnosis and criteria for treatment. *Liver Transplant Surg* 3:160, 1997.

85. Mortele KJ, Praet M, Van Vlierberghe H, et al: Focal nodular hyperplasia of the liver: Detection and characterization with plain and dynamic-enhanced MRI. *Abdom Imag* 27:700, 2002.

86. Ribeiro A, Burgart LJ, Nagorney DM, et al: Management of liver adenomatosis: Results with a conservative surgical approach. *Liver Transplant Surg* 4:388, 1998.

87. Charny CK, Jarnagin WR, Schwartz LH, et al: Management of 155 patients with benign liver tumours. *Br J Surg* 88:808, 2001.

88. Foster JH, Berman MM: The malignant transformation of liver cell adenomas. *Arch Surg* 129:712, 1994.

89. Descottes B, Glineur D, Lachachi F, et al: Laparoscopic liver resection of benign liver tumors. [erratum appears in *Surg Endosc* 17:668, 2003.] *Surg Endosc* 17:23, 2003.

90. Baer HU, Dennison AR, Mouton W, et al: Enucleation of giant hemangiomas of the liver. Technical and pathologic aspects of a neglected procedure. *Ann Surg* 216:673, 1992.

91. Gedaly R, Pomposelli JJ, Pomfret EA, et al: Cavernous hemangioma of the liver: Anatomic resection vs. enucleation. *Arch Surg* 134:407, 1999.

92. Terkivatan T, Vrijland WW, Den Hoed PT, et al: Size of lesion is not a criterion for resection during management of giant liver haemangioma. *Br J Surg* 89:1240, 2002.

93. Petri A, Hohn J, Hodi Z, et al: Pyogenic liver abscess—20 years' experience. Comparison of results of treatment in two periods. *Langenbecks Arch Surg* 387:27, 2002.

94. Lee KT, Wong SR, Sheen PC: Pyogenic liver abscess: An audit of 10 years' experience and analysis of risk factors. *Dig Surg* 18:459, 2001.

95. Alvarez Perez JA, Gonzalez JJ, Baldonedo RF, et al: Clinical course, treatment, and multivariate analysis of risk factors for pyogenic liver abscess. *Am J Surg* 181:177, 2001.

96. Lam YH, Wong SK, Lee DW, et al: ERCP and pyogenic liver abscess. *Gastrointest Endosc* 50:340, 1999.

97. Ch Yu S, Hg Lo R, Kan PS, et al: Pyogenic liver abscess: Treatment with needle aspiration. *Clin Radiol* 52:912, 1997.

98. Alvarez JA, Gonzalez JJ, Baldonedo RF, et al: Single and multiple pyogenic liver abscesses: Etiology, clinical course, and outcome. *Dig Surg* 18:283, 2001.

99. Sayek I, Onat D: Diagnosis and treatment of uncomplicated hydatid cyst of the liver. *World J Surg* 25:21, 2001.

100. Khuroo MS, Wani NA, Javid G, et al: Percutaneous drainage compared with surgery for hepatic hydatid cysts. *N Engl J Med* 337:881, 1997.

101. Sielaff TD, Taylor B, Langer B: Recurrence of hydatid disease. *World J Surg* 25:83, 2001.

102. Yorganci K, Sayek I: Surgical treatment of hydatid cysts of the liver in the era of percutaneous treatment. *Am J Surg* 184:63, 2002.

103. Hughes MA, Petri WA Jr.: Amebic liver abscess. *Infect Dis Clin North Am* 14:565, 2000.

104. Akgun Y, Tacyildiz IH, Celik Y: Amebic liver abscess: Changing trends over 20 years. *World J Surg* 23:102, 1999.

105. McGarr PL, Madiba TE, Thomson SR, et al: Amoebic liver abscess—results of a conservative management policy. *South Afr Med J* 93:132, 2003.

106. Fortner JG, Blumgart LH: A historic perspective of liver surgery for tumors at the end of the millennium. *J Am Coll Surg* 193:210, 2001.

107. Elliot JW: Surgical treatment of tumor of the liver with report of a case. *Ann Surg* 26:83, 1897.

108. Couinaud C: *Etudes anatomiques et chirurgales.* Paris: Mason, 1957, p 1.

109. Curley SA: Surgical management of hepatocellular carcinoma, in Curley SA (ed): *Liver Cancer.* M.D. Anderson Solid Tumor Oncology Series. New York: Springer-Verlag, 1998, p 28.

110. Lau H, Man K, Fan ST, et al: Evaluation of preoperative hepatic function in patients with hepatocellular carcinoma undergoing hepatectomy. *Br J Surg* 84:1255, 1997.

111. Kobayashi T, Kubota K, Imamura H, et al: Hepatic phenylalanine metabolism measured by the [13C]phenylalanine breath test. *Eur J Clin Invest* 31:356, 2001.

112. Meyer-Wyss B, Renner E, Luo H, et al: Assessment of lidocaine metabolite formation in comparison with other quantitative liver function tests. *J Hepatol* 19:133, 1993.

113. Hamming AW, Gallinger S, Greig PD, et al: The hippurate ratio as an indicator of functional hepatic reserve for resection of hepatocellular carcinoma in cirrhotic patients. *J Gastrointest Surg* 5:316, 2001.

114. Hwang EH, Taki J, Shuke N, et al: Preoperative assessment of residual hepatic functional reserve using 99mTc-DTPA-galactosyl-human serum albumin dynamic SPECT. *J Nucl Med* 40:1644, 1999.

115. Shiomi S, Iwata Y, Sasaki N, et al: Assessment of hepatic blood flow by PET with 15O water: Correlation between per-rectal portal scintigraphy with 99Tc(m)-pertechnetate and scintigraphy with 99Tc(m)-GSA. *Nucl Med Commun* 21:533, 2000.

116. Di Bisceglie AM, Carithers RL Jr., Gores GJ: Hepatocellular carcinoma. *Hepatology* 28:1161, 1998.

117. Anthony PP: Hepatocellular carcinoma: An overview. *Histopathology* 39:109, 2001.

118. Weiss L, Grundmann E, Torhorst J, et al: Haematogenous metastatic patterns in colonic carcinoma: An analysis of 1541 necropsies. *J Pathol* 150:195, 1986.

119. Bilimoria MM, Lauwers GY, Doherty DA, et al: Underlying liver disease, not tumor factors, predicts long-term survival after resection of hepatocellular carcinoma. *Arch Surg* 136:528, 2001.

120. Fong Y, Cohen AM, Fortner JG, et al: Liver resection for colorectal metastases. *J Clin Oncol* 15:938, 1997.

121. Resection of the liver for colorectal carcinoma metastases: A

121. multi-institutional study of indications for resection. Registry of Hepatic Metastases. *Surgery* 103:278, 1988.

122. Minagawa M, Makuuchi M, Torzilli G, et al: Extension of the frontiers of surgical indications in the treatment of liver metastases from colorectal cancer: Long-term results. *Ann Surg* 231:487, 2000.

123. Weber SM, Jarnagin WR, DeMatteo RP, et al: Survival after resection of multiple hepatic colorectal metastases. *Ann Surg Oncol* 7:643, 2000.

124. Poon RT, Fan ST, Lo CM, et al: Improving survival results after resection of hepatocellular carcinoma: A prospective study of 377 patients over 10 years. *Ann Surg* 234:63, 2001.

125. Grazi GL, Ercolani G, Pierangeli F, et al: Improved results of liver resection for hepatocellular carcinoma on cirrhosis give the procedure added value. *Ann Surg* 234:71, 2001.

126. Yanaga K, Nishizaki T, Yamamoto K, et al: Simplified inflow control using stapling devices for major hepatic resection. *Arch Surg* 131:104, 1996.

127. Ramacciato G, Balesh AM, Fornasari V: Vascular endostapler as aid to hepatic vein control during hepatic resections. *Am J Surg* 172:358, 1996.

128. Descottes B, Lachachi F, Sodji M, et al: Early experience with laparoscopic approach for solid liver tumors: Initial 16 cases. *Ann Surg* 232:641, 2000.

129. Cherqui D, Husson E, Hammoud R, et al: Laparoscopic liver resections: A feasibility study in 30 patients. *Ann Surg* 232:753, 2000.

130. Tuttle TM, Curley SA, Roh MS: Repeat hepatic resection as effective treatment for recurrent colorectal liver metastases. *Ann Surg Oncol* 4:125, 1996.

131. Imamura H, Kawasaki S, Miyagawa S, et al: Aggressive surgical approach to recurrent tumors after hepatectomy for metastatic spread of colorectal cancer to the liver. *Surgery* 127:528, 2000.

132. Nakajima Y, Ko S, Kanamura T, et al: Repeat liver resection for hepatocellular carcinoma. *J Am Coll Surg* 192:339, 2001.

133. Matsuda M, Fujii H, Kono H, et al: Surgical treatment of recurrent hepatocellular carcinoma based on the mode of recurrence: Repeat hepatic resection or ablation are good choices for patients with recurrent multicentric cancer. *J Hepatobiliary Pancreatic Surg* 8:353, 2001.

134. Kinoshita H, Sakai K, Hirohashi K, et al: Preoperative portal vein embolization for hepatocellular carcinoma. *World J Surg* 10:803, 1986.

135. Melendez J, Ferri E, Zwillman M, et al: Extended hepatic resection: A 6-year retrospective study of risk factors for perioperative mortality. *J Am Coll Surg* 192:47, 2001.

136. Vauthey JN, Chaoui A, Do KA, et al: Standardized measurement of the future liver remnant prior to extended liver resection: Methodology and clinical associations. *Surgery* 127:512, 2000.

137. Abdalla EK, Barnett CC, Doherty DA, et al: Extended hepatectomy in hepatobiliary malignancies with and without preoperative portal vein embolization. *Arch Surg* 137:675, 2002.

138. Kubota MK, Makuuchi M, Kusaka K, et al: Measurement of liver volume and hepatic functional reserve as a guide to decision-making in resectional surgery for hepatic tumors. *Hepatology* 26:1176, 1997.

139. Azoulay D, Castaing D, Smail A, et al: Resection of nonresectable liver metastases from colorectal cancer after percutaneous portal vein embolization. *Ann Surg* 231:480, 2000.

140. Urata K, Kawasaki S, Matsunami H, et al: Calculation of child and adult standard liver volume for liver transplantation. *Hepatology* 21:1317, 1995.

141. Nagino M, Kamiya J, Kanai M, et al: Right trisegment portal vein embolization for biliary tract carcinoma: Technique and clinical utility. *Surgery* 127:155, 2000.

142. Elias D, De Baere T, Roche A, et al: During liver regeneration following right portal embolization the growth rate of liver metastases is more rapid than that of the liver parenchyma. *Br J Surg* 86:784, 1999.

143. de Baere T, Roche A, Elias D, et al: Preoperative portal vein embolization for extension of hepatectomy indications. *Hepatology* 24:1386, 1996.

144. Imamura H, Shimada R, Kubota M, et al: Preoperative portal vein embolization: An audit of 84 patients. *Hepatology* 29:1099, 1999.

145. Shimamura T, Nakajima Y, Une Y, et al: Efficacy and safety of preoperative percutaneous transhepatic portal embolization with absolute ethanol: A clinical study. *Surgery* 121:135, 1997.

146. Kawasaki S, Makuuchi M, Miyagawa S, et al: Radical operation after portal embolization for tumor of hilar bile duct. *J Am Coll Surg* 178:480, 1994.

147. Wakabayashi H, Okada S, Maeba T, et al: Effect of preoperative portal vein embolization on major hepatectomy for advanced-stage hepatocellular carcinomas in injured livers: A preliminary report. *Surg Today* 27:403, 1997.

148. Elias D, Cavalcanti A, De Baere T, et al: Resultats carcinologiques a long terme des hepatectomies realisee apres embolisation portal selective. *Ann Chir* 53:559, 1999.

149. Abdalla EK, Hicks ME, Vauthey JN: Portal vein embolization: Rationale, technique and future prospects. *Br J Surg* 88:165, 2001.

150. McGahan JP, Brock JM, Tesluk H, et al: Hepatic ablation with use of radio-frequency electrocautery in the animal model. *J Vasc Intervent Radiol* 3:291, 1992.

151. Curley SA, Izzo F, Delrio P, et al: Radiofrequency ablation of unresectable primary and metastatic hepatic malignancies: Results in 123 patients. *Ann Surg* 230:1, 1999.

152. Curley SA, Izzo F, Ellis LM, et al: Radiofrequency ablation of hepatocellular cancer in 110 patients with cirrhosis. *Ann Surg* 232:381, 2000.

153. Curley SA: Radiofrequency ablation of malignant liver tumors. *Oncologist* 6:14, 2001.

154. Solbiati L, Ierace T, Tonolini M, et al: Radiofrequency thermal ablation of hepatic metastases. *Eur J Ultrasound* 13:149, 2001.

155. Siperstein A, Garland A, Engle K, et al: Local recurrence after laparoscopic radiofrequency thermal ablation of hepatic tumors. *Ann Surg Oncol* 7:106, 2000.

156. Wood TF, Rose DM, Chung M, et al: Radiofrequency ablation of 231 unresectable hepatic tumors: Indications, limitations, and complications. *Ann Surg Oncol* 7:593, 2000.

157. Siperstein AE, Berber E: Cryoablation, percutaneous alcohol injection, and radiofrequency ablation for treatment of neuroendocrine liver metastases. *World J Surg* 25:693, 2001.

158. Germer CT, Albrecht D, Roggan A, et al: Technology for in situ ablation by laparoscopic and image-guided interstitial laser hyperthermia. *Semin Laparosc Surg* 5:195, 1998.

159. Muralidharan V, Christophi C: Interstitial laser thermotherapy in the treatment of colorectal liver metastases. *J Surg Oncol* 76(Suppl):73, 2001.

160. Germer CT, Roggan A, Ritz JP, et al: Optical properties of native and coagulated human liver tissue and liver metastases in the near infrared range. *Lasers Surg Med* 23:194, 1998.

161. Sturesson C, Liu DL, Stenram U, et al: Hepatic inflow occlusion increases the efficacy of interstitial laser-induced thermotherapy in rat. *J Surg Res* 71:67, 1997.

162. Gilliams AR, Brokes J, Hare C: Follow-up of patients with metastatic liver lesions treated with interstitial laser therapy. *Br J Cancer* 76:31, 1997.

163. Giorgio A, Tarantino L, de Stefano G, et al: Interstitial laser photocoagulation under ultrasound guidance of liver tumors: Results in 104 treated patients. *Eur J Ultrasound* 11:181, 2000.

164. Mack MG, Straub R, Eichler K, et al: Percutaneous MR imaging-guided laser-induced thermotherapy metastases. *Abdom Imaging* 26:369, 2001.

165. Tabuse K, Katsumi M, Kobayashi Y, et al: Microwave surgery: Hepatectomy using a microwave tissue coagulator. *World J Surg* 9:136, 1985.

166. Seki T, Wakabayashi M, Nakagawa T, et al: Ultrasonically guided percutaneous microwave coagulation therapy for small hepatocellular carcinoma. *Cancer Res* 74:817, 1994.

167. Sato M, Watanabe Y, Ueda S, et al: Microwave coagulation therapy for hepatocellular carcinoma. *Gastroenterology* 110:1507, 1996.

168. Izumi N, Asahina Y, Noguchi O, et al: Risk factors for distant recurrence of hepatocellular carcinoma in the liver after complete coagulation by microwave or radiofrequency ablation. *Cancer Res* 91:949, 2001.

169. Nonami T, Takeuchi Y, Yasui M, et al: Regional adjuvant chemotherapy after partial hepatectomy for metastatic colorectal carcinoma. *Semin Oncol* 24:S6, 1997.

170. Lorenz M, Staib-Sebler E, Koch B, et al: The value of postoperative hepatic arterial infusion following curative liver resection. *Anticancer Res* 17:3825, 1997.

171. Ambiru S, Miyazaki M, Ito H, et al: Adjuvant regional chemotherapy after hepatic resection for colorectal metastases. *Br J Surg* 86:1025, 1999.

172. Kemeny N, Huang Y, Cohen AM, et al: Hepatic arterial infusion of chemotherapy after resection of hepatic metastases from colorectal cancer. *N Engl J Med* 341:2039, 1999.

173. Lau WY, Leung TW, Ho SK, et al: Adjuvant intra-arterial iodine-131-labelled lipiodol for resectable hepatocellular carcinoma: A prospective randomised trial. *Lancet* 353:797, 1999.

174. Adam R, Avisar E, Ariche A, et al: Five-year survival following hepatic resection after neoadjuvant therapy for non-resectable colorectal liver metastases. *Ann Surg Oncol* 8:347, 2001.

175. Scaife CL, Curley SA, Patt Y, et al: Feasibility of adjuvant hepatic arterial infusion (HAI) of chemotherapy following radiofrequency ablation (RFA) +/– resection in patients with hepatic metastasis from colorectal cancer. *Ann Surg Oncol* 10:348, 2003.

CHAPTER 31

Gallbladder and the Extrahepatic Biliary System

Margrét Oddsdóttir and John G. Hunter

ANATOMY

The Gallbladder

The gallbladder is a pear-shaped sac, about 7 to 10 cm long with an average capacity of 30 to 50 mL. When obstructed, the gallbladder can distend markedly and contain up to 300 mL.[1] The gallbladder is located in a fossa on the inferior surface of the liver that is in line with the anatomic division of the liver into right and left liver lobes. The gallbladder is divided into four anatomic areas: the fundus, the corpus (body), the infundibulum, and the neck. The fundus is the rounded, blind end that normally extends 1 to 2 cm beyond the liver's margin. It contains most of the smooth muscles of the organ, in contrast to the body, which is the main storage area and contains most of the elastic tissue. The body extends from the fundus and tapers into the neck, a funnel-shaped area that connects with the cystic duct. The neck usually follows a gentle curve, the convexity

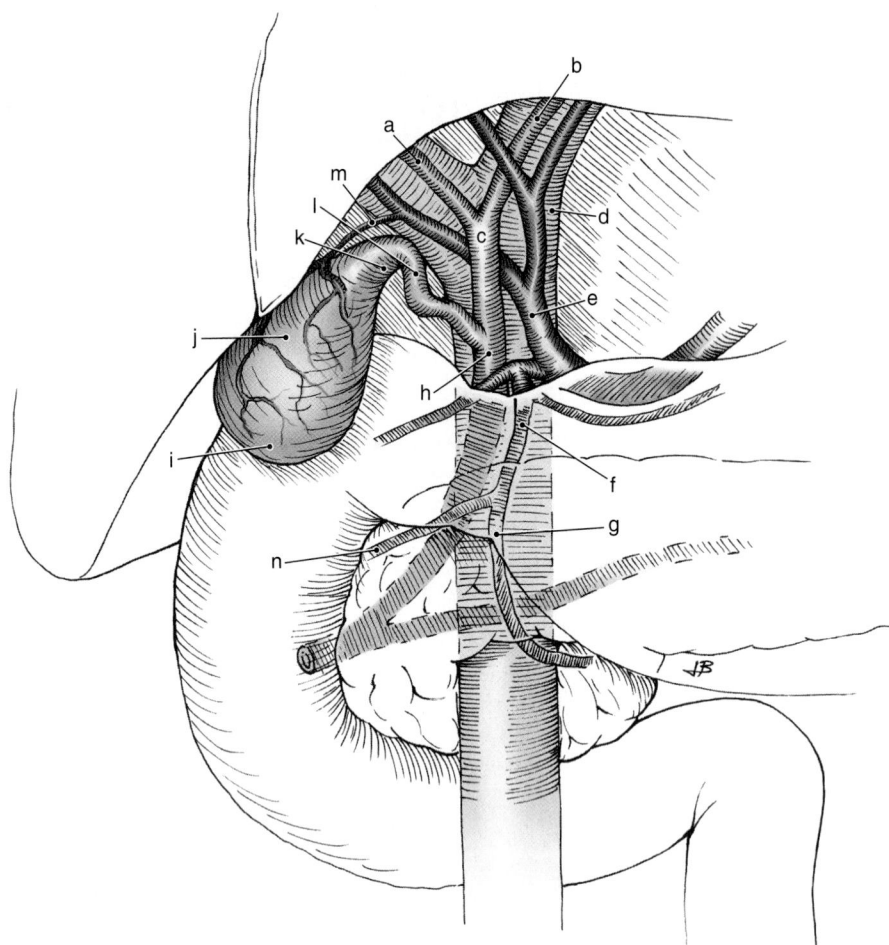

FIG. 31-1. Anterior aspect of the biliary anatomy. *a.* Right hepatic duct. *b.* Left hepatic duct. *c.* Common hepatic duct. *d.* Portal vein. *e.* Hepatic artery. *f.* Gastroduodenal artery. *g.* Right gastroepiploic artery. *h.* Common bile duct. *i.* Fundus of the gallbladder. *j.* Body of the gallbladder. *k.* Infundibulum. *l.* Cystic duct. *m.* Cystic artery. *n.* Superior pancreaticoduodenal artery. Note the situation of the hepatic bile duct confluence anterior to the right branch of the portal vein, and the posterior course of the right hepatic artery behind the common hepatic duct.

of which may be enlarged to form the infundibulum or Hartman's pouch. The neck lies in the deepest part of the gallbladder fossa and extends into the free portion of the hepatoduodenal ligament (Fig. 31-1).

The same peritoneal lining that covers the liver covers the fundus and the inferior surface of the gallbladder. Occasionally the gallbladder has a complete peritoneal covering, and is suspended in a mesentery off the inferior surface of the liver, and rarely it is embedded deep inside the liver parenchyma (an intrahepatic gallbladder).

The gallbladder is lined by a single, highly-folded, tall columnar epithelium that contains cholesterol and fat globules. The mucus secreted into the gallbladder originates in the tubuloalveolar glands found in the mucosa lining the infundibulum and neck of the gallbladder, but are absent from the body and fundus. The epithelial lining of the gallbladder is supported by a lamina propria. The muscle layer has circular longitudinal and oblique fibers, but without well-developed layers. The perimuscular subserosa contains connective tissue, nerves, vessels, lymphatics, and adipocytes. It is covered by the serosa except where the gallbladder is embedded in the liver. The gallbladder differs histologically from the rest of the gastrointestinal tract in that it lacks a muscularis mucosa and submucosa.

The cystic artery that supplies the gallbladder is usually a branch of the right hepatic artery (>90% of the time). The course of the cystic artery may vary, but it nearly always is found within the hepatocystic triangle, the area bound by the cystic duct, common hepatic duct, and the liver margin (triangle of Calot). When the cystic artery

reaches the neck of the gallbladder, it divides into anterior and posterior divisions. Venous return is carried either through small veins that enter directly into the liver, or rarely to a large cystic vein that carries blood back to the portal vein. Gallbladder lymphatics drain into nodes at the neck of the gallbladder. Frequently, a visible lymph node overlies the insertion of the cystic artery into the gallbladder wall. The nerves of the gallbladder arise from the vagus and from sympathetic branches that pass through the celiac plexus. The preganglionic sympathetic level is T8 and T9. Impulses from the liver, gallbladder, and the bile ducts pass by means of sympathetic afferent fibers through the splanchnic nerves and mediate the pain of biliary colic. The hepatic branch of the vagus nerve supplies cholinergic fibers to the gallbladder, bile ducts, and the liver. The vagal branches also have peptide-containing nerves containing agents such as substance P, somatostatin, enkephalins, and vasoactive intestinal polypeptide (VIP).[2]

The Bile Ducts

The extrahepatic bile ducts consist of the right and left hepatic ducts, the common hepatic duct, the cystic duct, and the common bile duct or choledochus. The common bile duct enters the second portion of the duodenum through a muscular structure, the sphincter of Oddi.[3]

The left hepatic duct is longer than the right and has a greater propensity for dilatation as a consequence of distal obstruction. The two ducts join to form a common hepatic duct, close to their emergence from the liver. The common hepatic duct is 1 to 4 cm in length and has a diameter of approximately 4 mm. It lies in front of

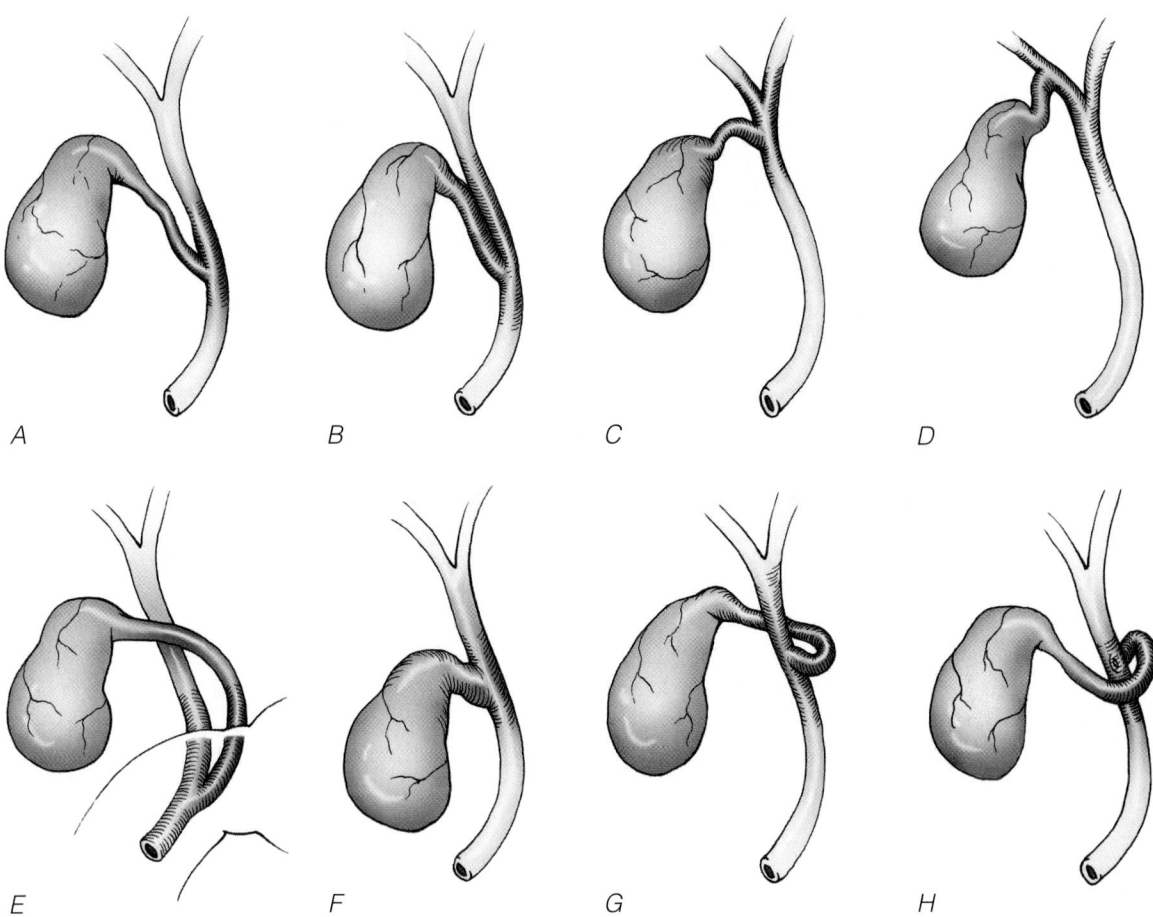

FIG. 31-2. Variations of cystic duct anatomy. *A*. Low junction between the cystic duct and common hepatic duct. *B*. Cystic duct adherent to the common hepatic duct. *C*. High junction between the cystic and the common hepatic duct. *D*. The cystic duct drains into right hepatic duct. *E*. Long cystic duct that joins the common hepatic duct behind the duodenum. *F*. Absence of the cystic duct. *G*. The cystic duct crosses posterior to the common hepatic duct and joins it anteriorly. *H*. The cystic duct courses anterior to the common hepatic duct and joins it posteriorly.

the portal vein and to the right of the hepatic artery. The common hepatic duct is joined at an acute angle by the cystic duct to form the common bile duct.

The length of the cystic duct is quite variable. It may be short or absent and have a high union with the hepatic duct, or long and run parallel, behind, or spiral to the main hepatic duct before joining it, sometimes as far as at the duodenum. Variations of the cystic duct and its point of union with the common hepatic duct are surgically important (Fig. 31-2). The segment of the cystic duct adjacent to the gallbladder neck bears a variable number of mucosal folds called the spiral valves of Heister. They do not have any valvular function, but may make cannulation of the cystic duct difficult.

The common bile duct is about 7 to 11 cm in length and 5 to 10 mm in diameter. The upper third (supraduodenal portion) passes downward in the free edge of the hepatoduodenal ligament, to the right of the hepatic artery and anterior to the portal vein. The middle third (retroduodenal portion) of the common bile duct curves behind the first portion of the duodenum and diverges laterally from the portal vein and the hepatic arteries. The lower third (pancreatic portion) curves behind the head of the pancreas in a groove, or traverses through it and enters the second part of the duodenum. There the pancreatic duct frequently joins it. The common bile duct runs obliquely downward within the wall of the duodenum for 1 to

2 cm before opening on a papilla of mucous membrane (ampulla of Vater), about 10 cm distal to the pylorus. The union of the common bile duct and the main pancreatic duct follows one of three configurations. In about 70% of people these ducts unite outside the duodenal wall and traverse the duodenal wall as a single duct. In about 20%, they join within the duodenal wall and have a short or no common duct, but open through the same opening into the duodenum. In about 10%, they exit via separate openings into the duodenum. The sphincter of Oddi, a thick coat of circular smooth muscle, surrounds the common bile duct at the ampulla of Vater (Fig. 31-3). It controls the flow of bile, and in some cases pancreatic juice, into the duodenum.

The extrahepatic bile ducts are lined by a columnar mucosa with numerous mucous glands in the common bile duct. A fibroareolar tissue containing scant smooth muscle cells surrounds the mucosa. A distinct muscle layer is not present in the human common bile duct. The arterial supply to the bile ducts is derived from the gastroduodenal and the right hepatic arteries, with major trunks running along the medial and lateral walls of the common duct (sometimes referred to as 3 o'clock and 9 o'clock). These arteries anastomose freely within the duct walls. The density of nerve fibers and ganglia increase near the sphincter of Oddi, but the nerve supply to the common bile duct and the sphincter of Oddi is the same as for the gallbladder.[1,2]

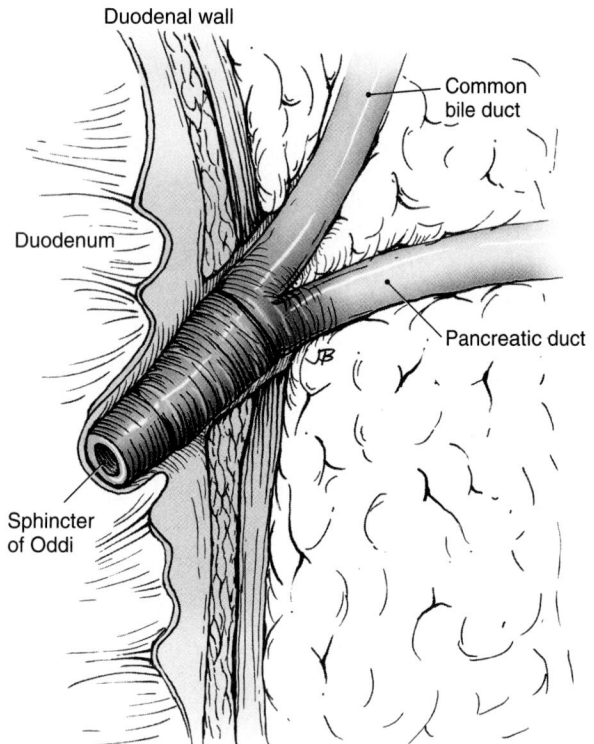

FIG. 31-3. The sphincter of Oddi.

Anomalies

The classic description of the extrahepatic biliary tree and its arteries applies only in about one third of patients.[4] The gallbladder may have abnormal positions, be intrahepatic, be rudimentary, have anomalous forms, or be duplicated. Isolated congenital absence of the gallbladder is very rare, with a reported incidence of 0.03%. Before the diagnosis is made, the presence of an intrahepatic bladder or anomalous position must be ruled out. Duplication of the gallbladder with two separate cavities and two separate cystic ducts has an incidence of about one in every 4000 persons. This occurs in two major varieties: the more common form in which each gallbladder has its own cystic duct that empties independently into the same or different parts of the extrahepatic biliary tree, and as two cystic ducts that merge before they enter the common bile duct. Duplication is only clinically important when some pathologic processes affect one or both organs. A left-sided gallbladder with a cystic duct emptying into the left hepatic duct or the common bile duct and a retrodisplacement of the gallbladder are both extremely rare. A partial or totally intrahepatic gallbladder is associated with an increased incidence of cholelithiasis.

Small ducts (of Luschka) may drain directly from the liver into the body of the gallbladder. If present, but not recognized at the time of a cholecystectomy, a bile leak with the accumulation of bile (biloma) may occur in the abdomen. An accessory right hepatic duct occurs in about 5% of cases. Variations of how the common bile duct enters the duodenum are described above.

Anomalies of the hepatic artery and the cystic artery are quite common, occurring in as many as 50% of cases.[5] In about 5% of cases there are two right hepatic arteries, one from the common hepatic artery and the other from the superior mesenteric artery. In about 20% of patients the right hepatic artery comes off the superior mesenteric artery. The right hepatic artery may course anterior to

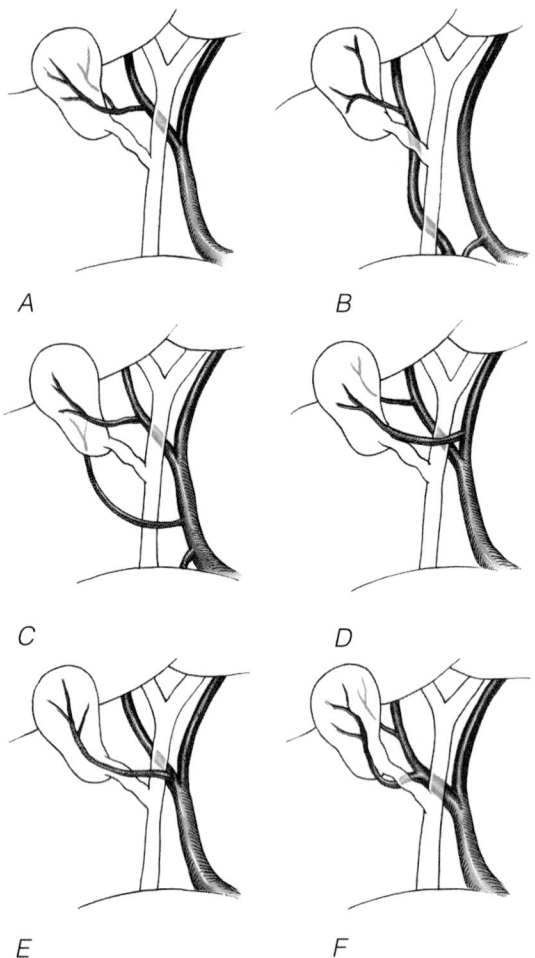

FIG. 31-4. Variations in the arterial supply to the gallbladder. A. The cystic artery from the right hepatic artery, about 80 to 90%. B. The cystic artery from the right hepatic artery (accessory or replacing) from the superior mesenteric artery, about 10%. C. Two cystic arteries, one from the right hepatic, the other from the common hepatic artery, rare. D. Two cystic arteries, one from the left hepatic artery, one from the right hepatic artery, rare. E. The cystic artery branching from the right hepatic artery and running anterior to the common hepatic duct, rare. F. Two cystic arteries arising from the right hepatic artery, rare.

the common duct. The right hepatic artery may be vulnerable during surgical procedures, in particular when it runs parallel to the cystic duct or in the mesentery of the gallbladder. The cystic artery arises from the right hepatic artery in about 90% of cases, but may arise from the left hepatic, common hepatic, gastroduodenal, or superior mesenteric arteries (Fig. 31-4).

PHYSIOLOGY

Bile Formation and Composition

The liver produces bile continuously and excretes it into the bile canaliculi. The normal adult consuming an average diet produces within the liver 500 to 1000 mL of bile a day. The secretion of bile is responsive to neurogenic, humoral, and chemical stimuli. Vagal stimulation increases secretion of bile, whereas splanchnic nerve stimulation results in decreased bile flow. Hydrochloric acid, partly digested proteins, and fatty acids in the duodenum stimulate the release of secretin from the duodenum that in turn increases bile production and bile flow. Bile flows from the liver through to the hepatic ducts, into the common hepatic duct, through the common bile duct, and finally into the duodenum. With an intact sphincter of Oddi, bile flow is directed into the gallbladder.

Bile is mainly composed of water, electrolytes, bile salts, proteins, lipids, and bile pigments. Sodium, potassium, calcium, and chlorine have the same concentration in bile as in plasma or extracellular fluid. The pH of hepatic bile is usually neutral or slightly alkaline, but varies with diet; an increase in protein shifts the bile to a more acidic pH. The primary bile salts, cholate and chenodeoxycholate, are synthesized in the liver from cholesterol. They are conjugated there with taurine and glycine, and act within the bile as anions (bile acids) that are balanced by sodium. Bile salts are excreted into the bile by the hepatocyte and aid in the digestion and absorption of fats in the intestines.[6] In the intestines, about 80% of the conjugated bile acids are absorbed in the terminal ileum. The remainder is dehydroxylated (deconjugated) by gut bacteria, forming secondary bile acids deoxycholate and lithocholate. These are absorbed in the colon, transported to the liver, conjugated, and secreted into the bile. Eventually, about 95% of the bile acid pool is reabsorbed and returned via the portal venous system to the liver, the so-called enterohepatic circulation. Five percent is excreted in the stool, leaving the relatively small amount of bile acids to have maximum effect.

Cholesterol and phospholipids synthesized in the liver are the principal lipids found in bile. The synthesis of phospholipids and cholesterol by the liver is in part regulated by bile acids. The color of the bile is due to the presence of the pigment bilirubin diglucuronide, which is the metabolic product from the breakdown of hemoglobin, and is present in bile in concentrations 100 times greater than in plasma. Once in the intestine, bacteria convert it into urobilinogen, a small fraction of which is absorbed and secreted into the bile.

Gallbladder Function

The gallbladder, the bile ducts, and the sphincter of Oddi act together to store and regulate the flow of bile. The main function of the gallbladder is to concentrate and store hepatic bile and to deliver bile into the duodenum in response to a meal.

Absorption and Secretion

In the fasting state, approximately 80% of the bile secreted by the liver is stored in the gallbladder. This storage is made possible because of the remarkable absorptive capacity of the gallbladder, as the gallbladder mucosa has the greatest absorptive power per unit area of any structure in the body. It rapidly absorbs sodium, chloride, and water against significant concentration gradients, concentrating the bile as much as tenfold and leading to a marked change in bile composition. This rapid absorption is one of the mechanisms that prevent a rise in pressure within the biliary system under normal circumstances. Gradual relaxation as well as emptying of the gallbladder during the fasting period also plays a role in maintaining a relatively low intraluminal pressure in the biliary tree.

The epithelial cells of the gallbladder secrete at least two important products into the gallbladder lumen: glycoproteins and hydrogen ions. The mucosal glands in the infundibulum and the neck of the gallbladder secrete mucus glycoproteins that are believed to protect the mucosa from the lytic action of bile and to facilitate the passage of bile through the cystic duct. This mucus makes up the colorless "white bile" seen in hydrops of the gallbladder resulting from cystic duct obstruction. The transport of hydrogen ions by the gallbladder epithelium leads to a decrease in the gallbladder bile pH.

The acidification promotes calcium solubility, thereby preventing its precipitation as calcium salts.[6]

Motor Activity

Gallbladder filling is facilitated by tonic contraction of the sphincter of Oddi, which creates a pressure gradient between the bile ducts and the gallbladder. During fasting the gallbladder does not simply fill passively. In association with phase II of the interdigestive migrating myenteric motor complex in the gut, the gallbladder repeatedly empties small volumes of bile into the duodenum. This process is mediated at least in part by the hormone motilin. In response to a meal, the gallbladder empties by a coordinated motor response of gallbladder contraction and sphincter of Oddi relaxation. One of the main stimuli to gallbladder emptying is the hormone cholecystokinin (CCK). CCK is released endogenously from the duodenal mucosa in response to a meal.[7] When stimulated by eating, the gallbladder empties 50 to 70% of its contents within 30 to 40 minutes. Over the following 60 to 90 minutes the gallbladder gradually refills. This is correlated with a reduced CCK level. Other hormonal and neural pathways also are involved in the coordinated action of the gallbladder and the sphincter of Oddi. Defects in the motor activity of the gallbladder are thought to play a role in cholesterol nucleation and gallstone formation.[8]

Neurohormonal Regulation

The vagus nerve stimulates contraction of the gallbladder, and splanchnic sympathetic stimulation is inhibitory to its motor activity. Parasympathomimetic drugs contract the gallbladder, whereas atropine leads to relaxation. Neurally mediated reflexes link the sphincter of Oddi with the gallbladder, stomach, and duodenum to coordinate the flow of bile into the duodenum. Antral distention of the stomach causes both gallbladder contraction and relaxation of the sphincter of Oddi.

Hormonal receptors are located on the smooth muscles, vessels, nerves, and epithelium of the gallbladder. CCK is a peptide that comes from epithelial cells of the upper gastrointestinal tract and is found in the highest concentrations in the duodenum. CCK is released into the bloodstream by acid, fat, and amino acids in the duodenum.[9] CCK has a plasma half-life of 2 to 3 minutes and is metabolized by both the liver and the kidneys. CCK acts directly on smooth muscle receptors of the gallbladder and stimulates gallbladder contraction. It also relaxes the terminal bile duct, the sphincter of Oddi, and the duodenum. CCK stimulation of the gallbladder and the biliary tree also is mediated by cholinergic vagal neurons. In patients who have had a vagotomy, the response to CCK stimulation is diminished and the size and the volume of the gallbladder are increased.

VIP inhibits contraction and causes gallbladder relaxation. Somatostatin and its analogues are potent inhibitors of gallbladder contraction. Patients treated with somatostatin analogues and those with somatostatinoma have a high incidence of gallstones, presumably due to the inhibition of gallbladder contraction and emptying. Other hormones such as substance P and enkephalin affect gallbladder motility, but the physiologic role is unclear.[7]

Sphincter of Oddi

The sphincter of Oddi regulates flow of bile (and pancreatic juice) into the duodenum, prevents the regurgitation of duodenal contents into the biliary tree, and diverts bile into the gallbladder. It is a complex structure that is functionally independent from the duodenal

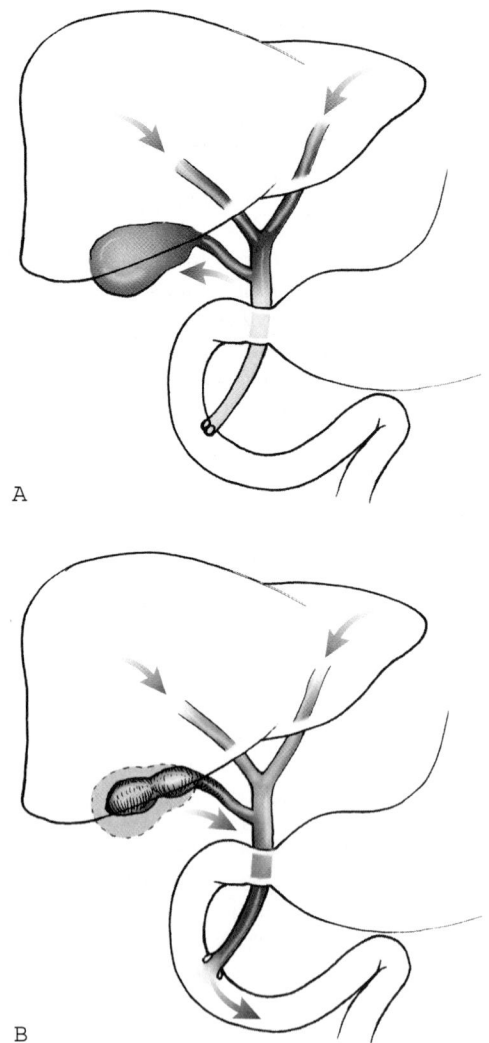

FIG. 31-5. *The effect of CCK on the gallbladder and the sphincter of Oddi. A. During fasting, with the sphincter of Oddi contracted and the gallbladder filling. B. In response to a meal, the sphincter of Oddi is relaxed and the gallbladder emptying.*

musculature and creates a high-pressure zone between the bile duct and the duodenum. The sphincter of Oddi is about 4 to 6 mm in length and has a basal resting pressure of about 13 mm Hg above the duodenal pressure. On manometry, the sphincter shows phasic contractions with a frequency of about four per minute and an amplitude of 12 to 140 mm Hg. The sphincter primarily controls the regulation of bile flow. Relaxation occurs with a rise in CCK, leading to diminished amplitude of phasic contractions and reduced basal pressure, allowing increased flow of bile into the duodenum (Fig. 31-5). During fasting, the sphincter of Oddi activity is coordinated with the periodic partial gallbladder emptying and an increase in bile flow that occurs during phase III of the migrating myoelectric complexes.[10]

DIAGNOSTIC STUDIES

A variety of diagnostic modalities are available for the patient with suspected disease of the gallbladder and the bile ducts. In 1924 the diagnosis of gallstones was improved significantly by the introduction of oral cholecystography by Graham and Cole. For decades it

was the mainstay of investigation for gallstones. In the 1950s biliary scintigraphy was developed, and later transhepatic and endoscopic retrograde cholangiography, allowing imaging of the biliary tract. Later ultrasonography, computed tomography (CT), and magnetic resonance imaging (MRI), vastly improved the ability to image the biliary tract.[11]

Blood Tests

When patients with suspected diseases of the gallbladder or the extrahepatic biliary tree are evaluated, a complete blood count (CBC) and liver function tests are routinely requested. An elevated white blood cell (WBC) count may indicate or raise suspicion of cholecystitis. If associated with an elevation of bilirubin, alkaline phosphatase, and aminotransferase, cholangitis should be suspected. Cholestasis, an obstruction to bile flow, is characterized by an elevation of bilirubin (i.e., the conjugated form), and a rise in alkaline phosphatase. Serum aminotransferases may be normal or mildly elevated. In patients with biliary colic, blood tests will typically be normal.

Ultrasonography

An ultrasound is the initial investigation of any patient suspected of disease of the biliary tree.[12] It is noninvasive, painless, does not submit the patient to radiation, and can be performed on critically ill patients. It is dependent upon the skills and the experience of the operator and it is dynamic (i.e., static images do not give the same information as those obtained during the ultrasound investigation itself). Adjacent organs can frequently be examined at the same time. Obese patients, patients with ascites, and patients with distended bowel may be difficult to examine satisfactorily with an ultrasound.

An ultrasound will show stones in the gallbladder with sensitivity and specificity of over 90%. Stones are acoustically dense and reflect the ultrasound waves back to the ultrasonic transducer. Because stones block the passage of sound waves to the region behind them, they also produce an acoustic shadow (Fig. 31-6). Stones also move with changes in position. Polyps may be calcified and reflect shadows, but do not move with change in posture. Some stones form a layer in the gallbladder; others a sediment or sludge. A thickened gallbladder wall and local tenderness indicate cholecystitis. The patient has acute cholecystitis if a layer of edema is seen within the wall of the gallbladder or between the gallbladder and the liver. When a stone obstructs the neck of the gallbladder, the gallbladder may become very large, but thin walled. A contracted, thick-walled gallbladder indicates chronic cholecystitis.

The extrahepatic bile ducts are also well visualized by ultrasound, except for the retroduodenal portion. Dilation of the ducts in a patient with jaundice establishes an extrahepatic obstruction as a cause for the jaundice. Frequently the site, and sometimes the cause of obstruction, can be determined by ultrasound. Small stones in the common bile duct frequently get lodged at the distal end of it, behind the duodenum, and are therefore difficult to detect. A dilated common bile duct on ultrasound, small stones in the gallbladder, and the clinical presentation allow one to assume that a stone or stones are causing the obstruction. Periampullary tumors can be difficult to diagnose on ultrasound, but beyond the retroduodenal portion, the level of obstruction and the cause may be visualized quite well. Ultrasound can be helpful in evaluating tumor invasion and flow in the portal vein, an important guideline for resectability of periampullary tumors.[13]

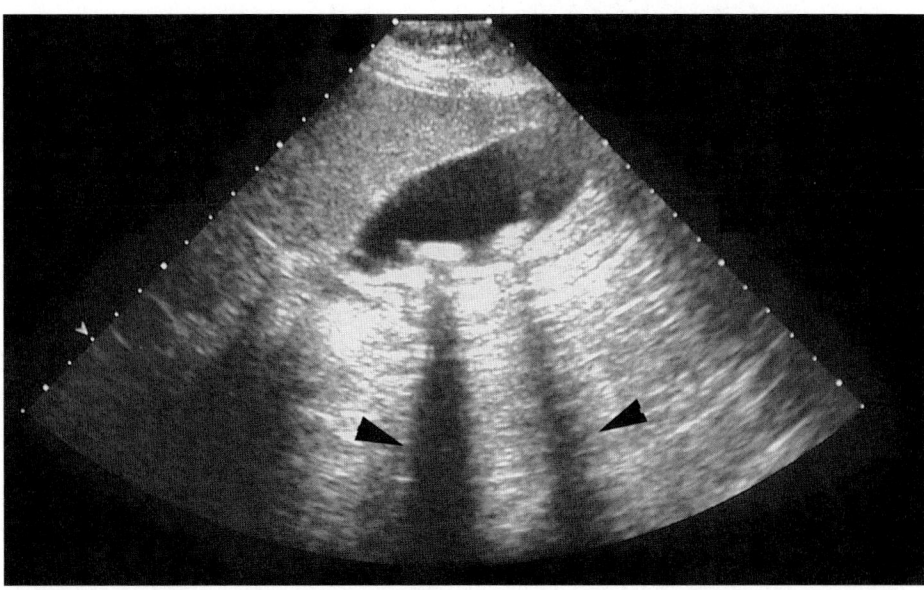

FIG. 31-6. An ultrasonogram of the gallbladder. Arrows indicate the acoustic shadows of stones in the gallbladder.

Oral Cholecystography

Once the diagnostic procedure of choice for gallstones, oral cholecystography has largely been replaced by ultrasonography. It involves oral administration of a radiopaque compound that is absorbed, excreted by the liver, and passed into the gallbladder. Stones are noted on a film as filling defects in a visualized, opacified gallbladder. Oral cholecystography is of no value in patients with intestinal malabsorption, vomiting, obstructive jaundice, and hepatic failure.

Biliary Radionuclide Scanning (HIDA Scan)

Biliary scintigraphy provides a noninvasive evaluation of the liver, gallbladder, bile ducts, and duodenum with both anatomic and functional information. ^{99m}-Technetium-labeled derivatives of dimethyl iminodiacetic acid (HIDA) are injected intravenously, cleared by the Kupffer cells in the liver, and excreted in the bile. Uptake by the liver is detected within 10 minutes, and the gallbladder, the bile ducts, and the duodenum are visualized within 60 minutes in fasting subjects. The primary use of biliary scintigraphy is in the diagnosis of acute cholecystitis, which appears as a nonvisualized gallbladder, with prompt filling of the common bile duct and duodenum. Evidence of cystic duct obstruction on biliary scintigraphy is highly diagnostic for acute cholecystitis. The sensitivity and specificity for the diagnosis is about 95% each. False-positive results are increased in patients with gallbladder stasis, as in critically ill patients and in patients receiving parenteral nutrition. Filling of the gallbladder and common bile duct with delayed or absent filling of the duodenum indicates an obstruction at the ampulla. Biliary leaks as a complication of surgery of the gallbladder or the biliary tree can be confirmed and frequently localized by biliary scintigraphy.[14]

Computed Tomography

Abdominal CT scans are inferior to ultrasonography in diagnosing gallstones. The major application of CT scans is to define the course and status of the extrahepatic biliary tree and adjacent structures. It is the test of choice in evaluating the patient with suspected malignancy of the gallbladder, the extrahepatic biliary system, or nearby organs, in particular the head of the pancreas. Use of CT scan is an integral part of the differential diagnosis of obstructive jaundice (Fig. 31-7). Spiral CT scanning provides additional staging information, including vascular involvement in patients with periampullary tumors.[15]

Percutaneous Transhepatic Cholangiography

An intrahepatic bile duct is accessed percutaneously with a small needle under fluoroscopic guidance. Once the position in a bile duct has been confirmed, a guidewire is passed and subsequently a catheter passed over the wire (Fig. 31-8). Through the catheter, a cholangiogram can be performed and therapeutic interventions done, such as biliary drain insertions and stent placements. Percutaneous transhepatic cholangiography (PTC) has little role in the management of patients with uncomplicated gallstone disease, but is particularly useful in patients with bile duct strictures and tumors, as it defines the anatomy of the biliary tree proximal to the affected segment. As with any invasive procedure, there are potential risks. For PTC these are mainly bleeding, cholangitis, bile leak, and other catheter-related problems.[14]

Magnetic Resonance Imaging

Available since the mid-1990s, MRI provides anatomic details of the liver, gallbladder, and pancreas similar to those obtained from CT. Using MRI with newer techniques and contrast materials, accurate anatomic images can be obtained of the bile ducts and the pancreatic duct. It has a sensitivity and specificity of 95 and 89%, respectively, at detecting choledocholithiasis.[16] If available, MRI with magnetic resonance cholangiopancreatography (MRCP) offers a single noninvasive test for the diagnosis of biliary tract and pancreatic disease[17] (Fig. 31-9).

Endoscopic Retrograde Cholangiography and Endoscopic Ultrasound

Using a side-viewing endoscope, the common bile duct can be cannulated and a cholangiogram performed using fluoroscopy (Fig. 31-10). The procedure requires intravenous sedation for the patient. The advantages of endoscopic retrograde cholangiography (ERC) include direct visualization of the ampullary region and direct access to the distal common bile duct, with the possibility of therapeutic intervention. The test is rarely needed for uncomplicated gallstone disease, but for stones in the common bile duct, in particular when associated with obstructive jaundice, cholangitis, or

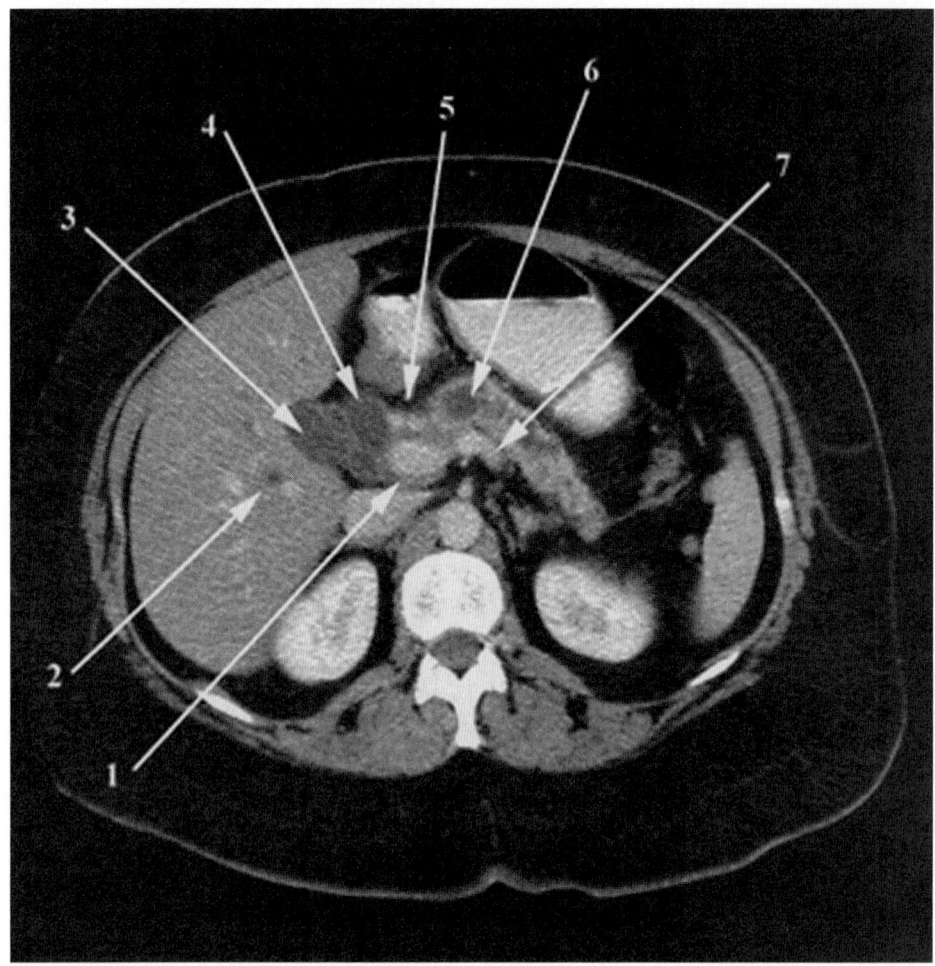

FIG. 31-7. CT scan of the upper abdomen from a patient with cancer of the distal common bile duct. The cancer obstructs the common bile duct as well as the pancreatic duct. 1. The portal vein. 2. A dilated intrahepatic bile duct. 3. Dilated cystic duct and the neck of the gallbladder. 4. Dilated common hepatic duct. 5. The bifurcation of the common hepatic artery into the gastroduodenal artery and the proper hepatic artery. 6. Dilated pancreatic duct. 7. The splenic vein.

gallstone pancreatitis, ERC is the diagnostic and often therapeutic procedure of choice. Once the endoscopic cholangiogram has shown ductal stones, sphincterotomy and stone extraction can be performed, and the common bile duct cleared of stones. In the hands of experts, the success rate of common bile duct cannulation and cholangiography is more than 90%. Complications of diagnostic ERC include pancreatitis and cholangitis, and occur in up to 5% of patients.[18]

An endoscopic ultrasound requires a special endoscope with an ultrasound transducer at its tip. The results are operator dependent, but offer noninvasive imaging of the bile ducts and adjacent structures. It is of particular value in the evaluation of tumors and their resectability. The ultrasound endoscope has a biopsy channel, allowing needle biopsies of a tumor under ultrasonic guidance. Endoscopic ultrasound also has been used to identify bile duct stones, and although it is less sensitive than ERC, the technique is less invasive.

GALLSTONE DISEASE

Prevalence and Incidence

Gallstone disease is one of the most common problems affecting the digestive tract. Autopsy reports have shown a prevalence of gallstones from 11 to 36%. The prevalence of gallstones is related to many factors, including age, gender, and ethnic background. Certain conditions predispose to the development of gallstones. Obesity, pregnancy, dietary factors, Crohn's disease, terminal ileal resection, gastric surgery, hereditary spherocytosis, sickle cell disease, and thalassemia are all associated with an increased risk of developing

gallstones.[8] Women are three times more likely to develop gallstones than men, and first-degree relatives of patients with gallstones have a twofold greater prevalence.[19]

Natural History

Most patients will remain asymptomatic from their gallstones throughout life. For unknown reasons some patients progress to a symptomatic stage, with biliary colic caused by a stone obstructing the cystic duct. Symptomatic gallstone disease may progress to complications related to the gallstones.[20] These include acute cholecystitis, choledocholithiasis with or without cholangitis, gallstone pancreatitis, cholecystocholedochal fistula, cholecystoduodenal fistula, cholecystoenteric fistula leading to gallstone ileus, and gallbladder carcinoma. Rarely, complication of gallstones is the presenting picture.

Gallstones in patients without biliary symptoms are commonly diagnosed incidentally on ultrasonography, CT scans, abdominal radiography, or at laparotomy. Several studies have examined the likelihood of developing biliary colic or developing significant complications of gallstone disease. Approximately 3% of asymptomatic individuals become symptomatic per year (i.e., develop biliary colic). Once symptomatic, patients tend to have recurring bouts of biliary colic. Complicated gallstone disease develops in 3 to 5% of symptomatic patients per year. Over a 20-year period, about two thirds of asymptomatic patients with gallstones remain symptom free.

Since few patients develop complications without previous biliary symptoms, prophylactic cholecystectomy in asymptomatic

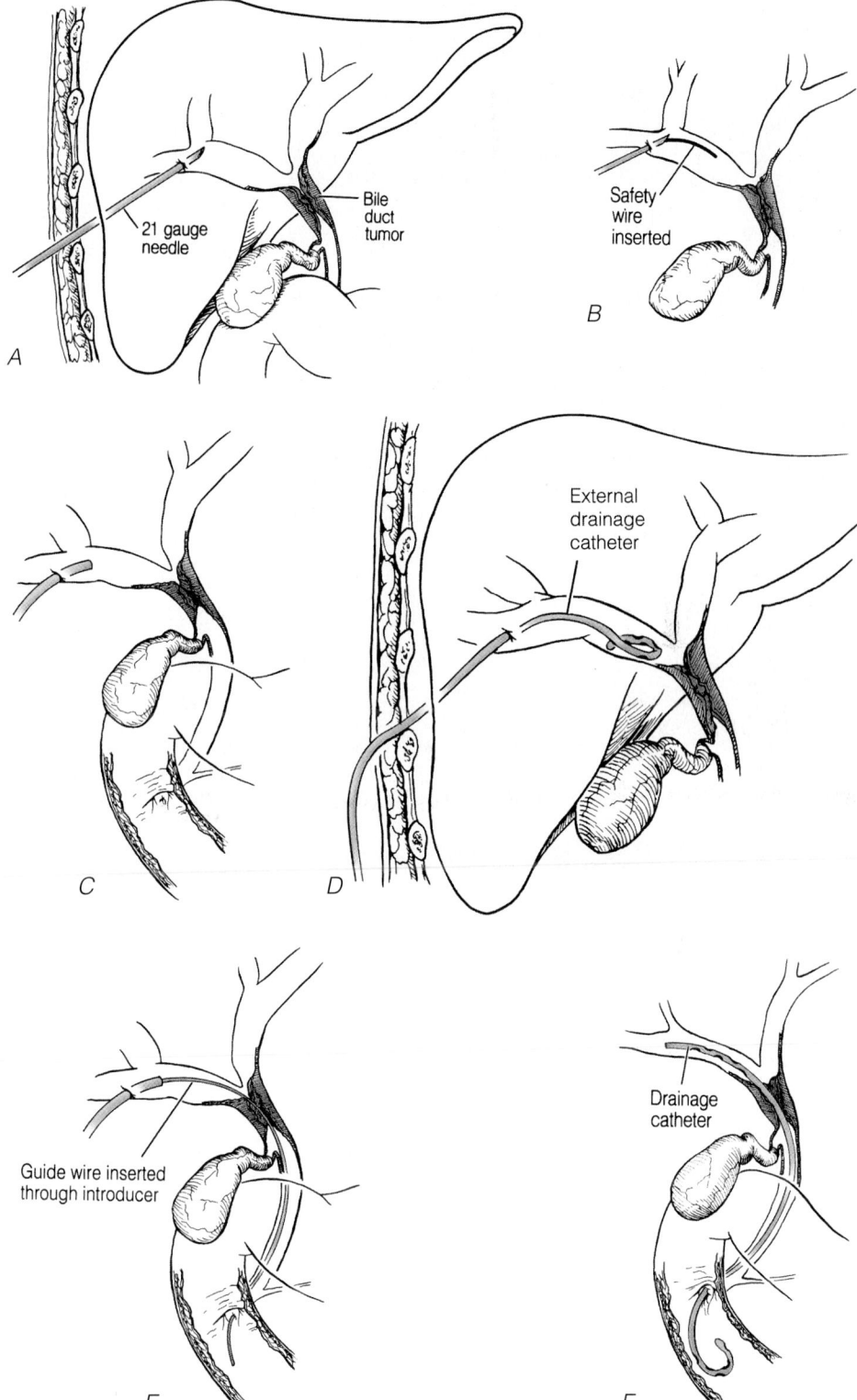

FIG. 31-8. Schematic diagram of percutaneous transhepatic cholangiogram (PTC) and drainage for an obstructing proximal cholangiocarcinoma. *A.* The dilated intrahepatic bile duct is entered percutaneously with a fine needle. *B.* A small guidewire is passed through the needle into the duct. *C.* A plastic catheter has been passed over the wire, and the wire is subsequently removed. A cholangiogram is performed through the catheter. *D.* An external drainage catheter in place. *E.* A long wire is placed via the catheter and advanced past the tumor and into the duodenum. *F.* An internal stent has been placed through the tumor.

persons with gallstones is rarely indicated. For elderly patients with diabetes, for individuals who will be isolated from medical care for extended periods of time, and in populations with increased risk of gallbladder cancer, a prophylactic cholecystectomy may be advisable. Porcelain gallbladder, a rare premalignant condition in which the wall of the gallbladder becomes calcified, is an absolute indication for cholecystectomy.

Gallstone Formation

Gallstones form as a result of solids settling out of solution. The major organic solutes in bile are bilirubin, bile salts, phospholipids, and cholesterol. Gallstones are classified by their cholesterol content as either cholesterol stones or pigment stones. Pigment stones can be further classified as either black or brown. In Western countries,

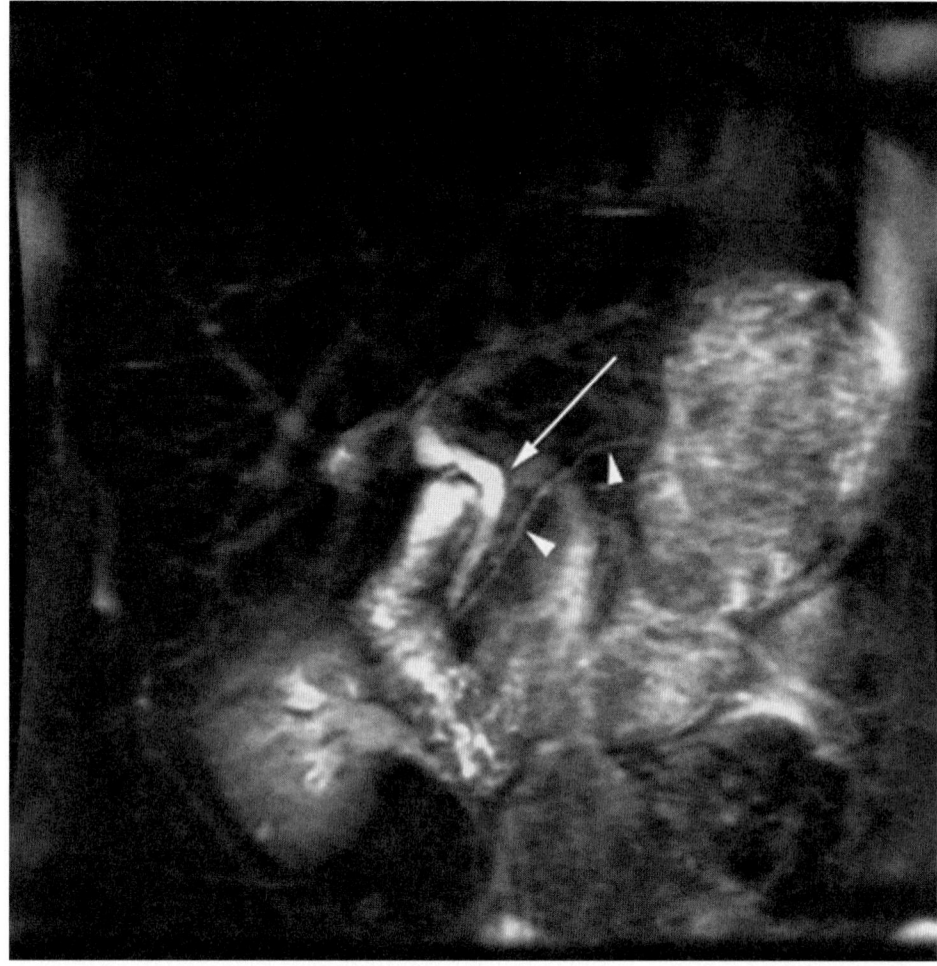

FIG.   31-9. Magnetic   resonance cholangiopancreatography   (MRCP). This view shows the course of the extrahepatic bile ducts (*arrow*) and the pancreatic duct (*arrowheads*).

about 80% of gallstones are cholesterol stones and about 15 to 20% are black pigment stones. Brown pigment stones account for only a small percentage. Both types of pigment stones are more common in Asia.

Cholesterol Stones

Pure chlolesterol stones are uncommon and account for less than 10% of all stones. They usually occur as single large stones with smooth surfaces. Most other cholesterol stones contain variable amounts of bile pigments and calcium, but are always more than 70% cholesterol by weight. These stones are usually multiple, of variable size, and may be hard and faceted or irregular, mulberry-shaped and soft (Fig. 31-11). Colors range from whitish yellow and green to black. Most cholesterol stones are radiolucent; less than 10% are radiopaque. Whether pure or of mixed nature, the common primary event in the formation of cholesterol stones is supersaturation of bile with cholesterol. Therefore high bile cholesterol levels and cholesterol gallstones are considered as one disease. Cholesterol is highly nonpolar and insoluble in water and bile. Cholesterol solubility depends on the relative concentration of cholesterol, bile salts, and lecithin (the main phospholipid in bile). Supersaturation almost always is caused by cholesterol hypersecretion rather than by a reduced secretion of phospholipid or bile salts.[2]

Cholesterol is secreted into bile as cholesterol-phospholipid vesicles. Cholesterol is held in solution by micelles, a conjugated bile salt-phospholipid-cholesterol complex, as well as by the cholesterol-phospholipid vesicles. The presence of vesicles and micelles in the same aqueous compartment allows the movement of lipids between the two. Vesicular maturation occurs when vesicular lipids are incorporated into micelles. Vesicular phospholipids are incorporated into micelles more readily than vesicular cholesterol. Therefore vesicles may become enriched in cholesterol, become unstable, and nucleate cholesterol crystals. In unsaturated bile, cholesterol enrichment of vesicles is inconsequential. In the supersaturated bile, cholesterol-dense zones develop on the surface of the cholesterol-enriched vesicles, leading to the appearance of cholesterol crystals. About one third of biliary cholesterol is transported in micelles, but the cholesterol-phospholipid vesicles carry the majority of biliary cholesterol[21] (Fig. 31-12).

Pigment Stones

Pigment stones contain less than 20% cholesterol and are dark because of the presence of calcium bilirubinate. Otherwise, black and brown pigment stones have little in common and should be considered as separate entities.

Black pigment stones are usually small, brittle, black, and sometimes spiculated. They are formed by supersaturation of calcium bilirubinate, carbonate, and phosphate, most often secondary to hemolytic disorders such as hereditary spherocytosis and sickle cell disease, and in those with cirrhosis. Like cholesterol stones, they almost always form in the gallbladder. Unconjugated bilirubin is much less soluble than conjugated bilirubin in bile. Deconjugation of bilirubin occurs normally in bile at a slow rate. Excessive levels of conjugated bilirubin, as in hemolytic states, lead to an increased

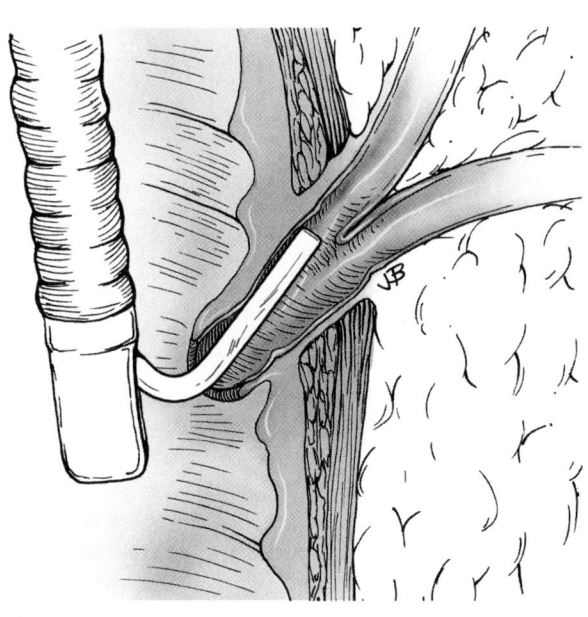

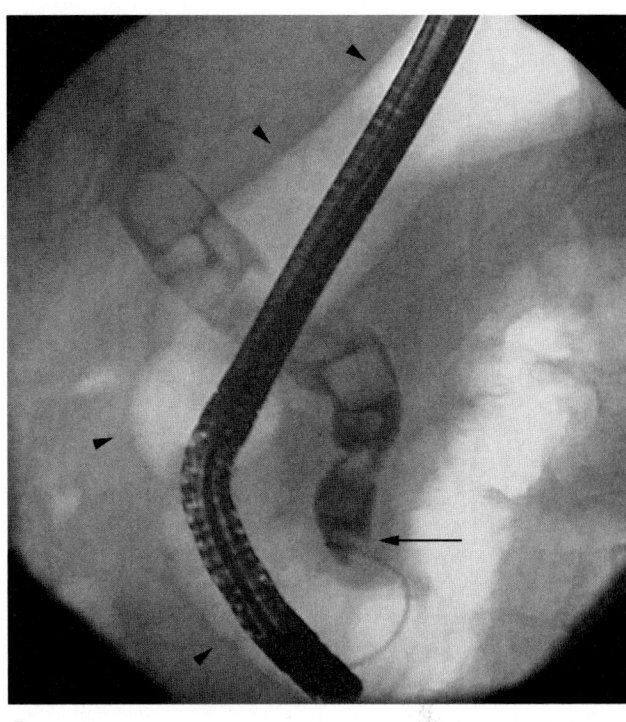

A   *B*

FIG. 31-10. Endoscopic retrograde cholangiography (ERC). *A. A schematic picture showing the side-viewing endoscope in the duodenum and a catheter in the common bile duct. B. An endoscopic cholangiography showing stones in the common bile duct. The catheter has been placed in the ampulla of vater (arrow). Note the duodenal shadow indicated with arrowheads.*

rate of production of unconjugated bilirubin. Cirrhosis may lead to increased secretion of unconjugated bilirubin. When altered conditions lead to increased levels of deconjugated bilirubin in bile, precipitation with calcium occurs. In Asian countries such as Japan, black stones account for a much higher percentage of gallstones than in the Western hemisphere.

Brown stones are usually less than 1 cm in diameter, brownish-yellow, soft, and often mushy. They may form either in the

gallbladder or in the bile ducts, usually secondary to bacterial infection caused by bile stasis. Precipitated calcium bilirubinate and bacterial cell bodies compose the major part of the stone. Bacteria such as *Escherichia coli* secrete beta-glucuronidase that enzymatically cleaves bilirubin glucuronide to produce the insoluble unconjugated bilirubin. It precipitates with calcium, and along with dead bacterial cell bodies, forms soft brown stones in the biliary tree.

Brown stones are typically found in the biliary tree of Asian populations and are associated with stasis secondary to parasite infection. In Western populations, brown stones occur as primary bile duct stones in patients with biliary strictures or other common bile duct stones that cause stasis and bacterial contamination.[2,22]

Symptomatic Gallstones

Chronic Cholecystitis

About two thirds of patients with gallstone disease present with chronic cholecystitis characterized by recurrent attacks of pain, often inaccurately labeled biliary colic. The pain develops when a stone obstructs the cystic duct, resulting in a progressive increase of tension in the gallbladder wall. The pathologic changes, which often do not correlate well with symptoms, vary from an apparently normal gallbladder with minor chronic inflammation in the mucosa, to a shrunken, nonfunctioning gallbladder with gross transmural fibrosis and adhesions to nearby structures. The mucosa is initially normal or hypertrophied, but later becomes atrophied, with the epithelium protruding into the muscle coat, leading to the formation of the so-called Aschoff-Rokitansky sinuses.

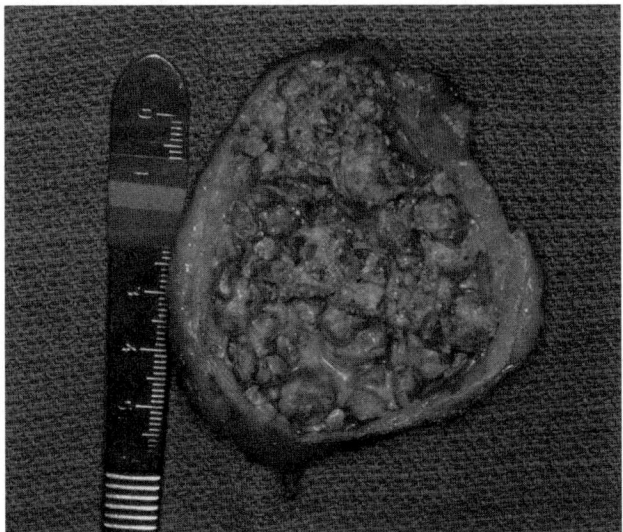

FIG. 31-11. *Gallbladder with cholesterol stones. Note the different shapes and sizes.*

Clinical Presentation. The chief symptom associated with symptomatic gallstones is pain. The pain is constant and increases in

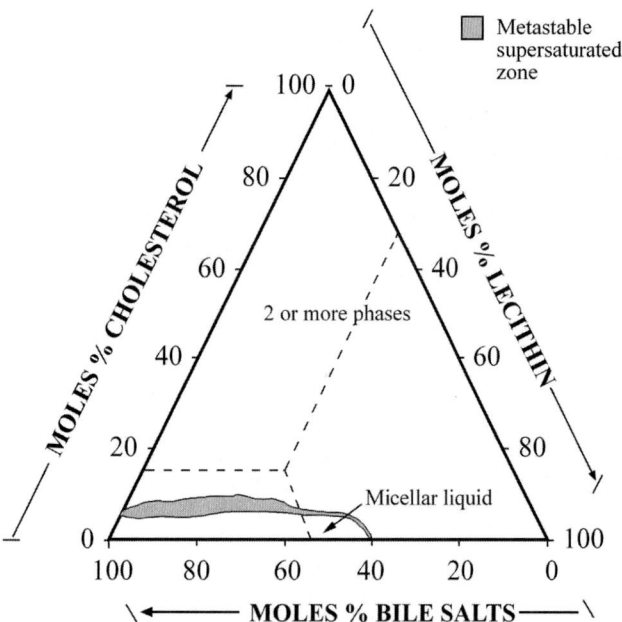

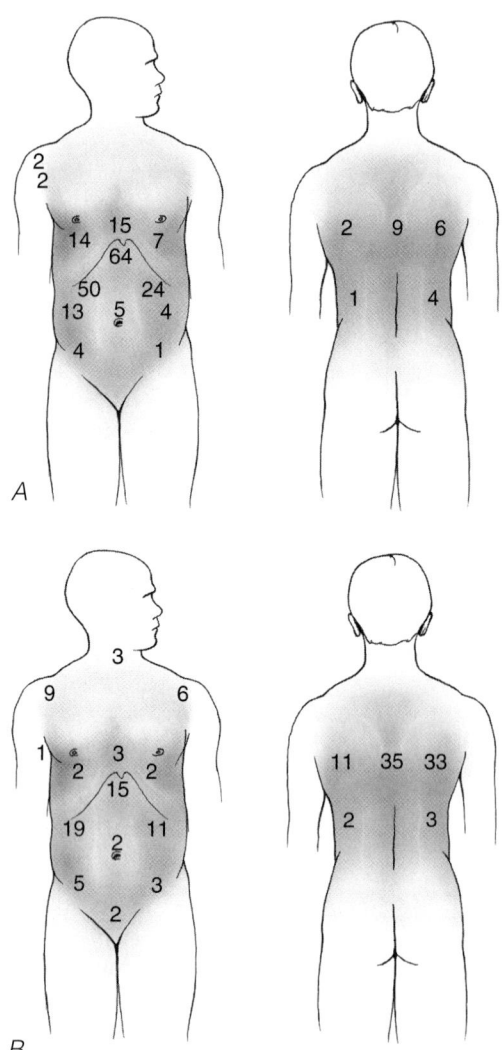

FIG. 31-12. The three major components of bile plotted on triangular coordinates. A given point represents the relative molar ratios of bile salts, lecithin, and cholesterol. The area labelled "micellar liquid" shows the range of concentrations found consistent with a clear micellar solution (single phase), where cholesterol is fully solubilized. The shaded area directly above this region corresponds to a metastable zone, supersaturated with cholesterol. Bile with a composition that falls above the shaded area has exceeded the solubilization capacity of cholesterol and precipitation of cholesterol crystals occurs. [Reproduced with permission from Holzbach RT: Pathogenesis and medical treatment of gallstones, in Slesinger MH, Fordtran JS (eds): Gastrointestinal Diseases. Philadelphia: WB Saunders, 1989, p 1360.]

FIG. 31-13. A. Sites of the most severe pain during an episode of biliary pain in 107 patients with gallstones (values add up to more than 100% because of multiple responses). The subxiphoid and right subcostal areas were the most common sites; note that the left subcostal area was not an unusual site of pain. B. Sites of pain radiation (%) during an episode of biliary pain in the same group of patients. [Reproduced with permission from Gunn A, Keddie N: Some clinical observations on patients with gallstones. Lancet 2:230, 2004.]

severity over the first half hour or so and typically lasts 1 to 5 hours. It is located in the epigastrium or right upper quadrant and frequently radiates to the right upper back or between the scapulae (Fig. 31-13). The pain is severe and comes on abruptly, typically during the night or after a fatty meal. It often is associated with nausea and sometimes vomiting. The pain is episodic. The patient suffers discrete attacks of pain, between which they feel well. Physical examination may reveal mild right upper quadrant tenderness during an episode of pain. If the patient is pain free, the physical exam is usually unremarkable. Laboratory values, such as white blood cell count and liver function tests, are usually normal in patients with uncomplicated gallstones.

Atypical presentation of gallstone disease is common. Association with meals is present in only about 50% of patients. Some patients report milder attacks of pain, but relate it to meals. The pain may be located primarily in the back or the left upper or lower right quadrant. Bloating and belching may be present and associated with the attacks of pain. In patients with atypical presentation, other conditions with upper abdominal pain should be sought out, even in the presence of gallstones. These include peptic ulcer disease, gastroesophageal reflux disease, abdominal wall hernias, irritable bowel disease, diverticular disease, liver diseases, renal calculi, pleuritic pain, and myocardial pain. Many patients with other conditions have gallstones.

When the pain lasts more than 24 hours, an impacted stone in the cystic duct or acute cholecystitis (see below) should be suspected. An impacted stone will result in what is called *hydrops of the gallbladder.* The bile gets absorbed, but the gallbladder epithelium continues to secrete mucus and the gallbladder becomes distended with

mucinous material. The gallbladder may be palpable, but usually is not tender. Hydrops of the gallbladder may result in edema of the gallbladder wall, inflammation, infection, and perforation. Although hydrops may persist with few consequences, early cholecystectomy is generally indicated to avoid complications.

Diagnosis. The diagnosis of symptomatic gallstones or chronic calculous cholecystitis depends on the presence of typical symptoms and the demonstration of stones on diagnostic imaging. An abdominal ultrasound is the standard diagnostic test for gallstones (see above).[23] Gallstones are occasionally identified on abdominal radiographs or CT scans. In these cases, if the patient has typical symptoms, an ultrasound of the gallbladder and the biliary tree should be added prior to surgical intervention. Stones diagnosed incidentally in patients without symptoms should be left in place as discussed previously. Occasionally, patients with typical attacks of biliary pain have no evidence of stones on ultrasonography.

Sometimes only sludge in the gallbladder is demonstrated on ultrasonography. If the patient has recurrent attacks of typical biliary pain and sludge is detected on two or more occasions, cholecystectomy is warranted. In addition to sludge and stones, cholesterolosis and adenomyomatosis of the gallbladder may cause typical biliary symptoms and may be detected on ultrasonography. Cholesterolosis is caused by the accumulation of cholesterol in macrophages in the gallbladder mucosa, either locally or as polyps. It produces the classic macroscopic appearance of a "strawberry gallbladder." Adenomyomatosis or cholecystitis glandularis proliferans is characterized on microscopy by hypertrophic smooth muscle bundles and by the ingrowths of mucosal glands into the muscle layer (epithelial sinus formation). Granulomatous polyps develop in the lumen at the fundus, and the gallbladder wall is thickened and septae or strictures may be seen in the gallbladder. In symptomatic patients, cholecystectomy is the treatment of choice for patients with these conditions.[24]

Management. Patients with symptomatic gallstones should be advised to have elective laparoscopic cholecystectomy. While waiting for surgery, or if surgery has to be postponed, the patient should be advised to avoid dietary fats and large meals. Diabetic patients with symptomatic gallstones should have a cholecystectomy promptly, as they are more prone to develop acute cholecystitis that is often severe. Pregnant women with symptomatic gallstones who cannot be managed expectantly with diet modifications can safely undergo laparoscopic cholecystectomy during the second trimester. Laparoscopic cholecystectomy is safe and effective in children as well as in the elderly. Cholecystectomy, open or laparoscopic, for patients with symptomatic gallstones offers excellent long-term results. About 90% of patients with typical biliary symptoms and stones are rendered symptom free after cholecystectomy. For patients with atypical symptoms or dyspepsia (flatulence, belching, bloating, and dietary fat intolerance) the results are not as favorable.

Acute Cholecystitis

Pathogenesis. Acute cholecystitis is secondary to gallstones in 90 to 95% of cases. Acute acalculous cholecystitis is a condition that typically occurs in patients with other acute systemic diseases (see acalculous cholecystitis section, below). In less than 1% of acute cholecystitis, the cause is a tumor obstructing the cystic duct. Obstruction of the cystic duct by a gallstone is the initiating event that leads to gallbladder distention, inflammation, and edema of the gallbladder wall. Why inflammation develops only occasionally with cystic duct obstruction is unknown. It is probably related to the duration of obstruction of the cystic duct. Initially, acute cholecystitis is an inflammatory process, possibly mediated by lysolecithin, a product of lecithin, as well as bile salts and platelet-activating factor. Secondary bacterial contamination is documented in over one half of patients undergoing early cholecystectomy for acute uncomplicated cholecystitis. In acute cholecystitis the gallbladder wall becomes grossly thickened and reddish with subserosal hemorrhages. Pericholecystic fluid often is present. The mucosa may show hyperemia and patchy necrosis. In severe cases, about 5 to 10%, the inflammatory process progresses and leads to ischemia and necrosis of the gallbladder wall. More frequently, the gallstone is dislodged and the inflammation resolves.[25]

When the gallbladder remains obstructed and secondary bacterial infection supervenes, an acute gangrenous cholecystitis develops and an abscess or empyema forms within the gallbladder. Rarely, perforation of ischemic areas occurs. The perforation is usually contained in the subhepatic space by the omentum and adjacent organs.

However, free perforation with peritonitis, intrahepatic perforation with intrahepatic abscesses, and perforation into adjacent organs (duodenum or colon) with cholecystoenteric fistula occur. When gas-forming organisms are part of the secondary bacterial infection, gas may be seen in the gallbladder lumen and in the wall of the gallbladder on abdominal radiographs and CT scans, an entity called an emphysematous gallbladder.

Clinical Manifestations. About 80% of patients with acute cholecystitis give a history compatible with chronic cholecystitis. Acute cholecystitis begins as an attack of biliary colic, but in contrast to biliary colic, the pain does not subside; it is unremitting and may persist for several days. The pain is typically in the right upper quadrant or epigastrium, and may radiate to the right upper part of the back or the interscapular area. It is usually more severe than the pain associated with uncomplicated biliary colic. The patient is often febrile, complains of anorexia, nausea, and vomiting, and is reluctant to move, as the inflammatory process affects the parietal peritoneum. On physical exam, focal tenderness and guarding are usually present in the right upper quadrant. A mass, the gallbladder and adherent omentum, is occasionally palpable; however, guarding may prevent this. A Murphy's sign, an inspiratory arrest with deep palpation in the right subcostal area, is characteristic of acute cholecystitis.

A mild to moderate leukocytosis (12,000 to 15,000 cells/mm^3) is usually present. However, some patients may have a normal WBC. A high WBC (above 20,000) is suggestive of a complicated form of cholecystitis such as gangrenous cholecystitis, perforation, or associated cholangitis. Serum liver chemistries are usually normal, but a mild elevation of serum bilirubin, less than 4 mg/mL, may be present along with mild elevation of alkaline phosphatase, transaminases, and amylase.[23] Severe jaundice is suggestive of common bile duct stones or obstruction of the bile ducts by severe pericholecystic inflammation secondary to impaction of a stone in the infundibulum of the gallbladder that mechanically obstructs the bile duct (Mirizzi's syndrome). In elderly patients and in those with diabetes mellitus, acute cholecystitis may have a subtle presentation resulting in a delay in diagnosis. The incidence of complications is higher in these patients, who also have approximately tenfold the mortality rate compared to that of younger and healthier patients.

The differential diagnosis for acute cholecystitis includes a peptic ulcer with or without perforation, pancreatitis, appendicitis, hepatitis, perihepatitis (Fitz-Hugh and Curtis syndrome), myocardial ischemia, pneumonia, pleuritis, and herpes zoster involving the intercostal nerve.

Diagnosis. Ultrasonography is the most useful radiologic test for diagnosing acute cholecystitis. It has a sensitivity and specificity of 95%. In addition to being a sensitive test for documenting the presence or absence of stones, it will show the thickening of the gallbladder wall and the pericholecystic fluid (Fig. 31-14). Focal tenderness over the gallbladder when compressed by the sonographic probe (sonographic Murphy's sign) also is suggestive of acute cholecystitis. Biliary radionuclide scanning (HIDA scan) may be of help in the atypical case. Lack of filling of the gallbladder after 4 hours indicates an obstructed cystic duct, and in the clinical setting of acute cholecystitis is highly sensitive and specific for acute cholecystitis. A normal HIDA scan excludes acute cholecystitis. CT scan is frequently performed on patients with acute abdominal pain. It demonstrates thickening of the gallbladder wall, pericholecystic fluid, and the presence of gallstones as well as air in the gallbladder wall, but is less sensitive than ultrasonography.

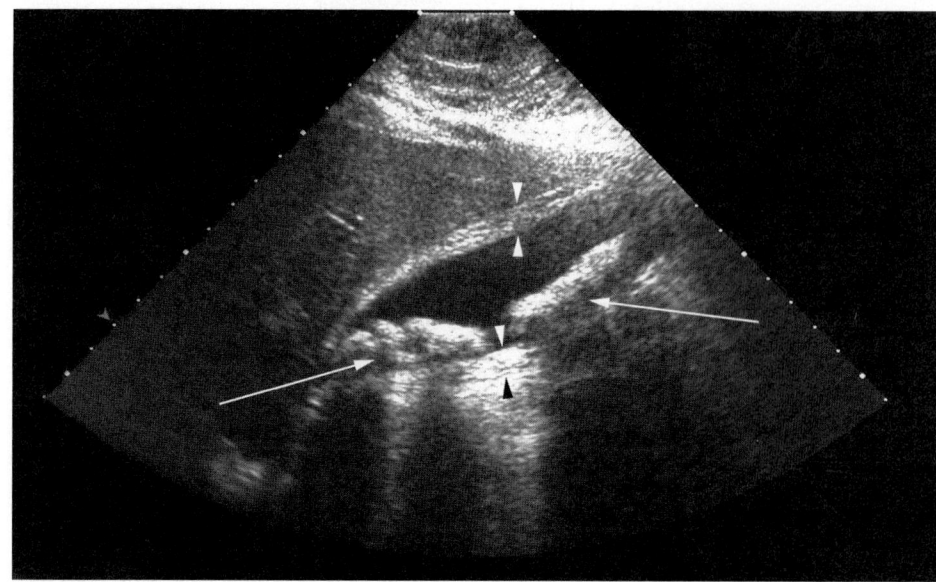

FIG. 31-14. Ultrasonography from a patient with acute cholecystitis. The arrowheads indicate the thickened gallbladder wall. There are several stones in the gallbladder (arrows) throwing acoustic shadows.

Treatment. Patients who present with acute cholecystitis will need intravenous fluids, antibiotics, and analgesia. The antibiotics should cover gram-negative aerobes as well as anaerobes. A third-generation cephalosporin with good anaerobic coverage or a second-generation cephalosporin combined with metronidazole are typical regimens. For patients with allergies to cephalosporins an aminoglycoside with metronidazole is appropriate. Although the inflammation in acute cholecystitis may be sterile in some patients, more than one half will have positive cultures from the gallbladder bile. It is difficult to know who is secondarily infected; therefore antibiotics have become a part of the management in most medical centers.

Cholecystectomy is the definitive treatment for acute cholecystitis.[26] The timing of cholecystectomy has been a matter of debate in the past. Early cholecystectomy performed within 2 to 3 days of the illness is preferred over interval or delayed cholecystectomy that is performed 6 to 10 weeks after initial medical treatment and recuperation. Several studies have shown that unless the patient is unfit for surgery, early cholecystectomy should be recommended as it offers the patient a definitive solution in one hospital admission, quicker recovery times, and an earlier return to work.[27]

Laparoscopic cholecystectomy is the procedure of choice for acute cholecystitis. The conversion rate to an open cholecystectomy is higher (10 to 15%) in the setting of acute cholecystitis than with chronic cholecystitis. The procedure is more tedious and takes longer than in the elective setting. However, when compared to the delayed operation, early operation carries a similar number of complications.

When patients present late, after 3 to 4 days of illness, or are for some reason unfit for surgery, they are treated with antibiotics with laparoscopic cholecystectomy scheduled for approximately 2 months later. Approximately 20% of patients will fail to respond to initial medical therapy and require an intervention. Laparoscopic cholecystectomy could be attempted, but the conversion rate is high and some prefer to go directly for an open cholecystectomy. For those unfit for surgery, a percutaneous cholecystostomy or an open cholecystostomy under local analgesia can be performed. Failure to improve after cholecystostomy usually is due to gangrene of the gallbladder or perforation. For these patients, surgery is unavoidable. For those who respond after cholecystostomy, the tube can be

removed once cholangiography through it shows a patent ductus cysticus. Laparoscopic cholecystectomy may then be scheduled in the near future.[28] For the occasional patient who will not tolerate surgery, the stones can be extracted via the cholecystostomy tube before its removal.

Choledocholithiasis

Common bile duct stones may be small or large, single or multiple, and are found in 6 to 12% of patients with stones in the gallbladder. The incidence increases with age. About 20 to 25% of patients above the age of 60 with symptomatic gallstones have stones in the common bile duct as well as in the gallbladder.[29] The vast majority of ductal stones in Western countries are formed within the gallbladder and migrate down the cystic duct to the common bile duct. These are classified as secondary common bile duct stones, in contrast to the primary stones that form in the bile ducts. The secondary stones are usually cholesterol stones, whereas the primary stones are usually of the brown pigment type. The primary stones are associated with biliary stasis and infection and are more commonly seen in Asian populations. The causes of biliary stasis that lead to the development of primary stones include biliary stricture, papillary stenosis, tumors, or other (secondary) stones.

Clinical Manifestations. Choledochal stones may be silent and often are discovered incidentally. They may cause obstruction, complete or incomplete, or they may manifest with cholangitis or gallstone pancreatitis. The pain caused by a stone in the bile duct is very similar to that of biliary colic caused by impaction of a stone in the cystic duct. Nausea and vomiting are common. Physical exam may be normal, but mild epigastric or right upper quadrant tenderness as well as mild icterus are common. The symptoms may also be intermittent, such as pain and transient jaundice caused by a stone that temporarily impacts the ampulla but subsequently moves away, acting as a ball valve. A small stone may pass through the ampulla spontaneously with resolution of symptoms. Finally the stones may become completely impacted, causing severe progressive jaundice. Elevation of serum bilirubin, alkaline phosphatase, and transaminases are commonly seen in patients with bile duct stones. However, in about one third of patients with common bile duct stones, the liver chemistries are normal.

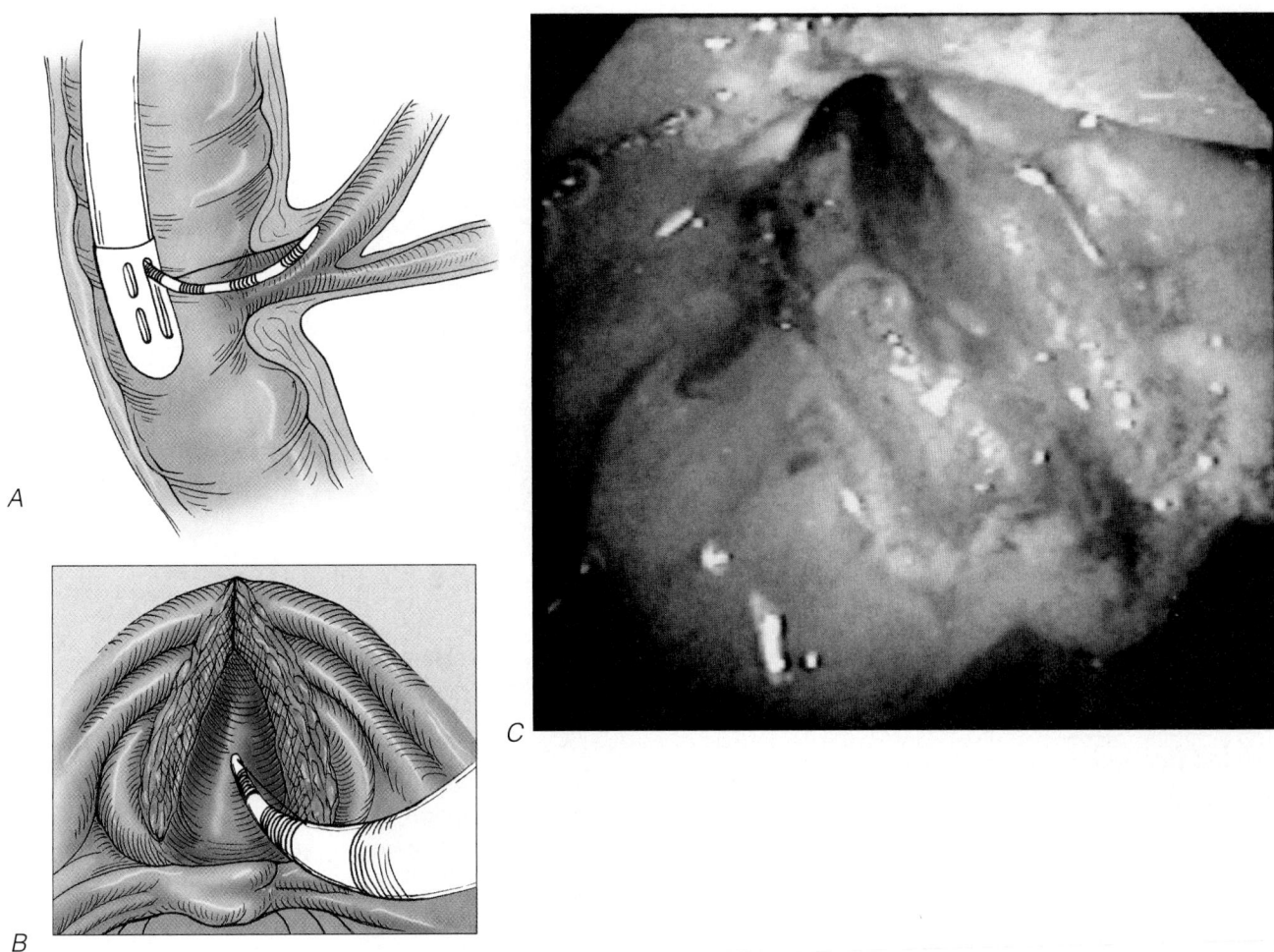

FIG. 31-15. *An endoscopic sphincterotomy. A. The sphincterotome in place. B. Completed sphinctero-tomy. C. Endoscopic picture of completed sphincterotomy.*

Commonly the first test, ultrasonography, is useful for documenting stones in the gallbladder (if they are still present), as well as determining the size of the common bile duct. As stones in the bile ducts tend to move down to the distal part of the common duct, bowel gas can preclude their demonstration on ultrasonography. A dilated common bile duct (>8 mm in diameter) on ultrasonography in a patient with gallstones, jaundice, and biliary pain is highly suggestive of common bile duct stones. Magnetic resonance cholangiography (MRC) provides excellent anatomic detail and has a sensitivity and specificity of 95 and 89%, respectively, at detecting choledocholithiasis.[17] Endoscopic cholangiography is the gold standard for diagnosing common bile duct stones. It has the distinct advantage of providing a therapeutic option at the time of diagnosis. In experienced hands, cannulation of the ampulla of Vater and diagnostic cholangiography are achieved in over 90% of cases, with associated morbidity of less than 5% (mainly cholangitis and pancreatitis). An endoscopic ultrasound is less sensitive, but can be done in nearly every patient without associated complications. PTC is rarely needed in patients with secondary common bile duct stones, but is frequently performed for both diagnostic and therapeutic reasons in patients with primary bile duct stones.

Treatment. For patients with symptomatic gallstones and suspected common bile duct stones, either preoperative endoscopic cholangiography or an intraoperative cholangiogram will document

the bile duct stones.[30] If an endoscopic cholangiogram reveals stones, sphincterotomy and ductal clearance of the stones is appropriate, followed by a laparoscopic cholecystectomy. An intraoperative cholangiogram at the time of cholecystectomy will also document the presence or absence of bile duct stones[31] (Fig. 31-15). Laparoscopic common bile duct exploration via the cystic duct or with formal choledochotomy allows the stones to be retrieved in the same setting (see next section). If the expertise and/or the instruments for laparoscopic common bile duct exploration are not available, a drain should be left adjacent to the cystic duct and the patient scheduled for endoscopic sphincterotomy the following day. An open common bile duct exploration is an option if the endoscopic method has already been tried or is for some reason not feasible. If a choledochotomy is performed, a T tube is left in place. Stones impacted in the ampulla may be difficult for both endoscopic ductal clearance as well as common bile duct exploration (open or laparoscopic). In these cases the common bile duct is usually quite dilated (about 2 cm in diameter). A choledochoduodenostomy or a Roux-en-Y choledochojejunostomy may be the best option for these circumstances.[32]

Retained or recurrent stones following cholecystectomy are best treated endoscopically (Fig. 31-16). If the stones were deliberately left in place at the time of surgery or diagnosed shortly after the cholecystectomy, they are classified as *retained*; those diagnosed months or years later are termed *recurrent*. If a common bile duct

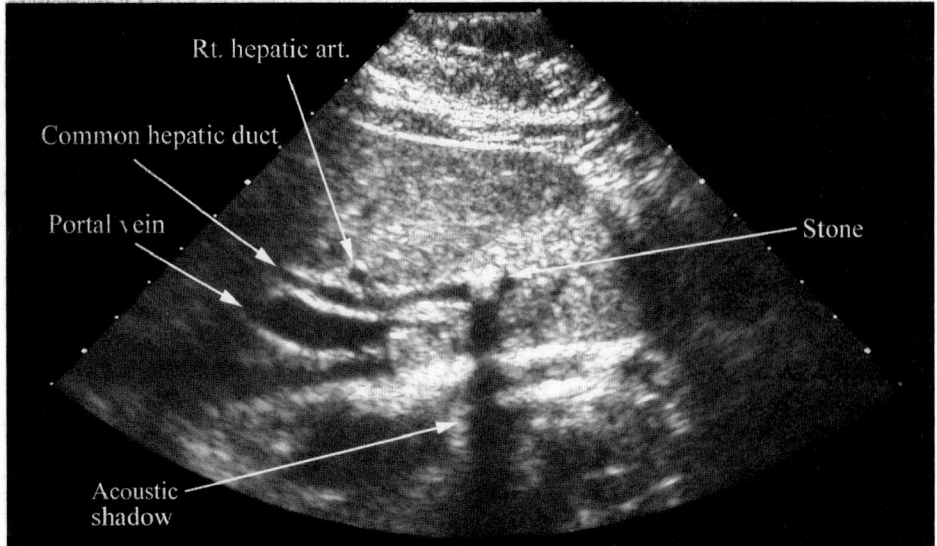

A

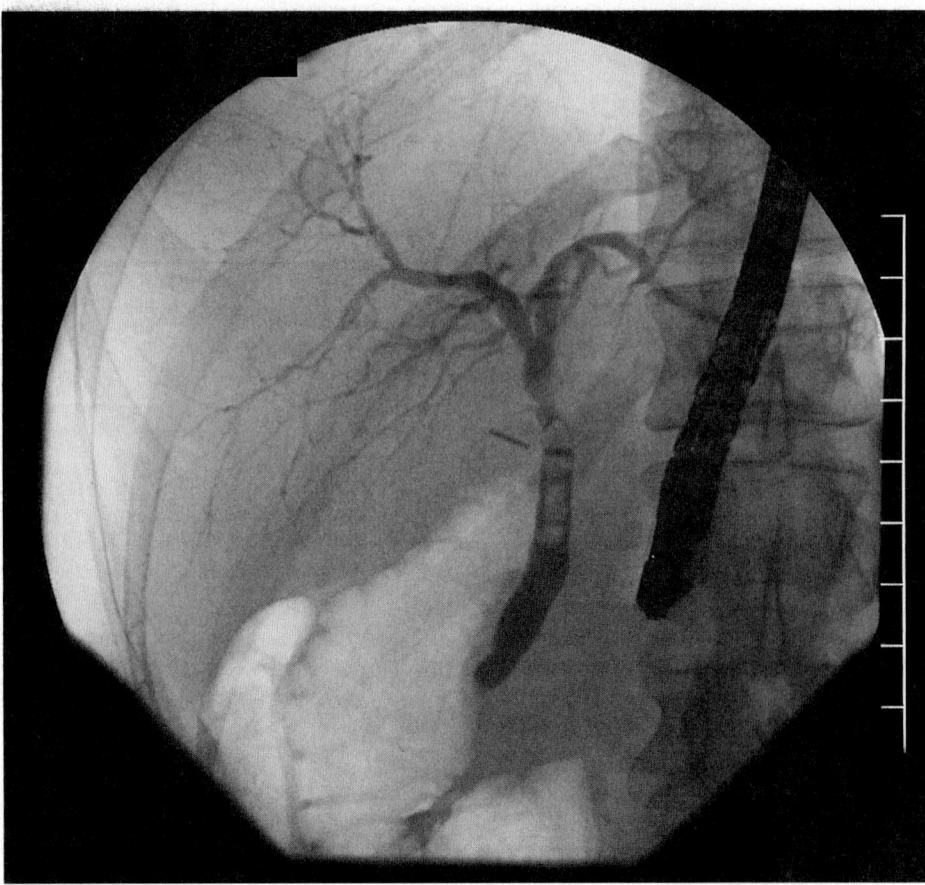

B

FIG. 31-16. Retained common bile duct stones. The patient presented 3 weeks after laparoscopic cholecystectomy. *A.* An ultrasound shows a normal or mildly dilated common bile duct with a stone. Note the location of the right hepatic artery anterior to the common hepatic duct (an anatomic variation). *B.* An ERC from the same patient shows multiple stones in the common bile duct. Only the top one showed on ultrasound, as the other stones lie in the distal common bile duct behind the duodenum.

exploration was performed and a T tube left in place, a T-tube cholangiogram is obtained prior to its removal. Retained stones can be retrieved either endoscopically or via the T-tube tract once it has matured (2 to 4 weeks). The T tube is then removed and a catheter passed through the tract into the common bile duct. Under fluoroscopic guidance the stones are retrieved with baskets or balloons.

Recurrent stones may be multiple and large. A generous endoscopic sphincterotomy will allow stone retrieval as well as spontaneous passage of retained and recurrent stones. Patients over the age of 70 presenting with bile duct stones should have their ductal stones cleared endoscopically. They do not need to be submitted for a cholecystectomy, as only about 15% will become symptomatic from their gallbladder stones, and such patients can be treated as the need arises by a cholecystectomy.

Cholangitis

Cholangitis is one of the two main complications of choledochal stones, the other being gallstone pancreatitis. Acute cholangitis is an ascending bacterial infection in association with partial or complete obstruction of the bile ducts. Hepatic bile is sterile, and bile in the bile ducts is kept sterile by continuous bile flow and by the presence of antibacterial substances in bile such as immunoglobulin. Mechanical hindrance to bile flow facilitates bacterial contamination. Positive bile cultures are common in the presence of bile duct stones as well as with other causes of obstruction. Biliary bacterial contamination alone does not lead to clinical cholangitis; the combination of both significant bacterial contamination and biliary obstruction is required for its development. Gallstones are the most common cause of obstruction in cholangitis; other causes are benign and malignant strictures, parasites, instrumentation of the ducts and indwelling stents, and partially obstructed biliary-enteric anastomosis. The most common organisms cultured from bile in patients with cholangitis include *Escherichia coli, Klebsiella pneumoniae, Streptococcus faecalis,* and *Bacteroides fragilis.*[33]

Clinical Presentation. Cholangitis may present as anything from a mild, intermittent, and self-limited disease to a fulminant, potentially life-threatening septicemia. The patient with gallstone-induced cholangitis is typically older and female. The most common presentation is fever, epigastric or right upper quadrant pain, and jaundice. These classic symptoms, well known as Charcot's triad, are present in about two thirds of patients. The illness may progress rapidly with septicemia and disorientation, known as Reynolds pentad (e.g., fever, jaundice, right upper quadrant pain, septic shock, and mental status changes). However, the presentation may be atypical, with little if any fever, jaundice, or pain. This occurs most commonly in the elderly, who may have unremarkable symptoms until they collapse with septicemia. Patients with indwelling stents rarely become jaundiced. On abdominal examination, the findings are indistinguishable from those of acute cholecystitis.[34]

Diagnosis and Management. Leukocytosis, hyperbilirubinemia, and elevation of alkaline phosphatase and transaminases are common, and when present, support the clinical diagnosis of cholangitis. Ultrasonography is helpful if the patient has not been diagnosed previously with gallstones, as it will document the presence of gallbladder stones, demonstrate dilated ducts, and possibly pinpoint the site of obstruction; however, rarely will it elucidate the cause. The definitive diagnostic test is ERC. In cases in which ERC is not available, PTC is indicated. Both ERC and PTC will show the level and the reason for the obstruction, allow culture of the bile, possibly allow the removal of stones if present, and drainage of the bile ducts with drainage catheters or stents. CT scanning and MRI will show pancreatic and periampullary masses, if present, in addition to the ductal dilatation.

The initial treatment of patients with cholangitis includes intravenous antibiotics and fluid resuscitation. These patients may require intensive care unit monitoring and vasopressor support. Most patients will respond to these measures. However, the obstructed bile duct must be drained as soon as the patient has been stabilized. About 15% of patients will not respond to antibiotics and fluid resuscitation, and an emergency biliary decompression may be required. Biliary decompression may be accomplished endoscopically, via the percutaneous transhepatic route, or surgically. The selection of

procedure should be based on the level and the nature of the biliary obstruction. Patients with choledocholithiasis or periampullary malignancies are best approached endoscopically, with sphincterotomy and stone removal, or by placement of an endoscopic biliary stent.[35] In patients in whom the obstruction is more proximal or perihilar, or when a stricture in a biliary-enteric anastomosis is the cause or the endoscopic route has failed, percutaneous transhepatic drainage is used. Where neither ERC nor PTC is possible, an emergent operation and decompression of the common bile duct with a T tube may be necessary and life-saving. Definitive operative therapy should be deferred until the cholangitis has been treated and the proper diagnosis established. Patients with indwelling stents and cholangitis usually require repeated imaging and exchange of the stent over a guidewire.

Acute cholangitis is associated with an overall mortality rate of approximately 5%. When associated with renal failure, cardiac impairment, hepatic abscesses, and malignancies, the morbidity and mortality rates are much higher.

Biliary Pancreatitis

Gallstones in the common bile duct are associated with acute pancreatitis. Obstruction of the pancreatic duct by an impacted stone or temporary obstruction by a stone passing through the ampulla may lead to pancreatitis. The exact mechanism by which the obstruction of the pancreatic duct leads to pancreatitis is still not clear. An ultrasonogram of the biliary tree in patients with pancreatitis is essential. If gallstones are present and the pancreatitis is severe, an ERC with sphincterotomy and stone extraction may abort the episode of pancreatitis. Once the pancreatitis has subsided, the gallbladder should be removed during the same admission. When gallstones are present and the pancreatitis is mild and self-limited, the stone has probably passed. For these patients a cholecystectomy and an intraoperative cholangiogram or a preoperative ERC is indicated.

Cholangiohepatitis

Cholangiohepatitis, also known as recurrent pyogenic cholangitis, is endemic to the Orient. It also has been encountered in the Chinese population in the United States as well as in Europe and Australia. It affects both sexes equally and occurs most frequently in the third and fourth decades of life. Cholangiohepatitis is caused by bacterial contamination (commonly *E. coli, Klebsiella* species, *Bacteroides* species, or *Enterococcus faecalis*) of the biliary tree, and often is associated with biliary parasites such as *Clonorchis sinensis, Opisthorchis viverrini,* and *Ascaris lumbricoides.* Bacterial enzymes cause deconjugation of bilirubin, which precipitates as bile sludge. The sludge and dead bacterial cell bodies form brown pigment stones. The nucleus of the stone may contain an adult *Clonorchis* worm, an ovum, or an ascarid. These stones are formed throughout the biliary tree and cause partial obstruction that contributes to the repeated bouts of cholangitis. Biliary strictures form as a result of recurrent cholangitis and lead to further stone formation, infection, hepatic abscesses, and liver failure (secondary biliary cirrhosis).[36]

The patient usually presents with pain in the right upper quadrant and epigastrium, fever, and jaundice. Recurrence of symptoms is one of the most characteristic features of the disease. The episodes may vary in severity, but without intervention will gradually lead to malnutrition and hepatic insufficiency. An ultrasound will detect stones in the biliary tree, pneumobilia from infection due to gas-forming organisms, liver abscesses, and occasionally strictures. The gallbladder may be thickened, but is inflamed in about 20%

of patients, and rarely contains stones. MRCP and PTC are the mainstays of biliary imaging for cholangiohepatitis. They can detect obstructions, define strictures and stones, and allow emergent decompression of the biliary tree in the septic patient. Hepatic abscesses may be drained percutaneously. The long-term goal of therapy is to extract stones and debris and relieve strictures. It may take several procedures and require a Roux-en-Y hepaticojejunostomy to establish biliary-enteric continuity. Occasionally, involved areas of the liver may offer the best form of treatment. Recurrences are common and the prognosis is poor once hepatic insufficiency has developed.[37]

OPERATIVE INTERVENTIONS FOR GALLSTONE DISEASE

Cholecystostomy

A cholecystostomy decompresses and drains the distended, inflamed, hydropic, or purulent gallbladder. It is applicable if the patient is not fit to tolerate an abdominal operation.[38] Ultrasound guided percutaneous drainage with a pigtail catheter is the procedure of choice. The catheter is inserted over a guidewire that has been passed through the abdominal wall, the liver, and into the gallbladder (Fig. 31-17). By passing the catheter through the liver, the risk of bile leak around the catheter is minimized.[39] The catheter can be removed when the inflammation has resolved and the patient's condition improved. The gallbladder can be removed later if indicated, usually by laparoscopy. Surgical cholecystostomy with a large catheter placed under local anesthesia is rarely required today.

Cholecystectomy

Cholecystectomy is the most common major abdominal procedure performed in Western countries. Carl Langenbuch performed the first successful cholecystectomy in 1882, and for over 100 years it was the standard treatment for symptomatic gallbladder stones. Open cholecystectomy was a safe and effective treatment for both acute and chronic cholecystitis. In 1987, laparoscopic cholecystectomy was introduced by Philippe Mouret in France and quickly revolutionized the treatment of gallstones. It not only supplanted open cholecystectomy, but also more or less ended attempts for noninvasive management of gallstones such as extracorporeal shock wave (ESWL) and bile salt therapy. Laparoscopic cholecystectomy

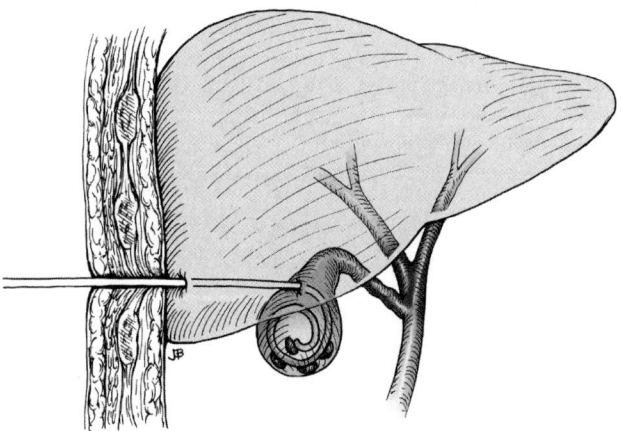

FIG. 31-17. *Percutaneous cholecystostomy. A pigtail catheter has been placed through the abdominal wall, the right lobe of the liver, and into the gallbladder.*

offers a cure for gallstones with a minimally-invasive procedure, minor pain and scarring, and early return to full activity. Today laparoscopic cholecystectomy is the treatment of choice for symptomatic gallstones.

Symptomatic gallstones are the main indication for cholecystectomy. Absolute contraindications for the procedure are uncontrolled coagulopathy and end-stage liver disease. Rarely, patients with severe obstructive pulmonary disease or congestive heart failure (e.g., cardiac ejection fraction <20%) may not tolerate pneumoperitoneum with carbon dioxide and require open cholecystectomy. Conditions formerly believed to be relative contraindications such as acute cholecystitis, gangrene and empyema of the gallbladder, biliary-enteric fistulae, obesity, pregnancy, ventriculoperitoneal shunt, cirrhosis, and previous upper abdominal procedures are risk factors for a potentially difficult laparoscopic cholecystectomy. When important anatomic structures cannot be clearly identified or when no progress is made over a set period of time, a conversion to an open procedure is usually indicated. In the elective setting, conversion to an open procedure is needed in about 5% of patients.[40] Emergent procedures may require more skill on the part of the surgeon, and be needed in patients with complicated gallstone disease; the incidence of conversion is 10 to 30%. Conversion to an open procedure is not a failure and the possibility should be discussed with the patient preoperatively.

Serious complications are rare. The mortality rate for laparoscopic cholecystectomy is about 0.1%. Wound infection and cardiopulmonary complication rates are considerably lower following laparoscopic cholecystectomy than are those for an open procedure, in which injury to the bile ducts is slightly more frequent (see section on injury to the biliary tract, below).[41]

Patients undergoing cholecystectomy should have a CBC and liver function tests preoperatively. Prophylaxis against deep venous thrombosis with either low molecular weight heparin or compression stockings is indicated. The patient should be instructed to empty their bladder before coming to the operating room. Urinary catheters are rarely needed. An orogastric tube is placed if the stomach is distended with gas, and is removed at the end of the operation.

Laparoscopic Cholecystectomy

The patient is placed supine on the operating table with the surgeon standing at the patient's left side. Some surgeons prefer to stand between the patient's legs while doing laparoscopic procedures in the upper abdomen. The pneumoperitoneum is created with carbon dioxide gas, either with an open technique or by closed needle technique. Initially, a small incision is made in the upper edge of the umbilicus. With the closed technique a special hollow insufflation needle (Veress needle) that is spring-loaded with a retractable cutting outer sheath is inserted into the peritoneal cavity and used for insufflation. Once an adequate pneumoperitoneum is established, a 10-mm trocar is inserted through the supraumbilical incision. With the open technique the supraumbilical incision is carried through the fascia and into the peritoneal cavity. A special blunt cannula (Hasson cannula) is inserted into the peritoneal cavity and anchored to the fascia. The laparoscope with the attached video camera is passed through the umbilical port and the abdomen inspected. Three additional ports are placed under direct vision (Fig. 31-18). A 10-mm port is placed in the epigastrium, a 5-mm port in the middle of the clavicular line, and a 5-mm port in the right flank, in line with the gallbladder fundus. Occasionally, a fifth port is required for better visualization in patients recovering from pancreatitis or those with semiacute cholecystitis, as well as in very obese patients.

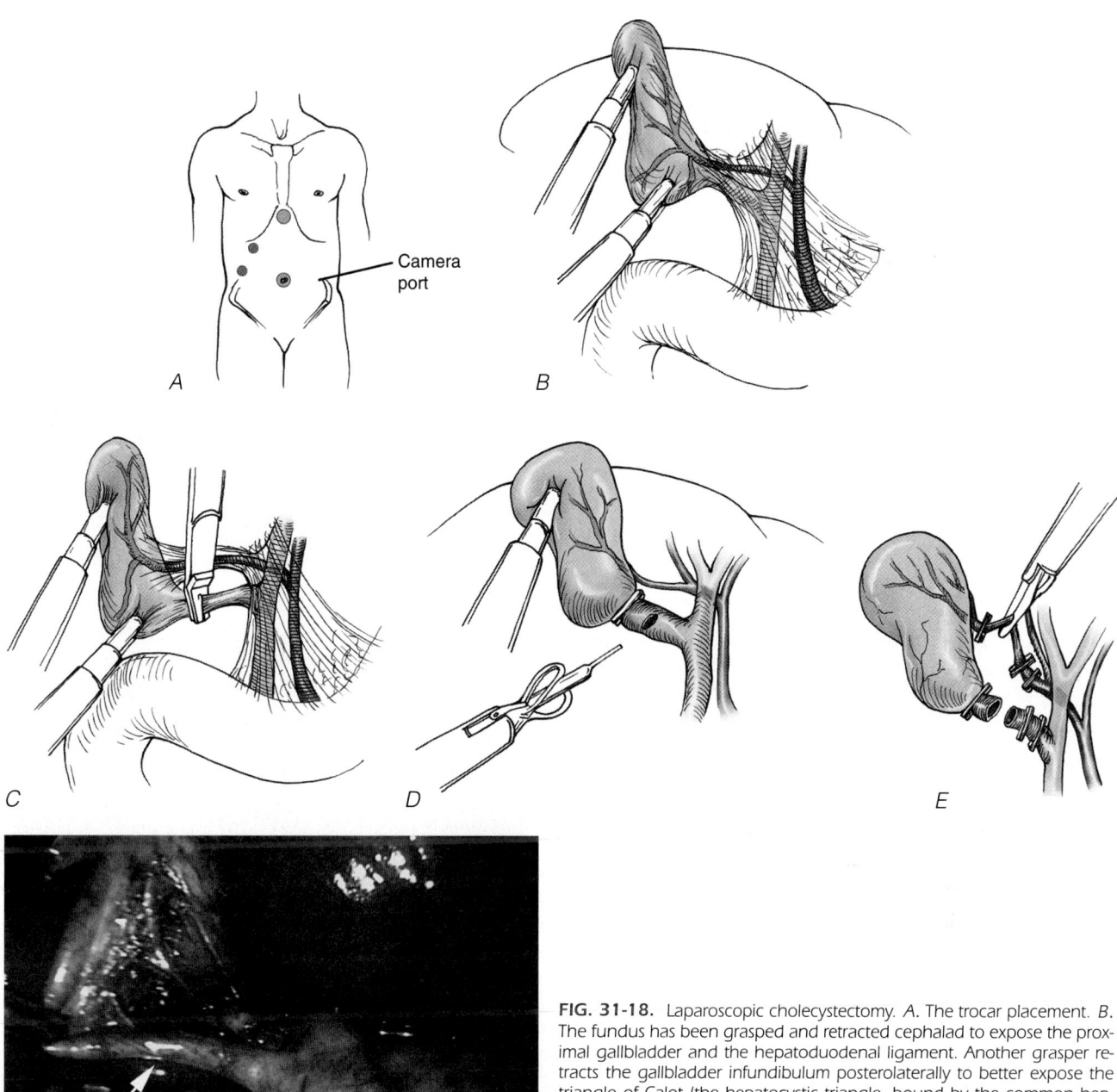

FIG. 31-18. Laparoscopic cholecystectomy. *A.* The trocar placement. *B.* The fundus has been grasped and retracted cephalad to expose the proximal gallbladder and the hepatoduodenal ligament. Another grasper retracts the gallbladder infundibulum posterolaterally to better expose the triangle of Calot (the hepatocystic triangle, bound by the common hepatic duct, cystic duct, and the liver margin). *C.* The triangle of Calot has been opened and the neck of the gallbladder and part of the cystic duct dissected free. A clip is placed on the cystic duct-gallbladder junction. *D.* A small opening has been made into the cystic duct and a cholangiogram catheter is inserted. *E.* The cystic duct has been divided and the cystic artery is being divided. *F.* An intraoperative picture showing a grasper pulling the infundibulum of the gallbladder laterally, exposing the triangle of Calot that has been dissected. The cystic artery can be seen crossing the dissected area upward and to the left.

Through the lateral-most port a grasper is used to grasp the gallbladder fundus. It is retracted over the liver edge upward and toward the patient's right shoulder to expose the proximal gallbladder and the hilar area. Through the midclavicular port a second grasper is used to grasp the gallbladder infundibulum and retract it laterally to expose the triangle of Calot. Prior to this, it may be necessary to take down any adhesions between the omentum, duodenum or colon, and the gallbladder. Most of the dissection is carried out through the epigastric port using a dissector, hook, or scissors. The dissection starts at the junction of the gallbladder and the cystic duct. A helpful anatomic landmark is the cystic artery lymph node. The peritoneum, fat, and loose areolar tissue around the gallbladder and the cystic duct-gallbladder junction is dissected off toward the bile duct. This is continued until the gallbladder neck and the proximal cystic duct are clearly identified. The next step is the identification of the cystic artery, which usually runs parallel to and somewhat behind the cystic duct. A hemoclip is placed on the proximal cystic duct. If an intraoperative cholangiogram is to be performed, a small incision is made on the anterior surface of the cystic duct, just proximal to the clip, and a cholangiogram catheter is passed into the cystic duct. Once the cholangiogram is completed, the catheter is removed and two clips are placed proximal to the incision, and the cystic duct is divided. A wide cystic duct may be too big for clips, requiring the placement of a pre-tied loop ligature to close. The cystic artery is then clipped and divided. Finally, the gallbladder is dissected out of the gallbladder fossa, using either a hook or scissors with electrocautery. Before the gallbladder is removed from the liver edge, the operative field is carefully searched for bleeding points and the placement of the clips on the cystic duct and cystic artery are inspected. The gallbladder is removed through the umbilical incision. The fascial defect and skin incision may need to be enlarged if the stones are large. If the gallbladder is acutely inflamed or gangrenous, or if the gallbladder is perforated, it is placed in a retrieval bag before it is removed from the abdomen. Any bile or blood that has accumulated during the procedure is sucked away, and if stones were spilled they are retrieved, placed inside a retrieval bag, and removed. If the gallbladder was severely inflamed, gangrenous, or if any bile or blood is expected to accumulate, a closed suction drain can be placed through one of the 5-mm ports and left underneath the right liver lobe close to the gallbladder fossa.

Open Cholecystectomy

The same surgical principles apply for laparoscopic and open cholecystectomies. Open cholecystectomy has become an uncommon procedure, usually performed either as a conversion from laparoscopic cholecystectomy or as a second procedure in patients who require laparotomy for another reason. After the cystic artery and cystic duct have been identified, the gallbladder is dissected free from the liver bed, starting at the fundus. The dissection is carried proximally toward the cystic artery and the cystic duct, that are then ligated and divided.

Intraoperative Cholangiogram or Ultrasound

The bile ducts are visualized under fluoroscopy by injecting contrast through a catheter placed in the cystic duct (Fig. 31-19A). Their size can then be evaluated, the presence or absence of common bile duct stones assessed, and filling defects confirmed, as the dye passes into the duodenum. Routine intraoperative cholangiography will detect stones in approximately 7% of patients, as well as outlining the anatomy and detecting injury[42,43] (Fig. 31-19B). A selective intraoperative cholangiogram can be performed when the patient has a history of abnormal liver function tests, pancreatitis, jaundice, a large duct and small stones, a dilated duct on preoperative ultrasonography, and if preoperative endoscopic cholangiography for the above reasons was unsuccessful. Laparoscopic ultrasonography is as accurate as intraoperative cholangiography in detecting common bile duct stones and it is less invasive; however, it requires more skill to perform and interpret.[44,45]

Choledochal Exploration

Common bile duct stones that are detected intraoperatively on intraoperative cholangiography or ultrasonography may be managed with laparoscopic choledochal exploration as a part of the laparoscopic cholecystectomy procedure. Patients with common bile duct stones detected preoperatively, but endoscopic clearance was either not available or unsuccessful, should also have their ductal stones managed during the cholecystectomy.

If the stones in the duct are small, they may sometimes be flushed into the duodenum with saline irrigation via the cholangiography

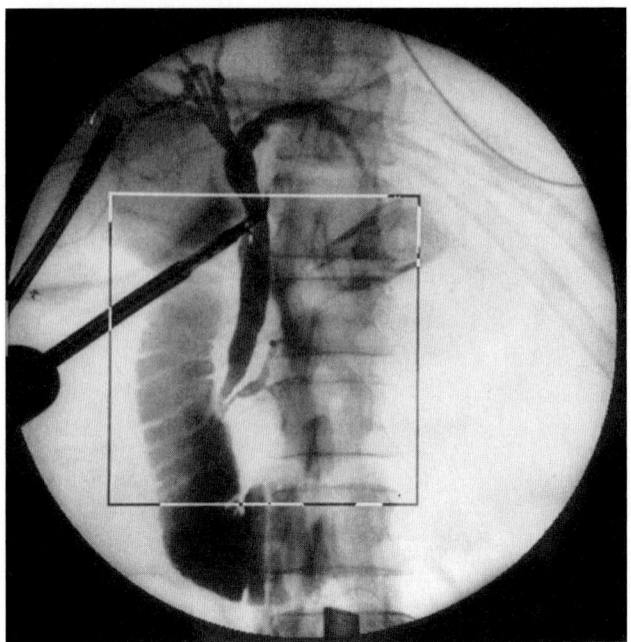

A

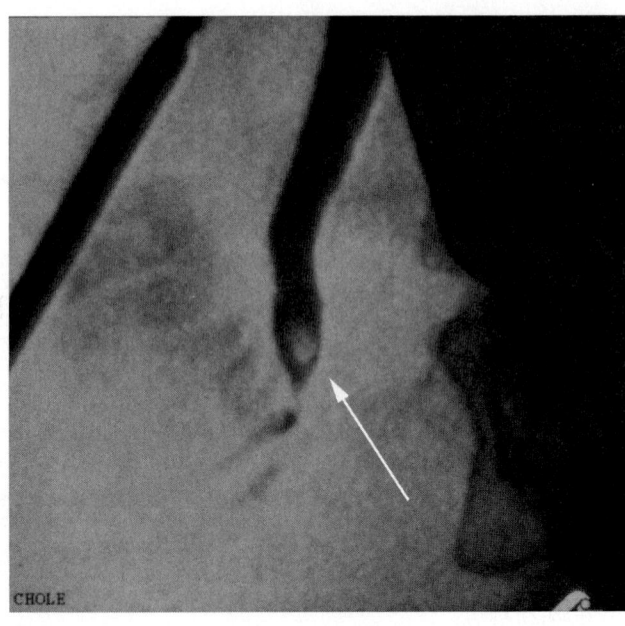

B

FIG. 31-19. *A.* An intraoperative cholangiogram. The bile ducts are of normal size, with no intraluminal filling defects. The left and right hepatic ducts are visualized; the distal common bile duct tapers down and the contrast empties into the duodenum. The grasper that holds the catheter and grasps the cystic duct stump partly projects over the common hepatic duct. *B.* An intraoperative cholangiogram showing common bile duct stone *(arrow).* A small amount of contrast has passed into the duodenum.

catheter after the sphincter of Oddi has been relaxed with glucagon. If irrigation is unsuccessful, a balloon catheter may be passed via the cystic duct and down the common bile duct, where it is inflated and withdrawn to retrieve the stones. The next attempt is usually made with a wire basket passed under fluoroscopic guidance to catch the stones (Fig. 31-20). If needed, a flexible choledochoscope is the next step. The cystic duct may have to be dilated to allow its

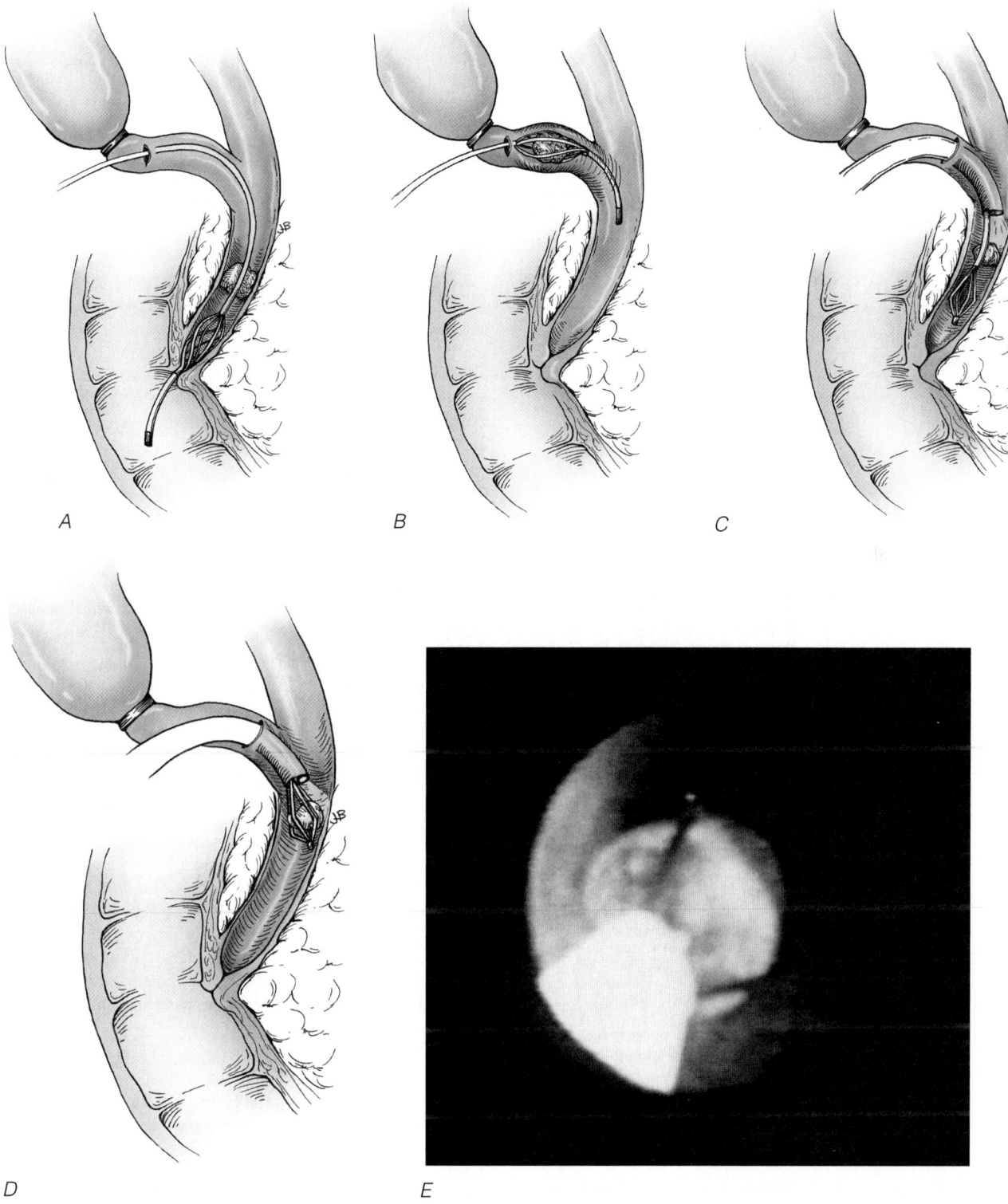

FIG. 31-20. Laparoscopic bile duct exploration. Laparoscopic choledochal exploration. *I.* Transcystic basket retrieval using fluoroscopy. *A.* The basket has been advanced past the stone and opened. *B.* The stone has been entrapped in the basket and together they are removed from the cystic duct. *II.* Transcystic choledochoscopy and stone removal. *C.* The basket has been passed through the working channel of the scope and the stone is entrapped under direct vision. *D.* Entrapped stone. *E.* A view from the choledochoscope. *III.* Choledochotomy and stone removal. *(Continued)*

passage. Once in the common bile duct, the stones may be caught into a wire basket under direct vision or pushed into the duodenum. When the duct has been cleared, the cystic duct is ligated and cut and the cholecystectomy completed. Occasionally a choledochotomy, an incision into the common bile duct itself, is necessary. The flexible choledochoscope is then passed into the duct for visualization and clearance of stones. The choledochotomy is sutured with a T tube left in the common bile duct with one end taken out through the

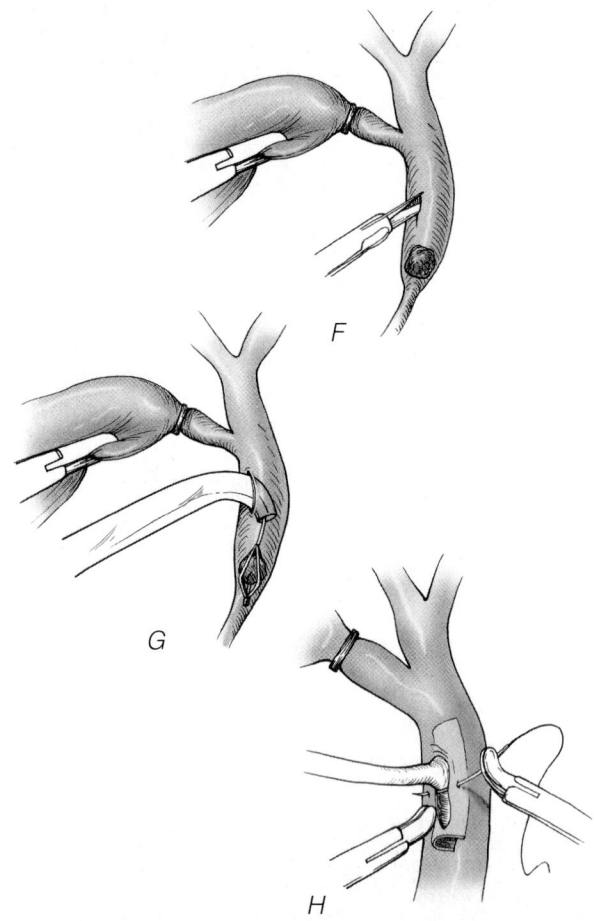

FIG. 31-20. *(continued)* F. A small incision is made in the common bile duct. G. The common bile duct is cleared of stones with choledochoscope guidance. H. A **T** tube is left in the common bile duct with one end taken out through the abdominal wall for decompression of the bile ducts.

abdominal wall for decompression of the bile ducts. By managing common bile duct stones at the time of the cholecystectomy, the patients can have all of their gallstone disease treated with one invasive procedure. It does, however, depend on the available surgical expertise.[46]

Choledochal Drainage Procedures

Rarely, when the stones cannot be cleared and/or when the duct is very dilated (larger than 1.5 cm in diameter), a choledochal drainage procedure is performed (Fig. 31-21). Choledochoduodenostomy is performed by mobilizing the second part of the duodenum (a Kocher maneuver) and anastomosing it side to side with the common bile duct.

A choledochojejunostomy is done by bringing up a 45-cm Roux-en-Y limb of jejunum and anastomosing it end to side to the choledochus.

Choledochojejunostomy, or more often a hepaticojejunostomy, also can be used to repair common bile duct strictures or as a palliative procedure for malignant obstruction in the periampullary region. If the common bile duct has been transected or injured, it can be managed by an end-to-end choledochojejunostomy.

Transduodenal Sphincterotomy

In the majority of cases, endoscopic sphincterotomy has replaced open transduodenal sphincterotomy. If an open procedure for common bile duct stones is being done in which the stones are impacted, recurrent, or multiple, the transduodenal approach may be feasible. The duodenum is incised transversely. The sphincter then is incised at the 11 o'clock position to avoid injury to the pancreatic duct. The impacted stones are removed as are large stones from the duct. There is no need to fully clear the duct of stones, as they can pass spontaneously through the cut sphincter.

OTHER BENIGN DISEASES AND LESIONS

Acalculous Cholecystitis

Acute inflammation of the gallbladder can occur without gallstones. Acalculous cholecystitis typically develops in critically ill patients in the intensive care unit. Patients on parenteral nutrition with extensive burns, sepsis, major operations, multiple trauma, or prolonged illness with multiple organ system failure are at risk for developing acalculous cholecystitis. The cause is unknown, but gallbladder distention with bile stasis and ischemia have been implicated as causative factors. Pathologic examination of the gallbladder wall reveals edema of the serosa and muscular layers, with patchy thrombosis of arterioles and venules.[47,48]

The symptoms and signs depend on the condition of the patient, but in the alert patient they are similar to acute calculous cholecystitis, with right upper quadrant pain and tenderness, fever, and leukocytosis. In the sedated or unconscious patient the clinical features are often masked, but fever and elevated white blood cell count, as well as elevation of alkaline phosphatase and bilirubin are indications for further investigation.

Ultrasonography is usually the diagnostic test of choice, as it can be done bedside in the intensive care unit. It can demonstrate the distended gallbladder with thickened wall, biliary sludge, pericholecystic fluid, and the presence or absence of abscess formation. Abdominal CT scan is as sensitive as ultrasonography and additionally allows imaging of the abdominal cavity and chest. A HIDA scan will not visualize the gallbladder. Acalculous cholecystitis requires urgent intervention. Percutaneous ultrasound- or CT-guided cholecystostomy is the treatment of choice for these patients, as they are usually unfit for surgery (see Fig. 31-17). If the diagnosis is uncertain, percutaneous cholecystostomy is both diagnostic and therapeutic. About 90% of patients will improve with the percutaneous cholecystostomy. However, if they do not improve, other steps, such as open cholecystostomy or cholecystectomy, may be required. If needed, cholecystectomy is performed after the patient has recovered from the underlying disease.

Biliary Cysts

Choledochal cysts are congenital cystic dilatations of the extrahepatic and/or intrahepatic biliary tree. They are rare—the incidence is between 1:100,000 and 1:150,000 in populations of Western countries—but are more commonly seen in populations of Eastern countries. Choledochal cysts affect females three to eight times more often than males. Although frequently diagnosed in infancy or childhood, as many as one half of the patients have reached adulthood when diagnosed. The cause is unknown. Weakness of the bile duct wall and increased pressure secondary to partial biliary obstruction are required for biliary cyst formation. More than 90% of patients have an anomalous pancreaticobiliary duct junction, with the pancreatic duct joining the common bile duct more than 1 cm proximal to the ampulla. This results in a long common channel that may allow free reflux of pancreatic secretions into the biliary tract, leading to inflammatory changes, increased biliary pressure, and cyst formation. Choledochal cysts are classified into five types

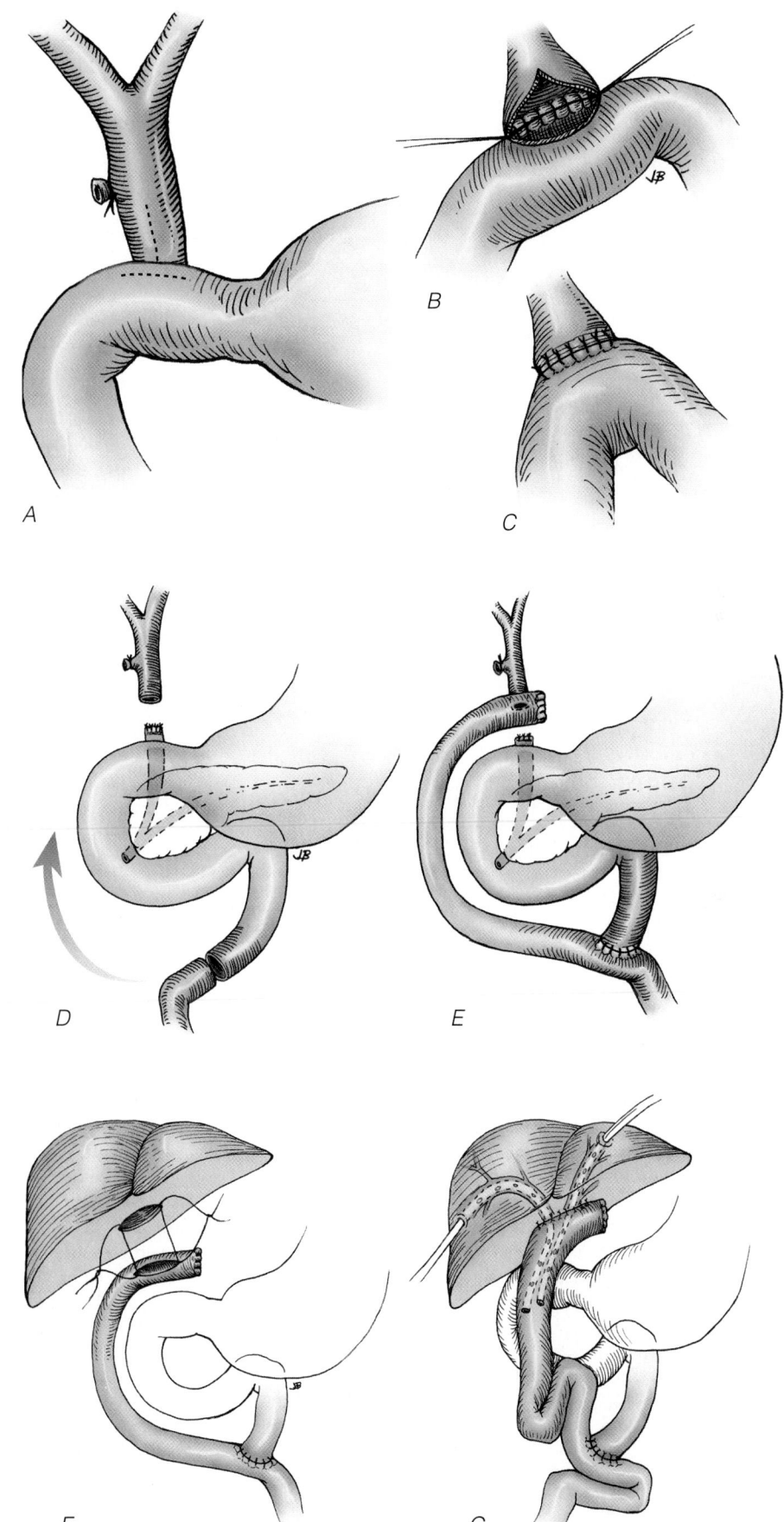

FIG. 31-21. Biliary enteric anastomoses. There are three types. *I.* Choledochoduodenostomy. *A.* The distal common bile duct is opened longitudinally, as is the duodenum. *B.* Interrupted sutures are placed between the common bile duct and the duodenum. *C.* Completed choledochoduodenostomy. *II.* Choledochojejunostomy. *D.* The common bile duct and small bowel are divided. *E.* A Roux-en-Y limb of jejunum is anastomosed to the choledochus. *III.* Hepaticojejunostomy. *F.* The entire extrahepatic biliary tree has been resected and the reconstruction done with a Roux-en-Y limb of jejunum. *G.* Percutaneous transhepatic stents are placed across hepaticojejunostomy.

Type I   Type II   Type III

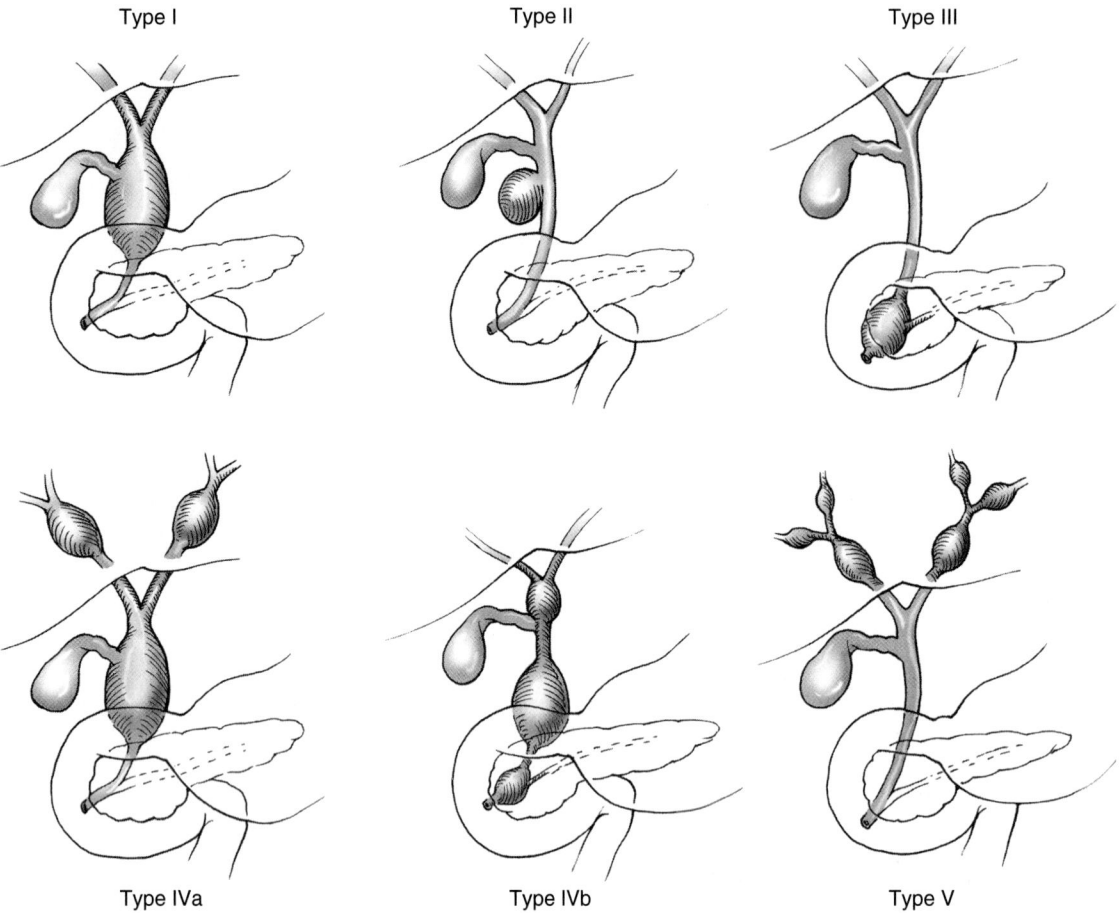

Type IVa   Type IVb   Type V

FIG. 31-22. Classification of choledochal cysts. Type I, fusiform or cystic dilations of the extrahepatic biliary tree, are the most common type, making up over 50% of all choledochal cysts. Type II, saccular diverticulum of an extrahepatic bile duct, is rare, comprising less than 5% of choledochal cysts. Type III, bile duct dilatations within the duodenal wall (choledochoceles), make up about 5% of choledochal cysts. Types IVa and IVb, multiple cysts, make up 5 to 10% of choledochal cysts. Type IVa affects both extrahepatic and intrahepatic bile ducts, while type IVb cysts affect the extrahepatic bile ducts only. Type V, intrahepatic biliary cysts, are very rare and make up only about 1% of choledochal cysts.

(Fig. 31-22). The cysts are lined with cuboidal epithelium and can vary in size from 2 cm in diameter to giant cysts.

Adults commonly present with jaundice or cholangitis. Less than one half of patients present with the classic clinical triad of abdominal pain, jaundice, and a mass. Ultrasonography or CT scanning will confirm the diagnosis, but endoscopic, transhepatic, or MRC is required to assess the biliary anatomy and to plan the appropriate surgical treatment. For types I, II, and IV, excision of the extrahepatic biliary tree, including cholecystectomy, with a Roux-en-Y hepaticojejunostomy are ideal. In type IV, additional segmental resection of the liver may be appropriate, particularly if intrahepatic stones, strictures, or abscesses are present, or if the dilatations are confined to one lobe. The risk of cholangiocarcinoma developing in choledochal cysts is as high as 15% in adults, and supports complete excision when they are diagnosed. For type III, sphincterotomy is recommended.[49]

Sclerosing Cholangitis

Sclerosing cholangitis is an uncommon disease characterized by inflammatory strictures involving the intrahepatic and extrahepatic biliary tree. It is a progressive disease that eventually results in secondary biliary cirrhosis. Sometimes, biliary strictures are clearly secondary to bile duct stones, acute cholangitis, previous biliary surgery, or toxic agents, and are termed secondary sclerosing cholangitis. However, primary sclerosing cholangitis is a disease entity of its own, with no known attributing cause. It is associated with ulcerative colitis in about two thirds of patients. Other diseases associated with sclerosing cholangitis include Riedel's thyroiditis and retroperitoneal fibrosis. Autoimmune reaction, chronic low-grade bacterial or viral infection, toxic reaction, and genetic factors have all been suggested to play a role in its pathogenesis. The human leukocyte antigen haplotypes HLA-B8, -DR3, -DQ2, and –DRw52A, commonly found in patients with autoimmune diseases, also are more frequently seen in patients with sclerosing cholangitis than in controls. Patients with sclerosing cholangitis are at risk for developing cholangiocarcinoma. Eventually 10 to 20% of the patients will develop cancer. Cholangiocarcinoma can present at any time during the disease process and does not correlate with the extent of sclerosing cholangitis or the development of liver failure, but frequently follows an aggressive course.

The mean age of presentation is 30 to 45 years and men are affected twice as commonly as women. The usual presentation is intermittent jaundice, fatigue, weight loss, pruritus, and abdominal pain. Symptoms of acute cholangitis are rare, without preceding biliary tract intervention or surgery. More than one half of patients are symptomatic when diagnosed. In several patients with ulcerative colitis, abnormal liver function tests found on routine testing lead to the diagnosis. The clinical course in sclerosing cholangitis is highly variable, but cyclic remissions and exacerbations are typical. However, some patients remain asymptomatic for years, while others progress rapidly with the obliterative inflammatory changes leading to secondary biliary cirrhosis and liver failure. In patients with associated ulcerative colitis, the course of each disease seems independent of the other. Colectomy for the colitis makes no difference to the course of primary sclerosing cholangitis. The median survival for patients with primary sclerosing cholangitis from the time of diagnosis ranges from 10 to 12 years, and most die from hepatic failure.[50]

The clinical presentation and elevation of alkaline phosphatase and bilirubin may suggest the diagnosis, but ERC, revealing multiple dilatations and strictures (beading) of both the intra- and extrahepatic biliary tree confirms it. The hepatic duct bifurcation is often the most severely affected segment. A liver biopsy may not be diagnostic, but is important to determine the degree of hepatic fibrosis and the presence of cirrhosis. Sclerosing cholangitis is followed by ERC and liver biopsies to provide appropriate management.

There is no known effective medical therapy for primary sclerosing cholangitis and no known curative treatment. Corticosteroids, immunosuppressants, ursodeoxycholic acid, and antibiotics have been disappointing. Biliary strictures can be dilated and stented either endoscopically or percutaneously. These measures have given short-term improvements in symptoms and serum bilirubin levels, and long-term improvements in only less than one half of the patients. Surgical management with resection of the extrahepatic biliary tree and hepaticojejunostomy has produced reasonable results in patients with extrahepatic and bifurcation strictures, but without cirrhosis or significant hepatic fibrosis.[51] In patients with sclerosing cholangitis and advanced liver disease, liver transplantation is the only option. It offers excellent results with overall 5-year survival as high as 85%. Primary sclerosing cholangitis recurs in 10 to 20% of patients and may require retransplantation.[52,53]

Stenosis of the Sphincter of Oddi

A benign stenosis of the outlet of the common bile duct is usually associated with inflammation, fibrosis, or muscular hypertrophy. The pathogenesis is unclear, but trauma from the passing of stones, sphincter motility disorders, and congenital anomalies have been suggested. Episodic pain of the biliary type with abnormal liver function tests is a common presentation. However, recurrent jaundice or pancreatitis also may play a role. A dilated common bile duct that is difficult to cannulate with delayed emptying of the contrast are useful diagnostic features. Ampullary manometry and special provocation tests are available in specialized units. If the diagnosis is well established, endoscopic or operative sphincterotomy will yield good results.[54]

Bile Duct Strictures

Benign bile duct strictures can have numerous causes. However, the vast majority are caused by operative injury, most commonly by laparoscopic cholecystectomy (see section on injury to the biliary

tract, below). Other causes include fibrosis due to chronic pancreatitis, common bile duct stones, acute cholangitis, biliary obstruction due to cholecystolithiasis (Mirizzi's syndrome), sclerosing cholangitis, cholangiohepatitis, and strictures of a biliary-enteric anastomosis. Bile duct strictures that go unrecognized or are improperly managed may lead to recurrent cholangitis, secondary biliary cirrhosis, and portal hypertension.[55]

Patients with bile duct strictures most commonly present with episodes of cholangitis. Less commonly, they may present with jaundice without evidence of infection. Liver function tests usually show evidence of cholestasis. An ultrasound or a CT scan will show dilated bile ducts proximal to the stricture, as well as provide some information about the level of the stenosis. MRC will also provide good anatomic information about the location and the degree of dilatation. In patients with intrahepatic ductal dilatation, a percutaneous transhepatic cholangiogram will outline the proximal biliary tree, define the stricture and its location, and allow decompression of the biliary tree with transhepatic catheters or stents (Fig. 31-23). An endoscopic cholangiogram will outline the distal bile duct. Treatment depends on the location and the cause of the stricture. Percutaneous or endoscopic dilatation and/or stent placement give good results

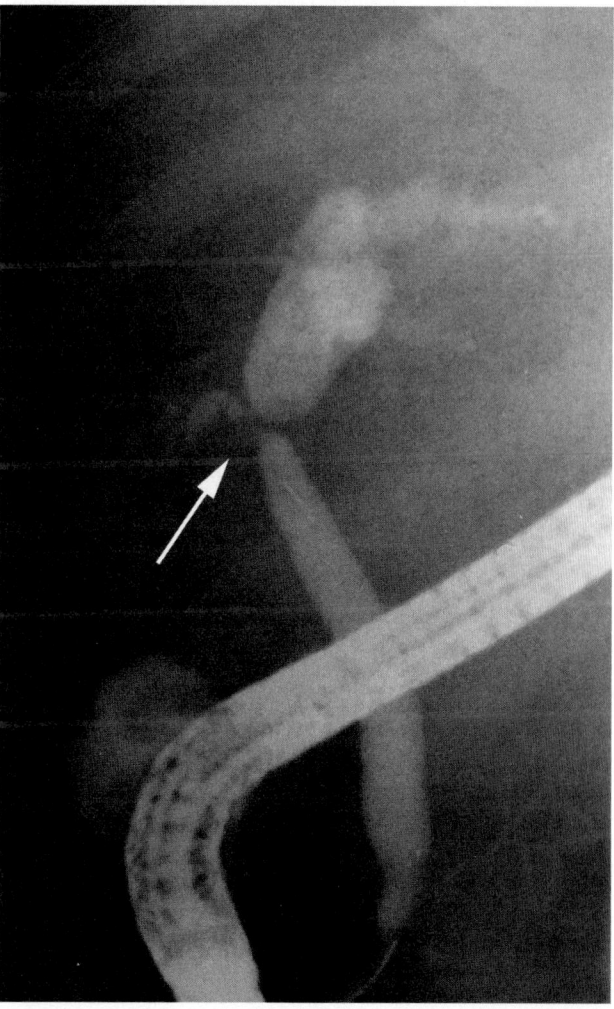

FIG. 31-23. An ERC showing stricture of the common hepatic duct (arrow). The patient had recently had a laparoscopic cholecystectomy; clips from the operation can be seen projected over the common bile duct.

in more than one half of patients. Surgery with Roux-en-Y chole-dochojejunostomy or hepaticojejunostomy is the standard of care with good or excellent results in 80 to 90% of patients.[56] Choledo-choduodenostomy may be a choice for strictures in the distal-most part of the common bile duct.

INJURY TO THE BILIARY TRACT

The Gallbladder

Injuries to the gallbladder are uncommon. Penetrating injuries are usually caused by gunshot wounds or stab wounds, and rarely by a needle biopsy procedure of the liver. Nonpenetrating trauma is extremely rare. These types of injury to the gallbladder include contusion, avulsion, laceration, rupture, and traumatic cholecystitis. The treatment of choice is cholecystectomy and the prognosis is directly related to the type and incidence of associated injury.

The Extrahepatic Bile Ducts

Penetrating trauma to the extrahepatic bile ducts is rare and is usually associated with trauma to other viscera. The great majority of injuries of the extrahepatic biliary duct system are iatrogenic, occurring in the course of laparoscopic or open cholecystectomies.[57] Less commonly, biliary injury is associated with common bile duct exploration, division or mobilization of the duodenum during gastrectomy, and dissection of the hepatic hilum during liver resections. The exact incidence of bile duct injury during cholecystectomy is unknown, but data suggest that during open cholecystectomy the incidence is relatively low (about 0.1 to 0.2%). However, the incidence during laparoscopic cholecystectomy, as derived from state and national databases, estimates the rate of major injury to be about 0.55%, and the incidence of minor injuries and bile leaks to be about 0.3%, a total of 0.85%. Limited view, difficult orientation and assessment of depth on a two-dimensional image, and the lack of tactile sensation and unusual manual skills that are needed have led to the rise in bile duct injury during laparoscopic cholecystectomy.[58]

A number of different factors are associated with bile duct injury during laparoscopic cholecystectomy. These include acute or chronic inflammation, obesity, anatomic variations, and bleeding. Surgical technique with inadequate exposure and failure to identify structures before ligating or dividing them are the most common cause of significant biliary injury. The bile ducts may be narrow and can be mistaken for the cystic duct. The cystic duct may run along side the common bile duct before joining it, leading the surgeon to the wrong place. Additionally, the cystic duct may enter the right hepatic duct, and the right hepatic duct may run aberrantly, coursing through the triangle of Calot and entering the common hepatic duct. A number of intraoperative technical factors have been implicated in biliary injuries. Excessive cephalad retraction of the gallbladder may align the cystic duct with the common bile duct, and the latter is then mistaken for the cystic duct and clipped and divided. The use of an angled laparoscope instead of an end-viewing one will help visualize the anatomic structures, in particular those around the triangle of Calot. An angled scope also will aid in the proper placement of clips. Careless use of electrocautery may lead to thermal injury. Dissection deep into the liver parenchyma may cause injury to intrahepatic ducts, and poor clip placement close to the hilar area or to structures not well visualized can result in a clip across a bile duct.[59,60]

The routine use of intraoperative cholangiography to prevent bile duct injury is controversial.[61] It may limit the extent of injury, but does not seem to prevent it. However, if a bile duct injury is suspected during cholecystectomy, a cholangiogram must be obtained to identify the anatomic features. It is important to check that the whole biliary system fills with contrast and to be sure there are no leaks.

Diagnosis

Only about 25% of major bile duct injuries (common bile duct or hepatic duct) are recognized at the time of operation. Most commonly, intraoperative bile leakage, recognition of the correct anatomy, and an abnormal cholangiogram lead to the diagnosis of a bile duct injury. Within the first postoperative month more than half of patients with injury have presented. The remainder present months or years later, with recurrent cholangitis or cirrhosis from a remote bile duct injury. In the early postoperative period, patients present either with progressive elevation of liver function tests due to an occluded or a stenosed bile duct, or with a bile leak from an injured duct. Bile leak, most commonly from the cystic duct stump, a transected aberrant right hepatic duct, or a lateral injury to the main bile duct usually presents with pain, fever, and a mild elevation of liver function tests. A CT scan or an ultrasound will show either a collection (biloma) in the gallbladder area or free fluid (bile) in the peritoneum (Fig. 31-24A). Bilious drainage through operatively placed drains or through the wounds is abnormal. An active leak and the site of the bile leak can be confirmed noninvasively with a HIDA scan. In patients with a surgical drain or a percutaneously-placed catheter, injection of water-soluble contrast media through the drainage tract (sinogram) can often define the site of leakage and the anatomy of the biliary tree.[62]

CT scan and ultrasound also are important in the initial evaluation of the jaundiced patient, as they can demonstrate the dilated part of the biliary tree proximal to the stenosis or obstruction, and may identify the level of the extrahepatic bile duct obstruction. In the jaundiced patient with dilated intrahepatic ducts, a percutaneous cholangiogram will outline the anatomy and the proximal extent of the injury and allow decompression of the biliary tree with catheter or stent placements. An endoscopic cholangiogram demonstrates the anatomy distal to the injury and may allow the placement of stents across a stricture to relieve an obstruction (see Fig. 31-23). MRI cholangiography, if available, provides an excellent, noninvasive delineation of the biliary anatomy both proximal and distal to the injury.

Management

The management of bile duct injuries depends on the type, extent, and level of injury, and the time of its diagnosis. Initial proper treatment of bile duct injury diagnosed during the cholecystectomy can avoid the development of a bile duct stricture. If a major injury is discovered and an experienced biliary surgeon is not available, an external drain and, if necessary, transhepatic biliary catheters are placed, and the patient is transferred to a referral center.[58]

Transected bile ducts smaller than 3 mm or those draining a single hepatic segment can safely be ligated. If the injured duct is 4 mm or larger, it is likely to drain multiple segments or an entire lobe, and thus needs to be reimplanted. Lateral injury to the common bile duct or the common hepatic duct, recognized at the time of surgery, is best managed with a T-tube placement. If the injury is a small incision in the duct, the T tube may be placed through it as if it were a formal choledochotomy. In more extensive lateral injuries the T tube should be placed through a separate choledochotomy and the injury closed over the T tube end to minimize the risk of subsequent stricture formation.

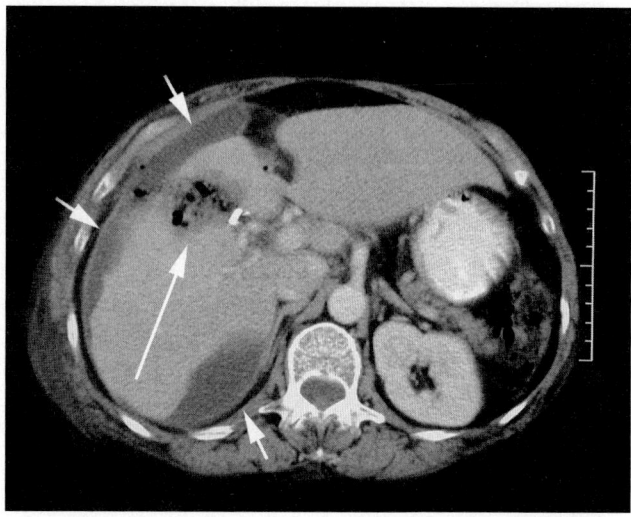

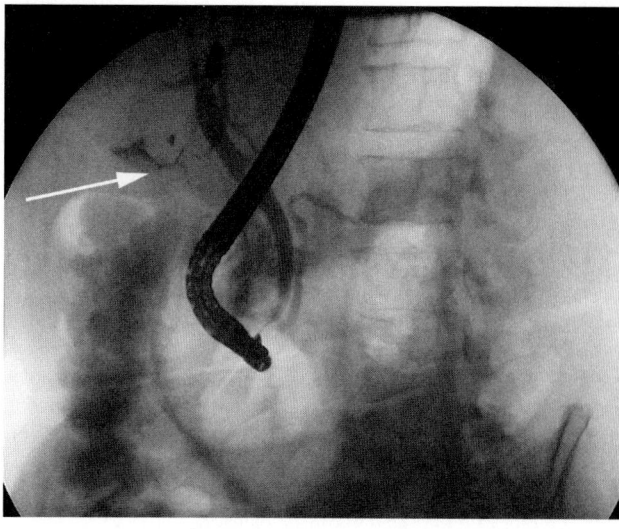

A   *B*

FIG. 31-24. *A. CT scan of a patient with bile leak after cholecystectomy. The short arrows indicate the intraperitoneal collections. Both air and bile is seen in the gallbladder bed (long arrow) as is a surgical clip. B. An ERC from the same patient showing a leak from the cystic duct stump (arrow). Note the filling of the pancreatic duct.*

Major bile duct injuries such as transection of the common hepatic or common bile duct are best managed at the time of injury. In many of these major injuries the bile duct has not only been transected, but a variable length of the duct removed. This injury usually requires a biliary enteric anastomosis with a jejunal loop. Either an end-to-side Roux-en-Y choledochojejunostomy, or more commonly a Roux-en-Y hepaticojejunostomy, should be performed. Transhepatic biliary catheters are placed through the anastomosis to stent it and to provide access to the biliary tract for drainage and imaging. Although rare, when the injury is to the distal common bile duct, a choledochoduodenostomy can be performed. If there is no or minimal loss of ductal length, a duct-to-duct repair may be done over a T tube that is placed through a separate incision. It is critical to perform a tension-free anastomosis to minimize the high risk of postoperative stricture formation.[51]

Cystic duct leaks can usually be managed with percutaneous drainage of intra-abdominal fluid collections followed by an endoscopic biliary stenting (see Fig. 31-24).

Major injuries diagnosed postoperatively require transhepatic biliary catheter placement for biliary decompression as well as percutaneous drainage of intra-abdominal bile collections, if any. When the acute inflammation has resolved 6 to 8 weeks later, operative repair is performed.

Patients with bile duct stricture from an injury or as a sequela of previous repair usually present with either progressive elevation of liver function tests or cholangitis. The initial management usually includes transhepatic biliary drainage catheter placement for decompression as well as for defining the anatomy and the location and the extent of the damage. These catheters will also serve as useful technical aids during subsequent biliary enteric anastomosis. An anastomosis is performed between the duct proximal to the injury and a Roux loop of jejunum. Balloon dilatation of a stricture usually requires multiple attempts and rarely provides adequate long-term relief. Self-expanding metal or plastic stents, placed either percutaneously or endoscopically across the stricture, can provide temporary drainage, and in the high-risk patient, permanent drainage of the biliary tree.

Outcome

Good results can be expected in 70 to 90% of patients with bile duct injuries.[63] The best results are obtained when the injury is recognized during the cholecystectomy and repaired by an experienced biliary tract surgeon. The operative mortality rate varies from 0 to almost 30% in various series, but commonly is about 5 to 8%. Common complications that are specific for bile duct repairs include cholangitis, external biliary fistula, bile leak, subhepatic and subphrenic abscesses, and hemobilia. Restenosis of a biliary enteric anastomosis occurs in about 10% of patients, and may manifest up to 20 years after the initial procedure. Approximately two-thirds of recurrent strictures become symptomatic within 2 years after repair. The more proximal strictures are associated with a lower success rate than are distal ones. The worst results are in patients with many operative revisions and in those who have evidence of liver failure and portal hypertension. However, previous repair does not preclude successful outcome of repeated attempts, particularly in patients with good liver function. Patients with deteriorating liver function are candidates for liver transplants.

TUMORS

Carcinoma of the Gallbladder

Cancer of the gallbladder is a rare malignancy that occurs predominantly in the elderly. It is an aggressive tumor, with poor prognosis except when incidentally diagnosed at an early stage after cholecystectomy for cholelithiasis. The overall reported 5-year survival rate is about 5%.[64]

Incidence

Gallbladder cancer is the fifth most common gastrointestinal malignancy in Western countries. However, it accounts for only 2 to 4% of all malignant gastrointestinal tumors, with about 5000 new cases diagnosed annually in the United States. It is two to three times more common in females than males, and the peak incidence is in the seventh decade of life. Its occurrence in random autopsy series is about 0.4%, but approximately 1% of patients undergoing cholecystectomy for gallstone disease are found incidentally to have gallbladder cancer. The incidence of gallbladder cancer is particularly high in native populations of the United States, Mexico, and Chile. The annual incidence in Native American females with gallstones approaches 75 per 100,000, compared with the overall incidence of gallbladder cancer of 2.5 cases per 100,000 residents in the United States.[65]

Etiology

Approximately 90% of patients with carcinoma of the gallbladder have gallstones. However, the 20-year risk of developing cancer for patients with gallstones is less than 0.5% for the overall population and 1.5% for high-risk groups. The pathogenesis has not been defined but is probably related to chronic inflammation. Larger stones (3 cm) are associated with a tenfold increased risk of cancer. The risk of developing cancer of the gallbladder is higher in patients with symptomatic than asymptomatic gallstones.

Polypoid lesions of the gallbladder are associated with increased risk of cancer, particularly in polyps larger than 10 mm.[66] The calcified "porcelain" gallbladder is associated with more than a 20% incidence of gallbladder carcinoma. These gallbladders should be removed, even if the patients are asymptomatic. Patients with choledochal cysts have an increased risk of developing cancer anywhere in the biliary tree, but the incidence is highest in the gallbladder. Sclerosing cholangitis, anomalous pancreaticobiliary duct junction, and exposure to carcinogens (azotoluene, nitrosamines) also are associated with cancer of the gallbladder.

Pathology

Between 80 and 90% of the tumors are adenocarcinomas. Squamous cell, adenosquamous, oat cell, and other anaplastic lesions occur rarely. The histologic subtypes of gallbladder adenocarcinomas include papillary, nodular, and tubular. Less than 10% are of the papillary type, but they are associated with an overall better outcome, as they are most commonly diagnosed while localized to the gallbladder. Cancer of the gallbladder spreads through the lymphatics, with venous drainage, and with direct invasion into the liver parenchyma. Lymphatic flow from the gallbladder drains first to the cystic duct node (Calot's), then the pericholedochal and hilar nodes, and finally the peripancreatic, duodenal, periportal, celiac, and superior mesenteric artery nodes. The gallbladder veins drain directly into the adjacent liver, usually segments IV and V, where tumor invasion is common (Fig. 31-25). The gallbladder wall differs histologically from the intestines in that it lacks a muscularis mucosa and submucosa. Lymphatics are present in the subserosal layer only. Therefore cancers invading but growing through the muscular layer have minimal risk of nodal disease. When diagnosed, about 25% of gallbladder cancers are localized to the gallbladder wall, 35% have regional nodal involvement and/or extension into adjacent liver, and approximately 40% have distant metastasis.[67]

Clinical Manifestations and Diagnosis

Signs and symptoms of carcinoma of the gallbladder are generally indistinguishable from those associated with cholecystitis and cholelithiasis. These include abdominal discomfort, right upper quadrant pain, nausea, and vomiting. Jaundice, weight loss, anorexia, ascites, and abdominal mass are less common presenting symptoms. More than one half of gallbladder cancers are not diagnosed before surgery. Common misdiagnoses include chronic cholecystitis, acute cholecystitis, choledocholithiasis, hydrops of

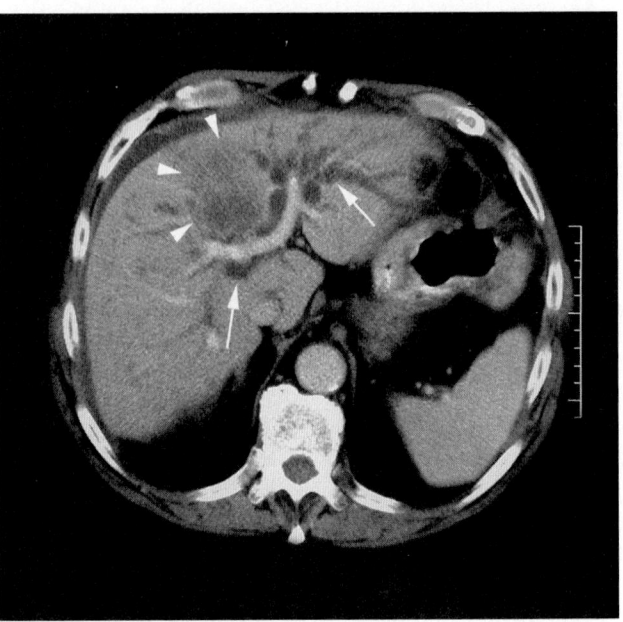

FIG. 31-25. *CT scan of a patient with gallbladder cancer. The image shown is from the level of the liver hilum. The portal vein is bifurcating into the left and right portal branch. The tumor has invaded segment IV of the liver (arrowheads) and obstructed the common hepatic duct, resulting in intrahepatic ductal dilatation (arrows).*

the gallbladder, and pancreatic cancer. Laboratory findings are not diagnostic, but if abnormal, are most often consistent with biliary obstruction. Ultrasonography often reveals a thickened, irregular gallbladder wall or a mass replacing the gallbladder. Ultrasonography may visualize tumor invasion of the liver, lymphadenopathy, and a dilated biliary tree. The sensitivity of ultrasonography in detecting gallbladder cancer ranges from 70 to 100%. CT scan may demonstrate a gallbladder mass or an invasion into adjacent organs. In addition, a spiral CT scans demonstrates the vascular anatomy. CT scan is a poor method for identifying nodal spread. In jaundiced patients a percutaneous transhepatic or endoscopic cholangiogram may be helpful to delineate the biliary tree, and typically shows a long stricture of the common bile duct. With newer MRI techniques, MRCP has evolved into a single noninvasive imaging method that allows complete assessment of biliary, vascular, nodal, hepatic, and adjacent organ involvement. If diagnostic studies suggest that the tumor is unresectable, a CT scan or ultrasound-guided biopsy of the tumor can be obtained.

Treatment

Surgery remains the only curative option for gallbladder cancer as well as for cholangiocarcinoma. However, palliative procedures for patients with unresectable cancer and jaundice or duodenal obstruction remain the most frequently performed surgery for gallbladder cancers. Today, patients with obstructive jaundice can frequently be managed with either endoscopic or percutaneously-placed biliary stents. There are no proven effective options for adjuvant radiation or chemotherapy for patients with gallbladder cancer.

The pathologic stage of gallbladder cancer determines the operative treatment for patients with localized gallbladder cancer. Patients without evidence of distant metastasis warrant exploration for tissue diagnosis, pathologic staging, and possible curative resection.

Tumors limited to the muscular layer of the gallbladder (T1), are usually identified incidentally, after cholecystectomy for gallstone

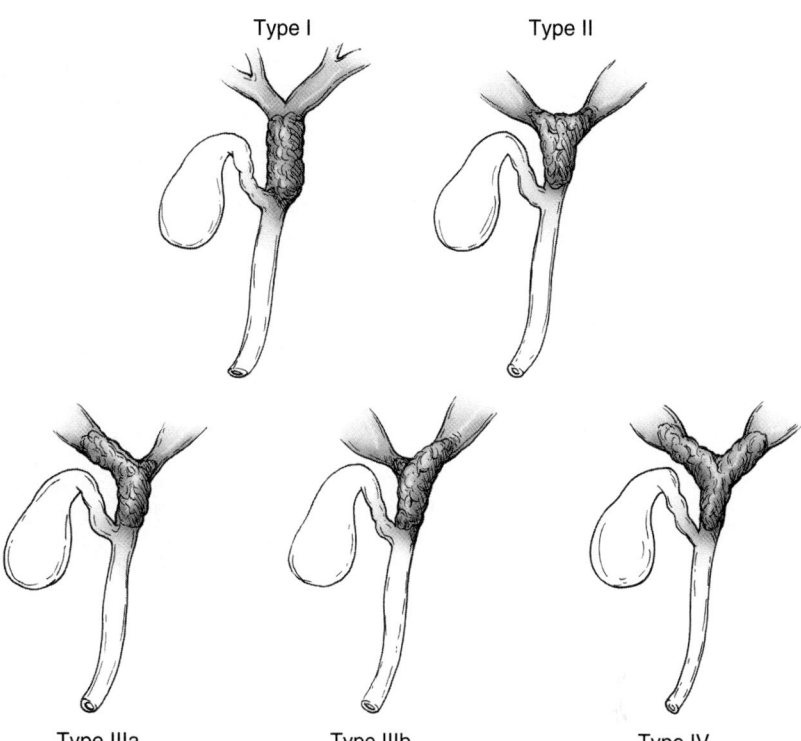

FIG. 31-26. Bismuth-Corlette classification of bile duct tumors.

Type I   Type II   Type IIIa   Type IIIb   Type IV

disease. There is near-universal agreement that simple cholecystectomy is an adequate treatment for T1 lesions and results in a near 100% overall 5-year survival rate. When the tumor invades the perimuscular connective tissue without extension beyond the serosa or into the liver (T2 tumors), an extended cholecystectomy should be performed.[68] That includes resection of liver segments IVB and V, and lymphadenectomy of the cystic duct, and pericholedochal, portal, right celiac, and posterior pancreatoduodenal lymph nodes. One half of patients with T2 tumors are found to have nodal disease on pathologic examination. Therefore, regional lymphadenectomy is an important part of surgery for T2 cancers.[69] For tumors that grow beyond the serosa or invade the liver or other organs (T3 and T4 tumors), there is a high likelihood of intraperitoneal and distant spread. If no peritoneal or nodal involvement is found, complete tumor excision with an extended right hepatectomy (segments IV, V, VI, VII, and VIII) must be performed for adequate tumor clearance. An aggressive approach in patients who will tolerate surgery has resulted in an increased survival for T3 and T4 lesions.

Prognosis

Most patients with gallbladder cancer have unresectable disease at the time of diagnosis. The 5-year survival rate of all patients with gallbladder cancer is less than 5%, with a median survival of 6 months.[70] Patients with T1 disease treated with cholecystectomy have an excellent prognosis (85 to 100% 5-year survival rate). The 5-year survival rate for T2 lesions treated with an extended cholecystectomy and lymphadenectomy compared with simple cholecystectomy is over 70% versus 25 to 40%, respectively. Patients with advanced but resectable gallbladder cancer are reported to have 5-year survival rates of 20 to 50%. However, the median survival for patients with distant metastasis at the time of presentation is only 1 to 3 months.

Recurrence after resection of gallbladder cancer occurs most commonly in the liver or the celiac or retropancreatic nodes. The prognosis for recurrent disease is very poor. Death occurs most commonly secondary to biliary sepsis or liver failure. The main goal of follow-up is to provide palliative care. The most common problems are pruritus and cholangitis associated with obstructive jaundice, bowel obstruction secondary to carcinomatosis, and pain.

Bile Duct Carcinoma

Cholangiocarcinoma is a rare tumor arising from the biliary epithelium and may occur anywhere along the biliary tree. About two-thirds are located at the hepatic duct bifurcation. Surgical resection offers the only chance for cure, however, many patients have advanced disease at the time of diagnosis. Therefore palliative procedures aimed to provide biliary drainage to prevent liver failure and cholangitis are often the only therapeutic possibilities. Most patients with unresectable disease die within a year of diagnosis.[71]

Incidence

The autopsy incidence of bile duct carcinoma is about 0.3%. The overall incidence of cholangiocarcinoma in the United States is about 1.0 per 100,000 people per year, with about 3000 new cases diagnosed annually. The male to female ratio is 1.3:1 and the average age of presentation is between 50 and 70 years.

Etiology

Risk factors associated with cholangiocarcinoma include primary sclerosing cholangitis, choledochal cysts, ulcerative colitis, hepatolithiasis, biliary-enteric anastomosis, and biliary tract infections with *Clonorchis* or in chronic typhoid carriers. Features common to most risk factors include biliary stasis, bile duct stones, and infection. Other risk factors associated with cholangiocarcinoma are liver flukes, dietary nitrosamines, Thorotrast, and exposure to dioxin.[72,73]

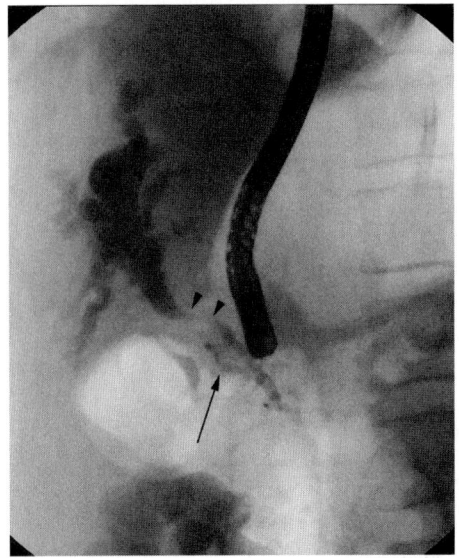

A

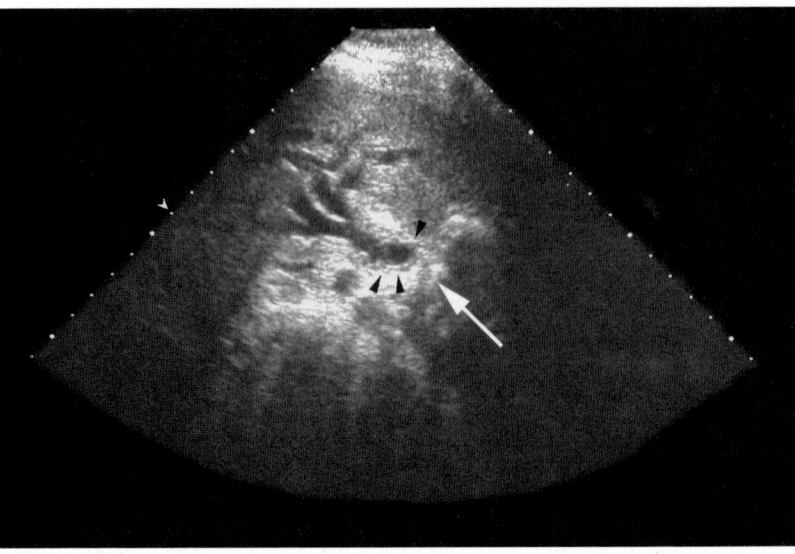

B

FIG. 31-27. *A.* An ERC from a patient with cancer of the common hepatic duct *(arrowheads)*. The common bile duct is of normal size as is the cystic duct *(arrow)*, but the proximal biliary tree is dilated. The gallbladder is not visualized because of tumor obstructing its neck. *B.* An ultrasound from the same patient showing dilated ducts and tumor obstructing the common hepatic duct *(arrow)*. The walls of the bile ducts adjacent to the obstruction are thickened by tumor infiltration *(arrowheads)*.

Pathology

Over 95% of bile duct cancers are adenocarcinomas. Morphologically they are divided into nodular (the most common type), scirrhous, diffusely infiltrating, or papillary. Anatomically they are divided into distal, proximal, or perihilar tumors. Intrahepatic cholangiocarcinomas occur, but they are treated like hepatocellular carcinoma, with hepatectomy when possible. About two-thirds of cholangiocarcinomas are located in the perihilar location. Perihilar cholangiocarcinomas, also referred to as Klatskin tumors, are further classified based on anatomic location by the Bismuth-Corlette classification (Fig. 31-26). Type I tumors are confined to the common hepatic duct, but type II tumors involve the bifurcation without involvement of the secondary intrahepatic ducts. Type IIIa and IIIb tumors extend into the right and left secondary intrahepatic ducts, respectively. Type IV tumors involve both the right and left secondary intrahepatic ducts.

Clinical Manifestations and Diagnosis

Painless jaundice is the most common presentation. Pruritus, mild right upper quadrant pain, anorexia, fatigue, and weight loss also may be present. Cholangitis is the presenting symptom in about 10% of patients, but occurs more commonly after biliary manipulation in these patients. Except for jaundice, physical examination is usually normal in patients with cholangiocarcinoma. Occasionally, asymptomatic patients are found to have cholangiocarcinoma while being evaluated for elevated alkaline phosphatase and gamma-glutamyltransferase levels.

The initial tests are usually ultrasound or CT scan. A perihilar tumor causes dilatation of the intrahepatic biliary tree, but normal or collapsed gallbladder and extrahepatic bile ducts distal to the tumor. Distal bile duct cancer leads to dilatation of the extra- and the intrahepatic bile ducts as well as the gallbladder. Ultrasound can establish the level of obstruction and rule out the presence of

bile duct stones as the cause of the obstructive jaundice (Fig. 31-27). It is usually difficult to visualize the tumor itself on ultrasound or on a standard CT scan. Either ultrasound or spiral CT can be used to determine portal vein patency. The biliary anatomy is defined by cholangiography. PTC defines the proximal extent of the tumor, which is the most important factor in determining resectability. ERC is used, particularly in the evaluation of distal bile duct tumors. For the evaluation of vascular involvement, celiac angiography may be necessary. With the newer types of MRI, a single noninvasive test has the potential of evaluating the biliary anatomy, lymph nodes, and vascular involvement, as well as the tumor growth itself.[74]

Tissue diagnosis may be difficult to obtain nonoperatively except in advanced cases. Percutaneous fine-needle aspiration biopsy, biliary brush or scrape biopsy, and cytologic examination have a low sensitivity in detecting malignancy. Patients with potentially resectable disease should therefore be offered surgical exploration based on radiographic findings and clinical suspicion.[75]

Treatment

Surgical excision is the only potentially curative treatment for cholangiocarcinoma. In the past 1 to 2 decades, improvements in surgical techniques have resulted in lower mortality and better outcome for patients undergoing aggressive surgical excision for cholangiocarcinoma.[76]

Patients should undergo surgical exploration if they have no signs of metastasis or locally unresectable disease. However, despite improvements in ultrasonography, CT scanning, and MRI, more than one half of the patients who are explored are found to have peritoneal implants, nodal or hepatic metastasis, or locally advanced disease that precludes resection. For these patients surgical bypass for biliary decompression and cholecystectomy to prevent the occurrence of acute cholecystitis should be performed.[77]

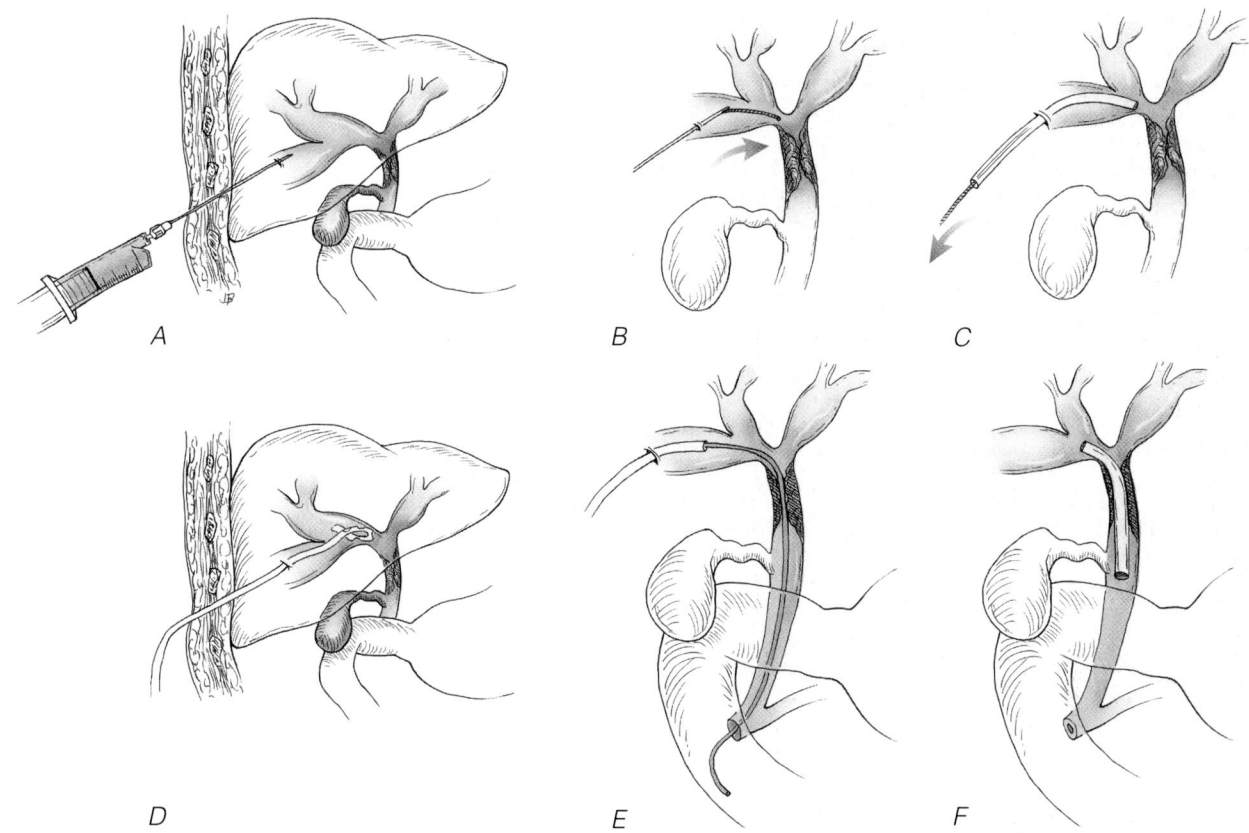

FIG. 31-28. Percutaneous transhepatic cholangiography and placement of a biliary drainage catheter. The catheter has been passed through tumor area (distal cholangiocarcinoma) obstructing the distal common bile duct, and into the duodenum.

For unresectable perihilar cholangiocarcinoma, Roux-en-Y cholangiojejunostomy to either segment II or III bile ducts or to the right hepatic duct can be performed.

For curative resection, the location and local extension of the tumor dictates the extent of the resection. Perihilar tumors involving the bifurcation or proximal common hepatic duct (Bismuth-Corlette type I or II) with no signs of vascular involvement are candidates for local tumor excision with portal lymphadenectomy, cholecystectomy, common bile duct excision, and bilateral Roux-en-Y hepaticojejunostomies. If the tumor involves the right or left hepatic duct (Bismuth-Corlette type IIIa or IIIb), right or left hepatic lobectomy, respectively, should also be performed. Frequently, resection of the adjacent caudate lobe is required because of direct extension into caudate biliary radicals or parenchyma.[75]

Distal bile duct tumors are more often resectable. They are treated with pylorus-preserving pancreatoduodenectomy (Whipple procedure). For patients with distal bile duct cancer found to be unresectable on surgical exploration, Roux-en-Y hepaticojejunostomy, cholecystectomy, and gastrojejunostomy to prevent gastric outlet obstruction should be performed.

Nonoperative biliary decompression is performed for patients with unresectable disease on diagnostic evaluation. Percutaneous placement of expandable metal stents or drainage catheters is usually the appropriate approach for proximal tumors. However, for distal bile duct tumors, endoscopic placement is often the preferred approach (Fig. 31-28). There is a significant risk of cholangitis with internal and external drainage, and stent occlusion is not uncommon.

However, although surgical bypass offers improved patency and fewer episodes of cholangitis, an operative intervention is not warranted in patients with metastatic disease.[78]

There is no proven role for adjuvant chemotherapy in the treatment of cholangiocarcinoma. Adjuvant radiation therapy has also not been shown to increase either quality of life or survival in resected patients. Patients with unresectable disease often are offered treatment with 5-fluorouracil alone or in combination with mitomycin C and doxorubicin, but the response rates are low, less than 10% and less than 30%, respectively. The combination of radiation and chemotherapy may be more effective than either treatment alone for unresectable disease, but no data from randomized trials are available. Giving chemoradiation to these patients can be difficult because of the high incidence of cholangitis. External beam radiation has not been shown to be an effective treatment for unresected disease. The use of interstitial (intraoperative) radiation, brachytherapy with iridium 192 via percutaneous or endoscopic stents, and combined interstitial and external beam radiation for unresectable cholangiocarcinoma has been reported with some encouraging results. However, no randomized, prospective trials have been reported.[75]

Prognosis

Most patients with perihilar cholangiocarcinoma present with advanced, unresectable disease. Patients with unresectable disease have a median survival between 5 and 8 months. The most common causes of death are hepatic failure and cholangitis. The overall

5-year survival rate for patients with resectable perihilar cholangio-carcinoma is between 10 and 30%, but for patients with negative margins it may be as high as 40%. The operative mortality for peri-hilar cholangiocarcinoma is 6 to 8%. Patients with distal cholangio-carcinoma are more likely to have resectable disease and improved prognosis compared to perihilar cholangiocarcinoma. The overall 5-year survival rate for resectable disease is 30 to 50%, and the median survival is 32 to 38 months.

The greatest risk factors for recurrence after resection are the presence of positive margins and lymph node–positive tumors. Therapy for recurrent disease is palliation of symptoms. Surgery is not recommended for patients with recurrent disease.[74]

References

1. Clemente CD: *Gray's Anatomy.* Philadelphia: Lea & Febiger, 1985, p 132.
2. Klein AS, Lillemoe KD, Yeo CJ, et al: Liver, biliary tract, and pancreas, in O'Leary JP (ed): *Physiologic Basis of Surgery.* Baltimore: Williams & Wilkins, 1996, p 441.
3. Scott-Conner CEH, Dawson DL: *Operative Anatomy.* Philadelphia: JB Lippincott Company, 1993, p 388.
4. Molmenti EP, Pinto PA, Klein J, et al: Normal and variant arterial supply of the liver and gallbladder. *Pediatr Transplant* 7:80, 2003.
5. Chen TH, Shyu JF, Chen CH, et al: Variations of the cystic artery in Chinese adults. *Surg Laparosc Endosc Percutan Tech* 10:154, 2000.
6. Boyer J: Bile secretion—models, mechanisms, and malfunctions. A perspective on the development of modern cellular and molecular concepts of bile secretion and cholestasis. *J Gastroenterol* 31:475, 1996.
7. Geoghegan J, Pappas TN: Clinical uses of gut peptides. *Ann Surg* 225:145, 1997.
8. Al-Jiffry BO, Shaffer EA, Saccone GT, et al: Changes in gallbladder motility and gallstone formation following laparoscopic gastric banding for morbid obesity. *Can J Gastroenterol* 17:169, 2003.
9. McDonnell CO, Bailey I, Stumpf T, et al: The effect of cholecystectomy on plasma cholecystokinin. *Am J Gastroenterol* 97:2189, 2002.
10. Yokohata K, Tanaka M: Cyclic motility of the sphincter of Oddi. *J Hepato-Biliary-Pancreatic Surg* 7:178, 2000.
11. Ahrendt SA: Biliary tract surgery. *Curr Gastroenterol Rep* 1:107, 1999.
12. Lee HJ, Choi BI, Han JK, et al: Three-dimensional ultrasonography using the minimum transparent mode in obstructive biliary diseases: Early experience. *J Ultrasound Med* 21:443, 2002.
13. Ralls PW, Jeffrey RB Jr., Kane RA, et al: Ultrasonography. *Gastroenterol Clin North Am* 31:801, 2002.
14. Wexler RS, Greene GS, Scott M: Left hepatic and common hepatic ductal bile leaks demonstrated by Tc-99m HIDA scan and percutaneous transhepatic cholangiogram. *Clin Nucl Med* 19:59, 1994.
15. Breen DJ, Nicholson AA: The clinical utility of spiral CT cholangiography. *Clin Radiol* 55:733, 2000.
16. Liu TH, Consorti ET, Kawashima A, et al: Patient evaluation and management with selective use of magnetic resonance cholangiography and endoscopic retrograde cholangiopancreatography before laparoscopic cholecystectomy. *Ann Surg* 234:33, 2001.
17. Magnuson TH, Bender JS, Duncan MD, et al: Utility of magnetic resonance cholangiography in the evaluation of biliary obstruction. *J Am Coll Surg* 189:63, 1999.
18. Washington M, Ghazi A: Complications of ERCP, in Scott-Conner CEH (ed): *The SAGES Manual.* New York: Springer-Verlag, 1999, p 516.
19. Nakeeb A, Comuzzie AG, Martin L, et al: Gallstones: Genetics versus environment. *Ann Surg* 235:842, 2002.
20. Brasca A, Berli D, Pezzotto SM, et al: Morphological and demographic associations of biliary symptoms in subjects with gallstones: Findings from a population-based survey in Rosario, Argentina. *Dig Liver Dis* 34:577, 2002.
21. Strasberg SM: The pathogenesis of cholesterol gallstones a review. *J Gastrointest Surg* 2:109, 1998.
22. Stewart L, Oesterle AL, Erdan I, et al: Pathogenesis of pigment gallstones in Western societies: The central role of bacteria. *J Gastrointest Surg* 6:891, 2002.
23. Trowbridge RL, Rutkowski NK, Shojania KG: Does this patient have acute cholecystitis? *JAMA* 289:80, 2003.
24. Fletcher DR: Gallstones. Modern management. *Aust Fam Physician* 30:441, 2001.
25. Strasberg SM: Cholelithiasis and acute cholecystitis. *Baillieres Clin Gastroenterol* 11:643, 1997.
26. Kiviluoto T, Siren J, Luukkonen P, et al: Randomised trial of laparoscopic versus open cholecystectomy for acute and gangrenous cholecystitis. *Lancet* 351:321, 1998.
27. Lo CM, Liu CL, Fan ST, et al: Prospective randomized study of early versus delayed laparoscopic cholecystectomy for acute cholecystitis. *Ann Surg* 227:461, 1998.
28. Chikamori F, Kuniyoshi N, Shibuya S, et al: Early scheduled laparoscopic cholecystectomy following percutaneous transhepatic gallbladder drainage for patients with acute cholecystitis. *Surg Endosc* 16:1704, 2002.
29. Ko C, Lee S: Epidemiology and natural history of common bile duct stones and prediction of disease. *Gastrointest Endosc* 56:S165, 2002.
30. Tranter S, Thompson M: Comparison of endoscopic sphincterotomy and laparoscopic exploration of the common bile duct. *Br J Surg* 89:1495, 2002.
31. Hamy A, Hennekinne S, Pessaux P, et al: Endoscopic sphincterotomy prior to laparoscopic cholecystectomy for the treatment of cholelithiasis. *Surg Endosc* 17:872, 2003.
32. Lilly MC, Arregui ME: A balanced approach to choledocholithiasis. *Surg Endosc* 15:467, 2001.
33. Lipsett PA, Pitt HA: Acute cholangitis. *Front Biosci* 8:S1229, 2003.
34. Lillemoe KD: Surgical treatment of biliary tract infections. *Am Surg* 66:138, 2000.
35. Rhodes M, Sussman L, Cohen L, et al: Randomised trial of laparoscopic exploration of common bile duct versus postoperative endoscopic retrograde cholangiography for common bile duct stones. *Lancet* 351:159, 1998.
36. Sperling RM, Koch J, Sandhu JS, et al: Recurrent pyogenic cholangitis in Asian immigrants to the United States: Natural history and role of therapeutic ERCP. *Dig Dis Sci* 42:865, 1997.
37. Thinh NC, Breda Y, Faucompret S, et al: Oriental biliary lithiasis. Retrospective study of 690 patients treated surgically over 8 years at Hospital 108 in Hanoi (Vietnam). *Medecine Tropicale* 61:509, 2001.
38. Byrne MF, Suhocki P, Mitchell RM, et al: Percutaneous cholecystostomy in patients with acute cholecystitis: Experience of 45 patients at a US referral center. *J Am Coll Surg* 197:206, 2003.
39. Akhan O, Akinci D, Ozmen MN: Percutaneous cholecystostomy. *Eur J Radiol* 43:229, 2002.
40. Khaitan L, Apelgren K, Hunter J, et al: A report on the Society of American Gastrointestinal Endoscopic Surgeons (SAGES) Outcomes Initiative: What have we learned and what is its potential? *Surg Endosc* 17:365, 2003.
41. Richards C, Edwards J, Culver D, et al: Does using a laparoscopic approach to cholecystectomy decrease the risk of surgical site infection? *Ann Surg* 237:358, 2003.
42. Flum DR, Dellinger EP, Cheadle A, et al: Intraoperative cholangiography and risk of common bile duct injury during cholecystectomy. *JAMA* 289:1639, 2003.
43. Hunter JG: Acute cholecystitis revisited: Get it while it's hot. *Ann Surg* 227:468, 1998.
44. Biffl W, Moore E, Offner P, et al: Routine intraoperative ultrasonography with selective cholangiography reduces bile duct complications during laparoscopic cholecystectomy. *J Am Coll Surg* 193:272, 2001.
45. Halpin VJ, Dunnegan D, Soper NJ: Laparoscopic intracorporeal ultrasound versus fluoroscopic intraoperative cholangiography: After the learning curve. *Surg Endosc* 16:336, 2002.

46. Barwood NT, Valinsky LJ, Hobbs MS, et al: Changing methods of imaging the common bile duct in the laparoscopic cholecystectomy era in Western Australia: Implications for surgical practice. *Ann Surg* 235:41, 2002.

47. Pelinka LE, Schmidhammer R, Hamid L, et al: Acute acalculous cholecystitis after trauma: A prospective study. *J Trauma-Injury Infect Crit Care* 55:323, 2003.

48. Ryu JK, Ryu KH, Kim KH: Clinical features of acute acalculous cholecystitis. *J Clin Gastroenterol* 36:166, 2003.

49. Lipsett PA, Pitt HA: Surgical treatment of choledochal cysts. *J Hepatobiliary Pancreat Surg* 10:352, 2003.

50. Ahrendt SA, Pitt HA, Nakeeb A, et al: Diagnosis and management of cholangiocarcinoma in primary sclerosing cholangitis. *J Gastrointest Surg* 3:357, 1999.

51. Ahrendt SA, Pitt HA, Kalloo AN, et al: Primary sclerosing cholangitis: Resect, dilate, or transplant? *Ann Surg* 227:412, 1998.

52. Goss JA, Shackleton CR, Farmer DG, et al: Orthotopic liver transplantation for primary sclerosing cholangitis. A 12-year single center experience. *Ann Surg* 225:472, 1997.

53. Ahrendt SA, Pitt HA: Surgical treatment for primary sclerosing cholangitis. *J Hepatobiliary Pancreat Surg* 6:366, 1999.

54. Linder JD, Klapow JC, Linder SD, et al: Incomplete response to endoscopic sphincterotomy in patients with sphincter of Oddi dysfunction: Evidence for a chronic pain disorder. *Am J Gastroenterol* 98:1738, 2003.

55. Lillemoe KD, Melton GB, Cameron JL, et al: Postoperative bile duct strictures: Management and outcome in the 1990s. *Ann Surg* 232:430, 2000.

56. Melton GB, Lillemoe KD: The current management of postoperative bile duct strictures. *Adv Surg* 36:193, 2002.

57. Archer SB, Brown DW, Smith CD, et al: Bile duct injury during laparoscopic cholecystectomy: results of a national survey. *Ann Surg* 234:549, 2001.

58. Ahrendt SA, Pitt HA: Surgical therapy of iatrogenic lesions of biliary tract. *World J Surg* 25:1360, 2001.

59. Strasberg SM: Avoidance of biliary injury during laparoscopic cholecystectomy. *J Hepato-Biliary-Pancreat Surg* 9:543, 2002.

60. Way LW, Stewart L, Gantert W, et al: Causes and prevention of laparoscopic bile duct injuries: Analysis of 252 cases from a human factors and cognitive psychology perspective [comment]. *Ann Surg* 237:460, 2003.

61. Flum DR, Flowers C, Veenstra DL: A cost-effectiveness analysis of intraoperative cholangiography in the prevention of bile duct injury during laparoscopic cholecystectomy. *J Am Coll Surg* 196:385, 2003.

62. Lee CM, Stewart L, Way LW: Postcholecystectomy abdominal bile collections. *Arch Surg* 135:538, 2000.

63. Melton GB, Lillemoe KD, Cameron JL, et al: Major bile duct injuries associated with laparoscopic cholecystectomy: Effect of surgical repair on quality of life. *Ann Surg* 235:888, 2002.

64. Grobmyer SR, Lieberman MD, Daly JM: Gallbladder cancer in the twentieth century: Single institution's experience. *World J Surg* 28:47, 2004.

65. Pandey M, Shukla VK: Diet and gallbladder cancer: A case-control study. *Eur J Cancer Prev* 11:365, 2002.

66. Csendes A, Burgos AM, Csendes P, et al: Late follow-up of polypoid lesions of the gallbladder smaller than 10 mm. *Ann Surg* 234:657, 2001.

67. Wagholikar G, Behari A, Krishnani N, et al: Early gallbladder cancer. *J Am Coll Surg* 194:137, 2002.

68. Bartlett DL, Fong Y, Fortner JG, et al: Long-term results after resection for gallbladder cancer. Implications for staging and management. *Ann Surg* 224:639, 1996.

69. Wakai T, Shirai Y, Hatakeyama K: Radical second resection provides survival benefit for patients with T2 gallbladder carcinoma first discovered after laparoscopic cholecystectomy. *World J Surg* 26:867, 2002.

70. Noshiro H, Chijiiwa K, Yamaguchi K, et al: Factors affecting surgical outcome for gallbladder carcinoma. *Hepato-Gastroenterol* 50:939, 2003.

71. Strasberg SM: Resection of hilar cholangiocarcinoma. *HPB Surg* 10:415, 1998.

72. Tocchi A, Mazzoni G, Liotta G, et al: Late development of bile duct cancer in patients who had biliary-enteric drainage for benign disease: A follow-up study of more than 1000 patients. *Ann Surg* 234:210, 2001.

73. Ahrendt SA, Rashid A, Chow JT, et al: p53 overexpression and K-ras gene mutations in primary sclerosing cholangitis-associated biliary tract cancer. *J Hepatobiliary Pancreat Surg* 7:426, 2000.

74. Ahrendt SA, Nakeeb A, Pitt HA: Cholangiocarcinoma. *Clin Liver Dis* 5:191, 2001.

75. Lillemoe KD, Cameron JL: Surgery for hilar cholangiocarcinoma: The Johns Hopkins approach. *J Hepatobiliary Pancreat Surg* 7:115, 2000.

76. Mulholland MW, Yahanda A, Yeo CJ: Multidisciplinary management of perihilar bile duct cancer. *J Am Coll Surg* 193:440, 2001.

77. Vollmer CM, Drebin JA, Middleton WD, et al: Utility of staging laparoscopy in subsets of peripancreatic and biliary malignancies [comment]. *Ann Surg* 235:1, 2002.

78. Strasberg SM: ERCP and surgical intervention in pancreatic and biliary malignancies. *Gastrointest Endosc* 56:S213, 2002.

CHAPTER 32

Pancreas

William E. Fisher, Dana K. Andersen, Richard H. Bell, Jr.,
Ashok K. Saluja, and F. Charles Brunicardi

ANATOMY AND PHYSIOLOGY

The pancreas is perhaps the most unforgiving organ in the human body, *leading most surgeons to avoid* even palpating it unless necessary. Situated deep in the center of the abdomen, the pancreas is surrounded by numerous important structures and major blood vessels. Therefore seemingly minor trauma to the pancreas can result in the release of pancreatic enzymes and cause life-threatening pancreatitis. Surgeons that choose to undertake surgery on the pancreas require a thorough knowledge of its anatomy. However, knowledge of the relationships of the pancreas and surrounding structures is also critically important for all surgeons to ensure that pancreatic injury is avoided during surgery on other structures.

Gross Anatomy

The pancreas is a retroperitoneal organ that lies in an oblique position, sloping upward from the C-loop of the duodenum to the splenic hilum (Fig. 32-1). In an adult, the pancreas weighs 75 to 100 g and is about 15 to 20 cm long. The fact that the pancreas is situated so deeply in the abdomen and is sealed in the retroperitoneum explains the poorly localized and sometimes ill-defined nature with which pancreatic pathology presents. Patients with pancreatic cancer without bile duct obstruction usually present after months of vague upper abdominal discomfort, or no antecedent symptoms at all. Due to its retroperitoneal location, pain associated with pancreatitis is often characterized as radiating through to the back.

Regions of the Pancreas

Surgeons typically describe the location of pathology within the pancreas in relation to four regions: the head, neck, body, and tail.

The head of the pancreas is nestled in the C-loop of the duodenum and is posterior to the transverse mesocolon. Just behind the head of the pancreas lie the vena cava, the right renal artery, and both renal veins. The neck of the pancreas lies directly over the portal vein. At the inferior border of the neck of the pancreas, the superior mesenteric vein joins the splenic vein and then continues toward the porta hepatis as the portal vein. The inferior mesenteric vein often joins the splenic vein near its junction with the portal vein. Sometimes the inferior mesenteric vein joins the superior mesenteric vein, or merges with the superior mesenteric portal venous junction to form a trifurcation (Fig. 32-2). The superior mesenteric artery lies parallel to and just to the left of the superior mesenteric vein. The uncinate process and the head of the pancreas wraps around the right side of the portal vein and end posteriorly near the space between the superior mesenteric vein and superior mesenteric artery. Venous branches draining the pancreatic head and uncinate process enter along the right lateral and posterior sides of the portal vein. There are usually no anterior venous tributaries, and a plane can usually be developed between the neck of the pancreas and the portal and superior mesenteric veins during pancreatic resection, unless the tumor is invading the vein anteriorly. The common bile duct runs in a deep groove on the posterior aspect of the pancreatic head until it passes through the pancreatic parenchyma to join the main pancreatic duct at the ampulla of Vater. The body and tail of the pancreas lie just anterior to the splenic artery and vein. The vein runs in a groove on the back of the pancreas and is fed by multiple fragile venous branches from the pancreatic parenchyma. These branches must be ligated in order to perform a spleen-sparing distal pancreatectomy. The splenic artery runs parallel to and just superior to the vein along the posterior superior edge of the body and tail

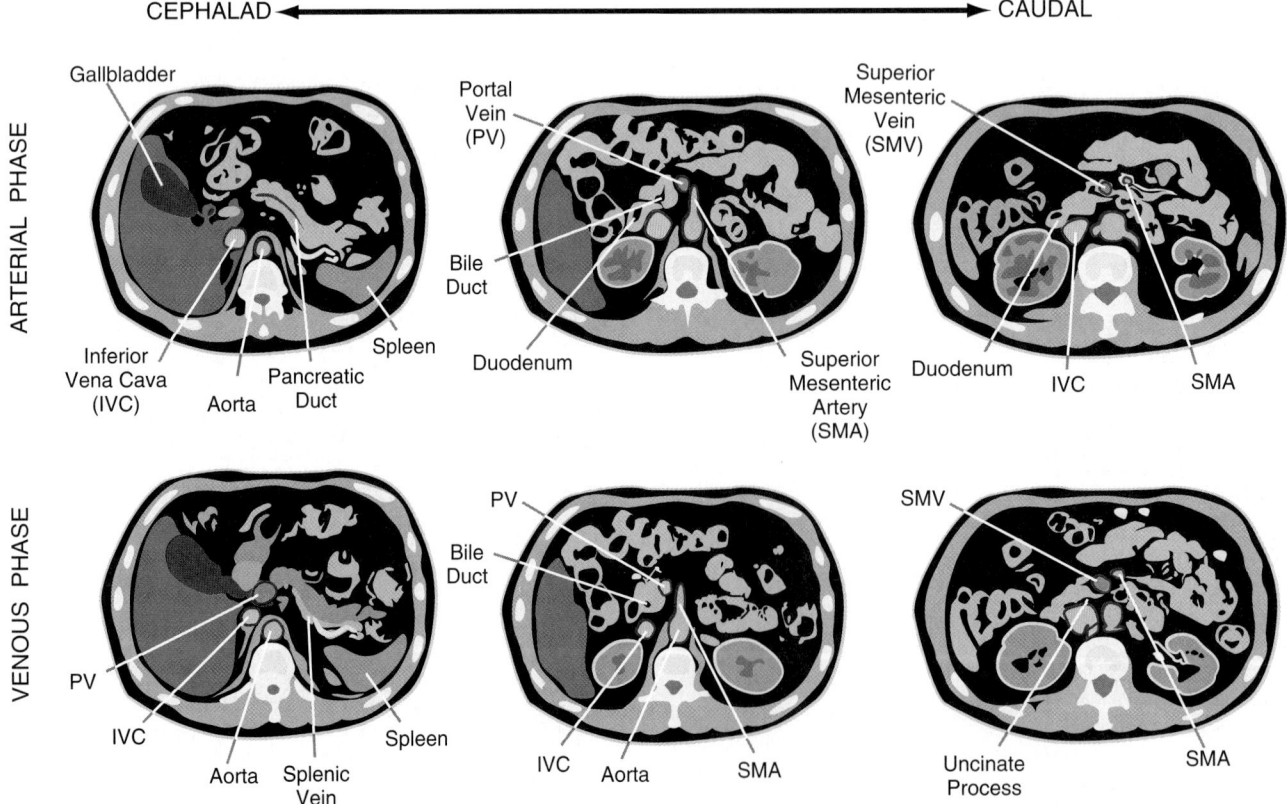

FIG. 32-1. *Pancreatic anatomy as seen on computed tomography. Knowledge of the relationship of the pancreas with surrounding structures is important to ensure that injury is avoided during abdominal surgery.*

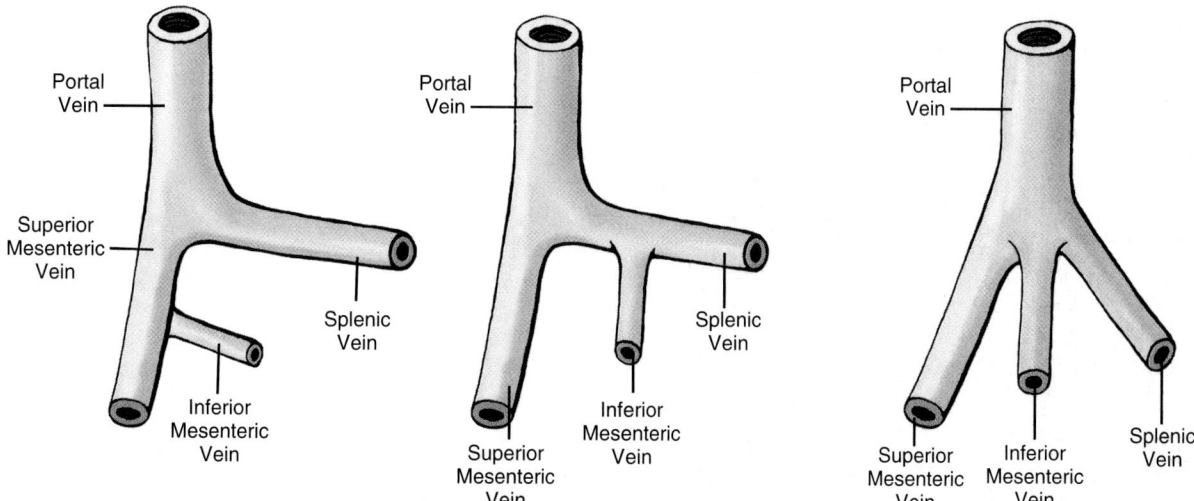

FIG. 32-2. *Variations in portal venous anatomy. The superior mesenteric vein joins the splenic vein and then continues toward the porta hepatis as the portal vein. The inferior mesenteric vein often joins the splenic vein near its junction with the portal vein, but sometimes joins the superior mesenteric vein; or the three veins merge as a trifurcation to form the portal vein.*

of the pancreas. The anterior surface of the body of the pancreas is covered by peritoneum. Once the gastrocolic omentum is divided, the body and tail of the pancreas can be seen along the floor of the lesser sac, just posterior to the stomach.

Pancreatic pseudocysts commonly develop in this area, and the posterior aspect of the stomach can form the anterior wall of the pseudocyst, allowing drainage into the stomach. The base of the transverse mesocolon attaches to the inferior margin of the body and tail of the pancreas. The transverse mesocolon often forms the inferior wall of pancreatic pseudocysts or inflammatory processes, allowing surgical drainage through the transverse mesocolon. The body of the pancreas overlies the aorta at the origin of the superior mesenteric artery. The neck of the pancreas overlies the vertebral body of L1 and L2, and blunt anteroposterior trauma can compress the neck of the pancreas against the spine, causing parenchymal and sometimes ductal injury. The neck divides the pancreas into approximately two equal halves. The small portion of the pancreas anterior to the left kidney is referred to as the tail, and is nestled in the hilum of the spleen near the splenic flexure of the left colon. Awareness of these anatomic relationships is important in order to avoid injury to the pancreatic tail during left colectomy or splenectomy.

Pancreatic Duct Anatomy

An understanding of embryology is required to appreciate the common variations in pancreatic duct anatomy. The pancreas is formed by the fusion of a ventral and dorsal bud. The duct from the smaller ventral bud, which arises from the hepatic diverticulum, connects directly to the common bile duct. The duct from the larger dorsal bud, which arises from the duodenum, drains directly into the duodenum. The duct of the ventral anlage becomes the duct of Wirsung, and the duct from the dorsal anlage becomes the duct of Santorini. With gut rotation, the ventral anlage rotates to the right and around the posterior side of the duodenum to fuse with the dorsal bud. The ventral anlage becomes the inferior portion of the pancreatic head and the uncinate process, while the dorsal anlage becomes the body and tail of the pancreas. The ducts from each anlage usually fuse together in the pancreatic head such that most of the pancreas drains through the duct of Wirsung, or main pancreatic duct, into the common channel formed from the bile duct and

pancreatic duct. The length of the common channel is variable. In about one third of patients the two ducts remain distinct to the end of the papilla, the two ducts merge at the end of the papilla in another one third, and in the remaining one third a true common channel is present for a distance of several millimeters. Commonly, the duct from the dorsal anlage, the duct of Santorini, persists as the lesser pancreatic duct, and sometimes drains directly into the duodenum through the lesser papilla just proximal to the major papilla. In approximately 30% of patients, the duct of Santorini ends as a blind accessory duct and does not empty into the duodenum.[1] In 10% of patients, the ducts of Wirsung and Santorini fail to fuse.[1] This results in the majority of the pancreas draining through the duct of Santorini and the lesser papilla, while the inferior portion of the pancreatic head and uncinate process drains through the duct of Wirsung and major papilla. This normal anatomic variant, which occurs in one out of 10 patients, is referred to as *pancreas divisum*. In a minority of these patients, the minor papilla can be inadequate to handle the flow of pancreatic juices from the majority of the gland. This relative outflow obstruction can result in pancreatitis and is sometimes treated by sphincteroplasty of the minor papilla (Fig. 32-3).

The main pancreatic duct is usually only 2 to 3 mm in diameter and runs midway between the superior and inferior borders of the pancreas, usually closer to the posterior than to the anterior surface. Pressure inside the pancreatic duct is about twice that in the common bile duct, which is thought to prevent reflux of bile into the pancreatic duct. The main pancreatic duct joins with the common bile duct and empties at the ampulla of Vater or major papilla, which is located on the medial aspect of the second portion of the duodenum. The muscle fibers around the ampulla form the sphincter of Oddi, which controls the flow of pancreatic and biliary secretions into the duodenum. Contraction and relaxation of the sphincter is regulated by complex neural and hormonal factors. When the accessory pancreatic duct or lesser duct drains into the duodenum, a lesser papilla can be identified approximately 2 cm proximal to the ampulla of Vater.

Vascular and Lymphatic Anatomy

The blood supply to the pancreas comes from multiple branches from the celiac and superior mesenteric arteries. The common

EMBRYOLOGY OF PANCREAS AND DUCT VARIATIONS

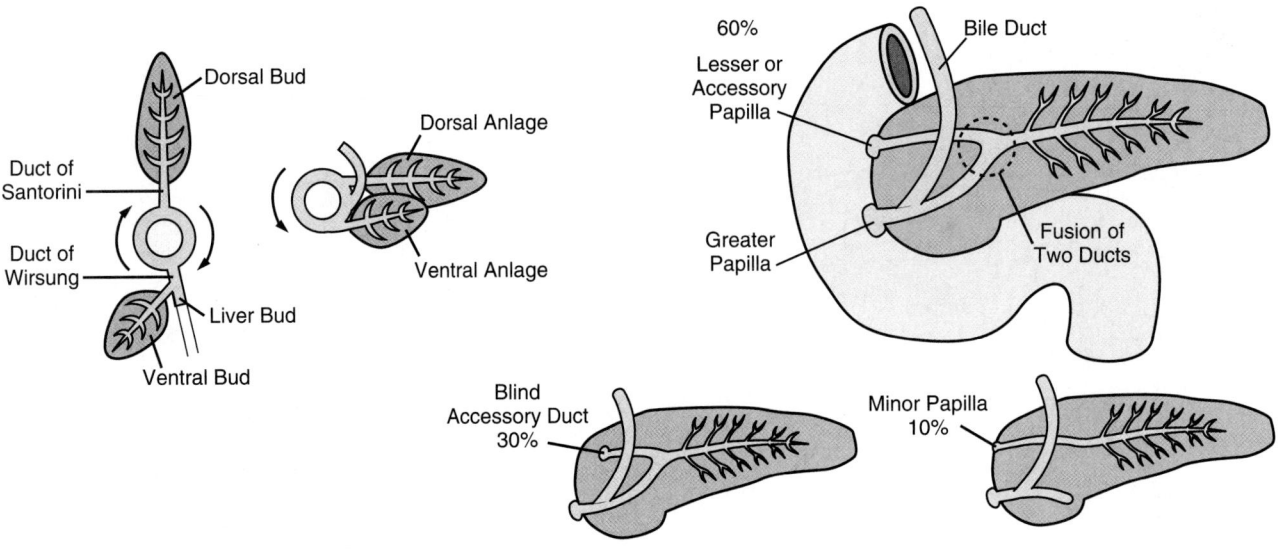

FIG. 32-3. Embryology of pancreas and duct variations. The duct of Wirsung from the ventral bud connects to the bile duct, while the duct of Santorini from the larger dorsal bud connects to the duodenum. With gut rotation, the two ducts fuse in most cases such that the majority of the pancreas drains through the duct of Wirsung to the major papilla. The duct of Santorini can persist as a blind accessory duct or drain through the lesser papilla. In a minority of patients, the ducts remain separate and the majority of the pancreas drains through the duct of Santorini, a condition referred to as pancreas divisum.

hepatic artery gives rise to the gastroduodenal artery before continuing toward the porta hepatis as the proper hepatic artery. The gastroduodenal artery becomes the superior pancreaticoduodenal artery as it passes behind the first portion of the duodenum and branches into the anterior and posterior superior pancreaticoduodenal arteries. As the superior mesenteric artery passes behind the neck of the pancreas, it gives off the inferior pancreaticoduodenal artery at the inferior margin of the neck of the pancreas. This vessel quickly divides into the anterior and posterior inferior pancreaticoduodenal arteries. The superior and inferior pancreaticoduodenal arteries join together within the parenchyma of the anterior and posterior sides of the head of the pancreas along the medial aspect of the C-loop of the duodenum to form arcades that give off numerous branches to the duodenum and head of the pancreas. Therefore it is impossible to resect the head of the pancreas without devascularizing the duodenum, unless a rim of pancreas containing the pancreaticoduodenal arcade is preserved. Variations in the arterial anatomy occur in one out of five patients. The right hepatic artery, common hepatic artery, or gastroduodenal arteries can arise from the superior mesenteric artery. In 15 to 20% of patients, the right hepatic artery will arise from the superior mesenteric artery and travel upwards toward the liver along the posterior aspect of the head of the pancreas (referred to as a "replaced right hepatic artery") (Fig. 32-4). During the Whipple procedure, it is important to look for this variation so the hepatic artery is recognized and injury is avoided. The body and tail of the pancreas are supplied by multiple branches of the splenic artery. The splenic artery arises from the celiac trunk and travels along the posterior-superior border of the body and tail of the pancreas toward the spleen. The inferior pancreatic artery arises from the superior mesenteric artery and runs to the left along the inferior border of the body and tail of the pancreas, parallel to the splenic artery. Three vessels run perpendicular to the long axis of the pancreatic body and tail and connect the splenic artery and inferior pancreatic artery. They are, from medial to lateral, the dorsal, great, and caudal

pancreatic arteries. These arteries form arcades within the body and tail of the pancreas, and account for the rich blood supply of the organ.

The venous drainage of the pancreas follows a pattern similar to that of the arterial supply. The veins are usually superficial to the arteries within the parenchyma of the pancreas. There is an anterior and posterior venous arcade within the head of the pancreas. The superior veins drain directly into the portal vein just above the neck of the pancreas. The posterior inferior arcade drains directly into the inferior mesenteric vein at the inferior border of the neck of the pancreas. The anterior inferior pancreaticoduodenal vein joins the right gastroepiploic vein and the right colic vein to form a common venous trunk, which enters into the superior mesenteric vein. Traction on the transverse colon during colectomy can tear these fragile veins, which then retract into the parenchyma of the pancreas, making control tedious. There are also numerous small venous branches coming from the pancreatic parenchyma directly into the lateral and posterior aspect of the portal vein. Venous return from the body and tail of the pancreas drains into the splenic vein (Fig. 32-5).

The lymphatic drainage from the pancreas is diffuse and widespread. The profuse network of lymphatic vessels and lymph nodes draining the pancreas provides egress to tumor cells arising from the pancreas. This diffuse lymphatic drainage contributes to the fact that pancreatic cancer often presents with positive lymph nodes and a high incidence of local recurrence after resection. Lymph nodes can be palpated along the posterior aspect of the head of the pancreas, where the mesenteric vein passes under the neck of the pancreas, and along the hepatic artery ascending into the porta hepatis. The pancreatic lymphatics also communicate with lymph nodes in the transverse mesocolon and mesentery of the proximal jejunum. Tumors in the body and tail of the pancreas often metastasize to these nodes and lymph nodes along the splenic vein and in the hilum of the spleen (Fig. 32-6).

ARTERIAL SUPPLY TO THE PANCREAS

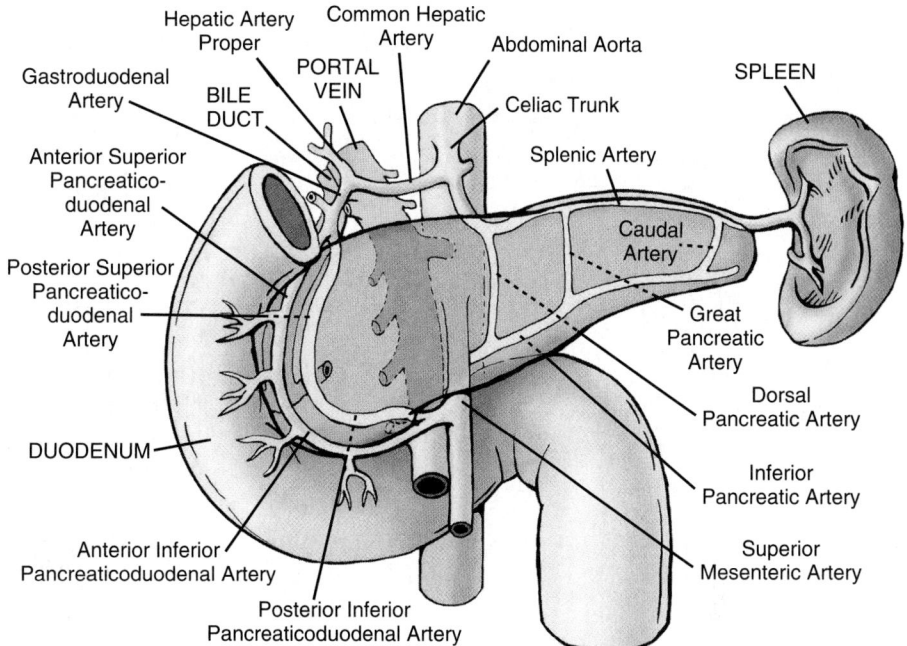

FIG. 32-4. Arterial supply to the pancreas. Multiple arcades in the head and body of the pancreas provide a rich blood supply. The head of the pancreas cannot be resected without devascularizing the duodenum unless a rim of pancreas containing the pancreaticoduodenal arcade is preserved.

Neuroanatomy

The pancreas is innervated by the sympathetic and parasympathetic nervous systems. The acinar cells responsible for exocrine secretion, the islet cells responsible for endocrine secretion, and the islet vasculature are innervated by both systems. The parasympathetic system stimulates endocrine and exocrine secretion and the sympathetic system inhibits secretion.[2] The pancreas is also innervated by neurons that secrete amines and peptides, such as somato-statin, vasoactive intestinal peptide (VIP), calcitonin gene-related peptide (CGRP), and galanin. The exact role of these neurons in pancreatic physiology is uncertain, but they do appear to affect both exocrine and endocrine function. The pancreas also has a rich supply of afferent sensory fibers, which are responsible for the intense pain associated with advanced pancreatic cancer, as well as acute and chronic pancreatitis. These somatic fibers travel superiorly to the celiac ganglia. Interruption of these somatic fibers can stop transmission of pain sensation (Fig. 32-7).

FIG. 32-5. Venous drainage from the pancreas. The venous drainage of the pancreas follows a pattern similar to the arterial supply, with the veins usually superficial to the arteries. Anterior traction on the transverse colon can tear fragile branches along the inferior border of the pancreas, which then retract into the parenchyma of the pancreas. Venous branches draining the pancreatic head and uncinate process enter along the right lateral and posterior sides of the portal vein. There are usually no anterior venous tributaries, and a plane can usually be developed between the neck of the pancreas and the portal and superior mesenteric veins.

VENOUS DRAINAGE FROM PANCREAS

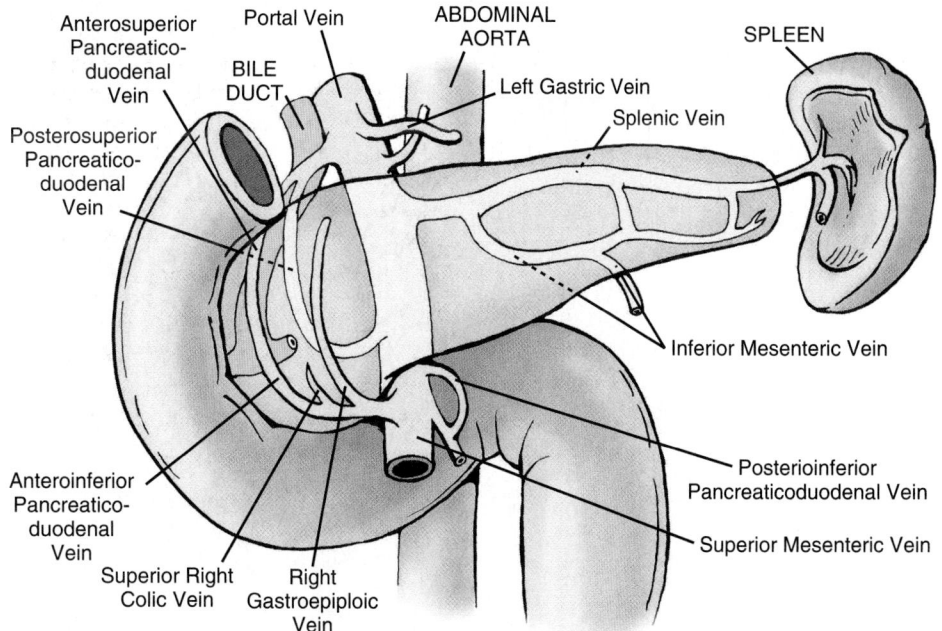

LYMPHATIC SUPPLY TO THE PANCREAS

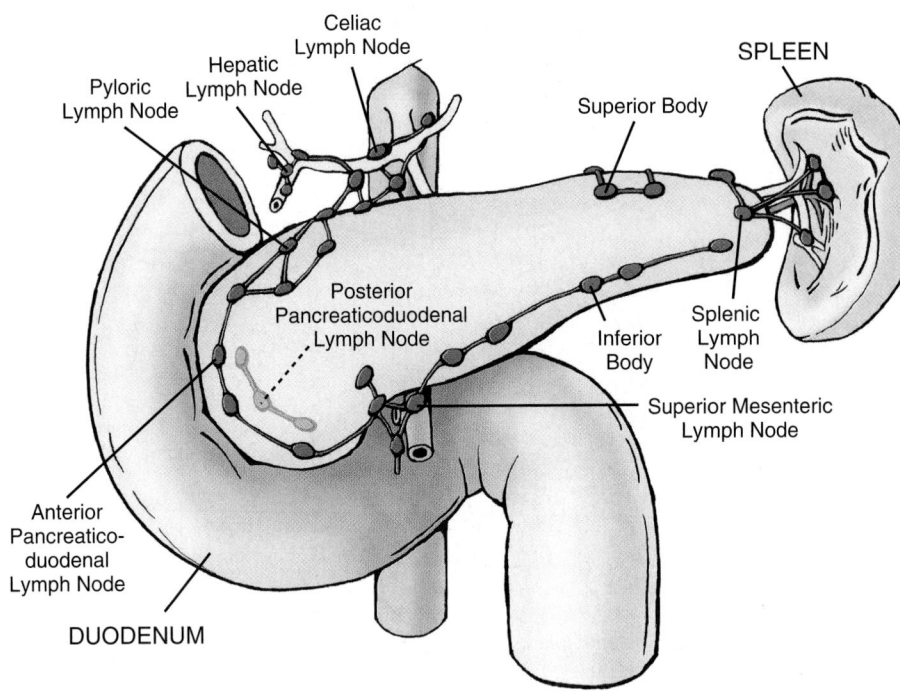

FIG. 32-6. Lymphatic supply to the pancreas. The lymphatic drainage from the pancreas is diffuse and widespread, which explains the high incidence of lymph node metastases and local recurrence of pancreatic cancer. The pancreatic lymphatics also communicate with lymph nodes in the transverse mesocolon and mesentery of the proximal jejunum. Tumors in the body and tail of the pancreas are often unresectable because they metastasize to these lymph nodes and to the hilum of the spleen. (*Reproduced with permission from Bell, Rikkers, Mulholland (eds): Atlas of Pancreatic Surgery, 1st ed. Philadelphia: Lippincott, Williams & Wilkins, 1996.*)

HISTOLOGY AND PHYSIOLOGY

The exocrine pancreas accounts for about 85% of the pancreatic mass; 10% of the gland is accounted for by extracellular matrix, and 4% by blood vessels and the major ducts, whereas only 2% of the gland is comprised of endocrine tissue. The endocrine and exocrine pancreas are sometimes thought of as functionally separate, but these different components of the organ are coordinated to allow an elegant regulatory feedback system for digestive enzyme and hormone secretion. This complex system regulates the type of digestion, its rate, and the processing and distribution of absorbed nutrients. This coordination is facilitated by the physical

INNERVATION OF THE PANCREAS

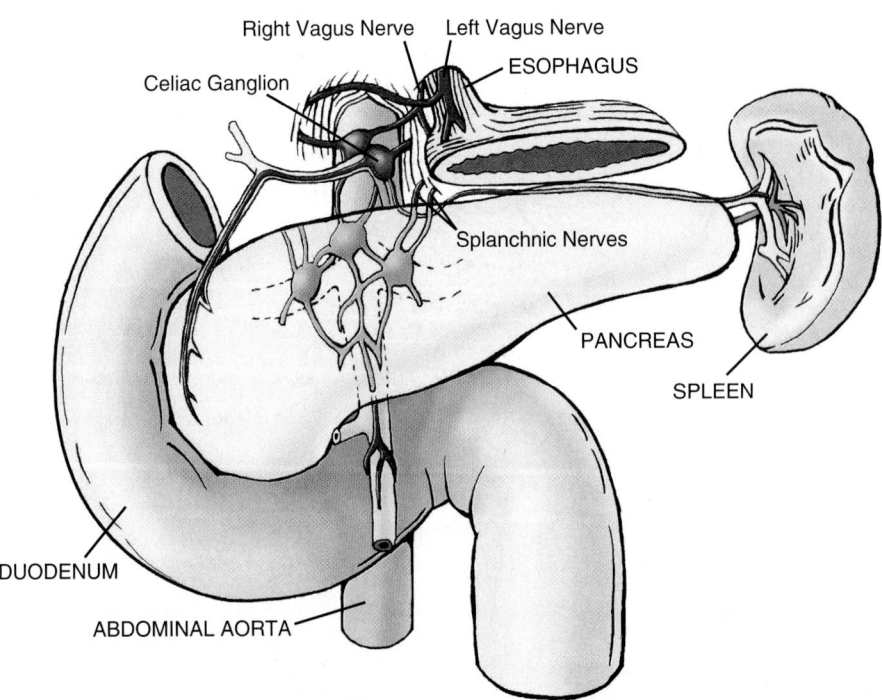

FIG. 32-7. Innervation of the pancreas. The pancreas has a rich supply of afferent sensory fibers that travel superiorly to the celiac ganglia. Interruption of these somatic fibers with a celiac plexus block can interfere with transmission of pancreatic pain. (*Reproduced with permission from Bell, Rikkers, Mulholland (eds): Atlas of Pancreatic Surgery, 1st ed. Philadelphia: Lippincott, Williams & Wilkins, 1996.*)

approximation of the islets and the exocrine pancreas, the presence of specific islet hormone receptors on the plasma membranes of pancreatic acinar cells, and the existence of an islet-acinar portal blood system.

Although patients can live without a pancreas when insulin and digestive enzyme replacement are administered, the loss of this islet-acinar coordination leads to impairments in digestive function. Although only approximately 20% of the normal pancreas is required to prevent insufficiency, in many patients undergoing pancreatic resection, the remaining pancreas is not normal, and pancreatic endocrine and exocrine insufficiency can develop with removal of smaller portions of the gland.

Exocrine Pancreas

The pancreas secretes approximately 500 to 800 mL per day of colorless, odorless, alkaline, isosmotic pancreatic juice. Pancreatic juice is a combination of acinar cell and duct cell secretions. The acinar cells secrete amylase, proteases and lipases, enzymes responsible for the digestion of all three food types: carbohydrate, protein, and fat. The acinar cells are pyramid-shaped, with their apices facing the lumen of the acinus. Near the apex of each cell are numerous enzyme-containing zymogen granules which fuse with the apical cell membrane (Fig. 32-8). Unlike the endocrine pancreas, where islet cells specialize in the secretion of one hormone type, individual acinar cells secrete all types of enzymes. However, the ratio

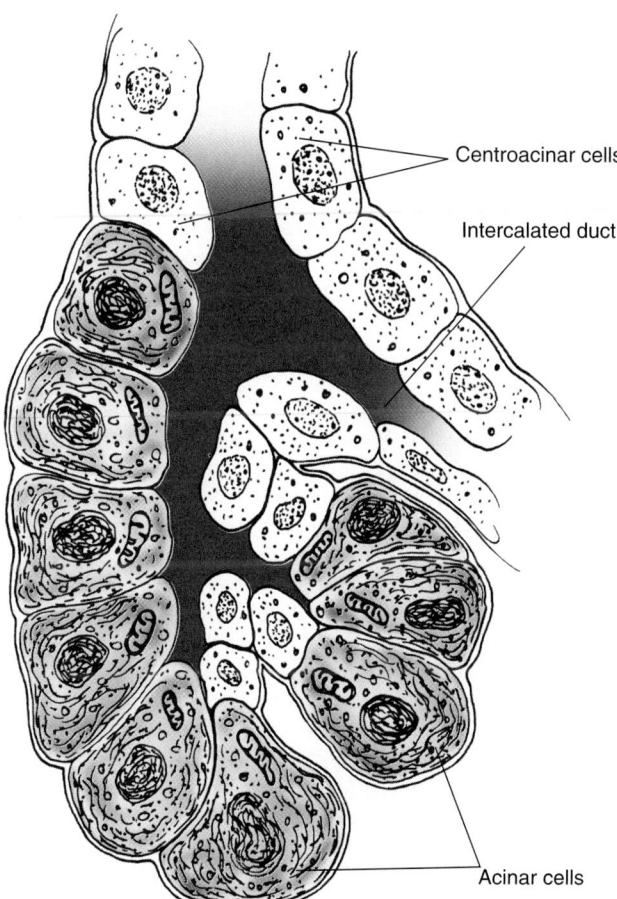

Centroacinar cells

Intercalated duct

Acinar cells

FIG. 32-8. *Acinar cell. Zymogen granules fuse with the apical membrane and release multiple enzymes to digest carbohydrates, proteins, and fat. (Reproduced with permission from O'Leary (ed): The Physiologic Basis of Surgery, 1st ed. Baltimore: Lippincott, Williams & Wilkins, 1993.)*

of the different enzymes released is adjusted to the composition of digested food through nonparallel regulation of secretion.

Pancreatic amylase is secreted in its active form and completes the digestive process already begun by salivary amylase. Amylase is the only pancreatic enzyme secreted in its active form, and it hydrolyzes starch and glycogen to glucose, maltose, maltotriose, and dextrins. These simple sugars are transported across the brush border of the intestinal epithelial cells by active transport mechanisms. Gastric hydrolysis of protein yields peptides that enter the intestine and stimulate intestinal endocrine cells to release cholecystokinin-releasing peptide (CCK-RP), cholecystokinin (CCK), and secretin, which then stimulate the pancreas to secrete enzymes and bicarbonate into the intestine.

The proteolytic enzymes are secreted as proenzymes that require activation. Trypsinogen is converted to its active form, trypsin, by another enzyme, enterokinase, which is produced by the duodenal mucosal cells. Trypsin in turn activates the other proteolytic enzymes. Trypsinogen activation within the pancreas is prevented by the presence of inhibitors that are also secreted by the acinar cells. A failure to express a normal trypsinogen inhibitor, pancreatic secretory trypsin inhibitor (PSTI) or *SPINK1*, is a cause of familial pancreatitis. Inhibition of trypsinogen activation ensures that the enzymes within the pancreas remain in an inactive precursor state and are activated only within the duodenum. Trypsinogen is expressed in several isoforms, and a missense mutation on the cationic trypsinogen, or *PRSS1*, results in premature, intrapancreatic activation of trypsinogen. This accounts for about two thirds of cases of hereditary pancreatitis. Chymotrypsinogen is activated to form chymotrypsin. Elastase, carboxypeptidase A and B, and phospholipase are also activated by trypsin. Trypsin, chymotrypsin, and elastase cleave bonds between amino acids within a target peptide chain, and carboxypeptidase A and B cleave amino acids at the end of peptide chains. Individual amino acids and small dipeptides are then actively transported into the intestinal epithelial cells. Pancreatic lipase hydrolyzes triglycerides to 2-monoglyceride and fatty acid. Pancreatic lipase is secreted in an active form. Colipase is also secreted by the pancreas and binds to lipase, changing its molecular configuration and increasing its activity. Phospholipase A2 is secreted by the pancreas as a proenzyme which becomes activated by trypsin. Phospholipase A2 hydrolyzes phospholipids, and as with all lipases, requires bile salts for its action. Carboxylic ester hydrolase and cholesterol esterase hydrolyze neutral lipid substrates like esters of cholesterol, fat-soluble vitamins, and triglycerides. The hydrolyzed fat is then packaged into micelles for transport into the intestinal epithelial cells, where the fatty acids are reassembled and packaged inside chylomicrons for transport through the lymphatic system into the bloodstream (Table 32-1).

The centroacinar and intercalated duct cells secrete the water and electrolytes present in the pancreatic juice. About 40 acinar cells are arranged into a spherical unit called an *acinus*. Centroacinar cells are located near the center of the acinus and are responsible for fluid and electrolyte secretion. These cells contain the enzyme carbonic anhydrase, which is needed for bicarbonate secretion. The amount of bicarbonate secreted varies with the pancreatic secretory rate, with greater concentrations of bicarbonate being secreted as the pancreatic secretory rate increases. Chloride secretion varies inversely with bicarbonate secretion such that the sum of these two remains constant. In contrast, sodium and potassium concentrations are kept constant throughout the spectrum of secretory rates[3] (Fig. 32-9). The hormone secretin is released from cells in the duodenal mucosa in response to acidic chyme passing through the pylorus into the duodenum. Secretin is the major stimulant for bicarbonate secretion,

Table 32-1
Pancreatic Enzymes

Enzyme	Substrate	Product
Carbohydrate		
Amylase (active)	Starch; glycogen	Glucose, maltose, maltotriose, dextrins
Protein		
Endopeptidases	Cleave bonds between amino acids	Amino acids, dipeptides
Trypsinogen (inactive) $\xrightarrow{\text{Enterokinase}}$ Trypsin (active)		
Chymotrypsinosin (inactive) $\xrightarrow{\text{Enterokinase}}$ Chymotrypsin (active)		
Proelastase (inactive) $\xrightarrow{\text{Enterokinase}}$ Elastase (active)		
Exopeptidases	Cleave amino acids from end of peptide chains	
Procarboxy peptidase A&B (inactive) $\xrightarrow{\text{Enterokinase}}$ Carboxypeptidase A&B (active)		
Fat		
Pancreatic lipase (active)	Triglycerides	2-Monoglycerides fatty acids
Phospholipase A_2 (inactive) $\xrightarrow{\text{Trypsin}}$ Phospholipase A_2 (active)	Phospholipase	
Cholesterol esterase	Neutral lipids	

which buffers the acidic fluid entering the duodenum from the stomach. CCK also stimulates bicarbonate secretion, but to a much lesser extent than secretin. CCK potentiates secretin-stimulated bicarbonate secretion. Gastrin and acetylcholine, both stimulants of gastric acid secretion, are also weak stimulants of pancreatic bicarbonate secretion.[4] Truncal vagotomy produces a myriad of complex effects on the downstream digestive tract, but the sum effect on the exocrine pancreas is a reduction in bicarbonate and fluid secretion.[5] The endocrine pancreas also influences the adjacent exocrine pancreatic secretions. Somatostatin, pancreatic polypeptide, and glucagon are all thought to inhibit exocrine secretion.

The acinar cells release pancreatic enzymes from their zymogen granules into the lumen of the acinus, and these proteins combine with the water and bicarbonate secretions of the centroacinar cells. The pancreatic juice then travels into small intercalated ducts.

Several small intercalated ducts join to form an interlobular duct. Cells in the interlobular ducts continue to contribute fluid and electrolytes to adjust the final concentrations of the pancreatic fluid. Interlobular ducts then join to form about 20 secondary ducts that empty into the main pancreatic duct. Destruction of the branching ductal tree from recurrent inflammation, scarring, and deposition of stones eventually contributes to destruction of the exocrine pancreas and exocrine pancreatic insufficiency. Although most pancreatic cancers are ductal adenocarcinomas and acinar cell tumors are rare, some studies implicate transdifferentiated acinar cells as the cells of origin. Other scientists are convinced that pancreatic cancer arises more frequently from cells adjacent to the islets, most probably reserve stem cells.[6] These cells are thought to be progenitor cells that can differentiate into endocrine or exocrine cells. The genetic mechanisms and signals involved in the normal differentiation process and abnormal transformation into pancreatic cancer cells is a major focus of current investigation.

Endocrine Pancreas

There are nearly one million islets of Langerhans in the normal adult pancreas. They vary greatly in size from 40 to 900 μm. Larger islets are located closer to the major arterioles and smaller islets are embedded more deeply in the parenchyma of the pancreas. Most islets contain 3000 to 4000 cells of four major types: alpha cells which secrete glucagon, beta cells which secrete insulin, delta cells which secrete somatostatin, and PP cells which secrete pancreatic polypeptide (Table 32-2).

Insulin is the best-studied pancreatic hormone. The discovery of insulin in 1920 by Frederick Banting, an orthopedic surgeon, and Charles Best, a medical student, was recognized with the awarding of the Nobel Prize in Physiology or Medicine. They produced diabetes in dogs by performing total pancreatectomy and then treated them with crude pancreatic extracts from dog and calf pancreata using techniques to prevent the breakdown of insulin by the proteolytic enzymes of the exocrine pancreas. Insulin was subsequently purified and found to be a 56-amino acid peptide with two chains, an alpha and a beta chain, joined by two disulfide bridges and a connecting peptide, or C-peptide. Proinsulin is made in the endoplasmic reticulum and then is transported to the Golgi complex, where it is packaged into granules and the C-peptide is cleaved off. There are

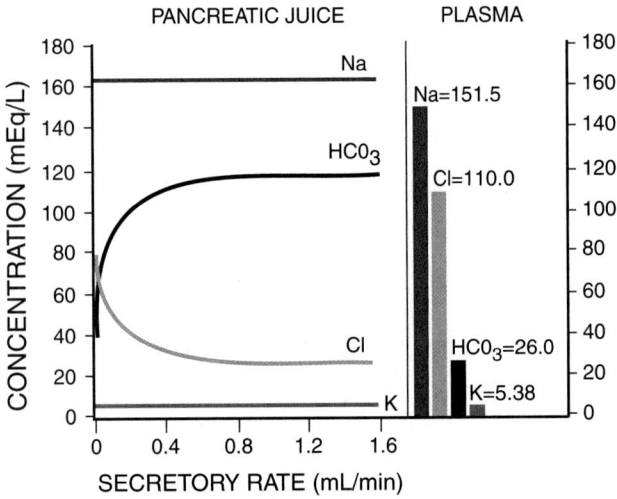

FIG. 32-9. Composition of pancreatic exocrine secretions. Greater concentrations of bicarbonate are secreted at higher secretory rates, and chloride secretion varies inversely with bicarbonate secretion. In contrast, sodium and potassium concentrations are independent of the secretory rate. (*Reproduced with permission from Davenport.[3]*)

Table 32-2
Pancreatic Islet Peptide Products

Hormones	Islet Cell	Functions
Insulin	β (beta cell)	Decreased gluconeogenesis, glycogenolysis, fatty acid breakdown and ketogenesis
		Increased glycogenesis, protein synthesis
Glucagon	α (alpha cell)	Opposite effects of insulin; increased hepatic glycogenolysis and gluconeogenesis
Somatostatin	δ (delta cell)	Inhibits gastrointestinal secretion
		Inhibits secretion and action of all gastrointestinal endocrine peptides
		Inhibits cell growth
Pancreatic polypeptide	PP (PP cell)	Inhibits pancreatic exocrine secretion and section of insulin
		Facilitates hepatic effect of insulin
Amylin (IAPP)	β (beta cell)	Counterregulates insulin secretion and function
Pancreastatin	β (beta cell)	Decreases insulin and somatostatin release
		Increases glucagon release
		Decreases pancreatic exocrine secretion

IAPP = islet amyloid polypeptide.

two phases of insulin secretion. In the first phase, stored insulin is released. This phase lasts about 5 minutes after a glucose challenge. The second phase of insulin secretion is a longer, sustained release due to ongoing production of new insulin. Beta cell synthesis of insulin is regulated by plasma glucose levels, neural signals, and the paracrine influence of other islet cells. The diagnosis of diabetes is made by using glucose tolerance tests. Oral glucose tolerance tests (OGTTs) and intravenous glucose tolerance tests (IVGTTs) are commonly used. Oral glucose not only enters the bloodstream, but also stimulates the release of enteric hormones such as gastric inhibitory peptide (GIP), glucagon-like peptide-1 (GLP-1), and CCK, that augment the secretion of insulin, and are therefore referred to as *incretins*. Therefore oral glucose is a more vigorous stimulus to insulin secretion than intravenous glucose. In the OGTT, the patient is fasted overnight and a basal glucose value is determined. Forty g/m^2 of glucose is given orally over 10 minutes. Blood samples are taken every 30 minutes for 2 hours. Normal values and criteria for diabetes vary by age, but essentially all values should be less than 200 mg/dL, and the 120-minute value should be less than 140 mg/dL.

Insulin secretion by the beta cell is also influenced by plasma levels of amino acids such as arginine, lysine, leucine, and free fatty acids. Glucagon, GIP, GLP-1, and CCK stimulate insulin release, while somatostatin, amylin, and pancreastatin inhibit insulin release.[7] Cholinergic fibers and beta sympathetic fibers stimulate insulin release, while alpha sympathetic fibers inhibit insulin secretion.

Insulin's function is to inhibit endogenous (hepatic) glucose production and to facilitate glucose transport into cells, thus lowering plasma glucose levels. Insulin also inhibits glycogenolysis, fatty acid breakdown and ketone formation, and stimulates protein synthesis. There is a considerable amount of functional reserve in insulin secretory capacity. If the remaining portion of the pancreas is healthy, about 80% of the pancreas can be resected without the patient becoming diabetic.[8] In patients with chronic pancreatitis, or other conditions in which much of the gland is diseased, resection of a smaller fraction of the pancreas can result in diabetes. Insulin receptors are dimeric, tyrosine kinase–containing transmembrane proteins that are located on all cells. Insulin deficiency (type I diabetes) results in an overexpression or upregulation of insulin receptors, which causes an enhanced sensitivity to insulin. Type II diabetes is associated with a downregulation of insulin receptors and

relative hyperinsulinemia, with resulting insulin resistance. Some forms of diabetes are associated with selected impairments of hepatic or peripheral insulin receptors, such as pancreatogenic diabetes or maturity-onset diabetes of the young (MODY).

Glucagon is a 29-amino-acid, single-chain peptide that promotes hepatic glycogenolysis and gluconeogenesis and counteracts the effects of insulin through its hyperglycemic action. Glucose is the primary regulator of glucagon secretion, as it is with insulin, but it has an inhibitory rather than stimulatory effect. Glucagon release is stimulated by the amino acids arginine and alanine. Gastric inhibitory peptide stimulates glucagon secretion at least in vitro, and GLP-1 inhibits glucagon secretion in vivo. Insulin and somatostatin inhibit glucagon secretion in a paracrine fashion within the islet. The same neural impulses that regulate insulin secretion also regulate glucagon secretion, so that the two hormones work together in a balance of actions to maintain glucose levels. Cholinergic and beta sympathetic fibers stimulate glucagon release, while alpha sympathetic fibers inhibit glucagon release.[9]

Although originally isolated from the hypothalamus, somatostatin is a peptide that is now known to have a wide anatomic distribution, not only in neurons but also in the pancreas, gut, and other tissues. It is a highly conserved peptide hormone, as it is found in lower vertebrates, and is now realized to be of fundamental importance in regulatory processes throughout the body. One gene encodes for a common precursor that is differentially processed to generate tissue-specific amounts of two bioactive products, somatostatin-14 and somatostatin-28. These peptides inhibit endocrine and exocrine secretion and affect neurotransmission, gastrointestinal and biliary motility, intestinal absorption, vascular tone and cell proliferation.

Five different somatostatin receptors have recently been cloned and the biologic properties of each are only now beginning to be unraveled.[10] All five are G-protein-coupled receptors with seven highly-conserved transmembrane domains and unique amino and carboxy termini. Phosphorylation sites located within the second and third intracellular loops and in the cytoplasmic C-terminal segment are thought to mediate receptor regulation. Although the naturally occurring peptides bind to all five receptors, somatostatin-28 is relatively selective for somatostatin receptor 5 (SSTR5). The hexapeptide and octapeptide analogs such as octreotide bind only to SSTR2, SSTR3, and SSTR5. These analogs have a longer serum half-life, and their potent inhibitory effect has been used clinically to treat both endocrine and exocrine disorders. For example, octreotide has been shown to decrease fistula output and speed the time it takes for enteric and pancreatic fistulas to close.[11]

Endocrine release of somatostatin occurs during a meal. The major stimulant is probably intraluminal fat. Acidification of the gastric and duodenal mucosa also releases somatostatin in isolated perfused organ preparations. Acetylcholine from the cholinergic neurons inhibits somatostatin release.

Current studies seek to determine whether each somatostatin receptor subtype is associated with one or more different G-proteins, and whether each subtype is coupled to multiple signaling pathways. Although these signal transduction pathways are just beginning to be understood, it is clear that individual somatostatin receptor subtypes are linked to multiple transmembrane effectors. What remains to be determined is which of these signaling mechanisms are important in different cell types for the various functions of somatostatin. It also appears that somatostatin receptors are dynamically regulated at the membrane in a time-dependent manner by ligand-dependent and -independent mechanisms.

Pancreatic polypeptide (PP) is a 36-amino-acid, straight-chain peptide discovered by Kimmel in 1968 during the process of insulin purification. Protein is the most potent enteral stimulator of PP release, closely followed by fat, whereas glucose has a weaker effect.[12,13] Hypoglycemia, whether or not it is insulin induced, strongly stimulates PP secretion through cholinergic stimulation.[14] Phenylalanine, tryptophan, and fatty acids in the duodenum stimulate PP release, probably by inducing CCK and secretin release. In the isolated perfused pancreas, insulin and GIP stimulate PP release, while glucagon and somatostatin inhibit it. Vagal stimulation of the pancreas is the most important regulator of PP secretion. In fact, vagotomy eliminates the rise in PP levels usually seen after a meal. This can be used as a test for the completeness of a surgical vagotomy, or for the presence of diabetic autonomic neuropathy.

PP is known to inhibit bile secretion, gallbladder contraction, and secretion by the exocrine pancreas. A number of studies suggest that PP's most important role is in glucose regulation through its regulation of hepatic insulin receptor gene expression. Deficiencies in PP secretion due to proximal pancreatectomy or severe chronic pancreatitis, are associated with diminished hepatic insulin sensitivity due to reduced hepatic insulin receptors.[15] These effects are reversed by PP administration.

In addition to the four main peptides secreted by the pancreas, there are a number of other peptide products of the islet cells, including amylin and pancreastatin, as well as neuropeptides such as VIP, galanin, and serotonin. Amylin or islet amyloid polypeptide (IAPP) is a 37-amino-acid polypeptide that was discovered in 1988. IAPP is predominantly expressed by the pancreatic beta cells, where it is stored along with insulin in secretory granules.[16] The function of IAPP seems to be the modulation or counterregulation of insulin secretion and function. Pancreastatin is a recently discovered pancreatic islet peptide product that inhibits insulin, and possibly somatostatin release, and augments glucagon release.[17,18] In addition to this effect on the endocrine pancreas, pancreastatin inhibits pancreatic exocrine secretion.[19]

INTRAISLET REGULATION

The beta cells are located in the central portion of each islet and make up about 70% of the total islet cell mass. The other cell types are located predominantly in the periphery. The delta cells are least plentiful, making up only 5%; the alpha cells make up 10%, and the PP cells make up 15%.[20] In contrast to the acinar cells that secrete the full gamut of exocrine enzymes, the islet cells seem to specialize in the secretion of predominantly one hormone. However, individual islets can secrete multiple hormones. For example, the beta cells secrete both insulin and amylin, which counterregulates the actions of insulin. In reality more than 20 different hormones are secreted by the islets, and the exact functions of this milieu are just beginning to be unraveled. There is diversity among the islets depending on their location within the pancreas. In general, islets located closer to major arterioles are larger than islets located more deeply in the parenchyma of the pancreas. The beta and delta cells are evenly distributed throughout the pancreas, but islets in the head and uncinate process (ventral anlage) have a higher percentage of PP cells and fewer alpha cells, whereas islets in the body and tail (dorsal anlage) contain the majority of alpha cells and few PP cells. This is clinically significant because pancreatoduodenectomy removes 95% of the PP cells in the pancreas. This may partially explain the higher incidence of glucose intolerance after the Whipple procedure than after distal pancreatectomy. In addition, chronic pancreatitis, which disproportionately affects the pancreatic head, is associated with PP deficiency and pancreatogenic diabetes.[21]

Control of islet secretion is complex and involves an interplay of neural signals, blood flow patterns, and autocrine, paracrine, and hormonal feedback loops. Although the pancreatic islets account for only 2% of the pancreatic mass, they receive about 20 to 30% of the pancreatic arteriolar flow. The manner in which the blood flows through an individual islet can affect islet function since the beta cells are located in the center and the other islet cells are located mostly in the periphery. Blood can flow into the center of the islet and then to the periphery, from the periphery to the center, or from one pole of the islet to the other. In rodents, in vivo microscopy has demonstrated blood flow from one pole to the other. In addition, sphincters at the feeding arteriole were observed regulating blood flow to the periphery or center of the islet as it passed from pole to pole. The sphincters are actually bulging endothelial cells of the afferent capillary. These sphincters seemed to be regulated by blood glucose concentrations, neural impulses, and nitric oxide. The predominant pattern of blood flow through the islets in the human pancreas is still conjectural. However, the peptide products of individual islet cells affect neighboring islet cells in a paracrine fashion. Recent experiments using isolated perfused pancreas and monoclonal antibodies to specific islet peptides have demonstrated that somatostatin from the delta cells inhibits insulin secretion from the beta cells, glucagon secretion from the alpha cells, and pancreatic polypeptide secretion from the PP cells. Somatostatin may have an important role in intraislet control of islet cell secretions[22] (Fig. 32-10). Islet hormone secretion is also regulated by endocrine feedback mechanisms. Insulin secretion, for example, is exquisitely sensitive to small increments in the arterial insulin concentration.

Although most of the blood supply to the exocrine pancreas comes directly from the pancreatic arterial flow, blood draining from the islet capillaries goes on to perfuse the exocrine pancreas. Perfusion of the acinar cells with venous blood from the islets allows the endocrine pancreas to influence the exocrine pancreas. For example, insulin release, stimulated by high levels of carbohydrates in the ingested meal is thought to promote an amylase-rich exocrine secretion which preferentially provides for digestion of starches and sugars.

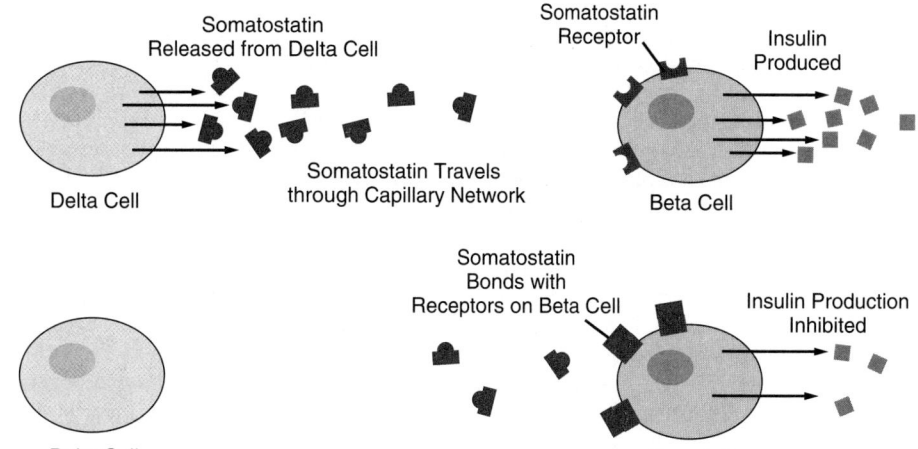

FIG. 32-10. Delta to beta cell axis. Somatostatin from the delta cells may play an important role in intraislet paracrine control of insulin secretion from the beta cells.

ACUTE PANCREATITIS

Definition and Incidence

Acute pancreatitis is an inflammatory disease of the pancreas that is associated with little or no fibrosis of the gland. It can be initiated by several factors including gallstones, alcohol, trauma, and infections, and in some cases it is hereditary. Very often patients with acute pancreatitis develop additional complications such as sepsis, shock, and respiratory and renal failure, resulting in considerable morbidity and mortality. Approximately 300,000 cases occur in the United States each year, 10 to 20% of which are severe, leading to over 3000 deaths. Pancreatitis is a contributing factor in an additional 4000 deaths annually and inflicts a heavy economic burden accounting for more than $2 billion in health costs annually in the U.S.[23] Despite the considerable amount of research underway relating to this disease, its pathophysiologic mechanisms remain incompletely understood. This can be attributed in part to the relative inaccessibility of clinical material for experimental studies, which has led to the development of several models of experimental pancreatitis with which its etiology, pathophysiology, and treatment regimens are being explored.

Etiolology

The etiology of acute pancreatitis is a complex subject because many different factors have been implicated in the causation of this disease, and sometimes there are no identifiable causes (Table 32-3). Two factors, biliary tract stone disease and alcoholism, account for 80 to 90 percent of the cases. The remaining 10 to 20 percent is accounted for either by idiopathic disease or by a variety of miscellaneous causes including trauma, surgery, drugs, heredity, infection and toxins.

Biliary Tract Disease

Although acute pancreatitis is documented in association with acalculous biliary tract disease, bile duct stones (choledocholithiasis) represent the most common form of associated biliary abnormality. The mechanism by which a gallstone may cause pancreatitis is not entirely clear, although gallstones have been implicated ever since Opie made the seminal observation in 1901 of two patients who died of acute pancreatitis with stones impacted in their ampulla of Vater.[24] This led him to propose the "common-channel hypothesis," in which a blockage below the junction of the biliary and pancreatic

ducts would cause bile to flow into the pancreas, which could then be damaged by the detergent action of bile salts.

Important objections to this theory include the anatomic reality that the majority of individuals have such a short common channel that a stone located there would block both the pancreatic and biliary ducts, effectively isolating the two systems. Furthermore, hydrostatic pressure in the biliary tract is lower than in the pancreas, a condition that would favor abnormal flow of pancreatic juice into the bile duct rather than in the opposite direction. These reservations are bolstered by the observation that in experimental animals the flow of normal bile through an unobstructed pancreatic duct does not result in acute pancreatitis (although *forceful* retrograde injection of bile into the pancreas causes injury similar to that of acute pancreatitis).

Another proposed mechanism of causation postulates that passage of a gallstone through the sphincter of Oddi renders it momentarily incompetent, permitting the reflux of duodenal juice containing activated digestive enzymes into the pancreatic ductal system. However, it is questionable whether the transit time through the

Table 32-3
Etiologies of Acute Pancreatitis

Alcohol
Biliary tract disease
Hyperlipidemia
Hereditary
Hypercalcemia
Trauma
   External
   Surgical
   Endoscopic retrograde cholangiopancreatography
Ischemia
   Hypoperfusion
   Atheroembolic
   Vasculitis
Pancreatic duct obstruction
   Neoplasms
   Pancreas divisum
   Ampullary and duodenal lesions
Infections
Venom
Drugs
Idiopathic

SOURCE: Reproduced with permission from Yeo CJ, Cameron JL: Exocrine pancreas, in Townsend CM et al (eds): *Sabiston's Textbook of Surgery.* New York: Lippincott Raven, 2000, p 1112.

sphincter of Oddi is long enough to cause sufficient incompetence. Finally, the observation remains that procedures designed to render the sphincter incompetent, such as sphincterotomy, do not routinely cause pancreatitis.

Therefore, although it is reasonable to dismiss an incompetent sphincter of Oddi as an etiologic factor in acute pancreatitis, it is not as simple to dismiss the role of gallstones. A clinical study showed that 88% of patients with acute pancreatitis passed gallstones in their feces within 10 days of the attack. This is in contrast to only 11% of gallstone patients who did not have pancreatitis, suggesting that the process of passing a gallstone may be linked to the development of acute pancreatitis.

This information justifies searching for a more likely causative factor than abnormal bile or duodenal juice backflow into the pancreas. A common phenomenon shared by gallstone disease and other conditions causing acute pancreatitis, such as helminthic infestation of the pancreatic duct or its blockage by tumors, is ductal hypertension resulting from ongoing exocrine secretion into an obstructed pancreatic duct. A simple mechanical explanation has been proposed whereby elevated intraductal pressure causes rupture of the smaller ductules and leakage of pancreatic juice into the parenchyma. Although the pancreatic duct fluid pH is maintained in the range of 8 to 9 by the secretion of bicarbonate, the interstitial pH of 7 within the pancreatic tissue favors activation of proteases when transductal extravasation of fluid occurs. While pancreatic ductal obstruction and hypertension are likely initiating factors in the etiology of acute pancreatitis, the mechanism by which ductal hypertension initiates pancreatic injury remains under investigation.[25] Although the mechanical factors which initiate the process are unclear, the *colocalization theory* of Steer and Saluja has gained acceptance as the cellular mechanism of acute pancreatitis.[26] In the normal pancreas, the inactive digestive zymogens and the lysosomal hydrolases are found separately in discrete organelles. However, in response to ductal obstruction, hypersecretion, or a cellular insult, these two classes of substances become improperly colocalized in a vacuolar structure within the pancreatic acinar cell. A cascade has been postulated in which trypsinogen colocalizes with cathepsin B to produce activated trypsin, which in turn activates the other digestive zymogens. These active digestive enzymes then begin autodigestion within the pancreatic acinar cells, leading to pancreatitis.

Alcohol

Although some patients show the symptoms of acute pancreatitis after little use or even a single exposure to alcohol, the disease commonly occurs in patients who have consumed alcohol for at least 2 years, and often much longer, up to 10 years. In a patient with an exposure history to ethanol and the total absence of other possible causative factors, a first attack of pancreatitis is considered alcohol-related acute pancreatitis. However, it is possible that a first attack of alcohol-related pancreatitis in the typical longstanding alcohol user is really the first manifestation of chronic pancreatitis. The disease can become recurrent with continued alcohol abuse. The nature of alcohol consumed (i.e., beer, wine, or hard liquor) is less significant than a daily intake of between 100 and 150 g of ethanol. Between 10 and 15% of individuals with this degree of alcohol intake go on to develop pancreatitis, while a similar proportion develop cirrhosis of the liver.

Ethanol can induce pancreatitis by several methods. The "secretion with blockage" mechanism is possible because ethanol causes spasm of the sphincter of Oddi, and more importantly, ethanol is a metabolic toxin to pancreatic acinar cells, where it can interfere with enzyme synthesis and secretion. The initial effect of ethanol is a brief secretory increase followed by inhibition. This can lead to elevation of enzyme proteins that can precipitate within the pancreatic duct. Calcium then can precipitate within this protein matrix, causing multiple ductal obstructions, while continued secretion can cause pressure buildup. Ethanol also increases ductal permeability, making it possible for improperly-activated enzymes to leak out of the pancreatic duct into the surrounding tissue. The inappropriate activation of trypsin by ethanol has been demonstrated in vitro. Ethanol also transiently decreases pancreatic blood flow, possibly causing focal ischemic injury to the gland.[27,28]

There is evidence that alcoholics who develop pancreatitis have a diet richer in protein and fat than those who do not. Ethanol can alter lipid metabolism and a transient hyperlipidemic state is sometimes seen during an attack of alcoholic pancreatitis, although the etiologic significance of this observation remains uncertain.

Tumors

A tumor should be considered in a nonalcoholic patient with acute pancreatitis who has no demonstrable biliary tract disease. Approximately 1 to 2% of patients with acute pancreatitis have pancreatic carcinoma, and an episode of acute pancreatitis can be the first clinical manifestation of a periampullary tumor. In both conditions, the pancreatitis possibly results from blockage of secreted juice and its upstream consequences.

Iatrogenic Pancreatitis

Acute pancreatitis can be associated with a number of surgical procedures, most commonly those performed on or close to the pancreas, such as pancreatic biopsy, biliary duct exploration, distal gastrectomy, and splenectomy. Acute pancreatitis is associated postoperatively with Billroth II gastrectomy and jejunostomy, in which increased intraduodenal pressure can cause backflow of activated enzymes into the pancreas. However, pancreatitis also can occur in association with surgery that employs low systemic perfusion, such as cardiopulmonary bypass and cardiac transplantation. Acute pancreatitis has been reported to be associated with severe hypothermia, and the hypothermia associated with cardiopulmonary bypass may be similarly causative. It also is possible that atheromatous emboli or ischemia may cause pancreatic injury. Most commonly, endoscopic retrograde cholangiopancreatography results in pancreatitis in 2 to 10% of patients, due to direct injury and/or intraductal hypertension.

Drugs

For practical reasons, it often is difficult to implicate a drug as the cause of pancreatitis. Many drugs can produce hyperamylasemia and/or abdominal pain, and a drug is considered suspect if the pancreatitis-like illness resolves with its discontinuation. Ethical considerations generally rule out rechallenge with the suspect drug, so the connection often remains vague. However, despite these limitations, certain drugs are known to be capable of causing acute pancreatitis. These include the thiazide diuretics, furosemide, estrogens, azathioprine, L-asparaginase, 6-mercaptopurine, methyldopa, the sulfonamides, tetracycline, pentamidine, procainamide, nitrofurantoin, dideoxyinosine, valproic acid, and acetylcholinesterase inhibitors.

Infections

Though mumps, coxsackievirus, and *Mycoplasma pneumoniae* are believed to be capable of inducing acute pancreatitis by infecting the acinar cells, none of these agents has been isolated from a diseased pancreas. The belief may have arisen from the observation that antibody titers to mumps and coxsackievirus are elevated in approximately 30% of patients with acute pancreatitis with no other identified cause. However, this elevation may be an anamnestic or nonspecific response to pancreatitis.

Hyperlipidemia

It has been suggested that lipase can liberate large amounts of toxic fatty acids into the pancreatic microcirculation. This could lead to endothelial injury, sludging of blood cells, and consequent ischemic states. Patients with types I and V hyperlipoproteinemia often experience attacks of abdominal pain that are thought to indicate episodes of acute pancreatitis. These episodes are frequently associated with marked hypertriglyceridemia and lactescent serum, and can be prevented by dietary modifications that restrict serum triglycerides.

Miscellaneous Causes

An episode of acute pancreatitis may be precipitated by several other factors. Hypercalcemic states arising from hyperparathyroidism can result in both acute and chronic pancreatitis; the mechanism most likely involves hypersecretion and the formation of calcified stones intraductally. Also implicated are infestations by *Ascaris lumbricoides* and the liver fluke *Clonorchis sinensis,* which is endemic to China, Japan, and Southeast Asia. These cause Oriental cholangitis, which is associated with cholangiocarcinoma obstructing the pancreatic duct. A dominant gene mutation following Mendelian inheritance is known to result in hereditary pancreatitis.[29] Recently Whitcomb and associates described several families from various parts of the world who have mutations in their cationic trypsinogen gene *PRSS1*, which results in pancreatitis.[30] Additionally, 20 to 45% of patients with pancreas divisum (unfused ducts of Wirsung and Santorini) develop pancreatitis, but the failure of procedures to improve drainage of the lesser papilla in reducing attacks of pancreatitis, as well as the observed lack of ductal dilatation in such patients, argues against pancreas divisum as an etiologic factor, rendering the role of this condition as yet unclear. Other implicated factors include azotemia, vasculitis, and the sting of the Trinidadian scorpion *Tityus trinitatis.* This scorpion's venom has been shown to cause neurotransmitter discharge from cholinergic nerve terminals, leading to massive production of pancreatic juice. Poisoning with antiacetylcholinesterase insecticides has a similar effect. Finally, no apparent cause can be ascribed to some episodes of acute pancreatitis, and these constitute the group referred to as "idiopathic pancreatitis." Some of these patients are eventually found to have gallstone-related pancreatitis, which calls for caution in labeling any episode "idiopathic."

Pathophysiology

Acute pancreatitis occurs in varying degrees of severity, the determinants of which are multifactorial. The generally prevalent belief today is that pancreatitis begins with the activation of digestive zymogens inside acinar cells which cause acinar cell injury. Recent

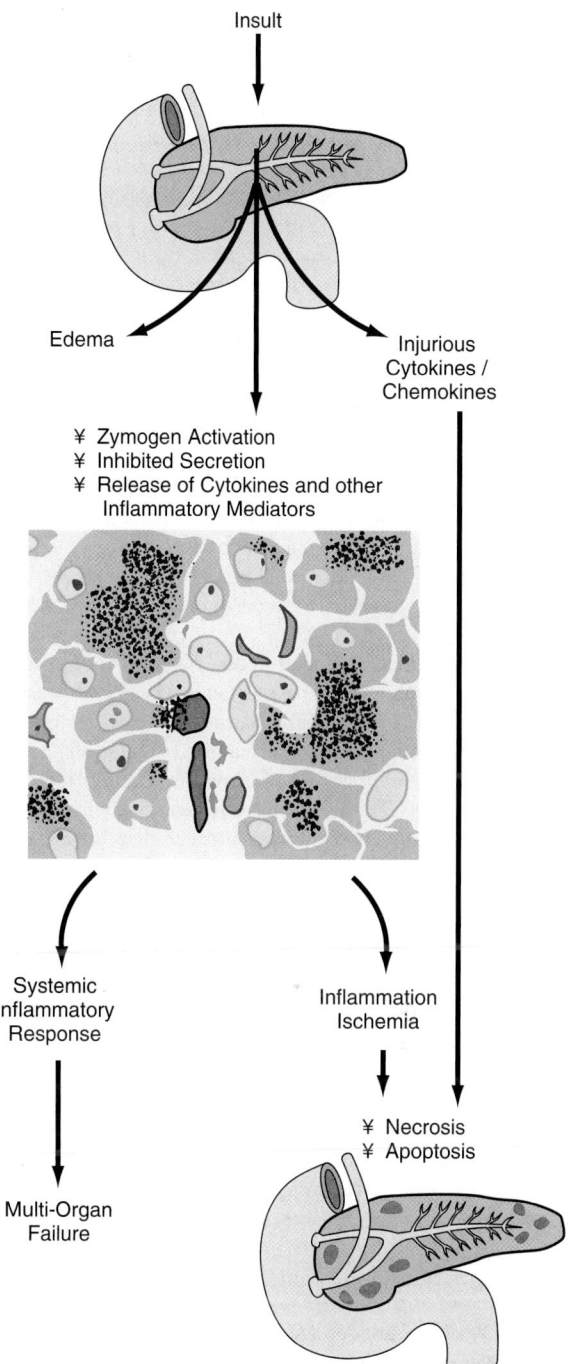

FIG. 32-11. Pathophysiology of acute pancreatitis.

studies suggest that the ultimate severity of the resulting pancreatitis may be determined by the events that occur subsequent to acinar cell injury.[31] These include inflammatory cell recruitment and activation, as well as generation and release of cytokines and other chemical mediators of inflammation (Fig. 32-11).

Initial Events Leading to the Onset of Pancreatitis

Under physiologic conditions, the pancreas synthesizes a large amount of protein. A majority of these proteins consist of digestive enzymes. Because the exocrine pancreas produces several enzymes that are potentially injurious to itself, it prevents autodigestion by intracellularly assembling the inactive precursors of these enzymes, called proenzymes or zymogens, which are then transported and secreted outside of the gland. Their activation occurs safely in the duodenum, where the brush-border enzyme enteropeptidase (or enterokinase) activates the trypsinogen, and the resulting trypsin then activates the other zymogens in a cascade reaction.

To further protect the pancreas from these potentially harmful digestive enzymes, they are segregated from the cytoplasmic space within acinar cells by being enclosed within membrane-bound organelles referred to as zymogen granules. Another layer of protection is provided by the synthesis of trypsin inhibitors, which are transported and stored along with the digestive enzyme zymogens. These are available to inhibit small amounts of prematurely-activated trypsinogen within pancreatic acinar cells. It is generally theorized that acute pancreatitis occurs when this process goes awry and the gland is injured by the erroneously-activated enzymes that it produces. There are three reasons for this theory: (1) the pancreas is digestible by the activated enzymes of the duodenum; (2) activated digestive enzymes are found within the pancreas during pancreatitis, and (3) the histology of pancreatitis is suggestive of a coagulative necrosis. However, the mechanism(s) of erroneous activation are not fully understood.

Using several different models, recent research has focused intensively on the etiology of the activation mechanism. It was seen that the synthesis and intracellular transport of digestive enzymes are not affected during the development of pancreatitis, but that the secretory output of enzymes of the pancreas is markedly reduced.[32] Very early in the development of the disease (shortly after the onset, but before morphologic or biochemical changes are apparent), digestive enzymes are localized in cytoplasmic vacuoles that also contain the lysosomal hydrolase cathepsin B, which is known to activate trypsinogen. Furthermore, intracellular trypsinogen activation was found synchronously with the colocalization phenomenon. Further support for this hypothesis is provided by recent findings that inhibition of cathepsin B activity by the highly specific inhibitor, CA-074me, protects against intra-acinar cell trypsinogen activation and pancreatitis in two different models of experimental pancreatitis.[33] These studies strongly suggest that trypsinogen is activated because it erroneously colocalizes in cytoplasmic vacuoles with cathepsin B. The opportunity is therefore created for autodigestion because when released into the cytoplasm, activated trypsin can cause injury, and can activate other proteases as well.

Factors Determining the Severity of Pancreatitis

Clinically, the severity of acute pancreatitis varies significantly. Some patients experience a mild form of the disease which is self-limiting, while others suffer a more severe and sometimes lethal attack. The factors determining the severity of pancreatitis are multifactorial, but their identification is of considerable therapeutic importance, since their manipulation may decrease the morbidity and mortality associated with the disease. It generally is believed that pancreatitis begins with the intrapancreatic activation of digestive enzyme zymogens, acinar cell injury, and activation of transcription factors such as nuclear factor-κB (NF-κB) and AP-1. This in turn leads to the production of proinflammatory factors, acinar cell necrosis, systemic inflammatory response syndrome, and distant organ dysfunction including lung injury that frequently manifests as the acute respiratory distress syndrome (ARDS). The ultimate severity of acute pancreatitis depends on the extent of the systemic inflammatory response, as well as several cytokines and chemokines

and their receptors that play a critical role in the activation and migration of inflammatory cells to the affected site.

In addition to the cells of the immune system such as the neutrophils, the pancreatic acinar cells are also a source of inflammatory mediators during pancreatitis. Over the past few years, the list of factors associated with pancreatitis and associated lung injury has grown rapidly to include tumor necrosis factor-α (TNF-α), monocyte chemotactic protein-1 (MCP-1), Mob1, interleukin-1β (IL-1β), platelet-activating factor (PAF), substance P, adhesion molecules (intercellular adhesion molecule-1 [ICAM-1] and selectins), interleukin-6 (IL-6), interleukin-8 (IL-8), interleukin-10 (IL-10), C5a, the CCR1 receptor and its ligands, granulocyte-macrophage colony-stimulating factor (GM-CSF), macrophage migration inhibitory factor (MIF), cyclooxygenase-2 (COX-2), prostaglandin E_1 (PGE$_1$), nitric oxide, and reactive oxygen species.[34] In addition, several recent studies have focused on the protective role played by heat shock proteins in pancreatitis.[35] The ultimate severity of pancreatitis and associated lung injury depends on the balance between the pro- and anti-inflammatory factors. Several therapeutic regimens aimed at reducing the inflammatory response have been tested and include anti–tumor necrosis factor-α antibody, interleukin-1 (IL-1) receptor antagonist, anti–ICAM-1 and anti-CD3 antibodies, interleukin-10 (IL-10), recombinant platelet activating factor acetylhydrolase (rPAF-AH), and the calcineurin antagonist FK506.

An alternate approach to prevent or reduce the severity of pancreatitis is to inhibit the two early events in pancreatitis, intrapancreatic trypsinogen and NF-κB activation. Agents that specifically prevent an increase in trypsin activity, either by inhibiting trypsinogen activation and colocalization (e.g., low doses of wortmannin, water immersion, and thermal stress), or inhibiting the cathepsin B activity (E64d or CA074me), have been successful in reducing the severity of pancreatitis in experimental rodent models. Prior thermal (and arsenite) stress and water immersion stress, which upregulate heat shock proteins 70 and 60, respectively, not only prevent cerulein-induced trypsinogen activation, but also inhibit cerulein-induced NF-κB activation in the pancreas and protect against pancreatitis.[36] These studies await verification in a clinical setting.

Diagnosis

The clinical diagnosis of pancreatitis is one of exclusion. The other upper abdominal conditions that can be confused with acute pancreatitis include perforated peptic ulcer, a gangrenous small bowel obstruction, and acute cholecystitis. Since these conditions often have a fatal outcome without surgery, urgent intervention is indicated in the small number of cases in which doubt persists.

All episodes of acute pancreatitis begin with severe pain, generally following a substantial meal. The pain is usually epigastric, but can occur anywhere in the abdomen or lower chest. It has been described as "knifing" or "boring through" to the back, and may be relieved by the patient leaning forward. It precedes the onset of nausea and vomiting, with retching often continuing after the stomach has emptied. Vomiting does not relieve the pain, which is more intense in necrotizing than in edematous pancreatitis. An episode of acute pancreatic inflammation in a patient with known chronic pancreatitis has the same findings.

On examination the patient may show tachycardia, tachypnea, hypotension, and hyperthermia. The temperature is usually only mildly elevated in uncomplicated pancreatitis. Voluntary and involuntary guarding can be seen over the epigastric region. The bowel sounds are decreased or absent. There are usually no palpable masses. The abdomen may be distended with intraperitoneal fluid. There may be pleural effusion, particularly on the left side.

With increasing severity of disease, the intravascular fluid loss may become life-threatening as a result of sequestration of edematous fluid in the retroperitoneum. Hemoconcentration then results in an elevated hematocrit. However, there also may be bleeding into the retroperitoneum or the peritoneal cavity. In some patients (about 1%), the blood from necrotizing pancreatitis may dissect through the soft tissues and manifest as a blueish discoloration around the umbilicus (Cullen's sign) or in the flanks (Grey Turner sign). The severe fluid loss may lead to prerenal azotemia with elevated blood urea nitrogen and creatinine levels. There also may be hyperglycemia, hypoalbuminemia, and hypocalcemia sufficient in some cases to produce tetany.

Serum Markers

Because pancreatic acinar cells synthesize, store, and secrete a large number of digestive enzymes (e.g., amylase, lipase, trypsinogen, and elastase), the levels of these enzymes are elevated in the serum of most pancreatitis patients. Because of the ease of measurement, serum amylase levels are measured most often. Serum amylase concentration increases almost immediately with the onset of disease and peaks within several hours. It remains elevated for 3 to 5 days before returning to normal. There is no significant correlation between the magnitude of serum amylase elevation and severity of pancreatitis; in fact, a milder form of acute pancreatitis is often associated with higher levels of serum amylase as compared with that in a more severe form of the disease.

It is important to note that hyperamylasemia can also occur as a result of conditions not involving pancreatitis. For example, hyperamylasemia can occur in a patient with small bowel obstruction, perforated duodenal ulcer, or other intra-abdominal inflammatory conditions. In contrast, a patient with acute pancreatitis may have a normal serum amylase level, which could be due to several reasons. In patients with hyperlipidemia, values might appear to be normal because of interference by lipids with chemical determination of serum amylase. In many cases, urinary clearance of pancreatic enzymes from the circulation increases during pancreatitis, therefore, urinary levels may be more sensitive than serum levels. For these reasons it is recommended that amylase concentrations also be mea-

sured in the urine. Urinary amylase levels usually remain elevated for several days after serum levels have returned to normal. In patients with severe pancreatitis associated with significant necrotic damage, the pancreas may not release large amounts of enzymes into the circulation. It is important to recognize that in patients with severe pancreatitis, frequent measurement of serum enzymes is not needed. Patients with alcoholic pancreatitis, in general, have a smaller increase in serum amylase levels.

Since hyperamylasemia can be observed in many extrapancreatic diseases, measuring pancreatic-specific amylase (p-amylase) rather than total amylase, which also includes salivary amylase (s-amylase), makes the diagnosis more specific (88 to 93%).

Other pancreatic enzymes also have been evaluated to improve the diagnostic accuracy of serum measurements. Specificity of these markers ranges from 77 to 96%, the highest being for lipase. Measurements of many digestive enzymes also have methodologic limitations and cannot be easily adapted for quantitation in emergency labs. Since serum levels of lipase remain elevated for a longer time than total or pancreatic amylase, it is the serum indicator of highest probability of the disease.

Ultrasound

Abdominal ultrasound examination is the best way to confirm the presence of gallstones in suspected biliary pancreatitis. It also can detect extrapancreatic ductal dilations and reveal pancreatic edema, swelling, and peripancreatic fluid collections (Fig. 32-12). However, in about 20% of patients, the ultrasound examination does not provide satisfactory results because of the presence of bowel gas, which may obscure sonographic imaging of the pancreas. A computed tomographic (CT) scan of the pancreas is more commonly used to diagnose pancreatitis (Fig. 32-13). CT scanning is used to distinguish milder (nonnecrotic) forms of the disease from more severe necrotizing or infected pancreatitis, in patients whose clinical presentation raises the suspicion of advanced disease.[37]

Assessment of Severity

An early discrimination between mild edematous and severe necrotizing forms of the disease is of the utmost importance in order

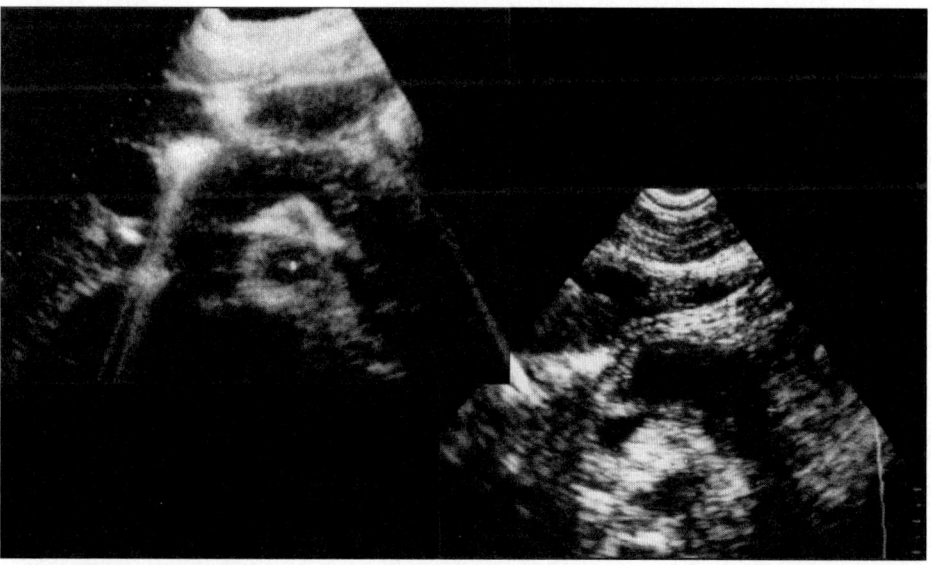

FIG. 32-12. *Ultrasound image of normal pancreas (left) and acute pancreatitis (right). Evidence of parenchymal edema and peripancreatic fluid accumulation is seen. (Courtesy of American Gastroenterological Association.)*

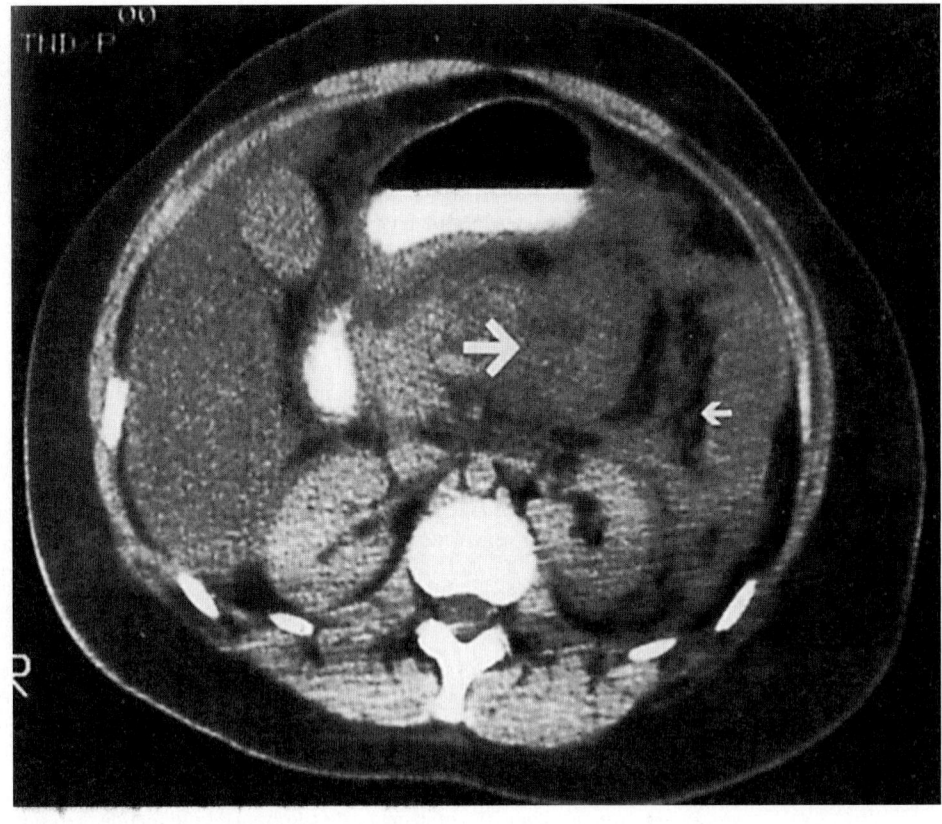

FIG. 32-13. Nonnecrotizing acute pancreatitis. The CT image reveals edema (swelling), but intact vascularization of the pancreas overall.

to provide optimal care to the patient. Several predictors of severity including early prognostic signs, serum markers, and CT scans are commonly used for this purpose.[38]

Early Prognostic Signs. In 1974, Ranson identified a series of prognostic signs for early identification of patients with severe pancreatitis.[39] Out of these 11 objective parameters, five are measured at the time of admission, whereas the remaining six are measured within 48 hours of admission (Table 32-4). Morbidity and mortality of the disease are directly related to the number of signs present. If the number of positive Ranson signs is less than two, the

mortality is generally zero; with three to five positive signs, mortality is increased to 10 to 20%. The mortality rate increases to more than 50% when there are more than seven positive Ranson signs. Although prognostic signs are useful in determining the severity of pancreatitis, there are several limitations to the value of these signs. One has to measure all 11 signs to achieve the best predictability of prognosis, and two full days are needed to complete the profile. A delay of 48 hours after admission merely for assessment may squander a valuable opportunity to prevent a complication during this time. It is important to realize that Ranson's prognostic signs are best used within the initial 48 hours of hospitalization and have not been validated for later time intervals. Although several investigators (Imrie, Banks, Agarwal-Pitchumoni, and others) have proposed modifications to simplify these prognostic criteria throughout the years since their inception, Ranson's original 11 signs are still the most commonly used.

Another set of criteria often used to assess the severity of pancreatitis is the *a*cute *p*hysiology *a*nd *c*hronic *h*ealth *e*valuation (APACHE-II) score. This grading system assesses severity on the basis of quantitative measures of abnormalities of multiple variables, including vital signs and specific laboratory parameters, coupled with the age and chronic health status of the patient. The main advantage of the APACHE-II scoring system is the immediate assessment of the severity of pancreatitis. A score of eight or more at admission is usually considered indicative of severe disease.[40]

Biochemical Markers

The ideal biochemical marker for prognosis of acute pancreatitis should not only have high specificity and sensitivity, but also should be able to discriminate between mild (edematous) and severe (necrotic) disease on admission. While serum enzymes such as

Table 32-4
Ranson's Prognostic Signs of Pancreatitis

Criteria for acute pancreatitis not due to gallstones	
At admission	*During the initial 48 h*
Age >55 y	Hematocrit fall >10 points
WBC >16,000/mm^3	BUN elevation >5 mg/dL
Blood glucose >200 mg/dL	Serum calcium <8 mg/dL
Serum LDH >350 IU/L	Arterial Po$_2$ <60 mm Hg
Serum AST >250 U/dL	Base deficit >4 mEq/L
	Estimated fluid sequestration >6 L
Criteria for acute gallstone pancreatitis	
At admission	*During the initial 48 h*
Age >70 y	Hematocrit fall >10 points
WBC >18,000/mm^3	BUN elevation >2 mg/dL
Blood glucose >220 mg/dL	Serum calcium <8 mg/dL
Serum LDH >400 IU/L	Base deficit >5 mEq/L
Serum AST >250 U/dL	Estimated fluid sequestration >4 L

AST = aspartate transaminase; BUN = blood urea nitrogen; LDH = lactate dehydrogenase; Po$_2$ = partial pressure of oxygen; WBC = white blood cell count.

SOURCE: Reproduced with permission from Ranson JHC: Etiological and prognostic factors in human acute pancreatitis: A review. *Am J Gastroenterol* 77:633, 1982.

amylase and lipase are helpful in the diagnosis of pancreatitis, these have no prognostic value. Several recent research studies have suggested additional markers that may have prognostic value, including acute phase proteins such as C-reactive protein (CRP), α_2-macroglobulin, PMN-elastase, α_1-antitrypsin, and phospholipase A_2. While CRP measurement is commonly available many of the others are not. Therefore, at this time CRP seems to be the marker of choice in clinical settings. The measurement of IL-6 has recently been shown to distinguish patients with mild or severe forms of the disease. However, these tests have to undergo large-scale evaluations before they can be recommended for routine use. Another prognostic marker under evaluation is urinary–trypsinogen activation peptide (TAP). TAP is a five- to seven-amino acid peptide that is released from the N-terminus of trypsinogen during its activation. In recent studies, Neoptolemos and colleagues have shown a good correlation between the severity of pancreatitis and concentrations of TAP in urine.[41] However, further testing and methodologic developments are needed before TAP can be used as a routine prognostic marker.

Computed Tomography Scan

Computed tomography (CT) scanning with bolus intravenous contrast has become the gold standard for detecting and assessing the severity of pancreatitis. While clinically mild pancreatitis is usually associated with interstitial edema, severe pancreatitis is associated with necrosis. In interstitial pancreatitis, the microcirculation of the pancreas remains intact, and the gland shows uniform enhancement on intravenous, contrast-enhanced CT scan (see Fig. 32-13). In necrotizing pancreatitis, however, the microcirculation is disrupted; therefore the enhancement of the gland on contrast-enhanced CT scan is considerably decreased (Fig. 32-14). The presence of air bubbles on a CT scan is an indication of infected necrosis or pancreatic abscess. Currently, intravenous (bolus), contrast-enhanced CT scanning is routinely performed on patients who are suspected of har-

boring severe pancreatitis, regardless of their Ranson's or APACHE scores.[42]

Treatment

The severity of acute pancreatitis covers a broad spectrum of illness, ranging from the mild and self-limiting to the life-threatening necrotizing variety. Regardless of severity, hospitalization of the patient with suspected acute pancreatitis for observation and diagnostic study is usually mandatory. Upon confirmation of the diagnosis, patients with moderate to severe disease should be transferred to the intensive care unit for observation and maximal support. The most important initial treatment is conservative intensive care with the goals of oral food and fluid restriction, replacement of fluids and electrolytes parenterally as assessed by central venous pressure and urinary excretion, and control of pain. In severe acute pancreatitis, or when signs of infection are present, most experts recommend broad-spectrum antibiotics (e.g., imipenem) and careful surveillance for complications of the disease (Table 32-5).

Mild Pancreatitis

Pancreatitis is classified as mild when the patient has no systemic complications, low APACHE-II scores and Ranson's signs, sustained clinical improvement, and when a CT scan rules out necrotizing pancreatitis. The treatment then is mostly supportive and has the important aim of *resting the pancreas* through restriction of oral food and fluids. Nasogastric suction and H_2-blockers have routinely been used in this connection, based on the reasoning that even the smallest amount of gastric acid reaching the duodenum could stimulate pancreatic secretion. However, these measures are of little value. The following secretion-inhibiting drugs have also been tried without notable success: atropine, calcitonin, somatostatin, glucagon, and fluorouracil.[43]

Pancreatitis is also an autodigestive process, and various protease-inhibiting drugs including aprotinin, gabexate mesylate, camostate, and phospholipase A_2 inhibitors, as well as fresh frozen

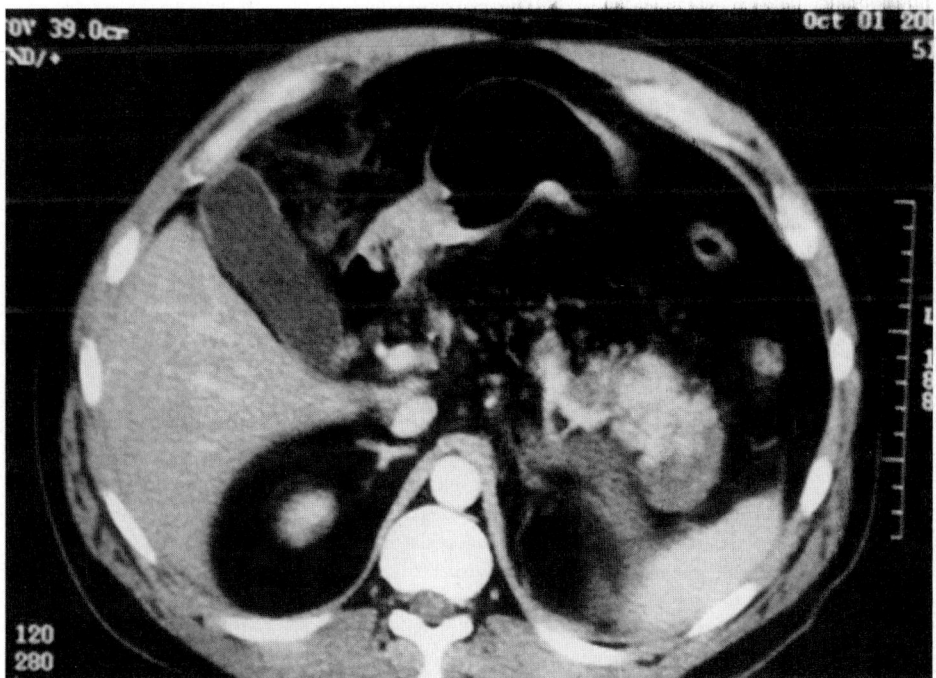

FIG. 32-14. Necrotizing (infected) acute pancreatitis. The CT image reveals areas of nonperfusion and the presence of gas in the region of severe necrosis, which indicates infection.

Table 32-5
Complications of Acute Pancreatitis

I. Local
  A. Pancreatic phlegmon
  B. Pancreatic abscess
  C. Pancreatic pseudocyst
  D. Pancreatic ascites
  E. Involvement of adjacent organs, with hemorrhage, thrombosis, bowel infarction, obstructive jaundice, fistula formation, or mechanical obstruction.
II. Systemic
  A. Pulmonary
    Pneumonia, atelectasis
    Acute respiratory distress syndrome
    Pleural effusion
  B. Cardiovascular
    Hypotension
    Hypovolemia
    Sudden death
    Nonspecific ST-T wave changes
    Pericardial effusion
  C. Hematologic
    Hemoconcentration
    Disseminated intravascular coagulopathy
  D. Gastrointestinal hemorrhage
    Peptic ulcer
    Erosive gastritis
    Portal vein or splenic vein thrombosis with varices
  E. Renal
    Oliguria
    Azotemia
    Renal artery/vein thrombosis
  F. Metabolic
    Hyperglycemia
    Hypocalcemia
    Hypertriglyceridemia
    Encephalopathy
    Sudden blindness (Purtscher's retinopathy)
  G. Central nervous system
    Psychosis
    Fat emboli
    Alcohol withdrawal syndrome
  H. Fat necrosis
    Intra-abdominal saponification
    Subcutaneous tissue necrosis

SOURCE: Reproduced with permission from Greenberger NJ, Toskes PP, Isselbacher KJ: Diseases of the pancreas, in *Harrison's Principles of Internal Medicine,* 2nd ed. New York: McGraw-Hill, 1987, p 1373.

plasma have been tested to prevent proteolysis, but with little success. Because a significant component of the patient's distress arises from the inflammatory aspect of pancreatitis, various methods have been tried to alleviate inflammation, including indomethacin and the prostaglandin inhibitors, but again, these have not proved to be of much value. Some recent studies examined a different strategy, namely the use of platelet-aggregating factor (PAF) antagonists such as PAF acetylhydrolase (PAF-AH) and Lexipafant. These showed promising results in experimental animals and in initial clinical studies, but did not live up to their promise in larger-scale clinical trials.[44]

The current principles of treatment are physiologic monitoring, metabolic support, and maintenance of fluid balance, which can become dangerously disturbed even in mild acute pancreatitis because of fluid sequestration, vomiting, and sudoresis. Because hypovolemia can result in pancreatic and other visceral ischemia, fluid balance should be assessed at least every 8 hours initially.

The severe pain of acute pancreatitis prevents the patient from resting, and results in ongoing cholinergic discharge, which stimulates gastric and pancreatic secretion. Therefore pain management is

of great importance. Administration of buprenorphine, pentazocine, procaine hydrochloride, and meperidine are all of value in controlling abdominal pain. Morphine is to be avoided, due to its potential to cause sphincter of Oddi spasm. Antibiotic therapy has not proved to be of value in the absence of signs or documented sources of infection.

Cautious resumption of oral feeding consisting of small and slowly increasing meals is permissible after the abdominal pain and tenderness have subsided, serum amylase has returned to normal, and the patient experiences hunger. This usually occurs within a week of the onset of an attack of mild acute pancreatitis. A low-fat, low-protein diet is advocated as the initial form of nutrition following an attack of acute pancreatitis.

Severe Pancreatitis

Pancreatitis can be classified as severe based on predictors such as APACHE-II scores and Ranson's signs, and any evidence that the condition is severe mandates care of the patient in the intensive care unit. Such evidence may take various forms, such as the onset of encephalopathy, a hematocrit over 50, urine output less than 50 mL/h, hypotension, fever, or peritonitis. Elderly patients with three or more Ranson's criteria should also be monitored carefully despite the absence of severe pain.[45]

Patients may develop ARDS, and many patients who die during the early stages of severe acute pancreatitis have this complication. Until recently, the lung injury has been thought to be caused by the systemic release of phospholipase A_2 and other enzymes that directly damage alveolar tissue and pulmonary capillaries. In addition, recent evidence implicates the cell adhesion molecule ICAM-1, neutrophils, PAF, substance P, and certain chemokines. The presence of ARDS usually requires assisted ventilation with positive end-expiratory pressure. The value of peritoneal lavage in removing enzyme-rich ascites remains unclear. It has been advocated in patients with deteriorating respiratory function and/or shock that is refractory to maximal management, but its effectiveness in reducing the mortality risk of severe acute pancreatitis remains unproven.

Acute pancreatitis may be accompanied by cardiovascular events such as cardiac arrhythmia, myocardial infarction, cardiogenic shock, and congestive heart failure. The conventional modalities of treatment apply in these cases in addition to the support described above.

Infections

Infection is a serious complication of acute pancreatitis and is the most common cause of death. It is caused most often by translocated enteric bacteria, and is seen commonly in necrotizing rather than interstitial pancreatitis. If there is an indication of infection (e.g., retroperitoneal air on CT scan), then a CT- or ultrasound-guided fine-needle aspiration should be performed for Gram's stain and culture of the fluid or tissue, and the indicated antibiotic therapy initiated. However, antibiotics alone may not be effective in infected necrosis, which has a mortality of nearly 50% unless débrided surgically (Fig. 32-15). The long-held opinion that antibiotic prophylaxis in necrotizing pancreatitis is of little use has been altered by recent studies showing a beneficial prophylactic effect with antibiotics such as metronidazole, imipenem, and third-generation cephalosporins.[46-48] Because *Candida* species are common inhabitants of the upper gastrointestinal tract, *Candida* sepsis

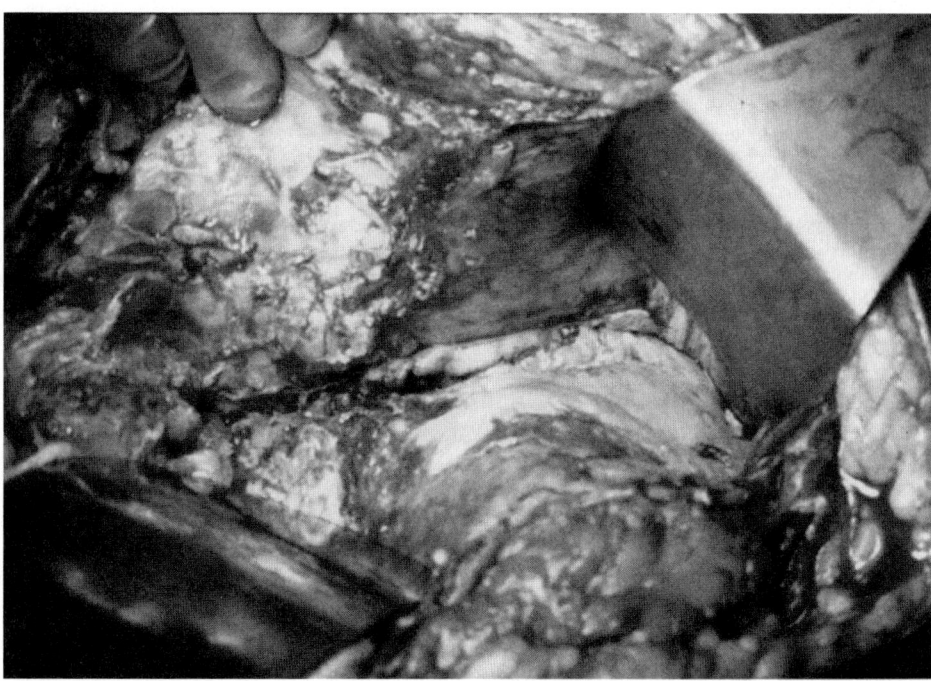

FIG. 32-15. Operative view of infected acute pancreatitis. Peripancreatic infection, characterized by mucopurulent exudate, extends far beyond the boundaries of the pancreas in the retroperitoneum.

and secondary fungal infection of pancreatic necrosis is a risk in severe disease. The role of empiric therapy with fluconazole in cases of severe acute pancreatitis is currently being investigated in large-scale clinical trials.

Sterile Necrosis

Patients with sterile necrosis have a far better prognosis than those with infected necrosis, with a reported mortality of near zero in the absence of systemic complications. However, others report mortality rates as high as 38% in patients with a single systemic complication.

Treatment of sterile necrotic pancreatitis falls into three degrees of aggressiveness. At one end of the scale is the patient with no systemic complications and no concerns about secondary infections, who can be managed with the supportive care described previously and be cautiously brought back to refeeding. The area of sterile necrosis may evolve into a chronic pseudocyst, or may resolve. An intermediate course is demonstrated by the patient who develops systemic complications, and in whom a secondary infection is suspected. A CT-guided, fine-needle aspiration then confirms or disproves infection, and in the latter instance the patient can be managed medically. The last and most serious condition is that of the patient who appears to be very ill, has high APACHE-II and Ranson's scores, and shows evidence of systemic toxicity including shock. Patients in this category have a poor chance of survival without aggressive débridement, and a decision may be made to proceed with exploration simply due to a relentless course of deterioration despite maximal medical therapy.[43] It must be emphasized that current opinion is against débridement in sterile necrosis unless it is accompanied by life-threatening systemic complications (Fig. 32-16).

Pancreatic Abscess

A pancreatic abscess occurs 2 to 6 weeks after the initial attack, in contrast to infected necrosis, which occurs in the first few hours or days. The mechanism of delayed infection is not clear, but the treatment consists of external drainage, whether established by surgical or by percutaneous catheter-based methods.

Nutritional Support

The guiding principle of resting the pancreas dictates that patients with acute pancreatitis not be fed orally until their clinical condition improves. This generally occurs in 3 to 7 days in patients with mild pancreatitis, but the situation in patients with severe pancreatitis is more complicated, requiring nutritional support for several weeks. This can be provided by total parenteral nutrition (TPN) or by enteral nutrition through a jejunal tube.[49] There is some debate regarding the preferred route, since TPN is known to result in early atrophy of the gut mucosa, a condition that favors transmigration of luminal bacteria, and intrajejunal feeding still stimulates pancreatic exocrine secretion through the release of enteric hormones. Recent animal studies and preliminary clinical trials on humans suggest that on balance, jejunal feeding may be superior to TPN.

Treatment of Biliary Pancreatitis

Gallstones are the most common cause of acute pancreatitis worldwide. Most patients pass the offending gallstone(s) during the early hours of acute pancreatitis, but have additional stones capable of inducing future episodes. This raises the question of the timing of surgical or endoscopic clearance of gallstones. The issue of when to intervene is controversial. Several studies have been aimed at resolving this controversy, but the issue is clouded by the fact that each position is open to some theoretical objection. Additional points of contention include varying inclusion criteria, years of observation of the studied groups, and a lack of uniformity regarding definitions. General consensus favors either urgent intervention (cholecystectomy) within the first 48 to 72 hours of admission, or briefly delayed intervention (after 72 hours, but during the initial hospitalization) to give an inflamed pancreas time to recover. Cholecystectomy and operative common duct clearance is probably the best treatment for otherwise healthy patients with obstructive pancreatitis. However, patients who are at high risk for surgical intervention are best

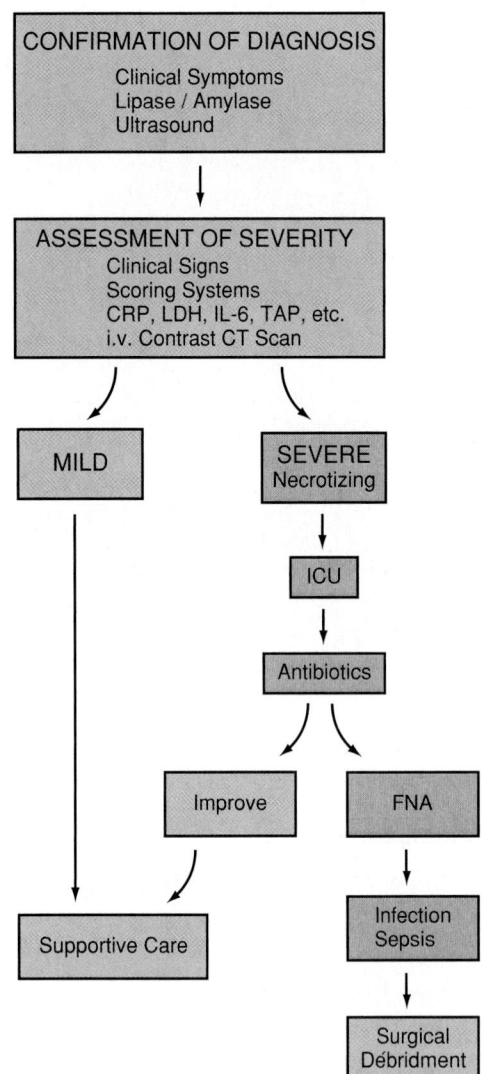

FIG. 32-16. *Algorithm for managing acute pancreatitis.*

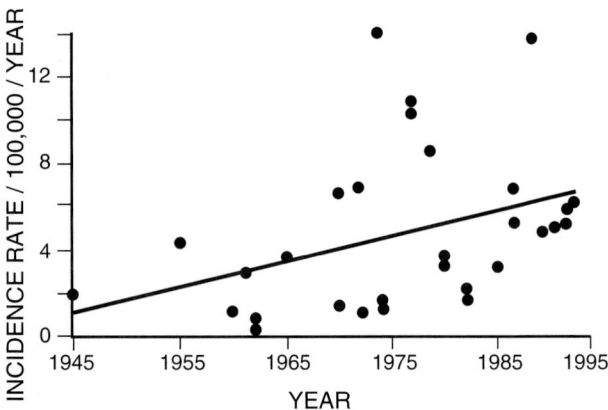

FIG. 32-17. *Incidence of chronic pancreatitis. The reported incidence of chronic pancreatitis has increased steadily over the past 50 years (Reproduced with permission from Worning.[53]).*

treated by endoscopic sphincterotomy, with clearance of stones by endoscopic retrograde cholangiopancreatography (ERCP).

In the case of acute biliary pancreatitis in which chemical studies suggest that the obstruction persists after 24 hours of observation, emergency endoscopic sphincterotomy and stone extraction is indicated. Routine ERCP for examination of the bile duct is discouraged in cases of biliary pancreatitis, as the probability of finding residual stones is low, and the risk of ERCP-induced pancreatitis is significant. Patients who are suspected of harboring a persistent impacted stone in the distal common bile duct or ampulla should have confirmation by radiologic imaging (CT, magnetic resonance cholangiopancreatography, or endoscopic ultrasonography) before intervention.

CHRONIC PANCREATITIS

Definition, Incidence, and Prevalence

Chronic pancreatitis is an incurable, chronic inflammatory condition that is multifactorial in its etiology, highly variable in its presentation, and a challenge to treat successfully. Autopsy studies indicate the prevalence to be as high as 5% in Scandinavia,[50]

although population studies suggest a prevalence that ranges from 5 to 27 persons per 100,000 population, with considerable geographic variation.[51,52] Differences in diagnostic criteria, regional nutrition, alcohol consumption, and medical access account for variations in the frequency of the diagnosis, but the overall incidence of the disease has risen progressively over the past 50 years[53] (Fig. 32-17).

Autopsy data are difficult to interpret because a number of changes associated with chronic pancreatitis, such as fibrosis, duct ectasia, and acinar atrophy, are also present in asymptomatic elderly patients.[54] Although the prevalence of chronic pancreatitis in patients with alcoholic cirrhosis and fatty liver ranges from 9 to 34%, the prevalence of chronic pancreatitis among known alcoholics is only 5 to 15%.[53,55,56]

Etiology

Worldwide, alcohol consumption and abuse is associated with chronic pancreatitis in up to 70% of cases (Table 32-6). In 1878, Freidreich proposed that "a general chronic interstitial pancreatitis may result from excessive alcoholism (drunkard's pancreas)."[59] Since that observation, numerous studies have shown that a causal relationship exists between alcohol and chronic pancreatitis, but the prevalence of this form of the disease in Western countries ranges widely, from 38 to 94%.[53] Other major causes worldwide include tropical (nutritional) and idiopathic disease, as well as hereditary causes.

Alcohol

There is a linear relationship between exposure to alcohol and the development of chronic pancreatitis.[60] The risk of disease is present in patients with even a low or occasional exposure to alcohol (1 to

Table 32-6
Etiology of Chronic Pancreatitis

Alcohol, 70%
Idiopathic (including tropical), 20%
Other, 10%
Hereditary
Hyperparathyroidism
Hypertriglyceridemia
Autoimmune pancreatitis
Obstruction
Trauma
Pancreas divisum

20 g/d), so there is no threshold level of alcohol exposure below which there is no risk of developing chronic pancreatitis. Furthermore, although the risk of disease is dose related, and highest in heavy (150 g/d) drinkers, fewer than 15% of confirmed alcohol abusers suffer from chronic pancreatitis.[61,62] In a study of 247 patients with fatal acute alcoholic pancreatitis, 53% of patients had no autopsy evidence of chronic pancreatitis.[63] However, the duration of alcohol consumption is definitely associated with the development of pancreatic disease. The onset of disease typically occurs between ages 35 to 40, after 16 to 20 years of heavy alcohol consumption. Recurrent episodes of acute pancreatitis are typically followed by chronic symptoms after 4 or 5 years.[64,65]

Although the pattern of disease presentation is well known in those alcohol users who develop pancreatic disease, the pathophysiology of alcohol-induced pancreatic disease is still an area of active investigation. In their 1946 classic study, Comfort, Gambill, and Baggenstoss proposed that chronic pancreatitis was the result of multiple episodes of acute inflammation, with residual and progressively increasing chronic inflammation.[66] Subsequently, other investigators proposed that initial acute inflammation was not necessarily linked to chronic changes in the pancreas,[67] and Kondo and associates showed that other, additional factors were necessary for repeated exposure to alcohol to cause chronic pancreatitis.[68] Regardless of the requirement for other predisposing or facilitative factors, the concept that multiple episodes (or a prolonged course) of pancreatic injury ultimately leads to chronic disease is widely accepted as the pathophysiologic sequence[65] (Fig. 32-18). Laboratory studies in rodents reveal that repeated episodes of acute–alcohol induced pancreatitis results in findings of chronic pancreatitis,[69,70] and the induction of severe acute pancreatitis by a single intraductal infusion of oleic acid reproducibly results in chronic pancreatitis in rats.[71]

Alcohol-associated chronic pancreatitis is less common in Japan and India, where a there is a lower per capita consumption of alcohol, and its incidence is otherwise quite variable with regard to geography, nutrition, and race.[67] Although alcohol exposure to the pancreatic ductal system, or elevated levels of alcohol in the bloodstream, has been shown to alter the integrity and function of pancreatic

ducts and acini directly,[72,73] most investigators believe that alcohol metabolites such as acetaldehyde, combined with oxidant injury, result in local parenchymal injury that is preferentially targeted to the pancreas in predisposed individuals. Repeated or severe episodes of toxin-induced injury activate a cascade of cytokines, which in turn induces pancreatic stellate cells to produce collagen and cause fibrosis (Fig. 32-19). It remains to be determined whether alcohol sensitizes the pancreas of susceptible individuals to another cause of acute inflammation, or whether genetic or other factors predispose to direct alcohol-related injury.[65]

Since the discovery of specific genetic mutations and deletions associated with hereditary pancreatitis (see below), many studies have been undertaken to determine whether specific genetic abnormalities are associated with alcoholic chronic pancreatitis.[74] No mutations of the major genetic abnormality associated with hereditary pancreatitis, the catatonic trypsinogen gene or *PRSS1*,[75] have been identified in patients with alcoholic chronic pancreatitis. A second genetic marker for hereditary pancreatitis, the pancreatic secretory trypsin inhibitor, or *SPINK1* gene, has also been studied. Mutations in *SPINK1* are observed in the general population, and Witt and colleagues found a 5.8% rate of *SPINK1* mutations in patients with alcoholic pancreatitis, compared to a 0.8% rate in the control population.[76] Studies which have examined some of the known polymorphisms and mutations of the cystic fibrosis transmembrane receptor (*CFTR*) gene have thus far failed to demonstrate an association with alcoholic chronic pancreatitis. Therefore, a dominant hereditary cofactor for alcoholic pancreatitis remains to be elucidated.

Alcohol may interfere with the intracellular transport and discharge of digestive enzymes, and may contribute to the colocalization of digestive enzymes and lysosomal hydrolase within acinar cells, leading to autodigestion[77,78] (see section on acute pancreatitis). A high-protein, low-bicarbonate, low-volume secretory output is seen after chronic alcohol exposure,[79] which may contribute to the precipitation of proteins in secondary ducts in the early stages of chronic pancreatitis.[80] Lithostathine, a protein found in pancreatic juice, inhibits the formation of calcium carbonate crystals,[81] and has been found to be decreased in the pancreatic duct fluid in alcoholic and nonalcoholic chronic pancreatitis patients[82] (see section on stone formation below). The zymogen membrane-associated protein GP2 is also found in protein precipitates within small ducts, and may contribute to small duct obstruction in chronic pancreatitis.[83] Calcium is complexed to protein plugs in small ductules, secondary ducts, and eventually in the main ductal system, which causes ductal cell injury and obstruction of the secretory system, which further promotes an inflammatory response.

Cigarette smoking has been strongly associated with chronic pancreatitis and with the development of calcific pancreatitis.[84] Studies on the role of smoking in the development of alcoholic pancreatitis have been conflicting, although the risk of cancer in chronic pancreatitis is increased significantly by smoking. In hereditary pancreatitis smoking has been found to lower the age of onset of carcinoma by about 20 years.[85] Smoking would therefore appear to be a definite risk factor for the late complications of alcoholic pancreatitis, if not an early cofactor.

Hyperparathyroidism

Hypercalcemia is a known cause of pancreatic hypersecretion,[104] and chronic hypercalcemia caused by untreated hyperparathyroidism is associated with chronic calcific pancreatitis.[105] Hypercalcemia is also a stimulant for pancreatic calcium secretion, which

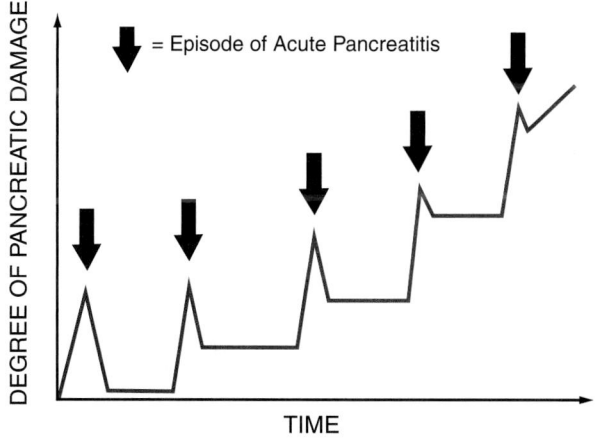

NECROSIS-FIBROSIS SEQUENCE

FIG. 32-18. "Multiple hit" theory of the etiology of acute pancreatitis. Multiple episodes of the acute pancreatitis cause progressively more organized inflammatory changes that ultimately result in chronic inflammation and scarring. (Reproduced with permission from Apte et al.[65]).

PATHOGENESIS OF ALCOHOLIC PANCREATIC FIBROSIS

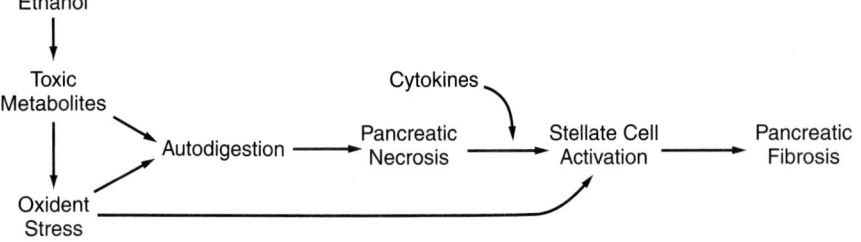

FIG. 32-19. Chemical pathogenesis of fibrosis in chronic pancreatitis. The relationship of cytokine release to the activation of pancreatic stellate cells (PSCs) illustrates pathways that are potential targets for therapeutic intervention.

contributes to calculus formation and obstructive pancreatopathy. The treatment is correction of the hyperparathyroidism and assessment of any additional endocrinopathies.

Hyperlipidemia

In addition to the risk of acute pancreatitis, hyperlipidemia and hypertriglyceridemia predispose women to chronic pancreatitis when they receive estrogen replacement therapy.[106] Fasting triglyceride levels less than 300 mg/dL are below the threshold for this to occur, and the mechanism of estrogen potentiation of hyperlipidemia-induced chronic pancreatitis is unknown. It is assumed that chronic changes occur after repeated subclinical episodes of acute inflammation. Aggressive therapy of hyperlipidemia is therefore important in peri- or postmenopausal patients who are candidates for estrogen therapy.

Classification

A major impediment to an accurate accounting of the frequency and severity of chronic pancreatitis has been the difficulty with which investigators and clinicians have struggled to identify a useful classification system. Multiple classification systems have been proposed. In 1963, Henri Sarles organized a symposium in Marceilles, France, and subsequent symposia were held in Cambridge (1983), Marseilles (1984), and Rome (1998). A current classification system, as delineated by Singer and Chari, is shown in Table 32-7.[57]

Chronic Calcifying (Lithogenic) Pancreatitis. This type is the largest subgroup in the current classification scheme, and includes patients with calcific pancreatitis of most etiologies. Although the majority of patients with calcific pancreatitis have a history of alcohol abuse, stone formation and parenchymal calcification can develop in a variety of etiologic subgroups; hereditary pancreatitis and tropical pancreatitis are particularly noteworthy for

the formation of stone disease. The clinician should therefore avoid the assumption that calcific pancreatitis confirms the diagnosis of alcohol abuse.

Chronic Obstructive Pancreatitis. This refers to chronic inflammatory changes which are caused by the compression or occlusion of the proximal ductal system by tumor, gallstone, posttraumatic scar, or inadequate duct caliber (as in pancreas divisum). In this category, the chronic pancreatitis may be clinically silent or present with exocrine or endocrine insufficiency, and the distribution of changes within the gland are uniformly distributed distal to the causative process.

Chronic Inflammatory Pancreatitis. This type is characterized by diffuse fibrosis and a loss of acinar elements with a predominant mononuclear cell infiltration throughout the gland.

Chronic Autoimmune Pancreatitis. This type is associated with a variety of illnesses with suspected or proven autoimmune etiology, such as Sjögren's syndrome.

Asymptomatic Pancreatic Fibrosis. This type is seen in some asymptomatic elderly patients, in tropical populations, or in asymptomatic alcohol users. There is diffuse perilobar fibrosis and a loss of acinar cell mass, but without a main ductular component.

A shortcoming of these clinical classification systems is the lack of histologic criteria of chronic inflammation, due to the usual absence of a biopsy specimen. The differentiation of recurrent acute pancreatitis from chronic pancreatitis with exacerbations of pain can be difficult to establish, and is not facilitated by the current system. Similarly, cystic fibrosis is known to cause fibrosis and acinar dysfunction, but is not included in the classification despite increasing evidence for its possible role in idiopathic chronic pancreatitis.[58] Therefore further refinements in the classification system for chronic pancreatitis are needed to allow a better prediction of its clinical course and a more accurate diagnosis of a likely etiologic agent.

Table 32-7
Classification of Chronic Pancreatitis

Chronic Calcific Pancreatitis	Chronic Obstructive Pancreatitis	Chronic Inflammatory Pancreatitis	Chronic Autoimmune Pancreatitis	Asymptomatic Pancreatic Fibrosis
Alcohol Hereditary Tropical Hyperlipidemia Hypercalcemia Drug-induced Idiopathic	Pancreatic tumors Ductal stricture Gallstone- or trauma-induced Pancreas divisum	Unknown	Associated with autoimmune disorders (e.g., primary sclerosing cholangitis) Sjögren's syndrome Primary biliary cirrhosis	Chronic alcoholic Endemic in asymptomatic residents in tropical climates

SOURCE: Reproduced with permission from Singer et al.[57]

Tropical (Nutritional) Pancreatitis. Tropical chronic pancreatitis is highly prevalent among adolescents and young adults raised in Indonesia, southern India, and tropical Africa.[86] Abdominal pain develops in adolescence, followed by the development of a brittle form of pancreatogenic diabetes. Parenchymal and intraductal calcifications are seen, and the pancreatic duct stones may be quite large.[87] Many of the patients appear malnourished, some present with extreme emaciation, and a characteristic cyanotic coloration of the lips may be seen.[88] In addition to protein-caloric malnutrition, toxic products of some indigenous foodstuffs may also contribute to the disease. Cassava root is a starch (the origin of tapioca) which is a staple in the diet throughout the Afro-Asian region where tropical pancreatitis is prevalent. Cassava contains toxic glycosides, which form hydrocyanic acid when mixed with (gastric) hydrochloric acid.[89] Hydrocyanic acid is reduced to thiocyanate, which blocks a variety of enzymes, including superoxide dismutase. The simultaneous deficiency of dietary trace elements such as zinc, copper, and selenium could retard the detoxification of cyanogens, and result in an increased susceptibility to free radical injury of the pancreas.

Clinically, tropical pancreatitis presents much like hereditary pancreatitis, and a familial pattern among cases is not unusual. Recently an association with mutations of the pancreatic secretory trypsin inhibitor (PSTI) or *SPINK1* gene in patients with tropical pancreatitis has been reported.[90,91] The accelerated deterioration of endocrine and exocrine function, the chronic pain due to obstructive disease, and the recurrence of symptoms despite decompressive procedures characterize the course of disease.[88] As immigrants from the tropical regions increasingly find their way to all parts of the world, an awareness of this severe form of chronic pancreatitis is helpful for those who treat patients with pancreatic disease.

Hereditary Pancreatitis. In 1952, Comfort and Steinberg reported a kindred of "hereditary chronic relapsing pancreatitis" after treating the proband, a 24-year-old woman, at the Mayo Clinic.[92] Subsequently, familial patterns of chronic, nonalcoholic pancreatitis have been described worldwide, and a familiar pattern has emerged. Typically, patients first present in childhood or adolescence with abdominal pain, and are found to have chronic calcific pancreatitis on imaging studies. Progressive pancreatic dysfunction is common, and many patients present with symptoms due to pancreatic duct obstruction. The risk of subsequent carcinoma formation is increased, reaching a prevalence in some series of 40%, but the age of onset for carcinoma is typically over 50 years.[93,94] The disorder is characterized by an autosomal dominant pattern of inheritance, with 80% penetrance and variable expression. The incidence is equal in both sexes. Whitcomb and colleagues,[95] and separately LeBodic and associates,[96] performed gene linkage analysis and identified a linkage for hereditary pancreatitis to chromosome 7q35. Subsequently, the region was sequenced, and revealed eight trypsinogen genes. Mutational analysis revealed a missense mutation resulting in an Arg to His substitution at position 117 of the cationic trypsinogen gene, or *PRSS1*, one of the primary sites for proteolysis of trypsin. This mutation prevents trypsin from being inactivated by itself or other proteases, and results in persistent and uncontrolled proteolytic activity and autodestruction within the pancreas.[97] The position 117 mutation of *PRSS1* and an additional mutation, now known collectively as the R122H and N291 mutations of *PRSS1*, account for about two thirds of cases of hereditary pancreatitis. Recently, Schneider and Whitcomb described a probable mutation in the anionic trypsinogen gene which may also be present in some cases.[98] Thus, hereditary pancreatitis results from one or more mutational defects which incapacitate an autoprotective process that normally prevents proteolysis within the pancreas.

Similarly, PSTI, also known as *SPINK1*, has been found to have a role in hereditary pancreatitis.[76] *SPINK1* specifically inhibits trypsin action by competitively blocking the active site of the enzyme. Witt and colleagues investigated 96 unrelated children with chronic pancreatitis in Germany and found a variety of *SPINK1* mutations in 23% of the patients.[76] Several studies have now confirmed an association of *SPINK1* mutations with familial and idiopathic forms of chronic pancreatitis, as well as tropical pancreatitis.[90,92,99,100] *SPINK1* mutations are common in the general population as well, and the frequency of these mutations varies in different cohorts of idiopathic chronic pancreatitis, from 6.4% in France[101] to 25.8% in the U.S.[99]

The cystic fibrosis transmembrane receptor (*CFTR*) gene contains over 4300 nucleotides, divided into 24 exons, which encode for a 1480-amino acid protein. Over 1000 polymorphisms have been reported, and many are common.[74] The severe *CFTR* mutation associated with the classic disease, F508, is rarely observed in chronic pancreatitis. But other minor *CFTR* mutations have been noted to be associated with chronic idiopathic pancreatitis in which the pulmonary, intestinal, and cutaneous manifestations of the disease are silent.[102,103] It is likely that many of the "idiopathic" forms of chronic pancreatitis, as well as some patients with the more common forms of the disease, will be found to have a genetic linkage or predisposition. The goal of this active area of research is to elucidate specific molecular abnormalities, and provide strategies for treatment and prevention.

Autoimmune Pancreatitis. A variant of chronic pancreatitis is a nonobstructive, diffusely infiltrative disease associated with fibrosis, a mononuclear cell (lymphocyte, plasma cell, or eosinophil) infiltrate, and an increased titer of one or more autoantibodies.[107] Compressive stenosis of the intrapancreatic portion of the common bile duct is frequently seen, along with symptoms of obstructive jaundice. Increased levels of serum beta-globulin or immunoglobulin G are also present. Steroid therapy is uniformly successful in ameliorating the disease, including any associated bile duct compression.[108] The differential diagnosis includes lymphoma, plasmacytoma ("pseudotumor" of the pancreas), and diffuse infiltrative carcinoma. Although the diagnosis is confirmed on pancreatic biopsy, presumptive treatment with steroids is usually undertaken, especially when clinical and laboratory findings support the diagnosis. Failure to obtain a cytologic specimen may lead to an unnecessary resectional procedure, and an untreated inflammatory component may cause sclerosis of the extrahepatic or intrahepatic bile ducts, with eventual liver failure.[109]

Chronic Obstructive Pancreatitis. Obstruction of the main pancreatic duct by inflammatory (posttraumatic) or neoplastic processes, including pseudocysts, intraductal mucin-secreting tumors, and ampullary and pancreatic tumors, can result in a form of chronic pancreatitis associated with diffuse fibrosis, dilated main and secondary pancreatic ducts, and acinar atrophy. The patient may have little in the way of pain symptoms, or may present with signs of exocrine insufficiency. Intraductal stone formation is rare, and both functional and structural abnormalities may improve when the obstructive process is relieved or removed. Trauma to the pancreas frequently results in duct injury and leakage, which may result in pseudocyst formation as well as local scar formation. Inadequately treated pancreatic trauma may result in persistent inflammatory changes in the distal gland.[110]

DUCT VARIATIONS

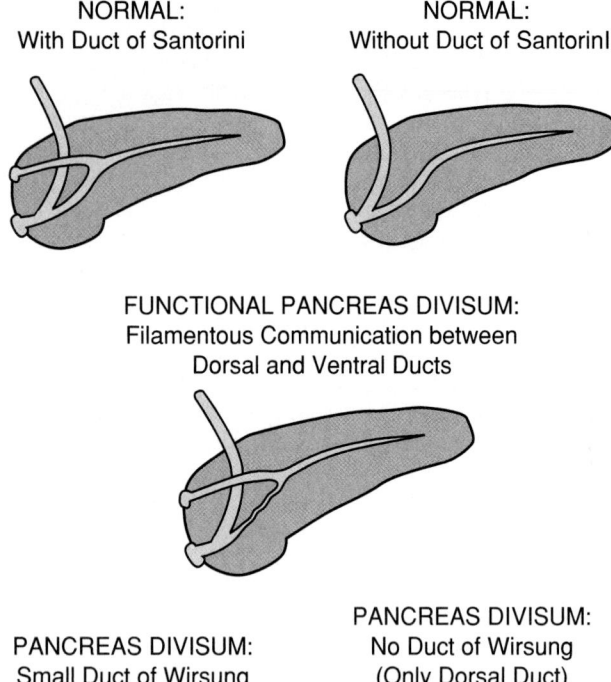

NORMAL:
With Duct of Santorini

NORMAL:
Without Duct of Santorinl

FUNCTIONAL PANCREAS DIVISUM:
Filamentous Communication between
Dorsal and Ventral Ducts

PANCREAS DIVISUM:
Small Duct of Wirsung

PANCREAS DIVISUM:
No Duct of Wirsung
(Only Dorsal Duct)

FIG. 32-20. *Pancreas divisum. Normal pancreatic duct anatomy and the variations of partial or complete pancreas divisum are shown. (Reproduced with permission from Warshaw.[112])*

Pancreas divisum represents a special case of obstructive pancreatitis. It is the most common congenital anomaly involving the pancreas and occurs in up to 10% of children. It is thought to predispose the pancreas to recurrent acute pancreatitis and chronic pancreatitis, due to functional obstruction of a diminutive duct of Santorini which fails to communicate with Wirsung's duct (Fig. 32-20). However, the classic picture of obstructive pancreatopathy with a dilated dorsal duct is unusual in pancreas divisum, so a decompressive operation or a lesser papilla sphincteroplasty is frequently not feasible or unsuccessful. Endoscopic stenting through the lesser papilla may result in temporary relief of symptoms, and this response would increase the possibility that a permanent surgical or endoscopic intervention will be successful. Although some authors emphasize the pathologic implications of pancreas divisum,[111,112] others express skepticism that it represents a true risk to pancreatic secretory capacity or contributes to the development of chronic pancreatitis.[113,114]

Idiopathic Pancreatitis. When a definable cause for chronic pancreatitis is lacking, the term "idiopathic" is used to categorize the illness. Not surprisingly, as diagnostic methods and clinical awareness of disease improve, fewer patients fall into the idiopathic category. Classically, the idiopathic group includes young adults and adolescents who lack a family history of pancreatitis, but who may represent individuals with spontaneous gene mutations encoding

for regulatory proteins in the pancreas. In addition, the idiopathic group has included a large number of older patients for whom no obvious cause of recurrent or chronic pancreatitis can be found.[115] However, because the prevalence of biliary calculi increases steadily with age, it is not surprising that as methods to detect biliary stone disease and microlithiasis have improved, a larger proportion of elderly "idiopathic" pancreatitis patients are found to have biliary tract disease.[116]

As noted in the section on hereditary pancreatitis above, an increasing number of mutations of the *CFTR* and *SPINK1* genes have been identified in association with idiopathic pancreatitis.[101–103] However, the role of genetic analysis in the management of these patients remains unclear, as guidelines have yet to be developed to allow physicians to use the data consistently. The clinical management of patients who harbor a minor *CFTR* mutation and chronic pancreatitis, for example, is still dictated by the manifestations of the pancreatitis. Any genetic counseling for the patient and his or her family has yet to be defined.[117]

Pathology

Histology

In early chronic pancreatitis, the histologic changes are unevenly distributed, and are characterized by induration, nodular scarring, and lobular regions of fibrosis (Fig. 32-21). As the disease progresses, there is a loss of normal lobulation, with thicker sheets of fibrosis surrounding a reduced acinar cell mass, and dilatation of ductular structures (Fig. 32-22). The ductular epithelium is usually atypical, and may display features of dysplasia, as evidenced by cuboidal cells with hyperplastic features, accompanied by areas of mononuclear cell infiltrates or patchy areas of necrosis. Cystic changes may be seen, but areas of relatively intact acinar elements and normal-appearing islets persist. In severe chronic pancreatitis, there is considerable replacement of acinar tissue by broad, coalescing areas of fibrosis, and the islet size and number are reduced (Fig. 32-23). Small arteries appear thickened and neural trunks become prominent.[118]

Tropical pancreatitis and hereditary pancreatitis are histologically indistinguishable from chronic alcoholic pancreatitis. In obstructive chronic pancreatitis, calculi are absent, although periacinar fibrosis and dilated ductular structures are prominent. In pancreatic lobular fibrosis seen in elderly subjects, small ducts are dilated, sometimes with small calculi trapped within. Hypertrophy of ductular epithelia is thought to cause this small-duct disease, which is accompanied by perilobular fibrosis.[119]

Fibrosis

A common feature of all forms of chronic pancreatitis is the perilobular fibrosis that forms surrounding individual acini, then propagates to surround small lobules, and eventually coalesces to replace larger areas of acinar tissue. The pathogenesis of this process involves the activation of pancreatic stellate cells (PSCs) that are found adjacent to acini and small arteries.[120] The extended cytoplasmic processes of PSCs encircle the acini, but appear quiescent in the normal gland, where they contain lipid vacuoles and cytoskeletal proteins. In response to pancreatic injury, the PSCs become activated and proliferate (similarly to hepatic stellate cells), lose their lipid vesicles, and transform into myofibroblast-like cells. These cells respond to proliferative factors such as transforming growth factor-β (TGF-β), platelet-derived growth factor (PDGF), and proinflammatory cytokines, and synthesize and secrete type I and III collagen and fibronectin. Recent studies indicate that vitamin A metabolites,

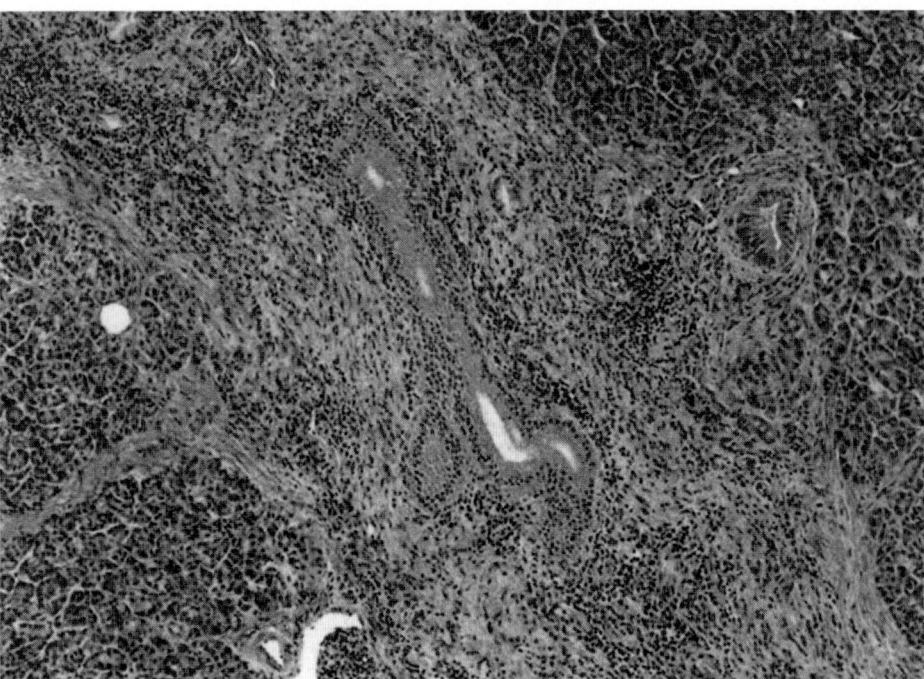

FIG. 32-21. Histology of early chronic pancreatitis. High-power microscopic (400x) histology of chronic pancreatitis shows an infiltration of mononuclear inflammatory cells throughout the interstitium of the pancreas, with little fibrosis. (*Courtesy of Dr. Rhonda Yantiss, Department of Pathology, University of Massachusetts Medical School.*)

similar to those present in quiescent PSCs, can inhibit the collagen production of activated cultured PSCs.[121] This raises the possibility that early intervention may be possible to interrupt or prevent the fibrosis resulting from ongoing activation of PSCs.

The overall pathogenic sequence proposed by Schneider and Whitcomb[122] whereby alcohol induces acute pancreatitis, and with ongoing exposure promotes the development of chronic fibrosis, is summarized in Fig. 32-24. Stellate cells surrounding the acinus are activated in acute pancreatitis, but may be inactivated by anti-inflammatory cytokines, and in the absence of further injury may revert to a quiescent state. The role of proinflammatory macrophages,

cytokines, and stellate cells in models of acute and chronic pancreatitis represent an important area of current research.

Stone Formation

Pancreatic stones are composed largely of calcium carbonate crystals trapped in a matrix of fibrillar and other material.[123] The fibrillar center of most stones contains no calcium, but a mixture of other metals. This suggests that stones form from an initial noncalcified protein precipitate, which serves as a focus for layered calcium carbonate precipitation. The same low-molecular-weight protein is

FIG. 32-22. Gross appearance of chronic pancreatitis. Areas of fibrosis and scarring are seen adjacent to other areas within the gland in which the lobar architecture is grossly preserved. A dilated pancreatic duct indicates the presence of downstream obstruction in this specimen removed from a patient with chronic pancreatitis. (*Courtesy of Dr. Rhonda Yantiss, Department of Pathology, University of Massachusetts Medical School.*)

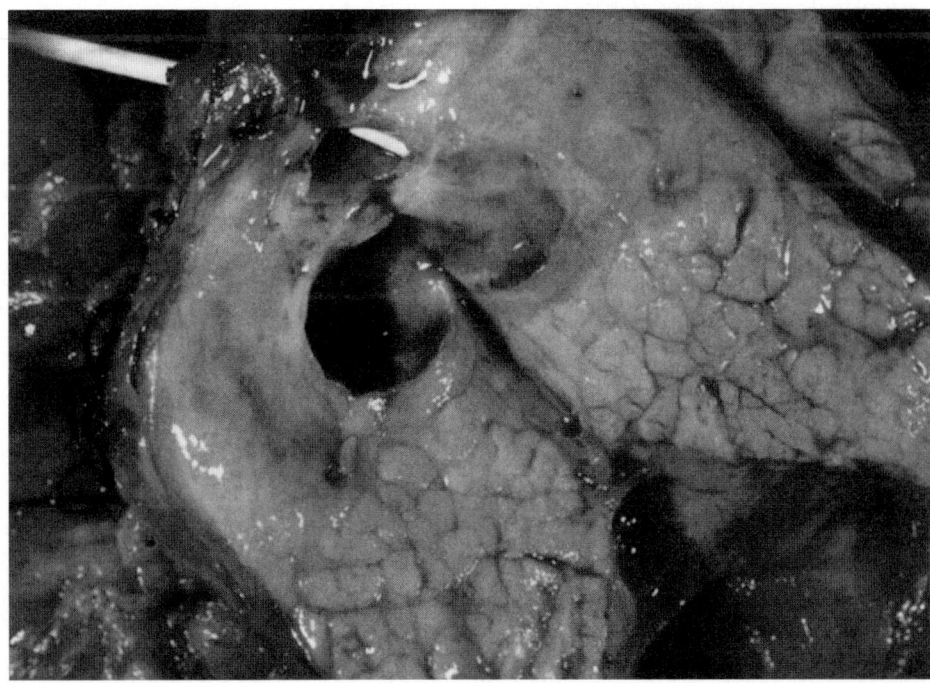

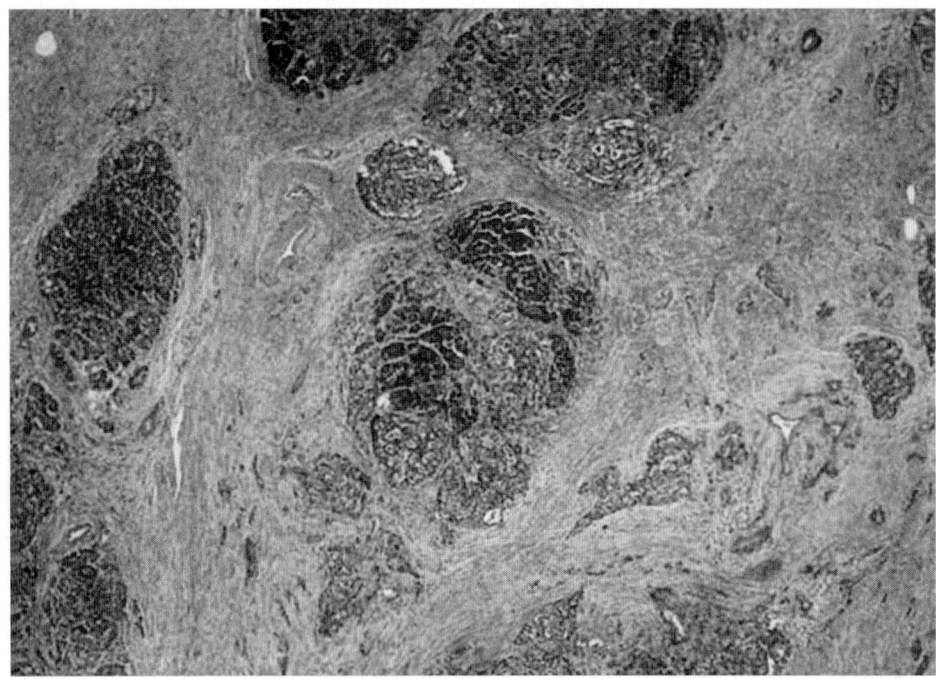

FIG. 32-23. Histology of severe chronic pancreatitis. High-power microscopic (400x) histologic appearance of advanced chronic pancreatitis shows extensive sheets of fibrosis and loss of acinar tissue, with preservation of islet tissue in scattered areas. *(Courtesy of Dr. Rhonda Yantiss, Department of Pathology, University of Massachusetts Medical School.)*

present in stones and protein plugs, and was initially named pancreatic stone protein, or PSP.[124] PSP comprises up to 14% of the protein content of mammalian pancreatic juice, and is secreted in four isoforms (PSP-S2, S3, S4, and S5), with molecular weights ranging from 16 to 20 kd. PSP was found to be a potent inhibitor of calcium carbonate crystal growth, and has subsequently been renamed lithostathine.[125] Independently, a 15-kd fibrillar protein isolated from the pancreas was named pancreatic thread protein, or PTP, and it has been shown to be homologous with lithostathine. Finally, a protein product of the *reg* gene, so named because it is expressed in association with regenerating islets in models of pancreatic injury, was isolated and called *reg* protein.[126] This also has been found to be homologous with lithostathine.[127] No overall homology has been found between lithostathine and other pancreatic proteins. The PSP/PTP/reg/lithostathine gene encodes for a 166-amino acid product that undergoes posttranslational modification to the S2 through S5 isoforms present in pancreatic juice. The protein is expressed in all rodents and mammals, both in the pancreas as well as in brain tissue, where it is found in particularly high concentrations in pyramidal neurons in Alzheimer's disease and Down's syndrome. It is also found in the renal tubules, which is consistent with its biologic action of preventing calcium carbonate precipitation.[127]

Calcium and bicarbonate ions are normally present in pancreatic juice in high concentration, and the solubility product of calcium carbonate is greatly exceeded under normal conditions. Microcrystals of calcium carbonate can be seen in normal pancreatic juice, but are usually clinically silent. Lithostathine is a potent inhibitor of calcium carbonate crystal formation, at a concentration of only 0.1 μmol/L. However, lithostathine concentrations in normal pancreatic juice are in the range of 20 to 25 μmol/L, so a constant suppression of calcium carbonate crystal formation is present in the normal pancreas.

In alcoholics and in patients with alcoholic chronic pancreatitis, lithostathine expression and secretion are dramatically inhibited[127-129] (Fig. 32-25). In addition, elevated levels of precipitated lithostathine in the duct fluid in chronic pancreatitis patients suggests that the availability of the protein may be further reduced by the action of increased proteases and other proteins present in the duct fluid of alcoholic patients. Increased pancreatic juice protein levels in alcoholic men are reversible by abstinence from alcohol,[130] so the availability and effectiveness of lithostathine may be restored in patients with early-stage disease by timely intervention. Nevertheless, calcific stone formation represents an advanced stage of disease, which can further promote injury or symptoms due to mechanical damage to duct epithelium or obstruction of the ductular network.

Duct Distortion

Although calcific stone disease is normally a marker for an advanced stage of disease, parenchymal and ductular calcifications do not always correlate with symptoms. Obstructing main duct stones are commonly observed and are thought to be an indication for endoscopic or surgical removal. The ball-valve effect of a stone in a secreting system produces inevitable episodes of duct obstruction, usually accompanied by pain. But some patients with complete duct obstruction have prolonged periods of painlessness. Ductular hypertension has been documented in patients with proximal stenosis of the main pancreatic duct, and prolonged ductular distention after secretin administration is taken as a sign of ductular obstruction.[131] Although calculus disease and duct enlargement appear together as late stages of chronic pancreatitis, controversy persists over whether they are associated, are independent events, or are causally related.

Radiology

Radiologic imaging of chronic pancreatitis assists in four areas: (1) diagnosis, (2) the evaluation of severity of disease, (3) detection of complications, and (4) assistance in determining treatment options.[132] With the advent of cross-sectional imaging techniques such as computed tomography (CT) and magnetic resonance imaging (MRI), the contour, content, ductal pattern, calcifications, calculi, and cystic disease of the pancreas are all readily discernible.

SAPE HYPOTHESIS

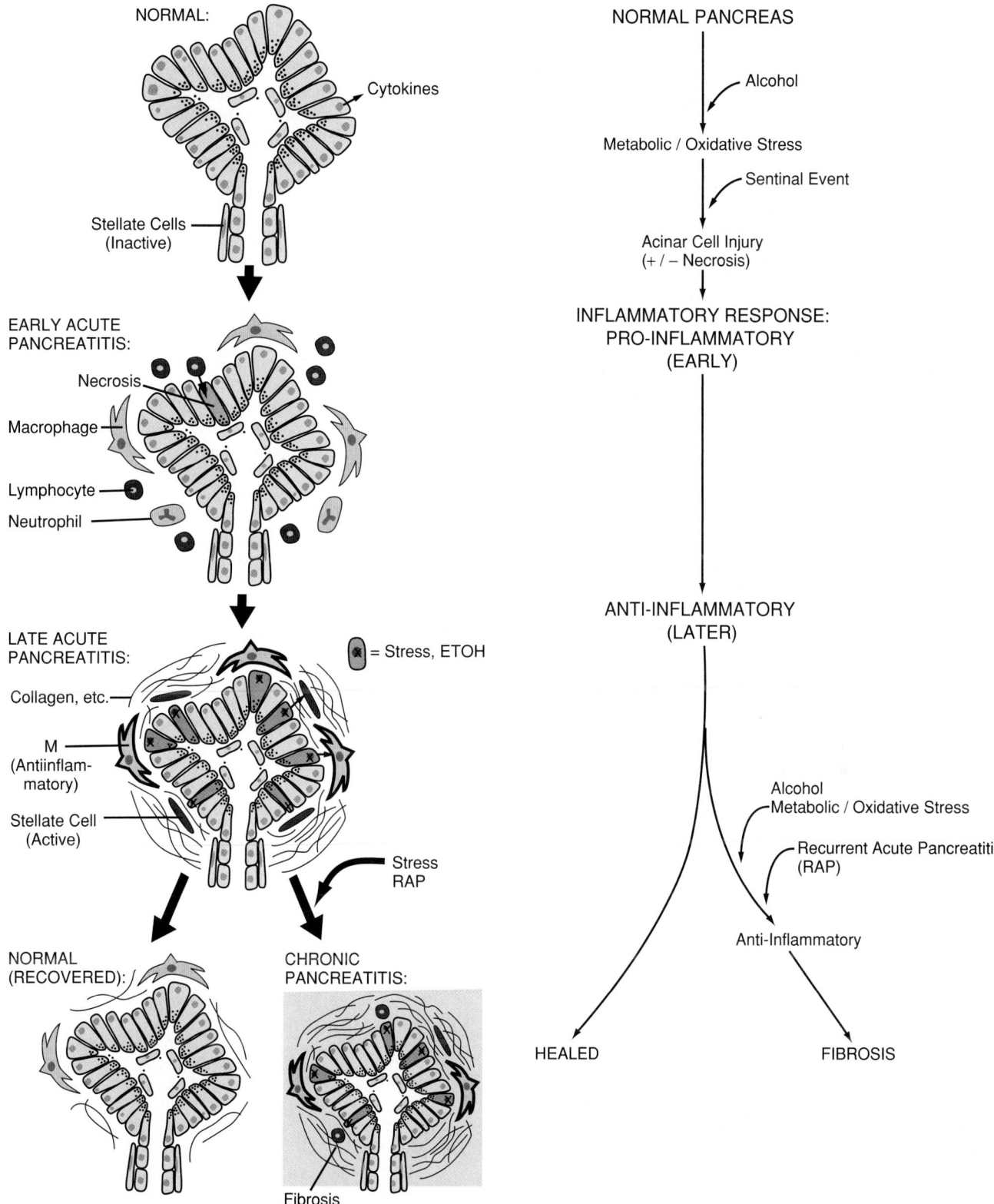

FIG. 32-24. The sentinel acute pancreatitis event (SAPE) hypothesis for the development of chronic pancreatitis. A critical episode of acute pancreatitis activates cytokine-induced transformation of pancreatic stellate cells (PSCs), which results in collagen production and fibrosis. (*Reproduced with permission from Whitcomb.[97]*)

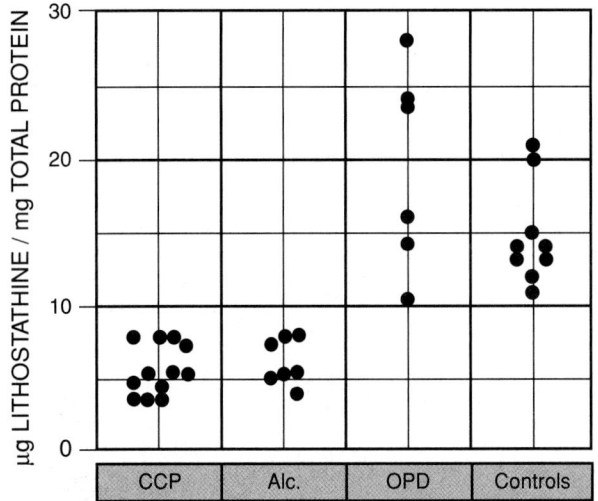

FIG. 32-25. *Lithostathine levels in chronic calcific pancreatitis (CCP) patients, patients with alcohol abuse (ALC), patients with other pancreatic disease (OPD), and controls. (Reproduced with permission from Goggin et al.[127])*

Transabdominal ultrasonography is frequently used as a screening method for patients with abdominal symptoms or trauma, and the extension of ultrasonic imaging to include endoscopic ultrasound (EUS) and laparoscopic ultrasound (LUS) have resulted in the highest-resolution images that are capable of detecting very small (<1 cm) abnormalities in the pancreas. EUS is now frequently employed as a preliminary step in the evaluation of patients with pancreatic disease, and magnetic resonance cholangiopancreatography (MRCP) is increasingly being used to select patients who are candidates for the most invasive imaging method, endoscopic retrograde cholangiopancreatography (ERCP). The staging of disease is important in the care of patients, and a combination of imaging methods is usually employed (Table 32-8).

Ultrasonography is frequently employed as an initial imaging method in patients with abdominal symptoms, and changes consistent with pancreatic duct dilatation, intraductal filling defects, cystic changes, and a heterogeneous texture are seen in chronic pancreati-

tis (Fig. 32-26). The sensitivity of transabdominal ultrasonography ranges from 48 to 96%, and is operator dependent.[133] However, the contour, texture, and ductal pattern are usually quite discernible, and it is a reliable method for periodic re-examination to determine the efficacy of treatment.

EUS has heavily impacted the evaluation and management of patients with chronic pancreatitis. Although it is more operator dependent and less widely available than transabdominal ultrasonography, EUS provides not only imaging capability, but adds the capacity to obtain cytologic and chemical samples of tissue and fluid aspirated with linear array monitoring (Fig. 32-27). EUS images obtained through a high-frequency (7.5- to 12.5-mHz) transducer are able to evaluate subtle changes in 2- to 3-mm structures within the pancreas, and can detect indolent neoplasms in the setting of chronic inflammation. Small intraductal lesions, intraductal mucus, cystic lesions, and subtle ductular abnormalities are recognizable by EUS (Table 32-9). This allows ERCP to be reserved for these patients who require therapeutic maneuvers, or for the evaluation of more complex problems. EUS is comparable to ERCP in the detection or advanced changes in chronic pancreatitis,[134] and may be more sensitive than ERCP in the detection of mild disease.[135]

CT scanning has affected the diagnosis of pancreatic disease more broadly than any other method. Prior to its widespread introduction in the early 1970s, pancreatic imaging was largely a matter of detecting the displacement of adjacent, contrast-filled viscera by mass lesions of the pancreas. Since the introduction of cross-sectional techniques, and with the advent of faster helical CT scanning and CT angiography, visualization of the nature, extent, location, and relative relationships of pancreatic structures and lesions is possible with great clarity. Duct dilatation, calculous disease, cystic changes, inflammatory events, and anomalies are all detectable with a resolution of 3 to 4 mm (Fig. 32-28). CT scanning has a false-negative rate of less than 10% for chronic pancreatitis, but early or mild chronic disease may go undetected by CT imaging. The earliest changes are dilatation of secondary ducts and heterogeneous parenchymal changes, which are detectable by EUS and ERCP. Another drawback of CT scanning is its lower sensitivity for detecting small neoplasms, which are seen with increased frequency in chronic pancreatitis, and may be invisible to all modalities except EUS.

Table 32-8
Cambridge Classification of Pancreatic Morphology in Chronic Pancreatitis

Classification	ERCP Findings	CT and US Findings
Normal	No abnormal SBDs	Normal gland size, shape; homogeneous parenchyma
Equivocal	MPD normal	One of the following: <3 abnormal SBDs; MPD 2–4 mm; gland enlarged <2 times normal size; heterogeneous parenchyma
Mild	MPD normal	Two or more of the following: <3 abnormal SBDs; MPD 2–4 mm; slight gland enlargement; heterogeneous parenchyma
Moderate	MPD changes SBD changes	Small cysts <10 mm; MPD irregularity focal acute pancreatitis; increased echogenicity of MPD walls; gland-contour irregularity

Severe	Any of the above changes plus one or more of the following:
	    Cysts <10 mm; intraductal filling defects; calculi;
	    MPD obstruction or stricture; severe MPD
	    irregularity; contiguous organ invasion	

CT = computed tomography; ERCP = endoscopic retrograde cholangiopancreatography; MPD = main pancreatic duct; SBD = side-branch duct; US = ultrasound.
SOURCE: Reproduced with permission from Freeney.[132]

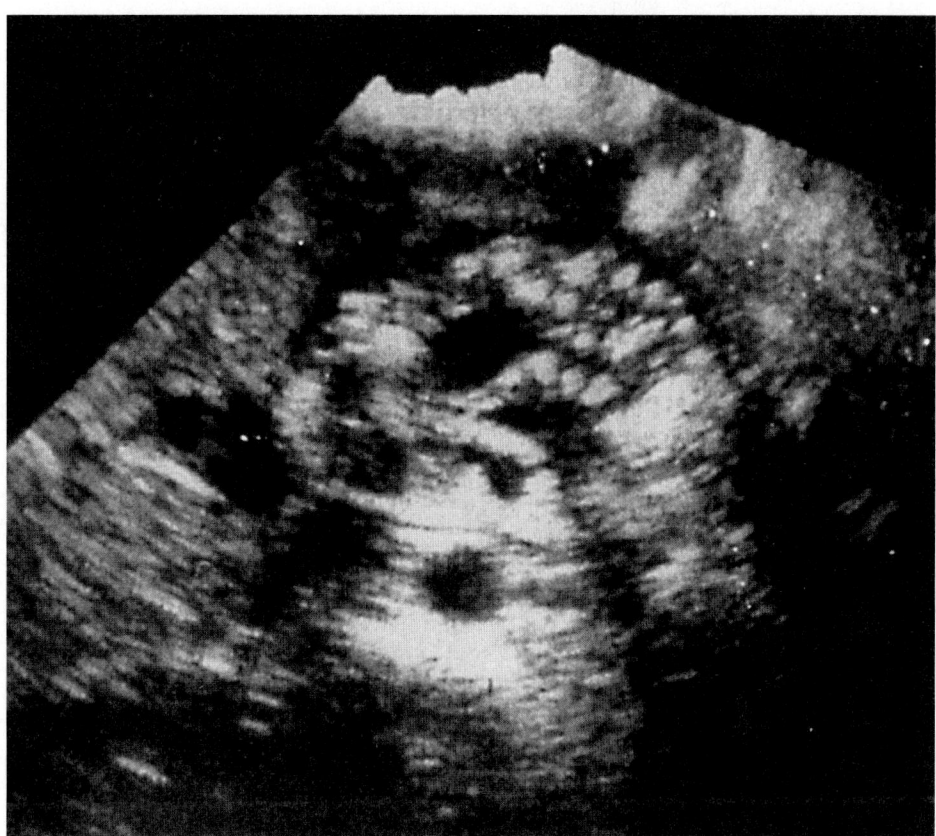

FIG. 32-26. Sonography in chronic pancreatitis. Transabdominal sonogram of patient with chronic pancreatitis demonstrates heterogeneity of the pancreatic parenchyma, dilated ductal systems, and cyst formation. (*Reproduced with permission from Bolondi et al.[133]*)

MRI, in both the cross-sectional mode and the coronally-oriented heavily weighted T2 or high spin ratio imaging (MRCP), that can disclose fluid-filled ducts and cystic lesions, have added greatly to the imaging options for chronic pancreatitis (Fig. 32-29). The resolution of cross-sectional MRI scanning is now approaching that of CT scanning, although the availability of MRI scanners and the complexity of the images produced have limited its large-scale use for routine imaging of the pancreas. MRCP has been shown to be an effective screening technique for disclosing ductal abnormalities that correlates closely with the contrast-filled ducts imaged by ERCP.[136] The advantages of MRCP include its noninvasive methodology, and its ability to image obstructed ducts that are not opacified

FIG. 32-27. Endoscopic ultrasound (EUS) of chronic pancreatitis. The EUS appearance of the parenchyma is heterogenous, and dilated ducts are seen, indicating early obstructive pancreatopathy. (*Courtesy of Dr. Mark Topazian, Division of Digestive Diseases, Department of Medicine, Mayo Clinic.*)

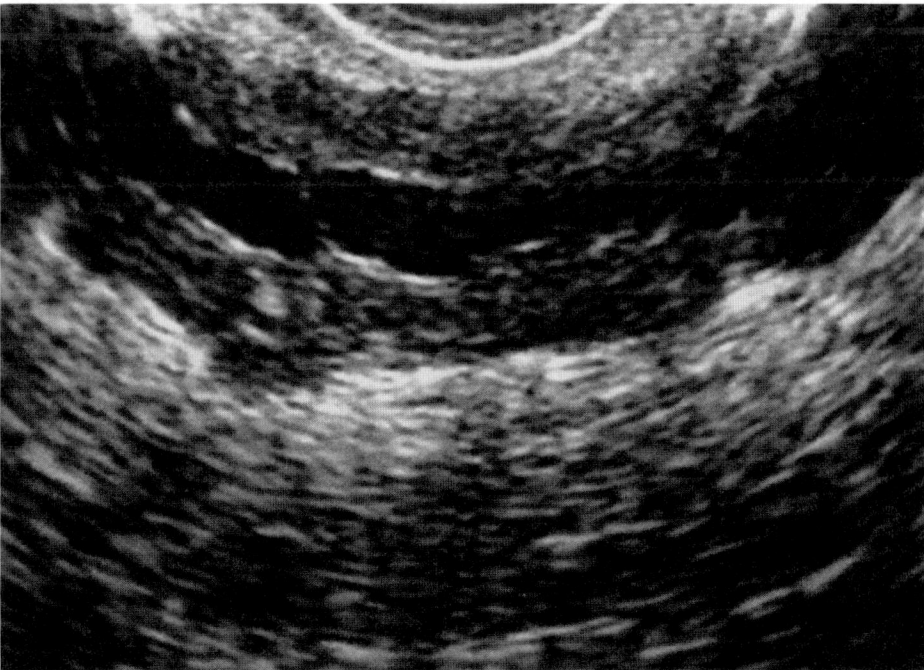

Table 32-9
Complications of Chronic Pancreatitis

Intrapancreatic complications
   Pseudocysts
      Duodenal or gastric obstruction
      Thrombosis of splenic vein
      Abscess
      Perforation
      Erosion into visceral artery
   Inflammatory mass in head of pancreas
      Bile duct stenosis
      Portal vein thrombosis
      Duodenal obstruction
   Duct strictures and/or stones
      Ductal hypertension and dilatation
   Pancreatic carcinoma
Extrapancreatic complications
   Pancreatic duct leak with ascites or fistula
   Pseudocyst extension beyond lesser sac into mediastinum,
      retroperitoneum, lateral pericolic spaces, pelvis, or adjacent viscera

by ERCP injection. It is therefore a useful screening study to detect duct abnormalities and to confirm the need for interventional procedures. Oral, intravenous, and intraductal contrast are unnecessary for MRCP, and its lack of ionizing radiation makes this the safest method to image the ductal system in high-risk patients.

ERCP is considered to be the gold standard for the diagnosis and staging of chronic pancreatitis. It also serves as a vehicle that enables other diagnostic and therapeutic maneuvers, such as biopsy or brushing for cytology, or the employment of stents to relieve obstruction or drain a pseudocyst (Fig. 32-30). Unfortunately, ERCP also carries a risk of procedure-induced pancreatitis that occurs in approximately 5% of patients.[137] Patients at increased risk include those with sphincter of Oddi dysfunction, and those with a previous history of post-ERCP pancreatitis. Post-ERCP pancreatitis occurs after uncomplicated procedures, as well as after those that require prolonged manipulation. Severe pancreatitis and deaths have occurred after ERCP. This method should be reserved for patients in whom the diagnosis is unclear despite the use of other imaging methods, or in whom a diagnostic or therapeutic maneuver is specifically indicated.

Newer imaging methods are being evaluated that detect changes in metabolic activity, instead of radiologic behavior, as a means to analyze abnormal tissue. The positron emission tomographic scan measures focal changes in nutrient (e.g., glucose) metabolism to detect focal changes in tissue behavior. This method has shown usefulness in the detection of occult neoplasms of the brain and lung, and evaluations are currently ongoing to assess its possible role in pancreatic imaging.

Presentation, Natural History, and Complications

Presenting Signs and Symptoms

Pain is the most common symptom of chronic pancreatitis. It is usually midepigastric in location, but may localize or involve either the left or right upper quadrant of the abdomen. Occasionally it is perceived in the lower mid-abdomen, but is frequently described as penetrating through to the back (Fig. 32-31). The pain is typically steady and boring, but not colicky. It persists for hours or days, and may be chronic with exacerbations caused by eating or drinking alcohol. Chronic alcoholics also describe a steady, constant pain that is temporarily relieved by alcohol, followed by a more severe recurrence hours later.[138,139]

Patients with chronic pancreatic pain typically flex their abdomen and either sit or lie with their hips flexed, or lie on their side in a fetal position. Unlike ureteral stone pain or biliary colic, the pain causes the patient to be still. Nausea or vomiting may accompany the pain, but anorexia is the most common associated symptom.

Pain from chronic pancreatitis has been ascribed to three possible etiologies. Ductal hypertension, due to strictures or stones, may predispose to pain that is initiated or exacerbated by eating. Chronic pain without exacerbation may be related to parenchymal disease or retroperitoneal inflammation with persistent neural involvement. Acute exacerbations of pain in the setting of chronic pain may be

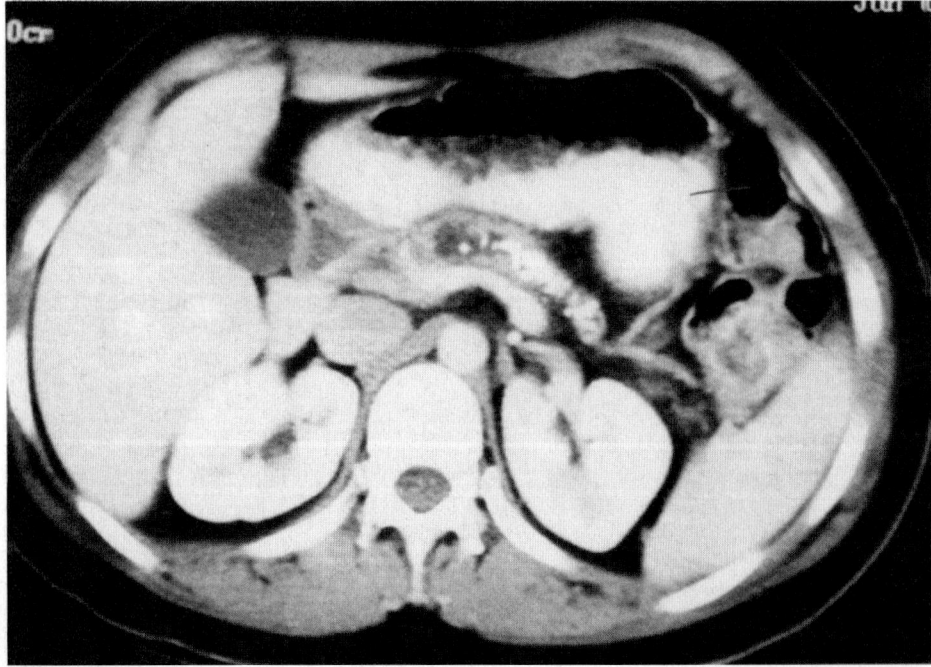

FIG. 32-28. CT imaging of chronic pancreatitis. A dilated pancreatic duct is seen, with evidence of intraductal stones and parenchymal calcification.

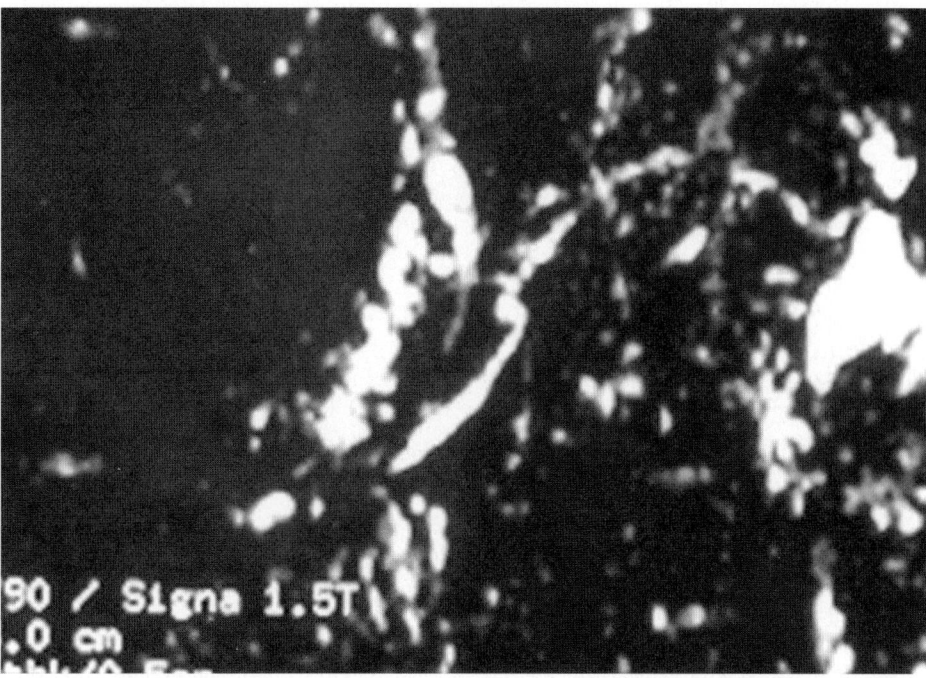

FIG. 32-29. Magnetic resonance cholangiopancreatography (MRCP) in chronic pancreatitis. A dilated pancreatic duct suggests obstructive pancreatopathy due to proximal scarring.

due to acute increases in duct pressure, or recurrent episodes of acute inflammation in the setting of chronic parenchymal disease. Nealon and Matin have described these various pain syndromes as being predictive of the response to various surgical procedures.[140] Pain that is found in association with ductal hypertension is most readily relieved by pancreatic duct decompression, through endoscopic stenting or surgical decompression.[139]

Ammann and colleagues also studied the pain patterns of patients with chronic pancreatitis and observed that the pain was commonly of relatively short (<10 days) duration, after which it was absent for long periods, or relentless or frequent, in which case it lasted for months.[141] Patients in the latter category frequently had other complications of pancreatitis, such as pseudocyst or duodenal compression.

FIG. 32-30. Pancreatic duct stenting. At ERCP, a stent is placed in the proximal pancreatic duct to relieve obstruction and reduce symptoms of pain. Pancreatic duct stents are left in place for only a limited time to avoid further inflammation.

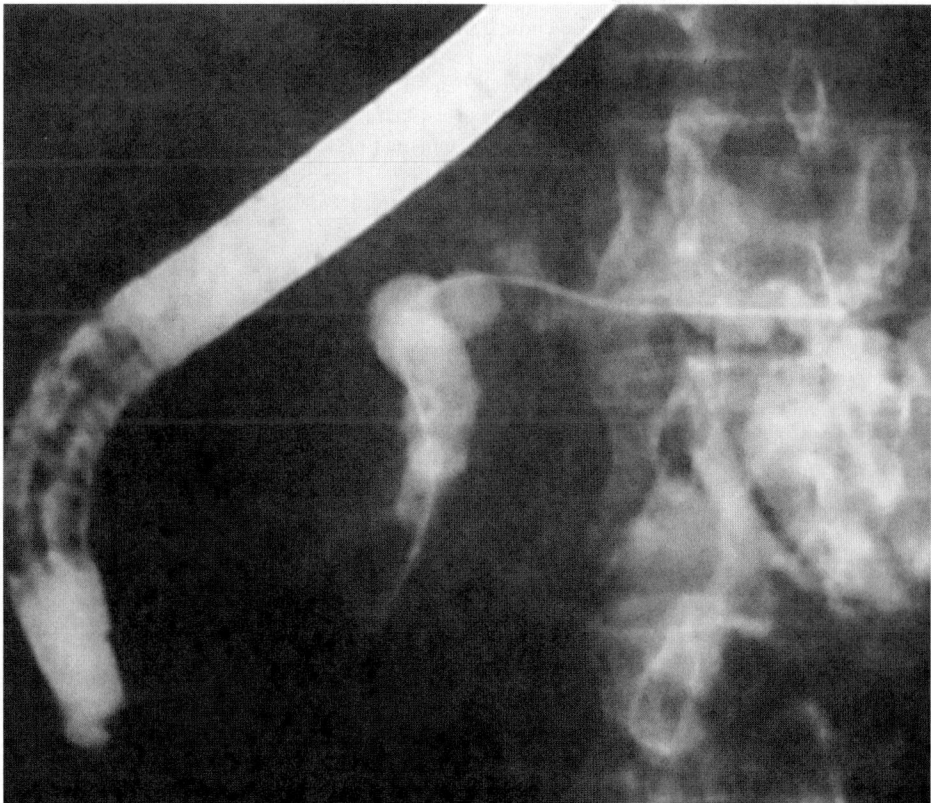

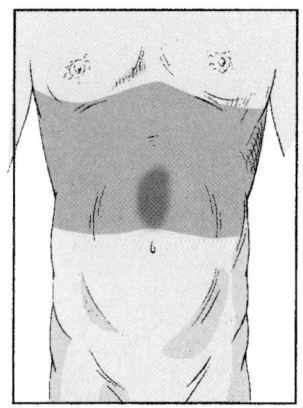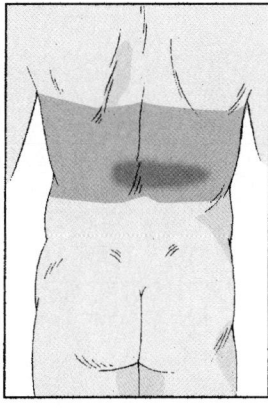

FIG. 32-31. Pain location in chronic pancreatitis. *(Reproduced with permission from Murayama et al.[138]).*

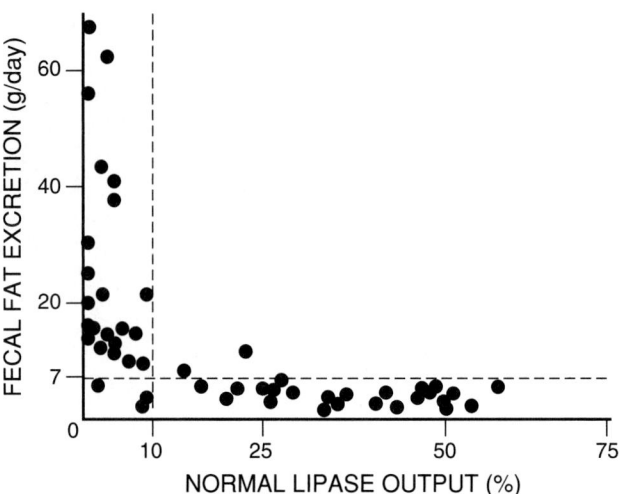

FIG. 32-32. Relationship of lipase output to fat malabsorption. Excess fecal fat appears when the pancreatic lipase output falls below 10% of normal secretory values. *(Reproduced with permission from DiMagno et al.[148]).*

The pain of chronic pancreatitis may decrease or disappear completely over a period of years, as symptoms of exocrine and endocrine deficiency become apparent.[142,143] This is referred to as "burned out" pancreatitis, and correlates with the progression of disease from a mild or moderate stage to severe destruction of the pancreas.[144] Despite the typical development of narcotic addiction, inability to work, and the sequelae of chronic illness, some physicians and some socialized health systems seek this outcome as a goal of therapy. To do so sentences the patient to a (shortened) lifetime of opioid use, prevents rehabilitation, and is a socioeconomic loss.

Although increased ductal pressure, and therefore parenchymal pressure, is thought to be the cause of pain in chronic obstructive pancreatitis,[145] the role of chronic inflammation per se, and the development of actual nerve damage in the diseased gland, are also thought to contribute to pain.[146] Chronic inflammation results in the infiltration of tissue by macrophages, which secrete prostaglandins and other nociceptive agents that cause chronic stimulation of afferent neural fibers. Inflammatory damage to the perineurial layers surrounding the unmyelinated pancreatic nerves, and a focal infiltration of inflammatory cells around nerves, suggest that neural fibers are a target for the cellular response to inflammation in the pancreas.[147]

Strategies to relieve pain are therefore based on three approaches: (1) reduce secretion and/or decompress the secretory compartment, (2) resect the focus of chronic inflammatory change, or (3) interrupt the transmission of afferent neural impulses through neural ablative procedures. A trial of antisecretory therapy or endoscopic duct damage may select those patients who will benefit preferentially from a decompressive procedure.

Malabsorption and Weight Loss

When pancreatic exocrine capacity falls below 10% of normal, diarrhea and steatorrhea develop[148] (Fig. 32-32). Patients describe a bulky, foul-smelling, loose (but not watery) stool that may be pale in color and float on the surface of toilet water. Frequently, patients will describe a greasy or oily appearance to the stool, or may describe an "oil slick" on the water's surface. In severe steatorrhea, an orange, oily stool is often reported.[50] As exocrine deficiency increases, symptoms of steatorrhea are often accompanied by weight loss. Patients may describe a good appetite despite weight loss, or diminished food intake due to abdominal pain.

In severe symptomatic chronic pancreatitis, anorexia or nausea may occur with or separate from abdominal pain. The combination of decreased food intake and malabsorption of nutrients usually results in chronic weight loss. As a result, many patients with severe chronic pancreatitis are below ideal body weight.

Lipase deficiency tends to manifest itself before trypsin deficiency,[149] so the presence of steatorrhea may be the first functional sign of pancreatic insufficiency. As pancreatic exocrine function deteriorates further, the secretion of bicarbonate into the duodenum is reduced, which causes duodenal acidification and further impairs nutrient absorption.[150]

Pancreatogenic Diabetes

The islets comprise only 2% of the mass of the pancreas, but they are preferentially conserved when pancreatic inflammation occurs. In chronic pancreatitis, acinar tissue loss and replacement by fibrosis is greater than the degree of loss of islet tissue, although islets are typically smaller than normal, and may be isolated from their surrounding vascular network by the fibrosis. With progressive destruction of the gland, endocrine insufficiency commonly occurs. Frank diabetes is seen initially in about 20% of patients with chronic pancreatitis, and impaired glucose metabolism can be detected in up to 70% of patients. In a study of 500 patients with predominantly alcoholic chronic pancreatitis, diabetes developed in 83% within 25 years of the clinical onset of chronic pancreatitis, and more than half of the diabetic patients required insulin treatment.[151] Ketoacidosis and diabetic nephropathy are relatively uncommon in pancreatogenic diabetes (Table 32-10), but retinopathy and neuropathy are seen to occur with a similar frequency as in idiopathic diabetes.[152]

Pancreatogenic diabetes is more common after surgical resection for chronic pancreatitis.[151] Distal pancreatectomy and Whipple procedures have a higher incidence of diabetes than do drainage procedures, and the severity of diabetes is frequently worse after partial pancreatectomy.[153]

The etiology and pathophysiology of pancreatogenic or type III diabetes is distinct from that of either insulin-dependent (type I) or non-insulin-independent (type II) diabetes. In pancreatogenic diabetes, due to the loss of functioning pancreatic tissue by disease or surgical removal, there is a global deficiency of all three glucoregulatory islet cell hormones: insulin, glucagon, and pancreatic polypeptide (PP). In addition, there is a paradoxical combination of enhanced peripheral sensitivity to insulin, and decreased hepatic sensitivity to insulin.[154] As a result, insulin therapy is frequently

Table 32-10
Types of Diabetes Mellitus

Parameter	Type I IDDM Juvenile Onset	Type II NIDDM Adult Onset	Type III Pancreatogenic Postoperative Onset
Ketoacidosis	Common	Rare	Rare
Hyperglycemia	Severe	Usually mild	Mild
Hypoglycemia	Common	Rare	Common
Peripheral insulin sensitivity	Normal or increased	Decreased	Increased
Hepatic insulin sensitivity	Normal	Normal or decreased	Decreased
Insulin levels	Low	High	Low
Glucagon levels	Normal or high	Normal or high	Low
Pancreatic polypeptide levels	High	High	Low
Typical age of onset	Childhood or adolescence	Adulthood	Any

IDDM = insulin-dependent diabetes mellitus; NIDDM = non-insulin-dependent diabetes mellitus.
SOURCE: Reproduced with permission from Slezak et al.[153]

difficult; patients are hyperglycemic when insulin replacement is insufficient (due to unsuppressed hepatic glucose production) or hypoglycemic when insulin replacement is barely excessive (due to enhanced peripheral insulin sensitivity and a deficiency of pancreatic glucagon secretion to counteract the hypoglycemia). This form of diabetes is referred to as "brittle" diabetes, and requires special attention.

Although the primary hormonal deficit is a loss of insulin secretory capacity, the additional deficiencies of glucagon and PP are pathognomonic for pancreatogenic diabetes. PP has recently been shown to be important in the regulation of insulin action.[155] The expression of the hepatic insulin receptor gene, and the subsequent availability and action of insulin receptors on hepatocyte membranes, are regulated by PP.[156,157] PP deficiency correlates with the severity of chronic pancreatitis, and impairments in the hepatic

action of insulin are reversed in PP-deficient chronic pancreatitis patients by administration of PP[158] (Fig. 32-33).

Because PP cells are predominantly located in the posterior head and uncinate process of the pancreas,[159] proximal pancreatectomy is invariably associated with profound PP deficiency. Seymour and associates studied a group of nondiabetic young men who had previously undergone various pancreatic resections for trauma, and showed that those who were PP deficient had a measurable loss of hepatic insulin sensitivity, and that this was reversed by PP administration[160] (Fig. 32-34). In addition, Hanazaki and colleagues showed that the addition of PP to insulin delivered via a pump in pancreatectomized dogs resulted in decreased insulin requirements

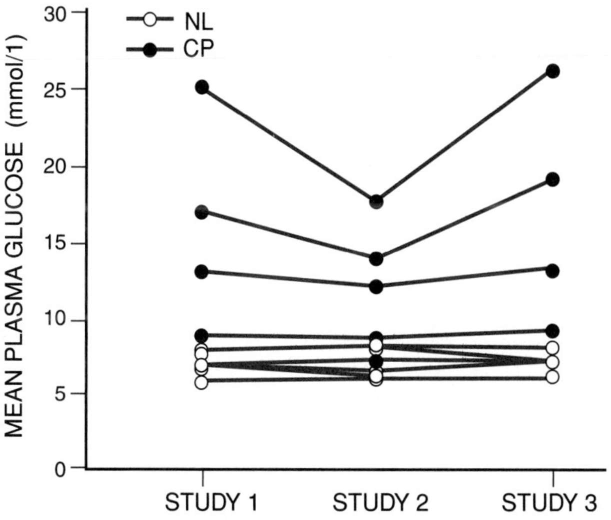

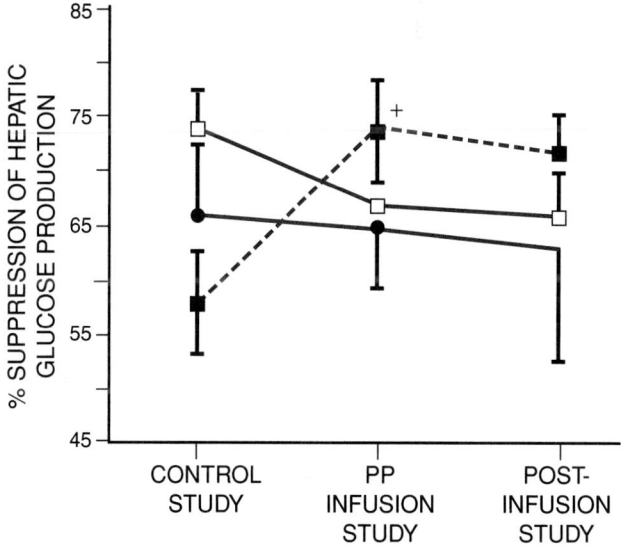

FIG. 32-33. Effect of pancreatic polypeptide (PP) replacement on plasma glucose levels. Main plasma glucose levels following ingestion of glucose (40 g/m² body surface area) before (study #1), immediately after (study #2) and 1 month after (study #3) an 8-hour infusion of bovine PP. NL represents normal control subjects (n = 6) and CP represents patients with chronic pancreatitis (n = 5), three of whom had an initial diabetic response. (Reproduced with permission from Brunicardi et al.[158]).

FIG. 32-34. Effect of PP infusion on insulin-induced suppression of hepatic glucose production. The percentage of suppression of hepatic glucose production (Rah) before (control study), during (PP infusion study) and 1 month after (postinfusion study) an 8-hour infusion of bovine PP, during a background infusion of insulin (0.25 mU/kg per minute). The results in normal subjects (open boxes), pancreatic resection patients with normal PP levels (closed symbols, solid line), and pancreatic resection patients with deficient PP levels (closed symbols, dashed line) are shown (+p < 0.02). (Reproduced with permission from Seymour et al.[160])

Table 32-11
Tests for Chronic Pancreatitis

I. Measurement of pancreatic products in blood
  A. Enzymes
  B. Pancreatic polypeptide
II. Measurement of pancreatic exocrine secretion
  A. Direct measurements
    1. Enzymes
    2. Bicarbonate
  B. Indirect measurement
    1. Bentiromide test
    2. Schilling test
    3. Fecal fat, chymotrypsin, or elastase concentration
    4. [^{14}C]-olein absorption
III. Imaging techniques
  A. Plain film radiography of abdomen
  B. Ultrasonography
  C. Computed tomography
  D. Endoscopic retrograde cholangiopancreatography
  E. Magnetic resonance cholangiopancreatography
  F. Endoscopic ultrasonography

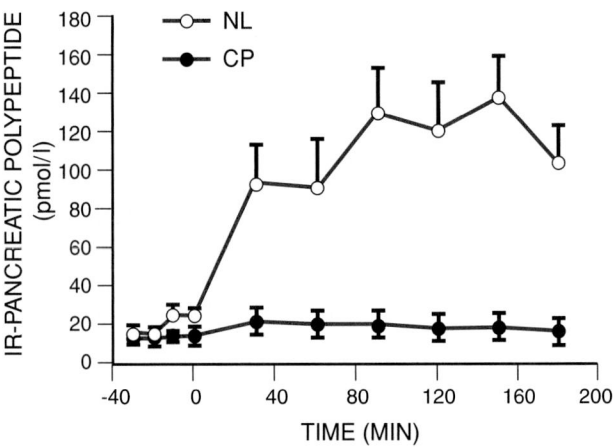

FIG. 32-35. Pancreatic polypeptide (PP) response to a test meal. Immunoreactive PP (IR-PP) responses in control subjects (NL, n = 6) and patients with severe chronic pancreatitis (CP) accompanied by PP deficiency (CP, n = 5) are shown. A test meal was administered at 0 minutes. Means ± SEM are shown. (Reproduced with permission from Brunicardi et al.[158]).

to achieve glucose control.[161] This suggests that the treatment of pancreatogenic diabetes may be improved by the use of PP or a PP receptor agonist.

Laboratory Studies

Unlike chronic liver disease or abnormalities of the upper and lower gastrointestinal tract, pancreatic disease presents a diagnostic challenge because a tissue biopsy and histologic confirmation of the type and stage of the disease process is almost never obtainable outside of the operating room. As a result, the diagnosis of chronic pancreatitis depends on the clinical presentation, a limited number of indirect measurements that correlate with pancreatic function, and selected imaging studies (Table 32-11).

The direct measurement of pancreatic enzymes (e.g., lipase and amylase) by blood test is highly sensitive and fairly specific in acute pancreatitis, but is seldom helpful in the diagnosis of chronic pancreatitis. The pancreatic endocrine product that correlates most strongly with chronic pancreatitis is the PP response to a test meal (Fig. 32-35). Severe chronic pancreatitis is associated with a blunted or absent PP response to feeding, but as with many other tests, a normal PP response does not rule out the presence of early disease.[162]

The measurement of pancreatic exocrine secretion requires aspiration of pancreatic juice from the duodenum after nutrient (Lundh test meal) or hormonal (cholecystokinin [CCK] or secretin) stimulation.[163,164] Direct aspiration of pancreatic juice by endoscopic cannulation of the duct has been proposed, but is not risk free, comfortable for the patient, or more sensitive than luminal intubation methods.[165]

Indirect tests of pancreatic exocrine function are based on the measurement of metabolites of compounds which are altered ("digested") by pancreatic exocrine products, and which can be quantified by serum or urine measurements. A commonly used indirect test is the bentiromide test, in which N-benzoyl-L-tyrosyl-p-aminobenzoic acid (NBT-PABA) is ingested by the subject, and the urinary excretion of the proteolytic metabolite PABA is measured. Free PABA is absorbed from the small intestine and excreted by the kidney in a linear correlation with the degree of chymotrypsin degradation of NBT-PABA.[166] Although the sensitivity of the test is as high as 100% in patients with severe chronic pancreatitis, it identifies only 40 to 50% of patients with mild disease.[167] Furthermore, reduced PABA excretion is found in patients with a variety of other

gastrointestinal, hepatic, and renal diseases. Therefore the test is of value not for the diagnosis of chronic pancreatitis, but for determining the extent of exocrine pancreatic insufficiency in patients with known disease.

Similarly, the absorption of vitamin B$_{12}$ is adversely affected by pancreatic exocrine insufficiency, and the recovery of urinary cobalamin correlates with the functional impairment. This method is referred to as the Schilling test, and has been modified by the addition of cobalamin binding agents such as intrinsic factor and R protein, which are differentially affected by exocrine secretion.[168] The test also is limited by poor sensitivity in patients with mild disease.

Fecal levels of chymotrypsin[169] and elastase[170] have been proposed as simpler, less expensive tests of exocrine function, and correlate well with loss of pancreatic function. As with other test methods, however, these tests lose their sensitivity in patients with mild to moderate chronic pancreatitis, and may be more sensitive for other causes of pancreatic dysfunction, including cystic fibrosis.

The quantification of stool fat has also been used as a measure of pancreatic lipase secretion, either through the direct measurement of total fecal fat levels while the subject consumes a diet of known fat content, or by the measurement of exhaled $^{14}CO_2$ after ingestion of [^{14}C]-triolein or [^{14}C]-olein. This so-called triolein breath test is less cumbersome than intubation methods, and avoids the necessity of stool collections and analysis, but also has a high false-negative rate.[171]

Radiologic imaging has become the principal method of diagnosis of chronic pancreatitis, with the codification of classification systems that correlate with proven disease. ERCP has been considered the most sensitive radiologic test for the diagnosis of chronic pancreatitis, with specific ERCP findings which are highly correlative with the degree or stage of chronic disease[172] (Table 32-12). CT scanning is sensitive for the diagnosis of chronic pancreatitis when calcification, duct dilatation, or cystic disease is present, but is not accurate in the absence of these findings. CT is helpful as a screening study to guide interventional therapy, or other diagnostic modalites.[132] EUS has recently become a more widely used study for the diagnosis of pancreatic disease, and offers the advantage of very-high-resolution images of the pancreatic parenchyma, the main and

Table 32-12
Cambridge Classification of Chronic Pancreatitis by Endoscopic Retrograde Cholangiopancreatography

Grade	Main Pancreatic Duct	Side Branches
Normal	Normal	Normal
Suggestive	Normal	<3 Abnormal
Mild	Normal	≥3 Abnormal
Moderate	Abnormal	>3 Abnormal
Severe	Abnormal plus at least one of the following: Large cavity Duct obstruction Dilation or duct irregularity Intraductal filing defects	

SOURCE: Reproduced with permission from Axon A: Endoscopic retrograde cholangiopancreatography in chronic pancreatitis: The Cambridge classification. *Radiol Clin North Am* 27:39, 1989.

secondary ductal systems, cystic lesions, and calcific changes.[173] Although operator dependent and invasive, the technique is far safer than ERCP, and in experienced hands is excellent for the diagnosis in moderate and severe stage disease[134] (Table 32-13). Most importantly, EUS is highly reliable in ruling out pancreatic carcinoma when EUS findings are normal.[174] Recent studies suggest that EUS may be more valuable than ERCP for the diagnosis of early chronic pancreatitis.[175]

Prognosis and Natural History

The prognosis for patients with chronic pancreatitis is dependent on the etiology of disease, the development of complications, and on the age and socioeconomic status of the patient. The influence of treatment is less evident in long-term studies, although the general absence of randomized, prospective trials clouds the issue of whether specific forms of therapy alter the long-term outlook for patients with the disease.[176]

Several studies have demonstrated that although symptoms of pain decrease over time in about half of the patients, this decline is also accompanied by a progression of exocrine and endocrine insufficiency.[142–144,177] In general, the likelihood of eventual pain relief is dependent upon the stage of disease at diagnosis, and the persistence of alcohol use in patients with alcoholic chronic pancreatitis. Miyake and colleagues found that pain relief was achieved in 60% of alcoholic patients who successfully discontinued drinking, but in only 26% who did not.[177]

Table 32-13
Endoscopic Ultrasound Features of Chronic Pancreatitis

Endoscopic Ultrasound Feature	Implication
Ductal changes	
Duct size >3 mm	Ductal dilation
Tortuous pancreatic duct	Ductal irregularity
Intraductal echogenic foci	Stones or calcification
Echogenic duct wall	Ductal fibrosis
Side-branch ectasia	Periductal fibrosis
Parenchymal changes	
Inhomogeneous echo pattern	Edema
Reduced echogenic foci (1–3 mm)	Edema
Enhanced echogenic foci	Calcifications
Prominent interlobular septae	Fibrosis
Lobular outer gland margin	Fibrosis, glandular atrophy
Large, echo-poor cavities (>5 mm)	Pseudocyst

SOURCE: Reproduced with permission from Catalano et al.[135]

The long-term survival of patients with chronic pancreatitis is less than for patients without pancreatitis. In an international multi-center study of over 2000 patients, Lowenfels and colleagues found that the 10- and 20-year survival rates for patients with chronic pancreatitis were 70 and 45%, respectively, compared to 93 and 65% for patients without pancreatitis.[178] The mortality risk was found to be 1.6-fold higher in patients who continued to abuse alcohol, compared to those who did not (Fig. 32-36). Continued alcohol abuse has a similar effect on the response to surgical treatment (Fig. 32-37), and results in a twofold increase in mortality over a 10- to 14-year follow-up period.[179]

In addition to progressive endocrine and exocrine dysfunction, and the risk of the specific complications outlined below, the other significant long-term risk for the patient with chronic pancreatitis is the development of pancreatic carcinoma.[180] There is a progressive, cumulative increased risk of carcinoma development in patients with chronic pancreatitis, which continues throughout the subsequent lifetime of the patient (Fig. 32-38). The incidence of carcinoma in patients with chronic pancreatitis ranges from 1.5 to 2.7%,[143,144] which is at least tenfold greater than that of patients of similar age seen in a hospital setting. In patients with advanced chronic pancreatitis referred for surgical therapy, the risk of indolent carcinoma can be over 10%.[181] The development of carcinoma

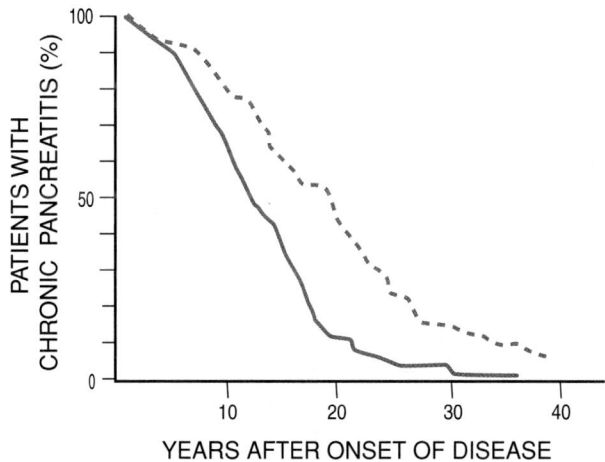

FIG. 32-36. Cumulative survival of patients with chronic pancreatitis. The overall survival rate for patients with chronic pancreatitis, with (*solid line*) or without (*dashed line*) continued alcohol abuse. (*Reproduced with permission from Lankisch.*[176])

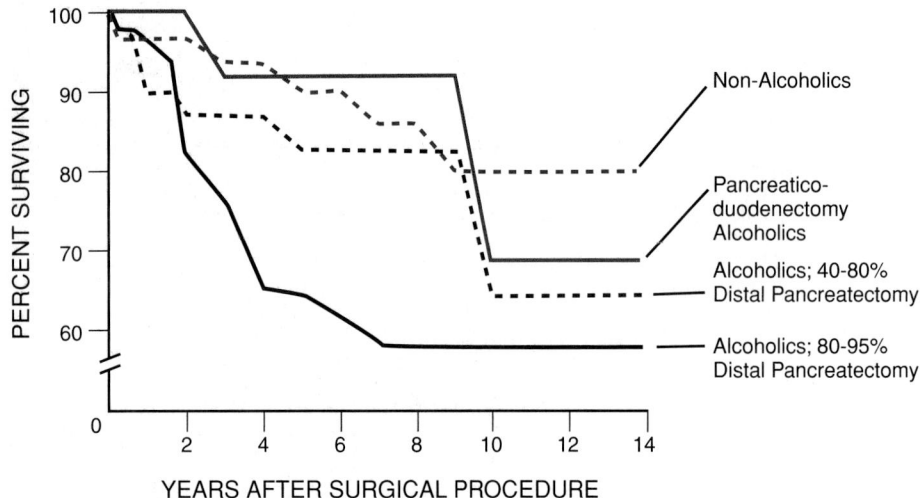

FIG. 32-37. Effect of alcohol use on survival after surgical procedures. The cumulative survival of patients with chronic pancreatitis following pancreaticoduodenectomy or distal pancreatectomy is shown for nonalcoholic and alcoholic patients. (*Reproduced with permission from Frey et al.[179]*)

in the setting of chronic pancreatitis is no doubt related to the dysregulation of cellular proliferation and tissue repair processes in the setting of chronic inflammation, as is seen throughout the alimentary tract and elsewhere. In the setting of chronic pancreatitis, carcinoma development can be especially cryptic, and the diagnosis of early-stage tumors is particularly difficult. Awareness of this risk justifies close surveillance for cancer in patients with chronic pancreatitis. Periodic measurement of tumor markers such as CA19-9, and periodic imaging of the pancreas with CT scan and EUS are necessary to detect the development of carcinoma in the patient with chronic pancreatitis.

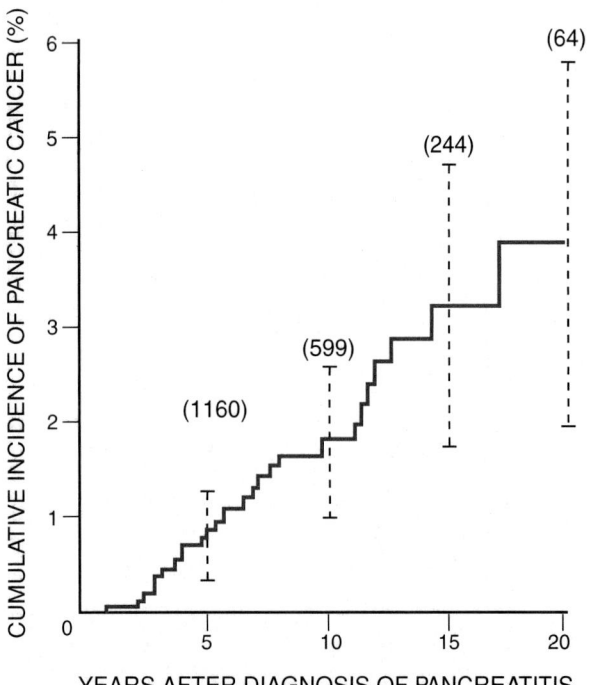

FIG. 32-38. Cumulative risk of pancreatic cancer in patients with chronic pancreatitis. The number of patients evaluated at different time intervals is shown in parentheses. (*Reproduced with permission from Lowenfels et al.[180]*)

Complications

Pseudocyst. A chronic collection of pancreatic fluid surrounded by a nonepithelialized wall of granulation tissue and fibrosis is referred to as a pseudocyst. Pseudocysts occur in up to 10% of patients with acute pancreatitis, and in 20 to 38% of patients with chronic pancreatitis, and thus they comprise the most common complication of chronic pancreatitis.[143,182,183] The identification and treatment of pseudocysts requires definition of the various forms of pancreatic fluid collections that occur (Table 32-14). In chronic pancreatitis, a pancreatic duct leak with extravasation of pancreatic juice results in a peripancreatic fluid collection (PFC). Over a period of 3 to 4 weeks, the PFC is sealed by an inflammatory reaction that leads to development of a wall of acute granulation tissue without much fibrosis. This is referred to as an acute pseudocyst. Acute pseudocysts may resolve spontaneously in up to 50% of cases, over a course of 6 weeks or longer.[182,183] Pseudocysts larger than 6 cm resolve less frequently than smaller ones, but may regress over a period of weeks to months. Pseudocysts are multiple in 17% of patients,[184] or may be multilobulated. They may occur intrapancreatically, or extend beyond the region of the pancreas into other cavities or compartments (Fig. 32-39).

Pseudocysts may become secondarily infected, in which case they become abscesses. They can compress or obstruct adjacent organs or structures, leading to superior mesenteric-portal vein thrombosis or splenic vein thrombosis.[185] They can erode into visceral arteries and cause intracystic hemorrhage or pseudoaneurysms (Fig. 32-40). They also can perforate and cause peritonitis or intraperitoneal bleeding.[186]

Pseudocysts usually cause symptoms of pain, fullness, or early satiety. Asymptomatic pseudocysts can be managed expectantly, and may resolve spontaneously or persist without complication.[183,188] Symptomatic or enlarging pseudocysts require treatment, and any presumed pseudocyst without a documented antecedent episode of acute pancreatitis requires investigation to determine the etiology of the lesion.[187] Although pseudocysts comprise roughly two thirds of all pancreatic cystic lesions, they resemble cystadenomas and cystadenocarcinoma radiographically. An incidentally discovered cystic lesion should be examined by EUS and aspirated to determine whether it is a true neoplasm or a pseudocyst.

The timing and method of treatment requires careful consideration.[188,189] Pitfalls in the management of pseudocysts

Table 32-14
Definitions of Pancreatic Fluid Collections

Term	Definition
Peripancreatic fluid collection	A collection of enzyme-rich pancreatic juice which occurs early in the course of acute pancreatitis, or which forms after a pancreatic duct leak; located in or near the pancreas, it lacks a well organized wall of granulation or fibrous tissue
Early pancreatic (sterile) necrosis	A focal or diffuse area of nonviable pancreatic parenchyma, typically occupying more than 30% of the gland, and containing liquefied debris and fluid
Late pancreatic (sterile) necrosis	An organized collection of sterile necrotic debris and fluid with a well-defined margin or wall within the normal domain of the pancreas
Acute pseudocyst	A collection of pancreatic juice enclosed within a perimeter of early granulation tissue, usually as a consequence of acute pancreatitis which has occurred within the preceding 3–4 weeks
Chronic pseudocyst	A collection of pancreatic fluid surrounded by a wall of normal granulation and fibrous tissue, usually persisting for more than 6 weeks
Pancreatic abscess	Any of the above in which gross purulence (pus) is present, with bacterial or fungal organisms documented to be present

SOURCE: Modified with permission from Baron et al.[189]

result from the incorrect (presumptive) diagnosis of a cystic neoplasm masquerading as a pseudocyst, a failure to appreciate the solid or debris-filled contents of a pseudocyst which appears to be fluid filled on CT scan, and a failure to document true adherence with an adjacent portion of the stomach before attempting transgastric internal drainage. Therefore the management of a pseudocyst, as with other treatment decisions regarding chronic pancreatitis, should involve the multidisciplinary evaluation and selection of any given treatment strategy. Surgeons, therapeutic endoscopists, and interventional radiologists together offer all the expertise necessary to obtain the best possible outcome for a patient with pseudocystic disease. The challenge is to select the best approach for each individual patient, and this requires dedicated and experienced representatives from each specialty to participate in the decision making.

If infection is suspected, the pseudocyst should be aspirated (not drained) by CT- or US-guided fine-needle aspiration, and the contents examined for organisms by Gram's stain and culture.[190] If

infection is present, and the contents resemble pus, external drainage is employed using either surgical or percutaneous techniques.

If the pseudocyst has failed to resolve with conservative therapy and symptoms persist, internal drainage is usually preferred to external drainage, to avoid the complication of a pancreaticocutaneous fistula. Pseudocysts communicate with the pancreatic ductal system in up to 80% of cases,[184,189] so external drainage creates a pathway for pancreatic duct leakage to and through the catheter exit site. Internal drainage may be performed with either percutaneous catheter-based methods (transgastric puncture and stent placement to create a cystogastrostomy), endoscopic methods (transgastric or transduodenal puncture and multiple stent placements, with or without a nasocystic irrigation catheter), or surgical methods (a true cystoenterostomy, biopsy of cyst wall, and evacuation of all debris and contents). Surgical options include a cystogastrostomy (Fig. 32-41), a Roux-en-Y cystojejunostomy, or a cystoduodenostomy. Cystojejunostomy is the most versatile method, and it can be applied to

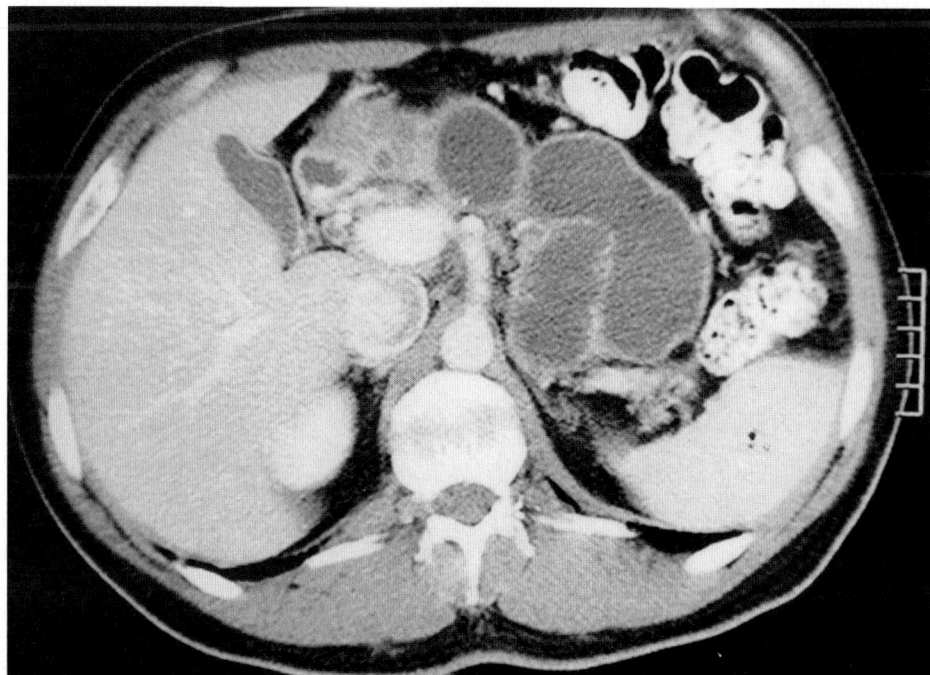

FIG. 32-39. Extensive pseudocyst disease. A CT scan in a patient with alcoholic chronic pancreatitis demonstrates multiloculated pseudocyst disease.

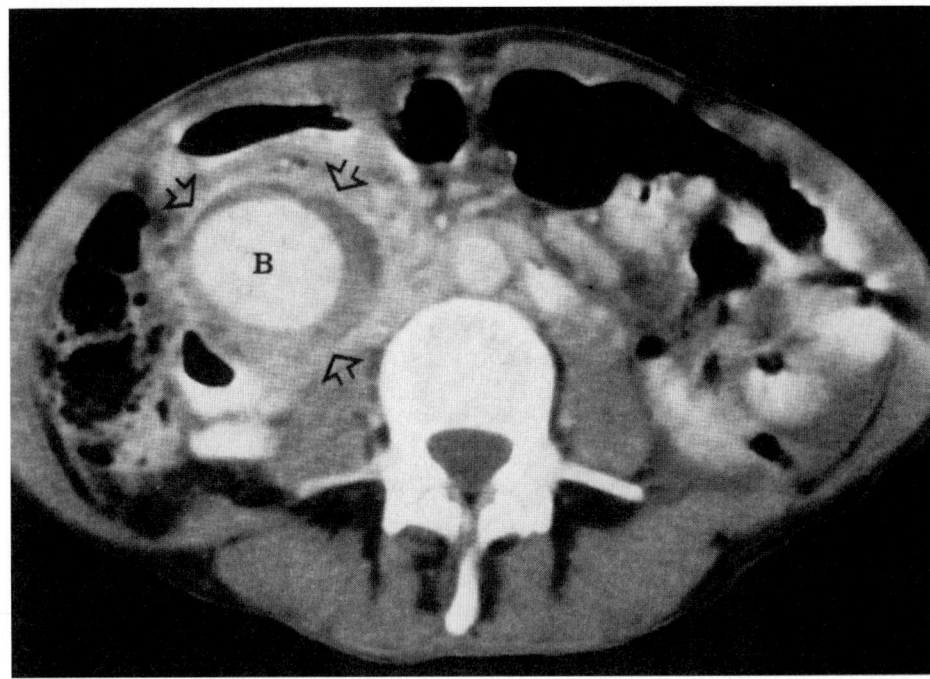

FIG. 32-40. Pseudoaneurysm of the gastroduodenal artery. A pseudocyst can erode into an adjacent artery, which results in contained hemorrhage otherwise known as a pseudoaneurysm. A contrast-injected CT scan reveals active bleeding (*B*) into a pseudocyst (*arrows*) as a result of this process. (*Reproduced with permission from Freeney.*[132])

pseudocysts that penetrate into the transverse mesocolon, the paracolic gutters, or the lesser sac. Cystogastrostomy can be performed endoscopically[191] (Fig. 32-42), laparoscopically,[192] or by a combined laparoscopic-endoscopic method.[193]

Because pseudocysts often communicate with the pancreatic ductal system, two newer approaches to pseudocyst management are based on main duct drainage, rather than pseudocyst drainage per se. Transpapillary stents inserted at the time of ERCP may be directed into a pseudocyst through the ductal communication itself (Fig. 32-43), or can be left across the area of suspected duct leakage to facilitate decompression and cyst drainage, analogous to the use of common bile duct stents in the setting of a cystic duct leak.[194,195] In a surgical series of patients with chronic pancreatitis, ductal dilatation, and a coexisting pseudocyst, Nealon and Walser showed that

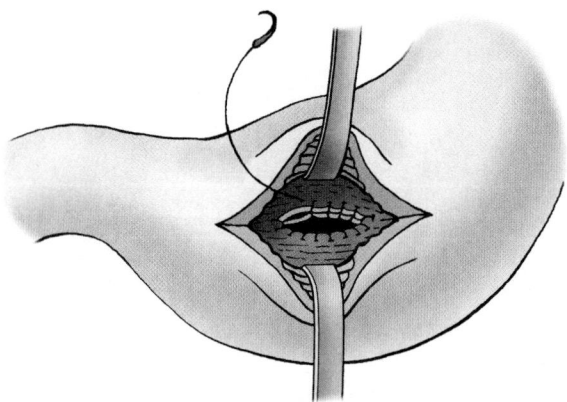

FIG. 32-41. Cystogastrostomy drainage of a retrogastric pancreatic pseudocyst. A larger opening is made through the common wall of a retrogastric pseudocyst, and a portion of the pseudocyst wall is submitted for histologic confirmation of the diagnosis. Suture reinforcement of the communication is performed to avoid the complication of bleeding. (*Reproduced with permission from Bell.*[192])

duct drainage alone, without a separate cystoenteric anastomosis, was as successful as a combined drainage procedure.[196] Furthermore, the "duct drainage only" group enjoyed a shorter hospital stay and fewer complications than the group who underwent a separate cystoenterostomy. These observations suggest that transductal drainage may be a safe and effective approach to the management of pseudocystic disease. The endoscopic approach seems logical in the treatment of postoperative or posttraumatic pseudocysts when duct disruption is documented, or in those patients with pseudocysts that communicate with the duct. Whether the technique will be as effective for chronic pseudocysts without demonstrable communication with the pancreatic duct remains open to investigation.

The complications of endoscopic or radiologic drainage of pseudocysts often require surgical intervention. Bleeding from the cystoenterostomy, and inoculation of a pseudocyst with failure of resolution and persistence of infection, may require surgical treatment. Bleeding risks may be lessened by the routine use of EUS in the selection of the site for transluminal stent placement.[194] Percutaneous and endoscopic treatment of pseudocysts requires large-bore catheters, multiple stents, and an aggressive approach to management for success to be achieved. Failure of nonsurgical therapy, with subsequent salvage procedures to remove infected debris and establish complete drainage, is associated with increased risks for complications and death.[197,198] The most experienced therapeutic endoscopists report a complication rate of 17 to 19% for the treatment of sterile pseudocysts, and deaths as a result of endoscopic therapy have occurred.[189] The use of endoscopic methods to treat sterile or infected pancreatic necrosis has a higher complication rate, and is indeed still controversial.[194] As Schutz and Leung state in a recent editorial, "pancreatic endotherapy is not for all, or even most, endoscopists . . . If removing bile duct stones is like riding a bicycle, then pancreatic endotherapy is equivalent to flying a fighter jet."[199]

Resection of a pseudocyst is sometimes indicated for cysts located in the pancreatic tail, or when a midpancreatic duct disruption

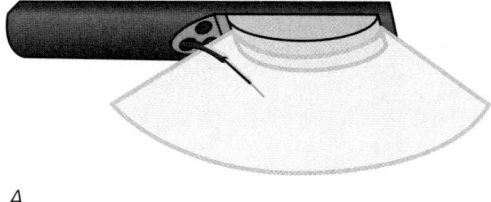

A

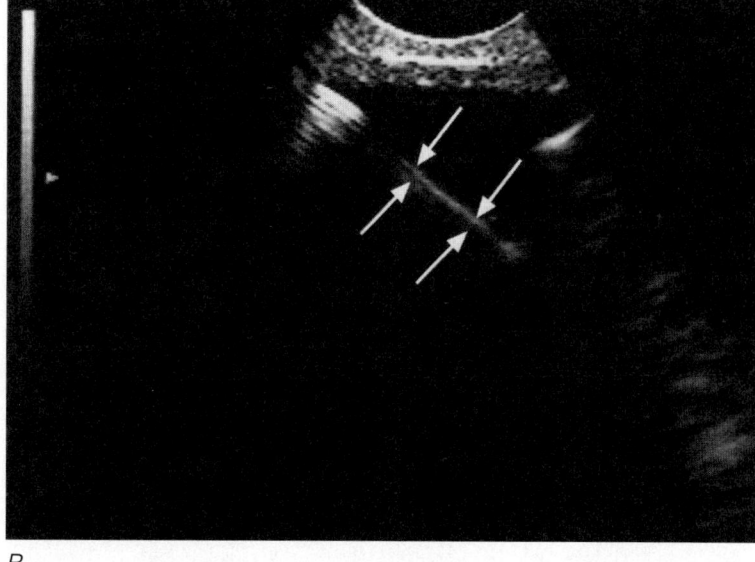

B

FIG. 32-42. *Technique of endoluminal cystogastrostomy. A. A diagram of the linear-array endoscopic ultrasound probe that incorporates a needle-knife within the field of the ultrasound scan. B. EUS image obtained showing extension of the needle-knife into the adjacent pseudocyst through the posterior gastric wall. (Reproduced with permission from Kozarek et al.[191])*

has resulted in a distally located pseudocyst. Distal pancreatectomy for removal of a pseudocyst, with or without splenectomy, can be a challenging procedure in the setting of prior pancreatitis. An internal drainage procedure of the communicating duct, or of the pseudocyst itself, should be considered when distal resection is being contemplated.

Pancreatic Ascites. When a disrupted pancreatic duct leads to pancreatic fluid extravasation that does not become sequestered as a pseudocyst, but drains freely into the peritoneal cavity, pancreatic ascites occurs. Occasionally, the pancreatic fluid tracks superiorly into the thorax, and a pancreatic pleural effusion occurs. Referred to as internal pancreatic fistulae, both complications are seen more often in patients with chronic pancreatitis, rather than after acute pancreatitis.[200–202] Pancreatic ascites and pleural effusion occur together in 14% of patients, and 18% have a pancreatic pleural effusion alone.[201]

Patients demonstrate the general demographics of chronic pancreatitis, and usually present with a subacute or recent history of progressive abdominal swelling despite weight loss. Pain and nausea are rarely present. The abdominal CT scan discloses ascites, and the presence of chronic pancreatitis or a partially collapsed pseudocyst (Fig. 32-44). Paracentesis or thoracentesis reveals noninfected fluid with a protein level greater than 25 g/L and a markedly elevated amylase level. Serum amylase may also be elevated, presumably from reabsorption across the parietal membrane. Serum albumin may be low, and patients may have coexisting liver disease. Paracentesis is therefore critical to differentiate pancreatic from hepatic ascites.

ERCP is most helpful to delineate the location of the pancreatic duct leak, and to elucidate the underlying pancreatic ductal anatomy. Pancreatic duct stenting may be considered at the time of ERCP, but if nonsurgical therapy is undertaken and then abandoned, repeat imaging of the pancreatic duct is appropriate to guide surgical treatment.

Antisecretory therapy with the somatostatin analog octreotide acetate, together with bowel rest and parenteral nutrition, is successful in more than half of patients.[203] Reapposition of serosal surfaces to facilitate closure of the leak is considered a part of therapy,

and this is accomplished by complete paracentesis. For pleural effusions, a period of chest tube drainage may facilitate closure of the internal fistula.[202,203] Surgical therapy is reserved for those who fail to respond to medical treatment. If the leak originates from the central region of the pancreas, a Roux-en-Y pancreaticojejunostomy is performed to the site of duct leakage (Fig. 32-45). If the leak is in the tail, a distal pancreatectomy may be considered, or an internal drainage procedure can be performed. The results of surgical treatment are usually favorable if the ductal anatomy has been carefully delineated preoperatively.

Pancreatic-Enteric Fistula. The erosion of a pancreatic pseudocyst into an adjacent hollow viscus can result in a pancreatic-enteric fistula. The most common site of communication is the transverse colon or splenic flexure. The fistula usually presents with evidence of gastrointestinal or colonic bleeding and sepsis. If the fistula communicates with the stomach or duodenum, it may close spontaneously or persist as a pancreatic-enteric fistula. When the fistula involves the colon, operative correction is usually required.[204]

Head-of-Pancreas Mass. In up to 30% of patients with advanced chronic pancreatitis, an inflammatory mass develops in the head of the pancreas.[205] The clinical presentation includes severe pain, and frequently includes stenosis of the distal common bile duct, duodenal stenosis, compression of the portal vein, and stenosis of the proximal main pancreatic duct (Table 32-15). In a series of 279 patients with chronic pancreatitis treated surgically at the University of Ulm in Germany, patients with pancreatic head enlargement represented half of the total group. The subgroup with pancreatic head enlargement appeared to have a lower incidence of endocrine and exocrine insufficiency, but a higher expression of epidermal growth factor and the c-erb B-2 protooncogene.[206] Mutations and polymorphisms of p53 were found in 3 and 8% of these patients, respectively, and a focus of ductular carcinoma was found in 3.7% of patients with pancreatic head enlargement. It was concluded that an accelerated transformation from hyperplasia to dysplasia exists in patients with pancreatic head enlargement, although the etiology

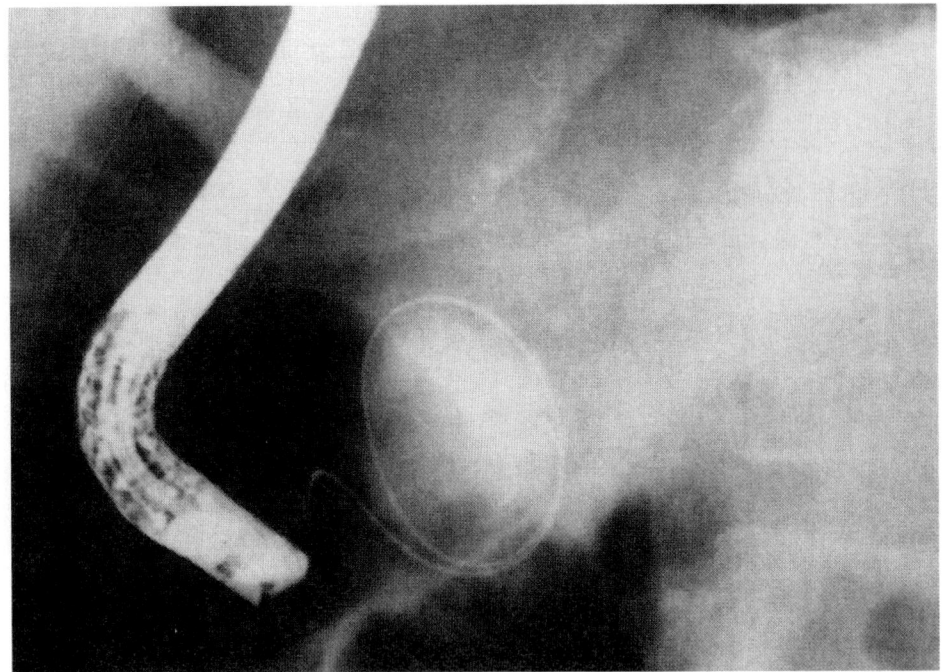

A

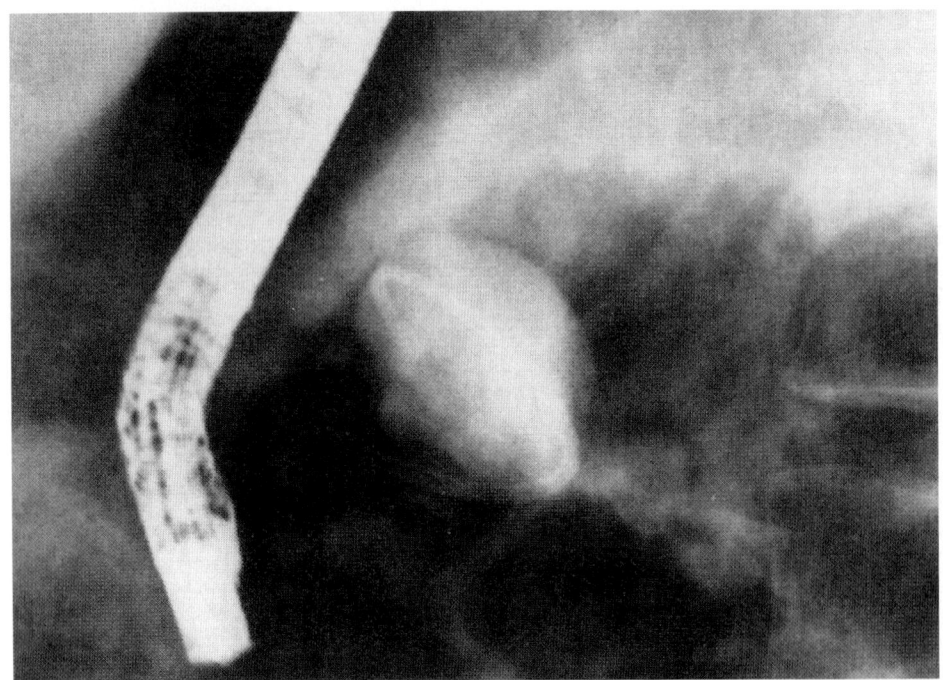

B

FIG. 32-43. Transpapillary drainage of a pancreatic pseudocyst. *A. Endoscopic passage of a flexible wire through the major papilla, through the pancreatic duct, and into a communicating pseudocyst. B. Placement of a stent over the wire into the pseudocyst with transpapillary drainage. (Reproduced with permission from Kozarek et al.[195])*

for this process remains unclear. Treatment in the majority of cases consisted of the duodenum-preserving pancreatic head resection, with good results.

Splenic and Portal Vein Thrombosis. Vascular complications of chronic pancreatitis are fortunately infrequent, because they are difficult to treat successfully. Portal vein compression and occlusion can occur as a consequence of an inflammatory mass in the head of the pancreas, and splenic vein thrombosis occurs in

association with chronic pancreatitis in 4 to 8% of cases.[207] Variceal formation can occur as a consequence of either portal or splenic venous occlusion, and splenic vein thrombosis with gastric variceal formation is referred to as left-sided or sinistral portal hypertension. Although bleeding complications are infrequent, the mortality risk of bleeding exceeds 20%. When gastroesophageal varices are caused by splenic vein thrombosis, the addition of splenectomy to prevent variceal hemorrhage is prudent when surgery is otherwise indicated to correct other problems.

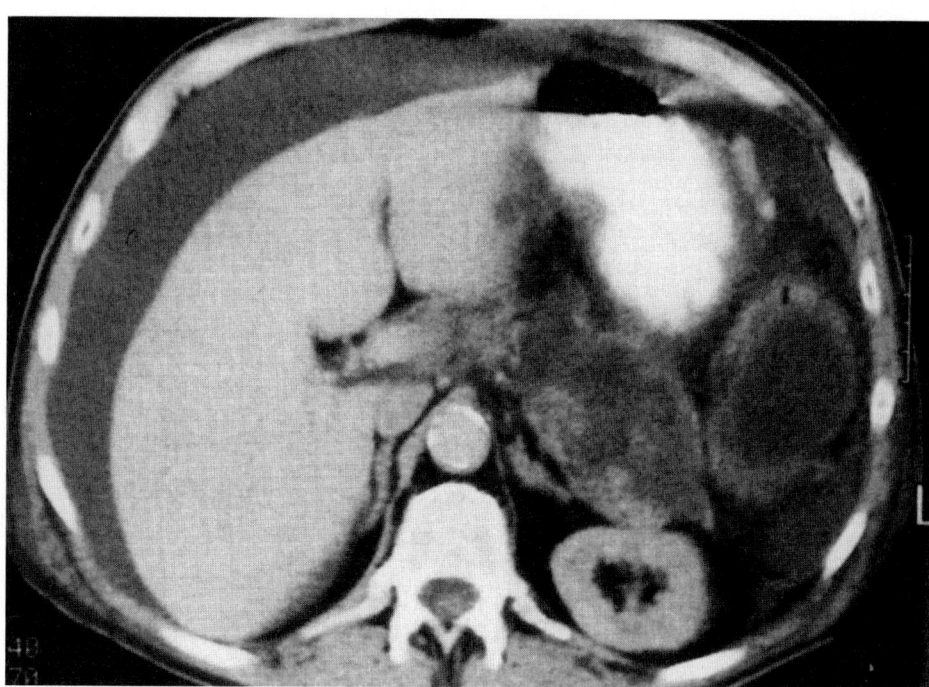

FIG. 32-44. Pancreatic ascites. CT scan of a patient with a ruptured pancreatic pseudocyst resulting in intraperitoneal pancreatic fluid. (*Reproduced with permission from Lipsett et al.*[200])

Treatment

Medical Therapy

The medical treatment of chronic or recurrent pain in chronic pancreatitis requires the use of analgesics, a cessation of alcohol use, oral enzyme therapy, and the selective use of antisecretory therapy.

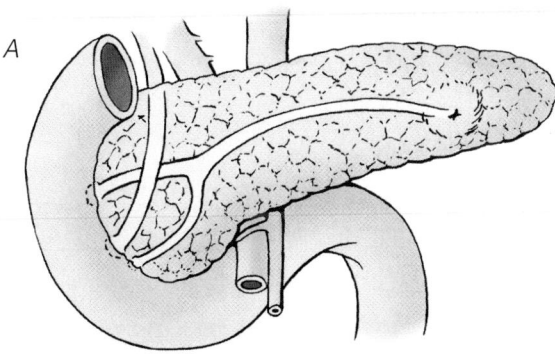

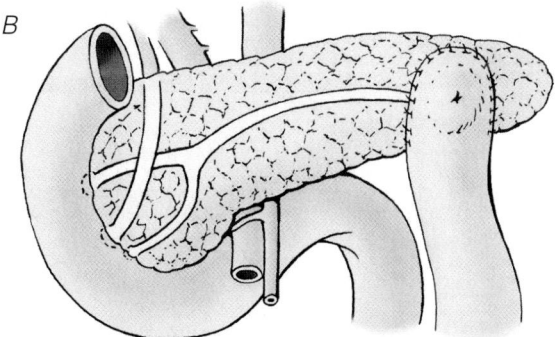

FIG. 32-45. Internal drainage for leaking pancreatic duct. A Roux-en-Y pancreaticojejunostomy is performed at the site of duct rupture to accomplish internal drainage of the pancreatic duct leak. (*Reproduced with permission from Cameron.*[202])

Interventional procedures to block visceral afferent nerve conduction or to treat obstructions of the main pancreatic duct are also an adjunct to medical treatment.

Analgesia. Oral analgesics are prescribed as needed, alone or with analgesia-enhancing agents such as gabapentin. Adequate pain control usually requires the use of narcotics, but these should be titrated to achieve pain relief with the lowest effective dose. Opioid addiction is common, and the use of long-acting analgesics by transdermal patch together with oral agents for pain exacerbations slightly reduces the sedative effects of high-dose oral narcotics.

It is essential for patients to abstain from alcohol. In addition to removing the causative agent, alcohol abstention results in pain reduction or relief in 60 to 75% of patients with chronic pancreatitis.[177,208] Despite this benefit, roughly half of alcoholic chronic pancreatitis patients continue to abuse alcohol.

Enzyme Therapy. Pancreatic enzyme administration serves to reverse the effects of pancreatic exocrine insufficiency, and may reduce or alleviate the pain experienced by patients. The choice of enzyme supplement, and the dose, should be selected based on whether malabsorption or pain (or both) are the indications

Table 32-15

Signs and Symptoms of Chronic Pancreatitis with and without a Pancreatic Head Mass

Signs and Symptoms	With Head Enlargement (n = 138) (%)	Without Head Enlargement (n = 141) (%)
Daily severe pain	67	40
Cholestasis	46	11
Slight to frequent pain	33	60
Duodenal obstruction	30	7
Diabetes mellitus	18	30
Vascular involvement	15	8

SOURCE: Reproduced with permission from Beger et al.[205]

Table 32-16
Pancreatic Enzyme Preparations

Name	Dose[a]	Lipase/Protease (USP Units)
Conventional (non-enteric-coated) compounds[b]		
Viokase	8 tablets each time	8000/30,000
Ku-Zyme HP	8 tablets each time	8000/30,000
Enteric-coated compounds[c]		
Creon 10	2–3 capsules each time	10,000/37,500
Creon 20	2–3 capsules each time	20,000/75,000
Pancrease MT 10	2–3 capsules each time	10,000/30,000
Pancrease MT 16	2–3 capsules each time	16,000/48,000

[a]The dosing schedule is before meals; can also take a dose at night if patient experiences pain.

[b]Conventional enzymes are the treatment of choice for pain relief. If no improvement occurs with conventional enzymes alone, add H_2-blockers or proton pump inhibitors to decrease peptic acid inhibition of the enzymes.

[c]Enteric-coated preparations are treatment of choice for steatorrhea. Acid-suppressive therapy should not be given with enteric-coated preparations.

USP = United States Pharmacopeia.

for therapy[209] (Table 32-16). Conventional (non-enteric-coated) enzyme preparations are partially degraded by gastric acid, but are available within the duodenal and jejunal regions to bind to cholecystokinin (CCK)-releasing peptide, and downregulate the release of CCK. This theoretically serves to reduce the enteric signal for pancreatic exocrine secretion, which reduces the pressure within a partially or completely obstructed pancreatic duct.[210,211] Enteric-coated preparations result in little to no pain relief, presumably due to their reduced bioavailability in the proximal gut.[212] Due to the loss of pancreatic enzymes by acid hydrolysis and proteolysis, relatively large doses are required to achieve effective levels of enzyme within the proximal small bowel. Enteric-coated preparations are protected from acid degradation, but are presumably not released in the critical proximal gut in sufficient quantity to inhibit the stimulus

for endogenous pancreatic enzyme secretion. Nonalcoholic patients may experience more effective pain relief than alcoholic patients,[209] but it is recommended that all patients with chronic pancreatitis pain begin a trial of non-enteric-coated enzyme supplements for 1 month. If pain relief is achieved, therapy is continued. If enzyme therapy fails, further investigation of the pancreatic ductal system by ERCP guides the therapy based on the presence or absence of large duct (obstructive) disease (Fig. 32-46).

Antisecretory Therapy Somatostatin administration has been shown to inhibit pancreatic exocrine secretion and CCK release.[213] The somatostatin analog octreotide acetate has therefore been investigated for pain relief in patients with chronic pancreatitis.[214,215] In a double-blind prospective randomized 4-week trial, 65% of patients who received 200 μg of octreotide acetate subcutaneously three times daily reported pain relief, compared with 35% of placebo-treated subjects. Patients who had the best results were patients with chronic abdominal pain, suggestive of obstructive pancreatopathy. However, in another trial that used a 3-day duration of treatment, no significant pain relief was observed.[216] None of the studies completed thus far have examined the sustained-release formulation of octreotide, and it remains unclear what subgroups of patients, or what dose of octreotide, might be beneficial in the treatment of pain. Anecdotal reports suggest that severe pain exacerbations in chronic pancreatitis can benefit from a combination of octreotide therapy and total parenteral nutrition, and trials are currently underway to assess the effectiveness of the sustained-release form of octreotide that requires only once-monthly administration.

Neurolytic Therapy. Celiac plexus neurolysis with alcohol injection has been an effective form of analgesic treatment in patients with pancreatic carcinoma. However, the use of radiologically- or endoscopically-guided celiac plexus blockade in chronic pancreatitis has been disappointing. Due to the risk of alcohol injury and the need for repeated injections, celiac plexus blockade in chronic

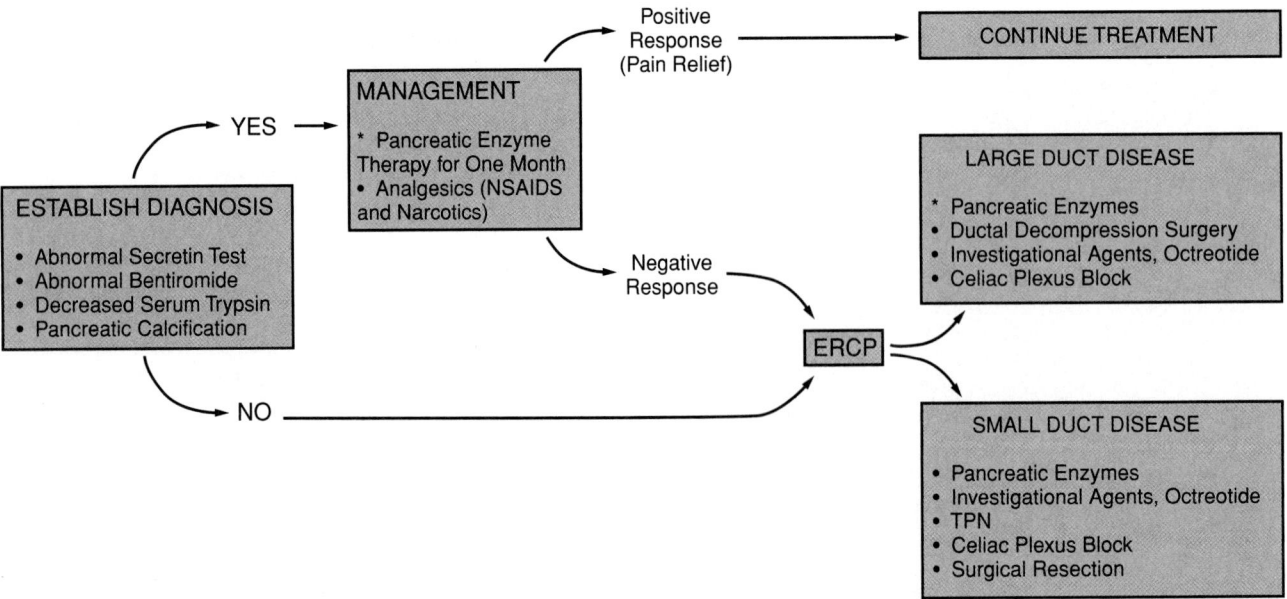

FIG. 32-46. Algorithm for the treatment of chronic pancreatitis pain. (*Reproduced with permission from Amann et al.[209]*) TPN = total parenteral nutrition; ERCP = endoscopic retrograde cholangiopancreatography.

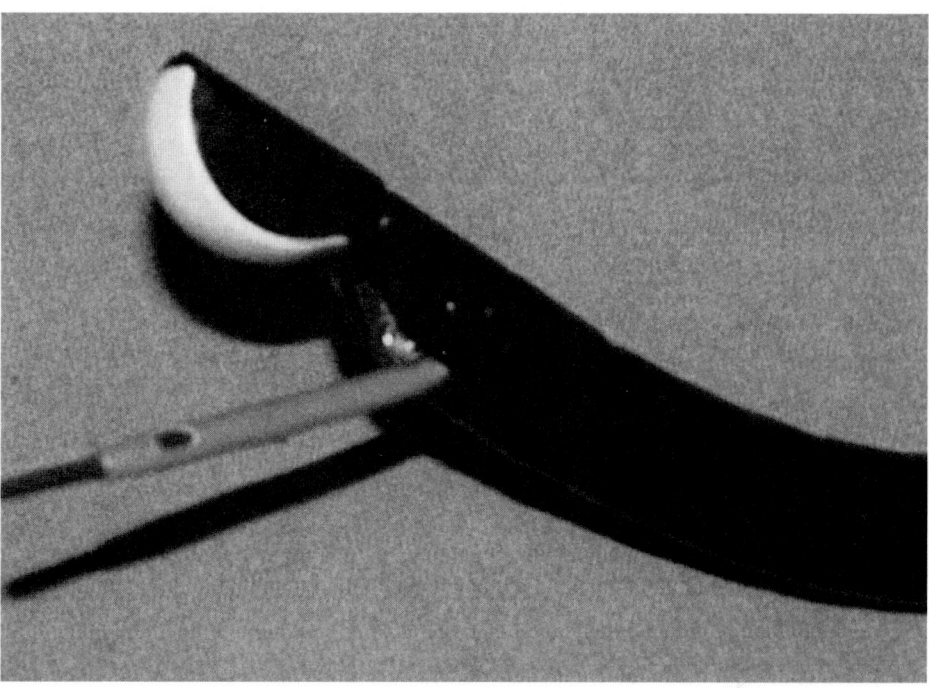

FIG. 32-47. Linear array ultrasound endoscope with a large working channel (model EG38UT; Pentax-Hitachi, Orangeburg, NY). This instrument allows ultrasound-guided endotherapy of pancreatic ductal and cystic abnormalities. *(Reproduced with permission from Giovannini M, et al: Endoscopic ultrasound-guided cystogastrostomy. Endoscopy 35:239, 2003.)*

pancreatitis has employed short-acting analgesics or other drugs rather than 50% alcohol. A recent trial of EUS-guided celiac plexus blockade revealed successful pain relief in 55% of patients, but the benefit lasted beyond 6 months in only 10% of patients.[217] The procedure therefore appears safe, but the effect is short lived in those patients who obtain pain relief.

Endoscopic Management

The techniques of endoscopic treatment of pancreatic duct obstruction, stone disease, pseudocyst formation, pancreatic duct leak, and for the diagnosis and management of associated pancreatic tumors have expanded greatly over the past 10 years. Newer endoscopes with expanded therapeutic capabilities have been introduced, and the role of EUS and EUS-guided needle and catheter insertion has expanded the ability of the therapeutic endoscopist in the diagnosis and treatment of chronic pancreatitis and its complications[218] (Fig. 32-47).

Pancreatic duct stenting is used for treatment of proximal pancreatic duct stenosis, decompression of a pancreatic duct leak, and for drainage of pancreatic pseudocysts that can be catheterized through the main pancreatic duct (Fig. 32-48). Pancreatic duct stents can

induce an inflammatory response within the duct, so prolonged stenting is usually avoided. Patients with sphincter of Oddi dyskinesia are at high risk for developing post-ERCP pancreatitis after biliary sphincterotomy, and a recent study demonstrated that the prophylactic placement of a pancreatic duct stent reduced the amylase level and development of pancreatitis after biliary sphincterotomy.[219]

Pancreatic duct leaks were seen in 37% of patients with acute pancreatitis, and pancreatic duct stenting appeared to facilitate the resolution of the leak.[220] Similarly, pancreatic duct stenting has been used to treat postsurgical pancreatic duct leaks and posttraumatic leaks.[221–223]

Pancreas divisum (see Fig. 32-3) is thought to cause pain and chronic pancreatitis due to functional or mechanical obstruction of the dorsal duct draining exclusively, or predominantly, through the lesser papilla. A recent study from Marseille reported good long-term results in 24 patients after minor papilla sphincterotomy and dorsal duct stenting.[224] The number of patients with chronic pain decreased from 83% before stenting to 29% after stenting, but pancreatitis or recurrent papillary stenosis occurred in 38%. Patients that responded best were those with intermittent pain, and this subset may be preferentially treated with endoscopic therapy.

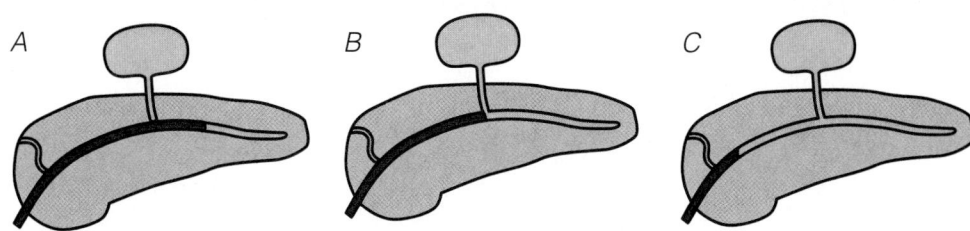

FIG. 32-48. Endoscopic decompression of a peripancreatic fluid collection through the pancreatic duct. Options for transpapillary placement include placement of the stent (*A*) beyond the point of duct disruption, (*B*) at the point of disruption, or (*C*) proximal to the point of duct disruption. Each of these locations may facilitate decompression of a peripancreatic fluid collection or pseudocyst caused by duct disruption, analogous to this successful treatment of a cystic duct leak by a common bile duct stent. *(Reproduced with permission from Hawes.[194])*

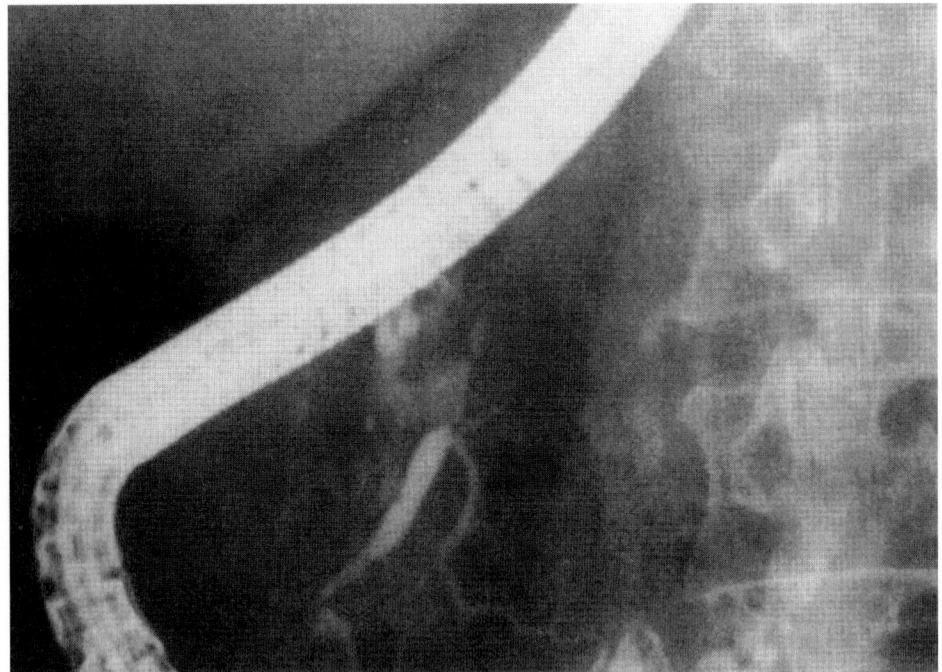

A

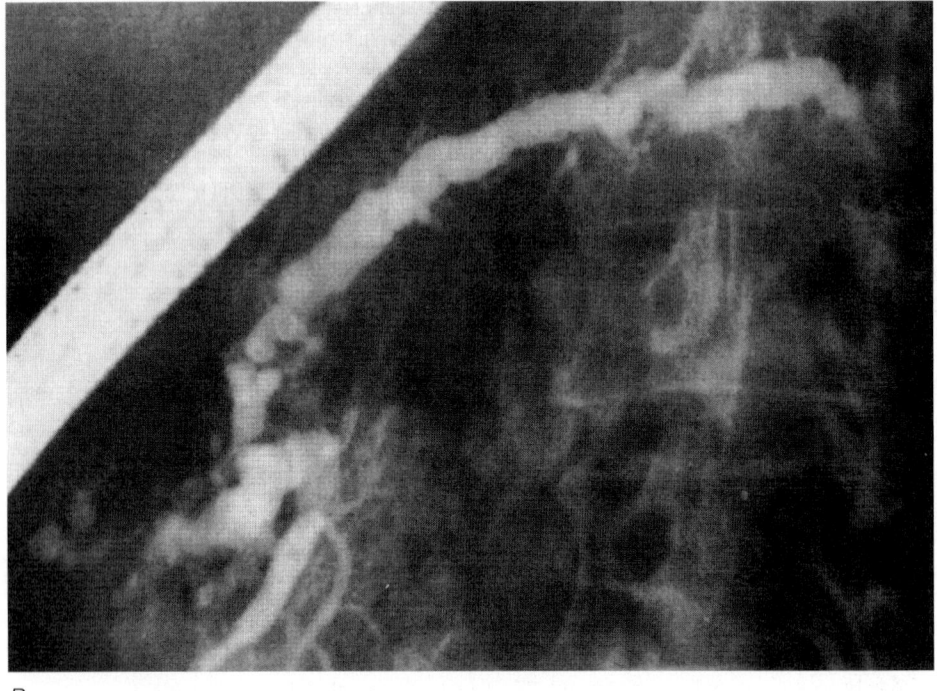

B

FIG. 32-49. Extracorporeal shock wave lithotripsy (ESWL) treatment of pancreatic duct stones. The ERCP images are shown (*A*) before and (*B*) after ESWL therapy of pancreatic duct obstruction due to calculus formation. (*Reproduced with permission from Kozarek et al.[227]*)

Idiopathic pancreatitis patients have been treated with endoscopic stenting, pancreatic duct sphincterotomy, and endoscopic stone removal with good results.[225,226] In a prospective randomized trial, 53% of idiopathic recurrent pancreatitis patients in the control group experienced continued episodes of pancreatitis, although only 11% of the treated patients had continued symptoms.[226]

Extracorporeal shock wave lithotripsy (ESWL) has been used for pancreatic duct stones, together with endoscopic stenting and stone removal.[227] A single ESWL session was used in 35 patients with pancreatic duct stones, together with 86 ERCP sessions to complete the stone removal process. After 2.4 years, 80% of patients had significant relief of symptoms (Fig. 32-49). However, due to the tendency for recurrent stone formation, the use of ESWL for long-term management of calcific pancreatitis remains uncertain.

Surgical Therapy

Indications and History. The traditional approach to surgical treatment of chronic pancreatitis and its complications has

Table 32-17

Effect of Surgical Drainage on Progression of Chronic Pancreatitis

Treatment Group	24-Month Evaluation
Operated ($n = 47$)	Mild to moderate 48 (87%); severe 6 (13%)
Nonoperated ($n = 36$)	Mild to moderate 8 (22%); severe 28 (78%)

Eighty-three patients with chronic pancreatitis were evaluated by exocrine, endocrine, nutritional, and ERCP studies, and all had mild to moderate disease and dilated pancreatic ducts. A Puestow-type duct decompression procedure was performed in 47 patients, and all subjects were restaged by the same methods 24 months later.

SOURCE: Reproduced with permission from Nealon et al.[228]

maintained that surgery should be considered only when the medical therapy of symptoms has failed. The role of surgery in the treatment of chronic pancreatitis, and its timing, is now based on the elucidation of pancreatic ductal disease. Nealon and Thompson published a landmark study in 1993 that showed that the progression of chronic obstructive pancreatitis could be delayed or prevented by pancreatic duct decompression.[228] No other therapy has been shown to prevent the progression of chronic pancreatitis, and this study demonstrated the role of surgery in the early management of the disease (Table 32-17). However, small-duct disease or the absence of a clear obstructive component are causes for caution. Major resections have a high complication rate, both early and late, in chronic alcoholic pancreatitis, and lesser procedures often result in symptomatic recurrence. So the choice of operation and the timing of surgery are based on each patient's pancreatic anatomy, the likelihood (or lack thereof) that further medical and endoscopic therapy will halt the symptoms of the disease, and the chance that a good result will be obtained with the lowest risk of morbidity and mortality. Finally, preparation for surgery should include restoration of protein-caloric homeostasis, abstinence from alcohol and tobacco, and a detailed review of the risks and likely outcomes, in order to establish a bond of trust and commitment between the patient and the surgeon.

Historically, the surgery for chronic pancreatitis before the second half of the twentieth century was a true demonstration of trial and error, with little anatomic information available prior to operation. Excellent results prior to CT scans and ERCP were either the result of serendipity, or due to the talent and creativity of the surgeon. In 1909, Coffey described a successful operation for chronic pancreatitis in which the pancreas was mobilized, skeletonized of the outer parenchyma, and then invaginated into a pouch made of small bowel.[229] In 1911, Link described an operation he devised on the spot, when a laparotomy in a young woman with abdominal pain revealed a fluctuant, obstructed pancreatic duct. After performing a dochotomy and evacuating multiple stones, he inserted a rubber tube, and exteriorized the pancreatostomy just above her navel[230] (Fig. 32-50). He later described the operation as having been a success for the next 30 years of the patient's life, during which the patient managed the care of the drainage tube without apparent problems.[231]

With the demonstration in 1942 by Priestly that total pancreatectomy was technically feasible,[232] and the report in 1946 by Whipple himself that proximal pancreatic resection was beneficial in patients with chronic pancreatitis,[233] the pendulum of surgical opinion swung toward resection as the operation of choice for chronic pancreatitis. By the mid-1950s, however, growing disappointment with

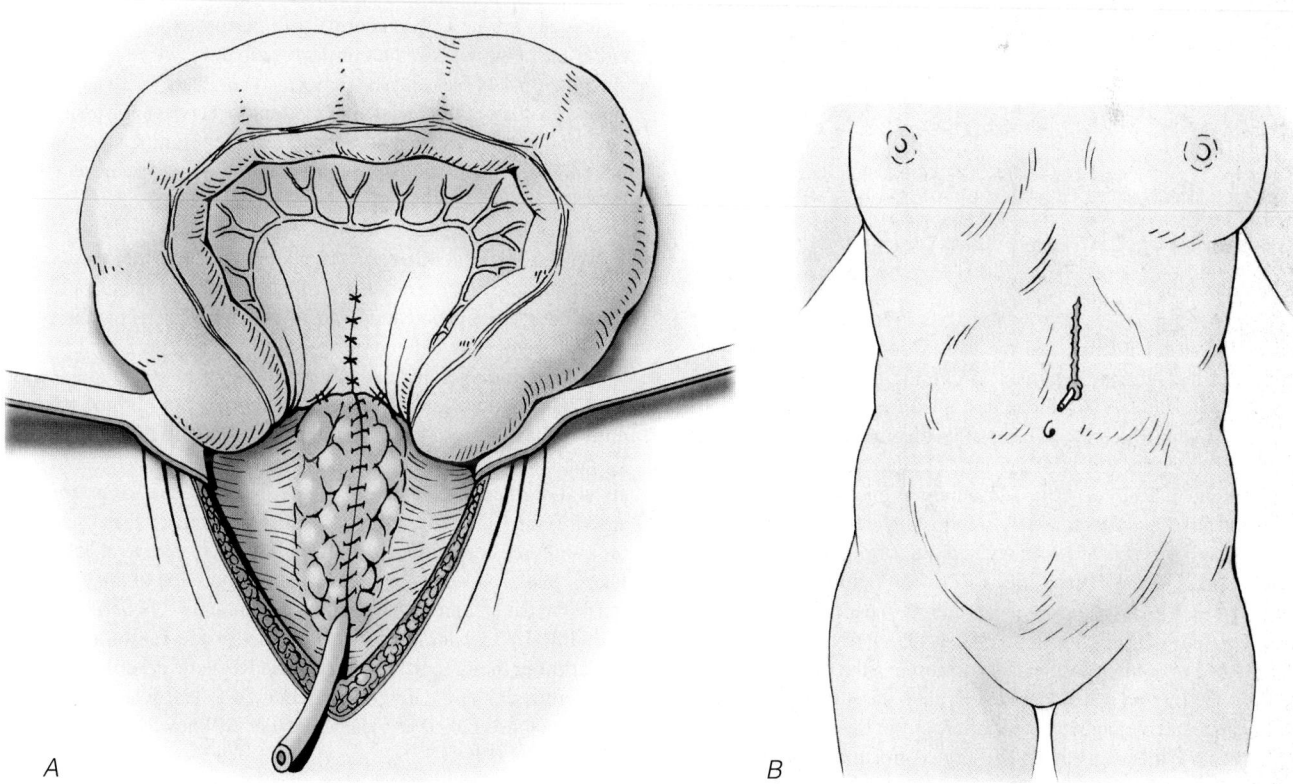

FIG. 32-50. Pancreatostomy for decompression of chronic calcific pancreatitis. *A.* Artist's rendering of Link's 1911 procedure in which a tube pancreatostomy was created to relieve symptoms of pancreatic duct obstruction. *B.* The cutaneous exit site of the pancreatostomy tube. (*Reproduced with permission from Link.*[230,231])

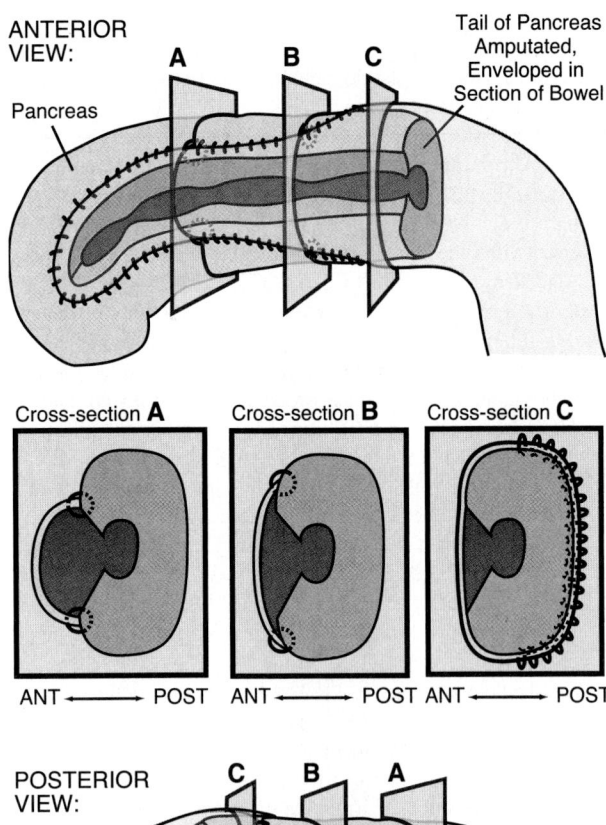

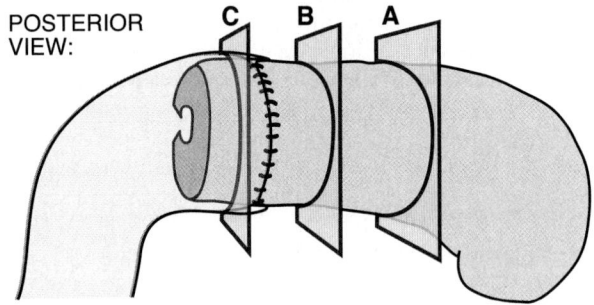

FIG. 32-51. Technique of pancreaticojejunal drainage originally described by Puestow and Gillesby. The distal pancreas was mobilized, the tail amputated, the duct opened longitudinally, and the pancreas was partially invaginated into a Roux-en-Y jejunal limb. (*Reproduced with permission from Puestow et al.[234]*)

the high risk of resection and the lack of long-term benefit overshadowed the surgical treatment of chronic pancreatitis. In 1954 Duval, and separately Zollinger, described the caudal pancreaticojejunostomy, in which the tail end of an obstructed pancreatic duct was anastomosed to a Roux-en-Y limb of jejunum. Two years later, Puestow and Gillesby described an ambitious operation in which the body and tail of the pancreas was mobilized, the tail amputated, and the duct and gland filleted open with drainage by invagination of the longitudinally opened gland into a Roux-en-Y limb of jejunum[234] (Fig. 32-51). Although conservative in terms of pancreatic resection, the operation was clearly formidable, despite Puestow's claim that no postoperative complications had occurred in the first 20 patients. In 1960, Partington and Rochelle described the side-to-side Roux-en-Y pancreaticojejunostomy variation of the Puestow procedure, which became the mainstay for the surgical treatment of obstructive pancreatopathy for the next 40 years.[235] Five years after Partington and Rochelle's report, Fry and Child described the 95% distal pancreatectomy as a more effective operation, and proposed that it was less morbid than the Whipple or total resection[236] (Fig. 32-52).

Proponents of resection and drainage procedures argued with passion, but these operations remained controversial until the 1970s, when the widespread adoption of ERCP and CT scans provided the ability to preoperatively diagnose obstructive and sclerotic disease, and this resulted in the rational selection of operative procedures. During this period, the major drawbacks to surgical therapy remained the approximately 20% incidence of recurrent disease, and the corresponding development of an inflammatory (or malignant) mass in the undrained pancreatic head (Fig. 32-53), or the high morbidity and mortality of major resectional procedures that seemed to predispose the patients to a cascade of metabolic problems.

In 1980, Beger described his experience with duodenum-preserving pancreatic head resection, and in 1987 Frey described his variation of the Partington and Rochelle variation of the Puestow procedure, in which the proximal pancreatic duct was opened completely, and the overlying parenchyma of the pancreatic head was conized, so as to allow a longitudinal pancreaticojejunostomy from duodenum to tail. As the twentieth century came to a close, the operative approach to obstructive pancreatopathy had become more proactive, and the surgery for small duct disease had become more cautious, while everyone waited for islet cell autotransplantation to become a practical reality.

Sphincteroplasty. The sphincter of Oddi and the pancreatic duct sphincter serve as gatekeepers for the passage of pancreatic juice into the duodenum (Fig. 32-54). Stenosis of either sphincter (sclerosing papillitis), due to scarring from pancreatitis or from the passage of gallstones, may result in obstruction of the pancreatic duct and chronic pain.[236] As gallstone pancreatitis became a popular diagnosis in the 1940s and 1950s, attention was focused on the ampullary region as a possible cause of chronic symptoms, and surgical sphincteroplasty was advocated. Although endoscopic techniques are now used routinely to perform sphincterotomy of either the common bile duct or pancreatic duct, a true (permanent) sphincteroplasty can only be performed surgically. Transduodenal sphincteroplasty with incision of the septum between the pancreatic duct and common bile duct appears to offer significant relief for patients with obstruction and inflammation isolated to this region[237] (Fig. 32-55).

Drainage Procedures. After the early reports of success with pancreatostomy for the relief of symptoms of chronic pancreatitis,[230] Cattell described pancreaticojejunostomy for relief of pain in unresectable pancreatic carcinoma.[239] Shortly thereafter Duval,[240] and separately Zollinger and associates,[241] described the caudal Roux-en-Y pancreaticojejunostomy for the treatment of chronic pancreatitis in 1954. The so-called Duval procedure was used for decades by some surgeons, but it almost invariably failed due to restenosis and segmental obstruction of the pancreas due to progressive scarring. In 1958, Puestow and Gillesby described these segmental narrowings and dilatations of the ductal system as a "chain of lakes," and proposed a longitudinal decompression of the body and tail of the pancreas into a Roux limb of jejunum.[234] Four of Puestow and Gillesby's 21 initial cases were side-to-side anastomoses, and 2 years after their report, Partington and Rochelle described a much simpler version of the longitudinal, or side-to-side Roux-en-Y pancreaticojejunostomy that became universally known as the Puestow procedure[235] (Fig. 32-56).

The effectiveness of decompression of the pancreatic duct is dependent on the extent to which ductal hypertension is the etiologic agent for the disease. Thus the diameter of the pancreatic duct is a surrogate for the degree of ductal hypertension, and the Puestow

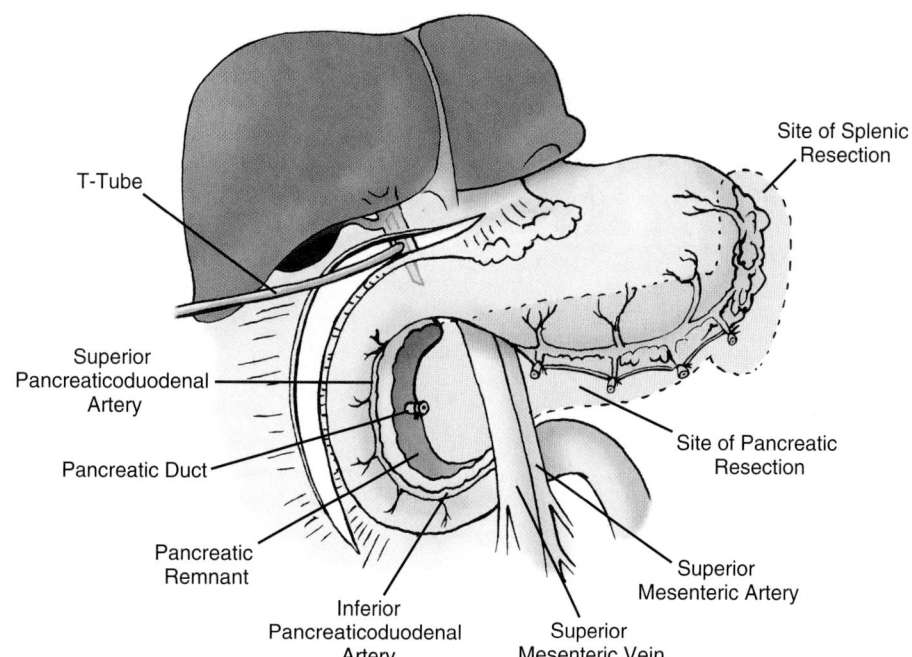

FIG. 32-52. Ninety-five percent (subtotal) distal pancreatectotomy. The spleen and distal pancreas are mobilized and removed, leaving a small rim of pancreatic tissue and an intact distal common bile duct. (*Reproduced with permission from Fry et al.[236]*)

procedure has been shown to be effective for pain relief when the maximum duct diameter exceeds 6 or 7 mm. Results are less impressive in glands with smaller caliber ducts, although Izbicki and associates have recently described good results with a conization method which allows a longitudinal decompression of more normal caliber ducts.[242]

Successful pain relief after the Puestow-type decompression procedure has been reported in 75 to 85% of patients for the first few years after surgery, but pain recurs in over 20% of patients after 5 years,[144] even in patients who are abstinent from alcohol. In 1987, Frey and Smith described the extended lateral

pancreaticojejunostomy with excavation of the pancreatic head down to the ductal structures[243] (Fig. 32-57). The Frey procedure provides thorough decompression of the pancreatic head as well as the body and tail of the gland, and a long-term follow-up suggested that improved outcomes are associated with this more extensive decompressive procedure. Frey and Amikura reported their results in 50 patients followed for over 7 years, and found complete or substantial pain relief in 87% of patients. There was no operative mortality, but 22% of patients developed postoperative complications.[244]

The degree and technique of pancreatic head decompression may be critical for good long-term pain relief. The Frey procedure opens

FIG. 32-53. Head-of-pancreas mass after Puestow procedure. The CT appearance of an inflammatory mass occupying the head of the pancreas, which developed 2 years after Puestow decompression of the body and tail of pancreas.

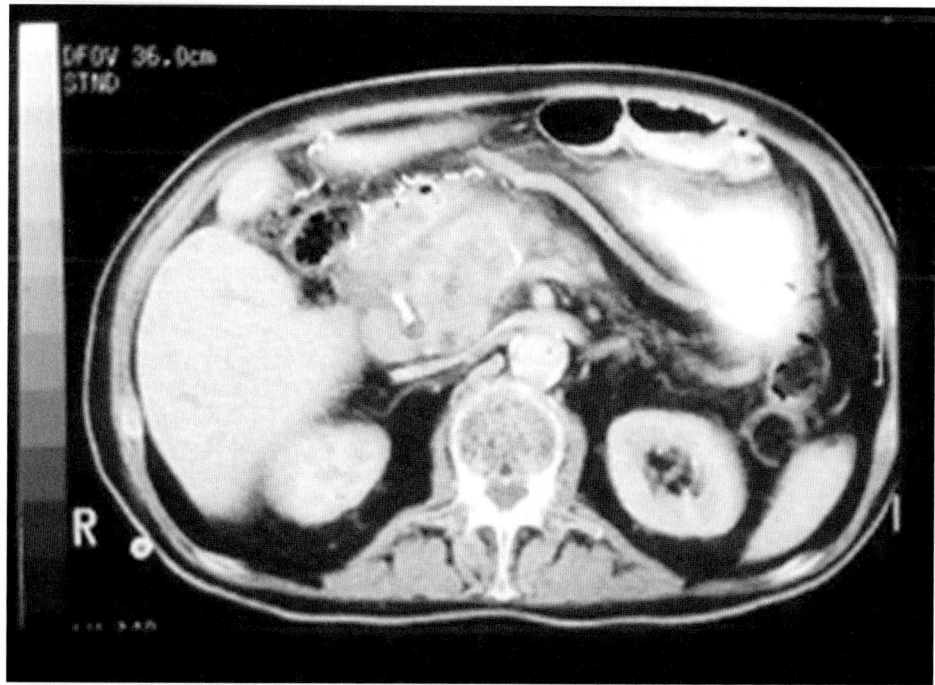

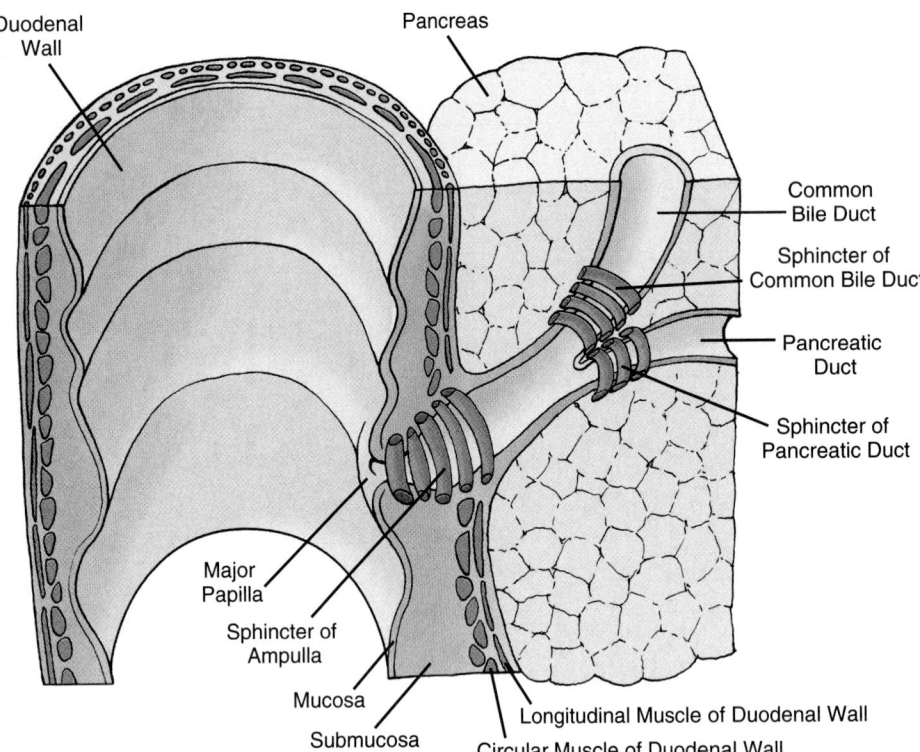

FIG. 32-54. Schematic diagram of the ampullary, biliary, and pancreatic duct sphincters. The point of merger of the bile duct and pancreatic duct is highly variable, and a true sphincter of the pancreatic duct may be poorly developed. [After Simeone DM: Gallbladder and biliary tract, in Yamada T et al (eds): Textbook of Gastroenterology, 4th ed. Philadelphia: Lippincott Williams & Wilkins, 2003, p 2173, with permission.]

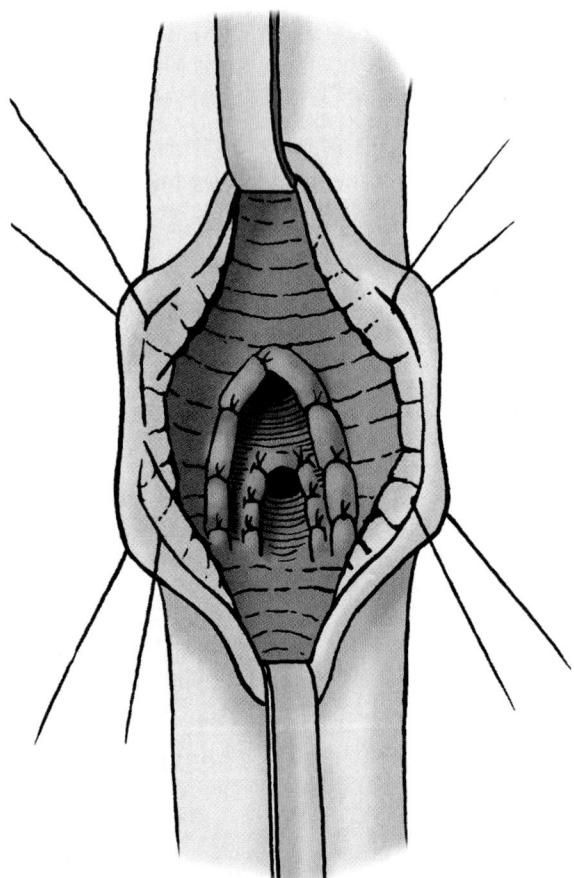

FIG. 32-55. Operative sphincteroplasty of the biliary and pancreatic duct. The ampullary and bile duct sphincters are divided, as is the pancreatic duct sphincter, with suture apposition of the mucosal edges of the incision. (Adapted with permission from Moody et al.[238])

the head of the gland down to the proximal ductal system, but was not described as a duct-removing procedure per se (Fig. 32-58). However, an actual excavation of the head of the pancreas, including the ductal system, may provide the best protection against recurrent stenosis, and the details of such a procedure, which also includes a single side-to-side Roux-en-Y pancreaticojejunostomy, have recently been described by Andersen and Topazian[245] (Fig. 32-59). This hybrid procedure combines the elements of a complete decompression of the pancreas with a limited form of pancreatic head resection. The advantages of such a procedure include its relatively low cost and early freedom from postoperative complications.

Resectional Procedures. For patients with focal inflammatory changes localized to the body and tail, or in whom no significant ductal dilatation exists, the technique of partial (40 to 80%) distal pancreatectomy has been advocated (Fig. 32-60). Although distal pancreatectomy is less morbid than more extensive resectional procedures, the operation leaves untreated a major portion of the gland, and is therefore associated with a significant risk of symptomatic recurrence.[139] It has been a more popular operation in British centers, where its success seems to be greater, perhaps due to the lower incidence of alcoholic chronic pancreatitis.[246] However, long-term outcomes reveal good pain relief in only 60% of patients, with completion pancreatectomy required for pain relief in 13% of patients.

In 1965, Fry and Child proposed the more radical 95% distal pancreatectomy, which was intended for patients with sclerotic (small duct) disease, and which attempted to avoid the morbidity of total pancreatectomy by preserving the rim of pancreas in the pancreaticoduodenal groove, along with its associated blood vessels and distal common bile duct[236] (see Fig. 32-52). The operation was found to be associated with pain relief in 60 to 77% of patients long term, but is accompanied by a high risk of brittle diabetes, hypoglycemic coma, and malnutrition.[247]

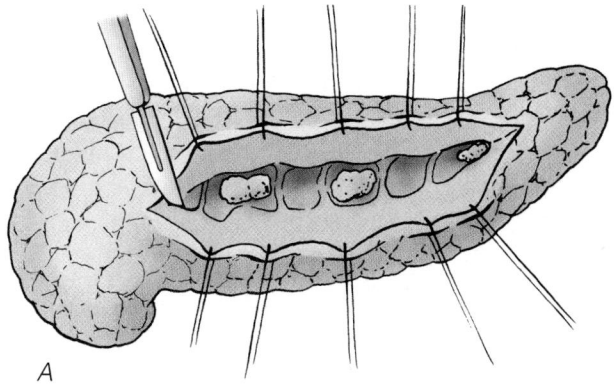

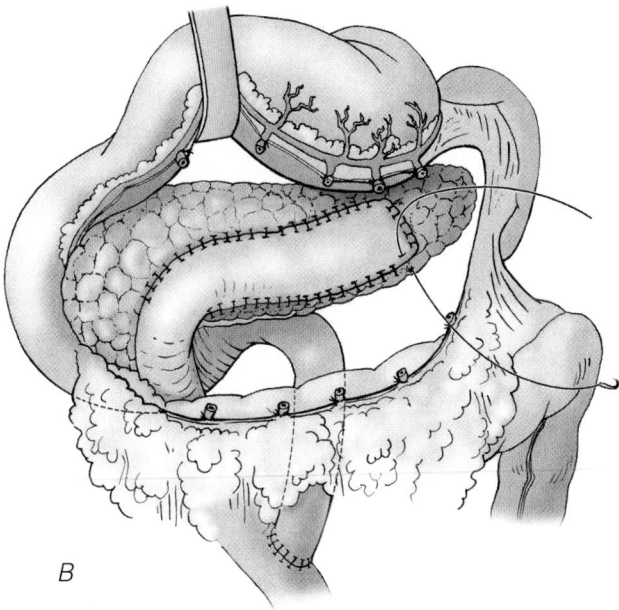

FIG. 32-56. *Longitudinal dichotomy in obstructing calcific pancreatitis. A longitudinal pancreatotomy typically discloses segmental stenosis of the pancreatic duct and the presence of intraductal calculi in a patient with chronic calcific pancreatitis (A). Following mobilization of a Roux limb of jejunum, a longitudinal pancreaticojejunostomy is performed to permit extensive drainage of the pancreatic duct system (B). This technique, described by Partington and Rochelle, is the typical method employed for the Puestow procedure. (Reproduced with permission from Partington et al.[235])*

Although the operation is seldom used today, there is great interest in combining this procedure with autologous islet transplantation (see below). Avoiding the metabolic consequences of subtotal or total pancreatectomy, while preserving the duodenum and distal bile duct, is an attractive surgical goal for the relief of nonobstructive pancreatic sclerosis.

In 1946, Whipple reported a series of five patients treated with either pancreaticoduodenectomy or total pancreatectomy for symptomatic chronic pancreatitis, with one operative death.[233] Subsequently, proximal pancreatectomy or pancreaticoduodenectomy, with or without pylorus preservation (Fig. 32-61), has been widely employed for the treatment of chronic pancreatitis.[140,204,248] In the three largest modern (circa 2000) series of the treatment of chronic pancreatitis by the Whipple procedure, pain relief 4 to 6 years after operation was found in 71 to 89% of patients. However, mortality

ranged from 1.5 to 3%, and major complications occurred in 25 to 38% of patients at the Johns Hopkins Hospital,[249] the Massachusetts General Hospital,[250] and the Mayo Clinic.[251] In follow-up, 25 to 48% of patients developed diabetes, and about the same percentage required exocrine therapy. Advocates of the Whipple procedure uniformly suggest that the high rate of symptomatic relief outweighs the metabolic consequences and the "acceptable" mortality risk of the procedure.

Beger and associates described the duodenum-preserving pancreatic head resection (DPPHR) in 1980[252] (Fig. 32-62), and published long-term results with DPPHR for the treatment of chronic pancreatitis in 1985,[253] and more recently in 1999.[254] In 388 patients who were followed for an average of 6 years after DPPHR, pain relief was maintained in 91%, mortality was less than 1%, and diabetes developed in 21% with 11% demonstrating a reversal of their preoperative diabetic status. These authors also compared the DPPHR procedure with the pylorus-sparing Whipple procedure in a randomized trial in 40 patients with chronic pancreatitis.[255] The mortality was zero in both groups, and the morbidity was also comparable. Pain relief (over 6 months) was seen in 94% of DPPHR patients, but in only 67% of Whipple patients. Furthermore, the insulin secretory capacity and glucose tolerance were noted to deteriorate in the Whipple group, but actually improved in the DPPHR patients.

The DPPHR requires the careful dissection of the gastroduodenal artery and the creation of two anastomoses (Fig. 32-63), and carries a similar complication risk as the Whipple procedure due to the risk of pancreatic leakage and intra-abdominal fluid collections. Izbicki and associates conducted a randomized trial comparing the Frey procedure with the DPPHR in patients with chronic pancreatitis, and confirmed a reduced morbidity of 9% after the Frey procedure, compared to 20% after DPPHR.[256] No significant differences were found in postoperative pain relief after the Frey or DPPHR (89 and 95%, respectively, over a mean follow-up of 1.5 years), nor were there any differences in the ability to return to work, or in endocrine or exocrine function postoperatively.

In a retrospective review of both the DPPHR and Frey procedures performed at Yale, Aspelund and associates found a 25% incidence of major complications after the DPPHR, but only a 16% incidence after Frey procedures performed for chronic pancreatitis.[181] During the same interval, major complications occurred after 40% of Whipple procedures, and new diabetes developed in 25% of Whipple patients. New diabetes occurred in only 8% of both DPPHR and Frey patients, during a follow-up period of 3 years, and preoperative diabetes improved in an equal number of DPPHR and Frey patients. These results corroborate the findings in the studies from Ulm and Hamburg, and suggest that duodenum-sparing pancreatic head resection, either in the form of the DPPHR (Beger) procedure or the Frey procedure, may provide better outcomes compared to the Whipple procedure for benign disease including chronic pancreatitis.

The decreased incidence of postoperative diabetes after the duodenum-sparing operations may be the result of a preserved beta-cell mass in the more conservative resections, and may also be due to the conservation of the pancreatic polypeptide–secreting cells localized to the posterior head and uncinate process.[153,160] Preservation of near-normal glucose metabolism and the avoidance of pancreatogenic diabetes is a significant benefit of the newer operative procedures.

Autotransplantation of Islets. Islet cell transplantation for the treatment of diabetes is an attractive adjunct to pancreatic surgery in the treatment of benign pancreatic disease, but problems due to

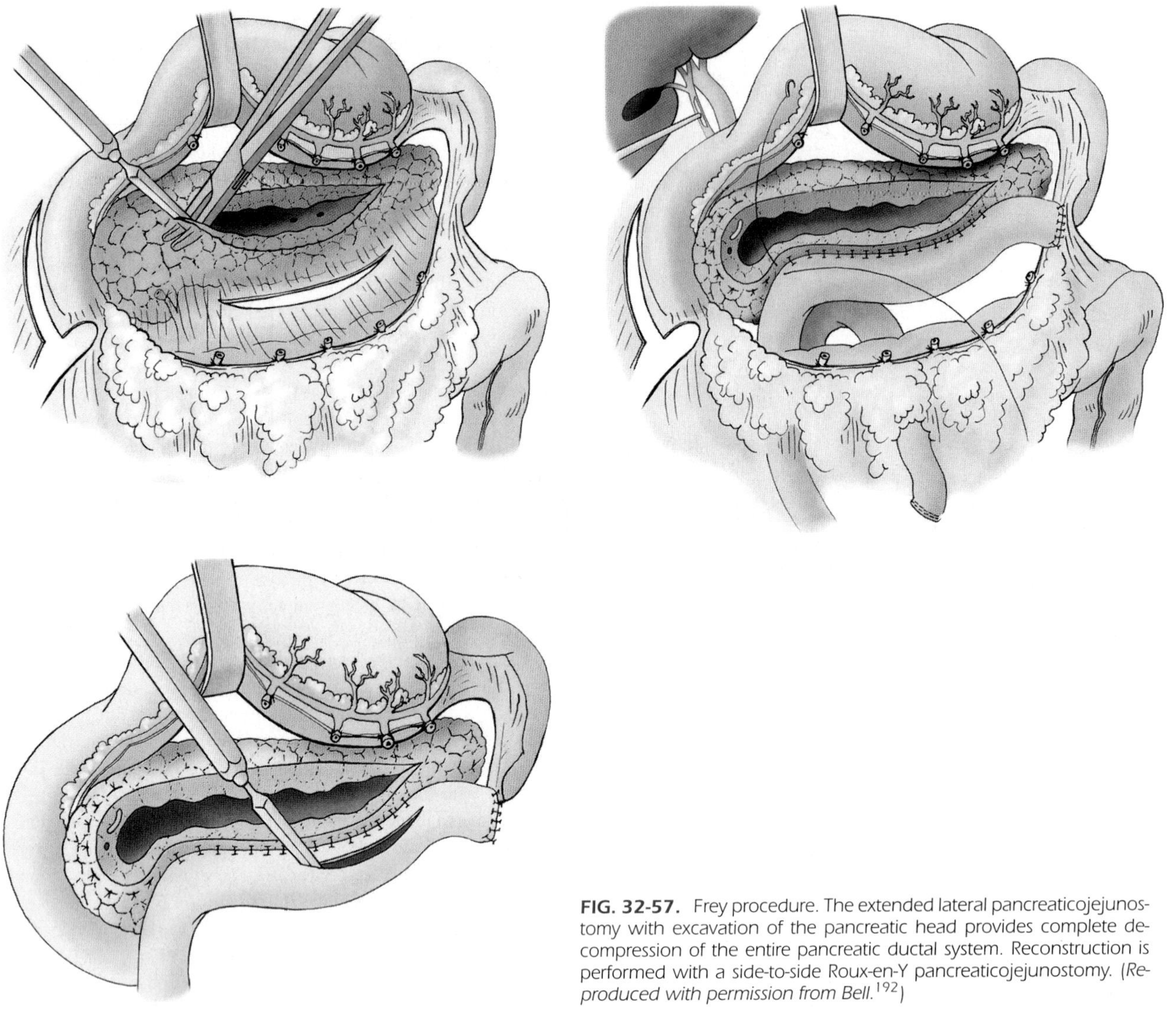

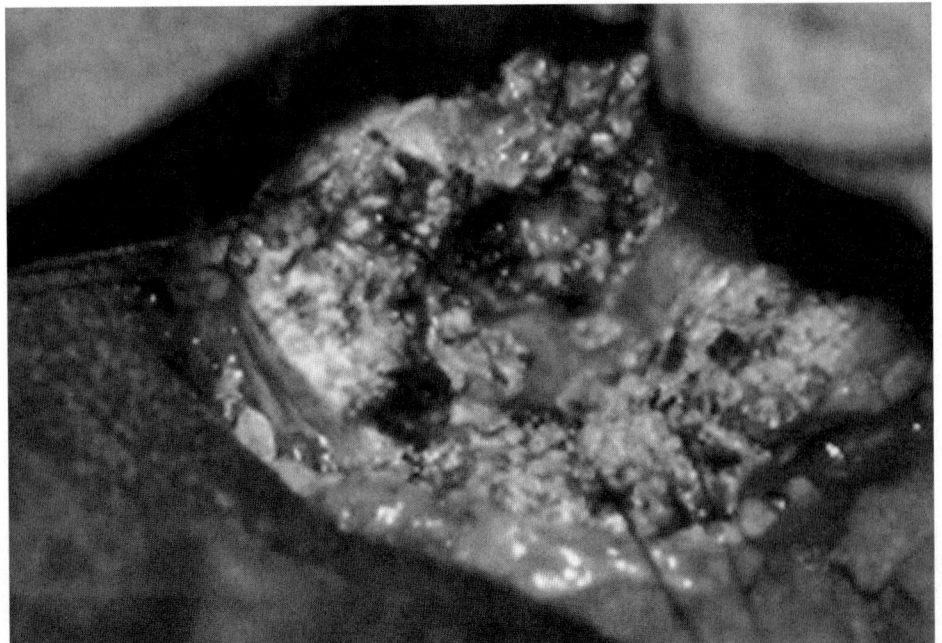

FIG. 32-57. Frey procedure. The extended lateral pancreaticojejunostomy with excavation of the pancreatic head provides complete decompression of the entire pancreatic ductal system. Reconstruction is performed with a side-to-side Roux-en-Y pancreaticojejunostomy. (*Reproduced with permission from Bell.*[192])

FIG. 32-58. Operative view of excavated head of the pancreas during the Frey procedure. The main pancreatic duct is opened widely down to the level of the ampulla, and the head of the pancreas is excavated in a conical fashion so as to allow complete decompression of the chronically obstructed and inflamed pancreatic ducts. (*Reproduced with permission from Aspelund et al.*[181])

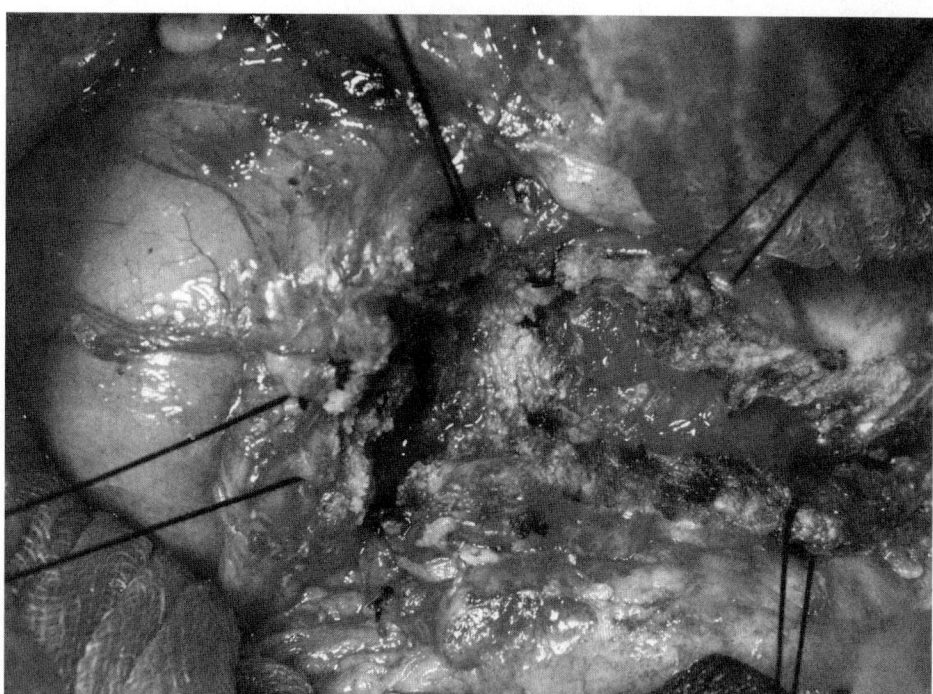

FIG. 32-59. Complete excavation of the pancreatic head and distal pancreatic dochotomy. A true excavation and removal of the proximal ductal system is combined with a distal pancreatic dochotomy in this resection-and-drainage version of the duodenum-preserving pancreatic head resection. Reconstruction is performed with a single side-to-side Roux-en-Y pancreaticojejunostomy. (*Reproduced with permission from Andersen et al.*[245])

FIG. 32-60. Distal (spleen-sparing) pancreatectomy. A distal pancreatectomy for chronic pancreatitis is usually performed with en-bloc splenectomy. In the presence of minimal inflammation, a spleen-sparing version can be performed, as shown here. (*Reproduced with permission from Bell.*[192])

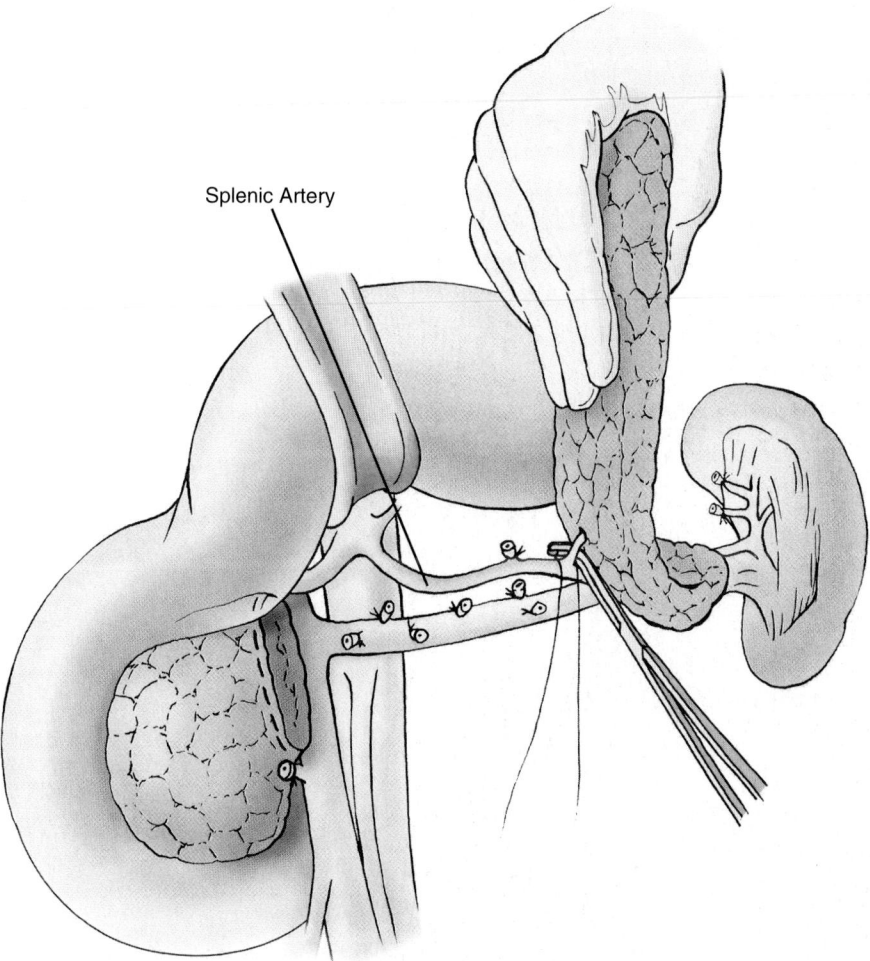

Splenic Artery

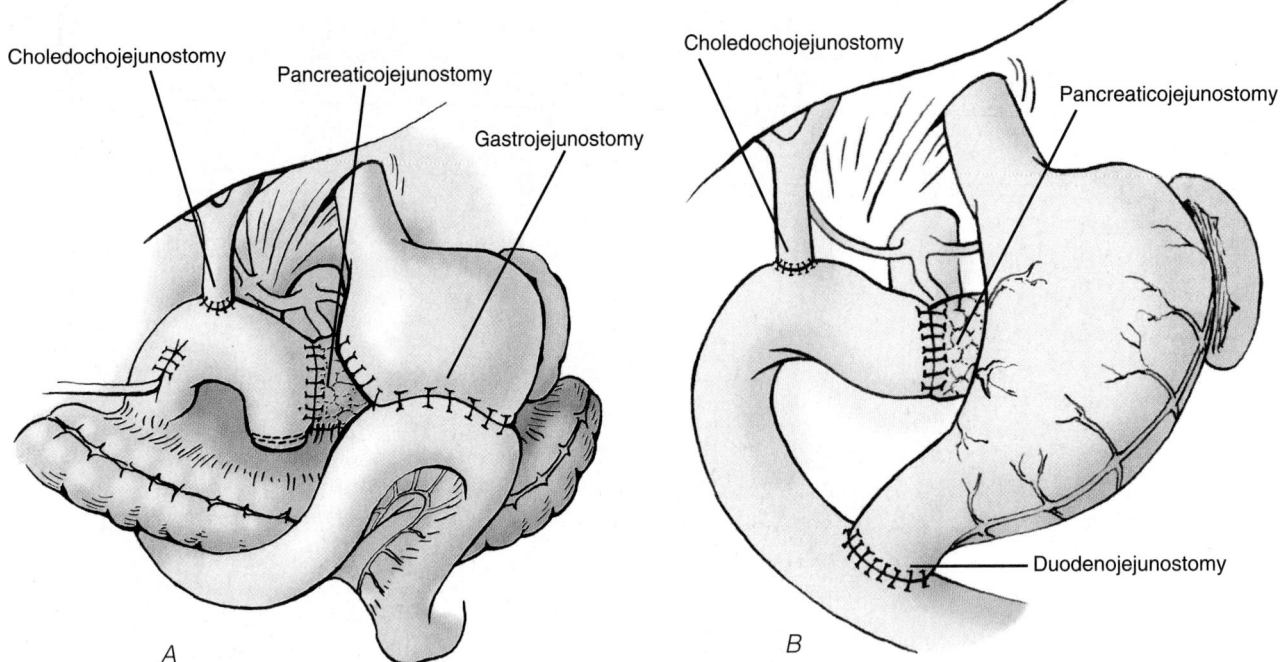

FIG. 32-61. The pancreaticoduodenectomy (Whipple procedure) can be performed either with the standard technique, which includes distal gastrectomy (*A*), or with preservation of the pylorus (*B*). The pylorus-sparing version of the procedure is used most commonly. [*Reproduced from Gaw JU, Andersen DK: Pancreatic surgery, in Wu GY, Aziz K, Whalen GF (eds): An Internist's Illustrated Guide to Gastrointestinal Surgery. Totowa, NJ: Humana Press, 2003, p 229, with permission.*]

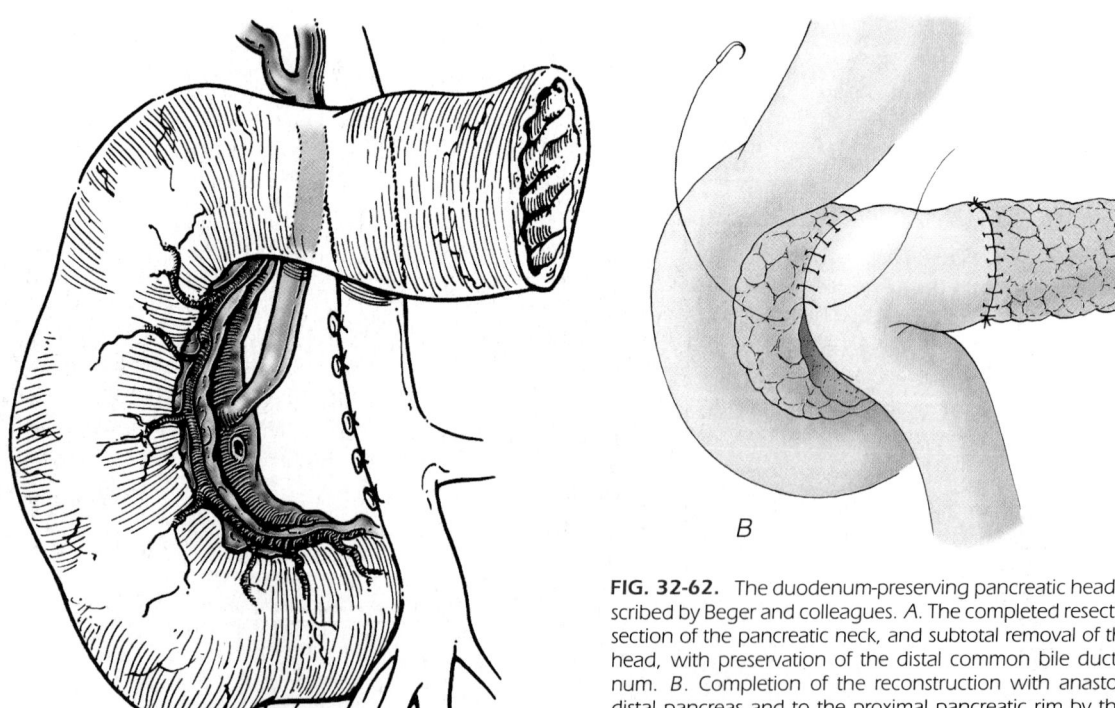

FIG. 32-62. The duodenum-preserving pancreatic head resection described by Beger and colleagues. *A.* The completed resection after transection of the pancreatic neck, and subtotal removal of the pancreatic head, with preservation of the distal common bile duct and duodenum. *B.* Completion of the reconstruction with anastomosis to the distal pancreas and to the proximal pancreatic rim by the same Roux limb of jejunum. (*Reproduced with permission from Bell.*[192])

rejection of allotransplanted islets have plagued this method since its initial clinical application in the early 1970s. However, despite the difficulties in recovering islets from a chronically inflamed gland, Najarian and associates demonstrated the utility of autotransplantation of islets in patients with chronic pancreatitis in 1980.[257] Subsequently, through refinements in the methods of harvesting and gland preservation, and through standardization of the methods by which islets are infused into the portal venous circuit for intrahepatic engraftment, the success of autotransplantation has steadily increased to achieve insulin independence in the majority of patients treated in recent series.[258,259] Although 2 to 3 million islets are required for successful engraftment in an allogeneic recipient, the autotransplant recipient can usually achieve long-term, insulin-independent status after engraftment of only 300,000 to 400,000 islets.[260] However, the ability to recover a sufficient quantity of islets from a sclerotic gland is dependent on the degree of disease present, so the selection of patients as candidates for autologous islet transplantation is important. As success with autotransplantation increases, patients with nonobstructive, sclerotic pancreatitis may be considered for resection and islet autotransplantation earlier in their course, as end-stage fibrosis bodes poorly for transplant success.[261] As the necessary expertise with islet transplantation becomes more widespread, this therapy may become routine in the treatment of chronic pancreatitis.

Denervation Procedures. In patients who have persistent and disabling pain, but who are poor candidates for resection or drainage procedures, a denervation procedure may provide symptomatic relief. As discussed above, neural ablation is a valid treatment strategy to block afferent sympathetic nociceptive pathways. In addition to direct infiltration of the celiac ganglia with long-acting analgesics or neurolytic agents,[262] a variety of true denervation procedures have been described for symptomatic relief in chronic pancreatitis. These include operative celiac ganglionectomy or splanchnicectomy,[263] transhiatal splanchnicectomy,[264] (Fig. 32-64), transthoracic splanchnicectomy with or without vagotomy,[265] and videoscopic transthoracic splanchnicectomy[266] (Fig. 32-65). Mallet-Guy demonstrated long-term pain relief in 83% of 215 patients treated with operative celiac splanchnicectomy,[263] and Michotey and associates claimed pain relief in all 14 patients treated with (transabdominal) transhiatal splanchnicectomy

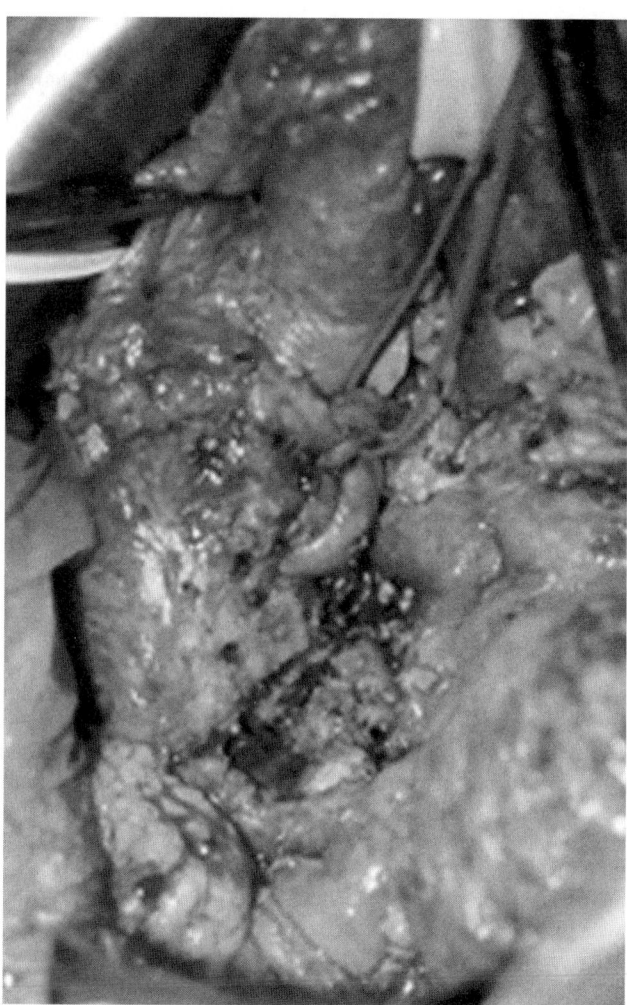

FIG. 32-63. Intraoperative view of the Beger procedure. The gastroduodenal artery is encircled by a vessel loop. Just below, the intrapancreatic portion of the common bile duct is exposed as it courses toward the ampulla. A rim of well-vascularized pancreatic tissue remains in the duodenal C-loop. Preservation of the posterior branch of the gastroduodenal artery is essential to preserve viability of these structures.

FIG. 32-64. Transhiatal splanchnicectomy. The transhiatal exposure of the right (A) and left (B) greater splanchnic nerves, reveals the splanchnic ganglia, the esophagus, the aorta, and the vertebral column. [Reproduced with permission from Klar E: Denervation procedures, in Beger HG et al (eds): The Pancreas. London: Blackwell Science, 1998, p 839.]

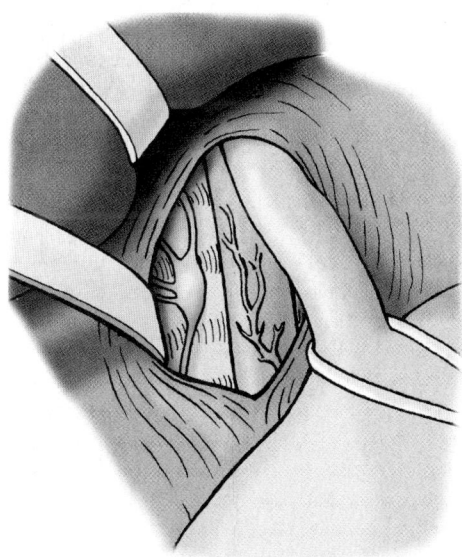

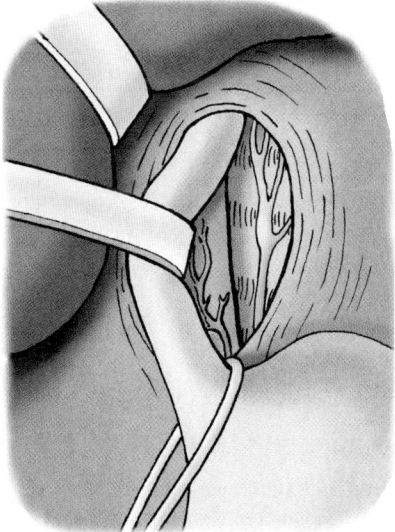

A

B

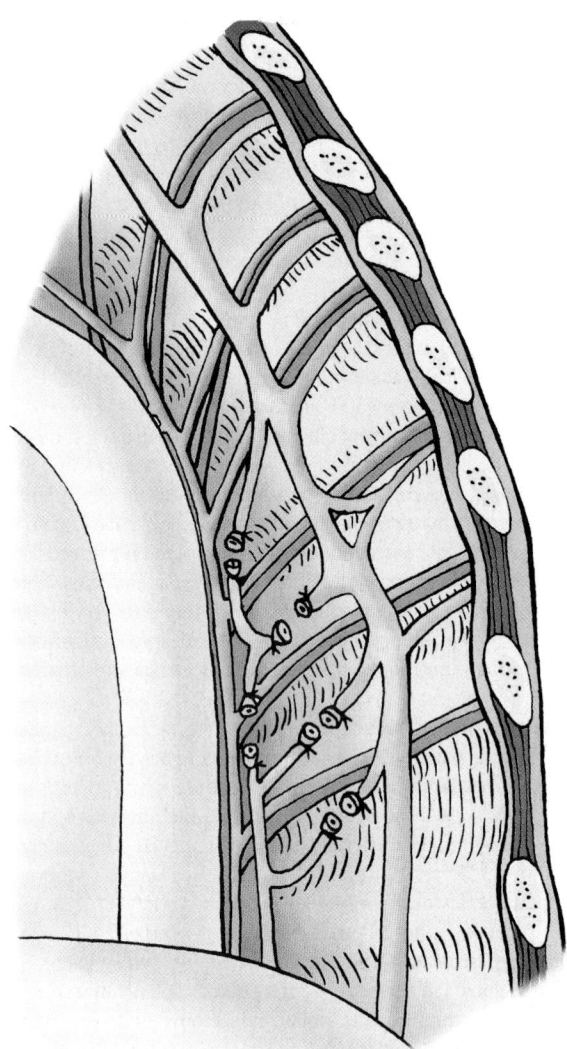

FIG. 32-65. *Anatomic landmarks for videoscopic transthoracic left splanchnicectomy. Diagram of the left plural cavity after clipping and division of the splanchnic nerves, showing the sympathetic chain, the intercostal vessels, and the aorta. [Reproduced with permission from Klar E: Denervation procedures, in Beger HG et al (eds): The Pancreas. London: Blackwell Science, 1998, p 839.]*

of the lower mediastinal sympathetic tracts,[264] but both of these approaches represent major abdominal procedures. For the patient who is a poor candidate for an abdominal procedure, the transthoracic ablation of the sympathetic chain, either on the left side alone[265] or bilaterally,[266] has been shown to result in pain relief in 60 to 66% of patients. The application of videoscopic techniques to thoracic splanchnicectomy has further reduced the risks and discomfort of these procedures in chronically-ill patients, and provides a valuable alternative to a direct attack on the pancreas.

PANCREATIC NEOPLASMS

Neoplasms of the Endocrine Pancreas

Neoplasms of the endocrine pancreas are relatively uncommon, but do occur with enough frequency (five cases per million population) that most surgeons will encounter them in an urban practice. The cells of the endocrine pancreas, or islet cells, originate

from neural crest cells, also referred to as amine precursor uptake and decarboxylation (APUD) cells. Multiple endocrine neoplasia (MEN) syndromes occur when these cells cause tumors in multiple sites. The MEN-1 syndrome involves pituitary tumors, parathyroid hyperplasia, and pancreatic neoplasms. Most pancreatic endocrine neoplasms are functional, secreting peptide products that produce interesting clinical presentations. Neoplasms of the endocrine pancreas that are not associated with excess hormone levels or a recognizable clinical syndrome are considered nonfunctional. Special immunohistochemical stains allow pathologists to confirm the peptide products being produced within the cells of a pancreatic endocrine tumor. However, the histologic characteristics of these neoplasms do not predict their clinical behavior, and malignancy is usually determined by the presence of local invasion and lymph node or hepatic metastases. Unfortunately, most pancreatic endocrine tumors are malignant, but the course of the disease is far more favorable than that seen with pancreatic exocrine cancer. The key to diagnosing these rare tumors is recognition of the classic clinical syndrome; confirmation is achieved by measuring serum levels of the elevated hormone. Localization of the tumor can be a challenging step, but once accomplished, the surgery is relatively straightforward. The goals of surgery range from complete resection, often accomplished with insulinomas, to controlling symptoms with debulking procedures, as is the case with most other pancreatic endocrine neoplasms. Unresectable disease in the liver is often addressed with chemoembolization.

As with pancreatic exocrine tumors, the initial diagnostic imaging test of choice for pancreatic endocrine tumors is a dynamic abdominal computed tomographic (CT) scan with fine cuts through the pancreas. Endoscopic ultrasound also can be valuable in localizing these tumors, which can produce dramatic symptoms despite their small (<1 cm) size. In contrast to pancreatic exocrine tumors, many of the endocrine tumors have somatostatin receptors that allow them to be detected by a radiolabeled octreotide scan. A radioactive somatostatin analog is injected intravenously, followed by whole-body radionuclide scanning. The success of this modality in localizing tumors and detecting metastases has decreased the use of older techniques such as angiography and selective venous sampling.

Insulinoma

Insulinomas are the most common pancreatic endocrine neoplasms and present with a typical clinical syndrome known as Whipple's triad. The triad consists of symptomatic fasting hypoglycemia, a documented serum glucose level less than 50 mg/dL, and relief of symptoms with the administration of glucose. Patients will often present with a profound syncopal episode and will admit to similar less severe episodes in the recent past. They also may admit to palpitations, trembling, diaphoresis, confusion or obtundation, and seizure, and family members may report that the patient has undergone a personality change. Routine laboratory studies will uncover a low blood sugar, the cause of all of these symptoms. The diagnosis is clinched with a monitored fast in which blood is sampled every 4 to 6 hours for glucose and insulin levels until the patient becomes symptomatic. Elevated C-peptide levels rule out the unusual case of surreptitious administration of insulin or oral hypoglycemic agents, because excess endogenous insulin production leads to excess C-peptide. Insulinomas are usually localized with CT scanning and endoscopic ultrasound (EUS). Technical advances in EUS have led to preoperative identification of more than 90% of insulinomas.[267] Visceral angiography with venous sampling is rarely required to accurately localize the tumor. Insulinomas are evenly distributed throughout the head, body, and tail of the pancreas.[268] Unlike most endocrine pancreatic tumors, the majority (90%) of insulinomas are benign and solitary, with only 10% malignant. They are typically cured by simple enucleation. However, tumors located close to the main pancreatic duct and large (>2 cm) tumors may require a distal pancreatectomy or pancreaticoduodenectomy. Intraoperative ultrasound is useful to determine the tumor's relation to the main pancreatic duct and guide intraoperative decision making. Enucleation of solitary insulinomas and distal pancreatectomy for insulinoma can be performed using a minimally-invasive technique.

Ninety percent of insulinomas are sporadic and 10% are associated with the MEN-1 syndrome. Insulinomas associated with the MEN-1 syndrome are more likely to be multifocal and have a higher rate of recurrence.

Gastrinoma

Zollinger-Ellison syndrome (ZES) is caused by a *gastrinoma,* an endocrine tumor that secretes gastrin, leading to acid hypersecretion and peptic ulceration. Many patients with ZES present with abdominal pain, peptic ulcer disease, and severe esophagitis. However, in the era of effective antacid therapy, the presentation can be less dramatic. While most of the ulcers are solitary, multiple ulcers in atypical locations that fail to respond to antacids should raise suspicion for ZES and prompt a work-up. Twenty percent of patients with gastrinoma have diarrhea at the time of diagnosis.

The diagnosis of ZES is made by measuring the serum gastrin level. It is important that patients stop taking proton pump inhibitors for this test. In most patients with gastrinomas, the level is greater than 1000 pg/mL. Gastrin levels can be elevated in conditions other than ZES. Common causes of hypergastrinemia include pernicious anemia, treatment with proton pump inhibitors, renal failure, G-cell hyperplasia, atrophic gastritis, retained or excluded antrum, and gastric outlet obstruction. In equivocal cases, when the gastrin level is not markedly elevated, a secretin stimulation test is helpful.

In 70 to 90% of patients, the primary gastrinoma is found in Passaro's triangle, an area defined by a triangle with points located at the junction of the cystic duct and common bile duct, the second and third portion of the duodenum, and the neck and body of the pancreas (Fig. 32-66). However, since gastrinomas can be

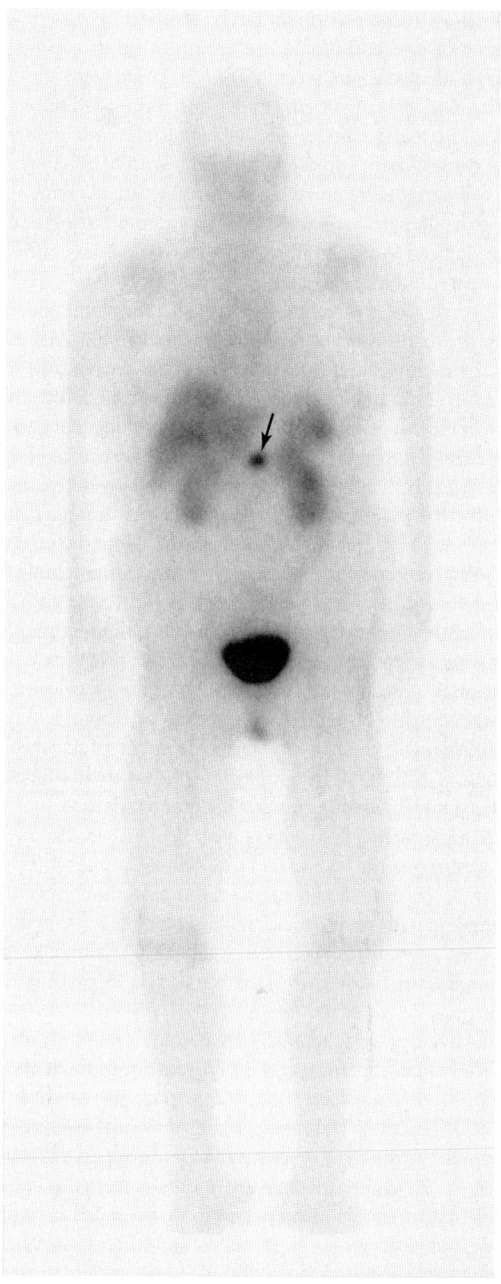

FIG. 32-67. Radionuclide octreotide scan demonstrating pancreatic endocrine tumor in the body of the pancreas (arrow).

found almost anywhere, whole-body imaging is required. The test of choice is somatostatin receptor (octreotide) scintigraphy in combination with CT (Fig. 32-67). The octreotide scan is more sensitive than CT, locating about 85% of gastrinomas and detecting tumors smaller than 1 cm. With the octreotide scan, the need for tedious and technically demanding selective angiography and measurement of gastrin gradients has declined. Endoscopic ultrasound is another new modality that assists in the preoperative localization of gastrinomas. It is particularly helpful in localizing tumors in the pancreatic head or duodenal wall, where gastrinomas are usually less than 1 cm in size. A combination of octreotide scan and EUS detects more than 90% of gastrinomas.

It is important to rule out MEN1 syndrome by checking serum calcium levels prior to surgery because resection of the

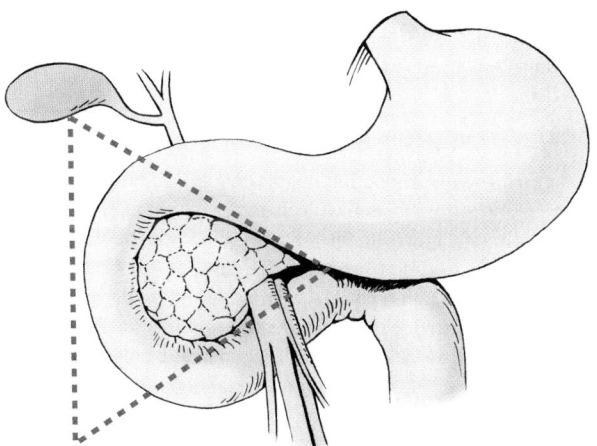

FIG. 32-66. Passaro's triangle. The typical location of a gastrinoma is described by this anatomic region, including the head of the pancreas, duodenum, and the lymphatic bed posterior and superior to the duodenum, as originally described by E. Passaro. (*Reproduced with permission from Bell.[192]*).

gastrinoma(s) in these patients rarely results in normalization of serum gastrin concentrations or a prolongation of survival. Only one fourth of gastrinomas occur in association with the MEN-1 syndrome. One half of patients with gastrinomas will have solitary tumors, while the remainder will have multiple gastrinomas. Multiple tumors are more common in patients with MEN-1 syndrome. Aggressive surgical treatment is justified in patients with sporadic gastrinomas. If patients have MEN-1 syndrome, the parathyroid hyperplasia is addressed with total parathyroidectomy and implantation of parathyroid tissue in the forearm.

Fifty percent of gastrinomas metastasize to lymph nodes or the liver, and are therefore considered malignant. Patients who meet criteria for operability should undergo exploration for possible removal of the tumor. Although the tumors are submucosal, a full-thickness excision of the duodenal wall is performed if a duodenal gastrinoma is found. All lymph nodes in Passaro's triangle are excised for pathologic analysis. If the gastrinoma is found in the pancreas and does not involve the main pancreatic duct, it is enucleated. Pancreatic resection is justified for solitary gastrinomas with no metastases. A highly-selective vagotomy can be performed if unresectable disease is identified or if the gastrinoma cannot be localized. This may reduce the amount of expensive proton pump inhibitors required. In cases in which hepatic metastases are identified, resection is justified if the primary gastrinoma is controlled and the metastases can be safely and completely removed. Debulking or incomplete removal of multiple hepatic metastases is probably not helpful, especially in the setting of MEN-1. The application of new modalities such as radiofrequency ablation seems reasonable, but data to support this approach are limited.[269] Postoperatively, patients are followed with fasting serum gastrin levels, secretin stimulation tests, octreotide scans, and CT scans. In patients found to have inoperable disease, chemotherapy with streptozocin, doxorubicin, and 5-fluorouracil is used. Other approaches such as somatostatin analogs, interferon, and chemoembolization also have been used in gastrinoma with some success.

Unfortunately, a biochemical cure is achieved in only about one third of the patients operated on for ZES. Despite the lack of success, long-term survival rates are good, even in patients with liver metastases. The 15-year survival rate for patients without liver metastases is about 80%, while the 5-year survival rate for patients with liver metastases is 20 to 50%. Pancreatic tumors are usually larger than tumors arising in the duodenum, and more often have lymph node metastases. In gastrinomas, liver metastases decrease survival rates, but lymph node metastases do not. The best results are seen after complete excision of small sporadic tumors originating in the duodenum. Large tumors associated with liver metastases, located outside of Passaro's triangle, have the worst prognosis.

VIPoma

In 1958, Verner and Morrison first described the syndrome associated with a pancreatic neoplasm secreting vasoactive intestinal polypeptide (VIP). The classic clinical syndrome associated with this pancreatic endocrine neoplasm consists of severe intermittent watery diarrhea leading to dehydration, and weakness from fluid and electrolyte losses. Large amounts of potassium are lost in the stool. The VIPoma syndrome is also called the WDHA syndrome due to the presence of *w*atery *d*iarrhea, *h*ypokalemia, and *a*chlorhydria. The massive (5 L/d) and episodic nature of the diarrhea associated with the appropriate electrolyte abnormalities should raise suspicion of the diagnosis. Serum VIP levels must be measured on multiple occasions because the excess secretion of VIP is episodic, and

single measurements might be normal and misleading. A CT scan localizes most VIPomas, although as with all islet cell tumors, EUS is the most sensitive imaging method. Electrolyte and fluid balance is sometimes difficult to correct preoperatively and must be pursued aggressively. Somatostatin analogs are helpful in controlling the diarrhea and allowing replacement of fluid and electrolytes. VIPomas are more commonly located in the distal pancreas and most have spread outside the pancreas. Palliative debulking operations can sometimes improve symptoms for a period, along with somatostatin analogs. Hepatic artery embolization also has been reported as a potentially beneficial treatment.[270]

Glucagonoma

Diabetes in association with dermatitis should raise the suspicion of a glucagonoma. The diabetes usually is mild. The classic necrolytic migratory erythema manifests as cyclic migrations of lesions with spreading margins and healing centers typically on the lower abdomen, perineum, perioral area, and feet. The diagnosis is confirmed by measuring serum glucagon levels, which are usually over 500 pg/mL. Glucagon is a catabolic hormone and most patients present with malnutrition. The rash associated with glucagonoma is thought to be caused by low levels of amino acids. Preoperative treatment usually includes control of the diabetes, parenteral nutrition, and octreotide. Like VIPomas, glucagonomas are more often in the body and tail of the pancreas and tend to be large tumors with metastases. Again, debulking operations are recommended in good operative candidates to relieve symptoms.

Somatostatinoma

Because somatostatin inhibits pancreatic and biliary secretions, patients with a somatostatinoma present with gallstones due to bile stasis, diabetes due to inhibition of insulin secretion, and steatorrhea due to inhibition of pancreatic exocrine secretion and bile secretion. Most somatostatinomas originate in the proximal pancreas or the pancreatoduodenal groove, with the ampulla and periampullary area as the most common site (60%). The most common presentations are abdominal pain (25%), jaundice (25%), and cholelithiasis (19%).[271] This rare type of pancreatic endocrine tumor is diagnosed by confirming elevated serum somatostatin levels, which are usually above 10 ng/mL. Although most reported cases of somatostatinoma involve metastatic disease, an attempt at complete excision of the tumor and cholecystectomy is warranted in fit patients.

Nonfunctioning Islet-Cell Tumors

Most pancreatic endocrine neoplasms do secrete one or more hormones and are associated with characteristic clinical syndromes. After insulinoma, however, the most common islet-cell tumor is the nonfunctioning islet-cell neoplasm. Because it is clinically silent until its size and location produce symptoms, it is usually malignant when first diagnosed. Some presumably nonfunctional pancreatic endocrine neoplasms stain positive for pancreatic polypeptide (PP), and elevated PP levels are therefore a marker for the lesion. Since clinical manifestations are absent, the tumors are usually large and metastatic at the time of diagnosis, unless they are detected serendipitously on CT scan or sonogram. Nonfunctioning islet-cell tumors are also seen in association with other multiple neoplasia syndromes, such as von Hippel-Lindau syndrome. The tumors grow slowly and 5-year survival is common, as opposed to pancreatic exocrine tumors, for which 5-year survival is extraordinarily rare.

Neoplasms of the Exocrine Pancreas

Epidemiology and Risk Factors

Cancer of the pancreas is the fifth leading cause of cancer death in the United States, with approximately 30,300 new cases and 29,700 deaths reported in 2002.[272] Despite its ubiquity, this disease is extremely difficult to treat, and its exact cause unknown. However, epidemiologic studies linking various environmental and host factors provide some clues. Recent discoveries using modern molecular biologic techniques have also improved our understanding of the causes of pancreatic cancer. The etiology of pancreatic cancer likely involves a complex interaction of genetic and environmental factors. Understanding these factors will become increasingly important as better diagnostic tools become available to screen populations at risk for developing pancreatic cancer.

A risk factor that is consistently linked to pancreatic cancer is cigarette smoking. Smoking increases the risk of developing pancreatic cancer by at least twofold due to the carcinogens in cigarette smoke.[273] Coffee and alcohol consumption have been investigated as possible risk factors, but the data are inconsistent. As in other gastrointestinal cancers, diets high in fat and low in fiber, fruits, and vegetables are thought to be associated with an increased risk of pancreatic cancer. Diabetes has been known to be associated with pancreatic cancer for many years. Pre-existing type II diabetes may increase the risk for development of pancreatic cancer.[274] The new onset of diabetes also can be an early manifestation of otherwise occult pancreatic cancer; evidence suggests that this phenomenon may be due to the secretion of a glucoregulatory peptide by the tumor cells. In fact, glucose intolerance is present in 80% of patients with pancreatic cancer, and approximately 20% have overt diabetes, a much greater incidence than would be expected to occur by chance. Thus the new onset of diabetes or a sudden increase in insulin requirement in an elderly patient with pre-existing diabetes should provoke concern for the presence of pancreatic cancer.

Recent epidemiologic studies have confirmed the fact that patients with chronic pancreatitis have an increased risk of developing pancreatic cancer.[275] Large, retrospective cohort studies of patients with pancreatitis have revealed up to a 20-fold increase in risk for pancreatic cancer. This increased risk seems to be independent of the type of pancreatitis, a finding consistent with the fact that most studies have shown little effect of alcohol ingestion per se on the risk of pancreatic carcinoma. The mechanisms involved in carcinogenesis in patients with pre-existing pancreatitis are unknown. However, the mutated K-*ras* oncogene, which is present in most cases of pancreatic cancer, has been detected in the ductal epithelium of some patients with chronic pancreatitis.

Genetics of Pancreatic Cancer

Pancreatic carcinogenesis involves the accumulation of multiple mutations. The K-*ras* oncogene is the most commonly mutated gene in pancreatic cancer, with approximately 90% of tumors having a mutation.[276] This prevalent mutation is present in precursor lesions and is therefore thought to occur early and be essential to pancreatic cancer development. K-*ras* mutations can be detected in DNA from serum, stool, pancreatic juice, and tissue aspirates of patients with pancreatic cancer, suggesting that the presence of this mutation may provide the basis for diagnostic testing in select individuals. The HER2/*neu* oncogene, homologous to the epidermal growth factor (EGF) receptor, is overexpressed in pancreatic cancers.[276] This receptor is involved in signal transduction pathways that lead to cellular proliferation. Multiple tumor suppressor genes

are deleted and/or mutated in pancreatic cancer, and include *p53*, *p16*, and *DPC4* (*Smad 4*), and in a minority of cases, *BRCA2*.[276] Most pancreatic cancers have three or more of the above mutations.

It is estimated that up to 10% of pancreatic cancers occur as a result of an inherited genetic predisposition. A family history of pancreatic cancer in a first-degree relative increases the risk of pancreatic cancer by about twofold.[276] Rare familial cancer syndromes that are associated with an increased risk of pancreatic cancer include BRCA2, the familial atypical multiple mole–melanoma (FAMM) syndrome, hereditary pancreatitis, familial adenomatous polyposis, hereditary nonpolyposis colorectal cancer (HNPCC), Peutz-Jeghers syndrome, and ataxia-telangiectasia.[277]

In addition to mutations in oncogenes and tumor suppressor genes, pancreatic cancers also are known to have aberrations in the expression of growth factors and their receptors. These growth factors include EGF, fibroblast growth factor (FGF), transforming growth factor-beta (TGF-β), insulin-like growth factor (IGF), hepatocyte growth factor (HGF), and vascular endothelial growth factor (VEGF)[278] (Fig. 32-68).

The fact that many gastrointestinal hormones and growth factors affect the growth of the normal exocrine pancreas suggests that these peptides also could affect the growth of pancreatic cancer. Studies in cell culture and laboratory animals suggest that somatostatin, vasoactive intestinal polypeptide, pancreatic polypeptide, peptide YY, and pancreastatin may inhibit pancreatic cancer cell growth, while other hormones such as cholecystokinin, gastrin, secretin, bombesin, EGF, FGF, IGF, and insulin may promote pancreatic cancer cell growth. Manipulation of these growth factors, their receptors, and secondary messengers may provide new clinical avenues to control the growth of pancreatic cancer.[278]

Pathology

The cell of origin for ductal pancreatic adenocarcinoma, the most common form of malignant pancreatic tumor, is unknown. Although it may seem intuitively obvious that pancreatic cancer arises from ductal cells, 95% of the pancreatic mass is comprised of acinar epithelium, which is known to dedifferentiate into a duct-like form under certain experimental conditions. Some animal models of pancreatic carcinogenesis suggest that cells within the islets of Langerhans are capable of transforming into ductal adenocarcinoma cells. It is quite possible that the cell of origin for pancreatic cancer is a pluripotent cell capable of differentiation along an endocrine or exocrine line. The molecular mechanisms and markers involved in normal pancreatic development are just beginning to be unraveled, and this information may shed some valuable light on the process of pancreatic carcinogenesis.

Pancreatic cancer does appear to arise through a stepwise progression of cellular changes, just as colon cancer progresses by stages from hyperplastic polyp to invasive cancer. Systematic histologic evaluation of areas surrounding pancreatic cancers has revealed the presence of precursor lesions which have been named pancreatic intraepithelial neoplasia (PanIN). Three stages of PanIN have been defined. These lesions demonstrate the same oncogene mutations and loss of tumor suppressor genes found in invasive cancers, the frequency of these abnormalities increasing with progressive cellular atypia and architectural disarray.[279] The ability to detect these precursor lesions in humans is an important goal of current pancreatic cancer research.

About two thirds of pancreatic adenocarcinomas arise within the head or uncinate process of the pancreas; 15% are in the body, and 10% in the tail, with the remaining tumors demonstrating

MOLECULAR BIOLOGY OF PANCREATIC CANCER

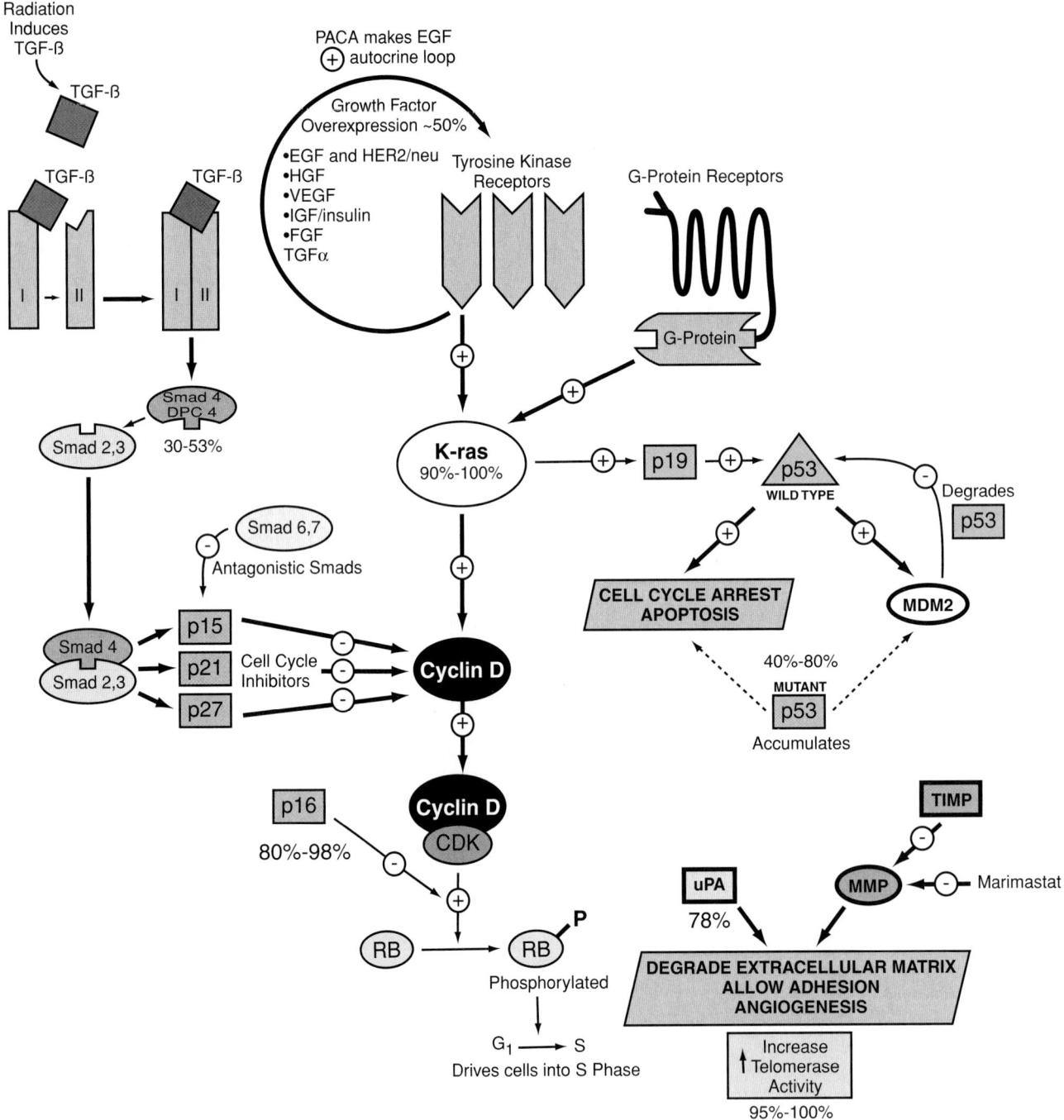

FIG. 32-68. Molecular biology of pancreatic cancer. Pancreatic carcinogenesis involves the accumulation of multiple mutations in oncogenes, tumor suppressor genes, and growth factor receptors. Most pancreatic cancers have three or more mutations.

diffuse involvement of the gland. Tumors in the pancreatic body and tail are generally larger at the time of diagnosis and therefore less commonly resectable. Tumors in the head of the pancreas are typically diagnosed earlier because they cause obstructive jaundice. Ampullary carcinomas, carcinomas of the distal bile duct, and peri-ampullary duodenal adenocarcinomas present in a similar fashion to pancreatic head cancer, but have a slightly better prognosis, probably

because early obstruction of the bile duct and jaundice leads to the diagnosis.

In addition to ductal adenocarcinoma, which makes up about 75% of nonendocrine cancers of the pancreas, there are a variety of less common types of pancreatic cancer. Adenosquamous carcinoma is a variant that has both glandular and squamous differentiation. The biologic behavior of this lesion is unfortunately no better than

Table 32-18
Staging of Pancreatic Cancer

Primary tumor (T)				
T1			Limited to pancreas, <2 cm	
T2			Limited to pancreas, >2 cm	
T3			Extension into duodenum or bile duct	
T4			Extension into portal vein, superior mesenteric vein, superior mesenteric artery, stomach, spleen, colon	
Regional lymph nodes (N)				
N0			No nodal metastases	
N1			Regional nodal metastases	
Distant metastases (M)				
M0			No distant metastases	
M1			Distant metastases (liver, lung)	

Stage	*T*	*N*	*M*	*Description*
I	1, 2	0	0	Tumor confined to pancreas
II	3	0	0	Tumor invades duodenum and/or bile duct outside pancreas; no lymph node involvement
III	1, 2, 3	1	0	Tumor has not spread beyond duodenum or bile duct, but includes regional lymph nodes
IVA	4	Any	0	Locally advanced tumor growing into blood vessels, stomach, spleen, and colon, with or without lymph node involvement
IVB	Any	Any	1	Distant metastases (liver, lungs) present

the typical ductal adenocarcinoma.[280] Acinar cell carcinoma is an uncommon type of pancreatic cancer that usually presents as a large tumor, often 10 cm in diameter or more, but the prognosis of patients with these tumors may be better than with ductal cancer.

Diagnosis and Staging

Exact pathologic staging of pancreatic cancer is important because it allows accurate quantitative assessment of results and comparisons between institutions. The *t*umor-*n*ode-*m*etastasis (TNM) staging of pancreatic cancer is shown in Table 32-18.

T1 lesions are smaller than 2 cm in diameter and are limited to the pancreas. T2 lesions also are limited to the pancreas, but are larger than 2 cm. T3 lesions extend into the duodenum or extrapancreatic bile duct. T4 lesions extend into the portal vein, superior mesenteric vein, superior mesenteric artery, stomach, spleen, or colon. T1 and T2 tumors with no lymph node involvement are considered stage I disease, while more extensive invasion, such as that associated with T3 tumors, indicates stage II disease. Any lymph node involvement indicates stage III disease. Stage IV disease is divided into patients with locally-advanced tumors (T4) without metastatic disease (stage IVA), and patients with metastases to distant sites such as the liver or lungs (stage IVB). In a review of national data covering the period from 1992 to 1999, only 16.6% of patients with pancreatic cancer presented with localized disease. Of patients presenting with disease confined to the pancreas, only 8% were still alive 5 years after diagnosis.[281]

The most critical deficit in the ability to treat pancreatic cancer effectively is the lack of tools for early diagnosis. The pancreas is situated deep within the abdomen, and the early symptoms of pancreatic cancer often are too vague to raise suspicion of the disease. Ultimately, the majority of patients present with pain and jaundice. On physical exam, weight loss is evident and the skin is icteric; a distended gallbladder is palpable in about one fourth of patients. More fortunate patients have tumors situated such that biliary obstruction and jaundice occurs early and prompts diagnostic tests.

Unfortunately, however, the vast majority of patients are not diagnosed until weight loss has occurred—a sign of advanced disease.

Although it is often taught that carcinoma of the pancreas presents with painless jaundice (to help distinguish it from choledocholithiasis), this aphorism is not accurate. Most patients do experience pain as part of the symptom complex of pancreatic cancer, and it is often the first symptom. Therefore awareness of the way pancreatic pain is perceived may help clinicians suspect pancreatic cancer. The pain associated with pancreatic cancer is usually perceived in the epigastrium, but can occur in any part of the abdomen and often, but not always, penetrates to the back. When questioned in retrospect, patients often recall mild and vague pain for many months before diagnosis. A low threshold for ordering a CT scan with "pancreatic protocol" should be maintained for elderly patients with unexplained, persistent, although vague, abdominal pain. As mentioned above, new-onset diabetes in an elderly patient, especially if combined with vague abdominal pain, should prompt a search for pancreatic cancer.

Unfortunately, at this time there is no sensitive and specific serum marker to assist in the timely diagnosis of pancreatic cancer. With jaundice, direct hyperbilirubinemia and elevated alkaline phosphatase are expected, but do not serve much of a diagnostic role other than to confirm the obvious. With longstanding biliary obstruction, the prothrombin time will be prolonged due to a depletion of vitamin K, a fat-soluble vitamin dependent on bile flow for absorption. CA19-9 is a mucin-associated carbohydrate antigen that can be detected in the serum of patients with pancreatic cancer. Serum levels are elevated in about 75% of patients with pancreatic cancer; however, CA19-9 is also elevated in about 10% of patients with benign diseases of the pancreas, liver, and bile ducts.[282] CA19-9 is thus neither sufficiently sensitive nor specific to allow an earlier diagnosis of pancreatic cancer. Despite the fact that many tumor markers, such as CA19-9, have been studied in an attempt to facilitate early diagnosis, there are still no effective screening tests for pancreatic cancer. Recently, microarray technology has been used to profile gene expression in pancreatic tumors, pancreatic cancer cell lines, chronic pancreatitis, and the normal pancreas. A review of the literature shows that there are more than 1000 genes that are differentially expressed in pancreatic tumors, and about 50 of these genes have been repeatedly reported by a number of different investigators using slightly different techniques.[283] The proteins encoded by these genes have potential for early detection of pancreatic cancer. Some of these genes would be expected to be expressed at the cell surface or in pancreatic juice and may be useful as biomarkers for pancreatic cancer. Immunocytochemistry using tissue microarrays and other experiments are underway to localize and quantify expression of these genes at the protein level in samples of human pancreatic cancer.

In patients presenting with jaundice, a reasonable first diagnostic imaging study is abdominal ultrasound. If bile duct dilation is not seen, hepatocellular disease is likely. Demonstration of cholelithiasis and bile duct dilation suggests a diagnosis of choledocholithiasis, and the next logical step would be endoscopic retrograde cholangiopancreatography (ERCP) to clear the bile duct. In the absence of gallstones, malignant obstruction of the bile duct is likely and a CT scan rather than ERCP would be the next logical step. For patients suspected of having pancreatic cancer who present without jaundice, ultrasound is not appropriate, and a CT scan should be the first test.

The current diagnostic and staging test of choice for pancreatic cancer is a dynamic contrast-enhanced spiral CT scan, and techniques are constantly improving (Fig. 32-69). The accuracy of CT scanning for predicting unresectable disease is 90 to 95 percent.[284] CT findings that indicate a tumor is unresectable include invasion of the hepatic or superior mesenteric artery, enlarged lymph nodes outside the boundaries of resection, ascites, distant metastases (e.g., liver), and distant organ invasion (e.g., colon). Invasion of the superior mesenteric vein or portal vein is not in itself a contraindication to resection as long as the veins are patent. In contrast, CT scanning is less accurate in predicting resectable disease. CT scanning will miss small liver metastases and predicting arterial involvement is sometimes difficult.

Currently, CT is probably the single most versatile and cost-effective tool for the diagnosis of pancreatic cancer. Abdominal MRI is rapidly evolving but currently provides essentially the same information as CT scanning. Positron emission tomography (PET) scanning is becoming more widely available and may help distinguish chronic pancreatitis from pancreatic cancer. EUS can be used to detect small pancreatic masses that could be missed by CT scanning, and is commonly used when there is a high suspicion for pancreatic cancer but no mass is identified by the CT scan. EUS has the added advantage of providing the opportunity for transluminal biopsy of pancreatic masses, although a tissue diagnosis prior to pancreaticoduodenectomy is not required. However, in specific patients a histologic diagnosis may be necessary such as for those in a neoadjuvant clinical trial or before chemotherapy in advanced tumors. EUS is a sensitive test for portal/superior mesenteric vein invasion, although it is somewhat less effective at detecting superior mesenteric artery invasion. When all of the current staging modalities are utilized, their accuracy in predicting resectability is reported to be about 80%, meaning that one in five patients brought to the operating room with the intent of a curative resection will be found at the time of surgery to have unresectable disease.[285]

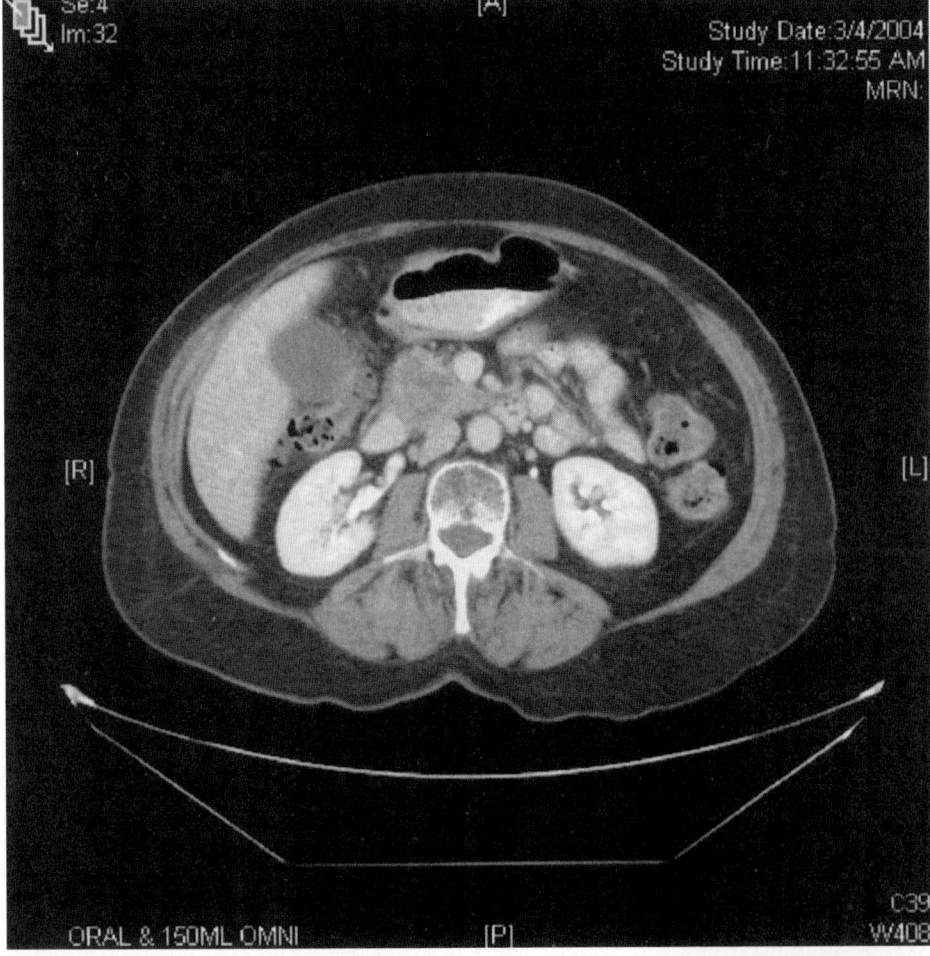

FIG. 32-69. CT scan demonstrating pancreatic cancer.

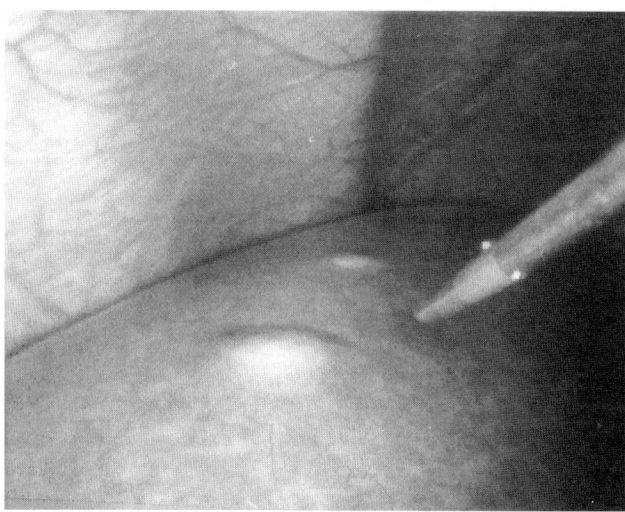

FIG. 32-70. *Diagnostic laparoscopy.*

In an attempt to avoid such futile laparotomies, several surgeons have advocated the use of preliminary laparoscopy for patients with disease felt to be resectable by imaging (Fig. 32-70). Diagnostic laparoscopy with the use of ultrasound is reported to improve the accuracy of predicting resectability to about 98%.[285] The technique involves more than simple visualization with the scope, and requires the placement of three ports and manipulation of the tissues. A general exploration of the peritoneal surfaces is carried out. The ligament of Treitz and the base of the transverse mesocolon are examined for tumor. The gastrocolic ligament is incised and the lesser sac is examined. The ultrasound probe is then used to examine the liver, porta hepatis, and the portal vein and superior mesenteric artery.

The percentage of patients in whom a positive laparoscopy helps avoid a nontherapeutic laparotomy varies from 10 to 30% in carcinoma of the head of the pancreas, but may be as high as 50% in patients with tumors in the body and tail of the gland. As the quality of CT scanning improves, the value of routine diagnostic laparoscopy decreases. However, the morbidity of diagnostic laparoscopy is less than that of laparotomy, and the procedure can be performed on an outpatient basis. Patients who are found to have

unresectable disease recover more rapidly than from a laparotomy and can receive palliative chemotherapy and radiation sooner. The potential immunosuppressive effects of a major surgical procedure also are avoided, as well as the negative psychologic impact of a major painful operation with little benefit.

Critics of the routine use of staging laparoscopy in pancreatic cancer argue that it unnecessarily increases operating room time in an already lengthy procedure. The overall cost of treatment is increased because approximately 80% of patients will proceed to an open laparotomy for resection. The use of laparoscopic techniques and ultrasound requires special expertise to obtain the reported level of accuracy. Finally, some surgeons recommend that patients should undergo laparotomy for a biliary and perhaps enteric bypass for palliation, believing endoscopic palliation to be inadequate. This concept is not supported by recent literature, which indicates that the failure rate after endoscopic stenting for unresectable disease is similar to the failure rate after open biliary bypass surgery. The endoscopist is successful in decompressing the bile duct in almost all cases. When large (10F) plastic stents are used, most patients do not require replacement for about 3 months. Metallic Wallstents last about 5 months on average and usually fail only with tumor ingrowth.[286] Keeping in mind that patients with unresectable pancreatic cancer usually live less than 1 year, the requirement for numerous stent changes is unlikely.

Diagnostic laparoscopy is possibly best applied to patients with pancreatic cancer on a selective basis. The routine use of diagnostic laparoscopy seems appropriate in centers offering clinical trials in which pretreatment biopsy and accurate staging are required. Diagnostic laparoscopy will also have a higher yield in patients with large tumors (>2cm), tumors located in the body or tail, patients with equivocal findings of metastasis or ascites on CT scan, and patients with other indications of advanced disease such as marked weight loss or markedly elevated CA19-9. An algorithm for the diagnosis, staging, and treatment of pancreatic cancer is shown in Fig. 32-71.

Palliative Surgery and Endoscopy

For the 85 to 90% of patients with pancreatic cancer who have disease that precludes surgical resection, appropriate and effective palliative treatment is critical to the quality of their remaining life. Because of the poor prognosis of the disease, it is not appropriate

DIAGNOSTIC AND TREATMENT ALGORITHM

FIG. 32-71. *Diagnostic and treatment algorithm for pancreatic cancer. If CT scan demonstrates a potentially resectable tumor, patients are offered participation in a clinical trial after histologic confirmation by CT or EUS-guided biopsy. If CT scan demonstrates resectable disease, diagnostic laparoscopy is used selectively in patients with tumors in the body/tail, equivocal findings of metastasis or CT scan, ascites, high CA19-9 or marked weight loss. Patients also have diagnostic laparoscopy if they elect to participate in a neoadjuvant clinical trial. In cases where no mass is demonstrated on CT scan, but suspicion of cancer remains, EUS or ERCP with brushings are performed and the CT may be repeated after an interval of observation.*

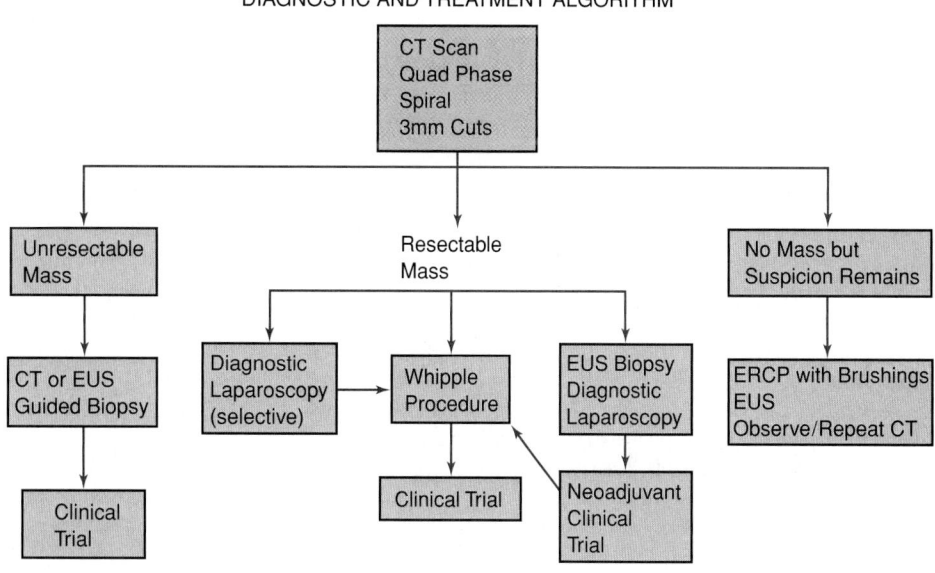

to employ invasive and toxic regimens in patients with extremely advanced disease and poor performance status. When patients do desire antineoplastic therapy, it is important to encourage them to enroll in clinical trials so that therapeutic advances can be made.

In general, there are three clinical problems in advanced pancreatic cancer that require palliation: pain, jaundice, and duodenal obstruction. The mainstay of pain control is oral narcotics. Sustained-release preparations of morphine sulfate are frequently used. Invasion of retroperitoneal nerve trunks accounts for the severe pain experienced by patients with advanced pancreatic cancer. A celiac plexus nerve block can control pain effectively for a period of months, although the procedure sometimes needs to be repeated. At the time of initial exploration for pancreatic cancer, it is a good practice to think about pain control and consider performing an intraoperative celiac block regardless of whether a resection is performed. The procedure is performed by injecting 50% alcohol directly into the tissues along the sides of the aorta just cephalad and posterior to the origin of the celiac trunk. This can be accomplished quite easily with either open surgery or laparoscopic surgery, and does not prolong the operation by more than a few minutes. If necessary, the procedure can be repeated postoperatively, either percutaneously or with use of endoscopic ultrasound guidance.

Jaundice is present in the majority of patients with pancreatic cancer, and the most troublesome aspect for the patient is the accompanying pruritus. Biliary obstruction may also lead to cholangitis, coagulopathy, digestive symptoms, and hepatocellular failure. In the past, surgeons traditionally performed a biliary bypass when unresectable disease was found at laparotomy. As many patients today already have a bile duct stent in place by the time of operation, it is not clear that operative biliary bypass is required. If an operative bypass is performed, choledochojejunostomy is the preferred approach. Although an easy procedure to perform, choledochoduodenostomy is felt to be unwise because of the proximity of the duodenum to tumor. Some have discouraged the use of the gallbladder for biliary bypass;[287] however, it is suitable as long as the cystic duct clearly enters the common duct well above the tumor.

Duodenal obstruction is usually a late event in pancreatic cancer and occurs in only about 20% of patients.[288] Therefore, in the absence of signs or symptoms of obstruction, such as nausea or vomiting, or a tumor that is already encroaching on the duodenum at the time of surgery, the routine use of prophylactic gastrojejunostomy when exploration reveals unresectable tumor is controversial. Although anastomotic leaks are uncommon, gastrojejunostomy is sometimes associated with delayed gastric emptying, the very symptom the procedure is designed to treat.

Whether performing both a biliary and enteric bypass or just a biliary bypass, the jejunum is brought anterior to the colon rather than retrocolic, where the tumor potentially would invade the bowel sooner. Some surgeons use a loop of jejunum with a jejunojejunostomy to divert the enteric stream away from the biliary-enteric anastomosis. Others use a Roux-en-Y limb with the gastrojejunostomy located 50 cm downstream from the hepaticojejunostomy (Fig. 32-72). Potential advantages of the defunctionalized Roux-en-Y limb include the ease with which it will reach up to the hepatic hilum, probable decreased risk of cholangitis, and easier management of biliary anastomotic leaks. If a gastrojejunostomy is performed, it should be placed dependently and posterior along the greater curvature to improve gastric emptying, and a vagotomy should not be performed. If patients are explored laparoscopically and found to have unresectable disease, palliation of jaundice can be achieved in a minimally-invasive fashion with ERCP and placement of a coated, expandable metallic endoscopic biliary stent

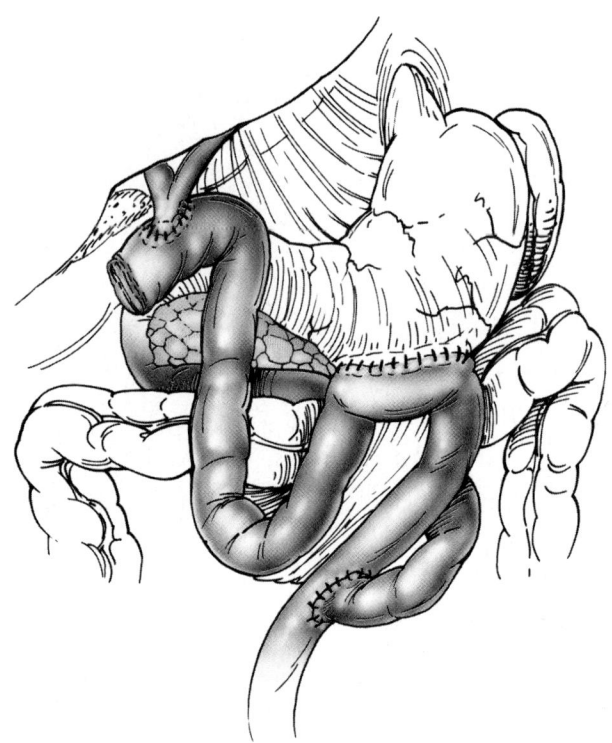

FIG. 32-72. Biliary-enteric bypass to palliate unresectable pancreatic cancer. (*Reproduced with permission from Bell, Rikkers, Mulholland (eds): Atlas of Pancreatic Surgery, 1st ed. Philadelphia: Lippincott, Williams & Wilkins, 1996.*)

(Fig. 32-73). Endoscopic stents are definitely not as durable as a surgical bypass. Recurrent obstruction and cholangitis is more common with stents and results in inferior palliation. However, this minimally-invasive approach is associated with considerably less initial morbidity and mortality than surgical bypass. Newer, expandable metallic Wallstents demonstrate improved patency and provide better palliation than plastic stents.

If an initial diagnostic laparoscopy reveals a contraindication to the Whipple procedure, such as liver metastases, it is not appropriate to perform a laparotomy simply to create a biliary bypass. In such a patient it is better to place an endoscopic stent. In contrast, if a laparotomy has already been performed as part of the assessment of resectability and the Whipple procedure is not possible, a surgical bypass is usually performed. However, if the patient has a functioning endoscopic stent already in place, it may be reasonable to forego surgical bypass.

Palliative Chemotherapy and Radiation

In patients with unresectable pancreatic cancer, gemcitabine results in symptomatic improvement, improved pain control and performance status, and weight gain.[289] However, survival is improved by only 1 to 2 months. Although these results may warrant treatment in patients who understand the benefits and risks, the lack of significant survival advantage should encourage physicians to refer motivated patients for experimental protocols such as gene therapy, since it is only through continued clinical research that more meaningful treatments for pancreatic cancer will be developed.

Surgical Resection: Pancreaticoduodenectomy

In a patient with appropriate clinical and/or imaging indications of pancreatic cancer, a tissue diagnosis prior to performing a

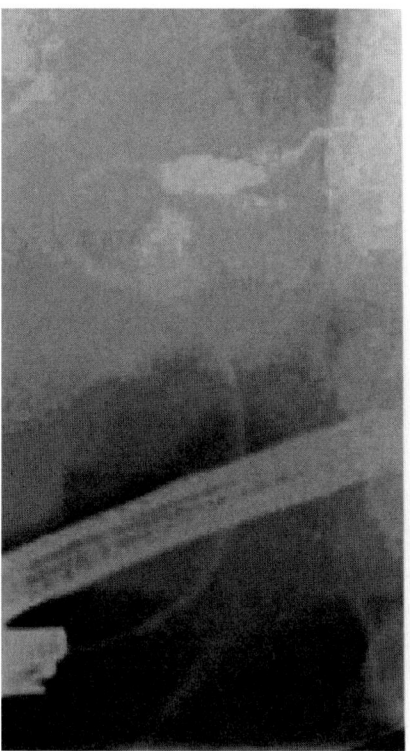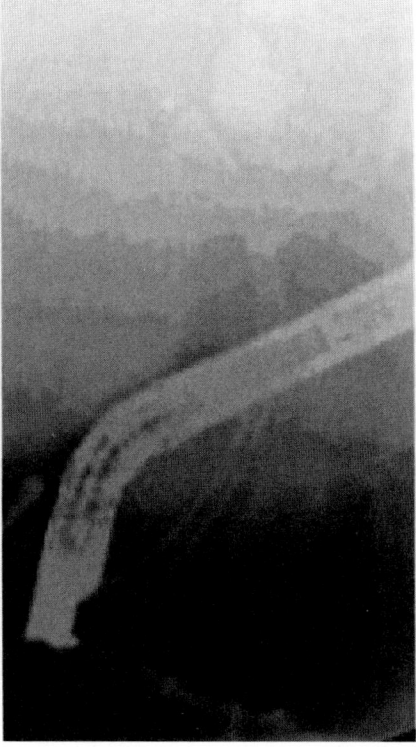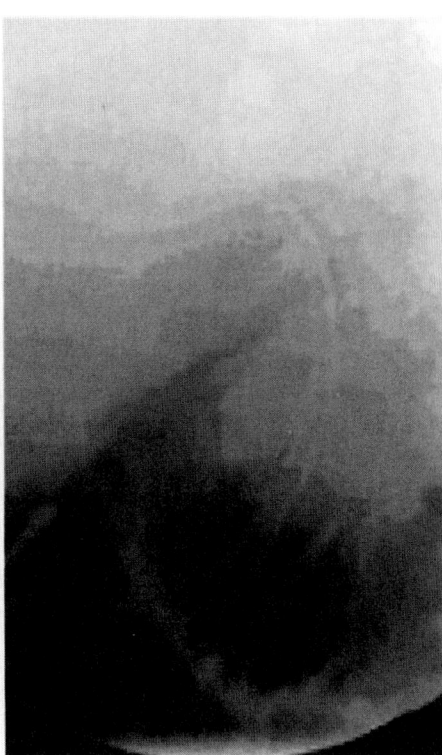

FIG. 32-73. Expandable metallic biliary stent.

pancreaticoduodenectomy is not essential. Although percutaneous CT-guided biopsy is usually safe, complications such as hemorrhage, pancreatitis, fistula, abscess, and even death can occur. Tumor seeding along the subcutaneous tract of the needle is uncommon. Likewise, fine-needle aspiration under endoscopic ultrasound guidance is safe and well tolerated. The problem with preoperative or even intraoperative biopsy is that many pancreatic cancers are not very cellular and contain a significant amount of fibrous tissue, so a biopsy may be misinterpreted as showing chronic pancreatitis if it does not contain malignant glandular cells. In the face of clinical and radiologic preoperative indications of pancreatic cancer, a negative biopsy should not preclude resection. In patients who are not candidates for resection because of metastatic disease, biopsy for a tissue diagnosis becomes important because these patients may be candidates for palliative chemotherapy and radiation therapy trials. It is especially important to make an aggressive attempt at tissue diagnosis prior to surgery in patients whose clinical presentation and imaging studies are more suggestive of alternative diagnoses such as pancreatic lymphoma or pancreatic islet-cell tumors. These patients might avoid surgery altogether in the case of lymphoma, or warrant an aggressive debulking approach in the case of islet-cell carcinoma.

Pancreaticoduodenectomy can be performed at a later date or immediately after and under the same anesthetic as the negative diagnostic laparoscopy with intraoperative ultrasound. The procedure can be performed through a midline incision from xiphoid to umbilicus or through a bilateral subcostal incision. The initial portion of the procedure is a continuation of the assessment of resectability. The steps are the same as those performed laparoscopically. The liver and visceral and parietal peritoneal surfaces are thoroughly assessed. The gastrohepatic omentum is opened and the celiac axis area is examined for enlarged lymph nodes. The base of the transverse mesocolon to the right of the middle colic vessels is examined for tumor involvement.

A Kocher maneuver is performed by dissecting behind the head of the pancreas. The superior mesenteric vein and artery are palpated for involvement. It also is important to assess for an aberrant right hepatic artery, which is present in 20% of patients. The aberrant artery arises from the superior mesenteric artery posterior to the pancreas, and ascends parallel and adjacent to the superior mesenteric and portal veins. The presence of an aberrant right hepatic artery is usually best ascertained by palpation on the back side of the hepatoduodenal ligament, where a prominent pulse will be felt next to the portal vein. The porta hepatis is examined. Enlarged or firm lymph nodes that can be swept down toward the head of the pancreas with the specimen do not preclude resection. If the assessment phase reveals no contraindications to the Whipple procedure (Table 32-19), the resection phase commences.

The hepatic artery is dissected and traced toward the porta hepatis. Small vessels in this area should be ligated with 3-0 or 4-0 silk ligatures to prevent bothersome hemorrhage later in the case that makes subsequent dissection more tedious. The gastroduodenal branch of the hepatic artery is identified. A test clamping is

Table 32-19
Findings at Exploration

Findings contraindicating resection
Liver metastases (any size)
Celiac lymph node involvement
Peritoneal implants
Invasion of transverse mesocolon
Hepatic hilar lymph node involvement

Findings not contraindicating resection
Invasion at duodenum or distal stomach
Involved peripancreatic lymph nodes
Involved lymph nodes along the porta hepatis that can
  be swept down with the specimen

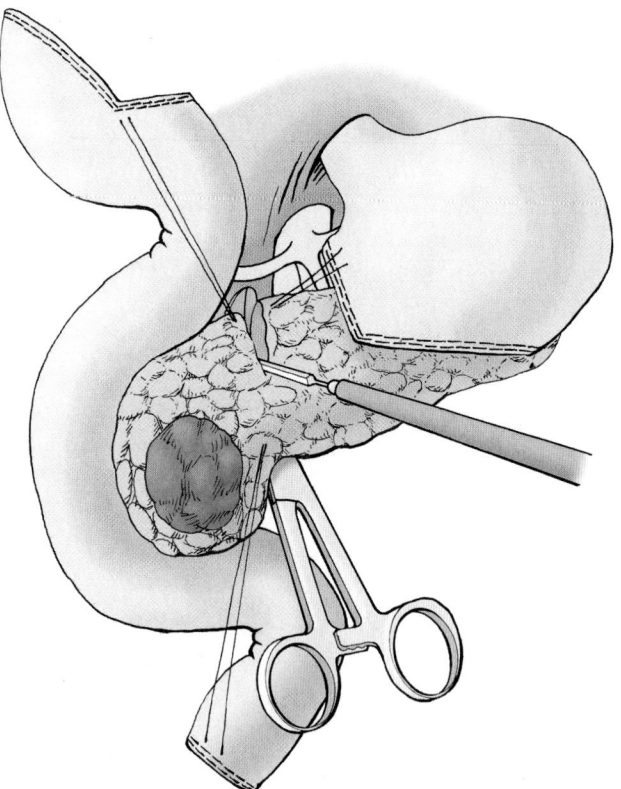

FIG. 32-74. Division of the pancreatic neck. The pancreatic neck is separated from the anterior surface of the portal vein and then divided. If there is no tumor involvement, the neck of the pancreas will separate from the vein easily. A large, blunt-tipped clamp is a safe instrument to use for this dissection. (*Reproduced with permission from Bell, Rikkers, Mulholland (eds): Atlas of Pancreatic Surgery, 1st ed. Philadelphia: Lippincott, Williams & Wilkins, 1996.*)

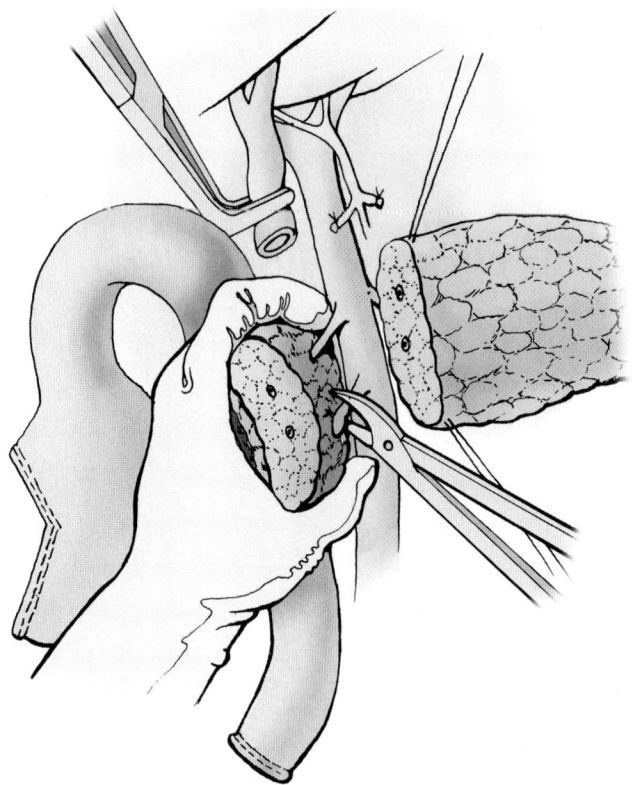

FIG. 32-75. Dissection of the pancreatic head and uncinate process. The pancreatic head and uncinate process are dissected off of the right lateral aspect of the superior mesenteric vein and portal vein by ligating the fragile venous branches. (*Reproduced with permission from Bell, Rikkers, Mulholland (eds): Atlas of Pancreatic Surgery, 1st ed. Philadelphia: Lippincott, Williams & Wilkins, 1996.*)

performed to assure that a strong pulse remains in the proper hepatic artery before division of the gastroduodenal artery. Once the gastroduodenal artery is divided, the hepatic artery is retracted medially and the common bile duct is retracted laterally to reveal the glistening anterior surface of the portal vein behind them. Dissection is performed only on the anterior surface of the vein. If there is no tumor involvement, the neck of the pancreas will separate from the vein easily. A large, blunt-tipped clamp is a safe instrument to use for this dissection (Fig. 32-74). The superior mesenteric vein is then identified running anterior to the third portion of the duodenum. Identification is facilitated by gentle inferior traction on the transverse mesocolon and tracing the middle colic vein retrograde. The tunnel under the neck of the pancreas can then be developed from inferior and superior.

The gallbladder is then mobilized from the liver, the cystic duct and artery are ligated, and the gallbladder is removed. The common hepatic duct is divided just above the entrance of the cystic duct, and the duct is dissected down to the superior margin of the duodenum. Inferior traction on the distal bile duct opens the plane to make visible the anterior portion of the portal vein (Fig. 32-75). Either the duodenum is divided 2 cm distal to the pylorus (pylorus-preserving pancreaticoduodenectomy) or the antrum is divided. The jejunum is divided beyond the ligament of Treitz and the mesentery is ligated until the jejunum can be delivered posterior to the superior mesenteric vessels from left to right. The pancreatic neck is divided anterior to the portal vein (see Fig. 32-74). The pancreatic head and uncinate process then are dissected off of the

right lateral aspect of the superior mesenteric vein, ligating the fragile branches draining the head and uncinate process into the portal vein (see Fig. 32-75). The uncinate process is then dissected off of the posterior aspect of the superior mesenteric artery. The wound is irrigated and meticulous hemostasis is assured at this point because the view of the portal vein area and retroperitoneum is more difficult after the reconstruction phase is completed.

The reconstruction involves anastomoses of the pancreas first, then the bile duct, and finally the duodenum or stomach. There are various techniques for the pancreatic anastomoses and all have equivalent outcomes. After the pancreatic anastomosis is completed, the choledochojejunostomy is performed about 10 cm down the jejunal limb from the pancreatic anastomosis. This is usually performed in an end-to-side fashion with one layer of interrupted sutures. The duodenojejunostomy or gastrojejunostomy is performed another 10 to 15 cm downstream from the biliary anastomosis, using a two-layer technique.

Variations and Controversies

The preservation of the pylorus has several theoretical advantages including prevention of reflux of pancreaticobiliary secretions into the stomach, decreased incidence of marginal ulceration, normal gastric acid secretion and hormone release, and improved gastric function. Patients with pylorus-preserving resections have appeared to regain weight better than historic controls in some studies. Return of gastric emptying in the immediate postoperative period may take longer after the pylorus-preserving operation, and it is controversial whether there is any significant improvement in long-term quality of life with pyloric preservation.[290-291]

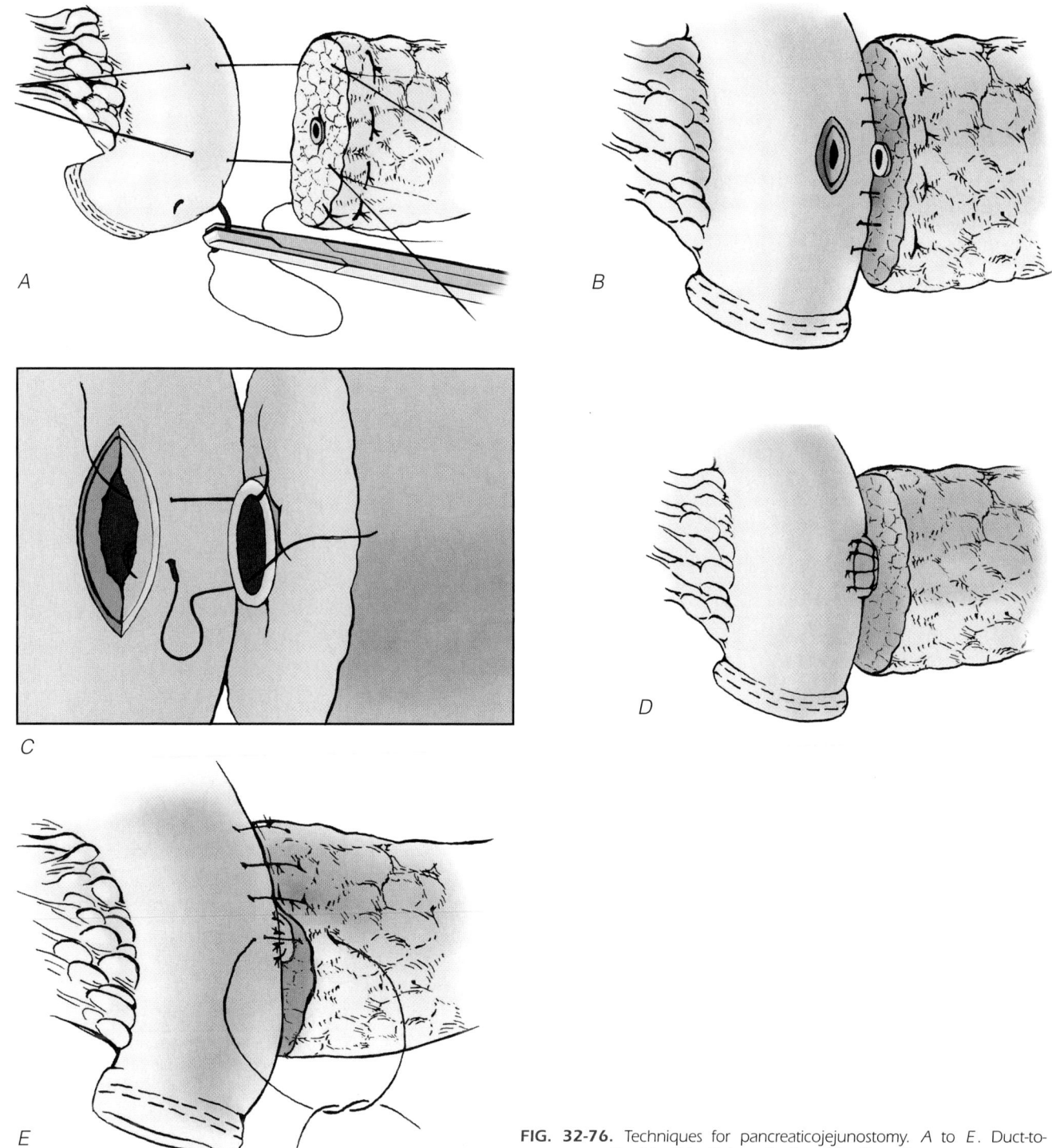

FIG. 32-76. Techniques for pancreaticojejunostomy. *A* to *E*. Duct-to-mucosa, end-to-side. *F* to *O*. Invagination. (*Continued*)

Techniques for the pancreaticojejunostomy include end-to-side or end-to-end and duct-to-mucosa sutures or invagination (Fig. 32-76). Pancreaticogastrostomy has also been investigated. Some surgeons use stents, fibrin glue to seal the anastomosis, or octreotide to decrease pancreatic secretions. No matter what combination of these techniques is used, the pancreatic leakage rate is always about 10%. Therefore the choice of techniques depends more on the surgeon's personal experience.

Traditionally, most surgeons place drains around the pancreatic and biliary anastomoses because the most dreaded complication of pancreaticoduodenectomy, disruption of the pancreaticojejunos-

tomy, cannot be avoided in 1 out of 10 patients. This complication can lead to the development of an upper abdominal abscess or can present as an external pancreatic fistula. Usually a pure pancreatic leak is controlled by the drains and will eventually seal spontaneously. Combined pancreatic and biliary leaks are cause for concern because bile will activate the pancreatic enzymes. In its most virulent form, disruption leads to necrotizing retroperitoneal infection, which can erode major arteries and veins of the upper abdomen, including the exposed portal vein and its branches or the stump of the gastroduodenal artery. Impending catastrophe is often preceded by a small herald bleed from the drain site. Such an event

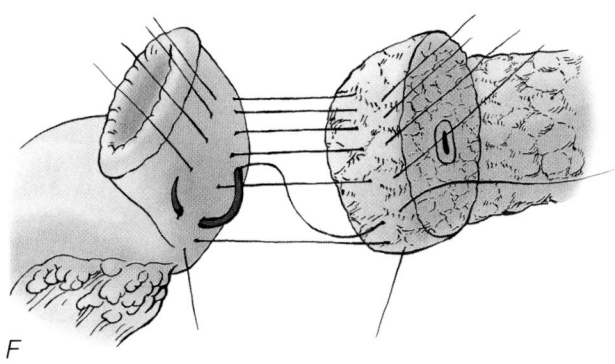

F

FIG. 32-76. *(continued)*

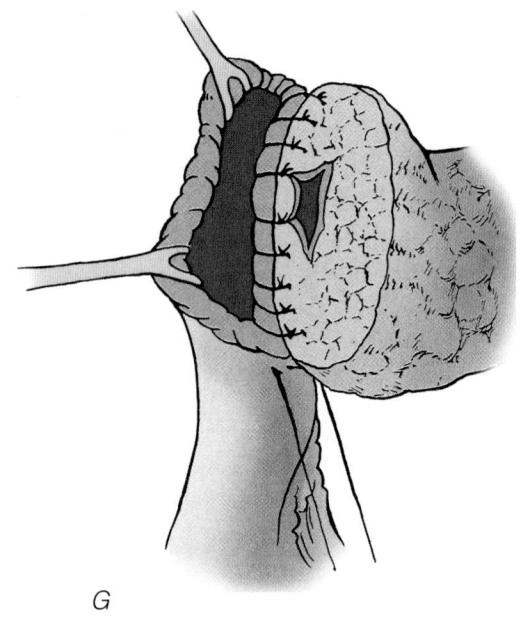

G

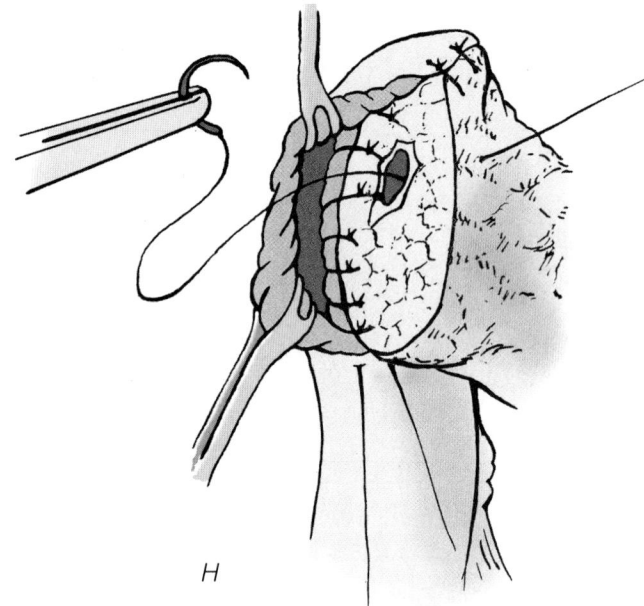

H

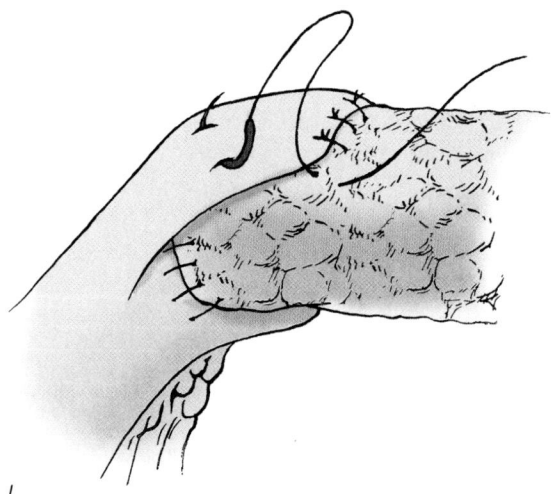

I

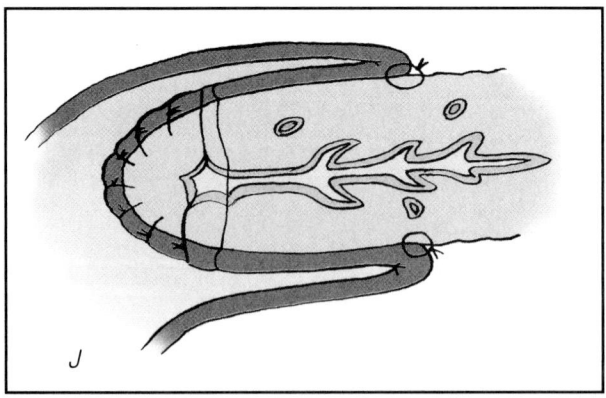

J

is an indication to return the patient to the operating room to widely drain the pancreaticojejunostomy and to repair the involved blood vessel. Open packing may be necessary to control diffuse necrosis and infection. Some recent studies have questioned the practice of routine drain placement after pancreaticoduodenectomy. These studies indicated that most pancreatic leaks can be managed with percutaneous drainage.[292] However, most surgeons continue to place drains near the pancreatic anastomosis.

Many patients with pancreatic cancer are malnourished preoperatively and suffer from gastroparesis in the immediate postoperative period. Some surgeons routinely place a feeding jejunostomy tube and gastrostomy tube in all pancreaticoduodenectomies,

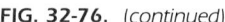

FIG. 32-76. *(continued)*

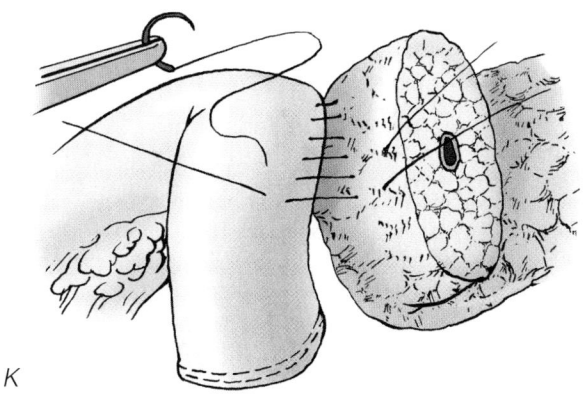

K

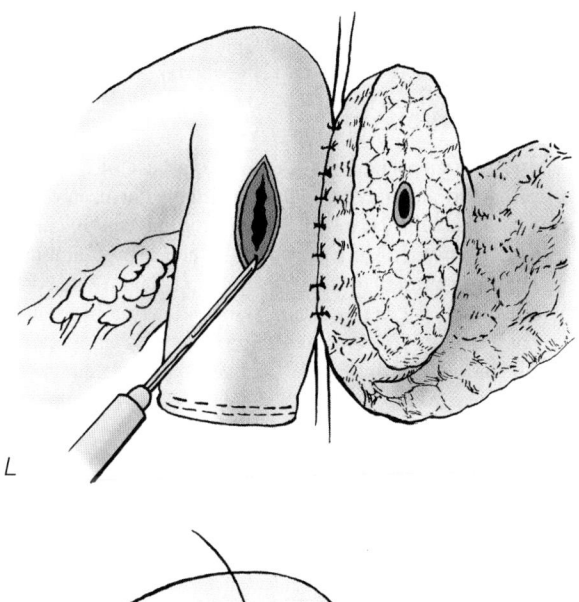

L

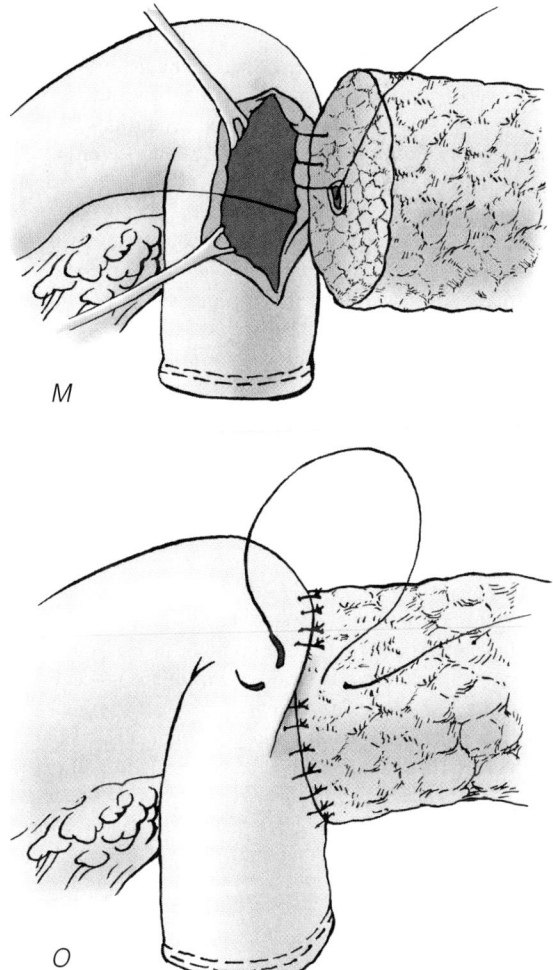

M

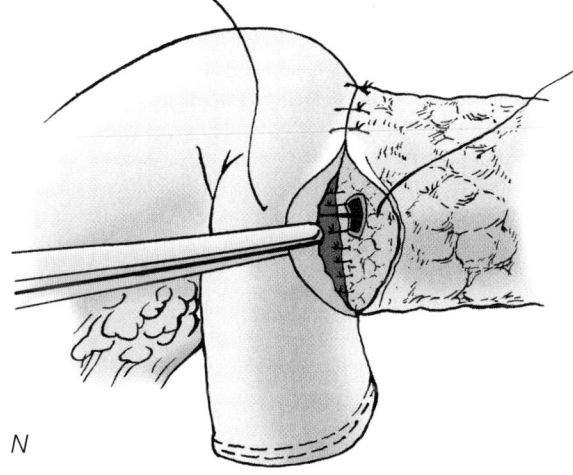

N

O

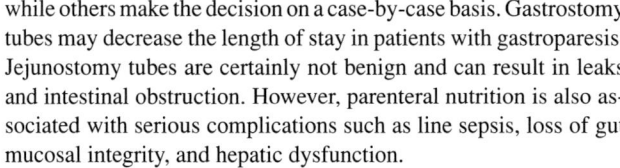

while others make the decision on a case-by-case basis. Gastrostomy tubes may decrease the length of stay in patients with gastroparesis. Jejunostomy tubes are certainly not benign and can result in leaks and intestinal obstruction. However, parenteral nutrition is also associated with serious complications such as line sepsis, loss of gut mucosal integrity, and hepatic dysfunction.

Because of the high incidence of direct retroperitoneal invasion and regional lymph node metastasis at the time of surgery, it has been argued that the scope of resection for pancreatic cancer should be enlarged to include a radical regional lymphadenectomy and

resection of areas of potential retroperitoneal invasion. The "radical pancreaticoduodenectomy" includes extension of the pancreatic resection to the middle body of the pancreas, segmental resection of the portal vein if necessary, resection of retroperitoneal tissue along the right perinephric area, and lymphadenectomy to the region of the celiac plexus. In the hands of experienced surgeons, these techniques are associated with greater blood loss but no increase in mortality; however, improved survival has not been demonstrated.[293] Total pancreatectomy has also been considered in the past. Although pancreatic leaks are eliminated, major morbidity from brittle diabetes and exocrine insufficiency outweigh any theoretical benefit.

Pancreatic cancer usually recurs locally after pancreaticoduodenectomy. Intraoperative radiotherapy (IORT) delivers a full therapeutic dose of radiation to the operative bed at the time of resection. Radiation to surrounding normal areas is minimized, but the radiation is delivered all in one setting, usually about 15 minutes, rather than in fractionated doses over time. IORT is best performed in a shielded, dedicated, operating room suite rather than by transporting the patient in the middle of an already long and complicated operation. IORT may improve local control and palliate symptoms after pancreaticoduodenectomy. However, IORT has not been shown to be superior to standard external beam radiation therapy, and further randomized trials are needed to determine how this modality should be utilized.[294]

Complications of Pancreaticoduodenectomy

The operative mortality rate for pancreaticoduodenectomy has decreased to less than 5% in "high volume" centers (where more than five cases per year are performed), suggesting that patients in rural areas would benefit from referral to large urban centers.[295,296] The most common causes of death are sepsis, hemorrhage, and cardiovascular events. Postoperative complications are unfortunately still very common, and include delayed gastric emptying, pancreatic fistula, and hemorrhage. Delayed gastric emptying is common after pancreaticoduodenectomy and is treated conservatively as long as complete gastric outlet obstruction is ruled out by a contrast study. Hemorrhage can occur either intraoperatively or postoperatively. Intraoperative hemorrhage typically occurs during the dissection of the portal vein. A major laceration of the portal vein can occur at a point in the operation at which the portal vein is not yet exposed. Temporary control of hemorrhage is generally possible in this situation by compressing the portal vein and superior mesenteric vein against the tumor with the surgeon's left hand behind the head of the pancreas. An experienced assistant is needed to divide the neck of the pancreas to the left of the portal vein and achieve proximal and distal control. Sometimes the vein can be sutured closed with minimal narrowing. Other times, a patch repair or segmental resection and interposition graft may be needed.

Postoperative hemorrhage can occur from inadequate ligature of any one of numerous blood vessels during the procedure. Hemorrhage can also occur due to digestion of retroperitoneal blood vessels due to a combined biliary-pancreatic leak. Uncommonly, a stress ulcer, or later a marginal ulcer, can result in gastrointestinal hemorrhage. Typically, a vagotomy is not performed when pancreaticoduodenectomy is performed for pancreatic cancer, but patients are placed on proton pump inhibitors.

Outcome and Value of Pancreaticoduodenectomy for Cancer

Survival figures indicate that few, if any, patients are cured indefinitely of pancreatic cancer with pancreaticoduodenectomy. The tumor tends to recur locally with retroperitoneal and regional lymphatic disease. In addition, most patients also develop hematogenous metastases, usually in the liver. Malignant ascites, peritoneal implants, and malignant pleural effusions are all common. Median survival after pancreaticoduodenectomy is about 12 to 15 months. Even long-term (5-year) survivors often eventually die due to pancreatic cancer recurrence. Although pancreaticoduodenectomy may be performed with the hope of the rare cure in mind, the operation more importantly provides better palliation than any other treatment, and is the only modality that offers any meaningful improvement in survival. If the procedure is performed without major complications,

many months of palliation are usually achieved. It is the surgeon's duty to make sure patients and their families have a realistic understanding of the true goals of pancreaticoduodenectomy.

Adjuvant Chemotherapy and Radiation

Small studies in the 1980s suggested that adjuvant chemotherapy with 5-fluorouracil combined with radiation improves survival by about 9 months after pancreatic resection for pancreatic adenocarcinoma.[297] Subsequent noncontrolled studies have reinforced that concept. However, a recent European multicenter trial concluded that there was no value to chemoradiotherapy, although the study suggested the possibility that chemotherapy alone might have survival benefit.[298] Remarkable results in adjuvant therapy have been reported by the Virginia Mason Clinic with combination S-Fu, cisplatinum, interferon-α and external beam radiation. Although the toxicity is high, the promising results have prompted larger confirmatory studies. Nevertheless, pending further study, it is typical in the United States for patients with acceptable functional status to receive adjuvant chemoradiotherapy after surgery.

Neoadjuvant Treatment

There are several potential advantages to the use of chemoradiation prior to an attempt at surgical resection. For example, it avoids the risk that adjuvant treatment is delayed by complications of surgery. Neoadjuvant treatment also may decrease the tumor burden at operation, increasing the rate of resectability and killing some tumor cells before they can be spread intraoperatively. Preoperative chemoradiation has been shown not to increase the perioperative morbidity or mortality of pancreaticoduodenectomy. It may even decrease the incidence of pancreatic fistula. Studies so far indicate that local or regional recurrence is decreased with this technique, but there is no proven survival advantage compared to traditional postoperative therapy.[299]

Gene Therapy

With recent developments in molecular biology techniques and the mapping of the entire human genome, gene therapy for pancreatic cancer has become a clinical reality. Several strategies are possible, including immunotherapeutic gene therapy, replacement of tumor suppressor gene function, inactivation of oncogenes, and suicide gene therapy.[300] With immunotherapeutic gene therapy, the goal is to assist the immune system in recognizing the cancer cells. Cancer cells have been forced to express cytokines that activate the immune system and that may have antitumor effects. Since pancreatic cancer is a disease with multiple genetic aberrations, inactivated tumor suppressor genes have been replaced and mutated oncogenes have been inactivated with gene therapy. In suicide gene therapy, a transgene is introduced which converts an inactive nontoxic drug into an active cytotoxic agent. The herpes simplex virus (HSV)-thymidine kinase system has been the most extensively studied.[300] Various delivery systems including viral vectors, liposomes, and protein-conjugated DNA exist. With each of these strategies and delivery systems, tumor cell–specific delivery would be extremely desirable, but awaits the discovery of tumor-specific promoters. Clinical trials involving gene therapy for pancreatic cancer are ongoing and offer hope for more meaningful treatment.

Management of Periampullary Adenomas

Benign villous adenomas of the ampullary region can be excised locally. This technique is applicable only for small tumors (approximately 2 cm or less) with no evidence of malignancy upon biopsy. A longitudinal duodenotomy is made and the tumor is excised with a

2- to 3-mm margin of normal duodenal mucosa. The edges of the bile duct and pancreatic duct are sewn to the duodenal wall as the excision progresses. A preoperative diagnosis of cancer is a contraindication to transduodenal excision and pancreaticoduodenectomy should be performed. Likewise, if final pathologic examination of a locally-excised tumor reveals invasive cancer, the patient should be returned to the operating room for a pancreaticoduodenectomy.

An important subset of patients are those with familial adenomatous polyposis (FAP), who develop periampullary or duodenal adenomas. These lesions have a high incidence of harboring carcinoma, and frequently recur unless the mucosa at risk is resected. A standard (not pylorus-sparing) Whipple is the procedure of choice in FAP patients with periampullary lesions.

Cystic Neoplasms of the Pancreas

Cystic epithelial tumors need to be excluded when patients present with a fluid-containing pancreatic lesion (Fig. 32-77). A variety of cystic neoplasms exist, and include benign serous cystic neoplasms, benign and malignant mucinous cystic neoplasms, and benign and malignant forms of intraductal papillary-mucinous neoplasms (IPMNs) (Table 32-20). IPMNs can present with a dilated pancreatic duct due to the production of mucin by the lesion. At ERCP or upper endoscopy, mucus may be seen extruding from a gaping ampullary orifice. This confirms the presence of an IPMN, and further investigation is warranted to localize the lesion. It is important to not assume that all fluid-filled pancreatic abnormalities represent pseudocysts, or that a dilated pancreatic duct repre-

sents only chronic pancreatitis. The presence of a solid component in a cystic lesion, septations within the cyst, and the absence of a clinical history of pancreatitis are factors that should alert the surgeon to the possible presence of a neoplasm. Even in the absence of these factors, presumed pseudocysts should be biopsied at the time of internal drainage to confirm the absence of malignancy, and dilated pancreatic ducts should be biopsied at the time of a decompression procedure to rule out a ductular neoplasm.

Cystic neoplasms with septations and/or irregular nodularity of the cyst wall are more suspicious for malignancy. In an effort to establish a preoperative diagnosis of malignancy, the cyst fluid can be

Table 32-20

World Health Organization Classification of Primary Tumors of the Exocrine Pancreas

A. Benign
  1. Serous cystadenoma (16%)
  2. Mucinous cystadenoma (45%)
  3. Intraductal papillary-mucinous adenoma (32%)
  4. Mature cystic teratoma
B. Borderline
  1. Mucinous cystic tumor with moderate dysplasia
  2. Intraductal papillary mucinous tumor with moderate dysplasia
  3. Solid pseudopapillary tumor
C. Malignant
  1. Ductal adenocarcinoma
  2. Serous/mucinous cystadenocarcinoma (29%)
  3. Intraductal mucinous papillary tumor

FIG. 32-77. Cystic epithelial tumor of the pancreas.

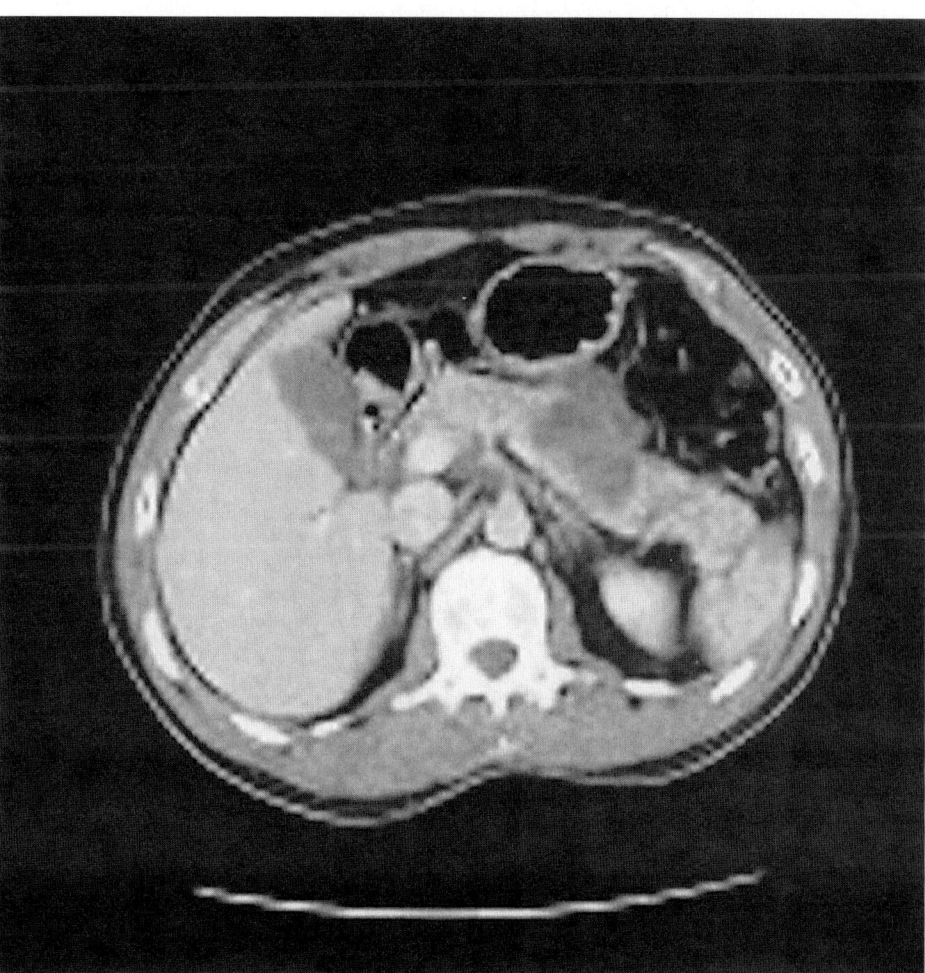

aspirated using EUS and analyzed. Cysts containing viscous fluid with a low amylase content and an elevated carcinoembryonic antigen level are more likely to be malignant. Cytologic examination of the aspirate also can be performed to aid in the diagnosis.

Cystic pancreatic lesions are usually resected if there is any concern regarding malignant potential. Enucleation of small cystic pancreatic neoplasms that are presumed to be benign may be a valid approach; the use of intraoperative ultrasound in such cases is helpful in avoiding injury to the main pancreatic duct and postoperative fistulas.[301] Laparoscopic distal pancreatectomy with or without splenic preservation may be employed for cystic lesions located in the tail of the pancreas.[302] With limited experience worldwide with laparoscopic pancreatic resection, caution is warranted before application of this technique to potentially malignant lesions.

Small cystic lesions in the head of the pancreas present a difficult challenge. Because of the morbidity and mortality risk of pancreaticoduodenectomy, a more conservative operative approach is attractive in a patient with a premalignant lesion such as a mucinous cystadenoma. The duodenum-preserving pancreatic head resections described earlier may offer a safer option when the lesion does not encroach on the duodenum and appears well delineated.

Pseudopapillary and Papillary-Cystic Neoplasms

An unusual form of exocrine neoplasm occurs predominantly in young women, and is characterized by a large, cystic or partially-cystic appearing lesion which contains frond-like papillary elements on histologic examination. Pseudopapillary and papillary-cystic neoplasms are usually benign, but may assume malignant (metastatic) behavior when they are discovered late in their course. Typically occurring in women from adolescence through the age of menopause, these lesions have been found to express estrogen and progesterone receptors in large numbers. Resection for cure is usually possible despite their typically large size.

Pancreatic Lymphoma

Lymphoma can affect the pancreas. Primary involvement of the pancreas with no disease outside the pancreas also occurs. The clinical presentation often is similar to pancreatic adenocarcinoma, with vague abdominal pain and weight loss. Identification of a large mass often involving the head and body of the pancreas should raise suspicion. Percutaneous or EUS-guided biopsy will confirm the diagnosis in most cases. If the diagnosis cannot be confirmed preoperatively, laparoscopic exploration and biopsy is indicated.[303] There is no role for resection in the management of pancreatic lymphoma. Endoscopic stenting to relieve jaundice followed by chemotherapy is the standard treatment, and long-term remission is often achieved.

References

1. Silen W: Surgical anatomy of the pancreas. *Surg Clin North Am* 44:1253, 1964.
2. Havel PJ, Taborsky GJ Jr.: The contribution of the autonomic nervous system to changes in glucagons and insulin secretion during hypoglycemic stress. *Endocr Rev* 10:332, 1989.
3. Davenport HW: Pancreatic secretion, in Davenport HN (ed): *Physiology of the Digestive Tract,* 5th *ed.* Chicago: Year Book Medical Publishers, 1982, p 143.
4. Valenzuela JE, Weiner K, Saad C: Cholinergic stimulation of human pancreatic secretion. *Dig Dis Sci* 31:615, 1986.
5. Konturek SJ, Becker HD, Thompson JC: Effect of vagotomy on hormones stimulating pancreatic secretion. *Arch Surg* 108:704, 1974.
6. Pour PM, Pandey KK, Batra SK: What is the origin of pancreatic adenocarcinoma? *Mol Cancer* 22:13, 2003.
7. Ebert R, Creutzfeldt W: Gastrointestinal peptides and insulin secretion. *Diabetes Metab Rev* 3:1, 1987.
8. Leahy JL, Bonner-Weir S, Weir GC: Abnormal glucose regulation of insulin secretion in models of reduced B-cell mass. *Diabetes* 33:667, 1984.
9. Brunicardi FC, Sun YS, Druck P, et al: Splanchnic neural regulation of insulin and glucagon secretion in the isolated perfused human pancreas. *Am J Surg* 153:34, 1987.
10. Yamada Y, Post SR, Wang K, et al: Cloning and functional characterization of a family of human and mouse somatostatin receptors expressed in brain, gastrointestinal tract and kidney. *Proc Natl Acad Sci USA* 89:251, 1992.
11. Voss M, Pappas T: Pancreatic fistula. *Curr Treat Options Gastroenterol* 5:345, 2002.
12. Feldman M, Richardson CT, Taylor IL, et al: Effect of atropine on vagal release of gastrin and pancreatic polypeptide. *J Clin Invest* 63:294, 1979.
13. Floyd JC, Fajans SS, Pek S: Regulation in healthy subjects of the secretion of human pancreatic polypeptide, a newly recognized pancreatic islet polypeptide. *Trans Assoc Am Physicians* 89:146, 1976.
14. Adrian TE, Bloom SR, Besterman HS, et al: Mechanism of pancreatic-polypeptide release in man. *Lancet* 1:161, 1977.
15. Seymour NE, Andersen DK: Pancreatic polypeptide and glucose metabolism, in Greeley GH (ed): *Gastrointestinal Endocrinology.* Totowa, NJ: Humana Press, 1999, p 321.
16. Westermark P, Wilander E, Westermark GT, et al: Islet amyloid polypeptide-like-immunoreactivity in the islet B-cells of type II (non-insulin-dependent) diabetic and non-diabetic individuals. *Diabetologia* 30:887, 1987.
17. Tatemoto K, Efendic S, Mutt V, et al: Pancreastatin, a novel pancreatic peptide that inhibits insulin secretion. *Nature* 324:476, 1986.
18. Efendic S, Tatemoto K, Mutt V, et al: Pancreastatin and islet hormone release. *Proc Nat Acad Sci USA* 84:7257, 1987.
19. Funakoshi A, Miyaska K, Nakamura R, et al: Inhibitory effect of pancreastatin on pancreatic exocrine secretin in the conscious rat. *Reg Peptides* 25:157, 1989.
20. Gorelick FS, Jamieson JD: Structure-function relationship of the pancreas, in Johnson LR (ed): *Physiology of the Gastrointestinal Tract.* New York: Raven Press, 1981, p 773.
21. Kennedy FP: Pathophysiology of pancreatic polypeptide secretion in human diabetes mellitus. *Diabetes Nutr Metab* 2:155, 1990.
22. Kleinman R, Ohning G, Wong H, et al: Regulatory role of intraislet somatostatin on insulin secretion in the isolated perfused human pancreas. *Pancreas* 9:172, 1994.
23. Saluja A, Bhagat L: Pancreatitis and associated lung injury: When MIF miffs. *Gastroenterol* 124:844, 2003.
24. Acosta JL, Ledesma CL: Gallstone migration as a cause for acute pancreatitis. *N Engl J Med* 290:484, 1974.
25. Lerch MM, Saluja AK, Runzi M, et al: Pancreatic duct obstruction triggers acute pancreatitis in the opossum. *Gastroenterology* 103:1768, 1993.
26. Steer ML, Saluja AK: Pathogenesis and pathophysiology of acute pancreatitis, in Beger HG, Warshaw AL, Buchler MW, et al (eds): *The Pancreas,* Vol. 2. London: Blackwell Science Ltd., 1998, p 383.
27. Schneider A, Whitcomb DC, Singer MV: Animal models in alcoholic pancreatitis—what can we learn? *Pancreatology* 2:189, 2002.
28. Apte MV, Wilson JS: Alcohol-induced pancreatic injury. *Best Pract Res Clin Gastroenterol* 17:593, 2002.
29. Whitcomb DC, Gorry MC, Preston RA, et al: Hereditary pancreatitis is caused by a mutation in the cationic trypsinogen gene. *Nat Genet* 14:141, 1996.
30. Whitcomb DC, Ulrich CD, Lerch MM, et al: Third International Symposium on Inherited Diseases of the Pancreas. *Pancreatology* 1:423, 2001.
31. Saluja AK, Steer ML: Pathophysiology of pancreatitis. Role of cytokines and other mediators of inflammation. *Digestion* 60:27, 1999.

32. Saluja A, Bhagat L: Experimental models of acute pancreatitis, in Johnson L (ed): *Encyclopedia of Gastroenterology.* San Diego, CA, Elsevier, 2004, p 111.

33. van Acker GJD, Saluja AK, Bhagat L, et al: The cathepsin B inhibitor CA-074 prevents intrapancreatic trypsinogen activation and reduces severity of pancreatitis. *Am J Physiol* 283:G794, 2003.

34. Makhija R, Kingsnorth AN: Cytokine storm in acute pancreatitis. *J Hepatobiliary Pancreat Surg* 9:401, 2002.

35. Bhagat L, Singh VP, Hietaranta AJ, et al: Heat shock protein 70 prevents secretagogue-induced cell injury in the pancreas by preventing intracellular trypsinogen activation. *J Clin Invest* 106:81, 2000.

36. Hietaranta AJ, Singh VP, Bhagat L, et al: Water immersion stress prevents caerulein-induced pancreatic acinar cell NF-κB activation by attenuating caerulein-induced intracellular Ca^{2+} changes. *J Biol Chem* 276:18742, 2001.

37. Kraft M, Lerch MM: Gallstone pancreatitis: When is endoscopic retrograde cholangiopancreatography truly necessary? *Curr Gastroenterol Rep* 5:125, 2003.

38. Werner J, Hartwig W, Uhl W, Muller C, Buchler MW: Useful markers for predicting severity and monitoring progression of acute pancreatitis. *Pancreatology* 3:115, 2003.

39. Ranson JHC: Acute pancreatitis: Surgical management, in Go VLW, DiMagno EP, Gardner JD, et al (eds): *The Pancreas: Biology, Pathophysiology, and Disease,* 2nd ed. New York: Raven Press, 1993, p 637.

40. Banks PA: Epidemiology, natural history, and predictors of disease outcome in acute and chronic pancreatitis. *Gastrointest Endosc* 56:S226, 2002.

41. Neoptolemos JP, Kemppainen EA, Mayer JM, et al: Early prediction of severity in acute pancreatitis by urinary trypsinogen activation peptide: A multicentre study. *Lancet* 355:1955, 2000.

42. Balthazar EJ: Complications of acute pancreatitis: Clinical and CT evaluation. *Radiol Clin North Am* 40:1211, 2002.

43. Loser CH, Folsch UR: Acute pancreatitis: Medical and endoscopic treatment, in Lankisch PG, DiMagno EP (eds): *Pancreatic Disease.* Berlin: Springer-Verlag, 1999, p 66.

44. Johnson CD, Kingsnorth AN, Imrie CW, et al: Double blind, randomized, placebo controlled study of a platelet activating factor antagonist, lexipafant, in the treatment and prevention of organ failure in predicted severe acute pancreatitis. *Gut* 48:62, 2001.

45. Banks PA: Medical management of acute pancreatitis and complications, in Go VLW, DiMagno EP, Gardner JD, et al (eds): *The Pancreas: Biology, Pathophysiology, and Disease,* 2nd ed. New York: Raven Press, 1993, p 593.

46. Runzi M, Layer P: Nonsurgical management of acute pancreatitis. Use of antibiotics. *Surg Clin North Am* 79:759, 1999.

47. Buchler P, Reber HA: Surgical approach in patients with acute pancreatitis. Is infected or sterile necrosis an indication—in whom should this be done, when, and why? *Gastroenterol Clin North Am* 28:661, 1999.

48. Clancy TE, Ashley SW: Current management of necrotizing pancreatitis. *Adv Surg* 36:103, 2002.

49. Imrie CW, Carter CR, McKay CJ: Enteral and parenteral nutrition in acute pancreatitis. *Best Pract Res Clin Gastroenterol* 16:391, 2002.

50. Skyhoj J, Olsen T: The incidence and clinical relevance of chronic inflammation in the pancreas in autopsy material. *Acta Pathol Microbiol Scand* 86:361, 1978.

51. Copenhagen Pancreatitis Study: An interim report from a prospective epidemiological multicenter study. *Scand J Gastroenterol* 16:305, 1981.

52. Worning H: Incidence and prevalence of chronic pancreatitis, in Beger HG, Buchler M, Ditschuneit H, Malfertheiner P (eds): *Chronic Pancreatitis.* Berlin: Springer-Verlag, 1990, p 8.

53. Worning H: Alcoholic chronic pancreatitis, in Beger HG et al (eds): *The Pancreas.* London: Blackwell-Sciences, 1998, p 672.

54. Zdankiewicz PD, Andersen DK: Pancreatitis in the elderly, in Rosenthal R, Katlic M, Zenilman ME (eds): *Principles and Practice of Geriatric Surgery.* New York: Springer-Verlag, 2001, p 740.

55. Pitchumoni M: Pathogenesis of alcohol-induced chronic pancreatitis: Facts, perceptions and misperceptions. *Surg Clin North Am* 81:379, 2001.

56. Strate T, Yekebas E, Knoefel W, et al: Pathogenesis of the natural course of chronic pancreatitis. *Eur J Gastroenterol Hepatol* 14:929, 2002.

57. Singer MV, Chari ST: Classification of chronic pancreatitis, in Beger HG et al (eds): *The Pancreas.* London: Blackwell-Science, 1998, p 665.

58. Cohn JA, Bornstein JD, Jowell PS: Cystic fibrosis mutations and genetic predisposition for idiopathic chronic pancreatitis. *Med Clin North Am* 84:621, 2000.

59. Freidreich N: Disease of the pancreas, in Ziemssen H (ed): *Cyclopedia of the Practice of Medicine.* New York: William Wood, 1878, p 549.

60. Durbec JP, Sarles H: Multicenter survey of the etiology of pancreatic disease: Relationship between the relative risk of developing chronic pancreatitis and alcohol, protein, and lipid consumption. *Digestion* 18:337, 1978.

61. Lankisch PG, Lowenfels AB, Maisonneuve P: What is the risk of alcoholic pancreatitis in heavy drinkers? *Pancreas* 24:411, 2002.

62. Dufour MC, Adamson MD:. The epidemiology of alcohol-induced pancreatitis. *Pancreas* 27:286, 2003.

63. Renner IG, Savage WT, Pantoja JL, et al: Death due to acute pancreatitis. *Dig Dis Sci* 30:1005, 1985.

64. Layer P, Yanamoto H, Kalthoff L, et al: The different courses of early- and late-onset idiopathic and alcoholic chronic pancreatitis. *Gastroenterol* 107:1481, 1994.

65. Apte MV, Wilson JS: Alcohol-induced pancreatic injury, in Singer MV (ed): Alcohol-related gastrointestinal disease. *Best Pract Res Clin Gastroenterol* 17:593, 2003.

66. Comfort HW, Gambill EE, Baggenstoss AH: Chronic relapsing pancreatitis: A study of 29 cases without associated disease of the biliary or gastrointestinal tract. *Gastroenterol* 6:239, 1946.

67. Ammann RW, Muelhaup B, Meyenberger C, et al: Alcoholic nonprogressive chronic pancreatitis: Prospective long-term study of a large cohort with alcoholic chronic pancreatitis (1976–1982). *Pancreas* 9:365, 1994.

68. Kondo T, Hayakawa T, Shibata T, et al: Aberrant pancreas is not susceptible to alcoholic pancreatitis. *Int J Pancreatol* 8:245, 1991.

69. Elsasser HP, Haake T, Grimmig M, et al: Repetitive cerulean-induced pancreatitis and pancreatic fibrosis in the rat. *Pancreas* 7:385, 1992.

70. Neuschwander-Terri BA, Burton FR, Presti ME, et al: Repetitive self-limited acute pancreatitis induces pancreatic fibrogenesis in the mouse. *Dig Dis Sci* 45:665, 2000.

71. Seymour NE, Turk JB, Laster MK, et al: In vitro hepatic insulin resistance in chronic pancreatitis in the rat. *J Surg Res* 45:450, 1989.

72. Niebergall-Roth E, Harder H, Singer MV: A review: Acute and chronic effects of ethanol and alcoholic beverages on pancreatic exocrine secretion in vitro and in vivo. *Alcoholism Clin Exp Res* 22:1570, 1998.

73. Steer ML, Glazer C, Manabe T: Direct effects of ethanol on exocrine secretion from the in vitro rabbit pancreas. *Dig Dis Sci* 24:769, 1979.

74. Hauck C, Schneider A, Whitcomb DC: Genetic polymorphisms in alcoholic pancreatitis, in Singer MV (ed): Alcohol related gastrointestinal disease. *Best Pract Res Clin Gastroenterol* 17:613, 2003.

75. Whitcomb DC, Gorry MC, Preston RA, et al: Hereditary pancreatitis is caused by a mutation in the cationic trypsinogen gene. *Nat Genet* 14:141, 1996.

76. Witt H, Luck W, Hennies HC, et al: Mutations in the gene encoding the serine protease inhibitor kazal type 1 are associated with chronic pancreatitis. *Nat Genet* 25:213, 2000.

77. Lerch MM, Albrecht E, Ruthenburger M, et al: Pathophysiology of alcohol-induced pancreatitis. *Pancreas* 27:291, 2003.

78. Gorelick F: Alcohol and zymogen activation in the pancreatic acinar cell. *Pancreas* 27:305, 2003.

79. Sahel J, Sarles H: Modifications of pure human pancreatic juice induced by chronic alcohol consumption. *Dig Dis Sci* 24:897, 1979.

80. Sarles H, Barnard JP, Chonson C: Pathogenesis and epidemiology of chronic pancreatitis. *Ann Rev Med* 40:453, 1989.

81. Yamedera K, Moriyama T, Makino I: Identification of immunoreactive pancreatic stone protein in pancreatic stone, pancreatic tissue, and pancreatic juice. *Pancreas* 5:255, 1990.

82. Multigner L, Sarles H, Lombardo D, et al: Pancreatic stone protein. I. Implications in stone formation during the course of chronic pancreatitis. *Gastroenterology* 89:381, 1985.

83. Freedman SD, Sakamoto K, Venu RP: GP2, the homologue to the renal cast protein uromodulin, is a major component of intraductal plugs in chronic pancreatitis. *J Clin Invest* 92:83, 1993.

84. Imoto M, DiMagno EP: Cigarette smoking increases the risk of pancreatic calcification in late-onset but not early-onset idiopathic chronic pancreatitis. *Pancreas* 21:115, 2000.

85. Lowenfels AB, Maisonneuve P, Whitcomb DC: Risk factors for cancer in hereditary pancreatitis. International Hereditary Pancreatitis Study Group. *Med Clin North Am* 84:565, 2000.

86. Shaper AG: Chronic pancreatic disease and protein malnutrition. *Lancet* 1:1223, 1960.

87. Mohan V, Pitchumoni CS: Tropical chronic pancreatitis, in Beger HG et al (eds): *The Pancreas*. London: Blackwell-Science, 1998, p 688.

88. GeeVarghese PJ: *Calcific Pancreatitis*. Bombay: Varghese Publishing House, 1985, p 1.

89. Pitchumoni CS, Jain NK, Lowenfels AB, et al: Chronic cyanide poisoning: A unifying concept for alcoholic and tropical pancreatitis. *Pancreas* 3:220, 1988.

90. Hassan Z, Mohan V, Ali L, et al: SPINK 1 is a susceptibility gene for fibrocalculous pancreatic diabetes in patients from the Indian subcontinent. *Am J Hum Genet* 71:964, 2002.

91. Schneider A, Suman A, Rossi L, et al: SPINK 1/PSTI mutations are associated with tropical pancreatitis and type II diabetes mellitus in Bangladesh. *Gastroenterology* 123:1026, 2002.

92. Comfort MW, Steinberg AG: Pedigree of a family with hereditary chronic relapsing pancreatitis. *Gastroenterology* 21:54, 1952.

93. Gross JB: Hereditary pancreatitis, in Go VLW, Gardner JD, Brooks FP et al (eds): *The Exocrine Pancreas: Biology, Pathophysiology, and Diseases*. New York: Raven Press, 1986, p 829.

94. Tomsik H, Gress TM, Adler G: Hereditary pancreatitis, in Beger HG et al (eds): *The Pancreas*. London: Blackwell-Science, 1998, p 355.

95. Whitcomb DC, Preston RA, Aston CE, et al: A gene for hereditary pancreatitis maps to chromosome 7q35. *Gastroenterology* 110:1975, 1996.

96. LeBodic LL, Bignon J-D, Raaguenes O, et al: The hereditary pancreatitis gene maps to the long arm of chromosome 7. *Hum Mol Genet* 5:549, 1996.

97. Whitcomb DC: Hereditary diseases of the pancreas, in Yamada T, Alpers DH, Laine L, Owyang C, Powell DC (eds): *Textbook of Gastroenterology*, 4th ed. Philadelphia: Lippincott Williams & Wilkins, 2002, p 2147.

98. Schneider A, Whitcomb DC: Anionic trypsinogen gene mutation in chronic pancreatitis. *Pancreas* 2004, (in press).

99. Pfutzer RH, Barmada MM, Brunskil APJ, et al: SPINK 1/PSTI polymorphisms act as disease modifiers in familial and idiopathic chronic pancreatitis. *Gastroenterology* 119:615, 2000.

100. Chen J-M, Mercier B, Audrezet M-P, Ferec C: Mutational analysis of the human pancreatic secretory inhibitor (PSTI) gene in hereditary and sporadic chronic pancreatitis. *J Med Genet* 37:67, 2000.

101. Chen J-M, Mercier B, Audrezet M-P, et al: Mutations of the pancreatic secretory trypsin inhibitor (PSTI) gene in idiopathic chronic pancreatitis. *Gastroenterology* 120:1061, 2001.

102. Cohn JA, Friedman KJ, Noone PG, et al: Relation between mutations of the cystic fibrosis gene and idiopathic pancreatitis. *N Engl J Med* 339:653, 1998.

103. Sharer N, Schwartz M, Malone G, et al: Mutations of the cystic fibrosis gene in patients with chronic pancreatitis. *N Engl J Med* 339:645, 1998.

104. Goebell H, Steffen C, Baltzel G, et al: Stimulation of pancreatic secretion of enzymes by acute hypercalcemia in man. *Eur J Clin Invest* 3:98, 1973.

105. Bess MA, Edis AJ, Van Heerden JA: Hyperparathyroidism and pancreatitis: Cause or casual association? *JAMA* 243:246, 1980.

106. Glueck CJ, Lang J, Hamer T, et al: Severe hypertriglyceridemia and pancreatitis when estrogen replacement therapy is given to hypertriglyceridemic women. *J Lab Clin Med* 123:59, 1994.

107. Yoshida K, Toki F, Takeuchi T, et al: Chronic pancreatitis caused by an autoimmune abnormality: Proposal of the concept of autoimmune pancreatitis. *Dig Dis Sci* 40:1561, 1995.

108. Ito T, Nakano I, Koyanagi S, et al: Autoimmune pancreatitis as a new clinical entity: Three cases of autoimmune pancreatitis with effective steroid therapy. *Dig Dis Sci* 42:1458, 1997.

109. Stathopoulos G, Nourmand AD, Weisenberg E, et al: Rapidly progressive sclerosing cholangitis following pancreatic pseudotumor formation. *J Clin Gastroenterol* 21:143, 1995.

110. Othersen HV, Moore FT, Boles ET: Traumatic pancreatitis and pseudocysts in childhood. *J Trauma* 8:535, 1968.

111. Cotton PB: Congenital anomaly of pancreas divisum as cause of obstructive pain and pancreatitis. *Gut* 21:105, 1980.

112. Warshaw AL: Pancreas divisum and pancreatitis, in Beger HG et al (eds): *The Pancreas*. London: Blackwell-Science, 1998, p 364.

113. Delhaye M, Engelholm L, Cremer M: Pancreas divisum: Congenital anatomic variant or anomaly? *Gastroenterology* 89:951, 1985.

114. Sugawa C, Walt AJ, Nunez DC, et al: Pancreas divisum: Is it a normal anatomic variant? *Am J Surg* 153:62, 1987.

115. Layer P, Kalthoff L, Clain JE, et al: Nonalcoholic chronic pancreatitis: Two diseases? *Dig Dis Sci* 30:980, 1985.

116. Ammann RW: Chronic pancreatitis in the elderly. *Gastroenterol Clin North Am* 19:905, 1990.

117. Cohen JA, Bornstein JD, Jowell PS: Cystic fibrosis mutations and genetic predisposition for idiopathic chronic pancreatitis. *Med Clin North Am* 84:621, 2000.

118. Kloppel G, Maillet B: Pathology of chronic pancreatitis, in Beger HG et al (eds): *The Pancreas*. London: Blackwell-Science, 1998, p 720.

119. Nagai H, Ohtsubo K: Pancreatic lithiasis in the aged. Its clinicopathology and pathogenesis. *Gastroenterology* 86:331, 1984.

120. Apte MV, Wilson JS: Stellate cell activation in alcoholic pancreatitis. *Pancreas* 27:316, 2003.

121. McCarrol JA, Phillips PA, Santucci N, et al: Vitamin A induces quiescence in culture-activated pancreatic stellate cells—potential as an antifibrotic agent? *Pancreas* 27:396, 2003.

122. Schneider A, Whitcomb DC: Hereditary pancreatitis: A model for inflammatory diseases of the pancreas. *Best Pract Res Clin Gastroenterol* 16:347, 2002.

123. Bockman DE, Kennedy RH, Multigner L, et al: Fine structure of the organic matrix of human pancreatic stones. *Pancreas* 1:204, 1986.

124. Guy O, Robles-Diaz G, Adrich Z, et al: Protein content of precipitates present in pancreatic juice of alcoholic subjects and patients with chronic calcifying pancreatitis. *Gastroenterology* 84:102, 1983.

125. Sarles H, Dagorn JC, Giorgi D, et al: Renaming pancreatic stone protein as "lithostathine." *Gastroenterology* 99:900, 1990.

126. Watanabe T, Yonekura H, Terazono K, et al: Complete nucleotide sequence of human *reg* gene and its expression in normal and tumoral tissues. The reg protein, pancreatic stone protein, and pancreatic thread protein are one and the same product of the gene. *J Biol Chem* 265:7432, 1990.

127. Goggin PM, Johnson CD: Pancreatic stones, in Beger HG et al (eds): *The Pancreas*. London: Blackwell-Science, 1998, p 711.

128. Giorgi D, Bernard JP, Rouquier S, Iovanna J, et al: Secretory pancreatic stone protein messenger RNA. Nucleotide sequence and expression in chronic calcifying pancreatitis. *J Clin Invest* 84:100, 1989.

129. Bernard JP, Barthet M, Gharib B, et al: Quantification of human lithostathine by high performance liquid chromatography. *Gut* 36:630, 1995.

130. Rinderknecht H, Renner IG, Koyama HH: Lysosomal enzymes in pure pancreatic juice from normal healthy volunteers and chronic alcoholics. *Dig Dis Sci* 24:180, 1979.

131. Warshaw AL, Simeone J, Schapiro RH, et al: Objective evaluation of ampullary stenosis with ultrasonography and pancreatic stimulation. *Am J Surg* 149:65, 1985.

132. Freeney PC: Radiology, in Beger HG et al (eds): *The Pancreas*. London: Blackwell-Science, 1998, p 728.

133. Bolondi L, Li Bassi S, Gaiani S, et al: Sonography of chronic pancreatitis. *Radiol Clin North Am* 27:815, 1989. Review.

134. Barish MA, Yucel EK, Soto JA, et al: MR cholangiopancreatography: Efficacy of three-dimensional turbo spin-echo technique. *AJR Am J Roentgenol* 165:295, 1995.

135. Catalano MF, Lahoti S, Geenen JE, et al: Prospective evaluation of endoscopic ultrasonography, endoscopic retrograde pancreatography, and secretin test in the diagnosis of chronic pancreatitis. *Gastrointest Endosc* ;48:11, 1998.

136. Kohl S, Glasbrenner B, Leadolter A: EUS in the diagnosis of early chronic pancreatitis: A prospective follow-up study. *Gastrointest Endosc* 55:507, 2002.

137. Freeman ML, DiSario JA, Nelson DB, et al: Risk factors for post-ERCP pancreatitis: A prospective, multicenter study. *Gastrointest Endosc* 54:425, 2001.

138. Murayama KM, Joehl RJ: Chronic pancreatitis, in Greenfield LJ, Mulholland M, Oldham KT, Zilewock GB, Lillenioe KD (eds): *Surgery. Scientific Principles and Practice*, 3rd ed. Philadelphia: Lippincott Williams & Wilkins, 2001, p 873.

139. Bradley EL III: Pancreatic duct pressure in chronic pancreatitis. *Am J Surg* 144:313, 1982.

140. Nealon WH, Matin S: Analysis of surgical success in preventing recurrent acute exacerbations in chronic pancreatitis. *Ann Surg* 233:793, 2001.

141. Ammann RW, Muellhaupt B: The natural history of pain in alcoholic chronic pancreatitis. *Gastroenterology* 116:1132, 1999.

142. Ammann RW, Akovbiantz A, Largiader F, et al: Course and outcome of chronic pancreatitis. Longitudinal study of a mixed medical-surgical series of 245 patients. *Gastroenterology* 86(5 Pt 1):820, 1984.

143. Girdwood AH, Marks IN, Bornman PC, et al: Does progressive pancreatic insufficiency limit pain in calcific pancreatitis with duct stricture or continued alcohol insult? *J Clin Gastroenterol* 3:241, 1981.

144. Lankisch PG, Lohr-Happe A, Otto J, et al: Natural course in chronic pancreatitis. Pain, exocrine and endocrine pancreatic insufficiency and prognosis of the disease. *Digestion* 54:148, 1993.

145. Bockman DE, Buchler M: Pain mechanisms, in Beger HG et al (eds): *The Pancreas*. London: Blackwell-Science, 1998, p 698.

146. Bockman DE, Buchler M, Malfertheiner P, et al: Analysis of nerves in chronic pancreatitis. *Gastroenterology* 94:1459, 1988.

147. Ebbehoj N, Borly L, Bulow J, et al: Pancreatic tissue fluid pressure in chronic pancreatitis. Relation to pain, morphology, and function. *Scand J Gastroenterol* ;25:1046, 1990.

148. DiMagno EP, Go VL, Summerskill WHJ: Relations between pancreatic enzyme outputs and malabsorption in severe pancreatic insufficiency. *N Engl J Med* 288:813, 1973.

149. DiMagno EP, Malagelada JR, Go VL: Relationship between alcoholism and pancreatic insufficiency. *Ann NY Acad Sci* 252:200, 1975.

150. Dutta SK, Russell RM, Iber FL: Influence of exocrine pancreatic insufficiency on the intraluminal pH of the proximal small intestine. *Dig Dis Sci* 24:529, 1979.

151. Malka D, Hammel P, Sauvanet A, et al: Risk factors for diabetes mellitus in chronic pancreatitis. *Gastroenterology* 119:1324, 2000.

152. Couet C, Genton P, Pointel JP, et al: The prevalence of retinopathy is similar in diabetes mellitus secondary to chronic pancreatitis with or without pancreatectomy and in idiopathic diabetes mellitus. *Diabetes Care* 8:323, 1985.

153. Slezak LA, Andersen DK: Pancreatic resection: Effects on glucose metabolism. *World J Surg* 25:452, 2000.

154. Kono T, Wang XP, Fisher WE, et al: Pancreatic polypeptide, in Martini L (ed): *Encyclopedia of Endocrine Disease*. San Diego, CA: Academic Press, 2004, (in press).

155. Seymour NE, Volpert AR, Lee EL, et al: Alterations in hepatocyte insulin binding in chronic pancreatitis: Effects of pancreatic polypeptide. *Am J Surg* 169:105, 1995.

156. Spector SA, Frattini JC, Zdankiewicz PD, et al: Insulin receptor gene expression in chronic pancreatitis: The effect of pancreatic polypeptide. *Surg Forum* 48:168, 1997.

157. Seymour NE: Insulin receptor gene expression in chronic pancreatitis. *Surg Forum* 48:168, 1997.

158. Brunicardi FC, Chaiken RL, Ryan AS, et al: Pancreatic polypeptide administration improves abnormal glucose metabolism in patients with chronic pancreatitis. *J Clin Endocrinol Metab* 81:3566, 1996.

159. Orci L: Macro- and micro-domains in the endocrine pancreas. *Diabetes* 31(6 Pt 1):538, 1982.

160. Seymour NE, Brunicardi FC, Chaiken RL, et al: Reversal of abnormal glucose production after pancreatic resection by pancreatic polypeptide administration in man. *Surgery* 104:119, 1988.

161. Hanazaki K, Nose Y, Brunicardi FC: Artificial endocrine pancreas. *J Am Coll Surg* 193:310, 2001.

162. Andersen DK: The role of pancreatic polypeptide in glucose metabolism, in Thompson JC (ed): *Gastrointestinal Endocrinology: Receptor and Post-Receptor Mechanisms*. San Diego, CA: Academic Press, 1990, p 333.

163. Gyr K, Agrawal NM, Felsenfeld O, et al: Comparison study of secretin and Lundh tests. *Am J Dig Dis* 20:506, 1975.

164. Somogyi I, Cintron M, Toskes P: Synthetic porcine secretin is highly accurate in pancreatic function testing in individuals with chronic pancreatitis. *Pancreas* 21:262, 2000.

165. Denver ME, Cotton PB: Pure pancreatic juice studies in normal subjects and patients with chronic pancreatitis. *Gut* 20:89, 1979.

166. Tanner AR, Fisher D, Smith CL: An evaluation of the one-day NBT-PABA/114C-PABA in the assessment of pancreatic exocrine insufficiency. *Digestion* 29:42, 1984.

167. Ammann RW, Buhler H, Pei P: Comparative diagnostic accuracy of four tubeless pancreatic function tests in chronic pancreatitis. *Scand J Gastroenterol* 17:997, 1982.

168. Brugge WR, Goff JS, Allen NC, et al: Development of a dual label Schilling test for pancreatic exocrine function based on the differential absorption of cobalamin malabsorption in pancreatic insufficiency. *J Clin Invest* 61:47, 1978.

169. Haverback BJ, Dyce BJ, Gutentag PJ: Measurement of trypsin and chymo-trypsin in stool: A diagnostic test for pancreatic exocrine function. *Gastroenterology* 44:588, 1986.

170. Gullo L, Ventrucci M, Tomasetti P, et al: Fecal elastase 1 determination in chronic pancreatitis. *Dig Dis Sci* 44:210, 1999.

171. Goff JS: Two-stage triolein breath test differentiates pancreatic insufficiency from other causes of malabsorption. *Gastroenterology* 83:44, 1982.

172. Axon ATR, Classen J, Cotton PB, et al: Pancreatography in chronic pancreatitis: International definitions. *Gut* 25:1107, 1984.

173. Brugge WR: The role of endoscopic ultrasound in pancreatic disorders. *Int J Pancreatol* 20:1, 1996.

174. Catanzaro A, Richardson S, Veloso H, et al: Long-term follow-up of patients with clinically indeterminate suspicion of pancreatic cancer and normal EUS. *Gastrointest Endosc* 58:836, 2003.

175. Kahl S, Glasbrenner B, Leodolter A, et al: EUS in the diagnosis of early chronic pancreatitis: A prospective follow up study. *Gastrointest Endosc* 55:507, 2002.

176. Lankisch PG: Prognosis, in Beger HG et al (eds): *The Pancreas*. London: Blackwell-Science, 1998, p 740.

177. Miyake H, Harada H, Kunichika K, et al: Clinical course and prognosis of chronic pancreatitis. *Pancreas* 2:378, 1987.

178. Lowenfels AB, Maisonneuve P, Cavallini G, et al: Prognosis of chronic pancreatitis: An international multicenter study. International Pancreatitis Study Group. *Am J Gastroenterol* 89:1467, 1994.

179. Frey CF, Child CG, Fry W: Pancreatectomy for chronic pancreatitis. *Ann Surg* 184:403, 1976.

180. Lowenfels AB, Maisonneuve P, Cavallini G, et al: Pancreatitis and the risk of pancreatic cancer. International Pancreatitis Study Group. *N Engl J Med* 328:1433, 1993.

181. Aspelund G, Topazian MD, Lee JH, et al: Improved results for benign disease with limited pancreatic head resection. *J Gastrointest Surg* 2004, (in press).

182. Sankaran S, Walt AJ: The natural and unnatural history of pancreatic pseudocysts. *Br J Surg* 62:37, 1975.

183. Yeo CJ, Bastidas JA, Lynch-Nyhan A, et al: The natural history of pancreatic pseudocysts documented by computed tomography. *Surg Gynecol Obstet* 170:411, 1990.

184. Goulet RJ, Goodman J, Schaffer R, et al: Multiple pancreatic pseudocyst disease. *Ann Surg* 199:6, 1984.

185. Vitas GJ, Sarr MG: Selected management of pancreatic pseudocysts: Operative versus expectant management. *Surgery* 111:123, 1992.

186. Warshaw AL, Jin GL, Ottinger LW: Recognition and clinical implications of mesenteric and portal vein obstruction in chronic pancreatitis. *Arch Surg* 122:410, 1987.

187. Pancreatitis: Pancreatic pseudocysts and their complications. *Gastroenterology* 73:593, 1977.

188. Warshaw AL, Rattner DW: Timing of surgical drainage for pancreatic pseudocyst. Clinical and chemical criteria. *Ann Surg* 202:720, 1985.

189. Baron TH, Harewood GC, Morgan DE, et al: Outcome differences after endoscopic drainage of pancreatic necrosis, acute pancreatic pseudocysts, and chronic pancreatic pseudocysts. *Gastrointest Endosc* 56:7, 2002.

190. Gerzof SG, Banks PA, Robbins AH, et al: Early diagnosis of pancreatic infection by computed tomography-guided aspiration. *Gastroenterology* 93:1315, 1987.

191. Kozarek RA, Brayko CM, Harlan J, et al: Endoscopic drainage of pancreatic pseudocysts. *Gastrointest Endosc* 31:322, 1985.

192. Bell RH Jr.: Atlas of pancreatic surgery, in Bell RH Jr., Rikkers LF, Mulholland MW (eds): *Digestive Tract Surgery. A Text and Atlas.* Philadelphia: Lippincott-Raven, 1996, p 963.

193. Park AE, Heniford BT: Therapeutic laparoscopy of the pancreas. *Ann Surg* 236:149, 2002.

194. Hawes RH: Endoscopic management of pseudocysts. *Rev Gastroenterol Disord* 3:135, 2003.

195. Kozarek RA, Ball TJ, Patterson DJ, et al: Endoscopic transpapillary therapy for disrupted pancreatic duct and peripancreatic fluid collections. *Gastroenterology* 100(5 Pt 1):1362, 1991.

196. Nealon WH, Walser E: Duct drainage alone is sufficient in the operative management of pancreatic pseudocyst in patients with chronic pancreatitis. *Ann Surg* 237:614, 2003.

197. Rao R, Fedorak I, Prinz RA: Effect of failed computed tomography-guided and endoscopic drainage on pancreatic pseudocyst management. *Surgery* 114:843, 1993.

198. Heider R, Meyer AA, Galanko JA, Behrns KE: Percutaneous drainage of pancreatic pseudocysts is associated with a higher failure rate than surgical treatment in unselected patients. *Ann Surg* 229:781, 1999.

199. Schutz SM, Leung JW: Pancreatic endotherapy for pseudocysts and fluid collections. *Gastrointest Endosc* 56:150, 2002.

200. Lipsett RA, Cameron JC: Internal pancreatic fistula. *Am J Surg* 163:216, 1992.

201. Uchiyama T, Suzuki T, Adachi A, et al: Pancreatic pleural effusion: A case report and review of 113 cases in Japan. *Am J Gastroenterol* 87:387, 1992.

202. Cameron JL: Chronic pancreatic ascites and pancreatic pleural effusions. *Gastroenterology* 74:134, 1987.

203. Lipsett PA, Cameron JL: Treatment of ascites and fistulas, in Beger HG et al (eds): *The Pancreas.* London: Blackwell-Science, 1998, p 788.

204. Yeo CJ, Cameron JL: Exocrine pancreas, in Townsend CM et al (eds): *Sabiston's Textbook of Surgery.* New York: Lippincott Raven, 2000, p 1112.

205. Beger HG, Schlosser W, Poch B, et al: Inflammatory mass in the head of the pancreas, in Beger HG et al (eds): *The Pancreas.* London: Blackwell-Science, 1998, p 757.

206. Friess H, Yamanaka Y, Buchler M, et al: A subgroup of patients with chronic pancreatitis overexpress the c-erb B-2 protooncogene. *Ann Surg* 220:183, 1994.

207. Sakorafas GH, Sarr MG, Farley DR, et al: The significance of sinistral portal hypertension complicating chronic pancreatitis. *Am J Surg* 179:129, 2000.

208. Trapnell JE: Chronic relapsing pancreatitis: A review of 64 cases. *Br J Surg* 66:471, 1979.

209. Amann ST, Toskes PP: Analgesic treatment, in Beger HG et al (eds): *The Pancreas.* London: Blackwell-Science, 1998, p 766.

210. Isaksson G, Ihse I: Pain reduction by an oral pancreatic enzyme preparation in chronic pancreatitis. *Dig Dis Sci* 28:97, 1983.

211. Ramo OJ, Puolakkainen PA, Seppala K, et al: Self-administration of enzyme substitution in the treatment of exocrine pancreatic insufficiency. *Scand J Gastroenterol* 24:688, 1989.

212. Halgreen H, Pedersen NT, Worning H: Symptomatic effect of pancreatic enzyme therapy in patients with chronic pancreatitis. *Scand J Gastroenterol* 21:104, 1986.

213. Hildebrand P, Ensinck JW, Gyr K, et al: Evidence for hormonal inhibition of exocrine pancreatic function by somatostatin 28 in humans. *Gastroenterology* 103:240, 1992.

214. Toskes PP, Forsmark CE, DeMeo MT, et al: A multicenter controlled trial of octreotide for pain of chronic pancreatitis. *Pancreas* 8:A774, 1993.

215. Toskes PP, Forsmark CE, DeMeo MT, et al: An open-label trial of octreotide for the pain of chronic pancreatitis. *Gastroenterology* 106:A326, 1994.

216. Malfertheiner P, Mayer D, Buchler M, et al: Treatment of pain in chronic pancreatitis by inhibition of pancreatic secretion with octreotide. *Gut* 36:450, 1995.

217. Gress F, Schmitt C, Sherman S, et al: Endoscopic ultrasound guided celiac plexus block for managing abdominal pain associated with chronic pancreatitis: A prospective single center experience. *Am J Gastroenterol* 96:409, 2001.

218. Mergener K, Kozarek RA: Therapeutic pancreatic endoscopy. *Endoscopy* 35:48, 2003.

219. Aizawa T, Ueno N: Stent placement in the pancreatic duct prevents pancreatitis after endoscopic sphincter dilation for removal of bile duct stones. *Gastrointest Endosc* 54:209, 2001.

220. Mergener K, Kozarek RA, Lau ST, et al: A pancreatic ductal leak should be sought to direct treatment in patients with acute pancreatitis. *Am J Surg* 181:411, 2001.

221. Mergener K, Kozarek RA, Costamagna G, et al: Endoscopic treatment of postsurgical external pancreatic fistulas. *Endoscopy* 33:317, 2001.

222. Canty TG Sr., Weinman D: Management of major pancreatic duct injuries in children. *J Trauma* 50:1001, 2001.

223. Kim HS, Lee DK, Kim IW, et al: The role of endoscopic retrograde pancreatography in the treatment of traumatic pancreatic duct injury. *Gastrointest Endosc* 54:49, 2001.

224. Heyries L, Barthet M, Delvasto C, et al: Long-term results of endoscopic management of pancreas divisum with recurrent acute pancreatitis. *Gastrointest Endosc* 55:376, 2002.

225. Gabbrielli A, Mutignani M, Pandolfi M, et al: Endotherapy of early onset idiopathic chronic pancreatitis: Results with long-term follow-up. *Gastrointest Endosc* 55:488, 2002.

226. Jacob L, Geenen JE, Catalano MF, et al: Prevention of pancreatitis in patients with idiopathic recurrent pancreatitis: A prospective non-blinded randomized study using endoscopic stents. *Endoscopy* 33:559, 2001.

227. Kozarek RA, Brandabur JJ, Ball TJ, et al: Clinical outcomes in patients who undergo extracorporeal shock wave lithotripsy for chronic calcific pancreatitis. *Gastrointest Endosc* 56:496, 2002.

228. Nealon WH, Thompson JC: Progressive loss of pancreatic function in chronic pancreatitis is delayed by main pancreatic duct decompression. A longitudinal prospective analysis of the modified Puestow procedure. *Ann Surg* 217:458, 1993.

229. Coffey RG: Pancreato-enterostomy and pancreatectomy. *Ann Surg* 1:1238, 1909.

230. Link G: Treatment of chronic pancreatitis by pancreatostomy. *Ann Surg* 53:768, 1911.

231. Link G: Long term outcome of pancreatostomy for chronic pancreatitis. *Ann Surg* 101:287, 1935.

232. Priestly JT, Comfort MW, Radcliffe J: Total pancreatectomy for hyperinsulinism. *Ann Surg* 119:211, 1944.

233. Whipple AO: Radical surgery for certain cases of pancreatic fibrosis associated with calcareous deposits. *Ann Surg* 124:991, 1946.

234. Puestow CB, Gillesby WJ: Retrograde surgical drainage of pancreas for chronic relapsing pancreatitis. *Arch Surg* 76:898, 1958.

235. Partington PF, Rochelle REL: Modified Puestow procedure for retrograde drainage of the pancreatic duct. *Ann Surg* 152:1037, 1960.

236. Fry WJ, Child CG III: Ninety-five percent distal pancreatectomy for chronic pancreatitis. *Ann Surg* 162:543, 1965.

237. Moody FG, Calabuig R, Vecchio R, et al: Stenosis of the sphincter of Oddi. *Surg Clin North Am* 70:1341, 1990.

238. Moody FG, Vecchio R, Calabuig R, et al: Transduodenal sphincteroplasty with transampullary septectomy for stenosing papillitis. *Am J Surg* 161:213, 1991.

239. Cattell RB: Anastomosis of the duct of Wirsung in palliative operation for carcinoma of the head of the pancreas. *Surg Clin North Am* 27:637, 1947.

240. Duval MK Jr.: Caudal pancreatico-jejunostomy for chronic relapsing pancreatitis. *Ann Surg* 140:775, 1954.

241. Zollinger RM, Keith LM Jr., Ellison EH: Pancreatitis. *N Engl J Med* 251:497, 1954.

242. Izbicki JR, Bloechle C, Broering DC, et al: Longitudinal V-shaped excision of the ventral pancreas for small duct disease in severe chronic pancreatitis: Prospective evaluation of a new surgical procedure. *Ann Surg* 227:213, 1998.

243. Frey CF, Smith GJ: Description and rationale of a new operation for chronic pancreatitis. *Pancreas* 2:701, 1987.

244. Frey CF, Amikura K: Local resection of the head of the pancreas combined with longitudinal pancreaticojejunostomy in the management of patients with chronic pancreatitis. *Ann Surg* 220:492, 1994.

245. Andersen DK, Topazian MD: Excavation of the pancreatic head: A variation on the theme of duodenum-preserving pancreatic head resection. *Arch Surg* 139:375, 2004.

246. Aldridge MC, Williamson RC: Distal pancreatectomy with and without splenectomy. *Br J Surg* 78:976, 1991.

247. Hess W: Surgical tactics in chronic pancreatitis, in Hess W, Berci G (eds): *Textbook of Bilio-Panacreatic Diseases,* Vol. 4. Padua, Italy: Piccin Nuova Libraria, 1997, p 2299.

248. Traverso LW, Longmire WP Jr.: Preservation of the pylorus in pancreaticoduodenectomy. *Surg Gynecol Obstet* 146:959, 1978.

249. Huang JJ, Yeo CJ, Sohn TA, et al: Quality of life and outcomes after pancreaticoduodenectomy. *Ann Surg* 231:890, 2000.

250. Sakorafas GH, Farnell MB, Nagorney DM: Pancreatico-duodenectomy for chronic pancreatitis. Long term results in 1105 patients. *Arch Surg* 135:517, 2000.

251. Jemenez RE, Fernandez-del Castillo C, Rattner DW, Chang Y, Warshaw AL: Outcome of pancreaticoduodenectomy with pylorus preservation or with antrectomy in the treatment of chronic pancreatitis. *Ann Surg* 231:293, 2000.

252. Beger HG, Witte C, Krautzberger W, et al: Experiences with duodenum-sparing pancreas head resection in chronic pancreatitis. *Chirurg* 51:303, 1980.

253. Beger HG, Krautzberger W, Bittner R, et al: Duodenum-preserving resection of the head of the pancreas in patients with severe chronic pancreatitis. *Surgery* 97:467, 1985.

254. Beger HG, Schlosser W, Friess HM et al: Duodenum-preserving head resection in chronic pancreatitis changes the natural course of the disease: A single-center 26-year experience. *Ann Surg* 230:512, 1999; discussion 519.

255. Buchler MW, Friess H, Muller MW, et al: Randomized trial of duodenum-preserving pancreatic head resection versus pylorus-preserving Whipple in chronic pancreatitis. *Am J Surg* 169:65, 1995.

256. Izbicki JR, Bloechle C, Knoefel WT, et al: Duodenum-preserving resection of the head of the pancreas in chronic pancreatitis. A prospective, randomized trial. *Ann Surg* 221:350, 1995.

257. Najarian JS, Sutherland DER, Baumgartner D, et al: Total or near total pancreatectomy and islet autotransplantation for treatment of chronic pancreatitis. *Ann Surg* 192:526, 1980.

258. Farney AC, Najarian JS, Nakhleh RE, et al: Autotransplantation of dispersed pancreatic islet tissue combined with total or near total pancreatectomy for treatment of chronic pancreatitis. *Surgery* 110:427, 1991.

259. Robertson RP, Lanz KJ, Sutherland DE, et al: Prevention of diabetes for up to 13 years by autoislet transplantation after pancreatectomy for chronic pancreatitis. *Diabetes* 50:47, 2001.

260. Rastellini C: Donor and recipient selection in pancreatic islet transplantation. *Curr Opin Organ Transplant* 7:196, 2002.

261. Robertson GS, Dennison AR, Johnson PR, et al: A review of pancreatic islet autotransplantation. *Hepatogastroenterology* 45:226, 1998.

262. Lillemoe KD, Cameron JL, Kaufman HS, et al: Chemical splanchnicectomy in patients with unresectable pancreatic cancer. A prospective randomized trial. *Ann Surg* 217:447, 1993.

263. Mallet-Guy P: Bilan de 215 operations nerveuses, splanchnicectomies ou gangliectomies coeliaqus gauches, pour pancreatite chronique et recidivante. *Lyon Chir* 76:361, 1980.

264. Michotey G, Sastre B, Argeme M, et al: Splanchnicectomy by Dubois' transhiatal approach. Technics, indications and results. Apropos of 25 nerve sections for visceral abdominal pain. *J Chir (Paris)* 120:487, 1983 [French].

265. Stone HH, Chauvin EJ: Pancreatic denervation for pain relief in chronic alcohol associated pancreatitis. *Br J Surg* 77:303, 1990.

266. Cuschieri A: Laparoscopic surgery of the pancreas. *J Roy Coll Surg Edinb* 39:178, 1994.

267. Richards ML, Gauger PG, Thompson NW, et al: Pitfalls in the surgical treatment of insulinoma. *Surgery* 132:1040, 2002; discussion 1049.

268. Howard TJ, Stabile BE, Zinner MJ, et al; Anatomic distribution of pancreatic endocrine tumors. *Am J Surg* 159:258, 1990.

269. Deol ZK, Frezza E, DeJong S, et al: Solitary hepatic gastrinoma treated with laparoscopic radiofrequency ablation. *JSLS* 7:285, 2003.

270. Case CC, Wirfel K, Vassilopoulou-Sellin R: Vasoactive intestinal polypeptide-secreting tumor (VIPoma) with liver metastases: Dramatic and durable symptomatic benefit from hepatic artery embolization, a case report. *Med Oncol* 19:181, 2002.

271. Tanaka S, Yamasaki S, Matsushita H, et al: Duodenal somatostatinoma: A case report and review of 31 cases with special reference to the relationship between tumor size and metastasis. *Pathol Int* 50:146, 2000.

272. Jemal A, Murray T, Samuels A, et al: Cancer statistics, 2003. *CA Cancer J Clin* 53:5, 2003.

273. Gold EB, Goldin SB: Epidemiology of and risk factors for pancreatic cancer. *Surg Oncol Clin North Am* 7:67, 1998.

274. Fisher WE: Diabetes: Risk factor for the development of pancreatic cancer or manifestation of the disease? *World J Surg* 25:503, 2001.

275. Lowenfels AB, Maisonneuve P, Cavallini G, et al: Pancreatitis and the risk of pancreatic cancer. International Pancreatitis Study Group. *N Engl J Med* 20:1433, 1993.

276. Jean ME, Lowy AM, Chiao PJ, et al: The molecular biology of pancreatic cancer, in Evans DB, Pisters PWT, Abbruzzese JL (eds): *M.D. Anderson Solid Tumor Oncology Series—Pancreatic Cancer.* New York: Springer-Verlag, 2002, p 15.

277. Berger DH, Fisher WE: Inherited pancreatic cancer syndromes, in Evans DB, Pisters PWT, Abbruzzese JL (eds): *M.D. Anderson Solid Tumor Oncology Series—Pancreatic Cancer.* New York: Springer-Verlag, 2002, p 73.

278. Fisher WE, Muscarella P, Boros LG, et al: Gastrointestinal hormones as potential adjuvant treatment of exocrine pancreatic adenocarcinoma. *Int J Pancreatol* 24:169, 1998.

279. Biankin AV, Kench JG, Dijkman FP, et al: Molecular pathogenesis of precursor lesions of pancreatic ductal adenocarcinoma. *Pathology* 35:14, 2003.

280. Wilentz RE, Hruban RH: Pathology of cancer of the pancreas. *Surg Oncol Clin North Am* 7:43, 1998.

281. Ries LAG, Eisner MP, Kosary CL, et al (eds): *SEER Cancer Statistics Review, 1975—2000*. Bethesda, MD: National Cancer Institute. http://seer.cancer.gov/csr/1975_2000, 2003.

282. Ritts RE, Pitt HA: CA 19-9 in pancreatic cancer. *Surg Oncol Clin North Am* 7:93, 1998.

283. Iacobuzio-Donahue CA, Maitra A, Olsen M, et al: Exploration of global gene expression patterns in pancreatic adenocarcinoma using cDNA microarrays. *Am J Pathol* 162:1151, 2003.

284. Squillaci E, Fanucci E, Sciuto F, et al: Vascular involvement in pancreatic neoplasm: A comparison between spiral CT and DSA. *Dig Dis Sci* 48:449, 2003.

285. Kim HJ, Conlon KC: Laparoscopic staging, in Evans DB, Pisters PWT, Abbruzzese JL (eds): *M.D. Anderson Solid Tumor Oncology Series—Pancreatic Cancer*. New York: Springer-Verlag, 2002, p 115.

286. Shah RJ, Howell DA, Desilets DJ, et al: Multicenter randomized trial of the spiral Z-stent compared with the Wallstent for malignant biliary obstruction. *Gastrointest Endosc* 57:830, 2003.

287. Watanapa P, Williamson RCN: Surgical palliation for pancreatic cancer: Developments during the past two decades. *Br J Surg* 79:8, 1992.

288. Singh SM, Reber HA: Surgical palliation for pancreatic cancer. *Surg Clin North Am* 69:599, 1989.

289. Casper ES, Green MR, Kelsen DP, et al: Phase II trial of gemcitabine (2′,2′-difluorodeoxycytidine) in patients with adenocarcinoma of the pancreas. *Invest New Drugs* 12:29, 1994.

290. Yamaguchi K, Kishinaka M, Nagai E, et al: Pancreatoduodenectomy for pancreatic head carcinoma with or without pylorus preservation. *Hepatogastroenterology* 48:1479, 2001.

291. Ohtsuka T, Yamaguchi K, Ohuchida J, et al: Comparison of quality of life after pylorus-preserving pancreatoduodenectomy and Whipple resection. *Hepatogastroenterology* 50:846, 2003.

292. Heslin MJ, Harrison LE, Brooks AD, et al: Is intra-abdominal drainage necessary after pancreaticoduodenectomy? *J Gastrointest Surg* 2:373, 1998.

293. Pedrazzoli S, DiCarlo V, Dionigi R, et al: Standard versus extended lymphadenectomy associated with pancreatoduodenectomy in the surgical treatment of adenocarcinoma of the head of the pancreas: A multicenter, prospective, randomized study. Lymphadenectomy Study Group. *Ann Surg* 228:508, 1998.

294. Sindelar WF, Kinsella TJ: Studies of intraoperative radiotherapy in carcinoma of the pancreas. *Ann Oncol* 10(Suppl):S226, 1999.

295. Birkmeyer JD, Finlayson SR, Tosteson AN, et al: Effect of hospital volume on in-hospital mortality with pancreaticoduodenectomy. *Surgery* 125:250, 1999.

296. Gordon TA, Bowman HM, Tielsch JM, et al: Statewide regionalization of pancreaticoduodenectomy and its effect on in-hospital mortality. *Ann Surg* 228:71, 1998.

297. Gastrointestinal Tumor Study Group: Further evidence of effective adjuvant combined radiation and chemotherapy following curative resection of pancreatic cancer. *Cancer* 59:2006, 1997.

298. Neoptolemos JP, Dunn JA, Stocken DD, et al: European Study Group for Pancreatic Cancer. Adjuvant chemoradiotherapy and chemotherapy in resectable pancreatic cancer: A randomised controlled trial. *Lancet* 10:1576, 2001.

299. Pisters PW, Abbruzzese JL, Janjan NA, et al: Rapid-fractionation preoperative chemoradiation, pancreaticoduodenectomy, and intraoperative radiation therapy for resectable pancreatic adenocarcinoma. *J Clin Oncol* 16:3843, 1998.

300. Yazawa K, Fisher WE, Brunicardi FC: Current progress in suicide gene therapy for cancer. *World J Surg* 26:783, 2002.

301. Kiely JM, Nakeeb A, Komorowski RA, et al: Cystic pancreatic neoplasms: Enucleate or resect? *J Gastrointest Surg* 7:890, 2003.

302. Obermeyer RJ, Fisher WE, Sweeney JF, et al: Laparoscopic distal pancreatectomy for serous oligocystic adenoma. *Surg Rounds* Vol. 423, 2003.

303. Boni L, Benevento A, Dionigi G, et al: Primary pancreatic lymphoma. *Surg Endosc* 16:1107, 2002-8. Epub 2002 May 03.

CHAPTER 33

Spleen

Adrian E. Park and Rodrick McKinlay

INTRODUCTION

Throughout history, a remarkable number of attributes and functions have been ascribed to the spleen. In writings dating back to the first century, the spleen has variously been described as the seat of laughter, the source of black bile giving rise to melancholy, and the locus of conflicting emotions. Thus a derivative meaning of the word "spleen" in English is "ill temper." Throughout the centuries the spleen also has been considered an impediment to fleetness of foot for both man and beast. Until modern times, however, removal of the spleen usually resulted in death of the patient.

Anecdotal reports of splenic surgery began to emerge in the sixteenth century. By the end of the eighteenth century, the vast majority of splenectomies performed were partial and not complete, and most cases requiring surgical attention were in patients who had suffered left upper quadrant stab wounds, resulting in partial or total splenic prolapse. Morgenstern,[1] in chronicling the history of splenectomy, pointed out that pre–nineteenth century splenectomy carried a mortality rate well in excess of 90%. By 1877 only 50 splenectomies had ever been performed, with an overall mortality rate of over 70%. Yet by 1900, large series of splenectomies were reported with an operative mortality rate that had already dropped to less than 40%, and when Moynihan[2] reported the Mayo Clinic experience with splenectomy in 1920, the accompanying mortality rate was 11%. Progress over the last 80 years has been somewhat less dramatic; the largest series of laparoscopic splenectomies report an overall mortality of 1% or less.[3,4]

EMBRYOLOGY AND ANATOMY

Consisting of an encapsulated mass of vascular and lymphoid tissue, the spleen is the largest reticuloendothelial organ in the body. Arising from the primitive mesoderm as an outgrowth of the left side of the dorsal mesogastrium, by the fifth week of gestation the spleen is evident in an embryo 8 mm long. The organ continues its differentiation and migration to the left upper quadrant, where it comes to rest with its smooth, diaphragmatic surface facing posterosuperiorly.[4]

The most common anomaly of splenic embryology is the accessory spleen. Present in up to 20% of the population, one or more accessory spleen(s) may occur in up to 30% of patients with hematologic disease. Over 80% of accessory spleens are found in the region of the splenic hilum and vascular pedicle. Other locations for accessory spleens in descending order of frequency are: the gastrocolic ligament, the tail of the pancreas, the greater omentum, the greater curve of the stomach, the splenocolic ligament, the small and large bowel mesentery, the left broad ligament in women, and the left spermatic cord in men (Fig. 33-1).[5,6]

The abdominal surface of the diaphragm separates the spleen from the lower left lung and pleura and the ninth to eleventh ribs. The visceral surface of the organ faces the abdominal cavity and

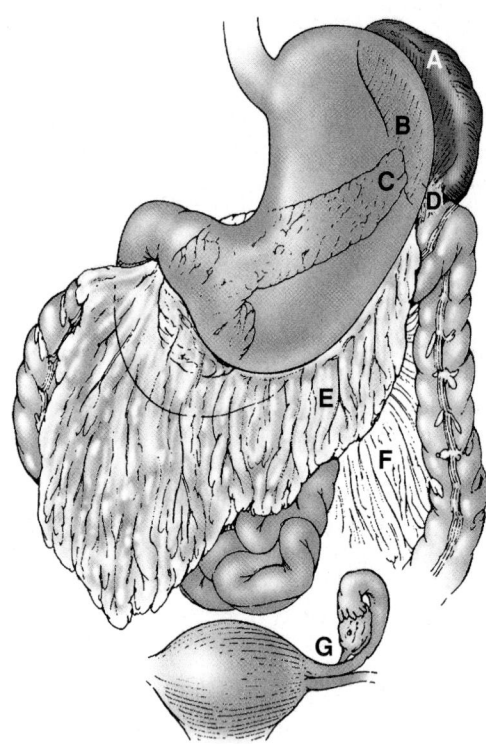

FIG. 33-1. Sites where accessory spleens are found in order of importance. A. Hilar region, 54%. B. Pedicle, 25%. C. Tail of pancreas, 6%. D. Splenocolic ligament, 2%. E. Greater omentum, 12%. F. Mesentery, 0.5%. G. Left ovary, 0.5%. (*Reprinted with permission from Poulin et al.[7]*)

contains gastric, colic, renal, and pancreatic impressions. Spleen size and weight vary with age and underlying pathologic conditions, but spleen size and weight diminish in the elderly. An average adult spleen is 7 to 11 cm in length and weighs 150 g (range 70 to 250 g). Within the surgical literature, splenomegaly is variably described as moderate, massive, and hyper, reflecting a lack of consensus among authors. Most authors would agree that "splenomegaly" would apply to organs weighing 500 mg or more and/or 15 cm or more in length. To be palpable below the left costal margin, a spleen must be at least double normal size.

The superior border of the spleen, which separates the diaphragmatic surface from the gastric impression of the visceral surface, often contains one or two notches, which can be pronounced when the spleen is greatly enlarged.

Of particular clinical relevance, the spleen is suspended in position by several ligaments and peritoneal folds to the colon (splenocolic ligament); the stomach (gastrosplenic ligament); the diaphragm (phrenosplenic ligament); and the kidney, adrenal gland, and tail of the pancreas (splenorenal ligament) (Fig. 33-2). Whereas the gastrosplenic ligament contains the short gastric vessels, the remaining ligaments are usually avascular, with rare exceptions, such as in a patient with portal hypertension. The relationship of the pancreas to the spleen also has important clinical implications. In cadaveric anatomic series, the tail of the pancreas has been demonstrated to lie within 1 cm of the splenic hilum 75% of the time and to actually abut the spleen in 30% of patients.

The spleen derives most of its blood from the splenic artery, the longest and most tortuous of the three main branches of the celiac artery. The splenic artery can be characterized by the pattern of its terminal branches. The *distributed type* of splenic artery is the most

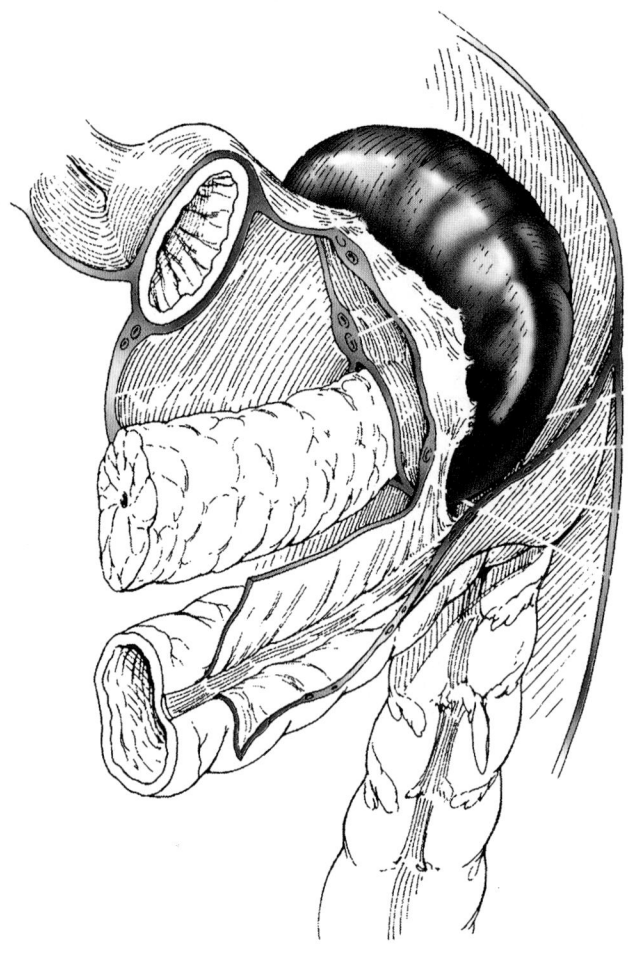

FIG. 33-2. Suspensory ligaments of the spleen. (*Reprinted with permission from Poulin et al.[7]*)

common (70%) and is distinguished by a short trunk with many long branches entering over three fourths of the medial surface of the spleen. The less common (30%) *magistral type* of splenic artery has a long main trunk dividing near the hilum into short terminal branches, which enter over 25 to 30% of the medial surface of the spleen. The spleen also receives some of its blood supply from the short gastric vessels, which are branches of the left gastroepiploic artery running within the gastrosplenic ligament. The splenic vein accommodates the major venous drainage of the spleen. It joins the superior mesenteric vein to form the portal vein.

When sectioned, the cut surface of a normal, freshly excised spleen is finely granular and predominantly dark red, but also contains whitish nodules liberally distributed across its expanse. This gross observation reflects the microstructure of the spleen. The splenic parenchyma is composed of two main elements: the red pulp, which constitutes approximately 75% of total splenic volume, and the white pulp. At the interface between the red and white pulp is the narrow marginal zone (Fig. 33-3).

The red pulp is comprised of large numbers of venous sinuses, which ultimately drain into tributaries of the splenic vein. The sinuses are surrounded and separated by a fibrocellular network, called the reticulum, consisting of collagen fibers and fibroblasts. Within this network or mesh lie splenic macrophages. These intersinusoidal regions appear as *splenic cords*. The venous sinuses are lined by long, narrow endothelial cells that are variably in close apposition

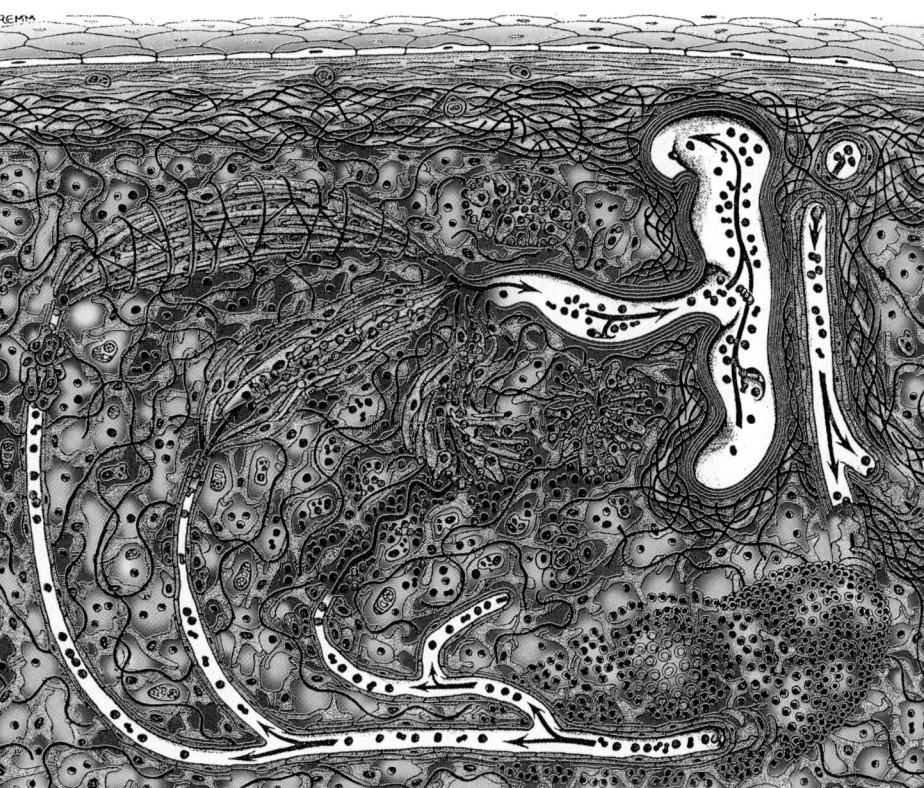

FIG. 33-3. The main features of splenic structure. The various elements are not drawn to scale, to enable representation on a single diagram. Note the capsule, trabeculae, reticular fibers and cells, the perivascular lymphatic aggregation (white pulp), and the ellipsoids, cell cords, and venous sinusoids of the red pulp. The "open" and "closed" theories of splenic circulation are illustrated. The venous sinusoids are shown in two states: (1) with their lining of "stave" cells (brown) in close apposition, and (2) with intercellular gaps (these have been overemphasized for clarity). (Reprinted with permission from Bannister LH: Haemolymphoid system, in: Gray's Anatomy, 38th ed. Edinburgh, UK: Churchill Livingstone, 1995, p 1438.)

to one another or separated by intercellular gaps in a configuration that is unique to the spleen. The red pulp serves as a dynamic filtration system, enabling macrophages to remove microorganisms, cellular debris, antigen/antibody complexes, and senescent erythrocytes from circulation.

Around the terminal millimeters of splenic arterioles, a *periarticular lymphatic sheath* replaces the native adventitia of the vessel. The sheath is comprised of T lymphocytes and intermittent aggregations of B lymphocytes or lymphoid follicles. When antigenically stimulated, the follicles, which are centers of lymphocyte proliferation, develop germinal centers. These regress as the stimulus or infection subsides. This white pulp, normally consisting of nodules 1 mm or less in size, can increase to several centimeters in size when nodules coalesce, as occurs with certain lymphoproliferative disorders. At the junction between the white and red pulp is the marginal zone, where lymphocytes are more loosely aggregated. Blood is delivered from this zone to the red pulp, where lymphocytes and locally produced immunoglobulins ultimately enter the systemic circulation.

PHYSIOLOGY AND PATHOPHYSIOLOGY

The spleen is contained by a capsule 1 to 2 mm thick. In humans, the capsule is rich in collagen and contains some elastin fibers. Many mammals have splenic capsules and trabeculae with abundant smooth muscle cells, which upon autonomic stimulation contract to expel large volumes of stored blood to the general circulation. Such spleens have been described as *storage spleens*. By contrast the human splenic capsule and trabeculae contain few or no smooth muscle cells and their function is largely related to immunologic protection; hence the human organ has been characterized as a *defense spleen*.[8]

Splenic function has historically been summarized as: (1) filtration, (2) host defense, (3) storage, and (4) cytopoiesis. Filtration and

immunologic function are the most important and dominant ones in the adult human. Total splenic inflow of blood is approximately 250 to 300 mL/min. Blood flows through successively tapering arteries to arterioles, traverses the white pulp, crosses the marginal zone, and enters the red pulp. At this point the rate of flow through the spleen can vary greatly. Animal studies measuring isotopically labeled blood transit times through the spleen have revealed three distinct velocities of flow. In humans, a fast or closed circulation, in which blood passes directly from arterioles into venous sinuses, and a slower or open circulation have long been recognized. It is via the slower circulation that most of the filtration function of the spleen occurs. In open circulation, blood percolates through the reticular space and splenic cords, gaining access to sinuses through the gaps or slits in the endothelial cell lining. Blood flows into and out of the venous sinuses through these gaps. The blood is thus exposed to extensive contact with splenic macrophages. There may also be temporary and unique adhesive contact between blood cells and components of the splenic cord, since plasma is not similarly slowed during its passage through these spaces. Further evidence of the selective slowing of blood cell flow versus plasma flow is the fact that the concentration of erythrocytes (hematocrit) within the spleen is twice that of the general circulation. It is likely that during this process of contact with splenic macrophages, the removal of cellular debris and senescent blood cells occurs.

The process by which the spleen removes erythrocyte inclusions, such as Heinz bodies (intracellular altered hemoglobin), without cell lysis while red blood cells travel through the spleen is not well understood. The spleen is the major site for clearance of damaged or aged red blood cells from the blood, but it also plays a role in the removal of abnormal white blood cells and platelets. During the 120-day life cycle of the erythrocyte, a minimum of 2 days is spent sequestered in the spleen. Approximately 20 mL of aged red blood cells are removed daily. There is evidence to suggest that as erythrocytes age, previously undetected antigens on their surfaces may attach to autoantibodies in the circulation; macrophages may then bind to the antibodies and initiate phagocytosis. It is also quite probable that multiple passages through the spleen and delayed transit through the congested and relatively hypoxic and acidotic environment of the splenic cords are detrimental over time to the erythrocyte. It is, however, interesting to note that splenectomized patients enjoy a normal red blood cell life span.

The spleen plays a significant though not indispensable role in host defense, contributing to both humoral and cell-mediated immunity. As discussed in the previous section, antigens are filtered in the white pulp and presented to immunocompetent centers within the lymphoid follicles. This gives rise to the elaboration of immunoglobulins (predominantly IgM). Following an antigen challenge, such an acute IgM response results in the release of opsonic antibodies from the white pulp of the spleen. Clearance of the antigen by the splenic and hepatic reticuloendothelial (RE) systems is then facilitated.

The spleen also produces the opsonins, tuftsin and properdin. Tuftsin, a likely stimulant to general phagocytic function in the host, appears to specifically facilitate clearance of bacteria.[9] It is circulating monocytes that are converted into fixed macrophages with the red pulp that account for the remarkable phagocytic activity of the spleen.

The spleen also appears to be a major source of the protein properdin, which is important in the initiation of the alternate pathway of complement activation. The splenic RE system is better able to clear bacteria that are poorly or inadequately opsonized from the circulation than is the hepatic RE system.[10] Encapsulated bacteria generally fit such a profile, hence the risk posed by pneumococcus and *Haemophilus influenzae* to an asplenic patient. There appears to be sufficient physiologic capacity within the complement cascade to withstand the loss of tuftsin and properdin production without increasing patient vulnerability postsplenectomy.[11]

In patients suffering chronic hemolytic disorders, splenic tissue may become permanently hypertrophied. The reticular spaces of the red pulp sometimes become distended with macrophages engorged with the products of erythrocyte breakdown. As a result the spleen may greatly enlarge (splenomegaly). Whereas splenomegaly alone is an uncommon indication for splenectomy, hypersplenism is one of the most common indications. Hypersplenism is defined as the presence of cytopenia (of one or more blood cell lines) in the context of normally responding bone marrow. Hypersplenism is cured or improved by splenectomy.

Disorders causing hypersplenism can be categorized as either (1) those in which increased destruction of abnormal blood cells occurs in an intrinsically normal spleen (e.g., hemolytic anemias), or (2) primary disorders of the spleen resulting in increased sequestration and destruction of normal blood cells (e.g., infiltrative disorders).

The life cycles of cellular elements in human blood vary widely. The normal half-life of a neutrophil in circulation is approximately 6 hours. The role of the spleen in the normal clearance of neutrophils is not well established. It is clear that hypersplenism may result in neutropenia by sequestration of normal white blood cells or the removal of abnormal ones. Platelets, on the other hand, generally survive in the circulation for 10 days. Under normal circumstances one third of the total platelet pool is sequestered in the spleen. Thrombocytopenia may result from excessive sequestration of platelets as well as accelerated platelet destruction in the spleen. Splenomegaly may result in sequestration of up to 80% of the platelet pool. The spleen may also contribute to the immunologic alteration of platelets, leading to thrombocytopenia in the absence of splenomegaly (e.g., idiopathic thrombocytopenic purpura [ITP]).

The immunologic functions of the spleen are consistent with those of other lymphoid organs. It is a site of blood-borne antigen presentation and the initiation of T and B lymphocyte activities involved in humoral and cellular immune responses. Alteration of splenic immune function often gives rise to antibody production, resulting in blood cell destruction.

Although the spleen contributes to the process of erythrocyte maturation, in adult humans there is little evidence of normal hematopoietic function. The spleen plays a minor role in hematopoiesis in the human fetus beginning in the fourth month, which can be reactivated in childhood if marrow capacity is exceeded. Splenic hematopoiesis giving rise to abnormal red blood cells is seen in adults with myeloproliferative disorders. As well, in response to some anemias, elements of the red pulp may revert to hematopoiesis.

EVALUATION OF SIZE AND FUNCTION

Imaging of the spleen is most frequently indicated to assess its size before elective splenectomy and to determine the degree of splenomegaly, if any. Other indications for splenic imaging include investigations of left upper quadrant pain, delineation of tumors or cysts of the spleen, characterization of splenic abscesses, and guidance for percutaneous procedures involving the spleen.[12,13]

Ultrasound (US) is the most cost-effective mode of splenic imaging for routine elective splenectomy. It is rapid, easy to perform, and does not expose the patient to ionizing radiation. The sensitivity of US for detecting textural lesions of the spleen is as high as 98% in experienced hands.[14] Computed tomography (CT) scanning affords a high degree of resolution and detail of the spleen as well. CT is useful for assessment of splenomegaly, identification of splenic lesions, and guidance for percutaneous procedures. The use of iodinated contrast material adds diagnostic clarity to CT imaging of the spleen.

Besides US and CT scan, plain radiography, magnetic resonance imaging (MRI), and radioscintigraphy can be used to image the spleen. Plain radiography is rarely used alone for splenic imaging, but can provide an outline of the spleen in the left upper quadrant or suggest splenomegaly by revealing displacement of adjacent air-filled structures, such as the stomach or splenic flexure of the colon. The spleen may also demonstrate calcifications. MRI is more expensive than CT scanning or US and offers no advantages in depicting anatomic abnormalities of the spleen.[15] Radioscintigraphy with ^{99m}Tc-sulfur colloid demonstrates splenic location and size. It may be especially helpful in locating accessory spleens following unsuccessful splenectomy for ITP. Although radiocolloid scans indicate the site of preferred sequestration of platelets in ITP, no conclusive outcome benefit has been shown for preoperative technetium scanning prior to splenectomy.[16] Damaged ^{99m}Tc-labeled red blood cells may be used to exclude or confirm abnormalities found by radiocolloid imaging.[17] Angiography typically yields little diagnostic information, but provides an effective therapeutic modality for embolizing bleeding splenic branches in trauma and has shown limited success in partial embolization for chronic ITP.[18] Some success has been reported with preoperative total splenic embolization for splenomegaly. The splenic index (SI) is a useful concept, initially proposed by Cools,[19] which expresses the size of the spleen as a volume in mL. The SI is obtained by multiplying the length, width, and height of the spleen as determined by a reliable imaging modality. Normal values for SI range from 120 mL to 480 mL. The normal ex vivo weight of the spleen is 150 g.[19] For patients more than 20 years old, no correlation has been identified between spleen size and age, gender, or body habitus.[20] Investigators have linked increased splenic index with a higher likelihood of bleeding esophageal varices in patients with cirrhosis.[21]

INDICATIONS FOR SPLENECTOMY

The conditions for which splenectomy is therapeutic may be classified according to their pathologic identity, including disorders of red blood cells, early cell lines (myeloproliferative disorders), white blood cells, platelets, and miscellaneous disorders and lesions (Table 33-1). The most common indication for splenectomy is trauma to the spleen, whether iatrogenic or otherwise. Splenectomy for traumatic rupture is addressed in Chap. 6. Historically the most common indication for elective splenectomy has been staging for Hodgkin's disease.[22] More recent data suggest that ITP is now the most frequent indication for splenectomy in the elective setting.[3,22] In descending order of frequency, other indications include hereditary spherocytosis, autoimmune hemolytic anemia, and thrombotic thrombocytopenic purpura.

Red Blood Cell Disorders

Acquired

Autoimmune Hemolytic Anemia (AIHA). The autoimmune hemolytic anemias are a set of disorders characterized by autoantibodies against antigens on red blood cells, which decrease the erythrocyte life span. AIHA is classified into "warm" or "cold" categories, based on the temperature at which the autoantibodies

Table 33-1
Indications for Splenectomy

1. Red cell disorders
   a. Congenital
      i. Hereditary spherocytosis
      ii. Hemoglobinopathies
         1. Sickle cell disease
         2. Thalassemia
         3. Enzyme deficiencies
   b. Acquired
      i. Autoimmune hemolytic anemia
      ii. Parasitic diseases
2. Platelet disorders
   a. Idiopathic thrombocytopenic purpura (ITP)
   b. Thrombotic thrombocytopenic purpura (TTP)
3. White cell disorders
   a. Leukemias
   b. Lymphomas
   c. Hodgkin's disease
4. Bone marrow disorders (myeloproliferative disorders)
   a. Myelofibrosis (myeloid metaplasia)
   b. Chronic myeloid leukemia (CML)
   c. Acute myeloid leukemia (AML)
   d. Chronic myelomonocytic leukemia (CMML)
   e. Essential thrombocythemia
   f. Polycythemia vera
5. Miscellaneous disorders and lesions
   a. Infections/abscess
   b. Storage diseases/infiltrative disorders
      i. Gaucher's disease
      ii. Niemann-Pick disease
      iii. Amyloidosis
   c. Felty's syndrome
   d. Sarcoidosis
   e. Cysts and tumors
   f. Portal hypertension
   g. Splenic artery aneurysm

SOURCE: Adapted from Hiatt, et al.[41]

exert their effect. Warm autoantibodies (IgG) bind erythrocytes at 37°C; cold agglutinins (typically IgM) cause erythrocytes to clump at cold temperatures; and a third type of autoantibody binds to red blood cell membranes in the cold, but activates the hemolytic cascade at 37°C, creating a syndrome known as paroxysmal cold hemoglobinuria.[24] For each of these types, the autoantibodies may be primary (idiopathic) or secondary (associated with an underlying disease or drug). Each type of anemia represents a characteristic clinical disorder, even though they are collectively referred to as autoimmune hemolytic anemia. Warm-antibody is the type of AIHA best treated by splenectomy.

Warm-Antibody AIHA. The incidence of warm-antibody AIHA is approximately 1:100,000.[24] More common among women, AIHA occurs at all ages, but is principally seen in mid-life. About one half of cases are idiopathic. Clinical findings include mild jaundice and symptoms and signs of anemia. Splenomegaly occurs in one third to one half of patients, sometimes enough to result in a palpable spleen on physical examination. Other physical findings may include pallor or slight jaundice. AIHA may develop acutely, with severe symptoms and signs, or gradually, with a relatively asymptomatic presentation. In acute disease, signs of congestive heart failure may be observed.

The diagnosis of AIHA is made by first demonstrating hemolysis, indicated by anemia, reticulocytosis, and the products of red blood cell destruction (bilirubin and related compounds) in the blood, urine, and stool. Once hemolysis has been shown, a direct Coombs' test is performed, in which a sample of the patient's blood is mixed with IgG antibody (Coombs' reagent). Agglutination represents a positive reaction, indicating the presence of IgG or complement bound to the red blood cell membrane. A positive direct Coombs' test confirms the diagnosis of AIHA and distinguishes autoimmune from other forms of hemolytic anemia.

Red blood cells are opsonized by autoantibodies and are destroyed, either directly within the circulation (intravascular hemolysis), or removed from the circulation by tissue macrophages located primarily in the spleen and to a lesser extent in the liver (extravascular hemolysis). Tissue macrophages in the spleen harbor receptors specific for the Fc portion of the autoantibody that facilitate clearance. The macrophages may ingest an opsonized red blood cell entirely or digest bits of the erythrocyte membrane via proteolytic enzymes, producing a spherocyte susceptible to hemolysis as it travels through the splenic circulation.

Treatment of AIHA depends on how severe it is and whether it is primary or secondary. Severe anemia (<4 g/dL), causing pulmonary edema, tachycardia, postural hypotension, dyspnea, and angina, demands red blood cell transfusion. Corticosteroids act as the mainstay of treatment for both primary and secondary forms of symptomatic, unstable AIHA. A dose of 1 to 2 mg/kg per day in divided doses is sufficient to start, and therapy should last until a response is noted by a rise in hematocrit and fall in reticulocyte count, which generally occurs within 3 weeks. Steroid therapy is more successful in producing a durable remission in children than in adults. Splenectomy is indicated for failure to respond to steroids, intolerance of steroid side effects, requirement for excessive steroid doses to maintain remission, or inability to receive steroids for other reasons. A favorable response to splenectomy can be expected in up to 80% of patients with warm-antibody AIHA.

Congenital

Hereditary Spherocytosis. Hereditary spherocytosis (HS) is a disorder of the red blood cell membrane resulting in hemolytic anemia, inherited primarily in an autosomal dominant fashion. With an estimated prevalence in Western populations of 1 in 5000, HS is the most common hemolytic anemia for which splenectomy is indicated.[25]

The underlying abnormality in HS is an inherited dysfunction or deficiency in one of the erythrocyte membrane proteins (spectrin, ankyrin, band 3 protein, or protein 4.2), which results in destabilization of the membrane lipid bilayer. This destabilization allows a release of lipids from the membrane, causing a reduction in membrane surface area and a lack of deformability, leading to sequestration and destruction of the spherocytic erythrocytes in the spleen.

Like HS, hereditary elliptocytosis (HE) results from genetic defects in skeletal membrane proteins. These defects permit elongation of the red blood cell as it circulates. Unlike HS, however, HE is usually a harmless trait, unless 50 to 90% of red blood cells are affected, in which case a clinical syndrome like HS may develop.

Most patients with HS are relatively asymptomatic, though rare fatal crises occur, usually in the setting of infection (e.g., parvovirus). Patients with typical forms of HS may have mild jaundice. Splenomegaly is usually present on physical examination. Laboratory examination reveals mild to moderate anemia, though patients with mild forms of the disease may have no anemia, and patients with severe forms may have hemoglobin levels as low as 4 to 6 g/dL. The mean corpuscular volume (MCV) is typically low to normal or slightly decreased. An elevated mean corpuscular hemoglobin concentration (MCHC), combined with an elevated erythrocyte distribution width, is an excellent predictor as a screening test. Other laboratory indicators of HS include evidence of rapid red blood cell destruction, such as an elevated reticulocyte count, elevated lactate dehydrogenase (LDH), and increased unconjugated bilirubin. Spherocytes are readily apparent on peripheral blood film.

Splenectomy is curative for typical forms of HS and serves as the sole mode of therapy.[24] Patients with severe disease usually show a dramatic clinical improvement, even though hemolysis may persist. Since HS may affect children, the timing of splenectomy is important in order to reduce the very small possibility of overwhelming postsplenectomy sepsis. Most authors recommend delaying the operation until the patient is between the ages of 4 and 6, unless the anemia and hemolysis accelerate.[23,25] Intractable leg ulcers represent an indication for early splenectomy, since they heal only after removal of the spleen.

Gallstones are more likely to develop in patients with HS, and over one half of patients with HS between the ages of 10 and 30 may have cholelithiasis.[26] Prophylactic cholecystectomy is recommended in children with cholelithiases at the time of splenectomy.[27]

Hemoglobinopathies. *Sickle cell disease* is an inherited chronic hemolytic anemia resulting from the mutant sickle cell hemoglobin (Hb S) within the red blood cell. It is inherited in an autosomal codominant fashion; persons who inherit an Hb S gene from one parent (heterozygous) are carriers, and those who inherit an Hb S gene from both parents (homozygous) have sickle cell anemia. The prevalence of sickle cell carriers is about 8 to 10% among African Americans in the United States, resulting in 4000 to 5000 newborns per year at risk for sickle cell disease. In western Africa, by contrast, approximately 120,000 newborns are at risk annually.[28]

The underlying abnormality in sickle cell disease is the mutation of adenine (A) to thymine (T) in the sixth codon of the beta-globin gene, resulting in the substitution of valine for glutamic acid as the sixth amino acid of the beta-globin chain. Mutant B chains included in the hemoglobin tetramer create Hb S. Deoxygenated Hb S is insoluble and becomes polymerized and sickled. The subsequent lack

of deformability of the red blood cell, in addition to other processes, results in microvascular congestion, which may lead to thrombosis, ischemia, and tissue necrosis. Intermittent painful episodes characterize the disorder.

Sequestration occurs in the spleen with resultant splenomegaly early in the course of the disease. In most patients subsequent infarction of the spleen and autosplenectomy occur at some later time.[23] The most frequent indications for splenectomy among patients with sickle cell disease are hypersplenism and acute sequestration crises, followed by splenic abscess.[29] The occurrence of one major acute sequestration crisis, characterized by rapid painful enlargement of the spleen and circulatory collapse, is generally considered sufficient grounds for splenectomy, as subsequent attacks occur in 40 to 50% of patients, with a mortality rate of 20%.[29] The incidence of acute sequestration crises is about 5% in children with sickle cell disease.[30] Approximately 3% of children with sickle cell disease ultimately require splenectomy.[30] Preoperative preparation includes special attention to adequate hydration and avoidance of hypothermia.

Splenectomy does not affect the sickling process, and therapy for sickle cell anemia largely remains palliative. Transfusions are indicated for anemia, for moderately severe episodes of the acute chest syndrome (i.e., a new infiltrate on chest radiograph associated with new symptoms, such as fever, cough, sputum production, or hypoxia[31]), and preoperatively before splenectomy. Patients sustaining stroke or a severe crisis may require hydration and an exchange transfusion, which may be performed manually or with automated apheresis equipment. In an exchange transfusion, the goal is typically to exchange a single volume of the patient's blood.[28] Hydroxyurea is an oral chemotherapeutic agent that upregulates fetal hemoglobin, which interferes with polymerization of Hb S, thus reducing the sickling process. Hydroxyurea has been shown to reduce the number of pain crises, the incidence of acute chest syndrome, and transfusion requirements in patients with sickle cell disease.[28]

Thalassemia. The thalassemias are a group of inherited disorders of hemoglobin synthesis prevalent among people of Mediterranean extraction, classified according to the hemoglobin chain affected (i.e., alpha, beta, or gamma). As a group they are the most common genetic diseases known arising from a single gene defect.[32,33] Most forms of thalassemia are inherited in mendelian recessive fashion from asymptomatic carrier parents. The incidence of thalassemia is between 2.5 and 15% in the so-called thalassemia belt extending along the shores of the Mediterranean, the Arabian Peninsula, Turkey, Iran, India, and southeastern Asia. However, thalassemias have been found in people of all ethnic origins.[32,34]

The primary defect in all forms of thalassemia is reduced or absent production of hemoglobin chains. Two significant consequences arise from this abnormality: (1) reduced functioning of hemoglobin tetramers, yielding hypochromia and microcytosis, and (2) unbalanced biosynthesis of individual alpha and beta subunits, resulting in insoluble red blood cells that cannot release oxygen normally and may precipitate with cell aging. Both underproduction of hemoglobin and the excess production of unpaired hemoglobin subunits contribute to the morbidity and mortality associated with thalassemia.

The diagnosis of thalassemia major (homozygous) is made by demonstrating hypochromic microcytic anemia associated with randomly distorted red blood cells and nucleated erythrocytes ("target cells") on peripheral blood smear.[6] Associated findings include an elevated reticulocyte count and white blood cell count. Because alpha chains are needed to form both fetal hemoglobin (Hb F) and adult hemoglobin (Hb A), alpha-thalassemia becomes symptomatic in utero or at birth. By contrast, beta-thalassemia becomes symptomatic at 4 to 6 months, since beta chains are only involved in adult hemoglobin synthesis.

The clinical spectrum of the thalassemias is wide. Heterozygous carriers of the disease are usually asymptomatic, but homozygous individuals typically present before 2 years of age with pallor, growth retardation, jaundice, and abdominal swelling due to liver and spleen enlargement. Other characteristics of thalassemia major include intractable leg ulcers, head enlargement, frequent infections, and a requirement for chronic blood transfusions. Untreated individuals usually die in late infancy or early childhood from severe anemia.[6]

Treatment for thalassemia consists of red blood cell transfusions to keep the hemoglobin count greater than 9 mg/dL, along with intensive parenteral chelation therapy with deferoxamine. Splenectomy is indicated for patients with excessive transfusion requirements (>200 mL/kg per year), discomfort due to splenomegaly, or painful splenic infarction.[6,35] A careful assessment of the risk:benefit ratio for splenectomy is essential, since infectious morbidity following splenectomy in patients with thalassemia is greater than in other patients undergoing splenectomy for hematologic indications.[36] This increase in infectious complications is likely due to coexisting immune deficiency, precipitated in large part by iron overload associated both with thalassemia itself and transfusions. When indicated, in rare circumstances splenectomy should be delayed until absolutely necessary, if possible after the age of 4 years.

Red Blood Cell Enzyme Deficiencies. Red blood cell enzyme deficiencies associated with hemolytic anemia may be classified into two groups: those needed to maintain a high ratio of reduced to oxidized glutathione in the red blood cell, such as glucose-6-phosphate dehydrogenase (G6PD) deficiency, and those involved in glycolytic pathways, such as pyruvate kinase (PK) deficiency.[6]

G6PD is an enzyme that reduces nicotinamide adenine dinucleotide phosphate (NADP) to NADP plus hydrogen (NADPH) in the glutathione pathway. This helps to maintain the balance of reduced to oxidized glutathione and protects the red blood cell from oxidative damage. Depending on the variant of G6PD deficiency, the clinical manifestation may be chronic hemolytic anemia, acute intermittent hemolytic episodes, or no hemolysis. Although hundreds of millions of people worldwide are affected by G6PD deficiency, most experience only moderate health risks and no reduction in longevity.[37] The diagnosis is established either by a fluorescent screening test or by spectrophotometric analysis of enzyme activity.[38] Therapy consists of avoidance of drugs known to precipitate hemolysis in G6PD patients and transfusions in cases of symptomatic anemia.[37] Splenectomy is not indicated in this disease.[6]

Although less common than G6PD deficiency overall, PK deficiency is the most common red blood cell enzyme deficiency to cause congenital chronic hemolytic anemia.[37] Its mechanism of action is unclear and PK deficiency affects people worldwide, with a slight preponderance among those of northern European or Chinese descent. The diagnosis is made either by a screening test (which may miss some forms of the disease)[35] or by detection of specific mutations at the cDNA or genomic level.[39] Clinical manifestations of the disease range widely, from transfusion-dependent severe anemia to well-compensated mild anemia.[40] Splenomegaly is common, and splenectomy in severe cases alleviates transfusion requirements.[6] As with other disorders causing hemolytic anemia in children, splenectomy should be delayed if possible to at least 4 years of age to reduce the risk of postsplenectomy infection.

Bone Marrow Disorders (Myeloproliferative Disorders)

The myeloproliferative disorders are characterized by an abnormal growth of cell lines in the bone marrow. They include chronic myeloid leukemia (CML), acute myeloid leukemia (AML), chronic myelomonocytic leukemia (CMML), essential thrombocythemia (ET), polycythemia vera (PV), and myelofibrosis, also known as agnogenic myeloid metaplasia (see the myelofibrosis section in this chapter). The common underlying problem leading to splenectomy in these disorders is symptomatic splenomegaly. Symptoms due to splenomegaly consist of early satiety, poor gastric emptying, heaviness or pain in the left upper quadrant, and even diarrhea. Hypersplenism, while usually associated with splenomegaly, is a distinct condition. Hypersplenism refers to the presence of one or more peripheral cytopenias in the presence of a normally compensating bone marrow, and can be corrected or improved by splenectomy.[41]

Splenomegaly can be treated by chemotherapeutic agents (busulfan, hydroxyurea, interferon-alpha) or low-dose radiation to achieve mild to moderate size reductions and some relief of symptoms, but discontinuing treatment may result in rapid splenic regrowth. Radiation has been used since 1903 to treat symptomatic splenomegaly, but today it is principally used in situations in which splenectomy is not an option. Radiation treatment typically consists of intermittent fractionated splenic irradiation in increasing dosages from 50 cGy to 100 cGy over several months.[42]

Chronic Myeloid Leukemia

CML is a disorder of the primitive pluripotent stem cell in the bone marrow, resulting in a significant increase in erythroid, megakaryotic, and pluripotent progenitors in the peripheral blood smear. The genetic hallmark is a transposition between the *bcr* gene on chromosome 9 and the *abl* gene on chromosome 22. CML accounts for 7 to 15% of all leukemias, with an incidence of 1.5 in 100,000 in the United States.[43] CML is frequently asymptomatic in the chronic phase, but symptomatic patients often present with the gradual onset of fatigue, anorexia, sweating, and left upper quadrant pain and early satiety secondary to splenomegaly. Enlargement of the spleen is found in roughly one half of patients with CML. Splenectomy is indicated to ease pain and early satiety.[44]

Acute Myeloid Leukemia

Like CML, AML involves the abnormal growth of stem cells in the bone marrow. Unlike CML, the clinical presentation is more rapid and dramatic in AML. The proliferation and accumulation of hematopoietic stem cells in the bone marrow and blood inhibit the growth and maturation of normal red blood cells, white blood cells, and platelets. Death usually results within weeks to months if AML remains untreated. The incidence of AML is approximately 9200 new cases each year in the United States, resulting in 1.2% of all cancer deaths.[45] Patients with other myeloproliferative disorders, such as polycythemia vera, primary thrombocytosis, or myeloid metaplasia, are at increased risk for leukemic transformation to AML. Presenting signs and symptoms of AML include a viral-like illness with fever, malaise, and frequently bone pain due to the expansion of the medullary space. Splenomegaly is modest but palpable on physical exam in up to 50% of patients.[46] Splenectomy is indicated in AML in the uncommon circumstance that left upper quadrant pain and early satiety become unbearable. Splenectomy in AML adds further risk of infection to patients immunocompromised by neutropenia and chemotherapy.

Chronic Myelomonocytic Leukemia

Like CML and AML, chronic myelomonocytic leukemia (CMML) is characterized by a proliferation of hematopoietic elements in the bone marrow and blood. CMML differs from CML in that it is associated with monocytosis in the peripheral smear ($>1 \times 10^3/mm^3$) and in the bone marrow. Splenomegaly occurs in one half of these patients, and splenectomy can result in symptomatic relief.

Essential Thrombocythemia

Essential thrombocythemia (ET) represents abnormal growth of the megakaryocyte cell line, resulting in increased levels of platelets in the bloodstream. The diagnosis is made after the exclusion of other chronic myeloid disorders, such as CML, PV, and myelofibrosis, that may also present with thrombocytosis.[47] Clinical manifestations of ET include vasomotor symptoms, thrombohemorrhagic events, recurrent fetal loss, and the transformation to myelofibrosis with myeloid metaplasia or acute myeloid leukemia. Hydroxyurea reduces thrombotic events in high-risk patients,[48] but does not alter transformation to myelofibrosis or leukemia. Splenomegaly occurs in one third to one half of patients with ET, and its presence may help to distinguish essential from secondary thrombocytosis. Splenectomy is not felt to be helpful in the early stages of ET, and is best reserved for the later stages of disease, in which myeloid metaplasia has developed.[47] Even in these circumstances, candidates should be chosen selectively, since significant bleeding has been reported to complicate splenectomy.

Polycythemia Vera

Polycythemia vera (PV) is a clonal, chronic, progressive myeloproliferative disorder characterized by an increase in red blood cell mass, frequently accompanied by leukocytosis, thrombocytosis, and splenomegaly. Patients affected by PV typically enjoy prolonged survival compared to others affected by hematologic malignancies, but remain at risk for transformation to myelofibrosis or AML. The disease is rare, with an annual incidence of 5 to 17 cases per million population.[49] Although the diagnosis may be discovered by routine screening laboratory tests in asymptomatic individuals, affected patients may present with any number of nonspecific complaints, including headache, dizziness, weakness, pruritus, visual disturbances, excessive sweating, joint symptoms, and weight loss.[50] Physical findings include ruddy cyanosis, conjunctival plethora, hepatomegaly, splenomegaly, and hypertension. The diagnosis is established by an elevated red blood cell mass ($>25\%$ of mean predicted value), thrombocytosis, leukocytosis, normal arterial oxygen saturation in the presence of increased red blood cell mass, splenomegaly, low serum erythropoietin (EPO) stores, and bone marrow hypercellularity.[50] Treatment should be tailored to the risk status of the patient and ranges from phlebotomy and aspirin to chemotherapeutic agents. As in ET, splenectomy is not helpful in the early stages of disease and is best reserved for late-stage patients in whom myeloid metaplasia has developed and splenomegaly-related symptoms are severe.[44]

Myelofibrosis (Agnogenic Myeloid Metaplasia)

The term *myelofibrosis* may be used to describe either the generic condition of fibrosis of the bone marrow (which may be associated with a number of benign and malignant disorders) or a specific, chronic, malignant hematologic disease associated with splenomegaly, red blood cell and white blood cell progenitors in the bloodstream, marrow fibrosis, and extramedullary hematopoiesis,

otherwise known as agnogenic myeloid metaplasia (AMM). AMM also can be referred to as myelosclerosis, idiopathic myeloid metaplasia, and osteosclerosis. Use of the term *myelofibrosis* in this chapter will be synonymous with AMM.

In AMM fibrosis of the bone marrow is believed to be a response to a clonal proliferation of hematopoietic stem cells. Marrow failure often ensues, but whether this failure is secondary to the fibrosis itself or to the malignant proliferation of cells is unknown.[50] The true incidence of AMM is unknown due to scant epidemiologic data, but one study from Minnesota estimated its incidence at 1.33 per 100,000 population in the United States.[51] Excessive radiation may play a role in the development of AMM, as persons within a 10,000-meter area of the atomic blasts in Japan, as well as those with a history of Thoratrast exposure, have been shown to exhibit a higher incidence of AMM.

Clinical manifestations of AMM most frequently relate to anemia, including fatigue, weakness, dyspnea on exertion, and palpitations. About 20% of patients, however, are asymptomatic and seek medical attention because of an enlarged spleen on physical exam or an abnormal blood smear.[50] Other clinical manifestations of AMM include bleeding, fever, weight loss, gout/renal stones, night sweats, and symptoms due to an enlarged spleen. Nearly all patients with AMM have splenomegaly, and two thirds have hepatomegaly, whereas 35% of patients have massive splenomegaly.[50]

The diagnosis is made by a careful examination of the peripheral blood smear and bone marrow. Nucleated red blood cells and immature myeloid elements in the blood are present in 96% of cases and strongly suggest the diagnosis. Teardrop poikilocytosis is another frequent finding. Care must be taken, however, to exclude a history of a primary neoplasm (such as lymphoma or adenocarcinoma of the stomach, lung, prostate, or breast) or tuberculosis, since patients with these conditions may develop secondary myelofibrosis.

Treatment depends on symptoms: asymptomatic patients are closely followed, while symptomatic patients undergo therapeutic intervention targeted toward their symptoms.[52] Splenomegaly-related symptoms are best treated with splenectomy. Although some chemotherapeutic agents (busulfan, hydroxyurea, interferon-alpha) and low-dose radiation can reduce splenic size, their discontinuation usually results in rapid splenic regrowth.

A thorough preoperative workup must precede splenectomy in patients with AMM. The candidate must possess acceptable cardiac, pulmonary, hepatic, and renal reserve for the operation. The coagulation system should be examined, including tests of coagulation factors V and VIII, fibrin split products, platelet count, and bleeding time. Low platelet counts may require adrenal steroids and/or platelet transfusion at the time of surgery. Splenectomy imparts durable, effective palliation for nearly all patients with AMM, though postoperative complications are more common in patients with AMM than in those with other hematologic indications.[6] In one series of splenectomies for patients with myeloid metaplasia with myelofibrosis, the most common complications were pneumonia and other bacterial infections (42%), cardiac events (19%), acute bleeding (15%), ileus (15%), and venous thrombosis (12%).[53]

White Blood Cell Disorders

Leukemias

Chronic Lymphocytic Leukemia (CLL). Chronic lymphocytic leukemia and hairy cell leukemia (HCL) are the two leukemias most amenable to treatment by splenectomy. The main characteristic of CLL is a progressive accumulation of long-lived but nonfunctional lymphocytes. Symptoms of CLL are nonspecific and include weakness, fatigue, fever without illness, night sweats, and frequent bacterial and viral infections. The most frequent finding is lymphadenopathy. Splenomegaly, when it occurs, may be massive or barely palpable below the costal margin. Splenectomy is indicated to improve cytopenias, and has been shown to be 75% effective in this regard in a combined group of patients with both CLL and nonmalignant Hodgkin's disease.[54] Splenectomy may thus facilitate chemotherapy in patients whose cell counts were prohibitively low prior to spleen removal. Palliative splenectomy also is indicated for symptomatic splenomegaly.

Hairy Cell Leukemia (HCL). Hairy cell leukemia is an uncommon blood disorder, representing only 2% of all adult leukemias. HCL is characterized by splenomegaly, pancytopenia, and large numbers of abnormal lymphocytes in the bone marrow. These lymphocytes contain irregular hair-like cytoplasmic projections identifiable on the peripheral smear. Most patients seek medical attention because of symptoms related to anemia, neutropenia, thrombocytopenia, or splenomegaly.[55] The most common physical finding is splenomegaly, which occurs in 80% of patients with HCL and is often palpable 5 cm below the costal margin. Many patients with HCL have few symptoms and require no specific therapy. Treatment is indicated for those with moderate to severe symptoms related to cytopenias, such as repeated infections or bleeding episodes, or to splenomegaly, such as pain or early satiety. Splenectomy does not correct the underlying disorder, but does return cell counts to normal in 40 to 70% of patients and alleviates pain and early satiety.[56,57] Newer chemotherapeutic agents (the purine analogues 2'-deoxycoformycin [2'-DCF] and 2-chlorodeoxyadenosine [2-CdA]) are able to induce durable complete remission in most patients.[58]

Lymphomas

Non-Hodgkin's Lymphoma (NHL). NHL encompasses all malignancies derived from the lymphoid system except classic Hodgkin's disease. NHL occurs in approximately 50,000 people annually in the United States, accounting for about 4% of all cancers.[59] A proliferation of any one of the three predominant lymph cell types—natural killer cells, T cells, or B cells—may be included in NHL. Because of the wide net cast by NHL, the clinical presentations of the disorders under its umbrella vary. The subentities of NHL may be clinically classified into nodal or extranodal, as well as indolent, aggressive, and very aggressive groups. Patients with indolent lymphomas may present with mild or no symptoms and seek medical attention for a swollen lymph node, whereas the aggressive and very aggressive lymphomas create easily noticeable symptoms, such as pain, swelling due to obstruction of vessels, fever, and night sweats. Surgical staging is no longer indicated for NHL, as the combination of history and physical examination, chest radiograph and abdominal/pelvic CT scan, biopsy of involved lymph nodes (including laparoscopically directed nodal and liver biopsies), and bone marrow biopsy is sufficient.[6] Splenomegaly exists in various, but not all, forms of NHL, and splenectomy is indicated for symptoms related to an enlarged spleen as well as to improve cytopenias.

Hodgkin's Disease (HD). HD is a disorder of the lymphoid system characterized by the presence of Reed-Sternberg cells, which actually form the minority of the Hodgkin's tumor. About 7500 new cases of HD are diagnosed annually in the United States, most commonly in men between the ages of 26 and 31.[60] More than 90% of patients with HD present with lymphadenopathy above the diaphragm.

Lymph nodes can become particularly bulky in the mediastinum, which may result in shortness of breath, cough, or obstructive pneumonia. Lymphadenopathy below the diaphragm is rare on presentation but can arise with disease progression. The spleen is often an occult site of spread, but massive splenomegaly is not common. In addition, large spleens do not necessarily signify involvement.

Four major histologic types exist: lymphocyte predominant, nodular sclerosis, mixed cellularity, and lymphocyte deplete. These histologic types, along with location of disease and symptomatology, influence survival for patients with HD. Stage I disease is limited to one anatomic region; stage II disease is defined by two or more contiguous or noncontiguous regions on the same side of the diaphragm; stage III disease involves disease on both sides of the diaphragm, but limited to lymph nodes, spleen, and Waldeyer's ring (the ring of lymphoid tissue formed by the lingual, palatine, and nasopharyngeal tonsils); and stage IV disease signifies involvement of the bone marrow, lung, liver, skin, gastrointestinal tract, and any organ or tissue other than the lymph nodes or Waldeyer's ring.[22]

The staging procedure for HD begins with a wedge biopsy of the liver, splenectomy, and the removal of representative nodes in the retroperitoneum, mesentery, and hepatoduodenal ligament. Staging for HD may be performed laparoscopically.[61] A laparoscopic core biopsy of the liver is performed under direct visualization, either using a Tru-cut needle percutaneously or by wedge resection with shears and cautery. Finally, an iliac marrow biopsy is generally included. In contrast to NHL outcomes, studies have concluded that surgical staging has altered clinical staging in as many as 42% of cases (26 to 37% upgraded, 7 to 15% downgraded).[6] Refinements of CT scanning and the more liberal use of chemotherapy for patients with HD have significantly reduced the indications for surgical staging of the disease. Current indications for surgical staging include clinical stage I or stage II with nodular sclerosing histology and no symptoms referable to HD.[6] Staging information affects treatment, as early-stage patients who have no splenic involvement may be candidates for radiotherapy alone. Those with splenic involvement generally require chemotherapy or multimodality therapy.

Platelet Disorders

Idiopathic Thrombocytopenic Purpura (ITP)

ITP, also called immune thrombocytopenic purpura, is an autoimmune disorder characterized by a low platelet count and mucocutaneous and petechial bleeding. The low platelet count stems from premature removal of platelets opsonized by antiplatelet IgG autoantibodies produced in the spleen. This clearance occurs through the interaction of platelet autoantibodies with Fc receptors expressed on tissue macrophages, predominantly in the spleen and liver. The estimated incidence of ITP is 100 persons per million annually, about one half of whom are children.[62] In adults, women are affected two to three times more often than men, whereas in children the sexes are affected equally.[63] Adult-onset and childhood-onset ITP are strikingly different in their clinical course and management.

Patients with ITP typically present with petechiae or ecchymoses, though some will experience major bleeding from the outset. Bleeding may occur from mucosal surfaces in the form of gingival bleeding, epistaxis, menorrhagia, hematuria, or even melena. The severity of bleeding frequently corresponds to the deficiency in platelets: patients with counts above 50,000/mm³ usually present with incidental findings; those with counts between 30,000 and 50,000/mm³ often have easy bruising; those with platelet counts between 10,000 and 30,000/mm³ may develop spontaneous petechiae or ecchymoses; and those with counts below 10,000/mm³ are at risk for internal bleeding.[62] The incidence of major intracranial hemorrhage is about 1%, usually occurring early in the disease course. The duration of the bleeding helps to distinguish acute from chronic forms of ITP. Children often present at a young age (peak age approximately 5 years) with sudden onset of petechiae or purpura several days to weeks after an infectious illness. In contrast, adults experience a more chronic form of disease with an insidious onset. Splenomegaly with ITP is uncommon in both adults and children, and its occurrence should prompt a search for a separate cause of thrombocytopenia. Up to 10% of children, however, will have a palpable spleen tip.[62]

Diagnosing ITP is based on exclusion of other possibilities in the presence of a low platelet count and mucocutaneous bleeding. Other diseases resulting in secondary forms of immune thrombocytopenic purpura, such as systemic lupus erythematosus, the antiphospholipid syndrome, lymphoproliferative disorders, HIV, and hepatitis C should be identified and treated when present. Additionally, a history of drug use known to cause thrombocytopenia, such as certain antimicrobials, anti-inflammatories, antihypertensives, and antidepressants, should be obtained. In addition to low platelets, laboratory findings characteristic of ITP consist of large, immature platelets (megathrombocytes) on peripheral blood smear. The bone marrow aspirate, when obtained, shows normal or increased megakaryocytes, characterized by degranulation and vacuolization of the cytoplasm. The indications for bone marrow aspiration are controversial; patients less than 60 years of age with typical presentations generally do not require it, but atypical cases or children about to receive corticosteroids are candidates. Platelet-associated antibody assays have been developed, but their appropriate place in the diagnostic workup is still being defined.

Adults generally require treatment at the time of presentation, since up to one half will present with counts below 10,000/mm^3.[64] The usual first line of therapy is oral prednisone at a dose of 1.0 to 1.5 mg/kg per day.[62] No consensus exists as to the optimal duration of steroid therapy, but most responses occur within the first 3 weeks. Response rates range from 50 to 75%, but relapses are common. Intravenous immunoglobulin, given at 1.0 g/kg per day for 2 to 3 days, is indicated for internal bleeding when counts remain below 5000/mm^3 or when extensive purpura exists.[62,64] Intravenous immunoglobulin is thought to impair clearance of IgG-coated platelets by competing for binding to tissue macrophage receptors.[65] An immediate response is common, but a sustained remission is not.[66] Splenectomy is indicated for failure of medical therapy, for prolonged use of steroids with undesirable effects, or for most cases of first relapse.[6] Prolonged use of steroids can be defined in various ways, but a persistent need for more than 10 to 20 mg/d for 3 to 6 months in order to maintain a platelet count above 30,000/mm^3 generally prompts referral for splenectomy.[62] Splenectomy provides a permanent response without subsequent need for steroids in 75 to 85% of the total number of patients undergoing splenectomy (see the "Splenectomy Outcomes" section of this chapter). Responses usually occur within the first postoperative week. Patients with extremely low platelet counts (<10,000/mm^3) should have platelets available for surgery, but should not receive them preoperatively. Once the splenic pedicle is ligated, platelets are given to those who continue to bleed.

In children with ITP, the course is self-limited, with durable and complete remission in over 70% of patients regardless of therapy. Because of the good prognosis without treatment, the decision to intervene is controversial and is largely pursued based on the fear of intracranial hemorrhage and untoward limitations on physical activity. The actual risk of intracranial hemorrhage is about 1%,

and it nearly always occurs in the setting of a platelet count below 20,000 mm^3.[67] Therefore children with typical ITP—and certainly those without hemorrhage—are managed principally by observation, with short-term therapy in select cases. Where therapy is indicated, intravenous immune globulin has been shown to shorten the duration of severe thrombocytopenia, and a short course of oral prednisone (4 mg/kg for 4 consecutive days) generally produces excellent results.[68] Splenectomy is reserved for failure of medical therapy in children who have had immune thrombocytopenic purpura for at least 1 year with symptomatic, severe thrombocytopenia. Urgent splenectomy may play a role in the rare circumstance of severe, life-threatening bleeding, in conjunction with aggressive medical therapy, for both children and adults.

Thrombotic Thrombocytopenic Purpura (TTP)

TTP is a serious disorder characterized by thrombocytopenia, microangiopathic hemolytic anemia, and neurologic complications. Abnormal platelet clumping occurs in arterioles and capillaries, reducing the lumen of these vessels and predisposing the patient to microvascular thrombotic episodes. The reduced lumen size also causes shearing stresses on erythrocytes, leading to deformed red blood cells subject to hemolysis. One aspect of hemolysis may be due to sequestration and destruction of erythrocytes in the spleen. Recent work has demonstrated that the underlying abnormality is likely related to the persistence of unusually large multimers of von Willebrand factor associated with platelet clumping in the patient's blood.[69]

TTP is a rare disorder, occurring in about 3.7 individuals per million,[70] but its dramatic clinical sequelae and favorable response to early therapy demand an understanding of its clinical presentation to bring about an early diagnosis. Clinical features of the disorder include petechiae, fever, neurologic symptoms, renal failure, and infrequently cardiac symptoms, such as heart failure or arrhythmias. Petechial hemorrhages in the lower extremities are the most common presenting sign. Along with fever, patients may experience flu-like symptoms, malaise, or fatigue. Neurologic changes range from generalized headaches to altered mental status, seizures, and even coma. Generally, however, the mere presence of petechiae and thrombocytopenia are sufficient to lead to the diagnosis of TTP and consideration of treatment.

The diagnosis is confirmed by the peripheral blood smear, which shows schistocytes, nucleated red blood cells, and basophilic stippling. Although other conditions such as tight aortic stenosis or prosthetic valves may result in schistocytes, these conditions are not generally accompanied by thrombocytopenia. TTP may be distinguished from autoimmune causes of thrombocytopenia, such as Evans syndrome (ITP and autoimmune hemolytic anemia) or systemic lupus erythematosus, by a negative Coombs' test.[69]

The first line of therapy for TTP is plasma exchange. This treatment has dramatically improved survival from less than 10% to about 90% since its implementation.[71] Plasma exchange consists of the daily removal of a single volume of the patient's plasma and its replacement with fresh-frozen plasma (FFP) until the correction of thrombocytopenia, anemia, and associated symptoms takes place. Therapy is then tapered over 1 to 2 weeks.[69] Splenectomy plays a key role for patients who relapse or require multiple plasma exchanges to control symptoms, and is generally well tolerated without significant morbidity.[72] Once the spleen is removed, patients typically do not relapse.[73] Platelet transfusions are not recommended in TTP, as severe clinical deterioration has been reported following their administration.[74]

Miscellaneous Disorders and Lesions

Infections and Abscesses

Abscesses of the spleen are uncommon, with an incidence of 0.14 to 0.7%, based on autopsy findings.[75] They occur more frequently in tropical locations, where they are associated with thrombosed splenic vessels and infarction in patients with sickle cell anemia. Five distinct mechanisms of splenic abscess formation have been described: (1) hematogenous infection; (2) contiguous infection; (3) hemoglobinopathy; (4) immunosuppression, including HIV and chemotherapy; and (5) trauma. The most common origins for hematogenous spread are infective endocarditis, typhoid fever, malaria, urinary tract infections, and osteomyelitis.[76] Presentation is frequently delayed, with most patients enduring symptoms for 16 to 22 days prior to diagnosis. Clinical manifestations include fever, left upper quadrant pain, leukocytosis, and splenomegaly in about one third of patients. The diagnosis is confirmed by ultrasound or CT scan, which has a 95% sensitivity and specificity. Upon discovery of a splenic abscess, broad-spectrum antibiotics should be started, with adjustment to more specific therapy based on culture results, and continued for 14 days. Splenectomy is the operation of choice, but percutaneous or open drainage are options for patients who cannot tolerate splenectomy.[6] Percutaneous drainage is successful for patients with unilocular disease.

Storage Diseases and Infiltrative Disorders

Gaucher's Disease. This is an inherited lipid storage disease characterized by the deposition of glucocerebroside in cells of the macrophage-monocyte system. The underlying abnormality is a deficiency in the activity of a lysosomal hydrolase. Abnormal glycolipid storage results in organomegaly, particularly hepato- and splenomegaly.[77] Patients with Gaucher's disease frequently experience symptoms related to splenomegaly—including early satiety and abdominal discomfort—and hypersplenism, including thrombocytopenia, normocytic anemia, and mild leukopenia. These latter findings occur as a result of excessive sequestration of formed blood elements in the spleen. Other symptoms in patients with Gaucher's disease include bone pain, pathologic fractures, and jaundice. Splenectomy alleviates hematologic abnormalities in patients with hypersplenism, but it does not correct the underlying disease process. Partial splenectomy has been shown to be effective in children to correct both hematologic problems and symptoms due to splenomegaly, without incurring the risk of overwhelming postsplenectomy sepsis. Children treated with partial splenectomy or splenectomy respond with improved growth rates.[78]

Niemann-Pick Disease. This is an inherited disease of abnormal lysosomal storage of sphingomyelin and cholesterol in cells of the macrophage-monocyte system. Four types of the disease (A, B, C, and D) exist, with unique clinical presentations. Types A and B result from a deficiency in lysosomal hydrolase, and are the forms most likely to demonstrate splenomegaly with its concomitant symptoms. Splenectomy has been reported to successfully treat symptoms of splenomegaly in these cases.[79]

Amyloidosis. Amyloidosis is a disorder of abnormal extracellular protein deposition. There are multiple forms of amyloidosis, each with its own individual clinical presentation, and the severity of disease may range from asymptomatic to multiorgan failure. Patients with primary amyloidosis, associated with plasma cell dyscrasia, have splenic involvement in about 5% of cases. Secondary amyloidosis, associated with chronic inflammatory conditions, also

may present with an enlarged spleen. Symptoms of splenomegaly are relieved by splenectomy. Removal of the spleen also has been reported to cure patients of factor X deficiency associated with primary amyloidosis.[80]

Felty's Syndrome

The triad of rheumatoid arthritis (RA), splenomegaly, and neutropenia is called *Felty's syndrome*. It exists in approximately 3% of all patients with RA, two thirds of which are women. Immune complexes coat the surface of white blood cells, leading to their sequestration and clearance in the spleen with subsequent neutropenia. This neutropenia ($<2000/mm^3$) increases the risk for recurrent infections and often drives the decision for splenectomy. The size of the spleen is variable, from nonpalpable in 5 to 10% of patients, to massive enlargement in others. The spleen in Felty's syndrome is four times heavier than normal. Corticosteroids, hematopoietic growth factors, methotrexate, and splenectomy have all been used to treat the neutropenia of Felty's syndrome. Responses to splenectomy have been excellent, with over 80% of patients showing a durable increase in white blood cell count. More than one half of patients who had infections prior to surgery did not have any infections after splenectomy.[81] Besides symptomatic neutropenia, other indications for splenectomy include transfusion-dependent anemia and profound thrombocytopenia.

Sarcoidosis

Sarcoidosis is an inflammatory disease of young adults, characterized by noncaseating granulomas in affected tissues. Signs and symptoms of the disease range in severity and typically are nonspecific, such as fatigue and malaise. Any organ system may be involved. The most commonly involved organ is the lung, followed by the spleen. Splenomegaly occurs in about 25% of patients. Massive splenomegaly (>1 kg) is rare.[82] Other affected areas include the lymph nodes, eyes, joints, liver, spleen, and heart. When splenomegaly occurs and causes symptoms related to size or hypersplenism, splenectomy effectively relieves symptoms and corrects hematologic abnormalities such as anemia and thrombocytopenia. Spontaneous splenic rupture has been reported in sarcoidosis.[83]

Cysts and Tumors

Splenic cysts are rare lesions. The most common etiology for splenic cysts worldwide is parasitic infestation, particularly echinococcal. Symptomatic parasitic cysts are best treated with splenectomy, though selected cases may be amenable to percutaneous aspiration, instillation of protoscolicidal agent, and reaspiration.[84] Nonparasitic cysts most commonly result from trauma and are called pseudocysts; however, dermoid, epidermoid, and epithelial cysts have been reported as well.[85,86] The treatment of nonparasitic cysts depends on whether or not they produce symptoms. Asymptomatic nonparasitic cysts may be observed with close ultrasound follow-up to exclude significant expansion. Patients should be advised of the risk of cyst rupture with even minor abdominal trauma if they elect nonoperative management for large cysts. Small symptomatic nonparasitic cysts may be excised with splenic preservation, and large symptomatic nonparasitic cysts may be unroofed. Both of these operations may be performed laparoscopically.[87]

Splenic cysts and lymphomas have similar anechoic appearances on ultrasound. However, an indistinct boundary is more typical of lymphoma and helps to distinguish between the two lesions.[88]

The most common primary tumor of the spleen is sarcomatous. Non-Hodgkin's lymphoma of the spleen is rare, but splenectomy imparts an excellent prognosis. Autopsy studies reveal an approximate 0.6% rate of tumor metastasis to the spleen, most of which are carcinomas.[89] Lung cancer is the most common tumor to spread to the spleen.

Portal Hypertension

Portal hypertension can result from numerous causes, but is usually due to cirrhosis. Splenomegaly and splenic congestion often accompany portal hypertension, resulting in sequestration and destruction of circulating cells in the spleen. Splenectomy, however, is not indicated for hypersplenism per se in patients with portal hypertension, since no correlation exists between the degree of pancytopenia and long-term survival in these patients.[6] In rare circumstances, in which splenectomy is required to reduce bleeding from esophageal varices exacerbated by thrombocytopenia, a concomitant splenorenal shunt should be performed to decompress the portal system.[6]

Portal hypertension secondary to splenic vein thrombosis is potentially curable with splenectomy. Patients with bleeding from isolated gastric varices in the presence of normal liver function tests, especially with a history of pancreatic disease, should be examined for splenic vein thrombosis and treated with splenectomy if positive.[90]

Splenic Artery Aneurysm

Although rare, splenic artery aneurysm (SAA) is the most common visceral artery aneurysm. Women are four times more likely to be affected than men. The aneurysm usually arises in the middle to distal portion of the splenic artery. The risk of rupture is between 3 and 9%; however, once rupture occurs, mortality is substantial (35 to 50%).[91] According to a recent series, mortality is significantly higher in patients with underlying portal hypertension (>50%) than in those without it (17%).[92] SAA is particularly worrisome when discovered during pregnancy, as rupture imparts a high risk of mortality to both mother (70%) and fetus (95%).[93] Most patients are asymptomatic and seek medical attention based on an incidental radiographic finding. About 20% of patients with SAA have symptoms of left upper quadrant pain.[94] Indications for treatment include presence of symptoms, pregnancy, intention to become pregnant, and pseudoaneurysms associated with inflammatory processes. For asymptomatic patients, size greater than 2 cm constitutes an indication for surgery.[91] Aneurysm resection or ligation alone is acceptable for amenable lesions in the mid-splenic artery, but distal lesions in close proximity to the splenic hilum should be treated with concomitant splenectomy. An excellent prognosis follows elective treatment. Splenic artery embolization has been used to treat SAA, but painful splenic infarction and abscess may follow.

PREOPERATIVE CONSIDERATIONS

Splenic Artery Embolization

The use of splenic artery embolization (SAE) as a preoperative technique became available with advances in angiographic technology. In the prelaparoscopic era, some surgeons recommended preoperative SAE for patients with complicated disease, such as massive splenomegaly, previous pancreatitis, gastric or pancreatic surgery, portal hypertension, varices, or uncorrectable thrombocytopenia.[94,95] Theoretical advantages of SAE include reduced operative blood loss from a devascularized spleen and reduced spleen size for easier dissection and removal. Potential disadvantages of the procedure, however, include acute left-sided pain (though usually of limited duration), pancreatitis, or other embolization-related complications.[96] Early in the laparoscopic era,

some authors recommended the use of SAE routinely for patients undergoing the laparoscopic approach, subsequently revising their recommendation to include patients with spleens larger than 20 cm.[98] Other reports have highlighted the utility of SAE in cases of portal hypertension followed by laparoscopic splenectomy.[99] The difficulty of left-sided pain resulting from embolization can be mitigated by performing the procedure under general anesthesia and immediately transporting the patient to the operating room for splenectomy.[100] Not all investigators use or recommend SAE, citing equivalent splenectomy-related blood loss and morbidity.[101] There is currently no consensus on the role of preoperative SAE for elective splenectomy.

Vaccination

Splenectomy imparts a small (<1 to 5%) but definite life-time risk of fulminant, potentially life-threatening infection (see section on "Overwhelming Postsplenectomy Infections" under "Splenectomy Outcomes" for further discussion on risk of infection). Therefore, when elective splenectomy is planned, vaccinations against encapsulated bacteria should be given at least 2 weeks before surgery to protect against such infection. The most common bacteria to cause serious infections in asplenic hosts are *Streptococcus pneumoniae*, *Haemophilus influenzae* type B, and meningococcus. Vaccinations are available for these bacteria and should be given. Other potential infectious bacterial sources include group A streptococci, *Capnocytophaga canimorsus* (related to dog bites), group B streptococci, *Enterococcus* species, *Bacteroides* species, *Salmonella* species, and *Bartonella* species.[102]

If the spleen is removed emergently (e.g., for trauma), vaccinations should be given as soon as possible following surgery, allowing at least 1 to 2 days for recovery. Booster injections of pneumococcal vaccine should be considered every 5 to 6 years regardless of the reason for splenectomy. In addition, annual influenza immunization is advisable. Splenectomized patients should maintain ongoing documentation and communication of immunization status.[103]

Deep Venous Thrombosis Prophylaxis

Deep venous thrombosis (DVT) is not uncommon following splenectomy, especially in cases involving splenomegaly and myeloproliferative disorders (MPD).[104] The risk of portal vein thrombosis (PVT) may be as high as 40% for patients with both splenomegaly and MPD. Postsplenectomy PVT typically presents with anorexia, abdominal pain, leukocytosis, and thrombocytosis. A high index of suspicion, early diagnosis with contrast-enhanced CT, and immediate anticoagulation are keys to successful treatment for PVT. Patients undergoing splenectomy should be treated with DVT prophylaxis, including sequential compression devices with subcutaneous heparin (5000 U).[105] No clear advantage for the use of low molecular weight heparin (LMWH) over low-dose unfractionated heparin has been established for the prevention of venous thromboembolism (VTE) for splenectomy.[106] Each patient's risk factors for DVT should be evaluated, and where elevated risk exists (obesity, history of prior VTE, known hypercoagulable state, age >60), a more aggressive antithrombotic regimen, including LMWH, may be pursued.

SPLENECTOMY TECHNIQUES

Patient Preparation

All patients undergoing elective splenectomy should be vaccinated at least 1 week preoperatively with polyvalent pneumococcal, meningococcal, and *Haemophilus* vaccines. Patients' potential need for transfusion of blood products must be assessed, and their preoperative coagulation status optimized. It is the authors' practice to type and screen normosplenic patients undergoing elective splenectomy. Anemic patients should be transfused to a hemoglobin of 10 g/dL prior to surgery. For more complex patients, including those with splenomegaly, at least 2 to 4 units of cross-matched blood should be available at the time of surgery. Thrombocytopenia may be transiently corrected with platelet transfusions. However, it is preferable that thrombocytopenic patients not be transfused prior to the day of surgery, and ideally not before the splenic artery has been ligated intraoperatively.

Patients who have been maintained on corticosteroid therapy preoperatively should receive parenteral corticosteroid therapy perioperatively. A bowel preparation is not routinely administered for patients undergoing elective splenectomy. All splenectomy patients do receive deep vein thrombosis (DVT) prophylaxis, as previously discussed. A first-generation cephalosporin is administered intravenously when the patient is brought to the operating room. After the patient has been endotracheally intubated, a nasogastric (NG) tube is inserted to decompress the stomach.

Open Splenectomy

Whereas laparoscopic surgery (LS) is increasingly accepted as the standard approach for normosplenic patients requiring splenectomy, open splenectomy (OS) is still widely practiced. The most common indication for OS remains traumatic rupture of the spleen. There are, however, several other clinical scenarios in which OS may be favored, such as in patients requiring splenectomy with massive splenomegaly, ascites, portal hypertension, multiple prior operations, extensive splenic radiation, or possible splenic abscess.

Open Splenectomy Technique

In preparation for OS, the patient is placed in the supine position. The surgeon is situated on the patient's right side. A midline incision is preferable for exposure of a ruptured or massively enlarged spleen or when abdominal access is needed for a staging laparotomy for Hodgkin's disease. Otherwise a left subcostal incision is preferred for most elective splenectomies. The incision parallels the left costal margin, lying two fingerbreadths below it. Rarely a thoracoabdominal incision may be required to gain access to a challenging or significantly enlarged spleen.

The spleen is mobilized by dividing ligamentous attachments, usually beginning with the splenocolic ligament (Fig. 33-4). For patients with significant splenomegaly it may be preferable to ligate the splenic artery in continuity along the superior border of the pancreas, once lesser sac access has been achieved either through the gastrosplenic or gastrohepatic attachments. This maneuver may serve several purposes: allowing for safer manipulation of the spleen and dissection of the splenic hilum, facilitating some shrinkage of the spleen, and providing an autotransfusion of erythrocytes and platelets. The spleen is further mobilized medially by incising its lateral peritoneal attachments, most notably the splenophrenic ligament. The short gastric vessels are then sequentially ligated and divided. Careful individual dissection and ligation of the short gastric vessels reduces the risk of their retraction and bleeding. Splenic hilar dissection follows. Whenever possible, care should be taken to dissect and individually ligate the splenic artery and vein (in that order) prior to dividing them. As noted in the previous discussion of splenic anatomy, the tail of the pancreas lies within 1 cm of the

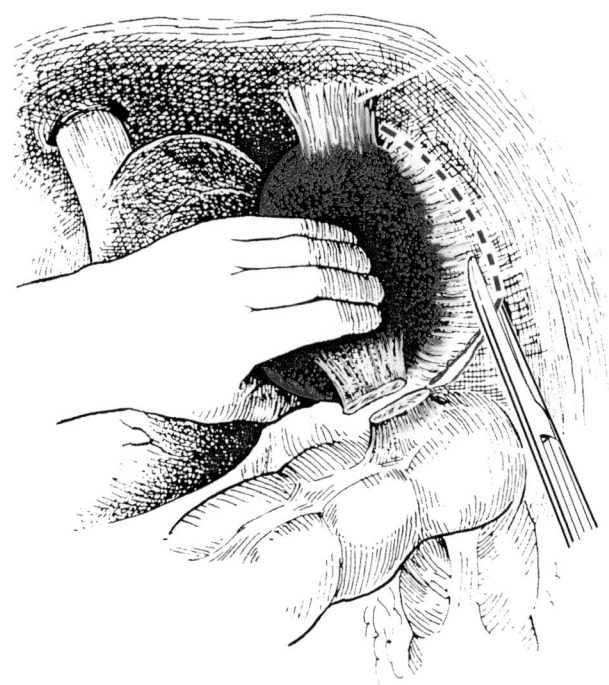

FIG. 33-4. The splenocolic ligament is divided at the beginning of open splenectomy.

splenic hilum in 75% of patients, therefore great care must be taken during hilar dissection to avoid injuring the pancreas.

Once the spleen is excised, the bed of dissection is irrigated, suctioned, and meticulously inspected to ensure hemostasis. The splenic bed is not routinely drained. When splenectomy has been performed for a hematologic disorder, a thorough search must be conducted for accessory spleens. The NG tube is removed at the completion of surgery in the operating room.

Laparoscopic Splenectomy

Since the mid-1990s LS has steadily supplanted OS as the approach of choice for most elective splenectomies. Initially case reports and thereafter large series of LS focused on its benefits to patients with normal-sized spleens. Subsequently a growing amount of literature has supported the role of LS, in appropriately expert and experienced hands, for patients with splenomegaly, multiple prior abdominal surgeries, morbid obesity, the need for concomitant procedures, or even pregnancy.

The earliest reports of LS detailed an anterior approach with the patient positioned supine or in the low lithotomy position on the operating table. Following the introduction of the lateral approach,[105] most LS procedures are now performed with the patient in the right lateral decubitus position (Fig. 33-5). Some authors advocate a midway "double access" technique in which the patient is in a 45 degree right lateral decubitus. This positioning facilitates the performance of concomitant surgery, such as laparoscopic cholecystectomy, more easily than with the lateral approach to LS. As with the anterior approach, the double access technique requires the placement of five or six trocars to perform LS. By contrast the lateral approach routinely involves the use of three or four trocars positioned as demonstrated in Fig. 33-5. An angled (30° or 45°) laparoscope (2 mm, 5 mm, or 10 mm) greatly facilitates the procedure. A further advantage of the lateral approach is exposure of the vital anatomy in a manner that

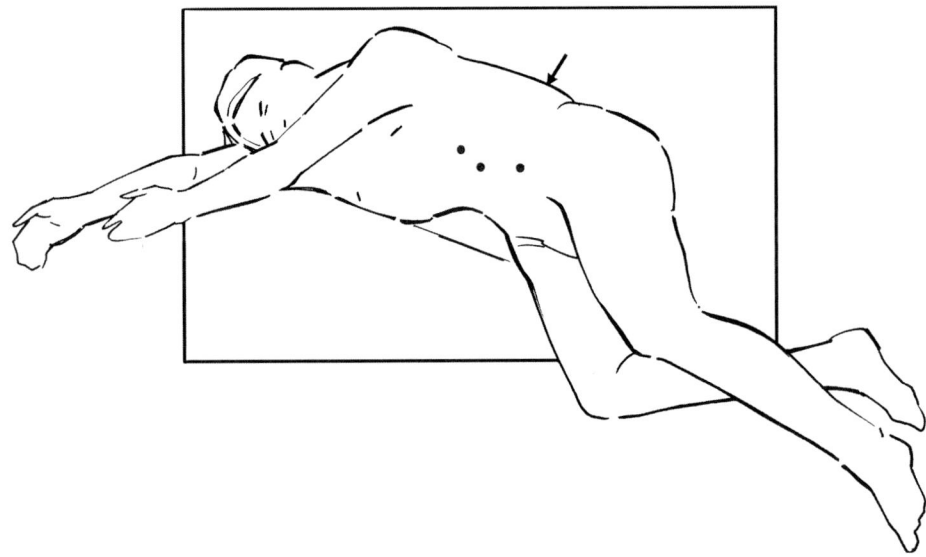

FIG. 33-5. Trocar positions for right lateral decubitus position in preparation for laparoscopic splenectomy.

allows for a more intuitive sequence of dissection, paralleling that of OS.

As with OS, the splenocolic ligament is divided, as are the lateral peritoneal attachments (Fig. 33-6), resulting in medial mobilization of the spleen. The short gastric vessels are divided by individual application of clips, the use of endovascular stapling cartridges, or more commonly by the use of hemostatic energy sources, such as ultrasonic dissection, diathermy, or radio frequency ablation. With the lower pole of the spleen gently retracted, the splenic hilum is then accessible to further applications of clips or an endovascular stapling device (Figs. 33-7 and 33-8). When possible, the splenic artery and vein are divided separately. However, mass hilar stapling is increasingly practiced with good long-term outcomes. Using the lateral approach with the spleen thus elevated, the surgeon easily visualizes the tail of the pancreas and avoids injury when placing the endovascular stapler.

Once excised, the spleen is placed in a durable nylon sac (Fig. 33-9), the neck of which is drawn through one of the 10-mm trocar sites (Fig. 33-10). The spleen is morcellated within the sac and extracted piecemeal; a blunt instrument should be used to disrupt and remove the spleen to avoid the risk of sac rupture, spillage of contents, and subsequent splenosis.

Hand-assisted LS has been suggested as a means by which LS can be more safely and expeditiously performed, particularly in patients with splenomegaly. Using this technique, the surgeon's left

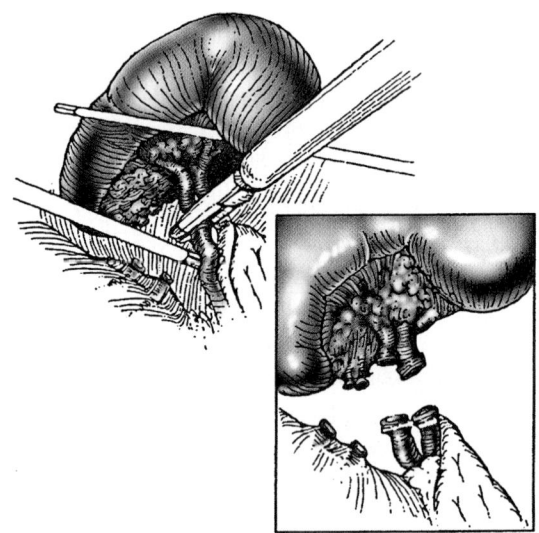

FIG. 33-7. Splenic artery and vein isolated and separately ligated and divided. (*Reprinted with permission from Park A, et al: Laparoscopic vs. open splenectomy. Arch Surg 134:1266, 1999.*)

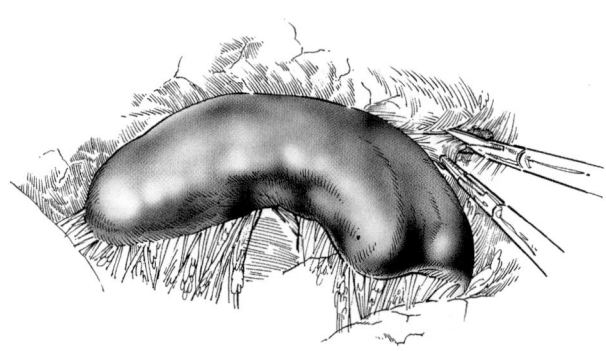

FIG. 33-6. Dividing the lateral peritoneal attachments.

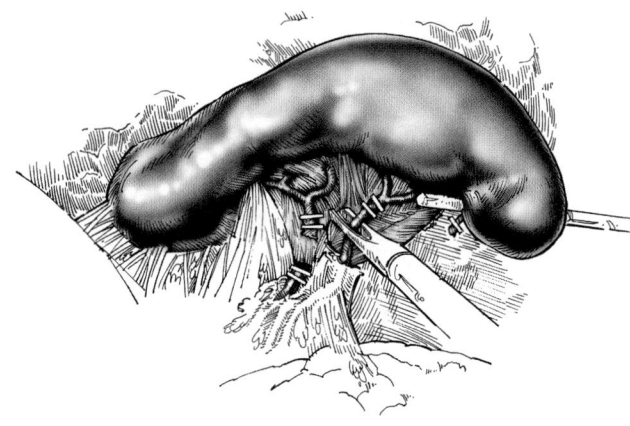

FIG. 33-8. Clipping the splenic hilum. When possible, the splenic artery and vein are divided separately.

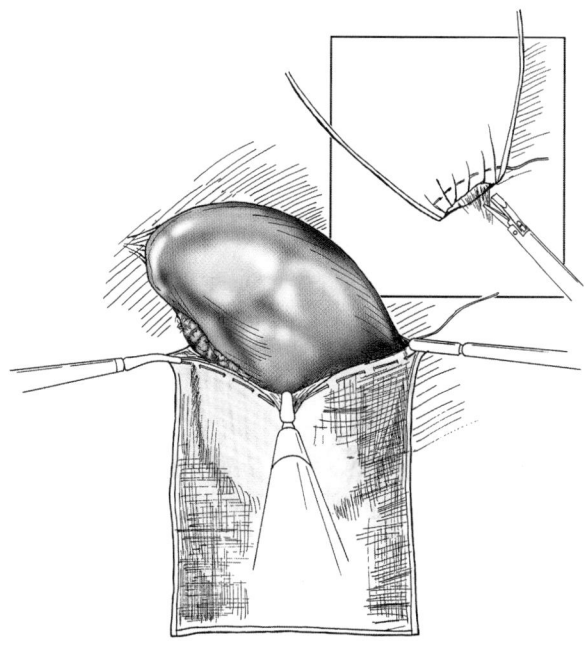

FIG. 33-9. *Enclosing the excised spleen in a nylon sac.*

hand is completely introduced into the peritoneal cavity (left-handed surgeons would insert their right hands). This maneuver allows for identification, retraction, and dissection of appropriate tissues by palpation under direct laparoscopic visualization. Clips, staples, and energy sources similar to those described previously are used to achieve hemostasis. The hand-access port is used to deliver the excised specimen. For removal of normal-sized spleens, the size of the incision required to admit the surgeon's hand may mitigate the advantages of this approach.

Partial Splenectomy

First reported in the early eighteenth century, the technique of partial splenectomy has been advocated and practiced more widely over the past few decades. It is particularly indicated in children, where possible, to minimize the risk of postsplenectomy sepsis. Certain lipid storage disorders leading to splenomegaly (e.g., Gaucher's disease) and some forms of traumatic (blunt and penetrating) splenic injury

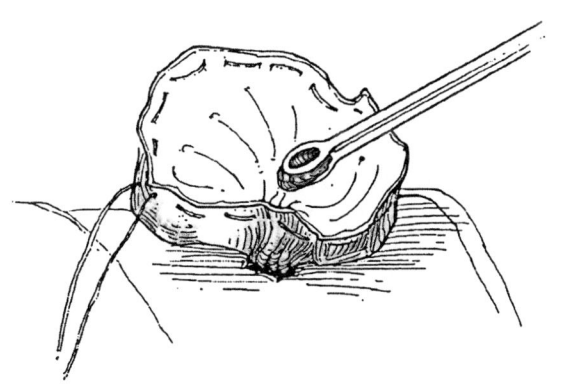

FIG. 33-10. *Morcellation and extraction of the spleen with the nylon sac extending through the 10-mm trocar site. (Reprinted with permission from Park A, et al: Laparoscopic vs. open splenectomy. Arch Surg 134:1266, 1999.)*

are amenable to partial splenectomy. The technique has been well described via an open approach as well as laparoscopically. The spleen must be adequately mobilized. Splenic hilar vessels attached to the targeted segment are ligated and divided. The devascularized segment of spleen is transected along an obvious line of demarcation. Bleeding from the cut surface of the spleen is usually limited and can be controlled by cauterization, argon coagulation, or application of direct hemostatic agents such as cellulose gauze and fibrin glue.

SPLENECTOMY OUTCOMES

Splenectomy results in characteristic changes to blood composition, including the appearance of Howell-Jolly bodies and siderocytes. Leukocytosis and increased platelet counts commonly occur following splenectomy as well. In patients with preoperative thrombocytopenia, platelet counts usually rise within 2 days, but may not peak for several weeks (see the "Hematologic Outcomes" section of this chapter). Similarly, the white blood cell count typically rises within 1 day after splenectomy, but may remain elevated for up to several months.

Complications

Complications of splenectomy may be classified as pulmonary, hemorrhagic, infectious, pancreatic, and thromboembolic. The most common complication is left lower lobe atelectasis, occurring in up to 16% of patients following OS.[107] Other pulmonary problems include pleural effusion and pneumonia, occurring in up to 10% of open splenectomy cases.[107] Hemorrhage usually occurs intraoperatively where it can be immediately addressed, but it occasionally presents as a subphrenic hematoma postoperatively. Transfusions have become less common with the advent of LS and depend on the indication for splenectomy. Across all elective indications, the need for transfusion arises in about 3 to 5% of cases.[3,107,108] Infectious complications include subphrenic abscess and wound infection. The placement of a drain in the left upper quadrant may be associated with postoperative subphrenic abscess and is therefore not routinely recommended. Pancreatic complications, including pancreatitis, pseudocyst, and pancreatic fistula, may result from intraoperative trauma to the pancreas, especially to the tail, during the dissection of the splenic hilum. Thromboembolic phenomena occur in 5 to 10% of patients undergoing splenectomy, and DVT prophylaxis is recommended routinely.[107] For patients with hemolytic anemia or myeloproliferative disorders and splenomegaly, the risk of DVT, particularly portal vein thrombosis, is significantly higher than for those without these underlying conditions.[104] Therefore, in addition to subcutaneous heparin and sequential compression devices, consideration should be given to low-dose anticoagulation therapy following surgery for such patients.

Hematologic Outcomes

The results of splenectomy may be appraised according to the level of hematologic response (e.g., rise in platelet and hemoglobin levels) for those disorders in which the spleen contributes to the hematologic problem. Hematologic responses may be divided into initial and long-term responses. For thrombocytopenia, the initial response is typically defined as a rise in platelet count within several days of splenectomy. A long-term response is defined as a platelet count greater than 150,000/mL more than 2 months after surgery without medications.[109] According to recently reported series, laparoscopic splenectomy is effective in providing a long-term platelet response

Table 33-2
Platelet Response Following Laparoscopic Splenectomy for Idiopathic Thrombocytopenic Purpura

Study (Lead Author)	N	Initial Response (%)	Long-Term Response (%)	Mean Follow-Up (m)
Szold et al[121]	104	NA	84	36
Katkhouda et al[3]	67	84	78	38
Trias et al[122]	48	NA	88	30
Tanoue et al[123]	35	83	79	36
Friedman et al[124]	31	NA	93	2
Stanton[125]	30	89	89	30
Fass et al[126]	29	90	80	43
Bresler et al[127]	27	93	88	28
Harold et al[128]	27	92	85	20
Lozano-Salazar et al[111]	22	89	88	15
Meyer et al[129]	16	NA	86	14
Watson et al[130]	13	100	83	60
Total/mean	**449**	**90**	**85**	**29**

in approximately 85% of individuals with ITP (Table 33-2). These results are consistent with the success of open splenectomy, which is associated with a long-term success rate of 65 to 90%.[110–113]

For chronic hemolytic anemias, a rise in hemoglobin levels to above 10 g/dL without the need for transfusion signifies a successful response to splenectomy. By this criterion, splenectomy has been reported to be successful in 60 to 80% of patients with chronic hemolytic anemia.[112,114] For the subset of patients with spherocytosis, the success rate is usually higher, ranging from 90 to 100%.[115]

The results of splenectomy may also be examined according to certain surgical and postsurgical characteristics, including the operative time, recovery time, and morbidity and mortality rates of the procedure, which tend to vary according to the hematologic indication (Tables 33-3 and 33-4).

To date, no prospective, randomized comparisons between laparoscopic and open splenectomy have been published. Numerous retrospective or case-controlled comparisons between LS and OS reveal that the laparoscopic approach typically results in longer operative times, shorter hospital stays, lower morbidity rates, similar blood loss, and similar mortality rates.[111,112,116–118] Although operating room charges are higher for LS, several studies have found that total cost to the patient is less with the laparoscopic procedure due to the reduced hospital stay.[112,116] The laparoscopic approach has emerged as the standard for nontraumatic, elective splenectomy.

Table 33-3
Splenectomy Results by Hematologic Indication

	ITP (n = 65)	TTP (n = 9)	Anemia (n = 11)	Malignancy (n = 43)
OR time (min)	134	127	171	170
EBL (mL)	126	161	271	380
LOS (days)	2.8	8.3	2.6	4.3
Conversions	0	0	0	5
Complications	7	0	0	8
Response	85%	89%	91%	74%

EBL = estimated blood loss; ITP = idiopathic thrombocytopenic purpura; LOS = length of hospital stay; OR = operating room; TTP = thrombotic thrombocytopenic purpura.

SOURCE: Data from Jaroszewski et al.[99]

Table 33-4
Splenectomy Results by Hematologic Indication

	ITP (n = 151)	TTP (n = 7)	Anemia (n = 40)	Malignancy (n = 28)
OR time (min)	128	146	149	165
EBL (mL)	137	96	116	238
LOS (days)	2.2	3.0	2.2	2.6
Conversions	3 (2%)	1 (14%)	1 (3%)	1 (4%)
Complications	14 (9%)	0	1 (3%)	3 (11%)

EBL = estimated blood loss; ITP = idiopathic thrombocytopenic purpura; LOS = length of hospital stay; OR = operating room; TTP = thrombotic thrombocytopenic purpura.

SOURCE: Data from A. Park, unpublished.

Overwhelming Postsplenectomy Infection (OPSI)

Regardless of technique or indication, splenectomy imparts a lifetime risk of severe infection to the patient. The true incidence of postsplenectomy sepsis remains unknown, with estimates varying between less than 1 and 5% during a patient's lifetime. A 30-year review of the relevant literature in English (1966–96) revealed an incidence of 3.2%.[36] Although the incidence of postsplenectomy infection was similar among children and adults, the mortality rate was higher for children (1.7 vs. 1.3%). The incidence and mortality rates were highest for patients with underlying hematologic conditions, such as thalassemia major (8.2% incidence rate and 5.1% mortality rate) and sickle cell disease (7.3% incidence rate and 4.8% mortality rate). However, much of the literature reporting OPSI and morbidity rates includes years before the widespread implementation of vaccinations, which occurred in the late 1970s and early 1980s. Substantial decreases in the incidence of OPSI among splenectomized children have been reported following the implementation of pneumococcal vaccine.[119]

The loss of the spleen's ability to filter and phagocytose bacteria and parasitized blood cells predisposes the patient to infection by encapsulated bacteria or parasites. Splenectomy also results in the loss of a significant source of antibody production. The most common source of infection reported in the literature is *Streptococcus pneumoniae*, accounting for 50 to 90% of cases. *Haemophilus influenzae* type B, meningococcus, and group A streptococci have reportedly accounted for an additional 25% of infections.[102] Protozoan infections invading the red blood cell, such as *Babesia microti* (resulting from tick bites) and malaria, occur more frequently in splenectomized individuals than in normal hosts.

OPSI is associated with pneumonia or meningitis in roughly one half of cases, but a substantial number of patients have no clear site of bacterial colonization. In these cases, a cryptic nasopharyngeal source is usually suspected. OPSI may begin with a relatively mild-appearing prodrome, including fever, malaise, myalgias, headache, vomiting, diarrhea, and abdominal pain. These symptoms may then progress rapidly to fulminant bacteremic septic shock, with accompanying hypotension, anuria, and disseminated intravascular coagulation. Of the patients who die as a result of OPSI, more than one half succumb within the first 48 hours of admission to the hospital.

Currently no tests exist that differentiate the small number of asplenic patients who will develop OPSI from the majority who will experience no infectious complications. However, some risk factors for the development of OPSI have been identified. These include the indication for splenectomy, overall immune status, and time interval from the date of surgery.[102] Patients undergoing splenectomy for hematologic indications carry a higher risk than those who undergo splenectomy for trauma. Individuals with compromised immune systems such as those with Hodgkin's disease or those taking chemotherapy or radiation therapy have a higher risk of OPSI than those who do not. OPSI usually develops within the first 2 years after splenectomy, especially in children.[120] Although diminished, a small risk remains after this initial 2-year period. Therefore patients and physicians must remain alert and take preventive measures for the rest of the patient's life. Such measures include wearing either a medical bracelet or carrying a laminated medical alert card, possessing a 5-day supply of stand-by antibiotics, and having readily available written advice for immunizations and stand-by antibiotics.[103]

Prudent immunoprophylaxis consists of pneumococcal, meningococcal, and *Haemophilus influenzae* type B vaccination at least 7 to 14 days before splenectomy or as soon as possible after surgery. In the case of pneumococcal vaccine, booster injections every 5 to 6 years should be considered. Annual influenza immunization is advisable. Antibiotic prophylaxis—usually a single daily dose of penicillin or amoxicillin—is recommended for asplenic children for the first 2 years after splenectomy.[102]

References

1. Morgenstern L: A history of splenectomy, in Hiatt JR, Phillips EH, Morgenstern L (eds): *Surgical Diseases of the Spleen.* Berlin-Heidelberg: Springer-Verlag, 1997, p 3.
2. Moynihan B: The surgery of the spleen. *Br J Surg* 8:307, 1920.
3. Katkhouda N, Hurwitz MG, Rivera RT, et al: Laparoscopic splenectomy: Outcome and efficacy in 103 consecutive patients. *Ann Surg* 228:1, 1998.
4. Morgenstern L, Skandalakis JE: Anatomy and embryology of the spleen, in Hiatt JR, Phillips EH, Morgenstern L (eds): *Surgical Diseases of the Spleen.* Berlin-Heidelberg: Springer-Verlag, 1997, p 15.
5. Poulin EC, Thibault C: The anatomical basis for laparoscopic splenectomy. *Can J Surg* 36:484, 1993.
6. Schwartz SI: Spleen, in Schwartz SI (ed): *Principles of Surgery: Specific Considerations,* 7th ed. New York: McGraw-Hill, 1999, p 1501.
7. Poulin EC, Schlachta CM, Mamaza J: Surgical anatomy. *Prob Gen Surg* 19:16, 2002.
8. Weiss L: Mechanisms of splenic clearance of the blood; a structural overview of the mammalian spleen, in Bowdler AJ (ed): *The Spleen. Structure, Function and Significance.* London: Chapman and Hall Medical, 1990, p 23.
9. Eichner ER: Splenic function: Normal, too much, and too little. *Am J Med* 66:311, 1979.
10. Frank EL, Neu HC: Postsplencetomy infection. *Surg Clin North Am* 61:135, 1981.
11. Hosea SW: Role of the spleen in pneumococcal infection. *Lymphology* 16:115, 1983.
12. Lucey BC, Boland GW, Maher MM, et al: Percutaneous nonvascular splenic intervention: A 10-year review. *Am J Roentgenol* 179:1591, 2002.
13. O'Malley ME, Wood BJ, Boland GW, et al: Percutaneous imaging-guided biopsy of the spleen. *Am J Roentgenol* 172:661, 1999.
14. Siniluoto TMJ, Tikkakoski TA, Lahde ST: Ultrasound or CT in splenic diseases? *Acta Radiol* 35:597, 1994.
15. Robertson F, Leander P, Ekberg O: Radiology of the spleen. *Eur Radiol* 11:80, 2001.
16. Radaelli F, Faccini P, Goldaniga M, et al: Factors predicting response to splenectomy in adult patients with idiopathic thrombocytopenic purpura. *Haematologica* 85:1040, 2000.
17. Armas RR: Clinical studies with spleen-specific radiolabeled agents. *Semin Nucl Med* 15:260, 1985.
18. Miyazaki M, Itoh H, Kaiho T, et al: Partial splenic embolization for the treatment of chronic idiopathic thrombocytopenic purpura. *Am J Roentgenol* 163:123, 1994.
19. Cools L, Osteaux M, Divano L, et al: Prediction of splenic volume by a simple CT measurement: A statistical study. *J Comp Assist Tomogr* 7:426, 1983.
20. Prassopoulos P, Daskalogiannaki M, Raissaki M, et al: Determination of normal splenic volume on computed tomography in relation to age, gender and body habitus. *Eur Radiol* 7:246, 1997.
21. Watanabe S, Hosomi N, Kitade Y, et al: Assessment of the presence and severity of esophagogastric varices by splenic index in patients with liver cirrhosis. *J Comput Assist Tomogr* 24:788, 2000.
22. Schwartz SI, Cooper RA Jr.: Surgery in the diagnosis and treatment of Hodgkin's disease. *Adv Surg* 6:175, 1972.
23. Schwartz SI: Role of splenectomy in hematologic disorders. *World J Surg* 20:1156, 1996.
24. Schwartz RS, Berkman EM, Silberstein LE: Autoimmune hemolytic anemias, in Hoffman R (ed): *Hematology: Basic Principles and Practice,* 3rd ed. New York: Churchill Livingstone, 2001, p 611.
25. Gallagher PG, Jarolim P: Red cell membrane disorders, in Hoffman R (ed): *Hematology: Basic Principles and Practice,* 3rd ed. New York: Churchill Livingstone, 2001, p 576.
26. Bates G, Brown C: Incidence of gallbladder disease in chronic hemolytic anemia (spherocytosis). *Gastroenterology* 21:104, 1952.
27. Sandler A, Winkel G, Kimura K, et al: The role of prophylactic cholecystectomy during splenectomy in children with hereditary spherocytosis. *J Pediatr Surg* 34:1077, 1999.
28. Embury SH, Vichinsky EP: Sickle cell disease, in Hoffman R (ed): *Hematology: Basic Principles and Practice,* 3rd ed. New York: Churchill Livingstone, 2001, p 510.
29. al-Salem AH, Qaisaruddin S, Nasserallah Z, et al: Splenectomy in patients with sickle-cell disease. *Am J Surg* 172:254, 1996.
30. Aquino VM, Norvell JM, Buchanan GR: Acute splenic complications in children with sickle cell–hemoglobin C disease. *J Pediatr* 130:961, 1997.
31. Vichinsky EP, Neumayr LD, Earles AN, et al: Causes and outcomes of the acute chest syndrome in sickle cell disease. National Acute Chest Syndrome Study Group. *N Engl J Med* 342:1855, 2000.
32. Forget BG: Thalassemia syndromes, in Hoffman R (ed): *Hematology: Basic Principles and Practice,* 3rd ed. New York: Churchill Livingstone, 2001, p 485.
33. Lo L, Singer ST: Thalassemia: Current approach to an old disease. *Pediatr Clin North Am* 49:1165, 2002.
34. Barrai I, Rosity A, Cappellozza G et al: Beta-thalassemia in the Po delta: Selection, geography and population structure. *Am J Hum Genet* 36:1121, 1984.
35. al Hawsawi ZM, Hummaida TI, Ismail GA: Splenectomy in thalassaemia major: Experience at Madina Maternity and Children's Hospital, Saudi Arabia. *Ann Trop Paediatr* 21:155, 2001.
36. Bisharat N, Omari H, Lavi I, et al: Risk of infection and death among post-splenectomy patients. *J Infect* 43:182, 2001.
37. Prchal JT, Gregg XT: Red cell enzymopathies, in Hoffman R (ed): *Hematology: Basic Principles and Practice,* 3rd ed. New York: Churchill Livingstone, 2001, p 561.
38. Beutler E: *Red Cell Metabolism: A Manual of Biochemical Methods,* 2nd ed. New York: Grune and Stratton, 1975, p 139.
39. Baronciani L, Beutler E: Analysis of pyruvate kinase mutations producing nonspherocytic hemolytic anemia. *Proc Natl Acad Sci USA* 90:4324, 1993.
40. Aizawa S, Kohdera U, Hiramoto M, et al: Ineffective erythropoiesis in the spleen of a patient with pyruvate kinase deficiency. *Am J Hematol* 74:68, 2003.
41. Hiatt JR, Phillips EH, Morgenstern L (eds): *Surgical Diseases of the Spleen.* Berlin-Heidelberg: Springer-Verlag, 1997, p 29.
42. McFarland JT, Kuzma C, Millard FE, et al: Palliative irradiation of the spleen. *Am J Clin Oncol* 26:178, 2003.
43. Morrison VA: Chronic leukemias. *CA Cancer J Clin* 44:353, 1994.
44. Mesa RA, Elliott MA, Tefferi A: Splenectomy in chronic myeloid leukemia and myelofibrosis with myeloid metaplasia. *Blood Rev* 14:121, 2000.

45. Parker SL, Tang T, Bolden S, Wingo PA: Cancer statistics. *CA Cancer J Clin* 47:5, 1997.

46. Miller KB, Daoust PR: Clinical manifestations of acute myeloid leukemia, in Hoffman R (ed): *Hematology: Basic Principles and Practice,* 3rd ed. New York: Churchill Livingstone, 2001, p 999.

47. Tefferi A, Murphy S: Current opinion in essential thrombocythemia: Pathogenesis, diagnosis, and management. *Blood Rev* 15:121, 2002.

48. Cortelazzo S, Finazzi G, Ruggeri M, et al: Hydroxyurea for patients with essential thrombocythemia and a high risk of thrombosis. *N Engl J Med* 332:1132, 1995.

49. Modan B: An epidemiological study of polycythemia vera. *Blood* 26:657, 1965.

50. Hoffman R: Polycythemia vera, in Hoffman R (ed): *Hematology: Basic Principles and Practice,* 3rd ed. New York: Churchill Livingstone, 2001, p 1130.

51. Mesa RA, Silverstein MN, Jacobsen SJ, et al: Population-based incidence and survival figures in essential thrombocythemia and agnogenic myeloid metaplasia. An Olmsted County Study, 1976–1995. *Am J Hematol* 61:10, 1999.

52. Mesa RA: Myelofibrosis with myeloid metaplasia: Therapeutic options in 2003. *Curr Hematol Rep* 2:264, 2003.

53. Akpek G, McAneny D, Weintraub L: Risks and benefits of splenectomy in myelofibrosis with myeloid metaplasia: A retrospective analysis of 26 cases. *J Surg Oncol* 77:42, 2001.

54. Delpero JR, Houvenaeghel G, Gastaut JA, et al: Splenectomy for hypersplenism in chronic lymphocytic leukaemia and malignant non-Hodgkin's lymphoma. *Br J Surg* 77:443, 1990.

55. Flandrin G, Sigaux F, Sebahoun G, et al: Hairy cell leukemia: Clinical presentation and follow-up in 211 patients. *Semin Oncol* 11:458, 1984.

56. Golomb HM, Vardiman JW: Response to splenectomy in 65 patients with hairy cell leukemia: An evaluation of spleen weight and bone marrow involvement. *Blood* 61:349, 1983.

57. Magee MJ, McKenzie S, Filippa DA, et al: Hairy cell leukemia durability of response to splenectomy in 26 patients and treatment of relapse with androgens in 6 patients. *Cancer* 56:2557, 1985.

58. Mey U, Strehl J, Gorschluter M, et al: Advances in the treatment of hairy cell leukemia. *Lancet Oncol* 4:86, 2003.

59. Van Beisin K, Cabanillas F: Clinical manifestations, staging, and treatment of Non-Hodgkin lymphoma, in Hoffman R (ed): *Hematology: Basic Principles and Practice,* 3rd ed. New York: Churchill Livingstone, 2001, p 1293.

60. Portlock CS, Glick J: Hodgkin disease: Clinical manifestations, staging, therapy, in Hoffman R (ed): *Hematology: Basic Principles and Practice,* 3rd ed. New York: Churchill Livingstone, 2001, p 1241.

61. Mazzarotto R, Boso C, Scarzello G, et al: Radiotherapy alone in the treatment of clinical stage I-IIA, nonbulky, Hodgkin's disease: Single institution experience on 73 patients staged with lymphangiography and laparoscopy. *Am J Clin Oncology* 25:149, 2002.

62. Cines DB, Blanchette VS: Immune thrombocytopenic purpura. *N Engl J Med* 346:995, 2002.

63. Sailer T, Weltermann A, Zoghlami C, et al: Mortality in severe, non-aggressively treated adult autoimmune thrombocytopenia. *Hematol J* 4:336, 2003.

64. McMillan R: Therapy for adults with refractory chronic immune thrombocytopenic purpura. *Ann Intern Med* 126:307, 1997.

65. Provan D, Newland A: Fifty years of idiopathic thrombocytopenic purpura (ITP): Management of refractory ITP in adults. *Br J Hematol* 188:933, 2002.

66. Huber MR, Kumar S, Tefferi A: Treatment advances in adult immune thrombocytopenic purpura. *Ann Hematol* 82:723, 2003.

67. Lilleyman JS: Intracranial haemorrhage in idiopathic thrombocytopenic purpura. *Arch Dis Child* 71:251, 1994.

68. Carcao MD, Zipursky A, Butchart S, et al: Short-course oral prednisone therapy in children presenting with acute immune thrombocytopenic purpura (immune thrombocytopenic purpura). *Acta Paediatr* (Suppl)424:71, 1998.

69. Nabhan C, Kwaan HC: Current concepts in the diagnosis and treatment of thrombotic thrombocytopenic purpura. *Hematol Clin North Am* 17:177, 2003.

70. Torok TJ, Holman RC, Chorba TL: Increasing mortality form thrombotic thrombocytopenic purpura in the United States—analysis of national mortality data, 1968–1991. *Am J Hematol* 50:84, 1995.

71. Bell WR, Braine HG, Ness PM, et al: Improved survival in thrombotic thrombocytopenic purpura–hemolytic uremic syndrome. Clinical experience in 108 patients. *N Engl J Med* 325:398, 1991.

72. Winslow GA, Nelson EW: Thrombotic thrombocytopenic purpura: Indications for and results of splenectomy. *Am J Surg* 170:558, 1995.

73. Veltman GA, Brand A, Leeksma OC, et al: The role of splenectomy in the treatment of relapsing thrombotic thrombocytopenic purpura. *Ann Hematol* 70:231, 1995.

74. Gordon LI, Kwaan HC, Rossi EC: Deleterious effects of platelet transfusions and recovery thrombocytosis in patients with thrombotic microangiopathy. *Semin Hematol* 24:194, 1987.

75. Phillips G, Radosevich M, Lipsett P: Splenic abscess: Another look at an old disease. *Arch Surg* 132:1331, 1997.

76. Chun C, Raff MJ, Contreras L, et al: Splenic abscess. *Medicine* 59:50, 1980.

77. Stone DL, Ginns EI, Krasnewich D, et al: Life-threatening splenic hemorrhage in two patients with Gaucher disease. *Am J Hematol* 64:140, 2000.

78. Rubin M, Yampolski I, Lambrozo R, et al: Partial splenectomy in Gaucher's disease. *J Pediatr Surg* 21:125, 1986.

79. Tassoni JP Jr., Fawaz KA, Johnston DE: Cirrhosis and portal hypertension in a patient with adult Niemann-Pick disease. *Gastroenterology* 100:567, 1991.

80. Boggio L, Green D: Recombinant human factor VIIa in the management of amyloid-associated factor X deficiency. *Br J Haematol* 112:1074, 2001.

81. Rashba EJ, Rowe JM, Packman CH: Treatment of the neutropenia of Felty syndrome. *Blood Rev* 10.177, 1996.

82. Xiao GQ, Zinberg JM, Unger PD: Asymptomatic sarcoidosis presenting as massive splenomegaly. *Am J Med* 113:698, 2002.

83. Nusair S, Kramer MR, Berkman N: Pleural effusion with splenic rupture as manifestations of recurrence of sarcoidosis following prolonged remission. *Respiration* 70:114, 2003.

84. Ammann RW, Eckert J: Cestodes. Echinococcus. *Gastroenterol Clin North Am* 25:655, 1996.

85. Nakao A, Saito S, Yamano T, et al: Dermoid cyst of the spleen: Report of a case. *Surg Today* 29:660, 1999.

86. John AK, Das KV, Vaidyanathan S: Partial splenectomy for splenic cyst: A case report and review of the literature. *Trop Gastroenterol* 23:148, 2002.

87. Comitalo JB: Laparoscopic treatment of splenic cysts. *JSLS* 5:313, 2001.

88. Ishida H, Konno K, Ishida J, et al: Splenic lymphoma: Differentiation from splenic cyst with ultrasonography. *Abdom Imaging* 26:529, 2001.

89. Lam KY, Tang V: Metastatic tumors to the spleen: A 25-year clinicopathologic study. *Arch Pathol Lab Med* 124:526, 2000.

90. Thavanathan J, Heughan C, Cummings TM: Splenic vein thrombosis as a cause of variceal hemorrhage. *Can J Surg* 35:649, 1992.

91. Messina LM, Shanley CJ: Visceral artery aneurysms. *Surg Clin North Am* 77:425, 1997.

92. Lee PC, Rhee RY, Gordon RY, et al: Management of splenic artery aneurysms: The significance of portal and essential hypertension. *J Am Coll Surg* 189:483, 1999.

93. Stanley JC, Zelenock GB: Splanchnic artery aneurysms, in Rutherford RB (ed): *Vascular Surgery,* 4th ed. Philadelphia: WB Saunders, 1995, p 1124.

94. Stanley JC, Thompson NW, Fry WJ: Splanchnic artery aneurysms. *Arch Surg* 101:689, 1970.

95. Hilleren DJ: Embolization of the spleen for the treatment of hypersplenism and in portal hypertension, in Kadir S (ed): *Current Practice of Interventional Radiology.* Philadelphia: BC Decker, 1991, p 494.

96. Kimura F, Ito H, Shimizu H, et al: Partial splenic embolization for the treatment of hereditary spherocytosis. *Am J Roentgenol* 181:1021, 2003.

97. Hiatt JR, Gomes AS, Machleder HI: Massive splenomegaly. Superior results with a combined endovascular and operative approach. *Arch Surg* 125:1363, 1990.

98. Poulin EC, Mamazza J: Laparoscopic splenectomy: Lessons from the learning curve. *Can J Surg* 41:28, 1998.

99. Jaroszewski DE, Schlinkert RT, Gray RJ: Laparoscopic splenectomy for the treatment of gastric varices secondary to sinistral portal hypertension. *Surg Endosc* 14:87, 2000.

100. Hickman MP, Lucas D, Novak Z: Preoperative embolization of the spleen in children with hypersplenism. *J Vasc Intervent Radiol* 3:647, 1992.

101. Farid H, O'Connell TX: Surgical management of massive splenomegaly. *Am Surg* 62:803, 1996.

102. Brigden ML, Pattullo AL: Prevention and management of overwhelming postsplenectomy infection—an update. *Crit Care Med* 27:836, 1999.

103. Davidson RN, Wall RA: Prevention and management of infections in patients without a spleen. *Clin Microbiol Infect* 7:657, 2001.

104. Winslow ER, Brunt LM, Drebin JA, et al: Portal vein thrombosis after splenectomy. *Am J Surg* 184:631, 2002.

105. Park AE, Gagner M, Pomp A: The lateral approach to laparoscopic splenectomy. *Am J Surg* 173:126, 1997.

106. Breddin HK: Low molecular weight heparins in the prevention of deep-vein thrombosis in general surgery. *Semin Thromb Hemost* 25(Suppl 3):83, 1999.

107. Ellison EC, Fabri PJ: Complications of splenectomy. Etiology, prevention, and management. *Surg Clin North Am* 63:1313, 1983.

108. Rosen M, Brody F, Walsh RM, et al: Outcome of laparoscopic splenectomy based on hematologic indications. *Surg Endosc* 16:272, 2002.

109. Difino SM, Lachant MA, Kirschner JJ: Adult idiopathic thrombocytopenic purpura: Clinical findings and response to therapy. *Am J Med* 69:430, 1980.

110. Mittelman M, Kyzer S, Zeidman A, et al: Splenectomy for haematological diseases—a single institution experience. *Haematologia (Budap)* 28:185, 1997.

111. Lozano-Salazar RR, Herrera MF, Vargas-Vorackova F, et al: Laparoscopic versus open splenectomy for immune thrombocytopenic purpura. *Laparoscopy* 176:366, 1998.

112. Glasgow RE, Yee LF, Mulhivill SJ: Laparoscopic splenectomy. The emerging standard. *Surg Endosc* 11:108, 1997.

113. Cordera F, Long KH, Nagtorney DM, et al: Open versus laparoscopic splenectomy for idiopathic thrombocytopenia purpura: Clinical and economic analysis. *Surgery* 134:45, 2003.

114. Bohner H, Tirier C, Rotzscher VM, et al: Indications for and results of splenectomy in different hematological disorders. *Langenbecks Arch Chir* 382:79, 1997.

115. Katkhouda N, Manhas S, Umbach TW: Laparoscopic splenectomy. *J Laparoendosc Adv Surg Tech* 11:383, 2001.

116. Friedman RL, Hiatt JR, Korman JL, et al: Laparoscopic or open splenectomy: Which approach is superior? *J Am Coll Surg* 185:49, 1997.

117. Watson DI, Conventry BJ, Chin T, et al: Laparoscopic versus open splenectomy for immune thrombocytopenic purpura. *Surgery* 121:18, 1997.

118. Park A, Marcaccio M, Sternbach M, et al: Laparoscopic vs open splenectomy. *Arch Surg* 134:1263, 1999.

119. Konradsen HB, Henrichsen J: Pneumococcal infections in splenectomized children are preventable. *Acta Paediatr Scand* 80:423, 1991.

120. Holdsworth RJ, Irving AD, Cuschieri A: Postsplenectomy sepsis and its mortality rate: Actual versus perceived risks. *Br J Surg* 78:1031, 1991.

121. Szold A, Kais H, Keidar A, et al: Chronic idiopathic thrombocytopenic purpura (ITP) is a surgical disease. *Surg Endosc* 16:155, 2002.

122. Trias M, Targarona EM, Espert JJ, et al: Impact of hematological diagnosis on early and late outcome after laparoscopic splenectomy: An analysis of 111 cases. *Surg Endosc* 14:556, 2000.

123. Tanoue K, Hashizume M, Morita M, et al: Results of laparoscopic splenectomy for immune thrombocytopenic purpura. *Am J Surg* 177:222, 1999.

124. Friedman RL, Fallas MJ, Carrol BJ, et al: Laparoscopic splenectomy for ITP. *Surg Endosc* 10:991, 1996.

125. Stanton CJ: Laparoscopic splenectomy for idiopathic thrombocytopenic purpura (ITP). A five-year experience. *Surg Endosc* 13:1083, 1999.

126. Fass SM, Hui TT, Lefor A, et al: Safety of laparoscopic splenectomy in elderly patients with idiopathic thrombocytopenic purpura. *Am Surg* 66:844, 2000.

127. Bresler L, Guerci A, Brunaud L, et al: Laparoscopic splenectomy for idiopathic thrombocytopenic purpura: outcome and long-term results. *World J Surg* 26:111, 2002.

128. Harold KL, Schlinkert RT, Mann DK, et al: Long-term results of laparoscopic splenectomy for immune thrombocytopenic purpura. *Mayo Clin Proc* 74:37, 1999.

129. Meyer G, Wichmann MW, Rau HG, et al: Laparoscopic splenectomy for idiopathic thrombocytopenic purpura. *Surg Endosc* 12:1348, 1998.

130. Watson DI, Conventry BJ, Chin T, et al: Laparoscopic versus open splenectomy for immune thrombocytopenic purpura. *Surgery* 121:18, 1997.

CHAPTER 34

Abdominal Wall, Omentum, Mesentery, and Retroperitoneum

Robert L. Bell and Neal E. Seymour

ABDOMINAL WALL

The abdominal wall is defined superiorly by the costal margins, inferiorly by the symphysis pubis and pelvic bones, and posteriorly by the vertebral column. It serves to support and protect abdominal and retroperitoneal structures, and its complex muscular functions enable twisting and flexing motions of the trunk. To gain surgical access to the abdominal cavity, an intimate knowledge of the arrangement of the muscles and aponeuroses of the abdominal wall is required.

Surgical Anatomy

The abdominal wall is an anatomically complex, layered structure with a segmentally derived blood supply and innervation (Fig. 34-1). It is mesodermal in origin and develops as bilateral migrating sheets, which originate in the paravertebral region and envelop the future abdominal area. The leading edges of these structures develop into the rectus abdominus muscles, which eventually meet in midline of the anterior abdominal wall. The muscle fibers of the rectus abdominus are arranged vertically and are encased within an aponeurotic sheath, the anterior and posterior layers of which are fused in the midline at the *linea alba.* The rectus abdominus has insertions on the symphysis pubis and pubic bones, on the anteroinferior aspects of the fifth and sixth ribs, as well as the seventh costal cartilage and the xiphoid process. The lateral border of the rectus muscles assumes a convex shape that gives rise to the surface landmark, the *linea semilunaris.* There are usually three tendinous intersections or inscriptions that cross the rectus muscles: one at the level of the xiphoid process, one at the level of the umbilicus, and one halfway between the xiphoid process and the umbilicus (see Fig. 34-1).

Lateral to the rectus sheath are three muscular layers with oblique fiber orientations relative to one another (Fig. 34-2). These layers derive from the laterally migrating mesodermal tissues during the sixth to seventh week of fetal development, prior to fusion of the developing rectus abdominus muscles in the midline. The external oblique muscle runs inferiorly and medially, arising from the margins of the lowest eight ribs and costal cartilages. The external oblique muscle originates laterally on the latissimus dorsi and serratus anterior muscles, as well as on the iliac crest. Medially it forms a tendinous aponeurosis, which is contiguous with the anterior rectus sheath. The *inguinal ligament* is the inferior-most edge of the external oblique aponeurosis, reflected posteriorly in the area between the anterior superior iliac spine and pubic tubercle. The internal oblique muscle lies immediately deep to the external oblique muscle and arises from the lateral aspect of the inguinal ligament, the iliac crest, and the thoracolumbar fascia. Its fibers course superiorly and medially and form a tendinous aponeurosis that contributes components to both the anterior and posterior rectus sheath. The lower medial and inferior-most fibers of the internal oblique course may fuse with the lower fibers of the transversus abdominis muscle (the *conjoined area*). The inferior-most fibers of the internal oblique muscle are contiguous with the cremasteric muscle in the inguinal canal. The transversus abdominis muscle is the deepest of the three lateral muscles, and, as its name implies, runs transversely from the bilateral lowest six ribs, the lumbosacral fascia, and the iliac crest to the lateral border of the rectus abdominus.

The complexities of the anterior and posterior aspects of the rectus sheath are best understood in their relationship to the *arcuate line* (semicircular line of Douglas), which lies roughly at the level of the anterior superior iliac spines (Fig. 34-3). Above the arcuate line, the anterior rectus sheath is formed by the external oblique aponeurosis and the external lamina of the internal oblique aponeurosis, while the posterior rectus sheath is formed by the internal lamina of the internal oblique aponeurosis, the transversus abdominis aponeurosis, and the transversalis fascia. Below the arcuate line, the anterior rectus sheath is formed by the external oblique aponeurosis, the laminae of the internal oblique aponeurosis, and the transversus

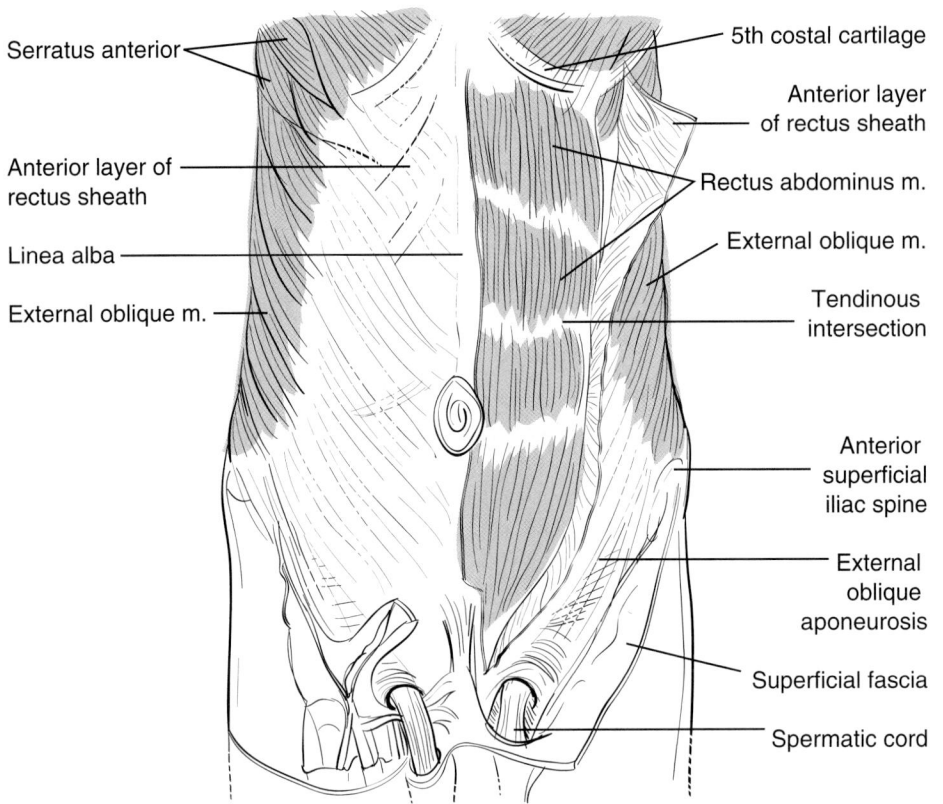

FIG. 34-1. Anterior abdominal wall. *Linea alba* is the midline aponeurotic demarcation between the bellies of the rectus abdominus muscles. The rectus abdominus muscle and its tendinous intersections on the left are shown deep to the reflected anterior rectus sheath. Segmental cutaneous nerve branches also are shown. *(Reproduced with permission from Moore KL, Dalley AF (eds): Clinically Oriented Anatomy, 4th ed. Philadelphia: Lippincott, Williams & Wilkins, 1999, p 181.)*

abdominis aponeurosis. There is no aponeurotic posterior covering of this lower portion of the rectus muscles, although the transversalis fascia remains a contiguous structure on the posterior aspect of the abdominal wall in this area as well.

The majority of the blood supply to the muscles of the anterior abdominal wall is derived from the superior and inferior epigastric arteries (Fig. 34-4). The superior epigastric artery arises from the internal thoracic artery, while the inferior epigastric artery arises from the external iliac artery. A collateral network of branches of the subcostal and lumbar arteries also contributes to the abdominal wall blood supply. The lymphatic drainage of the abdominal wall is predominantly to the major nodal basins in the superficial inguinal and axillary areas.

Innervation of the anterior abdominal wall is segmentally related to specific spinal levels. The motor nerves to the rectus muscles, the internal oblique muscles, and the transversus abdominis muscles run from the anterior rami of spinal nerves at the T6 to T12 levels. The overlying skin is innervated by afferent branches of the T4 to L1 nerve roots, with the nerve roots of T10 subserving sensation of the skin around the umbilicus (Fig. 34-5).

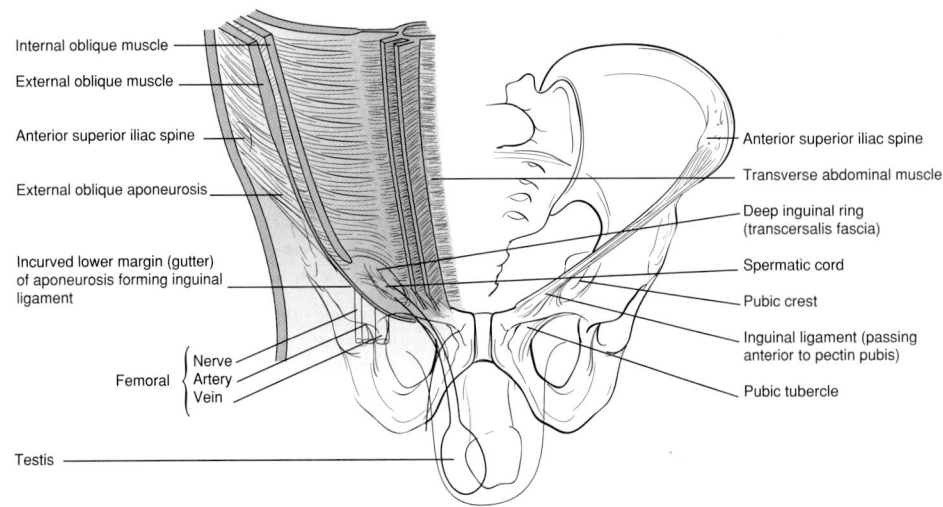

FIG. 34-2. The three muscular layers of the abdominal wall lateral to the rectus abdominus are the *external oblique, internal oblique,* and *transversus abdominus* muscles, shown here on the low abdomen, where the lower margin of the external oblique reflects posteriorly as the inguinal ligament. *(Reproduced with permission from Moore KL, Dalley AF (eds): Clinically Oriented Anatomy, 4th ed. Philadelphia: Lippincott, Williams & Wilkins, 1999, p 181.)*

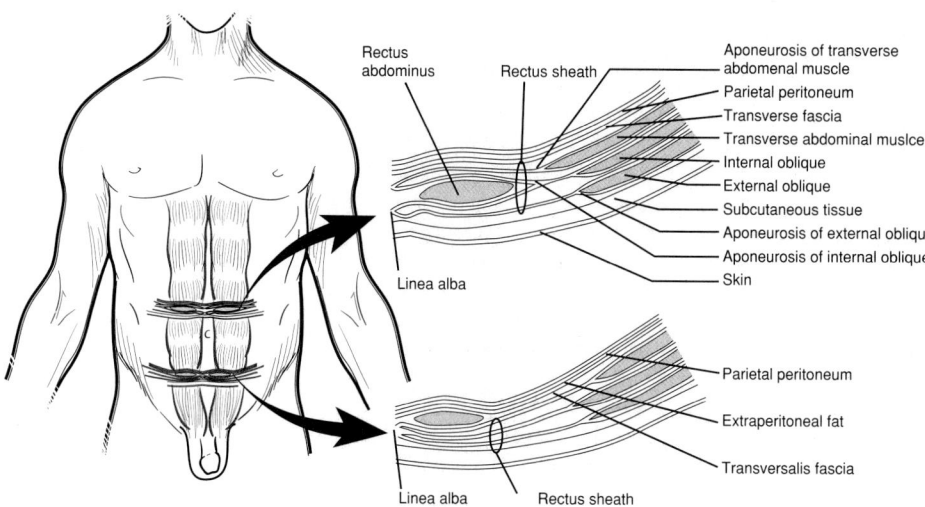

FIG. 34-3. Cross-sectional anatomy of the abdominal wall above and below the arcuate line of Douglas. The lower right abdominal wall segment shows clearly the absence of an aponeurotic covering of the posterior aspect of the rectus abdominus muscle inferior to the arcuate line. Superior to the arcuate line, there are both internal oblique and transversus abdominus aponeurotic contributions to the posterior rectus sheath. *(Reproduced with permission from Moore KL, Dalley AF (eds): Clinically Oriented Anatomy, 4th ed. Philadelphia: Lippincott, Williams & Wilkins, 1999, p 185.)*

Physiology

The rectus muscles, the external oblique muscles, and the internal oblique muscles work as a unit to flex the trunk anteriorly or laterally. Rotation of the trunk is achieved by the contraction of the external oblique muscle and the contralateral internal oblique muscle. For example, rotation of the trunk to the right is produced by contraction of the left external oblique muscle and the right internal oblique muscle. Additionally, all four muscles (i.e., rectus muscles, the external oblique muscles, the internal oblique muscle, and the transversus abdominis muscle) are involved in raising intra-abdominal pressure. If the diaphragm is relaxed when the abdominal musculature is contracted, the pressure exerted by the abdominal muscles results in expiration of air from the lungs or a cough if this contraction is forceful. Thus, these abdominal muscles are the primary muscles

of expiration. If the diaphragm is contracted when the abdominal musculature is contracted (*Valsalva maneuver*) the increased abdominal pressure aids in processes such as micturition, defecation, and childbirth.

Congenital Abnormalities

The layers of the anterior abdominal wall begin to form within the first several weeks after conception. Prominent in the early embryonic abdominal wall is a large central defect through which pass the vitelline (omphalomesenteric) duct and allantois. The vitelline duct connects the embryonic and fetal midgut to the yolk sac. During the sixth week of development, the abdominal contents grow too large for the abdominal wall to contain and the embryonic midgut herniates into the umbilical cord. While outside the confines of the developing abdomen, it undergoes a 270-degree counterclockwise rotation, and at the end of the twelfth week returns to the abdominal cavity. Defects in abdominal wall closure may lead to omphalocele or gastroschisis. In omphalocele, viscera protrude through an open umbilical ring and are covered by a sac derived from the amnion. In gastroschisis, the viscera protrude through a defect lateral to the umbilicus and no sac is present. These disorders are covered in greater depth in Chap. 38.

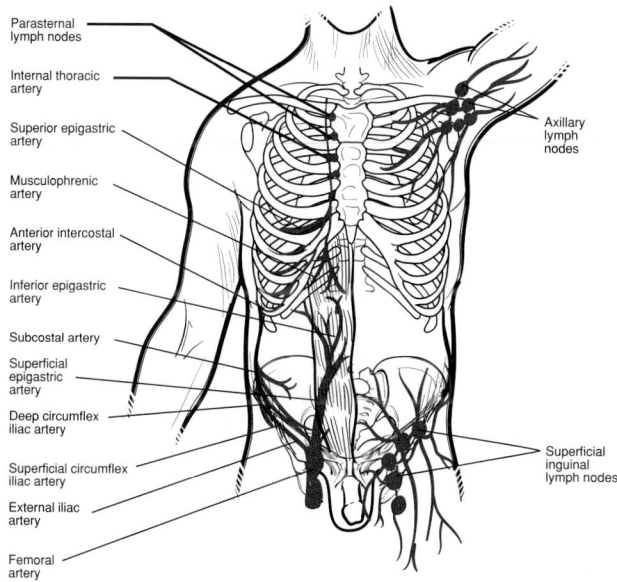

FIG. 34-4. The superior and inferior epigastric arteries form an anastomosing network of vessels in and around the rectus sheath, with collateralization to subcostal and lumbar vessels situated more laterally on the abdominal wall. Lymphatic drainage is via axially or inguinal nodal basins. *(Reproduced with permission from Moore KL, Dalley AF (eds): Clinically Oriented Anatomy, 4th ed. Philadelphia: Lippincott, Williams & Wilkins, 1999, p 86.)*

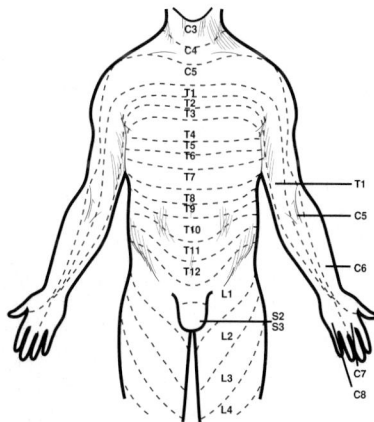

FIG. 34-5. Dermatomal sensory innervation of the abdominal wall. *(Reproduced with permission from Moore KL, Dalley AF (eds): Clinically Oriented Anatomy, 4th ed. Philadelphia: Lippincott, Williams & Wilkins, 1999, p 188.)*

During the third trimester, the vitelline duct regresses. Persistence of a vitelline duct remnant on the ileal border results in a *Meckel's diverticulum*. Complete failure of the vitelline duct to regress results in a *vitelline duct fistula*, which is associated with drainage of small intestinal contents from the umbilicus. If both the intestinal and umbilical ends of the vitelline duct regress into fibrous cords, a central *vitelline duct (omphalomesenteric) cyst* may occur. Persistent vitelline duct remnants between the gastrointestinal tract and the anterior abdominal wall may be associated with small intestinal volvulus in neonates. When diagnosed, vitelline duct fistulas and cysts should be excised along with any accompanying fibrous cord.

The urachus is a fibromuscular, tubular extension of the allantois that develops with the descent of the bladder to its pelvic position. Persistence of urachal remnants can result in cysts as well as fistulas to the urinary bladder, with drainage of urine from the umbilicus. These are treated by urachal excision and closure of any bladder defect that may be present.

Acquired Abnormalities

Rectus Abdominis Diastasis

Rectus abdominis diastasis (or diastasis recti) describes a clinically evident separation of the rectus abdominus muscle pillars, generally as a result of decreased tone of the abdominal musculature. The characteristic bulging of the abdominal wall in the epigastrium is sometimes mistaken for a ventral hernia, despite the fact that the midline aponeurosis is intact and no hernia defect is present. Diastasis may be congenital, as a result of a more lateral insertion of the rectus muscles to the ribs and costochondral junctions, but is more typically an acquired condition with advancing age, obesity, or following pregnancy. In the postpartum setting, rectus diastasis tends to occur in women of advanced maternal age, after multiple or twin pregnancies, or in women who deliver high-birth-weight infants. Diastasis is usually easily identified on physical examination (Fig. 34-6). Computed tomography (CT) scanning provides an accurate means of measuring the distance between the rectus pillars and will differentiate rectus diastasis from a true ventral hernia if clarification is required. Surgical correction of a severe rectus diastasis by plication of the anterior rectus sheath may be undertaken for

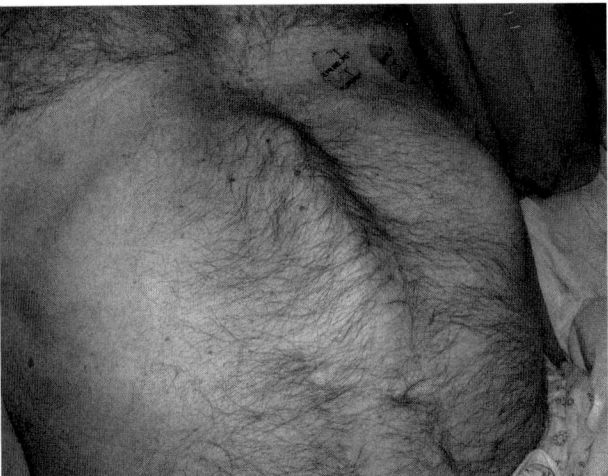

FIG. 34-6. Diastasis recti visible in the midepigastrium with Valsalva maneuver. The edges of the rectus abdominus muscle, rigid with voluntary contraction, are palpable the entire length of the bulging area. This should not be mistaken for a ventral hernia.

cosmetic indications, or if it is associated with disability of abdominal wall muscular function.

Rectus Sheath Hematoma

The terminal branches of the superior and inferior epigastric arteries course deep to the posterior aspect of the left and right rectus pillars and penetrate the posterior rectus sheath. Injury to these vessels or to any of the network of collateralizing vessels within the rectus sheath and muscles can result in a rectus sheath hematoma. Although there may be a history of significant blunt trauma, less-obvious events also have been reported to cause this condition, such as sudden contraction of the rectus muscles with coughing, sneezing, or any vigorous physical activity. Spontaneous rectus sheath hematomas have been described in the elderly and in those on anticoagulation therapy. Patients frequently describe the sudden onset of unilateral abdominal pain that may be confused with lateralized peritoneal disorders such as appendicitis. Below the arcuate line, a hematoma may cross the midline and cause bilateral lower quadrant pain.

History and physical examination alone may be diagnostic. Pain typically increases with contraction of the rectus muscles and a tender mass may be palpated. The ability to appreciate an intra-abdominal mass is ordinarily degraded with contraction of the rectus muscles. *Fothergill's sign* is a palpable abdominal mass that remains unchanged with contraction of the rectus muscles and is classically associated with rectus hematoma. A hemoglobin/hematocrit level and coagulation studies should be obtained. Abdominal ultrasonography may show a solid or cystic mass within the abdominal wall, depending on the chronicity of the bleeding event. Computed tomography is the most definitive study for establishing the correct diagnosis and excluding other intra-abdominal disorders. Magnetic resonance imaging (MRI) also has been employed for this purpose.

Specific treatment depends on the severity of the hemorrhage. Small, unilateral, and contained hematomas may be observed without hospitalization. Bilateral or large hematomas will likely require hospitalization, as well as potential resuscitation. The need for a red blood cell or coagulation factor transfusion is determined by the clinical circumstances. Reversal of warfarin (Coumadin) anticoagulation in the acute setting is frequently, but not always, necessary. Emergent operative intervention or angiographic embolization is required infrequently, but may be necessary if hematoma enlargement, free bleeding, or clinical deterioration occur. Surgical therapy consists of evacuation of the hematoma and ligation of any bleeding vessel identified. Mortality in this condition is rare, but has been reported in patients requiring surgical treatment and in the elderly.

Abdominal Wall Hernias

Hernias of the anterior abdominal wall, or *ventral* hernias, represent defects in the parietal abdominal wall fascia and muscle through which intra-abdominal or preperitoneal contents can protrude. Ventral hernias may be congenital or acquired. Acquired hernias may develop via slow architectural deterioration of the muscular aponeuroses or they may develop from failed healing of an anterior abdominal wall incision (*incisional hernia*). The most common finding is a mass or bulge on the anterior abdominal wall, which may increase in size with Valsalva. Ventral hernias may be asymptomatic or cause a considerable degree of discomfort, and generally enlarge over time. Physical examination reveals a bulge on the anterior abdominal wall that may reduce spontaneously, with recumbency, or with manual pressure. A hernia that cannot be reduced is described as *incarcerated* and will require emergent surgical correction. Incarceration of an intestinal segment may be accompanied by nausea, vomiting, and significant pain. Should the blood supply to the incarcerated bowel be compromised, the hernia is described as *strangulated*, and the localized ischemia may lead to infarction and perforation.

Primary ventral hernias (nonincisional) also are termed "true" ventral hernias. These are more properly named according to their anatomic location. *Epigastric* hernias are located in the midline between the xiphoid process and the umbilicus. They are generally small, may be multiple, and at elective repair, are usually found to contain omentum or a portion of the falciform ligament.

Umbilical hernias develop at the umbilical ring and may be present at birth or develop gradually during the life of the individual. Umbilical hernias are present in approximately 10% of all newborns and are more common in premature infants. Most congenital umbilical hernias close spontaneously by age 5 years. If closure does not occur by this time, elective surgical repair is usually advised. Adults with small, asymptomatic umbilical hernias may be followed clinically. Surgical treatment is offered if a hernia is observed to enlarge, is associated with symptoms, or if incarceration occurs. In the latter situation, emergent surgical treatment consisting of primary sutured repair is performed.

Spigelian hernias can occur anywhere along the length of the Spigelian line or zone—an aponeurotic band of variable width at the lateral border of the rectus abdominus. However, the most frequent location of these rare hernias is at or slightly above the level of the arcuate line. These are not always clinically evident as a bulge, and may come to medical attention because of pain or incarceration.

Patients with advanced liver disease, ascites, and umbilical hernia require special consideration. Enlargement of the umbilical ring usually occurs in this clinical situation as the result of increased intra-abdominal pressure from uncontrolled ascites. The first line of therapy is aggressive medical correction of the ascites with diuretics, dietary management, and paracentesis for tense ascites with respiratory compromise. These hernias usually are filled with ascitic fluid, but omentum or bowel may enter the defect after a large volume paracentesis. Uncontrolled ascites may lead to skin breakdown on the protuberant hernia and eventual ascitic leak, which can predispose the patient to bacterial peritonitis. Patients with refractory ascites may be candidates for transjugular intrahepatic portocaval shunting (TIPS), nonselective surgical portosystemic shunt, or liver transplantation. Umbilical hernia repair is best performed after the ascites is controlled.

Incisional hernias result from a healing failure of a prior abdominal wall surgical closure. Although estimates of incidence vary, careful investigation shows that they occur in at least 10 to 15% of all laparotomy incisions. Incisional hernias may be asymptomatic or present with pain, incarceration, or strangulation. Risk factors for the development of a ventral incisional hernia include postoperative wound infection, malnutrition, obesity, immunosuppression, and chronically increased intra-abdominal pressure.

Several techniques for the repair of ventral hernias have been described, including primary repair, open repair with mesh, and laparoscopic repair with mesh. Primary repair, even for small hernias (abdominal wall defects less than 3 cm), is associated with a high subsequent recurrence rate, often caused by failure to appreciate the multiple small defects that also are present. Investigators from the Netherlands prospectively compared primary and prosthetic mesh repairs in 200 patients with incisional hernias. After 3 years the cumulative recurrence rates for the primary suture and mesh repair groups were 43 and 24%, respectively. Identified risk factors for recurrence were primary suture repair, postoperative wound infection, prostatism, and surgery for abdominal aortic aneurysm. They concluded that mesh repair was superior to primary repair.

Open mesh repair of incisional hernias generally requires overlapping the prosthesis onto the anterior or posterior surfaces of intact abdominal wall fascia for a distance of at least 3 to 4 cm from defect edge. Peritoneum and hernia sac should be dissected away from all fascial defects. By one commonly performed method, a preperitoneal plane is developed to accommodate a large sheet of polypropylene or polyester (Mersilene) mesh. The mesh, which is isolated from peritoneal contents, is then secured to the fascia by using interrupted nonabsorbable sutures. Although polypropylene is an inert substance that induces no inflammatory response, eventual tissue ingrowth within the interstices of the mesh will result in dense attachment to whatever tissues it is in contact with. This effect is desired in a preperitoneal location, but when exposed to underlying bowel, the dense adhesions to mesh can lead to chronic abdominal pain, bowel obstruction, or fistulization. Polytetrafluoroethylene (PTFE) does not become incorporated into surrounding tissues in this way and does not induce dense adhesions to peritoneal structures such as intestine. It is therefore commonly used in intraperitoneal applications. New, commercially available prosthetic mesh materials make use of both polypropylene and PTFE on superficial and deep surfaces, respectively. Advantages to this type of prosthesis over either PTFE or polypropylene alone have not yet been established.

Minimally invasive repair of incisional hernias now is performed at least as frequently as open repair. The chief aim of laparoscopic repair is to reduce recurrence rates by eliminating the need for a large abdominal incision, when abdominal wall blood supply is already compromised. By this method, the entire undersurface of the wound can be examined, often revealing multiple defects that were not appreciated by physical examination. A recent multicenter trial has demonstrated a recurrence rate of only 3.4% over a mean follow-up time of 2 years. Of the recurrences noted, the vast majority were believed to be secondary to technical errors committed early in the surgeons' experience and were corrected during later cases.

The technique for laparoscopic repair generally involves laterally placed ports for midline defects and contralaterally placed ports for lateral defects. All adhesions to the anterior abdominal wall are divided, taking great care not to injure intestine either directly or with energy-delivery instruments. The contents of the hernia sac are completely reduced, but in contrast to open repairs, the sac itself is left in place. With the fascial edges of the hernia defect identified, an appropriate-size piece of PTFE or composite polypropylene/PTFE mesh is fashioned to allow sufficient overlap (i.e., 3 to 4 cm) onto healthy abdominal wall. After insertion into the abdomen, the prosthesis is fixed in place with transfascial sutures placed circumferentially around the mesh and spiral tacks according to surgeon preference (Fig. 34-7).

OMENTUM

Surgical Anatomy

The greater omentum and lesser omentum are fibrofatty aprons that provide support, coverage, and protection of peritoneal contents. These structures begin to develop during the fourth week of gestation. The greater omentum develops from the dorsal mesogastrium, which begins as a double-layered structure. The spleen develops in between the two layers, and later in development the two layers fuse, giving rise to the intraperitoneal spleen and the gastrosplenic ligament. The fused layers then hang from the greater curvature of the stomach and drape over the transverse colon, to which its posterior surface becomes fixed. The gastrocolic ligament and the gastrosplenic ligament are those segments of the greater omental

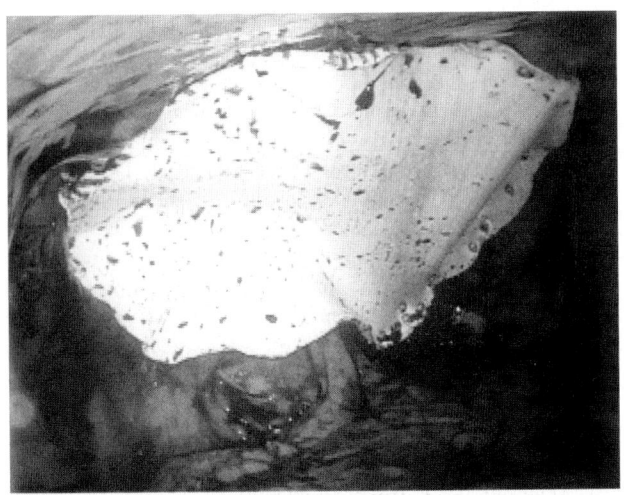

FIG. 34-7. Laparoscopic mesh placement for ventral incisional hernia.

apron that connect the named structures. In the adult, the greater omentum lies in between the anterior abdominal wall and the hollow viscera, and usually extends into the pelvis to the level of the symphysis pubis (Fig. 34-8).

The lesser omentum, otherwise known as the hepatoduodenal and hepatogastric ligaments, develops from the mesoderm of the septum transversum, which connects the embryonic liver to the foregut. The common bile duct, portal vein, and hepatic artery are located in the inferolateral margin of the lesser omentum, which also forms the anterior margin of the foramen of Winslow.

The blood supply to the greater omentum is derived from the right and left gastroepiploic arteries. The venous drainage parallels the arterial supply to a great extent with the left and right gastroepiploic veins ultimately draining into the portal system.

Physiology

In the early twentieth century, the British surgeon Rutherford Morison noted that the omentum tended to wall off areas of infection and limit the spread of intraperitoneal contamination. He termed the omentum the "abdominal policeman." Shortly after his description was published, several reports suggested intrinsic hemostatic characteristics of the omentum. In 1996, researchers from the Netherlands demonstrated that the concentration of tissue factor in omentum is over twice the amount per gram of that found in muscle. This facilitates activation of coagulation at sites of inflammation, ischemia, infection, or trauma within the peritoneal cavity.

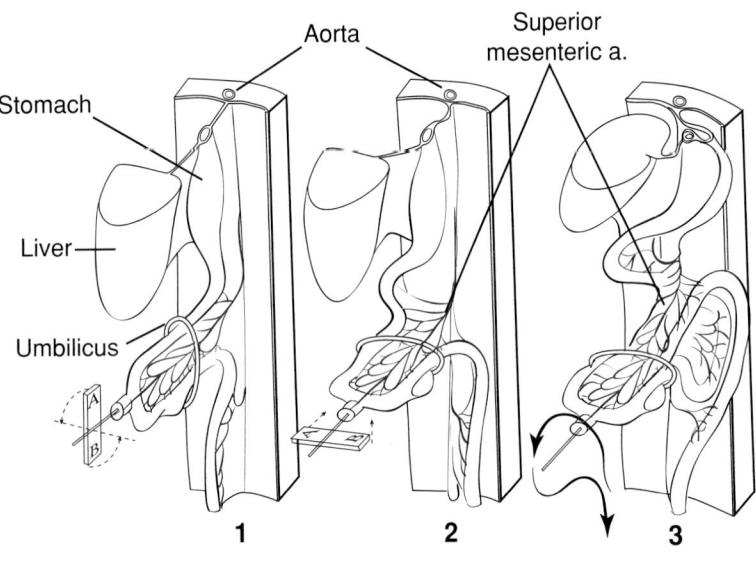

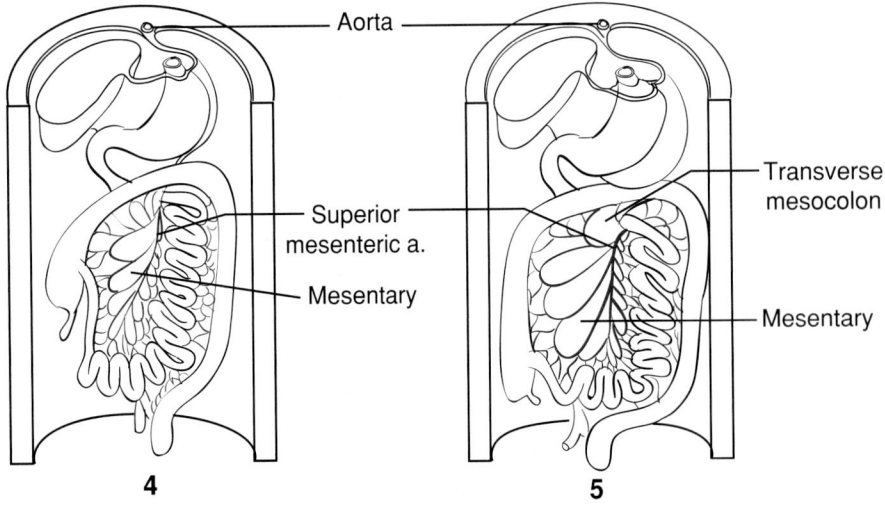

FIG. 34-8. Greater omentum draped over the small intestine. (*Reproduced with permission from Healy JE, Hodge J (eds): Surgical Anatomy, 2nd ed. Toronto: BC Decker, 1990, p 151.*)

The consequent local production of fibrin contributes to the ability of the omentum to adhere to areas of injury or inflammation.

Omental Infarction

Interruption of the blood supply to the omentum is a rare cause of an acute abdomen that may be secondary to torsion of the omentum around its vascular pedicle, thrombosis or vasculitis of the omental vessels, or omental venous outflow obstruction. Fewer than 100 cases have been reported in the literature, but the diagnosis is more likely to be made in male adults. Depending on the location of the infarcted omental tissue, this disease process may mimic appendicitis, cholecystitis, diverticulitis, perforated peptic ulcers, or ruptured ovarian cysts.

Patients typically present with localized right lower quadrant, right upper quadrant, or left lower quadrant pain. Although a mild degree of nausea may be present, patients do not usually have concomitant intestinal symptoms. Physical examination typically reveals a mild tachycardia and a low-grade temperature elevation. Abdominal examination may demonstrate a tender, palpable mass associated with guarding and rebound tenderness. The diagnosis is rarely made before abdominal imaging studies are obtained. Either abdominal computed tomography or ultrasonography will show a localized, inflammatory mass of fat density. Treatment of omental infarction depends on the certainty with which the diagnosis is made. In patients who are not toxic and whose abdominal imaging is convincing, supportive care is sufficient. However, many cases will be indistinguishable from suppurative appendicitis, cholecystitis, or diverticulitis. In these instances, laparoscopy has provided a great advance, providing access to an accurate diagnosis as well as treatment. Resection of the infarcted tissue results in rapid resolution of symptoms.

Omental Cysts

Cystic lesions of the omentum and mesentery are related disorders, likely resulting from lymphatic degeneration. Omental cysts are far less common than mesenteric cysts. Omental cysts may present as an asymptomatic abdominal mass, or it may cause abdominal pain or distention. Physical examination reveals a freely mobile intraabdominal mass. Both computed tomography and abdominal ultrasound reveal a well-circumscribed, cystic-mass lesion arising from the greater omentum. Treatment involves resection of all symptomatic omental cysts. Resection of these benign lesions is easily accomplished via laparoscopic techniques.

Omental Neoplasms

Primary tumors of the omentum are uncommon. Benign tumors of the omentum include lipomas, myxomas, and desmoid tumors. Because the omentum is derived from mesoderm, primary malignant tumors of the omentum are considered sarcomas. Liposarcomas, leiomyosarcomas, rhabdomyosarcomas, fibrosarcomas, and mesotheliomas have all been described. Metastatic tumors involving the omentum are quite common. Metastatic ovarian tumors have a high preponderance of omental involvement. Malignant tumors of the stomach, small intestine, colon, pancreas, biliary tract, uterus, and kidney may also metastasize to the omentum.

MESENTERY

Surgical Anatomy

The mesentery develops from mesenchyme that attaches the foregut, midgut, and hindgut to the posterior abdominal wall. During embryonic maturation, this mesenchyme forms the dorsal mesentery.

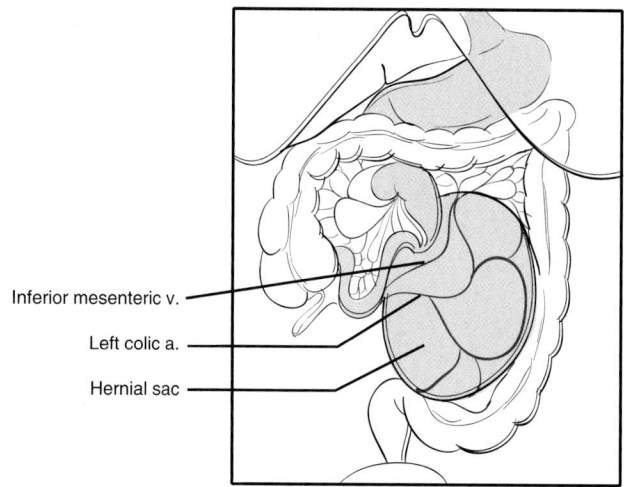

FIG. 34-9. Anatomic relationships of intestinal mesentery to the retroperitoneum following completion of intestinal rotation during fetal development. *(Reproduced with permission from Healey JE, Hodge J (eds): Surgical Anatomy, 2nd ed. Toronto: BC Decker, 1990, p 153.)*

In the region of the stomach, the dorsal mesentery becomes the greater omentum, whereas in the region of the jejunum and ileum the dorsal mesentery becomes the mesentery proper. In the region of the colon, the dorsal mesentery is known as the mesocolon. During embryonic development, after the 270-degree counterclockwise rotation of the herniated midgut, the reduced mesentery achieves its final fixation state. The segments at the duodenum, ascending colon, and descending colon become fixed to the retroperitoneum, whereas the small intestinal mesentery, transverse colon mesentery, and to a variable extent, the sigmoid colon mesentery remain mobile (Fig. 34-9). Rotational disorders of the intestine and its mesentery are discussed in Chap. 38.

The root of the small intestinal mesentery wall normally courses in an oblique direction, from the left upper quadrant at the ligament of Treitz to the right lower quadrant at the ileocecal valve and the fixed cecum. The small and large intestinal mesenteries serve as the major pathway for arterial, venous, lymphatic, and neural structures coursing to and from the bowel. Anatomic anomalies of the mesentery related to rotational disorders can lead to paraduodenal or mesocolic hernias, which can present as chronic or acute intestinal obstruction in children or adults.

Sclerosing Mesenteritis

Sclerosing mesenteritis, also referred to as mesenteric panniculitis or mesenteric lipodystrophy, is a rare chronic inflammatory and fibrotic process that involves a portion of the intestinal mesentery. There is no gender or race predominance, but sclerosing mesenteritis is most commonly diagnosed in individuals older than 50 years of age.

The etiology of this process is unknown, but its cardinal features are a nonneoplastic mesenteric mass and varying relative quantities of fibrosis and chronic inflammation on histologic examination. The mass may be up to 40 cm in diameter. Accordingly, patients typically present with symptoms of a mass lesion. Abdominal pain is the most frequent presenting symptom, followed by the presence of a nonpainful mass or intestinal obstruction.

Computed tomography of the abdomen will verify the presence of a mass lesion emanating from the mesentery. CT cannot distinguish sclerosing mesenteritis from a primary or secondary mesenteric tumor (Fig. 34-10). Surgical intervention is usually necessary, if only to establish a diagnosis and rule out malignancy (Fig. 34-11).

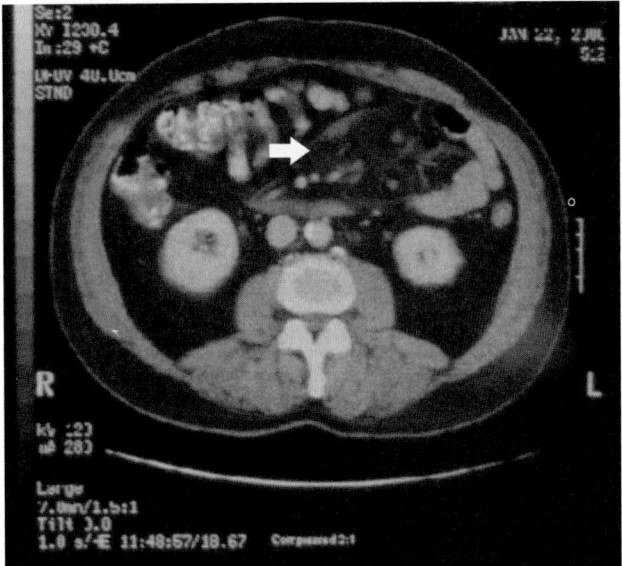

FIG. 34-10. CT scan of sclerosing mesenteritis (mesenteric lipodystrophy). This condition cannot easily be distinguished from a neoplasm of the mesentery on radiologic study. In this case, the study showed "fatty mesenteric tumor with involvement of mesenteric vessels," and mesenteric lipodystrophy only was demonstrated at exploration.

The extent of the disease process dictates the aggressiveness of the intervention, which may range from simple biopsy, to bowel and mesentery resection, to colostomy (in the cases of colonic obstruction).

Mesenteric Cysts

Cysts of the mesentery are benign lesions with an incidence of less than one in 100,000. Since its first description in 1507, approximately 1000 cases have been described in the literature. The etiology of such cysts remains unknown, but several theories regarding their development exist, including degeneration of the mesenteric lymphatics or simply arising as a congenital anomaly.

Mesenteric cysts may be asymptomatic or can cause symptoms of a mass lesion. Symptoms may be acute or chronic. Acute

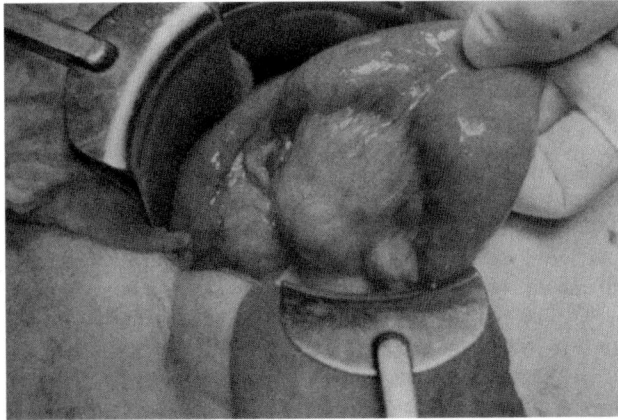

FIG. 34-11. Focal mesenteric lipodystrophy: Operative findings at the time of resection of what was believed to be a mesenteric tumor. This condition mimics a mesenteric neoplasm in its appearance, but may involve extensive segments of small intestinal mesentery, which is often the most significant item of information suggesting the actual diagnosis.

abdominal pain secondary to a mesenteric cyst is generally caused by rupture or torsion of the cyst or from acute hemorrhage into the cyst. Mesenteric cysts may also cause chronic intermittent abdominal pain secondary to compression of adjacent structures or spontaneous torsion followed by detorsion of the cyst. Mesenteric cysts can be the cause of nonspecific symptoms such as anorexia, nausea, vomiting, fatigue, and weight loss.

Physical examination may reveal a mass lesion that is mobile only from the patient's right to left or left to right (Tillaux's sign), in contrast to the findings with omental cysts, which should be freely mobile in all directions. Tillaux was the first to record this physical finding and, in 1850, the first to successfully remove a mesenteric cyst.

Computed tomography (Fig. 34-12), abdominal ultrasound, and magnetic resonance imaging all have been used to evaluate patients with mesenteric cysts. Each of the aforementioned imaging modalities reveal a cystic structure without a solid component in the central abdomen. These are generally unilocular, but may, on occasion, be multiple or multilocular. Irrespective of the imaging method used, it may be difficult to distinguish these cystic masses from rare solid mesenteric tumors with cystic components such as a cystic stromal tumor or mesothelioma. Mesenteric cystic lymphangioma may present as numerous, often large cysts in the setting of abdominal pain. These can be difficult to treat and almost invariably recur after excision.

When symptomatic, simple mesenteric cysts are surgically excised either openly or laparoscopically when feasible. Cyst unroofing or marsupialization is not recommended, as mesenteric cysts have a high propensity to recur after drainage alone. On rare occasions, adjacent mesentery may be densely adherent to the cyst or mesenteric vessels must be sacrificed in order to achieve complete excision, in which case segmental bowel resection is performed.

Mesenteric Tumors

Primary tumors of the mesentery are rare. Benign tumors of the mesentery include lipoma, cystic lymphangioma, and desmoid tumors. As described for omentum, primary malignant tumors of the mesentery are considered sarcomas. Liposarcomas, leiomyosarcomas, malignant fibrous histiocytomas, lipoblastomas, and lymphangiosarcomas have all been described. Metastatic small intestinal carcinoid in mesenteric lymph nodes may exceed the bulk of primary disease and compromise blood supply to the bowel. Treatment of mesenteric malignancies involves wide resection of the mass. Because of the proximity to the blood supply to the intestine, such resections may be technically unfeasible, or involve loss of substantial lengths of bowel.

RETROPERITONEUM

Surgical Anatomy

Although there are ectodermal, mesodermal, and endodermal contributions to the contents of the retroperitoneum, embryonic mesoderm predominates in the developing retroperitoneal space. From the *intermediate* mesoderm arise the organs of the urinary and genital systems. The *lateral plate* mesoderm eventually divides into two layers, the parietal layer and the visceral layer. These layers eventually become the pleura, pericardium, peritoneum, and retroperitoneum.

The retroperitoneum is defined as the space between the posterior envelopment of the peritoneum and the posterior body wall (Fig. 34-13). The retroperitoneal space is bounded superiorly by

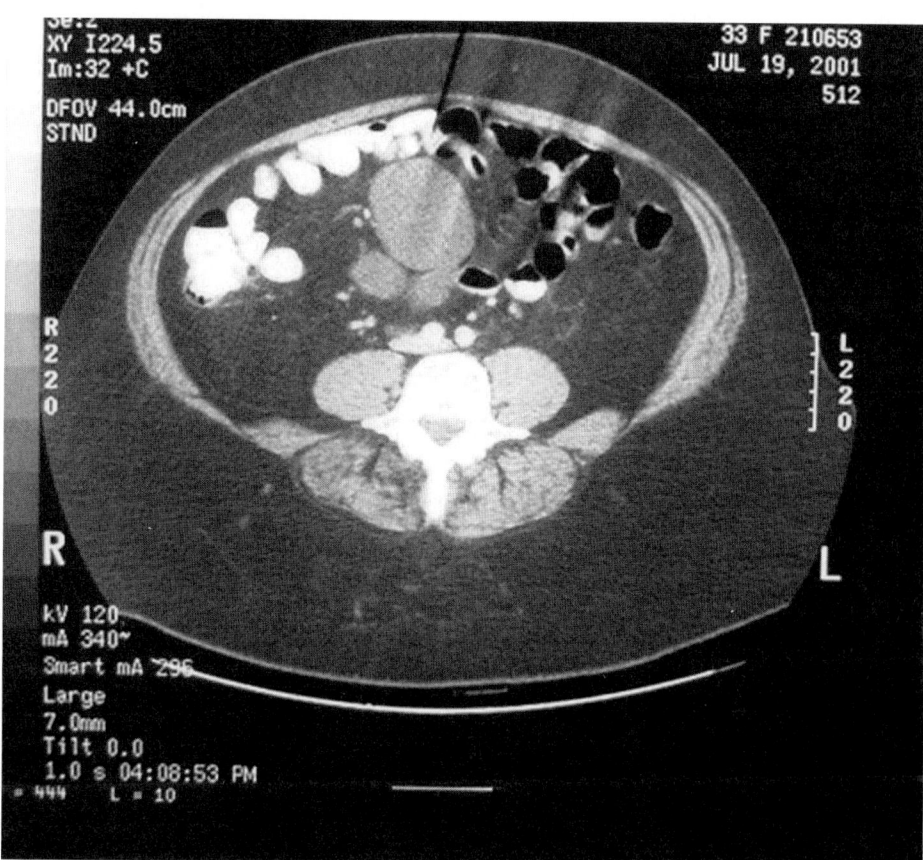

FIG. 34-12. *CT scan of a mesenteric cyst. Unilocular appearance without associated solid component strongly suggests the diagnosis of benign cyst.*

the diaphragm, posteriorly by the spinal column and iliopsoas muscles, and inferiorly by the levator ani muscles. Although technically bounded anteriorly by the posterior reflection of the peritoneum, the anterior border of the retroperitoneum is quite convoluted, extending into the spaces in between the mesenteries of the small and large intestine. Because of the rigidity of the superior, posterior, and inferior boundaries, and the compliance of the anterior margin, retroperitoneal tumors tend to expand anteriorly toward the peritoneal cavity. Table 34-1 lists the organs and structures that reside within the retroperitoneum.

Retroperitoneal Infections

The posterior reflection of the peritoneum limits the spread of most intra-abdominal infections into the peritoneum. Accordingly, the source of retroperitoneal infections is usually an organ contained within or abutting the retroperitoneum. Retrocecal appendicitis, perforated duodenal ulcers, pancreatitis, or diverticulitis may all lead to retroperitoneal infection with or without abscess formation. The substantial space and rather nondiscrete boundaries of the retroperitoneum allow some retroperitoneal abscesses to become quite large prior to diagnosis.

Patients with a retroperitoneal abscess usually present with pain, fever, and malaise. The site of the patient's pain may be variable and can include the back, pelvis, or thighs. Clinical findings can include tachypnea and tachycardia. Erythema may be observed around the umbilicus or flank. This is analogous to the ecchymosis seen in these locations after massive retroperitoneal hemorrhage (Cullen's sign or Grey Turner's sign, respectively.) A palpable flank or abdominal mass may be present. Laboratory evaluation usually reveals an elevated white blood cell count. The diagnostic imaging

modality of choice is CT, which may demonstrate stranding of the retroperitoneal soft tissues and/or a unilocular or multilocular collection (Fig. 34-14).

Management of retroperitoneal infections includes identification and treatment of the underlying condition, intravenous antibiotics, and drainage of all well-defined collections. While unilocular abscesses may be drained percutaneously under CT guidance, multilocular collections usually require operative intervention for adequate drainage. Because of the vastness of the retroperitoneal space, patients with retroperitoneal abscesses do not usually present until the abscess is advanced. Consequently, the mortality rate of retroperitoneal abscess, even when drained, has been reported to be as high as 25%, or even higher in rare cases of necrotizing fasciitis of the retroperitoneum.

Retroperitoneal Fibrosis

Retroperitoneal fibrosis is a class of disorders characterized by hyperproliferation of fibrous tissue in the retroperitoneum. This may be a primary disorder as in idiopathic retroperitoneal fibrosis, also known as Ormond's disease, or a secondary reaction to an inciting inflammatory process, malignancy, or medication. Idiopathic retroperitoneal fibrosis is a rare disorder, usually affecting 0.5 patients per 100,000 annually. Men are twice as likely to be affected as women, with no predilection for any particular ethnic group. The disease primarily affects individuals in the fourth to the sixth decades of life.

An allergic or autoimmune mechanism has been postulated for this condition. Circulating antibodies to ceroid, a lipoproteinaceous by-product of vascular atheromatous plaque oxidation, are present in more than 90% of patients with retroperitoneal fibrosis. The

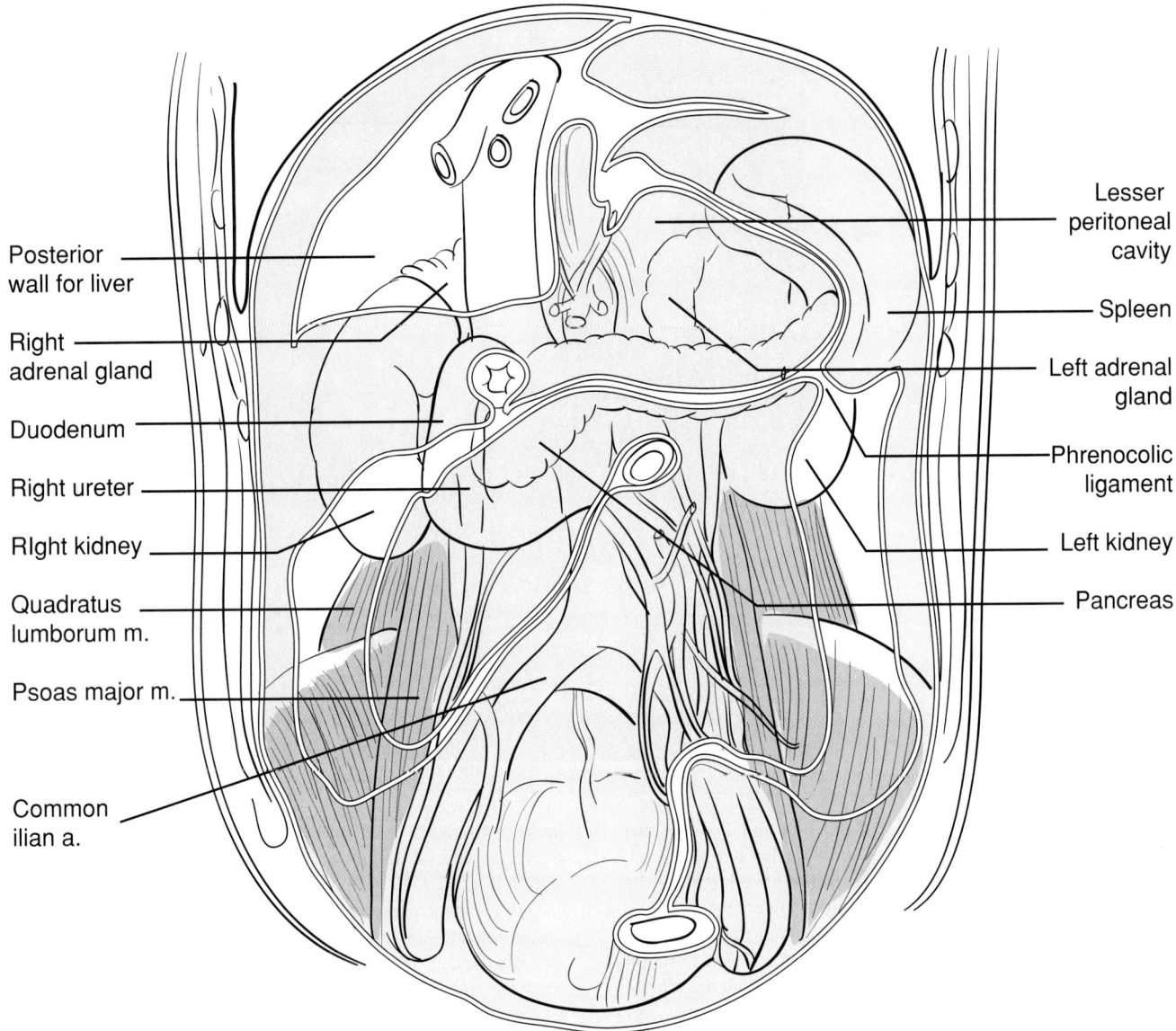

FIG. 34-13. Anatomy of the retroperitoneum. (*Reproduced with permission from Healey JE, Hodge J (eds): Surgical Anatomy, 2nd ed. Toronto: BC Decker, 1990, p 201.*)

relationship of this finding to the occurrence of fibrosis remains uncertain. The early inflammatory reaction is predominated by T-helper cells, plasma cells, and macrophages, but is subsequently replaced by collagen-synthesizing fibroblasts. Microscopically, the infiltrate is indistinguishable from the periadventitial involvement of aortic aneurysmal disease, Riedel's thyroiditis, sclerosing cholangitis, and Peyronie's disease. The fibrotic process begins in the retroperitoneum just below the level of the renal arteries. Fibrosis gradually expands, encasing the ureters, inferior vena cava, aorta,

mesenteric vessels, or sympathetic nerves. Bilateral involvement is noted in 67% of cases.

Retroperitoneal fibrosis may also occur secondary to a variety of inflammatory conditions or as an allergic reaction to a medication. This condition is known to occur in patients with abdominal aortic aneurysms, chronic pancreatitis, histoplasmosis, tuberculosis, or actinomycosis. It also is associated with a variety of malignancies (i.e., prostate, non-Hodgkin's lymphoma, sarcoma, carcinoid tumors, and gastric cancer) and autoimmune disorders (i.e.,

Table 34-1
Retroperitoneal Structures

Kidneys	Ureters	Bladder
Pancreas	Duodenum (D2 and D3)	Adrenal glands
Ascending colon	Descending colon	Rectum (upper two thirds)
Aorta	Inferior vena cava	Iliac vessels
Seminal vesicles	Vas deferens	Lymphatics (cysterna chyli)
Vagina (upper most)	Ovaries	Nerves (lumbar sympathetics)

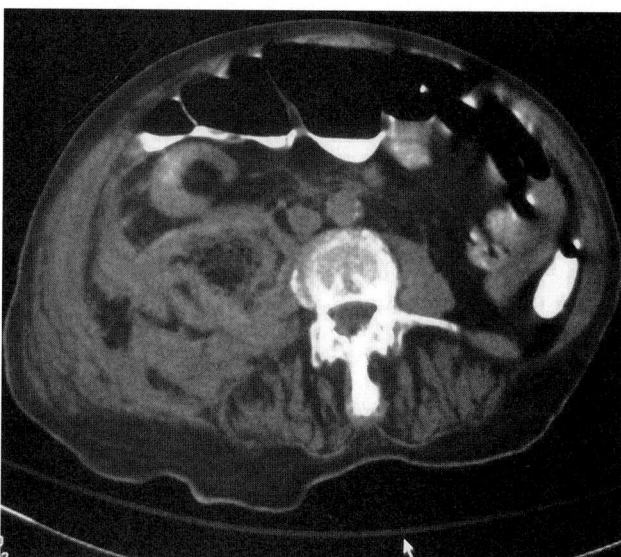

FIG. 34-14. CT scan of retroperitoneal abscess complicating complex, surgically treated retroperitoneal infection that had resulted from ampullary perforation at the time of endoscopic retrograde cholangiopancreatography. This pattern of infection may be difficult to treat and results in multiple interventions such as percutaneous drainage before resolution.

ankylosing spondylitis, systemic lupus erythematosus, Wegener's granulomatosis, and polyarteritis nodosa). The strongest case for a causal relationship between certain medications and retroperitoneal fibrosis is that of methysergide, a semisynthetic ergot alkaloid used in the treatment of migraine headaches. Other medications that have been linked to retroperitoneal fibrosis include beta blockers, hydralazine, and α-methyldopa. Entacapone, a relatively new medication that inhibits catechol-O-methyltransferase (COMT) and is used as an adjunct with levodopa in the treatment of Parkinson's disease, also has been implicated. The retroperitoneal fibrosis regresses upon discontinuation of these medications.

Presenting symptoms depend on the structure or structures affected by the fibrotic process. Initially, patients complain of the insidious onset of dull, poorly localized abdominal pain. Sudden-onset or severe abdominal pain may signify acute mesenteric ischemia. Other symptoms of retroperitoneal fibrosis may include unilateral leg swelling, intermittent claudication, oliguria, hematuria, or dysuria.

As with the patient's symptomatology, findings on physical examination vary with the retroperitoneal structure involved. Consequently, findings may include hypertension, the palpation of an abdominal or flank mass, lower-extremity edema (unilateral or bilateral), or diminished lower-extremity pulses (unilateral or bilateral). Laboratory evaluation may reveal an elevated blood urea nitrogen and/or creatinine levels. As with many autoimmune inflammatory processes, the erythrocyte sedimentation rate almost always is elevated in patients with retroperitoneal fibrosis.

Many imaging modalities have been used with various sensitivities to diagnose retroperitoneal fibrosis. Abdominal/lower extremity ultrasonography is the least-invasive imaging procedure, but is technician-dependent. It may be useful if iliocaval compressive or renal symptoms predominate. A lower-extremity ultrasound may show deep venous thrombosis, while abdominal ultrasonography may identify a mass lesion or hydronephrosis. Once the diagnostic procedure of choice, intravenous pyelography (IVP) is less

commonly used today. If the ureters are involved, IVP findings include ureteral compression, ureteral deviation toward the midline, and hydronephrosis.

Currently, the imaging procedure of choice for patients with retroperitoneal fibrosis is CT. Abdominal CT imaging will show the size and extent of the fibrotic process. If the patient has diminished renal function, the lack of intravenous contrast will reduce the distinction between retroperitoneal tissue planes. In this case, MRI is the procedure of choice. The signal intensity of the fibrotic process is discrete from muscle or fat. Additionally, MRI angiography will accurately assess the degree of iliocaval involvement. Once a mass lesion is identified, the mass should be biopsied to rule out a retroperitoneal malignancy. The specimen may be retrieved using image-guided techniques, laparoscopic retroperitoneal biopsy, or rarely, via laparotomy.

Once malignancy, drug-induced, and infectious etiologies are ruled out, treatment of the retroperitoneal fibrotic process is instituted. Corticosteroids, with or without surgery, is the mainstay of medical therapy. Surgical debulking, ureterolysis, or ureteral stenting is required in patients who present with moderate or massive hydronephrosis. All patients with iliocaval thrombosis will require at least 6 months of oral anticoagulation. Medical therapy is initiated with prednisone (60 mg every other day, for 2 months). Following this initial therapy, prednisone is gradually tapered off over the next 2 months. Therapeutic efficacy is assessed on the basis of patient symptomatology, erythrocyte sedimentation rate, and diagnostic imaging. Cyclosporine, tamoxifen, or azathioprine may be used to treat patients who are recalcitrant to the above regimen.

The overall prognosis in idiopathic retroperitoneal fibrosis is excellent, with 5-year survival rates of 90 to 100%. As long-term recurrences have been described, lifelong follow-up is warranted.

Bibliography

General References
Bendavid R, Abrahamson J, Arregui ME, et al (eds): *Abdominal Wall Hernias: Principles and Management,* 1st ed. New York: Springer-Verlag, 2001.
Nyhus LM, Condon RE (eds): *Hernia,* 4th ed. Philadelphia: J. B. Lippincott, 1995.
Skandalakis LJ, Colborn GL: Surgical anatomy of the abdominal wall, in Bendavid R (ed): *Prostheses and Abdominal Wall Hernias.* Austin, TX: RG Landes, 1994.
Zinner MJ, Schwartz SI, Ellis H (eds): *Maingot's Abdominal Operations,* 10th ed. Stamford, CT: Appleton and Lange, 1997.
Zuidema GD (ed): *Shackelford's Surgery of the Alimentary Tract,* 4th ed. Philadelphia: W. B. Saunders, 1996.

Abdominal Wall
Anthony T, Bergen PC, et al: Factors affecting recurrence following incisional herniorrhaphy. *World J Surg* 24:95, 2000.
Bendavid R: Composite mesh (polypropylene-e-PTFE) in the intraperitoneal position: A report of 30 cases. *Hernia* 1:5, 1997.
Edlow J, Juang P, et al: Rectus sheath hematoma. *Ann Emerg Med* 34:671, 1999.
Heniford BT, Park A, et al: Laparoscopic ventral and incisional hernia repair in 407 patients. *J Am Coll Surg* 190:645, 2000.
Hesselink VJ, Luijendijk R, et al: An evaluation of risk factors in incisional hernia recurrence. *Surg Gynecol Obstet* 176:228, 1993.
Klinger PJ, Wetcher G, et al: The use of ultrasound to differentiate rectus sheath hematoma from other acute abdominal disorders. *Surg Endosc* 13:1129, 1999.
Koehler RH, Voeller G: Recurrences in laparoscopic incisional hernia repairs: A personal series and review of the literature. *J Soc Laparoendo Surg* 2:221, 1998.

LeBlanc KA: Current consideration in laparoscopic incisional and ventral herniorrhaphy. *J Soc Laparoendo Surg* 4:131, 2000.

Luijendijk R, Hop W, et al: A comparison of suture repair with mesh repair for incisional hernia. *N Engl J Med* 343:392, 2000.

Mudge M, Hughes LE: Incisional hernia: A 10-year prospective study of incidence and attitudes. *Br J Surg* 72:70, 1985.

Park A, Birch DW, Lovrics P: Laparoscopic and open incisional hernia repair: A comparison study. *Surgery* 124:816, 1998.

Perry CW, Phillips BJ: Rectus sheath hematoma: Review of an uncommon surgical complication. *Hosp Physician* 37:35, 2001.

Ramshaw BJ, Esartia P, et al: Comparison of laparoscopic and open ventral herniorrhaphy. *Am Surg* 65:827, 1999.

Stoppa R, Ralaimiaramanana F, Henry X, et al: Evolution of large ventral incisional hernia repair: The French contribution to a difficult problem. *Hernia* 3:1, 1999.

Zainea GG, Jordan F: Rectus sheath hematomas: Their pathogenesis, diagnosis, and management. *Am Surg* 54:630, 1988.

Omentum

Beelen RHJ: The greater omentum: Physiology and immunological concepts. *Neth J Surg* 43:145, 1991.

Fukatsu K, Saito H, Han I, et al: The greater omentum is the primary site of neutrophil exudation in peritonitis. *J Am Coll Surg* 183:450, 1996.

Goldsmith HS (ed): *The Omentum: Research and Clinical Applications.* New York: Springer-Verlag, 2000.

Liebermann-Meffert D: The greater omentum. Anatomy, embryology, and surgical applications. *Surg Clin North* Am 80:275, 2000.

Liebermann-Meffert D, White H (eds): *The Greater Omentum. Anatomy, Physiology, Pathology, Surgery with an Historical Survey.* New York: Springer-Verlag, 1983.

Logmans A, Schoenmakers CHH, et al: High tissue factor concentration in the omentum, a possible cause of its hemostatic properties. *Eur J Clin Invest* 26:82, 1996.

Morison R: Remarks on some functions of the omentum. *Br Med J* 1:76, 1906.

O'Leary DP: Use of the greater omentum in colorectal surgery. *Dis Colon Rectum* 42:533, 1999.

Powers JC, Fitzgerald JF, McAlvanah MJ: The anatomical basis for the surgical detachment of the greater omentum from the transverse colon. *Surg Gynecol Obstet* 143:105, 1976.

Saborido BP, Romero CJ, et al: Idiopathic segmental infarction of the greater omentum as a cause of acute abdomen. Report of two cases and review of the literature. *Hepatogastroenterology* 48:737, 2001.

Schwartz RW, Reames M, et al: Primary solid neoplasms of the greater omentum. *Surgery* 109:543, 1990.

Sompayrac SW, Mindelzun RE, et al: The greater omentum. *Am J Roentgenol* 168:683, 1997.

Mesentery

Durst AL, Freund H, et al: Mesenteric panniculitis: Review of the literature and presentation of cases. *Surgery* 81:203, 1977.

Egozi EI, Ricketts RR: Mesenteric and omental cysts in children. *Am Surg* 63:287, 1997.

Emory T, Monihan J, et al: Sclerosing mesenteritis, mesenteric panniculitis, and mesenteric lipodystrophy. *Am J Surg Pathol* 21:392, 1997.

Genereau T, Bellin MF, et al: Demonstration of efficacy of combining corticosteroids and colchicine in two patients with idiopathic sclerosing mesenteritis. *Dig Dis Sci* 41:684, 1996.

Hebra A, Brown MF, et al: Mesenteric, omental and retroperitoneal cysts in children: A clinical study of 22 cases. *South Med J* 86:173, 1993.

Kelly JK, Hwang WS: Idiopathic retractile (sclerosing) mesenteritis and its differential diagnosis. *Am J Surg Pathol* 13:513, 1989.

Kurtz RJ, Heimann TM, et al: Mesenteric and retroperitoneal cysts. *Ann Surg* 203:109, 1986.

Kurzweg FT, Daron PB, et al: Mesenteric cysts. *Am J Surg* 40:462, 1974.

O'Brien MF, Winter DC, et al: Mesenteric cysts—A series of six cases with a review of the literature. *Ir J Med Sci* 168:233, 1999.

Ogden WW, Bradburn DM, Rives JD: Panniculitis of the mesentery. *Ann Surg* 151:659, 1960.

Ros PR, Olmsted WW, et al: Mesenteric and omental cysts: Histologic classification with imaging correlation. *Radiology* 164:327, 1987.

Shamiyeh A, Rieger R, Schrenk P, et al: Role of laparoscopic surgery in treatment of mesenteric cysts. *Surg Endosc* 13:937, 1999.

Takiff H, Calabria R, et al: Mesenteric cysts and intra-abdominal cystic lymphangiomas. *Arch Surg* 120:1266, 1985.

Retroperitoneum

Cerfolio RJ, Morgan AS, et al: Idiopathic retroperitoneal fibrosis: Is there a role for postoperative steroids? *Curr Surg* 47:423, 1990.

Gilkeson GS, Allen NB: Retroperitoneal fibrosis. A true connective tissue disease. *Rheum Dis Clin North Am* 22:23, 1996.

Higgins PM, Bennett-Jones DN, et al: Non-operative management of retroperitoneal fibrosis. *Br J Surg* 75:573, 1988.

Kardar AH, Kattan S, et al: Steroid therapy for idiopathic retroperitoneal fibrosis: Dose and duration. *J Urol* 168:550, 2002.

Koep L, Zuidema GD: The clinical significance of retroperitoneal fibrosis. *Surgery* 81:250, 1977.

Kottra JJ, Reed DN: Retroperitoneal fibrosis. *Radiol Clin North Am* 34:1259, 1996.

Marzano A, Trapani A, et al: Treatment of idiopathic retroperitoneal fibrosis using cyclosporine. *Ann Rheum Dis* 60:427, 2001.

Ormond JK: Bilateral ureteral obstruction due to envelopment and compression by an inflammatory process. *J Urol* 59:1072, 1948.

Pryor JP, Piotrowski E, et al: Early diagnosis of retroperitoneal necrotizing fasciitis. *Crit Care Med* 29:1071, 2001.

Rhee RY, Gloviczki P, et al: Iliocaval complications of retroperitoneal fibrosis. *Am J Surg* 168:179, 1994.

Uchida K, Okazaki K, et al: Case of chronic pancreatitis involving an autoimmune mechanism that extended to retroperitoneal fibrosis. *Pancreas* 26:92, 2003.

Woodburn KR, Ramsay G, et al: Retroperitoneal necrotizing fasciitis. *Br J Surg* 79:342, 1992.

CHAPTER 35

Soft Tissue Sarcomas

Janice N. Cormier and Raphael E. Pollock

INTRODUCTION

Incidence

Sarcomas are a heterogeneous group of tumors that arise predominantly from the embryonic mesoderm, but also can originate, as does the peripheral nervous system, from the ectoderm. In 2002, approximately 8300 new cases of soft tissue sarcoma were diagnosed in the United States.[1] These rare tumors account for less than 1% of cancers in adults and represent 7% of cancers in children.[2] Several distinct groups of sarcomas are recognized. Soft tissue sarcomas, the largest of these groups, is the focus of this chapter. Other groups include bone sarcomas (osteosarcomas and chondrosarcomas), Ewing's sarcomas, and peripheral primitive neuroectodermal tumors.

Soft tissue sarcomas can occur throughout the body and encompass more than 50 histiotypes (Table 35-1). Most primary soft tissue sarcomas originate in an extremity (59%); the next most common sites are the trunk (19%), retroperitoneum (13%), and head and neck (9%).[3] The most common histologic types of soft tissue sarcoma in adults (excluding Kaposi's sarcoma) are malignant fibrous histiocytoma (28%), leiomyosarcoma (12%), liposarcoma (15%), synovial sarcoma (10%), and malignant peripheral nerve sheath tumors (6%).[4,5] Rhabdomyosarcoma is the most common soft tissue sarcoma of childhood.[6]

Epidemiology

Except for malignant peripheral nerve sheath tumors in patients with neurofibromatosis, sarcomas do not seem to result from the progression or dedifferentiation of benign soft tissue tumors. Despite the variety of histologic subtypes, sarcomas have many common clinical and pathologic features. Overall the clinical behavior of most soft tissue sarcomas is similar and is determined by anatomic location (depth), grade, and size.[7] The dominant pattern of metastasis is hematogenous. Lymph node metastases are rare (<5%) except for a few histologic subtypes such as epithelioid sarcoma, rhabdomyosarcoma, clear-cell sarcoma, and angiosarcoma.[8]

Radiation Exposure

External radiation therapy is a well-established risk factor for soft tissue sarcoma. An eight- to 50-fold increase in the incidence of sarcomas has been reported among patients treated for cancer of the

Table 35-1
Relative Frequency of Histologic Subtypes of Soft Tissue Sarcoma

Histologic Subtypes	n	%
Malignant fibrous histiocytoma	349	28
Liposarcoma	188	15
Leiomyosarcoma	148	12
Unclassified sarcoma	140	11
Synovial sarcoma	125	10
Malignant peripheral nerve sheath tumor	72	6
Rhabdomyosarcoma	60	5
Fibrosarcoma	38	3
Ewing's sarcoma	25	2
Angiosarcoma	25	2
Osteosarcoma	14	1
Epithelioid sarcoma	14	1
Chondrosarcoma	13	1
Clear cell sarcoma	12	1
Alveolar soft part sarcoma	7	1
Malignant hemangiopericytoma	5	0.4

SOURCE: Reproduced with permission from Coindre et al.[4]

breast, cervix, ovary, testes, and lymphatic system.[9,10] In a review of 160 patients with postirradiation sarcomas, the most common histologic types were osteogenic sarcoma, malignant fibrous histiocytoma, angiosarcoma, and lymphangiosarcoma.[9] In that study, the risk of developing a sarcoma increased with higher radiation doses, and the median latency period was 10 years. Postirradiation sarcomas are usually diagnosed at advanced stages and generally have a poor prognosis.[10]

Occupational Chemicals

Exposure to some herbicides such as phenoxyacetic acids and wood preservatives containing chlorophenols has been linked to an increased risk of soft tissue sarcoma.[11,12] Several chemical carcinogens, including thorium oxide (Thoratrast), vinyl chloride, and arsenic, have been associated with hepatic angiosarcomas.

Trauma

Although patients with sarcomas often report a history of trauma, no causal relationship has been established. More often, a minor injury calls attention to a preexisting tumor that may be accentuated by an edema or a hematoma.

Chronic Lymphedema

In 1948, Stewart and Treves first described the association between chronic lymphedema after axillary dissection and subsequent lymphangiosarcoma.[13] Lymphangiosarcoma also has been described after filarial infections and in the lower extremities of patients with congenital or heritable lymphedema.[14]

Genetics

Specific inherited genetic alterations are associated with an increased risk of bone and soft tissue sarcomas. New developments in the field of molecular biology have led to better understanding of the basic cellular processes governed by oncogenes and tumor suppressor genes.

Oncogene Activation. Oncogenes are genes that can induce malignant transformation and tend to drive cells toward proliferation. Several oncogenes have been identified in association with soft tissue sarcomas, including *MDM2, N-myc, c-erbB2,* and members of the *ras* family. These oncogenes produce specific oncoproteins that either play a role in nuclear function and cellular signal transduction or function as growth factors or growth factor receptors. Amplification of these genes has been shown to correlate with adverse outcome in several soft tissue sarcomas.[15]

Cytogenetic analysis of soft tissue tumors has identified distinct chromosomal translocations that seem to encode for oncogenes associated with certain histologic subtypes. These specific genetic changes result in the in-frame fusion of genes and the fused product codes for the expression of oncoproteins that function as transcriptional activators or repressors.[16] The best characterized gene rearrangements are found in Ewing's sarcoma (*EWS—FLI-1* fusion), clear-cell sarcoma (*EWS—ATF1* fusion), myxoid liposarcoma (*TLS—CHOP* fusion), alveolar rhabdomyosarcoma (*PAX3—FHKR* fusion), desmoplastic small round-cell tumor (*EWS—WT1* fusion), and synovial sarcoma (*SSX—SYT* fusion).[17] The oncogenic potential of many of these genes has been demonstrated in vitro and in vivo.

Tumor Suppressor Genes. Tumor suppressor genes play a critical role in growth inhibition and can suppress growth in cancer cells. Inactivation of tumor suppressor genes (also known as *antioncogenes*) can occur through hereditary or sporadic mechanisms. The two genes that are most relevant to soft tissue tumors are the retinoblastoma (*Rb*) tumor suppressor gene and the *p53* tumor suppressor gene. Mutations or deletions in *Rb* can lead to development of retinoblastoma or sarcomas of soft tissue and bone. Mutations in the *p53* tumor suppressor gene are the most common mutations in human solid tumors and have been reported in 30 to 60% of soft tissue sarcomas.[18,19] Patients with germline mutations in the tumor suppressor gene *p53* (the Li-Fraumeni syndrome) have a high incidence of sarcomas. Mutant *p53* expression is thought to correlate with overall survival.[15] The *p53* mutation also has been used as a therapeutic molecule in gene therapy strategies.

Neurofibromatosis is a neurocutaneous condition of which two types exist. Neurofibromatosis type 1, also known as von Recklinghausen's disease, occurs in approximately 1 of every 3000 persons, and is due to various mutations in the *NF-1* tumor suppressor gene located on chromosome 17. Patients with neurofibromatosis type 1 have an estimated 3 to 15% additional lifetime risk of malignant disease which includes neurofibrosarcoma. Fifty percent of patients with neurofibrosarcomas have a mutation in *NF-1*.[20]

INITIAL ASSESSMENT

Clinical Presentation

Soft tissue sarcoma most commonly presents as an asymptomatic mass. The size at presentation is usually associated with the location of the tumor. Smaller tumors are generally located in the distal extremities, whereas tumors in the proximal extremities and retroperitoneum can grow quite large before becoming apparent. Often an extremity mass is discovered after a traumatic event that draws attention to a preexisting lesion. Soft tissue sarcomas often grow in a centrifugal fashion and compress surrounding normal structures. Infrequently, their impingement on bone or neurovascular bundles produces pain, edema, and swelling. Retroperitoneal soft tissue sarcoma almost always presents as a large asymptomatic mass. Infrequently, patients may present with obstructive gastrointestinal symptoms or neurologic symptoms related to compression of lumbar or pelvic nerves.

The differential diagnosis of a soft tissue mass includes benign lesions including lipomas, lymphangiomas, leiomyomas, and neuromas. In addition to sarcomas, other malignant lesions such as primary or metastatic carcinomas, melanomas, or lymphomas must be considered. Small lesions that have not changed for several years by clinical history may be closely observed. All other tumors should be considered for biopsy to establish a definitive diagnosis.

Diagnostic Imaging

Pretreatment radiologic imaging serves several purposes; it defines the local extent of a tumor, can be used to stage malignant disease, assists in percutaneous biopsy procedures, and aids in the diagnosis of soft tissue tumors (benign versus malignant or low grade versus high grade). Imaging studies also are crucial in monitoring tumor changes after treatment, especially preoperative chemotherapy or radiation therapy, and in detecting recurrences after surgical resection.[21]

Radiographs provide useful information on primary bone tumors but they are not useful in the evaluation of soft tissue sarcomas of the extremities unless underlying bone involvement from an adjacent soft tissue tumor is suspected.[21] Chest radiography should be performed for patients with primary sarcomas to assess for lung metastases. For patients with high-grade lesions or tumors larger than 5 cm (T2), computed tomography of the chest should be considered.

Computed tomography (CT) is the preferred technique for evaluating retroperitoneal sarcomas,[22] whereas magnetic resonance imaging (MRI) is often favored for soft tissue sarcomas of the extremities.[23,24] Both ultrasonography and computed tomography can assist in guiding fine-needle aspiration or core biopsy for initial diagnosis or at recurrence.

Ultrasonography

Ultrasonography may have a diagnostic role for patients who cannot undergo magnetic resonance imaging. Ultrasonography can also be a useful adjunct to magnetic resonance imaging when findings are indeterminate and for delineating adjacent vascular structures.[25]

Computed Tomography

Contrast-enhanced CT can assess the extent of soft tissue tumor burden and proximity of the tumor to vital structures. Computed tomography is the preferred imaging technique for evaluating retroperitoneal sarcomas.[22] Current CT techniques can provide a detailed survey of the abdomen and pelvis and delineate adjacent organs and vascular structures.[26] For extremity sarcomas, CT may be useful if MRI is not available or cannot be used. CT of the abdomen and pelvis should be done when histologic assessment of an extremity sarcoma reveals a myxoid liposarcoma, because this subtype is known to metastasize to the abdomen.[27]

Magnetic Resonance Imaging

MRI accurately delineates muscle groups and distinguishes among bone, vascular structures, and tumor. Sagittal and coronal views allow evaluation of anatomic compartments in three dimensions (Fig. 35-1A and B). Soft tissue sarcomas of the extremities usually present on MRI as heterogeneous masses. Their signal intensity tends to be equal to or slightly higher than that of adjacent skeletal muscle on T1-weighted images, and heterogeneous and high on T2-weighted images. Hemorrhagic and cystic or necrotic changes may be seen in the tumor.[23] Special MRI techniques, including magnetic resonance angiography, may be performed if adjacent vascular structures must be delineated.

MRI has supplanted CT as the imaging technique of choice for evaluation of soft tissue sarcomas of the extremities.[23,24] MRI is also valuable for assessing tumor recurrence after surgery (Fig. 35-2). A baseline image is usually obtained 3 months after surgery. Some clinicians believe that routine postoperative imaging of a primary extremity tumor site is not necessary for asymptomatic patients, whereas others advocate routine imaging every 6 months for the first 2 years, citing the difficulties in detecting early recurrence in scarred, irradiated tissue.[22]

MRI may be an important adjunct to cytologic analysis in distinguishing benign lesions such as lipomas, hemangiomas, schwannomas, neurofibromas, and intramuscular myxomas from their malignant counterparts.[21] In the setting of preoperative chemotherapy, contrast-enhanced T1-weighted MRIs can be used to evaluate intratumoral necrosis.

Biopsy Techniques

Fine-Needle Aspiration

Fine-needle aspiration is an acceptable method of diagnosing most soft tissue sarcomas, particularly when the results correlate closely with clinical and imaging findings.[28] However, fine-needle aspiration biopsy is indicated for primary diagnosis of soft tissue sarcomas only at centers where cytopathologists have experience with these types of tumors. Fine-needle aspiration biopsy is also the procedure of choice to confirm or rule out the presence of a metastatic focus or local recurrence. If tumor grading is essential for treatment planning, fine-needle aspiration biopsy is not the technique of choice.

Superficial lesions are often subjected to fine-needle aspiration biopsies in the clinic setting. Deeper tumors may require an interventional radiologist to perform the technique under sonographic or CT guidance. The technique generally involves the use of a 21- to 23-gauge needle that is introduced into the mass after appropriate cleansing of the skin and injection of local anesthetic. Negative pressure is applied, and the needle is pulled back and forth several times in various directions. After the negative pressure is released, the needle is withdrawn and the contents of the needle are used to prepare a smear.[29] A cytopathologist then examines the slides to determine whether sufficient diagnostic material is present. If insufficient diagnostic material is obtained, a core-needle biopsy should be performed.

Diagnostic accuracy rates for fine-needle aspiration biopsy of primary tumors range from 60 to 96%.[30] In general, the amount of material obtained from a fine-needle aspiration biopsy is small and diagnostic accuracy clearly depends on the experience of the cytopathologist.

Core-Needle Biopsy

Core-needle biopsy is a safe, accurate, and economical diagnostic procedure for diagnosing sarcomas. The tissue sample obtained from a core-needle biopsy is usually sufficient for several diagnostic tests such as electron microscopy, cytogenetic analysis, and flow cytometry. The reported complication rate for core-needle biopsy is less than 1%.[31]

CT guidance can enhance the positive yield rate of a core-needle biopsy by more accurately pinpointing the location of the tumor. Precise localization in the tumor mass is particularly important to avoid sampling nondiagnostic necrotic or cystic areas of the tumor.

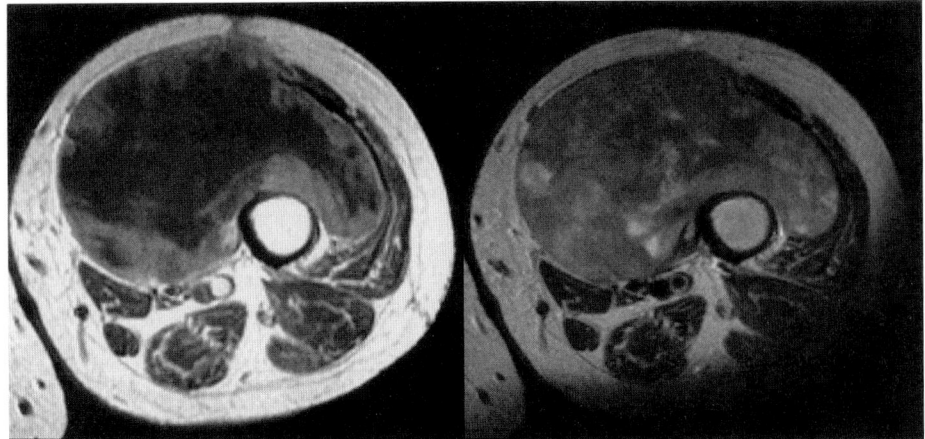

A

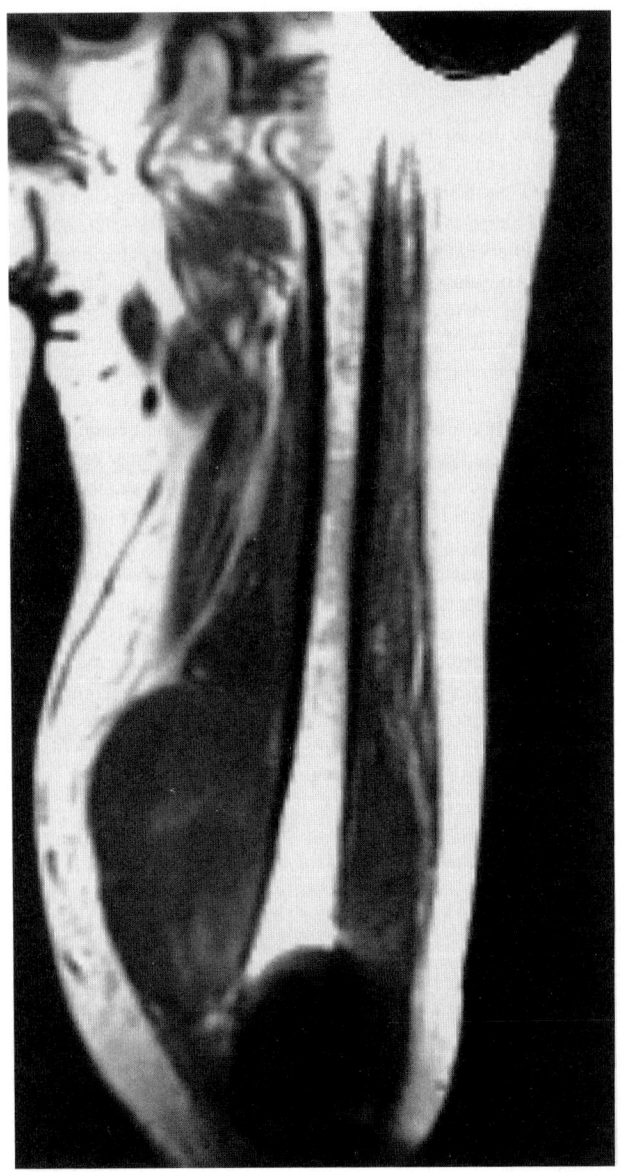

B

FIG. 35-1. *A.* A 77-year-old woman presented with T2 high-grade sarcoma of left thigh. MRI of the left lower extremity demonstrating a 12.6 x 9.7 x 15 cm thigh sarcoma. T1-weighted postcontrast image demonstrating nodular areas of peripheral enhancement with low signal centrally, which may represent hemorrhage and/or necrosis. The mass partially encases the femur (220°) and there is thinning of the anterior femoral cortex along most of the length of the mass, indicating bone involvement. *B.* Coronal image demonstrating the mass extending from the proximal to mid-diaphysis to just above the knee prosthesis.

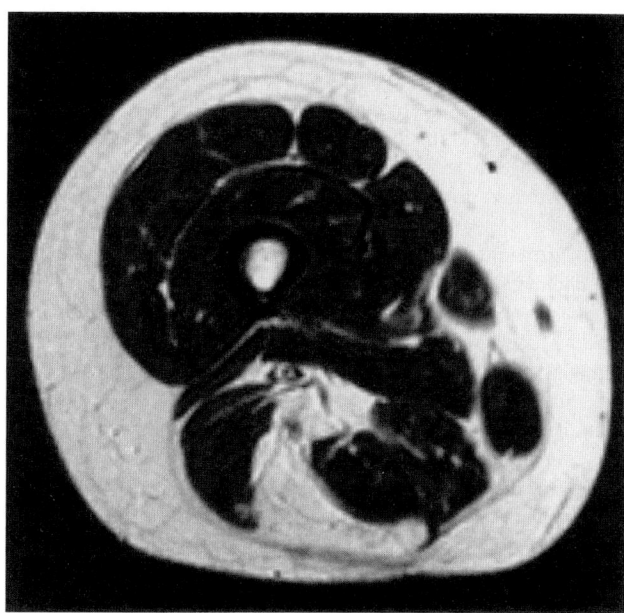

FIG. 35-2. A 48-year-old woman, 6 months status postexcision of an atypical lipomatous tumor of the right thigh. MRI of the thigh demonstrating a 4.8 x 4.5 cm recurrent lipomatous tumor in the posterior musculature of the right thigh.

CT guidance also permits access to tumors in otherwise inaccessible anatomic locations or near vital structures.

Dupuy and colleagues examined the accuracy of core-needle biopsy in 221 patients with musculoskeletal neoplasms.[31] Core-needle biopsy had an accuracy of 93% compared with the diagnosis given at the time of definitive treatment. Only 8% of patients had nondiagnostic or insufficient specimens.

Incisional Biopsy

Open biopsy is a reliable diagnostic method that allows adequate tissue to be sampled for definitive and specific histologic identification of bone or soft tissue sarcomas. When adequate tissue for diagnosis cannot be obtained by fine-needle aspiration biopsy or core biopsy, an incisional biopsy is indicated for deep tumors or for superficial soft tissue tumors larger than 3 cm. Because open biopsies may have complications, incisional biopsies are usually performed as a last resort when fine-needle aspiration or core biopsy specimens are nondiagnostic. Open biopsies should be performed only by surgeons experienced in the management of soft tissue sarcomas. In a series of 107 patients with soft tissue sarcomas, planned surgical

treatments had to be changed due to prior, poorly-oriented biopsies in 25% of the cases.[32] Other series have reported complications in up to 16% of open biopsies.[29]

An open biopsy ideally should be performed in a designated treatment center and by the surgeon who will perform the definitive surgery.[29] The biopsy incision should be oriented longitudinally along the extremity to allow a subsequent wide local excision that encompasses the biopsy site, scar, and tumor en bloc (Fig. 35-3). A poorly-oriented biopsy incision often mandates an excessively large surgical defect for a wide local excision, which in turn can result in a larger postoperative radiotherapy field to encompass all tissues at risk. Another mandate of surgical technique is that adequate hemostasis must be achieved at the time of biopsy to prevent dissemination of tumor cells into adjacent tissue planes by hematoma.

An incisional or open biopsy is the most reliable of the diagnostic methods, providing accurate histologic diagnosis and grading in more than 95% of soft tissue sarcomas. In addition, the amount of tissue obtained is often sufficient for additional diagnostic studies if necessary.[29]

Excisional Biopsy

Excisional biopsy can be performed for easily accessible (superficial) extremity or truncal lesions smaller than 3 cm. Excisional biopsy should not be done for lesions involving the hands and feet because definitive reexcision may not be possible after the biopsy. Excisional biopsy results have a 30 to 40% rate of recurrence when margins are positive or uncertain. Excisional biopsies rarely provide any benefit over other biopsy techniques and may cause postoperative complications that could ultimately delay definitive therapy.

Pathologic Classification

Some experts have suggested that pathologic classification of soft tissue sarcomas has more prognostic significance than does tumor grade when other pretreatment variables are taken into account (Fig. 35-4). Tumors with limited metastatic potential include desmoids, atypical lipomatous tumors (also called *well-differentiated liposarcoma*), dermatofibrosarcoma protuberans, and hemangiopericytomas. Tumors with an intermediate risk of metastatic spread usually have a large myxoid component and include myxoid liposarcoma, myxoid malignant fibrous histiocytoma, and extraskeletal chondrosarcoma. Among the highly aggressive tumors that have substantial metastatic potential are angiosarcomas, clear-cell sarcomas, pleomorphic and dedifferentiated liposarcomas, leiomyosarcomas, rhabdomyosarcomas, and synovial sarcomas.

FIG. 35-3. *A.* An appropriately placed surgical biopsy about the lateral aspect of the elbow. *B.* At the time of definitive tumor resection, the biopsy track is excised en bloc with the tumor specimen.

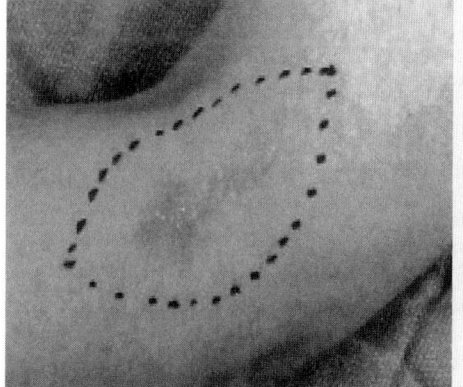

A

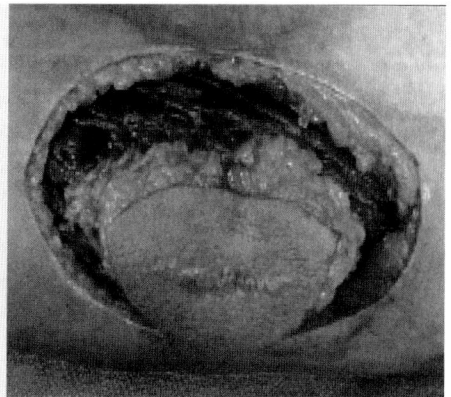

B

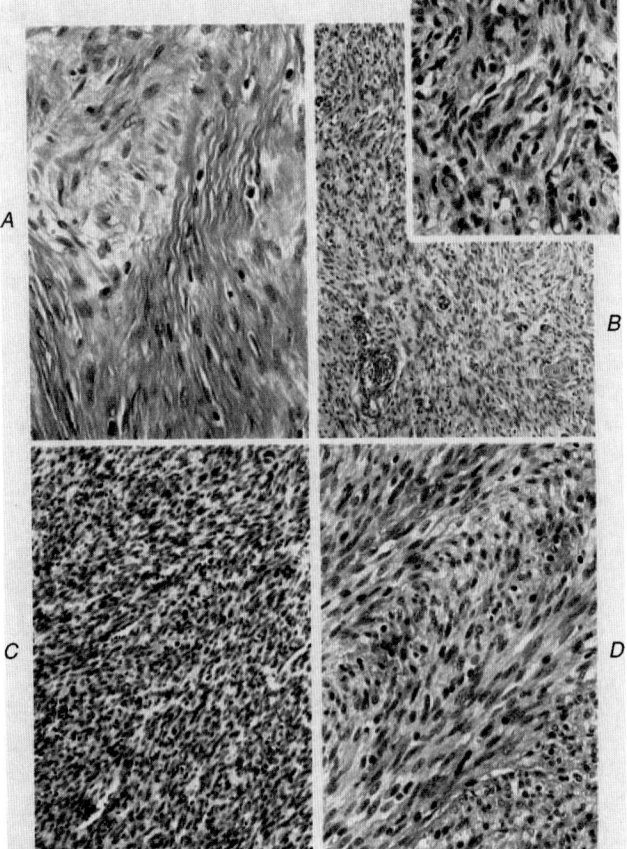

FIG. 35-4. Fibrous lesions. *A.* Desmoid fibromatosis, with bundles of elongated spindle-shaped cells surrounded by large amounts of collagen. *B.* Dermatofibrosarcoma protuberans, showing short intersecting fascicles of fibroblastic cells. Inset shows higher magnification (x400) with elongated fibroblasts exhibiting nuclear hyperchromasia and minimal pleomorphism. *C.* Infantile fibrosarcoma, showing densely packed short spindle-shaped neoplastic cells. *D.* Adult fibrosarcoma, with fibroblastic cells oriented in interlacing fascicles referred to as herringbone pattern.

Expert sarcoma pathologists disagree about the specific histologic diagnoses and the criteria for defining tumor grade in 25 to 40% of individual cases.[33–36] The high rate of discordance emphasizes the need for more objective molecular and biochemical markers to improve conventional histologic assessment.

Staging and Prognostic Factors

The current version of the American Joint Committee on Cancer staging criteria for soft tissue sarcomas relies on histologic grade, tumor size and depth, and the presence of distant or nodal metastases (Table 35-2).[37] This system does not apply to visceral sarcomas, Kaposi's sarcomas, dermatofibrosarcomas, or desmoid tumors.

Histologic Grade

Histologic grade remains the most important prognostic factor for patients with sarcomas. For an accurate determination of tumor grade, an adequate tissue sample must be appropriately fixed, stained, and reviewed by an experienced sarcoma pathologist. The features that define grade are cellularity, differentiation, pleomorphism, necrosis, and the number of mitoses. Tumor grade has been shown to predict the development of metastases and overall survival.[15,38] Coindre and associates found metastatic potentials of

5 to 10% for low-grade lesions, 25 to 30% for intermediate-grade lesions, and 50 to 60% for high-grade tumors.[38]

The number of grades varies according to the classification system used. The most commonly used classification systems, those of the National Cancer Institute[39] and the French Federation of Cancer Centers,[40] use three tumor grades. The National Cancer Institute system is based primarily on histologic tumor type, location, and the amount of necrosis. The French Federation of Cancer Centers system generates a score based on tumor differentiation, mitotic rate, and the amount of tumor necrosis. A comparative analysis of the two grading systems suggested that the French Federation of Cancer Centers system may have better prognostic capability predicting 5-year survival rates of 90%, 70%, and 40% for grade 1, 2, and 3 tumors, respectively.[40]

In the 2002 American Joint Committee on Cancer staging system, four tumor grades are designated: well differentiated (G1), moderately differentiated (G2), poorly differentiated (G3), and undifferentiated (G4). In this four-tiered system, grades 1 and 2 are considered "low grade" and grades 3 and 4 are considered "high grade."[37]

Tumor Size

Tumor size has long been recognized to be an important prognostic variable in soft tissue sarcomas. Sarcomas have classically been stratified into two groups on the basis of size; T1 lesions are 5 cm or smaller and T2 lesions are larger than 5 cm. Some authors have suggested that further stratification of patients on the basis of tumor size can provide more accurate prognostic information. For example, when 316 patients with soft tissue sarcomas were examined and grouped in four tumor-size subgroups (<5 cm, 5 to 10 cm, 10 to 15 cm, and >15 cm), each subgroup was found to have a different prognosis, and the respective 5-year survival rates were 84%, 70%, 50%, and 33%.[5]

The prognostic significance of anatomic tumor location with respect to its association with the investing fascia of the extremity or trunk was incorporated into the American Joint Committee on Cancer staging system in 1998.[41] Soft tissue sarcomas above the superficial investing fascia of the extremity or trunk are designated "a" lesions in the T score, whereas tumors invading or deep to the fascia as well as all retroperitoneal, mediastinal, and visceral tumors are designated "b" lesions.

Nodal Metastasis

Lymph node metastasis of soft tissue sarcomas is rare; less than 5% manifest nodal spread.[42] A few histologic subtypes, including rhabdomyosarcoma, epithelioid sarcoma, and malignant fibrous histiocytoma, have a higher incidence of nodal involvement. Nodal disease is designated as stage IV disease.

Distant Metastasis

Distant metastases occur most often in the lungs. Selected patients with pulmonary metastases may survive for long periods after surgical resection and chemotherapy. Other potential sites of metastasis include bone, the brain, and the liver. Visceral and retroperitoneal sarcomas have a higher incidence of liver and peritoneal metastases.

TREATMENT

Accurate preoperative histologic diagnosis is critical in choosing a primary treatment strategy for soft tissue sarcomas. Presentation

Table 35-2
American Joint Committee on Cancer

Primary Tumor (T)						
T1	Tumor ≤5 cm					
	T1a Superficial tumor					
	T1b Deep tumor					
T2	Tumor >5 cm					
	T2a Superficial tumor					
	T2b Deep tumor					
Regional Lymph Nodes (N)						
N0	No regional lymph node metastasis					
N1	Regional lymph node metastasis					
Distance Metastasis (M)						
M0	No distant metastasis					
M1	Distant metastasis					
Histologic Grade (G)						
G1	Well differentiated					
G2	Moderately differentiated					
G3	Poorly differentiated					
G4	Poorly differentiated or undifferentiated					
Stage Grouping						
Stage I	T1a, 1b, 2a, 2b		N0	M0	G1–2	G1
Stage II	T1a, 1b, 2a		N0	M0	G3–4	G2–3
Stage III	T2b		N0	M0	G3–4	G2–3
Stage IV	Any T		N1	M0	Any G	Any G
	Any T		N0	M1	Any G	Any G

SOURCE: Reproduced with permission from AJCC.[37]

with gross disease after incisional biopsy, core-needle biopsy, or fine-needle aspiration biopsy allows the treatment planning team the best opportunity to evaluate the tumor's proximity to vital structures and the likelihood of being able to perform surgical resection with negative histologic margins. In addition, the tumor can serve as a biologic marker of response if patients are to be enrolled in neoadjuvant treatment protocols.

In the past 2 decades, a multimodality treatment approach has improved survival and quality of life for patients with extremity sarcomas. For soft tissue sarcomas of the extremities, a multidisciplinary approach to management, including margin-negative resection plus radiotherapy to the tumor bed, has resulted in local control rates up to and exceeding 90%.[43] However, patients with abdominal sarcomas continue to have high rates of recurrence and poor overall survival.[44–46] The overall 5-year survival rate for all stages of soft tissue sarcomas is 50 to 60%. Most patients die of metastatic disease, which becomes evident within 2 to 3 years of initial diagnosis in 80% of cases.[2]

Surgery

Small (<5 cm) primary tumors with no evidence of distant metastatic disease are managed by local therapy consisting of surgery, alone or in combination with radiation therapy, when wide pathologic margins are limited because of anatomic constraints. The type of surgical resection is determined by several factors, including tumor location, tumor size, depth of invasion, involvement of nearby structures, need for skin grafting or autogenous tissue reconstruction, and the patient's performance status. In 1985, the National Institutes of Health developed a consensus statement recommending limb-sparing surgery for most patients with high-grade extremity sarcomas.[47] However, for patients whose tumor cannot be grossly resected with a limb-sparing procedure and

preservation of function (<5%), amputation remains the treatment of choice.[48]

Margin status after surgical resection has been shown to be an independent prognostic factor.[49,50] Patients with microscopically positive surgical margins have an increased risk of local failure; however, neither a positive surgical margin nor local failure has been shown to adversely affect overall survival.[51] These data should be factored into the management plan if achieving clear surgical margins requires amputation or substantial functional compromise of an extremity.[51]

Wide Local Excision

Wide local excision is the primary treatment strategy for extremity sarcomas. The goal of local therapy for extremity sarcomas is to resect the tumor with a 2-cm margin of surrounding normal soft tissue. The tumors are generally surrounded by a zone of compressed reactive tissue that forms a pseudocapsule, which may mistakenly guide resection (enucleation) by an inexperienced surgeon. Extensions of tumor that go beyond the pseudocapsule must be considered in planning surgery and radiotherapy. In some anatomic areas, negative margins cannot be attained because of the tumor's proximity to vital structures. The biopsy site or tract (if applicable) should also be included en bloc with the resected specimen.

Wide en bloc excision is seldom performed as a diagnostic procedure. When it is done for this purpose, the margin status is often not adequately evaluated in the pathologic assessment of the specimen. Unless detailed descriptions of the surgical procedure and the pathology specimen are provided, the margins should be classified as uncertain or unknown, a classification that carries the same prognosis as resection margins that are positive for tumor cells. In this setting, reexcision should be performed if possible to ensure negative margins.

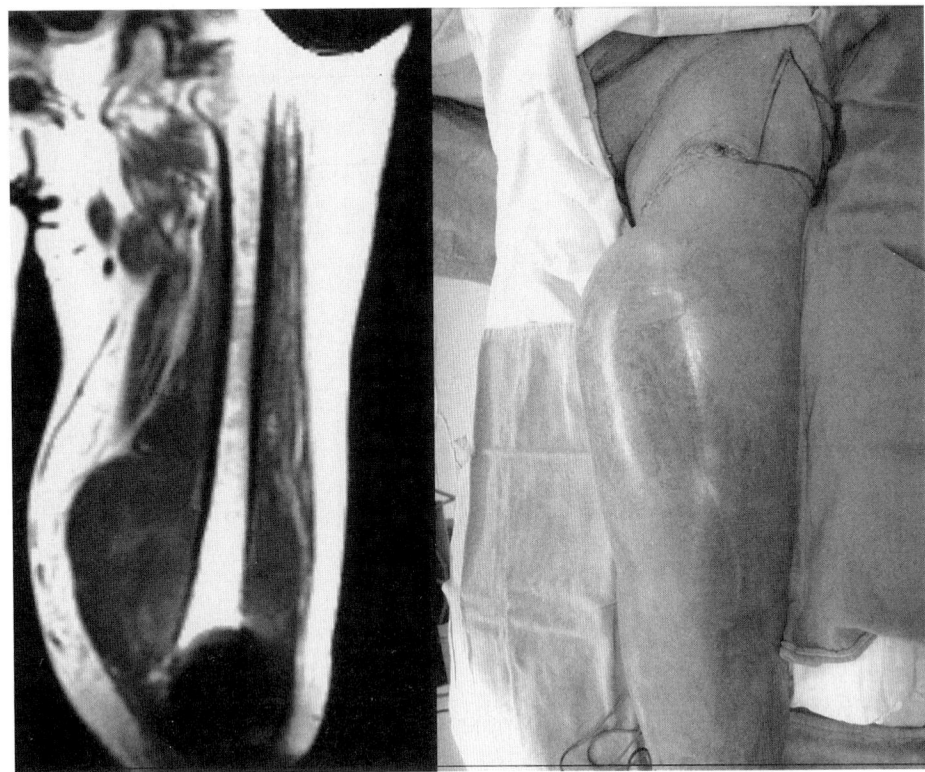

FIG. 35-5. Preparation for an above-knee amputation of a 12.6 cm distal thigh high-grade malignant fibrous histiocytoma.

Elective lymphadenectomy is rarely indicated for patients with soft tissue sarcomas. However, for patients with rhabdomyosarcoma or epithelioid sarcoma with suspicious clinical or radiologic findings, fine-needle aspiration biopsy of the lymph nodes should be considered. In these rare cases, lymph node dissection may be indicated for regional control of disease. A prospective trial is currently under way to evaluate the role of lymphatic mapping and sentinel lymph node biopsy in pediatric patients with extremity rhabdomyosarcomas.

The probability of local recurrence in the absence of appropriate surgery or combination treatment with surgery and radiation is greater than 50%. With modern surgical and radiotherapy techniques, rates of limb preservation and local control have improved. A currently reported local failure rate of 10% after appropriate treatment is typical for soft tissue sarcomas of the extremity. Karakousis and colleagues demonstrated that amputation was not required, even for patients with locally advanced tumors involving major vessels.[52] In their retrospective review of 21 patients, en bloc tumor resection with vascular reconstruction was performed safely, and rates of local recurrence and 5-year survival were similar to those for patients who did not require vessel resection.

Amputation

Amputation is the treatment of choice for patients with the rare 5% of tumors that cannot be grossly resected with a limb-sparing procedure and preservation of function (Fig. 35-5).[48] Historically, local excision of soft tissue sarcomas has resulted in local failure rates of 50 to 70%, even when a margin of normal tissue around the tumor was excised. As a consequence, radical resection or amputation has become the standard treatment. Because sarcomas usually spread along fascial planes or within muscle bundles, radical resection encompasses removal of all muscles in the involved compartment, along with nerves, vessels, and involved bone; hence this approach often requires amputation.

The addition of radiotherapy to less radical surgical resection has made limb salvage possible in many cases. A comparison of amputation versus limb-sparing surgery followed by adjuvant radiation therapy was performed at the National Cancer Institute between 1975 and 1981.[53] Forty-three patients were randomized; 27 to the limb-sparing group and 16 to the amputation group. The median follow-up was 4 years and 8 months. Four local recurrences were experienced in the limb-sparing group and none in patients in the amputation group. No statistical difference was noted in local recurrence or overall survival between the two groups. Potter and associates[54] later reviewed the entire National Cancer Institute experience with 123 patients treated with conservative surgery plus radiotherapy and 83 treated with amputation. The difference in local control was significant between groups, with a local failure rate of 8% in the surgery and adjuvant radiotherapy group and no recurrences in the amputation group. However, survival rates did not differ significantly between the groups. Several large single-institution studies also have reported favorable local control rates with conservative resection combined with radiation therapy.[55–58]

Isolated Regional Perfusion

Isolated regional perfusion is an investigational approach for treating extremity sarcomas. It has been attempted mainly as a limb-sparing alternative for patients with locally advanced soft tissue sarcomas or as a palliative treatment to achieve local control for patients with distant metastatic disease.

Isolated limb perfusion involves isolating the main artery and vein of the perfused limb from the systemic circulation. The choice of anatomic approach is determined by tumor site; external iliac vessels are used for thigh tumors, femoral or popliteal vessels for calf tumors, and axillary vessels for upper-extremity tumors. The vessels are dissected, and all collateral vessels are ligated. The vessels are then cannulated and connected to a pump oxygenator similar to that used in cardiopulmonary bypass. A tourniquet or Esmarch band is applied to the limb to achieve complete vascular isolation. For the lower limb, the Esmarch band is anchored at the anterior-superior iliac spine with the aid of a pin inserted into the pelvic bones. For the upper limb, the pin is anchored at the scapular and pectoral levels. Chemotherapeutic agents are then added to the perfusion circuit and circulated for 90 minutes. Systemic leakage from the perfused limb is monitored continuously by monitoring ^{99}Tc-radiolabeled human serum albumin injected into the perfusate. Radioactivity above the precordial area is recorded with a Geiger counter. The temperature of the perfused limb is maintained during the entire procedure by external heating and warming of the perfusate to 40°C. At the end of the procedure, the limb is washed out, the cannulas are extracted, and the blood vessels are repaired.

Despite a 40-year history of the use of isolated limb perfusion to treat extremity sarcomas, many questions remain to be answered. The choice of chemotherapeutic agent in the perfusion circuit, the benefits of hyperthermia, and the effectiveness of hyperthermic perfusion in the neoadjuvant or adjuvant setting remain to be elucidated. Studies published to date have involved heterogeneous patient groups and diverse chemotherapeutic agents. Despite these problems, favorable response rates ranging from 18 to 80% and overall 5-year survival rates of 50 to 70% have been reported.[59-62]

In 1974, McBride first reported results of 79 patients with extremity sarcomas who had been treated with isolated limb perfusion during the previous 14 years.[59] All patients had received melphalan and dactinomycin. The overall 5-year survival rate was 57% and only 13 patients had subsequent amputation for recurrent disease. Over the next 20 years, isolated perfusion of the extremity to treat sarcoma fell out of favor for several reasons, most notably, because improved survival and decreased local recurrence rates could be obtained with less radical therapy. Conservative surgical excision was combined with radiation therapy or neoadjuvant chemotherapy to provide limb-sparing options to patients who were previously thought to require amputation. In view of the encouraging results of combination therapy, it is difficult to justify the technically challenging and expensive isolated perfusion procedure.

In 1992, a report by Lienard and colleagues[63] revived interest in isolated limb perfusion as a therapy for extremity tumors. Those investigators reported a 100% response rate among patients with extremity melanomas and sarcomas when high-dose recombinant tumor necrosis factor-α plus interferon-gamma and melphalan were given in an isolated perfusion circuit. This report led to larger studies geared specifically to patients with sarcoma. The largest of these studies, the European Multicenter Study, was reported by Eggermont and associates in 1996.[62] In that study of 186 patients, the overall tumor response rate was 82%. The clinical and pathologic complete response rate was 29%. Although all patients entered in the study were candidates for amputation, the limb salvage rate was 82%.[62]

A similar study evaluated the role of hyperthermic isolated limb perfusion with tumor necrosis factor and melphalan for patients with extremity sarcomas. A complete response was seen in 26% of the patients, and an additional 30% had a partial response. Fourteen patients (32%) underwent amputation for progressive tumors, while the other 68% were able to undergo limb salvage surgery after isolated limb perfusion.[64] The inferior results in the U.S.-based studies are thought to be due to patient selection biases and the degree of pretreatment prior to limb perfusion.

Although melphalan has been reported to have minimal activity against soft tissue sarcomas when used as a systemic agent, it can produce significant responses with minimal toxicity when used in the limb perfusion circuit. Doxorubicin has been the most effective systemic agent for soft tissue sarcomas, but concerns about potential locoregional toxicity have limited its use in isolated limb perfusion. Rossi and associates[65] performed a phase II trial of hyperthermic isolated limb perfusion with doxorubicin for 23 patients with extremity sarcomas. They reported a limb salvage rate of 91% and acceptable rates of grade 3 and 4 systemic (4%) and locoregional toxicity (22%).

Radiation Therapy

In the 1970s, 50% of patients presenting with extremity sarcomas underwent amputation for local control of their tumors. Despite a local recurrence rate of less than 10% after radical surgery, large numbers of patients died of metastatic disease.[66] This realization prompted the development of local therapy involving conservative surgical excision combined with postoperative radiation therapy. These techniques offered local control rates of 78 to 91%.[55,67]

The evidence for adjunctive radiation therapy for patients eligible for conservative surgical resection comes from two randomized trials[68,69] and three large single-institution reports.[70-72] In a randomized trial by the National Cancer Institute, 91 patients with high-grade extremity tumors were treated with limb-sparing surgery followed by chemotherapy alone or radiation therapy plus adjuvant chemotherapy. A second group of 50 patients with low-grade tumors were treated with resection alone or resection with radiation therapy. The 10-year rate of local control for all patients receiving radiation therapy was 98%, compared with 70% for those not receiving radiation therapy ($p = 0.0001$).[68] Similarly, in a randomized trial from the Memorial Sloan-Kettering Cancer Center, 164 patients underwent observation or brachytherapy after conservative surgery. The 5-year local control rate for patients with high-grade tumors was 66% in the observation group and 89% in the brachytherapy group ($p = 0.003$).[69] No significant difference was observed between treatment groups for patients with low-grade tumors.[73]

Until recently, the standard treatment guidelines were to administer radiotherapy as an adjunct to surgery for all patients with intermediate or highly aggressive tumors of any size. However, in general, small tumors (≤ 5 cm) have not been associated with local recurrence, and radiation therapy may not be necessary. In a series of 174 patients reported by Geer and associates, postoperative radiation therapy did not improve 5-year local recurrence or survival rates for patients with small soft tissue sarcomas.[74] Karakousis and colleagues reported a 5-year local recurrence rate of 6% for 80 patients with extremity sarcomas treated with wide local excision and observation, a rate similar to that for 64 patients who underwent resection with more narrow surgical margins and adjuvant postoperative radiation.[75] These investigators argued that the high recurrence rates after less radical surgery were reported in the era before the use of preoperative MRI and improved surgical and pathologic techniques.

The optimal mode (external beam or brachytherapy) and timing (preoperative, intraoperative, or postoperative) have yet to be defined. External-beam radiation therapy can be delivered by photons or particle beams (electrons, protons, pions, or neutrons).[76] Conventional fractionation is usually 1.8 Gy to 2 Gy/d. Computed tomography is an integral part of radiation therapy. It is used to define the gross tumor volume and to estimate a margin of tissue at risk of microscopic tumor involvement. The optimal margin is not well defined; a radiation margin of 5 to 7 cm is standard, although some centers advocate wider margins for tumors larger than 15 cm.

At most institutions the typical preoperative dose is 50 Gy, given in 25 fractions.[76]

Postoperative radiation therapy planning is based on tumor grade, assessment of surgical margins, and institutional preferences. The entire surgical scar and drain sites should be included in the field so that a near-full dose is given to the superficial skin. Metallic clips placed in the tumor bed during surgery can help define the limits of the resection and aid in radiation therapy planning. Doses of 60 to 70 Gy are usually necessary for postoperative treatment.

No consensus exists on the optimal sequence of radiation therapy and surgery. The available data come largely from single-institution, nonrandomized studies. Proponents of preoperative radiation therapy cite several advantages. Multidisciplinary planning with radiation oncologists, medical oncologists, and surgeons is facilitated early in the course of therapy if the tumor is in place; moreover, lower doses of preoperative radiation can be delivered to an undisturbed tissue bed that may have improved tissue oxygenation.[77] In addition, Nielsen and colleagues[78] demonstrated that the size of preoperative radiation fields is smaller and the number of joints included on those fields is fewer than in postoperative radiation fields, which may result in improved functional outcome.

Critics of preoperative radiation therapy cite as deterrents the difficulty of pathologic assessment of margins and the increased rate of wound complications. However, plastic surgery techniques with advanced tissue transfer procedures are being used more often in these high-risk wounds, with better outcomes. In one study, the rate of healed wounds in a single-stage operation exceeded 90%.[79]

The only randomized comparison of preoperative and postoperative radiation therapy conducted to date was performed by the National Cancer Institute of Canada Clinical Trial Canadian Sarcoma Group.[80] This trial was designed to compare complications and the functional outcome of patients treated with preoperative and postoperative external-beam radiation therapy. The 190 patients were accrued from October 1994 to December 1997 and were randomized to receive preoperative radiotherapy (50 Gy) or postoperative radiotherapy (66 Gy). At a median follow-up of 3.3 years, wound complications had occurred in 35% of patients given preoperative radiotherapy and in 17% of patients given postoperative radiation therapy ($p = 0.01$). Both groups had achieved similarly high levels of local control and progression-free survival at 3 years.[80]

Brachytherapy involves the placement of multiple catheters in the tumor resection bed. The primary benefit of brachytherapy is the shorter overall treatment time of 4 to 6 days, compared with preoperative or postoperative radiation therapy regimens, which generally take 4 to 6 weeks.[81] Brachytherapy also produces less radiation scatter in critical anatomic regions (e.g., gonads or joints) and potentially improved function. A cost-analysis comparison of brachytherapy versus external-beam irradiation showed that costs were lower to undergo adjuvant irradiation with brachytherapy for soft tissue sarcomas.[82] Brachytherapy can also be used for recurrent disease previously treated with external-beam radiation. Guidelines established at the Memorial Sloan-Kettering Cancer Center recommend spacing the afterloading catheters in 1-cm increments and leaving a 2-cm margin around the surgical bed.[69] After adequate wound healing is established, usually after the fifth postoperative day, the catheters are loaded with seeds containing iridium-192 that deliver 42 to 45 Gy of radiation to the tumor bed over 4 to 6 days.[81] The primary disadvantage of brachytherapy is that it requires an extended inpatient stay and bedrest.

The utility of intraoperative radiation therapy for treating sarcoma is not well defined. The acceptable 5-year local control rates achieved with external-beam radiation therapy and brachytherapy for extremity tumors have reduced the enthusiasm for exploring alternative methods of treatment. Currently, intraoperative radiation therapy is primarily used at large centers to treat retroperitoneal sarcomas. At the time of surgical resection, intraoperative displacement of critical organs (e.g., bowel) allows treatment of the field at risk.

Local toxicity from radiation therapy varies depending on dose, field size, and timing (preoperative or postoperative). Wound complication rates of 16 to 37% have been reported for patients receiving preoperative radiation therapy, compared with 5 to 20% for patients receiving postoperative treatment.[83-87] With preoperative radiotherapy, the most frequent wound complications are delayed primary closure, dehiscence, ulceration, and cellulitis. Postoperative radiation treatment of free flaps is also often associated with wound complications, and patients should be warned that secondary surgical repair may be necessary. Rates of wound complications after brachytherapy are similar to those after postoperative radiation therapy if catheters are loaded after the fifth postoperative day.

Long-term effects of radiation therapy (those occurring more than 1 year after completion of therapy) are generally related to fibrosis, necrosis, edema, fracture, and contracture, all of which can cause substantial functional impairment. Variables associated with poorer functional outcome after radiation therapy include treatment of larger tumors, use of higher doses of radiation (>63 Gy), longer radiation fields (>35 cm), poor radiation technique, neural sacrifice, postoperative fractures, and wound complications.[76,88] The risks of edema and fracture are greater when tumors are in lower rather than upper extremities and should be discussed in detail with the patient.

Careful attention to the performance of radiation therapy rather than the choice of technique (preoperative versus postoperative versus brachytherapy) can substantially minimize long-term complications. Specific tactics to minimize posttreatment edema and maintain limb function for patients with extremity tumors include limiting radiation exposure to two-thirds of the circumference of the extremity, one half of joints, and one-half of the circumference of long bones.

Systemic Therapy

Systemic therapy generally is limited to patients with metastatic disease, those with small-cell sarcomas of any size, or those with large (≥5 cm) high-grade tumors or intermediate-grade tumors larger than 10 cm. However, despite improvements in local control rates, metastasis and death remain a significant problem for patients with high-risk soft tissue sarcomas. Patients considered at high risk of death from sarcoma include those presenting with metastatic disease and those presenting with localized sarcomas at nonextremity sites or sarcomas with intermediate- or high-grade histology larger than 5 cm (T2).[38,49] The treatment for patients with high-risk localized or metastatic disease often includes chemotherapy.

Results of conventional chemotherapy regimens have been poor for most patients with sarcoma. Sarcomas encompass a diverse group of cancers that vary greatly in natural history and response to treatment. As a group, sarcomas include histologic subtypes that are very responsive to cytotoxic chemotherapy and subtypes that are universally resistant to current agents. The most active chemotherapeutic agents for bone sarcomas are doxorubicin, methotrexate, cisplatin, and ifosfamide; reported single-agent response rates are 21 to 40% for osteosarcomas. For Ewing's sarcoma, doxorubicin, vincristine, cyclophosphamide, and ifosfamide have demonstrated response rates up to 90%.[89,90] Actinomycin D, vincristine, and VP-16 are active only in small-cell sarcomas, including Ewing's sarcoma, rhabdomyosarcoma, primitive neuroectodermal tumor, and neuroblastoma.

Only three drugs, doxorubicin, dacarbazine, and ifosfamide, have consistently demonstrated response rates of 20% or more for advanced soft tissue sarcomas. Doxorubicin and ifosfamide are the two most active agents, with consistently reported response rates of 20% or greater.[89,91,92] Both agents have demonstrated positive dose-response curves.[93,94] Response rates to ifosfamide have been reported to range from 20 to 60% in single-institution series using higher-dose regimens or in combination with doxorubicin.[94–98] For other tumors, the benefits of response in terms of long-term control of disease remain uncertain.

In the range of adult soft tissue sarcomas, a spectrum of chemosensitivity has been demonstrated for different histologic types. Demetri[99] classified synovial sarcoma, fibrosarcoma, and malignant fibrous histiocytoma as types that were highly sensitive to chemotherapy; liposarcoma and myxofibrosarcoma as having intermediate sensitivity to chemotherapy; and gastrointestinal stromal tumors, leiomyosarcoma, and chondrosarcoma as being highly resistant to chemotherapy. Considering the variability of responses, it is not surprising that no overall survival benefit has been demonstrated for all patients with soft tissue sarcoma who receive adjuvant systemic chemotherapy.

A major deterrent to the use of adjuvant chemotherapy has been the risk of adverse toxic effects in patients who do not respond to therapy. To optimize the use of doxorubicin and ifosfamide, investigators have tried to escalate the drug doses with combination regimens with the aim of maximizing tumor-cell kill. The ultimate goal is to achieve an incremental response rate and improve the quality of response sufficiently to influence survival. However, the limits to this approach are becoming apparent, even when treatment includes support with hematopoietic growth factors. The advent of growth factors like granulocyte colony-stimulating factor and granulocyte-macrophage colony-stimulating factor has helped minimize the morbidity related to neutropenia; however, dose-limiting thrombocytopenia continues to pose a challenge for treatment. Use of high-dose doxorubicin has been limited by myelotoxicity, epithelial toxicity, painful "hand-foot syndrome," and potentially severe cardiac toxicity.[99]

Integrating Multimodality Therapy

The primary objective of multimodality treatment is cure; when this endpoint is not possible, the goal is palliation of symptoms. Whenever possible, patients with a deep soft tissue mass should be referred, even before a biopsy is performed, to a tertiary treatment center that offers care by a team of specialists. Such multidisciplinary teams typically include oncologists from several disciplines (medicine, pediatrics [if applicable], surgery, and radiation therapy), as well as a pathologist, radiologist, and ancillary staff.

Adjuvant Chemotherapy

The use of adjuvant chemotherapy for soft tissue sarcomas remains controversial. The average 5-year disease-free survival rate for patients initially presenting with localized disease is only about 50%. More than a dozen individual randomized trials of adjuvant chemotherapy have failed to demonstrate improvement in disease-free patients and overall survival in patients with soft tissue sarcomas. However, several limitations of these individual trials may explain the lack of observed improvement. First, the

chemotherapy regimens used were suboptimal, relying on single-agent therapy (most commonly with doxorubicin) and insufficiently intensive dosing schedules. Second, the patient groups were not large enough to detect clinically significant differences in survival rates. Finally, most studies included patients at low risk of metastasis and death, namely those with small (<5 cm) and low-grade tumors.

The Sarcoma Meta-Analysis Collaboration analyzed 1568 patients from 14 trials of doxorubicin-based adjuvant chemotherapy to evaluate the effect of adjuvant chemotherapy on localized, resectable soft tissue sarcomas.[100] At a median follow-up of 9.4 years, doxorubicin-based chemotherapy significantly improved the time to local and distant recurrence and recurrence-free survival rates. However, the absolute benefit in overall survival for the sample was only 4%, which was not significant ($p = 0.12$). In subset analysis, patients with extremity tumors had a 7% benefit in survival ($p = 0.029$).[100]

Subsequent to this metaanalysis, additional randomized controlled trials of more modern (drugs, dose, and schedule) anthracycline/ifosfamide combinations for relatively small numbers of patients have yielded conflicting results. In an Italian cooperative trial, apparent improvement was seen in median disease-free and overall survival times in patients with high-risk extremity soft tissue sarcomas.[101] In that study, 104 patients with high-grade tumors 5 cm or larger were randomized to undergo definitive local therapy (surgery) versus local therapy plus adjuvant chemotherapy consisting of epirubicin (60 mg/m^2 per day on days 1 and 2) and ifosfamide (1.8 g/m^2 per day on days 1 to 5) for five cycles. At a median follow-up of almost 5 years, disease-free survival times were 16 months in the surgery-alone group and 48 months in the combined treatment group ($p = 0.04$). Similarly, overall survival times were 46 months versus 75 months ($p = 0.03$) for those treated with surgery versus surgery plus chemotherapy, respectively.[101] Other randomized studies have failed to confirm such benefit.[102,103] Interpretation of this literature is complex.[104] Because the evidence addressing treatment of stage III disease is inconclusive, considerable variation still exists in treatment standards.

Neoadjuvant (Preoperative) Chemotherapy

The rationale for using neoadjuvant and preoperative chemotherapy for soft tissue sarcomas is the belief that only 30 to 50% of patients will respond to standard (postoperative) chemotherapy. Neoadjuvant chemotherapy enables oncologists to identify patients whose disease responds to chemotherapy by assessing that response while the primary tumor is in situ. Patients whose tumors do not respond to short courses of preoperative chemotherapy are thus spared the toxic effects of prolonged postoperative or adjuvant chemotherapy.

Treatment approaches that combine systemic chemotherapy with radiosensitizers and concurrent external-beam radiation may improve disease-free survival by treating microscopic disease and enhancing the treatment of macroscopic disease. Concurrent chemoradiotherapy with doxorubicin-based regimens reportedly produces favorable local control rates for patients with sarcoma.[105] Since those findings were published, several groups have attempted to evaluate the optimal route of administration,[105–109] alternative chemotherapeutic agents,[83,110,111] and the toxicity of combined therapies.[112]

Theoretical advantages of concurrent treatment notwithstanding, use of concurrent local and systemic therapy decreases the total treatment time for patients with high-risk sarcoma. This decrease represents a substantial advantage over current sequential combined-method treatment approaches, for which the total duration of treatment for radiation, chemotherapy, surgery, and rehabilitation frequently exceeds 6 to 9 months.

SPECIAL SITUATIONS

Retroperitoneal Sarcomas

Fifteen percent of adult soft tissue sarcomas occur in the retroperitoneum. Most retroperitoneal tumors are malignant, and about one-third are soft tissue sarcomas. The most common sarcomas occurring in the retroperitoneum are liposarcomas, malignant fibrous histiocytomas, and leiomyosarcomas.[113] Most retroperitoneal sarcomas are liposarcomas or leiomyosarcomas. In contrast to extremity sarcomas, local recurrence and intra-abdominal spread are frequent patterns of relapse for retroperitoneal tumors.

Retroperitoneal sarcomas generally present as large masses; nearly 50% are larger than 20 cm at the time of diagnosis. They typically do not produce symptoms until they grow large enough to compress or invade contiguous structures. The differential diagnosis of a retroperitoneal tumor includes lymphoma, germ-cell tumors, and undifferentiated carcinomas. The work-up for a retroperitoneal mass begins with an accurate history that should exclude signs and symptoms associated with lymphoma (e.g., fever and night sweats). Complete physical examination, with particular attention to all nodal basins and testicular examination in men, is critically important. Laboratory assessment can be helpful; an elevated lactate dehydrogenase level may suggest lymphoma, and elevated beta-human chorionic gonadotropin levels or alpha-fetoprotein levels can indicate a germ cell tumor.

The overall prognosis for patients with retroperitoneal tumors is worse than that for patients with extremity sarcomas. Survival rates at 5 years are typically reported to be 40 to 50%. The best chance for long-term survival for patients with retroperitoneal sarcoma is achieved with a margin-negative resection. In one series,

the 5-year disease-free survival rate was 50% for patients who had margin-negative resection, compared with 28% for patients undergoing incomplete resection.[113] In the series reported by Lewis and associates,[114] about 75% of patients died of locally recurrent disease without distant metastasis.

Tumor stage at presentation, high histologic grade, unresectability, and grossly positive resection margins are strongly associated with increased rates of death from retroperitoneal sarcoma.[114] As is true for extremity lesions, tumor grade is a significant predictor of outcome for patients with retroperitoneal sarcoma. In the series reported by Jaques and colleagues,[115] patients with high-grade tumors (n = 65) had a median survival time of only 20 months, compared with 80 months for patients with low-grade tumors (n = 49).

Radiologic assessment should include CT of the abdomen and pelvis to define the extent of the tumor and its relationship to surrounding structures, particularly vascular structures (Fig. 35-6). Imaging should also encompass the liver for the presence of metastases, the abdomen for discontiguous disease, and the kidneys bilaterally for function. Thoracic CT is indicated to detect lung metastases. For patients presenting with an equivocal history, an unusual appearance of the mass, an unresectable tumor, or distant metastasis, CT-guided core-needle or laparoscopic biopsy is appropriate to obtain a sample for tissue diagnosis.

Complete surgical resection is the most effective treatment for primary or recurrent retroperitoneal sarcomas. However, these tumors often involve vital structures, precluding surgical resection. Even if surgical resection can be performed, the margins are often compromised because of anatomic constraints. In several retrospective assessments of patients with retroperitoneal sarcoma, complete surgical excision was achieved in only 40 to 60% of patients.[113,115] In an analysis of 500 patients with retroperitoneal soft tissue sarcomas treated at Memorial Sloan-Kettering Cancer Center, the median survival time for those who underwent complete resection was 103 months versus 18 months for

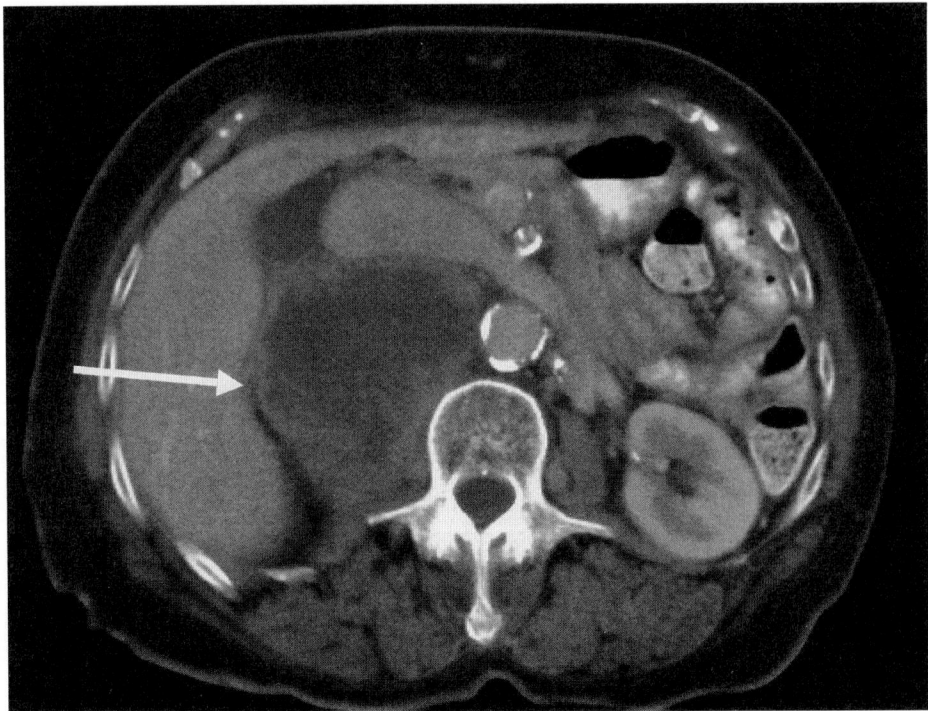

FIG. 35-6. A 77-year-old woman with retroperitoneal, pleomorphic high-grade sarcoma. CT scan of abdomen demonstrates a 9 x 6 cm mixed attenuation bilobed mass replacing the right psoas muscle and displacing the inferior vena cava anteriorly. There appears to be tumor thrombus within the inferior vena cava.

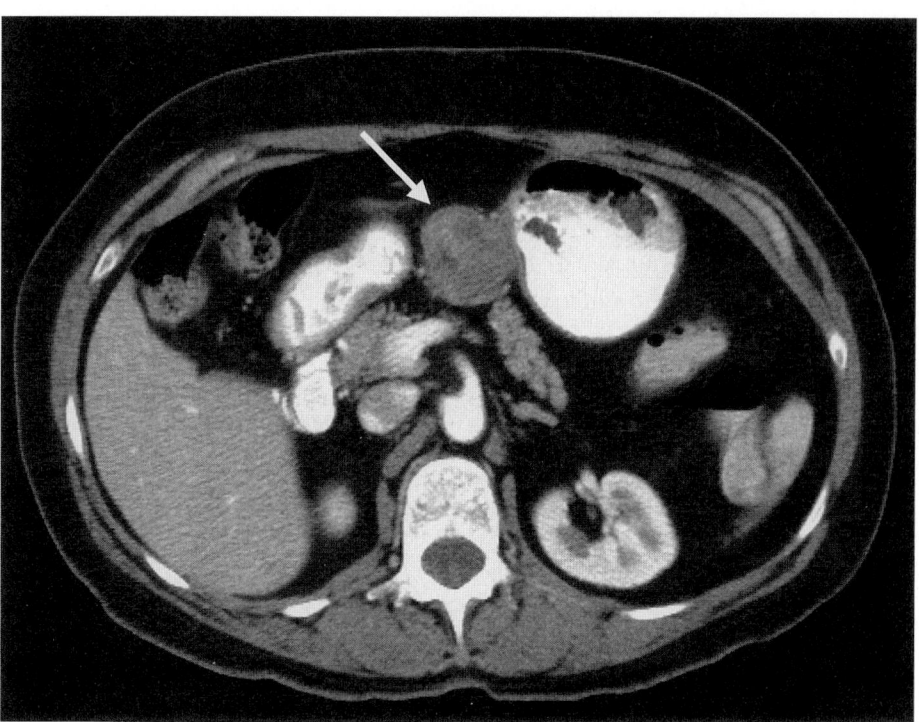

FIG. 35-7. A 66-year-old woman who presented with epigastric discomfort. Endoscopic biopsy revealed a low-grade gastrointestinal stromal tumor (GIST). CT scan of the abdomen demonstrating an exophytic 4 x 3.5 cm mass arising from the lesser curvature of the gastric antrum.

those who underwent incomplete resection, or observation without resection.[114]

Chemotherapy has not been shown to be effective against retroperitoneal sarcomas.[116] Protocols are ongoing at several centers to determine whether preoperative chemotherapy and radiation therapy have roles in treating these tumors.

Gastrointestinal Sarcomas

Gastrointestinal sarcomas, which account for only 0.1 to 3% of all gastrointestinal cancers, have presented a diagnostic and therapeutic dilemma for decades. The overall prognosis for patients with gastrointestinal sarcomas is poor. As is true for sarcomas at other sites, high histologic grade and large tumor size (>5 cm) have been shown to adversely affect prognosis. Regional recurrence in the peritoneum (sarcomatosis) is a common pattern of failure after surgical resection. The median survival time for patients after such recurrences is reported to range from 18 months to 2 years.

Patients with gastrointestinal sarcomas most often present with nonspecific gastrointestinal symptoms that are determined by the site of the primary tumor. In a series from Memorial Sloan-Kettering Cancer Center, early satiety and dyspepsia were noted in patients with upper gastrointestinal tumors, whereas tenesmus and changes in bowel habits were common in those with tumors of the lower gastrointestinal tract.[46] In a series of 80 patients with various smooth-muscle tumors of the gastrointestinal tract, Chou and associates[117] identified the most common presenting symptoms and signs as gastrointestinal bleeding (44%), abdominal mass (38%), and abdominal pain (21%). No patient presented with visceral perforation in either of these series, although other investigators have reported that 30 to 50% of gastrointestinal stromal tumors present as surgical emergencies with a perforated viscus or life-threatening bleeding.[118,119]

Establishing the diagnosis of a gastrointestinal sarcoma preoperatively is often difficult. Radiologic assessment, including CT of the abdomen or pelvis, is sometimes useful to determine the anatomic location, size, and extent of disease. Patients with localized disease frequently present with a large intra-abdominal mass but no radiographic evidence of the regional lymph node metastases that would be typical of an adenocarcinoma of comparable size and anatomic location (Fig. 35-7). In patients with advanced disease, CT may demonstrate disseminated intra-abdominal masses with or without concomitant ascites and possible invasion of tissue planes.

Endoscopy (esophagoduodenoscopy or colonoscopy) has become the mainstay for evaluating symptoms related to the gastrointestinal tract. For tumors involving the stomach, upper endoscopy with endoscopic ultrasonography and biopsy are important diagnostic tests used to distinguish adenocarcinoma from gastrointestinal stromal tumors. This distinction is clinically significant because the extent of resection (local excision versus gastrectomy) and the role of regional lymph node dissection differ for these two conditions.

For localized disease, the therapeutic benefit of radical excision (e.g., total gastrectomy) versus local excision has long been debated. Although prospective analyses have been done, several retrospective studies have failed to show significant survival differences according to the extent of surgical resection.[120–123] Based on published data and the primary pattern of distant (versus local) failure, the general recommendation is to perform a margin-negative resection with a 2- to 4-cm margin of normal tissue (Fig. 35-8). However, some cases may be technically challenging because of the tumor's anatomic location or size. For example, for gastric tumors located near the gastroesophageal junction, achieving adequate surgical margins may not be possible without a total or proximal subtotal gastrectomy. Similarly, large leiomyosarcomas arising from the stomach with invasion of adjacent organs should be resected together with the adjacent involved viscera en bloc.

Segmental bowel resection is the standard treatment for sarcomas of the small or large intestine. For the jejunum, ileum, and colon, the tumor is excised en bloc with the involved segment of intestine and its mesentery; radical mesenteric lymphadenectomy is not attempted.[124]

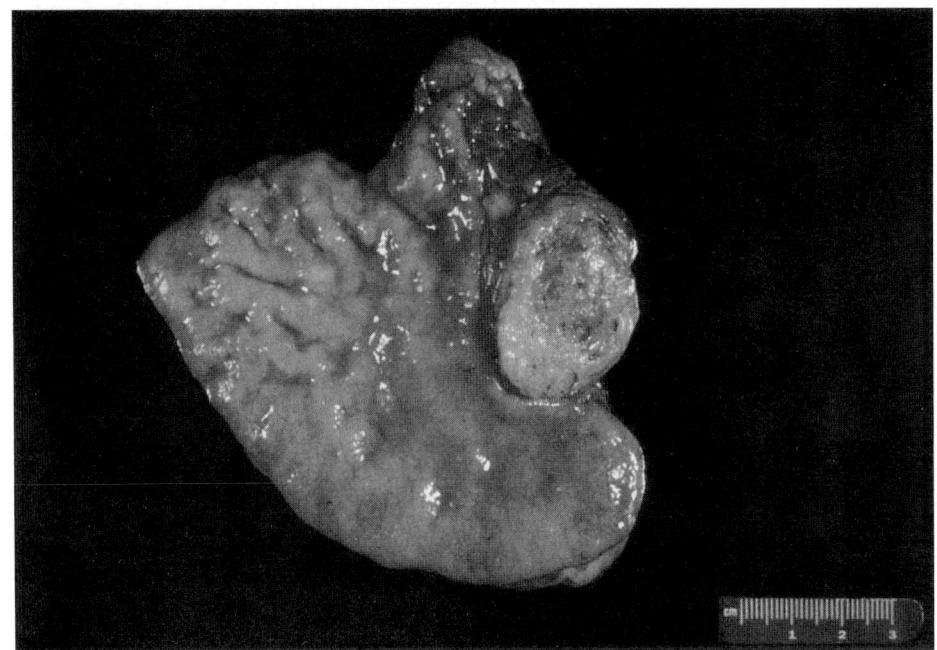

FIG. 35-8. Gross specimen of distal stomach with 5.0 x 4.5 cm submucosal mass in the lesser curvature of the stomach, which is 5 cm away from the proximal margin and 5 cm from the distal margin. Cross section of the mass revealed a well circumscribed, fish flesh–appearing mass that did not infiltrate to the overlying gastric mucosa and underlying serosa.[139]

For sarcomas originating in the rectum, the technique used for tumor resection is based on the anatomic location and size of the tumor. For small, low rectal lesions, it may be possible to achieve clear margins with a transanal excision. Large or locally invasive lesions may require more extensive operations for complete tumor extirpation.[125,126] Meijer and colleagues[126] reviewed the experience with 50 patients with primary colorectal sarcoma at Memorial Sloan-Kettering Cancer Center. In 32 cases, the primary tumor was located in the rectum, and 18 tumors involved the colon. Of the rectal lesions, 15 were treated with abdominoperineal resection and 12 were treated with local excision. Distant metastasis was the first recurrence in 11 of the 32 patients who underwent curative resection.[126]

Lymphatic spread is not the primary route of metastasis for gastrointestinal sarcomas; lymph node metastasis has been reported in 0 to 16% of cases.[120,121,124,127,128] Consequently, lymphadenectomy is not routinely performed as part of resection.

Gastrointestinal Stromal Tumors

Gastrointestinal stromal tumors (GISTs), which constitute the majority of gastrointestinal sarcomas, have distinctive immunohistochemical and genetic features. They are thought to arise from a pacemaker cell within the gastrointestinal tract known as the interstitial cell of Cajal.[129,130] The interstitial cells of Cajal and GIST cells express the hematopoietic progenitor cell marker CD34 and the growth factor receptor c-Kit (CD117).[129,131–134] c-Kit is a transmembrane glycoprotein receptor with an internal tyrosine kinase component which when activated triggers a cascade of intracellular signals regulating cell growth and survival.[135–138]

Surgery remains the primary treatment modality for both localized and locally advanced GISTs. Complete resection with negative margins, even of locally advanced tumors, is associated with improved survival.[44] The extent of surgery required to produce a complete resection does not seem to influence survival.[46] The 5-year survival rate for all patients with GISTs ranges from 20 to 44% and up to 75% for early-stage tumors that have been completely excised.[44] However, a more recent analysis of 200 patients by DeMatteo and colleagues noted a disease-specific survival rate of only 54% for patients in whom a grossly complete resection of primary GISTs had been achieved, and the median survival duration for patients with metastatic disease was only 20 months.[139]

c-Kit expression has emerged as an important defining feature of GISTs, the pathogenesis of which may be related to c-Kit mutations. Treatment with imatinib (Gleevec, ST1571), a selective c-Kit inhibitor, has resulted in impressive clinical responses in a large percentage of patients with advanced GISTs. Mutations of c-Kit are common in GISTs, and most of the mutations result from an inframe deletion or a point mutation in exon 11 (the juxtamembrane domain). These mutations, which occur predominantly in malignant GISTs,[140] lead to ligand-independent activation of the tyrosine kinase of c-Kit.[131,133,141] The resulting constitutive c-Kit tyrosine kinase activity has been shown to promote tumor growth in vitro and may be the key molecular pathway in the pathogenesis of GISTs.[131,141] Taniguchi and colleagues examined clinical outcomes in a series of 124 cases of GISTs, of which 71 (57%) had c-Kit mutations.[134] The patients with mutation-positive GISTs had a significantly higher recurrence rate (37 versus 11%) and a higher 5-year mortality rate (86 versus 49%) than did patients with no mutations. Imatinib has been shown to selectively inhibit c-Kit tyrosine kinase activity, resulting in decreased GIST cellular proliferation and increased induction of apoptosis.[142,143] These results provided the rationale for clinical trials of imatinib for patients with solid tumors that are dependent on the activity of wild-type or mutant c-Kit for proliferation.[142–144]

Until recently, there has been no effective therapy for advanced, unresectable GISTs. Traditional systemic chemotherapy regimens used for soft tissue sarcomas have not been effective against GISTs. In a prospective randomized trial of bolus versus infusional therapy with doxorubicin (60 mg/m^2) and dacarbazine (750 mg/m^2) for metastatic soft tissue sarcomas including GISTs, the overall response rate was 17%, and only 7% of patients with GISTs had a response.[145] Ifosfamide also has been ineffective against GISTs.[146,147]

Based on the treatment results from a single patient, a phase I study was initiated by the European Organization for Research and Treatment of Cancer Soft Tissue and Bone Sarcoma Group to test the safety and efficacy of imatinib.[148] The mechanism of action of imatinib is discussed further in the section on chemotherapeutic agents, later in this chapter. In that study, 19 (53%) of 36 patients with GISTs had confirmed partial responses, and only four patients had progressive disease. Investigators concluded that imatinib is safe and effective against GISTs.[148]

A multicenter, international trial was then begun in July of 2000 at four treatment centers: Dana-Farber Cancer Institute, Oregon Health Sciences University, Fox Chase Cancer Center, and University Hospital of Helsinki, Finland.[149] A total of 147 patients with unresectable or metastatic GISTs were randomized to receive one of two doses of imatinib (400 mg or 600 mg daily) for planned treatments of up to 24 months. Overall objective response was demonstrated in 79 patients (54%); all had partial responses and no significant difference was found between imatinib doses.[150] Fourteen percent of patients had disease progression. The toxicity profile was acceptable, with the predominant effects being gastrointestinal toxicity and periorbital edema, cramps, and fatigue. However, 21% of patients experienced serious adverse events (grade 3 or 4 toxicity) including gastrointestinal bleeding (5%), likely related to the rapid tumor response of mural lesions.

A phase III randomized intergroup trial was then performed to assess the clinical activity of imatinib at two dose levels for patients with unresectable or metastatic GISTs expressing the c-Kit tyrosine kinase.[151] Between December 15, 2000, and September 1, 2001, 746 patients were accrued and randomized to receive low-dose (400 mg/d) or high-dose (800 mg/d) imatinib. The primary endpoint of the trial was survival, and the outcome data are currently maturing. Preliminary toxicity data from 325 patients revealed a 23% incidence of grade 3 or 4 adverse events, including nausea and vomiting, gastrointestinal bleeding, abdominal pain, edema, fatigue, and rash. The European Organization for Research and Treatment of Cancer Soft Tissue and Bone Sarcoma Group in conjunction with the Italian Sarcoma Group and the Australasian Gastro-Intestinal Trials Group has accrued 753 patients with GISTs to another randomized phase III trial.[152] Response data from the trial are currently maturing.

Imatinib is the first effective systemic therapy for patients with metastatic or locally advanced GISTs. In February 2002, the U.S. Food and Drug Administration approved the use of imatinib to treat GIST. Initial results from clinical trials indicate that 54% of patients with GISTs respond to imatinib therapy and only 10 to 15% have progressive disease. However, little is known about the optimal length of treatment, the duration of benefit, or the long-term toxicity. Less than 4% of patients with GISTs have experienced serious adverse events with imatinib. Mild gastrointestinal toxicity is the most frequently reported adverse event, but gastrointestinal tract hemorrhage, presumably from rapid tumor necrosis, has also been reported. Thus all patients with GISTs treated on clinical protocols should be evaluated and followed by a team of medical professionals that includes a surgeon.

Pediatric Sarcomas

Soft tissue sarcomas account for 7 to 8% of all pediatric cancers, totaling approximately 600 new cases per year.[153] Associated with skeletal muscle, rhabdomyosarcomas are the most common soft tissue tumors among children younger than 15 years, and they can occur at any site that has striated muscle. These tumors generally

Table 35-3

Surgical-Pathologic Grouping of Soft Tissue Sarcoma (Intergroup Rhabdomyosarcoma Study Group)

Clinical Group	Definition
I	a. Localized, completely resected, confined to site of origin
	b. Localized, completely resected, beyond site of origin
II	a. Localized, grossly resected microscopic residual tumor
	b. Regional disease, involved lymph nodes, completely resected
	c. Regional disease, involved lymph nodes grossly resected with microscopic residual tumor
III	a. Local or regional grossly visible disease after biopsy only
	b. Grossly visible disease after >50% resection of primary tumor
IV	Distant metastases at diagnosis

present as a painless enlarging mass; about 30% arise in the head and neck region, 25% in the genitourinary system, and 20% in the extremities. About 15 to 20% of cases have metastasis at presentation, most commonly (40 to 50%) involving the lungs.[1] Several staging systems for rhabdomyosarcoma are available; that of the Intergroup Rhabdomyosarcoma Study Group is based on surgical-pathologic groupings (Table 35-3).

Rhabdomyosarcoma is classified as a small round-cell tumor that demonstrates muscle differentiation upon light microscopy and immunohistochemical analysis. Two primary histologic subtypes account for 90% of cases, an embryonal subtype (70%) and an alveolar subtype (20%). Alveolar rhabdomyosarcoma is associated with cytogenetic translocation [t(2:13)(q35:q14)] in 85 to 90% of cases and [t(1:13)(p36:q14)] in 10% of cases.[154] These translocations affect biologic activity at the levels of protein function and gene expression, affecting the control of cell growth, apoptosis, differentiation, and motility, ultimately contributing to tumorigenic behavior.[155] In contrast to the specific translocations found in alveolar rhabdomyosarcomas, most embryonal rhabdomyosarcomas have an allelic loss at chromosome 11p15.5[156] that is thought to affect tumor suppressor genes.[155] Both of these distinct molecular subtypes of rhabdomyosarcomas are thought to affect similar downstream targets, such as the p53 and Rb pathways.[155]

Complete surgical resection is the treatment of choice for rhabdomyosarcoma, when function and cosmesis can be preserved. Patients who are able to undergo a complete tumor resection with negative (group I) or microscopic surgical margins (group II) are able to undergo less intensive systemic therapy with overall survival rates approaching 90%.[157] Given the morbidity associated with resections at some anatomic sites, in particular the head and neck and genitourinary systems, surgery is often not undertaken. Recent findings suggest that chemotherapy can adequately control several such tumors without additional local therapy.[158] In the second International Society of Paediatric Oncology study of rhabdomyosarcoma (MMT84), the choice of local treatment was based on response to initial chemotherapy such that radical surgery and radiotherapy were avoided in 66% of patients. Among the patients who subsequently developed local relapse, the 5-year overall survival rate after salvage therapy was 46%.[157]

Unlike other soft tissue sarcomas, rhabdomyosarcomas have a high propensity for lymph node metastasis, with rates up to 20 to 30% for sites such as the extremities, paratesticular nodes, and prostate.[1] Lymph node sampling and more recently sentinel lymph node mapping have been used to evaluate regional node status in children with rhabdomyosarcoma.

In 1972, the Intergroup Rhabdomyosarcoma Study Committee was established to develop protocols for treating children with rhabdomyosarcomas. The chemotherapy regimens found to be the most active against rhabomyosarcomas have included vincristine, actinomycin D, and cyclophosphamide. Trials of various combinations including doxorubicin, ifosfamide, cisplatin, and etoposide have not demonstrated benefit.[157,159] Radiation therapy is given to most patients with microscopic residual disease (group II) after resection.

The prognosis for children with rhabdomyosarcoma is related to tumor site, surgical-pathologic grouping, and tumor histology.[160–162] The 5-year, disease-free survival rate for all patients has been reported as 65%. Disease-free survival by group (see Table 35-3) has been reported as 84%, 74%, 62%, and 23% for groups I, II, III, and IV, respectively.[1,162]

Recurrent Sarcomas

Up to 20% of patients with extremity sarcoma develop recurrent disease. The adequacy of surgical resection of sarcomas arising from any anatomic site is clearly related to local recurrence rates.[49] Patients with microscopically positive surgical margins are at increased risk of local recurrence. The effect of local treatment failure on survival and distant disease-free survival is controversial.[15] Many believe that recurrence is a harbinger of distant metastatic disease.

Recurrence can be detected on follow-up clinical examination or on imaging studies. Guidelines have been established for using MRI to distinguish recurrences from typical postsurgical changes. A discrete nodule with low signal intensity on T1-weighted images and higher signal intensity on T2-weighted images that enhances after administration of intravenous contrast is strongly suggestive of recurrence and should be sampled for biopsy.[163]

An isolated local recurrence should be treated aggressively with margin-negative resection. For patients with extremity sarcomas, this frequently requires amputation. However, some patients with recurrent extremity sarcoma can undergo function-preserving resection combined with additional radiation therapy, with or without chemotherapy, with acceptable rates of local control.[164–166] Nori and colleagues reported a local control rate of 69% among 40 patients with recurrent tumors treated with reexcision and brachytherapy to a median dose of 45 Gy.[164] In a similar series, limb-sparing conservative surgery was possible in 24 of 36 patients (66%), and the 5-year local recurrence-free survival rate was 72%.[165]

Retroperitoneal sarcomas recur locally in up to 60% of patients. These tumors also can spread diffusely throughout the abdominal cavity and recur as sarcomatosis. The preferred treatment for locally recurrent retroperitoneal tumors is surgical resection, if possible. In a large series of patients with retroperitoneal sarcoma treated at Memorial Sloan-Kettering Cancer Center, the investigators were able to resect recurrent tumors in 57% of patients having a first recurrence. However, the resection rate decreased to 20% after a second recurrence, and to 10% after a third.[114] In a retrospective analysis of 21 patients with an isolated locally-recurrent truncal or retroperitoneal sarcoma, Singer and associates reported that 67% were successfully treated with aggressive re-resection.[116]

Palliative Strategies

Most patients with soft tissue sarcomas present without evidence of distant metastases. The known risk factors for distant metastasis include tumor grade, histiotype, primary site, and size.

Metastases are present at diagnosis in 40 to 50% of patients with intermediate- or high-grade extremity sarcomas, as compared with only 5% in patients with low-grade sarcomas.

Most metastases to distant sites occur within 2 to 3 years of initial diagnosis. The pattern of recurrence is related to the anatomic site of the primary tumor. Patients with extremity sarcomas generally have recurrence as distant pulmonary metastases, whereas patients with retroperitoneal or intra-abdominal sarcomas tend to have local recurrences.[167] Other less common sites of metastasis include bone (7%), liver (4%),[54] and lymph nodes (<4%).[8] The incidence of lymph node involvement may be greater in cases of angiosarcoma, epithelioid sarcoma, synovial sarcoma, and rhabdomyosarcoma.[168] Myxoid liposarcoma of the extremity is known to metastasize to the abdomen and pelvis, and requires staging CT of these regions before definitive local therapy.[27]

The primary determinant of survival in patients with soft tissue sarcoma is development of distant metastases. Early recognition and treatment of recurrent, local, or distant disease can prolong survival. The ability of early detection of recurrence to improve overall survival depends on the availability of effective therapeutic interventions.[167] A few reports involving small numbers of patients have indicated that salvage after recurrent local disease is possible by performing radical reexcision with or without radiation therapy.[169] Similarly, several groups have reported that survival can be prolonged after resection of pulmonary metastases.[170] These limited data form the basis for the use of aggressive surveillance strategies for all patients with soft tissue sarcoma.

History and physical examination are the most useful components of follow-up in evaluating for local recurrence after definitive treatment. CT and MRI are useful for evaluating less accessible regions, such as the retroperitoneum, and in assessing equivocal changes on examination. Most recurrences of soft tissue sarcomas occur in the first 2 years after completion of therapy. Patients should be evaluated with a complete history and physical examination every 3 months and chest radiography every 6 months during the 2- to 3-year period of highest risk. Most experts recommend that the tumor site be evaluated every 6 months by performing MRI for extremity tumors or CT for intra-abdominal or retroperitoneal tumors. In some circumstances, ultrasonography can be used to assess recurrence of tumor in the extremities. Follow-up intervals can be lengthened to every 6 months, with annual imaging, for years 2 through 5. After 5 years, patients should be evaluated and undergo chest radiography annually.

Recurrence after surgery for abdominal soft tissue sarcomas is common. CT is useful for detecting recurrences at primary and distant anatomic sites in the abdomen and pelvis. After surgery, cross-sectional imaging every 3 to 6 months during the first 2 years and every 6 months for 3 years thereafter has been recommended. However, many experienced surgeons are advocating less aggressive imaging for asymptomatic patients, particularly after a second recurrence of retroperitoneal sarcoma. They argue that no evidence exists to suggest that survival is improved by earlier detection.[114]

Whooley and associates reviewed the efficacy of the surveillance strategy used at Roswell Park Cancer Institute for 174 patients with soft tissue sarcomas of the extremities.[167] Patients were evaluated every 3 months for the first 2 years, every 4 to 6 months during year

3, and every 6 months through year 5. Local recurrence occurred in 18% of patients at a median interval of 14 months, and all but one of the recurrences was detected by physical examination alone. Fifty-seven patients had distant recurrences (at a median of 18 months after treatment), of which 36 were asymptomatic and diagnosed by surveillance radiographic imaging. Those investigators determined that the positive predictive value of chest radiography in follow-up was 92%.[167] However, evaluation of the primary site by CT or MRI and routine laboratory assessment was ineffective in detecting recurrences. The authors of this report cautioned that their study did not conclusively demonstrate that CT and MRI should not be used. Rather, patient characteristics, location of the primary tumor, previous treatment, and physician familiarity with changes after surgery and radiation therapy should all be considered in determining the need for radiographic imaging.

Surgical Excision of Metastatic Sarcoma

The most common initial site of metastasis of soft tissue sarcomas is the lung. Selected patients with a limited number of pulmonary nodules (fewer than four), long disease-free intervals, and no endobronchial invasion may become long-term survivors after pulmonary resection; 15 to 40% of patients with complete resection of metastatic disease confined to the lung are long-term survivors.[167] In a retrospective multi-institutional study of 255 patients, the 5-year overall survival rate after metastasectomy was reported to be 38%.[170] Favorable prognostic factors in that study included microscopically free margins, age younger than 40 years, and grade I or II tumors.[170]

Chemotherapy for Metastatic Sarcoma

The only available treatment for most patients with metastatic disease is chemotherapy. Historically, response rates for patients with stage IV soft tissue sarcoma have been low. Several prognostic factors have been defined for patients undergoing chemotherapy, including performance status, previous response to chemotherapy, younger age, absence of hepatic metastases, low-grade tumors, and long disease-free interval.[171]

RESEARCH PERSPECTIVES

Experimental Therapeutics

In the emerging modern era of cancer treatment, it will become possible to design cancer therapies specifically targeted to the particular molecular mechanisms involved in a tumor's growth. As molecular techniques become more advanced, many potential pathways for therapeutic development are being elucidated. For example, fusion genes, which have been of interest in the molecular diagnosis and characterization of specific subtypes of soft tissue sarcomas, represent a potential target for treatment with antisense oligonucleotides.[17] In vitro studies have demonstrated that transfection with antisense expression plasmids can result in suppression of tumor cell growth.

Tumor suppressor genes that are critical in growth inhibition may provide an alternative pathway for therapeutic development. Mutations in p53 tumor suppressor genes have been reported in 30 to 40% of soft tissue sarcomas. Soft tissue sarcoma metastases can develop from clonal expansion of primary tumor cells bearing p53 mutations.[172] In vivo studies have demonstrated that the reintroduction of the wild-type p53 gene into sarcoma cells harboring a mutated p53 by means of adenoviral vectors can result in reduced

cell proliferation[173] and reduced tumor growth in severe combined immunodeficient mice.[174] The ability to transfer therapeutic genes such as those with wild-type p53 growth-regulatory functions into target cells may ultimately be a useful therapeutic modality for patients with soft tissue sarcomas. Virus-mediated gene transfer has been widely used in preclinical studies and clinical trials. An isolated limb perfusion model has been developed in rats to examine the effects of the site-specific gene delivery of adenovectors in the treatment of extremity sarcomas.[175,176]

The relationship between wild-type p53 expression and inhibition of sarcoma tumor growth is still not defined. Possible mechanisms include the ability of wild-type p53 overexpression to down-regulate vascular endothelial growth factor (VEGF), which is important in angiogenesis, and to activate apoptotic pathways.[17] Several experimental approaches based on these pathways that are being developed to treat tumors include neutralizing antibodies against VEGF[177] and suppression of angiogenesis by the transcriptional repression of VEGF expression.[178]

Chemotherapeutic Agents

Tyrosine kinases are enzymes that bind adenosine triphosphate (ATP) and transfer phosphates from ATP to the tyrosine residues on substrate proteins. These enzymes have long been considered attractive targets for selective pharmacologic inhibition because many human cancers display deregulated kinase pathways.[179] In the early 1980s, it was recognized that constitutively activated tyrosine kinase is important in the pathogenesis of chronic myelogenous leukemia (CML). The Bcr-Abl gene, which is the result of a reciprocal exchange of genetic material between chromosomes 9 and 22, was identified as the causative molecular abnormality in CML.[180] The genetic translocation was found to lead to the constitutive activation of a specific Bcr-Abl tyrosine kinase protein, resulting in the malignant expansion of myeloid cells, disruption of regulatory control by stromal cells, and inhibition of apoptosis.[179] In the late 1980s, Ciba-Geigy identified a series of compounds with kinase inhibitory activity and subsequently developed a compound, 4-[(4-methyl-1-piperazinyl)methyl]-N-[4-methyl-3-[[4-(3-pyridinyl)-2-pyrimidinyl]amino]-phenyl] benzamide-methanesulfonate, that specifically blocked the tyrosine kinase activity of ABL.[180,181] Formerly referred to as STI571 (signal transduction inhibitor 571), imatinib mesylate, marketed as Gleevec, selectively inhibits several structurally similar tyrosine kinases, including all Abl tyrosine kinases, the platelet-derived growth factor (PDGF) receptor, and the c-Kit tyrosine kinase.[142,144]

In preclinical studies, imatinib was found to selectively inhibit the proliferation of Bcr-Abl-expressing cell lines[182,183] and to eradicate leukemia cells in nude mice injected with Bcr-Abl–positive human leukemia cell lines.[184] In 1998, encouraging preclinical results led to clinical trials of imatinib for patients with CML. The results were impressive, with most patients demonstrating hematologic and cytogenetic remissions. Imatinib-induced Bcr-Abl tyrosine kinase inhibition in patients with CML represents the first example of a therapy that successfully targets molecular pathogenetic events.

In vitro studies confirmed that imatinib inhibits c-Kit at concentrations similar to those required for inhibition of Bcr-Abl and the PDGF receptor.[142,144] In a series of biochemical and cell-based assays performed at the Oregon Health Sciences University, imatinib was shown to selectively inhibit c-Kit tyrosine kinase activity, resulting in decreased GIST cellular proliferation and increased induction of apoptosis.[143] These results provided the rationale for extending clinical trials of imatinib to patients with solid tumors that are dependent on the activity of wild-type or mutant c-Kit for proliferation. Clinical trials of imatinib and other compounds are described further in the following paragraphs.

Clinical Trials

The rarity of soft tissue sarcomas creates a challenge for studying the effects of treatment. Collaborative efforts are required to accrue adequate numbers of patients for such studies.

Trials for Extremity and Truncal Soft Tissue Sarcoma

Radiation Therapy Oncology Group S-0120 Trial. The Radiation Therapy Oncology Group S-0120 Trial is an ongoing phase I/II trial of preoperative radiotherapy given with or without an antiangiogenesis compound (Sugen-5416; SU5416) in the management of low- and intermediate-grade soft tissue sarcoma of the extremities and trunk. The trial is designed to evaluate the possible synergistic mechanisms between the two types of therapy. The objectives of the study are to define the maximum tolerated dose of SU5416 that can be given with preoperative radiation, to assess whether SU5416 has quantitative antiangiogenic effects in vivo, and to assess clinical endpoints including disease-free survival, local recurrence, distant metastases, and overall survival rates in patients treated with radiation or with radiation combined with SU5416.

Trials for Retroperitoneal Soft Tissue Sarcoma

Radiation Therapy Oncology Group S-0124 Trial. The Radiation Therapy Oncology Group S-0124 Trial is an ongoing multicenter phase II trial of an innovative preoperative chemotherapy and radiation therapy approach to soft tissue sarcomas of the retroperitoneum. Patients with intermediate- or high-grade retroperitoneal sarcomas are given preoperative systemic therapy with doxorubicin and ifosfamide (up to four cycles), followed by preoperative external beam radiotherapy (45 to 50 Gy), and then surgical resection with an intraoperative or postoperative radiation boost. The objective of the trial is to assess the feasibility, toxicity, and complications of this multimodality treatment regimen.

Adjuvant Therapy Trials for Gastrointestinal Stromal Tumors

Given the promising results of imatinib therapy for metastatic or locally advanced GISTs, the logical next step is to study the efficacy of imatinib as adjuvant and neoadjuvant therapy to determine whether it can lower recurrence rates and prolong disease-specific survival after complete resection. The sections that follow discuss ongoing trials of adjuvant and neoadjuvant imatinib for patients with resectable GISTs.

Radiation Therapy Oncology Group S-01320 Trial. The Radiation Therapy Oncology Group S-01320 Trial is an ongoing phase II trial of neoadjuvant or adjuvant imatinib for patients with potentially resectable primary or recurrent GISTs. Patients with biopsy-proven, c-Kit–expressing GISTs are considered eligible if they have a potentially resectable primary tumor that is 5 cm or larger or a potentially resectable recurrent tumor that is 2 cm or larger. The accrual goal is 63 patients over approximately 2 years to ensure 50 evaluable patients. Patients will receive 600 mg/d of imatinib for 8 weeks and then undergo standard surgical resection with the objective of resecting all gross disease. Postoperatively, all patients who did not have progressive disease before surgery will resume imatinib therapy when they can tolerate oral medications.

Patients will remain in the study regardless of whether the surgery was curative or palliative, and will continue to receive imatinib until evidence of disease progression appears. The primary clinical objectives of the study are to determine the rate of disease recurrence at 2 years, to determine the rate of objective responses in patients given preoperative treatment, to assess the toxicity of postoperative imatinib, and to correlate tumor changes observed on positron-emission tomography with changes observed on conventional cross-sectional imaging. The secondary objective is to evaluate the biologic effects of imatinib on malignant GISTs to elucidate how the targeted molecular therapy works in vivo.

American College of Surgeons Oncology Group Z9000 Trial. The American College of Surgeons Oncology Group is sponsoring the Z9000 trial, a phase II study of adjuvant imatinib given after complete resection of high-risk primary GISTs. High-risk disease is defined as tumor size of at least 10 cm in maximum dimension or the presence of tumor rupture before or during surgery; intraperitoneal hemorrhage; or multifocal intraperitoneal tumors smaller than 5 cm. Within 8 weeks of surgery, eligible patients will be given imatinib at a dose of 400 mg/d for 1 year. The primary objective of the study is to determine whether patients with high-risk resected disease will have lower 2- and 5-year rates of recurrence and prolonged survival after treatment with imatinib as compared with historical control patients.

Phase III Trials. The American College of Surgeons Oncology Group also is sponsoring the Z9001 trial, a phase III randomized double-blind study of adjuvant imatinib versus placebo after complete resection of primary GISTs. Eligible patients will include those with a primary c-Kit–expressing GIST 3 cm or larger, tumor rupture before or during surgery, intraperitoneal hemorrhage, or 1 to 4 multifocal tumors. The patient must have a complete resection within 10 weeks before the initiation of imatinib therapy. The accrual goal is 100 eligible patients per year for 4 years, for a total of 380 evaluable patients.

Patients will be randomized to receive 400 mg/d imatinib or placebo for 1 year. If a patient in the imatinib group has a recurrence during the first year of treatment, the dose will be increased to 800 mg/d. If a patient in the placebo group has a recurrence at any time, imatinib will be started at 400 mg/d and may be increased to 800 mg/d. The primary objective is to ascertain whether patients with completely resected primary GISTs who receive imatinib have longer recurrence-free and disease-specific survival periods than do patients receiving placebo. Also important is to assess the toxicity of imatinib given as adjuvant therapy. The secondary objectives are to perform correlative analyses using tissue samples collected before and after treatment to define the genotype and phenotype of primary and recurrent tumors and to determine the effects and limitations of imatinib therapy.

The investigators in the Z9001 trial recognize that the crossover design may decrease the extent of any differences observed between the treatment groups. In addition, the availability of a higher dose has the potential to improve the survival duration for patients in the imatinib group. However, this design was believed to be necessary to encourage participation in the trial because of the great enthusiasm for imatinib despite its status as an experimental agent.

CONCLUSION

Soft tissue sarcomas are a family of rare tumors, constituting approximately 1% of adult malignancies. The etiology in the vast majority of patients is sporadic. The management of such diverse tumors is complex. Diagnosis by light microscopy is inexact. Molecular diagnosis, although still in its infancy, holds great promise for the future.

In spite of these confounding issues, the natural history of soft tissue sarcomas is well established. Approximately two-thirds of cases arise in the extremities, whereas the remaining one-third are distributed between the retroperitoneum, trunk, abdomen, and head and neck. The management algorithm for soft tissue sarcomas is complex and depends on tumor stage, site, and histology. The most common site of metastasis is the lungs, and it generally occurs within 3 years of diagnosis.

Progress is being made in understanding these tumors at the molecular level. It can be anticipated that molecular-based therapies will become increasingly incorporated into treatment strategies in the near future.

References

1. Herzog CE: Pediatric sarcomas, in Pollock RE (ed): *Soft Tissue Sarcomas*. Hamilton, Ontario: BC Decker Inc., 2002, p 337.
2. Pollock RE, Karnell LH, Menck HR, et al: The National Cancer Data Base report on soft tissue sarcoma. *Cancer* 78:2247, 1996.
3. Lawrence W Jr., Donegan WL, Natarajan N, et al: Adult soft tissue sarcomas. A pattern of care survey of the American College of Surgeons. *Ann Surg* 205:349, 1987.
4. Coindre JM, Terrier P, Guillou L, et al: Predictive value of grade for metastasis development in the main histologic types of adult soft tissue sarcomas: A study of 1240 patients from the French Federation of Cancer Centers Sarcoma Group. *Cancer* 91:1914, 2001.
5. Ramanathan RC, A'Hern R, Fisher C, et al: Modified staging system for extremity soft tissue sarcomas. *Ann Surg Oncol* 6:57, 1999.
6. Arndt CA, Crist WM: Common musculoskeletal tumors of childhood and adolescence. *N Engl J Med* 341:342, 1999.
7. Gaynor J, Tan C, Casper ES, et al: Refinement of clinicopathological staging for localized soft tissue sarcoma of the extremity: A study of 423 adults. *J Clin Oncol* 10:1317, 1992.
8. Fong Y, Coit DG, Woodruff JM, et al: Lymph node metastasis from soft tissue sarcoma in adults. Analysis of data from a prospective database of 1772 sarcoma patients. *Ann Surg* 217:72, 1993.
9. Brady MS, Gaynor JJ, Brennan MF: Radiation-associated sarcoma of bone and soft tissue. *Arch Surg* 127:1379, 1992.
10. Zahm SH, Fraumeni JF Jr.: The epidemiology of soft tissue sarcoma. *Semin Oncol* 24:504, 1997.
11. Hardell L, Sandstron A: A case-control study: Soft tissue sarcoma and exposure to phenoxyacetic acids or chlorophenols. *Br J Cancer* 39:711, 1979.
12. Smith AH, Pearce NE, Fisher DO: Soft tissue sarcoma and exposure to phenoxyherbicides and chlorophenols in New Zealand. *J Natl Cancer Inst* 73:1111, 1984.
13. Stewart FW, Treves N: Lymphangiosarcoma in post-mastectomy lymphedema. *Cancer* 1:64, 1948.
14. Muller R, Hajdu SI, Brennan MF: Lymphangiosarcoma associated with chronic filarial lymphedema. *Cancer* 59:179, 1987.
15. Levine EA: Prognostic factors in soft tissue sarcoma. *Semin Surg Oncol* 17:23, 1999.
16. Sorensen PH, Triche TJ: Gene fusions encoding chimaeric transcription factors in solid tumours. *Semin Cancer Biol* 7:3, 1996.
17. Vorburger SA, Hunt KK: Experimental approaches, in Pollock RE (ed): *Soft Tissue Sarcomas*. Hamilton, Ontario: BC Decker, 2002, p 375.
18. Latres E, Drobnjak M, Pollack D, et al: Chromosome 17 abnormalities and TP53 mutations in adult soft tissue sarcomas. *Am J Pathol* 145:345, 1994.
19. Hieken TJ, Das Gupta TK: Mutant p53 expression: A marker of diminished survival in well-differentiated soft tissue sarcoma. *Clin Cancer Res* 2:1391, 1996.
20. Karnes PS: Neurofibromatosis: A common neurocutaneous disorder. *Mayo Clin Proc* 73:1071, 1998.
21. Varma DG: Optimal radiologic imaging of soft tissue sarcomas. *Semin Surg Oncol* 17:2, 1999.
22. Heslin MJ, Smith JK: Imaging of soft tissue sarcomas. *Surg Oncol Clin North Am* 8:91, 1999.
23. Hanna SL, Fletcher BD: MR imaging of malignant soft-tissue tumors. *Magn Reson Imaging Clin North Am* 3:629, 1995.
24. Demas BE, Heelan RT, Lane J, et al: Soft-tissue sarcomas of the extremities: comparison of MR and CT in determining the extent of disease. *AJR Am J Roentgenol* 150:615, 1988.
25. Hodler J, Yu JS, Steinert HC, et al: MR imaging versus alternative imaging techniques. *Magn Reson Imaging Clin North Am* 3:591, 1995.
26. Storm FK, Mahvi DM: Diagnosis and management of retroperitoneal soft-tissue sarcoma. *Ann Surg* 214:2, 1991.
27. Pearlstone DB, Pisters PW, Bold RJ, et al: Patterns of recurrence in extremity liposarcoma: Implications for staging and follow-up. *Cancer* 85:85, 1999.
28. Kilpatrick SE, Geisinger KR: Soft tissue sarcomas: the usefulness and limitations of fine-needle aspiration biopsy. *Am J Clin Pathol* 110:50, 1998.
29. Ayala AG, Ro JY, Fanning CV, et al: Core needle biopsy and fine-needle aspiration in the diagnosis of bone and soft-tissue lesions. *Hematol Oncol Clin North Am* 9:633, 1995.
30. de Saint Aubain Somerhausen N, Fletcher CD: Soft-tissue sarcomas: An update. *Eur J Surg Oncol* 25:215, 1999.
31. Dupuy DE, Rosenberg AE, Punyaratabandhu T, et al: Accuracy of CT-guided needle biopsy of musculoskeletal neoplasms. *AJR Am J Roentgenol* 171:759, 1998.
32. Huvos AG: The importance of the open surgical biopsy in the diagnosis and treatment of bone and soft-tissue tumors. *Hematol Oncol Clin North Am* 9:541, 1995.
33. Singer S: New diagnostic modalities in soft tissue sarcoma. *Semin Surg Oncol* 17:11, 1999.
34. Shiraki M, Enterline HT, Brooks JJ, et al: Pathologic analysis of advanced adult soft tissue sarcomas, bone sarcomas, and mesotheliomas. The Eastern Cooperative Oncology Group (ECOG) experience. *Cancer* 64:484, 1989.
35. Presant CA, Russell WO, Alexander RW, et al: Soft-tissue and bone sarcoma histopathology peer review: The frequency of disagreement in diagnosis and the need for second pathology opinions. The Southeastern Cancer Study Group experience. *J Clin Oncol* 4:1658, 1986.
36. Alvegard TA, Berg NO: Histopathology peer review of high-grade soft tissue sarcoma: The Scandinavian Sarcoma Group experience. *J Clin Oncol* 7:1845, 1989.
37. American Joint Committee on Cancer: *Cancer Staging Manual*. New York: Springer, 2002, p 221.
38. Coindre JM, Terrier P, Bui NB, et al: Prognostic factors in adult patients with locally controlled soft tissue sarcoma. A study of 546 patients from the French Federation of Cancer Centers Sarcoma Group. *J Clin Oncol* 14:869, 1996.
39. Costa J, Wesley RA, Glatstein E, Rosenberg SA: The grading of soft tissue sarcomas. Results of a clinicohistopathologic correlation in a series of 163 cases. *Cancer* 53:530, 1984.
40. Guillou L, Coindre JM, Bonichon F, et al: Comparative study of the National Cancer Institute and French Federation of Cancer Centers Sarcoma Group grading systems in a population of 410 adult patients with soft tissue sarcoma. *J Clin Oncol* 15:350, 1997.
41. American Joint Committee on Cancer: *Cancer Staging Manual*, 5th ed. Philadelphia: Lippincott-Raven, 1998, p 139.
42. Mazeron JJ, Suit HD: Lymph nodes as sites of metastases from sarcomas of soft tissue. *Cancer* 60:1800, 1987.
43. Elias AD: The clinical management of soft tissue sarcomas. *Semin Oncol* 19:19, 1992.
44. Ng EH, Pollock RE, Munsell MF, et al: Prognostic factors influencing survival in gastrointestinal leiomyosarcomas. Implications for surgical management and staging. *Ann Surg* 215:68, 1992.

45. Ng EH, Pollock RE, Romsdahl MM: Prognostic implications of patterns of failure for gastrointestinal leiomyosarcomas. *Cancer* 69:1334, 1992.

46. Conlon KC, Casper ES, Brennan MF: Primary gastrointestinal sarcomas: Analysis of prognostic variables. *Ann Surg Oncol* 2:26, 1995.

47. National Institute of Health consensus development panel on limb-sparing treatment of adult soft tissue sarcoma and osteosarcomas, Vol. 3. Cancer Treatment Symposium, 1985, p 1.

48. Brennan MF, Casper ES, Harrison LB, et al: The role of multimodality therapy in soft-tissue sarcoma. *Ann Surg* 214:328, 1991.

49. Pisters PW, Leung DH, Woodruff J, et al: Analysis of prognostic factors in 1,041 patients with localized soft tissue sarcomas of the extremities. *J Clin Oncol* 14:1679, 1996.

50. Herbert SH, Corn BW, Solin LJ, et al: Limb-preserving treatment for soft tissue sarcomas of the extremities. The significance of surgical margins. *Cancer* 72:1230, 1993.

51. Tanabe KK, Pollock RE, Ellis LM, et al: Influence of surgical margins on outcome in patients with preoperatively irradiated extremity soft tissue sarcomas. *Cancer* 73:1652, 1994.

52. Karakousis CP, Karmpaliotis C, Driscoll DL: Major vessel resection during limb-preserving surgery for soft tissue sarcomas. *World J Surg* 20:345, 1996.

53. Rosenberg SA, Tepper J, Glatstein E, et al: The treatment of soft-tissue sarcomas of the extremities: Prospective randomized evaluations of (1) limb-sparing surgery plus radiation therapy compared with amputation and (2) the role of adjuvant chemotherapy. *Ann Surg* 196:305, 1982.

54. Potter DA, Glenn J, Kinsella T, et al: Patterns of recurrence in patients with high-grade soft-tissue sarcomas. *J Clin Oncol* 3:353, 1985.

55. Lindberg RD, Martin RG, Romsdahl MM, et al: Conservative surgery and postoperative radiotherapy in 300 adults with soft-tissue sarcomas. *Cancer* 47:2391, 1981.

56. Suit HD, Proppe KH, Mankin HJ, et al: Preoperative radiation therapy for sarcoma of soft tissue. *Cancer* 47:2269, 1981.

57. Abbatucci JS, Boulier N, de Ranieri J, et al: Radiotherapy as an integrated part of the treatment of soft tissue sarcomas. *Radiother Oncol* 2:115, 1984.

58. Leibel SA, Tranbaugh RF, Wara WM, et al: Soft tissue sarcomas of the extremities: Survival and patterns of failure with conservative surgery and postoperative irradiation compared to surgery alone. *Cancer* 50:1076, 1982.

59. McBride CM: Sarcomas of the limbs, results of adjuvant chemotherapy using isolation perfusion. *Arch Surg* 109:304, 1974.

60. Krementz ET, Carter RD, Sutherland CM, et al: Chemotherapy of sarcomas of the limbs by regional perfusion. *Ann Surg* 185:555, 1977.

61. Hoekstra HJ, Schraffordt Koops H, Molenaar WM, et al: Results of isolated regional perfusion in the treatment of malignant soft tissue tumors of the extremities. *Cancer* 60:1703, 1987.

62. Eggermont AM, Schraffordt Koops H, Klausner JM, et al: Isolated limb perfusion with tumor necrosis factor and melphalan for limb salvage in 186 patients with locally advanced soft tissue extremity sarcomas. The cumulative multicenter European experience. *Ann Surg* 224:756, 1996.

63. Lienard D, Ewalenko P, Delmotte JJ, et al: High-dose recombinant tumor necrosis factor alpha in combination with interferon gamma and melphalan in isolation perfusion of the limbs for melanoma and sarcoma. *J Clin Oncol* 10:52, 1992.

64. Fraker D, Alexander HR, Ross M: A phase II trial of isolated perfusion with high dose tumor necrosis factor and melphalan for unresectable extremity sarcomas. Society of Surgical Oncology Proceedings: Abstract #53, 1999.

65. Rossi CR, Vecchiato A, Foletto M, et al: Phase II study on neoadjuvant hyperthermic-antiblastic perfusion with doxorubicin in patients with intermediate or high grade limb sarcomas. *Cancer* 73:2140, 1994.

66. Sheen-Chen SM, Chou FF, Eng HL, et al: Gastric leiomyosarcoma: A clinicopathological review. *Eur J Surg* 160:681, 1994.

67. Suit HD, Russell WO: Radiation therapy of soft tissue sarcomas. *Cancer* 36:759, 1975.

68. Yang JC, Chang AE, Baker AR, et al: Randomized prospective study of the benefit of adjuvant radiation therapy in the treatment of soft tissue sarcomas of the extremity. *J Clin Oncol* 16:197, 1998.

69. Pisters PW, Harrison LB, Leung DH, et al: Long-term results of a prospective randomized trial of adjuvant brachytherapy in soft tissue sarcoma. *J Clin Oncol* 14:859, 1996.

70. Suit HD, Spiro I: Role of radiation in the management of adult patients with sarcoma of soft tissue. *Semin Surg Oncol* 10:347, 1994.

71. Barkley HT Jr., Martin RG, Romsdahl MM, et al: Treatment of soft tissue sarcomas by preoperative irradiation and conservative surgical resection. *Int J Radiat Oncol Biol Phys* 14:693, 1988.

72. Wilson AN, Davis A, Bell RS, et al: Local control of soft tissue sarcoma of the extremity: The experience of a multidisciplinary sarcoma group with definitive surgery and radiotherapy. *Eur J Cancer* 30A:746, 1994.

73. Pisters PW, Harrison LB, Woodruff JM, et al: A prospective randomized trial of adjuvant brachytherapy in the management of low-grade soft tissue sarcomas of the extremity and superficial trunk. *J Clin Oncol* 12:1150, 1994.

74. Geer RJ, Woodruff J, Casper ES, et al: Management of small soft-tissue sarcoma of the extremity in adults. *Arch Surg* 127:1285, 1992.

75. Karakousis CP, Emrich LJ, Rao U, et al: Limb salvage in soft tissue sarcomas with selective combination of modalities. *Eur J Surg Oncol* 17:71, 1991.

76. Wylie JP, O'Sullivan B, Catton C, et al: Contemporary radiotherapy for soft tissue sarcoma. *Semin Surg Oncol* 17:33, 1999.

77. Suit HD, Mankin HJ, Wood WC, et al: Preoperative, intraoperative, and postoperative radiation in the treatment of primary soft tissue sarcoma. *Cancer* 55:2659, 1985.

78. Nielsen OS, Cummings B, O'Sullivan B, et al: Preoperative and postoperative irradiation of soft tissue sarcomas: Effect of radiation field size. *Int J Radiat Oncol Biol Phys* 21:1595, 1991.

79. Langstein HN, Robb GL: Reconstructive approaches in soft tissue sarcoma. *Semin Surg Oncol* 17:52, 1999.

80. O'Sullivan B, Davis AM, Turcotte R, et al: Preoperative versus postoperative radiotherapy in soft-tissue sarcoma of the limbs: A randomised trial. *Lancet* 359:2235, 2002.

81. Harrison LB, Franzese F, Gaynor JJ, et al: Long-term results of a prospective randomized trial of adjuvant brachytherapy in the management of completely resected soft tissue sarcomas of the extremity and superficial trunk. *Int J Radiat Oncol Biol Phys* 27:259, 1993.

82. Janjan NA, Yasko AW, Reece GP, et al: Comparison of charges related to radiotherapy for soft-tissue sarcomas treated by preoperative external-beam irradiation versus interstitial implantation. *Ann Surg Oncol* 1:415, 1994.

83. Rhomberg W, Hassenstein EO, Gefeller D: Radiotherapy vs. radiotherapy and razoxane in the treatment of soft tissue sarcomas: Final results of a randomized study. *Int J Radiat Oncol Biol Phys* 36:1077, 1996.

84. Pollack A, Zagars GK, Goswitz MS, et al: Preoperative vs. postoperative radiotherapy in the treatment of soft tissue sarcomas: A matter of presentation. *Int J Radiat Oncol Biol Phys* 42:563, 1998.

85. Bujko K, Suit HD, Springfield DS, et al: Wound healing after preoperative radiation for sarcoma of soft tissues. *Surg Gynecol Obstet* 176:124, 1993.

86. Schray MF, Gunderson LL, Sim FH, et al: Soft tissue sarcoma. Integration of brachytherapy, resection, and external irradiation. *Cancer* 66:451, 1990.

87. Peat BG, Bell RS, Davis A, et al: Wound-healing complications after soft-tissue sarcoma surgery. *Plast Reconstr Surg* 93:980, 1994.

88. Stinson SF, DeLaney TF, Greenberg J, et al: Acute and long-term effects on limb function of combined modality limb sparing therapy for extremity soft tissue sarcoma. *Int J Radiat Oncol Biol Phys* 21:1493, 1991.

89. Seynaeva C, Verweij J: High-dose chemotherapy in adult sarcomas: No standard yet. *Semin Oncol* 26:119, 1999.

90. Antman KH: Chemotherapy of advanced sarcomas of bone and soft tissue. *Semin Oncol* 19:13, 1992.

91. Santoro A, Tursz T, Mouridsen H, et al: Doxorubicin versus CYVADIC versus doxorubicin plus ifosfamide in first-line treatment of advanced soft tissue sarcomas: A randomized study of the European Organization for Research and Treatment of Cancer Soft Tissue and Bone Sarcoma Group. *J Clin Oncol* 13:1537, 1995.

92. Benjamin RS, Legha SS, Patel SR, et al: Single-agent ifosfamide studies in sarcomas of soft tissue and bone: The M.D. Anderson experience. *Cancer Chemother Pharmacol* 31:S174, 1993.

93. O'Bryan RM, Baker LH, Gottlieb JE, et al: Dose response evaluation of adriamycin in human neoplasia. *Cancer* 39:1940, 1977.

94. Patel SR, Vadhan-Raj S, Papadopolous N, et al: High-dose ifosfamide in bone and soft tissue sarcomas: Results of phase II and pilot studies—dose-response and schedule dependence. *J Clin Oncol* 15:2378, 1997.

95. Nielsen OS, Judson I, van Hoesel Q, et al: Effect of high-dose ifosfamide in advanced soft tissue sarcomas. A multicentre phase II study of the EORTC Soft Tissue and Bone Sarcoma Group. *Eur J Cancer* 36:61, 2000.

96. Frustaci S, Buonadonna A, Romanini A, et al: Increasing dose of continuous infusion ifosfamide and fixed dose of bolus epirubicin in soft tissue sarcomas. A study of the Italian group on rare tumors. *Tumori* 85:229, 1999.

97. Palumbo R, Palmeri S, Antimi M, et al: Phase II study of continuous-infusion high-dose ifosfamide in advanced and/or metastatic pretreated soft tissue sarcomas. *Ann Oncol* 8:1159, 1997.

98. Buesa JM, Lopez-Pousa A, Martin J, et al: Phase II trial of first-line high-dose ifosfamide in advanced soft tissue sarcomas of the adult: A study of the Spanish Group for Research on Sarcomas (GEIS). *Ann Oncol* 9:871, 1998.

99. Demetri GD: Major developments in the understanding and treatment of soft-tissue sarcomas in adults. *Curr Opin Oncol* 10:343, 1998.

100. Tierney JF: Adjuvant chemotherapy for localised resectable soft-tissue sarcoma of adults: Meta-analysis of individual data. Sarcoma Meta-analysis Collaboration. *Lancet* 350:1647, 1997.

101. Frustaci S, Gherlinzoni F, De Paoli A, et al: Adjuvant chemotherapy for adult soft tissue sarcomas of the extremities and girdles: Results of the Italian randomized cooperative trial. *J Clin Oncol* 19:1238, 2001.

102. Petrioli R, Coratti A, Correale P, et al: Adjuvant epirubicin with or without ifosfamide for adult soft-tissue sarcoma. *Am J Clin Oncol* 25:468, 2002.

103. Brodowicz T, Schwameis E, Widder J, et al: Intensified adjuvant IFADIC chemotherapy for adult soft tissue sarcoma: A prospective randomized feasibility trial. *Sarcoma* 4:151, 2000.

104. Figueredo A, Bramwell VHC, Bell R, et al: Adjuvant chemotherapy following complete resection of soft tissue sarcoma in adults: A clinical practice guideline. *Sarcoma* 6:5, 2002.

105. Eilber F, Giuliano A, Huth J, et al: Neoadjuvant chemotherapy, radiation, and limited surgery for high grade soft tissue sarcoma of the extremity. Dordrecht, the Netherlands: Kluwer Academic Publishers, 1988, p 115.

106. Goodnight JE Jr., Bargar WL, Voegeli T, et al: Limb-sparing surgery for extremity sarcomas after preoperative intra-arterial doxorubicin and radiation therapy. *Am J Surg* 150:109, 1985.

107. Levine EA, Trippon M, Das Gupta TK: Preoperative multimodality treatment for soft tissue sarcomas [see comments]. *Cancer* 71:3685, 1993.

108. Wanebo HJ, Temple WJ, Popp MB, et al: Preoperative regional therapy for extremity sarcoma. A tricenter update. *Cancer* 75:2299, 1995.

109. Temple WJ, Temple CL, Arthur K, et al: Prospective cohort study of neoadjuvant treatment in conservative surgery of soft tissue sarcomas. *Ann Surg Oncol* 4:586, 1997.

110. Goffman T, Tochner Z, Glatstein E: Primary treatment of large and massive adult sarcomas with iododeoxyuridine and aggressive hyperfractionated irradiation. *Cancer* 67:572, 1991.

111. Sondak VK, Robertson JM, Sussman JJ: Preoperative idoxuridine and radiation for large soft tissue sarcomas: Clinical results with five-year follow-up. *Ann Surg Oncol* 5:106, 1998.

112. Pisters PW: Chemoradiation treatment strategies for localized sarcoma: Conventional and investigational approaches. *Semin Surg Oncol* 17:66, 1999.

113. Catton CN, O'Sullivan B, Kotwall C, et al: Outcome and prognosis in retroperitoneal soft tissue sarcoma. *Int J Radiat Oncol Biol Phys* 29:1005, 1994.

114. Lewis JJ, Leung D, Woodruff JM, et al: Retroperitoneal soft-tissue sarcoma: Analysis of 500 patients treated and followed at a single institution. *Ann Surg* 228:355, 1998.

115. Jaques DP, Coit DG, Hajdu SI, et al: Management of primary and recurrent soft-tissue sarcoma of the retroperitoneum. *Ann Surg* 212:51, 1990.

116. Singer S, Corson JM, Demetri GD, et al: Prognostic factors predictive of survival for truncal and retroperitoneal soft-tissue sarcoma. *Ann Surg* 221:185, 1995.

117. Chou FF, Eng HL, Sheen-Chen SM: Smooth muscle tumors of the gastrointestinal tract: Analysis of prognostic factors. *Surgery* 119:171, 1996.

118. Papagrigoriadis S, Papadopoulou P, Kolias V, et al: Gastrointestinal leiomyosarcomas: Experience of 14 cases and review of published reports. *Eur J Surg* 164:693, 1998.

119. Hansen CP: Leiomyosarcomas of the gastrointestinal tract. *Ann Chir Gynaecol* 83:13, 1994.

120. Grant CS, Kim CH, Farrugia G, et al: Gastric leiomyosarcoma. Prognostic factors and surgical management. *Arch Surg* 126:985, 1991.

121. Carson W, Karakousis C, Douglass H, et al: Results of aggressive treatment of gastric sarcoma. *Ann Surg Oncol* 1:244, 1994.

122. Bedikian AY, Khankhanian N, Valdivieso M, et al: Sarcoma of the stomach: clinicopathologic study of 43 cases. *J Surg Oncol* 13:121, 1980.

123. Sanders L, Silverman M, Rossi R, et al: Gastric smooth muscle tumors: Diagnostic dilemmas and factors affecting outcome. *World J Surg* 20:992, 1996.

124. Shiu MH, Farr GH, Egeli RA, et al: Myosarcomas of the small and large intestine: A clinicopathologic study. *J Surg Oncol* 24:67, 1983.

125. Horowitz J, Spellman JE Jr., Driscoll DL, et al: An institutional review of sarcomas of the large and small intestine. *J Am Coll Surg* 180:465, 1995.

126. Meijer S, Peretz T, Gaynor JJ, et al: Primary colorectal sarcoma. A retrospective review and prognostic factor study of 50 consecutive patients. *Arch Surg* 125:1163, 1990.

127. McGrath PC, Neifeld JP, Lawrence W Jr., et al: Gastrointestinal sarcomas. Analysis of prognostic factors. *Ann Surg* 206:706, 1987.

128. Lindsay PC, Ordonez N, Raaf JH: Gastric leiomyosarcoma: Clinical and pathological review of fifty patients. *J Surg Oncol* 18:399, 1981.

129. Kindblom LG, Remotti HE, Aldenborg F, et al: Gastrointestinal pacemaker cell tumor (GIPACT): Gastrointestinal stromal tumors show phenotypic characteristics of the interstitial cells of Cajal. *Am J Pathol* 152:1259, 1998.

130. Chan JK: Mesenchymal tumors of the gastrointestinal tract: A paradise for acronyms (STUMP, GIST, GANT, and now GIPACT), implication of c-kit in genesis, and yet another of the many emerging roles of the interstitial cell of Cajal in the pathogenesis of gastrointestinal diseases? *Adv Anat Pathol* 6:19, 1999.

131. Hirota S, Isozaki K, Moriyama Y, et al: Gain-of-function mutations of c-kit in human gastrointestinal stromal tumors. *Science* 279:577, 1998.

132. Sarlomo-Rikala M, Kovatich AJ, Barusevicius A, et al: CD117: A sensitive marker for gastrointestinal stromal tumors that is more specific than CD34. *Mod Pathol* 11:728, 1998.

133. Miettinen M, Sarlomo-Rikala M, Lasota J: Gastrointestinal stromal tumors: Recent advances in understanding of their biology [In Process Citation]. *Hum Pathol* 30:1213, 1999.

134. Taniguchi M, Nishida T, Hirota S, et al: Effect of c-kit mutation on prognosis of gastrointestinal stromal tumors. *Cancer Res* 59:4297, 1999.

135. Zsebo KM, Williams DA, Geissler EN, et al: Stem cell factor is encoded at the Sl locus of the mouse and is the ligand for the c-kit tyrosine kinase receptor. *Cell* 63:213, 1990.

136. Broudy VC: Stem cell factor and hematopoiesis. *Blood* 90:1345, 1997.

137. Yarden Y, Kuang WJ, Yang-Feng T, et al: Human proto-oncogene c-kit: A new cell surface receptor tyrosine kinase for an unidentified ligand. *EMBO J* 6:3341, 1987.

138. Williams DE, Eisenman J, Baird A, et al: Identification of a ligand for the c-kit proto-oncogene. *Cell* 63:167, 1990.

139. DeMatteo RP, Lewis JJ, Leung D, et al: Two hundred gastrointestinal stromal tumors: Recurrence patterns and prognostic factors for survival. *Ann Surg* 231:51, 2000.

140. Lasota J, Jasinski M, Sarlomo-Rikala M, et al: Mutations in exon 11 of c-Kit occur preferentially in malignant versus benign gastrointestinal stromal tumors and do not occur in leiomyomas or leiomyosarcomas. *Am J Pathol* 154:53, 1999.

141. Lux ML, Rubin BP, Biase TL, et al: KIT extracellular and kinase domain mutations in gastrointestinal stromal tumors. *Am J Pathol* 156:791, 2000.

142. Heinrich MC, Griffith DJ, Druker BJ, et al: Inhibition of c-kit receptor tyrosine kinase activity by STI571, a selective tyrosine kinase inhibitor. *Blood* 96:925, 2000.

143. Demetri GD: Targeting c-kit mutations in solid tumors: Scientific rationale and novel therapeutic options. *Semin Oncol* 28:19, 2001.

144. Buchdunger E, Cioffi CL, Law N, et al: Abl protein-tyrosine kinase inhibitor STI571 inhibits in vitro signal transduction mediated by c-kit and platelet-derived growth factor receptors. *J Pharmacol Exp Ther* 295:139, 2000.

145. Zalupski M, Metch B, Balcerzak S, et al: Phase III comparison of doxorubicin and dacarbazine given by bolus versus infusion in patients with soft-tissue sarcomas: A Southwest Oncology Group study. *J Natl Cancer Inst* 83:926, 1991.

146. Elias A, Ryan L, Sulkes A, et al: Response to mesna, doxorubicin, ifosfamide, and dacarbazine in 108 patients with metastatic or unresectable sarcoma and no prior chemotherapy. *J Clin Oncol* 7:1208, 1989.

147. Plaat BE, Hollema H, Molenaar WM, et al: Soft tissue leiomyosarcomas and malignant gastrointestinal stromal tumors: Differences in clinical outcome and expression of multidrug resistance proteins. *J Clin Oncol* 18:3211, 2000.

148. van Oosterom AT, Judson I, Verweij J, et al: Safety and efficacy of imatinib (STI571) in metastatic gastrointestinal stromal tumours: A phase I study. *Lancet* 358:1421, 2001.

149. Blanke CD, von Mehren M, Joensuu H, et al: Evaluation of the safety and efficacy of an oral molecularly-targeted therapy, STI571, in patients with unresectable metastatic gastrointestinal stromal tumors (GISTs) expressing C-KIT (CD117). *Proc Am Soc Clin Oncol* 20:1, 2001.

150. von Mehren M, Blanke C, Joensuu H, et al: High incidence of durable responses induced by imatinib mesylate (Gleevec) in patients with unresectable and metastatic gastrointestinal stromal tumors. *Proc Am Soc Clin Oncol* 21:1608, 2002.

151. Demetri G, Rankin C, Fletcher C, et al: Phase III dose-randomized study of imatinib mesylate (Gleevec, STI571) for GIST; intergroup S0033 early results. *Proc Am Soc Clin Oncol* 21:1651, 2002.

152. Casali PG, Verweij J, Zalcberg J, et al: Imatinib (Gleevec) 400 vs 800 mg daily in patients with gastrointestinal stromal tumors (GIST) a randomized phase III trial from the EORTC Soft Tissue and Bone Sarcoma Group, the Italian Sarcoma Group (ISC), and the Australasian Gastro-Intestinal Trials Group (AGITG). A toxicity report. *Proc Am Soc Clin Oncol* 21:1650, 2002.

153. Grovas A, Fremgen A, Rauck A, et al: The National Cancer Data Base report on patterns of childhood cancers in the United States. *Cancer* 80:2321, 1997.

154. Barr FG, Chatten J, D'Cruz CM, et al: Molecular assays for chromosomal translocations in the diagnosis of pediatric soft tissue sarcomas. *JAMA* 273:553, 1995.

155. Xia SJ, Pressey JG, Barr FG: Molecular pathogenesis of rhabdomyosarcoma. *Cancer Biol Ther* 1:97, 2002.

156. Scrable H, Witte D, Shimada H, et al: Molecular differential pathology of rhabdomyosarcoma. *Genes Chromosomes Cancer* 1:23, 1989.

157. Flamant F, Rodary C, Rey A, et al: Treatment of non-metastatic rhabdomyosarcomas in childhood and adolescence. Results of the second study of the International Society of Paediatric Oncology: MMT84. *Eur J Cancer* 34:1050, 1998.

158. Martelli H, Oberlin O, Rey A, et al: Conservative treatment for girls with nonmetastatic rhabdomyosarcoma of the genital tract: A report from the Study Committee of the International Society of Pediatric Oncology. *J Clin Oncol* 17:2117, 1999.

159. Crist WM, Anderson JR, Meza JL, et al: Intergroup rhabdomyosarcoma study—IV: Results for patients with nonmetastatic disease. *J Clin Oncol* 19:3091, 2001.

160. Maurer HM, Beltangady M, Gehan EA, et al: The Intergroup Rhabdomyosarcoma Study—I. A final report. *Cancer* 61:209, 1988.

161. Breneman JC, Lyden E, Pappo AS, et al: Prognostic factors and clinical outcomes in children and adolescents with metastatic rhabdomyosarcoma—a report from the Intergroup Rhabdomyosarcoma Study IV. *J Clin Oncol* 21:78, 2003.

162. Crist WM, Garnsey L, Beltangady MS, et al: Prognosis in children with rhabdomyosarcoma: A report of the intergroup rhabdomyosarcoma studies I and II. Intergroup Rhabdomyosarcoma Committee. *J Clin Oncol* 8:443, 1990.

163. Vanel D, Shapeero LG, De Baere T, et al: MR imaging in the follow-up of malignant and aggressive soft-tissue tumors: Results of 511 examinations. *Radiology* 190:263, 1994.

164. Nori D, Schupak K, Shiu MH, et al: Role of brachytherapy in recurrent extremity sarcoma in patients treated with prior surgery and irradiation [published erratum appears in *Int J Radiat Oncol Biol Phys* 21:1683, 1991] *Int J Radiat Oncol Biol Phys* 20:1229, 1991.

165. Midis GP, Pollock RE, Chen NP, et al: Locally recurrent soft tissue sarcoma of the extremities. *Surgery* 123:666, 1998.

166. Karakousis CP, Proimakis C, Rao U, et al: Local recurrence and survival in soft tissue sarcomas. *Ann Surg Oncol* 3:255, 1996.

167. Whooley BP, Mooney MM, Gibbs JF, et al: Effective follow-up strategies in soft tissue sarcoma. *Semin Surg Oncol* 17:83, 1999.

168. Hunt KK, Patel SR, Pollack A: Soft tissue sarcomas, in Torosian MH (ed): *Integrated Cancer Management: Surgery, Medical Oncology and Radiation Oncology*. Philadelphia: Marcel Dekker, Inc., 1999, p 394.

169. Singer S, Antman K, Corson JM, Eberlein TJ: Long-term salvageability for patients with locally recurrent soft-tissue sarcomas. *Arch Surg* 127:548, 1992.

170. van Geel AN, Pastorino U, Jauch KW, et al: Surgical treatment of lung metastases: The European Organization for Research and Treatment of Cancer-Soft Tissue and Bone Sarcoma Group study of 255 patients. *Cancer* 77:675, 1996.

171. Van Glabbeke M, van Oosterom AT, Oosterhuis JW, et al: Prognostic factors for the outcome of chemotherapy in advanced soft tissue sarcoma: an analysis of 2,185 patients treated with anthracycline-containing first-line regimens—a European Organization for Research and Treatment of Cancer Soft Tissue and Bone Sarcoma Group Study. *J Clin Oncol* 17:150, 1999.

172. Pollock RE, Lang A, Luo J, et al: Soft tissue sarcoma metastasis from clonal expansion of p53 mutated tumor cells. *Oncogene* 12:2035, 1996.

173. Pollock R, Lang A, Ge T, et al: Wild-type p53 and a *p53* temperature-sensitive mutant suppress human soft tissue sarcoma by enhancing cell cycle control. *Clin Cancer Res* 4:1985, 1998.

174. Milas M, Yu D, Lang A, et al: Adenovirus-mediated p53 gene therapy inhibits human sarcoma tumorigenicity. *Cancer Gene Ther* 7:422, 2000.

175. Milas M, Feig B, Yu D, et al: Isolated limb perfusion in the sarcoma-bearing rat: a novel preclinical gene delivery system. *Clin Cancer Res* 3:2197, 1997.

176. de Roos WK, de Wilt JH, van Der Kaaden ME, et al: Isolated limb perfusion for local gene delivery: Efficient and targeted adenovirus-mediated gene transfer into soft tissue sarcomas. *Ann Surg* 232:814, 2000.

177. Gerber HP, Kowalski J, Sherman D, et al: Complete inhibition of rhabdomyosarcoma xenograft growth and neovascularization requires blockade of both tumor and host vascular endothelial growth factor. *Cancer Res* 60:6253, 2000.

178. Zhang L, Yu D, Hu M, et al: Wild-type p53 suppresses angiogenesis in human leiomyosarcoma and synovial sarcoma by transcriptional suppression of vascular endothelial growth factor expression. *Cancer Res* 60:3655, 2000.

179. Savage DG, Antman KH: Imatinib mesylate—A new oral targeted therapy. *N Engl J Med* 346:683, 2002.

180. Goldman JM: Tyrosine-kinase inhibition in treatment of chronic myeloid leukemia. *Lancet* 355:1031, 2000.

181. Mauro MJ, O'Dwyer M, Heinrich MC, et al: STI571: A paradigm of new agents for cancer therapeutics. *J Clin Oncol* 20:325, 2002.

182. Druker BJ, Tamura S, Buchdunger E, et al: Effects of a selective inhibitor of the Abl tyrosine kinase on the growth of Bcr-Abl positive cells. *Nat Med* 2:561, 1996.

183. Deininger MW, Goldman JM, Lydon N, et al: The tyrosine kinase inhibitor CGP57148B selectively inhibits the growth of BCR-ABL-positive cells. *Blood* 90:3691, 1997.

184. le Coutre P, Mologni L, Cleris L, et al: In vivo eradication of human BCR/ABL-positive leukemia cells with an ABL kinase inhibitor. *J Natl Cancer Inst* 91:163, 1999.

CHAPTER 36

Inguinal Hernias

Robert J. Fitzgibbons, Jr., Charles J. Filipi, and Thomas H. Quinn

INTRODUCTION

References to the surgical treatment of an inguinal hernia date back to the first century; however, formal descriptions of hernia repairs did not appear until the fifteenth century. Castration with wound cauterization or hernia sac débridement with healing allowed by secondary intention were the most common operations. These early operations reflected a complete lack of understanding of the anatomy of the groin. Respectable physicians rarely recommended repair to their patients because the treatment was so brutal. In the early part of the eighteenth century, Sir Astley Cooper recommended a truss rather than surgery and felt that the only indication for operating on an inguinal hernia was strangulation.[1]

The latter part of the eighteenth century heralded dramatic changes as the anatomy of the groin became better understood. In 1881, a French surgeon, Lucas-Championnière, performed high ligation of an indirect inguinal hernia sac at the internal ring with primary closure of the wound. Edoardo Bassini (1844–1924) is considered the father of modern inguinal hernia surgery. By incorporating the developing disciplines of antisepsis and anesthesia with a new operation that included reconstruction of the inguinal floor along with high ligation of the hernia sac, he was able to substantially reduce morbidity. It is universally agreed that this concept was responsible for the advent of the modern surgical era of inguinal herniorrhaphy and is still valid today. The operation resulted in a recurrence rate one fifth of that which was generally accepted, and was considered the gold standard for inguinal hernia repair for most of the twentieth century.

Lotheissen, McVay, Halsted, Shouldice, and others described modifications of Bassini's repair in attempts to further reduce the recurrence rate and to avoid complications. Low recurrence rates have been achieved with these variations in the hands of expert surgeons. However, population-based studies have shown an unacceptably high recurrence rate of approximately 15% in general practice. In addition, these operations have been considered relatively painful because of the tension created by approximating tissues that are not naturally in apposition.

Although Bassini's principle of posterior wall reinforcement remains valid in surgical practice today, his operation has lost its popularity and is used only in selected cases in which the use of prosthetic material is contraindicated. This is because of the widespread acceptance of the concept of avoiding tension during herniorrhaphy, championed by Lichtenstein. Lichtenstein theorized that by using a mesh prosthesis to bridge the hernia defect rather than closing it with sutures, as with the Bassini repair and its modifications, tension is avoided, ostensibly resulting in a less painful operation. He also felt that the lack of tension reduced the incidence of suture pull-out, which would result in a lower recurrence rate. A Lichtenstein type operation has now become the method of choice in the United States.

Following the success of the tension-free concept, investigators focused on further reducing morbidity while still maintaining a low recurrence rate. Gilbert developed a technique of inverting the hernial sac and plugging the defect with a prosthetic mesh. This was further refined by Rutkow with the addition of an onlay patch over the triangle of Hesselbach to prevent development of a direct hernia. This operation is now referred to as the "plug and patch."

The preperitoneal space can also be used for repair of an inguinal hernia and has strong proponents because of the mechanical advantage gained from prosthesis placement behind the abdominal wall. Access to the preperitoneal space can be gained through a lower abdominal incision, transabdominally at the time of laparotomy or with the aid of laparoscopic guidance. Irrespective of the mode of entry to the preperitoneal space, a large prosthesis is used that extends far beyond the margins of the myopectineal orifice and envelops the visceral sac. This brief overview of the history of inguinal herniorrhaphy provides the background for a comprehensive look at the problem of inguinal herniation.

EPIDEMIOLOGY

Seventy-five percent of all abdominal wall hernias occur in the groin. Indirect hernias outnumber direct hernias by about 2:1, with femoral hernias making up a much smaller proportion. Right-sided groin hernias are more common than those on the left. The male:female ratio for inguinal hernias is 7:1. There are approximately 750,000 inguinal herniorrhaphies performed per year in the United States, compared to 25,000 for femoral hernias, 166,000 for umbilical hernias, 97,000 for incisional hernias, and 76,000 for miscellaneous abdominal wall hernias.[2]

Femoral hernias account for less than 10% of all groin hernias, but 40% of these present as emergencies with incarceration or strangulation. The mortality rate for emergency repair is higher than for elective repair. Femoral hernias are more common in older patients and in men who have previously undergone an inguinal hernia repair. Although the absolute number of femoral hernias in males and females is about the same, the incidence in females is four times that of males because of the lower overall frequency of groin hernia in women.[3]

Reliable figures concerning the incidence (new hernias per 100,000 per year) or the prevalence (percentage of the population affected at any given time) of groin hernias are not readily available. The variability in published reports is truly amazing given the frequency with which groin hernias affect the population and their associated socioeconomic impact. The major reason for this is the lack of objective criteria to consistently make an accurate diagnosis. Self-reporting by patients, audits of routine physical examinations, and insurance company databases are among the diverse sources from which such figures are derived, all of which are known to be notoriously inaccurate. Physician physical examination, even by trained surgeons, also is not dependable because of the difficulty differentiating between lipomas of the cord or a normal expansile bulge and a true groin hernia.

The prevalence of inguinal hernias in males is clearly age dependent. Congenital inguinal hernias are common in low birthweight individuals with a preponderance on the right side. In a study of male children with birthweight less than 1500 grams, 32% required a hernia operation by age 8.[4] For an adult male, the incidence increases steadily with age, and has been reported to approach 50% for men over the age of 75. Abramson and colleagues from Israel published a particularly helpful paper dealing with inguinal hernia epidemiology.[5] Four hundred fifty-five men with inguinal hernias were identified in subjects who were members of a settlement community from the early 1950s. The population was uniquely suited for study because of its heterogenicity related to the political realities in that country at the time. In addition to native-born Israelis, the group included substantial numbers of immigrant Europeans, Americans, Asians, and Africans. The patients were interviewed using a strictly standardized technique and then examined by a physician. Abramson reported the current prevalence rates (which excludes repaired hernias) and the lifetime prevalence rates (which includes repaired hernias) for various ages, the results of which are reproduced in Table 36-1. The overall current risk for a male to have an inguinal hernia was 18% and the lifetime risk was 24%. The lifetime risk for the development of bilaterality was 39% (age 25 to 34 = 31%, age 65 to 74 = 45%, age 75+ = 59%). Although the Abramson data are felt to be among the most reliable and are often referenced, again it must be noted that there is considerable variance in

Table 36-1
Inguinal Hernia Prevalence by Age

Age (Years)	25–34	35–44	45–54	55–64	65–74	75+
Current prevalence (%)	12	15	20	26	29	34
Lifetime prevalence (%)	15	19	28	34	40	47

Current = repaired hernias excluded; Lifetime = repaired hernias included.

the literature. For example, Akin and colleagues reviewed the files of 27,408 healthy adult male military recruits between 20 and 22 years of age who were examined to detect inguinal hernias.[6] Eight hundred eighty-five (3.2%) inguinal hernia cases were detected, which is substantially lower than that reported in the Abramson study.

NATURAL HISTORY

Risk factors that are useful in predicting complications in an adult patient with a groin hernia include old age, short duration, femoral hernia, and coexisting medical illness. In children, the risk factors are very young age, male sex, short duration, and right-sided hernia.[7] However, the question remains, "Just what is the *incidence* of a complication?" Surgeons are trained that all inguinal hernias should be repaired at diagnosis, even if asymptomatic, to prevent the complication of strangulation (see below) and that herniorrhaphy becomes more difficult the longer repair is delayed. The result is that it is difficult to find a whole group of patients with hernias that remain untreated. This makes it difficult to obtain an accurate picture of the natural history. The commonly quoted 4 to 6% lifetime risk for strangulation of an inguinal hernia is probably more the result of speculation than fact.[8] Incarceration and strangulation rates are also difficult to determine due to the lack of a uniform definition. For example, surgeon A might call an acutely painful, irreducible hernia a strangulated hernia and perform an emergency operation. Surgeon B, on the other hand, might see the same patient and use sedation and taxis, converting the event to elective.[9]

Some light can be shed on the subject by looking at patients with hernias from a time before inguinal herniorrhaphy was routinely performed. Records of patients from a Paris truss clinic (1880–1884) disclosed 242 episodes of hernia-related complications such as obstruction or strangulation in 8633 patients, for a probability of 0.0037 per patient per year.[10] Hernia prevalence data are also available from Colombia, South America, due to a 1-year government initiative to aggressively examine a stratified random sample of the civilian population to determine the frequency of common conditions such as inguinal hernia. By examining records years later from the hospitals in the city of Cali the probability of a hernia-related complication was found to be 0.0029 per year. Using life table analyses and the average of these two probabilities the lifetime risk of a hernia accident for an 18-year-old man is 0.272% or 1:368 patients. For a 72-year-old, it is 0.034% or 1:2941 patients.

Definitive data concerning other aspects of the natural history, such as the likelihood of progression (enlargement) and the difficulty of repair over time, are largely unavailable. Hair and colleagues provided some data concerning the likelihood of developing pain or incarceration by examining a prospectively maintained database of 699 patients.[9] Using Kaplan-Meier estimates, they were able to calculate that the probability of a patient developing pain by 10 years was 90%. However, this seemed to have minimal clinical significance because leisure activity was affected in only 29%, and only 13% of the employed patients had to take time off from work because of hernia-related symptoms. Similarly, the cumulative probability of a hernia becoming irreducible rose to 30% by 10 years, but only 10 patients in their series required an emergency operation and only two had to have strangulated hernia contents resected.

There are a large number of patients who either choose or are counseled by their primary care physician not to have their hernia repaired if it is not too bothersome. A better understanding of the natural history therefore becomes particularly important to identify subgroups that might be at greater risk for a complication. The United States Agency for Healthcare Related Quality of Life in conjunction with the American College of Surgeons are currently sponsoring a comprehensive clinical trial comparing a strategy of observation for asymptomatic patients with routine repair. It is hoped that these data will result in improved knowledge about the natural history. The natural history of symptomatic hernias cannot be studied with such a mechanism because of ethical considerations. However, waiting lists in health care systems where surgical correction is not immediately available are being examined to provide some information.

HERNIA ACCIDENT (INCARCERATION, BOWEL OBSTRUCTION, AND STRANGULATION)

An incarcerated hernia is by definition an irreducible hernia. However, this does not constitute a surgical emergency, as chronic states of incarceration are common because of the size of the neck of the hernia in relationship to its contents or because of adhesions to the hernia sac. The recommended treatment of an incarcerated hernia is surgical, but there is no urgency because there is no life-threatening complication present.

A patient with an incarcerated inguinal hernia exhibiting signs of a bowel obstruction or one who develops an acute incarceration that remains exquisitely tender represents a completely different clinical scenario. Unlike adhesive small bowel obstructions, partial small bowel obstructions are rare. Therefore most patients will have vomiting and absolute constipation (obstipation). In Western countries, groin hernia ranks third after adhesive obstruction and cancer as the most common cause of bowel obstruction. In other geographic areas, it remains the most prevalent. It is common for it to be overlooked on clinical examination, and therefore must be kept in mind in patients being evaluated for bowel obstruction.

Imaging studies are important in cases where there is the slightest question about the cause of the patient's obstructive pattern. This is because a distal intestinal obstruction secondary to another cause (e.g., adhesions) may result in distention of a coincidental nonobstructing groin hernia. Should the examiner focus attention exclusively on the hernia, the stage is set for disaster when the hernia is repaired and the real cause of the obstruction is missed. Plain roentgenograms of the abdomen will reveal the usual signs of an intestinal obstruction, such as dilated loops of bowel with air-fluid levels, absence of bowel gas distal to the obstruction, and bowel shadows in the region of the hernia. A lateral view is often useful to demonstrate this more clearly. Computed tomographic (CT) scans reliably demonstrate the hernia with characteristic features of obstruction, and should be considered if the clinical diagnosis is uncertain.

The initial treatment, in the absence of signs of strangulation, is taxis. Taxis is performed with the patient sedated and placed in the Trendelenburg position. The hernia sac neck is grasped with one hand, with the other applying pressure on the most distal part of the hernia. The goal is to elongate the neck of the hernia so that the contents of the hernia may be guided back into the abdominal cavity with a rocking movement. Mere pressure on the most distal part of the hernia causes bulging of the hernial sac around the neck that can occlude the neck and prevent its reduction (Fig. 36-1). Taxis should not be performed with excessive pressure. If the hernia is strangulated, gangrenous bowel might be reduced into the abdomen or perforated in the process. One or two gentle attempts should be made at taxis. If this is unsuccessful, the procedure should be abandoned. Rarely, the hernia together with its peritoneal sac and constricting neck may be reduced into the abdomen (reduction en masse). Reduction en masse of a hernia is defined as the displacement of a

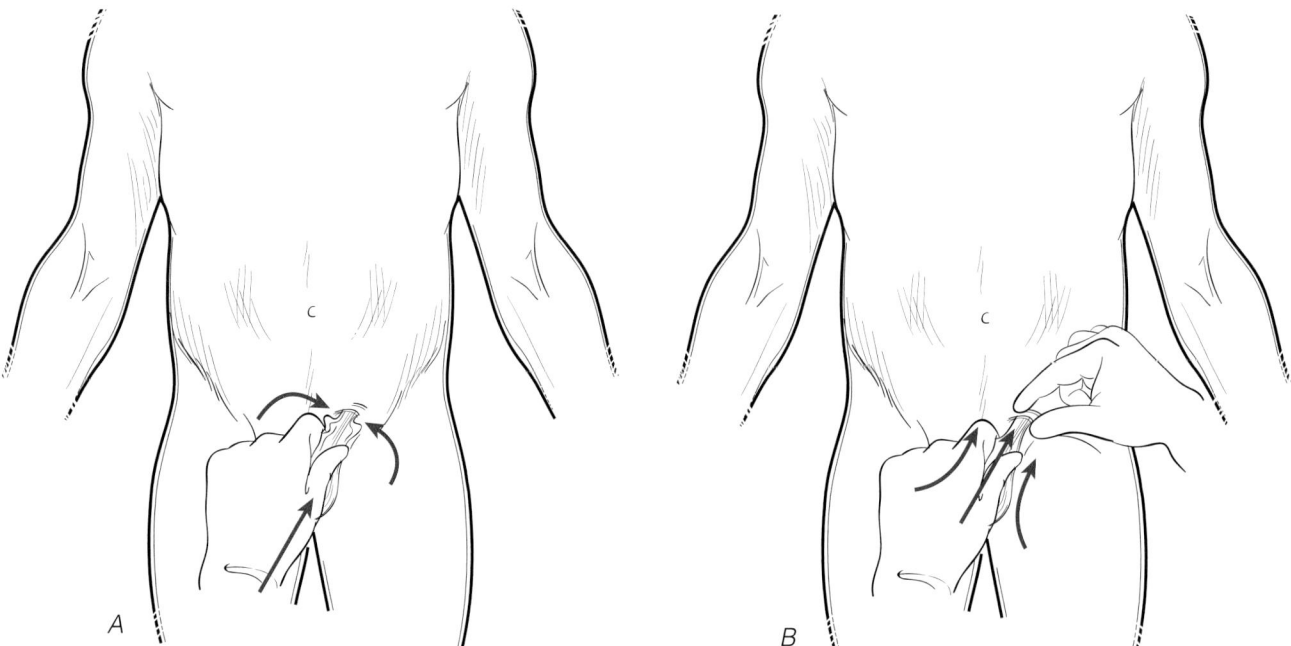

FIG. 36-1. The maneuver of taxis. A. Note that simple pressure on the hernia does not result in favorable distribution of pressure to reduce the hernia. B. By grasping the neck with the nondominant hand, the neck is elongated, making it easier to reduce incarcerated contents.

hernia mass without relief of incarceration or strangulation. This diagnosis must be considered in all cases of intestinal obstruction after apparent reduction of an incarcerated hernia. Laparoscopy can be both diagnostic and therapeutic and therefore is a particularly good option. Surgeon expertise may make laparotomy a better choice for some.[11]

The most significant complication of either acute incarceration or intestinal obstruction is strangulation. It is a serious, life-threatening condition because the hernia contents have become ischemic and nonviable. The clinical features of a strangulated obstruction are dramatic. In addition to the patient having developed an irreducible hernia and an intestinal obstruction, clinical signs indicate that strangulation has taken place. The hernia is tense and very tender, and the overlying skin may be discolored with a reddish or bluish tinge. There are no bowel sounds present within the hernia itself. The patient commonly has a leukocytosis with a left shift, and is toxic, dehydrated, and febrile. Arterial blood gases may reveal a metabolic acidosis.

Rapid resuscitation with intravenous fluids is essential, along with electrolyte replacement, antibiotics, and nasogastric suction. Urgent surgery is indicated once resuscitation has taken place. The initial surgical approach is to make an open inguinal hernia incision. If the bowel is viable, it is reduced into the abdominal cavity prior to repairing the hernia. The neck of the hernia is widened if any difficulty is encountered reducing the hernia. Although rare, the surgeon must be cognizant of the possibility that a nonviable abdominal organ may have been reduced into the abdominal cavity during the course of usual surgical maneuvers before it could be visualized. If such a suspicion is present, the entire gastrointestinal (GI) tract must be evaluated. If the bowel is found to be obviously gangrenous, more bowel must be pulled into the hernia so that viable bowel can be transected and the gangrenous portion removed. In the ideal situation, an end-to-end anastomosis is performed and the bowel is reduced into the abdominal cavity, followed by hernia repair. The slightest suspicion that the entire process cannot be

addressed from the groin mandates exploratory laparoscopy or laparotomy to unequivocally prove that all nonviable tissue has been resected. In the case of a femoral hernia, it is frequently necessary to incise the inguinal ligament anteriorly or the lacunar ligament medially to facilitate reduction.

ETIOLOGY

The cause of an inguinal hernia is far from completely understood, but it is undoubtedly multifactorial (Table 36-2). Familial predisposition plays a role.[5] There is increasing evidence that connective tissue disorders predispose to hernia formation by altering collagen formation. For example, lathyrism is associated with an increased incidence of inguinal hernia in animals, and lathyrogens can be

Table 36-2
Presumed Causes of Groin Herniation

Coughing
Chronic obstructive pulmonary disease
Obesity
Straining
    Constipation
    Prostatism
Pregnancy
Birthweight less than 1500 g
Family history of a hernia
Valsalva maneuvers
Ascites
Upright position
Congenital connective tissue disorders
Defective collagen synthesis
Previous right lower quadrant incision
Arterial aneurysms
Cigarette smoking
Heavy lifting
Physical exertion (?)

Table 36-3
Connective Tissue Disorders Associated with Groin Herniation

Osteogenesis imperfecta
Cutis laxa (congenital elastolysis)
Ehlers-Danlos syndrome
Hurler-Hunter syndrome
Marfan syndrome
Congenital hip dislocation in children
Polycystic kidney disease
Alpha$_1$-antitrypsin deficiency
Williams syndrome
Androgen insensitivity syndrome
Robinow syndrome
Serpentine fibula syndrome
Alport's syndrome
Tel Hashomer camptodactyly syndrome
Leriche's syndrome
Testicular feminization syndrome
Rokitansky-Mayer-Kuster syndrome
Goldenhar syndrome
Morris syndrome
Gerhardt syndrome
Menkes syndrome
Kawasaki disease
Pfannenstiel syndrome
Beckwith-Wiedemann syndrome
Rubenstein-Taybi syndrome
Alopecia-photophobia syndrome

used in the laboratory to produce hernias.[12] Cannon and Read used hydroxyproline concentration in the rectus sheath as a measure of collagen production to show it was decreased in patients with inguinal hernias. They pointed out the importance of defective collagen metabolism in cigarette smokers that causes hernia formation, and coined the term *metastatic emphysema*.[13] A higher prevalence of inguinal hernias is well known among patients suffering from certain congenital connective tissue disorders (Table 36-3). In children with congenital hip dislocation, inguinal hernia occurs five times more often in girls and three times more often in boys compared to children without this disease.[14] The role of physical exertion in the development of inguinal hernia is probably less important than is commonly believed. The cause-and-effect relationship between a specific lifting episode and the development of an inguinal hernia is present in less than 10% of patients, except in circumstances in which worker's compensation issues are involved.[15] In addition, athletes, even weightlifters, do not seem to have an excessive incidence of inguinal hernias.

Indirect Inguinal Hernias

The so-called "saccular theory" of indirect inguinal hernia formation proposed by Russell remains popular.[16] Russell's hypothesis that the "presence of a developmental diverticulum associated with a patent processus vaginalis, was *essential* in every case" is still valid in the minds of many surgeons today. Russell felt that increased intra-abdominal pressure might serve to further stretch and weaken the internal ring, allowing additional intra-abdominal organs to herniate through the orifice, but could not actually cause an indirect inguinal hernia. However, this does not explain all cases of indirect groin hernias. First, a patent processus vaginalis can be found at autopsy without clinical evidence of a hernia.[17] Second, there are patients with an obliterated processus vaginalis who have an abdominal wall defect lateral to the epigastric vessels.[18] Third, congenital structural malformations of the transversalis fascia and transversus abdominis aponeurosis can alter the strength and size of the internal inguinal ring. Denervation of the internal oblique muscle by adjacent inci-

sions (e.g., appendectomy) can also be associated with the eventual development of an indirect inguinal hernia.[19]

Excessive fatty tissue involving the cord or round ligament encountered by a surgeon during elective herniorrhaphy has traditionally been referred to as a lipoma of the cord. This term is unfortunate because it implies a neoplastic process, but a lipoma of the cord consists of normal fatty tissue. The reason for the term *lipoma* is that the fatty tissue can easily be separated from the cord structures and reduced into the preperitoneal space en masse, as if it were a tumor. A lipoma of the cord is important from a clinical standpoint for the following reasons: (1) it can cause hernia-type symptoms, although with less frequency than indirect hernias with a peritoneal sac; (2) it is often difficult to distinguish at physical examination from an indirect hernia with a peritoneal sac; and (3) it can be responsible for an unsatisfactory result because of an unchanged physical examination after elective inguinal herniorrhaphy, especially when a preperitoneal repair is utilized.[20] For the purposes of the large clinical trials referred to in other parts of this chapter, a lipoma of the cord was classified as an indirect hernia. There is no peritoneal sac by definition, because the contents of the indirect hernia (i.e., preperitoneal fat) come from the preperitoneal space rather than the abdominal cavity.

Direct Inguinal Hernias

Two major factors are felt to be important in the development of direct inguinal hernias. The first is increased intra-abdominal pressure associated with a variety of conditions listed in Table 36-2. The second factor is relative weakness of the posterior inguinal wall. An abnormally high-lying arch of the main body of the transversus abdominis muscle above the superior ramus of the pubis that results in a large area at risk has been incriminated (see anatomy section). Similarly, a limited insertion of the transversus abdominis muscle onto the pubis, weakness of the iliopubic tract, limited insertion of the iliopubic tract aponeurosis into Cooper's ligament, or a combination of these have been reported to contribute.[18]

Femoral Hernias

The size and shape of the femoral ring and increased intra-abdominal pressure are factors that contribute to the development of a femoral hernia. The femoral vein and the superior pubic ramus are the borders of the femoral ring laterally and inferiorly. These two structures are more or less constant and therefore are not a factor in the development of this hernia. The iliopubic tract anteriorly and medially accounts for the variability that allows the development of the hernia. The iliopubic tract normally inserts for a distance of 1 to 2 cm along the pectinate line between the pubic tubercle and the midportion of the superior pubic ramus. A femoral hernia can result if the insertion is less than 1 to 2 cm or if it is medially shifted. The net effect of either anatomic subtlety is to widen the femoral ring, predisposing to the hernia. Femoral hernias are particularly dangerous because of the rigid structures that make up the femoral ring. The slightest amount of edema at the ring can produce gangrenous changes of the sac contents, continuing distally into the femoral canal and thigh.

Femoral hernias that occur after inguinal herniorrhaphy either were missed during the original procedure or may even have been caused by the operation. It is often difficult to distinguish between the normal femoral plug of fatty lymphatic-connective tissue that resides in the femoral canal and a true femoral hernia. It has been suggested that the increased incidence of femoral hernias in laparoscopic herniorrhaphy series may be the result of this error. In the absence of clinical evidence of a femoral hernia, surgeons should

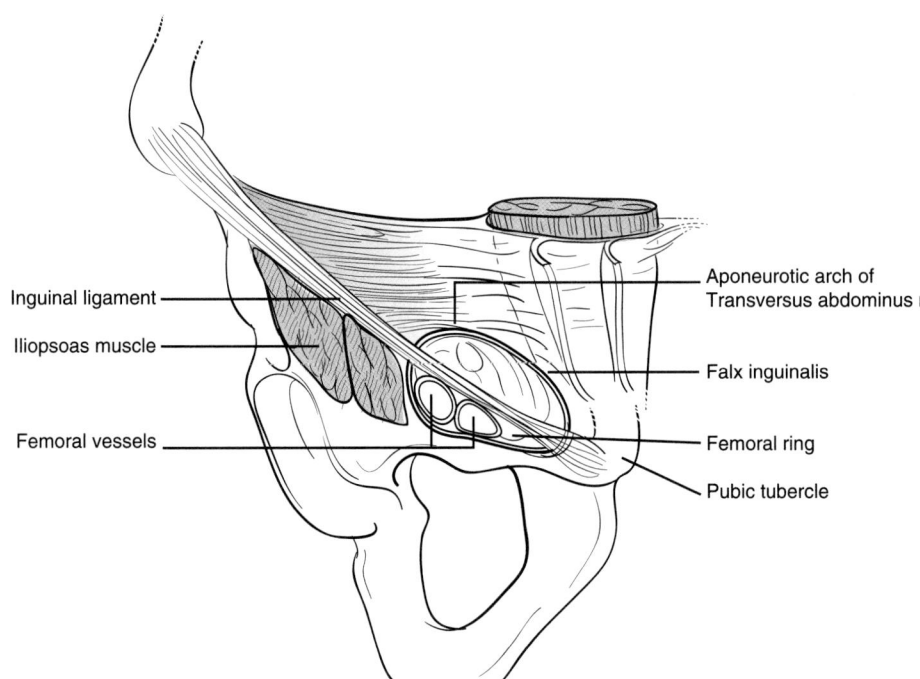

Inguinal ligament

Iliopsoas muscle

Femoral vessels

Aponeurotic arch of
Transversus abdominus m.

Falx inguinalis

Femoral ring

Pubic tubercle

FIG. 36-2. Anterior and posterior views of the myopectineal orifice of Fruchaud. The boundaries include the oblique muscles of the abdominal wall and transversus abdominis muscles superiorly, the rectus muscle and sheath medially, the iliopsoas muscle laterally, and by Cooper's ligament (pecten pubis) inferiorly. From an anterior perspective, the orifice is bisected by the inguinal ligament separating the femoral structures from the direct and indirect spaces. From the posterior prospective, the iliopubic tract bisects the same elements.

avoid manipulating the femoral pad, because inappropriate probing can compromise its protective effect and predispose the patient to development of a true femoral hernia.[21]

The Myopectineal Orifice of Fruchaud

Fruchaud's contribution to inguinal herniology was to examine the common anatomic etiology of direct, indirect, and femoral hernias, rather than to look at each individually. He popularized the use of the term *myopectineal orifice,* an area bound superiorly by the internal oblique and transversus abdominis muscles, medially by the rectus muscle and sheath, laterally by the iliopsoas muscle, and inferiorly by Cooper's ligament (pecten pubis) (Fig. 36-2). Critical anatomic landmarks such as the inguinal ligament, spermatic cord, and the femoral vessels are contained within this area. This funnel-shaped orifice is lined in its entirety by the transversalis fascia. Fruchaud's concept is that the fundamental cause of all groin hernia is failure of the transversalis fascia to retain the peritoneum. Thus if the hernia surgeon concentrates his or her efforts on restoring the integrity of the transversalis fascia, whether a groin hernia is direct, indirect, or femoral becomes irrelevant, because the abdominal wall defect does not need to be addressed. Fruchaud was René Stoppa's mentor and his influence led Stoppa to develop "la grande prothese de renforcement du sac visceral," that uses a large, permanent prosthesis that entirely replaces the transversalis fascia over Fruchaud's myopectineal orifice with a wide flap of surrounding tissue.[22] The giant prosthetic reinforcement of the visceral sac (GPRVS) popularized by Wantz in the United States was the direct result.

Sliding Inguinal Hernia

A *sliding inguinal hernia* is defined as any hernia in which part of the sac is the wall of a viscus. Approximately 8% of all groin hernias present with this finding, but the incidence is age related. It is rarely found in patients less than 30 years of age, but increases to 20% after the age of 70. On the right, the cecum, ascending colon, or appendix are most commonly involved, and on the left, the sigmoid

colon is involved. The uterus, fallopian tube, ovary, ureter, and bladder can be involved on either side. The sliding component is usually found on the posterolateral side of the internal ring. The importance of this condition has lessened considerably in the last several years with the realization that it is not necessary to resect hernia sacs, and that simple reduction into the preperitoneal space is sufficient. This eliminates the primary danger associated with sliding hernias, which is injury to the viscus during high ligation and sac excision.[23]

ANATOMY

The anatomy of the groin is best understood when observing from the approach used for the herniorrhaphy to be performed. For open operations, this means from the skin down through the deeper layers. For laparoscopic or preperitoneal operations, one should consider the anatomy from the abdominal cavity outward to the skin. Common to both perspectives is the bony skeleton of the pelvis, that is made up of the two large hip bones that are the anterior and lateral borders, and the sacrum and coccyx posteriorly (Fig. 36-3). Each hip bone is subdivided into the ilium, ischium, and pubis portions that join around the acetabulum (Fig. 36-4). The pelvis is best conceptualized in an upright human as a funnel attached to the lumbar vertebral column via the sacrum, with the spout or lower portion of the funnel tilting 50 to 60° backward. The top of the funnel consists of the iliac bones and the pubic bones, that form a complete circle with the sacrum. The pubic bones fuse in the anterior midline to form a symphysis, the pubic symphysis. The posterior or narrow end of the funnel is ringed by the coccyx, ischial tuberosities, and the superior rami of the pubic bones. This arrangement means that the anterior superior iliac spine and the pubic tubercle are on the same vertical axis in the upright position (Fig. 36-5A, B, and C). These bony structures are important to the hernia surgeon because of the various musculoaponeurotic and ligamentous structures that attach to them.

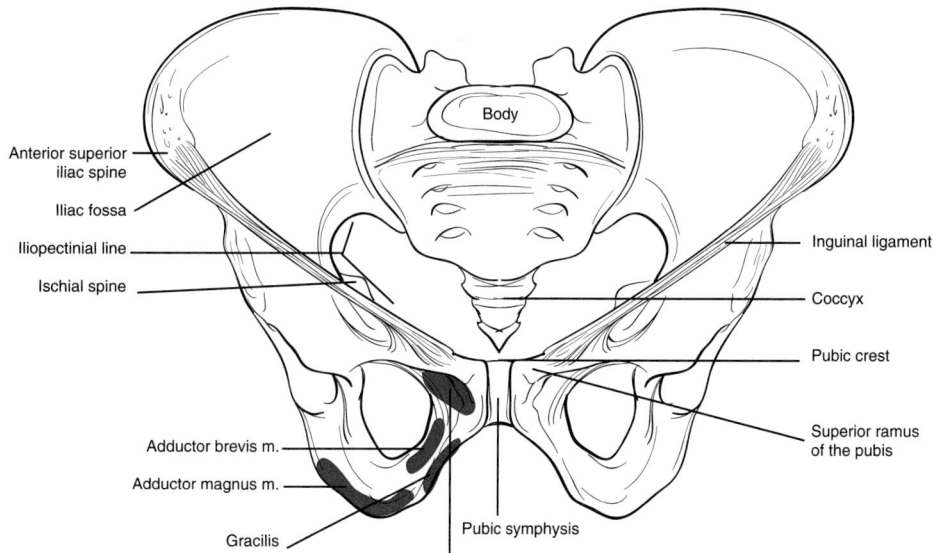

FIG. 36-3. The bony pelvis is made up of the two large hip bones that are the anterior and lateral borders, and the sacrum and coccyx posteriorly. The numbered shaded areas on the ischium and pubis correspond to the origins of some of the adductor muscles (adductor longus, adductor brevis, gracilis, and adductor magnus), which are important because of their prominence as a cause of obscure groin pain.

The Anterior Perspective (Open)

The skin of the lower anterior abdominal wall is innervated by anterior and lateral cutaneous branches of the ventral rami of the lower intercostal nerves, and from the ventral rami of the first and second lumbar nerves. These nerves course between the lateral flat muscles of the abdomen, and then enter the skin through the subcutaneous tissue.

The first layers encountered beneath the skin are Camper's and Scarpa's fascia in the subcutaneous tissue. The only significance of these layers is that they can be reapproximated when sufficiently developed, to provide another layer between a repaired inguinal floor and the outside. The major blood vessels of this superficial fatty layer are the superficial epigastric vessels and the superficial circumflex iliac vessels, which are branches of the femoral vessels.

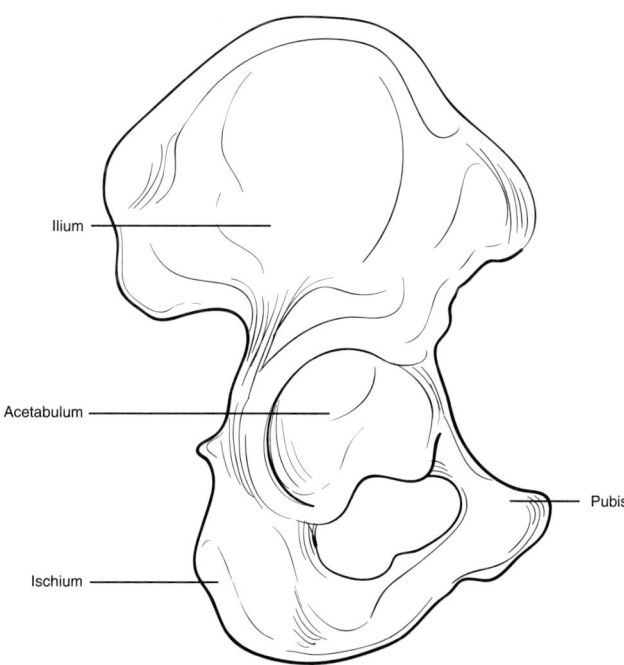

FIG. 36-4. The four major parts of the hip bone.

Fibrous tissue layers are of great importance to the hernia surgeon because of their ability to support sutures. *Fascia* and *aponeurosis* are terms commonly used to describe these fibrous structures, but are often confused and used interchangeably. For the purposes of this chapter, an aponeurosis is defined as the portion of a muscle containing no muscle fiber, that is usually present at insertion points. Muscle fibers are said to "give way" to the corresponding aponeurosis. Fascia, on the other hand, is the fibrous tissue that lines or envelops muscles.

The aponeurosis of the external oblique muscle is the next structure encountered as dissection proceeds through the abdominal wall. The muscle arises from the posterior aspects of the lower eight ribs and interdigitates with both the serratus anterior and the latissimus dorsi at its origin (see Fig. 36-5A). The posterior portion of the muscle is oriented vertically and inserts on the crest of the ilium. The anterior portion of the muscle courses inferiorly in an oblique direction toward the midline and pubis. The muscle fibers themselves are of no interest to the inguinal hernia surgeon until they form its aponeurosis, which occurs well above the inguinal region. The obliquely arranged anterior-inferior fibers of the aponeurosis of the external oblique muscle fold back onto themselves to form the inguinal ligament (synonyms: crural arch, fallopian arch, femoral arch, arcus inguinalis, fallopian ligament, Poupart ligament, and ligamentum inguinale). This structure attaches laterally to the anterior superior iliac spine. The medial insertion of the inguinal ligament in most individuals is dual. One portion inserts on the pubic tubercle and the pubic bone. The other portion is fan shaped and spans the distance between the inguinal ligament proper and the pectineal line of the pubis. This fan-shaped portion of the ligament is called the lacunar ligament (synonyms: Gimbernat ligament and ligamentum lacunare). It blends laterally with Cooper's (pectineal) ligament. The more medial fibers of the aponeurosis of the external oblique divide into a medial and a lateral crus to form the external or superficial inguinal ring, through which the spermatic cord or round ligament and branches of the ilioinguinal and genitofemoral nerves pass. The rest of the medial fibers insert into the linea alba after contributing to the anterior portion of the rectus sheath.

The internal spermatic vessels (pampiniform venous plexus and the testicular artery) and the genital branch of the genitofemoral nerve, a branch of the lumbar plexus, join the vas deferens at the

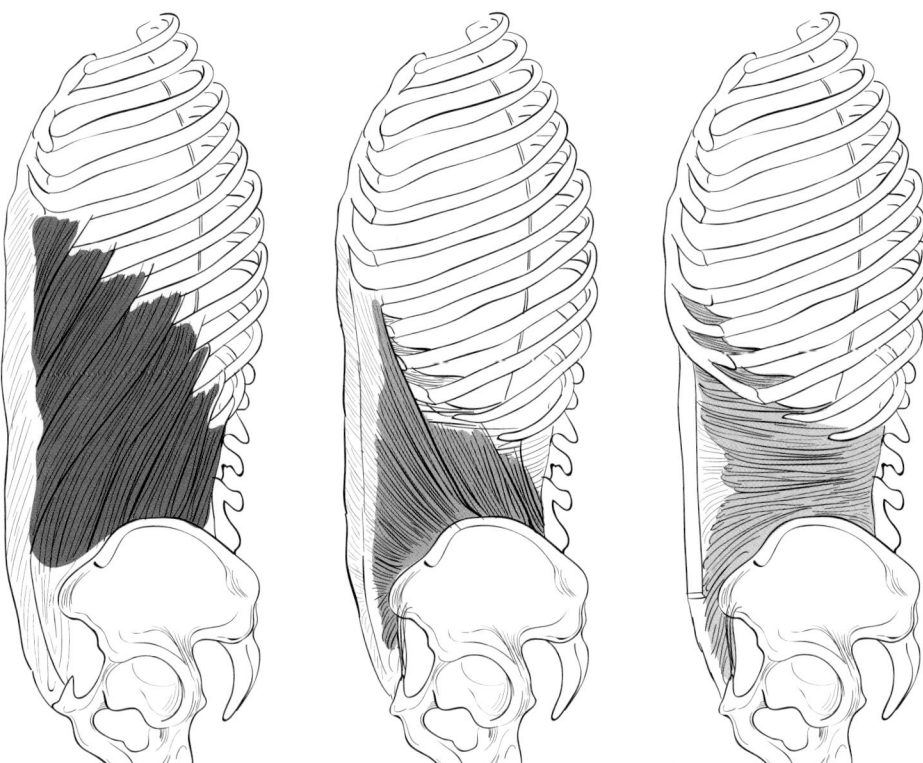

A *B* *C*

FIG. 36-5. *A. External oblique muscle. B. Internal oblique muscle. C. Transversus abdominis muscle.*

internal inguinal ring to begin the spermatic cord. The cord structures also include several investing layers. The innermost covering layer is the internal spermatic fascia. The middle covering layer is called the cremasteric fascia, and contains the cremasteric muscle bundles, both of which are derived from the internal abdominal oblique muscle and fascia. The outermost covering of the spermatic cord is the external spermatic fascia, which is continuous with the investing fascia of the external oblique muscle. The processus (tunica) vaginalis normally has atrophied and closed early in neonatal life. The structure is an invagination of peritoneum that results in fetal life, when the testicle that is attached to the peritoneum on its anterior surface descends retroperitoneally, pulling the peritoneum with it. Failure of this invagination to obliterate by natural processes (a patent processus vaginalis) is the sine qua non of a congenital indirect inguinal hernia.

The internal abdominal oblique muscle (see Fig. 36-5B) fibers fan out, following the shape of the iliac crest. The superior fibers course obliquely upward toward the distal ends of the lower three or four ribs, while the lower fibers orient themselves inferomedially toward the pubis to run parallel to the external oblique aponeurotic fibers. These fibers arch over the round ligament or the spermatic cord, forming the superficial part of the internal (deep) inguinal ring.

Important nerves lie in the space between the internal oblique muscle and the external oblique aponeurosis, and most surgeons feel these nerves must be respected if considerable postoperative morbidity is to be avoided (Fig. 36-6). The first lumbar nerve divides into the ilioinguinal and iliohypogastric nerves. These may divide within the psoas major muscle retroperitoneally or between the internal oblique and transversus abdominis muscles. The ilioinguinal nerve may communicate with the iliohypogastric nerve before innervating the internal oblique muscle. The ilioinguinal nerve then passes through the external inguinal ring to run with the spermatic cord, while the iliohypogastric nerve pierces the external oblique

to innervate the skin above the pubis. The cremaster muscle fibers, which are derived from the internal oblique muscle, are innervated by the genitofemoral nerve (L1, L2). The cutaneous responsibilities of these nerves are shown in Fig. 36-7. There can be considerable variability and overlap.

The transversus abdominis muscle (see Fig. 36-5C) arises from the inguinal ligament, the inner side of the iliac crest, the endoabdominal fascia, and the lower six costal cartilages and ribs, where it interdigitates with the lateral diaphragmatic fibers. The medial aponeurotic fibers of the transversus abdominis contribute to the rectus sheath and insert on the pecten pubis and the crest of the pubis, forming the falx inguinalis (Fig. 36-8). These fibers infrequently are joined by a portion of the internal oblique aponeurosis; only then is a true conjoined tendon formed.[18] Aponeurotic fibers of the transversus abdominis also form the structure known as the aponeurotic arch (see Fig. 36-8). It is theorized that the contraction of the transversus abdominis causes the arch to move downward toward the inguinal ligament, thereby constituting a shutter mechanism that reinforces the weakest area of the groin when intra-abdominal pressure is increased. The area beneath the arch varies. Many feel that a high arch resulting in a larger area devoid of muscle is a predisposing factor for a direct inguinal hernia.

The rectus abdominis muscle and sheath are important to the surgeon intent upon performing a Lichtenstein-type repair because the prosthesis should be securely anchored to this structure 2 cm medial to the pubic tubercle. It arises from the fifth to the seventh costal cartilages and inserts on the pubic symphysis and the pubic crest. The lateral edge of the muscle is demarcated by a slight depression in the aponeurotic fibers coursing toward the muscle; this depression is the semilunar line. The arcuate line of Douglas is formed at a variable distance between the umbilicus and the inguinal space because the fascia of the large, flat muscles of the abdominal wall contribute their aponeuroses to the anterior surface of the muscle,

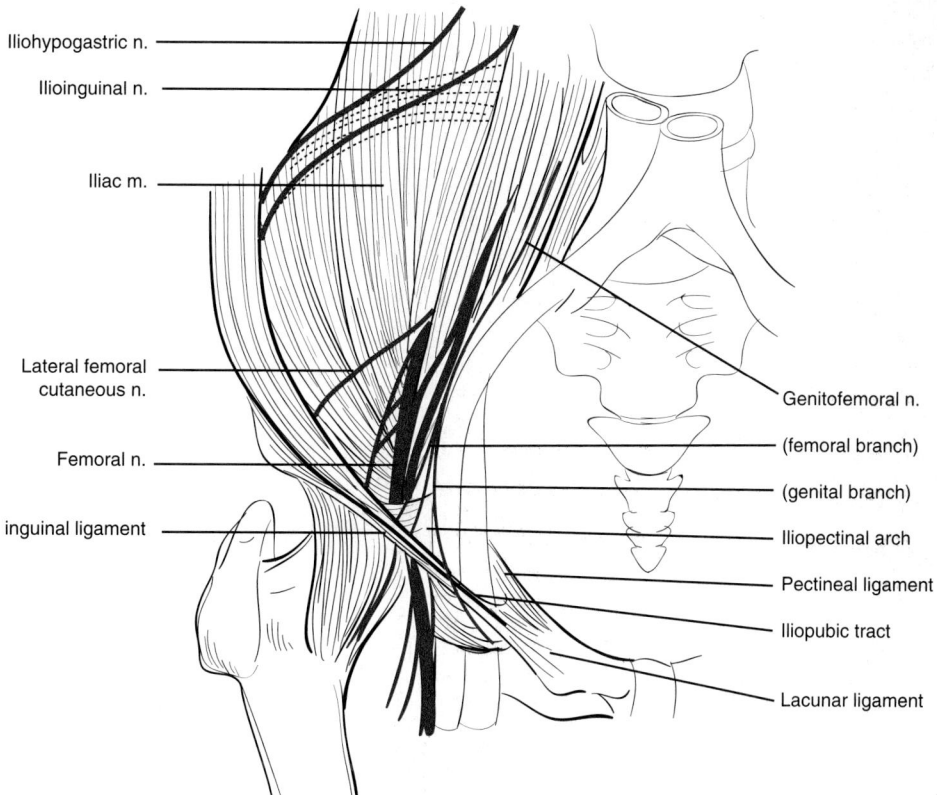

FIG. 36-6. This anterior-to-posterior view demonstrates the relationship of the five major nerves of the groin (ilioinguinal, iliohypogastric, genitofemoral, lateral femoral cutaneous, and femoral) to other anatomic landmarks.

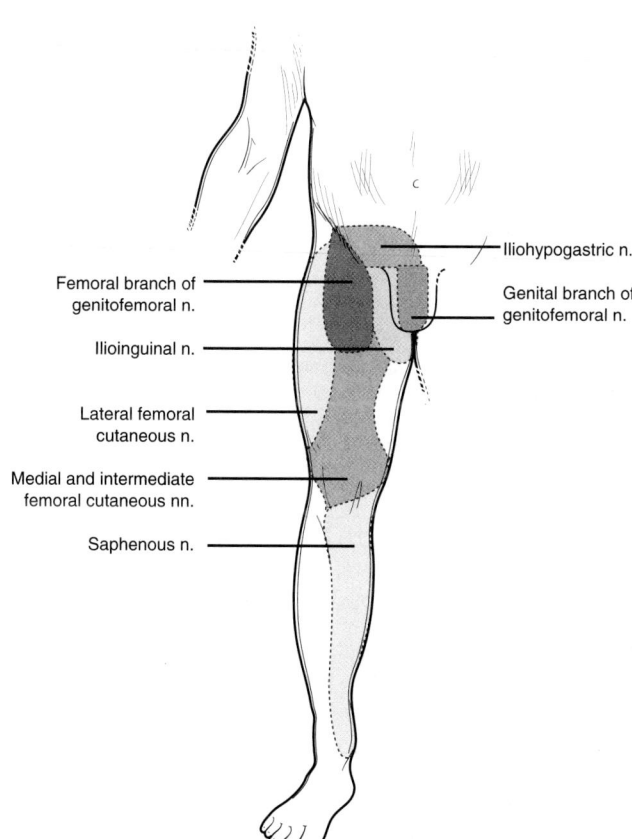

FIG. 36-7. Sensory distribution of the important nerves in the groin area.

leaving only transversalis fascia to cover the posterior surface of the rectus muscle. The pyramidalis muscle accompanies the rectus abdominis at its origin in a minority of individuals. It arises from the pubic symphysis and remains within the rectus sheath where it tapers to attach to the linea alba.

Hesselbach's inguinal triangle is the site of direct inguinal hernias. When described from the anterior aspect, the inguinal ligament forms the base of the triangle, the edge of the rectus abdominis is the medial border, and the inferior epigastric vessels are the superolateral border. It should be noted, however, that Hesselbach actually described Cooper's ligament as the base.

The endoabdominal fascia is the deep fascia covering the internal surface of the transversus abdominis, the iliacus, the psoas muscles, the obturator internus, and portions of the periosteum. It is a continuous sheet that extends throughout the extraperitoneal space, and is sometimes referred to as the "wallpaper" of the abdominal cavity. Commonly the fascia is subclassified according to the muscle covered by the fascia (e.g., iliac fascia).

For the surgeon, the transversalis fascia is perhaps the most commonly misunderstood structure in the literature devoted to groin hernia.[1] It was first described in detail by Cooper.[1] Since that time there has been considerable debate concerning its relative strength, its laminar structure (one layer or two), and its importance in a successful inguinal herniorrhaphy. The transversalis fascia is the structure that defines the anterior (superficial or skin side) wall of the preperitoneal space. It is actually a potential space because filmy, relatively avascular adhesions having the appearance of cotton candy during laparoscopic herniorrhaphy must be divided to create it at surgery.

The transversalis fascia is also important because it forms anatomic landmarks known as analogues or derivatives. The important transversalis fascia analogues for the hernia surgeon are the iliopectineal arch, the iliopubic tract, the crura of the deep inguinal

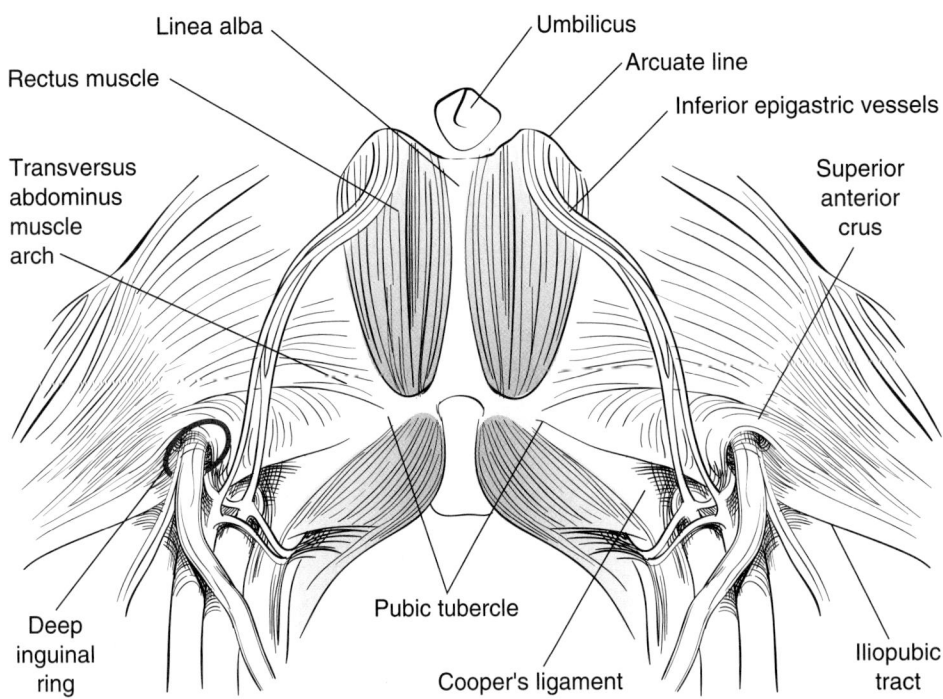

FIG. 36-8. *The transversalis fascia analogues from an abdominal perspective.*

Labels on figure: Linea alba, Umbilicus, Rectus muscle, Arcuate line, Inferior epigastric vessels, Transversus abdominus muscle arch, Superior anterior crus, Deep inguinal ring, Pubic tubercle, Cooper's ligament, Iliopubic tract

ring, and Cooper's (pectineal) ligament. The superior and inferior crura form a transversalis fascia sling, a "monk's hood"–shaped structure, around the deep inguinal ring. This sling has functional significance as the crura of the ring are pulled upward and laterally by the contraction of the transversus abdominis, resulting in a valvular action that helps to preclude indirect hernia formation (see Fig. 36-8). The iliopubic tract is the thickened band of the transversalis fascia that courses parallel to the more superficially located inguinal ligament. It is attached to the iliac crest laterally, and inserts on the pubic tubercle medially. The insertion curves inferolaterally for 1 to 2 cm along the pectinate line to blend with Cooper's (pectineal) ligament, ending at about the midportion of the superior pubic ramus. Cooper's ligament is actually a condensation of periosteum and is not a true analogue of the transversalis fascia.

Below the iliopubic tract are the critical anatomic elements that lead to the development of a femoral hernia. The iliopectineal arch (see Fig. 36-2A) separates the vascular compartment containing the femoral vessels from the neuromuscular compartment that contains the iliopsoas muscle, the femoral nerve, and the lateral femoral cutaneous nerve. The vascular compartment is invested by the femoral sheath, which has three subcompartments; the lateral, which contains the femoral artery and the femoral branch of the genitofemoral nerve; the middle, which contains the femoral vein; and the medial, the cone-shaped cul-de-sac known as the femoral canal. The femoral canal is normally a 1- to 2-cm blind pouch beginning at the femoral ring and extending to the level of the fossa ovalis (see Fig. 36-6). The femoral ring is bordered by the superior pubic ramus inferiorly and the femoral vein laterally. The iliopubic tract, with its curved insertion onto the pubic ramus, is the anterior and medial border. The canal normally contains preperitoneal fat, connective tissue, and lymph nodes, including Cloquet's node at its entrance, the femoral ring. Collectively these contents make up the femoral pad, a cushion for the femoral vein allowing expansion as might occur during a Valsalva maneuver, as well as a plug to prevent abdominal contents from entering the thigh. A femoral hernia exists when the blind end of the femoral canal becomes an opening (the femoral orifice) through which a peritoneal sac can protrude.

The Posterior Perspective (Laparoscopic)

An excellent view of the anterior abdominal wall can be obtained from a laparoscopic vantage point. Peritoneal folds are immediately obvious which correspond to important anatomic landmarks in the preperitoneal space (Fig. 36-9). The median umbilical fold extends from the umbilicus to the urinary bladder and covers the urachus, the usually fibrous remnant of the fetal allantois. The urachus may be patent for a variable distance in some patients. The medial umbilical fold is formed due to the presence of the underlying obliterated portion of the fetal umbilical artery. This cord-like structure, similar to the urachus, may be patent for a portion of its length. Indeed, the proximal portion of the artery normally supplies the superior vesicular arteries to the bladder. The lateral umbilical fold covers the inferior epigastric artery as it courses toward the posterior rectus sheath and enters it approximately at the level of the arcuate line.

Between the median and the medial ligaments, a depression usually exists called the supravesical fossa. This is the site of hernias of the same name. The fossa formed between the medial and the lateral ligaments is the medial fossa; it is the site of direct inguinal hernias. The lateral fossa is less well delineated than the other two. The lateral umbilical ligament and the rectus abdominis form the medial border of the fossa. There is no lateral border to this fossa, but rather the concavity slowly attenuates. The deep inguinal ring is located in the lateral fossa just lateral to the inferior epigastric vessels.

When the peritoneum is divided and the preperitoneal space entered, the key anatomic elements for a preperitoneal herniorrhaphy can be appreciated (Fig. 36-10). In the midline behind the pubis, the preperitoneal space is known as the space of Retzius, while laterally it is referred to as the space of Bogros. This space is important because many of the repairs that will be described later are performed in this area. Perhaps the single most important landmark is the inferior epigastric artery. This branch of the external iliac artery represents the primary blood supply to the deep anterior wall. Commonly an anastomotic vessel between the obturator vessels and the inferior epigastric vessels is present and can be seen arching over

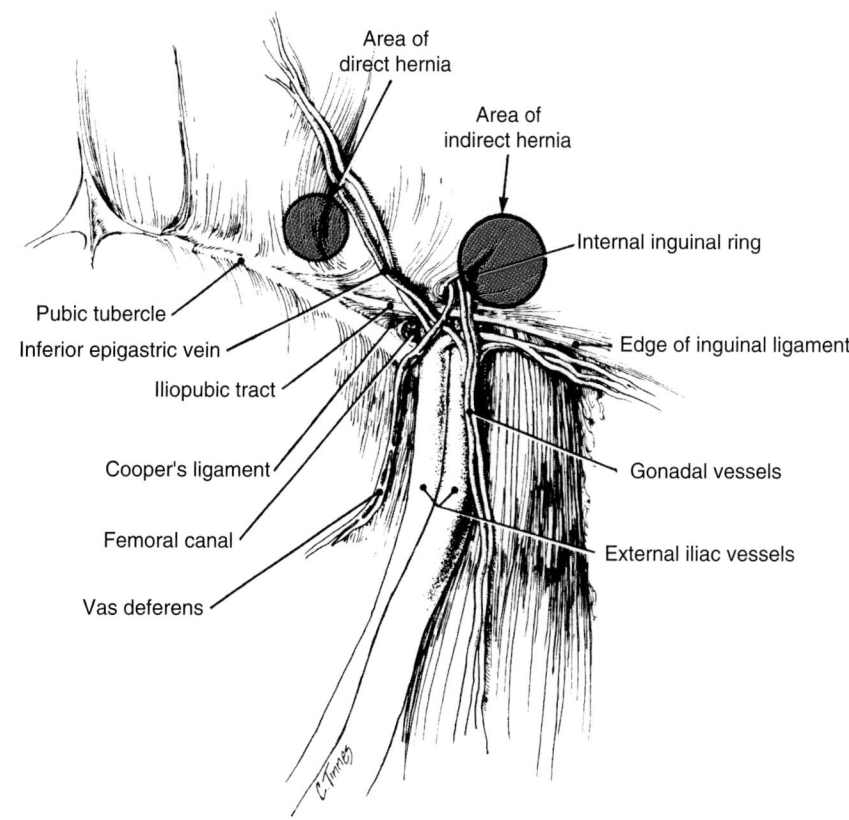

Area of
direct hernia

Area of
indirect hernia

Internal inguinal ring

Pubic tubercle

Inferior epigastric vein

Iliopubic tract

Edge of inguinal ligament

Cooper's ligament

Gonadal vessels

Femoral canal

External iliac vessels

Vas deferens

FIG. 36-9. *Peritoneal landmarks when looking at the groin from inside the abdomen.*

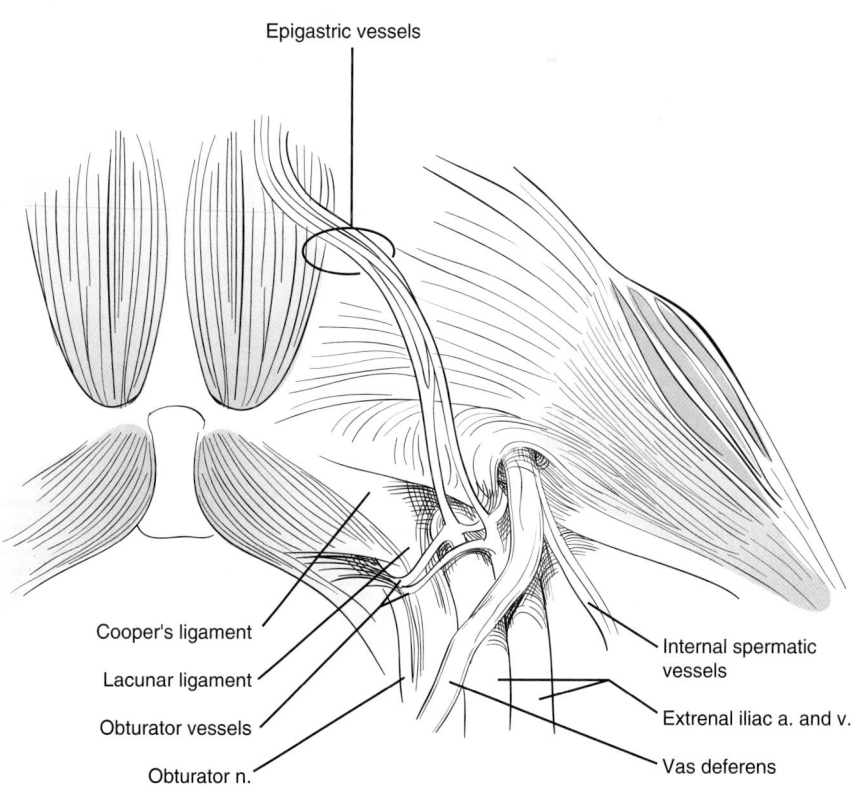

Epigastric vessels

Cooper's ligament

Lacunar ligament

Obturator vessels

Obturator n.

Internal spermatic vessels

Extrenal iliac a. and v.

Vas deferens

FIG. 36-10. *Important anatomic structures in the preperitoneal space.*

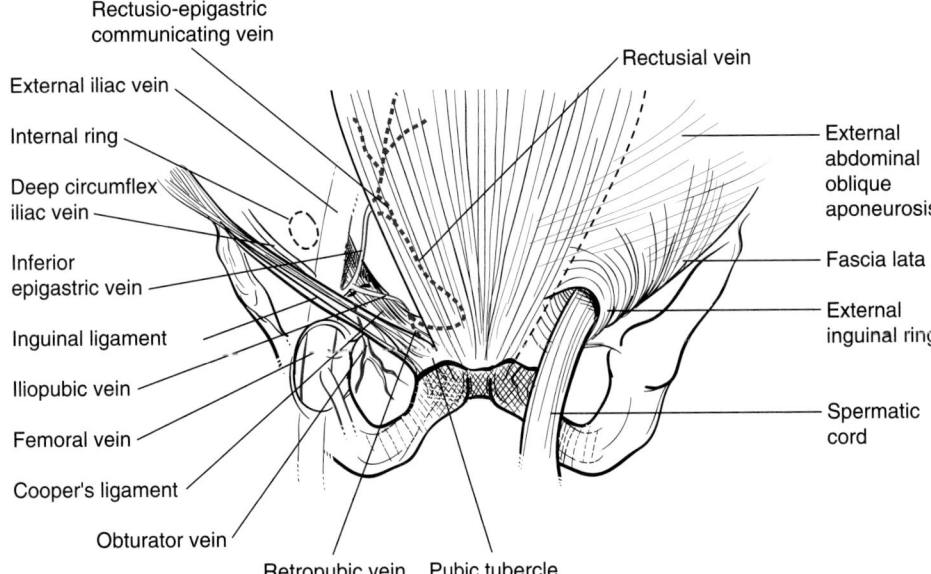

Rectusio-epigastric communicating vein

External iliac vein

Internal ring

Deep circumflex iliac vein

Inferior epigastric vein

Inguinal ligament

Iliopubic vein

Femoral vein

Cooper's ligament

Obturator vein

Retropubic vein   Pubic tubercle

Rectusial vein

External abdominal oblique aponeurosis

Fascia lata

External inguinal ring

Spermatic cord

FIG. 36-11. Important venous tributaries in the preperitoneal space of Bogros.

Cooper's ligament. Known as the corona mortis (death's crown), it is remarkable because of the significant hemorrhage that might occur if it is damaged during the course of either a preperitoneal or Cooper's ligament inguinal hernia repair. The veins in this area also can be troublesome since many, especially the iliopubic and obturator and their tributaries, may be larger than their accompanying arteries[24] (Fig. 36-11).

Other landmarks that require identification are the internal inguinal ring just lateral to the take-off of the inferior epigastric vessels, the internal spermatic artery and vein and the vas deferens, that join to form the spermatic cord just before entering the internal ring. The iliopubic tract, attached to the iliac crest laterally, crosses under the internal ring to make up its inferior border, and at the same time contributes to the anterior border of the femoral sheath, continuing to its insertion on the pubic tubercle. Cooper's ligament extends from the pubic tubercle inferolaterally along the pubic ramus, crossing under the femoral vessel. The femoral ring is readily visible from this viewpoint, being bordered by the femoral vein laterally, Cooper's ligament inferiorly, and the iliopubic tract superiorly. The inguinal ligament cannot be appreciated from this perspective as it is more superficial, but its downward and lateral extension, the lacunar (Gimbernat) ligament, can be seen from the insertion onto the pubic tubercle as it curves along the pubic ramus to become the medial border of the femoral ring.

The nerves traversing the preperitoneal space are prone to intraoperative injury if the surgeon is not cognizant of their location. Roots from the first four lumbar nerves, and in some the twelfth thoracic nerve, form the lumbar plexus. Five terminal branches of the plexus are at risk during preperitoneal herniorrhaphy: (1) the iliohypogastric nerve, (2) the ilioinguinal nerve, (3) the genitofemoral nerve, (4) the lateral femoral cutaneous nerve, and (5) the femoral nerve. The nerves form within or deep to the psoas major muscle, often ramifying with other nerves within or close to the muscle. The iliohypogastric and the ilioinguinal nerves were discussed in the anatomic section dealing with the anterior approach because they are more commonly seen from this perspective. Because they pierce the plane between the transversus abdominis and the internal abdominal oblique muscles before reaching the space that would usually be dissected during a preperitoneal herniorrhaphy, they are not visualized. However, they can be damaged when fastening a prosthesis if deep penetration of the fixation device occurs. The

genitofemoral nerve is the most anterior of the nerves encountered and is the most variable.[25] It may occur as a single trunk lying deep to the peritoneum and fascia on the anterior surface of the psoas muscle, or it may divide into its component genital and femoral branches within the muscle. The genital branch travels with the spermatic cord, entering at the deep inguinal ring; it ultimately innervates the cremaster muscle and the lateral scrotum. The femoral branch of the nerve innervates the skin of the proximal mid-thigh. The lateral femoral cutaneous nerve crosses the preperitoneal space lateral to the genitofemoral nerve and enters the thigh just beneath the iliopubic tract and the inguinal ligament. This nerve supplies sensory branches for the lateral side of the thigh (see Fig. 36-7). Both the genitofemoral and lateral femoral cutaneous nerves are readily identified lateral to the internal spermatic vessels when performing a preperitoneal herniorrhaphy. They usually enter the thigh below the iliopubic tract, but exceptions have been described.[26] The femoral nerve can be found immediately deep to the lateral aspect of the psoas muscle. Although not routinely encountered during a preperitoneal dissection, injuries have been reported.[27]

SYMPTOMS

Patients with groin hernias present with a wide range of clinical scenarios ranging from no symptoms to the life-threatening condition caused by strangulation of incarcerated hernia contents. Asymptomatic patients may have their hernias diagnosed at the time of a routine physical examination or seek medical attention because of a painless bulge in the groin. Indirect hernias are more likely to produce symptoms than direct hernias. Severe groin pain caused by groin strain is a problem because patients also commonly have a coincidental asymptomatic inguinal hernia, discovered because of the attention drawn by the groin strain. If the hernia is improperly determined to be the cause of the patient's pain, the stage is set for a postherniorrhaphy pain syndrome. Patient descriptions of discomfort with symptomatic hernias are highly variable. Many describe an annoying heavy feeling or dragging sensation that tends to get worse as the day wears on. The pain is commonly intermittent and radiation into the testicle is common. Others complain of a sharper pain that is either localized or diffuse. Patients with particularly severe pain may need to recline for a short period of time, or use other posture-altering techniques. Occasionally, patients must manually reduce the hernia to obtain relief. Although inguinal hernias tend to occur more frequently in heavy laborers, a history of sudden onset of pain after a specific lifting episode is unusual except in worker's compensation patients.

DIAGNOSIS

Physical Examination

Physical examination is the best way to determine the presence or absence of an inguinal hernia. The diagnosis may be obvious by simple inspection when a visible bulge is present. The differential diagnosis must be considered in questionable cases (Table 36-4). Nonvisible hernias require digital examination of the inguinal canal (Fig. 36-12). This is best done in both the lying and standing position. The examiner should place the tip of the index finger at the most dependent part of the scrotum and direct it into the external inguinal ring. The patient is then asked to strain. The ritual of having the patient cough is discouraged as it results in the overdiagnosis of a hernia because of the difficulty of differentiating a normal expansile bulge of muscle from a true hernia, especially in asthenic individuals.

Numerous authors have shown that the accuracy with which direct and indirect inguinal hernias can be distinguished clinically before surgery is low.[28,29,30] However, classic teaching is that an indirect hernia will push against the fingertip, whereas a direct hernia will push against the pulp of the finger. In addition, applying pressure over the mid-inguinal point (midway between the anterior superior iliac spine and the pubic tubercle, and just above the inguinal ligament) with the fingertip will control an indirect hernia and prevent it from protruding when the patient strains. A direct hernia will not be affected with this maneuver.

A femoral hernia presents as a swelling below the inguinal ligament and just lateral to the pubic tubercle. Femoral hernias are overdiagnosed because of the presence of a prominent femoral fat pad, a so-called femoral pseudohernia. Thin patients commonly have prominent bilateral bulges below the inguinal ligament medial to the femoral vessels. They are asymptomatic and disappear spontaneously when the patient assumes a supine position. Surgery is not indicated.[21]

Table 36-4
Differential Diagnosis of Groin Hernia

Malignancy
Lymphoma
Retroperitoneal sarcoma
Metastasis
Testicular tumor
Primary testicular
Varicocele
Epididymitis
Testicular torsion
Hydrocele
Ectopic testicle
Undescended testicle
Femoral artery aneurysm or pseudoaneurysm
Lymph node
Sebaceous cyst
Hidradenitis
Cyst of the canal of Nuck (female)
Saphenous varix
Psoas abscess
Hematoma
Ascites

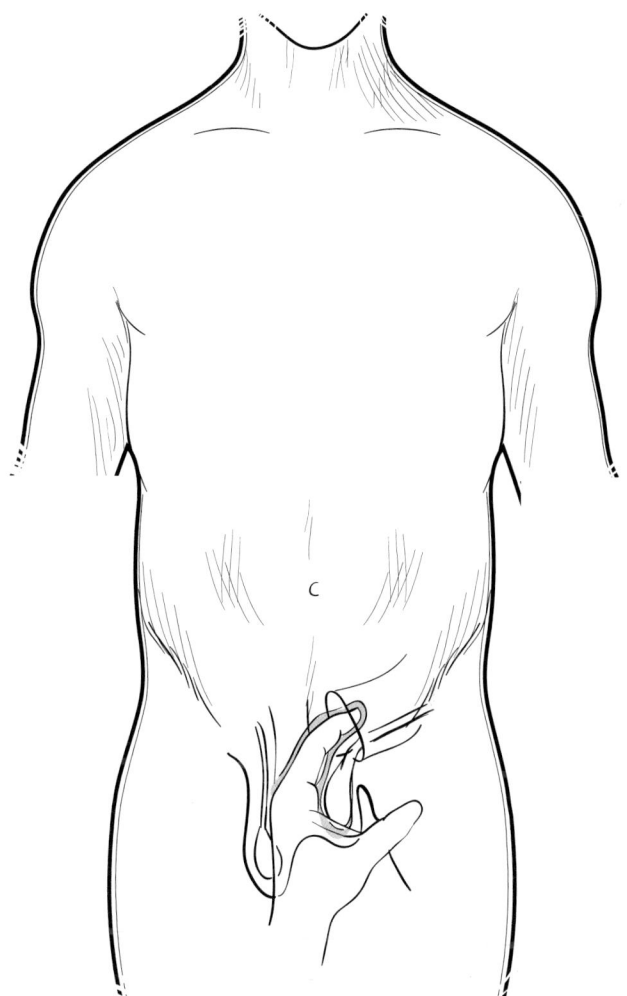

FIG. 36-12. *Digital examination of the inguinal canal.*

Radiologic Investigations

Radiologic investigation is sometimes warranted to correctly diagnose the cause of pain or a mass in the groin, as the physical examination can be equivocal. One radiologic diagnostic tool is herniography, which in some circumstances can help avoid unnecessary surgical exploration. Its major drawback is its invasiveness. Ultrasound is useful but is highly operator dependent. Cross-sectional imaging techniques are being employed with increasing frequency for the assessment of groin ailments. Hernias are visualized as abnormal ballooning of the anteroposterior diameter of the inguinal canal and/or simultaneous protrusion of fat or bowel within the inguinal canal. The development of fast imaging MRI scanners that allow dynamic imaging (i.e., imaging performed during straining) shows particular promise. Further refinement, with the fine tuning of the best weights for images and the addition of intraperitoneal contrast agents are forthcoming. Both MRI and CT may reveal other causes of groin pain because of their ability to visualize related structures in the groin. Van den Berg looked at a group of patients scheduled to undergo elective laparoscopic herniorrhaphy for either unilateral or bilateral inguinal hernias detected by physical examination. Blinded interpreters examined ultrasounds and MRI scans, looking not only at the affected side, but also the opposite side. Laparoscopy was considered the final means of determining the true groin pathology on either side. The sensitivity (percentage of patients with a correct positive diagnosis) and specificity (percentage of patients with a correct negative diagnosis) was 74.5 and 96.3% for physical examination, 92.7 and 81.5% for ultrasound, and 94.5 and 96.3% for MRI, respectively.[31]

CLASSIFICATION

Numerous authorities including Casten, Lichtenstein, Gilbert, Robbins and Rutkow, Bendavid, Nyhus, Schumpelick, and others have developed classification systems that bear their names. However, just as the number of inguinal herniorrhaphy procedures attests to the fact that the perfect one has yet to be described, so do the large number of classification schemes reflect the fact that most surgeons are not happy with any single classification.

The reason it is so difficult to develop a classification system that all surgeons can agree on is that in the final analysis, the physical examination represents an important component, and no one has been able to eliminate its subjectivity. The advent of laparoscopic herniorrhaphy has further compounded the issue because some of the measurements cannot be accomplished from the laparoscopic perspective. The Nyhus classification is listed in Table 36-5. It suffers from its dependence on subjective input, and does not address such factors as the size of the hernia defect, incarceration, strangulation, or patient comorbidities. Nevertheless, it enjoys the greatest degree of acceptance and may be the most useful for comparing laparoscopic procedures to open operations, although there are significant limitations. For example, a type I hernia is a source of confusion because a "normal internal ring" from a laparoscopic perspective is completely closed (i.e., the cord structures are completely covered by contiguous peritoneum). However, by definition no hernia exists. Therefore a subjective judgment must be made by the laparoscopic surgeon if there is unusual dilatation of the internal ring, and then a determination that a type II hernia is present. Another type I classification problem for laparoscopy is the small dimple at the internal ring, especially in a patient who clinically does not have a hernia. The natural history of these defects has yet to be determined. Many surgeons recommend routine repair in this situation, but caution must be exercised given the potential for postherniorrhaphy complications that may have lifelong effects (see complications section). Nevertheless, the Nyhus system has the least limitation in comparison to the other classification systems which require measuring the hernia defect size, because the defect is exaggerated by the pneumoperitoneum necessary for laparoscopy (see Table 36-5).

Table 36-5
Nyhus Classification System

Type I	Indirect hernia; internal abdominal ring normal; typically in infants, children, small adults
Type II	Indirect hernia; internal ring enlarged without impingement on the floor of the inguinal canal; does not extend to the scrotum
Type IIIA	Direct hernia; size is not taken into account
Type IIIB	Indirect hernia that has enlarged enough to encroach upon the posterior inguinal wall; indirect sliding or scrotal hernias are placed in this category because they are commonly associated with extension to the direct space; also includes pantaloon hernias
Type IIIC	Femoral hernia
Type IV	Recurrent hernia; modifiers A–D are sometimes added, which correspond to indirect, direct, femoral, and mixed, respectively

Table 36-6
Gilbert Classification System

Type 1	Small, indirect
Type 2	Medium, indirect
Type 3	Large, indirect
Type 4	Entire floor, direct
Type 5	Diverticular, direct
Type 6	Combined (pantaloon)
Type 7	Femoral

Perhaps the second most common classification system referenced in the literature is the one developed by Gilbert (Table 36-6). Type 1, 2, and 3 hernias are indirect. In type 1, the internal inguinal ring is normal. In type 2 hernias, the inguinal ring is dilated, but less than 4 cm. Type 3 hernias have the internal ring dilation measured at greater than 4 cm, commonly with encroachment on the direct space and medial displacement of the inferior epigastric vessels. Type 4 and 5 hernias are direct. There is extensive destruction of the inguinal floor with type 4 hernias, whereas in type 5 hernias there is a smaller defect of no more than 2 cm, without complete weakness of the direct space. The system was later modified by Rutkow and Robbins to include pantaloon hernias (direct and indirect combination), type 6, and femoral hernias, type 7.[32]

PREOPERATIVE CARE

Nonoperative Treatment

The term "watchful waiting" is used to describe this nonoperative treatment recommendation. It is only applicable in asymptomatic or minimally symptomatic hernias. Patients are counseled about the signs and symptoms of complications from their hernia so they might present promptly to their physician in case an adverse event takes place. Definitive data that this recommendation is safe are not available, and it is for this reason that surgical repair of all inguinal hernias at diagnosis is recommended. However, a randomized controlled trial is currently underway which should shed some light on this subject in the next few years.

A *truss* is a mechanical appliance consisting of a belt with a pad that is applied to the groin after spontaneous or manual reduction of a hernia. The purpose is twofold: to maintain reduction and to prevent enlargement. Whether either goal is achieved consistently is unknown, and it is doubtful that the incidence of hernia accidents is reduced. What is clear is that symptomatic relief is achieved in many patients. Most patients consider them cumbersome because of the complicated system of elastic, Velcro, straps, and/or springs usually required to make them effective. Some find them unacceptable because they are difficult to keep clean. Also, they are not without complications. Atrophy of the spermatic cord has been described, and the clinical experience of many surgeons is that an eventual hernia repair is made more difficult by the constant mechanical pressure in the groin area that renders the tissue more difficult to dissect due to atrophy and fibrosis. There are not enough valid studies to determine how effective trusses are and whether they are as effective as operative treatment in controlling symptoms.

Pneumoperitoneum

The establishment of a pneumoperitoneum in preparation for hernia surgery is an accepted practice for patients with "loss of domain."[33] The viscera protrude outside the confines of the abdominal cavity to the extent that replacement followed by hernia repair might cause respiratory embarrassment and/or an abdominal compartment syndrome. The object of the pneumoperitoneum is to stretch the abdominal wall preoperatively, increasing the amount of room in the peritoneal cavity. The term *progressive pneumoperitoneum* is more accurate because the therapy must be applied in successive sessions. The final decision to use pneumoperitoneum is most commonly based on a CT scan, which allows one to determine the degree of domain loss.[34,35]

The most dangerous aspect of pneumoperitoneum is the possibility of bowel or vascular injury. A safe technique of progressive pneumoperitoneum must avoid visceral injury, prevent herniation at the site of insufflation, and be able to be applied repeatedly over several weeks without undue risk of infection. The number of pneumoperitoneums varies, but the usual period is 15 to 30 days. Many techniques have been described. Some authorities favor daily needle punctures, but this increases the chance of visceral injury. The alternative is to place an indwelling catheter with a percutaneous needle introducer system or by minilaparotomy, but this increases the chance for infection. The introduction of laparoscopy into the practice of many general surgeons has increased the number of options. A Veress needle can be used repeatedly or a 5-mm cannula can

be left in place and used intermittently. A totally implanted system is shown in Fig. 36-13.

Although theoretically attractive, pneumoperitoneum is not always successful. The injected gas sometimes preferentially enters the hernia sac and distends it with minimal effect on the abdominal cavity. In addition, pneumoperitoneum has been shown to diminish lower extremity venous return. This could translate into a higher risk of thromboembolic complications. Deep venous thrombosis prophylaxis is prudent. It is unlikely there will ever be definitive pulmonary embolism incidence data because of the number of patients required to reach statistical significance.

ABDOMINAL WALL SUBSTITUTES

The modern era of herniorrhaphy has seen a progressive decrease in the recurrence rate due to improvement in surgical technique and prosthetics. It is apparent that the abdominal wall does not always heal satisfactorily after primary closure and that an irreducible percentage of recurrences are inevitable if one were to insist on pure tissue repairs. The only reasonable solution is the use of a structure that can bridge a defect in certain cases.

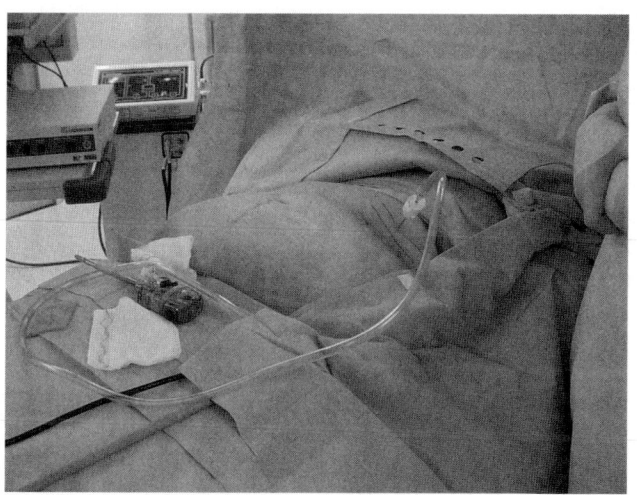

A

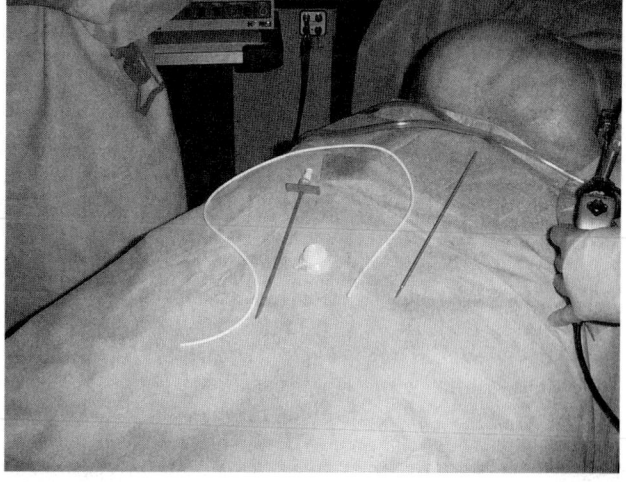

B

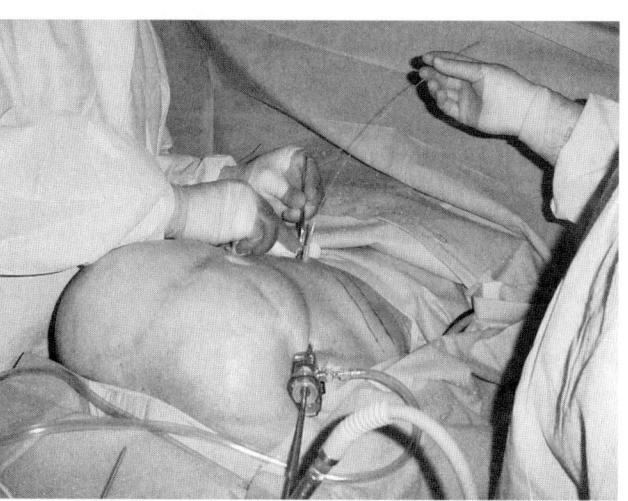

C

FIG. 36-13. A technique for pneumoperitoneum using laparoscopy. *A.* The lines in the left upper quadrant mark the left costal margin. A Veress needle has been introduced through the first interspace above (the ninth intercostal space). This alternate access site is especially useful when there has been extensive surgery near the midline, as might be seen in patients with ventral hernias. *B.* An implantable port and introducer system. *C.* The introducer system with guidewire in place.

Nonprosthetic Materials

Rotational flaps and relaxing incisions can be used but are not universally applicable. Free grafts of autologous tissue such as skin, fascia lata, pericardium, and periosteum, among others, have had phases of popularity, but harvesting tends to be time-consuming, there is increased pain because of the donor site, and unsightly scars are common. Homografts and xenografts of the same types of tissue failed because of fear of disease transmission and immunologic reactions, which may result in dissolution.[36]

Prosthetic Materials

The essential attributes of a suitable prosthesis have been delineated by Cumberland[37] (Table 36-7). It has now been proven that mesh herniorrhaphy can decrease the recurrence rate by approximately 50% when compared to non-mesh repairs.[38] However, this was not the early experience. The first prostheses used were metal, including silver wire, tantalum gauze, and stainless steel. These caused postoperative pain due to inflexibility, fragmentation, migration, infection, fistula formation, and difficulty in removal. The use of metal prostheses has largely been abandoned. Plastic prostheses such as polyvinyl (Ivalon), nylon, Silastic, Teflon, and carbon fibers were next tried with unsatisfactory results due to lack of resistance to infection, loss of elasticity, and decreasing strength caused by chemical degradation. The experience with these early prostheses led to a reluctance by surgeons to use foreign material. Foreign body reaction, infection, erosion into surrounding structures, rejection, increased incidence of postherniorrhaphy chronic groin pain, cost, and carcinogenesis remained a concern.

Now with nearly 50 years of continuous use of prosthetics it has become clear that the use of modern prostheses is safe and effective. Chronic postherniorrhaphy groin pain does occasionally occur after prosthetic repair and is relieved by prosthesis removal.[38] However, the overall incidence of chronic postherniorrhaphy groin pain is less with a prosthetic repair.[39] A theoretical concern is carcinogenesis, since sarcomatous transformation of soft tissue has been observed in laboratory animals after polypropylene implantation. However, there are no clinical data to suggest an increased incidence of malignancy in humans.[40] The materials that have emerged as suitable for routine use in hernia surgery that fulfill Cumberland's classic ideal characteristics (see Table 36-7) include polypropylene, either monofilament (Marlex, Prolene) or polyfilament (Surgipro); Dacron (Mersilene); and expanded polytetrafluoroethylene (e-PTFE; Gore-Tex). Absorbable prostheses such as those made of polyglactin are not durable and have no place in groin hernia surgery. The newer biologic prostheses made of human cadaver skin, porcine cross-linked dermal collagen, or porcine small-intestinal submucosa are more expensive and have no advantage over synthetic material for an uncomplicated hernia repair. However, they can be useful in infected groin wounds.[41]

Table 36-7
Description of the Ideal Prosthetic Material for Hernia Repair

It is not modified physically by tissue fluid
It is chemically inert
It does not cause inflammatory or foreign body reaction
It is not carcinogenic
It does not cause an allergic or hypersensitivity response
It is resistant to mechanical strain
It is pliable and therefore moldable
It is easily sterilized

ANESTHESIA FOR GROIN HERNIORRHAPHY

The type of anesthesia used for inguinal herniorrhaphy is highly variable, depending primarily on the personal preference of the surgeon. Laparoscopic herniorrhaphy is the exception as general endotracheal anesthesia is primarily mandated by the pneumoperitoneum. Epidural anesthesia has been used, especially in high-risk patients, but is rare. Open inguinal herniorrhaphy through a groin incision can be performed under local or regional anesthesia, which is one of the strongest arguments for open herniorrhaphy when compared to laparoscopic herniorrhaphy. Despite this, the best available evidence suggests that the majority of open herniorrhaphies are performed under a general anesthetic, with local and regional techniques finding their greatest popularity in specialty clinics. The perception about the frequency with which general anesthesia is used is a reflection of this, as it is these same specialty units that do most of the reporting. Nevertheless, local anesthesia, when used in adequate doses and far enough in advance of the initial incision, proves very effective when combined with the newer short-acting, amnesic, and anxiolytic agents such as propofol.

Most commonly used is 100 mL of 0.5% lidocaine with epinephrine, 0.25% bupivacaine with epinephrine, or a combination of the two, with or without sodium bicarbonate. The change in pH is commonly believed to decrease the pain of injection, while the rationale for combining the two local anesthetics is to obtain the best of both worlds with the use of the short-acting agent lidocaine with the longer-acting drug bupivacaine. However, the pharmacology is questionable. Several ongoing randomized controlled trials should settle the question. The epinephrine is optional and may be omitted in patients with a history of coronary artery disease. In an adult of normal size, the surgeon injects 70 mL of this solution prior to prepping and draping the patient. Ten milliliters is placed medial to the anterior superior iliac spine to block the ilioinguinal nerve, and the other 60 mL is used as a field block along the orientation of the planned incision in the subcutaneous and deeper tissues. Care is taken to inject into the areas of the pubic tubercle and Cooper's ligament, both of which can easily be identified by tactile sensation except in the very obese. Intradermal injection is unnecessary because by the time the surgeon is scrubbed and the patient draped, the anesthesia is complete. The remaining 30 mL is reserved for discretionary use during the procedure. With this technique, endotracheal intubation is avoided and the patient can be aroused from sedation at intervals to perform Valsalva maneuvers and test the repair.

Regional anesthesia in the form of spinal or epidural anesthesia also can be employed and is excellent, especially in experienced hands. If general anesthesia is used, a local anesthetic should be used at the end of the procedure as an adjunct to reduce immediate postoperative pain.

INGUINAL HERNIA REPAIRS

The inguinal herniorrhaphies described below should be considered representative of a group of operations. This is because numerous modifications of inguinal hernia repairs usually associated with a specific surgeon's name have been described over time. It is not practical to describe each one.

Open Anterior, Nonprosthetic

These types of procedures are sometimes referred to as "tension" repairs because the hernia defect is closed rather than bridged by a prosthesis. However, this term should not be used, as tension violates a surgical principle and would not knowingly be accepted.

Avoidance of tension in a nonprosthetic repair is accomplished by the use of a relaxing incision. A better name is "pure tissue repair."

Many principles and specific surgical maneuvers are common to all of these operations. In the interest of saving space, these common elements will be discussed before describing individual operations.

Initial Incision. Classically an oblique skin incision is made between the anterior superior iliac spine and the pubic tubercle. Many surgeons now use a more horizontally placed skin incision that follows the natural skin lines for cosmetic reasons. Regardless, it is deepened through Camper's and Scarpa's fascia and the subcutaneous tissue to expose the external oblique aponeurosis. This structure is incised medially down to and through the external inguinal ring. Bassini maintained that the external oblique aponeurosis incision should be as superior as possible, yet still allow the superficial external ring to be opened. This avoided having the reapproximation suture line directly over the suture line of the inguinal floor reconstruction. Whether this is significant is debatable.

Mobilization of the Cord Structures. The superior flap of the external oblique aponeurosis is bluntly dissected off the internal oblique muscle laterally and superiorly. The iliohypogastric nerve is identified at this time. It can be left in situ or freed from the surrounding tissue and isolated from the operative field by passing a hemostat under the nerve and grasping the upper flap of the external oblique aponeurosis. Routine division of this nerve along with the ilioinguinal nerve is practiced by some surgeons but not advised by most. The cord structures are then separated from the inferior flap of the external oblique aponeurosis by blunt dissection, exposing the shelving edge of the inguinal ligament and the iliopubic tract. The cord structures are lifted en masse with the fingers of one hand at the pubic tubercle so that the index finger can be passed underneath to meet the index finger of the other hand. Blunt dissection is used to complete mobilization of the cord structures and a Penrose drain is placed around them for retraction during the course of the procedure.

Division of the Cremaster Muscle. Complete division of the cremaster muscle, especially when dealing with an indirect hernia, has been common practice. The purpose is to facilitate sac identification and to lengthen the cord for better visualization of the inguinal floor. However, adequate exposure can usually be obtained by a longitudinal opening of the muscle, which lessens the likelihood of damage to cord structures and avoids the complication of testicular descent (see complications section). It is probably best not to divide the cremaster muscle unless the surgeon cannot obtain adequate visualization of the inguinal floor any other way.

High Ligation of the Sac. The term *high ligation of the sac* is used frequently as its historic significance has ingrained it in the description of most of the older operations. By convention, for this chapter, high ligation should be considered equivalent to reduction of the sac into the preperitoneal space without excision. Both methods work equally well and are highly effective. There is a perception among some surgeons that sac inversion will be associated with a decreased incidence of future adhesive complications and results in less pain because the richly innervated peritoneum is not incised. However, this has not been scrutinized by a randomized trial.[42] Sac inversion, in lieu of excision, does protect intra-abdominal viscera in cases of unrecognized incarcerated sac contents or a sliding hernia.

Management of Inguinal Scrotal Hernia Sacs. Complete excision of all indirect inguinal hernia sacs is felt to be important by some. The downside to this practice is an excessive rate of ischemic orchitis caused by trauma to the testicular blood supply,

especially the delicate venous plexuses that are easily disturbed. Testicular atrophy has been reported in up to 30%. A better approach is to divide indirect inguinal hernia sacs in the mid-inguinal canal, once one is confident that the hernia is not sliding, and there are no abdominal contents. The distal sac is not dissected but the anterior wall is opened as far distally as is convenient. Contrary to popular opinion in the urologic literature, this does not result in an excessive rate of postoperative hydrocele formation.

Relaxing Incision. A relaxing incision divides the anterior rectus sheath, extending from the pubic tubercle superiorly for a variable distance. Some surgeons prefer to "hockey stick" the incision laterally at the superior extent. The rectus muscle itself is strong enough to prevent future incisional herniation. The relaxing incision works by allowing the various components of the abdominal wall to displace laterally and inferiorly.

Wound Closure. The external oblique fascia is closed, serving to reconstruct the superficial (external) ring. The external ring must be loose enough to prevent strangulation of the cord structures, yet tight enough to avoid an inexperienced examiner from confusing a dilated ring with a recurrence. The later is sometimes referred to as an "industrial" hernia because historically it has at times been a problem during a pre-employment physical. Scarpa's fascia and the skin are closed to complete the operation.

Marcy

The Marcy repair is the simplest nonprosthetic repair performed today. Its main indication is in Nyhus type I indirect inguinal hernias where the internal ring is normal. It is appropriate for children and young adults in whom concern remains about the long-term effects of prosthetic material. The essential features of this operation are high ligation of the hernia sac plus narrowing of the internal ring. Displacing the cord structures laterally allows the placement of sutures through the muscular and fascial layers (Fig. 36-14).

Bassini

The major components of Bassini's "radical cure" are as follows:

1. Division of the external oblique aponeurosis over the inguinal canal through the external ring.
2. Division of the cremaster muscle lengthwise followed by resection so an indirect hernia is not missed, while simultaneously exposing the floor of the inguinal canal to more accurately assess for a direct inguinal hernia.
3. Division of the floor or posterior wall of the inguinal canal for its full length. This ensures adequate examination of the femoral ring from above and exposes the tissue layers that will be used for reconstructing the inguinal floor. By doing this, the surgeon is less likely to use the transversalis fascia alone for reconstruction, as it is the weakest layer of the posterior wall. This step was largely ignored when the operation was imported to North America, and this fact has been the cause of the inferior results with this procedure.
4. High ligation of an indirect sac.
5. Reconstruction of the posterior wall by suturing the transversalis fascia, the transversus abdominis muscle, the internal oblique muscle (Bassini's famous "triple layer") medially to the inguinal ligament laterally, and possibly the iliopubic tract. This step is suggested in drawings, but not clarified in original texts authored by Bassini.[43]

Following the initial dissection and reduction or ligation of the sac, attention turns to reconstructing the inguinal floor. Bassini began this part of the operation by opening the transversalis fascia (some prefer to use the term "posterior inguinal wall") from the

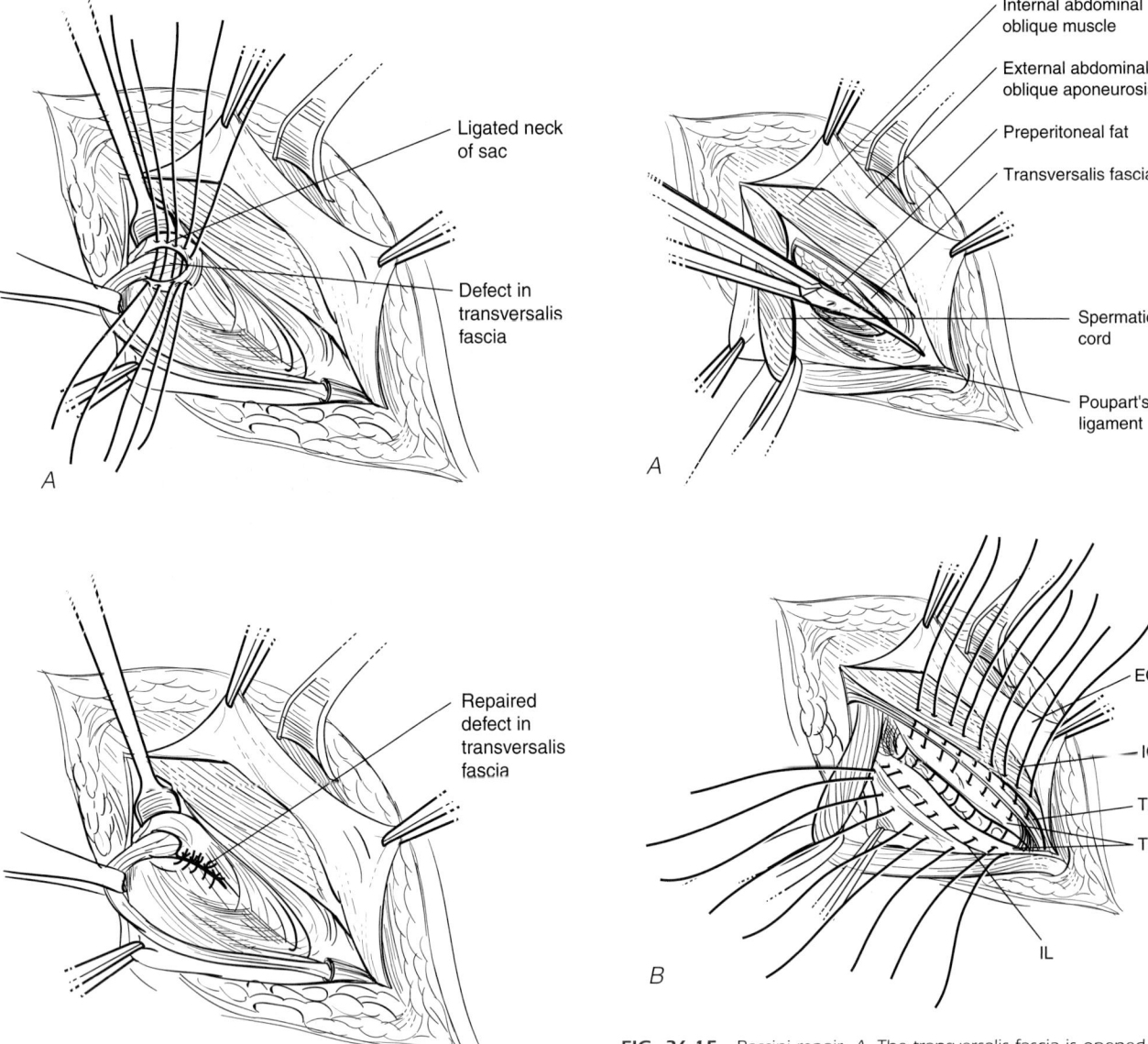

FIG. 36-14. Marcy repair. High ligation or reduction of the sac is followed by narrowing the internal ring by approximating the transversus abdominis muscle medial to the cord.

FIG. 36-15. Bassini repair. *A.* The transversalis fascia is opened from the internal inguinal ring to the pubic tubercle, exposing the preperitoneal fat. *B.* Reconstruction of the posterior wall by suturing the transversalis fascia (TF), the transversus abdominis muscle (TA), the internal oblique muscle (IO) (Bassini's famous "triple layer") medially to the inguinal ligament (IL) laterally. EO = external oblique aponeurosis.

internal inguinal ring to the pubic tubercle, exposing the preperitoneal fat, which was bluntly dissected away from the undersurface of the superior flap of the transversalis fascia (Fig. 36-15A). This allowed him to properly prepare the deepest structure in his famous triple layer (transversalis fascia, transversus abdominis muscle, and internal oblique muscle). The first stitch in the repair includes the triple layer superiorly and the periosteum of the medial side of the pubic tubercle along with the rectus sheath. Most surgeons now try to avoid the periosteum of the pubic tubercle to decrease the incidence of osteitis pubis. The repair is then continued laterally with nonabsorbable suture securing the triple layer to the reflected inguinal ligament (Poupart's ligament) (Fig. 36-15B). These sutures are continued until the internal ring has been closed on its medial side. A relaxing incision was not part of the original description but is commonly added now.

Bassini's operation as described above might better be considered a preperitoneal repair. However, it is traditionally grouped

with the open operations, primarily as it relates to the "Americanized" version of the procedure in which the floor is not opened. Concerns about injuries to neurovascular structures in the preperitoneal space as well as the bladder lead surgeons to abandon opening the inguinal floor, and thereby prevent proper development of the triple layer. In lieu of opening the floor, a forceps such as an Allis clamp is used to blindly grasp tissue, hoping to include the transversalis fascia and the transversus abdominis muscle. The layer is then sutured along with the internal oblique muscle to the reflected inguinal ligament as described above for Bassini's classic operation. The structure grasped in this modified procedure is sometimes referred to as the conjoined tendon, but this is not accurate due to the variability of what is grasped in the clamp; this is essentially a blind step. This imprecise approach almost certainly accounts for the inferior results achieved with this procedure in North America, resulting in the need for the development of better herniorrhaphies.

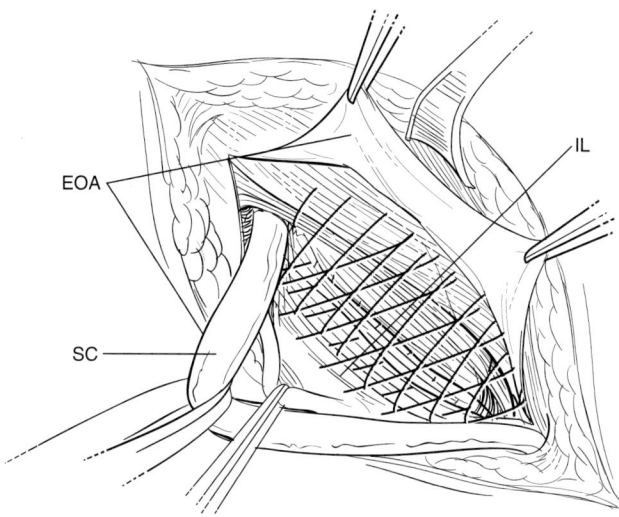

FIG. 36-16. *The Moloney darn. IL = inguinal ligament; EOA = external oblique aponeurosis; SC = spermatic cord.*

Moloney Darn

The procedure gets its name from the way a long nylon suture is repeatedly passed between the tissues to create a weave that one might consider similar to a mesh. The initial layer consists of a continuous nylon suture to oppose the usual elements of the abdominal wall medially (transversalis fascia and the transversus abdominis, rectus, and internal oblique muscles) to the inguinal ligament. This first suture is continued into the muscle about the cord, weaving in and out to form reinforcement around the cord, and is finally tied to the inguinal ligament on the lateral side of the cord (Fig. 36-16).

The darn is a second layer. The sutures may be made parallel or in a crisscross fashion, plicating well into the inguinal ligament below. The darn must be carried well over the medial edge of the inguinal canal. Once the darn is complete, the external oblique is closed over the cord structures. The rationale of the darn procedure is to form a meshwork of nonabsorbable suture that is well tolerated by the tissues. The interstices fill with fibrous connective tissue, producing a buttress across the weakened area of the inguinal canal.[44]

Shouldice

The Shouldice repair utilizes an initial approach that is similar to the Bassini repair, with particular importance placed upon freeing the cord from its surrounding adhesions, resection of the cremaster muscle, high dissection of the hernia sac, and division of the transversalis fascia. Continuous nonabsorbable suture is used to repair the floor. Traditionally, this has been monofilament steel wire. A continuous suture distributes tension evenly and prevents defects that could potentially occur between interrupted sutures, resulting in a recurrence. The repair is started at the pubic tubercle by approximating the iliopubic tract laterally to the undersurface of the lateral edge of the rectus muscle. The suture is continued laterally, approximating the iliopubic tract to the medial flap that is made up of the transversalis fascia and the internal oblique and transversus abdominis muscles (Fig. 36-17A). Eventually four suture lines are developed from the medial flap. The running suture is continued to the internal ring where the lateral stump of the cremaster muscle is picked up, forming a new internal ring. The direction of the suture is reversed back towards the pubic tubercle, approximating the

medial edge of the internal oblique and transversus abdominis muscle to Poupart's ligament and the wire is tied to itself (Fig. 36-17B). Thus there are two suture lines formed by the first suture. The second wire suture is started near the internal ring and approximates the internal oblique and transversus muscles to a band of external oblique aponeurosis superficial and parallel to the inguinal ligament, in effect creating a second artificial inguinal ligament. This forms the third suture line that ends at the pubic crest. The suture is then reversed and a fourth suture line is constructed in a similar manner, superficial to the third line. The cribiformis fascia is always incised in the thigh, parallel to the inguinal ligament, to make the inner side of the lower flap of the external oblique aponeurosis available for these multiple layers. This step is commonly omitted in general practice.

McVay Cooper's Ligament Repair

This operation is similar to the Bassini repair, except that Cooper's ligament instead of the inguinal ligament is used for the medial portion of the repair (Fig. 36-18). Interrupted sutures beginning at the pubic tubercle and continuing laterally along Cooper's ligament progressively narrow the femoral ring, and this constitutes its most common application (i.e., treatment of a femoral hernia). The last stitch to Cooper's ligament is known as a transition stitch and includes the inguinal ligament. The stitch has two purposes; to complete the narrowing of the femoral ring by approximating the inguinal ligament to Cooper's ligament as well as the medial tissue, and to provide a smooth transition or step-up to the inguinal ligament over the femoral vessel so that the repair can be continued laterally, identically to the Bassini repair. A relaxing incision should always be used given the considerable tension required to span such a large distance. This tension is felt by many to result in more pain than other herniorrhaphies, and predisposes to recurrence. For this reason, the operation is rarely chosen, with the notable exception of a femoral hernia in a patient with specific contraindications to the use of mesh (e.g., infection).

Miscellaneous Repairs

Several procedures have significant historical interest to the hernia surgeon including the Halsted operation with subcutaneous transplantation of the cord (Halsted I), the Ferguson operation, the Andrews operation, and the Halsted II (Ferguson-Andrews operation). However, since they are rarely used in clinical practice now, they will not be described in detail here. The Ferguson and Andrews operations are shown diagrammatically in Figs. 36-19 and 36-20.

Open Anterior, Prosthetic

Lichtenstein Tension-Free Hernioplasty

The initial steps of the Lichtenstein repair are similar to those of the Bassini repair. After the external oblique aponeurosis has been opened from just lateral to the internal ring through the external ring, the upper leaf is freed from the underlying anterior rectus sheath and internal oblique muscle aponeurosis in an avascular plane from a point at least 2 cm medial to the pubic tubercle to the anterior superior iliac spine laterally. Blunt dissection is continued in this avascular plane from lateral to the internal ring to the pubic tubercle along the inguinal ligament and iliopubic tract. Continuing this same motion, the cord, with its cremaster covering, is swept off the pubic tubercle and separated from the inguinal floor. The ilioinguinal nerve, external spermatic vessels, and the genital branch of the genitofemoral nerve all remain with the cord structures. The effect is to create a large space for the eventual placement of the

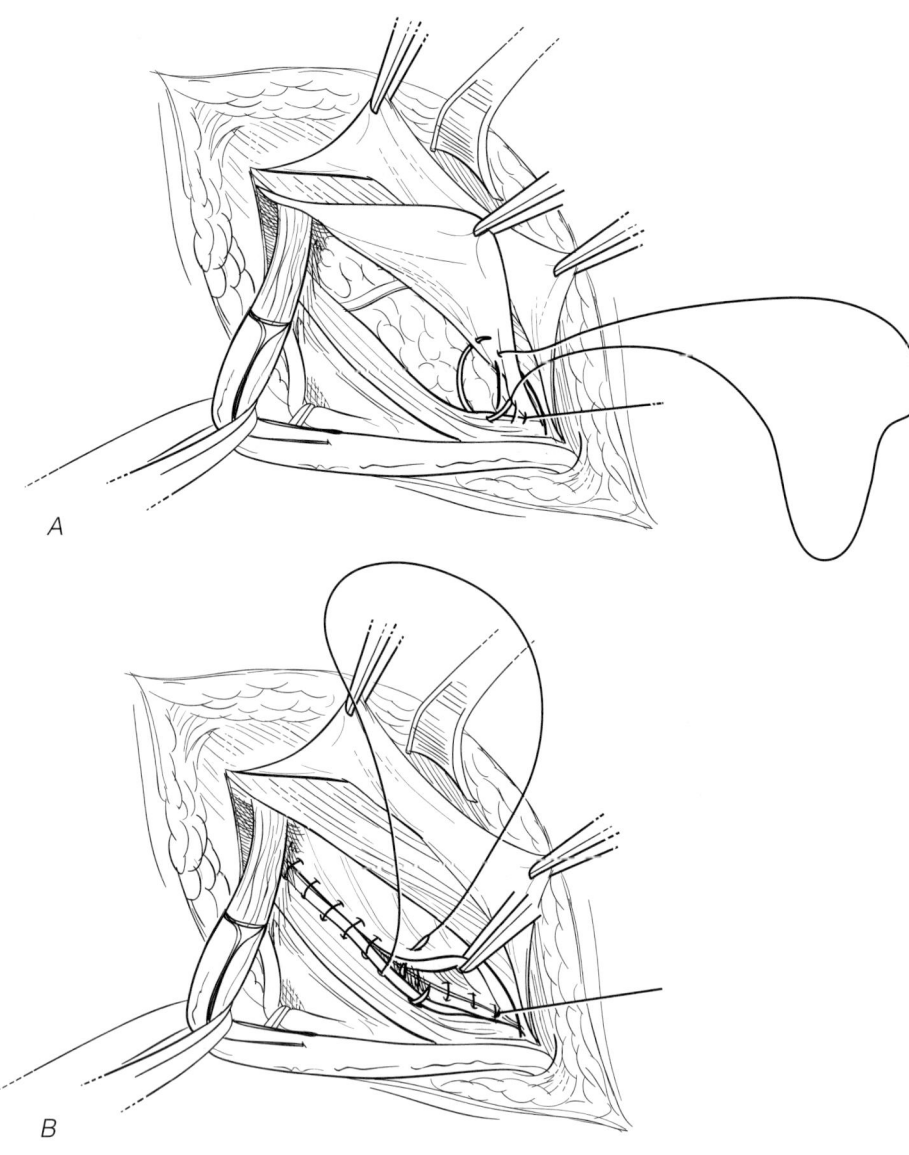

FIG. 36-17. The Shouldice repair. *A.* The iliopubic tract is sutured to the medial flap, which is made up of the transversalis fascia and the internal oblique and transversus abdominis muscles. *B.* This is the second of the four suture lines. After the stump of the cremaster muscle is picked up, the suture is reversed back toward the pubic tubercle, approximating the internal oblique and transversus muscles to the inguinal ligament. Two more suture lines will eventually be created suturing the internal oblique and transversus muscles medially to an artificially created pseudoinguinal ligament developed from superficial fibers of the inferior flap of the external oblique aponeurosis parallel to the true ligament.

prosthesis, and at the same time provide excellent visualization of the important nerves.

For indirect hernias, the cremaster muscle is incised longitudinally and the sac dissected free and reduced into the preperitoneal space. A theoretical criticism of this operation is that unless the inguinal floor is opened, an occult femoral hernia may be overlooked. However, an excessive incidence of missed femoral hernias has not been reported. In addition, it is possible to evaluate the femoral ring by entering the preperitoneal space through a small opening in the canal floor. Direct hernias are separated from the cord and other surrounding structures and reduced back into the preperitoneal space. Dividing the superficial layers of the neck of the sac circumferentially, which in effect opens the inguinal floor, usually facilitates reduction and aids in maintaining it while the prosthesis is being placed. This opening in the inguinal floor can also be used to palpate a femoral hernia. Suture can be used to invert the sac, but this adds no strength as the purpose is simply to allow the repair to proceed unencumbered by the sac continually protruding into the operative field.

A mesh prosthesis with a minimum size of 15 × 8 cm for an adult is positioned over the inguinal floor. The medial end is rounded

to correspond to the patient's anatomy and secured to the anterior rectus sheath a minimum of 2 cm medial to the pubic tubercle (Fig. 36-21). Either nonabsorbable or long-acting absorbable suture should be used. The wide overlap of the pubic tubercle is important as pubic tubercle recurrences are commonly seen with other operations. The suture is continued in a running locking fashion laterally, securing the prosthesis to either side of the pubic tubercle (not into it), and then the shelving edge of the inguinal ligament. The suture is tied at the internal ring.

A slit is made at the lateral end of the mesh creating two tails, a wide one (two thirds) above and a narrower (one third) below. The tails are positioned around the cord structures and placed beneath the external oblique aponeurosis laterally to about the anterior superior iliac spine, with the upper tail being placed on top of the lower. A single interrupted suture is used to secure the lower edge of the superior tail to the lower edge of the inferior tail, in effect creating a shutter valve at the internal ring. This step is considered crucial for the prevention of indirect recurrences that are occasionally seen when simple reapproximation of the tails is performed. Including the shelving edge of the inguinal ligament in this shutter valve stitch serves to buckle the mesh, medially over the direct

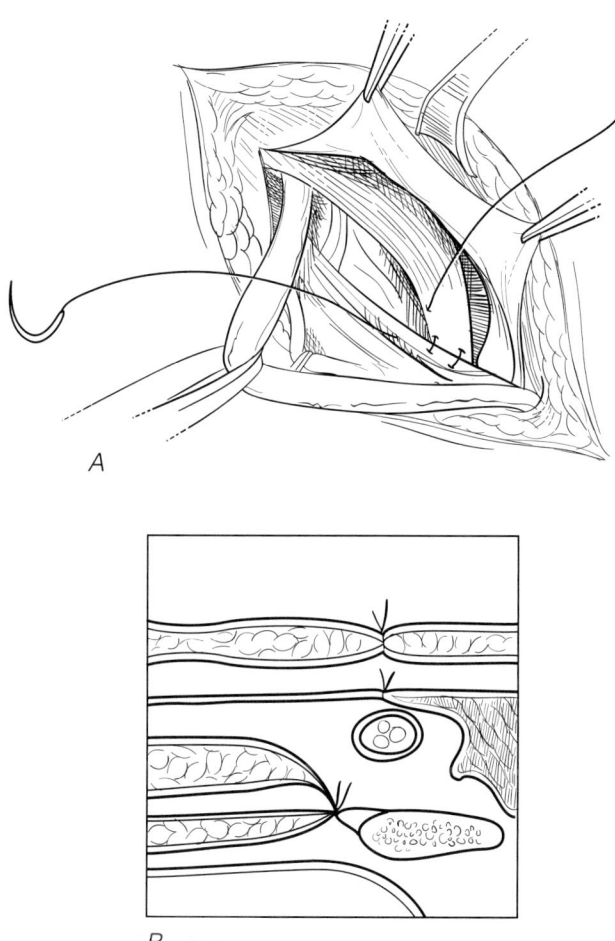

A

B

FIG. 36-18. McVay Cooper's ligament repair.

space, creating a dome-like effect that assures there is no tension, especially when the patient assumes an upright position. A few interrupted sutures are used to secure the superior and medial aspects of the prostheses to the underlying internal oblique muscle and rectus fascia. If the iliohypogastric nerve crosses up to the external oblique aponeurosis on the medial side, the prosthesis should be slit to accommodate it. The prosthesis can be trimmed in situ, but care should be taken to maintain sufficient laxity to account for the

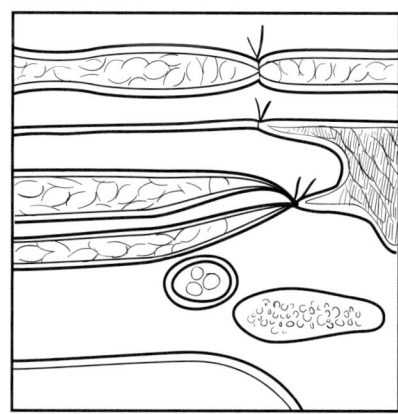

FIG. 36-19. Ferguson operation.

difference between the supine and upright positions, as well as the fact that mesh shrinkage will occur.

If a femoral hernia is present, the posterior surface of the mesh is sutured to Cooper's ligament after the inferior edge has been attached to the inguinal ligament. This closes the femoral canal. The wound is closed in layers.

Mesh Plug and Patch

The mesh plug technique was developed by Gilbert and then modified by Rutkow and Robbins, Millikan, and others.[45] The groin is entered through a standard anterior approach. The hernia sac is dissected away from surrounding structures and reduced back into the preperitoneal space. A flat sheet of polypropylene mesh is rolled up like a cigarette and held in place with suture. This plug is inserted in the defect and secured to either the internal ring for an indirect hernia, or the neck of the defect for a direct hernia, using interrupted sutures (Fig. 36-22A). The use of a prefabricated, commercially-available prosthesis that has the configuration of a flower is recommended by Rutkow and Robbins. The prosthesis is then individualized for each patient by removing some of the petals to avoid unnecessary bulk. This step is important, as rarely erosion into a surrounding structure such as the bladder has been reported. Millikan further modified the procedure by recommending that the inside petals be sewn to the ring of the defect.[46] For indirect hernias the inside petals are sewn to the internal oblique portion of the internal ring, which forces the outside of the prosthesis underneath the inner side of the defect, making it act like a preperitoneal underlay. For direct hernias, the inside petals are sewn to Cooper's ligament and the shelving edge of the inguinal ligament as well as the musculoaponeurotic ring of the defect superiorly, again forcing the outside of the mesh to act as an underlay. The patch portion of the procedure is optional, and involves placing a flat piece of polypropylene in the inguinal space, widely overlapping the plug in a fashion similar to the Lichtenstein procedure (Fig. 36-22B). The difference is that only one or two sutures, or perhaps no sutures, are used to secure the flat prosthesis to the underlying inguinal floor. Some surgeons place so many sutures that they have in effect performed a Lichtenstein operation on top of the plug. To the credit of its proponents, the plug and patch, in all of its varieties, has been skillfully presented and has rapidly become a popular repair. Not only is it fast, but it is also easy to teach, making it popular in both private and academic centers.[46]

Open Preperitoneal, Nonprosthetic

The preperitoneal space can be entered via either an anterior approach through the inguinal floor, or more commonly using the posterior. Read credits Annandale as the first surgeon to describe the anterior method for gaining access to the preperitoneal space in 1876.[47] As noted above, Bassini's operation is technically an anterior preperitoneal operation, although for practical reasons it is not discussed in that context. Cheatle and Henry first suggested the posterior approach to the preperitoneal space for repair of an inguinal hernia and it remained popular into the second half of the twentieth century, championed by such proponents as Nyhus. Today, these operations are of little more than historical significance, because it is now universally agreed that better results are obtained in this space when a prosthesis is used.[48,49]

Open Preperitoneal, Prosthetic

The key to preperitoneal prosthetic repairs is the placement of a large prosthesis in the preperitoneal space between the transversalis

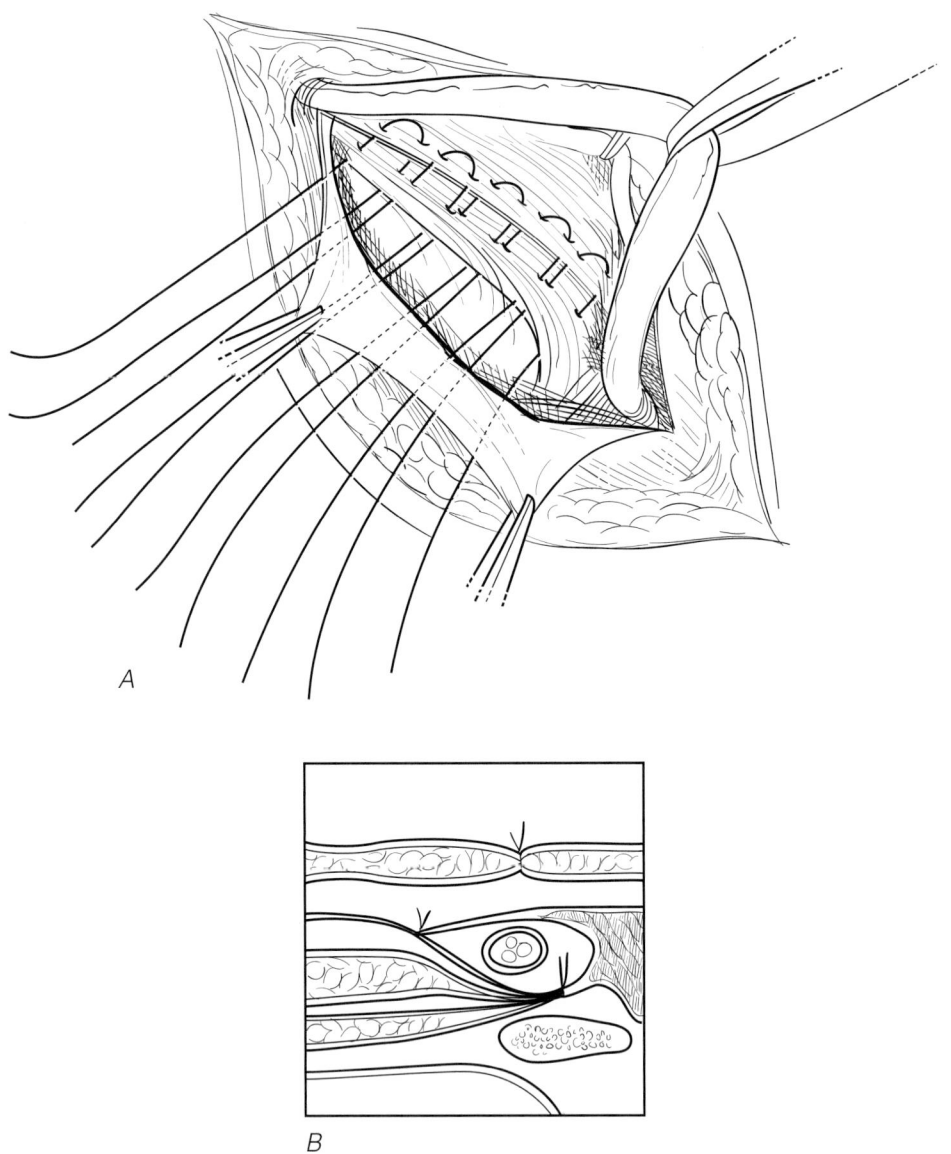

A

B

FIG. 36-20. Andrews operation.

fascia and the peritoneum, in effect replacing the transversalis fascia that has become deficient in its function of retaining the peritoneum (Fig. 36-23). The hernia defect itself may or may not be closed, depending on the preference of the surgeon. This is theoretically attractive because in contradistinction to an anterior repair, in which abdominal pressure might contribute to recurrence, the preperitoneal repair makes use of the abdominal pressure to help fix the prosthetic material against the abdominal wall, adding strength to the repair. The preperitoneal space can be entered from its anterior or posterior aspect. The major difference between the anterior and posterior approaches is that in the latter, the inguinal canal is not entered. Proponents point out that this avoids damage to the cremaster muscle and lessens the chance of cord injury. If an anterior approach is desirable, a groin incision is used because the space is entered directly through the inguinal floor. Either a lower midline, paramedian, or Pfannenstiel incision without opening the peritoneum can be used for the purposes of entering the preperitoneal space posteriorly, as originally popularized by Cheatle and later Henry; a technique which is now associated with their names.[50] The preperitoneal space can also be entered transabdominally as practiced by La Roque, using a laparotomy to repair an inguinal hernia, a

procedure that is only recommended if the laparotomy is being performed for another purpose.

The Anterior Approach

Read-Rives. This operation starts like a classic Bassini, including opening the inguinal floor. The inferior epigastric vessels are identified and the preperitoneal space completely dissected. The spermatic cord is parietalized by separating the ductus deferens from the spermatic vessels. A 12 × 16 cm piece of mesh is positioned in the preperitoneal space deep to the inferior epigastric vessels and secured with three sutures, one each to the pubic tubercle, Cooper's ligament, and the psoas muscle laterally. The transversalis fascia is closed over the prosthesis and the cord structures replaced. The rest of the closure is as described above for the Bassini repair.

The Posterior Approach

Wantz/Stoppa/Rives. These three procedures are grouped together under the heading of the giant prosthetic reinforcement of the visceral sac (GPRVS), because there are only minor variations between them. A lower midline, transverse, or Pfannenstiel incision

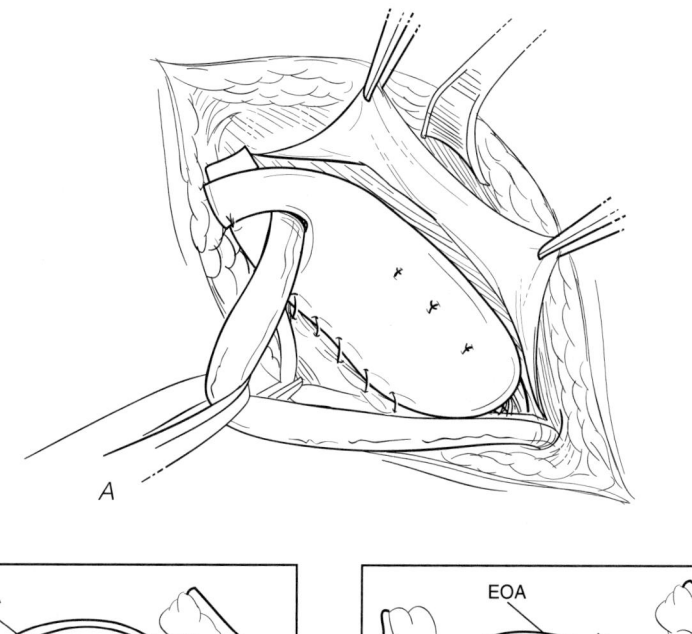

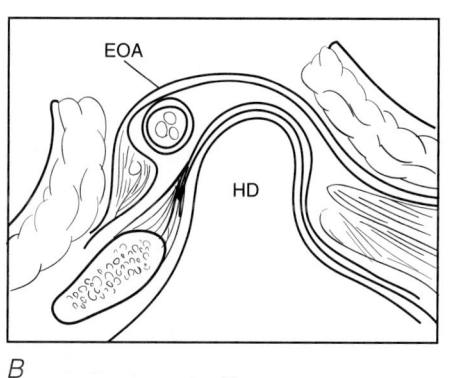

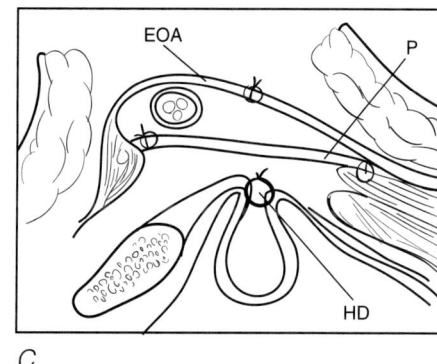

FIG. 36-21. *Lichtenstein tension-free hernioplasty. A. The medial border of the prosthesis has been sutured to the anterior rectus sheath 2 cm medial to the pubic tubercle. The same suture is continued in a running locking fashion to secure the inferior edge of the prosthesis to the inguinal ligament. A second suture is shown approximating the inferior surface of the superior tail to the inferior surface of the inferior tail and the inguinal ligament after the prosthesis was split laterally to accommodate the cord structures. B. and C. A lateral view of the repair. The hernia is reduced and the defect approximated merely for the convenience of keeping the hernia contents out of the inguinal canal during the repair. This adds no strength as the repair relies entirely on the overlying prosthesis. EOA = external oblique aponeurosis; P = prosthesis; HD = hernia defect.*

can be used according to surgeon preference. If a transverse incision is chosen, it should extend from the midline 8 to 9 cm in each direction laterally, and 2 to 3 cm below the level of the anterosuperior iliac spine, but above the internal ring.[51] The anterior rectus sheath and the oblique muscles are incised for the length of the skin incision. The lower flap of these structures is retracted inferiorly towards the pubis. The transversalis fascia is then incised along the lateral edge of the rectus muscle and the preperitoneal space entered. If a lower midline or Pfannenstiel incision is used, the fascia overlying the space of Retzius is opened without violating the peritoneum. A combination of blunt and sharp dissection is continued laterally, posterior to the rectus muscle and the inferior epigastric vessels. At this point the operation proceeds identically no matter which skin incision has been chosen. The preperitoneal space is completely dissected to a point lateral to the anterior superior iliac spine. The symphysis pubis, Cooper's ligament, and the iliopubic tract are identified. Inferiorly the peritoneum is generously dissected away from the vas deferens and the internal spermatic vessels to create a large pocket that will eventually accommodate a prosthesis without the possibility of roll-up (Figs. 36-24 and 25-C). The term *parietalization* of the spermatic cord, popularized by Stoppa, refers to the thorough dissection of the cord to provide enough length to move it laterally.

Direct hernia sacs are reduced during the course of the preperitoneal dissection. When reducing the peritoneum from a direct hernia defect, it is important to stay in the plane between the peritoneum and the transversalis fascia, allowing the latter structure to retract back into the hernia defect towards the skin. The transversalis fascia can be thin, and if it is inadvertently opened and incorporated with

the peritoneal sac during reduction, a needless and bloody dissection of the abdominal wall is the result. Indirect sacs are more difficult to deal with than direct sacs, as they can be adherent to the cord structures. Care must be taken to minimize trauma to the cord to prevent damage to the vas deferens or the blood supply to the testicle. A small sac should be mobilized from the cord structures and reduced back into the peritoneal cavity. A large sac may be difficult to mobilize from the cord without undue trauma if an attempt is made to remove the sac in its entirety. In this situation, the sac should be divided, leaving the distal sac in situ, with dissection of the proximal sac away from the cord structures (Fig. 36-25A and B). The division of the sac is most easily accomplished by opening it on the side opposite the cord structures. A finger can then be placed in the sac to facilitate its separation from the cord. Downward traction is then placed on the cord structures so that excessive amounts of fatty tissue (lipoma of the cord) can be separated and reduced into the preperitoneal space, to preclude the possibility of a pseudorecurrence when the fatty tissue is palpated during physical examination postoperatively.

Management of a direct abdominal wall defect varies somewhat. Rignault closes it loosely to avoid an unsightly early postoperative bulge.[52] Stoppa and Wantz usually leave it alone, but the transversalis fascia in the defect is occasionally plicated by suturing it to Cooper's ligament to prevent a seroma in the space previously occupied by the hernia contents.

The next step is the placement of the prosthesis. Dacron mesh is more pliable than polypropylene, and is therefore considered particularly suitable for this procedure as it conforms well to the preperitoneal space. For unilateral repairs, the size of the prosthesis

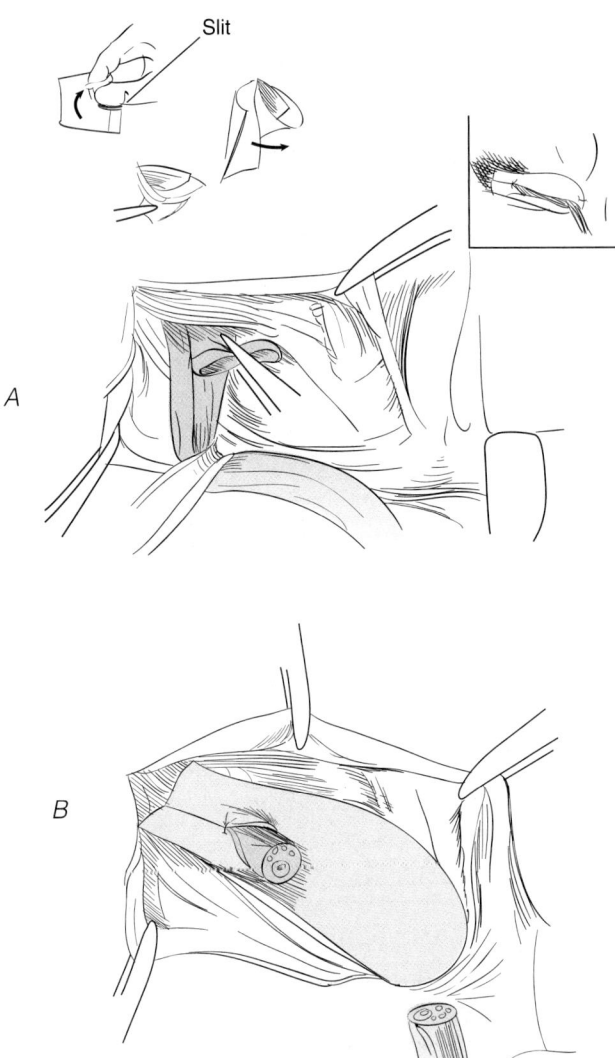

A

B

FIG. 36-22. *A.* The original Gilbert operation. A homemade plug (see insert) is fashioned and then inserted through the hernia defect into the preperitoneal space. The insert shows a 6–8 cm square polypropylene mesh which is being rolled around a partial slit in the mesh to form a cone. The plug is sometimes sutured to the ring of the hernia defect. *B.* A common modification is to place a flat sheet of mesh that overlaps significantly over the plug to cover the entire inguinal floor. The result then resembles a Lichtenstein-type repair on top of the plug, or a "Plugtenstein."

is approximately the distance between the umbilicus and the anterior superior iliac spine minus 1 cm for the width, with the height being approximately 14 cm. Wantz recommends an eccentric cut of the prosthesis, with the lateral side longer than the medial side, to achieve the best fit in the preperitoneal space. Because of his thorough parietalization of the cord structures, Stoppa believes that it is not necessary to split the prosthesis laterally to accommodate the cord structures. This avoids the keyhole defect created when the prosthesis is split, which has been incriminated in recurrences. Rignault, on the other hand, prefers a keyhole defect in the mesh to encircle the spermatic cord, believing that this provides the prosthesis with enough stability that the use of fixation sutures or tacks can be avoided. Minimizing fixation in this area is important because of the numerous anatomic elements in the preperitoneal space that can be inadvertently damaged during their placement. For Wantz's

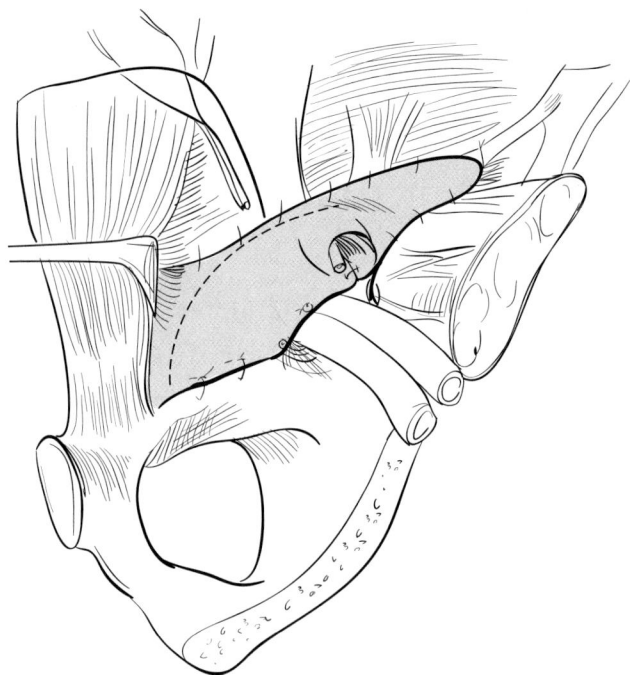

FIG. 36-23. Preperitoneal prosthetic hernia repair. Wide overlap of the myopectineal orifice with a large prosthetic patch is typical of a preperitoneal repair. In this case, the mesh has been "keyholed" to accommodate the cord structures. Other prefer parietalization with lateral displacement of the cord.

technique, three absorbable sutures are used to attach the superior border of the prosthesis to the anterior abdominal wall well above the defect (Fig. 36-26A to C). The three sutures are placed near the linea alba, semilunar line, and the anterior superior iliac spine from medial to lateral. A Reverdin suture needle facilitates this. Three long clamps are then placed on each corner and the middle of the

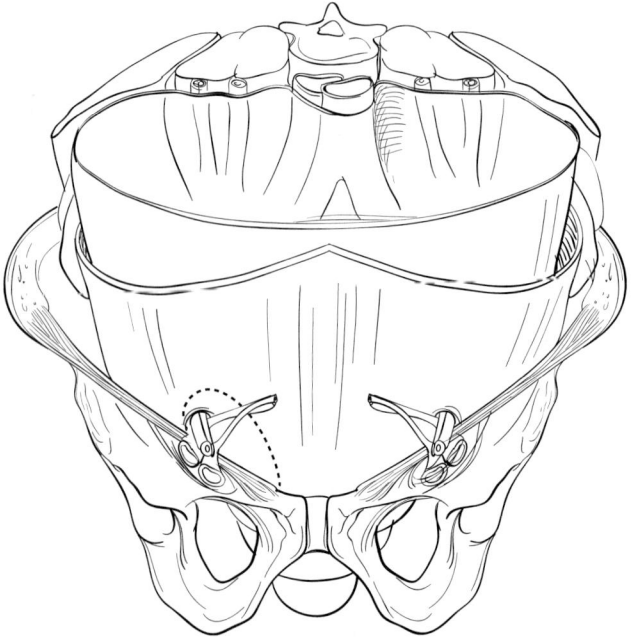

FIG. 36-24. Extensive dissection of the preperitoneal space on both sides will eventually accommodate the large prosthesis shown replacing the transversalis fascia.

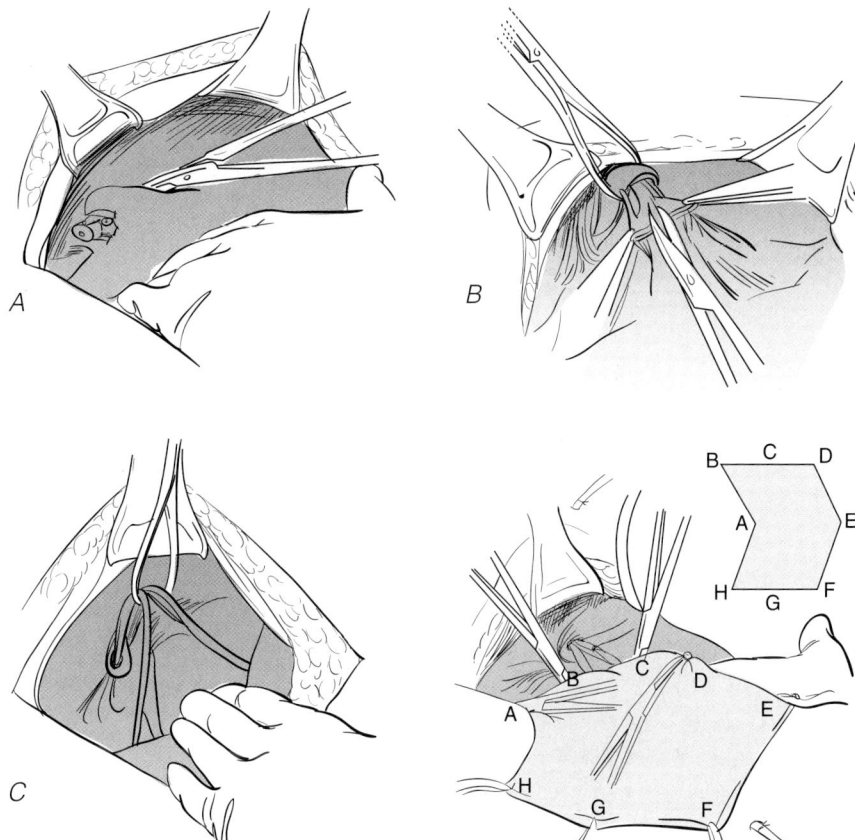

FIG. 36-25. *A.* A long indirect sac is isolated from the cord structures without disturbing the distal aspect. *B.* The sac is divided and the proximal end closed with sutures. *C.* After the sac has been further dissected proximally, the vas deferens and internal spermatic vessels are freed from the parietal peritoneum (Parietalization). *D.* Long clamps are attached at each of the lettered points on the prosthesis which will facilitate placement deep in the preperitoneal space. Point E will eventually end up near the umbilicus where the only suture in the repair will be placed from the prosthesis to the periumbilical fascia. Points B and H are particularly important because they correspond to the deepest penetration of the prosthesis laterally on either side. These clamps must be removed carefully to prevent roll-up.

inferior border of the prosthesis. The medial clamp is placed into the space of Retzius and held by an assistant. The middle clamp is positioned so that the mesh covers the pubic ramus, obturator fossa, and the iliac vessels, and is similarly held by the assistant. The lateral clamp is placed into the iliac fossa to cover the parietalized cord structures and the iliopsoas muscle. Care must be taken to prevent the prosthesis from rolling up as the clamps are removed (Fig. 36-27). Stoppa's technique is most often associated with one large prosthesis for bilateral hernias. The dimensions of this prosthesis are the distance between the two anterior superior iliac spines minus 2 cm for the width, and the height is equal to the distance between the umbilicus and the pubis. The prosthesis is cut in a chevron shape and eight clamps are positioned strategically around the prosthesis to facilitate placement into the preperitoneal space (Fig. 36-25D). The wound is closed in layers.

Nyhus/Condon (Iliopubic Tract Repair). The names Nyhus and Condon are firmly associated with this preperitoneal repair, especially in North America. The two authorities carried out extensive cadaver dissections and pointed out the importance of the iliopubic tract, which is why their operation is called the iliopubic tract repair. A transverse lower abdominal incision is made two fingerbreadths above the symphysis pubis. The anterior rectus sheath is opened on its lateral side to allow the rectus muscle to be retracted medially, and the two oblique and the transversus abdominis muscles are incised, exposing the transversalis fascia[53] (Fig. 36-28). A combination of sharp and blunt dissection inferiorly opens the preperitoneal space and exposes the posterior inguinal floor. Direct or indirect defects are repaired similarly after the peritoneal sac has been reduced or divided and closed proximally. The transverse

aponeurotic arch is sutured to the iliopubic tract inferiorly, occasionally including Cooper's ligament in the first few medial sutures. If the internal ring is particularly large, a suture is also placed lateral to the internal ring (Fig. 36-29). For femoral hernias the iliopubic tract is sutured to Cooper's ligament to close the canal (Fig. 36-30). Once the defect has been formally repaired, a tailored mesh prosthesis can be sutured to Cooper's ligament and the transversalis fascia for reinforcement. Initially this only was recommended for recurrent hernias, but with further patient follow-up it has now become routine for all hernias.

Kugel/Ugahary. These open preperitoneal prosthetic repairs were developed to compete with laparoscopic repairs by using a small (2 to 3 cm) skin incision, 2 to 3 cm above the internal ring.[54,55] Kugel locates this point by making an oblique incision one third lateral and two thirds medial to a point halfway between the anterosuperior iliac spine and the pubic tubercle. The incision is deepened through the external oblique fascia and the internal oblique muscle is bluntly spread. The transversalis fascia is opened vertically about 3 cm, but the internal ring is not violated. The preperitoneal space is entered and a blunt dissection performed. The inferior epigastric vessels are identified to assure that the dissection is into the correct plane. These vessels should be left adherent to the overlying transversalis fascia and retracted medially and anteriorly. The iliac vessels, Cooper's ligament, pubic bone, and hernia defect are identified by palpation. Most hernia sacs are simply reduced. The exception is large indirect sacs that are often divided to leave the distal sac in situ with proximal sac closure. Dr. Kugel feels that the cord structures must be thoroughly parietalized to allow adequate posterior dissection if recurrences are to be avoided. The

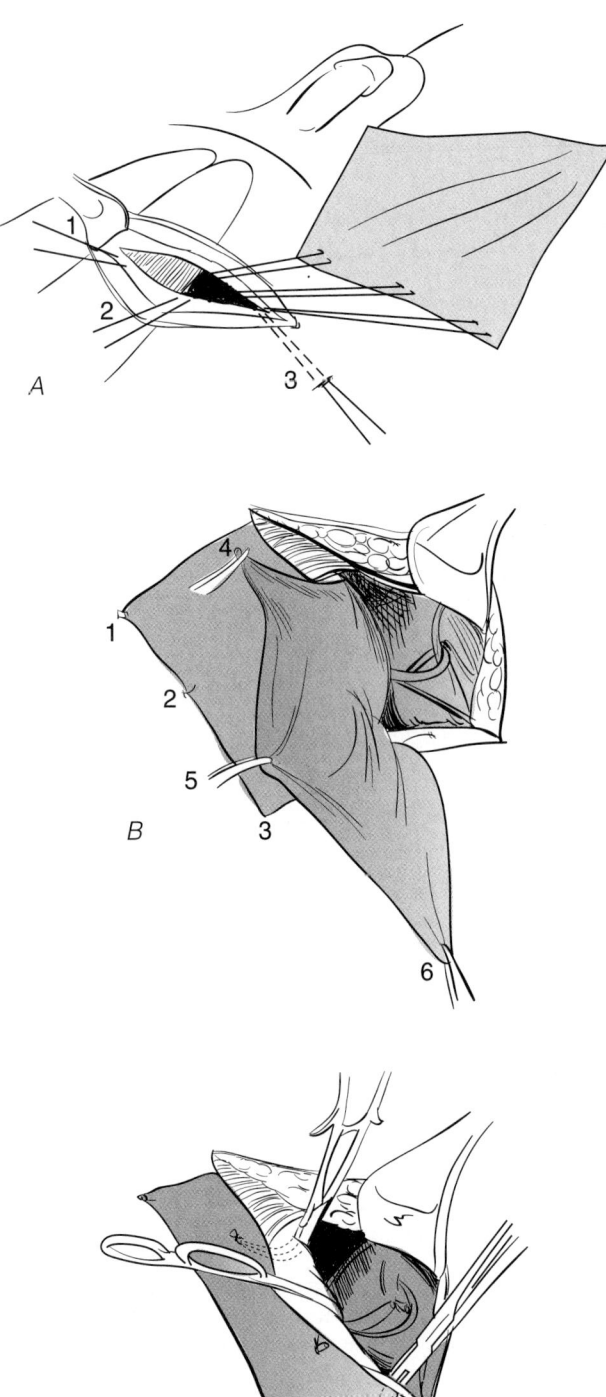

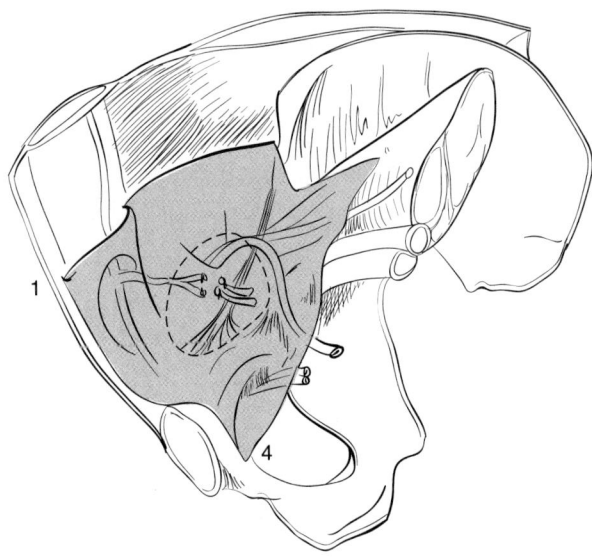

FIG. 36-27. Final appearance of Wantz's unilateral giant prosthetic reinforcement of the visceral sac (GPRVS).

prosthesis also has a slit on its anterior surface through which the surgeon places his or her finger to facilitate postioning.

Ugahary's operation is similar, but a special prosthesis is not required. Known as the gridiron technique, the preperitoneal space is prepared through a 3-cm incision in a manner similar to Kugel's. The space is held open using a narrow Langenbeck and two ribbon retractors. A 10 × 15 cm piece of polypropylene mesh is rolled onto a long forceps after the edges have been rounded and sutures placed to correspond to various anatomic landmarks. The rolled up mesh with forceps is introduced into the preperitoneal space and the mesh

FIG. 36-26. Wantz's unilateral preperitoneal repair. The prosthesis is (A) fixed to the anterior abdominal wall above the defect, and then long clamps (B and C) are used to drive the inferior border deep into the preperitoneal space. The clamps must be carefully removed to prevent the prosthesis from rolling up.

basis of the procedure is a specifically-designed, 8 × 12 cm prosthesis made of two pieces of polypropylene with a specially extruded single monofilament fiber located near its edge circumferentially. This allows the prosthesis to be deformed so that it can fit through the small incision. It then springs open to regain its normal shape, providing a wide overlap of the myopectineal orifice. The

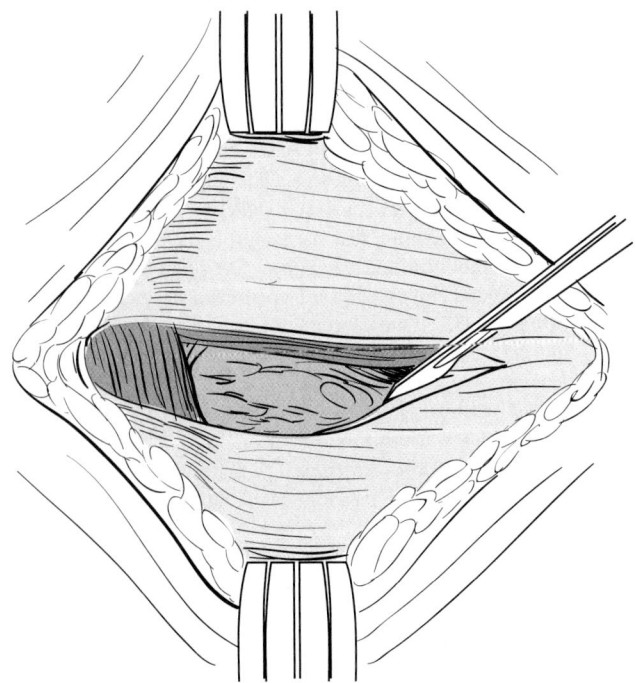

FIG. 36-28. Iliopubic tract repair. Initial incision. The lateral side of the anterior rectus sheath has been opened and the rectus muscle is visible. The external oblique, internal oblique, and the transversus abdominis muscles are incised to expose the transversalis fascia.

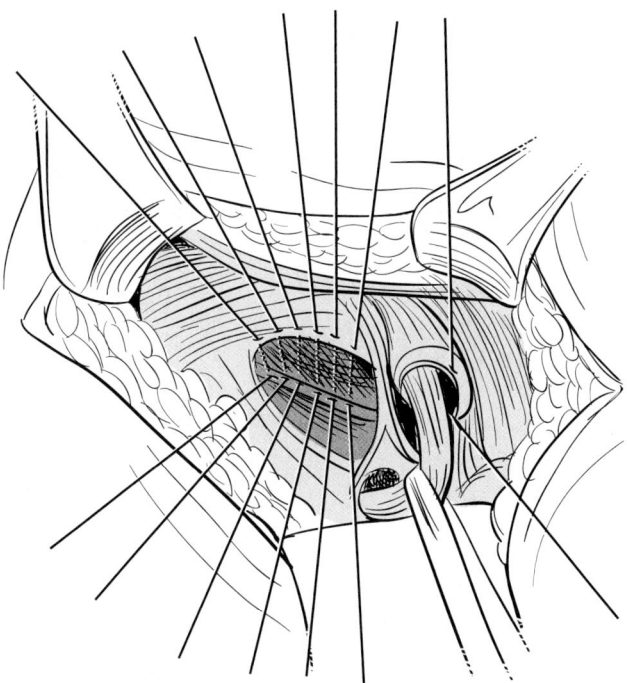

FIG. 36-29. Iliopubic tract repair. Direct hernia. The key to the repair is to suture the transverse aponeurotic arch to the iliopubic tract inferiorly. In this case, the internal ring is particularly large, so a suture is also placed lateral to the internal ring.

is unrolled using clamps and strategic movements of the ribbon retractors.

Both of these operations have been successful in experienced hands; however, considerable training is required to assure that the patch is properly positioned since it is placed blindly.

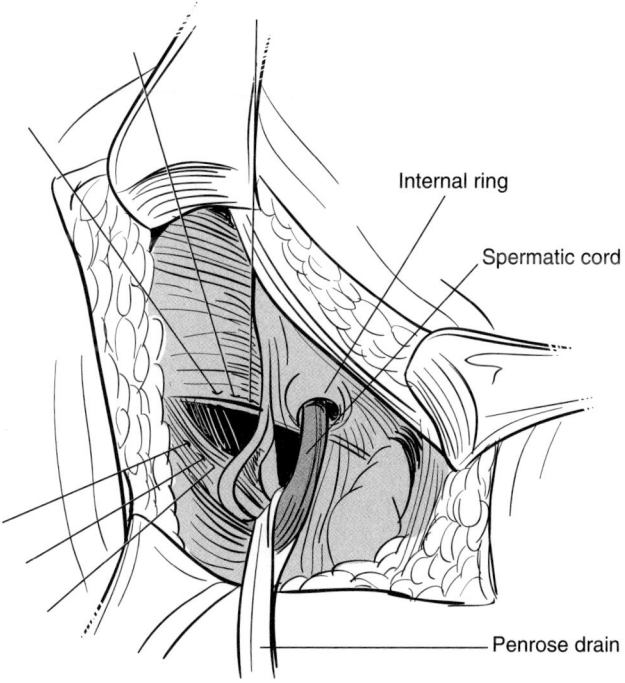

Internal ring

Spermatic cord

Penrose drain

FIG. 36-30. Iliopubic tract repair. Femoral hernia. The transverse aponeurotic arch remains the superior border, but Cooper's ligament instead of the iliopubic tract must be used inferiorly so the femoral canal is narrowed.

Combination Anterior and Preperitoneal, Prosthetic

The Bilayer Prosthetic Repair

This repair depends on a dumbbell-shaped device consisting of two flat pieces of polypropylene mesh connected by a cylinder of the same material. The purpose of this design is to allow the surgeon to take advantage of the presumed benefits of both the anterior and posterior approaches, since prosthetic material is placed in both the preperitoneal space and the inguinal canal. The initial steps are identical to those of a Lichtenstein procedure. Once the anterior space has been prepared, the preperitoneal space is entered through the hernia defect. Indirect hernias are reduced, and then a gauze sponge is used to bluntly develop the preperitoneal space through the internal ring. For direct hernias the transversalis fascia is opened and the space between this structure and the peritoneum is developed, again with a gauze sponge. The deep layer of the bilaminar prosthesis is deployed in the preperitoneal space, overlapping the direct and indirect spaces and Cooper's ligament. The superficial layer of the device occupies the open anterior space in a manner similar to Lichtenstein's. It is slit laterally or centrally to accommodate the cord structures, and then sutured using three or four interrupted sutures to the area of the pubic tubercle, the middle of the inguinal ligament, and the internal oblique muscle.

Laparoscopic Inguinal Herniorrhaphy

Laparoscopic inguinal herniorrhaphy was introduced in the late 1980s and early 1990s, at a time when many surgeons felt that most commonly performed abdominal procedures would eventually be adapted for laparoscopic methods. It was described by Ger in 1982, who pointed out its potential advantages such as less postoperative discomfort or pain, reduced recovery time allowing earlier return to full activity, easier repair of a recurrent hernia because the repair is performed in tissue that has not been previously dissected, the ability to treat bilateral hernias, the performance of a simultaneous diagnostic laparoscopy, the highest possible ligation of the hernia sac, and improved cosmesis.[56]

It is not universally accepted that these advantages have been achieved, and the operation remains controversial. Detractors point to the possibility of a laparoscopic accident resulting in a major complication such as bowel perforation or vascular injury, potential adhesive complications at sites where the peritoneum has been breached or prosthetic material has been placed, and the need for a general anesthetic. In addition, many surgeons are concerned about the expensive equipment needed, especially when dealing with an uncomplicated unilateral inguinal hernia. They argue that the open operation can be performed under local anesthesia on an outpatient basis, with minimal risk of intra-abdominal injury, at less cost. Nevertheless, it has been unequivocally proven that laparoscopic herniorrhaphy is superior to a open nonprosthetic operation in terms of the overall recurrence rate and decreased postoperative pain, and/or earlier return to normal activity, and/or improvement in the overall quality of life as measured by validated instruments.[57] In addition, with the exception of a study from Italy, the most commonly referenced randomized controlled trials that have compared an open tension-free operation to a laparoscopic one, have shown at least one statistically significant advantage for laparoscopic herniorrhaphy[58] (Table 36-8).

An extensive review of available data comparing laparoscopic herniorrhaphy with open herniorrhaphy was conducted by the Cochrane group in conjunction with the European Hernia

Table 36-8
Randomized Controlled Trials Comparing Open Tension-Free Hernia Repair to Laparoscopic Hernia Repair

Study	Intervention	Year	No. of Pts.	No. of Hernias	Follow-Up	Complications	Analgesic Use	Pain Score	Time to Recovery	Return to Work	Quality of Life	Comments
Andersson et al[90]	TEP vs. TFR	2003	168		1 w, 6 w, 1 y	NS	Yes	NS	Yes	Yes	NE	Long-term study
Douek et al[91]	TAPP vs. TFR	2003	403		5 y	NS	Yes		Yes	Yes	NE	
Bringman et al[92]	TEP vs. TFR vs. P&P	2003	299		20 m		NE	Yes	Yes	Yes	NE	Bilateral and recurrent only (Operating time less for laparoscopic hernia repair)
Mahon et al[93]	TAPP vs. TFR	2003	120		1 & 3 m				NE	Yes	?	
Colak et al[94]	TFR vs. TEP	2003	134		Short term	NS	NE	Yes	Yes	NE	NE	
Sarli et al[95]	TAPP vs. TFR	2001	43		24 h, 48 h, 7 d, long term	NE	Yes	Yes	NE	Yes	NE	Bilateral inguinal hernias (Cost higher for laparoscopic hernia repair)
Kumar et al[96]	TEP vs. TFR	1999	50		Short term	Yes	Yes		NE	NE	NE	Recurrent inguinal hernia only
Beets et al[97]	TAPP vs. GPRVS	1999	79	108	Mean = 34 m	NS	Yes	NE	Yes	Yes	NE	All index hernias recurrent (Operating time greater and recurrence rate higher for the TAPP repair), recurrence rate for TAPP
MRC Trial Group[98]	TAPP, TEP vs. mainly TFR	1999	928		1 w, 3 m, 1 y	Yes	NE	Yes	Yes	NE	NE	Three serious complications with laparoscopy (Operating time longer for laparoscopic hernia repair)
Picchio et al[58]	TAPP vs. TFR	1999	105		Short term	NE	NS	No	No	No	NE	Half the time
Khoury[99]	TEP vs. P&P	1998	45	315	1 w, q 4 m × 3 y	Less	Yes	NE	Yes	Yes	NE	
Heikkinen et al[100]	TEP vs. TFR	1998	45		Short term	NE	NE	NE	NE	NE	NE	All patients employed; (Overall cost less for laparoscopic hernia repair, cost higher for laparoscopic hernia repair)
Wellwood et al[101]	TAPP (gen) vs. TFR (local)	1998	400		d 1–7, 2 w, 1 & 3 m			Yes	Yes	Yes	Yes	
Wright et al[102]	Laparoscopic vs. TFR, Stoppa	1996	120		Short term	Yes	Yes	Yes	NE	NE	NE	One-half the hospital stay (Shorter hospital stay for laparoscopic hernia repair)
Payne et al[103]	TAPP vs. TFR	1994	100	100	1 w, ?		Yes		Yes	Yes	NE	

d = days; GPRVS = giant prosthetic reinforcement of the visceral sac; m = months; NE = not evaluated; NS = no significant difference; P&P = plug and patch; TAPP = transabdominal extraperitoneal repair; TEP = totally extraperitoneal repair; TFR = tension-free repair; w = weeks; y = year.

Trialists Collaboration.[59] The trialist group was particularly important because many of the principal investigators for the studies were brought together to update and clarify their data. Forty-one published reports dealing with 7161 hernia repairs were felt to be of suitable quality to allow meta-analysis. The analysis confirmed a significant advantage of the laparoscopic operation over the open nonprosthetic repairs in terms of pain, return to activity, and recurrence rate. However, there was no difference in recurrence rate when laparoscopy was compared with prosthetic tension-free repairs, and the laparoscopic operation took longer. Laparoscopic herniorrhaphy patients returned to work quicker and had less persisting pain and numbness. The laparoscopic operation cost more initially, but the difference was offset when the more rapid recovery was factored in. Operative complications were uncommon for both methods, but serious problems were more often seen in the laparoscopic group (visceral injury occurred in 8:2315 of the laparoscopic patients versus 1:2599 of the open repair group; for vascular injuries the respective rates were 7:2498 versus 5:2758). The analysis did not reach a firm conclusion whether the benefits of laparoscopy are worth the risk of a serious laparoscopic accident.[59] Definitive data concerning long-term problems with the laparoscopic approach such as trocar site hernia or adhesive bowel obstruction were not available for this review. However, the operation is now over 10 years old and the incidence does not seem excessive.

At present, the best indications for a laparoscopic inguinal herniorrhaphy are: (1) a recurrent hernia after a open repair because the operation is performed in normal, unscarred tissue, (2) bilateral hernias, as both sides can easily be repaired using the same small laparoscopic incisions, and (3) the presence of an inguinal hernia in a patient who requires a laparoscopy for another procedure (i.e., a laparoscopic cholecystectomy, assuming the Gram's stain of the bile is negative). The more contentious issue is the use of laparoscopy for the uncomplicated unilateral hernia. In 2001 a panel representing the prestigious National Institute for Clinical Excellence (NICE) in London issued guidelines that stated, "For repair of primary inguinal hernia, open [mesh] should be the preferred surgical procedure."[60] However, the recommendation has been criticized, because the 20-member panel included only one surgeon, expert testimony was obtained from only a single surgeon, and the conclusion was based primarily on cost to the National Health Service without regard to overall cost.

In summary, the issue of indications for laparoscopic herniorrhaphy remains unsettled and awaits the results of several large randomized trials. Until such data are available, all adult patients with inguinal hernias who are candidates for general anesthesia can be considered candidates for the laparoscopic inguinal hernia repair. Absolute contraindications include any sign of intra-abdominal infection or coagulopathy. Relative contraindications include intra-abdominal adhesions from previous surgery, ascites, or previous surgery in the space of Retzius because of the increased risk of bladder injury. Severe underlying medical illness is also a relative contraindication because of the added risk of general anesthesia. These patients are better suited for an open operation under local anesthesia. An incarcerated sliding scrotal hernia is a relative contraindication, especially when involving the sigmoid colon, due to the risk of perforation because of the traction needed to reduce it.

The two commonly performed laparoscopic herniorrhaphies, the transabdominal preperitoneal (TAPP) and the totally extraperitoneal (TEP), are modeled after the open preperitoneal operations described above. The major difference is that the preperitoneal space is entered through three trocar sites rather than a large open incision.

The ensuing radical dissection of the preperitoneal space with the placement of a large prosthesis is similar to the open preperitoneal operation.

Transabdominal Preperitoneal (TAPP) Procedure

Figure 36-31 demonstrates the operating room setup for the TAPP procedure. The surgeon stands on the opposite side of the table from the hernia. The first assistant stands opposite the surgeon. Three laparoscopic cannulae are placed in a horizontal plane with the umbilicus (Fig. 36-32). The sizes of the cannulae vary. A 10-mm cannula at the umbilicus allows the surgeon to use the larger 10-mm laparoscope and facilitates the introduction of a sufficiently sized mesh into the peritoneal cavity. The authors prefer an open technique for placement of the initial cannula to minimize the possibility of bowel injury. The two additional cannulae are placed just lateral to the rectus muscles. After an initial diagnostic laparoscopic procedure, pertinent anatomic landmarks including the median and medial umbilical ligaments, the bladder, the inferior epigastric vessels, the vas deferens, the spermatic vessels, the external iliac vessels, and the hernia defect are identified. An incision of the peritoneum is initiated at the medial umbilical ligament at least 2 cm above the hernia defect and extended laterally toward the anterior superior iliac spine. The preperitoneal space is exposed using a combination of blunt and sharp dissection, mobilizing the peritoneal flap inferiorly. The symphysis pubis, Cooper's ligament, the iliopubic tract, and the cord structures are identified. Direct hernia sacs are reduced during this dissection. Indirect sacs are more difficult to deal with, as they can be tenaciously adherent to the cord structures. The cord must be skeletonized, but care must be taken to minimize trauma to prevent damage to the vas deferens or the blood supply to the testicle (Fig. 36-33). A small sac should be reduced, but if it is large and/or extending into the scrotum, it may be divided. The proximal sac is then closed before reduction, and the distal sac is opened distally as far as possible on the side opposite the cord. The dissection of the cord structures is completed by removing excessive fatty tissue to prevent a pseudorecurrence caused by a "lipoma" of the cord. Finally, the peritoneal flap is dissected inferiorly well proximal to the divergence of the vas deferens and the internal spermatic vessels. This assures that the prosthesis will lie flat in the preperitoneal space and will not roll up when the peritoneum is closed.

Placement of the prosthesis is the next step. A large piece of mesh, 15 × 11 cm or greater, is introduced into the abdominal cavity through the umbilical cannula and is positioned over the myopectineal orifice so that it completely covers the direct, indirect, and femoral spaces. Some surgeons prefer to slit the mesh to accommodate the cord structures, while others prefer to simply place the prosthesis over them. Fixation of the mesh is controversial. If a large enough mesh is used, no staples are required, which avoids complications associated with the trauma related to the fixation device. Most surgeons fear the possibility of mesh shrinkage or migration, and therefore use staples, tacks, or biologic glue. The landmarks for fixing the prosthesis are the contralateral pubic tubercle and the symphysis pubis for the medial edge, Cooper's ligament or the tissue just above it for the inferior border, and the posterior rectus sheath and transversalis fascia at least 2 cm above the hernia defect superiorly. Staples or tacks are never placed below the iliopubic tract when lateral to the internal spermatic vessels, to minimize the chance of damage to the lateral cutaneous nerve of the thigh or the femoral branch of the genitofemoral nerve. The prosthesis extends

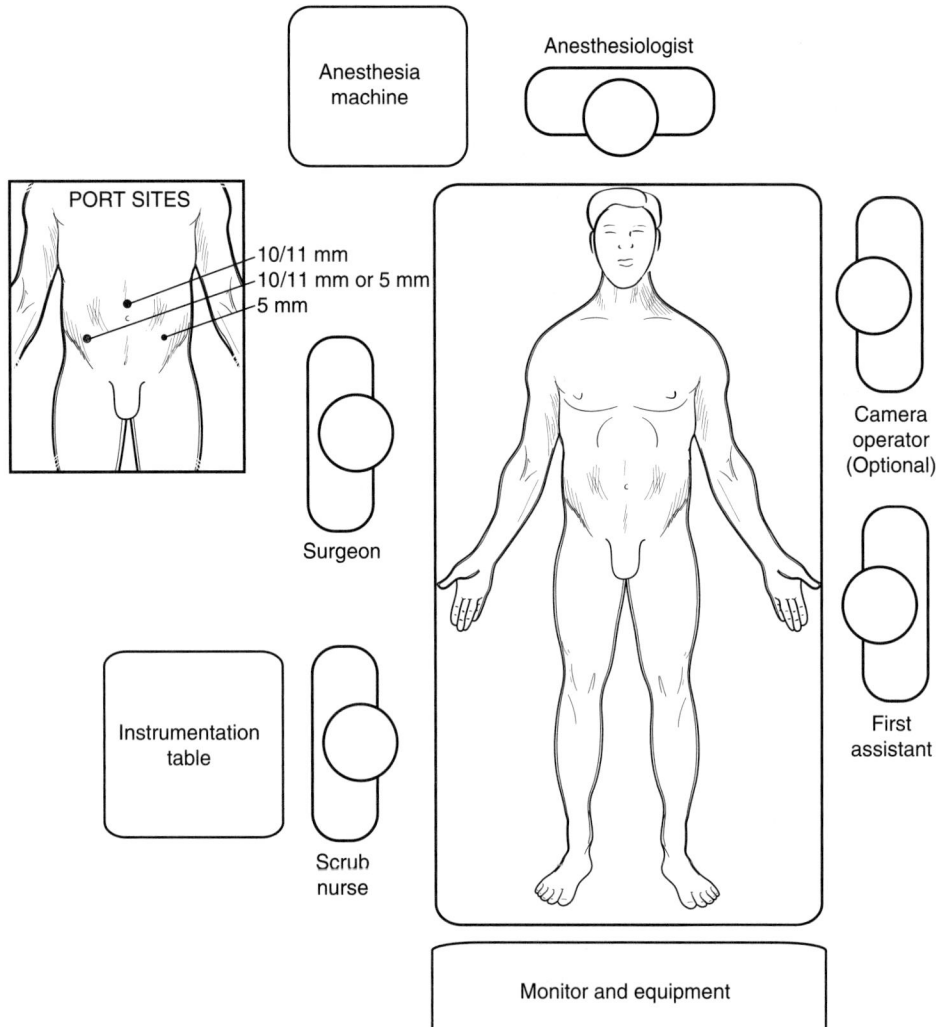

FIG. 36-31. Typical operating room set-up for a laparoscopic inguinal herniorrhaphy.

laterally to a point past the anterosuperior iliac spine to assure wide overlap. When closing the peritoneum, it is important to avoid gaps because small bowel has been known to find its way through them, resulting in a clinical bowel obstruction. It is sometime necessary to trim redundant mesh on the inferior border to prevent roll-up when the peritoneum is being closed.

Bilateral hernias can be repaired using two separate peritoneal incisions or one long transverse incision extending from one antero-superior iliac spine to the other on the opposite side. If two separate incisions are used (which avoids the theoretical problem that might occur if the patient has a patent urachus), the two preperitoneal spaces should be joined by dissecting behind the peritoneum and bladder in the space of Retzius so that a large prosthesis can be used in a manner similar to Stoppa's giant prosthetic reinforcement of the visceral sac (GPRVS).

Totally Extraperitoneal (TEP) Procedure

This operation is modeled after the Cheatle-Henry preperitoneal hernioplasties to address some of the major criticisms of the laparo-scopic TAPP procedure, namely the need to enter the peritoneal cavity and the attendant risk of injury to an intra-abdominal organ, intestinal obstruction secondary to adhesive complications, or trocar site herniation. The preperitoneal space is entered by establishing a plane of dissection outside of the peritoneal cavity between the posterior surface of the rectus muscle and the posterior rectus sheath and peritoneum. An incision is made at the umbilicus as if one were planning to perform open laparoscopy. The rectus sheath is opened on one side and the rectus muscle is retracted laterally. The space is enlarged by placing a blunt instrument blindly or using an operating laparoscope (a rigid laparoscope with a working channel). Once the surgeon is below the arcuate ligament, the preperitoneal space is entered and the dissection completed under direct vision. Two additional cannulas are placed in the midline, one approximately 5 cm above the symphysis pubis, and the other midway between the umbilicus and the symphysis pubis (Fig. 36-34). The operation then proceeds in an identical fashion to the TAPP procedure described above. Popular alternatives are to use a water- or air-filled balloon dissector (Figs. 36-35 and 36-36) to perform the preperitoneal dis-section, and to place the two accessory cannulae on either side of the umbilicus, similar to the TAPP procedure, instead of in the midline.

TAPP versus TEP. The Achilles heel of the TAPP procedure is the peritoneal closure. The peritoneum is frequently thin and tears easily once dissected, making it difficult to obtain complete cover-age of the prosthesis. This has resulted in major complications. The TEP procedure is more demanding than the TAPP initially because of the limited working space; however, once mastered, it completely eliminates the peritoneal closure step, making it faster. Most author-ities believe that a laparoscopic surgeon should be comfortable with

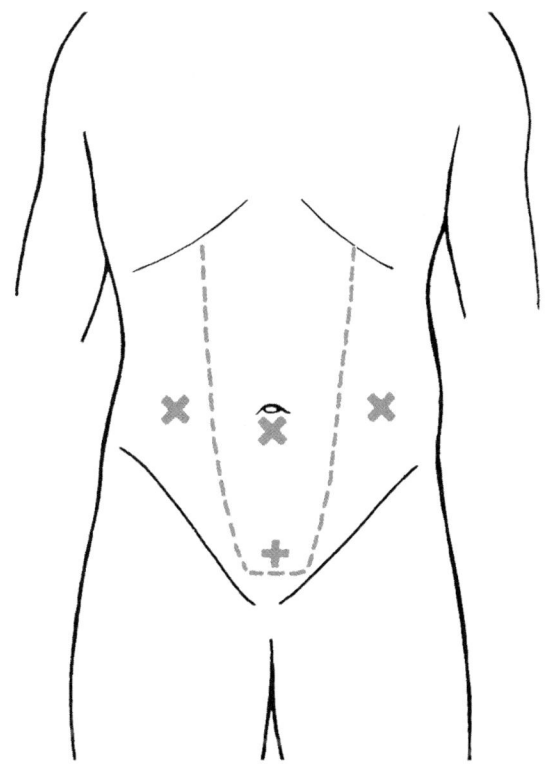

FIG. 36-32. *Laparoscopic cannula placement for a transabdominal preperitoneal (TAPP) or intraperitoneal onlay mesh (IPOM) herniorrhaphy.*

the TAPP herniorrhaphy before progressing to the TEP. The consequences of inadvertent breaches of the peritoneum, which are common with TEP, especially in patients with thin peritoneal tissue or those that have scar tissue associated with previous lower abdominal surgery, are as yet unknown. The peritoneal lacerations can be difficult to recognize because they are not in the visual field (Fig. 36-37). Intestinal obstruction secondary to bowel finding its way into the preperitoneal space has now been reported, so it has yet to be proven that the TEP procedure will actually substantially decrease the incidence of the major complication it was designed to prevent. At

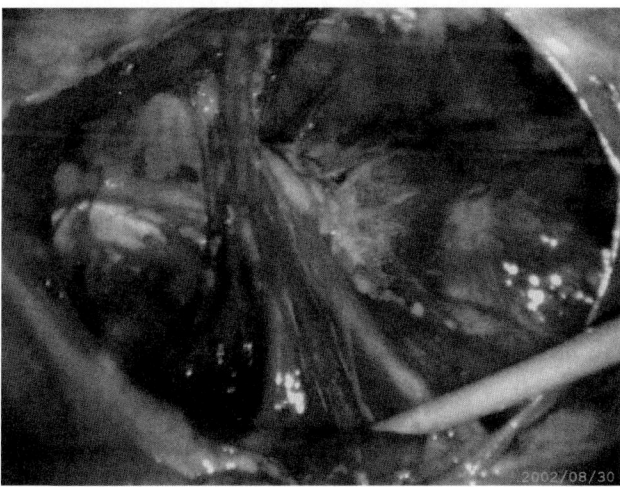

FIG. 36-33. *Completed preperitoneal dissection. Pertinent landmarks include the direct defect, the inferior epigastric vessels, the symphysis pubis, Cooper's ligament, the iliopubic tract, and the cord structures.*

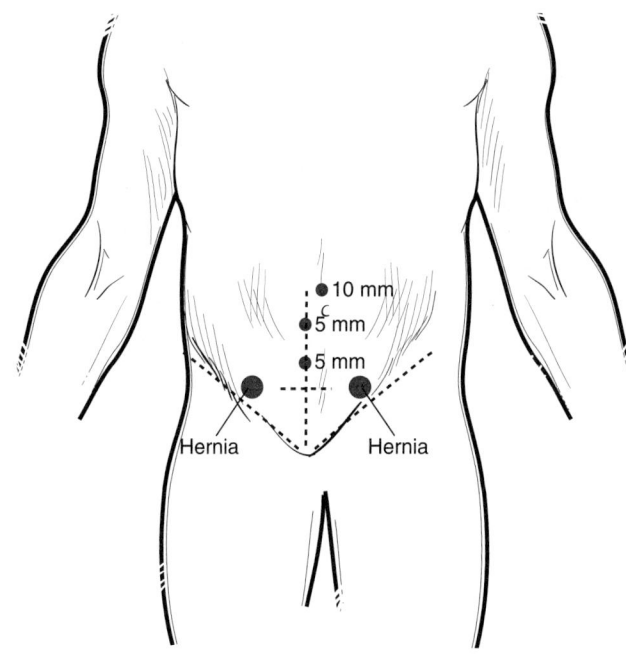

FIG. 36-34. *Laparoscopic cannula placement for a totally extraperitoneal (TEP) herniorrhaphy.*

the present time, the authors prefer the TEP procedure for smaller, simpler hernias, while patients with large hernias and those with previous lower abdominal incisions or any other complicating situation usually undergo a TAPP herniorrhaphy. The transabdominal preperitoneal operation is also the procedure of choice in a patient

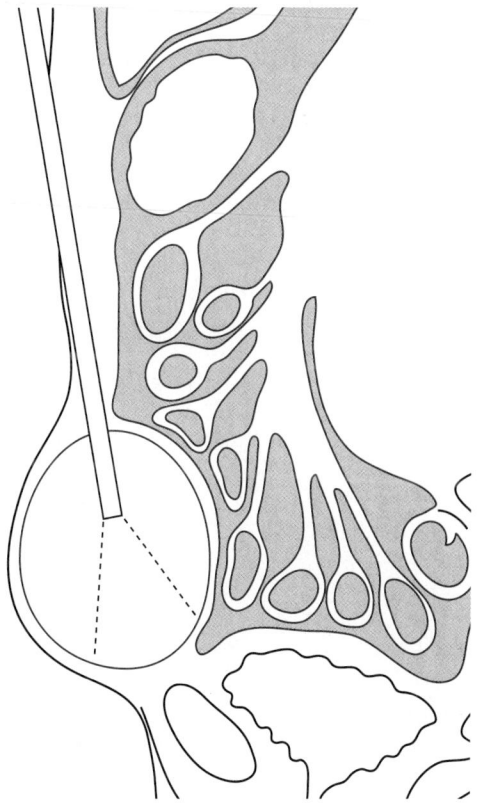

FIG. 36-35. *Balloon dissection of the preperitoneal space in a TEP herniorrhaphy.*

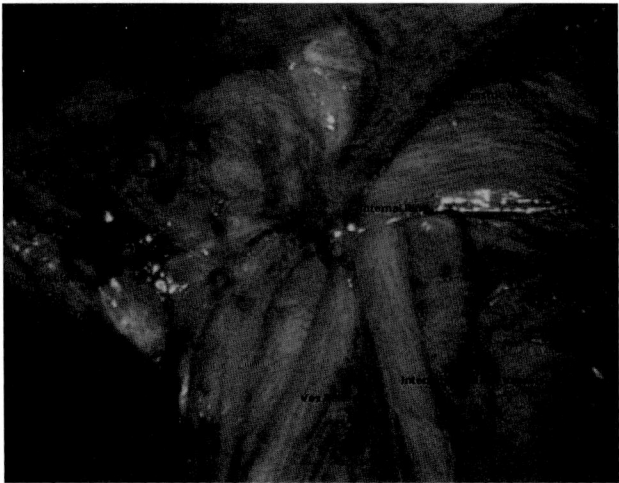

FIG. 36-36. Laparoscopic appearance of the preperitoneal space after TEP balloon dissection in a patient with a right recurrent direct inguinal hernia.

who has had a previous preperitoneal dissection (e.g., failed endoscopic herniorrhaphy or prostatic surgery), because of the difficulty of such a procedure and the need for wide exposure.

Intraperitoneal Onlay Mesh Procedure (IPOM)

The extensive dissection in the preperitoneal space required to perform either the TAPP or the TEP has limited the benefit of its minimally invasive nature especially when compared to other laparoscopic operations such as cholecystectomy, fundoplication, splenectomy and adrenalectomy. In fact, the considerable perioperative pain has caused some to suggest that the TEP or TAPP procedures should be called minimal-access surgery instead of minimally-invasive surgery. The basis of the IPOM repair is to place the prosthesis one layer deep to the preperitoneal space directly onto the peritoneum. Thus, no preperitoneal dissection is required and the hernia sac is undisturbed. Initial laparoscopy and accessory cannula placement is identical to those of the TAPP procedure. A

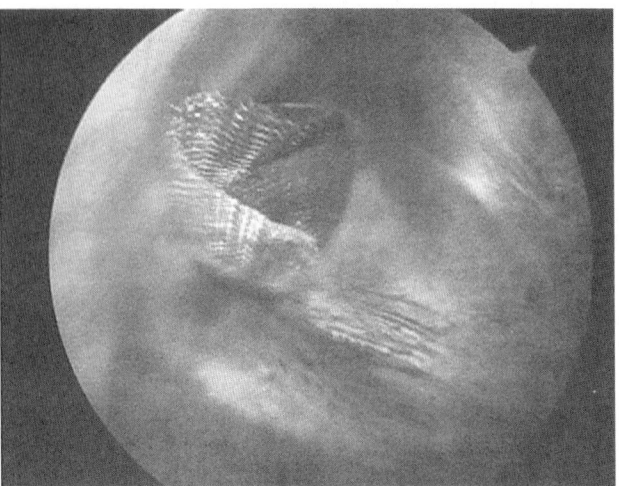

FIG. 36-37. Laparoscopic appearance of a peritoneal defect after a TEP hernia repair. This defect may have been difficult to see from a totally extraperitoneal perspective because it is located so far laterally outside the field of normal visualization.

large piece of prosthetic material is introduced into the peritoneal cavity and secured in place using staples, tacks, sutures, or a combination (Fig. 36-38). The landmarks for securing the prosthesis to the abdominal wall are identical to those of the TAPP or the TEP. This assures wide overlap of the defect and complete reinforcement of the entire inguinal floor. Some surgeons prefer to incise the peritoneum over Cooper's ligament, as they feel this aids in fixation of the prosthesis to this structure. The main concern, of course, is the possible development of complications from placing the prosthesis intraperitoneally, in contact with intra-abdominal organs. These include adhesion formation, visceral erosion with fistula formation, and infection and sepsis. It is these concerns that have made most surgeons feel that the IPOM should be considered an experimental procedure which has limited its use. Perhaps its best indication now is for the patient undergoing a laparoscopic herniorrhaphy for a failed previous preperitoneal repair. The risks associated with a difficult preperitoneal redissection might make the benefits worthwhile. Otherwise, until a completely inert prosthesis is developed, it should not be used in routine practice outside of highly controlled trials. Some authors feel that the use of expanded polytetrafluoroethylene (ePTFE) as an alternative to a mesh makes the operation more acceptable, but this remains unproven. A long term follow-up study of IPOM procedures using ePTFE was recently reported showing an unacceptable recurrence rate.[61] However, the ePTFE had been converted to a mesh using a skin graft expander which so changes the properties of ePTFE that it would be difficult to extrapolate to unaltered ePTFE.

Laparoscopic Surgery for a Failed Preperitoneal Repair

There are two groups of patients in whom a second preperitoneal dissection might be considered: (1) those with multiply-recurrent hernias where both spaces have already been dissected, and (2) those who insist on an endoscopic reoperative approach. The latter most commonly occurs when the herniorrhaphy on the recurrent side was laparoscopic and the patient has had a previous open repair on the opposite side.

Several groups have devised specific surgical strategies for approaching recurrent preperitoneal hernias laparoscopically.[62,63,64] The TAPP approach is almost always used, as it is too difficult to re-establish a preperitoneal working space and maintain peritoneal integrity. Generally, the old prosthesis is left in situ after the preperitoneal space is redissected, followed by completion of the coverage of the myopectineal orifice with a new prosthesis. If no hernia is evident from the laparoscopic vantage point, a pseudorecurrence consisting of a lipoma of the cord or an encapsulated seroma may account for the clinical findings. Medial recurrences, which are invariably near the pubic tubercle, are treated by opening the peritoneum at least 3 cm above the hernia defect, in unscarred tissue. Dissection proceeds medially and inferiorly, widely opening the space of Retzius to the opposite pubic tubercle. It is necessary to identify the opposite tubercle because this will assure sufficient overlap by a new prosthesis. By staying in unscarred tissue while identifying and freeing the bladder, one avoids injury to it, the major complication associated with this approach. After the space of Retzius is opened, dissection proceeds laterally across the ipsilateral pubic tubercle and the hernia defect. It is difficult to separate the peritoneum from the old prosthesis, but nevertheless this is relatively safe, because there are no significant structures in harm's way until the internal ring is reached. A new prosthesis is fastened in place after sufficient overlap is achieved. Lateral recurrences are more difficult because of the scarring at the internal ring caused by

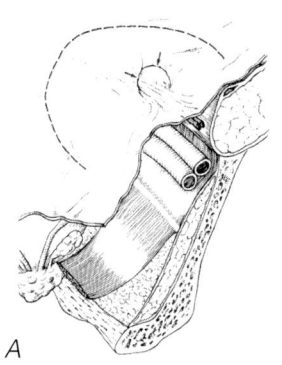
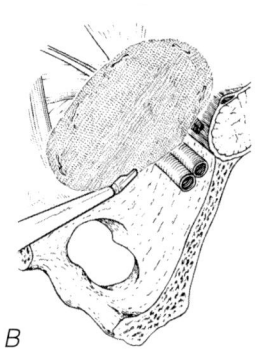
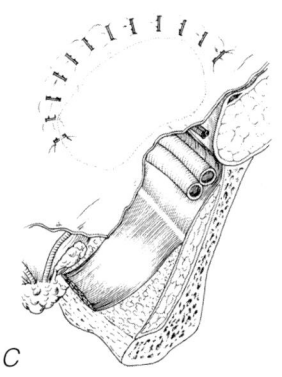

FIG. 36-38. Placement of mesh for an IPOM herniorrhaphy. *A.* The mesh is brought over the indirect defect. *B.* The mesh properly positioned. *C.* Completed IPOM procedure.

the old prosthesis and the recurrent sac. It is probably best to open the preperitoneal space above the hernia defect and get behind the previous prosthesis so that an en bloc mobilization of peritoneum and prosthesis from the transversalis fascia can be accomplished.[63] Dividing the inferior epigastric vessels facilitates this. The identification and mobilization of the lateral hernia sac can then be safely done after separation of the cord structures. A new mesh is then slit and positioned around the cord in the opposite direction of the original. A second un-slit mesh is placed over the first, again reinforcing the entire myopectineal orifice. Finally, the prosthesis must be covered. Peritoneum is best, but at times it can be so shredded that an omental flap is necessary.

COMPLICATIONS OF GROIN HERNIA REPAIRS

To facilitate discussion of complications the authors prefer to divide the complications into those related to the herniorrhaphy itself, those related to laparoscopy, and those that are general to any operation (Table 36-9).

Recurrence

Historically, the recurrence rate has been the exclusive yardstick for comparing different types of hernia repairs. However, two factors have surfaced that have served to decrease the importance of recurrence. The first is the better ability to measure quality of life, which has resulted in a realization by surgeons that the incidence of postherniorrhaphy sequelae such as chronic groin pain occurs more frequently than one might have anticipated. Just how "successful" is a hernia repair that is not associated with a recurrence, yet the patient sustains a chronic postoperative syndrome which alters lifestyle? The second factor decreasing the importance of the recurrence rate is the development of the newer tension-free approaches that have brought the recurrence rate down to an essentially irreducible number (i.e., less than 1%) in experienced hands. Nevertheless, hernia recurrences will continue to be seen because a recurrence rate of 1% still translates into a relatively large number because of the size of the denominator. In addition, experienced surgeons do not perform all herniorrhaphies, and therefore technical misadventures may result in a higher recurrence rate in some groups of patients.

A recurrent hernia usually presents as a bulge with a cough impulse. Occasionally pain only brings the possibility of recurrence to the doctor's attention. In this situation, a consistent definition of a recurrent hernia does not exist because of the difficulty in differentiating a lipoma of the cord, seroma, or an expansile bulge of the internal oblique muscle from a true hernia recurrence. For the purposes of reporting results, the authors do not believe that a hernia should be classified as recurrent unless there is a visible bulge or

there is unequivocal evidence of a hernia by an imaging modality such as ultrasound, CT scan, or MRI.

The general principle for managing recurrent hernias depends on the original repair. The logical approach is to perform the herniorrhaphy in the space that has not been dissected. If the patient had a previous open repair, then a preperitoneal repair is best. On the other hand, if the index operation was a preperitoneal one, then a repair which is performed in the open inguinal space is best.

Chronic Groin Pain

Various groin pain syndromes may develop, usually from scar tissue, reaction to prosthetic material, or involvement of a nerve in staples or suture material during repair of the hernia. Chronic postherniorrhaphy groin pain, which is defined as pain lasting more than 3 months, occurs with greater frequency than was previously thought. The incidence in recent studies ranges form 0 to 53%. A critical review of studies published between the years 1987 and 2000 suggested the overall incidence to be about 25%, with 10% fitting a definition of moderate or severe[65] (Table 36-10). There are predictors of the development of a postoperative groin pain syndrome (Table 36-11). However, it occurs without regard to the type of repair performed, and is difficult to categorize because patients' descriptions of their pain are so heterogeneous. The difficulty is magnified several fold if workman's compensation issues are involved. Nevertheless, an attempt should be made to assign patients to one of two types: (1) nociceptive pain that is caused by tissue damage and is further subdivided into somatic and visceral, and (2) neuropathic, which means direct nerve damage. Somatic pain is the most common and is usually caused by damage to ligaments, tendons, and muscles. Osteitis pubis and a new syndrome which includes various tendinitides involving the adductor mechanism of the hip called adductor tenoperiostitis (ATP) (formerly grouped under the heading of adductor strain) are part of this group. Visceral pain refers to that which is related to a specific visceral function such as urination or ejaculation (see dysejaculation syndrome section below). The principles for assessing and treating patients with nociceptive pain are similar to those used for patients who present with groin pain but do not have an obvious hernia. This is discussed further below.

Neuropathic groin pain is caused by damage to a nerve in the groin region and may be due to partial or complete division, stretching, contusion, crushing, suturing, or electrocautery. The nerves that are usually involved are the ilioinguinal nerve, iliohypogastric nerve, both the genital and femoral branches of the genitofemoral nerve, and the lateral femoral cutaneous nerve of the thigh. The first two are especially prone to injury during an open herniorrhaphy, while the latter are more likely damaged during laparoscopy. The genital and femoral branches of the genitofemoral nerve and the lateral

Table 36-9

Complications of Groin Hernia Repairs

Recurrence
Chronic groin pain
  Nociceptive
    Somatic
    Visceral
  Neuropathic
    Iliohypogastric
    Ilioinguinal
    Genitofemoral
    Lateral cutaneous
    Femoral
Cord and testicular
  Hematoma
  Ischemic orchitis
  Testicular atrophy
  Dysejaculation
  Division of vas deferens
  Hydrocele
  Testicular descent
Bladder injury
Wound infection
Seroma
Hematoma
  Wound
  Scrotal
  Retroperitoneal
Osteitis pubis
Prosthetic complications
  Contraction
  Erosion
  Infection
  Rejection
  Fracture
Laparoscopic
  Vascular injury
    Intra-abdominal
    Retroperitoneal
    Abdominal wall
    Gas embolism
  Visceral injury
    Bowel perforation
    Bladder perforation
  Trocar site complications
    Hematoma
    Hernia
    Wound infection
    Keloid
  Bowel Obstruction
    Trocar or peritoneal closure site hernia
    Adhesions
  Miscellaneous
    Diaphragmatic dysfunction
    Hypercapnia
General
  Urinary
  Paralytic ileus
  Nausea and vomiting
  Aspiration pneumonia
  Cardiovascular and respiratory insufficiency

Table 36-10

Classification of Chronic Postherniorrhaphy Groin Pain and Pain Descriptors

Mild pain
  Occasional pain or discomfort
  Does not limit activity
  Return to prehernia lifestyle
Moderate pain
  Prevents return to normal preoperative activities, such as sports
    and lifting
Severe pain
  Incapacitating
  Interferes with activities of daily living

Postherniorrhaphy groin pain descriptors
  Stinging
  Throbbing
  Burning
  Tender
  Stabbing
  Numbness
  Cleaving
  Dull
  Dull aching
  Pounding
  Tiring
  Sickening
  Punishing
  Shooting
  Pricking
  Constricting
  Tearing
  Sharp
  Pulling
  Drilling
  Tingling
  Pins and needles
  Radiating
  Irritating
  Frightful

is extremely rare and is almost always the result of a gross technical misadventure. Its rarity is fortunate because of the severe associated morbidity.

The classic presentation is with pain and/or paresthesia in the distribution of one of the major nerves. The most common patient

Table 36-11

Factors Predicting the Development of a Chronic Postherniorrhaphy Groin Pain Syndrome

Definite
  Recurrent hernia
  Preoperative pain
  Absence of a visible bulge
  Young age
  High early pain scores
  Numbness
  Delayed onset
  More than 4 weeks to return to work
  Workman's compensation involved
Probable
  Preoperative psychological state
  Chronic pain after other surgeries
Not predictive
  Surgical technique
  Gender
  Hernia anatomy
  Postoperative morbidity

cutaneous nerve of the thigh are most at risk when the surgeon staples below the iliopubic tract when lateral to the internal spermatic vessels. A burning, tingling pain along the lateral aspect of the thigh in the distribution of the lateral femoral cutaneous nerve is known as *meralgia paresthetica,* and is due to entrapment of that nerve; the affected skin area may be hyperesthetic and/or pruritic, and patients may complain of the tactile hallucination of a sensation of small insects creeping under the skin (formication). A femoral nerve injury descriptors of the pain are tearing, throbbing, stabbing, shooting, numbness, dullness, pulling, and tugging. The patients are difficult to assess because the overlap and interdigitation of the nerves as well as the variability of the pain descriptors make precise identification of the involved nerve confounding. The onset is often delayed and pain is aggravated by ambulation, stooping, hyperextension of hip, and sexual intercourse. It is commonly relieved by a recumbent position and/or flexion of the hip and thigh. Reassurance and conservative treatment with anti-inflammatory medications and local nerve blocks are preferred initially, as commonly the symptoms will resolve spontaneously. The only exception might be the patient who complains of severe pain immediately (i.e., in the recovery room) after the procedure. This patient may be best treated by immediate re-exploration before scar tissue develops. Otherwise, the authors scrupulously avoid surgery before 1 year to allow the possibility of spontaneous resolution. When groin exploration is required, neurectomy and neuroma excision are performed. The results are often less than satisfying.

Cord and Testicles

Bleeding can occur, producing a scrotal hematoma. This is usually the result of delayed bleeding from the cremasteric, internal spermatic, or branches of the inferior epigastric vessels. Although this complication can be quite disabling, conservative treatment with reassurance is the best course of action. Evacuation is rarely required. Ischemic orchitis is defined as postoperative inflammation of the testicle occurring within 1 to 5 days after surgery. It occurs in about 1% of primary hernioplasties, but is much more common with operations performed for recurrent hernias.[66] The patient develops enlargement of the testicle that can be excruciatingly painful. A low-grade fever is common and examination discloses an enlarged, hard mass associated with the testicle. The etiology of this complication is not completely understood, but most authorities feel it is caused by thrombosis of the veins draining the testicle secondary to extensive dissection of the spermatic cord. Management consists of supportive care only, with scrotal support and anti-inflammatory agents, as the condition is usually self limiting. Antibiotics and steroids have been used but their value is unproven. Significant short-term complications such as abscess formation are extremely rare. Surgical decompression by opening the external inguinal ring or actually incising the capsule of the testicle is of historic interest only.

The feared long-term complication of ischemic orchitis is testicular atrophy. This occurrence, however, is quite unpredictable, as most patients who develop this complication do not have a history of testicular problems associated with the index herniorrhaphy. Likewise, most patients who develop ischemic orchitis after a herniorrhaphy, or any other testicular complication for that matter, go on to recover without testicular atrophy. The possibility of developing testicular atrophy increases dramatically with the need to repair a recurrent hernia, and is progressive with each successive re-repair of a recurrence. It is generally accepted that testicular complications can be decreased by division of large inguinal-scrotal sacs rather than excision leaving the distal sac open in situ.[67]

The dysejaculation syndrome is defined as a burning, searing, painful sensation occurring just before, during, and/or after ejaculation. It is probably caused by a stenotic lesion in the vas deferens. The condition is commonly self-limiting so the initial treatment is expectant. Infertility after bilateral inguinal herniorrhaphy is a rare

but potentially devastating complication. It has been observed with both tension-free and nonprosthetic repairs. It has been suggested that it may occur more frequently in the future because of the routine use of mesh prostheses in hernia repair, and therefore demands vigilance on the part of surgeons and such cases should be reported. It should be emphasized that this is speculation without supporting clinical data. Therefore at the present time the authors do not believe that informed consent concerning infertility should be any different between mesh and nonmesh repairs. Should the vas deferens actually be transected during herniorrhaphy, reanastomosis should be attempted if fertility is an issue.

Hydroceles occasionally develop after inguinal herniorrhaphy, but the cause is not known and therefore taking preventive measures is not possible. The urologic literature suggests that the practice of leaving an indirect inguinal sac in situ rather than removing it should be incriminated, but this is not accepted by most experienced hernia surgeons. The treatment is the same as for any other hydrocele. Testicular descent is a complication believed to be related to complete division of the cremaster muscle, but the occurrence is variable. The cord structures lose their tethering effect, allowing the testicle to descend into the most dependent portion of the scrotum. Due to the elasticity of the scrotum, time and gravity cause it to elongate, prompting complaints from patients. Few hernia surgeons now routinely completely divide the cremaster muscle, so it is hoped that this will become a rare phenomenon. At the Shouldice Clinic, where routine division of the cremaster muscle is practiced, the medial cremasteric stump is anchored with suture near the pubic tubercle to prevent this complication.

Bladder Injury

Bladder injury is unusual when the herniorrhaphy is performed in the open anterior space. The exception might be a sliding hernia which contains the bladder. The bladder is at much greater risk with a preperitoneal operation whether open or laparoscopic. It is most commonly seen in patients with previous surgery in the space of Retzius. Previous surgery in this space (i.e., a prostate operation) should be considered a relative contraindication to preperitoneal hernia repair. Bladder injuries are best treated by two-layer repair with absorbable suture, followed by extended indwelling Foley catheter drainage until a cystogram confirms bladder integrity (i.e., 10 to 14 days).

Wound Infection

The groin appears to be a protected area, as wound infection after inguinal herniorrhaphy occurs in less than 5% of patients.[68] It is not clear why the rate is so much lower than for other abdominal wall hernia repairs such as an incisional. However, a word of caution is in order as the infection rate may be underestimated due to late presentation. For example, in a study from the United Kingdom, the median interval between repair and presentation was 4 months (range, 2 weeks to 39 months).[69] Nevertheless, the low rate of infection calls into question the need for prophylactic antibiotics, a practice much more common in North America than the rest of the world. A recent meta-analysis conducted by the Cochrane group showed no evidence that prophylactic administration of antibiotics for elective inguinal hernia repair reduced infection rates. Infection with a nonprosthetic repair is treated as any other wound infection, with open drainage and dressing changes, with or without oral or intravenous antibiotics depending on signs of extensive local cellulitis or systemic sepsis. The initial approach is the same for a prosthetic repair. However, prosthesis removal is also commonly required. In general, ePTFE prostheses almost always have to be removed, but mesh prostheses can occasionally be salvaged with conservative treatment. The late recurrence rate is much higher after a postoperative wound infection.

Seroma

This localized accumulation of serum is common with the use of synthetic mesh in hernia repairs, and is probably a physiologic reaction to the foreign body. Indeed, some surgeons routinely place suction drains for a few days after extensive prosthetic repair such as the GPRVS, although this is controversial. The practice of actively treating seromas with repeated aspirations should be discouraged, as it has been found that this is not necessary and that the fluid eventually resorbs. The concern about repeated aspiration is bacterial contamination of the prosthesis; therefore aspiration is performed for symptomatic relief only. Fluid collections in the scrotum also are common, especially when a large inguinoscrotal sac is completely mobilized. These too will usually resolve spontaneously.

Hematoma

Wound hematomas are common after inguinal herniorrhaphy, but usually are self-limiting. If large, the patient should be returned to the operating room for evacuation and control of the offending vessel. Scrotal hematomas are discussed above (see cord and testicular complications). A retroperitoneal hematoma associated with the herniorrhaphy itself and not related to a laparoscopic accident is caused by injury to the rich plexus of veins or the corona mortis in the vicinity of Cooper's ligament. Injuries to the deep circumflex artery or branches of the external iliac vessels may also be the cause. The retroperitoneal space is quite expansile, so these can be associated with significant blood loss. Expectant treatment is recommended even when severe because of the morbidity associated with a retroperitoneal dissection. A paralytic ileus may develop. Urgent arteriography is mandatory with formal vascular repair if injury to a major vessel such as the external iliac or femoral artery is suspected because of symptoms suggesting leg ischemia.

Osteitis Pubis

For hernia surgeons, the term *osteitis pubis* has become synonymous with pain caused by the placement of staples or sutures through the periosteum of the pubis. In fact, this painful inflammatory condition of the symphysis pubis and surrounding muscle fascia was first described in athletes, and continues to be a source of considerable disability, most often caused by repeated traumatic or exertional stresses on the fascia and joint.[70] Since it has also been described in sedentary patients and pregnancy, it is important to rule this out as being the cause of the preoperative groin symptoms. Plain roentgenograms, bone scans, and MRI have a role in the diagnosis. Regardless of the cause, the initial treatment is conservative, including anti-inflammatory medication and local therapeutic modalities such as cryomassage, heat, ultrasound, or electric stimulation. Physical therapy involving strengthening the abdominal and hip muscles and improving range of motion of the hip, particularly of the muscles of internal rotation, also may be helpful. Corticosteroid injection is commonly employed, but the value has not been conclusively proven. Surgical exploration with an attempt to find and remove an offending suture or staple should be the last resort. When surgery is being considered, it is wise to involve a consultant with expertise in wedge resection of the symphysis, curettage, or arthrodesis should nothing be found, as these have been used with variable success.

Prosthetic Complications

A detailed discussion of prosthetic complications is not necessary here because most of the information has already been included in the sections on prosthetic materials, wound infection, and cord and testicular complications. Shrinkage of polypropylene as well other meshes should be considered by surgeons when performing prosthetic repairs. Sufficient overlap anticipating a 20% contracture is accepted by most.[71] The decrease in size is felt to be due to scarification of the recipient's tissue, which causes the mesh to contract as scar tissue develops. Intestinal obstruction or fistulization is possible by erosion, especially if there is physical contact between intestine and the prosthesis. Intra-abdominal placement of a mesh prosthesis should be avoided in favor of ePTFE or perhaps a biologic prosthesis whenever possible. Local erosion into the cord structures has also been reported. Rejection because of an allergic response is possible, but extremely rare. What patients term "rejection" in their histories usually is the result of infection.

Laparoscopic Complications

Vascular Injury

Injury to vessels residing in the retroperitoneum is the most feared complication, as the associated mortality rate is significant. These usually occur during initial access to the abdomen or preperitoneal space in the case of a TEP repair. A Veress needle injury is most common, but is less serious and may be self-limiting. On the other hand, a trocar injury usually is associated with major disruption of the involved vessel, resulting in immediate life-threatening hemorrhage. Vessel injuries due to trocar injury are usually transmural due to the relatively large size of the trocar point. When recognized, the trocar and cannula should be left in place to tamponade the vessel and a formal vascular repair through an open laparotomy undertaken. Mortality due to retroperitoneal injury secondary to trocar insertion ranges from 9 to 36%, even with rapid identification and attempted repair. There is no place for laparoscopic management of a suspected major vascular injury. Immediate laparotomy is essential with tamponade of the injury until appropriate instrumentation and personnel are assembled. Proper vascular isolation and repair can then be accomplished, avoiding potential mortality. Mesenteric and omental vessel injuries can also be dangerous and should be treated the same as a retroperitoneal injury. However, if hemorrhage is not brisk and the patient is stable, these may be controlled laparoscopically.

Injuries to vessels of the abdominal wall also occur, but are less serious. The inferior epigastric vessels are at greatest risk, especially when performing a TAPP procedure. They can be avoided by careful secondary trocar placement under direct vision. The best method for control is to use one of the disposable or reusable trocar site fascial closure devices to suture-ligate the bleeding vessel. The use of full-thickness abdominal sutures or a Foley catheter for balloon tamponade is of historic interest only.

Although not strictly a vascular complication, gas embolism occurs with intravascular insufflation. It is an uncommon complication, apparently unique to the Veress needle technique, with an incidence of 0.003%. The decline in the incidence of gas embolism over the last 40 years is largely due to advances in electrocautery and laser systems (i.e., avoiding gas cooling), and better regulation of the pneumoperitoneal pressure by sensor control. Careful attention to tests confirming proper peritoneal placement will continue to keep this complication at a low incidence.

Visceral Injury

Visceral injury is rare with laparoscopic herniorrhaphy compared to general laparoscopy because surgeons tend to use an open operation in a high-risk patient (e.g., anticipated significant abdominal adhesions). Bowel injury is the most significant because it often goes unnoticed at the time of insult. The mortality rate is high when these patients present with peritonitis and sepsis several days after surgery.

If it is suspected that the Veress needle has been placed in the bowel because bile is aspirated, the needle should be left in place and another placement made with a second needle. After the second trocar has been carefully placed, the location of the tip of the first needle should be identified and the injury assessed. Leaving the first needle in place facilitates the identification of the damaged site for repair. If the bowel is damaged by the initial trocar, transmural injury is probable. Due to its size, the trocar point often causes lateral tear injuries requiring formal repair. If the skill of the laparoscopist is sufficient, the injury may be repaired laparoscopically. More commonly the tear requires either a minilaparotomy or full laparotomy.

Bladder injury with peritoneal access is rare but possible. It usually is the result of a distended bladder. Less commonly, it is associated with congenital bladder abnormalities. Again, the most common offender is the Veress needle, followed by the initial trocar. When bladder injury occurs, it is usually obvious. Urine is withdrawn into the syringe or blood and gas distend the drainage bag if the patient is catheterized. If the Veress needle is the offending instrument, the needle is left in place and a second attempt at access with a sterile needle can be made after decompression of the bladder. If minor injury is confirmed, it is treated conservatively with a postoperative indwelling catheter. When the injury is caused by a trocar, formal two-layer bladder repair with absorbable suture is recommended. Rarer still is the disruption of a patent urachus. When the bladder is fully decompressed, the patent urachus is devoid of urine. Thus, this complication usually presents late, with a urine leak through the umbilical incision. It may also be manifest by generalized peritonitis.

Routine preoperative catheterization of all patients undergoing laparoscopic herniorrhaphy is controversial. Emptying the urinary bladder by preoperative catheterization has the advantages of enlarging the working space and reducing the risk of bladder injury. However, the overall incidence of bladder injury is rare, and studies have demonstrated a higher incidence of urinary tract complications in patients with routine catheterization.[72] In addition, preoperative catheterization with removal of the catheter at the end of operation has not been found to reduce the incidence of urinary retention.[73] Many surgeons choose to avoid routine catheterization in favor of immediate voiding before entering the operating theater, except in unusual circumstances such as a history of bladder outlet obstruction or prostatism.

Trocar Site Complications

Hematoma formation is relatively uncommon and is caused by disruption of small nutrient vessels of the abdominal wall muscle or the preperitoneal fatty tissue. Careless introduction of secondary trocars can result in hematoma if the inferior epigastric vessels are lacerated. Umbilical trocar site hernias occur about 1% of the time after laparoscopic herniorrhaphy, and the incidence is about

the same for secondary trocar sites, varying in relation to the size of the cannula.[74] It is hoped that this complication will lessen now that most surgeons routinely close any trocar defect larger than 5 mm. There are now numerous disposable and reusable devices that facilitate trocar site closure available to surgeons. The incidence of umbilical wound infection is reported to be about 2%, which is no different than that seen in general laparoscopy, so infection is equally likely whether the open or closed technique is used. Unsightly scars at cannula insertion sites can develop, especially in patients who form keloids, and are not unique to herniorrhaphy. Particularly distressing for patients are prominent scars that occur at sites where towel clips were used for abdominal wall elevation, as they tend to be very noticeable. Towel clips should not be used for elevation of the skin in patients with a history of keloid scar formation.

Bowel Obstruction

This complication is almost unheard of with an open groin herniorrhaphy and its association with the laparoscopic approach is perhaps the most significant argument against the procedure made by opponents of the TAPP approach. Indeed, the major advantage of the TEP procedure is the theoretical avoidance of this problem. The complication was frequent in the developmental stages of the laparoscopic procedure because inadequate peritoneal closure over the prosthesis allowed bowel to migrate into the preperitoneal space, resulting in obstruction. Bowel obstruction related to trocar site hernia is discussed above in the section on trocar site hernias. The incidence of bowel obstruction has greatly diminished because of better technique. The frequency of delayed bowel obstruction related to adhesions because of the intra-abdominal nature of the procedure has yet to be determined, but would appear to be extremely low, as very few reports have appeared.

Miscellaneous Complications

Diaphragmatic dysfunction has been reported with other laparoscopic procedures as well as herniorrhaphy. It manifests as phrenic nerve palsy and is usually transient, but has been known to require a short period of mechanical ventilation. Stretching because of the pneumoperitoneum probably causes it. Hypercapnia is the result of inadequate compensatory ventilation, given the fact that the vast majority of laparoscopies are performed using carbon dioxide as the insufflating agent.

General Complications

One of the most common complications of elective herniorrhaphy is urinary retention. It has important socioeconomic implications because it often results in an unscheduled admission. Contributing factors include choice of anesthetic agent, postoperative pain, use of opiates for analgesia, pre-existing bladder outlet obstruction, and intraoperative overhydration leading to bladder distension. The highest incidence is with general anesthesia, followed by regional and local.[75] In addition, there appears to be a subgroup of healthy, young, muscular men who are also affected.[76] Treatment is repeated bladder catheterizations until normal voiding resumes. Some surgeons prefer an indwelling Foley catheter to allow for early discharge of the patient. The catheter is then removed later in the outpatient area. Urologic consultation should be reserved for persistent cases and is not needed initially.

Paralytic ileus can be seen with either the open or the laparoscopic procedure, but is more common with the latter. The occurrence of this complication is unpredictable, just as its etiology is unclear. Treatment is symptomatic with spontaneous resolution the rule. Nasogastric decompression is occasionally needed. Nausea and vomiting can be seen with patients who are unusually sensitive to pain medications. The complication is frequent with laparoscopy, as nausea and vomiting is a known side effect in a fixed percentage of patients undergoing laparoscopy for any reason. Again, the treatment is symptomatic with appropriate adjustment of pain medications.

Aspiration pneumonia and cardiorespiratory complications occur at about the same rate as for any other operative procedure. Prevention by careful preoperative assessment looking for underlying medical illness is the best approach. The complication may be lessened by local anesthesia, but this view is not universally shared by anesthesiologists, as some favor a completely anesthetized patient with a controlled airway as opposed to a partially sedated patient breathing on his or her own. Local anesthesia is commonly employed in specialty hernia centers, but its use in general practice is less common.

GROIN HERNIAS IN WOMEN

Groin hernias are much less common in women than in men. Less than 10% of all elective inguinal hernia repairs are performed in women.[77] Nevertheless, given the overall frequency of the condition, the absolute number is still significant. Femoral hernias are ten times more common in women than in men (10% in women versus 1% in men), giving rise to the false notion that it is the most common groin hernia; in fact, indirect hernias are much more common. Direct hernias are rare, almost to the point of being reportable. Occult inguinal hernias are a significant problem in women because the skin of the labium majus does not allow easy examination of the inguinal canal. There is insufficient skin redundancy to invert and allow the examining finger to directly palpate the inguinal floor. The extensive differential diagnosis of groin pain (see Table 36-4) makes the definitive diagnosis of an occult hernia difficult.

The indications for surgery are similar in men and women. There is no place for a strategy of watchful waiting for femoral hernias, as the incidence of incarceration and/or strangulation is far too high to justify such a recommendation. The choice of procedure is largely left to the surgeon based on experience and training. Resection of the round ligament simplifies many of the repairs because complete closure of the internal ring is then possible. Groin hernias become evident during pregnancy in 1 in 1000 to 3000 pregnancies. These are best managed expectantly and repaired after gestation is complete.

GROIN PAIN IN PATIENTS WITHOUT AN OBVIOUS HERNIA (SPORTSMAN'S HERNIA)

There are a variety of conditions that cause groin pain in the absence of an obvious inguinal hernia. These have significant economic consequences in professional athletes, thus the name "sportsman's hernia." Hockey, soccer, and American-style football players are particularly prone to this injury, but it also occurs in nonathletes. Athletic pubalgia and groin disruption are other names commonly used to describe this condition. The literature dealing with this subject can be confusing because some authors include the entire spectrum of groin pain etiologies under the heading of sportsman's hernia, while others restrict use of the term to the subset of patients who have an

Table 36-12
Conditions Associated with Chronic Groin Pain

Occult hernia (herniography only)
Muscle injury
Adductor strains
Tendon injury
Iliopsoas bursitis
Osteitis pubis
Pelvic stress fractures
Snapping hip syndrome
Lumbosacral disorders
Connective tissue disease
Nerve entrapment
Hip disorders
    Synovitis
    Avascular necrosis
    Osteoarthritis
    Legg-Calvé-Perthes disease
    Slipped femoral capital epiphysis
    Osteochondritis dissecans or avascular necrosis of the femoral head
    Acetabular labral tears
Prostatitis
Epididymitis
Nephrolithiasis
Urinary tract infection
Lymphadenitis
Intra-abdominal pathology
History of a previous herniorrhaphy

occult hernia detected either by an imaging modality or found at diagnostic surgical exploration.

Most patients give a history of gradual onset of pain over a 1 to 6 month period. Only about 10% have sudden-onset pain related to a specific incident. The differential diagnosis of this condition is extensive, making a correct diagnosis difficult (Table 36-12). Physical examination is occasionally helpful, especially when the pain is localized to a specific anatomic structure such as the pubic tubercle or an adductor tendon. More commonly, the pain is vague and the examination severely compromised by the tenderness, which makes adequate palpation difficult. CT, ultrasonography, herniography, laparoscopy, and MRI all have their place in the evaluation of these patients. MRI has emerged as the most beneficial study because of its ability to differentiate between muscle tear, osteitis pubis, bursitis, and stress fracture. The incidence of the various causes of groin pain varies widely from series to series. For example, in some series, an occult hernia was the most common cause of pain, while in others it was rarely reported as a source of pain. Overall, strain of the adductor muscle complex (the adductor longus, brevis, and magnus, and gracilis muscles) is the most common.

In the absence of a specifically correctable surgical lesion, conservative management consisting of rest, anti-inflammatory agents, ice, and specific stretching and strengthening exercises is used first. Other conservative measures such as pulsed radiofrequency, cryotherapy, and even acupuncture have been reported with varying degrees of success. Patients who fail conservative management will commonly come to surgery. Tenotomy of an adductor tendon is highly successful in the properly selected patient. Groin exploration is most rewarding when a specifically correctable lesion such as a torn external oblique aponeurosis with or without ilioinguinal nerve entrapment is found. More commonly, a nonspecific deficiency of the posterior wall of the inguinal canal that includes an occult hernia is found, and a variety of modified Bassini-type inguinal floor reconstructions have been proposed. Laparoscopic and prosthetic repairs have also been used. A consistent staging system to describe the pathology is lacking, and there is no consensus concerning the best procedure for patients with this difficult-to-treat condition. Given the level of discomfort endured by some of these patients, as well as the fact that many are high-profile athletes, there is significant potential for hucksterism in the treatment of this condition.[78,79]

PEDIATRIC HERNIAS

Most inguinal hernias in children are indirect, related to a persistent patent processus vaginalis. Approximately 1 to 5% of children are born with or develop an inguinal hernia. However, the incidence rises in preterm infants and those with low birth weights (13% of babies born before 32 weeks and 30% of babies with a birth weight less than 1000 g).[80] Overall, right-sided hernias are twice as common as left-sided hernias, and about 10% of hernias diagnosed at birth are bilateral, but this varies greatly on the basis of numerous risk factors, the most important of which is age. The right-sided predominance is felt by most authorities to be related to the later descent of the right testicle during gestation.[81,82] There are several conditions which predispose a child to develop an inguinal hernia. (Table 36-13)

Infants or children may present with a mass in the groin or scrotum. The diagnosis may seem obvious, but one must be careful to differentiate the mass from other cord and testicular abnormalities such as a hydrocele, undescended testicle, varicocele, or even a testicular tumor. Commonly, no hernia is able to be demonstrated when the patient presents to the surgeon. Some surgeons rely on the so-called "silk glove sign," which reflects the way the hernia sac feels as it is palpated over the cord structures. The finding is controversial and there is some evidence that what is actually being felt is a hypertrophied cremaster muscle.[83] Overall, the diagnosis commonly hinges on the observation of the referring physician or a parent. Most surgeons feel that the risk:benefit ratio favors this as an acceptable indication for operation when the source seems reliable, rather than taking the chance of incurring a strangulation.

Incarceration is a more serious problem in the pediatric patient than the adult, with large series reporting rates of up to 20%. The patient presents with a hard, tender groin mass. Seventy-five to eighty percent of these can be successfully reduced, so the initial treatment consists of sedation, Trendelenburg position, ice packs, and gentle taxis. A reasonable attempt at conservative management of an incarcerated pediatric hernia before proceeding to emergency surgery is

Table 36-13
Conditions Associated with an Increased Incidence of Pediatric Hernia

Family history
Undescended testis
Hypospadias/epispadias
Ventriculoperitoneal shunt
Peritoneal dialysis
Cryptorchism
Prematurity
Other abdominal wall defect
Cystic fibrosis
Ascites
Intersex conditionsp
Connective tissue disorders
Hunter-Hurler syndrome
Ehlers-Danlos syndrome

in the patient's best interest, because the complication rate compared to elective herniorrhaphy is increased 20-fold, including irreversible abnormalities such as testicular infarction or atrophy. If no progress is made within 6 hours, or the patient exhibits signs of peritonitis or systemic toxicity, immediate operation is appropriate.

Most pediatric inguinal hernias are repaired using the principle of high ligation of the sac. The external oblique aponeurosis is opened for a short distance beginning at the external ring and proceeding laterally. The sac is then gently dissected away from the cord structures proximally until the internal ring is reached, then the sac is twisted, suture ligated, and amputated. If the sac extends into the scrotum, it can be divided, leaving the distal sac in situ. Care must be taken to exclude abdominal contents such as the tube and ovary before the suture ligation. Occasionally a Marcy repair of the internal ring is added if the structure is unusually large.

Exploration of the opposite groin remains controversial. As an alternative, ultrasound examination has become popular at some centers, but is largely dependent on the expertise of the ultrasonographer.[84,85] The size of the internal ring and the presence of bowel or fluid in the spermatic cord are diagnostic criteria indicative of a positive exam. Another alternative is laparoscopy using either a rigid or a flexible endoscope through the contralateral hernia sac. The accuracy is high for properly trained laparoscopists, such that it is considered the gold standard in studies using both ultrasonography and laparoscopy. The disadvantage of laparoscopy is high cost and potential intra-abdominal complications.[86,87,88]

SPECIAL SITUATIONS

Ascites

An inguinal hernia in a patient with ascites should be approached differently. Malnutrition, coagulopathy, increased abdominal pressure, and the risk of an ascitic leak make treatment more dangerous. Incarceration and strangulation are rare in patients with ascites, possibly because of a protective effect provided by the widening of the hernia orifice secondary to pressure from the fluid.[89] Erosion of the skin is also rare in the groin, especially when compared to umbilical hernias in the same population. For these reasons, elective repair is not recommended for these patients. Operation should be reserved for only the most symptomatic, and then only after vigorous attempts to control the ascites have been made. A femoral hernia represents an exception to this rule, as the incidence of incarceration is higher than in other groin hernias.

Named Inguinal Hernia Syndromes

Eponyms are commonly related to the specific organs that are involved with the hernia, especially if there is a facet of the treatment of that organ that is controversial. For example, in 1735, Claudius Amyand removed the appendix of an 11-year-old boy through a groin incision. The anatomically correct name for this condition is an appendicocele. Nevertheless, the presence of an appendix in a hernia sac is commonly referred to as Amyand's hernia. An Amyand's hernia involving a noninflamed appendix raises controversy regarding removal versus reduction of the appendix. Similarly, a Littré's hernia is a femoral hernia with a Meckel's diverticulum. A list of named groin hernia syndromes is provided in Table 36-14.

Table 36-14
Named Groin Hernia Syndromes

Hernia Name	Definition
Appendicocele	The vermiform appendix in a hernial sac
Béclard	A hernia through the opening for the saphenous vein
Bilocular femoral	A femoral hernia with two sacs, the first being in the femoral canal, and the second passing through a defect in the superficial fascia and appearing immediately beneath the skin
Cecal	A hernia containing cecum
Complete	An indirect inguinal hernia in which the contents extend into the tunica vaginalis
Cloquet	A femoral hernia perforating the aponeurosis of the pectineus and insinuating itself between this aponeurosis and the muscle, lying therefore behind the femoral vessels
Cooper	Synonym for bilocular femoral hernia
Cremnocele	A protrusion of intestine into the labium majus
External femoral	A hernia that passes beneath the inguinal ligament and the iliopubic tract but lateral to the femoral vessels
Extrasaccular	Synonym for sliding inguinal hernia
Hernia en bissac	A complicated hernia having a double sac, one part in the inguinal canal, the other projecting from the internal inguinal ring in the subperitoneal tissues; synonym for properitoneal inguinal hernia
Hey	Synonym for bilocular femoral hernia
Hesselbach's	Synonym for external femoral hernia
Inguinoscrotal	An inguinal hernia descending into the scrotum
Intrailiac	An interstitial hernia projecting from the internal inguinal ring
Krönlein	Synonym for hernia en bissac or properitoneal inguinal hernia
Labial	Hernia through the canal of Nuck (female)
Lacunar ligament	Synonym for Laugier hernia
Laugier	Hernia passing through an opening in the lacunar ligament
Littré	A hernia containing a Meckel's diverticulum
Malgaigne	Infantile inguinal hernia prior to the descent of the testis
Obturator	Hernia through the obturator foramen
Paraperitoneal	A vesical herniation in which only a part of the protruded organ is covered by the peritoneum of the sac
Parasaccular	Synonym for sliding inguinal hernia
Pectineal	Synonym for Cloquet hernia
Prevascular	A femoral hernia in which the intestine is in front of the blood vessels
Properitoneal inguinal	Synonym for hernia en bissac
Retropubic	Projecting downward, in the subperitoneal tissues, from the internal inguinal ring
Serafini's	The hernia sac passes behind the femoral vessels inside the sheath of the femoral vein
Velpeau	Synonym for prevascular; the term has also been used as a synonym for a Laugier hernia
Vesicle	Protrusion of a segment of the bladder through the abdominal wall or into the inguinal canal and into the scrotum

References

1. Cooper A: *The Anatomy and Surgical Treatment of Abdominal Hernia.* Philadelphia: Lee and Blanchard, 1804, p 26.
2. Rutkow IM: Epidemiologic, economic, and sociologic aspects of hernia surgery in the United States in the 1990s. *Surg Clin North Am* 78:941, 1998.
3. McIntosh A, Hutchinson A, Roberts A, et al: Evidence-based management of groin hernia in primary care—a systematic review. *Fam Pract* 17:5, 442.
4. Kitchen WH, Doyle LW, Ford GW: Inguinal hernia in very low birth-weight children: a continuing risk to age 8 years. *J Paediatr Child Health* 27:300, 1991.
5. Abramson JH, Gofin J, Hopp C, et al: The epidemiology of inguinal hernia. A survey in western Jerusalem. *J Epidemiol Community Health* 32:59, 1978.
6. Akin ML, Karakaya M, Batkin A, et al: Prevalence of inguinal hernia in otherwise healthy males of 20 to 22 years of age. *J R Army Med Corps* 143:101, 1997.
7. Rai S, Chandra SS, Smile SR: A study of the risk of strangulation and obstruction in groin hernias. *Aust N Z J Surg* 68:650, 1998.
8. Report of a working party convened by the Royal College of Surgeons of England: Clinical guidelines on the management of groin hernia in adults. London: Royal College of Surgeons of England, 1993.
9. Hair A, Paterson C, Wright D, et al: What effect does the duration of an inguinal hernia have on patient symptoms? *J Am Coll Surg* 193:125, 2001.
10. Neuhauser D: Elective inguinal herniorrhaphy versus truss in the elderly, in Bunker JP, Barnes BA, Mosteller F (eds): *Costs Risks, and Benefits of Surgery.* New York: Oxford University Press, 1977, p 223.
11. Kaiwa Y, Namiki K, Matsumoto H: Laparoscopic relief of reduction en masse of incarcerated inguinal hernia. *Surg Endosc* 17:352, 2003.
12. Wirtschafter ZT, Bentley JP: Hernias as a collagen maturation defect. *Ann Surg* 160:852, 1964.
13. Cannon DJ, Read RC: Metastatic emphysema: A mechanism for acquiring inguinal herniation. *Ann Surg* 194:270, 1981.
14. Uden A, Lindhagen T: Inguinal hernia in patients with congenital dislocation of the hip. A sign of general connective tissue disorder. *Acta Orthop Scand* 59:667, 1988.
15. Smith GD, Crosby DL, Lewis PA: Inguinal hernia and a single strenuous event. *Ann R Coll Surg Engl;* 78:367, 1996.
16. Russell RH: The saccular theory of hernia and the radical operation. *Lancet* 3:1197, 1906.
17. Hughson W: The persistent or performed sac in relation to oblique inguinal hernia. *Surg Gynecol Obstet* 41:610, 1925.
18. Condon RE: The anatomy of the inguinal region and its relation to the groin hernia, in Nyhus LM, Condon RE (eds): *Hernia,* 3rd ed. Philadelphia: JP Lippincott, 1989, p 18.
19. Arnbjornsson E: Development of right inguinal hernia after appendectomy. *Am J Surg* 143:174, 1982.
20. Lilly MC, Arregui ME: Lipomas of the cord and round ligament. *Ann Surg* 235:586, 2002.
21. Bendavid R: Femoral pseudo-hernias. *Hernia* 6:141, 2002.

22. Stoppa RE: The midline preperitoneal approach and prosthetic repair of groin hernias, in Fitzgibbons Jr. RJ, Greenburg AG (eds): *Nyhus and Condon's Hernia,* 5th ed. Philadelphia: Lippincott Williams & Wilkins, 2002, p 199.

23. Bendavid R: Sliding hernias. *Hernia* 6:137, 2002.

24. Bendavid R: The space of Bogros and the deep inguinal venous circulation. *Surg Gynecol Obstet* 174:355, 1992.

25. Annibali R, Quinn TH, Fitzgibbons RJ Jr.: Anatomy of the inguinal region from the laparoscopic perspective: critical areas for laparoscopic hernia repair, in Bendavid R (ed): *Prostheses and Abdominal Wall Hernias.* Austin, TX: Landes Publishing, 1994, p 82.

26. Rosenberger RJ, Loeweneck H, Meyer G: The cutaneous nerves encountered during laparoscopic repair of inguinal hernia: new anatomical findings for the surgeon. *Surg Endosc* 14:731, 2000.

27. Annibali R, Quinn TH, Fitzgibbons RJ Jr.: Avoiding nerve injury during laparoscopic hernia repair: critical areas for staple placement, in Arregui ME, Nagan RF (eds): *Inguinal Hernia: Advances or Controversies?* Oxford: Radcliffe Medical Press, 1994, p 41.

28. Ralphs DN, Brain AJ, Grundy DJ, et al: How accurately can direct and indirect inguinal hernias be distinguished? *Br Med J* 280:1039, 1980.

29. Cameron AE: Accuracy of clinical diagnosis of direct and indirect inguinal hernia. *Br J Surg* 81:250, 1994.

30. Kark A, Kurzer M, Waters KJ: Accuracy of clinical diagnosis of direct and indirect inguinal hernia. *Br J Surg* 81:1081, 1994.

31. van den Berg JC, de Valois JC, Go PM, Rosenbusch G: Detection of groin hernia with physical examination, ultrasound, and MRI compared with laparoscopic findings. *Invest Radiol* 34:739, 1999.

32. Zollinger RM Jr.: Classification of ventral and groin hernias, in Fitzgibbons RJ Jr., Greenburg AG (eds): *Nyhus and Condon's Hernia,* 5th ed. Philadelphia: Lippincott Williams & Wilkins, 2002, p 71.

33. Toniato A, Pagetta C, Bernante P, et al: Incisional hernia treatment with progressive pneumoperitoneum and retromuscular prosthetic hernioplasty MR. *Langenbecks Arch Surg* 387:246, 2002.

34. Fitzgibbons R, Schmid S, Santoscoy R, et al: Open laparoscopy for laparoscopic cholecystectomy. *Surg Laparosc Endosc* 1:216, 1991.

35. Nordestgaard AG, Bodily KC, Osborne RW, et al: Major vascular injuries during laparoscopic procedures. *Am J Surg* 169:543, 1995.

36. Read RC: Prosthesis in abdominal wall hernia surgery in prosthesis and abdominal wall hernias, in Bendavid R (ed): TITLE?. Austin, TX: RG Landes Co, 1994, p 2.

37. Cumberland VH: A preliminary report on the use of a prefabricated nylon weave in the repair of ventral hernia. *Med J Aust* 1:143, 1952.

38. Heise CP, Starling JR: Mesh inguinodynia: a new clinical syndrome after inguinal herniorrhaphy? *J Am Coll Surg* 187:514, 1998.

39. EU Hernia Trialists Collaboration: Repair of groin hernia with synthetic mesh: meta-analysis of randomized controlled trials. *Ann Surg* 235:322, 2002.

40. Ghadimi BM, Langer C, Becker H. The carcinogenic potential of biomaterials in hernia surgery. *Chirurg* 73:833, 2002.

41. Franklin ME Jr., Gonzalez JJ Jr., Michaelson RP, et al: Preliminary experience with new bioactive prosthetic material for repair of hernias in infected fields. *Hernia* 6:171, 2002.

42. Smedberg SGG, Broome AEA, Gullmo A: Ligation of the hernia sac? *Surg Clin North Am* 64:299, 1984.

43. Castrini G, Pappalardo G, Trentino P, et al: The original Bassini technique in the surgical treatment of inguinal hernia. *Int Surgery* 71:141, 1986.

44. Lifschutz H: The inguinal darn. *Arch Surg* 121:717, 1986.

45. Gilbert AI: Sutureless repair of inguinal hernia. *Am J Surg* 163:331, 1992.

46. Millikan KW, Cummings B, Doolas A: A prospective study of mesh plug hernioplasty. *Am Surg* 67:285, 2001.

47. Reed RC: Annandale's role in the development of preperitoneal groin herniorrhaphy. *Hernia* 1:111, 1997.

48. Cheatle GL: An operation for the radical cure of inguinal and femoral hernia. *Br Med J* 2:68, 1920.

49. Henry AK: Operation for femoral hernia by a midline extraperitoneal approach, with a preliminary note on the use of this route for reducible inguinal hernia. *Lancet* 1:531, 1936.

50. Rutkow IM: A selective history of groin herniorrhaphy in the 20th century. *Surg Clin North Am* 73:395, 1993.

51. Waantz GE, Fischer E: Unilateral giant prosthetic reinforcement of the visceral sac, in Fitzgibbons RJ Jr., Greenburg AG (eds): *Nyhus and Condon's Hernia,* 5th ed. Philadelphia: Lippincott Williams & Wilkins, 2002, p 219.

52. Rignault DP: Properitoneal prosthetic inguinal hernioplasty through a Pfannenstiel approach. *Surg Gynecol Obstet* 163:465, 1986.

53. Nyhus LM: Iliopubic tract repair of inguinal and femoral hernia. The posterior (preperitoneal) approach. *Surg Clin North Am* 73:487, 1993.

54. Kugel RD: Minimally invasive, nonlaparoscopic, preperitoneal, and sutureless, inguinal herniorrhaphy. *Am J Surg* 178:298, 1999.

55. Ugahary F: The gridiron hernioplasty, in Bendavid R, Abrahamson J, Arregui M, Flament JB, Phillips EH (eds): *Hernias of the Abdominal Wall: Principles and Management.* New York: Springer-Verlag, 2001, p 407.

56. Ger R: The management of certain abdominal herniae by intraabdominal closure of the neck of the sac. Preliminary communication. *Ann R Coll Surg Engl* 64:342, 1982.

57. The EU Hernia Trialists Collaboration: Laparoscopic compared with open methods of groin hernia repair: systematic review of randomized controlled trials. *Br J Surg* 87:860, 2000.

58. Picchio M, Lombardi A, Zolovkins A, et al: Tension-free laparoscopic and open hernia repair: randomized controlled trial of early results. *World J Surg* 23:1004, 1999; discussion 1008.

59. McCormack K, Scott NW, Go PM, Ross S, Grant AM; EU Hernia Trialists Collaboration. Laparoscopic techniques versus open techniques for inguinal hernia repair. *Cochrane Database Syst Rev* 1:CD001785, 2003.

60. National Institute for Clinical Excellence (NICE): Guidance on the use of laparoscopic surgery for inguinal hernia. London: NICE, 2001 (Technology appraisal guidance no. 18).

61. Kingsley D, Vogt DM, Nelson MT, et al: Laparoscopic intraperitoneal onlay inguinal herniorrhaphy. *Am J Surg* 176:548, 1998.

62. Felix EL: A unified approach to recurrent laparoscopic hernia repairs. *Surg Endosc* 15:969, 2001.

63. Leibl BJ, Schmedt CG, Kraft K, et al: Recurrence after endoscopic transperitoneal hernia repair (TAPP): causes, reparative techniques, and results of the reoperation. *J Am Coll Surg* 190:651, 2000.

64. Knook MTT, Weidema WE, Stassen LPS, et al: Laparoscopic repair of recurrent inguinal hernias after endoscopic herniorrhaphy. *Surg Endosc* 13:1145, 1999.

65. Poobalan AS, Bruce J, Smith WC, et al: A review of chronic pain after inguinal herniorrhaphy. *Clin J Pain* 19:48, 2003.

66. Bendavid R: Complications of groin hernia surgery. *Surg Clin North Am* 78:1089, 1998.

67. Wantz GE: Testicular atrophy as a risk inguinal hernioplasty. *Surg Gynecol Obstet* 154:570, 1982.

68. Sanchez-Manuel FJ, Seco-Gil JL: Antibiotic prophylaxis for hernia repair. *Cochrane Database Syst Rev* 2:CD003769, 2003.

69. Taylor SG, O'Dwyer PJ: Chronic groin sepsis following tension-free inguinal hernioplasty. *Br J Surg* 86:562, 1999.

70. Rodriguez C, Miguel A, Lima H, et al: Osteitis pubis syndrome in the professional soccer athlete: A case report. *J Athl Train* 36:437, 2001.

71. Amid PK: How to avoid recurrence in Lichtenstein tension-free hernioplasty. *Am J Surg* 184:259, 2002.

72. Liu SK, Rassai H, Krasner C, et al: Urinary catheter in laparoscopic cholecystectomy: is it necessary? *Surg Laparosc Endosc Percutan Tech* 9:184, 1999.

73. Haskell DL, Sunshine B, Heifetz CJ: A study of bladder catheterization with inguinal hernia operations. *Arch Surg* 109:378, 1974.

74. Voitk AJ, Tsao SG: The umbilicus in laparoscopic surgery. *Surg Endosc* 15:878, 2001.

75. Jensen P, Mikkelsen T, Kehlet H: Postherniorrhaphy urinary retention—effect of local, regional, and general anesthesia: A review. *Reg Anesth Pain Med* 27:612, 2002.

76. Condon RE, Nyhus LM: Complications of groin hernia, in Condon RE, Nyhus LM (eds): *Hernia,* 4th ed. Philadelphia: Lippincott, 1995, p 269.

77. Bendavid R: Femoral hernias in females: Facts, figures and fallacies, in Bendavid R (ed): *Prostheses and Abdominal Wall Hernias.* Austin, TX: Landes Publishing, 1994, p 82.

78. Fon LJ, Spence RA: Sportsman's hernia. *Br J Surg* 87:545, 2000.

79. Polglase AL, Frydman GM, Farmer KC: Inguinal surgery for debilitating chronic groin pain in athletes. *Med J Aust* 155:674, 1992.

80. Kurkchubasche AG, Tracy TF: Unique features of groin hernia repair in infants and children, in Fitzgibbons RJ Jr., Greenburg AG (eds): *Nyhus and Condon's Hernia,* 5th ed. Philadelphia: Lippincott Williams & Wilkins, 2002, p 435.

81. Skinner MA, Grosfeld JL: Inguinal and umbilical hernia repair in infants and children. *Surg Clin North Am* 73:439, 1993.

82. Rowe MI, Copelson LW, Clatworthy HW: The patent processus vaginalis and the inguinal hernia. *J Pediatr Surg* 4:102, 1969.

83. Brisson P, Patel H, Feins N: Cremasteric muscle hypertrophy accompanies inguinal hernias in children. *J Pediatr Surg* 34:1320, 1999.

84. Chen KC, Chu CC, Chou TY, et al: Ultrasonography for inguinal hernias in boys. *J Pediatr Surg* 34:1890, 1999.

85. Erez I, Rathause V, Vacian I, et al: Preoperative ultrasound and intraoperative findings of inguinal hernias in children: A prospective study of 642 children. *J Pediatr Surg* 37:865, 2002.

86. Gardner TA, Ostad M Mininber DT: Diagnostic flexible peritoneoscopy: assessment of the contralateral internal inguinal ring during unilateral herniorrhaphy. *J Pediatr Surg* 33:1486, 1998.

87. Yerkes EB, Brock JW, Holcomb GW, et al: Laparoscopic evaluation for a contralateral patent processus vaginalis: part III. *Urology* 51:480, 1998.

88. Rescoria FJ, West KW, Engum SA, et al: The "other side" of pediatric hernias: the role of laparoscopy. *Am Surg* 63:690, 1997.

89. Hurst RD, Butler BN, Soybel DI, et al: Management of groin hernias in patients with ascites. *Ann Surg* 216:696, 1992.

90. Andersson B, Hallen M, Leveau P, Bergenfelz A, Westerdahl J: Laparoscopic extraperitoneal inguinal hernia repair versus open mesh repair: a prospective randomized controlled trial. *Surgery* 133:464, 2003.

91. Douek M, Smith G, Oshowo A, Stoker DL, Wellwood JM: Prospective randomised controlled trial of laparoscopic versus open inguinal hernia mesh repair: five year follow up. *BMJ* 326:1012, 2003.

92. Bringman S, Ramel S, Heikkinen TJ, et al: Tension-free inguinal hernia repair: TEP versus mesh-plug versus Lichtenstein: a prospective randomized controlled trial. *Ann Surg* 237:142, 2003.

93. Mahon D, Decadt B, Rhodes M: Prospective randomized trial of laparoscopic (transabdominal preperitoneal) vs. open (mesh) repair for bilateral and recurrent inguinal hernia. *Surg Endosc* 2003, Jun 17.

94. Colak T, Akca T, Kanik A, et al: Randomized clinical trial comparing laparoscopic totally extraperitoneal approach with open mesh repair in inguinal hernia. *Surg Laparosc Endosc Percutan Tech* 13:191, 2003.

95. Sarli L, Iusco DR, Sansebastiano G, Costi R: Simultaneous repair of bilateral inguinal hernias: a prospective, randomized study of open, tension-free versus laparoscopic approach. *Surg Laparosc Endosc Percutan Tech* 11:262, 2001.

96. Kumar S, Nixon SJ, MacIntyre IM: Laparoscopic or Lichtenstein repair for recurrent inguinal hernia: one unit's experience. *J R Coll Surg Edinburgh* 44:301, 1999.

97. Beets GL, Dirksen CD, Go PM, et al: Open or laparoscopic preperitoneal mesh repair for recurrent inguinal hernia? A randomized controlled trial. *Surg Endosc* 13:323, 1999.

98. No authors listed: Laparoscopic versus open repair of groin hernia: a randomised comparison. The MRC Laparoscopic Groin Hernia Trial Group. *Lancet* 354:185, 1999.

99. Khoury N: A randomized prospective controlled trial of laparoscopic extraperitoneal hernia repair and mesh-plug hernioplasty: a study of 315 cases. *J Laparoendosc Adv Surg Tech A* 8:367, 1998.

100. Heikkinen TJ, Haukipuro K, Koivukangas P, et al: A prospective randomized outcome and cost comparison of totally extraperitoneal endoscopic hernioplasty versus Lichtenstein hernia operation among employed patients. *Surg Laparosc Endosc* 8:338, 1998.

101. Wellwood J, Sculpher MJ, Stoker D, et al: Randomised controlled trial of laparoscopic versus open mesh repair for inguinal hernia: outcome and cost. *BMJ* 317:103, 1998.

102. Wright DM, Kennedy A, Baxter JN, et al: Early outcome after open versus extraperitoneal endoscopic tension-free hernioplasty: a randomized clinical trial. *Surgery* 119:552, 1996.

103. Payne JH Jr., Grininger LM, Izawa MT, et al: Laparoscopic or open inguinal herniorrhaphy? A randomized prospective trial. *Arch Surg* 129:973, 1994; discussion 979.

CHAPTER 37

Thyroid, Parathyroid, and Adrenal

Geeta Lal and Orlo H. Clark

Thyroid

HISTORICAL BACKGROUND

Goiters (from the Latin *guttur,* throat), defined as an enlargement of the thyroid, have been recognized since 2700 B.C. even though the thyroid gland was not documented as such until the Renaissance period. In 1619, Hieronymus Fabricius ab Aquapendente recognized that goiters arose from the thyroid gland. The term thyroid gland (Greek *thyreoeides,* shield-shaped) is, however, attributed to Thomas Wharton in his *Adenographia* (1656). In 1776, the thyroid was classified as a ductless gland by Albrecht von Haller and was thought to have numerous functions ranging from lubrication of the larynx to acting as a reservoir for blood to provide continuous flow to the brain, to beautifying women's necks. Burnt seaweed was considered to be the most effective treatment for goiters.

The first accounts of thyroid surgery for the treatment of goiters were given by Roger Frugardi in 1170. In response to failure of medical treatment, two setons were inserted at right angles into the goiter and tightened twice daily until the goiter separated. The open wound was treated with caustic powder and left to heal. However, thyroid surgery continued to be hazardous with prohibitive mortality rates (>40%) until the latter half of the nineteenth century, when advances in general anesthesia, antisepsis, and hemostasis enabled surgeons to perform thyroid surgery with significantly reduced mortality and morbidity rates. The most notable thyroid surgeons were Emil Theodor Kocher (1841–1917) (Fig. 37-1) and C. A. Theodor Billroth (1829–1894), who performed thousands of operations with increasingly successful results. However, as more patients survived thyroid operations, new problems and issues became apparent. After total thyroidectomy, patients (particularly children) became myxedematous with cretinous features. Kocher used the term "cachexia strumipriva" to describe this condition and initially wrongly attributed it to operative tracheal trauma, giving rise to chronic asphyxia. Felix Semon suggested that myxedema was secondary to the loss of thyroid function, a view originally treated

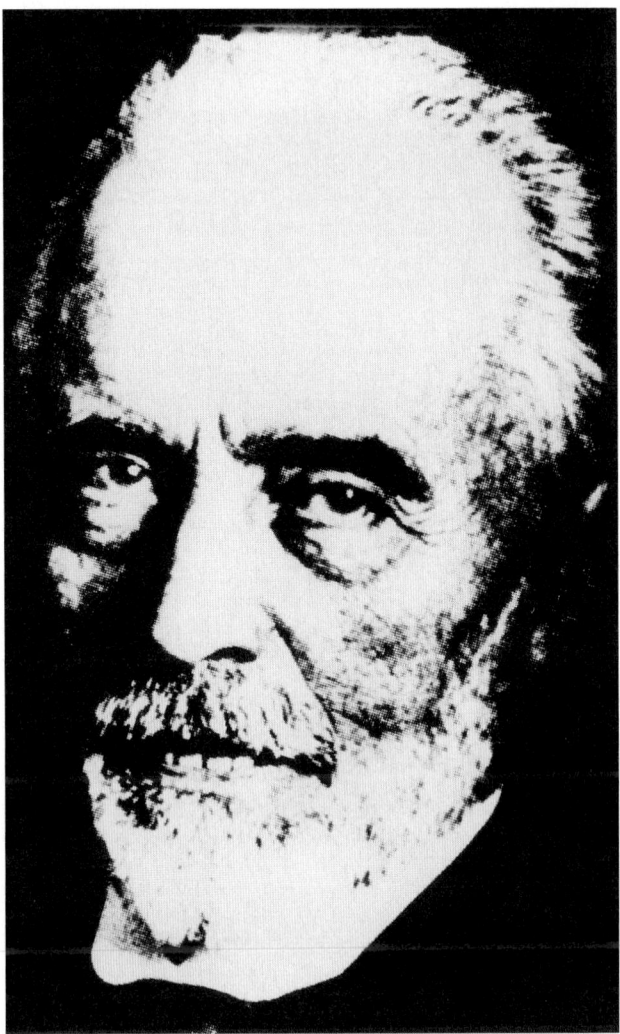

FIG. 37-1. Emil Kocher is considered the father of thyroid surgery. He won the Nobel Prize in medicine, in 1909, in recognition of his work on the thyroid gland.

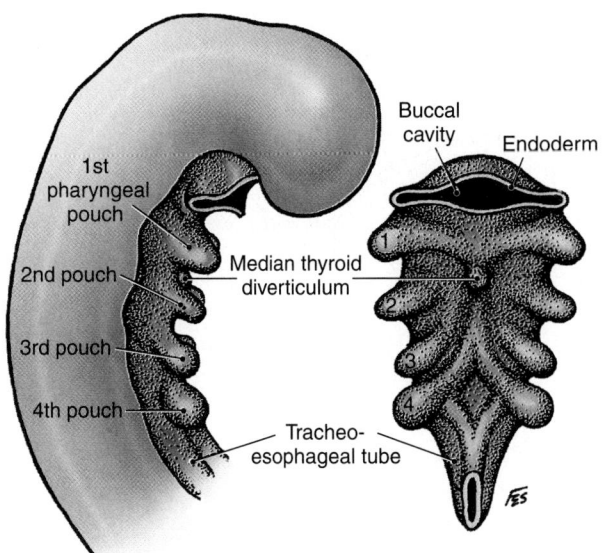

FIG. 37-2. Thyroid embryology. Early development of the median thyroid anlage as a pharyngeal pouch. [*Reproduced with permission from Embryology and developmental abnormalities, in Cady B, Rossi R (eds): Surgery of the Thyroid and Parathyroid Glands. W.B. Saunders, 1991, p. 6.*]

with some skepticism. Myxedema was first effectively treated in 1891 by George Murray, who used a subcutaneous injection of an extract of sheep's thyroid; later, Edward Fox demonstrated that oral therapy was equally effective.

William Halsted was the first surgeon to suggest that outcomes were dependent upon operative technique. Kocher was extremely neat and precise, operating slowly in a bloodless field and often removed the entire thyroid. His patients developed myxedema but rarely suffered laryngeal nerve damage or postoperative tetany. Billroth, however, worked rapidly and with less concern for hemorrhage. He often removed the parathyroid glands but left more thyroid tissue, therefore, encountering significant postoperative hypoparathyroidism but rarely myxedema. In 1909, Kocher was awarded the Nobel Prize for medicine in recognition "for his works on the physiology, pathology, and surgery of the thyroid gland."

EMBRYOLOGY

The thyroid gland arises as an outpouching of the primitive foregut around the third week of gestation. It originates at the base of the tongue in the vicinity of the foramen cecum. Endoderm cells in the floor of the pharyngeal anlage thicken to form the medial thyroid anlage (Fig. 37-2) that descends in the neck anterior to structures that form the hyoid bone and larynx. During its descent, the anlage remains connected to the foramen cecum via an epithelial-lined tube known as the thyroglossal duct. The epithelial cells making up the anlage give rise to the thyroid follicular cells. Paired lateral anlages originate from the fourth branchial pouch and fuse with the median anlage at approximately the fifth week of gestation. The lateral anlages are neuroectodermal in origin (ultimobranchial bodies) and provide the calcitonin producing parafollicular or C cells, which come to lie in the superoposterior region of the gland. Thyroid follicles are initially apparent by 8 weeks and colloid formation begins by the 11th week of gestation.

DEVELOPMENTAL ABNORMALITIES

Thyroglossal Duct Cyst and Sinus

Thyroglossal duct cysts are the most commonly encountered congenital cervical anomalies. During the fifth week of gestation, the thyroglossal duct lumen starts to obliterate and the duct disappears by the eighth week of gestation. Rarely, the thyroglossal duct may persist in whole, or in part. Thyroglossal duct cysts may occur anywhere along the migratory path of the thyroid, although 80% are found in juxtaposition to the hyoid bone. They are usually asymptomatic, but occasionally become infected by oral bacteria, prompting the patient to seek medical advice. Thyroglossal duct sinuses result from infection of the cyst secondary to spontaneous or surgical drainage of the cyst and are accompanied by minor inflammation of the surrounding skin. Histologically, thyroglossal duct cysts are lined by pseudostratified ciliated columnar epithelium and squamous epithelium with heterotopic thyroid tissue present in 20% of cases.

The diagnosis is usually established by observing a 1- to 2-cm, smooth, well-defined midline neck mass that moves upward with protrusion of the tongue. Routine thyroid imaging is not necessary,

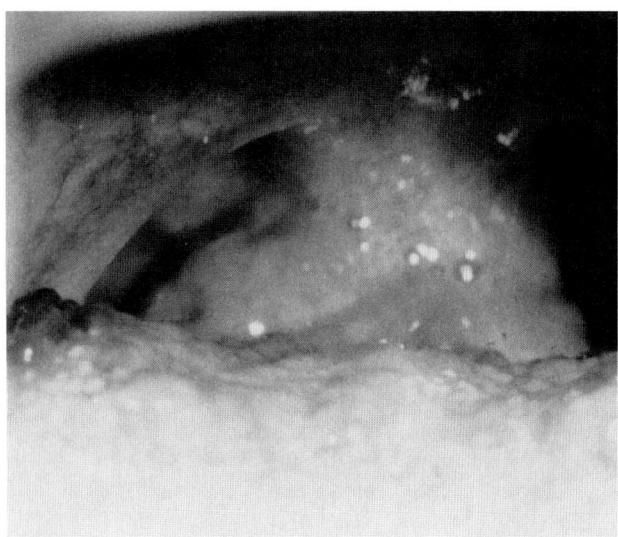

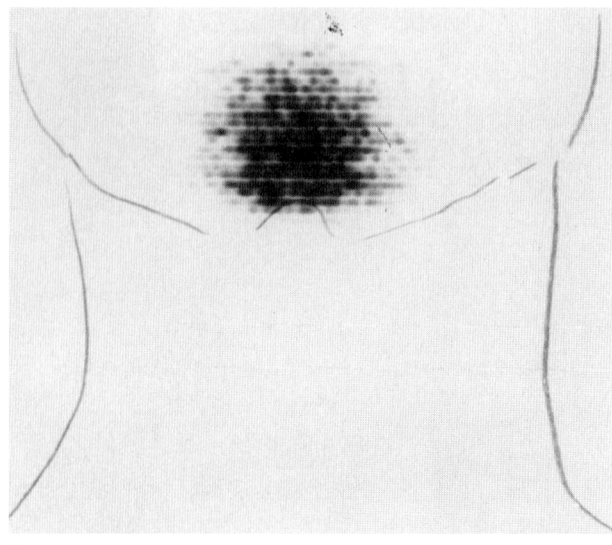

A   *B*

FIG. 37-3. *A. A large lingual thyroid is located at the posterior aspect of the tongue. B. Radioactive iodine scan of the same patient showing all the activity above the hyoid bone and no activity in the neck.*

although thyroid scintigraphy and ultrasound have been performed to document the presence of normal thyroid tissue in the neck. Treatment involves the "Sistrunk operation," which consists of en bloc cystectomy and excision of the central hyoid bone to minimize recurrence.[1] Approximately 1% of cysts are found to contain cancer that is usually papillary (85%). Squamous, Hürthle cell, and anaplastic cancers also have been reported, but are rare. Medullary thyroid cancers are, however, not found in thyroglossal duct cysts.

Lingual Thyroid

A lingual thyroid represents a failure of the median thyroid anlage to descend normally and may be the only thyroid tissue present (Fig. 37-3). Intervention becomes necessary for obstructive symptoms such as choking, dysphagia, airway obstruction, and hemorrhage. Many of these patients develop hypothyroidism. Medical treatment options include administration of exogenous thyroid hormone to suppress thyroid-stimulating hormone (TSH) and radioactive iodine ablation followed by hormone replacement. Surgical excision is rarely needed, but if required, should be preceded by an evaluation of normal thyroid tissue in the neck to avoid inadvertently rendering the patient hypothyroid.

Ectopic Thyroid

Normal thyroid tissue may be found anywhere in the central neck compartment, including the esophagus, trachea, and anterior mediastinum. Thyroid tissue has been observed adjacent to the aortic arch, in the aortopulmonary window, within the upper pericardium, and in the interventricular septum. Often, "tongues" of thyroid tissue are seen to extend off the inferior poles of the gland and are particularly apparent in large goiters. Thyroid tissue situated lateral to the carotid sheath and jugular vein, previously termed "lateral aberrant thyroid," almost always represents metastatic thyroid cancer in lymph nodes, and not remnants of the lateral anlage that had failed to fuse with the main thyroid, as previously suggested by Crile. Even if not readily apparent on physical examination or

ultrasound imaging, the ipsilateral thyroid lobe contains a focus of papillary thyroid cancer, which may be microscopic.

Pyramidal Lobe

Normally, the thyroglossal duct atrophies, although it may remain as a fibrous band. In approximately 50% of individuals, the distal end that connects to the thyroid persists as a pyramidal lobe projecting up from the isthmus, lying just to the left or right of the midline. In the normal individual the pyramidal lobe is not palpable, but in disorders resulting in thyroid hypertrophy (e.g., Graves' disease, diffuse nodular goiter, or lymphocytic thyroiditis), the pyramidal lobe is usually enlarged and palpable.

THYROID ANATOMY

Figure 37-4 depicts the anatomic relations of the thyroid gland and surrounding structures. The adult thyroid gland is brown in color and firm in consistency, and is located posterior to the strap (sternothyroid and sternohyoid) muscles. The normal thyroid gland weighs approximately 20 g, but gland weight varies with body weight and iodine intake. The thyroid lobes are located adjacent to the thyroid cartilage and connected in the midline by an isthmus which is typically located just inferior to the cricoid cartilage. A pyramidal lobe, which represents the most caudal end of the thyroglossal duct, is found in approximately 50% of individuals having thyroid operations. The thyroid lobes extend to mid-thyroid cartilage superiorly and lie adjacent to the carotid sheaths and sternocleidomastoid muscles laterally. The strap muscles (sternohyoid, sternothyroid and superior belly of the omohyoid) are located anteriorly and are innervated by the ansa cervicalis (ansa hypoglossi). The thyroid gland is enveloped by a loosely connecting fascia that is formed from the partition of the deep cervical fascia into anterior and posterior divisions. The true capsule of the thyroid is a thin, densely adherent fibrous layer that sends out septa that invaginate into the gland, forming pseudolobules. The thyroid capsule is condensed into the posterior suspensory or Berry's ligament near the cricoid cartilage and upper tracheal rings.

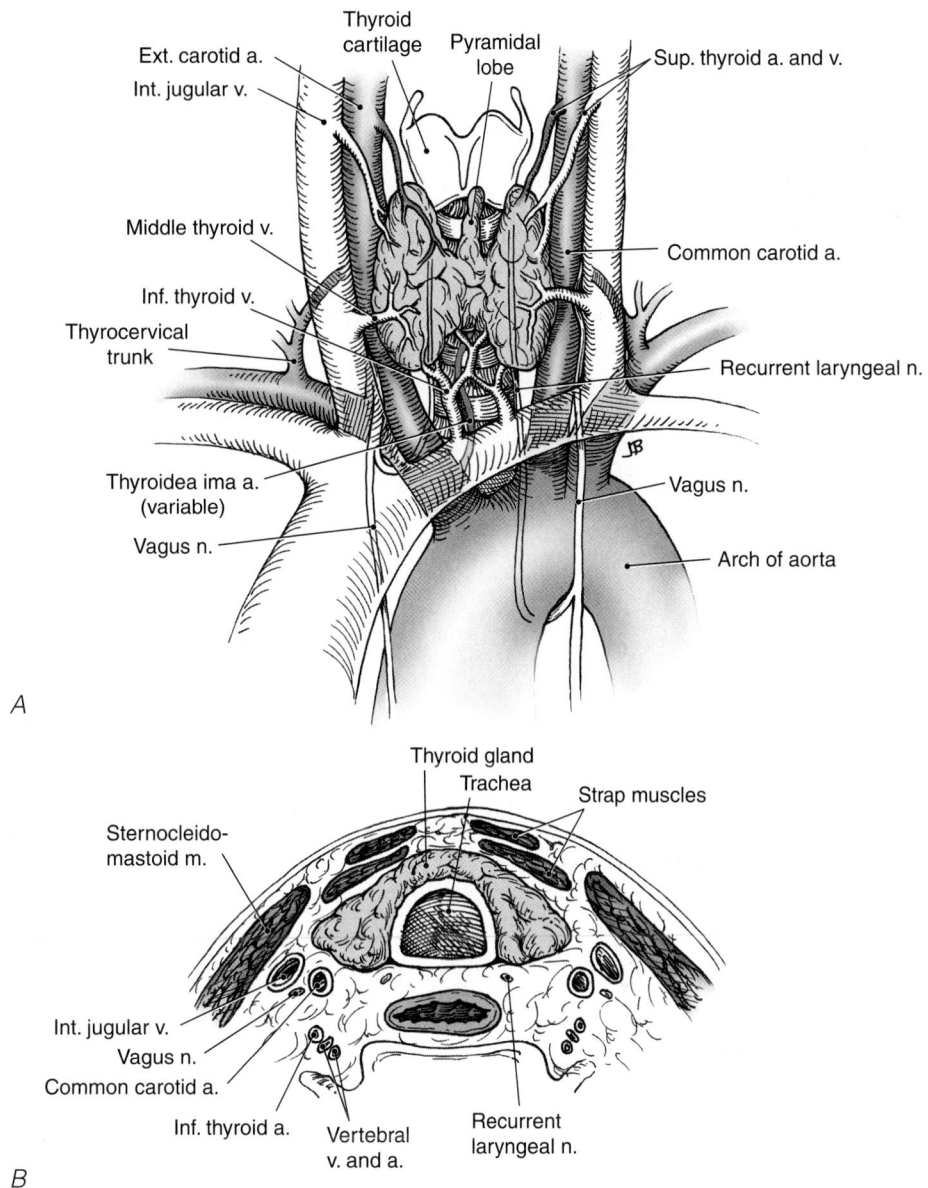

FIG. 37-4. Anatomy of the thyroid gland and surrounding structures, viewed anteriorly (A) and in cross section (B).

Blood Supply

The thyroid gland is well vascularized by two major sets of arteries. The superior thyroid arteries arise from the ipsilateral external carotid arteries and divide into anterior and posterior branches at the apices of the thyroid lobes. The inferior thyroid arteries are derived from the thyrocervical trunk shortly after their origin from the subclavian arteries. The inferior thyroid arteries travel upward in the neck posterior to the carotid sheath to enter the thyroid lobes at their midpoint. A thyroidea ima artery arises directly from the aorta or innominate in 1 to 4% of individuals, to enter the isthmus or replace a missing inferior thyroid artery. The inferior thyroid artery is intimately associated with the recurrent laryngeal nerve (RLN), necessitating identification of the RLN before the arterial branches can be ligated. Venous drainage of the thyroid gland occurs via multiple small surface veins, which coalesce to form three sets of veins—the superior, middle, and inferior thyroid veins. The superior thyroid veins run with the superior thyroid arteries bilaterally. The middle vein or veins are the least consistent. The superior and middle veins

drain directly into the internal jugular veins, the inferior veins often form a plexus, which drains into the brachiocephalic veins.

Nerves

The left RLN arises from the vagus nerve where it crosses the aortic arch, loops around the ligamentum arteriosum and ascends medially in the neck within the tracheoesophageal groove. The right RLN arises from the vagus at its crossing with the right subclavian artery. The nerve passes posterior to the artery before ascending in the neck, its course being more oblique than the left RLN. Along their course in the neck, the RLNs may branch, and pass anterior, posterior or interdigitate with branches of the inferior thyroid artery (Fig. 37-5). The right RLN may be nonrecurrent in 0.5 to 1% of individuals and is often associated with a vascular anomaly in this situation.[2] Nonrecurrent left RLNs are rare, but have been reported in patients with situs inversus and a right-sided aortic arch. The RLN may branch in its course in the neck, and identification of a small nerve should alert the surgeon to this possibility. Identification of the nerves or

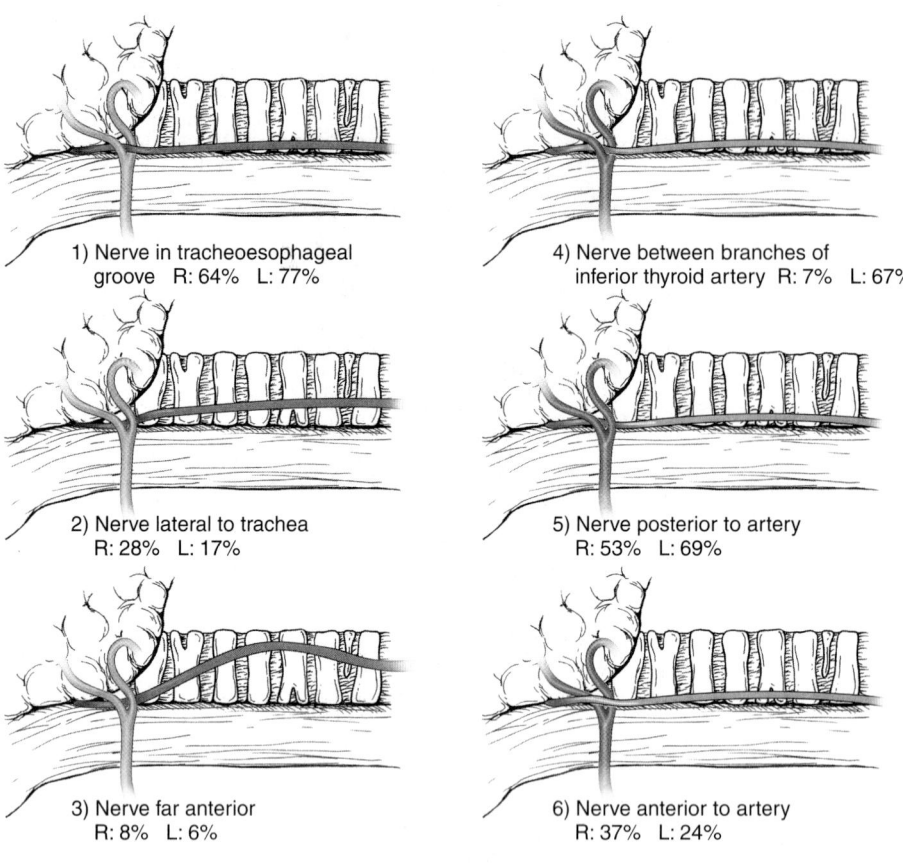

1) Nerve in tracheoesophageal
groove   R: 64%   L: 77%

2) Nerve lateral to trachea
R: 28%   L: 17%

3) Nerve far anterior
R: 8%   L: 6%

4) Nerve between branches of
inferior thyroid artery   R: 7%   L: 67%

5) Nerve posterior to artery
R: 53%   L: 69%

6) Nerve anterior to artery
R: 37%   L: 24%

7) Artery absent   R: 3%   L: 1%

FIG. 37-5. Relationship of RLN to the inferior thyroid artery. The superior parathyroid is characteristically dorsal to the plane of the nerve, whereas the inferior gland is ventral to the nerve.

their branches often necessitates mobilization of the most lateral and posterior extent of the thyroid gland, the tubercle of Zuckerkandl, at the level of the cricoid cartilage. The last segments of the nerves often course below the tubercle and are closely approximated to the ligament of Berry. Branches of the nerve may traverse the ligament in 25% of individuals, and are particularly vulnerable to injury at this junction. The recurrent laryngeal nerves terminate by entering the larynx posterior to the cricothyroid muscle.

The RLNs innervate all the intrinsic muscles of the larynx, except the cricothyroid muscles, which are innervated by the external laryngeal nerves. Injury to one RLN leads to paralysis of the ipsilateral vocal cord, which comes to lie in the paramedian or the abducted position. The paramedian position results in a normal, but weak voice, whereas the abducted position leads to a hoarse voice and an ineffective cough. Bilateral RLN injury may lead to airway obstruction, necessitating emergency tracheostomy, or loss of voice. If both cords come to lie in an abducted position, air movement can occur, but the patient has an ineffective cough and is at increased risk of repeated respiratory tract infections from aspiration.

The superior laryngeal nerves also arise from the vagus nerves. After their origin at the base of the skull, these nerves travel along the internal carotid artery and divide into two branches at the level of the hyoid bone. The internal branch of the superior laryngeal nerve is sensory to the supraglottic larynx. Injury to this nerve is rare in thyroid surgery, but its occurrence may result in aspiration. The external branch of the superior laryngeal nerve lies on the inferior pharyngeal constrictor muscle and descends alongside the superior thyroid vessels before innervating the cricothyroid muscle. Cernea

and associates[3] proposed a classification system to describe the relationship of this nerve to the superior thyroid vessels (Fig. 37-6). The type 2a variant, in which the nerve crosses below the tip of the thyroid superior pole, occurs in up to 20% of individuals and places the nerve at a greater risk of injury. Therefore, the superior pole vessels should not be ligated en masse, but should be individually divided, low on the thyroid gland, and dissected lateral to the cricothyroid muscle. This nerve also has been called the Amelita Galla Curci or "high note" nerve after the opera singer. Injury to this nerve leads to inability to tense the ipsilateral vocal cord and hence difficulty "hitting high notes," projecting the voice, and voice fatigue during prolonged speech.

Sympathetic innervation of the thyroid gland is provided by fibers from the superior and middle cervical sympathetic ganglia. The fibers enter the gland with the blood vessels and are vasomotor in action. Parasympathetic fibers are derived from the vagus nerve and reach the gland via branches of the laryngeal nerves.

Parathyroid Glands

The embryology and anatomy of the parathyroid glands is discussed in detail in the parathyroid gland section of this chapter (see under "Parathyroid"). Most individuals have four parathyroid glands, which derive their blood supply primarily from branches of the inferior thyroid artery. Generally, parathyroid glands can be found within 1 cm of the junction of the inferior thyroid artery and the RLN. The superior glands are usually located dorsal to the RLN, whereas the inferior glands are usually found ventral to the RLN (Fig. 37-7).

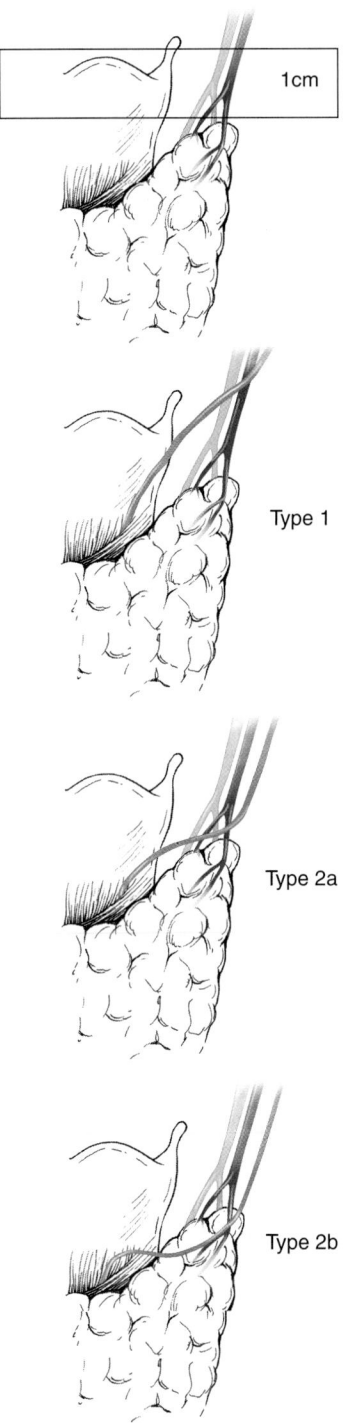

FIG. 37-6. *Relationship of the external branch of the superior laryngeal nerve and superior thyroid artery originally described by Cernea and associates. In type 1 anatomy, the nerve crosses the artery ≥1 cm above the superior aspect of the thyroid lobe. In type 2 anatomy, the nerve crosses the artery <1 cm above the thyroid pole (2a) or below (2b) it. (Reproduced with permission from Bliss RD, et al: Surgeons' approach to the thyroid gland: Surgical anatomy and the importance of technique. World J Surg 24(8):893, 2000.)*

Lymphatic System

The thyroid gland is endowed with an extensive network of lymphatics. Intraglandular lymphatic vessels connect both thyroid lobes through the isthmus and also drain to perithyroidal structures and

lymph nodes. Regional lymph nodes include pretracheal, paratracheal, perithyroidal, recurrent laryngeal nerve, superior mediastinal, retropharyngeal, esophageal, and upper, middle, and lower jugular chain nodes. These lymph nodes can be classified into seven levels, as depicted in Fig. 37-8. The central compartment includes nodes located in the area between the two carotid sheaths, whereas nodes lateral to the vessels are present in the lateral compartment. A thorough knowledge of these lymph node regions is needed for the adequate management of patients with thyroid cancers that have a predilection for lymph node metastases, such as papillary and medullary thyroid cancer. Thyroid cancers may metastasize to any of these regions, although metastases to submaxillary nodes (level I) are rare (<1%).

THYROID HISTOLOGY

Microscopically, the thyroid is divided into lobules that contain 20 to 40 follicles (Fig. 37-9). There are roughly 3×10^6 follicles in the adult male thyroid gland. The follicles are spherical and average 30 μm in diameter. Each follicle is lined by cuboidal epithelial cells and contains a central store of colloid secreted from the epithelial cells under the influence of the pituitary hormone, TSH. The second group of thyroid secretory cells is the C cells or parafollicular cells, which contain and secrete the hormone calcitonin. They are found as individual cells or clumped in small groups in the interfollicular stroma and located in the upper poles of the thyroid lobes.

THYROID PHYSIOLOGY

Iodine Metabolism

The average daily iodine requirement is 0.1 mg, which can be derived from foods such as fish, milk, and eggs, or as additives in bread or salt. In the stomach and jejunum, iodine is rapidly converted to iodide and absorbed into the bloodstream, from where it is distributed uniformly throughout the extracellular space. Iodide is actively transported into the thyroid follicular cells by an ATP-dependent process. In fact, the thyroid is the storage site of greater than 90% of the body's iodine content and accounts for one-third of the plasma iodine loss. The remaining plasma iodine is cleared via renal excretion.

Thyroid Hormone Synthesis, Secretion, and Transport

The synthesis of thyroid hormone consists of several steps[4] (Fig. 37-10). The first step, iodide trapping, involves active (ATP-dependent) transport of iodide across the basement membrane of the thyrocyte via an intrinsic membrane protein, the Na^+/I^- symporter (NIS). Thyroglobulin (Tg) is a large (660-kDa) glycoprotein, which is present in thyroid follicles and has four tyrosyl residues. The second step in thyroid hormone synthesis involves oxidation of iodide to iodine and iodination of tyrosine residues on Tg, to form monoiodotyrosines (MITs) and diiodotyrosines (DITs). Both processes are catalyzed by thyroid peroxidase. The recently identified protein pendrin is thought to mediate iodine efflux at the apical membrane.[5] The third step leads to coupling of two DIT molecules to form tetraiodothyronine or thyroxine (T_4), and one DIT molecule with one MIT molecule to form 3,5,3'-triiodothyronine (T_3) or reverse 3,3',5'-triiodothyronine (rT_3). When stimulated by TSH, thyrocytes form pseudopodia, that encircle portions of cell membrane containing thyroglobulin, which, in turn, fuse with enzyme-containing lysosomes. In the fourth step, thyroglobulin is

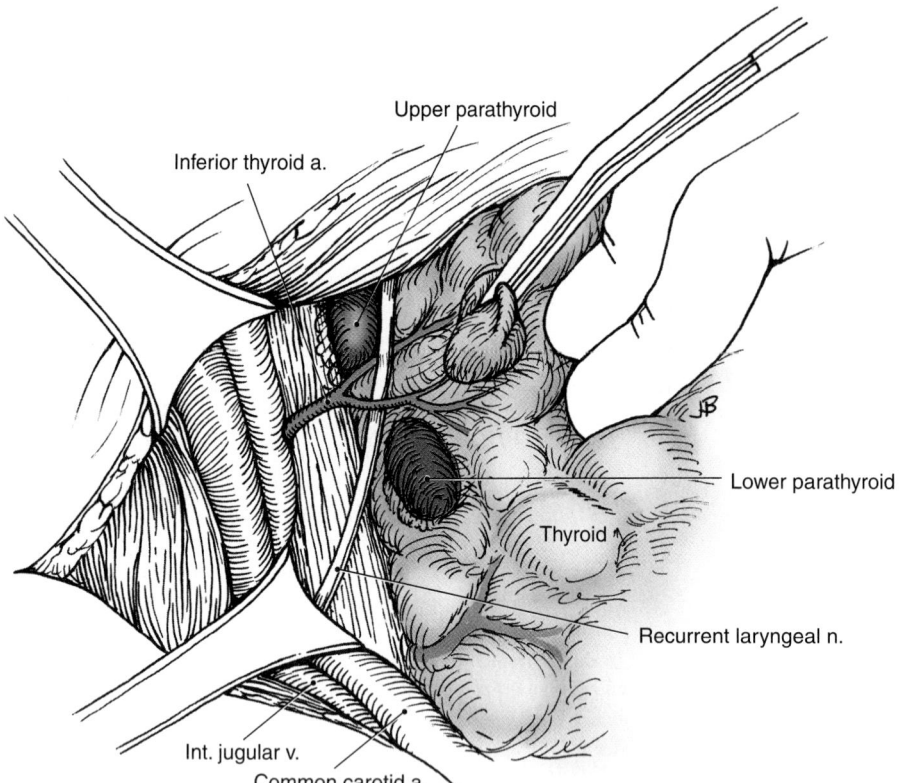

Upper parathyroid

Inferior thyroid a.

Lower parathyroid

Thyroid

Recurrent laryngeal n.

Int. jugular v.

Common carotid a.

FIG. 37-7. Relationship of the parathyroids to the RLN.

hydrolyzed to release free iodothyronines (T_3 and T_4) and mono- and diiodotyrosines. The latter are deiodinated in the fifth step to yield iodide, which is reused in the thyrocyte. Figure 37-11 illustrates the structures of the thyroid hormone precursors, T_4 and T_3.

In the euthyroid state, T_4 is produced and released entirely by the thyroid gland, whereas only 20% of the total T_3 is produced by the thyroid. Most of the T_3 is produced by peripheral deiodination (removal of 5'-iodine from the outer ring) of T_4 in the liver, muscles, kidney, and anterior pituitary, a reaction that is catalyzed by 5'-monodeiodinase. Some T_4 is converted to rT_3, the metabolically inactive compound, by deiodination of the inner ring of T_4. In conditions such as Graves' disease, toxic multinodular goiter, or a stimulated thyroid gland, the proportion of T_3 released from the thyroid may be dramatically elevated. Thyroid hormones are transported in serum bound to carrier proteins such as thyroxine-binding globulin (TBG), thyroxine-binding prealbumin (TBPA), and albumin. Only a small fraction (0.02%) of thyroid hormone (T_3 and T_4) is free (unbound) and is the physiologically active component. T_3 is the more potent of the two thyroid hormones, although its circulating plasma level is much lower than that of T_4. T_3 is less-tightly bound to protein in the plasma than is T_4, and so it enters tissues more readily. T_3 is three to four times more active than T_4 per unit weight, with a half-life of about 1 day, compared to approximately 7 days for T_4.

The secretion of thyroid hormone is controlled by the hypothalamic–pituitary–thyroid axis (Fig. 37-12). The hypothalamus produces a peptide, the thyrotropin-releasing hormone (TRH), which stimulates the pituitary to release TSH or thyrotropin. TRH reaches the pituitary via the portovenous circulation. TSH, a 28-kDa glycopeptide, mediates iodide trapping, secretion, and release of thyroid hormones, in addition to increasing the cellularity and vascularity of the thyroid gland. The TSH receptor belongs to a family of G-protein-coupled receptors that have seven transmembrane-spanning domains and utilize cAMP in the signal-transduction pathway. TSH secretion by the anterior pituitary also is regulated via a negative feedback loop by T_4 and T_3. Because the pituitary has the ability to convert T_4 to T_3, the latter is thought to be more important in this feedback control. T_3 also inhibits the release of TRH.

The thyroid gland also is capable of autoregulation, which allows it to modify its function independent of TSH. As an adaptation to low iodide intake, the gland preferentially synthesizes T_3 rather than T_4, thereby increasing the efficiency of secreted hormone. In situations of iodine excess, iodide transport, peroxide generation, synthesis, and secretion of thyroid hormones are inhibited. Excessively large doses of iodide may lead to initial increased organification, followed by suppression, a phenomenon called the Wolff-Chaikoff effect. Epinephrine and human chorionic gonadotrophin (hCG) hormones stimulate thyroid hormone production. Thus, elevated thyroid hormone levels are found in pregnancy and in gynecologic malignancies such as hydatidiform mole. In contrast, glucocorticoids inhibit thyroid hormone production. In severely ill patients, peripheral thyroid hormones may be reduced, without a compensatory increase in TSH levels, the sick-euthyroid low T_3 syndrome.

Thyroid Hormone Function

Free thyroid hormone enters the cell membrane by diffusion or by specific carriers and is carried to the nuclear membrane by binding to specific proteins. T_4 is deiodinated to T_3 and enters the nucleus via active transport, where it binds to the thyroid hormone receptor. The T_3 receptor is similar to the nuclear receptors for glucocorticoids, mineralocorticoids, estrogens, vitamin D, and retinoic acid. In humans, two types of T_3 receptor genes (α and β) are located on chromosomes 3 and 17. Thyroid receptor expression depends

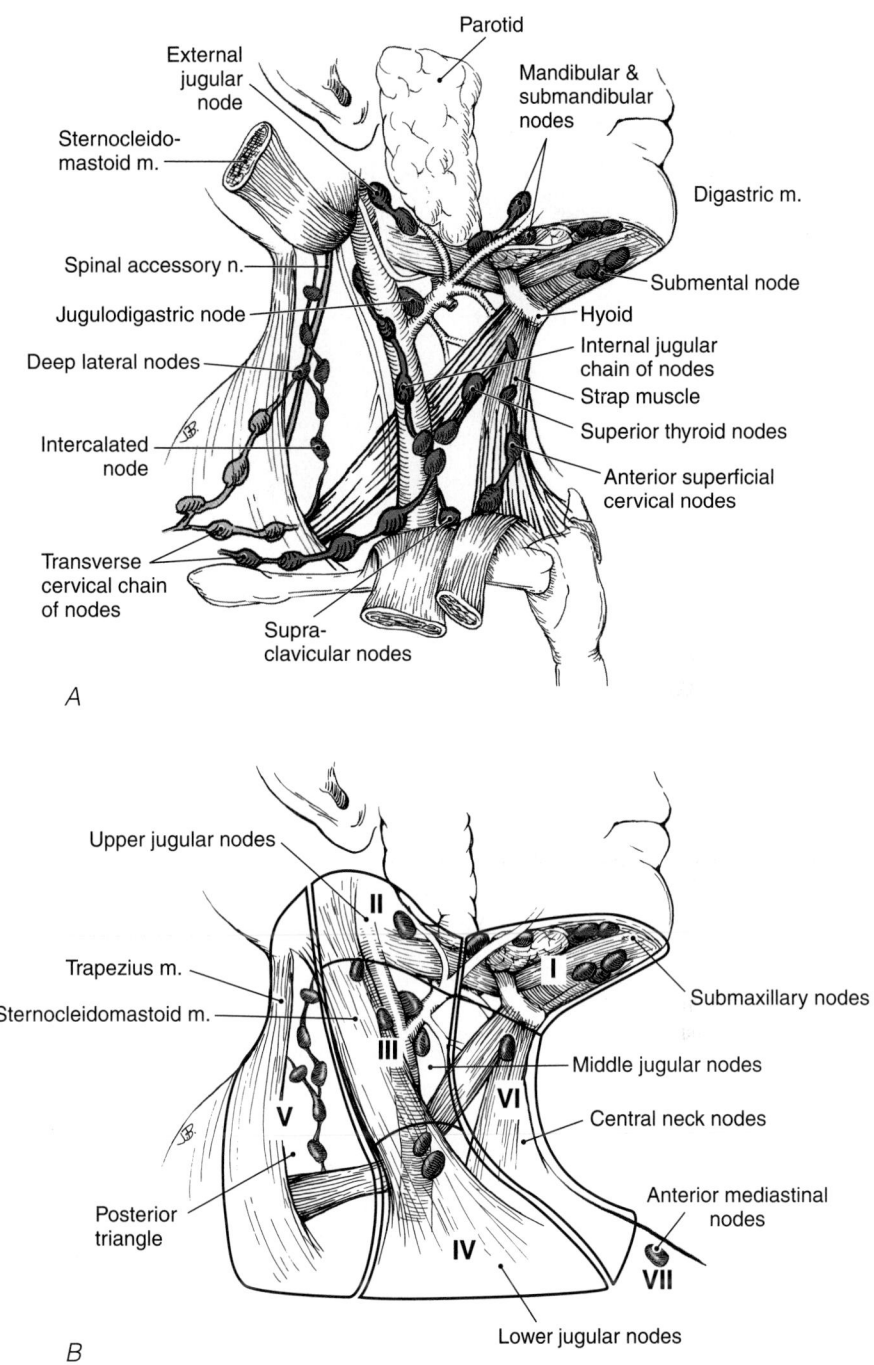

FIG. 37-8. Lymph nodes in the neck. The strap muscles have been divided to better show the various nodal basins in *A*. The lymph nodes can be divided into seven regions as shown in *B*.

upon peripheral concentrations of thyroid hormones and is tissue specific—the α form is abundant in the central nervous system, whereas the β form predominates in the liver. Each gene product has a ligand-independent, aminoterminal domain; a ligand-binding, carboxyterminal domain; and centrally located DNA-binding regions. Binding of thyroid hormone leads to the transcription and translation of hormone-responsive specific genes.

Thyroid hormones affect almost every system in the body. They are important for fetal brain development and skeletal maturation. T_3 increases oxygen consumption, basal metabolic rate and heat production by stimulation of Na^+/K^+ ATPase in various tissues. It also has a positive inotropic and chronotropic effect on the heart

by increasing transcription of the Ca^{2+} ATPase in the sarcoplasmic reticulum and increasing levels of beta-adrenergic receptors and concentration of G proteins. Myocardial α receptors are decreased and actions of catecholamines are amplified. Thyroid hormones are responsible for maintaining the normal hypoxic and hypercapnic drive in the respiratory center of the brain. They also increase gastrointestinal motility, leading to diarrhea in hyperthyroidism and constipation in hypothyroidism. Thyroid hormones also increase bone and protein turnover and the speed of muscle contraction and relaxation. They also increase glycogenolysis, hepatic gluconeogenesis, intestinal glucose absorption, and cholesterol synthesis and degradation.

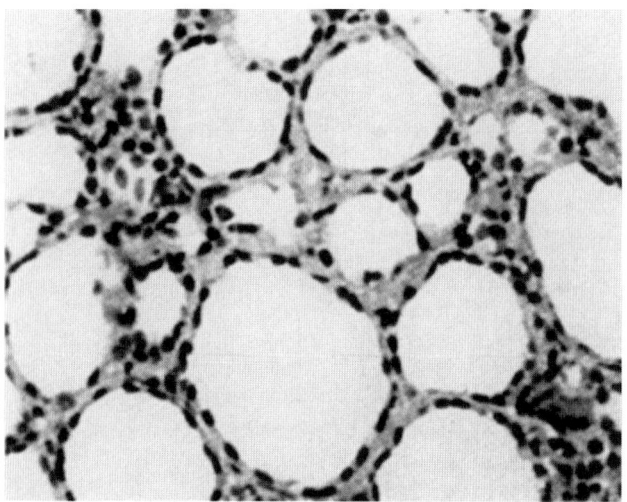

FIG. 37-9. Normal thyroid histology: follicular cells surround colloid.

EVALUATION OF PATIENTS WITH THYROID DISEASE

Tests of Thyroid Function

A multitude of different tests are available to evaluate thyroid function. No single test is sufficient to assess thyroid function in all situations and the results must be interpreted in the context of the patient's clinical condition,[6] TSH is the only test necessary in most patients with thyroid nodules that clinically appear to be euthyroid.

Serum TSH

The tests for serum TSH (normal 0.5 to 5 μU/mL) are based on the principle that monoclonal TSH antibodies are bound to a solid matrix and bind serum TSH. A second monoclonal antibody binds to a separate epitope on TSH and is labeled with radioisotope, enzyme or fluorescent tag. Therefore, the amount of serum TSH is proportional to the amount of bound secondary antibody (immunometric assay). Older radioimmunoassays for TSH were able to detect elevated TSH levels in hypothyroidism, but were not sensitive enough to detect suppressed levels of TSH characteristic of hyperthyroidism. Newer, second-generation, "sensitive" TSH assays can measure levels less than 0.1 μU/mL and third-generation or "supersensitive or ultrasensitive" assays can detect TSH levels as low as 0.01 μU/mL. Serum TSH levels reflect the ability of the anterior pituitary to detect free T_4 levels. There is an inverse relationship between the free T_4 level and the logarithm of the TSH concentration—small changes in free T_4 lead to a large shift in TSH levels. Thus, the ultrasensitive TSH assay has become the most sensitive and specific test for the diagnosis of hyper- and hypothyroidism and for optimizing T_4 replacement and suppressive therapy.

Total T_4 and Total T_3

Total T_4 (reference range: 55 to 150 nmol/L) and T_3 (reference range: 1.5 to 3.5 nmol/L) levels are measured by radioimmunoassay and measure both the free and bound components of the hormones. Total T_4 levels reflect the output from the thyroid gland, whereas T_3 levels in the nonstimulated thyroid gland are more indicative of peripheral thyroid hormone metabolism and are, therefore, not generally suitable as a general screening test. Total T_4 levels are increased not only in hyperthyroid patients, but also in those

A Major signaling pathways regulating thyroid cell growth and function

B Key steps in thyroid hormone synthesis

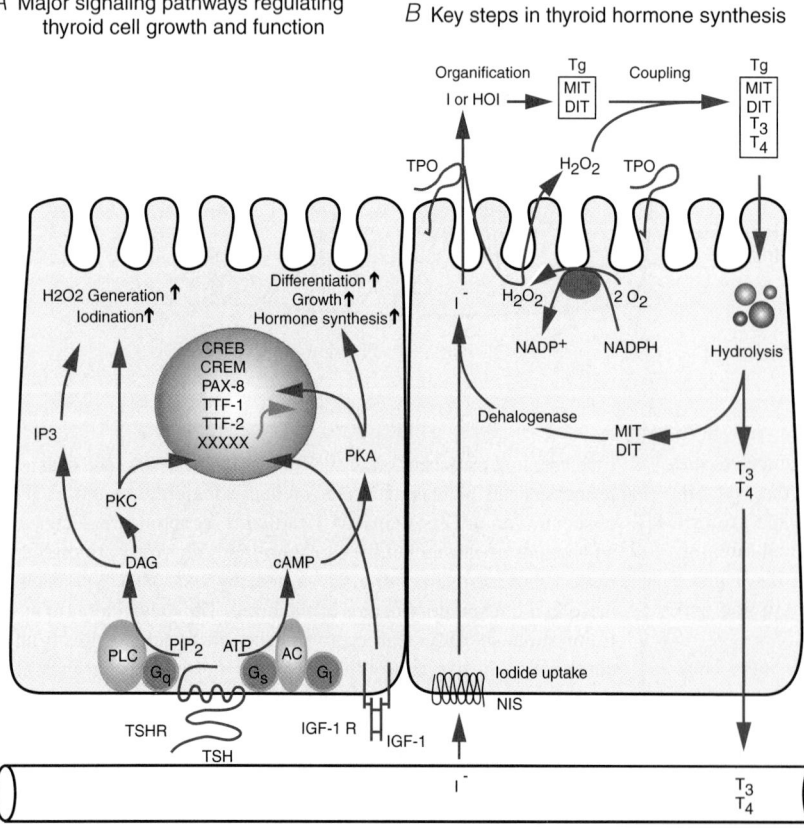

FIG. 37-10. Thyroid follicular cell showing the major signaling pathways involved in thyroid cell growth and function (A) and key steps in thyroid hormone synthesis (B). The basal membrane of the cell in contact with the circulation and its apical surface contacts the thyroid follicle. Thyroid hormone synthesis is initiated by the binding of TSH to the TSH receptor, a G-protein coupled transmembrane receptor, on the basal membrane. Activation leads to an increase in cAMP, phosphorylation of protein kinase A (PKA), and activation of target cytosolic and nuclear proteins. The protein kinase C (PKC) pathway is stimulated at higher doses of TSH. Iodide is actively transported into the cell via the Na/I symporter (NIS) and flows down an electrical gradient to the apical membrane. There, thyroid peroxidase (TPO) oxidizes iodide and iodinated tyrosyl residues on thyroglobulin (Tg) in the presence of peroxide (H_2O_2). Mono- and diiodotyrosine (MIT, DIT) residues are also coupled to form T_4 and T_3 by TPO. Thyroglobulin carrying T_4 and T_3 is then internalized by pinocytosis and digested in lysosomes. Thyroid hormone is released into the circulation, while MIT and DIT are deiodinated and recycled. CREB = cAMP response element binding protein; CREM = cAMP response element modulator; DAG = diacylglycerol; IGF-1 = insulin-like growth factor; IP3 = inositol-3-phosphate; PLC = phospholipase C. (Reproduced with permission from Kopp P, p 114.[4])

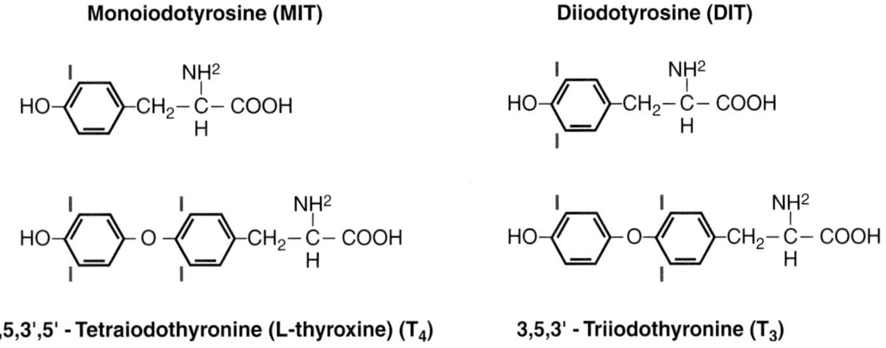

FIG. 37-11. Molecular structure of iodotyrosines and iodothyronines formed during the synthesis of thyroid hormones. In the initial steps, monoiodotyrosines (MITs) and diiodotyrosines (DITs) are formed. Tetraiodothyronine (T_4) is formed by the coupling of two DIT molecules and triiodothyronine (T_3) is formed by a similar reaction between an MIT and a DIT molecule. [*Reproduced with permission from Hurley J: Benign thyroid disease, in Randolph G (ed): Surgery of the Thyroid and Parathyroid Glands. W.B. Saunders, 2003.*]

Monoiodotyrosine (MIT)

Diiodotyrosine (DIT)

3,5,3',5' - Tetraiodothyronine (L-thyroxine) (T_4)

3,5,3' - Triiodothyronine (T_3)

patients with elevated thyroglobulin levels secondary to pregnancy, estrogen/progesterone use, or congenital diseases. Similarly, total T_4 levels decrease in hypothyroidism and in patients with decreased thyroglobulin levels caused by anabolic steroid use and by protein-losing disorders such as nephrotic syndrome. Individuals with these latter disorders may be euthyroid if their free T_4 levels are normal. Measurement of total T_3 levels is important in clinically hyperthyroid patients with normal T_4 levels, who may have T_3 thyrotoxicosis. As discussed previously, total T_3 levels are often increased in early hypothyroidism.

Free T_4 and Free T_3

These radioimmunoassay-based tests are a sensitive and accurate measurement of biologically active thyroid hormone. Free T_4 (reference range: 12 to 28 pmol/L) estimates are not performed as a routine screening tool in thyroid disease. Use of this test is confined

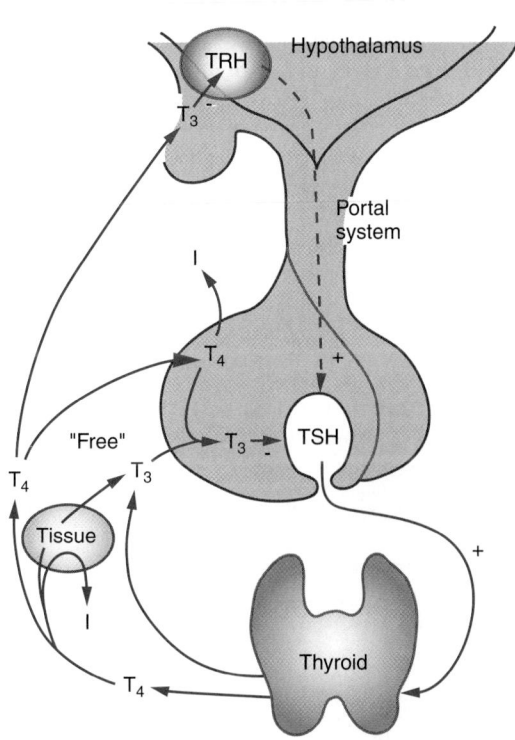

FIG. 37-12. Hypothalamic–pituitary–thyroid hormone axis. In both the hypothalamus and pituitary, T_3 is primarily responsible for inhibition of TRH and TSH secretion. (*Reproduced with permission from Greenspan F: The thyroid gland, in Greenspan F, Gardner D (eds): Basic and Clinical Endocrinology. Appleton and Lange, 2000, p. 217.*)

to cases of early hyperthyroidism in which total T_4 levels may be normal but free T_4 levels are raised. In patients with end-organ resistance to T_4 (Refetoff syndrome), T_4 levels are increased, but TSH levels usually are normal. Free T_3 (reference range: 3 to 9 pmol/L) is most useful in confirming the diagnosis of early hyperthyroidism, in which levels of free T_4 and free T_3 rise before total T_4 and T_3. Free T_4 levels may also be measured indirectly using the T_3 resin-uptake test. If free T_4 levels are increased, fewer hormone-binding sites are available for binding radiolabeled T_3 that has been added to the patient's serum. Therefore, more T_3 binds with an ion-exchange resin and the T_3 resin uptake is increased.

Thyrotropin-Releasing Hormone

This test is useful to evaluate pituitary TSH secretory function and is performed by administering 500 μg of TRH intravenously and measuring TSH levels after 30 and 60 minutes. In a normal individual, TSH levels should increase at least 6 μIU/mL from the baseline. This test was also previously used to assess patients with borderline hyperthyroidism, but has largely been replaced by sensitive TSH assays for this purpose.

Thyroid Antibodies

Thyroid antibodies include antithyroglobulin (anti-Tg), antimicrosomal or antithyroid peroxidase (anti-TPO) and thyroid-stimulating immunoglobulin (TSI). Anti-Tg and anti-TPO antibody levels do not determine thyroid function; instead, they indicate the underlying disorder, usually an autoimmune thyroiditis. Approximately 80% of patients with Hashimoto's thyroiditis have elevated thyroid antibody levels, but levels may also be increased in patients with Graves' disease, multinodular goiter, and, occasionally, with thyroid neoplasms.

Serum Thyroglobulin

Thyroglobulin is not normally released into the circulation in large amounts, but increases dramatically in destructive processes of the thyroid gland, such as thyroiditis or overactive states such as Graves' disease and toxic multinodular goiter. The most important use for serum thyroglobulin levels is in monitoring patients with differentiated thyroid cancer for recurrence, particularly after total thyroidectomy and radioactive iodine ablation.

Thyroid Imaging

Radionuclide Imaging

Both iodine-123 (^{123}I) and iodine-131 (^{131}I) are used to image the thyroid gland. The former emits low-dose radiation, has a half-life of 12 to 14 hours, and is used to image lingual thyroids or goiters.

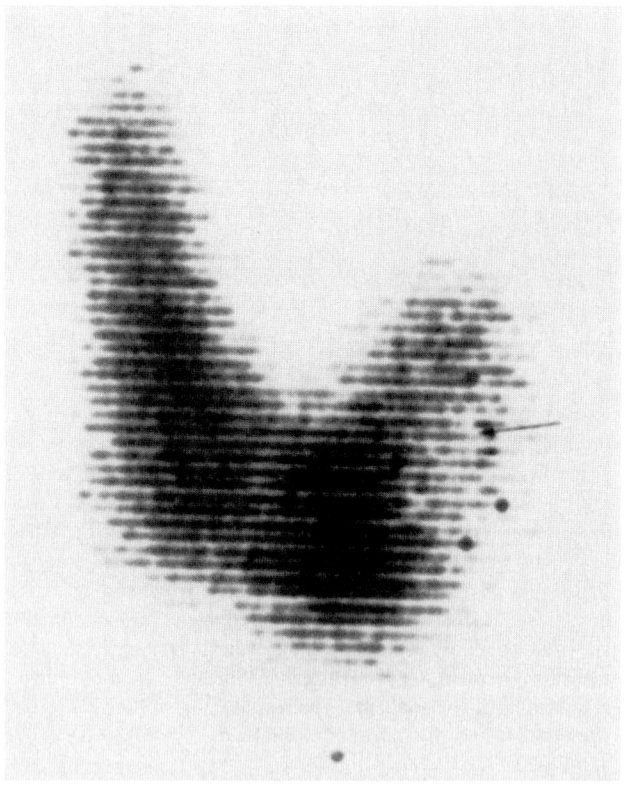

FIG. 37-13. Radioactive iodine scan of the thyroid with the arrow showing an area of decreased uptake, a cold nodule.

In contrast, ^{131}I use leads to higher-dose radiation exposure and has a half-life of 8 to 10 days. Therefore, this isotope is used to screen and treat patients with differentiated thyroid cancers for metastatic disease. The images provide information not only about the size and shape of the gland, but also the distribution of functional activity. Areas that trap less radioactivity than the surrounding gland are termed "cold" (Fig. 37-13), whereas areas that demonstrate increased activity are termed "hot." The risk of malignancy is higher in "cold" lesions (15 to 20%) than in "hot" or "warm" lesions (<5%). Technetium-99m (^{99m}Tc) pertechnetate is taken up by the thyroid gland and also used for thyroid evaluation. This isotope is taken up by the mitochondria, but is not organified. It also has the advantage

of having a shorter half-life and minimizes radiation exposure. It is particularly sensitive for nodal metastases. More recently, ^{18}F-fluorodeoxyglucose positron emission tomography (FDG PET) has been used to screen for metastases in patients with thyroid cancer, in whom other imaging studies are negative.[7] However, this technique is expensive and not widely available.

Ultrasound

Ultrasound is an excellent, noninvasive and portable imaging method for studying the thyroid gland, and it has the added advantage of no radiation exposure. It is helpful in the evaluation of thyroid nodules, distinguishing solid from cystic ones, and providing information about size and multicentricity. Ultrasound also can be used to assess for cervical lymphadenopathy (Fig. 37-14) and to guide fine-needle aspiration (FNA) biopsy. However, it cannot be used to image thyroid tissue outside the neck (e.g., to assess the extent of a substernal goiter).

CT/MRI Scan

These studies provide excellent imaging of the thyroid gland and adjacent nodes, and are particularly useful in evaluating the extent of large, fixed or substernal goiters and their relationship to the airway and vascular structures. Noncontrast CT scans should be obtained in patients who are likely to require subsequent radioactive iodine therapy.

BENIGN THYROID DISORDERS

Hyperthyroidism

The clinical manifestations of hyperthyroidism result from an excess of circulating thyroid hormone. Table 37-1 lists the conditions from which hyperthyroidism can arise. It is important to distinguish disorders such as Graves' disease and toxic nodular goiters that result from increased production of thyroid hormone from those disorders that lead to release of stored hormone from injury to the thyroid gland (thyroiditis) or from other non-thyroid gland–related conditions. The former disorders lead to an increase in radioactive iodine uptake (RAIU), whereas the latter group is characterized by low RAIU. Of these disorders, Graves' disease, toxic multinodular goiter, and solitary toxic nodule are most relevant to the surgeon and discussed in detail below. Thyroiditis is described in a later section.

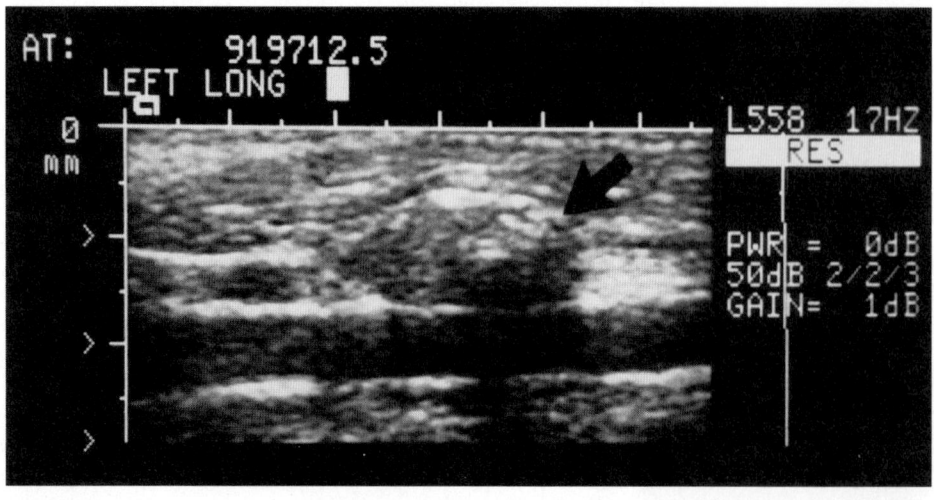

FIG. 37-14. Thyroid ultrasound showing a lymph node along the carotid artery.

Table 37-1
Differential Diagnosis of Hyperthyroidism

Increased hormone synthesis (increased RAIU)	Release of preformed hormone (decreased RAIU)
Graves' disease (diffuse toxic goiter)	Thyroiditis—acute phase of Hashimoto's thyroiditis, subacute thyroiditis
Toxic multinodular goiter	Factitious (iatrogenic) thyrotoxicosis
Plummer's disease (toxic adenoma)	"Hamburger thyrotoxicosis"
Drug induced—amiodarone, iodine (Jodbasedow)	
Thyroid cancer	
Struma ovarii	
Hydatidiform mole	
TSH-secreting pituitary adenoma	

RAIU = radioactive iodine uptake.

Graves' Disease

Although originally described by the Welsh physician Caleb Parry in a posthumous article in 1825, the disease is known as Graves' disease after Robert Graves, an Irish physician who described three patients in 1835. Graves' disease is by far the most common cause of hyperthyroidism in North America, accounting for 60 to 80% of cases. It is an autoimmune disease of unknown cause with a strong familial predisposition, female preponderance (5:1), and peak incidence between the ages of 40 and 60 years. Graves' disease is characterized by thyrotoxicosis, diffuse goiter, and extrathyroidal conditions, including ophthalmopathy, dermopathy (pretibial myxedema), thyroid acropachy, gynecomastia, and other manifestations.

Etiology, Pathogenesis, and Pathology. The exact etiology of the initiation of the autoimmune process in Graves' disease is unknown. However, conditions such as the postpartum state, iodine excess, lithium therapy, and bacterial and viral infections have been suggested as possible triggers. Genetic factors also play a role, because haplotyping studies indicate that Graves' disease is associated with certain human leukocyte antigen (HLA) haplotypes—HLA-B8 and HLA-DR3 and HLADQA1*0501 in white patients—whereas HLA-DRB1*0701 is protective. Polymorphisms of the cytotoxic T-lymphocyte antigen 4 (*CTLA-4*) gene also have been associated with Graves' disease development.[8] Once initiated, the process causes sensitized T-helper lymphocytes to stimulate B lymphocytes, which produce antibodies directed against the thyroid hormone receptor (TRAbs). TSI or antibodies (TSAbs) that stimulate the TSH receptor, as well as TSH-binding inhibiting immunoglobulins (TSIIs) or antibodies (TBIAs) have been described. The thyroid-stimulating antibodies stimulate the thyrocytes to grow and synthesize excess thyroid hormone, which is a hallmark of Graves' disease. Graves' disease is also associated with other autoimmune conditions such as type I diabetes mellitus, Addison's disease, pernicious anemia, and myasthenia gravis.

Macroscopically, the thyroid gland in patients with Graves' disease is diffusely and smoothly enlarged, with a concomitant increase in vascularity. Microscopically, the gland is hyperplastic, and the epithelium is columnar with minimal colloid present. The nuclei exhibit mitosis, and papillary projections of hyperplastic epithelium are common. There may be aggregates of lymphoid tissue, and vascularity is markedly increased.

Clinical Features. The clinical manifestations of Graves' disease can be divided into those occurring in any patient with hyperthyroidism and those specific to Graves' disease. Symptoms common to most patients with hyperthyroidism include heat intolerance, increased sweating and thirst, and weight loss despite adequate caloric intake. Symptoms of increased adrenergic stimulation include palpitations, nervousness, fatigue, emotional lability, hyperkinesis, and tremors. The most common gastrointestinal symptoms include increased frequency of bowel movements and diarrhea. Female patients often develop amenorrhea, decreased fertility, and an increased incidence of miscarriages. Children experience rapid growth with early bone maturation, whereas older patients present with cardiovascular complications such as atrial fibrillation and congestive heart failure.

On physical examination, weight loss and facial flushing may be evident. The skin may be warm and moist and African American patients often note darkening of their skin. Tachycardia or atrial fibrillation is present, with cutaneous vasodilation leading to a widening of the pulse pressure and a rapid falloff in the transmitted pulse wave (collapsing pulse). A fine tremor, muscle wasting, and proximal muscle group weakness with hyperactive tendon reflexes are often present.

Approximately 50% of patients with Graves' disease also develop clinically evident ophthalmopathy (Fig. 37-15). Eye

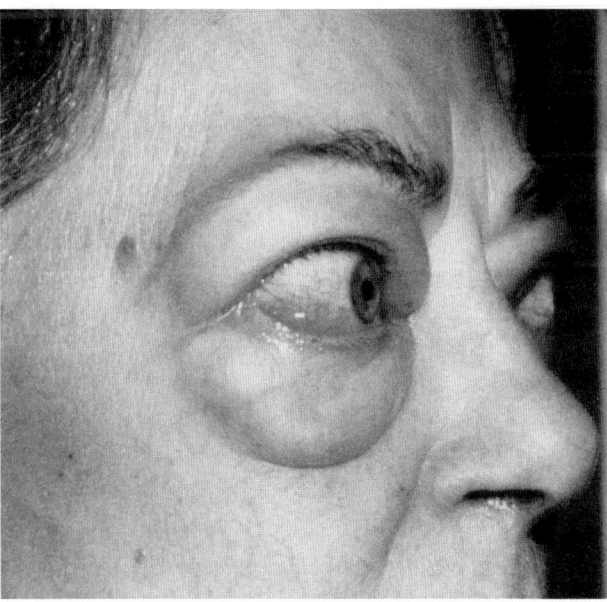

FIG. 37-15. Graves' ophthalmopathy. This patient demonstrates exophthalmos, proptosis, periorbital swelling, congestion, and edema of the conjunctiva.

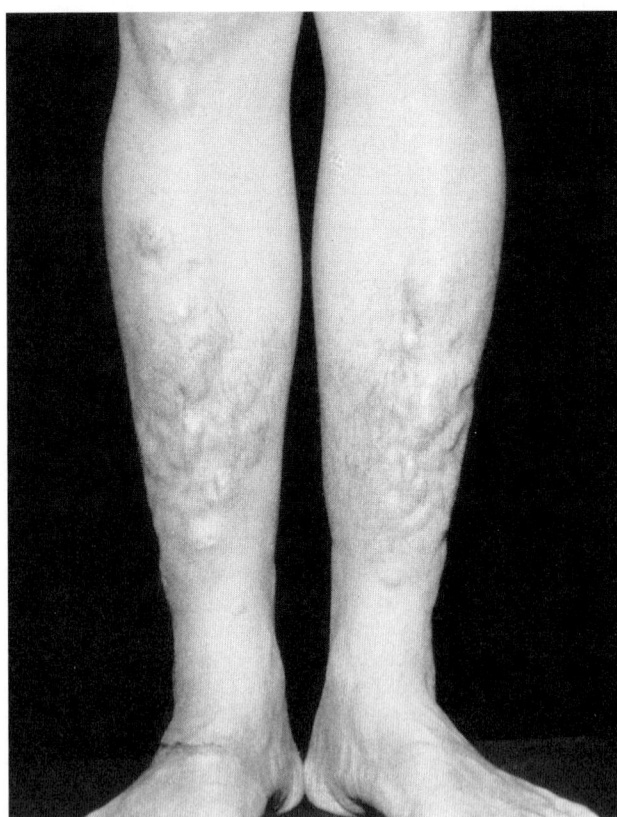

FIG. 37-16. Pretibial myxedema may be found in 3 to 5% of patients with Graves' disease.

symptoms include lid lag (von Graefe's sign), spasm of the upper eyelid revealing the sclera above the corneoscleral limbus (Dalrymple's sign), and a prominent stare as a consequence of catecholamine excess. True infiltrative eye disease results in periorbital edema, conjunctival swelling and congestion (chemosis), proptosis, limitation of upward and lateral gaze (from involvement of the inferior and medial recti muscles, respectively), keratitis, and even blindness as a result of optic nerve involvement. The etiology of Graves' ophthalmopathy is not completely known; however, orbital fibroblasts and muscles are thought to share a common antigen with thyrocytes, the TSH receptor. Ophthalmopathy results from inflammation caused by cytokines released from sensitized killer T lymphocytes and cytotoxic antibodies. Dermopathy occurs in 1 to 2% of patients and is characterized by deposition of glycosaminoglycans leading to thickened skin in the pretibial region and dorsum of the foot (Fig. 37-16). Gynecomastia is common in young men. Rare bony involvement leads to subperiosteal bone formation and swelling in the metacarpals (thyroid acropachy). Onycholysis or separation of fingernails from their beds, is a more commonly observed finding. On physical exam, the thyroid is usually diffusely and symmetrically enlarged, as evidenced by an enlarged pyramidal lobe. There may be an overlying bruit or thrill and loud venous hum in the supraclavicular space.

Diagnostic Tests. The diagnosis of hyperthyroidism is made by a suppressed TSH with or without an elevated free T_4 or T_3 level. If eye signs are present, other tests are generally not needed. However, in the absence of eye findings, an ^{123}I uptake and scan should be performed. An elevated uptake, with a diffusely enlarged gland confirms the diagnosis of Graves' disease and helps to differentiate

it from other causes of hyperthyroidism. If free T_4 levels are normal, free T_3 levels should be determined as they are often elevated in early Graves' or Plummer's disease (T_3 toxicosis). Anti-Tg and anti-TPO antibodies are elevated in up to 75% of patients, but are not specific. Elevated thyroid-stimulating hormone receptor (TSH-R) or TSAb are diagnostic of Graves' disease and are increased in approximately 90% of patients. MRI scans of the orbits are useful in evaluating Graves' ophthalmopathy.

Treatment. Graves' disease may be treated by any of three treatment modalities: antithyroid drugs, thyroid ablation with radioactive ^{131}I, and thyroidectomy.[9] The choice of treatment depends upon several factors, including the age of the patient, the severity of the disease, the size of the gland, any coexistent pathology, associated ophthalmopathy, patient's preferences, and desire for pregnancy.

Antithyroid Drugs. Antithyroid medications are generally administered in preparation for radioactive iodine ablation or surgery. The medications commonly used are propylthiouracil (PTU, 100 to 300 mg three times daily) and methimazole (10 to 30 mg three times daily). Methimazole has a longer half-life and can be dosed once daily. Both drugs reduce thyroid hormone production by inhibiting the organic binding of iodine and the coupling of iodotyrosines (mediated by thyroid peroxidase). In addition, PTU also inhibits the peripheral conversion of T_4 to T_3, making it useful for the treatment of thyroid storm. Both drugs can cross the placenta, inhibiting fetal thyroid function, and are excreted in breast milk, although PTU has a lower risk of transplacental transfer. Methimazole is also associated with congenital aplasia, therefore PTU is more preferred in pregnant and breast-feeding women. Side effects of treatment include reversible granulocytopenia, skin rashes, fever, peripheral neuritis, polyarteritis, vasculitis, and, rarely, agranulocytosis and aplastic anemia. Patients should be monitored for these possible complications and should always be warned to stop PTU or methimazole immediately and to seek medical advice, should they develop a sore throat or fever. Treatment of agranulocytosis involves admission to the hospital, discontinuing the drug and broad-spectrum antibiotic therapy. Surgery should be postponed until the granulocyte count reaches 1000 cells/m³.

The dose of antithyroid medication is titrated as needed in accordance with TSH and T_4 levels. Most patients have improved symptoms in 2 weeks and become euthyroid in about 6 weeks. Some physicians use the block–replace regimen by adding thyroxine (0.05 to 0.10 mg) to prevent hypothyroidism and to suppress TSH secretion, because a few studies suggest that this reduces recurrence rates. The length of therapy is debated. Treatment with antithyroid medications is associated with a high relapse rate when these drugs are discontinued, with 40 to 80% of patients developing recurrent disease after a 1- to 2-year course. Patients with small glands are less likely to recur so that treatment for curative intent is reserved for patients with small, nontoxic goiters (<40 g), mildly elevated thyroid hormone levels, and rapid decrease in gland size with antithyroid medications.

The catecholamine response of thyrotoxicosis can be alleviated by administering beta-blocking agents. These drugs have the added effect of decreasing the peripheral conversion of T_4 to T_3. Propranolol is the most commonly prescribed medication in doses of about 20 to 40 mg four times daily. Higher doses are sometimes required because of increased clearance of the medication.

Radioactive Iodine Therapy. Radioactive iodine (RAI; ^{131}I) forms the mainstay of Graves' disease treatment in North America. The major advantages of this form of treatment are the avoidance of a surgical procedure and its concomitant risks, reduced overall treatment costs, and ease of treatment. Antithyroid drugs are given until the patient is euthyroid and then discontinued to maximize drug uptake. The ^{131}I dose is calculated after a preliminary scan, and usually consists of 8 to 12 mCi administered orally. However, RAI is associated with the progressive development of hypothyroidism (over 70% at 11 years), requiring lifelong thyroxine replacement therapy. It is also more often associated with progression of Graves' ophthalmopathy. After standard treatment with RAI, most patients become euthyroid within 2 months. Unfortunately, only approximately 50% of patients treated with RAI are euthyroid 6 months after treatment, and the remaining are still hyperthyroid or already hypothyroid.[10] After 1 year, approximately 2.5% of patients develop hypothyroidism each year. RAI also has been documented to lead to progression of Graves' ophthalmopathy (33% after RAI as compared to 16% after surgery), and ophthalmopathy is more common in smokers. Although there is no evidence of long-term problems with infertility, and overall cancer incidence rates are unchanged, there is a small increased risk of nodular goiter, thyroid cancer,[11] and hyperparathyroidism[12] in patients who have been treated with RAI. Therapy may also precipitate cardiac arrhythmias and arrest, particularly in elderly patients. Lastly, patients treated with RAI have an unexplained increase in their overall cardiovascular mortality rates when compared to the general population.

Consequently, RAI therapy is most often used in older patients with small or moderate-size goiters, in patients who have relapsed after medical or surgical therapy, and in patients in whom antithyroid drugs or surgery are contraindicated. Absolute contraindications to RAI include women who are pregnant or breast-feeding. Relative contraindications include young patients (especially children and adolescents), patients with thyroid nodules, and patients with ophthalmopathy. The higher the initial dose of ^{131}I, the earlier the onset and the higher the incidence of hypothyroidism. Women of childbearing age are advised to wait at least 1 year after RAI before attempting to conceive.

Surgical Treatment. In North America, surgery is recommended when RAI is contraindicated, as in patients who (1) have confirmed cancer or suspicious thyroid nodules, (2) are young, (3) are pregnant or desire to conceive soon after treatment, (4) have allergies to antithyroid medications, (5) have large goiters causing compressive symptoms, and (6) are reluctant to undergo RAI therapy. Relative indications for thyroidectomy include patients, particularly smokers, with moderate to severe Graves' ophthalmopathy, patients who desire rapid control of hyperthyroidism with a chance of being euthyroid, and patients who demonstrate poor compliance with antithyroid medications. The goal of thyroidectomy for Graves' disease should be the complete and permanent control of the disease with minimal morbidity related to RLN injury or hypoparathyroidism. Patients should be rendered euthyroid before operation with antithyroid drugs that should be continued up to the day of surgery. Lugol's iodide solution or supersaturated potassium iodide (SSKI) should also be administered preoperatively—3 drops twice daily beginning 10 days preoperatively—to reduce vascularity of the gland and decrease the risk of precipitating thyroid storm. The major action of iodine in this situation is to inhibit release of thyroid hormone.

The extent of thyroidectomy to be performed is controversial and is determined by the desired outcome (risk of recurrence versus euthyroidism) and surgeon experience. Patients with coexistent thyroid cancer, and those patients who refuse RAI therapy, who have severe ophthalmopathy, or who have life-threatening reactions to antithyroid medications, such as vasculitis, agranulocytosis, or liver failure, should undergo total or near-total thyroidectomy, which can

be performed with minimal morbidity by an experienced thyroid surgeon. Ophthalmopathy has been demonstrated to stabilize or improve in most patients after total thyroidectomy, presumably from removal of the antigenic stimulus. A subtotal thyroidectomy, leaving a 4- to 7-g remnant, is recommended for all remaining patients. Remnants smaller than 3 g are associated with a 2 to 10% recurrence rate, but a high (>40%) rate of hypothyroidism. During subtotal thyroidectomy, 1 to 2 g of remnant tissue may be left on each side (bilateral subtotal thyroidectomy), or a total lobectomy can be performed on one side with a subtotal thyroidectomy on the other side (Hartley-Dunhill procedure), which these authors prefer. Results are similar with either procedure,[13] but the latter procedure is theoretically associated with fewer complications and requires reentering only one side of the neck should recurrence require reoperation. Most studies, however, show no difference in the rates of complications with either approach. Recurrent thyrotoxicosis is usually managed by radioiodine treatment. Long-term follow-up should be maintained for all patients, with clinical review and yearly TSH measurement to detect the possible late onset of hypothyroidism or recurrent hyperthyroidism.

Toxic Multinodular Goiter

Toxic multinodular goiters usually occur in individuals older than 50 years of age, who often have a prior history of a nontoxic multinodular goiter. Over several years, enough thyroid nodules become autonomous to cause hyperthyroidism. The presentation is often insidious in that hyperthyroidism may only become apparent when patients are placed on low doses of thyroid hormone suppression for the goiter. Some patients have T_3 toxicosis, whereas other patients have apathetic hyperthyroidism, atrial fibrillation, or congestive heart failure. Hyperthyroidism can also be precipitated by iodide-containing drugs such as contrast media and the antiarrhythmic agent amiodarone (Jodbasedow phenomenon). Symptoms and signs of hyperthyroidism are similar to Graves' disease, but are less severe and extrathyroidal manifestations are absent.

Diagnostic Studies. Blood tests are similar to Graves' disease with a suppressed TSH level and elevated free T_4 or T_3 levels. RAI uptake is also increased, showing multiple nodules with increased uptake and suppression of the remaining gland.

Treatment. Hyperthyroidism must be adequately controlled as described above. Surgical resection is the preferred treatment method for patients with toxic multinodular goiter, with subtotal thyroidectomy being the standard procedure. Remnant size is not as crucial a concern because these patients require thyroid hormone suppression to prevent recurrence of the goiter. The Hartley-Dunhill procedure is preferred over a bilateral subtotal thyroidectomy for the reasons outlined earlier. Care must be taken in identifying the RLN, which may be found laterally on the thyroid (rather than posterior) or stretched anteriorly over a nodule. Total thyroidectomy may sometimes be necessary if no normal thyroid tissue is present posteriorly.

RAI therapy is reserved for elderly patients who represent very poor operative risks, provided there is no airway compression from the goiter and thyroid cancer is not a concern. However, because uptake is less than in Graves' disease, larger doses of RAI often are needed to treat the hyperthyroidism. Furthermore, RAI-induced thyroiditis has the potential to cause swelling and acute airway compromise, and leaves the goiter intact, with the possibility of recurrent hyperthyroidism.

Plummer's Disease (Toxic Adenoma)

Hyperthyroidism from a single hyperfunctioning nodule typically occurs in younger patients who note recent growth of a long-standing nodule along with the symptoms of hyperthyroidism. Most toxic adenomas are characterized by somatic mutations in the TSH receptor gene; G-protein-stimulating gene (*gsp*) mutations occur less commonly.[14] Most hyperfunctioning or autonomous thyroid nodules have attained a size of at least 3 cm before hyperthyroidism occurs. Physical examination usually reveals a solitary thyroid nodule without palpable thyroid tissue on the contralateral side. RAI scanning shows a "hot" nodule with suppression of the rest of the thyroid gland. These nodules are rarely malignant. Smaller nodules may be managed with antithyroid medications and RAI, but rarely cause hyperthyroidism. Surgery (lobectomy and isthmusectomy) is recommended to treat young patients and those with larger nodules.

Thyroid Storm

Thyroid storm is a condition of hyperthyroidism accompanied by fever, central nervous system agitation or depression, cardiovascular dysfunction that may be precipitated by infection, surgery, or trauma. Occasionally, thyroid storm may result from amiodarone administration. This condition was previously associated with high mortality rates, but can be appropriately managed in an ICU setting. Beta blockers are given to reduce peripheral T_4-to-T_3 conversion and to decrease the hyperthyroid symptoms. Oxygen supplementation and hemodynamic support should be instituted. Nonaspirin compounds can be used to treat pyrexia, and Lugol's iodine or sodium ipodate (intravenously) should be administered to decrease iodine uptake and thyroid hormone secretion. PTU therapy blocks the formation of new thyroid hormone and reduces peripheral conversion of T_4 to T_3, and corticosteroids help to prevent adrenal exhaustion. Corticosteroids also block hepatic thyroid hormone conversion.

Hypothyroidism

Deficiency in the circulating levels of thyroid hormone leads to hypothyroidism, and, in neonates, to cretinism, which is characterized by neurologic impairment and mental retardation. Hypothyroidism may also be associated with deafness (Pendred's syndrome)[4] and Turner's syndrome. Table 37-2 lists conditions that cause hypothyroidism.

Clinical Features

Failure of thyroid gland development or function in utero leads to cretinism and characteristic facies similar to those of children with Down syndrome and dwarfism. Failure to thrive and severe mental retardation are often present. Immediate testing and treatment with thyroid hormone at birth can lessen the neurologic and intellectual deficits. Hypothyroidism developing in childhood or adolescence results in delayed development and may also lead to abdominal distention, umbilical hernia, and rectal prolapse. Mental performance tends to be diminished with the onset of hypothyroidism after 6 months of age, but severe retardation is uncommon. In adults, symptoms in general are nonspecific; they include tiredness, weight gain, cold intolerance, constipation, and menorrhagia. Patients with severe hypothyroidism or myxedema develop characteristic facial features as a consequence of the deposition of glycosaminoglycans in the subcutaneous tissues, leading to facial and periorbital puffiness. The skin becomes rough and dry and often develops a yellowish hue from reduced conversion of carotene to vitamin A. Hair becomes dry and brittle, and severe hair loss may occur. There also is a characteristic loss of the outer two-thirds of the eyebrows. An enlarged tongue may impair speech, which is already slowed, in keeping with the impairment of mental processes. Untreated dementia may lead to myxedema madness. Patients may also have nonspecific abdominal pain accompanied by distention and constipation. Libido and fertility are impaired in both sexes. Cardiovascular changes in hypothyroidism include bradycardia, cardiomegaly, pericardial effusion, reduced cardiac output, and pulmonary effusions. Cardiac failure is uncommon. When hypothyroidism occurs as a result of pituitary failure, features of hypopituitarism such as pale, waxy skin, loss of body hair, and atrophic genitalia may be present.

Laboratory Findings

Hypothyroidism is characterized by low circulating levels of T_4 and T_3. Raised TSH levels are found in primary thyroid failure, whereas secondary hypothyroidism is characterized by low TSH levels that do not increase following TRH stimulation. Thyroid autoantibodies are present and are highest in patients with autoimmune disease (Hashimoto's thyroiditis, Graves' disease), although they are also elevated in patients with nodular goiter and thyroid neoplasms. Other findings include anemia, hypercholesterolemia, and decreased voltage with flattening or inversion of T waves on electrocardiogram. Comatose patients with myxedema also have hyponatremia and CO_2 retention.

Treatment

Thyroxine is the treatment of choice and is administered in dosages varying from 50 to 200 μg per day, depending upon patient's size and condition. Starting doses of 100 μg of thyroxine daily are well tolerated; however, elderly patients and those with coexisting heart disease and profound hypothyroidism should be started on a considerably lower dose such as 25 to 50 μg daily because of associated hypercholesterolemia and atherosclerosis. The dose can be slowly increased over weeks to months to attain a euthyroid state. A baseline ECG should always be obtained in patients with severe hypothyroidism prior to treatment. Patients are instructed to take tablets in the morning, usually without other medications, or at mealtime to assure good absorption. Thyroxine dosage is titrated against clinical response and TSH levels, which should return to normal. The management of patients with subclinical hypothyroidism (normal T_4, slightly raised TSH) is controversial. Evidence suggests that patients with subclinical hypothyroidism and increased antithyroid antibody levels should be treated because they will subsequently develop hypothyroidism. Patients who present with myxedema coma, in contrast to the patients with mild to moderate hypothyroidism, require an initial emergency treatment with large doses of

Table 37-2
Causes of Hypothyroidism

Primary (increased TSH levels)
Hashimoto's thyroiditis
RAI therapy for Graves' disease
Postthyroidectomy
Excessive iodine intake
Subacute thyroiditis
Medications: antithyroid drugs, lithium
Rare: iodine deficiency, dyshormonogenesis
Secondary (decreased TSH levels)
Pituitary tumor
Pituitary resection or ablation
Tertiary
Hypothalamic insufficiency
Resistance to thyroid hormone

intravenous thyroxine (300 to 400 μg), and careful monitoring in an ICU setting.

Thyroiditis

Thyroiditis is defined as an inflammatory disorder of the thyroid gland and is usually classified into acute, subacute, and chronic forms, each associated with a distinct clinical presentation and histology. Chronic and subacute thyroiditis is usually managed medically, but surgical treatment is occasionally needed.

Acute (Suppurative) Thyroiditis

The thyroid gland is inherently resistant to infection as a consequence of its extensive blood and lymphatic supply, high iodide content, and fibrous capsule, but infectious agents can seed it (1) via the hematogenous or lymphatic route; (2) via direct spread from persistent pyriform sinus fistulae or thyroglossal duct cysts; (3) as a result of penetrating trauma to the thyroid gland; or (4) as a result of immunosuppression. *Streptococcus* and anaerobes account for about 70% of cases, but *Escherichia coli, Pseudomonas aeruginosa, Haemophilus influenzae, Eikenella corrodens, Corynebacterium, and Coccidiomycosis* species also have been cultured.[15]

Acute suppurative thyroiditis is more common in children and is often preceded by an upper respiratory tract infection or otitis media. It is characterized by severe neck pain radiating to the jaws or ear, fever, chills, odynophagia, and dysphonia. Rarely, complications such as systemic sepsis, tracheal or esophageal rupture, jugular vein thrombosis, laryngeal chondritis or perichondritis and sympathetic trunk paralysis may result.

The diagnosis is established by leukocytosis on blood tests and FNA biopsy for Gram's stain, culture, and cytology. CT scans may help to delineate the extent of infection. A persistent pyriform sinus fistula should always be suspected in children with recurrent acute thyroiditis. A barium swallow demonstrates the anomalous tract with 80% sensitivity. Treatment consists of parenteral antibiotics and drainage of abscesses. Patients with pyriform sinus fistulae require complete resection of the sinus tract, including the area of the thyroid where the tract terminates, in order to prevent recurrence.

Subacute Thyroiditis

Subacute thyroiditis can occur in either the painful or painless forms. Although the exact etiology is unknown, painful thyroiditis is thought to be viral in origin or result from a postviral inflammatory response. Genetic predisposition may also play a role, as manifested by its strong association with the HLA-B35 haplotype. One model of pathogenesis suggests that viral or thyroid antigens, when presented by macrophages in the context of HLA-B35, stimulate cytotoxic T lymphocytes and damage thyroid follicular cells.

Painful thyroiditis most commonly occurs in 30- to 40-year-old women and is characterized by the sudden or gradual onset of neck pain, which may radiate toward the mandible or ear. History of a preceding upper respiratory tract infection can often be elicited. The gland is enlarged, exquisitely tender, and firm. The disorder classically progresses through four stages. An initial hyperthyroid phase, caused by release of thyroid hormone, is followed by a second, euthyroid phase. The third phase, hypothyroidism, occurs in approximately 20 to 30% of patients and is followed by resolution and return to the euthyroid state in greater than 90% of patients. A few patients develop recurrent disease.

In the early stages of the disease, TSH is decreased, and thyroglobulin, T_4 and T_3 levels are elevated as a result of the release of preformed thyroid hormone from destroyed follicles. Erythrocyte

sedimentation rate (ESR) is typically greater than 100 mm/h. RAIU is also decreased (<2% at 24 hours), even in euthyroid patients, because of the release of thyroid hormones with TSH suppression from destruction of the thyroid parenchyma. Painful thyroiditis is self-limited and therefore, treatment is primarily symptomatic. Aspirin and other nonsteroidal anti-inflammatory drugs (NSAIDs) are used for pain relief, but steroids may be indicated in more severe cases. Short-term thyroid replacement may be needed after the hyperthyroid phase and may shorten the duration of symptoms. Thyroidectomy is reserved for the rare patient who has a prolonged course not responsive to medical measures or for recurrent disease.

Painless thyroiditis is considered to be autoimmune in origin and may occur sporadically or in the postpartum period; the latter typically occurs at about 6 weeks after delivery in women with high TPO antibody titers in early pregnancy.[16] This timing is thought to coincide with a decrease in the normal immune tolerance of pregnancy and consequent rebound elevation of antibody titers. Silent thyroiditis can also develop after therapeutic doses of external beam radiation or after drugs such as interferon-α.

Painless thyroiditis is also more common in women and usually occurs between 30 and 60 years of age. Physical examination demonstrates a normal sized or minimally enlarged, slightly firm, nontender gland. Laboratory tests and RAIU are similar to those in painful thyroiditis, except for a normal ESR. The clinical course also parallels painful thyroiditis. Specific treatment is sometimes required in patients with symptoms and includes beta blockers and thyroid hormone replacement. Thyroidectomy or RAI ablation is only indicated for the rare patient with recurrent, disabling episodes of thyroiditis.

Chronic Thyroiditis

Lymphocytic (Hashimoto's) Thyroiditis. This disorder was first described by Hashimoto, in 1912, as *struma lymphomatosa*—a transformation of thyroid tissue to lymphoid tissue—and is the most common inflammatory disorder of the thyroid and the leading cause of hypothyroidism.

Etiology, Pathogenesis, and Pathology. Hashimoto's thyroiditis is an autoimmune process that is thought to be initiated by the activation of CD4+T (helper) lymphocytes with specificity for thyroid antigens. Once activated, T cells can recruit cytotoxic CD8+T cells to the thyroid. Hypothyroidism results not only from the destruction of thyrocytes by cytotoxic T cells, but also from autoantibodies, which lead to complement fixation and killing by natural killer cells or block the TSH receptor. Antibodies are directed against the three main antigens—Tg (60%), TPO (95%), the TSH-R (60%)[17]—and less commonly against the sodium/iodine symporter (25%). Apoptosis (programmed cell death) is also implicated in the pathogenesis of Hashimoto's thyroiditis. Chronic thyroiditis is also associated with increased intake of iodine and administration of medications such as interferon-α, lithium, and amiodarone. Support for an inherited predisposition includes an increased incidence of thyroid autoantibodies in first-degree relatives of patients with Hashimoto's thyroiditis, as compared to controls, and by the occurrence of the autoantibodies and hypothyroidism in patients with specific chromosomal abnormalities such as Turner's syndrome and Down syndrome. Associations with HLA-B8, DR3, and DR5 haplotypes of the major histocompatibility complex also have been described.

On gross examination, the thyroid gland is usually mildly enlarged throughout and has a pale, gray-tan cut surface that is granular, nodular, and firm. On microscopic examination, the gland is diffusely infiltrated by small lymphocytes and plasma cells, and occasionally shows well-developed germinal centers. Thyroid follicles are smaller than normal with reduced amounts of colloid and increased interstitial connective tissue. The follicles are lined by Hürthle or Askanazy cells, which are characterized by abundant eosinophilic, granular cytoplasm.

Clinical Presentation. Like other autoimmune diseases, Hashimoto's thyroiditis is also more common in women (male: female ratio 1:10 to 20) between the ages of 30 and 50 years. The most common presentation is that of a minimally or moderately enlarged firm gland discovered on routine physical examination or the awareness of a painless anterior neck mass, although 20% of patients present with hypothyroidism, and 5% present with hyperthyroidism (hashitoxicosis). In classic goitrous Hashimoto's thyroiditis, physical examination reveals a diffusely enlarged, firm gland, which is also lobulated. An enlarged pyramidal lobe is often palpable. Thyroid-associated ophthalmopathy is rare in patients with chronic autoimmune thyroiditis.

Diagnostic Studies. When Hashimoto's thyroiditis is suspected clinically, an elevated TSH, reduced T_4 and T_3 levels, and the presence of thyroid autoantibodies confirm the diagnosis. FNA biopsy is indicated in patients who present with a solitary suspicious nodule or a rapidly enlarging goiter. Thyroid lymphoma is a rare but well-recognized, ominous complication of chronic autoimmune thyroiditis, and has a prevalence 80 times higher than expected frequency in this population than in a control population without thyroiditis.[18]

Treatment. Thyroid hormone replacement therapy is indicated in overtly hypothyroid patients, with a goal of maintaining normal TSH levels. The management of patients with subclinical hypothyroidism (normal T_4 and elevated TSH) is controversial. Because these patients do progress to overt hypothyroidism, treatment is generally recommended, especially for male patients and those with TSH greater than 10 mU/L.[19] Treatment is also indicated in euthyroid patients to shrink large goiters. Surgery may occasionally be indicated for suspicion of malignancy or for goiters causing compressive symptoms or cosmetic deformity.

Riedel's Thyroiditis. This rare variant of thyroiditis, also known as Riedel's struma or invasive fibrous thyroiditis, is characterized by the replacement of all or part of the thyroid parenchyma by fibrous tissue, which also invades into adjacent tissues. The etiology of this disorder is controversial and it has been reported to occur in patients with other autoimmune diseases, such as pernicious anemia and Graves' disease. This association, coupled with the presence of lymphoid infiltration and response to steroid therapy, suggests a primary autoimmune etiology. Riedel's thyroiditis also is associated with other focal sclerosing syndromes, including mediastinal, retroperitoneal, periorbital, and retro-orbital fibrosis, and sclerosing cholangitis, suggesting that it may in fact be a primary fibrotic disorder.

The disease occurs predominantly in women between the ages of 30 and 60 years. It typically presents as a painless, hard anterior neck mass, which progresses over weeks to years to produce symptoms of compression including dysphagia, dyspnea, choking, and hoarseness. Patients may present with symptoms of hypothyroidism and hypoparathyroidism as the gland is replaced by fibrous tissue. Physical examination reveals a hard, "woody" thyroid gland with fixation to surrounding tissues. The diagnosis needs to be confirmed by open thyroid biopsy, because the firm and fibrous nature of the gland renders FNA biopsy inadequate.

Surgery is the mainstay of the treatment. The chief goal of operation is to decompress the trachea by wedge excision of the thyroid isthmus and to make a tissue diagnosis. More extensive resections are not advised because of the infiltrative nature of the fibrotic

Table 37-3
Etiology of Nontoxic Goiter

Endemic: iodine deficiency, dietary goitrogens
Medications: iodide, amiodarone, lithium
Thyroiditis: subacute, chronic
Familial: hormonal dysgenesis from enzyme defects
Resistance to thyroid hormone
Neoplasm

process that obscures usual landmarks and structures. Hypothyroid patients are treated with thyroid hormone replacement. Some patients who remain symptomatic have been reported to experience dramatic improvement after treatment with corticosteroids and tamoxifen.[20]

Goiter

Any enlargement of the thyroid gland is referred to as a goiter. Table 37-3 lists the causes of nontoxic goiters. Most nontoxic goiters are thought to result from TSH stimulation secondary to inadequate thyroid hormone synthesis and other paracrine growth factors.[21] The thyroid gland enlarges in order to maintain the patient in a euthyroid state. Goiters may be diffuse, uninodular, or multinodular. Familial goiters resulting from inherited deficiencies in enzymes necessary for thyroid hormone synthesis may be complete or partial. The former leads to cretinism, whereas the latter leads to mild hypothyroidism, elevated TSH, and a goiter, although patients may be euthyroid. At least five different enzyme deficiencies have been described affecting steps such as iodine transport, oxidation, coupling, and deiodination. The term endemic goiter refers to the occurrence of a goiter in a significant proportion of individuals in a particular geographic region. In the past, dietary iodine deficiency was the most common cause of endemic goiter. This condition has largely disappeared in North America as a consequence of routine use of iodized salt and iodination of fertilizers, animal feeds, and preservatives. However, in areas of iodine deficiency, such as Central Asia, South American, and Indonesia, up to 90% of the population have goiters. Other dietary goitrogens that may participate in endemic goiter formation include kelp, cassava, and cabbage. In many sporadic goiters, no obvious cause can be identified.

Elevated TSH levels induce diffuse thyroid hyperplasia, followed by focal hyperplasia resulting in nodules that may or may not concentrate iodine, colloid nodules, or microfollicular nodules. The TSH-dependent nodules progress to become autonomous, possibly related to activation of the TSH receptor gene, and, less commonly to the *gsp* proto-oncogene.

Clinical Features

Most patients with nontoxic goiters are asymptomatic, although patients often complain of a pressure sensation in the neck, particularly with motion. As the goiters become very large (Fig. 37-17), compressive symptoms, such as dyspnea and dysphagia, ensue. Patients also describe having to clear their throats frequently (catarrh). Dysphonia from recurrent laryngeal nerve injury is rare, except when malignancy is present. Obstruction of venous return at the thoracic inlet from a substernal goiter results in a positive Pemberton's sign—facial flushing and dilatation of cervical veins upon raising the arms above the head (Fig. 37-18). Sudden enlargement of nodules or cysts because of hemorrhage may cause acute pain. Physical examination may reveal a soft, diffusely enlarged gland (simple goiter) or nodules of various size and consistency in case of a multinodular goiter. Deviation of the trachea may be apparent.

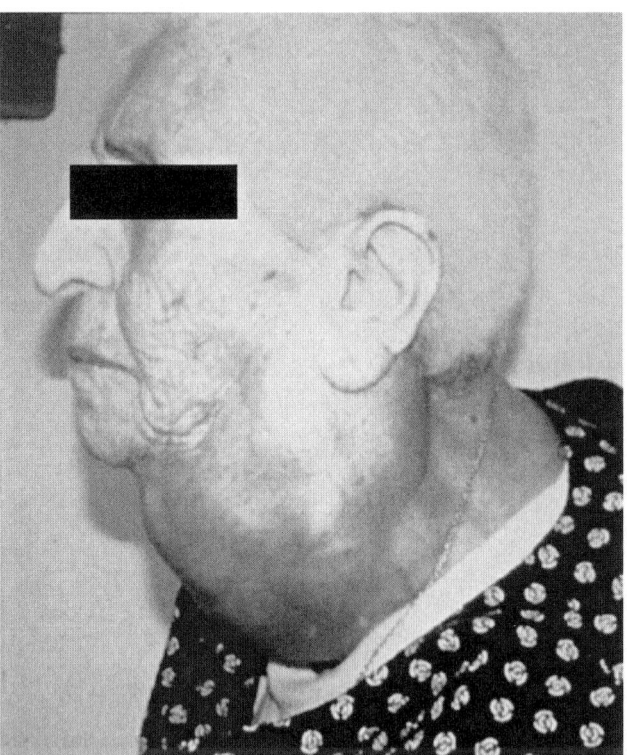

FIG. 37-17. Elderly patient with a multinodular goiter.

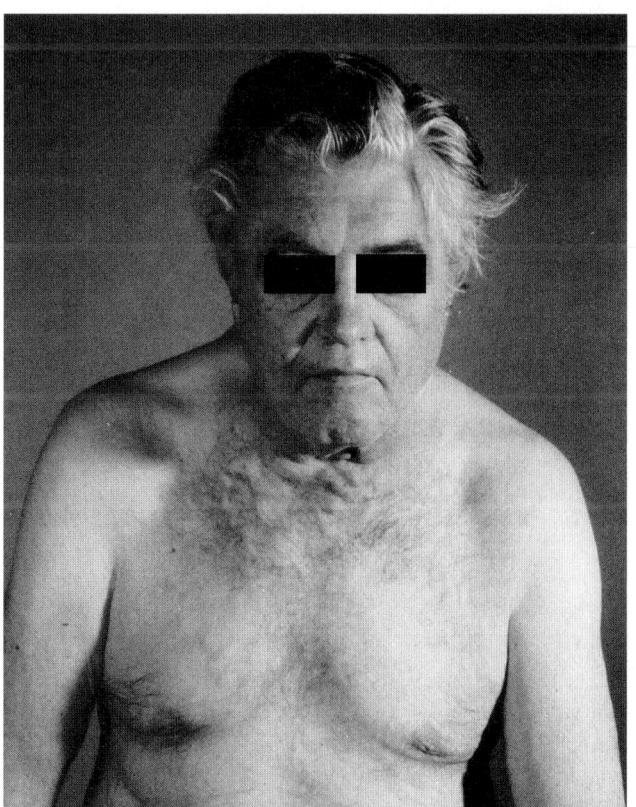

FIG. 37-18. Retrosternal extension of a large goiter may result in impeded flow in the superior vena cava, leading to dilated veins over the chest wall. This may become more prominent when the patient raises his arms above the head (Pemberton's sign).

Diagnostic Tests

Patients are usually euthyroid with normal TSH and low-normal or normal free T_4 levels. If some nodules develop autonomy, patients have suppressed TSH levels or become hyperthyroid. RAI uptake often shows patchy uptake with areas of hot and cold nodules. FNA biopsy is recommended in patients who have a dominant nodule or one that is painful or enlarging, as carcinomas have been reported in 5 to 10% of multinodular goiters. CT scans are helpful to evaluate the extent of retrosternal extension and airway compression (Fig. 37-19).

Treatment

Most euthyroid patients with small, diffuse goiters do not require treatment. Some physicians give patients with large goiters exogenous thyroid hormone to reduce the TSH stimulation of gland growth; this treatment may result in a decrease and/or stabilization of goiter size. Endemic goiters are treated by iodine administration. Surgical resection is reserved for goiters that (1) continue to increase despite T_4 suppression, (2) cause obstructive symptoms, (3) have substernal extension, (4) are suspected to be malignant or are proven malignant by FNA biopsy, and (5) are cosmetically unacceptable. Subtotal thyroidectomy is the treatment of choice and patients require lifelong T_4 therapy to prevent recurrence.

SOLITARY THYROID NODULE

Solitary thyroid nodules are present in approximately 4% of individuals in the United States, whereas thyroid cancer has a much lower incidence of 40 new cases per 1 million. Hence, the majority of thyroid nodules are benign and do not require removal. Therefore, it is of utmost importance to determine which patients with solitary thyroid nodule would benefit from surgery.

History

Details regarding the nodule, such as time of onset, change in size, and associated symptoms, such as pain, dysphagia, dyspnea, or choking, should be elicited. Pain is an unusual symptom and when present, should raise suspicion for intrathyroidal hemorrhage in a benign nodule, thyroiditis, or malignancy. Patients with medullary thyroid cancer may complain of a dull, aching sensation. A history of hoarseness is worrisome because it may be secondary to malignant involvement of the recurrent laryngeal nerves. Most importantly, patients should be questioned regarding risk factors for malignancy, such as exposure to ionizing radiation and family history of thyroid and other malignancies associated with thyroid cancer.

External Beam Radiation

Low-dose therapeutic radiation has been used to treat conditions such as tinea capitis (6.5 cGy), thymic enlargement (100 to 400 cGy), enlarged tonsils and adenoids (750 cGy), acne vulgaris (200 to 1500 cGy), and other conditions, such as hemangioma and scrofula. Radiation (approximately 4000 cGy) is also an integral part of the management of patients with Hodgkin's disease. It is now known that a history of exposure to low-dose ionizing radiation to the thyroid gland places the patient at increased risk for developing thyroid cancer. The risk increases linearly from 6.5 to 2000 cGy, beyond which the incidence declines as the radiation causes destruction of the thyroid tissue. The risk is maximum 20 to 30 years after exposure, but these patients require lifelong monitoring. During the more recent nuclear fallout from Chernobyl in 1986, ^{131}I release was accompanied by a marked increase in the incidence

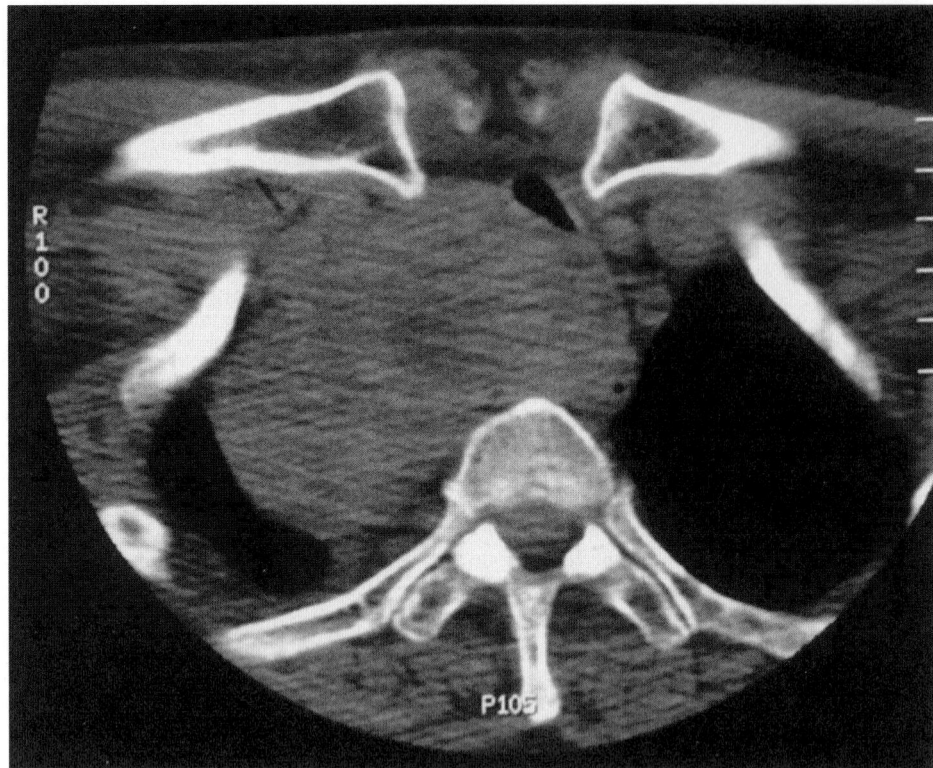

FIG. 37-19. CT scan demonstrating retrosternal extension and consequent tracheal deviation and compression of a large goiter.

of both benign and malignant thyroid lesions first noted within 4 years of exposure, particularly in children.[22] Most thyroid carcinomas following radiation exposure are papillary and some of these cancers with a solid type of histology and presence of RET/PTC (RET protein/papillary thyroid cancer) translocations appear to be more aggressive, with a higher incidence of local invasion, multifocality, lymph node metastases, and a higher stage at presentation. There is a 40% chance that patients presenting with a thyroid nodule and a history of radiation have thyroid cancer. Of those patients who have thyroid cancer, the cancer is located in the dominant nodule in 60% of patients, but is in another nodule in the thyroid gland in the remaining 40% of patients.

Family History

A family history of thyroid cancer is a risk factor for the development of both medullary and nonmedullary thyroid cancer.[23] Familial medullary thyroid cancers occur in isolation or in association with other tumors as part of multiple endocrine neoplasia type

2 (MEN2) syndromes. Nonmedullary thyroid cancers can occur in association with other known familial cancer syndromes such as Cowden's syndrome, Werner's (adult progeroid) syndrome, and familial adenomatous polyposis (Table 37-4). Nonmedullary thyroid cancers also can occur independently of these syndromes. Candidate loci that predispose to these tumors have been identified, but they account for only a small proportion of families.

Physical Examination

Thyroid masses move with swallowing and failure to observe the patient swallowing may lead one to miss a large substernal goiter. The thyroid gland is best palpated from behind the patient and with the neck in mild extension. The cricoid cartilage is an important landmark, because the isthmus is situated just below it. Nodules that are hard, gritty, or fixed to surrounding structures, such as to the trachea or strap muscles, are more likely to be malignant. The cervical chain of lymph nodes should be assessed as well as the nodes in the posterior triangle. One should examine the patient for

Table 37-4
Familial Cancer Syndromes Causing Nonmedullary Thyroid Cancer

Syndrome	Gene	Manifestation	Thyroid Tumor
Cowden's syndrome	PTEN	Intestinal hamartomas, benign and malignant breast tumors	FTC, rarely PTC and Hürthle cell tumors
FAP	APC	Colon polyps and cancer, duodenal neoplasms, desmoids	PTC
Werner's syndrome	WRN	Adult progeroid syndrome	PTC, FTC, anaplastic cancer

FAP = familial adenomatous polyposis; FTC = follicular thyroid cancer; PTC = papillary thyroid cancer.

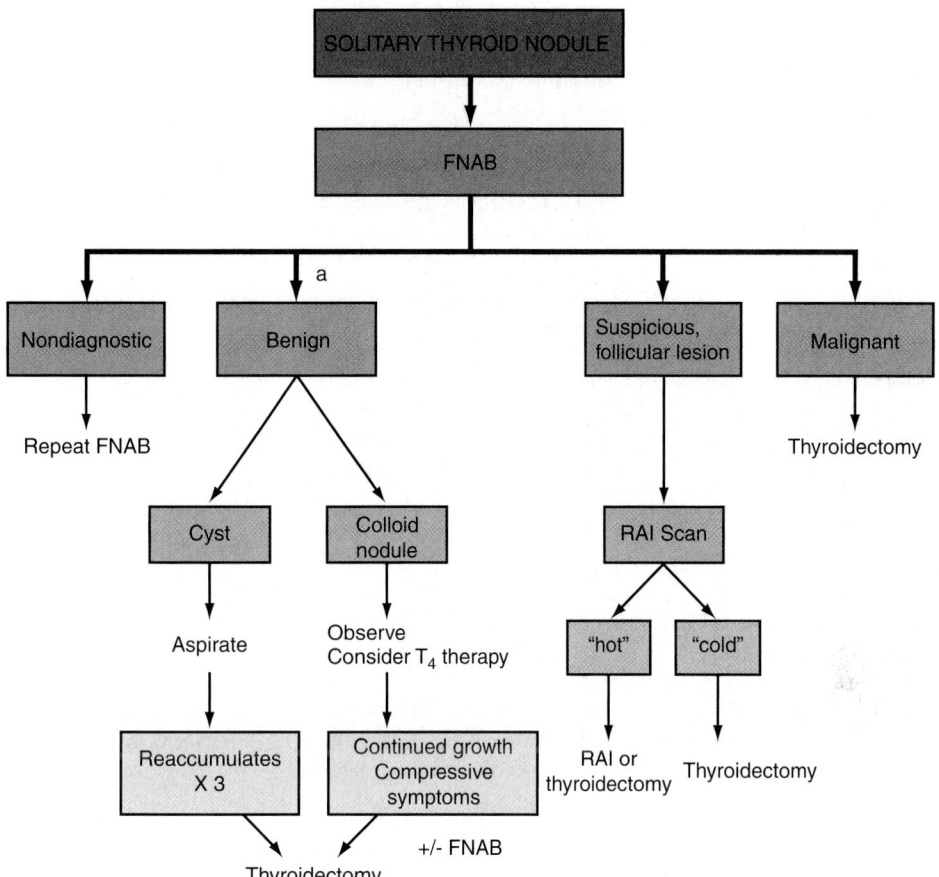

FIG. 37-20. *Management of a solitary thyroid nodule.[a] (Except in patients with a history of external radiation exposure or a family history of thyroid cancer). FNAB = fine-needle aspiration biopsy; RAI = radioactive iodine.*

a Delphian node and pyramidal lobe situated just above the thyroid isthmus and cricoid cartilage.

Diagnostic Tests

Figure 37-20 shows an algorithm for the work-up of a solitary thyroid nodule.

Fine-Needle Aspiration Biopsy

This procedure has become the single most important test in the evaluation of patients with thyroid masses and can be performed with or without ultrasound guidance.[24] Ultrasound guidance is recommended for nodules that are difficult to palpate and for complex, solid cystic nodules that recur after the initial aspiration. A 23-gauge needle is inserted into the thyroid mass, and several passes are made while aspirating the syringe. After releasing the suction on the syringe, the needle is withdrawn and the cells are immediately placed on prelabeled dry glass slides; some are immersed in a 70% alcohol solution, while the others are air dried. A sample of the aspirate is also placed in a 90% alcohol solution for cytospin or cell pellet. The slides are stained by Papanicolaou (Pap) or Wright's stains and examined under the microscope. If a bloody aspirate is obtained, the patient should be repositioned in a more upright position and the biopsy repeated with a finer (25- to 30-gauge) needle.

After FNA biopsy, the majority of nodules can be categorized into the following groups: benign (65%), suspicious (20%), malignant (5%), and nondiagnostic (10%). The incidence of false-positive results is approximately 1% and false-negative results occur in approximately 3% of patients. If a biopsy is reported as nondiagnostic, it should usually be repeated. Bloody FNA biopsy may also be

reported as nondiagnostic and often indicates a follicular neoplasm. Benign lesions include cysts and colloid nodules. The risk of malignancy in this setting is less than 3%. The risk of malignancy in the setting of a suspicious cytology is anywhere from 10 to 20%. Most of these lesions are follicular or Hürthle cell neoplasms. In this situation, diagnosis of malignancy relies on demonstrating capsular or vascular invasion, features that cannot be determined via FNA biopsy. FNA biopsy is also less reliable in patients who have a history of head and neck irradiation or a family history of thyroid cancer, because of a higher likelihood of multifocal lesions. There is little or no value in repeating an FNA biopsy for a follicular or Hürthle cell lesion, but repeat FNA biopsy can be useful for patients when the cytology has some abnormalities that suggest a papillary thyroid cancer, but not enough to make this diagnosis.

Laboratory Studies

Most patients with thyroid nodules are euthyroid. Determining the blood TSH level is helpful. If a patient with a nodule is found to be hyperthyroid, the risk of malignancy is approximately 1%. Serum Tg levels cannot differentiate benign from malignant thyroid nodules unless the levels are extremely high, in which case metastatic thyroid cancer should be suspected. Thyroglobulin levels are, however, useful in following patients who have undergone total thyroidectomy for thyroid cancer and also for serial evaluation of patients undergoing nonoperative management of thyroid nodules. Serum calcitonin levels should be obtained in patients with medullary thyroid cancer or a family history of medullary thyroid cancer (MTC) or MEN2. All patients with MTC should be tested for RET oncogene mutations and have a 24-hour urine collection with measurement of levels of vanillylmandelic acid (VMA), metanephrine, and catecholamine to rule out a coexisting pheochromocytoma. Approximately 10% of patients with familial MTC and MEN2A have de novo *RET* mutations, so that their children are at risk for thyroid cancer.

Imaging

Ultrasound is helpful for detecting nonpalpable thyroid nodules, for differentiating solid from cystic nodules, and for identifying adjacent lymphadenopathy. It also provides a noninvasive and inexpensive method of following the size of suspected benign nodules diagnosed by FNA biopsy. CT and MRI are unnecessary in the routine evaluation of thyroid tumors, except for large, fixed, or substernal lesions. Scanning the thyroid with ^{123}I or ^{99m}Tc is rarely necessary, unless evaluating patients for "hot" or autonomous thyroid nodules. Thyroid scanning is currently recommended in the assessment of thyroid nodules only in patients who have follicular thyroid nodules on FNA biopsy and a suppressed TSH.

Management

Malignant tumors are treated by thyroidectomy, as discussed later in the section, "Thyroid Surgery." Simple thyroid cysts resolve with aspiration in approximately 75% of cases, although some require a second or third aspiration. If the cyst persists after three attempts at aspiration, unilateral thyroid lobectomy is recommended. Lobectomy is also recommended for cysts greater than 4 cm in diameter and for complex cysts with solid and cystic components, because the latter have a higher incidence of malignancy (15%). When FNA biopsy is used in complex nodules, the solid portion should be sampled. If a colloid nodule is diagnosed by FNA biopsy, patients should still be observed with serial ultrasound and Tg measurements. If the nodule enlarges, repeat FNA biopsy is often indicated. Although controversial, L-thyroxine in doses sufficient to maintain a serum TSH level between 0.1 and 1.0 μU/mL may also be administered. Approximately 50% of these nodules decrease in size in response to the TSH suppression of this regimen, and others may not continue to grow, but it is most effective for nodules smaller than 3 cm. One should not cause marked TSH suppression because this increases the risk of osteoporosis and cardiac arrhythmias. Thyroidectomy should be performed if a nodule enlarges on TSH suppression, causes compressive symptoms, or for cosmetic reasons. An exception to this general rule is the patient who has had previous irradiation of the thyroid gland or who has a family history of thyroid cancer. In these patients total or near-total thyroidectomy is recommended because of the high incidence of thyroid cancer ($\geq$40%) and decreased reliability of FNA biopsy in this setting.

MALIGNANT THYROID DISEASE

In the United States, thyroid cancer accounts for less than 1% of all malignancies (2% of women and 0.5% of men). Thyroid cancer is responsible for six deaths per 1 million persons annually. Most patients present with a palpable swelling in the neck, which initiates assessment through a combination of history, physical examination, and FNA biopsy.

Molecular Genetics of Thyroid Tumorigenesis

Cancer-predisposing genes can be classified into broad functional groups. Proto-oncogenes may encode growth factors, growth factor receptors and hormones, intracellular transducer proteins, transcription factors, and cell-cycle regulatory proteins. Oncogenes arise from proto-oncogenes by various mechanisms such as somatic point mutations, amplification, and gene rearrangements, and lead to their constitutive activation or overexpression. Thus, mutated oncogenes lead to a gain of function in a dominant fashion. In contrast, tumor-suppressor genes normally act as barriers to cell proliferation and growth. Mutations in these genes, therefore, lead to uncontrolled growth and proliferation. However, two hits are usually needed for this. An initial mutation event inactivates one copy of the gene and the second event inactivates the remaining allele via various mechanisms which include mutations, deletions, chromosomal rearrangements or mitotic recombination. Thus, tumor-suppressor genes are functionally recessive.

As Table 37-5 depicts, several oncogenes and tumor-suppressor genes are involved in thyroid tumorigenesis.[25] The RET

Table 37-5

Oncogenes and Tumor-Suppressor Genes Involved in Thyroid Tumorigenesis

Gene	Function	Tumor
Oncogenes		
RET	Membrane receptor with tyrosine kinase activity	Sporadic and familial MTC, PTC (RET/PTC rearrangements)
MET	Same	Overexpressed in PTC
TRK1	Same	Activated in some PTC
TSH-R	Linked to heterotrimeric G protein	Hyperfunctioning adenoma
Gsα (gsp)	Signal transduction molecule (GTP binding)	Hyperfunctioning adenoma, follicular adenoma
ras	Signal-transduction protein	Follicular adenoma and carcinoma, PTC
PAX8/PPARγ 1	Oncoprotein	Follicular adenoma, follicular carcinoma
Tumor suppressors		
p53	Cell-cycle regulator, arrests cells in G$_1$, induces apoptosis	Dedifferentiated PTC, FTC, anaplastic cancers
p16	Cell-cycle regulator, inhibits cyclin-dependent kinase	Thyroid cancer cell lines
PTEN	Protein tyrosine phosphatase	Follicular adenoma and carcinoma

FTC = follicular thyroid cancer; MTC = medullary thyroid cancer; PTC = papillary thyroid cancer.

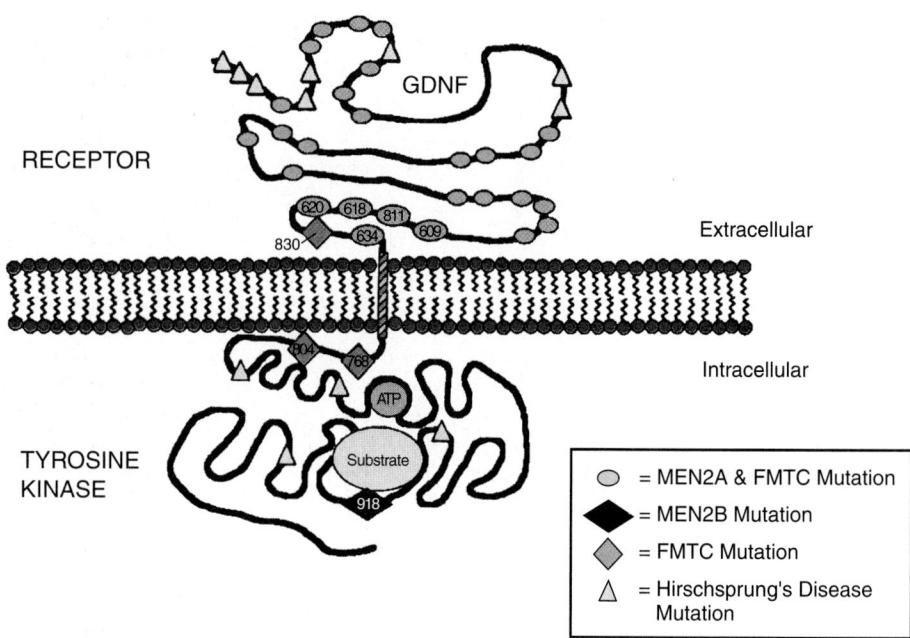

FIG. 37-21. *Structure of the RET tyrosine kinase receptor. MEN2A, MEN2B, familial medullary thyroid cancer (FMTC), and Hirschsprung's disease result from germline mutations in the RET proto-oncogene. The extracellular domain binds the ligand glial-derived neurotrophic factor (GDNF) and contains 28 cysteine residues. Mutations in cysteine residues at codons 609, 611, 618, 620, and 634, which are in the juxtamembrane region of the receptor, are associated with MEN2A and FMTC. The ATP binding site is located intracellularly near the site, which binds the substrate for the tyrosine kinase catalytic domain. Mutations at codon 918 (Met to Thr) alter the substrate binding pocket located in the intracellular region and cause MEN2B. FMTC is associated with mutations at codons 768 and 804. [Reproduced with permission from Wells S, Franz C: Medullary carcinoma of the thyroid. World J Surg 24(8):954, 2000.]*

RECEPTOR

GDNF

Extracellular

Intracellular

TYROSINE
KINASE

ATP

Substrate

○ = MEN2A & FMTC Mutation
◆ = MEN2B Mutation
◇ = FMTC Mutation
△ = Hirschsprung's Disease Mutation

proto-oncogene (Fig. 37-21) plays a significant role in the pathogenesis of thyroid cancers. It is located on chromosome 10 and encodes a receptor tyrosine kinase, which binds several growth factors such as glial-derived neurotrophic factor (GDNF) and neuturin. The RET protein is expressed in tissues derived from the embryonic nervous and excretory systems. Therefore, RET disruption can lead to developmental abnormalities in organs derived from these systems, such as the enteric nervous system (Hirschsprung's disease) and kidney. Germline mutations in the RET proto-oncogene are known to predispose to MEN2A, MEN2B, and familial medullary thyroid cancers; and somatic mutations have been demonstrated in tumors derived from the neural crest, such as MTCs (30%) and pheochromocytomas. The tyrosine kinase domain of RET can fuse with other genes by rearrangement. These fusion products also function as oncogenes and have been implicated in the pathogenesis of PTCs. At least 15 RET/PTC rearrangements have been described and appear to be early events in tumorigenesis. Young age and radiation exposure seem to be independent risk factors for the development of RET/PTC rearrangements. Up to 70% of papillary cancers in children exposed to the radiation fallout from the 1986 Chernobyl disaster carry RET/PTC rearrangements, the most common being RET/PTC1 and RET/PTC3. As previously mentioned, RET/PTC3 is associated with a solid type of papillary thyroid cancer that appears to present at a higher stage and to be more aggressive.[26] Other tyrosine kinase receptor groups, such as *trk* and *met,* also have been implicated in thyroid tumorigenesis.

Receptor tyrosine kinase pathways are proximally regulated by three guanosine phosphatase-binding proteins known as *ras* (H, N, and K). Mutated *ras* oncogenes have been identified in up to 40% of thyroid follicular adenomas and carcinomas, multinodular goiters, and papillary and anaplastic carcinomas. They are believed to be an early mutation. Mutations in the TSH-R can occur in up to 80% of toxic adenomas, but also occur in hyperfunctioning nodules of multinodular goiters, and rarely in thyroid cancers. Mutations of the *gsp* oncogene also commonly occur in toxic thyroid adenomas, but are less common than *TSH-R* mutations.

The *p53* gene is a tumor-suppressor gene encoding a transcriptional regulator, which causes cell-cycle arrest, allowing repair of damaged DNA, thus helping to maintain genomic integrity. Mutations of *p53* are rare in PTCs, but are common in undifferentiated thyroid cancers and thyroid cancer cell lines. Other cell-cycle regulators and tumor suppressors, such as *p15* and *p16,* are mutated more commonly in thyroid cancer cell lines than in primary tumors. An oncogene resulting from the fusion of the DNA binding domain of the thyroid transcription factor *PAX8* gene to the peroxisome proliferator-activated receptor gamma 1 (*PPARγ1*) has been noted to play an important role in the development of follicular neoplasms, including follicular cancers.[27]

Specific Tumor Types

Papillary Carcinoma

Papillary carcinoma accounts for 80% of all thyroid malignancies in iodine-sufficient areas and is the predominant thyroid cancer in children and individuals exposed to external radiation. Papillary carcinoma occurs more often in women, with a 2:1 female:male ratio; the mean age at presentation is 30 to 40 years. Most patients are euthyroid and present with a slow-growing painless mass in the neck. Dysphagia, dyspnea, and dysphonia are usually associated with locally advanced invasive disease. Lymph node metastases are common, especially in children and young adults, and may be the presenting complaint. The so-called "lateral aberrant thyroid" almost always denotes a cervical lymph node that has been invaded by metastatic cancer. Suspicion of thyroid cancer often originates through physical examination of the patient and a review of the patient's history. Diagnosis is established by FNA biopsy of the thyroid mass or lymph node. Distant metastases are uncommon at initial presentation, but may ultimately develop in up to 20% of patients. The most common sites are the lungs, followed by bone, liver, and brain.

Pathology. On gross examination, PTCs are generally hard and whitish and remain flat on sectioning with a blade, in contrast to normal tissue or benign nodular lesions that tend to bulge. Macroscopic calcification, necrosis, or cystic change may be apparent. Histologically, papillary carcinomas may exhibit papillary

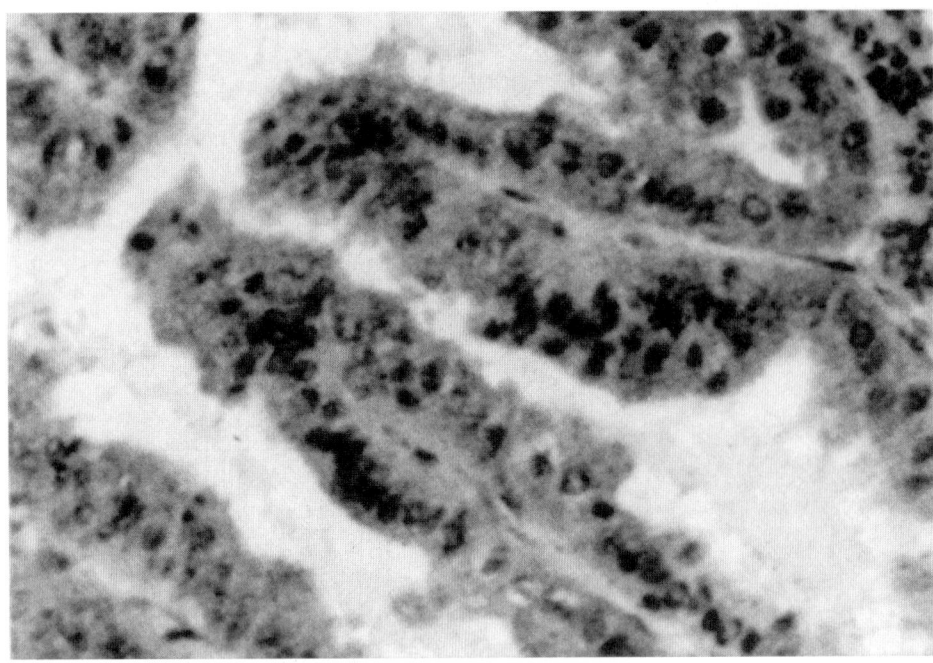

FIG. 37-22. Histomicrograph of a papillary thyroid cancer (H and E stain).

projections (Fig. 37-22), a mixed pattern of papillary and follicular structures, or a pure follicular pattern (follicular variant). The diagnosis is established by characteristic cellular features. Cells are cuboidal with pale, abundant cytoplasm, "grooving," crowded nuclei, and intranuclear cytoplasmic inclusions, leading to the designation of *Orphan Annie* nuclei (Fig. 37-23), which allows diagnosis by FNA biopsy. Psammoma bodies, which are microscopic, calcified deposits representing clumps of sloughed cells, may be present. Mixed papillary–follicular tumors and follicular variant of papillary carcinoma are classified as papillary carcinomas because they act biologically as papillary carcinomas. Multifocality is common in papillary carcinoma and may be present in up to 85% of cases on microscopic examination. Multifocality is associated with

an increased risk of cervical nodal metastases and these tumors may rarely invade adjacent structures such as the trachea, esophagus, and recurrent laryngeal nerves. Other variants of papillary carcinoma include tall cell, insular, columnar, diffuse sclerosing, clear cell, trabecular, and poorly differentiated types. These variants account for approximately 1% of all papillary carcinomas and are generally associated with a worse prognosis.

Macroscopically, there are three recognized forms of PTC, each based on the size and extent of the primary disease. Minimal or occult/microcarcinoma tumors originally included papillary cancers up to 1.5 cm in diameter. They now are defined as tumors of 1 cm or less in size with no evidence of local invasiveness through the thyroid capsule or angioinvasion, and are not associated with lymph node metastases. They are nonpalpable and usually are incidental findings at operative, histologic, or autopsy examination. Occult papillary thyroid cancer is present in 2 to 36% of thyroid glands removed at autopsy. The recurrence rate in patients with tumors 1.5 cm or smaller after removal is approximately 5% and the mortality rate approximately 0.5%. Intrathyroidal tumors are confined to the thyroid gland, with no evidence of extrathyroid invasion. Extrathyroidal tumors invade through the thyroid capsule and/or into adjacent structures. All types of primary thyroid cancers can be associated with lymph node metastases and invasion into intrathyroidal blood vessels or occasionally distant metastases. Long-term prognosis is better for patients with intrathyroidal lesions.

Prognostic Indicators. In general, patients with PTC have an excellent prognosis with a greater than 95% 10-year survival rate. Several prognostic indicators have been incorporated into various staging systems, which enable patients to be stratified into low-risk and high-risk groups. Unfortunately, all of these classification systems rely on data that is not available preoperatively.

In 1987, Hay and associates,[28] at the Mayo Clinic, proposed the AGES scoring system, which incorporates *a*ge, histologic *g*rade, *e*xtrathyroidal invasion and metastases, and tumor *s*ize to predict the risk of dying from papillary cancer. Low-risk patients are young, with well-differentiated tumors, no metastases, and small primary lesions, whereas high-risk patients are older, with poorly

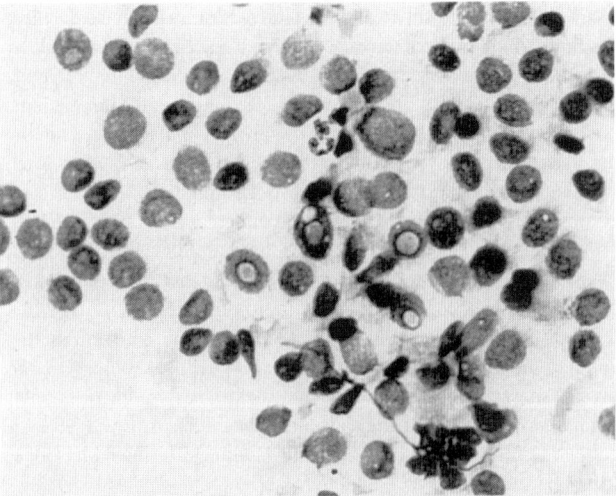

FIG. 37-23. Fine-needle aspiration biopsy specimen from a papillary thyroid cancer showing typical intranuclear cytoplasmic inclusions (Wright's stain) in the center of the slide. [*Reproduced with permission from Abele J, Tressler P: Fine needle aspiration thyroid nodule, in Clark O (ed): Endocrine Surgery of the Thyroid and Parathyroid Glands. C. V. Mosby, 1985, p. 343.*]

differentiated tumors, local invasion, distant metastases, and large primary lesions. The MACIS scale is a more sophisticated postoperative system modified from the AGES scale. This scale incorporates distant *m*etastases, *a*ge at presentation, *c*ompleteness of original surgical resection, extrathyroidal *i*nvasion, and *s*ize of original lesion (in centimeters) and classifies patients into four risk-groups based on their scores. Cady proposed the AMES system[29] to classify differentiated thyroid tumors into low- and high-risk groups using *a*ge (men <40 years, women <50 years), *m*etastases, *e*xtrathyroidal spread, and *s*ize of tumors (<or >5 cm). Another classification system is the TNM system, (*t*umor, *n*odal status, *m*etastases; Table 37-6), used by most medical centers in North America.[30] A simplified system by DeGroot and associates[31] uses four groups: class I (intrathyroidal), class II (cervical nodal metastases), class III (extrathyroidal invasion), and class IV (distant metastases) to determine prognosis.

Several molecular and genetic markers, such as tumor DNA aneuploidy, decreased cAMP response to TSH, increased epidermal growth factor binding, presence of N-*ras* and *gsp* mutations, overexpression of c-*myc*, and presence of *p53* mutations, are also associated with a worse prognosis.

Surgical Treatment. Most authors agree that patients with high-risk tumors (judged by any of the classification systems discussed above) or bilateral tumors should undergo total or near-total thyroidectomy. When patients are found to have a minimal papillary thyroid carcinoma in a thyroid specimen removed for other reasons, unilateral thyroid lobectomy and isthmusectomy is usually considered to be adequate treatment, unless the tumor has evidence of angioinvasion, multifocality, or positive margins. The optimal surgical strategy in the majority of patients with low-risk (small, unilateral) cancers remains controversial. The focus of the debate centers around outcome data and risks associated with either lobectomy or total thyroidectomy in this group of patients.

Proponents of total thyroidectomy argue that the procedure (1) enables one to use RAI to effectively detect and treat residual thyroid tissue or metastatic disease; (2) makes the serum Tg level a more sensitive marker of recurrent or persistent disease; (3) eliminates the contralateral occult cancers as sites of recurrence (because up to 85% of tumors are multifocal); (4) reduces the risk of recurrence and improves survival; (5) decreases the 1% risk of progression to undifferentiated or anaplastic thyroid cancer; and (6) reduces the need for reoperative surgery with its attendant risk of increased complication rates.[32]

Investigators that favor lobectomy argue that (1) total thyroidectomy is associated with a higher complication rate than lobectomy; (2) recurrence in the remaining thyroid tissue is unusual (5%) and most are curable by surgery; (3) tumor multicentricity seems to have little prognostic significance; and (4) patients who have undergone lesser procedures, such as lobectomy, still have an excellent prognosis.

However, it is known that a significant proportion (33 to 50%) of patients who develop a recurrence die from their disease,[33] and even though the data are retrospective, long-term, follow-up studies suggest that recurrence rates are lowered, and some, but not all, investigations suggest that survival is improved in patients undergoing near-total or total thyroidectomy (Fig. 37-24).[31,34–36] In addition, diminished survival is noted in patients with so-called low-risk disease (mortality rates of 5% at 10 to 20 years) and it is not possible to accurately risk stratify patients preoperatively. Given the above, it is recommended that even patients with low-risk tumors undergo total or near-total thyroidectomy, provided complication rates are low (<2%).

Table 37-6
TNM Classification of Thyroid Tumors

Papillary or Follicular Tumors	
Stage	*TNM*
Younger than age 45 Years	
I	Any T, Any N, M0
II	Any T, Any N, M1
Age 45 Years and older	
I	T1, N0, M0
II	T2, N0, M0
III	T3, N0, M0; T1-3, N1a, M0
IVA	T4a, N0-1a, M0; T1-4a, N1b, M0
IVB	T4b, Any N, M0
IVC	Any T, any N, M1

Medullary Thyroid Cancer	
Stage	*TNM*
I	T1, N0, M0
II	T2-3, N0, M0
III	T1-3, N1a, M0
IVA	T4a, N0-1a, M0; T1-4a, N1b, M0
IVB	T4b, any N, M0
IVC	Any T, Any N, M1

Anaplastic Cancer	
Stage	*TNM*
IVA	T4a, Any N, M0
IVB	T4b, Any N, M0
IVC	Any T, Any M, M1

Definitions:
Primary tumor (T)

TX	Primary tumor cannot be assessed
T0	No evidence of primary tumor
T1	Tumor ≤2 cm in diameter, limited to thyroid
T2	Tumor >2 cm but <4 cm in diameter, limited to thyroid
T3	Tumor >4 cm in diameter, limited to thyroid, or any tumor with minimal extrathyroidal invasion
T4a	Any size tumor extending beyond capsule to invade subcutaneous soft tissue, larynx, trachea, esophagus, or recurrent laryngeal nerve, or intrathyroidal anaplastic cancer
T4b	Tumor invading prevertebral fascia, or encasing carotid artery or mediastinal vessels, or extrathyroidal anaplastic cancer

Regional lymph nodes (N) include central, lateral, cervical, and upper mediastinal nodes

Nx	Regional lymph nodes cannot be assessed
N0	No regional lymph node metastasis
N1	Regional lymph node metastasis
N1a	Metastases to level VI (pretracheal, paratracheal, and prelaryngeal/Delphian lymph nodes)
N1b	Metastases to unilateral, bilateral, or contralateral cervical or superior mediastinal lymph nodes

Distant metastasis (M)

MX	Distant metastases cannot be assessed
M1	No distant metastasis

SOURCE: Reproduced with permission from *AJCC Cancer Staging Manual*, 6th ed. New York: Springer-Verlag, 2002.

Consequently, most patients with thyroid nodules should have FNA biopsy performed. When PTC is diagnosed, the definitive operation can be done without confirming the diagnosis by frozen section during the operation. Patients with a nodule that may be papillary cancer should be treated by thyroid lobectomy, isthmusectomy, and removal of any pyramidal lobe or adjacent lymph nodes. If intraoperative frozen-section examination of a lymph node or of the primary tumor confirms carcinoma, completion of total or near-total thyroidectomy should be performed. If a definitive diagnosis

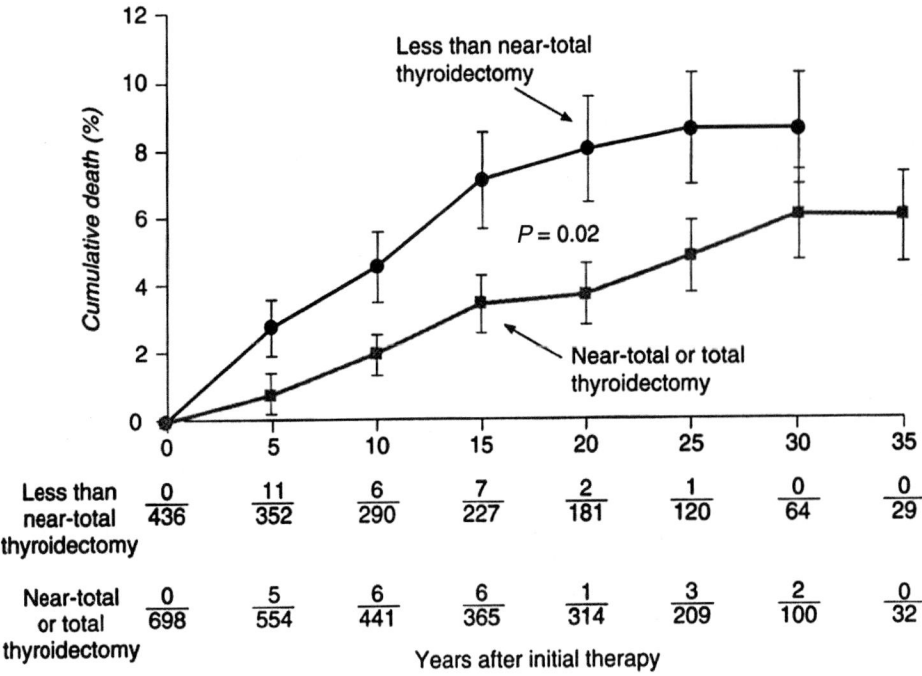

FIG. 37-24. Improved survival in patients with papillary or follicular thyroid cancer following total or near-total thyroidectomy as compared to those who underwent less than near-total thyroidectomy. (*Reproduced with permission from Mazzaferri E, et al, p. 424.[34]*)

cannot be made, or if the surgeon is concerned about the viability of the parathyroid glands or the status of the RLN, the operation should be terminated. When final histology confirms carcinoma, completion of total thyroidectomy is usually performed. For patients who have minimal papillary thyroid cancers confined to the thyroid gland without angioinvasion, no further operative treatment is recommended.

During thyroidectomy, enlarged ipsilateral central neck nodes should be removed. Lymph node metastases in the lateral neck in patients with papillary carcinoma usually should be managed with modified radical or functional neck dissection as described later under "Neck Dissection for Nodal Metastases." Dissection of the posterior triangle and suprahyoid dissection are usually not necessary unless there is extensive metastatic disease in levels 2, 3, and 4, but should be performed when appropriate.[37] Prophylactic neck node dissection is not necessary in patients with PTC, because these cancers do not appear to metastasize systemically from lymph nodes and micrometastases appear to be ablated with RAI therapy.

Follicular Carcinoma

Follicular carcinomas account for 10% of thyroid cancers and occur more commonly in iodine-deficient areas. The overall incidence of this tumor is declining in the United States, probably as a result of iodine supplementation and improved histologic classification. Women have a higher incidence of follicular cancer, with a female:male ratio of 3:1, and a mean age at presentation of 50 years. Follicular cancers usually present as solitary thyroid nodules, occasionally with a history of rapid size increase, and long-standing goiter. Pain is uncommon, unless hemorrhage into the nodule has occurred. Unlike papillary cancers, cervical lymphadenopathy is uncommon at initial presentation (approximately 5%), although distant metastases may be present. In less than 1% of cases, follicular cancers may be hyperfunctioning, leading patients to present with signs and symptoms of thyrotoxicosis. FNA biopsy is unable to

distinguish benign follicular lesions from follicular carcinomas.[38] Therefore, preoperative diagnosis of cancer is difficult unless distant metastases are present. Large follicular tumors (>4 cm) in older men are more likely to be malignant.

Pathology. Follicular carcinomas are usually solitary lesions, the majority of which are surrounded by a capsule. Histologically, follicles are present, but the lumen may be devoid of colloid. Architectural patterns depend on the degree of differentiation demonstrated by the tumor. Malignancy is defined by the presence of capsular and vascular invasion (Fig. 37-25). Minimally-invasive tumors

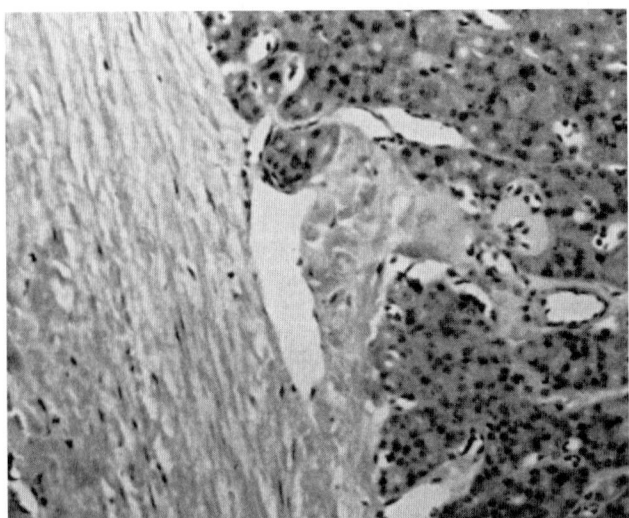

FIG. 37-25. H and E stained section from a microfollicular thyroid carcinoma showing capsular invasion. [*Reproduced with permission from Abele J, Tressler P: Fine needle aspiration thyroid nodule, in Clark O (ed): Endocrine Surgery of the Thyroid and Parathyroid Glands. C. V. Mosby, 1985, p. 335.*]

appear grossly encapsulated but have evidence of microscopic invasion through the tumor capsule and/or invasion into small- to medium-size vessels (venous caliber) in or immediately outside the capsule, but not within the tumor.[39] On the other hand, widely invasive tumors demonstrate evidence of large-vessel invasion and/or broad areas of tumor invasion through the capsule. They may, in fact, be unencapsulated. It is important to note that there is a wide variation of opinion among clinicians and pathologists with respect to the above definitions. Tumor infiltration and invasion, as well as tumor thrombus within the middle thyroid or jugular veins, may be apparent at operation.

Surgical Treatment and Prognosis. Patients diagnosed by FNA biopsy as having a follicular lesion should undergo thyroid lobectomy because at least 80% of these patients will have benign adenomas. Some surgeons recommend total thyroidectomy in older patients with follicular lesions larger than 4 cm because of the higher risk of cancer in this setting (50%). Intraoperative frozen-section examination usually is not helpful, but should be performed when there is evidence of capsular or vascular invasion, or when adjacent lymphadenopathy is present. Total thyroidectomy should be performed when thyroid cancer is diagnosed. There is debate among experts about whether patients with minimally-invasive follicular cancers should undergo completion thyroidectomy because the prognosis is so good in these patients. A diagnosis of frankly invasive carcinoma necessitates completion of total thyroidectomy primarily so that ^{131}I can be used to detect and ablate metastatic disease. Total thyroidectomy in patients with angioinvasion is also recommended. Prophylactic nodal dissection is unwarranted because nodal involvement is infrequent, but in the unusual patient with nodal metastases, therapeutic neck dissection is recommended. The cumulative mortality from follicular thyroid cancer is approximately 15% at 10 years and 30% at 20 years. Poor long-term prognosis is predicted by age older than 50 years at presentation, tumor size larger than 4 cm, higher tumor grade, marked vascular invasion, extrathyroidal invasion, and distant metastases at the time of diagnosis.

Hürthle Cell Carcinoma

Hürthle cell carcinomas account for approximately 3% of all thyroid malignancies. Under the World Health Organization classification, Hürthle cell carcinomas are considered to be a subtype of follicular thyroid cancer. Like follicular cancers, Hürthle cell cancers are characterized by vascular or capsular invasion, and therefore cannot be diagnosed by FNA biopsy. Tumors contain sheets of eosinophilic cells packed with mitochondria, which are derived from the oxyphilic cells of the thyroid gland. Hürthle cell tumors also differ from follicular carcinomas in that they are more often multifocal and bilateral (approximately 30%), usually do not take up RAI (approximately 5%), are more likely to metastasize to local nodes (25%) and distant sites, and are associated with a higher mortality rate (approximately 20% at 10 years). Hence, they are considered to be a separate class of tumors by some surgeons.

Management is similar to that of follicular neoplasms, with lobectomy and isthmusectomy being sufficient surgical treatment for unilateral Hürthle cell adenomas. When Hürthle cell neoplasms are found to be invasive on intraoperative, frozen-section, or definitive paraffin-section histology, then total thyroidectomy should be performed. These patients should also undergo routine central neck node removal, similar to patients with MTC, and modified radical neck dissection when lateral neck nodes are palpable. Although RAI scanning and ablation usually are ineffective, they probably should be considered for ablation of any residual normal thyroid

tissue and, occasionally, for ablation of tumors, because there is no other good therapy.[40] Redifferentiating therapies, such as retinoic acid and PPARγ agonists, may prove useful in the future.

Postoperative Management of Differentiated Thyroid Cancer

Treatment

Thyroid Hormone. Thyroxine is necessary not only as replacement therapy in patients after total or near-total thyroidectomy, but has the additional effect of suppressing TSH and reducing the growth stimulus for any possible residual thyroid cancer cells. TSH suppression reduces tumor recurrence rates, particularly in young patients with papillary and follicular thyroid cancer. Thyroxine should be administered to ensure that the patient remains euthyroid, with circulating TSH levels at about 0.1 μU/L in low-risk patients, or less than 0.1 μU/mL in high-risk patients. The risk of tumor recurrence must be balanced with the side effects associated with prolonged TSH suppression, including osteopenia and cardiac problems, particularly in older patients.

Thyroglobulin Measurement. Thyroglobulin levels in patients who have undergone total thyroidectomy should be below 2 ng/mL when the patient is taking T_4, and below 5 ng/mL when the patient is hypothyroid. A Tg level above 2 ng/mL is highly suggestive of metastatic disease or persistent normal thyroid tissue, especially if it increases when TSH levels increase when the patient is hypothyroid during preparation for RAI scanning.[41] Approximately 95% of patients with persistent or recurrent thyroid cancer of follicular cell origin will have Tg levels higher than 2 ng/mL. Thyroglobulin and anti-Tg antibody levels should be measured initially at 6-month intervals and then annually if the patient is clinically disease free. High-risk patients should also have an ultrasound of the neck and CT or MRI scan of the neck and mediastinum for early detection of any persistent or recurrent disease.

Radioiodine Therapy. The issue of whether RAI therapy offers any benefit to patients with differentiated thyroid cancer remains controversial in the absence of prospective, randomized controlled trials. Some experts advise routine RAI scan and therapy for all patients except those with occult or minimally-invasive tumors, whereas others treat only high-risk patients. Long-term cohort studies by Mazzaferri and Jhiang and DeGroot and associates demonstrate that postoperative RAI therapy reduces recurrence (Fig. 37-26) and provides a small improvement in survival, even in low-risk patients.[31,34] Although screening with radioactive iodine is more sensitive than chest x-ray or CT scanning for detecting metastases, it is less sensitive than Tg measurements for detecting metastatic disease in most differentiated thyroid cancers except Hürthle cell tumors, because only 5 to 10% of the latter take up RAI. Screening and treatment are facilitated by the removal of all normal thyroid tissue, which effectively competes for iodine uptake. Metastatic differentiated thyroid carcinoma can be detected and treated by ^{131}I in approximately 75% of patients. Multiple studies show that RAI effectively treats more than 70% of lung micrometastases that are detected by RAI scan in the presence of a normal chest x-ray, whereas the success rates drop to less than 10% with pulmonary macrometastases. Early detection, therefore, appears to be very important to improve prognosis.

Generally, T_4 therapy should be discontinued for approximately 6 weeks prior to scanning with [131]I. Patients should receive T_3 during this time period to decrease the period of hypothyroidism. T_3 has a shorter half-life than T_4 (1 day vs. 1 week) and needs to be

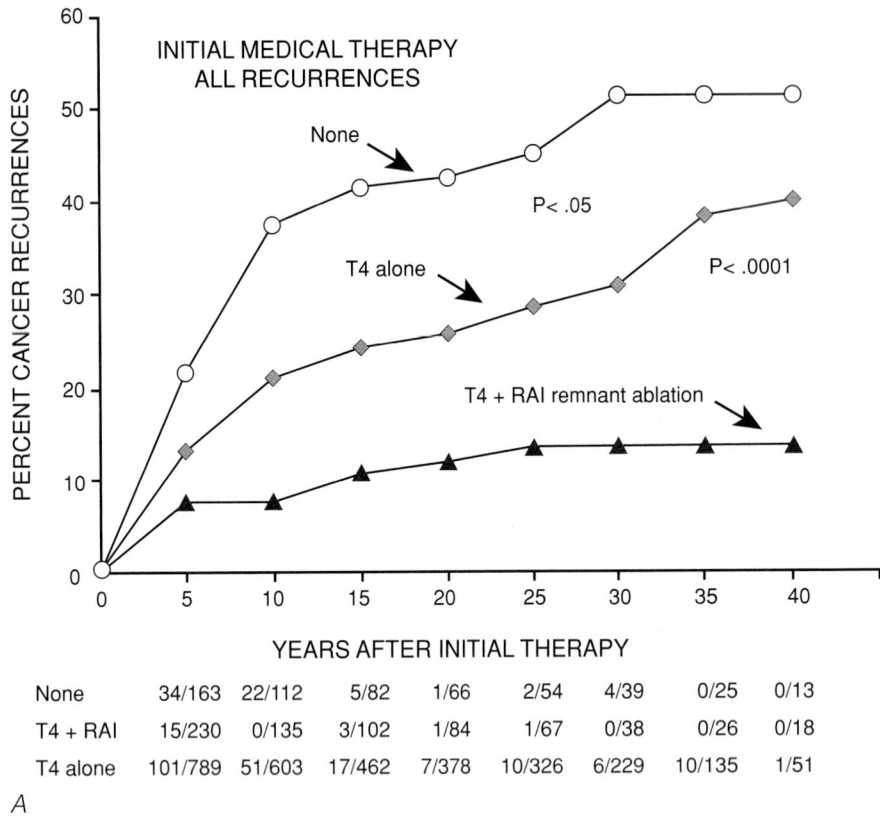

None	34/163	22/112	5/82	1/66	2/54	4/39	0/25	0/13
T4 + RAI	15/230	0/135	3/102	1/84	1/67	0/38	0/26	0/18
T4 alone	101/789	51/603	17/462	7/378	10/326	6/229	10/135	1/51

A

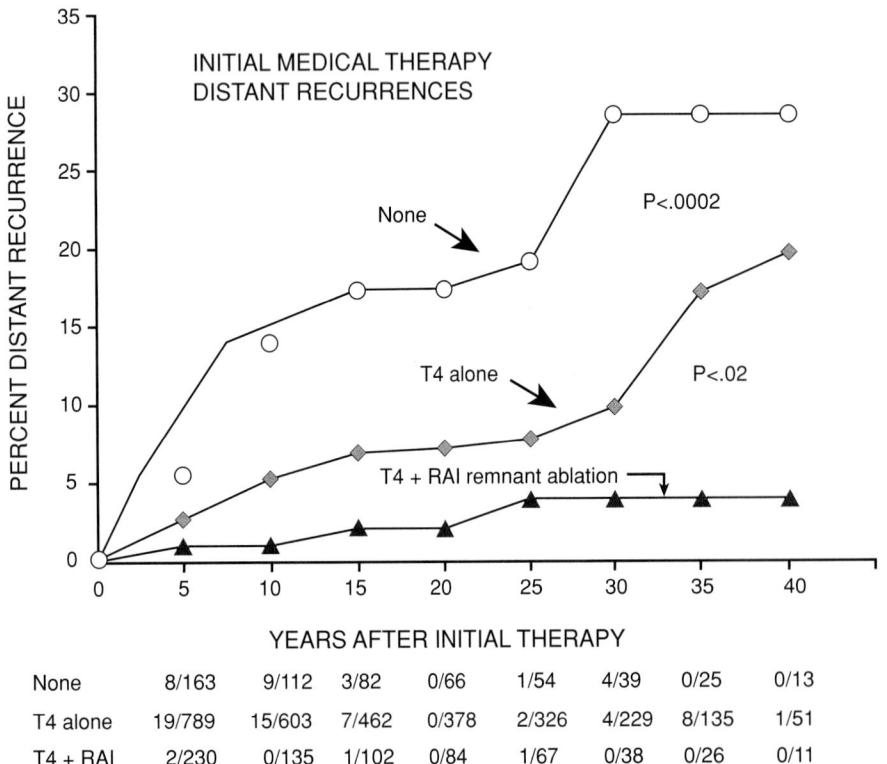

None	8/163	9/112	3/82	0/66	1/54	4/39	0/25	0/13
T4 alone	19/789	15/603	7/462	0/378	2/326	4/229	8/135	1/51
T4 + RAI	2/230	0/135	1/102	0/84	1/67	0/38	0/26	0/11

B

FIG. 37-26. Tumor recurrence at a median of 16.7 years after thyroid surgery. The numerator is the number of patients with recurrence and the denominator is the number of patients in each time interval. The p-values are derived from log-rank statistical analysis of 40-year life-table data. The figure shows that all recurrences (*A*) and distant metastases (*B*) were reduced in patients who received RAI in addition to T_4 therapy. (*Reproduced with permission from Mazzaferri E, Kloos R: Current approaches to primary therapy for papillary and follicular thyroid cancer. J Clin Endocrinol Metab 86:1453, 2001.*)

discontinued for 2 weeks to allow TSH levels to rise prior to treatment. A low-iodine diet is also recommended during this 2-week period. The usual protocol involves administering a screening dose of about 2 mCi of ^{131}I and measuring uptake 24 hours later. After a total thyroidectomy, this value should be less than 1%. A "hot" spot in the neck after initial screening usually represents residual normal tissue in the thyroid bed. If there is significant uptake, then a therapeutic dose of ^{131}I should be administered to patients (low-risk patients: 30 to 100 mCi; high-risk patients: 100 to 200 mCi). If patients have an elevated Tg level, but negative RAI scan, some physicians recommend treating with 100 mCi of ^{131}I and repeating the scan 1 to 2 weeks later. Approximately one-third of these patients demonstrate uptake on posttreatment imaging and Tg levels usually decrease in these patients, documenting therapeutic benefit. Others recommend omitting the scanning dose altogether to minimize thyrocyte "stunning" and subsequent requirement for higher treatment doses. Patients with previously positive scans and patients with serum thyroglobulin levels greater than 2 ng/mL usually need another ^{131}I treatment after 6 to 12 months until one or two negative scans are obtained. The follow-up scan can be done after hormone withdrawal or after recombinant TSH. The maximum dose of radioiodine that can be administered at one time without performing dosimetry is approximately 200 mCi with a cumulative dose of 1000 to 1500 mCi. Up to 500 mCi can be given with proper pretreatment dosimetry. Table 37-7 lists the complications of RAI therapy.

Other Imaging. If RAI scans are negative, but Tg levels remain elevated, other imaging studies such as neck ultrasound, MRI scan, and FDG-PET scans may be considered.

External Beam Radiotherapy and Chemotherapy. External beam radiotherapy is occasionally required to control unresectable, locally invasive or recurrent disease[42] and to treat metastases in support bones to decrease the risk of fractures. It also is of value for the treatment and control of pain from bony metastases when there is minimal or no RAIU. Single and multidrug chemotherapy has been used with little success in disseminated thyroid cancer. Adriamycin and Taxol are the most frequently used agents.

Medullary Carcinoma

MTCs account for about 5% of thyroid malignancies and arise from the parafollicular or C cells of the thyroid, which, in turn,

are derived from the ultimobranchial bodies.[43] These cells are concentrated superolaterally in the thyroid lobes, which is where MTC usually develops. C cells secrete calcitonin, a 32-amino-acid polypeptide that functions to lower serum calcium levels. In some animals, especially those that lay eggs with shells, calcitonin is a significant regulator of calcium metabolism, but in humans, it has only minimal physiologic effects.

Most MTCs occur sporadically. However, approximately 25% occur within the spectrum of several inherited syndromes such as familial medullary thyroid cancer, MEN2A, and MEN2B. All these variants are known to result secondary to germline mutations in the RET proto-oncogene. The syndromes are also characterized by genotype–phenotype correlations, with specific mutations leading to particular clinical manifestations. Table 37-8 outlines the salient clinical and genetic features of these syndromes. Figure 37-27 shows some of the clinical features of MEN2B patients.

Patients with MTC often present with a neck mass that may be associated with palpable cervical lymphadenopathy (15 to 20%). Local pain or aching is more common in patients with these tumors, and local invasion may produce symptoms of dysphagia, dyspnea, or dysphonia. Distant blood-borne metastases to the liver, bone (frequently osteoblastic), and lung occur later in the disease. The female:male ratio is 1.5:1. Most patients present between 50 and 60 years of age, although patients with familial disease present at a younger age. Medullary thyroid tumors secrete not only calcitonin and carcinoembryonic antigen (CEA), but also other peptides such as calcitonin gene-related peptide (CGRP), histaminadases, prostaglandins E_2 and $F_{2\alpha}$, and serotonin. Patients with extensive metastatic disease frequently develop diarrhea, which may result from increased intestinal motility and impaired intestinal water and electrolyte flux. Approximately 2 to 4% of patients develop Cushing's syndrome as a result of ectopic production of adrenocorticotropic hormone (ACTH).

Pathology. MTCs are typically unilateral (80%) in patients with sporadic disease, and multicentric in familial cases, with bilateral tumors occurring in up to 90% of familial patients. Familial cases are also associated with C-cell hyperplasia (Fig. 37-28), which is considered a premalignant lesion. Microscopically, tumors are composed of sheets of infiltrating neoplastic cells separated by collagen and amyloid. Marked heterogeneity is present; cells may be polygonal or spindle-shaped. The presence of amyloid is a diagnostic finding, but immunohistochemistry for calcitonin is more

Table 37-7
Complications of Radioactive Iodine Therapy (^{131}I) and Doses at Which They Are Observed

Acute	*Long-Term*
Neck pain, swelling, and tenderness	Hematologic
Thyroiditis (if remnant present)	Bone marrow suppression (>500 mCi)
Sialadenitis (50–450 mCi), taste dysfunction	Leukemia (>1000 mCi)
Hemorrhage (brain metastases)	Fertility
Cerebral edema (brain metastases, 200 mCi)	Ovarian/testicular damage, infertility
Vocal cord paralysis	Increased spontaneous abortion rate
Nausea and vomiting (50–450 mCi)	Pulmonary fibrosis
Bone marrow suppression (200 mCi)	Chronic sialadenitis, nodules, taste dysfunction
	Increased risk of cancer
	Anaplastic thyroid cancer
	Gastric cancer
	Hepatocellular cancer
	Lung cancer
	Breast cancer (>1000 mCi)
	Bladder cancer
	Hypoparathyroidism

Table 37-8
Clinical and Genetic Features of Medullary Thyroid Cancer Syndromes

Syndrome	Manifestations	Ret Mutations
MEN2A	MTC, pheochromocytoma, primary hyperparathyroidism, lichen planus, amyloidosis	Exon 10: codons 609, 611, 618, 620 Exon 11: codon 634 (more commonly associated with pheochromocytoma and primary hyperparathyroidism
MEN2B	MTC, pheochromocytoma, marfanoid habitus, mucocutaneous ganglioneuromatosis	exon 16: codon 918
Familial MTC	MTC	Codons 609, 611, 618, 620, and 634 Codons 768, 790, 791, or 804 (rare)
MEN2A and Hirschsprung's disease	MTC, pheochromocytoma, primary hyperparathyroidism, Hirschsprung's disease	Codons 609, 618, 620

commonly used as a diagnostic tumor marker. These tumors also stain positively for CEA and CGRP.

Diagnosis. The diagnosis of MTC is established by history, physical examination, raised serum calcitonin or CEA levels, and FNA cytology of the thyroid mass. Attention to family history is important because approximately 25% of patients with MTC have familial disease. Because it is not possible to distinguish sporadic from familial disease at initial presentation, all new patients with MTC should be screened for *RET* point mutations, pheochromocytoma (24-hour urinary levels of VMA, catecholamine, and metanephrine), and hyperparathyroidism (serum calcium). It is important to rule out a coexisting pheochromocytoma to avoid precipitating a hypertensive crisis and death. Screening of patients with familial MTC for *RET* point mutations has largely replaced using provocation testing with pentagastrin or calcium-stimulated calcitonin levels to make the diagnosis. Calcitonin and CEA are used to identify patients with persistent or recurrent MTC. Calcitonin is a more sensitive tumor marker, but CEA is a better predictor of prognosis.

Treatment. If patients are found to have a pheochromocytoma, this must be operated on first. These tumors are generally (>50%) bilateral. Total thyroidectomy is the treatment of choice for patients with MTC because of the high incidence of multicentricity, the more aggressive course, and ^{131}I therapy is not usually effective. The central compartment nodes are frequently involved early in the disease process, so that a bilateral central neck node dissection should be routinely performed. In patients with palpable cervical nodes or involved central neck nodes, ipsilateral or bilateral, modified radical neck dissection is recommended. Similarly, patients with tumors larger than 1.5 cm should undergo ipsilateral prophylactic modified radical neck dissection, because greater than 60% of these patients have nodal metastases. Approximately 30% of these patients will also have contralateral nodal metastases. In the case of locally recurrent or metastatic disease, tumor debulking is advised, not only to ameliorate symptoms of flushing and diarrhea, but also to decrease risk of death from recurrent central neck or mediastinal disease. External beam radiotherapy is controversial, but is recommended for patients with unresectable residual or recurrent tumor. There is no effective chemotherapy regimen. Radiofrequency ablation done laparoscopically appears promising in the palliative treatment of liver metastases larger than 1.5 cm. Tumors that express c-*kit* may also respond to tyrosine kinase inhibitors such as Gleevec.

In patients who have hypercalcemia at the time of thyroidectomy, only obviously enlarged parathyroid glands should be removed. The other parathyroid glands should be preserved and marked in patients

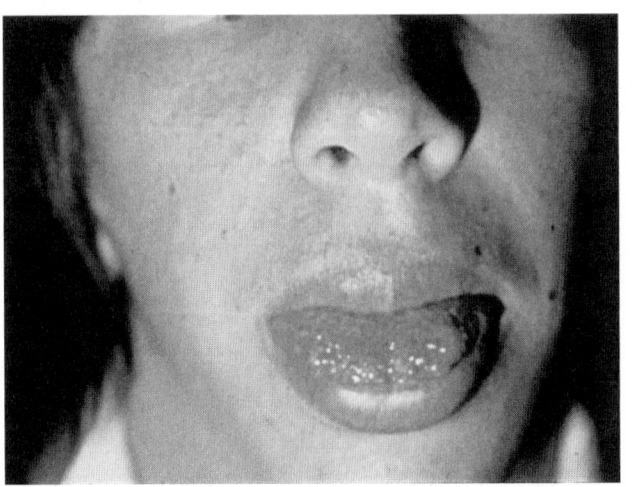

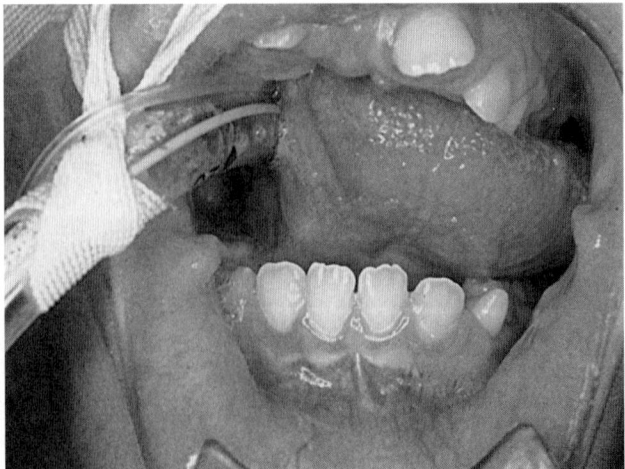

A   *B*

FIG. 37-27. Features of MEN2B: thickened lips (*A*) and mucosal neuromas (*A* and *B*).

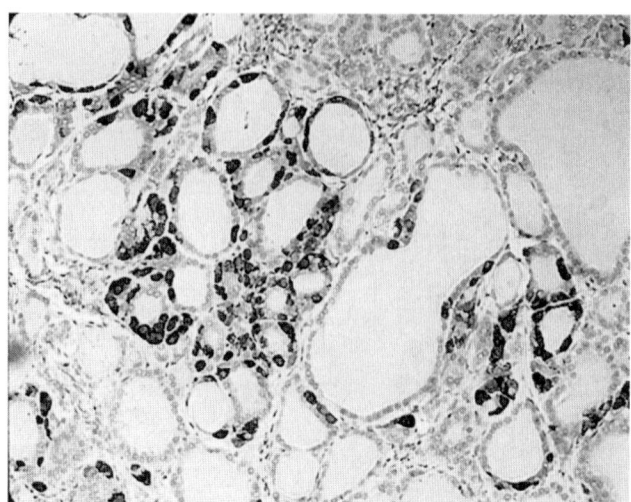

FIG. 37-28. C-cell hyperplasia, often found in patients with hereditary forms of medullary thyroid cancer.

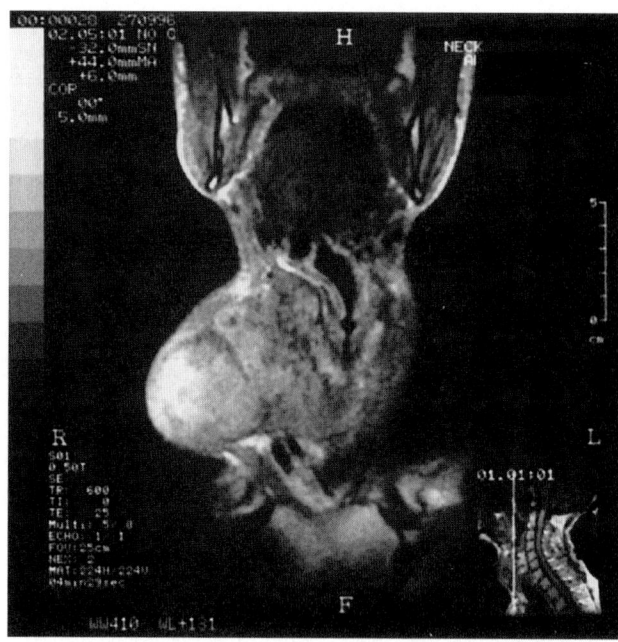

FIG. 37-29. MRI scan of a patient with anaplastic thyroid cancer.

with normocalcemia as only approximately 20% of patients with MEN2A develop hyperparathyroidism. When a normal parathyroid cannot be maintained on a vascular pedicle, it should be removed, biopsied to confirm that it is a parathyroid, and then autotransplanted to the forearm of the nondominant arm in MEN2A patients and in the sternocleidomastoid muscle in other patients.

Total thyroidectomy is indicated in RET mutation carriers once the mutation is confirmed. The procedure should be performed before age 6 years in MEN2A patients and prior to age 1 year in MEN2B patients.[44] Central neck dissection can be avoided in children who are *RET* positive and calcitonin negative with a normal ultrasound examination. When the calcitonin is increased or the ultrasound suggests a thyroid cancer, a prophylactic central neck dissection is indicated.

Postoperative Follow-Up and Prognosis. Prognosis is related to disease stage. The 10-year survival rate is approximately 80% but decreases to 45% in patients with lymph node involvement. Survival also is significantly influenced by disease type. It is best in patients with non-MEN familial MTC, followed by patients with MEN2A, and then by patients with sporadic disease. Prognosis is the worst (35% at 10 years) in patients with MEN2B. Patients with tumors that stain poorly for calcitonin and with a heterogeneous distribution of calcitonin do worse than patients in whom calcitonin staining is increased and homogeneous. Performing prophylactic surgery in *RET* oncogene mutation carriers not only improves survival rates, but also renders most patients calcitonin free.

Anaplastic Carcinoma

Anaplastic carcinoma accounts for approximately 1% of all thyroid malignancies in the United States and is declining in incidence. Women are more commonly affected, and the majority of tumors present in the seventh and eighth decades of life. The typical patient has a long-standing neck mass, which rapidly enlarges and may be painful. Associated symptoms, such as dysphonia, dysphagia, and dyspnea, are common. The tumor is large and may be fixed to surrounding structures or may be ulcerated (Fig. 37-29). Lymph nodes usually are palpable at presentation. Evidence of metastatic spread also may be present. Diagnosis is confirmed by FNA biopsy revealing characteristic giant and multinucleated cells. Incisional biopsy

is occasionally needed to confirm the diagnosis and isthmusectomy is performed to alleviate tracheal compression.

Pathology. On gross inspection, anaplastic tumors are firm and whitish in appearance. Microscopically, sheets of cells with marked heterogeneity are seen. Cells may be spindle-shaped, polygonal, or large, multinucleated cells. Foci of more differentiated thyroid tumors, either follicular or papillary, may be seen, suggesting that anaplastic tumors arise from more well-differentiated tumors. One should confirm that the tumor is not an MTC or a small-cell lymphoma because the prognosis varies considerably.

Treatment and Prognosis. This tumor is one of the most aggressive thyroid malignancies, with few patients surviving 6 months beyond diagnosis. All forms of treatment have been disappointing. If anaplastic carcinoma presents as a resectable mass, thyroidectomy may lead to a small improvement in survival, especially in younger individuals. Combined radiation and chemotherapy in an adjuvant setting in patients with resectable disease has been associated with prolonged survival.[45] Tracheostomy may be needed to alleviate airway obstruction.

Lymphoma

Lymphomas account for less than 1% of thyroid malignancies and most are of the non-Hodgkin's B-cell type. Although the disease can arise as part of a generalized lymphomatous condition, most thyroid lymphomas develop in patients with chronic lymphocytic thyroiditis.[18] Chronic antigenic lymphocyte stimulation has been suggested to result in lymphocyte transformation. Patients usually present with symptoms similar to those of patients with anaplastic carcinoma, although the rapidly enlarging neck mass often is painless. Patients may present with acute respiratory distress. The diagnosis usually is suggested by FNA biopsy, although needle-core or open biopsy may be necessary for definitive diagnosis. Staging studies should be obtained to assess the extent of extrathyroidal spread.

Treatment and Prognosis. Patients with thyroid lymphoma respond rapidly to chemotherapy (CHOP—cyclophosphamide, doxorubicin, vincristine, and prednisone), which is also associated with improved survival. Combined treatment with radiotherapy and chemotherapy is often recommended. Thyroidectomy and nodal resection are used to alleviate symptoms of airway obstruction in patients who do not respond quickly to the above regimens, or in patients who have completed the regimen prior to diagnosis. Prognosis depends on the histologic grade of the tumor and whether the lymphoma is confined to the thyroid gland or is disseminated. The overall 5-year survival rate is about 50%; patients with extrathyroidal disease have markedly lower survival rates. Although there are no prospective studies, similar remission rates have been reported for patients who underwent diagnostic biopsy plus adjuvant therapy alone (85%), when compared to debulking surgery plus adjuvant therapy. These findings support the argument for chemotherapy and radiotherapy for most patients.

Metastatic Carcinoma

The thyroid gland is a rare site of metastases from other cancers, including kidney, breast, lung, and melanoma.[46] Clinical examination and a review of the patient's history often suggest the source of the metastatic disease, and FNA biopsy usually provides definitive diagnosis. Resection of the thyroid, usually lobectomy, may be helpful in many patients, depending on the status of their primary tumor.

THYROID SURGERY

Preoperative Preparation

Patients with any recent or remote history of altered phonation or prior neck surgery should undergo vocal cord assessment by direct or indirect laryngoscopy prior to thyroidectomy. Patients with hyperthyroidism must be prepared as described earlier. Prophylactic antibiotics are not used routinely.

Conduct of Thyroidectomy

Thyroidectomy is performed under general anesthesia. The patient is positioned supine, with a sandbag between the scapulae. The head is placed on a donut cushion and the neck is extended to provide maximal exposure. A Kocher transverse collar incision, typically 4 to 5 cm in length, is placed in or parallel to a natural skin crease 1 cm below the cricoid cartilage (Fig. 37-30). Longer incisions may be needed in patients with large tumors, in patients with a short, fat neck or whose neck cannot be extended, and in patients with low-lying thyroid glands. The subcutaneous tissues and platysma are incised sharply and subplatysmal flaps are raised superiorly to the level of the thyroid cartilage and inferiorly to the suprasternal notch (Fig. 37-31). Towels are placed along the skin edges and a self-retaining retractor is also applied. The strap muscles are divided in the midline along the entire length of the mobilized flaps and the thyroid gland is exposed. On the side to be approached first, the sternohyoid muscles are separated from the underlying sternothyroid muscle by blunt dissection until the internal jugular vein and ansa cervicalis nerve are identified. The strap muscles rarely need to be divided to gain exposure to the thyroid gland. If this maneuver is necessary, the muscles should be divided high in order to preserve their innervation by branches of the ansa cervicalis. If there is evidence of direct tumor invasion into the strap muscles, the portion of involved muscle should be resected en bloc with the thyroid gland. The sternothyroid muscle is then dissected off the underlying thyroid by a combination of sharp and blunt dissection, thus exposing

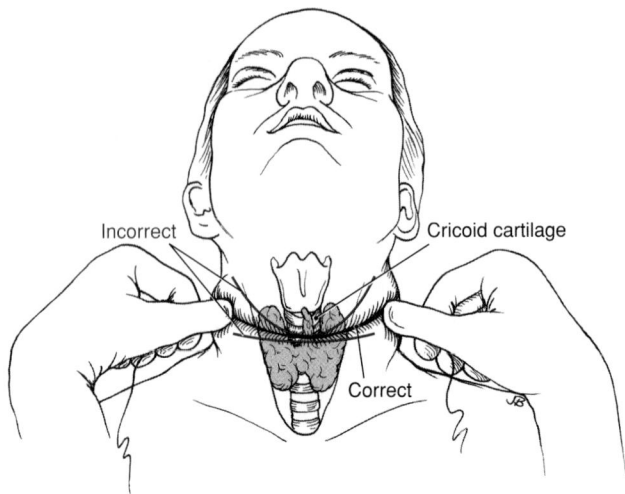

FIG. 37-30. Conduct of thyroidectomy: correct placement of thyroidectomy incision.

the middle thyroid veins. The thyroid lobe is retracted medially and anteriorly and the lateral tissues are swept posterolaterally using a peanut sponge. The middle thyroid veins are ligated and divided (Fig. 37-32). Attention is then turned to the midline where Delphian nodes and the pyramidal lobe are identified. The fascia just cephalad to the isthmus is divided. The superior thyroid pole is identified by retracting the thyroid first inferiorly and medially, and then the upper pole of the thyroid is mobilized caudally and laterally. The dissection plane is kept as close to the thyroid as possible and the superior pole vessels are individually identified, skeletonized, ligated, and divided low on the thyroid gland, to avoid injury to the external branch of the superior laryngeal nerve (Fig. 37-33). Once these vessels are divided, the tissues posterior and lateral to the superior pole can be swept from the gland, to reduce the risk of damaging vessels supplying the upper parathyroid.

The recurrent laryngeal nerve should then be identified. The course of the right RLN is more oblique than the left RLN. The nerves can be most consistently identified at the level of the cricoid cartilage. The parathyroids can usually be identified within 1 cm of the crossing of the inferior thyroid artery and the RLN. The upper parathyroid is dorsal to the RLN, whereas the lower parathyroid is anterior to it. If not present in this location, the lower glands may be found in the thyrothymic ligament or the upper thymus. The lower pole of the thyroid gland should be mobilized by gently sweeping all tissues dorsally. The inferior thyroid vessels are dissected, skeletonized, ligated, and divided as close to the surface of the thyroid gland as possible, to minimize devascularization of the parathyroids (extracapsular dissection) or injury to the RLN. Any structure that could be the RLN should not be divided. The RLN is most vulnerable to injury in the vicinity of the ligament of Berry. The nerve often passes through this structure, along with small crossing arterial and venous branches (Fig. 37-34). Any bleeding in this area should be controlled with gentle pressure before carefully identifying the vessel and ligating it. Use of the electrocautery should be avoided in proximity to the RLN. Once the ligament is divided, the thyroid can be separated from the underlying trachea by sharp dissection. The pyramidal lobe, if present, must be dissected in a cephalad direction to above the level of the notch in the thyroid cartilage or higher in continuity with the thyroid gland. If a lobectomy is to be performed, the isthmus is divided flush with the trachea on the contralateral side

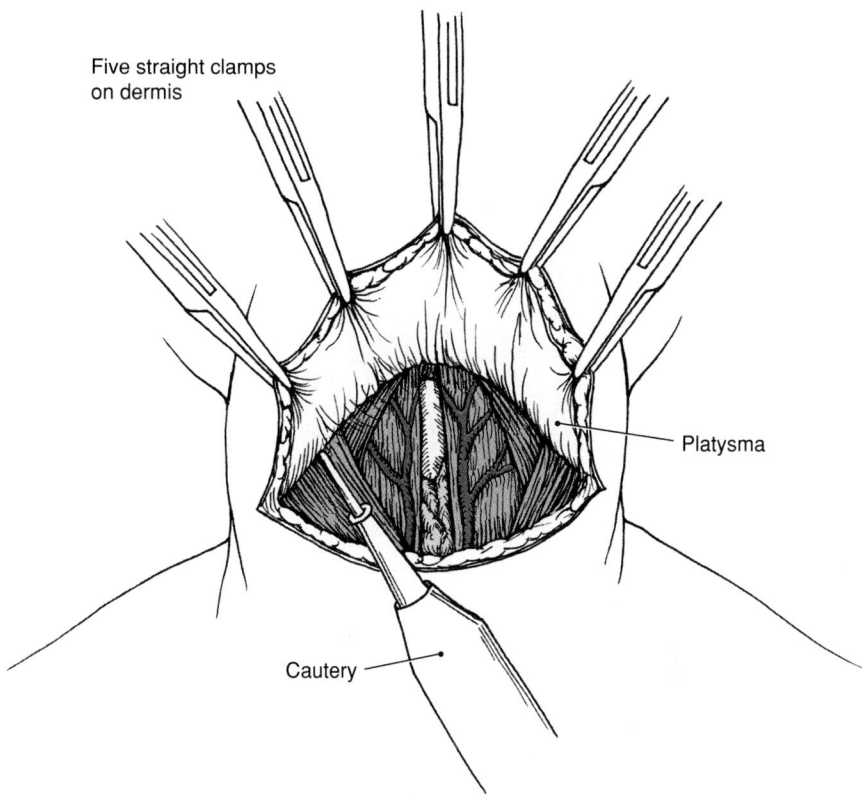

FIG. 37-31. Conduct of thyroidectomy: raising subplatysmal flaps.

and suture ligated. The procedure is repeated on the opposite side for a total thyroidectomy.

Parathyroid glands that are located anteriorly on the surface of the thyroid, cannot be dissected from the thyroid with a good blood supply, or have been inadvertently removed during the thyroidectomy, should be resected, confirmed as parathyroid tissue by frozen section, divided into 1-mm fragments, and reimplanted into individual pockets in the sternocleidomastoid muscle. The sites should be marked with silk sutures and a clip. If a subtotal thyroidectomy is

to be performed, once the superior pole vessels are divided and the thyroid lobe mobilized anteriorly, the thyroid lobe is cross-clamped with a Mayo clamp, leaving approximately 4 g of the posterior portion of the thyroid. The thyroid remnant is suture ligated, taking care to avoid injury to the recurrent laryngeal nerve. Routine drain placement is rarely necessary. After adequate hemostasis is obtained, the strap muscles are reapproximated in the midline using absorbable sutures. The platysma is approximated in a similar fashion. The skin can be closed with subcuticular sutures or clips.

FIG. 37-32. Conduct of thyroidectomy: dissection of middle thyroid vein.

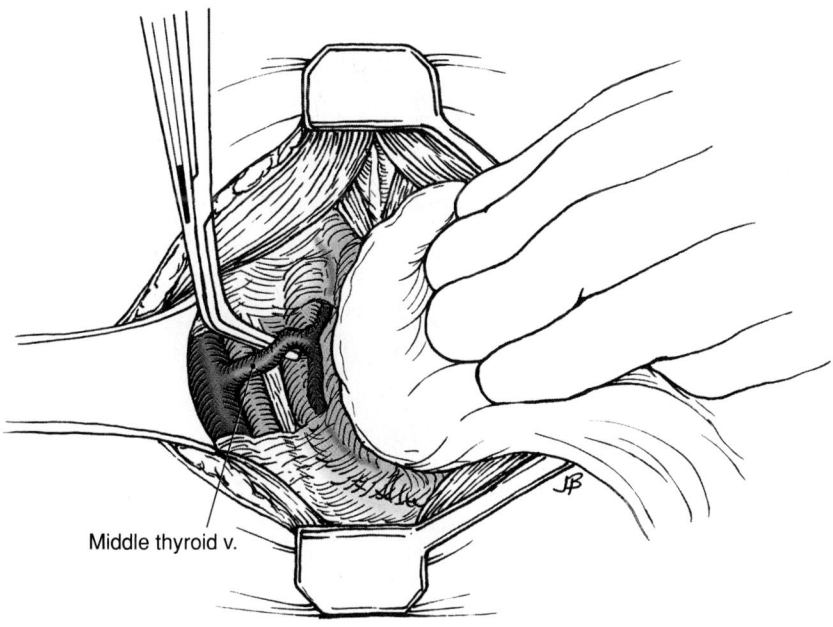

Middle thyroid v.

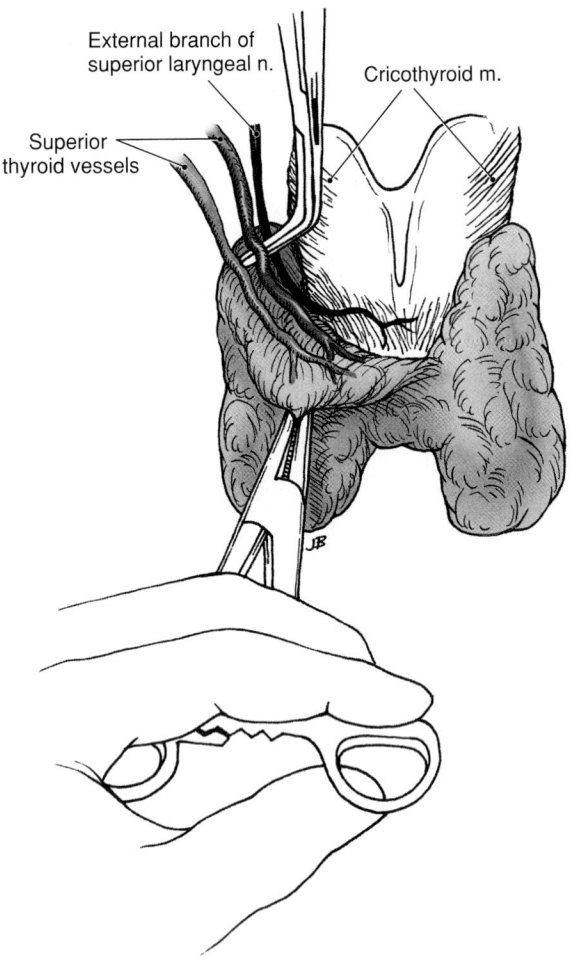

FIG. 37-33. Dissection of the superior pole vessels, which should be individually ligated.

Several approaches to minimally-invasive thyroidectomy, such as video-assisted thyroidectomy and endoscopic thyroidectomy via axillary incisions, have been proposed. These methods are feasible, but clear benefits over the "traditional" open approach have not been established.

Surgical Removal of Intrathoracic Goiter

Large cervical goiters may extend partially into the chest. A goiter is considered mediastinal if at least 50% of the thyroid tissue is located intrathoracically. Mediastinal goiters can be primary or secondary. Primary mediastinal goiters constitute approximately 1% of all mediastinal goiters and arise from accessory (ectopic) thyroid tissue located in the chest. These goiters are supplied by intrathoracic blood vessels and do not have any connection to thyroid tissue in the neck. The vast majority of mediastinal goiters are, however, secondary mediastinal goiters that arise from downward extension of cervical thyroid tissue along the fascial planes of the neck and derive their blood supply from the superior and inferior thyroid arteries. Virtually all intrathoracic goiters can be removed via a cervical incision.[47] Patients who have invasive thyroid cancers, have had previous thyroid operations and may have developed parasitic mediastinal vessels, or have primary mediastinal goiters with no thyroid tissue in the neck, may require a median sternotomy for removal. The chest, however, should be prepared in most cases, in the event it is necessary to perform a median sternotomy to control mediastinal bleeding or to completely remove an unsuspected invasive cancer. The goiter is approached by a neck incision as described above. The superior pole vessels and the middle thyroid veins are identified and ligated first. Early division of the isthmus helps with subsequent mobilization of the substernal goiter from beneath the sternum. Placement of large 1-0 or 2-0 sutures deep into the goiter, when necessary, helps deliver it. The goiter is delivered into the neck through a combination of traction and blunt dissection. In patients in whom thyroid cancer is suspected or demonstrated in an intrathoracic gland, attempts should be made to avoid rupture of the

FIG. 37-34. Conduct of thyroidectomy: dissection at the ligament of Berry. Note the small artery and vein within the ligament and the RLN coursing laterally.

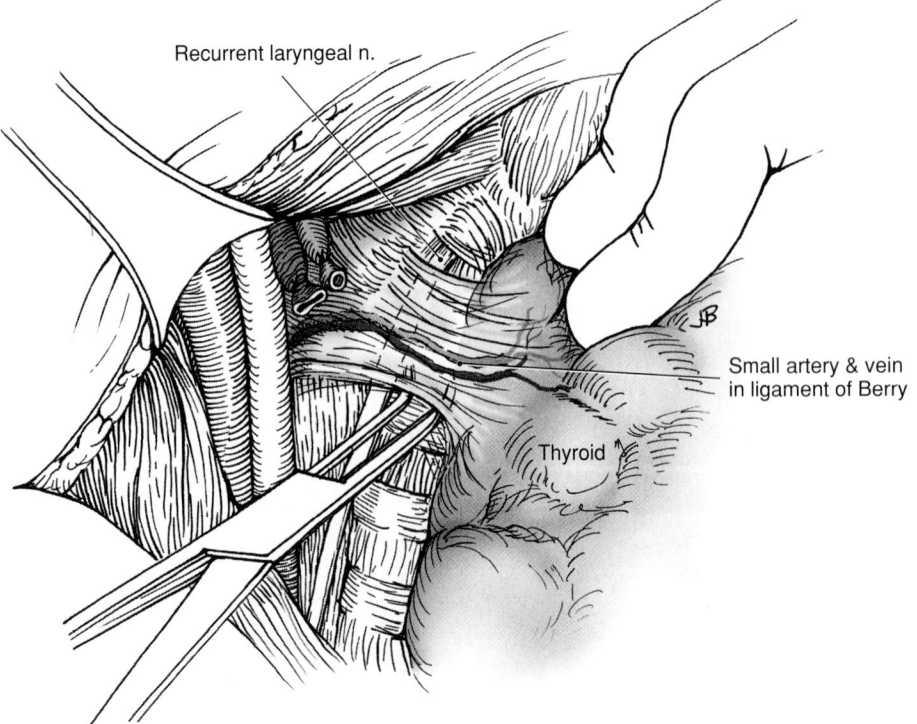

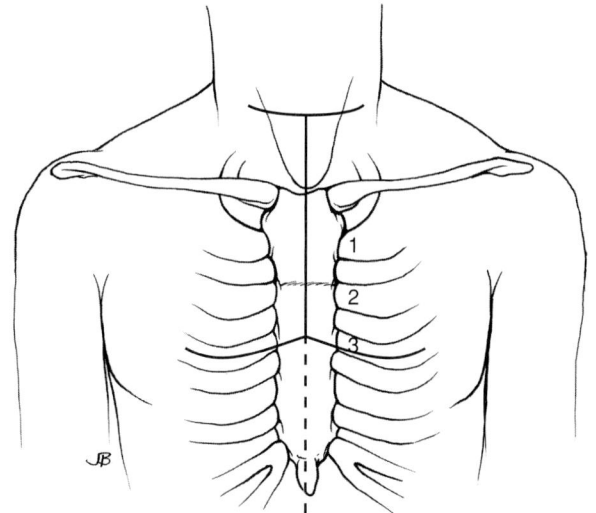

FIG. 37-35. Conduct of thyroidectomy: incisions for a partial sternotomy.

thyroid capsule. When sternotomy is indicated, the sternum usually should be divided to the level of the third intercostal space and then laterally on one side at the space between the third and fourth ribs (Fig. 37-35). Median sternotomy provides excellent exposure of the upper mediastinum and lower neck.

Neck Dissection for Nodal Metastases

Central compartment (medial to the carotid sheath) lymph nodes are frequently involved in patients with papillary, medullary, and Hürthle cell carcinomas, and should be removed at the time of thyroidectomy, preserving the recurrent laryngeal nerves and parathyroid glands. Central neck dissection is particularly important in patients with medullary and Hürthle cell carcinoma because of the high frequency of microscopic tumor spread and because these tumors cannot be ablated with ^{131}I. An ipsilateral modified radical neck dissection is indicated in the presence of palpable cervical lymph nodes or prophylactically in patients with medullary carcinoma when the thyroid lesion is larger than 1.5 cm.

A modified radical (functional) neck dissection can be performed via the cervical incision used for thyroidectomy, which can be extended laterally (Fig. 37-36A) to the anterior margin of the trapezius muscle (MacFee extension). The procedure involves removal of all fibrofatty tissue along the internal jugular vein (levels II, III, and IV) and the posterior triangle (level V). In contrast to a radical neck dissection, the internal jugular vein, the spinal accessory nerve, the cervical sensory nerves, and the sternocleidomastoid muscle are preserved unless they are adherent to or invaded by tumor. The procedure begins by opening the plane between the strap muscles medially and the sternocleidomastoid muscle laterally. The anterior belly of the omohyoid muscle is retracted laterally and the dissection is carried posteriorly until the carotid sheath is reached. The internal jugular vein is retracted medially with a vein retractor and the fibrofatty tissue and lymph nodes are dissected away from it by a combination of sharp and blunt dissection. The lateral dissection is carried along the posterior border of the sternocleidomastoid muscle, removing the tissue from the posterior triangle. The deep dissection plane is the anterior scalenus muscle, the phrenic nerve, the brachial plexus, and the medial scalenus muscle. The phrenic nerve is preserved on the scalenus anterior muscle, as are the cervical sensory nerves in most patients (Fig. 37-36B). Dissection along

the spinal accessory nerve superiorly is most important because this is a frequent site of metastatic disease.

Complications of Thyroid Surgery

Nerves, parathyroids, and surrounding structures are all at risk of injury during thyroidectomy.[48] Injury to the RLN may occur by severance, ligation, or undue traction, but should occur in less than 1% of patients undergoing thyroidectomy by experienced surgeons. Whether the nerves should be routinely identified was controversial, but the current consensus indicates that the RLN should be identified at some point during the procedure in most patients. The RLN is most vulnerable to injury during the last 2 to 3 cm of its course, but also can be damaged if the surgeon is not alert to the possibility of nerve branches and nonrecurrent nerves, particularly on the right side. If the injury is recognized intraoperatively, most surgeons advocate primary reapproximation of the perineurium using nonabsorbable sutures. Approximately 20% of patients are at risk of injury to the external branches of the superior laryngeal nerve, especially if superior pole vessels are ligated en masse. Intraoperative RLN and external laryngeal nerve monitoring techniques are now being used to minimize these nerve injuries. The cervical sympathetic trunk is at risk of injury in the rare scenario of retroesophageal goiter extension and might result in Horner's syndrome. Transient hypocalcemia (from surgical injury or inadvertent removal of parathyroid tissue) has been reported in up to 50% of cases, but permanent hypoparathyroidism occurs less than 2% of the time. Postoperative hypocalcemia is more likely in patients who undergo concomitant thyroidectomy and neck dissection. Postoperative hematomas or bleeding may also complicate thyroidectomies, and rarely necessitate emergency reoperation to evacuate the hematoma. Bilateral vocal cord dysfunction can require immediate reintubation. Seromas may need aspiration to relieve patient discomfort. Wound cellulitis and infection, and injury to surrounding structures, such as the carotid artery, jugular vein, and esophagus, are infrequent.

Parathyroid
HISTORICAL BACKGROUND

In 1849, the curator of the London Zoological Gardens, Sir Richard Owen, provided the first accurate description of the normal parathyroid gland after autopsy examination of an Indian rhinoceros that had been given to the zoo by the government of India. In 1879, Anton Wölfler documented that tetany occurred after total thyroidectomy in a patient operated on by C.A. Theodor Billroth. However, human parathyroids were not grossly and microscopically described until 1879, when they were described by Ivar Sandström, a medical student in Uppsala, Sweden. He suggested that these glands be named the *glandulae parathyroideae*, although their function was not known.

The association of hyperparathyroidism and the bone disease osteitis fibrosa cystica (described by von Recklinghausen) was recognized in 1903. Calcium measurement became possible in 1909, and the association between serum calcium levels and the parathyroid glands was established. The first successful parathyroidectomy was performed in 1925 by Felix Mandl on a 38-year-old man who had severe bone pain secondary to advanced osteitis fibrosa cystica (Fig. 37-37). The patient's condition dramatically improved after the operation, and he lived for another 7 years before dying of recurrent hyperparathyroidism or renal failure. One year later, the first parathyroid operation was performed at the Massachusetts General Hospital. Edward Churchill, assisted by an

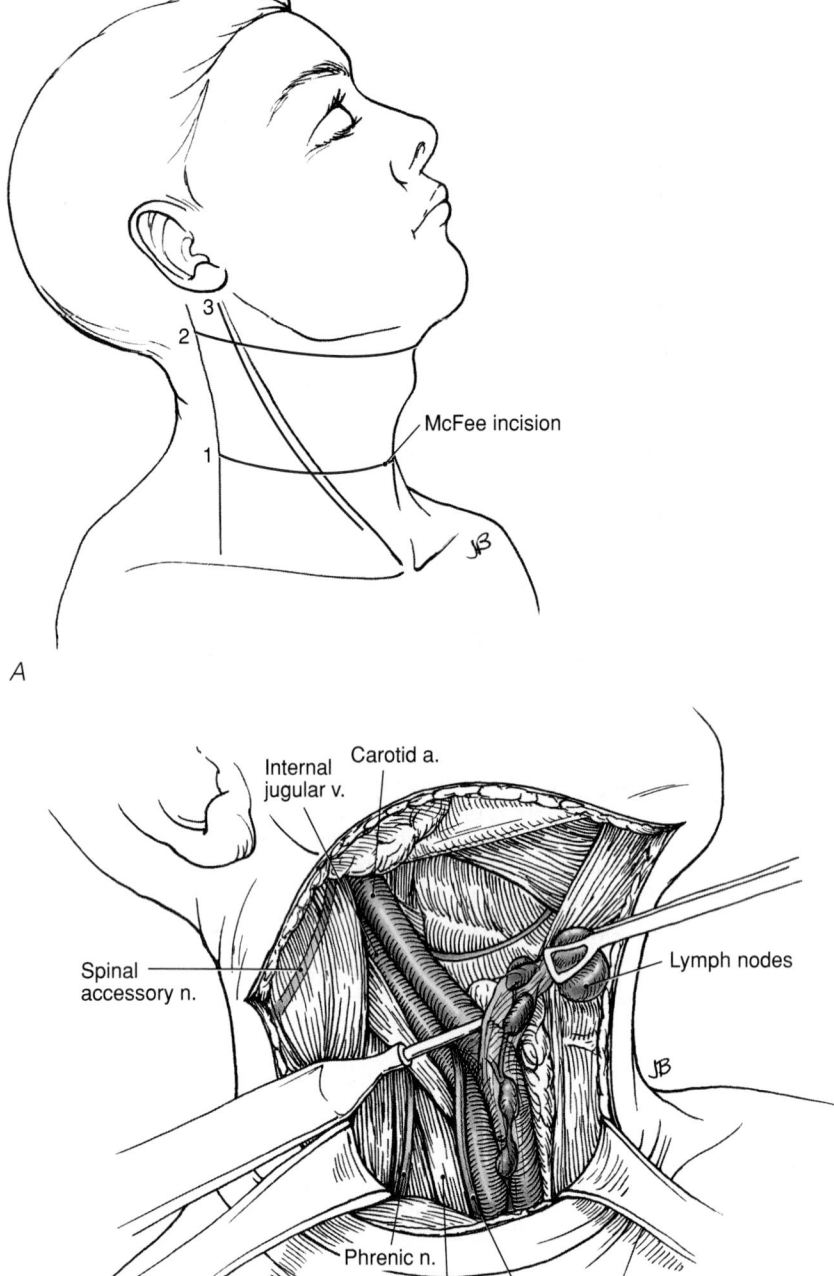

A

B

FIG. 37-36. *A.* Conduct of thyroidectomy: incisions for modified radical neck dissection. *B.* Conduct of thyroidectomy: anatomic relations of structures identified during a modified radical neck dissection.

intern named Oliver Cope, operated for the seventh time on the famous sea captain Charles Martell (Fig. 37-38) for severe primary hyperparathyroidism. Although no abnormalities had been found during previous operations, which included total thyroidectomy, an ectopic adenoma was found substernally. However, Captain Martell died 6 weeks later, likely as a consequence of laryngeal spasm and complications of renal stones and ureteral obstruction. The first successful parathyroidectomy for hyperparathyroidism in the United States was performed on a 56-year-old woman in 1928 by Isaac Y. Olch at the Barnes Hospital in St. Louis, Missouri. At operation, a parathyroid adenoma was found attached to the left lower lobe of the thyroid gland. Postoperatively the patient developed life-threatening tetany. Although she recovered and lived for many years, she did require lifelong supplemental calcium.

EMBRYOLOGY

In humans, the superior parathyroid glands are derived from the fourth branchial pouch, which also gives rise to the thyroid gland. The third branchial pouches give rise to the inferior parathyroid

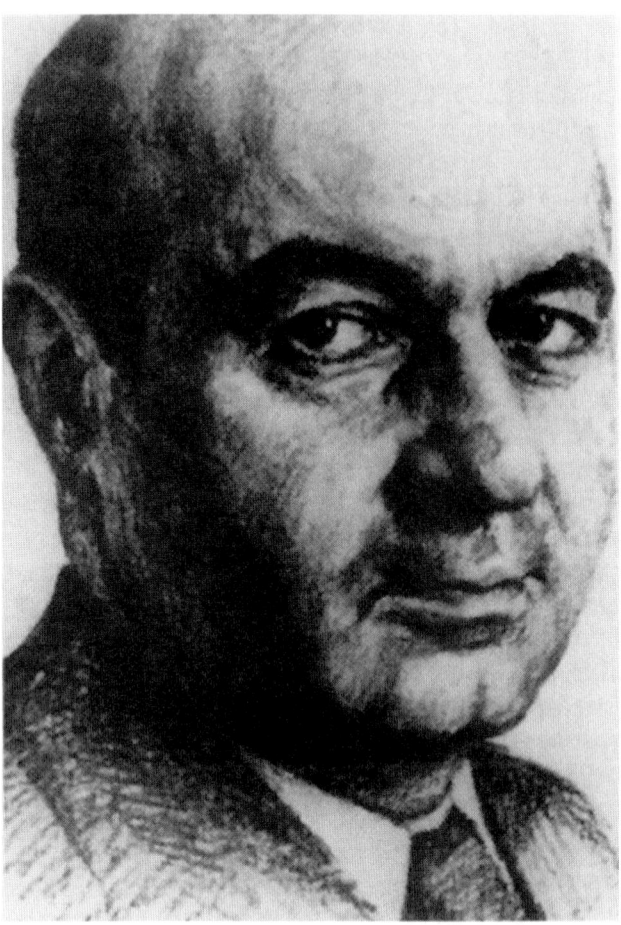

FIG. 37-37. Felix Mandl. *[Reproduced with permission from Organ C: History of parathyroid surgery. J Am Coll Surg 191(3):292, 2000.]*

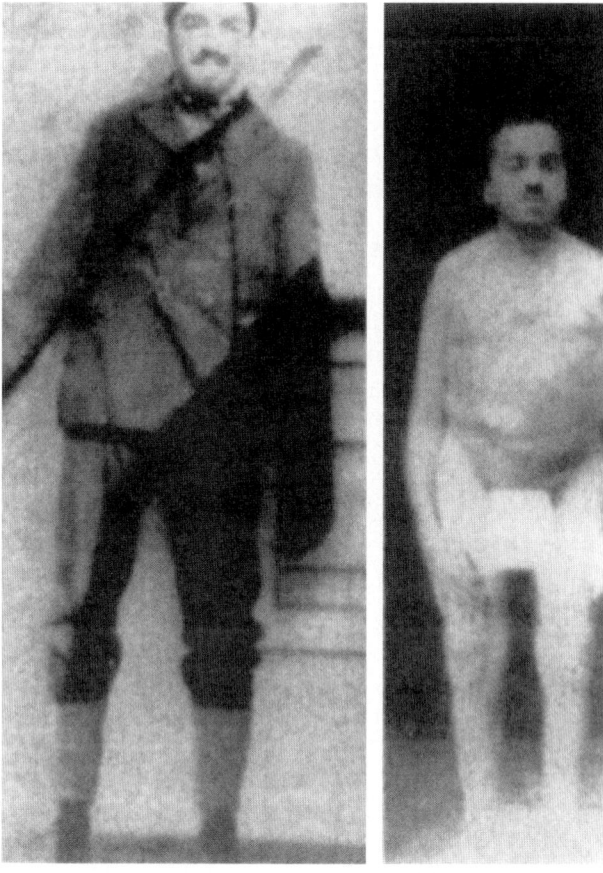

FIG. 37-38. Captain Charles Martell before and after development of the complications of primary hyperparathyroidism. *[Reproduced with permission from Organ C: History of parathyroid surgery. J Am Coll Surg 191(3):293, 2000.]*

glands and the thymus (Fig. 37-39). The parathyroids remain closely associated with their respective branchial pouch derivatives. The position of normal superior parathyroid glands is more consistent, with 80% of these glands being found near the posterior aspect of the upper and middle thyroid lobes, at the level of the cricoid cartilage.[49] Approximately 1% of normal upper glands may be found in the paraesophageal or retroesophageal space. Enlarged superior glands may "descend by gravity" in the tracheoesophageal groove and come to lie caudal to the inferior glands. Truly ectopic superior parathyroid glands are rare, but may be found in the middle or posterior mediastinum, commonly in the aortopulmonary window.[49] As the embryo matures, the thymus and inferior parathyroids migrate together caudally in the neck. The most common location for inferior glands is within a distance of 1 cm from a point centered where the inferior thyroid artery and recurrent laryngeal nerve cross.[49] Approximately 15% of inferior glands are found in the thymus. The position of the inferior glands, however, tends to be more variable as a consequence of their longer migratory path. Undescended inferior glands may be found near the skull base, angle of the mandible, or superior to the superior parathyroid glands, along with an undescended thymus. The frequency of intrathyroidal glands varies in the literature from 0.5 to 3%, with some authors considering upper glands to be more likely to occur in this location because of the close embryologic association of the upper glands and the lateral thyroid

anlage. Intrathyroidal parathyroid glands account for about 8% of patients with persistent hyperparathyroidism.

ANATOMY AND HISTOLOGY

Most patients have four parathyroid glands. The superior glands are usually dorsal to the RLN at the level of the cricoid cartilage, whereas the inferior parathyroid glands are located ventral to the nerve. Normal parathyroid glands are gray and semitransparent in newborns, but appear golden-yellow to light-brown in adults. Parathyroid color depends on numerous factors, including cellularity, fat content, and vascularity. Moreover, they are often embedded in and sometimes difficult to discern from surrounding fat. Normal parathyroid glands are located in loose tissue or fat and are ovoid. Figure 37-40 shows the variable parathyroid shapes. They measure 5 to 7 mm in size and weigh approximately 40 to 50 mg each. The parathyroid glands usually derive most of their blood supply from branches of the inferior thyroid artery, although branches from the superior thyroid artery supply at least 20% of upper glands. Branches from the thyroidea ima, and vessels to the trachea, esophagus, larynx, and mediastinum may also be found. The parathyroid glands drain ipsilaterally by the superior, middle, and inferior thyroid veins.

Akerstrom and associates,[49] in an autopsy series of 503 cadavers, found four parathyroid glands in 84% of cases. Supernumerary glands were present in 13% of patients, most commonly in the

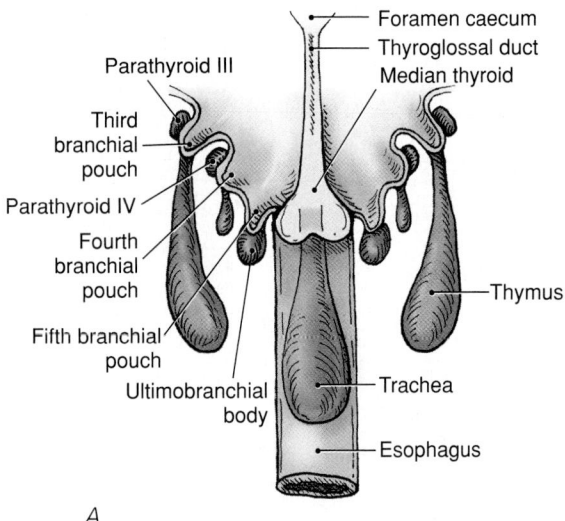

A

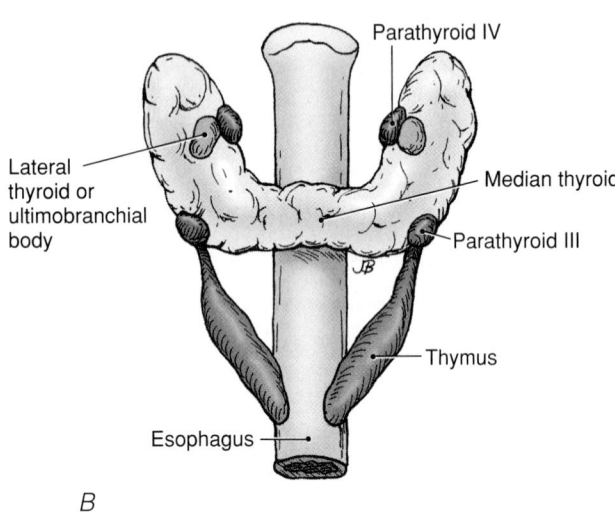

B

FIG. 37-39. Parathyroid embryology. The above demonstrates a schematic view of the pharynx of an 8- to 10-mm embryo (*A*) and locations of the thyroid, parathyroid, and thymic tissues in a 13- to 14-mm embryo (*B*). The lower parathyroids are derived from the third branchial pouch and migrate with the thymus, whereas the upper parathyroids are derived from the fourth branchial pouch and lie in close proximity to the ultimobranchial bodies. (*Reproduced with permission from Henry J: Applied embryology of the thyroid and parathyroid glands in Randolph G: Surgery of the Thyroid and Parathyroid Glands. W.B. Saunders, 2003.*)

thymus. Only 3% of patients had less than four glands. Similar results were obtained in other dissection studies of 428 human subjects by Gilmour who reported a 6.7% incidence of supernumerary glands.[50]

Histologically, parathyroid glands are composed of chief cells and oxyphil cells arranged in trabeculae, within a stroma composed primarily of adipose cells (Fig. 37-41). The parathyroid glands of infants and children are composed mainly of chief cells, which produce parathyroid hormone (PTH). Acidophilic, mitochondria-rich oxyphil cells are derived from chief cells, can be seen around

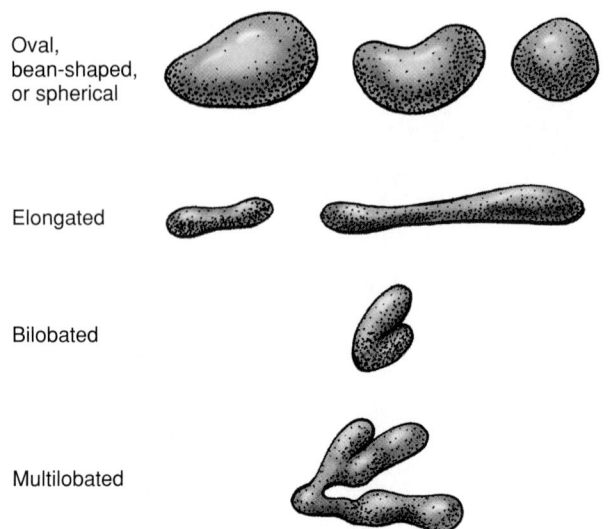

FIG. 37-40. Shapes of parathyroid glands. (*Reproduced with permission from Akerstrom G, et al, p 15.[49]*)

puberty, and increase in numbers in adulthood. A third group of cells, known as water-clear cells, also are derived from chief cells, are present in small numbers, and are rich in glycogen. Although most, but not all, oxyphil and water-clear cells retain the ability to secrete PTH, their functional significance is unknown.

PARATHYROID PHYSIOLOGY AND CALCIUM HOMEOSTASIS

Calcium is the most abundant cation in human beings, and has several crucial functions. Extracellular calcium levels are 10,000-fold higher than intracellular levels and both are tightly controlled. Extracellular calcium is important for excitation–contraction coupling in muscle tissues, synaptic transmission in the nervous system, coagulation, and secretion of other hormones. Intracellular calcium is an important second messenger regulating cell division, motility, membrane trafficking, and secretion. Calcium is absorbed from the

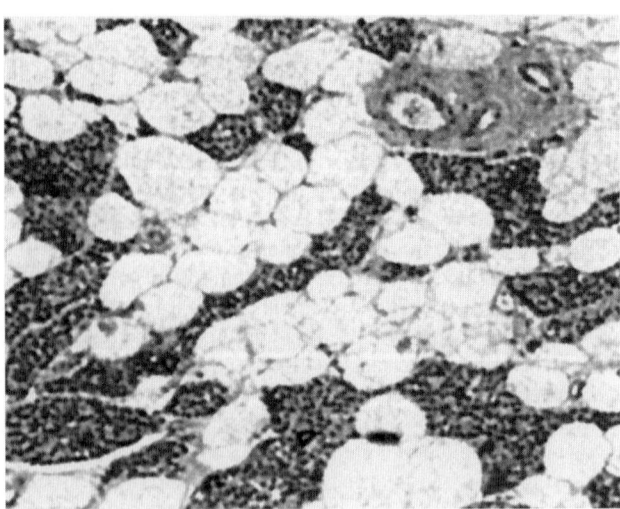

FIG. 37-41. Normal parathyroid histology showing chief cells interspersed with adipose cells.

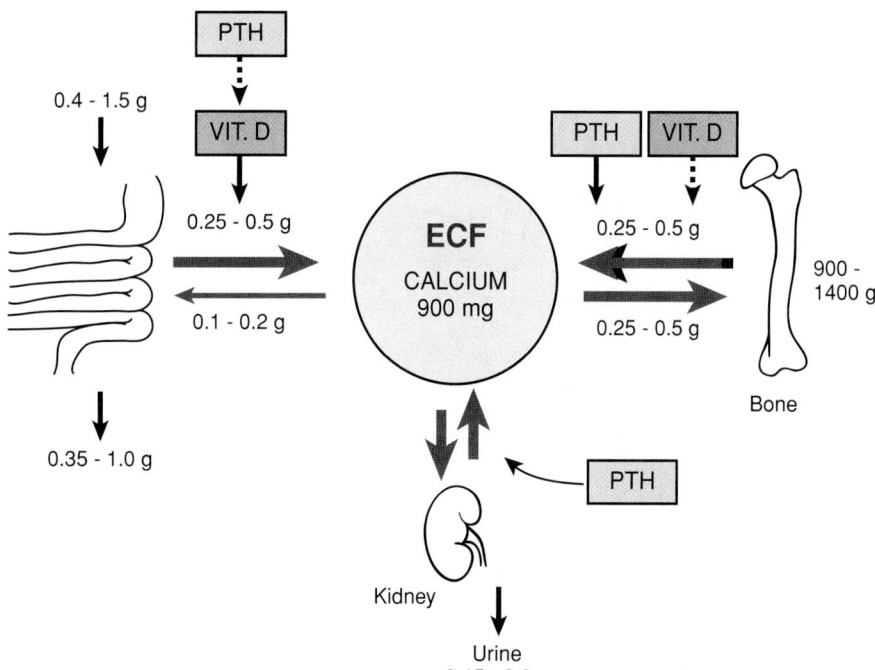

FIG. 37-42. Calcium balance and fluxes in a normal human. *Solid arrows* depict a direct effect whereas *dashed arrows* depict an indirect effect. The thickness of the arrows is representative of the magnitude of the flux. [*Reproduced with permission from Bruder J, et al: Mineral metabolism, in Felig P, Frohman L (eds): Endocrinology and Metabolism. McGraw-Hill, 2001, p. 1081.*]

small intestine in its inorganic form. Figure 37-42 depicts calcium fluxes in the steady state.

Extracellular calcium (900 mg) accounts for only 1% of the body's calcium stores, the majority of which is sequestered in the skeletal system. Approximately 50% of the serum calcium is in the ionized form, which is the active component. The remainder is bound to albumin (40%) and organic anions such as phosphate and citrate (10%). The total serum calcium levels range from 8.5 to 10.5 mg/dL (2.1 to 2.6 mmol/L) and ionized calcium levels range from 4.4 to 5.2 mg/dL (1.1 to 1.3 mmol/L). Both concentrations are tightly regulated. The total serum calcium level must always be considered in its relationship to plasma protein levels, especially serum albumin. For each gram per deciliter of alteration of serum albumin above or below 4.0 mg/dL, there is a 0.8 mg/dL increase or decrease in protein-bound calcium, and thus in total serum calcium levels. Total, and particularly ionized, calcium levels are influenced by various hormone systems.

Parathyroid Hormone

The parathyroid cells rely on a G-protein-coupled membrane receptor designated the calcium-sensing receptor (CASR), to regulate PTH secretion by sensing extracellular calcium levels (Fig. 37-43).[51] PTH secretion also is stimulated by low levels of 1,25-dihydroxy vitamin D, catecholamines, and hypomagnesemia. The PTH gene is located on chromosome 11. PTH is synthesized in the parathyroid gland as a precursor hormone, preproparathyroid hormone, which is cleaved first to proparathyroid hormone and then to the final 84-amino-acid PTH. Secreted PTH has a half-life of 2 to 4 minutes. In the liver, PTH is metabolized into the active N-terminal component and the relatively inactive C-terminal fraction. The C-terminal component is excreted by the kidneys and accumulates in chronic renal failure.

PTH functions to regulate calcium levels via its actions on three target organs, the bone, kidney, and gut. PTH increases the resorption of bone by stimulating osteoclasts and promotes the release

of calcium and phosphate into the circulation. At the kidney, calcium is primarily absorbed in concert with sodium in the proximal convoluted tubule, but fine adjustments occur more distally. PTH acts to limit calcium excretion at the distal convoluted tubule via an active transport mechanism. PTH also inhibits phosphate reabsorption (at the proximal convoluted tubule) and bicarbonate reabsorption. It also inhibits the Na^+/H^+ antiporter, which results in a mild metabolic acidosis in hyperparathyroid states. PTH and hypophosphatemia also enhance 1-hydroxylation of 25-hydroxyvitamin D, which is responsible for its indirect effect of increasing intestinal calcium absorption.

Calcitonin

Calcitonin is produced by thyroid C cells and functions as an antihypercalcemic hormone by inhibiting osteoclast-mediated bone resorption. Calcitonin production is stimulated most dramatically by calcium and pentagastrin, and also by catecholamines, cholecystokinin, and glucagon. It produces hypocalcemia, when administered intravenously to experimental animals. At the kidney, calcitonin increases phosphate excretion by inhibiting its reabsorption. Calcitonin plays a minimal, if any, role in the regulation of calcium levels in humans. However, it is very useful as a marker of medullary thyroid cancer and in treating acute hypercalcemic crisis.

Vitamin D

Vitamin D refers to vitamin D_2 and vitamin D_3, both of which are produced by photolysis of naturally occurring sterol precursors. Vitamin D_2 is available commercially in pharmaceutical preparations, whereas vitamin D_3 is the most important physiologic compound and is produced from 7-dehydrocholesterol, which is found in the skin. Vitamin D is metabolized in the liver to its primary circulating form, 25-hydroxy vitamin D. Further hydroxylation in the kidney results in 1,25-dihydroxy vitamin D, which is the most metabolically active form of vitamin D. Vitamin D stimulates the absorption of calcium and phosphate from the gut and the resorption of calcium from the bone.

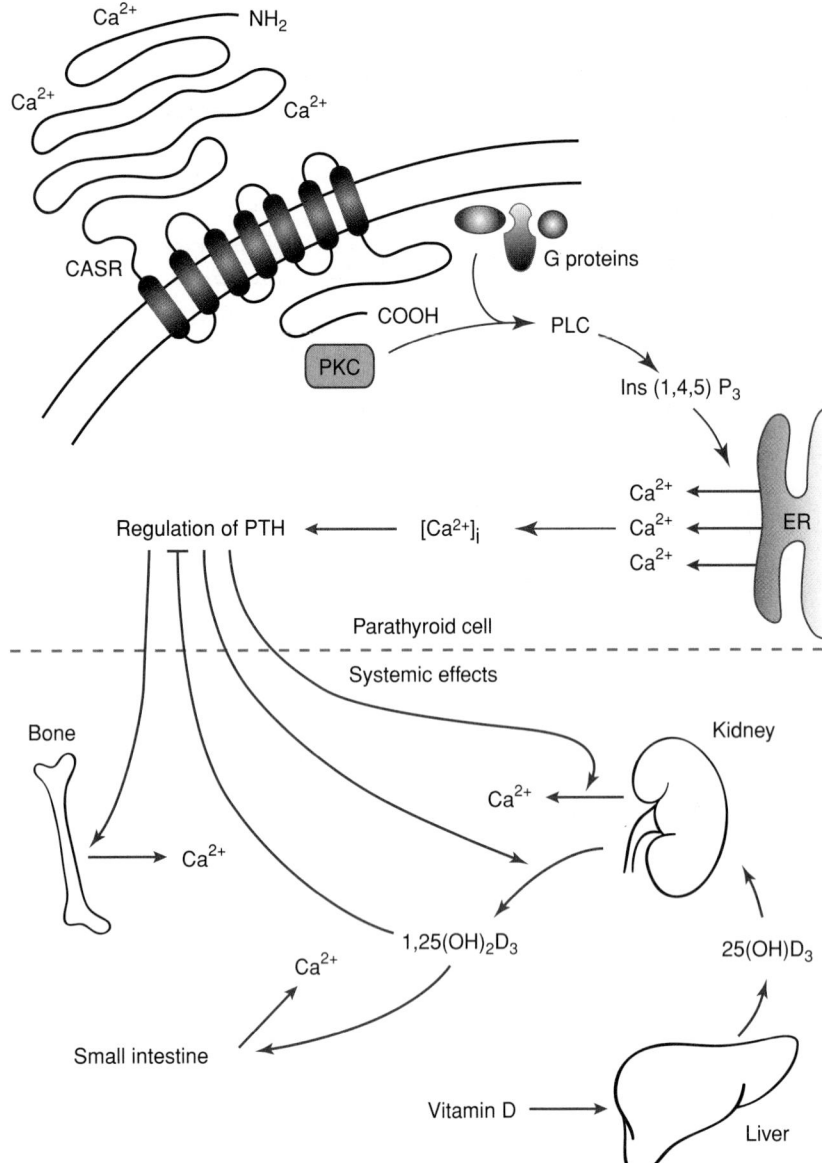

FIG. 37-43. *Regulation of calcium homeostasis. The calcium-sensing receptor (CASR) is expressed on the surface of the parathyroid cell and senses fluctuations in the concentration of extracellular calcium. Activation of the receptor is thought to increase intracellular calcium levels, which, in turn, inhibit PTH secretion via posttranslational mechanisms. Increased PTH secretion leads to an increase in serum calcium levels by increasing bone resorption and enhancing renal calcium reabsorption. PTH also stimulates renal 1α-hydroxylase activity, leading to an increase in 1,25-dihydroxy vitamin D, which also exerts a negative feedback on PTH secretion. (Reproduced with permission from Carling T, p 54.[51])*

HYPERPARATHYROIDISM

Hyperfunction of the parathyroid glands may be classified as primary, secondary, or tertiary. Primary hyperparathyroidism (PHPT) arises from increased PTH production from abnormal parathyroid glands and results from a disturbance of normal feedback control exerted by serum calcium. Elevated PTH levels may also occur as a compensatory response to hypocalcemic states resulting from chronic renal failure or gastrointestinal malabsorption of calcium. This state is referred to as secondary hyperparathyroidism (HPT) and can be reversed by correction of the underlying problem, (e.g., kidney transplantation for chronic renal failure). However, chronically stimulated glands may occasionally become autonomous, resulting in persistence or recurrence of hypercalcemia after successful renal transplantation, resulting in tertiary HPT.

Primary Hyperparathyroidism

PHPT is a common disorder, affecting 100,000 individuals annually in the United States. PHPT occurs in 0.1 to 0.3% of the general population and is more common in women (1:500) than in men (1:2000). Increased PTH production leads to hypercalcemia via increased gastrointestinal absorption of calcium, increased production of vitamin D_3 and reduced renal calcium clearance. PHPT is characterized by increased parathyroid cell proliferation and PTH secretion which is independent of calcium levels.

Etiology

The exact cause of PHPT is unknown, although exposure to low-dose therapeutic ionizing radiation and familial predisposition account for some cases. Various diets and intermittent exposure to sunshine may also be related. Other causes include renal leak of calcium and declining renal function with age, as well as alteration in the sensitivity of parathyroid glands to suppression by calcium. The latency period for development of PHPT after radiation exposure is longer than that for the development of thyroid tumors, with most cases occurring 30 to 40 years after exposure. Patients who have been exposed to radiation have similar clinical presentations and calcium levels when compared to patients without a history of radiation exposure. However, the former tend to have higher PTH levels and a higher incidence of concomitant thyroid neoplasms. Lithium therapy has been known to shift the set-point for PTH secretion in parathyroid cells, thereby resulting in elevated PTH levels and mild hypercalcemia. Lithium stimulates the growth of abnormal parathyroid glands in vitro, and in susceptible patients in vivo.[52] PHPT results from the enlargement of a single gland or parathyroid adenoma in approximately 80% of cases, multiple adenomas or hyperplasia in 15 to 20% of patients and parathyroid carcinoma in 1% of patients. Existence of two enlarged glands or double adenomas is supported by biochemical (calcium and PTH), intraoperative PTH, molecular, and histologic data. This entity is less common in younger patients, but accounts for up to 10% of older patients with primary HPT. It should be emphasized that when more than one abnormal parathyroid gland is identified preoperatively or intraoperatively, the patient has hyperplasia (all glands abnormal) until proven otherwise.

Genetics

Although most cases of PHPT are sporadic, PHPT does occur within the spectrum of a number of inherited disorders such as MEN1, MEN2A, isolated familial HPT, and familial HPT with jaw-tumor syndrome. All of these syndromes are inherited in an autosomal dominant fashion. Primary HPT is the earliest and most common manifestation of MEN1[53] and develops in 80 to 100% of patients by age 40 years. These patients are also prone to pancreatic neuroendocrine tumors and pituitary adenomas, and less commonly to adrenocortical tumors, lipomas, skin angiomas, and carcinoid tumors of the bronchus, thymus, or stomach. Approximately

50% of patients develop gastrinomas, which are often multiple and metastatic at diagnosis. Insulinomas develop in 10 to 15% of cases, whereas many patients have nonfunctional pancreatic endocrine tumors. Prolactinomas occur in 10 to 50% of MEN1 patients and constitute the most common pituitary lesion. MEN1 has been shown to result from germline mutations in the *MEN1* gene, a tumor-suppressor gene located on chromosome 11q12-13 (Fig. 37-44) that encodes menin, a protein that is postulated to interact with the transcription factor JunD in the nucleus. Most *MEN1* mutations result in a nonfunctional protein, but, unfortunately, are scattered throughout the translated nine exons of the gene. This makes presymptomatic screening for mutation carriers difficult. *MEN1* mutations also have been found in kindreds initially suspected to represent isolated familial HPT. Hyperparathyroidism develops in approximately 20% of patients with MEN2A and is generally less severe. MEN2A is caused by germline mutations of the *RET* proto-oncogene located on chromosome 10. In contrast to MEN1, genotype–phenotype correlations have been noted in this syndrome in that individuals with mutations at codon 634 are more likely to develop HPT. Patients with the familial HPT with jaw-tumor syndrome have an increased predisposition to parathyroid carcinoma. This syndrome maps to a tumor-suppressor locus *HRPT2*, on chromosome 1. Patients belonging to isolated hyperparathyroidism kindreds also appear to demonstrate linkage to *HRPT2*.

Approximately 25 to 40% of sporadic parathyroid adenomas and some hyperplastic parathyroid glands have loss of heterozygosity at 11q13, the site of the *MEN1* gene.[54] The parathyroid adenoma 1 oncogene (*PRAD1*), which encodes cyclin D1, a cell-cycle control protein, is overexpressed in approximately 18% of parathyroid

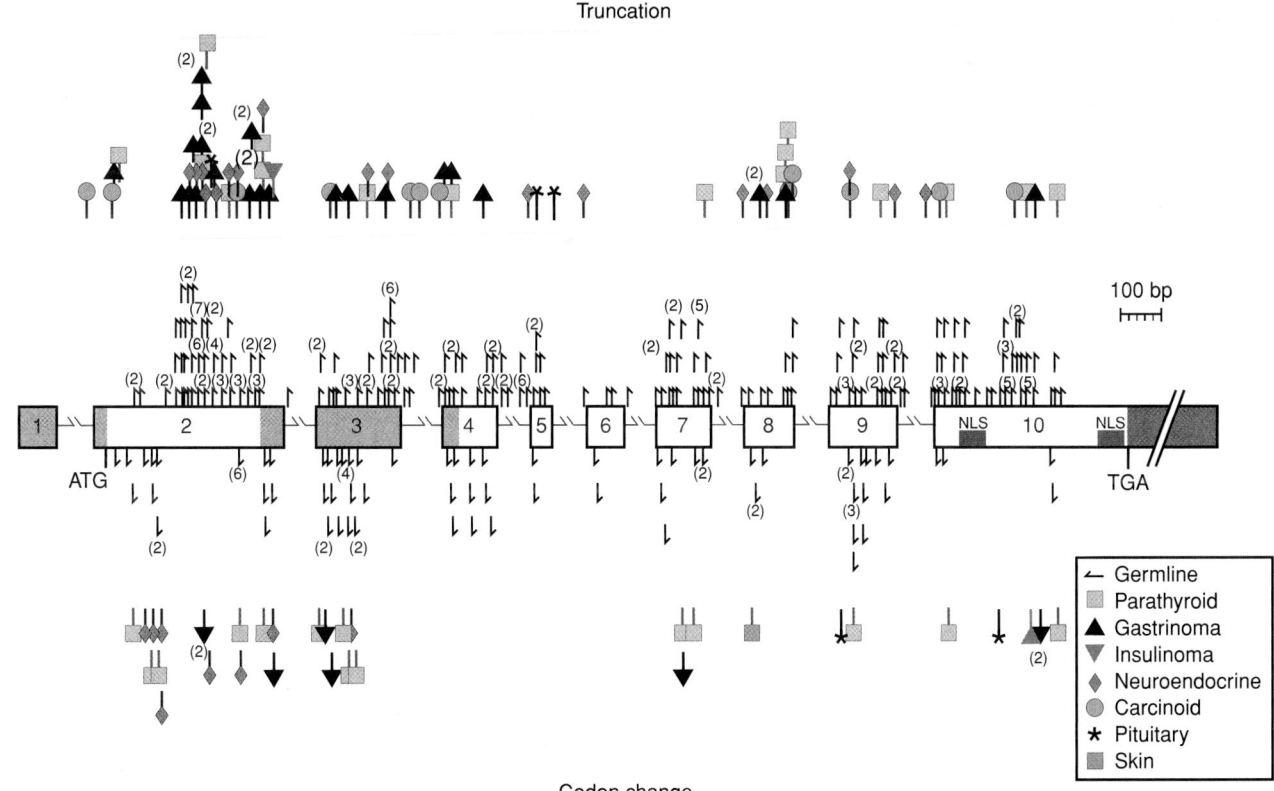

FIG. 37-44. Schematic structure of the *MEN1* or *MENIN* gene, which encodes a 610-amino-acid protein, menin. (*Reproduced with permission from Schussheim D, et al: Multiple endocrine neoplasia type 1: New clinical and basic findings. Trends Endocrinol Metab 12:175, 2001.*)

adenomas. This results from a rearrangement on chromosome 11 that places the *PRAD1* gene under the control of the PTH promoter. Other chromosomal regions deleted in parathyroid adenomas and possibly reflecting loss of tumor-suppressor genes include 1p, 6q, and 15q, whereas amplified regions suggesting oncogenes have been identified at 16p and 19p. Sporadic parathyroid cancers are characterized by uniform loss of the tumor-suppressor gene *RB,* which is involved in cell-cycle regulation and 60% of parathyroid cancers have *HRPT2* mutations. These alterations are rare in benign parathyroid tumors and may have implications for diagnosis. The *p53* tumor-suppressor gene is also inactivated in a subset (30%) of parathyroid carcinomas.

Clinical Manifestations

Patients with PHPT formerly presented with the "classic" pentad of symptoms (i.e., kidney stones, painful bones, abdominal groans, psychic moans, and fatigue overtones). With the advent and widespread use of automated blood analyzers in the early 1970s, there has been an alteration in the "typical" patient with PHPT, who is more likely to be minimally symptomatic or asymptomatic. Currently, most patients present with weakness, fatigue, polydipsia, polyuria, nocturia, bone and joint pain, constipation, decreased appetite, nausea, heartburn, pruritus, depression, and memory loss. In keeping with these nonspecific findings, patients with PHPT also tend to score lower than healthy controls when assessed by general multidimensional health assessment tools, such as the Medical Outcomes Study Short-Form Health Survey (SF-36),[55,56] and by other specific questionnaires, such as those designed by Pasieka and associates.[57] Furthermore, these symptoms and signs improve in most, but certainly not all, patients after parathyroidectomy. Truly "asymptomatic" PHPT appears to be rare. Complications of HPT are described below.

Renal Disease. Approximately 80% of patients with PHPT have some degree of renal dysfunction or symptoms. Kidney stones were previously found in up to 80% of patients, but now occur in approximately 20 to 25%. The calculi are typically composed of calcium phosphate or oxalate. In contrast, primary HPT is found to be the underlying disorder in only 3% of patients presenting with nephrolithiasis. Nephrocalcinosis, which refers to renal parenchymal calcification, is found in fewer than 5% of patients and is more likely to lead to renal dysfunction. Chronic hypercalcemia can also impair concentrating ability, thereby resulting in polyuria, polydipsia, and nocturia. The incidence of hypertension is variable, but has been reported to occur in up to 50% of patients with PHPT. Hypertension appears to be more common in older patients and seems to correlate with the magnitude of renal dysfunction, and, in contrast to other symptoms or metabolic complications, is least likely to improve after parathyroidectomy.

Bone Disease. Bone disease, including osteopenia, osteoporosis, and osteitis fibrosa cystica, is found in approximately 15% of patients with PHPT. Increased bone turnover can usually be determined by documenting an elevated blood alkaline phosphatase level. Advanced PHPT and/or vitamin D deficiency leads to osteitis fibrosa cystica, a condition that previously was more common, but which now occurs in less than 5% of patients. It is characterized by pathognomonic radiologic findings, which are best seen on x-rays of the hands that demonstrate subperiosteal resorption (most apparent on the radial aspect of the middle phalanx of the second and third fingers), bone cysts, and tufting of the distal phalanges (Fig. 37-45). The skull may also be affected and appears mottled

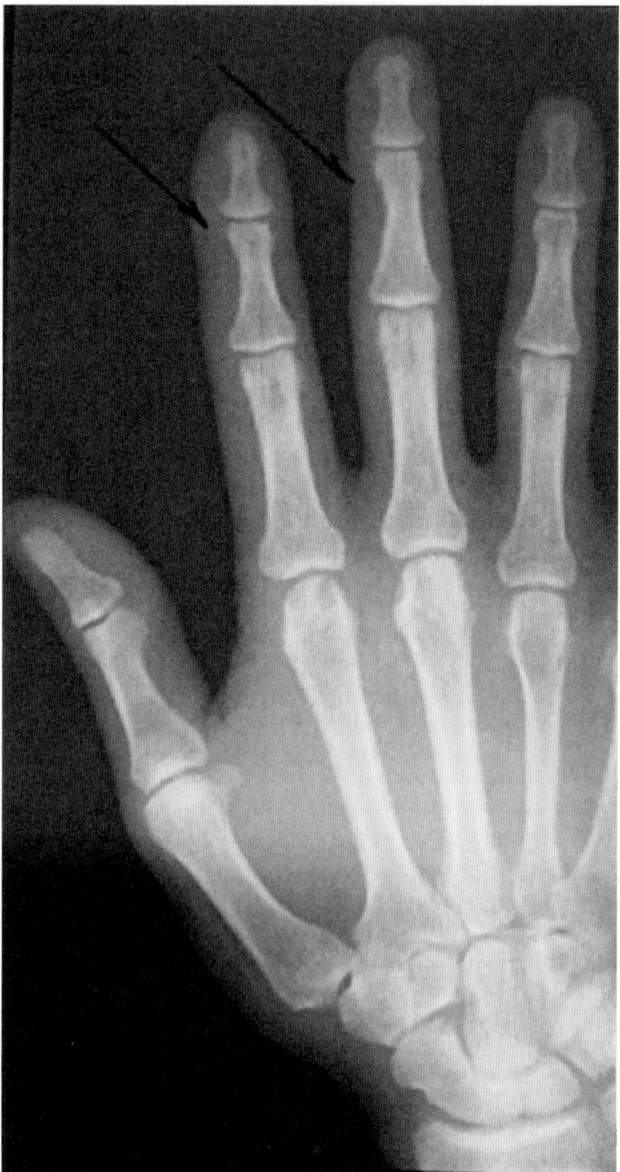

FIG. 37-45. X-rays of the hand showing subperiosteal bone resorption most apparent along the radial aspect of the middle phalanx, which is characteristic of osteitis fibrosa cystica.

(salt and pepper) with a loss of definition of the inner and outer cortices. Brown or osteoclastic tumors and bone cysts may also be present. Severe bone disease, resulting in bone pain and tenderness and/or pathologic fractures, is rarely presently observed. However, reductions of bone mineral density (BMD) with osteopenia and osteoporosis are more common. Patients with normal serum alkaline phosphatase levels almost never have clinically apparent osteitis fibrosa cystica. Hyperparathyroidism typically results in a loss of bone mass at sites of cortical bone, such as the radius and relative preservation of cancellous bone such as that located at the vertebral bodies. Patients with PHPT, however, may also have osteoporosis of the lumbar spine (trabecular bone) that improves dramatically following parathyroidectomy. Fractures also occur more frequently in patients with PHPT and the incidence of fractures decreases beginning 1 year after parathyroidectomy. Bone disease correlates with blood PTH and vitamin D levels.

Gastrointestinal Complications. PHPT has been associated with peptic ulcer disease. In experimental animals, hypergastrinemia has been shown to result from PTH infusion into blood vessels supplying the stomach, independent of its effects on serum calcium. An increased incidence of pancreatitis also has been reported in patients with PHPT, although this appears to occur only in patients with profound hypercalcemia ($Ca^{2+} \geq 12.5$ mg/dL). Patients with PHPT also have an increased incidence of cholelithiasis, presumably as a consequence of an increase in biliary calcium, which leads to the formation of calcium bilirubinate stones.

Neuropsychiatric Manifestations. Severe hypercalcemia may lead to various neuropsychiatric manifestations such as florid psychosis, obtundation, or coma. Other findings, such as depression, anxiety, and fatigue, are more commonly observed in patients with only mild hypercalcemia. The etiology of these symptoms is unknown. Studies demonstrate that levels of certain neurotransmitters (monoamine metabolites 5-hydroxyindoleacetic acid [5-HIAA] and homovanillic acid [HVA]) are reduced in the cerebrospinal fluid of patients with primary HPT when compared to controls. Electroencephalogram abnormalities also occur in patients with primary and secondary HPT and normalize following parathyroidectomy.

Other Features. Primary HPT can also lead to fatigue and muscle weakness, which is prominent in the proximal muscle groups. Although the exact etiology of this finding is unknown, muscle biopsy studies show that weakness results from a neuropathy, rather than from a primary myopathic abnormality. Patients with HPT also have an increased incidence of chondrocalcinosis and pseudogout, with deposition of calcium pyrophosphate crystals in the joints. Calcification at ectopic sites such as blood vessels, cardiac valves, and skin, also has been reported, as has hypertrophy of the left ventricle independent of the presence of hypertension.[58] Several large studies from Europe also suggest that PHPT is associated with increased death rates from cardiovascular disease and cancer, even in patients with mild HPT,[59] although this finding was not substantiated in North American patients.[60]

Physical Findings

The neck should be examined for evidence of masses and/or lymphadenopathy. Parathyroid tumors are seldom palpable, except in patients with profound hypercalcemia. A palpable neck mass in a patient with PHPT is more likely to be thyroid in origin or a parathyroid cancer. Patients may also demonstrate evidence of band keratopathy, a deposition of calcium in Bowman's membrane just inside the iris of the eye. This condition is generally caused by chronic eye diseases such as uveitis, glaucoma, and trauma, but may also occur in the presence of conditions associated with high calcium or phosphate levels. Fibro-osseous jaw tumors, or the presence of familial disease in patients with PHPT and jaw-tumors, if present, should alert the physician to the possibility of parathyroid carcinoma.

Differential Diagnosis

Hypercalcemia may be caused by a multitude of conditions (Table 37-9). PHPT and malignancy account for more than 90% of all cases of hypercalcemia. PHPT is more common in the outpatient setting, whereas malignancy is the leading cause of hypercalcemia in hospitalized patients. PHPT can virtually always be distinguished from other diseases causing hypercalcemia by a combination of history, physical examination, and appropriate laboratory investigations.

Table 37-9
Differential Diagnosis of Hypercalcemia

Hyperparathyroidism
Malignancy—hematologic (multiple myeloma), solid tumors (caused by PTHrP)
Endocrine diseases—hyperthyroidism, addisonian crisis, VIPoma
Granulomatous diseases—sarcoidosis, tuberculosis, berylliosis, histoplasmosis
Milk–alkali syndrome
Drugs—thiazide diuretics, lithium, vitamin A or D intoxication
Benign familial hypocalciuric hypercalcemia
Paget's disease
Immobilization

PTHrP = parathyroid hormone-related protein; VIPoma = vasoactive intestinal peptide-secreting tumor.

Hypercalcemia associated with malignancy can be thought of as including three distinct syndromes. Although bone metastases may cause hypercalcemia, patients with solid tumors of the lung, breast, kidney, head and neck, and ovary often have humoral hypercalcemia of malignancy without any associated bony metastases. In addition, hypercalcemia also can be associated with hematologic malignancies such as multiple myeloma. Humoral hypercalcemia of malignancy is known to be mediated primarily by parathyroid hormone-related peptide (PTHrP), which also plays a role in the hypercalcemia associated with bone metastases and multiple myeloma.[61]

Thiazide diuretics cause hypercalcemia by decreasing renal clearance of calcium. This corrects in normal patients within days to weeks after discontinuing the diuretic but patients with PHPT continue to be hypercalcemic. Thiazide diuretics can, therefore, exacerbate underlying PHPT and were formerly used to unmask primary HPT in patients with borderline hypercalcemia. Benign familial hypocalciuric hypercalcemia (BFHH) is a rare autosomal dominant condition with nearly 100% penetrance and results from inherited heterozygous mutations in the CASR gene located on chromosome 3. Homozygous germline mutations at this locus result in neonatal hypercalcemia, a condition that can rapidly prove fatal. Patients with BFHH have lifelong hypercalcemia, which is not corrected by parathyroidectomy. Hypercalcemia is also found in approximately 10% of patients with sarcoidosis secondary to increased 25-hydroxy vitamin D 1-hydroxylase activity in lymphoid tissue and pulmonary macrophages, which is not subject to inhibitory feedback control by serum calcium. Thyroid hormone also has bone-resorption properties, thus causing hypercalcemia in thyrotoxic states, especially in immobilized patients. Hemoconcentration appears to be an important factor in the hypercalcemia associated with adrenal insufficiency and pheochromocytoma, although the latter patients may have associated parathyroid tumors (MEN2A) and some pheochromocytomas are known to secrete PTHrP. Other endocrine lesions, such as vasoactive intestinal peptide-secreting tumors (VIPomas), may be associated with hypercalcemia because of the increased secretion of PTHrP. Milk–alkali syndrome requires the ingestion of large quantities of calcium with an absorbable alkali such as that used in the treatment of peptic ulcer disease with antacids. Ingestion of large quantities of vitamins D and A are infrequent causes of hypercalcemia.

Diagnostic Investigations

Biochemical Studies. The presence of an elevated serum calcium and intact PTH (iPTH) or two-site PTH levels establishes the diagnosis of PHPT with virtual certainty. These sensitive PTH

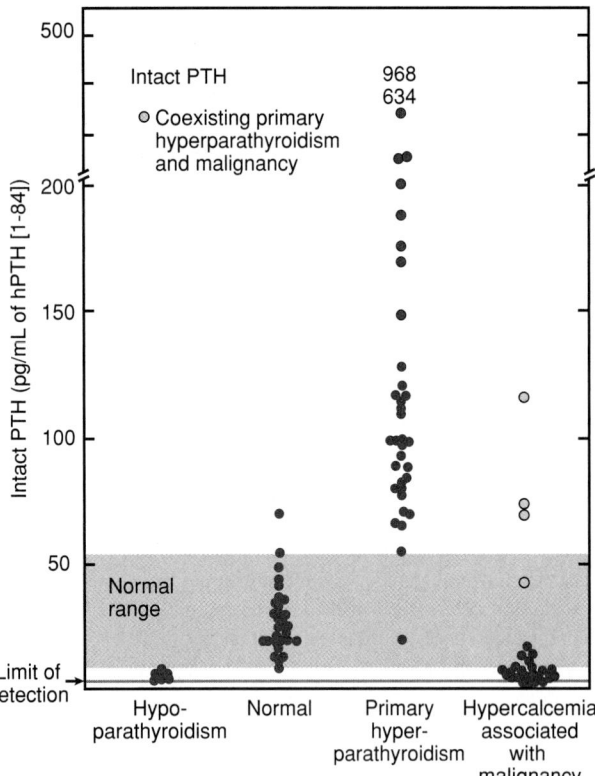

FIG. 37-46. Intact PTH measurement allows differentiation between the various causes of hypercalcemia. (*Reproduced with permission from Endres D, et al: Measurement of parathyroid hormone. Endocrinol Metab Clin North Am 18:622, 1989.*)

assays employ immunoradiometric or immunochemiluminescent techniques, and can reliably distinguish primary HPT from other causes of hypercalcemia. Furthermore, they do not cross-react with PTHrP (Fig. 37-46). In patients with metastatic cancer and hypercalcemia, iPTH levels help to determine whether the patient also has concurrent PHPT. Although rare, a patient with hypercalcemia may have a tumor that secretes PTH. FNA biopsy of such a tumor for PTH levels or selective venous catheterization of the veins draining such tumors can help clarify the diagnosis.

Patients with PHPT also typically have decreased serum phosphate (approximately 50%) and elevated 24-hour urinary calcium concentrations (approximately 60%). A mild hyperchloremic metabolic acidosis is also present (80%), thereby leading to an elevated chloride:phosphate ratio (>33). Urinary calcium levels need not be measured routinely, except in patients who have not had previously documented normocalcemia, or who have a family history of hypercalcemia, in order to rule out BFHH. The biochemical profile of BFHH is similar to primary HPT, except that the hypercalcemia is mild and PTH levels are high-normal or only slightly elevated. However, 24-hour urinary calcium excretion is characteristically low (<100 mg/d). Furthermore, the serum calcium to creatinine clearance ratio is usually less than 0.01 in patients with BFHH, whereas it is typically greater than 0.02 in patients with primary hyperparathyroidism. Table 37-10 lists other biochemical features of PHPT. Elevated levels of alkaline phosphatase may be found in approximately 10% of patients with PHPT and are indicative of high-turnover bone disease. These patients are prone to developing postoperative hypocalcemia as a consequence of bone hunger. Blood urea nitrogen and creatinine levels should be obtained to

Table 37-10
Biochemical Features of Primary Hyperparathyroidism

Serum Tests	Alteration
Calcium	Increased, except in normocalcemic primary hyperparathyroidism
Intact PTH	Increased or inappropriately high
Chloride	Increased or high normal
Phosphate	Decreased or low normal
Chloride:phosphate ratio	Increased (usually >33)
Magnesium	Unchanged or decreased (in patients with osteitis fibrosa cystica)
Uric acid	Normal or increased
Alkaline phosphatase	Normal or increased (in the presence of bone disease)
Acid–base status	Mild hyperchloremic metabolic acidosis
Calcium:creatinine clearance ratio	>0.02 (vs. <0.01 in BFHH)
1,25-dihydroxy vitamin D	Normal or increased
Urine Tests	
24-Hour urinary calcium	Normal or increased

determine the extent of damage to the kidneys. Serum and urine protein electrophoresis may be necessary to exclude multiple myeloma.

Occasionally, patients present with normocalcemic PHPT caused by vitamin D deficiency, a low serum albumin, excessive hydration, a high phosphate diet, or a low normal blood calcium set-point. These patients have increased total PTH levels with or without increased blood ionized calcium levels and must be distinguished from patients with renal leak hypercalciuria who also have increased PTH levels as a result of excessive calcium loss in the urine. This can be accomplished by administering thiazide diuretics. In patients with idiopathic hypercalciuria, the urinary calcium level falls, and the secondary increase in the blood PTH level also decreases to normal, whereas patients with normocalcemic hyperparathyroidism continue to have elevated urine calcium and blood PTH levels, and may in fact become hypercalcemic.

Radiologic Tests. In patients with profound hypercalcemia or PHPT associated with vitamin D deficiency, hand and skull x-rays may demonstrate osteitis fibrosa cystica, as outlined earlier. However, given the altered clinical presentation of most patients with PHPT, routine hand x-rays are only recommended in patients with an elevated bone alkaline phosphatase level. Bone mineral density studies using dual-energy absorptiometry are, however, being increasingly used to assess the effects of PHPT on bone. Abdominal ultrasound examination is used selectively to document renal stones. Parathyroid localization studies are not used to confirm the diagnosis of PHPT, but rather to aid in identifying the location of the offending gland(s), as discussed below.

Treatment

Rationale for Parathyroidectomy and Guidelines for Operative Treatment. Most authorities agree that patients who have developed complications such as kidney stones, osteoporosis, or renal dysfunction, have the "classic" symptoms of PHPT, or who are younger than age 50 years, should undergo parathyroidectomy. However, the treatment of patients with asymptomatic PHPT has been the subject of controversy, partly because there is little agreement on what constitutes an "asymptomatic" patient. At the National Institutes of Health (NIH) consensus conference in 1990,

Table 37-11

Indications for Parathyroidectomy in Patients with Asymptomatic Primary HPT (1990 NIH Consensus Conference Guidelines)

At initial evaluation:
  Markedly increased serum calcium
  Episode of life-threatening hypercalcemic episode
  Reduced creatinine clearance
  Kidney stones on abdominal x-rays
  Markedly elevated 24-hour urinary calcium excretion ($\geq$400 mg/d)
  Substantially decreased bone mass
  Age <50 years
Development of any of the following during follow-up:
  Typical skeletal, renal, or gastrointestinal symptoms
  Serum calcium >1–1.6 mg/dL above upper normal range
  A >30% decline in creatinine clearance
  Urinary calcium >400 mg/d
  Bone mass reduced to <2 SD below age-, gender-, and race-matched controls
  Unwillingness or inability to undergo continued follow-up

"asymptomatic" PHPT was defined as "the absence of common symptoms and signs of PHPT, including no bone, renal, gastrointestinal, or neuromuscular disorders." The panel advocated nonoperative management of these patients with mild PHPT based on observational studies, which suggested relative stability of biochemical parameters over time.[62] This was further substantiated by more recent work, including the study by Silverberg and associates.[63] In their cohort of 52 patients with asymptomatic HPT followed without surgery, levels of serum and urinary calcium, PTH, alkaline phosphatase, and vitamin D metabolites remained relatively stable over a 10-year period in most patients. However, the consensus panel considered certain patients to be candidates for surgery, as summarized in Table 37-11.[64] These guidelines were recently reassessed at a second workshop on asymptomatic primary HPT held at the NIH in 2002.[65] The guidelines are essentially unchanged except for those relating to parathyroidectomy. It is now recommended for patients with smaller elevations in serum calcium levels (<1 mg/dL above the upper limit of normal) and if bone mineral density measured at any of three sites (radius, spine, or hip) is greater than 2.5 SD below those of gender- and race-matched, but not age-matched, controls (i.e., peak bone density or T-score [rather than Z-score] <2.5). The panel still recommends exercising caution in using neuropsychologic abnormalities, cardiovascular disease, gastrointestinal symptoms, menopause, and elevated serum or urine indices of increased bone turnover as sole indications for parathyroidectomy. Lastly, it is important to note that in the previously mentioned cohort studies, a significant proportion of patients were either lost to follow-up or experienced progression of disease requiring surgery. Silverberg and associates reported development of a new indication for surgery in 14 of 52 (27%) of their asymptomatic patients, and because approximately 50% of their patients were initially treated surgically, overall, approximately 75% of patients were treated surgically.[63]

Successful parathyroidectomy results in resolution of osteitis fibrosa cystica, improved bone mineral density,[63] decreased formation of new renal stones,[63] increased muscle strength, and decreased left ventricular hypertrophy. In addition, it also improves peptic ulcer disease and a number of the nonspecific manifestations of PHPT such as fatigue, polydipsia, polyuria and nocturia, bone and joint pain, constipation, nausea, and depression in most, but not all, patients. This also has been demonstrated using symptom questionnaires and various standardized general quality of life

assessments such as SF-36,[56] and a specific parathyroidectomy assessment of symptoms scale.[57] The results were similar in a randomized controlled trial[55] of patients with mild PHPT. The increased death rate in patients with PHPT appears to be reversible by successful parathyroidectomy.[66] Lastly, parathyroidectomy can be accomplished with greater than a 95% success rate with minimal morbidity, even in elderly patients, and is the only curative treatment option for PHPT. Although a number of medical therapies such as bisphosphonates and calcimimetics (modifiers of the sensitivity of the calcium-sensing receptor) show promise in the treatment of patients with PHPT, these therapies are experimental, long-term outcome data is lacking, and their routine use is not advocated at this time. Previous investigations also document that parathyroidectomy is more cost-effective than medical follow-up within 5 years of initial treatment. Therefore, it is recommended that parathyroidectomy should be offered to virtually all patients except those in whom the operative risks are prohibitive.

Unfortunately, to date, there are no definitive criteria to indicate which patients with mild PHPT will have progressive disease. Therefore, patients who do not undergo surgery should undergo routine follow-up consisting of biannual calcium measurements and annual measurements of bone mineral density and serum creatinine.[65]

Preoperative Localization Tests. It is important to emphasize that the diagnosis of PHPT is a metabolic one and that localization studies should not be used to make or confirm it. Several localization studies currently are used to identify the location of the enlarged gland(s) and may be classified into noninvasive or invasive modalities. These studies have variable performance characteristics, which, in turn, vary with experience and institutional experience. Table 37-12 outlines the features of various localization studies.

Most endocrine surgeons agree that localization studies are mandatory and invaluable prior to any redo-parathyroid surgery, but their utility prior to initial neck exploration continues to be controversial. However, the last decade has seen the introduction and widespread use of various localization tests, including intraoperative PTH. These studies have permitted surgeons to perform more limited operations, some of them under local anesthesia. These "minimally-invasive" procedures include unilateral and focused neck exploration, radio-guided parathyroidectomy, and several endoscopic or video-assisted approaches.[67] Thus, the use of localization studies has been shown to be associated with lower morbidity rates (hypoparathyroidism and recurrent laryngeal nerve injury) and decreased operative times, reduced duration of hospital stay, and improved cosmetic outcomes, while maintaining success rates similar to those obtained with traditional bilateral neck explorations. Some studies also show that use of localization studies may be more cost-effective.

There also is little consensus on which localization studies should be used. The performance characteristics of these studies vary with institutional and radiologist experience and are discussed in Table 37-12. [99m]Technetium-labeled sestamibi (Fig. 37-47) is the most widely used and accurate modality, with a sensitivity greater than 80% for detection of parathyroid adenomas.[68] Sestamibi, also known as Cardiolite, was initially introduced for cardiac imaging and is concentrated in mitochondria-rich tissue. It was subsequently noted to be useful for parathyroid localization because of the delayed washout of the radionuclide from hypercellular parathyroid tissue when compared to thyroid tissue. Sestamibi scans are generally complemented by neck ultrasound (Fig. 37-48), which can identify adenomas with greater than 75% sensitivity in experienced centers, and is most useful in identifying intrathyroidal parathyroids.

Table 37-12
Parathyroid Localization Studies

Study	Advantages	Disadvantages
Preoperative, noninvasive		
^{99m}Technetium-sestamibi scan	Allows planar and 3D SPECT imaging	False-positive tests because of thyroid nodules, lymphadenopathy; false-negative study more common with multiple abnormal parathyroids
Ultrasound	Identification of juxta- and intrathyroidal tumors; relatively inexpensive	False-positive results because of thyroid nodules, lymph nodes, esophageal lesions; false-negatives result from substernal, ectopic, and undescended tumors
CT scan	Localization of ectopic (mediastinal) glands	Not useful for juxta- or intrathyroidal glands; false-positives from lymph nodes; relatively high cost; radiation exposure; requires intravenous contrast; interference from shoulders and metallic clips
MRI scan	Localization of ectopic tumors; no radiation exposure; no intravenous contrast; no metal clip artifact;	Expensive; false-positives from lymph nodes and thyroid nodules; cannot be used in claustrophobic patients
Preoperative, invasive		
FNA biopsy	Helpful for distinguishing parathyroid tumor from lymphadenopathy	Experienced cytologist needed
Angiogram	Provides a road map for selective venous sampling; treatment of mediastinal tumors by embolization	Expensive; experienced radiologist needed; neurologic complications
Venous sampling	Useful to lateralize tumor in equivocal cases	Expensive; experienced radiologist needed
Intraoperative		
PTH assay	Immediate confirmation of tumor removal	Expensive

Single-photon emission computed tomography (SPECT), when used with planar sestamibi, has particular utility in the evaluation of ectopic parathyroid adenomas, such as those located deep in the neck or in the mediastinum. Specifically, SPECT can indicate whether an adenoma is located in the anterior or posterior mediastinum (aortopulmonary window), thus enabling the surgeon to modify the operative approach accordingly.[69] CT and MRI scans are less sensitive than sestamibi scans, but are helpful in localizing mediastinal glands. Intraoperative parathyroid hormone was initially introduced in 1993, and is used to determine the adequacy of parathyroid resection (Fig. 37-49).[70] According to one commonly used criterion, when the PTH falls by 50% or more in 10 minutes after removal of a parathyroid tumor, as compared to the highest preremoval value, the test is considered positive and the operation is terminated.

Although preoperative localization studies and intraoperative PTH have become widely used since their inception, the literature is lacking in studies directly comparing procedures performed with and without these studies. Furthermore, localization studies, including intraoperative PTH, are less sensitive and accurate when they are most necessary, such as in the presence of multiple gland parathyroid disease. Long-term outcome data and cost-effectiveness studies are needed before routine use of localization studies can be recommended; however, they should be used if a focused approach or reoperation is planned.[65]

Operative Approaches

Unilateral parathyroid exploration was first carried out using intraoperative staining of a biopsy from the normal parathyroid gland with Sudan black dye to rule out a double adenoma. Initially, the choice of side to be explored was random, but the introduction of preoperative localization studies has enabled a more directed approach. In contrast, the focused approach identifies only the enlarged parathyroid gland and no attempts are made to locate other normal parathyroid glands. Unilateral neck explorations have several advantages over bilateral neck exploration, including reduced operative times and complications, such as injury to the recurrent laryngeal nerve and hypoparathyroidism.[71] However, most existing studies comparing the two approaches are retrospective and do not analyze the results on an intention-to-treat basis. A recent randomized trial attempted to address these deficiencies but the study was underpowered. Another argument against a unilateral exploration is the risk of missing another adenoma on the opposite side of the neck. The incidence of double adenomas has been reported to range from 0 to 10%, with an increased incidence in elderly patients. Upper

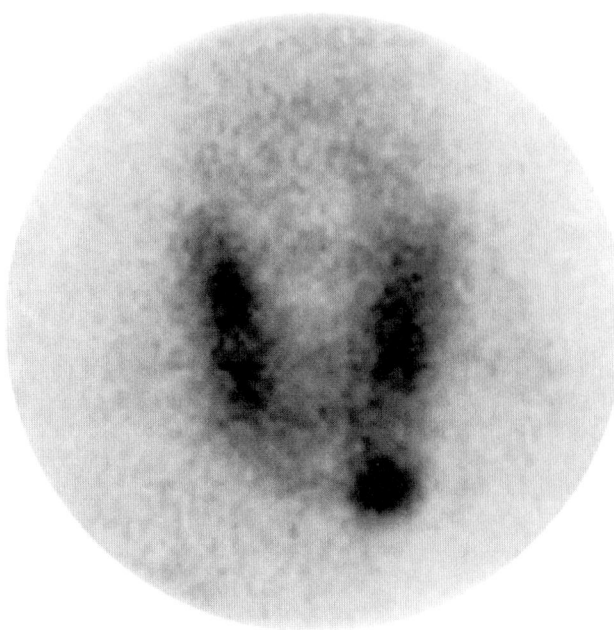

FIG. 37-47. Sestamibi scan in a patient with PHPT showing persistent uptake, suggesting a left lower hypercellular parathyroid gland.

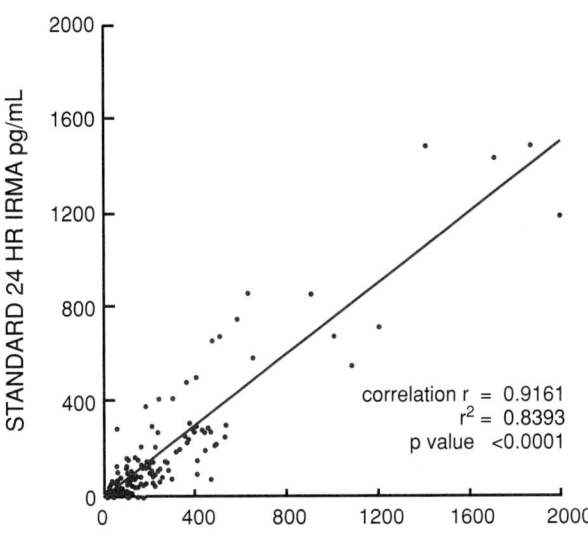

FIG. 37-49. Correlation of the 10-minute incubation time quick PTH assay with the 24-hour immunoradiometric assay (IRMA) PTH assay from 138 paired intraoperative samples from 38 patients undergoing parathyroidectomy. [*Reproduced with permission from Irvin G, et al: Clinical usefulness of an intraoperative "quick parathyroid hormone" assay. Surgery 111(6):1020, 1993.*]

parathyroid glands appear to be involved more frequently than lower glands. The risk of missing a second adenoma is higher in populations with a higher incidence of multiple adenomas, such as those with familial HPT, MEN syndromes, and the elderly. Another difficulty inherent with unilateral exploration is the inability to discern whether the combination of an abnormal gland and a normal gland on the initial side constitute a single adenoma or asymmetric hyperplasia. These issues will only be resolved by a large, prospective, multicenter study or by improved molecular analytic techniques.

Radio-guided parathyroidectomy takes advantage of the ability of parathyroid tumors to retain sestamibi and uses a hand-held gamma probe to guide the identification of the offending gland. Although many studies demonstrated the feasibility of this technique, it is rarely used now, largely because it offers little advantage over preoperative sestamibi scans and is associated with increased operative times.[72] Like preoperative scanning, it also has reduced accuracy in the presence of multiglandular disease. Similarly, although various videoscopic and video-assisted techniques of parathyroidectomy

FIG. 37-48. Neck ultrasound in a patient with PHPT showing a left lower parathyroid adenoma.

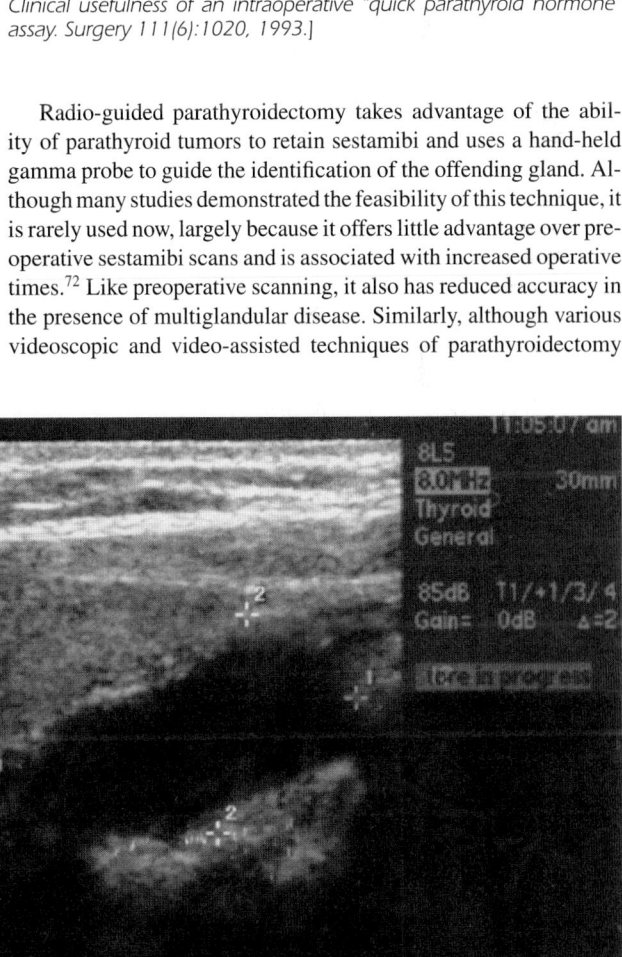

currently are in use, they are also associated with increased operating times, often require more personnel, are expensive, and have, in general, not been useful for patients with multiglandular disease or a large thyroid mass, or in patients who have had previous neck surgery and irradiation. Their greatest utility has been in patients with tumors at ectopic sites, such as the mediastinum.

The recommended practice involves obtaining both a sestamibi scan and neck ultrasound in patients with PHPT. Studies show that if both studies independently identify the same enlarged parathyroid gland, and no other gland, it is indeed the abnormal gland in approximately 95% of cases. These patients with sporadic PHPT are candidates for a focused neck exploration. A standard bilateral neck exploration is planned if parathyroid localization studies or intraoperative parathyroid hormone are not available; if the localizing studies fail to identify any abnormal parathyroid gland, or identify multiple abnormal glands, in patients with a family history of PHPT, MEN1, or MEN2A; or if there is a concomitant thyroid disorder that requires bilateral exploration. In addition, finding a minimally abnormal parathyroid gland on the side indicated by localization studies during focal exploration should prompt a bilateral exploration or at least the identification of a normal parathyroid gland on the same side. In patients with MEN1, hyperparathyroidism should be corrected prior to treatment of gastrinomas, because gastrin levels decline after parathyroidectomy.

Conduct of Parathyroidectomy (Standard Bilateral Exploration)

An experienced parathyroid surgeon with a thorough knowledge of parathyroid anatomy and embryology and meticulous technique is crucial for the best surgical results. The procedure is usually performed under general anesthesia. The patient is positioned supine on the operating table with the neck extended and the arms tucked on either side. The neck is prepped and draped with sterile drapes. For a bilateral exploration, the neck is explored via a 3- to 4-cm incision just caudal to the cricoid cartilage. The initial dissection and exposure is similar to that used for thyroidectomy. After the strap muscles are separated in the midline, one side of the neck is chosen for exploration. During a thyroidectomy, blood vessels are dissected and ligated as close to the thyroid surface as possible, so as to preserve the blood supply to the parathyroids. In contrast, the dissection during a parathyroidectomy is maintained lateral to the thyroid, making it easier to identify the parathyroid glands and not disturb their blood supply.

Identification of the Parathyroid Glands. A bloodless field is important to enable identification of parathyroid glands. The middle thyroid veins are ligated and divided, thus enabling medial and anterior retraction of the thyroid lobe. This may be facilitated by a peanut sponge or placement of 2-0 silk sutures into the thyroid substance. The space between the carotid sheath and thyroid is then opened by gentle sharp and blunt dissection, from the cricoid cartilage superiorly to the thymus inferiorly and the RLN is identified. Approximately 85% of the parathyroid glands are found within 1 cm of the junction of the inferior thyroid artery and recurrent laryngeal nerves. The upper parathyroid glands are usually superior to this junction and dorsal (posterior) to the nerve, whereas the lower glands are located inferior to the junction and ventral (anterior) to the recurrent nerve. Because parathyroid glands are partly surrounded by fat, any fat lobule at typical parathyroid locations should be explored, because the normal or abnormal parathyroid gland may be concealed in the fatty tissue. The thin fascia overlying a "suspicious" fat lobule should be incised using a sharp, curved hemostat

and scalpel. This maneuver often causes the parathyroid gland to "pop" out. Alternatively, gentle, blunt peanut sponge dissection between the carotid sheath and the thyroid gland often reveals a "float" sign, suggesting the site of the abnormal parathyroid gland.

Parathyroid tissue can be confused with normal or brown fat tissue, thyroid nodules, lymph nodes, and ectopic thymus. Lymph nodes are generally light beige to whitish-gray in color, and appear glassy, whereas thyroid nodules are generally more vascular, firm, dark or reddish-brown in color, and have a more variegated appearance. Normal parathyroids are light beige and only slightly darker or more brown than adjacent fat. Intraoperatively, a suspicious nodule may be aspirated using a fine needle attached to a syringe containing 1 mL of saline. Very high PTH levels in the aspirate are diagnostic in the intraoperative identification of parathyroid glands.[73] Several characteristics, such as size (>7 mm), weight, and color, are used to distinguish normal from hypercellular parathyroid glands. Hypercellular glands are generally darker, more firm, and more vascular than normocellular glands. An intraoperative density test was developed to take advantage of the fact that hypercellular glands sink in saline solutions because of their low fat content, whereas normal parathyroid glands float, but few surgeons use this test today. Because no single method is 100% reliable, the parathyroid surgeon must rely on experience, and sometimes a good pathologist, to help distinguish normal from hypercellular glands. Although several molecular studies have shown utility in distinguishing parathyroid adenomas from hyperplasia, this determination must also be made by the surgeon intraoperatively by documenting the presence of a normal parathyroid gland.

Location of Parathyroid Glands. The majority of lower parathyroid glands are found in proximity to the lower thyroid pole (Fig. 37-50A). If not found at this location, the thyrothymic ligament and thymus should be mobilized as follows: The thymus extends into the mediastinum as a tongue of tissue that is sometimes indistinguishable from the perithymic fat, except that it is slightly firmer with more discrete margins. The upper end is gently grasped with a right-angle clamp and the distal portion is bluntly dissected from perithymic fat with a peanut sponge. One can then "walk down" the thymus with successive right-angle clamps (Fig. 37-50B). Applying light tension along with a "twisting" motion helps to free the upper thymus. The carotid sheath should also be opened from the bifurcation to the base of the neck if the parathyroid tumor cannot be found. If these maneuvers are unsuccessful, an intrathyroidal gland should be sought by using intraoperative ultrasound, incising the thyroid capsule on its posterolateral surface, or by performing an ipsilateral thyroid lobectomy and "bread-loafing" the thyroid lobe. Preoperative or intraoperative ultrasonography can be useful for identifying intrathyroidal parathyroid glands. Rarely, the third branchial pouch may maldescend and be found high in the neck (undescended parathymus), anterior to the carotid bulb, along with the missing parathyroid gland. Upper parathyroid glands are more consistent in position and are usually found near the junction of the upper and middle thirds of the gland, at the level of the cricoid cartilage (Fig. 37-50C). Ectopic upper glands may be found in the carotid sheath, tracheoesophageal groove, in the retroesophageal, or in the posterior mediastinum. Figure 37-51 shows the locations of ectopic upper and lower parathyroid glands. Every attempt must be made to identify all four glands. Treatment depends upon the number of abnormal glands.

A single adenoma is presumed to be the cause of a patient's primary HPT if only one parathyroid tumor is identified and the other parathyroid glands are normal, a situation present in approximately

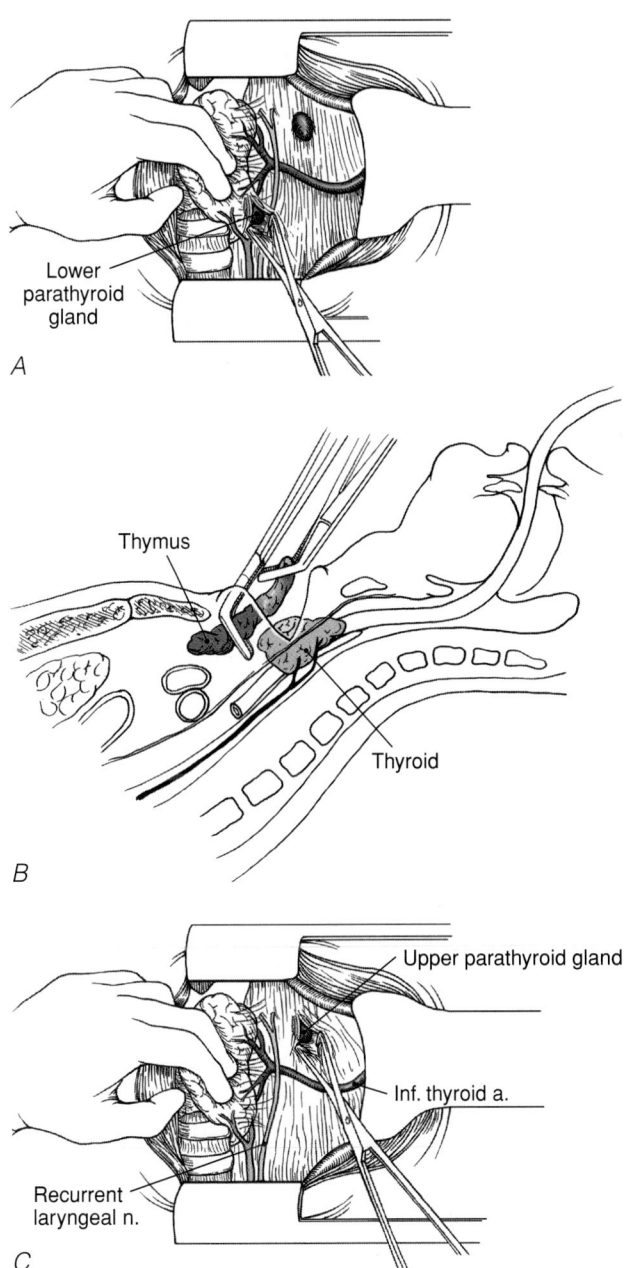

Lower parathyroid gland

A

Thymus

Thyroid

B

Upper parathyroid gland

Inf. thyroid a.

Recurrent laryngeal n.

C

FIG. 37-50. Conduct of parathyroidectomy: *A*. Exposure of the lower parathyroid gland near the inferior pole of the thyroid gland and anterior to the RLN. *B*. A thymectomy may be necessary if the lower parathyroid cannot be found in its usual location, or if the patient has familial PHPT or secondary HPT. *C*. Exposure of the upper parathyroid gland near the insertion of the RLN at the level of the cricothyroid muscle.

80% of patients with PHPT. Adenomas typically have an atrophic rim of normal parathyroid tissue, but this characteristic may be absent. The adenoma is dissected free of surrounding tissue, taking care to stay immediately adjacent to the tumor, without fracturing it. This is accomplished by both blunt and sharp dissection. The vascular pedicle is clamped, divided, and ligated. Care should be taken to not rupture the parathyroid gland, thereby decreasing the risk of parathyromatosis. If there is any question about the presumed normal glands, one of them should be biopsied and examined by frozen section.

If two abnormal and two normal glands are identified, the patient has double adenomas. Triple adenomas are present if three glands are abnormal and one is normal. Multiple adenomas are more common in older patients with an incidence of up to 10% in patients more than 60 years old. The abnormal glands should be excised, provided the remaining glands are confirmed as such, thus excluding asymmetric hyperplasia, after biopsy and frozen section.

If all parathyroid glands are enlarged or hypercellular, patients have parathyroid hyperplasia, which has been shown to occur in approximately 15% of patients in various series. These glands are often lobulated, usually lack the rim of normal parathyroid gland seen in adenomas, and may be variable in size. It is often difficult to distinguish multiple adenomas from hyperplasia with variable gland size. Hyperplasia may be of the chief cell (more common), mixed, or clear-cell type. Patients with hyperplasia may be treated by subtotal parathyroidectomy or by total parathyroidectomy and autotransplantation, with the choice of procedure being determined by rates of recurrence, postoperative hypocalcemia, and failure rates of autotransplanted tissue. Initial studies demonstrated equivalent cure rates and postoperative hypocalcemia for the two techniques, with the latter having the added advantage of avoiding recurrence in the neck. However, subtotal parathyroidectomy is preferred because autotransplanted tissue may fail to function in approximately 5% of cases.

All four parathyroid glands are identified and carefully mobilized. For patients with hyperplasia, a titanium clip is placed across the most normal gland, leaving a 50-mg remnant and taking care to avoid disturbing the vascular pedicle, and resecting the gland with a sharp scalpel. The authors' preference, if possible, is to subtotally resect an inferior gland, which is more easily accessible in case of recurrence because of its anterior location with respect to the recurrent laryngeal nerve. The resected parathyroid tissue is confirmed by frozen section or PTH assay. If the remnant appears to be viable, the remaining glands are resected. If there is any question as to the viability of the initially subtotally resected gland, another gland is chosen for subtotal resection and the initial remnant is removed. Bilateral upper cervical thymectomy is also routinely performed because supernumerary glands occur in up to 20% of patients. Whenever multiple parathyroids are resected, it is preferable to cryopreserve tissue, so that it may be autotransplanted should the patient become hypoparathyroid. Parathyroid tissue is usually transplanted into the nondominant forearm. A horizontal skin incision is made overlying the brachioradialis muscle a few centimeters below the antecubital fossa. Pockets are made in the belly of the muscle and one to two pieces of parathyroid tissue, measuring 1 mm each, are placed into each pocket. Twelve to 14 pieces are transplanted. Autotransplanted tissue also has been reported to function when transplanted into fat.

Indications for Sternotomy

Generally, a median sternotomy is performed to locate a missing gland only after a complete search has been conducted in the neck. A bilateral upper thymectomy also has been performed. A sternotomy is not usually recommended at the initial operation, unless the calcium level is greater than 13 mg/dL. Rather, it is preferred to biopsy the normal glands and subsequently close the patient's neck and obtain localizing studies, if they were not obtained previously. Intraoperative PTH assay during the operation from large veins may be helpful. Using selective venous catheterization postoperatively may also be needed when noninvasive localization studies are negative, equivocal, or conflicting.

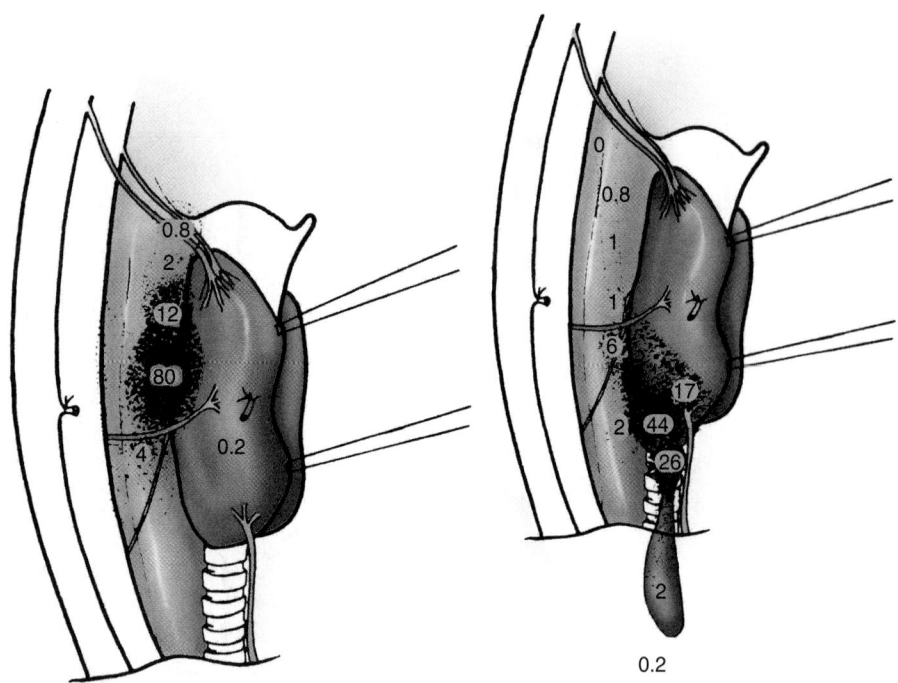

FIG. 37-51. Location of ectopic upper and lower parathyroid glands. The numbers represent the percentages of glands found in the different locations. (Reproduced with permission from Akerstrom G, et al, p 15.[49])

Lower parathyroid glands tend to migrate into the anterior mediastinum in the thymus or perithymic fat and can usually be approached via a cervical incision. A sternotomy is needed to deliver these tumors in approximately 5% of cases. Generally, the gland can be approached by a partial sternotomy to the third intercostal space. The midline sternotomy can be extended to the left or right side as required. Upper glands tend to migrate to the posterior mediastinum in the tracheoesophageal groove, and, therefore require a complete sternotomy for exposure. Mediastinal glands may also be found in the aortopulmonary window, pericardium, or attached to the ascending aorta, aortic arch, or its branches. Tumors identified in the aortopulmonary window are ideal for attempted removal via a thoracoscopic approach.

Special Situations

Parathyroid Carcinoma. Parathyroid cancer accounts for approximately 1% of the cases of PHPT. It may be suspected preoperatively by the presence of severe symptoms, serum calcium levels greater than 14 mg/dL, significantly elevated PTH levels (five times normal), and a palpable parathyroid gland. Local invasion is most common; approximately 15% of patients have lymph node metastases and 33% have distant metastases at presentation. Intraoperatively, parathyroid cancer is suggested by the presence of a large, gray-white to gray-brown parathyroid tumor that is adherent to or invasive into surrounding tissues such as muscle, thyroid, recurrent laryngeal nerve, trachea, or esophagus. Enlarged lymph nodes also may be present. Accurate diagnosis necessitates histologic examination, which reveals local tissue invasion, vascular or capsular invasion, trabecular or fibrous stroma, and frequent mitoses.

Treatment of parathyroid cancer consists of bilateral neck exploration, with en bloc excision of the tumor and the ipsilateral thyroid lobe. Modified radical neck dissection is recommended in the presence of lymph node metastases. Prophylactic neck dissection is not advised because it is associated with an increased risk of complications and does not appear to have a significant impact on survival. If the diagnosis is made postoperatively, a decision must

be made regarding the adequacy of initial surgery based on a review of operative notes, pathology reports, localization studies, and calcium and PTH levels. If any question exists, histologic review by another experienced pathologist can be helpful. Additional procedures can then be performed accordingly. Reoperation is indicated for locally recurrent or metastatic disease because uncontrolled hypercalcemia is the major cause of death in these patients, but is associated with significant morbidity. Radiation and chemotherapy can be considered in patients with unresectable disease. Bisphosphonates and calcimimetic drugs may also be effective in long-term palliation.

Familial HPT. PHPT is usually sporadic, but may occur as a component of various inherited syndromes such as MEN1 and MEN2A. Inherited primary hyperparathyroidism also can occur as isolated familial hyperparathyroidism (non-MEN), or familial hyperparathyroidism with jaw tumors. The diagnosis of familial HPT is known or suspected in approximately 85% of patients preoperatively. Furthermore, patients with hereditary hyperparathyroidism generally have a higher incidence of multiglandular disease, supernumerary glands, and recurrent or persistent disease. Therefore, these patients warrant a more aggressive approach and are not candidates for various focused surgical approaches described previously.

It is recommended to obtain a preoperative sestamibi scan and ultrasound in patients with inherited hyperparathyroidism to identify potential ectopic glands. A standard bilateral neck exploration is performed, along with a bilateral cervical thymectomy, regardless of the results of localization studies. Both subtotal parathyroidectomy and total parathyroidectomy with autotransplantation are appropriate, and parathyroid tissue should also be cryopreserved. If an adenoma is found in patients with familial HPT, the adenoma and the ipsilateral normal parathyroid glands are resected. The normal appearing glands on the contralateral side are biopsied and marked, so that only one side of the neck will need to be explored in the event of recurrence. In patients with MEN1, as previously mentioned, hypercalcemia should be treated prior to treatment of gastrinoma, because gastrin levels often decline in these patients following parathyroidectomy. Patients with MEN2A require total thyroidectomy and central neck dissection for prevention/treatment of MTC, a procedure that places the parathyroids at risk. Moreover, HPT is less aggressive in these patients. Hence, only abnormal parathyroid glands need to be resected at neck exploration. The other normal parathyroid glands should be marked with a clip.

Neonatal HPT. Infants with neonatal HPT present with severe hypercalcemia, lethargy, hypotonia, and mental retardation. This disorder is associated with homozygous mutations in the CASR gene. Urgent total parathyroidectomy (with autotransplantation and cryopreservation) and thymectomy is indicated. Subtotal resection is associated with high recurrence rates.

Parathyromatosis. Parathyromatosis is a rare condition characterized by the finding of multiple nodules of hyperfunctioning parathyroid tissue throughout the neck and mediastinum, usually following a previous parathyroidectomy. The true etiology of parathyromatosis is not known. It is postulated to arise either from overgrowth of congenital parathyroid rests (ontogenous parathyromatosis) or seeding at surgery from rupture of parathyroid tumors or subtotal resection of hyperplastic glands. Parathyromatosis represents a rare cause of persistent or recurrent HPT[74] and can be identified intraoperatively. Aggressive local resection of these deposits can result in normocalcemia, but is rarely curative. Some studies suggest that these patients have low-grade carcinoma because of invasion into muscle and other structures distant from the resected parathyroid tumor.

Postoperative Care and Follow-Up

Patients are reexamined 2 weeks postoperatively, at which time the wound is checked and blood work (calcium, phosphate, and PTH levels) is obtained. Patients who have undergone parathyroidectomy are advised to undergo calcium level checks annually. Recurrence rates are rare (less than 1%), except in patients with familial hyperparathyroidism. Recurrence rates of 15% at 2 years and 67% at 8 years have been reported for MEN1 patients.

Persistent and Recurrent Hyperparathyroidism

Persistence is defined as hypercalcemia that fails to resolve after parathyroidectomy and is more common than recurrence, which refers to HPT occurring after an intervening period of at least 6 months of biochemically documented normocalcemia.[75] The most common causes for both these states include ectopic parathyroids, unrecognized hyperplasia, supernumerary glands, subtotal resection of a parathyroid tumor, parathyroid cancer, and parathyromatosis. More rare causes include parathyroid carcinoma, missed adenoma in a normal position, incomplete resection of an abnormal gland, and an inexperienced surgeon. The most common sites of ectopic parathyroid glands in patients with persistent or recurrent HPT are paraesophageal (28%), mediastinal (26%), intrathymic (24%), intrathyroidal (11%), carotid sheath (9%), and high cervical or undescended (2%) (Fig. 37-52).

Once the diagnosis of persistent or recurrent HPT is suspected, it should be confirmed by the necessary biochemical tests. In particular, a 24-hour urine collection should be performed to rule out BFHH. If this is not helpful, a urine calcium to creatinine ratio of less than 0.01 is confirmatory for BFHH. In redo parathyroid surgery, the

FIG. 37-52. Anatomic location of ectopic thyroid glands. Numbers represent number of glands found in each location with a total of 54. (*Reproduced with permission from Shen W, et al: Re-operation for persistent or recurrent primary hyperparathyroidism. Arch Surg 131:864, 1996.*)

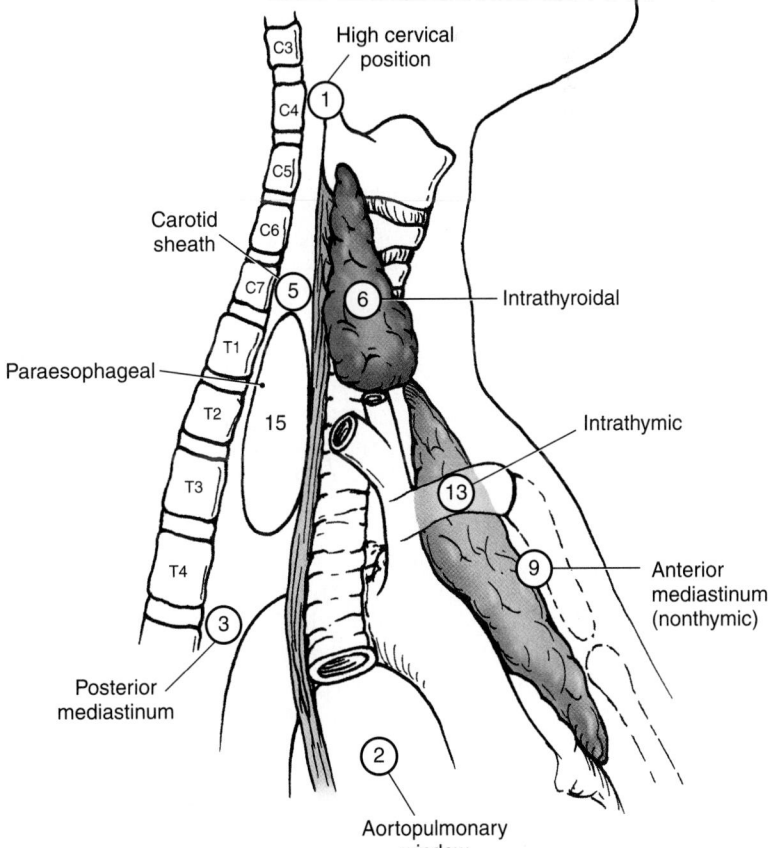

glands are more likely to be in ectopic locations and postoperative scarring tends to make the procedure more technically demanding. Cure rates are generally lower (80 to 90% as compared with 95 to 99% for initial operation) and risk of injury to RLNs and permanent hypocalcemia are higher. Therefore, an evaluation of severity of HPT and the patient's anesthetic risk (using the American Society of Anesthesiology classification of physical status or the Goldman cardiac index) is important. High-risk patients whose tumors cannot be identified by localization studies may benefit from nonoperative management such as calcimimetic drugs or angiographic embolization. Although the latter approach is associated with significant complications and has not gained widespread acceptance, it may be helpful for poor-risk patients with ectopic glands in the mediastinum.

Preoperative localization studies are routinely performed. Noninvasive studies, such as a sestamibi scan, ultrasound, and MRI (with gadolinium contrast), are recommended and reportedly have a combined accuracy of approximately 85% for these studies in cases of persistent or recurrent HPT. If these studies are negative or equivocal, highly selective venous catheterization for PTH levels is performed, which increases the accuracy to 95%. Previous operative notes and pathology reports should be carefully reviewed and reconciled with the information obtained from localization studies prior to any neck reexploration. Figure 37-53 shows an algorithm for the treatment of patients with recurrent and persistent HPT.

Generally, these patients are approached with a focused exploration with intraoperative PTH measurement to reduce the risk of complications. This is because reoperations are inherently more difficult as a consequence of extensive scarring from previous surgery. The lateral approach is usually used to identify the recurrent laryngeal nerve more easily. Parathyroid tissue is cryopreserved routinely. If localizing studies suggest a gland in the anterior mediastinum, it can usually be removed via the previous cervical incision. If this is unsuccessful, or if the gland is located in the posterior or middle mediastinum, a median sternotomy is performed. A thoracoscopic approach may also be used, as previously discussed.

Hypercalcemic Crisis

Patients with primary HPT may occasionally present acutely with nausea, vomiting, fatigue, muscle weakness, confusion and a decreased level of consciousness; a complex referred to as *hypercalcemic crisis*. This condition is thought to result from severe hypercalcemia from uncontrolled PTH secretion, worsened by polyuria, dehydration, and reduced kidney function, and may occur with other conditions causing hypercalcemia. Calcium levels are markedly elevated and may be as high as 16 to 20 mg/dL. Parathyroid glands tend to be large or multiple, and the tumor may be palpable. Patients with parathyroid cancer or familial HPT are more likely to present with hyperparathyroid crisis.

FIG. 37-53. *Management of recurrent and persistent HPT.*

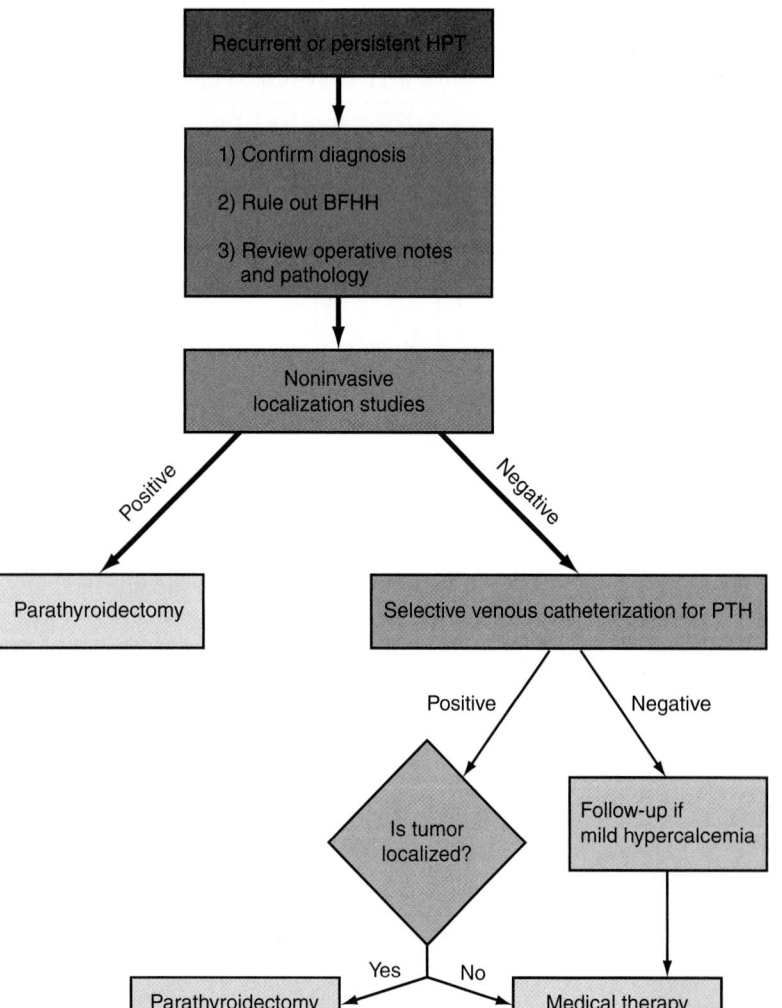

Table 37-13
Medications Used to Treat Hypercalcemia

Medication	Dosage and Administration	Mechanism Onset of Action and Duration	Side Effects
Bisphosphonates (pamidronate)	60–90 mg IV over 4–24 hours	Inhibits osteoclastic bone resorption; rapid onset, (2–3 days)	May cause local pain and swelling, low-grade fever, lymphopenia, electrolyte abnormalities
Calcitonin	4 IU/Kg SC/IM	Inhibits osteoclast function, augments renal calcium excretion; onset of action in hours; but short-lived, therefore not useful as sole therapy	Transient nausea and vomiting, abdominal cramps, flushing, and local skin reaction
Mithramycin (Plicamycin)	25 μg/kg per day IV for 3–4 days	Inhibits osteoclast RNA secretion; rapid onset of action (12 hours); peaks at 48–72 hours and lasts days to several weeks	May cause renal, hepatic, and hematologic complications, nausea and vomiting
Gallium nitrate	200 mg/m^2 BSA per day IV for 5 days	Reduces urinary calcium excretion; onset of action delayed (5–7 days)	Nephrotoxicity, nausea, vomiting, hypotension, anemia, hypophosphatemia
Glucocorticoids	Hydrocortisone 100 mg IV q8h	Delayed onset of action (7–10 days); useful for hematologic malignancies, sarcoidosis, vitamin D intoxication, hyperthyroidism	Hypertension, hyperglycemia

BSA = body surface area.

Treatment consists of therapies to lower serum calcium levels followed by surgery to correct hyperparathyroidism.[76] The mainstay of therapy involves rehydration with a 0.9% saline solution to keep urine output greater than 100 mL/h. Once urine output is established, diuresis with furosemide is begun. Furosemide works by increasing renal calcium clearance, but should not be used without adequate rehydration and salt loading. If these methods are unsuccessful, other drugs, as outlined in Table 37-13, can be used to lower serum calcium levels. Occasionally, in life-threatening cases, hemodialysis may be of benefit.

Secondary Hyperparathyroidism

Secondary HPT commonly occurs in patients with chronic renal failure but may also occur in those with hypocalcemia secondary to inadequate calcium or vitamin D intake, or malabsorption. The pathophysiology of HPT in chronic renal failure is complex and is thought to be related to hyperphosphatemia (and resultant hypocalcemia), deficiency of 1,25-dihydroxy vitamin D as a result of loss of renal tissue, low calcium intake, decreased calcium absorption, and abnormal parathyroid cell response to extracellular calcium or vitamin D in vitro and in vivo.[77] Patients are generally hypocalcemic or normocalcemic. Aluminum hydroxide, which was often used as a phosphate binder, contributes to the osteomalacia observed in this disease. These patients are generally treated medically with a low-phosphate diet, phosphate binders, adequate intake of calcium and 1,25-dihydroxyvitamin D, and a high-calcium, low-aluminum dialysis bath. Calcimimetics control parathyroid hyperplasia and osteitis fibrosa cystica associated with secondary HPT in animal studies, and decrease plasma PTH and total and ionized calcium levels in humans.

Surgical treatment is indicated and recommended for patients with bone pain, pruritus, and (1) a calcium-phosphate product ≥70, (2) Ca greater than 11 mg/dL with markedly elevated PTH, (3) calciphylaxis, (4) progressive renal osteodystrophy, and (5) soft-tissue calcification and tumoral calcinosis. Calciphylaxis is a rare, limb- and life-threatening complication of secondary HPT characterized by painful (sometimes throbbing), violaceous and mottled lesions, usually on the extremities, which often become necrotic and progress to nonhealing ulcers, gangrene, sepsis, and death.

Patients should undergo routine dialysis the day prior to surgery to correct electrolyte abnormalities, especially in serum potassium levels. Localizations studies are unnecessary but can identify ectopic parathyroid glands. A bilateral neck exploration is indicated. The parathyroid glands in secondary HPT are characterized by asymmetric enlargement and nodular hyperplasia. These patients may be treated by subtotal resection, leaving about 50 mg of the most normal parathyroid gland or total parathyroidectomy and autotransplantation of parathyroid tissue into the brachioradialis muscle of the nondominant forearm. Upper thymectomy is usually performed because 15 to 20% of patients have one or more parathyroid glands situated in the thymus or perithymic fat.

Benefits of Parathyroidectomy in Secondary Hyperparathyroidism

Bone and joint pain improve in approximately 75% of patients who undergo parathyroidectomy. Pruritus and malaise also improve in most, but not all, patients. Parathyroidectomy also improves bone mineral density,[78] sexual function, and survival in patients with secondary HPT.

Tertiary Hyperparathyroidism

Tertiary hyperparathyroidism is seen most commonly in patients with long-standing renal dysfunction who undergo successful renal transplantation. Generally, renal transplantation is an excellent method of treating secondary HPT, but some patients develop autonomous parathyroid gland function and tertiary HPT. Tertiary HPT can cause problems similar to PHPT, such as pathologic fractures, bone pain, renal stones, peptic ulcer disease, pancreatitis, and mental status changes. The transplanted kidney is also at risk.

Operative intervention is indicated for symptomatic disease or if autonomous PTH secretion persists for more than 1 year after a successful transplant. All parathyroid glands should be identified. The traditional surgical management of these patients consisted of subtotal or total parathyroidectomy with autotransplantation.

However, more recent studies[79] suggest that these patients derive similar benefit from excision of only obviously enlarged glands, while avoiding the higher risks of hypocalcemia associated with the former approach. It is recommended that all parathyroid glands be identified. If one gland is distinctly abnormal and others minimally abnormal, the abnormal gland and the more-normal gland on the same side should be resected with the remaining parathyroids marked. If all the glands are abnormal, a subtotal parathyroidectomy should be performed with upper thymectomy.

COMPLICATIONS OF PARATHYROID SURGERY

Parathyroidectomy can be accomplished successfully in greater than 95% of patients with minimal mortality and morbidity, provided the procedure is performed by a surgeon experienced in parathyroid surgery. General complications include bleeding and wound complications such as seromas and infection. Wound infections are rare. Specific complications include transient and permanent vocal cord palsy and hypoparathyroidism. The latter is more likely to occur in patients who undergo four-gland exploration with biopsies, subtotal resection with an inadequate remnant, or total parathyroidectomy with a failure of autotransplanted tissue. Furthermore, hypocalcemia is more likely to occur in patients with high turnover bone disease as evidenced by elevated preoperative alkaline phosphatase levels. Vocal cord paralysis and hypoparathyroidism are considered permanent if they persist for more than 6 months. Fortunately, these complications are rare, occurring in approximately 1% of patients undergoing surgery by experienced parathyroid surgeons.

Patients with symptomatic hypocalcemia or those with calcium levels less than 8 mg/dL are treated with oral calcium supplementation (up to 1 to 2 g every 4 hours). 1,25-Dihydroxy vitamin D (Rocaltrol 0.25 to 0.5 μg bid) may also be required, particularly in patients with severe hypercalcemia and elevated serum alkaline phosphatase levels preoperatively and with osteitis fibrosa cystica. Intravenous calcium supplementation is rarely needed, except in cases of severe, symptomatic hypocalcemia. Caution should be exercised in its administration because extravasation from the vein can cause extensive tissue necrosis.

HYPOPARATHYROIDISM

Table 37-14 lists the conditions that can cause hypocalcemia. The parathyroid glands may be congenitally absent in the DiGeorge syndrome, which also is characterized by lack of thymic development, and, therefore, a thymus-dependent lymphoid system.[80] Hyperparathyroidism in pregnant women can lead to hypoparathyroidism in neonates from suppression of fetal parathyroid tissue. By far, the most common cause of hypoparathyroidism is thyroid surgery, particularly total thyroidectomy with a concomitant central neck dissection. Patients often develop transient hypocalcemia as a result of bruising or damage to the vascular supply of the glands; permanent hypoparathyroidism is rare. Hypoparathyroidism may also occur after parathyroid surgery, which is more likely if patients have parathyroid hyperplasia and undergo a subtotal resection or total parathyroidectomy with parathyroid autotransplantation. Parathyroid tissue should be cryopreserved in any patient who could develop hypoparathyroidism, but is only needed in approximately 2% of patients.

Acute hypocalcemia results in decreased ionized calcium and increased neuromuscular excitability. Patients initially develop circumoral and fingertip numbness and tingling. Mental symptoms

Table 37-14
Conditions Causing Hypocalcemia

Hypoparathyroidism
  Surgical
  Neonatal
  Familial
  Heavy metal deposition
  Magnesium depletion
Resistance to the action of PTH
  Pseudohypoparathyroidism
  Renal failure
  Medications—calcitonin, bisphosphonates, mithramycin
Failure of normal 1,25-dihydroxy vitamin D production
Resistance to the action of 1,25-dihydroxy vitamin D
Acute complex formation or deposition of calcium
  Acute hyperphosphatemia
  Acute pancreatitis
  Massive blood transfusion (citrate overload)
  "Hungry bones"

include anxiety, confusion, and depression. Physical examination reveals positive Chvostek's sign (contraction of facial muscles elicited by tapping on the facial nerve anterior to the ear) and Trousseau's sign (carpopedal spasm, which is elicited by occluding blood flow to the forearm with a blood pressure cuff for 2 to 3 minutes). Tetany, which is characterized by tonic–clonic seizures, carpopedal spasm, and laryngeal stridor, may prove fatal and should be avoided. Most patients with postoperative hypocalcemia can be treated with oral calcium and vitamin D supplements. Intravenous calcium infusion is rarely required.

Adrenal

HISTORICAL BACKGROUND

Eustachius provided the first accurate anatomic account of the adrenals in 1563. The anatomic division of the adrenals into the cortex and medulla was described much later, by Cuvier in 1805. Subsequently, Thomas Addison described the features of adrenal insufficiency, which still bear his name. DeCreccio provided the first description of congenital adrenal hyperplasia occurring in a female pseudohermaphrodite in 1865. Pheochromocytomas were first identified by Frankel in 1885, but were not named as such until 1912 by Pick, who noted the characteristic chromaffin reaction of the tumor cells. Adrenaline was identified as an agent from the adrenal medulla that elevated blood pressure in dogs and was subsequently named epinephrine in 1897. The first successful adrenalectomies for pheochromocytoma were performed by Roux, in Switzerland, and Charles Mayo, in the United States.

In 1932, Harvey Cushing described 11 patients who had moon facies, truncal obesity, hypertension, and other features of the syndrome that now bears his name. Although several individuals prepared adrenocortical extracts to treat adrenalectomized animals, cortisone was first synthesized by Kendall. Aldosterone was identified in 1952, and the syndrome resulting from excessive secretion of this mineralocorticoid was first described in 1955 by Conn.

EMBRYOLOGY

The adrenal glands are two endocrine organs in one; an outer cortex and an inner medulla, each with distinct embryologic, anatomic, histologic, and secretory features. The cortex originates around the fifth week of gestation from mesodermal tissue near the gonads on

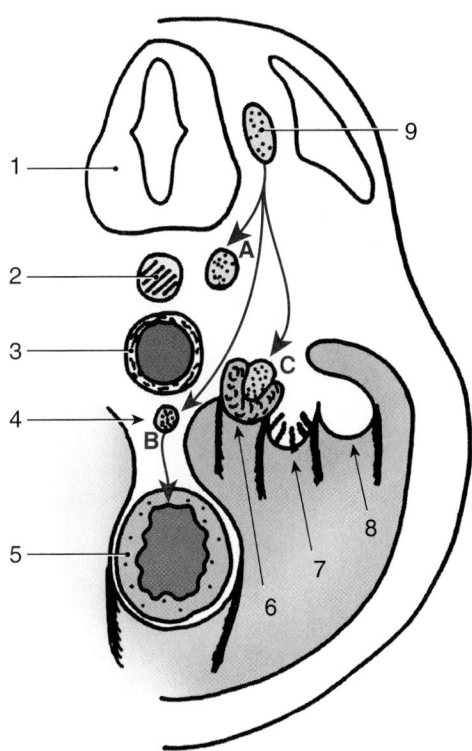

FIG. 37-54. *Cross section of the embryo depicting adrenal development. (1) Neural tube, (2) chorda, (3) aorta, (4) base of the mesentery, (5) digestive tube, (6) adrenal cortex, (7) undifferentiated gonad, (8) mesonephros, (9) neural crest. Cells migrate from the neural crest to form the ganglia of the sympathetic trunk (A), sympathetic plexi (B), and the adrenal medulla and paraganglia (C). (Reproduced with permission from Avisse C, et al: Surgical anatomy and embryology of the adrenal glands. 80:414, 2000.)*

the adrenogenital ridge (Fig. 37-54). Therefore, ectopic adrenocortical tissue may be found in the ovaries, spermatic cord, and testes. The cortex differentiates further into a thin, definitive cortex and a thicker, inner fetal cortex. The latter is functional and produces fetal adrenal steroids by the eighth week of gestation, but undergoes involution after birth, resulting in a decrease in adrenal weight during the first three postpartum months. The definitive cortex persists after birth to form the adult cortex over the first 3 years of life. In contrast, the adrenal medulla is ectodermal in origin and arises from the neural crest. At around the same time as cortical development, neural crest cells migrate to the para-aortic and paravertebral areas and toward the medial aspect of the developing cortex to form the medulla. Most extra-adrenal neural tissue regresses, but may persist at several sites. The largest of these is located to the left of the aortic bifurcation near the inferior mesenteric artery origin and is designated as the organ of Zuckerkandl. Adrenal medullary tissue may also be found in neck, urinary bladder, and para-aortic regions. Several factors are involved in adrenal development and include insulin-like growth factor 2, gastric inhibitory peptide (GIP), and the dosage-sensitive, sex-reversal adrenal hypoplasia (*DAX1*) gene.

ANATOMY

The adrenal glands are paired, retroperitoneal organs located superiorly and medially to the kidneys at the level of the eleventh ribs. The normal adrenal gland measures $5 \times 3 \times 1$ cm and weighs 4 to 5 g. The right gland is pyramidal shaped and lies in close proximity

to the right hemidiaphragm, liver, and inferior vena cava. The left adrenal is closely associated with the aorta, spleen, and tail of the pancreas. Each gland is supplied by three groups of vessels: the superior adrenal arteries derived from the inferior phrenic artery, the middle adrenal arteries derived from the aorta, and the inferior adrenal arteries derived from the renal artery. Other vessels originating from the intercostal and gonadal vessels may also supply the adrenals. These arteries branch into about 50 arterioles to form a rich plexus beneath the glandular capsule and require careful dissection, ligation, and division during adrenalectomy. In contrast to the arterial supply, each adrenal is usually drained by a single, major adrenal vein. The right adrenal vein is usually short and drains into the inferior vena cava, whereas the left adrenal vein is longer and empties into the left renal vein after joining the inferior phrenic vein. Accessory veins occur in 5 to 10% of patients; on the right, these vessels may drain into the right hepatic vein or the right renal vein; on the left, accessory veins may drain directly into the left renal vein. Figure 37-55 depicts the anatomic relationships of the adrenals and surrounding structures.

The adrenal cortex appears yellow because of its high lipid content and accounts for approximately 80 to 90% of the gland's volume. Histologically, the cortex is divided into three zones: zona glomerulosa, zona fasciculata, and zona reticularis. The outer area of the zona glomerulosa consists of small cells and is the site of production of the mineralocorticoid hormone aldosterone. The zona fasciculata is made up of larger cells, which often appear foamy because of multiple lipid inclusions, whereas the zona reticularis cells are smaller. These latter zones are the site of production of glucocorticoids and adrenal androgens. The adrenal medulla constitutes up to 10 to 20% of the gland's volume and is reddish-brown in color. It produces the catecholamine hormones epinephrine and norepinephrine. The cells of the adrenal medulla are arranged in cords and are polyhedral in shape. They are often referred to as chromaffin cells because they stain specifically with chromium salts.

ADRENAL PHYSIOLOGY

Cholesterol, derived from the plasma or synthesized in the adrenal, is the common precursor of all steroid hormones derived from the adrenal cortex. Cholesterol is initially cleaved within mitochondria to 5-δ-pregnenolone, which, in turn, is transported to the smooth endoplasmic reticulum where it forms the substrate for various biosynthetic pathways leading to steroidogenesis (Fig. 37-56).

Mineralocorticoids

The major adrenal mineralocorticoid hormones are aldosterone, 11-deoxycorticosterone (DOC), and cortisol. Cortisol has minimal effects on the kidney because of hormone degradation. Aldosterone secretion is regulated primarily by the renin–angiotensin system (Fig. 37-57). Decreased renal blood flow, decreased plasma sodium and increased sympathetic tone, all stimulate the release of renin from juxtaglomerular cells. Renin, in turn, leads to the production of angiotensin I from its precursor angiotensinogen. Angiotensin I is cleaved by pulmonary angiotensin-converting enzyme (ACE) to angiotensin II, which is not only a potent vasoconstrictor, but also leads to increased aldosterone synthesis and release. Hyperkalemia is another potent stimulator of aldosterone synthesis, whereas ACTH, pituitary pro-opiomelanocortin (POMC), and antidiuretic hormone (ADH) are weak stimulators.

Aldosterone is secreted at a rate of 50 to 250 μg/d (depending on sodium intake) and circulates in plasma chiefly as a complex

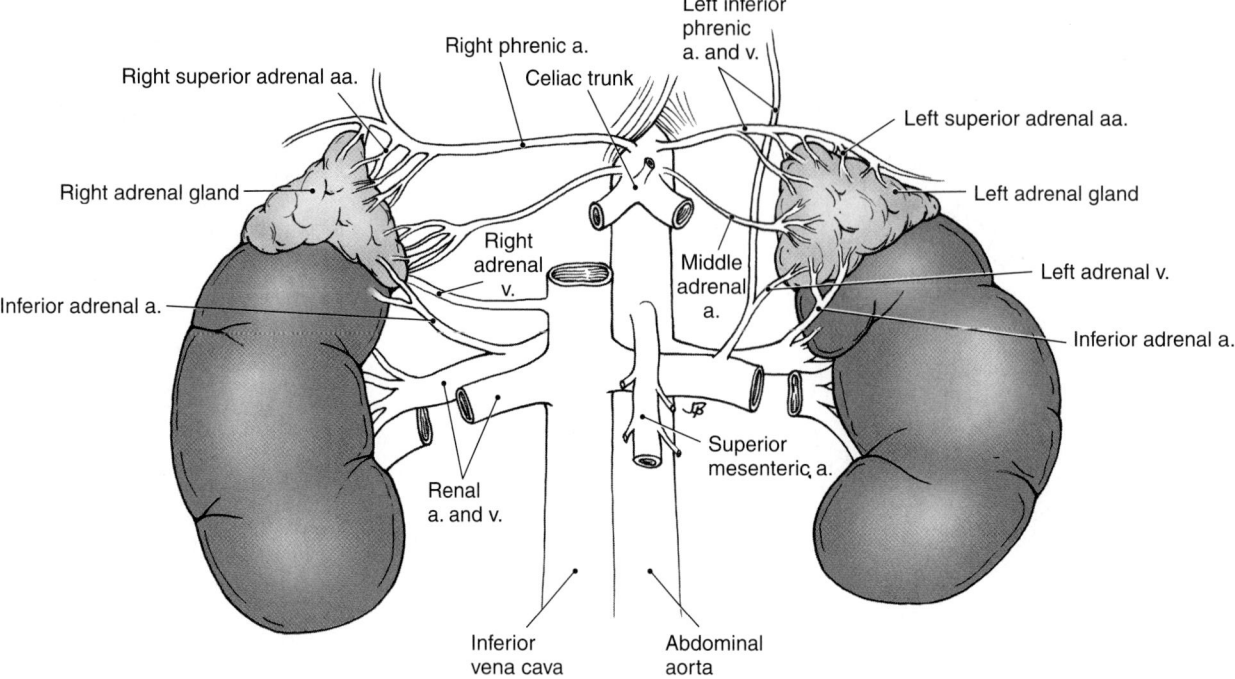

FIG. 37-55. Anatomy of the adrenals and surrounding structures.

with albumin. Small amounts of the hormone bind to corticosteroid-binding globulin (CBG), and approximately 30 to 50% of secreted aldosterone circulates in a free form. The hormone has a half-life of only 15 to 20 minutes and is rapidly cleared via the liver and kidney.

A small quantity of free aldosterone is also excreted in the urine. Mineralocorticoids cross the cell membrane and bind to cytosolic receptors. The receptor–ligand complex is subsequently transported into the nucleus where it induces the transcription and translation of

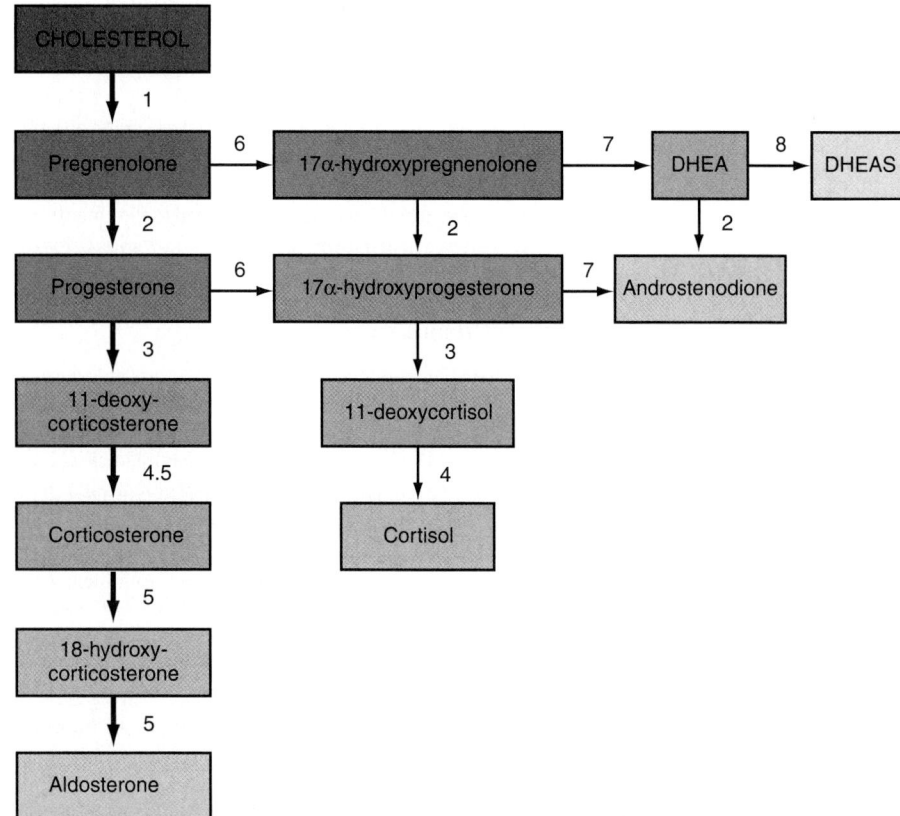

FIG. 37-56. Synthesis of adrenal steroids. The enzymes involved are (1) p450scc (cholesterol side chain cleavage), (2) 3β-hydroxysteroid dehydrogenase, (3) p450c21 (21β-hydroxylase), (4) p450c11 (11β-hydroxylase), (5) p450c11AS (aldosterone synthase), (6) p450c17 (17α-hydroxylase activity), (7) p450c17 (17,20-lyase/desmolase activity), and (8) sulfokinase. DHEAS = dehydroepiandrosterone sulfate.

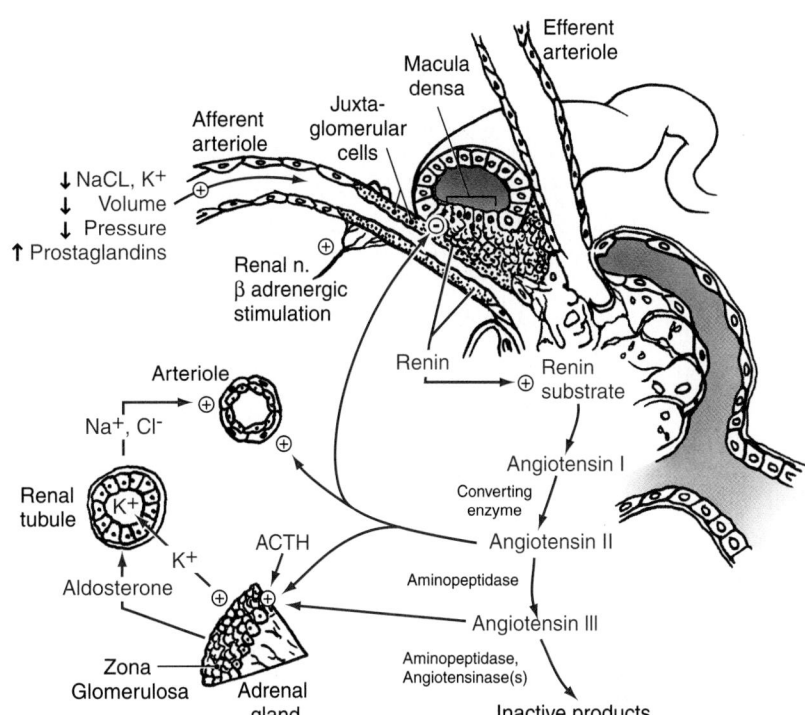

FIG. 37-57. The renin–angiotensin system. *[Reproduced with permission from Hsueh W, et al: Endocrinology of hypertension, in Felig P, Frohman L (eds): Endocrinology and Metabolism. McGraw-Hill, 2001, p 558.]*

specific responsive genes. Aldosterone functions mainly to increase sodium reabsorption and potassium and hydrogen ion excretion at the level of the renal distal convoluted tubule. Less commonly, aldosterone increases sodium absorption in salivary glands and gastrointestinal mucosal surfaces.

Glucocorticoids

The secretion of cortisol, the major adrenal glucocorticoid, is regulated by ACTH secreted by the anterior pituitary, which in turn, is under the control of corticotrophin-releasing hormone (CRH) secreted by the hypothalamus. ACTH is a 39-amino-acid protein, which is derived by cleavage from a larger precursor, POMC. ACTH is further cleaved into α-melanocyte-stimulating hormone (MSH) and corticotropin-like intermediate peptide. ACTH not only stimulates the secretion of glucocorticoids, mineralocorticoids, and adrenal androgens, but is trophic for the adrenal glands. ACTH secretion may be stimulated by pain, stress, hypoxia, hypothermia, trauma, and hypoglycemia. ACTH secretion fluctuates, peaking in the morning and reaching nadir levels in the late afternoon. Thus, there is a diurnal variation in the secretion of cortisol with peak cortisol excretion also occurring in the early morning and declining during the day to its lowest levels in the evening (Fig. 37-58). Cortisol controls the secretion of both CRH and ACTH via a negative-feedback loop.

FIG. 37-58. Diurnal variation in cortisol levels as determined by half-hourly sampling in a 16-year-old woman. *(Reproduced with permission from Krieger DT, et al: Characterization of the normal temporal pattern of corticosteroid levels. J Clin Endocrinol Metab 32:269, 1971.)*

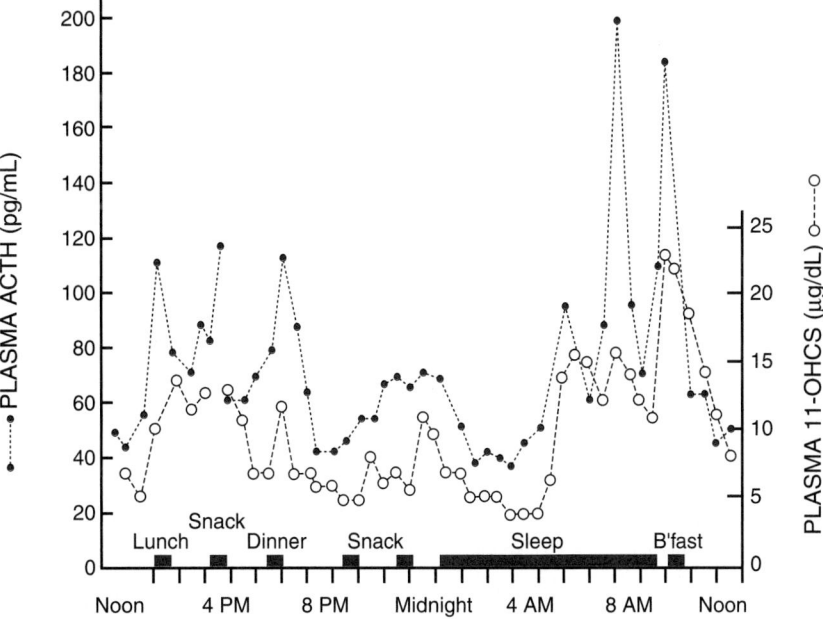

Table 37-15
Functions of Glucocorticoid Hormones

Function/System	Effects
Glucose metabolism	Increases hepatic glycogen deposition, and gluconeogenesis; decreases muscle glucose uptake and metabolism
Protein metabolism	Decreases muscle protein synthesis; increased catabolism
Fat metabolism	Increases lipolysis in adipose tissue
Connective tissue	Inhibition of fibroblasts, loss of collagen, thinning of skin, striae formation
Skeletal system	Inhibits bone formation; increases osteoclast activity; potentiates the action of PTH
Immune system	Increases circulation polymorphonuclear cells; decreases numbers of lymphocytes, monocytes and eosinophils; reduces migration of inflammatory cells to sites of injury
Cardiovascular system	Increases cardiac output and peripheral vascular tone
Renal system	Sodium retention, hypokalemia, hypertension via mineralocorticoid effect; increases glomerular filtration via glucocorticoid effects
Endocrine system	Inhibits TSH synthesis and release, decreases TBG levels, decreases conversion of T_4 to T_3

A similar mechanism leads to the inhibition of CRH secretion by ACTH.

Cortisol is transported in plasma bound primarily to CBG (75%) and albumin (15%). Approximately 10% of circulating cortisol is free and is the biologically active component. The plasma half-life of cortisol is 60 to 90 minutes and is determined by the extent of binding and rate of inactivation. Cortisol is converted to di- and tetrahydrocortisol and cortisone metabolites in the liver and the kidney. The majority (95%) of cortisol and cortisone metabolites are conjugated with glucuronic acid in the liver, thus facilitating their renal excretion. A small amount of unmetabolized cortisol is excreted unchanged in the urine.

Glucocorticoid hormones enter the cell and bind cytosolic steroid receptors. The activated receptor–ligand complex is then transported to the nucleus where it stimulates the transcription of specific target genes via a "zinc finger" DNA-binding element. Cortisol also binds the mineralocorticoid receptor with an affinity similar to aldosterone. However, the specificity of mineralocorticoid action is maintained by the production of 11β-hydroxysteroid dehydrogenase, an enzyme that inactivates cortisol to cortisone in the kidney. As Table 37-15 outlines, glucocorticoids have important functions in intermediary metabolism, but also affect growth and development and the connective tissue, immune, cardiovascular, renal, and central nervous systems.

Sex Steroids

Adrenal androgens are produced in the zona fasciculata and reticularis from 17-hydroxypregnenolone in response to ACTH stimulation. The adrenal androgens include dehydroepiandrosterone (DHEA) and its sulfated counterpart (DHEAS), androstenedione, and small amounts of testosterone and estrogen. Adrenal androgens are weakly bound to plasma albumin. They exert their major effects by peripheral conversion to the more potent testosterone and dihydrotestosterone, but also have weak intrinsic androgen activity. Androgen metabolites are conjugated as glucuronides or sulfates and excreted in the urine.

During fetal development, adrenal androgens promote the formation of male genitalia. In normal adult males, the contribution of adrenal androgens is minimal; however, they are responsible for the development of secondary sexual characteristics at puberty. Adrenal androgen excess leads to precocious puberty in boys and virilization, acne, and hirsutism in girls and women.

Catecholamines

Catecholamine hormones (epinephrine, norepinephrine, and dopamine) are produced both in the central and sympathetic nervous system and in the adrenal medulla. The substrate tyrosine is converted to catecholamines via a series of steps as shown in Fig. 37-59. Phenylethanolamine-N-methyltransferase, which converts norepinephrine to epinephrine, is only present in the adrenal medulla and the organ of Zuckerkandl. Therefore, the primary catecholamine produced can be used to distinguish adrenal medullary tumors from those situated at extra-adrenal sites. The catecholamines are stored

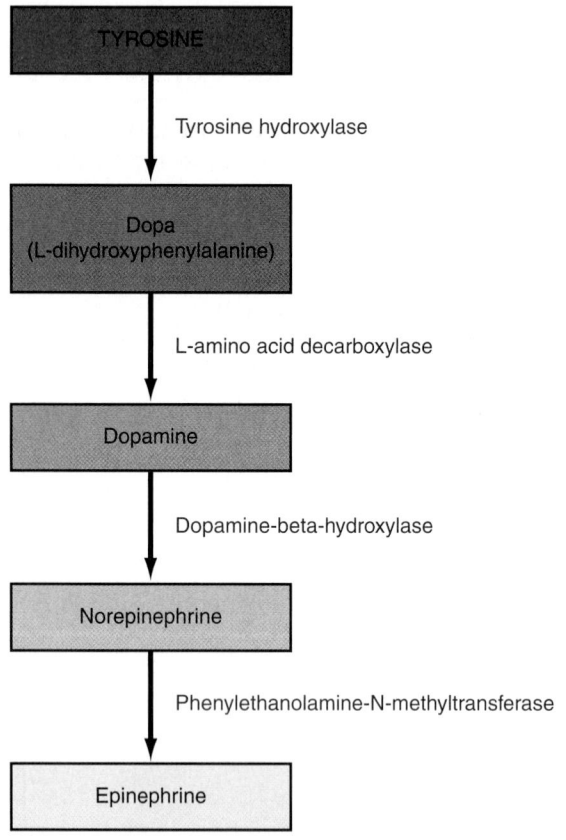

FIG. 37-59. Synthesis of catecholamines.

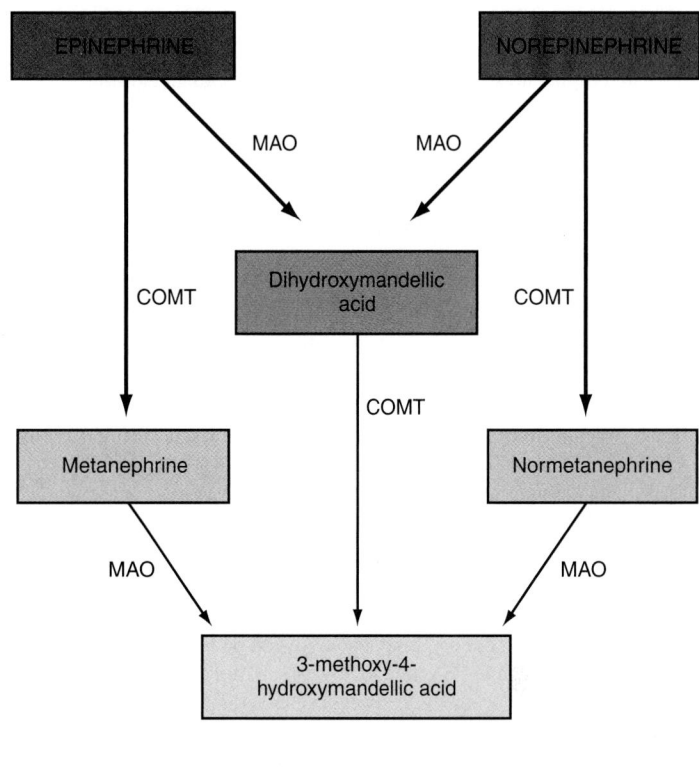

FIG. 37-60. *Metabolism of catecholamine hormones.*

MAO Monoamine oxidase   **COMT** Catechol *O*-methyltransferase

in granules in combination with other neuropeptides, ATP, calcium, magnesium and water-soluble proteins called chromogranins. Hormonal secretion is stimulated by various stress stimuli and mediated by the release of acetylcholine at the preganglionic nerve terminals. In the circulation, these proteins are bound to albumin and other proteins. Catecholamines are cleared by several mechanisms including reuptake by sympathetic nerve endings, peripheral inactivation by catechol-*O*-methyltransferase (COMT) and monoamine oxidase (MAO), and direct excretion by the kidneys. Metabolism of catecholamines occurs primarily in the liver and kidneys, and leads to the formation of metabolites such as metanephrines, normetanephrines, and vanillylmandelic acid which may undergo further glucuronidation or sulfation prior to being excreted in the urine (Fig. 37-60).

Adrenergic receptors are transmembrane-spanning molecules, which are coupled to G-proteins. They may be subdivided into α and β subtypes, which are localized in different tissues, have varying affinity to various catecholamines, and mediate distinct biologic effects (Table 37-16). The receptor affinities for α receptors are epinephrine > norepinephrine >> isoproterenol; for β_1 receptors: isoproterenol > epinephrine = norepinephrine; and for β_2 receptors: isoproterenol > epinephrine >> norepinephrine.

DISORDERS OF THE ADRENAL CORTEX

Hyperaldosteronism (Conn's Syndrome)

Hyperaldosteronism may be secondary to stimulation of the renin–angiotensin system from renal artery stenosis and to low-flow states such as congestive heart failure and cirrhosis. Hyperaldosteronism resulting from these conditions is reversible by treatment of the underlying cause. Primary hyperaldosteronism results from autonomous aldosterone secretion, which, in turn, leads to suppression

of renin secretion. Primary aldosteronism usually occurs in individuals between the ages of 30 and 50 years and accounts for 1% of cases of hypertension. Primary hyperaldosteronism is usually associated with hypokalemia; however, more patients with Conn's syndrome are being diagnosed with normal potassium levels. Most cases result from a solitary functioning adrenal adenoma (approximately 70%) and idiopathic bilateral hyperplasia (30%). Adrenocortical

Table 37-16
Catecholamine Hormone Receptors and the Effects They Mediate

Receptor	Tissue	Function
α_1	Blood vessels	Contraction
	Gut	Decreased motility, increased sphincter tone
	Pancreas	Decreased insulin and glucagon release
	Liver	Glycogenolysis, gluconeogenesis
	Eyes	Pupil dilation
	Uterus	Contraction
	Skin	Sweating
α_2	Synapse (sympathetic)	Inhibits norepinephrine release
	Platelet	Aggregation
β_1	Heart	Chronotropic, inotropic
	Adipose tissue	Lipolysis
	Gut	Decreased motility, increased sphincter tone
	Pancreas	Increased insulin and glucagon release
β_2	Blood vessels	Vasodilation
	Bronchioles	Dilation
	Uterus	Relaxation

carcinoma and glucocorticoid suppressible hyperaldosteronism are rare, each accounting for less than 1% of cases.[81] Glucocorticoid-suppressible hyperaldosteronism is an autosomal dominant form of hypertension in which aldosterone secretion is abnormally regulated by ACTH. This condition is caused by recombinations between linked genes encoding closely related isozymes, 11β-hydroxylase (CYP11B1) and aldosterone synthase (CYP11B2), and generating a dysregulated chimeric gene with aldosterone synthase activity.[82]

Symptoms and Signs

Patients typically present with hypertension, which is long-standing, moderate to severe, and may be difficult to control despite multiple-drug therapy. Some authors report that patients may be hypertensive for a mean of 7 to 11 years prior to diagnosis. Other symptoms include muscle weakness, polydipsia, polyuria, nocturia, headaches, and fatigue. Weakness and fatigue are related to the presence of hypokalemia

Diagnostic Studies

Laboratory Studies. Hypokalemia is a common finding and hyperaldosteronism must be suspected in any hypertensive patient who presents with coexisting spontaneous hypokalemia (K <3.2 mmol/L), or hypokalemia (<3 mmol/L) while on diuretic therapy, despite potassium replacements. However, it is important to note that up to 40% of patients with a confirmed aldosteronoma were normokalemic preoperatively.[83] Once the diagnosis is suspected, further tests are necessary to confirm the diagnosis. Prior to testing, patients must have adequate sodium and potassium replacements. Antihypertensive medications should be held, if possible, and spironolactone, beta blockers, ACE inhibitors, and angiotensin II receptor blockers should be avoided. Patients with primary hyperaldosteronism have an elevated plasma aldosterone concentration (PAC) level with a suppressed plasma renin activity (PRA); a PAC:PRA ratio of 25 to 30:1 is strongly suggestive of the diagnosis. False-positive results can occur, particularly in patients with chronic renal failure. Patients with primary hyperaldosteronism also fail to suppress aldosterone levels with sodium loading. This test can be performed by performing a 24-hour urine collection for cortisol, sodium, and aldosterone after 5 days of a high-sodium diet, or, alternatively, by giving the patient a load of 2 L of saline while in the supine position, 2 to 3 days after being on a low-sodium diet. Plasma aldosterone levels less than 8.5 ng/mL or a 24-hour urine aldosterone less than 14 μg after saline loading essentially rules out primary hyperaldosteronism.

Once the biochemical diagnosis is confirmed, further evaluation should be directed at determining which patients have a unilateral aldosteronoma versus bilateral hyperplasia, because surgery is almost always curative for the former, but usually not the latter. No biochemical studies can make this distinction with 100% sensitivity, thus radiologic studies are necessary.

Radiologic Studies. CT scans with 0.5 cm cuts in the adrenal area can localize aldosteronomas with a sensitivity of 90%. A unilateral 0.5- to 2-cm adrenal tumor with a normal-appearing contralateral gland confirms an aldosteronoma in the presence of appropriate biochemical parameters. MRI scans are less sensitive, but more specific, particularly if opposed-phase chemical-shift images are obtained. MRI scans also have increased utility in pregnant patients, and in patients who are unable to tolerate intravenous contrast. If adrenal hyperplasia is suspected, the algorithm depicted in Fig. 37-61 is useful. Selective venous catheterization, adrenal vein sampling for aldosterone, is 95% sensitive and 90% specific in

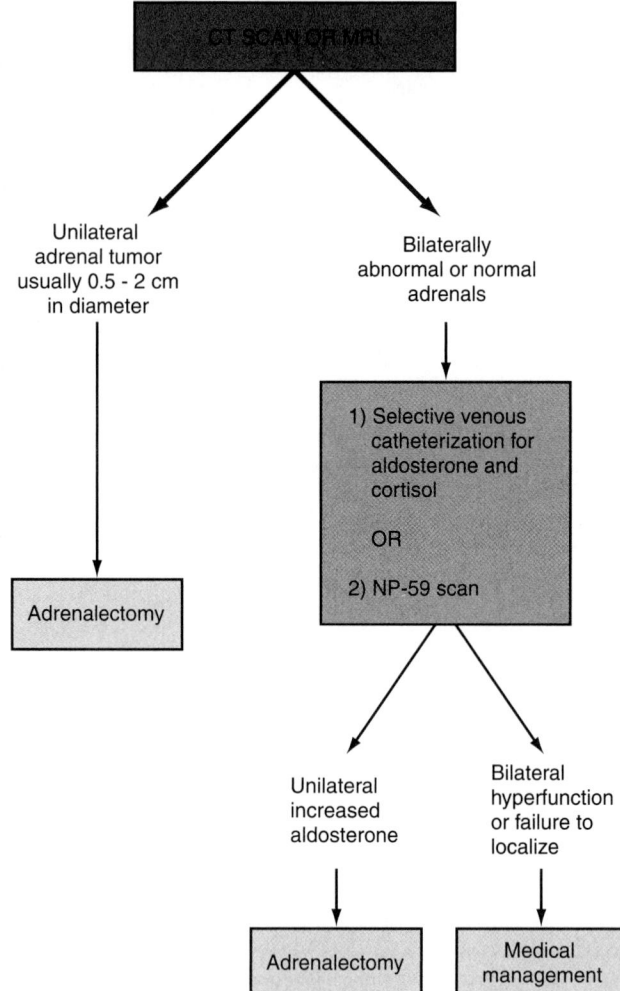

FIG. 37-61. *Management of an adrenal aldosteronoma.*

localizing the aldosteronoma. In this procedure, the adrenal veins are cannulated and blood samples for aldosterone and cortisol are obtained from both adrenal veins and the vena cava after ACTH administration.[84] Measurement of cortisol levels is necessary to confirm proper placement of the catheters in the adrenal veins. A greater than fourfold difference in the aldosterone:cortisol ratios between the adrenal veins indicates the presence of a unilateral tumor. Some investigators use this study routinely, but it is invasive, requires an experienced interventional radiologist, and can lead to adrenal vein rupture in approximately 1% of cases. Therefore, most groups advocate use of this modality selectively in ambiguous cases, when the tumor cannot be localized, and in patients with bilateral adrenal enlargement to determine whether there is unilateral or bilateral increased secretion of aldosterone. Scintigraphy with [131]I-6β-iodomethyl noriodocholesterol (NP-59) may also be used for the same purpose. Like cholesterol, this compound is taken up by the adrenal cortex, but unlike cholesterol, it remains in the gland without undergoing further metabolism. Adrenal adenomas appear as "hot" nodules with suppressed contralateral uptake, whereas hyperplastic glands show bilaterally increased uptake.

Treatment

Preoperatively, control of hypertension and adequate potassium supplementation (to keep K >3.5 mmol/L) are important. Patients are generally treated with spironolactone (an aldosterone antagonist), amiloride (a potassium-sparing diuretic that blocks sodium channels in the distal nephron), nifedipine (a calcium channel blocker), or captopril (an ACE inhibitor). Unilateral tumors producing aldosterone are best managed by adrenalectomy, either by a laparoscopic approach (preferred) or via a posterior open approach. If a carcinoma is suspected, because of the large size of the adrenal lesion or mixed hormone secretion, an anterior transabdominal approach is preferred to permit adequate determination of local invasion and distal metastases. Only 20 to 30% of patients with hyperaldosteronism secondary to bilateral adrenal hyperplasia benefit from surgery, and, as mentioned, selective venous catheterization is useful to predict which patients will respond. For the other patients, medical therapy with spironolactone, amiloride, or triamterene is the mainstay of management, with adrenalectomy reserved for patients with the most refractory cases. Glucocorticoid-suppressible hyperaldosteronism is treated by administering exogenous dexamethasone at doses of 0.5 to 1 mg daily. Treatment with spironolactone and other above-mentioned medications may help decrease glucocorticoid requirements in this condition and avoid symptoms of Cushing's syndrome.

Postoperatively, some patients experience transient hypoaldosteronism requiring mineralocorticoids for up to 3 months. Rarely, acute Addison's disease may occur 2 to 3 days after unilateral adrenalectomy. Adrenalectomy is greater than 90% successful in improving hypokalemia and approximately 70% successful in correcting the hypertension. Patients who respond to spironolactone therapy, and those with a shorter duration of hypertension with minimal end-organ (renal) damage, are more likely to achieve improvement in hypertension, whereas male patients, those older than age 50 years, and those with multiple adrenal nodules are least likely to benefit from adrenalectomy.

Cushing's Syndrome

As previously mentioned, Cushing described patients with a peculiar fat deposition, amenorrhea, impotence (in men), hirsutism, purple striae, hypertension, diabetes, and other features that constitute the syndrome (Fig. 37-62). He also recognized that several of these patients had basophilic tumors of the pituitary gland and concluded that these tumors produced hormones, which caused adrenocortical hyperplasia, thus resulting in the manifestations of the syndrome. Today, the term Cushing's syndrome refers to a complex of symptoms and signs resulting from hypersecretion of cortisol, regardless of etiology. In contrast, Cushing's disease refers to a pituitary tumor, usually an adenoma, which leads to bilateral adrenal hyperplasia and hypercortisolism. Cushing's syndrome (endogenous) is a rare disease, affecting 10 in 1 million individuals. It is more common in adults, but may occur in children. Women are more commonly affected than men (male:female ratio 1:8). Although most individuals have sporadic disease, Cushing's syndrome may be found in MEN1 families and can result from ACTH-secreting pituitary tumors, primary adrenal neoplasms, or an ectopic ACTH-secreting carcinoid tumor (more common in men) or bronchial adenoma (more common in women).

Cushing's syndrome may be classified as ACTH-dependent or ACTH-independent (Table 37-17). The most common cause of hypercortisolism is exogenous administration of steroids. However, approximately 70% of cases of endogenous Cushing's syndrome are caused by an ACTH-producing pituitary tumor. Primary adrenal sources (adenoma, hyperplasia, and carcinoma) account for approximately 20% of cases and ectopic ACTH-secreting tumors account

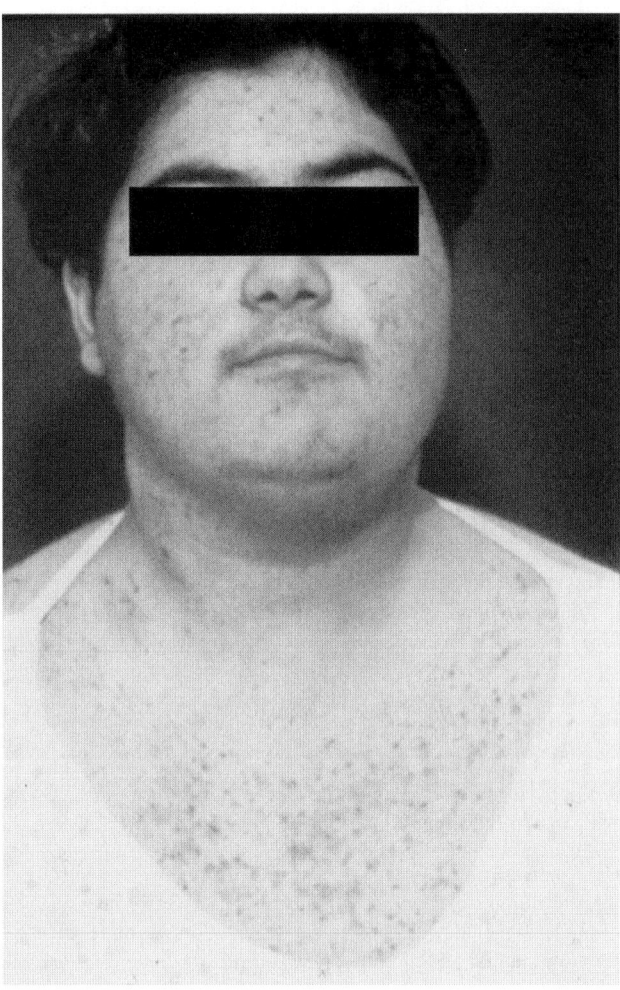

FIG. 37-62. Some characteristic features of Cushing's syndrome: moon facies, hirsutism, and acne.

for less than 10% of cases. CRH may also be secreted ectopically in bronchial carcinoid tumors, pheochromocytomas, and other tumors. These patients are difficult to distinguish from those with ectopic ACTH production, but can be diagnosed by determining CRH levels.[85] Patients with major depression, alcoholism, pregnancy, chronic renal failure, or stress may also have elevated cortisol

Table 37-17
Etiology of Cushing's Syndrome

ACTH-dependent (70%)
Pituitary adenoma or Cushing's disease (~70%)
Ectopic ACTH production[a] (~10%)
Ectopic CRH production (<1%)
ACTH-independent (20–30%)
Adrenal adenoma (10–15%)
Adrenal carcinoma (5–10%)
Adrenal hyperplasia—pigmented micronodular cortical hyperplasia or gastric inhibitory peptide-sensitive macronodular hyperplasia (5%)
Other
Pseudo-Cushing's syndrome
Iatrogenic—exogenous administration of steroids

[a] From small-cell lung tumors, pancreatic islet cell tumors, medullary thyroid cancers, pheochromocytomas, and carcinoid tumors of the lung, thymus, gut, pancreas, and ovary.

levels and symptoms of hypercortisolism. However, these manifestations resolve with treatment of the underlying disorder and these patients are deemed to have pseudo-Cushing's syndrome.

Primary adrenal hyperplasia may be micronodular, macronodular, or massively macronodular. Adrenal hyperplasia resulting from ACTH stimulation is usually macronodular (3-cm nodules). Primary pigmented nodular adrenocortical disease is a rare cause of ACTH-independent Cushing's syndrome, which is characterized by the presence of small (<5 mm), black adrenal nodules. Primary pigmented nodular adrenocortical disease may be associated with Carney complex (atrial myxomas, schwannomas, and pigmented nevi) and is thought to be immune related.

Symptoms and Signs

Table 37-18 lists the classic features of Cushing's syndrome. Early diagnosis of this disease requires a thorough knowledge of these manifestations, coupled with a high clinical suspicion. In some patients, symptoms are less pronounced and may be more difficult to recognize, particularly given their diversity and the absence of a single defining symptom or sign. Progressive truncal obesity is the most common symptom, occurring in up to 95% of patients. This pattern results from the lipogenic action of excessive corticosteroids centrally and catabolic effects peripherally, along with peripheral muscle wasting. Fat deposition also occurs in unusual sites, such as the supraclavicular space and posterior neck region, leading to the so-called buffalo hump. Purple striae are often visible on the protuberant abdomen. Rounding of the face secondary to thickening of the facial fat leads to moon facies, and thinning of subcutaneous tissue leads to plethora. There is an increase in fine hair growth on the face, upper back, and arms, although true virilization is more commonly seen with adrenocortical cancers. Endocrine abnormalities include glucose intolerance, amenorrhea, and decreased libido or impotence. Large, purple striae on the abdomen or proximal extremities are most reliable for making the diagnosis. In children, Cushing's syndrome is characterized by obesity and stunted growth. Patients with Cushing's disease may also present with headaches, visual field defects, and panhypopituitarism. Hyperpigmentation of the skin, if present, suggests an ectopic ACTH-producing tumor with high levels of circulating ACTH.

Diagnostic Tests

The aims of diagnostic tests in the evaluation of patients suspected of having Cushing's syndrome are twofold: to confirm the presence of Cushing's syndrome and to determine its etiology (Fig. 37-63).

Table 37-18
Features of Cushing's Syndrome

System	Manifestation
General	Weight gain—central obesity, buffalo hump, supraclavicular fat pads
Integumentary	Hirsutism, plethora, purple striae, acne, ecchymosis
Cardiovascular	Hypertension
Musculoskeletal	Generalized weakness, osteopenia
Neuropsychiatric	Emotional lability, psychosis, depression
Metabolic	Diabetes or glucose intolerance, hyperlipidemia
Renal	Polyuria, renal stones
Gonadal	Impotence, decreased libido, menstrual irregularities

Laboratory Studies. The secretion of cortisol is episodic and has a diurnal variation, therefore a single measurement of the plasma cortisol level is unreliable in diagnosing Cushing's syndrome. Cushing's syndrome is characterized by elevated glucocorticoid levels that are not suppressible by exogenous hormone administration and loss of diurnal variation. This phenomenon is used to screen patients using the overnight low-dose dexamethasone suppression test. In this test, 1 mg of a synthetic glucocorticoid (dexamethasone) is given at 11 P.M. and plasma cortisol levels are measured at 8 A.M. the following morning. Physiologically normal adults suppress cortisol levels less than 3 μg/dL, whereas most patients with Cushing's syndrome do not. False-negative results may be obtained in patients with mild disease, therefore some authors consider the test positive only if cortisol levels are suppressed to less than 1.8 μg/dL. False-positive results can occur in up to 3% of patients with chronic renal failure, depression, or those taking medications such as phenytoin, which enhance dexamethasone metabolism. In patients with a negative test, but a high clinical suspicion, the classic low-dose dexamethasone (0.5 mg every 6 hours for 8 doses, or 2 mg over 48 hours) suppression test or urinary cortisol measurement should be performed. Measurement of elevated 24-hour urinary cortisol levels is a very sensitive (95 to 100%) and specific (98%) modality of diagnosing Cushing's syndrome, and is particularly useful for identifying patients with pseudo-Cushing's syndrome. A urinary free cortisol excretion of less than 100 μg/dL (in most laboratories) rules out hypercortisolism. Recently, salivary cortisol measurements using commercially available kits also have demonstrated superior sensitivity in diagnosing Cushing's syndrome.[86] However, they are not used routinely.

Once a diagnosis is established, further testing is aimed at determining the cause, i.e., ACTH-dependent or ACTH-independent Cushing's syndrome. This is best accomplished by measurement of plasma ACTH levels using immunoradiometric assay (normal 10 to 100 pg/mL). Elevated ACTH levels are found in patients with adrenal hyperplasia as a result of Cushing's disease (15 to 500 pg/mL) and those with CRH-secreting tumors, but the highest levels are found in patients with ectopic sources of ACTH (>1000 pg/mL). In contrast, ACTH levels are characteristically suppressed (<5 pg/mL) in patients with primary cortisol-secreting adrenal tumors. The high-dose dexamethasone suppression test is used to distinguish between the causes of ACTH-dependent Cushing's syndrome (pituitary vs. ectopic). The standard test (2 mg dexamethasone every 6 hours for 2 days) or the overnight test (8 mg) may be used, with 24-hour urine collections for cortisol and 17-hydroxy steroids performed over the second day. Failure to suppress urinary cortisol by 50% confirms the diagnosis of an ectopic ACTH-producing tumor. Patients suspected of having ectopic tumors should also undergo testing of serum calcitonin levels (to rule out MTC) and urine for catecholamines. Bilateral petrosal vein sampling also is helpful for determining whether the patient has Cushing's disease or ectopic Cushing's syndrome.

The CRH test also is helpful in determining the etiology of Cushing's syndrome. Ovine CRH (1 μg/kg) is administered intravenously, followed by serial measurements of ACTH and cortisol at 15-minute intervals for 1 hour. Patients with a primary adrenal cause of hypercortisolism exhibit a blunted response (ACTH peak <10 pg/mL), whereas those with ACTH-dependent Cushing's syndrome demonstrate a higher elevation of ACTH (>30 pg/mL). CRH stimulation also can enhance the usefulness of petrosal vein sampling, as described in the next section. Patients with pituitary tumors have a higher peak ACTH than those with ectopic ACTH-producing tumors.

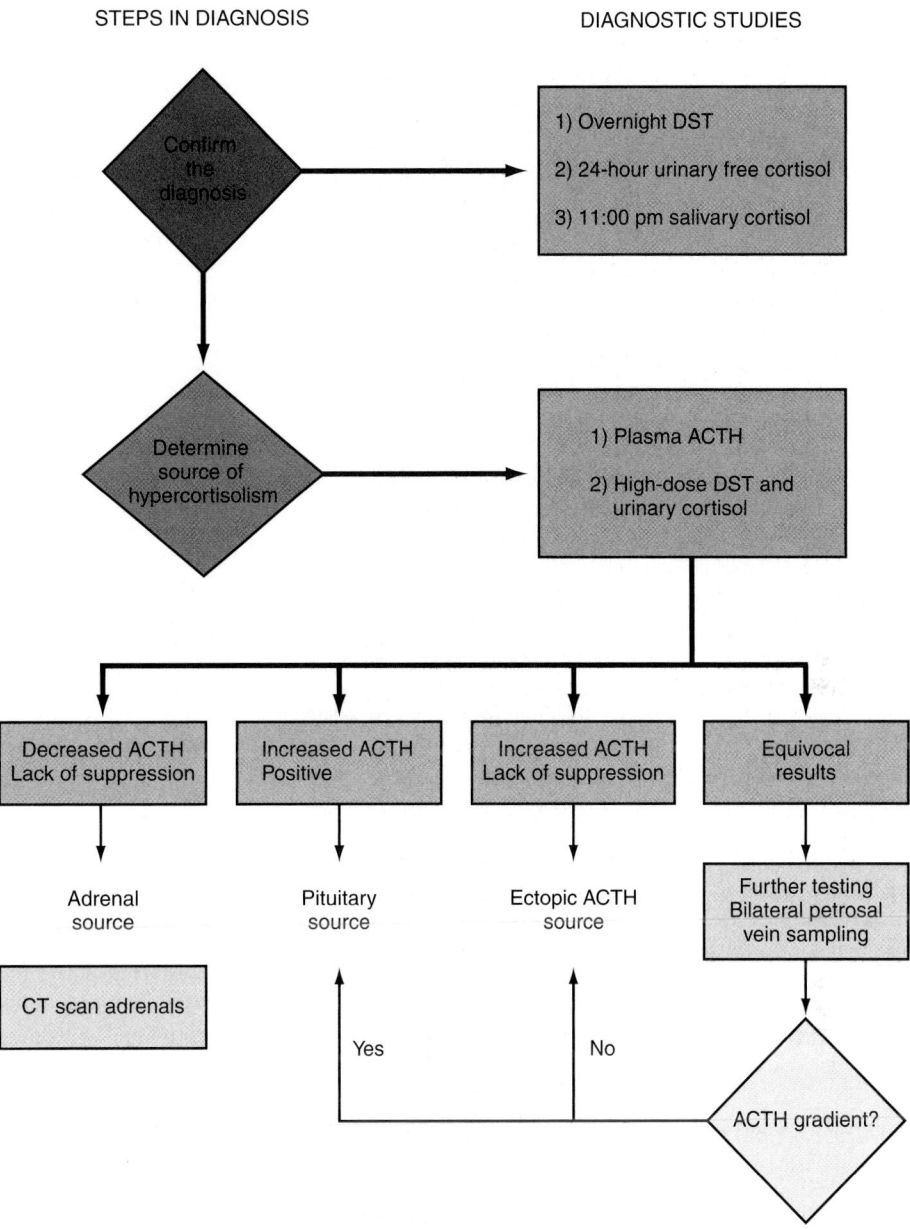

STEPS IN DIAGNOSIS

DIAGNOSTIC STUDIES

Confirm the diagnosis

1) Overnight DST

2) 24-hour urinary free cortisol

3) 11:00 pm salivary cortisol

Determine source of hypercortisolism

1) Plasma ACTH

2) High-dose DST and urinary cortisol

Decreased ACTH Lack of suppression

Increased ACTH Positive

Increased ACTH Lack of suppression

Equivocal results

Adrenal source

Pituitary source

Ectopic ACTH source

Further testing Bilateral petrosal vein sampling

CT scan adrenals

Yes

No

ACTH gradient?

FIG. 37-63. Diagnosis of Cushing's syndrome using the dexamethasone suppression test.

Radiologic Studies. CT and MRI scans of the abdomen can identify adrenal tumors with 95% sensitivity. They are also helpful in distinguishing adrenal adenomas from carcinomas, as discussed in a subsequent section. MRI scans of the adrenals are also useful for this purpose and have the added advantage of allowing assessment of vascular anatomy. Adrenal adenomas appear darker than the liver on T2-weighted imaging. Radioscintigraphic imaging of the adrenals using NP-59 also can be used to distinguish adenoma from hyperplasia. Adrenal adenomas show increased uptake of NP-59 with suppression of uptake in the contralateral gland, whereas hyperplastic glands demonstrate bilateral uptake. Reports suggest that "cold" adrenal nodules are more likely to be cancerous, although this distinction is not absolute. NP-59 scanning is most useful in identifying patients with adrenal source of hypercortisolism and primary pigmented micronodular hyperplasia.

Thin-section CT scans are only 22% sensitive at identifying pituitary tumors. Contrast-enhanced MRI scans of the brain are better (sensitivity 33 to 67%), although small microadenomas may still escape detection. Inferior petrosal sinus sampling for ACTH before and after injection of CRH has been helpful in this regard, and has a sensitivity approaching 100%. In this study, catheters are placed in both internal jugular veins and a peripheral vein. A ratio of petrosal to peripheral vein ACTH level of greater than 2 in the basal state and greater than 3 after CRH stimulation is diagnostic of a pituitary tumor.

In patients suspected of having an ectopic tumor producing ACTH, CT or MRI scans of the chest and anterior mediastinum should be performed first, followed by imaging of the neck, abdomen, and pelvis if the initial studies are negative.

Treatment

Unilateral laparoscopic adrenalectomy is the treatment of choice for patients with adrenal adenomas. Open adrenalectomy is reserved for large tumors (≥6 cm) or those suspected to be adrenocortical cancers. Bilateral adrenalectomy is curative for primary adrenal hyperplasia.

The treatment of choice in patients with Cushing's disease is transsphenoidal excision of the pituitary adenoma, which is successful in 80% of patients. Pituitary irradiation has been used for patients with persistent or recurrent disease after surgery. However, it is associated with a high rate of panhypopituitarism and some patients develop visual deficits. This has led to increased use of stereotactic radiosurgery, which uses CT guidance to deliver high doses of radiotherapy to the tumor (photon or gamma knife). Patients who fail to respond to either treatment are candidates for pharmacologic therapy with adrenal inhibitors such as ketoconazole, metyrapone, or aminoglutethimide, or bilateral adrenalectomy. Several series have reported the safety and effectiveness of bilateral laparoscopic adrenalectomy in this setting.

Patients with ectopic ACTH production are best managed by treating the primary tumor, including recurrences, if possible. Medical adrenalectomy with metyrapone, aminoglutethimide, and mitotane, or bilateral adrenalectomy has been used to palliate patients with unresectable disease. Bilateral laparoscopic adrenalectomy, as used for recurrent or persistent Cushing's disease has also been shown to be safe and effective in the management of patients with Cushing's disease whose ectopic ACTH-secreting tumor cannot be localized.

Patients undergoing surgery for a primary adrenal adenoma-secreting glucocorticoids require preoperative and postoperative steroids because of suppression of the contralateral adrenal gland. These patients are also at increased predisposition for infectious complications and thromboembolic complications, the latter because of a hypercoagulable state resulting from an increase in clotting factors, such as factor VIII and von Willebrand factor complex, and by impaired fibrinolysis. Duration of steroid therapy is determined by the ACTH stimulation test. Exogenous steroids may be needed for up to 2 years, but are needed indefinitely in patients who have undergone bilateral adrenalectomy. This latter group of patients also may require mineralocorticoid replacement therapy. Typical replacement doses include hydrocortisone (10 to 20 mg q A.M. and 5 to 10 mg q P.M.) and fludrocortisone (0.05 to 0.2 mg/d q A.M.).

Adrenocortical Cancer

Adrenal carcinomas are rare neoplasms with a worldwide incidence of 2 per 1 million. These tumors have a bimodal age distribution, with an increased incidence in children and in adults in the fourth and fifth decades of life. Functioning tumors are more common in women, whereas men are more likely to develop nonfunctioning carcinomas. The majority are sporadic, but adrenocortical carcinomas also occur in association with germline mutations of *p*53 (Li-Fraumeni syndrome) and *MENIN* (multiple endocrine neoplasia 1) genes. Loci on 11p (Beckwith-Wiedemann syndrome), 2p (Carney complex), and 9q have also been implicated.

Symptoms and Signs

Approximately 50% of adrenocortical cancers are nonfunctioning.[87] The remaining secrete cortisol (30%), androgens (20%), estrogens (10%), aldosterone (2%), or multiple hormones (35%). Patients with functioning tumors often present with the rapid onset of Cushing's syndrome accompanied by virilizing features. Nonfunctioning tumors more commonly present with an enlarging abdominal mass and abdominal pain. Rarely, weight loss, anorexia, and nausea may be present.

Diagnostic Tests

Diagnostic evaluation of these patients begins with measurement of serum electrolyte levels to rule out hypokalemia—an overnight 1-mg dexamethasone suppression test and a 24-hour urine collection for cortisol, 17-ketosteroids, and catecholamines (to rule out pheochromocytomas).

CT and MRI scans are used to image these tumors. The size of the adrenal mass on imaging studies is the single most important criterion to help diagnose malignancy. In the series reported by Copeland and associates, 92% of adrenal cancers were greater than 6 cm in diameter.[88] CT imaging characteristics suggesting malignancy include tumor heterogeneity, irregular margins and the presence of hemorrhage and adjacent lymphadenopathy or liver metastases (Fig. 37-64). Moderately bright signal intensity on T2-weighted images (adrenal mass:liver ratio 1.2:2.8), significant lesion enhancement, and slow washout after injection of gadolinium contrast also indicate malignancy, as does evidence of local invasion into surrounding structures such as the liver, blood vessels (inferior vena cava), and distant metastases. Once adrenal cancer is diagnosed, CT scans of the chest and pelvis should be performed for staging. Table 37-19 depicts the tumor–node–metastasis (TNM) staging system for adrenocortical carcinoma. Most patients present with advanced disease; up to 70% of patients present with stage III or IV disease.

Pathology

Most adrenocortical cancers are large, weighing between 100 and 1000 g. On gross examination, areas of hemorrhage and necrosis are often evident. Microscopically, cells are hyperchromatic and typically have large nuclei and prominent nucleoli. It is very difficult to distinguish benign adrenal adenomas from carcinomas by histologic examination alone. Other criteria supporting malignancy include invasion, distant metastases, the presence of aneuploidy, increased mitotic figures and production of androgens and 11-deoxysteroids.

Treatment

The most important predictor of survival in patients with adrenal cancer is the adequacy of resection. Patients who undergo complete resection have 5-year actuarial survival rates ranging from 32 to 48%, whereas median survival is less than 1 year in those undergoing incomplete excision. Therefore, adrenocortical carcinomas are treated by excision of the tumor en bloc, with any contiguously involved lymph nodes or organs, such as the diaphragm, kidney, pancreas, liver, or inferior vena cava. This is best accomplished by open adrenalectomy via a generous subcostal incision or a thoracoabdominal incision (on the right side). The incisions should permit wide exposure, minimize chances of capsule rupture and tumor spillage and allow vascular control of the aorta, inferior vena cava, and renal vessels, as needed.

Mitotane or *o*,*p*-DDD or 1,1-dichloro-2-(*o*-chlorophenyl)-2-(*p*-chlorophenyl) ethane, which is a derivative of the insecticide DDT, has adrenolytic activity and has been used in the adjuvant setting and for the treatment of unresectable or metastatic disease. However, the therapeutic effectiveness is conflicting and consistent improvement in survival rates are lacking. Moreover, the drug is associated with significant gastrointestinal and neurologic side effects, particularly at the effective doses of 2 to 6 g/d. The routine use of this medication awaits evaluation in controlled trials. Determination of blood mitotane levels is helpful to ascertain whether therapeutic and nontoxic

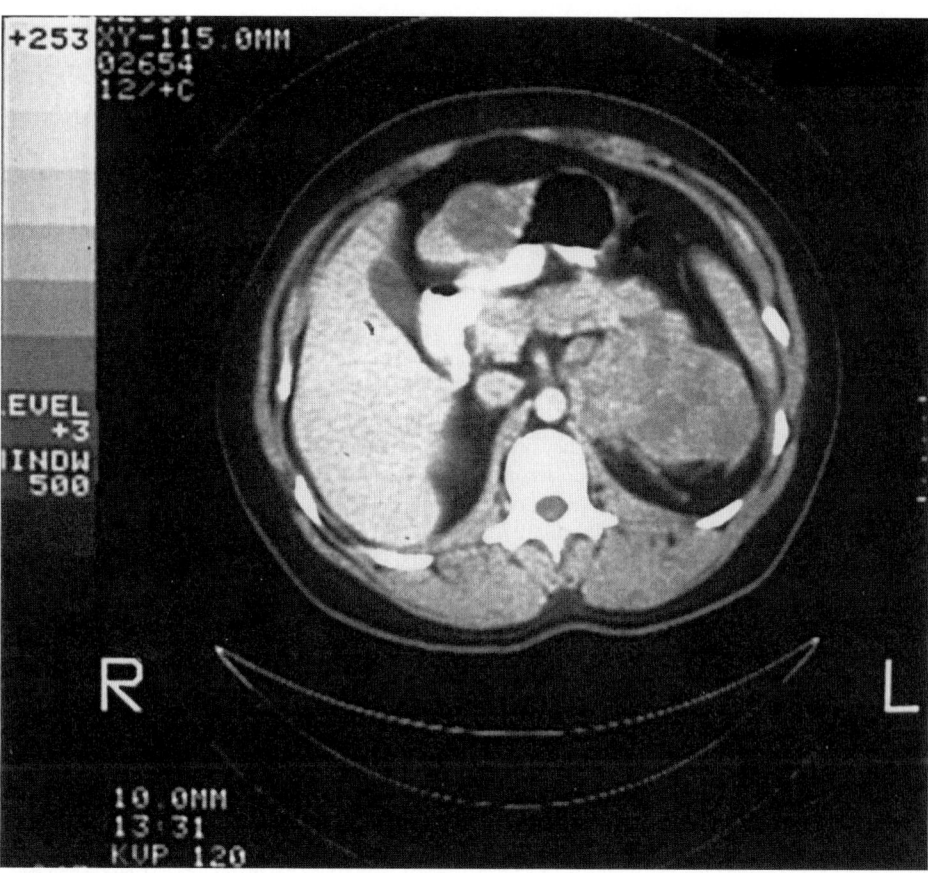

FIG. 37-64. CT scan of the abdomen showing a left adrenocortical cancer with synchronous liver metastasis.

levels are present.[89] Adrenocortical tumors commonly metastasize to the liver, lung, and bone.

Surgical debulking is recommended for isolated, recurrent disease and has been demonstrated to prolong survival. Systemic chemotherapeutic agents used in this tumor include etoposide, cisplatin, doxorubicin, and, more recently, paclitaxel, but consistent responses are rare, possibly as a consequence of the expression of the multidrug resistance gene (*MDR-1*) in tumor cells. In vitro data indicate that mitotane may be able to reverse this resistance when combined with various chemotherapeutic agents. Suramin, a growth factor inhibitor, has shown minimal partial response rates. Adrenocortical cancers are also relatively insensitive to conventional

external beam radiation therapy. However, this modality is used in the palliation of bony metastases. Ketoconazole, metyrapone, or aminoglutethimide may also be useful in controlling steroid hypersecretion.

Sex Steroid Excess

Adrenal adenomas or carcinomas that secrete adrenal androgens lead to virilizing syndromes. While women with virilizing tumors develop hirsutism, amenorrhea, infertility, and other signs of masculinization, such as increased muscle mass, deepened voice, and temporal balding, men with these tumors are more difficult to diagnose and hence usually present with disease in advanced stages. Children with virilizing tumors have accelerated growth, premature development of facial and pubic hair, acne, genital enlargement, and deepening of their voice. Feminizing adrenal tumors are less common and occur in men in the third to fifth decades of life. These tumors lead to gynecomastia, impotence, and testicular atrophy. Women with these tumors develop irregular menses or dysfunctional uterine bleeding. Vaginal bleeding may occur in postmenopausal women. Girls with these tumors experience precocious puberty with breast enlargement and early menarche.

Diagnostic Tests

Virilizing tumors produce excessive amounts of the androgen precursor, DHEA, which can be measured in plasma or urine as 17-ketosteroids. Patients with feminizing tumors also have elevated urinary 17-ketosteroids, in addition to increased estrogen levels. Androgen-producing tumors are often associated with production of other hormones such as glucocorticoids.

Table 37-19
TNM Staging for Adrenocortical Cancer

Stage	TNM Class
I	T1, N0, M0
II	T2, N0, M0
III	T3, N0, M0
	T1-2, N1, M0
IV	T3-4, N1, M0
	Any T, Any N, M1

Primary tumor (T): T1, size ≤5 cm without local invasion; T2 size >5 cm without local invasion; T3, any size with local invasion but no involvement of adjacent organs; T4, any size with involvement of adjacent organs.

Nodes (N): N0, no involvement of regional nodes; N1, positive regional lymph nodes.

Metastasis (M): M0, no known distal metastases; M1, distant metastases present.

SOURCE: Reproduced with permission from *AJCC Cancer Staging Manual*, 6th ed. New York: Springer-Verlag, 2002.

Treatment

Virilizing and feminizing tumors are treated by adrenalectomy. Malignancy is difficult to diagnose histologically, but is suggested by the presence of local invasion, recurrence, or distal metastases. Adrenolytic drugs, such as mitotane, aminoglutethimide, and ketoconazole, may be useful in controlling symptoms in patients with metastatic disease.

Congenital Adrenal Hyperplasia

Congenital adrenal hyperplasia (CAH) refers to a group of disorders that result from deficiencies, or complete absence, of enzymes involved in adrenal steroidogenesis. 21-Hydroxylase (CYP21A2) deficiency is the most common enzymatic defect, accounting for more than 90% of cases of CAH. This deficiency prevents the production of 11-deoxycortisol and 11-deoxycorticosterone from progesterone precursors. Deficiency of glucocorticoids and aldosterone leads to elevated ACTH levels and overproduction of adrenal androgens and corticosteroid precursors such as 17-hydroxyprogesterone and Δ^4-androstenedione. These compounds are converted to testosterone in the peripheral tissues, thereby leading to virilization. Complete deficiency of 21-hydroxylase presents at birth with virilization, diarrhea, hypovolemia, hyponatremia, hyperkalemia, and hyperpigmentation. Partial enzyme deficiency may present at birth or later with virilizing features. These patients are less prone to the salt-wasting that characterizes complete enzyme deficiency. 11β-Hydroxylase deficiency is the second most common form of congenital adrenal hyperplasia and leads to hypertension (from 11-deoxycorticosterone accumulation), virilization, and hyperpigmentation. Other enzyme deficiencies include 3β-hydroxydehydrogenase and 17-hydroxylase deficiency. Congenital adrenal lipoid hyperplasia is the most severe form of CAH, which is caused by cholesterol desmolase deficiency. It leads to the disruption of all steroid biosynthetic pathways, thus resulting in a fatal salt-wasting syndrome in phenotypic female patients.

Diagnostic Tests

The particular enzyme deficiency can be diagnosed by karyotype analysis and measurement of plasma and urinary steroids. The most common enzyme deficiency, absence of 21-hydroxylase, leads to increased plasma17-hydroxyprogesterone and progesterone levels, because these compounds cannot be converted to 11-deoxycortisol and 11-deoxycorticosterone, respectively. 11β-Hydroxylase deficiency is the next most common disorder and results in elevated plasma 11-deoxycorticosterone and 11-deoxycortisol. Urinary 17-hydroxyprogesterone, androgens, and 17-ketosteroids are also elevated. The dexamethasone suppression test (2 to 4 mg divided qid for 7 days) can be used to distinguish adrenal hyperplasia from neoplasia. CT, MRI, and iodocholesterol scans are generally used to localize the tumors.

Treatment

Patients with CAH have traditionally been managed medically, with cortisol and mineralocorticoid replacement to suppress the hypothalamic–pituitary–adrenal axis. However, the doses of steroids required are often supraphysiologic and lead to iatrogenic hypercortisolism. More recently, bilateral laparoscopic adrenalectomy has been proposed as an alternative treatment for this disease and has been successfully performed in a limited number of patients for various forms of CAH.[90]

DISORDERS OF THE ADRENAL MEDULLA

Pheochromocytomas

Pheochromocytomas are rare tumors with prevalence rates ranging from 0.3 to 0.95% in autopsy series, and approximately 1.9% in series using biochemical screening. They can occur at any age with a peak incidence in the fourth and fifth decades of life, and have no gender predilection, although they tend to occur more frequently in female children. Extra-adrenal tumors, also called functional paragangliomas, may be found at sites of sympathetic ganglia in the organ of Zuckerkandl, neck, mediastinum, abdomen, and pelvis. Pheochromocytomas are often called the "10% tumor," because 10% are bilateral, 10% are malignant, 10% occur in pediatric patients, 10% are extra-adrenal, and 10% are familial.

Pheochromocytomas occur in families with MEN2A and MEN2B, in approximately 50% of patients. Both syndromes are inherited in an autosomal dominant fashion and are caused by germline mutations in the *RET* proto-oncogene. Another familial cancer syndrome with an increased risk of pheochromocytomas includes von Hippel-Lindau disease, which also is inherited in an autosomal dominant manner. This syndrome also includes retinal angioma, hemangioblastomas of the central nervous system, renal cysts, and carcinomas, pancreatic cysts, and epididymal cystadenomas. The incidence of pheochromocytomas in the syndrome is approximately 14%, but varies depending on the series. The gene causing von Hippel-Lindau disease has been mapped to chromosome 3p and is a tumor-suppressor gene. Pheochromocytomas are also included within the tumor spectrum of neurofibromatosis type 1 and other neuroectodermal disorders (Sturge-Weber syndrome and tuberous sclerosis), Carney's syndrome (gastric epithelioid leiomyosarcoma, pulmonary chondroma, and extra-adrenal paraganglioma), and, rarely, in the MEN1 syndrome. Familial pheochromocytomas may also rarely occur without other associated disorders.

Symptoms and Signs

Headache, palpitations, and diaphoresis constitute the "classic triad" of pheochromocytomas. Symptoms such as anxiety, tremulousness, paresthesias, flushing, chest pain, shortness of breath, abdominal pain, nausea, vomiting, and others are nonspecific and may be episodic in nature. Cardiovascular complications, such as myocardial infarction and cerebrovascular accidents, may ensue.[91] These symptoms can be incited by a range of stimuli including exercise, micturition, and defecation. The most common clinical sign is hypertension. In fact, pheochromocytomas are one of the few curable causes of hypertension and are found in 0.1 to 0.2% of hypertensive patients. The hypertension related to this tumor may be paroxysmal with intervening normotension, sustained with paroxysms, or sustained hypertension alone. Sudden death may occur in patients with undiagnosed tumors who undergo other operations or biopsy.

Diagnostic Tests

Biochemical Studies. Pheochromocytomas are diagnosed by testing 24-hour urine samples for catecholamines and their metabolites, as well as by determining plasma metanephrine levels. Urinary metanephrines are 98% sensitive and are also highly specific for pheochromocytomas, whereas vanillylmandelic acid (VMA) measurements are slightly less sensitive and specific. False-positive VMA tests may result from ingestion of caffeine, raw fruits or medications (alpha-methyl dopa). Fractionated urinary catecholamines (norepinephrine, epinephrine, and dopamine) are also sensitive but less specific for pheochromocytomas. Because extra-adrenal sites lack phenylethanolamine-*N*-methyltransferase, these tumors secrete norepinephrine, whereas epinephrine is the main hormone secreted from adrenal pheochromocytomas.

Many physiologic and pathologic states can alter the levels of plasma catecholamines. Hence, they are often thought to be less accurate than urinary tests. Both epinephrine and norepinephrine should be measured because tumors often secrete one or the other hormone. Sensitivities of 85% and specificities of 95% have been reported using cutoff values of 2000 pg/mL for norepinephrine and 200 pg/mL for epinephrine. Provocative tests may rarely be necessary if the results of the basal urinary and plasma measurements are borderline. A threefold increase or stimulated level of greater than 2000 pg/mL 1 to 3 minutes after the administration of 1 to 2 mg of glucagon intravenously suggests a pheochromocytoma, with an 80% sensitivity and 100% specificity. Clonidine is an agent that suppresses neurogenically mediated catecholamine excess but not secretion from pheochromocytomas. A normal clonidine suppression test is defined by a decrease of basal catecholamine levels of less than 500 pg/mL within 2 to 3 hours after an oral dose of 0.3 mg of clonidine. Provocative tests can be associated with mortality and significant morbidity and are rarely used. Chromogranin A is a monomeric, acidic protein that is stored in the adrenal medulla and released along with catecholamine hormones. It has been reported to have a sensitivity of 83% and a specificity of 96% and is useful in conjunction with catecholamine measurement for diagnosing pheochromocytomas. Recent studies have shown that plasma metanephrines are the most reliable tests to identify pheochromocytomas, with sensitivity approaching 100%.[92]

Radiologic Studies. These are useful to localize tumors 3 cm in diameter and to assess the extent of spread once the diagnosis has been made with biochemical tests. CT scans are 85 to 95% sensitive and 70 to 100% specific for pheochromocytomas (Fig. 37-65A). The scans should be performed without contrast to minimize the risk of precipitating a hypertensive crisis and should image the region from the diaphragm to the aortic bifurcation so as to image the organ of Zuckerkandl. However, CT scans do not provide functional information and cannot definitively diagnose pheochromocytomas. MRI scans are 95% sensitive and almost 100% specific for pheochromocytomas because these tumors have a characteristic appearance on T2-weighted images or after gadolinium. MRI is also the study of choice in pregnant women as there is no risk of radiation exposure. Metaiodobenzylguanidine (MIBG) is taken up and concentrated by vesicles in the adrenal medullar cells because its structure is similar to norepinephrine. Normal adrenal medullary tissue does not take up MIBG. Consequently, ^{131}I radiolabeled MIBG is useful for localizing pheochromocytomas (Fig. 37-65B), especially those in ectopic positions. This test has a reported sensitivity of 77 to 89% and a specificity ranging from 88 to 100%.

Treatment

The medical management of pheochromocytomas is aimed chiefly at blood pressure control and volume repletion. Alpha blockers such as phenoxybenzamine are started 1 to 3 weeks before surgery at doses of 10 mg twice daily, which may be increased to 300 to 400 mg/d. Patients who perspire are not adequately blocked and the dose should be increased. Other alpha blockers such as prazosin, and other classes of drugs, such as ACE inhibitors and calcium channel blockers, are also useful. Beta blockers, such as propranolol at doses of 10 to 40 mg every 6 to 8 hours, often need to be added preoperatively in patients who have persistent tachycardia and arrhythmias. Beta blockers should only be instituted after adequate alpha blockade and hydration in order to avoid the effects of unopposed alpha stimulation, i.e., hypertensive crisis and congestive heart failure. Patients should also be volume repleted preoperatively in order to avoid postoperative hypotension, which ensues with the loss of vasoconstriction after tumor removal.

Adrenalectomy is the treatment of choice. The chief goal of surgery is to resect the tumor completely with minimal tumor manipulation or rupture of the tumor capsule. Surgery should be performed with both noninvasive and invasive monitors, including an arterial

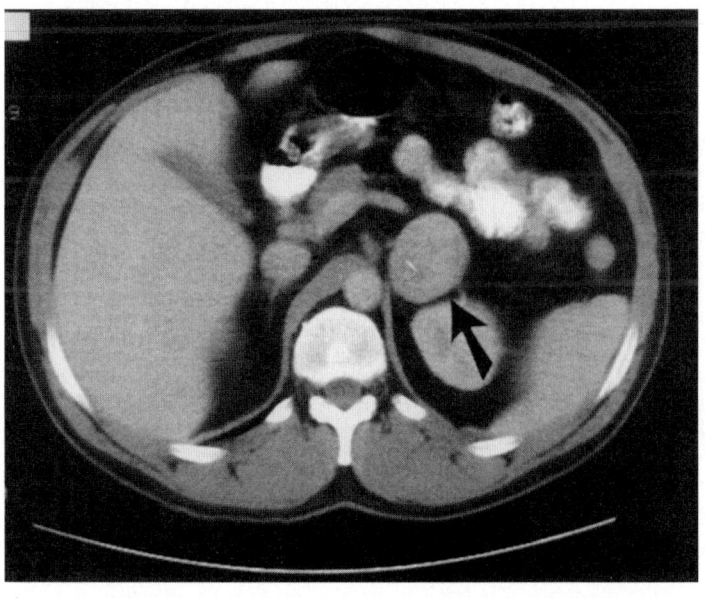

A

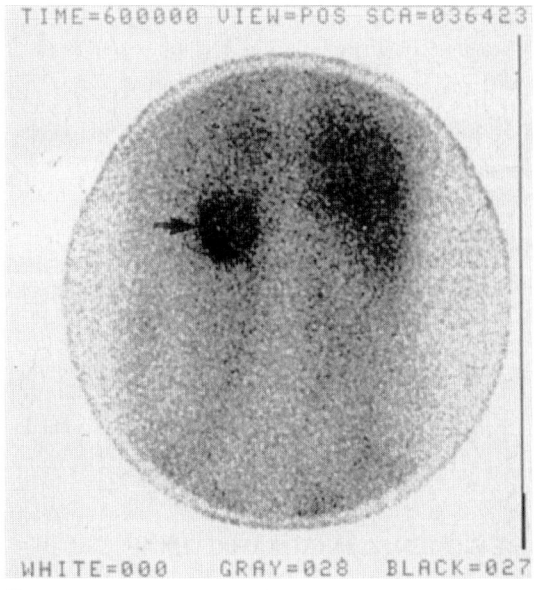

B

FIG. 37-65. *A.* A left-sided pheochromocytoma imaged by a CT scan of the abdomen and (*B*) a metaiodobenzylguanidine scan viewed posteriorly.

line and central venous lines. In patients with congestive heart failure or underlying coronary artery disease, Swan-Ganz catheters may be necessary. Stress must be avoided during anesthesia induction, and use of inhaled agents such as isoflurane and enflurane are preferred because they have minimal cardiac depressant effects. The common medications used for intraoperative blood pressure control include nitroprusside, nitroglycerin, and phentolamine. Intraoperative arrhythmias are best managed by short-acting beta blockers such as esmolol. Adrenalectomy was usually performed via an open anterior approach to facilitate detection of bilateral tumors, extra-adrenal lesions, or metastatic lesions. However, many pheochromocytomas less than 5 cm in diameter are currently safely resected laparoscopically, provided the principles discussed earlier are observed. Postoperatively, these patients are prone to hypotension because of loss of adrenergic stimulation and consequent vasodilatation, and therefore need large-volume resuscitation.

Hereditary Pheochromocytomas

Inherited pheochromocytomas tend to be multiple and bilateral. Generally, unilateral adrenalectomy is recommended in the absence of obvious lesions in the contralateral adrenal gland, because the high incidence of an addisonian crisis in patients undergoing bilateral adrenalectomy. For patients with tumors in both adrenal glands, cortical-sparing subtotal adrenalectomy may preserve adrenocortical function and avoid the morbidity of bilateral total adrenalectomy.[93] Laparoscopic subtotal adrenalectomy provides short-term clinical results comparable to total adrenalectomy, with reduced surgical morbidity. However, these patients remain at risk for recurrent pheochromocytoma, which has been reported in 20% of patients with von Hippel-Lindau disease a median of 40 months after partial adrenalectomy, and in 33% of MEN2 patients followed for 54 to 88 months after surgery. Autotransplantation of adrenocortical tissue after total adrenalectomy may be another option for these patients and removes the risk of recurrence. However, the transplanted cortical tissue rarely provides full function and steroid replacement is usually required.

Malignant Pheochromocytoma

Approximately 12 to 29% of pheochromocytomas are malignant and associated with decreased survival. There are no definitive histologic criteria defining malignant pheochromocytomas. Traditionally, malignancy is usually diagnosed when there is evidence of invasion into surrounding structures or distant metastases. The most common sites for metastatic disease are bone, liver, regional lymph nodes, lung, and peritoneum. The brain, pleura, skin, and muscles may also occasionally be involved. However, capsular and vascular invasion may be seen in benign lesions as well. Given this difficulty defining malignancy clinically (in the absence of metastatic disease), a number of other features, such as DNA ploidy, tumor size, and necrosis, neuropeptide Y mRNA expression and serum neuron-specific enolase expression have been studied. Malignant pheochromocytomas are more likely to express p53 and bcl-2, and have activated telomerase.[94]

THE ADRENAL INCIDENTALOMA

An adrenal lesion discovered during imaging performed for unrelated reasons is referred to as an incidentaloma. This definition excludes tumors discovered on imaging studies performed during the course of evaluating symptoms of hormone hypersecretion or

Table 37-20
Differential Diagnosis of Adrenal Incidentaloma

Functioning Lesions	Nonfunctioning Lesions
Benign	*Benign*
Aldosteronoma	Cortical adenoma
Cortisol-producing adenoma	Myelolipoma
Sex-steroid-producing adenoma	Cyst
Pheochromocytoma	Ganglioneuroma
	Hemorrhage
Malignant	*Malignant*
Adrenocortical cancer	Metastasis
Malignant pheochromocytoma	

staging patients with known cancer. The incidence of these lesions identified by CT scans ranges from 0.4 to 4.4%.

Differential Diagnosis

The differential diagnosis includes a multitude of lesions that are listed in Table 37-20. Nonfunctional cortical adenomas account for the majority (36 to 94%) of adrenal incidentalomas in patients without a history of cancer.[95] In a series of patients from the Mayo Clinic, no nonfunctional lesion progressed to cause clinical or biochemical abnormalities. However, other studies indicate that a proportion (5 to 20%) of patients with apparently nonfunctioning cortical adenomas have underlying, subtle abnormalities of glucocorticoid secretion and a rare, benign-appearing incidentaloma is a cancer.

By definition, patients with incidentalomas do not have clinically overt Cushing's syndrome, but subclinical Cushing's syndrome is estimated to occur in approximately 8% of patients. This disorder is characterized by subtle features of cortisol excess, which are manifested by weight gain, skin atrophy, facial fullness, diabetes, and hypertension. On laboratory examination, there is loss of normal diurnal variation in cortisol secretion, autonomous cortisol secretion and resistance to suppression by dexamethasone, even though total cortisol produced and 24-hour urinary cortisol levels may be normal.[96] Examination of the natural history of subclinical Cushing's syndrome indicates that although most patients of this disorder remain asymptomatic, some do progress to clinically evident Cushing's syndrome. Furthermore, cases of postoperative adrenal crisis from unrecognized suppression of the contralateral adrenal have been reported, making preoperative identification of this condition imperative. This is important to emphasize because these patients are often discharged within 24 hours after laparoscopic adrenalectomy.

The adrenal is a common site of metastases of lung and breast tumors, melanoma, renal cell cancer, and lymphoma. In patients with a history of nonadrenal cancer and a unilateral adrenal mass, the incidence of metastatic disease has been reported to range from 32 to 73%. Myelolipomas are benign, biochemically nonfunctioning lesions composed of elements of hematopoietic and mature adipose tissue, which are rare causes of adrenal incidentaloma. Other, less-commonly encountered lesions include adrenal cysts, ganglioneuromas, and hemorrhage.

Diagnostic Investigations

The diagnostic work-up of an adrenal incidentaloma is aimed at identifying patients who would benefit from adrenalectomy; that is, patients with functioning tumors and those at increased risk of being malignant. It is particularly important to identify patients with subclinical Cushing's disease.

It is not necessary for asymptomatic patients whose imaging studies are consistent with obvious cysts, hemorrhage, myelolipomas, or diffuse metastatic disease to undergo additional investigations. All other patients should be tested for underlying hormonally active tumors by (1) low-dose (1 mg) overnight dexamethasone suppression test or 24-hour urine cortisol to rule out subclinical Cushing's syndrome; (2) a 24-hour urine collection for catecholamines, metanephrines, vanillylmandelic acid, or plasma metanephrine to rule out pheochromocytoma; and (3) in hypertensive patients, serum electrolytes, plasma aldosterone, and plasma renin to rule out an aldosteronoma. Confirmatory tests can be performed based on the results of the initial screening studies.

Determination of the malignant potential of an incidentaloma is more complicated. As discussed earlier, the risk of malignancy in an adrenal lesion is related to its size. Lesions greater than 6 cm in diameter have an approximate risk of malignancy of approximately 35%.[88] However, this size cutoff is not absolute because adrenal carcinomas have also been reported in lesions smaller than 6 cm.

This has led to increased use of the imaging characteristics of incidentalomas to predict malignancy. Benign adrenal adenomas tend to be homogenous and well-encapsulated, and to have smooth and regular margins. They also tend to be hypoattenuating lesions (<10 Hounsfield units) on CT scanning. In contrast, adrenal cancers tend to be hyperattenuating (>18 Hounsfield units), inhomogeneous, have irregular borders and may show evidence of local invasion or adjacent lymphadenopathy. On MRI T2-weighted imaging, adenomas demonstrate low signal intensity when compared to the liver (adrenal mass:liver ratio less than 1.4), whereas carcinomas and metastases have moderate intensity (mass:liver ratio 1.2:2.8). Pheochromocytomas are extremely bright with mass:liver ratios greater than 3. Unfortunately, the ranges overlap and signal intensity is not 100% reliable for determining the nature of the lesion. Therefore, other features, such as enhancement of the lesion with gadolinium contrast, have been proposed. Radionuclide imaging with NP-59 (^{131}I-6β-iodomethyl-19-norcholesterol) also has been used to distinguish between various adrenal lesions, with some investigators suggesting that uptake of NP-59 was 100% predictive of a benign lesion (adenoma), whereas absence of imaging was 100% predictive of a nonadenomatous lesion. However, the technique has not gained widespread acceptance because patients need to be given cold iodine 1 week before the study to prevent thyroid uptake, imaging needs to be delayed by 5 to 7 days after administration of the contrast, and false-positive and false-negative results occur.

FNA biopsy has gained widespread use for the diagnosis of many endocrine lesions, but cannot be used to distinguish adrenal adenomas from carcinomas. This being said, FNA biopsy is useful in the setting of a patient with a history of cancer and a solitary adrenal mass. The positive predictive value of FNA biopsy in this situation has been shown to be almost 100%, although false-negative rates of up to 33% have been reported. Biopsies are usually performed under CT guidance and appropriate testing to rule out pheochromocytomas should be undertaken prior to the procedure in order to avoid precipitating a hypertensive crisis.

Management

An algorithm for the management of patients with incidentally discovered adrenal tumors is shown in Fig. 37-66. Patients with functional tumors, as determined by biochemical testing, or with obviously malignant lesions, should undergo adrenalectomy. Operative intervention also is advised in patients with subclinical Cushing's

syndrome with suppressed plasma ACTH levels and elevated urinary cortisol levels because these patients are at high risk for progression to overt Cushing's syndrome.[96] Adrenalectomy should also be considered in patients with normal ACTH and urinary free cortisol if they are younger than 50 years old or have recent weight gain, hypertension, diabetes, or osteopenia.

For nonfunctional lesions that do not meet any of the above criteria, the risk of malignancy or malignant potential needs to be balanced with operative morbidity and mortality. Lesions larger than 6 cm, or those with suspicious features on imaging studies such as heterogeneity, irregular capsule, or adjacent nodes, should be treated by adrenalectomy because of the increased prevalence of malignancy in this group. Nonoperative therapy, with close periodic follow-up is advised for lesions less than 4 cm in diameter with benign imaging characteristics. However, the management of lesions 4 to 6 cm in size with benign imaging features remains controversial; i.e., this group of patients can be treated with observation or surgery. Recommendations from various groups of endocrine surgeons regarding this "intermediate" group of patients are variable, with some advising adrenalectomy for tumors at cutoff sizes of 3, 4, or 5 cm. However, several important points must be considered in the management of these patients. First, size criteria for malignancy are not definitive and are derived from a selected series of patients. Second, the actual size of adrenal tumors can be underestimated by at least 1 cm by modalities such as CT scans, because tumors are larger in a cephalocaudal axis. Third, the natural history of incidentalomas is variable and depends on the underlying diagnosis, age of the study population, and the size of the mass. Older patients are more likely to have nonfunctioning adenomas. Existing data in terms of the long-term behavior of these nonfunctional lesions, although limited, indicates that malignant transformation is uncommon. Furthermore, tumors that increase in size by at least 1 cm over a 2-year follow-up period, and those with subtle hormonal abnormalities, were more likely to enlarge. Overt hormone overproduction is more likely in tumors greater than 3 cm and those with increased NP-59 uptake.[97] Surgeons are more likely to operate on a 40-year-old patient with a 4-cm lesion, while electing to follow an 80-year-old patient with a similar lesion but multiple concurrent comorbidities. The current recommendation of these authors concerning size threshold for adrenalectomy is 3 to 4 cm in young patients with no comorbidity, and 5 cm in older patients with significant comorbidity.

Lesions that grow during follow-up are also treated by adrenalectomy. Myelolipomas generally do not warrant adrenalectomy unless there is concern regarding malignancy, which is rare, or bleeding into the lesion, which is more likely in myelolipomas greater than 4 cm in size. When indicated, laparoscopic adrenalectomy is the procedure of choice for this lesion. Resection of solitary adrenal metastases in patients with a history of nonadrenal cancer, especially nonsmall-cell lung and renal cancers, has been demonstrated to lead to prolonged patient survival. Suspected adrenal metastases may also be resected for diagnosis or for palliation, if large and symptomatic.

ADRENAL INSUFFICIENCY

Adrenal insufficiency may be primary, resulting from adrenal disease, or secondary, as a result of a deficiency of ACTH (Table 37-21). The most commonly encountered causes of primary adrenal insufficiency are autoimmune disease, infections, and metastatic deposits.[98] Spontaneous adrenal hemorrhage can occur in patients

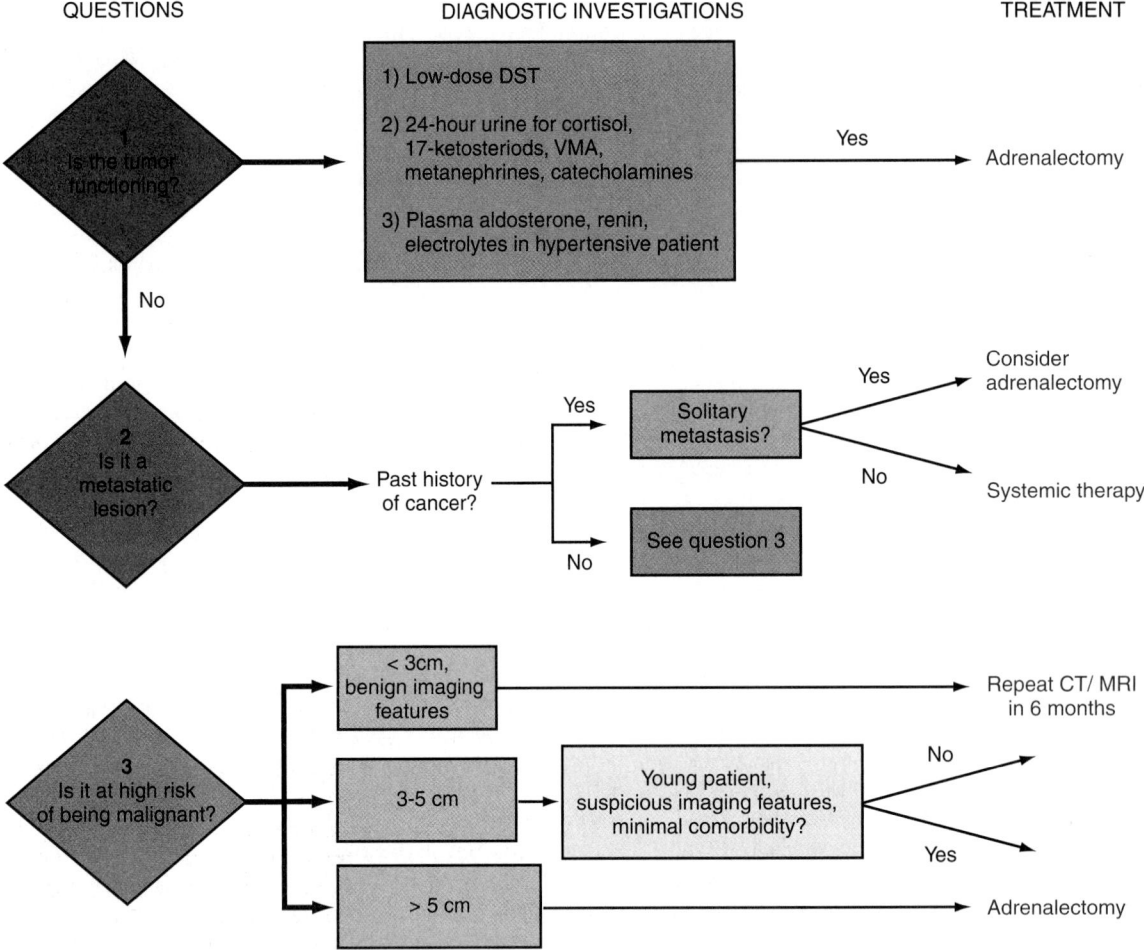

FIG. 37-66. *Management algorithm for an adrenal incidentaloma.*

with fulminant meningococcal septicemia, and in this context is referred to as the Waterhouse-Friderichsen syndrome. It can also occur secondary to trauma, severe stress, infection, and coagulopathies. Exogenous glucocorticoid therapy with suppression of the adrenal glands is the most common cause of secondary adrenal insufficiency when the steroids are discontinued.

Symptoms and Signs

Acute adrenal insufficiency should be suspected in stressed patients with any of the relevant risk factors. It may mimic sepsis and presents with fever, nausea, vomiting, lethargy, mild abdominal pain, or severe hypotension. Chronic adrenal insufficiency, such as that occurring in patients with metastatic tumors, may be more subtle.

Table 37-21
Etiology of Adrenal Insufficiency

Primary	*Secondary*
Autoimmune (autoimmune polyglandular disease types I and II)	Exogenous glucocorticoid therapy
Infectious: TB, fungi, CMV, HIV	Bilateral adrenalectomy
Hemorrhage—spontaneous (Waterhouse-Friderichsen syndrome) and secondary to stress, trauma, infections, coagulopathy, or anticoagulants	Pituitary or hypothalamic tumors
Metastases	Pituitary hemorrhage (postpartum Sheehan's syndrome)
Infiltrative disorders: amyloidosis, hemochromatosis	Transsphenoidal resection of pituitary tumor
Adrenoleukodystrophy	
Congenital adrenal hyperplasia	
Drugs: ketoconazole, metyrapone, aminoglutethemide, mitotane	

Symptoms include fatigue, salt-craving, weight loss, nausea, vomiting, abdominal pain, and diarrhea. These patients may appear hyperpigmented from secretion of large quantities of CRH and ACTH, with an increase in MSH side products.

Diagnostic Studies

Characteristic laboratory findings include hyponatremia, hyperkalemia, eosinophilia, mild azotemia, and fasting or reactive hypoglycemia. The peripheral blood smear may demonstrate eosinophilia in approximately 20% of patients. Adrenal insufficiency is diagnosed by the ACTH stimulation test. ACTH (250 μg) is infused intravenously, and cortisol levels are measured at 0, 30, and 60 minutes. Peak cortisol levels less than 20 μg/dL suggest adrenal insufficiency. ACTH levels also enable one to distinguish primary from secondary causes. High ACTH levels with low plasma cortisol levels are diagnostic of primary adrenal insufficiency.

Treatment

Treatment measures should begin based on clinical suspicion alone, even before test results are obtained or the patient is unlikely to survive. Management includes volume resuscitation with at least 2 to 3 L of a 0.9% saline solution or 5% dextrose in saline solution. Blood should be obtained for electrolyte (decreased Na^+ and increased K^+), glucose (low), and cortisol (low) levels, ACTH (increased in primary and decreased in secondary), and quantitative eosinophilic count. Dexamethasone (4 mg) should be administered intravenously. Hydrocortisone (100 mg IV every 6 hours) may also be used, but it interferes with testing of cortisol levels. Once the patient has been stabilized, underlying conditions, such as infection, should be sought, identified, and treated. The ACTH stimulation test should be performed to confirm the diagnosis. Glucocorticoids can then be tapered to maintenance doses (oral hydrocortisone 15 to 20 mg in the morning and 10 mg in the evening). Mineralocorticoids (fludrocortisone 0.05 to 0.1 mg daily) may be required once the saline infusions are discontinued.

ADRENAL SURGERY

Choice of Procedure

Adrenalectomy may be performed via an open or laparoscopic approach. In either approach, the gland may be approached anteriorly, laterally, or posteriorly via the retroperitoneum. The choice of approach depends on the size and nature of the lesion and expertise of the surgeon. Laparoscopic adrenalectomy has rapidly become the standard procedure of choice for the excision of most benign-appearing adrenal lesions less than 6 cm in diameter. The role of laparoscopic adrenalectomy in the management of adrenocortical cancers is controversial. The data with respect to local tumor recurrence and intra-abdominal carcinomatosis from laparoscopic adrenalectomy for malignant adrenal tumors that were not appreciated as such, preoperatively or intraoperatively, are conflicting. Although laparoscopic adrenalectomy appears to be feasible and safe for solitary adrenal metastasis[99] (provided there is no local invasion and the tumor can be resected intact), open adrenalectomy is the safest option for suspected or known adrenocortical cancers and malignant pheochromocytomas. Technical considerations and institutional experience rather than absolute tumor size usually determine the size threshold for laparoscopic resection. Hand-assisted laparoscopic adrenalectomy may provide a bridge between laparoscopic adrenalectomy and conversion to an open procedure. There have been no randomized trials directly comparing open versus laparoscopic adrenalectomy. However, studies have shown that laparoscopic adrenalectomy is associated with decreased blood loss, postoperative pain and narcotic use, reduced length of hospital stay, and faster return to work.

Laparoscopic Adrenalectomy

The procedure is performed under general anesthesia. Arterial lines are used routinely and central lines are necessary in patients in whom massive fluid shifts are anticipated, for example, those with large, active pheochromocytomas. A nasogastric tube, Foley catheter, and sequential compression devices are recommended. Routine preoperative antibiotics are not needed, except in patients with Cushing's syndrome, who are more prone to perioperative infections.

The adrenals can be removed laparoscopically via a transabdominal (anterior or lateral) or retroperitoneal (lateral or posterior) approach. The anterior transabdominal approach offers the advantage of a conventional view of the abdominal cavity and allows a bilateral adrenalectomy to be performed without the necessity of repositioning the patient. The lateral approach is preferred by most laparoscopic surgeons and uses gravity to aid retraction of surrounding organs. Patients, however, need to be repositioned for a bilateral procedure.

Lateral Transabdominal Approach

The patient is placed in the lateral decubitus position and the operating table is flexed at the waist to open the space between the lower rib cage and the iliac crest. The surgeon and assistant both stand on the same side, facing the front of the patient. After pneumoperitoneum is created, four 10-mm trocars are placed between the mid-clavicular line medially and the anterior axillary line laterally, 1 to 2 fingerbreadths below the costal margin (Fig. 37-67). A 30-degree laparoscope is inserted through the second port.

For a right adrenalectomy, a fan retractor is inserted through the most medial port to retract the liver. An atraumatic grasper and an L-hook cautery are inserted via the two lateral ports for the dissection. The right triangular ligament is divided and the liver is rotated medially (Fig. 37-68A). Rarely, the hepatic flexure of the colon may need mobilization during a right adrenalectomy. The right kidney is identified visually and by palpation with an atraumatic grasper. The adrenal gland is identified on the superomedial aspect of the kidney. Gerota's fascia is incised with the hook cautery. Dissection of the adrenal is started superomedially and then proceeds inferiorly, dissecting around the adrenal in a clockwise manner. The peri-adrenal tissues are grasped or moved with a blunt grasper to facilitate circumferential dissection. Although early identification of the adrenal vein is helpful to facilitate mobilization and prevent injury, it can be dissected whenever it is safe to do so. The right adrenal vein is identified at its junction with the inferior vena cava, ligated with clips and divided using endoscopic scissors. There may be a second adrenal vein on the right. Generally, two clips are left on the vena cava side. Early ligation of the adrenal vein makes it easier to mobilize the gland, but may make subsequent dissection more difficult because of venous congestion. The arterial branches to the adrenal gland can be electrocoagulated, if small, or clipped and divided.

For a left adrenalectomy, the fan retractor is used to retract the spleen. The splenic flexure is mobilized early and the lateral attachments to the spleen and the tail of the pancreas are divided using the electrocautery (see Fig. 37-68B). Gravity allows the spleen and the pancreatic tail to fall medially. The remainder of the dissection proceeds similar to that described for the right adrenal. In addition to the adrenal vein, the inferior phrenic vein, which joins the left

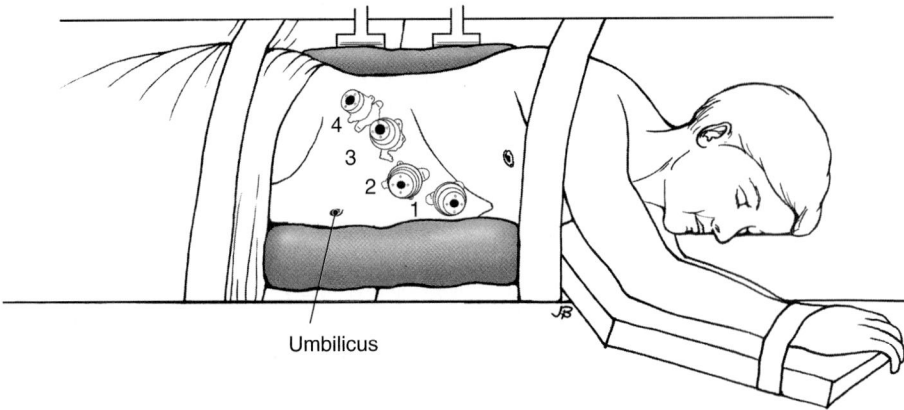

Umbilicus

FIG. 37-67. Positioning of the patient and placement of trocars for a laparoscopic adrenalectomy. Four trocars are placed from the mid-clavicular to the anterior axillary line.

adrenal vein medially, also needs to be dissected, doubly clipped, and divided. Once the dissection is complete, the area of the adrenal bed can be irrigated and suctioned. A drain is rarely necessary. The gland is placed in a nylon specimen bag, which is brought out via one of the ports after morcellation, if necessary.

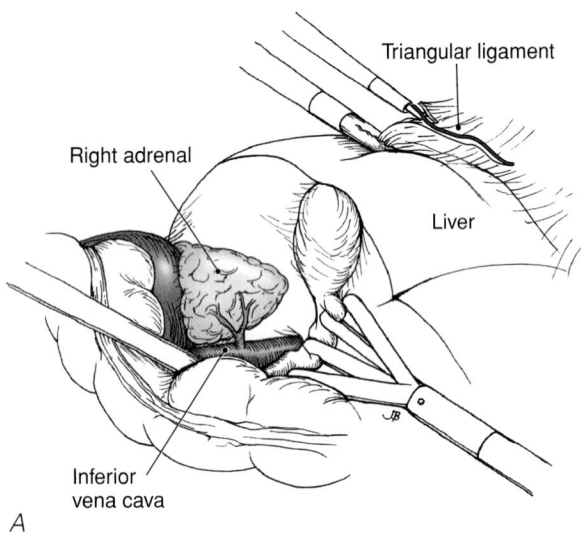

Triangular ligament

Right adrenal

Liver

Inferior vena cava

A

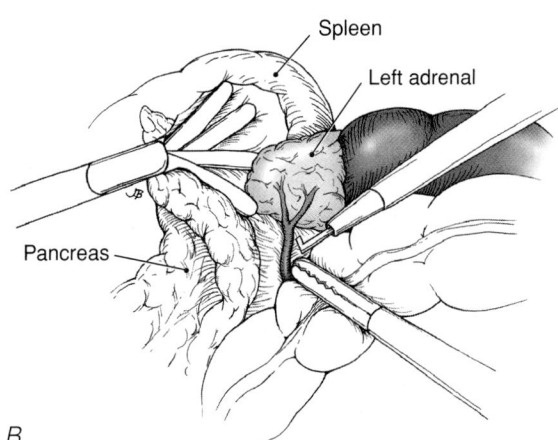

Spleen

Left adrenal

Pancreas

B

FIG. 37-68. Technique of laparoscopic adrenalectomy. Exposure of the right adrenal is facilitated by division of the triangular ligament (A) and dissection and reflection of the spleen and tail of the pancreas aids in identifying the left adrenal (B).

Posterior Retroperitoneal Approach

The retroperitoneal approach provides more direct access to the adrenal gland and avoids abdominal adhesions in patients who have had previous abdominal surgery. Furthermore, bilateral adrenalectomy can be performed without repositioning the patient. Intraoperative ultrasound is helpful for identifying the adrenal but the dissection and exposure is more difficult because the working space is limited. This makes vascular control difficult and also renders it unsuitable for large (>5 cm) lesions.

The patient is placed in the prone-jackknife position and the operating table is flexed at the waist to open the space between the posterior costal margin and the pelvis. Palpation is used to identify the position of the twelfth rib. Percutaneous ultrasound is performed to determine the outline of the underlying kidney and adrenal. When done laparoscopically, the surgeon stands on the side of the adrenal to be removed and the assistant stands on the opposite side. A 1.5-cm incision is placed 2 cm inferior and parallel to the twelfth rib, laterally at the level of the inferior pole of the kidney. Gerota's space is entered under direct vision by using a 12-mm direct-viewing trocar with a zero-degree laparoscope through the muscle layers of the posterior abdominal wall. Alternatively, blunt dissection with the surgeon's finger also can identify the space behind Gerota's fascia. The trocar is then replaced by a dissecting balloon, which is manually inflated using a hand pump under direct vision through the laparoscope. A 12-mm trocar is then reinserted into this space and carbon dioxide is insufflated to 12 to 15 mm Hg pressure. The zero-degree laparoscope is replaced by a 45-degree laparoscope. Two additional 5- or 10-mm trocars are placed, one each on either side of the first port. Laparoscopic ultrasound is then used to help locate the adrenal gland and vessels. The adrenal dissection is begun at the superior pole and then proceeds to the lateral and inferior aspect. The medial dissection is usually performed last and the vessels are identified and divided as described in the previous section.

Open Adrenalectomy

Open adrenalectomy may be performed via four approaches, each with specific advantages and disadvantages. The anterior approach allows examination of the abdominal cavity and resection of bilateral tumors via a single incision. The posterior approach avoids the morbidity of a laparotomy incision, especially in patients with cardiopulmonary disease and those prone to wound complications (Cushing's syndrome) and avoids abdominal adhesions in patients who have undergone previous abdominal surgery. Recovery time is also quicker and hospitalization shorter. However, the retroperitoneal exposure is difficult, particularly in obese patients and the small working space makes it unsuitable for tumors greater than 6 cm in diameter. The lateral approach is best for obese patients and for large tumors because it provides a bigger working space. The thoracoabdominal approach is most useful for en bloc resection of large (>10 cm), malignant lesions. However, it is associated with significant morbidity and should be used selectively.

Anterior Approach

The adrenals may be removed via a midline incision or bilateral subcostal incision (Fig. 37-69). The former allows adequate infraumbilical exposure for examination of extra-adrenal tumors, whereas the latter provides better superior and lateral exposure. For the right side, the hepatic flexure of the colon is mobilized inferiorly, the triangular ligament is incised to retract the liver, and a Kocher maneuver is used to mobilize the duodenum anteriorly and expose the adrenal gland and the inferior vena cava (Fig. 37-70A). Gerota's fascia is incised and the gland is freed of surrounding fibrofatty tissue. The lateral and superior surfaces are usually mobilized first. Then, the short, right adrenal vein is dissected, ligated, and divided, taking care not to injure the hepatic veins and inferior vena cava.

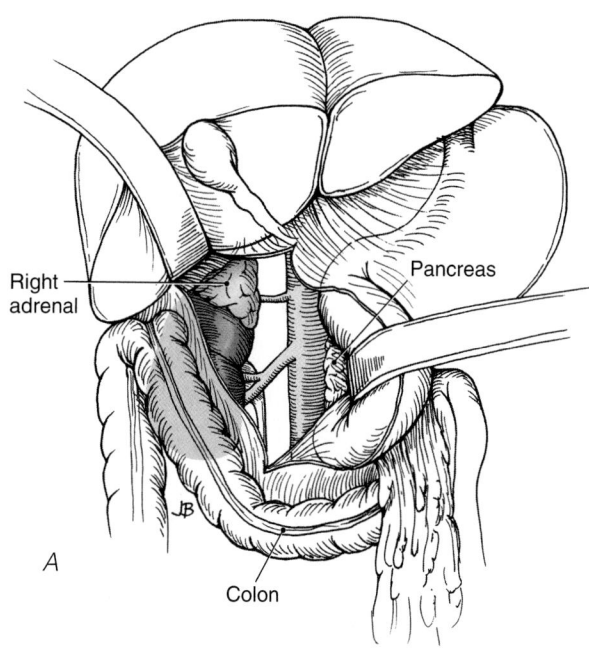

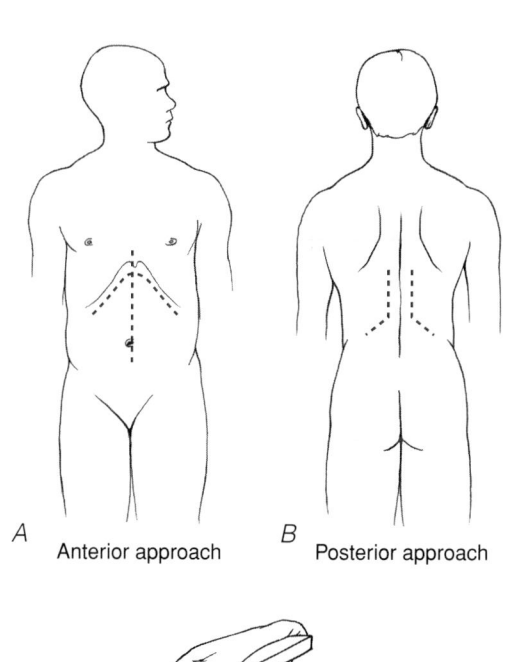

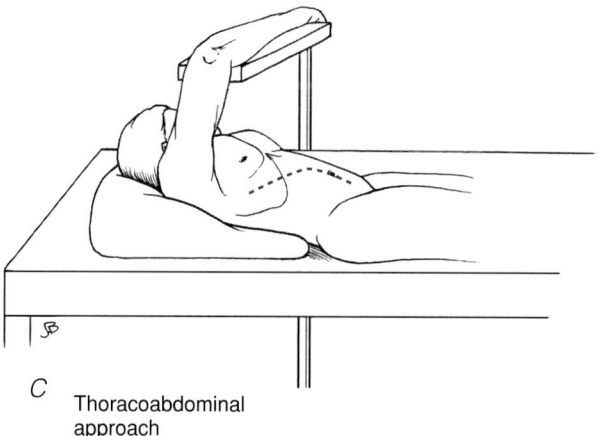

FIG. 37-69. *Incisions for open adrenalectomy: anterior approach (A), posterior approach (B), and thoracoabdominal approach (C).*

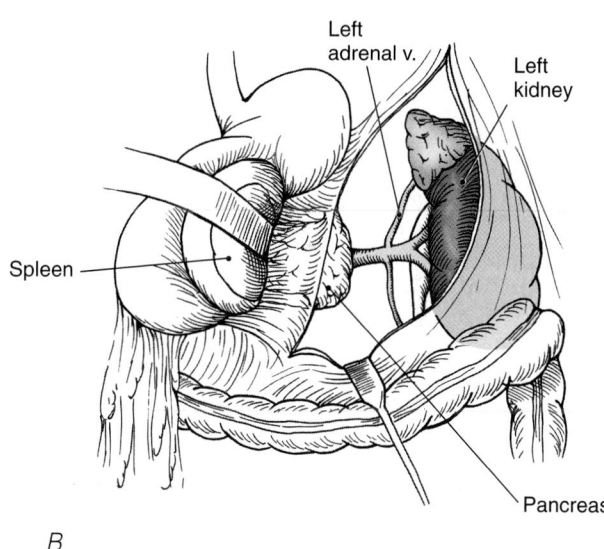

FIG. 37-70. Technique of open adrenalectomy: *A.* Exposure of the right adrenal is facilitated by a Kocher maneuver to mobilize the duodenum and upward retraction of the liver. *B.* The left adrenal can be exposed by medial visceral rotation of the spleen and pancreas.

On the left side, the adrenal is located cephalad to the pancreatic tail and just lateral to the aorta. For large tumors, the adrenal is best approached by medial visceral rotation to mobilize the spleen, colon, and pancreas toward the midline (see Fig. 37-70B). An alternative approach is to enter the lesser sac by division of the gastrocolic ligament. The pancreas is mobilized superiorly by incision of its inferior peritoneal attachments, thus exposing the left kidney and adrenal. The gland is then mobilized as on the right side.

Posterior Approach

The patient is placed prone on the operating table, similar to the laparoscopic approach. A hockey stick or curvilinear incision may be used, and extended through the latissimus dorsi and sacrospinous fascia. The twelfth rib is generally excised at its base and the eleventh rib is retracted superiorly to reveal the pleura and the lateral arcuate ligament of the liver on the right side. The pleura is also mobilized cephalad and the adrenal and kidney are identified. The superior aspect of the gland is dissected first, and the superior vessels are identified and ligated. This prevents superior retraction of the adrenal gland. The remainder of the gland is then dissected and the adrenal gland and tumor removed. The resulting space is generally filled with perinephric fat and closed in layers. If the pleura is entered, a red-rubber catheter may be placed in the chest and removed after a Valsalva maneuver, once the chest is closed. If structural lung injury has occurred, a chest tube is needed. After closure of the muscle layers, the patient is given positive pressure and the catheter is removed. A chest x-ray is obtained postoperatively to rule out a pneumothorax.

Lateral Approach

The patient is placed in a lateral position with the table flexed and an incision is made between the eleventh and twelfth ribs or subcostally. The dissection is then done as indicated previously.

Complications of Adrenal Surgery

General complications associated with laparoscopic adrenalectomy include wound and infection, urinary tract infections, and deep vein thrombosis. Patients with Cushing's syndrome are more prone to infectious (incisional and intra-abdominal abscess) and thrombotic complications. Specific complications arising from the creation of pneumoperitoneum include injury to various organs from Veress needle and trocar insertion, subcutaneous emphysema, pneumothorax, and hemodynamic compromise. Excessive retraction and dissection may lead to bleeding from injury to the inferior vena cava and renal vessels, or from injury to surrounding organs, such as the liver, pancreas, spleen, and stomach. Postoperative hemodynamic instability may be evident in patients with pheochromocytomas and patients are at risk of adrenal insufficiency after bilateral adrenalectomy and sometimes after unilateral adrenalectomy (unrecognized Cushing's syndrome or, very rarely, Conn's syndrome). Long-term morbidity results mainly from injury to nerve roots during trocar insertion, which can lead to chronic pain syndromes or muscle weakness, although this is more of an issue in case of open procedures.

Approximately 30% of patients who undergo bilateral adrenalectomy for Cushing's disease are at risk of developing Nelson's syndrome from progressive growth of the preexisting pituitary tumor. This leads to increased ACTH levels, hyperpigmentation, visual field defects, headaches, and extraocular muscle palsies. Transsphenoidal pituitary resection is the initial mode of therapy,[100] and external beam radiotherapy is used in patients with residual tumor or extrasellar invasion.

References

1. Dedivitis RA, Camargo DL, Peixoto GL, et al: Thyroglossal duct: A review of 55 cases. *J Am Coll Surg* 194:274, 2002.
2. Pisanu A, Pili S, Uccheddu A: Non-recurrent inferior laryngeal nerve. *Chir Ital* 54:7, 2002.
3. Cernea CR, Ferraz AR, Nishio S, et al: Surgical anatomy of the external branch of the superior laryngeal nerve. *Head Neck* 14:380, 1992.
4. Kopp P: Pendred's syndrome and genetic defects in thyroid hormone synthesis. *Rev Endocr Metab Disord* 1:109, 2000.
5. Yoshida A, Taniguchi S, Hisatome I, et al: Pendrin is an iodide-specific apical porter responsible for iodide efflux from thyroid cells. *J Clin Endocrinol Metab* 87:3356, 2002.
6. Bouknight AL: Thyroid physiology and thyroid function testing. *Otolaryngol Clin North Am* 36:9, 2003.
7. Khan N, Oriuchi N, Higuchi T, et al: PET in the follow-up of differentiated thyroid cancer. *Br J Radiol* 76:690, 2003.
8. Vaidya B, Oakes EJ, Imrie H, et al: CTLA4 gene and Graves' disease: Association of Graves' disease with the CTLA4 exon 1 and intron 1 polymorphisms, but not with the promoter polymorphism. *Clin Endocrinol (Oxf)* 58:732, 2003.
9. Streetman DD, Khanderia U: Diagnosis and treatment of Graves disease. *Ann Pharmacother* 37:1100, 2003.
10. Hagen F, Ouelette RP, Chapman EM: Comparison of high and low dosage levels of I-131 in the treatment of thyrotoxicosis. *N Engl J Med* 277:559, 1967.
11. Singer RB: Long-term comparative cancer mortality after use of radioiodine in the treatment of hyperthyroidism, a fully reported multicenter study. *J Insur Med* 33:138, 2001.
12. Cundiff JG, Portugal L, Sarne DH: Parathyroid adenoma after radioactive iodine therapy for multinodular goiter. *Am J Otolaryngol* 22:374, 2001.
13. Muller PE, Bein B, Robens E, et al: Thyroid surgery according to Enderlen-Hotz or Dunhill: A comparison of two surgical methods for the treatment of Graves' disease. *Int Surg* 86:112, 2001.
14. Krohn K, Paschke R: Somatic mutations in thyroid nodular disease. *Mol Genet Metab* 75:202, 2002.
15. Brook I: Microbiology and management of acute suppurative thyroiditis in children. *Int J Pediatr Otorhinolaryngol* 67:447, 2003.
16. Ando T, Davies TF: Clinical review 160: Postpartum autoimmune thyroid disease: The potential role of fetal microchimerism. *J Clin Endocrinol Metab* 88:2965, 2003.
17. Orgiazzi J, Madec AM, Ducottet X: The role of stimulating, function-blocking and growth-blocking anti-TSH receptor antibodies (TRAbs) in GD, Hashimoto's disease and in atrophic thyroiditis. *Ann Endocrinol (Paris)* 64:31, 2003.
18. Pasieka JL: Hashimoto's disease and thyroid lymphoma: Role of the surgeon. *World J Surg* 24:966, 2000.
19. Owen PJ, Lazarus JH: Subclinical hypothyroidism: The case for treatment. *Trends Endocrinol Metab* 14:257, 2003.
20. De M, Jaap A, Dempster J: Tamoxifen therapy in steroid-resistant Riedel's disease. *Scott Med J* 47:12, 2002.
21. Knudsen N, Laurberg P, Perrild H, et al: Risk factors for goiter and thyroid nodules. *Thyroid* 12:879, 2002.
22. Williams D: Cancer after nuclear fallout: Lessons from the Chernobyl accident. *Nat Rev Cancer* 2:543, 2002.
23. Hemminki K, Li X: Familial risk of cancer by site and histopathology. *Int J Cancer* 103:105, 2003.
24. Morgan JL, Serpell JW, Cheng MS: Fine-needle aspiration cytology of thyroid nodules: How useful is it? *Aust N Z J Surg* 73:480, 2003.
25. Segev DL, Umbricht C, Zeiger MA: Molecular pathogenesis of thyroid cancer. *Surg Oncol* 12:69, 2003.
26. Nikiforov YE: RET/PTC rearrangement in thyroid tumors. *Endocr Pathol* 13:3, 2002.
27. Cheung L, Messina M, Gill A, et al: Detection of the PAX8-PPAR gamma fusion oncogene in both follicular thyroid carcinomas and adenomas. *J Clin Endocrinol Metab* 88:354, 2003.
28. Hay ID, Grant CS, Taylor WF, et al: Ipsilateral lobectomy versus bilateral lobar resection in papillary thyroid carcinoma: A retrospective analysis of surgical outcome using a novel prognostic scoring system. *Surgery* 102:1088, 1987.
29. Cady B, Rossi R: An expanded view of risk-group definition in differentiated thyroid carcinoma. *Surgery* 104:947, 1988.
30. *AJCC Cancer Staging Manual*, 6th ed. New York: Springer-Verlag, 2002.
31. DeGroot LJ, Kaplan EL, McCormick M, et al: Natural history, treatment, and course of papillary thyroid carcinoma. *J Clin Endocrinol Metab* 71:414, 1990.
32. Kebebew E, Clark OH: Differentiated thyroid cancer: "Complete" rational approach. *World J Surg* 24:942, 2000.

33. Cady B, Sedgwick CE, Meissner WA, et al: Risk factor analysis in differentiated thyroid cancer. *Cancer* 43:810, 1979.

34. Mazzaferri EL, Jhiang SM: Long-term impact of initial surgical and medical therapy on papillary and follicular thyroid cancer. *Am J Med* 97:418, 1994.

35. Hay ID, Grant CS, Bergstralh EJ, et al: Unilateral total lobectomy: Is it sufficient surgical treatment for patients with AMES low-risk papillary thyroid carcinoma? *Surgery* 124:958, 1998.

36. Mazzaferri EL, Massoll N: Management of papillary and follicular (differentiated) thyroid cancer: New paradigms using recombinant human thyrotropin. *Endocr Relat Cancer* 9:227, 2002.

37. Sivanandan R, Soo KC: Pattern of cervical lymph node metastases from papillary carcinoma of the thyroid. *Br J Surg* 88:1241, 2001.

38. Haigh PI: Follicular thyroid carcinoma. *Curr Treat Options Oncol* 3:349, 2002.

39. Thompson LD, Wieneke JA, Paal E, et al: A clinicopathologic study of minimally invasive follicular carcinoma of the thyroid gland with a review of the English literature. *Cancer* 91:505, 2001.

40. Lopez-Penabad L, Chiu AC, Hoff AO, et al: Prognostic factors in patients with Hürthle cell neoplasms of the thyroid. *Cancer* 97:1186, 2003.

41. Mazzaferri EL, Robbins RJ, Spencer CA, et al: A consensus report of the role of serum thyroglobulin as a monitoring method for low-risk patients with papillary thyroid carcinoma. *J Clin Endocrinol Metab* 88:1433, 2003.

42. Kim TH, Yang DS, Jung KY, et al: Value of external irradiation for locally advanced papillary thyroid cancer. *Int J Radiat Oncol Biol Phys* 55:1006, 2003.

43. Clayman GL, el-Baradie TS: Medullary thyroid cancer. *Otolaryngol Clin North Am* 36:91, 2003.

44. Brandi ML, Gagel RF, Angeli A, et al: Guidelines for diagnosis and therapy of MEN type 1 and type 2. *J Clin Endocrinol Metab* 86:5658, 2001.

45. Pasieka JL: Anaplastic thyroid cancer. *Curr Opin Oncol* 15:78, 2003.

46. Giuffrida D, Ferrau F, Pappalardo A, et al: Metastasis to the thyroid gland: A case report and review of the literature. *J Endocrinol Invest* 26:560, 2003.

47. Hedayati N, McHenry CR: The clinical presentation and operative management of nodular and diffuse substernal thyroid disease. *Am Surg* 68:245, 2002.

48. Fewins J, Simpson CB, Miller FR: Complications of thyroid and parathyroid surgery. *Otolaryngol Clin North Am* 36:189, 2003.

49. Akerstrom G, Malmaeus J, Bergstrom R: Surgical anatomy of human parathyroid glands. *Surgery* 95:14, 1984.

50. Gilmour JR: The gross anatomy of the parathyroid glands. *J Pathol* 46:133, 1938.

51. Carling T: Molecular pathology of parathyroid tumors. *Trends Endocrinol Metab* 12:53, 2001.

52. Awad SS, Miskulin J, Thompson N: Parathyroid adenomas versus four-gland hyperplasia as the cause of primary hyperparathyroidism in patients with prolonged lithium therapy. *World J Surg* 27:486, 2003.

53. Skogseid B: Multiple endocrine neoplasia type 1. *Br J Surg* 90:383, 2003.

54. Arnold A, Shattuck TM, Mallya SM, et al: Molecular pathogenesis of primary hyperparathyroidism. *J Bone Miner Res* 17:N30, 2002.

55. Talpos GB, Bone HG 3rd, Kleerekoper M, et al: Randomized trial of parathyroidectomy in mild asymptomatic primary hyperparathyroidism: Patient description and effects on the SF-36 health survey. *Surgery* 128:1013, 2000.

56. Sheldon DG, Lee FT, Neil NJ, et al: Surgical treatment of hyperparathyroidism improves health-related quality of life. *Arch Surg* 137:1022, 2002.

57. Pasieka JL, Parsons LL, Demeure MJ, et al: Patient-based surgical outcome tool demonstrating alleviation of symptoms following parathyroidectomy in patients with primary hyperparathyroidism. *World J Surg* 26:942, 2002.

58. Nappi S, Saha H, Virtanen V, et al: Left ventricular structure and function in primary hyperparathyroidism before and after parathyroidectomy. *Cardiology* 93:229, 2000.

59. Vestergaard P, Mollerup CL, Frokjaer VG, et al: Cardiovascular events before and after surgery for primary hyperparathyroidism. *World J Surg* 27:216, 2003.

60. Wermers RA, Khosla S, Atkinson EJ, et al: Survival after the diagnosis of hyperparathyroidism: A population-based study. *Am J Med* 104:115, 1998.

61. Deftos LJ: Hypercalcemia in malignant and inflammatory diseases. *Endocrinol Metab Clin North Am* 31:141, 2002.

62. Scholz DA, Purnell DC: Asymptomatic primary hyperparathyroidism: 10-Year prospective study. *Mayo Clin Proc* 56:473, 1981.

63. Silverberg SJ, Shane E, Jacobs TP, et al: A 10-year prospective study of primary hyperparathyroidism with or without parathyroid surgery. *N Engl J Med* 341:1249, 1999.

64. Anonymous: Proceedings of the NIH Consensus Development Conference on diagnosis and management of asymptomatic primary hyperparathyroidism. Bethesda, Maryland, October 29–31, 1990. *J Bone Miner Res* 6:S1, 1991.

65. Bilezikian JP, Potts JT Jr., El-Hajj Fuleihan G, et al: Summary statement from a workshop on asymptomatic primary hyperparathyroidism: A perspective for the 21st century. *J Clin Endocrinol Metab* 87:5353, 2002.

66. Hedback G, Oden A: Increased risk of death from primary hyperparathyroidism—An update. *Eur J Clin Invest* 28:271, 1998.

67. Sosa JA, Udelsman R: Minimally invasive parathyroidectomy. *Surg Oncol* 12:125, 2003.

68. Fujii H, Kubo A: Sestamibi scintigraphy for the application of minimally invasive surgery of hyperfunctioning parathyroid lesions. *Biomed Pharmacother* 56:7s, 2002.

69. Banzo I, Pena FJ, Allende RH, et al: MIBI SPECT and radioguided surgery in the accurate location of a posterior mediastinal parathyroid adenoma. *Clin Nucl Med* 28:584, 2003.

70. Proctor MD, Sofferman RA: Intraoperative parathyroid hormone testing: What have we learned? *Laryngoscope* 113:706, 2003.

71. Udelsman R, Donovan PI, Sokoll LJ: One hundred consecutive minimally invasive parathyroid explorations. *Ann Surg* 232:331, 2000.

72. Perrier ND, Ituarte PH, Morita E, et al: Parathyroid surgery: Separating promise from reality. *J Clin Endocrinol Metab* 87:1024, 2002.

73. Perrier ND, Ituarte P, Kikuchi S, et al: Intraoperative parathyroid aspiration and parathyroid hormone assay as an alternative to frozen section for tissue identification. *World J Surg* 24:1319, 2000.

74. Lentsch EJ, Withrow KP, Ackermann D, et al: Parathyromatosis and recurrent hyperparathyroidism. *Arch Otolaryngol Head Neck Surg* 129:894, 2003.

75. Wells SA Jr., Debenedetti MK, Doherty GM: Recurrent or persistent hyperparathyroidism. *J Bone Miner Res* 17:N158, 2002.

76. Ziegler R: Hypercalcemic crisis. *J Am Soc Nephrol* 12:S3, 2001.

77. Llach F, Velasquez Forero F: Secondary hyperparathyroidism in chronic renal failure: Pathogenic and clinical aspects. *Am J Kidney Dis* 38:S20, 2001.

78. Chou FF, Lee CH, Shu K, et al: Improvement of sexual function in male patients after parathyroidectomy for secondary hyperparathyroidism. *J Am Coll Surg* 193:486, 2001.

79. Nichol PF, Starling JR, Mack E, et al: Long-term follow-up of patients with tertiary hyperparathyroidism treated by resection of a single or double adenoma. *Ann Surg* 235:673, 2002.

80. Marx SJ: Hyperparathyroid and hypoparathyroid disorders. *N Engl J Med* 343:1863, 2000.

81. Auchus RJ: Aldo is back: Recent advances and unresolved controversies in hyperaldosteronism. *Curr Opin Nephrol Hypertens* 12:153, 2003.

82. Jackson RV, Lafferty A, Torpy DJ, et al: New genetic insights in familial hyperaldosteronism. *Ann N Y Acad Sci* 970:77, 2002.

83. Stewart PM: Mineralocorticoid hypertension. *Lancet* 353:1341, 1999.

84. Espiner EA, Ross DG, Yandle TG, et al: Predicting surgically remedial primary aldosteronism: Role of adrenal scanning, posture testing, and adrenal vein sampling. *J Clin Endocrinol Metab* 88:3637, 2003.

85. Raff H, Findling JW: A physiologic approach to diagnosis of the Cushing syndrome. *Ann Intern Med* 138:980, 2003.

86. Putignano P, Toja P, Dubini A, et al: Midnight salivary cortisol versus urinary free and midnight serum cortisol as screening tests for Cushing's syndrome. *J Clin Endocrinol Metab* 88:4153, 2003.

87. Ng L, Libertino JM: Adrenocortical carcinoma: Diagnosis, evaluation and treatment. *J Urol* 169:5, 2003.

88. Copeland PM: The incidentally discovered adrenal mass. *Ann Intern Med* 98:940, 1983.

89. Baudin E, Pellegriti G, Bonnay M, et al: Impact of monitoring plasma 1,1-dichlorodiphenildichloroethane (*op'*-DDD) levels on the treatment of patients with adrenocortical carcinoma. *Cancer* 92:1385, 2001.

90. Gmyrek GA, New MI, Sosa RE, et al: Bilateral laparoscopic adrenalectomy as a treatment for classic congenital adrenal hyperplasia attributable to 21-hydroxylase deficiency. *Pediatrics* 109:E28, 2002.

91. Pederson LC, Lee JE: Pheochromocytoma. *Curr Treat Options Oncol* 4:329, 2003.

92. Lenders JW, Pacak K, Walther MM, et al: Biochemical diagnosis of pheochromocytoma: Which test is best? *JAMA* 287:1427, 2002.

93. Sackett WR, Bambach CP: Bilateral subtotal laparoscopic adrenalectomy for phaeochromocytoma. *Aust N Z J Surg* 73:664, 2003.

94. Kanauchi H, Wada N, Clark OH, et al: Apoptosis regulating genes, bcl-2 and bax, and human telomerase reverse transcriptase messenger RNA expression in adrenal tumors: Possible diagnostic and prognostic importance. *Surgery* 132:1021, 2002.

95. Brunt LM, Moley JF: Adrenal incidentaloma. *World J Surg* 25:905, 2001.

96. Reincke M: Subclinical Cushing's syndrome. *Endocrinol Metab Clin North Am* 29:43, 2000.

97. Libe R, Dall'Asta C, Barbetta L, et al: Long-term follow-up study of patients with adrenal incidentalomas. *Eur J Endocrinol* 147:489, 2002.

98. Arlt W, Allolio B: Adrenal insufficiency. *Lancet* 361:1881, 2003.

99. Kebebew E, Siperstein AE, Clark OH, et al: Results of laparoscopic adrenalectomy for suspected and unsuspected malignant adrenal neoplasms. *Arch Surg* 137:948, 2002.

100. Kelly PA, Samandouras G, Grossman AB, et al: Neurosurgical treatment of Nelson's syndrome. *J Clin Endocrinol Metab* 87:5465, 2002.

CHAPTER 38

Pediatric Surgery

David J. Hackam, Kurt Newman, and Henri R. Ford

INTRODUCTION

In his 1953 classic textbook titled *The Surgery of Infancy and Childhood,* Dr. Robert E. Gross summarized the essential challenge of pediatric surgery: "Those who daily operate upon adults, even with the greatest of skill, are sometimes appalled—or certainly are not at their best—when called upon to operate upon and care for a tiny patient. Something more than diminutive instruments or scaled-down operative manipulations are necessary to do the job in a suitable manner." To this day, surgical residents often approach the pediatric surgical patient with a mix of fear and anxiety. Nonetheless, they generally complete their pediatric surgical experience with a clear sense of the enormous ability of children to tolerate large operations, and with a true appreciation for the precision required in their care, both in the operating room and during the perioperative period. The specialty has evolved considerably in its ability to care for the smallest of patients with surgical disorders, so that in utero surgery is now an option in certain circumstances. Similarly, our understanding of the pathophysiology of the diseases that pediatric surgeons face has increased greatly to the point where our focus has shifted from an understanding of anatomy and physiology to an appreciation of the molecular or cellular pathways that regulate tissue growth and differentiation. There are few specialties in all of medicine that provide the opportunity to intervene in such a positive manner in such a wide array of diseases, and to receive the most heartfelt appreciation possible—that of a parent whose child's life has forever been improved.

GENERAL CONSIDERATIONS

Fluid and Electrolyte Balance

In managing the pediatric surgical patient, an understanding of fluid and electrolyte balance is critical, as the margin between dehydration and fluid overload is small. Several surgical diagnoses, such as gastroschisis or short-gut syndrome, are characterized by a predisposition to fluid loss. Others require judicious restoration of intravascular volume in order to prevent cardiac failure, as in patients with congenital diaphragmatic hernia and associated pulmonary hypertension. It is important to realize that the infant's physiologic day is approximately 8 hours in duration. A careful assessment of the individual patient's fluid balance tally—showing fluid intake and output fluid for the previous 8 hours—will prevent dehydration or fluid overload. Clinical signs of dehydration include tachycardia and reduced urine output as well as a depressed fontanelle, lethargy, and poor feeding. Fluid overload is often manifested by the onset of new oxygen requirements, respiratory distress, tachypnea, and tachycardia.

The infant is born with a surplus of body water, which is normally excreted by the end of the first week of life. At birth, fluid requirements are 65 mL/kg (750 mL/m^2) and increase to 100 mL/kg (1000 mL/m^2) by the end of the first week. Daily maintenance fluids for most children can be estimated using the formula: 100 mL/kg for the first 10 kg plus 50 mL/kg for 11 to 20 kg plus 25 mL/kg for each additional kilogram of body weight thereafter. Because intravenous fluid orders are written as milliliters per hour, this can be conveniently converted to 4 mL/kg per hour up to 10 kg by adding 2 mL/kg per hour for 11 to 20 kg, and 1 mL/kg per hour for each additional kilogram of body weight thereafter. For example, a 26-kg child has an estimated maintenance fluid requirement of $(10 \times 4)+(10 \times 2) + (6 \times 1) = 66$ mL/h in the absence of massive fluid losses or shock. Fluid for maintenance is generally provided as 5% dextrose in one quarter normal saline. For short-term intravenous therapy, the administration of 5 mEq/kg per day of sodium and 2 mEq/kg per day of potassium will satisfy the daily need. Fluid and electrolyte losses secondary to protracted vomiting or diarrhea are corrected by modifying this formula according to the measured losses. In infants the normal serum osmolarity is between 280 and 290 mmol/L. Newborns have the ability to concentrate their urine well by the fifth day of life; thus urine concentration as well as output must be considered when ordering intravenous fluids postoperatively. If the child has a significant ongoing fluid loss (e.g., from a nasogastric tube), it is best to properly replace that loss with IV fluids at least every 4 hours. A typical replacement formula is $D_5 \frac{1}{2}$ normal saline +20 mEq KCl/L. Whatever the formula used to calculate fluid replacement for the infant or small child, the optimal strategy is to analyze serum electrolytes and fluid losses and to replace the appropriate constituents precisely.

Acid-Base Equilibrium

Acute metabolic acidosis usually implies inadequate tissue perfusion, and is a serious disorder in children. Potentially life-threatening causes that are specific for the pediatric population must be sought, including intestinal ischemia from necrotizing enterocolitis (in the neonate), midgut volvulus, or incarcerated hernia. Other causes include chronic bicarbonate loss from the gastrointestinal tract or an acid accumulation as in chronic renal failure. Respiratory acidosis implies hypoventilation, the cause of which should be apparent. Treatment of acute metabolic acidosis should be aimed at restoring tissue perfusion by addressing the underlying abnormality first. For severe metabolic acidemia where the serum pH is less than 7.25, sodium bicarbonate should be administered using the following guideline: base deficit × weight in kilograms × 0.5 (in newborns). The last factor in the equation should be 0.4 for smaller children, and 0.3 for older children. The dose should be diluted to a concentration of 0.5 mEq/mL because full-strength sodium bicarbonate is hyperosmolar. One half the corrective dose is given, and the serum pH is measured again. During cardiopulmonary resuscitation (CPR), one half the corrective dose can be given as an intravenous bolus and the other half given slowly intravenously.

Respiratory alkalosis is usually caused by hyperventilation, which is readily correctable. Metabolic alkalosis most commonly implies gastric acid loss, as in the child with pyloric stenosis or overaggressive diuretic therapy. In the child with gastric fluid loss, IV fluids of 5% dextrose, 0.5% normal saline, and 20 mEq KCl/L usually correct the alkalosis.

Blood Volume and Blood Replacement

Criteria for blood transfusion in infants and children remain poorly defined. The decision to transfuse a critically-ill pediatric patient may depend on a number of clinical features that include the patient's age, primary diagnosis, the presence of ongoing bleeding, coagulopathy, hypoxia, hemodynamic compromise, lactic acidosis, and cyanotic heart disease, as well as overall severity of illness. A recent survey of transfusion practices among pediatric intensivists showed that the baseline hemoglobin levels that would prompt them to recommend a red blood cell (RBC) transfusion ranged from 7 to 13 g/dL. Patients with cyanotic heart disease are often transfused to higher hemoglobin values, although the threshold for transfusion in this population remains to be defined. To decrease the need for transfusion, other strategies have been considered. Studies in both critically-ill adults and neonates have shown that administration of erythropoietin decreases RBC transfusion requirements. In general terms, there is a trend toward an avoidance of the use of RBC products whenever possible, as current studies suggest that lower hemoglobin concentrations are well tolerated by many groups of patients, and that administration of RBCs may have unintended negative consequences.

A useful guideline for estimation of blood volume for the infant is 85 mL/kg of body weight. When packed red blood cells (PRBC) are utilized, the transfusion requirement is calculated as 10 mL/kg, which roughly is equivalent to a 500-mL transfusion for a 70-kg

adult. At the authors' institution, the following formula is used to determine the volume of blood in mL:

(target hematocrit − current hematocrit) × weight (kg) × 80/65

= blood volume

In the child, coagulation deficiencies may rapidly assume clinical significance after extensive blood transfusion. It is advisable to have fresh frozen plasma and platelets available if more than 30 mL/kg have been transfused. Plasma is given in a dose of 10 to 20 mL/kg, and platelets are given in a dose of 1 unit/5 kg. Each unit of platelets consists of 40 to 60 mL of fluid, and platelets can be spun down to a platelet "button" for infants who require restricted fluid administration. Following transfusion of PRBC to neonates, with tenuous fluid balance, a single dose of a diuretic (such as furosemide 1 mg/kg) may help to facilitate excretion of the extra fluid load.

Hyperalimentation and Nutrition

The nutritional requirements of the surgical neonate must be met in order for the child to grow and to heal surgical wounds. If inadequate protein and carbohydrate calories are given, the child may not only fail to recover from surgery, but may also exhibit growth failure and impaired development of the central nervous system. Neonates that are particularly predisposed to protein-calorie malnutrition include those with gastroschisis, intestinal atresia, or intestinal insufficiency from other causes such as necrotizing enterocolitis. The protein and caloric requirements for the surgical neonate are shown in Table 38-1.

Nutrition can be provided via either the enteral or parenteral routes. Whenever possible, the enteral route is preferred, because it not only promotes the growth and function of the gastrointestinal system, but also ensures that the infant learns how to feed. There are various enteral feeding preparations available, which are outlined in Table 38-2. The choice of formula is based upon the clinical state of the individual child. Pediatric surgeons are occasionally faced with situations in which oral feeding is not possible. This problem can be seen in the extremely premature infant who has not yet developed the feeding skills, or in the infant with concomitant craniofacial abnormalities that impair sucking. In these instances, enteral feeds can be administered using either a nasojejunal or a gastrostomy tube.

When the gastrointestinal tract cannot be used because of mechanical, ischemic, inflammatory, or functional disorders, parenteral alimentation must be given. When an extended period of parenteral nutrition is required, central venous catheters are placed. Peripheral intravenous alimentation can be given, utilizing less concentrated but greater volumes of solutions. To prevent the development of trace metal deficiencies, supplemental copper, zinc, and iron are provided to patients receiving long-term total parenteral nutritional (TPN) support.

Table 38-1
Nutritional Requirements for the Pediatric Surgical Patient

Age	Calories (kcal/kg per day)	Protein (g/kg per day)
0 to 6 months	100–120	2
6 months–1 year	100	1.5
1 year–3 years	100	1.2
4 years–6 years	90	1
7 years–10 years	70	1
11 years–14 years	55	1
15 years–18 years	45	1

Table 38-2
Formulas for Pediatric Surgical Neonates

Formula	kcal/mL	Protein (g/mL)	Fat (g/mL)	Carbohydrate (g/mL)
Human Milk	0.67	0.011	0.04	0.07
Milk Based				
Enfamil 20	0.67	0.015	0.038	0.069
Similac 20	0.67	0.015	0.036	0.072
Soy Based				
Prosobee	0.67	0.02	0.036	0.07
Isomil	0.67	0.018	0.037	0.068
Special				
Pregestimil	0.67	0.019	0.028	0.091
Alimentum	0.67	0.019	0.038	0.068
Preterm				
Enfamil Premature	0.80	0.024	0.041	0.089

A major complication of long-term TPN is the development of liver failure. This is characterized by cholestatic liver disease that eventually progresses to end-stage hepatic fibrosis. To prevent this major complication, concomitant enteral feedings must be instituted, and the gastrointestinal tract should be used as soon as possible. In instances in which proximal stomas are in place, continuity of the gastrointestinal tract should be restored as soon as possible. Where intestinal insufficiency is associated with dilation of the small intestine, tapering or intestinal lengthening procedures may be beneficial. Other strategies to minimize the development of TPN-related liver disease include avoidance of infection by meticulous catheter care, aggressive treatment of any infection, and early cycling of parenteral nutrition to include a period during the day when parenteral nutrition is not given.

Venous Access

Obtaining reliable vascular access in an infant or child is a major responsibility of the pediatric surgeon. The goal should always be to place the catheter in the least invasive, least risky, and least painful manner, and in a location that is most accessible and facilitates use of the catheter without complications for as long as needed. In infants, the general approach of these authors is to place a central venous catheter using a cutdown approach, either in the antecubital fossa, external jugular vein, facial vein, or proximal saphenous vein. If the internal jugular vein is used, placing a purse-string suture at the venotomy is recommended, if possible, to prevent venous occlusion. In infants over 2 kg and in older children, percutaneous access of the subclavian, internal jugular, or femoral veins is possible in most cases, and central access is achieved using the Seldinger technique. The catheters are tunneled to an exit site separate from the venotomy site. Regardless of whether the catheter is placed by a cutdown approach or percutaneously, a chest x-ray to confirm central location of the catheter tip and to exclude the presence of a pneumothorax or hemothorax is mandatory. When discussing the placement of central venous catheters with parents, it is important to note that the complication rate for central venous lines in children is high. The incidence of catheter-related sepsis or infection approaches 10% in many series. Superior or inferior vena caval occlusion is a significant risk, particularly in the smallest premature patients.

Thermoregulation

Careful regulation of the ambient environment of infants and children is crucial, as these patients are extremely thermolabile. Premature infants are particularly susceptible to changes in environmental

temperature. Because they are unable to shiver and lack stores of fat, their potential for thermogenesis is impaired. This is compounded by the administration of anesthetic and paralyzing agents. Since these patients lack adaptive mechanisms to cope with the environment, the environment must be regulated. Attention to heat conservation during transport of the infant to and from the operating room is essential. Transport units incorporating heating units are necessary for premature infants. In the operating room, the infant is kept warm by the use of overhead heating lamps, a heating blanket, warming of inspired gases, and coverage of the extremities and head with occlusive materials. During abdominal surgery, extreme care is taken to avoid wet and cold drapes. All fluids used to irrigate the chest or abdomen must be warmed to body temperature. Constant monitoring of the child's temperature is critical in a lengthy procedure, and the surgeon should continuously communicate with the anesthesiologist regarding the temperature of the patient. The development of hypothermia in infants and children can result in cardiac arrhythmias or coagulopathy. These potentially life-threatening complications can be avoided by careful attention to thermoregulation.

Pain Control

Despite previously held beliefs to the contrary, it has now been definitively established that neonates experience pain. Therefore, any procedure that is performed on a neonate must be accompanied by the provision of adequate analgesia. There is a range of pain management options that can improve the child's well being, as well as the parents' sense of comfort. The use of a pacifier, which may be dipped in sucrose, has been shown to decrease crying time and neonatal pain scores after minor procedures. For situations in which more pain is expected, intravenous narcotic agents should be used. Morphine and fentanyl have an acceptable safety margin and can be administered judiciously to neonates and children. A recent randomized trial of neonates on ventilators showed that the use of a morphine infusion decreased the incidence of intraventricular hemorrhage by 50%. Additional analgesic modalities include the use of topical anesthetic ointment (e.g., EMLA [eutectic mixture of local anesthetics] cream), and the use of regional anesthesia, such as caudal blocks for hernias, or epidural infusion for thoracic surgery. In the postoperative period, patient-controlled analgesia (PCA) is another excellent method of pain control. By ensuring that the pediatric surgical patient has adequate analgesia, the surgeon ensures that the patient receives the most humane and thorough treatment, and provides important reassurance to all other members of the health care team and to the family that pain control is a high priority.

NECK MASSES

The management of neck masses in children is determined by their location and the length of time that they have been present. Neck lesions are found either in the midline or lateral compartments. Midline masses include thyroglossal duct remnants, thyroid masses, thymic cysts, or dermoid cysts. Lateral lesions include branchial cleft remnants, cystic hygromas, vascular malformations, salivary gland tumors, torticollis, and lipoblastoma (a rare benign mesenchymal tumor of embryonal fat occurring in infants and young children). Enlarged lymph nodes and rare malignancies such as rhabdomyosarcoma can occur either in the midline or laterally.

Lymphadenopathy

The most common cause of a neck mass in a child is an enlarged lymph node, which typically can be found laterally or in the midline.

The patient is usually referred to the pediatric surgeon for evaluation after the mass has been present for several weeks. A detailed history and physical examination often helps determine the likely etiology of the lymph node, and the need for excisional biopsy. Enlarged tender lymph nodes are usually the result of a bacterial infection (*Staphylococcus* or *Streptococcus*). Treatment of the primary cause (e.g., otitis media or pharyngitis) with antibiotics often is all that is necessary. However, when the involved nodes become fluctuant, incision and drainage are indicated. More chronic forms of lymphadenitis, including infections with tuberculosis, atypical mycobacteria, as well as cat-scratch fever, are determined based on serologic findings and excisional biopsy. The lymphadenopathy associated with infectious mononucleosis can be diagnosed based on serology. When the neck nodes are firm and fixed, and others also are present in the axillae or groin, or the history suggests the presence of a hematologic malignancy, excisional biopsy is indicated. In these cases, a chest radiograph must be obtained to evaluate whether a mediastinal mass also is present. The presence of a large mediastinal mass should be identified preoperatively, as this may cause airway compression when muscle relaxants are administered. Under these cirumstances, tissue should be obtained under local anesthesia. The tissue is sent to pathology fresh for evaluation.

Thyroglossal Duct Remnants

Pathology and Clinical Manifestations

The thyroid gland buds off the foregut diverticulum at the base of the tongue in the region of the future foramen cecum at 3 weeks of embryonic life. As the fetal neck develops, the thyroid tissue becomes more anterior and caudad until it rests in its normal position. The "descent" of the thyroid is intimately connected with the development of the hyoid bone. Residual thyroid tissue left behind in the migration may persist and subsequently present in the midline of the neck as a thyroglossal duct cyst. The mass is most commonly appreciated in the 2- to 4-year-old child when the baby fat disappears and irregularities in the neck become more readily apparent. Usually the cyst is encountered in the midline at or below the level of the hyoid bone, and moves up and down with swallowing or with protrusion of the tongue. Occasionally it presents as an intrathyroidal mass. Most thyroglossal duct cysts are asymptomatic. If the duct retains its connection with the pharynx, infection may occur, and the resulting abscess will necessitate incision and drainage, occasionally resulting in a salivary fistula. Submental lymphadenopathy and midline dermoid cysts can be confused with a thyroglossal duct cyst. Rarely, midline ectopic thyroid tissue masquerades as a thyroglossal duct cyst, and may represent the patient's only thyroid tissue. Therefore, if there is any question regarding the diagnosis or if the thyroid gland cannot be palpated in its normal anatomic position, it is advisable to obtain a nuclear scan to confirm the presence of a normal thyroid gland. Although rarely the case in children, in adults the thyroglossal duct may contain thyroid tissue that can undergo malignant degeneration. The presence of malignancy in a thyroglossal cyst should be suspected when the cyst grows rapidly, or when the ultrasound demonstrates a complex anechoic pattern or the presence of calcification.

Treatment

If the cyst presents with an abscess, treatment should consist of drainage and antibiotics. Following resolution of the inflammation, resection of the cyst in continuity with the central portion of the hyoid bone and the tract connecting to the pharynx, in addition to ligation at the foramen cecum (the Sistrunk operation) is curative. Lesser operations result in unacceptably high recurrence rates, and

recurrence is more frequent following infection. According to a recent review, factors predictive of recurrence included more than two infections prior to surgery, age under 2 years, and inadequate initial operation.

Branchial Cleft Anomalies

Paired branchial clefts and arches develop early in the fourth gestational week. The first cleft and the first, second, third, and fourth pouches give rise to adult organs. The embryologic communication between the pharynx and the external surface may persist as a fistula. A fistula is seen most commonly with the second branchial cleft, which normally disappears, and extends from the anterior border of the sternocleidomastoid muscle superiorly, inward through the bifurcation of the carotid artery, and enters the posterolateral pharynx just below the tonsillar fossa. The branchial cleft remnants may contain small pieces of cartilage and cysts, but internal fistulas are rare. A second branchial cleft sinus is suspected when clear fluid is noted draining from the external opening of the tract at the anterior border of the lower third of the sternocleidomastoid muscle. Rarely, branchial cleft anomalies occur in association with biliary atresia and congenital cardiac anomalies, an association that is referred to as Goldenhar's complex.

Treatment

The treatment is surgical, and complete removal of the cyst and tract is necessary for cure. Dissection of the sinus tract is facilitated by passing a fine lacrimal duct probe through the external opening into the tract and utilizing it as a guide for dissection. Injection of a small amount of methylene blue dye into the tract also may be useful. A series of two or sometimes three small transverse incisions in a "stepladder" fashion is preferred to a long oblique incision in the neck, which is cosmetically undesirable. Branchial cleft cysts can present as abscesses. In these cases, initial treatment includes incision and drainage with a course of antibiotics to cover *Staphylococcus* and *Streptococcus* species, followed by excision of the cyst after the infection resolves.

Cystic Hygroma

Etiology and Pathology

Cystic hygroma (lymphangioma) occurs as a result of sequestration or obstruction of developing lymph vessels in approximately 1 in 12,000 births. Although the lesion can occur anywhere, the most common sites are in the posterior triangle of the neck, axilla, groin, and mediastinum. The cysts are lined by endothelium and filled with lymph. Occasionally unilocular cysts occur, but more often there are multiple cysts infiltrating the surrounding structures and distorting the local anatomy. A particularly troublesome variant of cystic hygroma is that which involves the tongue, floor of the mouth, and structures deep in the neck. Adjacent connective tissue may show extensive lymphocytic infiltration. The mass may be apparent at birth or may appear and enlarge rapidly in the early weeks or months of life as lymph accumulates; most present by age 2 years (Fig. 38-1A). Extension of the lesion into the axilla or mediastinum occurs about 10% of the time and can be demonstrated preoperatively by chest x-ray, ultrasound (US), or computed tomographic (CT) scan. Cystic hygromas occasionally contain nests of vascular tissue. These poorly supported vessels may bleed and produce rapid enlargement and discoloration of the hygroma. Infection within the cysts, usually caused by *Streptococcus* or *Staphylococcus,* may occur. In the neck this can cause rapid enlargement, which may result in airway compromise. Rarely, it may be necessary to carry out percutaneous aspiration of a cyst to relieve respiratory distress.

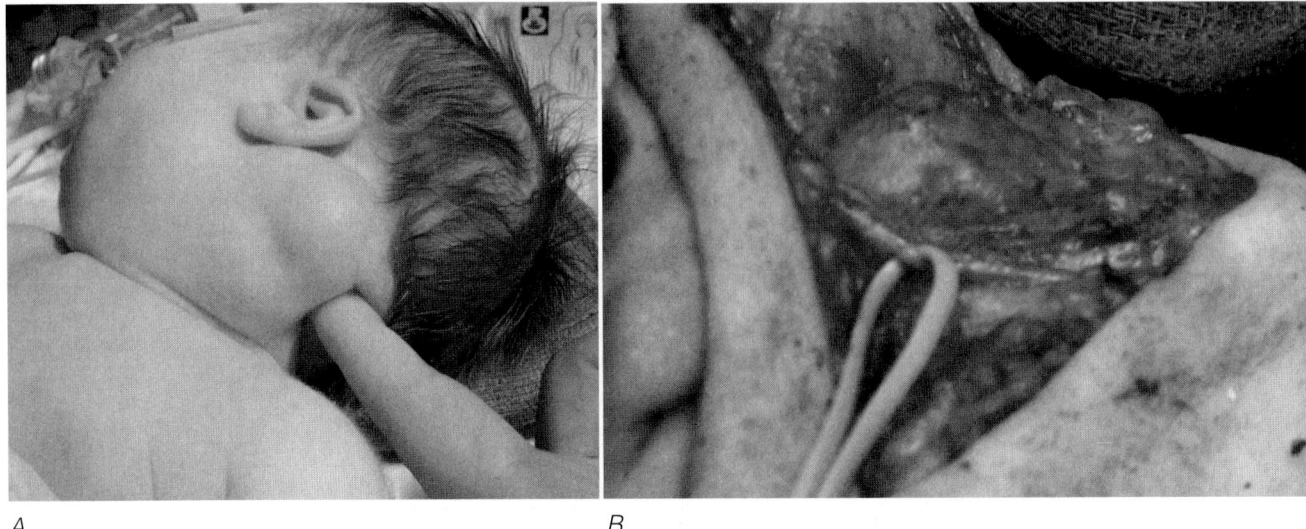

A   *B*

FIG. 38-1. *A.* Left cervical cystic hygroma in a 2-day-old baby. *B.* Intraoperative photograph showing a vessel loop around the spinal accessory nerve.

The diagnosis of cystic hygroma by prenatal US before 30 weeks' gestation has detected a "hidden mortality," as well as a high incidence of associated anomalies, including abnormal karyotypes and hydrops fetalis. Occasionally, very large lesions can cause obstruction of the fetal airway. Such obstruction can result in the development of polyhydramnios by impairing the ability of the fetus to swallow amniotic fluid. In these circumstances, the airway is usually markedly distorted, which can result in immediate airway obstruction unless the airway is secured at the time of delivery. Orotracheal intubation or urgent emergency tracheostomy while the infant remains attached to the placenta, the *ex utero intrapartum technique* (EXIT) procedure, may be necessary to secure the airway.

Treatment

Surgical excision is the treatment of choice for cystic hygromas. Total removal may not be possible because of the extent of the hygroma and its proximity to, and intimate relationship with, adjacent nerves, muscles, and blood vessels (see Fig. 38-1B). Radical ablative surgery is not indicated for this lesion. Conservative excision and unroofing of remaining cysts is advised, with repeated partial excision of residual hygroma if necessary, preserving all adjacent crucial structures. Postoperative wound drainage is important and is best accomplished by closed-suction technique. Fluid may accumulate beneath the surgically-created flaps in the area from which the hygroma was excised, requiring multiple needle aspirations. Injection of sclerosing agents (OK-432 or bleomycin) with favorable results has been reported. OK-432 is composed of a lyophilized mixture of group A *Streptococcus pyogenes,* and has been used in neonates without systemic toxicity. The use of these agents has not been widely adopted.

Torticollis

The presence of a lateral neck mass in infancy in association with rotation of the head toward the opposite side of the mass indicates the presence of congenital torticollis. This lesion results from fibrosis of the sternocleidomastoid muscle. The mass may be palpated in the affected muscle in approximately two-thirds of cases. Histologically, the lesion is characterized by the deposition of collagen

and fibroblasts around atrophied muscle cells. In the majority of cases, physical therapy is of benefit. Rarely surgical transection of the affected muscle can be curative, if needed.

RESPIRATORY SYSTEM

Congenital Diaphragmatic Hernia

Pathology

During formation of the diaphragm, the pleural and coelomic cavities remain in continuity by means of the pleuroperitoneal canal. The posterolateral communication is the last to be closed by the developing diaphragm. Failure of diaphragmatic development leaves a posterolateral defect known as a Bochdalek hernia. This anomaly is encountered more commonly on the left (80 to 90%). Incomplete development of the posterior diaphragm allows the abdominal viscera to fill the chest cavity. The abdominal cavity is small and underdeveloped and remains scaphoid after birth. Both lungs are hypoplastic, with decreased bronchial and pulmonary artery branching. Lung weight, lung volume, and deoxyribonucleic acid (DNA) content also are decreased, but these findings are more striking on the ipsilateral side. In many instances, evidence suggests that a paucity of surfactant is present, which compounds the degree of respiratory insufficiency. Amniocentesis with karyotyping may show chromosomal defects, especially trisomy 18 and 21. Associated anomalies, once thought to be uncommon, are identified in 40% of these infants, and most commonly involve the heart, brain, genitourinary system, craniofacial structures, or limbs.

Prenatal ultrasonography is successful in making the diagnosis of congenital diaphragmatic hernia (CDH) as early as 15 weeks' gestation. Ultrasound findings include herniated abdominal viscera, abnormal anatomy of the upper abdomen, and mediastinal shift away from the herniated viscera (Fig. 38-2). Accurate prenatal prediction of outcome for fetuses who have CDH is difficult. A useful index of severity for patients with left CDH is the lung-to-head ratio (LHR), which is the product of the length and the width of the right lung at the level of the cardiac atria divided by the head circumference (all measurements in millimeters). An LHR value of less than 1.0 is

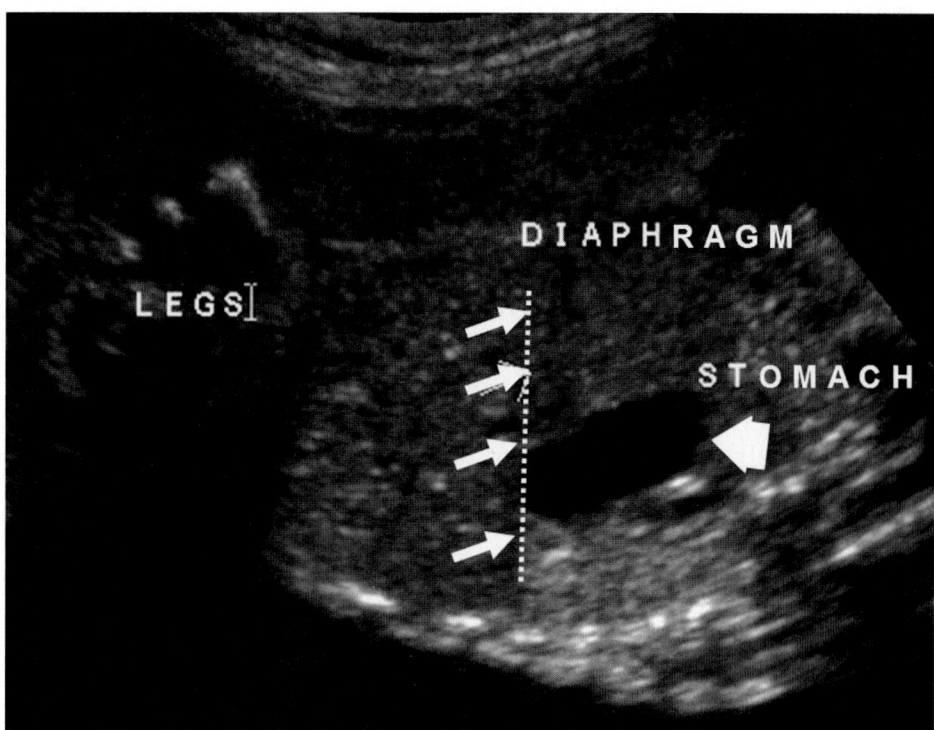

FIG. 38-2. Prenatal ultrasound of a fetus with a congenital diaphragmatic hernia. Arrows point to the location of the diaphragm. Arrowhead points to the stomach, which is in the thoracic cavity.

associated with a poor prognosis, whereas an LHR greater than 1.4 predicts a more favorable outcome.

Following delivery, the diagnosis of CDH is made by chest x-ray (CXR) (Fig. 38-3). The differential diagnosis includes congenital cystic adenomatoid malformation, in which the intrathoracic loops of bowel may be confused with multiple lung cysts. The vast majority of infants with CDH develop immediate respiratory distress, which is due to the combined effects of three factors. First, the air-filled bowel in the chest compresses the mobile mediastinum, which shifts to the opposite side of the chest, compromising air exchange in the contralateral lung. Second, pulmonary hypertension develops. This phenomenon results in persistent fetal circulation, with resultant decreased pulmonary perfusion and impaired gas exchange. Finally, the lung on the affected side is often markedly hypoplastic, such that it is essentially nonfunctional. Varying degrees of pulmonary hypoplasia on the opposite side may compound these effects. As a result, neonates with CDH are extremely sick, and the overall mortality in most series is approximately 60 to 70%.

Treatment

Many infants are symptomatic at birth due to hypoxia, hypercarbia, and metabolic acidosis. Prompt cardiorespiratory stabilization is mandatory. It is interesting that the first 24 to 48 hours after birth are often characterized by a period of relative stability, with high Pao_2 (partial pressure of arterial oxygen) levels and relatively good perfusion. This has been termed the "honeymoon period," and is often followed by progressive cardiorespiratory deterioration in the majority of patients. In the past, correction of the hernia was felt to be a surgical emergency, and these patients underwent surgery shortly after birth. It is now accepted that the presence of persistent pulmonary hypertension that results in right-to-left shunting across the open foramen ovale or the ductus arteriosus, and the degree of pulmonary hypoplasia, are the leading causes of cardiorespiratory insufficiency. Therefore, current management is directed toward

preventing or reversing the pulmonary hypertension, and minimizing barotrauma while optimizing oxygen delivery. To achieve this goal, infants are placed on mechanical ventilation using relatively low or "gentle" settings that prevent overinflation of the noninvolved lung. $Paco_2$ (partial arterial pressure of carbon dioxide) levels in the range of 50 to 60 mm Hg or higher are acceptable, as long as the pH remains 7.25 or greater. If these objectives cannot be achieved using conventional ventilation, high-frequency oscillatory ventilation (HFOV) may be employed to avoid the injurious effects of conventional tidal volume ventilation. Echocardiography is used to assess the degree of pulmonary hypertension and to identify the presence of a coexisting cardiac anomaly. To minimize the degree of pulmonary hypertension, inhaled nitric oxide may be used. In certain patients, this agent significantly improves pulmonary perfusion, as manifested by improved oxygenation. Nitric oxide is administered into the ventilation circuit, and is used in concentrations up to 40 parts per million. Correction of acidosis using bicarbonate solution may minimize the degree of pulmonary hypertension. As the degree of pulmonary hypertension becomes hemodynamically significant, right-sided heart failure develops and systemic perfusion is impaired. Administration of excess intravenous fluid will compound the degree of cardiac failure, and lead to marked peripheral edema. Inotropic support using epinephrine is therefore useful in optimizing cardiac contractility and maintaining mean arterial pressure.

Infants with CDH who remain severely hypoxic despite maximal ventilatory care may be candidates for treatment of their respiratory failure by extracorporeal membrane oxygenation (ECMO). Venovenous or venoarterial bypass is used. Venovenous bypass is established with a single cannula through the internal jugular vein, with blood removed from and infused into the right atrium by separate ports. Venoarterial bypass is used preferentially by some centers because it provides the cardiac support that is often needed. The right atrium is cannulated by means of the internal jugular vein and the aortic arch through the right common carotid artery. As much

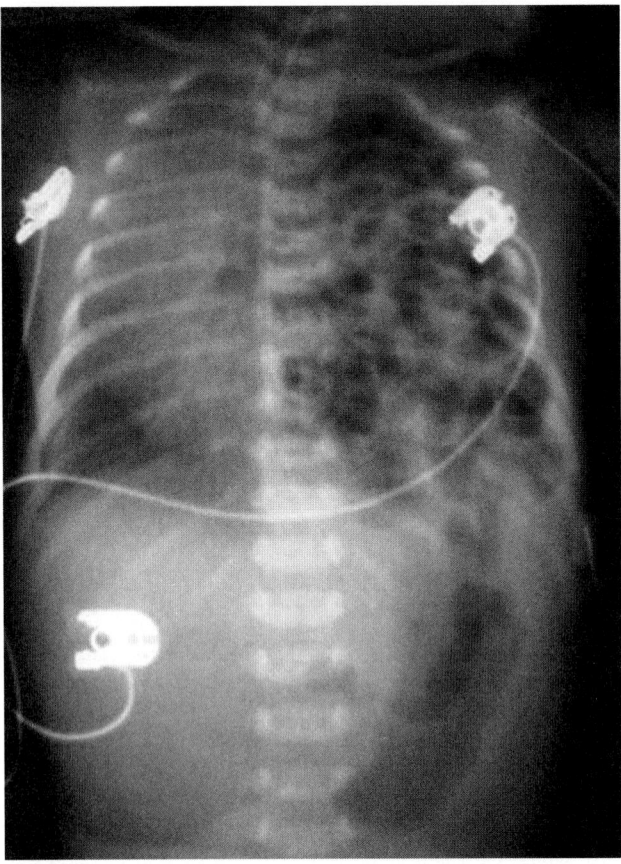

FIG. 38-3. Chest x-ray showing a left congenital diaphragmatic hernia.

of the cardiac output is shunted through the membrane oxygenator as needed to provide oxygenated blood to the infant and remove carbon dioxide. The infant is maintained on bypass until the pulmonary hypertension is reversed and lung function, as measured by compliance, is improved. This is usually seen within 7 to 10 days, but in some infants it may take up to 3 weeks to occur. The use of ECMO is associated with significant risk and because patients require systemic anticoagulation, bleeding complications are the most significant. They may occur intracranially or at the site of cannula insertion, and can be life threatening. Systemic sepsis is a significant problem, and may necessitate decannulation. Criteria for placing infants on ECMO include the presence of normal cardiac anatomy by echocardiography, the absence of fatal chromosome anomalies, and the expectation that the infant would die without ECMO. Traditionally, a threshold of weight greater than 2.5 kg and gestational age greater than 34 weeks has been used to select patients for ECMO, although success has been achieved at weights as low as 1.8 kg. It is important to emphasize that although ECMO may salvage a population of neonates with refractory pulmonary hypertension, the use of this technique remains controversial. A strategy that does not involve the use of ECMO, but instead emphasizes the use of permissive hypercapnia and the avoidance of barotrauma, may provide equal overall outcome in patients with CDH. This likely reflects the fact that mortality is related to the degree of pulmonary hypoplasia and the presence of congenital anomalies, neither of which are correctable by ECMO.

The timing of diaphragm repair is controversial. In patients that are not placed on ECMO, most surgeons perform repair once the hemodynamic status has been optimized. In neonates that are on bypass, some surgeons perform early repair on bypass; others wait until the infant's lungs are fully recovered, repair the diaphragm, and discontinue bypass within hours of surgery. Still others repair the diaphragm only after the infant is off bypass. Operative repair of the diaphragmatic hernia is best accomplished by an abdominal approach. Through a subcostal incision, the abdominal viscera are withdrawn from the chest, exposing the defect in the diaphragm. Care must be taken when reducing the spleen and liver, as bleeding from these structures can be fatal. The anterior margin is often apparent, while the posterior muscular rim is attenuated. If the infant is heparinized on bypass, minimal dissection of the muscular margins is performed. Electrocautery is used liberally to minimize postoperative bleeding. Most infants who require ECMO support prior to hernia repair have large defects, often lacking the medial and posterior margins. Prior to the availability of ECMO therapy, most of these infants died. About three fourths of infants repaired on bypass require prosthetic material to patch the defect, suturing it to the diaphragmatic remnant or around ribs or costal cartilages for large defects. If there is adequate muscle for closure, a single layer of nonabsorbable horizontal mattress suture is used to close the defect. Just before the repair is complete, a chest tube may be positioned in the thoracic cavity. We tend to reserve the use of chest tubes for patients who are repaired on ECMO, as these patients are at risk for developing a hemothorax, which can significantly impair ventilation. Anatomic closure of the abdominal wall may be impossible after reduction of the viscera. Occasionally a prosthetic patch of GoreTex or Surgisis may be sutured to the fascia and facilitate closure. The patch can be removed at a later time and the ventral hernia can be closed at that time or subsequently.

If the diaphragm has been repaired on ECMO, weaning and decannulation are accomplished as soon as possible. All infants are ventilated postoperatively to maintain preductal arterial oxygenation of 80 to 100 mm Hg. Very slow weaning from the ventilator is necessary to avoid recurrent pulmonary hypertension. Oscillation ventilation may be switched to conventional ventilation as part of the process of weaning.

Congenital Lobar Emphysema

Congenital lobar emphysema (CLE) is a condition manifested during the first few months of life as a progressive hyperexpansion of one or more lobes of the lung. It can be life threatening in the newborn period, but in the older infant it causes less respiratory distress. Air entering during inspiration is trapped in the lobe; on expiration, the lobe cannot deflate and progressively overexpands, causing atelectasis of the adjacent lobe or lobes. This hyperexpansion eventually shifts the mediastinum to the opposite side and compromises the other lung. CLE usually occurs in the upper lobes of the lung (left greater than right), followed next in frequency by the right middle lobe, but it also can occur in the lower lobes. It is caused by intrinsic bronchial obstruction from poor bronchial cartilage development or extrinsic compression. Approximately 14% of children with this condition have cardiac defects, with an enlarged left atrium or a major vessel causing compression of the ipsilateral bronchus.

Symptoms range from mild respiratory distress to full-fledged respiratory failure, with tachypnea, dyspnea, cough, and late cyanosis. These symptoms may be stable or they may progress rapidly or result in recurrent pneumonia. Occasionally, infants with CLE present with failure to thrive, which likely reflects the increased work associated with the overexpanded lung. Diagnosis is made by chest x-ray, which shows a hyperlucent affected lobe with adjacent

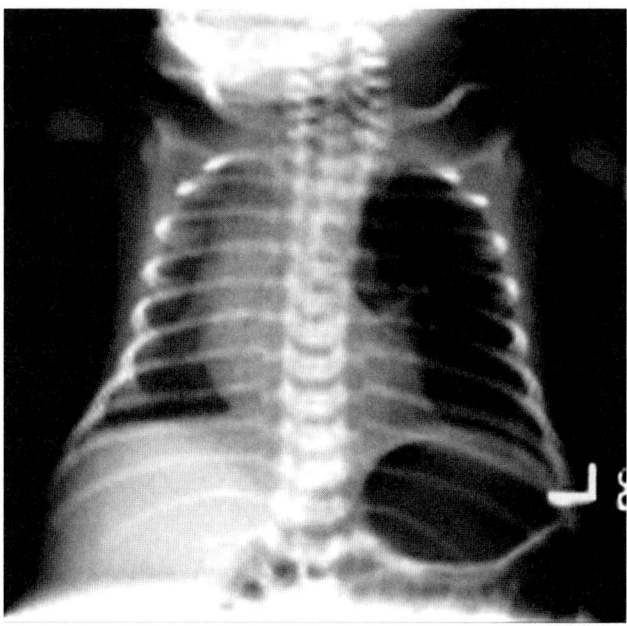

FIG. 38-4. Congenital lobar emphysema of the left upper lobe in a 2-week-old boy. Mediastinal shift is present.

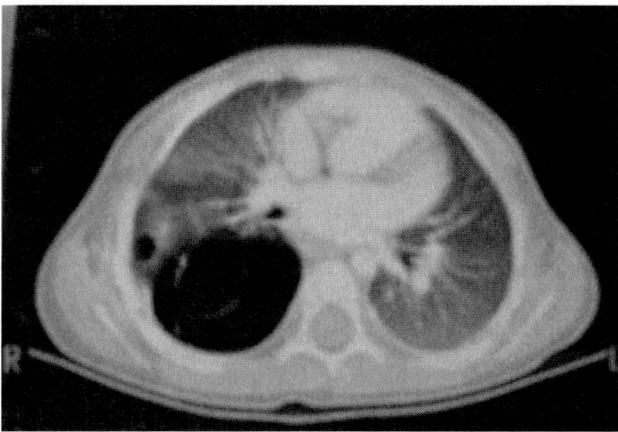

FIG. 38-5. CT scan of the chest showing a congenital cystic adenomatoid malformation of the left lower lobe.

lobar compression and atelectasis with varying degrees of shift of the mediastinum to the opposite side and compression of the contralateral lung (Fig. 38-4). If definitive diagnosis is unclear by chest x-ray, CT scan may be helpful. Unless foreign body or mucus plugging is suspected as a cause of hyperinflation, bronchoscopy is not advisable because it can produce more air trapping and cause life-threatening respiratory distress in a stable infant. Treatment is resection of the affected lobe. Unless symptoms necessitate earlier surgery, resection can usually be performed after the infant is several months of age. The prognosis is excellent.

Congenital Cystic Adenomatoid Malformation

This malformation consists of cystic proliferation of the terminal airway, producing cysts lined by mucus-producing respiratory epithelium, and elastic tissue in the cyst walls without cartilage formation. There may be a single cyst with a wall of connective tissue containing smooth muscle. Cysts may be large and multiple (type I), smaller and more numerous (type II), or they may resemble fetal lung without macroscopic cysts (type III). Most congenital cystic adenomatoid malformation (CCAM) occurs in the left lower lobe. However, this lesion can occur in any lobe and may occur in both lungs simultaneously. In the left lower lobe, type I may be confused at birth with a congenital diaphragmatic hernia. Clinical symptoms may range from none at all to severe respiratory failure at birth. The cyst(s), whether single or multiple, can produce air trapping and may be confused with congenital lobar emphysema pneumatoceles or even pulmonary sequestrations. They also can be involved with repeated infections and produce fever and cough in older infants and children. The diagnosis often can be made by CXR. In certain cases US or CT scan may be definitive (Fig. 38-5). Prenatal US may suggest the diagnosis. In the newborn period, US may also be useful, especially to distinguish between CCAM and congenital diaphragmatic hernia. Resection is curative and may need to be performed urgently in the infant with severe respiratory distress. Lobectomy is usually required (Fig. 38-6). Prognosis is excellent.

Pulmonary Sequestration

Pulmonary sequestration is uncommon and consists of a mass of lung tissue, usually in the left lower chest, occurring without the usual connections to the pulmonary artery or tracheobronchial tree, yet with a systemic blood supply from the aorta. There are two kinds of sequestration. Extralobar sequestration is usually a small area of nonaerated lung separated from the main lung mass, with a systemic blood supply, that is located immediately above the left diaphragm. It is commonly found in cases of congenital diaphragmatic hernia. Intralobar sequestration more commonly occurs within the parenchyma of the left lower lobe, but can occur on the right. There is no major connection to the tracheobronchial tree, but a secondary connection may be established, perhaps through infection or via adjacent intrapulmonary shunts. The blood supply is systemic from the aorta, is often multiple vessels, and frequently originates below the diaphragm (Fig. 38-7). Venous drainage of both types can be systemic or pulmonary. The cause of sequestration is unknown, but most probably involves an abnormal budding of the developing lung that picks up a systemic blood supply and never becomes connected with the bronchus or pulmonary vessels. Extralobar sequestration is asymptomatic and is usually discovered incidentally on CXR. If the

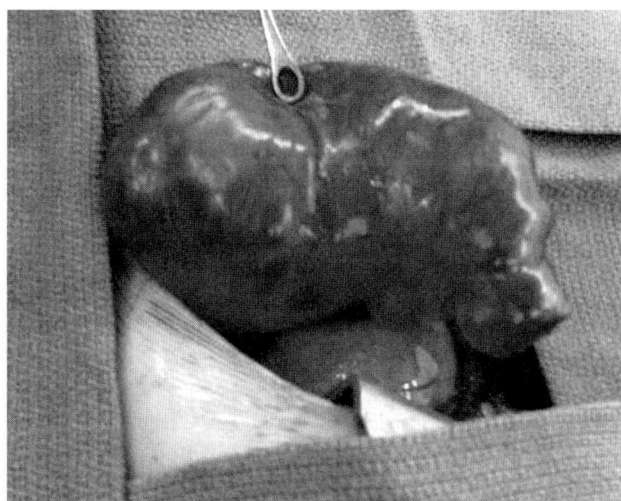

FIG. 38-6. Intraoperative photograph showing the left lower lobe congenital cystic adenomatoid malformation seen in Fig. 38-5.

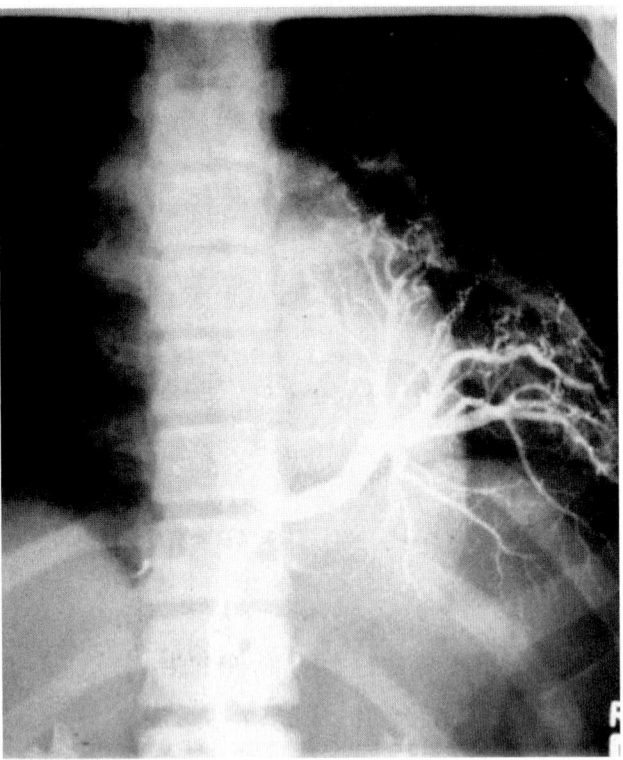

FIG. 38-7. Arteriogram showing large systemic artery supply to intralobar sequestration of the left lower lobe.

diagnosis can be confirmed (e.g., by CT scan), resection is not necessary. Diagnosis of intralobar sequestration, on the other hand, is usually made after repeated infections manifested by cough, fever, and consolidation in the posterior basal segment of the left lower lobe. Increasingly the diagnosis is being made in the early months of life by US, and color Doppler often can be helpful in delineating the systemic arterial supply. Removal of the entire left lower lobe is usually necessary since the diagnosis often is made late after multiple infections. Occasionally the sequestered part of the lung can be removed segmentally. Prognosis is excellent.

Bronchogenic Cyst

Bronchogenic cysts can occur anywhere along the respiratory tract from the neck to the lung parenchyma. They can present at any age. Histologically, they are hamartomatous, and usually consist of a single cyst lined with respiratory epithelium containing cartilage and smooth muscle. They are probably embryonic rests of foregut origin that have been pinched off from the main portion of the developing tracheobronchial tree, and are closely associated in causation with other foregut duplication cysts arising from the esophagus. Bronchogenic cysts may be seen on prenatal US, but are discovered most often incidentally on postnatal CXR. Although they may be completely asymptomatic, bronchogenic cysts may produce symptoms, depending on their anatomic location. In the paratracheal region of the neck they can produce airway compression and respiratory distress. In the lung parenchyma, they may become infected and present with fever and cough. In addition they may cause obstruction of the bronchial lumen with distal atelectasis and infection. They may also cause mediastinal compression. Rarely, rupture of the cyst can occur. CXR usually shows a dense mass, and CT scan or magnetic resonance imaging (MRI) delineates the precise anatomic

location of the lesion. Treatment consists of resection of the cyst, which may need to be undertaken in emergency circumstances for airway or cardiac compression. Resection can be performed either as an open procedure or using a thoracoscopic approach.

Bronchiectasis

Bronchiectasis is an abnormal and irreversible dilatation of the bronchi and bronchioles associated with chronic suppurative disease of the airways. These children usually will have an underlying congenital pulmonary anomaly, cystic fibrosis, or immunologic deficiency. Bronchiectasis also can result from chronic infection secondary to a neglected bronchial foreign body. The symptoms include a chronic cough, often productive of purulent secretions, recurrent pulmonary infection, and hemoptysis. The diagnosis is suggested by a CXR that shows increased bronchovascular markings in the affected lobe. Chest CT delineates bronchiectasis with excellent resolution. The preferred treatment for bronchiectasis is medical, consisting of antibiotics, postural drainage, and bronchodilator therapy, since many children with the disease show signs of airflow obstruction and bronchial hyperresponsiveness. Lobectomy or segmental resection is indicated for localized disease that has not responded appropriately to medical therapy. In severe cases, lung transplantation may be required to replace the terminally-damaged, septic lung.

Foreign Bodies

The inherent curiosity of children, and their innate propensity to place new objects into their mouths to fully explore them, places them at great risk for aspiration. Aspirated objects can be found either in the airway or in the esophagus, and in both cases the results can be life threatening.

Airway Ingestion

Aspiration of foreign bodies most commonly occurs in toddlers. Peanuts are the most common object that is aspirated, although other materials (e.g., popcorn) may also be involved. A solid foreign body often will cause air trapping, with hyperlucency of the affected lobe or lung seen especially on expiration. Oil from a peanut is irritating and may cause pneumonia. Delay in diagnosis can lead to atelectasis and infection. The most common anatomic location for a foreign body is the right main stem bronchus or the right lower lobe. The child usually will cough or choke while eating, but may then become asymptomatic. Total respiratory obstruction with tracheal foreign body may occur; however, respiratory distress is usually mild if present. A unilateral wheeze is often heard on auscultation. This wheeze often leads to an inappropriate diagnosis of asthma, and may delay the correct diagnosis for some time. CXR will show a radiopaque foreign body, but in the case of nuts, seeds, or plastic toy parts, the only clue may be nondeflation of the affected lobe on an expiratory film or fluoroscopy. Bronchoscopy confirms the diagnosis and allows removal of the foreign body. It can be a simple procedure or it may be extremely difficult, especially with a smooth foreign body that cannot be grasped easily, or one that has been retained for some time. The rigid bronchoscope should be used in all cases, and utilization of the optical forceps facilitates grasping the inhaled object. Epinephrine may be injected into the mucosa when the object has been present for a long period of time, which minimizes bleeding. Bronchiectasis may be seen as an extremely late phenomenon after repeated infections of the poorly aerated lung, and may require partial or total resection of the affected lobe.

Esophagus Ingestion

The most common foreign body found in the esophagus is a coin, followed by small toy parts. Toddlers are most commonly affected. The coin is retained in the esophagus at one of three locations: the cricopharyngeus, the area of the aortic arch, or the gastroesophageal junction; all areas of normal anatomic narrowing. Symptoms are variable depending on the anatomic position of the foreign body and the degree of obstruction. There is often a relatively asymptomatic period after ingestion. The initial symptoms are gastrointestinal and include dysphagia, drooling, and vomiting. The longer the foreign body remains in the esophagus, the greater the incidence of respiratory symptoms, which include cough, stridor, and wheezing. These findings may be interpreted as signs of upper respiratory infections. Objects that are present for a long period of time—particularly in children who have underlying neurologic impairment—may manifest as chronic dysphagia. The CXR is diagnostic in the case of a coin. A contrast swallow may be required for nonradiopaque foreign bodies. Coins lodged within the upper esophagus for less than 24 hours may be removed using Magill forceps. For all other situations, the treatment is by esophagoscopy, rigid or flexible, and removal of the foreign body. In the case of sharp foreign bodies such as open safety pins, extreme care is required on extraction to avoid injury to the esophagus. Rarely, esophagotomy is required for removal, particularly of sharp objects. Diligent follow-up is required after removal of foreign bodies, especially batteries, which can cause strictures, and sharp objects, which can injure the underlying esophagus.

ESOPHAGUS

Esophageal Atresia and Tracheoesophageal Fistula

Esophageal atresia (EA) and tracheoesophageal fistula (TEF) are among the most gratifying pediatric surgical conditions to treat. In the distant past, nearly all infants born with EA or TEF died. In 1939 Ladd and Leven achieved the first successful repair by ligating the fistula, placing a gastrostomy, and reconstructing the esophagus at a later time. Subsequently, Dr. Cameron Haight in Ann Arbor, Michigan, performed the first successful primary anastomosis for esophageal atresia, which remains the current approach for treatment of this condition. Despite the facts that there are several common varieties of this anomaly, and the underlying cause remains obscure, a careful approach consisting of meticulous perioperative care and attention to the technical detail of the operation can result in an excellent prognosis in most cases.

Anatomic Varieties

The five major varieties of EA and TEF are shown in Fig. 38-8. The most commonly seen variety is EA with distal TEF (type C), which occurs in approximately 75–85% of the cases in most series. The next most frequent is pure EA (type A), occurring in 8 to 10% of patients, followed by TEF without EA (type E). This occurs in 5–8% of cases, and also is referred to as an H-type fistula, based on the anatomic similarity to that letter (Fig. 38-9). EA with fistula between both proximal and distal ends of the esophagus and trachea (type D) is seen in approximately 1–2% of cases, and type B, EA with TEF between proximal segments of esophagus and trachea, is seen in approximately 1% of all cases.

Etiology and Pathologic Presentation

The esophagus and trachea share a common embryologic origin. They typically divide into separate tubes by approximately the thirty-sixth day of gestation. Failure of this occurrence can result in the spectrum of anomalies seen in Fig. 38-8. Recent studies have shed light on some of the molecular mechanisms underlying this condition. Mice deficient in the Sonic-hedgehog signaling pathway develop a phenotype that includes esophageal atresia-tracheoesophageal fistula (EA-TEF), suggesting a role for this molecule in the pathogenesis of the anomaly in humans. In support of this theory, Sonic-hedgehog transcripts were absent in human esophageal samples obtained from infants with TEF. Similarly,

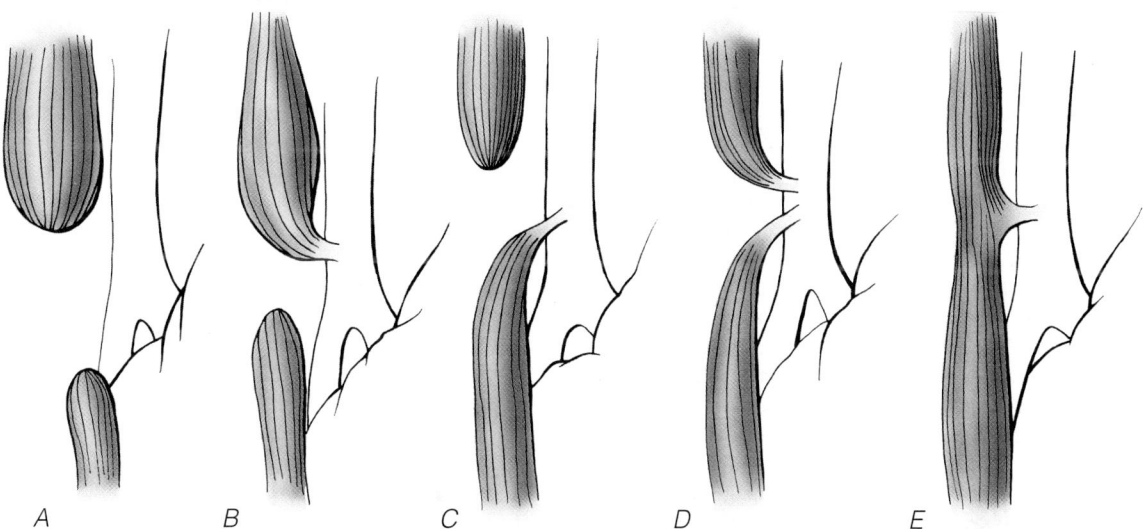

FIG. 38-8. The five varieties of esophageal atresia and tracheoesophageal fistula. *A.* Isolated esophageal atresia. *B.* Esophageal atresia with tracheoesophageal fistula between proximal segments of esophagus and trachea. *C.* Esophageal atresia with tracheoesophageal fistula between distal esophagus and trachea. *D.* Esophageal atresia with fistula between both proximal and distal ends of esophagus and trachea. *E.* Tracheoesophageal fistula without esophageal atresia (H-type fistula).

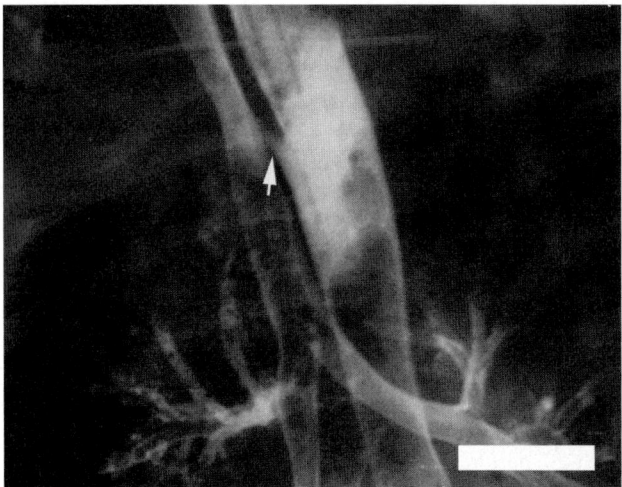

FIG. 38-9. Barium esophagram showing H-type tracheoesophageal fistula (*arrow*).

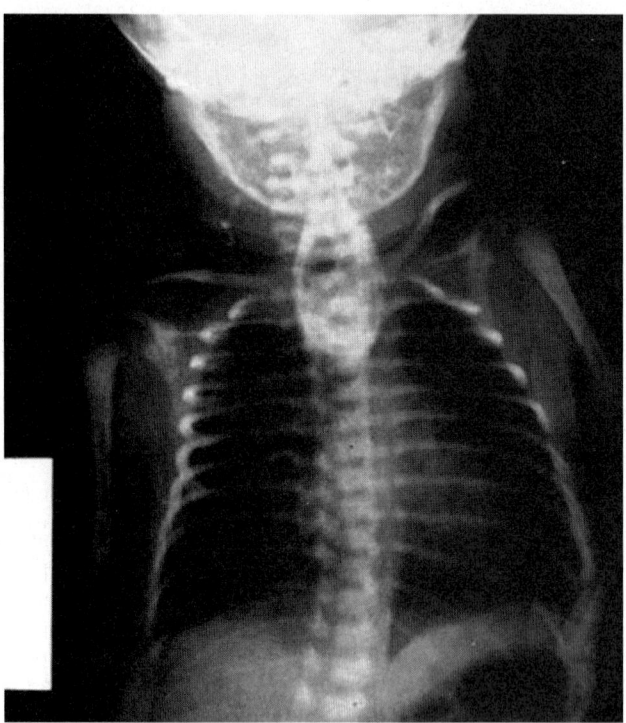

FIG. 38-10. Type C esophageal atresia with tracheoesophageal fistula. Note the catheter that is coiled in the upper pouch, and the presence of gas below the diaphragm, which confirms the presence of the tracheoesophageal fistula.

tissue obtained from the fistula tract was found to express thyroid transcription factor one (TTF-1) and fibroblast growth factor (FGF-10), suggesting that the fistula is of respiratory origin. Although a genetic basis for EA-TEF has not been definitively established, reports indicate that this anomaly may occur in several generations of the same family. Twin studies also demonstrate the presence of esophageal atresia in sets of dizygotic twins.

Other congenital anomalies frequently occur in association with EA-TEF. These defects are known by the acronyms VATER or VACTERRL syndrome, which refers to *v*ertebral (missing vertebra) and *a*norectal (imperforate anus) anomalies, *c*ardiac defects (severe congenital cardiac disease), *t*racheoesophageal fistula, *r*enal anomalies (renal agenesis and renal anomalies), and *r*adial *l*imb hyperplasia. In nearly 20% of infants born with esophageal atresia, some variant of congenital heart disease is present.

Clinical Presentation

The anatomic variant of infants with EA-TEF predicts the clinical presentation. When the esophagus ends either as a blind pouch or as a fistula into the trachea (as in types A, B, C, or D), infants present with excessive drooling, followed by choking or coughing immediately after feeding. As a result, aspiration occurs through the fistula tract. As the neonate coughs and cries, air is transmitted through the fistula into the stomach, resulting in abdominal distention. As the abdomen distends, it becomes increasingly more difficult for the infant to breathe. This leads to further atelectasis, which compounds the pulmonary dysfunction. In patients with type C and D varieties, the regurgitated gastric juice passes through the fistula, where it collects in the trachea and lungs and leads to a chemical pneumonitis, which further exacerbates the pulmonary status. In many instances, the diagnosis is actually made by the nursing staff, who attempt to feed the baby and notice the accumulation of oral secretions.

The diagnosis of esophageal atresia is confirmed by the inability to pass an orogastric tube into the stomach (Fig. 38-10). The dilated upper pouch may occasionally be seen on a plain chest radiograph. If a soft feeding tube is used, the tube will coil in the upper pouch, which provides further diagnostic certainty. An important alternative diagnosis that must be considered when an orogastric tube does not enter the stomach is that of an esophageal perforation. This problem can occur in infants after traumatic insertion of a nasogastric or

orogastric tube. In this instance, the perforation classically occurs at the level of the piriform sinus, and a false passage is created which prevents the tube from entering the stomach. Whenever there is any diagnostic uncertainty, a contrast study will confirm the diagnosis of EA and occasionally document the TEF. The presence of a TEF can be demonstrated clinically by finding air in the gastrointestinal tract. This can be proven at the bedside by percussion of the abdomen, and confirmed by obtaining a plain abdominal radiograph. Occasionally, a diagnosis of EA-TEF can be suspected prenatally on ultrasound evaluation. Typical features include failure to visualize the stomach and the presence of polyhydramnios. These findings reflect the absence of efficient swallowing by the fetus.

In a child with esophageal atresia, it is important to identify whether coexisting anomalies are present. These include cardiac defects in 38%, skeletal defects in 19%, neurologic defects in 15%, renal defects in 15%, anorectal defects in 8%, and other abnormalities in 13%. Examination of the heart and great vessels with echocardiography is important to exclude cardiac defects, as these are often the most important predictors of survival in these infants. The echocardiogram also demonstrates whether the aortic arch is left sided or right sided, which may influence the approach to surgical repair. Vertebral anomalies are assessed by plain radiography, and a spinal ultrasound is obtained if any are detected. A patent anus should be confirmed clinically. The kidneys in a newborn may be assessed clinically by palpation. An ultrasound of the abdomen will demonstrate the presence of renal anomalies, which should be suspected in the child who fails to make urine. The presence of extremity anomalies is suspected when there are missing digits, and confirmed by plain radiographs of the hands, feet, forearms, and legs. Rib anomalies may also be present. These may include the presence of a thirteenth rib.

Initial Management

The initial treatment of infants with esophageal atresia-tracheoesophageal fistula includes attention to the respiratory status, decompression of the upper pouch, and appropriate timing of surgery. Because the major determinant of poor survival is the presence of other severe anomalies, a search for other defects including congenital cardiac disease is undertaken in a timely fashion. The initial strategy after the diagnosis is confirmed is to place the neonate in an infant warmer with the head elevated at least 30 degrees. A sump catheter is placed in the upper pouch on continuous suction. Both of these strategies are designed to minimize the degree of aspiration from the esophageal pouch. When saliva accumulates in the upper pouch and is aspirated into the lungs, coughing, bronchospasm, and desaturation episodes can occur, which may be minimized by ensuring the patency of the sump catheter. Intravenous antibiotic therapy is initiated, and warmed electrolyte solution is administered. Where possible, the right upper extremity is avoided as a site to start an intravenous line, as this location may interfere with positioning of the patient during the surgical repair.

The timing of repair is influenced by the stability of the patient. Definitive repair of the EA-TEF is rarely a surgical emergency. If the child is hemodynamically stable and is oxygenating well, definitive repair may be performed within 1 to 2 days after birth. This allows for a careful determination of the presence of coexisting anomalies and for selection of an experienced anesthetic team.

Management in the Preterm Infant

The ventilated, premature neonate with EA-TEF and associated hyaline membrane disease represents a patient who may develop severe pulmonary disease. TEF can worsen the fragile pulmonary status as a result of recurrent aspiration through the fistula, and of increased abdominal distention, which impairs lung expansion. Moreover, the elevated airway pressure that is required to ventilate these patients can worsen the clinical course by forcing air through the fistula into the stomach, thereby exacerbating the degree of abdominal distention and compromising lung expansion. In this situation, the first priority is to minimize the degree of positive pressure needed to adequately ventilate the child. This can be accomplished using HFOV. If the gastric distention becomes severe, a gastrostomy tube should be placed. This procedure can be performed at the bedside under local anesthetic, if necessary. The dilated, air-filled stomach can easily be accessed through an incision in the left upper quadrant of the abdomen. Once the gastrostomy tube is placed, and the abdominal pressure is relieved, the pulmonary status can paradoxically worsen. This is because the ventilated gas may pass preferentially through the fistula, which is the path of least resistance, and bypass the lungs thereby worsening the hypoxemia. To correct this problem, the gastrostomy tube may be placed under water seal, elevated, or intermittently clamped. If these maneuvers are to no avail, ligation of the fistula may be required. This procedure can be performed in the neonatal intensive care unit if the infant is too unstable to be transported to the operating room. These interventions allow for the infant's underlying hyaline membrane disease to improve, for the pulmonary secretions to clear, and for the infant to reach a period of stability so that definitive repair can be performed.

Primary Surgical Correction

In a stable infant, definitive repair is achieved through performance of a primary esophagoesophagostomy. The infant is brought to the operating room, intubated, and placed in the lateral decubitus position with the right side up in preparation for a right posterolateral thoracotomy. If a right-sided arch was determined previously by echocardiography, consideration is given to performing the repair through the left chest, although most surgeons believe that the repair can be performed safely from the right side as well. Bronchoscopy may be performed to exclude the presence of additional, upper pouch fistulae in cases of esophageal atresia (i.e., differentiation of types B, C, and D), and identification of a laryngeotracheoesophageal cleft.

The operative technique for primary repair is as follows (Fig. 38-11). A retropleural approach is generally used, as this technique prevents widespread contamination of the thorax if a postoperative anastomotic leak occurs. The sequence of steps includes:

1. Mobilization of the pleura to expose the structures in the posterior mediastinum.
2. Division of the fistula and closure of the tracheal opening.
3. Mobilization of the upper esophagus sufficiently to permit an anastomosis without tension, and to determine whether a fistula is present between the upper esophagus and the trachea. Forward pressure by the anesthesia staff on the sump drain in the pouch can greatly facilitate dissection at this stage of the operation. Care must be taken when dissecting posteriorly to avoid violation of either the lumen of the trachea or esophagus.
4. Mobilization of the distal esophagus. This needs to be performed judiciously to avoid devascularization, since the blood supply to the distal esophagus is segmental from the aorta. Most of the esophageal length is obtained from mobilizing the upper pouch, since the blood supply travels via the submucosa from above.
5. Performing a primary esophagoesophageal anastomosis. Most surgeons perform this procedure in a single layer using 5-0 sutures. If there is excess tension, the muscle of the upper pouch can be circumferentially incised without compromising blood supply to increase its length. Many surgeons place a transanastomotic feeding tube in order to institute feeds in the early postoperative period.
6. A retropleural drain is placed, and the incision is closed in layers.

Postoperative Course

The postoperative management strategy of patients with EA-TEF is influenced to a great degree by the preference of the individual surgeon and the institutional culture. Many surgeons prefer not to leave the infants intubated postoperatively, to avoid the effects of positive pressure on the site of tracheal closure. However, it may not be possible in babies with preoperative lung disease either from prematurity or pneumonia, or when there is any cord edema. When a transanastomotic tube is placed, feeds are begun slowly in the postoperative period. Some surgeons institute parenteral nutrition for several days, using a central line. The retropleural drain is assessed daily for the presence of saliva, indicating an anastomotic leak. Many surgeons obtain a contrast swallow 1 week after repair to assess the caliber of the anastomosis and to determine whether a leak is present. If there is no leak, feedings are started.

Complications of Surgery

Anastomotic leakage occurs in 10 to 15% of patients, and may be seen either in the immediate postoperative period, or after several days. Early leakage is manifested by a new pleural effusion, pneumothorax, and sepsis, and requires immediate exploration. In these circumstances, the anastomosis may be completely disrupted, possibly due to excessive tension. Revision of the anastomosis may be possible. If not, cervical esophagostomy and gastrostomy placement is required, with a staged procedure to reestablish esophageal continuity. Anastomotic leakage that is detected after several days usually heals without intervention, particularly if a retropleural approach is used. Under these circumstances, broad-spectrum antibiotics, pulmonary toilet, and optimization of nutrition are important. After

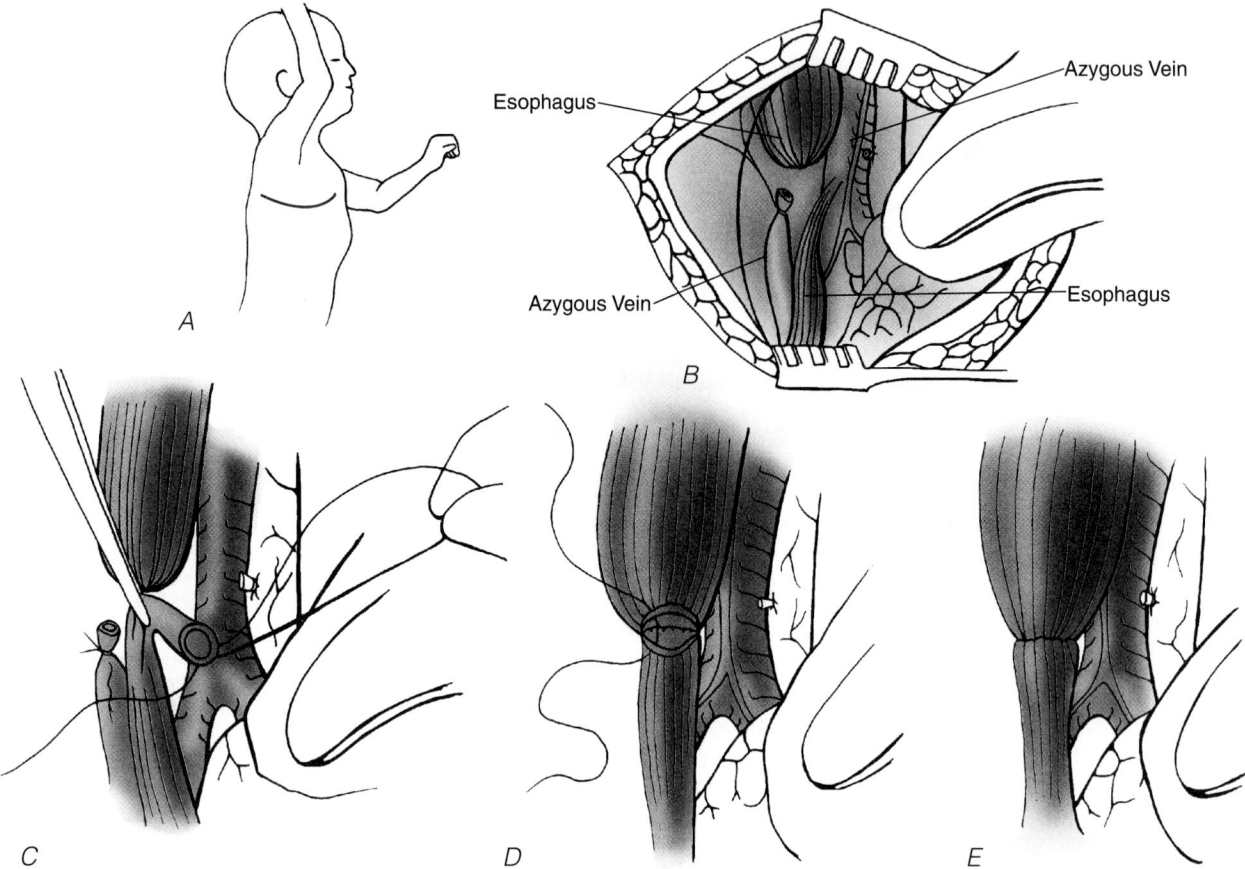

FIG. 38-11. *Primary repair of type C tracheoesophageal fistula. A. Right thoracotomy incision. B. Azygos vein transected, proximal and distal esophagus demonstrated, and fistula identified. C. Tracheoesophageal fistula transected and defect in trachea closed. D. End-to-end anastomosis between proximal and distal esophagus (posterior row). E. Completed anastomosis.*

approximately a week or so, a repeat esophagram should be performed, at which time the leakage may have resolved.

Strictures are not infrequent (10 to 20%), particularly if a leak has occurred. A stricture may become apparent at any time, from the early postoperative period to months or years later. It may present as choking, gagging, or failure to thrive, but often becomes clinically apparent with the transition to eating solid food. A contrast swallow or esophagoscopy is confirmatory, and simple dilatation is usually corrective. Occasionally, repeated dilatations are required. These may be performed in a retrograde fashion, during which a silk suture is placed into the oropharynx and delivered from the esophagus through a gastrostomy tube. Tucker dilators are then tied to the suture and passed in a retrograde fashion from the gastrostomy tube and delivered out of the oropharynx. Increasing sizes are used, and the silk is replaced at the end of the procedure, where it is taped to the side of the face at one end, and to the gastrostomy tube at the other.

"Recurrent" tracheoesophageal fistula may represent a missed upper pouch fistula or a true recurrence. This may occur after an anastomotic disruption, during which the recurrent fistula may heal spontaneously. Otherwise, reoperation may be required. Recently, the use of fibrin glue has been successful in treating recurrent fistulas, although long-term follow-up is lacking.

Gastroesophageal reflux commonly occurs after repair of EA-TEF, potentially due to alterations in esophageal motility

and the anatomy of the gastroesophageal junction. The clinical manifestations of such reflux are similar to those seen in other infants with primary gastroesophageal reflux disease (GERD). A loose antireflux procedure, such as a Nissen fundoplication, is used to prevent further reflux, but the child may have feeding problems after antireflux surgery as a result of the innate dysmotility of the distal esophagus. The fundoplication may be safely performed laparoscopically in experienced hands, although care should be taken to ensure that the wrap is not excessively tight.

Special Circumstances

Patients with type E TEFs (also called H-type) most commonly present beyond the newborn period. Presenting symptoms include recurrent chest infections, bronchospasm, and failure to thrive. The diagnosis is suspected using barium esophagography, and confirmed by endoscopic visualization of the fistula. Surgical correction is generally possible through a cervical approach, and requires mobilization and division of the fistula. Outcome usually is excellent.

Patients with duodenal atresia and EA-TEF may require urgent treatment due to the presence of a closed obstruction of the stomach and proximal duodenum. In stable patients, treatment consists of repair of the esophageal anomaly and correction of the duodenal atresia if the infant is stable during surgery. If not, a staged approach should be utilized, consisting of ligation of the fistula and placement of a gastrostomy tube. Definitive repair can then be performed at a later time.

Primary esophageal atresia (type A) represents a challenging problem, particularly if the upper and lower ends are too far apart for an anastomosis to be created. Under these circumstances, treatment strategies include placement of a gastrostomy tube and performing serial bougienage to increase the length of the upper pouch. Occasionally, when the two ends cannot be brought safely together, esophageal replacement is required, using either a gastric pull-up or colon interposition (see below).

Outcome

Various classification systems have been utilized to predict survival in patients with EA-TEF and to stratify treatment. A system devised by Waterston in 1962 was used to stratify neonates based on birth weight, the presence of pneumonia, and the identification of other congenital anomalies. In response to advances in neonatal care, the surgeons from the Montreal Children's Hospital proposed a new classification system in 1993. In the Montreal experience only two characteristics independently affected survival: preoperative ventilator dependence and associated major anomalies. Pulmonary disease as defined by ventilator dependence, appeared to be more accurate than pneumonia. When the two systems were recently compared, the Montreal system more accurately identified children at highest risk. Spitz and colleagues recently analyzed risk factors in infants with EA-TEF who died. Two criteria were found to be important predictors of outcome: birth weight less than 1500 g and the presence of major congenital cardiac disease. A new classification for predicting outcome in esophageal atresia was therefore proposed as follows: group I: birth weight $\geq$1500 g, without major cardiac disease, survival 97% (283 of 293); group II: birth weight <1500 g, or major cardiac disease, survival 59% (41 of 70); and group III: birth weight <1500 g, and major cardiac disease, survival 22% (2 of 9).

In general, surgical correction of EA-TEF leads to a satisfactory outcome with nearly normal esophageal function in most patients. Overall survival rates of greater than 90% have been achieved in patients classified as stable, in all the various staging systems. Unstable infants have an increased mortality (40 to 60% survival) because of potentially fatal associated cardiac and chromosomal anomalies or prematurity. However, the use of a staged procedure also has increased survival, even in these high-risk infants.

Corrosive Injury of the Esophagus

Injury to the esophagus after ingestion of corrosive substances most commonly occurs in toddlers. Both strong alkalies and strong acids produce injury by liquefaction or coagulation necrosis, and since all corrosive agents are extremely hygroscopic, the caustic substance will cling to the esophageal epithelium. Subsequent strictures occur at the anatomically narrowed areas of the esophagus, cricopharyngeus, midesophagus, and gastroesophageal junction. A child who has swallowed an injurious substance may be symptom free, but usually will be drooling and unable to swallow saliva. The injury may be restricted to the oropharynx and esophagus, or may extend to include the stomach. There is no effective immediate antidote. Diagnosis is by careful physical examination of the mouth, and endoscopy with a flexible or rigid esophagoscope. It is important to endoscope only to the first level of the burn in order to avoid perforation. Early barium swallow may delineate the extent of the mucosal

injury. It is important to realize that the esophagus may be burned without evidence of injury to the mouth. Although previously used routinely, steroids have not been shown to alter stricture development or modify the extent of injury. Therefore they are no longer part of the management of caustic injuries. Antibiotics are administered during the acute period.

The extent of injury is graded endoscopically as mild, moderate, or severe (grade I, II, or III). Circumferential esophageal injuries with necrosis have an extremely high likelihood of stricture formation. These patients should undergo placement of a gastrostomy tube once clinically stable. A string should be inserted through the esophagus, either immediately or during repeat esophagoscopy several weeks later. When established strictures are present (usually after 3 to 4 weeks), dilatation is performed. Retrograde dilatations are safest, using graduated dilators brought through the gastrostomy and advanced into the esophagus via the transesophageal string. For less severe injuries, dilatation may be attempted in antegrade fashion by either graded bougies or balloons. Management of esophageal perforation during dilation should include antibiotics, irrigation, and closed drainage of the thoracic cavity to prevent systemic sepsis. When recognition is delayed or if the patient is systemically ill, esophageal diversion may be required, with staged reconstruction at a later time.

Although the native esophagus can be preserved in most cases, severe stricture formation that does not respond to dilation is best managed by esophageal replacement. The most commonly used options for esophageal substitution are the colon (right colon or transverse/left colon) and the stomach (gastric tubes or gastric pull-up). Pedicled or free grafts of the jejunum are less commonly used. The right colon is based on a pedicle of the middle colic artery, and the left colon on a pedicle of the middle colic or left colic artery. Gastric tubes are fashioned from the greater curvature of the stomach, based on the pedicle of the left gastroepiploic artery. When the entire stomach is used, as in gastric pull-up, the blood supply is provided by the right gastric artery. The neoesophagus may transverse: (1) subinternally, (2) through a transthoracic route, or (3) through the posterior mediastinum to reach the neck. A feeding jejunostomy is placed at the time of surgery, and tube feedings are instituted once the postoperative ileus has resolved. In a recent review of patients treated by gastric pull-up, long-term outcome was good. Complications included esophagogastric anastomotic leak (n = 15; 36%), which uniformly resolved without intervention, and stricture formation (n = 20; 49%), which responded to a course of dilation. Long-term follow-up has shown that all methods of esophageal substitution can support normal growth and development, and the children enjoy reasonably normal eating habits. Because of the potential for late complications such as ulceration and stricture, follow-up into adulthood is mandatory, but complications appear to diminish with time.

Gastroesophageal Reflux

Gastroesophageal reflux (GER) occurs to some degree in all children, and refers to the passage of gastric contents into the esophagus. By contrast, GERD describes the situation in which reflux is symptomatic. Typical symptoms include failure to thrive, bleeding, stricture formation, reactive airway disease, aspiration pneumonia, or apnea. Failure to thrive and pulmonary problems are particularly common in infants with GERD, whereas strictures and esophagitis are more common in older children and adolescents. GERD is particularly problematic in neurologically-impaired children.

Clinical Manifestations

Because all infants experience occasional episodes of GER to some degree, care must be taken before a child is labeled as having pathologic reflux. A history of repeated episodes of vomiting that interferes with growth and development, or the presence of apparent life-threatening events, are required before the diagnosis of GERD can be made. In older children, esophageal bleeding, stricture formation, severe heartburn, or the development of Barrett's esophagus unequivocally connote pathologic reflux or GERD. In neurologically-impaired children, vomiting due to GER must be distinguished from chronic retching.

The work-up of patients suspected of having GERD includes documentation of the episodes of reflux and evaluation of the anatomy. A barium swallow should be performed as an initial test. This will determine whether there is obstruction of the stomach or duodenum (due to duodenal webs or pyloric stenosis), and will determine whether malrotation is present. The frequency and severity of reflux should be assessed using a 24-hour pH probe study. Although this test is poorly tolerated, it provides the most accurate determination that GERD is present. Esophageal endoscopy with biopsies may identify the presence of esophagitis, and is useful to determine the length of intra-abdominal esophagus and the presence of Barrett's esophagus. Some surgeons obtain a radioisotope "milk scan" to evaluate gastric emptying, although there is little evidence to show that this test changes management when a diagnosis of GERD has been confirmed using the above modalities.

Treatment

Most patients with GERD are treated initially by conservative means. In the infant, propping up the baby and thickening the formula with rice cereal are generally recommended. Some authors prefer a prone head-up position. In the infant unresponsive to position and formula changes and the older child with severe GERD, medical therapy is based on gastric acid reduction with an H_2-blocking agent and/or a proton pump inhibitor. Medical therapy is successful in most neurologically normal infants and younger children, many of whom will outgrow their need for medications. In certain patients, however, medical treatment does not provide symptomatic relief, and surgery is therefore indicated. The least invasive surgical option includes the placement of a nasojejunal or gastrojejunal feeding tube. Because the stomach is bypassed, food contents do not enter the esophagus, and symptoms are often improved. However, as a long-term remedy, this therapy is associated with several problems. The tubes often become dislodged, acid reflux still occurs, and bolus feeding is generally not possible. Fundoplication provides definitive treatment for GER and is highly effective in most circumstances. The fundus may be wrapped around the distal esophagus either 360°C (i.e., Nissen), or to lesser degrees (i.e., Thal). At present, the standard approach in most children is to perform these procedures laparoscopically whenever possible. In children with feeding difficulties and in infants under 1 year of age, a gastrostomy tube should be placed at the time of surgery. Early postoperative complications include pneumonia and atelectasis, often due to inadequate pulmonary toilet and pain control, which leads to abdominal splinting. Late postoperative complications include wrap breakdown with recurrent reflux, which may require repeat fundoplication, and dysphagia due to a wrap that is too tight, which generally responds to dilation. These complications are more common in children with neurologic impairment. The keys to successful surgical management of patients with GERD include careful patient selection and meticulous operative technique.

GASTROINTESTINAL TRACT

Hypertrophic Pyloric Stenosis

Clinical Manifestations

Timely diagnosis and treatment of infants with hypertrophic pyloric stenosis (HPS) is extremely gratifying. It is one of the few instances in surgery in which a relatively simple operation can have such a dramatic long-term effect. HPS occurs in approximately 1 in 300 live births, and classically presents in a first-born male between 3 and 6 weeks of age. However, children outside of this age range also are commonly seen, and the disease is by no means restricted to either males or first-born children. The cause of HPS has not been determined. Studies have shown that HPS is found in several generations of the same family, suggesting a familial link. Administration of erythromycin in early infancy has been linked to the subsequent development of HPS, although the cause is unclear.

Infants with HPS present with nonbilious vomiting that becomes increasingly projectile over the course of several days to weeks. Eventually, the infant develops an almost complete gastric outlet obstruction, and is no longer able to tolerate even clear liquids. Despite the recurrent emesis, the child normally has a voracious appetite, leading to a cycle of feeding and vomiting that invariably results in severe dehydration if left untreated. Jaundice may occur in association with HPS, although the reason for this is unclear. Particularly perceptive caregivers will mention that their infant is passing less flatus, which provides a further clue that gastric outlet obstruction is complete.

Infants with HPS develop a hypochloremic, hypokalemic metabolic alkalosis. The urine pH level is high initially, but eventually drops because hydrogen ions are preferentially exchanged for sodium ions in the distal tubule of the kidney as the hypochloremia becomes severe. The diagnosis of pyloric stenosis usually can be made on physical examination by palpation of the typical "olive" in the right upper quadrant, and the presence of visible gastric waves on the abdomen. When the olive cannot be palpated, ultrasound can diagnose the condition accurately in 95% of patients. Criteria for ultrasound diagnosis include a channel length of over 16 mm and pyloric thickness over 4 mm.

Treatment

Pyloric stenosis is never a surgical emergency, although dehydration and electrolyte abnormalities may present a medical emergency. Fluid resuscitation with correction of electrolyte abnormalities and metabolic alkalosis is essential before induction of general anesthesia for surgery. For most infants, fluid containing 5% dextrose and 0.45% saline with added potassium of 2 to 4 mEq/kg given at a rate of approximately 150 to 175 mL/kg for 24 hours will correct the underlying deficit. It is important to ensure that the child has an adequate urine output (>1 mL/kg per hour) as further evidence that rehydration has occurred. After resuscitation, a Fredet-Ramstedt pyloromyotomy is performed (Fig. 38-12). It may be performed using an open or laparoscopic approach. The open pyloromyotomy is performed through either an umbilical or a right upper quadrant transverse abdominal incision. The former route is cosmetically more appealing, although the transverse incision provides easier access to the antrum and pylorus. In recent years, the laparoscopic approach has gained great popularity. Whether done through an open or laparoscopic approach, the operation involves splitting the pyloric muscle until the submucosa is seen bulging upward. The incision begins at the pyloric vein of Mayo and extends onto the gastric antrum; it typically measures between 1 and 2 cm

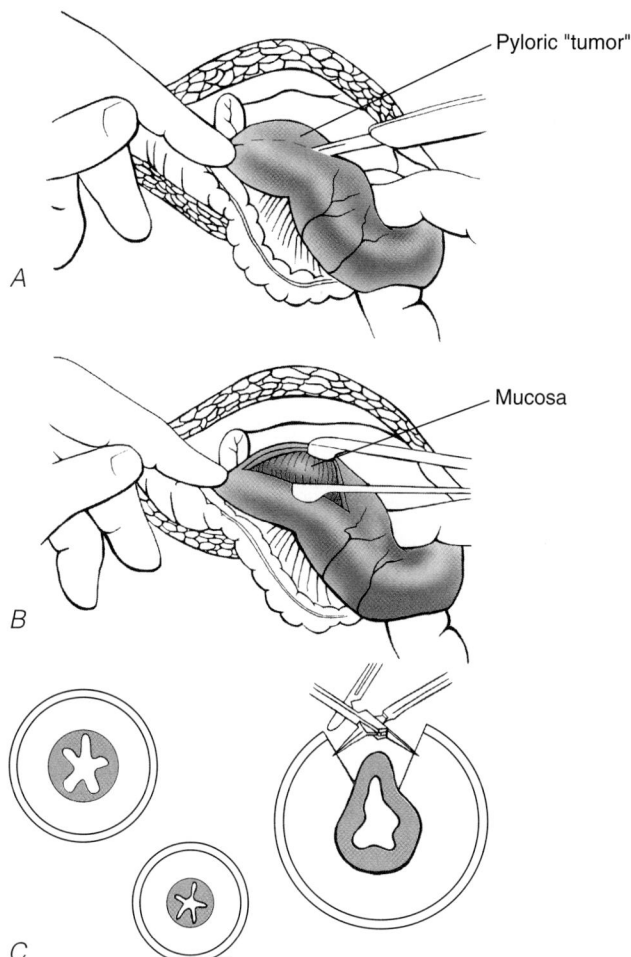

FIG. 38-12. Fredet-Ramstedt pyloromyotomy. A. Pylorus delivered into wound and seromuscular layer incised. B. Seromuscular layer separated down to the submucosal base to permit herniation of mucosa through the pyloric incision. C. Cross section demonstrating hypertrophied pylorus, depth of incision, and spreading of muscle to permit mucosa to be herniated through the incision.

in length. Postoperatively, intravenous fluids are continued for several hours, after which Pedialyte followed by formula or breast milk are offered, and are gradually increased to 60 mL every 3 hours. Most infants can be discharged home within 24 to 48 hours following surgery. Recently, several authors have shown that ad lib feeds are safely tolerated by the neonate and result in a shorter hospital stay.

The complications of pyloromyotomy include perforation of the mucosa (1 to 3%), bleeding, wound infection, and recurrent symptoms due to inadequate myotomy. When perforation occurs, the mucosa is repaired with a stitch that is placed to tack the mucosa down and reapproximate the serosa in the region of the tear. A nasogastric tube is left in place for 24 hours. The outcome is generally good.

Intestinal and Rectal Disorders in the Newborn

The cardinal symptom of intestinal obstruction in the newborn is bilious emesis. Prompt recognition and treatment of neonatal intestinal obstruction can truly be life saving. Intestinal obstruction can be thought of as either proximal or distal to the ligament of Treitz. Proximal obstruction presents as bilious vomiting, with minimal

abdominal distention. In cases of complete obstruction, there may be a paucity of gas, and no distal air will be seen on the supine and upright films of the abdomen. In this case, the diagnosis of malrotation and midgut volvulus must be excluded. Distal obstruction presents with abdominal distention and bilious emesis. The physical examination will determine whether the anus is patent. Calcifications on the abdominal plain film may indicate meconium peritonitis; pneumatosis and/or free abdominal air indicates necrotizing enterocolitis, with or without intestinal perforation. A contrast enema will show whether there is a microcolon indicative of jejunoileal atresia or meconium ileus. If a microcolon is not present, the diagnoses of Hirschsprung's disease, small left colon syndrome, or meconium plug syndrome should be considered. In all cases of intestinal obstruction, it is vital to obtain abdominal films in the supine and upright (lateral decubitus) views. This is the only way to assess the presence of air-fluid levels or free air, and to characterize the obstruction as proximal or distal. Moreover, it is important to realize that in the absence of contrast, it is difficult to determine whether a loop of dilated bowel is part of the small or large intestine, as the neonatal bowel lacks typical features, such as haustra or plicae circulares, that characterize these loops in older children or adults. For this reason, care must be taken to ensure that a complete prenatal history is obtained, to perform a thorough physical examination, and to judiciously determine the need for further contrast studies versus immediate abdominal exploration.

Duodenal Obstruction

Whenever the diagnosis of duodenal obstruction is entertained, malrotation and midgut volvulus must be excluded. This topic is covered in further detail below. Other causes of duodenal obstruction include duodenal atresia, duodenal web, stenosis, annular pancreas, or duodenal duplication cyst. Duodenal obstruction is easily diagnosed on prenatal ultrasound, which demonstrates the fluid-filled stomach and proximal duodenum as two discrete cystic structures in the upper abdomen. Associated polyhydramnios is common and presents in the third trimester. In 85% of infants with duodenal obstruction, the entry of the bile duct is proximal to the level of obstruction, such that vomiting is bilious. Abdominal distention is typically not present because of the proximal level of obstruction. In those infants with obstruction proximal to the bile duct entry, the vomiting is nonbilious. The classic finding on abdominal radiography is the "double bubble" sign, which represents the dilated stomach and duodenum (Fig. 38-13). In association with the appropriate clinical picture, this finding is sufficient to confirm the diagnosis of duodenal obstruction. However, if there is any uncertainty, particularly when a partial obstruction is suspected, a contrast upper gastrointestinal series is diagnostic.

Treatment. An orogastric tube is inserted to decompress the stomach and duodenum and the infant is given intravenous fluids to maintain adequate urine output. If the infant appears ill, or if abdominal tenderness is present, a diagnosis of malrotation and midgut volvulus should be considered, and surgery should not be delayed. Typically, the abdomen is soft and the infant is stable. Under these circumstances, the infant should be evaluated thoroughly for other associated anomalies. Approximately one-third of newborns with duodenal atresia have associated Down syndrome (trisomy 21). Patients then should be evaluated for associated cardiac anomalies. Once the work-up is complete and the infant is stable, the patient is taken to the operating room and the abdomen is entered through a transverse right upper quadrant supraumbilical incision under general endotracheal anesthesia. Associated anomalies should be sought

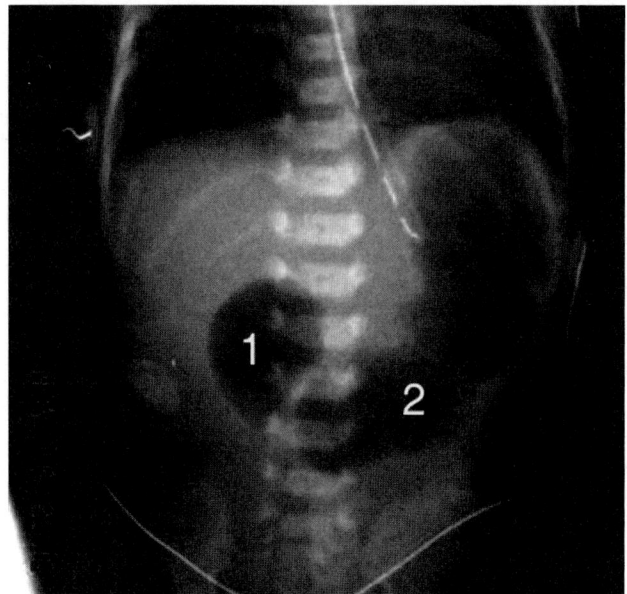

FIG. 38-13. *Abdominal x-ray showing "double bubble" sign in a newborn infant with duodenal atresia. The two "bubbles" are numbered.*

at the time of the operation. These include malrotation, anterior portal vein, a second distal web, and biliary atresia. The surgical treatment of choice for duodenal obstruction due to duodenal stenosis or atresia or annular pancreas is a duodenoduodenostomy. This procedure can be most easily performed using a proximal transverse-to-distal longitudinal (diamond-shaped) anastomosis. In cases in which the duodenum is extremely dilated, the lumen may be tapered using a linear stapler with a large Foley catheter (≥24F) in the duodenal lumen. It is important to emphasize that an annular pancreas is never divided. Treatment of duodenal web includes vertical duodenotomy, excision of the web, oversewing of the mucosa, and closing the duodenotomy horizontally. Gastrostomy tubes are not placed routinely. Recently reported survival rates exceed 90%. Late complications from repair of duodenal atresia occur in approximately 12 to 15% of patients, and include megaduodenum, intestinal motility disorders, and gastroesophageal reflux.

Intestinal Atresia

Obstruction due to intestinal atresia can occur at any point along the intestinal tract. Most cases are believed to be caused by in utero mesenteric vascular accidents leading to segmental loss of the intestinal lumen. The incidence of intestinal atresia has been estimated to be between 1 in 2000 to 1 in 5000 live births, with equal representation of the sexes. Infants with jejunal or ileal atresia present with bilious vomiting and progressive abdominal distention. The more distal the obstruction, the more distended the abdomen becomes, and the greater the number of obstructed loops on upright abdominal films (Fig. 38-14).

In cases in which the diagnosis of complete intestinal obstruction is ascertained by the clinical picture and the presence of staggered air-fluid levels on plain abdominal films, the child can be brought to the operating room after appropriate resuscitation. In these circumstances, there is little extra information to be gained by performing a barium enema. By contrast, when there is diagnostic uncertainty, or when distal intestinal obstruction is apparent, a barium enema is useful to establish whether a microcolon is present, and to diagnose the presence of meconium plugs, small left colon syndrome,

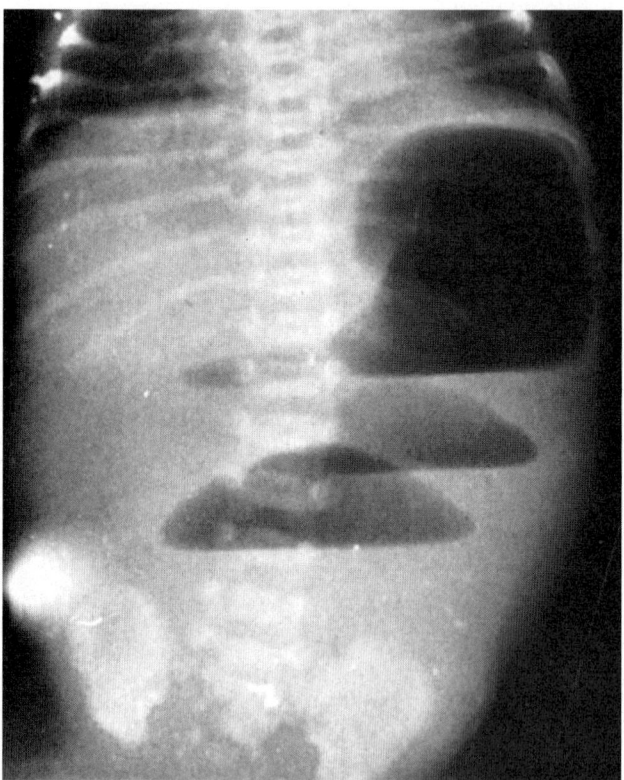

FIG. 38-14. *Intestinal obstruction in the newborn, showing several loops of distended bowel with air-fluid levels. This child has jejunal atresia.*

Hirschsprung's disease, or meconium ileus. Judicious use of barium enema is therefore required in order to safely manage neonatal intestinal obstruction, based on an understanding of the expected level of obstruction.

Surgical correction of the small intestinal atresia should be performed urgently. At laparotomy, one of several types of atresia will be encountered. In type I there is a mucosal atresia with intact muscularis. In type 2 the atretric ends are connected by a fibrous band. In type 3A the two ends of the atresia are separated by a V-shaped defect in the mesentery. Type 3B is an "apple-peel" deformity or "Christmas tree" deformity, in which the bowel distal to the atresia receives its blood supply in a retrograde fashion from the ileocolic or right colic artery (Fig. 38-15). In type 4 atresia, there are multiple atresias with a "string of sausage" or "string of beads" appearance. Disparity in lumen size between the proximal distended bowel and the small diameter of collapsed bowel distal to the atresia has lead to a number of innovative techniques of anastomosis. However, under most circumstances, an anastomosis can be performed using the end-to-back technique, in which the distal, compressed loop is "fish-mouthed" along its antimesenteric border. The proximal distended loop can be tapered as described above. Because the distended proximal bowel rarely has normal motility, the extremely dilated portion should be resected prior to performing the anastomosis.

Occasionally the infant with intestinal atresia will develop ischemia or necrosis of the proximal segment secondary to volvulus of the dilated, bulbous, blind-ending proximal bowel. Under these conditions, an end ileostomy and mucus fistula should be created, and the anastomosis should be deferred to another time, after the infant stabilizes.

and complete infarction of the midgut occur unless the problem is promptly corrected surgically.

Presentation and Management. Midgut volvulus can occur at any age, though it is seen most often in the first few weeks of life. Bilious vomiting is usually the first sign of volvulus, and all infants with bilious vomiting must be evaluated rapidly to ensure that they do not have intestinal malrotation with volvulus. The child with irritability and bilious emesis should raise particular suspicions for this diagnosis. If left untreated, vascular compromise of the midgut initially causes bloody stools, but eventually results in circulatory collapse. Additional clues to the presence of advanced ischemia of the intestine include erythema and edema of the abdominal wall, which progresses to shock and death. It must be reemphasized that the index of suspicion for this condition must be high, since abdominal signs are minimal in the early stages. Abdominal films show a paucity of gas throughout the intestine with a few scattered air-fluid levels (Fig. 38-16). When these findings are present, the patient should undergo immediate fluid resuscitation to ensure adequate perfusion and urine output, followed by prompt exploratory laparotomy.

Often the patient will not appear ill, and the plain films may suggest partial duodenal obstruction. Under these conditions, the patient may have malrotation without volvulus. This is best diagnosed by an upper GI series that shows incomplete rotation with the duodenojejunal junction displaced to the right. The duodenum may have a corkscrew shape indicating volvulus, or complete duodenal obstruction, with the small bowel loops entirely in the right side of the abdomen. Barium enema may show a displaced cecum, but this

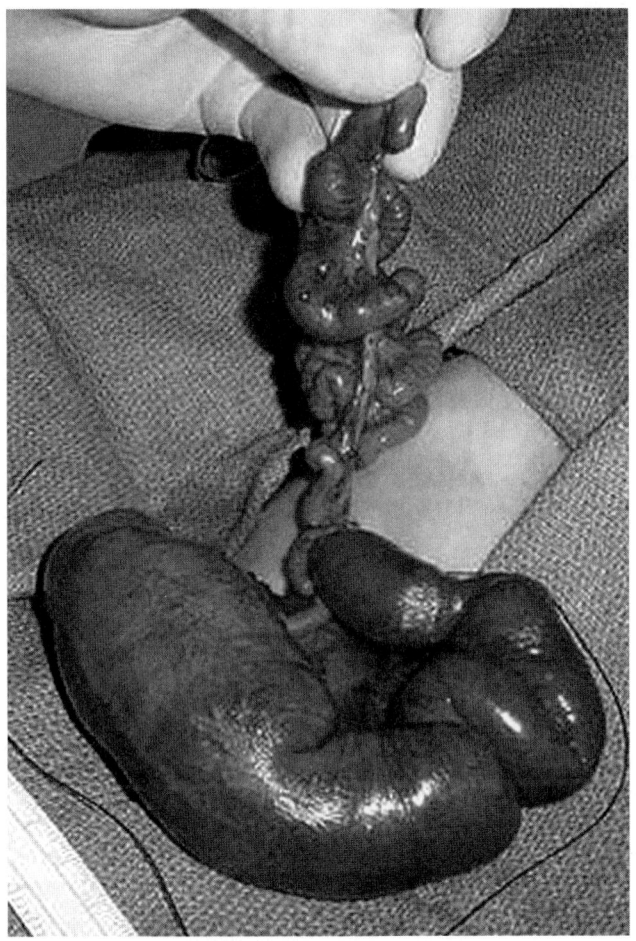

FIG. 38-15. Operative photograph of newborn with "Christmas tree" type of ileal atresia.

Malrotation and Midgut Volvulus

Embryology. During the sixth week of fetal development, the midgut grows too rapidly to be accommodated in the abdominal cavity, and it therefore prolapses into the umbilical cord. Between the tenth and twelfth week, the midgut returns to the abdominal cavity, undergoing a 270 degree counterclockwise rotation around the superior mesenteric artery. Because the duodenum also rotates caudal to the artery, it acquires a C-loop which traces this path. The cecum rotates cephalad to the artery, which determines the location of the transverse and ascending colon. Subsequently, the duodenum becomes fixed retroperitoneally in its third portion and at the ligament of Treitz, while the cecum becomes fixed to the lateral abdominal wall by peritoneal bands. The takeoff of the branches of the superior mesenteric artery elongates and becomes fixed along a line extending from its emergence from the aorta to the cecum in the right lower quadrant. If rotation is incomplete, the cecum remains in the epigastrium, but the bands fixing the duodenum to the retroperitoneum and cecum continue to form. This results in (Ladd's) bands extending from the cecum to the lateral abdominal wall and crossing the duodenum, which creates the potential for obstruction. The mesenteric takeoff remains confined to the epigastrium, resulting in a narrow pedicle suspending all the branches of the superior mesenteric artery and the entire midgut. A volvulus may therefore occur around the mesentery. This twist not only obstructs the proximal jejunum, but also cuts off the blood supply to the midgut. Intestinal obstruction

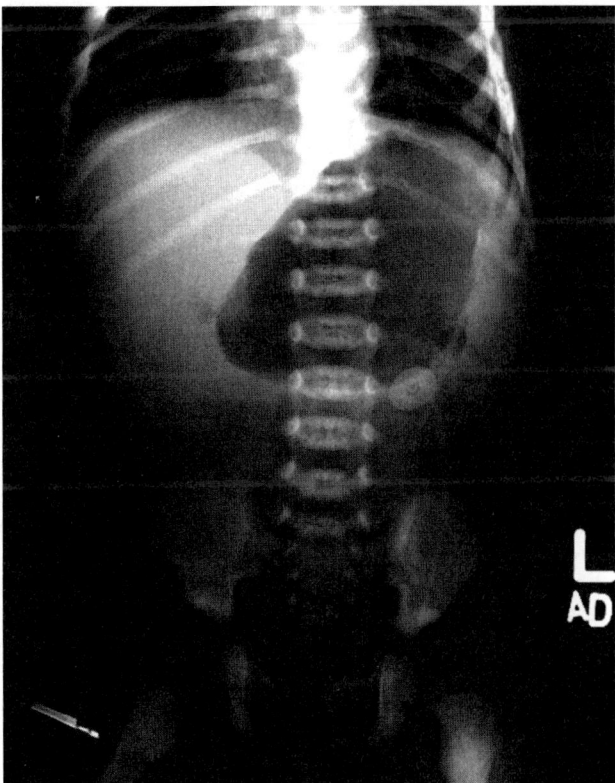

FIG. 38-16. Abdominal x-ray of a 10-day-old infant with bilious emesis. Note the dilated proximal bowel and the paucity of distal bowel gas, characteristic of a volvulus.

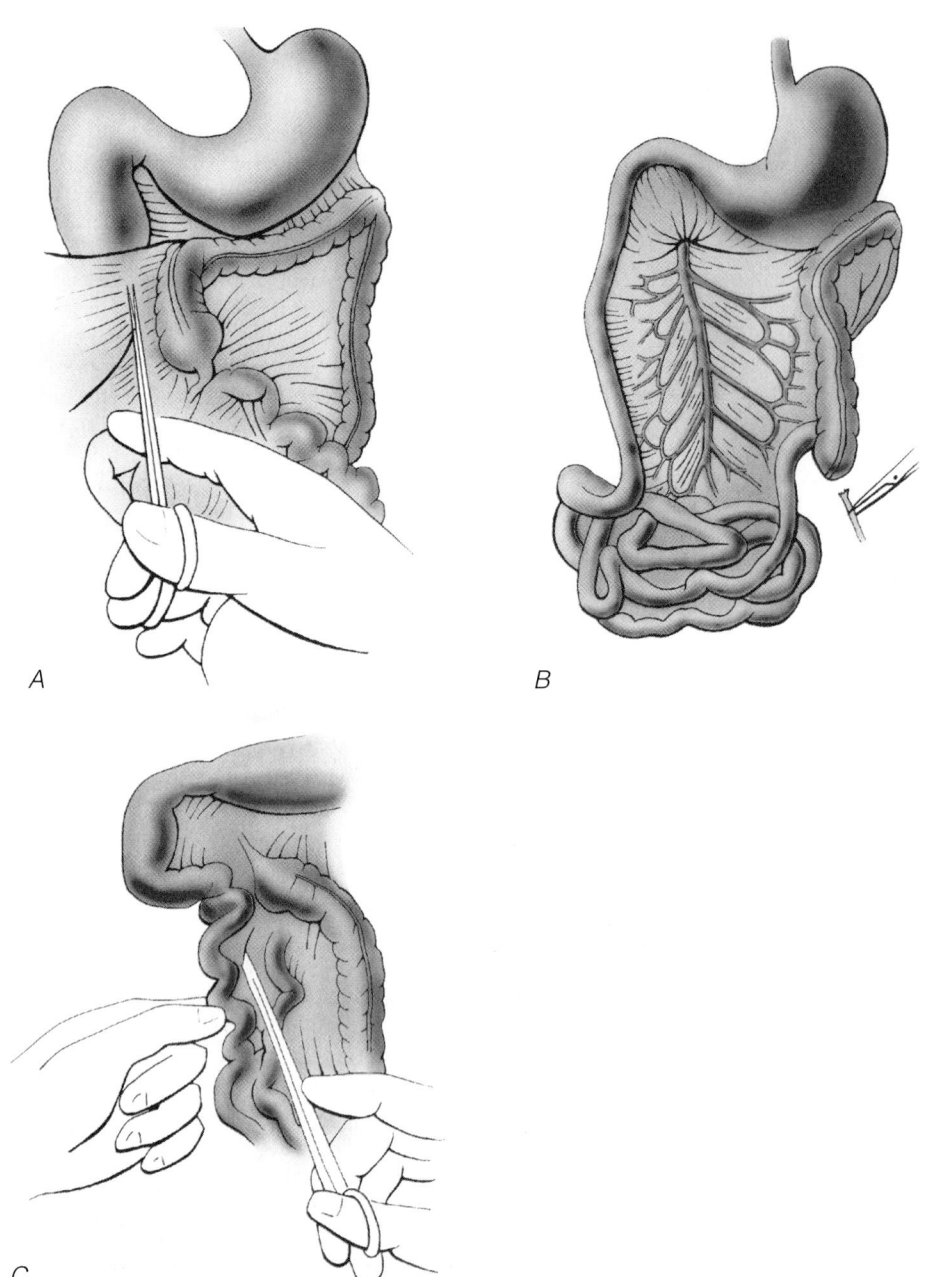

FIG. 38-17. Ladd's procedure for malrotation. *A.* Lysis of cecal and duodenal bands. *B.* Broadening the mesentery. *C.* Appendectomy.

sign is unreliable, especially in the small infant in whom the cecum is normally in a somewhat higher position than in the older child.

When volvulus is suspected, early surgical intervention is mandatory if the ischemic process is to be avoided or reversed. Volvulus occurs clockwise, and it is therefore untwisted counterclockwise. This can be remembered using the memory aid "turn back the hands of time." Subsequently, Ladd's procedure is performed. This operation does not correct the malrotation, but does broaden the narrow mesenteric pedicle to prevent volvulus from recurring. This procedure is performed as follows (Fig. 38-17): The bands between the cecum and the abdominal wall and between the duodenum and terminal ileum are divided sharply to splay out the superior mesenteric artery and its branches. This maneuver brings the straightened duodenum into the right lower quadrant and the cecum into the left lower quadrant. The appendix is removed to avoid diagnostic errors in later life. No attempt is made to suture the cecum or duodenum in

place. With advanced ischemia, reduction of the volvulus without the Ladd's procedure is accomplished, and a second-look procedure 24 to 36 hours later will often show some vascular recovery. A transparent plastic silo may be placed to facilitate constant evaluation of the intestine, and to plan for the timing of reexploration. Frankly necrotic bowel can then be resected conservatively. With early diagnosis and correction, the prognosis is excellent. However, diagnostic delay can lead to mortality or to short gut syndrome, requiring intestinal transplantation.

A subset of patients with malrotation will demonstrate chronic obstructive symptoms. These symptoms may result from Ladd's bands across the duodenum, or occasionally from intermittent volvulus. Symptoms include intermittent abdominal pain and intermittent vomiting that may occasionally be bilious. Infants with malrotation may demonstrate failure to thrive, and they may be diagnosed initially as having gastroesophageal reflux disease. Surgical correction using Ladd's procedure as described above can prevent volvulus from occurring and improve symptoms in many instances.

Meconium Ileus

Pathogenesis and Clinical Presentation. Infants with cystic fibrosis have characteristic pancreatic enzyme deficiencies and abnormal chloride secretion in the intestine that result in the production of viscous, water-poor meconium. Meconium ileus occurs when this thick, highly viscous meconium becomes impacted in the ileum and leads to high-grade intestinal obstruction. Meconium ileus can be either uncomplicated, in which case there is no intestinal perforation, or complicated, in which case prenatal perforation of the intestine has occurred or vascular compromise of the distended ileum develops. Antenatal ultrasound may reveal the presence of intra-abdominal or scrotal calcifications, or distended bowel loops. These infants present shortly after birth with progressive abdominal distention and failure to pass meconium with intermittent bilious emesis. Abdominal radiographs show dilated loops of intestine. Because the enteric contents are so viscous, air-fluid levels do not form, even when obstruction is complete. Small bubbles of gas become entrapped in the inspissated meconium in the distal ileum, where they produce a characteristic "ground glass" appearance on radiograph.

The diagnosis of meconium ileus is confirmed by a contrast enema, which typically demonstrates a microcolon. In patients with uncomplicated meconium ileus, the terminal ileum is filled with pellets of meconium. In patients with complicated meconium ileus, intraperitoneal calcifications form, producing an eggshell pattern on plain abdominal x-ray.

Management. The treatment strategy depends on whether the patient has complicated or uncomplicated meconium ileus. Patients with uncomplicated meconium ileus can be treated nonoperatively. Dilute water-soluble contrast is advanced through the colon into the dilated portion of the ileum under fluoroscopic control. Since these contrast agents act partially by absorbing fluid from the bowel wall into the intestinal lumen, maintaining adequate hydration of the infant during this maneuver is extremely important. The enema may be repeated at 12-hour intervals over several days until all the meconium is evacuated. Failure to reflux the contrast into the dilated portion of the ileum signifies the presence of an associated atresia or complicated meconium ileus, and thus warrants exploratory laparotomy. If surgical intervention is required because of failure of contrast enemas to relieve obstruction, operative irrigation with a dilute contrast agent, the mucolytic N-acetylcysteine, or saline through a purse-string suture may be successful. Alternatively, resection of the distended terminal ileum is performed and the meconium pellets are flushed from the distal small bowel. At this point, ileostomy and mucous fistula may be created from the proximal and distal ends, respectively. Alternatively, a Bishop-Koop anastomosis may be fashioned, or an end-to-end anastomosis may be performed (Fig. 38-18).

Necrotizing Enterocolitis

Clinical Features. Necrotizing enterocolitis (NEC) is the most common and lethal gastrointestinal disorder affecting the intestine of the stressed, preterm neonate. Over 25,000 cases of NEC are reported annually, and the overall mortality ranges between 10 and 50%. Advances in neonatal care such as surfactant therapy, as well as improved methods of mechanical ventilation, have resulted in increasing numbers of low-birth-weight infants surviving neonatal hyaline membrane disease. An increasing proportion of survivors of neonatal respiratory distress syndrome will therefore be at risk

for developing NEC. Consequently, it is estimated that NEC soon will surpass respiratory distress syndrome as the principal cause of death in the preterm infant.

Multiple risk factors have been associated with the development of NEC. These include prematurity, initiation of enteral feeding, bacterial infection, intestinal ischemia resulting from birth asphyxia, umbilical artery cannulation, persistence of a patent ductus arteriosus, cyanotic heart disease, and maternal cocaine abuse. Nonetheless, the mechanisms by which these complex interacting etiologies lead to the development of the disease remain undefined. The only consistent epidemiologic precursors for NEC are prematurity and enteral alimentation, representing the commonly encountered clinical situation of a stressed infant who is fed enterally. Of note, there is some debate regarding the importance of enteral alimentation in the pathogenesis of NEC. A prospective randomized study showed no increase in the incidence of NEC despite an aggressive feeding strategy, and up to 10% of infants with NEC have never received any form of enteral nutrition.

The indigenous intestinal microbial flora have been postulated to play a central role in the pathogenesis of NEC. Bacterial colonization may be a prerequisite for the development of this disease, as oral prophylaxis with vancomycin or gentamicin reduced the incidence of NEC. The importance of bacteria in the pathogenesis of NEC is further supported by the finding that NEC occurs in episodic waves that can be abrogated by infection control measures, and the fact that NEC usually develops at least 10 days postnatally, when the GI tract is colonized by coliforms. Common bacterial isolates from the blood, peritoneal fluid, and stool of infants with advanced NEC include *Escherichia coli, Enterobacter, Klebsiella,* and occasionally, coagulase-negative *Staphylococcus* species.

NEC may involve single or multiple segments of the intestine, most commonly the terminal ileum, followed by the colon. The gross findings in NEC include bowel distention with patchy areas of thinning, pneumatosis, gangrene, or frank perforation. The microscopic features include the appearance of a "bland infarct" characterized by full-thickness necrosis.

Pathogenesis. The exact mechanisms that lead to the development of NEC remain incompletely understood. However, current thinking suggests that in the setting of an episode of perinatal stress, such as respiratory distress syndrome, the premature infant suffers a period of intestinal hypoperfusion. This is followed by a period of reperfusion, and the combination of ischemia and reperfusion lead to mucosal injury. The damaged intestinal mucosa can then be readily breached by indigenous microorganisms that translocate across it. The translocated bacteria then initiate an inflammatory cascade that involves the release of various proinflammatory mediators, which in turn may be responsible for further epithelial injury and the systemic manifestations of NEC. It is postulated that maintenance of the gut barrier is essential for the protection of the host against NEC, and that impairment of the mechanisms that normally repair the damaged mucosal barrier may facilitate propagation of the mucosal injury, and thus NEC.

Clinical Manifestations. Infants with NEC present with a spectrum of disease. In general, the infants are premature and may have sustained one or more episodes of stress, such as birth asphyxia, or they may have congenital cardiac disease. The clinical picture of NEC has been characterized by Bell and colleagues as progressing from a period of mild illness to that of severe, life-threatening sepsis. Although not all infants progress through the various "Bell stages," this classification scheme provides a useful format to describe the

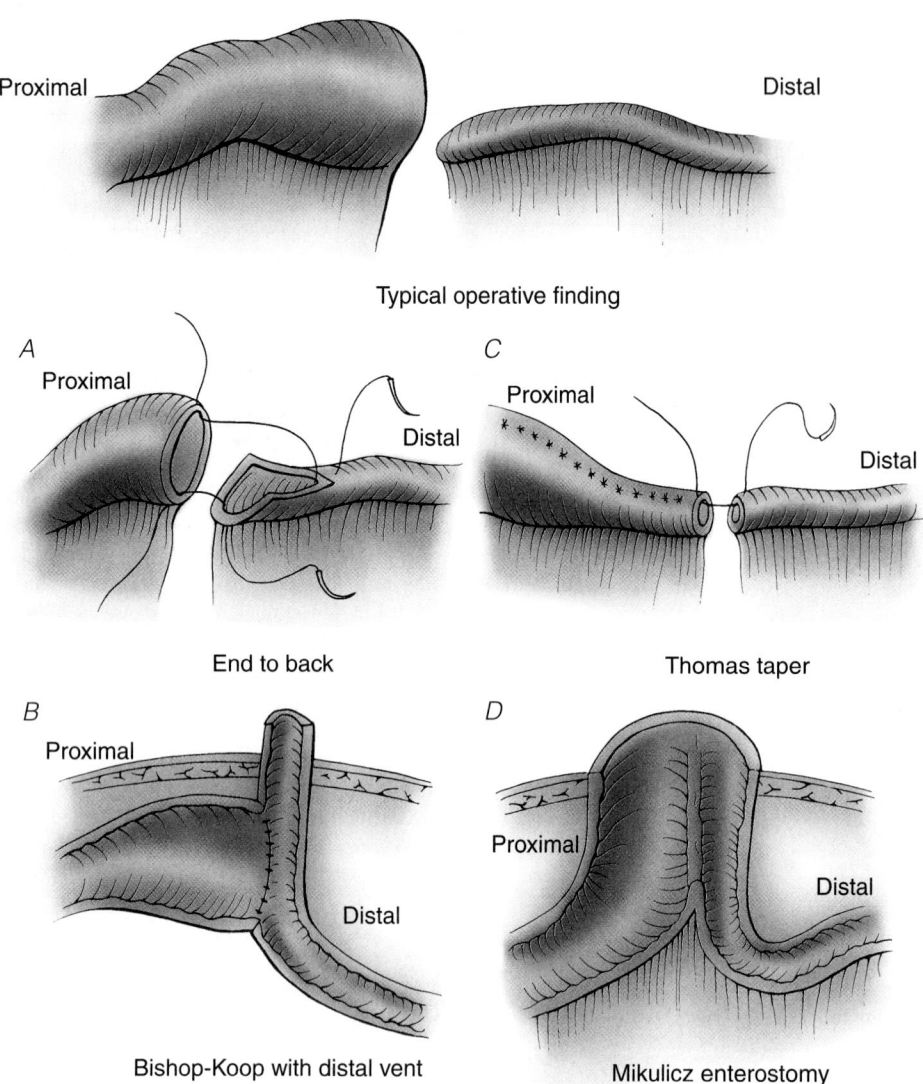

Typical operative finding

A

End to back

B

Bishop-Koop with distal vent

C

Thomas taper

D

Mikulicz enterostomy

FIG. 38-18. Techniques of intestinal anastomosis for infants with small bowel obstruction. *A.* The end-to-back distal limb has been incised, creating a "fishmouth" to enlarge the lumen. *B.* Bishop-Koop anastomosis. The proximal distended limb is joined to the side of the distal small bowel, which is vented by a "chimney" to the abdominal wall. *C.* Tapering. A portion of the antimesenteric wall of the proximal bowel is excised, with longitudinal closure to minimize disparity in the limbs. *D.* A Mikulicz double-barreled enterostomy is constructed by suturing the two limbs together, and then exteriorizing the double stoma. The common wall can be crushed with a special clamp to create a large stoma. The stoma can be closed in an extraperitoneal manner.

clinical picture associated with the development of NEC. In the earliest stage (Bell stage I), infants present with formula intolerance. This is manifested by vomiting or by finding a large residual volume from a previous feeding in the stomach at the time of the next feeding. Following appropriate treatment, which consists of bowel rest and intravenous antibiotics, many of these infants will not progress to more advanced stages of NEC. These infants are colloquially described as suffering from "NEC scare," and represent a population of neonates that are at risk of developing more severe NEC if a more prolonged period of stress supervenes.

Infants with Bell stage II have established NEC that is not immediately life threatening. Clinical findings include abdominal distention and tenderness, bilious nasogastric aspirate, and bloody stools, which indicate the development of intestinal ileus and mucosal ischemia. Abdominal examination may reveal a palpable mass indicating the presence of an inflamed loop of bowel, diffuse abdominal tenderness, cellulitis, and edema of the anterior abdominal wall. The infant may appear systemically ill, with decreased urine output, hypotension, tachycardia, and noncardiac pulmonary edema. Hematologic evaluation reveals either leukocytosis or leukopenia, an increase in the number of bands, and thrombocytopenia. An increase in the blood urea nitrogen and plasma creatinine levels may be found, which signify the development of renal dysfunction. The

diagnosis of NEC may be confirmed by abdominal radiography. The pathognomonic radiographic finding in NEC is pneumatosis intestinalis, which represents invasion of the ischemic mucosa by gas-producing microbes (Fig. 38-19). Other findings include the presence of ileus or portal venous gas. The latter is a transient finding that indicates the presence of severe NEC with intestinal necrosis. A fixed loop of bowel may be seen on serial abdominal radiographs, which suggests the possibility that a diseased loop of bowel, potentially with a localized perforation, is present. Although these infants are at risk of progressing to more severe disease, with timely and appropriate treatment, they often recover.

Infants with Bell stage III have the most advanced form of NEC. Abdominal radiographs often demonstrate the presence of pneumoperitoneum, indicating that intestinal perforation has occurred. These patients may develop a fulminant course with progressive peritonitis, acidosis, sepsis, disseminated intravascular coagulation, and death.

Treatment. In all infants suspected of having NEC, feedings are discontinued, a nasogastric tube is placed, and broad-spectrum parenteral antibiotics are given. The infant is resuscitated, and inotropes are administered to maintain perfusion as needed. Intubation and mechanical ventilation may be required to maintain

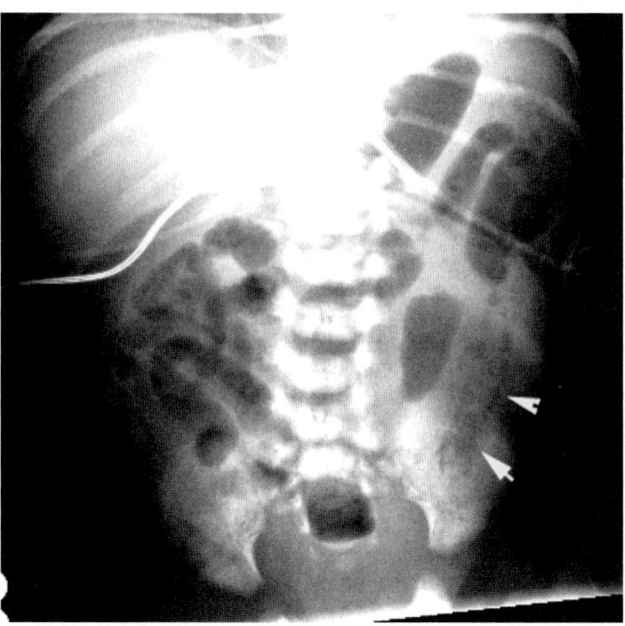

FIG. 38-19. *Abdominal radiograph of infant with necrotizing entero-colitis. Arrows point to area of pneumatosis intestinalis.*

oxygenation. Total parenteral nutrition is started. Subsequent treatment may be influenced by the particular stage of NEC that is present. Patients with Bell stage I are closely monitored, and generally remain NPO (nil per OS; nothing by mouth) and on intravenous antibiotics for 7 to 10 days prior to reinitiating enteral nutrition. After this time, providing the infant fully recovers, feedings may be reinitiated.

Patients with Bell stage II disease merit close observation. Serial physical examinations are performed to search for the development of diffuse peritonitis, a fixed mass, progressive abdominal wall cellulitis, or systemic sepsis. If infants fail to improve after several days of treatment, consideration should be given to exploratory laparotomy. Paracentesis may be performed, and if the Gram's stain demonstrates multiple organisms and leukocytes, perforation of the bowel should be suspected, and patients should be treated as Bell stage III patients.

In the most severe form of NEC (Bell stage III), patients have definite intestinal perforation, or have not responded to nonoperative therapy. Two schools of thought direct further management. One group favors exploratory laparotomy. At laparotomy, frankly gangrenous or perforated bowel is resected, and the intestinal ends are brought out as stomas. When there is massive intestinal involvement, marginally viable bowel is retained and a second-look procedure is carried out after the infant stabilizes (24 to 48 hours). Patients with extensive necrosis at the second-look may be managed by placing a proximal diverting stoma, resecting bowel that is definitely not viable, and leaving questionably viable bowel behind distal to the diverted segment. When the intestine is viable except for a localized perforation without diffuse peritonitis, and if the infant's clinical condition permits, intestinal anastomosis may be performed either proximal or distal to the divided segment. In cases in which the diseased, perforated segment cannot be safely resected, drainage catheters may be left in the region of the diseased bowel, and the infant is allowed to stabilize.

An alternative approach to the management of infants with perforated NEC involves drainage of the peritoneal cavity. This may be performed under local anesthesia at the bedside, and can be an effective means of stabilizing the desperately-ill infant by relieving increased intra-abdominal pressure and allowing ventilation. When successful, this method also allows for drainage of perforated bowel by establishing a controlled fistula. Approximately one-third of infants treated with drainage alone survive without requiring additional operations. Infants that do not respond to peritoneal drainage alone after 48 to 72 hours should undergo laparotomy. This procedure allows for the resection of frankly necrotic bowel and diversion of the fecal stream. As well, laparotomy may allow for more effective drainage.

Outcome. Survival in patients with NEC is dependent on the stage of disease, the extent of prematurity, and the presence of associated comorbidities. Survival by stage has recently been shown to be approximately 85%, 65%, and 35% percent for stages I, II, and III, respectively. Strictures develop in 20% of medically or surgically treated patients, and a contrast enema is mandatory before reestablishing intestinal continuity. If all other factors are favorable, the ileostomy is closed when the child weighs between 2 and 2.5 kg. At the time of stoma closure, the entire intestine should be examined to search for areas of NEC. Patients that developed massive intestinal necrosis are at risk of developing short-gut syndrome, particularly when the total length of the viable intestinal segment is below 40 cm. These patients require TPN to provide adequate calories for growth and development, and may develop TPN-related cholestasis and hepatic fibrosis. In a significant number of these patients, transplantation of the liver and small bowel may be required.

Intussusception

Intussusception is the leading cause of intestinal obstruction in the young child. It refers to the condition whereby a segment of intestine becomes drawn into the lumen of the more proximal bowel. The process usually begins in the region of the terminal ileum, and extends distally into the ascending, transverse, or descending colon. Rarely, an intussusception may prolapse through the rectum.

The cause of intussusception is not clear, although current thinking suggests that hypertrophy of the Peyer's patches in the terminal ileum from an antecedent viral infection acts as the starting point. Peristaltic action of the intestine then causes the bowel distal to this point to invaginate into itself. Idiopathic intussusception occurs in children between the ages of approximately 6 and 24 months. Beyond this age group, one should consider the possibility that a pathologic starting point may be present. These include polyps, malignant tumors such as lymphoma, enteric duplication cysts, or Meckel's diverticulum. Such intussusceptions are rarely reduced by air or contrast enema, and thus the starting point is identified when operative reduction of the intussusception is performed.

Clinical Manifestations. Since intussusception is frequently preceded by a gastrointestinal viral illness, the onset may not be easily determined. Typically, the infant develops paroxysms of crampy abdominal pain and intermittent vomiting. Between attacks, the infant may act normally, but as symptoms progress, increasing lethargy develops. Bloody mucus ("currant-jelly" stool) may be passed per rectum. Ultimately, if reduction is not accomplished, gangrene of the intussusceptum occurs, and perforation may ensue. On physical examination, an elongated mass is detected in the right upper quadrant or epigastrium, with an absence of bowel in the right lower quadrant (Dance's sign). The mass may be seen on plain abdominal x-ray, but is more easily demonstrated on air or contrast enema.

Treatment. Patients with intussusception should be assessed for the presence of peritonitis and for the severity of systemic illness. Following resuscitation and administration of intravenous antibiotics, the child is assessed for suitability to proceed with radiographic versus surgical reduction. In the absence of peritonitis, the child should undergo radiographic reduction. If peritonitis is present, or if the child appears systemically ill, urgent laparotomy is indicated.

In the stable patient, the air enema is both diagnostic and often curative. It constitutes the preferred method of diagnosis and nonoperative treatment of intussusception. Air is introduced with a manometer, and the pressure that is administered is carefully monitored. Under most instances, this should not exceed 120 mm Hg. Successful reduction is marked by free reflux of air into multiple loops of small bowel, and symptomatic improvement as the infant suddenly becomes pain free. Unless both of these signs are observed, it cannot be assumed that the intussusception is reduced. If reduction is unsuccessful, and the infant remains stable, the infant should be brought back to the radiology suite for a repeat attempt at reduction after a few hours. This strategy has improved the success rate of nonoperative reduction in many centers. In addition, hydrostatic reduction with barium may be useful if pneumatic reduction is unsuccessful. The overall success rate of radiographic reduction varies based on the experience of the center, and is typically between 60 and 90%.

If nonoperative reduction is successful, the infant may be given oral fluids after a period of observation. Failure to reduce the intussusception mandates surgery. Two approaches are used. In an open procedure, exploration is carried out through a right lower quadrant incision, delivering the intussuscepted mass into the wound. Reduction usually can be accomplished by gentle distal pressure, where the intussusceptum is gently milked out of the intussuscipiens (Fig. 38-20). Care should be taken not to pull the bowel out, as this can cause damage to the bowel wall. The blood supply to the appendix often is compromised, and appendectomy is performed. If the bowel is frankly gangrenous, resection and primary anastomosis is performed. In experienced hands, laparoscopic reduction may be performed, even in very young infants. This is performed using a 5-mm laparoscope placed in the umbilicus, and two additional 5-mm ports in the left and right lower quadrants. The bowel is inspected, and if it appears to be viable, reduction is performed by milking the

bowel or using gentle traction, although this approach is normally discouraged during manual reduction. Atraumatic bowel graspers allow the bowel to be handled without injuring it.

Intravenous fluids are continued until the postoperative ileus subsides. Patients are started on clear liquids and their diet is advanced as tolerated. Of note, recurrent intussusception occurs in 5 to 10% of patients, independent of whether the bowel is reduced radiographically or surgically. Patients present with recurrent symptoms in the immediate postoperative period. Treatment involves repeat air enema, which is successful in most cases. In patients who experience three or more episodes of intussusception, the presence of a pathologic starting point should be suspected and carefully evaluated using contrast studies. After the third episode of intussusception, many pediatric surgeons will perform an exploratory laparotomy to reduce the bowel and to resect a pathologic starting point if identified.

Appendicitis

Presentation. Correct diagnosis of appendicitis in children can be one of the most humbling and challenging tasks facing the pediatric surgeon. The classic presentation is known to all students and practitioners of surgery: generalized abdominal pain that localizes to the right lower quadrant, followed by nausea, vomiting, fever, and localized peritoneal irritation in the region of McBurney's point. When children present in this manner, there should be little diagnostic delay. The child should be made NPO, administered intravenous fluids and broad-spectrum antibiotics, and brought to the operating room for an appendectomy. However, children often do not present in this manner. The coexistence of viral syndromes, and the inability of young children to describe the location and quality of their pain, often results in diagnostic delay. As a result, children with appendicitis often present with perforation, particularly those who are under 5 years of age. Perforation increases the length of hospital stay, and makes the overall course of the illness significantly more complex.

Diagnosis of Appendicitis in Children. Controversy exists regarding the role of radiographic studies in the diagnosis of acute appendicitis. Because children have less periappendiceal fat than adults, CT scanning is less reliable in making the diagnosis. In addition, radiation exposure resulting from the CT scan may potentially have long-term adverse effects. Likewise, ultrasonography is neither sufficiently sensitive nor specific to accurately make the diagnosis of appendicitis, although it is useful for excluding ovarian causes of abdominal pain. Therefore the diagnosis of appendicitis remains largely clinical, and each clinician should develop their own threshold to operate or to observe the patient. A reasonable practice guideline is as follows: when the diagnosis is clinically apparent, appendectomy should obviously be performed with minimal delay. Localized right lower quadrant tenderness associated with low-grade fever and leukocytosis in boys should prompt surgical exploration. In girls, ovarian or uterine pathology must also be considered. When there is diagnostic uncertainty, the child may be observed, rehydrated, and reassessed. In girls of menstruating age, an ultrasound may be obtained to exclude ovarian pathology (i.e., cysts, torsion, or tumor). If all studies are negative yet the pain persists, and the abdominal findings remain equivocal, diagnostic laparoscopy may be employed to determine the etiology of the abdominal pain. The appendix should be removed even if it appears to be normal, unless another pathologic cause of the abdominal pain is definitively identified and the appendectomy would substantially increase morbidity.

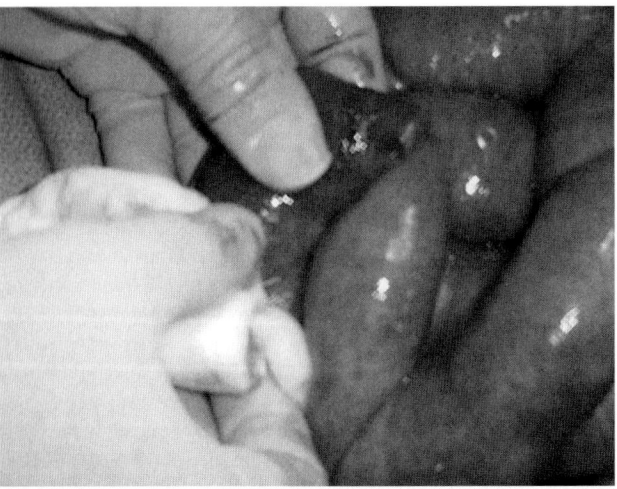

FIG. 38-20. Open reduction of intussusception, showing how the bowel is milked backward to relieve the obstruction.

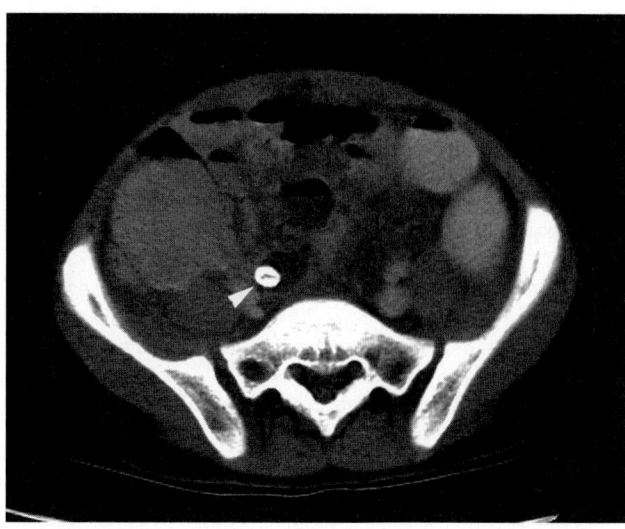

FIG. 38-21. CT scan of the abdomen showing the presence of a ruptured appendix with pelvic fluid and a fecalith (*arrow*).

Management of the Child with Perforated Appendicitis. The signs and symptoms of perforated appendicitis can closely mimic those of gastroenteritis, and include abdominal pain, vomiting, and diarrhea. Alternatively, the child may present with symptoms of intestinal obstruction. An abdominal mass may be present in the lower abdomen. When the symptoms have been present for more than 4 or 5 days and an abscess is suspected, it is reasonable to obtain a CT study of the abdomen and pelvis with intravenous, oral, and rectal contrast in order to visualize the appendix and the presence of an associated abscess, phlegmon, or fecalith (Fig. 38-21).

An individualized approach is necessary for the child who presents with perforated appendicitis. When there is evidence of generalized peritonitis, intestinal obstruction, or systemic toxicity, the child should undergo appendectomy. This should be delayed only for as long as is required to ensure adequate fluid resuscitation and administration of broad-spectrum antibiotics. The operation can be performed through a laparotomy or through a laparoscopic approach. One distinct advantage of the laparoscopic approach is that it provides excellent visualization of the pelvis and all four quadrants of the abdomen. At the time of surgery, adhesions are gently lysed, abscess cavities are drained, and the appendix is removed. Drains are seldom used, and the skin incisions can be closed primarily. If a fecalith is identified outside the appendix on CT scan, every effort should be made to retrieve it and to remove it along with the appendix, if at all possible. Often, the child in whom symptoms have been present for more than 4 or 5 days will present with an abscess cavity without evidence of generalized peritonitis. Under these circumstances, it is appropriate to perform image-guided percutaneous drainage of the abscess, followed by broad-spectrum antibiotic therapy. The inflammation will generally subside within several days, and the appendix can be safely removed on an outpatient basis 6 to 8 weeks later. If the child's symptoms do not improve, or if the abscess is not amenable to percutaneous drainage, then laparoscopic or open appendectomy and abscess drainage is required. Patients who present with a phlegmon in the region of a perforated appendix may be managed in a similar manner. In general, children who are younger than 4 or 5 years of age do not respond as well to an initially nonoperative approach, because their bodies do not localize or isolate the inflammatory process. Thus these patients are more likely to require early surgical intervention. Patients who have had

symptoms of appendicitis for no more than 4 days should probably undergo early appendectomy, since the inflammatory response is not as excessive during the initial period and the procedure can be performed safely.

Intestinal Duplications

Duplications represent mucosa-lined structures that are in continuity with the gastrointestinal tract. Although they can occur at any level in the gastrointestinal tract, these inguinal anomalies are found most commonly in the ileum within the leaves of the mesentery. Duplications may be long and tubular, but usually are cystic masses. In all cases, they share a common wall with the intestine. Symptoms associated with enteric duplication cysts include recurrent abdominal pain, emesis from intestinal obstruction, or hematochezia. Such bleeding typically results from ulceration in the duplication, or in the adjacent intestine if the duplication contains ectopic gastric mucosa. On examination, a palpable mass is often identified. Children may also develop intestinal obstruction. Torsion may produce gangrene and perforation.

The ability to make a preoperative diagnosis of enteric duplication cyst usually depends on the presentation. CT, ultrasonography, and technetium pertechnetate scanning can be helpful. Occasionally, a duplication is seen on small bowel follow-through or barium enema. In the case of short duplications, resection of the cyst and adjacent intestine with end-to-end anastomosis can be performed in a straightforward fashion. If resection of long duplications would compromise intestinal length, multiple enterotomies and mucosal stripping in the duplicated segment will allow the walls to collapse and become adherent. An alternative method is to divide the common wall using the Endo-GIA stapler, forming a common lumen. Patients with duplications who undergo complete excision without compromise of the length of remaining intestine have an excellent prognosis.

Meckel's Diverticulum

A Meckel's diverticulum is a remnant of a portion of the embryonic omphalomesenteric (vitelline) duct. It is located on the antimesenteric border of the ileum, usually within 60 cm of the ileocecal valve (Fig. 38-22). It may be found incidentally at surgery or may present with inflammation, masquerading as appendicitis. Perforation of a Meckel's diverticulum may occur if the outpouching becomes impacted with food, leading to distention and necrosis.

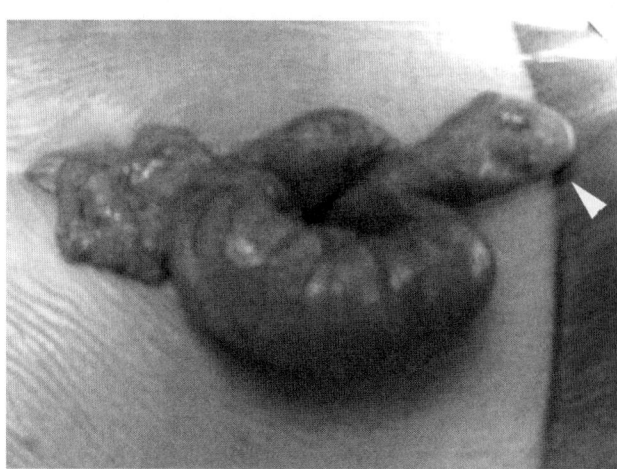

FIG. 38-22. Operative photograph showing the presence of a Meckel's diverticulum (*arrow*).

Occasionally, bands of tissue extend from the Meckel's diverticulum to the anterior abdominal wall, and these may represent starting points around which internal hernias may develop. This is an important cause of intestinal obstruction in the older child who has a scarless abdomen. Similarly to duplications, ectopic gastric mucosa may produce ileal ulcerations that bleed and lead to the passage of maroon-colored stools. Pancreatic mucosa may also be present. Diagnosis may be made by technetium pertechnetate scans when the patient presents with bleeding. Treatment is surgical. If the base is narrow and there is no mass present in the lumen of the diverticulum, a wedge resection of the diverticulum with transverse closure of the ileum can be performed. A linear stapler is especially useful in this circumstance. When a mass of ectopic tissue is palpable, if the base is wide, or when there is inflammation, it is preferable to perform a resection of the involved bowel and end-to-end ileoileostomy.

Mesenteric Cysts

Mesenteric cysts are similar to duplications in their location within the mesentery. However, they do not contain any mucosa or muscular wall. Chylous cysts may result from congenital lymphatic obstruction. Mesenteric cysts can cause intestinal obstruction or may present as an abdominal mass. The diagnosis may be made by abdominal ultrasound or CT. Treatment involves surgical excision. This may require resection of the adjacent intestine, particularly for extensive, multicystic lesions. In cases in which complete excision is not possible due to the close proximity to vital structures, partial excision or marsupialization should be performed.

Hirschsprung's Disease

Pathogenesis. In his classic textbook titled *Pediatric Surgery,* Dr. Orvar Swenson—who is eponymously associated with one of the classic surgical treatments for Hirschsprung's disease—described this condition as follows: "...congenital megacolon is caused by a malformation in the pelvic parasympathetic system which results in the absence of ganglion cells in Auerbach's plexus of a segment of distal colon. Not only is there an absence of ganglion cells, but the nerve fibers are large and excessive in number, indicating that the anomaly may be more extensive than the absence of ganglion cells." This description of Hirschsprung's disease is as accurate today as it was nearly 50 years ago, and summarizes the essential pathologic features of this disease: absence of ganglion cells in Auerbach's plexus and hypertrophy of associated nerve trunks. The cause of Hirschsprung's disease remains incompletely understood, although current thinking suggests that the disease results from a defect in the migration of neural crest cells, which are the embryonic precursors of the intestinal ganglion cell. Under normal conditions, the neural crest cells migrate into the intestine from cephalad to caudad. The process is completed by the twelfth week of gestation, but the migration from midtransverse colon to anus takes 4 weeks. During this latter period, the fetus is most vulnerable to defects in migration of neural crest cells. This may explain why most cases of aganglionosis involve the rectum and rectosigmoid. The length of the aganglionic segment of bowel is therefore determined by the most distal region that the migrating neural crest cells reach. In rare instances, total colonic aganglionosis may occur.

Recent studies have shed light on the molecular basis for Hirschsprung's disease. Patients with Hirschsprung's disease have an increased frequency of mutations in several genes, including *GDNF,* its receptor *Ret,* or its coreceptor *Gfra-1.* Moreover, mutations in these genes also lead to aganglionic megacolon in mice, which provides the opportunity to study the function of the encoded proteins. Initial investigations indicate that *GDNF* promotes the survival, proliferation, and migration of mixed populations of neural crest cells in culture. Other studies have revealed that *GDNF* is expressed in the gut in advance of migrating neural crest cells, and is chemoattractive for neural crest cells in culture. These findings raise the possibility that mutations in the *GDNF* or *Ret* genes could lead to impaired neural crest migration in utero, and the development of Hirschsprung's disease.

Clinical Presentation. The incidence of sporadic Hirschsprung's disease is 1 in 5000 live births. There are reports of increased frequency of Hirschsprung's disease in multiple generations of the same family. Occasionally, such families have mutations in the genes described above, including the *Ret* gene. Because the aganglionic colon does not permit normal peristalsis to occur, the presentation of children with Hirschsprung's disease is characterized by a functional distal intestinal obstruction. In the newborn period, the most common symptoms are abdominal distention, failure to pass meconium, and bilious emesis. Any infant who does not pass meconium beyond 48 hours of life must be investigated for the presence of Hirschsprung's disease. Occasionally, infants present with a dramatic complication of Hirschsprung's disease called enterocolitis. This pattern of presentation is characterized by abdominal distention and tenderness, and is associated with manifestations of systemic toxicity that include fever, failure to thrive, and lethargy. Infants are often dehydrated, and demonstrate a leukocytosis or increase in circulating band forms on hematologic evaluation. On rectal examination, forceful propulsion of foul-smelling liquid feces is typically observed, and represents the accumulation of stool under pressure in an obstructed distal colon. Treatment includes rehydration, systemic antibiotics, nasogastric decompression, and rectal irrigations while the diagnosis of Hirschsprung's disease is being confirmed. In children that do not respond to nonoperative management, a decompressive stoma is required. It is important to ensure that this stoma is placed in ganglion-containing bowel, which must be confirmed by frozen section at the time of stoma creation.

In approximately 20% of cases, the diagnosis of Hirschsprung's disease is made beyond the newborn period. These children have severe constipation, which has usually been treated with laxatives and enemas. Abdominal distention and failure to thrive may also be present at diagnosis.

Diagnosis. The definitive diagnosis of Hirschsprung's disease is made by rectal biopsy. Samples of mucosa and submucosa are obtained at 1 cm, 2 cm, and 3 cm from the dentate line. This can be performed at the bedside in the neonatal period without anesthesia, as samples are taken in bowel that does not have somatic innervation, and is thus not painful to the child. In older children, the procedure should be performed using intravenous sedation. The histopathology of Hirschsprung's disease is the absence of ganglion cells in the myenteric plexuses, increased acetylcholinesterase-positive nerve fibers, and the presence of hypertrophied nerve bundles.

It is important to obtain a barium enema in children in whom the diagnosis of Hirschsprung's disease is suspected. This test may demonstrate the location of the transition zone between the dilated ganglionic colon and the distal constricted aganglionic rectal segment. The authors' practice is to obtain this test before instituting rectal irrigations, so the difference in size between the proximal and distal bowel is preserved. Although the barium enema can only suggest, but cannot reliably establish the diagnosis of Hirschsprung's disease, it is useful in excluding other causes of distal intestinal obstruction. These include small left colon syndrome (as occurs in infants of diabetic mothers), colonic atresia, meconium plug syndrome, or the unused colon observed in infants after the administration of magnesium or tocolytic agents. The barium enema in total colonic aganglionosis may show a markedly shortened colon. Some surgeons have found the use of rectal manometry helpful, particularly in older children, although it is relatively inaccurate.

Treatment. The diagnosis of Hirschsprung's disease requires surgery in all cases. The classic surgical approach consisted of a multiple stage procedure. This included a colostomy in the newborn period, followed by a definitive pull-through operation after the child weighed over 10 kg. There are three viable options for the definitive pull-through procedure that are currently used. Although individual surgeons may advocate one procedure over another, studies have demonstrated that the outcome after each type of operation is similar. For each of these procedures, the principles of treatment include confirming the location in the bowel where the transition zone between ganglionic and aganglionic bowel exists, resecting the aganglionic segment of bowel, and performing an anastomosis of ganglionated bowel to either the anus or a cuff of rectal mucosa (Fig. 38-23).

Recently it has been shown that a primary pull-through procedure can be performed safely, even in the newborn period. This approach follows the same treatment principles as a staged procedure, and saves the patient from an additional surgical procedure. Many surgeons perform the intra-abdominal dissection using the laparoscope. This approach is especially useful in the newborn period, as this provides excellent visualization of the pelvis. In children with significant colonic distention, it is important to allow for a period of decompression using a rectal tube if a single-stage pull-through is to be performed. In older children with an extremely distended, hypertrophied colon, it may be prudent to perform a colostomy to allow the bowel to decompress prior to performing a pull-through procedure. However, it should be emphasized that there is no upper age limit for performing a primary pull-through.

Of the three pull-through procedures performed for Hirschsprung's disease, the first is the original Swenson procedure. In this operation, the aganglionic rectum is dissected in the pelvis and removed down to the anus. The ganglionic colon is then anastomosed to the anus via a perineal approach. In the Duhamel procedure, dissection outside the rectum is confined to the retrorectal space, and the ganglionic colon is anastomosed posteriorly just above the anus. The anterior wall of the ganglionic colon and the posterior wall of the aganglionic rectum are anastomosed using a stapler. Although both of these procedures are extremely effective, they are limited by the possibility of damage to the parasympathetic nerves that are adjacent to the rectum. To circumvent this potential problem, Soave's procedure involves dissection entirely within the rectum. The rectal mucosa is stripped from the muscular sleeve, and the ganglionic colon is brought through this sleeve and anastomosed to the anus. This operation may be performed completely from below. In all cases, it is critical to determine the level at which ganglionated bowel exists. Most surgeons believe that the anastomosis should be performed at least 5 cm from the point at which ganglion cells begin. This avoids performing a pull-through in the transition zone, which is associated with a high incidence of complications due to inadequate emptying of the pull-through segment. Up to one-third of patients who undergo a transition zone pull-through will require a reoperation.

The main complications of all procedures include postoperative enterocolitis, constipation, and anastomotic stricture. As mentioned,

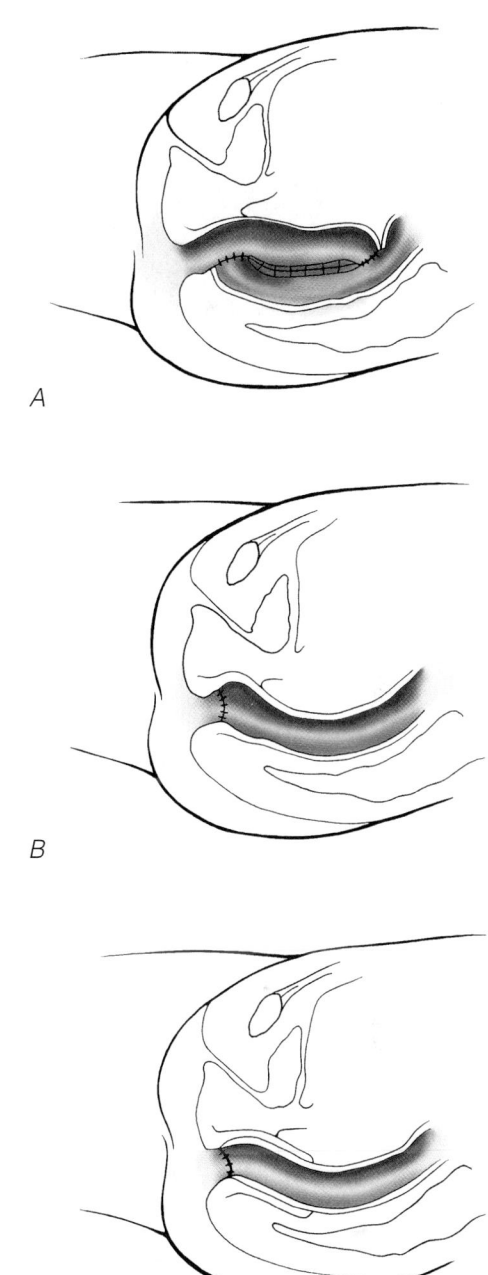

FIG. 38-23. The three operations for surgical correction of Hirschsprung's disease. A. The Duhamel procedure leaves the rectum in place and brings ganglionic bowel into the retrorectal space. B. The Swenson procedure is a resection with end-to-end anastomosis performed by exteriorizing bowel ends through the anus. C. The Soave operation is performed by endorectal dissection and removal of mucosa from the aganglionic distal segment and bringing the ganglionic bowel down to the anus within the seromuscular tunnel.

long-term results with the three procedures are comparable and generally excellent in experienced hands. These three procedures also can be adapted for total colonic aganglionosis, in which case the ileum is used for the pull-through segment.

Anorectal Malformations

Anatomic Description. Anorectal malformations describe a spectrum of congenital anomalies that include imperforate anus and

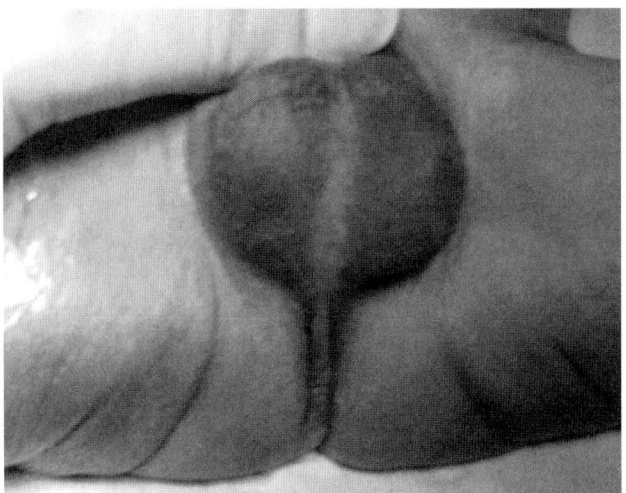

FIG. 38-24. Low imperforate anus in a male. Note the well developed buttocks. The perineal fistula was found at the midline raphe.

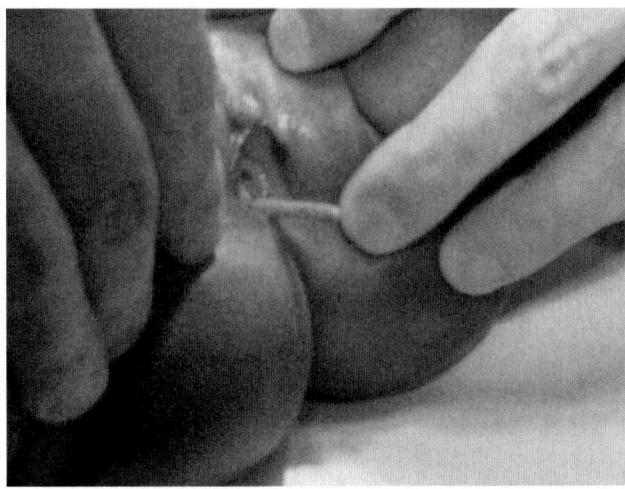

FIG. 38-25. Imperforate anus in a female. A catheter has been placed into the fistula, which is in the vestibule of the vagina.

persistent cloaca. Anorectal malformations occur in approximately 1 in 5000 live births and affect males and females almost equally. The embryologic basis includes failure of descent of the urorectal septum. The level to which this septum descends determines the type of anomaly that is present, which subsequently influences the surgical approach.

In patients with imperforate anus, the rectum fails to descend through the external sphincter complex. Instead, the rectal pouch ends blindly in the pelvis, above or below the levator ani muscle. In most cases, the blind rectal pouch communicates more distally with the genitourinary system or with the perineum through a fistulous tract. Traditionally, anatomic description of imperforate anus has been characterized as either "high" or "low," depending on whether the rectum ends above the levator ani muscle complex or partially descends through this muscle (Fig. 38-24). Based upon this classification system, in male patients with high imperforate anus, the rectum usually ends as a fistula into the membranous urethra. In females, high imperforate anus often occurs in the context of a persistent cloaca. In both males and females, low lesions are associated with a fistula to the perineum. In males, the fistula connects with the median raphe of the scrotum or penis. In females, the fistula may end within the vestibule of the vagina, which is located immediately outside the hymen, or at the perineum.

Because this classification system is somewhat arbitrary, Peña proposed a classification system that specifically and unambiguously describes the location of the fistulous opening. In males the fistula may communicate with: (1) the perineum (cutaneous perineal fistula); (2) the lowest portion of the posterior urethra (rectourethral bulbar fistula); (3) the upper portion of the posterior urethra (rectourethral prostatic fistula); or (4) the bladder neck (rectovesicular fistula). In females, the urethra may open onto the perineum between the female genitalia and the center of the sphincter (cutaneous perineal fistula), or into the vestibule of the vagina (vestibular fistula) (Fig. 38-25). In both sexes, the rectum may end in a completely blind fashion (imperforate anus without fistula). In rare cases, patients may have a normal anal canal, yet there may be total atresia or severe stenosis of the rectum.

The most frequent defect in males is imperforate anus with rectourethral fistula, followed by rectoperineal fistula, then rectovesical fistula or recto–bladder neck. In females, the most frequent defect is the rectovestibular defect, followed by the cutaneous perineal

fistula. The third most common defect in females is the persistent cloaca. This lesion represents a wide spectrum of malformations in which the rectum, vagina, and urinary tract meet and fuse into a single common channel. On physical examination, a single perineal orifice is observed, and is located at the place where the urethra normally opens. Typically, the external genitalia are hypoplastic.

Associated Malformations. Approximately 60% of patients have an associated malformation. The most common is a urinary tract defect, which occurs in approximately 50% of patients. Skeletal defects also are seen, and the sacrum is most commonly involved. Spinal cord anomalies, especially a tethered cord, are common, particularly in children with high lesions. Gastrointestinal anomalies occur, most commonly esophageal atresia. Cardiac anomalies may be noted, and occasionally patients present with a constellation of defects as part of the VACTERRL syndrome (*v*ertebral [missing vertebra] and *a*norectal anomalies, *c*ardiac defects [severe congenital cardiac disease], *t*racheo*e*sophageal fistula, *r*enal anomalies [renal agenesis and renal anomalies], and *r*adial *l*imb hyperplasia).

Management of Patients with Imperforate Anus. Patients with imperforate anus are usually stable, and the diagnosis is readily apparent. Despite the obstruction, the abdomen is initially not distended, and there is rarely any urgency to intervene. The principles of management center around diagnosing the type of defect that is present (high versus low), and evaluating the presence of associated anomalies. It may take up to 24 hours before the presence of a fistula on the skin is noted, and thus it is important to observe the neonate for some time before definitive surgery is undertaken. All patients should therefore have an orogastric tube placed and be monitored for the appearance of meconium in or around the perineum, or in the urine. Investigation for associated defects should include an ultrasound of the abdomen to assess for the presence of urinary tract anomalies. Other tests should include an echocardiogram and spinal radiographs. An ultrasound of the spine should be performed to look for the presence of a tethered cord. To further classify the location of the fistula as either high or low, a lateral abdominal radiograph can be obtained with a radiopaque marker on the perineum. By placing the infant in the inverted position, the distance between the most distal extent of air in the rectum and the perineal surface can be measured. However, this study is imprecise.

The surgical management of infants with imperforate anus is determined by the anatomic defect. In general, when a low lesion is present, only a perineal operation is required, without a colostomy. Infants with a high lesion require a colostomy in the newborn period, followed by a pull-through procedure at approximately 2 months of age. When a persistent cloaca is present, the urinary tract needs to be carefully evaluated at the time of colostomy formation to ensure that normal emptying can occur, and to determine whether the bladder needs to be drained by means of a vesicostomy. If there is any doubt about the type of lesion, it is safer to perform a colostomy rather than jeopardize the infant's long-term chances for continence by performing an injudicious perineal operation.

The type of pull-through procedure favored by most pediatric surgeons today is the posterior sagittal anorectoplasty (PSARP) procedure, as described by Peña and DeVries. This involves dividing the levator ani and external sphincter complex in the midline posteriorly, and bringing down the rectum after sufficient length is achieved. The muscles are then reconstructed and sutured to the rectum. The outcome of 1192 patients who had undergone this procedure was recently reviewed by Peña and Hong. Seventy-five percent of patients were found to have voluntary bowel movements, and nearly 40% were considered totally continent. As a rule, patients with high lesions demonstrate an increased incidence of incontinence, whereas those with low lesions are more likely to be constipated.

JAUNDICE

Approach to the Jaundiced Infant

Jaundice is present during the first week of life in 60% of term infants and 80% of preterm infants. There is usually accumulation of unconjugated bilirubin, but there may also be deposition of direct bilirubin. During fetal life, the placenta is the principal route of elimination of unconjugated bilirubin. In the newborn infant, bilirubin is conjugated through the activity of *glucuronosyltransferase*. In the conjugated form, bilirubin is water soluble, which results in its excretion into the biliary system, then into the gastrointestinal tract. Newborns have a relatively high level of circulating hemoglobin, and relative immaturity of the conjugating machinery. This results in a transient accumulation of bilirubin in the tissues, which is manifested as jaundice. Physiologic jaundice is evident by the second or third day of life, and usually resolves within approximately 5 to 7 days. By definition, jaundice that persists beyond 2 weeks is considered pathologic.

Pathologic jaundice may be due to biliary obstruction, increased hemoglobin load, or to liver dysfunction. The work-up of the jaundiced infant therefore should include a search for the following possibilities: (1) obstructive disorders, including biliary atresia, choledochal cyst, and inspissated bile syndrome; (2) hematologic disorders, including ABO incompatibility, Rh incompatibility, and spherocytosis; (3) metabolic disorders, including alpha$_1$-antitrypsin deficiency, galactosemia, or pyruvate kinase deficiency; and (4) congenital infection, including syphilis and rubella.

Biliary Atresia

Pathogenesis

The most important surgical cause of jaundice in the newborn period is biliary atresia. The incidence of this disease is approximately 1 in 20,000. This disease is characterized by an obliterative process of the extrahepatic bile ducts, and is associated with hepatic fibrosis. The etiology is unknown. In the classic textbook *Abdominal*

Surgery of Infancy and Childhood, Ladd and Gross described the cause of biliary atresia as an "... arrest of development during the solid stage of bile duct formation." More recent evidence suggests an acquired basis for this disease, and studies in both animals and humans have implicated a role for the immune system and systemic viral infections in its pathogenesis.

Clinical Presentation

Jaundice, a constant finding, is usually present at birth or shortly thereafter, but may go undetected or may be regarded as physiologic until the child is 2 or 3 weeks old. The infant demonstrates acholic, grey-appearing stools, secondary to obstructed bile flow. Infants with biliary atresia also manifest progressive failure to thrive, and if untreated, progress to develop stigmata of liver failure and portal hypertension, particularly splenomegaly and esophageal varices. The obliterative process involves the common duct, cystic duct, one or both hepatic ducts, and the gallbladder, in a variety of combinations. Approximately 25% of patients have coincidental malformations often associated with polysplenia, and may include intestinal malrotation, preduodenal portal vein, and intrahepatic vena cava.

Diagnosis

Generally, a combination of investigations is required in order to ascertain the diagnosis of biliary atresia, as no single test is sufficiently sensitive or specific. In many centers the nuclear medicine scan using technetium-99m (^{99m}Tc) iminodiacetate (DISIDA), performed after pretreatment of the patient with phenobarbital, has proven to be an accurate and reliable study. If radionuclide appears in the intestine, extrahepatic bile duct patency is ensured and the diagnosis of biliary atresia is excluded. If radiopharmaceutical is normally concentrated by the liver but not excreted despite treatment with phenobarbital, and the metabolic screen, particularly alpha$_1$-antitrypsin determination, is normal, the presumptive diagnosis is biliary atresia. An ultrasound may be performed to assess for the presence of other causes of biliary tract obstruction, including choledochal cyst. The presence of a gallbladder is also evaluated, although it is important to emphasize that the presence of a gallbladder does not exclude the diagnosis of biliary atresia. In approximately 10% of patients, the distal biliary tract is patent and a gallbladder may be visualized, even though the proximal ducts are atretic. It is worth noting that the intrahepatic bile ducts are never dilated in the patient with biliary atresia. A percutaneous liver biopsy may at times differentiate biliary atresia from neonatal hepatitis. When these tests point to a diagnosis of biliary atresia, surgical exploration is warranted. At surgery a cholangiogram is performed, using the gallbladder as a conduit. This demonstrates the anatomy of the biliary tree, determines whether extrahepatic bile duct atresia is present, and evaluates whether there is distal bile flow into the duodenum. The cholangiogram may demonstrate hypoplasia of the extrahepatic biliary system. This condition is associated with hepatic parenchymal disorders that cause severe intrahepatic cholestasis, including alpha$_1$-antitrypsin deficiency and arteriohepatic dysplasia (Alagille's syndrome).

The presentation of biliary atresia closely mimics that of *inspissated bile syndrome.* This term is applied to patients with normal biliary tracts who have persistent obstructive jaundice. Increased viscosity of bile and obstruction of the canaliculi are implicated as causes. The condition has been seen in infants receiving parenteral nutrition, but it is also encountered in conditions associated with hemolysis, or in cystic fibrosis. In some instances, no etiologic factors can be defined. *Neonatal hepatitis* may present in a fashion

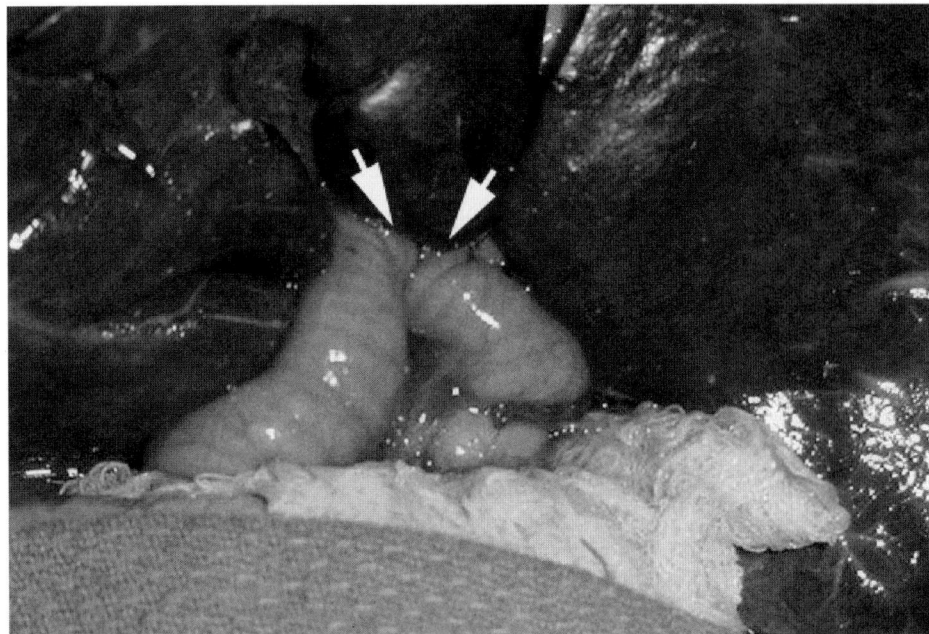

FIG. 38-26. Operative photograph showing the Kasai portoenterostomy. Arrows denote site of the anastomosis. Note the engorged liver.

similar to biliary atresia. This disease is characterized by persistent jaundice due to acquired biliary inflammation without obliteration of the bile ducts. There may be a viral etiology, and the disease is usually self-limited.

Treatment

If the intraoperative cholangiogram confirms the presence of biliary atresia, then surgical correction should be immediately undertaken. The most effective surgical treatment for biliary atresia is the portoenterostomy, as described by Kasai. The purpose of this procedure is to promote bile flow into the intestine. The procedure is based on Kasai's observation that the fibrous tissue at the porta hepatis invests microscopically patent biliary ductules, that in turn communicate with the intrahepatic ductal system (Fig. 38-26). Transecting this fibrous tissue, which is invariably encountered cephalad to the bifurcating portal vein, opens these channels and establishes bile flow into a surgically constructed intestinal conduit, usually a Roux-en-Y limb of jejunum (Fig. 38-27). Some authors believe that an intussuscepted antireflux valve is useful in preventing retrograde bile reflux, although the data suggest that it does not impact outcome. A liver biopsy is performed at the time of surgery to determine the degree of hepatic fibrosis that is present. The likelihood of surgical success is increased if the procedure is accomplished before the infant attains the age of 8 weeks. Although the outlook is less favorable for patients after the twelfth week, it is reasonable to proceed with surgery even beyond this point, as the alternative is certain liver failure. It is noteworthy that a significant number of patients do have favorable outcomes when operated on at this time.

Bile drainage is anticipated when the operation is carried out early; however, bile flow does not necessarily imply cure. Approximately one-third of patients remain symptom free after portoenterostomy, the remainder require liver transplantation due to progressive liver failure. Independent risk factors that predict failure of the procedure include bridging liver fibrosis at the time of surgery and postoperative cholangitic episodes. A recent review of the data of the Japanese Biliary Atresia Registry (JBAR), which includes

the results of 1381 patients, showed that the 10-year survival rate without transplantation was 53%; with transplantation the rate was 66.7%. A common postoperative complication is cholangitis. There is no effective strategy to completely eliminate this complication, and the effectiveness of long-term prophylactic antibiotics has not been fully resolved.

Choledochal Cyst

Classification

The term *choledochal cyst* refers to a spectrum of congenital biliary tract disorders that were previously grouped under the name "idiopathic dilation of the common bile duct." After the classification system proposed by Alonso-Lej, five types of choledochal cyst were described. A type I cyst is characterized by fusiform dilatation of the bile duct. This is the most common type and is found in 80 to 90% of cases. A type II choledochal cyst appears as an isolated diverticulum protruding from the wall of the common bile duct. The cyst may be joined to the common bile duct by a narrow stalk. Type III choledochal cysts arise from the intraduodenal portion of the common bile duct and are also known as choledochoceles. Type IVA cysts consist of multiple dilatations of the intrahepatic and extrahepatic bile ducts. Type IVB choledochal cysts are multiple dilatations involving only the extrahepatic bile ducts. Type V (Caroli's disease) consists of multiple dilatations limited to the intrahepatic bile ducts.

Choledochal cysts are most appropriately considered the predominant feature in a constellation of pathologic abnormalities that can occur within the pancreatobiliary system. Frequently associated with choledochal cyst is an anomalous junction of the pancreatic and common bile ducts. The etiology of choledochal cyst is controversial. Babbit proposed an abnormal pancreatic and biliary duct junction, with the formation of a common channel into which pancreatic enzymes are secreted. This process results in weakening of the bile duct wall by gradual enzymatic destruction, leading to dilatation, inflammation, and finally cyst formation. Not all patients with choledochal cysts demonstrate an anatomic common channel, which raises questions regarding the accuracy of this model.

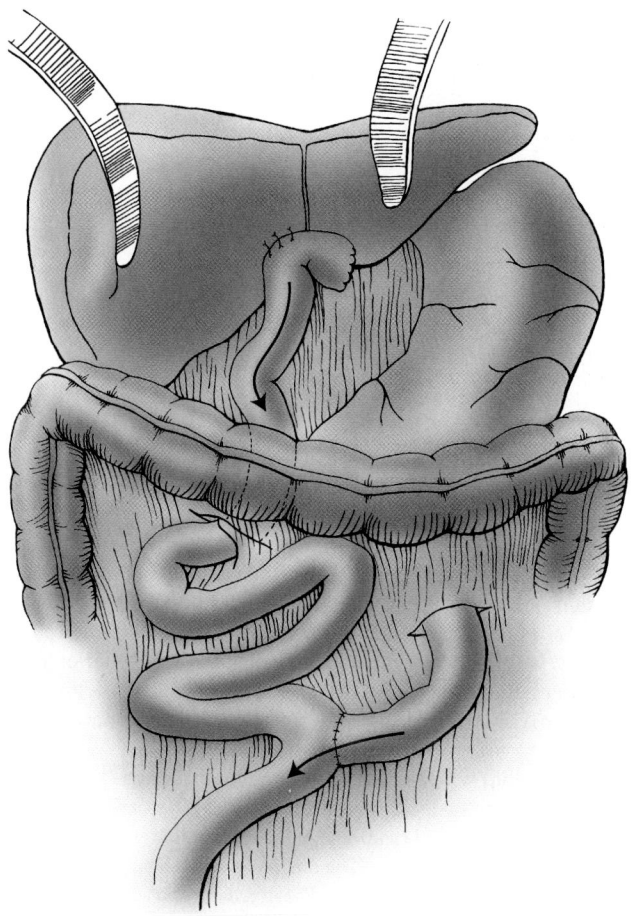

FIG. 38-27. Schematic illustration of the Kasai portoenterostomy for biliary atresia. An isolated limb of jejunum is brought to the porta hepatis and anastomosed to the transected ducts at the liver plate.

Clinical Presentation

Choledochal cysts are more common in females than in males (4:1). Typically these present in children beyond the toddler age group. The classic symptom triad consists of abdominal pain, mass, and jaundice. However, this complex is actually encountered in fewer than half of the patients. The more usual presentation is that of episodic abdominal pain, often recurring over the course of months or years, and generally is associated with only minimal jaundice that may escape detection. If the condition is not recognized, the patient develops cholangitis, which may lead to the development of cirrhosis and portal hypertension. Choledochal cysts can present in the newborn period, when the symptoms are similar to those of biliary atresia. Often neonates will have an abdominal mass at presentation.

Diagnosis

A choledochal cyst is frequently diagnosed in the fetus at a screening prenatal ultrasound. In the older child or adolescent, abdominal ultrasonography may reveal a cystic structure arising from the biliary tree. CT scan will confirm the diagnosis. These studies will demonstrate the dimensions of the cyst and define its relationship to the vascular structures in the porta hepatis, as well as the intrahepatic ductal configuration. Endoscopic retrograde cholangiopancreatography (ERCP) is reserved for patients in whom confusion remains after evaluation by less-invasive imaging modalities. Magnetic resonance cholangiopancreatography may provide a more

detailed depiction of the anatomy of the cyst, and its relationship to the bifurcation of the hepatic ducts and the pancreas.

Treatment

The cyst wall is composed of fibrous tissue and is devoid of mucosal lining. As a result, the treatment of choledochal cysts is surgical excision followed by biliary-enteric reconstruction. There is no role for internal drainage by cystenterostomy, which leaves the cyst wall intact and leads to the inevitable development of cholangitis. Rarely, choledochal cyst can lead to the development of a biliary tract malignancy. This provides a further rationale for complete cyst excision.

Resection of the cyst requires circumferential dissection. The posterior plane between the cyst and portal vein must be carefully dissected to accomplish removal. The pancreatic duct, which may enter the distal cyst, is vulnerable to injury during distal cyst excision, but this can be avoided by avoiding entry into the pancreatic parenchyma. In cases in which the pericystic inflammation is extremely dense, it may be unsafe to attempt complete cyst removal. In this instance, it is reasonable to dissect within the posterior wall of the cyst, which allows the inner lining of the back wall to be dissected free from the outer layer that directly overlies the portal vascular structures. The lateral and anterior cyst, as well as the internal aspect of the back wall, is removed, yet the outer posterior wall remains behind. Cyst excision is accomplished, and the proximal bile duct is anastomosed to the intestinal tract.

The prognosis for children who have undergone complete excision of a choledochal cyst is excellent. Complications include anastomotic stricture, cholangitis, and intrahepatic stone formation. These complications may develop a long time after surgery has been completed.

DEFORMITIES OF THE ABDOMINAL WALL

Embryology

The abdominal wall is formed by four separate embryologic folds—cephalic, caudal, and right and left lateral folds—each of which is composed of somatic and splanchnic layers. Each of the folds develops toward the anterior center portion of the celomic cavity, joining to form a large umbilical ring that surrounds the two umbilical arteries, the vein, and the yolk sac or omphalomesenteric duct. These structures are covered by an outer layer of amnion, and the entire unit composes the umbilical cord. Between the fifth and tenth weeks of fetal development, the intestinal tract undergoes rapid growth outside the abdominal cavity within the proximal portion of the umbilical cord. As development is completed, the intestine gradually returns to the abdominal cavity. Contraction of the umbilical ring completes the process of abdominal wall formation.

Failure of the cephalic fold to close results in sternal defects such as congenital absence of the sternum. Failure of the caudal fold to close results in exstrophy of the bladder, and in more extreme cases, exstrophy of the cloaca. Interruption of central migration of the lateral folds results in omphalocele. Gastroschisis, originally thought to be a variant of omphalocele, probably results from a fetal accident in the form of intrauterine rupture of a hernia of the umbilical cord.

Umbilical Hernia

Failure of the umbilical ring to close results in a central defect in the linea alba. The resulting umbilical hernia is covered by normal umbilical skin and subcutaneous tissue, but the fascial defect allows

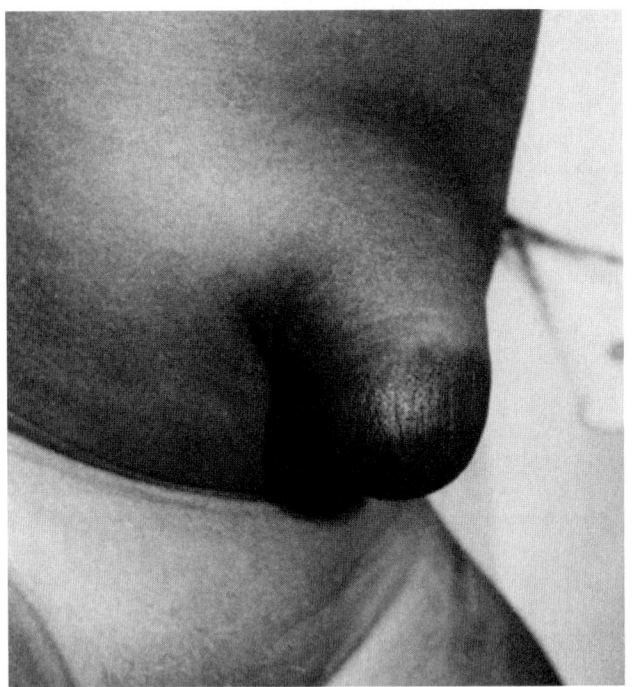

FIG. 38-28. Umbilical hernia in a 1-year-old female.

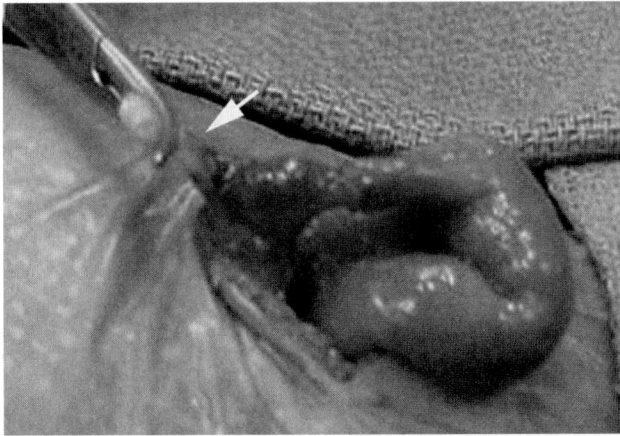

FIG. 38-29. Patent vitelline duct. Note the communication between the umbilicus and the small bowel at the site of a Meckel's diverticulum.

protrusion of abdominal contents. Hernias less than 1 cm in size at the time of birth usually will close spontaneously by 4 years of age. Sometimes the hernia is large enough that the protrusion is disfiguring and disturbing to both the child and the family. In such circumstances early repair may be advisable (Fig. 38-28).

Umbilical hernias are generally asymptomatic protrusions of the abdominal wall. They are generally noted by parents or physicians on physical examination, and present for a surgical opinion out of concerns for possible incarceration. Although incarceration rarely is seen in an umbilical hernia, it can happen. Children present with abdominal pain, bilious emesis, and a tender, hard mass protruding from the umbilicus. This constellation of symptoms mandates immediate exploration and repair of the hernia. More commonly, the child is asymptomatic and treatment is governed by the size of the defect, the age of the patient, and the concern that the child and family have regarding the cosmetic appearance of the abdomen. When the defect is small and spontaneous closure is likely, most surgeons will delay surgical correction until 4 or 5 years of age. If closure does not occur by this time, it is reasonable to repair the hernia. If a younger child has an extremely large hernia, or if the family or child is bothered by the cosmetic appearance, then repair is indicated.

Repair of uncomplicated umbilical hernia is performed under general anesthesia as an outpatient procedure. A small curving incision that fits into the skin crease of the umbilicus is made, and the sac is dissected free from the overlying skin. The fascial defect is repaired with permanent or long-lasting absorbable interrupted sutures that are placed in a transverse plane. The skin is closed using subcuticular sutures.

Patent Urachus

During the development of the celomic cavity, there is free communication between the urinary bladder and the abdominal wall through the urachus, which exits adjacent to the omphalomesenteric duct. Persistence of this tract results in a communication between the bladder and the umbilicus. The first sign of a patent urachus is moisture or urine flow from the umbilicus. Recurrent urinary tract infection can result. The urachus may be partially obliterated, with a remnant remaining beneath the umbilicus in the extraperitoneal position as an isolated cyst that may be identified by ultrasound. Such a cyst usually presents as an inflammatory mass inferior to the umbilicus. Initial treatment is drainage of the infected cyst, followed by cyst excision as a separate procedure once the inflammation has resolved.

In the child with a persistently draining umbilicus, a diagnosis of patent urachus should be considered. The differential diagnosis includes an umbilical granuloma, which generally responds to local application of silver nitrate. The diagnosis of patent urachus is confirmed by umbilical exploration. The urachal tract is excised and the bladder is closed. A patent vitelline duct also may present with umbilical drainage. In this circumstance, there is a communication with the small intestine, often at the site of a Meckel's diverticulum (Fig. 38-29). Treatment includes umbilical exploration with resection of the involved bowel.

Omphalocele

Clinical Presentation

Omphalocele refers to a congenital defect of the abdominal wall in which the bowel and solid viscera are covered by peritoneum and amniotic membrane (Fig. 38-30). The umbilical cord inserts into the sac. The abdominal wall defect can measure 4 cm or more in diameter. The incidence is approximately 1 in 5000 live births, and it occurs in association with special syndromes such as exstrophy of the cloaca (vesicointestinal fissure), the Beckwith-Wiedemann constellation of anomalies (macroglossia, macrosomia, hypoglycemia, visceromegaly, and omphalocele), and Cantrell's pentalogy (lower thoracic wall malformations [cleft sternum], ectopia cordis, epigastric omphalocele, anterior midline diaphragmatic hernia, and cardiac anomalies). The size of the defect may be very small, or large enough that it contains most of the abdominal viscera. There is a 60 to 70% incidence of associated anomalies, especially cardiac (20 to 40% of cases) and chromosomal abnormalities. Chromosomal anomalies are more common in children with smaller defects. Omphalocele is associated with prematurity (10 to 50% of cases) and intrauterine growth restriction (20% of cases).

Treatment

Immediate treatment of an infant with omphalocele consists of attending to the vital signs and maintaining the body temperature. The omphalocele should be covered with saline-soaked gauze and

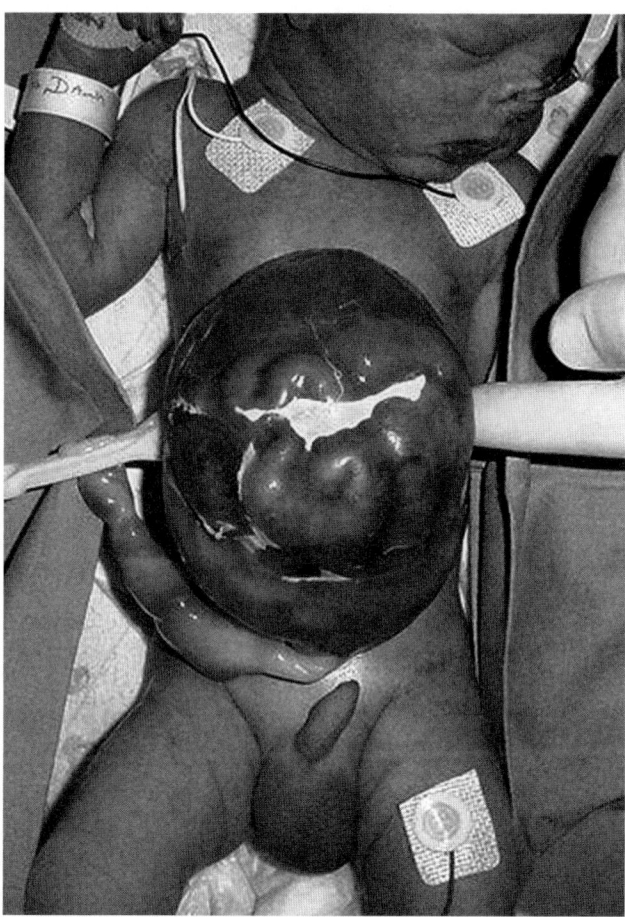

FIG. 38-30. *Giant omphalocele in a newborn male.*

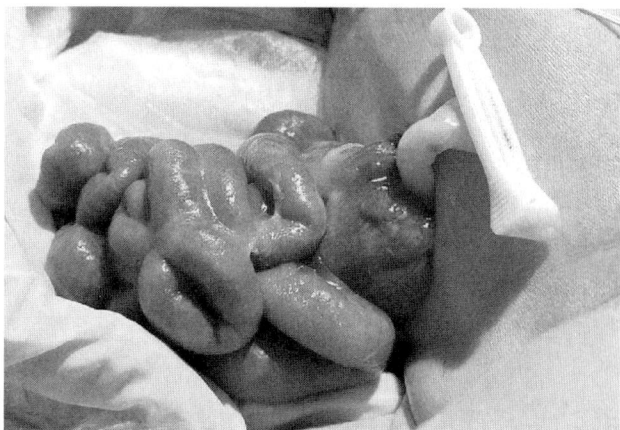

FIG. 38-31. *Gastroschisis in a newborn. Note the location of the umbilical cord, and the edematous, thickened bowel.*

the trunk should be wrapped circumferentially. No pressure should be placed on the omphalocele sac in an effort to reduce its contents, as this maneuver may increase the risk of rupture of the sac, or may interfere with abdominal venous return. Prophylactic antibiotics should be administered in case of rupture. Whenever possible, a primary repair of the omphalocele should be undertaken. This involves resection of the omphalocele membrane and closure of the fascia. A layer of prosthetic material may be required to achieve closure.

Occasionally, an infant will have a giant omphalocele (defect greater than 7 cm in diameter) that cannot be closed primarily because there is simply no room to reduce the viscera into the abdominal cavity (see Fig. 38-30). Other infants may have associated congenital anomalies that complicate surgical repair. Under these circumstances, a nonoperative approach can be used. The omphalocele sac can be treated with desiccating substances such as povidone-iodine. It typically takes 2 to 3 months before reepithelialization occurs. In the past, mercury compounds were used, but have been discontinued because of associated systemic toxicity.

Gastroschisis

Clinical Presentation

Gastroschisis represents a congenital defect characterized by a defect in the anterior abdominal wall through which the intestinal contents freely protrude. Unlike the omphalocele, there is no overlying sac and the size of the defect is much smaller (<4 cm). The abdominal wall defect is located at the junction of the umbilicus and normal skin, and is almost always to the right of the umbilicus

(Fig. 38-31). The umbilicus becomes partly detached, allowing free communication with the abdominal cavity. The appearance of the bowel provides some information with respect to the in utero timing of the defect. The intestine may be normal in appearance, suggesting that the rupture occurred relatively late during the pregnancy. More commonly, however, the intestine is thick, edematous, discolored, and covered with exudate, implying a more long-standing process.

Unlike infants born with omphalocele, associated anomalies seen with gastroschisis consist mostly of intestinal atresia. This defect can readily be diagnosed on prenatal ultrasound (Fig. 38-32). There is no advantage to performing a cesarean section over a vaginal delivery. Even though the thickness of the peel on the surface of the bowel indicates that a shorter gestational time would be less injurious, there is no benefit to early versus late delivery.

Treatment

All infants born with gastroschisis require urgent surgical treatment. In many instances, the intestine can be returned to the abdominal cavity, and a primary surgical closure of the abdominal wall is performed. Techniques that facilitate primary closure include mechanical stretching of the abdominal wall, thorough orogastric suctioning with foregut decompression, rectal irrigation, and evacuation of all meconium. Care must be taken to prevent increased abdominal

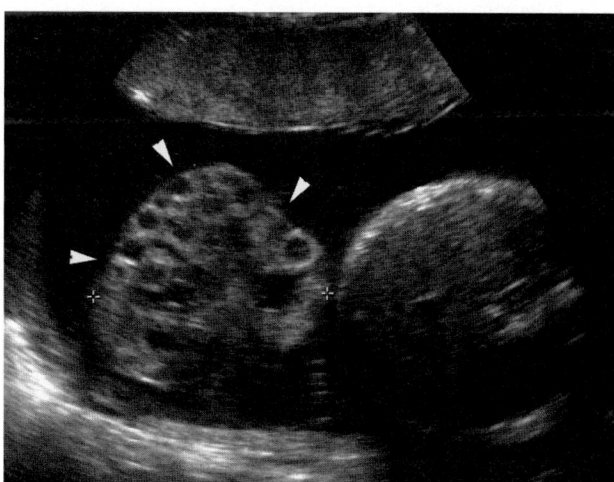

FIG. 38-32. *Prenatal ultrasound of a fetus at 30 weeks' gestation with a gastroschisis. Arrows point to the bowel outside within the amniotic fluid.*

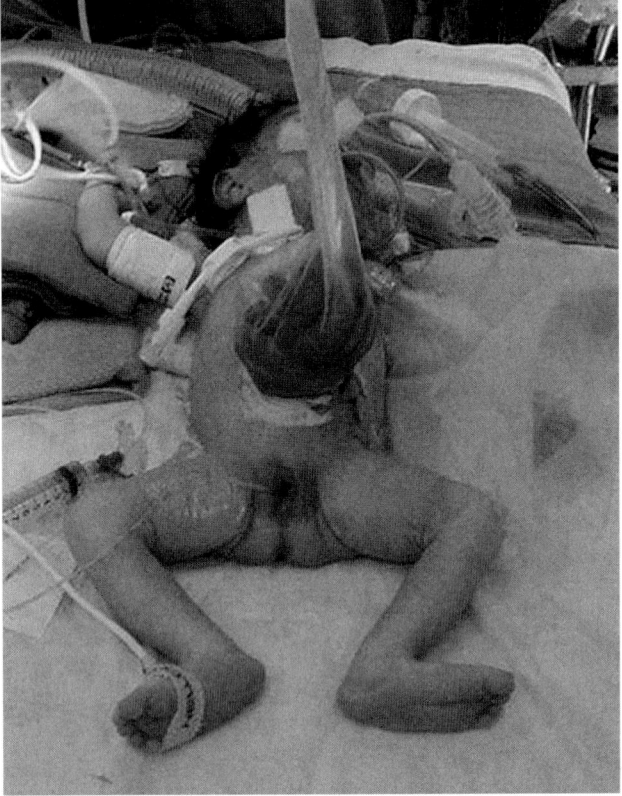

FIG. 38-33. *Use of a silo with a gastroschisis to allow the bowel wall edema to resolve and to facilitate closure of the abdominal wall.*

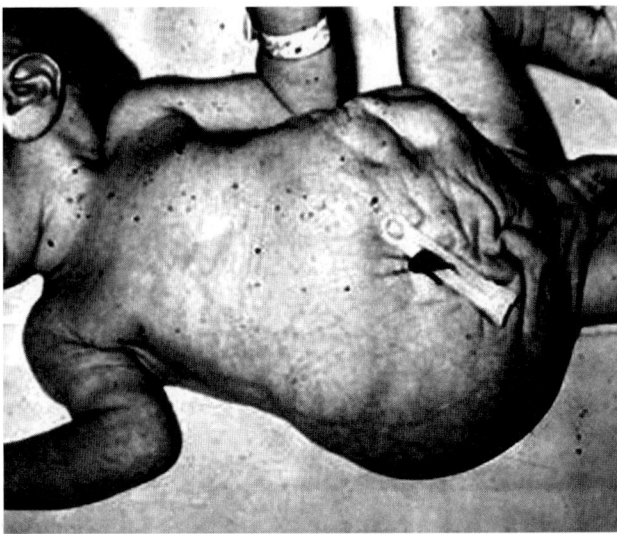

FIG. 38-34. *Eagle-Barrett (prune-belly) syndrome. Notice the lax, flaccid abdomen.*

pressure during the reduction, which would lead to compression of the inferior vena cava, respiratory dysfunction, and result in abdominal compartment syndrome. To avoid this complication, it is helpful to monitor the bladder or airway pressure during reduction. In infants whose intestine has become thickened and edematous, it may be impossible to reduce the bowel into the peritoneal cavity in the immediate postnatal period. Under such circumstances, a plastic spring-loaded silo can be placed onto the bowel and secured beneath the fascia. The silo covers the bowel and allows for graduated reduction on a daily basis as the edema in the bowel wall decreases (Fig. 38-33). Surgical closure can usually be accomplished within approximately 1 week. A prosthetic piece of material (e.g., GoreTex or Surgisis) may be required to bring the edges of the fascia together. If an atresia is noted at the time of closure, it is prudent to reduce the bowel at the first operation, then to return after several weeks once the edema has resolved to correct the atresia. Intestinal function does not typically return for several weeks in patients with gastroschisis. This is especially true if the bowel is thickened and edematous. As a result, these patients will require central line placement and institution of total parenteral nutrition in order to grow.

Prune-Belly Syndrome

Clinical Presentation

Prune-belly syndrome refers to a disorder that is characterized by a constellation of symptoms including extremely lax lower abdominal musculature, dilated urinary tract including the bladder, and bilateral undescended testes (Fig. 38-34). The term *prune-belly syndrome* appropriately describes the wrinkled appearance of the anterior abdominal wall that characterizes these patients. Prune-belly

syndrome is also known as Eagle-Barrett syndrome and the triad syndrome, because of the three major manifestations. The incidence is significantly higher in males. Patients manifest a variety of comorbidities. The most significant is that of pulmonary hypoplasia, which can lead to death in the most severe cases. Skeletal abnormalities include dislocation or dysplasia of the hip and pectus excavatum.

The major genitourinary manifestation in prune-belly syndrome is ureteral dilation. The ureters are typically long and tortuous, and become more dilated distally. Ureteric obstruction is rarely present, and the dilation is thought to be caused by decreased smooth muscle and increased collagen in the ureters. Approximately 80% of individuals will have some degree of vesicoureteral reflux, which can predispose to urinary tract infection. Despite the marked dilatation of the urinary tract, most children with prune-belly syndrome have adequate renal parenchyma for growth and development. Factors associated with the development of long-term renal failure include the presence of abnormal kidneys on ultrasound or renal scan and persistent pyelonephritis.

Treatment

Despite the ureteric dilation, there is currently no role for ureteric surgery unless an area of obstruction develops. The testes are invariably intra-abdominal and bilateral orchiopexy can be performed in conjunction with abdominal wall reconstruction at 6 to 12 months of age. Despite orchiopexy, fertility in a boy with prune-belly syndrome is unlikely, as spermatogenesis over time is insufficient. Deficiencies in the production of prostatic fluid and a predisposition toward retrograde ejaculation contribute to infertility. Abdominal wall repair is accomplished through an abdominoplasty, which typically requires a transverse incision in the lower abdomen extending into the flanks.

Inguinal Hernia

An understanding of the management of pediatric inguinal hernias is a central component of modern pediatric surgical practice. Inguinal hernia repair represents one of the most common operations performed in children. The presence of an inguinal hernia in a child is an indication for surgical repair. Surgery to repair an inguinal hernia is termed a *herniorrhaphy*, because it involves closing off the patent processus vaginalis. This is in contrast with the *hernioplasty* that is performed in adults, which requires reconstruction of the inguinal floor.

Embryology

In order to understand how to diagnose and treat inguinal hernias in children, it is critical to understand the embryologic origin. It is useful to describe these events to the parents, who are often under the misconception that the hernia was somehow caused by their inability to console their crying child, or the child's high activity level. Inguinal hernia results from a failure of closure of the processus vaginalis, a finger-like projection of the peritoneum that accompanies the testicle as it descends into the scrotum. Closure of the processus vaginalis normally occurs a few months prior to birth. This explains the high incidence of inguinal hernias in premature infants. When the processus vaginalis remains completely patent, a communication persists between the peritoneal cavity and the groin, resulting in a hernia. Partial closure can result in entrapped fluid, which results in the presence of a hydrocele. A *communicating hydrocele* refers to a hydrocele that is in communication with the peritoneal cavity, and can therefore be thought of as a hernia. Using the classification system that is typically applied to adult hernias, all congenital hernias in children are by definition indirect inguinal hernias. Children also present with direct inguinal and femoral hernias, although these are much less common.

Clinical Manifestations

Inguinal hernias occur more commonly in males than females (10:1), and are more common on the right side than the left. Infants are at high risk for incarceration of an inguinal hernia because of the narrow inguinal ring. Patients most commonly present with a groin bulge that is noticed by the parents as they change the diaper (Fig. 38-35). Older children may notice the bulge themselves. On examination, the cord on the affected side will be thicker, and pressure on the lower abdomen usually will display the hernia on the affected side. The presence of an incarcerated hernia is manifested by a firm bulge that does not spontaneously resolve, and may be associated with fussiness and irritability in the child. The infant that has a strangulated inguinal hernia will manifest an edematous, tender bulge in the groin, occasionally with overlying skin changes. The child will eventually develop intestinal obstruction, peritonitis, and systemic toxicity.

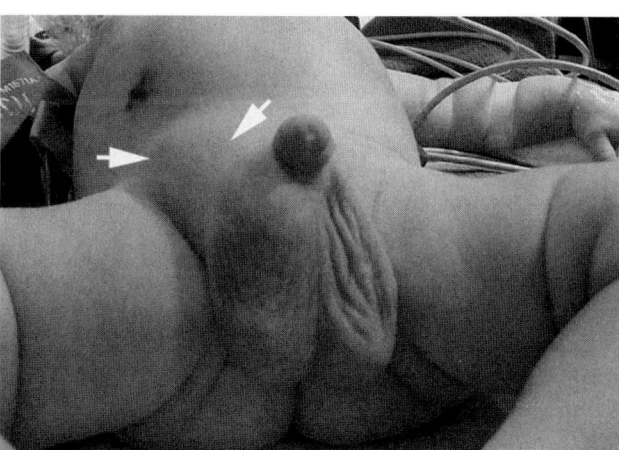

FIG. 38-35. *Right inguinal hernia in a 4-month-old male. The arrows point to the bulge in the right groin.*

Usually an incarcerated hernia can be reduced. Occasionally this may require light sedation. Gentle pressure is applied on the sac from below in the direction of the internal inguinal ring. Following reduction of the incarcerated hernia, the child may be admitted for observation, and herniorrhaphy is performed within the next 24 hours to prevent recurrent incarceration. Alternatively, the child may be scheduled for surgery at the next available time slot. If the hernia cannot be reduced, or if evidence of strangulation is present, emergency surgery is necessary. This may require a laparotomy and bowel resection.

When the diagnosis of inguinal hernia is made in an otherwise normal child, operative repair should be planned. Spontaneous resolution does not occur and therefore a nonoperative approach can never be justified. An inguinal hernia in a female frequently contains an ovary rather than intestine. Although the gonad usually can be reduced into the abdomen by gentle pressure, it often prolapses in and out until surgical repair is carried out. In some patients, the ovary and fallopian tube constitute one wall of the hernial sac (sliding hernia), and in these patients the ovary can be reduced effectively only at the time of operation. If the ovary is irreducible, prompt hernia repair is indicated to prevent ovarian torsion or strangulation.

When a hydrocele is diagnosed in infancy and there is no evidence of a hernia, observation is proper therapy until the child is older than 12 months. If the hydrocele has not disappeared by 12 months, invariably there is a patent processus vaginalis, and operative hydrocelectomy with excision of the processus vaginalis is indicated. When the first signs of a hydrocele are seen after 12 months of age, the patient should undergo elective hydrocelectomy, which in a child is always performed through a groin incision. Aspiration of hydroceles is discouraged, since almost all without a patent processus vaginalis will resorb spontaneously, and those with a communication to the peritoneum will recur and require operative repair eventually.

Surgical Repair

The repair of a pediatric inguinal hernia can be extremely challenging, particularly in the premature child with incarceration. A small incision is made in a skin crease in the groin directly over the internal inguinal ring. Scarpa's fascia is seen and divided. The external oblique muscle is dissected free from overlying tissue, and the location of the external ring is confirmed. The external oblique aponeurosis is then opened along the direction of the external ring. The undersurface of the external oblique is then cleared from surrounding tissue. The cremasteric fibers are separated from the cord structures and hernia sac, and then are elevated into the wound. Care is taken not to grasp the vas deferens. The hernia sac then is dissected up to the internal ring and doubly suture ligated. The distal part of the hernia sac is opened widely to drain any hydrocele fluid. When the hernia is very large and the patient very small, tightening of the internal inguinal ring or even formal repair of the inguinal floor may be necessary, although the vast majority of children do not require any treatment beyond high ligation of the hernia sac.

Controversy exists regarding the role for exploration of an asymptomatic opposite side in a child with an inguinal hernia. Several reports indicate that frequency of a patent processus vaginalis on the side opposite the obvious hernia is approximately 30%, although this figure decreases with increasing age of the child. Management options include never exploring the opposite side or to explore only under certain conditions, such as in premature infants or in patients in whom incarceration is present. The opposite side may be explored laparoscopically. To do so, a blunt 4-mm trocar is placed into the hernia sac of the affected side. The abdominal cavity is insufflated, and the 4-mm 70 degree camera is placed through the trocar such that the opposite side is visualized. The status of the processus vaginalis on the opposite side can be visualized. However, the presence of a patent processus vaginalis by laparoscopy does not always imply the presence of a hernia.

Several authors have now reported a completely laparoscopic approach in the management of inguinal hernias in children. This technique requires insufflation through the umbilicus, and the placement of an extraperitoneal suture to ligate the hernia sac. Proponents of this procedure emphasize the fact that no groin incision is used and there is a decreased chance of injuring cord structures. The long-term results of this technique remain to be established.

Inguinal hernias in children recur in less than 1% of patients, and recurrences usually result from missed hernia sacs at the first procedure, a direct hernia, or a missed femoral hernia. All children should have local anesthetic administered either by caudal injection or by direct injection into the wound. Spinal anesthesia in preterm infants decreases the risk of postoperative apnea when compared with general anesthesia.

GENITALIA

Undescended Testis

Embryology

The term *undescended testicle* (cryptorchidism) refers to the interruption of the normal descent of the testis into the scrotum. The testicle may reside in the retroperineum, in the internal inguinal ring, in the inguinal canal, or even at the external ring. The testicle begins as a thickening on the urogenital ridge in the fifth to sixth week of embryologic life. In the seventh and eighth months the testicle descends along the inguinal canal into the upper scrotum, and with its progress the processus vaginalis is formed and pulled along with the migrating testicle. At birth, approximately 95% of infants have the testicle normally positioned in the scrotum.

A distinction should be made between the undescended testicle and the ectopic testicle. By definition, an ectopic testis is one that has passed through the external ring in the normal pathway, and then has come to rest in an abnormal location overlying the rectus abdominis or external oblique muscle, the soft tissue of the medial thigh, or behind the scrotum in the perineum. A congenitally absent testicle results from failure of normal development or an intrauterine accident leading to loss of blood supply to the developing testicle.

Clinical Presentation

The incidence of undescended testes is approximately 30% in preterm infants, and 1 to 3% at term. For diagnosis, the child should be examined in the supine position, where visual inspection may reveal a hypoplastic or poorly rugated scrotum. A unilateral undescended testicle usually can be palpated in the inguinal canal or in the upper scrotum. Occasionally, the testicle will be difficult or impossible to palpate, indicating either an abdominal testicle or congenital absence of the gonad. If the testicle is not palpable in the supine position, the child should be examined with his legs crossed while seated. This maneuver diminishes the cremasteric reflex and facilitates identification of the location of the testicle.

It is now established that cryptorchid testes demonstrate an increased predisposition to malignant degeneration. In addition, fertility is decreased when the testicle is not in the scrotum. For these reasons, surgical placement of the testicle in the scrotum (orchidopexy) is indicated. It should be emphasized that this procedure does improve the fertility potential, although fertility is never normal. Similarly, the testicle is still at risk of malignant change, although its location in the scrotum facilitates potentially earlier detection of a testicular malignancy. Other reasons to consider orchidopexy include the risk of trauma to the testicle located at the pubic tubercle, an increased incidence of torsion, and the psychologic impact of an empty scrotum in a developing male. The reason for malignant degeneration is not established, but the evidence points to an inherent abnormality of the testicle that predisposes it to incomplete descent and malignancy, rather than malignancy as a result of an abnormal environment.

Treatment

Males with bilateral undescended testicles are often infertile. When the testicle is not within the scrotum, it is subjected to a higher temperature, resulting in decreased spermatogenesis. Mengel and coworkers studied 515 undescended testicles by histology and demonstrated a decreasing presence of spermatogonia after 2 years of age. Consequently it is now recommended that the undescended testicle be surgically repositioned by 2 years of age. Despite orchidopexy, the incidence of infertility is approximately two times higher in men with unilateral orchidopexy compared to men with normal testicular descent.

The use of chorionic gonadotropin occasionally may be effective in patients with bilateral undescended testes, suggesting that these patients are more apt to have a hormone deficiency than children with unilateral undescended testicle. If there is no testicular descent after a month of endocrine therapy, operative correction should be undertaken. A child with unilateral cryptorchidism should have surgical correction of the problem. The operation is typically performed through a combined groin and scrotal incision. The cord vessels are fully mobilized, and the testicle is placed in a dartos pouch within the scrotum. An inguinal hernia often accompanies a cryptorchid testis. This should be repaired at the time of orchidopexy.

Patients with a nonpalpable testicle present a challenge in management. The current approach involves laparoscopy to identify the location of the testicle. If the spermatic cord is found to traverse the internal ring, or the testis is found at the ring and can be delivered into the scrotum, a groin incision is made and an orchidopexy is performed. If an abdominal testis is identified that is too far to reach the scrotum, a two-staged Fowler-Stephens approach is used. In the first stage, the testicular vessels are clipped laparoscopically. The orchidopexy then is performed through the groin approximately 6 months later, after which time collateral flow supplies the testicle. It is preferable to preserve the testicular vessels whenever possible. When the testicle is within 1 or 2 cm from the ring, its blood supply may be preserved by mobilizing the testicular vessels up to the renal hilum, then releasing the peritoneal attachments. This often provides sufficient length to allow an orchidopexy to be performed through the groin.

Some patients who have an absent testis are greatly bothered by this anatomic deficiency. Prostheses of all sizes are now available, and can be simply inserted into the scrotum, achieving normal appearance and a normal structure for palpation. Any patient who has an undescended testicle corrected surgically should be examined yearly by the surgeon until his mid-teenage years. At that time, the individual should be thoroughly informed about the possibility of malignant degeneration, and be instructed in self-examination, which should be carried out at least twice a year for life.

Vaginal Anomalies

Surgical diseases of the vagina in children are either congenital or acquired. Congenital anomalies include a spectrum of diseases that include simple defects (imperforate hymen) to more complex forms of vaginal atresia, including distal, proximal, and most severe, complete. These defects are produced by abnormal development of müllerian ducts and/or urogenital sinus. The diagnosis is made most often by physical examination. Secretions into the obstructed vagina produce hydrocolpos, which may present as a large, painful abdominal mass. The anatomy may be defined using ultrasound. Pelvic MRI provides the most thorough and accurate assessment of the pelvic structure. Treatment is dependent on the extent of the defect. For an imperforate hymen, division of the hymen is curative. More complex forms of vaginal atresia require mobilization of the vaginal remnants and creating an anastomosis at the perineum. Laparoscopy can be extremely useful in mobilizing the vagina, in draining hydrocolpos, and in evaluating the internal genitalia. Complete vaginal atresia requires the construction of skin flaps or the creation of a neovagina using a segment of colon.

The most common acquired disorder of the vagina is the straddle injury. This often occurs as young girls fall on blunt objects that cause a direct injury to the perineum. Typical manifestations include vaginal bleeding and inability to void. Unless the injury is extremely superficial, patients should be examined in the operating room, where the lighting is optimal and sedation can be administered. Vaginal lacerations are repaired using absorbable sutures, and the proximity to the urethra should be carefully assessed. Prior to discharge, it is important that patients be voiding spontaneously. In all cases of vaginal trauma, it is essential that the patient be assessed for the presence of sexual abuse.

Ovarian Cysts and Tumors

Pathologic Classification

Ovarian cysts and tumors may be classified as non-neoplastic or neoplastic. Non-neoplastic lesions include cysts (e.g., simple, follicular, inclusion, paraovarian, or corpus luteum), endometriosis, and inflammatory lesions. Neoplastic lesions are classified based on the three primordia that contribute to the ovary: mesenchymal components of the urogenital ridge, germinal epithelium overlying the urogenital ridge, and germ cells migrating from the yolk sac. The most common variety is germ cell tumors. Germ cell tumors are classified based on the degree of differentiation and the cellular components involved. The least differentiated tumors are the dysgerminomas, which share features similar to the seminoma in males. Although these are malignant tumors, they are extremely sensitive to radiation and chemotherapy. The most common lesions are the teratomas, which may be mature, immature, or malignant. The degree of differentiation of the neural elements of the tumor determines the degree of immaturity. The sex cord stromal tumors arise from the mesenchymal components of the urogenital ridge. These include the granulosa-thecal cell tumors and the Sertoli-Leydig cell tumors. These tumors often produce hormones that result in precocious puberty or hirsutism, respectively. Although rare, epithelial tumors do occur in children. These include serous and mucinous cystadenomas.

Clinical Presentation

Children with ovarian lesions usually present with abdominal pain. Other signs and symptoms include a palpable abdominal mass, evidence of urinary obstruction, symptoms of bowel obstruction,

and endocrine imbalance. The surgical approach depends on the appearance of the mass at operation (i.e., whether it is benign-appearing or is suspicious for malignancy). In the case of a simple ovarian cyst, surgery depends on the size of the cyst and the degree of symptoms it causes. In general, large cysts (over 4 to 5 cm) should be resected, as they are unlikely to resolve, may be at risk of torsion, and may mask an underlying malignancy. Resection may be performed laparoscopically, and ovarian tissue should be spared in all cases.

Surgical Management

For ovarian lesions that appear malignant, it is important to obtain tumor markers including alpha-fetoprotein (teratomas), lactate dehydrogenase (dysgerminoma), beta human chorionic gonadotropin (choriocarcinoma), and CA-125 (epithelial tumors). Although the diagnostic sensitivity of these markers is not always reliable, they provide material for postoperative follow-up and indicate the response to therapy. When a malignancy is suspected, the patient should undergo a formal cancer operation. This procedure is performed through either a midline incision or a Pfannenstiel approach. Ascites and peritoneal washings should be collected for cytologic study. The liver and diaphragm are inspected carefully for metastatic disease. An omentectomy is performed if there is any evidence of tumor present. Pelvic and para-aortic lymph nodes are biopsied and the primary tumor is resected completely. Finally, the contralateral ovary is carefully inspected, and if a lesion is seen, it should be biopsied. Dysgerminomas and epithelial tumors may be bilateral in up to 15% of cases. It is occasionally possible to preserve the ipsilateral fallopian tube. More radical procedures are not indicated.

Ovarian Cysts in the Newborn

An increasing number of ovarian cysts are being detected by prenatal ultrasonography. In the past, surgical excision was recommended for all cysts greater than 5 cm in diameter because of the perceived risk of ovarian torsion. More recently, it has become apparent from serial US examinations that many of these lesions will resolve spontaneously. Therefore asymptomatic simple cysts may be observed, and surgery can be performed only when they fail to decrease in size or become symptomatic. Typically, resolution occurs by approximately 6 months of age. A laparoscopic approach may be utilized. By contrast, complex cysts of any size require surgical intervention at presentation.

Ambiguous Genitalia

Embryology

Normal sexual differentiation occurs in the sixth fetal week. In every fetus, wolffian (male) and müllerian (female) ducts are present until the onset of sexual differentiation. Normal sexual differentiation is directed by the sex-determining region of the Y chromosome (SRY). This is located on the distal end of the short arm of the Y chromosome. SRY provides a genetic switch that initiates gonadal differentiation in the mammalian urogenital ridge. Secretion of müllerian inhibiting substance (MIS) by the Sertoli cells of the seminiferous tubules results in regression of the müllerian duct, the anlagen of the uterus, fallopian tubes, and the upper vagina. The result of MIS secretion therefore is a phenotypic male. In the absence of SRY in the Y chromosome, MIS is not produced, and the müllerian duct derivatives are preserved. Thus the female phenotype prevails.

In order for the male phenotype to develop, the embryo must have a Y chromosome, the SRY must be normal without point mutations or deletions, testosterone and MIS must be produced by the differentiated gonad, and the tissues must respond to these hormones. Any disruption of the orderly steps in sexual differentiation may be reflected clinically as variants of the intersex syndromes.

These may be classified as (1) true hermaphroditism (with ovarian and testicular gonadal tissue), (2) male pseudohermaphroditism (testicles only), (3) female pseudohermaphroditism (ovarian tissue only), and (4) mixed gonadal dysgenesis (usually underdeveloped or imperfectly formed gonads).

True Hermaphroditism

This represents the rarest form of ambiguous genitalia. Patients have both normal male and female gonads, with an ovary on one side and a testis on the other. Occasionally, an ovotestis is present on one or both sides. The majority of these patients have a 46,XX karyotype. Both the testis and the testicular portion of the ovotestis should be removed.

Male Pseudohermaphroditism

This condition occurs in infants with an XY karyotype, but deficient masculinization of the external genitalia. Bilateral testes are present, but the duct structures differentiate partly as phenotypic females. The causes include inadequate testosterone production due to biosynthetic error, inability to convert testosterone to dihydrotestosterone due to 5-alpha-reductase deficiency, or deficiencies in androgen receptors. The latter disorder is termed *testicular feminization syndrome*. Occasionally, the diagnosis in these children is made during routine inguinal herniorrhaphy in a phenotypic female at which time testes are found. The testes should be resected due to the risk of malignant degeneration, although this should be performed only after a full discussion with the family has occurred.

Female Pseudohermaphroditism

These children commonly have congenital adrenal hyperplasia. They have a 46,XX karyotype, but have been exposed to excessive androgens in utero. Common enzyme deficiencies include 21-hydroxylase, 11-hydroxylase, and 3-beta hydroxysteroid dehydrogenase. These deficiencies result in overproduction of intermediary steroid hormones, which result in masculinization of the external genitalia of the XX fetus. These patients are unable to synthesize cortisol. In 90% of cases, deficiency of 21-hydroxylase causes adrenocorticotropic hormone (ACTH) to stimulate the secretion of excessive quantities of adrenal androgen, which masculinizes the developing female (Fig. 38-36). These infants are prone to salt loss, and require cortisol replacement. Those with mineralocorticoid deficiency also require fludrocortisone replacement.

Mixed Gonadal Dysgenesis

This syndrome is associated with dysgenetic gonads and retained müllerian structures. The typical karyotype is mosaic, usually 45XO,46XY. A high incidence of malignant tumors occur in the dysgenetic gonads, most commonly gonadoblastoma. Therefore they should be removed.

Management

In the differential diagnosis of patients with intersex anomalies, the following diagnostic steps are necessary: (1) evaluation of the genetic background and family history; (2) assessment of the anatomic structures by physical examination, ultrasound and/or MRI; (3) chromosome studies; (4) determination of biochemical factors in serum and urine to evaluate the presence of an enzyme

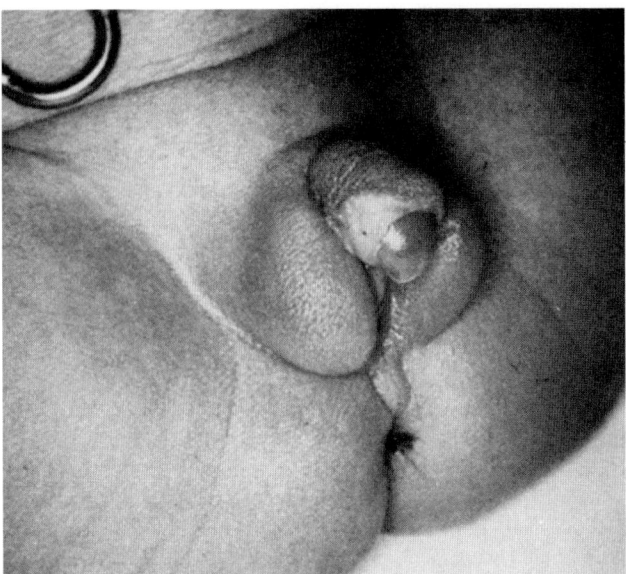

FIG. 38-36. *Ambiguous genitalia manifest as enlarged clitoris and labioscrotal folds in a baby with the adrenogenital syndrome.*

defect; and (5) laparoscopy for gonadal biopsy and further evaluation of the anatomy. Treatment should include correction of electrolyte and volume losses in cases of congenital adrenal hyperplasia, and replacement of hormone deficiency. Surgical assignment of gender is controversial, and must take into account considerations of the anatomy as well as the psychosocial effects involved. In most instances, female gender is assigned. There are those who believe that anatomy and endocrine studies may not be sufficiently reliable to accurately assign a particular gender, and that pre- and postnatal hormones have a significant impact on gender identity. In general terms, surgical reconstruction should be performed after a full workup, and with the involvement of pediatric endocrinologists, pediatric plastic surgeons, and ethicists with expertise in gender issues and the family. This approach will serve to reduce the anxiety associated with these disorders, and will help to ensure the normal physical and emotional development of these patients.

PEDIATRIC MALIGNANCY

Cancer is the second leading cause of death in children after trauma, and accounts for approximately 11% of all pediatric deaths in the United States. Several features distinguish pediatric from adult cancers, including the presence of tumors that are predominantly seen in children, such as neuroblastoma and germ cell tumors, and the favorable response to chemotherapy observed for many pediatric solid malignancies, even in the presence of metastases.

Wilms' Tumor

Clinical Presentation

Wilms' tumor is the most common primary malignant tumor of the kidney in children. There are approximately 500 new cases annually in the United States, and most are diagnosed between 1 and 5 years with the peak incidence at age 3. Advances in the care of patients with Wilms' tumor have resulted in an overall cure rate of roughly 90%, even in the presence of metastatic spread. The tumor usually develops in otherwise healthy children, as an asymptomatic mass in the flank or upper abdomen. Frequently, the mass is discovered by a parent while bathing or dressing the child. Other symptoms include hypertension, hematuria, obstipation, or weight loss. Occasionally the mass is discovered following blunt abdominal trauma.

Genetics

Wilms' tumor can arise from both germline and somatic mutations, and can occur in the presence or absence of a family history. Nearly 97% of Wilms' tumors are sporadic in that they occur in the absence of a heritable or congenital cause or risk factor. When a heritable risk factor is identified, the affected children often present at an earlier age, and are frequently bilateral. Most of these tumors are associated with germline mutations. It is well established that there is a genetic predisposition to Wilms' tumor in the WAGR syndrome, which consists of *W*ilms' tumour, *a*niridia, *g*enitourinary abnormalities, and mental *r*etardation. In addition, there is an increased incidence of Wilms' tumor in certain overgrowth conditions, particularly Beckwith-Wiedemann syndrome and hemihypertrophy. The WAGR syndrome has been shown to result from the deletion of one copy each of the Wilms' tumor gene, *WT1,* and the adjacent aniridia gene, *PAX6,* on chromosome 11p13. Beckwith-Wiedemann syndrome is an overgrowth syndrome that is characterized by visceromegaly, macroglossia, and hyperinsulinemic hypoglycemia. It arises from mutations at the 11p15.5 locus. There is evidence to suggest that analysis of the methylation status of several genes in the 11p15 locus could predict the individual risk to the development of Wilms' tumor. Importantly, most patients with Wilms' tumor do not have mutations at these genetic loci.

Surgical Treatment

Before operation, all patients suspected of Wilms' tumor should undergo abdominal and chest CT scanning. These studies characterize the mass, identify the presence of metastases, and provide information on the opposite kidney (Fig. 38-37). CT scanning also indicates the presence of nephrogenic rests, which are precursor lesions to Wilms' tumor. An abdominal ultrasound should be performed to detect the presence of renal vein or vena caval extension.

The management of patients with Wilms' tumor has been carefully evaluated within the context of large studies involving thousands of patients. These studies have been coordinated by the National Wilms' Tumor Study Group (NWTSG) in North America and the International Society of Paediatric Oncology (SIOP), mainly involving European countries. Significant differences in the approach to patients that present with Wilms' tumor have been highlighted by these studies. NWTSG supports a strategy of surgery followed by chemotherapy in most instances, whereas the SIOP approach is to shrink the tumor using preoperative chemotherapy. There are instances in which preoperative chemotherapy is supported by both groups, including the presence of bilateral involvement or inferior vena cava involvement that extends above the hepatic veins, and involvement of a solitary kidney by Wilms' tumor. The NWTSG proponents argue that preoperative therapy in other instances results in a loss of important staging information, and therefore places patients at higher risk for recurrence; alternatively it may lead to overly aggressive treatment in some cases. However, the overall survival rates are no different between the NWTSG and SIOP approaches.

The goals of surgery include complete removal of the tumor. It is crucial to avoid tumor rupture or injury to contiguous organs. A sampling of regional lymph nodes should be included, and all suspicious nodes should be sampled. Typically a transverse abdominal incision is made, and a transperitoneal approach is used. The opposite side is carefully inspected to ensure that there is no disease present. A radical nephroureterectomy is then performed with control of the renal pedicle as an initial step. If there is spread above the hepatic veins, an intrathoracic approach may be required. If bilateral disease is encountered, both lesions are biopsied, and chemotherapy is administered, followed by a nephron-sparing procedure.

Chemotherapy

Following nephroureterectomy for Wilms' tumor, the need for chemotherapy and/or radiation therapy is determined by the histology of the tumor and the clinical stage of the patient (Table 38-3). Essentially, patients who have disease confined to one kidney that is totally removed surgically receive a short course of chemotherapy, and can expect a 97% 4-year survival rate, with tumor relapse rare after that time. Patients with more advanced disease or with unfavorable histology receive more intensive chemotherapy and radiation. Even in stage IV, cure rates of 80% are achieved. The survival rates are worse in the small percentage of patients considered to have unfavorable histology. The major chemotherapeutic agents are

Table 38-3
Staging of Wilms' Tumor

Stage I: Tumor limited to the kidney and completely excised.

Stage II: Tumor that extends beyond the kidney, but is completely excised. No residual tumor is apparent at or beyond the margins of excision. The tumor was biopsied or there was local spillage of tumor confined to the flank. In the National Wilms' Tumor Study 5 (NWTS-5), tumors with evidence of invasion of vessels in the renal sinus (without any other reason to classify as stage II) were classified as stage II vs. the stage I classification given in NWTS-1 through 4.

Stage III: Residual tumor confined to the abdomen. Lymph nodes in the renal hilum, the periaortic chains, or beyond contain tumor. Diffuse peritoneal contamination by the tumor, such as by spillage of tumor beyond the flank before or during surgery, or by tumor growth that has penetrated through the peritoneal surface. Implants are found on the peritoneal surfaces. Tumor extends beyond the surgical margins either microscopically or grossly. Tumor is not completely resectable because of local infiltration into vital structures.

Stage IV: Hematogenous metastases.

Stage V: Bilateral renal involvement.

SOURCE: Reproduced with permission from D'Angio GJ, Breslow N, Beckwith JB, et al: Treatment of Wilms' tumor. Results of the Third National Wilms' Tumor Study. *Cancer* 64:349, 1989.

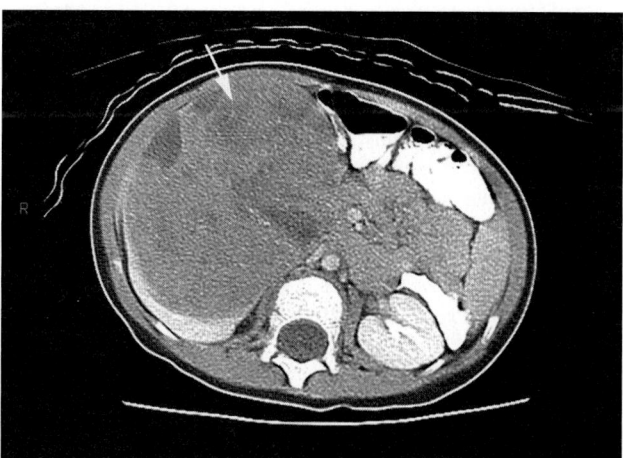

FIG. 38-37. *Wilms' tumor of the right kidney (arrow) in a 3-year-old girl.*

dactinomycin and vincristine, with the addition of doxorubicin for more advanced stages.

Neuroblastoma

Clinical Presentation

Neuroblastoma is the third most common pediatric malignancy, and accounts for approximately 10% of all childhood cancers. The vast majority of patients have advanced disease at the time of presentation, and unlike Wilms' tumor, the overall survival is less than 30%. Over 80% of cases present before the age of 4 years, and the peak incidence is at 2 years of age. Neuroblastomas arise from the neural crest cells and show different levels of differentiation. The tumor originates most frequently in the adrenal glands, posterior mediastinum, neck, or pelvis, but can arise in any sympathetic ganglion.

Two-thirds of these tumors are first noted as an asymptomatic abdominal mass. The tumor may cross the midline, and a majority of patients will already show signs of metastatic disease. Occasionally, children may present with pain from the tumor mass or to bone pain from metastases. Proptosis and periorbital ecchymosis may occur due to the presence of retrobulbar metastasis. Because they originate in paraspinal ganglia, neuroblastomas may invade through neural foramina and compress the spinal cord, causing muscle weakness or sensory changes. Rarely, children may have severe watery diarrhea due to the secretion of vasoactive intestinal polypeptide by the tumor, or with paraneoplastic neurologic findings including cerebellar ataxia or opsoclonus/myoclonus.

Diagnostic Evaluation

Since these tumors derive from the sympathetic nervous system, catecholamines and their metabolites will be produced at increased levels. These include elevated levels of serum catecholamines (dopamine and norepinephrine) or urine catecholamine metabolites (vanillylmandelic acid [VMA] or homovanillic acid [HVA]). Measurement of VMA and HVA in serum and urine aids in the diagnosis and in monitoring adequacy of future treatment and recurrence. The minimum criterion for a diagnosis of neuroblastoma is based on one of the following findings: (1) an unequivocal pathologic diagnosis made from tumor tissue by light microscopy (with or without immunohistology, electron microscopy, or increased levels of serum catecholamines or urinary catecholamine metabolites); and (2) the combination of bone marrow aspirate or biopsy containing unequivocal tumor cells and increased levels of serum catecholamines or urinary catecholamine metabolites as described above.

The patient should be evaluated by abdominal CT scan, which usually shows displacement and occasionally obstruction of the ureter of an intact kidney (Fig. 38-38). Prior to the institution of therapy, a complete staging work-up should be performed. This includes radiograph of the chest, bone marrow biopsy, and radionuclide scans to search for metastases. Any abnormalities on chest x-ray should be followed up with CT of the chest.

Prognostic Indicators

A number of biologic variables have been studied in children with neuroblastoma. An open biopsy is required in order to provide tissue for this analysis. Hyperdiploid tumor DNA is associated with a favorable prognosis, and N-myc amplification is associated with a poor prognosis regardless of patient age. The Shimada classification describes tumors as having either favorable or unfavorable histology based on the degree of differentiation, the mitosis-karyorrhexis

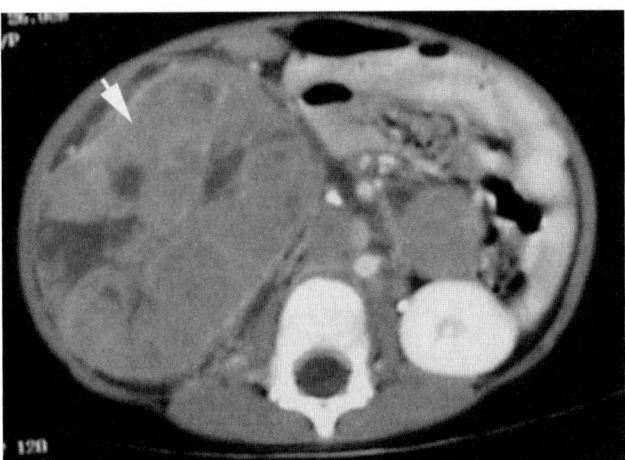

FIG. 38-38. Abdominal neuroblastoma arising from the right retroperitoneum (*arrow*).

index, and the presence or absence of schwannian stroma. In general, children of any age with localized neuroblastoma and infants younger than 1 year of age with advanced disease and favorable disease characteristics have a high likelihood of disease-free survival. By contrast, older children with advanced-stage disease have a significantly decreased chance for cure despite intensive therapy. For example, aggressive multiagent chemotherapy has resulted in a 2-year survival rate of approximately 20% in older children with stage IV disease. Neuroblastoma in the adolescent has a worse long-term prognosis, regardless of stage or site, and in many cases, a more prolonged course.

Surgery

The goal of surgery is complete resection. However, this is often not possible due to the extensive locoregional spread of the tumor at the time of presentation. Under these circumstances, a biopsy is performed and preoperative chemotherapy is provided based on the stage of the tumor. After neoadjuvant treatment has been administered, surgical resection is performed. The principal goal of surgery is to obtain at least a 95% resection, without compromising major structures. Abdominal tumors are approached through a transverse incision. Thoracic tumors may be approached through a posterolateral thoracotomy or through a thoracoscopic approach. These may have an intraspinal component.

Neuroblastoma in Infants

Spontaneous regression of neuroblastoma has been well described in infants, especially in those with stage 4S disease. Regression generally occurs only in tumors with a near triploid number of chromosomes that also lack N-myc amplification and loss of chromosome 1p. Recent studies indicate that infants with asymptomatic, small, low-stage neuroblastoma detected by screening may have tumors that spontaneously regress. These patients may be observed safely without surgical intervention or tissue diagnosis.

Rhabdomyosarcoma

Rhabdomyosarcoma is a primitive soft tissue tumor that arises from mesenchymal tissues. The most common sites of origin include the head and neck (36%), extremities (19%), genitourinary tract (21%), and trunk (9%), although the tumor can arise virtually anywhere.

Table 38-4
Staging of Rhabdomyosarcoma

Stage 1: Localized disease involving the orbit or head and neck (excluding parameningeal sites), or genitourinary region (excluding bladder/prostate sites), or biliary tract (favorable sites).

Stage 2: Localized disease of any other primary site not included in the stage 1 category (unfavorable sites). Primary tumors must be ≤5 cm in diameter, and there must be no clinical regional lymph node involvement by tumor.

Stage 3: Localized disease of any other primary site. These patients differ from stage 2 patients by having primary tumors >5 cm and/or regional node involvement.

Stage 4: Metastatic disease at diagnosis.

SOURCE: Reproduced with permission from Lawrence W Jr., Gehan EA, Hays DM, et al: Prognostic significance of staging factors of the UICC staging system in childhood rhabdomyosarcoma: A report from the Intergroup Rhabdomyosarcoma Study (IRS-II). *J Clin Oncol* 5:46, 1987; and Lawrence W Jr., Anderson JR, Gehan EA, et al: Pretreatment TNM staging of childhood rhabdomyosarcoma: A report of the Intergroup Rhabdomyosarcoma Study Group. Children's Cancer Study Group. Pediatric Oncology Group. *Cancer* 80:1165, 1997.

The clinical presentation of the tumor depends on the site of origin. The diagnosis is confirmed with incisional or excisional biopsy after evaluation by MRI, CT scans of the affected area and the chest, and bone marrow biopsy. The tumor grows locally into surrounding structures and metastasizes widely to lung, regional lymph nodes, liver, brain, and bone marrow. The staging system for rhabdomyosarcoma is based on the tumor-node-metastasis (TNM) system, as established by the Soft Tissue Sarcoma Committee of the Children's Oncology Group (Table 38-4). Surgery is an important component of the staging strategy, and involves biopsy of the lesion and evaluation of lymphatics. Primary resection should be undertaken when complete excision can be performed without causing disability. If this is not possible, the lesion is biopsied and intensive chemotherapy is administered. It is important to plan the biopsy so that it does not interfere with the subsequent resection. After the tumor has decreased in size, resection of gross residual disease should be performed. Radiation therapy is effective in achieving local control when microscopic or gross residual disease exists following initial treatment. Patients with completely resected tumors of embryonal histology do well without radiation therapy, but radiation therapy benefits patients with stage 1 tumors with alveolar or undifferentiated histology.

Prognosis

The prognosis for rhabdomyosarcoma is related to the site of origin, resectability, presence of metastases, number of metastatic sites, and histopathology. Primary sites with more favorable prognoses include the orbit and nonparameningeal head and neck, paratestis and vagina (nonbladder, nonprostate genitourinary), and the biliary tract. Patients with tumors under 5 cm in size have improved survival compared to children with larger tumors, while children with metastatic disease at diagnosis have the poorest prognosis. Tumor histology influences prognosis, and the embryonal variant is favorable, while the alveolar subtype has an unfavorable prognosis.

Teratoma

Teratomas are tumors composed of tissue from all three embryonic germ layers. They may be benign or malignant, may arise in any part of the body, and are usually found in midline structures. Thoracic teratomas usually present as an anterior mediastinal mass. Ovarian teratomas present as an abdominal mass, often with symptoms of torsion, bleeding, or rupture. Retroperitoneal teratomas may present as a flank or abdominal mass.

Mature teratomas usually contain well-differentiated tissues and are benign, while immature teratomas contain varying degrees of immature neuroepithelium or blastemal tissues. Immature teratomas can be graded from 1 to 3, based on the amount of immature neuroglial tissue present. Tumors of higher grade are more likely to have foci of yolk sac tumor. Malignant germ cell tumors usually contain frankly neoplastic tissues of germ cell origin (i.e., yolk sac carcinoma, embryonal carcinoma, germinoma, or choriocarcinoma). Yolk sac carcinomas produce alpha-fetoprotein, while choriocarcinomas produce beta human chorionic gonadotropin (bHCG), resulting in elevation of these substances in the serum, which can serve as tumor markers. In addition, germinomas also can produce elevation of serum bHCG, but not to the levels associated with choriocarcinoma.

Sacrococcygeal Teratoma

Sacrococcygeal teratoma usually presents as a large mass extending from the sacrum in the newborn period. Diagnosis may be established by prenatal ultrasound. In fetuses with evidence of hydrops and a large sacrococcygeal teratoma, prognosis is poor; thus prenatal intervention has been advocated in such patients. The mass may be as small as a few centimeters in diameter or as massive as the size of the infant (Fig. 38-39). The tumor has been classified based on the location and degree of intrapelvic extension. Lesions with growth predominantly into the presacral space often present later in childhood. The differential diagnosis consists of neural tumors, lipoma, and myelomeningoceles.

Most tumors are identified at birth and are benign. Malignant yolk sac tumor histology occurs in a minority of these tumors. Complete resection of the tumor as early as possible is essential. The rectum and genital structures are often distorted by the tumor, but usually can be preserved in the course of resection. Perioperative complications of hypothermia and hemorrhage can occur with massive tumors and may prove lethal. This is of particular concern

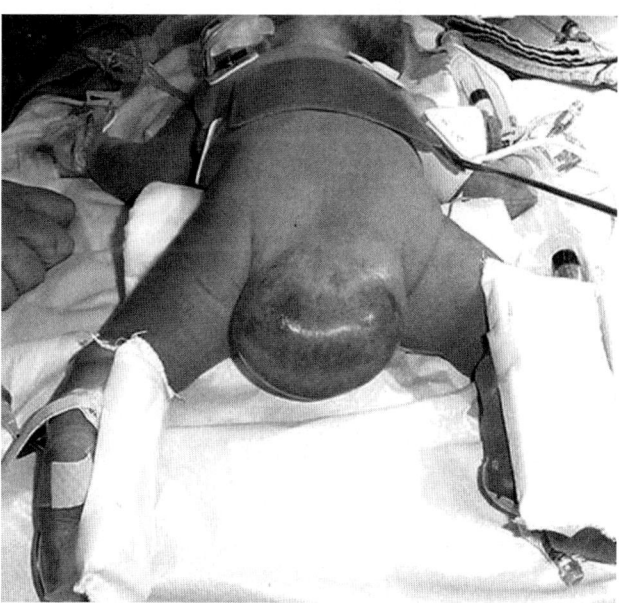

FIG. 38-39. *Sacrococcygeal teratoma in a 2-day-old boy.*

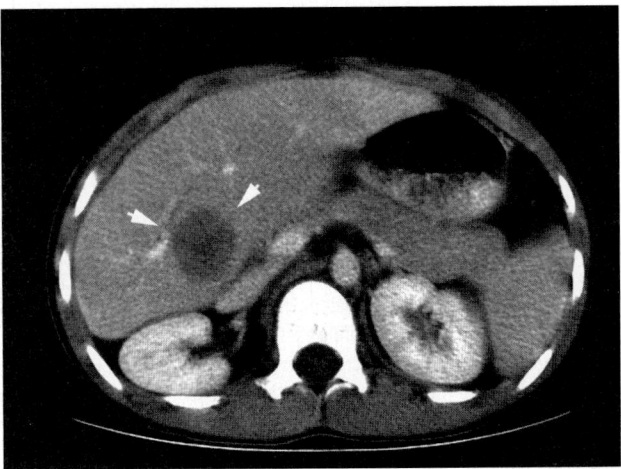

FIG. 38-40. CT scan of the abdomen showing a hepatocellular carcinoma in a 12-year-old boy.

in small preterm infants with large tumors. The cure rate is excellent if the tumor is excised completely. The majority of patients who develop recurrent disease are salvageable with subsequent platinum-based chemotherapy.

Liver Tumors

More than two-thirds of all liver tumors in children are malignant. There are two major histologic subgroups: hepatoblastoma and hepatocellular carcinoma. The age of onset of liver cancer in children is related to the histology of the tumor. Hepatoblastoma is the most common malignancy of the liver in children, with most of these tumors diagnosed before 4 years of age. Hepatocellular carcinoma is the next most common, with a peak age incidence between 10 and 15 years. Malignant mesenchymomas and sarcomas are much less common, but constitute the remainder of the malignancies. The finding of a liver mass does not necessarily imply that a malignancy is present. Nearly 50% of all masses are benign, and hemangiomas are the most common lesions.

Most children with a liver tumor present with an abdominal mass that is usually painless, which the parents note while changing the child's clothes or while bathing the child. The patients are rarely jaundiced, but may complain of anorexia and weight loss. Most liver function tests are normal. Alpha-fetoprotein levels are elevated in 90% of children with hepatoblastomas, but are increased much less commonly in other liver malignancies. Radiographic evaluation of these children should include an abdominal CT scan to identify the lesion and to determine the degree of local invasiveness (Fig. 38-40). For malignant-appearing lesions, a biopsy should be performed unless the lesion can be completely resected easily. Hepatoblastoma is most often unifocal, while hepatocellular carcinoma is often extensively invasive or multicentric. If a hepatoblastoma is completely removed, the majority of patients survive, but only a minority of patients have lesions amenable to complete resection at diagnosis.

A staging system based on postsurgical extent of tumor and surgical resectability is shown in Table 38-5. The overall survival rate for children with hepatoblastoma is 70%, but is only 25% for hepatocellular carcinoma. Children diagnosed with stage I disease and II hepatoblastoma have a cure rate of greater than 90%, compared to 60% for stage III and approximately 20% for stage IV. In children diagnosed with hepatocellular carcinoma, those with stage I have a good outcome, whereas stages III and IV are usually fatal. The

Table 38-5
Staging of Pediatric Liver Cancer

Stage I: No metastases, tumor completely resected.

Stage II: No metastases, tumor grossly resected with microscopic residual disease (i.e., positive margins); or tumor rupture or spillage at the time of surgery.

Stage III: No distant metastases, tumor unresectable or resected with gross residual tumor, or positive lymph nodes.

Stage IV: Distant metastases regardless of the extent of liver involvement.

SOURCE: Reproduced with permission from Douglass E, Ortega J, Feusner J, et al: Hepatocellular carcinoma (HCA) in children and adolescents: Results from the Pediatric Intergroup Hepatoma Study (CCG 8881/POG 8945). *Proc Am Soc Clin Oncol* 13: A-1439, 420, 1994.

fibrolamellar variant of hepatocellular carcinoma may have a better prognosis.

Surgery

The abdominal CT scan usually will determine the resectability of the lesion, although occasionally this can only be determined at the time of exploration. Complete surgical resection of the tumor is the primary goal and is essential for cure. For tumors that are unresectable, preoperative chemotherapy should be administered to reduce the size of the tumor and improve the possibility for complete removal. Chemotherapy is more successful for hepatoblastoma than for hepatocellular carcinoma. Areas of locally invasive disease, such as the diaphragm, should be resected at the time of surgery. For unresectable tumors, liver transplantation has recently been used with some success. The fibrolamellar variant of hepatocellular carcinoma may have a better outcome with liver transplant than other hepatocellular carcinomas.

TRAUMA IN CHILDREN

Injury is the leading cause of death among children older than 1 year. In fact, trauma accounts for almost half of all pediatric deaths, more than cancer, congenital anomalies, pneumonia, heart disease, homicide, and meningitis combined. Death from unintentional injury accounts for 65% of all injury deaths in children younger than 19 years. From 1972 to 1992, motor vehicle collisions were the leading cause of death in people aged 1 to 19 years, followed by homicide or suicide (predominantly with firearms) and drowning. Each year, approximately 20,000 children and teenagers die as a result of injury in the United States. For every child who dies from an injury, it is calculated that 40 others are hospitalized and 1120 are treated in emergency departments. An estimated 50,000 children acquire permanent disabilities each year, most of which are the result of head injuries. Thus the problem of pediatric trauma continues to be one of the major threats to the health and well-being of children.

Specific considerations apply to trauma in children that influence management and outcome. These relate to the mechanisms of injury, the anatomic variations in children compared to adults, and the physiologic responses.

Mechanisms of Injury

Most pediatric trauma is blunt. Penetrating injuries are seen in the setting of gun violence, falls onto sharp objects, or penetration by glass after falling through windows. Age and gender significantly influence the patterns of injury. Male children younger than 18 years are exposed to contact sports and drive motor vehicles. As a result, they have a different pattern of injury than younger children, characterized by higher injury severity scores. In the infant and toddler age group, falls are a common cause of severe injury. Injuries in the home are extremely common. These include falls, near-drownings, caustic ingestion, and nonaccidental injuries.

Initial Management

The goals of managing the pediatric trauma patient are similar to those of adults, and follow Advanced Trauma Life Support guidelines as established by the American College of Surgeons. Airway control is the first priority. In a child, respiratory arrest can proceed quickly to cardiac arrest. It is important to be aware of the anatomic differences between the airway of the child and the adult. The child has a shorter neck, smaller and anterior larynx, floppy epiglottis, short trachea, and large tongue. The child's fifth digit can provide an estimate of the size of the correct endotracheal tube. Alternatively, the formula (age in years + 16)/4 may be used. It is important to use uncuffed endotracheal tubes in children younger than 8 years in order to minimize tracheal trauma. After evaluation of the airway, breathing is assessed. It is important to consider that gastric distention from aerophagia can severely compromise respirations. A nasogastric tube should therefore be placed early in the resuscitation. Pneumothorax or hemothorax should be treated promptly. When evaluating the circulation, it is important to recognize that tachycardia is usually the earliest measurable response to hypovolemia. Other signs of impending hypovolemic shock in children include changes in mentation, delayed capillary refill, skin pallor, and hypothermia. Intravenous access should be rapidly obtained once the patient arrives in the trauma bay. The first approach should be to use the antecubital fossae. If this is not possible, a cutdown into the saphenous vein at the groin can be performed quickly and safely. Intraosseous cannulation can provide temporary access in infants until intravenous access is established. Percutaneous neck lines should generally be avoided. Blood is drawn for cross-match and evaluation of liver enzymes, lipase, amylase, and hematologic profile, after the intravenous lines are placed.

In patients who show signs of volume depletion, a 20-mL/kg bolus of saline or lactated Ringer's solution should be promptly given. If the patient does not respond to three boluses, blood should be transfused (10 mL/kg). The source of bleeding should be established. Common sites include the chest, abdomen, pelvis, extremity fractures, or large scalp wounds. These should be carefully sought. Care is taken to avoid hypothermia by infusing warmed fluids and by using external warming devices.

Evaluation of Injury

All patients should receive an x-ray of the cervical spine, chest, and abdomen with pelvis. All extremities that are suspicious for fracture should also be evaluated by x-ray. Screening blood work that includes aspartate aminotransferase and alanine aminotransferase, and amylase/lipase is useful for the evaluation of liver and pancreatic injuries. Significant elevation in these tests requires further evaluation by CT scanning. The child with significant abdominal tenderness and a mechanism of injury that could cause intra-abdominal injury should undergo abdominal CT scanning using intravenous and oral contrast in all cases. There is a limited role for diagnostic peritoneal lavage (DPL) in children as a screening test. However, it can be useful in the child that is brought emergently to the operating room for management of significant intracranial hemorrhage. At the time of craniotomy, a DPL can be performed concurrently to identify abdominal bleeding. Although abdominal ultrasound is

extremely useful in the evaluation of adult abdominal trauma, it has not been widely accepted in the management of pediatric injury. In part this relates to the widespread use of nonoperative treatment for most solid-organ injuries, which would result in a positive abdominal ultrasound scan.

Injuries to the Central Nervous System

The central nervous system (CNS) is the most commonly injured organ system, and CNS injury is the leading cause of death among injured children. In the toddler age group, nonaccidental trauma is the most common cause of serious head injury. Findings suggestive of abuse include the presence of retinal hemorrhage on funduscopic evaluation, intracranial hemorrhage without evidence of external trauma (indicative of a shaking injury), and fractures at different stages of healing on skeletal survey. In older children, CNS injury occurs most commonly after falls and bicycle and motor vehicle collisions. The initial head CT scan can often underestimate the extent of injury in children. Criteria for head CT scan include any loss of consciousness or amnesia to the trauma, or inability to assess the CNS status as in the intubated patient. Patients with mild, isolated head injury (Glasgow Coma Scale [GCS] score 14 to 15) and negative CT scans can be discharged if their neurologic status is normal after 6 hours of observation. Young children and those in whom there is multisystem involvement should be admitted to the hospital for a period of overnight observation. Any change in the neurologic status warrants neurosurgical evaluation and repeat CT scanning. In patients with severe head injury (GCS score 8 or less), urgent neurosurgical consultation is required. These patients are evaluated for intracranial pressure monitoring, and for the need to undergo craniotomy.

Thoracic Injuries

The pediatric thorax is pliable due to incomplete calcification of the ribs and cartilages. As a result, blunt chest injury commonly results in pulmonary contusion, although rib fractures are rare. Diagnosis is made by chest radiograph, and may be associated with severe hypoxia requiring mechanical ventilation. Pulmonary contusion usually resolves with careful ventilator management and judicious volume resuscitation. Children who have sustained massive blunt thoracic injury may develop traumatic asphyxia. This is characterized by cervical and facial petechial hemorrhages or cyanosis associated with vascular engorgement and subconjunctival hemorrhage. Management includes ventilation and treatment of coexisting CNS or abdominal injuries. Penetrating thoracic injuries may result in damage to the lung, or to major disruption of the bronchi or great vessels.

Abdominal Injuries

In children, the small rib cage and minimal muscular coverage of the abdomen can result in significant injury after seemingly minor trauma. The liver and spleen in particular are relatively unprotected, and are often injured after direct abdominal trauma. Duodenal injuries are usually the result of blunt trauma, which may arise from child abuse or injury from a bicycle handlebar. Duodenal hematomas usually resolve without surgery. Small intestinal injury usually occurs in the jejunum in the area of fixation by the ligament of Treitz. These injuries are usually caused by rapid deceleration while the child is restrained by a lap belt. There may be a hematoma on the anterior abdominal wall caused by a lap belt, the so-called "seat belt sign" (Fig. 38-41A). This should alert the caregiver to the possibility

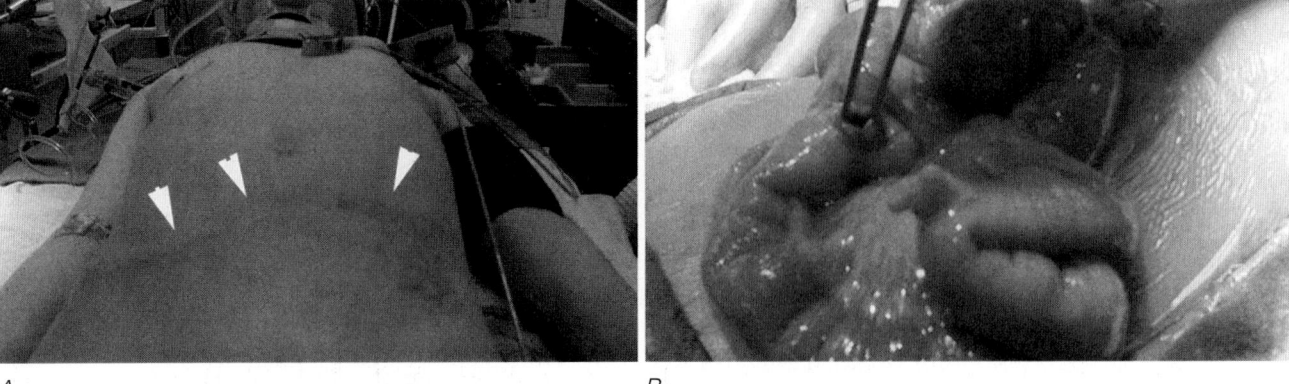

A   *B*

FIG. 38-41. Abdominal CT scan of patient that sustained a lap belt injury. A. Bruising is noted across the abdomen from the lap belt. B. At laparotomy, a perforation of the small bowel was identified.

of an underlying small bowel injury (Fig. 38-41B), as well as to a potential lumbar spine injury (Chance fracture).

The spleen is injured relatively commonly after blunt abdominal trauma in children. The extent of injury to the spleen is graded (Table 38-6), and the management is governed by the injury grade. Current treatment involves a nonoperative approach in most cases, even for grade IV injuries, providing the patient is hemodynamically stable. This approach avoids surgery in most cases. All patients should be placed in a monitored unit, and type-specific blood should be available for transfusion. When nonoperative management is successful, as it is in most cases, an extended period of bedrest is prescribed. This optimizes the chance for healing, and minimizes the likelihood of reinjury. A typical guideline is to keep the children on extremely restricted activity for 2 weeks longer than the grade of spleen injury (i.e., a child with a grade IV spleen injury receives 6 weeks of restricted activity). In children that have an ongoing fluid requirement, or when a blood transfusion is required, exploration should not be delayed. At surgery the spleen can often be salvaged. If a splenectomy is performed, prophylactic antibiotics and immunizations should be administered to protect against overwhelming postsplenectomy sepsis. The liver also is commonly injured after blunt abdominal trauma. A grading system is used to characterize hepatic injuries (Table 38-7), and nonoperative management is usually successful (Fig. 38-42). Recent data have shown that associated injuries are more significant predictors of outcome in children with liver injuries than the actual injury grade. Criteria for

surgery are similar to those for splenic injury and primarily involve hemodynamic instability. The intraoperative considerations in the management of massive hepatic injury are similar in children and adults. Renal contusions may occur after significant blunt abdominal trauma. Nonoperative management is usually successful, unless patients are unstable due to active renal bleeding. It is important to confirm the presence of a normal contralateral kidney at the time of surgery.

FETAL INTERVENTION

One of the most exciting developments in the field of pediatric surgery has been the emergence of fetal surgery. The performance of a fetal intervention is justified when a defect is present that would cause devastating consequences to the infant if left uncorrected. For the vast majority of congenital anomalies, postnatal surgery is the preferred modality. However, in specific circumstances, fetal surgery may offer the best possibility for a successful outcome. The decision to perform a fetal intervention requires careful patient selection, as well as a multidisciplinary center that is dedicated to the surgical care of the fetus and the mother. Patient selection is dependent in part on highly accurate prenatal imaging, which includes ultrasound and MRI. At the present time, fetal surgery is performed at a few centers in North America, although this number is increasing.

Significant risks may be associated with the performance of a fetal surgical procedure, to both the mother and the fetus. From the maternal viewpoint, open fetal surgery may lead to uterine bleeding due to the uterine relaxation required during the procedure. The

Table 38-6
Grading of Splenic Injuries

Grade I: Subcapsular hematoma, <10% surface area capsular tear, <1 cm in depth.
Grade II: Subcapsular hematoma, nonexpanding, 10–50% surface area; intraparenchymal hematoma, nonexpanding, <2 cm in size; capsular tear, active bleeding, 1–3 cm size, does not involve trabecular vessel.
Grade III: Subcapsular hematoma, >50% surface area or expanding; intraparenchymal hematoma, >2 cm in size or expanding; laceration >3 cm in depth or involving trabecular vessels.
Grade IV: Ruptured intraparenchymal hematoma with active bleeding; laceration involving segmental or hilar vessels producing major devascularizatrion (>25% of spleen).
Grade V: Shattered spleen; hilar vascular injury that devascularizes spleen.

Table 38-7
Liver Injury Grading System

Grade I: Capsular tear <1 cm in depth.
Grade II: Capsular tear 1–3 cm in depth, <10 cm length.
Grade III: Capsular tear >3 cm in depth.
Grade IV: Parenchymal disruption 25–75% of hepatic lobe or 1–3 Couinaud segments.
Grade V: Parenchymal disruption >75% of hepatic lobe or >3 Couinaud segments within a single lobe; injury to retrohepatic vena cava.

SOURCE: Reproduced with permission from Moore EE, Cogbill TH, Malangoni MA, et al: Organ injury scaling. *Surg Clin North Am* 75:293, 1995.

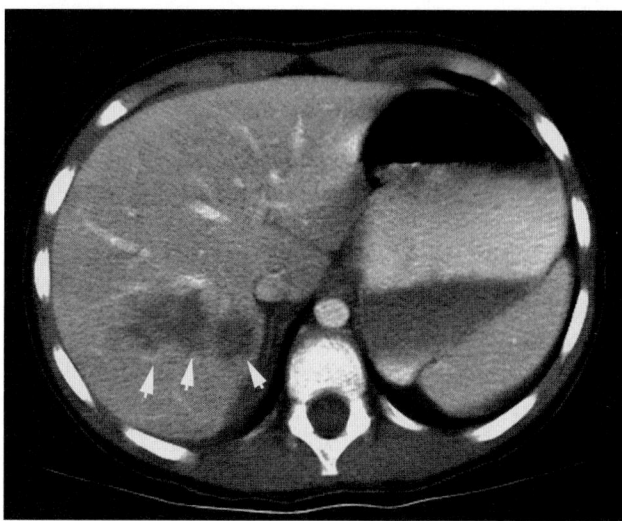

FIG. 38-42. *Abdominal CT scan of a child demonstrating a grade III liver laceration (arrows).*

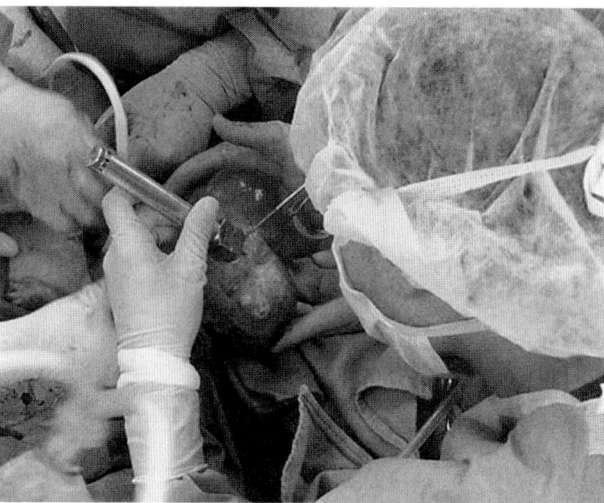

FIG. 38-43. *The EXIT (ex-utero intrapartum treatment) procedure in a baby at 34 weeks' gestation with a large cervical teratoma. Intubation is performed while the fetus is on placental support.*

long-term effects on subsequent pregnancies remain to be established. For the fetus, in utero surgery carries the risk of premature labor and amniotic fluid leakage. As a result, these procedures are performed only when the expected benefit of fetal intervention outweighs the risk to the fetus of standard postnatal care.

Surgery for Lower Urinary Tract Obstruction

Lower urinary tract obstruction refers to a group of diseases characterized by obstruction of the distal urinary system. Common causes include the presence of posterior urethral valves and urethral atresia, as well as other anomalies of the urethra and bladder. The pathologic effects of lower urinary tract obstruction lie in the resultant massive bladder distention that occurs, which can lead to reflux hydronephrosis. This may result in oligohydramnios, and cause limb contractures, facial anomalies (Potter facies), and pulmonary hypoplasia. Carefully selected patients with lower urinary tract obstruction may benefit from vesicoamniotic shunting. By relieving the obstruction and improving renal function, fetal growth and lung development may be preserved.

Fetal Surgery for Congenital Diaphragmatic Hernia

Given the high mortality associated with the most severe cases of CDH, tremendous efforts have been undertaken to determine whether fetal intervention could improve the outcome of this disease. In 1990, Harrison and colleagues reported the first open fetal repair for CDH. The high morbidity of the open technique led to the development of fetal tracheal occlusion as a therapeutic approach. This was based on the observation that tracheal occlusion could lead to increased lung growth and reduction of the intrathoracic viscera in animal models. Tracheal occlusion can be achieved in utero by placement of clips that are removed at the time of delivery. Despite initial enthusiasm for this approach, a recent randomized trial that compared fetal tracheal occlusion with standard postnatal care for left-sided CDH showed no improvement in survival for patients treated with tracheal occlusion.

Fetal Surgery for Myelomeningocele

Myelomeningocele refers to a spectrum of anomalies in which portions of the spinal cord are uncovered by the spinal column. This leaves the neural tissue exposed to the injurious effects of the amniotic fluid, as well as to trauma from contact with the uterine wall. Nerve damage ensues, resulting in varying degrees of lower extremity paralysis, as well as bowel and bladder dysfunction. Initial observations indicated that the extent of injury progressed throughout the pregnancy, which provided the rationale for fetal intervention. The current in utero approach for the fetus with myelomeningocele has focused on obtaining coverage of the exposed spinal cord. Initial results have shown a decrease in the development of obstructive hydrocephalus requiring ventriculoperitoneal shunting. A National Institutes of Health–sponsored trial is currently underway, in which patients are randomized to receive either in utero coverage of the spinal cord or standard postnatal care. The effects of the treatment approach on neurologic function can then be determined.

The Ex-Utero Intrapartum Treatment Procedure

The EXIT procedure is utilized in circumstances in which an airway obstruction is predicted at the time of delivery, due to the presence of a large neck mass such as a cystic hygroma or teratoma (Fig. 38-43), or congenital tracheal stenosis. The success of the procedure is dependent on the maintenance of uteroplacental perfusion for a sufficient duration to secure the airway. To achieve this, deep uterine relaxation is obtained during a cesarean section under general anesthesia. Uterine perfusion with warmed saline also promotes relaxation and blood flow to the placenta. On average, between 20 and 30 minutes of placental perfusion can be achieved. The fetal airway is secured either by placement of an orotracheal tube, or performance of a tracheostomy. Once the airway is secured, the cord is cut, and a definitive procedure may be performed to relieve the obstruction postnatally.

Bibliography

Ahuja AT, King AD, et al: Thyroglossal duct cysts: Sonographic appearances in adults. *Am J Neuroradiol* 20:579, 1999.

Andersen B, Kallehave F, et al: Antibiotics versus placebo for prevention of postoperative infection after appendicectomy. *Cochrane Database Syst Rev* 2:CD001439.

Anderson KD, Rouse TM, et al: A controlled trial of corticosteroids in children with corrosive injury of the esophagus. *N Engl J Med* 323:637, 1990.

Azarow K, Messineo A, et al: Congenital diaphragmatic hernia—a tale of two cities: The Toronto experience. *J Pediatr Surg* 32:395, 1997.

Billmire D, Vinocur C, et al: Malignant mediastinal germ cell tumors: An intergroup study. *J Pediatr Surg* 36:18, 2001.

Bohn D: Congenital diaphragmatic hernia. *Am J Respir Crit Care Med* 166:911, 2002.

Boloker J, Bateman DA, et al: Congenital diaphragmatic hernia in 120 infants treated consecutively with permissive hypercapnea/spontaneous respiration/elective repair. *J Pediatr Surg* 37:357, 2002.

Bouchard S, Johnson MP, et al: The EXIT procedure: Experience and outcome in 31 cases. *J Pediatr Surg* 37:418, 2002.

Branstetter BF, Weissman JL, et al: The CT appearance of thyroglossal duct carcinoma. *Am J Neuroradiol* 21:1547, 2000.

Bratton S, Annich G: Packed red blood cell transfusions for critically ill pediatric patients: When and for what conditions? *J Pediatr* 142:95, 2003.

Breneman JC, Lyden E, et al: Prognostic factors and clinical outcomes in children and adolescents with metastatic rhabdomyosarcoma—A report from the Intergroup Rhabdomyosarcoma Study IV. *J Clin Oncol* 21:78, 2003.

Bruner JP, Tulipan N, et al: Fetal surgery for myelomeningocele and the incidence of shunt-dependent hydrocephalus. *JAMA* 282:1819, 1999.

Chertin B, De Caluwé D, et al: Is contralateral exploration necessary in girls with unilateral inguinal hernia? *J Pediatr Surg* 38:756, 2003.

Cohen J, Schanen NC: Branchial cleft anomaly, congenital heart disease, and biliary atresia: Goldenhar complex or Lambert syndrome? *Genet Couns* 11:153, 2000.

Cohn SL, London WB, et al: MYCN expression is not prognostic of adverse outcome in advanced-stage neuroblastoma with nonamplified MYCN. *J Clin Oncol* 18:3604, 2000.

Coppes MJ, Haber DA, et al: Genetic events in the development of Wilms' tumor. *N Engl J Med* 331:586, 1994.

Cotterill SJ, Pearson ADJ, et al: Clinical prognostic factors in 1277 patients with neuroblastoma: Results of The European Neuroblastoma Study Group Survey 1982–1992. *Eur J Cancer* 36:901, 2000.

Crystal P, Hertzanu Y, et al: Sonographically guided hydrostatic reduction of intussusception in children. *J Clin Ultrasound* 30:343, 2002.

Dunn J, Fonkalsrud E, et al: Simplifying the Waterston's stratification of infants with tracheoesophageal fistula. *Am Surg* 65:908, 1999.

Ferrari A, Bisogno G, et al: Paratesticular rhabdomyosarcoma: Report from the Italian and German Cooperative Group. *J Clin Oncol* 20:449, 2002.

Freedman AL, Johnson MP, et al: Long-term outcome in children after antenatal intervention for obstructive uropathies. *Lancet* 354:374, 1999.

Geisler DP, Jegathesan S, et al: Laparoscopic exploration for the clinically undetected hernia in infancy and childhood. *Am J Surg* 182:693, 2001.

Georgeson K: Laparoscopic-assisted pull-through for Hirschsprung's disease. *Semin Pediatr Surg* 11:205, 2002.

Georgeson K: Results of laparoscopic antireflux procedures in neurologically normal infants and children. *Semin Laparosc Surg* 9:172, 2002.

Gollin GA, Abarbanell AA, et al: Peritoneal drainage as definitive management of intestinal perforation in extremely low-birth-weight infants. *J Pediatr Surg* 38:1814, 2003.

Gorsler C, Schier F: Laparoscopic herniorrhaphy in children. *Surg Endosc* 17:571, 2003.

Guthrie S, Gordon P, et al: Necrotizing enterocolitis among neonates in the United States. *J Perinatol* 23:278, 2003.

Hackam DJ, Filler R, et al: Enterocolitis after the surgical treatment of Hirschsprung's disease: Risk factors and financial impact. *J Pediatr Surg* 33:830, 1998.

Hackam DJ, Potoka D, et al: Utility of radiographic hepatic injury grade in predicting outcome for children after blunt abdominal trauma. *J Pediatr Surg* 37:386, 2002.

Hackam DJ, Reblock K, et al: The influence of Down's syndrome on the management and outcome of children with Hirschsprung's disease. *J Pediatr Surg* 38:946, 2003.

Hackam DJ, Superina R, et al: Single-stage repair of Hirschsprung's disease: A comparison of 109 patients over 5 years. *J Pediatr Surg* 32:1028, 1997.

Harrison MR: Fetal surgery: Trials, tribulations, and turf. *J Pediatr Surg* 38:275, 2003.

Harrison MR, Keller RL, et al: A randomized trial of fetal endoscopic tracheal occlusion for severe fetal congenital diaphragmatic hernia. *N Engl J Med* 349:1916, 2003.

Harrison MR, Sydorak RM, et al: Fetoscopic temporary tracheal occlusion for congenital diaphragmatic hernia: Prelude to a randomized, controlled trial. *J Pediatr Surg* 38:1012, 2003.

Hedrick H, Flake A, et al: History of fetal diagnosis and therapy: Children's Hospital of Philadelphia experience. *Fetal Diagn Ther* 18:65, 2003.

Hirschl RB, Philip WF, et al: A prospective, randomized pilot trial of perfluorocarbon-induced lung growth in newborns with congenital diaphragmatic hernia. *J Pediatr Surg* 38:283, 2003.

Johnson MP, Sutton LN, et al: Fetal myelomeningocele repair: Short-term clinical outcomes. *Am J Obstet Gynecol* 189:482, 2003.

Kalapurakal J, Li S, et al: Influence of radiation therapy delay on abdominal tumor recurrence in patients with favorable histology Wilms' tumor treated on NWTS-3 and NWTS-4: A report from the National Wilms' Tumor Study Group. *Int J Radiat Oncol Biol Phys* 57:495, 2003.

Kamata S, Ishikawa S, et al: Prenatal diagnosis of abdominal wall defects and their prognosis. *J Pediatr Surg* 31:267, 1996.

Katzenstein HM, Krailo MD, et al: Hepatocellular carcinoma in children and adolescents: Results from the Pediatric Oncology Group and the Children's Cancer Group Intergroup Study. *J Clin Oncol* 20:2789, 2002.

Kim HB, Lee PW, et al: Serial transverse enteroplasty for short bowel syndrome: A case report. *J Pediatr Surg* 38:881, 2003.

Konkin D, O'hali W, et al: Outcomes in esophageal atresia and tracheoesophageal fistula. *J Pediatr Surg* 38:1726, 2003.

Langer J, Durrant A, et al: One-stage transanal Soave pullthrough for Hirschsprung disease: A multicenter experience with 141 children. *Ann Surg* 238:569, 2003.

Levitt MA, Ferraraccio D, et al: Variability of inguinal hernia surgical technique: A survey of North American pediatric surgeons. *J Pediatr Surg* 37:745, 2002.

Lintula H, Kokki H, et al: Single-blind randomized clinical trial of laparoscopic versus open appendicectomy in children. *Br J Surg* 88:510, 2001.

Lipshutz G, Albanese C, et al: Prospective analysis of lung-to-head ratio predicts survival for patients with prenatally diagnosed congenital diaphragmatic hernia. *J Pediatr Surg* 32:1634, 1997.

Little D, Rescorla F, et al: Long-term analysis of children with esophageal atresia and tracheoesophageal fistula. *J Pediatr Surg* 38:852, 2003.

Marianowski R, Ait Amer JL, et al: Risk factors for thyroglossal duct remnants after Sistrunk procedure in a pediatric population. *Int J Pediatr Otorhinolaryngol* 67:19, 2003.

Maris JM, Weiss MJ, et al: Loss of heterozygosity at 1p36 independently predicts for disease progression but not decreased overall survival probability in neuroblastoma patients: A Children's Cancer Group Study. *J Clin Oncol* 18:1888, 2000.

Meyers RL, Book LS, et al: High-dose steroids, ursodeoxycholic acid, and chronic intravenous antibiotics improve bile flow after Kasai procedure in infants with biliary atresia. *J Pediatr Surg* 38:406, 2003.

Miyano T, Yamataka A, et al: Hepaticoenterostomy after excision of choledochal cyst in children: A 30-year experience with 180 cases. *J Pediatr Surg* 31:1417, 1996.

Molik KA, West KW, et al: Portal venous air: The poor prognosis persists. *J Pediatr Surg* 36:1143, 2001.

Moss R, Dimmitt R, et al: A meta-analysis of peritoneal drainage versus laparotomy for perforated necrotizing enterocolitis. *J Pediatr Surg* 36:1210, 2001.

Moyer V, Moya F, et al: Late versus early surgical correction for congenital diaphragmatic hernia in newborn infants. *Cochrane Database Syst Rev* 3:CD001695, 2002.

Nadler E, Stanford A, et al: Intestinal cytokine gene expression in infants with acute necrotizing enterocolitis: Interleukin-11 mRNA expression inversely correlates with extent of disease. *J Pediatr Surg* 36:1122, 2001.

Neville HL, Andrassy RJ, et al: Lymphatic mapping with sentinel node biopsy in pediatric patients. *J Pediatr Surg* 35:961, 2000.

Nio M, Ohi R, et al: Five- and 10-year survival rates after surgery for biliary atresia: A report from the Japanese Biliary Atresia Registry. *J Pediatr Surg* 38:997, 2003.

Olutoye OO, Coleman BG, et al: Prenatal diagnosis and management of congenital lobar emphysema. *J Pediatr Surg* 35:792, 2000.

Ortega JA, Douglass EC, et al: Randomized comparison of cisplatin/vincristine/fluorouracil and cisplatin/continuous infusion doxorubicin for treatment of pediatric hepatoblastoma: A report from the Children's Cancer Group and the Pediatric Oncology Group. *J Clin Oncol* 18:2665, 2000.

Panesar J, Higgins K, et al: Nontuberculous mycobacterial cervical adenitis: A ten-year retrospective review. *Laryngoscope* 113:149, 2003.

Pedersen A, Petersen O, et al: Randomized clinical trial of laparoscopic versus open appendicectomy. *Br J Surg* 88:200, 2001.

Pena A, Guardino K, et al: Bowel management for fecal incontinence in patients with anorectal malformations. *J Pediatr Surg* 33:133, 1998.

Poenaru D, Laberge J, et al: A new prognostic classification for esophageal atresia. *Surgery* 113:426, 1993.

Potoka DA, Schall LC, et al: Risk factors for splenectomy in children with blunt splenic trauma. *J Pediatr Surg* 37:294, 2002.

Potoka D, Schall L, et al: Improved functional outcome for severely injured children treated at pediatric trauma centers. *J Trauma* 51:824, 2001.

Powers CJ, Levitt MA, et al: The respiratory advantage of laparoscopic Nissen fundoplication. *J Pediatr Surg* 38:886, 2003.

Pritchard-Jones K: Controversies and advances in the management of Wilms' tumour. *Arch Dis Child* 87:241, 2002.

Puapong D, Kahng D, et al: Ad libitum feeding: Safely improving the cost-effectiveness of pyloromyotomy. *J Pediatr Surg* 37:1667, 2002.

Quinton AE, Smoleniec JS: Congenital lobar emphysema—the disappearing chest mass: Antenatal ultrasound appearance. *Ultrasound Obstet Gynecol* 17:169, 2001.

Rosen NG, Hong AR, et al: Rectovaginal fistula: A common diagnostic error with significant consequences in girls with anorectal malformations. *J Pediatr Surg* 37:961, 2002.

Rothenberg S: Laparoscopic Nissen procedure in children. *Semin Laparosc Surg* 9:146, 2002.

Samuel M, McCarthy L, et al: Efficacy and safety of OK-432 sclerotherapy for giant cystic hygroma in a newborn. *Fetal Diagn Ther* 15:93, 2000.

Sandler A, Ein S, et al: Unsuccessful air-enema reduction of intussusception: Is a second attempt worthwhile? *Pediatr Surg Int* 15:214, 1999.

Schier F, Montupet P, et al: Laparoscopic inguinal herniorrhaphy in children: A three-center experience with 933 repairs. *J Pediatr Surg* 37:395, 2002.

Section on Hematology/Oncology: Guidelines for the pediatric cancer center and role of such centers in diagnosis and treatment. *Pediatrics* 99:139, 1997.

Shamberger R, Guthrie K, et al: Surgery-related factors and local recurrence of Wilms tumor in National Wilms Tumor Study 4. *Ann Surg* 229:292, 1999.

Shimada H, Ambros I, et al: The International Neuroblastoma Pathology Classification (the Shimada system). *Cancer* 86:364, 1999.

Simons SHP, van Dijk M, et al: Routine morphine infusion in preterm newborns who received ventilatory support: A randomized controlled trial. *JAMA* 290:2419, 2003.

Soffer SZ, Rosen NG, et al: Cloacal exstrophy: A unified management plan. *J Pediatr Surg* 35:932, 2000.

Spitz L, Kiely E, et al: Oesophageal atresia: At-risk groups for the 1990s. *J Pediatr Surg* 29:723, 1994.

Strauss RA, Balu R, et al: Gastroschisis: The effect of labor and ruptured membranes on neonatal outcome. *Am J Obstet Gynecol* 189:1672, 2003.

Suzuki N, Tsuchida Y, et al: Prenatally diagnosed cystic lymphangioma in infants. *J Pediatr Surg* 33:1599, 1998.

Teich S, Barton D, et al: Prognostic classification for esophageal atresia and tracheoesophageal fistula: Waterston versus Montreal. *J Pediatr Surg* 32:1075, 1997.

Teitelbaum D, Coran A: Reoperative surgery for Hirschsprung's disease. *Semin Pediatr Surg* 12:124, 2003.

Thibeault DW, Olsen SL, et al: Pre-ECMO predictors of nonsurvival in congenital diaphragmatic hernia. *J Perinatol* 22:682, 2002.

Tolia V, Wureth A, et al: Gastroesophageal reflux disease: Review of presenting symptoms, evaluation, management, and outcome in infants. *Dig Dis Sci* 48:1723, 2003.

Tulipan N, Sutton L, et al: The effect of intrauterine myelomeningocele repair on the incidence of shunt-dependent hydrocephalus. *Pediatr Neurosurg* 38:27, 2003.

Wenzler D, Bloom D, et al: What is the rate of spontaneous testicular descent in infants with cryptorchidism? *J Urol* 171:849, 2004.

Wildhaber B, Coran A, et al: The Kasai portoenterostomy for biliary atresia: A review of a 27-year experience with 81 patients. *J Pediatr Surg* 38:1480, 2003.

Wilson J, Lund D, et al: Congenital diaphragmatic hernia—a tale of two cities: The Boston experience. *J Pediatr Surg* 32:401, 1997.

Urology

Hyung L. Kim and Arie Belldegrun

The Penis
   Hypospadias
   Phimosis
   Paraphimosis
The Testicle
   Testicular Torsion
   Hydrocele

ANATOMY

The Kidney and Ureter

The organs of the urinary system, which include the kidney, ureter, and bladder, are located in the retroperitoneum.[1-3] The kidneys are paired organs surrounded by perirenal fat and Gerota's fascia (Fig. 39-1). The superior aspect of the kidney is contained within the lower thoracic cavity at the level of the tenth rib. The posterior aspect of the kidney lies against the quadratus lumborum, and the renal hilum lies against the psoas muscle. The upper pole of the right kidney abuts the liver. Anteriorly, the right kidney is adjacent to the duodenum and hepatic flexure of the colon. The left kidney is bounded anteriorly by the splenic flexure.

The blood supply to the kidney comes from the renal artery. The right and left renal arteries come off the aorta just inferior to the takeoff of the superior mesenteric artery. The right renal artery passes posterior to the inferior vena cava. The renal veins are anterior to the renal arteries and drain into the inferior vena cava. The renal artery and vein are anterior to the renal pelvis and proximal ureter at the level of the renal hilum. In the kidney, the arteries are end-arteries, while the veins anastomose freely. The left

adrenal vein and left gonadal vein drain into the left renal vein, while on the right, these same vessels drain directly into the vena cava.

The urine formed in the kidney drains into the collecting system and passes into the renal pelvis. The renal pelvis drains urine into the bladder through the ureter. Ureteral peristalsis originates from pacemaker cells located in the collecting system of the kidney. Along the course of the ureter in the retroperitoneum, the ureteral lumen is relatively narrower at the ureteral pelvic junction, at the pelvic brim where the ureter crosses the common iliac vessels and at the ureteral vesical junction. In patients passing a kidney stone, these areas represent common sites of impaction.

Adrenal Gland

The adrenal glands are endocrine organs that lie superomedial to the kidneys. They are surrounded by the perirenal fat and contained within Gerota's fascia. The right adrenal gland is positioned posterolateral to the inferior vena cava and tends to be more superior in relation to the left adrenal gland. The arterial blood supply to the adrenal glands is provided primarily by the inferior phrenic artery. On the right, the primary venous drainage is directly to the inferior vena cava. On the left, the primary venous drainage is to the left renal vein.

Bladder and Urethra

The bladder is a hollow, muscular organ adapted for storing and expelling urine. When it is empty, it lies posterior to the pubic symphysis in the pelvis and is extraperitoneal. The dome of the bladder is covered with peritoneum, and when the bladder is full, it can

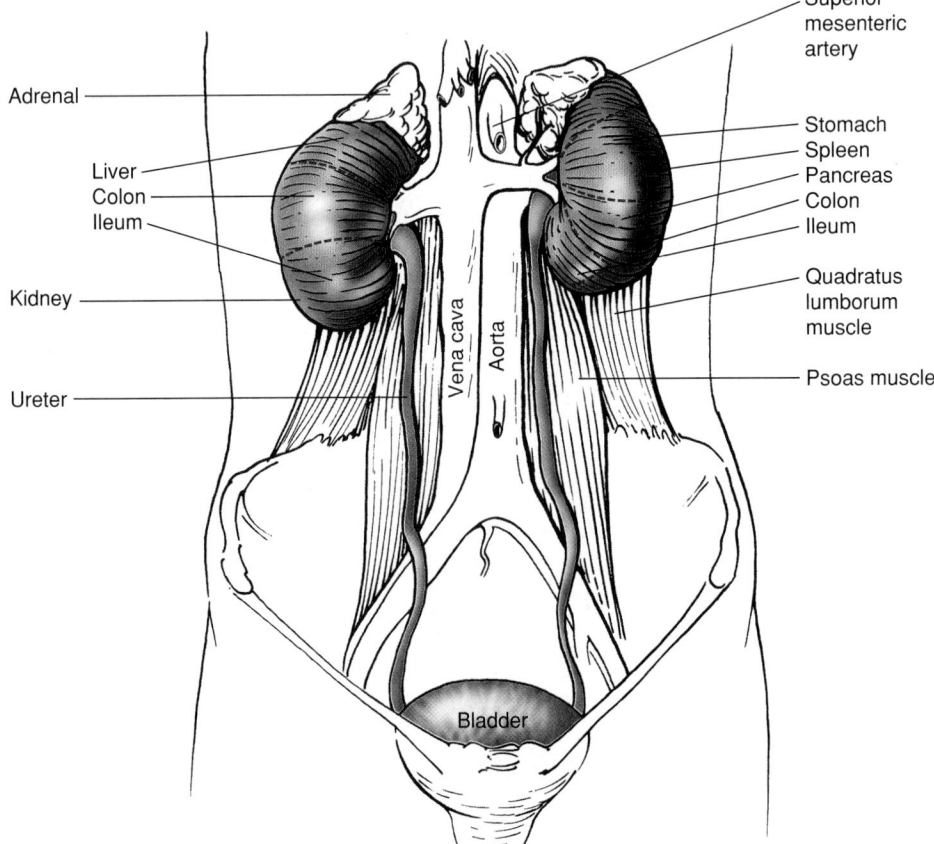

FIG. 39-1. Relations of the kidneys, ureters, and bladder. Anterior regions of the kidney labeled with adjacent organs.

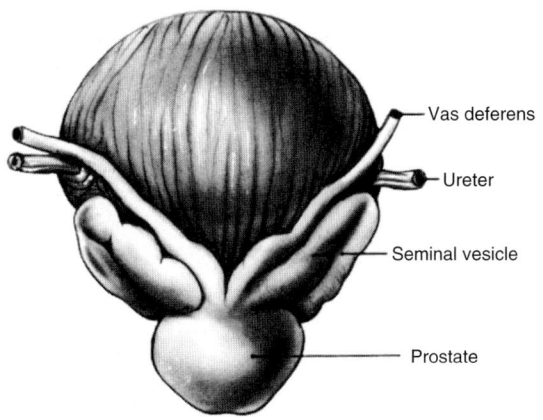

FIG. 39-2. *Relations of the prostate, seminal vesicles, and bladder.*

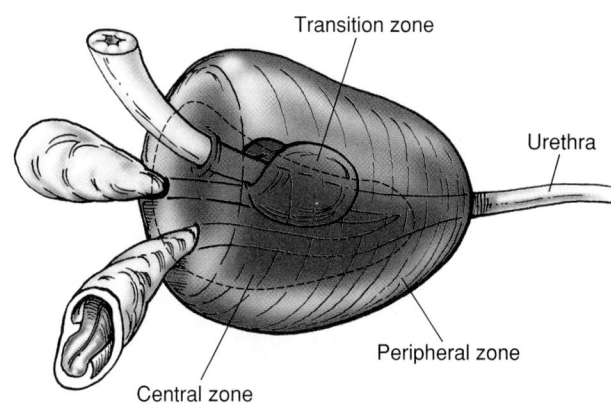

FIG. 39-3. *Zonal anatomy of the prostate.*

rise into the abdomen and is palpable on physical examination. The normal bladder can store approximately 350 to 450 mL. The muscularis propria, also referred to as the bladder detrusor, forms the muscular wall of the bladder. Close to the urethra, the muscle fibers become organized into three layers: an inner longitudinal, middle-circular, and outer-longitudinal. The arterial blood supply to the bladder comes from the superior, middle, and inferior vesical arteries, which are all branches of the internal iliac artery. The venous return from the bladder drains into the internal iliac vein.

In men, urinary continence is maintained by the internal and external sphincters. The internal sphincter, composed of smooth muscle, is formed by the middle circular layer of the bladder wall as it invests the prostate gland. Contraction of this sphincter during ejaculation prevents retrograde ejaculation by directing the semen toward the urethral meatus. The external sphincter surrounds the urethra at the level of the distal prostate gland and is composed of both smooth and striated muscle fibers.

In women, the continence mechanism is quite different. There is no internal sphincter and the middle circular layer of the bladder muscularis, which is prominent in the male bladder neck, is not found. Continence is maintained by the resistance provided by the coaptation of the urethral mucosa and the external striated sphincter surrounding the distal two-thirds of the urethra.

Prostate and Seminal Vesicle

The prostate gland and the seminal vesicles are part of the male reproductive system (Fig. 39-2). Secretions from these two organs make up part of the male semen. The prostate surrounds the proximal urethra. The gland can be divided into several zones (Fig. 39-3). Most prostate cancers form in the peripheral zone. The central zone surrounds the ejaculatory ducts as they empty into the urethra at the verumontanum. Benign prostatic hyperplasia (BPH) is caused by enlargement of the transition zone surrounding the urethra. BPH, which is common in the elderly population, can lead to increased urinary resistance and voiding symptoms.

Testis and Epididymis

The volume of an average testis is approximately 20 mL (Fig. 39-4). The testicles have two important functions: androgen and sperm production. The Leydig cells in the testis produce testosterone. The Sertoli cells support the maturation of spermatogenic cells into sperm. The Sertoli cells are also responsible for establishing a blood–testis barrier.

The testicles are surrounded by several fascial layers that are embryologically derived from the same layers comprising the anterior abdominal wall (Fig. 39-5). The external spermatic fascia

FIG. 39-4. *Testis, epididymis, and vas deferens.*

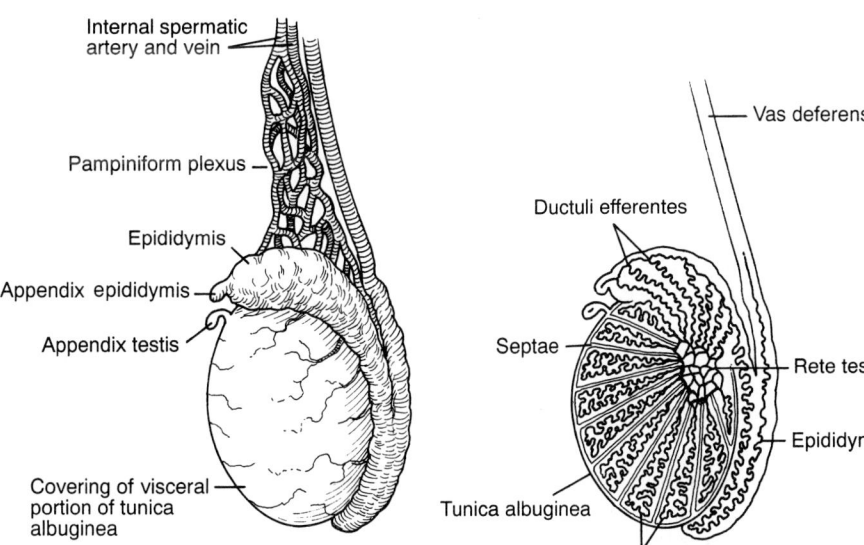

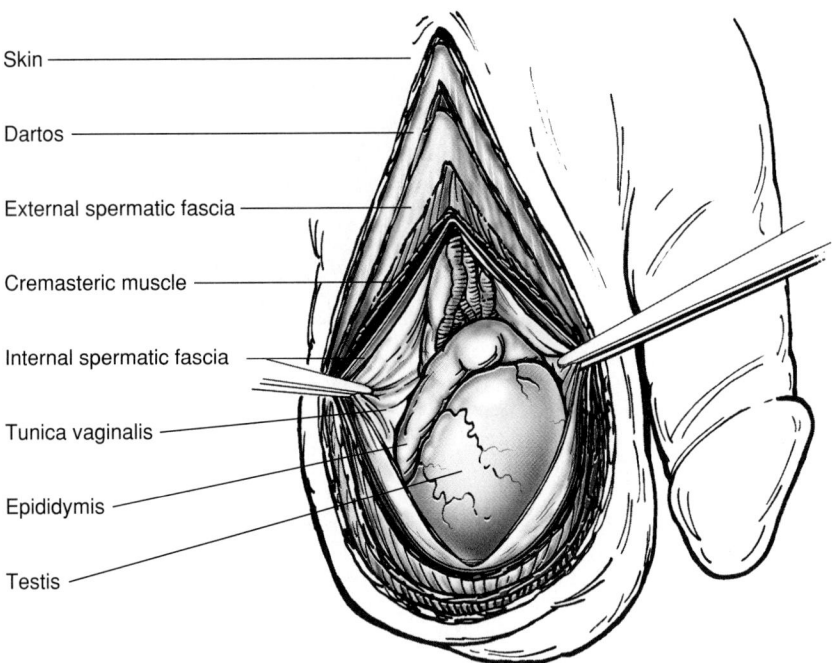

Skin

Dartos

External spermatic fascia

Cremasteric muscle

Internal spermatic fascia

Tunica vaginalis

Epididymis

Testis

FIG. 39-5. The testicle and its surrounding layers.

is analogous to the external oblique. The cremasteric muscle envelops the spermatic cord and is analogous to the internal oblique and transversus abdominis. The internal spermatic fascia is analogous to the transversalis fascia. The visceral and parietal layers of the tunica vaginalis testis represent peritoneum that surrounded the testicle during its descent into the scrotum.

The blood supply to the testicles is provided by three arteries: gonadal, cremasteric, and vasal. The gonadal artery branches directly from the aorta. The cremasteric artery branches from the inferior epigastric artery, and the vasal artery branches from the superior vesical artery. The venous drainage from the testicles forms the pampiniform plexus at the level of the spermatic cord. At the internal inguinal ring, the pampiniform plexus coalesces to form the gonadal vein, which drains into the inferior vena cava on the right and into the renal vein on the left.

The epididymis is located on the posterolateral aspect of the testis. Spermatogenesis occurs in the seminiferous tubules of the testes. Mature sperm is conducted by the efferent ducts into the epididymis where they are stored. Under sympathetic stimulation, the sperm is conducted along the vas deferens during a process termed *emission.* The vas deferens is joined by the seminal vesicle to form the ejaculatory duct. The semen that is deposited into the urethra is carried along the urethra under somatic enervation during ejaculation.

Penis

The penis is formed by three corpora bodies: two corpora cavernosa and a corpus spongiosum (Fig. 39-6). The corpus spongiosum surrounds the male urethra. The three corpora bodies are covered by the tunica albuginea. The next layer, going outward toward the skin, is Buck's fascia. Buck's fascia splits dorsally to envelop the neurovascular structures and splits ventrally to surround the corpora spongiosum. The superficial dartos fascia is just underneath the skin and is contiguous with the Colles fascia in the perineum and the Scarpa fascia in the abdominal wall. The base of the penis is supported by suspensory ligaments that attach to the linea alba and pubic symphysis.

The common penile artery is the terminal branch of the internal pudendal artery. It divides into three branches that supply blood to the penis. The cavernous arteries supply the corpora cavernosa. The bulbourethral branch supplies the glans, urethra, and corpus spongiosum. The dorsal arteries run in the neurovascular bundle enveloped by Buck's fascia and supply the corpus spongiosum and urethra. Venous drainage from the penis is provided by the dorsal and cavernous veins, which join to form the internal pudendal vein. Sensory innervation is carried by the dorsal nerves that run with the dorsal vessels. Autonomic innervation is provided by the cavernous nerves that pierce the tunica albuginea to innervate the smooth muscles found in the corpora cavernosa.

SIGNS AND SYMPTOMS

Symptoms Related to Voiding

Symptoms related to voiding can be broadly categorized as irritative or obstructive. Specific irritative symptoms include dysuria, frequency, and urgency. These symptoms generally imply inflammation of the urethra, prostate, or bladder. Although irritative voiding symptoms are commonly caused by infection, they can also be caused by malignancy, and in patients with symptoms that persist after treatment with appropriate antibiotics, malignant processes such as transitional cell carcinoma must be ruled out. In symptomatic patients with no specific etiology, the diagnosis of interstitial cystitis or chronic nonbacterial prostatitis is often made. The pathophysiology of both these processes is poorly understood and results of available treatments are often unsatisfactory.

Specific obstructive voiding symptoms include a weak urinary stream, urgency, frequency, hesitancy, intermittency, nocturia, and sense of incomplete emptying. Hesitancy refers to a delay in initiating a urinary stream and intermittency refers to repeated starting and stopping of the urine stream during voiding. The most common cause of obstructive voiding in men is benign prostatic hyperplasia.

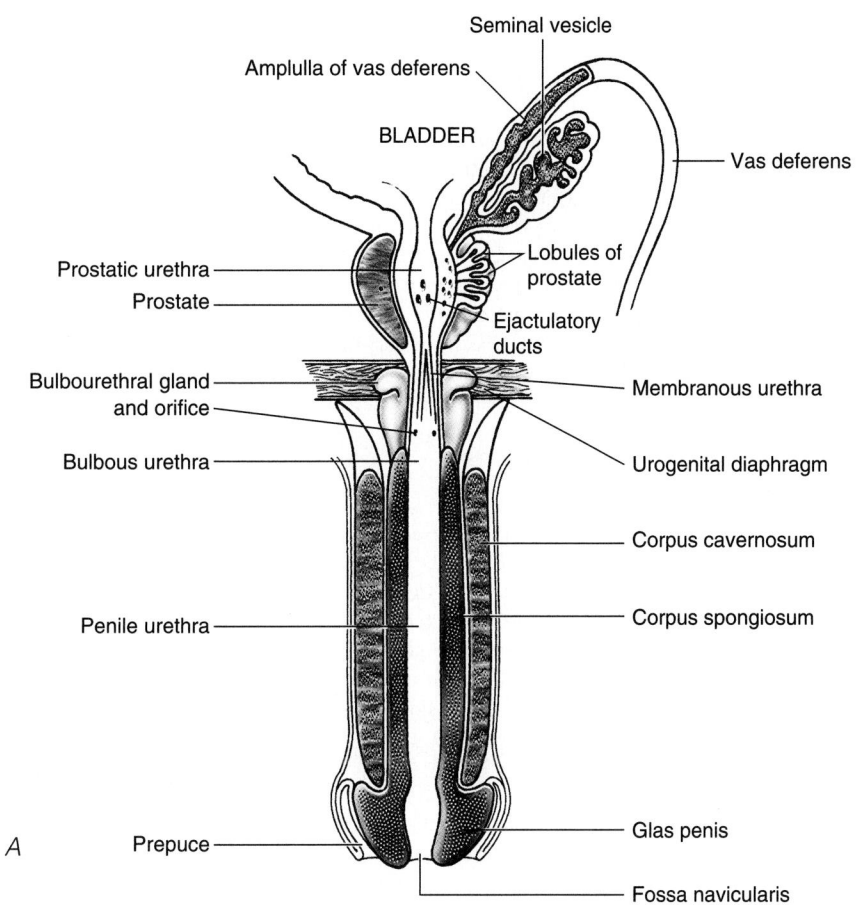

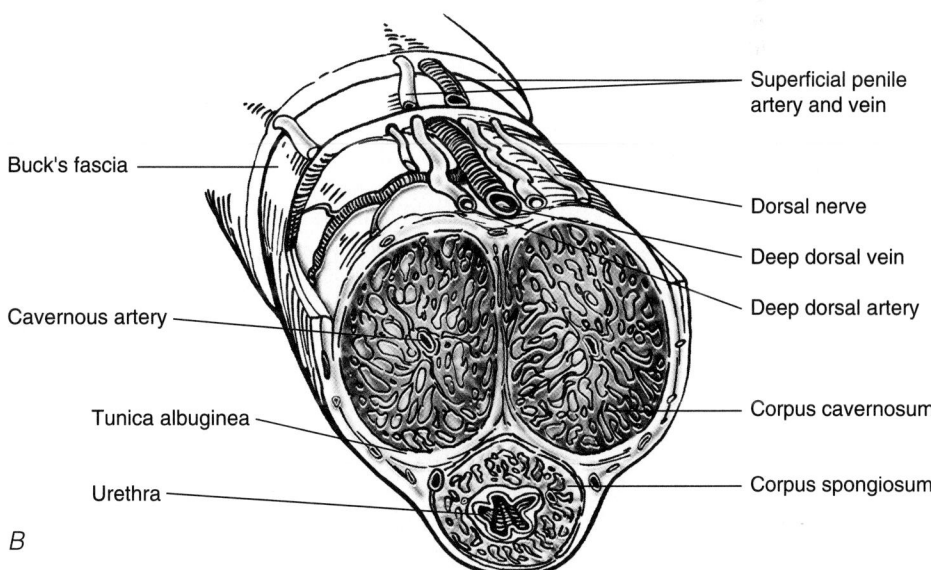

FIG. 39-6. *(A)* Longitudinal and *(B)* cross-sectional anatomy of the penis. *(A is reproduced with permission from Schwartz's Textbook of General Surgery, 6th ed. New York: McGraw-Hill, 1994, p. 1728.)*

Urethral strictures may also obstruct the bladder outlet and are often secondary to trauma, urethritis or previous instrumentation of the bladder.

Urinary Incontinence

Urinary incontinence can be categorized as stress, urge, total, and overflow. Stress incontinence refers to incontinence associated with an increase in intra-abdominal pressure. Patients often report leakage of urine when coughing, laughing, or during physical exertion. Stress incontinence is secondary to a decrease in the resistance provided by the urinary continence mechanisms and generally implies an anatomic disorder, such as an iatrogenic injury to the external sphincter in a male or prolapse of the bladder in a female. Urge incontinence is secondary to an involuntary contraction of the bladder and is accompanied by a sudden sense of needing to void. Urge incontinence may be secondary to inflammation and irritation of the bladder, or it may result from neurologic disorders such as a stroke or spinal cord injury.

Total incontinence refers to a continuous leakage of urine and implies a fistula between the skin or vagina and the urinary tract, proximal to the sphincter mechanism. Women with a vesicovaginal fistula secondary to malignancy or trauma will complain of continuous leakage of urine. Overflow incontinence is secondary to an obstruction of the lower urinary tract. As urine builds up in the bladder, the intravesical pressure increases and overcomes the resistance provided by the urinary sphincter. All patients at risk for urinary tract obstruction who develop new-onset incontinence should be checked for urinary retention by postvoid bladder ultrasound or catheterization of the bladder.

Hematuria

Patients with gross or microscopic hematuria, in the absence of obvious evidence of a urinary tract infection, need to be evaluated with upper and lower tract studies. On microscopic examination of the urine, more than five red blood cells per high power field in spun urine or more than two red blood cells per high power field in unspun urine is considered significant microscopic hematuria. Because hematuria can be intermittent, even a single documented episode of significant microscopic hematuria warrants a complete evaluation. The upper tract, which includes the kidney and ureter, should be evaluated with an intravenous pyelogram, CT scan, or retrograde pyelogram. The CT scan should be performed with intravenous contrast and delayed images should be obtained once the excreted contrast has filled the upper tract collecting system. The lower tract, which includes the bladder and urethra, should be evaluated by cystoscopy.

The differential diagnosis for hematuria includes malignancies, infections, kidney stones, and trauma. Malignancies of the kidney and bladder classically present with painless hematuria. Patients with gross painless hematuria should be considered to have a urinary tract malignancy until proven otherwise. Infections involving the bladder or urethra are generally associated with symptoms of irritative voiding. Pyelonephritis is a clinical diagnosis based on findings of irritative voiding symptoms, fever, and flank pain. Kidney stones are associated with a colicky pain. The localization of the pain depends on the level of obstruction by the stone. An obstruction at the ureteropelvic junction will cause flank pain while obstruction of the lower ureter can produce colicky pain referred to the lower abdomen or groin.

Other Findings

Other complaints and findings related to the urinary system include urethral discharge, hematospermia, and pneumaturia. Urethral discharge is a common complaint that usually results from infection with *Neisseria gonorrhoeae* or *Chlamydia trachomatis*. The discharge is often associated with dysuria. Hematospermia refers to blood in the ejaculated semen and is caused by inflammation of seminal vesicles or prostate. As a general rule, hematospermia is self-limiting and does not require further evaluation or treatment. Pneumaturia refers to air in the voided urine. The finding of pneumaturia can be confirmed by having the patient void in a tub with the urethral meatus submerged. Pneumaturia may result from recent instrumentation of the bladder or from a fistula between the urinary tract and the intestine.

PHYSICAL EXAMINATION

Examination of the Penis, Scrotum, and Testis

The physical examination of a male patient should be performed with the patient standing and the physician seated on a stool. Initially, the skin of the penis, scrotum, and the surrounding inguinal region should be visually inspected. The testicles should be palpated for masses or tenderness and the size of the testicles should be noted. The epididymis can be palpated on the posterolateral surface of the testicles. Any nodules should be noted and an effort should be made to determine if palpable lesions are associated with the testis or the epididymis. The vas deferens can be felt by gently compressing the scrotum above the testicles.

Hydroceles represent a buildup of fluid between the two layers of the tunica vaginalis. If the testicles are enlarged by a hydrocele, the presence of a hydrocele sac can be confirmed by transilluminating the sac with a penlight. Varicoceles may be palpable in the scrotum and represent dilated veins, which are analogous to varicose veins found on the leg. The penis should be gently massaged to express any urethral discharge. The penile shaft and urethra should be palpated along the length of the penis. Any nodules or fibrotic plaques on the corporal bodies should be noted.

Prostate Exam

The prostate is examined with the patient leaning over an examination bench and resting on his elbows. Alternatively, the patient can be lying in a lateral decubitus position. Initially, the anus and surrounding area is visually inspected. Using lubrication, the index finger is gently inserted into the rectum. The prostate is palpated, and any nodules, indurations or asymmetry should be noted. Although the seminal vesicle is too far to reach in most men, they may occasionally be palpable just above the prostate. Having the patient Valsalva will often bring the prostate closer to the anus and facilitate the exam.

LABORATORY EXAMINATION

Examination of the Urine

In the patient with urologic complaints, urinalysis is a simple, but powerful tool. The proper collection of the urine sample is critical. Ideally, the urine sample is collected by sterilely catheterizing the bladder. However, this is not always practical, and a clean midstream catch is usually adequate, especially in men. In women, an abnormal urinalysis may need to be confirmed with a catheterized specimen to rule out possible contamination by the vaginal flora. In children, urine can be collected by placing a urine collection bag over the urethral meatus; however, urine specimen for bacterial culture may need to be obtained by catheterization or suprapubic aspiration.

The complete urinalysis includes testing with a dipstick impregnated with an array of chemical reagents and a microscopic examination of urinary sediments obtained by centrifugation.[1,2] A reasonable approach to urinalysis is to reserve the microscopic examination for patients with abnormalities detected using the dipstick. Most standard dipsticks will test for urinary pH, specific gravity, protein, glucose, ketones, bilirubin, urobilinogen, hemoglobin, leukocytes, and nitrites. The dipstick analysis relies on color changes produced by chemical reactions with substances in the urine, and, therefore, any medications taken by the patient that changes the color of the urine, such as phenazopyridine (Pyridium), will interfere with the test. Usually the urine pH will reflect the pH of the serum. Exceptions to this rule occur in patients with renal tubular acidosis or a urinary tract infection involving a urea-splitting organism.

The specific gravity of the urine reflects the hydration status of the patient and the concentrating ability of the kidney. Proteinuria detected on dipstick may indicate intrinsic renal pathology or the presence of excess protein in the serum. Persistent proteinuria determined using a dipstick should be confirmed by a 24-hour urine collection for protein. Testing for urinary glucose and ketones is useful in screening for diabetes. Urinary glucose will usually be detected when serum glucose levels are greater than 180 mg/dL. A small amount of urobilinogen can normally be detected in the urine. However, a positive test for bilirubin and high levels of urobilinogen may indicate liver disease or hemolysis. Presence of hemoglobin, myoglobin, and red blood cells in the urine can produce a positive result on dipstick tests for blood. Therefore, a positive dipstick test should be confirmed by microscopy.

A positive urinalysis for leukocytes and nitrites suggests inflammation, which is most commonly caused by a bacterial infection. The dipstick tests for leukocyte esterase, which is an enzyme found in neutrophils. The urine may be positive for leukocytes in the presence of both hematuria and pyuria. Therefore, suspected pyuria should be confirmed by microscopic examination of the urine. Normal urine does not contain nitrites. However, in the presence of urea-splitting organisms, urinary nitrates are converted to nitrites, which can be detected by the dipstick test. Urea-splitting bacteria include the *Proteus, Klebsiella, Pseudomonas, Enterococcus,* and *Morganella* species. This list does not include *Escherichia,* which is the most common cause of urinary infections.

Urine Culture

It is important to keep in mind that the urinalysis results may be normal in patients with a urinary tract infection. A urine culture is the most definitive test for symptomatic patients. Greater than 10^5 organisms/mL of urine is consistent with a urinary tract infection. However, in patients who have irritative voiding symptoms, such as frequency and dysuria, 100 organisms/mL of a known urinary pathogen is sufficient evidence of a bacterial infection. In patients with recurrent or resistant infections, it may be important to identify the organism and test for antibiotic sensitivities by using a urine culture. Some urinary pathogens, such as *Neisseriae, Mycobacteria,* and anaerobes, require special culture techniques and a local laboratory should be consulted regarding the specific requirements.

Tests of Kidney Function

Several simple tests can be used to estimate kidney function. Urine-specific gravity can be measured in the office by using a dipstick. As renal function decreases, the ability of the kidney to concentrate urine decreases. This is reflected by a proportional change in specific gravity. However, specific gravity is also dependent on hydration status, and with a progressive decrease in renal function, the specific gravity does not decrease below approximately 1.015. Serum creatinine level is a better approximation of kidney function. Creatinine is an end-product of muscle creatine metabolism and is excreted by the kidney. Serum creatinine levels are less affected by hydration status. However, creatinine does not reflect early loss of renal function, as serum creatinine levels remain in the normal range until approximately 50% of the kidney function is lost.

The best measure of kidney function that does not involve infusion of exogenous substances is the endogenous creatinine clearance rate. Creatinine clearance is defined as the volume of plasma from which creatinine is completely removed per unit of time and is a clinical approximation of the glomerular filtration rate (GFR) and renal function. Creatinine clearance is calculated from a 24-hour urine collection according to the following formula:

$$\text{Clearance} = UV/P$$

In this formula, U and P represent the urine and plasma concentrations of creatinine, respectively, and V represents the urine flow rate. Normal creatinine clearance is 90 to 110 mL/min.

The gold standard for measuring GFR involves infusing and measuring the clearance of inulin. Inulin is an ideal substance for measuring GFR because it is completely filtered by the kidney without being secreted or reabsorbed by the tubules. In contrast, creatinine is secreted in small amounts by the proximal tubule. Therefore, creatinine clearance will slightly overestimate GFR at all levels of kidney function. This effect is most pronounced when kidney function is severely compromised, where creatinine clearance can overestimate GFR by as much as 1.5- to twofold.

RADIOLOGIC STUDIES OF THE URINARY SYSTEM

Imaging of Kidney and Ureter

With recent improvements in computed tomography (CT) technology, CT scans have become the study of choice for general imaging of the kidney and ureter.[1,2] The primary advantage of a CT scan is the amount of information it provides. On a CT scan, kidney stones that are radiolucent on plain x-ray are readily visible (Fig. 39-7). Uptake of contrast by the renal parenchyma during the nephrogram phase of the CT scan provides a rough estimate of the kidney function. A comparison of the uptake of contrast by each kidney provides an estimate of the differential function between the right and left kidneys. After the contrast is excreted by the kidney into the collecting system, the collecting system can be evaluated for subtle filling defects and hydronephrosis. The CT scan also allows for evaluation of other organ systems in the abdomen and pelvis.

CT scans are useful when renal or ureteral malignancy is suspected. When a CT scan is performed for evaluation of hematuria, the study should be performed with and without IV contrast, and delayed images should be obtained after the contrast has been excreted into the renal pelvis and ureter. Renal cell carcinomas classically appear as solid, enhancing masses. The degree of enhancement can be determined by comparing the images with and without contrast. Transitional cell tumors of the renal pelvis and ureter often present as filling defects on delayed images. Transitional cell tumors in the kidney and ureter can obstruct the collecting system and hydronephrosis may be seen. When a CT scan is performed for evaluation of malignancy, oral contrast should be given. This will facilitate delineation of any pathologically enlarged lymph nodes in the retroperitoneum and pelvis.

Although CT scan is the study of choice in most settings, an intravenous pyelogram (IVP) is a better test when the primary goal is to evaluate the collecting system. To obtain an IVP, radiologic contrast is infused and a series of plain x-rays are taken of the abdomen and pelvis. The diameter and contour of the renal pelvis is readily appreciated on IVP, and congenital anomalies of the ureter and renal pelvic filing defects are easily seen. When an IVP is not

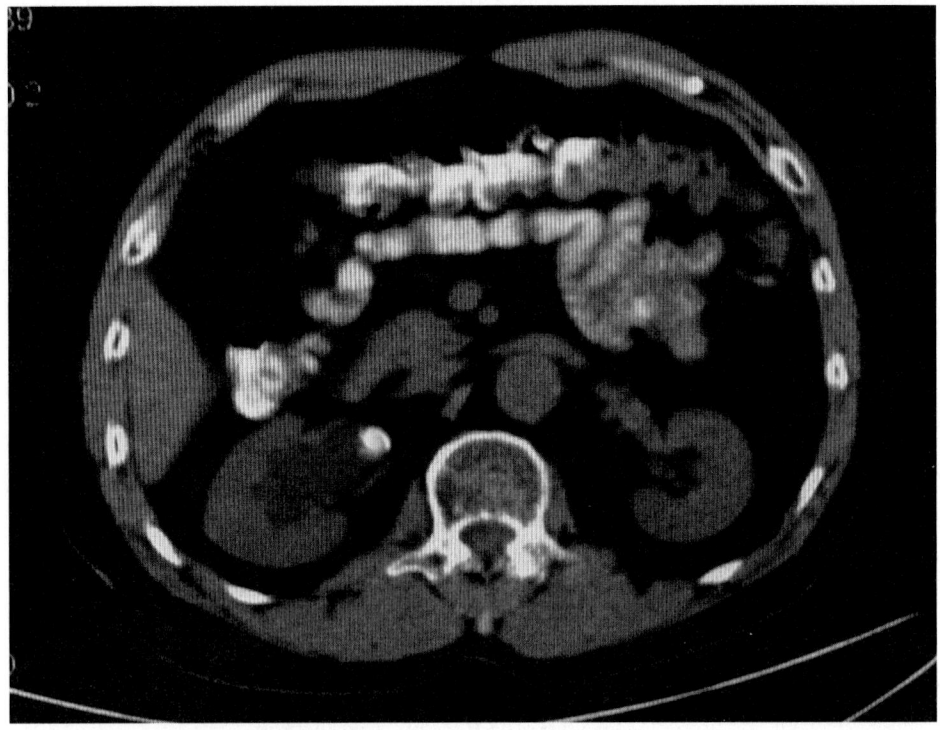

A

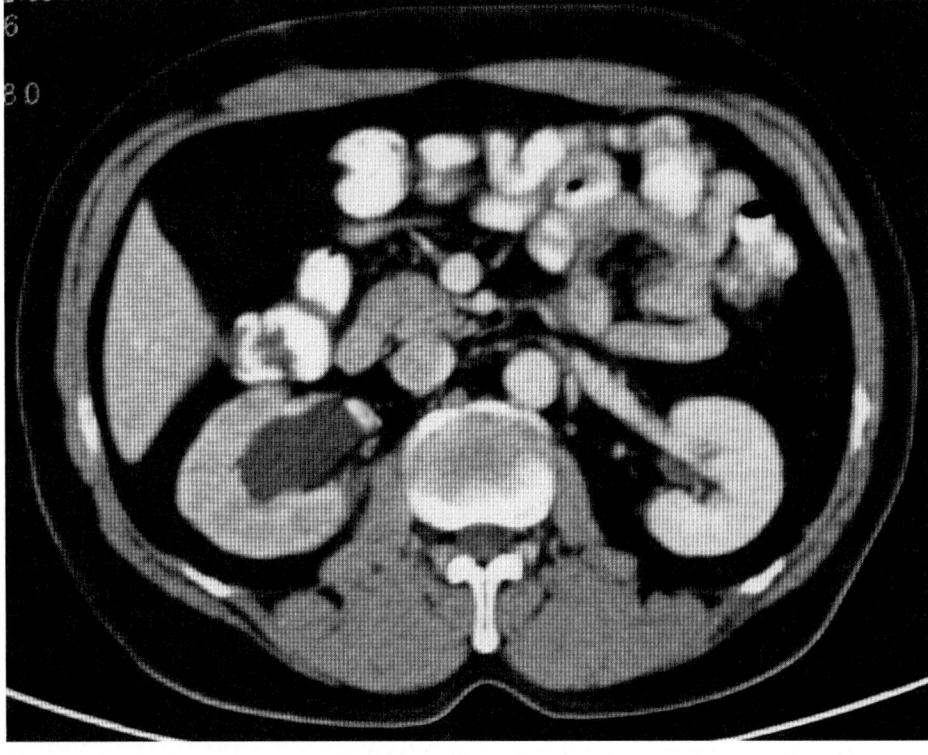

B

FIG. 39-7. *(A)* CT scan performed without IV contrast and *(B)* CT scan performed with IV contrast. A urinary stone is visible at the level of the (right) ureteropelvic junction, causing hydronephrosis. Following administration of contrast, there is a delay in uptake of contrast by the right kidney, suggesting a decrease in renal function. The right renal function is expected to return to normal after relief of urinary obstruction of limited duration.

diagnostic, or if the patient is allergic to IV contrast, a retrograde pyelogram can be performed (Fig. 39-8). A magnetic resonance image (MRI) obtained with contrast medium such as gadolinium can generally be used in place of a CT scan when renal insufficiency or contrast allergy prohibits the use of CT contrast.

A retrograde pyelogram is performed by visualizing the ureteral orifice through a cystoscope and cannulating the ureters with a 6 to 8 F catheter. Radiologic contrast is injected through the catheter and the collecting system is visualized in real-time by fluoroscopy. At the time of the procedure, a urine sample or a saline

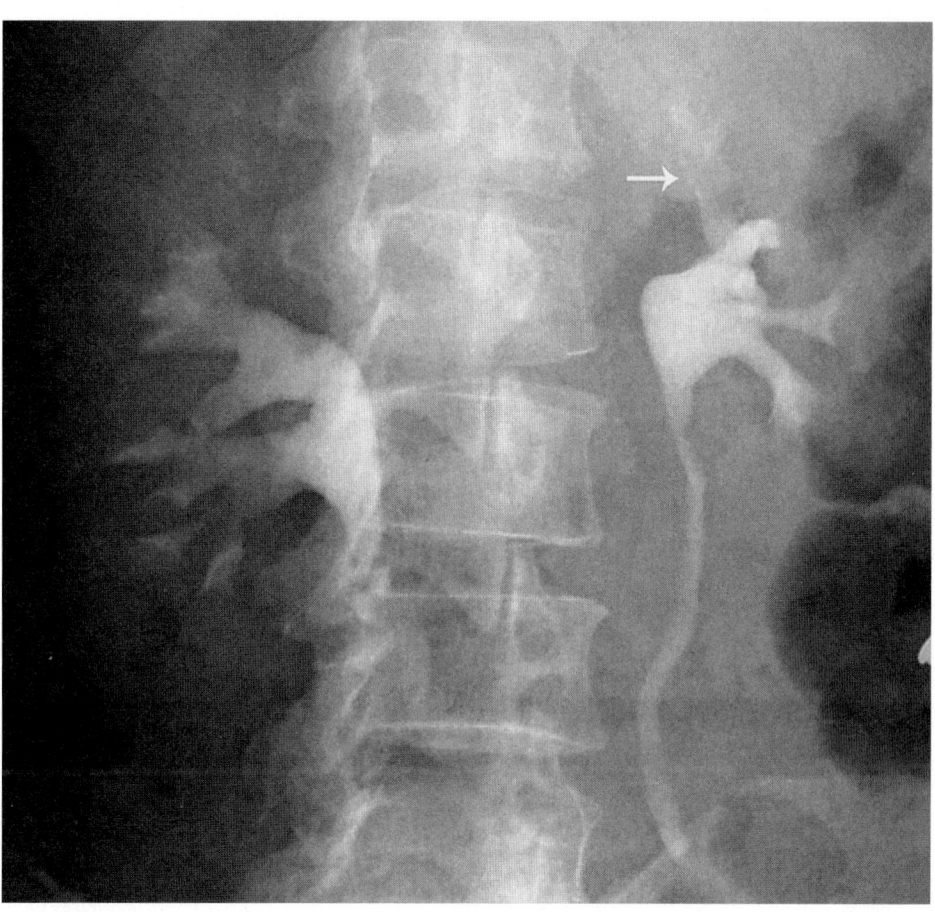

FIG. 39-8. Retrograde pyelogram. A filling defect, suspicious for a transitional cell carcinoma, is present in the left renal pelvis (*arrow*).

wash sample from the upper tract can be collected through the ureteral catheter and sent for cytology or culture. Urine collected from each of the upper tracts may allow for localization of malignancy or infection to the right or left side. The primary disadvantage to performing a retrograde pyelogram is that it is an invasive procedure, which is usually performed in the operating room under anesthesia.

The least-invasive imaging modality for the kidney is a renal ultrasound. Many common renal pathologies have a characteristic appearance on ultrasound. Kidney stones are identified as a hyperechoic lesion associated with hypoechoic "shadowing" behind the stone (Fig. 39-9). On ultrasound, fluid is hypoechoic, therefore renal cysts and hydronephrosis are readily identified. Renal masses appear as hyperechoic lesions and generally warrant further evaluation with a CT scan. In the pediatric population, a renal ultrasound is the first screening test obtained when a congenital abnormality of the urinary system is suspected.

Imaging of the Bladder and Urethra

A urethrogram should be performed when a urethral stricture or a traumatic urethral disruption is suspected (Fig. 39-10). A Foley catheter is inserted just beyond the tip of the meatus and the catheter balloon is inflated with approximately 0.5 mL of fluid. Radiologic contrast is injected in a retrograde fashion and a plain x-ray is taken. Alternatively, the urethra is visualized during the injection using fluoroscopy.

An antegrade urethrogram can also be performed during a voiding cystourethrogram (VCUG). For a VCUG, a small-diameter catheter is inserted into the bladder and a cystogram is obtained.

The patient is then asked to void the contrast and a urethrogram is taken. In the pediatric population, a VCUG is most commonly performed to rule out ureteral reflux or a posterior urethral valve. In adults, a cystogram is most commonly performed to rule out a bladder perforation in a trauma patient.

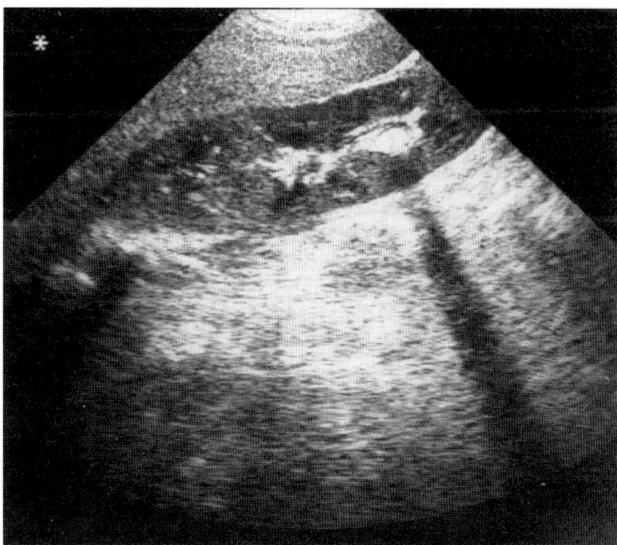

FIG. 39-9. Renal ultrasound demonstrating a urinary stone. The urinary stone is a hyperechoic lesion creating a hypoechoic "shadow" distally.

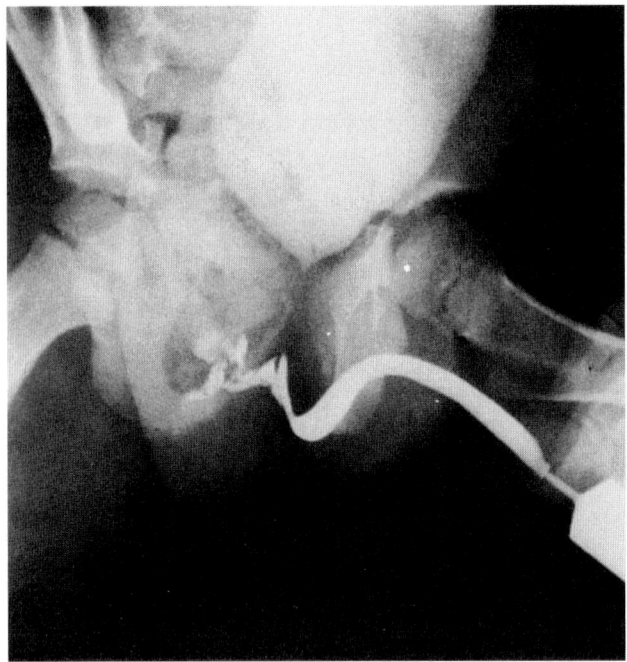

FIG. 39-10. Retrograde urethrogram. The urethrogram obtained following blunt trauma to the pelvis demonstrates a urethra disruption where extravasation of radiologic contrast is seen.

Testicular Ultrasound

A testicular ultrasound is most commonly performed to evaluate testicular pain or a palpable lesion noted on physical examination. The differential diagnoses for acute testicular pain include testicular torsion, epididymal orchitis, and scrotal abscess. On Doppler ultrasound, the absence of blood flow is consistent with a testicular torsion, while increased blood flow suggests epididymal orchitis. For palpable lesions of the testicle, an ultrasound is well suited for distinguishing between solid and cystic lesions. Solid masses in the testicle or in the epididymis should be considered a malignancy until proven otherwise and an orchiectomy should be performed to make a definitive diagnosis.

Renal Scan

A renal scan is a nuclear medicine study used to determine renal function and evaluate drainage of the renal pelvis and ureter (Fig. 39-11). After intravenous administration of a radioactive tracer, the kidneys are imaged. Depending on the indications for the study, different tracers are used. If the primary purpose of the study is to image the renal cortex to detect parenchyma scarring, which is often seen in pediatric patients following an episode of pyelonephritis, technetium-99m dimercaptosuccinic acid (DMSA) is used. This tracer is bound to the proximal tubule and is slowly excreted, a property that makes it an ideal agent for visualizing the kidney cortex.

Technetium-99m diethylenetriamine-pentaacetic acid (DTPA) is excreted following glomerular filtration and can be used to determine the GFR DTPA also can be used to evaluate the drainage of the collecting system. Once DTPA is excreted into the renal pelvis, Lasix can be given and the half-life ($T_{1/2}$) of the tracer activity is measured. A high $T_{1/2}$ (greater than 20 minutes) is consistent with an obstruction. The third agent, technetium-99m mercaptoacetyltriglycine (MAG-3), is both filtered by the glomeruli and secreted by the tubules. Therefore, it is well suited for imaging the renal cortex,

estimating differential renal function, and evaluating drainage of the renal pelvis.

BENIGN PROSTATIC HYPERPLASIA

Etiology

BPH refers to the stromal and epithelial proliferation in the prostate gland that may eventually result in voiding symptoms. BPH occurs primarily in the transition zone of the prostate gland (see Fig. 39-3). In autopsy studies, histologic evidence of BPH is rare in men who are younger than 40 years of age; however, it can be found in approximately 70% of men in their seventies, and in nearly all men in their nineties.[4] Although androgen production is required for BPH to occur, androgen merely plays a permissive role in the development of BPH. The precise hormonal, autocrine, and paracrine factors involved in stimulating BPH are unknown.

Natural History

Patients with BPH can present with both obstructive and irritative voiding symptoms, which are often referred to collectively as lower urinary tract symptoms (LUTS). Patients may complain of a decreased urinary stream, frequency, nocturia, urgency, hesitancy, intermittency, and a sense of incomplete emptying. Although these symptoms are certainly related to a bladder outlet obstruction secondary to an enlarged prostate, other, less-clearly defined factors are involved. This is underscored by several studies documenting that there is a minimal relationship between the degree of symptoms, the size of the prostate, and the degree of urethral obstruction.[5,6] Therefore, treatment should primarily be dictated by the patient's symptoms and the extent to which the patient is bothered by the symptoms, rather than merely the size of the prostate gland.

Without treatment, the symptoms of BPH tend to wax and wane over the short-term; however, with long-term follow-up, the common trend is toward a worsening of symptoms. As the transition zone of the prostate enlarges and becomes progressively more obstructive, the bladder initially undergoes compensatory hypertrophy. As long as the hypertrophied bladder is able to generate enough pressure to overcome the increased outlet resistance, the patient is able to void to completion. However, as the bladder outlet resistance continues to increase, the bladder may not be able to generate enough pressure to overcome the outlet resistance. Persistent bladder outlet obstruction and increasing postvoid urinary residuals lead to a decompensated bladder characterized by a thin bladder wall, large capacity, and poor contractility. Without intervention, potential sequelae of a decompensated bladder include urinary retention requiring emergent catheterization, upper tract dilation, and renal failure.

The differential diagnosis for a patient presenting with LUTS includes urinary tract infection, prostatitis, bladder stones, urethral stricture, and neurogenic bladder. The work-up for LUTS should include a thorough voiding history. The symptoms can be quantified by having the patient fill out an international prostate symptom score (I-PSS) questionnaire (Table 39-1). This questionnaire has been validated as a useful means for assessing and following symptoms resulting from BPH.[7] Treatment is recommended for an I-PSS greater than 7. A digital rectal exam and a focused neurologic exam should be performed because symptoms such as urgency and frequency may be signs of a neurologic disorder.[8] A urinalysis should be obtained in all patients and a urine culture should be obtained in patients with dysuria or abnormal urinalysis.

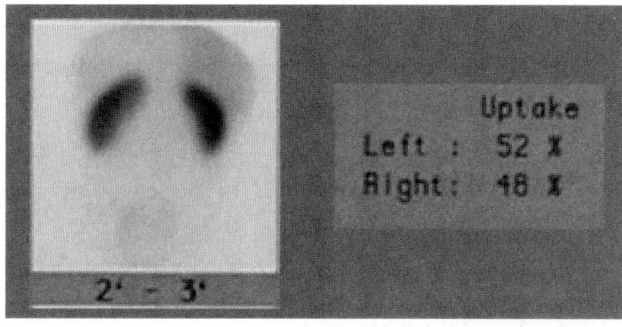

A

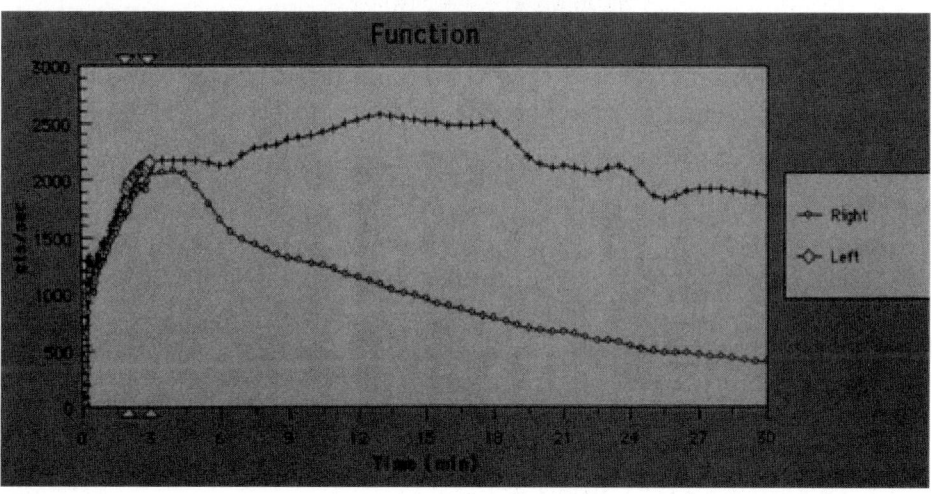

B

FIG. 39-11. *A.* Renal scan in a patient with a ureteropelvic junction obstruction. Renal scan obtained using technetium-99m mercaptoacetyltriglycine (MAG-3). A quantitative assessment of uptake of MAG-3 by the renal parenchyma approximately 2 minutes following injection suggests that the differential functions of the left and right kidneys are 52 and 48%, respectively. *B.* Following administration of Lasix, the $T_{1/2}$ for the washout of the nucleotide in the renal pelvis of the right kidney is 9 minutes and 30 seconds; however, the nucleotide never washes out of the left kidney. $T_{1/2} > 20$ minutes is consistent with obstruction.

In patients presenting with urinary retention or severe voiding symptoms, a check of serum creatinine levels to evaluate renal function is reasonable.

Other studies can be more selectively obtained in patients with voiding symptoms. Cystoscopy should be performed for patients who also present with hematuria or when a urethral stricture is suspected. For patients with a very poor stream, or for patients complaining of a sense of incomplete emptying, a postvoid residual should be measured by ultrasound or by catheterization. A renal ultrasound should be performed in patients with an elevated creatinine. For select patients, a pressure-flow study may be necessary. A decrease in urinary flow may result from bladder outlet obstruction or from failure of the bladder to effectively contract. To distinguish between the two, a small-diameter catheter can be inserted into the bladder to transduce bladder pressures during voiding. High bladder pressure and low flow rates are consistent with obstruction. Low bladder pressure and low flow rates suggest a neurogenic bladder that is unable to effectively contract.

Medical Therapy

BPH is not always progressive. Patients with mild symptoms can be managed by watchful waiting. Patients with more severe symptoms should be treated based on the degree of bother. Absolute indications for treatment include urinary retention, bladder stones, upper tract dilation, and renal failure. Relative indications for treatment include large postvoid residuals, hematuria, and recurrent urinary tract infections. There are two components to the bladder outlet obstruction resulting from BPH: mechanical and dynamic. The mechanical component refers to the urethral compression resulting from the enlarged prostate. The dynamic component refers to the smooth muscles in the urethra and prostatic stroma that contract and further obstruct the bladder outlet.[9]

The smooth muscles at the bladder outlet are under alpha$_1$-adrenergic innervation. The first line therapy for BPH is an alpha blocker, which targets the dynamic component of the bladder outlet obstruction. Three alpha blockers that are available in the United States for the treatment of BPH are terazosin, doxazosin, and tamsulosin.[10] Terazosin and doxazosin are selective for alpha$_1$-adrenoceptors, which are found in the prostate, as well as in the vascular endothelium and central nervous system. Both terazosin and doxazosin significantly lower blood pressure, especially in men with clinical hypertension. Therefore, terazosin and doxazosin are good choices in the approximately 30% of men with BPH who also have clinical hypertension. The most common side effects with these two medications are dizziness and orthostatic hypertension. Both medications should be titrated up over 1 to 2 weeks to their target dose.

Tamsulosin is the newest alpha blocker. It is selective for the α_{1a}-adrenoceptor subtype, which is predominately found in the prostate.[11] Its effect on blood pressure is clinically insignificant, and its primary advantage is that it does not need to be titrated. It can be started at its effective dose. Retrograde ejaculation, which refers to the passage of semen into the bladder during ejaculation, and rhinitis are more common with tamsulosin than with the less specific alpha$_1$-blockers. Although the side-effect profiles differ slightly between the alpha blockers, all three alpha blockers appear to be equally effective for the treatment of BPH.

Table 39-1
International Prostate Symptom Score (I-PSS) Questionnaire

	Not At All	Under 1/5 the Time	Under 1/2 the Time	1/2 Time	Over 1/2 the Time	Almost Always	Your Score
1. Incomplete Emptying Over the last month, how often have you had a sensation of not emptying your bladder completely after you finish urinating?	0	1	2	3	4	5	
2. Frequency Over the last month, how often have you had to urinate again less than two hours after you finished urinating?	0	1	2	3	4	5	
3. Intermittency Over the last month, how often have you found you stopped and started again several times when you urinated?	0	1	2	3	4	5	
4. Urgency Over the last month, how often have you found it difficult to postpone urination?	0	1	2	3	4	5	
5. Weak Stream Over the last month, how often have you had a weak urinary stream?	0	1	2	3	4	5	
6. Straining Over the last month, how often have you had to push or strain to begin urination?	0	1	2	3	4	5	

	None	1 Time	2 Times	3 Times	4 Times	5+ Times	Your Score
7. Nocturia Over the last month, how many times did you most typically get up to urinate from the time you went to bed at night until the time you got up in the morning?	0	1	2	3	4	5	
Total I-PSS Score							

	Delighted	Pleased	Mostly Satisfied	Mixed	Mostly Dissatisfied	Unhappy	Terrible	Your Score
Quality of Life Due to Urinary Symptoms If you were to spend the rest of your life with your urinary condition just the way it is now, how would you feel about that?	0	1	2	3	4	5	6	

Patients in urinary retention require emergent catheterization and the catheter should be left in place for at least 24 hours to allow the acutely distended bladder to remain decompressed. Tamsulosin may be preferred for previously untreated patients who present in acute urinary retention. Before attempting catheter removal, tamsulosin can be started at the therapeutic dose without need for titration.

Other common medical therapies for BPH include saw palmetto and finasteride.[12,13] Saw palmetto is derived from the American dwarf palm tree and is sold in the United States as an herbal supplement. In several randomized, controlled studies, saw palmetto improved symptoms and urinary flow rates. Multiple studies have shown that saw palmetto is safe with no significant adverse effects; however, the precise mechanism of action is not known.

Finasteride is commonly used for the treatment of BPH as well as for the treatment of hair loss. Development of prostatic hyperplasia requires the presence of androgen, and more specifically, dihydrotestosterone. Finasteride is a 5α-reductase inhibitor, and it blocks the conversion of testosterone to dihydrotestosterone. Finasteride is effective in decreasing the risk of urinary retention and hematuria in men with very large prostate glands. However, finasteride has no proven benefit in men with LUTS and smaller prostate glands.

Surgical Management

Surgery should be recommended for patients who continue to be bothered by their symptoms or who experience urinary retention despite medical therapy. Surgery should also be recommended for patients with upper tract dilation, renal insufficiency secondary to BPH, or bladder stones. Surgery for BPH is most commonly performed endoscopically; however, if the prostate gland is greater than 80 to 100 g, an open prostatectomy should be performed.

The standard endoscopic procedure for BPH is a transurethral resection (TUR) of the prostate. TUR is performed with a nonhemolytic fluid such as 1.5% glycine. Saline cannot be used because electrolytes in the irrigation fluid will dissipate the electric current used to resect the prostate. During the resection some of the irrigation fluid is absorbed through venous channels in the prostate. If enough fluid is absorbed, TUR syndrome may develop from the resulting hypervolemia and dilutional hyponatremia. Patients with TUR syndrome may experience hypertension, bradycardia, nausea, vomiting, visual disturbance, mental status changes, and even seizures. During the procedure and the postoperative period, patients should be monitored for evidence of TUR syndrome, which occurs in approximately 2% of patients. Patients with evidence of TUR syndrome should be treated with diuretics, and electrolyte imbalances should be corrected.

Following a TUR, patients are hospitalized overnight for continuous bladder irrigation. The hematuria is usually minimal by the following day, and the bladder irrigation can be stopped. If the urine remains clear or light pink while off irrigation, the catheter can be removed and the patient discharged from the hospital. Although TURs are associated with minimal morbidity, bleeding can occasionally be significant. In an attempt to further minimize the morbidity of BPH surgery, other technologies for ablating the prostate have been advocated. These newer technologies use lasers or produce thermal ablation by using radiofrequency or microwave energy.[14] Most studies have concluded that while these newer options are slightly less morbid than a TUR, they are also less effective than TUR in relieving the BPH-related obstruction.

UROLOGIC ONCOLOGY

Renal Cell Carcinoma

Epidemiology

Each year more than 30,000 new cases of renal cell carcinoma are diagnosed in the United States, resulting in approximately 12,000 deaths.[15] With the increased use of ultrasonography and CT scanning, incidental detection of early renal cell carcinoma has accounted, at least in part, for a 3% increase in incidence each year since the 1970s.[16] However, the mortality rate for renal cell carcinoma also has been increasing, suggesting that other factors are involved. Currently, renal cell carcinoma represents approximately 3% of all malignancies. The male:female ratio is approximately 3:2. At the time of diagnosis, approximately one-third of patients have metastatic disease.

Presentation and Prognosis

Before the widespread use of radiologic studies, patients often presented with advance disease with findings of a palpable mass, flank pain, and hematuria. Today, most renal tumors are incidentally discovered on ultrasounds and CT scans performed for unrelated disorders.[17] Patients with renal cell carcinoma also can present with paraneoplastic manifestations such as anemia, hepatic dysfunction (Stauffer syndrome), cachexia, polycythemia, and hypercalcemia. Paraneoplastic findings result from soluble substances released by the tumor or by immune cells in response to the tumor. Paraneoplastic findings resulting from localized disease resolve following a nephrectomy.

Well-established predictors of prognosis include stage, grade, and performance status. Renal cell carcinomas can be staged according to the tumor–node–metastasis (TNM) staging criteria proposed by the American Joint Committee on Cancer. Tumor grade is determined by using the Fuhrman grading system, which categorizes nuclear grade. Performance status is determined by the patient's ability to provide self-care and perform normal, day-to-day activities. Other reported indicators of poor prognosis include cachexia, anemia, hypercalcemia, and sarcomatoid histologic features.

Work-Up

All patients with a history of gross or microscopic hematuria should undergo a cystoscopy and an upper tract imaging study such

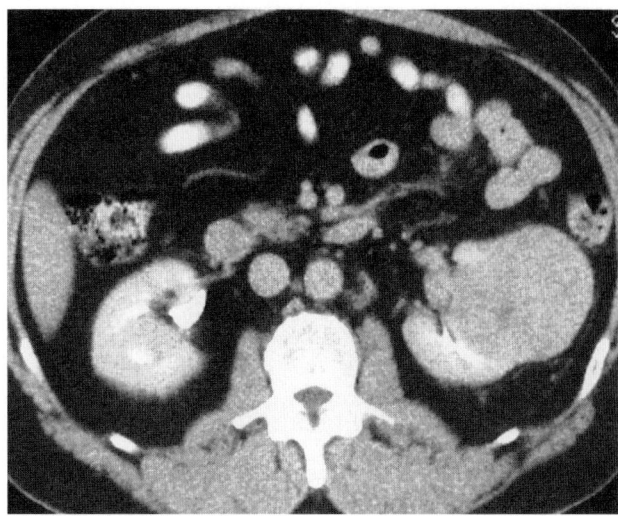

FIG. 39-12. CT scan with IV contrast demonstrating an enhancing, solid mass of the left kidney.

as a CT scan, MRI, or renal ultrasound. A solid, enhancing mass in the kidney has a 90% chance of being a renal cell carcinoma (Fig. 39-12). Except in select cases, a renal biopsy is unnecessary. A renal biopsy is associated with a high false-negative rate because of potential sampling error and difficulty interpreting the pathology from a biopsy sample. Therefore, a negative or nondiagnostic biopsy does not obviate the need for surgical removal of the mass. A biopsy may be helpful in patients with a history of another primary malignancy or in patients with metastatic disease in whom the primary site is unknown. In these patients, a biopsy is performed to determine whether the renal mass is a primary tumor or a metastatic deposit.

A simple cyst in the kidney is a common, benign finding. However, a complex cyst may harbor a malignant tumor (Fig. 39-13). Several features of a renal cyst are suggestive of a malignant

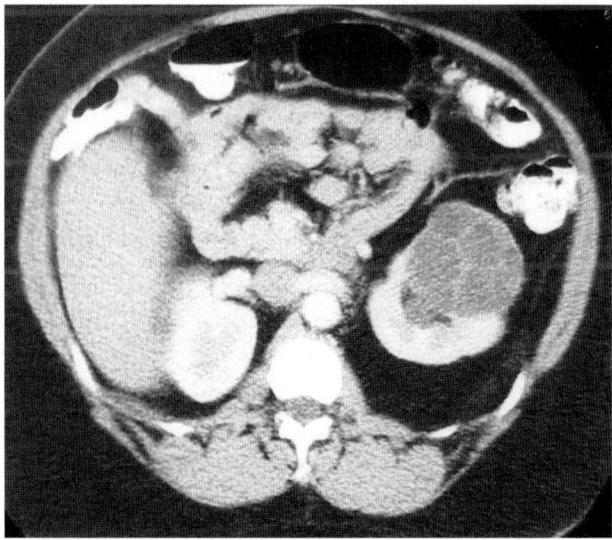

FIG. 39-13. CT scan with IV contrast demonstrating a complex left renal cyst. A complex cyst may harbor a malignancy. Features of a renal cyst suggestive of a malignant component include multiple septations, irregular cyst walls, calcifications, and walls or septations that enhance with IV contrast on CT scan.

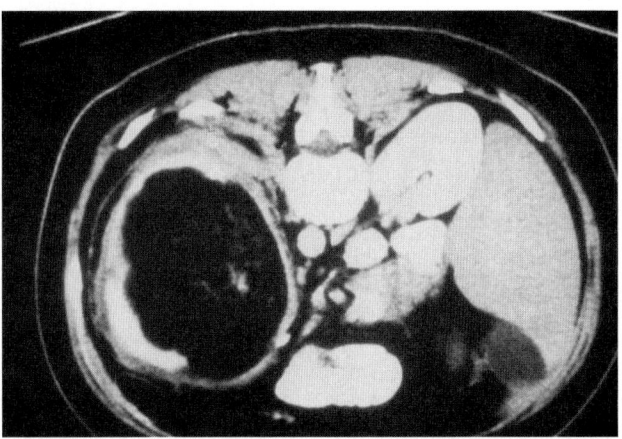

FIG. 39-14. *CT scan demonstrating an angiomyolipoma of the right kidney. The fatty component has a characteristic dark appearance on CT scan. Angiomyolipomas can usually be diagnosed by radiologic criteria alone and a histologic diagnosis is not necessary.*

component. These features include multiple septations, irregular cyst wall, calcifications, and wall or septations that enhance with IV contrast on CT or MRI.

The most common benign tumors in the kidney are oncocytomas and angiomyolipomas. Oncocytomas do not have a characteristic radiologic appearance and the diagnosis is made histologically following a nephrectomy. Angiomyolipomas are benign lesions common in patients with tuberous sclerosis. They have a characteristic appearance on CT scan, and nephrectomy is generally not necessary to confirm the diagnosis (Fig. 39-14). Large angiomyolipomas, however, have a high risk of bleeding and embolization should be considered for lesions larger than 4 cm.

Several histologic subtypes of renal cell carcinoma have been defined. Approximately 80% of renal cell carcinomas are clear cell tumors and approximately 75% of sporadic clear cell tumors have a mutation of the von Hippel-Lindau (VHL) gene found on chromosome 3.[18] The papillary subtype represents 10 to 15% of renal cell carcinomas and is associated with activation of the MET proto-oncogene or cytogenetic abnormalities involving chromosomes 7 and 17.[19]

Both clear cell and papillary subtypes are thought to arise from the proximal tubules of the nephron. Chromophobe and collecting duct subtypes represent most of the remaining renal cell carcinomas and both are thought to arise from the distal tubules and collecting duct of the nephron. Stage for stage, there is no consensus on the prognostic significance of these four subtypes. However, medullary cell carcinoma is a rare subtype that occurs in younger patients with sickle cell trait and is uniformly associated with a poor prognosis. Sarcomatoid lesions in a tumor also suggest a poor prognosis; however, this lesion is not considered a separate subtype.

All patients with a renal mass should undergo a metastatic workup that includes liver function tests, chest x-ray, and imaging of the abdomen and pelvis with a CT scan or MRI. The CT scan or MRI should be performed with and without IV contrast. If there is any suspicion of renal vein or inferior vena cava involvement by a tumor thrombus, a vena cavagram or MR angiogram with coronal sections should be performed to evaluate the extent of caval involvement. Patients with metastatic lesions on imaging of the chest, abdomen, and pelvis should undergo a bone scan and a head CT as well.

Treatment

The standard treatment for localized renal cell carcinoma remains a radical nephrectomy. The classic radical nephrectomy involves removal of the kidney, the ipsilateral adrenal gland, and all the fat contained within Gerota's fascia. However, it has been shown that if there is no evidence of adrenal involvement by the tumor on the CT scan, the adrenal gland can be spared. A radical nephrectomy can be performed using either an open or a laparoscopic approach. The laparoscopic approach is associated with less postoperative pain and a more rapid return to normal activities. For a radical nephrectomy, a laparoscopic procedure is now the standard of care.

For tumors less than 4 cm in size, a partial nephrectomy is an equally effective option for cancer control.[20] It is preferred in patients who are at risk for renal insufficiency secondary to conditions such as hypertension, recurrent stone disease, or diabetes. When performing a partial nephrectomy, meticulous attention needs to be paid to preventing bleeding and urine leaks, and this is most effectively accomplished by an open surgical approach (Fig. 39-15). Although laparoscopic partial nephrectomies have been reported, an open surgical procedure remains the standard of care when performing a partial nephrectomy.

Another option for a small renal lesion (less than 3 cm in diameter) is laparoscopic cryoablation.[21] The tumor is mobilized laparoscopically and cryoprobes that deliver argon gas or liquid nitrogen are inserted into the tumor. Usually a double freeze–thaw cycle is used to ablate the tumor. Although follow-up is limited, early reports suggest that cryotherapy is an effective treatment for small, peripheral lesions.

Metastatic renal cell carcinoma is resistant to radiation and standard chemotherapies. There are several important principles to guide the treatment of metastatic disease. Any metastatic lesion to the central nervous system can become rapidly symptomatic and should be addressed by the radiation oncologist and neurosurgeon prior to initiating any further treatment. Patients with a relatively good prognosis, as determined by a good performance status and a limited number of metastatic sites, are candidates for a cytoreductive nephrectomy and interleukin-2 or interferon-based immunotherapy. The combination of neoadjuvant nephrectomy and immunotherapy represents the current standard of care for patients with metastatic renal cell carcinoma.[22,23]

Approximately 75% of patients treated for localized renal cell carcinoma are cured of their disease. For patients with metastatic disease, the response rates for treatment with immunotherapy range from 10 to 20% and the median survival is 12 to 17 months.[24,25] However, it is important to point out that with immunotherapy durable responses lasting as long as 10 years are achieved in approximately 5 to 7% of patients.

Bladder Cancer

Epidemiology

In the United States, approximately 56,000 new cases of bladder cancer are diagnosed each year, resulting in approximately 13,000 deaths.[15,26,27] Bladder cancer represents 7% of all newly diagnosed cancers in men and 2% of all newly diagnosed cancers in women. Following prostate cancer, it is the most common genitourinary cancer in men. Bladder cancer is approximately 2.5 times more common in men than in women, and is more common in whites than in African American and Hispanic populations. The median age at diagnosis is 68 years and the incidence increases directly with

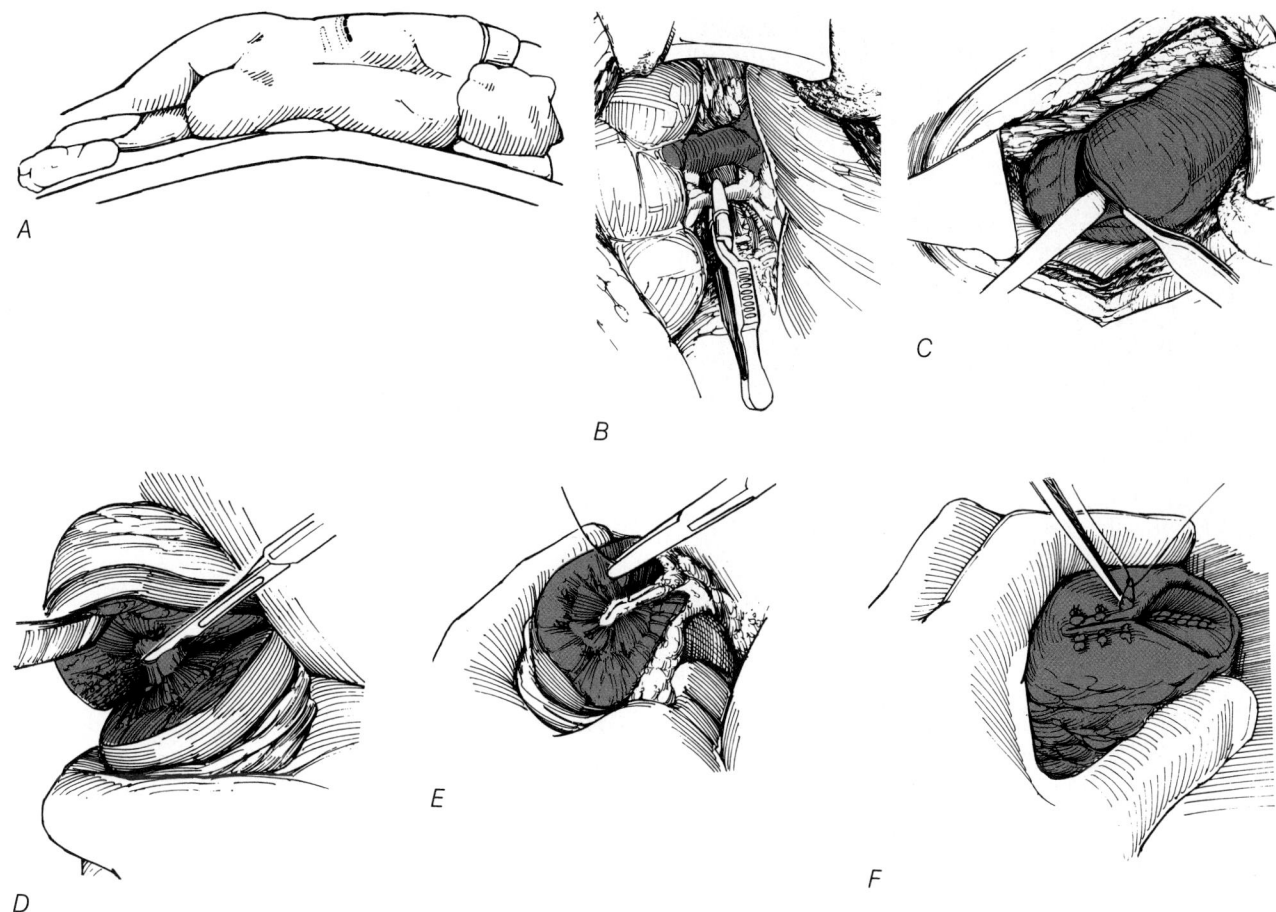

FIG. 39-15. Partial nephrectomy. *A.* The patient is placed in a flank position. *B.* The kidney should be cooled with ice before clamping the artery with a bulldog clamp. *C.* The tumor is sharply excised with a margin of normal tissue. *D.* The collecting system is identified and divided if necessary. *E.* The collecting system and bleeding vessels are meticulously oversewn with absorbable sutures. *F.* The capsule is closed and covered with fat.

age. The majority of patients with bladder cancer have superficial disease, which is associated with long-term survival. Therefore, there is a cohort of 300,000 to 400,000 patients with bladder cancer in the United States at all times.

In Western countries, more than 90% of bladder cancers are transitional cell carcinomas, approximately 5% are squamous cell carcinomas, and less than 2% are adenocarcinomas. In the developing countries, 75% of bladder cancers are squamous cell carcinomas and most of these are secondary to *Schistosoma haematobium* infection. Squamous cell carcinomas of the bladder in the United States are associated with chronic inflammation caused by chronic indwelling Foley catheters and bladder stones. There is no convincing evidence for a hereditary factor in the development of bladder cancer. Although most of the following discussion applies to bladder cancer in general, the primary focus is on transitional cell carcinoma (TCCa).

TCCa is strongly linked to environmental exposures. Smoking accounts for more than 50% of bladder cancers, and 2-naphthylamine and 4-aminobiphenyl are likely the most significant carcinogens found in cigarette smoke that lead to TCCa. The development of bladder cancer also has been associated with industrial exposure to aromatic amines in dyes, paints, solvents, leather dust, inks, combustion products, rubber, and textile. Prior radiation treatments to the pelvis and acrolein, a urinary metabolite of

cyclophosphamide, increase the risk of bladder cancer. However, coffee and artificial sweeteners are not believed to increase the risk of bladder cancer in humans.

Presentation

The classic presentation of bladder cancer is painless hematuria. Eighty-five percent of patients with bladder cancer present with hematuria.[28] Hematuria, whether gross or microscopic, requires a urologic evaluation. Microscopic hematuria as a result of bladder cancer may be intermittent, therefore, bladder cancer cannot be ruled out with a repeat negative urinalysis. Persistent, irritative voiding symptoms may be a result of carcinoma in situ (CIS) or muscle-invasive bladder cancer. Therefore, irritative voiding symptoms that do not resolve with treatment for a urinary tract infection require further evaluation. A urologic work-up for hematuria includes cystoscopy and radiographic imaging of the upper urinary tract as previously discussed.

Work-Up

At the time of clinic cystoscopy, a bladder wash for cytology can be sent. Bladder cytology is 95% accurate for diagnosing high-grade tumors and CIS, however, its accuracy for diagnosing low-grade carcinoma is only 10 to 50%. Newer assays for the detection and surveillance of TCCa in voided urine include the BTA-Stat,

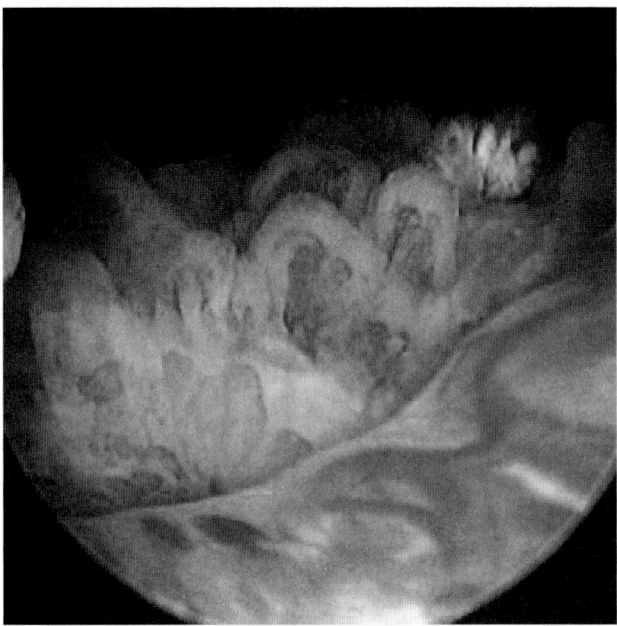

FIG. 39-16. *Cystoscopic image of a papillary bladder lesion suspicious for a transitional cell carcinoma.*

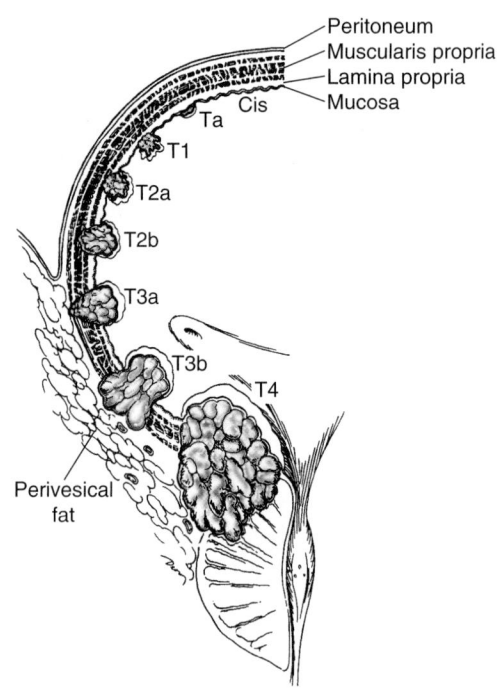

FIG. 39-17. *Staging of bladder cancer. T stage determined by depth of invasions: Cis = carcinoma in situ; Ta = mucosa; T1 = lamina propria; T2a = superficial bladder muscle; T2b = deep bladder muscle; T3a = perivesical fat (microscopic); T3b = perivesical fat (gross); T4 = adjacent structures such as prostate, rectum, or pelvic sidewall.*

NMP-22, and FDP tests.[29] However, because of high false-positive rates and high false-negative rates, it is unlikely that these tests will obviate the need for cystoscopy. Patients with an abnormal cystoscopic exam or suspicious bladder wash cytology should be further evaluated with an operating room cystoscopy (Fig. 39-16). In the operating room, all suspicious lesions should be endoscopically biopsied. Blood effluxing from either ureteral orifice should be further investigated with a retrograde pyelogram and possibly ureteroscopy.

Both tumor grade and stage correlate independently with prognosis. Transitional cell cancer is most commonly graded on a scale between 1 and 3, representing well, moderate, and poorly differentiated tumors. The TNM system, developed by the International Union Against Cancer and the American Joint Committee on Cancer Staging, is used to stage bladder cancer (Fig. 39-17). Tumors that involve the bladder mucosa (Ta and CIS) or lamina propria (T1) are considered superficial cancers. CIS is a unique designation that signifies a flat, high-grade tumor confined to the mucosa, and CIS generally implies a higher risk of recurrence following treatment. Tumors that invade the muscular layer of the bladder wall (T2) or beyond (T3 and T4) are considered muscle invasive.

Approximately 25% of patients with bladder cancer have muscle-invasive disease at the time of diagnosis.[28] Patients with muscle-invasive bladder cancer should undergo a metastatic work-up, which includes a CT scan of the abdomen and pelvis, chest x-ray, serum chemistries, and liver function tests. If the patients are asymptomatic with normal calcium and alkaline phosphatase, bone scans are unnecessary. Approximately 15% of all patients have metastatic disease at the time of initial presentation.[30] The life expectancy for most patients with overt metastatic disease is less than 2 years; however, approximately 25% of patients with only limited regional lymph node metastases discovered during cystectomy and pelvic lymph node dissection may survive beyond 5 years.[31,32]

Treatment of Superficial Bladder Cancer (Ta, T1, CIS)

Most superficial bladder cancers are adequately treated by endoscopic resection and fulguration of the bladder tumor. No further metastatic work-up is indicated if the pathology confirms a low-grade, superficial TCCa. However, bladder cancer is considered a polyclonal, field-change defect and continued surveillance is mandatory. In other words, the underlying genetic changes that resulted in the bladder cancer have occurred in the entire urothelium, making the entire urothelium susceptible to future tumor formation. The risk of recurrence following the treatment of superficial bladder cancer is approximately 70% within 5 years.[33]

The risk of disease progression, defined as a subsequent increase in tumor grade or stage, depends on the initial tumor grade. The risk of progression for TCCa grades I, II, and III is 10 to 20%, 19 to 37%, and 33 to 67%, respectively.[34] Carcinoma in situ alone or in association with Ta or T1 papillary tumor carries a poorer prognosis, with a recurrence rate of 63 to 92%. Other risk factors for recurrence and progression include tumor size, grade, and interval to recurrence. The high rate of disease recurrence and progression in superficial bladder cancer underscores the need for careful follow-up. Patients with a history of superficial TCCa should undergo surveillance with cystoscopy and bladder wash cytology every 3 months for 2 years. If they are disease free during this period, the follow-up intervals can be gradually increased.

Intravesical therapy is effective for patients with high-risk, superficial TCCa in reducing the risk of recurrence.[35] The most effective intravesical therapy is bacille Calmette-Guérin (BCG), which is a live, attenuated strain of *Mycobacterium bovis*. BCG is recommended for carcinoma in situ, T1 tumors, and high-risk Ta tumors (large, high-grade, recurrent or multifocal tumors). The beneficial effects of intravesical BCG is thought to be mediated by a non-specific immune cytokine response. Because BCG is a live, attenuated organism, it can cause tuberculosis-like symptoms if it is absorbed into the bloodstream. Contraindications for BCG treatment include active hematuria, immunodeficiency, and active urinary tract infection. BCG therapy reduces recurrence and some studies suggest it may reduce the risk of progression as well.

Other forms of adjuvant therapy for superficial bladder cancer include intravesical triethylenethiophosphoramide (thiotepa), mitomycin C, doxorubicin, and epirubicin. Although these agents can increase the time to disease recurrence, there is no evidence that any of these intravesical chemotherapies can prevent disease progression. With treatment, superficial bladder cancer has a good prognosis with 5-year survival rates of 82 to 100%.

Treatment of Muscle-Invasive Bladder Cancer (T2, T3, T4)

The gold standard for organ-confined, muscle-invasive bladder cancer (T2 and T3) is radical cystoprostatectomy in men and anterior pelvic exenteration in women. In men, radical cystectomy involves the removal of the bladder, prostate, and pelvic lymph nodes. A total urethrectomy also is performed if the urethral margin is positive. In women, a classic anterior pelvic exenteration includes the removal of the bladder, urethra, uterus, ovaries, and anterior vaginal wall. However, in a female patient, if the bladder neck margin is negative, the urethra and anterior vaginal wall may be spared. With treatment, the 5-year survival rates for pathologic T2, T3, T4a, and N+ tumors are 63 to 80%, 19 to 57%, 0 to 36%, and 15 to 44% respectively.[36]

After cystectomy, the urine is diverted using segments of bowel. The various types of urinary diversions can be separated into continent and incontinent diversions. The most commonly performed incontinent diversion is the ileal conduit. A small segment of ileum is taken out of continuity with the GI tract while maintaining its mesenteric blood supply. The ureters are anastomosed to one end of the conduit and the other end is brought out to the abdominal wall as a stoma. The urine continuously collects in an external collection device worn over the stoma.

There are two commonly performed continent urinary diversions. An Indiana pouch is a urinary reservoir created from detubularized right colon and an adjacent limb of terminal ileum (Fig. 39-18). The terminal ileum is plicated and brought to the abdominal wall, creating a catheterizable stoma. The native ileocecal valve provides the continence mechanism. The Indiana pouch is emptied by clean intermittent catheterization of the stoma four to six times per day. An orthotopic neobladder is a similar reservoir that is connected to the urethra (Fig. 39-19). Various segments of intestine, including small and large bowel, may be used in constructing the orthotopic neobladder. The orthotopic neobladder most closely restores the natural storage and voiding function of the native bladder. Patients have volitional control of urination and void by Valsalva maneuver.

In certain centers, a bladder preserving strategy for T2-T3 TCCa is applied using a combination of external beam radiation, chemotherapy and endoscopic resection.[37] This approach has resulted in comparable survival rates when compared to radical surgery; however, its widespread application has been limited by the complexity of the protocol, associated toxicity, and a high treatment-related mortality rate. The mortality rate in the two largest U.S. series with the longest follow-up is 4 to 5%. In comparison, the mortality rate for most modern cystectomy series is 1 to 2%. In addition, a significant number of patients ultimately require a salvage cystectomy, which is associated with increased morbidity when compared to primary cystectomy. In some series local recurrence of bladder cancer is as high as 50 to 60% despite completion of bladder preserving therapy.

Transitional cell carcinoma is considered a chemosensitive cancer. The standard treatment of metastatic bladder cancer is MVAC, which is a combination of methotrexate, vinblastine, Adriamycin, and cisplatin. MVAC has an objective response rate of approximately 70% and a complete response rate of approximately 20%. However, long-term survival is rare, and with MVAC therapy, the 2-year survival is approximately 20%. At many centers, MVAC has been replaced by a combination of gemcitabine and cisplatin, which appears to produce comparable response rates with fewer toxic effects. As many as 50% of patients with clinically localized disease have micrometastases, and present with overt metastatic disease within 5 years of cystectomy. Therefore, chemotherapy also is advocated in the adjuvant setting for high-risk, localized disease.

Prostate Cancer

Epidemiology

Prostate cancer is the most common cancer in men and the second most common cause of cancer-related death in the United States. Each year, approximately 189,000 cancers are diagnosed, representing approximately 30% of all cancers diagnosed in men, and approximately 30,000 deaths results from prostate cancer.[15] It is estimated that in the United States, one in six men will be diagnosed with prostate cancer during their lifetime. Since the widespread use of screening prostate-specific antigen (PSA) in the late 1980s, the incidence of prostate cancer has dramatically increased; however, after about 1990, the death rate from prostate cancer has been declining. It is often suggested that this decline in prostate cancer mortality has resulted from increased screening and early detection of prostate cancer.

Family history, race, and environmental factors determine the risk of prostate cancer. Approximately 15 to 25% of patients diagnosed with prostate cancer report having at least one blood relative with the same diagnosis.[38,39] Men with a father or a brother with prostate cancer are twice as likely to develop prostate cancer when compared with men with no family history. The risk of prostate cancer is directly related to the number of affected family members and if three first-degree relatives are affected, the relative risk may be as high as 11. In the United States, the risk of prostate cancer is also related to race. African Americans have a higher incidence of prostate cancer than do whites, while Hispanics and Asians have a lower incidence than whites. Environmental factors also affect the risk of prostate cancer. There is scientific evidence suggesting that the risk of prostate cancer can be lowered by a low-fat diet, as well as by various nutritional supplements including lycopene, vitamin E, and selenium.[40]

Prostate Cancer Screening

Until prostate cancer metastasizes or becomes locally advanced, it does not generally cause symptoms. Most prostate cancers are diagnosed based on an elevated PSA or an abnormal digital rectal examination (DRE) of the prostate. PSA is a serine protease that is synthesized by the prostate epithelium and is elevated in prostate cancer. A PSA greater than 4 ng/mL is considered abnormal. Approximately 25% of patients with a PSA greater than 4 ng/mL will have a positive prostate biopsy, which establishes the diagnosis of prostate cancer. Approximately 50% of patients with both an elevated PSA and an abnormal DRE will have a biopsy positive for prostate cancer.

Both BPH and prostate cancer increase serum PSA. Therefore, in an effort to improve the accuracy of PSA for predicting prostate cancer, several variations of the PSA test have been proposed, including age-specific PSA (higher normal PSA ranges for older age groups), PSA density (PSA/size of prostate measured on ultrasound), PSA

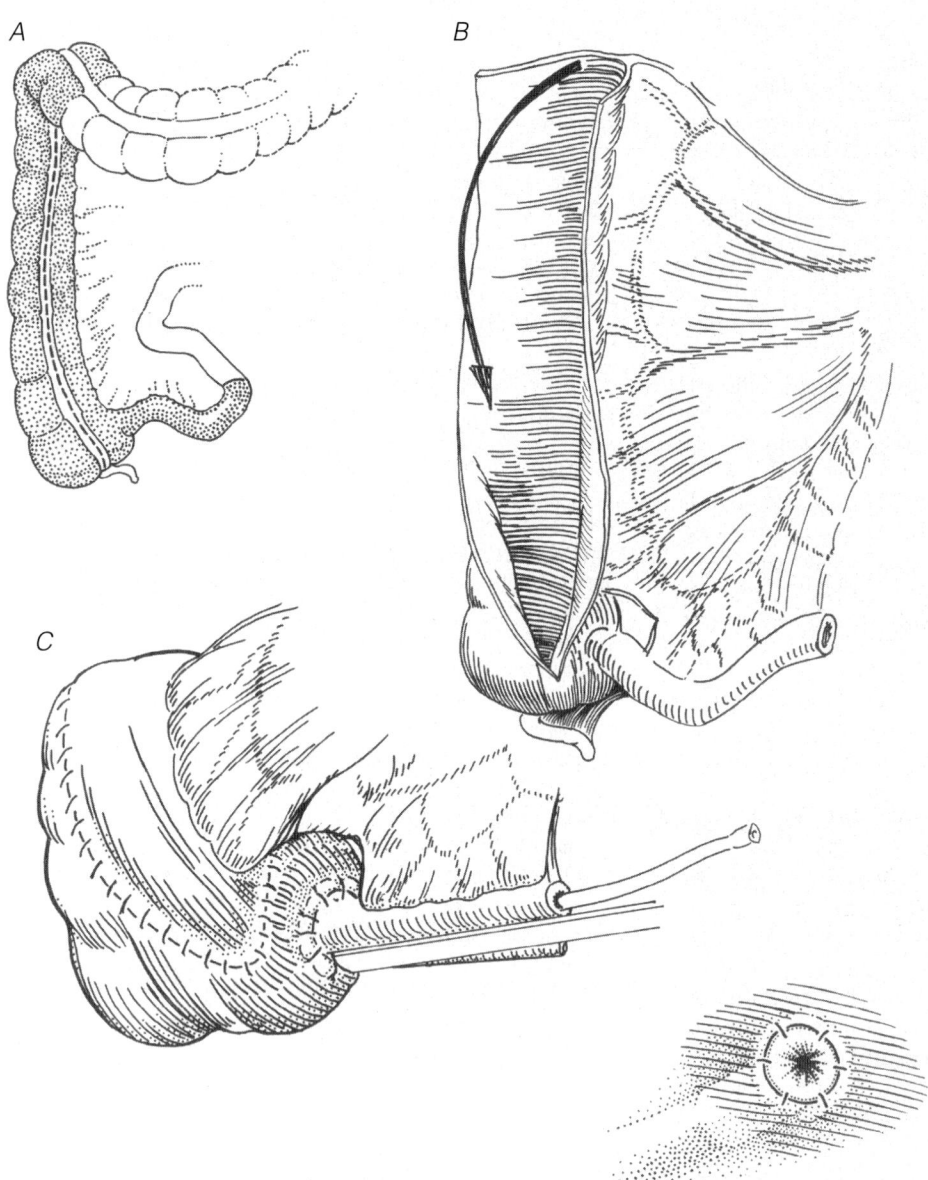

FIG. 39-18. Indiana pouch. *A.* An ileocecal segment is used to construct a continent reservoir that is emptied by periodic catheterization. *B.* The ileocecal segment is detubularized and *(C)* fashioned into a pouch. The terminal ileum is plicated and brought to the abdominal wall, creating a catheterizable stoma. [*Reproduced with permission from Carroll PR: Urinary diversion and bladder substitution, in Tanagho E, McAninch J (eds): Smith's General Urology, 14th ed. Norwalk, CT: Appleton & Lange, 1995, p 457.*]

velocity (change in PSA/year), and percent-free PSA (free PSA/total PSA). The rationale for using percent-free PSA is based on the observation that a lower fraction of serum PSA is free and not bound to serum proteins in men with prostate cancer than in men with BPH.

The American Cancer Society recommends offering annual prostate cancer screening to men starting at 50 years of age who have at least a 10-year life expectancy. Additionally, the society recommends offering PSA screening at 45 years of age in African American men and in men with a family history of prostate cancer. However, the value of screening is debated within the medical community, and this debate is reflected by the conflicting guidelines published by several medical and health care organizations.[41] Randomized prospective studies are currently being conducted to address the role of prostate cancer screening.

Several issues contribute to the controversy regarding annual screening. PSA testing has a relatively low positive predictive value, resulting in a high number of "unnecessary" prostate biopsies. Based on autopsy studies, approximately 30% of men older than 50 years of

age have histologic prostate cancer; however, only a small fraction of these men will actually die from prostate cancer or even progress to clinically symptomatic disease. Prostate cancer often has a long and indolent course and occurs in older men, and as a result, many men with histologic prostate cancer eventually die of other, unrelated causes. Finally, the morbidity, such as incontinence and impotence, associated with the available treatments can significantly impact quality of life.

Work-Up

Despite the controversy surrounding prostate cancer screening, it is important to point out that most cancers detected as a result of an elevated PSA or abnormal DRE are clinically significant cancers that should be treated in men with at least a 10-year life expectancy. The diagnosis of prostate cancer is made by biopsy. Using transrectal ultrasound guidance, the biopsy needles are directed at the peripheral zones where prostate cancer tends to develop. Prostate cancer is graded by the pathologist using the Gleason system. The two most predominant histologic patterns of the prostate cancer are assigned

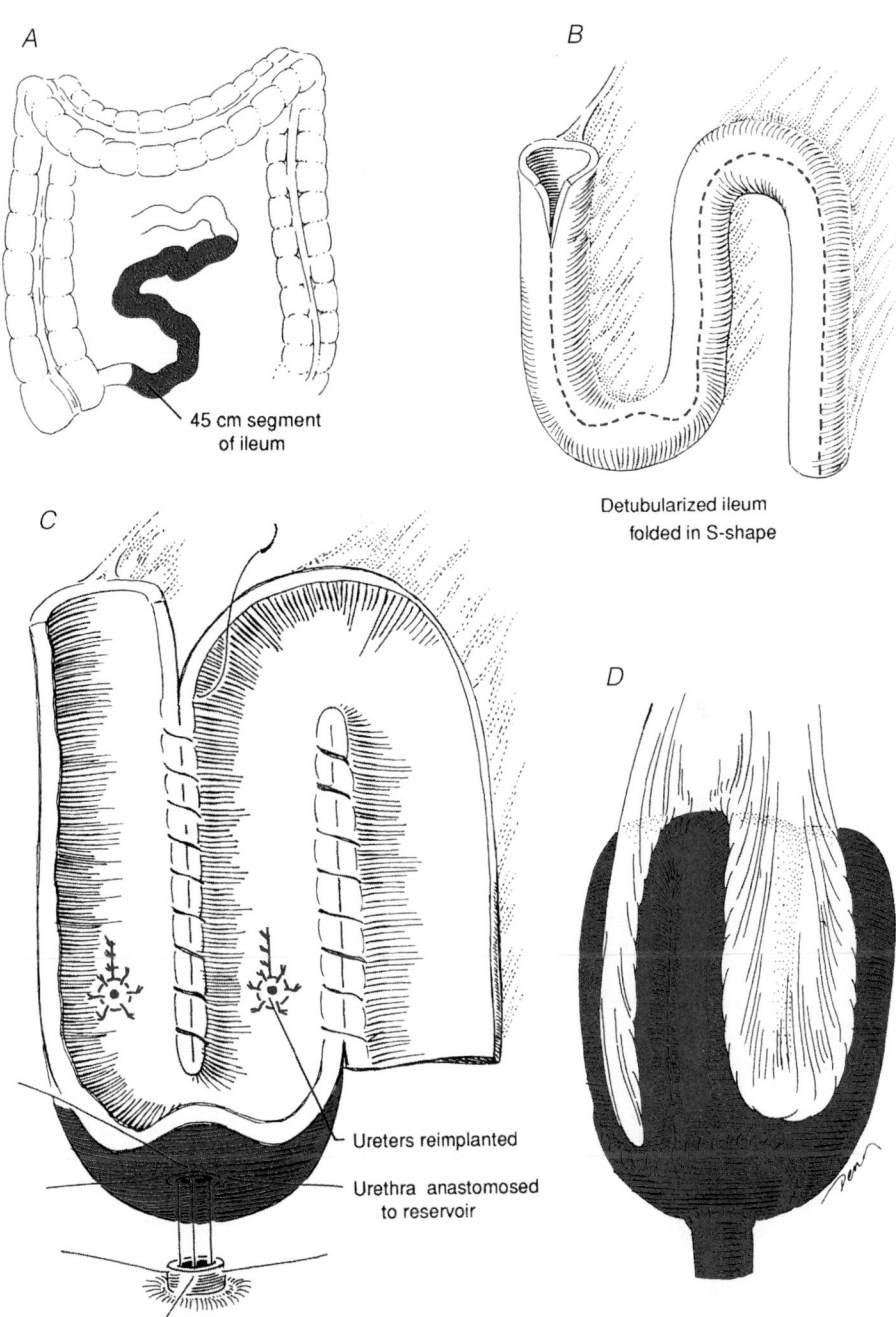

FIG. 39-19. Orthotopic neobladder. *A and B. A continent reservoir is created by detubularizing a segment of ileum, (C) fashioning the bowel into a pouch, and (D) anastomosing the neobladder to the urethra. [Reproduced with permission from Carroll PR: Urinary diversion and bladder substitution, in Tanagho E, McAninch J (eds): Smith's General Urology, 14th ed. Norwalk, CT: Appleton & Lange, 1995, p 457.]*

a Gleason grade, on a scale from 1 to 5. The two Gleason grades are added to give a Gleason score, on a scale from 2 to 10.

Tumors with Gleason scores of 8 to 10 are considered high-grade tumors, and tumors with Gleason scores of 5 to 7 are considered intermediate-grade tumors. High-grade prostatic intraepithelial neoplasia (PIN) is considered a premalignant lesion that may indicate the presence of adjacent cancer. Given the possibility for sampling error, the presence of PIN in a biopsy that is negative for prostate cancer is an indication for repeating the biopsy; a repeat biopsy will be positive for prostate cancer in approximately 40% of cases.

Prostate cancer is most commonly staged using the TNM system. The most common sites of metastasis for prostate cancer are the axial bones and pelvic lymph nodes. For the majority of patients diagnosed with prostate cancers, no formal metastatic work-up is

necessary. However, a PSA greater than 20 ng/mL or a PSA greater than 10 ng/mL in a patient with a Gleason score 8 to 10 tumor is associated with an increased risk of metastatic disease, and a bone scan and pelvic CT scan should be performed. In addition, any patient complaining of bone pain should undergo a bone scan.

Treatment

Localized Prostate Cancer. Prostate cancer tends to progress slowly and have a long, natural history. Therefore, treatment for localized prostate cancer is generally offered to patients with at least a 10-year life expectancy. Patients with high-grade tumors (Gleason score of 8 to 10) may represent an exception to this rule; without treatment, they are at a significantly higher risk of developing symptomatic disease and dying from their disease. Therefore, in these patients, curative therapy should be considered regardless of life expectancy. The treatment options for localized prostate cancer can be broadly categorized as involving surgery or radiation therapy.

The most commonly performed surgical procedure is a radical retropubic prostatectomy (RRP) (Fig. 39-20). A pelvic lymph node dissection is generally performed for staging purposes at the time of surgery. The most significant complications associated with surgery are urinary incontinence and erectile dysfunction, which occur in approximately 5 to 10% and 14 to 30% of cases, respectively.[42,43] During RRP, care should be taken to avoid injuring the urinary sphincter located just distal to the apex of the prostate. The neurovascular bundles that run along the posterolateral border of the prostate contain the cavernous nerves, which are responsible for erectile function. Care should be taken to separate the neurovascular bundle from the prostate and preserve it during surgery. Other less frequently employed surgical options include perineal radical prostatectomy and cryotherapy.

Options for radiation therapy include external radiation therapy (XRT) and brachytherapy. With most XRT protocols, 60 to 80 Gy is delivered by conformal radiotherapy. The primary genitourinary side effects following XRT include frequency, dysuria, hematuria, and decreased bladder capacity. The primary gastrointestinal side effects include diarrhea, rectal pain, and rectal bleeding. The sexual dysfunction following XRT develops gradually and 40 to 50% of previously potent men are impotent 5 years following treatment. Brachytherapy involves the percutaneous placement of radioactive seeds into the prostate. Although the side effects associated with brachytherapy are generally less severe than those associated with XRT, brachytherapy is less effective than XRT for treatment of high-risk prostate cancer.

There are currently no definitive studies demonstrating that surgery or XRT provides better cancer control. Although brachytherapy appears effective based on initial results treating patients with favorable prognosis, long-term follow-up is not yet available. In several studies, including several phase III studies, long-term use of androgen-ablative therapy in conjunction with XRT improves survival. However, studies assessing the role of neoadjuvant androgen-ablative therapy before RRP demonstrate no added benefit when compared to RRP alone.

Metastatic Prostate Cancer. The first-line therapy for metastatic prostate cancer is androgen-ablative hormone therapy. Since Charles Huggins won the Nobel Prize in 1966 for discovering the therapeutic effects of androgen ablation on metastatic prostate cancer, the fundamental principles for treating metastatic prostate cancer have not changed. Androgen-ablation is accomplished by performing bilateral orchiectomies or by administering gonadotropin-releasing hormone (GnRH) agonist. Testosterone synthesis by the Leydig cell in the testicles is stimulated by luteinizing hormone (LH) from the pituitary. The release of LH requires a pulsatile discharge of GnRH. Therefore, a constant GnRH stimulation paradoxically results in inhibition of LH and testosterone. Nonsteroidal antiandrogens such as flutamide and bicalutamide are often added to block the low levels of androgens produced by the adrenal medulla.

Testis Cancer

Testicular cancer is the most common cancer in men between the ages of 20 and 35 years.[15,44] There are approximately 7000 new cases and 400 deaths related to testis cancer per year. For more than 90% of patients, testicular cancer is curable. Any patient with a solid testicular mass, which has been confirmed on ultrasound, is considered

to have testicular cancer until proven otherwise, and should undergo a radical orchiectomy to make a definitive diagnosis. Prior to surgery, serum markers for testicular cancer should be obtained. The two markers used in routine clinical practice are human chorionic gonadotropin (hCG) and follicle-stimulating hormone (FSH).

When performing a radical orchiectomy, the surgery should be performed by an inguinal approach rather than a scrotal approach. The metastatic spread of testicular cancer is ordered and predictable. The primary metastatic landing sites for left and right testicular cancers are the para-aortic and the interaortocaval nodes in the retroperitoneum, respectively. The lymphatic drainage of the scrotum, on the other hand, is to the inguinal nodes. If the scrotum is surgically violated by performing a scrotal orchiectomy, metastatic spread to both the retroperitoneal and the inguinal nodes becomes possible. Following an orchiectomy for localized germ cell tumor, hCG (half-life of 5 to 7 days) and FSH (half-life of 24 to 36 hours) levels that were elevated before surgery should normalize.

The diagnosis of testicular cancer is made based on the pathology of the orchiectomy specimen. Approximately 95% of testicular cancers are germ cell tumors, while approximately 4% of testicular cancers are nongerm cell tumors such as Leydig cell tumors and Sertoli cell tumors. Germ cell tumors are further classified as seminomas and nonseminomas.[45] For clinically localized seminomas, the standard of care is to treat the retroperitoneum with radiation to prevent nodal recurrence, although observation and close follow-up are also reasonable.[46] For clinically localized nonseminomas that are at high risk for recurrence,[47] the options include a prophylactic retroperitoneal lymph node dissection, two cycles of prophylactic chemotherapy or observation with very close follow-up. Patients electing observation should understand that there is a 30% risk of retroperitoneal recurrence. The treatment of metastatic germ cell tumor generally involves chemotherapy. Most chemotherapy protocols employ a combination of bleomycin, etoposide and *cis*-platinum.

Penile Cancer

Penile cancer is rare in the United States, representing less than 1% of all tumors in men.[15] However, in certain regions of Africa and South America, penile cancer represents 10 to 20% of all malignancies. The majority of penile malignancies are squamous cell carcinomas. The diagnosis is made on biopsy. The primary lesion should be completely resected, whenever possible, to prevent the morbidities associated with local invasion. Penile cancer spreads in a predictable pattern to the inguinal lymph nodes and then to the pelvic lymph nodes.[48] Patients who present with enlarged pelvic lymph nodes on CT scan should undergo a diagnostic pelvic lymph node dissection.[49,50] Pathologically confirmed pelvic lymph node metastasis should be further treated with chemotherapy, and no further surgical therapy is indicated.

For patients without involvement of pelvic lymph nodes, the inguinal lymph nodes are evaluated. However, primary penile tumors often have an infectious component that can result in enlargement of the inguinal lymph nodes. Therefore, following resection of the primary tumor, the patient should be treated with antibiotics for 6 weeks before evaluating the inguinal nodes. Following antibiotic therapy, patients with palpable inguinal lymph nodes should undergo an inguinal lymph node dissection. In addition, all patients with high-grade primary penile tumors or primary tumors invading the corporal bodies should undergo an inguinal lymph node dissection regardless of whether the nodes are palpable or not. Approximately one-third of patients with disease in the inguinal nodes are cured following an inguinal node dissection.

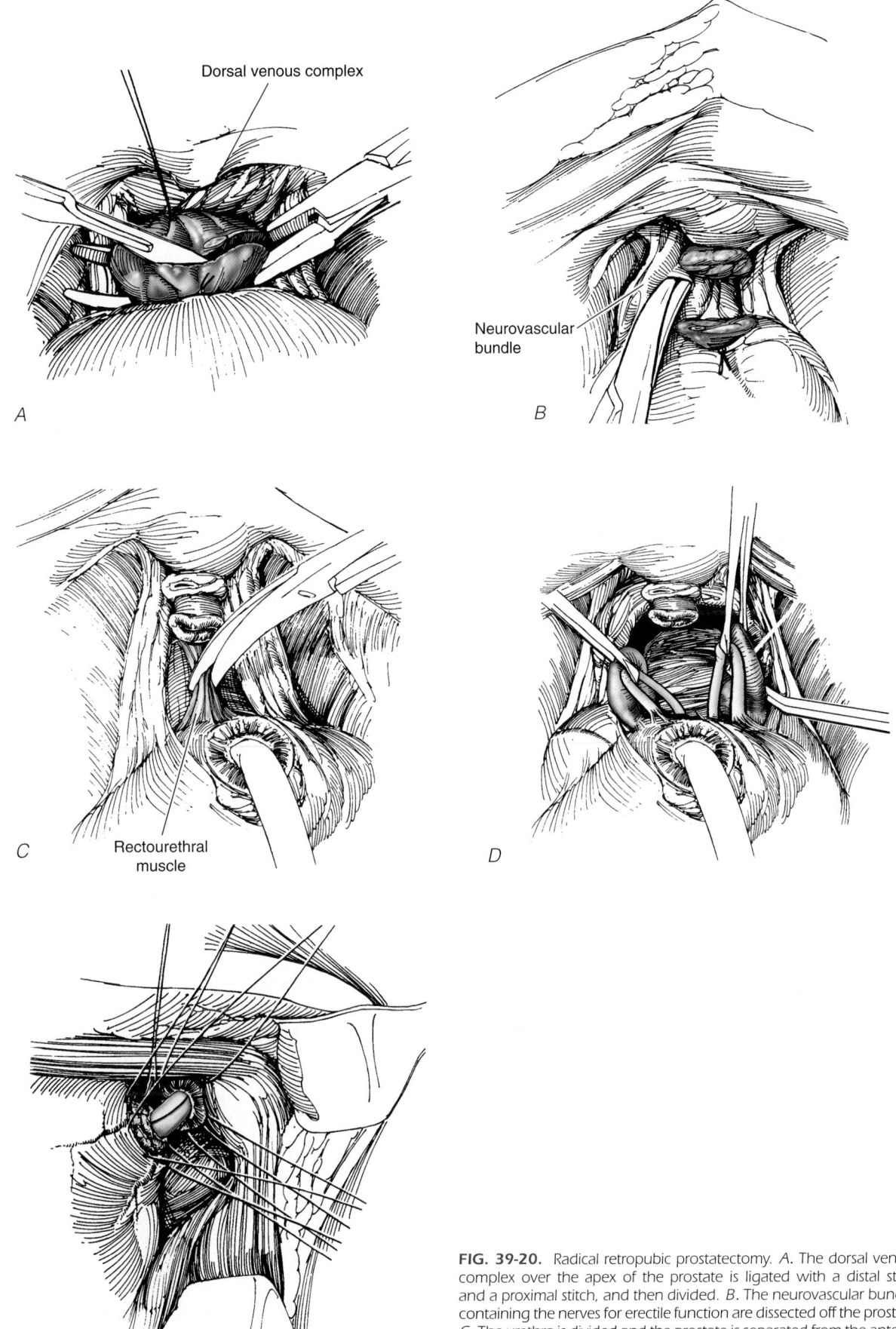

Dorsal venous complex

A

Neurovascular
bundle

B

Rectourethral
muscle

C

D

E

FIG. 39-20. Radical retropubic prostatectomy. *A.* The dorsal venous complex over the apex of the prostate is ligated with a distal stitch and a proximal stitch, and then divided. *B.* The neurovascular bundles containing the nerves for erectile function are dissected off the prostate. *C.* The urethra is divided and the prostate is separated from the anterior rectum. *D.* The vasa deferentia are divided and the seminal vesicles are dissected and removed with the specimen. *E.* The bladder neck is reanastomosed to the distal urethral stump.

1539

UROLOGIC INFECTIONS

Cystitis

Cystitis is inflammation of the bladder mucosa and is usually caused by bacterial organisms. *E. coli* is the most common cause of urinary tract infection (UTI), including cystitis. Other common causative organisms include *Proteus, Klebsiella, Enterococcus,* and *Staphylococcus saprophyticus.* Women are at a higher risk for UTI than men because their urethra is shorter. Fecal flora contaminating the vaginal mucosa can ascend through the female urethra. Certain bacterial factors, such as type 1 pili found on some strains of *E. coli,* mediate adhesion and are more likely to cause UTI.[51] In addition, certain host factors such as vaginal pH, can promote vaginal colonization and UTI.[52]

Symptoms of cystitis include urinary frequency, urgency, and dysuria. Uncomplicated cystitis does not generally cause fevers or leukocytosis. Patients with voiding symptoms can be worked up with a urinalysis. However, a urine culture provides a more definitive diagnosis of a UTI than a urinalysis. Important considerations when obtaining a urine culture have been previously discussed in this chapter. Bacterial UTI in women should be treated with 3 days of antibiotics. In men, bacterial UTI should be treated with 7 days of antibiotics and younger men should be evaluated for correctable structural anomalies with an IVP or CT scan with IV contrast, and a cystoscopy.

Asymptomatic bacteriuria occurs in approximately 30% of elderly nursing home residents and in 5% of sexually active women. Asymptomatic bacteriuria is the rule in patients with chronic indwelling Foley catheters. Most asymptomatic bacteriuria does not need to be treated. However, asymptomatic patients with urea-splitting organisms should be treated with antibiotics. Pregnant women with bacteriuria should also be treated as they are at an increased risk for developing pyelonephritis.

Pyelonephritis

Pyelonephritis refers to inflammation of the renal parenchyma and collecting system. It is a clinical diagnosis that is made based on the presence of fever, flank pain, and infected urine. Older patients and young children may present with less-specific symptoms such as mental status changes, abdominal discomfort, and low-grade fevers. The most common causative agents are gram-negative bacteria such as *E. coli, Proteus, Pseudomonas,* and *Klebsiella.* Most bacterial agents gain access to the urinary system through the urethra and ascend to the kidney. Therefore, women are generally more susceptible to UTI and pyelonephritis because of the shorter urethra in females compared to males.

Patients presenting with signs and symptoms of pyelonephritis should have a urine culture and serial blood cultures. The results of the urine culture may not be available for 48 hours; therefore, a urinalysis can be used to support a presumptive diagnosis of pyelonephritis. Healthy adults with no significant comorbidities can be treated as an outpatient; however, most patients diagnosed with pyelonephritis are admitted to the hospital. Broad-spectrum IV antibiotics, such as ampicillin and gentamicin, should be started until the results of the urine culture are available and a more selective antibiotic can be identified. When patients are afebrile, they can be discharged on oral antibiotics. Uncomplicated pyelonephritis should be treated for a total of 14 days while pyelonephritis associated with structural or functional abnormalities should be treated for 21 days.

In patients being treated for pyelonephritis, after 24 hours of antibiotic therapy, the urine should be sterile and leukocytosis should be minimal. However, patients often continue to have periodic fever spikes for several days after initiating treatment. This is believed to be a result of resolving inflammation in the kidney rather than an active infection. With appropriate treatment, the magnitude of each subsequent fever spike should decrease. In most patients, no radiologic studies are initially necessary. However, if there is no clinical improvement following 2 to 3 days of treatment, a CT scan with IV contrast should be obtained. Patients with renal insufficiency or allergy to IV contrast can have an MRI, a renal ultrasound, or a CT scan without contrast.

In select patients with pyelonephritis, the upper tracts should be imaged at the time of presentation. In selecting patients for early radiologic study, the most important principle to keep in mind is that an obstructed and infected urinary system is a surgical emergency that requires prompt intervention to establish drainage. Therefore, the upper tracts should be studied in any patient with a history of kidney stones, anatomic abnormalities such as a ureteropelvic junction obstruction, or malignancies that may cause extrinsic compression of the urinary system. Options for emergently draining an obstructed kidney include percutaneous nephrostomy tube placement and cystoscopic placement of a ureteral stent. Bladder outlet obstruction causing bilateral hydronephrosis can be relieved by the placement of a Foley catheter.

Other findings on CT scan and MRI may require surgical intervention. Small renal and perirenal abscesses (Fig. 39-21) can be conservatively managed with antibiotics in clinically stable patients.[53] However, if there is inadequate clinical improvement or if the abscess is large, the infectious collection should be immediately drained. Drainage is preferably accomplished percutaneously. Emphysematous pyelonephritis is often seen in older diabetic patients and represents a medical emergency (Fig. 39-22). Air bubbles produced by gas-forming organisms can be seen in the renal parenchyma on x-ray or CT scan. Emphysematous pyelonephritis should be promptly treated with percutaneous drainage; if there is no evidence of clinical improvement, an urgent nephrectomy should be performed.[54]

In adult patients, there is no permanent sequela following successful treatment of pyelonephritis. However, pyelonephritis in an infant kidney that is still developing can be devastating.

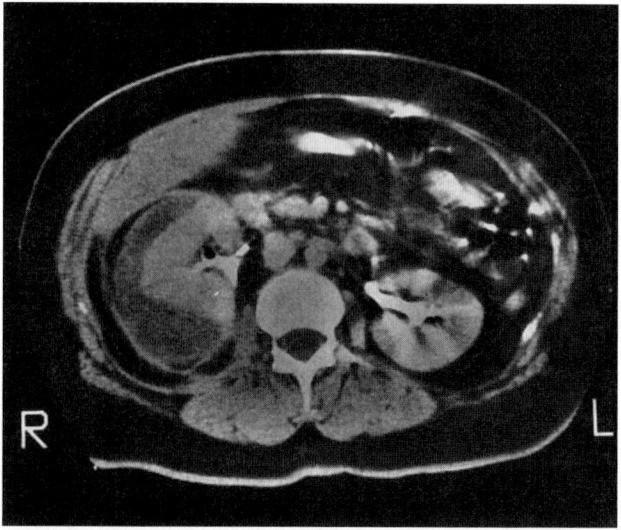

FIG. 39-21. Right perirenal abscess. CT scan of a 40-year-old patient presenting with fever, chills, and flank pain. Patient improved on antibiotics after the perirenal collection was drained percutaneously.

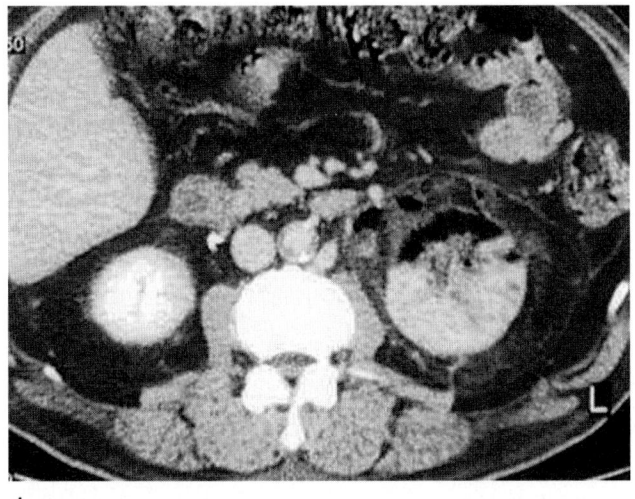

A

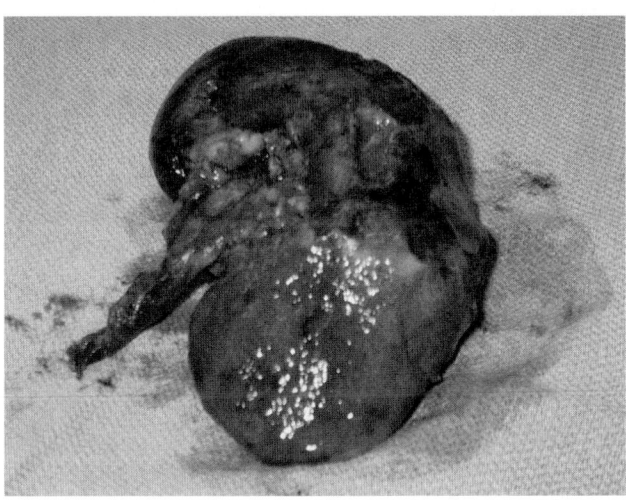

B

FIG. 39-22. Emphysematous pyelonephritis. *A.* CT scan of a 52-year-old diabetic patient presenting with sepsis. Note the air in parenchyma formed by gas-producing organisms. *B.* Picture of kidney following emergent nephrectomy.

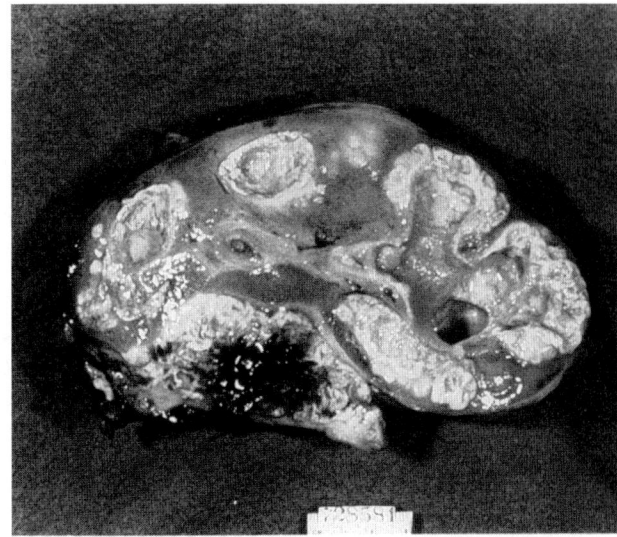

A

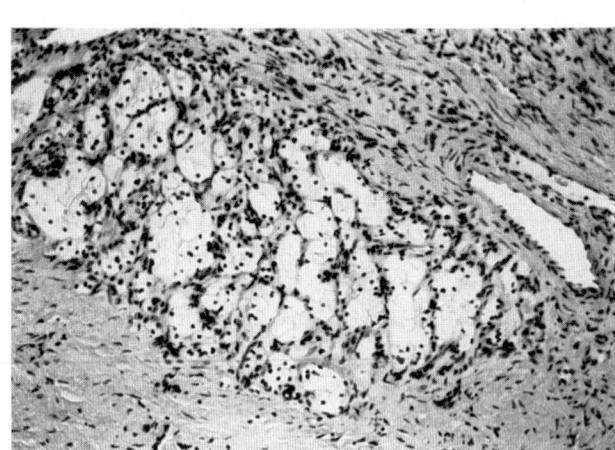

B

FIG. 39-23. Xanthogranulomatous pyelonephritis. *A.* Note excrescences surrounding calyces (grossly yellow). *B.* Micrograph showing clear cells, which are lipid-laden macrophages that may resemble clear cell renal cell carcinoma. A stone is often present in the kidney in cases of xanthogranulomatous pyelonephritis.

Pyelonephritis can lead to permanent parenchymal scarring and loss of renal function.[55] The most common abnormality resulting in pyelonephritis in infants and children is ureteral reflux. Ureteral reflux can carry an infectious organism from the bladder to the kidney, and severe reflux can cause hydronephrosis and urinary stasis. Therefore, pediatric patients with cystitis or pyelonephritis should be worked up with a renal ultrasound and a voiding cystourethrogram. Any pediatric patient at risk for pyelonephritis should be treated with long-term antibiotic prophylaxis.

Xanthogranulomatous Pyelonephritis

Xanthogranulomatous pyelonephritis (XGP) is a rare form of chronic pyelonephritis. The presumptive diagnosis of XGP is made on CT scan or MRI based on the presence of calcification and large cystic lesions replacing the majority of the parenchyma in patients with chronic flank pain and low-grade fevers. A nephrectomy should be performed to rule out a malignant process. Following the nephrectomy, a definitive diagnosis of XGP is made histologically by the presence of inflammatory cells and large lipid-laden macrophages (Fig. 39-23).

Fungal Infections

Most fungal infections of the urinary tract are opportunistic infections. They tend to occur in debilitated or immunocompromised patients. *Candida* is responsible for the vast majority of fungemia and funguria. Risk factors for fungal infection include immunosuppression, diabetes, antibiotic use, steroid therapy, and long-term use of urinary catheters.[56] On cystoscopy, affected areas may appear as white patches on the bladder wall. Upper tract radiographic studies such as CT scan and IVP may demonstrate a fungal mass.

For patients with fungal UTI, treatment is based on whether the infection is simple or complex. Simple fungal infections are diagnosed by a urine culture positive for more than 10^5 organisms/mL and are confined to the bladder. Simple fungal infections may be asymptomatic or they may cause irritable voiding symptoms such as dysuria and frequency. These infections are usually managed successfully by stopping any antibiotics, or removing urinary catheters and temporarily instituting intermittent catheterizations. Infections that do not resolve with these simple measures may require bladder irrigation with amphotericin B (50 mg/L of water administered at 42 mL/h).[57,58]

Complex fungal infections refer to infections involving the upper urinary tract or infections resulting in positive blood cultures. Complex fungal infections should be treated with IV antifungal agents. If fungal balls are present in the upper urinary tract, the effected kidney should be treated by percutaneously removing the fungal ball and directly irrigating the renal pelvis with amphotericin B. The gold standard for complex fungal infections is IV amphotericin B. Amphotericin B binds the ergosterol component of fungal cell walls and disrupts the cellular membrane. The half-life of amphotericin B is 15 days and resistance is unusual. Systemic effects, such as rigors, chills, and fevers, associated with treatment can be minimized by premedicating with steroid, meperidine, ibuprofen, and dantrolene.

Prostatitis

Prostatitis is a common disease that accounts for approximately 8% of urology-related office visits. Prostatitis is diagnosed in men who complain of pain and discomfort that generally localizes to the perineal region.[59] Although the term implies an inflammation of the prostate gland, often there is no clinical or histologic evidence of inflammation. Based on the clinical presentation, prostatitis can be categorized as acute or chronic. Acute prostatitis refers to a bacterial infection of the prostate that leads to system findings such as fever, chills, and leukocytosis. Chronic prostatitis includes all other forms of prostatitis associated with local symptoms. The most common causes of bacteria prostatitis are the same organisms in the fecal flora that are responsible for urinary tract infections, and include *E. coli*, *Proteus*, *Klebsiella*, and *Pseudomonas*.

Patients with acute prostatitis are febrile and often complain of frequency, urgency, dysuria and a decreased urinary stream. Occasionally, patients may even present in shock with tachycardia and hypotension. On physical exam, the prostate is extremely tender to palpation, and the digital exam should be performed gently to prevent shedding bacteria into the blood stream. Laboratory exam will reveal an elevated white blood cell count and urinalysis and urine culture findings will be consistent with a bacterial infection. The treatment for acute bacterial prostatitis is similar to the treatment for pyelonephritis. Usually the treatment is initiated with broad-spectrum IV antibiotics. When patients are afebrile and hemodynamically stable, treatment can continue with oral antibiotics for a total of 3 weeks.

Chronic prostatitis can be subdivided into bacterial and non-bacterial prostatitis. Classically, chronic, bacterial prostatitis is characterized by recurrent urinary tract infections by the same organism. Treatment involves 30 days of antibiotic therapy with a fluoroquinolone or trimethoprim/sulfamethoxazole. Patients with local symptoms of prostatitis without a history of urinary tract infections can be assumed to have nonbacterial prostatitis. Nonbacterial prostatitis represents the vast majority of all cases of prostatitis and can be a very frustrating problem for both the patient and the treating physician. The etiology is poorly understood and a variety of treatments, including alpha blockers, antibiotics, anticholinergics, and benzodiazepines, have been used with inconsistent and modest results.

URINARY INCONTINENCE

Urinary incontinence refers to unintended leakage of urine from the bladder. It is estimated that in the United States, more than 17 million

men and women suffer from urinary incontinence. The vast majority of patients treated for urinary incontinence are women past middle-age. In the elderly population, approximately 50% of nursing home residents suffer from urinary incontinence. Approximately $26 billion is spent annually in the United States for management of this problem.[60]

Normal Voiding Physiology

Urinary storage occurs in the bladder when there is a coordinated relaxation of the bladder wall muscle, and contraction of the urinary sphincter. Stimulation of beta-adrenergic receptors in the bladder leads to relaxation of the bladder wall. Contraction of the smooth and striated muscles in the urinary sphincter result from alpha-adrenergic and cholinergic stimulation. Conversely, voiding occurs when there is a coordinated contraction of the bladder smooth muscle and relaxation of the urinary sphincter. Bladder wall contraction is mediated by the cholinergic receptors. Nitric oxide stimulates the nonadrenergic noncholinergic pathway, resulting in relaxation of the urinary sphincter.

Normal voiding is coordinated by the pontine micturition center in the brain stem. Patients with neurologic insults affecting the brain stem or spinal column may suffer from a form of uncoordinated voiding known as detrusor–sphincter dyssynergia, where the bladder and sphincter contract at the same time during voiding, leading to high intravesical pressures. Neuronal connections from higher centers of the brain to the pontine micturition center regulate voluntary control of micturition. All disorders affecting the upper tract such as strokes and spinal cord injuries can lead to involuntary bladder contractions.

As discussed in the section on urinary signs and symptoms, incontinence can be categorized as stress, urge, total, and overflow. A thorough history, including a history of voiding complaints, urologic diseases, obstetric events, and neurologic diseases should be obtained. Urinary tract infections can lead to urinary incontinence and should be ruled out. A focused neurologic exam should be performed, noting any sensory or motor deficits and decrease in anal tone. If overflow incontinence is suspected, a postvoid urinary residual should be checked by catheterization or bladder ultrasound. In female patients, a pelvic exam should be performed with the patient in stirrups. Prolapse of any pelvic structures should be noted. The patient should be asked to bare down to assess for stress incontinence or rotational descent of the bladder and proximal urethra. Rotational descent can be quantified with a "Q-tip test." A lubricated cotton swab is inserted into the urethra and the patient is asked to bear down. If the angle of the cotton swab changes by more than 30 degrees, the patient is considered to have significant urethral descent.

Urodynamics

Multiple categories of urinary incontinence may often coexist. For example, a patient may have both urge and stress incontinence. To better delineate the components of incontinence, a urodynamics test may be performed.[61] To perform the test, a small catheter, usually 7F, with multiple channels is inserted into the bladder to allow simultaneous filling of the bladder and transducing of intraluminal pressures. There are four primary components to urodynamics testing. The first component is cystometry, which involves measuring detrusor pressures at various bladder volumes. Detrusor pressure, which is generated by the bladder wall, is calculated as the pressure measured in the bladder lumen minus the intra-abdominal pressure measured by a catheter in the rectum. As the bladder fills,

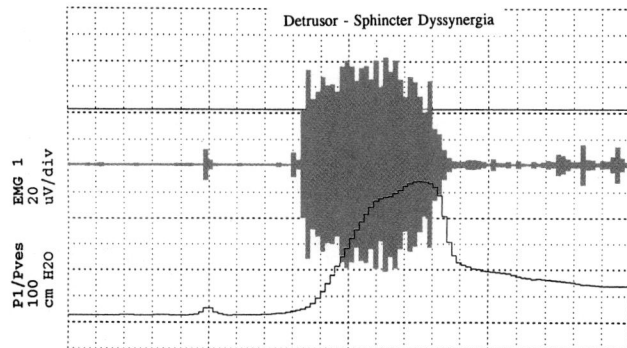

FIG. 39-24. Urodynamic study demonstrating detrusor–external sphincter dyssynergia. Note the hyperactivity of the external sphincter (large black area) while the patient is voiding. The resulting outlet resistance can produce hydronephrosis and ultimately diminish renal function.

involuntary detrusor contractions are recorded and the bladder sensory function is assessed by noting when the patient feels the need to void. After filling the bladder, the patient is asked to void and evidence of detrusor–external sphincter dyssynergia is noted by monitoring external sphincter contractions by electromyography (Fig. 39-24).

The second component of urodynamics is a pressure-flow study to assess for bladder outlet obstruction. A decreased urinary flow rate may result from either bladder outlet obstruction or a poorly contracting bladder. Therefore, both vesical pressure and maximum urinary flow rate are simultaneously measured to assess the bladder outlet. The third component is a urethral pressure study to assess the resistance provided by the urinary sphincter. To perform a urethral pressure study, the bladder is filled to 150 to 200 mL. The patient is asked to Valsalva and the abdominal pressure that produces urinary leakage is noted as the Valsalva leak point pressure. A Valsalva leak point pressure less than 60 mm H_2O is consistent with intrinsic sphincter deficiency. The fourth component to urodynamics is videourodynamics. The bladder is filled with radiographic contrast and the bladder is imaged in real time on a fluoroscopic screen. The relationship between the bladder, the urethra, and various pelvic landmarks can be noted, and the status of the bladder neck can be assessed during rest, Valsalva, and voiding.

Stress Urinary Incontinence

Stress urinary incontinence occurs with increase in intra-abdominal pressure associated with activities such as coughing, laughing, or exercise.[62] In women, stress incontinence can result from loss of urethral support, intrinsic sphincter deficiency or a combination of the two. The loss of urethral support can lead to rotational descent of the bladder. This leads to a change in the normal angle between the urethra and proximal bladder.[63] The relationship between these two structures is important for proper functioning of the urinary sphincter. In addition, a lax urethral support can lead to poor transmission of intra-abdominal pressure, which normally helps to coapt the urethral mucosa and form a water-tight seal.

A variety of conditions contribute to the structural changes associated with stress incontinence. Labor and childbirth have long been associated with the development of stress continence.[64] Prolonged labor, number of childbirths, and use of delivery forceps have all been linked to subsequent development of stress incontinence—the most important mechanism appears to be partial disruption of the innervation to the pelvic floor musculature.[65] Other factors associated

with the development of stress incontinence include aging, pelvic surgery, trauma, hypoestrogenic states, and neurologic conditions that result in denervation of the urinary sphincter. In men, stress incontinence is most commonly caused by intrinsic sphincter deficiency following radical prostate surgery or transurethral prostate resection.

Mild stress incontinence may be improved by conservative measures such as using estrogen supplements in postmenopausal women, pelvic floor exercises, and timed voiding. However, the most effective treatment options for stress incontinence involve surgery. In female patients, a urethral sling procedure can be performed to increase urethral resistance and to correct mild to moderate degrees of urethral prolapse. A variety of sling techniques have been described, however most procedures involve placing a sling material around the urethra and tacking the material to the rectus fascia.[66] In male patients with stress incontinence, the most effective procedure is an artificial urinary sphincter. The artificial sphincter has three components. A fluid-filled sphincter is placed around the bulbar urethra, a pump is placed in the scrotum and a reservoir is placed in the prevesical space. The sphincter increases urethral resistance and helps prevent incontinence. When the patient wishes to void, he opens the sphincter by compressing the pump in his scrotum and moving fluid from the sphincter to the reservoir.

Urge Incontinence

An overactive bladder is characterized by involuntary detrusor contractions. If these involuntary contractions generate sufficient pressure to overcome the urethral resistance, urinary incontinence results. Two terms distinguish the etiology of overactive bladders. Involuntary bladder contractions secondary to an upper tract neurologic insult, such as a stroke or spinal cord injury, is referred to as detrusor hyperreflexia. Involuntary contractions resulting from irritation of the bladder itself is termed detrusor instability. Common causes of detrusor instability include urinary tract infections, bladder prolapse, stress incontinence and bladder outlet obstruction. When possible, the underlying etiology for an overactive bladder should be addressed. For example, if stress incontinence is the primary problem, the urge incontinence will resolve in more than half of patients after surgical treatment for stress incontinence.

The vast majority of patients with overactive bladders do not have a clearly identifiable cause and symptomatic treatment is employed. Anticholinergics are effective, particularly when combined with timed voiding. Various biofeedback programs are effective for motivated patients with milder symptoms. A permanent sacral nerve stimulator can be implanted to inhibit bladder contractions and help prevent urinary incontinence.

Total Incontinence

Total incontinence refers to continuous leakage of urine and implies that a fistula exists between the urinary tract and the skin or vagina.[67] In industrialized countries, the most common cause of a vesicovaginal fistula is routine pelvic surgery such as vaginal hysterectomies, which account for approximately 75% of cases. In developing countries, the major cause of vesicovaginal fistulas is birth trauma. Other causes include malignancy, inflammatory bowel disease, and urinary tuberculosis. The diagnosis can be confirmed by instilling dye into the bladder and evaluating the color of the draining vaginal fluid. Cystoscopy and vaginoscopy can be performed to localize the fistula.

The treatment generally involves surgical repair; however, if a fistula is identified immediately following the responsible iatrogenic injury, a trial of conservative management with catheter drainage of the bladder is reasonable. The principles for surgical repair are the same as for repair of fistulas in other parts of the body. A tension-free closure with multiple, nonoverlapping lines of closure is critical to the success of the repair. When possible, vascularized tissue should be interposed between the layers of closure.

Overflow Incontinence

Overflow incontinence, often termed *false incontinence,* is secondary to urinary retention, resulting either from an obstruction or an atonic bladder. Patients with new onset of urinary incontinence should be catheterized or have a bladder ultrasound to check for a postvoid residual. If the urinary retention is secondary to bladder outlet obstruction, the cause of the obstruction should be addressed.

Urinary retention following pelvic surgery is usually temporary and resolves following several days of catheter drainage or intermittent catheterization. Spinal cord injury above the level of the sacrum can result in a hyperreflexic bladder. However, during the immediate 6 to 8 weeks following the injury, there is a period of bladder atony, termed *spinal shock.* Other causes of an atonic bladder include diabetes, sacral spinal cord injury, and pernicious anemia. If long-term management is required for an atonic bladder, clean, intermittent catheterization is a safe and effective option.

TRAUMA

Kidney and Ureter

Approximately 10% of traumas involve the urologic system, most commonly the kidneys. The best study for evaluating the kidneys is a helical abdominal CT scan with IV contrast. A CT scan should be performed for all penetrating traumas. For adult patients with blunt trauma, a CT scan should be obtained in patients with gross hematuria, or with microscopic hematuria and systolic blood pressure less than 90 mm Hg at any point during the transport and resuscitation.[68] Approximately one-third of renovascular injuries present with complete absence of hematuria, and, therefore, mechanism of injury and associated clinical findings, such as flank contusions and lower rib fractures, should also prompt a CT scan.[69,70] Pediatric patients are able to maintain blood pressure despite an almost 50% loss of circulating volume. Therefore, hypotension is a poor indicator for radiologic work-up. All pediatric patients with gross hematuria should have a CT scan, and all pediatric patients with microscopic hematuria and potential renal trauma based on the mechanism of injury should have a CT scan.

The most commonly applied staging system for renal injury was developed by the American Association for the Surgery of Trauma (Table 39-2 and Fig. 39-25). Approximately 95% of renal traumas are grade 1. Approximately 98% of renal injuries can be managed nonoperatively. The only absolute indications for surgical management of a renal injury are persistent bleeding resulting in hemodynamic instability or an expanding perirenal hematoma. Relative indications for surgical management include major urinary extravasation, vascular injury, and devitalized parenchymal tissue. Studies show that even large urinary extravasations will resolve with conservative management.[71] Smaller vascular injuries resulting in devitalized tissue also can be managed without surgery; however, if the amount of devitalized tissue exceeds 20% of the renal tissue, surgical management leads to quicker resolution of the injury and to fewer subsequent complications.[72]

Patients managed nonoperatively should be placed on bedrest until resolution of gross hematuria. After resuming ambulation, the

Table 39-2

Staging System for Renal Injury Developed by the American Association for the Surgery of Trauma

Grade	Description of Injury
1	Contusion or nonexpanding subcapsular hematoma No laceration
2	Nonexpanding perirenal hematoma Cortical laceration <1 cm deep without extravasation
3	Cortical laceration >1 cm without urinary extravasation
4	Laceration: through corticomedullary junction into collecting system *or* Vascular: segmental renal artery or vein injury with contained hematoma
5	Laceration: shattered kidney *or* Vascular: renal pedicle injury or avulsion

SOURCE: From Moore EE, Shackford SR, Pachter HL, et al: Organ & injury scaling: Spleen, liver, and kidney. *J Trauma* 29:1664, 1989.

patient should be carefully monitored for recurrence of gross hematuria, which requires reinstitution of bedrest. Surgical exploration should be performed following CT staging when possible. If the patient requires immediate exploration for hemodynamic instability and a CT scan cannot be performed, a one-shot intravenous pyelogram (1 mL/kg of body weight of 30% contrast administered 10 minutes before x-ray) should be performed intraoperatively to evaluate the kidneys and confirm the presence of a functioning contralateral kidney. Surgical exploration should be performed through a midline approach. The renal vessels should be identified and controlled prior to opening Gerota's fascia, in order to allow the vessels to be rapidly occluded if massive bleeding is encountered. Injuries to the collecting system should be repaired by a watertight closure. Devitalized tissue should be excised and meticulous hemostasis should be obtained by ligating open segmental vessels. If bleeding cannot be controlled or only minimal vitalized tissue remains, a nephrectomy should be performed.

Ureteral injuries are rare, with the majority of injuries resulting from penetrating trauma. The diagnosis of ureteral injuries can be challenging as they often present without hematuria. Ureteral injuries are often discovered during radiographic work-up or abdominal exploration for related injuries. If a ureteral injury is suspected, an intravenous pyelogram, a retrograde pyelogram, or a contrast CT scan should be obtained. When performing a CT scan, delayed images should be obtained after the contrast has entered the collecting system. Surgical repair depends on the level of injury and the length of the injured segment. Important principles for surgical repair include a tension-free, water-tight closure after widely débriding the injured segment. For coverage of large ureteral defects, interposition of intestinal segments or bladder flaps may be required to achieve a tension-free repair. The adventitia surrounding the ureter should be carefully preserved to maintain the tenuous, ureteral blood supply.

Bladder

Hematuria, gross or microscopic, is the hallmark of bladder injury. The vast majority of bladder injuries are found in patients with pelvic fractures.[73,74] More than 90% of patients diagnosed with bladder injury have a pelvic fracture and approximately 10% of pelvic fractures are associated with bladder ruptures. Therefore, radiographic imaging should be obtained in all patients with hematuria and pelvic

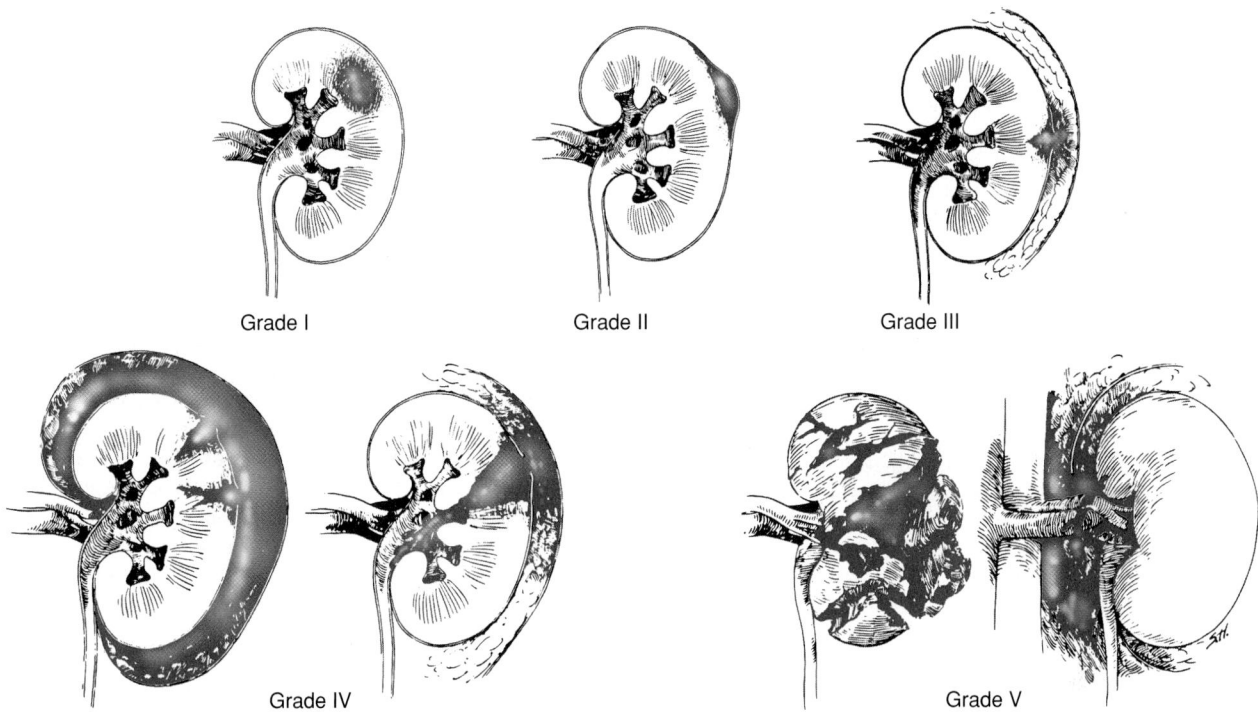

Grade I   Grade II   Grade III

Grade IV   Grade V

FIG. 39-25. Grading for renal trauma.

fractures, or in patients with penetrating trauma to the pelvis and lower abdomen. Rarely, bladder injury can occur in the absence of a pelvic fracture. Therefore, radiographic imaging also should be considered if pelvic contusions or urethral injuries are present.

A retrograde cystogram is the most accurate test for ruling out a bladder rupture. When performing a retrograde cystogram, it is critical to adequately distend the bladder (400 mL or 40 cm H_2O) and obtain a postdrainage film to look for extravasation of contrast. An alternative study is a CT cystogram, which can be obtained at the same time the abdomen and pelvis are imaged for related injuries. The management of bladder injury depends on the site of rupture. Extraperitoneal ruptures can usually be managed conservatively with prolonged catheter drainage; however, intraperitoneal ruptures should be explored and surgically repaired.

Urethra

Patients with urethral injury resulting from trauma classically present with blood at the meatus and inability to void. Other potential findings include a perineal hematoma (Fig. 39-26) and a "high-riding" prostate on digital rectal exam. If any of these findings are present, a retrograde urethrogram should be performed before attempting to catheterize the bladder. To perform a retrograde urethrogram, a small Foley catheter is placed just inside the meatus and the Foley balloon is inflated with 1 to 2 mL of water. Lateral decubitus films are taken while 30 to 50 mL of radiographic contrast is gently injected through the catheter. When feasible, performing the study under fluoroscopy is preferred. Urethral injuries are categorized as posterior or anterior injuries.

Posterior Urethra

Trauma to the posterior urethral, which includes the prostatic and membranous urethra, occurs in the context of pelvic fractures. The statistics are similar to that of bladder trauma.[75] More than 90% of

posterior urethral injuries occur in patients with a pelvic fracture and approximately 10% of pelvic fractures are associated with urethral injuries.

Although a suprapubic tube provides effective urinary drainage without risking further disruption of the urethra, a urethral Foley should be placed across the injury when possible. If the disruption

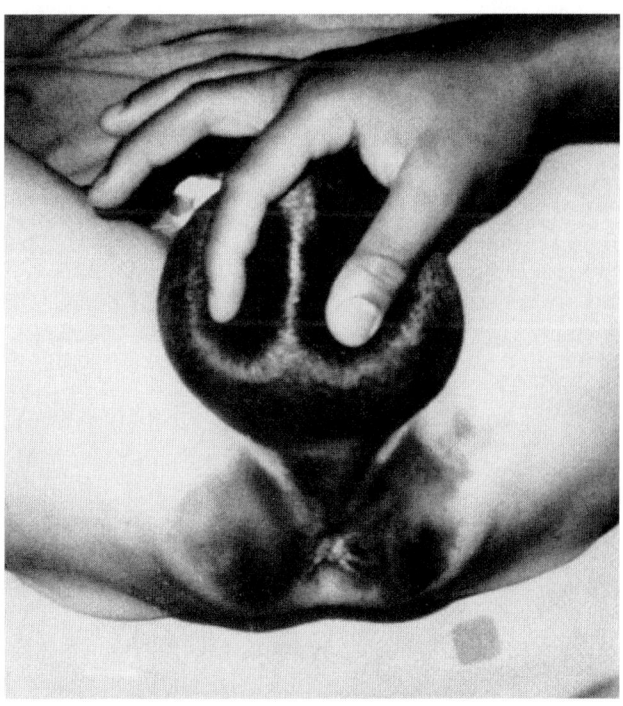

FIG. 39-26. Perineal hematoma contained by Colles' fascia.

is only partial, this can be accomplished by placing a guidewire into the bladder by using a flexible cystoscope, or even a flexible ureteroscope, and placing a catheter over the wire. If complete urethral disruption is present, two flexible cystoscopes, inserted through the meatus as well as through a suprapubic cystostomy, can be used to align the urethra.[76] A guidewire can be placed across the aligned urethra to permit insertion of a Foley catheter. Early urethral alignment can often obviate the need for formal, surgical repair of the urethra. If a completely disrupted urethra cannot be aligned, a definitive repair should be performed in 4 to 6 months. Early exploration following pelvic trauma should not be performed in order to avoid disrupting the pelvic hematoma and causing additional bleeding.

Anterior Urethra

The anterior urethra includes the bulbous and penile urethral. Anterior urethral traumas are usually isolated injuries that most commonly result from a straddle injury. Anterior urethral injury can also occur as a result of direct trauma to the penis. Pelvic fractures are rare in patients with anterior urethral injuries. More distal injuries are contained by Buck's fascia and resulting hematomas dissect along the penile shaft (Fig. 39-27). More proximal injuries to the anterior urethra may be contained by Colles' fascia and produce a perineal hematoma.

The treatment of choice for most blunt and penetrating injuries is immediate exploration, débridement, and direct repair. An exception is an anterior urethral injury resulting from a high-velocity gunshot, which should be managed with a suprapubic cystostomy and delayed repair after clear demarcation of injured tissues.

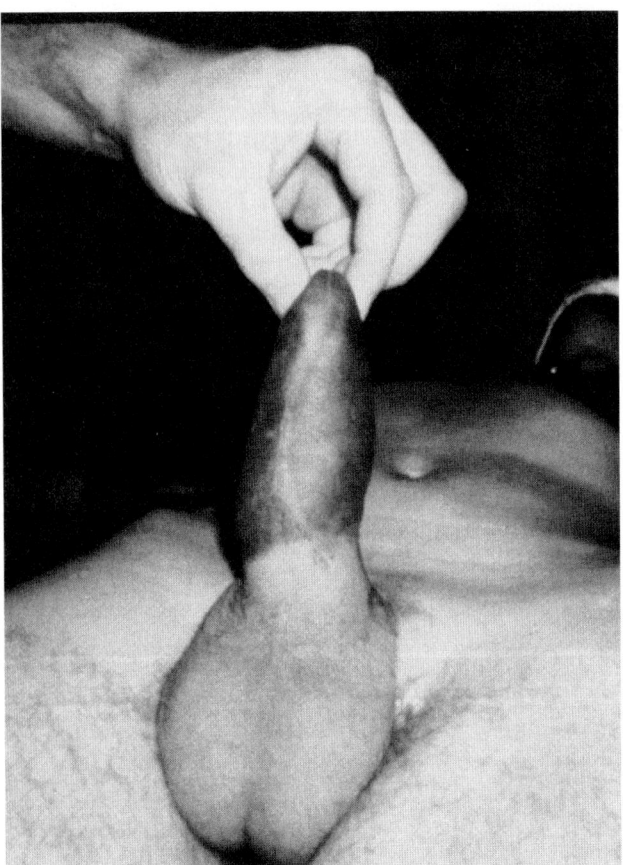

FIG. 39-27. Rupture of a corporal body contained by Buck's fascia.

Proximal injuries to the anterior urethra can be approached through a perineal incision, and more distal injuries can be approached by making a circumferential, subcoronal incision and degloving the penis.

Penis

Penetrating injuries to the penis are rare. Injuries to the penile corporal should be repaired by closing ruptures of the tunica albuginea. Blunt or penetrating penile injuries resulting from an accident should be evaluated with a urethrogram. Urethral injuries should be managed as described in the section on urethral trauma.

Penile fractures represent a traumatic rupture of the tunica albuginea. Most penile fractures occur during sexual intercourse with the woman on top of the man. The erect penis slips out of the vagina and is bent against the pubis and perineum. Patients describe a cracking sound followed by immediate loss of penile rigidity and onset of penile swelling. Patients providing such a history should be immediately explored in the operating room using a circumferential, subcoronal incision to deglove the penis. Generally, no further radiologic work-up is needed. In cases where the history and physical examination is equivocal, a cavernosogram and a urethrogram can be performed.

The most common cause of penile amputations is self-mutilation. When possible, reimplantation should be attempted. Reattachment can be attempted following up to 6 hours of warm ischemia. During surgery, the structures that should be reapproximated include the urethra, the corporal bodies, the dorsal artery and vein, and the dorsal nerves. In cases of self-mutilation, psychiatric consultation is essential to prevent further injury and to control the psychiatric illness.

Testis

The most common causes of testicular injury are assaults and sports injuries. Blunt trauma to the scrotum can disrupt the vessels surrounding the testicles and result in a hematocele. Small traumatic hematoceles do not require surgical intervention. An ultrasound should be performed to confirm that the testicles are intact. Rupture of the testicle itself is rare and requires immediate exploration and surgical repair. The testicles should be immediately explored with no need for an ultrasound if physical findings such as a large hematocele, large hematoma, or gross disruption of the testicular wall are found, suggesting testicular rupture. At the time of surgery, the hematoma should be evacuated and the tunica albuginea should be closed. Penetrating scrotal injuries should be explored, and amputated testicles can often be successfully reimplanted when warm ischemia time is less than 6 hours.

STONE DISEASE

Etiology

Stone disease is one of the most common urologic diseases, affecting one in eight white men by age 70 years.[77,78] Stone disease is most common in 20- to 40-year-olds and is three times more common in men than in women. The prevalence of urinary tract stone disease has been estimated at 2 to 3%. For patients developing a stone, the risk of recurrent stone formation within 5 years may be as high as 50%.[79] Therefore, successful treatment of stone disease not only involves management of the acute stone, but also long-term medical management to prevent future stone formation.

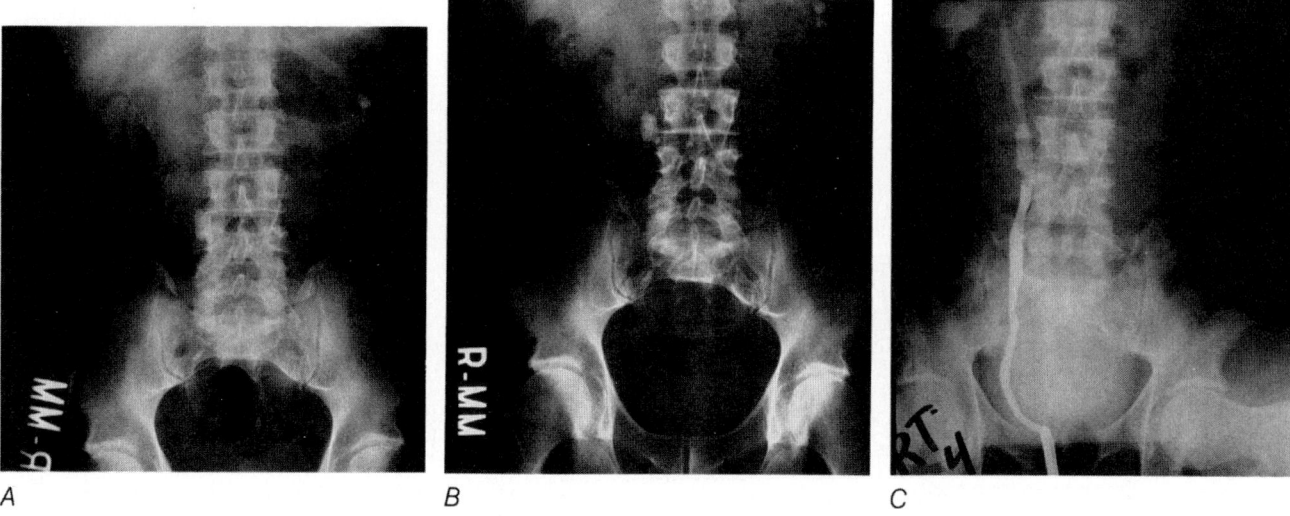

A   B   C

FIG. 39-28. *A. Plain x-ray of a large, right ureteral stone somewhat obscured by the spinal column. B. Oblique view of the same patient clearly reveals the large stone in the right midureter. C. A retrograde pyelogram was performed to better define the anatomy of the urinary collecting system.*

Acute Kidney Stone

Presentation

An acute stone is defined as a urinary stone obstructing the kidney or ureter, and causing symptoms. The classic symptoms of an obstructing kidney stone include colicky flank pain and hematuria, often accompanied by nausea and vomiting. If the stone moves down the ureter, the pain may localize to the ipsilateral lower abdomen. A stone impacted in the distal, intramural ureter may produce pain referred to the inguinal and perineal areas. On physical exam, costovertebral angle tenderness can usually be appreciated. The hematuria accompanying stone disease may be microscopic or gross. However, approximately 15% of acute renal stones present without hematuria. Patients with a superimposed urinary tract infection may present with fever and irritative voiding symptoms. Patients with an infected urinary system and a completely impacted stone may even present with signs and symptoms of sepsis.

Radiologic Work-Up

The diagnosis of a urinary stone can be confirmed radiologically. A plain x-ray of the abdomen and pelvis is the simplest test to obtain (Fig. 39-28); however, radiolucent stones, such as uric acid stones and cystine stones, may not be visualized, and stool in the colon may make it difficult to identify smaller stones in the ureter. The test of choice at most centers for diagnosing an acute stone is a noncontrast, helical CT scan (see Fig. 39-7). All stones, regardless of composition, are visualized on CT scan with the exception of a small percentage of indinavir stones. Indinavir stones form in HIV-positive patients treated with the protease inhibitor indinavir sulfate. Urinary stones can also be diagnosed using intravenous pyelograms and renal ultrasounds (see Fig. 39-9). Both of these modalities, as well as CT scans, are well suited for evaluating the degree of hydronephrosis resulting from an obstructive stone.

Management

The majority of renal stones will pass spontaneously. Only 10% of patients presenting with an acute renal stone require hospital admission. Patients with any of the following presentations should be managed as an inpatient: intractable pain, severe nausea with inability to tolerate oral intake, urinary infection, or renal insufficiency. All other patients can be managed on an outpatient basis. Patients with urinary stones usually present for medical attention as a result of pain, making pain relief a priority. Intramuscular injections of meperidine or morphine are effective. Oral narcotics should be prescribed as necessary. Hydration should be encouraged to promote passage of the stone and patients should be instructed to filter their urine. Retrieved stones can be analyzed for chemical composition.

Patients with obstructing stones and no evidence of urinary infection can safely be given up to 4 weeks to spontaneously pass their stone. No detectable renal damage occurs within 4 weeks of even complete ureteral obstruction. However, in the presence of a urinary infection, emergent intervention is indicated. A percutaneous nephrostomy tube or a ureteral stent should be placed to establish drainage of the obstructed urinary system. Following treatment of the urinary infection, the stone can be treated electively. Stones 4 to 5 mm in diameter have at least a 40 to 50% chance of passing spontaneously; however, stones greater than 6 mm in diameter have less than 5% chance of passing. Therefore, patients with larger stones should be considered for early intervention.

Surgical Management. The least-invasive treatment option for renal stones is extracorporeal shock wave lithotripsy (ESWL) (Fig. 39-29). Shock waves are generated outside the body and focused on the stone. The shock waves harmlessly propagate through intervening tissue and attain sufficient intensity to fragment the stone only when it reaches the calculus. The stone is placed in the focal point of the shock waves by using ultrasound or fluoroscopy. ESWL has a 50 to 80% overall stone-free rate when treating stones less than 3 cm. Smaller stones are associated with a higher success rate, and residual stones can be retreated. Extremely hard stones, such as cystine stones, calcium phosphate stones, and calcium oxalate monohydrate stones, are relatively resistant to fragmentation by ESWL.

Endoscopic options for the surgical treatment of upper tract stone disease include retrograde ureteroscopy and percutaneous nephroscopy. Selection of the specific approach depends on the size

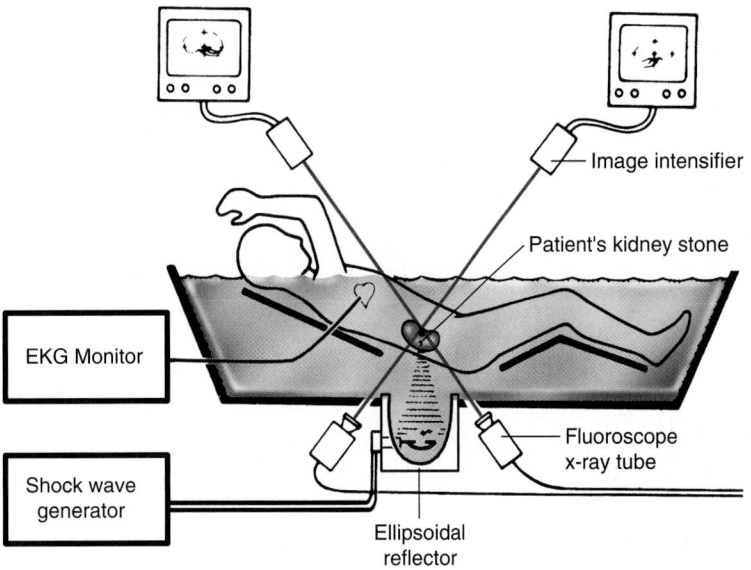

FIG. 39-29. Extracorporeal shock wave lithotripsy. Shock waves are generated extracorporeally and are focused on the stone by the ellipsoidal reflector.

and location of the stone. For example, a large stone filling multiple renal calyces is best treated using a percutaneous approach to directly access the kidney through the flank. The scopes used through a percutaneous flank incision are shorter and larger in diameter compared to a ureteroscope. Thus, larger and more powerful instruments can be inserted through the working port to fragment the stone. A distal ureteral stone, on the other hand, is easily accessed in a retrograde fashion by ureteroscopy. The scope is inserted through the urethra, into the bladder, and up the ureter. Retrograde ureteroscopy represents a less-invasive approach when compared to percutaneous nephroscopy.

Once the stone is endoscopically visualized through a nephroscope or a ureteroscope, small stones can be snared and removed with a number of specialized instruments, such as a stone basket or a three-prong grasper. Larger stones can be fragmented intracorporeally by using a variety of energies, including laser, ultrasound, or mechanical force. Energy is applied to the stone through the working port of the scope and the stone is fragmented under direct vision.

Medical Management

Stone Composition

If the stone is available, it should be analyzed to determine its composition. Calcium oxalate stones are the most common stones found in patients in the United States. Hypercalciuria, which can lead to urinary stone formation, can result from increased resorption of bone as a consequence of hyperparathyroidism, from primary calcium loss by the kidney, or from pathologically increased absorption of calcium in the jejunum (Table 39-3). Hyperoxaluria occurs in patients with chronic diarrhea or inflammatory bowel disease.

Table 39-3
Classification of Hypercalciuria

Type	Serum Calcium	Fasting Urine Calcium	Urine Calcium After Loading
Resorptive	Increased	Increased	Increased
Absorptive	Normal	Normal	Increased
Renal leak	Normal	Increased	Increased

Fatty stools in these patients result in saponification of intestinal calcium. Intestinal oxalate that is unbound to calcium is available for absorption and is eventually excreted by the kidney. An increase in urinary oxalate may also result from excess vitamin C ingestion and primary hyperoxaluria. Primary hyperoxaluria is caused by an enzymatic defect in the liver. The second most common calcium-based stones are calcium phosphate stones, which most often occur in patients with distal (type I) renal tubular acidosis.

Not all urinary stones are calcium based. Struvite stones are usually composed of magnesium, ammonium, and phosphate; however, they may also be composed of carbonate apatite. Struvite stones form in alkaline urine resulting from urinary infections with nitrate-reducing bacteria such as *Proteus, Pseudomonas,* or *Klebsiella* species. They are usually large stones that fill multiple calyces (Fig. 39-30). Uric acid stones, on the other hand, form in acidic urine with a pH level less than 5.5. Medical therapy to alkalinize the urine will dissolve uric acid stones and can circumvent the need for surgical intervention. Pure uric acid stones are radiolucent and are associated with gout, myeloproliferative diseases, and administration of chemotherapy. Cystine stones are faintly radiopaque on plain film. They occur in patients with primary cystinuria, which is inherited as an autosomal recessive disorder. Patients with primary cystinuria also have increased urinary loss of ornithine, arginine, and lysine.

Medical Treatment

Without medical treatment, more than half of all patients with a history of stone disease will have recurrent stones within 5 years.[79,80] Patients with kidney stones and the following characteristics are at a high risk for recurrence and should undergo a metabolic work-up: prior history of stone disease, family history of stone disease, chronic urinary tract infections, inflammatory bowel disease, gout, bone disease, and nephrocalcinosis. The need for an extensive work-up and treatment in first-time stone formers is controversial. However, all patients with a history of stone disease should be instructed to make several lifestyle changes that reduce the risk of stone formation.[81] Patients should drink enough water to produce at least 2 L of urine per day. They should limit protein and salt intake, and should not ingest excessive amounts of vitamin C. However, they should not limit calcium intake because several studies show that

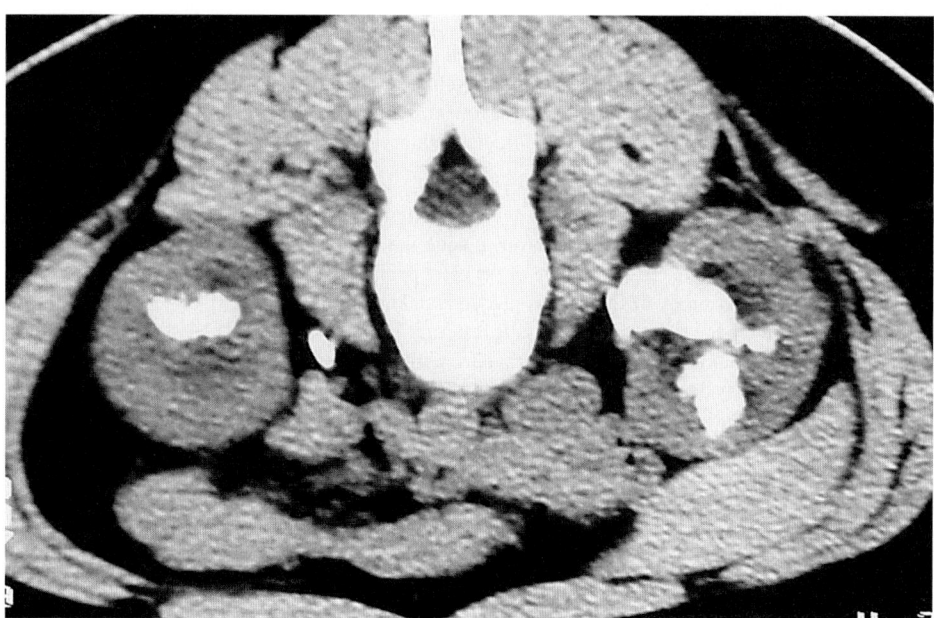

FIG. 39-30. Bilateral staghorn calculi seen on CT scan. Staghorn calculi extend into multiple calyces and are most commonly struvite stones, composed of magnesium, ammonium, and phosphate.

higher calcium diets are associated with a reduced risk of stone formation.

The metabolic work-up should be performed after at least 1 month following an acute stone episode. A simple evaluation, which can be performed in all patients with a history of stone disease, includes radiologic imaging such as a CT scan or IVP, complete blood count, serum chemistries, urinalysis, and urine culture. Patients with abnormalities on this simplified evaluation, or patients at higher risk for recurrent stone disease, should be further evaluated with a 24-hour urine collection for calcium, oxalate, magnesium, phosphorus, uric acid, and creatinine. Based on the specific metabolic abnormality, directed therapy can be prescribed. However, more empiric therapy simply based on 24-hour urinary calcium appears to be equally effective. Patients with normal levels of urinary calcium can be treated with potassium citrate, which acts as an inhibitor for stone formation in the urine. Thiazide diuretics, which decrease urinary calcium excretion, can be added in patients with increased urinary calcium.

SEXUAL DYSFUNCTION

Erectile Dysfunction

Erectile dysfunction is defined as the inability to maintain an erection sufficient for sexual performance. The prevalence of erectile dysfunction increases with age. According to the Massachusetts Male Aging Study, which surveyed 1709 men, the prevalence of complete erectile dysfunction is approximately 5% in 40-year-old men and 15% in 70-year-old men.[82] Moderate erectile dysfunction was found in 17% of 40-year-old men and 34% of 70-year-old men. Some have estimated that as many as one in four men will suffer from erectile dysfunction by the age of 65 years. Risk factors for erectile dysfunction in the general population include age, diabetes mellitus, heart disease, and hypertension.

Normal erections occur in response to parasympathetic innervation received from the cavernous nerve, and involve arterial dilation and relaxation of the smooth muscles of the corpora cavernosa. The venules in the corpora cavernosa become passively compressed by the engorging sinusoids, resulting in the trapping of blood. Nitric oxide is the major neurotransmitter responsible for erections. Nitric oxide results in increased production of cyclic adenosine monophosphate (cAMP) and cyclic guanosine monophosphate (cGMP), which are important secondary transmitters mediating relaxation of corporal smooth muscles.[83] Detumescence occurs when phosphodiesterases break down cAMP and cGMP.[84]

Evaluation of erectile dysfunction starts with a detailed history, including medical and psychosexual history, and physical examination. Basic diagnostic tests should be obtained to assess risk factors for erectile dysfunction such as fasting glucose, glycosylated hemoglobin, lipid profile, and testosterone levels. Other diagnostic tests to consider include serum prolactin, luteinizing hormone, thyroid-stimulating hormone, complete blood count, and urinalysis. All abnormal findings should be further evaluated. For example, in patients with decreased serum testosterone, the hypothalamic–pituitary–gonadal axis should be evaluated with luteinizing hormone and follicle-stimulating hormone levels. Patients with endocrine disorders resulting in decreased testosterone levels may have decreased sexual interest; however, they do not, in general, have erectile failure.

For patients with no treatable disorders identified on initial evaluation, a therapeutic trial can be offered. Oral drugs, such as sildenafil, inhibit cGMP phosphodiesterases and are effective in 60 to 70% of patients.[85] These drugs are, however, contraindicated in patients with severe cardiac disease and in patients taking nitrates such nitroglycerin or amyl nitrate. Patients with erectile dysfunction resulting from neurogenic and vasogenic causes may benefit from treatment with phosphodiesterase inhibitors; however, patients who have had both cavernous nerves excised during radical retropubic prostatectomy will not respond. Such patients might respond to intracavernous injections. The most commonly used agent for intracavernous injections is prostaglandin E_1, which stimulates cAMP synthesis. Other treatment options include vacuum erection devices and surgical implantation of a penile prosthesis.

For younger patients with potentially correctable causes of erectile dysfunction, or for patients who wish to know the specific etiology of their erectile dysfunction, more specialized studies can be performed. As an example, a patient with arteriogenic impotence caused by a focal arterial stenosis following blunt trauma is a candidate for surgical revascularization. Studies that can delineate the etiology of erectile dysfunction include further psychiatric evaluation, nocturnal penile tumescence/rigidity assessment, penile angiography, cavernosography, and neurophysiologic testing.

Peyronie's Disease

Peyronie's disease results from a dense fibrous plaque that forms on the tunica albuginea, causing a curvature of the erect penis.[86–88] Although the precise etiology of the fibrous plaque is unknown, it is believed that the plaque represents scar tissue resulting from microscopic tears of the tunica albuginea that form during intercourse. Very dense plaques may be appreciated on physical exam. However, in most patients, the flaccid penis is normal on examination and the penile curvature is only noted in the erect penis.

Peyronie's disease has an acute phase and a chronic phase. The acute phase is associated with pain and inflammation as the plaque is forming. During the acute phase, medical therapy with p-aminobenzoic acid, vitamin E, colchicines, or tamoxifen may be modestly successful. Once the pain subsides and the plaque is stable, patients with mild curvatures that do not interfere with intercourse should be observed. Surgical correction should be considered if the penile curvature interferes with sexual intercourse. Patients with Peyronie's disease and erectile dysfunction can be treated with a penile implant. Patients with normal erection can be treated either by plicating the tunica albuginea on the outside of the Peyronie's curvature or by grafting a patch onto the inside of the Peyronie's curvature.

Priapism

Priapism refers to an erection that is unrelated to sexual activity or persists beyond sexual activity. Priapism can be classified as low-flow (ischemic) or high-flow (nonischemic). The two forms of priapism can be distinguished by assessing the blood gas drawn from the penile corpora. The blood gas from a normal penis that is erect or a penis affected by high-flow priapism is similar to an arterial blood gas. However, in low-flow priapism, the blood gas will be similar to that of venous blood. Low-flow priapism results from venous occlusion. It is associated with severe pain. It is essentially a compartment syndrome of the penis and should be treated as a medical emergency. Most priapisms are idiopathic; however, specific causes of low-flow priapism include sickle cell disease, pelvic tumors, leukemia, spinal cord injury, penile injections for erectile dysfunction, antidepressants, and antipsychotics, especially chlorpromazine.

The management of low-flow priapism should be dictated by the duration of the priapism. Within 36 hours of onset of low-flow priapism, intracorporal irrigation with an alpha-adrenergic agonist may be effective. A variety of protocols exist. One example of a protocol for intracorporal irrigation involves diluting 5 mg of phenylephrine in 500 mL of normal saline and repeatedly aspirating 20 mL of blood and injecting 20 to 30 mL of the phenylephrine solution through a 21-gauge butterfly needle.

If this is ineffective, or if the priapism has been present for more than 36 hours, a distal shunt should be performed under anesthesia. A commonly performed distal shunt is the Winter shunt,[89] in which a biopsy needle is inserted through the penile glans into the corpora cavernosa to create a shunt (Fig. 39-31). If this procedure is unsuccessful, a more proximal shunting procedure, between the corpora cavernosum and the corpora spongiosum, should be performed. The rationale for these shunting procedures is that the glans of the penis

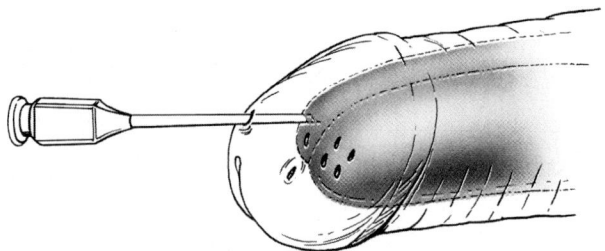

FIG. 39-31. Winter shunt. A biopsy needle is inserted through the penile glans into the corpora cavernosum. A shunt is created between the corpora cavernosum, which is affected by a veno-occlusive process in priapism, and the glans, which is unaffected.

and the corporal spongiosum are flaccid during priapism and unaffected by the veno-occlusive process. Therefore, a shunt will allow the occluded blood in the corpora cavernosa to drain.

Priapism resulting from sickle cell disease or leukemia should initially be managed medically. Patients with sickle cell disease tend to have recurrence of priapism, and, therefore, a trial of conservative therapy directed at preventing additional sickling is warranted. Medical therapy should include hydration, oxygenation, and alkalinization. Transfusions or exchange transfusions should be considered. Patients with leukemia should be promptly treated with chemotherapy rather than surgery.

High-flow priapism is generally painless, and because tissue ischemia is not a feature, treatment is less urgent. Nonischemic priapism results from an arterial-venous fistula that is most commonly secondary to trauma. The diagnosis of high-flow priapism can be confirmed by color Doppler ultrasound. The arterial-venous fistula can be identified by angiography and selectively embolized. If this fails, the fistula can be surgically ligated.

Infertility

Approximately 15% of couples are unable to conceive within 1 year.[90–92] Of couples treated for infertility, approximately 20% of cases are a result of a male factor and 30 to 40% of cases are a result of a combination of male and female factors. It is important to keep in mind that 1% of men being evaluated for infertility have a serious underlying medical condition, such as testicular cancer. The initial evaluation should start with a thorough reproductive and sexual history. Couples trying to conceive should ideally have intercourse every other day, starting about 6 days before the predicted date of ovulation. Medications that have antiandrogen effects (i.e., spironolactone, ketoconazole, cimetidine, and tetracycline) or that impair spermatogenesis (i.e., tetracycline, erythromycin, and nitrofurantoin) should be stopped. Many commercial lotions and lubrications impair sperm motility and should not be used during intercourse. It is also important to keep in mind that spermatogenesis may be impaired for up to 3 months following a febrile illness.

During the physical exam the patient should be assessed for signs of abnormalities associated with infertility. Gynecomastia may be a sign of an endocrine disorder. Eunuchoid body habitus may suggest Klinefelter's syndrome. The scrotal contents should be carefully examined. The normal testicular volume in white men is 20 mL or approximately 4 × 3 cm. The vas deferens is absent in cystic fibrosis. The spermatic cord should be examined with and without a Valsalva maneuver for presence of varicoceles. Clinically detected varicoceles are the most common abnormality in men treated for infertility, and surgical repair leads to improved semen quality in approximately two-thirds of patients, doubling the chances of

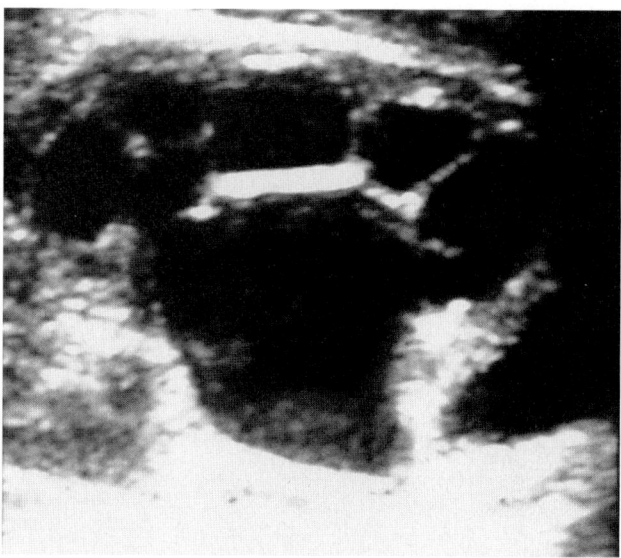

FIG. 39-32. Renal ultrasound in a newborn demonstrating significant hydronephrosis.

conception. However, there is no evidence that repair of subclinical varicoceles detected on ultrasound or venography improves pregnancy rates.

The next step in the evaluation is a semen analysis. The specimen should be obtained following at least 3 days of abstinence and examined within 1 to 2 hours of collection. At least two specimens collected several weeks apart should be examined. The ejaculate is evaluated for volume, sperm count, and motility and morphology of the sperm. Low ejaculatory volume may be caused by retrograde ejaculation into the bladder or obstruction of the vas deferens. The hypothalamic-pituitary axis should be evaluated in patients with oligospermia (less than 5 to 10 million sperm/mL); men with primary hypogonadism should undergo chromosomal study. Patients who are azoospermic or who have severe oligospermia may have testicular failure or obstructed vas deferens.

Further work-up following a semen analysis might include a vasogram and testicular biopsy. A vasogram will detect strictures

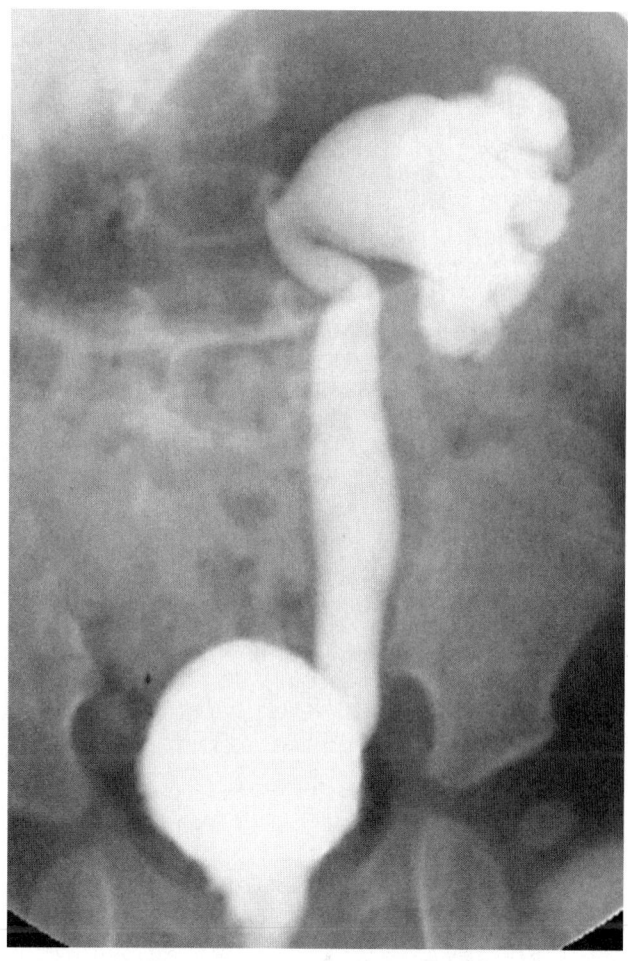

FIG. 39-34. Voiding cystourethrogram. This VCUG in an infant demonstrates grade IV ureteral reflux on the left.

of the vas deferens and ejaculatory duct. At the time of testicular biopsy, sperm can be retrieved for use with assisted reproductive techniques. During the evaluation of the male partner, all correctible causes of infertility should be identified and treated. If treatment is not possible or the treatment is unsuccessful, assisted reproductive techniques such as intracytoplasmic sperm injection can be tried with a 20 to 30% success rate per cycle.

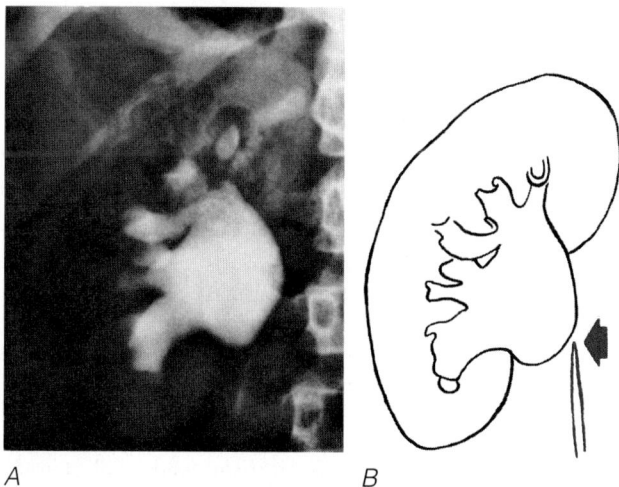

A   *B*

FIG. 39-33. *A.* Hydronephrosis resulting from a ureteropelvic junction obstruction. *B.* Site of stenosis (*arrow*).

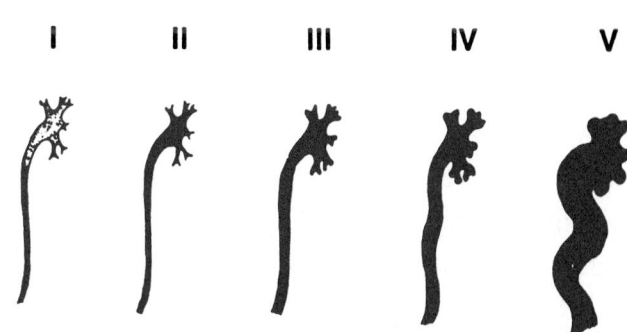

FIG. 39-35. The grading system adopted by the International Reflux Study in Children. The urinary system is represented in brown. (*Reproduced with permission from Arant BS Jr: Vesicoureteral reflux and renal injury. Am J Kidney Dis 10:491, 1991.*)

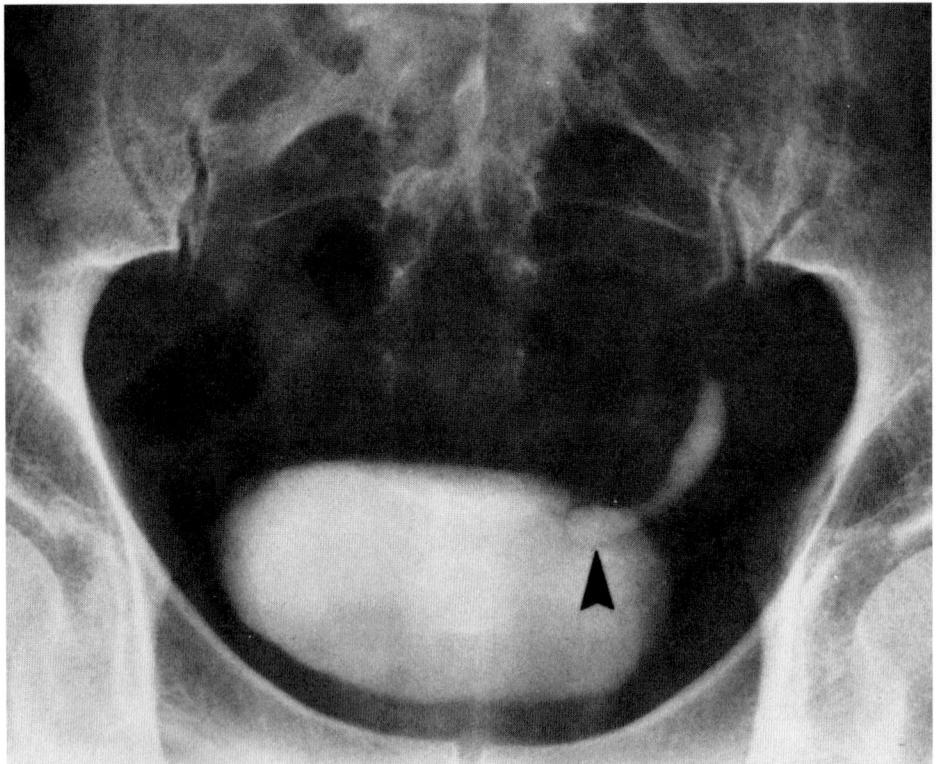

A

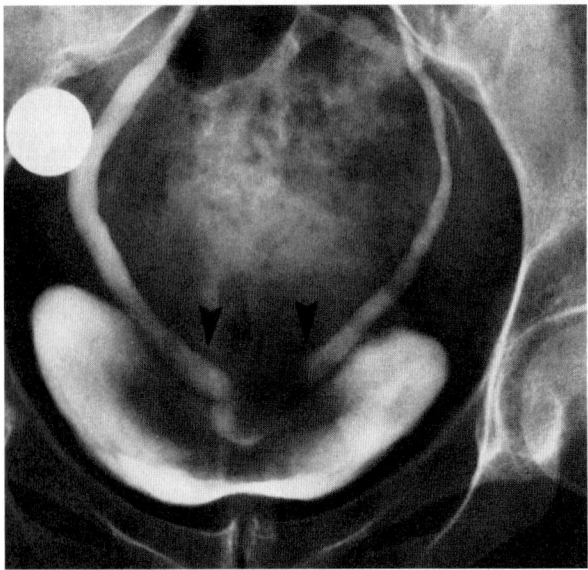

B

FIG. 39-36. Ureterocele. *A.* Left ureterocele *(arrow)*. *B.* Bilateral ureteroceles *(arrows)*.

PEDIATRIC UROLOGY

Hydronephrosis

Hydronephrosis, or dilation of the upper urinary tract, may signify a congenital anomaly with the potential for adversely impacting renal function. Fetal hydronephrosis is diagnosed in 1 of 500 routine prenatal ultrasounds.[93] The majority of fetal hydronephrosis resolves by birth or within the first year of life. Fetal intervention is rarely necessary, and should only be considered in cases of bilateral hydronephrosis and severe oligohydramnios. Following birth,

severe hydronephrosis may be appreciated as a palpable abdominal mass.

In cases of bilateral hydronephrosis, a renal ultrasound (Fig. 39-32) and a VCUG should be obtained shortly after birth. For unilateral hydronephrosis, both studies can be obtained electively at approximately 1 month of life. Because neonates with hydronephrosis are at a higher risk for pyelonephritis, all neonates diagnosed with unilateral or bilateral hydronephrosis should be started on antibiotic prophylaxis (i.e., amoxicillin, 10 mg/kg per 24 hours). Pyelonephritis during the first year of life, when the

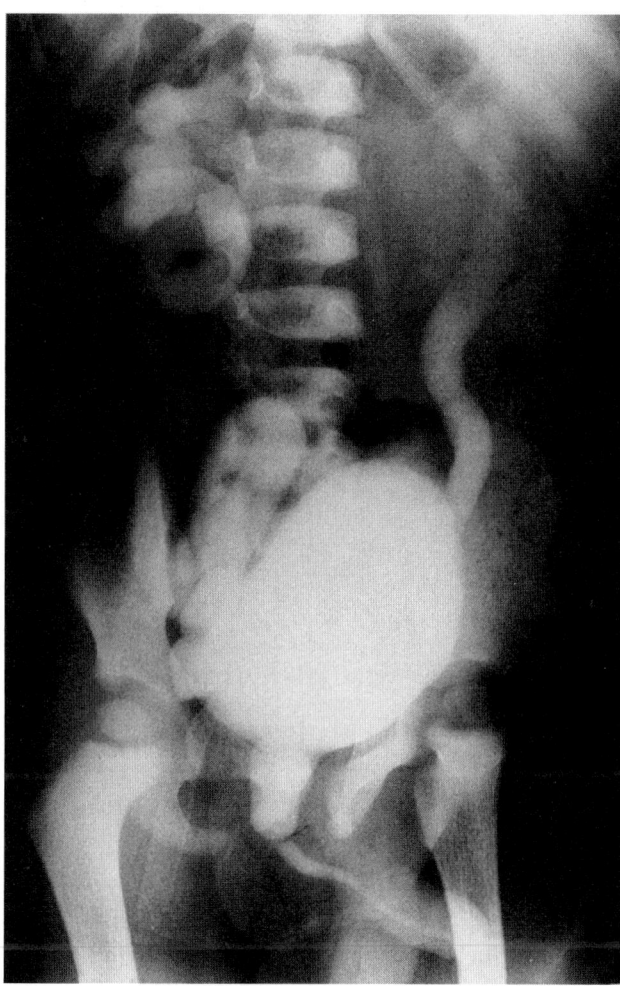

FIG. 39-37. *Posterior urethral valve. The urethral is seen bulging proximal to the urethral valve. Bilateral ureteral reflux is seen in this voiding cystourethrogram (VCUG).*

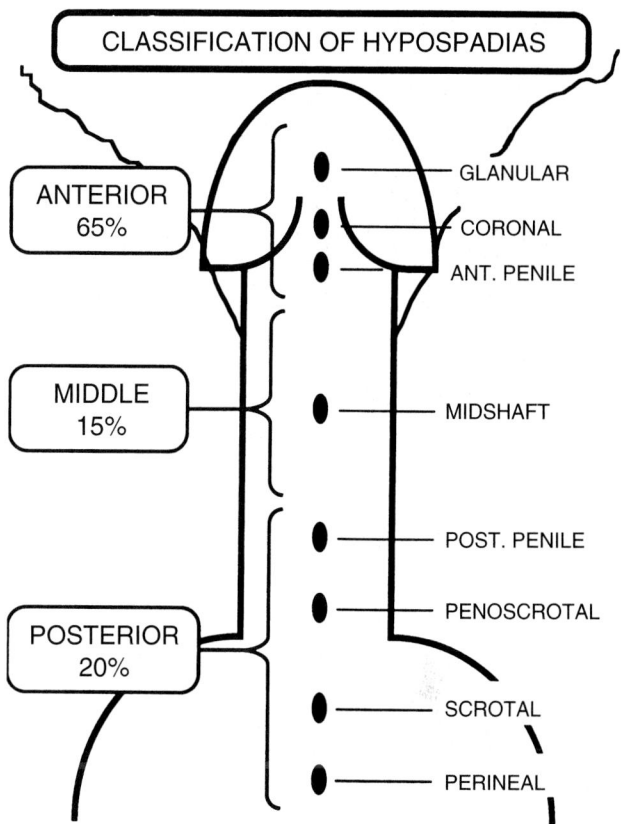

FIG. 39-38. *Classification of hypospadias and frequency by location of hypospadias.*

kidney is still immature, leads to permanent deterioration in renal function.

Ureteropelvic Junction Obstruction

Ureteropelvic junction (UPJ) obstruction is the most common cause of hydronephrosis in neonates (Fig. 39-33). The precise etiology is poorly defined. UPJ obstructions may result from abnormal development of the smooth muscle at the UPJ. In some cases, an aberrant lower pole vessel crosses the UPJ, possibly resulting in extrinsic compression. Most neonates are asymptomatic, while older children present with symptoms, such as flank or abdominal pain.

Initial evaluation should include a renal ultrasound and a VCUG to rule out coexisting reflux. If a UPJ obstruction is suspected, a nuclear renal scan should be performed to assess differential function in the right and left kidneys, and to assess renal pelvic drainage by timing the washout of nuclear isotope following Lasix administration (see Fig. 39-11). Mild to moderate hydronephrosis resulting from a UPJ obstruction can be safely observed and will usually resolve by 2 years of age. Antibiotic prophylaxis should be continued until the UPJ obstruction resolves completely.

Surgical repair should be performed for a UPJ obstruction associated with severe hydronephrosis, diminished renal function, high-grade obstruction or breakthrough infections while on antibiotic prophylaxis. The most commonly performed surgical repair is a dismembered pyeloplasty. The dyskinetic segment of the collecting system at the UPJ is resected, and the ureter and renal pelvis are brought over any crossing vessels that may be present and then anastomosed. The ureter in older patients may readily accommodate endoscopic instruments and a UPJ obstruction may be incised using either a percutaneous or a ureteroscopic approach. Kidneys with minimal function may best be treated with a simple nephrectomy.

Vesicoureteral Reflux

Vesicoureteral reflux is the second most common cause of hydronephrosis and may be found in as many as 70% of infants presenting with a urinary tract infection.[94–97] For vesicoureteral reflux detected after birth, there is a female preponderance, with 85% of cases diagnosed in females. Vesicoureteral reflux is often an inherited anomaly. It is ten times more common in whites than in blacks and up to 45% of siblings of children with reflux also have reflux.[98] Primary reflux is a congenital anomaly caused by a deficiency of the longitudinal bladder muscle surrounding the intramural portion of the ureter. Secondary reflux results from bladder outlet obstruction and an increase in intravesical pressure. Secondary reflux is corrected by addressing the underlying bladder outlet obstruction.

Infants with hydronephrosis on prenatal ultrasound, history of a urinary tract infection, or siblings diagnosed with reflux should be evaluated for primary reflux. Vesicoureteral reflux is diagnosed by demonstrating ureteral reflux on VCUG (Fig. 39-34). The degree of reflux can be graded according to the International Classification

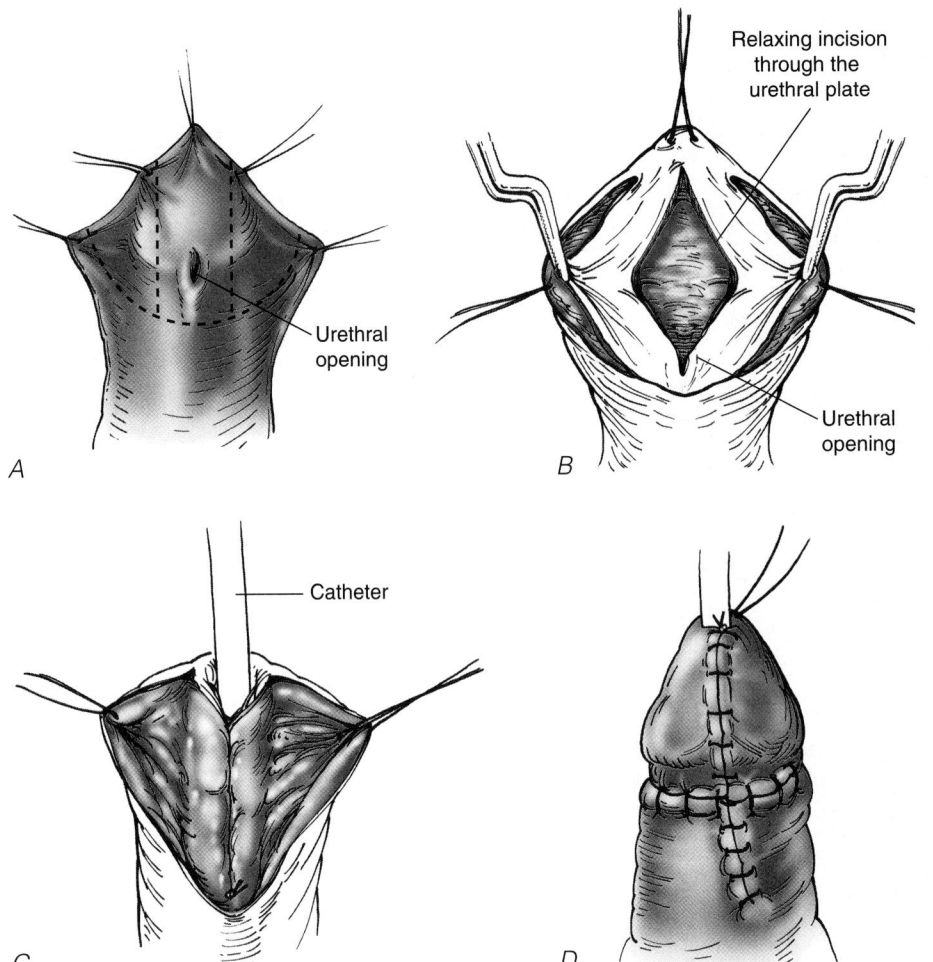

FIG. 39-39. Tabularized incised plate urethroplasty. *A* and *B*. The two critical steps to this procedure involve a "relaxing" incision of the urethral plate distal to the hypospadias opening and (*C, D*) tubularization of the "relaxed" urethral plate.

System devised in 1981 by the International Reflux Study Committee (Fig. 39-35). As the infant bladder grows and the bladder wall thickens, most low-grade refluxes resolve.[99,100] Approximately 85% of all grades I and II reflux will spontaneously resolve, while 30 to 40% of grades III and IV reflux and 9% of grade V reflux will resolve. Given that some high-grade reflux will eventually resolve, it is reasonable to conservatively follow children with reflux, regardless of the grade. However, it is critical that patients managed conservatively are maintained on antibiotic prophylaxis.

Surgical repair should be performed in all patients with a breakthrough infection while on antibiotic prophylaxis. Although there is some controversy surrounding this issue, most practitioners recommend surgical correction before the onset of puberty for girls with persistent reflux. The rationale for this recommendation is based on the reasoning that after the cessation of longitudinal growth, the likelihood of spontaneous resolution of reflux is small, and during pregnancy, reflux places women at a higher risk of pyelonephritis and miscarriage. Boys are at a lower risk of infection secondary to reflux. Therefore, most practitioners recommend stopping antibiotic prophylaxis after early childhood and continuing to observe persistent reflux.

The gold standard for intervention is an open surgical reimplant of the ureter into the bladder. Another option involves cystoscopically injecting a bulking agent, such as collagen or a synthetic material. The bulking agent is injected submucosally with the goal of increasing resistance at the ureteral orifice and preventing reflux.

Ureterocele

A ureterocele is a cystic dilation of the distal ureter associated with a stenotic ureteral opening (Fig. 39-36).[101–106] Ureteroceles occur four times more frequently in girls than in boys and occur almost exclusively in whites. Approximately 80% are associated with the upper-pole moiety of a duplicated ureter. If a duplicated urinary collection system is present, the upper-pole ureter inserts more caudally and medially in relation to the lower-pole ureter. Ureteroceles with the orifice in the bladder trigone are considered orthotopic, while ureteroceles with the orifice distal to the bladder neck are considered ectopic.

The majority of neonatal ureteroceles are diagnosed postnatally during work-up prompted by prenatal hydronephrosis. After birth, the ureterocele can be seen on both ultrasound and VCUG. A VCUG is performed to better localize the ureterocele and evaluate for reflux. It is not uncommon for a ureterocele to distort the bladder and produce ureteral reflux in the contralateral ureter or the ipsilateral lower pole moiety of a duplicated ureter.

The findings associated with a ureterocele vary based on the location of the ureterocele and size of the ureteral opening. If a duplicated ureter is present, 65% of the ureters to the lower-pole

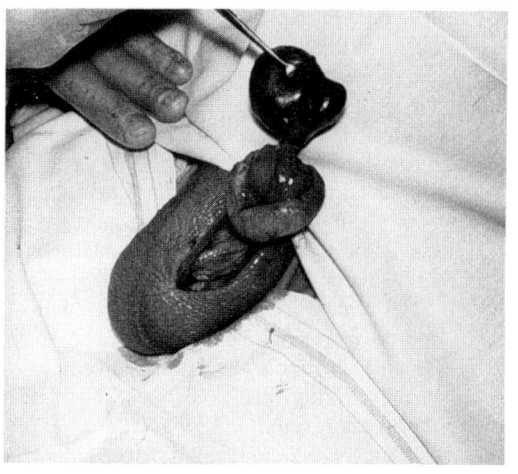

A

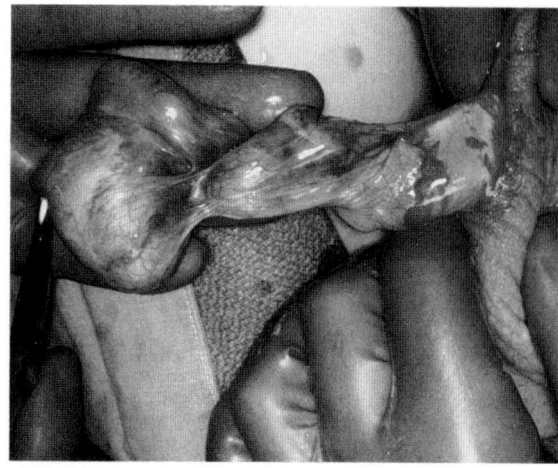

B

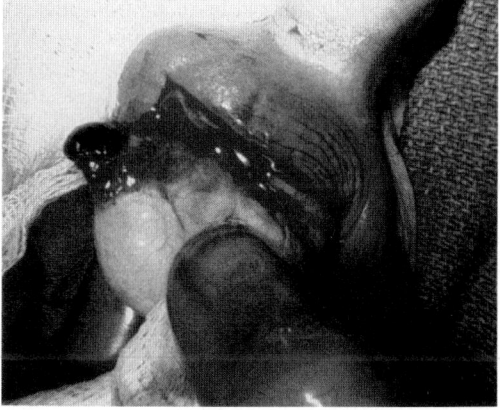

C

FIG. 39-40. Testicular torsion. *A.* In intravaginal torsion, the tunica vaginalis is opened to demonstrate the torsion. *B.* In extravaginal torsion, both layers of the tunica vaginalis twist with the cord. *C.* Torsion of the appendix testis.

kidney will reflux. An orthotopic ureterocele usually produces ipsilateral hydronephrosis; however, a large, orthotopic ureterocele may obstruct the contralateral ureter and produce bilateral hydronephrosis. An ectopic ureterocele can obstruct the urethra, resulting in bladder outlet obstruction and may also produce bilateral hydronephrosis. Ureteroceles associated with a single collecting system are generally less obstructive and usually found incidentally in adult patients. These ureteroceles in adults rarely require intervention.

In the pediatric population, the treatment depends on the clinical presentation. It is not uncommon for infants with undiagnosed ureteroceles to present with urosepsis. Such patients need to be emergently treated by endoscopically incising the ureterocele and establishing ureteral drainage. Uninfected neonates can be electively treated with endoscopic incision. Following this procedure, approximately 25% will develop reflux and may require a secondary procedure, such as ureteral reimplantation.

Infants presenting after 1 year of age with a ureterocele will have had long-standing obstruction and are less likely to have functioning renal tissue draining into the affected ureter. Treatment for such patients should be individualized, and reconstructive procedures should be performed with the goal of establishing drainage, preventing reflux and decreasing risk of future urinary infections.

Posterior Urethral Valve

Posterior urethral valves are obstructive urethra lesions usually diagnosed in male newborns and infants. The valves are thin, membranous folds located in the prostatic urethra. Posterior urethra valves are the most common cause of bilateral hydronephrosis detected on prenatal ultrasound. The test of choice to confirm the diagnosis following birth is a VCUG (Fig. 39-37). Older children with undiagnosed posterior urethral valve often present with urinary incontinence. The first step in treatment involves endoscopic ablation of the valve. A Foley catheter should be placed in the bladder until the procedure can be performed. Depending on the degree of obstruction, patients with posterior valves are at high risk of renal failure, and renal function should be closely monitored.

The Penis

Hypospadias

Hypospadias results from incomplete fusion of the urethral plate during development of the male penis. Hypospadias occurs in one in 300 males. The risk for hypospadias is increased by history of maternal estrogen or progestin use during pregnancy. Hypospadias are classified by the location of the urethral opening (Fig. 39-38).

Approximately 70% of hypospadias occur on the corona or distal shaft of the penis. Neonates with a hypospadias are not at increased risk for having other congenital abnormalities of the urinary tract. However, penoscrotal or perineal hypospadias may represent an intersex disorder and evaluation should include a karyotype. An intersex work-up is also indicated if a hypospadias and an undescended testicle are noted.

For psychologic reasons, the hypospadias should be repaired before 2 years of age. Newborns diagnosed with a hypospadias should not be circumcised. The foreskin may be needed for future corrective surgery. The goals of surgical treatment include correction of any penile curvature, moving the urethral opening to the tip of the glans, and producing a cosmetically satisfactory result. A very effective procedure for correction of distal hypospadias is tabularized incised plate urethroplasty (Fig. 39-39). The two critical steps to this procedure involve a "relaxing" incision of the urethral plate distal to the hypospadias opening and tubularization of the "relaxed" urethral plate. Repair of more proximal hypospadias defects may require use of skin grafts. For example, the penile skin or the foreskin can be mobilized on a pedicle of dartos fascia and used either as an onlay or a tubularized graft.

Phimosis

Phimosis is the inability to retract the foreskin past the glans of the penis. In most neonates, a physiologic phimosis exists. By 3 years of age, 90% of males are able to retract their foreskin. Forceful retraction of the foreskin is not recommended. If a phimosis continues to exist at 4 or 5 years of age, a topical corticosteroid cream can be applied to the foreskin three to four times daily for 6 weeks.[107] This will allow the foreskin to be easily retracted in approximately two-thirds of cases. If the phimosis is resistant to topical steroid therapy, or if the patient requires treatment for balanitis, circumcision should be considered.

Paraphimosis

Paraphimosis occurs when the foreskin that has been retracted past the glans of the penis cannot be reduced to its normal position. Constriction of the distal penis by the foreskin leads to venous congestion and swelling, making reduction of the foreskin even more difficult. As swelling and edema worsen, arterial supply to the glans may be compromised, resulting in ischemia, and even necrosis of the glans. Paraphimosis should be reduced emergently. A variety of techniques have been described. However, in most cases, simply squeezing the glans to reduce the swelling and forcefully reducing the foreskin is successful.

The Testicle

Testicular Torsion

Testicular torsion occurs when the testicle rotates and strangulates its blood supply at the level of the spermatic cord. Testicular torsion is a medical emergency that requires prompt surgical attention. Torsion occurring in the neonatal and prenatal period is extravaginal—the testicle and both layers of the tunica vaginalis rotate. Testicular torsion in neonates may not produce symptoms and is usually only noted after the testicle has atrophied. Torsion in children and young adults is intravaginal—the testicle and the inner layer of the tunica vaginalis rotate (Fig. 39-40).

Intravaginal torsion is most common in 12- to 18-year-olds, with peak incidence at age 13 years. In patients at risk for intravaginal torsion, the tunica attaches higher up on the spermatic cord (bell clapper deformity) and the cremasteric muscle inserts

obliquely on the cord. As a result, the testicle has a horizontal lie when the patient is standing. It is believed that contraction of the cremasteric muscle initiates the characteristic rotation seen in torsion. From the examining physician's perspective, the patient's left testicle rotates counterclockwise and the right testicle rotates clockwise.

Adolescents presenting with testicular torsion complain of severe pain. The differential diagnosis includes epididymo-orchitis and torsion of the appendix testis. Epididymo-orchitis is rare in adolescents and is accompanied by pyuria. Torsion of the appendix testis produces a more focal area of pain and often a bluish discoloration can be appreciated in the scrotum over the testicular appendage. When evaluating a patient with torsion, manual detorsion can be attempted. If this fails, the patient should be immediately taken to the operating room.

Surgery performed within 4 to 6 hours of onset of pain has better than a 90% testicular salvage rate. Therefore, unless the evidence for a competing diagnosis is overwhelming, surgery should not be delayed by diagnostic studies. At the time of surgery, an orchiopexy should be performed by fixing the testicle to the scrotal wall at three different points. The anatomic predisposition to torsion affects both testicles; therefore, the contralateral testicle should be similarly repaired. In select cases where the diagnosis is uncertain and testicular torsion is unlikely, Doppler ultrasound or nuclear scintigraphy can be performed to more definitively rule out testicular torsion.

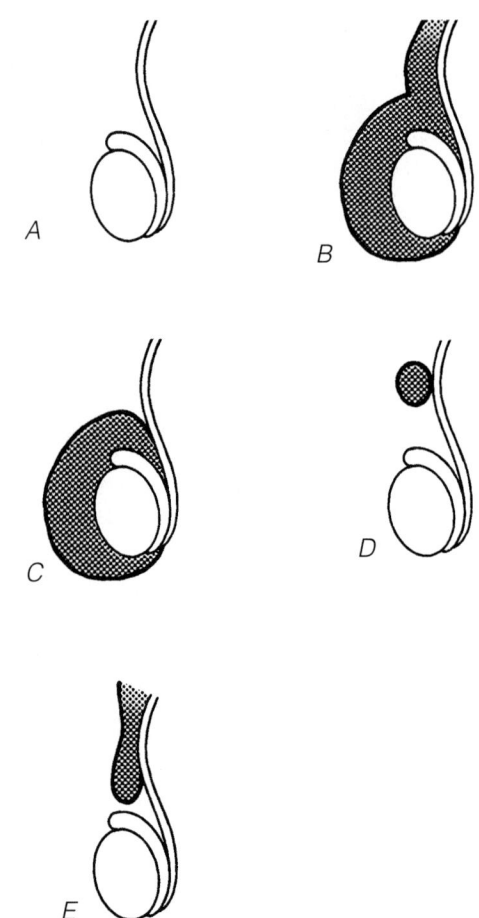

FIG. 39-41. Differential diagnosis of scrotal fluid collections. *A.* Normal. *B.* Communicating hydrocele. *C.* Noncommunicating hydrocele. *D.* Noncommunicating inguinal hydrocele. *E.* Hernia.

Hydrocele

In infants, hydroceles are fluid collections within the tunica vaginalis or processus vaginalis (Fig. 39-41). During development, the testicles are enveloped by a double layer of peritoneum, which becomes the tunica vaginalis. With normal development, the processus vaginalis, which connects the tunica vaginalis with the peritoneum, becomes obliterated. If the process vaginalis persists, peritoneal fluid can track into the space surrounding the testicles, creating a communicating hydrocele. If bowel tracks down the same space, an indirect inguinal hernia is the result. If the processus vaginalis obliterates and traps fluid in the tunica vaginalis, a noncommunicating hydrocele is the result.

Surgical repair is reserved for tense hydroceles that may interfere with testicular circulation or large hydroceles that may cause discomfort. Communicating hydroceles in newborns should generally be observed. Spontaneous closure of the processus vaginalis and resolution of the hydrocele is common; however, hydroceles that persist beyond the first year of life are unlikely to resolve. In pediatric patients, the surgery should be performed through an inguinal incision. The processus vaginalis should be ligated and the distal hydrocele sac should be excised. In adults, hydroceles most commonly form as a consequence of local inflammation and the process vaginalis is almost never patent. Consequently, surgery is performed through a scrotal incision. The hydrocele sac is decompressed and then either plicated or excised to prevent recurrence.

References

1. Walsh PC, Retik AB, Vaughan ED, et al (eds): *Campbell's Urology,* 8th ed. Philadelphia: W.B. Saunders, 2002.
2. Tanagho EA, McAninch JW (eds): *Smith's General Urology,* 16th ed. New York: McGraw-Hill, 2003.
3. Marshall FF (eds): *Textbook of Operative Urology.* Philadelphia: W.B. Saunders, 1996.
4. Berry SJ, Coffey DS, Walsh PC, et al: The development of human benign prostatic hyperplasia with age. *J Urol* 132:474, 1984.
5. Bosch JL, Kranse R, van Mastrigt R, et al: Reasons for the weak correlation between prostate volume and urethral resistance parameters in patients with prostatism. *J Urol* 153:689, 1995.
6. Steele GS, Sullivan MP, Sleep DJ, et al: Combination of symptom score, flow rate and prostate volume for predicting bladder outflow obstruction in men with lower urinary tract symptoms. *J Urol* 164:344, 2000.
7. O'Leary MP, Barry MJ, Fowler FJ Jr.: Hard measures of subjective outcomes: Validating symptom indexes in urology. *J Urol* 148:1546, 1992.
8. McConnell JD, Barry MJ, Bruskewitz RC, et al: *Benign Prostatic Hyperplasia: Diagnosis and Treatment. Clinical Practice Guideline, No. 8.* Rockville, MD: Agency for Health Care Policy and Research, Public Health Service, U.S. Department of Health and Human Services. 1994.
9. Shapiro E, Hartanto V, Lepor H: The response to alpha blockade in benign prostatic hyperplasia is related to the percent area density of prostate smooth muscle. *Prostate* 21:297, 1992.
10. Djavan B, Marberger M: A meta-analysis on the efficacy and tolerability of alpha$_1$-adrenoceptor antagonists in patients with lower urinary tract symptoms suggestive of benign prostatic obstruction. *Eur Urol* 36:1, 1999.
11. Lepor H: Phase III multicenter placebo-controlled study of tamsulosin in benign prostatic hyperplasia. Tamsulosin Investigator Group. *Urology* 51:892, 1998.
12. Marks LS, Partin AW, Epstein JI, et al: Effects of a saw palmetto herbal blend in men with symptomatic benign prostatic hyperplasia. *J Urol* 163:1451, 2000.
13. Marberger MJ: Long-term effects of finasteride in patients with benign prostatic hyperplasia: A double-blind, placebo-controlled, multicenter study. PROWESS Study Group. *Urology* 51:677, 1998.
14. Pomer S, Dobrowoloski ZF: The therapy of benign prostatic hyperplasia using less-invasive procedures: The current situation. *BJU Int* 89:773, 2002.
15. Jemal A, Murray T, Samuels A, et al: Cancer statistics, 2003. *CA Cancer J Clin* 53:5, 2003.
16. Pantuck AJ, Zisman A, Belldegrun AS: The changing natural history of renal cell carcinoma. *J Urol* 166:1611, 2001.
17. Tsui KH, Shvarts O, Smith RB, et al: Renal cell carcinoma: Prognostic significance of incidentally detected tumors. *J Urol* 163:426, 2000.
18. Gnarra JR, Tory K, Weng Y, et al: Mutations of the VHL tumour suppressor gene in renal carcinoma. *Nat Genet* 7:85, 1994.
19. Zbar B, Tory K, Merino M, et al: Hereditary papillary renal cell carcinoma. *J Urol* 151:561, 1994.
20. Uzzo RG, Novick AC: Nephron sparing surgery for renal tumors: Indications, techniques and outcomes. *J Urol* 166:6, 2001.
21. Gill IS, Novick AC, Meraney AM, et al: Laparoscopic renal cryoablation in 32 patients. *Urology* 56:748, 2000.
22. Mickisch GH, Garin A, van Poppel H, et al: Radical nephrectomy plus interferon-alfa-based immunotherapy compared with interferon alfa alone in metastatic renal-cell carcinoma: A randomised trial. *Lancet* 358:966, 2001.
23. Flanigan RC, Salmon SE, Blumenstein BA, et al: Nephrectomy followed by interferon alfa-2b compared with interferon alfa-2b alone for metastatic renal-cell cancer. *N Engl J Med* 345:1655, 2001.
24. Figlin RA: Renal cell carcinoma: Management of advanced disease. *J Urol* 161:381, 1999.
25. Fisher RI, Rosenberg SA, Fyfe G: Long-term survival update for high-dose recombinant interleukin-2 in patients with renal cell carcinoma. *Cancer J Sci Am* 6(Suppl 1):S55, 2000.
26. Cohen SM, Johansson SL: Epidemiology and etiology of bladder cancer. *Urol Clin North Am* 19:421, 1992.
27. Johansson SL, Cohen SM: Epidemiology and etiology of bladder cancer. *Semin Surg Oncol* 13:291, 1997.
28. Varkarakis MJ, Gaeta J, Moore RH, et al: Superficial bladder tumor. Aspects of clinical progression. *Urology* 4:414, 1974.
29. Lokeshwar VB, Soloway MS: Current bladder tumor tests: Does their projected utility fulfill clinical necessity? *J Urol* 165:1067, 2001.
30. Kaye KW, Lange PH: Mode of presentation of invasive bladder cancer: Reassessment of the problem. *J Urol* 128:31, 1982.
31. Lerner SP, Skinner DG, Lieskovsky G, et al: The rationale for en bloc pelvic lymph node dissection for bladder cancer patients with nodal metastases: Long-term results. *J Urol* 149:758, 1993.
32. Stein JP, Cai J, Groshen S, et al: Risk factors for patients with pelvic lymph node metastases following radical cystectomy with en bloc pelvic lymphadenectomy: Concept of lymph node density. *J Urol* 170:35, 2003.
33. Lutzeyer W, Rubben H, Dahm H: Prognostic parameters in superficial bladder cancer: An analysis of 315 cases. *J Urol* 127:250, 1982.
34. Carroll P (ed): *Urothelial Carcinoma Cancers of the Bladder Ureter and Renal Pelvis,* 14th ed. Norwalk, CT: Appleton and Lange, 1995.
35. Malmstrom PU, Wijkstrom H, Lundholm C, et al: 5-Year follow-up of a randomized prospective study comparing mitomycin C and bacillus Calmette-Guérin in patients with superficial bladder carcinoma. Swedish-Norwegian Bladder Cancer Study Group. *J Urol* 161:1124, 1999.
36. Schoenberg M: Management of invasive and metastatic bladder cancer, in Walsh PC, Retik AB, Vaughan ED, et al (eds): *Campbell's Urology,* 8th ed. Philadelphia: W.B. Saunders, 2002, p. 2803.
37. Kim HL, Steinberg GD: The current status of bladder preservation in the treatment of muscle invasive bladder cancer. *J Urol* 164:627, 2000.
38. Carter BS, Bova GS, Beaty TH, et al: Hereditary prostate cancer: Epidemiologic and clinical features. *J Urol* 150:797, 1993.
39. Kim HL, Steinberg GD: New insights and candidate genes and their implications for care of patients with hereditary prostate cancer. *Curr Urol Rep* 1:9, 2000.

40. Moyad MA: Selenium and vitamin E supplements for prostate cancer: Evidence or embellishment? *Urology* 59:9, 2002.

41. Kim HL, Benson DA, Stern SD, et al: Practice trends in the management of prostate disease by family practice physicians and general internists: An Internet-based survey. *Urology* 59:266, 2002.

42. Walsh PC, Marschke P, Ricker D, et al: Patient-reported urinary continence and sexual function after anatomic radical prostatectomy. *Urology* 55:58, 2000.

43. Catalona WJ, Carvalhal GF, Mager DE, et al: Potency, continence and complication rates in 1,870 consecutive radical retropubic prostatectomies. *J Urol* 162:433, 1999.

44. Prow DM: Germ cell tumors: Staging, prognosis, and outcome. *Semin Urol Oncol* 16:82, 1998.

45. Donohue JP: Selecting initial therapy. Seminoma and nonseminoma. *Cancer* 60:490, 1987.

46. Warde P, Jewett MA: Surveillance for stage I testicular seminoma. Is it a good option? *Urol Clin North Am* 25:425, 1998.

47. Shahidi M, Norman AR, Dearnaley DP, et al: Late recurrence in 1263 men with testicular germ cell tumors: Multivariate analysis of risk factors and implications for management. *Cancer* 95:520, 2002.

48. Cabanas RM: An approach for the treatment of penile carcinoma. *Cancer* 39:456, 1977.

49. McDougal WS, Kirchner FK Jr., Edwards RH, et al: Treatment of carcinoma of the penis: The case for primary lymphadenectomy. *J Urol* 136:38, 1986.

50. Culkin DJ, Beer TM: Advanced penile carcinoma. *J Urol* 170:359, 2003.

51. Jacobson SH, Kallenius G, Lins LE, et al: P-fimbriae receptors in patients with chronic pyelonephritis. *J Urol* 139:900, 1988.

52. Stamm WE, Raz R: Factors contributing to susceptibility of postmenopausal women to recurrent urinary tract infections. *Clin Infect Dis* 28:723, 1999.

53. Dalla Palma L, Pozzi-Mucelli F, Ene V: Medical treatment of renal and perirenal abscesses: CT evaluation. *Clin Radiol* 54:792, 1999.

54. Rathod KR, Narlawar RS, Garg A, et al: Percutaneous conservative management of emphysematous pyelonephritis. *J Postgrad Med* 47:66, 2001.

55. Smellie JM: Urinary tract infection, vesicoureteric reflux, and renal scarring. *Semin Urol* 4:82, 1986.

56. Wainstein MA, Graham RC Jr., Resnick MI: Predisposing factors of systemic fungal infections of the genitourinary tract. *J Urol* 154:160, 1995.

57. Wise GJ, Kozinn PJ, Goldberg P: Amphotericin B as a urologic irrigant in the management of noninvasive candiduria. *J Urol* 128:82, 1982.

58. Kauffman CA, Vazquez JA, Sobel JD, et al: Prospective multicenter surveillance study of funguria in hospitalized patients. The National Institute for Allergy and Infectious Diseases (NIAID) Mycoses Study Group. *Clin Infect Dis* 30:14, 2000.

59. Drach GW, Fair WR, Meares EM, et al: Classification of benign diseases associated with prostatic pain: Prostatitis or prostatodynia? *J Urol* 120:266, 1978.

60. Wagner TH, Hu TW: Economic costs of urinary incontinence in 1995. *Urology* 51:355, 1998.

61. Schafer W, Abrams P, Liao L, et al: Good urodynamic practices: Uroflowmetry, filling cystometry, and pressure-flow studies. *Neurourol Urodyn* 21:261, 2002.

62. Dupont MC, Albo ME, Raz S: Diagnosis of stress urinary incontinence. An overview. *Urol Clin North Am* 23:407, 1996.

63. Carey MP, Dwyer PL: Position and mobility of the urethrovesical junction in continent and in stress incontinent women before and after successful surgery. *Aust N Z J Obstet Gynaecol* 31:279, 1991.

64. Groutz A, Gordon D, Keidar R, et al: Stress urinary incontinence: Prevalence among nulliparous compared with primiparous and grand multiparous premenopausal women. *Neurourol Urodyn* 18:419, 1999.

65. Snooks SJ, Setchell M, Swash M, et al: Injury to innervation of pelvic floor sphincter musculature in childbirth. *Lancet* 2:546, 1984.

66. Govier FE, Kobashi K: Pubovaginal slings: A review of the technical variables. *Curr Opin Urol* 11:405, 2001.

67. Symmonds RE: Incontinence: Vesical and urethral fistulas. *Clin Obstet Gynecol* 27:499, 1984.

68. Carroll PR, McAninch JW: Operative indications in penetrating renal trauma. *J Trauma* 25:587, 1985.

69. Cass AS: Renovascular injuries from external trauma. Diagnosis, treatment, and outcome. *Urol Clin North Am* 16:213, 1989.

70. Santucci RA, McAninch JW: Diagnosis and management of renal trauma: Past, present, and future. *J Am Coll Surg* 191:443, 2000.

71. Matthews LA, Smith EM, Spirnak JP: Nonoperative treatment of major blunt renal lacerations with urinary extravasation. *J Urol* 157:2056, 1997.

72. Husmann DA, Gilling PJ, Perry MO, et al: Major renal lacerations with a devitalized fragment following blunt abdominal trauma: A comparison between nonoperative (expectant) versus surgical management. *J Urol* 150:1774, 1993.

73. Cass AS, Luxenberg M: Features of 164 bladder ruptures. *J Urol* 138:743, 1987.

74. Cass AS: The multiple injured patient with bladder trauma. *J Trauma* 24:731, 1984.

75. Mayher BE, Guyton JL, Gingrich JR: Impact of urethral injury management on the treatment and outcome of concurrent pelvic fractures. *Urology* 57:439, 2001.

76. Moudouni SM, Patard JJ, Manunta A, et al: Early endoscopic realignment of post-traumatic posterior urethral disruption. *Urology* 57:628, 2001.

77. Johnson CM, Wilson DM, O'Fallon WM, et al: Renal stone epidemiology: A 25-year study in Rochester, Minnesota. *Kidney Int* 16:624, 1979.

78. Marshall V, White RH, De Saintonge MC, et al: The natural history of renal and ureteric calculi. *Br J Urol* 47:117, 1975.

79. Bek-Jensen H, Tiselius HG: Stone formation and urine composition in calcium stone formers without medical treatment. *Eur Urol* 16:144, 1989.

80. Zerwekh JE, Reed-Gitomer BY, Pak CY: Pathogenesis of hypercalciuric nephrolithiasis. *Endocrinol Metab Clin North Am* 31:869, 2002.

81. Coe FL, Parks JH, Asplin JR: The pathogenesis and treatment of kidney stones. *N Engl J Med* 327:1141, 1992.

82. Johannes CB, Araujo AB, Feldman HA, et al: Incidence of erectile dysfunction in men 40 to 69 years old: Longitudinal results from the Massachusetts male aging study. *J Urol* 163:460, 2000.

83. Ignarro LJ, Bush PA, Buga GM, et al: Nitric oxide and cyclic GMP formation upon electrical field stimulation cause relaxation of corpus cavernosum smooth muscle. *Biochem Biophys Res Commun* 170:843, 1990.

84. Soderling SH, Bayuga SJ, Beavo JA: Identification and characterization of a novel family of cyclic nucleotide phosphodiesterases. *J Biol Chem* 273:15553, 1998.

85. Montorsi F, Salonia A, Deho F, et al: Pharmacological management of erectile dysfunction. *BJU Int* 91:446, 2003.

86. Davis CJ Jr.: The microscopic pathology of Peyronie's disease. *J Urol* 157:282, 1997.

87. Brock G, Hsu GL, Nunes L, et al: The anatomy of the tunica albuginea in the normal penis and Peyronie's disease. *J Urol* 157:276, 1997.

88. Gholami SS, Gonzalez-Cadavid NF, Lin CS, et al: Peyronie's disease: A review. *J Urol* 169:1234, 2003.

89. Winter CC: Cure of idiopathic priapism: New procedure for creating fistula between glans penis and corpora cavernosa. *Urology* 8:389, 1976.

90. Spira A: Epidemiology of human reproduction. *Hum Reprod* 1:111, 1986.

91. Thonneau P, Marchand S, Tallec A, et al: Incidence and main causes of infertility in a resident population (1,850,000) of three French regions (1988–1989). *Hum Reprod* 6:811, 1991.

92. Niederberger CS: Understanding the epidemiology of fertility treatments. *Urol Clin North Am* 29:829, 2002.

93. Helin I, Persson PH: Prenatal diagnosis of urinary tract abnormalities by ultrasound. *Pediatrics* 78:879, 1986.

94. Smellie JM, Normand C: Reflux nephropathy in childhood, in Kincaid-Smith P (ed): *Reflux Nephropathy*. New York: Masson Publishing, 1979, p. 14.

95. Scott JE, Stansfeld JM: Ureteric reflux and kidney scarring in children. *Arch Dis Child* 43:468, 1968.

96. Smellie JM, Normand IC: Clinical features and significance of urinary tract infection in children. *Proc R Soc Med* 59:415, 1966.

97. Mor Y, Leibovitch I, Zalts R, et al: Analysis of the long-term outcome of surgically corrected vesico-ureteric reflux. *BJU Int* 92:97, 2003.

98. Noe HN: The long-term results of prospective sibling reflux screening. *J Urol* 148:1739, 1992.

99. Edwards D, Normand IC, Prescod N, et al: Disappearance of vesicoureteric reflux during long-term prophylaxis of urinary tract infection in children. *Br Med J* 2:285, 1977.

100. Medical versus surgical treatment of primary vesicoureteral reflux: Report of the International Reflux Study Committee. *Pediatrics* 67:392, 1981.

101. Monfort G, Guys JM, Coquet M, et al: Surgical management of duplex ureteroceles. *J Pediatr Surg* 27:634, 1992.

102. Mandell J, Blyth BR, Peters CA, et al: Structural genitourinary defects detected in utero. *Radiology* 178:193, 1991.

103. Rickwood AM, Reiner I, Jones M, et al: Current management of duplex-system ureteroceles: Experience with 41 patients. *Br J Urol* 70:196, 1992.

104. Shekarriz B, Upadhyay J, Fleming P, et al: Long-term outcome based on the initial surgical approach to ureterocele. *J Urol* 162:1072, 1999.

105. Cooper CS, Andrews JI, Hansen WF, et al: Antenatal hydronephrosis: Evaluation and outcome. *Curr Urol Rep* 3:131, 2002.

106. Coplen DE: Management of the neonatal ureterocele. *Curr Urol Rep* 2:102, 2001.

107. Monsour MA, Rabinovitch HH, Dean GE: Medical management of phimosis in children: Our experience with topical steroids. *J Urol* 162:1162, 1999.

CHAPTER 40

Gynecology

Gregory P. Sutton, Robert E. Rogers, William W. Hurd, and Martina F. Mutone

Radical Hysterectomy (Modified from Okabayashi)
Resection of Ovarian Cancer
Vaginal Procedures
Hysterectomy
Pessaries
Injuries Associated with Pelvic Surgery

ANATOMY

External Genitalia (Vulva)

The vulva is bounded by the symphysis pubis anteriorly, the anal sphincter posteriorly, and the ischial tuberosities laterally (Fig. 40-1). The *labia majora* form the cutaneous boundaries of the lateral vulva and represent the female homologue of the male scrotum. The labia majora are fatty folds covered by hair-bearing skin in the adult. They fuse anteriorly with the anterior prominence of the *symphysis pubis*, the *mons veneris*. Posteriorly, the labia majora meet in a structure that blends with the perineal body and is referred to as the *posterior commissure*.

Adjacent and medial to the labia majora are the *labia minora*, smaller folds of connective tissue covered laterally by non-hair-bearing skin and medially by vaginal mucosa. The anterior fusion of the labia minora forms the *prepuce of the clitoris;* posteriorly, the labia minora fuse in the *fossa navicularis,* or posterior fourchette. The term *vestibule* refers to the area medial to the labia minora bounded by the fossa navicularis and the clitoris. Both the urethra and the vagina open into the vestibule. The clitoris lies superior to the urethral meatus; the male homologue is the penis.

Skene's glands lie lateral and inferior to the urethral meatus and occasionally harbor pathogens such as *Neisseria gonorrhoeae.* Cysts, abscesses, and neoplasms may arise in these glands.

Musculature of the Pelvic Floor

The *levator ani* muscles (Fig. 40-2) form the muscular floor of the pelvis. These muscles include, from anterior to posterior, bilaterally, the *pubococcygeus, puborectalis, iliococcygeus,* and *coccygeus* muscles. The first two of these muscles contribute fibers to the fibromuscular perineal body. The *urogenital hiatus* is bounded laterally by the pubococcygeus muscles and anteriorly by the *symphysis pubis*. It is through this muscular defect that the urethra and vagina pass, and it is the focal point for the study of disorders of pelvic support such as cystocele, rectocele, and uterine prolapse.

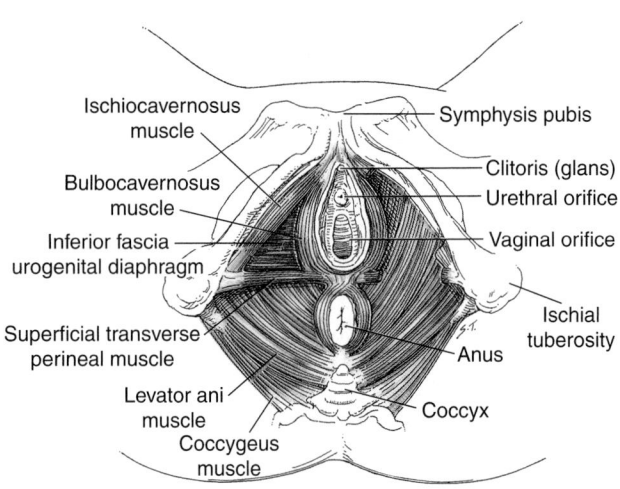

FIG. 40-2. Inferior view of perineal and pelvic muscles.

Distal or cauded to the levator ani muscles, or *levator sling* is the *perineal membrane*. This structure is bounded by the ischial tuberosities inferolaterally and by the pubic arch superiorly. Lateral to the perineal membrane are the *ischiocavernosus* muscles. These structures parallel and are attached to the inferior rami of the symphysis pubis and, like the *bulbocavernosus* muscles, contain erectile tissue that becomes engorged during sexual arousal. The bulbocavernosus muscles arise in the inferoposterior border of the *symphysis pubis* and around the distal vagina before inserting into the perineal body.

The *transverse perinei* muscles arise from the inferior rami of the symphysis just anterior to the pubic tuberosities and insert medially into the perineal body, lending muscle fibers to this structure as well.

Internal Genitalia

Figure 40-3 provides an overhead view of the internal genitalia. The central uterus and cervix are suspended by the lateral fibrous cardinal, or *Mackenrodt's, (uterosacral) ligaments,* which insert into the paracervical fascia medially and into the muscular sidewalls of the pelvis laterally. Posteriorly, the uterosacral ligaments provide

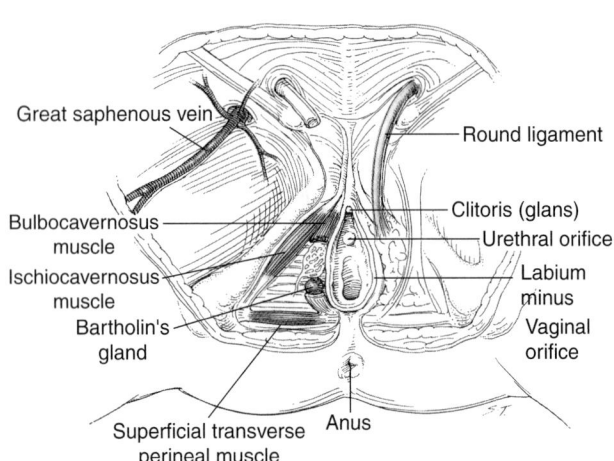

FIG. 40-1. The external anatomy of the vulva.

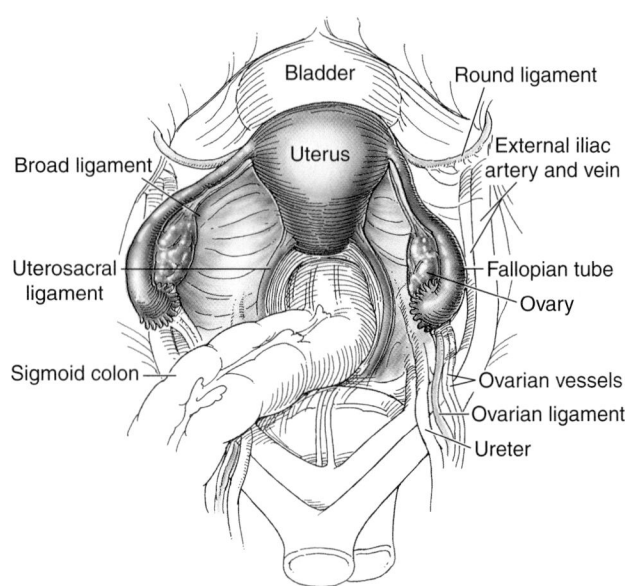

FIG. 40-3. Internal pelvic anatomy from above.

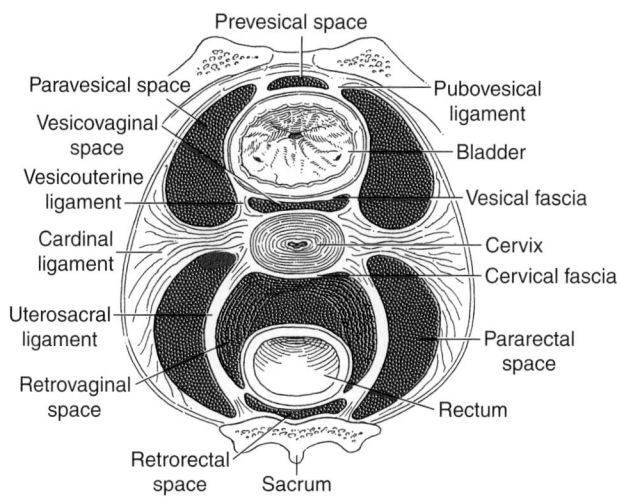

FIG. 40-4. *The avascular spaces of the female pelvis.*

support for the vagina and cervix as they course from the sacrum lateral to the rectum and insert into the paracervical fascia.

The bilateral fallopian tubes arise from the upper lateral *cornua* of the uterus and course posterolaterally and anterior to the ovaries. Each widens in the distal third, or *ampulla.* The ovaries are attached to the uterine cornu by the *proper ovarian ligaments.* These fibrous bands are analogous to the gubernaculum testis in the male and continue laterally from the uterus as the *round ligaments.* These structures exit the pelvis through the internal inguinal ring and course through the inguinal canal (canal of Nuck) and external inguinal ring to the subcutaneous tissue of the mons veneris. They insert into the connective tissue of the labia majora. The ovaries are seemingly suspended from the lateral pelvis by their vascular pedicles, the *infundibulopelvic ligaments.* The peritoneum enfolding the *adnexa* (tube, round ligament, and ovary) is referred to as the *broad ligament,* although it is no more ligamentous than the peritoneum overlying the ovarian artery and vein.

The peritoneal recesses in the pelvis anterior and posterior to the uterus are referred to as the *anterior* and *posterior cul-de-sacs.* The latter is also called the *pouch* or *cul-de-sac of Douglas.*

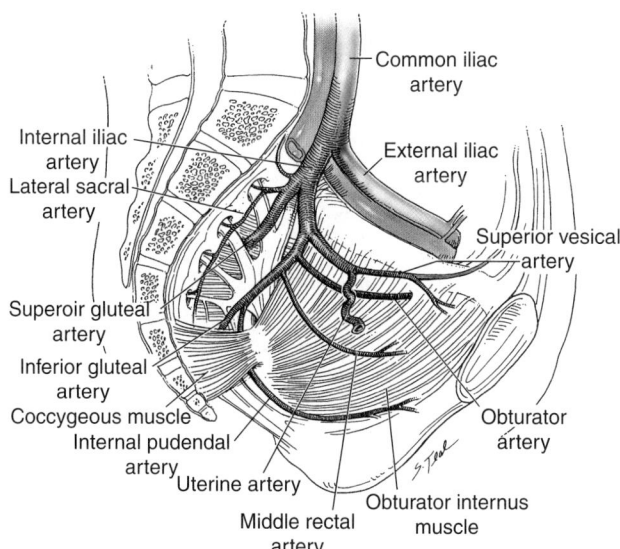

FIG. 40-5. *The muscles and vasculature of the pelvis.*

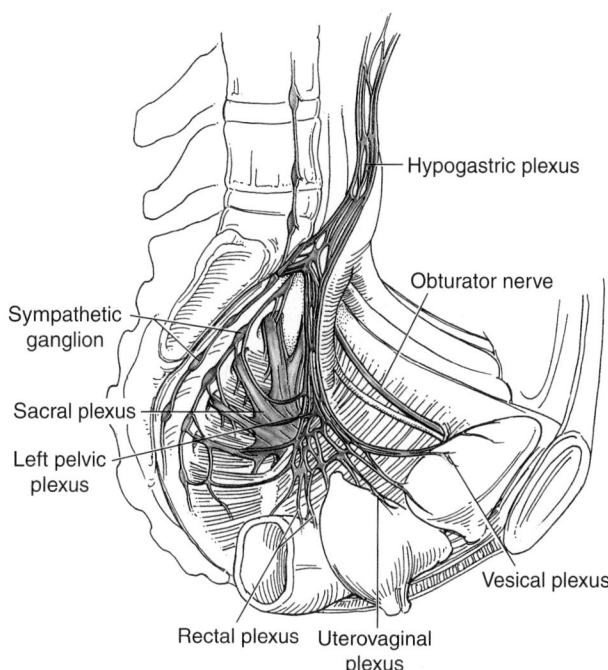

FIG. 40-6. *The nerve supply of the female pelvis.*

On transverse section (Fig. 40-4), several avascular, and therefore important, surgical planes, can be identified. These include the lateral paravesical and pararectal spaces, and, from anterior to posterior, the retropubic or prevesical space of Retzius and the vesicovaginal, rectovaginal, and retrorectal or presacral spaces. The pelvic brim demarcates the obstetric, or true, from the false pelvis contained within the iliac crests.

The muscles of the pelvic sidewall (Fig. 40-5) include the iliacus, the psoas, and the obturator; with the exception of the middle sacral artery, which originates at the aortic bifurcation, the blood supply arises from the internal iliac arteries. The internal iliac, or hypogastric, arteries divide into anterior and posterior branches. The latter supply lumbar and gluteal branches and give rise to the pudendal arteries. From the anterior division of the hypogastric arteries arise the obturator, uterine, superior, and middle vesical arteries.

The nerve supply to the pelvis is composed of the sciatic, obturator, and femoral nerves (Fig. 40-6). Sympathetic fibers course along the major arteries and parasympathetics form the superior and inferior pelvic plexus.

The ureters enter the pelvis as they cross the distal common iliac arteries laterally and then course inferior to the ovarian arteries and veins until they cross under the uterine arteries just lateral to the cervix. After traveling around to the cervix, the ureters course downward and medially over the anterior surface of the vagina before entering the base of the bladder.

DIAGNOSIS

Gynecologic History

The gynecologic evaluation includes a general history with special emphasis on the function of the reproductive system. The history should include the purpose of the visit; present illness; menstrual and reproductive history, as well as medical, surgical, obstetric, emotional, social, family, and sexual history, including note of any high-risk sexual practices or sexually transmitted disease. Medications, allergies, family planning, and a systems review should also be included.

The gynecologic history should include the patient's age, date of her last menstrual period (LMP), the number of pregnancies, the number of deliveries, and the number of abortions. Gravidity, parity, and abortions are frequently indicated as G-P-A. The patient's menstrual history should include her age at the onset of menses, menstrual interval (time from the beginning of one period until the beginning of the next), number of days of flow, and some description in regard to the amount of flow (light, moderate, or heavy). The examiner should inquire as to when the patient's last cervical cytology was obtained, and, in patients older than 35 years of age, the date of the patient's last mammogram should be noted. A description of the patient's current and recent contraceptive methods should be listed. The age of the patient at the time of her last menstrual period is recorded in postmenopausal patients.

Physical Examination

The initial evaluation and the presurgical work-up of a patient should include a general physical examination that includes a description of the patient's height, weight, nutritional status, blood pressure, head and neck (including thyroid), heart, lungs, and lymph nodes.

The gynecologic portion of the examination should document an examination of the breasts, the abdomen, and the pelvis. The pelvic examination is performed on all female patients with a pelvic complaint or on the occasion of their annual gynecologic examination. The patient is examined with her legs comfortably placed in stirrups on an examination table. A good light is essential. Instruments should be warm. Vaginal specula of several sizes must be available.

The external genitalia are inspected, noting the distribution and condition of the pubic hair. The glans clitoris, labia, urethral meatus, and the vaginal introitus are evaluated. The condition of the perineum is noted. The anus and perianal area are inspected.

The speculum is inserted into the vagina, and the vaginal walls and cervix are studied. A cervical cytology is taken at this time. The speculum is removed, and a bimanual examination of the pelvis is performed (Fig. 40-7). The Bartholin, urethral, and suburethral

areas are palpated. The vaginal walls are palpated. The cervix is examined, and its consistency, shape, mobility, and tenderness to motion are noted. The uterus and adnexa are evaluated by pressing them between two fingers of the vaginal hand and a hand placed on the lower abdomen. The size, shape, mobility, and tenderness of these organs are noted. After the bimanual examination, a rectovaginal examination should be performed. The middle finger is inserted into the rectum while the index finger is inserted into the vagina. This important maneuver allows the physician to evaluate the posterior surface of the uterus as well as the rectovaginal septum and uterosacral ligaments (Fig. 40-8).

Diagnostic Procedures

Cervical Cytology

An annual cervical cytology (Papanicolaou [Pap] smear) and pelvic examination should be scheduled for all women who are or who have been sexually active or who have reached 18 years of age. After a woman has had three or more consecutive, satisfactory, annual cytologic examinations with normal findings, the Pap test may be performed less frequently on a low-risk woman at the discretion of her physician (ACOG Committee Opinion Number 186, September 1997).

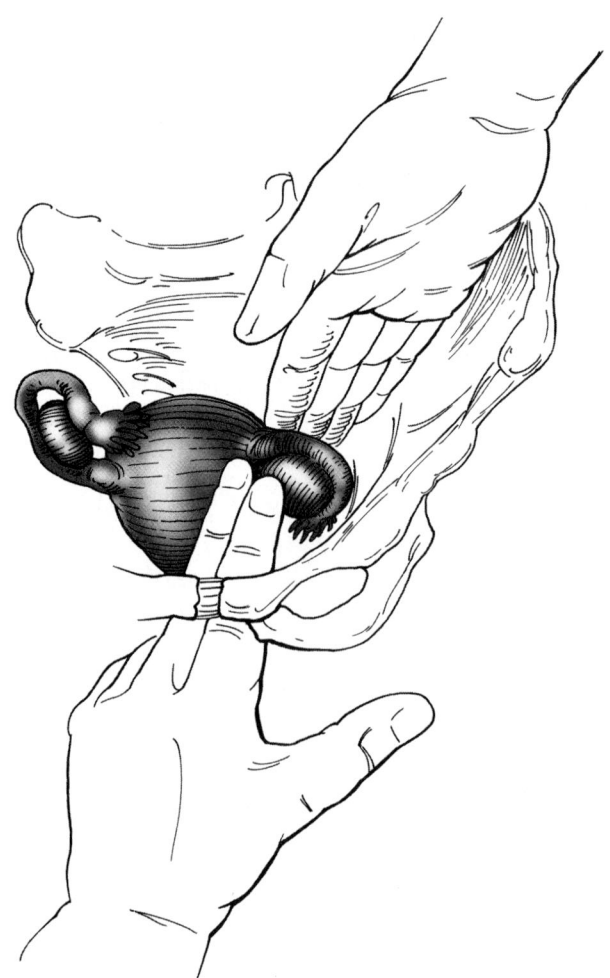

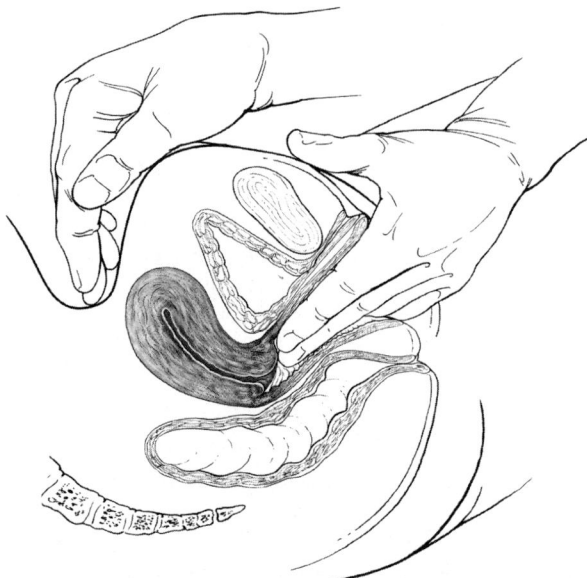

FIG. 40-7. *Bimanual abdominovaginal palpation of the uterus.*

FIG. 40-8. *Bimanual abdominovaginal palpation of the adnexa.*

Table 40-1
The Bethesda Classification for the Classification of Pap Smear Abnormalities

Adequacy of the specimen	*Epithelial cell abnormalities*
Satisfactory for evaluation	Squamous cell
Satisfactory for evaluation but limited by . . . (specify)	Atypical squamous cells of undetermined significance
Unsatisfactory . . . (specify)	Low-grade squamous intraepithelial lesion encompassing human papillomavirus
General categorization	
Within normal limits	High-grade squamous intraepithelial lesion encompassing moderate dysplasia, severe dysplasia, carcinoma in situ
Benign cellular changes: see descriptive diagnosis	
Epithelial cell abnormality: see descriptive diagnosis	Squamous cell carcinoma
Descriptive diagnosis	Glandular cell
Benign cellular changes	Endometrial cells, cytologically benign in postmenopause
Trichomonas vaginalis	
Fungus organisms	Atypical glandular cells of undetermined significance
Predominence of coccobacilli	
Consistent with *Actinomyces* sp.	Endocervical adenocarcinoma
Consistent with herpes simplex virus	Endometrial adenocarcinoma
Reactive changes	Extrauterine adenocarcinoma
Changes associated with inflammation	*Adenocarcinoma, NOS*
Atrophy with inflammation	*Other malignant neoplasms (specify)*
Radiation	*Hormonal evaluation (applies to vaginal smears only)*
Intrauterine contraceptive device	
	Hormonal pattern compatible with age and history
	Hormonal pattern incompatible with age and history
	Hormonal evaluation not possible due to . . . (specify)

SOURCE: From the International Federation of Gynecology and Obstetrics.

After removal of the uterus and cervix for benign disease, the Pap test is not required as a part of the periodic examination. Except in emergency situations, all women who are having a gynecologic surgical procedure should have had a recent cervical cytologic evaluation. Cervical cytologic specimens are obtained at the time of pelvic examination. The cervix is exposed, and the external cervix is scraped with a suitable spatula. The material is placed on a slide expeditiously fixed with any of the fixatives favored by the cytology laboratory that serves the practice. A sample of endocervical cells is then collected, either with a cotton-tipped applicator or with one of the specialized cytologic brushes. This specimen is then placed on a slide and fixed in the manner of the previous specimen.

The practitioner should expect a report from the laboratory in the format of the Bethesda classification (Table 40-1) for cervical cytologic reporting. The Bethesda system for reporting cervical cytologic diagnoses was developed in 1988 and improved in 1991; it replaced the original Papanicolaou reporting system and provides a uniform format for cytopathology reports.

All cytologic reports must be studied carefully to determine whether further evaluation or treatment is indicated (Fig. 40-9). Atypical smears or smears with severe inflammation should be repeated generally in 3 months. Persistent (two or more consecutive) atypical smears should be evaluated with colposcopic examination. All smears that indicate dysplasia or neoplasia should be investigated with colposcopy.

Colposcopy is a specialized technique that allows evaluation of the cervix under magnification, enabling the practitioner to do directed biopsies of abnormal areas. In many cases, the endocervical canal, which is not directly visible to the colposcopist, is biopsied with a small curette at the time of colposcopic evaluation. Colposcopic examination is important to define the severity and size of a cervical lesion. The colposcopic examination following abnormal cervical cytology will preempt cone biopsy and allow office treatment of cervical dysplasia in most patients. Colposcopy may find a lesion too large for the ablative procedure that was planned and indicate another approach. When an endocervical lesion is found, the biopsy indicates a lesser lesion than cytologic report, or the biopsy is indicative of microinvasion of the cervix, a cone biopsy is indicated.

Office Tissue Biopsy

Biopsy of suspicious lesions of the vulva, vagina, cervix, and uterus should be obtained in the office. Vulvar biopsy is obtained by infiltrating the biopsy site with a small amount of 1% lidocaine using a 27-gauge needle. Adequate biopsies can be obtained using a dermatologic skin punch to the vulvar skin and rotating it slightly. The biopsy then is separated from its base with thumb forceps and a pair of fine scissors. Any bleeding from the biopsy site is controlled with a silver nitrate stick.

Biopsy of vaginal lesions is accomplished under local anesthesia. A 25-gauge needle is helpful to reach lesions in the middle or upper vagina. Most lesions of the vaginal wall can be obtained through the use of specialized cervical biopsy forceps or laryngeal biopsy forceps.

Biopsy of the cervix does not require anesthesia. Specialized cervical biopsy punches, such as the Kevorkian or Tischler type, are used. The endocervical canal may be sampled with an endocervical curette such as the Kevorkian or Duncan endocervical curette.

Biopsy of the endometrial cavity is an office procedure. It is essential to be assured that the patient is not pregnant before performing this procedure. A number of instruments are currently available for this biopsy. The Novak endometrial biopsy curette has been

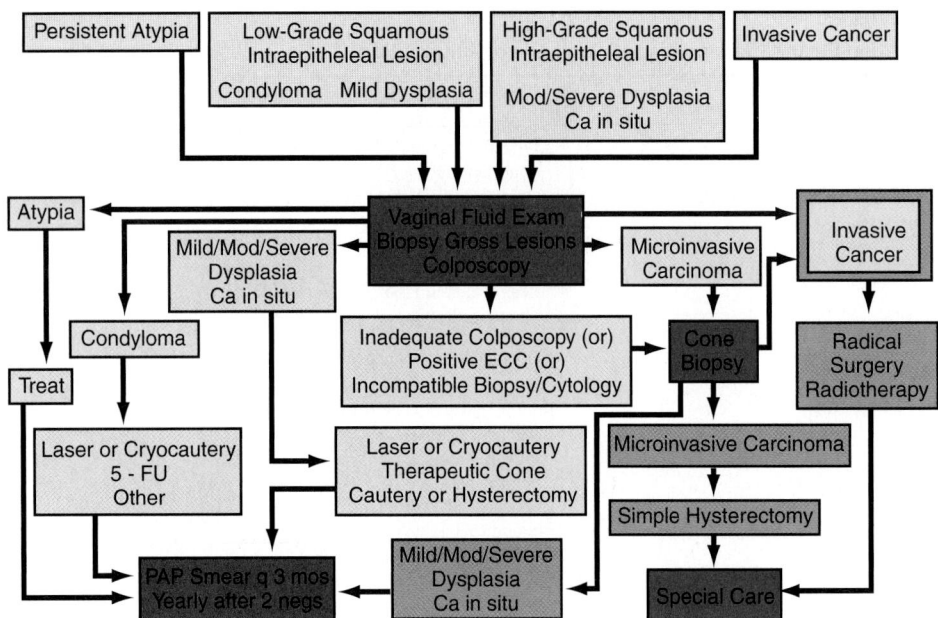

FIG. 40-9. The management of abnormal cytologic findings.

replaced largely by sampling devices such as the Pipelle endometrial biopsy instrument or the Vabra suction instrument; these instruments have the advantages of being narrow in caliber, fitting more comfortably into the cervical os, and being entirely disposable.

Vaginal Discharge

The patient's complaint of abnormal vaginal discharge should be investigated. Vaginal secretions that appear abnormal or have a foul odor must be studied. The pH of the vagina, which is normally between 3.8 and 4.4, may be an aid to diagnosis. A vaginal pH of 4.9 or more indicates either a bacterial or protozoal infection. The pH is obtained by dipping a pH tape in the vaginal secretions collected in the vaginal speculum.

Vaginal fluid is collected for study by using a cotton-tipped applicator and transferring the sections to a small test tube containing a few drops of saline. The "wet mount" is prepared by placing a small amount of the saline suspension on a microscopic slide with a cover slip and examining it under magnification. The examiner may note motile trichomonads, indicative of *Trichomonas vaginalis;* characteristic "clue cells," indicative of bacterial vaginosis; or pus cells, which may be indicative of a variety of vaginal, cervical, and uterine problems, such as gonorrhea, chlamydial, or other bacterial infections.

After the initial microscopic examination, a drop of 10% potassium hydroxide is placed on the specimen, and the vaginal material is evaluated again. Potassium hydroxide has the ability to lyse cellular material and enable the practitioner to appreciate the presence of mycelia characteristic of *Candida* vaginitis.

Cultures

Vaginal and cervical cultures are most useful for the detection of sexually transmitted disease. While the diagnosis of gonorrhea might be suspected when gram-negative intracellular *diplococci* are found on a vaginal smear stained by Gram's stain, culture should be obtained to prove the infection. Gonorrhea is cultured on a chocolate agar plate and incubated in a reduced oxygen atmosphere. Cultures are most conveniently collected on a Thayer-Martin medium in a bottle containing a carbon dioxide atmosphere.

Chlamydial infection is suggested by the finding of a characteristic thick, yellow mucus (mucopus) in the cervical canal. Mucopus should be collected with a calcium alginate–tipped swab and sent to the laboratory in transport media specifically designated for *Chlamydia.* Some laboratories are now offering urine tests for gonorrhea and *Chlamydia* using the ligase chain reaction (LCR). This test offers improved sensitivity and specificity for gonorrhea and *Chlamydia.*

Pregnancy Tests

A number of pregnancy tests are available for use in the office. These tests measure increased amounts of the beta subunit of human chorionic gonadotropin (hCG) in urine. These urine tests are very sensitive and specific, measuring hCG as low as 50 mIU/mL. Serum tests are even more accurate and sensitive, and have an advantage in that they can be quantitated to give an hCG level. Serial hCG levels are helpful in circumstances where it is important to determine that hCG levels are increasing or decreasing, such as in the management of threatened abortion, ectopic pregnancy, or trophoblastic disease.

Abnormal Bleeding

After the first menstrual period (menarche), cyclic bleeding is considered the norm but is subject to great variation. Menstrual interval varies from 21 to 45 days (time from the beginning of one menstrual period until the beginning of another). Menstrual duration varies from 1 to 7 days. The menstrual flow is a subjective assessment and varies from light to heavy. Some women experience bleeding at midcycle at the time of ovulation. Abnormal genital bleeding falls into six categories.

Bleeding Associated with Pregnancy

The availability of extremely sensitive pregnancy tests has made it possible to confirm pregnancy in the early days of gestation. Although bleeding can occur in up to 25% of all normally pregnant women, this symptom must be considered a threatened abortion until the bleeding is otherwise clarified. In the presence of threatened abortion, the pregnancy test is positive, the cervix is closed, and the uterus is generally consistent with the history of gestation. An abortion is considered inevitable when the cervix is dilated and fetal tissue appears at the cervical os. Abortion is incomplete after a portion of the products of conception has been expelled; it is considered complete after all the products of conception have been expelled. Inevitable and incomplete abortion is generally treated by dilatation and curettage.

Ectopic pregnancy must be considered in any patient with a positive pregnancy test, pelvic pain, and abnormal uterine bleeding. Approximately 20% of patients with ectopic pregnancy have no bleeding, but others might complain of vaginal spotting or, occasionally, of hemorrhage.

Gestational trophoblastic disease also causes abnormal bleeding associated with a positive pregnancy test. Most gestational trophoblastic disease is represented by hydatidiform mole. Molar pregnancy is suggested when the uterus is larger than would be expected from the history of gestation, vaginal bleeding, and the passage of grape-like tissue from the vagina. Quantitative gonadotropin levels are almost always greater than expected for the age of gestation. Gestational trophoblastic disease must be differentiated from normal pregnancy. Ultrasound examinations and knowing quantitative gonadotropin levels are helpful in diagnosis.

Dysfunctional Uterine Bleeding

This type of bleeding abnormality is characterized by irregular menses with occasional extended intervals of amenorrhea. When bleeding does occur after one of these periods of amenorrhea, it tends to be extremely heavy. The combination of a period of amenorrhea and extremely heavy bleeding occasionally suggests spontaneous abortion. In the majority of instances, the problem is secondary to failure to ovulate. Evaluation of these patients should include a pregnancy test, which should be negative. Endometrial sampling usually reveals a nonsecretory or proliferative endometrium. In the presence of extremely heavy bleeding, dilatation and curettage is occasionally required, but in most instances, the condition can be managed with cyclic estrogen/progesterone treatment.

Trauma

The bleeding associated with genital trauma may be diagnosed secondary to a history of rape or genital injury. In the presence of genital bleeding secondary to trauma, the lesion must be evaluated carefully and repaired in the operating room under anesthesia if necessary.

In infants and premenarchal patients, the vaginal canal should be examined carefully for foreign bodies.

Bleeding Secondary to Neoplasm

Tumors, both benign and malignant, involving the genital tract from the vulva to the ovary, can produce abnormal bleeding. The most important tool in diagnosis is a meticulous pelvic examination that includes visualization of the vulva, vagina, and cervix, and careful bimanual examination of the uterus, tubes, and ovaries. Lesions of the vulva, vagina, and cervix that produce bleeding should be biopsied to exclude malignancy.

The most common cause of abnormal bleeding in reproductive-age women are leiomyomas (fibroids). Leiomyomas are almost always benign and are a common cause of heavy noncyclic bleeding (menometrorrhagia). Dilatation and curettage is helpful in diagnosing submucous uterine tumors. Pelvic ultrasound and other forms of pelvic imaging are helpful in the diagnosis of uterine fundal tumors. The bleeding associated with tumors of the fallopian tube and ovary

is generally scanty and is almost always associated with a palpable pelvic mass.

Bleeding from Infection

Bleeding is an uncommon symptom of pelvic inflammation. It is associated most often with inflammatory conditions of the vulva, vagina, and cervix. On rare occasions, patients with endometriosis and acute pelvic inflammatory disease have vaginal bleeding.

Bleeding of a Nongenital Etiology

Genital bleeding can be associated with coagulopathy secondary to the use of systemic anticoagulants, clotting disorders, or blood dyscrasias.

Pain

Pelvic pain and abdominal pain are common gynecologic complaints. Pain associated with menses is the most common office complaint. Cyclic pain limited to that period just before or with the onset of menses is referred to as *dysmenorrhea.* Pain occurring without a demonstrable pathologic lesion is referred to as *primary dysmenorrhea* and is a common feature of ovulatory menstrual cycles. This condition is usually treated satisfactorily with simple analgesics. In some cases producing periodic disability, the use of ovarian suppression with oral contraceptives may be considered. *Secondary dysmenorrhea* is commonly associated with endometriosis, cervical stenosis, and pelvic inflammation. Acute pelvic pain must be studied carefully. It may have its origin in abnormal pregnancy, benign or malignant neoplasia, or a variety of nongynecologic diseases. Pregnancy disorders include threatened abortion, inevitable abortion, incomplete abortion, and ectopic pregnancy.

Neoplasms cause acute pain through degeneration of a myoma or torsion of a myoma or ovarian neoplasm. The spontaneous rupture of an ovarian cyst can produce severe pelvic pain. Pain associated with pelvic malignancy is a late symptom and generally follows other opportunities to diagnose this condition.

Common causes of acute pain are salpingitis and endometriosis. Pain secondary to inflammatory conditions is associated with fever and other evidence of infection in most cases. Pelvic infection secondary to *C. trachomatis* is the exception to this rule. The possibility of a nongynecologic condition as the cause of pain must be always considered. Appendicitis and other acute gastrointestinal problems are also causes of acute pelvic and abdominal pain. Patients with severe abdominal and pelvic pain should be evaluated for urinary problems such as renal and ureteral stones as well as inflammatory conditions of the bladder.

In women in the reproductive age group, a differential diagnosis commonly involves appendicitis, ectopic pregnancy, and salpingitis. Readily available, rapidly performed, sensitive, and accurate pregnancy tests have made it possible to quickly exclude the possibility of pregnancy in many situations. Bilateral low abdominal pain increased by movement of the cervix and associated with fever and leukocytosis most often indicates acute pelvic inflammatory disease. Right abdominal pain and tenderness at McBurney's point, associated with a history of gastrointestinal symptoms, on most occasions, will indicate appendicitis. In many cases it may not be possible to make a definitive diagnosis in the office, and some form of exploratory operation may be required. Direct visualization of the pelvis can be carried out with a laparoscope. Acute appendicitis, ruptured tuboovarian abscess, torsion of a tube or ovary, or an ectopic gestation may indicate celiotomy. The finding of pelvic inflammation in most cases will dictate medical treatment.

Pelvic Mass

The finding of a pelvic tumor is a common event in reproductive-age women. At one time, pelvic examination was the only tool for detection and diagnosis of pelvic tumors, but with increasingly sensitive imaging devices, the surgeon is called to evaluate masses that in the past escaped detection. The clinician must be aware that several physiologic conditions cause enlargement of pelvic organs. Pregnancy should be considered in all cases of uterine enlargement in reproductive-age women. Ovarian enlargement, as a result of ovulation and corpus luteum hematomas, produces masses that are easily palpable and that may persist for several weeks. In addition to a carefully performed pelvic examination, abdominal and vaginal ultrasonography is a useful tool. No imaging method will always distinguish between benign and malignant disease, however.

Pelvic ultrasonography, computed tomography (CT), and magnetic resonance imaging (MRI) all provide clues to the origin of pelvic tumors. Uterine enlargement may suggest pregnancy, uterine myomata, adenomyosis, or malignancy, such as endometrial cancer or sarcoma. Tubal tumors may represent a tubal pregnancy, inflammatory conditions of the tube and hydrosalpinx formation, or a primary fallopian tumor. Ovarian enlargement may suggest endometriosis, ectopic pregnancy, tuboovarian abscess, or benign or malignant tumor of the ovary. The decision to operate is predicated on the patient's age, clinical presentation, and character and clinical course of the mass. If the differential diagnosis points to a strong possibility of ovarian malignancy, the patient should be explored under conditions that will allow for the treatment of a pelvic cancer.

INFECTIONS

Vulvar and Vaginal Infections

Vulvar, perineal, and perianal itching and burning are symptoms that may indicate an inflammatory condition. The area is subject to most of the infections that involve skin on any other part of the body. Vulvar infection may be primary on the vulva or can originate in the vagina.

Mycotic Infection

The most common cause of vulvar pruritus is candidal vulvovaginitis. The infection is most common in patients who are diabetic, pregnant, or on antibiotics. The majority of cases are caused by *C. albicans,* although other species may be incriminated. The most prominent symptom is itching; burning of the skin, dysuria, and dyspareunia are also common. Diagnosis is confirmed by examination of the vaginal secretions and recognition of the characteristic pseudomycelia. The condition is treated by the topical application of any one of a number of azole preparations. Intravaginal agents include a number of azole creams generally used over a 3- to 7-day period. Systemic treatment is possible through the oral use of fluconazole 150 mg tablet in a single dose.

Parasitic Infections

Pin worms (*Enterobius vermicularis*), which are common in young girls, cause vulvitis. Diagnosis is made by finding the adult worms or recognizing the ova on microscopic examination of perianal material collected on adhesive tape. A number of antihelmintic agents are available; mebendazole therapy is commonly used.

Trichomonas vaginalis causes primarily a vaginal infection, but the copious vaginal discharge causes secondary vulvitis. The patient complains of heavy, foul-smelling discharge. Diagnosis is made by recognizing the motile flagellates on microscopic examination. Treatment consists of metronidazole 250 mg given three times daily for 7 days.

The vulvar skin is a frequent site for infestation by *Phthirus pubis* (crab lice) and *Sarcoptes scabiei* (scabies, itch mites). The primary symptom of both these infestations is severe pruritus. The adult and immature forms are recognized on close inspection of the skin. Treatment consists of a lindane compound, available for medical use as Kwell. The use of this agent is contraindicated in pregnancy.

Bacterial Infections

Many bacteria attack the vulvovaginal region; on occasion, bacteria, considered normal inhabitants of the genital tract, cause symptoms. The streptococci and staphylococci are the most common offenders.

Bacterial vaginosis is the most common bacterial pathogen. The vaginal discharge found with this condition is not unlike that found with trichomonal vaginitis. The discharge is thin and gray-green in color. The patient complains of a foul, fishy, or "dead mouse" odor. Diagnosis is made by microscopic study of the vaginal secretions to identify characteristic "clue cells." The condition is treated with metronidazole 500 mg orally every 12 hours for 1 week. Metronidazole and clindamycin topical creams are also effective.

Viral Infections

A number of viral infections affect the vulva and vagina, the most common of these being *condyloma acuminatum*. The causative organism is the human papillomavirus. This infection has increased dramatically in the past 20 years. The lesions are characteristic wart-like growths that begin as single lesions but can grow to huge confluent lesions that distort the normal structures. The lesions enlarge rapidly in pregnancy. Diagnosis is suspected on the basis of appearance and confirmed by biopsy. Treatment depends on the destruction of the lesions with caustic agents, cryocautery, laser ablation, or electrocautery. Some large lesions could require surgical removal.

Herpes simplex infection causes painful vesicles followed by ulceration of the vulva, vagina, or cervix. Initial infection is usually widespread, but recurrent infection usually involves a single lesion. Cytologic evaluation of lesions in the vagina is helpful; culture is confirmatory for herpes infection. Once a patient is infected, there is a tendency for the lesions to recur at various intervals for the life of the patient. The attacks may be aborted and the interval between attacks lengthened through the use of acyclovir 400 mg orally three times daily for 7 to 10 days. Active infection in pregnancy carries the risk of newborn infection if the patient delivers vaginally. Cesarean section is recommended in patients in labor with vulvar or vaginal ulceration as a result of herpes simplex infection.

Molluscum contagiosum causes groups of small pruritic nodules with an umbilicated center. The lesions are treated by ablation by cautery, curettage, or corrosive medication.

Pelvic Inflammatory Disease

While pelvic inflammatory disease is basically a medical problem, it has profound surgical implications. It is estimated that there are approximately 1.5 million cases of pelvic inflammatory disease in the United States each year. This condition produced approximately 350,000 hospital admissions and could be responsible for more than 100,000 surgical procedures annually. The condition might produce infertility in 10% of the cases that occur; 3% or more of patients will have ectopic pregnancy, and chronic pain is a problem in many others.

Pelvic inflammatory disease is largely limited to sexually active females. Several factors have been recognized as placing the patient at risk: age younger than 20 years, multiple sexual partners, nulliparity, and previous pelvic inflammatory disease.

Pelvic inflammatory disease is classified as *acute* or *chronic*. The most common organisms that produce the condition are *N. gonorrhoeae* and *Chlamydia,* but numerous other organisms have been incriminated. Diagnosis of pelvic inflammatory disease is based on clinical findings. The classic signs include fever, lower abdominal pain with pelvic tenderness, and purulent vaginal discharge. Some patients, however, will have minimal or absent symptomatology, particularly in the presence of a chlamydial infection. The lack of symptoms does not preclude pelvic inflammatory disease and tubal damage. Those patients who present with an acute illness must be studied thoroughly to rule out the possibility of acute appendicitis, ectopic pregnancy, gastrointestinal obstruction or perforation, and urinary stones.

In patients requiring further study, laparoscopy, pelvic ultrasonography, and pelvic CT scanning may be helpful in confirming a diagnosis. When pelvic inflammatory disease is present, laparoscopy will confirm it by finding tubal edema, erythema, and exudate. The presence of a tuboovarian abscess can be confirmed in this manner. Various imaging techniques, such as ultrasound and CT scanning, may also confirm a pelvic abscess.

Treatment

Empiric antibiotic treatment of sexually active women who have even minimal symptoms of pelvic inflammatory disease is indicated if no other cause for the symptoms is found. Women with pelvic inflammatory disease can be treated as inpatients or outpatients, depending on the severity of their disease. Patients with evidence of peritonitis, high fever, or suspected tuboovarian abscess should be admitted to the hospital for observation and intravenous antibiotics. Some specialists believe that all women with pelvic inflammatory disease should be admitted to the hospital for more intensive care, which may preserve fertility.

The Centers for Disease Control (CDC) recommends one of the following oral regimens: ofloxacin 400 mg orally twice a day for 14 days or levofloxacin 500 mg orally once daily for 14 days with or without metronidazole 500 mg orally twice daily for 14 days.

Follow-up of patients treated on an ambulatory basis should be carried out within 48 to 72 hours. If there is no improvement in the patient, she should be admitted for intravenous antibiotics.

Recommendations from the CDC for parenteral treatment include cefotetan 2.0 g IV every 12 hours or cefoxitin 2 g IV every 6 hours plus doxycycline 100 mg orally or IV every 12 hours. This regimen is continued for at least 24 hours after the patient shows clinical improvement. Doxycycline 100 mg orally twice daily is given to complete a total of 14 days of therapy.

It is now known that the use of broad-spectrum antibiotics, which must include an antibiotic with anaerobic activity, will result in cures of some pelvic abscesses. Some patients may require surgery for persistent abscess or chronic pelvic pain.

Surgical Therapy

Surgery becomes necessary under the following conditions: (1) the intraperitoneal rupture of a tuboovarian abscess; (2) the persistence of a pelvic abscess despite antibiotic therapy; and (3) chronic pelvic pain.

At one time, total abdominal hysterectomy with bilateral salpingo-oophorectomy was considered the procedure of choice when surgery for pelvic inflammatory disease was required. The availability of good antibiotics and a better understanding of the pathophysiology of the disease allow less-radical surgery. In young women whose reproductive goals have not been achieved, especially in the presence of unilateral disease, a unilateral salpingo-oophorectomy may be more appropriate than total hysterectomy with removal of both ovaries and fallopian tubes.

The rupture of a tuboovarian abscess is a true surgical emergency. Physical findings are frequently nonspecific. Rupture is most frequently associated with a sudden severe increase in abdominal pain. A shock-like state commonly accompanies rupture. Leukocyte counts are not necessarily increased, and some patients are afebrile. In the days before surgical intervention for this problem was common, mortality approached 100%. With prompt surgical intervention and intensive medical management, the mortality rate today is less than 5%.

The patient with a ruptured abscess must be explored promptly through an adequate incision. Hysterectomy and oophorectomy are commonly indicated. Operation may be technically difficult because of the distortion and edema secondary to the inflammatory process. Before the extirpation of any pelvic organ, adhesions must be lysed and normal structures, such as ureters and the large and small bowel, identified. At the conclusion of the procedure, the abdomen should be liberally irrigated. If the uterus is removed, the vaginal cuff should be left open for drainage. Patients should be treated with high-dose intravenous antibiotics. Because abdominal wound infection is extremely common in these patients, the rectus fascia should be closed securely with a mass closure of the Smead-Jones type. The skin and subcutaneous tissue can be closed but frequently are left open for later delayed closure.

ENDOMETRIOSIS

Endometriosis is one of the most common conditions encountered by the pelvic surgeon. It has been estimated that endometriosis will be demonstrated in approximately 20% of all laparotomies in women in the reproductive age group. Although the condition occurs in teenage women, it is found most often in the third and fourth decades of life. Endometriosis persists into the postreproductive years.

The exact cause of endometriosis is unknown, but the most common theory is that it is initiated by retrograde menstruation. The theory is supported by the fact that it is extremely common in women who have congenital anomalies of the lower reproductive tract that would favor menstrual reflux. The most common of these anomalies is an imperforate hymen.

The most common lesions of endometriosis can be recognized as bluish or black lesions, sometimes raised, sometimes puckered, giving them a "gunpowder burn" appearance. Some lesions are white or yellow, but these are less common. The disease is found most commonly on the ovary, and in many cases will involve both ovaries. Other involved organs can include the uterosacral ligaments, the peritoneal surfaces of the deep pelvis, the fallopian tubes, rectosigmoid, and a number of distant sites, including the skin or even the lungs, diaphragm, and nasopharynx.

While many patients are asymptomatic even with widespread endometriosis, others have severe pain, particularly dysmenorrhea, and dyspareunia. Other signs and symptoms depend on the location and depth of endometriotic implants. Infertility and abnormal bleeding are common problems.

The complaint of pain is common, and in most cases, is characteristic of the disease. Pain is associated most often with the menstrual period, characteristically beginning before the flow starts and ending when bleeding is complete. Deep pelvic dyspareunia is commonly associated with this disease, particularly in those individuals with implants involving the uterosacral ligaments or the rectovaginal septum.

The finding of a pelvic mass and tender nodularity of the uterosacral ligament strongly suggests endometriosis. The mass usually represents an ovarian endometrioma, often referred to as a "chocolate cyst" because of its dark-brown fluid contents. Endometriomas are found in approximately one-third of women with endometriosis and are often bilateral. Endometriotic involvement of the skin, mucous membranes, or peritoneum is characteristically a bluish discoloration, which will bleed or cause discomfort at the time of menstruation.

Although endometriosis may be suspected on the basis of clinical findings and the patient's history, the definitive diagnosis is made visually, usually with the aid of a laparoscope. Biopsy may be helpful in atypical cases. Medical management of this condition should not be started without a confirmed diagnosis. Laparoscopy offers the best diagnostic opportunity for this disease.

Treatment

Choices of treatment include expectant management only, medical management, and surgery. Patients with minimal endometriosis who are asymptomatic can be cared for through simple observation and management with cyclic oral contraceptives and simple analgesia. The medical management of this condition involves the use of a number of agents in several pharmacologic classes. Progestins have been used for the management of endometriosis for many years. Medroxyprogesterone acetate is given orally. The agent is used in doses of 10 mg two to three times daily and frequently provides symptomatic relief.

Pseudomenopause is currently the most common medical treatment for endometriosis. The most common medications used today for this purpose are the gonadotropin-releasing hormone agonists (GnRHa). These agents produce a suppression of ovarian function by suppression of both follicle-stimulating hormone and luteinizing hormone as a result of continuous stimulation of pituitary GnRH receptors. These agents have low toxicity, and while they reliably produce the hypoestrogenic effects of hot flashes and vaginal atrophy, these symptoms are generally well tolerated. They can be given by depot injection or daily nasal spray. Because bone loss is also a result of hypoestrogenism, it is recommended that the treatment not be continued for more than 6 months.

In the past, medications were used to create a pseudomenopause. These agents suppress pituitary gonadotropins by negative hypothalamic feedback. The resulting ovarian suppression produces endometrial atrophy and regression of ectopic endometrium. Along with vasomotor symptoms and vaginal atrophy, this medication has many other symptoms, including weight gain, muscle cramps, and signs of androgen excess, including oily skin, acne, and hirsutism. For this reason, it has been replaced largely by either GnRHa or progestin therapy for the medical treatment of endometriosis.

All these medical therapies have been well documented to result in temporary relief in patients with symptomatic endometriosis. In some patients, the effects can be relatively long lasting, but complete, permanent regression of endometriosis is rare with medical therapy. Although these treatments are used widely to enhance fertility, there is little evidence that medical therapy actually increases pregnancy rates compared with expectant therapy.

Conservative surgical therapy for endometriosis has become much more common with the advancement of laparoscopic surgery. At the time of initial diagnosis, superficial endometrial implants can be ablated with electrocautery or laser, and ovarian endometriomas can be removed. This approach appears to result in short-term enhancement of fertility and may give substantial temporary pain relief. In some cases of severe pain, deep retroperitoneal endometriosis implants can be removed either by laparoscopy or laparotomy with good results. However, as with medical therapy, conservative surgical treatment for endometriosis is palliative rather than curative in most patients.

The approach to ovarian endometriomas deserves special consideration. These "chocolate cysts" cannot be treated effectively medically. In general, even large endometriomas can be drained and the cyst lining removed laparoscopically. Although it was recommended in the past to close the ovary with several layers of absorbable sutures, it appears that this approach tends to increase postoperative adhesion formation. For this reason, it is recommended that after hemostasis is achieved, the ovary should be left open to close spontaneously. Other methods to minimize adhesion formation include atraumatic handling of the tissues and the use of a cellulose-adhesion barrier (Interceed) over the surgical site. Several series document pregnancy of approximately 50% rates following conservative operation.

Extirpative surgery is the only permanent treatment for symptomatic endometriosis. Patients with symptomatic endometriosis whose reproductive goals have been achieved may have no interest in preserving their reproductive potential. In these circumstances, extirpation of the endometriosis, along with the patient's fallopian tubes, ovaries, and uterus, may be the best choice. If extirpative surgery has been chosen, removal of all ovarian tissue has been advocated in the past to prevent the stimulation of residual endometriosis or the development of the residual ovary syndrome. In younger patients, a normal ovary may be spared in some cases. If total hysterectomy with bilateral salpingo-oophorectomy is required, replacement hormone therapy is indicated and recurrence is uncommon. To minimize the risk of recurrent endometriosis, it is recommended that replacement hormones include daily estrogen combined with a progestin such as medroxyprogesterone acetate, 2.5 mg given orally.

ECTOPIC PREGNANCY

Ectopic pregnancy affects a large number of women of reproductive age in this country. The incidence of this condition has increased dramatically over the last two decades. Because of improvements in diagnostic and therapeutic approaches, however, maternal mortality has declined over the same period of time.

Women in the reproductive age group have an increased risk of ectopic pregnancy as they age. Women in the last 10 years of their reproductive life have more than three times the risk of women in the first 10 years of reproductive life. Black and Hispanic women have a higher risk than white women. A history of salpingitis is common in women with ectopic pregnancy. Sterilization protects against ectopic pregnancy, but when sterilization methods fail, the risk of tubal implantation is increased.

The most common complaint of patients with ectopic pregnancy is pain, frequently associated with irregular vaginal bleeding. Approximately 80% of affected women will recall a missed menstrual period. Physical findings include abdominal tenderness on cervical motion and adnexal tenderness on bimanual pelvic examination. An adnexal mass may be palpated in approximately 50% of patients. As a result of the intraperitoneal bleeding, some patients present in shock.

The most helpful laboratory examination is measurement of the beta subunit of hCG (beta-hCG). Modern-day testing, with a sensitivity of 50 mIU/mL or less, enables the surgeon to confirm the pregnant state in almost all patients at risk for ectopic pregnancy. Once the physician is assured that the patient is pregnant, it must be determined that the pregnancy is in the uterus. Pelvic ultrasonography, particularly when performed with a vaginal transducer, is proving important in differentiating uterine gestations from ectopic gestations.

If the patient's condition is not emergent, the serum level of beta-hCG at 24- to 48-hour intervals is followed. In a normally implanted pregnancy, hCG levels will double every 2 days in early pregnancy, enabling the surgeon to separate normally implanted pregnancies from those with impending abortion or those located in an ectopic site.

Ultrasonic evaluation of the pelvis is increasingly important. The vaginal probe enables the clinician to determine whether the developing pregnancy is in the uterus or in the tube at a time when the hCG levels are barely more than 1000 mIU/mL. Significant intraperitoneal hemorrhage also can be visualized by vaginal ultrasound. However, culdocentesis remains an expedient means to determine the presence of hemoperitoneum in an emergency situation. In those patients who do not desire to continue the pregnancy, curettage of the uterus with examination of the tissue can be diagnostic. In the event that fetal tissue is not found, a diagnostic laparoscopy is usually required in the symptomatic patient for definitive diagnosis. In the presence of hemodynamic instability or significant intraperitoneal bleeding that precludes adequate visualization of the pelvis, immediate laparotomy is indicated.

Treatment

Once a diagnosis of ectopic pregnancy has been established, several choices are available for treatment.

Laparoscopic Procedures

The laparoscope has been an important diagnostic tool for the last several decades, but only recently has it become the standard approach for treatment. Linear salpingostomy is the treatment of choice for ectopic pregnancies less than 4 cm in diameter that occur in the distal third (ampullary) segment of the tube. To aid in hemostasis, the mesentery below the involved tubal segment is infiltrated with a dilute vasopressin solution. The tube may then be opened in its long axis along the antimesenteric side with either a laser or a unipolar cutting cautery. The conceptus is then aspirated, and any bleeding is electrocoagulated with bipolar cautery. Closing the tube is not necessary because the tube closes spontaneously in almost every case. If hemostasis cannot be achieved, coagulation of a portion of the mesosalpinx just below the segment may be required. Partial or total salpingectomy is indicated when the pregnancy is located in the isthmic portion of the tube. Bipolar electrocoagulation is used to desiccate a short segment of fallopian tube on either side of the pregnancy, and the pregnancy and tubal segment are removed together. Larger ectopic pregnancies are managed by total salpingectomy because adequate hemostasis is difficult to achieve without extensive tubal damage. For this procedure, the mesosalpinx is

serially coagulated with bipolar cautery and transected with scissors. When the uterotubal junction is reached, the tube is desiccated with bipolar cautery, and the entire tube and pregnancy are removed with the aid of a specimen bag and a large port.

Abdominal Operation

In those cases in which the surgeon has elected to perform a laparotomy, the same treatment options exist that were available laparoscopically. In a patient who desires future pregnancy, every attempt should be made to preserve a functional fallopian tube. If linear salpingostomy cannot be performed, consideration should be given to midsegment resection. Midsegment resection invariably shortens the tube but preserves the fimbria, which allows later reanastomosis. Salpingectomy should be reserved for those patients who have completed their reproductive goals, for those patients in whom salpingostomy has failed, and for those patients whose tube has been so completely destroyed by the ectopic gestation that it cannot be salvaged.

Medical Therapy

A relatively new approach to ectopic pregnancy is the use of methotrexate. Conservative criteria for treatment of ectopic pregnancy with methotrexate include serum beta-hCG levels less than 3500 IU/L and vaginal ultrasound that reveals the tubal pregnancy to be less than 3.5 cm in diameter with no visible fetal cardiac motion and no sign of hemoperitoneum. In this situation, studies show that administration of intramuscular methotrexate will result in complete resolution of the ectopic pregnancy in 96% of the cases. Subsequent tubal patency on the affected side can be documented in approximately 85% of the patients so treated. The risk of rupture and intraperitoneal hemorrhage must be made clear to the patient. In these cases, surgical management can be lifesaving. To what degree methotrexate treatment of ectopic pregnancy will replace definitive surgery has yet to be established.

PELVIC FLOOR DYSFUNCTION

Pelvic Organ Prolapse

Female pelvic floor dysfunction is common. It includes many clinical conditions, the most prevalent of which are pelvic organ prolapse and urinary incontinence. The muscles and connective tissues that comprise the pelvic floor and support the pelvic organs can be injured directly or indirectly by neuropathy. Different manifestations of pelvic floor dysfunction often coexist in the same patient owing to shared risk factors. Race, collagen metabolism, vaginal delivery, chronic constipation, chronic lung disease, and smoking are among the factors thought to be associated with the development of pelvic floor dysfunction. The percentage of women who have undergone at least one surgical operation for prolapse or incontinence by age 80 years is 11.1%, and of those nearly 30% undergo reoperation for recurrence of symptoms.

The word "prolapse" is a Latin derivative, meaning "to slip or fall." Pelvic organ prolapse is the descent of the pelvic organs into or through the vagina because of deficient support of the vaginal walls. The various types of pelvic support defects seldom occur as isolated problems. Consequently, labels such as "cystocele," "rectocele," and "enterocele" can be misleading to both patients and practitioners because of their implication that a specific organ has lost support rather than the vaginal vault itself. The standardization report of the International Continence Society in 1996 named

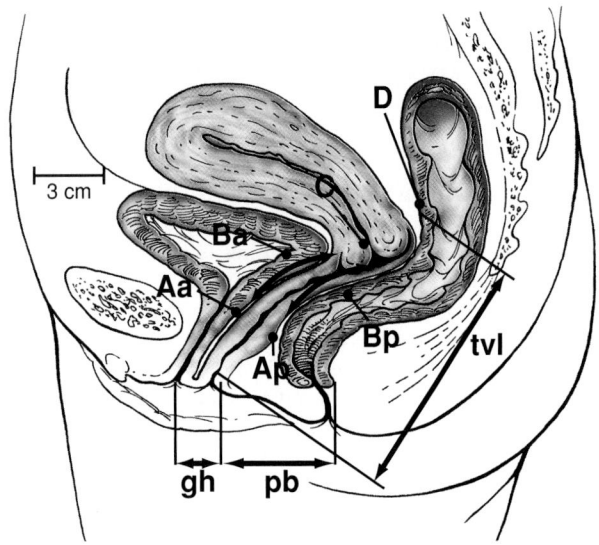

FIG. 40-10. Six sites (points Aa, Ba, C, D, Bp, and Ap), genital hiatus (gh), perineal body (pb), and total vaginal length (tvl) used for pelvic organ support quantitation.

"anterior vagina," "posterior vagina," and "vaginal apex" as reference points in the description of pelvic organ prolapse. This terminology, known as the Pelvic Organ Prolapse Quantification (POP-Q) system, quantifies prolapse according to the positions of those reference points relative to the hymen. The POP-Q has replaced the arbitrary grading systems that have been used in the past, improving the quality of description of the examination findings and facilitating communication among practitioners. It is easily learned and reliable. Measurements are taken at maximum Valsalva, preferably in the sitting or standing position. Figure 40-10 represents the locations of the reference points on the vaginal walls, as well as two external measurements and the vaginal depth. Figure 40-11A is a diagrammatic representation of normal and complete prolapse using the standardized system. Figure 40-11B depicts how predominantly anterior or posterior vaginal prolapse is quantified. Figure 40-11C shows the staging system. Most reconstructive operations are performed for Stage II or greater prolapse. A majority of vaginally parous women have stage II prolapse; most of these are asymptomatic and do not require surgery.

Patients with symptomatic pelvic organ prolapse report pelvic pressure and heaviness or a bulge protruding through the vagina. These symptoms are most often worst at the end of the day, or after prolonged physical activity or standing. Patients may report difficulty with bowel or bladder emptying, which requires them to push the prolapsed tissue back in manually. Obstructed voiding may occur, predisposing to urinary tract infection, urinary frequency and urgency, or, in rare cases, hydroureter and hydronephrosis. Because of shared risk factors, many patients with prolapse also have urinary incontinence. However, the relationship between urinary incontinence and prolapse is complex. Advanced prolapse may be associated with paradoxical continence, in which obstruction of the urethra by the prolapse masks symptoms of stress incontinence which would otherwise occur because of a defective urethral closure mechanism. Many patients with varying degrees of prolapse report generalized pelvic discomfort or backache. However, these symptoms are common and multifactorial and may not be a direct result of prolapse.

Reconstructive surgery is indicated for cases of stage II or greater prolapse from which the patient is symptomatic, whether from

discomfort, irritation, or disturbance of bowel and bladder function. Not all patients with prolapse require surgery. It is important to carefully define which of the patient's symptoms can be reasonably expected to improve with an operation. Certain patients may prefer to avoid surgery or be inappropriate surgical candidates; for those, a pessary trial is often recommended. A pessary trial may also help, when a patient's symptoms are disproportionate to her physical findings, to identify which symptoms are attributable to prolapse. Some patients with mild prolapse may achieve relief with a physical therapy program. Patients with chronic constipation often experience significant improvement after instituting a high-fiber diet. The reconstructive pelvic surgeon must recognize pelvic organ prolapse as a quality-of-life issue. This means that surgical goals and outcomes are measured not only by restoration of anatomy, but by relief of specific symptoms with which the patient presents.

Urinary Incontinence

Urinary incontinence is defined as involuntary leakage of urine. It may be subdivided into several conditions. Stress urinary incontinence is leakage of urine on exertion or effort, or with sneezing or coughing, which can be objectively demonstrated. It results from a dynamic urethral closure mechanism that is insufficient to overcome increases in abdominal pressure. Urge incontinence, by contrast, is characterized by urine leakage that is accompanied or immediately preceded by urgency. Urge incontinence is thought to result from inappropriate activation of the micturition reflex ("overactive bladder"). Stress incontinence, but not urge incontinence, is amenable to surgical therapy. However, the symptom of stress incontinence is not specific, and may occur in patients with incontinence caused by other bladder disorders.

A baseline physical examination for a patient complaining of urinary incontinence includes a standing stress (cough) test, pelvic examination—including prolapse staging and evaluation for pelvic mass—urinalysis, and postvoid residual determination. Urethral mobility may be evaluated using the cotton swab (Q-Tip) test. A sterile cotton swab lubricated with local anesthetic gel is inserted to the urethrovesical junction. The angle of the swab relative to the floor is measured at rest and at maximum Valsalva maneuver. Urethral hypermobility is defined as an excursion of 30 degrees or greater. Urethral hypermobility often serves as a focus for repair in continence operations. It is important to note, however, that urethral hypermobility is not specific for, nor causative of, urinary incontinence.

A patient presenting with symptoms and objective confirmation of stress urinary incontinence, with a normal pelvic examination, prolapse of stage II or less, a normal urinalysis, normal postvoid residual, and urethral hypermobility may be a candidate for surgical therapy. However, many patients have factors that complicate their condition. These include a history of previous incontinence or prolapse surgery; prolapse greater than stage II; elevated postvoid residual or abnormal voiding function; urinary urgency, frequency, or symptoms of urge incontinence; hematuria; neurologic disease; and previous pelvic radiation or radical pelvic surgery. Those patients should undergo complex urodynamic studies and evaluation by a pelvic floor specialist prior to consideration of an incontinence operation.

Stress urinary incontinence may be treated conservatively or surgically. Conservative management before surgery for most patients is recommended by the National Institute of Health's Agency for Health Care Policy and Research. Two of the most commonly used conservative treatments are pelvic floor physical therapy and a continence ring or dish. Patients are frequently instructed to perform

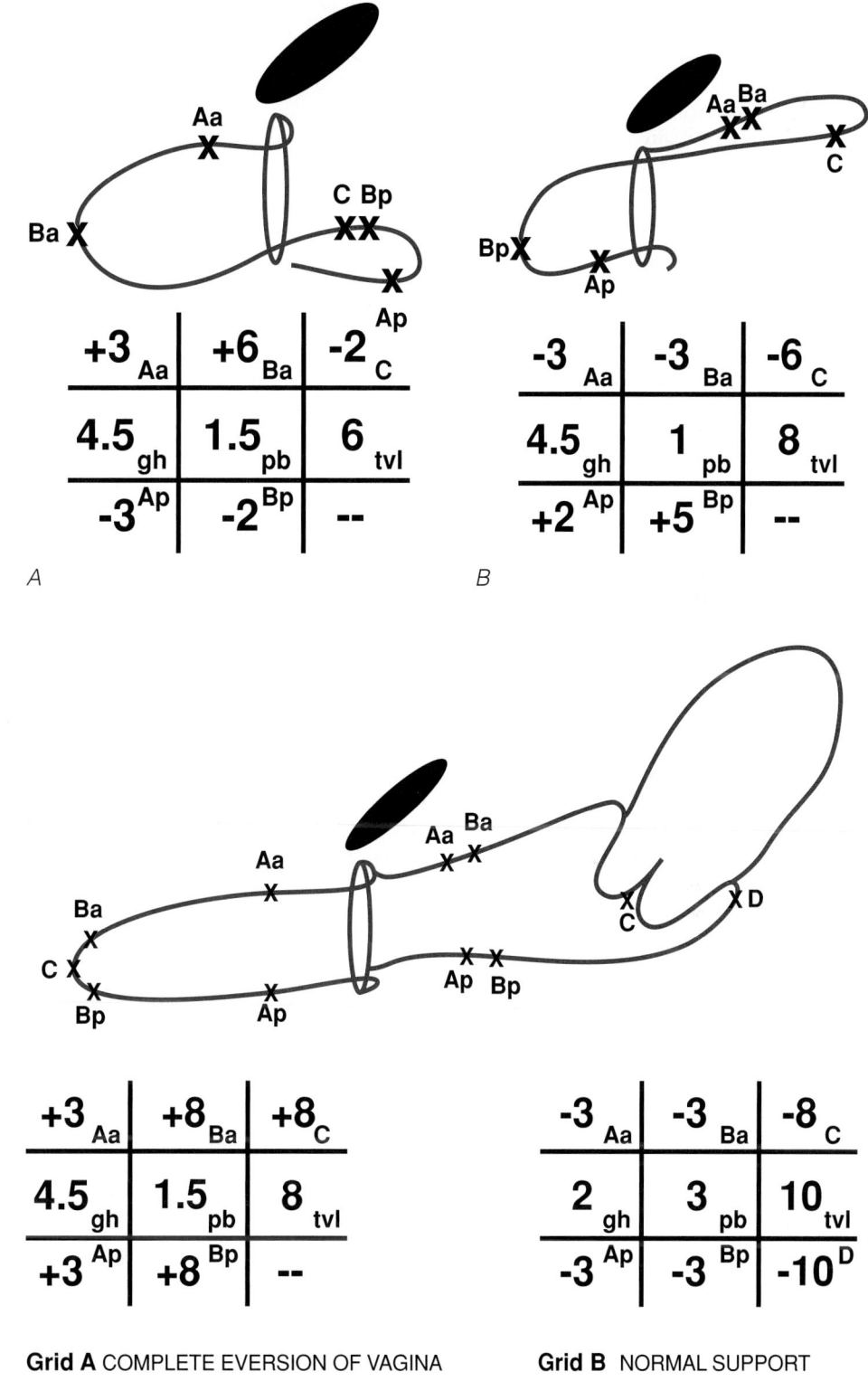

FIG. 40-11. *A.* Diagram of normal and complete prolapse using the standardized system. *B.* Quantification of anterior or posterior vaginal prolapse. *C.* Staging system for quantifying anterior and posterior vaginal prolapse.

pelvic muscle exercises, or "Kegels," to treat pelvic floor dysfunction. However, brief verbal instruction in exercise technique may be inadequate. Physical therapy for incontinence emphasizes strengthening of the pelvic floor muscles, often in concert with bladder retraining, urge deferment techniques, and education in lower urinary tract function. A continence dish is a flexible latex or silicone device worn intravaginally in order to mechanically obstruct the urethra. Estrogen supplementation and alpha-adrenergic medications have been advocated for the treatment of stress incontinence, but their efficacy remains unproven.

Continence is a dynamic, complex function which surgery attempts to restore by compensatory means. The goal of a continence operation is to improve the ability of the urethra to close with increases in abdominal pressure, yet avoid impairing voiding function. Surgical treatments for urinary incontinence have been performed since the beginning of the twentieth century, pioneered by Howard Kelly and other gynecologic surgeons. Hundreds of different of operations have been developed, a fact that testifies to the difficulty of consistently achieving satisfactory and long-lasting outcomes.

SURGERY FOR PELVIC ORGAN PROLAPSE

Many factors are important in determining which reconstructive operation is optimal for a given patient. Vaginal, abdominal, and laparoscopic approaches have been used. The most popular operation for uterovaginal prolapse has historically been vaginal hysterectomy with colporrhaphy. It may be combined with procedures designed to support the vaginal apex, such as uterosacral or sacrospinous ligament suspension. The abdominal approach to prolapse includes suspension of the vaginal apex to the sacrum using synthetic mesh. Many variations of each operative technique have been described. Surgical decisions are often based on case series and expert opinions which may not have universal applicability. There are few controlled studies in the literature reporting on standardized techniques that include meaningful outcome comparisons and long-term follow-up. Those that have been published suggest that failure rates for vaginal reconstruction may be twice as high with the vaginal route as with the abdominal route. The preponderance of the vaginal route is therefore being challenged.

In patients with an intact uterus, hysterectomy accompanies prolapse repair. Hysterectomy itself is not treatment for uterovaginal prolapse, which is caused by defective anatomic support structures. However, most prolapse repairs cannot be performed effectively with the uterus in place. An exception is the LeFort partial colpocleisis, which obviates the need for hysterectomy. Prolapse surgery is best reserved for the patient who has completed childbearing. Removal of the ovaries is performed according to age-appropriate indications.

Vaginal Procedures

Colporrhaphy

The oldest type of vaginal reconstructive operation is colporrhaphy. Widely used in the mid-nineteenth century, these procedures involved destroying or removing parts of the vaginal epithelium and reapproximating the edges to reduce vaginal caliber. Modern-day colporrhaphy, also known as "anterior repair" or "posterior repair," involves excision of vaginal epithelium and as such differs little from the original techniques. Anterior colporrhaphy begins with incision of the anterior vaginal epithelium in a midline sagittal direction. The epithelium is sharply dissected away from the underlying vaginal muscularis. Although many surgical descriptions refer to plication of the "endopelvic" or "pubocervical" fascia, such structures have not been shown to exist as histologically distinct layers. The vaginal muscularis is plicated with interrupted delayed absorbable stitches, following which the epithelium is trimmed and reapproximated. The vaginal canal is shortened and narrowed proportionate to the amount of removed epithelium. Posterior colporrhaphy is performed in a similar manner, often including the distal pubococcygeus muscles in the plication. In addition to the vaginal shortening and neuropathy, which may be induced by these dissections, levator plication is associated with a significant risk of postoperative dyspareunia. These factors influence the selection of appropriate patients for colporrhaphy procedures.

Sacrospinous Fixation

Sacrospinous ligament suspension of the vaginal vault was introduced in the United States in 1971. The sacrospinous ligament is used as a unilateral fixation point for the vaginal apex. The procedure begins with entry into the rectovaginal space, usually by incising the posterior vaginal wall at its attachment to the perineal body. The space is developed to the level of the vaginal apex. The rectal pillar is penetrated to gain access to the pararectal space. The sacrospinous ligament is found embedded in, and continuous with, the coccygeus muscle which extends from the ischial spine to the lateral surface of the sacrum. A long-ligature carrier is used to place a nonabsorbable monofilament suture two fingerbreadths medial to the ischial spine, through the substance of the ligament-muscle complex rather than around it, in order to minimize the risk of injury or entrapment of the pudendal neurovascular bundle. Other structures at risk of injury in this area include the inferior gluteal neurovascular bundle, lumbosacral plexus, and sciatic nerve. Two stitches are placed, the free ends of which are sewn to the undersurface of the vaginal cuff. After reapproximation of the proximal vaginal epithelium, the sacrospinous stitches are tied to firmly approximate the vagina to the ligament without suture bridging. The remainder of the epithelial incision is then closed.

Uterosacral Ligament Suspension

Like sacrospinous fixation, suspension of the vaginal apex to the uterosacral ligaments may be performed immediately following vaginal hysterectomy or applied to posthysterectomy vaginal vault prolapse. This approach is based on the original description of posterior culdoplasty by McCall in 1957. The procedure is based on the concept that the natural superior, or level I, support structures for the vagina are the uterosacral ligaments. The repair is designed to restore those attachments and to bring the ligaments together in the midline to occlude the posterior cul-de-sac. When using the uterosacral ligaments for repair of prolapse, it is important to recall that these structures are not "ligaments" in the true sense of the word, but rather condensations of smooth muscle, collagen, and elastin. The integrity and strength of these structures may vary greatly from patient to patient. The uterosacral ligaments are exposed with an intraperitoneal approach. Studies suggest the strongest part of the ligament is the proximal third. The repair uses the middle third of the ligament, which allows firm tissue-to-tissue approximation to the vagina and does not divert the ureter medially. Delayed absorbable or permanent suture is used, keeping in mind that permanent suture material must be buried beneath the vaginal epithelium, within the muscularis and away from the lumen. Several support stitches are placed, such that the lateral-most portion of the vaginal cuff is attached to the distal-most part of the ligament and the medial cuff to the proximal ligament. Many variations on the technique of uterosacral vault suspension have been described. Ancillary repair of anterior or posterior wall prolapse may be performed concurrently. Intraoperative evaluation of the lower urinary tract is important to confirm the absence of ureteral compromise.

Colpocleisis

Colpocleisis is the term applied to a class of vaginal prolapse operations that involve removal of part or all of the vaginal epithelium. These procedures do not correct any anatomic defect, but rather obliterate the vaginal vault, leaving the external genitalia unchanged. Colpocleisis is reserved for patients who are elderly, who do not wish to retain coital ability, and for whom there is good reason not to perform a more extensive reconstructive operation. The main benefits of colpocleisis operations are their simplicity, speed, and high efficacy.

The LeFort colpocleisis technique, done for complete uterovaginal prolapse, requires preoperative screening of the cervix and endometrium for malignancy. The procedure involves denudation of a rectangular portion of vaginal epithelium on both the anterior and posterior walls using sharp dissection, followed by suture reapproximation of the exposed submucosal surfaces. The uterus is left in situ. Lateral drainage canals remain for drainage of uterine secretions. By contrast, total colpocleisis involves hysterectomy (if applicable), followed by excision of the entire anterior and posterior epithelium. Successive purse-string sutures through the vaginal muscularis are used to reduce the prolapsed organs to above the level of the levator plate. In both partial and total colpocleisis, the pubococcygeus muscles may be plicated together in the rectovaginal space, together with a wide perineorrhaphy. Because the bladder neck is displaced posteriorly by the repair, placing the patient at risk for postoperative stress incontinence, a concomitant procedure to stabilize the urethrovesical junction is recommended. This may involve plication of the anterior vaginal muscularis (Kelly plication), pubourethral ligament plication, or a sling procedure, depending on preoperative urodynamic findings.

Abdominal Procedures

Sacral Colpopexy

Pelvic reconstructive surgery by the abdominal approach has as its main advantage the use of graft material for support of the vaginal apex. The natural apical support structure, the cardinal–uterosacral ligament complex, is often damaged and attenuated. The use of graft material to compensate for defective vaginal support structures is well described. Suspension of the vaginal vault to the anterior surface of the sacrum using graft material was first reported in 1962. As noted earlier, apical support defects rarely exist in isolation. Therefore, the sacral colpopexy may be modified to include the anterior and posterior vaginal walls, as well as the perineal body, in the suspension.

Abdominal sacral colpoperineopexy begins with the attachment of graft material to the perineal body. The rectovaginal space is opened, as with a posterior colporrhaphy, carrying the dissection laterally to the crura of the pubococcygeus muscles and opening the posterior cul-de-sac peritoneum. An allograft or xenograft trimmed to the appropriate dimensions is anchored to the levator ani muscles bilaterally and the perineal body distally, using delayed absorbable or permanent monofilament suture in interrupted fashion. The vaginal epithelium is then reapproximated and a perineorrhaphy constructed. Synthetic mesh is not used in the distal rectovaginal space because of its propensity for erosion into the distal vagina, particularly underneath the suture line. Laparotomy is then performed and the graft is retrieved. A rigid stent is placed into the vagina to facilitate its dissection from the overlying bladder and to allow the graft material to be spread evenly over its surface. A strip of synthetic mesh is fixed to the remainder of the posterior vaginal wall directly and another to the anterior wall. The peritoneum overlying the presacral area is opened, extending to the posterior cul-de-sac. Retracting the sigmoid colon medially, the anterior surface of the sacrum is skeletonized. Two to four permanent sutures are placed through the anterior longitudinal ligament in the midline, starting at the S2 level and proceeding distally. The sutures are passed through both leaves of the graft at the appropriate location which supports the vaginal vault under no tension. The peritoneum is then closed with an absorbable running suture. Retroperitoneal

placement is important to minimize the risk of graft adherence to abdominal viscera. The most dangerous potential complication of sacral colpopexy is life-threatening sacral hemorrhage. Sacral osteomyelitis has also been reported.

SURGERY FOR STRESS URINARY INCONTINENCE

There is a multitude of studies addressing the efficacy of different surgical procedures for urinary incontinence. The interpretation of this literature is often difficult, owing to the lack of standardized definitions. Diagnostic entities such as "stress incontinence," "intrinsic sphincter deficiency," and "voiding dysfunction" have no set criteria. The same surgical procedures are often performed with a variety of modifications unique to each operator. In addition, outcome criteria, particularly the definition of "cure," are not uniformly defined. As a result, adequate comparison of results among patients with a given procedure, or among procedures, is difficult.

The choice of an incontinence operation for a given patient may depend in part on her symptoms. Intrinsic sphincter deficiency (ISD) is a term applied to a subset of stress-incontinent patients who have particularly severe symptoms, including urine leakage with minimal exertion. This condition is often recognized clinically as the "low pressure" or "drainpipe" urethra. The urethral sphincter mechanism in these patients is severely damaged, limiting coaptation of the urethra. There are no set specific or objective criteria that define ISD, although urodynamic criteria are often used to support it.

In cases of uncomplicated stress incontinence accompanied by urethral hypermobility, retropubic colposuspension is most commonly used. In the presence of intrinsic sphincter deficiency, success rates with colposuspension may be less than 50%. Therefore, ISD with urethral hypermobility is best treated with suburethral sling procedures. ISD may also exist without urethral hypermobility, often when the urethra is fixed and scarred from multiple previous operations or from radiation therapy. In such cases, suburethral slings, periurethral bulk injections, or, rarely, artificial sphincters are used. The need to perform concurrent operations with incontinence surgery, most often reconstructive operations for prolapse, may also direct the type of procedure performed and whether it is done by the abdominal or vaginal route.

Standard surgical procedures used to correct stress incontinence share a common feature: partial urethral obstruction that achieves urethral closure under stress. Despite older literature to the contrary, this objective does not require that the bladder neck be "elevated to a high retropubic location." Many types of operations, in fact, achieve their surgical objectives without changing the anatomic position of the urethra. Incontinence operations fall into one of three categories: needle suspension, retropubic urethropexy, and suburethral sling. Anterior vaginal wall plication, or anterior colporrhaphy, is no longer advocated for the surgical treatment of stress incontinence.

Needle Suspension

The transvaginal needle suspension was first described in 1959 by Pereyra. Variations on this technique include the Stamey, Gittes, and Raz procedures. After an anterior colpotomy is made, the vaginal epithelium is dissected and mobilized to the level of the descending pubic rami. The space of Retzius is entered bilaterally using a blunt clamp or closed heavy Mayo scissors to penetrate the perineal membrane along the inferior aspect of the descending pubic ramus. Through a small transverse suprapubic incision a long, angled needle is passed through the rectus fascia through the space of Retzius to bring up the ends of a suture that has been secured to the periurethral vaginal muscularis. Variations exist with regard to the way in which suture is attached to the periurethral tissue as well as the method of abdominal wall fixation. Long-term studies of needle procedures have shown evidence of steadily increasing failure rates, likely a result of suture pullout from the periurethral vaginal tissue.

Retropubic Colposuspension

The first retropubic colposuspension was described in 1949 and modified in 1961. From an abdominal approach, the space of Retzius is approached extraperitoneally, allowing the bladder to be mobilized from the surrounding adipose tissue and lateral pelvis. Overlying fat and blood vessels in the area of the vesical neck are cleared away.

Marshall-Marchetti-Krantz (MMK) Procedure

Permanent suture is placed lateral to the urethra bilaterally and tied to the periosteum of the pubic ramus or perichondrium of the symphysis pubis. The surgical objective is to appose the urethra to (or within 1 to 2 cm of) the posterior surface of the symphysis pubis. Osteitis pubis (a rare, but serious, potential complication that can result from trauma and devascularization of the symphysis), as well as suture pullout from the symphysis, prompted the search for improved techniques.

Burch Procedure

Of the many descriptions, the most quoted is that of Tanagho in 1976. Two pairs of large-caliber delayed-absorbable suture are placed through the periurethral vaginal wall, one pair at the midurethra and one at the urethrovesical junction. Each stitch is then anchored to the ipsilateral Cooper's (iliopectineal) ligament. With the operator's nondominant hand placed vaginally, the distal and then proximal sutures are tied to give preferential support to the urethrovesical junction relative to the anterior vaginal wall without overcorrection. Specifically, two fingerbreadths of space between the urethra and pubic bone are recommended. Long-term outcome studies up to 10 years have shown cure rates of 80 to 85% for the Burch procedure. With all retropubic colposuspensions, the anterior displacement of the vagina is associated with a 7 to 20% risk of postoperative enterocele. Therefore, concurrent obliteration of the posterior cul-de-sac is advised.

Suburethral Sling

Suburethral sling procedures for stress incontinence have been in use since the beginning of the twentieth century. The early techniques involved the use of gracilis muscle, pyramidalis muscle, and rectus fascia flaps. A variety of organic and synthetic graft materials have been used to construct suburethral slings. Synthetic materials fell out of favor after a high incidence of postoperative urinary retention and urethral damage were found to be associated with their use. Currently, the most commonly used sling materials include autografts (rectus fascia) and processed cadaveric allografts (fascia lata). The procedure is performed by a combined abdominovaginal approach, using a small transverse suprapubic skin incision. The anterior vaginal epithelium is incised in the midline from the midurethra to just proximal to the urethrovesical junction, as identified by the bulb of an indwelling urethral catheter. The epithelium is dissected from the underlying muscularis using sharp dissection bilaterally. The space of Retzius is entered using a blunt clamp or closed heavy Mayo scissors to penetrate the perineal membrane along the inferior aspect of the descending pubic ramus. Maintenance of the proper angle of penetration is important to minimize

the risk of injury to the obturator neurovascular bundle or ilioinguinal nerve laterally, and urethra or bladder medially. A Bozeman clamp or long-angled ligature carrier is used to perforate the rectus fascia two fingerbreadths superior to the pubic bone just medial to the pubic tubercle, and the instrument is guided along the back of the pubic bone through the space of Retzius and into the vaginal incision to retrieve one arm of the sling. After bringing up the other side of the sling, and confirming the absence of urinary tract injury, the sling arms are fixed in place such that a sterile cotton swab placed to the urethrovesical junction is 5 to 10 degrees from the horizontal. Most often the sling arms are sutured to the rectus fascia, although procedures using pubic bone anchors also have been described. The base of the sling is positioned at the urethrovesical junction. Cure rates for the many different types of sling procedures described in the literature range from 75 to 95%. Slings are associated with higher complication rates than most other incontinence procedures, most frequently involving voiding dysfunction, urinary retention, new-onset urge incontinence, and foreign-body erosion.

Tensionless Sling

The tension-free vaginal tape (TVT) procedure was introduced in 1996. It is a modified sling that uses a strip of polypropylene mesh. Unlike traditional sling procedures, the mesh is positioned at the midurethra, not the urethrovesical junction, and is not sutured or otherwise fixed into place. Advantages of TVT include the ability to perform the procedure under local anesthesia and on an outpatient basis. Through an anterior vaginal wall incision, small subepithelial tunnels are made bilaterally to the descending pubic rami using sharp dissection. A specialized conical metal needle coupled to a handle is used to drive one end of the sling through the perineal membrane, space of Retzius, and through one of two small suprapubic stab incisions. After bringing up the other end of the tape through the other side, the bladder is filled and intraoperative cough testing is used to set the position of the mesh relative to the undersurface of the urethra. The 5-year cure rate of TVT for stress incontinence is 85%. Risks of the procedure include visceral injury from blind introduction of the needle, voiding dysfunction, and delayed erosion of mesh into the bladder or urethra.

Collagen

Bulking agent injection is indicated for patients with urodynamically proven stress incontinence that meets criteria for intrinsic sphincter deficiency but is negative for urethral hypermobility by cotton swab testing. Polytetrafluoroethylene (PTFE) was first used as a periurethral bulking agent in the early 1970s, following which glutaraldehyde cross-linked (GAX) bovine dermal collagen was introduced in 1991, and has since become the most widely used injectable. Use of other materials, including silicone polymers (Macroplastique) and carbon-coated zirconium beads (Durasphere), also has been described. Anesthesia for injection is easily obtained by using intraurethral 2% lidocaine jelly and/or transvaginal injection of the periurethral tissues with 5 mL of 1% lidocaine. A transurethral or periurethral technique may be used, using a 30 degree operating female cystourethroscope to directly visualize the injection. The material is injected underneath the urethral mucosa at the bladder neck and proximal urethra, usually at the 4 and 8 o'clock positions, until mucosal apposition is seen. Prior to injection, patients must demonstrate a negative reaction to a collagen skin test. The long-term cure rate is 20 to 30%, with an additional 50 to 60% of patients demonstrating improvement. Repeat injections are frequently necessary because of migration and dissolution of the collagen material.

Surgical Complications

The most common complication of incontinence surgery is voiding dysfunction. Complete urinary retention may be transient or permanent, depending on the procedure and the way it is performed. There is also a spectrum of voiding difficulties related to partial urethral obstruction. Because of the 1 to 3% risk of injury to bladder or ureters, intraoperative evaluation of the urinary tract is recommended whenever incontinence surgery is performed. Other potential complications include urinary tract infection, retropubic hemorrhage or abscess, intestinal tract injury, ilioinguinal or other nerve injury, enterocele formation, foreign-body complications caused by graft materials, and inflammatory or infectious processes involving the pubic bones.

BENIGN TUMORS

Ovarian Tumors

Nonneoplastic Cysts

By definition, a cystic enlargement of the ovary should be at least 2.5 cm in diameter to be termed a *cyst*.

Follicular Cysts. These are unruptured, enlarged graafian follicles. They grossly resemble true cystomas. They can rupture, causing acute peritoneal irritation, undergo torsion and infarction of the ovary or infarction of the tube and ovary, or spontaneously regress.

Corpus Luteum Cysts. These cysts may become as large as 10 to 11 cm. They can rupture and lead to severe hemorrhage and, occasionally, to vascular collapse from blood loss. The symptoms and physical findings of these cysts mimic those of ectopic pregnancy, and they are occasionally associated with delayed menses and spotting.

Endometriomas. These account for most "chocolate cysts" and are cystic forms of endometriosis of the ovary.

Wolffian Duct Remnants. These are not ovarian cysts but often cannot be distinguished clinically from tumors of the ovary. They are small unilocular cysts. Occasionally, they enlarge and can twist and infarct. In most instances, they are incidental findings at laparotomy and cause no difficulties or symptoms.

Müllerian Duct Remnants. These can appear as paraovarian cysts or as small cystic swellings at the fimbriated end of the fallopian tube (hydatids of Morgagni).

Nonfunctioning Tumors

Cystadenomas. Serous cystadenomas appear as cysts within translucent walls containing clear fluid and lined by simple ciliated epithelium. They frequently are on a pedicle and may undergo torsion leading to pain and infarction. When encountered surgically, they are adequately treated by simple salpingo-oophorectomy. Many fluid-containing cystic tumors of the ovary are also accompanied by papillary projections and are known as *papillary serous cystadenomas*. Because of epithelial variation in these tumors, it is often difficult to be sure where they fit in the spectrum of benign to malignant disease. A similar problem of malignant potential exists for the *mucinous cystadenoma,* which is a cystic tumor containing sticky, gelatinous material. These mucinous tumors are less likely to be malignant than the serous cystadenomas. Approximately 20% of the serous tumors and 5% of the mucinous tumors are bilateral. It is not always possible to be sure by gross inspection whether cystic tumors with solid components are benign or malignant. It is usually necessary to excise the involved ovary completely, even though there is no definite evidence of malignancy. The malignant potential of the cystadenoma is then determined by histologic examination. Some cystadenomas are classified as borderline tumors, or tumors of low malignant potential. These (grade 0) carcinomas usually are associated with an excellent prognosis and, if they are unilateral, may be treated by unilateral adnexectomy for women in their reproductive years. Frozen-section examination of the tumor at the time of surgical intervention is necessary to determine the proper course of therapy for patients in the reproductive age group. The opposite ovary should be inspected.

Occasionally, a condition known as *pseudomyxoma peritonei* is encountered; this is a locally infiltrating tumor composed of multiple cysts containing thick mucin. These tumors arise either from ovarian mucinous cystadenomas or from mucoceles of the appendix, both of which commonly coexist. Histologically, they are benign, but by local spread and infiltration they compromise surrounding vital structures. Localized tumors should be excised completely, if possible. Both ovaries and the appendix are removed, even though they grossly appear to be normal.

Mature Teratoma. These germ cell tumors are thought to arise from the totipotential germ cells of the ovary. The tumors often contain calcified masses, and, occasionally, either teeth or pieces of bone can be seen on abdominal radiographs. Mature teratomas occur at any age but are more frequent in patients between 20 and 40 years old. They are benign dermoid cysts. The occasional solid teratoma is usually malignant (immature teratoma).

If a teratoma (dermoid) is encountered in a young woman, it is preferable to shell it out from the ovarian stroma, preserving functioning tissue in the affected ovary. Usually these cysts contain ectodermal, mesodermal, and endodermal tissues, in addition to a thick, greasy, fatty material. If this material is spilled during surgery, a chemical peritonitis may result; therefore, it is important to remove these tumors intact. The opposite ovary should be inspected, but no further operative procedure is performed if the opposite ovary appears normal. In approximately 12% of patients, these tumors are bilateral. In patients of childbearing age, some functional ovarian tissue should be preserved. Immature teratomas are treated as other malignant germ cell tumors, with conservative resection and appropriate adjuvant chemotherapy.

Brenner Tumor. These are rare epithelial tumors that usually do not secrete hormones. Histologically, the epithelial elements are similar to Walthard rests and are believed to arise from them. These tumors occur primarily in later life and have a small malignant potential. Simple oophorectomy is usually sufficient therapy, and the prognosis is excellent.

Meigs' Syndrome. This pertains to ascites with hydrothorax, seen in association with benign ovarian tumors with fibrous elements, usually fibromas. It is more common to see fluid accumulation with ovarian fibromas that are more than 6 cm in size. The cause of the condition is unknown, but the ascitic fluid may originate from the tumor, as a result of lymphatic obstruction of the ovary. Frequently, this clinical picture is encountered with other ovarian tumors, especially ovarian malignancies, which can produce a cytologically benign pleural effusion; in such cases, it is termed a *pseudo-Meigs' syndrome.* Meigs' syndrome can be cured by excising the fibroma.

Functioning Tumors

Granulosa Cell.

Theca Cell Tumor. Pure theca cell tumors (thecomas) are benign, but those with granulosa cell elements may be malignant. It is often impossible to predict their behavior from the histologic features, and prolonged follow-up is necessary in order to judge the nature. Usually, granulosa cell tumors elaborate estrogen, but some of these tumors have no hormone production. In young girls, they are characteristically manifested by isosexual precocity, and in elderly women, they are sometimes associated with postmenopausal bleeding or endometrial carcinoma. The tumor can occur at all ages from childhood to the postmenopausal period, but it is most common in later life, with maximal occurrence between the ages of 40 and 60 years. If the tumor is discovered in the reproductive years and confined to one ovary without signs of surface spread or dissemination, a simple oophorectomy may be sufficient therapy. If it is discovered in later life, removal of both ovaries with the uterus is indicated. These tumors produce inhibin, which may be measured in the peripheral circulation.

Sertoli-Leydig Cell Tumors (Arrhenoblastomas).

These rare, but potentially malignant, tumors are associated with androgen output and masculinization. Rarely, they elaborate estrogen. They usually occur in the reproductive age group and appear to contain tubular structures as well as Leydig-type cells. In young patients with a single involved ovary, unilateral oophorectomy is adequate therapy, provided there is no extension of the tumor. For older patients or for those with bilateral involvement, total hysterectomy and bilateral salpingo-oophorectomy are performed.

Struma Ovarii.

This term refers to the presence of grossly detectable thyroid tissue in the ovary, usually as the predominant element in dermoid cysts. This tissue occasionally may produce the clinical picture of hyperthyroidism and is rarely malignant.

Uterine Tumors

Leiomyomas

Uterine leiomyomas are the most common benign tumor in the female pelvis. It is estimated that up to 50% of all women at some time in their life have one or more of these uterine tumors. The tumor is never seen before menarche, it grows during reproductive life, and it generally regresses following menopause. The tumors significantly complicate pregnancy by virtue of their rapid growth secondary to the response to pregnancy hormones.

Many leiomyomas are asymptomatic; when they do produce symptoms, they cause pain, abnormal uterine bleeding, infertility, ureteral obstruction, bladder distortion, and pressure symptoms secondary to the enlarged uterus.

Uterine leiomyomata are subject to a number of degenerative changes, including calcification, necrosis (occasionally with liquefaction), fatty degeneration, and, occasionally, sarcomatous change. Malignant degeneration occurs in less than 1% of all tumors. Uterine myomas may be found in a number of locations within the uterus (Fig. 40-12). The most common location is intramural, but tumors frequently are found just below the peritoneum and occasionally as a pedunculated mass attached to the uterus. Other tumors grow into the endometrial cavity, where they are pedunculated on occasion, prolapsing through the cervix.

Treatment. Most symptomatic tumors can be managed expectantly. When symptoms indicate surgical treatment, consideration must be given to the age of the patient, the number of children she desires, the patient's age, and her reaction to possible loss of

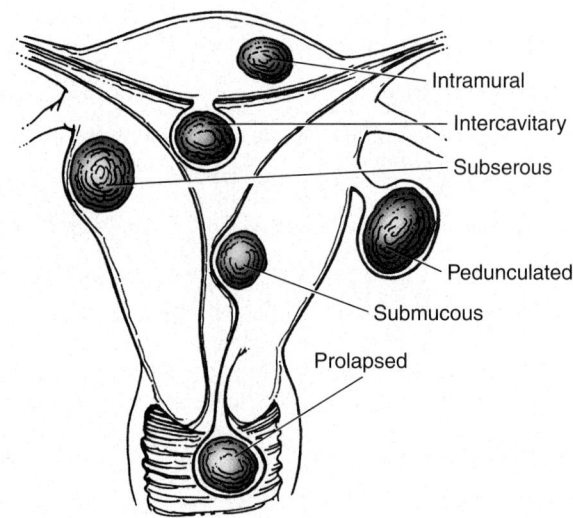

FIG. 40-12. *Types of uterine myomas.*

reproductive and menstrual function. Surgery should be fitted to the needs and desires of the patient. Therapeutic options may include myomectomy, total abdominal hysterectomy, or transvaginal hysterectomy.

Pedunculated myomas are the easiest to remove because the stalk of the tumor is simply ligated or coagulated and the tumor separated from the uterus. Pedunculated tumors in the endometrial cavity often can be removed with the operative hysteroscope. Similarly, tumors projecting from the external wall of the uterus into the peritoneal cavity can be removed laparoscopically by ligating the tumor pedicle and then morcellating the tumor intraperitoneally for removal or removing the tumor through a cul-de-sac incision.

Most myomectomies will be performed transabdominally. The most common indication for abdominal myomectomy is the presence of myomas that cause pain, bleeding, or infertility in a patient who continues to desire pregnancy. Before performing myomectomy, the patient must be evaluated completely and counseled about the risk of operation. Blood loss associated with myomectomy frequently exceeds that of hysterectomy. The patient should be advised of the possibility of hysterectomy in the event that myomectomy cannot be effectively performed. It is wise to set aside two or more units of autologous blood for possible operative use. The patient's tubal status should be evaluated with a hysterosalpingogram, and the patient's sexual partner should be evaluated with a semen analysis. In the presence of a very large tumor, chemoreduction of the tumor is currently being performed using a GnRHa, such as nafarelin, given by nasal inhalation for a period of 3 months, or leuprolide acetate given intramuscularly every month for 2 months. These agents will cause the tumor to regress in size, and in most cases, provide for less blood loss at the time of operation.

Adenomyosis

Adenomyosis is a growth of endometrial tissue in the myometrium of the uterus and is sometimes referred to as *endometriosis of the uterine corpus*. The condition occurs primarily during reproductive years and leads to a thickening of the myometrial wall with subsequent uterine enlargement. Adenomyosis usually occurs in women who have had a number of pregnancies. Occasionally, patients with adenomyosis will complain of dysmenorrhea, and some present with increased uterine bleeding and heavy menstrual flow. However, a number of patients with adenomyosis in hysterectomy specimens have been asymptomatic. Therefore, the association of adenomyosis with heavy menstrual bleeding and dysmenorrhea is questionable.

Polyps

Endometrial polyps can occur at any time after puberty. A *polyp* is a local hyperplastic growth of endometrial tissue that usually causes postmenstrual or postmenopausal bleeding or staining, which is cured by polyp removal or curettage. The polyps are usually benign, but cases of adenocarcinoma of the endometrium arising in a polyp have been reported.

Cervical Lesions

Cervical polyps cause the same symptoms as endometrial polyps. Because they are often quite small and are visible at the external os, they often can be removed as an outpatient procedure followed by cauterization of the base of the polyp. Nabothian cysts are mucous inclusion cysts of the cervix. They are occasionally associated with chronic inflammation and can be removed easily with a cautery. They are harmless, usually asymptomatic, and generally do not require surgery.

During reproductive years, the portio of the cervix is covered primarily with glycogenated squamous epithelium, and columnar epithelium is normally found centrally near the external os in most women. This exposed columnar epithelium, termed *ectropion* or *eversion,* is usually bright red. Unless accompanied by inflammation and a purulent discharge (cervicitis), it requires no treatment. During adult life, the columnar epithelium is usually replaced by squamous metaplasia, and this physiologic process occurs in the transformation zone at the interface of squamous and columnar epithelium. After menopause, the squamous columnar junction is usually in the endocervical canal.

Vulvar Lesions

The term *leukoplakia* is often used for any white patch of the vulva; it is properly reserved for areas that show histologically atypical epithelial activity. These alterations may precede the development of malignant changes. In many instances, chronically irritated and itchy white areas of the vulva will show sclerosing atrophy of the skin *(lichen sclerosus).* Lichen sclerosus is a pruritic lesion that does not appear to be premalignant. Hyperplastic lesions termed *hypertrophic dystrophies* are found that may be benign (epithelial hyperplasia) or that may show atypia, in which case dysplastic changes can be observed. The pruritic symptoms can be helped by topical application of corticosteroids. Testosterone or clobetasol ointment also has been beneficial, especially for the atrophic changes of lichen sclerosus.

Noninvasive malignant change of the surface squamous epithelium of the vulva occurs in the same way as that described for the cervix. Carcinoma in situ of the vulva both histologically and clinically behaves like carcinoma in situ of the cervix. The changes are confined to the squamous elements of the vulva, and the condition is sometimes referred to as *Bowen's disease.* In certain instances, the apocrine glandular elements of the vulva are involved in association with an intensely pruritic area. Histologically, large, foamy Paget's cells are seen, similar to those noted in the breast, although invasive carcinoma occasionally can accompany Paget's cells. Bowen's disease, and usually Paget's disease, are considered part of the carcinoma in situ complex of the vulva; they are adequately treated by wide local surgical excision (simple vulvectomy). The laser also is used to treat these lesions locally.

MALIGNANT TUMORS

Ovarian Tumors

Ovarian Carcinoma

Ovarian carcinomas are divided histologically into epithelial, germ cell, and stromal malignancies. The majority of the 27,000 or more cases of ovarian cancer diagnosed annually in the United States are of the epithelial type. The median age at diagnosis for epithelial ovarian cancer is 61 years, and the overall 5-year survival rate for epithelial cancers is 37%. Approximately 15,000 women die of this disease in the United States annually.

Although the etiology of ovarian cancer is uncertain, approximately 5% of patients with epithelial tumors come from families where one or more first-degree relatives also have the disease. In such families, prophylactic oophorectomy may be considered at the completion of childbearing, especially if specific BRCA1 or BRCA2 mutations are identified. Testing for these mutations is now readily available in the United States. Primary peritoneal carcinomatosis has been reported in women who have undergone prophylactic surgery, however. Life-long screening with CA 125 levels, pelvic examination, and vaginal ultrasonography of women from affected families is important.

Table 40-2 outlines the International Federation of Gynecology and Obstetrics (FIGO) staging system for ovarian cancer. Early lesions are largely asymptomatic, and advanced tumors may produce only nonspecific symptoms such as early satiety, abdominal distention, and vague gastrointestinal symptoms. Although an annual

Table 40-2
FIGO (1986) Staging System for Ovarian Cancer

Stage	Characteristic
I	Growth limited to the ovaries
IA	Growth limited to one ovary; no ascites; no tumor on the external surfaces, capsule intact
IB	Growth limited to both ovaries; no ascites; no tumor on the external surfaces, capsule intact
IC	Tumor either stage IA or stage IB but with tumor on the surface of one or both ovaries, or with capsule ruptured, or with ascites containing malignant cells or with positive peritoneal washings
II	Growth involving one or both ovaries on pelvic extension
IIA	Extension or metastases to the uterus or tubes
IIB	Extension to other pelvic tissues
IIC	Tumor either stage IIA or IIB with tumor on the surface of one or both ovaries, or with capsule(s) ruptured, or with ascites containing malignant cells or with positive peritoneal washings
III	Tumor involving one or both ovaries with peritoneal implants outside the pelvis or positive retroperitoneal or inguinal nodes; superficial liver metastases equals stage III; tumor is limited to the true pelvis but with histologically verified malignant extension to small bowel or omentum
IIIA	Tumor grossly limited to the true pelvis with negative nodes but with histologically confirmed microscopic seeding of abdominal peritoneal surfaces
IIIB	Tumor of one or both ovaries; histologically confirmed implants of abdominal peritoneal surfaces, none exceeding 2 cm in diameter; nodes negative
IIIC	Abdominal implants greater than 2 cm in diameter or positive retroperitoneal or inguinal nodes
IV	Growth involving one or both ovaries with distant metastases; if pleural effusion is present, there must be positive cytologic test results to allot a case to stage IV; parenchymal liver metastases equals stage IV

SOURCE: From the International Federation of Gynecology and Obstetrics.

pelvic examination is valuable in detecting early ovarian cancer, efforts to establish other cost-effective screening programs using serum markers such as CA 125 and vaginal ultrasound examination are being developed. Vaginal ultrasound is a promising technology that is not presently cost-effective in mass screening programs, because the yield is no more than 1 ovarian cancer per 1000 asymptomatic postmenopausal women screened. Currently, the more than 70% of women with epithelial cancer have stage III tumors at the time of diagnosis. Widespread peritoneal dissemination, omental involvement, and ascites are the rule, rather than the exception, in these women.

Treatment. In general, therapy for epithelial ovarian cancer consists of surgical resection and appropriate staging followed by adjuvant radiation or chemotherapy. Women with low-grade early stage (IA or IB) cancers who have undergone appropriate surgical staging may be treated with surgery without adjuvant therapy. If the lesion is bilateral (stage IB), abdominal hysterectomy and bilateral salpingo-oophorectomy are sufficient. It is in the limited group of patients with unilateral histologic grade 1 or 2 lesions that fertility can be preserved by performing adnexectomy and staging biopsies without removing the uterus or contralateral ovary and fallopian tube. In all other patients (stage IA, grade 3, and stage IC and above), appropriate initial surgery includes bilateral salpingo-oophorectomy, abdominal hysterectomy if the uterus has not been removed on a prior occasion, appropriate staging, and tumor resection.

Staging. Staging indicates surgical resection or biopsy of all potential areas of tumor spread. Thorough staging is imperative in determining appropriate treatment for patients with ovarian cancer. Among patients whose cancer is confined to one or both ovaries at the time of gross inspection, occult metastases can be identified by careful surgical staging in one-third. If staging is improperly performed and adjuvant therapy omitted in patients whose tumors are apparently confined to the ovary, 35% will suffer preventable relapse.

Epithelial ovarian cancers disseminate along peritoneal surfaces and by lymphatic channels. The first site of spread is the pelvic peritoneum. Later the abdominal peritoneal surfaces and diaphragms are involved. The omentum is a common site for metastases, as are both the para-aortic and pelvic lymph nodes. Because the abdominal cavity in its entirety is not accessible through a transverse pelvic incision, it is paramount that surgery for ovarian malignancies be performed through a full-length midline abdominal incision. After the peritoneal cavity is entered, the visceral and parietal surfaces are inspected for metastatic disease, and any suspicious areas are biopsied. If ascites is present, it should be aspirated and heparinized. Cytologic evaluation for metastatic cells or clusters is then performed. If no ascites is found, peritoneal washings with balanced salt solution or lactated Ringer's solution are obtained from the abdominal cavity and submitted for cytologic evaluation after centrifugation and fixation.

Appropriately staged patients with histologic grade 1 or grade 2 tumors confined to one or both ovaries (stage IA or IB) require no postoperative therapy. Five-year survival in this group of patients exceeds 90%.

Those patients who have stage I, grade 3 lesions, stage IC tumors (malignant peritoneal washings, rupture of tumor, surface excrescences, or ascites), or stage II cancers that are completely resected may be treated equally well with systemic chemotherapy, radiotherapy of the whole abdomen, or a single instillation of intraperitoneal radioactive chromic phosphate. Five-year survival approaches 75% in this group of patients.

Women with stages III and IV disease require systemic chemotherapy with cisplatin or carboplatin, generally in combination with a taxane such as paclitaxel. Survival at 5 years in such patients may exceed 20%, although this rate drops as low as 10% at 10 years.

Survival in advanced ovarian cancer is influenced by a number of factors, such as patient age, the histologic type and grade of the lesion, the presence or absence of ascites, and the type of chemotherapy employed. Of prime importance in advanced-stage disease, however, is the volume of tumor remaining after the initial surgical procedure. Many patients with stages III and IV ovarian cancer have diffuse peritoneal, retroperitoneal, diaphragmatic, and mesenteric metastases that resist complete surgical resection. It is often possible, however, to remove large amounts of peritoneal tumor by entering the retroperitoneal spaces and freeing the disease-laden surfaces from the underlying viscera.

It is widely accepted that patients in whom little or no residual disease remains after initial operation, on average, live longer than those in whom a great deal of tumor remains unresected. The terms *debulking* and *cytoreduction* indicate aggressive surgical removal of ovarian cancer. When disease remaining after surgical resection consists of nodules or plaques less than 1 to 2 cm in diameter, the surgical effort is termed *optimal,* and when a larger volume of residual disease remains, the surgical removal is termed *suboptimal.* Because of the survival advantage, every effort should be made to resect as much disease at the time of diagnostic laparotomy as is possible. Because many patients with advanced ovarian cancer are elderly and nutritionally depleted, surgical enthusiasm must be tempered by proper preoperative evaluation and support with appropriate central monitoring and hyperalimentation where indicated. Occasionally, it is more prudent to obtain confirmation of the diagnosis, treat with systemic chemotherapy, and then perform definitive surgery when the tumor has diminished in size and the patient has been nutritionally resuscitated.

Resection of nodules involving the small or large bowel is warranted if the exercise results in complete removal of all observed disease. Such procedures are probably not indicated if tumor remains at other sites. After surgical extirpation of the tumor, patients with suboptimal ovarian cancers must be treated with chemotherapy. Approximately 80% of these tumors will respond to platinum-based combination therapy; 40% of all patients will experience a complete response, or complete resolution of tumor identified on physical examination or radiographic or serologic study.

Resection of Advanced Ovarian Cancer. When advanced ovarian carcinoma is discovered at the time of exploratory laparotomy, the first reaction is often one of resignation. There has been a tendency to perform a diagnostic biopsy and close the abdomen without further surgical intervention. In experienced hands, however, successful reduction of tumor volume to nodules 2 cm or less is possible in at least 50% of women with advanced ovarian cancer. If the primary surgeon is incapable of obtaining such results, the patient should be referred to one with sufficient expertise in this area. Survival following chemotherapy is inversely related to the volume of residual disease at the time of primary surgery.

Several techniques ensure adequate resection. First, most ovarian cancer is found on peritoneal surfaces and not invading viscera. A retroperitoneal approach thus facilitates mobilization of the involved mesothelium. The lateral aspects of the paracolic gutters may be incised and dissection carried medially to undermine tumors in these locations. The ovarian artery and vein should be identified at this point and securely ligated before division. Once the blood supply to the main body of the ovarian tumor is secured, the adnexa may be mobilized more easily. It is often useful to dissect the ureter from the underlying pelvic peritoneum and retract it laterally with a vessel loop. This allows access to the lateral pelvic peritoneum. Tumor nodules on anterior and posterior cul-de-sac peritoneum may be resected by developing planes in the retroperitoneal spaces and isolating the disease from the underlying bladder, sigmoid colon, and ureters. Opening the pararectal and paravesical spaces facilitates this dissection and also allows access to the uterine vessels, which then may be clamped, ligated, and divided. When the hysterectomy and adnexectomy are complete, the omentum may be resected.

Disease on the right diaphragm may be resected by transecting the falciform ligament and retracting the liver inferiorly. If it serves to remove all remaining tumor, splenectomy may be performed. Resection of small and large bowel may be performed if the operation removes all residual disease. Use of the ultrasound aspirator and argon beam coagulator have resulted in an increased ability to completely remove tumors, including those that are implanted on the serosal surfaces and mesentery of the bowel. With diligence it is often possible to remove all appreciable disease with these instruments.

"Second-Look" Operations

"Second-Look" Laparotomy. Ovarian cancer often defies diagnosis because it does not produce symptoms and is detectable neither radiographically nor serologically, even in relatively advanced stages. The assessment of ovarian cancer during and after therapy is similarly difficult. Although CT or MRI may identify masses as small as 2 to 3 cm in diameter, neither technique can reliably detect smaller masses, much less the miliary spread so often identified in advanced ovarian cancer.

CA 125 is more sensitive than radiographic or magnetic scanning, but is also associated with a number of false-positive results and may not be elevated in patients with mucinous tumors. In addition, approximately half of patients with advanced ovarian cancer whose CA 125 levels normalize during chemotherapy harbor viable and clinically undetectable disease. Radiolabeled monoclonal antibodies raised against epithelial tumor surface antigens may be more sensitive than traditional methods but remain to be proven effective.

The practice of performing exploratory surgery following chemotherapy originated during a time when alkylating agents were used almost exclusively. Because acute nonmyelocytic leukemia is associated with prolonged administration of such agents, a "second-look" operation was performed at an interval of 12 to 24 months following primary surgery so that treatment could be stopped in women with no disease. Presently, the duration of postoperative combination chemotherapy is often only 5 to 6 months, and the risk of leukemia is very low. In approximately 20 to 30% of patients who receive such treatment, no cancer will be identified at the time of a second operation. These patients have an excellent long-term prognosis. In women who have persistent microscopic disease, the prognosis is also favorable, and in those with persistent gross tumors, the prognosis is relatively poor.

Second-look surgery is currently used primarily as a research tool. New treatment regimens can be evaluated quickly by performing a second-look operation, because the findings at such an operation reflect the ultimate clinical outcome and hence the value of the treatment regimen. Second-look surgery is also valuable in determining when therapy can be discontinued and when

further treatment is indicated. There is no known survival benefit from second-look surgery.

If a tumor is identified and can be resected, a Tenckhoff catheter may be placed, through which intraperitoneal chemo- or immunotherapy may be given. If no visible disease is present, a silicone drain can be inserted for the postoperative administration of radioactive chromic phosphate. Although the morbidity of second-look surgery is very low, there is no place for this type of operation in patients who wish or who can physiologically tolerate no further treatment at the conclusion of primary combination chemotherapy. Nor is there any reason to reexplore such a patient without the ability or intention to perform a thorough, deliberate staging procedure that can guide subsequent therapy.

Other Secondary Operations. Surgical resection of tumor after chemotherapy or at the time of relapse is termed *secondary cytoreduction.* In the occasional patient who undergoes diagnostic biopsy only before the administration of chemotherapy, early reexploration may be termed *interval cytoreduction.* There is evidence that the surgical removal of an extensive tumor is facilitated by the administration of one or two courses of combination chemotherapy. In patients with a massive tumor burden, this approach may not only be safer, but also might result in a more successful tumor resection before the completion of chemotherapy. It also promotes the early administration of intraperitoneal chemotherapy.

The importance of secondary cytoreduction is not clearly established. In patients with relapsing ovarian cancer, the prognosis depends in part on the extent of the tumor and in part on the type of response to previous therapy. Also important is the interval between primary therapy and relapse. In those who completely responded to platinum combination treatment and who have a disease-free period exceeding 2 years, resumption of platinum-based chemotherapy is very effective. Paclitaxel therapy may be effective in similar situations. It is in such patients that surgical removal of the recurrent tumor is likely to be the most beneficial.

Palliative Surgery. In most cases of advanced ovarian cancer, death is associated with bowel dysfunction or frank obstruction. Although invasion of the small bowel and colon is unusual, growth of the tumor adjacent to the bowel leads to mesenteric compromise and dysfunction usually heralded by distention, nausea, and vomiting. When bowel obstruction occurs early in the clinical course of ovarian cancer, particularly if it occurs before the administration of chemotherapy, surgical intervention is warranted and should be aggressive. Resection or bypass of the involved bowel is indicated; colonic resection also may be indicated. It is important to perform adequate radiographic studies preoperatively so that obstructed small bowel is not decompressed into a compromised colon.

When bowel obstruction occurs after chemotherapy, the prognosis is unfavorable. Women who develop such difficulties have a limited survival following surgical correction. Surgery is often difficult to perform because of an extensive tumor. Laparotomy may be complicated by intestinal injury or fistula. Often the best approach in these patients is the use of a percutaneous or endoscopically positioned gastrostomy tube and intravenous fluids or conservative nutritional support. Such a procedure may limit the length of hospitalization and allow the patient to remain in a supportive home environment for a greater period of time.

Laparoscopy in Ovarian Cancer. At present, our ability to resect large ovarian cancers successfully using laparoscopic equipment is limited. In the past, efforts to perform second-look procedures through the laparoscope were ineffective when compared with laparotomy. However, with the advent of new equipment and techniques, the role of laparoscopy in the staging and treatment of ovarian malignancies may be expanding. Several investigators have developed successful methods of performing both pelvic and para-aortic lymphadenectomies using endoscopic equipment. In addition, ultrasonographic and serologic criteria are evolving that will allow the surgeon to more successfully distinguish between benign and malignant neoplasms of the ovary. Caution must be exercised when dealing with potentially malignant unresected ovarian tumors using the laparoscope.

Tumors of Low Malignant Potential

These are epithelial tumors of malignant potential intermediate between benign lesions and frank malignancies. Histologically, most are of the serous type. Although these tumors may be associated with epithelial budding, atypia, mitoses, and stratification, they are distinguished from invasive cancers microscopically by lack of stromal invasion. The median age of diagnosis is approximately 10 years younger than that of patients with epithelial cancers. The vast majority occur in stage I and have a favorable prognosis. Surgery should include abdominal hysterectomy and bilateral salpingo-oophorectomy unless fertility is to be preserved in patients with unilateral lesions. These patients may undergo unilateral salpingo-oophorectomy. Ovarian cystectomy or nonextirpative resections commonly result in recurrences.

Patients with stages III and IV lesions have 5-year survival rates that approach 85% after complete surgical resection. There is little evidence that either chemotherapy or radiotherapy administered after surgery improves survival; on the other hand, deaths from chemotherapy-induced leukemia are not uncommon.

Germ Cell Tumors

These tumors occur in women in the first three decades of life and typically grow rapidly, producing symptoms of distention and abdominal fullness. Torsion may occur, producing an acute abdomen. Most are unilateral, and all have a tendency to spread to the para-aortic lymph nodes, as well as throughout the peritoneal cavity. Although they are similar in many ways to testicular cancer in the male, there are some differences.

Dysgerminoma, the female equivalent of testicular seminoma, is composed of pure, undifferentiated germ cells. It is bilateral in 10 to 15% of patients and is occasionally associated with elevated levels of hCG or lactate dehydrogenase (LDH). It is the most common ovarian malignancy diagnosed during pregnancy. Patients bearing dysgerminomas should undergo appropriate staging at the time of the primary resection but need not undergo hysterectomy (if fertility is to be preserved) or removal of the opposite ovary if it is normal in appearance. Secondary operations solely for staging purposes are unwarranted. Adjuvant therapy is unnecessary unless there is evidence of extraovarian spread. Either radiotherapy encompassing the whole abdomen or systemic chemotherapy can be given to patients with metastases. This tumor is exquisitely sensitive to either type of treatment, and the cure rate exceeds 90% even in patients with metastases. Chemotherapy has the advantage of preserving ovarian function, whereas radiotherapy results in ovarian failure.

The other germ cell tumors, in order of frequency, are immature teratoma; endodermal sinus, or "yolk sac," tumor; mixed tumors; embryonal carcinomas; and choriocarcinomas. The first may be associated with elevated levels of alpha-fetoprotein (AFP). Elevated AFP levels are found in all patients with endodermal sinus tumors and mixed tumors that contain this component. Embryonal carcinomas are associated with abnormal levels of both AFP and hCG, and choriocarcinomas secrete hCG.

These tumors are invariably unilateral but may spread by peritoneal, hematogenous, or lymphatic routes. Surgical therapy involves unilateral oophorectomy and appropriate staging. Except for those with completely resected stage I, grade 1 immature teratomas and those with stage I dysgerminoma, all patients with germ cell tumors require systemic chemotherapy. Three courses of a platinum and etoposide-containing combination suffice in those patients whose tumors are completely resected. Cure rates in these patients approach 90%. In women with incompletely resected nondysgerminomatous germ cell tumors, cure may still be expected in more than 50%, but prolonged chemotherapy may be necessary. These tumors are *not* sensitive to radiotherapy.

Carcinoma of the Cervix

Carcinoma of the cervix accounts for about 16,000 cases and 5000 deaths annually in the United States. Risk factors include multiple sexual partners, early age at first intercourse, and early first pregnancy. DNA related to that found in the human papillomavirus has been identified in cervical dysplasia and carcinoma in situ, both precursor lesions, as well as in invasive cancers and lymph node metastases. Cigarette smoking is highly associated with an increased risk of cervical cancer and may impair the activity of T lymphocytes.

In no other cancer has widespread screening had as profound an impact on mortality as it has in carcinoma of the cervix. Georges Papanicolaou developed the cytologic smear that bears his name in 1943. Since then, screening programs have dramatically reduced the rate of invasive cervical cancer in countries where this test is widely available. Use of the Papanicolaou (Pap) smear has shifted the frequency of cervical abnormalities toward the premalignant intraepithelial diseases, dysplasia, and carcinoma in situ. Although there are histologic grades of dysplasia leading to carcinoma in situ, all intraepithelial lesions are noninvasive and can be treated successfully using conservative methods.

Eighty percent of all cervical cancers are squamous cell in type and arise from the squamocolumnar junction of the cervix. This epithelial transition zone is found on the face of the cervix or ectocervix in adolescence, and, through a process of squamous metaplasia, gradually moves into the endocervical canal as menopause is passed. Dysplasia represents a disordered metaplasia and gives rise to epithelial cells that contain increased mitotic rates and nuclear atypia and that lack appropriate maturation within the epithelium. Identification and eradication of intraepithelial lesions before invasion can occur are the goals of cervical cancer screening.

The remainder of cervical malignancies arise in the endocervical canal and are either adenocarcinomas or adenosquamous carcinomas. Although adenocarcinomas are very similar in their clinical behavior to squamous cancers, there is some evidence that adenosquamous cancers are more aggressive. Other rare histologic varieties associated with poor prognosis are neuroendocrine small cell carcinomas and clear cell cancers. The latter are frequently associated with maternal exposure to diethylstilbestrol.

Staging

Cervical cancers spread predominantly by lymphatic channels. The first lymph nodes involved are those in the tissues immediately lateral to the cervix. This region is referred to as the *paracervical* or *parametrial area*. The next lymph nodes to be involved, in order, are those in the obturator fossa, the internal and external iliac chain, the common iliac chain, and the para-aortic lymph nodes. Direct vaginal extension may occur. The lymph nodes in the presacral area may be

Table 40-3
FIGO Staging System for Cervical Cancer

Stage	Characteristic
0	Carcinoma in situ
I	The carcinoma is strictly confined to the cervix (extension to the corpus should be disregarded)
IA	Preclinical carcinomas of the cervix; that is, those diagnosed only by microscopy
IA$_1$	Minimal microscopically evident stromal invasion
IA$_2$	Lesions detected microscopically that can be measured. The upper limit of the measurement should not show a depth of invasion of more than 5 mm taken from the base of the epithelium, either surface or glandular, from which it originates, and a second dimension, the horizontal spread, must not exceed 7 mm. Larger lesions should be staged as IB
IB	Lesions of greater dimensions than Stage IA$_2$ whether seen clinically or not. Preformed space involvement should not alter the staging but should be specifically recorded so as to determine whether it should affect treatment decisions in the future
IB$_1$	Tumor size no greater than 4 cm
IB$_2$	Tumor size greater than 4 cm
II	Involvement of the vagina but not the lower third, or infiltration of the parametria but not out to the sidewall
IIA	Involvement of the vagina but no evidence of parametrial involvement
IIB	Infiltration of the parametria but not out to the sidewall
III	Involvement of the lower third of the vagina or extension to the pelvic sidewall
IIIA	Involvement of the lower third of the vagina but not out to the pelvic sidewall if the parametria are involved
IIIB	Involvement of one or both parametria out to the sidewall
III (urinary)	Obstruction of one or both ureters on intravenous pyelogram (IVP) without the other criteria for stage III disease
IV	Extension outside the reproductive tract
IVA	Involvement of the mucosa of the bladder or rectum
IVB	Distant metastasis or disease outside the true pelvis

SOURCE: From the International Federation of Gynecology and Obstetrics.

involved in early stage lesions, and the supraclavicular lymph nodes are the most common site of distant nodal metastases.

FIGO staging for cervical cancer is based on clinical examination, intravenous pyelography, and chest radiography. CT or MRI findings do not affect the clinical stage. Table 40-3 illustrates the FIGO staging system. Note that the presence of hydronephrosis connotes stage IIIB even if there is no clinical evidence of extracervical spread. Except for selected patients with stage IVA lesions and those with distant metastases, all patients with stage IIB cancer and above are treated primarily with radiotherapy in the United States.

Treatment

Intraepithelial or Preinvasive Disease. Abnormal Pap smears must be evaluated by colposcopy and biopsy. Colposcopy is the examination of the cervix with a low-power (x10 to 50) microscope after application of dilute acetic acid to the cervix. The acid solution is mucolytic and serves to desiccate the epithelium, a process that brings out subtle epithelial patterns referred to as white epithelium, punctation, mosaicism, and abnormal vasculature. Abnormal areas must undergo mechanical biopsy or wide excision with

a wire loop electrode and are examined histologically. If loop excision is not performed, the endocervical canal should be curetted to exclude epithelial abnormalities in this area, which is difficult to visualize colposcopically.

Once the diagnosis of an intraepithelial process is made and stromal invasion excluded, local therapy can be performed. If there are abnormal cells on the endocervical curettage specimen, a diagnostic cone biopsy or loop electrosurgical excision procedure (LEEP) is indicated to exclude the possibility of an invasive or microinvasive lesion in the endocervical canal.

Cervical intraepithelial neoplasia is treated in a number of ways. In general, the larger the lesion and the higher the grade of dysplasia, the greater the failure rate. Similarly, more aggressive therapy yields lower failure rates at increased risk of complications. The most definitive treatment for cervical intraepithelial neoplasia is vaginal or abdominal hysterectomy. This operation is associated with a rate of subsequent dysplasia at the vaginal apex of 1 to 2%. This major operation is usually reserved, however, for patients with extensive or high-grade lesions, those with recurrent disease after conservative treatment, those in whom adequate follow-up is unlikely, and those with other indications for hysterectomy, such as prolapse, abnormal uterine bleeding, pain, or a pelvic mass. Cervical cone biopsy is curative in most cases of cervical intraepithelial neoplasia. In patients in whom the surgical margins of the cone specimen are uninvolved, the risk of recurrence is less than 5%. If the surgical margins are involved, half of such patients will develop recurrent disease. This is an outpatient procedure and associated with few serious risks. It may, however, require general anesthesia.

More conservative methods of treating cervical intraepithelial neoplasia include wire loop excision, laser vaporization, and cryosurgery. Loop excision can be done under local anesthesia (paracervical block) in the outpatient setting. The advantage of loop excision is that it removes the diseased area and provides a diagnostic biopsy specimen. The main disadvantage is the relatively large amount of cervical stroma that is taken with the involved epithelium. In cases of cervical intraepithelial neoplasia confined to the ectocervix, such deep excision is probably unnecessary.

Laser vaporization is usually performed with a carbon dioxide laser, but other laser instruments may be used. The ectocervical transformation zone is ablated to a depth of about 7 mm to ensure the removal of endocervical glandular epithelium. This is a convenient outpatient procedure that results in a clearly visible squamocolumnar junction at the site of treatment. Risks of bleeding and infection are small. Cryotherapy is an inexpensive outpatient procedure that produces a frostbite injury to the ectocervical epithelium. When the cervix reepithelializes, the dysplasia generally does not recur. This is a simple technique that should not be applied to patients with endocervical lesions. The main disadvantage of cryotherapy is obliteration of the squamocolumnar junction, making subsequent colposcopic examination somewhat difficult. In patients with very localized mild dysplasias or low-grade cervical intraepithelial neoplasia, local excision or electrocautery may be sufficient to eradicate the disease.

Microinvasive Cervical Cancer. FIGO (see Table 40-3) subdivides microinvasive cancers into those with "early" invasion (stage IA$_1$) and those in which the tumor measurements are less than 5 mm in thickness and 7 mm in lateral extent (stage IA$_2$). This aspect of the FIGO staging system for cervical cancer fails to distinguish adequately between stages IA$_2$ and IB, however, because both may have occult lymph node metastases requiring regional therapy.

Many prefer the original system of the Society of Gynecologic Oncologists, in which stage IA (microinvasive) tumors may invade to no more than 3 mm and must lack capability of lymphatic space invasion. Stage IB includes all other cancers clinically confined to the cervix, even if they cannot be visualized on examination. The advantage of this system is that it clearly divides stage I cancer into two treatment groups. Few patients with stage IA cervical cancer have metastases to the lymph nodes. Simple, or extrafascial, hysterectomy without lymphadenectomy is therefore adequate therapy. Five-year survival rates approach 100% in these patients. In exceptional patients, cervical cone biopsy or electrosurgical excision may be sufficient treatment, provided close surveillance is possible.

Early Invasive Cervical Cancer (Stages IB and IIA). Stages IB and IIA tumors are associated with a risk of pelvic lymph node metastases of 10 to 15% and a risk of spread to the para-aortic nodes of about 5%. Treatment must include the regional lymph nodes in these patients. Radical hysterectomy with pelvic lymphadenectomy or definitive radiotherapy is effective treatment in this stage cancer. Prognosis with either modality depends on the size of the primary lesion, the presence or absence of lymph–vascular space involvement, spread to the regional lymph nodes, and status of the surgical margins.

Women with stage IB$_2$ cervical cancers (exceeding 4 cm in diameter), especially those endocervical primaries that distend the cervix circumferentially, may require a combination of radiotherapy and surgery. These large endocervical tumors are referred to as "barrel" lesions and are refractory to surgery or radiotherapy alone. Isodose curves from cesium sources may not encompass the entire tumor (Fig. 40-13). Cure rates with either treatment may be as low as 50%.

One current approach to these tumors is the administration of pelvic radiotherapy followed by a cesium implant and subsequent simple hysterectomy. This technique may reduce the number of patients who have persistent invasive cancer in the cervix after radiotherapy and consequently improve survival.

Stage IB$_1$ lesions and early stage IIA cancers may be treated successfully with radical hysterectomy and pelvic lymphadenectomy. This operation was pioneered by John Clark in 1895. Radical surgery was transiently eclipsed by the first use of radium in the treatment of cervical cancer by Sjögren and Stenbeck in 1899, and subsequent establishment of the first radium hospital in Stockholm, Sweden, in 1910.

Radical surgery reemerged in the treatment of early carcinoma of the cervix with the advent of the Pap smear and increased diagnosis of early stage tumors in young women. Because early cervical cancer so rarely spreads to the ovaries, radical hysterectomy need not include oophorectomy. Ovarian preservation is one of the strongest arguments for the use of surgery over radiotherapy, because the latter inevitably results in the premature loss of ovarian function.

Locally Advanced Carcinoma of the Cervix (Stages IIB to IVA). These cancers are treated primarily with radiotherapy, with cisplatin as a radiosensitizer. Treatment consists of a combination of external therapy to the pelvis (teletherapy) from a high-energy source such as a linear accelerator and a local dose delivered to the cervix and parametrial tissue (brachytherapy) using a cesium applicator such as a Fletcher-Suite tandem and ovoids (Fig. 40-14). Combination therapy is essential because doses adequate to control cervical tumors exceeding about 1 cm in diameter cannot be given using teletherapy alone. Bladder and rectal tolerances are approximately 6000 rads; higher doses can only be attained by combination therapy. The addition of cisplatin as a weekly radiosensitizer has resulted in improved survival with no apparent increase in toxicity when compared with radiation alone.

Cure rates for stage IIB cervical cancers approach 65%, and those for stage IIIB approach 35%. Because the risk of pelvic sidewall

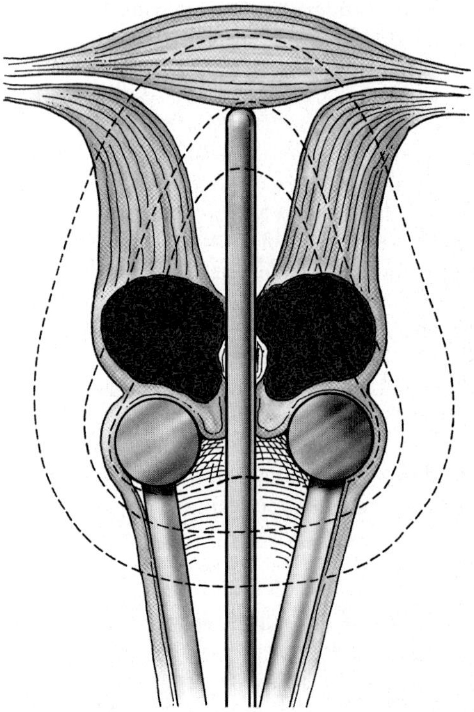

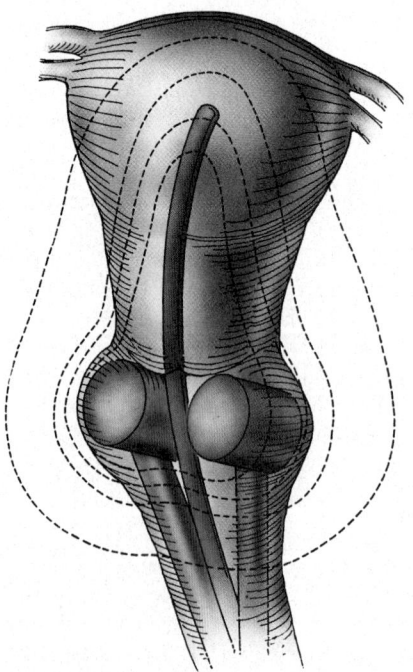

FIG. 40-13. Radiotherapeutic isodose curves superimposed on a large stage IB "barrel" lesion of the cervix. The upper margins of the tumor may receive an inadequate dose of radiotherapy.

FIG. 40-14. Fletcher-Suite tandem and paired ovoids. Hollow applicators that can be placed in the uterus and vagina and "afterloaded" once the appropriate position and dosimetry are established.

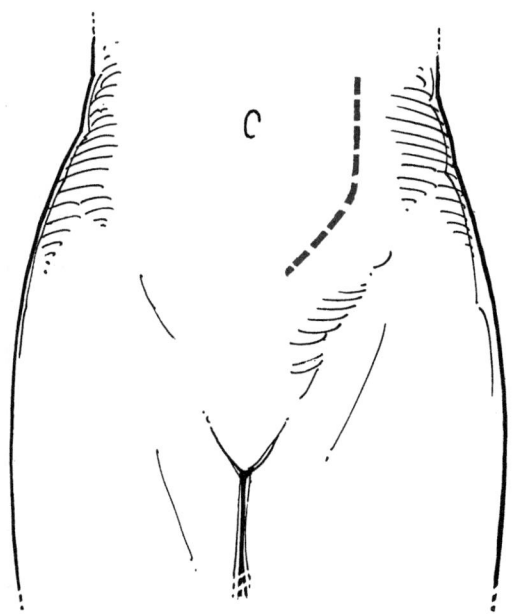

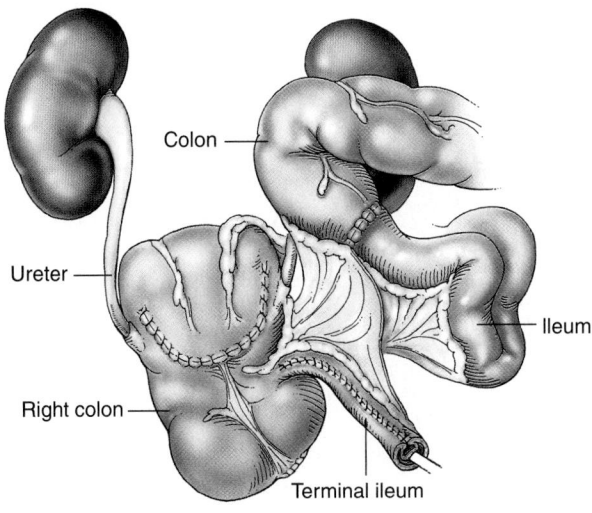

FIG. 40-16. Indiana continent urinary reservoir based on the right colon and terminal ileum. The ileum is plicated to preserve continence.

FIG. 40-15. "Hockey stick" incision used for retroperitoneal para-aortic lymph node dissection in cases of locally advanced cervical cancer.

lymph node involvement increases with advancing stage, the dose of radiotherapy to this area is advanced with increasing stage. When para-aortic metastases are present in either stage, survival is significantly impaired. Survival for patients with stage IIB carcinoma of the cervix and para-aortic metastases is poorer than that for those with stage IIIB disease and negative para-aortic lymph nodes. Gross para-aortic lymph node metastases may be detected by CT, MRI, lymphangiography, or PET scanning. Microscopic nodal metastases are best detected by retroperitoneal common iliac and para-aortic lymphadenectomy, a relatively simple procedure performed through a "hockey stick" or paramedian incision (Fig. 40-15). The fascial layers are divided, sparing the peritoneum, which is reflected medially to expose the lymph node–bearing areas overlying the major blood vessels. Laparoscopic staging and pelvic and para-aortic lymph node dissection may be used by appropriately trained surgeons.

The finding of metastases in the common iliac or para-aortic chain indicates the need for extended-field radiotherapy encompassing these areas in addition to the pelvis. Even with such therapy, 5-year survival rates are low, seldom exceeding 20%. Many consider the presence of para-aortic lymph node metastases to be an indicator of systemic disease, although supraclavicular metastases are present in fewer than 25% of such patients.

Recurrent Cervical Cancer. As a rule, patients who develop local recurrences after primary surgical therapy are treated most effectively with external and internal beam radiotherapy. Although those with lymph node failures may not be curable in this setting, those with vaginal recurrences often can be saved with such an approach. Patients who suffer recurrences at sites distant from the pelvis may be treated with palliative local radiotherapy or chemotherapy with limited success.

Women who develop recurrent cancer following primary radiotherapy are generally not candidates for curative therapy. If, however, the recurrent lesion is small, the interval to failure is a year or more, and the lesion is unaccompanied by symptoms such as back or leg pain or edema, surgical resection may be possible. Because

radiotherapy results in fibrosis of the connective tissues surrounding the cervix, radical hysterectomy is impractical. The risk of vesicovaginal or rectovaginal fistulas approaches 50%. In addition, surgical margins may be compromised by limited resection in such a situation.

Most gynecologic oncologists prefer to perform pelvic exenteration in such circumstances. Often, an anterior exenteration with en bloc removal of the bladder, cervix, uterus, and upper vagina is feasible. These operations require urinary diversion. Because of radiation exposure, however, an ileal conduit may be associated with urinary leakage from ureteroileal anastomoses. The preferred method of diversion in these patients is the creation of a sigmoid urostomy or transverse colon conduit. Other surgical options include a Koch pouch or the Indiana reservoir (Fig. 40-16), both of which provide a means of urinary continence without an external appliance.

In the case of extensive local recurrences, sigmoid resection may be required in addition to removal of the bladder. A total pelvic exenteration is performed. The sigmoid colon may be brought to the skin as a colostomy or reanastomosed to the rectal stump. Pelvic exenterations may be subclassified as supralevator or infralevator depending on whether this muscular diaphragm is broached (Fig. 40-17). Supralevator exenterations are generally associated with less operative morbidity. An infralevator exenteration is required if the tumor involves the middle or lower third of the vagina or the vulva. Vaginal reconstruction in these extensive procedures with gracilis or rectus abdominis myocutaneous flaps is highly satisfactory (Figs. 40-18 and 40-19).

In general, about half the patients thought to be candidates for pelvic exenteration are found to have intraperitoneal spread or nodal metastases at the time of exploratory laparotomy, and, in most centers, do not undergo resection. Laparoscopy may be a useful way of excluding such patients from laparotomy. Of the remaining patients in whom surgery is possible, 30 to 50% will develop a second, nearly always fatal, recurrence after surgery. This complex operation should thus be undertaken only in carefully selected patients.

Endometrial Cancer

Endometrial cancer is the most common female genital malignancy, accounting for 34,000 cases annually in the United States. It is a

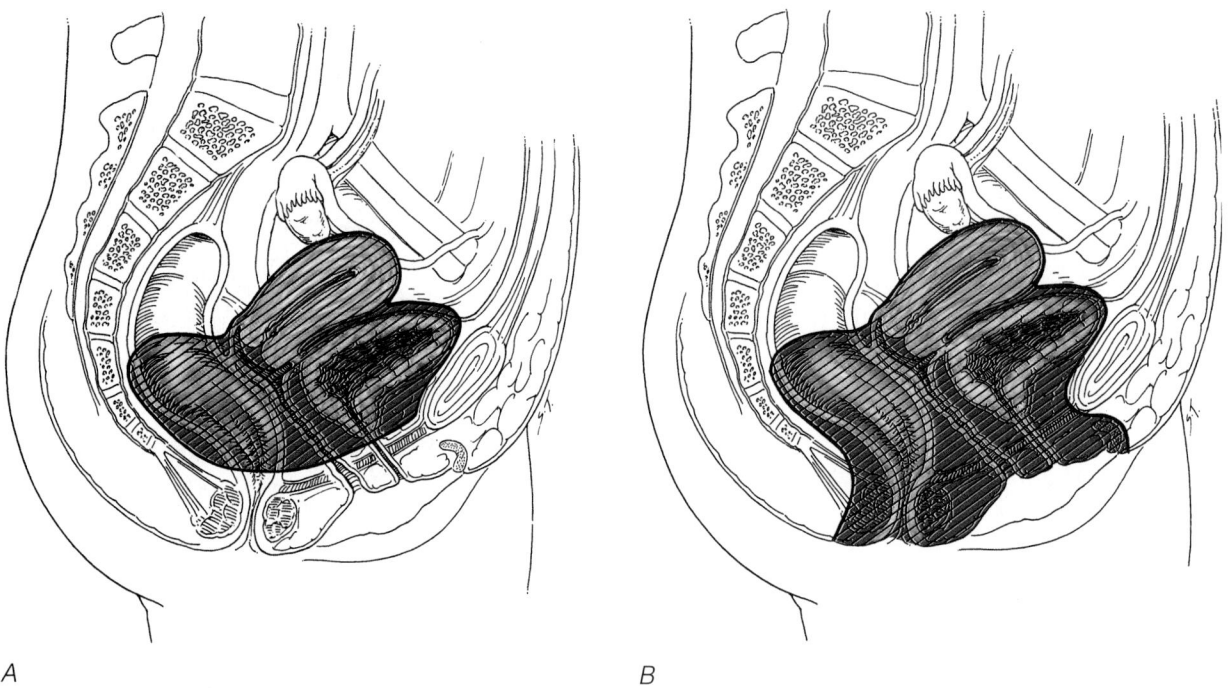

A   *B*

FIG. 40-17. Pelvic exenteration may be limited to the supralevator space (*A*) or can extend below the levator ani muscle (shaded area) (*B*).

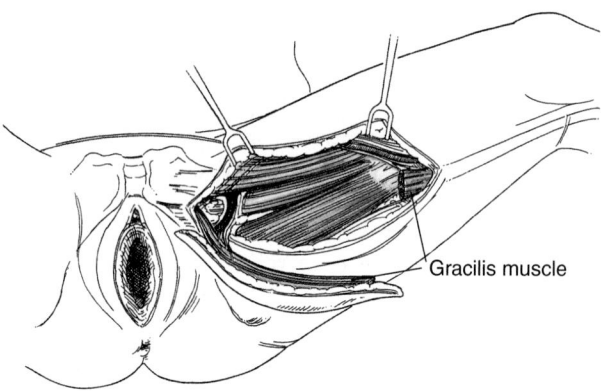

Gracilis muscle

FIG. 40-18. Development of gracilis myocutaneous flaps.

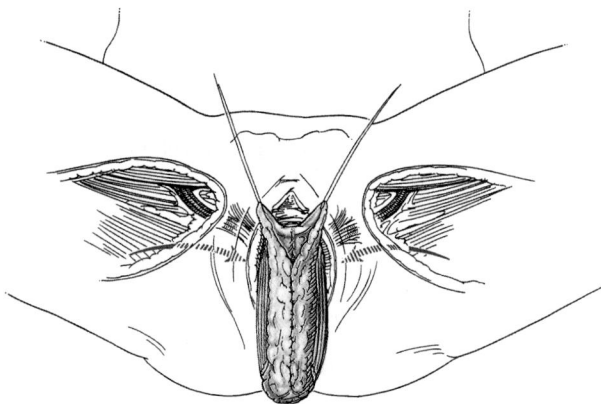

FIG. 40-19. Rotation of the flaps inferomedially and creation of a neo-vaginal tube that is rotated into the pelvic defect.

highly treatable cancer, with approximately only 6000 deaths reported each year.

Risk factors for endometrial cancer include obesity, diabetes mellitus, hypertension, low parity, early menarche, and late menopause. Prolonged or unopposed exposure to estrogens is implicated in the genesis of endometrial cancer and its precursor, endometrial hyperplasia. Women who take estrogens in the menopausal years are known to have a sixfold increase in the risk of endometrial cancer if progestational agents are not taken as well. There is also an increase in the incidence of endometrial lesions in women with a history of chronic anovulation (Stein-Leventhal syndrome) and in those with estrogen-producing ovarian stromal neoplasms, such as granulosa cell tumors, and in those who take tamoxifen.

Endometrial hyperplasia may be divided into classifications of simple and complex, depending on the microscopic architecture, and into those with or without atypia. These hyperplasias are thought to be estrogen-dependent. Atypical complex hyperplasias are most likely to give rise to frank adenocarcinomas. They occur in women at an average age that is 5 to 10 years younger than those with frank carcinomas. Simple hysterectomy is the preferred method of treatment for the hyperplasias. In women with underlying health problems that preclude surgical therapy, therapy with progestational agents such as megestrol or medroxyprogesterone acetate may be used with success. Careful monitoring with endometrial biopsy or curettage or vaginal ultrasound is required in these patients, however.

Both endometrial hyperplasia and carcinoma are often heralded by abnormal perimenopausal or postmenopausal uterine bleeding. This symptom accounts for the early detection and relative curability of these neoplasms.

Treatment

Endometrial cancer is staged according to the FIGO criteria detailed in Table 40-4. Many patients have stage I disease and can be

Table 40-4
FIGO (1988) Staging System for Endometrial Cancer

Stages	Characteristics
IA G123	Tumor limited to endometrium
IB G123	Invasion to <1/2 myometrium
IC G123	Invasion to >1/2 myometrium
IIA G123	Endocervical glandular involvement only
IIB G123	Cervical stromal invasion
IIIA G123	Tumor invades serosa or adnexae or positive peritoneal cytology
IIIB G123	Vaginal metastases
IIIC G123	Metastases to pelvic or para-aortic lymph nodes
IVA G123	Tumor invasion bladder and/or bowel mucosa
IVB	Distant metastases including intra-abdominal and/or inguinal lymph node

Histopathology—Degree of Differentiation
Cases should be grouped by the degree of differentiation of the adenocarcinoma:

G1	5% or less of a nonsquamous or nonmorular solid growth pattern
G2	6%–50% of a nonsquamous or nonmorular solid growth pattern
G3	More than 50% of a nonsquamous or nonmorular solid growth pattern

Notes on Pathologic Grading
Notable nuclear atypia, inapppropriate for the architectural grade, raises the grade of a grade I or grade II tumor by I.
In serous adenocarcinomas, clear cell adenocarcinomas, and squamous cell carcinomas, nuclear grading takes precedence.
Adenocarcinomas with squamous differentiation are graded according to the nuclear grade of the glandular component.

Rules Related to Staging
Because corpus cancer is now surgically staged, procedures previously used for determination of stages are no longer applicable, such as the finding of fractional D&C to differentiate between stage I and II. It is appreciated that there may be a small number of patients with corpus cancer who will be treated primarily with radiation therapy. If that is the case, the clinical staging adopted by FIGO in 1971 would still apply but designation of that staging system would be noted.
Ideally, width of the myometrium should be measured along with the width of tumor invasion.

managed successfully with abdominal hysterectomy and bilateral salpingo-oophorectomy. Adjuvant radiotherapy may be required, primarily to reduce the risk of vaginal recurrence. This can be given preoperatively with external therapy or a Fletcher-Suite implant or intrauterine packing (Heyman's or Simon's capsules). Some clinicians prefer to deliver radiotherapy postoperatively after the uterus has been evaluated thoroughly. Either external beam therapy or vaginal cesium may be used.

Pelvic lymph node metastases occur in about 12% of patients with endometrial cancer apparently confined to the uterus. Lymph node metastases have a significant negative impact on survival. Risk factors associated with lymph node spread include high histologic grade (grade 2 or 3), low levels of progesterone receptor, deep myometrial or lymphatic channel invasion, spread to the adnexa, endocervical extension, and unusual histologic variants, such as papillary serous or clear cell carcinomas. It may be unnecessary to perform lymph node sampling in patients with grade 1 adenocarcinomas confined to the endometrium or the inner one-third of myometrium. Other patients should have pelvic and para-aortic lymph nodes sampled at the time of hysterectomy. Therapeutic lymphadenectomy is not advocated; sampling of the external and internal iliac and obturator areas, as well as of the common iliac and para-aortic lymph nodes, is sufficient for patients with endometrial cancer. Those with a high likelihood of spread to pelvic lymph nodes (grade 3, the outer one-third myometrial or uterine serosal involvement, and those with high-risk histologic subtypes) should undergo sampling of the common iliac and para-aortic lymph nodes, because these areas lie outside the usual fields of pelvic radiotherapy. Patients with papillary serous tumors may present with metastases in the abdominal cavity or omentum much as those with ovarian epithelial tumors; omentectomy, diaphragmatic, and peritoneal biopsies should be obtained.

Another important element of staging endometrial cancer is the evaluation of peritoneal lavage fluid for the presence of malignant cells. Approximately 12% of patients are found to have malignant peritoneal cytology; one-half have other evidence of extrauterine spread of the disease, but the remainder have no other associated risk factors. Malignant peritoneal cytology increases the risk for intra-abdominal failure and treatment for this finding deserves consideration. If external beam radiotherapy is not used, intraperitoneal radioactive chromic phosphate may be of benefit.

Vaginal hysterectomy is occasionally useful in patients with early endometrial cancer when lymph node metastases are thought to be unlikely. This operation is particularly well suited for massively obese parous patients in whom an abdominal incision would be prohibitively difficult.

It is unnecessary to perform radical surgery in women with endometrial cancer even if there is spread to the cervix (stage II). Although lymphatic spread is important, these cancers also may be disseminated by hematogenous or peritoneal routes. Radical surgery has never been shown to improve survival in comparison with simple hysterectomy and adjuvant radiotherapy. Simple, extrafascial, or complete abdominal hysterectomy is demonstrated in (Fig. 40-20) and contrasted with radical hysterectomy. It is critical to remove the ovaries in women undergoing surgery for endometrial cancer because 5% harbor occult metastases. Additionally, the source of estrogen secretion in premenopausal women with endometrial cancer should be removed.

In patients with large stage IIB and III lesions, consideration is generally given to preoperative pelvic radiotherapy, because surgery may be otherwise difficult or impossible. These tumors should receive appropriate surgical staging or thorough radiographic evaluation if primary radiotherapy is used.

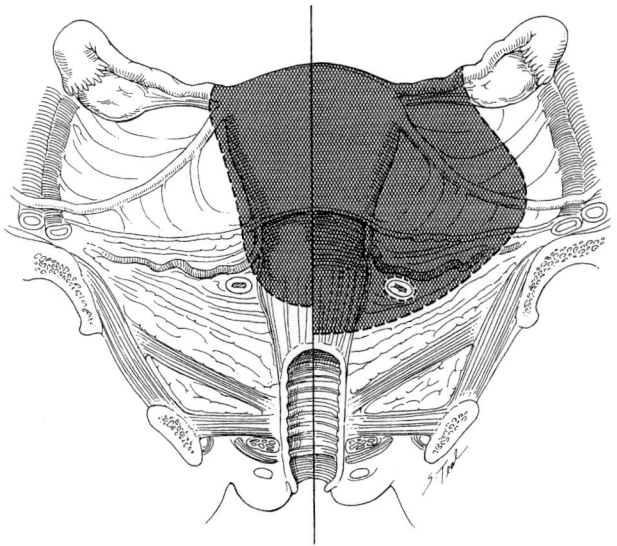

FIG. 40-20. Extent of simple (extrafascial) hysterectomy (*left*) as compared with radical hysterectomy (*right*).

Pelvic exenteration is rarely necessary in the treatment of patients with endometrial cancer unless it occurs following full irradiation for a preexisting cervical cancer. However, such cases are rare.

Radiotherapy alone may be the treatment of choice in patients at excessive risk for operative intervention. Radiotherapy alone produces results inferior to those of surgery or surgery and adjuvant radiotherapy, however; therefore patients treated without hysterectomy should be selected carefully. Advanced or recurrent endometrial cancer is responsive to progestin or tamoxifen therapy in 30% of unselected patients. Lesions that are well differentiated contain higher levels of progesterone receptor and respond more frequently. Only 10% of poorly differentiated cancers respond to hormonal treatment. Local radiotherapy or chemotherapy with paclitaxel, doxorubicin, platinum compounds, or combinations may be of benefit in some cases as well.

Vulvar Cancer

Vulvar cancer accounts for approximately 5% of all gynecologic cancers. Although uncommon histologic types such as malignant melanoma and adenocarcinoma of the Bartholin's gland occur, more than 90% of vulvar malignancies are squamous carcinomas.

Epidemiologic risk factors include older age, smoking, previous intraepithelial or invasive squamous cancer of the cervix or vagina, chronic vulvar dystrophy (often associated with diabetes mellitus), and immunocompromise (organ-transplant recipients, systemic lupus erythematosus). Human papillomavirus-like DNA has been identified in both preinvasive and invasive squamous carcinomas of the vulva. Although the etiology of this cancer is not well understood, it is likely that the human papillomavirus plays an important role, especially in younger women.

Spread of squamous carcinoma of the vulva is primarily via the lymphatics of the vulva. Lesions arising in the anterior aspect of the vulva drain preferentially to the inguinal lymph nodes, and posterior lesions may drain directly to the lymph nodes of the pelvis.

Stanley Way of Great Britain identified five main groups of lymphatic drainage of carcinoma of the vulva (Fig. 40-21): (1) the superficial inguinal lymph nodes, which lie in the subcutaneous tissue overlying the inguinal ligament; (2) the deep inguinal lymph nodes, which lie along the course of the round ligament in the inguinal canal; (3) the superficial femoral lymph nodes, grouped around the saphenous vein just superficial to the fossa ovalis, with efferents to the deep femoral lymph nodes; (4) the deep femoral lymph nodes, including the most cephalad lymph node of Cloquet or Rosenmüller; and (5) the external iliac lymph nodes.

Because the lymph node of Cloquet receives efferents from the inguinal region and the vulva and drains into the medial portion of the external iliac chain, it is an important sentinel in the route of spread of vulvar lesions to the pelvic lymph nodes. There are also direct lymphatic connections between the clitoris and Cloquet's node.

The 1988 FIGO staging system for vulvar cancer (Table 40-5) is currently accepted. This system requires surgical evaluation of the inguinal lymph nodes and provides a schema in which prognosis and therapy are closely linked with stage.

Treatment

Historically, the single-stage en bloc "extended" radical vulvectomy championed in Great Britain by Way, and in the United States by Friedrich Taussig, was used to treat all vulvar neoplasms (Fig. 40-22). In this operation, wide margins of skin and subcutaneous tissue around the primary tumor are removed together with underlying lymphatic structures in the groins and the labia majora and minora and clitoris in the vulva. Also removed are the proximal saphenous vein and its tributaries, the superficial circumflex iliac, superficial external pudendal, and superficial inferior epigastric veins.

The deep inguinal lymph nodes are removed by opening the external oblique fascia overlying the inguinal canal; most of the round ligament is removed at the same time.

Pelvic lymphadenectomy is easily performed by opening the transversalis fascia below the inguinal ligament and exposing the

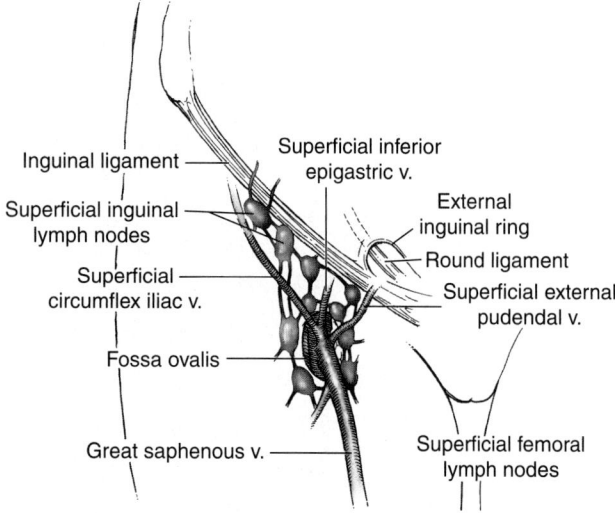

FIG. 40-21. Lymphatic drainage of the vulva delineated by Stanley Way.

Table 40-5
FIGO Staging of Vulvar Cancer

Stage 0	
Tis	Carcinoma in situ, intraepithelial carcinoma.
Stage I	
T1 N0 M0	Tumor confined to the vulva and/or perineum—2 cm or less in greatest dimension. No nodal metastasis.
Stage IA	≤1 mm invasion + other criteria
Stage IB	>1 mm invasion + other criteria
Stage II	
T2 N0 M0	Tumor confined to the vulva and/or perineum—more than 2 cm in greatest dimension. No nodal metastasis.
Stage III	
T3 N0 M0	Tumor of any size with
T3 N1 M0	1) adjacent spread to the lower urethra and/or the vagina, or the anus, and/or
T1 N1 M0	2) unilateral regional lymph node metastasis.
T2 N1 M0	
Stage IV A	
T1 N2 M0	Tumor invades any of the following:
T2 N2 M0	Upper urethra, bladder mucosa, rectal mucosa, pelvic bone, and/or bilateral regional node metastasis.
T3 N2 M0	
T4 Any N M0	
Stage IV B	
Any T, Any N, M1	Any distant metastasis, including pelvic lymph nodes.

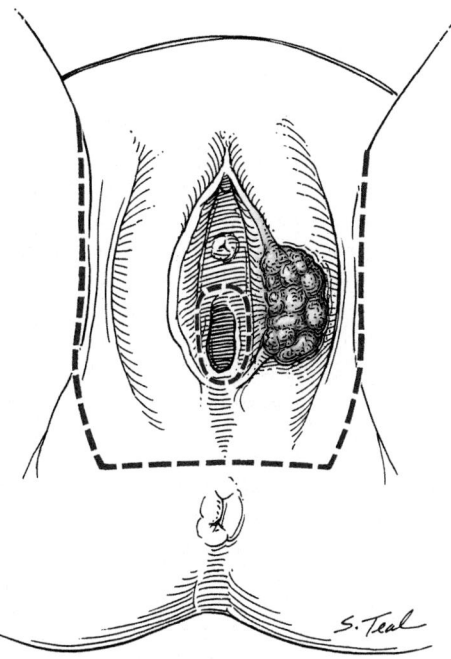

FIG. 40-22. En bloc radical vulvectomy outlined by Way and Taussig.

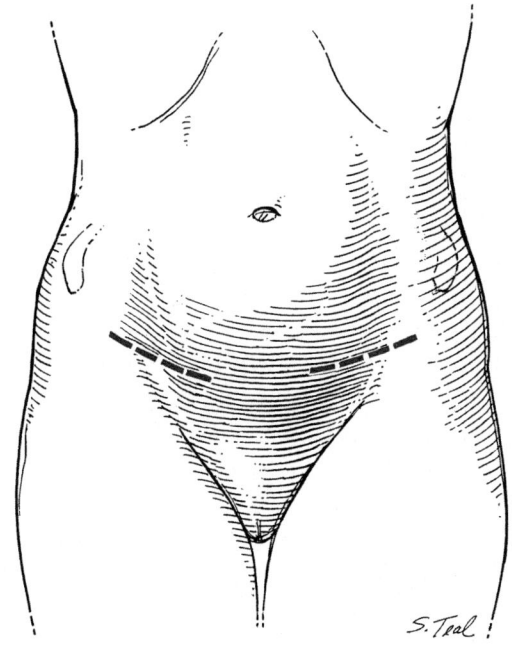

FIG. 40-23. Radical vulvectomy and inguinal lymphadenectomy through separate incisions.

external iliac vessels in the retroperitoneal space medial to the psoas muscle. Pelvic lymphadenectomy is probably not indicated in vulvar cancer except in those patients found to have grossly enlarged pelvic lymph nodes on preoperative CT or MRI. Patients with inguinal node metastases are best treated with inguinal and pelvic radiotherapy following resection of the inguinal lymph nodes. In the case of large vulvar primaries or suspicious inguinal lymph nodes, this approach yields better survival rates than those obtained when pelvic lymphadenectomy alone is performed.

Because extended radical vulvectomy is associated with long hospital stays and significant morbidity from wound breakdown and infectious complications, there has been a long-standing interest in more conservative surgery for early vulvar cancer. The first efforts to this end were made in the 1960s. Several investigators introduced the concept of radical vulvectomy and inguinal lymphadenectomy through separate incisions. This approach not only reduces hospital time but also results in fewer major wound complications. This approach, illustrated in Fig. 40-23, has been widely embraced by gynecologic oncologists. Because inguinal node metastases are the result of an embolic process rather than infiltration or direct extension, the approach is rational. Early concerns regarding recurrence in the skin bridge between the vulvar and groin incisions have been largely allayed by experience with this approach. Recurrence in the skin bridge is usually associated with preexisting large inguinal metastases.

Another area of progress in the surgical management of vulvar carcinoma has been the use of conservative surgery for early lesions of the vulva. Although specific criteria vary, most investigators recognize that squamous cancers of the vulva less than 2 cm in diameter and no more than 1 mm thick, and that are of histologic grade 1 or 2, are associated with a very small risk of inguinal metastases. Such lesions are adequately treated with deep, wide excision, provided skin margins of 1 cm are obtained and the dissection is carried to the level of the superficial transverse perineal muscles. Inguinal lymphadenectomy can be omitted in such patients.

In patients with intermediate lesions located on the labium minus or majus that do not cross the midline or involve midline structures such as the clitoris, perineal body, or perianal area, modified hemivulvectomy and ipsilateral inguinal lymphadenectomy have been used successfully. This approach should be considered if the primary lesion is less than 2 cm in diameter and 5 mm or less in thickness. Lymph node metastases are uncommon in this group of patients and the groin nodes may be evaluated by frozen section at the time of surgery. Sentinal lymph node biopsy is being evaluated in vulvar cancer. While it was once believed that superficial inguinal lymph nodes (Fig. 40-24) were "sentinel," it has been demonstrated that vulvar cancer often involves the deep femoral lymph nodes primarily as well. A conservative groin incision (Fig. 40-25) can also be used to sample these lymph nodes. If "sentinel" lymph nodes are free of tumor, the risk of involvement of other groin or pelvic lymph nodes is probably small. Figure 40-26 depicts the outlines of the modified

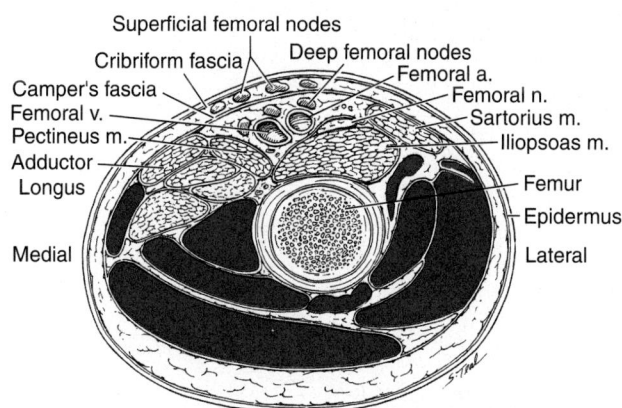

FIG. 40-24. Superficial inguinal lymphadenectomy.

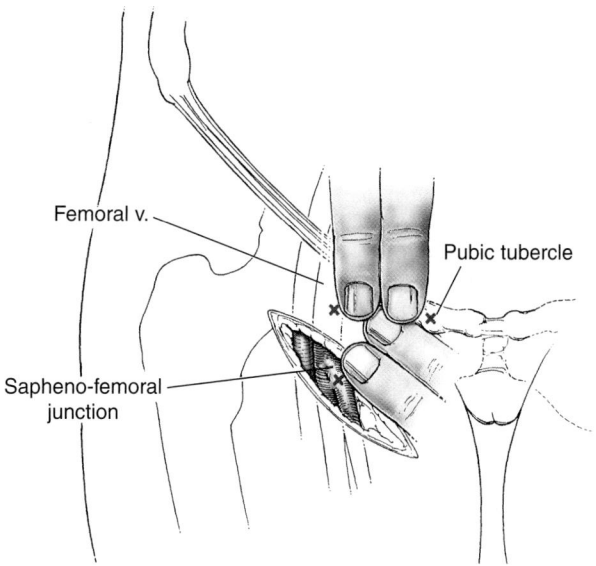

FIG. 40-25. Incision recommended for superficial inguinal lymphadenectomy.

radical hemivulvectomy. This excision site may be closed primarily with good results.

Another controversial area in the management of squamous carcinomas of the vulva is that of the patient with locally advanced disease. When extensive vulvar cancer involves more than the distal urethra, the vagina or rectovaginal septum, or the anal musculature, ultraradical surgery may be required. Anterior, posterior, or total pelvic exenteration may be necessary to resect such lesions successfully. The presence of fixed, matted, or ulcerating inguinal lymph nodes presents another problem that may require extensive surgical excision. Following such extirpative procedures, reconstruction of the vulva and groins is accomplished using myocutaneous flaps

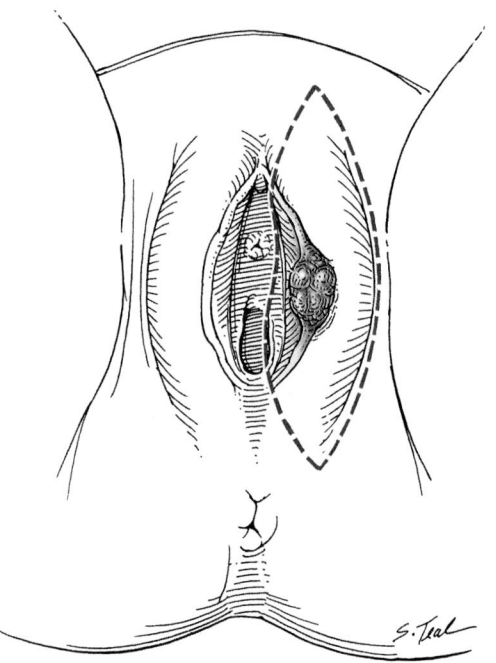

FIG. 40-26. Extent of modified radical hemivulvectomy for stages I and II squamous cancer of the vulva.

based on the gracilis, sartorius, or tensor fasciae latae muscles. Approximately 50% of patients are cured by such surgical procedures.

In recent years, such locally advanced lesions of the vulva also have been treated successfully with external beam radiotherapy combined with radiosensitizing drugs such as cisplatin. At the completion of combination therapy, the areas of involvement are excised widely or biopsied. This approach is associated with results as good as or better than those achieved with ultraradical surgery and generally results in less morbidity. The need for urinary and fecal diversion is also obviated.

Uncommon Vulvar Tumors

Melanoma. Traditional surgical therapy for malignant melanoma of the vulva has included en bloc radical vulvectomy and inguinofemoral lymphadenectomy. It is now known that lesions less than 1 mm thick or Clark level II lesions may be treated conservatively with wide local excision. The value of inguinofemoral lymphadenectomy is controversial in lesions of greater depth, although primary surgical cure is occasionally achieved in patients with microscopic nodal metastases. Melanomas of the urethra or vagina are usually diagnosed in advanced stages and may require pelvic exenteration for successful management.

Intraepithelial Disease. Intraepithelial disease (Bowen's disease, bowenoid papulosis, vulvar intraepithelial neoplasia, carcinoma in situ) may be treated successfully by removing the involved epithelium. Characteristically, this is a raised, velvety lesion with sharply demarcated borders that may contain gray, brown, or red pigmentation. Removal is accomplished by simple vulvectomy, where the plane of dissection is limited to the epithelium, or by wide excision. In the case of diffuse intraepithelial disease, a so-called skinning vulvectomy and split-thickness skin graft may be required. This approach is associated with prolonged hospital stays, however, and should be reserved for exceptional cases. Also effective in the treatment of intraepithelial disease are the carbon dioxide laser and the electrosurgical loop.

Paget's disease is an unusual epithelial or invasive process characterized by the presence of distinct "Paget cells" in the involved epithelium. Grossly, the lesion is confluent, raised, red, and waxy in appearance. This lesion also can be excised widely, although the microscopic extent of the disease may exceed the visible margins. Intravenous fluorescein dye and ultraviolet light highlight areas that cannot be detected by the naked eye, and this assists in excision. Frozen-section examination of the surgical margins also is helpful but time-consuming. Paget's disease is occasionally associated with an underlying invasive adenocarcinoma; careful pelvic examination and proctoscopy are indicated in patients with this process.

Bartholin's gland carcinoma represents less than 1% of all vulvar malignancies and may be squamous carcinoma, adenocarcinoma, or adenosquamous or adenoid cystic carcinoma. Hemivulvectomy with dissection of the ischiorectal fossa and resection of involved contiguous structures is indicated. Because of the risk of inguinofemoral metastases, groin lymphadenectomy should accompany the vulvar operation.

GYNECOLOGIC OPERATIONS

Dilatation and Curettage

At one time dilatation of the cervix and curettage of the endometrial cavity was among the most common surgical procedures performed in this country. Simple office biopsy and medical means of dealing with abnormal bleeding have largely replaced the need for diagnostic dilatation and curettage.

In some cases curettage is necessary for the relief of profuse uterine hemorrhage. It is indicated for removal of endometrial polyp or therapeutic termination of pregnancy and for retained placental tissue following abortion or obstetric delivery.

The patient is placed on the operating table in a lithotomy position, and the vagina and cervix are prepared as for any vaginal operation. The cervix is grasped on the anterior lip with a tenaculum. The cervix is gently pulled toward the outlet of the vagina. Some traction on the cervix is necessary to reduce the angulation between the cervical canal and the uterine cavity. A sound is inserted into the uterine cavity, and the depth of the uterus is noted. The cervical canal is then systematically dilated beginning with a small cervical dilator. Most operations can be performed after the cervix is dilated to accommodate a number 8 or 9 Hegar dilator or its equivalent. Dilatation is accomplished by firm, constant pressure with a dilator directed in the axis of the uterus (Fig. 40-27).

After the cervix is dilated to admit the curette, the endocervical canal should be curetted and the sample submitted separate from the endometrial curettings. The endometrial cavity is then systemically scraped with a uterine curette. The curettings are collected on a small piece of gauze or Telfa. The curettings are then placed in the fixative. After the uterus has been thoroughly curetted, a ureteral stone forceps may be used to explore the endometrial cavity, searching for polyps or pedunculated neoplasms. When the procedure is complete, the tenaculum is removed; the tenaculum site is evaluated for bleeding, and, if the puncture sites are bleeding, they are treated with a small amount of silver nitrate.

The major complication of dilatation and curettage is perforation of the uterus. Perforation is diagnosed when the operator finds no resistance to a dilator or curette at a point where the operator normally would expect it. Perforation generally is treated in an expectant manner. The patient should be watched for several hours for signs of hemorrhage and be warned of the possibility of pelvic infection. A falling hematocrit and other signs of intraperitoneal bleeding indicate the need for laparotomy and control of the bleeding site. Any infection following dilatation and curettage should be treated with antibiotics.

Uterine curettage is often required for incomplete abortion in the first or second trimester of pregnancy. Dilatation of the cervix in these cases is invariably present. Curettage of the postabortal uterus must be approached carefully because the uterus is extremely soft and perforation can occur with very little warning. Using the largest curette available is a safer choice than a small curette, which tends to cause perforation with less pressure. In the postabortal uterus, the endometrial cavity must be scraped thoroughly until the distinctive gritty feeling of curette against muscle is felt.

In recent years, suction curettage for incomplete abortion, hydatid mole, and therapeutic abortion has become popular. Suction machines fitted with cannulas that vary from 4 to 12 mm in diameter evacuate the uterus in less time and save blood loss. Most of these

FIG. 40-27. Dilatation and curettage of the uterus. *A.* Technique for uterine curettage; *B.* Common duct stone searcher; *C.* Introduction of Randall stone forceps into the endometrial cavity.

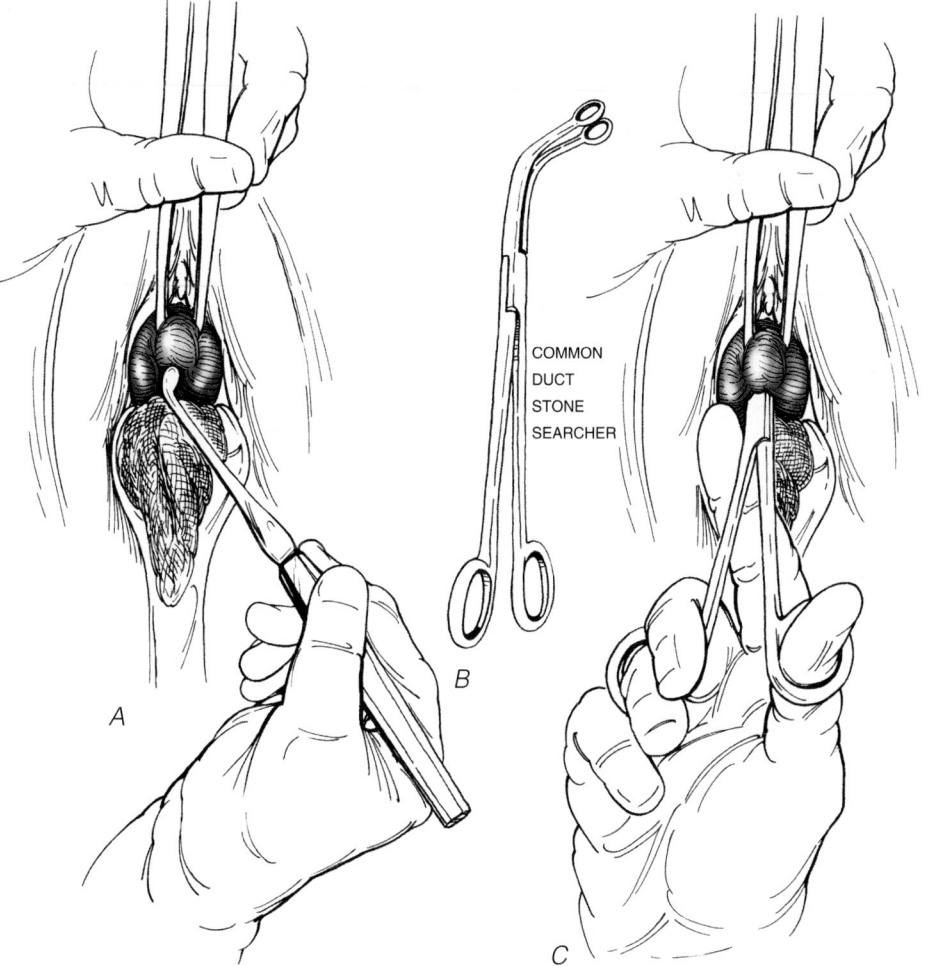

COMMON
DUCT
STONE
SEARCHER

A

B

C

procedures are accomplished under sedation and paracervical block. Following the curettage, the uterine cavity is explored with a placental forceps or sponge forceps to remove any loose tissue within the cavity. Uterine perforation continues to be a concern when curettage is carried out for incomplete abortion. Perforation of the puerperal uterus is a much more serious problem because the organ is much more vascular than the nonpregnant uterus.

Postoperative bleeding should be modest if the curettage has been complete. Some operators control bleeding with the use of uterotonic agents such as vasopressin and prostaglandin-17α.

Endoscopic Surgery

Endoscopic surgery, including both laparoscopy and hysteroscopy, has assumed a major role in gynecology. Laparoscopy, once used almost exclusively for diagnostic purposes and for tubal ligation, is now being applied to almost every kind of gynecologic procedure. Hysteroscopy has found an expanded role from purely diagnostic to removal of intrauterine pathology and ablation of the endometrium for abnormal uterine bleeding. Although the limits of what is possible continue to be defined, the relative safety of some of these techniques in general use remains uncertain.

Laparoscopy

Laparoscopy was developed more than 25 years ago as a diagnostic tool and was soon adapted to perform tubal sterilization techniques. From the beginning, a few intrepid gynecologists used this approach for much more, including lysis of pelvic adhesions, treatment of endometriosis, and removal of ectopic tubal pregnancies. Slowly the role of the laparoscope expanded for conservative surgery and for removal of diseased tissue. More recently, laparoscopic approaches were developed for hysterectomy and gynecologic oncologic procedures. Ongoing research and experience continue to

establish which of these approaches represent real advantages to the patients.

General Techniques for Laparoscopy

Placement of the Veress Needle and Primary Trocar. The standard method for gynecologic laparoscopy remains the serial placement through the umbilicus of a retractable-pointed Veress needle for insufflation, followed by a sharp 5- or 10-mm primary trocar and sleeve. For decades, reusable instruments were standard. Today, disposable instruments are more commonly used despite continued concerns regarding both cost and safety.

When placing the Veress needle through the anterior abdominal wall, the goal is to minimize the risk of preperitoneal placement while avoiding retroperitoneal vessel injury by the use of proper placement techniques. In patients who are of normal weight or who are overweight but not obese (i.e., less than 200 lb), instruments are placed through the umbilicus toward the pelvis. After the sacral prominence is palpated, the abdominal wall is elevated by grasping the skin and subcutaneous tissue midway between the symphysis pubis and the umbilicus in an effort to maximize the distance between the umbilicus and major vessels. The Veress needle is inserted through the base of the umbilicus at 45 degrees from horizontal.

In the obese patient (>200 lb), the thickness of the abdominal wall requires an alteration of the approach for inserting the Veress needle. If the needle is placed through the base of the umbilicus at 45 degrees, it may not reach the peritoneal cavity (Fig. 40-28). For this reason, it has been suggested that the Veress needle be placed at near 90 degrees from horizontal. To minimize the risk of vascular injury, the umbilicus should be elevated (i.e., supported to avoid depression), and a standard length Veress needle should be used and checked for location as described previously. Following insufflation, a primary 5- or 10-mm trocar is also inserted at near 90 degrees from horizontal.

FIG. 40-28. *Changes in the anterior abdominal wall anatomy with weight.*

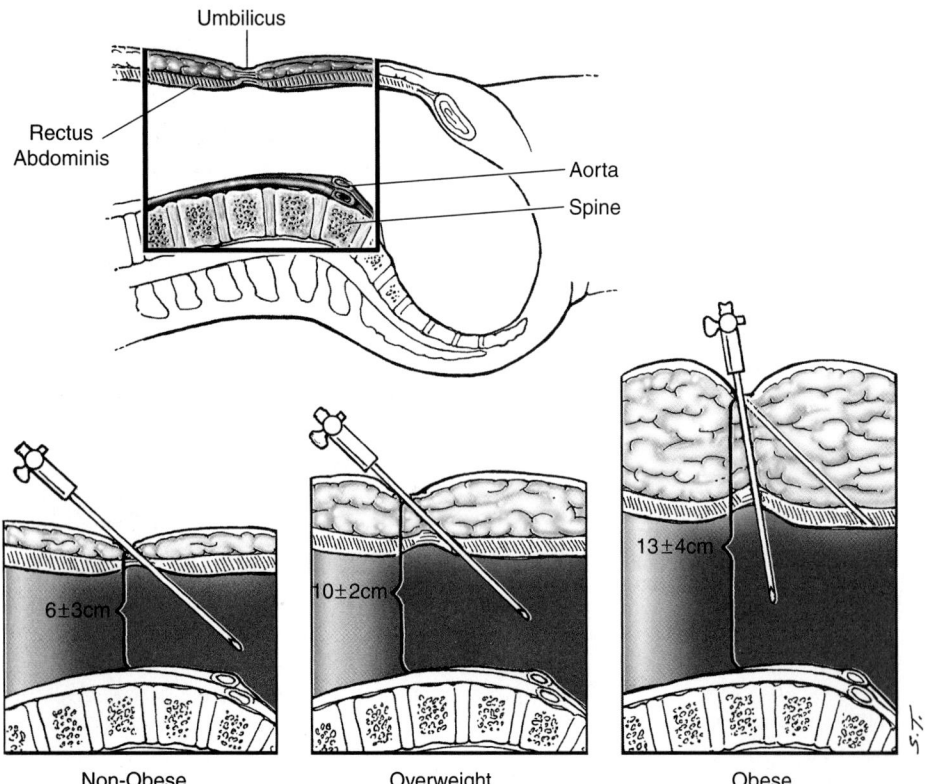

Umbilicus

Rectus Abdominis

Aorta

Spine

6±3cm
Non-Obese

10±2cm
Overweight

13±4cm
Obese

Alternatively, open laparoscopic techniques continue to be refined and more widely applied. For these techniques, the anterior rectus fascia is incised with a scalpel, the peritoneal cavity is entered bluntly, and a blunt-tipped trocar is placed into the peritoneal cavity. Pneumoperitoneum is maintained at the site of entry either by sutures or by mechanisms built into the sleeves such as balloons or fascial threads. Although once reserved for patients with previous surgery, many laparoscopists use an open technique exclusively to avoid the risk of major retroperitoneal injury and to minimize the risk of bowel injury associated with closed techniques.

Placement of Secondary Trocars. As laparoscopic techniques advanced, the need for secondary trocars increased dramatically. After transillumination to locate the superficial vessels, an attempt is made to laparoscopically locate the inferior epigastric vessels. Secondary trocars are placed under laparoscopic visualization either 3 to 4 cm above the symphysis pubis in the midline, or 8 cm above the symphysis pubis approximately 8 cm lateral to the midline. This location approximates McBurney's point on the right side of the abdomen. At the end of the procedure, the sleeves are removed and the sites observed for signs of hemorrhage. Any trocar site larger than 5 mm should be closed with a full-thickness suture (to include both the anterior and posterior rectus abdominus fascia) to prevent herniation through the defect.

Power Instruments. Scissors and sutures have long been used for laparoscopic dissections and vessel ligation. However, because of the limitations of laparoscopy, including decreased depth perception and limited field of vision, innovative instruments have been developed for laparoscopic use both for tissue cutting and for vessel occlusion. Initially, unipolar electrosurgery was the only power instrument available, but because of concern about inadvertent damage to adjacent organs, other techniques were developed. Bipolar electrosurgery is excellent for hemostasis but has limited cutting ability. Laser, which can be aimed or placed in the proper location before activation, offers precision and some degree of hemostasis. Recently, an ultrasonic scalpel was developed that avoids both the smoke and char associated with other power techniques. Although the safety of these different instruments appears to be reasonably comparable, the difference in cost is dramatic and remains a significant concern.

Methods for Large-Vessel Occlusion. As techniques to remove tissue with significant blood supplies (e.g., adnexa, uterus) were developed, methods to effectively divide and occlude major vessels also were developed. Laparoscopic suture ligation, using either intra- or extracorporeal knot tying, is relatively slow and technically difficult. For this reason, four alternative approaches are now widely applied. Pretied loops, linear stapling devices, bipolar electrocautery, and ultrasonic coagulating shears are all reasonably expeditious and effective, although cases of delayed bleeding have been reported. Once again, differences in cost remain an important consideration.

Laparoscopic Procedures

Diagnostic Laparoscopy. This common procedure involves the placement of a 5- or 10-mm lens through an intraumbilical port, often with a 5-mm port placed above the symphysis for manipulation. Pelvic organs are closely inspected in a systematic fashion for signs of disease, and if tubal patency is an issue, a dilute dye solution is injected transcervically (chromopertubation). Biopsies can be obtained if malignancy is suspected.

Tubal Sterilization Procedures. As in diagnostic laparoscopy, a one- or two-port technique can be used. Tubes are occluded in the mid-isthmic section (approximately 3 cm from the cornua) using clips, elastic bands, or bipolar electrosurgery. With electrosurgery, approximately 2 cm of tube should be desiccated. Pregnancy rates after any of these techniques have been reported in the range of 3 per 1000 women.

Lysis of Adhesions. Pelvic adhesions usually are related to previous surgery, endometriosis, or infection, the latter of which can be either genital (i.e., pelvic inflammatory disease) or extragenital (e.g., ruptured appendix) in origin. Adhesions can be associated with decreased fertility or pain and can be lysed mechanically with scissors or any of the power techniques discussed above. Some degree of adhesion re-formation is unavoidable, and residual intrinsic tubal damage continues to interfere with fertility in most patients.

Adhesion re-formation can be minimized by achieving good hemostasis using discrete application of electrosurgery. Postoperatively, intraperitoneal solutions are used commonly to "hydrofloat" the adnexal structures, but controlled studies of their efficacy have been disappointing. Barrier methods have been shown to decrease adhesion formation in both animal and human studies but have not been demonstrated to improve outcome in terms of either subsequent pregnancies or pain relief.

Fulguration of Endometriosis. Conservative laparoscopic treatment of endometriosis increases fertility and often helps with pelvic pain. This condition and the various approaches to treatment were considered earlier in this chapter (see "Endometriosis").

Treatment of Ectopic Pregnancy. Laparoscopy has established itself as the primary treatment approach for ectopic pregnancies, a condition considered earlier in this chapter (see "Ectopic Pregnancy, Treatment").

Ovarian Cystectomy. The laparoscopic removal of ovarian cysts less than 6 cm in diameter in premenopausal women has become common. Using a multiple-port technique, the peritoneal cavity is inspected for signs of malignancy, including ascites, peritoneal or diaphragmatic implants, and liver involvement. In the absence of signs of malignancy, pelvic washings are obtained, and the ovarian capsule is excised with scissors or a power instrument. The cyst is shelled out carefully and placed in a bag, intact if possible. The bag opening is brought through the lower port incision along with the 10-mm port. The cyst is then drained and the cyst wall removed. Hemostasis of the ovary is achieved with bipolar electrosurgery, but the ovary is usually not closed, because this may increase postoperative adhesion formation. Except in the obvious cases of simple cysts, endometriomas, or dermoid cysts, the cyst wall should be sent for frozen section to verify the absence of the malignancy. If malignancy is detected, immediate definitive surgery, usually by laparotomy, is recommended. All cyst walls are sent for permanent section and pathologic diagnosis.

In many cases the cyst will rupture prior to removal. This is always the case with an endometrioma that contains "chocolate" fluid. On rupture, the cyst contents are thoroughly aspirated, and the cyst wall is removed and sent for pathologic evaluation. The peritoneal cavity is copiously rinsed with Ringer's lactate solution. This is especially important when a dermoid cyst is ruptured, because the sebaceous material can cause a chemical peritonitis unless all the visible oily substance is carefully removed.

Although malignancies are not commonly encountered using these guidelines, there is concern that rupture may worsen the patient's prognosis. Data are accumulating that suggest that cyst rupture may not alter prognosis. At the same time, laparoscopies in patients with ovarian malignancies are associated with an apparent high risk of port-site metastases. Based on conventional wisdom, every effort should be made to remove ovarian cysts without intraperitoneal spillage. When a malignancy is diagnosed, definitive surgical treatment should not be delayed.

Ovarian cysts larger than 6 cm and those discovered in post-menopausal women also can be removed laparoscopically. Because of the increased risk of malignancy associated with these situations, laparotomy is more commonly used. Laparoscopy may be a reasonable alternative in select patients if standard methods for staging are used in conjunction with appropriate frozen-section evaluation and expedient definitive therapy when indicated.

Removal of Adnexa. Occasionally, all or part of an adnexa must be removed. This may be the case with a large tubal pregnancy, a large hydrosalpinx, or when a small but growing cyst is found in a postmenopausal woman. Using a multiple-port technique, the vascular supply to the tissue is first desiccated with bipolar cautery and then divided with scissors. Alternatively, the ovarian vessels in the infundibulopelvic ligament can first be occluded with one of the techniques described earlier (see "Methods for Large-Vessel Occlusion"). Special care should be taken to identify and avoid the ureter, which lies retroperitoneally as it crosses the ovarian vessels and courses along the ovarian fossa (see Fig. 40-3).

Once the adnexa has been excised and hemostasis is achieved, attention is turned to removing the tissue from the peritoneal cavity. Small specimens can be removed using a retrieval bag via a 12-mm port. The port is removed with the sack, and the fascial incision is enlarged, if required.

For larger specimens, the opening of the sack is exposed outside the abdomen while the specimen remains in the abdomen. A cyst can be aspirated, and the remaining specimen can be removed piecemeal, taking care not to allow intraperitoneal spillage.

In difficult cases, the specimen can be removed via a colpotomy incision. For this procedure, a 12-mm port is placed through the posterior cul-de-sac under direct visualization. A retrieval sack is placed through the port, and the port and specimen in the sack are removed together. The distensible peritoneum and vaginal wall will allow the removal of a large specimen through a relatively small defect, which can then be closed with a running suture vaginally. Prophylactic antibiotics may decrease the risk of infection.

Myomectomy. Uterine leiomyomas are often approachable via the laparoscope. Hemostasis is assisted by intrauterine injection of dilute vasopressin (10 U in 50 mL) at the site of incision. Pedunculated leiomyomas can be excised at the base using scissors or a power instrument. Intramural leiomyomas require deep dissection into the uterine tissue, which must be closed subsequently with laparoscopic suturing techniques. Because myomectomies are associated with considerable postoperative adhesion formation, barrier techniques are used to decrease adhesion formation.

Removing the specimen can be difficult. In general, morcellation is required, and power morcellators have been developed that significantly expedite this technique. Although leiomyomas of any size or location technically can be removed laparoscopically, it is yet to be proven that either menorrhagia or infertility, the two most common indications for myomectomy, are as effectively treated laparoscopically as they are by laparotomy.

Hysterectomy. Laparoscopy was first used to restore normal anatomy prior to vaginal hysterectomy. More recently, laparoscopy has been used to perform some or all of the actual hysterectomy to avoid laparotomy in patients with known pelvic adhesions, endometriosis, or in whom the uterus is enlarged by leiomyoma. Although multiple variations in technique exist, there are three basic laparoscopic approaches for hysterectomy: laparoscopic-assisted vaginal hysterectomy (LAVH), laparoscopic hysterectomy (LH), and laparoscopic supracervical hysterectomy (LSH). While basic techniques for each of these methods have become somewhat standardized, the indications and relative risk for each remain controversial.

The technically simplest, and probably the most widely applied, is the LAVH. For this procedure, a multiple-port approach is used to survey the peritoneal cavity, and any pelvic adhesions are lysed. The round ligaments are then occluded and divided, and the uterovesical peritoneum is incised. Next, the proximal uterine blood supply is occluded and divided. When the ovaries are removed, the infundibulopelvic ligaments (containing the ovarian vessels) are divided. If the ovaries are conserved, the utero-ovarian ligament and blood vessels are divided and occluded. In some cases, the posterior cul-de-sac is also incised laparoscopically. The remainder of the case is performed vaginally, including dissection of the bladder from the anterior uterus, ligation of the uterine vessels, removal of the specimen, and closure of the vaginal cuff.

A LH differs from an LAVH in that almost the entire hysterectomy is performed laparoscopically. This procedure is used for the indications listed above and also when lack of uterine descent makes the vaginal approach impossible.

LH is begun in a manner identical to LAVH. But after the proximal uterine blood supply is divided, the bladder is dissected from the anterior uterus. This is followed by a retroperitoneal dissection in which the ureter is identified along its entire pelvic course and the uterine vessels are selectively occluded and divided. The uterosacral ligaments are likewise divided and the posterior cul-de-sac incised. The specimen is removed vaginally, and the vaginal cuff is closed. The drawback to this approach is the reported increased risk of bladder and ureter injuries as compared to both abdominal and vaginal approach for hysterectomy.

The third common laparoscopic approach is the LSH. This procedure has been advocated for all benign indications for hysterectomy. Technically, it is begun in a manner identical to the first two approaches. However, after the proximal vessels are divided and the bladder is dissected from the anterior uterus, the ascending branches of the uterine arteries are occluded and the entire uterine fundus is removed from the cervix. The endocervix is either cauterized or cored out with a special instrument. The fundus is then morcellated and removed through a 12-mm abdominal port or through a special transcervical morcellator. The end result is an intact cervix and cuff, with no surgical dissection performed near the uterine artery and adjacent ureter. This approach avoids both a large abdominal incision and a vaginal incision. According to its advocates, this approach minimizes operating time, recovery time, and risk of both infection and ureteral injury. LSH has yet to be widely applied, in part out of concern for the subsequent risk of developing cancer in the residual cervical stump.

Oncologic Procedures. As techniques developed, it became apparent that laparoscopy also could be applied to oncologic procedures. In addition to the treatment of potentially malignant ovarian cysts, the laparoscopic approach also has been used for "second-look" and staging procedures, including peritoneal washes and biopsy, partial omentectomy, and pelvis and periaortic lymphadenectomy. If positive nodes are discovered, treatment options often do not include laparotomy, and thus major surgery can be avoided without compromising patient prognosis. Laparoscopic approaches have been developed for definitive procedures, notably laparoscopically-assisted radical vaginal hysterectomy.

A guiding principle is that the same care must be rendered laparoscopically that would be performed by laparotomy with the same or less risk of complications. Until the relative risk of complications and effect on prognoses have been established for these approaches compared with laparotomy, application of the laparoscopic approach in gynecologic oncology will remain highly controversial.

Risks of Laparoscopy. The many unique aspects of laparoscopy contribute to the distinctive complications associated with this approach.

Gas Embolism. Because pressurized CO_2 is used routinely to insufflate the abdomen for laparoscopy, gas embolization continues to be a rare but serious complication. This is related most commonly to misplacement of the Veress needle used for insufflation prior to primary trocar insertion. If the tip of the needle inadvertently enters the aorta or its branches, temporary distal arterial occlusion will result. Because CO_2 is quickly absorbed, no serious sequelae have been reported as a result of arterial embolization, but arterial bleeding from this injury can be serious.

In contrast, inadvertent insufflation of the inferior vena cava or any of its venous branches can be fatal. Massive CO_2 embolism can result in partial or complete pulmonary arterial obstruction. This serious complication can be avoided in most cases by careful determination of Veress needle location prior to insufflation. Techniques for this include (1) ensuring lateral mobility of the needle because retroperitoneal penetration will prevent this; (2) aspirating through the needle with a syringe to detect intravascular placement; and (3) use of the "hanging drop test," in which a drop of saline placed on the hub of the needle is pulled into the hub of the needle when the abdominal wall is elevated to verify intraperitoneal placement. If any of these tests is not reassuring, the needle should be removed and replaced into the peritoneal cavity.

When CO_2 embolism is encountered, swift recognition and treatment can be lifesaving. Removal of the needle and placement of the patient in left lateral decubitus position are the first steps. In the presence of extreme hypotension, external cardiac massage has been suggested to break up large bubbles. Definitive treatment of this condition is central line placement and aspiration of the gas from the right-sided heart chambers and pulmonary vasculature.

Injury to Abdominal Wall Vessels. Abdominal wall vessel injuries have become more common with the development of more complicated operative laparoscopic procedures that use lateral trocar placement and larger trocars. These vessels include the inferior ("deep") epigastric vessels, the superficial epigastric vessels, and the superficial circumflex iliac vessels (Fig. 40-29). Injury to the inferior epigastric artery can result in life-threatening hemorrhage. Injury to these or other vessels can result in significant hematoma or postoperative blood loss if unrecognized.

The primary methods to avoid vessel injury are knowledge of the vessels at risk and visualization of them prior to trocar placement when possible. The superficial vessels often can be seen and avoided by transillumination of the abdominal wall with the laparoscope. This is especially true in light-skinned and thin women. In contrast, the larger inferior epigastric vessels cannot be seen by transillumination because of their deeper location. But these vessels often can be seen laparoscopically and avoided as they course along the peritoneum between the lateral umbilical fold of the bladder and the insertion of the round ligament into the inguinal canal.

Because the vessels may not be visible in some patients either by transillumination or laparoscopically, it is important to know their most likely location and place lateral trocars accordingly. Although the traditional location used for lateral trocar placement was approximately 5 cm from the midline, a safer location may be 8 cm or more above the symphysis pubis and 8 cm from the midline, because both the superficial and inferior epigastric arteries are located approximately 5.5 cm from the midline (see Fig. 40-29).

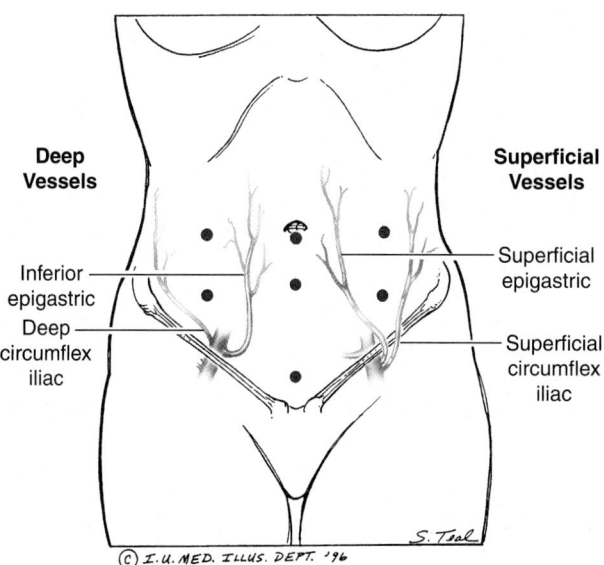

FIG. 40-29. *Location of anterior abdominal wall blood vessels.*

Anatomic variation and anastomoses between vessels make it impossible to know the exact location of all the abdominal wall vessels. For this reason, other strategies also should be used to avoid vessel injury, including the use of trocars with conical tips rather than pyramid tips, and the use of the smallest trocars possible lateral to the midline.

Injury to Retroperitoneal Major Vessels. Injury to major retroperitoneal vessels is one of the least common but most serious complications of the closed laparoscopic technique, occurring in approximately 3 per 10,000 laparoscopies. This includes both vessel perforation by the Veress needle with intravascular insufflation and vessel laceration by the 5- or 10-mm primary trocar.

Theoretically, the blind placement of sharp instruments through the umbilicus aimed toward the pelvis should rarely, if ever, result in vessel injury because both the aorta and the inferior vena cava bifurcate near level of the umbilicus. Unfortunately, in many patients the aortic bifurcation is at or below the level of the umbilicus, and in most patients the left common iliac vein crosses the midline below the umbilicus. The margin of error may be small, especially in thin patients, where the anteroposterior distance from the umbilicus to the retroperitoneal vessels may be as little as 2 to 3 cm (see Fig. 40-28).

The primary strategy to minimize the risk of vessel injury is to vary the angle of insertion based on the weight of the patient (see "Placement of the Veress Needle and Primary Trocar"). An alternative strategy to avoid the risk is the exclusive use of an open technique. Although techniques for open laparoscopy have been available for years, the majority of gynecologic laparoscopic procedures are performed using a closed rather than an open technique. Because of the potential advantage of laparoscopy in terms of patient recovery time, complications, and cost, new techniques and instruments continue to be developed and evaluated.

Intestinal Injury. Another potentially serious complication of laparoscopic surgery is injury to either small or large intestines. An unrecognized bowel injury may occur at the time of trocar insertion, especially if the patient has had previous abdominal procedures that often result in bowel adhesions to the anterior abdominal wall peritoneum. To minimize the risk of bowel injury in patients who have undergone previous laparotomy, many gynecologic surgeons recommend the use of an open technique.

Other factors that appear to alter the risk of bowel injury include establishment of pneumoperitoneum prior to trocar placement and the type of primary trocar used. Placing the primary trocar without establishing a pneumoperitoneum appears to increase the risk of bowel injury threefold. The extreme sharpness of disposable trocars makes insertion through the anterior abdominal wall easier, but also has the potential to increase the risk of bowel injury. In one series, the risk of bowel injury with disposable trocars was approximately three times that previously reported for reusable trocars. Although the majority of disposable trocars have automatically extending shields designed to decrease the risk of inadvertent injury to these structures, no study has examined the relative safety of disposable versus reusable trocars.

Another laparoscopic risk to bowel is thermal injuries that may occur when power sources are used, such as electrocautery or laser. Regardless of the cause, major bowel injuries usually become obvious during surgery. However, because of the limited field of view, some bowel injuries may not be seen during surgery. These injuries usually manifest 1 to 3 days after surgery, well after the patient has been released following these primarily outpatient procedures.

Urologic Injuries. Bladder injury is an uncommon laparoscopic injury, most commonly occurring as a result of retroperitoneal perforation during lower trocar placement or during sharp dissection of the bladder from the lower uterine segment during hysterectomy. The latter of these two situations is usually recognized intraoperatively; the first sign of the former may be postoperative hematuria or lower-port incisional drainage. Once diagnosed, large defects require layered closure, whereas smaller defects usually close spontaneously within days or weeks with the aid of transurethral catheter drainage.

Ureteral injury may occur as a result of any procedure that requires dissection or ligation of sidewall vessels, such as removal of an adnexa, because the ureter is adjacent to the pelvic peritoneum in the area of the ovarian fossa (see Fig. 40-3). This complication also has been reported after fulguration of endometriosis on the pelvic sidewall.

Another common cause of ureteral injury is hysterectomy, because the ureter is often located less than 2 cm from the cervix. This type of injury appears to be increased during laparoscopic hysterectomy when compared to abdominal or vaginal hysterectomy, apparently because of the modification of the standard techniques required for the laparoscopic approach.

Ureteral injuries, including complete ligation, partial resection, or thermal injuries, usually will manifest within hours to days of surgery. Complete obstruction most often manifests as flank pain, whereas the first sign of transection may be symptoms of intra-abdominal irritation caused by urine leakage. Transperitoneal thermal injuries resulting from fulguration of endometriosis may be similar to those after transection, but the appearance of symptoms may be delayed several days until tissue necrosis occurs.

Incisional Herniation. Incisional hernias after laparoscopy were rare prior to the use of large secondary ports (>5 mm) lateral to the midline. In recent times, incisional hernias have become a well-appreciated problem. A small peritoneal defect below the rectus abdominis muscle can allow bowel to become entrapped beneath the anterior rectus abdominis fascia. For this reason, closure of both the anterior and posterior layers of the rectus abdominus fascia is recommended whenever trocars greater than 5 mm are used. Special needles have been developed for this purpose.

Hysteroscopy

Hysteroscopy, like laparoscopy, has gained widespread support as a very useful technique for both diagnosis and treatment of intrauterine pathology and for ablation of the endometrium as an alternative to hysterectomy for the treatment of abnormal uterine bleeding.

General Hysteroscopic Techniques

Type of Instruments. Hysteroscopes can be divided into the categories of diagnostic, operative, and hysteroresectoscope. The lens for all three is identical. This is usually a fiberoptic lens and light source with an outside diameter of 3 mm and an objective lens that is offset up to 30 degrees from the long axis of the instrument. In contrast, the sleeves for the three types of hysteroscopes vary considerably. The diagnostic sleeve usually has an external diameter of 5 mm and a single-direction flow. Because outflow is limited, bleeding may impede a clear intrauterine view.

The operative sleeve, with an external diameter usually less than 10 mm, has a flow-through design with separate channels for input and outflow of distention media. A separate channel is available for placement of fine operating instruments.

The final type of sleeve is the hysteroresectoscope. This is also of a flow-through design and has an integral unipolar resecting loop identical to a urologic resectoscope. The loop can be replaced with a roller bar for endometrial ablation.

Distention Media and Pumps. Several distention media have found widespread use for hysteroscopy. For diagnostic hysteroscopy, CO_2 gives excellent clarity. Although it is extremely safe in general use, fatal gas embolisms have been reported when CO_2 was used after cervical dilatation or intrauterine surgery. To minimize this risk, CO_2 should be used for diagnostic hysteroscopy only with specifically designed pumps that are relatively high pressure (80 to 90 mm Hg) and low flow. More importantly, the use of CO_2 should be avoided after cervical dilatation or any uterine instrumentation.

For operative hysteroscopy, one of the first fluid media used was 32% dextran and 70% dextrose. This syrup-like substance is usually introduced by hand with a large syringe. The advantage is simplicity and low cost. The view is excellent in the absence of bleeding. The disadvantage is the difficulty in completely removing the substance from the instruments. If this solution is allowed to dry in critical movable points, the instrument may "freeze up," and it is very difficult to remove. In addition, intravascular intravasation can result in pulmonary edema.

More recently, aqueous solutions with pressure-controlled pumps have been used. For operative hysteroscopy, where electrosurgery is not being used, it is safest to use a balanced salt solution, such as Ringer's lactate. Moderate fluid intravasation will be of no consequence in a healthy individual. However, intravasation of larger volumes can result in fluid overload, especially in a patient with any cardiac compromise. To minimize this risk, the use of a fluid-medium pump is recommended rather than gravity or a pressure cuff. This allows the maximal pressure to be limited to approximately 80 mm Hg to prevent excess intravasation of distention media.

When electrosurgery is used for hysteroresectoscope excision of leiomyomas or roller-blade endometrial ablation, a nonconducting solution such as glycine must be used. Significant vascular intravasation can cause hyponatremia, potentially resulting in cerebral edema, coma, or even death. For this reason, protocols must be followed rigorously to detect and treat significant intravasation whenever these solutions are used. Intraoperatively, differences in distention medium input and output should be calculated every 15 minutes. If the difference is greater than 500 mL, a diuretic should be given. If the difference is greater than 1000 mL, the procedure also should be terminated. Whenever significant intravasation is suspected, serum sodium level should be checked immediately postoperatively and a few hours later because later hyponatremia, presumably due to transperitoneal absorption, has been reported.

Hysteroscopic Procedures

Diagnostic Hysteroscopy. This common procedure is often performed prior to uterine curettage to identify any focal abnormalities such as an endometrial polyp or a malignancy. This procedure is usually performed in the operating room with either general or regional anesthesia, although it has been performed by some as an office procedure with minimal analgesia.

After determining the position of the uterus, the anterior cervix is grasped with a tenaculum and traction placed to straighten the cervical canal. The lens and diagnostic sleeve are placed into the cervix, and distention medium is introduced with a pressure of 80 to 90 mm Hg. The hysteroscope is advanced slowly and carefully toward the fundus, using tactile and visual cues to avoid perforation. The entire uterine cavity is inspected, and any abnormal anatomy is documented. As the hysteroscope is withdrawn, the uterocervical junction and the endocervix are examined.

Directed Endometrial Biopsy. If a focal abnormality of the endometrium is observed, directed biopsy may be more accurate than a simple uterine curettage. The cervix is dilated to allow passage of an 8- to 10-mm flow-through operating hysteroscope, and a balanced salt solution is used for distention. Once the hysteroscope is positioned in the uterine cavity, the area of interest is biopsied under direct visualization.

Polypectomy. If an intrauterine polyp is discovered, the base of the polyp is incised with hysteroscopic scissors, and the polyp is grasped with grasping forceps. The hysteroscope, sleeve, and polyp are removed simultaneously, because most polyps will not fit through the operating channel. Extremely large polyps may have to be removed piecemeal. Any residual base of the polyp may be removed with biopsy forceps.

Uterine Septum Resection. A septum may be resected with scissors, electrosurgery, or laser. Scissors are used most commonly in light of the minimal vascularity of septa and the decreased potential for bowel injury should inadvertent uterine perforation occur. An operating hysteroscope is placed into the uterine cavity, which will appear to be two tubular structures rather than the broad uterine fundus usually encountered. The septum is then evenly divided across the fundus. If scissors are used, rather than a power cutting instrument, the presence of bleeding indicates that the level of resection is shifting from the avascular septum to the vascular myometrium. After surgery, no special device is placed in the uterus because intrauterine synechiae formation is uncommon.

Removal of Intrauterine Synechiae. Intrauterine synechiae are almost always associated with previous uterine curettage, especially when performed in the immediate postpartum period. These synechiae may result in amenorrhea or infertility.

The removal of synechiae is performed in a manner similar to that described above for a uterine septum, with some differences. The first is that the anatomy, and thus the visual cues for location of normal uterine wall, are completely unpredictable from patient to patient. Preoperative hysterosalpingography is usually very helpful. Findings can vary from a few small synechiae to complete obliteration of the cavity.

In difficult cases, simultaneous transabdominal ultrasound is extremely helpful in guiding the direction and limits of hysteroscopic resection. Standby laparoscopy should be available in the event of perforation, which is a significant risk in these patients. However, once pneumoperitoneum is achieved, abdominal ultrasound is no longer possible.

Following surgery, some type of intrauterine splint, such as an intrauterine device or a balloon catheter, is often placed to avoid synechia re-formation. Patients are usually placed on estrogen supplementation for a month and prophylactic antibiotics until the intrauterine splint is removed 1 to 2 weeks later.

Intrauterine Myomectomy. Pedunculated or submucosal leiomyoma can be removed safely hysteroscopically with subsequent improvement in both abnormal uterine bleeding and infertility. Because myoma tissue is relatively dense, a power cutting instrument is required. The choices are either laser or, more commonly, electrosurgery. For argon or Nd:YAG laser, a fiber is placed through the operating channel of the operating hysteroscope, and a balanced salt solution is used for distention. When electrosurgery is used via a hysteroresectoscope, an electrolyte-free solution, such as glycine or sorbitol, must be used because a balanced salt solution will dissipate the current and prevent cutting. Use of an electrolyte-free solution requires a thorough understanding of the potential risk and prevention of hyponatremia, because fatal complications have been reported with its use (see "Fluid Overload and Hyponatremia" below).

Both pedunculated and submucosal fibroids are shaved into small pieces with either the laser fiber or the hysteroresectoscope. In the case of a pedunculated fibroid, the urge to simply transect the stalk as a first step should be resisted unless the fibroid is 10 mm or less in size. Fibroids that are larger than this are difficult to remove in one piece without excessive cervical dilatation. Morcellation is much easier when the stalk is still attached for stability.

When the field of view is obscured by multiple pieces of tissue, the hysteroresectoscope is removed and the tissue collected in the urologic pouch. The hysteroscope is replaced in the uterus, and the procedure is repeated until the pedunculated fibroid and its stalk are completely removed, or the submucosal fibroid is shaved flush to the adjacent wall of the uterine cavity. After surgery, some gynecologists will treat the patient with estrogen or place an intrauterine splint as described above (see "Removal of Intrauterine Synechiae" above).

Endometrial Ablation. A common treatment for abnormal uterine bleeding in the absence of endometrial hyperplasia is ablation of the endometrium. In the recent past, this was performed with an operative hysteroscope using a laser fiber or with a resectoscope using an electrosurgical "roller barrel." As described previously for myoma resection, a balanced salt solution is used for laser resection, and an electrolyte-free solution is used for electrosurgery. For both techniques, the endometrium is destroyed down to the myometrium in a systematic fashion starting at the cornua and ending in the lower uterine segment. Electrosurgery has been used for resection of the endometrium with a loop electrode as well as for ablation. Both loop resection and laser ablation may have a somewhat greater chance of subsequent amenorrhea, but both appear to be technically more difficult with a greater risk of perforation than the more widely applied roller-barrel electrosurgical ablation.

More recently, hysteroscopic endometrial ablation has been widely supplanted by balloon thermal ablation. For this procedure, a probe with attached balloon is blindly placed into the uterus. Heated saline is circulated in the balloon to coagulate the endometrium. Balloon ablation requires less technical skill and appears to have less risk of complication than the hysteroscopic approaches.

Both hysteroscopic and balloon ablation techniques result in amenorrhea in approximately half the patients and decreased menstruation in another third of the patients over the first year of therapy. However, a large portion of these patients subsequently will require another ablative procedure for bleeding or a hysterectomy for residual bleeding or dysmenorrhea.

A theoretical risk of endometrial ablation is the delay of vaginal bleeding if the patient subsequently develops an endometrial malignancy. However, after more than a decade of widespread application of these techniques, this has not manifested as a significant risk. Nevertheless, the long-term risk of this problem remains uncertain and patients undergoing this procedure should be aware of this.

Risks of Hysteroscopy

Gas Embolism. Gas embolism has been reported when using CO_2 for distention after intrauterine surgery. It is recommended that CO_2 not be used for any operative procedure or after significant dilation of the cervix. If symptoms of massive gas embolism occur during diagnostic hysteroscopy, the procedure should be stopped and the patient treated as described above (see "Risks of Laparoscopy, Gas Embolism" above).

Fluid Overload and Hyponatremia. During operative hysteroscopy, significant intravasation of distention medium can occur through venous channels opened during surgery or transperitoneally as a result of any fluid forced through the tubes. Symptomatic fluid overload has been reported with all fluid distention media, including 32% dextran 70 in dextrose. The volume of distention medium introduced through the operating hysteroscope or hysteroresectoscope should always be compared with the volume retrieved using a urologic collection drape. When using a balanced salt solution (e.g., Ringer's lactate), symptomatic fluid overload is treated effectively with diuretics.

When electrolyte-free solutions are used for electrosurgery, the potential exists for serious and even fatal hyponatremia, even without significant fluid overload. Electrolyte-free solutions should not be used for hysteroscopy when electrosurgery is not required. When these solutions are used, careful monitoring of fluid balance should be performed every 15 minutes to detect intravasation.

Uterine Perforation and Bowel Injury. Uterine perforation is a common risk of uterine dilation prior to hysteroscopy. If it is not possible to distend the uterine cavity when the hysteroscope is placed in the uterus, perforation should be suspected. If no sharp instrument or power source has been placed through the defect, expectant outpatient management is appropriate.

Occasionally, perforation will occur during resection of a septum or leiomyoma or other operative procedures. If any chance of bowel injury exists, laparoscopy to evaluate contiguous bowel for injury is a reasonable precaution.

Intrauterine Synechia. The formation of adhesions between the anterior and posterior uterine walls, referred to as *synechiae,* is an uncommon complication after intrauterine surgery.

Although intrauterine devices, intrauterine catheters, and high-dose estrogen therapy have been advocated to decrease the risk of this complication, the efficacy of these treatments remains uncertain.

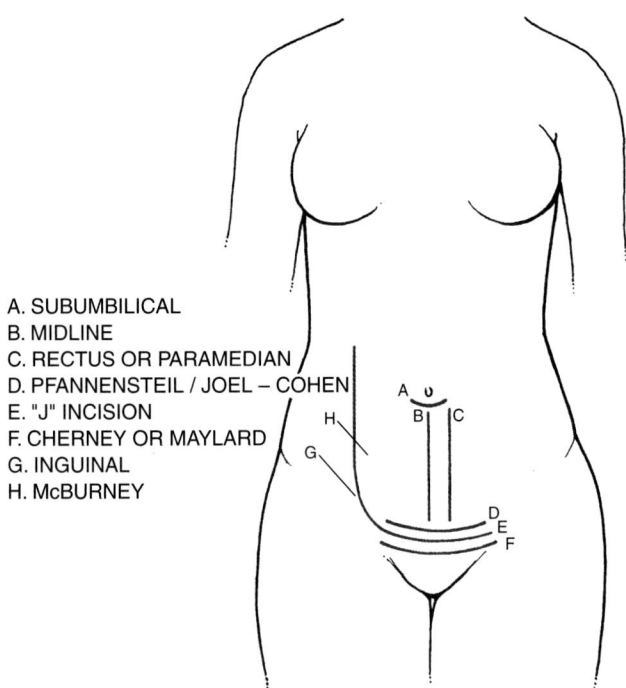

A. SUBUMBILICAL
B. MIDLINE
C. RECTUS OR PARAMEDIAN
D. PFANNENSTEIL / JOEL – COHEN
E. "J" INCISION
F. CHERNEY OR MAYLARD
G. INGUINAL
H. McBURNEY

FIG. 40-30. Incisions useful for pelvic surgery.

Abdominal Procedures

Incisions

The pelvic surgeon must consider a number of factors before beginning a pelvic operation. The most important requirement is that the incision provides adequate exposure for the anticipated procedure. Pelvic surgery is performed through vertical and transverse incisions. Figure 40-30 shows the majority of the incisions used in pelvic surgery. The midline incision is the most useful. It is simple and tends to bleed less than incisions made off the midline. The midline incision provides excellent exposure of the pelvis, and, when necessary, the entire abdomen is accessible for operation. This incision is more susceptible to hernia formation and is somewhat more uncomfortable than the transverse incision. The resulting scar occasionally is thicker than incisions made along Langer's lines, resulting in a less-desirable cosmetic result.

Transverse incisions are used more often by a pelvic surgeon because the entire incision is centered over the area of operative interest. The incisions are more comfortable postoperatively and heal with a lower incidence of dehiscence or hernia formation. The most common transverse incision is the Pfannenstiehl incision (Fig. 40-31). The skin is incised transversely approximately 2 cm above the symphysis pubis, and the incision is taken down to the rectus fascia, which is entered transversely. The rectus fascia is dissected bluntly away from the underlying rectus muscles in both a superior and inferior direction. The rectus muscles are separated in the midline, and the peritoneum is opened in the vertical midline.

The Maylard incision carries with it the advantages of a transverse incision but affords more exposure of the pelvis than that provided by the Pfannenstiehl. The skin is incised transversely approximately 2 cm above the symphysis pubis, and the rectus fascia is opened transversely but not separated from the underlying rectus muscles. The rectus muscles are cut directly under the fascial incision, and several small bleeders in the body of the rectus muscles are clamped and coagulated. The epigastric artery and vein located just

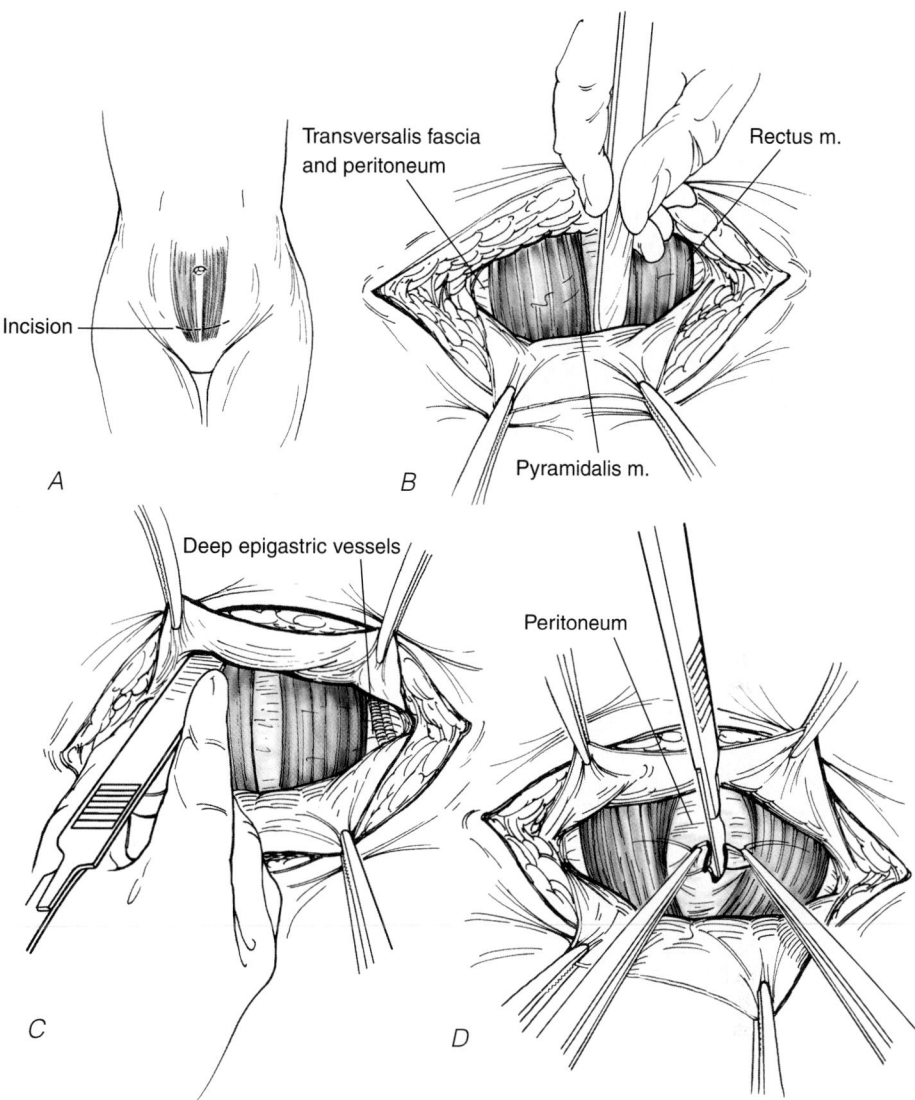

Incision

Transversalis fascia
and peritoneum

Rectus m.

Pyramidalis m.

A

B

Deep epigastric vessels

Peritoneum

C

D

FIG. 40-31. Pfannenstiehl incision
(see text for description).

below the lateral edge of the rectus muscles are ligated and cut; the peritoneum is then opened transversely to afford good visualization and access to the entire pelvis.

The Cherney incision provides the advantages of a transverse incision and all the visibility provided by the Maylard incision. The incision is made in the transverse direction in the lower abdomen approximately 2 cm above the symphysis, the rectus fascia is opened transversely, the lower portion of the rectus sheath is dissected free of the rectus muscle, and the insertion of the rectus muscles on the symphysis pubis is visualized. The tendon of the rectus muscle is then cut free of the symphysis pubis, and the muscle is allowed to retract upward. The peritoneum is opened transversely. This incision is repaired by simply sewing the rectus tendon to the lower aspect of the rectus sheath just above the symphysis before closing the rectus sheath at the completion of the operation.

All the incisions used in pelvic surgery have advantages as well as disadvantages. The pelvic surgeon should anticipate the need for surgical exposure in the upper abdomen and in such cases choose a vertical incision. The Pfannenstiehl incision is suitable for most operations for benign disease in the pelvis, but if wide pelvic or upper abdominal exposure is needed, the Maylard or Cherney incisions provide better operative exposure.

Hysterectomy for Benign Disease

The abdomen is entered through an appropriate incision. The upper abdomen is examined for evidence of extrapelvic disease, and a suitable retractor is placed in the abdominal wound. The self-retaining bowel is packed out of the pelvis and held in place with a retractor. The uterus is grasped at either cornu with Kocher clamps and pulled up into the wound (Fig. 40-32A). The round ligament is identified and suture ligated and cut (Fig. 40-32B). If the ovaries are to be removed, the peritoneal incision is extended from the round ligament lateral to the infundibulopelvic ligament for approximately 2.5 cm. The retroperitoneal space is bluntly opened. The ureter is identified on the medial leaf of the broad ligament. The infundibulopelvic ligament is isolated, clamped, and cut, and the suture ligated. A similar procedure is carried out on the opposite side.

In the event that the ovaries are not to be removed, after ligating the round ligament, an avascular area in the broad ligament is chosen and the broad ligament bluntly fractured with a finger, producing an opening below the ovarian ligament and fallopian tube (see Fig. 40-32C). The fallopian tube and ovarian ligament are clamped, cut, and ligated.

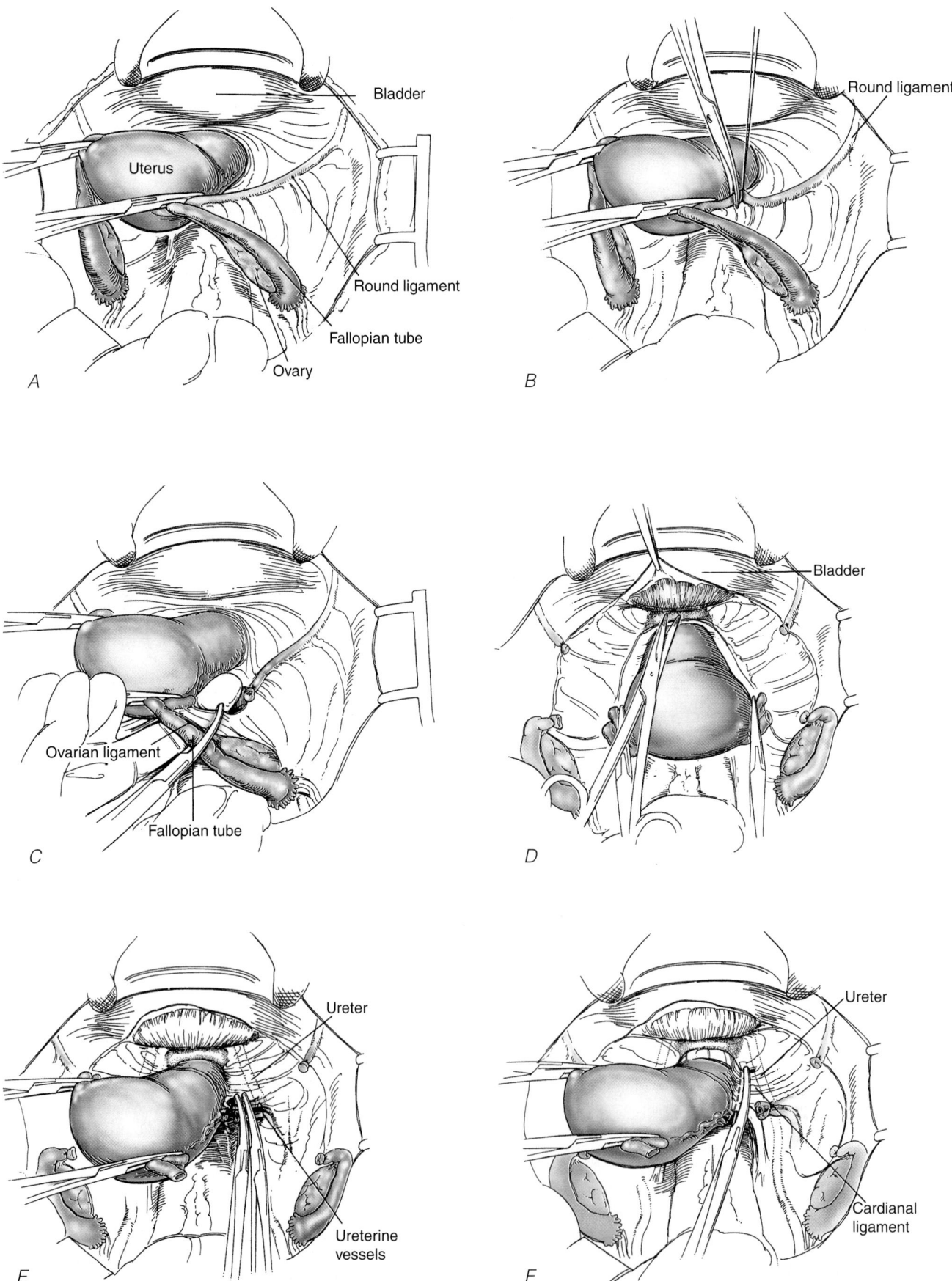

FIG. 40-32. *Hysterectomy. A.* The uterus grasped at the cornua. *B.* The round ligament is cut. *C.* The ovarian ligament and fallopian tube are isolated. *D.* The bladder is mobilized. *E.* The uterine vessels are clamped. *F.* The cardinal ligaments are clamped. *(Continued)*

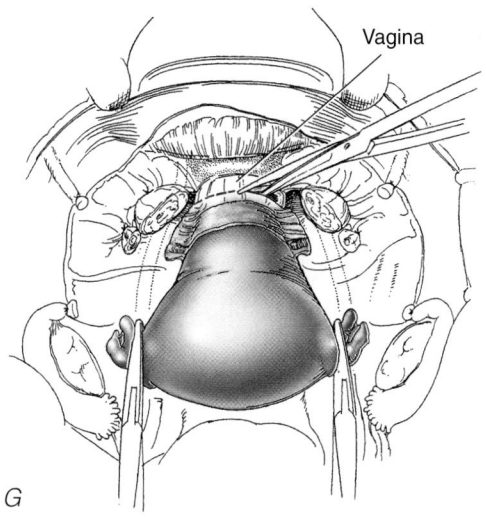

Vagina

G

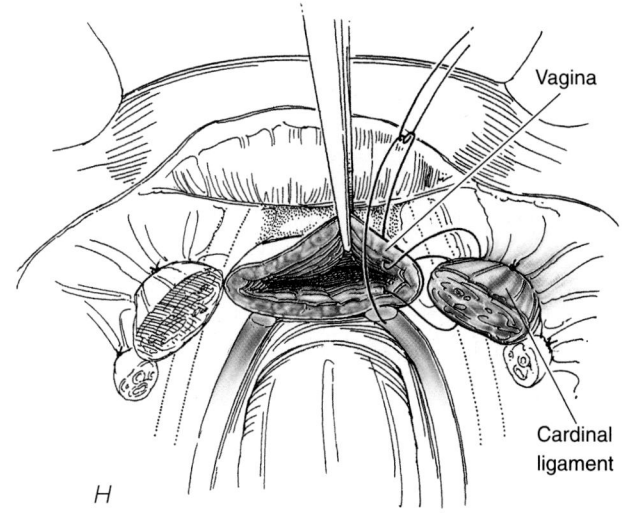

Vagina

Cardinal
ligament

H

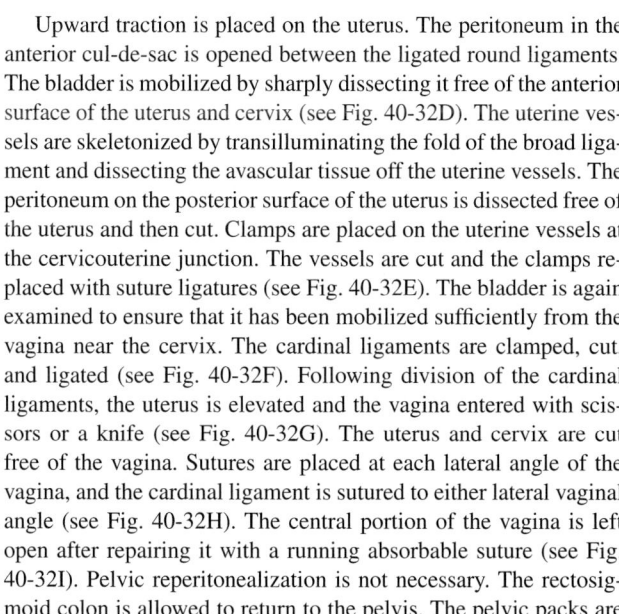

Vagina

© *I.U. MED.ILLUS. DEPT. '92*

I

FIG. 40-32. *(continued) G.* The vagina is entered. *H.* The cardinal ligaments are sutured to the vagina. *I.* The vagina is "closed open."

Upward traction is placed on the uterus. The peritoneum in the anterior cul-de-sac is opened between the ligated round ligaments. The bladder is mobilized by sharply dissecting it free of the anterior surface of the uterus and cervix (see Fig. 40-32D). The uterine vessels are skeletonized by transilluminating the fold of the broad ligament and dissecting the avascular tissue off the uterine vessels. The peritoneum on the posterior surface of the uterus is dissected free of the uterus and then cut. Clamps are placed on the uterine vessels at the cervicouterine junction. The vessels are cut and the clamps replaced with suture ligatures (see Fig. 40-32E). The bladder is again examined to ensure that it has been mobilized sufficiently from the vagina near the cervix. The cardinal ligaments are clamped, cut, and ligated (see Fig. 40-32F). Following division of the cardinal ligaments, the uterus is elevated and the vagina entered with scissors or a knife (see Fig. 40-32G). The uterus and cervix are cut free of the vagina. Sutures are placed at each lateral angle of the vagina, and the cardinal ligament is sutured to either lateral vaginal angle (see Fig. 40-32H). The central portion of the vagina is left open after repairing it with a running absorbable suture (see Fig. 40-32I). Pelvic reperitonealization is not necessary. The rectosigmoid colon is allowed to return to the pelvis. The pelvic packs are removed and the small bowel is allowed to return to the pelvis. The omentum is placed over the bowel and under the abdominal wound. The abdominal wound is closed in an appropriate manner. In some circumstances, uterine myomata interfere with the operative procedure and myomectomy or supracervical hysterectomy might be accomplished before removing the cervix.

Myomectomy

Myomectomy should be performed through an incision that will allow good visibility of the pelvis. Hemostasis for the procedure is aided by the placement of a Penrose drain (Fig. 40-33A) around the base of the uterus and pulled through small perforations in the broad ligament lateral to the uterine blood supply on either side. This "uterine tourniquet" is held in place with a clamp.

Further hemostasis may be obtained by placing bulldog or rubber-shod clamps on the infundibulopelvic ligament in order to control the utero-ovarian blood supply. When possible, the uterine incision should be made in the anterior surface of the uterus in order to reduce the incidence of postoperative adhesions. An incision is made through the uterine musculature (see Fig. 40-33B) into the

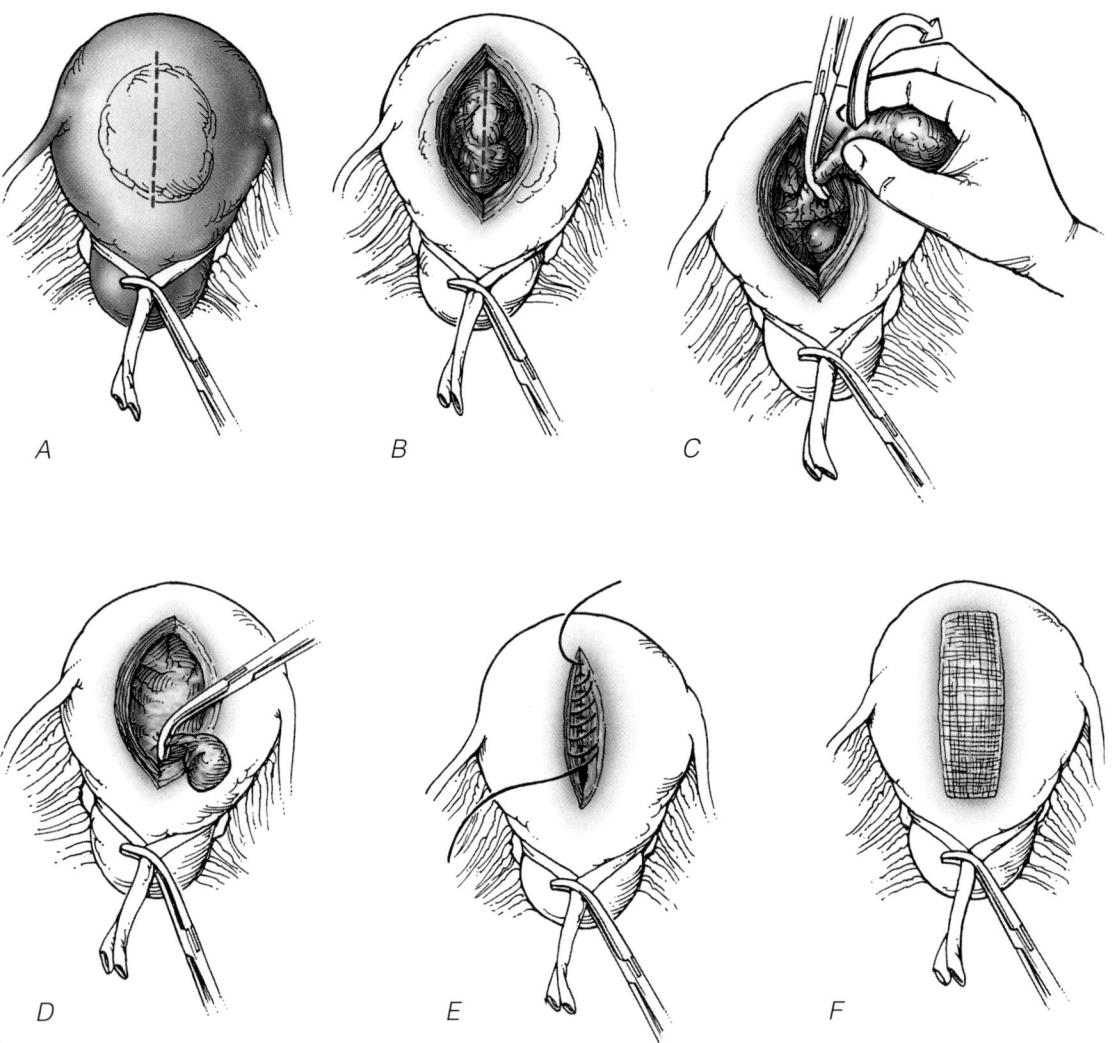

FIG. 40-33. Myomectomy. *A.* Hemostatic "tourniquet" in place before myomectomy. *B.* Uterine incision for myomectomy. *C.* Removal of myoma. *D.* Several myomas may be removed through a single incision. *E.* The uterine wound is closed with absorbable suture. *F.* The uterine wound covered with mesh to retard adhesions.

myoma. The pseudocapsule surrounding the tumor is identified and the tumor is bluntly dissected out with scissors, a knife handle, or a finger. After the tumor is freed of its lateral attachments, it can be twisted to expose a pedicle that frequently contains its major blood supply (see Fig. 40-33C). On occasion, several myomas may be removed through a single incision (see Fig. 40-33D). The uterine wounds are closed with absorbable sutures to obliterate the dead space and provide hemostasis (see Fig. 40-33E). The uterine serosa is closed with a 000 absorbable suture placed subserosally if possible. A patch of Interceed to cover the uterine incision may prevent adhesion formation(Fig. 40-33F).

Radical Hysterectomy (Modified from Okabayashi)

The patient is placed in a modified lithotomy position with legs in obstetric stirrups, hips abducted 45 degrees and flexed 15 degrees. The peritoneal cavity is entered through a Maylard incision (Fig. 40-34A) after ligating and dividing the inferior epigastric vessels (Fig. 40-34B). The Maylard incision permits unequaled exposure of structures on the lateral pelvic sidewall. Access to the retroperitoneum is obtained by dividing the round ligaments (Fig. 40-34C).

A U-shaped incision is carried from one lateral abdominal gutter to the other, including the peritoneum of the bladder reflection (Fig. 40-34D). The pararectal and paravesical spaces are opened using blunt digital or instrument dissection, and narrow rigid retractors are placed to maintain exposure (Fig. 40-34E). Pelvic lymphadenectomy is performed by removing lymph nodes from the external, internal, and common iliac vessels (Fig. 40-34F), as well as the obturator fossa (Fig. 40-34G). If there are no pelvic lymph node metastases, para-aortic lymph node sampling is unnecessary. Isolation of the superior vesicle artery by lateral retraction brings the uterine artery into view; this vessel is skeletonized and clipped at its origin from the anterior division of the internal iliac artery (Fig. 40-34H). The branches of the posterior division are generally not visualized at the time of radical hysterectomy. Next, the structures inferior to the uterine artery in the cardinal ligament are clamped and divided (Fig. 40-34I); freeing the cervix and upper vagina from the lateral pelvic sidewall. A linear stapling device may expedite this portion of the procedure.

At this point, the proper ovarian ligaments and the proximal fallopian tubes may be transected between clamps (see Fig. 40-34J). After the ovarian vessels are mobilized, the ovaries may be marked

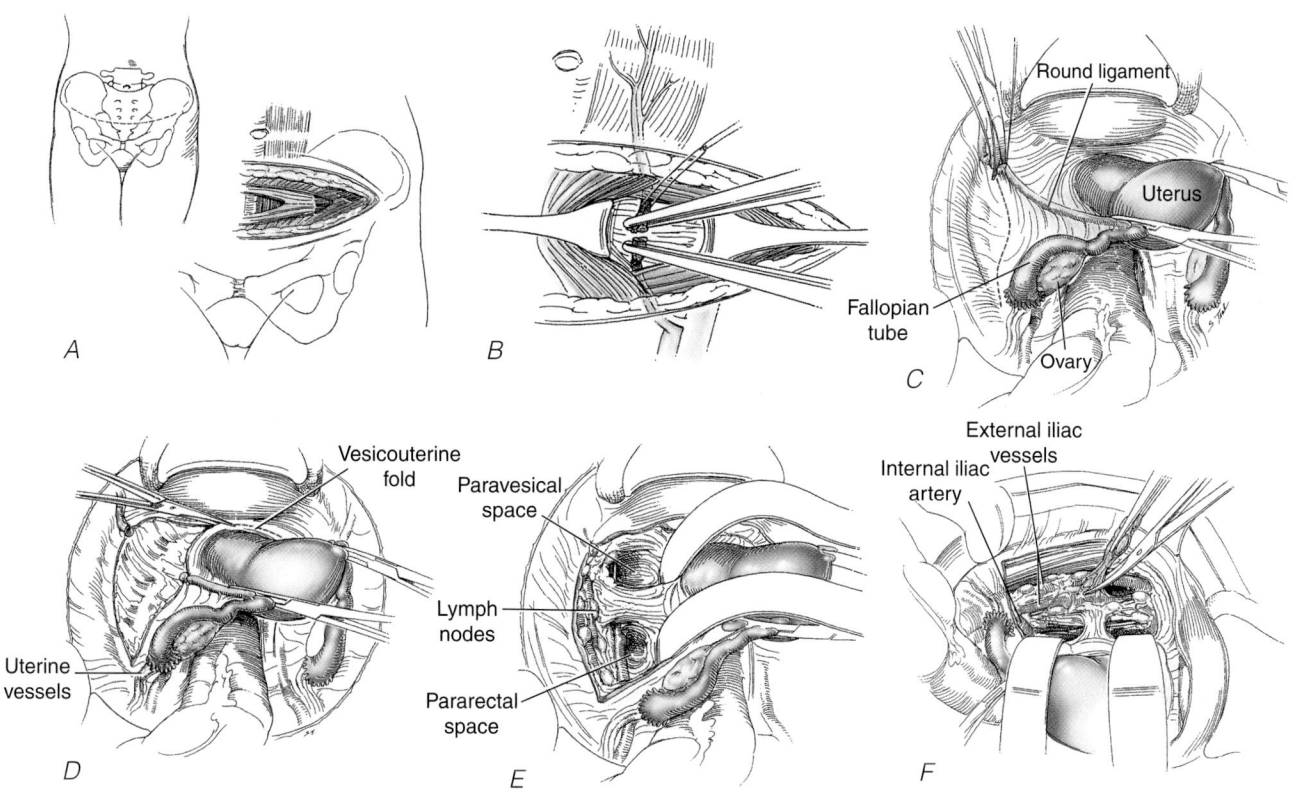

FIG. 40-34. *Radical hysterectomy. A. Exposure of the inferior epigastric vessels before transection of the rectus muscles. B. Ligation of the inferior epigastric vessels before transection of the rectus muscles. C. Ligation and division of the round ligaments opens the pelvic retroperitoneum. D. First peritoneal incision lateral to the ovarian vessels and across the vesicouterine fold. E. Narrow malleable retractors (Indiana retractors) are placed into the paravesical and pararectal spaces to provide excellent access to the lateral pelvic sidewall and pelvic lymph nodes. F. Pelvic lymphadenectomy (external and internal iliac vessels). (Continued)*

with vascular clips and suspended in the lateral abdominal gutters above the pelvic brim. This measure protects the ovaries if postoperative pelvic radiotherapy is to be given. The ureters are carefully detached from the posterior leaves of the broad ligament for a short distance and retracted laterally (Fig. 40-34K) before the posterior cul-de-sac is entered and the rectovaginal space developed bluntly (see Fig. 40-34L); the uterosacral ligaments are divided. Upward traction on the uterus facilitates dissection of the bladder inferiorly away from the underlying cervix and upper vagina. The ureters are freed from their investment in the paracervical tissue, allowing the bladder and ureters to be displaced inferolaterally, exposing the upper vagina and paravaginal tissues. The tissues are clamped and cut, taking care to remove a 3- to 4-cm "cuff" of vagina with the cervix (see Fig. 40-34M). The vagina is closed, a suprapubic catheter is inserted, and the abdominal incision is repaired.

Radical hysterectomy is associated with 85 to 90% cure rates in patients without lymph node, parametrial, or marginal involvement, and with 65 to 70% cure rates in those with spread to the regional nodes. The primary morbidity is bladder denervation, which occurs to some extent in almost all women undergoing this procedure. Generally, loss of bladder sensation is the only deficit, although inability to void is not uncommon in the immediate postoperative period. Rectal dysfunction may result in difficult defecation. Ureterovaginal fistulas occur in approximately 1% of all patients in recent studies.

Postoperative external beam radiotherapy may be elected if nodal metastases, positive surgical margins, or parametrial tissue

involvement is found. Because bladder and ureteral complications are more common in women undergoing postoperative radiotherapy, surgical candidates must be chosen with care.

Resection of Ovarian Cancer

Radical or modified radical hysterectomy is indicated in the treatment of epithelial ovarian cancer only if peritoneal tumor nodules obliterate the posterior cul-de-sac or extend to the retroperitoneal spaces. Generally, extrafascial (simple or conservative) hysterectomy (see Fig. 40-20) suffices in the resection of these tumors.

When hysterectomy and salpingo-oophorectomy are completed, the infracolic omentum should be removed by reflecting the fatty organ superiorly, isolating and dividing the right and left gastroepiploic vessels, and dissecting through the avascular posterior leaf before isolating and dividing the vessels in the anterior leaf of the omentum. If the omentum contains a large amount of disease, the gastrocolic omentum should be removed by isolating and dividing the short gastric vessels along the greater curvature of the stomach. In cases of extensive omental involvement, care must be taken not to injure the spleen, stomach, or transverse colon. Generous peritoneal biopsies should be obtained from the right hemidiaphragm, both lateral abdominal gutters, and the anterior and posterior peritoneum of the pelvis.

If gross intraperitoneal tumor is completely resected, the lymph nodes should be evaluated. The left para-aortic lymph nodes may be exposed by reflecting the sigmoid colon medially. These lymph

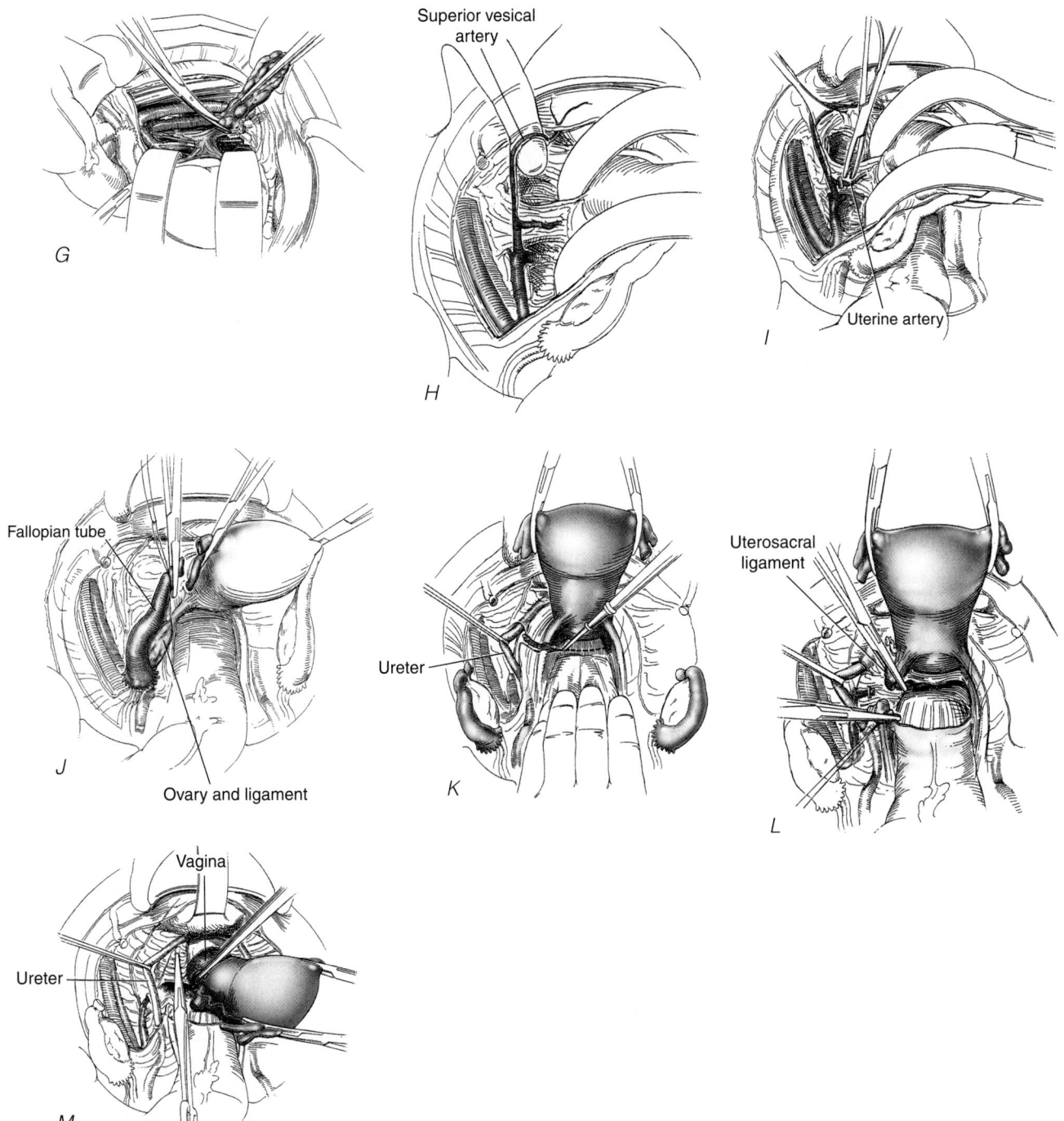

FIG. 40-34. *(continued) G.* Pelvic lymphadenectomy (obturator fossa). *H.* Development of the uterine and superior vesical arteries. *I.* The uterine artery has been clipped and divided near its origin. *J.* The proper ovarian ligament and proximal fallopian tube is clamped and divided if the ovary is to be preserved. *K.* The ureters have been detached from the posterior peritoneum of the broad ligament and are retracted laterally. The rectovaginal space is developed using blunt finger dissection. *L.* Transection of the uterosacral ligaments. *M.* Clamps are placed on the lateral vagina, taking care to remove 3 to 4 cm of the upper vagina.

nodes should be liberally sampled, keeping in mind that the primary venous drainage of the left ovary is the left renal vein and that of the right ovary is the inferior vena cava at the level of the renal vein. Metastases are more common above than below the inferior mesenteric artery. The right para-aortic lymph nodes may be sampled transperitoneally or by mobilizing the ileocecal area and reflecting it superiorly.

Pelvic lymph node sampling is also an important aspect of surgical staging in ovarian cancer and is completed by removing lymph nodes from the distribution of the external and internal iliac vessels and obturator space above the level of the obturator nerve. This part of the staging procedure is facilitated by first opening the paravesical and pararectal spaces as described for radical hysterectomy above. Lymph node sampling is primarily a diagnostic procedure in the

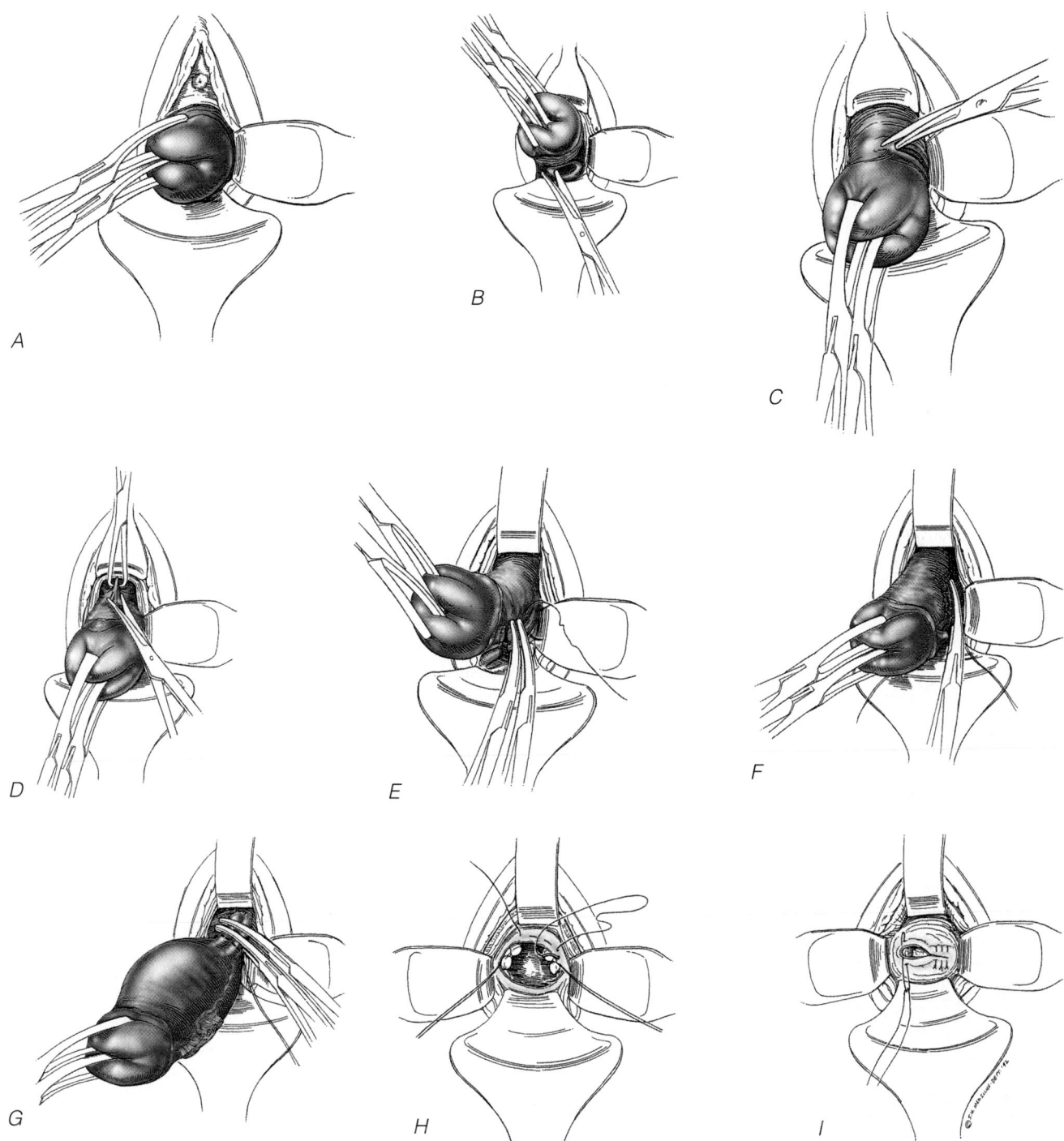

FIG. 40-35. Vaginal hysterectomy. *A.* Traction is placed on the uterus. *B.* The posterior cul-de-sac is entered. *C.* The vaginal mucosa is circumcised. *D.* The anterior cul-de-sac is entered. *E.* The uterosacral ligaments are clamped. *F.* The uterosacral ligaments are tied. *G.* The fallopian tube, round ligament, and ovarian ligament are ligated. *H.* The peritoneum is closed. *I.* The vaginal mucosa is closed.

management of early ovarian cancers. There is little evidence that complete lymphadenectomy is therapeutic in patients with advanced and unresected disease.

Vaginal Procedures

Hysterectomy

The removal of the uterus through the vagina is preferred in many cases of myoma, uterine prolapse, intraepithelial neoplasia,

and uterine bleeding disorders. Patients are more comfortable and operative time, hospital stay, and recovery time are shorter than in cases of abdominal operation. Vaginal hysterectomy is an acceptable approach in those patients in whom the uterus descends, the bony pelvis allows vaginal operation, the uterine tumors are small enough to permit vaginal removal, and the patient is amenable to vaginal operation. In the presence of large myomas, pretreatment with a GnRHa will allow vaginal operation that would have been impossible previously.

The patient is placed in a high lithotomy position, and the pelvis is examined under anesthesia. This examination should confirm previous findings and provide assurance that the operation is possible through the vaginal route. The bladder is not catheterized before operation unless it is greatly distended. A weighted vaginal speculum is placed in the posterior vagina, and the cervix is grasped with a tenaculum and pulled in the axis of the vagina (Fig. 40-35A). The posterior cul-de-sac is identified and entered with scissors (Fig. 40-35B). Mayo scissors are used to circumcise the cervix, and the mucosa is cut down to the pubocervical-vesical fascia (Fig. 40-35C). The vaginal mucosa and the bladder are sharply and bluntly dissected free of the cervix and the lower portion of the uterus. Care must be taken not to injure the bladder.

When the peritoneum of the anterior cul-de-sac is identified, it is entered with the scissors, and a retractor is placed in the defect (see Fig. 40-35D). The uterosacral ligaments are identified, doubly clamped, cut, and doubly ligated (see Fig. 40-35E). The second ligature is held long. Serial clamps are placed on the parametrial structures above the uterosacral ligament; these pedicles are cut, and the clamps are replaced with ties (see Fig. 40-35F). At the cornu of the uterus, the tube, round ligament, and suspensory ligament of the ovary are doubly clamped and cut (see Fig. 40-35G). The procedure is carried out on the opposite side, and the uterus is removed. The first clamp is replaced with a free tie; the second clamp is replaced with a suture ligature that is transfixed. The second suture ligature is held long. The pelvis is inspected for hemostasis; all bleeding must be meticulously controlled at this point.

The pelvic peritoneum is closed with a running purse-string suture incorporating those pedicles which were held (see Fig. 40-35H). This exteriorizes those areas which might tend to bleed. The sutures attached to the ovarian pedicles are cut. The vagina may be closed with interrupted mattress stitches, incorporating the uterosacral ligaments into the corner of the vagina with each lateral stitch (see Fig. 40-35I). The vaginal cuff is inspected again for hemostasis. In most cases, no vaginal packing is required. A catheter is left in the bladder until the patient has fully awakened and is ambulatory.

On occasion, the uterus, which is initially too large to remove vaginally, may be reduced in size by morcellation (Fig. 40-36). After the uterine vessels have been clamped and ligated, serial wedges are taken from the central portion of the uterus in order to reduce the uterine mass. This procedure will allow the vaginal delivery of even very large uterine leiomyomas.

Pessaries

The vaginal pessary has been used since ancient times. It involves placing a plastic or rubber device into the vagina to support the vaginal apex and the vaginal walls. The device is finding little use in modern gynecology. When pessaries are used, they should be removed at least every 4 weeks. They produce discomfort secondary to pelvic pressure, and vaginal ulceration secondary to pressure necrosis is common.

Injuries Associated with Pelvic Surgery

Intestinal Injury. Adhesion formation is the most common antecedent to enterotomy at the time of pelvic operation. When lysis of adhesions is carefully carried out, this complication should occur rarely. Injuries to the small bowel range from serosal tears to through-and-through lacerations. Serosal tears are usually oversewn with a 4-0 nonabsorbable suture. Injuries to the lumen of the bowel are generally repaired using single- or double-layer closure; a single layer of 4-0 absorbable suture followed by an outer layer of

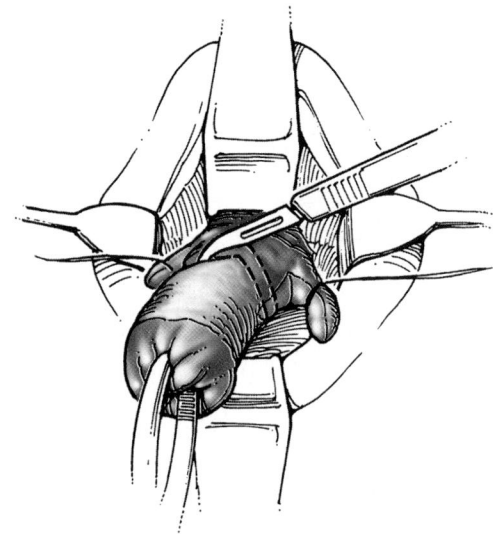

FIG. 40-36. Uterine morcellation through the vagina.

interrupted nonabsorbable suture is effective. Lacerations that are extensive or involve multiple areas should be treated by resecting the injured segment.

Injury to the colon may occur during an operation to remove a left adnexal mass. When this injury occurs in a prepared colon, it is primarily repaired in a two-layer closure similar to that used in a small bowel repair. Large injuries may require resection of a segment of the colon.

Injury to the unprepared large bowel is a significant problem. A small wound that is promptly recognized may be treated primarily with a single- or double-layer closure. The patient should be treated with intraoperative and postoperative antibiotics to cover both anaerobic and aerobic organisms. A major injury to unprepared large bowel will require colostomy in most cases.

Ureteral Injury. Ureteral injury at the time of pelvic surgery is uncommon and largely preventable. The ureters are at highest risk when the infundibulopelvic ligament is clamped for removal of an ovary and when the uterine arteries or cardinal ligaments are clamped during the course of hysterectomy. In most cases, visualization or palpation of the ureter before placing a hemostatic clamp will avoid this complication. The ureter is at highest risk in the course of pelvic operation for endometriosis, pelvic inflammatory disease, and pelvic neoplasia. The surgery for most of these conditions allows the dissection of the ureter beginning at the pelvic brim with meticulous exposure down to and through the operative field. Transection of the ureter high in the pelvis may allow primary reanastomosis of the ureter. Ureteral injuries near the bladder generally require ureteral reimplantation into the bladder.

Bladder Injury. The pelvic surgeon must be constantly aware of the proximity of the bladder to the cervix and the anterior portion of the uterine fundus. The bladder must be dissected carefully free of the cervix at the time of hysterectomy. Hemostasis should be meticulous, and large clamps and ligatures should be avoided to prevent devitalization of the bladder wall. Operative entry into the bladder should be recognized immediately. If there is any question about the integrity of the bladder at the time of hysterectomy, a dilute solution of methylene blue will detect the defect and allow for closure.

Bladder injuries must be fully visualized in preparation for repair irrespective of whether they were produced by vaginal or abdominal operation. The surgeon must ascertain that the wound does not involve the ureter and that the resulting repair will not compromise ureteral function. At either extent of the bladder laceration, 4-0 polyglycolic acid sutures are placed and held for retraction. The suture does not enter the lumen of the bladder. Once the bladder injury is delineated by the two initial sutures, the wound is closed with 4-0 interrupted polyglycolic acid suture in a running mattress stitch in order to strengthen the first layer and to remove any tension produced by the initial closure. An indwelling catheter should remain in the bladder for 5 to 7 days or until microscopic hematuria has disappeared. Some pelvic surgeons test their repair with a small amount of sterile milk. Milk is preferred to methylene blue or indigo carmine because it will not stain the tissue, allowing subsequent testing.

Bibliography

Baggish MS, Sze EH: Endometrial ablation: A series of 568 patients treated over an 11-year period. *Am J Obstet Gynecol* 174:908, 1966.

Copeland LJ: *Textbook for Gynecology*. St. Louis: CV Mosby, 1993.

Herbst AL, Michell D, et al: *Comprehensive Gynecology*, 2d ed. St. Louis: CV Mosby, 1992.

Hoskins WJ, Perez. CA, Young RC (eds): *Gynecologic Oncology*. Philadelphia: JB Lippincott, 1992.

Hurd WW, Bude RO, et al: The location of abdominal wall blood vessels in relationship to abdominal landmarks apparent at laparoscopy. *Am J Obstet Gynecol* 171:642, 1994.

Kurman RJ: *Blaustein's Pathology of the Female Genital Tract*, 4th ed. New York: Springer-Verlag, 1994.

Lee RH: *Atlas of Gynecologic Surgery*. Philadelphia: WB Saunders, 1992.

Nichols DH: *Gynecologic and Obstetric Surgery*. St Louis: CV Mosby, 1993.

Rubin SC, Sutton GP (eds): *Ovarian Cancer*, 2nd ed. New York: McGraw-Hill, 2002.

Saidi MH, Sadler RK, et al: Diagnosis and management of serious urinary complications after major operative laparoscopy. *Obstet Gynecol* 87:272, 1996.

Shingleton HM, Fowler WC, et al (eds): *Gynecologic Oncology*. Philadelphia: WB Saunders, 1996.

Singer A, Monaghan JM: *Lower Genital Tract Precancer*. Boston: Blackwell Scientific, 1994.

Speroff L, Glass RH, Kase NG: *Clinical Gynecologic Endocrinology and Infertility*, 5th ed. Baltimore: Williams and Wilkins, 1994.

Steege JF: Laparoscopic approach to the adnexal mass. *Clin Obstet Gynecol* 37:392, 1994.

Thompson JD, Rock JA (eds): *TeLinde's Operative Gynecology*, 7th ed. Philadelphia: JB Lippincott, 1992.

CHAPTER 41

Neurosurgery

Michael L. Smith and M. Sean Grady

Neurologic surgery is a discipline of medicine and the specialty of surgery that provides the operative and nonoperative management (i.e., prevention, diagnosis, evaluation, treatment, critical care, and rehabilitation) of disorders of the central, peripheral, and autonomic nervous systems, including their supporting structures and vascular supply; the evaluation and treatment of pathologic processes that modify the function or activity of the nervous system, including the hypophysis; and the operative and nonoperative management of pain. As such, neurologic surgery encompasses the treatment of adult and pediatric patients with disorders of the nervous system. These disorders include those of the brain, meninges, skull and skull base, and their blood supply, including surgical and endovascular treatment of disorders of the intracranial and extracranial vasculature supplying the brain and spinal cord; disorders of the pituitary gland; disorders of the spinal cord, meninges, and vertebral column, including those that may require treatment by fusion, instrumentation, or endovascular techniques; and disorders of the cranial and spinal nerves throughout their distribution.

An accurate history is the first step toward neurologic diagnosis. A history of trauma or of neurologic symptoms is of obvious interest, but general constitutional symptoms also are important. Neurologic disease may have systemic effects, while diseases of other symptoms may affect neurologic function. The patient's general medical ability to withstand the physiologic stress of anesthesia and surgery should be understood. A detailed history from the patient and/or family, along with a reliable physical examination will clarify these issues.

NEUROANATOMY

An understanding of neuroanatomy is the foundation of comprehensive neurologic examination and diagnosis. Salient features will be considered, from cephalad to caudad. The cerebral hemispheres (or telencephalon) consist of the cerebral cortex, underlying white matter, the basal ganglia, hippocampus, and amygdala. The cerebral cortex is the most recently evolved part of the nervous system. Its functions are mapped to discrete anatomic areas. The frontal areas are involved in executive function, decision making, and restraint of emotions. The motor strip, or precentral gyrus, is the most posterior component of the frontal lobes, and is arranged along a homunculus with the head inferior and lateral to the lower extremities superiorly and medially. The motor speech area (Broca's area) lies in the left posterior inferior frontal lobe in almost all right-handed people and in up to 90% of left-handed people. The parietal lobe lies between the central sulcus anteriorly and the occipital lobe posteriorly. The postcentral gyrus is the sensory strip, also arranged along a homunculus. The rest of the parietal lobe is involved with awareness of one's body in space and relative to the immediate environment, body orientation, and spatial relationships. The occipital lobes are most posterior. The visual cortex is arrayed along the apposing medial surfaces of the occipital lobes. The left occipital lobe receives and integrates data from the left half of each retina. A left occipital lesion would therefore result in inability to see objects right of center. The temporal lobes lie below the sylvian fissures. The hippocampus, amygdala, and lower optic radiations (Meyer's loops) are important components of the temporal lobe. They are involved in memory, emotion, and visual pathways, respectively. The receptive speech area (Wernicke's area) lies in the area of the posterior superior temporal lobe and the inferior parietal lobe, usually on the left. The basal ganglia include the caudate, putamen, and the globus pallidus. Basal ganglia structures are involved with modulation of movement via inhibition of motor pathways.

Lying deep to the cerebral hemispheres is the diencephalon, which includes the thalamus and hypothalamus. The thalamus is a key processor and relay circuit for most motor and sensory information going to or coming from the cortex. The hypothalamus, at the base of the brain, is a key regulator of homeostasis, via the autonomic and neuroendocrine systems.

The brain stem consists of the midbrain (mesencephalon), pons (metencephalon), and medulla (myelencephalon). Longitudinal fibers run through the brain stem, carrying motor and sensory information between the cerebral hemispheres and the spinal cord. The corticospinal tract is the major motor tract, while the medial lemniscus and the spinothalamic tracts are the major sensory tracts. The nuclei of cranial nerves III through XII are also located within the brain stem. These nerves relay the motor, sensory, and special sense functions of the eye, face, mouth, and throat. The cerebellum arises from the dorsal aspect of the brain stem. It integrates somatosensory, vestibular, and motor information for coordination and timing of movement. Midline, or vermian, lesions lead to truncal ataxia. Lateral, or hemispheric, lesions lead to tremor and dyscoordination in the extremities.

The ventricular system is a cerebrospinal fluid (CSF)-containing contiguous space inside the brain, continuous with the subarachnoid space outside the brain. The paired lateral ventricles consist of temporal, occipital, and frontal horns, as well as the main body. CSF travels from each lateral ventricle through the foramina of Monroe to the third ventricle, located between the left and right thalami. CSF then drains through the cerebral aqueduct to the fourth ventricle in the brain stem. The foramen of Magendie (midline) and paired foramina of Luschka (lateral) drain to the subarachnoid space. Choroid plexus creates the CSF, mostly in the lateral ventricles. The average adult has an approximate CSF volume of 150 mL and creates approximately 500 mL per day.

The spinal cord starts at the bottom of the medulla and extends through the spinal canal down to approximately the first lumbar vertebra. Motor tracts (efferent pathways) continue from the brain stem down via the lateral and anterior corticospinal tracts to anterior horn cells, and then exit via ventral nerve roots. Sensory information (afferent pathways) enters via dorsal nerve roots, travels up the dorsal columns (proprioception and fine touch) or the spinothalamic tract (pain and temperature) and into the brain stem. Paired nerves exit the spinal cord at each level. There are 31 pairs: 8 cervical, 12 thoracic, 5 lumbar, 5 sacral, and 1 coccygeal.

The dorsal and ventral nerve roots at each level fuse to form mixed motor-sensory spinal nerves and spread through the body to provide innervation to muscles and sensory organs. The C5–T1 spinal nerves intersect in the brachial plexus and divide to form the main nerve branches to the arm, including the median, ulnar, and radial nerves. The L2–S4 spinal nerves intersect in the lumbosacral plexus and divide to form the main nerve branches to the leg, including the common peroneal, tibial, and femoral nerves.

The principal motor tract is the corticospinal tract. It is a two-neuron path, with an upper motor neuron and a lower motor neuron. The upper motor neuron cell body is in the motor strip of the cerebral cortex. The axon travels through the internal capsule to the brain stem, decussates at the brain stem–spinal cord junction, and travels down the contralateral corticospinal tract to the lower motor neuron in the anterior horn at the appropriate level. The lower motor neuron axon then travels via peripheral nerves to its target muscle. Damage to upper motor neurons results in hyperreflexia and mild atrophy. Damage to lower motor neurons results in flaccidity and significant atrophy.

The two major sensory tracts are three-neuron paths. The fine touch and proprioception signals ascend ipsilaterally via the dorsal column, synapse and decussate in the lower medulla, travel up the contralateral medial lemniscus to the second synapse in the thalamus, and then ascend to the sensory cortex. The pain and temperature fibers synapse in the dorsal horn of the spinal cord at their entry level, decussate, and travel up the contralateral spinothalamic tracts to the thalamus. The second synapse occurs in the thalamus, and the output ascends to the sensory cortex.

The nervous system is composed of the somatic nervous system and the autonomic nervous system (ANS). The motor and sensory tracts described so far compose the former. The latter carries messages for homeostasis and visceral regulation from the central nervous system (CNS) to target structures such as arteries, veins, the heart, sweat glands, and the digestive tract.[1] CNS control of the ANS arises particularly from the hypothalamus and the nucleus of the tractus solitarius. The ANS is divided into the sympathetic, parasympathetic, and enteric systems. The sympathetic system drives the "fight or flight" response, and uses epinephrine to increase heart rate, blood pressure, blood glucose, and temperature, and to dilate the pupils. It arises from the thoracolumbar spinal segments. The parasympathetic system promotes the "rest and digest" state, and uses acetylcholine to maintain basal metabolic function under nonstressful circumstances. It arises from cranial nerves III, VII, IX, and X, and from the second to fourth sacral segments. The enteric nervous system controls the complex synchronization of the digestive tract, especially the pancreas, gallbladder, and small and large bowels. It can run autonomously, but is under the regulation of the sympathetic and parasympathetic systems.

NEUROLOGIC EXAMINATION

The neurologic examination is divided into several components and is generally done from head to toe. First assess mental status. A patient may be awake, lethargic (will follow commands and answer questions, but then returns to sleep), stuporous (difficult to arouse at all), or comatose (no purposeful response to voice or pain). Cranial nerves may be thoroughly tested in the awake patient, but pupil reactivity, eye movement, facial symmetry, and gag are the most relevant when mental status is impaired. Motor testing is based on maximal effort of major muscle groups in those able to follow commands, while assessing for amplitude and symmetry of movement to deep central pain may be all that is possible for stuporous patients. Table 41-1 details scoring for motor assessment tests. Characteristic motor reactions to pain in patients with depressed mental status include withdrawal from stimulus, localization to stimulus, flexor (decorticate) posturing, extensor (decerebrate) posturing, or no reaction (in order of worsening pathology). Figure 41-1 diagrams the clinical patterns of posturing. This forms the basis of determining the Glasgow Coma Scale motor score, as detailed in Table 41-2. Light touch, proprioception, temperature, and pain testing may be useful in awake patients but is often impossible without good cooperation. It is critical to document sensory patterns in spinal cord injury patients. Muscle stretch reflexes should be checked. Often comparing left to right or upper extremity to lower extremity reflexes for symmetry is the most useful for localizing a lesion. Check for ankle-jerk clonus or up-going toes (the Babinski test). Presence of either is pathologic and signifies upper motor neuron disease.

Diagnostic Studies

Plain Films

Plain x-rays of the skull may demonstrate fractures, osteolytic or osteoblastic lesions, or pneumocephaly (air in the head). The use of skull plain films has decreased given the rapid availability and significantly increased detail of head computed tomography (CT) scans. Plain films of the cervical, thoracic, and lumbar spine are used to assess for evidence of bony trauma or soft-tissue swelling suggesting fracture. Spinal deformities and osteolytic or osteoblastic

Table 41-1
Motor Scoring System

Grade	Description
0	No muscle contraction
1	Visible muscle contraction without movement across the joint
2	Movement in the horizontal plane, unable to overcome gravity
3	Movement against gravity
4	Movement against some resistance
5	Normal strength

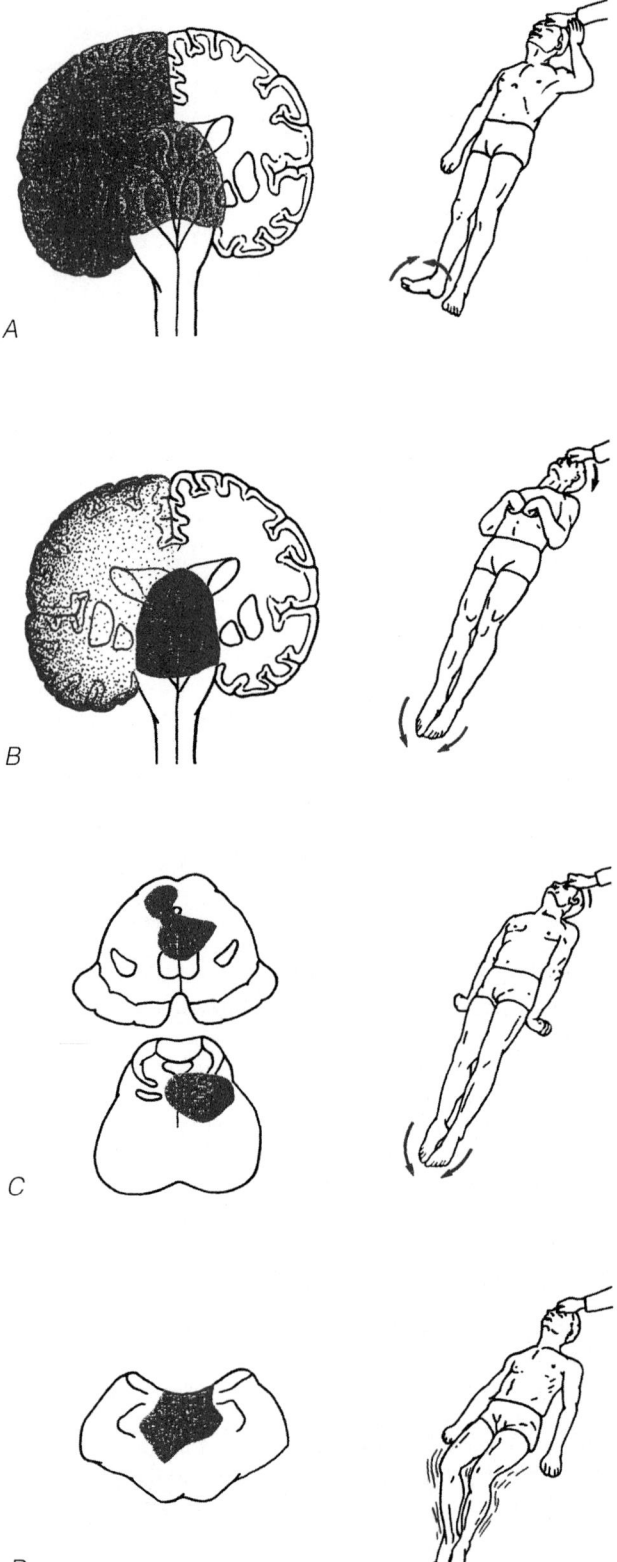

FIG. 41-1. Patterns of motor responses associated with various lesions. *A.* Left hemispheric lesion with right hemiplegia and left localization. *B.* Deep cerebral/thalamic lesion with bilateral flexor posturing. *C.* Midbrain or pontine lesion with bilateral extensor posturing. *D.* Medullary lesion with general flaccidity. [*Adapted with permission from: Rengachary SS, Duke DA: Impaired consciousness, in Rengachary SS, Wilkins RA (eds): Principles of Neurosurgery. London: Wolfe Publishing Ltd., 1994, p 3.10.*]

pathologic processes also will be apparent. The shoulder girdle usually poses problems in visualizing the cervicothoracic junction clearly.

Computed Tomography

The noncontrast CT scan of the head is an extremely useful diagnostic tool in the setting of new focal neurologic deficit, decreased mental status, or trauma. It is rapid and almost universally available in hospitals in the United States. Its sensitivity allows for the detection of acute hemorrhage. A contrast-enhanced CT scan will help show neoplastic or infectious processes. In the current era, contrast CT is generally used for those patients who cannot undergo magnetic resonance imaging (MRI) scanning due to pacemakers or metal in the orbits. Fine-slice CT scanning of the spine is helpful for defining bony anatomy and pathology, and is usually done after an abnormality is seen on plain films, or because plain films are inadequate (especially to visualize C7 and T1 vertebrae). Finally, high-speed multislice scanners, combined with timed-bolus contrast injections, allow CT-angiography (CT-A). A thin-slice axial scan is obtained during the passage of contrast through the cerebral arteries and reconstructed in 3-D to assess for vascular lesions. CT-A does not reliably detect lesions, such as cerebral aneurysms, less than 3 mm across, but can provide detailed morphologic data of larger lesions. Newer, multislice scanner technology is approaching the resolution of conventional angiography.

Magnetic Resonance Imaging

MRI provides excellent imaging of soft tissue structures in the head and spine. It is a complex and evolving science. Several of the most clinically useful MRI sequences are worth describing. T1 sequences made before and after gadolinium administration are useful for detecting neoplastic and infectious processes. T2 sequences facilitate assessment of neural compression in the spine by the presence or absence of bright T2 CSF signals around the cord or nerve roots. Diffusion-weighted images (DWI) can detect ischemic stroke earlier than CT. Fine-slice time-of-flight (TOF) axial images can be reformatted in three dimensions to build MRI-angiograms (MR-A) and MRI-venograms (MR-V). MR-A can detect stenosis of the cervical carotid arteries or intracranial aneurysms greater than 3 mm in diameter. MR-V can assess the sinuses for patency or thrombosis.

Angiography

Transarterial catheter-based angiography remains the gold standard for evaluation of vascular pathology of the brain and spine. The current state of the art is biplanar imaging to reduce dye load and facilitate interventional procedures. Digital subtraction technologies minimize bony interference in the resultant images. Bilateral carotid arteries and bilateral vertebral arteries may be injected and followed through arterial, capillary, and venous phases for a complete cerebral angiogram.

Electromyography and Nerve Conduction Studies

Electromyography and nerve conduction studies (EMG and NCS) are useful for assessing the function of peripheral nerves. EMG records muscle activity in response to a proximal stimulation of the motor nerve. NCS records the velocity and amplitude of the nerve action potential. EMG/NCS is typically performed approximately 4 weeks after an acute injury, as nerves distal to the injury continue to transmit electrical impulses normally until degeneration of the distal nerve progresses.

Table 41-2
The Glasgow Coma Scale (GCS) Score[a]

Motor Response (M)		Verbal Response (V)		Eye-Opening Response (E)	
Obeys commands	6	Oriented	5	Opens spontaneously	4
Localizes to pain	5	Confused	4	Opens to speech	3
Withdraws from pain	4	Inappropriate words	3	Opens to pain	2
Flexor posturing	3	Unintelligible sounds	2	No eye opening	1
Extensor posturing	2	No sounds	1		
No movement	1				

[a] Add the three scores to obtain the Glasgow Coma Scale score, which can range from 3 to 15. Add "T" after the GCS if intubated and no verbal score is possible. For these patients, the GCS can range from 2T to 10T.

Invasive Monitoring

There are several methods of monitoring intracranial physiology. The three described here are bedside intensive care unit (ICU) procedures and allow continuous monitoring. All three involve making a small hole in the skull with a hand-held drill. They are generally placed in the right frontal region to minimize the neurologic impact of possible complications, such as hemorrhage. The most reliable monitor, *always*, is an alert patient with a reliable neurologic exam. If a reliable neurologic exam is not possible due to the presence of brain injury, sedatives, or paralytics, and there is active and unstable intracranial pathology, then invasive monitoring is required.

External Ventricular Drain (EVD). An EVD is also known as a ventriculostomy. A perforated plastic catheter is inserted into the frontal horn of the lateral ventricle. An uninterrupted fluid column through a rigid tube allows transduction of intracranial pressure (ICP). CSF also can be drained to reduce ICP or sampled for laboratory studies.

Intraparenchymal Fiberoptic Pressure Transducer. This device is commonly referred to as a "bolt." Again, a small hole is drilled in the skull. A threaded post locks securely into the skull and holds the fiberoptic catheter in place. A bolt allows ICP monitoring only, but is smaller and less invasive than a ventriculostomy, and may be associated with fewer complications, although the data are not clear.

Brain Tissue Oxygen Sensors. The brain tissue oxygen sensor is a recent development. The device is screwed into the skull in the same manner as the bolt; however, the sensor catheter is an electrochemical oxygen–tension sensitive membrane. A single bolt can be designed to accept a pressure sensor, oxygen sensor, and brain temperature sensor. Patients with severe brain injury due to trauma or aneurysmal hemorrhage may benefit from placement of these three sensors and a ventriculostomy to drain CSF for control of ICP. This requires two twist-drill holes, which may be adjacent or on opposite sides of the head.

NEUROLOGIC AND NEUROSURGICAL EMERGENCIES

Raised Intracranial Pressure

ICP normally varies between 4 and 14 mm Hg. Sustained ICP levels above 20 mm Hg can injure the brain. The Monro-Kellie doctrine states that the cranial vault is a rigid structure, and therefore the total volume of the contents determines ICP. The three normal contents of the cranial vault are brain, blood, and CSF. The brain's contents can expand due to swelling from traumatic brain injury (TBI), stroke, or reactive edema. Blood volume can increase by extravasation to form a hematoma, or by reactive vasodilation in a hypoventilating, hypercarbic patient. CSF volume increases in the setting of hydrocephalus. Figure 41-2 demonstrates classic CT findings of hydrocephalus. Addition of a fourth element, such as a tumor or abscess, will also increase ICP. The pressure-volume curve depicted in Fig. 41-3 demonstrates a compensated region with a small $\Delta P/\Delta V$, and an uncompensated region with large $\Delta P/\Delta V$. In the compensated region, increased volume is offset by decreased volume of CSF and blood.

Increased ICP can injure the brain in several ways. Focal mass lesions cause shift and herniation. Temporal lesions push the uncus medially and compress the midbrain. This is known as uncal herniation. The posterior cerebral artery passes between the uncus and

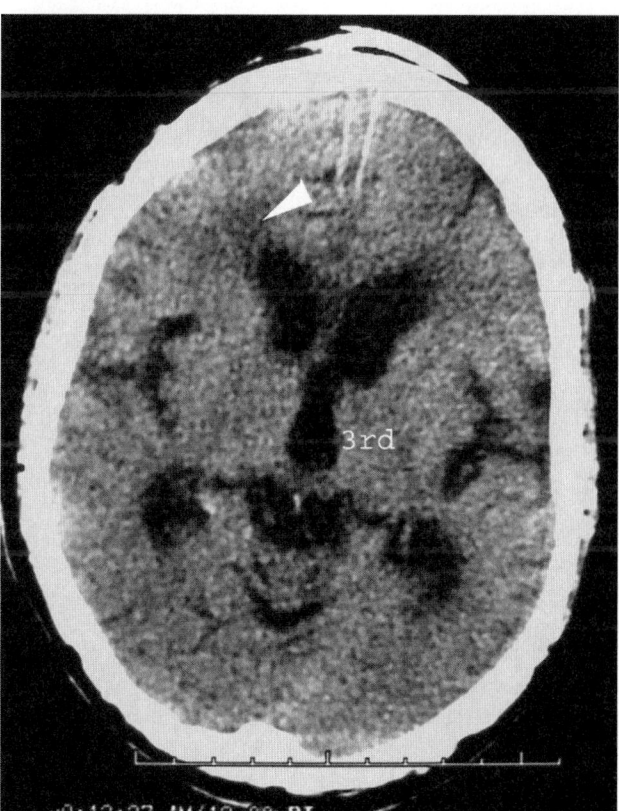

FIG. 41-2. Head CT scan demonstrating hydrocephalus. The third ventricle (*3rd*) is widened and rounded, the anterior horns of the lateral ventricles are plump, and pressure-driven flow of CSF into brain parenchyma adjacent to the ventricles is seen (*arrowhead*). This is known as transependymal flow of CSF.

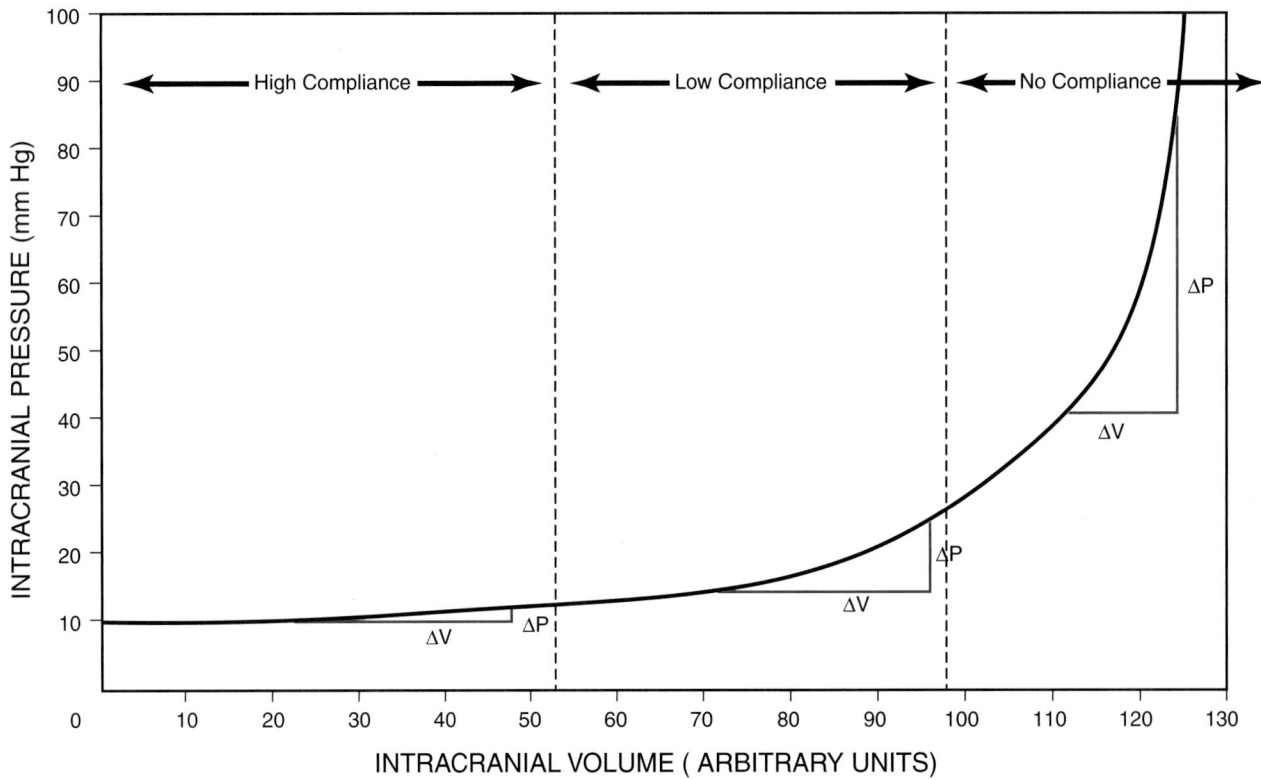

FIG. 41-3. Pressure-volume curve demonstrating the effect of changing the volume of intracranial contents on ICP. Note the compensated zone, with little change of pressure with change of volume, and the uncompensated zone, with significant change of pressure with change of volume. [*Adapted with permission from Rengachary SS, Duke DA: Increased intracranial pressure, cerebral edema, and brain herniation, in Rengachary SS, Wilkins RA (eds): Principles of Neurosurgery. London: Wolfe Publishing Ltd., 1994, p 2.3.*]

midbrain and may be occluded, leading to occipital infarct. Masses higher up in the hemisphere can push the cingulate gyrus under the falx cerebri. This is known as subfalcine herniation. The anterior cerebral artery branches run along the medial surface of the cingulate gyrus and may be occluded, leading to medial frontal and parietal infarcts. Diffuse increases in pressure in the cerebral hemispheres can lead to central, or transtentorial, herniation. Increased pressure in the posterior fossa can lead to upward central herniation or downward tonsillar herniation through the foramen magnum. Uncal, transtentorial, and tonsillar herniation can cause direct damage to the very delicate brain stem. Figure 41-4 diagrams patterns of herniation.

Patients with increased ICP, also called intracranial hypertension (ICH), will often present with headache, nausea, vomiting, and progressive mental status decline. Cushing's triad is the classic presentation of ICH: hypertension, bradycardia, and irregular respirations. This triad is usually a late manifestation. Focal neurologic deficits may also be present if there is a focal mass lesion causing the problem. Patients with these symptoms should have a head CT as soon as possible.

Initial management of ICH includes airway protection and adequate ventilation. A bolus of mannitol up to 1 g/kg causes free water diuresis, increased serum osmolality, and extraction of water from the brain. The effect is delayed by about 20 minutes and has a transient benefit. Driving serum osmolality above 300 mOsm/L is of indeterminate benefit and can have deleterious cardiovascular side effects, such as hypovolemia that leads to hypotension and decreased brain perfusion. Cases of ICH usually need rapid neurosurgical evaluation. Ventriculostomy or craniotomy may be needed for definitive decompression.

It is critical to note that lethargic or obtunded patients often have decreased respiratory drive. This causes the partial pressure of arterial carbon dioxide ($Paco_2$) to increase, resulting in cerebral vasodilation and worsening of ICH. This cycle causes a characteristic "crashing patient," who rapidly loses airway protection, becomes apneic, and herniates. Emergent intubation and ventilation to reduce $Paco_2$ to roughly 35 mm Hg can reverse the process and save the patient's life.

Brain Stem Compression

Disease in the posterior fossa (brain stem and cerebellum) requires special consideration. The volume of the posterior fossa is small. Hemorrhage or stroke in the posterior fossa causes mass effect and can rapidly kill the patient in two ways. Occlusion of the fourth ventricle causes acute obstructive hydrocephalus, leading to raised ICP, herniation, and then death. The mass effect can also lead directly to brain stem compression (Fig. 41-5). Symptoms of brain stem compression include progressive obtundation and hypertension, followed rapidly by brain death. A patient with evidence of either or both needs emergent neurosurgical evaluation for possible ventriculostomy and suboccipital craniectomy (removal of the bone covering the cerebellum). This situation is especially critical, as expeditious decompression can lead to significant functional recovery of patients who present near brain death.

Stroke

Patients who present with acute focal neurologic deficits for whom the time of onset of symptoms can be clearly defined (i.e., when the patient was last seen in a normal state of health) must be evaluated

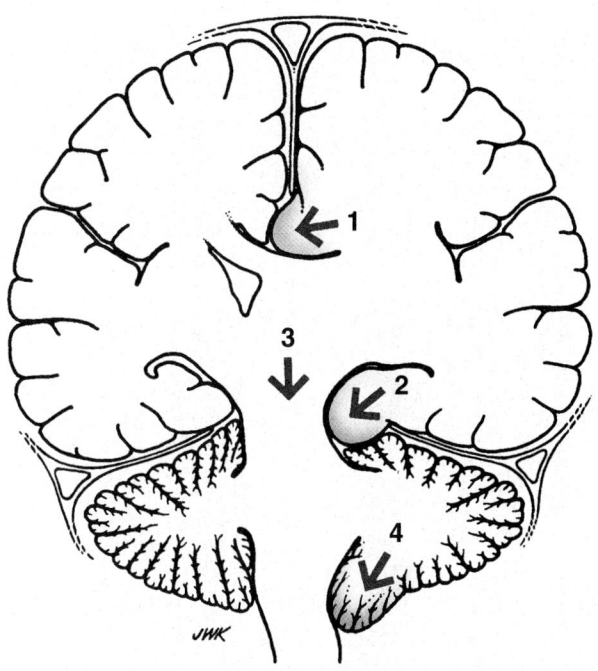

FIG. 41-4. *Schematic drawing of brain herniation patterns. 1. Subfalcine herniation. The cingulate gyrus shifts across midline under the falx cerebri. 2. Uncal herniation. The uncus (medial temporal lobe gyrus) shifts medially and compresses the midbrain and cerebral peduncle. 3. Central transtentorial herniation. The diencephalon and midbrain shift caudally through the tentorial incisura. 4. Tonsillar herniation. The cerebellar tonsil shifts caudally through the foramen magnum. [Adapted with permission from Cohen DS, Quest DO: Increased intracranial pressure, brain herniation, and their control, in Rengachary SS, Wilkins RA (eds): Principles of Neurosurgery, 2nd ed. London: Wolfe Publishing Ltd., 1996, p 345.]*

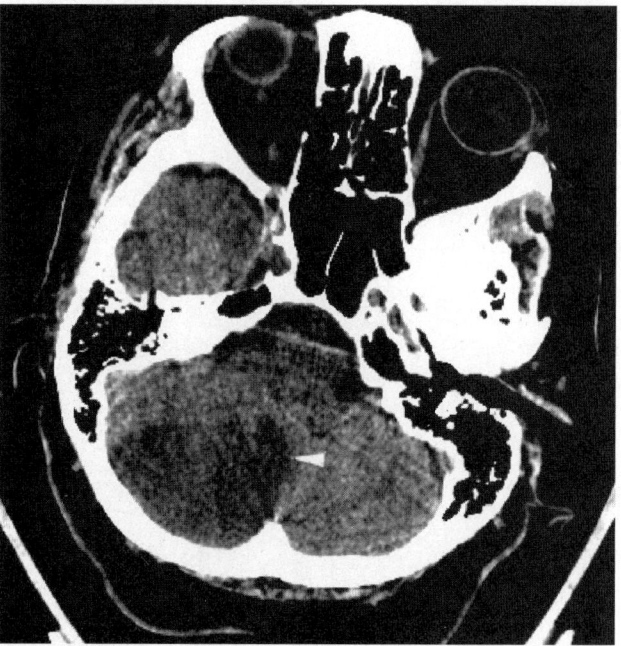

FIG. 41-5. *Maturing cerebellar stroke seen as a hypodense area in the right cerebellar hemisphere on head CT in a patient with rapidly progressing obtundation 2 days after the initial onset of symptoms. Swelling of the infarcted tissue causes posterior fossa mass effect. The fourth ventricle is obliterated and not visible, and the brain stem is being compressed.*

as rapidly as possible. An emergent head CT scan should be done. This is often normal, because CT changes from ischemic stroke may take up to 24 hours to appear (Fig. 41-6). A patient with a clinical diagnosis of acute stroke less than 3 hours old, without hemorrhage on CT, may be a candidate for thrombolytic therapy with tissue plasminogen activator (tPA).

Seizure

A seizure is defined as uncontrolled neuronal electrical activity. New-onset seizure often signifies an irritative mass lesion in the brain. Tumors commonly present with seizure. Patients with traumatic intracranial hemorrhage are at risk for seizure. A seizing patient is at risk for neural damage if the seizure is not stopped, as well as airway and ventilation problems. Any patient with new-onset seizure should have imaging of the brain, such as a head CT scan, after the seizure is controlled and the patient resuscitated.

TRAUMA

Trauma is the leading cause of death in children and young adults; however, incidences of death and disability from trauma have been slowly decreasing. This is partly attributable to increased awareness of the importance of using seat belts and bicycle and motorcycle helmets. However, trauma remains a major cause of morbidity and mortality, and can affect every major organ system in the body. The three main areas of neurosurgic interest in trauma are TBI, spine and spinal cord injury (SCI), and peripheral nerve injury.

Head Trauma

Glasgow Coma Scale (GCS) Score

The initial assessment of the trauma patient includes the primary survey, resuscitation, secondary survey, and definitive care. Neurosurgical evaluation begins during the primary survey with the determination of the GCS score (usually referred to simply as the GCS) for the patient. The GCS is determined by adding the scores of the best responses of the patient in each of the three categories. The motor score ranges from 1 to 6, verbal from 1 to 5, and eyes from 1 to 4. The GCS therefore ranges from 3 to 15, as detailed in Table 41-2.

Scalp Injury

Blunt or penetrating trauma to the head can cause injury to the densely vascularized scalp, and significant blood loss can occur. Direct pressure initially controls the bleeding, allowing close inspection of the injury. If a simple laceration is found, it should be copiously irrigated and closed primarily. If the laceration is short, a single-layer percutaneous suture closure will suffice. If the laceration is long or has multiple arms, the patient may need débridement and closure in the operating room, with its superior lighting and wider selection of instruments and suture materials. Careful reapproximation of the galea will provide a more secure closure and better hemostasis. Blunt trauma can also cause crush injury with subsequent tissue necrosis. These wounds require débridement and consideration of advancement flaps to cover the defect.

Skull Fractures

The usual classification system for bone fractures may be applied to the skull. Characterization may be done using skull x-rays or head CT.[2] A closed fracture is covered by intact skin. An open, or compound, fracture is associated with disrupted overlying skin. The

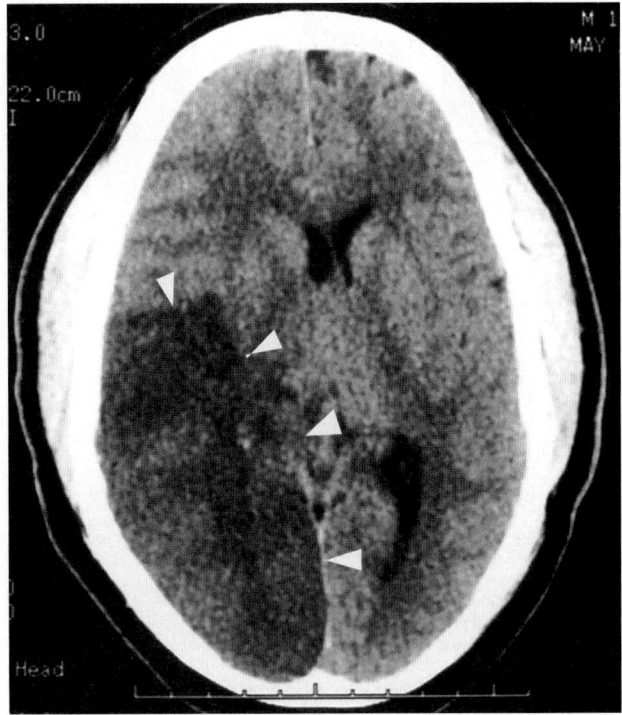

A

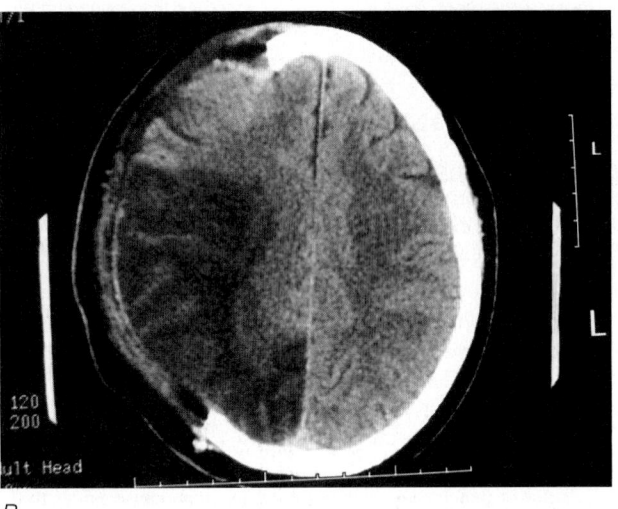

B

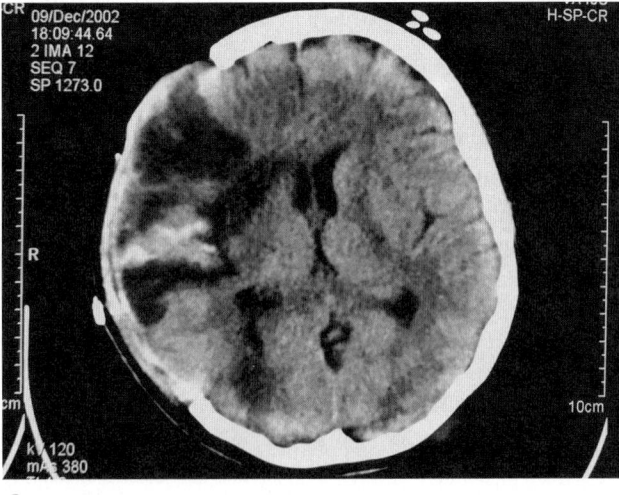

C

FIG. 41-6. *A.* Head CT scan of a patient with a 4-day-old stroke that occluded the right middle cerebral and posterior cerebral arteries. The infarcted tissue is the hypodense (dark) area indicated by the arrowheads. The patient presented with left-sided weakness and left visual field loss, but then became less responsive, prompting this head CT. Note the right-to-left midline shift. *B.* Same patient status postdecompressive right hemicraniectomy. Note the free expansion of swollen brain outside the normal confines of the skull. *C.* Patient with a right middle cerebral artery ischemic stroke with areas of hemorrhagic conversion, seen as hyperdense (bright) areas within the infarcted tissue. This patient also required hemicraniectomy for severe mass effect. Note the lack of midline shift postoperatively.

fracture lines may be single (linear); multiple and radiating from a point (stellate); or multiple, creating fragments of bone (comminuted). Closed skull fractures do not normally require specific treatment. Open fractures require repair of the scalp. Skull fractures in general indicate that a significant amount of force was transmitted to the head, and should increase the suspicion for intracranial injury. Fractures that cross meningeal arteries can cause rupture of the artery and subsequent epidural hematoma formation.

Depressed skull fractures may result from a focal injury of significant force. The inner and outer cortices of the skull are disrupted, and a fragment of bone is pressed in toward the brain in relation to adjacent intact skull. The fragment may overlap the edge of intact bone, or may plunge completely below the level of adjacent normal skull. The inner cortex of the bone fragments often has multiple sharp edges that can lacerate dura, brain, and vessels. Craniotomy is required to elevate the fracture, repair dural disruption, and obtain

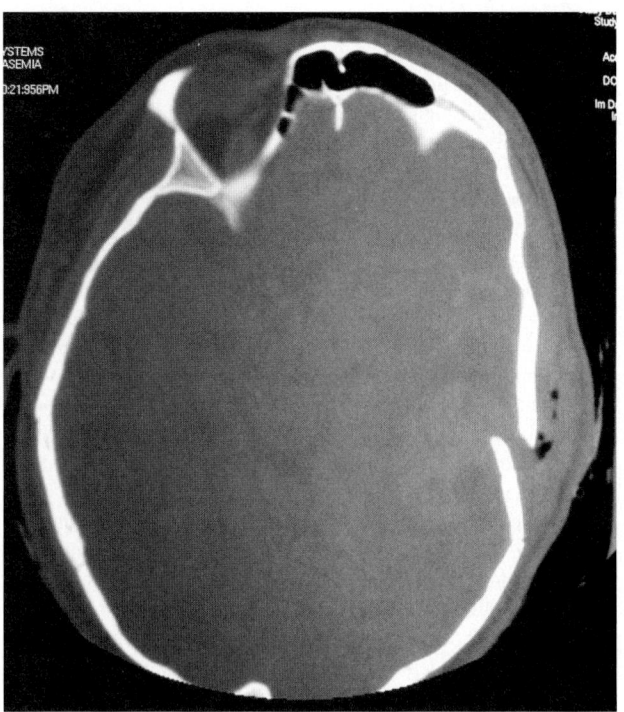

A

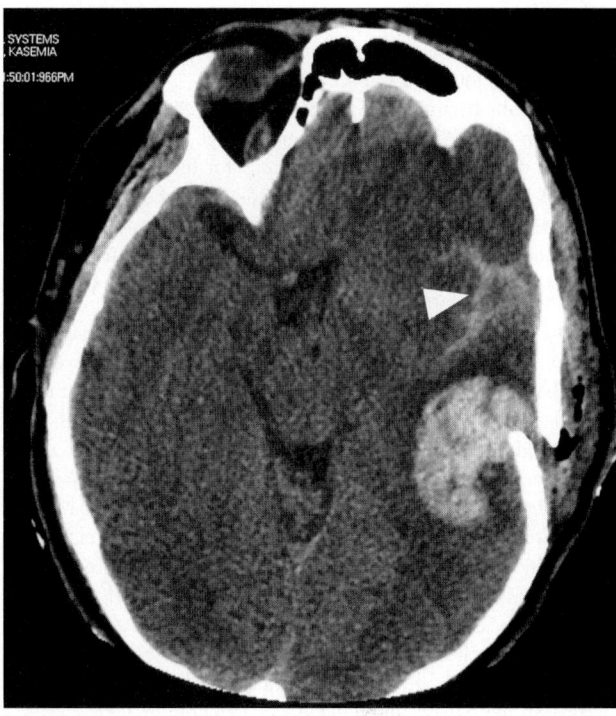

B

FIG. 41-7. *A.* Bone-window axial head CT of a patient who presented aphasic after being struck with the bottom of a beer bottle. CT demonstrates a depressed skull fracture in the left posterior temporoparietal area. *B.* Brain-window axial head CT demonstrating intraparenchymal hematoma caused by laceration of cortical vessels by the edge of the fractured bone. Arrowhead indicates traumatic subarachnoid hemorrhage in the sylvian fissure.

hemostasis in these cases (Fig. 41-7). Fractures overlying dural venous sinuses require restraint. Surgical exploration can lead to life-threatening hemorrhage from the lacerated sinus.

Fractures of the skull base are common in head-injured patients, and they indicate significant impacts. They are generally apparent on routine head CT, but should be evaluated with dedicated fine-slice coronal-section CT scan to document and delineate the extent of the fracture and involved structures. If asymptomatic, they require no treatment. Symptoms from skull base fractures include cranial nerve deficits and CSF leaks. A fracture of the temporal bone, for instance, can damage the facial or vestibulocochlear nerve, resulting in vertigo, ipsilateral deafness, or facial paralysis. A communication may be formed between the subarachnoid space and the middle ear, allowing CSF drainage into the pharynx via the eustachian tube or from the ear (otorrhea). Extravasation of blood results in ecchymosis behind the ear, known as Battle's sign. A fracture of the anterior skull base can result in anosmia (loss of smell from damage to the olfactory nerve), CSF drainage from the nose (rhinorrhea), or periorbital ecchymoses, known as raccoon eyes.

Copious clear drainage from the nose or ear makes the diagnosis of CSF leakage obvious. Often, however, the drainage may be discolored with blood or small in volume if some drains into the throat. The halo test can help differentiate. Allow a drop of the fluid to fall on an absorbent surface such as a facial tissue. If blood is mixed with CSF, the drop will form a double ring, with a darker center spot containing blood components surrounded by a light halo of CSF. If this is indeterminate, the fluid can be sent to the lab for beta-transferrin testing. Beta-transferrin testing will only be positive if CSF is present.

Many CSF leaks will heal with elevation of the head of the bed for several days. A lumbar drain can augment this. A lumbar drain is a catheter placed in the lumbar CSF cistern to decompress the cranial vault and allow the defect to heal by eliminating normal hydrostatic pressure. There is no proven efficacy of antibiotic coverage for preventing meningitis in patients with CSF leaks.

Traumatic cranial neuropathies are generally managed conservatively, with documentation of the extent of impairment and signs of recovery. Patients with traumatic facial nerve palsies may benefit from a course of steroids, although their benefit is unproven. Patients with facial nerve palsy of abrupt onset, who do not respond to steroids within 48 to 72 hours may be considered for surgical decompression of the petrous portion of the facial nerve. Patients may also present with delayed-onset facial nerve palsy. Again, steroids are employed and surgery is considered, with mixed results.

Closed Head Injury

Closed head injury (CHI) is the most common type of TBI, and a significant cause of morbidity and mortality in the United States. There are two important factors that affect the outcome in CHI and TBI in general. The initial impact causes the *primary injury*, defined as the immediate injury to neurons from transmission of the force of impact. The long, delicate axons of the neurons can shear as the different areas of the brain through which they pass accelerate and decelerate at different speeds. Prevention strategies, such as wearing helmets, remain the best means to decrease disability from primary injury. Subsequent neuronal damage due to the sequelae of trauma is referred to as *secondary injury*. Hypoxia, hypotension, hydrocephalus, intracranial hypertension, and intracranial hematoma are all mechanisms of secondary injury. The focus of basic research into brain trauma, critical care medicine, and neurosurgical intervention is to decrease the effects of secondary injury.

The Brain Trauma Foundation released, with the approval of the American Association of Neurological Surgeons, an updated summary of management recommendations for brain-injured patients in 2000. The guidelines standardize the care of these patients with the hope of improving outcomes. Some of the common patterns of CHI, including concussion, contusion, and diffuse axonal injury, are discussed below.

Initial Assessment. The initial evaluation of a trauma patient remains the same whether or not the primary surveyor suspects head injury. The first three elements of the ABCDs of resuscitation, *a*irway, *b*reathing, and *c*irculation, must first be assessed and stabilized. Hypoxia and hypotension worsen outcome in TBI (due to secondary injury), so cardiopulmonary stabilization is critical. Patients who cannot follow commands require intubation for airway protection and ventilatory control. The fourth element, assessment of the D, for *d*isability, is undertaken next. Motor activity, speech, and eye opening can be assessed in a few seconds and a GCS assigned.

An efficient way for the primary surveyor to assess disability and ascertain the status of the three components of the GCS follows. Approach the patient and enter his or her field of view. Observe whether the patient visually orients to you. Clearly command: "Tell me your name." Then ask the patient to lift up two fingers on each side sequentially, and wiggle the toes. A patient not responsive to these prompts should be assessed for response to deep central painful stimulus, with a firm, twisting pinch of the sensitive skin above the clavicle. Watch for eye opening and movement of the extremities, whether purposeful or reflex. Assess the verbal response. The motor, verbal, and eye-opening scores may be correctly assigned using this rapid examination, and an initial assessment of the probability of significant head injury made. Also take note of any external signs of head injury, including bleeding from the scalp, nose, or ear, or deformation of the skull or face.

Medical Management. Several medical steps may be taken to minimize secondary neuronal injury and the systemic consequences of head injury. Patients with a documented closed head injury should receive a 17-mg/kg phenytoin loading dose, followed by 1 week of therapeutic maintenance phenytoin, typically 300 to 400 mg/d. Phenytoin prophylaxis has been shown to decrease the incidence of early posttraumatic seizures. There is no evidence to support longer-term use of prophylactic antiepileptic agents. Blood glucose levels should be closely monitored by free blood sugar checks and controlled with sliding scale insulin. Fevers should also be evaluated and controlled with antipyretics, as well as source-directed therapy when possible. Hyperglycemia and hyperthermia are toxic to injured neurons, and so contribute to secondary injury. Head-injured patients have an increased prevalence of peptic ulceration and gastrointestinal (GI) bleeding. Peptic ulcers occurring in patients with head injury or high ICP are referred to as Cushing's ulcers, and may be related to hypergastrinemia. Ulcer prophylaxis should be used. Compression stockings or athrombic pumps should be used when the patient cannot be mobilized rapidly.

Classification. Head injury can be classified as mild, moderate, or severe. For patients with a history of head trauma, classification is as follows: severe head injury if the GCS is 3 to 8, moderate head injury if the GCS is 9 to 12, and mild head injury if the GCS is 13 to 15. Many people present to emergency rooms and trauma bays

with a history of head trauma, so a triage system must be employed to maximize resource utilization while minimizing the chance of missing occult or progressing injuries.

Head trauma patients who are asymptomatic; who have only headache, dizziness, or scalp lacerations or abrasions; or who did not lose consciousness have a low risk for intracranial injury and may be discharged home without a head CT scan.[3,4] Head-injured patients who are discharged should be sent home with reliable family or friends who can observe the patient for the first postinjury day. Printed discharge instructions, which describe monitoring for confusion, persistent nausea, weakness, or speech difficulty, should be given to the caretaker. The patient should return to the emergency department for evaluation of such symptoms.

Patients with a history of altered or lost consciousness, amnesia, progressive headache, skull or facial fracture, vomiting, or seizure have a moderate risk for intracranial injury and should undergo prompt head CT. If the CT is normal, and the neurologic exam has returned to baseline (excluding amnesia of the event), then the patient can be discharged to the care of a responsible adult, again with printed criteria for returning to the ER. Otherwise the patient must be admitted for a 24-hour observation period.

Patients with depressed consciousness, focal neurologic deficits, penetrating injury, depressed skull fracture, or changing neurologic exam have a high risk for intracranial injury. These patients should undergo immediate head CT and admission for observation or intervention as needed.

Concussion. A concussion is temporary neuronal dysfunction after nonpenetrating head trauma. The head CT is normal, and deficits resolve over minutes to hours. Definitions vary; some require transient loss of consciousness, while others include patients with any alteration of mental status. Memory difficulties, especially amnesia of the event, are very common. Concussions may be graded. One method is the Colorado Medical Society system. Head trauma patients with confusion only are grade 1, patients with amnesia are grade 2, and patients who lose consciousness are grade 3. Studies have shown that the brain remains in a hypermetabolic state for up to a week after injury. The brain is also much more susceptible to injury from even minor head trauma in the first 1 to 2 weeks after concussion. This is known as second-impact syndrome, and patients should be informed that even after mild head injury they might experience memory difficulties or persistent headaches.[5]

Contusion. A contusion is a bruise of the brain, and occurs when the force from trauma is sufficient to cause breakdown of small vessels, and extravasation of blood into the brain. The contused areas appear bright on CT scan, as seen in Fig. 41-8. The frontal, occipital, and temporal poles are most often involved. The brain sustains injury as it moves in relation to rough bony surfaces. Contusions themselves rarely cause significant mass effect as they represent small amounts of blood in injured parenchyma rather than coherent blood clots. Edema may develop around a contusion, causing mass effect. Contusions may also enlarge, or develop a true hematoma, especially during the first 24 hours. Contusions may also be seen in brain tissue opposite the site of impact. This is known as a contre coup injury. These contusions result from deceleration of the brain against the skull.

Diffuse Axonal Injury. Diffuse axonal injury is caused by damage to axons throughout the brain, due to rotational acceleration and then deceleration. Axons may be completely disrupted and then retract, forming axon balls. Small hemorrhages can be seen in more

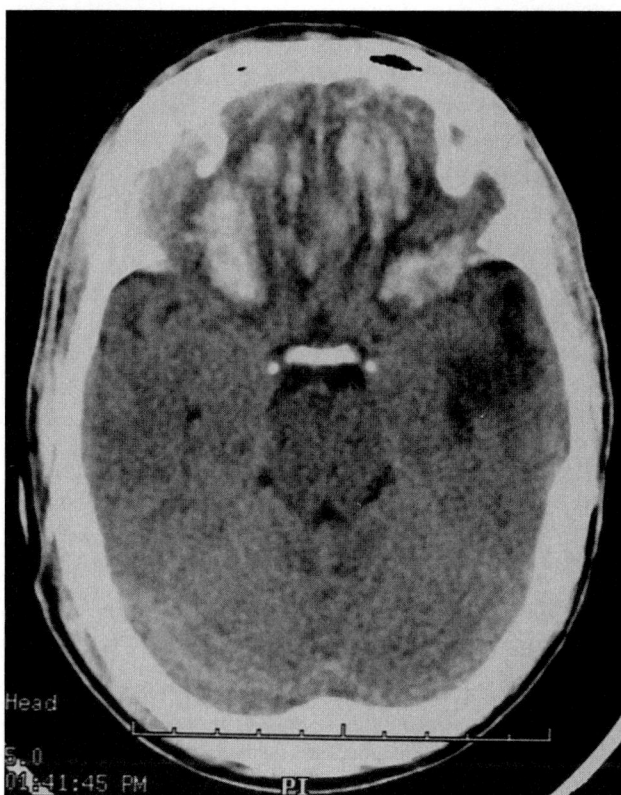

FIG. 41-8. *Severe bilateral contusions in the basal aspect of the frontal lobes, caused by the brain moving over the rough, irregular skull base during sudden cranial acceleration.*

severe cases, especially on MRI. Hemorrhage is classically seen in the corpus callosum and the dorsolateral midbrain.

Penetrating Injury. These are complex and must be evaluated individually. The two main subtypes are missile injury (e.g., due to bullets or fragmentation devices) and nonmissile injury (e.g., due to knives or ice picks). Some general principles do apply. If available, skull x-rays and CT scans are useful in assessing the nature of the injury. Cerebral angiography must be considered if the object passes near a major artery or dural venous sinus. Operative exploration is necessary to remove any object extending out of the cranium, as well as for débridement, irrigation, hemostasis, and definitive closure. Small objects contained within brain parenchyma are often left in place to avoid iatrogenic secondary brain injury. Antibiotics are given to decrease the chances of meningitis or abscess formation. High-velocity missile injuries (from high-powered hunting rifles or military weapons) are especially deadly, because the associated shock wave causes cavitary tissue destruction of an area that is much larger than the projectile itself. Projectiles that penetrate both hemispheres or traverse the ventricles are almost universally fatal.

Traumatic Intracranial Hematomas

The various traumatic intracranial hematomas contribute to death and disability secondary to head injury. Hematomas can expand rapidly and cause brain shifting and subsequent herniation. Emergent neurosurgical evaluation and intervention are often necessary.

Epidural Hematoma. Epidural hematoma (EDH) is the accumulation of blood between the skull and the dura. EDH usually results from arterial disruption, especially of the middle meningeal artery. The dura is adherent to bone and some pressure is required to dissect between the two. EDH has a classic three-stage clinical presentation that is probably seen in only 20% of cases. The patient is initially unconscious from the concussive aspect of the head trauma. The patient then awakens and has a lucid interval while the hematoma subclinically expands. As the volume of the hematoma grows, the decompensated region of the pressure-volume curve is reached, the ICP increases, and the patient becomes lethargic and herniates. Uncal herniation from an EDH classically causes ipsilateral third nerve palsy and contralateral hemiparesis.

On head CT the clot is bright, biconvex (lentiform), and has a well-defined border that usually respects cranial suture lines. The clot generally forms over the convexities, but may rarely occur in the posterior fossa as well.

Open craniotomy for evacuation of the congealed clot and hemostasis is indicated for EDH, except in selected cases of asymptomatic clots that are less than 1 cm in maximum thickness, seen in patients with a negative neurologic examination. Prognosis after successful evacuation is better for epidural hematoma than subdural hematoma. EDHs are associated with lower-energy trauma with less resultant primary brain injury. Good outcomes may be seen in 85 to 90% of patients, with rapid CT scan and intervention.

Acute Subdural Hematoma. An acute subdural hematoma (SDH) is the result of an accumulation of blood between the arachnoid membrane and the dura. Acute SDH usually results from venous bleeding, usually from tearing of a bridging vein running from the cerebral cortex to the dural sinuses. The bridging veins are subject to stretching and tearing during acceleration/deceleration of the head, because the brain shifts in relation to the dura, which firmly adheres to the skull. Elderly and alcoholic patients are at higher risk for acute SDH formation after head trauma due to the greater mobility of their atrophied brains within the cranial vault.

On head CT scan, the clot is bright or mixed-density, crescent-shaped (lunate), may have a less distinct border, and does not cross the midline due to the presence of the falx. Most SDHs are over the cerebral hemispheres, but they may also layer on the tentorium or be interhemispheric.

Open craniotomy for evacuation of the clot is indicated for any acute SDH more than 1 cm in thickness, or smaller hematomas that are symptomatic. Symptoms may be as subtle as a contralateral pronator drift, or as dramatic as coma. Smaller hematomas may stabilize and eventually reabsorb, or become chronic SDHs. Nonoperatively managed patients require frequent neurologic exams until stabilization of the clot if proven by serial head CT scans.

The prognosis for functional recovery is significantly worse for acute SDH than EDH, because it is associated with greater primary injury to brain parenchyma from high-energy impacts. Prompt recognition and intervention minimizes secondary injury. Elderly patients, patients with low admission GCS, or high postoperative ICP do poorly, with as few as 5% attaining functional recovery.[6]

Chronic Subdural Hematoma. Chronic SDH is a collection of blood breakdown products that is at least 3 weeks old. Acute hematomas are bright white (hyperdense) on CT scan for approximately 3 days, after which they fade to isodensity with brain, and then to hypodensity after 2 to 3 weeks. A true chronic SDH will be as dark as CSF on CT. Traces of white are often seen due to small hemorrhages into the collection. These small bleeds may expand the collection enough to make it symptomatic. This is referred to as acute-on-chronic SDH. Figure 41-9 demonstrates the CT

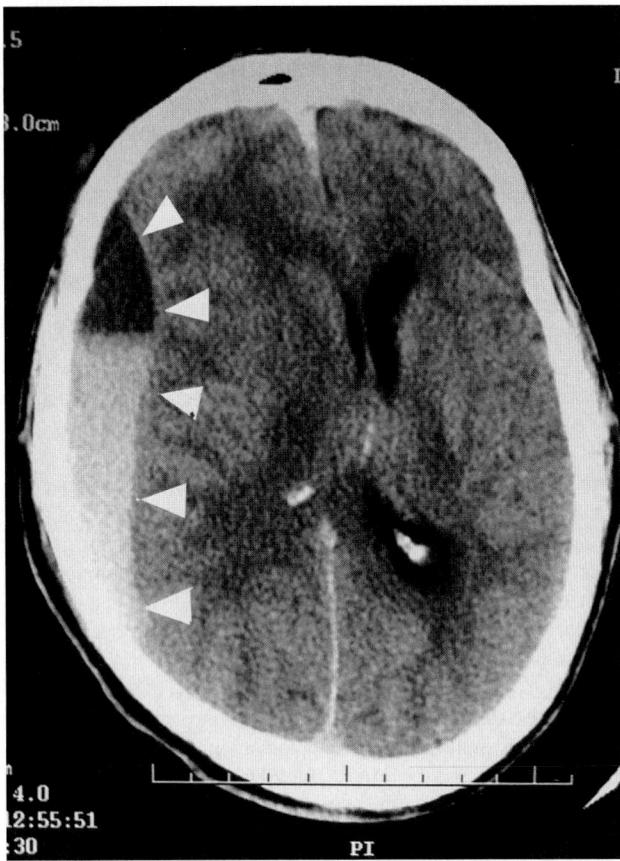

FIG. 41-9. Head CT scan of an elderly patient with progressing left hemiplegia and lethargy, demonstrating an acute-on-chronic subdural hematoma. History revealed that the patient sustained a fall 4 weeks prior to presentation. Arrowheads outline the hematoma. The acute component is slightly denser, and is seen as the hyperdense area in the dependent portion.

appearance of an acute-on-chronic SDH. Vascularized membranes form within the hematoma as it matures. These membranes may be the source of acute hemorrhage.

Chronic SDHs often occur in patients without a clear history of head trauma, as they may arise from minor trauma. Alcoholics, the elderly, and patients on anticoagulation are at higher risk for developing chronic SDH. Patients may present with headache, seizure, confusion, contralateral hemiparesis, or coma.

A chronic SDH thicker than 1 cm, or any symptomatic SDH should be surgically drained. Unlike acute SDH, which consists of a thick, congealed clot, chronic SDH typically consists of a viscous fluid, with a texture and the dark brown color reminiscent of motor oil. As such, a simple burr hole can effectively drain most chronic SDHs. There remains controversy about the optimum treatment of chronic SDH, but most authorities agree that burr hole drainage should be attempted first, to obviate the risks of formal craniotomy. A single burr hole placed over the dependent edge of the collection can be made, and the space copiously irrigated until the fluid is clear. A second, more anterior, burr hole can then be placed if the collection does not drain satisfactorily due to containment by membranes. The procedure is converted to open craniotomy if the SDH is too congealed for irrigation drainage, the complex of membranes prevents effective drainage, or persistent hemorrhage occurs that cannot be reached with bipolar cautery through the burr hole. The required surgical prepping and draping are always performed

to allow simple conversion to craniotomy, and the incisions and burr holes placed to allow easy incorporation into question mark–shaped craniotomy flaps.

There are various strategies to prevent reaccumulation of blood. Subdural or subgaleal drains may be left in place for 1 to 2 days. Mild hydration and bedrest with the head of bed flat may encourage brain expansion. High levels of inspired oxygen may help draw nitrogen out of the cavity. Regardless of the strategy used, follow-up head CT scans are required immediately postoperatively and approximately 1 month later to document resolution.

Intraparenchymal Hemorrhage. Isolated hematomas within the brain parenchyma are more often associated with hypertensive hemorrhage or arteriovenous malformations. Bleeding may occur in a contused area of brain. Mass effect from developing hematomas may present as delayed neurologic deficit. Delayed traumatic intracerebral hemorrhage is most likely to occur within the first 24 hours. Patients with contusion on the initial head CT scan should be reimaged 24 hours after the trauma to document stable pathology.

Vascular Injury

Trauma to the head or neck may cause damage to the carotid or vertebrobasilar systems. In general usage, dissection refers to violation of the vessel wall intima. Blood at arterial pressure can then open a plane between the intima and media, within the media, or between the media and adventitia. The newly created space within the vessel wall is referred to as the false lumen. Tissue or organs supplied by traumatically-dissected vessels may subsequently be injured in several ways. Expansion of the hematoma within the vessel wall can lead to narrowing of the true vessel lumen and reduction or cessation of distal blood flow. Slow-flowing or stagnant blood within the false lumen exposed to thrombogenic vessel wall elements may thrombose. Pieces of thrombus may then detach and cause distal embolic arterial occlusion. Also, the remaining partial-thickness vessel wall may rupture, damaging adjacent structures.

Traumatic dissection may occur in the carotid artery (anterior circulation) or the vertebral or basilar arteries (posterior circulation). Dissections may be extradural or intradural. Intradural dissection can present with subarachnoid hemorrhage, whereas extradural dissection cannot.

Traditional angiography remains the basis of diagnosis and characterization of arterial dissection. Angiographic abnormalities include stenosis of the true lumen, visible intimal flaps, and the appearance of contrast in the false lumen. Four-vessel cerebral angiography should be performed when suspicion of dissection exists.

Patients with documented arterial dissection should be anticoagulated with heparin and then warfarin to prevent thromboembolic stroke. Trauma patients often have concomitant absolute or relative contraindications to anticoagulation, complicating management. Warfarin may be discontinued when the angiogram normalizes, or after several months. Consider surgical intervention for persisting embolic disease and for vertebral dissections presenting with subarachnoid hemorrhage. Surgical options include vessel ligation and bypass grafting. Interventional radiology techniques include stenting and vessel occlusion. Occlusion techniques depend on good collateral circulation to perfuse the vascular territory previously supplied by the occluded vessel.

Carotid Dissection. Carotid dissection may result from neck extension combined with lateral bending to the opposite side, or trauma from an incorrectly placed shoulder belt tightening across the neck in a motor vehicle accident. Extension/bending stretches the carotid over the bony transverse processes of the cervical vertebrae, while seat belt injuries cause direct trauma. Symptoms of cervical carotid dissection include contralateral neurologic deficit from brain ischemia, headache, and ipsilateral Horner's syndrome from disruption of the sympathetic tracts ascending from the stellate ganglion into the head on the surface of the carotid artery. The patient may complain of hearing or feeling a bruit.

Traumatic vessel wall injury to the portion of the carotid artery running through the cavernous sinus may result in a carotid-cavernous fistula (CCF). This creates a high-pressure, high-flow pathophysiologic blood flow pattern. CCFs classically present with pulsatile proptosis (the globe pulses outward with arterial pulsation), retro-orbital pain, and decreased visual acuity or loss of normal eye movement (due to damage to cranial nerves III, IV, and VI as they pass through the cavernous sinus). Symptomatic CCFs should be treated to preserve eye function. Fistulae may be closed by balloon occlusion using interventional neuroradiology techniques. Fistulae with wide necks are difficult to treat and may require total occlusion of the parent carotid artery.

Vertebrobasilar Dissection. Vertebrobasilar dissection may result from sudden rotation or flexion/extension of the neck, chiropractic manipulation, or a direct blow to the neck. Common symptoms are neck pain, headache, and brain stem stroke or subarachnoid hemorrhage. Treatment is as described above.

Brain Death

Brain death occurs when there is an absence of signs of brain stem function or motor response to deep central pain in the absence of pharmacologic or systemic medical conditions that could impair brain function.

Clinical Examination. A neurologist, neurosurgeon, or intensivist generally performs the clinical brain death exam. Two exams consistent with brain death 12 hours apart, or one exam consistent with brain death followed by a consistent confirmatory study is generally sufficient to declare brain death (see below). Hospital regulations and local laws regarding documentation should be followed closely.

Establish the absence of complicating conditions before beginning the exam. The patient must be normotensive, euthermic, and oxygenating well. The patient may not be under the effects of any sedating or paralytic drugs.

Documentation of no brain stem function includes the following: nonreactive pupils; lack of corneal blink, oculocephalic (doll's eyes), or oculovestibular (cold calorics) reflexes; and loss of drive to breathe (apnea test). The apnea test demonstrates no spontaneous breathing even when Pa_{CO_2} is allowed to rise above 60 mm Hg.

Deep central painful stimulus is provided by forceful twisting pinch of the sensitive skin above the clavicle. Pathologic responses such as flexor or extensor posturing are not compatible with brain death. Spinal reflexes to peripheral pain, such as triple flexion of the lower extremities, are compatible with brain death.

Confirmatory Studies. Confirmatory studies are performed after a documented clinical exam consistent with brain death. A study consistent with brain death may obviate the need to wait 12 hours for a second exam. This is especially important when the patient is a potential organ donor, as brain dead patients often have progressive hemodynamic instability. Lack of cerebral blood flow consistent with brain death may be documented by cerebral angiography or technetium radionuclide study. A "to-and-fro" pattern

on transcranial Doppler (TCD) ultrasonography indicates no net forward flow through the cerebral vasculature, consistent with brain death. An electroencephalogram (EEG) documenting electrical silence has been used, but is generally not favored because there is often artifact or noise on the recording. This can confuse the situation and be especially difficult for families to understand.

Spine Trauma

The spine is a complex biomechanic and neural structure. The spine provides structural support for the body as the principal component of the axial skeleton, while protecting the passing spinal cord and nerve roots. Trauma may fracture bones or cause ligamentous disruption. Often bone and ligament damage occur together. Damage to these elements reduces the strength of the spine and may cause the spine to be unstable. This compromises both its structural support function and its ability to protect neural elements. Spine trauma may occur with or without neurologic injury. Neurologic injury from spine trauma is classified as either incomplete, if there is some residual motor or sensory neurologic function below the level of the lesion, or complete, if there is no residual neurologic function below the level of the lesion, as assessed by clinical exam.[7] A patient with complete neurologic dysfunction persisting 24 hours after injury has a very low probability of return of function in the involved area.

Neurologic injury from spine trauma may occur immediately or in delayed fashion. Immediate neurologic injury may be due to direct damage to the spinal cord or nerve roots from penetrating injuries, especially from stab wounds or gunshots. Blunt trauma may transfer sufficient force to the spine to cause acute disruption of bone and ligament and lead to subluxation, which is shift of one vertebral element in relation to the adjacent level. Subluxation decreases the size of the spinal canal and neural foramina, and causes compression of the cord or roots. Such neural impingement can also result from propulsion of bone fragments into the canal during a fracture. Transection, crush injury, and cord compression impairing perfusion are mechanisms leading to spinal cord injury. Delayed neurologic injury may occur during transportation or examination of a patient who is not properly immobilized.

The Mechanics of Spine Trauma

Trauma causes a wide variety of injury patterns in the spine due to its biomechanic complexity. A mechanistic approach facilitates an understanding of the patterns of injury, as there are only a few types of forces that can be applied to the spine. Although these forces are discussed individually, they often occur in combination. Several of the most common injury patterns are then presented to illustrate the clinical results of these forces and combinations of forces applied at pathologically high levels.

Flexion/Extension. Bending the head and body forward into a fetal position flexes the spine. Flexion loads the spine anteriorly (the vertebral bodies) and distracts the spine posteriorly (the spinous process and interspinous ligaments). High flexion forces occur during front-end motor vehicle collisions, and backward falls when the head strikes first. Arching the neck and back extends the spine. Extension loads the spine posteriorly and distracts the spine anteriorly. High extension forces occur during rear-end motor vehicle collisions (especially if there is no headrest), frontward falls when the head strikes a first, or diving into shallow water.

Compression/Distraction. Force applied along the spinal axis (axial loading) compresses the spine. Compression loads the spine anteriorly and posteriorly. High compression forces occur when a falling object strikes the head or shoulders, or when landing on the feet, buttocks, or head after a fall from height. A pulling force in line with the spinal axis distracts the spine. Distraction unloads the spine anteriorly and posteriorly. Distraction forces occur during a hanging, when the chin or occiput strikes an object first during a fall, or when a passenger submarines under a loose seat belt during a front-end motor vehicle collision.

Rotation. Force applied tangential to the spinal axis rotates the spine. Rotation depends on the range of motion of intervertebral facet joints. High rotational forces occur during off-center impacts to the body or head or during glancing automobile accidents.

Patterns of Injury

Certain patterns of injury resulting from the forces described above or from combinations of those forces occur commonly and should be recognized during plain film imaging of the spine. Always completely evaluate the spine. A patient with a spine injury at one level is at significant risk for additional injuries at other levels.

Cervical. The cervical spine is more mobile than the thoracolumbar spine. Stability comes primarily from the multiple ligamentous connections of adjacent vertebral levels. Disruption of the cervical ligaments can lead to instability in the absence of fracture. The mass of the head transmits significant forces to the cervical spine during abrupt acceleration or deceleration, increasing risk for injury.

Jefferson Fracture. Jefferson's fracture is a bursting fracture of the ring of C1 (the atlas) due to compression forces. There are usually two or more fractures through the ring of C1. The open-mouth odontoid view may show lateral dislocation of the lateral masses of C1. The rule of Spence states that 7 mm or greater combined dislocation indicates disruption of the transverse ligament. The transverse ligament stabilizes C1 with respect to C2. Jefferson fractures dislocated less than 7 mm are usually treated with a rigid collar, while those dislocated 7 mm or greater are usually treated with a halo vest. Surgical intervention is not indicated.

Odontoid Fractures. The odontoid process, or dens, is the large ellipse of bone arising anteriorly from C2 (the axis) and projecting up through the ring of C1 (the atlas). Several strong ligaments connect the odontoid to C1 and to the base of the skull. Odontoid fractures usually result from flexion forces. Odontoid fractures are classified as type I, II, or III. A type I fracture involves the tip only. A type II fracture passes through the base of the odontoid process. A type III fracture passes through the body of C2. Types I and II are considered unstable and should be externally immobilized by a halo vest or fused surgically. Surgery is often undertaken for widely displaced fractures (poor chance of fusing) and for those that fail external immobilization. Type III fractures usually fuse with external immobilization only.

Hangman's Fracture. Traditionally considered a hyperextension/distraction injury from placement of the noose under the angle of the jaw, hangman's fractures may also occur with hyperextension/compression, as with diving accidents, or hyperflexion. Its definition is bilateral C2 pars interarticularis fracture. The pars interarticularis is the bone between superior and inferior facet joints. The bony connection between C1 and C3 is lost. Hangman's fractures heal well with external immobilization. Surgery is indicated if there is spinal cord compression or after failure of external immobilization.

Jumped Facets—Hyperflexion Injury. The facet joints of the cervical spine slope forward, and the facet from the level above can slide up and forward over the facet from the level below if the joint capsule is torn. Hyperflexion/rotation can cause a unilateral jumped facet, whereas straight hyperflexion leads to bilateral jumped facets. Patients with a unilateral injury are usually neurologically intact, while those with bilateral injury usually have spinal cord damage. The anteroposterior diameter of the spinal canal decreases more with bilateral injury, leading to spinal cord compression (Fig. 41-10).

Thoracolumbar. The thoracic spine is significantly stabilized by the rib cage. The lumbar spine has comparatively very large vertebrae. Thus the thoracolumbar spine has a higher threshold for injury than the cervical spine. The three-column model is useful for categorizing thoracolumbar injuries. The anterior longitudinal ligament and the anterior half of the vertebral body constitute the anterior column. The posterior half of the vertebral body and the posterior longitudinal ligament constitute the middle column. The pedicles, facet joints, laminae, spinous processes, and interspinous ligaments constitute the posterior column.

Compression Fracture. This is a compression/flexion injury causing failure of the anterior column only. It is stable and not associated with neurologic deficit, although the patient may still have significant pain (Fig. 41-11).

Burst Fracture. This is a pure axial compression injury causing failure of the anterior and middle columns. It is unstable, and perhaps half of patients have neurologic deficit due to compression of the cord or cauda equina from bone fragments retropulsed into the spinal canal.

Chance Fracture. This is a flexion-distraction injury causing failure of the middle and posterior columns. It is typically unstable and is often associated with neurologic deficit.

Fracture-Dislocation. This is failure of the anterior, middle, and posterior columns caused by flexion/distraction, shear, or compression forces. Neurologic deficit can result from retropulsion of middle column bone fragments into the spinal canal, or from subluxation causing decreased canal diameter (Fig. 41-12).

Initial Assessment and Management

The possibility of a spine injury must be considered in all trauma patients. A patient with no symptoms referable to neurologic injury, a normal neurologic exam, no neck or back pain, and a known mechanism of injury unlikely to cause spine injury is at minimal risk for significant injury to the spine. Victims of moderate or severe trauma, especially those with injuries to other organ systems, usually fail to meet these criteria or cannot be assessed adequately. The latter is often due to impaired sensorium or significant pain. Because of the potentially catastrophic consequences of missing occult spine instability in a neurologically intact patient, a high level of clinical suspicion should govern patient care until completion of clinical and radiographic evaluation.

The trauma patient should be kept on a hard flat board with straps and pads used for immobilization. A hard cervical collar is kept in place. These steps minimize forces transferred through the spine, and therefore decrease the chance of causing dislocation, subluxation, or neural compression during transport to the trauma bay. The patient is then moved from the board to a flat stretcher. The primary survey and resuscitation are completed. Physical exam and initial x-rays follow.

For the exam, approach the patient as described in the section on neurologic examination earlier in this chapter. Evaluation for spine or spinal cord injury is easier and more informative in awake

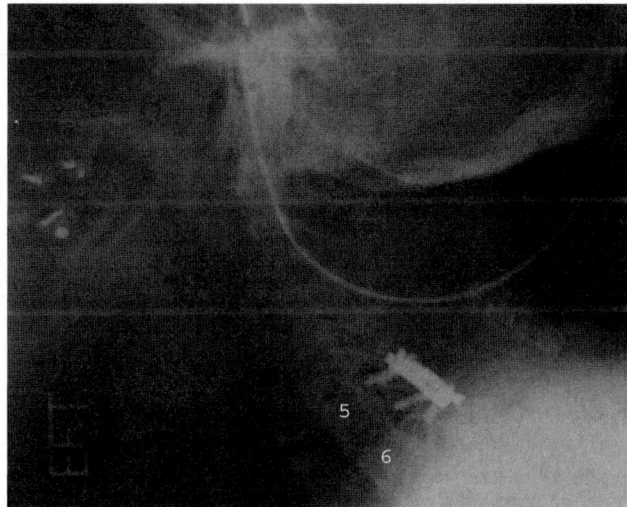

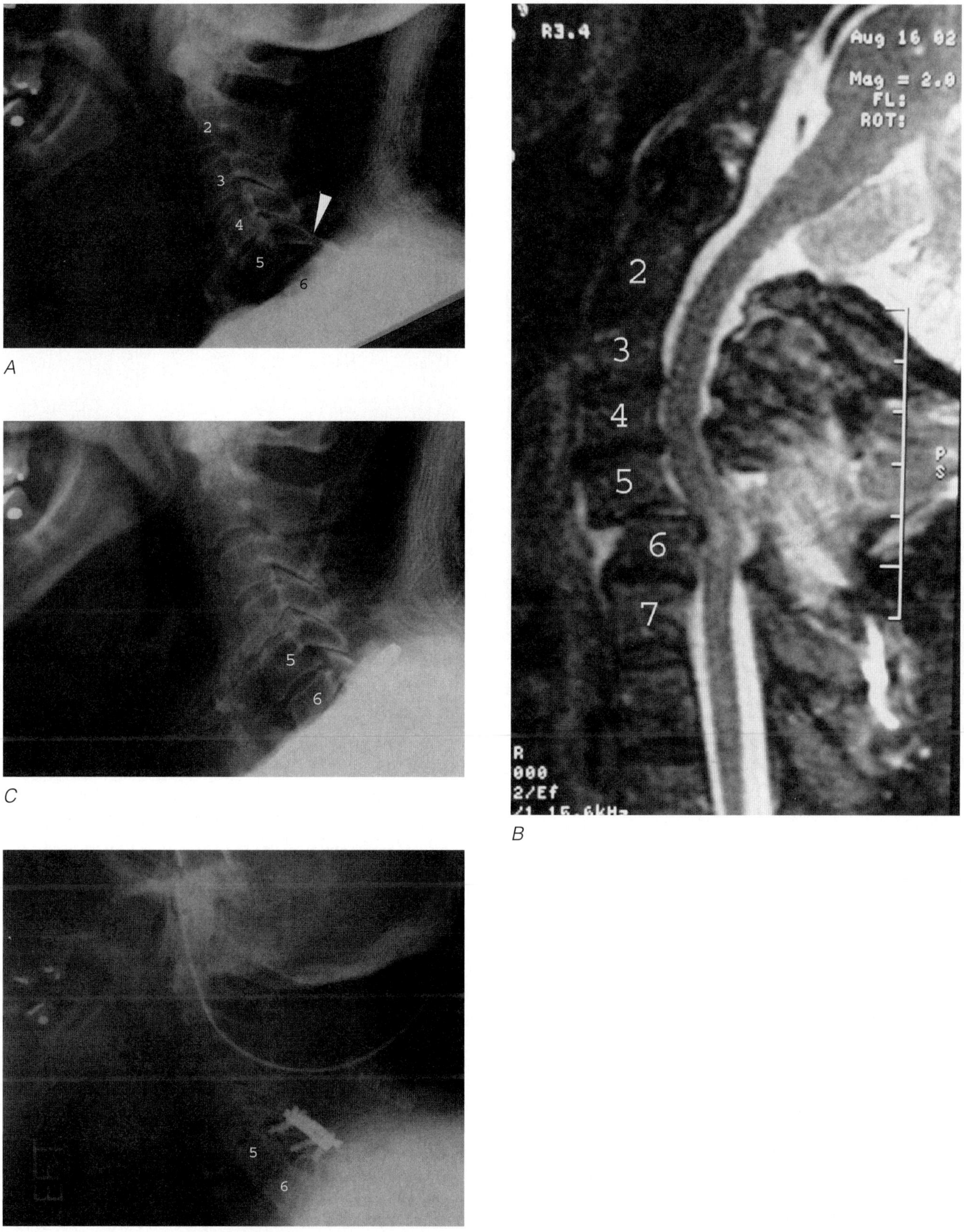

FIG. 41-10. *A.* Lateral cervical spine x-ray of an elderly woman who struck her head during a backward fall. Arrowhead points to jumped facets at C5–C6. Note the anterior displacement of the C5 body with respect to the C6 body. *B.* Sagittal T2-weighted MRI of the same patient, revealing compromise of the spinal canal and compression of the cord. Note the bright signal within the cord at the level of compression, indicating spinal cord injury. *C.* Lateral cervical spine x-ray of same patient after application of cervical traction and manual reduction. Note restoration of normal alignment. *D.* Lateral cervical spine x-ray after posterior cervical fusion to restabilize the C5–C6 segment of the spine.

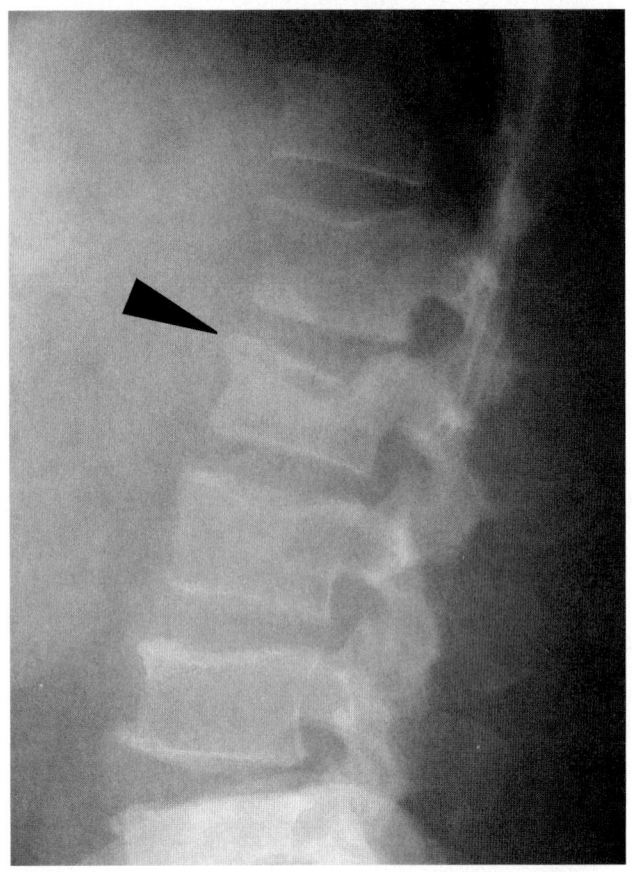

A

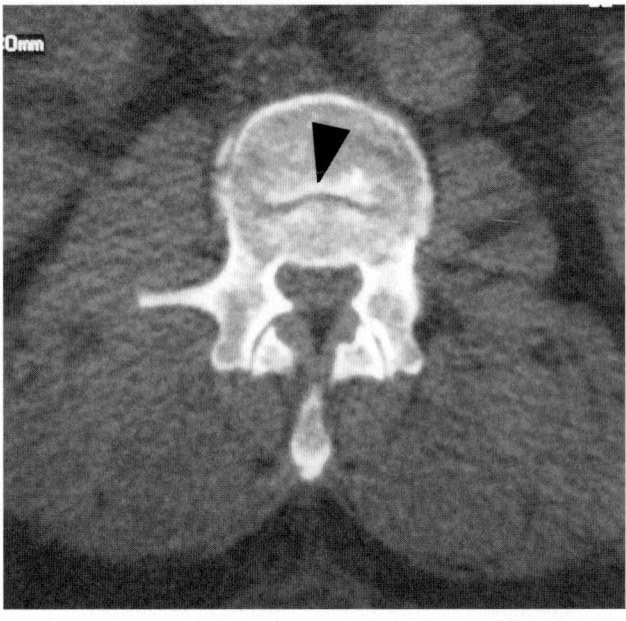

B

FIG. 41-11. *A.* Lateral lumbar spine x-ray showing a compression fracture of L2. Note the posterior wall of the vertebral body has retained normal height and alignment. *B.* Axial CT scan through the same fracture. Arrowhead demonstrates a transverse discontinuity in the superior endplate of the L2 body.

patients. If the patient is awake, ask if he or she recalls details of the nature of the trauma, and if there was loss of consciousness, numbness, or inability to move any or all limbs. Assess motor function by response to commands or pain, as appropriate. Assess pinprick, light touch, and joint position if possible. Determining the anatomically lowest level of intact sensation can pinpoint the level of the lesion along the spine. Test sensation in an ascending fashion, as the patient will be better able to note when he or she first feels the stimulus, rather than when he or she can no longer feel it. Document muscle stretch reflexes, lower sacral reflexes (i.e., anal wink and bulbocavernosus), and rectal tone.

American Spinal Injury Association Classification. The American Spinal Injury Association (ASIA) provides a method of classifying patients with spine injuries. The classification indicates completeness and level of the injury and the associated deficit. A form similar to that shown in Fig. 41-13 should be available in the trauma bay and completed for any spine injury patient. The association also has worked to develop recommendations and guidelines to standardize the care of SCI patients in an effort to improve the quality of care.

Neurologic Syndromes

Penetrating, compressive, or ischemic cord injury can lead to several characteristic presentations based on the anatomy of injury. The neurologic deficits may be deduced from the anatomy of the

long sensory and motor tracts and understanding of their decussations (Fig. 41-14). Four patterns are discussed. First, injury to the entire cord at a given level results in anatomic or functional cord transection with total loss of motor and sensory function below the level of the lesion. The typical mechanism is severe traumatic vertebral subluxation reducing spinal canal diameter and crushing the cord. Second, injury to half the cord at a given level results in Brown-Sequard syndrome, with loss of motor control and proprioception ipsilaterally, and loss of nociception and thermoception contralaterally. The typical mechanism is a stab or gunshot wound. Third, injury to the interior of the cord results in central cord syndrome, with upper extremity worse than lower extremity weakness and varying degrees of numbness. The typical mechanism is transient compression of the cervical cord by the ligamentum flavum buckling in posteriorly during traumatic neck hyperextension. This syndrome occurs in patients with preexisting cervical stenosis. Fourth, injury to the ventral half of the cord results in anterior cord syndrome, with paralysis and loss of nociception and thermoception bilaterally. The typical mechanism is acute disc herniation or ischemia from anterior spinal artery occlusion.

Studies

Anteroposterior (AP) and lateral plain films provide a rapid survey of the bony spine. Plain films detect fractures and dislocations well. Adequate visualization of the lower cervical and upper thoracic spine is often impossible because of the shoulder girdle. Complete

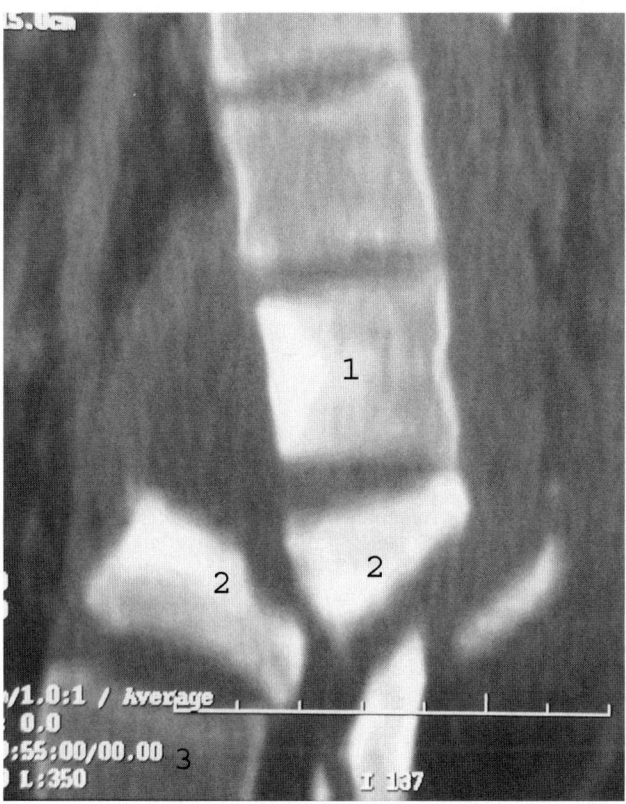

FIG. 41-12. Sagittal reconstruction of an axial fine-slice CT scan through the lumbar spine demonstrating a severe fracture-dislocation through the body of L2.

plain film imaging of the cervical spine includes an open-mouth odontoid view to assess the odontoid and the lateral masses of C1. Fine-slice CT scan with sagittal and coronal reconstructions provides good detail of bone anatomy, and is good for characterizing fractures seen on plain films, as well as visualizing C7–T1 when not well seen on plain films. MRI provides the best soft tissue imaging. Canal compromise from subluxation, acute disc herniations, or ligamentous disruption is clearly seen. MRI also may detect damage to the spinal cord itself, including contusions or areas of ischemia.

Definitive Management

Spinal-Dose Steroids. The National Acute Spinal Cord Injury Study (NASCIS) I and II papers provide the basis for the common practice of administering high-dose steroids to patients with acute spinal cord injury. A 30-mg/kg IV bolus of methylprednisolone is given over 15 minutes, followed by a 5.4-mg/kg per hour infusion begun 45 minutes later. The infusion is continued for 23 hours if the bolus is given within 3 hours of injury, or for 47 hours if the bolus is given within 8 hours of injury. The papers indicate greater motor and sensory recovery at 6 weeks, 6 months, and 1 year after acute spinal cord injury in patients who received methylprednisolone.[8,9] However, the NASCIS trial data have been extensively criticized, as many argue that the selection criteria and study design were flawed, making the results ambiguous. Patients who receive such a large corticosteroid dose have increased rates of medical and ICU complications, such as pneumonias, which have a deleterious affect on outcome. A clear consensus on the use of spinal-dose steroids does not exist.[10] A decision to use or not use spinal-dose steroids may be dictated by local or regional

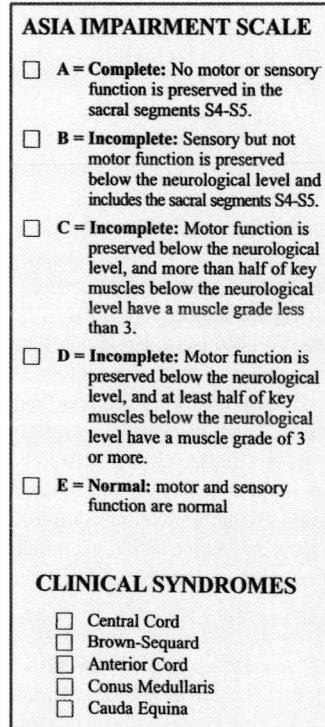

A

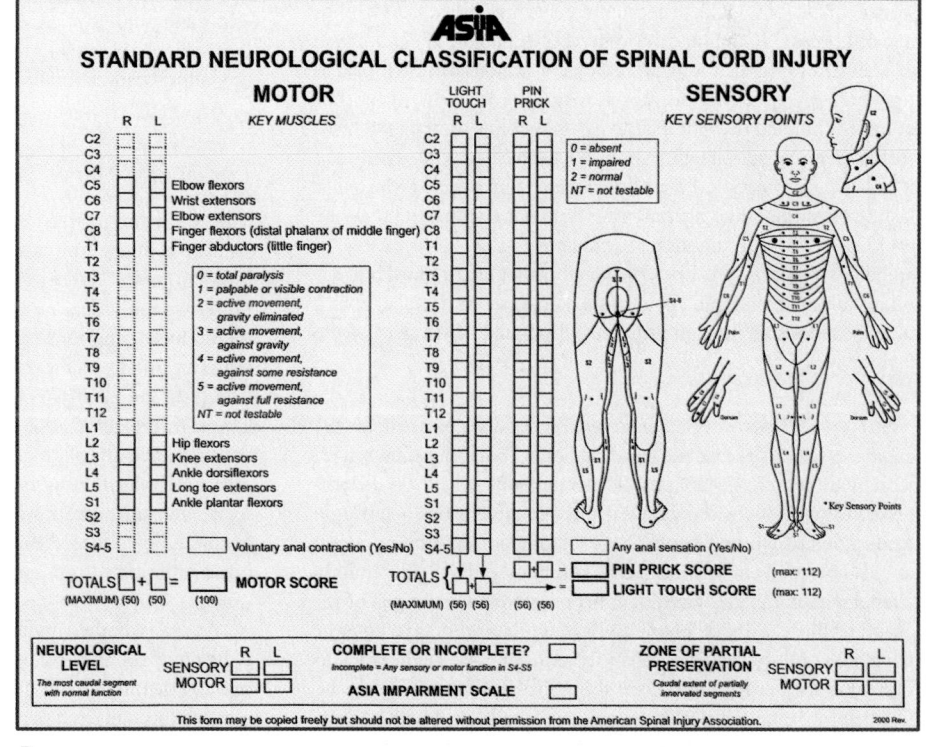

B

FIG. 41-13. The American Spinal Injury Association system for categorizing spinal cord injury patients according to level and degree of neurologic deficit.

SPINAL CORD SYNDROMES

Dorsal column
(touch, vibration)

Corticospinal tract
(upper motor)

Anterior horn
(lower motor)

Spinothalmic tract
(pain, temperature)

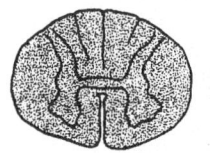

Transection

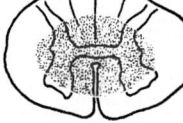

Central cord

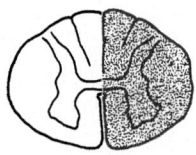

Brown-Sequard

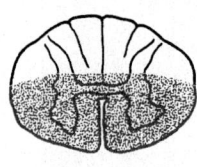

Anterior spinal a.

FIG. 41-14. Spinal cord injury patterns. (*Adapted with permission from Hoff J, Boland M: Neurosurgery, from Schwartz's Textbook of General Surgery, 7th ed. New York: McGraw-Hill, 1999, p 1837.*)

practice patterns, especially given the legal liability issues surrounding spinal cord injury. Patients with gunshot injuries or nerve root (cauda equina) injury, as well as those on chronic steroid therapy, who are pregnant, or who are less than 14 years old were excluded from the NASCIS studies, and should not receive spinal-dose steroids.

Orthotic Devices. Rigid external orthotic devices can stabilize the spine by decreasing range of motion and minimizing stress transmitted through the spine. Commonly used rigid cervical orthotics include Philadelphia and Miami-J collars. Cervical collars are inadequate for C1, C2, or cervicothoracic instability. Cervicothoracic orthoses (CTOs) brace the upper thorax and the neck, improving stabilization over the cervicothoracic region. Minerva braces improve high cervical stabilization by bracing from the upper thorax to the chin and occiput. Halo-vest assemblies provide the most external cervical stabilization. Four pins driven into the skull lock the halo ring in position. Four posts arising from a tight-fitting rigid plastic vest immobilize the halo ring. Lumbar stabilization may be provided by thoracolumbosacral orthoses (TLSOs). A variety of companies manufacture lines of spinal orthotics. A physician familiar with the technique should fit a halo-vest. Assistance from a trained orthotics technician improves fitting and adjustment of the other devices.

Surgery. Neurosurgical intervention has two goals. First is the decompression of the spinal cord or nerve roots in patients with incomplete neurologic deficits. These patients should be decompressed expeditiously, especially if there is evidence of neurologic deterioration over time. Second is the stabilization of injuries judged too unstable to heal with external orthotics only. Spine trauma patients with complete neurologic deficit, without any signs of recovery, or those without any neurologic deficits who have bony or ligamentous injury requiring open fixation, may be medically stabilized before undergoing surgery. Surgical stabilization may be indicated for some injuries that would eventually heal with conservative treatment. Surgical stabilization can allow early mobilization, aggressive nursing care, and physical therapy. Solid surgical stabilization may also allow a patient to be managed with a rigid cervical collar who would otherwise require halo-vest immobilization.

Continued Care

Regional spinal cord injury centers with nurses, respiratory therapists, pulmonologists, physical therapists, physiatrists, and neurosurgeons specifically trained in caring for these patients may improve outcomes. Frequently encountered ICU issues include hypotension and aspiration pneumonia. Chronically, prevention and treatment of deep venous thrombosis, autonomic hyperreflexia, and decubitus ulcer formation are important. Patients with high cervical cord injuries (C4 or above) will often be terminally ventilator dependent. Many patients with cervical or high thoracic cord injuries require prolonged ventilatory support until the chest wall becomes stiff enough to provide resistance for diaphragmatic breathing. Patients should be transferred to spinal cord injury rehabilitation centers after stabilization of medical and surgical issues.

Peripheral Nerve Trauma

The peripheral nervous system extends throughout the body and is subject to injury from a wide variety of traumas. Peripheral nerves transmit motor and sensory information between the CNS and the body. An individual nerve may have pure motor, pure sensory, or mixed motor and sensory functions. The key information-carrying structure of the nerve is the axon. The axon transmits information from the neuronal cell body and may measure from less than 1 mm to greater than 1 m in length. Axons that travel a significant distance are often covered with myelin, which is a lipid-rich, electrically-insulating sheath formed by Schwann cells. Myelinated axons transmit signals much more rapidly than unmyelinated axons, because the voltage shifts and currents that define action potentials effectively jump from gap to gap over the insulated lengths of the axon.

Axons, whether myelinated or unmyelinated, travel through a collagenous connective tissue known as endoneurium. Groups of axons and their endoneurium form bundles known as fascicles. Fascicles run through a tubular collagenous tissue known as perineurium. Groups of fascicles are suspended in mesoneurium. Fascicles and their mesoneurium run through another tubular collagenous tissue known as epineurium. The epineurium and its contents form the nerve.

There are four major mechanisms of injury to peripheral nerves. Nerves may be lacerated, stretched, compressed, or contused. Knives, passing bullets, or jagged bone fractures may lacerate nerves. Adjacent expanding hematomas or dislocated fractures may stretch nerves. Expanding hematomas, external orthoses such as casts or braces, or blunt trauma over a superficial nerve may compress or crush nerves. Shock waves from high-velocity bullets may contuse nerves. These mechanisms of injury cause damage to the various anatomic components of the nerve. The patterns of damage are categorized below.

Certain nerve segments are particularly vulnerable to injury. The following four characteristics make a nerve segment more vulnerable: proximity to a joint, superficial course, passage through a confined space, and being fixed in position.

Types of Injury

The traditional classification system for peripheral nerve injury is the Seddon classification. Seddon described three injury patterns: neurapraxia, axonotmesis, and neurotmesis, as defined below. The Seddon classification provides a simple, anatomically-based approach to peripheral nerve injury.

Neurapraxia. Neurapraxia is defined as the temporary failure of nerve function without physical axonal disruption. Axon degeneration does not occur. Return of normal axonal function occurs over hours to months, often in the 2- to 4-week range.

Axonotmesis. Axonotmesis is the disruption of axons and myelin. The surrounding connective tissues, including endoneurium, are intact. The axons degenerate proximally and distally from the area of injury. Distal degeneration is known as wallerian degeneration. Axon regeneration within the connective tissue pathways can occur, leading to restoration of function. Axons regenerate at a rate of 1 mm per day. Significant functional recovery may occur for up to 18 months. Scarring at the site of injury from connective tissue reaction can form a neuroma and interfere with regeneration.

Neurotmesis. Neurotmesis is the disruption of axons and endoneurial tubes. Peripheral collagenous components, such as the epineurium, may or may not be intact. Proximal and distal axonal degeneration occurs. The likelihood of effective axonal regeneration across the site of injury depends on the extent of neuroma formation and on the degree of persisting anatomic alignment of the connective tissue structures. For instance, an injury may damage axons, myelin, and endoneurium, but leave perineurium intact. In this case the fascicle sheath is intact, and appropriate axonal regeneration is more likely to occur than if the sheath is interrupted.

Management of Peripheral Nerve Injury

The sensory and motor deficits should be accurately documented. Deficits are usually immediate. Progressive deficit suggests a process such as an expanding hematoma, and may need early surgical exploration. Clean, sharp injuries may also benefit from early exploration and reanastomosis. Most other peripheral nerve injuries should be observed. Electromyography and nerve conduction studies (EMG/NCS) should be done 3 to 4 weeks postinjury if deficits persist. Axon segments distal to the site of injury conduct action potentials normally until wallerian degeneration occurs, so EMG/NCS before 3 weeks is not informative. Continue observation if function improves. Explore the nerve surgically if no functional improvement occurs over 3 months. If intraoperative electrical testing reveals conduction across the injury, continue observation. In the absence of conduction, the segment should be resected and end-to-end primary anastomosis attempted. Anastomoses under tension will not heal, so a nerve graft may be needed to bridge the gap between the proximal and distal nerve ends. The sural nerve is often harvested, as it carries only sensory fibers and leaves a minor deficit when harvested. The connective tissue structures of the nerve graft may provide a pathway for effective axonal regrowth across the injury.

Patterns of Injury

Brachial Plexus. The brachial plexus may be injured in a variety of ways. Parturition or a motorcycle accident can lead to plexus injury due to dislocation of the glenohumeral joint. Attempting to arrest a fall with one's hands can lead to a stretch injury of the plexus due to abrupt movement of the shoulder girdle. A lung apex tumor, known as a Pancoast tumor, can cause compression injury to the plexus. There are many patterns of neurologic deficits possible with injury to the various components of the brachial plexus, and understanding them all would require extensive neuroanatomic discussion. Two well-known eponymous syndromes are Erb's palsy and Klumpke's palsy. Injury high in the plexus to the C5 and C6 roots resulting from glenohumeral dislocation causes Erb's palsy with the characteristic "bellhop's tip" position. The arm hangs at the side, internally rotated. Hand movements are not affected. Injury low in the plexus, to the C8 and T1 roots, resulting from stretch or compression injury, causes Klumpke's palsy with the characteristic "claw hand" deformity. There is weakness of the intrinsic hand muscles, similar to that seen with ulnar nerve injury.

Radial Nerve. The radial nerve courses through the axilla, and then laterally and posteriorly in the spiral groove of the humerus. Improper crutch use can cause damage to the axillary portion. The section of the nerve traversing the spiral groove can be damaged by humerus fractures or pressure from improper positioning during sleep. This classically occurs when the patient is intoxicated and is called "Saturday night palsy." The key finding is wrist drop (i.e., weakness of hand and finger extensors). Axillary (proximal) injury causes tricep weakness in addition to wrist drop.

Common Peroneal Neuropathy. The common peroneal nerve forms the lateral half of the sciatic nerve (the medial half being the tibial nerve). It receives contributions from L4, L5, S1, and S2. It emerges as a separate nerve in the popliteal fossa and wraps laterally around the fibular neck, after which it splits to form the deep peroneal nerve and the superficial peroneal nerve. The superficial, fixed location at the fibular neck makes the nerve susceptible to compression. The classic cause of traumatic peroneal neuropathy is crush injury from a car bumper striking the lateral aspect of the leg at the level of the knee. Symptoms of common peroneal neuropathy include foot drop (weakness of the tibialis anterior) and numbness over the anterolateral surface of the lower leg and dorsum of the foot. Surgical exploration of this lesion is typically unsatisfying. Rare cases may be due to compressive fibers or adhesions that may be lysed, with the possibility of return of function.

CEREBROVASCULAR DISEASE

Cerebrovascular disease is the most frequent cause of new rapid-onset, nontraumatic neurologic deficit. It is a far more common etiology than seizures or tumors. Vascular structures are subject to a variety of chronic pathologic processes which compromise vessel wall integrity. Diabetes, high cholesterol, high blood pressure, and smoking are risk factors for vascular disease. These conditions can lead to vascular damage by such mechanisms as atheroma deposition causing luminal stenosis, endothelial damage promoting thrombogenesis, and weakening of the vessel wall resulting in aneurysm formation or dissection. These processes may coexist. For instance, a vessel may contain an atheromatous plaque that significantly decreases lumen diameter, and also have compromised endothelium over the plaque, providing the opportunity for thrombus formation, which can lead to acute total occlusion of the remaining lumen. Aneurysms and dissection often occur in atheromatous vessels. Specific patterns of disease relevant to the cerebrovascular system are atheromatous and thrombotic carotid occlusion, brain ischemia due to embolus from a proximal source, vessel wall breakage leading to hemorrhage, and rupture of abnormal, thin-walled structures, specifically aneurysms and arteriovenous malformations.

Ischemic Diseases

Ischemic stroke accounts for approximately 85% of acute cerebrovascular events. Symptoms of acute ischemic stroke vary based on the functions of the neural tissues supplied by the occluded vessel, and the presence or absence of collateral circulation. The circle of Willis provides extensive collateral circulation, as it connects the right and left carotid arteries to each other and each to the vertebrobasilar system. Patients with complete occlusion of the carotid artery proximal to the circle of Willis may be asymptomatic if the blood flow patterns can shift and provide sufficient circulation to the ipsilateral cerebral hemisphere from the contralateral carotid and the basilar artery. However, the anatomy of the circle of Willis is highly variable. Patients may have a hypoplastic or missing communicating artery, both anterior cerebral arteries supplied by one carotid, or the posterior cerebral artery supplied by the carotid rather than the basilar. Similarly, one vertebral artery is often dominant, and the other hypoplastic. These variations may make disease in a particular vessel more neurologically devastating than in a patient with full collateral circulation. Occlusion distal to the circle of Willis generally results in stroke in the territory supplied by the particular artery.

Neurologic deficit from occlusive disease may be temporary or permanent. A patient with sudden-onset focal neurologic deficit that resolves within 24 hours has had a transient ischemic attack (TIA). If the deficit resolves between 24 hours and 1 week, then the patient has had a reversible ischemic neurologic deficit (RIND). A patient with permanent deficits has had a cerebrovascular accident (CVA). CVA is a commonly used, but vague term. Some prefer the term *completed stroke*.

Thrombotic Disease

The most common area of neurologically significant vessel thrombosis is the carotid artery in the neck. Disease occurs at the carotid bifurcation. Thrombosis of a carotid artery chronically narrowed by atheroma can lead to acute carotid occlusion. As discussed above, this may or may not cause symptoms. The more common concern is thromboembolus. Intracranial arterial occlusion by local thrombus formation may occur, but is considered rare compared to embolic occlusion.

Management

Complete occlusion of the carotid artery without referable neurologic deficit requires no treatment. A patient with new neurologic deficit and an angiographically demonstrated complete carotid occlusion contralateral to the symptoms should be considered for emergency carotid endarterectomy.[11] Surgery should not be performed on obtunded or comatose patients, and should be done within

2 hours of symptom onset. This time restriction significantly reduces the number of candidates.

Embolic Disease

Emboli causing strokes may originate in the left atrium due to atrial fibrillation, on a hypokinetic left ventricular wall segment, or in valvular vegetations, an atheromatous aortic arch, or stenosed carotid bifurcations, or from the systemic venous system in the presence of a right-to-left shunt, such as a patent foramen ovale. The majority of emboli enter the anterior (carotid) circulation rather than the posterior (vertebrobasilar) circulation. Characteristic clinical syndromes result from embolic occlusion of the various vessels.

Common Types of Strokes

Anterior Cerebral Artery Stroke. The ACA supplies the medial frontal and parietal lobes, including the motor strip, as it courses into the interhemispheric fissure. ACA stroke results in contralateral leg weakness.

Middle Cerebral Artery Stroke. The MCA supplies the lateral frontal and parietal lobes and the temporal lobe. MCA stroke results in contralateral face and arm weakness. Dominant-hemisphere MCA stroke causes language deficits. Proximal MCA occlusion causing ischemia and swelling in the entire MCA territory can lead to significant intracranial mass effect and midline shift (see Fig. 41-6).

Posterior Cerebral Artery Stroke. The PCA supplies the occipital lobe. PCA stroke results in a contralateral homonymous hemianopsia (see Fig. 41-6).

Posterior Inferior Cerebellar Artery Stroke. The PICA supplies the lateral medulla and the inferior half of the cerebellar hemispheres. PICA stroke results in nausea, vomiting, nystagmus, dysphagia, ipsilateral Horner's syndrome, and ipsilateral limb ataxia. The constellation of symptoms resulting from PICA occlusion is referred to as lateral medullary syndrome or Wallenberg's syndrome.

Management

Ischemic stroke management has two goals: reopen the occluded vessel and maintain blood flow to borderline ischemic tissues on the border of the vascular territory. This bordering tissue is referred to as the ischemic penumbra. The first goal, reopening the vessel, may be attempted with recombinant tPA.[12] tPA administration within 3 hours of the onset of neurologic deficit improves outcome at 3 months. Obtain a head CT immediately in the setting of suspected ischemic stroke to differentiate ischemic from hemorrhagic stroke. Intracranial hemorrhage, major surgery in the previous 2 weeks, gastrointestinal or genitourinary hemorrhage in the previous 3 weeks, platelet count $<100,000/\mu L$, and systolic blood pressure (SBP) >185 mm Hg are among the contraindications to tPA therapy. The neurology stroke team should be called while taking the patient to head CT.

Patients not eligible for tPA require hemodynamic optimization and neurologic monitoring. Admit such patients to the ICU stroke service for blood pressure management and frequent neurologic checks. Allow the blood pressure to run high to maximize cerebral perfusion. SBP more than 180 mm Hg may require treatment. Give normal saline solution without glucose (which could injure neurons in the penumbra), and aim for normovolemia. A stroke patient who worsens clinically should undergo repeat head CT to evaluate for hemorrhage or significant mass effect from swelling. Swelling typically peaks 3 to 5 days after the stroke. Significant swelling from an MCA stroke or cerebellar stroke may be life threatening and require hemicraniectomy or suboccipital craniectomy, respectively, as described in the section on neurosurgical emergencies, earlier in this chapter.

Hemorrhagic Diseases

Intracranial hemorrhage (ICH) from abnormal or diseased vascular structures accounts for approximately 15% of acute cerebrovascular events. Hypertension and amyloid angiopathy account for most intraparenchymal hemorrhages, although arteriovenous malformations (AVMs), aneurysms, venous thrombosis, tumors, hemorrhagic conversion of ischemic infarct, and fungal infections may also be the cause. The term *intracranial hemorrhage* is frequently used to mean intraparenchymal hemorrhage, and will be used here. ICH causes local neuronal injury and dysfunction, and can also cause global dysfunction due to mass effect if of sufficient volume. AVM or aneurysm rupture results in subarachnoid hemorrhage (SAH), because the major cerebral and cortical blood vessels travel between the pia and the arachnoid membrane, in the subarachnoid space. SAH can cause immediate concussive-like neuronal dysfunction by exposure of the brain to intra-arterial pressure pulsations during the hemorrhage, and can cause delayed ischemia from cerebral arterial vasospasm.

Patients presenting with ICHs that do not follow typical patterns should undergo angiography or MRI to evaluate for possible underlying lesions, such as AVM or tumor.

Patients who suffer a hemorrhagic stroke are more likely to present lethargic or obtunded than those who suffer an ischemic stroke. Depressed mental status results from brain shift and herniation secondary to mass effect from the hematoma. Ischemic stroke does not cause mass effect acutely, therefore patients are more likely to present with normal consciousness and a focal neurologic deficit. Hemorrhagic strokes tend to present with a relatively smooth onset of symptoms as the hematoma expands, rather than the immediately maximal symptoms caused by ischemic stroke. Table 41-3 provides a listing of relative incidences of ICH by anatomic distribution.

Hypertension

Hypertension increases the relative risk of ICH by approximately fourfold, likely due to chronic degenerative vasculopathy. Hypertensive hemorrhages often present in the basal ganglia, thalamus, or pons, and result from breakage of small perforating arteries that branch off of much larger parent vessels (Fig. 41-15).

Most hypertensive hemorrhages should be medically managed. The hematoma often contains intact, salvageable axons because the blood dissects through and along neural tracts, and surgical clot evacuation destroys these axons. Factors that indicate that surgery may be appropriate include superficial clot location, young age, nondominant hemisphere, rapid deterioration, and significant mass effect. Most studies fail to show overall improved outcomes. Medical management includes moderate blood pressure control, normalizing platelet and clotting function, phenytoin, and electrolyte management. Intubate patients who cannot clearly follow commands, to prevent aspiration and hypercarbia. Follow and document the neurologic exam and communicate with the family regarding appropriateness for rehabilitation versus withdrawal of care.

Amyloid Angiopathy

The presence of pathologic amyloid deposition in the media of small cortical vessels compromises vessel integrity, predisposes to more superficial (lobar) hemorrhages, and may cause multiple hemorrhages over time.

The superficial location of amyloid hemorrhages may make surgical evacuation less morbid than for typical deep hypertensive hemorrhages. Approach medical management and family counseling similarly to patients with hypertensive hemorrhages.

Cerebral Aneurysm

An aneurysm is focal dilatation of the vessel wall, and is most often a balloon-like outpouching, but may also be fusiform. Aneurysms usually occur at branch points of major vessels [e.g., internal carotid artery (ICA) bifurcation], or at the origin of smaller vessels (e.g., posterior communicating artery or ophthalmic artery). Approximately 85% of aneurysms arise from the anterior circulation (carotid) and 15% from the posterior circulation (vertebrobasilar). Table 41-4 shows the percentage distribution of cerebral aneurysms by location. Aneurysms are thin-walled and at risk for rupture. The major cerebral vessels, and therefore aneurysms, lie in the subarachnoid space. Rupture results in SAH. The aneurysmal tear may be small and seal quickly or not. SAH may consist of a thin layer of blood in the CSF spaces, or thick layers of blood around the brain and extending into brain parenchyma, resulting in a clot with mass effect. The meningeal linings of the brain are sensitive, so SAH usually results in a sudden, severe "thunderclap" headache. A patient will classically describe "the worst headache of my life." Presenting neurologic symptoms may range from mild headache to coma to sudden death. The Hunt-Hess grading system categorizes patients clinically (Table 41-5).

Patients with symptoms suspicious for SAH should have a head CT immediately. Acute SAH appears as a bright signal in the fissures and CSF cisterns around the base of the brain, as shown in Fig. 41-16. CT is rapid, noninvasive, and approximately 95% sensitive. Patients with suspicious symptoms but negative head CT should

Table 41-3
Anatomic Distribution of Intracranial Hemorrhages (ICHs) and Correlated Symptoms

% of ICHs	Location	Classic Symptoms
50%	Basal ganglia (putamen, globus pallidus), internal capsule	Contralateral hemiparesis
15%	Thalamus	Contralateral hemisensory loss
10–20%	Cerebral white matter (lobar)	Depends on location (weakness, numbness, partial loss of visual field)
10–15%	Pons	Hemiparesis; may be devastating
10%	Cerebellum	Lethargy or coma due to brain stem compression and/or hydrocephalus
1–6%	Brain stem (excluding pons)	Often devastating

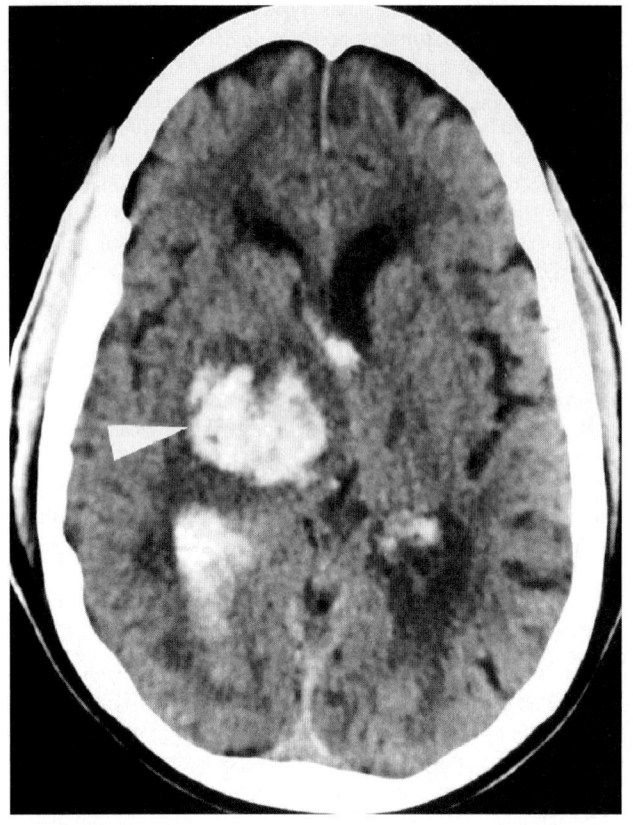

A

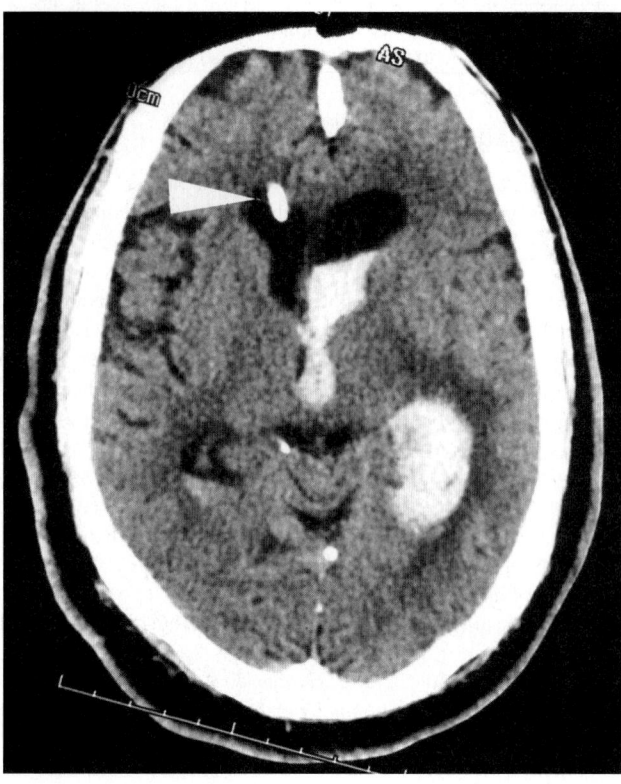

B

FIG. 41-15. *A.* Head CT scan of a patient with left-sided weakness and progressive lethargy reveals a right basal ganglia hemorrhage. The blood clot is bright white. Hypodensity around the clot represents cerebral edema. There is blood within the ventricular system. *B.* Another patient with intraventricular extension of a basal ganglia hemorrhage. The patient developed right-sided weakness and then lethargy. Head CT indicated hydrocephalus. A ventriculostomy was placed for CSF drainage (*arrowhead* indicates cross-sectional view of the catheter entering the anterior horn of the right lateral ventricle).

undergo lumbar puncture. A lumbar puncture (LP) with xanthochromia and high red blood cell (RBC) counts (usually 100,000/mL), which do not decrease between tubes 1 and 4, is consistent with SAH. Negative CT and LP essentially rules out SAH. Patients diagnosed with SAH require four-vessel cerebral angiography within 24 hours to assess for aneurysm or other vascular malformation. Catheter angiography remains the gold standard for assessing the patient's cerebral vasculature, relevant anomalies, and presence, location, and morphology of the cerebral aneurysms. Parts A and B of Fig. 41-17 demonstrate the typical digital subtraction angiographic (DSA) view of a cerebral aneurysm. Part C shows the anatomy of

the circle of Willis in a simplified graphic representation to assist in visualizing the locations of various cerebral aneurysms.

SAH patients should be admitted to the neurologic ICU. Hunt-Hess grade 4 and 5 patients require intubation and hemodynamic monitoring and stabilization. The current standard of care for ruptured aneurysms requires early aneurysmal occlusion. There are two options for occlusion. The patient may undergo craniotomy with microsurgical dissection and placement of a titanium clip across

Table 41-4
Prevalence of Cerebral Aneurysm by Location

Prevalence (%)	Aneurysm Location (Vernacular Name)
Anterior circulation 85%	30% Anterior communicating artery (A-Comm) 25% Posterior communicating artery (P-Comm) 20% Middle cerebral artery bifurcation (MCA) 10% Other
Posterior circulation 15%	10% Basilar artery, most frequently at the basilar tip 5% Vertebral artery, usually at the posterior inferior cerebellar artery (PICA)

Table 41-5
The Hunt-Hess Clinical Grading System for Subarachnoid Hemorrhage

Hunt-Hess Grade	Clinical Presentation
0	Asymptomatic; unruptured aneurysm
1	Awake; asymptomatic or mild headache; mild nuchal rigidity
2	Awake; moderate to severe headache, cranial nerve palsy (e.g., CN III or IV), nuchal rigidity
3	Lethargic; mild focal neurologic deficit (e.g., pronator drift)
4	Stuporous; significant neurologic deficit (e.g., hemiplegia)
5	Comatose; posturing

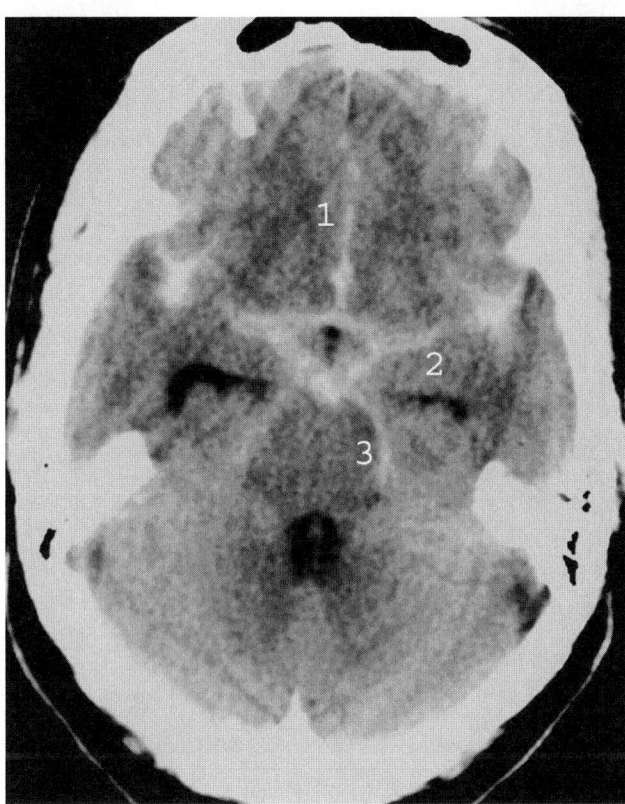

FIG. 41-16. *Head CT scan of a patient who experienced a sudden, severe headache. Subarachnoid hemorrhage is visible as hyperdense signal in the interhemispheric fissure (number 1), bilateral sylvian fissures (number 2 shows the left fissure), and in the ambient cisterns around the midbrain (number 3). This gives the classic five-pointed-star appearance of SAH. Visible temporal tips of the lateral ventricles indicate hydrocephalus.*

the aneurysm neck to exclude the aneurysm from the circulation and reconstitute the lumen of the parent vessel. The second option is to take the patient to the interventional neuroradiology suite for endovascular placement of looped titanium coils inside the aneurysm dome. The coils support thrombosis and prevent blood flow into the aneurysm. Factors favoring craniotomy and clipping include young age, good medical condition, and broad aneurysm necks. Factors favoring coiling include old or medically-frail patients and narrow aneurysm necks. Clipping results in a more definitive cure, because coils can move and compact over time, requiring repeat angiograms and placement of additional coils. The decision to clip or coil is complex and should be fully explored. The International Subarachnoid Aneurysm Trial (ISAT) researchers suggested that endovascular occlusion resulted in better outcomes for certain types of cerebral aneurysms, although this trial was marred by poor selection and randomization techniques, and the validity of its conclusions have been questioned.[13] Debate also continues regarding optimal care for unruptured intracranial aneurysms.[14]

SAH patients often require 1 to 3 weeks of ICU care after aneurysm occlusion for medical complications that accompany neurologic injury. In addition to routine ICU concerns, SAH patients are also at risk for cerebral vasospasm. In vasospasm, cerebral arteries constrict pathologically and can cause ischemia or stroke from 4 to 21 days after SAH. Current vasospasm prophylaxis includes maintaining hypertension and mild hypervolemia to optimize perfusion, and administering nimodipine, a calcium channel blocker that may decrease the incidence and degree of spasm. Neurointerventional

options for treating symptomatic vasospasm are intra-arterial papaverine and balloon angioplasty.

Aneurysmal SAH has an approximate mortality rate of 50% in the first month. Approximately one-third of survivors returns to pre-SAH function, and the remaining two-thirds have mild to severe disability. Most require rehabilitation after hospitalization.

Arteriovenous Malformations

AVMs are abnormal, dilated arteries and veins without an intervening capillary bed. The nidus of the AVM contains a tangled mass of vessels, but no neural tissue. AVMs may be asymptomatic or present with SAH or seizures. Small AVMs present with hemorrhage more often than large AVMs, which tend to present with seizures. Headache, bruit, or focal neurologic deficits are less common symptoms. AVMs hemorrhage at an average rate of 2 to 4% a year. Figure 41-18 demonstrates the angiographic appearance of an AVM in arterial and venous phases.

There are several management differences for SAH due to AVM versus aneurysm. Definitive therapy for the AVM is usually delayed 3 to 4 weeks to allow the brain to recover from acute injury. There is less risk of devastating early rebleeding from AVMs, and vasospasm is less relevant. Adjacent brain may be hyperemic after removal of the high-flow arteriovenous (A-V) shunt, so hypertension and hypervolemia are not beneficial. Three therapeutic modalities for AVMs are currently in common use: microsurgical excision, endovascular glue embolization, and stereotactic radiosurgery. AVMs that are large, near eloquent cortex, or that drain to deep venous structures are considered high grade and more difficult to surgically resect without causing significant neurologic deficit. Radiosurgery can treat these lesions, although it is limited to lesions less than 3 cm in diameter and has a 2-year lag time (i.e., the AVM may bleed in the interval). Embolization reduces flow through the AVM. It is usually considered adjunctive therapy, but may rarely be the sole treatment for deep, inaccessible lesions.

TUMORS OF THE CENTRAL NERVOUS SYSTEM

A wide variety of tumors affect the brain and spine. Primary benign and malignant tumors arise from the various elements of the CNS, including neurons, glia, and meninges. Tumors metastasize to the CNS from many primary sources. Presentation varies widely depending on relevant neuroanatomy. Prognosis depends on histology and anatomy. Modern brain tumor centers utilize team approaches to CNS tumors, as patients may require a combination of surgery, radiation therapy, chemotherapy, stereotactic radiosurgery, and research protocol enrollment. Tumors affecting the peripheral nervous system are discussed in the peripheral nerve section.

Intracranial Tumors

Intracranial tumors are brain tumors that cause mass effect, dysfunction or destruction of adjacent neural structures, swelling, abnormal electrical activity, or a combination of these. Supratentorial tumors commonly present with focal neurologic deficit, such as contralateral limb weakness or visual field deficit, or headache or seizure. Infratentorial tumors often cause increased ICP, due to hydrocephalus due to compression of the fourth ventricle, leading to headache, nausea, vomiting, or diplopia. Cerebellar hemisphere or brain stem dysfunction can lead to ataxia, nystagmus, or cranial nerve palsies. Infratentorial tumors rarely cause seizures.

All patients with symptoms concerning for brain tumor should undergo MRI with and without gadolinium. Initial management of a

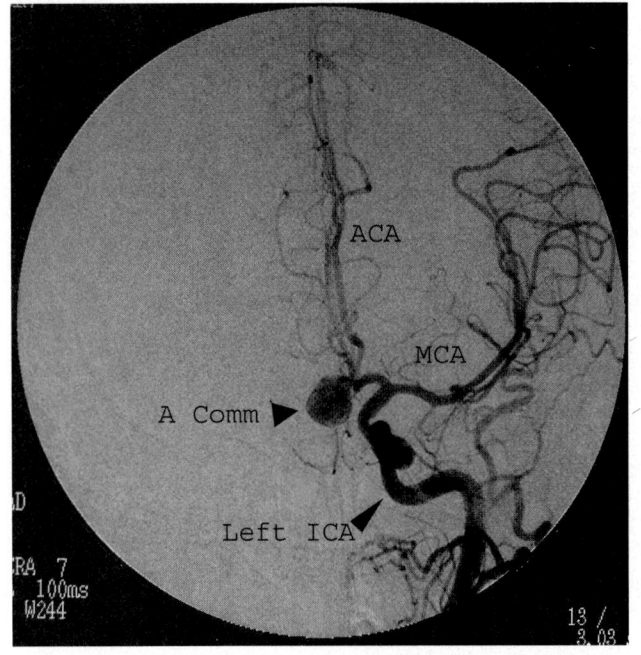

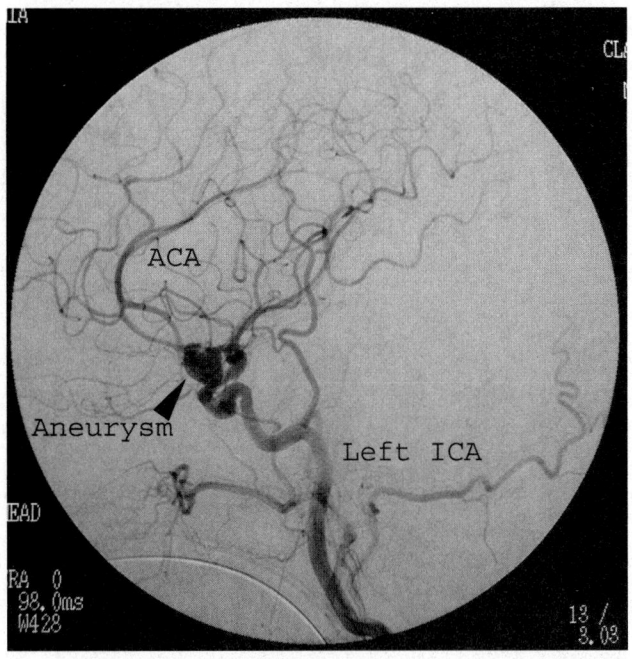

A

B

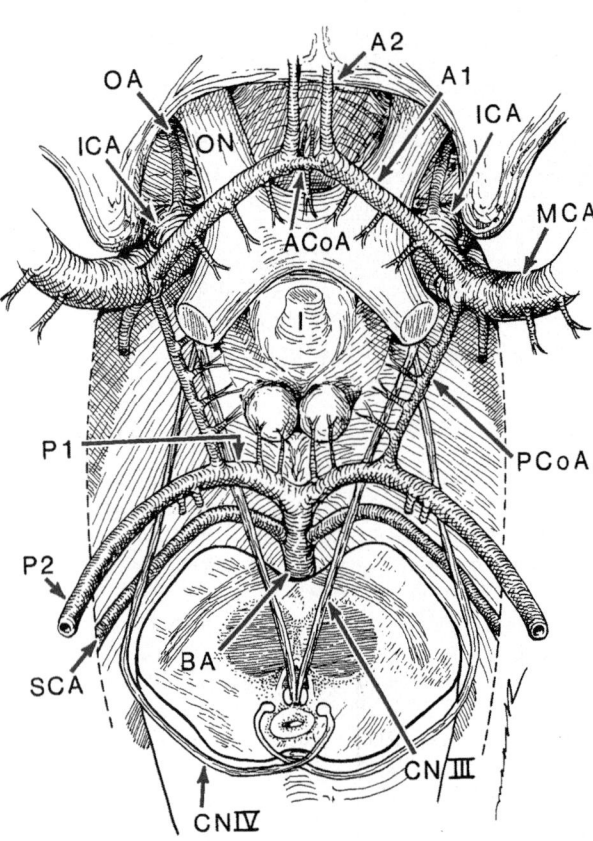

C

FIG. 41-17. *A.* Anteroposterior view after injection of contrast dye in the left internal carotid artery demonstrates a 13-mm diameter anterior communicating artery aneurysm (labeled *A Comm*). The left internal carotid, middle carotid, and anterior cerebral arteries are clearly seen. *B.* Lateral view of the same injection again demonstrates the aneurysm. *C.* Figure depicting the anatomy of the circle of Willis in relation to key structures on the base of the brain. ACoA = anterior communicating artery; A1 = first section of anterior cerebral artery (ACA), before ACoA; A2 = second section of ACA, after ACoA; BA = basilar artery; CN III = third cranial nerve (oculomotor nerve); CN IV = fourth cranial nerve (trochlear nerve); I = infundibulum (the attachment of the pituitary stalk); ICA = internal cerebral artery; MCA = middle cerebral artery; OA = ophthalmic artery; ON = optic nerve; PCoA = posterior communicating artery; P1 = first section of posterior cerebral artery (PCA), before the PCoA; P2 = second section of the PCA, after the PCoA; SCA = superior cerebellar artery. *(Reproduced with permission from Diagnostic Cerebral Angiography, Osborn.)*

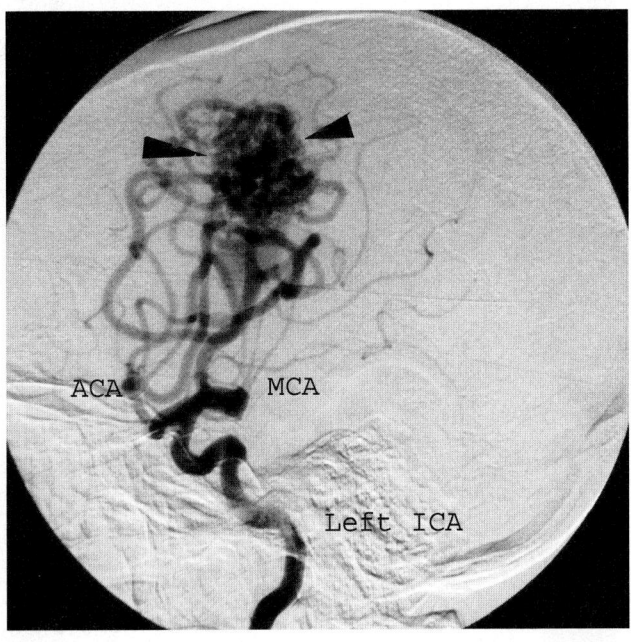

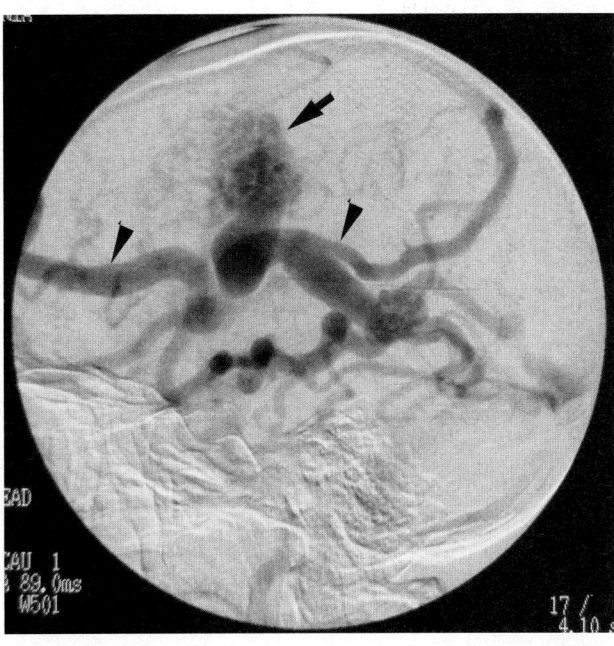

FIG. 41-18. *A.* Lateral view after injection of contrast dye in the left internal carotid artery demonstrates a 3 × 4 cm left frontal arteriovenous malformation indicated by arrowheads. This image was taken 1.06 seconds after dye injection, and is referred to as an arterial phase image. *B.* Same view taken 4.10 seconds after dye injection, providing a venous phase image. The arrow points to the AVM nidus. The arrowheads indicate two pathologically enlarged draining veins.

patient with a symptomatic brain tumor generally includes dexamethasone (if edema is present) and phenytoin (supratentorial tumors only). Patients with significant weakness, lethargy, or hydrocephalus should be admitted for observation until definitive care is administered.

Metastatic Tumors

Prolonged cancer patient survival and improved CNS imaging have increased the likelihood of diagnosing cerebral metastases. The sources of most cerebral metastases are (in decreasing frequency) the lung, breast, kidney, GI tract, and melanoma. Lung and breast cancers account for more than half of cerebral metastases. Metastatic cells usually travel to the brain hematogenously and frequently seed the gray-white junction. Other common locations are the cerebellum and the meninges. The latter leads to carcinomatous meningitis, also known as leptomeningeal carcinomatosis. MRI pre– and post–contrast administration is the study of choice for evaluation. Figure 41-19 demonstrates bilateral cerebellar metastases. Metastases are often very well circumscribed, round, and multiple. Such findings should instigate a metastatic work-up, including CT scan of the chest, abdomen, and pelvis, and a bone scan.

Management depends on the primary tumor, tumor burden, patient's medical condition, and location and number of metastases. The patient's and family's beliefs regarding aggressive care must be considered. Craniotomy may benefit patients with one or two accessible metastases and should be discussed. Studies do not support craniotomy unless all detectable metastases can be resected. Surgery should be followed by whole brain radiation therapy. Surgery plus radiation therapy increases average survival from 1 month to 8 months. Recent data suggest stereotactic radiosurgery (e.g., gamma knife) may be applied to multiple metastases in one session with improved outcome.

Glial Tumors

Glial cells provide the anatomic and physiologic support for neurons and their processes in the brain. The several types of glial cells give rise to distinct primary CNS neoplasms.

Astrocytomas

Astrocytoma is the most common primary CNS neoplasm. The term *glioma* is often used to refer to astrocytomas specifically, excluding other glial tumors. Astrocytomas are graded from I to IV. Grades I and II are referred to as low-grade astrocytoma, grade III as anaplastic astrocytoma, and grade IV as glioblastoma multiforme (GBM). Prognosis varies significantly between grades I/II, III, and IV, but not between I and II. Median survival is 8 years after diagnosis with a low-grade tumor, 2 to 3 years with an anaplastic astrocytoma, and roughly 1 year with a GBM. GBMs account for almost two-thirds of all astrocytomas, anaplastic astrocytomas account for two-thirds of the rest, and low-grade astrocytomas the remainder. Figure 41-20 demonstrates the typical appearance of a GBM.

The great majority of astrocytomas infiltrate adjacent brain. Juvenile pilocytic astrocytomas and pleomorphic xanthoastrocytoma are exceptions. These are circumscribed, low grade, and associated with good prognosis. Histologic features associated with higher grade include hypercellularity, nuclear atypia, and endovascular hyperplasia. Necrosis is present only with GBMs; it is required for the diagnosis.

Gross total resection should be attempted for suspected astrocytomas. Motor cortex, language centers, deep or midline structures, or brain stem location may make this impossible without unacceptable, devastating neurologic deficit. These may require stereotactic needle biopsy. Gross total resection followed by radiation therapy improves survival for all grades, although radiation therapy may be delayed

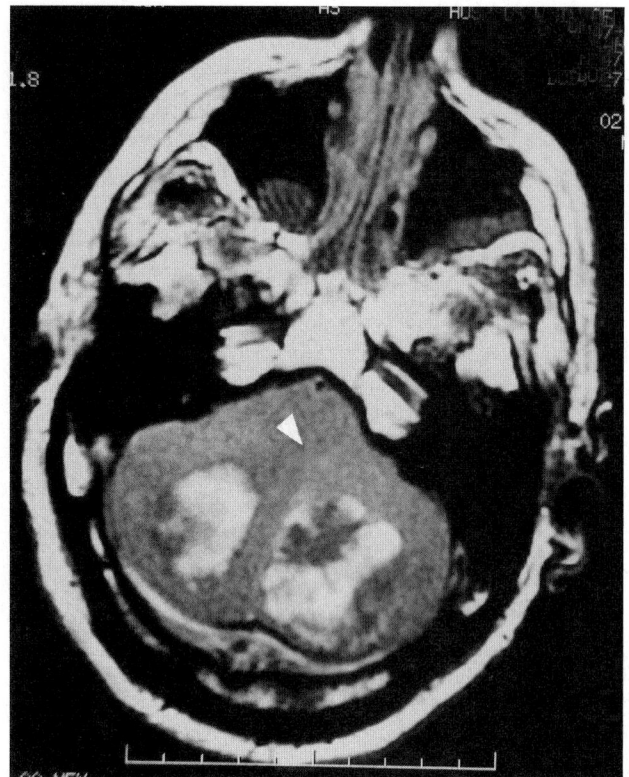

A

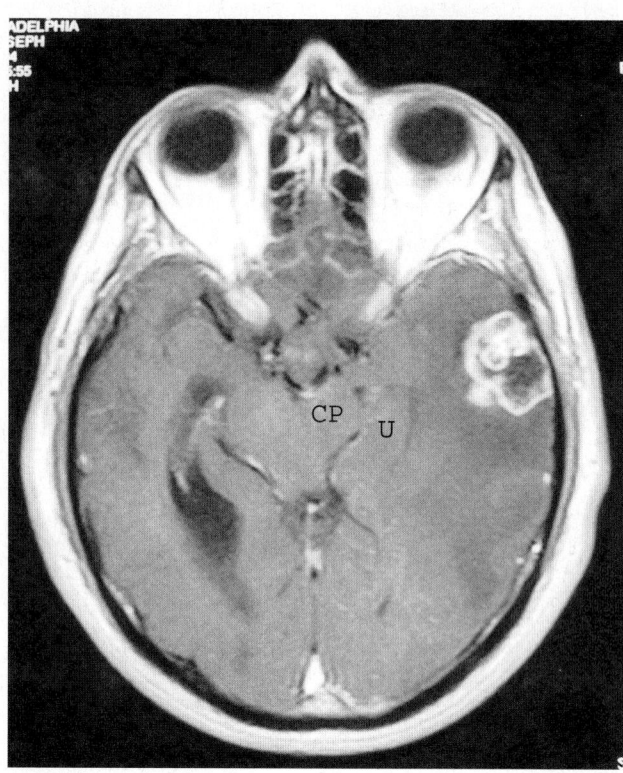

B

FIG. 41-19. *A.* Precontrast T1-weighted axial MRI demonstrating bilateral hemorrhagic cerebellar metastases. Patient presented with ataxia and then lethargy progressing to deep coma. This patient has total effacement of the fourth ventricle and severe brain stem compression. The fourth ventricle CSF space should be at the tip of the arrowhead. Patient recovered to normal mental status after emergent posterior fossa craniotomy. *B.* Postcontrast T1-weighted axial MRI demonstrating a ring-enhancing lesion in the lateral left temporal lobe with moderate edema. The uncus (U) is compressing the left cerebral peduncle (CP) and displacing the brain stem to the right.

until recurrence in low-grade tumors. Chemotherapy may be considered, but is of limited efficacy so far. There are various ongoing research studies for GBM adjuvant therapy; these should be discussed with the patient and family. Other options are carmustine-containing wafers for local chemotherapy (Gliadel) and Iotrex-containing balloons for conformal radiation brachytherapy (Glia-Site), both placed in the resection cavity at the time of surgery. Adjuvant therapy remains marginally effective; survival has changed little over the last several decades.

Oligodendroglioma

Oligodendroglioma accounts for approximately 10% of gliomas. They often present with seizures. Calcifications and hemorrhage on CT or MRI suggest the diagnosis. Oligodendrogliomas are also graded from I to IV; grade portends prognosis. Prognosis is better overall than for astrocytomas. Median survival ranges from 2 to 7 years for highest and lowest grade tumors, respectively. Aggressive resection improves survival. Many oligodendrogliomas will respond to procarbazine, lomustine (CCNU), vincristine (PCV) chemotherapy. Radiation has not been clearly shown to prolong survival.

Ependymoma

The lining of the ventricular system consists of cuboidal/columnar ependymal cells from which ependymomas may arise. Two-thirds of adult ependymomas are infratentorial, while most

pediatric ependymomas are supratentorial. Supratentorial ependymomas arise from the lateral or third ventricles. The infratentorial tumors arise from the floor of the fourth ventricle (i.e., off the back of the brain stem). The most common symptoms are headache, nausea, vomiting, or vertigo, secondary to increased ICP from obstruction of CSF flow through the fourth ventricle. The tumors may grow out the foramina of Luschka to form a cerebellopontine angle (CPA) mass, or may spread through the CSF to form "drop mets" in the spinal cord. Two main histologic subtypes are papillary ependymomas and anaplastic ependymomas, the latter characterized by increased mitotic activity and areas of necrosis. Gross total resection is often impossible because the tumor arises from the brain stem. The goal of surgery is maximal resection without injuring the very delicate brain stem. Suboccipital craniotomy and midline separation of the cerebellar hemispheres allows access to tumors in the fourth ventricle. Postoperative radiation therapy significantly improves survival. Patients with CSF spread documented by lumbar puncture or contrast MRI should also have whole-spine radiation plus focused doses to visualized metastases.

Choroid Plexus Papilloma

The choroid plexus is composed of many small vascular tufts covered with cuboidal epithelium. It represents part of the interface between blood and brain. The choroid cells create CSF from blood and release it into the ventricular system. Choroid plexus papillomas

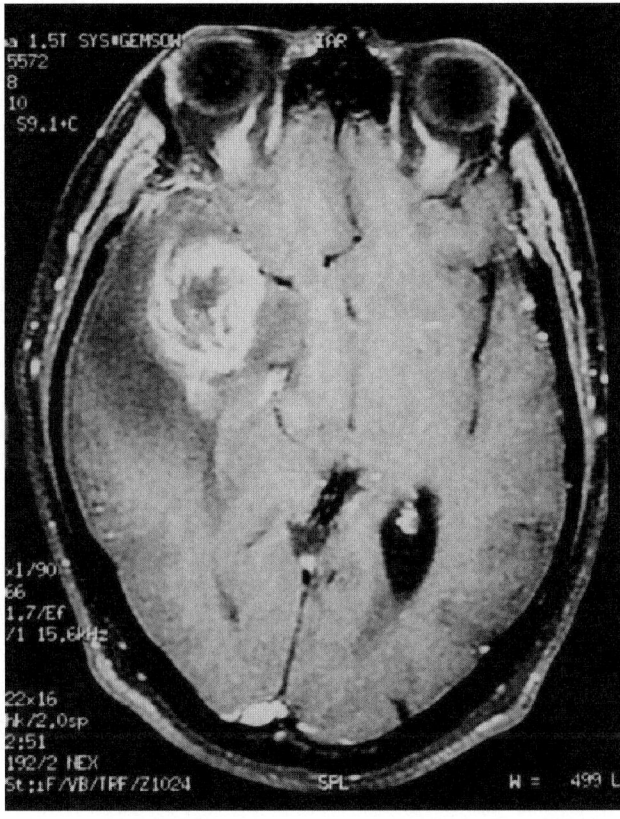

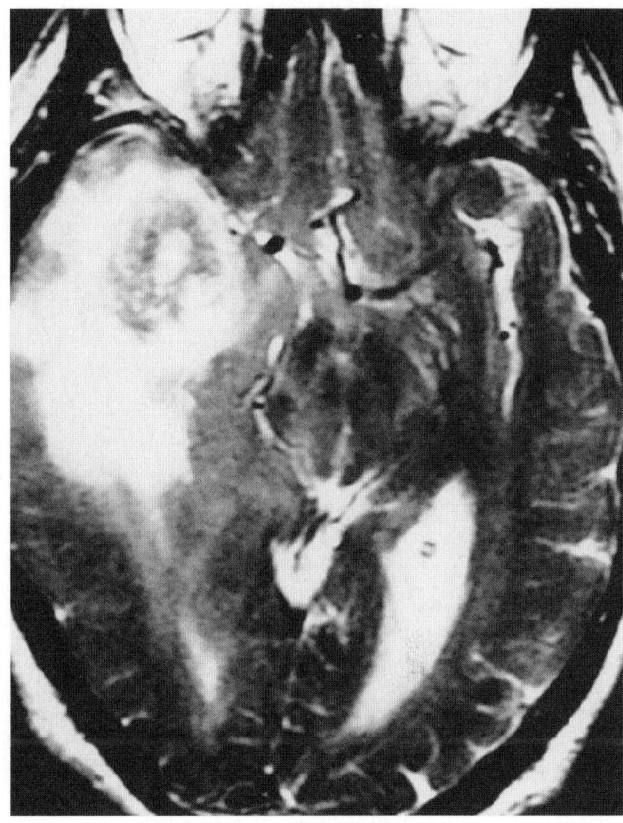

A   B

FIG. 41-20. *A. Postcontrast T1-weighted axial MRI demonstrating a ring-enhancing lesion in the anteromedial right temporal lobe with central necrosis (dark area) consistent with glioblastoma multiforme. B. T2-weighted axial MRI with extensive bright signal signifying peritumoral edema seen with GBMs.*

and choroid plexus carcinomas (rare, mostly pediatric) may arise from these cells. Papillomas usually occur in infants (usually supratentorial in the lateral ventricle), but also occur in adults (usually infratentorial in the fourth ventricle). Papillomas are well circumscribed and vividly enhance due to extensive vasculature. Like ependymomas, adult choroid plexus papillomas usually present with symptoms of increased ICP. Treatment is surgical excision. Total surgical excision is curative; recurrent papillomas should be re-resected. Do not use radiation or chemotherapy for papillomas. Radiation is adjunctive to aggressive surgery for carcinomas, but results are poor regardless.

Neural Tumors and Mixed Tumors

Neural and mixed tumors are a diverse group that includes tumors variously containing normal or abnormal neurons and/or normal or abnormal glial cells. Primitive neuroectodermal tumors (PNETs) arise from bipotential cells, capable of differentiating into neurons or glial cells.

Medulloblastoma

PNETs are the most common medulloblastomas. Most occur in the first decade of life, but there is a second peak around age 30. Medulloblastoma is the most common malignant pediatric brain tumor. They are usually midline. Most occur in the cerebellum and present with symptoms of increased ICP. Histologic characteristics include densely packed small round cells with large nuclei and scant cytoplasm. They are generally not encapsulated, frequently

disseminate within the CNS, and should undergo surgical resection followed by radiation therapy and chemotherapy.

Ganglioglioma

Ganglioglioma is a mixed tumor in which both neurons and glial cells are neoplastic. They occur in the first three decades of life, often in the medial temporal lobe, as circumscribed masses that may contain cysts or calcium and may enhance. The presenting symptom is usually a seizure, due to the medial temporal location. Patients have a good prognosis after complete surgical resection.

Neural Crest Tumors

Multipotent neural crest cells develop into a variety of disparate cell types, including smooth muscle cells, sympathetic and parasympathetic neurons, melanocytes, Schwann cells, and arachnoid cap cells. They migrate in early development from the primitive neural tube throughout the body.

Miscellaneous Tumors

Meningioma

Meningiomas are derived from arachnoid cap cells of the arachnoid mater. They appear to arise from the dura mater grossly and on MRI, and so are commonly referred to as dural-based tumors. The most common intracranial locations are along the falx (Fig. 41-21), the convexities (i.e., over the cerebral hemispheres), and the sphenoid wing. Less common locations include the foramen

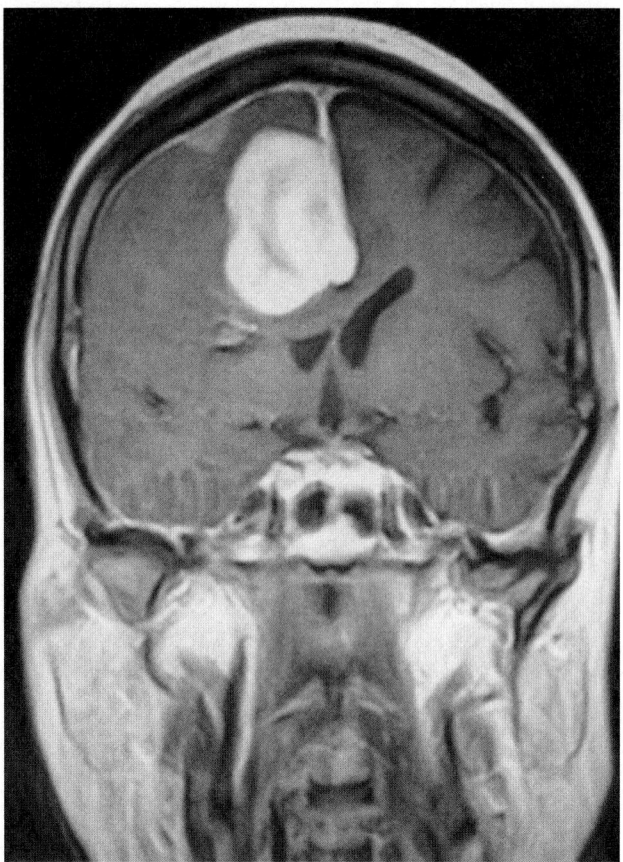

FIG. 41-21. Postcontrast T1-weighted coronal MRI demonstrating a brightly enhancing lesion arising from the falx cerebri with moderate edema and mass effect on the right lateral ventricle. This is a falcine meningioma. Note also the small separate meningioma arising from the dura over the cerebral convexity.

magnum, olfactory groove, and inside the lateral ventricle. Most are slow growing, encapsulated, benign tumors. Aggressive atypical or malignant meningiomas may invade adjacent bone or into the cortex. Previous cranial irradiation increases the incidence of meningiomas. Approximately 10% of patients with a meningioma have multiple meningiomas. Total resection is curative, although involvement with small perforating arteries or cranial nerves may make total resection of skull base tumors impossible without significant neurologic deficit. Small, asymptomatic meningiomas can be followed until symptomatic or significant growth is documented on serial imaging studies. Atypical and malignant meningiomas may require postoperative radiation. Patients may develop recurrences from the surgical bed or distant de novo tumors.

Vestibular Schwannoma (Acoustic Neuroma)

Vestibular schwannomas arise from the superior half of the vestibular portion of the vestibulocochlear nerve (cranial nerve VIII) (Fig. 41-22). They most commonly present with progressive hearing loss, tinnitus, or balance difficulty. Large tumors may cause brain stem compression and obstructive hydrocephalus. Bilateral acoustic neuromas are pathognomonic for neurofibromatosis type 2, a syndrome resulting from chromosome 22 mutation. NF-2 patients have an increased incidence of spinal and cranial meningiomas and gliomas.

Vestibular schwannomas may be treated with microsurgical resection or with conformal stereotactic radiosurgery (gamma knife

or linear accelerator technology). The main complication with treatment is damage to the facial nerve (cranial nerve VII), which runs through the internal auditory canal with the vestibulocochlear nerve. Risk of facial nerve dysfunction increases with increasing tumor diameter.

Pituitary Adenoma

Pituitary ademomas arise from the anterior pituitary gland (the adenohypophysis). Tumors less than 1 cm diameter are microadenomas; larger tumors are macroadenomas. Pituitary tumors may be functional (i.e., secrete endocrinologically active compounds at pathologic levels) or nonfunctional (i.e., secrete nothing or inactive compounds). Functional tumors are often diagnosed when quite small, due to endocrine dysfunction. The most common endocrine syndromes are Cushing's disease due to adrenocorticotropic hormone (ACTH) secretion, Forbes-Albright syndrome due to prolactin secretion, and acromegaly due to growth hormone secretion. Nonfunctional tumors commonly present when larger due to mass effect. Figure 41-23 demonstrates a large pituitary adenoma. Common symptoms include visual field deficits due to compression of the optic chiasm, or panhypopituitarism due to compression of the gland. Hemorrhage into a pituitary tumor causes abrupt symptoms of headache, visual disturbance, decreased mental status, and endocrine dysfunction. This is known as pituitary apoplexy. Pituitary tumors should be decompressed surgically to eliminate symptomatic mass effect and/or to attempt endocrine cure. Prolactinomas usually shrink with dopaminergic therapy. Consider surgery for prolactinomas with persistent mass effect or endocrinologic dysfunction in spite of adequate dopamine agonist therapy. Most pituitary tumors are approached through the nose by the transsphenoidal approach. Endoscopic sinus surgery techniques may be helpful and are increasingly being used.

Hemangioblastoma

Hemangioblastomas occur almost exclusively in the posterior fossa. Twenty percent occur in patients with von Hippel-Lindau (VHL) disease, a multisystem neoplastic disorder. Other tumors associated with VHL are renal cell carcinoma, pheochromocytoma, and retinal angiomas. Many appear as cystic tumors with an enhancing tumor on the cyst wall known as the mural nodule. Surgical resection is curative for sporadic (non-VHL associated) tumors. Pathology reveals abundant thin-walled vascular channels, so internal debulking may be bloody. En bloc resection of the mural nodule alone, leaving the cyst wall, is sufficient.

Lymphoma

CNS lymphoma may arise primarily in the CNS or secondary to systemic disease. Recent increasing incidence may be due to increasing numbers of immunocompromised people in the transplant and AIDS populations. Presenting symptoms include mental status changes, headache due to increased ICP, and cranial nerve palsy due to lymphomatous meningitis (analogous to carcinomatous meningitis). Many are hyperdense on CT scan due to their dense cellularity, and most enhance. Surgical excision has little role. Diagnosis is often made by stereotactic needle biopsy. Subsequent treatment includes steroids, whole brain radiation, and chemotherapy. Intrathecal methotrexate chemotherapy is an option.

Embryologic Tumors

Embryologic tumors result from embryonal remnants that fail to involute completely or differentiate properly during development.

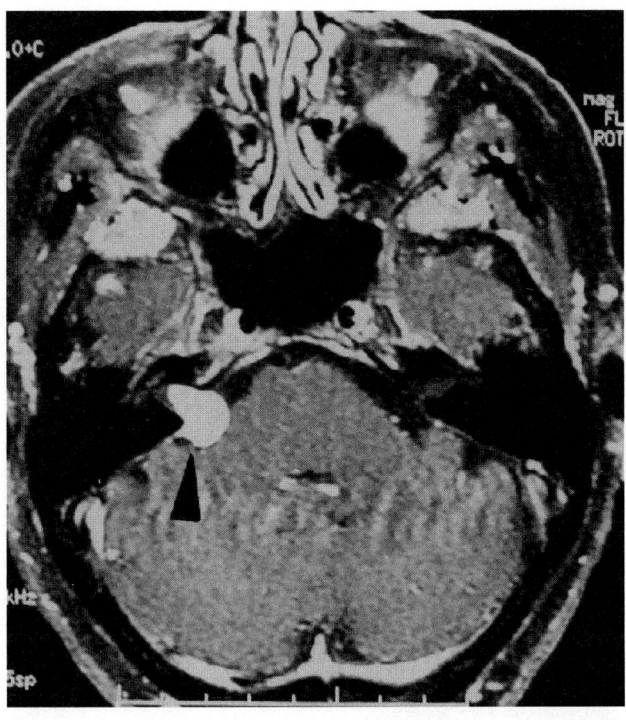 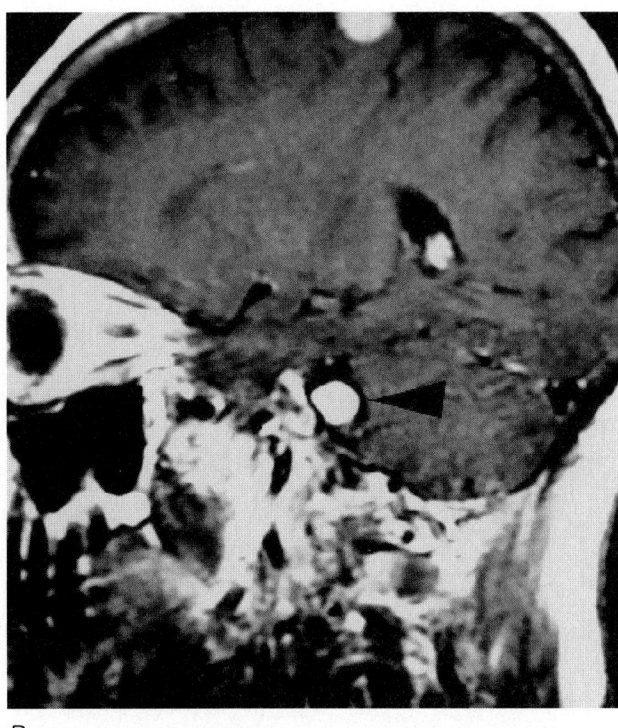

A *B*

FIG. 41-22. *A.* Postcontrast T1-weighted axial MRI demonstrating a brightly enhancing mass on the right vestibular nerve with an enhancing tail going into the internal auditory canal (*arrowhead*). Pathology demonstrated vestibular schwannoma. *B.* Postcontrast T1-weighted sagittal MRI of the same lesion, indicated by the arrowhead. Note small incidental meningioma at the top of the scan.

Craniopharyngioma

Craniopharyngiomas are benign cystic lesions that occur most frequently in children. There is a second peak of occurrence around 50 years of age. All pediatric, and half of adult craniopharyngiomas calcify. Symptoms result from compression of adjacent structures, especially the optic chiasm. Pituitary or hypothalamic dysfunction or hydrocephalus may develop. Treatment is primarily surgical. Excision is easier in children, as the tumor is usually soft and suckable. Adult tumors are often firm and adherent to adjacent vital structures. Visual loss, pituitary endocrine hypofunction, diabetes insipidus, and cognitive impairment from basal frontal injury may result from incautious resection.

Epidermoid

These are cystic lesions with stratified squamous epithelial walls from trapped ectodermal cell rests that grow slowly and linearly by desquamation into the cyst cavity. The cysts contain keratin, cholesterol, and cellular debris (Fig. 41-24). They occur most frequently in the cerebellopontine angle and may cause symptoms due to brain stem compression. Recurrent bouts of aseptic meningitis may occur due to release of irritating cyst contents into the subarachnoid space (Mollaret's meningitis). Treatment is surgical drainage and removal of cyst wall. Intraoperative spillage of cyst contents leads to severe chemical meningitis and must be avoided by containment and aspiration.

Dermoid

Dermoids are less common than epidermoids. They contain hair follicles and sebaceous glands in addition to a squamous epithelium.

Dermoids are more commonly midline structures and are associated with other anomalies than are epidermoids. They may be traumatic, as from a lumbar puncture that drags skin structures into the CNS. Bacterial meningitis may occur when associated with a dermal sinus tract to the skin. Treatment of symptomatic lesions is surgical resection, again with care to control cyst contents.

Teratoma

Teratomas are germ cell tumors that arise in the midline, often in the pineal region (the area behind the third ventricle, above the midbrain and cerebellum). They contain elements from all three embryonal layers: ectoderm, mesoderm, and endoderm. Teratomas may contain skin, cartilage, GI glands, and teeth. Teratomas with more primitive features are more malignant, while those with more differentiated tissues are more benign. Surgical excision may be attempted. Prognosis for malignant teratoma is very poor.

Spinal Tumors

A wide variety of tumors affect the spine. Approximately 20% of CNS tumors occur in the spine. The majority of spinal tumors are histologically benign, unlike cranial tumors. Understanding the two major spinal concepts facilitates understanding of the effects of spinal tumors. The two concepts are spinal stability and neural compression. Destruction of bones or ligaments can cause spinal instability, and lead to deformities such as kyphosis or subluxation and possible subsequent neural compression. Tumor growth in the spinal canal or neural foramina can cause direct compression of the spinal cord or nerve roots and cause loss of function. Anatomic categorization provides the most logical approach to these tumors. The various tumors present in characteristic locations. An understanding

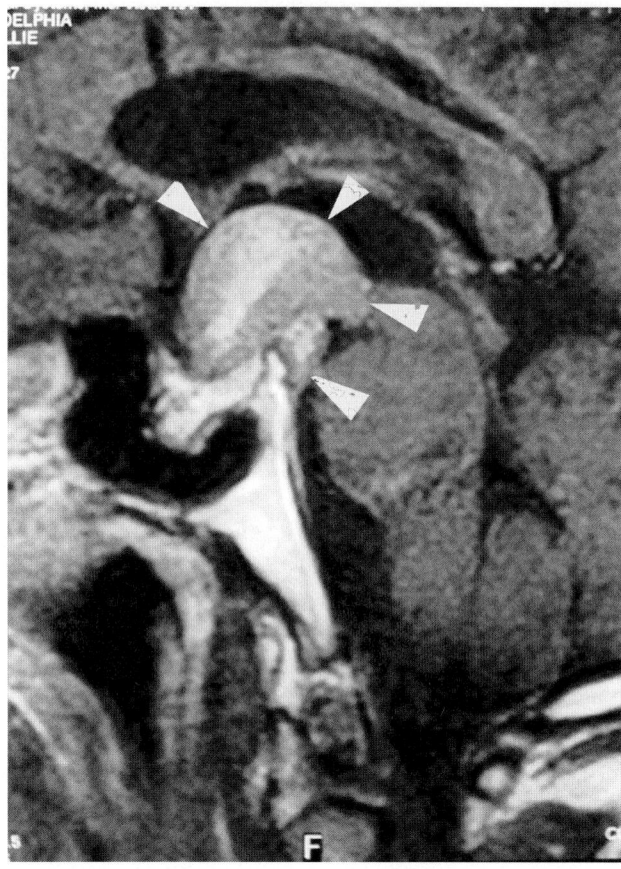

FIG. 41-23. Postcontrast T1-weighted sagittal MRI demonstrating a large sellar/suprasellar lesion involving the third ventricle superiorly, and abutting the midbrain and pons posteriorly. The patient presented with progressive visual field and acuity loss. Pathology and lab work revealed a nonfunctioning pituitary adenoma.

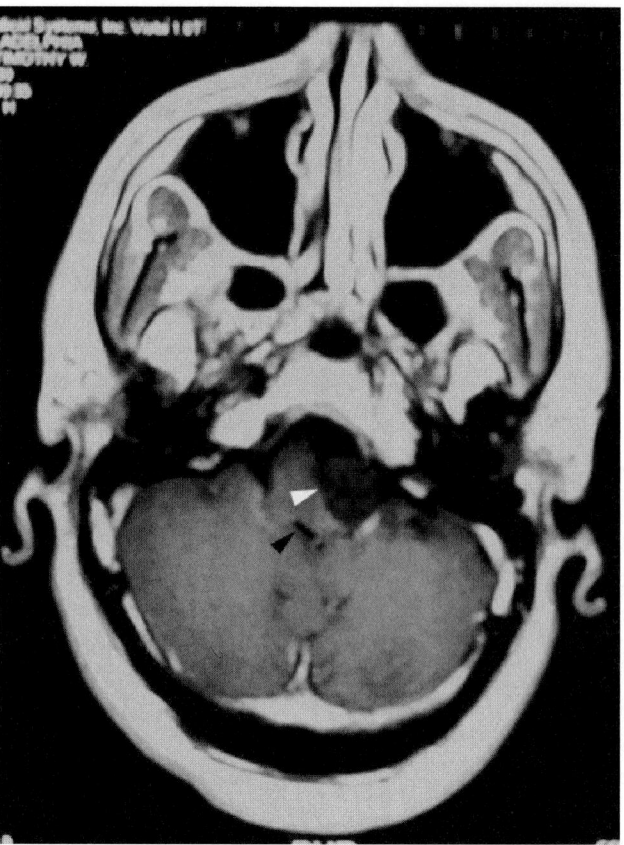

FIG. 41-24. Postcontrast T1-weighted axial MRI demonstrating a nonenhancing mass in the left cerebellopontine angle with brain stem compression. White arrowhead indicates interface of tumor and brain stem. Black arrowhead indicates deformed fourth ventricle. Pathology revealed epidermoid tumor.

of the anatomy leads to an understanding of the clinical presentation and possible therapeutic options.

Extradural Tumors

Extradural tumors comprise 55% of spinal tumors. This category includes tumors arising within the bony structures of the vertebrae and in the epidural space. Destruction of the bone can lead to instability and fractures, leading to pain and/or deformity. Epidural expansion can lead to spinal cord or nerve root compression with radiculopathy or myelopathy, respectively.

Metastatic Tumors. Metastatic tumors are the most common extradural tumors. Spinal metastases most commonly occur in the thoracic and lumbar vertebral bodies because the greatest volume of red bone marrow is found therein. The most common primary tumors are lymphoma, lung, breast, and prostate. Other sources include renal, colon, thyroid, sarcoma, and melanoma. Most spinal metastases create osteolytic lesions. Osteoblastic, sclerotic lesions suggest prostate cancer in men and breast cancer in women. Patients with progressing neurologic dysfunction or debilitating pain should undergo urgent surgery or radiation therapy. Preoperative neurologic function correlates with postoperative function. Patients may lose function over hours. These patients should be given high-dose intravenous dexamethasone, taken immediately to MRI, and then to the operating room or radiation therapy suite. Indications for surgery include failure of radiation therapy, spinal instability, recurrence after radiation therapy, and the need for diagnosis in cases of unknown primary tumors. Most cases with significant bone involvement require both decompression and fusion. Bony fusion usually takes 2 to 3 months. Prognosis governs operative decisions. Surgery is unlikely to improve quality of life for patients with a life expectancy of 3 months or less, but is likely to improve quality of life for patients with life expectancy of 6 months or more. Benefit for patients with 3 to 6 months life expectancy is unclear and requires frank discussion with the patient and family. Patients who are unlikely to tolerate general anesthesia, are already completely paralyzed, or who have very radiosensitive tumors such as myeloma and lymphoma, should generally not be offered surgery.

Primary Tumors. Hemangiomas are benign tumors found in 10% of people at autopsy. They occur in the vertebral bodies of the thoracolumbar spine and are frequently asymptomatic. They are often vascular and may hemorrhage, causing pain or neurologic deficit. Large hemangiomas can destabilize the body and predispose to fracture. Osteoblastic lesions include osteoid osteoma and osteoblastoma. The latter tends to be larger and more destructive. Aneurysmal bone cysts are nonneoplastic, expansile, lytic lesions containing thin-walled blood cavities which usually occur in the lamina or spinous processes of the cervicothoracic spine. They may cause pain or sufficiently weaken the bone to lead to fracture.

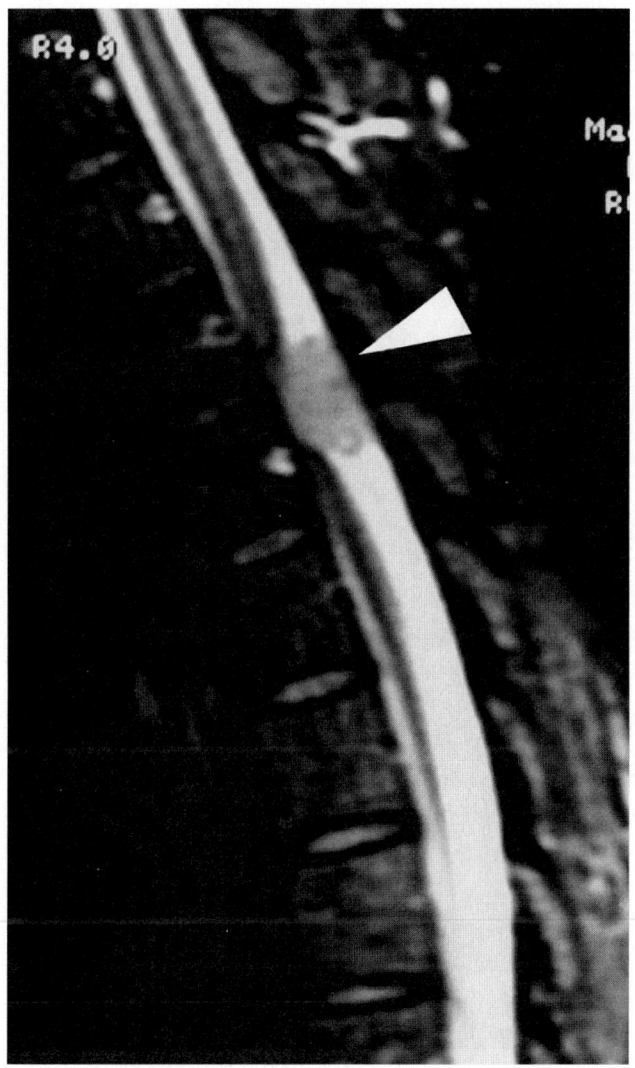

FIG. 41-25. T2-weighted sagittal MRI of the midthoracic spine demonstrating a well-encapsulated tumor arising from the dura posteriorly and compressing the spinal cord. The patient presented with worsening gait and lower extremity spasticity. Pathology demonstrated meningioma.

Cancers arising primarily in the bony spine include Ewing's sarcoma, osteosarcoma, chondrosarcoma, and plasmacytoma.

Intradural Extramedullary Tumors

Intradural extramedullary tumors comprise 40% of spinal tumors and arise from the meninges or nerve root elements. They may compress the spinal cord, causing myelopathy, or the nerve roots, causing radiculopathy. All of the most common intradural extramedullary tumors are typically benign, slow growing, and well circumscribed. Rare benign epidural masses include arachnoid cysts, dermoids, and epidermoids. Rare malignant epidural tumors include metastases and high-grade gliomas.

Meningioma. Meningiomas arise from the arachnoid mater. They appear to be dural based and enhance on MRI. An enhancing "dural tail" may be seen. They occur most commonly in the thoracic spine (Fig. 41-25), but also arise in the cervical and lumbar regions. Some spinal meningiomas grow into the epidural space. Growth causes cord compression and progressive myelopathy with hyperreflexia, spasticity, and gait difficulties. Surgical excision is the treatment of choice. The surgeon often finds a clean margin between the tumor and dura, and between the tumor and spinal cord, allowing en bloc resection without damage to the cord.

Schwannoma. Schwannomas are derived from peripheral nerve sheath Schwann cells. They are benign, encapsulated tumors that almost never undergo malignant degeneration. Two-thirds are entirely intradural, one-sixth are entirely extradural, and one-sixth have the classic dumbbell shape from intradural and extradural components. Symptoms result from radiculopathy, often presenting as pain, or myelopathy. Symptomatic lesions should be surgically resected. The parent nerve root can usually be preserved. Patients with multiple schwannomas likely have neurofibromatosis type 2 (NF-2). Resect symptomatic lesions in NF-2 patients.

Neurofibroma. Neurofibromas tend to be more fusiform and grow within the parent nerve, rather than forming an encapsulated mass off the nerve, as with schwannomas. They are benign but not encapsulated. They present similarly to schwannomas and the two may be difficult to differentiate on imaging. Salvage of the parent nerve is more challenging with neurofibromas. Thoracic and high cervical nerve roots may be sacrificed with minimal deficit, to improve likelihood of total resection. Patients with multiple neurofibromas likely have neurofibromatosis type 1, also known as von Recklinghausen's neurofibromatosis. Resection for symptomatic lesions should be offered.

Intramedullary Tumors

Intramedullary tumors comprise 5% of spinal tumors. They arise within the parenchyma of the spinal cord. Common presenting symptoms are local or radicular pain, sensory loss, weakness, or sphincter dysfunction. Patients with such symptoms should undergo MRI of the entire spine with and without enhancement.

Ependymoma. Ependymomas are the most common intramedullary tumors in adults. There are several histologic variants. The myxopapillary type occurs in the conus medullaris or the filum terminale in the lumbar region and has the best prognosis after resection. The cellular type occurs more frequently in the cervical cord. Many spinal ependymomas have cystic areas and may contain hemorrhage. Surgical removal can improve function. A distinct tumor margin often exists, allowing safer excision. Postoperative radiation therapy after subtotal resection may prolong disease control.

Astrocytoma. Astrocytomas are the most common intramedullary tumors in children, although they also occur in adults. They may occur at all levels, although more often in the cervical cord. The tumor may interfere with the CSF-containing central canal of the spinal cord, leading to a dilated central canal, referred to as syringomyelia, or simply syrinx. Spinal astrocytomas are usually low grade, but complete excision is rarely possible due to the nonencapsulated, infiltrative nature of the tumor. As such, patients with astrocytomas fare worse overall than patients with ependymomas.

Other Tumors. Other types of rare tumors include high-grade astrocytomas, dermoids, epidermoids, teratomas, hemangiomas, hemangioblastomas, and metastases. Patients usually present with pain. Prognosis depends generally on preoperative function and the histologic characteristics of the lesion.

SPINE

The spine is a complex structure subject to a wide variety of pathologic processes, including degeneration, inflammation, infection, neoplasia, and trauma. Please refer to the sections on trauma, tumor, and infection for discussions of how these processes impact the spine. General concepts relevant to the spine, as well as some common patterns of disease and operative interventions, are presented.

The spine consists of a series of stacked vertebrae, intervening discs, and longitudinal ligaments. The vertebrae consist of the vertebral body anteriorly and the pedicles, articular facets, laminae, and spinous processes posteriorly. The intervertebral discs have two components. The tough, fibrous ring that runs around the outer diameter of the two adjacent vertebral bodies is known as the annulus fibrosus. The spongy material inside the ring of the annulus is known as the nucleus pulposus. The annulus and the nucleus provide a cushion between adjacent vertebral bodies, absorb forces transmitted to the spine, and allow some movement between the vertebral bodies. The ligaments stabilize the spine by limiting the motion of adjacent vertebrae.

Two concepts critical to understanding the mechanics and pathologic processes affecting the spine are stability and neural compression.

Stability

The spinal column is the principal structural component of the axial spine, and it must bear significant loads. The vertebrae increase in size from the top to the bottom of the spine, correlating with the increased total loads the more caudal elements of the spine must bear. The cervical spine is the most mobile. Cervical stability depends greatly on the integrity of the ligaments that run from level to level. The thoracic spine is the least mobile, due to the stabilizing effect of the rib cage. The lumbar spine has relatively massive vertebrae, supports heavy loads, and has intermediate mobility. The sacral spine is fused together and has no intrinsic mobility. The load borne by the lumbar spine is transmitted to the sacrum, and then the pelvis through the sacroiliac joints. The coccyx is the inferiormost segment of the spine and has no significant contribution to load bearing or to mobility.

A stable spine is one that can bear normally experienced forces resulting from body mass, movement, and muscle contraction, while maintaining normal structure and alignment. An unstable spine will shift or sublux under these forces. The determinants of spinal stability vary throughout the cervical, thoracic, and lumbar portions. In elementary form, stability depends on the structural integrity of the hard, bony elements of the vertebral column, as well as the tensile integrity and secure attachments of the supporting ligamentous structures. Plain x-rays and CT scans have good sensitivity for detecting bony defects such as fractures or subluxation. MRI better detects disruption of the soft tissues, including ligaments and intervertebral discs. Specific patterns of abnormalities seen on imaging studies may lead to a diagnosis of, or high suspicion of, spinal instability.

A common form of nontraumatic spinal instability is lumbar spondylolisthesis (i.e., forward slippage of a lumbar vertebra with relation to the next lower vertebra on which it rests). This results from congenital or degenerative disruption of the pars interarticularis, the critical bridge of bone that spans adjacent facet joints. In the setting of a so-called pars defect, there is no solid bony connection between the adjacent vertebrae. This makes the spine unstable and can lead to slippage. Patients typically present with severe low

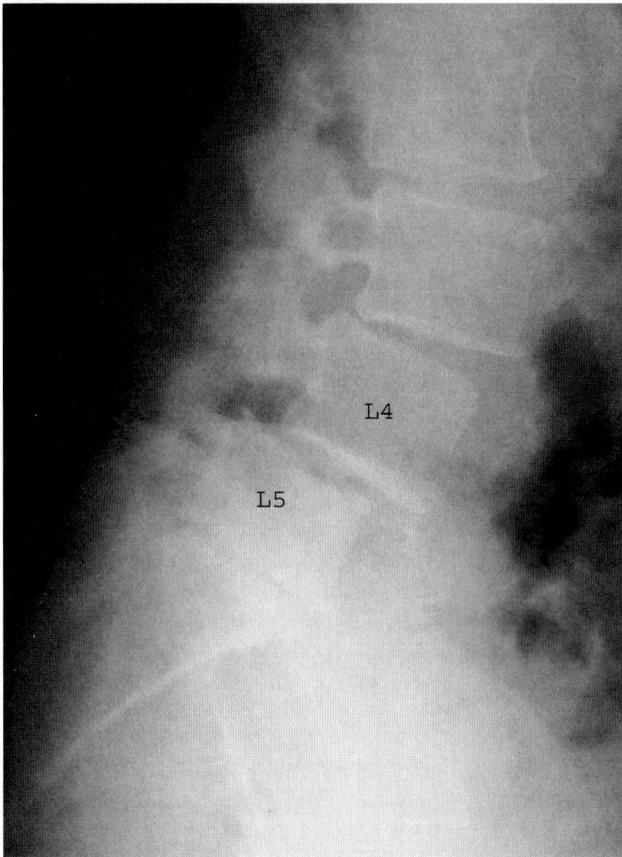

FIG. 41-26. *Lateral lumbar spine x-ray demonstrates a 25% anterior slippage of L4 on L5 due to a defect in the L4 pars interarticularis. This is called spondylolisthesis.*

back pain that is exacerbated with movement and load bearing (mechanical low back pain). Figure 41-26 demonstrates an L4 and L5 spondylolisthesis.

Neural Compression

Besides providing a stable central element of the body's support structure, the spine must also protect the spinal cord as it descends in the central canal, and the nerve roots as they pass from the central canal out the neural foramina to form the peripheral nervous system. In a healthy spine, the spinal cord and nerve roots are suspended in CSF, free of mechanical compression. Pathologic processes that can lead to impingement on the CSF spaces and neural compression include hypertrophic degenerative changes in the intervertebral discs and facet joints, expanding epidural masses such as tumors or abscesses, and slippage of adjacent vertebral bodies with respect to each other (i.e., subluxation). Subluxation may be due to trauma that exceeds the spine's load-bearing capabilities and leads to structural failure, or chronic structural degradation by degenerative disease, infection, or tumor. Subluxation reduces the cross-sectional area of the central canal and the neural foramina (see Fig. 41-10B). Reduced central canal area can lead to myelopathy. Reduced neural foraminal area can lead to radiculopathy.

Myelopathy

Compression of the spinal cord causes disturbance of cord function, known as myelopathy. Myelopathy may be secondary to the direct effects of compression, cord ischemia due to reduced

Table 41-6
Cervical Disc Herniations and Symptoms by Level

Level	Frequency	Root Injured	Reflex	Weakness	Numbness
C4–C5	2%	C5		Deltoid	Shoulder
C5–C6	19%	C6	Biceps	Biceps brachii	Thumb
C6–C7	69%	C7	Triceps	Wrist extensors (wrist drop)	Second and third digits
C7–T1	10%	C8		Hand intrinsics	Fourth and fifth digits

SOURCE: Adapted with permission from Greenberg MS: *Handbook of Neurosurgery,* 4th ed: Greenberg Graphics, 1997, Chap. 10.2, p 199.

perfusion, or pathologic changes due to repeated cord trauma. These mechanisms lead to demyelination of the corticospinal tracts, which are long descending motor tracts. Corticospinal tract damage leads to upper motor neuron signs and symptoms, including hyperreflexia, spasticity, and weakness. These mechanisms also cause damage to the dorsal columns, which carry ascending proprioception, vibration, and two-point discrimination information. Loss of proprioception makes fine motor tasks and ambulation difficult.

Radiculopathy

Compression of the nerve roots causes disturbance of root function, known as radiculopathy. Characteristic features of radiculopathy include lower motor neuron signs and symptoms (hyporeflexia, atrophy, and weakness) and sensory disturbances such as numbness, tingling sensations (paresthesias), burning sensations (dysesthesias), and shooting pain. Myelopathy and radiculopathy often present together in diseases that involve the central canal and the neural foramina. This can lead to lower motor neuron dysfunction at the level of disease, and upper motor neuron dysfunction below that level.

Patterns of Disease

Cervical Radiculopathy

The cervical nerve roots exit the central canal above the pedicle of the same-numbered vertebra and at the level of the higher adjacent intervertebral disc. So, for example, the C6 nerve root passes above the C6 pedicle at the level of the C5–C6 discs. The cervical nerve roots may be compressed acutely by disc herniation, or chronically by hypertrophic degenerative changes of the discs, facets, and ligaments. Table 41-6 summarizes the effects of various disc herniations. Most patients with acute disc herniations will improve without surgery. Nonsteroidal anti-inflammatory drugs or cervical traction may help alleviate symptoms. Patients whose symptoms do not resolve or who have significant weakness should undergo decompressive surgery. The two main options for nerve root decompression are anterior cervical discectomy and fusion (ACDF) and posterior cervical foraminotomy (keyhole foraminotomy). ACDF allows more direct access to and removal of the pathology (anterior to the nerve root), but requires fusion. Figure 41-27 demonstrates a C6–C7 ACDF. Keyhole foraminotomy allows decompression without requiring fusion, but may be less effective for removing the pathology.

Cervical Spondylotic Myelopathy

The term *spondylosis* refers to diffuse degenerative and hypertrophic changes of the discs, intervertebral joints, and ligaments, that cause spinal stenosis. Spinal cord dysfunction (myelopathy) due to cord compression from cervical spinal degenerative disease is therefore referred to as cervical spondylotic myelopathy, or CSM.

CSM classically presents with spasticity and hyperreflexia due to corticospinal tract dysfunction, upper extremity weakness and atrophy from degeneration of the motor neurons in the anterior horns of the spinal gray matter, and loss of lower extremity proprioception due to dorsal column injury. Figure 41-28 demonstrates typical findings. Patients complain of difficulty buttoning shirts, using utensils, and ambulating. Spondylosis is usually diffuse, so the usual treatment for CSM is multilevel (usually C3–C7) cervical laminectomy, although patients with disease localized over one to three levels may be candidates for anterior decompression and fusion. Figure 41-29 demonstrates the postoperative appearance of a vertebral corpectomy and fusion for CSM. Thorough cervical laminectomy decompresses the cord posteriorly. Patients often have slow recovery due to the extensive chronic changes in the cervical cord, and may benefit from rehabilitation programs. The other disease that classically presents with combined upper and lower motor neuron symptoms is amyotrophic lateral sclerosis (ALS). Care must be taken to avoid offering cervical laminectomy to a patient with undiagnosed ALS. Two findings help differentiate CSM from ALS: cranial nerve dysfunction such as dysphagia (never caused by cervical spine disease) and sensory disturbance (not found in ALS).

Thoracic Disc Herniation

Thoracic disc herniation accounts for less than 1% of herniated discs. They may present with radicular pain or sensory or motor changes in the lower extremities, due to cord compression. A posterior approach via midline incision and laminectomy should be avoided because of the high incidence of cord injury from manipulation and retraction. Anterior approaches via thoracotomy minimize risk to the cord and allow excellent access to the disc. The radicular arteries running from the aorta to the thoracic cord should be spared when possible, to avoid ischemia.

Lumbar Radiculopathy

Lumbar nerve roots exit the thecal sac, pass over the higher adjacent disc space, and exit the canal under the pedicle of the same-numbered vertebra. Therefore, the L5 nerve root passes over the L4–L5 disc space and exits under the L5 pedicle (Fig. 41-30). Lumbar discs may herniate with or without a history of trauma or straining. They normally cause pain lancing down the leg (Table 41-7). Most acute herniated lumbar discs improve symptomatically without surgery. Surgery is indicated for symptoms persisting more than 6 to 8 weeks, progressive motor deficit (e.g., foot drop), or for patients with incapacitating pain not manageable with analgesics. Discectomy is performed using a midline incision, partial removal of the overlying laminae (hemilaminectomy or laminotomy), identification of the thecal sac and nerve root, and extraction of disc fragments. Free-floating disc fragments may be found. Often, however, the herniated disc material is still contained within the annulus, and so the annulus must be incised and the disc space curetted.

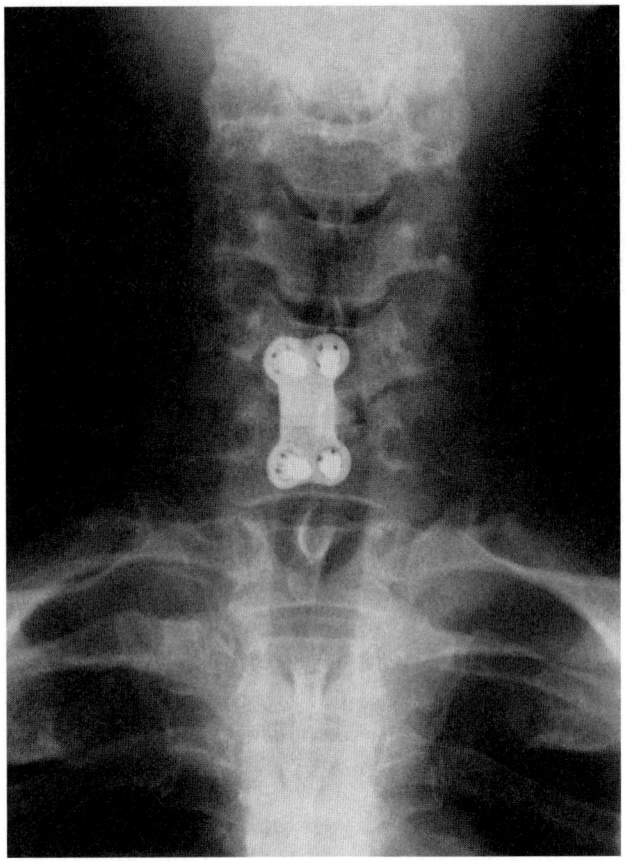

A

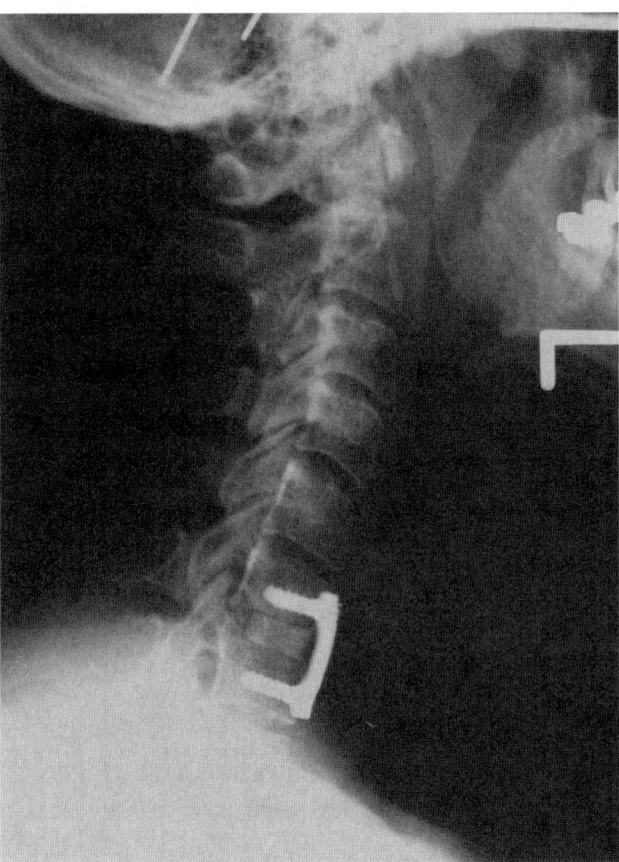

B

FIG. 41-27.   *A. Anteroposterior cervical spine x-ray showing the position of an anterior cervical plate used for stabilization after C6–C7 discectomy. Patient presented with right triceps weakness and dysesthesias in the right fifth digit. MRI revealed a right paracentral C6–C7 herniated disc compressing the exiting C7 nerve root. B. Lateral cervical spine x-ray of the same patient clearly demonstrates the position of the plate and screws. The allograft bone spacer placed in the drilled-out disc space is also apparent.*

After lumbar discectomy, approximately two-thirds of patients will have complete relief of pain, and up to 85% will have significant improvement.

Neurogenic Claudication

Neurogenic claudication is characterized by low back and leg pain that occurs while walking and is relieved by stopping, leaning forward, or sitting. It is normally caused by degenerative lumbar stenosis causing compression of the cauda equina. Neurogenic claudication must be distinguished from vascular claudication. Vascular claudication pain tends to resolve quickly with cessation of walking without need to change position, be in a stocking distribution rather than a dermatomal distribution, and be associated with cold, pale feet. Patients typically have a normal neurologic exam. Patients with neurogenic claudication have a slowly progressive course and may be surgical candidates when their pain interferes with their lifestyle. The usual surgery is an L3 to L5 lumbar laminectomy to decompress the nerve roots.

Cauda Equina Syndrome

Cauda equina syndrome is due to compression of the cauda equina and may result from massive disc herniation, epidural hematoma, epidural abscess, tumor, or subluxation from trauma. Patients with cauda equina compression often present with urinary

retention, saddle anesthesia, or progressing leg weakness. Saddle anesthesia is numbness in the perineum, genitals, buttocks, and upper inner thighs. Patients with suspected cauda equina syndrome should undergo immediate MRI of the lumbar spine to evaluate for a surgical lesion. Mass lesions should be removed urgently via laminectomy to preserve sphincter function and ambulation.

Spine Fusion Surgery

Patients whose spines have been destabilized by disease or by surgical intervention require fusion to restore stability. Fusion procedures lock adjacent vertebrae together. Fusion occurs when the body forms a solid mass of bone incorporating the adjacent vertebrae, eliminating normal intervertebral movement. Stabilization and immobilization promote bony fusion. Internal instrumentation and external orthoses are often used to stabilize and immobilize the spinal segment being fused.

Spinal Instrumentation

Internal fixation devices for spinal segmental immobilization have been developed for all levels of the spine. Most spinal instrumentation constructs have two elements. The first element is a device that solidly attaches to the vertebral bodies. Options include wires wrapped around laminae or spinous processes, hooks placed under the lamina or around the pedicles, or screws placed in the pedicles or

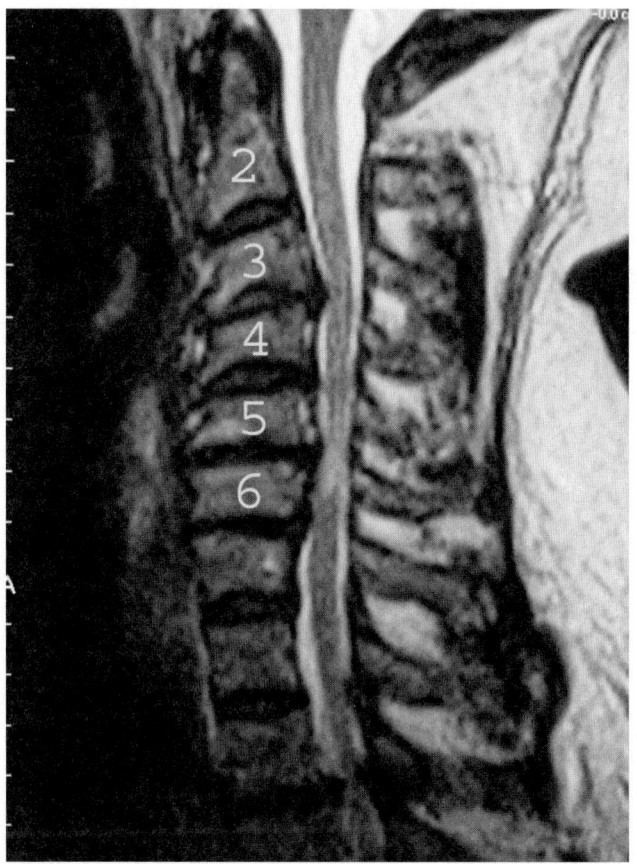

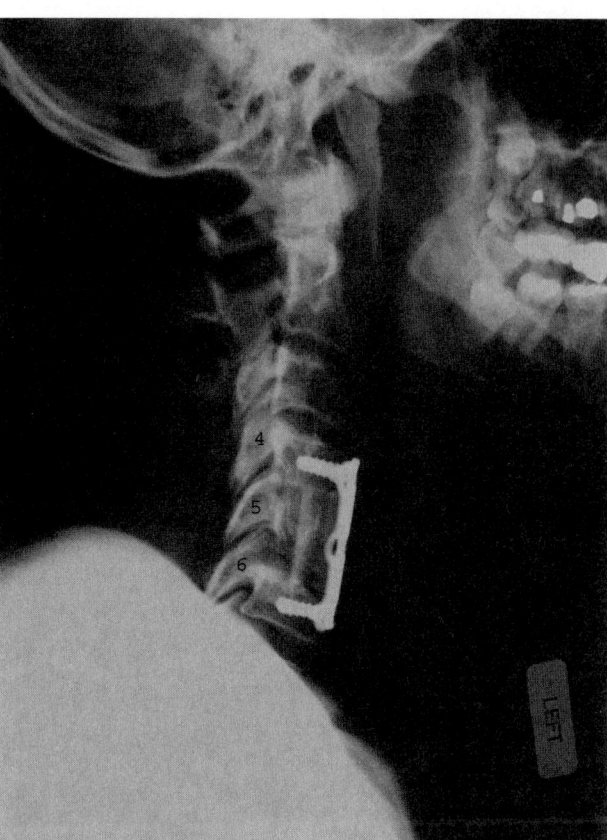

FIG. 41-28. T2-weighted sagittal MRI of the cervical spine showing multilevel degenerative changes causing spinal stenosis that is worst at C5–C6. Note the bright signal within the cord at that level, consistent with myelopathy.

FIG. 41-29. Lateral cervical spine x-ray status post C5 corpectomy for CSM. This involves removal of the C4–C5 disc, C5 vertebral body, and C5–C6 disc, decompressing at two levels. A bone strut is visible bridging C4 to C6. The plate and screws stabilize the segments.

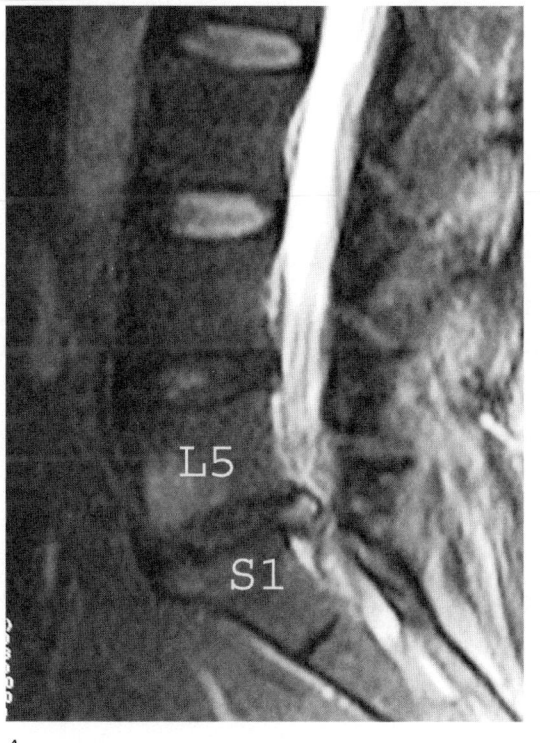

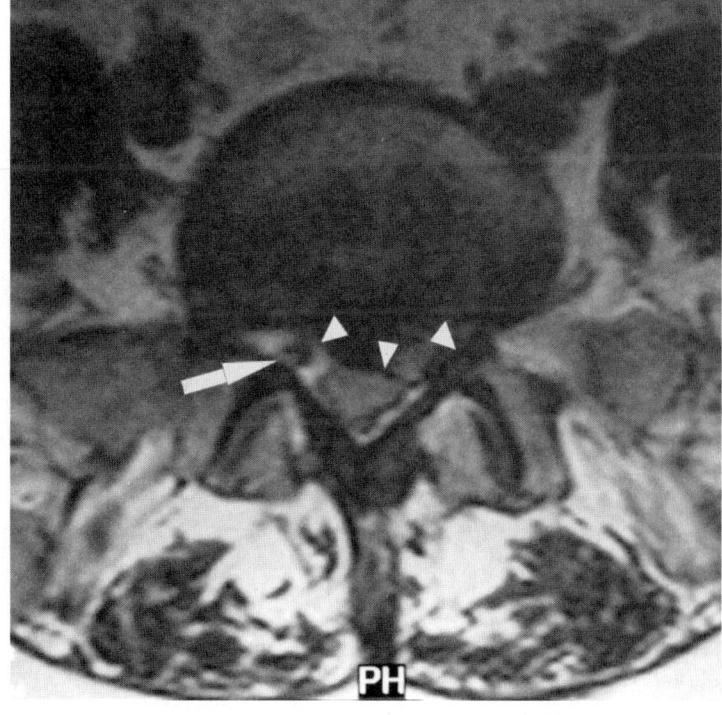

A   *B*

FIG. 41-30. *A.* T2-weighted sagittal MRI shows an L5–S1 disc herniation causing significant canal compromise and displacement of nerve roots. *B.* T2-weighted axial MRI of the same patient shows the large left paracentral disc herniation at L5–S1. Arrowheads delineate the extent of the herniation. The arrow indicates the right S1 nerve root passing through free of compression. The left S1 nerve root is under severe compression and is not seen.

Table 41-7
Lumbar Disc Herniations and Symptoms by Level

Level	Frequency	Root Injured	Reflex	Weakness	Numbness
L3–L4	5%	L4	Patellar	Quadriceps	Anterior thigh
L4–L5	45%	L5		Tibialis anterior (foot drop)	Great toe
L5–S1	50%	S1	Achilles	Gastrocnemius	Lateral foot

SOURCE: Adapted with permission from Greenberg MS: *Handbook of Neurosurgery,* 4th ed: Greenberg Graphics, 1997, Chap. 10.2, p 183.

the vertebral bodies. The second element is a device that traverses vertebral segments. Options include rods and plates that lock directly to the wires, hooks, or screws at each vertebral level. Spinal instrumentation devices are available for anterior and posterior fusion in the cervical, thoracic, and lumbar regions. Most modern spinal instrumentation devices are made of titanium to minimize problems with future MRI scanning (Fig. 41-31). All spinal instrumentation constructs will eventually fail by loosening or breaking if bony fusion does not occur.

Arthrodesis

Arthrodesis refers to the obliteration of motion or instability by incorporating the relevant components into a solid mass of bone.

Arthrodesis must occur in any fused segment to have long-term stability. Failure of arthrodesis results in failed fusion, often in the form of a fibrous nonunion. The rates of successful fusion are higher in the cervical spine than the lumbar spine. Arthrodesis requires ingrowth of new bone formed by the patient's osteoblasts across the unstable defect. Inserting graft material, such as autograft or allograft, into the defect provides a bridge for osteoblasts and promotes fusion. The term *autograft* refers to the patient's own bone, often harvested from the iliac crest. Iliac crest bone graft is a source of both cortical and cancellous bone. Cortical bone provides structural support, while cancellous bone provides a matrix for bony ingrowth. The term *allograft* refers to sterilized bone from human tissue banks. Allografts also may be cortical, cancellous, or both.

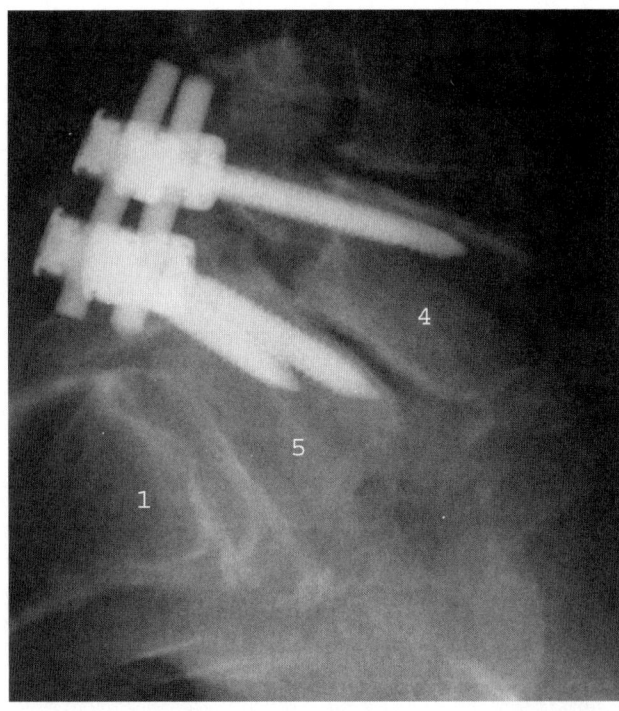

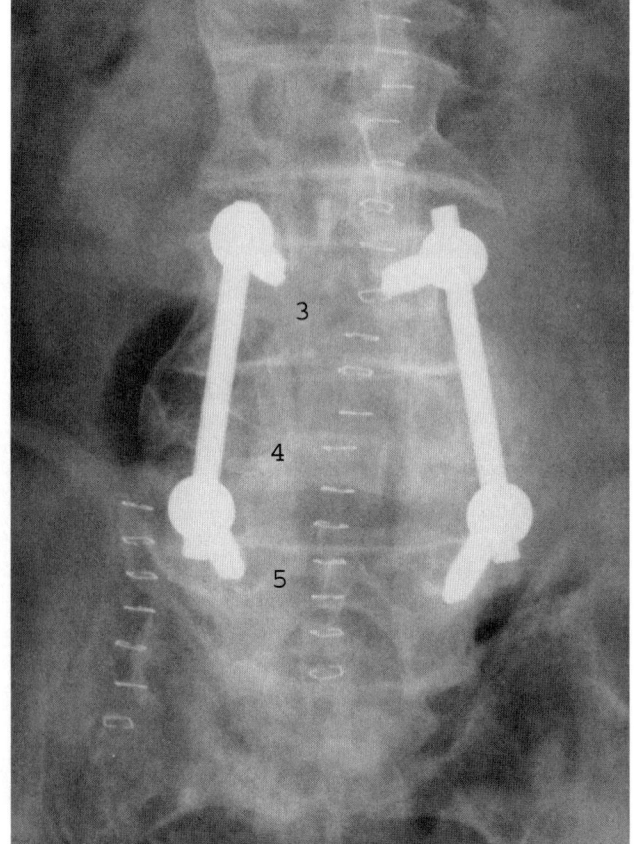

A   *B*

FIG. 41-31. *A.* Lateral lumbar spine x-ray showing pedicle screws and connecting rods used to stabilize L4 with respect to L5. This instrumentation was placed as part of a fusion operation to stabilize progressive L4–L5 spondylolisthesis with intractable low back pain. *B.* Anteroposterior lumbar spine x-ray showing L3 to L5 instrumentation with pedicle screws and connecting rods. The patient had previously sustained an L4 burst fracture. Note the significant loss of height of the L4 body compared to adjacent levels. The small row of staples to the right delineates the incision over the iliac crest used to harvest cancellous bone as a nonstructural osteoinductive autograft fusion designed to induce formation of a solid bone bridge from L3 to L5 (arthrodesis).

Allograft lacks the array of osteoinductive endogenous compounds intrinsic to autograft, although supplemental products such as demineralized bone matrix paste can be added to encourage new bone formation. Other techniques for increasing the rates of successful fusion are being developed, including the integration of osteoinductive bone morphogenetic proteins, known as BMPs, into the fusion constructs.

PERIPHERAL NERVE

Common pathologic processes that compromise function of the peripheral nervous system include mechanical compression, ischemia, inflammation, and neoplasia.

Peripheral Nerve Tumors

Most peripheral nerve tumors are benign and grow slowly. Significant pain increases the likelihood that the patient has a malignant tumor. Treatment for peripheral nerve tumors is surgical resection to establish diagnosis and evaluate for signs of malignancy. These tumors have various degrees of involvement with that parent nerve. Some can be resected with minimal or no damage to the nerve. Tumors that grow within the nerve often contain functioning fascicles. Total excision of these tumors requires sacrifice of the parent nerve. The choice of subtotal resection, nerve preservation, and observation, versus total resection with nerve sacrifice depends on tumor histology and the functions of the parent nerve.

Schwannoma

Schwannomas are the most common peripheral nerve tumors, also referred to as neurilemomas or neurinomas. Most occur in the third decade of life. These benign tumors arise from Schwann cells, which form myelin in peripheral nerves. The most characteristic presentation is a mass lesion with point tenderness and shooting pains on direct palpation. Spontaneous or continuous pain suggests malignancy. They tend to grow slowly and eccentrically on the parent nerve. The eccentric location and discrete encapsulated nature of these tumors often allow total resection without significant damage to the parent nerve. Subtotal resection and observation is reasonable for schwannomas entwined in important nerves, as the incidence of malignant transformation is extremely low.

Neurofibroma

Neurofibromas arise within the nerve and tend to be fusiform masses, unlike schwannomas, which tend to grow out of the nerve. Neurofibromas often present as a mass that is tender to palpation. They usually lack the shooting pains characteristic of schwannomas. Neurofibromas are often difficult to resect completely without sacrifice of the parent nerve. Neurofibromas have a higher incidence of malignant transformation, so patients with known residual tumors require close observation. Patients with von Recklinghausen's neurofibromatosis often have multiple neurofibromas. These patients should be offered resection for symptomatic tumors. They also have a higher risk of malignant degeneration, up to 10%. Malignant neurofibromas have the histologic characteristics of sarcoma.

Malignant Nerve Sheath Tumors

Malignant nerve sheath tumors include solitary sarcomas, degenerated neurofibromas, and neuroepitheliomas. Patients with malignant peripheral nerve tumors typically complain of constant pain, rather than pain only on palpation, and are more likely to have motor and sensory deficits in the distribution of the parent nerve. Treatment for these tumors is radical excision. This often requires sacrifice of the parent nerve. Invasion of nearby soft tissues may occur and necessitate wide resection or amputation in an attempt to prevent systemic metastasis.

Entrapment Neuropathies

Entrapment neuropathy is neurologic dysfunction in nerves passing through a pathologically small, fixed space. Nerve dysfunction may result directly from chronic, repetitive pressure on the nerve, or from ischemic damage due to impaired perfusion.[15] Entrapment causing dysfunction of nerve signaling may cause numbness, paresthesias, weakness, or muscle atrophy. By far the two most common sites of entrapment neuropathy are the ulnar nerve at the medial aspect of the elbow and the median nerve at the wrist. Electomyography and nerve conduction studies (EMG/NCS) usually demonstrate slowing across the entrapped segment of nerve. Mechanical peripheral nerve disorders resulting from trauma (brachial plexus disruption, radial nerve damage from humerus fractures, and common peroneal nerve crush injuries) are discussed in the section on trauma.

Ulnar Neuropathy

The ulnar nerve has contributions from the C7, C8, and T1 nerve roots, arises from the medial cord of the brachial plexus, and supplies most of the intrinsic hand muscles (interossei and third and fourth lumbricals), and sensation to the fourth and fifth digits. It passes posteriorly to the medial epicondyle at the elbow in the condylar groove. This segment is superficial and subject to external compression and repetitive minor impacts. Patients with ulnar entrapment at the elbow present with numbness and tingling in the medial palm and the fourth and fifth digits. Motor deficits include weakness and wasting of the intrinsic hand muscles. Treatment for symptomatic ulnar entrapment neuropathy is surgical exploration and incision of the fibrous aponeurotic arch that overlies the nerve. A 6-cm curvilinear incision between the medial epicondyle and the olecranon allows exploration of up to 10 cm of nerve and lysis of compressive tissues.

Carpal Tunnel Syndrome

The median nerve has contributions from the C5 to T1 nerve roots, arises from the medial and lateral cords of the brachial plexus, and supplies the muscles of wrist and finger flexion and sensation to the palmar aspect of the first, second, and third digits. The median nerve passes through the carpal tunnel in the wrist, lying superficial to the four deep and four superficial flexor tendons. The transverse carpal ligament is a tough, fibrous band that forms the roof of the carpal tunnel. The ligament attaches to the pisiform and hamate medially and the trapezium and scaphoid laterally. Patients complain of numbness and tingling in the supplied digits, clumsiness, and worsening with sleep or repetitive wrist movement. Patients may notice wasting of the thenar eminence. Treatment for symptomatic carpal tunnel syndrome unresponsive to splinting, analgesics, and rest is surgical division of the flexor retinaculum. This often provides prompt relief of pain symptoms and slow recovery of numbness and strength.

Autoimmune and Inflammatory Disorders

These are not surgical diseases, but merit brief mention as they are included in the differential diagnosis for new-onset weakness. Their characteristic presentations help distinguish them from weakness due to structural lesions.

Guillain-Barré Syndrome

Guillain-Barré syndrome is an acute inflammating demyelinating polyradiculopathy often occurring after viral infection, surgery, inoculations, or mycoplasma infections. Patients classically present with weakness ascending from the legs to the body, arms, and even cranial nerves. Symptoms usually progress over 2 to 4 weeks and then resolve. Care is supportive. Respiratory weakness may require ventilatory support.

Myasthenia Gravis

Myasthenia gravis is an autoimmune process in which antibodies form to the acetylcholine receptors of muscles, leading to fluctuating weakness. Most patients have either thymic hyperplasia or thymoma. The most common symptoms are diplopia, ptosis, dysarthria, and dysphagia. More severe cases have limb or respiratory involvement. Weakness worsens with repetitive movement. Treatment is with acetylcholinesterase inhibitors and possible thymectomy.

Eaton-Lambert Syndrome

Autoimmune process with antibodies to the presynaptic calcium channels. This is a paraneoplastic syndrome most commonly associated with oat cell carcinoma. Patients have weakness of proximal limb muscles that improves with repetitive movement. This diagnosis must prompt oncologic evaluation.

INFECTION

Central nervous system infections of interest to neurosurgeons include those that cause focal neurologic deficit due to mass effect, require surgical aspiration or drainage because antibiotic therapy alone is insufficient, cause mechanical instability of the spine, or occur after neurosurgical procedures.

Cranial

Osteomyelitis

The skull is highly vascular and resistant to infections. Osteomyelitis of the skull may develop by contiguous spread from pyogenic sinus disease or from contamination by penetrating trauma. *Staphylococcus aureus* and *S. epidermidis* are the most frequent causative organisms. Patients usually present with redness, swelling, and pain. Contrast head CT aids diagnosis and shows the extent of involved bone, along with associated abscesses or empyema. Osteomyelitis treatment entails surgical débridement of involved bone followed by 2 to 4 months of antibiotics. Craniotomy wound infections are a special concern because performing a craniotomy creates a devascularized free bone flap susceptible to infection and not penetrated by antibiotics. These wounds must be débrided and the bone flaps removed and discarded. Subsequent care involves appropriate antibiotic therapy, observation for signs of recurrent infection off antibiotics, and return to the OR for titanium or methylmethacrylate cranioplasty 6 to 12 months later.

Subdural Empyema

Subdural empyema is a rapidly progressive pyogenic infection. The subdural space lacks significant barriers to the spread of the infection, such as compartmentalization or septations. Subdural empyema usually occurs over the cerebral convexities. Potential infectious sources include sinus disease, penetrating trauma, and otitis. Streptococci and staphylococci are the most frequently found organisms. Presenting symptoms include fever, headache, neck stiffness, seizures, or focal neurologic deficit. Neurologic deficit results from inflammation of cortical blood vessels, leading to thrombosis and stroke. The most common deficit is contralateral hemiparesis. Patients with suggestive symptoms should undergo rapid contrast CT scan. Lumbar puncture frequently fails to yield the offending organism and risks herniation due to mass effect. Typical treatment is wide hemicraniectomy, dural opening, and lavage. The pus may be thick or septated, making burr hole drainage or small craniotomy insufficient. Patients then require 1 to 2 months of antibiotics. Subdural empyema has 10 to 20% mortality and common chronic sequelae, including seizure disorder and residual hemiparesis. However, many patients make a good recovery.

Brain Abscess

Brain abscess is encapsulated infection within the brain parenchyma. It may spread hematogenously in patients with endocarditis or intracardiac or intrapulmonary right-to-left shunts, by migration from the sinuses or ear, or via direct seeding by penetrating trauma. Disorganized cerebritis often precedes formation of the organized, walled-off abscess. Patients may present with nonspecific symptoms such as headache, nausea, or lethargy, or with focal neurologic deficit such as hemiparesis. Alternatively, patients may present in extremis if the abscess ruptures into the ventricular system. Abscesses appear as well-demarcated, ring-enhancing, thin-walled lesions on CT scan and MRI, and often have associated edema and mass effect. Patients require antibiotic therapy after needle aspiration or surgical evacuation. Antibiotic therapy without surgical evacuation may be considered for patients with small, multiple, or critically located abscesses. Abscesses that cause mass effect, decreased mental status, are large, or that fail to decrease in size after a week of antibiotics, should be evacuated. Nonsurgical management still requires aspiration or biopsy for organism culture and sensitivities. Blood and CSF cultures rarely give definitive diagnosis. Removal of an encapsulated abscess significantly shortens the length of antibiotic therapy required to eliminate all organisms. Common chronic sequelae after successful treatment include seizures or focal neurologic deficit.

Spine

Pyogenic Vertebral Osteomyelitis

Pyogenic vertebral osteomyelitis is a destructive bacterial infection of the vertebrae, usually of the vertebral body. Vertebral osteomyelitis frequently results from hematogenous spread of distant disease, but may occur as an extension of adjacent disease, such as psoas abscess or perinephric abscess. *S. aureus* and *Enterobacter* spp. are the most frequent etiologic organisms. Patients usually present with fever and back pain. Diabetics, IV drug abusers, and dialysis patients have increased incidence of vertebral osteomyelitis. Epidural extension may lead to compression of the spinal cord or nerve roots with resultant neurologic deficit. Osteomyelitis presents a lytic picture on imaging and must be distinguished from neoplastic disease. Adjacent intervertebral disc involvement occurs frequently with pyogenic osteomyelitis, but rarely with neoplasia. Plain films and CT help assess the extent of bony destruction or deformity such as kyphosis. MRI shows adjacent soft tissue or epidural disease. Most cases can be treated successfully with antibiotics alone, although the organism must be isolated to steer antibiotic choice. Blood cultures may be positive. Surgical intervention may be required for débridement when antibiotics alone fail, or for stabilization and fusion in the setting of instability and deformity.

Tuberculous Vertebral Osteomyelitis

Tuberculous vertebral osteomyelitis, also known as Pott's disease, occurs most commonly in underdeveloped countries and in immunocompromised people. Several features differentiate tuberculous osteomyelitis from bacterial osteomyelitis. The infection is indolent and symptoms often progress slowly over months. Tuberculosis rarely involves the intervertebral disc. The involved bodies may have sclerotic rather than lytic changes. Multiple nonadjacent vertebrae may be involved. Diagnosis requires documentation of acid-fast bacilli. Treatment involves long-term antimycobacterial drugs. Patients with spinal instability or neural compression from epidural inflammatory tissue should undergo débridement and fusion as needed.

Discitis

Primary infection of the intervertebral disc space, or discitis, is most commonly secondary to postoperative infections. Spontaneous discitis occurs more commonly in children. *S. epidermidis* and *S. aureus* account for most cases. The primary symptom is back pain. Other signs and symptoms include radicular pain, fevers, paraspinal muscle spasm, and localized tenderness to palpation. Many cases will resolve without antibiotics. Antibiotics are generally given for positive blood or biopsy cultures or persistent constitutional symptoms. Most patients will have spontaneous fusion across the involved disc and do not need débridement or fusion.

Epidural Abscess

Epidural abscesses may arise from or spread to the adjacent bone or disc, so distinguishing between vertebral osteomyelitis or discitis and a spinal epidural abscess may be difficult. The most common presenting signs and symptoms are back pain, fever, and tenderness to palpation of the spine. The most significant risk of epidural abscess is weakness progressing to paralysis due to spinal cord or nerve root damage. Cord and root damage may be due to direct compression or to inflammatory thrombosis resulting in venous infarction. *S. aureus* and *Streptococcus* spp. are the most common organisms. The source may be hematogenous spread, local extension, or operative contamination. MRI best demonstrates the epidural space and degree of neural compromise. Patients with suspected spinal epidural abscess should undergo surgical débridement for decompression and diagnosis, followed by culture-directed antibiotic therapy. Relative contraindications to surgery include prohibitive comorbidities or total lack of neurologic function below the involved level. Patients with no neurologic deficits and an identified organism may be treated with antibiotics alone and very close observation. This is controversial, however, because these patients can undergo rapid and irreversible neurologic decline. Most epidural abscesses can be accessed via laminectomy without fusion. Collections predominantly anterior to the cervical or thoracic cord may require anterior approach and fusion.

FUNCTIONAL NEUROSURGERY

Epilepsy Surgery

Seizures result from uncontrolled neuronal electrical activity. Seizures may result from irritative lesions in the brain, such as tumors or hematomas, or from physiologic or structural abnormalities. Seizures may involve a part of the brain (focal) or the entire brain (generalized). Focal seizures may be associated with normal consciousness (simple) or decreased consciousness (complex). All generalized seizures cause loss of consciousness. Focal seizures may secondarily generalize. Patients with multiple unprovoked seizures over time have epilepsy. Epilepsy categorization depends on such factors as type of seizures, electroencephalographic (EEG) findings, associated syndromes, and identifiable etiologies. All patients with unexplained seizures (i.e., no obvious cause such as head trauma or alcohol withdrawal) or epilepsy require thorough neurologic evaluation, including imaging to evaluate for a mass lesion. Antiepileptic drugs (AEDs) form the first line of therapy for epilepsy, initially as monotherapy, then as combination therapy. Epilepsy patients who have failed satisfactory trials of several AED combination regimens may be candidates for surgical intervention. Lack of seizure control or patient intolerance of the medications may constitute failure. Epilepsy surgery can decrease the frequency of seizures by resection of the electrical source of the seizures, or decrease the severity of seizures by severing white matter tracts through which the abnormal electrical activity spreads. Three types of epilepsy surgery are discussed. Epilepsy surgery appears to be extremely underutilized, given the relatively low risk of the procedures, and the crippling social and economic effects of uncontrolled or partially controlled epilepsy.[16] Patients with symptoms, imaging abnormalities, and EEG analysis compatible with a specific seizure focus are most likely to have good results from epilepsy surgery.

Anterior Temporal Lobectomy

Medial temporal lobe structural abnormalities can lead to complex partial seizures (CPS). Many patients with CPS have poor seizure control on medications. Patients with CPS may have significant reduction in seizure frequency or cessation of seizures after resection of the anterior temporal lobe. The amygdala and the head of the hippocampus are removed as part of the lobectomy. Resection may be taken back approximately 4.5 cm from the temporal tip in the language-dominant hemisphere, and 6 cm from the temporal tip in the language nondominant hemisphere, with low risk of significant deficits.[17] Two main risks of anterior temporal lobectomy are memory problems and visual problems. Removal of the hippocampus in a patient with an atrophied or nonfunctional contralateral hippocampus causes a global memory deficit. Interruption of the optic radiations, which carry visual signals from the contralateral superior visual quadrants of both eyes, causes a contralateral superior quadrantanopia, known as a "pie in the sky" field deficit.

Corpus Callosotomy

Patients with generalized seizures, atonic seizures associated with drop attacks, or absence seizures, who are found to have bilaterally coordinated pathologic cortical discharges on EEG, and who fail AED therapy may be candidates for corpus callosotomy. The corpus callosum is a large white matter tract that connects the cerebral hemispheres. Loss of consciousness requires simultaneous seizure activity in both hemispheres. Focal or partial seizures may spread via the corpus callosum to the contralateral hemisphere, causing generalization and loss of consciousness. Division of the corpus callosum can interrupt this spread. Patients may have decreased numbers of seizures and/or fewer episodes of lost consciousness. Usually only the anterior half or two-thirds of the corpus callosum is divided, as more extensive division increases the risk of disconnection syndrome. Patients with disconnection syndrome are unable to match objects in the opposite visual hemifields, to identify objects held in one hand with the other hemifield, and to write with the left hand or name objects held in the left hand (in left hemisphere–dominant patients).

Hemispherectomy

Children with intractable epilepsy, structural anomalies in one hemisphere, and contralateral hemiplegia, may have improved seizure control after resection of the hemisphere (anatomic hemispherectomy) or disruption of all connections to the hemisphere (functional hemispherectomy). Functional hemispherectomy is often preferred over anatomic hemispherectomy because of the high incidence of complications such as hematoma formation and ventriculoperitoneal shunt dependence associated with the latter.

Deep Brain Stimulators

Patients with essential tremor and medically refractory Parkinson's disease have abnormal activity in the nuclei of the basal ganglia. The basal ganglia are extrapyramidal structures that modulate and regulate signals in the corticospinal (pyramidal) tracts. Abnormal extrapyramidal activity leads to the loss of the normal modulation of movement and thus the clinical manifestations of the diseases. Fine electrical leads placed in these deep basal ganglia nuclei and connected to pulse generators modify the pathologic signals. The pulse generators are usually placed in the chest in a manner similar to cardiac pacemakers. Connector wires travel from the generators in the subcutaneous space up the neck and in the subgaleal space in the head, to connect the pulse generators to the electrical leads. Proper lead placement is accomplished with stereotactic guidance. A frame is rigidly locked to the patient's head and an MRI is obtained with the frame in place. Calculation of the coordinates of the millimeter-sized deep brain nuclei in relation to the three-dimensional space defined by the fixed frame allows accurate targeting, and the fine electrical leads are placed within the desired nuclei (Fig. 41-32). Postoperatively the pulse generators can be interrogated and adjusted with hand-held, transcutaneous, noninvasive devices as needed for symptom control.

Essential Tremor

Essential tremors are action tremors of 4 to 8 Hz rhythmic oscillation that often affect one arm or the head. Essential tremor often

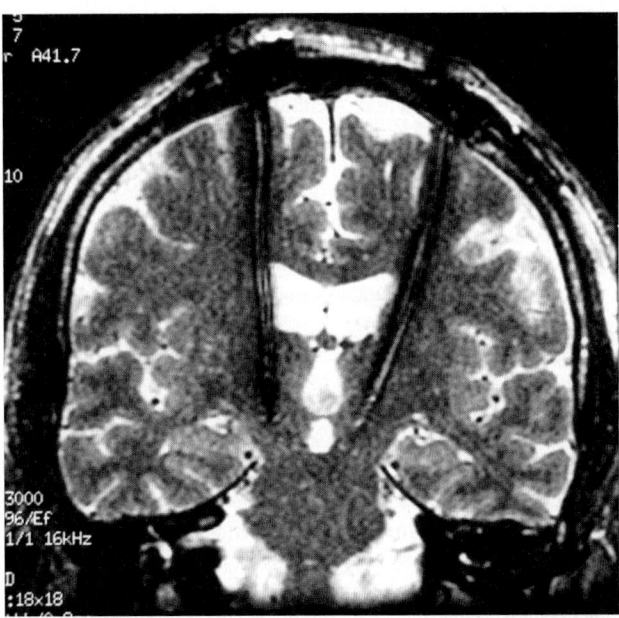

FIG. 41-32. Fast spin echo coronal MRI demonstrating position of deep brain stimulator leads in the subthalamic nuclei bilaterally. The electrodes appear thick and wavy due to magnetic susceptibility artifact.

starts in the third or fourth decade of life, and increases in frequency and amplitude with age. Beta blockers decrease symptoms. Patients with poor medical control and significant functional impairment can benefit significantly from placement of a deep brain stimulator in the contralateral ventrointermediate nucleus (VIN) of the thalamus. Placement of VIN stimulators for essential tremors appears to result in durable symptom control with good postoperative neuropsychologic outcomes in properly selected patients.[18,19]

Parkinson's Disease

Parkinson's disease is a progressive disorder characterized by rigidity, bradykinesia, and resting tremor, due to loss of dopamine-secreting neurons in the substantia nigra and locus ceruleus. It is also known as paralysis agitans. Dopaminergic agents such as levodopa/carbidopa and anticholinergic agents such as amantadine and selegiline form the basis of medical therapy. Patients with poor medical control or significant drug side effects may benefit significantly from placement of bilateral deep brain stimulators in the subthalamic nuclei (STN) or globus pallidus pars interna (GPi). Debate continues regarding the relative efficacy of each target.[20] A blinded trial is currently underway through the Veteran's Administration Parkinson's Disease Research, Education, and Clinical Centers (PADRECCs) comparing outcomes with STN and GPi stimulation. Deep brain stimulation seems to provide durable symptom relief with good postoperative neuropsychologic function in properly selected patients.[21]

Trigeminal Neuralgia

Trigeminal neuralgia, also known as tic douloureux, is characterized by repetitive, unilateral, sharp and lancinating pains in the distribution of one of the three branches of cranial nerve V, the trigeminal nerve. The patient may describe a "trigger point," an area on the face that elicits the pain when touched. A current leading etiologic hypothesis for trigeminal neuralgia is irritation and pulsatile compression of the root entry zone of the nerve by an artery in the posterior fossa, usually a loop of the superior cerebellar artery. The pain is excruciating and can be debilitating. Medical therapy, including carbamazepine and amitriptyline, may reduce the frequency of events. Options for medically refractory cases include percutaneous injection of glycerol into the path of the nerve, peripheral transection of the nerve branches, stereotactic radiosurgery, and microvascular decompression (MVD).

MVD involves performing a small posterior fossa craniotomy on the side of the symptoms, retraction of the cerebellar hemisphere, and exploration of cranial nerve V. If an artery is found near the nerve, the vessel is freed of any adhesions and nonabsorbable material is placed between the nerve root and the artery. MVD remains the first definitive management option because stereotactic radiosurgery is associated with a high incidence of facial numbness.[22]

STEREOTACTIC RADIOSURGERY

The term *stereotactic radiosurgery* (SRS) refers to techniques that allow delivery of high-dose radiation that conforms to the shape of the target and has rapid isodose fall-off, minimizing damage to adjacent neural structures. The two most common devices used for conformal SRS for intracranial lesions are the LINAC (linear accelerator) and the gamma knife. LINAC delivers a focused beam of x-ray radiation from a port that arcs partway around the patient's head. Linear accelerators are commonly used to provide fractionated radiation for lesions outside the CNS. They are found in most radiation oncology departments. SRS can be performed with these existing units, after upgrades to the software and collimators. The gamma knife delivers approximately 200 focused beams of gamma radiation from cobalt sources through a specially designed colander-like helmet. Gamma knife units are used only for intracranial disease and cost up to $5 million; thus they are most appropriate in high patient–volume centers. There is ongoing debate in the literature regarding the two technologies.[23–25] Both continue to evolve, allowing more precise and complex isodose conformation to complex lesions. Most lesions can be treated equally well with either technology. Lesions abutting the medulla or the spinal cord should not be treated with SRS, because these structures do not tolerate the radiation dose delivered to structures within millimeters of the target. Also, medullary or spinal cord compression can result from swelling of the lesion after the radiosurgery dose, resulting in devastating neurologic deficit.

Arteriovenous Malformations

SRS has been found to be an effective stand-alone therapy for AVMs up to 3 cm in diameter. SRS is best for lesions that are difficult to access surgically due to high likelihood of postoperative neurologic deficit. SRS is not effective for lesions larger than 3 cm. Effective obliteration and elimination of the risk of hemorrhage takes 2 years. There is an approximately 2% annual incidence of hemorrhage during this 2-year period.[26] Thus surgical excision remains the preferred therapeutic modality, with SRS reserved for cases deemed very high-risk for surgery due to location or patient factors.[27] Some patients with large AVMs who undergo surgery will have unresectable residual lesions. SRS may be used as an effective adjunctive therapy in these patients.

Vestibular Schwannomas

SRS has been introduced as a therapeutic alternative to microsurgical resection for vestibular schwannomas up to 2.5 cm in maximum diameter. SRS provides high rates of tumor growth arrest and possible reduction in size with low rates of facial nerve palsy. Patients with functional ipsilateral hearing preprocedure may be more likely to retain functional hearing postprocedure than with microsurgery. The limitations of SRS include inability to treat tumors larger than 2.5 cm, the possibility of radiation-induced malignant transformation of these benign tumors, and lack of long-term follow-up. SRS centers are accumulating experience with these tumors and accumulating data on long-term results.[28,29] The indications for microsurgery and SRS will continue to evolve. Either approach should be undertaken at a high-volume center, as studies show the patient outcomes improve with increased surgeon experience.[30]

Intracranial Metastases

Patients with solitary or multiple intracranial metastases may be treated primarily with SRS.[31] Patients have improved survival after SRS compared to no treatment or whole-brain radiation therapy (WBRT), and similar survival to patients undergoing total surgical resection. Patients with lesions greater than 3 cm in diameter or evidence of intracranial hypertension should undergo surgical decompression rather than SRS. Some studies show improved survival with up to seven intracranial masses. Patients with multiple intracranial masses have almost zero long-term survival, and most will die of their intracranial disease. Patients with intracranial metastases live 3 to 6 months on average with medical care and WBRT. This can be extended to 9 to 16 months with SRS or surgery, depending on tumor type, age, and patient condition.[32]

CONGENITAL AND DEVELOPMENTAL ANOMALIES

Dysraphism

Dysraphism describes defects of fusion of the neural tube involving the neural tube itself, or overlying bone or skin. Dysraphism may occur in the spine or the head. Neural tube defects are among the most common congenital abnormalities. Prenatal vitamins, especially folic acid, reduce the incidence of neural tube defects.

Spina Bifida Occulta

Spina bifida occulta is congenital absence of posterior vertebral elements. The spinous process is always missing, the laminae may be missing to various degrees, but the underlying neural tissues are not involved. Spina bifida occulta is found in 25% of the general population, and is asymptomatic unless associated with other developmental abnormalities.

Spina Bifida with Myelomeningocele

Spina bifida with myelomeningocele describes congenital absence of posterior vertebral elements with protrusion of the meninges through the defect, and underlying neural structural abnormalities. Common findings are weakness and atrophy of the lower extremities, gait disturbance, urinary incontinence, and deformities of the foot. Myelomeningoceles arising from the high lumbar cord usually cause total paralysis and incontinence, while those arising from the sacral cord may have only clawing of the foot and partial urinary function. Myelomeningocele patients often have hydrocephalus and a Chiari II malformation, an abnormal downward herniation of the cerebellum and brain stem through the foramen magnum. Patients with abnormal protrusion of meninges through the bony defect without abnormalities of the underlying neural tissue have a meningocele. Most of these patients are neurologically normal.

Encephalocele

Herniation of brain encased in meninges through the skull that forms an intracranial mass is referred to as encephalocele. Herniation of meninges without brain tissue is referred to as a meningocele. Most occur over the convexity of the skull. More rarely, the tissue protrudes through the skull base into the sinuses. Treatment involves excision of the herniated tissue and closure of the defect. Most patients with encephaloceles and meningoceles have impaired cognitive development. Patients with greater amounts of herniated neural tissue tend to have more severe cognitive deficits.

Craniosynostosis

Craniosynostosis is the abnormal early fusion of a cranial suture line with resultant restriction of skull growth in the affected area and compensatory bulging at the other sutures. Skull growth occurs at the cranial sutures for the first 2 years of life, at the end of which the skull has achieved over 90% of its eventual adult size. Fusion of the sagittal suture, or sagittal synostosis, results in a boat-shaped head, known as scaphocephaly. Unilateral coronal synostosis results in ipsilateral forehead flattening and outward deviation of the orbit, known as plagiocephaly. The contralateral normal forehead appears to bulge by comparison. Bilateral coronal synostosis results in a broad, flattened forehead, known as brachycephaly, and is often associated with maxillary hypoplasia and proptosis. Unilateral or bilateral lambdoid synostosis results in flattening of the occiput. Occipital flattening can result from abnormal suture fusion (synostosis), or from physical remolding of the skull caused by always

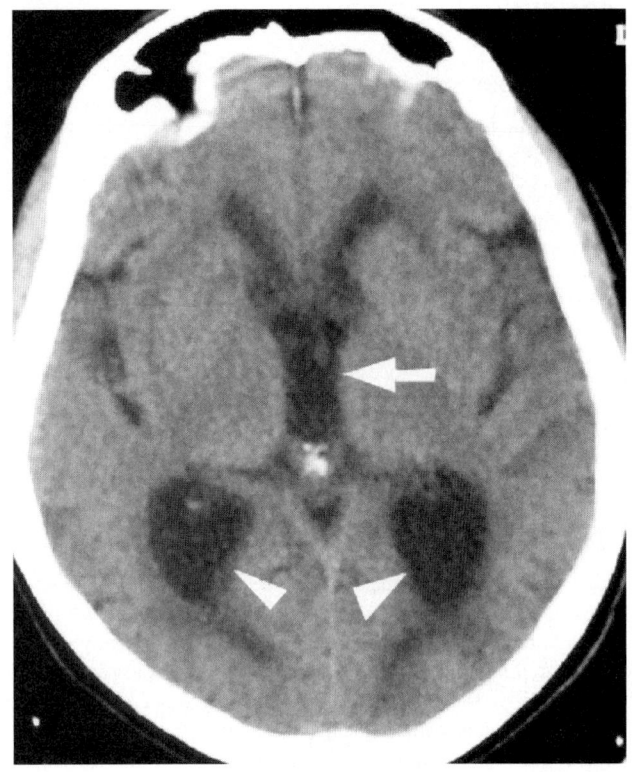

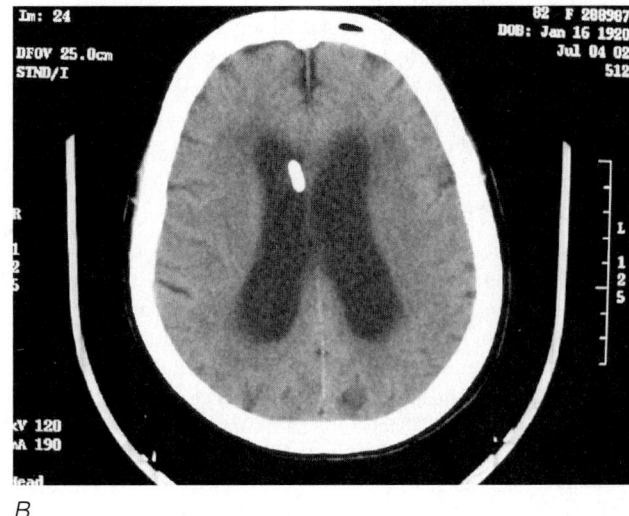

A   *B*

FIG. 41-33. *A.* Axial head CT scan revealing dilated ventricular system. Note dilated atria of the lateral ventricles *(arrowheads)* and rounded third ventricle *(arrow)*. The large size of the ventricles and lack of transependymal flow indicate a chronic process (contrast to Fig. 41-2). The patient has normal-pressure hydrocephalus, and had improved ambulation after placement of a ventriculoperitoneal shunt. *B.* Higher cut from same scan showing ventricular catheter in place in the frontal horn of the right lateral ventricle.

placing the baby in the supine position for sleep (known as positional plagiocephaly). Placing the baby in the prone position or tilted onto the contralateral side may restore near-normal skull shape in most cases of lambdoid synostosis, avoiding surgery. Treatment for synostoses in general is surgical, involving resection of the fused suture, or more complex reconstructive techniques for severe or refractory cases.

Hydrocephalus

Excess CSF in the brain that results in enlarged ventricles is known as hydrocephalus. The adult forms approximately 500 mL of CSF per day, much of it in the lateral ventricles. CSF flows from the ventricles to the subarachnoid space, and is then absorbed into the venous blood through the arachnoid granulations. Hydrocephalus may be classified as communicating or obstructive (outlined below), and congenital or acquired. Congenital lesions associated with or causing hydrocephalus include stenosis of the cerebral aqueduct, Chiari malformations, myelomeningoceles, and intrauterine infections. Acquired hydrocephalus may result from occlusion of arachnoid granulations by meningitis or subarachnoid hemorrhage, or occlusion of CSF pathways by adjacent tumors (Fig. 41-33).

Communicating Hydrocephalus

Obstruction at the level of the arachnoid granulations constitutes communicating hydrocephalus. This usually causes dilation of the lateral, third, and fourth ventricles equally. The most common causes in adults are meningitis and subarachnoid hemorrhage. Hydrocephalus may be transient after subarachnoid hemorrhage,

with reestablishment of normal CSF absorption after the protein content of the CSF returns to normal and the granulations reopen.

Obstructive Hydrocephalus

Obstruction of CSF pathways is known as obstructive hydrocephalus. Ventricles proximal to the obstruction dilate, while those distal to the obstruction remain normal in size. Typical patterns include dilation of the lateral ventricles due to a colloid cyst occluding the foramen of Monro, dilation of the lateral and third ventricles due to a tectal (midbrain) glioma or pineal region tumor occluding the cerebral aqueduct, or dilation of the lateral and third ventricles with obliteration of the fourth ventricle by an intraventricular tumor of the fourth ventricle. Obstructive hydrocephalus may present precipitously and require urgent shunting to prevent herniation.

Chiari I Malformation

Chiari I malformation is the caudal displacement of the cerebellar tonsils below the foramen magnum, and may be seen as an incidental finding on MRI scans in asymptomatic patients. Symptomatic patients usually present with headache, neck pain, or symptoms of myelopathy, including numbness or weakness in the extremities. The brain stem and lower cranial nerves are normal in Chiari I malformations. Chiari II malformations are more severe and involve caudal displacement of the lower brain stem and stretching of the lower cranial nerves. Symptomatic patients may be treated with suboccipital craniectomy to remove the posterior arch of the foramen magnum, along with removal of the posterior ring of C1. Removal of these bony structures relieves the compression of the cerebellar

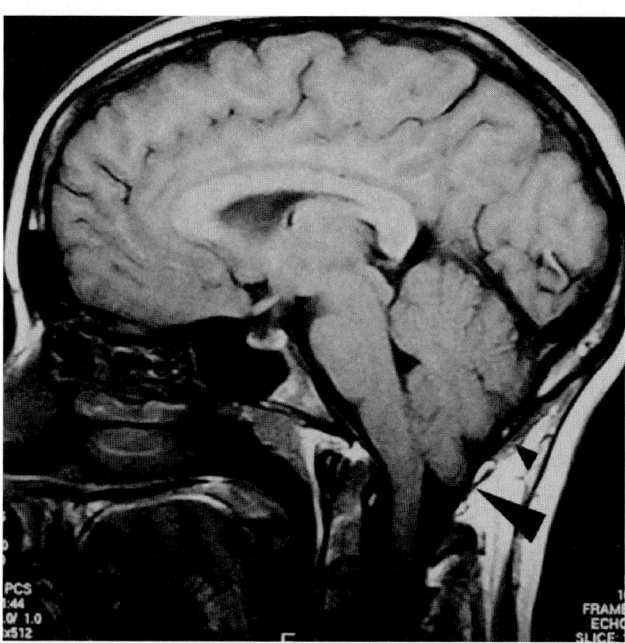

FIG. 41-34. T1-weighted sagittal MRI of a patient with a Chiari I malformation. The large arrowhead points to the cerebellar tonsils. The small arrow points to the posterior arch of the foramen magnum.

tonsils and cervicomedullary junction, and may allow reestablishment of normal CSF flow patterns. Figure 41-34 demonstrates typical MRI appearance of a Chiari I malformation.

References

1. Kandel E, Schwartz J, Jessell T: *Principles of Neural Science*, 3rd ed. New York: Elsevier, 1991, p. 961.
2. Masters SJ, McClean PM, Aracarese JS, et al: Skull x-ray examination after head trauma. *N Engl J Med* 316:84, 1987.
3. Stein SC, Ross SE: The value of CT scans in patients with low-risk head injuries. *Neurosurgery* 26:638, 1990.
4. Ingebrigsten R, Romner B: Routine early CT scan is cost-saving after minor head injury. *Acta Neurol Scand* 93:207, 1996.
5. Kelly JP, Nichols JS, Filley CM: Concussion in sports: Guidelines for the prevention of catastrophic outcome. *JAMA* 266:2867, 1991.
6. Howard MA, Gross AS, Dacey RG, et al: Acute subdural hematomas: An age-dependent clinical entity. *J Neurosurg* 71:856, 1989.
7. Maynard FM, Bracken MB, Creasey G, et al: International Standards for Neurological and Functional Classification of Spinal Cord Injury. American Spinal Injury Association. *Spinal Cord* 35:266, 1997.
8. Bracken MB, Shepard MJ, Collins WF, et al: A randomized, controlled trial of methylprednisolone or naloxone in the treatment of acute spinal cord injury. *N Engl J Med* 322:1405, 1990.
9. Bracken MB, Shepard MJ, Collins WF, et al: Methylprednisolone or naloxone treatment after acute spinal cord injury: 1-Year follow up data. *J Neurosurg* 76:23, 1992.
10. Hugenholts H, Cass DE, Dvorak MF, et al: High-dose methylprednisolone for acute closed spinal cord injury—only a treatment option. *Can J Neurol Sci* 29:227, 2002.
11. North American Symptomatic Carotid Endarterectomy Trial Collaborators: Beneficial effects of carotid endarterectomy in symptomatic patients with high-grade carotid stenosis. *N Engl J Med* 325:445, 1991.
12. The National Institute of Neurologic Disorders and Stroke rt-PA Stroke Study Group: Tissue plasminogen activator for acute ischemic stroke. *N Engl J Med* 333:1581, 1995.
13. Monylneux A, Kerr R, Stratton I, et al: International Subarachnoid Aneurysm Trial (ISAT) of neurosurgical clipping versus endovascular coiling in 2143 patients with ruptured intracranial aneurysms: A randomised trial. *Lancet* 360:1267, 2002.
14. Raftopoulos C, Goffette P, Vaz G, et al: Surgical clipping may lead to better results than coil embolization: Results from a series of 101 consecutive unruptured intracranial aneurysms. *Neurosurgery* 52:1280, 2003.
15. Dawson D, Hallett M, Wilbourn A: *Entrapment Neuropathies*, 3rd ed. Baltimore: Lippincott-Raven, 1999, Chap 2, p 4.
16. Benbadis S, Heriaud L, Tatum WO, et al: Epilepsy surgery, delays and referral patterns—are all your epilepsy patients controlled? *Seizure* 12:167, 2003.
17. Rausch R, et al: Early and late cognitive changes following temporal lobe surgery for epilepsy. *Neurology* 60:9551, 2003.
18. Rehncrona S, et al: Long-term efficacy of thalamic deep brain stimulation for tremor: Double-blind assessments. *Move Disord* 18:163, 2003.
19. Fields J, Troster AI, Woods SP, et al: Neuropsychologic and quality of life outcomes 12 months after unilateral thalamic stimulation for essential tremor. *J Neurol Neurosurg Psychiatry* 74:305, 2003.
20. Krause M, Fogel W, Heck A, et al: Deep brain stimulators for the treatment of Parkinson's disease: Subthalamic nucleus versus globus pallidus internus. *J Neurol Neurosurg Psychiatry* 70:464, 2001.
21. Perozzo P, Rissone M, Bergamoasco B, et al: Deep brain stimulation of the subthalamic nucleus in Parkinson's disease: Comparison of pre- and post-operative neuropsychologic evaluation. *J Neurol Sci* 193:9, 2001.
22. Kondo A: Microvascular decompression surgery for trigeminal neuralgia. *Stereotactic and Functional Neurosurgery* 77:187, 2001.
23. Suh J, Barnett GH, Miller DW, et al: Successful conversion from a linear accelerator-based program to a gamma knife radiosurgery program: The Cleveland Clinic experience. *Stereotactic and Functional Neurosurgery* 72(Suppl 1):159, 1999.
24. Konigsmaier H, de Pauli-Ferch B, Hackl A, et al: The costs of radiosurgical treatment: Comparison between gamma knife and linear accelerator. *Acta Neurochir* 140:1101, 1998.
25. Bova J, Goetsch S: Modern linac [linear accelerator] radiosurgery systems have rendered the gamma knife obsolete. *Med Phys* 28:1839, 2001.
26. Karlsson B, Lax I, Soderman M: Risk for hemorrhage in the 2-year latency period following gamma-knife radiosurgery for AVM. *Int J Radiation Oncol Biol Phys* 49:1045, 2001.
27. Pan D, Guo WY, Chung WY, et al: Gamma knife radiosurgery as a single treatment modality for large cerebral AVMs. *J Neurosurg* 93:113, 2000.
28. Regis J, Pellet W, Delsanti C, et al: Functional outcome after gamma knife surgery or microsurgery for vestibular schwannomas. *J Neurosurg* 97:1091, 2002.
29. Shim M, Ueki K, Kurita H, et al: Malignant transformation of a vestibular schwannoma after gamma knife radiosurgery. *Lancet* 360:309, 2002.
30. Elsmore A, Mendoza N: The operative learning curve for vestibular schwannoma excision via the retrosigmoid approach. *Br J Neurosurg* 16:448, 2002.
31. Gerosa M, Nicolato A, Foroni R, et al: Gamma knife radiosurgery for brain metastases: A primary therapeutic option. *J Neurosurg* 97:515, 2002.
32. Pollock B, Brown PD, Foote RL, et al: Properly selected patients with multiple brain metastases may benefit from aggressive treatment of their intracranial disease. *J Neurooncol* 61:73, 2003.

Orthopaedics

Dempsey Springfield

Heel Pain
Hallux Valgus
Lesser-Toe Deformity
Stress Fractures
Arthritis
Ankle Instability
Diabetic Foot
Interdigital Neuroma
Tarsal Tunnel Syndrome

Pediatric Disorders

Developmental Dysplasia of the Hip
Slipped Capital Femoral Epiphysis
Legg-Calvé-Perthes Disease
Talipes Equinovarus
Metatarsus Adductus
Tarsal Coalition
Blount Disease
Osgood-Schlatter Disease

Nicolas Andry coined the word from which the English word orthopaedics is derived when he wrote a book titled *L'Ortho'edie* in 1741. Orthopaedics is derived from the two Greek words Andry chose: *orthos,* meaning straight or free from deformity, and *pais,* meaning child. Since that time orthopaedics has expanded to include the evaluation and treatment of all musculoskeletal injury and disorders. Until the later half of the twentieth century, orthopaedics was predominately the nonoperative treatment of fractures, treatment of musculoskeletal infections (often tuberculosis), and polio. As we enter the twenty-first century, orthopaedic surgery includes the replacement of degenerated joints, operative fixation of fractures, arthroscopic repair of torn meniscus, rotator cuffs, and a whole host of other intra-articular abnormalities. Musculoskeletal research laboratories have found means of stimulating the body to make new bones and soon cartilage production will be accomplished. Gene therapies for a variety of musculoskeletal diseases are on the horizon. Orthopaedics is a dynamic field and orthopaedic surgeons treat both sexes and all ages of patients with a wide variety of skeletal, ligamentous, and muscular problems. Orthopaedics are involved in the management of a newborn's dislocated hip, a teenager's curved spine, an athlete's injury knee, a motor vehicle accident victim, an adult's worn-out joint, and an elderly woman's fracture hip.[1-5]

The musculoskeletal system is a complex biomechanical organ. It is constantly responding to the demands of the patient. Bone is in constant turnover. It atrophies when not used, and hypertrophies when stressed. Overall bone mass is increased until some time between 30 and 35 years of age, after which there is an overall decrease of bone as a consequence of more resorption than production. Bone can heal without leaving a scar. Articular cartilage is a special material because it has properties that people have not been able to reproduce. It is a wonderful shock absorber, yet when sliding with another surface of articular cartilage bathed in normal synovial fluid, the constant of friction is a fraction of that found with ice-on-ice. Unfortunately, upon reaching adulthood, the ability to generate new articular cartilage ceases and as it wears out or is injured, it is not replaced. Repair fibrocartilage, metal, and plastic are the materials currently substituted for articular cartilage. Skeletal muscle accounts for almost 50% of the body's weight making it the single largest tissue mass in the human body. There is one basic structural unit in muscle fiber; however, the arrangement of these fibers varies depending on a particular muscle's function. Muscle fibers are either parallel or oblique with oblique fibers existing in various configurations.

SKELETAL GROWTH AND PHYSIOLOGY

The skeletal system is initially formed as cartilage with the exception of the craniofacial bones and clavicle. These bones do not have a cartilaginous analogue and are formed directly from membranous tissue. The process of bone formation without an intermediate cartilage form is called *intramembranous bone formation.* The majority of an adult's bone is formed by intramembranous bone formation because diaphyseal bone grows circumferentially by the apposition of bone by the surrounding periosteum without cartilage being produced. *Enchondral ossifications* is the formation of bone through the initial formation of a cartilage model that then becomes bone. The skeletal system is formed in utero as cartilage; however, prior to birth, some of these prebone structures are well on their way to bone formation. This happens first in the *middle of the diaphysis,* known as the primary center of ossification. Later, at the secondary ossification center, bone will begin to form at the ends of the prebone structures. The secondary center of ossification has articular cartilage surrounding it on the side facing the joint and epiphyseal cartilage on the side facing the primary ossification center. The bone grows in length through the epiphyseal growth plate, which produces cartilage that undergoes enchondral ossification (Fig. 42-1).

The epiphyseal growth plate is made up of proliferating cartilage cells that eventually die. After the cartilage cells die, osteoblasts line the calcified cartilage matrix previously produced by the chondrocytes, thus forming bone. The epiphyseal growth plate is divided into zones. The number of zones often varies in the literature dependent upon the author; however, a general consensus specifies five zones. The first zone is the resting or reserve zone, followed by the proliferative zone, the maturation zone, the degeneration zone, and the zone of calcification. The zones of maturation, degeneration, and calcification are often referred to as the *hypertrophic zone.* The initial bone formed consists of spicules of bone with a calcified cartilaginous core and is called the *primary spongiosa.* The calcified cartilage will be removed entirely as the bone continues to remodel. The area of the bone with the primary spongiosa is called the *metaphysis.* This bone remodels to become the narrower diaphysis (Fig. 42-2). The initial bone formed during this process is referred to as *woven bone.* This bone is unorganized both grossly and microscopically. As it remodels and matures, it becomes *lamellar bone.* It can be either cortical bone with a blood supply and a Haversian system, or trabecular bone, which does not have a Haversian system (Fig. 42-3).

Bone is produced by osteoblasts, which become osteocytes once they are trapped within a matrix of bone. Osteoclasts are multinucleated cells that have the capability of resorbing bone. Osteoblast and osteocytes are recognized under the microscope by the matrix they produce. Chondrocytes are cells responsible for making cartilage and live within the cartilage matrix. (Use of the term chondroblast for the cartilage-producing cells lining a surface of cartilage production is appropriate, but rarely used.)

Bone remodels constantly, primarily under the influence of a mechanical load. During the first 30 years of life, a person's overall skeletal mass perpetually increases; however, after 30 years of age, overall skeletal mass decreases, with women experiencing a period of accelerated loss just after menopause (Fig. 42-4). The more bone an individual has acquired by age 30, the less likely she or he are to develop osteoporosis.

GROWTH PLATE

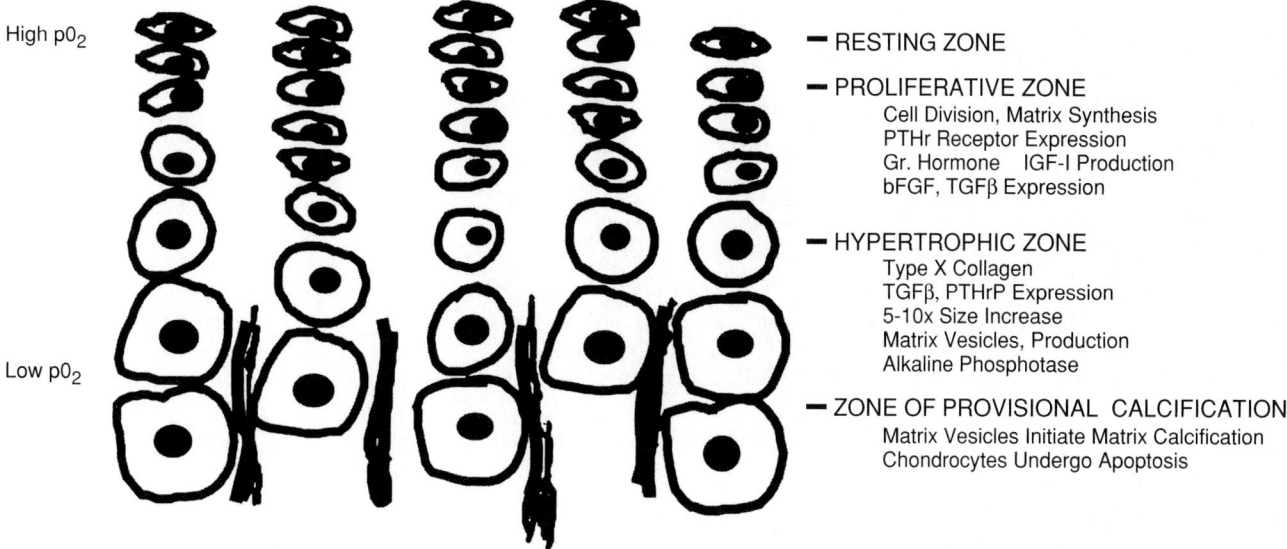

- RESTING ZONE

- PROLIFERATIVE ZONE
    Cell Division, Matrix Synthesis
    PTHr Receptor Expression
    Gr. Hormone   IGF-I Production
    bFGF, TGFβ Expression

- HYPERTROPHIC ZONE
    Type X Collagen
    TGFβ, PTHrP Expression
    5-10x Size Increase
    Matrix Vesicles, Production
    Alkaline Phosphotase

- ZONE OF PROVISIONAL CALCIFICATION
    Matrix Vesicles Initiate Matrix Calcification
    Chondrocytes Undergo Apoptosis

High pO$_2$

Low pO$_2$

FIG. 42-1. *Structure and function relationships of the growth plate. Calcified cartilage bars form scaffold for osteoblasts to deposit new bone; osteoclast-like cells reabsorb calcified cartilage through remodelling.*

Osteoporosis is defined as a loss of bone per unit of volume. A more strict definition is bone with a bone mineral density (BMD) as measured by a dual-energy x-ray absorptiometry (DEXA) scan of more than 2.5 below the norm. The norm is based on a series of

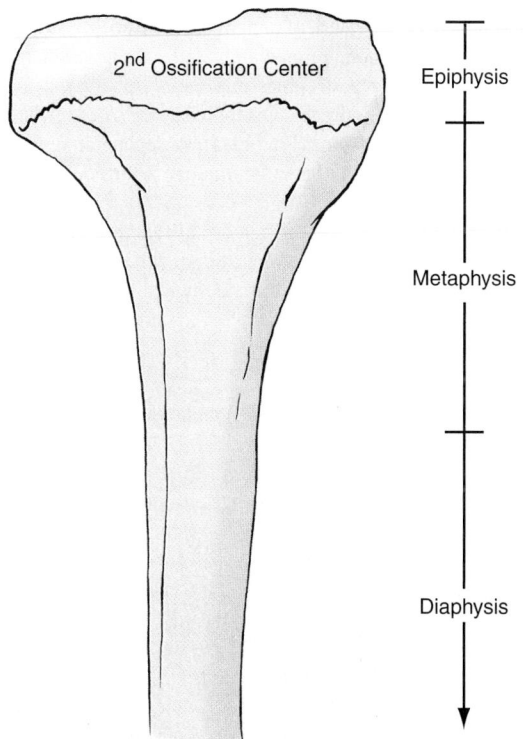

FIG. 42-2. *Long bones have three sections. The end is the epiphysis or secondary ossification center, the adjacent area is the metaphysis, and the middle of the bone is the diaphysis. The metaphysis is broader than the diaphysis, has a thin cortex, and is composed of primarily cancellous bone.*

bone mineral density analyses done on healthy women who were at the peak bone mass. *Osteomalacia* (disorder in adults) and rickets (disorder in children) are the inadequate mineralization of bone. *Osteopenia* is the term used to describe the radiographic appearance of a bone with less density than expected. Osteoporosis should be prevented by having young persons, especially women, take adequate amounts of calcium and vitamin D, as well as exercise to build their skeletal system to its maximum. Osteomalacia is treated by restoring a normal calcium metabolism. Abnormal calcium metabolism may be caused by a congenital disorder, dietary abnormalities, gastrointestinal disorders, by-pass surgery, parathyroid dysfunction, or renal disease.

JOINT ANATOMY AND PHYSIOLOGY

A *diarthrodial joint* is one in which a complete separation between the connecting parts is present. The diarthrodial joint contains synovial fluid, which lubricates the two articular cartilage-covered surfaces that rub against one another. Articular cartilage is unique in that its coefficient of friction between the two articular surfaces with normal synovial fluid is estimated to be 10 times less than that which exists between two blocks of ice. This allows free movement with little wear of the articular surfaces.

The amount of articular cartilage achieved upon completing growth (mid-teenage years) is the total amount a person will possess for the remainder of life. Once damaged, it cannot be replaced. Repair cartilage (fibrocartilage) can look similar and even have similar (not identical) properties, but does not have the mechanical properties to withstand the high demands placed on a joint surface. Additionally, fibrocartilage wears out within a few years when it is subjected to the forces experienced across a normal joint. Research continues in an effort to better understand cartilage in order to replace damaged portions before the entire joint is destroyed.

Articular cartilage is composed of hyaline cartilage, which is between 60 and 80% water. The remaining composition consists of macromolecules—collagen, proteoglycans, and noncollagenous

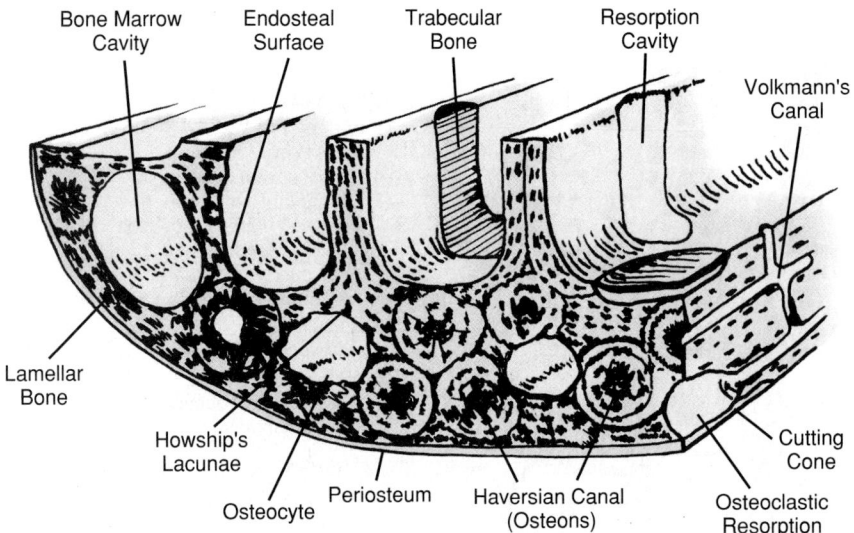

FIG. 42-3. The cellular and structural organization of bone.

proteins—which are all composed of amino acids and sugars. Type II collagen accounts for approximately 95% of the collagen in articular cartilage. There are three major proteoglycans in articular cartilage that are all polysaccharide chains with a protein core. The two larger proteoglycans are referred to as aggrecans, which, along with water, fill the interfibrillar spaces and give cartilage its mechanical properties. One contains mainly chondroitin sulfate and the other mainly keratin sulfate. A smaller one contains mainly dermatan sulfate.

Articular cartilage is organized into four zones or layers; superficial or gliding, middle or transitional, deep or radial, and calcified. Each has its own organization, collagen and proteoglycan contents, and function. Disruption of any layer causes the articular cartilage to malfunction. There are many other minor proteins in articular cartilage that are critical to the normal function of the cartilage.

The extremely limited healing ability of cartilage is in direct contrast to that of bone. Bone has the capacity to not only heal after an injury but the ability to heal without a scar. Cartilage does not heal. An injury to articular cartilage will be followed by a response of the chondrocytes, but the response is limited and will not heal any injury. If the injury, including a laceration, is superficial and does not include the underlying subchondral bone, there will be no clinical evidence of healing. If the injury includes the subchondral bone it will bleed, thus producing a healing response; however, the restorative cartilage made is not identical to the original articular cartilage and does not function in the same manner because it wears too quickly and does not hold up to the type of stresses normally experienced by a joint.

Degenerative arthritis or *osteoarthritis* is the wearing away of articular cartilage. It can occur secondary to an injury, from malalignment leading to abnormal forces, from numerous conditions that interfere with the synovial lining from doing its job, or for no apparent reason. Idiopathic or osteoarthritis of old age is the most common form. The hallmark of degenerative arthritis is a loss of articular cartilage. The bone immediately under the articular cartilage (subchondral bone) hypertrophies and the peripheral cartilage responds to produce osteophytes. Osteophytes are osteocartilaginous at the periphery of the joint (Fig. 42-5). A degenerative pattern is seen as the end stage of the inflammatory arthritides such as in rheumatoid arthritis.

The synovium is critical to the normal function of the joint as it provides synovial fluid, which surrounds the joint that is necessary to maintain the extremely low coefficient of friction between

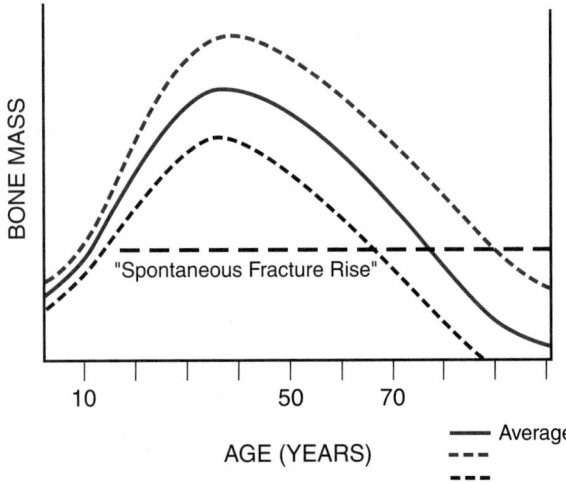

FIG. 42-4. Until the age of 30 to 35 years bone mass increases, but from then on it decreases. For women there is an acceleration of loss associated with menopause.

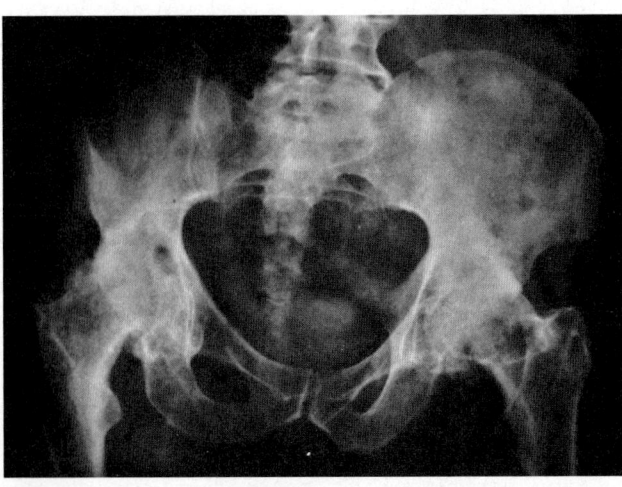

FIG. 42-5. Bilateral osteoarthritis of the hips showing marked osteophyte formation, sclerosis, acetabular cysts, obliteration of joint space, and partial subluxation.

Table 42-1
Synovial Fluid Analysis

Clinical Example	Normal	Noninflammatory (Osteoarthrosis)	Inflammatory (Rheumatoid)	Septic (Bacterial)
Color	Clear	Clear yellow	Opalescent yellow	Turbid yellow to green
Viscosity	High	High	Low	Low
WBC/mm^3	200	200–2000	200–100,000	>100,000
% PMM leukocytes	<25%	<25%	>50%	>75%
Culture	Negative	Negative	Negative	Positive
Mucin clot	Firm	Firm	Friable	Friable
Glucose (% of serum glucose)	100%	100%	50–75%	<50%
Total protein	Normal	Normal	Elevated	Elevated

the articular surfaces. The synovial fluid also contains the nutrients needed for chondrocytes in the articular cartilage to survive. It is a dialysate of blood and contains hyaluronate and glycosaminoglycan. The hyaluronate is a long-chain with a weight of 1 to 2 million daltons. Normal synovial fluid is viscous, slightly yellow, and has no white blood cells, erythrocytes, or clotting factors. However, a traumatic or nonspecific reactive synovitis produces synovial fluid with decreased viscosity that can contain as many as 10,000 white blood cells. A synovitis associated with an inflammatory, noninfectious condition can have a white blood cell count of up to 50,000. Synovial fluid associated with an infectious process will usually have a white blood cell count of over 50,000 (Table 42-1).

Joints are stabilized by a combination of ligaments and muscles that cross the joint. These ligaments are subject to injury when stretched, resulting in a sprain. The degree of the injury is usually reflected in the severity of the local swelling and pain. Ligaments heal as does other collagenous tissue. Often the ligaments need surgical repair to assure that they are properly tensioned. Otherwise, persistent joint laxity occurs, which leads to early degeneration of the joint. Ligaments tend to shorten if held in their shortest position.

This is especially true if they have been injured. This shortening accounts for the joint stiffness observed after prolonged immobilization. Proper positioning of joints to keep the major ligaments at their maximal length during prolonged immobilization produces the least amount of joint stiffness and allows the quickest return to function once the immobilization device is discontinued.

Ligaments alone cannot continuously keep a joint stable. If the muscles that cross the joint do not act to maintain joint stability (i.e., secondary to paralysis) the ligaments will be stretched and the joint will become lax.

MUSCLE ANATOMY AND PHYSIOLOGY

Muscle is the single largest tissue mass in the body. It makes up almost half of body's total weight. Myofibers, consisting of the contractile elements, are bundled together into fibers. A number of fibers are bundled together to make up a fascicle, and numerous fascicles are arranged in a variety of patterns to make up a muscle. The fascicles are structurally arranged depending on the function of the muscle (Fig. 42-6).

FIG. 42-6. Organization of skeletal muscle from the microscopic to the macrostructural level. [*Reproduced with permission from Simon SR (ed): Orthopaedic Basic Science. Rosemont, IL: American Academy of Orthopaedic Surgeons, 1994, p. 91.*]

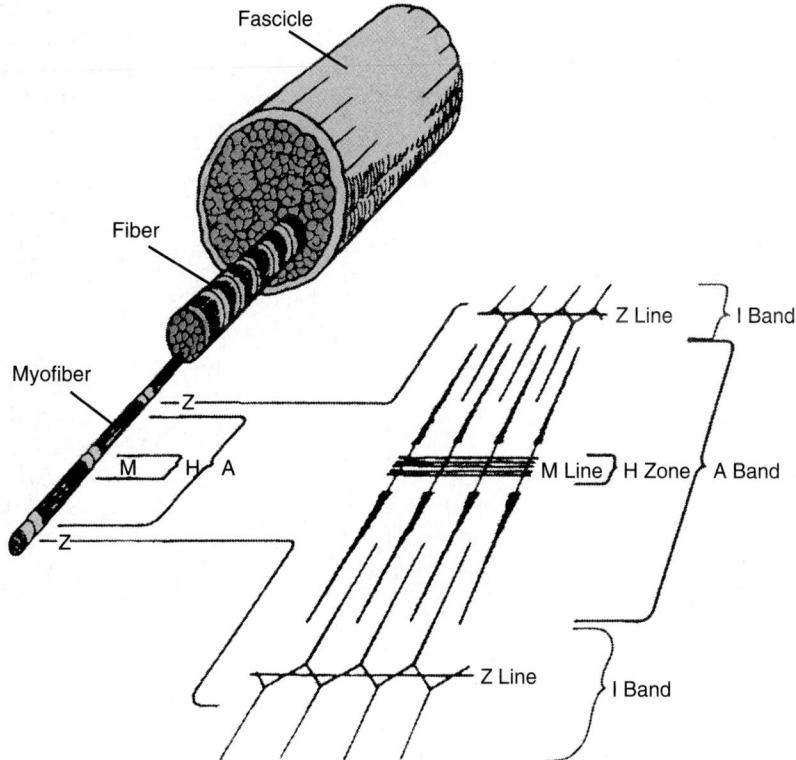

At the nerve's point of entry into the muscle, the nerve cell axon branches so that each fiber has a single nerve terminal. That terminal is called a motor end plate. The motor unit is made up of all fibers innervated by a single nerve axon. These are not necessarily adjacent fibers. The electrical impulse from the nerve stimulates a release of calcium; the increase in calcium causes the release of acetylcholine, which then diffuses across the synapsis, depolarizing the cell and the muscle contracts. Any alteration in the levels of calcium, acetylcholine, and medicines that affect these has an effect on muscle function. For example, myasthenia gravis leads to quick fatigue of muscle because there is inadequate acetylcholine. Hypercalcemia can lead to overexcitation of muscle and constant muscular contraction.

There are two groups of muscle fiber types. Type I is a slow-twitch muscle fiber. Its speed of contraction is slow, its strength on contraction is low, and it has a high fatigue resistance. Type II is a fast-twitch fiber. There are three subcategories of type II fibers. Type IIA has fast speed and high strength of contraction but is fatigable. Type IIB contacts even faster and stronger, but is more fatigable than Type IIA. Type IIC is composed of specialized, fast-twitch fibers found mainly in the jaw muscles. There is a considerable variation in the percentage of fiber types among humans; however, a mere determination of the percentage of fiber types does not accurately predict function as there are too many other variables. Therefore, percentage fiber types are not predictive.

Another important anatomic consideration is the gross direction of the muscle fibers. The architectural arrangement determines the specific function of the muscle. Fibers are either parallel or oblique. Oblique fibers are arranged in various fashions, sorting them into categories of pennate, bipennate, or multipennate. Some muscles have complex arrangements.

The origin of a muscle is usually its more proximal end, while the insertion is the more distal end. Most muscles cross only one joint and therefore have an action pertaining only to that joint. Some muscles (e.g., biceps in the upper extremity, sartorius, rectus femoris, gracilis, the hamstrings, and gastrocnemius in the lower extremity) cross two joints and act on both. When examining an extremity, it is often possible to distinguish between joint contracture and muscle contracture by changing the position of one joint while testing the motion of the other. If the range of motion does not change with a change in position of the other joint, the contracture is in the effected joint and not caused by contracted muscles.

Direct injuries to muscle usually heal with little functional loss. Disruption of the muscle at the musculotendinous junction may need repair; however, this remains controversial. Atrophy of muscle occurs quickly when the muscle is not used and changes are seen even after only 2 weeks of disuse. Biopsy of the muscle should be done only after consultation with a pathologist so the best muscle is chosen; this is commonly the muscle in the earliest stages of a disorder.

BASIC BIOMECHANICS

Basic knowledge of biomechanics makes understanding the musculoskeletal system easier. It also aids in determining the mechanisms of injury, how to correct deformed fractures and dislocated joints, and to figure out where to place fixation devices. Even the use of braces is improved when the surgeon understands the mechanics of the musculoskeletal system. Disturbances in gait are explained and their cause understood by analyzing gait with biomechanical principles.

Every muscle works through a lever arm principle. The length of the lever arm often changes as the body part moves and the strength

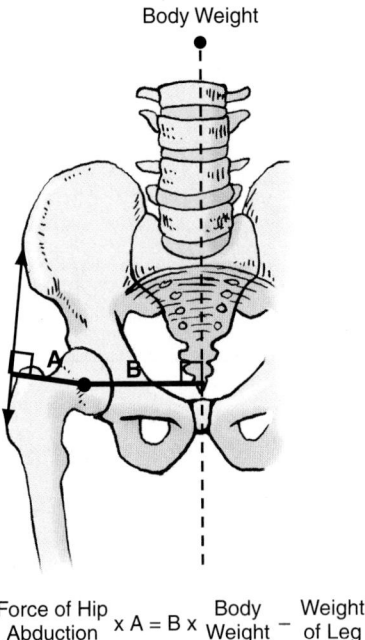

Body Weight

$$\text{Force of Hip Abduction} \times A = B \times \text{Body Weight} - \text{Weight of Leg}$$

FIG. 42-7. Any change in the distance between the greater trochanter and the center of the femoral head changes the force required to balance the body weight.

of a muscle's action can be improved or impaired by changing the lever arm. The force required to move an object depends on the lever arm's length. The relationship is not linear but exponential, with the force requirement decreasing or increasing by the square of the distance, depending on whether the lever arm length is increased or decreased. This is most often observed in the hip. The abductors originate from the iliac wing and insert on the greater trochanter (Fig. 42-7).

The concept of fatigue failure is important in understanding the musculoskeletal system. All parts of the musculoskeletal system are subjected to cyclic loads. Millions of steps are taken each year and each step loads and unloads the musculoskeletal system. Fatigue failure results when the cyclic loads cause the material to fail. A common example of this is the typical way one would break a metal coat hanger. By bending it back and forth multiple times it fails. Bones are subject to fatigue failure. This type of fracture is often called a stress fracture and is most commonly seen when an increase in intensity or duration occurs over a 3- or 4-week time period. The bone can respond to cyclic loads and become stronger if the loads are not beyond their physiologic capacity. Metal implants also are subject to similar fatigue fracture. The properties of the metal and the structure of the implant both influence the fatigue strength of the implants.

Stress is the force per unit area. *Strain* is a measure of deformity. The properties of any material are often expressed using a stress–strain curve (Fig. 42-8). The area under the curve is the amount of energy that the object can absorb. The steepness of the early part of the curve indicates how stiff a material is. Generally it is found that the steeper the line, the stiffer the material. The straight-line aspect of that curve is the elastic portion, while the portion of the curve to the left is the plastic portion curve. Those materials with limited plasticity are considered brittle, while those with large plasticity are considered ductile.

Stress risers are defects or structural aspects of a material that concentrate forces at a point and increase the risk of failure of that material. Bone stress risers are usually holes in the bone, either

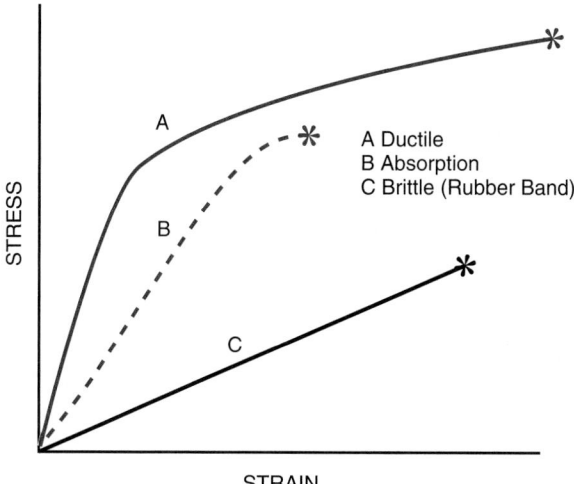

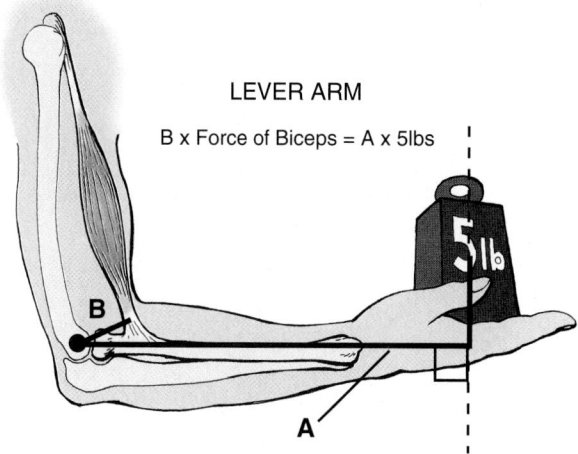

FIG. 42-8. This is a classic stress-strain curve depicting a material's properties. The straight portion of the graph is elastic deformation, the curved portion is plastic deformation, and the end of the curve is the material's failure point. The area under the curve is the energy the material can absorb before failure. Materials that have a long curved portion of the graph are ductile, while those with no curved portion are brittle.

FIG. 42-10. The biceps muscle with its insertion to the bicipital tuberosity of the radius has a short lever arm when compared to the length of the forearm that is the lever arm for the weight in the hand. The biceps force must be much greater than the weight of the ball because of the difference between the two lever arms.

caused by a tumor or, more commonly, a drill. Anytime a drill hole is made in a bone, it produces a stress riser. The larger the hole, the more the forces are concentrated and the greater the risk for failure (fracture) (Fig. 42-9). One of the more common clinical situations illustrating this phenomenon is when screws are removed from drill holes. Plates and screws are often removed from a bone after the fracture heals. Those holes are stress risers until the bone can remodel to accommodate the increased forces at the edge of the hole. The accommodation takes 6 to 8 weeks, during which time the patient must protect the bone from fracture with reduced activities and crutches if it is in a bone of the lower extremity.

Knowledge of lever arms is also important for understanding some of the principles related to how the musculoskeletal system works, as well as some of the fixation systems. The concepts relate to those of basic engineering or elementary physics. A force will tend to rotate an object about some axis. The perpendicular distance between that axis and the point of application of the force is the length of the lever arm (Fig. 42-10). The amount of force needed to move the object or to counteract a force tending to move the object in the opposite direction is dependent on the length of the lever arm. An everyday application of this principle is found on a playground where the central axis of a seesaw is adjustable so that children of different weights can balance and counterbalance; the longer the lever, the less force necessary to rotate the object or counteract rotation. The effect of length is the square of the distance. A common clinical situation where this effect is seen is in the hip. When standing on one leg, the body weight creates a force that tends to rotate the body, employing the hip abductor muscles of the leg on the ground to balance the body with an axis of the hip joint (Fig. 42-11). If the perpendicular distance from the point of contact between the femoral head and acetabulum is reduced, the hip abductor muscles must pull harder to balance the body. If they cannot pull hard enough, the patient must lean his or her torso toward the side with the leg on the ground. This produces a limp that is called a *gluteus medius limp* and a sign called a *Trendelenburg* (Fig. 42-12). The concept of lever arms is important with the use of internal fixation devices. Long lever arms mean the fixation device or construct will be subject to higher torsion than will the constructs with shorter lever arms. In general, shorter lever arm constructions are better than longer lever arm constructions.

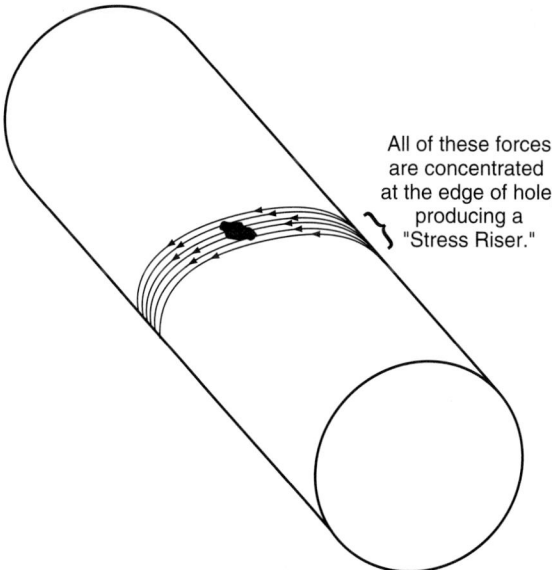

FIG. 42-9. A stress riser is a hole or defect in a material that produces a concentration of forces. This increases the risk of the material failing under conditions that without the stress riser would not lead to failure of the material.

TUMORS OF THE MUSCULOSKELETAL SYSTEM

General Considerations

Primary tumors of the musculoskeletal system are rare. The histogenetic type of the tumor is dependent on the tissue of origin. In addition, specific types of lesions tend to occur in particular bones

OFFSET TROCHANTER

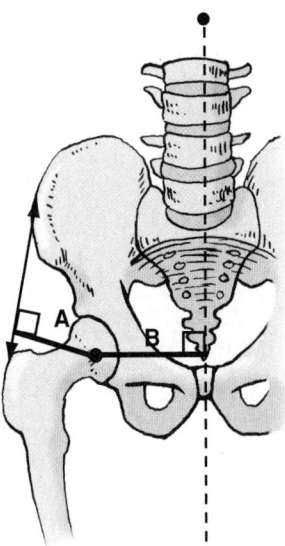

FIG. 42-11. *The lever arms around the hip joint. By making "A" longer, the force of abduction does not have to be as great as with the shorter "A." This also reduces forces exerted across the hip joint.*

or areas of bones, usually in areas of maximal growth or remodeling. Giant cell tumors (osteoclastomas) occur near the growth plate, where a high level of resorption takes place as part of remodeling; osteosarcomas occur in the metaphysis, where new bone formation is

POSITIVE TRANDELENBERG
SIGN/GAIT

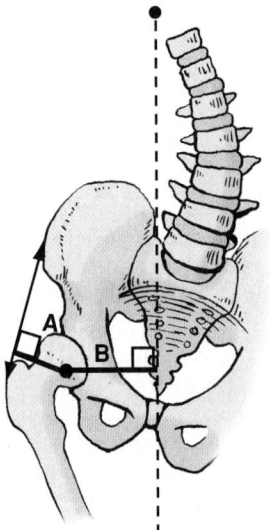

FIG. 42-12. *A Trendelenburg limp occurs when the abductors of the hip cannot balance the weight of the body. The patient shifts the weight toward the weakened abductors of the hip to reduce the length of the lever arm, allowing the weakened abductors to balance the forces. When force of hip abduction is reduced the patient must lean toward the weak muscles to move the center of body weight closer to the center of the femoral head to shorten lever arm "B." This also reduces the force across the femoral head and is a means of giving relief to a painful hip joint.*

maximal; cartilage tumors involve the metaphysis near the growth plate, and round cell tumors occur in the metaphyseal/diaphyseal bone marrow (Fig. 42-13). These neoplastic processes are thought to represent a derangement of normal growth and bone remodeling functions, which become uncontrolled.

Etiology. The cause of most bone and soft-tissue neoplasms is unknown, but recent molecular biology studies promise to elucidate these mechanisms, with identification of specific genetic mutations and chromosomal aberrations in some tumors, derangements of tumor suppressor gene function, and expression of oncogenes. Most histogenetic tumor types have variable levels of aggressiveness and occur in benign and malignant forms. Table 42-2 illustrates the range of incidence and histogenesis of musculoskeletal neoplasms. The biologic behavior of tumors can vary, as reflected by the pathologic grade of the tumor. While various grading systems exist for different tumors, in general the simplified system adopted by the Musculoskeletal Tumor Society reflects overall gross behavior differences, with benign, low-grade malignant, and high-grade malignant forms.

Characteristics. Musculoskeletal neoplasms are characterized by initial centrifugal growth from a single focus, pseudoencapsulation (formation of a zone of reactive tissue around the expanding lesion, which in malignant lesions can be focally invaded by the tumor), and a tendency to respect anatomic boundaries early in the evolution of the lesion. These tumors thus tend to spread along fascial planes and tend to remain contained in anatomic compartments, a crucial characteristic in strategies for staging and surgical treatment of these lesions. Anatomic compartments include bones, muscle compartments, joints, skin and subcutaneous tissue, and in some cases, major neurovascular sheaths.

Metastasis. Metastasis of malignant musculoskeletal neoplasms is associated with a poor prognosis. Metastases are most often pulmonary, although some tumors tend also to involve regional lymph nodes, and bony metastases also occur. Brain and visceral metastases are unusual, generally occurring only in terminal end-stage disseminated disease.

Staging. The most widely used staging system for musculoskeletal neoplasms, shown in Table 42-3, has been applied to both soft-tissue and bone lesions. Benign lesions are graded as latent, active, or aggressive. Malignant lesions are staged on the basis of whether they are high grade (stage II) or low grade (stage I), and intracompartmental (A) or extracompartmental (B). Metastatic tumors are all stage III regardless of local extent and have a dismal prognosis. This staging system has shown great value in predicting survival (Fig. 42-14).

Clinical Manifestations. Patients typically present with a history of pain that is often worse at night and usually is not activity related. A mass or swelling may be present, but constitutional symptoms (weight loss, fevers, night sweats, malaise) usually are absent, except in cases with disseminated disease. Lesions adjacent to joints can cause effusion, contractures, and pain with motion. Soft-tissue tumors often are painless unless there is involvement of neurovascular structures. Compression of veins or lymphatics in a limb can cause distal edema, and larger masses exhibit a pattern of overlying venous distention. Malignant soft-tissue masses can be firm and fixed to subcutaneous tissue, muscle, or bone, and usually are nontender. Local warmth is evident because malignant lesions induce local angiogenesis. Patients may also present with a pathologic fracture as a manifestation of benign or malignant intraosseous

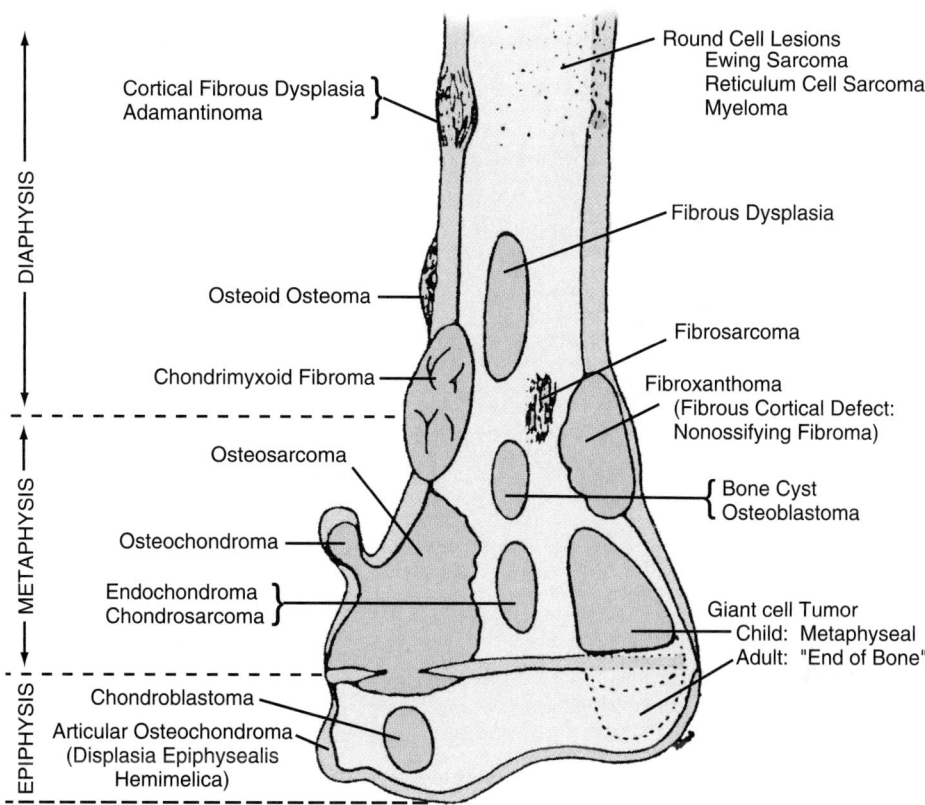

FIG. 42-13. Composite diagram demonstrating the most common sites of specific primary bone tumors. (*Reproduced with permission from Madewell et al: Radiol Clin North Am 1991.*)

lesions, with bone destruction and subsequent mechanical failure. Pain on weight bearing is an ominous clinical symptom that often indicates an impending fracture.

Evaluation should include a thorough history and physical examination of the affected region, with attention to joint, muscle, neurologic, and vascular structures. Examination of regional and distant lymph nodes is essential, as are pulmonary and abdominal examinations to assess the possibility of metastatic disease.

Radiographic Findings. The plain radiograph is the single most useful study in differential diagnosis of bone lesions. Considerations include the following:

Table 42-2
Incidence of Bone Tumors (After Dahlin)

Histology	Benign	% Cases	Malignant	% Cases
Hemopoietic (28%)			Myeloma	24.7
			Lymphoma	3.1
Chondrogenic (27%)	Osteochondroma	12.0	Primary chondrosarcoma	8.7
	Enchondroma	4.3		
	Chondroblastoma	0.7	Secondary chondrosarcoma	0.8
	Chondromyxoid fibroma	0.6		
Osteogenic (25%)	Osteoid osteoma	2.5	Osteosarcoma	9.9
	Osteoblastoma	0.7	Chondroblastic osteosarcoma	6.0
			Fibroblastic osteosarcoma	4.6
			Parosteal osteosarcoma	0.9
Unknown origin (12%)	Giant cell tumor	4.8	Ewing's sarcoma	6.2
			Giant cell tumor	0.5
			Adamantinoma	0.2
Fibrogenic (4%)	Fibroma	1.5	Fibrosarcoma	2.5
Notochordal (3.5%)			Chordoma	3.5
Vascular (0.8%)	Hemangioma	0.6	Hemangioendothelioma	0.1
	Hemangiopericytoma	0.1		
Lipogenic (0.1%)	Lipoma	0.1		
Neurogenic (<1%)	Neurilemmoma	<0.1		

Table 42-3
Surgical Staging System for Musculoskeletal Tumors (After Enneking)

Stage	Characteristics	Metastases
Benign		
1	Latent	No
2	Active	No
3	Aggressive	No
Malignant		
IA	Low grade; intracompartmental	No
IB	Low grade; extracompartmental	No
IIA	High grade; intracompartmental	No
IIB	High grade; extracompartmental	No
III	Low or high grade; intra or extracompartmental	Yes

SOURCE: Modified from Enneking WF, Gearen PF, 1986, with permission.

1. Evidence of matrix production (bone formation, calcification)
2. Pattern of growth (permeative, geographic, moth-eaten, loculated, expansile, exophytic)
3. Presence of bony reaction to the lesion (periosteal reaction, sclerotic margination)
4. Zone of transition between the host bone and lesion (narrow or well marginated versus wide or poorly defined)
5. Age of the patient
6. Bone involved (flat bone, long bone, skull, vertebrae, acral bone)
7. Location within the bone (epiphyseal, metaphyseal, diaphyseal)
8. Associated soft-tissue mass, clinical symptoms
9. Presence of solitary versus multiple lesions

Using these criteria, an accurate differential diagnosis can be formulated in most cases. Infection (osteomyelitis) must always be considered given its highly variable radiographic appearance. Metabolic, inflammatory, dysplastic, traumatic, congenital, and degenerative conditions also are always considered. Soft-tissue lesions are better evaluated by MRI than any other type of radiographic study.

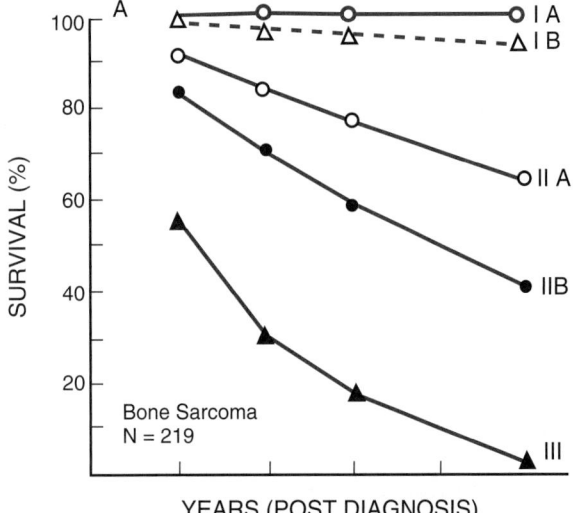

FIG. 42-14. Survival of patients with bone sarcomas according to surgical stage. (Modified with permission from Enneking WF, Gearen PF: Fibrous dysplasia of the femoral neck: Treatment by cortical bone grafting. J Bone Joint Surg Am 68:1415, 1986.)

Diagnostic Evaluation. Routine laboratory studies include complete blood count and differential; erythrocyte sedimentation rate; serum alkaline phosphatase, calcium, and phosphate levels, renal and liver function studies, and urinalysis. If multiple myeloma is within the differential diagnostic possibilities, determination of serum protein level or immunoelectrophoresis should also be performed. In most instances of primary tumors the majority of these studies are normal. The alkaline phosphatase level may be elevated in osteosarcoma, and the blood count and erythrocyte sedimentation rate are helpful in excluding infection. Further staging studies vary according to the location of the lesion, diagnostic possibilities, age of the patient, and likelihood of malignancy. A bone scan almost always is indicated to assess the activity and extent of the primary lesion as well as to exclude the presence of other lesions. With soft-tissue tumors bone scan is reserved for lesions close to bone or suspected of malignancy. For suspected malignant lesions, other recommended studies include chest radiograph (or preferably CT scan) and abdominal CT scan to exclude metastatic disease. A diagnostic staging algorithm is shown in Fig. 42-15.

Biopsy. For lesions with a radiographically benign appearance, imaging studies of the lesion usually are unnecessary, and the appropriate next step is tissue diagnosis by biopsy. For any potentially malignant lesion, three-dimensional imaging studies (CT or, preferably, MRI) before biopsy are recommended to fully assess the extent of the lesion and to plan the biopsy procedure, minimizing potential contamination of compartments, which could compromise subsequent definitive surgery. Depending on the experience of the surgeon and pathologist, needle or trocar biopsy is appropriate for the majority of soft-tissue and bone tumors. General principles of the biopsy procedure include the following:

1. Biopsy incisions should always be longitudinal on extremities.
2. Needle biopsy tracts and incisional biopsy should be placed so that they can be excised en bloc at the time of resection.
3. Radiographic localization should be done to ensure accuracy.
4. Frozen-section examination should be done to be sure that adequate tissue has been obtained.
5. Cultures and appropriate microbiologic studies should be performed.
6. The bone biopsy cortical window should be as small as possible and oval in shape to minimize the risk of pathologic fracture.
7. Central or necrotic areas should be avoided; biopsy at the periphery of the lesion is most helpful.
8. Exposure of any major neurovascular structures should be avoided.
9. Hemostasis must be obtained to prevent hematoma, which could seed other compartments; for bone lesions suspected of malignancy, the biopsy site should be plugged with methacrylate cement to prevent hematoma.
10. Tourniquet use is helpful for intraoperative accuracy of dissection.
11. Use of a drain with its tract in line with the biopsy incision and near it will facilitate later en bloc resection.
12. Contamination of any uninvolved compartment must be avoided.
13. In general, the surgeon providing definitive treatment should also perform the biopsy whenever possible; this would usually involve a tertiary care referral center.

Treatment. In the treatment of benign and nonmetastatic malignant musculoskeletal tumors the primary goal is eradication of the disease; preservation of limb function is an important but secondary consideration. Long-term results have improved dramatically in the past two decades, and the treatment approach for malignant lesions has changed, with a shift away from amputations and toward limb salvage procedures. The specific treatment varies with the lesion but usually includes a combination of serveral modalities: surgery, chemotherapy, and radiotherapy. Benign lesions usually are

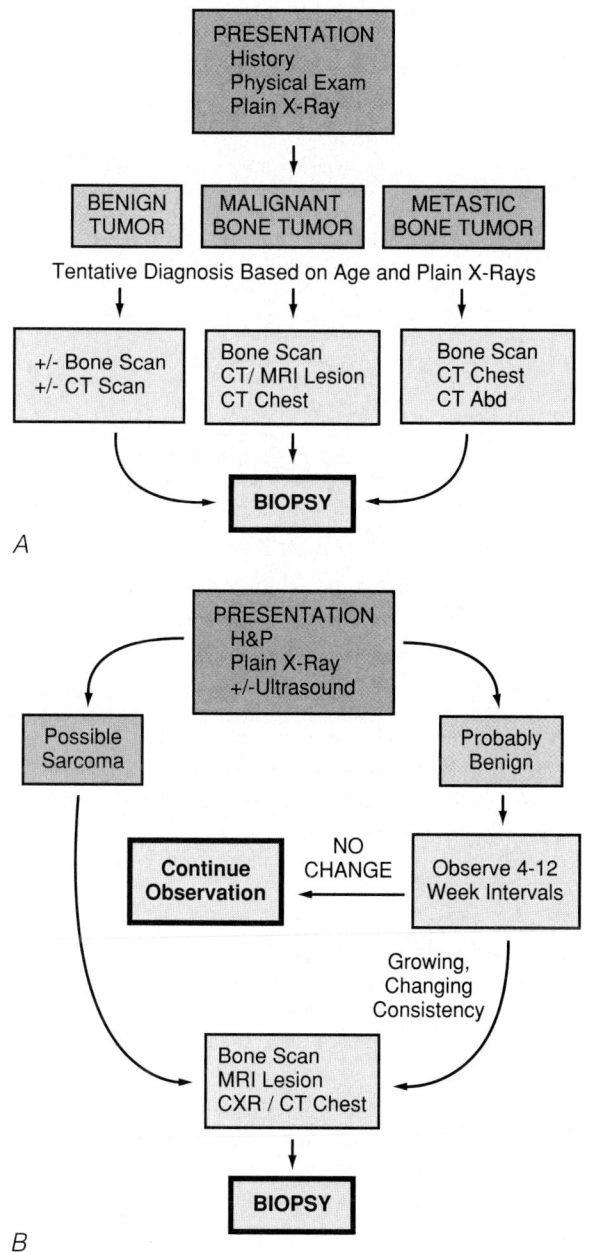

A

B

FIG. 42-15. Staging algorithms for (A) bone tumors and (B) soft-tissue tumors. [*Modified with permission from Kasser JR (ed): Orthopaedic Knowledge Update 5. Rosemont, IL: American Academy of Orthopaedic Surgeons, 1996, p. 136.*]

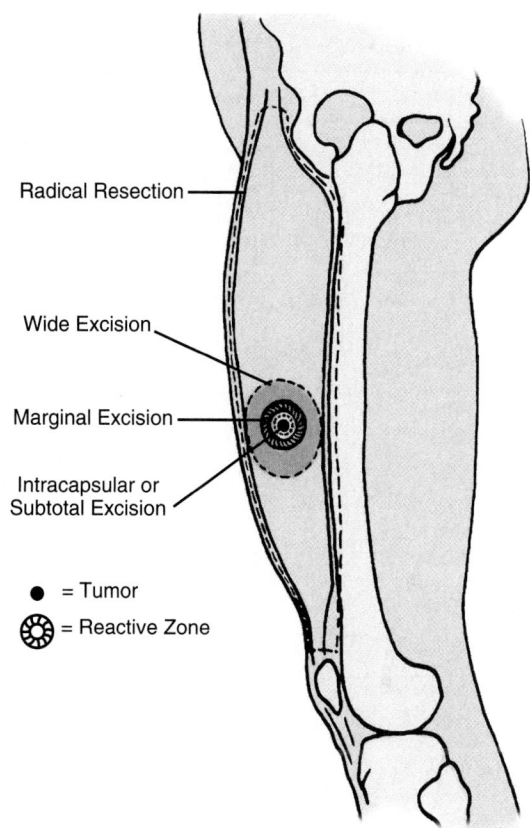

FIG. 42-16. Definitions of surgical margins for bone and soft-tissue sarcomas. (*Modified with permission from Enneking WF, Gearen PF: Fibrous dysplasia of the femoral neck: Treatment by cortical bone grafting. J Bone Joint Surg Am 68:1415,1986.*)

2. Marginal: removal through the reactive zone of the tumor; may leave microscopic residual in malignant tumors.

3. Wide: removal with some normal tissue beyond reactive zone in all directions.

4. Radical: complete removal of all compartments (bone, muscle, joint) involved with the tumor or its reactive zone.

These surgical procedure definitions are summarized in Fig. 42-16. For benign stage I or stage II lesions, intralesional or marginal excision is adequate, while stage III aggressive lesions require marginal to wide resection for cure. Low-grade (stage I) malignant tumors can be treated with wide surgical resection, with a high probability of local control. High-grade (stage II) malignant lesions can be treated by radical surgical excision, or wide excision plus adjuvant treatment, with comparable low recurrence rates (5 to 10%). In the treatment of tumors with similar margins the result of amputation versus resection are also comparable, forming the basis for the predominance of limb salvage surgery in recent years.

Technological advances also have contributed to this change in treatment approach, given the availability of custom computer-designed prosthetic implants, which can replace all or part of a bone or joint; osteochondral allografts; new limb lengthening techniques; and microvascular techniques for free tissue transfers of bone and soft tissue. Amputation may still be necessary for tumors in which involvement of major neurovascular structures or multiple compartments precludes resection with preservation of useful limb function. Specific treatment and adjuvant therapies vary according to the histogenetic tumor type and grade, and are summarized in Table 42-4.

treated surgically. For malignant tumors the primary treatment usually is surgery, with chemotherapy or radiotherapy as a secondary (adjuvant) treatment. Commonly used chemotherapeutic agents include doxorubicin, methotrexate, cyclophosphamide, ifosfamide, vincristine, and actinomycin D. Radiation treatment may be given preoperatively, postoperatively, or by implantation of catheters at operation followed by postoperative loading with short-range isotopes (brachytherapy). Effective doses for control of microscopic disease are generally in the range of 50 to 60 Gy.

Surgical Procedures. Surgical procedures used in treatment of tumors are defined as follows:

1. Intralesional: leaves microscopic and macroscopic residual, as in curettage of a benign lesion.

Table 42-4
Treatments for Musculoskeletal Tumors

Tumor	Chemotherapy	Radiation	Surgery
Osteoid osteoma	No	No	Excision
Osteoblastoma	No	No	Curettage or resection and bone graft
Osteosarcoma	Neoadjuvant and postoperative	No	Wide to radical resection with limb salvage or amputation
Secondary osteosarcoma	If patient can tolerate	Palliative only	Radical resection or amputation
Parosteal osteosarcoma	No	No	Wide surgical resection and reconstruction or wide amputation
Osteochondroma	No	No	Simple excision; all cartilage cap must be removed
Enchondroma	No	No	Curettage and bone graft
Parosteal chondroma	No	No	Marginal to wide resection and bone grafting
Chondroblastoma	No	No	Curettage and bone graft
Chondromyxoid fibroma	No	No	Aggressive curettage or marginal to wide excision and grafting
Chondrosarcoma	No	May be useful as adjuvant for high-grade lesions	Wide or radical surgical resection and reconstruction or amputation
Fibroma	No	No	Curettage/grafting
Fibrosarcoma	Adjuvant systemic may improve survival	Yes	Wide to radical resection
Ewing's sarcoma	Yes	Yes	Adjuvant surgery (wide to marginal resection) improves outcome
Unicameral cyst	Steroid injection	No	Curettage and bone graft for latent cysts or with steroid failure
Aneurysmal cyst	No	In unresectable cases	Curettage or marginal excision and grafting
Giant cell tumor	No	Only unresectable cases	Curettage, followed by cementation or cryotherapy
Soft tissue sarcoma	Controversial as adjuvant; does benefit in metastatic disease	Yes—preoperative, postoperative or brachytherapy	Wide resection or amputation and radiation
Metastatic carcinoma	Yes	Yes	Internal fixation of fractures or impending fractures or joint replacement

Prognosis. Malignant musculoskeletal tumors remain serious and life-threatening diseases, although the prognosis has improved significantly over the past two decades. For stage II lesions 5-year survival rates range from 40 to 80%, while for stage I lesions 5-year survival rates are in the 70 to 90% range. Local control rates of 90% or better can be anticipated in the majority of tumor types. Local recurrence of benign lesions varies with stage and tumor type.

Given that the major problem in the treatment of skeletal malignancies remains late metastatic disease, further scientific advantages in this area are needed. Recent research has identified multiple drug resistance gene expression in patients treated with chemotherapy whose tumors become resistant to the drugs. These genes lead to the production of an ATPase (P-glycoprotein) that pumps a wide variety of drugs out of the tumor cells, maintaining sublethal intracellular levels. Other mechanisms of drug and radiation resistance also exist. Experimental pharmacologic approaches to the enhancement of chemotherapeutic effectiveness by inhibiting these resistance mechanisms are currently under study and show promise for improving outcomes of sarcoma treatment. Other experimental methods of metastatic sarcoma treatment under investigation include the use of immunotherapy, in which the patient's immune system is sensitized to tumor antigens, and bone marrow transplantation, in which high-intensity chemotherapy is followed by the reintroduction of autologous marrow obtained in advance.

Specific Musculoskeletal Tumors

Bone-Forming Tumors

Osteoma. This small, sessile benign body tumor occurs most often in the skull and neither causes symptoms nor requires

treatment. It consists of an abnormal excrescence of surface bone. Similar lesions occur posttraumatically on the femur in the area of the adductor magnus insertion (rider's bone), or in relation to the medial collateral ligament of the knee (Pellegrini-Stieda lesion).

Osteoid Osteoma. This benign bone-forming lesion primarily affects patients under 30 years of age and has a male preponderance. Patients present with local pain, which can be quite severe and is often relieved by aspirin. Radiographically, a small (less than 1 cm) lucent lesion (nidus) is seen, typically surrounded by marked reactive sclerosis (Fig. 42-17). Sometimes areas of radiodensity are seen within the lucent lesion, corresponding histologically to disorganized woven bone formation. The lesion gradually regresses over a period of 5 to 10 years, but most patients are unable to tolerate the symptoms and opt for surgical resection of the lesion, which usually is curative if the entire nidus is removed.

Osteoblastoma. Osteoblastoma is a benign bone-forming tumor affecting primarily children and young adults. Any bone may be involved, but the spine, particularly its posterior elements, is most often affected. The lesions are expansile and have a mixed lytic and blastic radiographic appearance. Patients usually present with pain, and treatment involves marginal resection or curettage and bone grafting if resection is not feasible without excessive morbidity. Histologically, vascular stroma, woven bone formation, giant cells, and osteoid may be present, and differentiation from osteoid osteoma is based on clinical and radiographic criteria (i.e., a lesion greater than 1 cm in diameter, without reactive cortical sclerosis) rather than histology. Cellular lesions can easily be confused with osteosarcoma, and careful evaluation by a qualified pathologist is essential to avoid misdiagnosis.

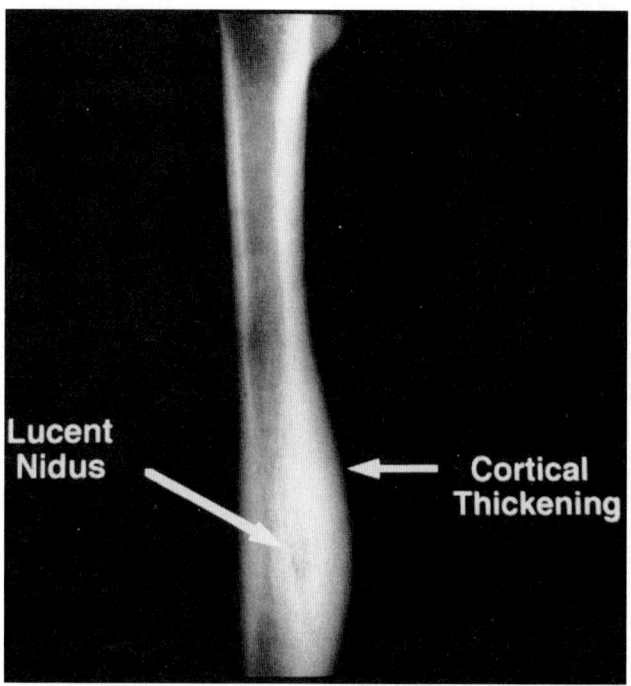

FIG. 42-17. *Osteoid osteoma of the femoral shaft, with reactive cortical thickening and radiolucent nidus representing the tumor.*

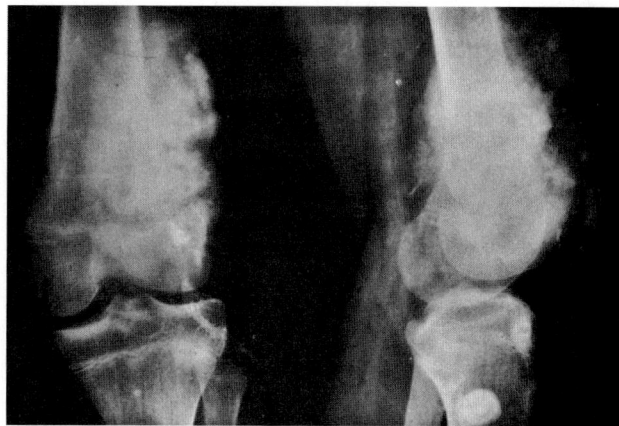

FIG. 42-18. *Osteogenic sarcoma of the femur. The films show characteristic bone destruction, soft-tissue mass, new bone formation, and sclerosis limited to the metaphysic of the lower femur.*

Osteosarcoma (Osteogenic Sarcoma). Osteosarcoma is the most common primary bone malignancy apart from multiple myeloma, although it is nonetheless a rare disease (incidence 2.8/1,000,000). Patients 10 to 25 years of age are most often affected, and the most common sites are areas of maximal bone growth (distal femur—52%; proximal tibia—20%; proximal humerus—9%). Usually the lesions are metaphyseal. Although any bone can be involved, the disease seldom occurs in the small bones of the distal extremities and in the spine. This disease has a number of variants:, (1) "classic" central or medullary high-grade osteosarcoma; (2) periosteal osteosarcoma; (3) parosteal osteosarcoma; (4) osteosarcoma secondary to malignant degeneration of Paget's disease, fibrous dysplasia, or radiation; and (5) telangiectatic osteosarcoma.

Osteosarcoma exhibits a blastic radiographic appearance in most cases because of the neoplastic woven bone formation. The periosteum may be raised off the bone by the tumor mass, causing a fusiform swelling with reactive periosteal bone at the periosteal margins (Codman's triangle). The malignant bone formation may have a sunburst appearance (Fig. 42-18), with invasion into adjacent compartments. Pathologic fractures can occur but are unusual.

Histologically, the tumor consists of small pleomorphic spindle cells, with osteoid and woven bone formation, and there is often cartilage formation as well. Cartilage formation is a prominent feature of periosteal and parosteal variants of osteosarcoma. Telangiectatic variants are lytic and expansible, resembling an aneurysmal bone cyst, and have prominent vascular spaces and relatively sparse bone formation.

Patients present with pain that often is nocturnal and a mass or swelling. Metastatic spread usually is pulmonary, and evaluation of the chest by CT is necessary. Serum alkaline phosphatase levels may be markedly elevated, but laboratory studies are otherwise usually negative. Evaluation also should include bone scan to rule out bone metastases, and CT or, preferably, MRI of the region for surgical planning. Most osteosarcomas present as stage IIB lesions.

Osteosarcoma is not particularly sensitive to radiation, but it does typically respond well to combination chemotherapy. Depending on the extent and location of the lesion, treatment typically involves wide surgical resection or amputation, usually after preoperative (neoadjuvant) chemotherapy. Bone resected in limb salvage operations can be reconstructed by custom prosthetic replacement, arthrodesis, or allografting (Fig. 42-19). Results of combination chemotherapy with resection are better than even radical surgical amputation without adjuvant therapy, with 50 to 70% 5-year survival rates and usually better than 90% local control (compared with a 20% 5-year survival rate with radical surgery alone). Pathologic fracture, with contamination of all compartments, can preclude limb salvage surgery. Chemotherapy is continued after surgery for 1 year. Prosthetic designs that can be periodically lengthened by a minor surgical procedure allow limb salvage even in relatively young children with osteosarcoma, in whom progressive limb length discrepancy might otherwise be a severe problem. Preoperative intra-arterial chemotherapy and radiotherapy have been used instead of neoadjuvant systemic chemotherapy, and results appear to be comparable.

Parosteal Osteosarcoma. These tumors occur in a slightly older age group and start adjacent to the periosteum rather than in the bone. The posterior aspect of the femur and proximal humerus and tibia are the most frequent sites. The tumor tends to be well circumscribed and slow-growing and metastasizes only late, usually to the lungs. Histologically, bland spindle cells with woven bone formation, fibrous stroma, and focal cartilage formation are the typical characteristics. These lesions are not sensitive to adjuvant treatments and are treated by wide surgical resection and appropriate reconstruction, or by amputation. Prognosis is significantly better than for conventional high-grade osteosarcoma.

Secondary Osteosarcoma. In older patients, osteosarcoma can arise secondary to a chronic predisposing condition. The most common of these is Paget's disease (malignant degeneration reported in 1 to 10% of cases), but osteosarcoma also has been reported in fibrous dysplasia, and rarely with chronic osteomyelitis. As many as 5 to 10% of patients subjected to high-intensity radiation therapy for other cancers (sarcoma, lymphoma, etc.) may develop secondary sarcomas 10 to 20 years later, of which one type is osteosarcoma. Secondary osteosarcomas invariably are high-grade aggressive tumors, and prognosis is poor, with a tendency for early metastasis. Most patients in this age group are unable to tolerate the toxicity of

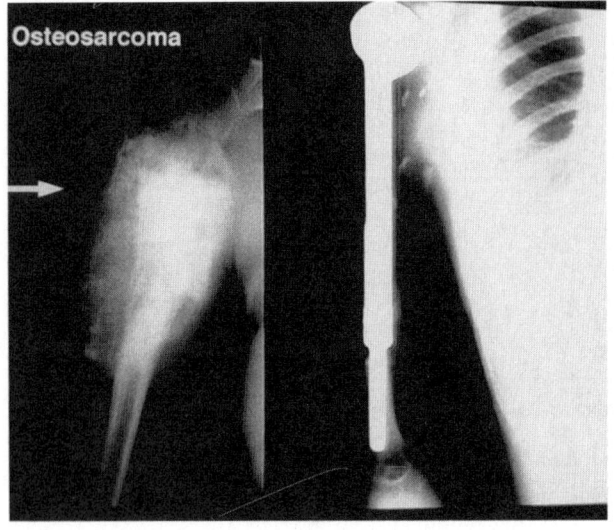

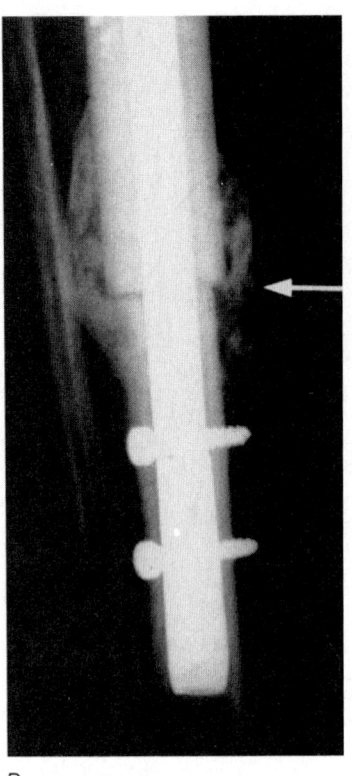

FIG. 42-19. *A.* Osteosarcoma of the proximal humerus treated by custom prosthetic replacement. *B.* Osteosarcoma of the proximal tibia treated by resection and an intercalary allograft arthrodesis. Note the incorporation of the allograft at the junction with the host bone. The allograft arthrodesis was internally fixed using an interlocking intramedullary nail.

intensive chemotherapy, and the usual treatment consists of surgical resection or amputation.

Cartilaginous Tumors

Osteochondroma (Exostosis). This lesion is a common exophytic benign lesion that occurs during childhood, usually in the metaphyses of the long bones (Fig. 42-20). It is thought to result from an aberrant fragment of the growth plate that is left behind and undergoes spontaneous growth. The lesions have a bony base with a cartilaginous cap, from which the growth occurs as it does in normal growth plates during childhood. A multiple hereditary form occurs and was discussed earlier. There is a familial condition called multiple hereditary exostosis in which patients have

FIG. 42-20. Osteochondroma of the tibia. *A.* Plain film x-ray demonstrates a benign appearance, with trabecular bone within the base and calcification in the cartilaginous cap. *B.* CT scan shows a thin cartilage cap, which rules out malignant transformation.

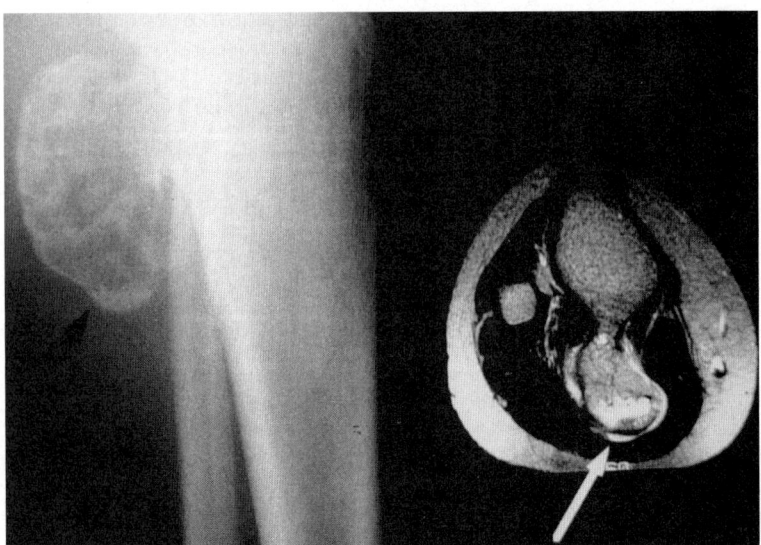

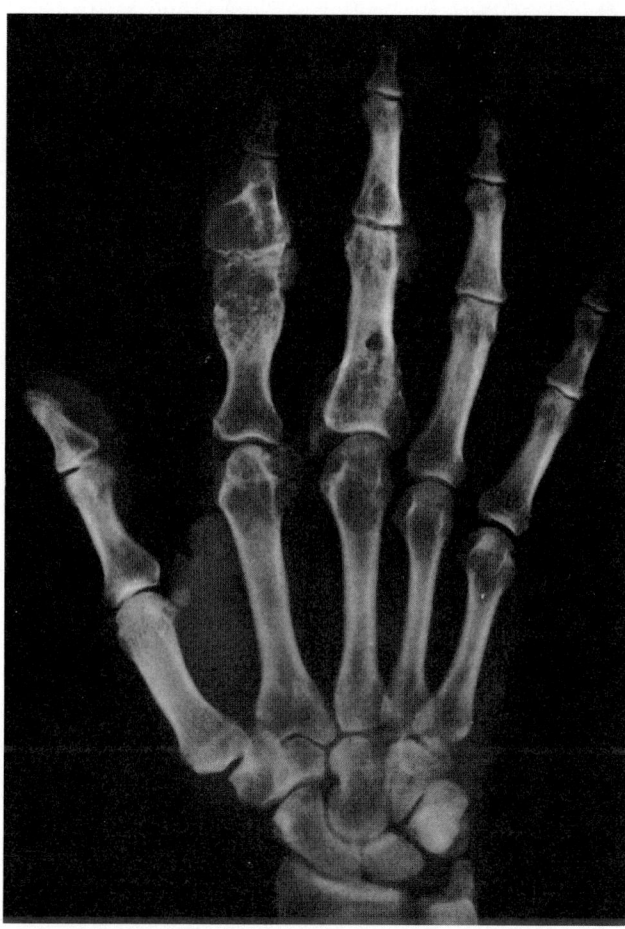

FIG. 42-21. Multiple enchondromas of the hand.

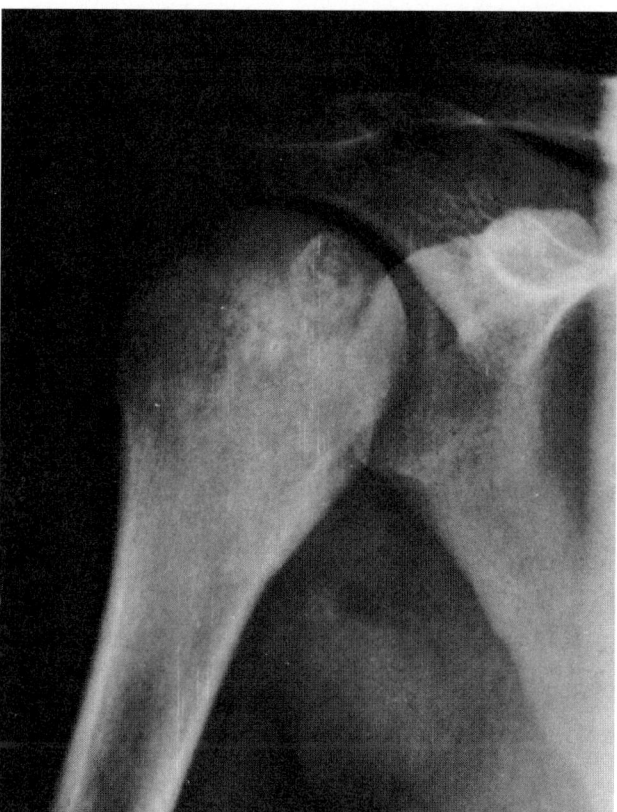

FIG. 42-22. Benign chondroblastoma (Codman's tumor) of the humerus.

many osteochondroma. It has a variable penetrance. The lesions may cause pain from impingement on tendons, nerves, or muscle and frequently require surgical excision. Growth of the lesion, while not of concern in children, may indicate malignant transformation in adults. A cartilaginous cap thickness of more than 1 cm (assessed by CT or MRI) should arouse suspicion of malignancy. In solitary lesions the risk of malignant degeneration is less than 1%, while in multiple lesions it may be as high as 15%. Marginal to wide excision of benign or malignant lesions usually is curative if all the cartilage is removed.

Enchondroma. Enchondromas are intramedullary cartilage lesions, often exhibiting calcification and expansion of the bone. The small bones of the hands and feet are commonly involved, but long bone involvement also occurs (Fig. 42-21). The disease occurs in solitary and multiple forms. Patients may present with pain or pathologic fracture. The usual treatment is intralesional resection (curettage) and bone grafting. The most serious concern is the possibility of malignant degeneration, and careful sampling at the time of biopsy is necessary to exclude the possibility of chondrosarcoma.

Parosteal Chondroma. This is a rare benign cartilage lesion arising subperiosteally, often in the humerus or small bones of the hand or foot. The lesions are somewhat more aggressive than enchondromas and are prone to local recurrence. Accordingly, marginal or wide resection and bone grafting is indicated and is curative in the majority of cases.

Chondroblastoma. This is one of the few epiphyseal tumors and occurs most often in the first and second decades of life, when the growth plate is still open. Patients present with pain, joint effusions, or contractures, and radiographs show a lytic lesion with calcifications in the epiphysis (Fig. 42-22). The lesion is composed of chondroblasts, cartilage, giant cells, and vascular stroma. Treatment is by curettage and bone grafting and is often challenging because of the intra-articular location of the lesions. A rare malignant epiphyseal cartilage tumor in older adults, clear cell chondrosarcoma, probably represents the malignant degenerative counterpart of chondroblastoma.

Chondromyxoid Fibroma. This rare metaphyseal tumor affects children and young adults, typically arising in the femur or tibia. The lesion is benign, but it exhibits aggressive local behavior, with a high propensity for local recurrence and spread. The radiographic appearance is primarily geographic and lytic with occasional calcifications; an expansile or multilocular appearance with a relatively well-defined zone of transition between the tumor and host bone also is found. Histologic examination reveals a lobular configuration with three components: cellular fibroblastic areas, chondroid areas, and myxoid areas with typical stellate tumor cells. Treatment is by wide or marginal resection and bone graft reconstruction, although aggressive curettage with grafting also has been associated with satisfactory results.

Chondrosarcoma. Chondrosarcoma can be primary or secondary (as discussed above) and affects a broad age range (age 20 to 60 years). The pelvis, femur, tibia, and other long bones can be involved, and lesions closer to the axial skeleton are more likely to be malignant. Intramedullary calcifications are usually evident. Differential diagnosis includes bone infarction and enchondroma. Features of cortical destruction and pain are important indicators

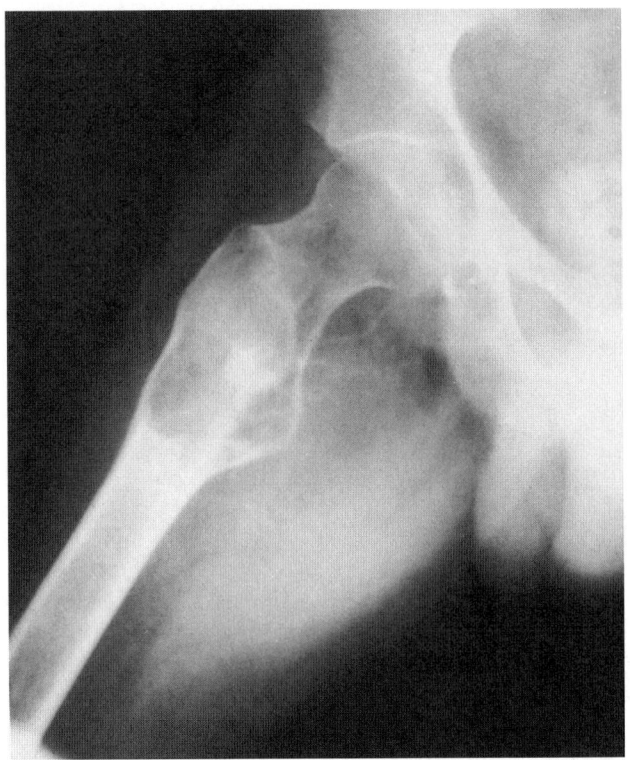

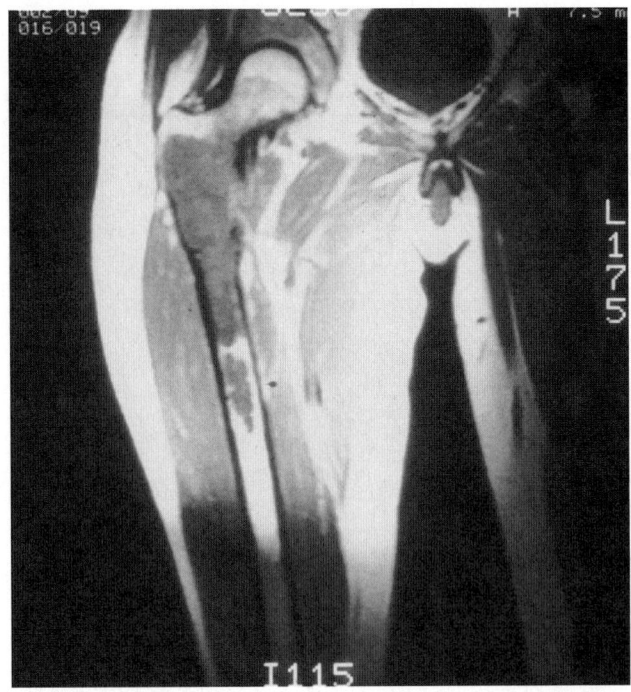

A

B

FIG. 42-23. *A. Plain radiograph of proximal femur with primary chondrosarcoma demonstrating lucency and calcification in lesion. B. MRI shows marrow destruction and extension of lesion through cortex into soft tissues medially.*

of possible malignancy (Fig. 42-23). The tumors are graded as low, intermediate, or high grade of malignancy on the basis of cytologic features and presence of matrix production. Lower-grade lesions can be treated by wide resection, but with high-grade lesions metastatic disease is frequent and the prognosis is poor. Limb salvage surgery often is feasible, but adjuvant treatments are not particularly helpful since these lesions tend to be resistant to chemotherapy and radiotherapy.

Fibrous Lesions

Fibroma. Small intracortical fibrous lesions, referred to as fibrous cortical defects, are common incidental radiographic findings in the long bone metaphyses of children and tend to disappear spontaneously at skeletal maturity. Larger variants, which can progressively enlarge into the medullary cavity and occasionally cause pathologic fractures, are referred to as *non-ossifying fibromas.* The tumor consists of bland fibroblastic and histiocytic cells, with osteoclasts and cholesterol clefts from lipid-laden macrophages. A variant of this tumor that ossifies occurs in the mandible (ossifying fibroma). In larger or symptomatic lesions, curettage and bone grafting is indicated, and recurrences after this treatment are uncommon.

Desmoid. This is a rare aggressive fibrous tumor of bone that is analogous to its soft-tissue counterpart, aggresive fibromatosis. Marginal to wide resection is indicated rather than curettage because of the tendency for local recurrence. With aggressive fibromatosis of soft tissues, local invasiveness causes frequent and progressively problematic recurrences after surgical treatment. The lesions do not metastasize and have been treated with wide surgical resection or radiation treatment, with local control rates of approximately

50%. Significantly better results have been obtained by marginal to wide local resection in conjunction with moderate-dose (45 to 55 Gy) radiation therapy. Systemic therapy with methotrexate also has been reported to control or cause regression of aggressive fibromatosis.

Fibrosarcoma. Primary fibrosarcoma of bone is rare and is characterized by a geographic lytic radiographic appearance with cortical destruction and associated soft-tissue mass (Fig. 42-24). Some of these lesions are better classified as malignant fibrous histiocytomas, with a mixed cell population. The tumors are moderately radiosensitive, and adjuvant chemotherapy can be effective in improving survival rates. Surgery consists of wide or radical resection and reconstruction rather than amputation, often in conjunction with adjuvant radiation treatment. These tumors also arise as secondary lesions in fibrous dysplasia and Paget's disease and after radiation treatment for other cancers.

Cystic Lesions

Unicameral (Solitary) Bone Cyst. This lesion occurs in children in the metapysis of the long bones adjacent to the growth plate, most often the humerus or femur, although the radius, calcaneus, and tibia also can be affected. Usually the lesions are painless and may present with a pathologic fracture as the initial manifestation of the disease. The lesions are lytic, expansile, and well marginated (Fig. 42-25), and may be found in the diaphysis in older children as a result of continued growth of the growth plate away from the lesion. In young children fractures heal, but the lesions usually recur, causing recurrent fractures during childhood. The cyst fluid contains high levels of bone resorptive cytokines, presumably

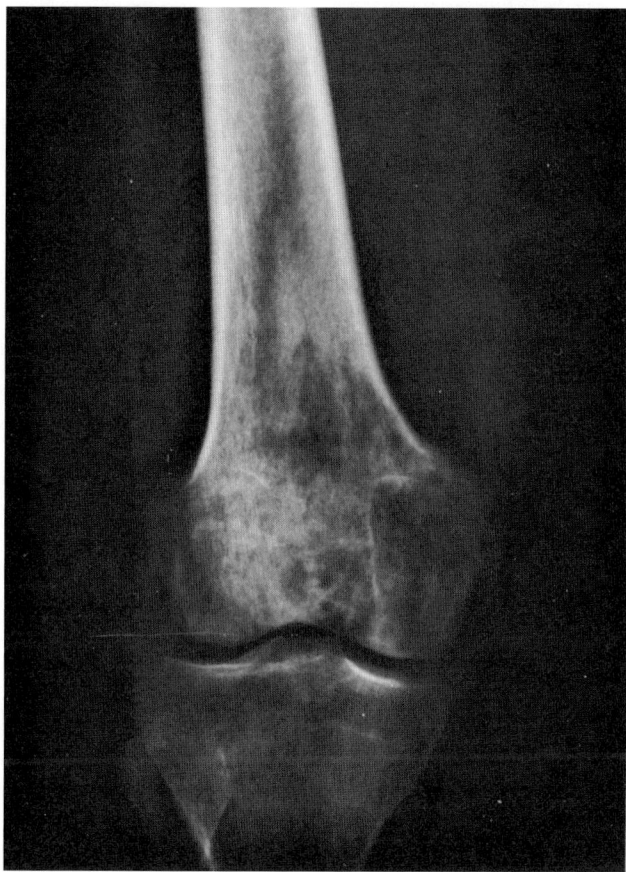

FIG. 42-24. Fibrosarcoma of the lower femur. The films show a lytic lesion, apparently of medullary origin, on the distal end of the femur. The lesion is destroying cortex. There is no evidence of sclerosis and new bone formation or any definite soft-tissue mass.

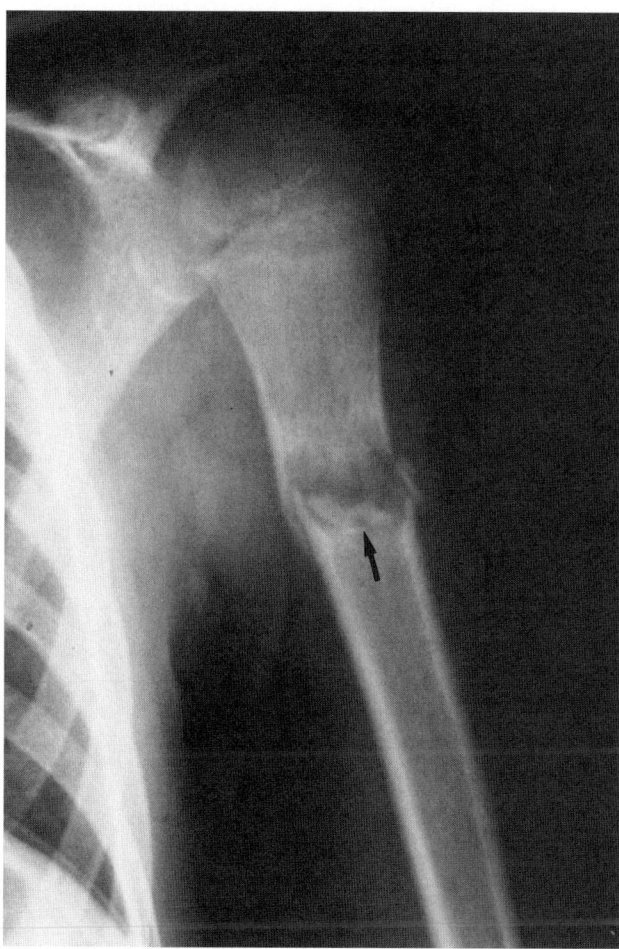

FIG. 42-25. Unicameral bone cyst presenting with pathologic fracture. Note "fallen fragment sign" from a fracture fragment that has fallen through the fluid-filled cyst to the bottom of the cavity (arrow).

produced by the living tissue and accounting for the aggressive bone resorption in these lesions. At skeletal maturity the cysts tend gradually to disappear. In older children and young adults, the lesions become latent (stage I) and do not progress. Recurrence rates in active (stage II) lesions in younger children after surgical treatment (curettage and bone grafting) average 50%. Partial or complete healing of the majority of these lesions has been obtained after intraosseous injection of methylprednisolone, currently the preferred treatment (70 to 90% effective with up to three sequential injections). In older children or adults with latent cysts, curettage and bone grafting is effective, and steroid injections appear to have little effect.

Aneurysmal Bone Cyst. This tumor, found most often in children or young adults, consists of a cystic lesion with large vascular spaces, characterized by aggressive, expansile lysis of bone. The tumor is composed of fibrous tissue, vascular spaces with a lining resembling endothelium, giant cells, and reactive bone formation at the periphery. Aneurysmal cysts can arise as a secondary degenerative vascular lesion within another primary benign or malignant bone tumor, such as giant cell tumor or chondroblastoma; however, about half are thought to represent primary lesions. Because recurrence is relatively frequent with simple curettage, local resection with bone grafting is preferable. Embolization has been used successfully in unresectable spinal or pelvic lesions, as has intermediate-dose radiation treatment. Preoperative embolization of large lesions is helpful in decreasing the risk of hemorrhage.

Round Cell Tumors

Ewing's Sarcoma. Ewing's sarcoma is a highly malignant primary bone tumor of children (age range 5 to 15 years) that tends to arise in the diaphyses of long bones. The spine and pelvis also may be primary sites. The radiographic appearance usually is that of an aggressive lesion, with a permeative pattern of bone lysis and periosteal reaction (Fig. 42-26). Often there is an associated large soft-tissue mass, and patients have systemic symptoms (fever, weight loss) in addition to local pain, which tends to be worse at night. A soft-tissue variant of Ewing's sarcoma, primitive neuroectodermal tumor (PNET), occurs as well, usually exhibiting evidence of neural differentiation immunohistochemically. Differential diagnosis includes osteomyelitis, lymphoma, and eosinophilic granuloma.

Diagnostic evaluation includes chest and abdominal CT scans and bone scan to rule out metastases. Treatment consists of a combination of local radiation therapy and systemic chemotherapy. Five-year survival rates with this approach are around 50%. A multimodality treatment that uses adjuvant surgery (wide or marginal resection) has resulted in 5-year survival rates of 75%. In young children amputation may be necessary because of the severe compromise of bone growth that can result from the effect of the required levels of radiation on the growth plates.

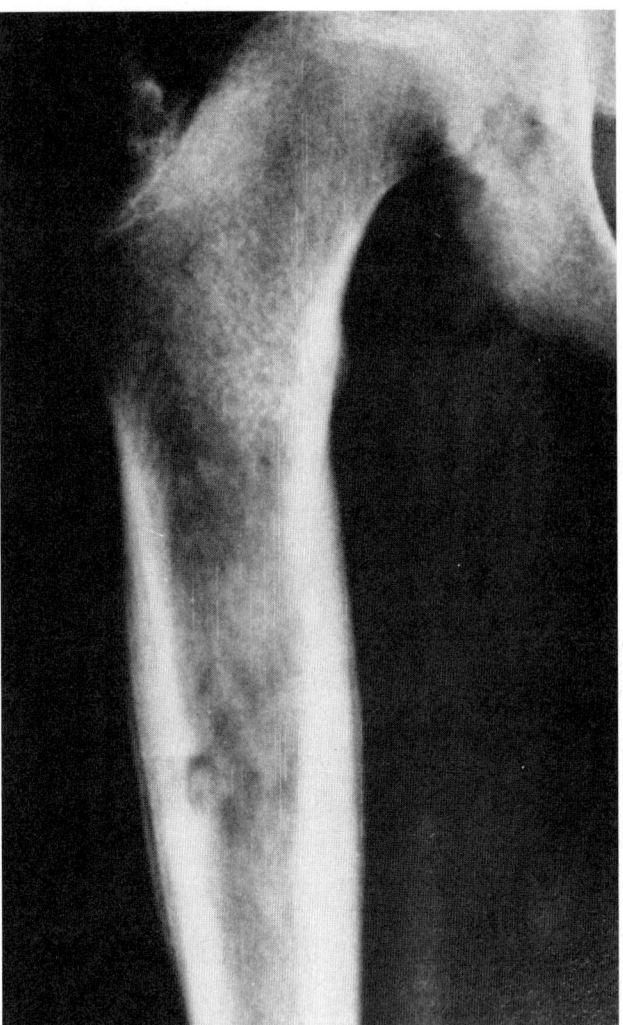

FIG. 42-26. Ewing's sarcoma involving the proximal femur. Note permeative nature of lesion and periosteal reaction.

Histiocytic Lymphoma (Reticulum Cell Sarcoma). This tumor occurs in patients 20 to 40 years of age, usually affecting the diaphyses of long bones. Its radiographic appearance is similar to that of Ewing's sarcoma, with permeation, periosteal reaction, and frequently a large associated soft-tissue mass. Pathologic fracture may occur. A significant proportion of patients present with or develop regional or distant lymph node involvement. Treatment consists of radiation to the local lesion in conjunction with systemic chemotherapy. If feasible, resection of the primary tumor improves survival and decreases the risk of local recurrence.

Other Tumors

Giant Cell Tumor (Osteoclastoma). These tumors arise in the epiphyses of young adults, most commonly in the proximal tibia, distal femur, proximal femur, and distal radius. Characteristically the lesion is radiographically purely lytic, well circumscribed, and occasionally expansile with cortical destruction. The lesion often extends to the subchondral surface and can even invade the joint (Fig. 42-27). Although usually benign, a malignant variant occurs in a small proportion of cases, and even the benign lesions are stage III tumors, with local aggressive behavior and a high tendency to recur after surgical treatment. Patients usually present with pain, and pathologic fracture may occur. The tumor consists of monocytic stromal cells, vascular tissue, and sheets of large, multinucleated osteoclast-like cells. The key feature in differentiating these tumors from other tumors that can contain large numbers of giant cells (eosinophilic granuloma, brown tumor of hyperparathyroidism, aneurysmal bone cyst, chondroblastoma, osteoblastoma, nonossifying fibroma) is that the oval nuclei of the monocytic stroma resemble those of the giant cells, suggesting a common origin. The most common cause of malignant giant cell tumors is prior radiation therapy for a benign giant cell tumor, which was a former mode of treatment and can be associated with malignant recurrence in up to 10 percent of cases. Because of this radiation is no longer used in the treatment of giant cell tumors except in dire circumstances (such as unresectable lesions in the spine with threat of neurologic deficit).

The most common treatment of a giant cell tumor, curettage of the lesion, is associated with recurrences in 25 to 50% of cases.

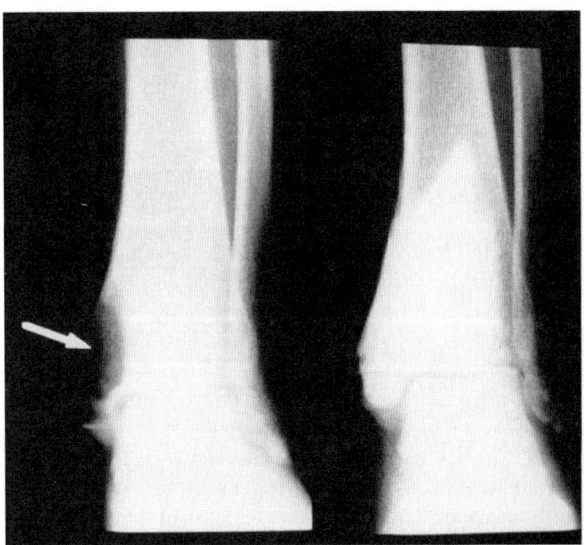
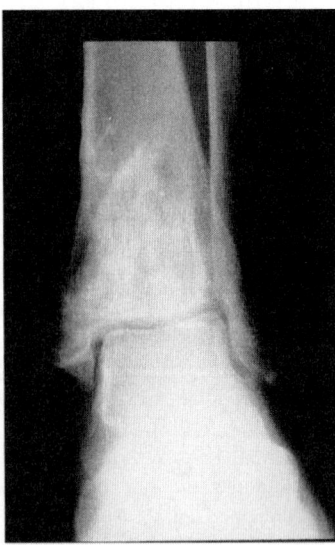

A   *B*   *C*

FIG. 42-27. Giant cell tumor of the tibia. *A.* Note the epiphyseal location and well-delineated margins. *B.* The lesion was treated by curettage and menthyl methacrylate cementation. *C.* To prevent degeneration of the articular cartilage of the ankle joint from the abnormal stress transfer, 2 years later the cement was removed and the defect bone grafted.

Alternative treatments therefore have included wide resection (usually reserved for recurrent cases) and adjuvant local treatments such as cryotherapy with liquid nitrogen or phenol and, most recently, filling the defect with methyl methacrylate. The lowest recurrence rates have been with cryotherapy and methyl methacrylate cementation. Cementation causes a thermal kill of tissue within several millimeters of the margin in bone as a result of the exothermic reaction that occurs during polymerization of the cement. If local recurrence occurs after cementation, it is readily detectable radiographically as a lucency next to the cement. With bone grafting, remodeling changes in the graft can obscure signs of recurrence. Because these are epiphyseal lesions, the presence of cement next to the articular cartilage may predispose to cartilage degeneration, and in young patients, some advise removal of the cement and bone grafting after 2 years if the patient remains free of recurrence. Given an incidence of joint degeneration of only 15 to 20% in long-term follow-up studies, the indications for cement removal are controversial. Control of the lesion with this treatment approach has been successful in 90% of cases.

Vascular Tumors

Hemangioma. Hemangiomas of bone often are noted in the spine as an incidental finding. These benign lesions are characterized by endothelial vascular spaces, and because they typically do not cause symptoms management usually is simply observation. A more aggressive lesion is the hemangioendothelioma, which can occur in bone or in the soft tissues and generally is characterized as a low-grade malignancy. In bone the lesions appear cystic and well marginated, with increased local perfusion on bone scan or angiography. Occasionally lesions occur in several bones. Treatment is with wide local resection, although curettage with radiotherapy has been successful in some cases.

Angiosarcoma. Angiosarcoma is a highly malignant sarcoma of the bone or soft tissues. The prognosis of this lesion is poor, with early hematogenous spread to the lungs the rule. Amputation or radical resection in nonmetastatic cases is appropriate.

Tumors Arising from Included Tissues

Adamantinoma. Adamantinoma is a rare epithelial tumor occurring in the jaw and occasionally in the tibia or fibula of young adults. The tumor, although malignant, is slow growing and presents with pain and a lytic, multiloculated or bubbly radiographic appearance. The diaphyseal portion of the bone tends to be involved. Treatment is with wide resection or amputation, and adjuvant therapies have not been shown to be effective. Metastasis to the lungs occurs in about 50 percent of cases.

Chordoma. This rare, low-grade malignant neoplasm arises in the sacrococcygeal or occipitocervical area and is thought to develop from embryonic remnants of the notochord. Sixty percent of cases occur in the sacrum or coccyx (Fig. 42-28). Patients present with a mass, neurologic symptoms, or pain. The lesions are slow growing and occur usually in older adults. Differential diagnosis includes plasmacytoma, giant cell tumor, and metastatic carcinoma. The tumor is composed of cords and nests of cells resembling chondrocytes, with typical highly vacuolated "basket" or physaliferous cells. The stroma consists of a basophilic, mucoid, or myxoid ground substance. The location makes wide resection difficult and causes significant morbidity, but without treatment the lesion is uniformly fatal, with late pulmonary metastases. The lesions are not responsive to radiotherapy or chemotherapy, and surgical

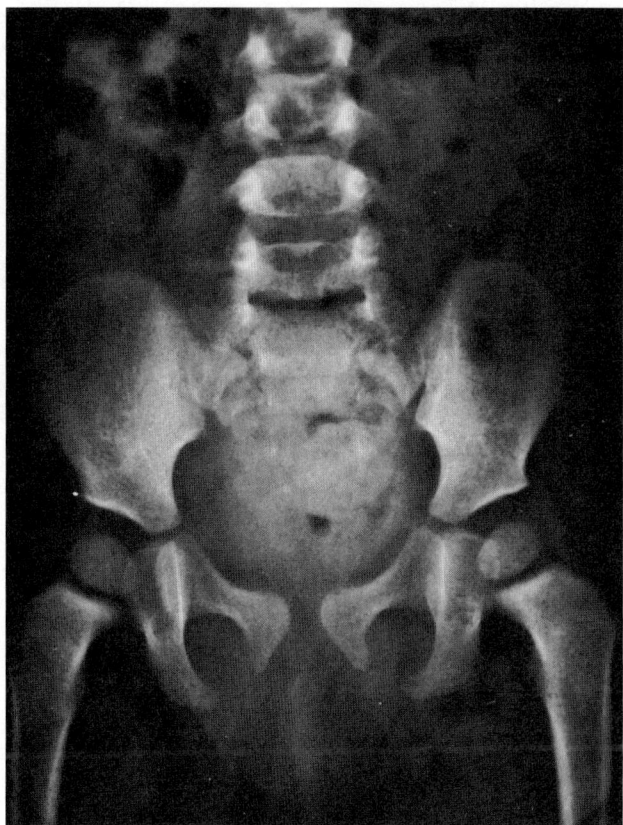

FIG. 42-28. Chordoma destroying the coccyx of a child.

resection is the treatment of choice. Some recent evidence suggests that this tumor may be somewhat responsive to proton beam irradiation.

Soft-Tissue Sarcoma

Soft-tissue sarcomas are more than twice as common as malignant primary bone tumors. Malignant fibrous histiocytoma is the most common type, but a wide variety of other histogenetic types exist, including fibrosarcoma, liposarcoma, malignant nerve sheath tumors (neurofibrosarcoma or malignant schwannoma), rhabdomyosarcoma, synovial sarcoma, lymphoma, PNET, and extraskeletal chondrosarcoma. In general these lesions occur in patients over 50 years of age, and the treatment is similar for all tumors despite the differences in histogenesis. Soft-tissue sarcomas are as a rule somewhat sensitive to radiation. While chemotherapy has proved beneficial in controlling disease in patients with metastasis and prolonging their survival, its role as an adjuvant therapy is controversial, with the majority of recent data indicating only minimal efficacy in improving outcome. Exceptions to this include rhabdomyosarcoma, PNET, and lymphoma.

Treatment usually involves appropriate staging followed by a combination of surgery and radiation therapy. Achieving wide to radical surgical margins is necessary, and in most cases can be accomplished by a limb salvage operation. MRI is essential in treatment planning and in assessment of local compartment involvement (Fig. 42-29). Radiation therapy may be administered preoperatively or postoperatively by brachytherapy or external beam irradiation. With this approach 90 to 95% local control can be anticipated, but a significant proportion of patients (about one-third) succumb to later metastatic disease. In selected cases of soft-tissue and other

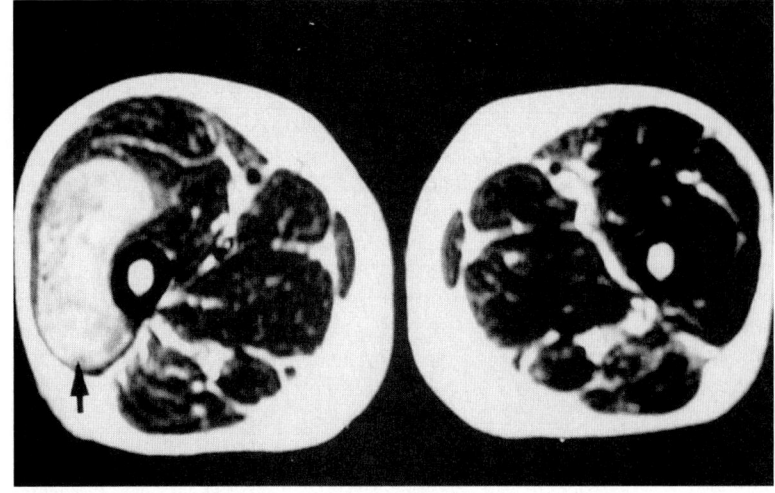

FIG. 42-29. MRI demonstrating soft-tissue sarcoma of the thigh (malignant fibrous histiocytoma) with involvement of the vastus lateralis muscle. Note the tendency to spread along, rather than to traverse, anatomic boundaries such as the anterior compartment fascia and periosteum.

sarcomas, resection of pulmonary metastases has led to cures in approximately 30% of those treated.

Metastatic Bone Tumors

Carcinomas often metastasize to the skeleton, and metastatic lesions are much more common than primary bone lesions in general orthopaedic practice. The five primary cancers with a strong propensity to metastasize to bone are those originating in the breast, prostate, lung, kidney, and thyroid. Multiple myeloma, although technically a primary bone tumor, also must be considered in this group because of its similar age distribution (patients over age 50 years), radiographic presentation, and orthopaedic problems and treatment (pathologic fractures). Over 90% of patients with metastatic breast or prostate carcinoma have at least microscopic bone involvement.

The axial skeleton, including the skull, thoracic spine, ribs, lumbar spine, and pelvis, is most commonly involved. The proximal long bones, particularly the humerus and femur, also are affected frequently. Acral (distal) metastases are uncommon and are almost always secondary to lung carcinoma when they do occur. The predilection of particular tumors for bone, and for particular regions of specific bones, is thought to be caused by cytokines, local growth factors, or matrix components that attract and support growth of these lesions in specific areas. Lesions can be blastic (breast, prostate), lytic (breast, lung, myeloma, kidney, thyroid), or mixed (breast, lung) in radiographic appearance. Blastic or sclerotic lesions are less prone to pathologic fractures.

Patients with multiple lesions may have elevated alkaline phosphatase levels and occasionally are hypercalcemic, a result of secretion of PTH-like protein by some tumors, or more frequently, secondary to massive osteolysis by the tumor cells. The presenting complaint usually is pain in the affected area. Patients with spinal lesions may present with neurologic deficit or back pain. The major orthopaedic problem is that of fracture or impending fracture, with resulting functional disability and pain.

The mainstay of treatment of metastatic disease is radiation therapy, which often controls symptomatic lesions with relatively moderate doses (35 Gy). Larger lesions (larger than 3 cm in a weight-bearing bone), lesions that progress despite radiation, lesions that involve more than one-third of the cortex, and lesions that present with pain on weight bearing (impending fractures) should be internally fixed prophylactically. Fractures are treated surgically if the patient is able to tolerate the procedure medically, since aggressive

mobilization significantly improves quality of life. Newer prosthetic implants for joint reconstruction and fracture fixation allow stabilization in the majority of cases (Figs. 42-30 and 42-31). Bracing or casting is rarely successful for pathologic fractures, since pain control remains a persistent problem, and fractures usually will not heal by closed means if irradiated because of the suppression of callus formation by radiation therapy. Exceptions include spinal fractures, which respond to bracing and radiation treatment, but if neurologic deficit occurs they require surgical decompression and internal fixation either anteriorly or posteriorly. If large areas of bone are destroyed, stabilization often necessitates filling the defect with methyl methacrylate cement to supplement hardware fixation. The goals of treatment are maintenance or restoration of function and pain relief, since carcinoma metastatic to the bones is essentially always incurable. Rarely, a solitary metastasis is amenable to

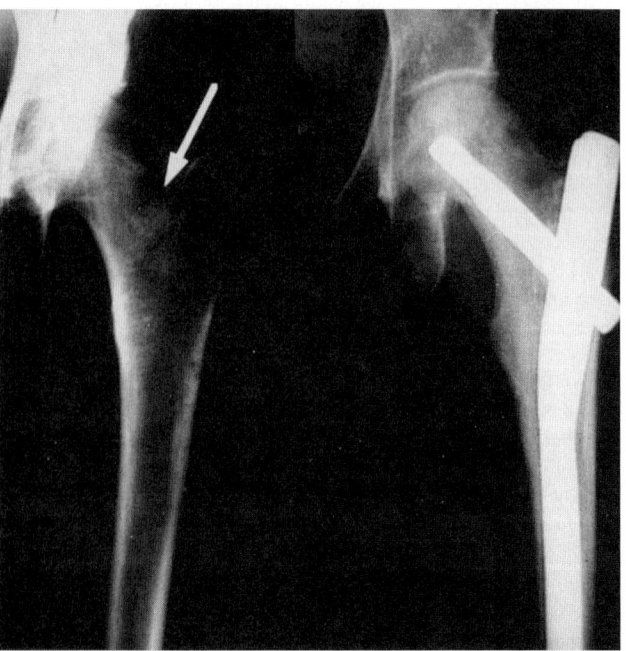

FIG. 42-30. Impending fracture of the proximal femur from metastatic breast carcinoma. Internal fixation using an intramedullary device (Zickel nail) with subsequent radiation therapy allows local control of the tumor and healing of the fracture.

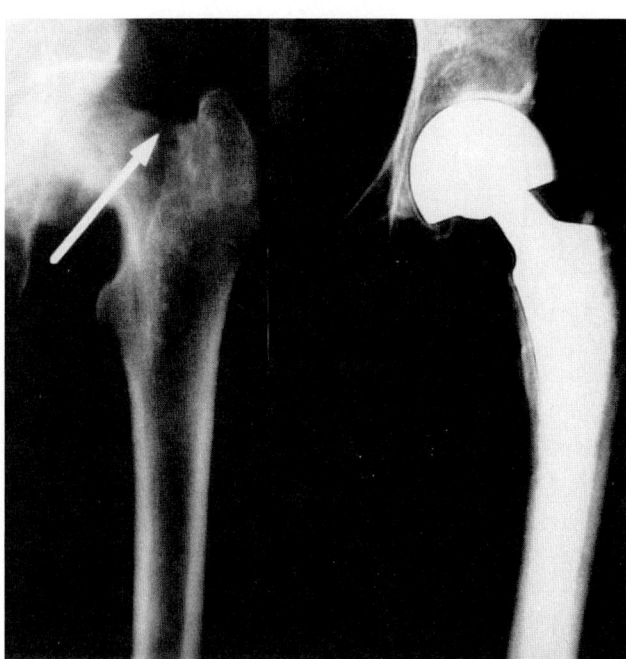

FIG. 42-31. Pathologic fracture of the femoral neck, treated by femoral head excision and endoprosthetic hip replacement. In cases with acetabular involvement, the acetabulum must also be replaced.

curative resection if the primary tumor has been removed; this situation can occur with renal cell carcinoma. Resection or amputation is also considered for pain relief or control of bulky, fungating lesions. Experimental treatments under investigation for metastatic disease, including immunotherapy and bone marrow transplantation, may offer future alternatives to current palliative treatment approaches.

EVALUATION OF THE MUSCULOSKELETAL SYSTEM

History and Physical Examination

Collecting a thorough history and performing a physical examination is the foremost priority when examining a patient who has a musculoskeletal condition. The physical examination is concentrated on the musculoskeletal system, including its neurologic aspects, but a complete general examination is also important. The patient's chief complaint should direct the nature of history taking. Because the most common complaint is pain, it is important to note its location, duration, its intensity, how long it lasts, what makes it worse, what makes it better, and what they do to relieve it. It is also important to know what past treatments have been employed and their results. In conjunction with a past medical and familial history, a social history is often important for conditions of the musculoskeletal system because many problematic musculoskeletal system conditions are a result of the patient's occupation or hobby. In addition, decisions about treatment should take the patient's expectations and physical requirements into consideration.

The initial aspect of the physical examination is to observe the patient's general condition. The patient should be wearing a minimal amount of clothing. Observe how the patient moves about, examining their gait pattern. An antalgic gait indicates pain. Its feature is marked by a shortened period of time with the extremity bearing weight. A Trendelenburg gait or gluteus medius limp is caused by malfunction of the hip abductor mechanism. A positive indicator for

Trendelenburg's sign is if the patient leans toward the affected side when the opposite extremity is raised off the floor (see Fig. 42-12). The following questions may help to elucidate additional musculoskeletal dysfunctions: Is the alignment of the lower extremities symmetric? Do the upper extremities move symmetrically? Does the patient stand straight? Additionally, the patient's range of motion of all joints should be measured and areas of interest palpated. Joints should be inspected for effusion. A check of the vascular supply and a neurologic examination should also be performed.

Virtually all patients with musculoskeletal complaints should have plain radiographs. The minimum is two views taken perpendicular to one another. Once these have been examined, a differential diagnosis can be made which usually includes only a few conditions. Additional diagnostic tests may be needed before a treatment plan can be finalized.

The evaluation of a patient who has sustained acute trauma requires a slightly different approach, which involves collecting a detailed summary of the events of the injury. The following questions may be helpful in this effort: What was the patient doing when the patient was injured? Was the twist internal rotation or external rotation? Can the patient estimate the height from which the patient fell? Was the patient a pedestrian, cyclist, or passenger in or driver of an automobile? Was the patient wearing a seatbelt? Did the patient lose consciousness? Was the patient ejected from the vehicle? Answers to questions such as these can provide clues to the degree of injury and indicate possible associated injuries that should be looked for.

The measurement of joint motion is important and can be ascertained with the help of a goniometer. Figure 42-32 describes certain conventions used to describe range of motion. Comparing the affected side to the unaffected side is useful. In general, 0 degrees is the neutral anatomic position. Movements into the plane anterior to the body are *flexion* and movements into the plane posterior to the body are *extension*. Rotation (internal and external), abduction, and adduction are also important indicators to the measurement of motion. In general, flexion and extension are maintained longer than rotation, abduction, and adduction. Loss of motion can be from pathology intrinsic or extrinsic to the joint. For example, a patient with loss of flexion, rotation, and abduction in the hip might have degenerative disease of the hip joint or the patient might have muscular contractures. A careful analysis of the patient should distinguish between intrinsic and extrinsic causes.

An examination for muscle atrophy should be performed. If found, a determination should be made concerning whether it is secondary to nerve damage, disuse, or direct muscle damage. Muscle strength should be tested on a reliable scale that is frequently used (Table 42-5).

Joint stability is important and ligaments are examined by stressing the joint in various directions. The knee, shoulder, elbow, and ankle are all joints commonly associated with injuries that lead to ligamentous disruption. The specifics for each of these joints are described in their respective sections.

The vascular supply to the extremity should be determined. If the patient has good pulses of the dorsalis pedis, posterior tibial, radial, and ulnar arteries, significant vascular injury or arterial disease is unlikely. Those patients without peripheral pulses should be examined more thoroughly to determine the status of the vascular supply. Edema should be noted if present.

Radiology

After physical examination, plain radiographs are the single-most important diagnostic tool for evaluating a patient with a complaint

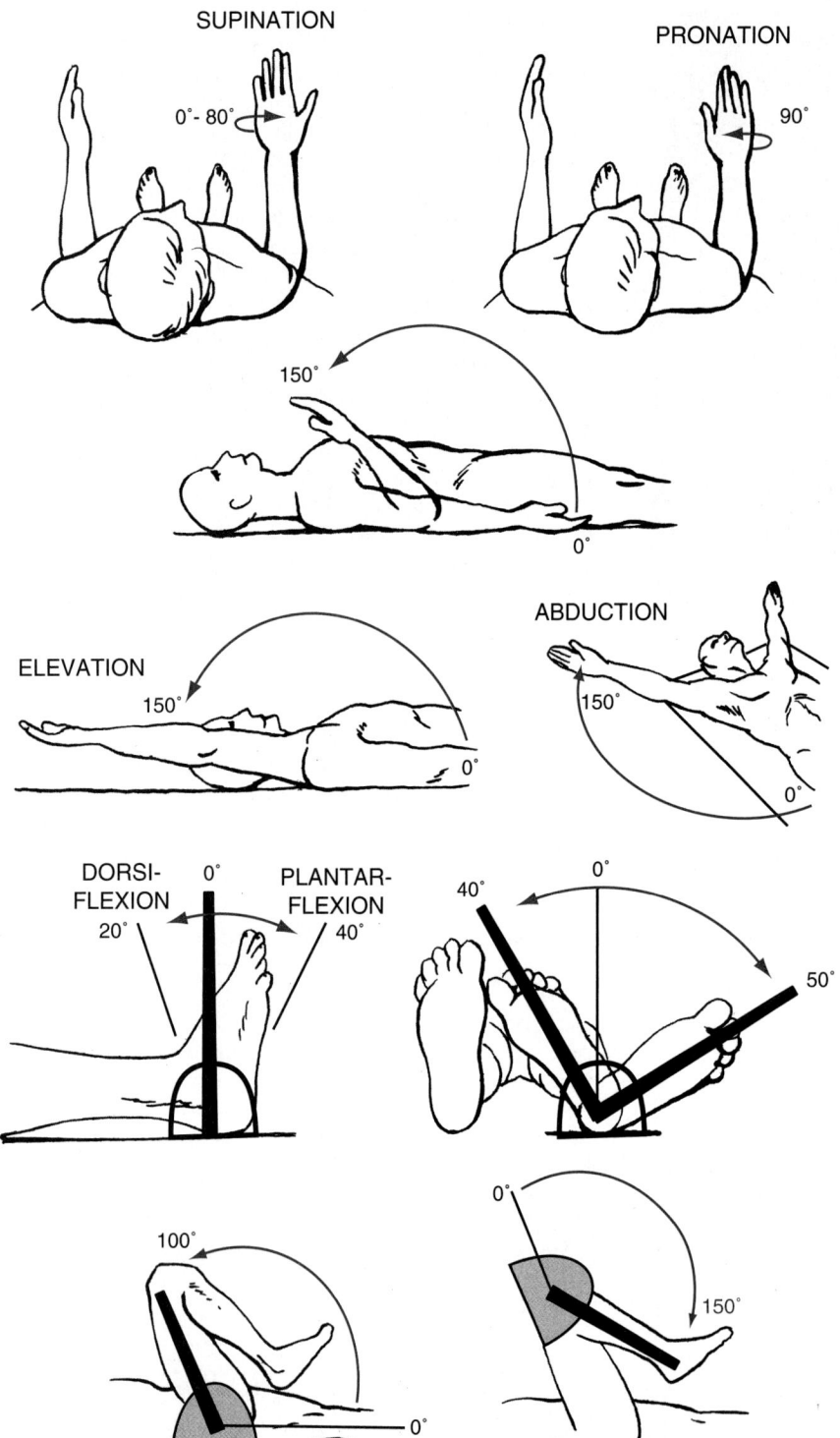

FIG. 42-32. Range of motion (ROM) is measured in degrees. Each joint has a normal range and when examining a patient with a joint or extremity disorder, the involved joint's ROM should be measured and recorded.

Table 42-5
Muscle Strength Testing

0	No contraction
1	Trace contraction
2	Active movement, no gravity
3	Active movement against gravity
4	Mild weakness
5	Normal strength

related to the musculoskeletal system. Before obtaining a computerized tomography (CT scan) or a magnetic resonance image (MRI), a plain radiograph should always be taken. A minimum of two views at right angles to one another should be obtained. Obliques are often useful to visualize certain aspects of the skeletal anatomy. The quality of the radiograph is important; the bone should be clearly seen and the soft tissues, although visible, should not interfere with visualization of the bone.

There are a few anatomic areas that are known to be troublesome on plain radiographs. Seeing C7 on the lateral can be difficult and it is important when evaluating a patient with neck pain to be sure it is visible. This can be done by having the patient's arms pulled down while the lateral view is taken or by taking a "swimmer's" view. Patients with a dislocated shoulder will not want their shoulder moved and obtaining a lateral view can be difficult. For an anterior dislocation this usually is not a problem because the dislocation can be easily appreciated on the anteroposterior (AP) view. Unfortunately, for a posterior dislocation, the AP view can fail to show the dislocation, and it may be missed if the lateral view is not also obtained. A lateral or equivalent view of the shoulder should always be obtained. A "scapular lateral" view can be taken without the patient having to move the arm. Because nondisplaced fractures of the distal humerus in children can be particularly difficult to appreciate, radiographs of the opposite elbow are usually taken when a child has an elbow injury without an obvious fracture. Fractures of the carpal navicular often are not displaced and cannot be seen on the initial radiographs. For a patient with a wrist injury and pain, but no obvious fracture, it is recommended to treat the patient as if the patient has a fractured carpal navicular and repeat a radiograph in 10 to 14 days because the fracture is usually visible then. Patients with low back pain, especially young patients, may have an injury or abnormality of the pars. The pars is seen best with an oblique view of the lumbar spine. These are suggested for any patient with persistent lower back pain whose AP and lateral views are normal. Nondisplaced fractures of the femoral neck are often not visible on plain radiographs. Because these fractures should be internally stabilized as soon as possible, immediate diagnosis is necessary. An MRI of the femoral neck is the best method to use in the elderly patient who has fallen and has hip pain but whose plain radiograph does not show an apparent fracture. Whenever evaluating a patient with ankle pain, three views of the ankle should be obtained. The usual AP and lateral views should be taken in addition to a "mortise" view (Fig. 42-33). Combined, these three views allow for better assessment of the relationship between the distal fibula and tibia.

All aspects of the image need to be examined and it is recommended that a routine method be used to review the film. Often it is best to initially ignore the most obvious abnormality while carefully searching other aspects of the radiograph in an effort to discover more subtle ones. Specifically, examination of the soft tissues often shows abnormal densities, calcification, or ossification. The bone's medullary canal and cortex should be examined and subtle periosteal reactions should be looked for. Specific conditions relating to the joint should also be suspected such as thinning of the radiolucency of the joint that indicates loss of articular cartilage, thickening of the subchondral bone that indicates degenerative joint disease, the presence of osteophytes (Fig. 42-34), or an incorrect alignment.

When examining a bone with a fracture, it is important to look at all parts of the bone (i.e., a fracture at the periphery of the film can be easily missed). Remember that adjacent joints may be damaged and should be examined with both a physical examination and radiographs. The specifics of the fracture should be noticed and recorded in the patient's record and can include whether the fracture is simple or comminuted; whether it is a spiral, oblique, or transverse; its location in the bone; and whether it is diaphyseal, metaphyseal, or intra-articular (Fig. 42-35). In children, it should be noted whether the fracture crosses the growth plate. The answers to these questions are critical in deciding what treatment is needed. For most musculoskeletal abnormalities further radiographic evaluations are not needed.

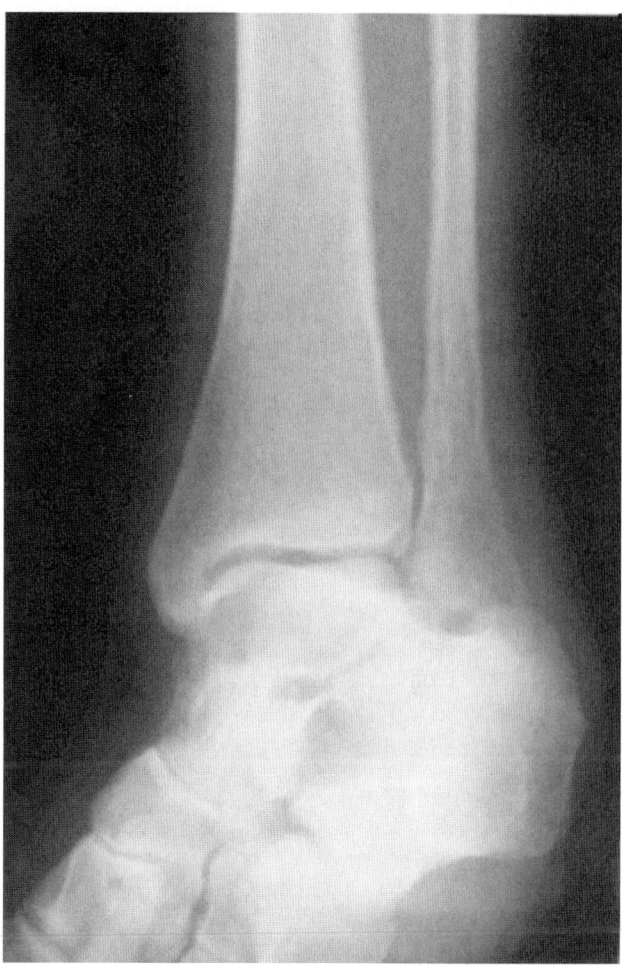

FIG. 42-33. A mortise view of a normal ankle. This view allows visualization of the relationship between the distal tibia and fibula.

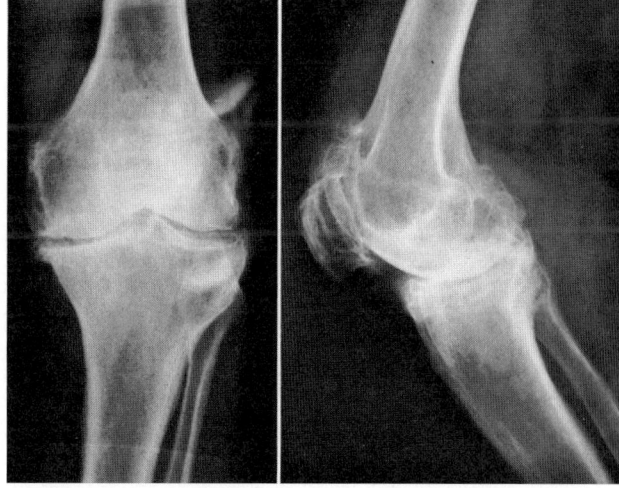

FIG. 42-34. Primary osteoarthritis of the knee. AP and lateral radiographs showing varus deformity of the knee with joint space narrowing and osteophyte production on medial, lateral, and posterior aspects of the tibia, on anterior aspects of the femoral condyles, and on upper and lower poles of the patella. There is minimal cyst formation and sclerosis of subchondral bone of the medial joint space.

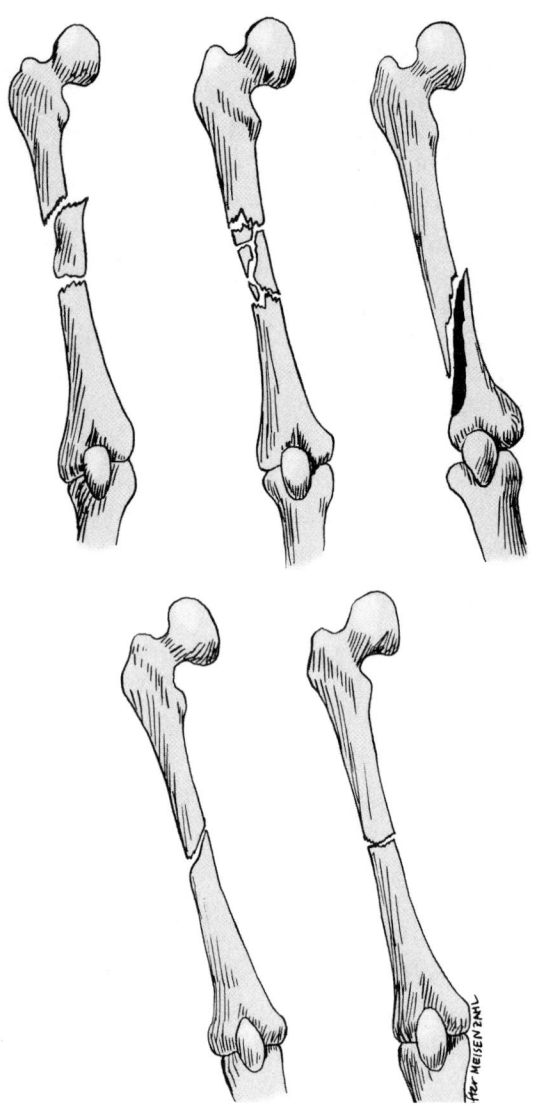

FIG. 42-35. *Types of fracture. Top row:* Segmental, comminuted, and spiral; *bottom row:* oblique and transverse.

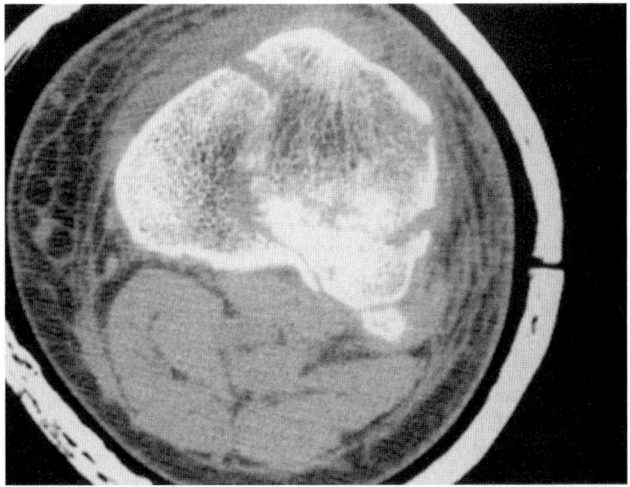

FIG. 42-36. *CAT image of a proximal tibial fracture. The details of the fracture are more easily seen with a CT scan. This improves preoperative surgical planning.*

Ultrasound can be used for musculoskeletal conditions but is not commonly obtained. Advances in ultrasound technology have allowed examination of tendons and ligaments in real time, but are dependent on the technical expertise of the person performing the examination.

Nuclear studies are often used to evaluate the skeletal system. Technetium-99 (^{99}Tc) bone scans are the most commonly used study. The ^{99}Tc is tagged to phosphorus, which attaches itself to the bone. The amount of ^{99}Tc attached to the bone is directly related to bone formation. Therefore, any reactivity of the bone is seen as a "hot" spot. The patient is injected with the ^{99}Tc and approximately 2 hours later images are taken. The scan is sensitive but not specific. Indium (In) scans are used primarily to determine if there is an infection. White blood cells from the patient are tagged with In and injected into the patient. Because the tagged white blood cells concentrate at the site of an infection, the scan has a "hot" spot. Thallium scans are also occasionally used to identify soft-tissue inflammatory lesions.

Computed axial tomography (CAT) is the best method to use for visualizing the details of bone and calcifications. It is often used to evaluate fractures, especially comminuted ones and those involving an articular surface (Fig. 42-36). Three-dimensional reconstructions can be done to better evaluate the injury. CT is useful in the evaluation of patients with suspected herniated nucleus pulposus, although MRI is probably better.

MRI is most valuable for the examination of soft tissues. It is particularly valuable in examining the soft tissue around joints. Torn ligaments and meniscus can usually be seen on an MRI (Fig. 42-37). It is also an excellent means of examining the soft tissues of the extremities and the spine. The spinal canal is visible and damage to the spinal cord can be seen easily.

Diagnostic Injections

Frequently an injection of Novocain with or without corticosteroids is useful for the evaluation of patients with pain. By anesthetizing a bursa or joint and reexamining the patient, it is possible to determine if one or the other is a source of pain. The most common site for this injection when evaluating a patient with shoulder pain is the

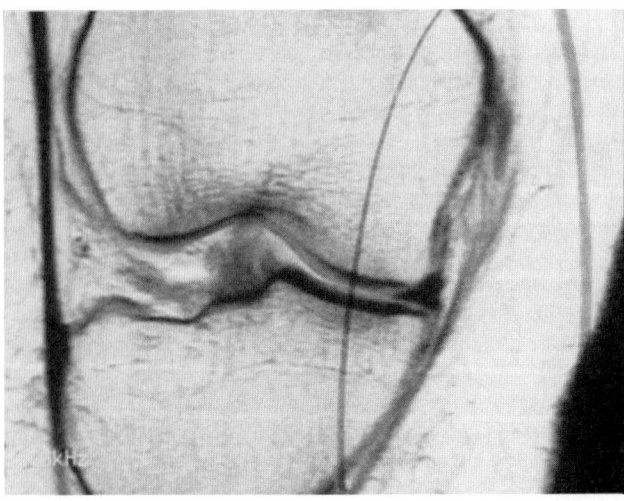

FIG. 42-37. *Coronal MRI image of a knee. The meniscus is easily seen as a dark (no signal) triangular structure between the femoral condyle and tibia. The medial collateral ligament is disrupted. MRI is a valuable tool to evaluate injuries to the soft tissues of the extremities.*

subacromial bursa. If the pain is relieved postinjection, a diagnosis of subacromial bursitis can be made. When suspicion is high for subacromial bursitis prior to injection, corticosteroid is added to the Novocain to simultaneously treat the bursitis. Other bursae and joints can be injected in a similar fashion. Usually only 1 mL is needed and should be performed in sterile conditions.

DISORDERS OF THE MUSCULOSKELETAL SYSTEM

Osteomyelitis

Osteomyelitis is an infection of the bone that most commonly occurs secondary to an open wound with an associated or compound fracture. However, osteomyelitis also can occur spontaneously, presumably as a consequence of circulating bacteria in the bloodstream, and is known as *hematogenous osteomyelitis*.[6] Hematogenous osteomyelitis is an infection that predominantly occurs in children. The most common causative organism is *Staphylococcus*, but any bacteria can produce osteomyelitis. Less-common infectious agents include viruses, fungi, and mycobacteria. Osteomyelitis is divided into "acute" and "chronic" categories. Although the time limits delineating one category from the other are somewhat arbitrary, as a rule, infections up to 3 months' duration are termed acute, while those enduring longer than 3 months are termed chronic. Some authors include a third category, "subacute," for patients who exhibit symptoms that endure longer than 3 months but who have not developed extensive necrotic bone. In general, acute osteomyelitis is associated with systemic findings of an infection with fever, malaise, elevated white blood cell count, erythrocyte sedimentation rate (ESR), and C-reactive protein (CRP). The site of the infection is tender and the patient often does not want to move the extremity involved. Patients with chronic osteomyelitis are usually not systemically sick. They are more likely to have a draining sinus, necrotic bone (a sequestrum) surrounded by reactive bone (an involucrum) (Fig. 42-38). Acute osteomyelitis is usually successfully treated with an aspiration of the pus, occasionally an open débridement, and systemic antibiotics. Chronic osteomyelitis treatment requires débridement of all necrotic bone and soft tissue and often a soft-tissue procedure for definitive coverage with long-term therapy (3 months or more) of antibiotics. However, even with these treatments, relapse is common.

Hematogenous osteomyelitis is often associated with an infection within a joint, or *pyarthrosis*. Joint infections can also occur without bone involvement and should be recognized and treated as soon as possible to reduce damage to the articular cartilage (Fig. 42-39).

Pyogenic Arthritis

With early diagnosis of septic arthritis and appropriate treatment, the prognosis for maintenance of normal joint function is excellent. The lysosomal enzymes released from white cells in the joint, however, can permanently destroy the articular cartilage and lead to progressive degenerative change if inadequately treated. Joint infections can result from hematogenous spread from septicemia, direct infection from adjacent traumatic wounds or surgery, or extension of an adjacent metaphyseal osteomyelitis.

Staphylococcus aureus and hemolytic streptococci are the two most common organisms that cause pyogenic arthritis. Gonococcal and coliform organisms, *Hemophilus influenzae* (in infants), pneumococci, meningococci, and *Brucella* are other causative agents. With the advent of widespread *H. influenzae* vaccination in children,

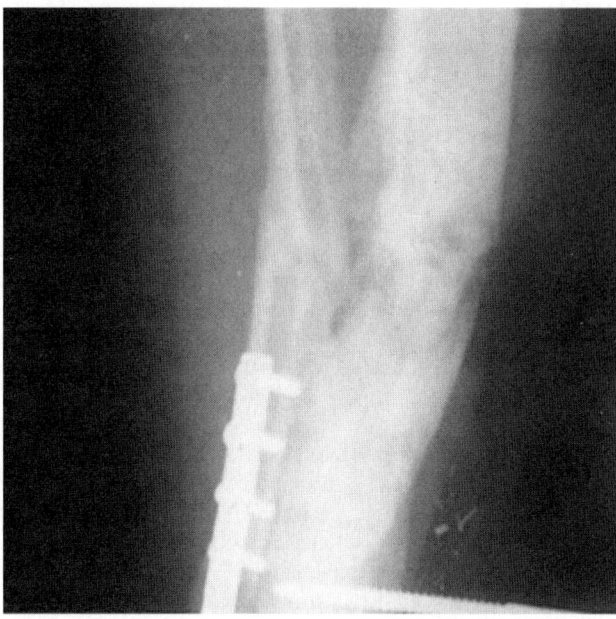

FIG. 42-38. AP radiograph of a patient with chronic osteomyelitis. The patient had a compound (open) fracture of his tibia treated with an open reduction and internal fixation. He has developed a chronic infection. The plate that was on his tibia has been removed. The bone is denser than normal and the medullary canal cannot be seen well, which suggest that there is sequestered (necrotic) bone that needs to be débrided if the infection is to be controlled.

the incidence of infections because of this organism has dramatically declined.

Septic arthritis occurs in children and adults and is more common in debilitated patients or those undergoing steroid therapy or immunologic suppression.

In patients with hematogenous spread from bacteremia several joints may be involved. Complaints include fever, pain and swelling in the affected joint, chills, and malaise. Elevation of the white blood count and erythrocyte sedimentation rate are common. The

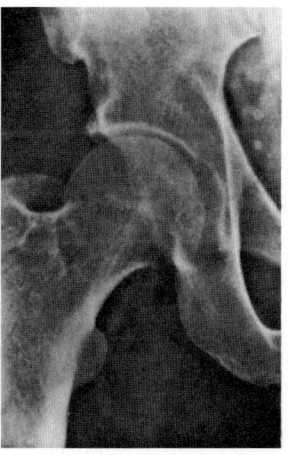 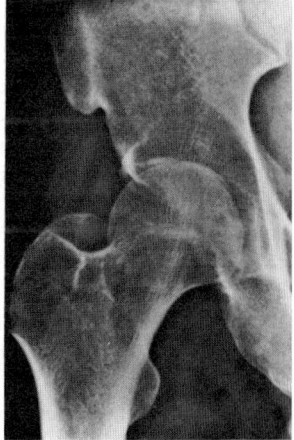

A   *B*

FIG. 42-39. Pyogenic hip joint. *A.* AP radiograph of hip joint taken 48 h after onset of acute hip pain associated with minor hip injury. Joint space is normal, and no bone changes are seen. *B.* Three and one-half weeks later there is complete loss of joint space with no bone changes. Cartilage destruction was a result of Haemophilus influenzae septic arthritis.

affected joint(s) are swollen, tender, erythematous, warm to touch, and painful during range-of-motion maneuvers. The physical findings vary greatly and often depend on the virulence of the organism; indolent infections present with a nearly normal examination.

Radiographs reveal effusion. In more advanced infections, erosions and joint space narrowing occur as consequences of the destruction of the articular cartilage (Fig. 42-39). With chronic infection or a large abscess, subluxation of the joint also may be evident. Diagnosis is made by aspiration of the joint with culture, Gram stain, and analysis of the synovial fluid. The presence of organisms and an elevated white cell count in the fluid are diagnostic. The white cell count in the fluid may range from $25,000/mm^3$ to more than $200,000/mm^3$, usually with a high percentage (greater then 90%) of leukocytes.

Treatment. In the presence of an elevated synovial white cell count and other signs and symptoms of septic arthritis, antibiotic therapy is started empirically, usually with coverage for *S. aureus* (cephalosporin), streptococci (cephalosporin or a penicillin), and, in children, *H. influenzae* (ampicillin).

Controversy exists as to whether surgical drainage, arthroscopic drainage, or repeated daily aspiration represents the best treatment option. Generally it is agreed that for hip infections, which can result in rapid destruction and secondary osteonecrosis and can be difficult to aspirate, emergent surgical drainage is indicated. Chronic infections with loculation or thick purulence also require surgical drainage. In chronic infections removal of hypertrophic infected synovium can be advantageous. For the knee, arthroscopic drainage may be appropriate. Shoulder and ankle infections can be managed either by sequential aspiration or surgical drainage. In general, patients who undergo surgical drainage undergo defervescence and improve clinically more rapidly. Depending on the organism, intravenous antibiotic therapy is indicated for 2 to 4 weeks. If the septic arthritis results from extension from an adjacent osteomyelitis, intravenous antibiotic therapy for 6 weeks or longer is needed. Early joint motion is encouraged to restore nutrition to the articular cartilage and prevent stiffness.

For cases in which articular cartilage destruction progresses despite treatment, late secondary degenerative arthritis can result. Options for treatment when symptoms are severe include arthrodesis, resection arthroplasty, and, in rare cases, joint replacement arthroplasty.

Compound fractures with contamination and devascularized bone will lead to osteomyelitis if not cleaned and the necrotic bone débrided. The initial management of all open fractures is to wash out the wound in the operating room, débride all necrotic tissue (especially necrotic bone), and stabilize the fracture. Broad-spectrum antibiotics are used initially until either the wound is successfully closed or a specific bacterium is grown. If an organism is identified the antibiotic of choice is the one most effective for that organism. The initial débridement is critical and repeated débridements are usually needed to completely clean a wound. After the wound begins to heal and there is no evidence of necrotic tissue or active infection, the wound may be closed. This can be accomplished with primary closure, but more often requires a local muscle pedicle flap closure or tissue transfer.[7] If the initial wound is managed correctly, chronic osteomyelitis is almost always prevented.

Hematogenous osteomyelitis is a relative emergency and should be diagnosed and treated as soon as possible. Early in the course of the disease, within the first 24 to 72 hours, an aspiration of the infected bone and antibiotics is usually successful. If diagnosis occurs later, or if the infection involves a joint (especially the hip joint), operative drainage is usually necessary. Patients usually present to an emergency room with fever and a history of disuse of the effected extremity. Very young children will have a pseudoparalysis. The effected bone is tender and occasionally swollen and red. The child will have an elevated white blood cell count, CRP, and ESR. The initial plain radiograph may be normal or there can be subtle periosteal reaction. If there is a visible periosteal reaction, the infection is more than 5 to 7 days old. A ^{99}Tc bone scan will show increased activity at the site of the infection and an MRI will show extensive edema in the affected bone and surrounding soft tissue.

The mechanism of hematogenous osteomyelitis in children is thought to be a result of the rich but sluggish blood supply on the metaphyseal side of the growth plate. It is postulated that bacteria in the bloodstream are deposited in the metaphysis near the growth plate. These bacteria proliferate to produce an abscess, which enlarges, destroys bone, and eventually penetrates the cortex to produce a subperiosteal abscess. Most patients do not present for treatment until the infection penetrates the cortex.

If the patient received treatment early in the course of the infection the bone usually resorbs the limited amount of necrotic bone and repairs itself. If the infection is left untreated, the amount of necrotic bone may be so large that it is not resorbed and is left surrounded by pus. This bone is called a *sequestrum*. The viable bone then will produce a new, reactive bone that tends to surround the necrotic sequestrum. This is called an *involucrum*. Left untreated, the infection will eventually spontaneously drain through the skin. In the United States, this degree of chronic osteomyelitis is rarely seen but it is not uncommon in underdeveloped countries.

Arthritis

There are a variety of pathways by which a joint is transformed from an efficient, mobile, low-friction, shock-absorbing, and energy-conserving structure to one that is painful and stiff. One common pathway involves greater or lesser degrees of destruction of articular cartilage.

Chondrocytes, or cartilage cells, lie embedded within their own environment of extracellular hydrated matrix. They receive nutrition via diffusion from the synovial fluid through the matrix and there are no vascular or neural elements present. The chondrocyte receives all of the input required for the maintenance of the extracellular matrix, as well as the cell's intracellular activities from biomechanical modulations of its tissue. During mechanical loading, matrix molecule and ion fluxes occur. As such, the chondrocyte often has been described as a link between physical and chemical life processes.

Articular cartilage can be divided into four zones. The superficial zone is composed of several layers of flattened cells. These cells respond readily to irritation and appear to have macrophage-like functions. The next two zones are the middle and deep zones. The major population of chondrocytes is found here. The chondrocytes at the deeper layers produce almost all of the components necessary for extracellular matrix; type II collagen, proteoglycans, glycoproteins, hyaluronate, and degradative enzymes (metalloproteinases). The deepest zone has chondrocytes found within an extracellular matrix, which has calcified. This zone forms a transition to the subchondral bone. The calcified zone prevents the diffusion of nutrients from bone into cartilage and also provides the mechanical link to the bone for load transmission. The *tidemark* is a thin, acellular line visible with histologic staining that divides noncalcified and calcified cartilage.

The extracellular matrix is vital and has a compound structure. Type II collagen fibers form gothic arches with apex at the joint surface. Considerable amounts of water bind directly to the collagen as well as to the hydrophilic macromolecular aggregates of proteoglycans, glycoproteins, and hyaluronate. The arches of collagen keep the water-rich aggregates in place and as load is applied, the water content is released into the joint. This allows for joint lubrication and low friction. With cyclic loading and unloading there is a constant flow of water and ions in and out, as well as an inflow of nutrients and an elimination of waste products. Proteoglycans are the most important water-binding molecules.

Lacerations or other superficial injuries to articular cartilage layers do not heal. The chondrocyte and matrix activity in response to such injury is brief and inadequate. With acute injury there can be some increase in chondrocyte activity. However, the presence of proinflammatory enzymes causes a downregulation of all matrix syntheses. A deep (to the bone) injury will cause bleeding and hematoma formation with subsequent fibrin clot. This leads to the formation of some elements of inadequate repair, including type I collagen as in fibrocartilage, which is not designed for cyclic loading. Many attempts to surgically repair articular cartilage defects produce this fibrocartilage.

The irreversible loss of proteoglycans is the transition to permanent changes in the articular cartilage. Because most of the biomechanical behavior of articular cartilage depends upon this, many changes follow including loss of water, softening and fibrillation of the cartilage occur, and a cessation of type II collagen synthesis. Degradative enzymes cleave to the collagen and the complex fiber network is lost because of an inadequate repair mechanism, which lacks the biomechanical function required. The low-friction capacity of the joint is lost and wear rates increase as the typical, specific features of the arthritic joint emerge. The process can be initiated by a primary inflammatory problem, a mechanical overload caused by trauma, deformity, or malalignment, by crystal deposition, or by infection.

Osteoarthritis

Osteoarthritis (OA) is the most common form of arthritis, with up to 40 million people in the United States having been diagnosed with it. Also known as degenerative joint disease, OA and has been generally considered to be noninflammatory. Some prefer to refer to this disease as osteoarthrosis, changing the suffix -itis to -osis to emphasize the noninflammatory degenerative nature of this aliment. In fact, the same cytokines and interleukins seen in inflammatory arthritis are also seen in osteoarthritis, although in lesser quantity. Theories of etiology include both primary biomechanical, or primary biochemical effects and secondary biomechanical-derived effects leading to a gradual loss of articular cartilage. Many patients do not have a clearly identifiable source for their OA. Other patients may demonstrate problems such as chronic instability, malalignment, prior injury, crystalline disease, past history of meniscectomy, or excessive and repetitive loading. A genetic predisposition is present in some patients. The knee is the most commonly affected joint. Radiographic evidence of OA is common by age 40 years, but clinically significant osteoarthritis is less common until about age 60 years when it is estimated that about 1 in 4 of the general population has pain and/or disability related to OA.

Typical findings on a radiographic examination reveal loss of articular cartilage shown by "joint narrowing" especially on weight-bearing films (see Fig. 42-34). Osteophytes and subchondral cysts are common radiographic findings.

Physical examination reveals pain upon walking (an antalgic gait pattern) or motion of the involved joint. Patients have some degree of limitation of motion, pain and/or crepitus with that motion. Usually there is an effusion in the joint.

The initial treatment includes activity modification weight reduction if indicated, the use of a cane for lower-extremity problems, and nonsteroidal anti-inflammatory and nonnarcotic analgesic medications if required. Patients should be encouraged to maintain their joint motion and muscular strength. If they cannot do this on their own, they should be referred to a physical therapist. Rarely, an intra-articular corticosteroid injection can be used for an acutely painful joint, but it is only a temporary solution. The potential value of nutritional supplements or intra-articular injections of synthetic hyaluronate are currently controversial and the subject of prospective randomized trials.

Surgical options are based on the dramatic success of joint replacement to relieve pain and restore function to the arthritic joint. Improved wear-resistant plastic socket liners or alternate bearing surfaces of metal-on-metal or ceramic may prove successful to safely extend the indication for joint replacement to younger arthritic patients. However, for joints with malalignment or osteotomy, realigning the weight-bearing mechanical forces through the arthritic joint may be an important temporizing procedure. Arthroscopic removal of a torn meniscus in an arthritic knee can relieve mechanical symptoms of painful clicking or locking. For areas of focal articular cartilage loss direct transplantation of cores of the patient's own cartilage from an available donor site, or else, delayed implantation after passage through cell culture may prove valuable to preserve the natural joint.

Rheumatoid Arthritis

Rheumatoid arthritis is the most common form of inflammatory arthritis (Fig. 42-40). It is an apparent autoimmune response that involves synovium, articular cartilage, and soft tissue. The joints of the hand are most commonly involved, but wrists, feet, knees, and hips are frequently affected. This disease is often symmetric, i.e., both knees and both hands. Patients frequently suffer from morning stiffness. Subcutaneous nodules may be palpated, especially at the proximal ulna. The rheumatoid arthritis (RA) factor is positive in approximately 80% of patients.

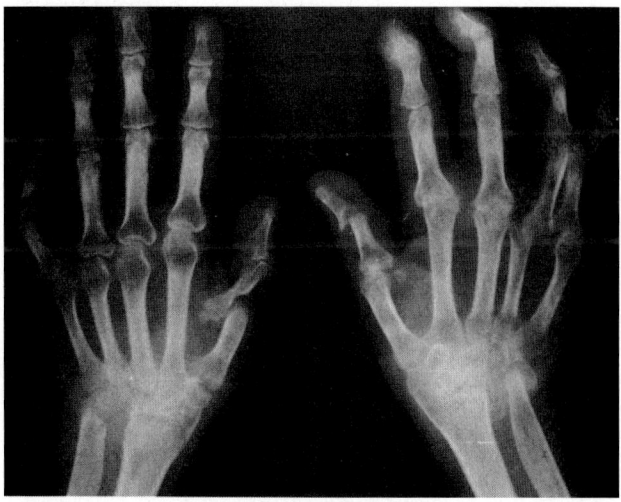

FIG. 42-40. *Radiographic changes in rheumatoid arthritis: severe destruction of radiocarpal articulation with subluxation and ulna deviation at the wrist; loss of ulnar styloid bilaterally; dislocation of the proximal interphalangeal joint of the left thumb and dislocation of the right fourth and fifth finger metacarpophalangeal joints and left metacarpophalangeal joint; diffuse joint space narrowing of many interphalangeal joints.*

Typical radiographs show loss of articular cartilage, osteopenia, and periarticular erosions (see Fig. 42-40). A typical hip deformity of the femoral protruding medially into the pelvis (protrusio acetabulum) is not uncommon. These patients can have vasculitis, pericarditis, and pulmonary involvement.

Treatment is initially medical and often by a rheumatologist. A variety of medications are available that can either relieve symptoms or possibly alter the course of the disease (disease-modifying agents). Intra-articular cortisone injections can be a benefit in an acute flair.

For those with persistent joint damage, total joint replacement is the most beneficial method to relieve pain and disability and to restore function. When endotracheal intubation is a possibility it is wise to obtain cervical spine radiographs. Instability of the cervical spine is not rare and this should be checked prior to the manipulations required for anesthetic intubation.

Patients with systemic lupus erythematoid (SLE) may have a rheumatoid arthritis-like syndrome. However, many also develop osteonecrosis as a result of the common treatment of their disease with corticosteroids. MRI is useful in making the diagnosis of osteonecrosis.

Miscellaneous Arthritides

Ankylosing spondylitis predominantly effects males. The predominant feature is joint pain and restricted motion, with the spine usually having the most involvement. An early physical examination finding is restricted chest expansion. These patients usually have a positive HLA-B27 titer in their serum.

Lyme disease is a tick-borne (deer tick, *Ixodes dammini*) illness caused by the spirochete *Borrelia burgdorferi*. Affected patients may have intermittent attacks of swelling in one or more large joints, accompanied by a characteristic skin rash (erythema chronicum migrans) that often precedes the arthritis. The knee is the most effected joint. A serum Lyme titer is diagnostic. Treatment includes tetracycline, penicillin, or erythromycin.

Gout results from abnormalities in the metabolism of urate that cause deposition of urate crystals in joints, kidneys, and musculoskeletal soft tissues. When deposited in the synovium, the urate crystals may cause an acute inflammatory reaction. The patient often presents with acute onset of pain, swelling, and erythema of a single joint. The most commonly affected joint is the first metatarsophalangeal (MP) joint of the foot. The patient has elevated serum uric acid levels and urate crystals are seen on an analysis of the joint fluid. The crystals are long and thin. Colchicine has been used since the days of Hippocrates. A 0.65 mg dose is given orally every 1 to 2 hours until the pain subsides or diarrhea begins. For less-painful episodes, nonsteroidal anti-inflammatory medication can be used. Patients with gout should be treated to lower their serum urate levels.

Calcium pyrophosphate deposition disease (CPPD or pseudogout) is also an inflammatory synovial disorder caused by crystals. The crystals of CPPD are calcium pyrophosphate. The presentation is similar to gout but usually not as painful. Calcifications are often seen in the cartilage or meniscus. The crystals can be seen on analysis of the joint fluid. They are short and rectangular. Nonsteroidal anti-inflammatory medication is usually sufficient treatment.

Patients with inflammatory bowel disease may show an inflammatory arthritis typical of large joints such as the hip or knee. Five to 10% of patients with psoriasis will develop psoriatic arthritis. This typically involves small joints such as the hands or feet, but can also involve the spine.

Infectious Arthritis

Infectious arthritis, also known as septic arthritis or pyarthrosis, is relatively uncommon. It is most often seen in patients younger than age 5 years or older than age 80 years. However, both morbidity and mortality rates can be relatively high. The knee and hip are the joints most typically infected. *Staphylococcus aureus*, streptococci, and gonococci are the organisms most typically involved. Viruses, mycobacteria, fungal agents, and Lyme disease are other causes. Early diagnosis and treatment limits joint destruction and preserves function. Demonstrating organisms in a synovial fluid using Gram's stain or culture helps to establish a definitive diagnosis. Early joint drainage and lavage are the mainstays of treatment, followed by intravenous antibiotics. Hematogenous seeding during a transient or persistent bacteremia is believed to be the most common mechanism in septic arthritis. This can also occur from direct inoculation during a surgical procedure or an intra-articular injection. Septic arthritis can also occur from a direct extension of infection from an adjacent area such as a cellulitis or osteomyelitis. When an organism enters the joint it causes an acute inflammatory synovitis with release of the various proinflammatory enzymes, cytokines, tumor necrosis factor alpha, interleukin-1, and proteases. This leads to the inevitable destruction of cartilage.

The American College of Rheumatology defines septic arthritis as a synovial fluid aspirate that demonstrates a minimum of 50,000 white blood cells (WBC) per high-powered field and at least 80% neutrophils on differential count. In patients with previous total joint replacements, much lower counts can be diagnostic.

Risk factors are both systemic and local and include age older than 80 years, diabetes, intravenous (IV) drug abuse, indwelling catheters, and a compromised immune status. Rheumatoid arthritis predisposes to the latter formation of septic arthritis. After a total joint replacement there is a risk (by virtue of the foreign material present) of infection from hematogenous spread.

S. aureus is the most common organism. Gonococcus should be suspected if there is a history of sexual activity. The definitive diagnosis of septic arthritis is established by aspiration of the joint and demonstrating organisms in the synovial fluid either by Gram's stain or by culture. Lidocaine should be avoided prior to the aspiration because it has antibacterial properties and can interfere with recovery of a positive culture. If tuberculosis or a fungal agent is suspected, a synovial membrane biopsy and culture may be required to establish the diagnosis.

The exact mechanism that leads to destruction of the joint is unclear. There is marked proliferation of the synovial lining. This synovial reaction is most likely the cause of articular cartilage damage. If the articular cartilage is spared, the joint is usually able to regain near-normal function.

Prompt initiation of the appropriate antibiotic is mandatory. The joint needs to be drained of the fluid and débrided. This can be accomplished by an open arthrotomy but an arthroscopic lavage and débridement often proves effective. This may need to be repeated. If the joint has significant articular damage as a consequence of the infection, pain and disability usually result.

TRAUMA

Initial Assessment

The initial evaluation of the injured patient should be geared toward identifying life-threatening injuries. Injuries to the chest, head, abdomen, and major vessels may require emergent treatment and take precedence over most musculoskeletal injuries. Patients suffering multiple injuries often have suffered severe trauma and can be hemodynamically unstable from skeletal injuries alone. Orthopaedic and trauma surgeons should be particularly alert to this when major pelvic injuries are present. In this scenario, the orthopaedist must work in tandem with the trauma surgeon to stabilize and treat the patient. Patients in shock must be treated aggressively with volume replacement. Unstable pelvic fractures often require some type of stabilization to control hemorrhage. Persistent shock, despite fluid resuscitation and stabilization of the pelvic fracture, is an indicator of possible arterial bleeding. Occult arterial bleeding requires emergency arteriography and embolization.

The trauma surgeon, in conjunction with the orthopaedic surgeon, should make the assessment of skeletal injuries. Evaluation of all open injuries, long-bone fractures, and spinal injuries is imperative. This evaluation should be made as soon as possible, especially in an unstable patient. The patient should not be mobilized until appropriate radiographs of the spine have been taken and evaluated. Anterior and posterior radiographs of the cervical spine are the minimal requirement. The extremities need to be evaluated for neurovascular compromise, soft-tissue and bony injuries, and ligamentous injuries. Sensory and motor examinations, including peripheral pulses and capillary refill, should be evaluated and carefully documented. It is helpful to have a trauma check-off list for quick documentation. Often, this task is left to the most junior person on the team and can result in poor documentation.

Injured extremities need to be splinted for soft-tissue management and mobilization of the patient. Skeletal traction should be considered for long-bone fractures when the patients are not going directly to the operating room, but femur fractures in multiply-injured patients require stabilization as soon as possible. A prospective randomized study has shown that this decreases morbidity and mortality; however, this type of prospective evaluation has not been done for other long-bone fractures. The trauma surgeon, orthopaedist, and anesthesiologist must work together to determine the best treatment for the patient. Sometimes this will include surgical fixation of all fractures immediately; at other times, this may require staged procedures. Delaying treatment of some fractures for a fresh surgical team experienced in orthopaedic trauma is sometimes in the best interest of the patient. This is especially true of complex intra-articular fractures, which require special instrumentation and a prolonged operation.

Open Fractures

An open fracture is defined as any fracture that is exposed to the outside environment. This can result from a penetrating injury that has caused a fracture or from a displaced fragment of bone that has violated the skin. Open fractures are often caused by high-energy injuries and associated injuries should be sought.

The early goals of treatment should include immediate irrigation and débridement combined with skeletal stabilization to prevent infection and to facilitate soft-tissue healing. Vascular injuries, larger wounds, greater comminution, and soft-tissue loss are all associated with increased risk of osteomyelitis.[8] Once osteomyelitis has been established, it may be extremely difficult to eradicate. Therefore, early treatment should include aggressive and immediate débridement of the wound and fracture site in an operative environment and intravenous antibiotic therapy. Repeat intraoperative débridement is recommended when significant soft-tissue damage or contamination is present. Primary closure of wounds is controversial. Open wounds with fractures are classified to indicate the degree of damage and allow easy communication of injury level

Table 42-6
Grading of Open Wounds

Type I	Low energy, <1 cm
Type II	Modest energy, >1 cm
Type III	High energy, usually >10 cm
A	No vascular involvement
B	Vascular injury

(Table 42-6). Low-grade, open wounds are often closed and sometimes not emergently débrided. This remains controversial and should not be the standard for surgeons inexperienced in dealing with open fractures. Higher-grade, open wounds will need surgical evaluation by a plastic surgeon as soon as possible. The orthopaedic surgeon and the plastic surgeon must work together to achieve soft-tissue closure, to prevent infection, and to achieve bony union. Ultimately, a prolonged course of rehabilitation will be necessary to ensure the best possible function for these patients.

Goals of Treatment of Musculoskeletal Injuries

When treating the trauma patient, it is important to keep treatment goals in perspective. The patient and surgeon must have realistic patient goals. In the severely multiply-injured patient, the initial goal is to preserve life. If this goal is achieved, the next and equally important goal is to preserve function. Often, the goal of the trauma surgeon is to preserve life; however, for the orthopaedic surgeon, the goal is to preserve function. Sometimes these goals can lead to conflict between surgical services. This disparity in treatment goals becomes glaringly evident when the trauma surgeon quickly spends crucial minutes obtaining hemostasis in an emergent laparotomy. This is in contrast to the orthopaedic traumatologist who spends hours piecing together a complex, comminuted intra-articular fracture. On the one hand, the trauma surgeon is preserving life, and on the other hand the orthopaedic surgeon realizes that there may be only one chance to preserve function by reconstructing a joint. Of course, these complex reconstructions must be performed in a hemodynamically stable patient. The trauma surgeon must coordinate care on the patient and be the team leader. This important role must not be given to any surgical subspecialist. The orthopaedic traumatologists' goal is to preserve mobility—the ability to use one's extremities. All treating physicians need to remind patients that their quality of life may be changed forever. Patients with severe musculoskeletal injuries, including neurologic and soft-tissue damage, will certainly experience a change in their quality of life.

In patients with an isolated extremity injury, immediate life-threatening problems are not commonly present. Therefore, the decision-making process in regard to preservation of function concerning these types of injuries, weighted against issues of morbidity and expense to the patient, should take the wishes of the patient into consideration.

Principles of Treatment

To achieve the goal of restoring function to the patient with a musculoskeletal injury, the extent of the injury must first be determined. This was discussed earlier under "Initial Assessment." Complete examination of the injured extremity is performed by physical exam and imaging. Imagery is done with routine radiographs supplemented by CT scan or MRI. Sometimes an image fluoroscopy is used for immediate diagnostic evaluation of the extremity.

The first principle of treatment involves reduction of the fracture. If a fracture is truly nondisplaced, then no reduction is necessary. For displaced fractures and dislocations, a reduction maneuver is usually performed. For dislocations, it is recommended to reduce the joint anatomically. For extra-articular fractures, this is often unnecessary. Guidelines for determining what an adequate reduction is exist as a range of parameters; however, these parameters may differ among surgeons. In general, lower extremities require more precise reduction. Intra-articular fractures require an almost anatomic reduction. Joint dislocations are best treated with anatomic reductions.

The second principle of treatment is to maintain the reduction. Some dislocations are inherently stable after reduction and no external maintenance of reduction is necessary. The patient is cautioned against certain activities that may risk re-dislocation or loss of reduction. However, with skeletal fractures, stabilization is usually required. Variability exists in determining what an acceptable means of stabilization is. There is an arsenal of treatment methods available to the orthopaedic surgeon, including internal fixation and external fixation. External fixation includes casts or skeletal external fixation with percutaneous pins and external fixators. Internal fixation includes screw fixation, plate fixation, intramedullary fixation, and other types of metals or absorbable materials for fixation. In some cases, a suture fixation is all that is necessary. Surgeons with different training can successfully treat the same fracture by totally different, but equally acceptable, methods. It is important to remember that the goal of treatment is function and how the reduction is maintained is simply a means to the end.

Achieving skeletal union does not equate to successful function. Often, only half of the battle is won by healing the fracture. The other half of the battle is composed of physical rehabilitation and patient motivation. The duration of rehabilitation is often longer than the time to union. In some cases, physical rehabilitation can be started immediately after skeletal stabilization, especially when internal fixation is used. The ability to rehabilitate earlier is often used as an indication for early internal fixation of fractures. Other variables, such as the surgeon's technical ability, the patient's motivation, and the patient's ability to comply with treatment protocols, will factor into the decision making of how a fracture is treated and what results can be achieved. All of these variables make algorithm-type treatment of orthopaedic injuries very difficult to employ. It is best to use the principles and to prescribe treatment that is familiar to the surgeon and the institution. Different institutions will have different treatment protocols that are successful for their patient population.

The current milieu of hospital and insurance company administrative scrutiny requires surgeons to justify treatment methods as being both treatment- and cost-effective. Physicians ultimately must keep treatment goals and patient care at the forefront and are key in determining whether new technology is, indeed, beneficial to the patients' treatment or is superfluous.

Terminology

It is useful for surgeons of all disciplines to understand some basic orthopaedic terminology. Orthopaedic surgeons use different terms to facilitate communication. Understanding these concepts and terms will help the physician communicate with the orthopaedist. A fracture is determined to be *open* when the fracture communicates with the outside environment. Fortunately, most fractures are *closed* and the soft-tissue envelope is intact. However, the internal soft-tissue injury can be quite variable and attempts have been made to classify the soft-tissue injury with closed fractures. The orthopaedic surgeon is aware that there are *low-energy* closed fractures and *high-energy* closed fractures. High-energy closed fractures are generally more difficult to treat because they tend to be

more "displaced." *Displacement* is defined as fracture ends that are no longer contiguous. The authors describe displacement based on the distal segment. The distal segment can be medial or lateral on an anteroposterior radiograph. The distal segment can be anterior or posterior on a lateral radiograph.

Fractures are often "angulated." *Angulation* is described by the vertex of the angulation. The authors measure angulation by the deviation from normal alignment. If the vertex points anterior, then "anterior angulation" is present. Anterior and posterior angulation can be seen on lateral radiographs. Anterior/posterior radiographs can show "varus" or "valgus" angulation. If the fracture has a vertex that points medially, the fracture is in "valgus." If the vertex points laterally, the fracture is in "varus."

Rotational malalignment is sometimes difficult to determine on plain radiographs. Often this is quite evident by the clinical appearance of the extremity. If the distal portion of the extremity is rotated externally, then "external rotation" is present. Conversely, if the distal portion of the extremity is rotated internally, the fracture is described as being "internally rotated." Radiographically, a joint should be viewed from above and below to see the rotational alignment. This visualization of the joints, above and below the fracture, also is necessary to determine if there has been a joint injury associated with the fracture.

If a long bone is displaced 100%, it is said that "shortening" of the fracture has occurred. Shortening can be seen on either anterior/posterior or lateral radiographs. The amount of shortening will not change from AP to lateral radiographs. However, two radiographs in planes 90 degrees to each other are necessary to visualize translation and angulation.

This terminology is essential in describing postreduction radiographs. The orthopaedic surgeon must carefully document and observe the radiographic alignment of fractures as they heal. Each follow-up visit is an opportunity for the orthopaedic surgeon to intervene in the treatment protocol. Fractures treated with plaster often have the most ability to change position from one visit to the next. The orthopaedic surgeon must be adept in determining which fractures are at the highest risk to displace and may benefit from an alternate type of treatment. The orthopaedic surgeon must determine which method of treatment he or she is most comfortable with. Managing a fracture with cast immobilization can prove more difficult than a fracture treated with internal fixation. The orthopaedic surgeon must have the experience to know the natural history of different fractures. Fractures are more apt to displace based on their soft-tissue injury, location, pattern, and quality of treatment. The surgeon must have knowledge and experience to give the best advice as to whether a reduction is in acceptable position. The orthopaedic surgeon must know the healing time that may be involved for that fracture. Then, the orthopaedic surgeon must use the proper methods of maintaining that reduction until the fracture is healed. Rarely are fractures allowed to proceed to a fibrous nonunion; however, sometimes this may be the best treatment for the patient.

Pelvic Fractures

The pelvic rim is composed of the innominate bones and sacrum. It provides protection for the pelvic viscera, attachment of muscles, and the transmission of weight-bearing forces from the lower extremities. This ring is held together by some of the strongest ligaments in the body. Injuries to the pelvic ring should be differentiated between the low-energy, stable fractures and the high-energy, life-threatening injuries. The former are commonly seen in elderly osteoporotic patients who may have sustained isolated fractures of the pubic rami or nondisplaced fractures of the acetabuli or sacrum from a fall. These fractures usually do not have disruption of the pelvic ring or weight-bearing segments and are considered stable.

High-energy injuries are the result of automobile collisions, pedestrians and cyclists being struck by motor vehicles, or falls from significant heights. These injuries are caused by direct crush, either from the anterior or lateral direction or vertical shear, or combinations of rotational stress on the iliac wings. Patients with this type of injury should be sent or transferred to a capable trauma center as soon as possible. A team approach in the successful management of major pelvic injuries includes a trauma-trained general surgeon, an orthopaedic surgeon, a skilled interventional radiology team, and an urologist.

The initial role of the orthopaedic surgeon is to help determine whether the patient has a mechanically unstable pelvic injury. This type of injury can cause or contribute to hemodynamic instability. If hemodynamic instability occurs and other causes of blood loss have been ruled out, stabilization of the pelvis combined with possible arteriography and embolization can be life saving.

Initial evaluation of pelvic injuries includes an AP radiograph (Fig. 42-41). Further imaging includes inlet and outlet views. Associated acetabular fractures and lumbar spine injuries require 45-degree oblique (Judet) views and AP and lateral radiographs of the lumbosacral spine. Most pelvic injuries will also need a CT scan with 3-mm cuts to evaluate a posterior injury to the pelvis. A CT scan is best used for evaluation of the sacrum and sacroiliac joints.

There are two major classifications for pelvic fractures. Tile classified pelvic fractures based on the stability of the fracture.[9,10] Type A fractures were stable; type B fractures were rotationally unstable but vertically stable; and type C fractures were rotationally and vertically unstable. Burgess and Young classified pelvic fractures according to the mechanism of injury: lateral compression, anterior-posterior compression, and vertical shear or combined mechanism injuries.[11]

It is essential in the treatment of pelvic fractures to recognize the unstable injury and to treat the patient for potential shock, if it is not already present. Initial stabilization of the patient and assessment of all associated injuries are essential. If the patient is already in shock and does not respond to standard volume replacement, stabilization of the pelvis can help significantly to contain hemorrhage and stabilize the patient for further diagnostic evaluation. Stabilization of the pelvis can consist of formal application of an external fixator, emergent application of a pelvic fixator clamp, or simple pelvic binders. There are commercially available pelvic binders for such treatment. However, application of a sheet tied around the pelvis can suffice temporarily.

Continued, unexplained blood loss despite fracture stabilization and aggressive resuscitation is an indication for angiography. Early recognition of potential arterial bleeding should include early notification of the interventional radiology team. Angiography and embolization may be required in up to 20% of anterior-posterior injuries, vertical shear injuries, and combined mechanical injuries. Surgical exploration with ligation of bleeding sites and packing of the retroperitoneal space is most common in European centers and fraught with danger. The space is packed and the packing is changed every 2 to 3 days. In general, opening of the retroperitoneal space is not recommended. It is important for the trauma surgeon to recognize there are possible pitfalls.

Definitive treatment of the mechanically unstable pelvic injury with an external fixator is contraindicated and is associated with a high failure rate. In patients who are hemodynamically stable, an emergent external fixator is not required. Atomic and definitive fixation with open reduction and internal fixation should improve the outcome.

Isolated fractures occurring in elderly patients from a single fall are treated by bed rest for a few days until acute symptoms subside. The patient is then gradually mobilized and weight bearing is allowed as it is tolerated. Because the anterior structures are not contributing to the weight-bearing arch, there is no problem of pelvic

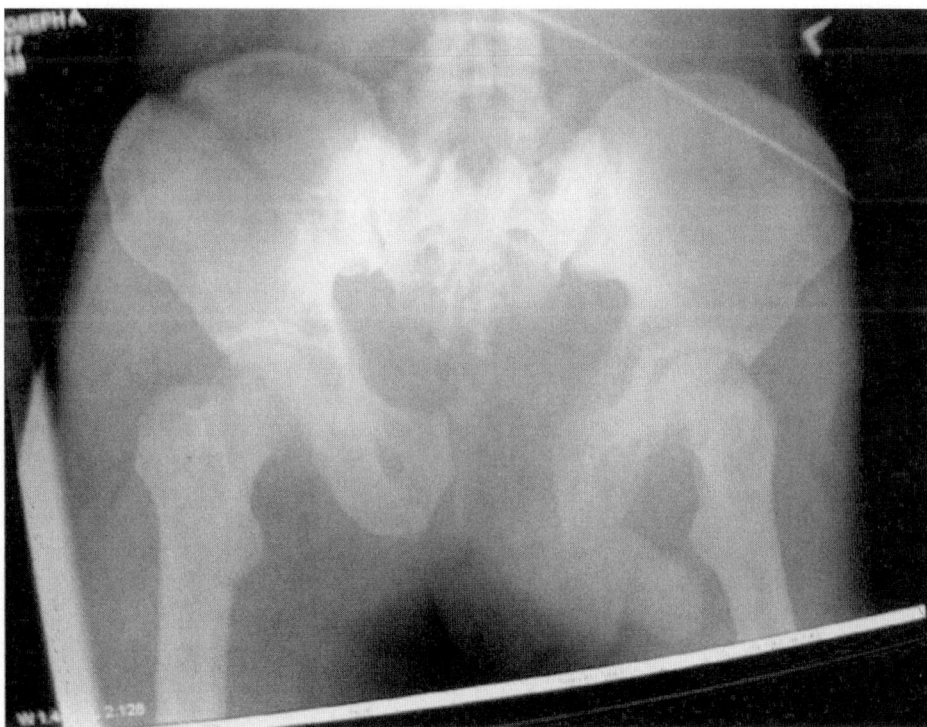

FIG. 42-41. AP radiograph of a patient with a fractured pelvis. There is widening of the symphysis pubis and a displaced fracture of the right ilium.

instability. Complications to be prevented and treated are deep vein thrombosis, urinary retention, and ileus.

Isolated fractures of the iliac wing are usually the result of a direct blow to the iliac crest. If the major portion of the iliac wing is intact, weight bearing will not be affected. Fractures of the coccyx occur from a direct fall onto the coccyx. These fractures are treated with cushions and avoidance of pressure on the coccyx. Fractures of the sacrum may occur from direct trauma. Most fractures are stable and impacted and can be treated with weight bearing as tolerated. Neurologic compromise may be present and is associated with poor outcomes. Unstable fractures are best treated with internal fixation.

All patients with pelvic fractures, whether stable or unstable, should be made aware of potential loss of function. Loss of function may occur from pelvic malunion, pain, and complications from the injury. It is common for these patients to have persistent pain despite minimally displaced fractures. The etiology of this pain is not well understood.

Acetabular Fractures

Acetabular fractures are a subset of pelvic fractures that involve the acetabulum. These intra-articular fractures may result in posttraumatic arthritis of the hip and are sometimes associated with hip dislocations, which are discussed in the next section.

Thorough evaluation of acetabulum fractures requires 45-degree oblique views (Judet views) of the pelvis to assess the integrity of the anterior and posterior columns and the anterior and posterior walls. In addition, CT-scans are helpful in fully delineating fracture patterns and demonstrating the presence of intra-articular bony fragments. Acetabular fractures were classified by Letournel into 10 types.[12] There are five simple acetabular fractures: posterior wall, posterior column, anterior wall, anterior column, and transverse fractures. There are five complex fracture types: T-shaped; posterior wall and posterior column; transverse and posterior wall; anterior

with posterior hemitransverse; and both column fractures. This classification integrates pelvic anatomy and fracture biomechanics into useful clinical material that allows the surgeon to correctly approach these difficult fractures. The classification is useful for determining treatment but is not predictive in prognosis.

Nondisplaced or minimally displaced fractures are determined after complete evaluation of the radiographs and acetabular CT scans. Radiographs should be taken with traction removed and preferably with stress applied. Any degree of incongruence involving the weight-bearing surface of the acetabulum is unacceptable and is an indication for surgical treatment.

Nondisplaced fractures may be treated with a period of traction followed by progressive weight bearing. An alternative treatment would be immediate nonweight bearing on that acetabulum fracture. A complication of this strategy would be displacement of the fracture. Healing of the joint surface with anatomic restoration has been shown to result in excellent long-term results. The amount of residual articular displacement affects the development of posttraumatic arthritis. Studies show that 2 mm of intra-articular displacement of fractures and incongruous hip reduction, marginal impaction greater than 2 mm, and intra-articular debris accelerate the development of arthritis.

Hip Dislocation

Dislocation of the hip is often caused by a force applied to the femur and can be associated with fractures of the acetabulum or femoral head (Fig. 42-42). The most common mechanism of injury is motor vehicles accidents. Force applied to an abducted hip can result in anterior dislocation, while striking the knee on a car dashboard with the hip flexed and adducted, results in posterior dislocations. Posterior dislocations are often associated with a fracture of the posterior wall of the acetabulum. Direct trauma to the greater trochanter from a lateral direction can result in medial wall fractures or central acetabular fractures/dislocations.

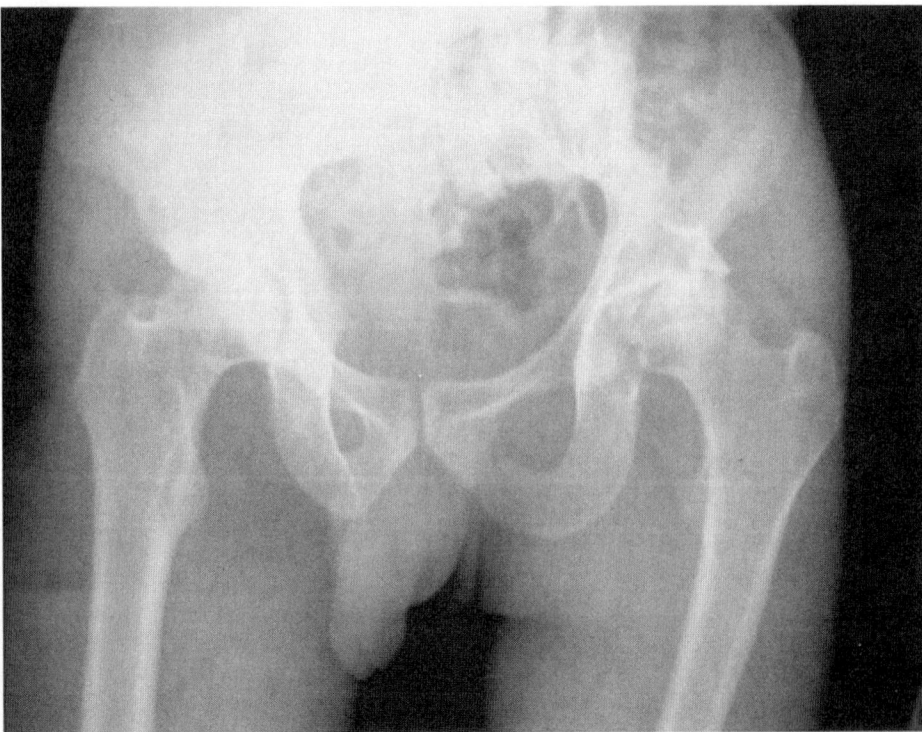

FIG. 42-42. AP radiograph of a patient with a fracture-dislocation of the left hip. The femoral head is not within the acetabulum and there is fragmentation of the acetabulum. A CT scan is indicated to better evaluate this injury.

Thorough evaluation of hip dislocations often requires Judet radiographic views and additional CT scans. Similar to patients with pelvic fractures, these patients may have other major injuries and careful evaluation of the chest, abdomen, spine, and neurologic status is necessary. Prompt reduction of hip dislocations is essential in minimizing the incidence of osteonecrosis of the femoral head.

Anterior Hip Dislocations

Anterior hip dislocations resulting from forced abduction or anterior-posterior force to an abducted thigh are much less common than posterior dislocation (10 to 15% of all hip dislocations). Femoral head fractures may occur in a significant percentage of these cases and late osteonecrosis may occur in approximately 10%. There is an incidence of late posttraumatic arthritis with these dislocations. The patient often presents with the lower extremity abducted and externally rotated. Closed reduction is possible under adequate sedation by longitudinal traction and subsequent flexion and internal rotation. Postreduction radiographs and CT scan are essential to evaluate the quality of the reduction. Intra-articular fragments or inadequate reduction are an indication for arthrotomy and open reduction. Postreduction treatment is usually followed by early mobilization and protective weight bearing for 6 weeks.

Posterior Hip Dislocations

Posterior hip dislocations are often associated with posterior wall fractures. The presence of a significant fracture impairs stability of the dislocation after reduction is achieved. The patient often presents with the lower extremity adducted, internally rotated, and flexed. However, once the hip has been completely dislocated posteriorly, it may appear shortened and externally rotated. Sometimes the femoral head or acetabular fractures are associated with this dislocation. Sciatic nerve injuries are present in up to 15% of posterior hip dislocations. Closed reduction is usually accomplished by longitudinal traction, followed by gentle abduction and external rotation. Stability of the reduction should be determined at the time of closed reduction. If the reduction is unstable and associated with a posterior wall fracture, open reduction and internal fixation is indicated. A postreduction CT scan is indicated to rule out the presence of intra-articular fragments. The timing of reduction is associated with the incidence of late osteonecrosis of the femoral head. Osteonecrosis of the femoral head has been reported to range from 10 to 50% and is often delayed for several years following the injury.[13] Stable reductions can be started on protective weight bearing immediately. The patient is cautioned against excessive flexion and internal rotation of the hip. Patients who receive internal fixation are usually treated with non-weight-bearing or toe-touch weight-bearing therapy for approximately 6 weeks. Long-term complications include osteonecrosis, formation of heterotopic ossification, and posttraumatic arthritis. Most sciatic nerve injuries are neurapraxias and 60 to 80% of the patients with these injuries will recover to some degree. Although full recovery of strength is unusual, good function can be achieved in 60 to 80% of patients.

Femur Fractures

The mortality and morbidity of proximal femur fractures has significantly improved with modern methods of treatment. However, a proximal femur fracture still represents a major challenge to the health care system with the increasing age of the population. These fractures generally occur in the seventh and eighth decades of life. Femoral neck and intertrochanteric fractures occur with approximately equal frequency and similar epidemiology. Osteoporosis is a major contributing factor to hip fractures. An increasing awareness of this disease accompanied by new methods of treatment may facilitate the prevention of proximal femur fractures. This is extremely significant in light of the high mortality rate of hip fractures in the elderly, which have been reported to be as high as 50% in the first year.

Femoral Neck Fractures

Femoral neck fractures are most commonly related to falls. The patient most often complains of pain in the groin or thigh and is unable to bear weight on the injured extremity. The lower extremity appears shortened and externally rotated. Most attempts at motion, especially rotational motion, cause severe pain. The diagnosis is confirmed by anteroposterior and lateral radiographs of the hip. A careful physical examination is necessary to rule out other injuries to the patient.

The most widely used classification of femoral neck fractures is the Garden classification (Fig. 42-43).[14] Type I fractures are incomplete fractures with valgus impaction. Type II fractures are complete without displacement. Type III fractures are complete fractures with partial displacement. Type IV fractures are complete fractures with total displacement. This classification is useful in determining prognosis and treatment.

The undisplaced type I and type II fractures can sometimes be difficult to diagnose. Some patients may have surprisingly little pain and are even able to bear weight. Usually, internal rotation of the hip causing pain and ecchymosis over the greater trochanter should raise suspicion of an undisplaced fracture. A bone scan or MRI should be performed in any patient with unexplained hip pain and negative radiographs after a fall. Types III and IV fractures can be easily diagnosed on plain radiographs. These fractures are at risk for nonunion, malunion, and osteonecrosis.

The femoral head has a precarious blood supply. The majority of the blood supply comes in through the neck and through the subcapital epiphyseal vessels that run in the inferior capsule. The small contribution in patients can come from the artery of the ligamentum teres. Disruption of the blood supply often occurs with displaced

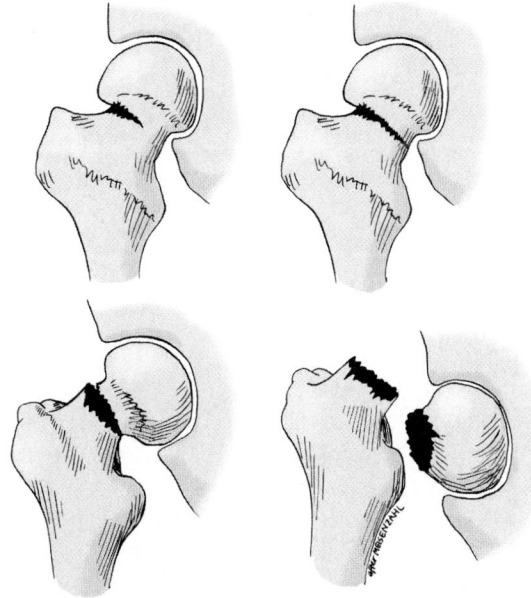

FIG. 42-43. *Types of subcapital fracture in Garden classification (see text).*

femoral neck fractures. In elderly patients, surgical treatment allows early mobilization and significantly decreased mortality and morbidity. Early fixation of fractures has been associated with a decreased incidence of osteonecrosis but should not preclude adequate medical evaluation and clearance prior to surgery.

Internal fixation is indicated in nondisplaced fractures. This allows early weight bearing and prevents possible future displacement of the fracture. The treatment of displaced femoral neck fractures is more controversial. Recent studies indicate that the best functional outcome and the least number of repeat operations are performed when these patients are treated with initial total hip replacement. Classical treatment of these fractures has been divided between hemiarthroplasty and internal fixation. Hemiarthroplasty can be performed either with bipolar hip replacements or unipolar hip replacements. Unipolar hip replacements articulate between a metal prosthetic surface and the acetabular cartilage. Bipolar hip replacements have a second articulation between an inner bearing of metal and polyethylene. The advantage of bipolar hip replacements is controversial and some studies indicate that there is relatively little advantage in using a bipolar hip replacement. Total hip replacement surgery includes replacing the acetabular cartilage with a prosthesis. Total hip replacements can be fixed in the bone with either a press-fit or cemented application. Careful technique and preparation of the bone should lead to prosthetic life span of greater than 10 years.

Displaced femoral neck fractures can also be treated with reduction and internal fixation. This method of treatment is often reserved for younger, more active, individuals. This method of treatment results in possible nonunion, malunion, and osteonecrosis. These complications are avoided when arthroplasty is used in conjunction with resection of the fracture.

Postoperatively, patients are mobilized as rapidly as possible. Because of the high incidence of probable embolic disease in elderly patients after hip fracture, some form of preoperative prophylaxis is indicated. Treatment may include low-dose aspirin, Warfarin,

antiembolism stockings, pneumatic compression devices, and low molecular weight heparin. The patient should bear only partial weight until the fracture is healed, usually within 4 to 6 months. If a prosthesis has been used, the patient usually can begin weight bearing as tolerated with ambulatory aids. These patients must be cautioned against possible dislocation. Patients with hemiarthroplasty may complain of groin pain. These patients also must be cautioned against possible infection and dislocation in the future.

Intertrochanteric and Subtrochanteric Fractures

These fractures occur in the elderly and are related to falls, and after significant trauma in younger individuals. In general, these are mechanically less stable than femoral neck fractures. The instability of these fractures is related to the comminution of the posteromedial cortex in the area of the calcar and lesser trochanter (Fig. 42-44). This results in a varus deformity of the proximal femur. Patients present with an inability to bear weight, shortening, external rotation of the lower extremity, and often swelling or ecchymosis about the hip. These patients may have more significant blood loss related to the hip fracture.

Nondisplaced fractures can be much more difficult to diagnose based on initial clinical and radiographic evaluation. Similar to patients with femoral neck fractures, these patients may report hip pain with weight bearing or certain movements. Further diagnostic testing for an occult fracture can include a bone scan, MRI, or CT scan. The bone scan is most reliable 72 hours after the fracture. An MRI is more expensive, but accurate within hours after injury.

The classification of intertrochanteric fractures by Evans was based on the ability to achieve and maintain an anatomic reduction. Most surgeons will find it more useful to define these fracture patterns as either stable or unstable. An unstable fracture pattern will tend to displace and collapse into varus. Stable fractures will generally resist compressive loads and heal with minimal displacement.

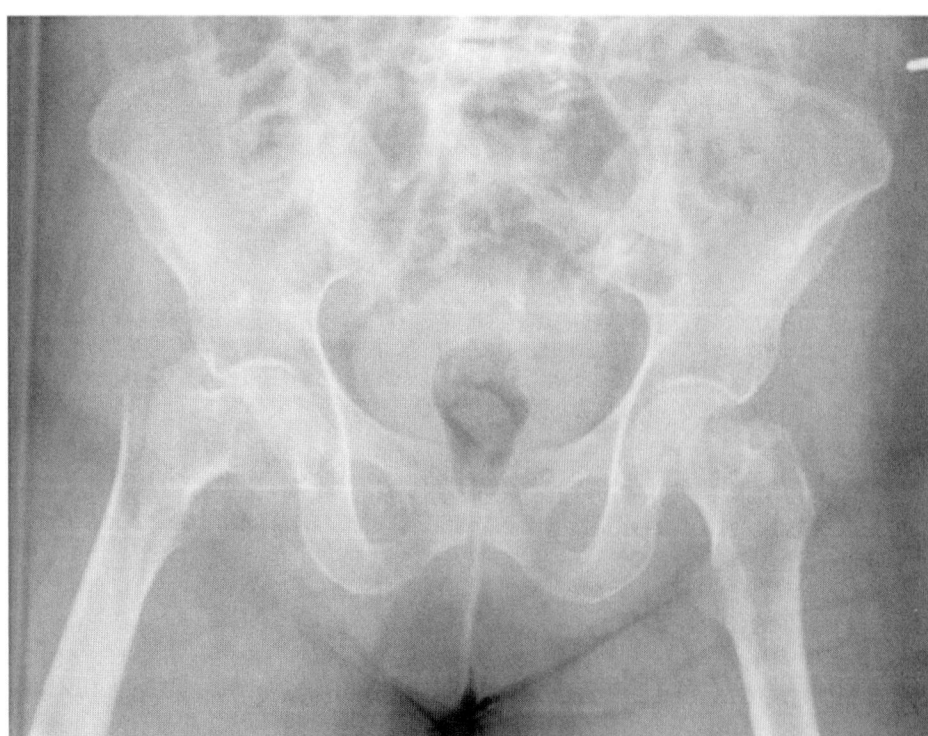

FIG. 42-44. AP radiograph of a patient with an intertrochanteric fracture of the right femur. There is minimal displacement. Internal fixation is indicated so the patient can be mobilized.

Subtrochanteric femur fractures occur more distally below the level of the lesser trochanter. These fractures occur within 5 cm of the lesser trochanter. Below this level, the fracture is considered a femoral shaft fracture. The subtrochanteric region of the proximal femur is a high stress area. These fractures tend to be more unstable and require stronger implants to resist varus deformity and implant failure.

Classically, the sliding hip screw with a side plate continues to be the preferred implant for most stable and unstable intertrochanteric hip fractures. Nonetheless, failures with this implant remain common with unstable intertrochanteric hip fractures. For this reason, modifications to the side plate have been advocated in an attempt to decrease treatment failures. Modifications include proximal extension of the side plate to achieve better fixation of the proximal fragment. The Medoff sliding plate allows additional impaction of the sliding screw in the axis of the shaft. A percutaneous compression plate allows percutaneous application of a side plate with two sliding hip screws to achieve rotational stability of the proximal fragment. Position and type of hip screw also has been found to be important in the fixation of these fractions. The location of the screw in the femoral has been shown to be an important variable in the strength of the bone implant construct. Modifications of the screw with deeper threads or wires that extend out of the screw have been used to improve the fixation of the screw within the femoral head.

More recently, fixed-angle sliding screws that incorporate an intramedullary nail to gain purchase to the shaft have been used to fix these fractures. The implant itself acts as a buttress against excessive fracture collapse and shaft medialization in unstable fracture patterns. These devices can be inserted percutaneously and offer potentially smaller insult to the fracture zone as well as to the patient. The intramedullary implants can be locked distally to prevent implant subsidence within the femoral canal. Several studies have been done comparing the efficacy of intramedullary fixation to extramedullary plate fixation of these fractures. The conclusion is that either treatment is generally successful when surgeons have been properly trained in their use. Plate fixation has a slight advantage in prospective randomized studies.

Finally, calcar-substituting hemiarthroplasty or total joint arthroplasty remain surgical options in patients with severely fragmented or pathologic peritrochanteric fractures. However, the risk of a major surgical insult for these frequently debilitated patients must be considered. Arthroplasty is usually reserved for salvage of treatment failures.

Postoperative treatment is very similar to that of femoral neck fractures. The amount of weight the patient bears on the implants should be decided by the treating surgeon. Often, weight bearing as-tolerated can be started immediately. Prophylaxis of deep vein thrombosis is a standard part of the postoperative treatment. Perioperative antibiotics are used, usually for 24 to 48 hours following surgery. Patients with hip fractures often require prolonged physiotherapy. These patients are often transferred to either acute rehabilitation units or to subacute rehabilitation centers. These patients often lose some ability to ambulate and may require ambulatory aids to assist with their ambulation.

Fractures of the Femoral Shaft

Femoral shaft fractures may occur at any age from severe violence (Fig. 42-45). However, these injuries may occur from less severe, direct torsional stress. Multiply-injured trauma patients require evaluation of any associated injuries of the head, abdomen, and chest. These patients present with instability of the lower extremity, pain

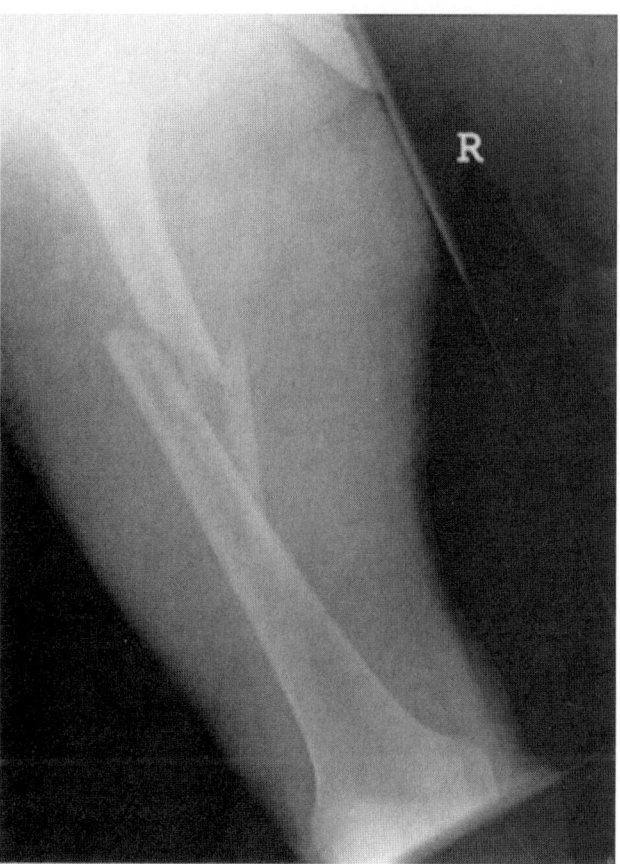

FIG. 42-45. AP radiograph of a patient with a minimally comminuted fracture of the femur. This can be treated closed with traction but is more often treated with internal fixation. It can be internally fixed with a plate or intramedullary rod. An intramedullary rod is more often used.

with motion, external rotational deformity, and shortening of the affected lower extremity. A complete neurovascular examination is essential because there may be injury to the sciatic or femoral nerve or femoral artery. Open femur fractures are associated with a 10% incidence of limb-threatening vascular injury. Associated femoral neck fractures or knee ligament injuries occur in approximately 5% of patients and must be intentionally looked for. Any signs of distal ischemia should be evaluated by vascular surgeons and is indication for immediate vascular exploration. Arteriography can be done in the operating room to save precious time.

Femoral shaft fractures are classified by their location (proximal third, middle third, and distal third), geometry of the fracture line, degree of comminution, and severity of the soft-tissue injury. Winquist devised a classification system to describe fracture comminution (Table 42-7).[15]

Table 42-7
Winquist Classification of Femoral Fractures

Type I	Minimal or no comminutation
Type II	Less than 50% of cortex comminuted
Type III	More that 50% of cortex comminuted
Type IV	Complete loss of cortical integrity

SOURCE: Reproduced with permission from Winquist RA, Hansen ST Jr.: Comminuted fractures of the femoral shaft treated by intramedullay nailing. *Orthop Clin North Am* 11:633, 1980.

Femoral shaft fractures were historically treated in traction. This method had several disadvantages, such as shortening, rotational malunion, and knee stiffness. Traction is now mostly used as a temporizing measure until patients are stable enough to undergo definitive surgical stabilization.

The gold standard of treatment of these fractures is reamed, locked, antegrade intramedullary nailing performed through a closed technique. Opening of the fracture site is associated with increased infection and nonunion. Reaming of the femoral canal is associated with better union rates. Antegrade application of the nail from the trochanteric side of the femur is the traditional method. Recently, trauma surgeons have used a retrograde insertion of the nail for certain fracture types. These fractures can include a more distal fracture, bilateral fractures, ipsilateral femoral shaft and tibia fracture, ipsilateral femoral shaft, and femoral neck fractures. Locking of the femoral nail helps prevent shortening of the extremity and rotational deformity. Locking of the femoral nails does not increase the rates of nonunion.

Femoral shaft fractures, by virtue of the surrounding muscle mass, often heal well. Studies show that union rates of greater than 95% can be achieved with the above methods. Plating of femoral shaft fractures is reserved for special indications. These may include patients with open physes, multiply-injured patients, and patients who for some reason cannot be placed on a fracture table. The timing of fracture stabilization is extremely important. The benefits of early stabilization of femoral shaft fractures in multiply-injured patients are well established. Bone and associates demonstrated, in a prospective, randomized series, that early femoral shaft stabilization in patients with an Injury Severity Score (ISS) greater than 18, leads to decreases in the incidence of adult respiratory distress syndrome (ARDS) and pulmonary complications and in length of stay in intensive care units.[15a] No pulmonary complications occurred in the less-severely injured group (ISS less than 18). Patients who underwent immediate stabilization spent fewer days in the hospital and incurred lower costs. Patients with isolated femoral shaft fractures do not have increased morbidity with delayed stabilization of their fractures.

Complications of treating femoral shaft fractures include infection (<1%), delayed union, nonunion, malunion, compartment syndrome, neurologic injury, and heterotopic ossification. Nonunion is more common in patients with a history of smoking and diabetes.

Distal Femur Fractures

Distal femoral fractures occur in all age groups as a result of a variety of injuries. Older patients with osteoporotic bone may suffer this fracture from simple falls. Younger patients usually require higher-energy injuries, such as a motor vehicle accident, pedestrian injury, or falls from heights, to suffer supracondylar femur fractures. Patients usually present with pain, swelling, and deformity. Simple nondisplaced fractures may present only with a knee effusion. Supracondylar fractures are intra-articular fractures because of the large extension of the suprapatellar pouch of the knee. Even these fractures, which may be nonarticular, may result in scarring within the suprapatellar pouch and knee stiffness. Intracondylar fractures, by definition, involve the articular cartilage of the distal femur. Knee stiffness and posttraumatic arthritis is a major late complication of these fractures. The most widely accepted classification for these fractures is the AO classification by Mueller. Type A fractures are extra-articular; type B fractures are partially articular; and type C fractures are intra-articular. These fractures are further subdivided based on location and combination.

Successful treatment of these fractures involves four major principles: (1) anatomic reduction of the fracture fragments, particularly intra-articular reduction; (2) preservation of the blood supply to the fracture fragments; (3) stable internal fixation; and (4) early, active, pain-free motion. Treatment is generally surgical for most of these fractures. Occasionally, a nondisplaced fracture is stable enough to be treated nonoperatively in a cast-brace. The majority of displaced fractures, including nondisplaced intra-articular fractures are treated with surgery. There are a variety of surgical methods available to the orthopaedic surgeon for stabilizing these fractures. All of these methods take into account the principles that were previously described. Classically, these fractures were treated with anatomic reduction of the articular fragments and reattachment of the articular fragments to the femoral shaft with a lateral plate. Occasionally, the combination is so severe that a second medial plate may be necessary. More recently, it has been recognized that anatomic reduction of the metaphyseal fragments is unnecessary and may be undesirable because of the periosteal stripping necessary to achieve it. Currently, methods of inserting these plates percutaneously are being explored. Restoration of the articular segments to the shaft also can be achieved through a retrograde intramedullary rod. These rods are similar to the antegrade nails but are locked distally at the knee and proximally through freehand methods. If the retrograde nail is short enough, it can be similarly locked through a jig attached to the nail distally.

The most current technology for fixation of these difficult fractures includes modification of the lateral side plates. These side plates now have threaded holes to lock in the screws at fixed angles. The pull-out strength of these locking plates is greatly improved. Postoperatively, patients treated with internal plate or rod fixation are started on early range-of-motion therapy without weight bearing. Complications include infection, nonunion, malunion, knee stiffness, and posttraumatic arthritis.

Occasionally, some of these fractures may be so osteoporotic that reconstruction is impossible. When this is the case, a distal femoral endoprosthetic replacement can be used. Prosthetic replacement allows immediate weight bearing, early knee motion, and possibly better functional outcomes.

A patient with open growth plate fractures may have growth abnormalities. Absolute anatomic reductions are valuable in reducing this complication. The Salter-Harris classification system groups fractures through the growth plate into five types. Type I is through the growth plate; type II is through the growth plate with extension into the metaphysis; type III is through the growth plate with extension into the epiphysis; type IV crosses the growth plate; and type V is a crush of the growth plate. The higher the type, the greater the risk of a growth abnormality. All growth plates can sustain fractures, but the most common site is the distal femur.

Patella Fractures

Patella fractures are usually caused by direct trauma to the patella but may also occur as a result of avulsion forces on the patella (Fig. 42-46). This happens when the knee experiences sudden forced flexion while the quadriceps muscle is actively contracting. Fractures are classified by their geometry and location. The more common fractures are transverse secondary to avulsion forces; comminuted or stellate fractures may be caused by direct trauma. The patella functions as an integral part of the extensor mechanism and displacement of the patella usually is an indication that the extensor retinaculum has been interrupted. Disruption of the extensor retinaculum will make active extension of the knee impossible. Similar

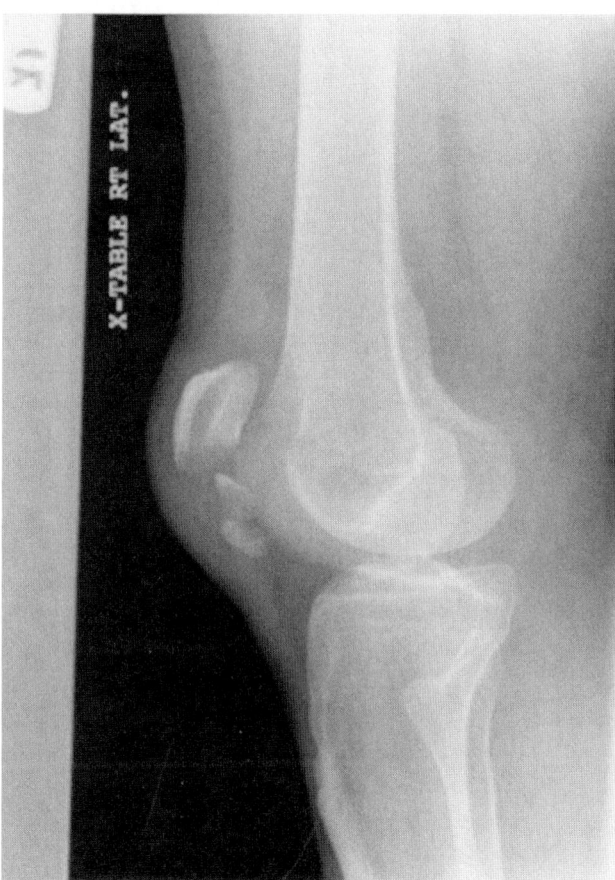

FIG. 42-46. *Lateral radiograph of a patient with a fracture patella. The inferior pole of the patella is comminuted and displaced. Internal fixation is indicated if the patient cannot actively extend the knee.*

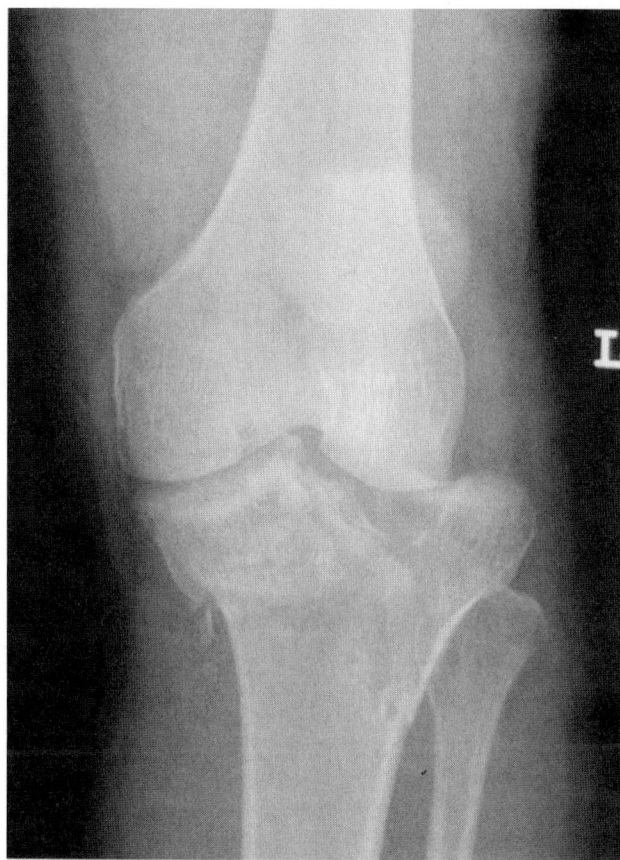

FIG. 42-47. *AP radiograph of a patient with a comminuted tibial plateau fracture. This injury is usually treated with an open reduction and internal fixation.*

soft-tissue disruptions of either the quadriceps tendon or patellar tendon may result from a similar mechanism of injury and present with lack of active extension. These injuries usually present with tenderness and a palpable defect over the ruptured tendon. The treatment of the soft-tissue injuries is surgical repair. The treatment of patella fractures is to restore the extensor mechanism and reconstruct the articular surface of the patella.

Nondisplaced fractures of the patella require immobilization in extension. This can be accomplished with a plaster cylinder cast or knee immobilizer. Immobilization of 6 to 8 weeks should allow healing and prevent separation of the fragments. Radiographs need to be obtained at 7 to 10 days to be certain that displacement has not occurred. The patient may bear weight with the knee in extension when using crutches.

Displaced fractures require open reduction and internal fixation. The goal of treatment is to restore the articular surface and repair the fragments securely enough to start early range-of-motion therapy. Usually protected weight bearing with the knee in extension is started postoperatively. The patient is also allowed to do active and passive range-of-motion exercises to the knee.

Grossly comminuted fractures may require excision of some of the fragments and repair of the soft tissue to the bony surface. In this case, early range-of-motion exercise is usually postponed for 6 to 8 weeks. This treatment by partial patellectomy is associated with atrophy and weakness of the quadriceps mechanism. In addition, long-term follow-up studies demonstrate significant patellofemoral osteoarthritis in the majority of patients treated with partial

patellectomy. For these reasons, patella fractures should be reconstructed whenever possible.

Complications of patella fractures include nonunion, malunion, and symptomatic hardware. Nonunions may not be symptomatic and would need no treatment. Symptomatic nonunions should be treated with revision surgery using established fracture fixation techniques. Symptomatic hardware is usually treated with removal of hardware after the fracture has completely healed.

Tibial Plateau Fractures

Tibial plateau fractures involve the articular surface of the proximal tibia. These fractures occur when the knee experiences a varus or valgus force, with or without a combined action or compression force (Fig. 42-47).[16] The force causes failure of the bone or ligaments, but rarely both within the same compartment. Lateral plateau fractures are the most common followed by bicondylar and finally medial fractures. Lateral plateau fractures usually occur from a force directed from the lateral side with a resultant valgus force. The amount of force and degree of osteopenia determines the magnitude of depression, displacement, and combination. Typically, younger patients have split-type fractures. Elderly patients with osteopenia usually have split-depression fractures.

The principles of treatment are to restore the articular surface, maintain alignment of the articular surface with the rest of the leg, and to resume early range-of-motion exercise. These goals are best accomplished with internal fixation of the fracture. The challenge for the orthopaedic surgeon is to achieve these goals with avoidance of the severe complications that can occur with this fracture.

Surgical indications for treatment have changed from the historical indication of greater than 10 degrees of instability and greater than 10 mm of joint depression. With improved surgical treatment options, articular step-off of greater than 3 mm or a widening of greater than 5 mm are indicators for surgery. Instability of greater than 5 degrees or angulation of greater than 5 degrees should also be treated surgically. Any bony avulsions of the cruciate ligaments should be repaired at the time of internal fixation. The menisci should be repaired and saved whenever possible.

Nonsurgical treatment consists of short-term immobilization with a long leg cast followed by bracing or immediate cast-bracing with delayed weight bearing. The non-weight-bearing period should last approximately 8 weeks and full weight bearing should be deferred for 3 months. If loss of reduction occurs during the nonsurgical period, surgical intervention is recommended to prevent malunion and unacceptable alignment.

Possible surgical treatment options include plating versus external fixation. Plating for unicondylar plateau fractures with anatomic reduction of the articular surface is the treatment of choice. Double plating for bicondylar fractures risks soft-tissue compromise. This may result in the need for soft-tissue coverage such as gastrocnemius or soleus flap. The timing of plating is critical to achieving a satisfactory result. Bicondylar fractures are often associated with large soft-tissue contusions and excessive swelling. Definitive reconstruction should be delayed until the soft-tissue envelope has stabilized and swelling is minimal. During this period of time, the patient can be treated in a splint, skeletal calcaneal traction, or spanning external fixator. These are temporary treatment options which may involve prolonged hospitalization. This need for hospitalization may alter the surgeon's treatment plan in favor of treatment of temporizing external fixation and splinting.

Procedures have been devised to try to preserve the soft tissue envelope. Anatomic reduction of the articular surface was obtained with screw fixation. Often these screws can be placed percutaneously, however a formal open reduction of the articular surface is performed when necessary. The articular surface is reattached to the shaft by using a hybrid external fixator. Proximally, the fixator includes small K-wires placed under tension, distally. Classic half pins are employed; thus, the name hybrid external fixator. When possible, the proximal pins can be substituted with classic half pins if the fragments are large enough. The use of this type of treatment has resulted in a significant decrease in wound complications.

Fair to poor results occur in approximately 18 to 32% of fractures treated by limited internal fixation and external fixation. Posttraumatic arthritis and deep infections still occur, but are rare. More commonly, with the use of hybrid external fixators, pin tract infections and septic arthritis are possible. Tibial plateau fractures may lead to degenerative arthritis resulting from instability, malalignment, articular incongruity, or initial articular insult. Arthritic changes can take 5 to 7 years to develop, so patients need to be counseled as to this potential problem. Preservation of the menisci is important and correlates with better results. Uniformly good to excellent results do not occur even with newer and less-invasive techniques. Because of the potential for significant complications, patients who sustain complex fractures of the tibial plateau should be informed of the severity of their injury and potential for poor outcome regardless of the method of fracture treatment.

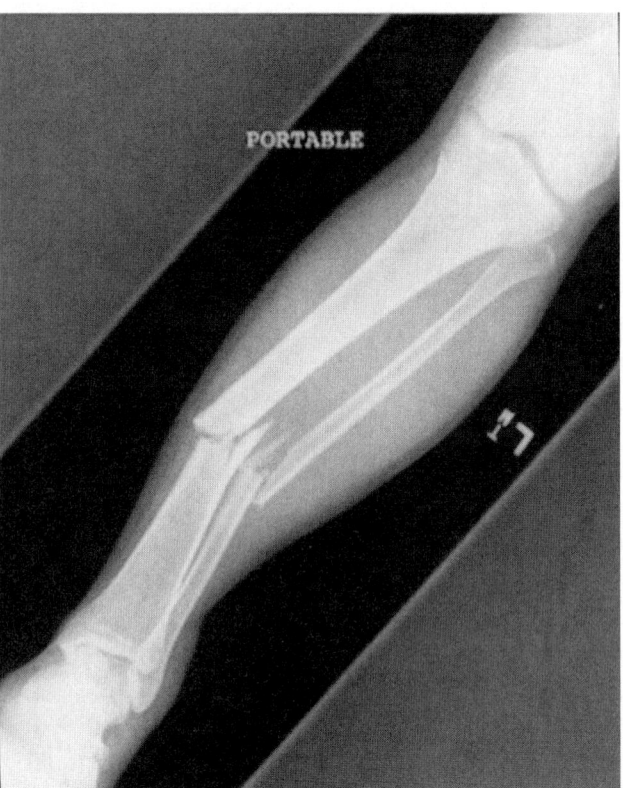

FIG. 42-48. AP radiograph of a patient with a fractured tibia and fibula. There is minimal comminution and valgus angulation. This injury can be treated with a closed reduction and long-leg cast or with intramedullary fixation.

Tibial Shaft Fractures

Tibia shaft fractures result from direct traumas such as motor vehicle accidents, sport injuries, and falls (Fig. 42-48).[17] All age groups are affected and approximately 30% of fractures are open injuries. The high incidence of open fractures is a result of the subcutaneous position of the bone. Nondisplaced fractures may present with localized pain and swelling, and an inability to bear weight, but lack obvious deformity. Displaced or angulated fractures are easily diagnosed on physical examination. The physician must perform a careful neurovascular examination of the extremity with a special concern to any signs or symptoms of compartment syndrome. There is no significant difference in the rate of healing of tibial fractures according to the location of the fracture, plane of the fracture, or treatment of the fracture. Rate of healing appears to be more a relationship with the severity of the trauma. Fractures caused by high-energy trauma with open wounds, such as those associated with automobile accidents, have the longest rate of healing.

Classification of tibial fractures is geared more to the severity of the injury. Open fractures are most commonly classified by the Gustilo and Anderson classification.[13] However, the intraobserver agreement of the Gustilo classification for open fractures is relatively low at 60%. The orthopaedic community still needs a better classification for tibia shaft fractures, especially open fractures.

Treatment options vary widely and should be discussed with regard to open versus closed injuries. Closed tibia fractures, in general, can be treated successfully with closed reduction and cast immobilization. The cast is usually changed to a fracture brace sometime during treatment. Indications for cast treatment are usually limited to fractures with no more than 12 mm of initial shortening. Sometimes severe soft-tissue injury or pending compartment syndrome makes casting impossible. Other special considerations are segmental fractures, ipsilateral limb injury, multitrauma, intra-articular extension, and bilateral tibial fractures. Although, cast treatment is still possible in these situations, most authors recommend surgical stabilization of the tibia. This indication is also extended to higher-energy, closed tibia fractures with greater displacement and more instability. There are few prospective randomized studies comparing closed, displaced tibia shaft fractures treated with surgery to nonoperative treatment. Most indications for surgical treatment of closed tibia fractures remain relative and generally are at the discretion of the treating orthopaedic surgeon. Surgical treatment consists of reamed or nonreamed nailing of the fracture. These fractures also can be successfully treated with plates and screws. Reamed intramedullary nailing has higher rates of union, but has an increased risk of compartment syndrome.

Management of open tibia fractures remains a challenge to the orthopaedic surgeon. These fractures are usually the result of high-energy, direct trauma and there may be associated trauma elsewhere in the body. In some cases, the limb is so severely traumatized that salvage of the limb may be impossible. Scoring systems have been devised to try to help the surgeon make this difficult decision of initial, immediate amputation. The most important criteria are the severity of muscle damage, severity and timing of vascular injury, and the absence of plantar sensation.

Stabilization of open tibia fractures can be performed with internal fixation or external fixation. External fixation has long been the standard of care for open tibia fractures. The main benefit has been to limit any further devascularization of the leg while providing needed stability. However, studies comparing external fixation with intramedullary nailing conclude that intramedullary nailing gives better results. Intramedullary nailing can be performed either reamed or nonreamed. Nonreamed nailing has been touted as less invasive and at potentially less risk of infection. Prospective randomized studies have not been able to confirm this hypothesis. Because of the ability to statically lock tibia nails quite proximal and distal, nailing has now been extended to the proximal and distal segments of the tibia. Extended applications of tibial nailing is certainly more challenging for the treating orthopaedic surgeon. However, with proper technique, good to excellent results can be obtained.

Complications of intramedullary nailing include knee pain, malalignment, nonunion, and compartment syndrome. External fixation can result in malunion and nonunion. Plate fixation may result in a nonunion and compartment syndrome. Finally, cast treatment is most commonly associated with malunion and delayed union.

In summary, intramedullary nailing is increasingly important in the treatment of both closed and open tibia shaft fractures. When compared to the nonsurgical treatment of displaced closed fractures, intramedullary nailing shows improved results. Because of these improved results, extension of the indications of reamed intramedullary nailing has now included its use in both proximal and distal fractures of the tibial shaft.

Ankle Injury

Injuries to the ankle are common. The majority are ankle sprains that need temporary rest and completely heal with no residual consequences. There are more significant ligament injuries that occur to the ankle that can present like a simple ankle sprain. These more significant ligament injuries need to be treated with at least immobilization in a cast, and sometimes with surgery to allow maximum recovery. The patients with ankle fractures can be treated with a

reduction and cast immobilization or open reduction and internal fixation. The patients also should have physical therapy after their injury has healed to regain their motion, strength, and ankle proprioception.

The mechanism of injury can suggest what tissues may be injured. Almost all ankle sprains are caused by inversion of the ankle with axial loading. This means the ankle is turned in and the weight is placed on the lateral aspect of the foot. This leads to injuries to the lateral ligaments. Depending on the degree of injury, the patient can sustain a strain, sprain, or complete disruption of the lateral ligaments. The degree of swelling and ecchymosis is directly correlated with the degree of ligamentous injury and is a simple means of determining the significance of the injury. If there is concern that the ligaments are completely torn and that the ankle is unstable, stress radiographs can be taken to evaluate the stability of the ankle. When stress radiographs are taken, both ankles need to be examined because the amount of stability is variable. Injuries leading to completely torn lateral ligament are not common. When the degree of the ligamentous injury is in question the initial management should be immobilization in a cast with a reassessment after the swelling and acute pain has subsided.

The description of the injury that leads to an ankle fracture is a combination of the position the ankle was in and the direction of the force when the injury occurred, i.e., supination–eversion, supination–adduction, pronation–eversion, or pronation–abduction.[18] When the ankle is in pronation, the medial malleolus fractures on the deltoid ligament tears, the tibiofibular syndesmosis fails, and the fibula fractures (Fig. 42-49). When the ankle is in supination, the fibula usually fails without disruption of the

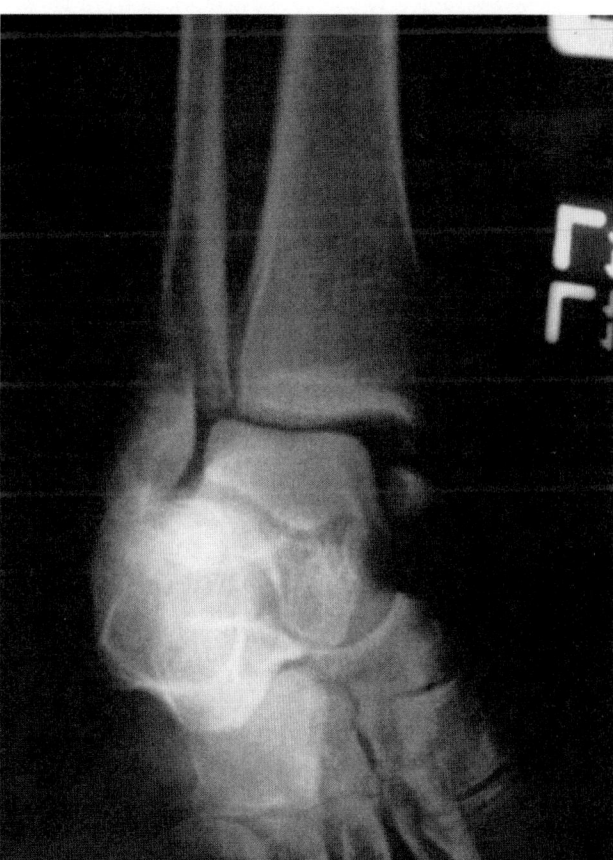

FIG. 42-49. *AP radiograph of a patient with a bimalleolar fracture.*

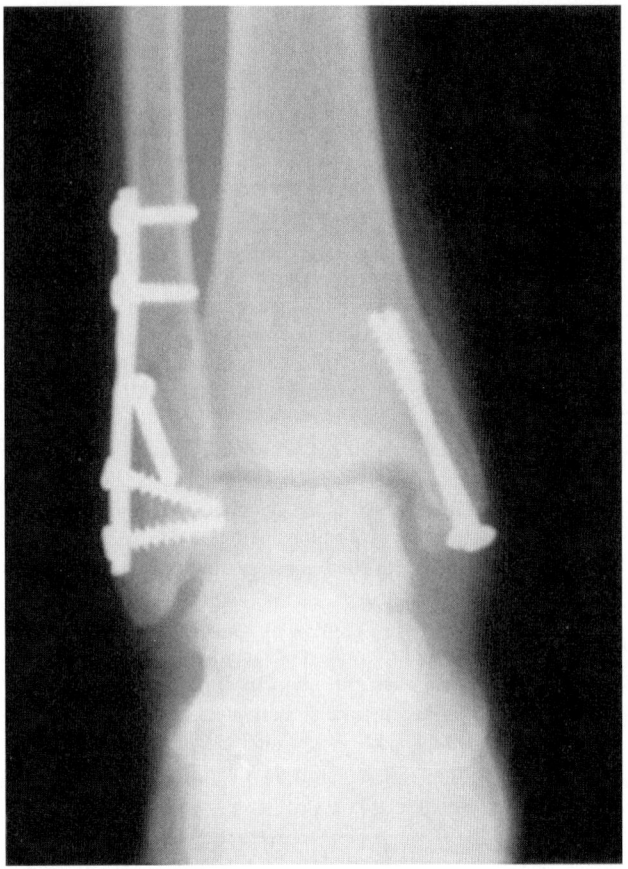

FIG. 42-50. AP radiograph of a patient who has an open reduction and internal fixation of the bimalleolar ankle fracture.

tibiofibular syndesmosis and the medial malleolar fractures on the deltoid ligament tears. When treating this injury with a closed procedure, it is important to reverse the direction of the injury and hold the ankle in the opposition position.

The distal fibula is attached to the distal tibia by the tibiofibular syndesmosis. This structure is important for normal ankle function. When torn, it needs to be allowed to heal. The fibula should be held in its anatomic position in relation to the distal tibia. If the patient has internal fixation, a screw can be used to hold the fibula in place. If closed treatment is elected, care should be taken to be sure the reduction of the fibula is anatomic. Radiographs of the ankle should always include the usual anterior-posterior and lateral views, as well as a mortis view. This is obtained by internally rotating the ankle 10 to 15 degrees and taking a second anterior-posterior view. This view allows one to see the relationship between the distal tibia and fibula (see Fig. 42-33).

In general, ankle fractures that can be easily reduced and held with the foot in an anatomic position can be treated with a closed procedure. The patient is initially placed in a long-leg cast. This can be shortened to a well-molded short-leg cast after 3 to 4 weeks. Patients whose fracture cannot be reduced, or cannot be held reduced without placing the foot in an extreme position, should have open reduction and internal fixation (Fig. 42-50).

The fibula is most often internally fixed with a plate, while the medial malleolus is held with one or two screws. If the deltoid ligament is torn but the talus reduces anatomically with reduction and fixation of the lateral malleolus, no surgery treatment of the deltoid is needed. If the reduction of the talus within the ankle mortis

is not anatomic, the medial side of the ankle should be opened to remove any tissue that is preventing the reduction.

Talus

The talus is at risk of sustaining a fracture. Fortunately these fractures are uncommon and are usually the result of major trauma. The most common fracture location is through the neck of the talus. The degree of displacement is both prognostically important and indicates the best treatment. The classification system used most commonly is that of Hawkins.[19] There are four types of displacement in this classification system. Type I is a nondisplaced fracture, which can be treated nonoperatively with cast immobilization. In type I, the patient has less than a 10% risk of developing osteonecrosis of the talar head. The other types are all displaced fractures. Type II is associated with a subtalar dislocation; type III is associated with a subtalar and ankle dislocation; and type IV is associated with subtalar, ankle, and talonavicular dislocation. These fractures usually need internal fixation and the risk of osteonecrosis increases from approximately 35% for type II to 100% with type IV. Prolonged nonweight bearing until the talus has a chance to revascularize is the treatment for the osteonecrosis.

Calcaneus

Fractures of the calcaneus are common. They usually are caused by falls from heights. They may be associated with a lumbar fracture. The patient will have marked swelling of the hindfoot and usually cannot bear weight. The treatment depends on the amount of displacement and the expectations of the patient. Those with minimal displacement are treated closed. Any displacement of an articular fragment involving the subtalar joint should be reduced. Böhler angle is a radiographic measurement indicating the amount of displacement. It is the angle measured between a line across the calcaneal tuberosity and a line across the anterior and posterior subtalar joint (Fig. 42-51). The normal angle is between 25 and 40 degrees.

Midfoot Injury

Dislocations between the tarsal bones and proximal metatarsals are a more common injury than is realized. They are often seen after what seems to be a minor injury. The patient complains of pain in the

TYPES OF CALCANEUS FRACTURES

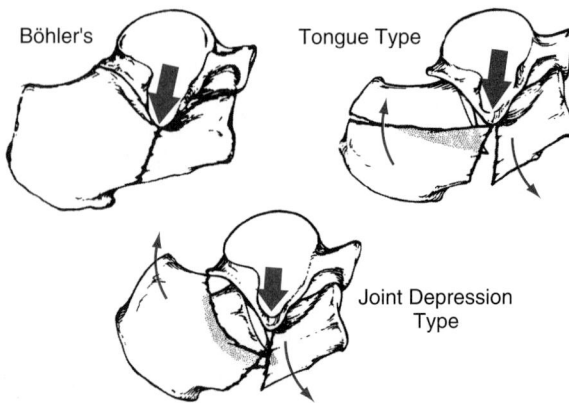

FIG. 42-51. Types of calcaneus fractures. Böhler angle is flattened in fractures involving the subtalar joint. (*Modified with permission from Rockwood CA, Green DP, Bucholz RW: Rockwood and Green's Fractures in Adults, 1991.*)

midfoot and there is swelling. The plain radiographic findings are subtle and one has to suspect the injury to make the diagnosis. Often, it can be treated closed, but open reduction and internal fixation is indicated if the closed reduction is not anatomic or cannot be held reduced.

Metatarsal Fractures

Fractures of the metatarsals are usually a result of direct trauma (e.g., dropping a heavy object on the dorsum of the foot). These are easily treated by nonweight bearing for 4 to 6 weeks, followed by gradual resumption of activities.

An exception is the base of the fifth metatarsal. There are two types of fractures at this site. Avulsion injuries occur when the peroneus brevis muscle pulls off the bone with a fragment of the bone. This can be treated closed and will be healed within 6 weeks. Bone union is not necessary for normal function. A Jones fracture is a fracture to the proximal fifth metatarsal through the metaphysic or proximal diaphysis. This injury has an increased risk of delayed union or nonunion. Often, internal fixation is recommended immediately and should be used if the bone is not united within 3 months.

Toes

Fractures of the phalanges of the toes are very common. Treatment is almost always only taping to the adjacent toe. If the great toe has a displaced fracture, pin fixation may be indicated.

Clavicle

Fractures of the clavicle occur in adults and children. More than 80% occur in the middle third of the clavicle, and almost all of the remainder occur in the distal third of the clavicle (Fig. 42-52). The most common causes are a direct blow to the clavicle, a fall on the shoulder, or a fall on an outstretched arm. Clavicle fractures are often seen in patients with multiple injuries and should be specifically looked for in this situation because they can be easily missed. Swelling and tenderness are usually found at the fracture site and pain is associated with shoulder motion. Associated neurovascular injuries can occur, but are uncommon.

Fractures that occur in the middle third of the clavicle are treated by placing the injured arm in a sling. In the past, a "figure-of-eight" splint was used but it is uncomfortable and is no longer felt to be needed. The patient should start to move the shoulder as soon as pain allows, usually within a few days to a week, to reduce the risk of developing restricted shoulder motion. Healing usually occurs in about 6 to 8 weeks with return to full function in about 3 months. Children will heal the fracture faster and start using their arm earlier than an adult. Nonunion is rare.

Distal-third clavicle fractures are less common and require more care. They are classified into three types based on the location of the fracture relative to the coracoclavicular ligaments. Type I fractures occur between the coracoclavicular and coracoacromial ligaments. As long as the coracoclavicular ligaments are not disrupted, this type of distal clavicle fracture is stable and is treated with a sling similar to middle-third clavicle fractures. Type II fractures occur medial to the coracoclavicular ligaments. The muscle attachments to the medial fragment pull it superiorly, while the weight of the shoulder girdle and arm pull the distal fragment inferiorly. The amount of displacement may lead to a nonunion, but the management of this type of clavicle fracture is controversial. Those who recommend nonoperative treatment believe that initial operative treatment does not always result in a satisfactory outcome, and even if a nonunion develops, it is usually not symptomatic or can be treated. Those who advocate operative treatment believe the management of the symptomatic nonunion is so difficult that it is better to treat all of the fractures initially with an anatomic reduction and internal fixation. Type III fractures involve the articular surface of the acromioclavicular joint. They are managed nonoperatively as long as there is not gross displacement. If the patient develops subsequent symptomatic acromioclavicular degenerative disease and pain, resection of the distal clavicle can be performed.

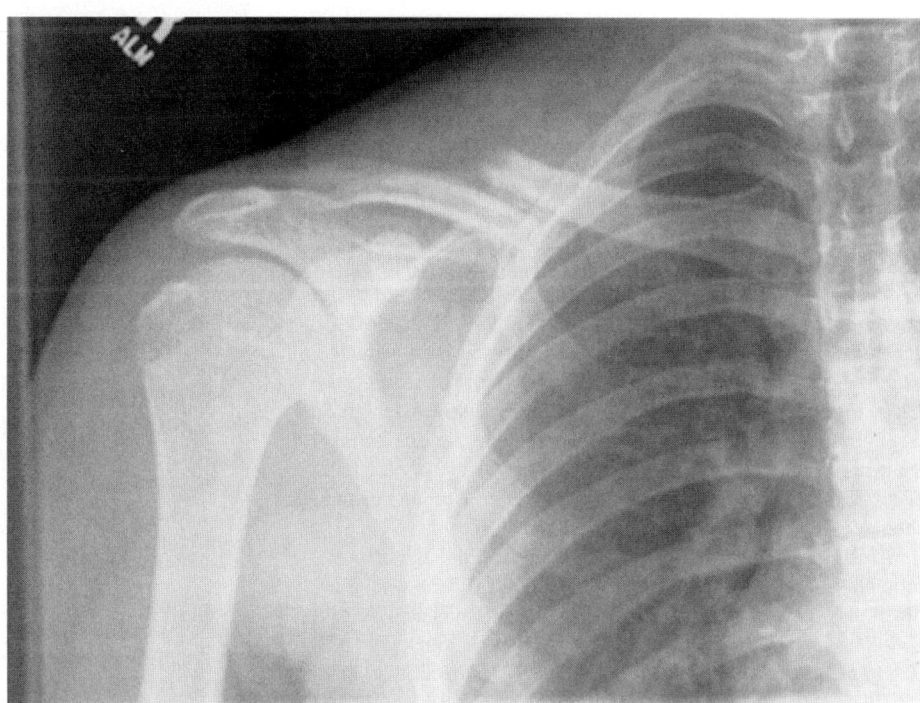

FIG. 42-52. AP radiograph of a patient with a fracture clavicle. As usual there is elevation of the medial fragment and shortening of the clavicle. This fracture will heal and the function will be excellent with closed treatment. The patient can be treated with a sling.

Acromioclavicular Separation

The mechanism of injury of the acromioclavicular (AC) joint is usually direct trauma to the acromion with a fall onto the shoulder. The patient presents with pain, swelling, and tenderness at the AC joint. Shoulder motion also causes pain. Direct pressure on the distal clavicle often demonstrates the instability of the joint.

Acromioclavicular injuries are classified by anatomic relationships between the acromion and clavicle. The displacement is caused by injuries to the ligaments that stabilize the AC joint. These include the capsule of the AC joint and the coracoclavicular ligaments. The Rockwood classification has six types of AC separations.[20] This classification system helps to describe the anatomic injury and determine treatment. A type I AC separation has no displacement of the distal clavicle. The AC joint capsule is stretched or torn, but the coracoclavicular ligaments are intact. A type II AC separation has an elevated distal clavicle but without complete dislocation of the joint. These patients have a complete tear of the AC capsule and stretching of the coracoclavicular ligaments. A type III AC separation has total displacement of the distal clavicle from the acromion. These patients have complete disruption of the AC joint capsule and coracoclavicular ligaments. Types IV, V, and VI are uncommon variations of AC joint separations and do not warrant further discussion here.

All AC joint separations can be treated nonoperatively. The more active the patient and the more displaced the more likely the patient will benefit from an open reduction and internal fixation. Type I injuries are treated with a sling for a few days to 2 weeks, depending on the symptoms. Early range of motion to the shoulder is important to reduce the risk of shoulder stiffness. Type II injuries are usually treated nonoperatively, as are type I injuries. These patients are more likely to have pain in the joint after the injury has healed and are more likely to need surgery than a patient with a type I injury. Those patients with persistent pain are operated on later. The treatment of type III injuries is more controversial. Unless the skin over the end of the clavicle is at risk of being damaged by the underlying distal clavicle, surgery is not required. In athletes, especially those who perform a throwing motion, operative reduction and internal fixation is usually recommended because this treatment is the most likely to provide optimal functional results. There are numerous surgical techniques used to stabilize the AC joint and the technical aspects are not discussed in this text. Types IV, V, and VI are all treated by surgical methods.

Anterior Shoulder Dislocation

The glenohumeral joint is the most commonly dislocated large joint in the body. The humerus can dislocate anteriorly, posteriorly, or inferiorly relative to the glenoid. Anterior dislocations are by far the most common, accounting for more than 95% of cases. They generally occur after an indirect trauma with the arm abducted, externally rotated, and extended. Anterior dislocations often cause a tear in the glenoid labrum (Bankart lesion) and also can cause a compression fracture of the posterolateral aspect of the humeral head by the glenoid rim (Hill-Sachs lesion). When one of these occur, the patient usually develops recurrent dislocations of their shoulder.[21]

Patients present with a painful shoulder held in slight external rotation and abduction. Physical examination may show squaring off of the shoulder with loss of the deltoid prominence, as well as fullness anteriorly, where the humeral head is situated. There is minimal active motion of the shoulder. A neurovascular exam should be performed. Sensation over the lateral deltoid region must be assessed, because the axillary nerve is the most common nerve injured. Anteroposterior, scapular Y, and axillary radiographs are obtained. Radiographs will demonstrate the anterior dislocation and any associated fractures of the proximal humerus or glenoid.

Reduction of the dislocated shoulder should be performed expeditiously. Narcotic analgesics and sedatives are usually necessary to facilitate reduction. Numerous reduction maneuvers have been described, but two of the more commonly used are the Stimson technique and the Hippocratic technique. The Stimson technique involves placing the patient prone with the involved arm hanging off the side of the table (Fig. 42-53). Traction is applied by hanging weights from the patient's wrist. The patient must relax. Usually the shoulder reduces quickly, but it may take 15 minutes before the tensed shoulder muscles fatigue and allow the shoulder to reduce. In the Hippocratic technique, longitudinal traction is applied with the arm slightly abducted. Countertraction is applied in the axillary region, either with one's foot as originally described by Hippocrates or by an assistant holding onto a sheet wrapped around the patient's chest. If the reduction cannot be obtained, closed or possibly open reduction may be required in the operating room. This is particularly true with chronic dislocations. Radiographs are repeated after reduction to ensure the shoulder is reduced and to evaluate for fractures.

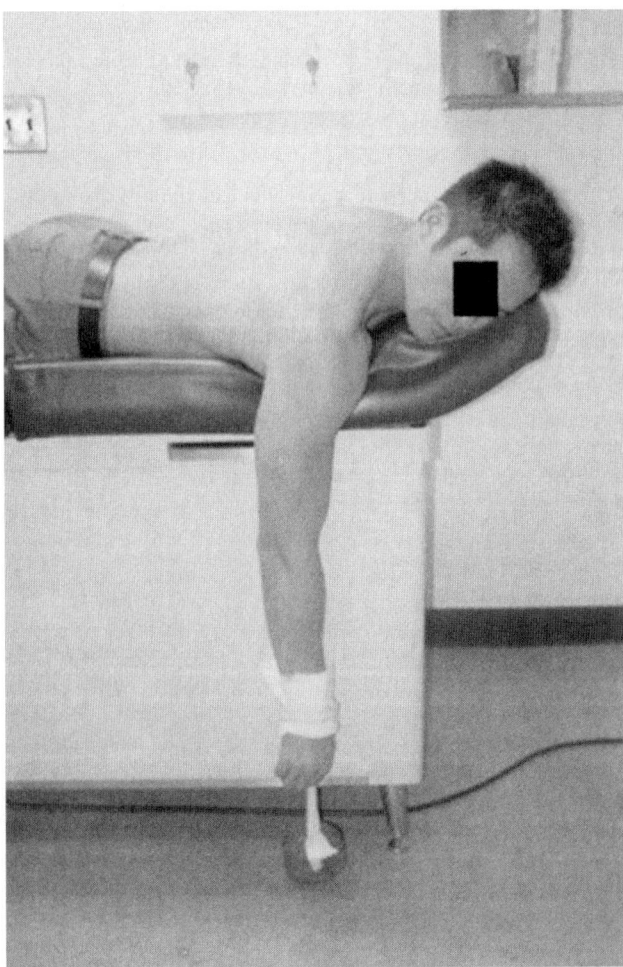

FIG. 42-53. This is a clinical photograph of the Stimson method of a closed reduction of an anterior dislocated shoulder. The patient is given mild sedation. Five to 10 pounds of weight are hung from the wrist and the patient is asked to relax. Within a few minutes the shoulder should reduce with minimal trauma and almost no pain.

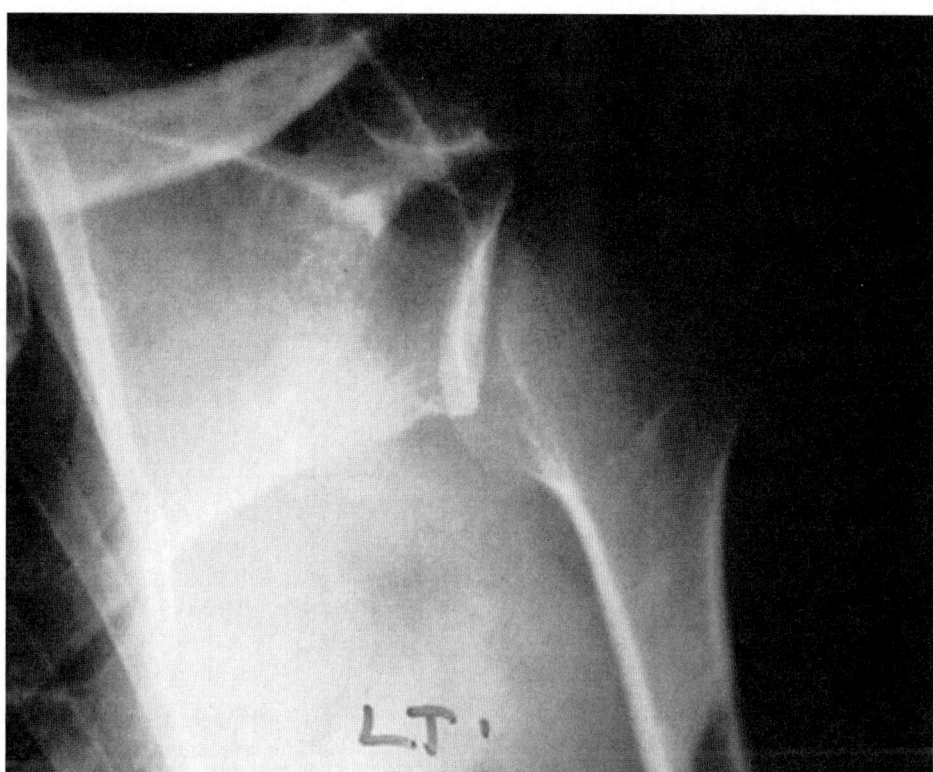

FIG. 42-54. AP radiograph of a patient with a posterior dislocation of the shoulder. This dislocation is frequently missed. The patient holds the arm internally rotated and resists external rotation. The injury is often caused by an electrical shock or seizure.

The patient is immobilized in a sling and swathe. Older patients are prone to develop shoulder stiffness so passive range-of-motion, along with isometric exercises, is begun in 1 to 2 weeks. Rotator cuff tears are a common associated injury after shoulder dislocation in elderly patients. Slow progress with rehabilitation in this group should prompt one to evaluate for a cuff tear, because surgical cuff repair may be beneficial. Young patients are at risk for redislocation so they are kept immobilized from 3 to 4 weeks. Redislocation is the most common complication after shoulder dislocation. The age of the patient is the most important factor, with recurrence rates as high as 80 to 90% in patients younger than age 20 years, and as low as 10 to 15% in patients older than age 40 years. Young athletes in contact sports are at particularly high risk for redislocation and arthroscopic stabilization with repair of the Bankart lesion should be considered after a shoulder dislocation in this select population.

Chronic Dislocation

If a shoulder joint has been dislocated for a few days, it becomes much harder to reduce by closed techniques. Open reduction is the only means to reduce the shoulder joint in this circumstance. However, this procedure may be extremely difficult, particularly if several weeks have elapsed from the time of injury. The dislocation causes the anatomy to be distorted and the neurovascular structures may be bound down in scar tissue. In elderly patients with low functional demands and minimal pain with a chronic shoulder dislocation, conservative treatment leaving the shoulder joint dislocated may be the best option.

Posterior Shoulder Dislocation

Posterior shoulder dislocations can occur as a result of direct trauma to the anterior humerus or indirectly from seizures or electric shock. Patients present with pain, the shoulder held in internal rotation, and adduction. The injury is frequently not recognized in the emergency room. Physical findings include a prominent coracoid process, fullness of the posterior shoulder, and limited external rotation and elevation of the shoulder. Anteroposterior, scapular Y, and axillary radiographs are obtained. The dislocation may be missed on the anteroposterior radiograph (Fig. 42-54), because the findings are subtle. The standard axillary view best demonstrates the dislocation (Fig. 42-55), but may be difficult to obtain because of the patient's

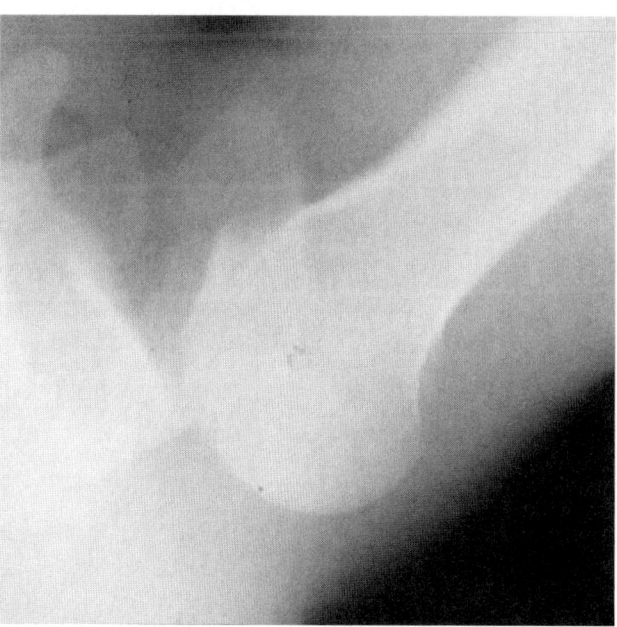

FIG. 42-55. Axillary view of the patient in Fig. 42-54. This view demonstrates the posterior position of the humeral head with respect to the glenoid.

discomfort with shoulder abduction. In this case, a modified axillary view, such as the Velpeau axillary lateral view, should be obtained. Associated fractures, including a reverse Hill-Sachs lesion (compression fracture of the anteromedial humeral head caused by the posterior glenoid rim), should be noted on the radiographs.

Reduction is performed using the Hippocratic technique with longitudinal traction. After the reduction is obtained and confirmed with repeat radiographs, the shoulder is immobilized for 3 to 4 weeks in a shoulder spica cast, with the shoulder in neutral rotation and slight abduction and extension.

Proximal Humerus Fractures

Proximal humerus fractures are common in the elderly population and generally occur from a fall on an outstretched hand. They occur less commonly in young adults, but are often more serious with associated injuries such as shoulder dislocation because of the higher forces required to fracture nonosteoporotic bone. Patients present with pain, swelling, and tenderness about the shoulder and have difficulty with active motion. Three orthogonal radiographic views of the shoulder best demonstrate the displacement of the fracture. These consist of an anteroposterior view, a scapular Y view, and axillary view. The location(s) of the fracture can be categorized as anatomic neck, surgical neck, greater tuberosity, and lesser tuberosity. Displacement of the fracture fragments can be explained by the muscular forces that are applied to them. In surgical neck fractures, the shaft tends to displace anteromedially because of the pull of the pectoralis major. Greater tuberosity fractures are displaced superiorly and posteriorly by the attached supraspinatus, infraspinatus, and teres minor (Fig. 42-56). Lesser tuberosity fragments are displaced medially by the subscapularis. The Neer classification

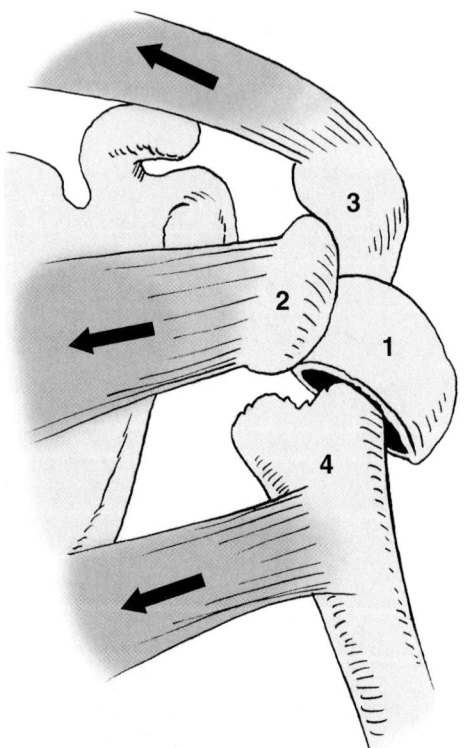

FIG. 42-56. This illustrates how the muscular attachments of the proximal humerus displace the fragments of a four-part humeral head fracture. The muscles are the deforming forces that make holding the fragments in their proper place difficult.

is most commonly used and is subdivided by the number of displaced fracture fragments. A two-part fracture is any fracture with one major fragment displaced from the remainder of the humerus. Similarly, three- and four-part fractures describe fractures with two and three displaced major fragments, respectively. Displacement requiring reduction is defined as that which is greater than 1 cm or has an angulation of more than 45 degrees.

Minimally displaced fractures are treated with immobilization followed by early range of motion. Closed reduction is attempted on displaced two-part surgical neck fractures, but if an adequate reduction cannot be obtained or maintained, surgical reduction and fixation is performed. Displaced greater tuberosity fractures usually require surgery as they may impinge on the undersurface of the acromion when the shoulder is elevated and block elevation as well as external rotation. Displaced three-part fractures are usually treated with closed reduction and percutaneous pin fixation, while four-part fractures are often treated with humeral head prostheses because of the high incidence of osteonecrosis of the humeral head. To minimize shoulder stiffness, early postoperative passive range-of-motion exercise is begun if adequate stability was obtained with surgery.

Humeral Shaft Fractures

Fractures of the humeral shaft can be the result of either direct or indirect trauma. Patients present with pain, swelling, and difficulty moving the shoulder and elbow. Examination reveals swelling and tenderness of the arm with crepitus and motion at the fracture site. A careful neurovascular examination must be performed. Radial nerve palsies are commonly associated injuries, particularly with fractures of the middle third of the humerus.[22] Most of these are neuropraxias that resolve spontaneously within 3 to 4 months and therefore do not require operative nerve exploration.

A vast majority of humeral shaft fractures can be treated nonoperatively. A U-shaped plaster coaptation splint is commonly used initially. This is frequently converted to a humeral functional brace after 1 to 2 weeks, allowing better early range-of-motion exercises of the shoulder and elbow.[23] A large amount of fracture displacement can be tolerated because of the mobility of the shoulder. Acceptable limits of 30 degrees of varus, 20 degrees of anterior-posterior angulation, and 3 cm of shortening have been proposed. Operative stabilization of humeral shaft fractures is recommended in certain cases including inability to obtain an adequate alignment with a splint or brace, open fracture, floating elbow (fractures of humerus and radius/ulna), fracture with vascular injury, polytrauma, and pathologic fracture. Fracture fixation can be done with compression plate, intramedullary rod, or external fixation.

Elbow Fractures

Olecranon and distal humerus fractures are generally pure bone injuries with intact ligaments, barring iatrogenic injury (Fig. 42-57). Open reduction and rigid internal fixation is recommended in the adult. The tension-band technique has been reliable for olecranon fractures, while plates and screws are used to restore and maintain the normal, complex anatomy of the distal humerus. In general, early mobilization is also desirable to minimize loss of motion. In children with supracondylar fractures, closed reduction can almost always be done. Those with minimal initial displacement can be treated in a cast; however, those with complete displacement (unstable supracondylar fractures) are best treated with percutaneous fixation after the closed reduction (Fig. 42-58).

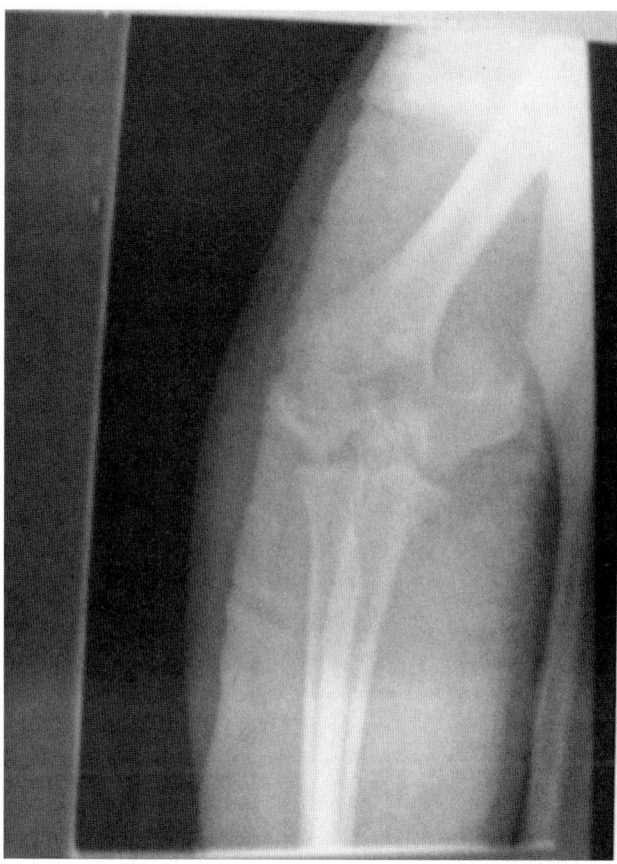

FIG. 42-57. AP radiograph of a patient with a comminuted distal humeral intra-articular fracture. This fracture should be treated with open reduction and internal fixation.

In the adult fracture, dislocations and fractures are frequently associated with ligament injuries that may include coronoid fractures, radial head fractures, and Monteggia fractures of the proximal ulna with a concomitant radial head dislocation. If left untreated, this ligamentous injury can lead to long-term instability. Proper treatment to restore stability may require ligament repair or reconstruction in addition to fixation of the fracture. If stability cannot be restored with a surgical repair because of massive trauma or bone destruction, an articulated external fixator permits early motion while maintaining the elbow in a reduced position. Radial head fractures may be unreconstructable as a consequence of comminution; replacement arthroplasty with either silicone or metallic implants is recommended, along with reconstruction or repair of the collateral ligaments.

Complications of elbow fracture treatment include infection, neurovascular injury, stiffness, and heterotopic ossification (Fig. 42-59). Significant posttraumatic stiffness rarely responds to conservative treatment and therapy, but good results can be obtained by radical capsulectomy, excision of any heterotopic ossification, and, if necessary, recontouring of the distal humerus and/or proximal ulna. This surgery cannot also be performed arthroscopically, with equivalent results and less morbidity. Simple manipulation under anesthesia is not indicated because of its association with ulnar nerve injury caused by compression in the cubital tunnel.

Forearm Fractures

The radius and ulna are the two bones of the forearm. Motor vehicle accidents, sports injuries, falls, or direct blows to the forearm may cause a fracture to one or both of these bones. The fracture may or may not have a significant associated soft-tissue or joint injury. Fractures of both bones of the forearm are described by their location (proximal, midshaft, or distal), by the amount of displacement

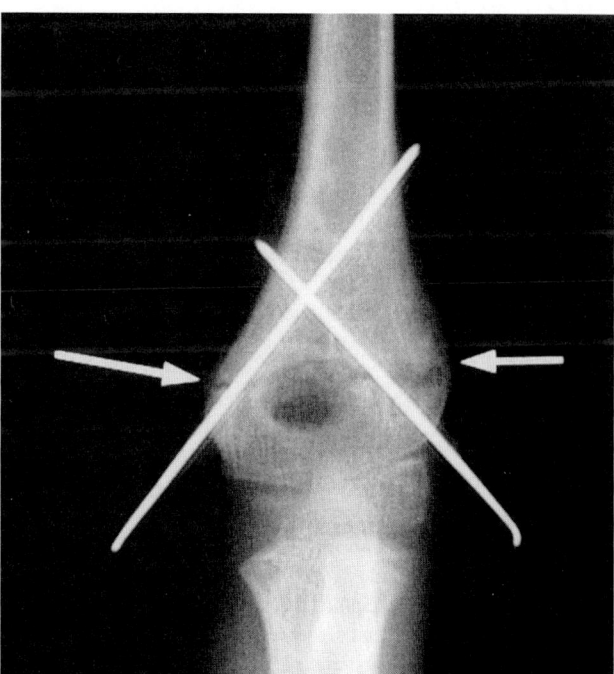

FIG. 42-58. Supracondylar fracture of the humerus with closed reduction and percutaneous pin fixation.

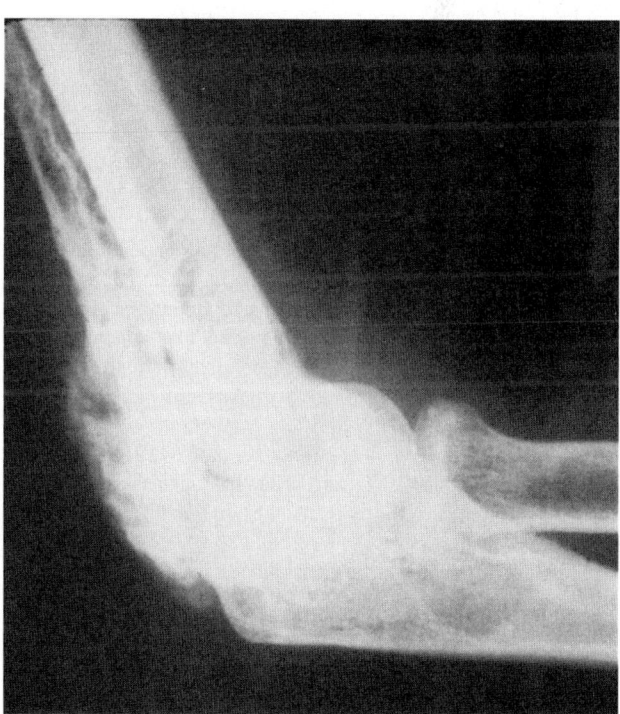

FIG. 42-59. Lateral radiograph of a patient who dislocated the elbow and developed heterotopic ossification. This caused severe restriction of motion and was treated with surgical excision.

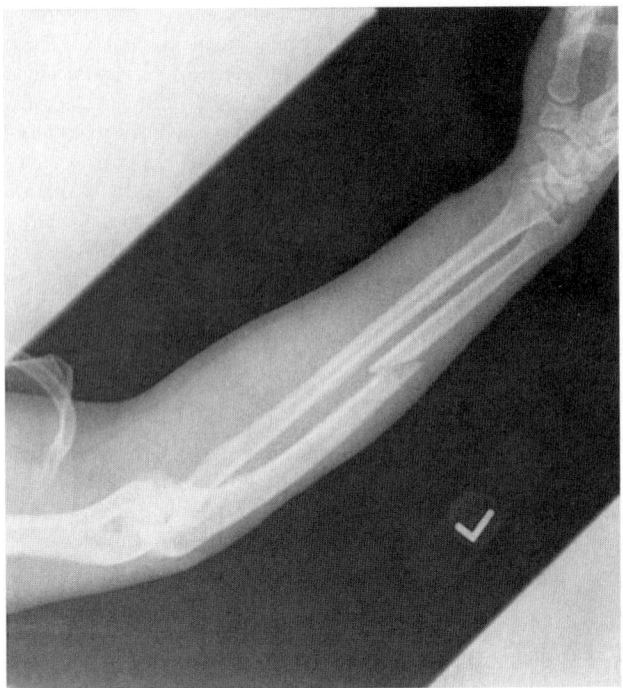

FIG. 42-60. Lateral radiograph of a patient with a Monteggia fracture. The ulna is displaced and the radius is not broken, therefore there should be an injury to either the elbow or wrist. Usually with the displaced fracture of the ulna, the radial head dislocates at the elbow.

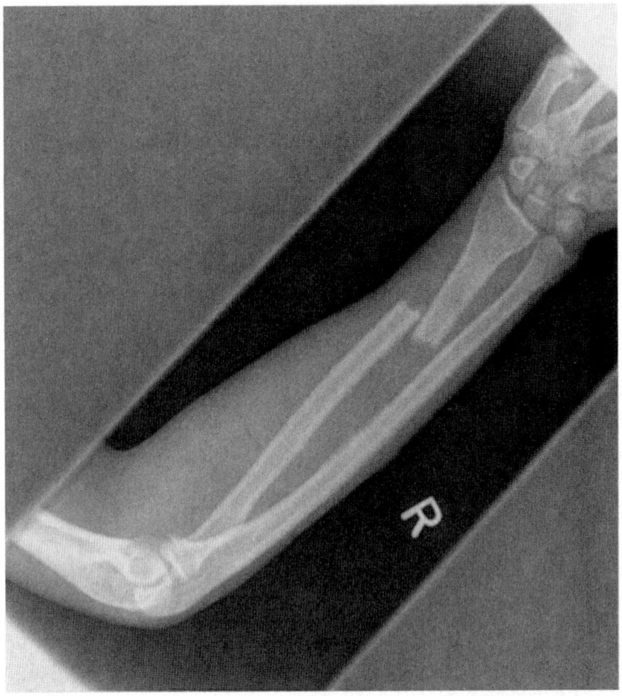

FIG. 42-61. Lateral radiograph of a patient with a Galeazzi fracture. This is essentially the reverse of a Monteggia fracture. The fracture of the radius is displaced and the distal ulna is dislocated.

(minimal, moderate, or complete), the degree of angulation, the extent of comminution, and whether the fracture is open (compound) or closed.

A fracture of the ulna with an associated dislocation of the radial head was first described by Monteggia in 1814 (before radiographs were discovered) and is now known as a Monteggia fracture (Fig. 42-60).[24] A fracture in the distal third of the radius with an associated dislocation of the distal radioulnar joint is called a Galeazzi fracture after the physician who, in 1934, described this combination of injuries (Fig. 42-61).[25] An isolated fracture of the ulna is called a "nightstick" fracture because being hit by a nightstick was a common mechanism of injury.

Rotation of the forearm is crucial to the proper positioning and function of the hand, and is therefore important in activities of daily living (ADL). Normally, the radius rotates around the fixed ulna. The ability of the radius to rotate around the ulna depends on the normal shape of each bone. The ulna is relatively straight while the radius is bowed. Restoration of this normal anatomy after fracture is imperative for a return to full function. A deformity in the proximal forearm has a relatively greater effect of forearm rotation when compared to the more distal deformity. Therefore, management should restore the normal anatomy and hold the bones in this position until the fractures heal.

Individuals with displaced or angulated fractures of the forearm will present with pain, swelling, and deformity. The neurovascular status of the forearm and hand should be determined. Anteroposterior and lateral radiographs are usually all that are needed to demonstrate the fractures. The elbow and wrist should be examined and both should be seen on the radiographs to look for fractures or dislocations in one of these joints. In cases of suspected injury to the proximal or distal radioulnar joints, a CT scan may be of value. While displacement, angulation, and shortening are easily seen on

routine radiographs, rotational alignment is not easily determined. If, on the anteroposterior view, the radial styloid (lateral) and bicipital tuberosity (medial) are both evident and prominent, rotational alignment is present in the supinated radius. In the lateral view, the coronoid process of the ulna points anteriorly and the ulna styloid posteriorly. Recognizing a dislocation of the radial head from its normal articulation with the humeral capitellum can be difficult. A line perpendicular to the articular surface and through the central position of the radial head should bisect the capitellum. This relationship should be seen on all projections if the radial head is anatomically located.

Generally, forearm fractures are treated with a closed manipulation and cast immobilization for children and open reduction and internal fixation in adults. It is generally true that the younger the patient, the greater the remodeling potential and the less need for an immediate anatomic reduction. In addition, the thicker periosteum seen in children usually remains intact or partially intact and makes it easier to reduce and hold the reduction compared to those in adults. A unique feature of immature bones is the capacity to undergo plastic deformation without breaking and to sustain an incomplete fracture called a "greenstick" fracture.

To reduce a displaced, angulated, both-bone forearm fracture requires anesthesia or sedation. The forearm is manipulated to reduce the displacement and the arm is placed in a long-arm cast. The more proximal the fracture the more the patient's forearm should be placed in supination. A midshaft fracture is placed in neutral rotation and a distal forearm fracture is immobilized in mild pronation. They are kept in a long-arm cast for at least 6 weeks. Callus should be visible before removing the cast. The cross section of the cast should be oval with the anteroposterior distance being less than the medial to lateral distance. This maintains the interosseous distance and helps hold the reduction.

Plastically displaced bones are reduced by gradual, sustained force to straighten the bent bone. Greenstick fractures are completed so that they can be properly aligned. Both types of fractures are held in a long-arm cast. In children, bringing the ulna out to length and correcting the angulation reduces the Monteggia fracture. This reduces the radial head in almost all cases. The patient is then placed in a long-arm cast with the elbow flexed to at least 100 degrees and the forearm in a semisupinated position. Galeazzi fractures in children are usually stable after a closed reduction of the radius and can be held in a long-arm cast with the forearm supinated and wrist neutral.

Displaced, both-bone forearm fractures in adults are usually unstable and are best treated with open reduction and internal fixation. Malunion and delayed union rates are unacceptably high with closed treatments. In addition, the length of immobilization is such that prolonged stiffness occurs. This dramatically lengthens the period of disability. Compression plating with 3.5-mm plates is the most accepted form of internal fixation. Both bone forearm fractures are fixed with two plates, one on each bone (Fig. 42-62). Plate fixation of the bony fracture in an adult with a Monteggia fracture or Galeazzi fracture is recommended and usually reduces the joint dislocation.

Distal Radius Fractures

Fractures of the distal radius are among the most common fractures encountered in children and in adults. There is a bimodal peak of incidence occurring in later childhood and after the sixth decade of life. Fractures in males contribute a greater number to the earlier peak, while fractures in females predominate in the later years. The most common mechanism of injury in both children and adults is a lower-energy fall from ground level onto an outstretched hand with the wrist extended. Fractures that do occur from higher-energy injuries have varying degrees of comminution, may occur in any age group, and have a higher incidence of associated injuries. Anteroposterior, lateral, and possibly oblique radiographs are usually all that are needed to assess distal radius fractures. In the presence of comminution and intra-articular involvement, a CT scan may be of use to assess the status of the radiocarpal, and especially the radioulnar, joints. Patients with distal radius fractures present with pain, swelling, and deformity. Examination must include a neurologic assessment prior to and after reduction of the fracture.

Even though numerous newer classification schemes have been introduced, eponyms have endured as the most common way of referring to these fractures in adults, and thus are reviewed here. They usually communicate location and direction of displacement, but do not aid in determining the type of treatment nor prognosis. The Colles-Pouteau fracture denotes a fracture of the distal radial metaphysis with dorsal displacement of the distal fragment and is by far the most common fracture of the distal radius (Fig. 42-63).[26] In contrast, the direction of displacement of the Smith-Goyrand metaphyseal fracture is volar. A dorsal articular marginal fracture (the volar portion of the articular surface is still intact to the shaft of the radius) is referred to as a Barton's fracture. In a volar Barton's fracture (also referred to as Letenneur's fracture), the articular fracture is volar or anterior. A fracture of the radial styloid is referred to as a Hutchinson's or Chauffeur's fracture.

Numerous, more recent fracture classifications have been developed, but no one classification scheme has gained wide acceptance over the others. These classifications have delineated whether the fractures are intra-articular or extra-articular, have differing fracture patterns, the presence and location of comminution, associated ulnar styloid fracture, and have sought to predict the degree of stability and determine the best course of treatment and prognosis.

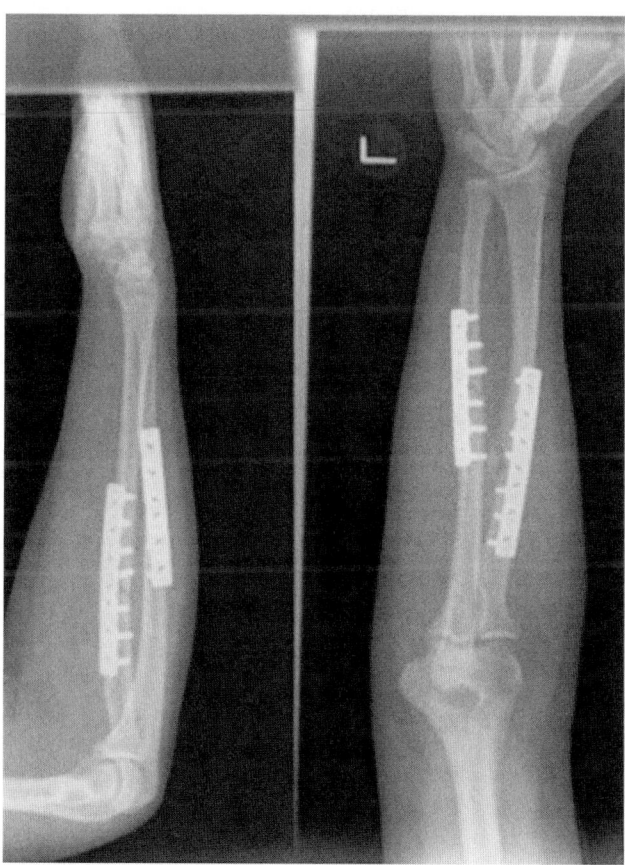

FIG. 42-62. AP and lateral radiographs of a patient who had open reduction and internal fixation of a both-bone fracture. Plate fixation is used so there is sufficiently rigid fixation that the patient can use the arm while it is healing.

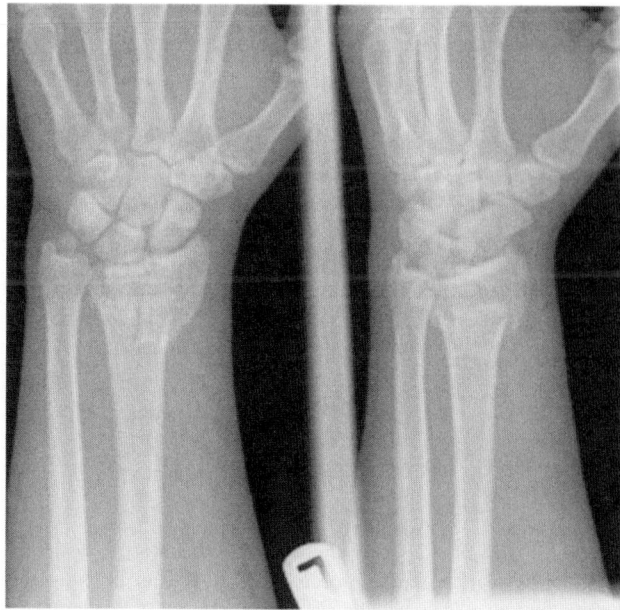

FIG. 42-63. AP and oblique radiograph of a patient with a comminuted distal radial fracture. This is the so-called Colles-Pouteau fracture. It is most often seen in patients with osteoporosis.

In children, the distal radius fractures are grouped into metaphyseal (more common) and physeal fractures. The metaphyseal fractures may be complete or incomplete (buckle or torus fracture). The physeal fractures are described according to the Salter-Harris classification. The majority of these fractures in children are treated by closed means. Buckle fractures are treated in plaster for 4 weeks. Angulated and/or displaced fractures are manipulated and kept in a cast for 6 weeks. Because of an intact periosteum on one side of the metaphyseal fracture, traction prior to manipulation may be of little help, and, in fact, may be counterproductive in completely displaced fractures. If at least 2 years of growth remain, up to 20 degrees of angulation may be accepted because remodeling will occur. Similarly, even "bayonet apposition" (side-to-side alignment of the fracture fragments) in the absence of severe angulation or rotatory deformity will remodel without residual functional deficits. Physeal injuries are reduced by gentle distraction and manipulation avoiding repeated attempts and possible further physeal injury. Unstable, severely displaced, and angulated metaphyseal or physeal fractures may necessitate closed or open reduction accompanied by internal fixation (usually smooth K-wires) or external fixation in order to prevent loss of reduction.

The aim of treatment of distal radius fractures in adults is to restore the general alignment of the distal radius and ulna, avoiding radial shortening of greater than 3 to 5 mm, residual angulation greater than 10 to 15 degrees, and articular incongruity of greater than 2 to 3 mm. The degree of residual deformity accepted will depend on the age and functional needs of the individual patient. The majority of these fractures are extra-articular or have a minimally displaced, intra-articular component, and are treated successfully by closed reduction followed by 6 weeks of protection in a cast, splint, or brace. Closed reduction is obtained by finger-trap traction followed by manipulation and application of the splint of choice, usually under hematoma-block local anesthesia. Fractures with severe shortening, angulation, and comminution are usually unstable and require some form of fixation. Displaced intra-articular fractures such as volar Barton's or radial styloid fractures are also unstable and require some form of fixation in order to restore articular congruity. Fixation may be obtained by internal fixation (pins, wires, screws, or plates), by percutaneous fixation (pins or external fixation), or by varying combinations of each method. Arthroscopically assisted fracture reduction and augmentation with bone graft or cement materials also have been used.

The most common complications of this method of reduction include malunion, nerve injury, tendon injury, stiffness, and reflex sympathetic dystrophy. If a malunion causes pain and significant limitation of motion and function, an osteotomy may be used to correct this situation. Early and tardy nerve symptoms, most commonly median nerve/carpal tunnel syndrome, can be treated by the appropriate release. Tendons might be entrapped, requiring a release, or ruptured, requiring a repair or transfer. Finger stiffness and pain, whether associated with swelling in the early postfracture period or as part of a reflex sympathetic dystrophy, require early and aggressive intervention by the occupational therapist.

Spinal Injuries

Injuries to the spinal column are potentially the most devastating of orthopaedic injuries. They occur most often after high-energy trauma such as motor vehicle accidents and falls from significant heights.[27,28] Initial stabilization of potential spinal injuries at the scene of the accident is done with rigid backboard to protect the thoracic and lumbar spine and with a rigid cervical collar to immobilize the cervical spine. All patients with high-energy injuries should be presumed to have spine injuries until proven otherwise.

Spine fractures, dislocations, and fracture/dislocations are caused by falls, major trauma, and diving accidents. The location of the fracture can be predicted by the mechanism of the injury. Diving accidents cause injuries to the cervical spine. This is one of the most common causes of paralysis. Often, patients present with a history of diving into water that was too shallow. Injuries to the thoracic spine, especially to the lower thoracic/upper lumbar spine, are usually a result of major trauma from an automobile accident or when a pedestrian is struck by a car. Lower lumbar injuries are more likely a result of a fall, with the patient landing on his or her feet or buttocks. Common combinations of injuries are calcaneal fractures with a lumbar burst fracture.

There are general categories of fractures. The most important initial differential is whether the patient has or does not have neurologic injury. The next differential is whether the spine is stable or unstable. Any neurologic injury indicates that the spine is unstable. Differentiation should be made between those injuries that are acutely unstable, meaning that there is a risk that the spine will displace with minimal movement, as opposed to chronic instability, which means that over time the spine will slowly displace. Both acutely unstable and chronically unstable spines need to be stabilized. This is usually done via an operation.

To determine whether the spine is stable it is useful to think of the spine as being composed of three columns: the anterior, middle, and posterior (Fig. 42-64). The anterior column is the vertebral body. The middle column is the posterior cortex of the vertebral body and posterior longitudinal ligament. The posterior column is the facet joints and posterior processes. As a general rule, if two or more of these columns are injured, the spine is considered unstable. If only one column is injured, it is unusual for the spine to be unstable. Although stable and unstable bone injuries will heal and the spine will become stable, ligament injuries are more prone to result in chronic instability and need surgical stabilization more often than do bone injuries.

Initial management of trauma patients must follow the Advanced Trauma Life Support (ATLS) protocol and focus on airway, breathing, and circulation. An examination for possible spine injuries can be performed subsequent to this. All patients should be carefully log-rolled and the spinous processes along the entire spine palpated for tenderness. A rapid, but thorough neurologic examination should be performed. In patients with severe spinal cord injuries, it is important to determine whether the injury is complete (with total motor and sensory loss) or incomplete. The prognosis for complete spinal cord injuries is worse with no return of functional strength below the level of injury. The presence of rectal tone, perianal sensation, or great toe flexor activity indicates that the injury is incomplete with sacral sparing and that the prognosis for recovery of nerve function is better. An absent bulbocavernosus reflex (anal sphincter contraction after pressure is applied to the glans penis or the clitoris or after gently tugging on the Foley catheter) indicates that spinal shock is present. Determination of whether a seemingly complete neurologic deficit is actually so cannot be made until spinal shock has resolved, which nearly always occurs within 24 hours.

A lateral cervical spine radiograph is part of the initial "trauma series" that is obtained on all multitrauma patients (Fig. 42-65). The radiograph must include the entire cervical spine from the occiput to the first thoracic vertebra. Inability to obtain a proper lateral radiograph necessitates additional views, such as swimmer's view, to visualize the lower cervical spine or a CT scan. Other views of the cervical spine that should be obtained after the patient is sufficiently

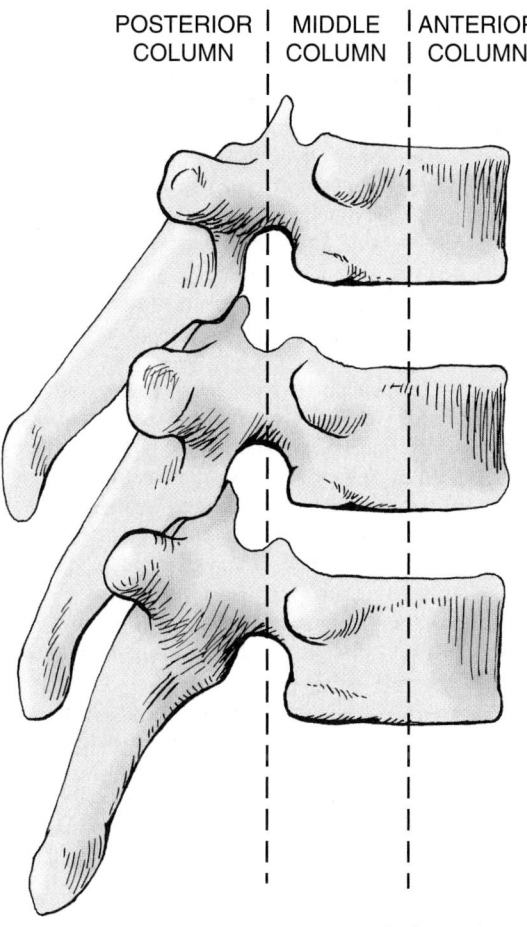

POSTERIOR | MIDDLE | ANTERIOR
COLUMN | COLUMN | COLUMN

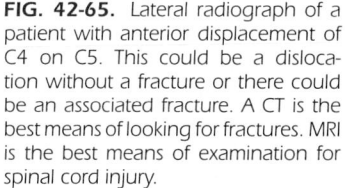

FIG. 42-64. *The spine can be thought of as three columns. Two of three can maintain stability.*

resuscitated and stabilized are the AP and open-mouth odontoid views. Anteroposterior, lateral thoracic spine, and lumbar spine radiographs are obtained in all unconscious or mentally-impaired patients, and in conscious, alert patients with pain and/or tenderness in those regions.

Patients with neurologic injuries seen within 24 hours of their injury are started on 30 mg/kg methylprednisolone, then 5.4 mg/kg per hour for 24 hours. Although there is some controversy as to its efficacy, most believe the steroid improves the chance of recovery.[29] Patients with spinal cord injuries may also have neurogenic shock with hypotension and bradycardia secondary to disruption of sympathetic outflow.

Cervical Spine

The treatment of cervical spine injuries is dictated by the degree of instability of the injury, the likelihood of healing, and the presence of spinal cord compression causing nerve injury. Stable injuries without nerve deficit can generally be treated with a cervical orthosis or a halo vest. The halo vest provides better immobilization than a cervical orthosis and is therefore preferred when there is a risk of instability. However, the halo vest does not completely restrict cervical motion and thus is not sufficient in patients with grossly unstable injuries. These types of patients require operative internal stabilization.

The likelihood of healing an injury also influences treatment decisions. For example, distractive flexion injuries to the cervical spine treated with a halo vest have been reported to have late instability in more than 60% of patients. One may therefore select early operative stabilization or for halo vest treatment followed by flexion-extension radiographs to assess for instability, with late operative stabilization if residual instability is present.

The presence of spinal cord compression with incomplete nerve injury generally necessitates operative decompression of the spine to facilitate recovery and prevent further damage to the cord. In cases of complete spinal cord injury, decompression may allow for

FIG. 42-65. *Lateral radiograph of a patient with anterior displacement of C4 on C5. This could be a dislocation without a fracture or there could be an associated fracture. A CT is the best means of looking for fractures. MRI is the best means of examination for spinal cord injury.*

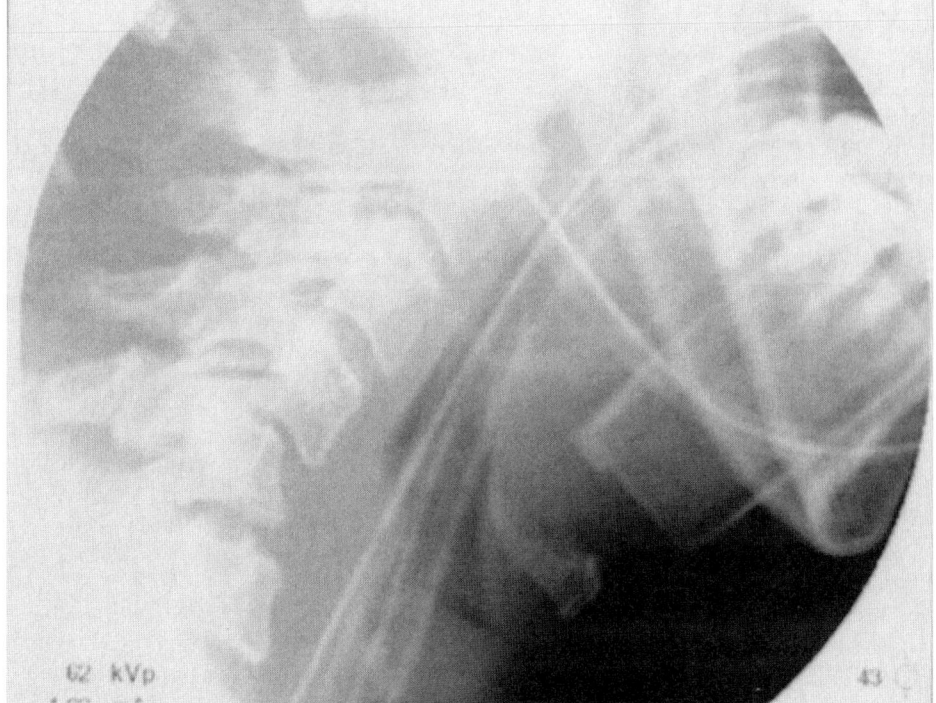

recovery of the nerve roots at the level of injury although there is usually little functional recovery distally.

Spinal cord injury is more common with lower cervical spine fractures than with upper cervical spine fractures. One reason for this is that there is more canal space for the spinal cord in the upper cervical spine with the spinal cord occupying one-third of the space in this region, as opposed to half of the canal space in the lower cervical spine.

Atlas fractures are axial loading injuries and are generally stable injuries without spinal cord injury. They can usually be treated with a rigid cervical orthosis or a halo vest. However, widely displaced lateral masses indicate that the transverse ligament has been torn, and the fracture is reduced with halo traction for several weeks prior to halo vest application.

Odontoid fractures are a relatively common injury and are classified into three types based on the location of the fracture. Type I, a fracture of the tip of the odontoid process, is generally a stable pattern that can be treated with cervical collar immobilization. Type II is a fracture through the base of the odontoid and is the most common type. The nonunion rate with nonoperative treatment is approximately 30%. The treatment is controversial and options include halo vest immobilization and surgical management with posterior C1-C2 arthrodesis or anterior internal fixation. Type III denotes a fracture through the body of C2 and has a higher rate of union than does a type II fracture because of the broad area of cancellous bone at the fracture site. It is treated with halo vest immobilization.

Traumatic spondylolisthesis of C2, also known as hangman's fracture, is a bilateral C2 pars interarticularis fracture. Minimally displaced fractures can be treated with cervical collar immobilization. Halo traction followed by halo vest immobilization is used for moderately displaced fractures. Severely displaced fractures with unilateral or bilateral facet dislocations are generally treated with open reduction followed by posterior stabilization of the facet dislocation and halo vest immobilization of the pars fracture.

Fractures of the lower cervical spine are classified according to the direction of the force applied and the position of cervical spine. Distractive flexion injuries are the most common pattern of lower cervical spine injuries and are commonly caused by a sudden deceleration in a motor vehicle. This can result in unilateral or bilateral facet dislocations. A unilateral facet dislocation results in a 25% anterior subluxation of the superior vertebral body relative to the inferior one. A bilateral facet dislocation causes a 50% subluxation. Closed reduction of the dislocation is attempted with traction while carefully monitoring the patient's neurologic status. After closed reduction, a unilateral facet dislocation can be managed in a halo vest while a bilateral dislocation, being more unstable, is treated with operative posterior stabilization. If an open reduction is necessary, an MRI should be obtained first to determine the presence of a herniated disc that may compress the cord after reduction.

Vertical compression injuries from direct blows to the top of the head, most often a diving injury, can result in burst fractures, which are compression fractures of the vertebral body with displacement into the spinal canal. Neurologic injury is common. These injuries are unstable and are treated with anterior decompression of the spinal canal followed by anterior or posterior stabilization.

Most injuries are adequately seen on plain radiographs, but CT scans are often used to better appreciate the details of the bone fragments (Fig. 42-66). For patients with neurologic injury an MRI is useful because the spinal cord and soft tissues within the canal can be visualized (Fig. 42-67).

As a rule, stabilization is done posteriorly (Fig. 42-68). Anterior stabilization is indicated when there is extensive anterior injury and is almost always combined with posterior stabilization. The instrumentation available for spine fixation has dramatically improved over the past decade, allowing much better fixation of the spine. In turn, more patients undergo internal fixation, reducing the use of halo and cast fixation.

JOINT REPLACEMENT SURGERY

Total joint arthroplasty is one of the major medical successes of the twentieth century. Total hip arthroplasty was first popularized in the early 1960s by Sir John Charnley and represents a major milestone

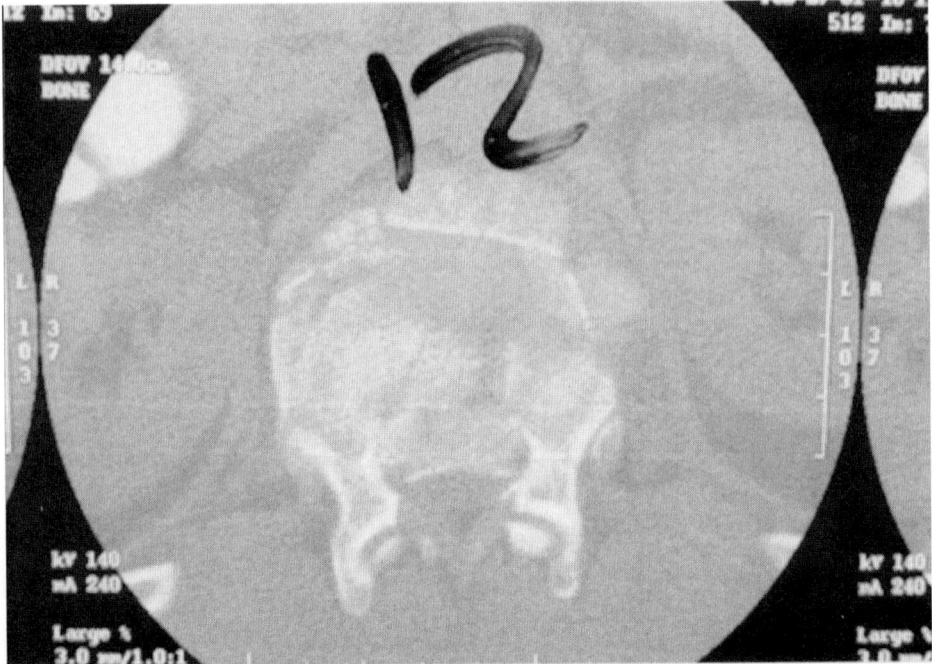

FIG. 42-66. Axial CT scan of a patient with a fractured lumbar vertebra. The fragmentation of the vertebral body is seen, as is the displacement of a fragment into the spinal canal. If the patient has abnormal neurologic findings, this fragment probably should be removed from the spinal canal.

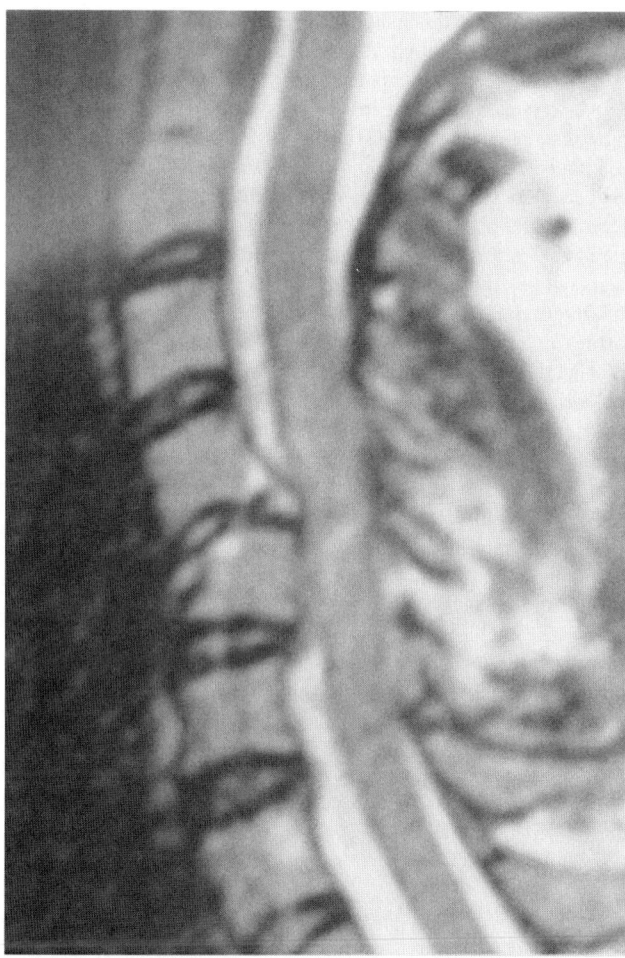

FIG. 42-67. *Sagittal MRI of the spine of a patient with neurologic loss after an automobile accident. The bone injury is seen with the displaced fragments shown to be pushing on the spinal cord. The pressure should be relieved if there is evidence of only a partial neurologic injury.*

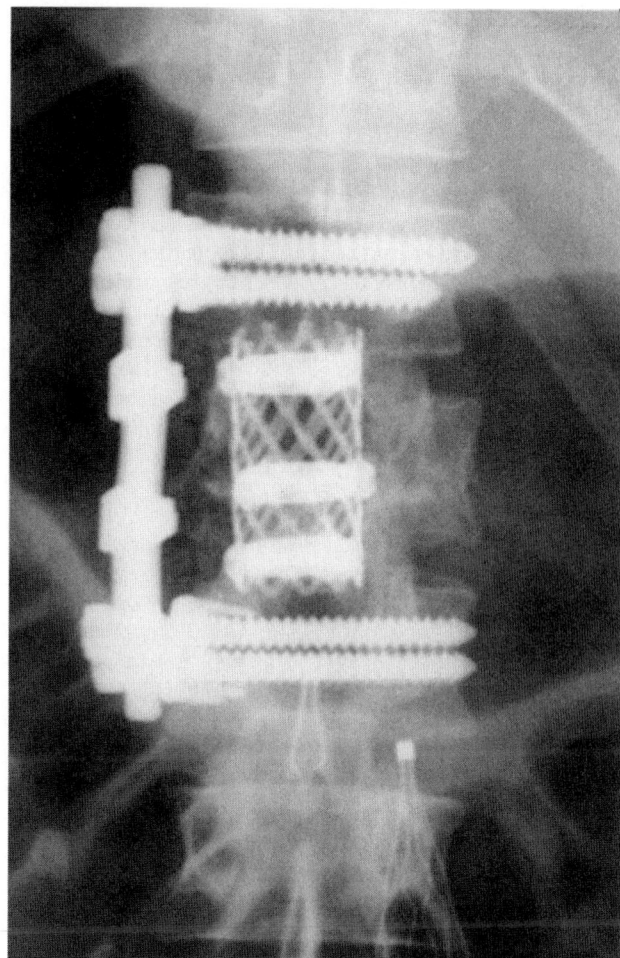

FIG. 42-68. *AP radiograph of a patient who has had an anterior decompression of an injury to T12. The wire cage is filled with bone graft. This is an exception because this patient had surgery anteriorly only.*

in orthopaedic surgery.[30] John Insall, an American surgeon, was largely responsible for the current techniques used in modern knee replacement and designed one of the most frequently used knee implants in the world. Today, more than 350,000 hips and knees are replaced annually in the United States alone, at an estimated cost of more than $2.5 billion. Most joint replacements are performed in patients older than 65 years of age. With the graying demographics of the population, the number of procedures is expected to increase significantly.

Total Hip Replacement

Pain and progressive disability in the face of failed conservative measures constitute the primary indication for total hip replacement and provide the basis for the most successful outcomes. Prior to the successful advent of joint replacement these patients were condemned to a downward spiral of limited function and ultimate immobility. Total hip replacement is indicated in patients with deterioration of the hip joint, which may result from a number of causes, including degenerative arthritis, rheumatoid arthritis, osteonecrosis, ankylosing spondylitis, postinfectious arthritis, benign and malignant bone tumors of the hip joint, and hip fractures.

Active infection, abductor muscle loss, progressive neurologic disease, and neurotrophic joints are specific contraindications to

total hip replacement. In the presence of active infection, implantation of any foreign implant will lead to persistence of that infection and preclude the longevity of any form of implant fixation. The abductor muscles provide stability of the prosthetic hip joint and their loss leads to the increased likelihood of recurrent dislocations. In some instances, such as the resection of a tumor about the hip, the abductor loss is only a relative contraindication in considering hip reconstruction. Neuropathic joints and progressive neurologic conditions usually lead to early loosening as a consequence of repetitive trauma and recurrent dislocation caused by muscle imbalance.

In the early history of hip replacement, age was an overwhelming consideration in patient selection. With general uncertainty surrounding long-term implant survival and efficacy, elderly patients were considered the primary candidates for total hip arthroplasty. Younger patients were considered contraindicated. With increasing data on the long-term success of total hip arthroplasty, the indications have continued to expand to younger and more active patients. The surgeon must, however, educate these young patients about the limitations of the procedure. High-intensity athletics, heavy lifting, and high activity levels can lead to premature implant failure. Younger, more active patients and manual laborers must modify their activity levels to a more moderate sedentary lifestyle to ensure the ultimate success and long-term survival of their joint implants.

The classic technique for fixation of the hip implant as described by Sir John Charnley involved the use of an acrylic bone cement, polymethylmethacrylate (PMMA), for fixation of the femoral and acetabular implants. Early reports revealed excessive failures of the femoral fixation with an associated development of large periprosthetic radiolucency on plain radiographs. This process was initially thought to be a reaction to the acrylic bone cement and was termed *cement disease*. Significant research directed at these failures elucidated the root cause: particles generated from motion of prosthetic interfaces. These motions may include the movement of the prosthetic head against the polyethylene, the motion between the modular taper of a femoral head and stem, or the motion between a modular acetabular shell and its polyethylene liner. These particles lead to macrophage and giant cell release of prostaglandin (PG) E_2 collagenase and other humoral factors, resulting in bone absorption. This process is known as osteolysis and continues to be the major factor leading to the failure of total hip replacement.

The concept of failure caused by "cement disease" lead to innovations in the late 1970s and early 1980s that improved cement fixation and provided alternative methods of component fixation without cement. Today, two types of fixation are employed: cement and cementless (Fig. 42-69). Cementless fixation is based on the use of a porous material that allows bone grow into the prosthesis. Roughened surfaces and biologically active coatings promote ingrowth of bone as a fixation method. For fixation of the acetabular component, cementless fixation is used in most healthy patients undergoing primary total hip replacement. Cemented fixation is used primarily in elderly patients (currently those older than 70 years of age), and in patients where ingrowth is unlikely, such as those with significant prior irradiation to the pelvis. For fixation of the femoral component, both cemented and cementless stems are employed. In patients older than age 65 years, and in patients with compromised bone stock as a result of metastatic disease, cemented fixation remains the gold standard. In young patients (those younger than 65 years of age), those more than 25% of their ideal body weight, and those with excellent bone stock, cementless fixation offers a long-lasting biologic alternative.

The major complications associated with total hip arthroplasty include infection, thromboembolism, heterotopic ossification, and dislocation. Infection is the most devastating consequence after total hip arthroplasty. The incidence of infection was 3.2% a decade ago; however, modern advances in surgical technique, the use of body-exhaust suits during surgery, and perioperative antibiotics have reduced the rate to 0.5 to 1% for primary total hip replacement. Thromboembolism is the most common complication following total hip arthroplasty and the leading cause of postoperative morbidity. The incidence of deep venous thrombosis, depending on how hard one looks, ranges from 8 to 70% with the occurrence of fatal pulmonary embolus, and from 1 to 2% in patients who are not given prophylaxis for thromboembolism. Many patients with

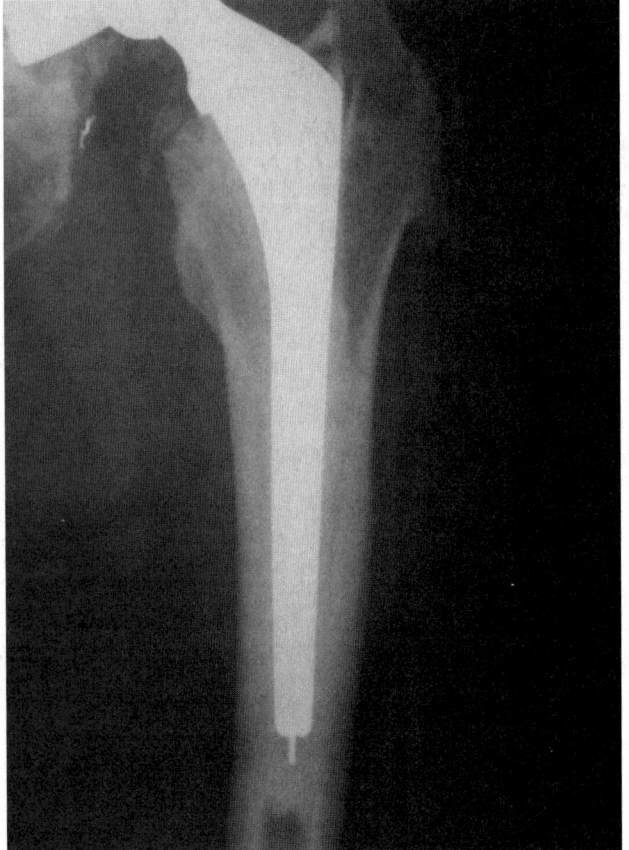
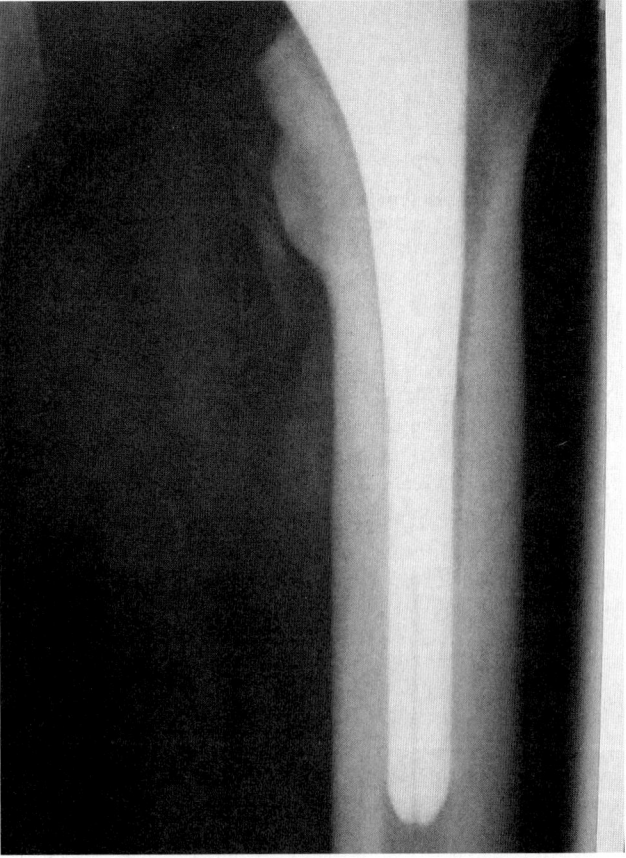

A *B*

FIG. 42-69. *A. Femoral stems can be secured to the bone with PMMA. Barium is put in the PMMA so it can be seen on the radiograph. B. Femoral stems can be implanted without cement. This prosthesis has a coating that allows bone to grow into it and secure the stem to the bone.*

a deep vein thrombosis have no complaints or abnormal physical findings, but the presence of calf tenderness (Homans' sign), low-grade fever, fatigue, tachycardia, and diaphoresis are of particular concern. The classic presentation of pulmonary embolus consists of shortness of breath, pleuritic chest pain, and mental status changes, but often the complaints are much more subtle and it is important to always be aware of the risk of a pulmonary embolus in a patient who has had hip or knee surgery. Multiple methods of postoperative prophylaxis (aspirin, warfarin, heparin, support hose, and sequential compression devices) are employed to lessen the incidence of deep vein thrombosis and pulmonary embolism. Heterotopic ossification is another common complication of total hip arthroplasty with an incidence of 0.6 to 62%. Although the etiology is unknown, heterotopic ossification formation has been associated with hypertrophic arthritis, posttraumatic arthritis, ankylosing spondylitis, diffuse idiopathic skeletal hyperostosis, prolonged surgical time, and trauma to the soft tissues at the time of surgery. Another complication following total hip arthroplasty is dislocation with rates reported from 1 to 3%. Adherence to the postoperative regimen of restricted motion is essential in lessening dislocation rates. Restriction of motion is continued for at least 6 weeks because this allows time for healing of the soft tissues that surround the implant.

Despite the success of total hip arthroplasty, relatively short-term implant survival rates in active, young patients and in heavy laborers make its use in these groups problematic. As previously stated, the presence of an active infection is a contraindication to total hip arthroplasty. For patients in these situations, alternatives to hip arthroplasty include hip arthrodesis, hip osteotomies, and resection arthroplasty. Arthrodesis is favored in young arthritic patients with unilateral disease with a normal lumbar spine and ipsilateral knee. A return to manual labor and high activity is expected with full relief of pain. Femoral osteotomy is commonly used when there is a localized defect that can be redirected to non-weight-bearing areas of the joint. The best results are achieved in young, thin patients with near normal range of motion and focal defects. Resection arthroplasty is primarily reserved as a salvage procedure for the patient with continued hip pain after an infection. It is best for the patient with limited functional demands.

Total Knee Replacement

The evolution of total knee replacement in its current form has progressed significantly over the past 30 years. Disappointing results were seen with various early techniques including soft tissue interposition, joint resection, and the interposition of acrylic and metal. Gunston and others expanded on these early ideas to develop metal runners, which articulated with polyethylene attached to the tibial plateau. These early designs evolved into today's implants, which resurface the distal femur and articulate with a polyethylene surface that is attached to the tibia. Most commonly, the patella is also resurfaced with a dome-shaped implant made of high-density polyethylene. Fixation of the implants to the bone surfaces is either achieved with acrylic bone cement or by bone ingrowth into a roughened or coated prosthesis. Today, cemented knee replacements are the most commonly performed because of the excellent results achieved in long-term clinical studies.

Several current studies show survivorship of total knee replacements to be approximately 93% at 10 years (Fig. 42-70). Additionally, patients were able to regain function and maintain motion of the knee. It is important to note, however, that postoperative range of motion closely relates to preoperative range of motion. Although

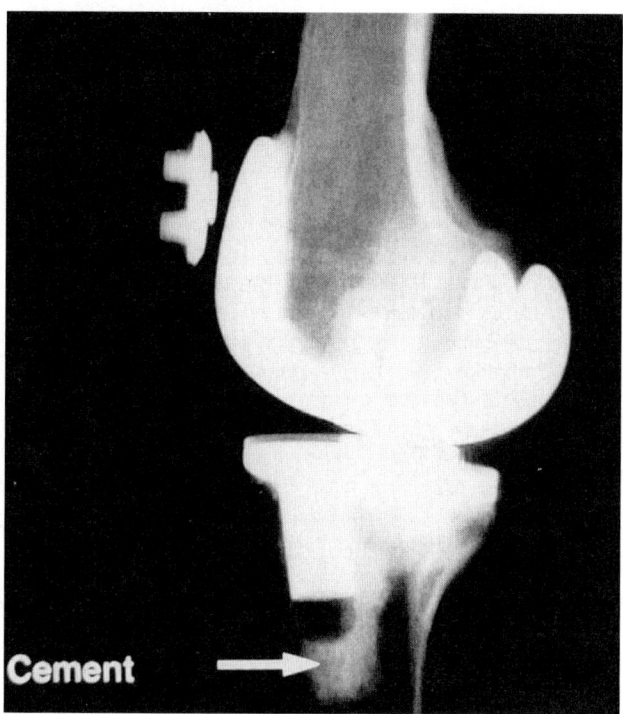

FIG. 42-70. Lateral radiograph of a total knee arthroplasty.

commonly used, continuous passive motion machines and postoperative manipulation and physical therapy of the knee do not affect long-term range of motion. Functionally, 90 degrees of motion is required to arise from a chair without the use of the upper extremities. Postoperative recovery after total knee replacement must therefore not only achieve pain relief and ambulatory capacity, but also good range of motion in order to obtain a satisfactory result.

Local complications specific to total knee arthroplasty include fractures of the patella and femur, patellofemoral pain and dislocation, peroneal nerve palsy, skin breakdown, and postoperative stiffness. In resurfacing the patella, the lateral geniculate artery may be sacrificed resulting in an avascular patella. Additionally, overaggressive resurfacing may lead to a thin patella. Both instances increase the risk of fracture. Minimally displaced fractures may be treated with immobilization. Displaced fractures may require component removal with subsequent patellectomy or open reduction with internal fixation. Osteopenia and intraoperative notching of the femur can predispose to fracture of the femur above the femoral implant. This injury usually requires either complete knee revision or open treatment of the fracture. Improper positioning of the patellar or femoral components may lead to postoperative pain and dislocation of the patella. In addition to careful intraoperative component positioning, this complication may be avoided with attention to soft-tissue releases to ensure proper patellofemoral tracking with knee motion. Peroneal nerve injury may occur during surgery as a consequence of excessive force from retractors or with correction of significant valgus deformities of the knee. Patients who have had prior operative procedures through different skin incisions may have breakdown of the skin in areas that bridge these different sites. To minimize the risk of this complication, skin bridges should be at least 4 cm. To maintain good motion, a structured postoperative rehabilitation program is essential. Some patients, because of pain, scarring, or incomplete rehabilitation, may have poor postoperative range of motion. Early in the postoperative phase of total knee replacement, poor motion is treated with a return to the operating room for manipulation of the knee under anesthesia. The patient then continues with physical therapy to retain this motion. Special attention is directed to pain control during this period to allow the patient maximum benefit from physical therapy.

As in other types of joint replacement, infection and deep venous thrombosis are significant systemic complications. Infection rates have been reported at 1 to 2% and represent several thousand cases given that 200,000 total knee arthroplasties are performed annually in the United States alone. Infection presents a formidable challenge to the surgeon because of prolonged treatment and additional surgical procedures, long-term antibiotic therapy, and diminished functional outcomes. Deep venous thrombosis occurs in approximately 50% of unilateral cases and in as many as 75% of bilateral cases without prophylaxis. Unlike deep vein thrombosis following total hip arthroplasty in which clots occur mainly in the calf veins, life-threatening emboli generally occur in the pelvis following total hip arthroplasty. However, these clots may propagate and involve the proximal femoral vein and pelvic veins.

Despite the indicated successes of total knee arthroplasty, younger patients continue to present a difficult challenge and often require alternate treatments. Osteotomy of the tibia or femur is often used to transfer weight-bearing load to an uninvolved tibiofemoral joint surface when there is unicompartmental disease. This procedure is most commonly done at the proximal tibia for medial compartmental disease but may also be performed at the distal femur in lateral compartment disease. The knee should have limited deformity of less than 15 degrees in the valgus or varus planes with no instability or subluxation. The best results are achieved in young patients who are not overweight and who have good bone stock. This procedure is used primarily as a temporizing measure to gain 5 to 10 years before total joint arthroplasty is performed.

Arthrodesis provides another surgical alternative for the management of young patients with unstable degenerative knees, the management of septic arthritis with extensive destruction of the joint, and in neuropathic joints. Arthrodesis and resection arthroplasty may be employed in patients with failed total knee replacement in which prosthetic implantation is not an option.

SHOULDER DISORDERS

Rotator Cuff and Biceps Tendon

The rotator cuff consists of four muscles: the supraspinatus, infraspinatus, teres minor, and subscapularis. All insert onto the tuberosities of the humeral head. The primary function of the rotator cuff is to provide dynamic stabilization of the glenohumeral joint by depressing the humeral head into the glenoid cavity. The rotator cuff separates the subacromial bursa from the glenohumeral joint. The acromion covers the bursa and can contribute to local problems (Fig. 42-71). Tears of the rotator cuff, either partial or complete, are common in individuals older than age 40 years and increase with each subsequent decade. Patients with rotator cuff pathology present with pain (especially at night), weakness, and difficulties with the activities of daily living, particularly overhead motions. On physical examination, they have limited shoulder abduction because of pain. It is important to rule out referred pain from cervical spine pathology. Plain radiographs are indicated, but MRI is the most useful means of evaluating the rotator cuff.

The biceps muscle has two heads—a long and short. The long head tendon is intra-articular. It originates on the supraglenoid tubercle of the glenoid and lies between the lesser and greater tuberosities

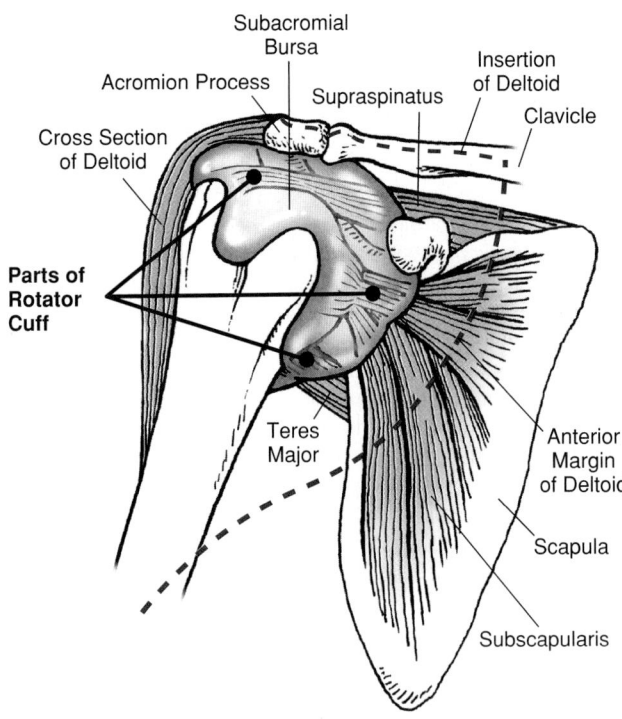

FIG. 42-71. *The subacromial bursa. This bursa is often inflamed and produces shoulder pain and limited shoulder motion.*

of the humeral head. The long head can be inflamed and can be a source of shoulder pain. Rupture of the long head of the biceps can lead to the characteristic "Popeye" deformity of the arm. This is caused by the muscle bunching in the upper arm. This is treated in young, active patients, but not in older patients.

Frozen Shoulder

Patients with adhesive capsulitis or "frozen section" present with shoulder pain and limited motion. Because the scapula moves on the chest wall, patients often do not appreciate how limited their motion is. Careful examination reveals complete loss of motion at the glenohumeral joint. Most often this occurs after a short period of immobilization of the shoulder. Other patients have no inciting event. Diabetics have a higher incidence of adhesive capsulitis than do nondiabetics. Physical therapy is the mainstay of treatment and it often takes up to 1 year to regain full motion.[31] Rarely is surgical intervention necessary.

Glenohumeral Instability

Glenohumeral instability is a spectrum of disorders, which can vary in severity (subluxation to complete dislocation), direction (anterior, posterior, or multidirectional), and duration (acute, recurrent, or chronic).[21] An acute, traumatic, anterior dislocation is the most common instability situation. The risk of developing recurrent subluxation or dislocations is inversely proportional to age, with those patients who have their first acute dislocation before they are 20 years of age having more than an 80% incidence of recurrence. Recurrent instability is most often caused by a tear of the anterior labrum off the anterior glenoid, the so-called Bankart lesion (Fig. 42-72). Most patients who have repeated dislocations of their shoulder require surgical repair. Posterior dislocations more often are caused by a seizure or a fall in an elderly patient. This dislocation is often missed by the unsuspecting physician. The patient holds the arm

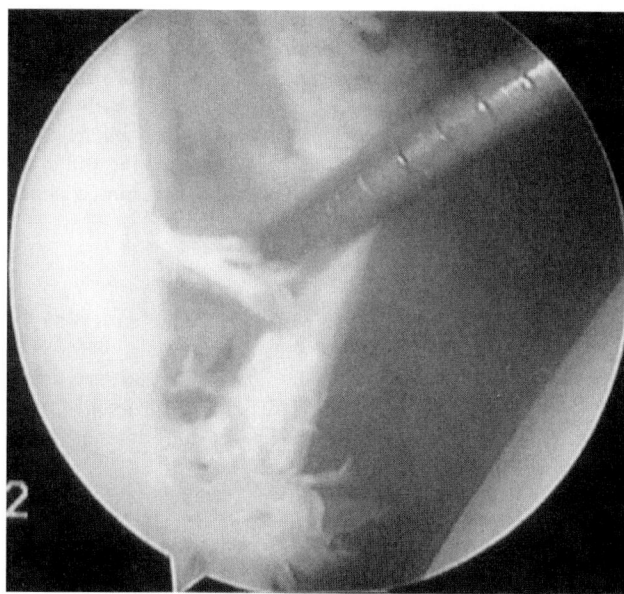

FIG. 42-72. An arthroscopic view of a torn anterior glenoid labrum. This is the classic Bankart lesion that is associated with recurrent anterior dislocations of the shoulder. A traumatic anterior shoulder dislocation causes it.

internally rotated and the usual anterior bulge of the humeral head is not present. A careful neurovascular examination, especially of the axillary nerve, should be done for all patients with a shoulder dislocation. Plain radiographs in two plains at right angles to each other (anteroposterior and lateral or axillary view) are necessary to evaluate the patient's shoulder joint.

Patients with multidirectional instability usually have not sustained trauma and multi-directional instability is most often is seen in young athletes with lax ligaments. These patients rarely benefit from surgery and are treated with muscular strengthening.

Glenohumeral Arthritis

Arthritis of the shoulder joint occurs less often than arthritis of the hip or knee. Idiopathic osteoarthritis is the most common cause of shoulder degeneration; however, other arthritic conditions can produce shoulder damage (e.g., rheumatoid, septic, posttraumatic, and rotator cuff deficiency arthropathy). Pain, weakness, limited motion in all planes of motion, and crepitus are common complaints. If conservative measures such as heat, activity modifications, and nonsteroidal anti-inflammatory medications (NSAIDs) do not produce relief, total shoulder arthroplasty may be indicated.[32]

The acromioclavicular joint often is subject to osteoarthritis and commonly is a result of prior trauma. The patient complains of shoulder pain with abduction and movements of the arm across the body. The joint is tender to palpation. Resection of the distal clavicle often is performed for this disorder.

ELBOW DISORDERS

The elbow is a complex joint allowing flexion and extension as well as pronation and supination of the forearm. A normal elbow has 180 degrees of extension or a few degrees of hyperextension and flexion to 15 degrees. Complete supination should allow the palm to be flat with the elbow at the side, and full pronation is 180 degrees from that point. Flexion extension requires both the proximal ulna and radius to articulate freely with the distal humerus. With pronation/supination the radius rotates at its proximal articulation while the distal ulna and hand rotate around the distal radius.

Epicondylitis most often affects the lateral epicondyle; however, the incidence of medial epicondylitis has increased with the popularity of golf. Lateral epicondylitis has been considered a tendinopathy of the extensor carpi radialis longus (ECRB) origin. Release or repair of the ECRB tendinous origin has had mixed results (when splinting or with cortisone injection) and when combined with activity modification, is unsuccessful. However, recent findings during arthroscopy suggest "lateral epicondylitis" may comprise different pathologic conditions, which may be amenable to arthroscopic treatment. Medial epicondylitis is even less well understood and treatment is controversial.

Another common, nontraumatic elbow condition is ulnar nerve compression (cubital tunnel syndrome), which is caused by compression of the ulnar nerve in the cubital tunnel or proximal flexor carpi ulnaris muscle, and causes pain and dysesthesias in the little and ulnar border of the ring fingers. If severe, weakness and atrophy of the ulnar-innervated intrinsic muscles of the hand may occur causing Froment's, Wartenberg's, or Jeanneau's signs. If splinting the elbow in extension at night is not curative, ulnar nerve neurolysis and transposition anterior to the medial epicondyle, in either a subcutaneous or submuscular position, is recommended. Compression of the radial nerve or posterior interosseous nerve beneath the supinator muscle is much less common than ulnar nerve compression. The vague forearm aching and pain associated with this syndrome may respond to neurolysis, but electrodiagnostic studies, unlike cubital tunnel syndrome, are not diagnostic.

Rupture of the distal biceps tendon attachment to the bicipital tuberosity of the proximal radius may occur as a consequence of a chronic, degenerative tendinopathy. Treatment may be conservative or surgical repair may be performed. If treated conservatively, the patient can expect good flexion strength, but notable weakness of supination and aching with heavy use. Repair, using either a one- or two-incision technique, can restore full, asymptomatic function, but should be performed acutely to avoid permanent contracture and the need for an interposition graft.

Joint surface congruity and collateral ligaments on the medial (medial ulnar collateral ligament) and lateral (lateral ulnar collateral ligament) sides of the elbow impart stability. Elbow injuries may be broadly classified as pure bone, ligament, or bone and ligament injuries. Simple elbow dislocations rupture the collateral ligaments but are usually stable after closed reduction and early mobilization minimizes stiffness. Even though a normal elbow has approximately 165 degrees of flexion-extension, functional range of motion is from 25 to 125 degrees of flexion. However, an elbow injury easily leads to significant loss of motion and elbow stiffness is less-well tolerated than that affecting any other major joint because inability to reach the mouth and head or to perform perineal care is a major functional deficit.

The incidence of arthritis in the elbow is less than that in other major joints, but the morbidity can be profound. Rheumatoid disease can affect the elbow and synovectomy, either arthroscopic or open, is helpful. Radial head resection has traditionally improved pain and motion, but may accelerate the progression of arthritis by removing the secondary restrain to valgus stress. Elbow replacement arthroplasty, using a semiconstrained "floppy hinge" implant, provides good results and acceptable longevity in low-demand patients.

In younger patients, osteoarthritis, or posttraumatic arthritis, is a difficult problem as such patients are not candidates for total elbow arthroplasty because high demands are associated with implant loosening and/or failure as a consequence of prosthetic wear. Aggressive arthroscopic débridement, osteophyte removal, and contracture release have proven valuable, although long-term studies are lacking. Interposition arthroplasty, with or without distraction using an external fixator, may be necessary in younger patients with severe joint destruction. Osteoarthritis in the elderly patient is not common but can be successfully treated with a total elbow replacement. Elbow arthrodesis is poorly tolerated and is a last resort for the failed or infected arthroplasty patient with an unsatisfactory flail elbow.

SPINE DISORDERS

The construction of the musculoskeletal system is centered around the spine with its central nervous core and associated ligaments, muscles, and intervertebral discs. Anatomically, the spine is divided into cervical, thoracic, lumbar, and sacral areas. The special functional requirements of each area are served by the anatomic structural arrangement unique to the segment.

The cervical spine provides the attachment for the head to the body and requires mobility in all directions in order to place the head in positions most advantageous for the use of the various sensory receptors. It is composed of seven vertebrae, the lower five of similar construction. The upper two vertebrae—the atlas and axis—are modified in shape to provide increased flexion and extension of the head (atlas-cranial motion) and increased rotation of the head and neck (atlas-axis motion).

The thoracic spine, composed of 12 vertebrae of similar shape, serves as the attachment for the ribs. Individual vertebral motion is limited by these fixed anterior structures. The sagittal alignment of the vertebrae in kyphosis enhances the bellows action of the lungs, which are contained within the chest.

The lumbar spine consists of five vertebrae connecting the thoracic spine to the pelvis. There is motion between each segment resulting in an appreciable amount of motion for the entire lumbar spine. The range of motion in flexion and extension is enhanced by a large contribution from the hips.

The sacrum consists of five fused vertebrae. It is locked between the two ilia of the pelvis and forms an integral part of the pelvic ring.

The spinal column serves to encase and protect the spinal cord and peripheral nerve roots. The degree of functional disability resulting from an insult to the spinal column is magnified if the neural structures are also involved. The spinal cord extends from the first cervical vertebra to the twelfth thoracic or first lumbar vertebra. The terminal aspect of the spinal cord is called the *conus medullaris*. From this area emerge the multiple nerve roots supplying motor and sensory function to the lower extremities known as the *cauda equina*.

The spine is subject to all of the same disorders that afflict the rest of the musculoskeletal system; however, only the most common problems are discussed in this chapter.

Low Back Pain

Pain in the lumbar area and buttock is one of the most common complaints heard in medicine. The majority of adults will have at least one episode of low back pain during their life, and many adults have recurrent episodes. Most instances of low back pain will not have a specific diagnosis and the cause is generally muscular strain and spasm. More significant abnormalities need to be excluded when a patient with low back pain is evaluated. The most important spinal diagnosis to exclude is a neoplasia; however it is also the least likely cause. Patients with aortic aneurysms and pancreatic cancer can present with low back pain and these diagnoses must be considered. Degenerative arthritis is a more common cause of low back pain, but a delay in making this diagnosis is not significant. Herniated disc with nerve compression is a relatively common cause of back pain associated with leg pain and should be recognized from the patient's history and physical examination.

The initial evaluation includes the taking of a history to determine how the pain started, how long it has persisted, how severe it is, what makes it worse, and what makes it better. The abdomen should be examined. The patient's back is examined for tenderness, masses, muscular spasm, alignment, and motion. A neurologic examination should be done and a rectal examination is recommended. If no abnormalities are noted, except decreased motion and muscular spasm, the patient can be treated with a few days of rest and mild pain medication. If pain persists, a more complete evaluation is indicated.

Patients with a herniated disc without compression of a nerve root do not need specific treatment. They present with low back pain and virtually all will improve with nonoperative care. Those with compression of a nerve root will have pain that is distributed in the dermatome of the compressed nerve root (Fig. 42-73). The patient usually has a positive straight-leg-raise test. Initially, nonoperative

HERNIATED NUCLEUS PULPOSUS

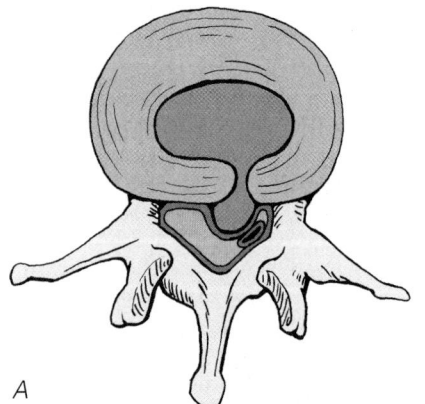
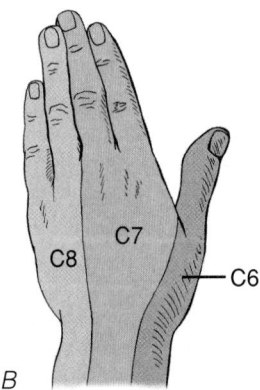
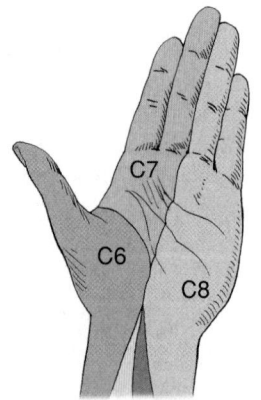
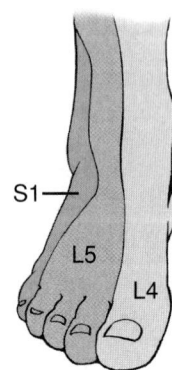

A   *B*

FIG. 42-73. *A. Axial view of herniated nucleus pulposis compressing a nerve root. B. Each nerve root level has a corresponding level of sensory innervation. Abnormalities with the nerve roots are reflected in changes over the distribution of that nerve's dermatome.*

treatment is recommended, and most patients will have relief. Those with persistent pain or recurrent pain should undergo disc removal.

Discitis is an infection of the disc. This is not uncommon is children but is unusual in adults unless they are immunosuppressed or IV drug users. These patients will have unremitting back pain. On a radiograph there will be a loss of disc height; however, this may not be apparent until sometime after the patient has sought medical treatment.

Degenerative arthritis occurs in the elderly, and typically can be managed with physical therapy and anti-inflammatory medication. Some patients will develop spinal stenosis as a result of compromise of the spinal canal. These patients may require decompression.

Another common cause of back pain, although usually seen more in the mid-back than in the lower back, is a compression fracture. Most compression fractures occur in osteoporotic bone and are caused by minimal trauma (Fig. 42-74). Compression fractures can occur in patients with normal bone and are usually caused by significant trauma. However, the most common scenario is an elderly female who complains of acute onset back pain after a minor fall or automobile accident. There will be anterior wedging of a mid-thoracic vertebra. These patients are treated nonoperatively, usually with an extension brace.

Neck Pain

Like low back pain, neck pain is common. Usually it occurs after a minor injury and is often referred to as "whiplash." The usual patient has pain in the neck without a radicular component, loss of motion, and muscular spasm.

Anteroposterior and lateral plain radiographs should be taken. The alignment should be normal and care should be taken to look for fractures or dislocations. If there is any doubt, a CT scan of the cervical spine is indicated.

Those patients with a fracture or dislocation may need surgical stabilization. The guidelines for management of these patients are beyond the scope of this text. Patients without fracture or dislocation are treated with a soft cervical collar, rest, and pain medication. The patient should be instructed that when he or she lays supine, the neck should be in extension. Those patients with radicular pain or a neurologic deficit need to be more thoroughly evaluated. An MRI is the best examination for these patients.

Alignment Disorders

The spine is normally straight in the anteroposterior plane with a cervical and lumbar lordosis and thoracic kyphosis in the lateral plane (Fig. 42-75). In a normal spine the foramen magnum is directly over the body of S1. When there is a curve in the anteroposterior plane, the patient has a scoliosis (Fig. 42-76). The type of scoliosis is described by its location in the spine, degree of curve, direction of curve, and underlying cause. If the malalignment is in the lateral plane, it can be caused by excessive or insufficient kyphosis or lordosis. If the malalignment does not alter the position of the foramen magnum over S1, the curve is said to be compensated, but is uncompensated if the foramen magnum is not over S1. Treatment depends on the degree of curve, loss of compensation, and cause.

MUSCLE AND TENDON INJURIES

The most commonly injured muscles in the lower extremity are the hamstrings, quadriceps, and gastrocnemius. Injuries to these muscles either originate from a direct blow or, more typically, from a sudden eccentric contraction (acute lengthening of muscle as it is trying to shorten). This, in turn, ruptures muscle fibers. In severe cases, a defect in the muscle can be palpated; however, in most cases there is no gross defect. A well-defined sequence of events then occurs: bleeding, damage to muscle cells, and an inflammatory response that leads to a repair. Scar tissue then forms, ultimately leaving the muscle stiffer (less elastic) and more prone to reinjury. Treatment, therefore, involves controlling the pain and inflammation acutely and stretching as the muscle heals to try to keep it at its normal resting length. In severe cases where there is a disruption in the muscle tissue, both remodeled muscle tissue and postinjury muscle strength are improved by suturing the torn muscle tissue together.

Another sequence of events that can be spawned from a quadriceps contusion is myositis ossificans (MO). Myositis ossificans is also called heterotopic bone formation. The majority of patients with MO will recover full function and can be successfully treated nonoperatively. Rarely, a patient will have persistent loss of motion and need the ectopic bone removed. This should not be done until 1 year or more after the injury. A careful history should be taken with someone who has ossification within a muscle, because MO histologically resembles osteosarcoma, and an incorrect diagnosis either way can be disastrous.

Tendinitis and bursitis are commonly caused by overuse, trauma, or through compensation for another injured area. The presence of a bursa is a normal. It is a thin fluid-filled sac with a lining of blood vessels and nerve endings. Bursa occur in any area that has soft tissue repetitively rubbing over a bony prominence. Once irritated, they swell and become painful. The most common sites to develop bursitis around the knee are overlying the patella and the patella tendon (prepatella bursitis), at the anteromedial aspect of the proximal tibia where the pes anserine tendons (sartorius,

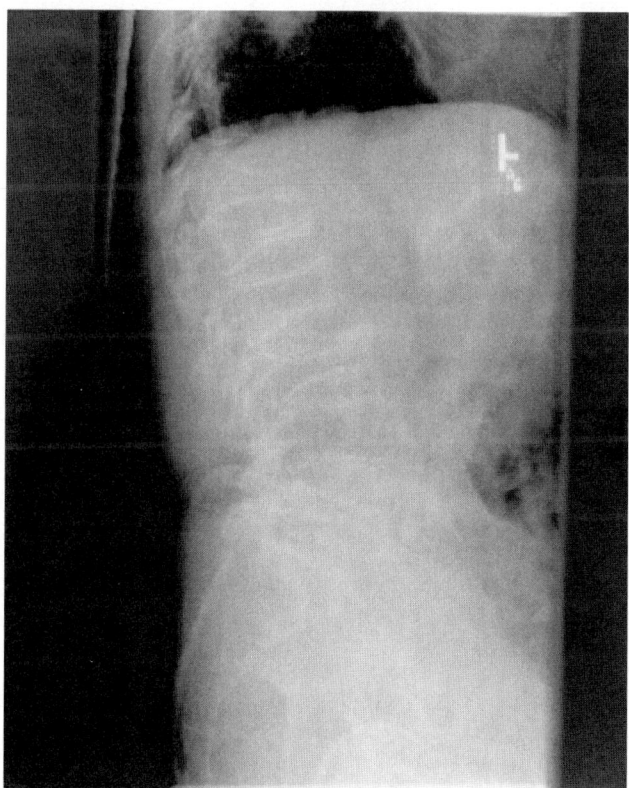

FIG. 42-74. Lateral radiograph of a patient with severe osteoporosis and multiple compression fractures of her lumbar spine.

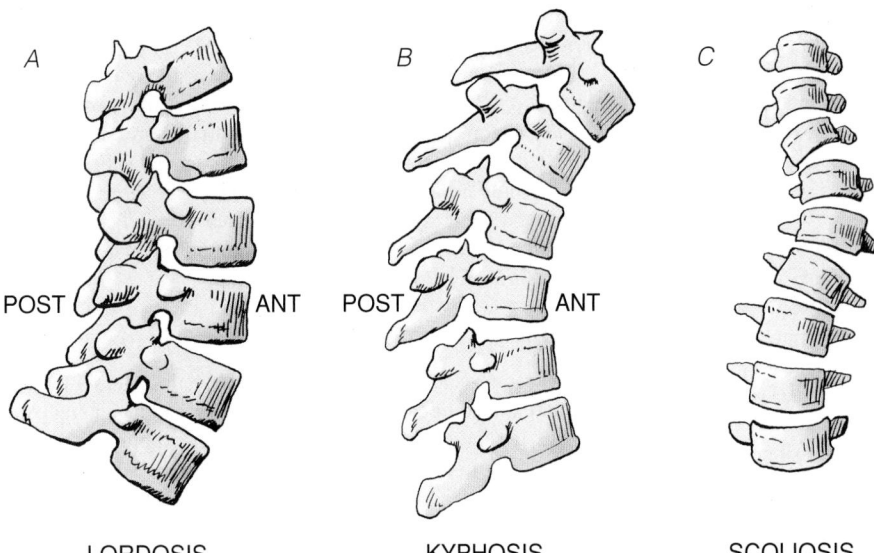

LORDOSIS
(Lateral View)

KYPHOSIS
(Lateral View)

SCOLIOSIS
(Anterior View)

FIG. 42-75. From a lateral view, the normal spine is curved. The cervical spine is in lordosis, the thoracic spine in kyphosis, and the lumbar spine in lordosis. In a normal spine, these curves balance so the head is directly over the sacrum.

gracilis, and semitendinosus) insert (pes anserine bursitis), and at the posteromedial corner of the tibia where the semimembranosus inserts (semimembranosus bursitis). Other common sites of bursitis are the bursa inferior to the acromion (subacromial bursa), the bursa over the greater trochanter of the femur (greater trochanter bursa), and the bursa over the olecranon (olecranon bursa).

Initial treatment involves decreasing the inflammation through icing, anti-inflammatory medication, and removing the offending

insult. With the patella, in particular, it is important to avoid pressure through kneeling or bumping the knee. If this fails, the next step is to use a cortisone injection, aspirating the bursa first, if necessary. Finally, if conservative treatment fails, an excision of the bursa can be performed.

Tendinitis typically occurs from overuse. Endurance sports, such as running and cycling and power sports such as basketball, volleyball, and racquet sports are most frequently involved. The tendons

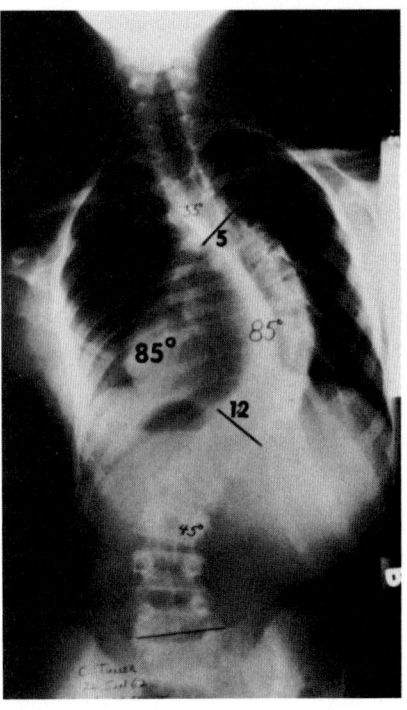

A

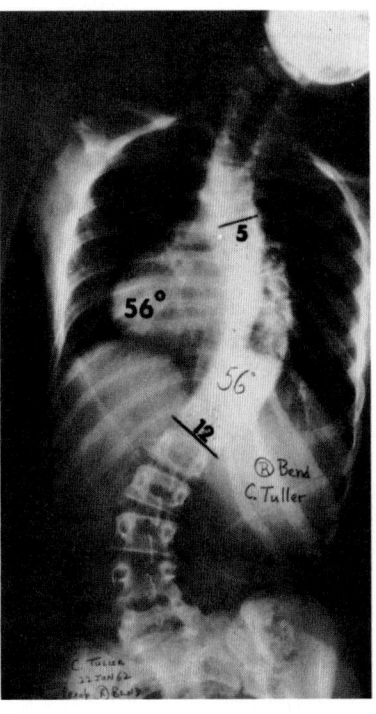

B

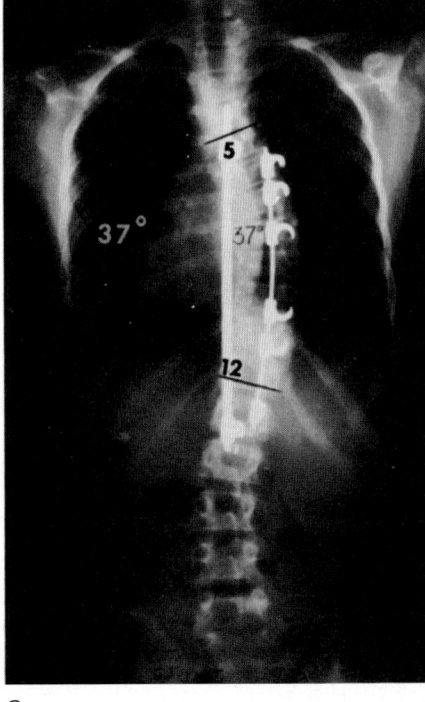

C

FIG. 42-76. Idiopathic scoliosis treated by Goldstein technique of Harrington rod and massive bone graft. *A.* An 85-degree right thoracic primary curve between T5 and T12. *B.* Lateral bend to the right corrects curve to 56 degrees. *C.* Postoperative correction after Harrington rod instrumentation and bone grafting with massive autogenous cancellous bone. The curve is corrected to 37 degrees and fusion to T1 is performed.

are injured by cumulative microtrauma where there is a failed adaptation of the cells and extracellular matrix to repetitive activities at submaximal load. Essentially the microinjuries are unable to heal themselves quickly enough, leading to fatigue of the tendon and, finally, to symptomatic injury. At the knee, the hamstring tendons are most commonly involved and iliotibial band friction syndrome is the most common cause of lateral-based knee pain in runners. The iliotibial band repetitively rubs over the lateral femoral epicondyle, causing both a bursitis and a tendinitis. Other common sites for tendinitis are the biceps tendon (both proximal and distal), common wrist extenders (tennis elbow), the abductor pollicis longus (de Quervain's disease), Achilles tendon, and posterior tibial tendon.

Treatment is focused on calming the inflammation and pain. Ice and rest are the initial modalities. Anti-inflammatory medications are usually prescribed. As the pain subsides, stretching of all tight structures and the use of modalities such as ultrasound and electrical stimulation may be beneficial. Rarely is surgical intervention required. When needed, surgical procedures include tendon sheath débridement (for tenosynovitis), tendon-relaxing incisions or lengthening, or tendon advancement.

The Athletic Knee

The knee is a commonly injured joint. These injuries occur predominantly in young, healthy athletes and are the major focus of most "sports medicine" orthopaedic surgeons. The majority of these injuries are of the ligaments or cartilage. Fractures about the knee are discussed with other typical traumatic injuries to the musculoskeletal system.

The nonoperatively treated injuries are typically the "sprains and strains"; overuse injuries leading to tendinitis or bursitis, muscle contusions, and milder ligament sprains. The surgical injuries tend to involve the anterior cruciate ligament (ACL), the menisci, and the articular cartilage (chondral injuries).

Meniscal Injuries

Each knee has a medial and lateral meniscus. These are C-shaped fibrocartilage rings, triangular in cross-section, that serve as shock absorbers and secondary restraints to the ligaments. The lateral meniscus is more circular than the medial meniscus, but less-well attached to the capsule, particularly posteriorly. Because the medial meniscus is more constrained, it is subjected to higher forces and tears more frequently than the lateral meniscus. The peripheral 25% of the meniscus is vascularized, thus making it amenable to repair. The inner 75% has no blood supply, will not repair a tear, and requires resection if torn and symptomatic. A twisting or hyperflexion event is the usual cause of tears in the athletic population; however, in older individuals, tears may occur without a defined moment, presumably via a cumulative microtraumatic degenerative mechanism.

People with symptomatic tears may recall hearing a pop or tear and then the development of swelling. They complain of pain at the involved joint line, a sense of catching or locking, and often have difficulty with deep flexion. Typically, they cannot squat. On exam there is tenderness over the joint line, particularly posteromedially or laterally, there is pain with hyperflexion (pressure is being placed on the posterior horns) and the McMurray test is positive. This test involves maximum flexion, followed by internal or external rotation and circumduction as the knee is brought into extension. The torn meniscus is being trapped and then tugged. A positive test involves both pain and an audible click or clunk. Further confirmation of a tear can be made with greater than 90% accuracy with an MRI.[33]

The tear (a white line on a T2-weighted MRI) must reach the surface of the meniscus either above or below to be considered clinically significant. Signal changes within the meniscus not touching an articular surface are considered degenerative in nature, are within the meniscus, and cannot be seen or probed during an arthroscopic examination. There is no satisfactory treatment for a degenerative meniscus except removal, which leads to degenerative arthritis.

An arthroscopic repair or trimming is the treatment of choice for symptomatic meniscal tears. This procedure uses a fiberoptic camera in a pencil-thin cannula and biting and motorized shaving instruments of similar diameter. The joint in its entirety can be evaluated and any meniscal or chondral damage repaired. Arthroscopy is typically performed through two or three one-fourth-inch incisions called *portals*. Repair of a peripherally torn meniscus is beneficial. If successful, the normal biomechanics of the joint are maintained. Without a normal meniscus the biomechanics are altered and the joint damaged. Meniscal repair can be performed using sutures and small accessory medial or lateral incisions, or it can be performed completely arthroscopically by using bioabsorbable implants. Total meniscectomies performed in the era before arthroscopy have taught that over a period of 10 to 20 years, knees without a meniscus develop arthritis.[34] The benefit of arthroscopy is that if the meniscal tear is not repairable, the least amount possible can be resected and the remaining meniscus contoured and smoothed so as to maintain its shock absorbing and stabilizing function. Twelve-year follow-up has shown minimal degenerative changes in knees having undergone arthroscopic partial meniscectomies.

Occasionally, a meniscus will tear peripherally and the central torn segment will flip over and stick in the notch of the knee. This is called a *bucket-handle tear*. The bucket handle often "locks" the knee, preventing extension. This is considered a semi-urgent situation requiring surgery. In the older individual with a meniscal tear, particularly in a patient with mild arthritis seen on the radiograph, an attempt at conservative treatment with physical therapy, and possibly a cortisone injection, can be done and should be considered. The younger, more active patient with a longer life expectancy should have the meniscus repaired.

Ligament Injuries

The ACL and posterior cruciate ligament (PCL) are the central pivots to the knee. The ACL provides anterior translation restraint and anterolateral rotatory stability, while the PCL provides mostly posterior translation restraint. They also act as secondary restraints for the collateral ligaments (medial collateral ligament [MCL] and lateral collateral ligament [LCL]), which provide valgus and varus control.

A patient presenting with knee pain after a twisting injury or a varus or valgus torque to his or her knee with immediate swelling and who reports hearing a pop should be evaluated for a ligament sprain. If the effusion is tense and painful, the knee should be aspirated. Often, more than 100 mL of blood can be withdrawn. The examination should include assessing the tibial step-off at 90 degrees of flexion. This is the amount of tibia protruding anterior to the femur viewed from the medial side. Normally there should be a step-off of 1 cm. No step-off indicates posterior translation of the tibia and a PCL injury. An anterior, then posterior deforming force should be applied to the tibia (an anterior drawer and posterior drawer test, respectively). Increased motion compared to the opposite side indicates an ACL or PCL injury. Varus and valgus stress should then be applied both in full extension and 30 degrees of flexion. Thirty degrees of flexion isolates the collateral ligament, and gapping of more than 1 cm indicates a complete rupture (grade 3) of

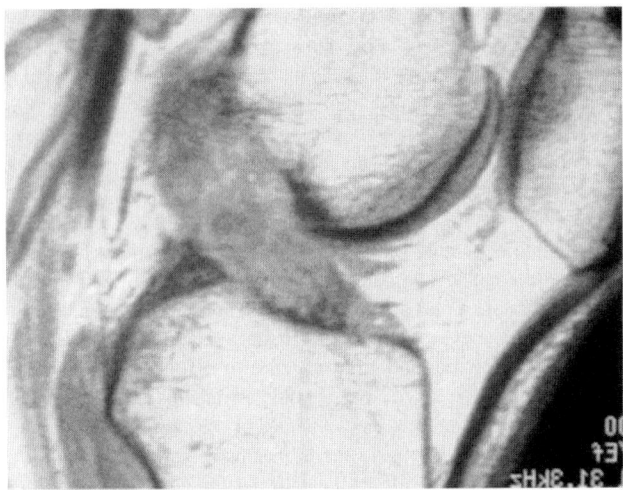

FIG. 42-77. *Sagittal view of an MRI from a patient with a torn anterior cruciate ligament. The intermediate, fuzzy signal running diagonally from the posterior femur to the tibial plateau is the torn ACL. A normal ACL is a black structure.*

the collateral ligament. Mild opening is considered grade 2 (partial tearing of the fibers). Pain, but no opening, is considered grade 1 (strain of the fibers but no tearing). Any gapping with the knee in full extension usually indicates the involvement of one of the cruciate ligaments, as well as the collateral ligament. The ACL can be further tested for with a "pivot-shift test." An axial and valgus load is applied to the extended knee. As it is flexed upward, a "clunk" is felt at 30 degrees when the anteriorly subluxed tibia reduces. An MRI of the knee demonstrates the cruciate tear (Fig. 42-77).

The PCL can be further assessed with the "sag test" and the "quadriceps active test." In the former, the heel is supported with both the hip and knee flexed to 90 degrees. Without a PCL, the tibia can be seen to sag posteriorly on the femur. Without a PCL, the foot is held firmly on the examining table and with the hip and knee flexed and the patient is asked to try to slide the foot forward. The tibia can be seen to move forward from a posteriorly subluxed position under the force of the quadriceps. Finally, posterolateral complex (LCL, popliteus, popliteofibular, and arcuate ligaments) insufficiency can be evaluated with "external rotation test." With the patient supine and the knees flexed to 30 degrees, the feet are externally rotated. If the involved foot rotates 10 degrees or more than the opposite foot, the test is considered positive. If the external rotation increases still further at 90 degrees, PCL involvement is indicated as well.

Anterior Cruciate Ligament

The ACL, although less frequently injured than the MCL, is the most notorious ligament in regard to injury in the world of sports. Pivoting, sharp decelerating, being clipped, or falling backward while skiing will typically cause injury to the ACL. The injury is extremely painful and usually swells immediately. Within a few weeks the pain subsides and the swelling resolves. Once torn, the ligament cannot heal, even if sewn together, and therefore the ligament must be recreated by using other tissue. Most activities of daily living can be done without difficulty with a torn ACL.[35] However, a quick turn or step off a curb may cause the knee to buckle. For those individuals exhibiting functional instability or a desire to return to high-demand sports (football, basketball, soccer, tennis, or skiing), an ACL reconstruction should be considered.

The reconstruction is done by replacing the ACL. The most common graft sources are the central third of the patella tendon, the hamstring tendons, or an allograft tendon. Synthetic materials have been tried in the past without much success and cause tremendous inflammatory responses when they break down. Bone tunnels are created in the tibia and femur to recreate the origin and insertion of the ACL in the joint, and the graft is fixated with an interference screw within the tunnel or sutures tied over a post. A complete functional recover is expected, although the knee will not return to normal and continues to have measurable abnormalities.

Posterior Cruciate Ligament

The PCL is typically injured with greater trauma than that required for an ACL injury such as a dashboard injury sustained while driving in which the tibia is posteriorly displaced on the femur or the knee is hyperextended. Unless an individual exhibits instability, isolated PCL injuries can be treated conservatively. Many people participate in high-demand sports such as football without a PCL. There is some long-term risk for the development of patellofemoral and medial compartment arthritis with chronic PCL instability. When reconstructed, it is done with a similar procedure to that of the ACL.[36]

Collateral Ligaments

The LCL is rarely injured; however, when it is, the posterolateral complex is often injured as well, and both require repair. Acute repair within the first 2 weeks following injury provides for a much better repair. Repair later than 2 weeks following injury is plagued by retracted tissue that has scarred down, leaving their identification and subsequent repair impossible. Chronic tears require reconstruction with allograft tissue, hamstring tendons, or iliotibial band.

The MCL is often injured and almost always heals without surgical intervention. It is surrounded by a vascular bed of muscular tissue that enhances healing. Typically, 6 weeks of protection from valgus stress in a hinged, range-of-motion knee brace is required. The MCL scars quickly and prolonged immobilization can cause loss of motion, especially with extension. In rare instances of wide opening with an isolated grade 3 tear or in conjunction with an ACL or PCL tear, the MCL requires surgical repair. As with the LCL, the best results are obtained when a primary repair is done within the first 2 to 3 weeks.

The Dislocated Knee

This condition can be a limb-threatening injury. It usually occurs with high-speed vehicular trauma or with a fall from heights, but can also happen in sporting activities, typically a contact sport. Usually the ACL, PCL, and one of the collateral ligaments are disrupted. There is a high incidence of popliteal artery, tibial nerve, and peroneal nerve injury; therefore, close attention should be paid to the neurovascular status during evaluation of a dislocated knee. An angiogram should be considered in all cases of knee dislocation. Intimal tears of the artery may not be evident for several days. In younger individuals, knee dislocations should be treated with surgery within the first 2 to 3 weeks. In older or sedentary individuals, 6 weeks of immobilization may provide sufficient stability. However, in these cases it is understood that range of motion is being sacrificed.

Articular Cartilage Injuries

Articular cartilage does not repair well. Although considerable metabolic activity takes place in chondrocytes, they possess extremely limited ability to heal an injury. Partial thickness lacerations will remain permanently without any repair process. If an injury penetrates the entire depth of the cartilage to expose bone, the bleeding from the bone will allow a healing response and the production of cartilage. Unfortunately, the cartilage produced in this situation is fibrocartilage and not articular cartilage. The fibrocartilage is insufficient to replace articular cartilage and wears out quickly.

For this reason, it is always best to save as much articular cartilage. Therefore, whenever any cartilaginous body has been knocked loose it should be replaced into the defect if possible. The current methods available to repair defects in articular cartilage are all of limited success. The simplest method is a drilling of the subchondral bone to stimulate the production of fibrocartilage. The knee is moved as much as possible during the repair process to stimulate the production of cartilage. Cartilage plugs can be taken from one part of the knee (areas exposed to less weight bearing) and placed into the defective area. Finally, cartilage cells can be removed from the knee and cultured to establish a pool of chondrocytes that can then be placed in the defect. It is expected that they will then produce articular cartilage to completely repair the defect. There is some promise to this method, but it has yet to be perfected.

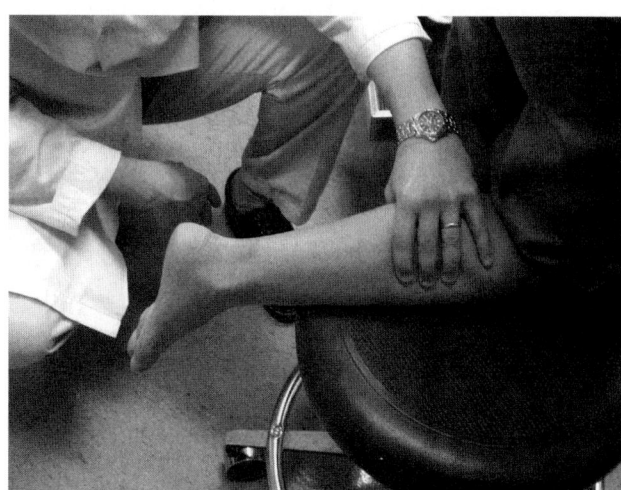

FIG. 42-78. *Before compression of the calf muscle with the knee flexed and the patient relaxed, the foot is in neutral.*

FOOT AND ANKLE DISORDERS

Tendon Disorders

Tendon disorders of the foot and ankle are common problems, with chronic tendinosis, tendinitis, and frank rupture of the Achilles tendon constituting the majority.[37] The Achilles tendon is the most commonly affected and tendinosis, or a chronic partial tear of the Achilles tendon, presents with thickening of the tendon and pain with palpation. MRI shows degeneration within the tendon and thickening. Tendinitis of the Achilles tendon also presents with pain and inflammation around the tendon. MRI shows fluid around the tendon within the paratenon surrounding the tendon. Tendinosis and tendinitis are treated nonsurgically with NSAIDs, gentle stretching, bracing, and a heel lift. Steroid injections should be avoided in this area because of the risk of rupture of the tendon.

History and physical examination easily diagnose complete rupture of the tendon. Patients report a feeling of being struck in the back of the leg and an inability to ambulate following the injury. It is unusual for a patient with a ruptured Achilles tendon to have had tendinitis of the Achilles tendon. The Thompson test is useful in diagnosing a complete Achilles tendon rupture. This is performed with the patient prone and knees flexed to 90 degrees. The calf is then squeezed on both the affected and normal leg. The normal side will show plantar flexion of the foot with calf compression, while the affected side will not. Absence of plantar flexion is a positive indicator for a disrupted tendon (Fig. 42-78). Nonsurgical treatment of a ruptured Achilles tendon consists of casting the ankle in slight plantar flexion or functional bracing. Surgery is often recommended to repair the ruptured tendon, however, wound complications are common.

Peroneal tendinitis is a common cause of lateral ankle pain following an inversion injury.[38] Symptoms include lateral ankle swelling and pain with resisted eversion of the ankle. Tenderness to palpation is seen over the area just posterior to the distal fibula, and pain may be elicited with passive inversion. MRI is often helpful in imaging the peroneal tendons. Nonsurgical treatment includes rest, a stirrup ankle support, NSAIDs, and physical therapy. Surgery may include direct repair of the tendon and tenodesis to the adjacent peroneal tendon, as well as tendon transfer.

Posterior tibial tendon insufficiency, often referred to as the adult acquired flat foot, has three distinct stages and presents with pain along the medial side of the ankle and progressive flattening of the longitudinal arch. In stage I, there is swelling and pain along the medial side of the ankle; however, the foot alignment remains normal. In stage II, the posterior tibial tendon and the ligaments supporting the arch begin to stretch, allowing lowering of the longitudinal arch. The heel drifts into valgus and the forefoot abducts; however, the deformity is still flexible. In stage III of posterior tibial tendon insufficiency, arthritis of the hindfoot develops and the hindfoot remains fixed in valgus. At this stage, patients often report pain on the lateral aspect of the ankle, which is caused by impingement between the calcaneus and fibula. Stage IV occurs with long-standing deformity and consists of tilting of the talus within the mortise of the ankle. Radiographs are useful in assessing the position of the foot and ankle and determining the presence of arthritic changes. MRI is very helpful in assessment of the integrity of the posterior tibial tendon. Nonsurgical treatment consists of braces and orthoses, NSAIDs, and cast immobilization. Physical therapy does not usually help in this condition. Surgical treatment consists of tendon transfer with calcaneal osteotomy or lateral column lengthening. Often, an Achilles tendon lengthening is combined with these procedures. For patients with arthritic changes, selective arthrodesis of the hindfoot is necessary.

Heel Pain

Plantar heel pain, most often caused by plantar fasciitis, is one of the most common problems seen in the foot. Patients report severe pain with the first step after arising from sleep or after prolonged periods of sitting. The pain usually subsides after a few minutes of walking and often recurs later in the day after prolonged standing or walking. Usually plantar fasciitis is atraumatic in onset. Examination reveals point tenderness along the medial origin of the plantar fascia on the calcaneus. Heel cord contracture is often present. Approximately 40% of patients with plantar fasciitis will also have evidence of compression of the first branch of the lateral plantar nerve. Imaging studies should be used to eliminate other causes of heel pain such as a calcaneal stress fracture or insertional Achilles tendinitis. Treatment consists of plantar fascia and heel cord stretching, padding, custom-molded orthoses, NSAIDs, and a night splint to maintain passive stretch on the Achilles tendon and fascia. Cortisone injection can help relieve pain and inflammation.

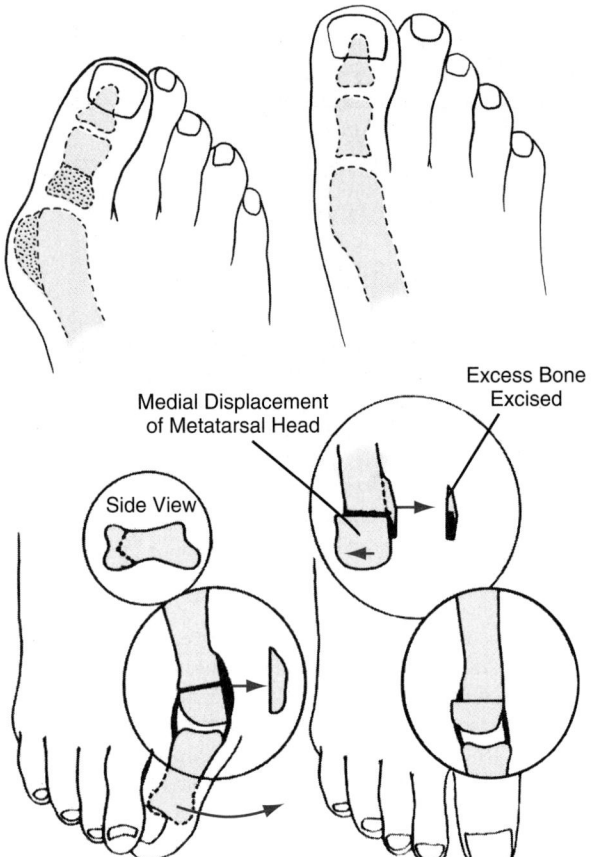

Medial Displacement of Metatarsal Head

Excess Bone Excised

Side View

CHEVRON OSTEOTOMY FOR HALLUX VALGUS

FIG. 42-79. Keller arthroplasty. A. Exostosis and proximal phalangectomy carried out through dorsal medial incision. B. A patient with a bunion. The prominence off the medial metatarsal head is often called an exostosis but it is not neoplastic tissue; it is a reactive process.

Surgery is rarely necessary and consists of releasing a portion of the plantar fascia along with decompression of the lateral plantar nerve.

Hallux Valgus

Hallux valgus is commonly known as a bunion. The great toe is deviated toward the second toe. The angle between the first metatarsal and proximal phalanges of the great toe is a valgus angle (Fig. 42-79). The common causes of hallux valgus are genetic predisposition combined with improper shoes. Many patients will not have symptoms and do not need treatment. Others complain of pain over the medial eminence and difficulty fitting shoes. Lesser toe deformities often accompany hallux valgus as the migration of the great toe pushes the lateral toes out of proper alignment. As the hallux rotates, the sesamoid complex subluxes lateral to the first metatarsal head. Treatment of hallux valgus consists of wider toe box shoes, shoe orthoses, and surgical correction. The indication for surgical correction is continued pain, even with nonoperative treatment. Surgery for this condition includes removal of the medial eminence with a corrective osteotomy of the first metatarsal to decrease the angle between the first and second metatarsals. Often, it is necessary to perform lesser-toe correction along with the hallux valgus procedure.

Lesser-Toe Deformity

Hammertoes are caused by an imbalance between the intrinsic and extrinsic musculature of the foot. The toe extends at the metatarsophalangeal joint and flexes at the proximal interphalangeal (PIP) joint. The patient may experience discomfort over the plantar aspect of the metatarsal, as well as the dorsal part of the PIP joint. Patients with a peripheral neuropathy may develop ulceration and osteomyelitis. Nonsurgical treatment consists of high toe box shoes with a soft, leather upper, as well as splints and padding. Surgical correction is an alternative. The contractures at both the metatarsophalangeal joint and the PIP joints are released and bony resection is done. This is often performed in conjunction with a hallux valgus procedure.

Stress Fractures

Stress fracture, or fatigue fracture of the metatarsals, is a common cause of forefoot pain. Most commonly affected are the second and third metatarsals. Athletes and dancers commonly suffer this problem, along with patients with underlying bone disorders. Symptoms consist of swelling and warmth in the foot, with point tenderness over the affected metatarsal. Radiographs are often negative initially; however, the healing fracture is usually evident by the third week of symptoms. Treatment consists of supportive shoes and temporary cessation of the activity that led to the fatigue fracture. Surgery is rarely necessary.

Arthritis

Degenerative arthritis can affect all areas of the foot and ankle. It often occurs posttrauma and is seen most frequently in the midfoot at the tarsometatarsal articulation. Diagnosis is made upon physical examination along with radiographic narrowing of the midfoot joints. Nonoperative treatment consists of orthotic inserts and a rocker bottom sole to decrease stress to the affected areas. Surgical treatment may include resection of osteophytes or arthrodesis of the midfoot joints.

Arthritis of the hallux metatarsophalangeal joint, known as hallux rigidus, causes stiffness and pain with motion of the great toe. Patients report pain with walking and difficulty with shoes because of painful osteophytes. Nonsurgical treatment includes orthotic inserts, a rocker sole, anti-inflammatory medications, and steroid injections. Surgical procedures for hallux rigidus include joint débridement, arthrodesis, resection arthroplasty, and joint replacement.

Hindfoot arthritis can occur as a result of long-standing acquired flat foot, calcaneal fracture, tarsal coalition, and rheumatoid arthritis. Nonsurgical modalities include bracing and orthoses, NSAIDs, and steroid injection. Surgical procedures often include arthrodesis of one or more of the hindfoot joints.

Ankle arthritis is most often posttraumatic in origin and is easily seen on plain radiographs. Nonoperative treatments include NSAIDs, bracing, and injections. Surgical treatment of ankle arthritis is of significant interest recently, with cartilage replacement techniques and ankle replacement gaining popularity. The mainstay of treatment for ankle arthritis continues to be arthrodesis. Inflammatory arthritis can affect any area of the foot and ankle.

Ankle Instability

Fifteen percent of patients with an ankle sprain will develop chronic instability of the ankle requiring treatment. Usually an inversion injury causes damage to the lateral ligament complex, including the anterior talofibular and calcaneofibular ligaments. Patients report pain and swelling on the lateral aspect of the ankle, often associated with feelings of "giving way" or weakness of the ankle. Physical examination consists of the anterior drawer test and inversion stress test. Stress radiographs help confirm the diagnosis. If intra-articular or tendinous pathology is suspected, an MRI can confirm or rule out these abnormalities. Most patients improve with physical therapy consisting of peroneal muscle strengthening along with a stirrup ankle support. There are many surgical procedures described for repair of the lateral ligament complex. Most popular are the Broström anatomic ligament repair and several weave procedures using the peroneus brevis tendon.

Diabetic Foot

Diabetes commonly affects the foot and can lead to devastating complications, including amputation.[39] Diabetes is the most common cause of neuropathy leading to loss of protective sensation on the plantar aspect of the foot. Charcot arthropathy is a form of arthritis seen in the neuropathic foot and leads to severe deformity (Fig. 42-80). The combination of deformity with a lack of protective sensation leads to pressure ulceration and infection. This can develop into osteomyelitis, and often requires bony resection or amputation. Patients with neuropathy as a consequence of diabetes should be treated with protective shoes consisting of a soft orthoses and accommodative shoes with a soft, leather upper. Pressure relief may be obtained with bracing and shoe modifications. In those patients with deformity not treatable with shoe modifications, surgery is necessary. The goals of surgery are resection of bony prominences, as well as restoration of normal foot architecture. Surgical débridement should remove all necrotic tissue while producing a stable, plantigrade foot. Correction of the deformity can be successful given the patient has adequate circulation. Preoperative vascular evaluation is often necessary. Adequate glucose control promotes healing of ulcerations, as well as surgical wounds.

Interdigital Neuroma

Interdigital neuroma is often called a Morton neuroma. The patient's symptoms are a burning or tingling in the plantar aspect of the forefoot radiating into the toes. It most often occurs in the third web space and may be seen between the second and third toes. There are several theories to explain the etiology, including compression of

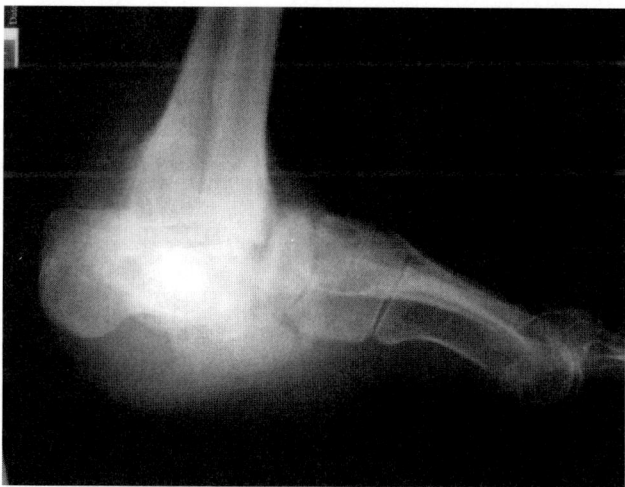

FIG. 42-80. *Lateral radiograph of an ankle with a destructive arthritis caused by a neuropathic condition. This occurs in the ankle and foot as a consequence of diabetes mellitus, in the knee as a consequence of syphilis, and in the shoulder as a consequence of syringomyelia.*

the plantar interdigital nerve by the intermetatarsal ligament, compression from narrow shoes, and inflammation of the intermetatarsal bursa. Diagnosis is made from history and findings on examination of pain with pressure applied to the planter surface in the affected web space while applying a compressive force on the metatarsals. MRI also can be helpful in making the diagnosis. Treatment consists of shoe modifications, padding, steroid injections, and surgical resection of the affected nerve.

Tarsal Tunnel Syndrome

Tarsal tunnel syndrome occurs with compression of the tibial nerve as it passes beneath the flexor retinaculum of the ankle. Patients present with vague symptoms, usually consisting of numbness and tingling on the plantar aspect of the foot. A positive Tinel's sign is present over the tibial nerve; however, sensation is usually preserved. Examination should also include the lower spine to rule out a radiculopathy as the source for the symptoms. MRI is often helpful to rule out a space-occupying lesion within the tarsal canal causing compression of the nerve. Tumors, varicose veins, and subtalar joint osteophytes are common causes of pressure on the tibial nerve. Electromyogram studies may be helpful in confirming the diagnosis, but are not always positive in this disorder. Other causes of neuropathy should also be explored as the source of neuritic pain. Nonsurgical treatment consists of supportive shoes, custom-molded orthoses, medication for neuritis, and physical therapy. Surgery includes release of the flexor retinaculum without manipulation of the tibial nerve. Space-occupying lesions should be removed along with release of the retinacular ligament.

PEDIATRIC DISORDERS

Developmental Dysplasia of the Hip

Developmental dysplasia of the hip (DDH) is a spectrum of disorders involving degrees of instability of the hip and underdevelopment of the acetabulum (socket).[40,41] The term used in the past was *congenital dislocation of the hip*, but this is currently out of favor. The disorder is usually diagnosed shortly after birth because all newborns are screened for the condition by physical examination and, in some areas, by ultrasonography. DDH can present in the toddler, although controversy exists as to whether these cases represent missed diagnoses.

The left hip is more commonly afflicted, probably because of intrauterine positioning. Bilateral cases are more common than cases involving the right side alone. DDH is more common in females, first-born children, breech presentation, and those with a family history of the disorder. The American Academy of Pediatrics recommends ultrasound screening of all female breech babies.

The physical examination consists of two provocative maneuvers: the Ortolani test and the Barlow test. The Ortolani maneuver attempts to relocate a dislocated or subluxed hip. The Barlow maneuver attempts to dislocate or subluxate a reduced, but unstable hip. In addition, the child is inspected for unequal skin folds and apparent limb length discrepancy. Children older than 3 or 4 months of age may no longer have instability, rendering the Ortolani and Barlow tests negative; however, limited hip abduction will be present. Toddlers who develop hip dysplasia, or in whom the diagnosis was missed, present with a Trendelenburg, or "waddling," gait.

The treatment of DDH depends on the age of the child at the time of diagnosis. In children up to 3 or 4 months of age, a cloth brace known as the Pavlik harness is worn full-time for 6 to 8 weeks (Fig. 42-81). The harness positions the hips in such a way that the

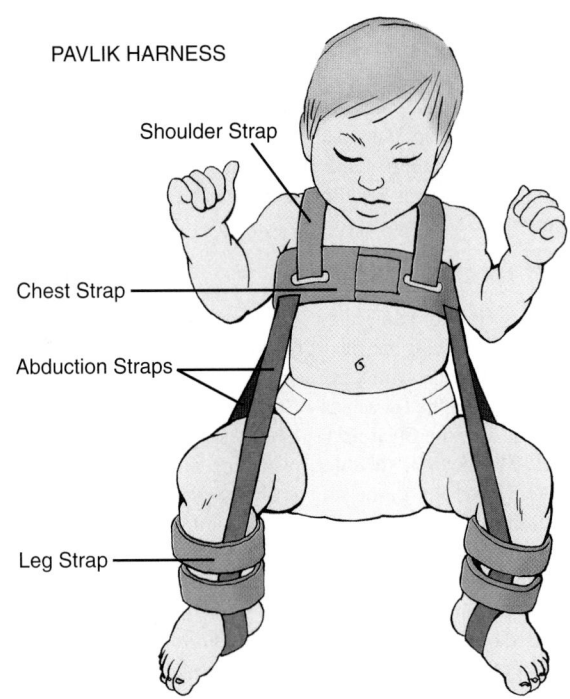

PAVLIK HARNESS

Shoulder Strap

Chest Strap

Abduction Straps

Leg Strap

FIG. 42-81. Pavlik harness used to treat newborns with hip dysplasia. (*Reproduced with permission from http://www.musckids.com/ health_library/orthopaedics/images/1harnessff.gif.*)

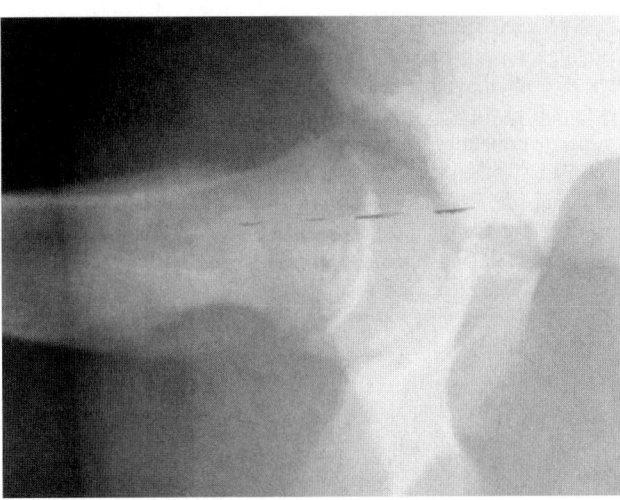

FIG. 42-82. Lateral radiograph of a patient with a slipped capital femoral epiphysis. The displacement is more obvious on a frog-leg lateral view of the hip joint. A line drawn in the middle of the femoral neck bisects the femoral head when it is in the proper position.

baby is able to kick through a stable range of motion while the ligaments and capsule tighten and the acetabulum deepens. The progress of treatment is followed with physical exam and either ultrasonography or plain radiographs, depending on the child's age. The Pavlik harness is successful in 95% of cases and has a very low complication rate. Children who have persistent instability after 3 weeks of bracing, or who present when they are older than 3 to 4 months of age, often require spica cast immobilization.

A closed reduction of the hip under general anesthesia may be necessary if bracing is not effective. The reduction is confirmed with an arthrogram and a spica cast is worn for several months until the acetabular development is normal. Patients older than approximately 1 year of age, or for whom a closed reduction does not reduce the hip, require an open reduction of the hip, often with reconstructive procedures of the proximal femur, acetabulum, or both. A spica cast is worn postoperatively for about 12 weeks. Untreated DDH can lead to degenerative joint disease early in life. Properly treated DDH, particularly in infancy, should have no permanent consequence.

Slipped Capital Femoral Epiphysis

A slipped capital femoral epiphysis (SCFE) is a developmental disorder in which there is dissociation between the epiphysis and metaphysis of the proximal femur.[42] The term is a misnomer because the epiphysis is fixed in the acetabulum and it is the metaphysis, along with the rest of the femur, that slips. In the vast majority of slips, the epiphysis is posteromedial with respect to the metaphysis (Fig. 42-82). A SCFE usually occurs during the adolescent growth spurt and is bilateral in about one-third of cases. Sixty to 65% of patients are above the 90th percentile for weight.

Patients usually present with pain and a limp. The extremity is usually rotated externally and the time spent on the leg is less than the unaffected leg. The gait produced from this shortened time on the leg is called an antalgic gait and is an indication of pain

with weight bearing. The pain is frequently in the thigh or knee despite the pathology being at the hip. The physical exam is most remarkable for limitation of internal rotation of the hip. Radiographs are usually diagnostic and are used to grade the severity of the slip. Occasionally, an MRI is needed to visualize a very early SCFE or "preslip." SCFEs are classified as acute if symptoms have been present for less than 3 weeks, and chronic or acute-on-chronic if there has been a recent exacerbation. They are also classified as stable or unstable depending on whether the patient can bear weight. Acute, unstable slips require emergent treatment.

The treatment of virtually all SCFEs is to stabilize the slip with one partially-threaded, cannulated screw. Reducing the slippage is contraindicated because it damages the blood supply to the epiphysis and may cause osteonecrosis of the femoral head. Occasionally, a reconstructive osteotomy is required to improve the mechanics of the joint.

Legg-Calvé-Perthes Disease

Legg-Calvé-Perthes disease (LCP) is defined as idiopathic osteonecrosis of the proximal femoral epiphysis. It occurs between the ages of 2 and 12 years with a peak incidence between 5 and 7 years of age. This corresponds to the period when the blood supply to the epiphysis is discreet. LCP is three to five times more common in males than in females, and is bilateral in 10 to 20% of cases.

Although idiopathic, the pathogenesis is thought to involve a period of ischemia followed by revascularization. After revascularization, creeping substitution of the necrotic bone renders the epiphysis structurally vulnerable. Symptoms occur once the subchondral bone collapses.

Patients with LCP present with pain in the groin, thigh, or knee. They may have an antalgic or a Trendelenburg gait. Plain radiographs and MRI help to classify the degree of head involvement, which has prognostic significance (Fig. 42-83).[43,44]

There are two main principles in treating LCP: maintaining range of motion of the hip and ensuring containment of the epiphysis. Range of motion is maintained with physical therapy. Occasionally, short periods of traction are required to alleviate a reactive synovitis. In cases where there is greater head involvement, particularly of the lateral epiphysis, there is a tendency for the bone to extrude

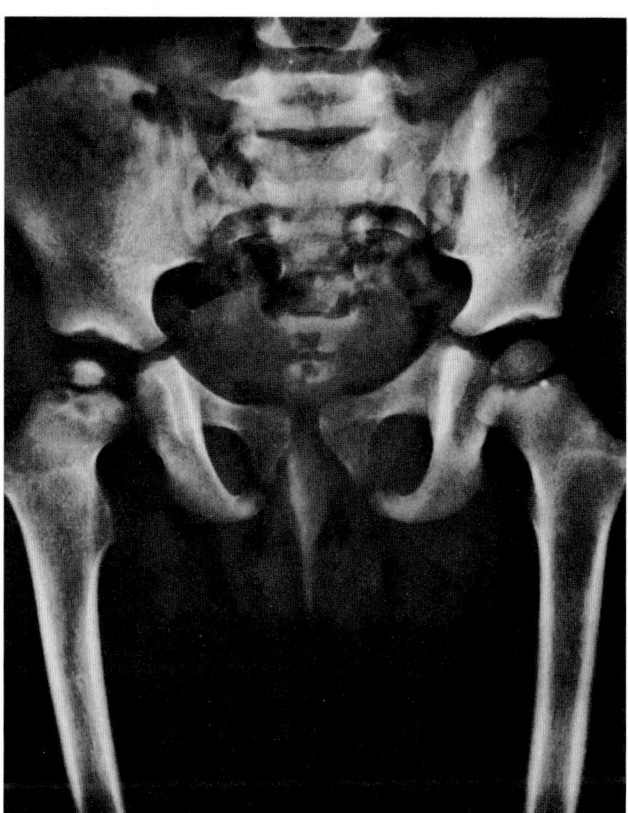

FIG. 42-83. *AP radiograph of a patient with Legg-Calvé-Perthes disease of the right femoral head. This patient's femoral head is small and denser than normal.*

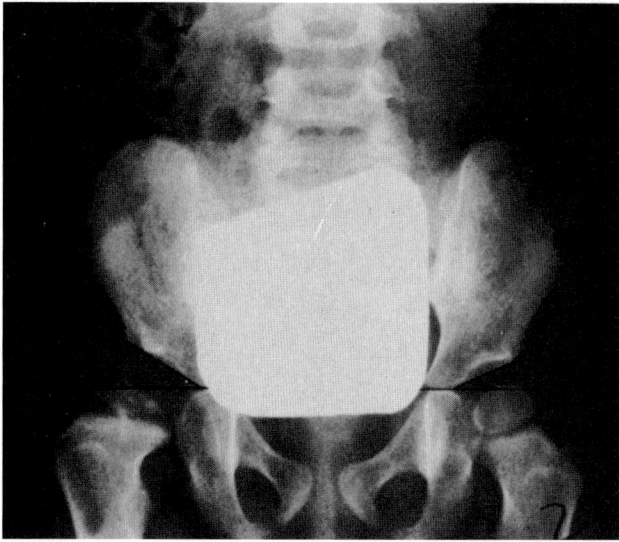

A

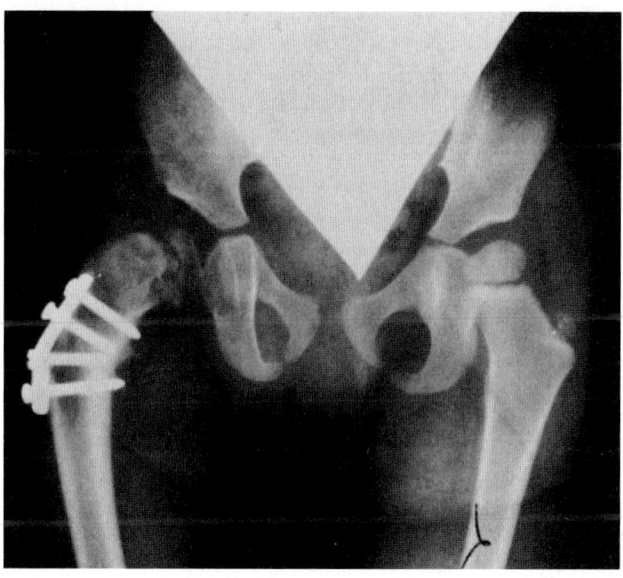

B

FIG. 42-84. *A. AP pelvic radiograph with LCP involving the right femoral head. B. A varus osteotomy was done to contain the femoral head within the acetabulum.*

laterally from the acetabulum. This leads to an incongruous joint. Containment of the extrusion can be accomplished with either a brace or with surgery. Various braces have been designed to hold the hip in abduction while allowing a free range of motion. Surgery to contain the head can be with a proximal femoral varus osteotomy or an innominate pelvic osteotomy such as a Salter (Fig. 42-84). The results of each are comparable. Distraction of the joint during the healing phase using an external fixator currently is being investigated.

The outcome of LCP is somewhat dependent on the morphology of the hip once the disease has run its course. Hips that are spherical and congruent do better than those that are aspherical and incongruent. Long-term studies show that most patients who had LCP are asymptomatic into their sixth decade of life. The most important prognostic factor is age at the time of diagnosis. Patients younger than 6 years of age have the best prognoses; those older than 8 years of age have the worst.

Talipes Equinovarus

Talipes equinovarus (TEV) is referred to as "clubfoot." TEV is an idiopathic congenital deformity of the foot in which there is equinus at the ankle joint, varus and medial rotation at the subtalar joint, and adduction of the midfoot and forefoot.[45] It occurs in 1 to 2 individuals per 1000 live births and is bilateral in 50% of cases (Fig. 42-85).

TEV can be roughly classified as postural, anatomic, or teratologic. The postural clubfoot is thought to be a result of intrauterine molding and it is easily correctable. The teratologic clubfoot is associated with generalized neuromuscular conditions such as myelodysplasia or arthrogryposis. The teratologic clubfoot is rare, rigid, and more resistant to correction. The remainder of this section discusses the anatomic clubfoot.

Although the exact cause of anatomic TEV is unknown, there is clearly a genetic component. A higher incidence of TEV exists in first-degree relatives of patients with TEV than in the general population.

Clinical classification systems exist to assess the severity of the deformity. These are based on the rigidity of the foot and the presence and depth of skin creases posteriorly and medially. On plain radiographs, Kite's talocalcaneal angle is measured on the anteroposterior projection. A normal angle is between 20 and 40 degrees and is lower with TEV. Similarly, the talocalcaneal angle on the lateral projection, normally 35 to 55 degrees, is lower.

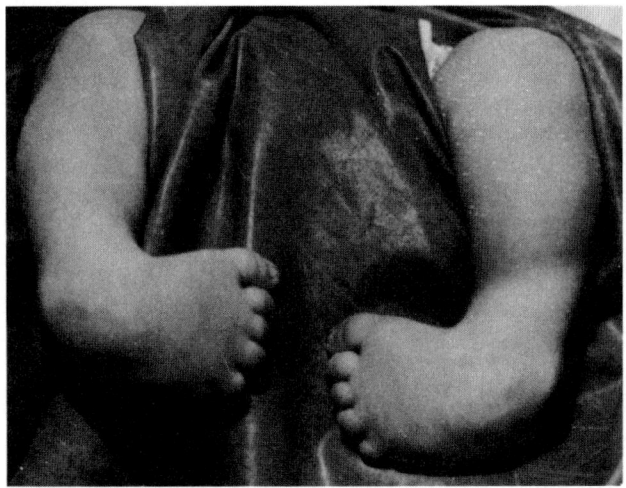

FIG. 42-85. Characteristic deformities of talipes equinovarus, or club-foot.

Treatment of TEV begins at the time of diagnosis, which should be immediately after birth, and initially consists of serial manipulations followed by casting in a sequentially corrected position.[46] The closed treatment of a clubfoot requires that the manipulations be done carefully to prevent causing other deformities. Manipulation is the key; the cast holds the foot between manipulations. Initially, the foot is gently stretched. The talonavicular joint is reduced first, then the heel varus is corrected, then the forefoot adduction, and, finally, the external rotation. Each is addressed at every manipulation. Only after these deformities are corrected is the tight heel cord (Achilles tendon) addressed. Often it is released with a percutaneous technique.

The indication for operative treatment is incomplete correction with serial manipulation. Surgery is delayed until the patient is older than 4 months of age and consists of a posteromedial soft-tissue release with pinning of the subtalar and talonavicular joints. After 6 weeks, the postoperative cast is changed and the pins removed.[47,48]

The results of TEV treatment tend to be excellent. Affected feet are generally one-half to one shoe size smaller, although a supple, plantigrade foot is usually achieved. For severe recurrence or late diagnosis, a bony salvage procedure, such as an osteotomy or fusion, can be done.

Metatarsus Adductus

Metatarsus adductus (MA) is differentiated from talipes equinovarus because these patients have a normal midfoot and hindfoot. Ordinarily, the lateral border of the foot is straight; in MA, the lateral border curves inward at the tarsal-metatarsal joints, producing a bean-shaped foot.

Metatarsus adductus is classified as mild, moderate, or severe depending on which toe is intersected by a line drawn up the center of the heel. If the line intersects the third toe, then the MA is considered mild. If it intersects the fourth toe, it is moderate; if it intersects lateral to the forth toe, it is severe. Mild MA never requires treatment because there is no functional problem and minimal cosmetic concern. The treatment of moderate and severe MA depends on whether the deformity is supple.

If the MA is passively correctable or corrects reflexively when stroking the lateral border of the foot then no treatment other than stretching by the parent is required. Eighty-five percent of feet with

MA correct spontaneously. If correction has not been achieved by 6 months of age, corrective casts or straight-last shoes can be worn.

If the MA is rigid, then stretching by the parent is tried until 3 months of age. In general, after 1 year of age corrective casts or shoes will not improve the position. Multiple metatarsal osteotomies are only indicated in the severe foot with functional impairment or skin embarrassment.

Tarsal Coalition

A tarsal coalition is an abnormal congenital connection between two or more tarsal bones. The calcaneonavicular and talocalcaneal joints are most commonly affected. Tarsal coalition is bilateral in 50 to 60% of patients. The cause is a failure of differentiation and segmentation during embryogenesis and is likely to be genetic. Tarsal coalition is estimated to occur in 1 to 3% of the population, and can be asymptomatic. When symptoms occur, they usually do so in early adolescence, when the coalition begins to ossify. Symptoms consist of activity-related foot and ankle pain associated with a fairly inflexible flat foot.

Plain radiographs may be sufficient to visualize the coalition, particularly when special oblique projections are used. When plain radiographs are not diagnostic, CT and MRI can be used. CT is best for bony coalitions and MRI is best for cartilaginous or fibrous coalitions.

Treatment is indicated only for symptomatic patients. Patients are initially treated with cast immobilization followed by custom-fitted orthotics. Serial treatments may be required throughout adolescence. Surgical treatment is indicated for patients with persistent pain not responsive to immobilization alone. Excision of the coalition with interposition of fat or wax to prevent recurrence is the treatment of choice. Salvage procedures, such as triple arthrodesis, are reserved for patients with arthritis or coalitions that are not resectable.

Blount Disease

Infants born with physiologic genu varum (bow legs) of about 20 degrees have a characteristic of Blount disease.[49] Ordinarily, the bowing gradually straightens until about the age of 3 years, at which time progressive genu valgum (knock-knees) develops. Maximum valgus occurs by the 5 years of age and gradually straightens to physiologic genu valgum (about 3 to 5 degrees) by the age of 7 years.

Infantile Blount disease is a disorder of toddlers in which the physiologic genu varum becomes progressive, damaging the anteromedial physis of the proximal tibia. As the bowing continues, increasing pressure on the anteromedial physis inhibits growth medially, which perpetuates the bowing.

Infantile Blount disease is diagnosed between the ages of 18 and 24 months. Affected children are generally early walkers who are above the 80th percentile for weight. Clinically, patients present with increasingly bowed legs and lateral instability of the knee evidenced by a thrust during single-leg stance of gait. Because the anterior portion of the medial physis is more affected than the posterior portion, these patients tend also to have increased internal tibial torsion.

Radiographs are used to measure the metaphyseal-diaphyseal angle (MDA) of Drennan.[50] A measurement of greater than 11 to 16 degrees in the 18- to 24-month-old infant is predictive of progression. Classification systems of severity exist and depend on the extent of medial depression of the physis.[51]

Patients with significant genu varum but a normal MDA are simply observed at 6- to 8-week intervals. Patients with an abnormal

MDA and lateral instability are treated with bracing. The brace is designed to apply three-point pressure to the extremity to provide a valgus force, which unloads the medial physis. Controversy exists as to whether the brace should be worn full-time, only during weight bearing, or while sleeping. Bracing is effective in reversing the progression in approximately 50% of cases, which reversal can be observed within 3 to 6 months.

Patients who either progress despite brace treatment or recur following treatment should have a proximal tibial osteotomy to restore the physiologic valgus alignment. An oblique osteotomy is made in the proximal metaphysis. Rotation at the osteotomy site corrects both the varus and torsion.

Adolescent Blount disease is a similar entity that occurs during the adolescent growth spurt. The MDA as an indicator of the significance of the genu valgum in adolescents has not been established. Adolescent Blount disease does not respond to bracing. The treatment is a proximal tibial osteotomy to realign the mechanical axis of the knee. These osteotomies are stabilized with an external fixator to accommodate the generally large size of the patient.

Osgood-Schlatter Disease

Growth cartilage that serves as the origin or insertion of a tendon is called an *apophysis*. If the muscle associated with the tendon becomes tight, the tendon pulls with excessive force on the apophysis, which becomes inflamed. This condition is known as *traction apophysitis*. Traction apophysitis can occur at virtually any apophysis and affects different apophyses at different ages. The most common location is the tibial tubercle where the condition is known by the eponym Osgood-Schlatter disease (OSD).

OSD is caused by a tight quadriceps and is typically seen in patients 12 to 14 years old. Patients with OSD complain of activity related pain very specifically at the tibial tubercle. The pain can be severe and may also occur after prolonged sitting. On physical exam, the tubercle is prominent and tender and the quadriceps are tight. Stretching of the quadriceps generally reproduces the pain. In unilateral cases, radiographs should be obtained to rule out occult lesions. The treatment is activity modification as dictated by the symptoms and physical therapy to stretch the quadriceps.

Other areas of traction apophysitis include, but are not limited to, the calcaneus (Sever's disease), inferior pole of the patella (Sinding-Larsen-Johansson disease), anterior inferior iliac spine, and base of the fifth metatarsal.

ACKNOWLEDGMENT

This chapter was co-written by members of the Leni and Peter W. May Department of Orthopaedics at the Mount Sinai School of Medicine; Evan Flatow, MD and Professor; Michael Hausman, MD and Professor; Roger Levy, MD and Professor; Sheldon Lichtblau, MD; Elton Strauss, MD and Associate Professor; Edward Yang, MD and Associate Professor; Richard Ghillani, MD and Assistant Professor; James Gladstone, MD and Assistant Professor; Judith Levine, MD and Assistant Professor; Michael Parks, MD and Assistant Professor; Steven Weinfeld, MD and Assistant Professor; and Randy Rosier, Professor and Chairman, Department of Orthopaedics, University of Rochester Medical Center.

Bibliography

Bucholz RW, Heckman JD, Kasser JR, et al: *Rockwood, Green, Wilkins' Fractures,* 5th ed. Philadelphia: Lippincott, Williams, and Wilkins, 2001.

Canale ST: *Campbell's Operative Orthopaedics*, 10th ed. St. Louis: Mosby, 2003.

Canale ST, Beaty JH: *Operative Pediatric Orthopaedics*, 2nd ed. St. Louis: Mosby, 1995.

Chapman MW, et al: *Chapman's Orthopaedic Surgery*, 3rd ed. Philadelphia: Lippincott, Williams, and Wilkins, 2000.

Fitzgerald RH, Kaufer H, Malkani AL: *Orthopaedics*. St. Louis: Mosby, 2002.

Herring JA: *Tachdjian's Pediatric Orthopaedics*, 3rd ed. St. Louis: Mosby, 2002.

Morrissy RT, Weinstein SL: *Atlas of Pediatric Orthopaedic Surgery*, 3rd ed. Philadelphia: Lippincott, Williams, and Wilkins, 2000.

Nordin M, Frankel VH: *Basic Biomechanics of the Musculoskeletal System*. Philadelphia: Lea and Febiger, 1989.

Reider B: *The Orthopaedic Physical Examination*. St. Louis: Mosby, 1999.

Simon SR: *Orthopaedic Basic Science*. Rosemont, IL: American Academy of Orthopaedic Surgeons, 1994.

References

1. Enneking WF, Spanier SS, et al: A system for the surgical staging of musculoskeletal sarcoma. *Clin Orthop* 153:106, 1980.
2. Mankin HJ, Mankin DJ, et al: The hazards of the biopsy, revisited. Members of the musculoskeletal tumor society. *J Bone Joint Surg Am* 78:656, 1996.
3. Simon MA: Current concepts review: Limb salvage for osteosarcoma. *J Bone Joint Surg Am* 70:307, 1988.
4. Simon MA, Finn HA: Diagnostic strategy for bone and soft-tissue tumors. *J Bone Joint Surg Am* 75:622, 1993.
5. Yasko AW, Lane JM: Current concepts review: Chemotherapy for bone and soft-tissue sarcoma of the extremities. *J Bone Joint Surg Am* 73:1263, 1991.
6. Trueta J: Acute hematogenous osteomyelitis: Its pathology and treatment. *Bull Hosp Jt Dis* 14:5, 1953.
7. Weiland AJ, Moore FR, Daniel RK: The efficacy of free tissue transfer in the treatment of osteomyelitis. *J Bone Joint Surg Am* 66:181, 1984.
8. Gustilo RB, Anderson JT: Prevention of infection in the treatment for one thousand and twenty-five open fractures of long bones. *J Bone Joint Surg Am* 58:453, 1976.
9. Tile M: Acute pelvic fracture: I. Causation and classification. *J Am Acad Orthop* 4:143, 1996.
10. Tile M: Acute pelvic fracture: II. Principles of management. *J Am Acad Orthop* 4:152, 1996.
11. Burgess AR, Eastridge BJ, Young JWR, et al: Pelvic ring disruptions: Effective classification system and treatment protocols. *J Trauma* 30:848, 1990.
12. Letournel E: Acetabulum fractures: Classification and management. *Clin Orthop* 151:81, 1980.
13. Shin SS: Circulatory and vascular changes in the hip flowing traumatic hip dislocation. *Clin Orthop* 140:255, 1979.
14. Garden RS: Malreduction and avascular necrosis in subcapital fractures of the femur. *J Bone Joint Surg Br* 53:183, 1971.
15. Winquist RA, Hansen ST, Clawson K: Close intramedullary nailing of femoral fractures: A report of five hundred and twenty cases. *J Bone Joint Surg Am* 66:259, 1984.
15a. Bone LB, Johnson KD, Weigelt J, et al: Early vs. delayed stabilization of femoral fractures: A prospective randomized study. *J Bone Joint Surg* 71:336, 1989.
16. Schatzker J, McBroom R, Bruce D: The tibial plateau fracture: The Toronto experience 1968–1975. *Clin Orthop* 138:94, 1979.
17. Nicoll EA: Fractures of the tibial shaft: A survey of 705 cases. *J Bone Joint Surg Br* 46:373, 1964.
18. Lauge-Hansen N: Fractures of the ankle. II. Combined experimental-surgical and experimental-roentgenologic investigations. *Arch Surg* 60:957, 1950.
19. Hawkins LG: Fractures of the neck of the talus. *J Bone Joint Surg Am* 52:991, 1970.

20. Rockwood CA, Matsen FA: *The Shoulder*, 2nd ed. Vol. 1. Philadelphia: WB Saunders, 1998, p. 495.

21. Silliman JF, Hawkins RJ: Classification and physical diagnosis of instability of the shoulder. *Clin Orthop* 291:7, 1993.

22. Holstein A, Lewis GB: Fractures of the humerus with radial nerve paralysis. *J Bone Joint Surg Am* 45:1382, 1963.

23. Sarmiento A, Kinman PB, Galvin EG, et al: Functional bracing of fractures of the shaft of the humerus. *J Bone Joint Surg Am* 59:596, 1977.

24. Ring D, Jupiter JB, Simpson NS: Monteggia fractures in adults. *J Bone Joint Surg Am* 80:1733, 1998.

25. Mikic ZDJ: Galeazzi fracture-dislocations. *J Bone Joint Surg Am* 57:1071, 1975.

26. Colles A: On the fracture of the carpal extremity of the radius. *Edin Med Surg J* 182, 1814.

27. Vaccaro AR: *Fractures of the Cervical, Thoracic, and Lumbar Spine.* New York: Marcel Dekker, 2003.

28. Cotler JM, Silveri CP, An HS, et al: *Surgery of Spinal Trauma.* Philadelphia: Lippincott Williams and Wilkins, 2000.

29. Hugenholtz H, Cass DE, Dvorak MF, et al: High-dose methylprednisolone for acute closed spinal cord injury—Only a treatment option. *Can J Neurol Sci* 29:227, 2002.

30. Charnley J: *Low Friction Arthroplasty: Theory and Practice.* London: Churchill-Livingstone, 1979.

31. Goldberg BA, Scarlet MM, Harryman DT II: Management of the stiff shoulder. *J Orthop Sci* 4:462, 1999.

32. Neer CS II: *Shoulder Reconstruction.* Philadelphia: WB Saunders, 1990.

33. Mackenzie R, Palmer CR, Lomas DJ, et al: Magnetic resonance imaging of the knee: Diagnostic performance studies. *Clin Radiol* 51:251, 1996.

34. Fairbank TJ: Knee joint changes after meniscectomy. *J Bone Joint Surg Br* 30:664, 1948.

35. Shirakura K, Terauchi M, Kizuki S, et al: The natural history of untreated anterior cruciate ligaments tears in recreational athletes. *Clin Orthop* 317:227, 1995.

36. Harner CD, Hoher J: Current concepts: Evaluation and treatment of posterior cruciate ligament injuries. *Am J Sports Med* 26:471, 1998.

37. Krause Jo, Brodsky JW: Peroneus brevis tendon tears: Pathophysiology, surgical reconstruction, and clinical results. *Foot Ankle Int* 19:271, 1998.

38. Saltzman C, Teursch DS: Achilles tendon injuries. *J Am Acad Orthop Surg* 6:316, 1998.

39. Caputo GM, Cavanagh PR, Ulbrecht JS, et al: Current concepts: Assessment and management of foot disease in patients with diabetes. *N Engl J Med* 331:854, 1994.

40. Weinstein SL, Mubarak SJ, Wenger DR: Developmental hip dysplasia and dislocation. Part I. *J Bone Joint Surg Am* 85:1824, 2003.

41. Weinstein SL, Mubarak SJ, Wenger DR: Developmental hip dysplasia and dislocation. Part II. *J Bone Joint Surg Am* 85:2024, 2003.

42. Crawford AH: Current concepts review: Slipped capital femoral epiphysis. *J Bone Joint Surg Am* 70:1422, 1988.

43. Catterall A: The natural history of Perthes' disease. *J Bone Joint Surg Br* 53:37, 1971.

44. Herring JS, Neustadt JB, William JJ, et al: The lateral pillar classification of Legg-Calvé-Perthes disease. *J Pediatr Orthop* 12:143, 1992.

45. Cummings RJ, Davidson RS, Armstrong PF, et al: Congenital clubfoot. *J Bone Joint Surg Am* 84:290, 2002.

46. Lichtblau S: A medial and lateral release operation for clubfoot: A preliminary report. *J Bone Joint Surg Am* 55:1377, 1973.

47. Turco VJ: Surgical correction of the resistant clubfoot: One-stage posteromedial release with internal fixation: A preliminary report. *J Bone Joint Surg Am* 53:477, 1971.

48. Ponseti IV: *Congenital Clubfoot. Fundamentals for Treatment.* Oxford: Oxford University Press, 1996.

49. Blount WP: Tibia vara, osteochondrosis deformans tibiae. *J Bone Joint Surg* 19:1, 1937.

50. Levine AM, Drennan JC: Physiological bowing and tibia vara. The metaphyseal-diaphyseal angle in the measurement of bowleg deformities. *J Bone Joint Surg Am* 64:1159, 1982.

51. Langenskiold A: Tibia vara (osteochondrosis deformans tibiae): A survey of 23 cases. *Acta Chir Scand* 103:1, 1952.

Surgery of the Hand and Wrist

Clayton A. Peimer

Philosophically, physiologically, and anatomically, the interaction of hand and brain uniquely identify *Homo sapiens*. Throughout history humankind's progress is measured through the evolution of a strong and mobile upper limb with an independently opposable thumb and the cognitive powers to use them. The balance, precision, and specialization of the hand give it a central functional and communicative role. The goal of surgical treatment of the injured, diseased, or dysfunctional hand is to retain maximum useful part length; independent, stable motion; and unimpaired mobility of sensate parts.

GENERAL CONSIDERATIONS

Examination

Prior records and diagnostic images in addition to the verbal interview may precisely define the extent, limitations, and duration of the patient's disorder and the clinical course. The history should include information of relevant systemic diseases such as diabetes, atherosclerosis, neurologic and psychiatric disorders, and other serious diseases or chronic problems.

The examiner should use the patient's normal anatomy—the contralateral, uninvolved limb—to observe for differences in alignment, contour, and symmetry. Observing the hand and forearm at rest in pronation and in supination should reveal any swelling, masses, erythema, ulceration, atrophy, anhidrosis, or excoriations (Fig. 43-1). The reproducibility of the patient's active participation in the examination process is important. Responses (physical and verbal) should be consistent; repeated efforts, such as in grip testing, should produce similar values. Accurate recording of detailed information by the examiner is important (Fig. 43-2).

Light palpation provides information concerning excessive or absent sweating associated with anxiety or insensibility in particular

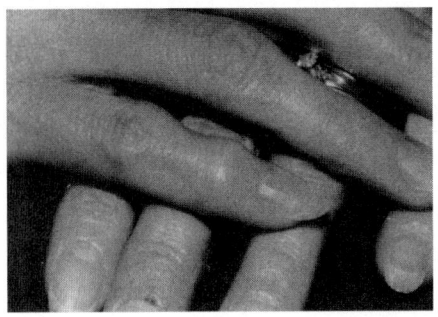 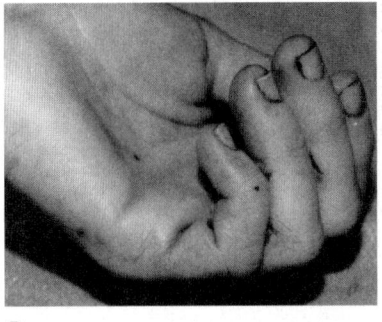 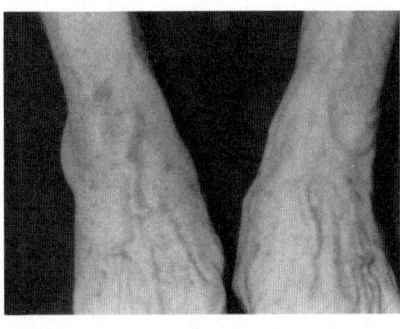

A *B* *C*

FIG. 43-1. Interruption of normal symmetry and comparison with a known normal render abnormal physical findings more apparent. *A.* Heberden's nodes are strikingly apparent in monarticular degenerative arthritis of the distal interphalangeal joint in the small finger of this woman with youthful, symmetrical, and aesthetically attractive hands. *B.* Interruption of the normal, progressive flexion cascade by absent distal interphalangeal joint flexion in the middle and ring fingers strongly suggested the diagnosis in this woman, who had lacerated the flexor digitorum profundus tendon in both fingers. *C.* Ulnar wrist synovitis due to rheumatoid arthritis is more evident in the wrist on the left when compared side-by-side with the uninvolved wrist.

zones, nerve distributions, dermatomes, or body parts. Variations in skin contour, texture, color, temperature, capillary refill, and hair characteristics offer information regarding circulation, nerve supply, masses, and joint swelling. Abnormal, injured, and scarred soft tissues can restrain joint motion, produce skin blanching with attempted active function, or cause visible dimpling of adherent deep structures, such as injured, repaired, or adherent tendons.

The nails and eponychial and paronychial cuticular tissues often mirror systemic disease as well as acute and chronic injury. Nails have a limited range of biologic responses. Splitting and fissuring, onycholysis and onychorrhexis may reflect loss of nail adherence to the bed matrix after trauma, aging, or malnutrition. The transverse post-traumatic nail crease that parallels the proximal nail fold and advances with growth (Beau's line) represents a single alteration of nail metabolism at the time of trauma. This finding is common after injury, but does not mean a poor prognosis. Multiple transverse grooves (Mee's lines) can occur with diseases such as Hodgkin's disease, malaria, and psoriasis, and are normal in the latter part of pregnancy. Pigmented longitudinal bands may occur commonly in darker-skinned individuals, but also in melanoma, glomus tumor, and carpal tunnel syndrome. Nail bed pigmentation can be found with systemic sepsis, subungual infection, and benign and malignant tumors (Fig. 43-3).

Motion should be recorded with a small goniometer and strength with a dynamometer. Simple line drawings may be used to record sites of injury, swelling, part loss, or dysfunction, and can precisely record and communicate findings (Fig. 43-4).

Imaging Studies

Diagnostic imaging includes traditional roentgenography, single- and multiple-phase technetium bone scans, computed tomography (CT), and magnetic resonance imaging (MRI) scans. Most patients should have plain radiographs in posteroanterior, lateral, and one or both oblique projections. Radiographs provide information with intermediate sensitivity, high specificity, and reasonable cost. Diagnoses can be missed if only specialized and expensive evaluations such as CT, MRI, or scintigraphic bone scans are used.

The x-ray beam *must* be centered on the part in question. Requesting an x-ray "of the hand" may be too general—and tangential—for diagnosing a problem in a specific finger. The physician evaluating

the imaging studies should receive the history, physical findings, and a working differential diagnosis (Fig. 43-5).

SURGICAL PRINCIPLES

Pre- and Postoperative Preparation and Principles

Skin Preparation

Detergents and solutions assist in mechanically débriding skin, and also mechanically decrease the microfloral population; however, all can irritate skin, and each has limitations.

Alcohols work primarily through the denaturation of proteins and produce the most rapid reduction in microbial counts. They work against most gram-positive and gram-negative organisms. Alcohols are not sporicidal, but are active against many fungi and tuberculosis; they also act against some viruses, including human immunodeficiency virus (HIV) and cytomegalovirus. Alcohols do not have persistent effects.

Hexachlorophene is bactericidal through cell wall destruction, and is especially active against gram-positive cocci. It is minimally effective against gram-negative, viral, and fungal organisms. This agent is potentially toxic systemically when absorbed, and is not recommended for open wounds.

Iodophors, iodine complexes that irritate the skin less than the iodine/alcohol tinctures, are effective against a broad spectrum of gram-positive and gram-negative bacteria, fungi, viruses, and mycobacteria by cell wall penetration and oxidation. Iodophors have almost immediate onset of action, and residual activity declines quickly. Because the iodophors can cause skin irritation, tissue damage, and allergic reactions in some patients, these solutions are not recommended for chronic use on open wounds, as additional tissue irritation may make the wound more susceptible to late infection.

Chlorhexidine gluconate is a broad-spectrum antibacterial that is effective against many viruses, with limited activity against fungi and the tubercle bacillus. The time of onset of action is intermediate, and residual bactericidal action continues for several hours. Chlorhexidine gluconate alcohol-based solution may provide the added benefit of rapid onset and residual activity with minimal toxicity.

Name:

Hospital Number:

Date:

Major Hand: Right/Left

Symptomatic Hand: Right/Left

		ACTIVE MOTION									SENSIBILITY			
		MP		PIP		DIP		Distance From PULP to MPL (cm)		Pinprick		2-Point (mm) static/moving	
		Right	Left	Right	Left	Right	Left	Right	Left	Right	Left	Right	Left
THUMB	Extension												
	Flexion												
INDEX	Extension												
	Flexion												
MIDDLE	Extension												
	Flexion												
RING	Extension												
	Flexion												
LITTLE	Extension												
	Flexion												

		Right	Left
WRIST	D.F.		
	P.F.		
	R.D.		
	U.D.		
THUMB	ABD		
	ADD		
	PRO		
	SUP		
PINCH (KG/LBS/PSI)			
GRIP (KG/LBS/PSI)			

		Right	Left
FOREARM	Pronation		
	Supination		
ELBOW	Extension		
	Flexion		
CIRCUMFERENCE (CM) 10 CM FROM EPICONDYLE OR AT MPL	Biceps		
	Forearm		
	Palm		

NOTE:

1. 0° = STRAIGHT LINE (FULL EXTENSION). Other figures refer to angles from full extension. Thus 30/70 = lacks 30° of extension and flexes to 70°; 40/40 =ankylosed in 40° of flexion.

2. Passive motion, when different from active, is noted in parenthesis.

3. Motions not recorded are considered normal.

A

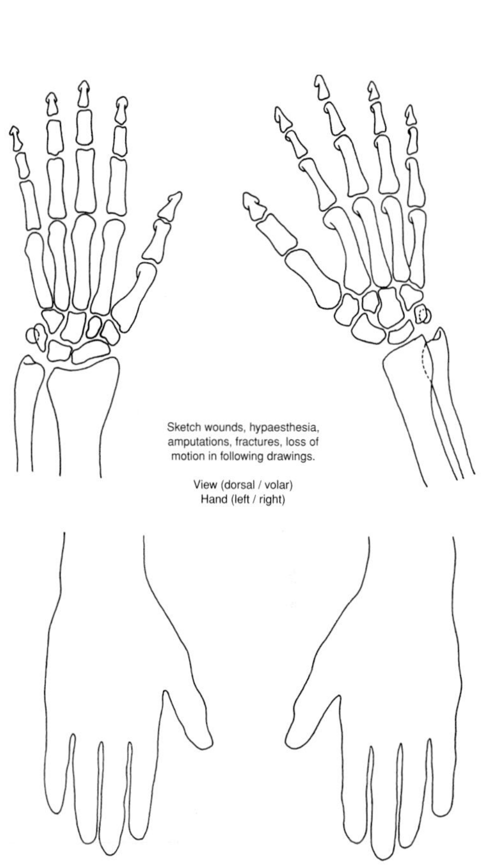

Sketch wounds, hypaesthesia, amputations, fractures, loss of motion in following drawings.

View (dorsal / volar)
Hand (left / right)

B

FIG. 43-2. *A* and *B*. Preprinted sheets for recording data from the history and physical examination can be tailored to the individual surgeon's practice to facilitate documentation.

Chloroxylenol or *parachlorometaxylenol* (PCMX) is active through destruction of microbial cell walls. It has intermediate onset and good activity against gram-positive organisms, but only fair activity against gram-negatives, fungi, mycobacterial species, and viruses. It is not toxic and rarely causes skin irritation. It may be a good choice in many situations.

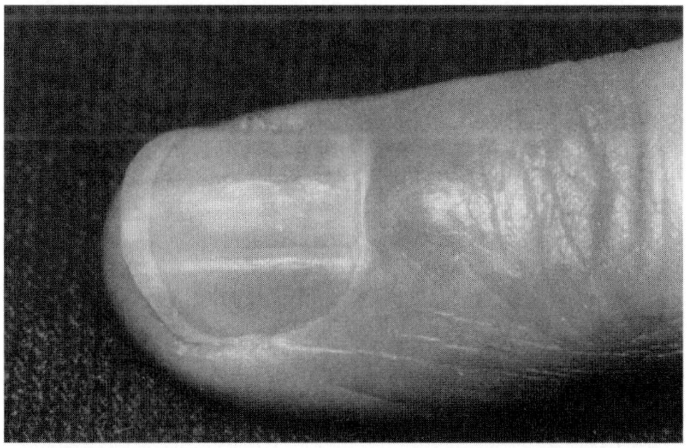

Hair Removal. While the conventional wisdom is that routine hair removal eliminates a potential wound contaminant, most studies reveal that hair removal is not a benign procedure, and that close skin shaving increases the risk of postoperative wound infection, with risk rising as the time between the shave and the surgical procedure increases. In a case in which the presence of hair would interfere with wound closure or tissue and skin manipulation, the use of electric clippers or depilatories is preferable, and hair removal should be done at the start of the procedure rather than hours before.

Anesthesia

Regional anesthesia for upper limb surgery offers effective pain control and the avoidance of mental confusion or other side effects from sedatives and general anesthesia (Fig. 43-6). Regional anesthesia is not risk-free or always fully satisfactory; systemic and local reactions may be serious, and appropriate monitoring is mandatory. Forearm or axillary tourniquets are used for most hand surgery, but patients are not often able to tolerate continuous pneumatic

FIG. 43-3. The combination of a firm, translucent swelling of the proximal nail fold with a furrow of the nail distally is characteristic of a pedunculated ganglion (mucous cyst) from the distal interphalangeal joint that has produced chronic pressure on the nail matrix.

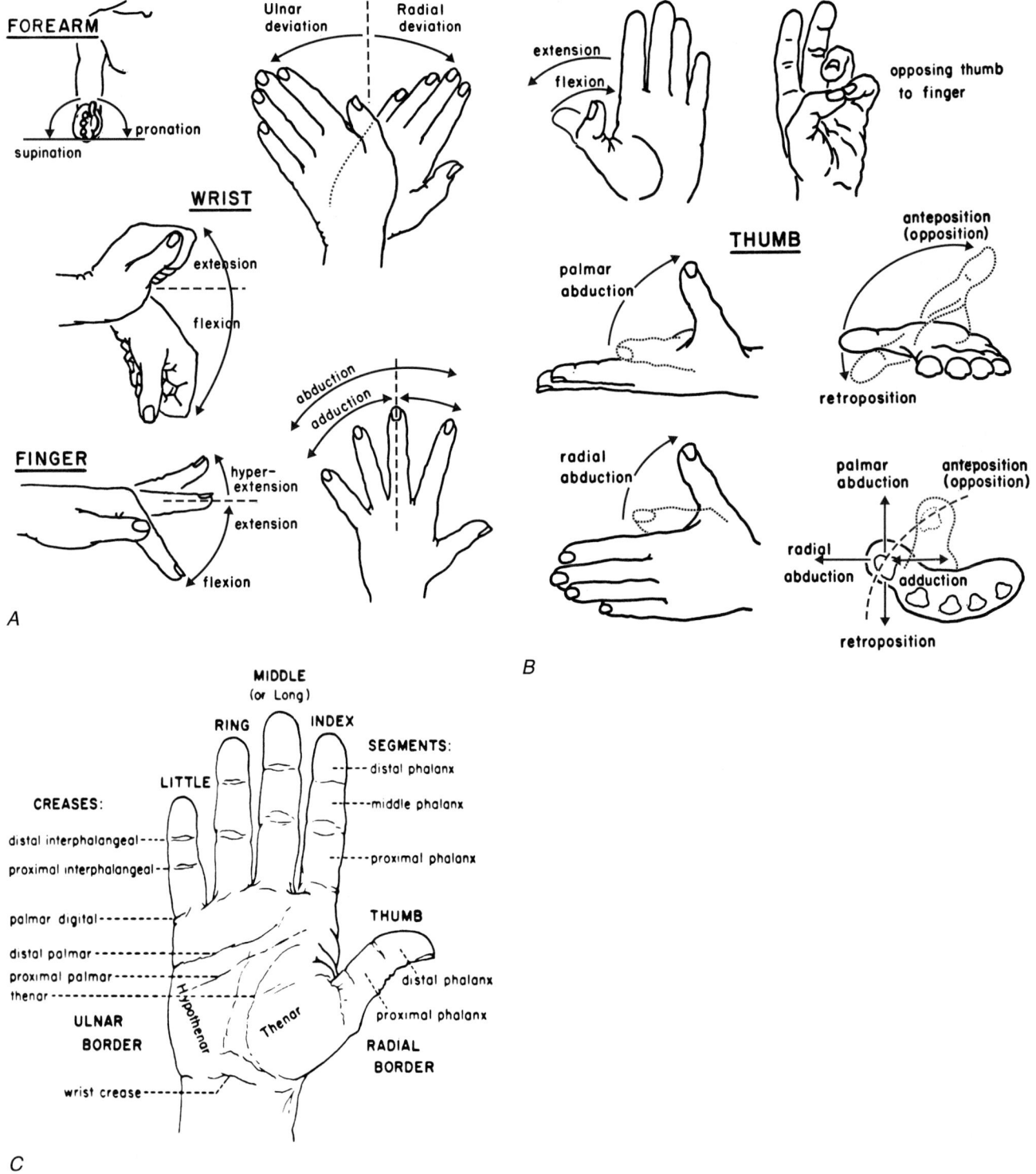

FIG. 43-4. *A* and *B*. Common terminology used in describing hand mobility. *C*. The anatomy of the volar surface of the hand. *(Reproduced with permission from American Society for Surgery of the Hand: The Hand: Examination and Diagnosis, 3rd ed. New York: Churchill-Livingstone, 1990.)*

tourniquet applications for more than 30 minutes without intravenous (IV) sedation. Isolated peripheral blocks have more limited usefulness.

Distal peripheral blocks in the upper extremity should be done *without* epinephrine added to the anesthetic solution. The injection technique is based on infiltration of anesthetic around the nerve

and not directly into nerve substance. Although inadvertent needle entry into nerves is common, without epinephrine in the injection solution and with the use of a fine-gauge needle, it should present no problem. Should a patient complain of paresthesias, the needle is withdrawn and redirected. Intraneural injection with epinephrine-containing solutions may result in extended intraneural ischemia,

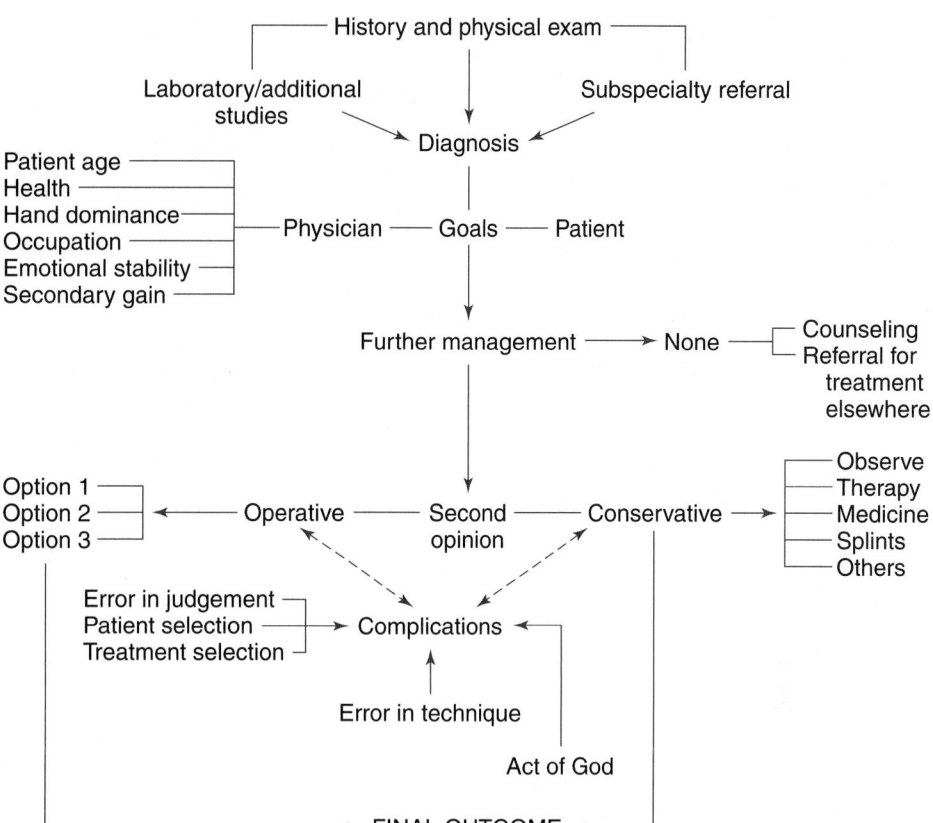

FIG. 43-5. Flow chart providing a graphic summary of the decision-making process. Note that both patient and physician play a necessary role in this process. Also note that a similarity in the goals and expectations of both patient and physician is central to this process.

and secondary permanent fibrosis, as well as peripheral vascular compromise, particularly in the digital end-arterial circulation.

Ulnar Nerve Block. Proximal block is among the more useful peripheral techniques (Fig. 43-7). The ulnar nerve is palpated just posterior to the medial epicondyle and injected with 5 to 8 mL of 1% mepivacaine hydrochloride without epinephrine via a 23- to 26-gauge needle. The nerve should not be pinned to the epicondyle with the needle; intense paresthesias elicited from neural perforation warrant immediate needle withdrawal and redirection.

The ulnar nerve at the wrist is in the volar flexor compartment located dorsal to the flexor carpi ulnaris tendon, and just ulnar to the ulnar artery; both nerve and artery are dorsal to the tendon. The dorsal cutaneous branch of the ulnar nerve has already branched 4 to 8 cm proximal to the ulnar styloid process. Initially deep to the flexor carpi ulnaris tendon, it courses dorsally to exit on its dorsal edge distal to the ulnar styloid process, where it can be blocked separately (Fig. 43-8). A fine-gauge needle is inserted into the skin just dorsal and ulnar to the flexor carpi ulnaris tendon; the needle is aimed palmarward and distally, toward the ring finger and Guyon's canal. The skin concavity for needle entry is just dorsal to the flexor carpi ulnaris tendon, and is easily palpated and visualized during

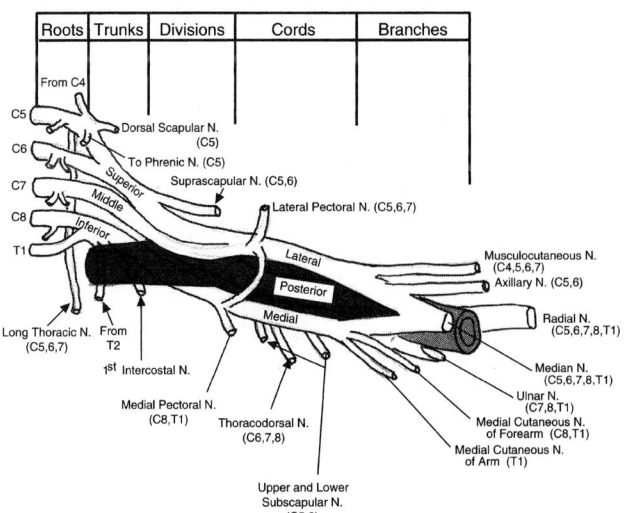

FIG. 43-6. The brachial plexus. Organization of the roots, trunks, divisions, and cords, as well as root origins of peripheral nerves.

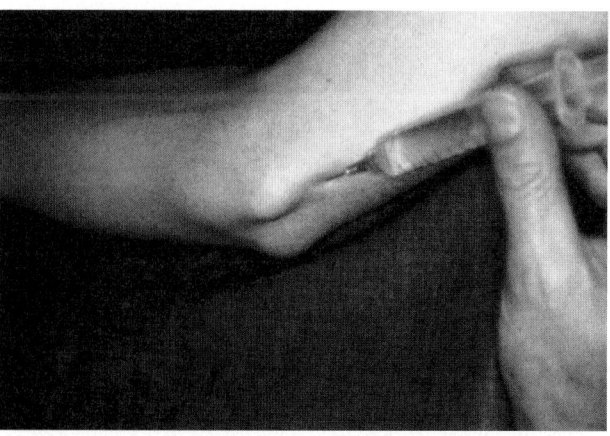

FIG. 43-7. The ulnar nerve is blocked at the elbow with 5 to 8 mL of local anesthetic without epinephrine. A fine-gauge needle is used, aiming distally with care being taken to avoid impaling the nerve.

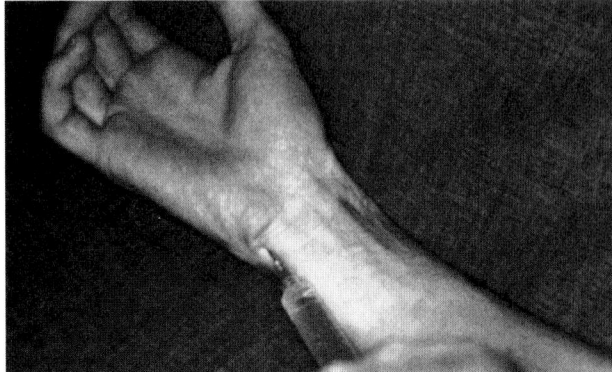

A

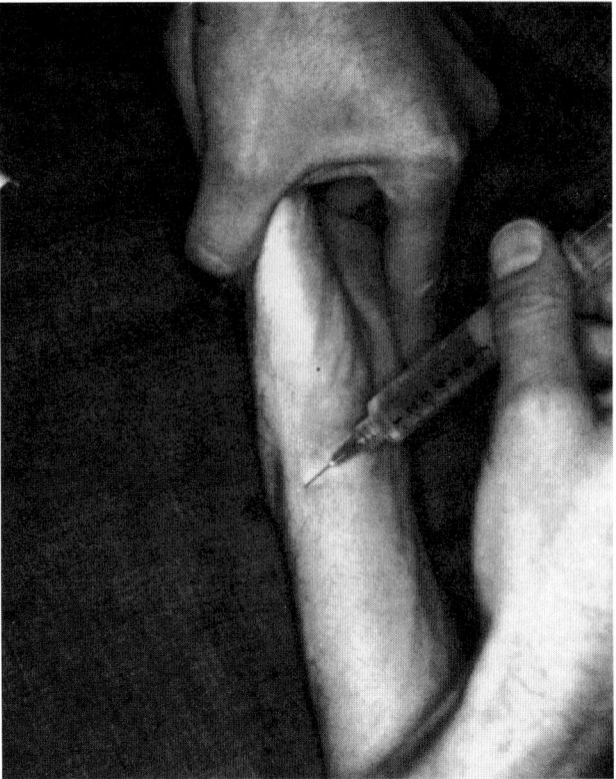

B

FIG. 43-8. *A. The ulnar nerve is blocked at the wrist with needle entry* dorsal *to the flexor carpi ulnaris tendon, aiming toward the ring finger in the plane of the palm. Aspiration serves to prevent needle placement in the more radially located ulnar artery during injection. B. Subcutaneous block of the dorsal branch is done at the ulnar styloid process.*

active wrist flexion and ulnar deviation. Aspiration before injection avoids intra-arterial injection. After needle entry, paresthesias may be elicited, and 5 mL of anesthetic is injected. The dorsal branch of the ulnar nerve is blocked with an additional subcutaneous infiltration of 2 to 3 mL after first pulling the needle proximally, and then redirecting it subcutaneously, dorsal and distal to the ulnar styloid.

Radial Nerve Block. The radial nerve is located between the lateral edge of the biceps and the anterior border of the triceps muscles; motor and sensory components can be anesthetized with injection approximately 4 cm proximal to the lateral epicondyle,

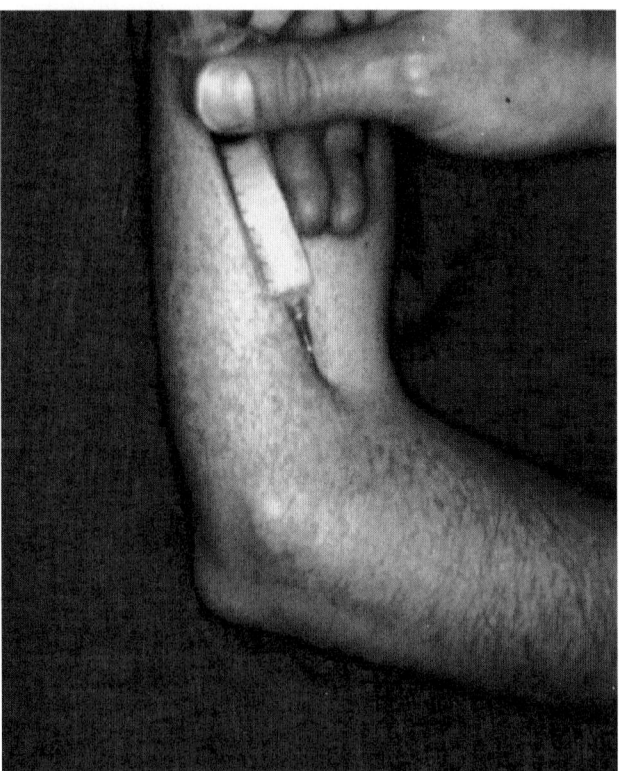

FIG. 43-9. *Radial nerve block is done 4 cm proximal to the lateral epicondyle by eliciting paresthesias in the intermuscular groove between the lateral border of the biceps brachialis and brachioradialis muscles.*

where the nerve lies on the humerus in this intermuscular space (Fig. 43-9). The needle is aimed distally and inserted; paresthesias confirm needle and nerve location. The needle is then withdrawn slightly and 7 to 10 mL of anesthetic is injected, with another 2 to 3 mL of anesthetic infiltrated in the subcutaneous plane, which also blocks the lateral antebrachial cutaneous nerve.

The purely sensory superficial radial nerve emerges at the dorsal edge of the brachioradialis tendon 4 to 6 cm proximal to the radial styloid process. As it courses distally, the nerve divides into multiple terminal branches. Subcutaneous anesthetic infiltration at the styloid process of the radius with a total of 6 to 8 mL of anesthetic effectively blocks the superficial radial nerve in this region (Fig. 43-10).

Median Nerve Block. Blocking the median nerve is considerably more difficult in the region of the elbow, where it is rather deep, than at the wrist, where it is superficial. At the elbow, the median nerve is posterior and ulnar to the brachial artery. A fine hypodermic needle is introduced from a location medial to the palpated brachial artery, aiming distally. After aspiration, 8 to 10 mL of anesthetic is injected. If intense paresthesias are elicited, the needle is withdrawn slightly before injection (Fig. 43-11).

The median nerve becomes progressively more superficial as it approaches the wrist, where it lies in the most palmar and radial quadrant of the carpal canal. Proximal to the canal, the nerve is located dorsal and slightly radial to the palmaris longus tendon, but ulnar to the flexor carpi radialis tendon (i.e., between the two tendons). Proper technique avoids both the canal contents and the nerve. The most consistent and comfortable skin portal is about 2 to 3 cm proximal to the wrist crease. The needle is aimed 30 to 45 degrees dorsal and distal, toward the third web space (Fig. 43-12). Injecting 6 to 8 mL of anesthetic consistently blocks the median nerve. The

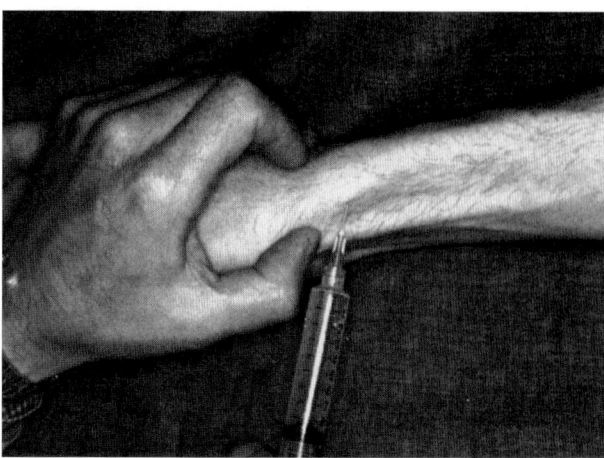

FIG. 43-10. *Superficial (sensory) radial nerve block at the wrist is done by subcutaneous infiltration at the styloid process of the radius and along the dorsum of the wrist.*

palmar cutaneous branch of the median and lateral antebrachial cutaneous nerves can be blocked with another 2 to 3 mL of anesthetic injected subcutaneously, aiming more superficially and 45 degrees radially from the same entry point.

Digital Nerve Block. The fingers receive their sensory supply from the common digital nerve branches of the median and ulnar nerves. Digital anesthesia can be achieved by injecting the anesthetic into the looser web tissues about the common digital nerves, which is preferable to a ring block in the base of the finger. The so-called ring block technique risks vascular compromise from volume compression when a solution is injected circumferentially about the base of the finger. Digital anesthetic solution must *not* include epinephrine, because resulting digital vessel spasm may compromise finger circulation.

Anesthetic is injected retrograde from the web, advancing about 1 cm proximally into the palm, where 2 mL of anesthetic is injected after aspiration. The needle can be withdrawn and turned into the dorsal subcutaneous tissues of the web to ensure anesthesia of the dorsal branch of the digital nerve with another 1 to 2 mL of anesthetic. The technique is repeated on the opposite side of the finger or sequentially in several digits as needed. No more than 5 to 7 mL total of anesthetic solution should be injected for any one finger with this technique (Fig. 43-13).

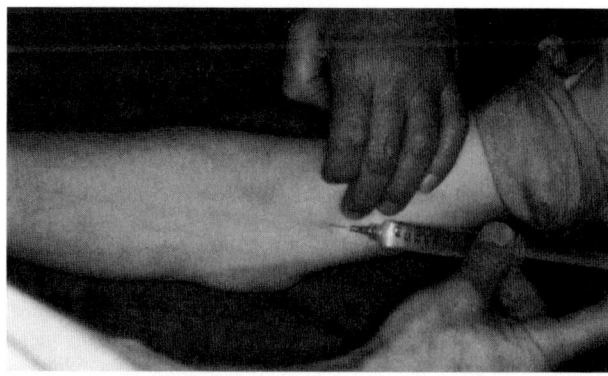

FIG. 43-11. *Proximal median nerve block is performed just above the intercondylar line, ulnar and posterior to the palpable brachial artery (index finger).*

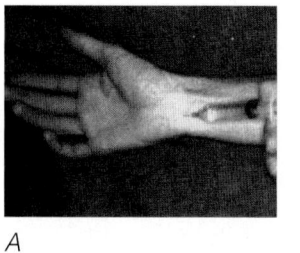

A

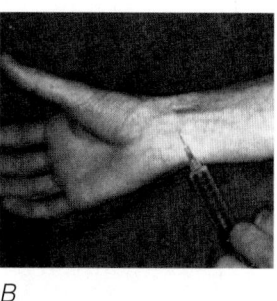

B

FIG. 43-12. *A. Median nerve injection at the carpal tunnel is accomplished from a point 3 cm proximal to the transverse carpal ligament, aiming toward the third ray and slightly dorsal in order to stay within the carpal canal and avoid impaling the nerve. B. Additional subcutaneous infiltration is done to block the palmar cutaneous and lateral antebrachial cutaneous nerve branches.*

Flexor Sheath Block. Single-digit anesthesia can also be achieved with injection of 2 mL of anesthetic directly into the flexor sheath. A fine hypodermic needle is introduced into the flexor tendon from the palmar side at the level of the distal palm or metatarsophalangeal flexion crease. Rapid onset of anesthesia can be achieved. This method has the advantage of a single injection, but the disadvantage of sometimes failing to completely anesthetize the dorsal divisions of the proper digital nerves.

Tourniquet

The use of tourniquets dates to Roman times, but the device acquired its name from surgical application in eighteenth-century France, from the verb *tourner,* meaning "to turn." Hand surgery is routinely performed using an axillary or forearm pneumatic

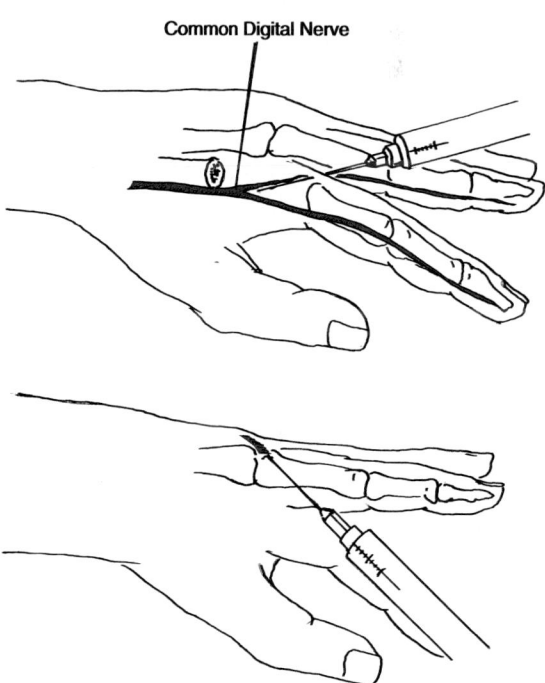

Common Digital Nerve

FIG. 43-13. *For intermetacarpal digital block, the needle is introduced into the web space, aimed in a proximal and palmar direction, and advanced for a distance of 1 cm. After aspiration, 1 to 2 mL of anesthetic is injected around the common digital nerve. The needle is withdrawn, and an additional 1 to 2 mL is infiltrated in the web and about the dorsum of the metacarpal metaphysis.*

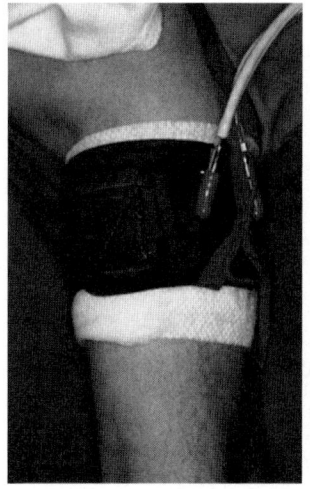 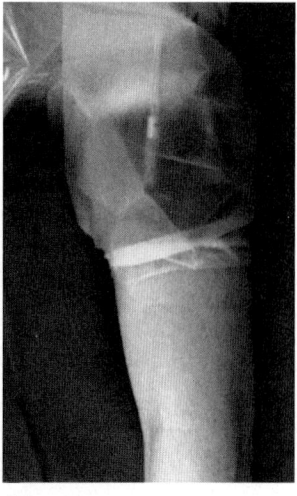

A   B

FIG. 43-14. *A. Padding beneath an axillary tourniquet. B. Occlusive drape distal to both tourniquet and padding to prevent wicking of antiseptic solution beneath the cuff.*

tourniquet. Fingertip procedures can be done using a digital tourniquet made from a $1/4$-inch rubber drain hose or with a finger cut from a sterile surgical glove; the tip of the finger sleeve is pierced, placed over the patient's finger and rolled proximally; simultaneously exsanguinating and achieving a tourniquet effect. In the absence of proximal anesthetic blockade or sedation, the maximum tourniquet time a patient will tolerate is 30 to 60 minutes.

Except in the presence of infections and suspected aggressive and malignant tumors, the arm is exsanguinated before tourniquet application; limb elevation may be used for partial exsanguination. Covering the arm with a fabric stockinette before elastic bandage exsanguination reduces skin shear; this may be important in patients with delicate skin, those with connective tissue diseases, and those who are on steroids. Axillary and forearm tourniquet cuffs are best applied over cast padding. Nonsterile pneumatic tourniquets should be draped away from the operative field with an occlusive plastic tape or draped distal to the cuff to prevent wicking of antiseptic solution during extremity preparation and risking subjacent chemical irritation (Fig. 43-14).

Pneumatic tourniquet pressures of 225 to 250 mm Hg for adults and 200 mm Hg in children are adequate. Patients with large or obese arms require higher pressures and larger cuffs, as do hypertensive patients, in whom tourniquet pressure should be 100 mm Hg over systolic blood pressure. Tourniquet time is limited by the most oxygen-sensitive extremity cells, muscle cells, and their most oxygen-sensitive organelles, the mitochondria. Continuous tourniquet application should not exceed 3 hours to avoid irreversible mitochondrial changes. In cases in which longer tourniquet times are required, the tourniquet should be deflated after the wound has been dressed temporarily, and left deflated for at least 10 minutes per hour of prior inflation. Tourniquet complications involve not only ischemia in labile distal tissues, but also ischemia and direct injury to skin, nerves, and muscles located immediately beneath tourniquets. Assuming operative tourniquet times greater than 30 minutes, at tourniquet deflation, tissues show reactive hyperemia driven by the tourniquet-induced hypoxia that is directly proportional to the time of tourniquet use. This hyperemia may complicate hemostasis if the surgeon tries to immediately close the skin.

The tourniquet is deflated before wound closure; deflation should be immediately followed by 7 to 10 minutes of direct, moderate wound pressure before electrocautery is used, unless there is a significantly bleeding vessel. To avoid hematoma, the wound is closed when an acceptably dry field has been achieved. If oozing persists, a suction drain is used to keep dead spaces empty.

Incisions and Exposures

Skin incisions can be linear, curved, or angled, and may be oriented in longitudinal or transverse directions relative to the limb. Ideally, elective wounds are placed to lie in and about the soft-tissue skin creases. Hand incisions are not made perpendicular to joint creases, so iatrogenic contracture and unsightly scars are prevented (Fig. 43-15).

A sterile skin-marking pen is used to draw out the incisions before the skin is opened. Cross-hatch markings of the incision at regular intervals assist in realigning the skin edges for closure (Fig. 43-16). Angles, pedicles, and turns in incisions should not be so narrow as to risk vascular compromise by creating a narrow skin peninsula.

Dressings and Splints

The hand dressing is an intrinsic part of the surgical procedure. The dressing and splint are as important to the outcome of the operation as the cutting and suturing techniques. Application of dressings and splints should not be delegated without supervision by the responsible surgeon. A poorly applied dressing may destroy or disrupt the intended effect of the operation.

The bottom layer of the dressing should be conforming, nonocclusive, and preferably nonadherent, such as Xeroform or Adaptic. Dressing sponges may be dry or moistened for contour. When interdigital dressings are appropriate, a single gauze pad is folded, not twisted, between fingers. The involved fingers or the entire hand is then overwrapped loosely with a Kerlix or a similar type of bulky rolled gauze. Padded dorsal or volar splints are applied to maintain the desired positions of the operated parts.

The generic position for hand immobilization includes splinting the wrist at about 30 degrees of extension, the metacarpophalangeal joints at 70 degrees flexion, the interphalangeal joints at 0 to 5 degrees flexion, and with wide palmar abduction of the thumb metacarpal if the thumb needs to be included. The splint is extended to the fingertips, and care is taken to avoid compressing the dressing and splint too tightly and risking circulatory compromise. Fingertips should be exposed and visible for circulation checks. Hand and arm elevation is encouraged for comfort and to minimize edema during the first several postinjury and postoperative days. With or without a sling, when the patient is supine, sitting, or walking, the hand is kept at or above the level of the heart and above the elbow.

Postoperative Hand Therapy

Hand therapy is begun early and depends on the specific diagnosis, procedure, and patient. Operative goals include minimizing the time of immobilization, enhancing internal stabilization with minimal invasion, and allowing early mobilization of skin, joints, and tendons.

Exercises appropriate for the condition and surgery performed are prescribed, and a therapist instructs the patient in doing these exercises. Exercises should be gentle, never painful, but should take the patient to the limit of potential motion at that time. The therapy program should emphasize soft-tissue mobilization and a decrease in edema. When doing therapy for the hand, mobility in the

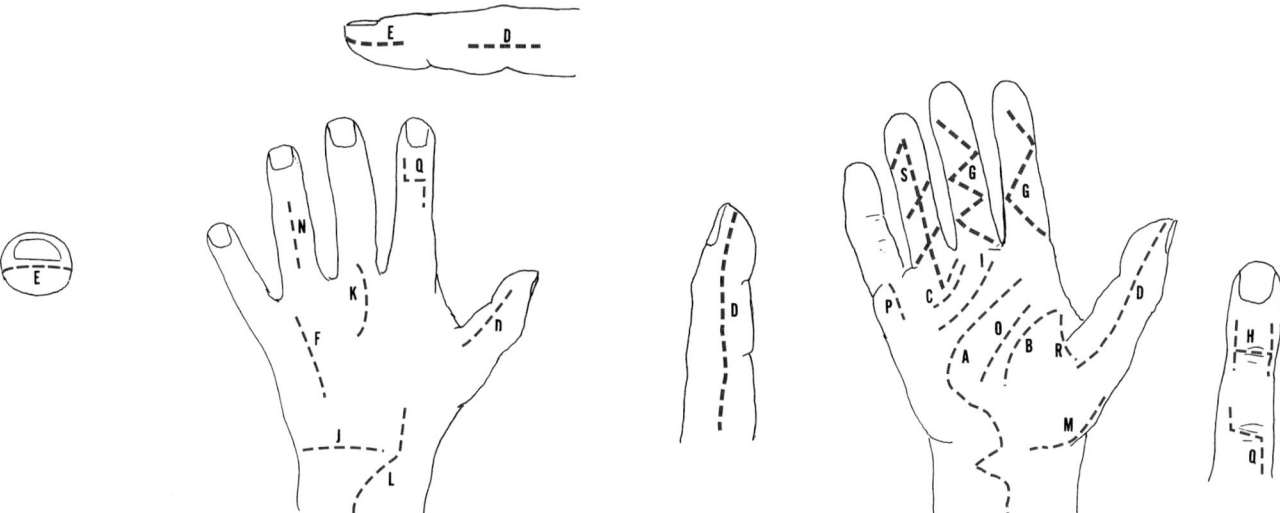

FIG. 43-15. Common palmar and dorsal incisions in the hand. *A.* Incision opening the palm or draining the midpalmar space parallels flexion creases, exposes by triangular flap, enters between median and ulnar nerve supplies, and may be extended through the ulnar side of the carpal ligament up the forearm. Curve-crossing creases in wrist avoid contracture. *B.* Drainage for the thenar space parallels the thenar crease, and must not sever the thenar motor nerve. Pedicles between it and the palmar incision must be wide enough to nourish intermediate skin. *C.* Drainage of collar button abscess. Avoid the digital nerve. *D.* Midaxial incisions in digits spare nerves and vessels and do not cause flexion contractures. *E.* Drainage for pulp abscess posterior to the tactile surface should sever the vertical fat columns and not cause tenosynovitis by opening the flexor sheath. *F.* Dorsal incisions over the second and fourth web spaces for decompressing dorsal and volar interosseous compartments. *G.* Both modifications of Bruner's zigzag volar digital incisions for flexor tendon surgery. *H.* H-type incision for distal interphalangeal joint débridement or fusion. The terminal extensor tendon may be transected and repaired. *I.* Incision along the distal palmar crease to expose the palmar fascia. *J.* Transverse incisions parallel wrinkles, thus avoiding conspicuous keloid formation. *K.* Curvilinear incision on the radial side of metacarpophalangeal joints for isolated interphalangeal joint synovectomy or extensor centralization. *L.* Approach to the dorsal wrist. The central axis of the incision is moved radialward or ulnarward for approach to the various dorsal wrist compartments. *M.* A Wagner incision to approach the carpometacarpal joint of the thumb. Care is taken to avoid crossing branches of the dorsoradial sensory nerve. The abductor pollicis brevis is reflected palmarward/ulnarward. *N.* Straight dorsal incision for approach to the proximal interphalangeal (PIP) joint. The elasticity and redundancy of skin over the dorsal PIP joints, coupled with the great power of the flexor mechanism eliminates concerns regarding contracture across a joint crease. *O.* Approach to the midpalm. *P.* Longitudinal incision over the A1 pulley for trigger finger release. Care is taken to avoid crossing the flexion creases. Incision is made midline on the tendon, avoiding the neurovascular bundles on either side. *Q.* Incision exposing the extensor tendon central slip. *R.* Short transverse incision for release of trigger thumb. *S.* The McGregor incision, sometimes used in Dupuytren's contracture surgery. After contracture release, flaps are interposed to gain length and avoid linear incisions across flexion creases.

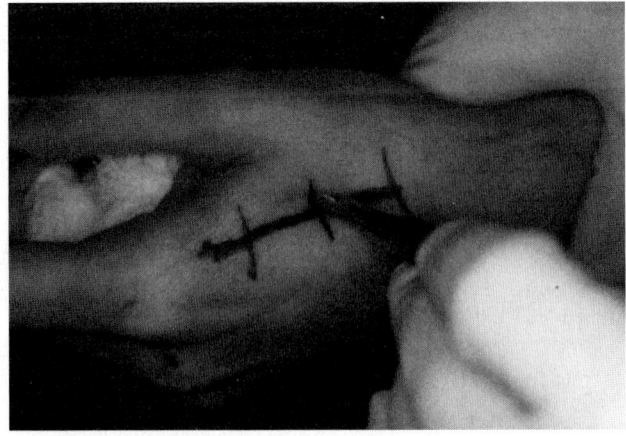

FIG. 43-16. Preincision marking and scoring the skin for easier, more accurate alignment of wound edges at closure.

forearm, elbow, and shoulder should be included, especially in older patients. The use of whirlpools is limited to patients with special needs, such as those with burns and those whose wounds require periodic débridement. Heating the tissues is rarely if ever done acutely; ice is often more appropriate for posttraumatic conditions. Use of warm water or paraffin baths is reserved for chronic conditions of systemic inflammation and periarticular stiffness. After injury, tissue swelling often increases proportionally to heat, worsening the prospects of rehabilitation in those swollen parts.

TRAUMA

It is estimated that one-third of musculoskeletal trauma occurs to the upper limb. The annual economic impact from diminished or lost hand and upper extremity function annually reaches billions of dollars in the United States. The best care is delivered initially, when tissues are fresh and potentially can be salvaged, revascularized, and directly repaired; are without the burdens of secondary scar tissue after delayed healing; and to avoid osteoarticular degeneration or infection. It is in the acute situation that success is greatest in achieving a potentially functional and aesthetically satisfactory result.

Skeletal Trauma

Forearm and Wrist

The forearm is a two-bone musculotendinous unit with complex biomechanical interactions. The osteoarticular and ligamentous connections of radius, ulna, interosseous membrane, and proximal and distal radioulnar joints allow the wide variety of possible hand positions and force transfers. The disruption of any one part of this anatomic and mechanical construct should cause the physician to search for less obvious injuries elsewhere. Most suboptimal outcomes after forearm fractures can be related to failure to recognize injury to a proximal or distal region, often at the radioulnar joints, or failure to appreciate progressive loss of initial reduction after treatment. Severe neurovascular problems are uncommon, but when present, may be related to acute vascular compromise from trauma, immobilization, or compartment syndrome.

The distal radius forms a biconcave articular surface to seat the proximal row of carpal bones, the scaphoid, lunate, and triquetrum. The radius articulates distally not only with the carpals, but also with the ulna. The restoration of length and congruent relationships of these several bones must be considered after trauma. The traumatized limb usually can be easily compared to native preinjury state with radiographs of the opposite side (Figs. 43-17 and 43-18).

Distal radius fractures have been variously classified, but a guide that integrates assessment of fracture patterns and treatment is useful (Table 43-1). Because there are many variations of fracture patterns in the distal radius, this system simplifies common characteristics and suggests treatment for each generic type of fracture. The treatment for a specific patient should be based not only on the pattern, but also on age, hand dominance, occupation, social needs, cognitive and psychosocial factors, and living arrangements.

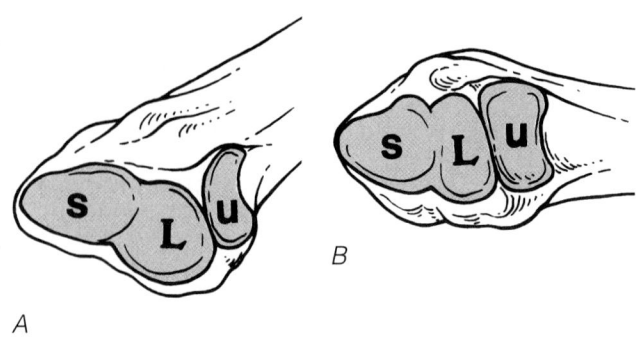

FIG. 43-18. *A and B. The articular surface of the distal radius demonstrates articular facets for the scaphoid (S), the lunate (L), and the ulnar head in the sigmoid notch (U).*

Radiographically and functionally, radius fractures are stable or unstable, displaced or nondisplaced, and with or without involvement of the radiocarpal and/or radioulnar articular surfaces. The condition of surrounding soft tissues and the presence of associated injury in other regions of the hand, forearm, and elbow affect the decision-making process. Because these fractures most commonly occur from a sudden impact on an outstretched hand (a fall or vehicular accident), they result in a bending moment with the load through the radius metaphysis, and associated neurovascular injuries, particularly to the median nerve at the carpal canal, are common. There may be an associated avulsion fracture of the ulnar styloid process, but the distal radioulnar joint (DRUJ) does not become unstable without a significant fracture of the ulna and attached ligaments.

The radius is more commonly displaced dorsally, as in classic Colles' fracture, with impaction, proximal displacement, and dorsal angulation of its distal articular surface. In such cases, the dorsal cortex of the distal fragment is comminuted, and this has significantly negative prognostic implications for postreduction bone stability when managed entirely by external manipulation and cast or splint fixation (Fig. 43-19). Less frequently, a flexion or bending moment occurs, creating palmar displacement (Barton's/Smith's fractures). When intra-articular, either of these volar fracture patterns

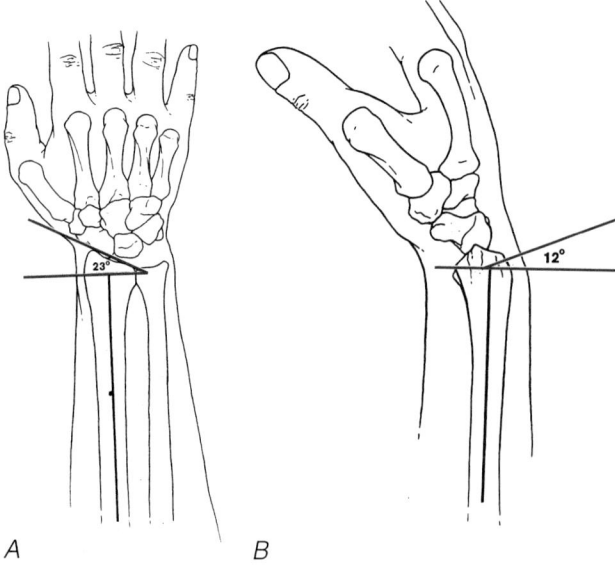

FIG. 43-17. *A. This illustration of an anteroposterior view of the distal radius demonstrates its normal angle of inclination of 23 degrees in relationship to the long axis of the radius. B. A lateral view demonstrates the normal palmar tilt of 12 degrees of the lunate fossa in its orientation with the long axis of the radius.*

Table 43-1

Classification and Treatment of Distal Radius Fractures

Classification of Radius Fracture	Treatment Preference
I. Nonarticular, nondisplaced	Cast immobilization
II. Nonarticular, displaced	
A. Reducible, stable	Cast immobilization
B. Reducible, unstable	Percutaneous pins
C. Irreducible	Open reduction/external fixation
III. Articular, nondisplaced	Cast immobilization with or without percutaneous pins
IV. Articular, displaced	Closed reduction
A. Reducible, stable	Percutaneous pins (Kirschner wires) with or without external fixation
B. Reducible, unstable	Closed reduction/external fixation, with or without percutaneous pins, with or without bone graft
C. Irreducible	Open reduction/external fixation with percutaneous pins
D. Complex	Open reduction/external plate fixation with bone graft (with or without percutaneous pins)

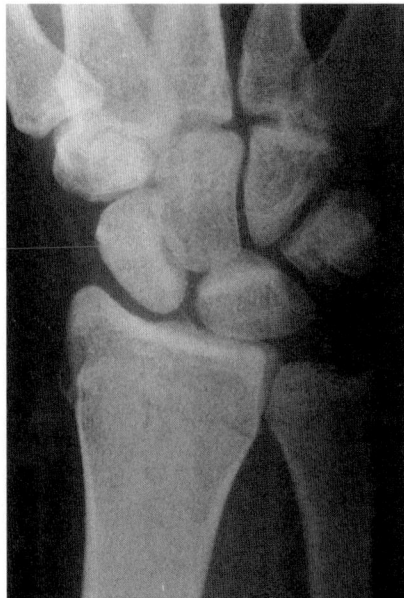

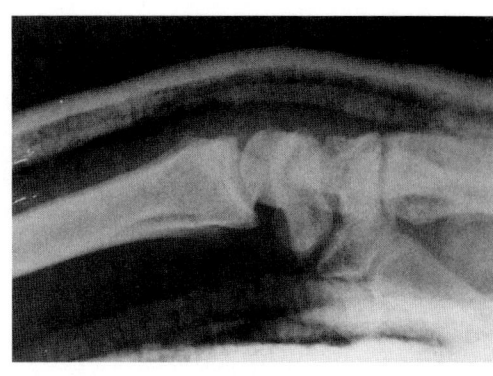

B

A

FIG. 43-19. *A and B. This radiograph demonstrates a nonarticular, nondisplaced (type I) inherently stable fracture of the distal radius.*

may have associated primary or secondary radiocarpal subluxation, but this problem is more often associated with the volar lip variant, the Smith's type III or Barton's fracture pattern.

Even nondisplaced fractures without comminution potentially misalign during the healing process as resorption and bone remodeling occur at the fracture site. Maintaining length and alignment during healing is important, and patients should be observed every 10 to 15 days with examination and x-rays if in casts or splints. This injury may be associated with significant swelling. It is the preference of this author to never initially use circular cast immobilization; cast immobilization should be delayed until initial swelling has subsided. A sugar-tong forearm and wrist splint may be applied that maintains bone length and alignment while simultaneously controlling forearm rotation without a rigid circumferential shell (Fig. 43-20).

The displaced dorsal fragment can be reduced comfortably under fracture block anesthesia, with or without addition of intravenous or intramuscular sedation. After sterile skin preparation, a 22-gauge needle is introduced obliquely into the fracture site via overlying skin. Aspiration will reveal when the needle is within the fracture hematoma; 6 to 8 mL of 1% mepivacaine or lidocaine without epinephrine can be injected to produce anesthesia in 5 to 10 minutes. The typical fracture, with dorsal displacement and angulation from an extension vector, can be disengaged and reduced by distraction applied by allowing the arm to hang from finger traps placed on the index and middle fingers, with the arm itself serving as a counterweight for about 5 to 10 minutes. A dorsal-to-palmar force is applied by the surgeon over the distal fragment at the area of displacement after the fragments have been thus disimpacted. The wrist is immobilized in neutral forearm rotation with only slight wrist flexion and minimal ulnar deviation to avoid causing secondary compression of the median nerve. The sugar-tong splint is applied. The width of the padded plaster should allow adequate space for tissue swelling. The dorsal and palmar edges of the splint should therefore not touch each other. For most adults, a 3-inch plaster width is adequate, but in large individuals, 4-inch plaster may be needed, which is applied over generous soft-tissue padding. After reduction and splint application, x-rays are obtained to record the reduction. If fracture realignment is incomplete, or if significant intra-articular

misalignment (>2 mm step/gap) and osteoarticular incongruity remains, repeated manipulative reduction or an alternate method of fixation needs to be considered.

Patients should have a neurovascular examination before manipulative reduction, and their median nerve sensory status should be assessed again after the application of the plaster splint. Fracture position and neurovascular status must be followed carefully.

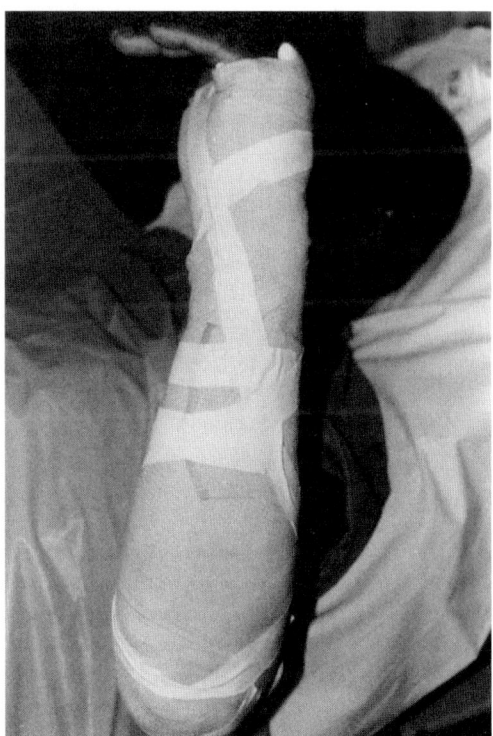

FIG. 43-20. *Application of sugar-tong splint. The splint can be wrapped with a gently applied elastic bandage, after which full flexion of the metacarpophalangeal joints must be demonstrated.*

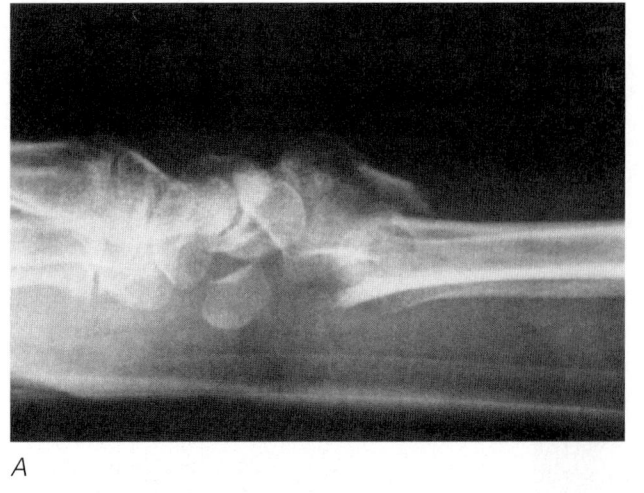

A

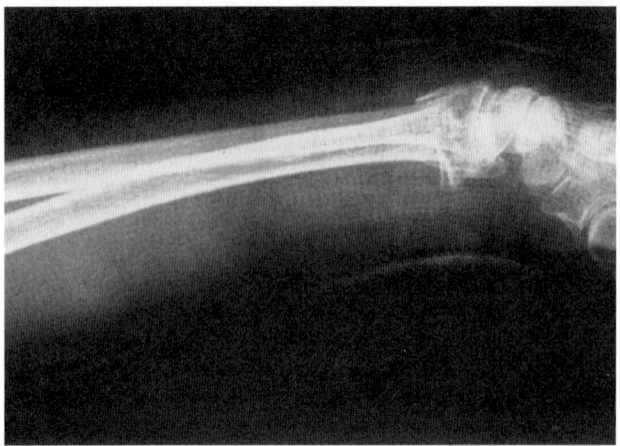

B

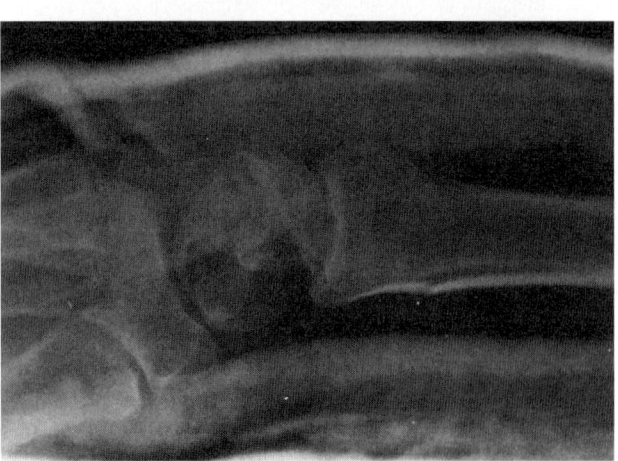

C

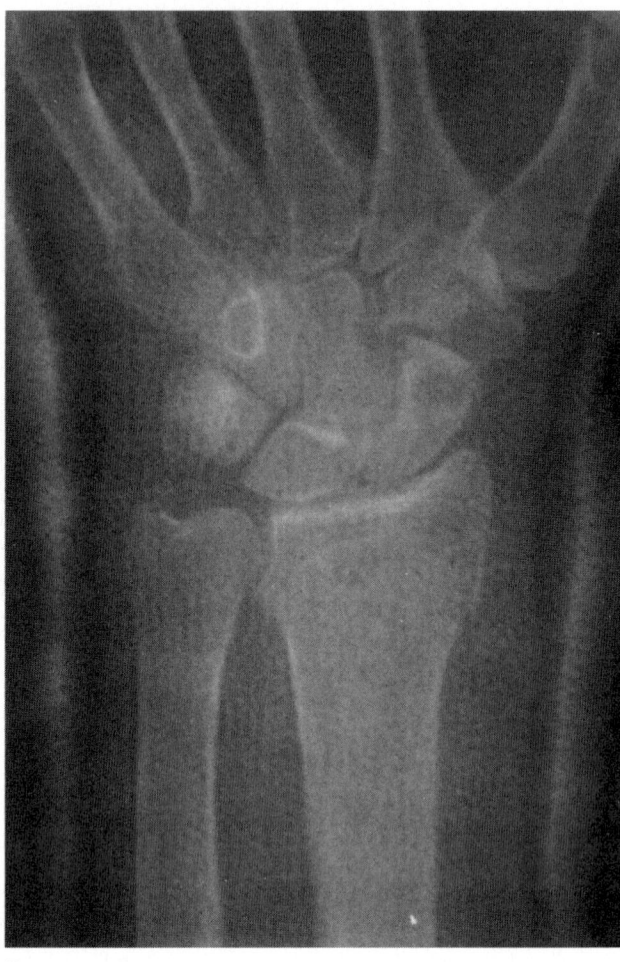

D

FIG. 43-21. *A* and *B*. A type II, displaced but stable, extra-articular fracture of the distal radius has been treated with closed reduction and application of a sugar-tong splint. *C* and *D*. Ten days later a conversion has been made to a long arm cast, and x-rays demonstrate maintenance of length and alignment.

After 7 to 10 days, the patient has repeat x-rays. Elevation and digital motion will have significantly diminished swelling in many cases, and the splint may be replaced with a circular cast. Some circumstances may dictate snugging the splint with a replacement circular gauze overwrap and delaying cast application an additional week or two. In young patients, a long arm cast may be preferable; in older patients, the risk of elbow stiffness is significant, and prolonged immobilization of that joint is not advisable. Elevation of the

hand plus finger mobilization and a therapy program that is directed to the entire upper limb, including the shoulder, is started at this time. When the splint is changed into a cast, x-rays are obtained again after cast application. Radiographs are repeated every 1 to 2 weeks to monitor healing and observe for collapse, angulation, and displacement (Fig. 43-21). Most casts can be removed about 6 weeks after trauma, when radiographs demonstrate obvious new bone formation and the fracture region is relatively nontender. If no

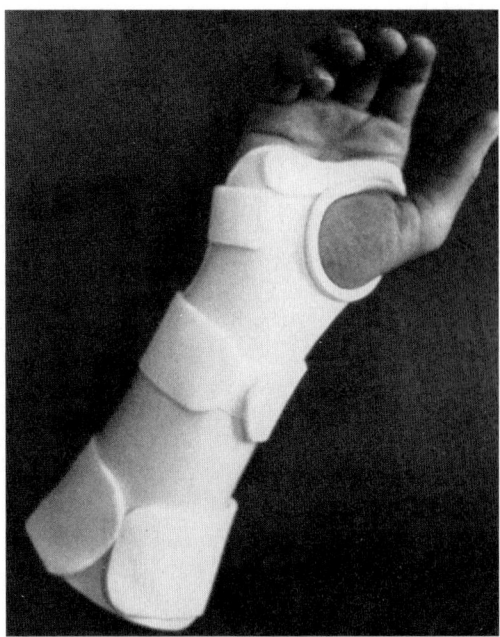

FIG. 43-22. A removable thermoplastic splint with Velcro fasteners is molded to the palmar aspect of the patient's hand and wrist. This provides support between periods of active range-of-motion exercise in the initial mobilization period.

motion or significant pain is elicited at the fracture site, cast immobilization may be discontinued. Therapists can fabricate a custom thermoplastic resting/protective splint and active motion exercises can begin (Fig. 43-22). The custom splint can generally be discontinued after another 2 to 4 weeks, depending on patient comfort and progress in rehabilitation. Motion exercises for the hand and wrist are continued and followed by progressive strengthening, increasing activities of daily living, and return to function.

Unstable fractures of the distal radius are treated with percutaneous or open fracture pinning under fluoroscopic monitoring. Many of these fractures also require an external fixation device to prevent progressive collapse and loss of alignment at the comminuted fracture line. When fractures are significantly impacted, areas of obvious bone loss within the submetaphyseal region are evident after reduction, and require bone graft or bone substitute to prevent delayed union or nonunion. Management by open reduction, with the combination of external and internal fixation with plates and screws, is appropriate for the more severe subgroup with articular incongruity and significant comminution where length and alignment cannot be maintained. More often these are younger patients whose injuries are the result of high-impact trauma, such as those sustained in vehicular accidents and mishaps with heavy machinery; however, patients having fragment-specific internal fixation can be mobilized within days of surgery, and are seen to both regain better motion earlier and overall compared to other methods (Figs. 43-23, 43-24, and 43-25). Increasingly, however, primary internal fixation with the new fragment-specific (TriMed) low-profile plates and screws is being used via small incisions and fluoroscopic control to stabilize fragments, allow early rehabilitation and independence, and avoid the complications of (what the Swiss often call) "cast disease."

Carpal Bone Fractures. The eight carpal bones have a large proportion of their surfaces covered with articular cartilage, a fact that has two clinical implications. First, the limited periosteal attachments offer a tenuous blood supply; after fracture one or more of the fragments is potentially at risk for avascular necrosis. Second, most carpal fractures are by definition intra-articular injuries. The displaced fracture often needs surgical repair to avoid secondary arthritis from joint surface incongruity. The pattern of carpal fracture or fracture dissociation may not be clearly discernible on standard posteroanterior and lateral radiographs, and oblique views, carpal tunnel projection, and other views may be necessary. If imaging information is nondiagnostic or equivocal, CT scans (sometimes needing three-dimensional reconstruction) will demonstrate the fractures

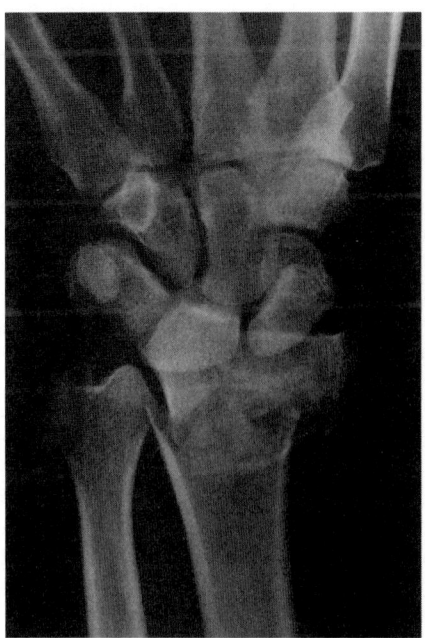
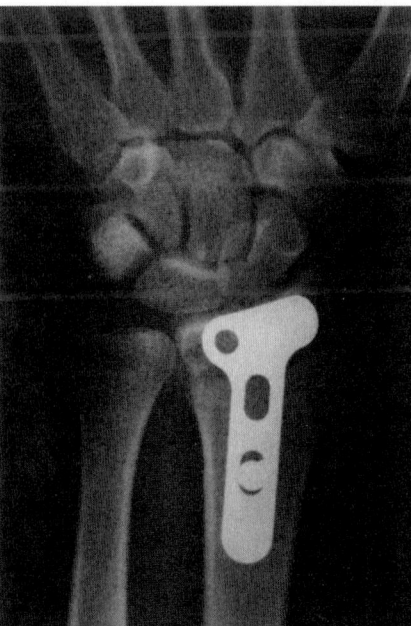
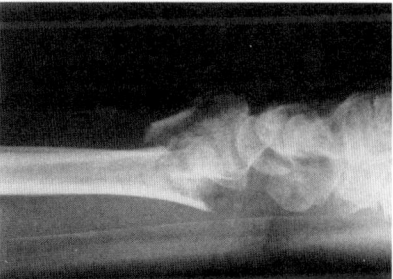
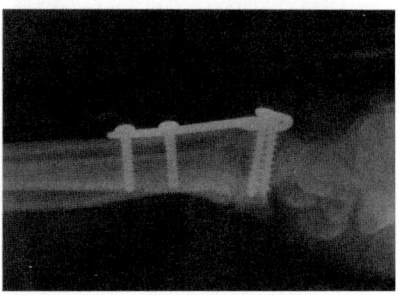

FIG. 43-23. Radiographs of this unstable displaced fracture demonstrate return of length, angle or inclination, and palmar tilt using this dorsal buttress plate.

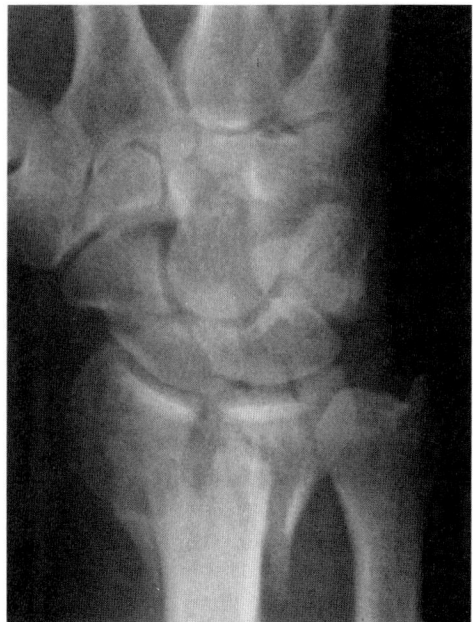

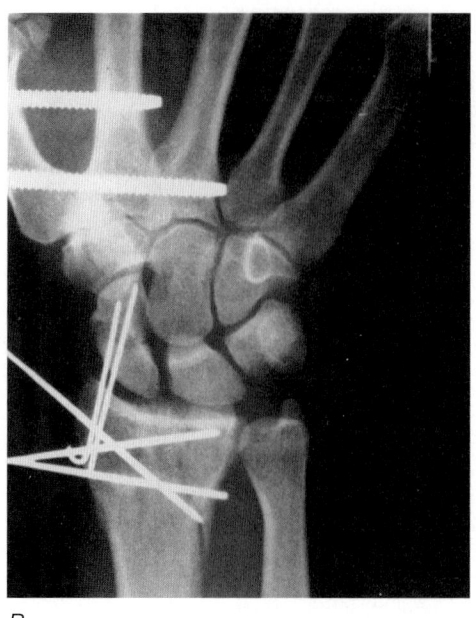

A

B

FIG. 43-24. *A.* A comminuted unstable intra-articular fracture of the distal radius is seen combined with a transverse fracture of the scaphoid waist. *B.* The scaphoid fracture has been anatomically fixed with two Kirschner wires, and the distal radius fracture has been managed with a combination of external fixation, internal fixation, and bone grafting.

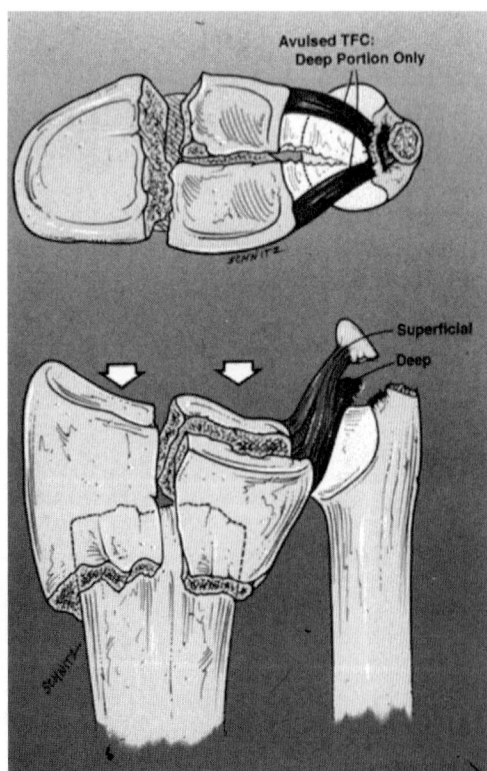

FIG. 43-25. Both insertions of the triangular fibrocartilage (the styloid and foveal insertions) may be severely damaged when plain x-rays reveal a displaced ulnar styloid fracture through its base. The clinician must thoroughly appreciate the magnitude of soft-tissue injury when assessing x-rays after wrist trauma.

and fragment positions. When there is doubt about the presence of a fracture, a frequent problem with injuries about the radial side of the carpus, especially the scaphoid, the use of technetium bone scan 72 hours after trauma is diagnostic. MRI scanning is also extremely sensitive in delineating the presence of a carpal fracture (but is somewhat more expensive).

Scaphoid Fracture. Nearly two-thirds of all carpal fractures are of the scaphoid. This injury occurs most often in males aged 15 to 30 years. Scaphoid fractures occur most commonly through the middle third of the waist or at the juncture of the middle and proximal poles. Diagnosis requires clinical and imaging information. After a fall on the outstretched hand, the patient's wrist is tender at the anatomic snuffbox, the hollow between the thumb extensor tendons on the radial aspect of the wrist, just dorsal and distal to the styloid process of the radius. Pain is elicited and symptoms reproduced with direct pressure over the tuberosity of the scaphoid at the palmar base of the thenar eminence and with passive wrist motion. Routine radiographs in posteroanterior, lateral, and oblique views, along with a posteroanterior projection in ulnar deviation of the wrist to elongate the scaphoid, helps to visualize the fracture. If initial radiographs are normal but the history and physical examination suggest the possibility of scaphoid fracture, continuous immobilization in a thumb spica splint or cast is advised. Repeat radiographs in 2 to 3 weeks, MRI scan, or technetium bone scan after 72 hours, will make the diagnosis.

Fracture configuration (Fig. 43-26) and location affect stability and lability of the fractured bone's blood supply. The proximal pole of the scaphoid is supplied from vessels entering the distal two-thirds. Fracture of the proximal one-third or a smaller fragment risks avascularity in the small proximal fragment, resulting in nonunion and secondary arthrosis. Nondisplaced scaphoid fractures treated with adequate immobilization have a union rate of 90 to 95%. Displaced fractures, defined as ≥1.0 mm displacement, are

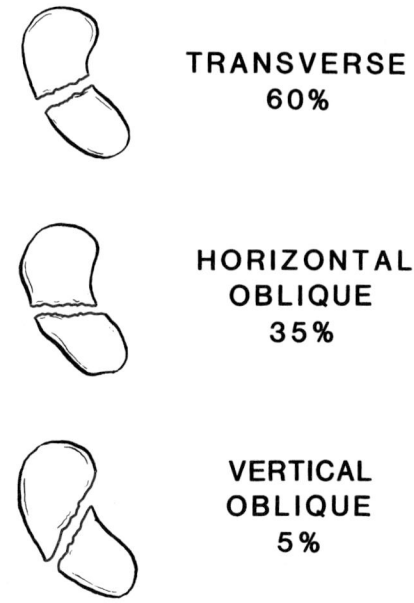

TRANSVERSE
60%

HORIZONTAL
OBLIQUE
35%

VERTICAL
OBLIQUE
5%

FIG. 43-26. *Russe's classification of scaphoid fractures.*

associated with avascular necrosis and nonunions in half of patients if not reduced and stabilized operatively. Scaphoid fracture fragment displacement of 2.0 mm or more should raise suspicion of an associated intercarpal ligament injury, such as transscaphoid perilunate instability, or subluxation.

In the treatment of the nondisplaced, stable scaphoid fracture, one study demonstrated decreased time to union and decreased incidence of delayed and nonunion when long-arm (above-elbow) thumb spica casts were used for the first 6 weeks, followed by a short-arm spica cast for approximately 6 weeks. Immobilization of the wrist in slight flexion and radial deviation relaxes the volar radioscaphoid ligament. The thumb metacarpophalangeal joint needs to be included in the cast, at least during the initial 6 weeks. Open reduction and internal fixation can be done most effectively with an interfragmentary lag compression screw for all displaced fractures. The screw technique is more stable and allows earlier mobilization.

The use of percutaneous compression screws for immediate internal stabilization of the acute but nondisplaced fracture is increasingly popular. Recent experience suggests a more rapid course and decreased acute and long-term disability without a significant increase in complications. Interfragmentary screw technique for this bone is technically demanding, but rewarding for the patient when properly executed. For individuals whose livelihood or lifestyle depends on hand use and rapid recovery of wrist mobility, internal fixation has compelling advantages and lower risks than long-term immobilization.

When immediate postinjury imaging does not clearly demonstrate the presence of fracture, immobilization and additional imaging information by standard radiographs in 2 weeks, or MRI scan or bone scan after 3 days, are necessary to make the diagnosis. Fracture displacement is unacceptable, and 1 to 2 mm of malposition, angulation, or any intercarpal collapse should prompt open repair. Less than 5% of nondisplaced fractures result in nonunion (defined as absence of x-ray evidence of healing 4 to 6 months after injury); however, there is a 50% nonunion rate for displaced fractures.

Other Carpal Fractures. The *lunate* most commonly fractures secondary to idiopathic avascular necrosis or lunatomalacia (Kienböck's disease) without a history of acute trauma. The lunate is seen as more radiodense on posteroanterior projection radiographs. Mild radiodensity, however, is not uncommon after carpal injuries, and should not be acutely confused with Kienböck's disease. However, simple, acute lunate fractures are uncommon. They should be treated with immobilization when nondisplaced; open treatment is required when displaced or with intercarpal misalignment.

Fractures of the *capitate* are uncommon. The proximal pole, like that of the scaphoid, receives its blood supply from vessels that enter distally. Capitate neck fractures are therefore at potential risk for avascular necrosis. When avascular necrosis occurs, usually it is incomplete (i.e., temporary). Capitate head collapse is uncommon.

Isolated fractures of the *trapezium* and *trapezoid* are uncommon. Injuries to these bones are often associated with intra-articular fractures of the base of the first metacarpal. Open reduction is often necessary, with internal fixation by Kirschner wires or small compression screws.

Fractures of the *pisiform* are usually secondary to a direct blow to the hypothenar eminence. The fractured pisiform is best seen in carpal tunnel projection radiographs or CT scan. Excision may be required, and is symptomatically curative for displaced fractures, nonunion, malunion, and secondary arthritis. There are two types of fracture of the *hamate:* those involving the body and those of the hamulus (hook). Fractures of the body of the hamate are difficult to diagnose on plain radiographs; imaging may require several oblique projections, or even better, CT scan. The patient may have pain referred to the dorsal hand or wrist with fractures of the body or hook. Most fractures of the body of the hamate heal with immobilization for 4 to 6 weeks. Fractures of the hamulus are more common, and usually are the result of a direct force transmitted into the base of the palm from a grasped object. The palm is tender to direct pressure over the hamate, but sometimes the discomfort is reported as being dorsal with such a maneuver or with use. Secondary ulnar neuropathy in the distal third of Guyon's canal may be present. Late flexor tendon ruptures (little and ring finger flexors) have been reported, especially in those whose undiagnosed palmar pain syndrome is treated [sic] with repeated steroid injections. Routine radiographs and carpal tunnel views may be negative; CT scan will make this diagnosis evident. The acute hook fracture should be expected to heal in a short-arm cast (4+ weeks); displaced fractures and symptomatic nonunions are most efficiently treated by excision of the hamulus and smoothing of the fracture base, but taking care to visualize and protect the deep motor branch of the ulnar nerve, which courses radially around the distal edge of the hamulus as it goes dorsally into the mid-palm.

Carpal Dislocations and Intercarpal Instability. The radiocarpal and intercarpal articulations are not inherently stable on the basis of their osseous anatomy; it is the integration of osteoligamentous support that secures these bones for the complex kinematics of wrist function (Fig. 43-27). Most carpal dislocations are caused by an acute axial load and wrist hyperextension. The first of a sequence of dislocations occurs at the midcarpal joint, with dorsal displacement of the capitate. When the capitate displaces, the scaphoid must fracture or its ligaments tear (i.e., either must occur), allowing it to rotate "into flexion" from a relatively horizontal position (as seen on the lateral x-ray) to become vertical, with the now untethered proximal pole rotating dorsally. This situation is called *dorsal perilunate dislocation* (Figs. 43-28, 43-29, and 43-30). These are serious and unstable intra-articular injuries, with or without associated scaphoid fracture or triquetral fractures and/or triquetrolunate separation, which require careful realignment, most all by open reduction with internal fixation. Direct trauma to the median nerve from impact

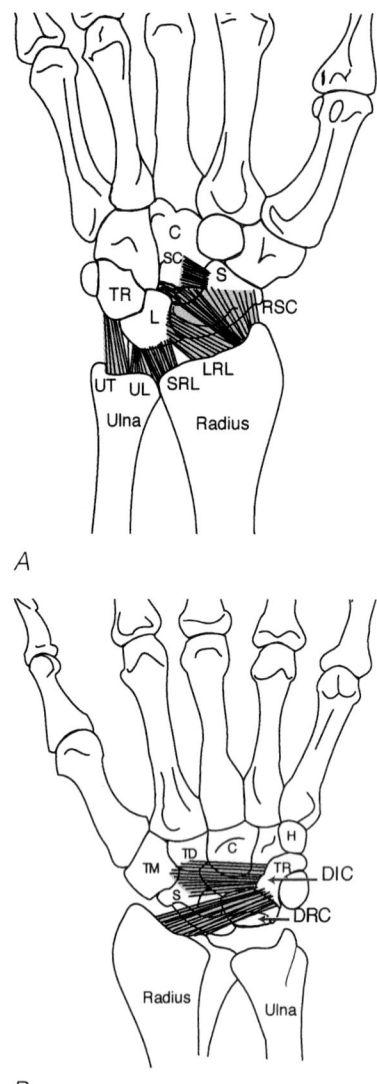

A

B

FIG. 43-27. Ligamentous anatomy of the wrist. *A.* Palmar wrist ligaments. LRL = long radiolunate; RSC = radioscaphocapitate; SC = scaphocapitate; SRL = short radiolunate; UL = ulnolunate; UT = ulnotriquetral. The space between the LRL and SRL is where the radioscapholunate ligament (ligament of Testut), now known to be a neurovascular pedicle, enters the radiocarpal joint. Carpals: C = capitate; L = lunate; S = scaphoid; TR = triquetrum. *B.* Dorsal wrist ligaments. DIC = dorsal intercarpal; DRC = dorsal radiocarpal. Carpals: C = capitate; H = hamate; S = scaphoid; TD = trapezoid; TM = trapezium; TR = triquetrum.

and by secondary stretching from dorsal displacement of the carpus, or from blood and swelling within the carpal tunnel, should be elucidated by neurovascular examination and pressure measurement in the latter case. Carpal instabilities of all types should be treated aggressively definitively to prevent chronic instability and dysfunction (Fig. 43-31).

Metacarpal Fractures. Because of their subcutaneous location and relatively rigid proximal articulations, the metacarpals represent one-third of hand and wrist fractures. Failure to reconstitute the metacarpals may lead to finger misalignment, pain, and permanent functional deficits. Complications from extensive surgical exposure for plate fixation can be high, and the risk of additional injury must be weighed against outcomes expected with conservative measures and percutaneous K-wire fixation. Functional misalignment

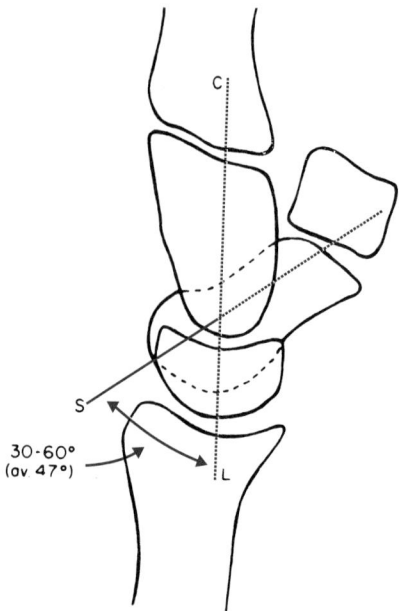

FIG. 43-28. Lateral wrist view demonstrates a normal scapholunate angle of 30 to 60 degrees. The capitolunate angle should be less than 30 degrees. Here both lunate and capitate axes are coaxial.

must be corrected, and stabilized fractures (no matter what the method) allow immediate therapy to prevent and minimize stiffness.

Whether internal or external immobilization is used is immaterial, as long as bone length, rotation, and articular relationships are

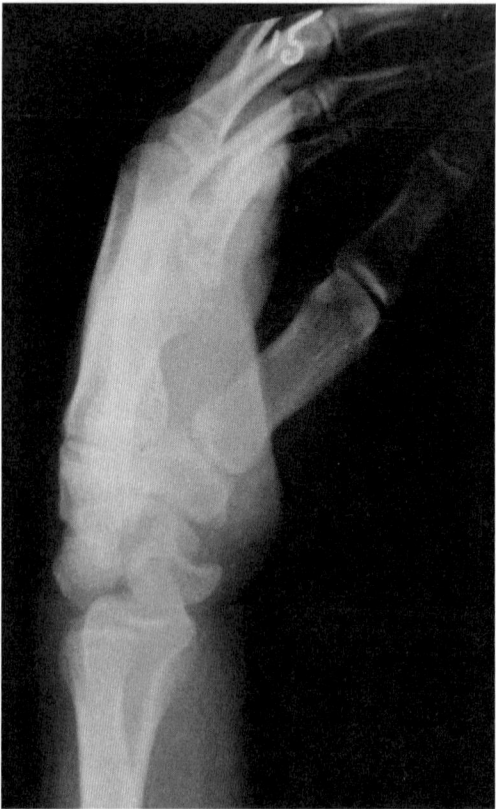

FIG. 43-29. Lateral radiograph of a dorsal perilunate dislocation.

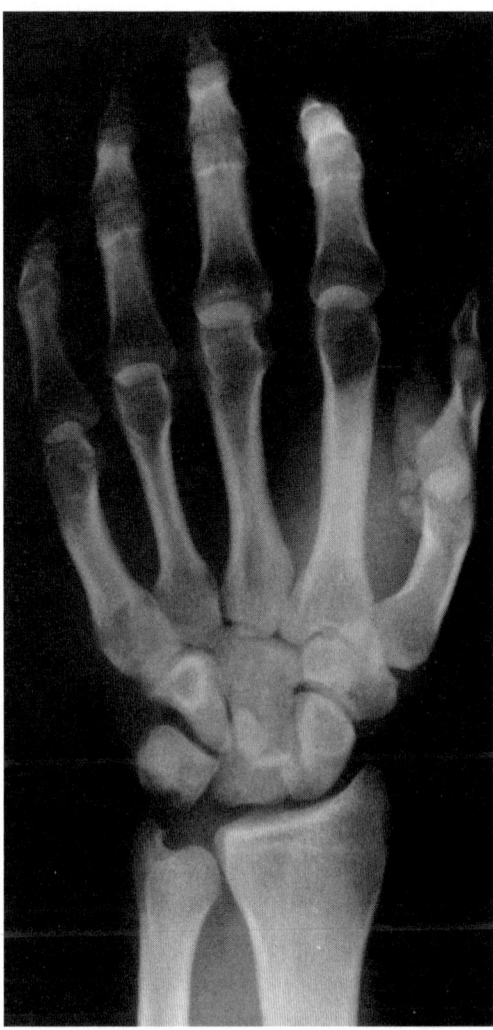

FIG. 43-30. *Anteroposterior radiograph of a dorsal perilunate dislocation.*

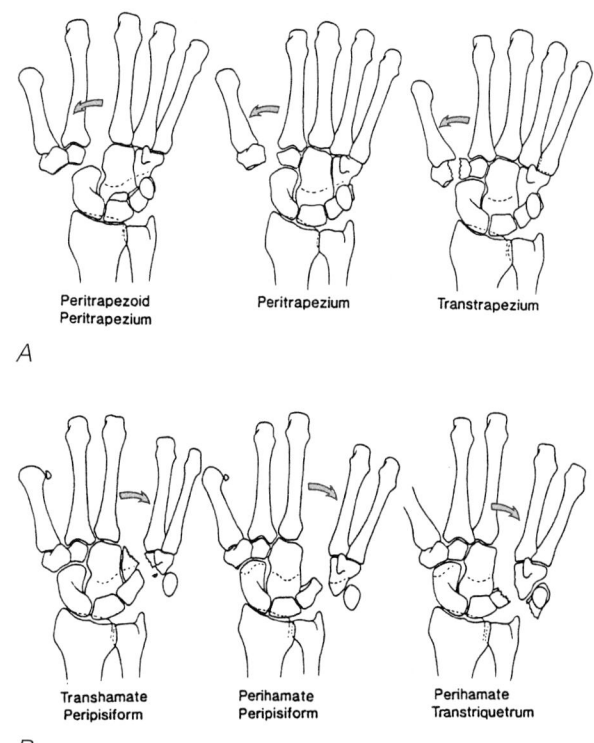

FIG. 43-31. *The most common types of axial disruption of the carpus. A. Axial-radial disruption. B. Axial-ulnar disruption. (Modified with permission from Garcia-Elias M, Dobyns JH, Cooney WP, et al: Traumatic axial dislocations of the carpus. J Hand Surg 14A:449, 1989.)*

preserved, and soft-tissue management and therapy techniques can be instituted rapidly.

The second and third metacarpals form a rigid longitudinal arch because of their convexity dorsally. There also is a dynamic transverse arch based on the mobile carpometacarpal articulations of the thumb opposing those of the ring and little fingers. The thenar and hypothenar muscles dynamize these arches, allowing precision and strength in hand use. Because of stable proximal and distal ligamentous support, isolated fractures of the central (third and fourth) metacarpals are less likely to shorten, rotate, and angulate. Spiral and oblique fractures that shorten and displace will by definition also rotate. Metacarpal shortening also may occur from comminution and with bone loss or angular deformity. Midshaft angulation produces a more serious finger deformity due to the longer lever arm than with distal metacarpal (neck) fractures (Fig. 43-32).

Pain and swelling are the hallmarks of metacarpal fractures, as the looser dorsal tissues allow large amounts of edema fluid and fracture hematoma to accumulate. The bony prominence of an angulated fracture apex is always located dorsally because of the pull of the interosseous (intrinsic) muscles. A skin laceration most often connotes an open fracture and mandates surgical débridement. This is critically important in metacarpal fractures from tooth impact, as in a fight, which results in a contaminated puncture wound at the fracture site or at the metacarpophalangeal joint. Patients with human or animal bites require surgical irrigation of the fracture site or joint plus high-dose IV antibiotics.

Rotational alignment of the figures after metacarpal fracture is best assessed with the finger(s) flexed at the metacarpophalangeal joint(s), because this tightens the collateral ligaments and links or locks the finger's position to the distal portion of the fractured metacarpal. With an uncooperative juvenile or an unconscious

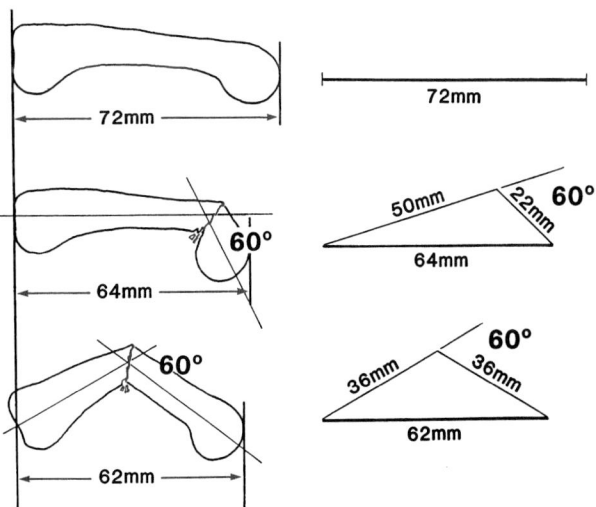

FIG. 43-32. *The effect of location of a metacarpal fracture on shortening. Sixty-degree angulation of a midshaft fracture will produce more shortening than an equivalent angulation at the metacarpal neck.*

patient, the wrist can be passively flexed and extended, with the resulting extrinsic flexor and extensor effect (tenodesis) on digital alignment observed. Malrotation produces a degree of visible digital overlap in flexion. Malrotation and radial-ulnar angulation interferes with hand function and requires correction.

Fractures of the metacarpal heads are less common, and are usually the result of direct trauma. The second and fifth metacarpals are the most commonly traumatized, with a 3:1 male predominance. As these are intra-articular injuries a step-off ≥ 1.0 mm is significant. Unstable fractures may be fixed with pins, screws, or plates.

The metacarpal neck is the most common fracture site. As with other displaced and angulated fractures, the cortex on the concavity at the angulated side usually is comminuted. The normal pull of the intrinsic muscles further flexes the head (distal) fragment, making it difficult to maintain reduction. The degree of angulation and the specific metacarpal involved determines the best treatment for the fracture. As the second and third carpometacarpal joints are rigid, no more than 10 to 15 degrees of palmar angulation of the distal fragment is acceptable. Considerably more angulation (30 to 50 degrees) can be functionally and aesthetically acceptable in the neck region of the fourth and fifth metacarpals. Closed reduction may be effected through the combination of direct and counterpressure applied with the finger flexed (Fig. 43-33). The hand must *not* be immobilized in the position depicted for manipulative reduction. If fracture comminution prevents maintenance of realignment, open reduction may be necessary, but internal fixation is required. In short, metacarpal shaft fractures should be protected when position and angulation are acceptable, but repaired when they are not. Spiral and oblique fractures rotate and displace because of the normal forces of the extrinsic flexor and extensor tendons and the hand intrinsics. Those that are not initially displaced or rotated must be carefully observed. Internal fixation allows for rapid soft-tissue mobilization, and when fixation is needed, percutaneous K-wire technique, local block anesthesia, and fluoroscopic monitoring are highly effective. Some of these fractures require open reduction (Figs. 43-34, 43-35, and 43-36).

Intra-articular carpometacarpal fracture-dislocations are of functional significance in the mobile fourth and fifth metacarpal-hamate saddle joints, in which periarticular tendon insertions favor

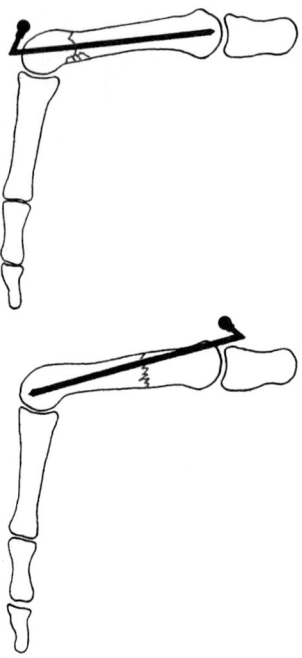

FIG. 43-34. Two methods for percutaneous or open intramedullary fixation of metacarpal fractures.

displacement (Figs. 43-37 and 43-38). Reduction is best maintained with (percutaneous) internal fixation. Some require open reduction and fixation to restore accurate osteoarticular alignment.

Delayed union and nonunions of closed metacarpal injuries are most uncommon. Bone consolidation should eventually be discernible by radiographs within 12 to 16 weeks. Immobilization of the hand for several months seriously risks compromising function; usually, only 3 or 4 weeks of immobilization is adequate. Nonunions may be associated with inadequate immobilization, loss of bone substance, infection, or disruption of blood supply. Digital impairment results from tendon adhesions directly over a fracture site, secondary small-joint contractures from prolonged immobilization, or scarring of traumatized intrinsic muscles. Simultaneous skeletal stabilization and small-joint mobilization should be achieved to optimize outcome.

Phalangeal Fractures. The goal of phalangeal fracture treatment is restoration of anatomy, bone healing, and functional recovery. Dysfunctional angulation and rotation are not acceptable. Stabilized fracture anatomy must allow rapid mobilization. Each method of fracture care has relative advantages and risks. Less-invasive methods may offer less stability, but they inflict less soft-tissue damage. An algorithm for care is outlined in Fig. 43-39. When operation is required, the least traumatic method should be used to avoid violation of gliding tendon and joint structures when possible. The patient's active participation in a rehabilitation program with custom splinting and home exercises is critical for recovery of function. Proximal interphalangeal joint motion, particularly extension, can be difficult to regain if an injured, swollen finger is immobilized in flexion for a long period. Scar tissue can tether the extensor tendons or prevent the flexors from gliding, impairing grasp and manipulation, and preventing return to preinjury employment.

When K-wires are used, they may be buried and then retrieved in the office under local anesthesia after about 4 weeks, as sufficient fracture healing usually has occurred by then, despite the delayed appearance of interfragmentary callus on radiographs. When

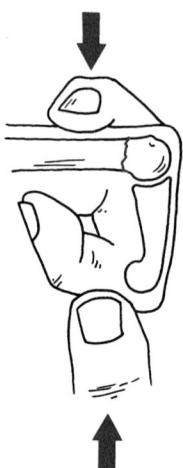

FIG. 43-33. The Jahss "90–90" maneuver for reduction of metacarpal neck fractures. Dorsally directed force along the proximal phalanx (*arrows*) serves to reduce neck angulation, while rotational control is gained via tightening of collateral ligaments in metacarpophalangeal flexion.

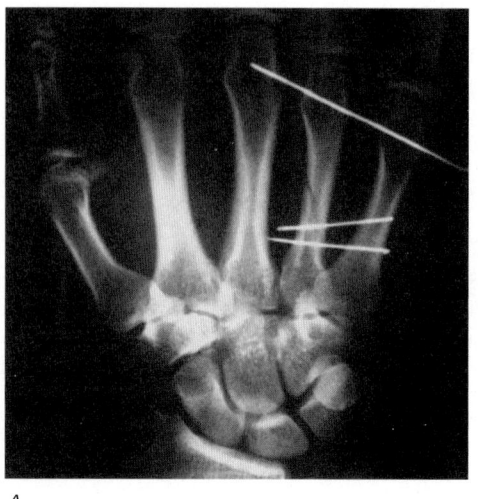

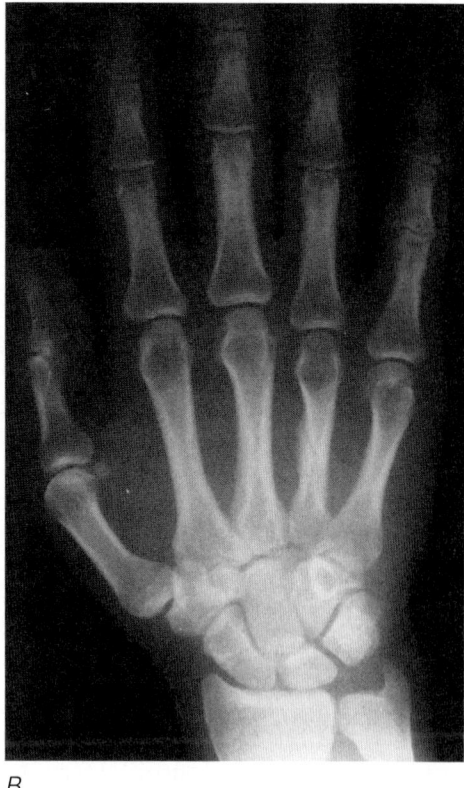

FIG. 43-35. *A.* Percutaneous fixation of short oblique metacarpal shaft fracture. Fixation of both the proximal and distal shaft fragments is recommended for stability in fractures of the fourth and fifth metacarpal shafts. *B.* Uneventful healing at 6 weeks.

Kirschner wires are left outside the skin, as in all juveniles, pins must be capped and cared for meticulously. Screws and plates usually are not removed unless symptomatic, and more than 12 months after fracture healing. Intra-articular fractures need accurate reduction; many require internal fixation.

Finger Ligament Injuries

Metacarpophalangeal Joint. Metacarpophalangeal (MP) joint dislocations can be managed by closed means through gentle reduction and splinting under local anesthesia. Rarely, significant residual collateral ligament instability in a particular finger is present, making surgical repair necessary. Patients with acute collateral injuries may have a malrotated finger (Fig. 43-40), because of rotation about the uninjured, intact ligament. The ruptured ligament region is swollen and tender. Evaluation by gentle passive stress should be done with the MP joint in flexion—a position in which the collateral ligaments are normally tight. Some perform simultaneous radiographic evaluation during this passive stress. Patients with

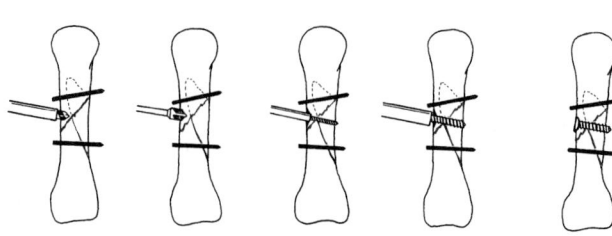

FIG. 43-36. Steps for placement of provisional Kirschner wires and interfragmentary screws.

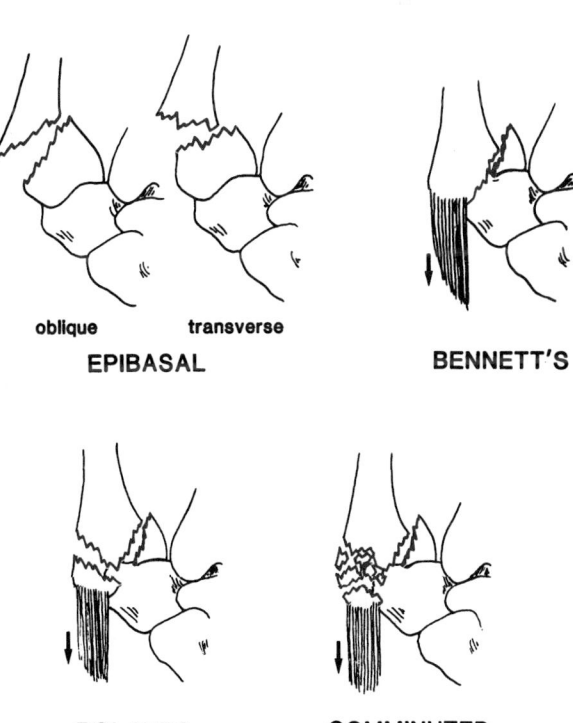

FIG. 43-37. Four different types of metacarpal base fractures.

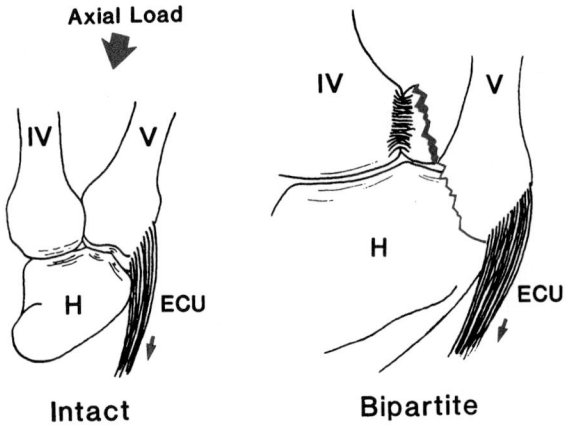

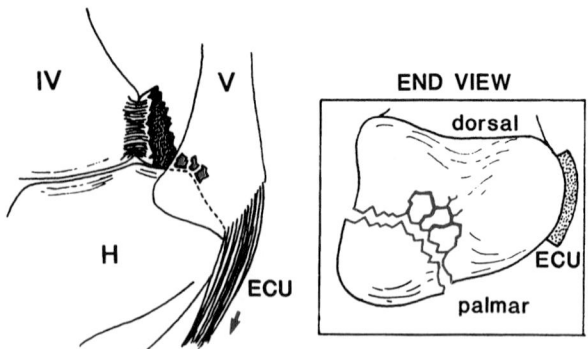

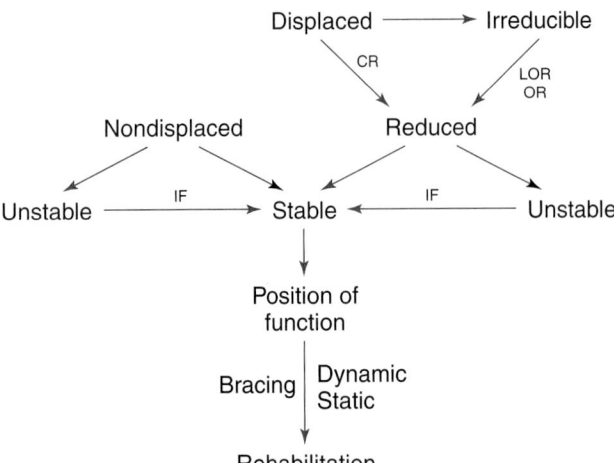

FIG. 43-38. Types of fifth carpometacarpal fracture-dislocations. A bipartite fracture-dislocation, which results from a dorsally directed load on the fifth metacarpal shaft, leaves a minor fragment attached to the fourth metacarpal by the intermetacarpal ligaments. The comminuted fracture-dislocation is a result of axial loading, and the radial facet of the hamate causes a variable degree of central impaction of the fifth metacarpal base.

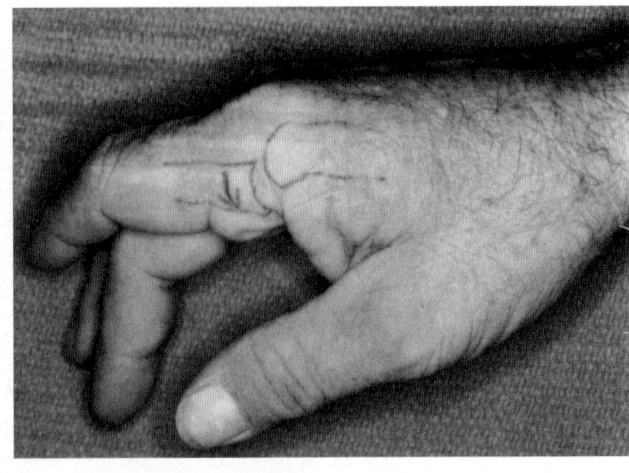

A

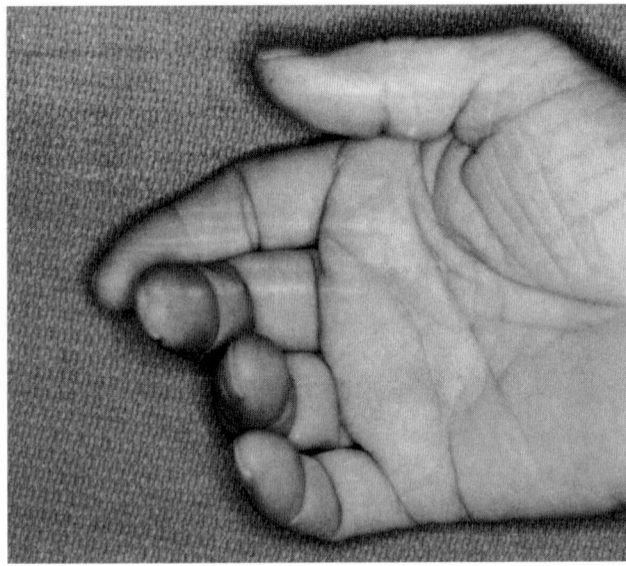

B

FIG. 43-40. Rupture of the radial collateral ligament of the index finger MP joint. *A.* Rupture of the radial collateral ligament allows the radial base of the proximal phalanx to subluxate palmarward and to rotate around the remaining ulnar collateral ligament. *B.* The rotation at the base of the proximal phalanx becomes magnified over the length of the digit, causing the index finger to overlap the long finger.

extreme discomfort who cannot tolerate soft-tissue stress in order to evaluate joint stability can be better examined after 1.0 mL of local anesthetic agent is injected into the joint. Dorsal MP dislocations that are irreducible are almost exclusively in a border finger, and are characterized by dimpling of the palmar skin over a prominent metacarpal head. Interposed soft tissues can prevent joint reduction. In these cases surgical treatment is required (Fig. 43-41).

Thumb MP joint injuries result from axial load plus angular displacement. Such injuries often occur when the patient jams the thumb into an object while falling. Disruption of the ulnar collateral ligament of the thumb is called *gamekeeper's thumb*, although the term was originally applied only to chronic ulnar collateral instability. A large number of these injuries are caused by jamming the thumb. Collateral laxity at the thumb MP joint is highly dysfunctional and painful, and may later lead to late arthritis. After plain radiographs fail to detect the presence of intra-articular fractures,

FIG. 43-39. Phalangeal fracture management algorithm. CR = closed reduction; IF = internal fixation; LOR = limited open reduction; OR = open reduction.

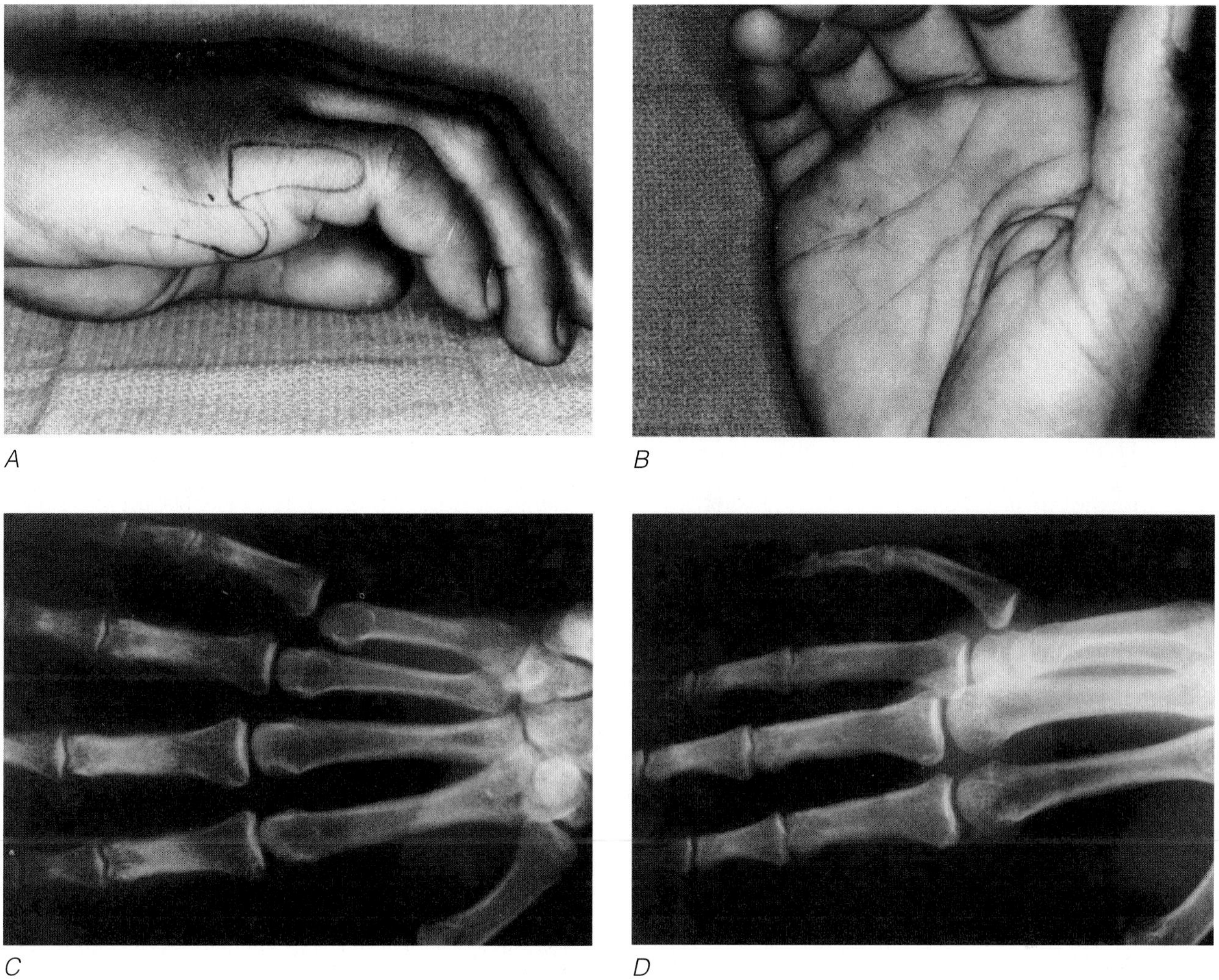

A

B

C

D

FIG. 43-41. Dorsal complex (irreducible) dislocation of the MP joint. *A.* The proximal phalanx rests in bayonet apposition on the dorsal aspect of the metacarpal head. The resulting digital deformity is subtle. *B.* A palmar skin dimple (outlined here with small radiating marks) is a pathognomonic sign of a complex dislocation. *C.* The anteroposterior x-ray demonstrates joint-space widening and subtle subluxation. *D.* An oblique film clearly demonstrates the dorsal dislocation.

the thumb is carefully examined in about 30 degrees of MP flexion, gently and progressively stressing the suspect collateral ligament (Fig. 43-42). Radiographs may be obtained simultaneously (Fig. 43-43); the stress radiograph is best performed by the examining physician. Treatment of incomplete collateral ligament injuries without associated instability is best done closed, with cast immobilization for approximately 3 weeks, followed by custom-splint immobilization. Soreness may persist for several months. Complete disruption of the ulnar or radial collateral ligament of the thumb MP joint should be repaired and protected by temporary pin fixation of the joint, an approach which is most likely to give a better result and a shorter period of disability than secondary (tendon graft) ligament reconstruction.

Proximal Interphalangeal Joint. The tightly congruent osteoarticular contours of the proximal interphalangeal (PIP) joint make restoration of stable alignment of disrupted or displaced structures essential, allowing safe institution of early mobilization. Stiffness, rather than instability, is the common and disabling result that must be avoided after trauma in the region of the PIP joint. Most dorsal and lateral PIP dislocations can be treated by closed reduction

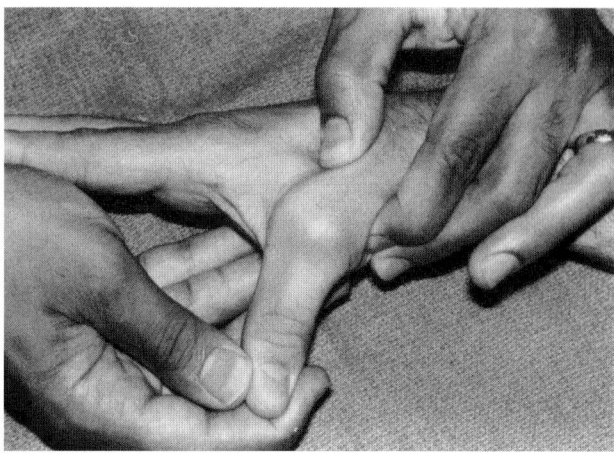

FIG. 43-42. Laxity of 30 degrees more than the uninjured thumb measured in neutral and 30 degrees of flexion are strongly suggestive of a complete ulnar collateral ligament tear. There is no "endpoint" to the radial deviation of the phalanx.

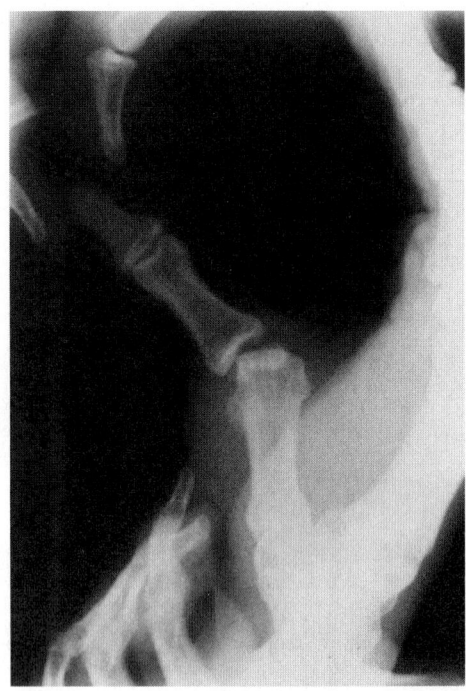

FIG. 43-43. Stress x-ray of a thumb with a complete ulnar collateral ligament tear demonstrates marked instability of the ulnar side of the MP joint and radial deviation of the proximal phalanx.

and should be stable. Immobilization for 10 to 15 days allows the patient to recover from the acute posttraumatic effects before a protected mobilization program is started, with compressive wrapping and buddy tapes to an adjacent finger. Joints without an actual history of displacement, deformity, or reduction by patient, coach, trainer, or physician may still have considerable swelling and stiffness if not remobilized early. Dislocations with fractures are more likely to be unstable (Figs. 43-44 and 43-45). Postoperative immobilization that inadvertently stresses an osteoarticular fragment results in posttraumatic instability (Fig. 43-46). The combination of joint surface impaction and ligament disruption has the worst prognosis (Fig. 43-47), and such fracture-dislocations have an ultimate outcome that is often unsatisfactory.

Palmar (Volar) Proximal Interphalangeal Joint Dislocations.
With volar PIP joint dislocations, the middle phalanx is displaced

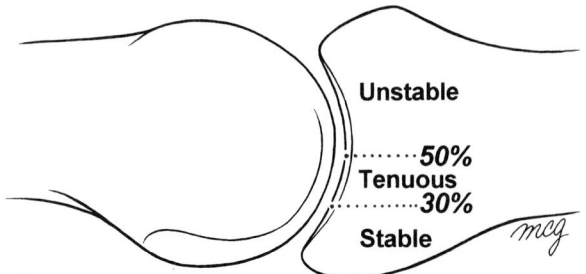

FIG. 43-44. Classification of PIP fracture-dislocations. Stable (type I) injuries involve less than 30% of the articular surface and demonstrate no instability on stress testing. Tenuous (type II) injuries involve 30 to 50% of the articular surface, but reduction can be maintained with 30 degrees or less of joint flexion. All fracture-dislocations that involve 50% or more of the articular surface are unstable. Fractures with 30 to 50% joint surface involvement that will only stay reduced with more than 30 degrees of flexion are also classified as unstable.

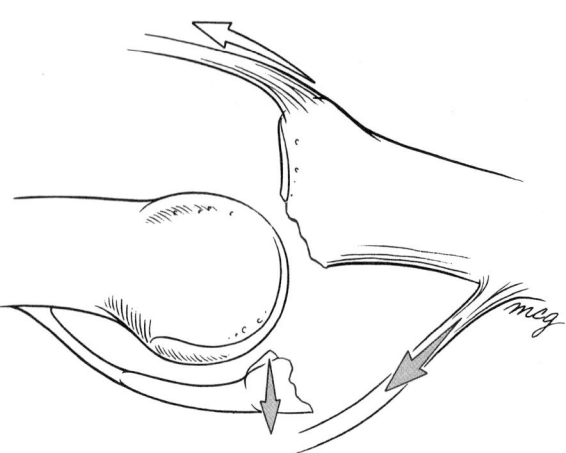

FIG. 43-45. Unstable fracture-dislocation of the PIP joint. The slope of the remaining dorsal articular surface, the pull of the central tendon, and the angulatory moment created by the distal insertion of the flexor digitorum superficialis tendon combine to cause dorsal subluxation of the middle phalanx. The mechanical buttress provided by the volar lip of the middle phalanx is the only support that counteracts these forces. Restoring this buttress is the primary treatment goal for unstable PIP fracture-dislocations.

palmarward, many times resulting in serious instability (rather than stiffness). This PIP dislocation results from the combination of axial load and palmar vectors, most often during sports (Fig. 43-48). Often unrecognized, this injury has associated disruptions of the central slip of the extensor tendon and one collateral ligament. Closed reduction and pinning, or open reduction for the irreducible variant, with early supervised postoperative therapy is the rule.

Distal Interphalangeal Joint. The distal interphalangeal (DIP) joint must be comfortable and stable for precision pinch and power grip. Ideally, rehabilitation after DIP joint trauma restores a pain-free and stable arc of motion, but this is not always possible. Some compromise between stability, motion, and symptoms may be necessary; functional alignment in near extension and DIP joint stability are critical to regaining a useful hand. Collateral ligament injuries and dorsal or palmar dislocations may occur at this level. Stable joints for which closed reduction is possible need not be pinned. Percutaneous fixation under fluoroscopic guidance, with maintenance of pin fixation for 5 to 6 weeks, is a useful adjunct, because it allows the rest of the hand to be rapidly mobilized. It is preferable to bury pins in adults and to remove them in the office using local anesthesia.

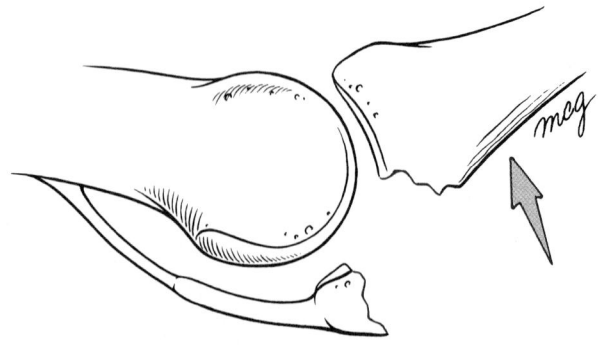

FIG. 43-46. Palmar plate avulsion fracture. Noncomminuted volar lip fractures are caused by forceful hyperextension of the PIP joint.

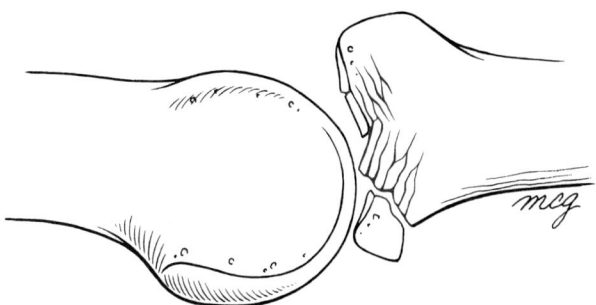

FIG. 43-47. *Impaction shear PIP joint fracture-dislocation. Longitudinal loading with the PIP joint slightly flexed or extended causes extensive comminution of the articular surface and impaction of osteochondral fragments into the metaphyseal bone. By definition, the dorsal cortex and some portion of the dorsal articular surface remain intact.*

Swelling and discomfort that decreases in intensity over 3 to 6 months may persist after DIP and PIP injury in most patients. Functional recovery of mobility and power occurs more slowly than most patients perceive it should. Protection during sports and similar activities may be needed for more than 6 months, and this should be explained to patients early on. The sooner a patient understands, the more likely they are to accept their role in recovery.

Fingertip Injuries. Conservative treatments such as healing by secondary intention for fingertip amputations may prolong recovery and may result in painful scarring or deformity if tissue loss is significantly >1 cm. The requirements for satisfactory outcome after fingertip amputation are: (1) maintenance of functional finger length (additional shortening during or as a complication of treatment should be avoided); (2) the residual tip/pulp requires a resistant and resilient character like normal palmar skin; (3) sensibility should be maintained to avoid "blinding" the finger; and (4) bone support under the nail is needed to minimize beaking deformity. Achieving all of these targets simultaneously may be impossible, and choices or tradeoffs may be necessary. Anatomy and function in conjunction with the type and level of injury in each patient should be considered (Figs. 43-49 and 43-50).

Which finger is injured and how it was injured influence treatment. For the thumb, every reasonable effort must be made to restore a sensate and durable pulp. Requirements for sensibility are more critical in the index and middle fingers, but they also are significant in the ulnar pulp of the small finger. Amputations can be clean and sharp, but the common crush-avulsion may have extensive trauma to surrounding skin, soft tissue, and neurovascular tissue that requires débridement, and in some cases, staging of the closure. Treatment of partial amputations, crush injuries, and partial devascularizing injuries should be directed toward preserving soft tissues.

Distal phalangeal fractures, including bursting or tuft fractures, are frequently associated with crush trauma and nail bed disruption or lacerations. Nail bed injuries are not always obvious, and subungual hematoma may be the only sign of nail bed injury. Nail bed injuries should be repaired to prevent permanent late nail deformity. Nail bed repairs usually are done with fine, 6-0 absorbable suture. After repair, the nail that was removed is replaced beneath the cuticle to splint (stent) the bed (Figs. 43-51 and 43-52). Surgical treatments used to treat fingertip amputations are listed below.

Bone Shortening and Primary Closure. Performed under local or regional anesthesia, bone shortening and primary closure consists of débriding enough bone so the skin can be closed without tension with a few 5-0 sutures. Thorough débridement of contaminated,

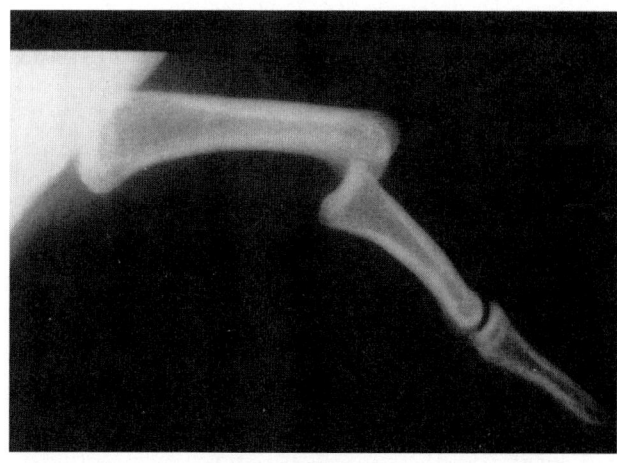

A

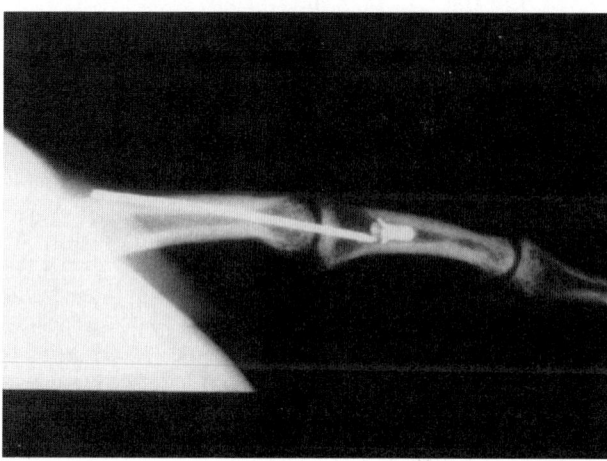

B

FIG. 43-48. *Volar dislocation of the PIP joint. A. Lateral radiograph demonstrates the palmar subluxation of the middle phalanx. The rotational component of the injury is recognized by observing a true lateral view of one bone (in this case the middle phalanx), and an oblique view of the opposite joint member (here the proximal phalanx). B. Reducible volar dislocations can be managed with closed reduction and percutaneous pin fixation. If surgical repair of the central tendon is elected, suture repair usually is not feasible, because the tendon typically avulses directly off of the bone. The tendon can be secured with a pullout wire, or as in this case, a Mitek suture.*

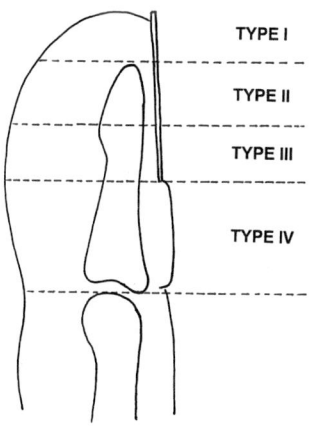

FIG. 43-49. *Transverse amputations; classification into four types.*

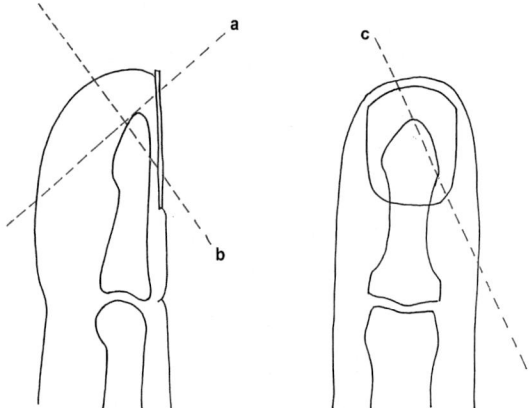

FIG. 43-50. Oblique defects. (a) Volar oblique. (b) Dorsal oblique. (c) Lateral oblique.

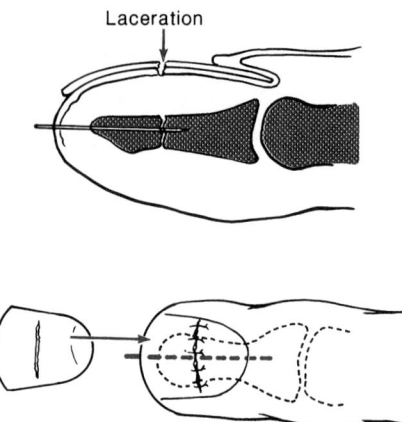

FIG. 43-52. Unstable fractures of the distal phalanx require reduction and Kirschner wire fixation. Care is taken to properly align the dorsal cortex of the bone. The nail bed laceration is repaired, and the nail is replaced as a stent for the injury, as well as to provide a conforming surface for the healing nail bed.

devitalized tissues is required to afford coverage with soft tissues of normal sensibility, and a well-padded fingertip is not painful. However, the cost is some bone length and at least a portion of the fingernail. Inadequate bone resection produces a fingertip with unpadded bone, resulting in pain during grasping.

Composite Pulp Reattachment. Reapplication of the "composite" of skin and pulp, or skin, pulp, and bone, can be done when the mass of the amputated part is very small. This choice should be reserved for young children. It is best to débride any residual bone. At the least, superficial necrosis of the reapplied part should be expected. In most situations, this is a temporary biologic dressing.

Skin Grafting. Grafts offer coverage for skin defects. They are not time consuming and theoretically can be applied to a wide range of fingertip amputations. The major drawbacks are sensory loss in the graft area and the lack of padding if the graft is applied over unpadded bone and periosteum on prehensile surfaces.

The aesthetics of the graft are affected primarily by the donor site. The best functional and cosmetic result for the pulp surface is achieved in all races with full- or split-thickness grafts taken from the glabrous skin at the hypothenar eminence. The defect covered with skin graft should be a skin defect, and the recipient bed must have adequate native padding. Skin graft will not satisfactorily protect bone, regardless of the skin donor source. Skin graft to the palm from any area other than glabrous skin produces a result that is relatively hyperpigmented. Split grafts are usually inadequate for surfaces subject to pressure and friction. Toe-to-finger and foot

instep-to-hand pulp skin grafting can be performed, but the short-term disadvantages are obvious compared to the use of hypothenar skin.

Local Flaps. Local tissue transfer from more proximally on the injured finger affords vascularized, padded, and often sensate tissues. Coverage is by advancement, transposition, or rotation (Figs. 43-53 and 43-54).

Regional and Distant Flaps. Cross-finger, thenar, and other heterodigital flaps have been used since the early part of the twentieth century, generally for more extensive pulp loss and otherwise uncoverable bone and tendon (Fig. 43-55). These flaps have the advantage of retaining finger length, but carry the risk of posttraumatic deformity or dysfunction in an adjacent donor finger. Great care must be taken to avoid dysfunction from immobilization of the injured and the donor parts because of nonphysiologic positioning during flap healing before pedicle detachment. Such flaps usually are not sensate.

Replantation and Microvascular Neurosensory Flaps. Microsurgical advances have made finger- and hand-part reattachment possible, and allowed reconstruction by composite neurovascular pulp tissue from toes, with or without joints and tendons. Isolated single-digit amputation in the adult usually is not suitable for replantation, especially if proximal to the PIP joint, because the functional and aesthetic recovery does not justify the morbidity and costs of the replantation procedure. Multiple digit amputations, subtotal hand amputations, amputations in the upper limb proximal to the hand, and most pediatric-age amputations should be evaluated for replantation or primary composite microvascular reconstruction (Fig. 43-56).

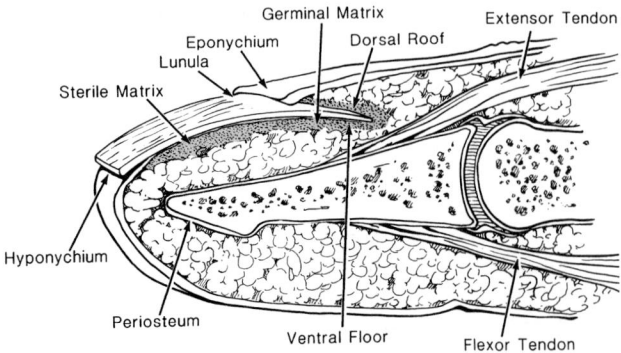

FIG. 43-51. The pertinent anatomy of the nail bed includes the distal phalanx, nail bed, nail plate, and surrounding soft tissue.

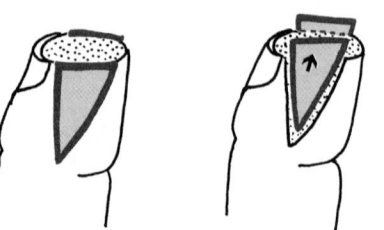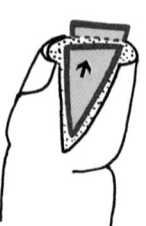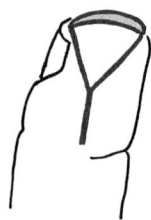

FIG. 43-53. Kutler's flap.

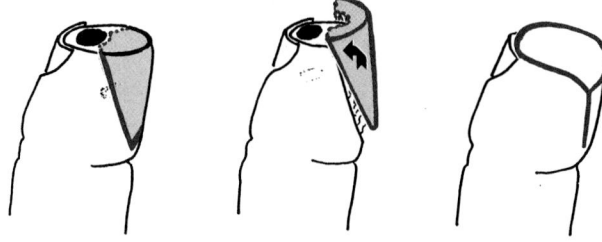

FIG. 43-54. *V-Y advancement flap (Tranquilli-Leali).*

Soft-Tissue Trauma

Tendon Injuries

Flexor Tendons. Flexor mechanism injuries in the hand and fingers are no longer treated by late reconstruction in the vast majority, because direct primary and delayed primary tendon repairs achieve good to excellent results. Satisfactory results are reported in 75 to 98% of patients in various series; nonetheless flexor tendon repair and functional rehabilitation is still a considerable challenge.

Flexor tendons are not difficult to repair, but achieving good function of repaired tendons is daunting, particularly in zones in which multiple tendons of different excursion are in juxtaposition. Tendons must glide, and simultaneously they are restrained by ligaments, such as within the digital sheath and within the carpal tunnel. This remains the core of the problem. The critical operative principle in tendon repair is to achieve near-perfect anatomic alignment of the tendon ends. There should be no gaps at the repair site, and "bunching" of the repair zone should be avoided in order to permit the repaired tendon(s) to glide within a sheath or pulley system. Repairs are now done with multistrand, nonreactive intratendinous "core" suture, plus epitendon stitching to appose the cut surfaces. The zones of the flexor tendons are defined by the number of tendons, restraints, and pulleys, and the presence or absence of synovial membrane at that specific anatomic level (Figs. 43-57 and 43-58).

In the diagnosis of tendon disruption, the patient often presents with an open wound and loss of active motion. Observing the part at rest (Fig. 43-59), along with active, separate evaluations of the flexor digitorum profundus and flexor digitorum superficialis tendons (Fig. 43-60) confirms this diagnosis. A high level of suspicion should be maintained with injuries that produce loss of active flexion

or extension when x-rays do not show skeletal disruption. Tendon avulsions may occur without attached bone, and can be diagnosed clinically only if the examiner is suspicious. Closed, isolated flexor profundus avulsion is most common in the ring finger; the DIP joint will not flex, but the PIP joint does, often with pain. For primary or delayed primary repair to be effective, early diagnosis is essential (Figs. 43-61 and 43-62).

Partial tendon lacerations, up to approximately one-third of the tendon's cross-sectional area, do not present serious risk of rupture, but the lacerated edge may catch on a nearby pulley, producing posttraumatic triggering. Lacerations involving 30 to 50% of the tendon's cross-sectional area may be treated by epitendinous suture alone. Division of greater than 50% should be treated surgically as though division were complete. Flexor mechanism salvage by graft and staged reconstructions, or with posttraumatic tenolysis or grafting, is beyond the scope of this text. Secondary tenolysis should be reserved for those patients whose fingers have achieved a stable local biologic state greater than 3 to 4 months after trauma, where tissues are no longer edematous, and maximum passive joint mobilization has been achieved. Critically, the patient must be willing to have a second operation and attendant therapy for the possible additional recovery.

Extensor Tendons. The superficial location of the extensor tendons on the dorsum of the fingers and hand make them vulnerable to injury, especially when the fingers are flexed. Trauma comes from lacerations, crush impacts, abrasions, and bites. Extensor tendon injuries are more common than flexor injuries, and may be treated too casually in an emergency department.

Extensor dysfunction may result in loss of active flexion from scar tethering as well as from diminished active extension. The extensor system is more intricate and complex than the flexor system due to the multilevel interconnections of the *extrinsic* digital extensor tendons from the forearm muscles, and the *intrinsic* tendons, in which muscles and tendons are entirely in the hand. The two sets of tendons collaborate to flex the metacarpophalangeal joints and extend the interphalangeal joints. Because excursion of the extensor mechanism is limited over the finger joints, preservation of tendon length is critical to maintain and restore tendon balance.

The flexor tendons are thick, round, cord-like structures with spiraling fibers. The extensor tendons are thin and flat, and the longitudinal fibers of the extensors do not hold sutures well. The limited amount of soft tissues about these tendons also makes repairs prone to adherence and scarring.

The brachioradialis and extensor carpi radialis longus are innervated by the radial nerve, and the extensor carpi radialis brevis and extensor carpi ulnaris muscles by the deep (posterior interosseous) branch of the radial nerve. This branch of the radial nerve innervates all proper and common thumb and digital extensors. The tendons cross the wrist through six (pulley) compartments, serving to extend the wrist and the MP and interphalangeal (IP) joints. These six tendon tunnels at the wrist are defined by reflections of the extensor retinaculum into the dorsal cortex of the radius and wrist capsule, and limit the vector effect of the digital extensors at the wrist joint by maintaining their proximity to the center of axis of wrist motion (i.e., bowstringing is prevented). Extrinsic digital extensor tendons elevate/extend the proximal phalanx. This means that they extend the MP joint via the aponeurotic sagittal fibers that reach around the lateral sides of the phalanx to insert on the palmar margin of the bone, flexor sheath, and volar plate, thereby lifting the metacarpal via a broad palmar attachment, rather than at a single attachment point dorsally. The extrinsic extensor tendon is the only MP joint

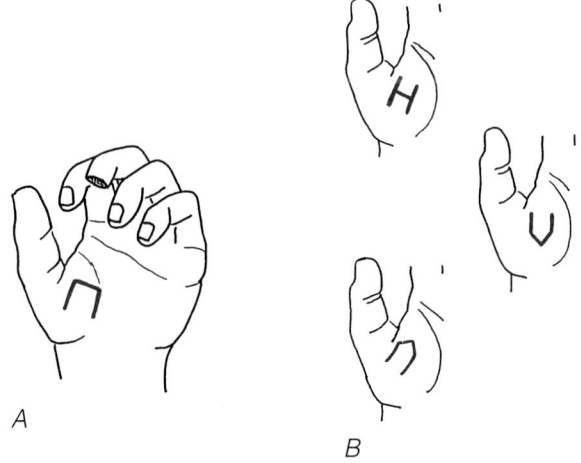

FIG. 43-55. *Thenar flap. A. Classic outline with a proximal pedicle. B. Modification by Smith (top), Dellon (middle), and Melone (bottom).*

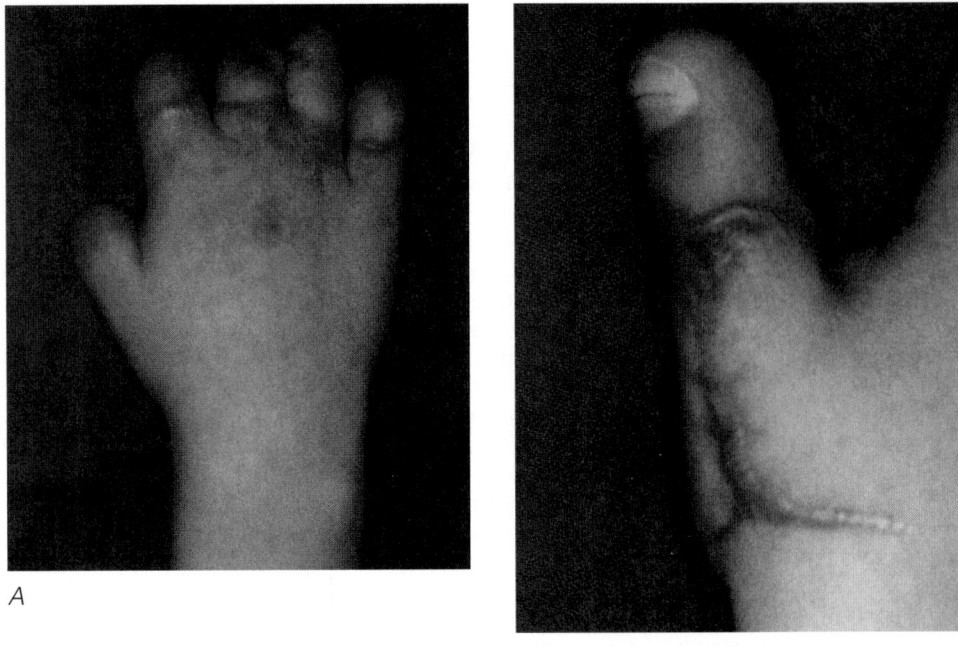

A

B

FIG. 43-56. *A.* Traumatic amputation of all fingers in a 3-year-old child. *B.* Reconstruction with a free partial transfer from the great toe.

extensor. Distally, the intrinsic and extrinsic tendons together form the dorsal tendon apparatus in the fingers (Fig. 43-63).

The intrinsic tendons arise from the four dorsal and three palmar interosseous muscles. There also are three thenar, three hypothenar, and four lumbrical muscles. The group serves as the primary independent metacarpophalangeal joint flexors and as IP joint extensors. The MP joint flexor fibers course distally from a palmar position, sending their transverse aponeurosis dorsally to insert on the lateral

edges of the extrinsic extensor tendon in the proximal third of the proximal phalanx (see Fig. 43-63). The direct distal continuation of the intrinsic tendon is the lateral band that continues to reach a position dorsal to the center of axis of PIP motion before crossing over the distal third of the proximal phalanx, thereby making it an extensor for both IP joints. At the distal metaphysis of the proximal phalanx and the base of the middle phalanx, the extrinsic and intrinsic tendons converge to become conjoined extensors. The central slip inserts into the dorsal lip of the middle phalanx as its direct extensor, but the conjoined lateral bands run along the dorsolateral edge of the PIP joint to then converge distally over the middle phalanx to become the terminal tendon that inserts into the dorsal lip of the distal phalanx, functioning as this last joint's only extensor.

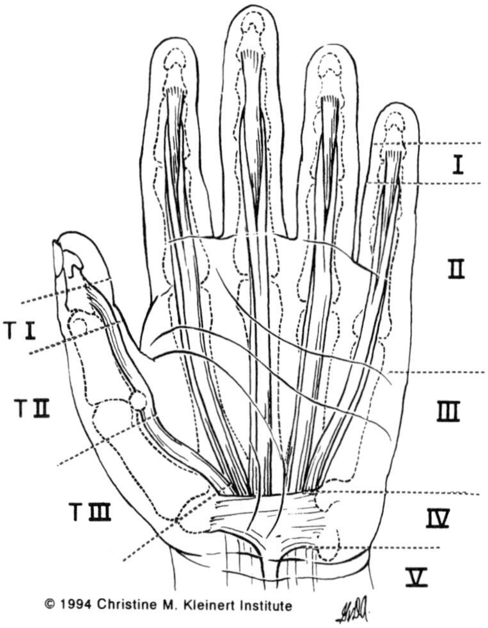

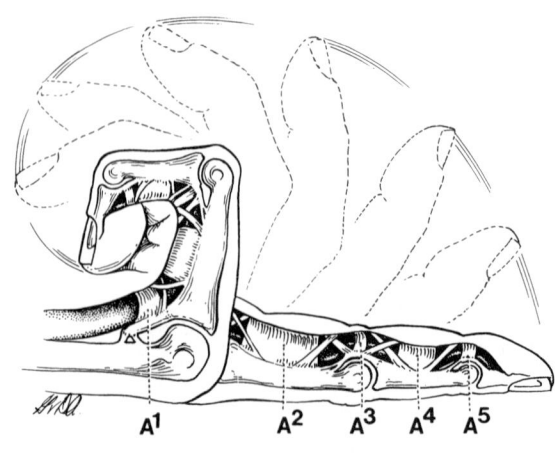

FIG. 43-57. The five flexor tendon zones in the hand and the three zones in the thumb. ©1994 Christine M. Kleinert Institute.

FIG. 43-58. The annular pulley system. ©1992 Kleinert, Kutz and Associates Hand Care Center.

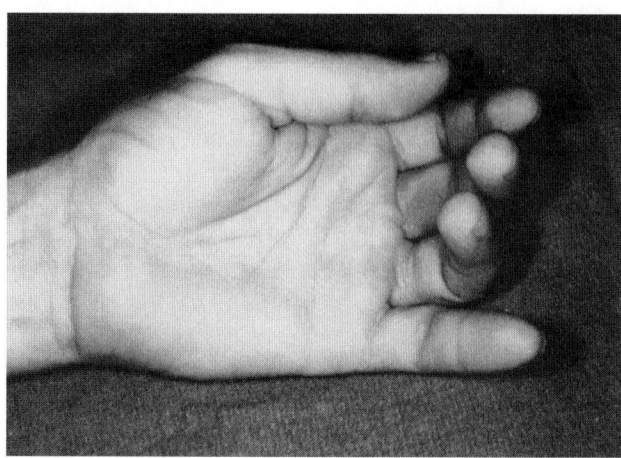

FIG. 43-59. *The normal cascade of flexion is disrupted in the injured hand.*

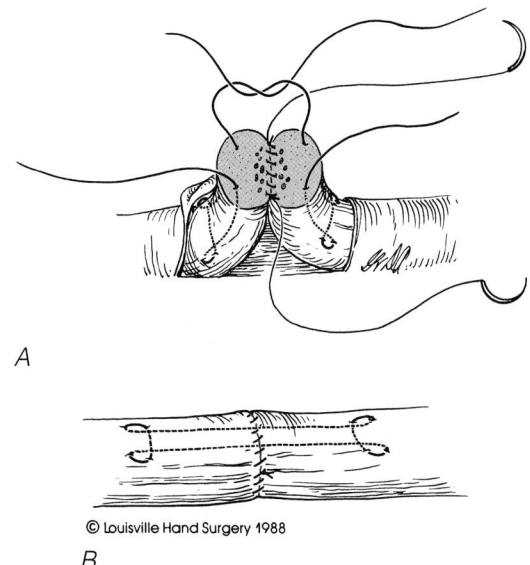

© Louisville Hand Surgery 1988

B

FIG. 43-61. *A. Débrided tendon ends are aligned and sutured. A permanent core suture is placed so as not to disturb tendon vessels in the volar aspect. B. The completed repair.* ©1988 Louisville Hand Surgery.

Because of the normal dorsolateral position of the lateral bands, in certain direct injuries to the dorsum of the finger at the PIP joint, the lateral bands may subluxate volarly, both failing to extend the PIP joint and hyperextending the terminal joint. This is called the *boutonnière deformity*. When the terminal tendon insertion at the DIP joint is avulsed or transected, the distal joint droops and the secondary proximal and dorsal retraction of the lateral bands produces gradual hyperextension at the proximal interphalangeal level. This latter deformity is known as *mallet* or *baseball finger;* it may progress to a *swan-neck deformity* when secondary PIP hyperextension is added.

The type of injury and the results of surgery vary because of the structural and functional differences in the extensor system from fingertip to forearm. Extensor tendon characteristics have been categorized by eight anatomic zones; the four zones with odd numbers overlie joints, and the four with even numbers are the tendon segments between the joints (Fig. 43-64). General recommendations for repair methods are illustrated in Fig. 43-65.

Zone 1 (Mallet Finger and Late Secondary Swan-Neck Deformity). Terminal tendon injury may occur by avulsion with

or without an attached bone fragment, and by transection from laceration or crush (Figs. 43-66 and 43-67). Closed injuries are most successfully treated by closed means; open injuries also may be well treated by extension splinting. Open or closed injuries that include fracture of the joint surface with secondary palmar subluxation of the distal phalanx require reduction and internal fixation in neutral extension to restore DIP joint congruence and proper tendon relationships, and to permit almost immediate joint plus hand rehabilitation while protecting the repaired tendon and joint, and making wound care easier. Otherwise, the terminal (DIP) joint is rarely pinned. Splints that immobilize the DIP articulation in extension (for 6 to 8 weeks) but leave the PIP joint unrestrained are usually preferred (Fig. 43-68).

Zone 2. Zone 2 is the area over the middle phalanx where the lateral bands unite to form the terminal tendon. The lateral bands are connected proximally by the thin triangular ligament. Injuries in this area usually are from laceration with resultant mallet deformity. Direct repair and terminal joint pinning for 6 to 8 weeks is appropriate for open cases; closed splinting for closed injuries without significant fracture is equally effective.

Zone 3 (Boutonnière). Zone 3 is the area over the PIP joint where the central slip and lateral bands interconnect. Injury may be closed or open and may include avulsion of the central slip, with or without a dorsal bone fragment. The latter injuries require accurate reduction of the joint, bone, and contiguous tendon mechanism. Pinning the PIP joint in extension for about 3 to 4 weeks allows early rehabilitation of the other joints. Untreated, this boutonnière deformity progresses to a fixed PIP joint flexion contracture with secondary hyperextension of the terminal joint. Closed splint or percutaneous pin management may be equally effective for the pure tendon injuries (Fig. 43-69).

Zone 4. The dorsum of the proximal phalanx is covered entirely by the confluent extrinsic extensor tendon and by the two lateral bands arising from tendons of intrinsic muscles. Because of this local anatomy, most tendon injuries in zone 4 are functionally partial and the cut tendon ends do not retract significantly. Only direct inspection can confirm this diagnosis. If interphalangeal joint

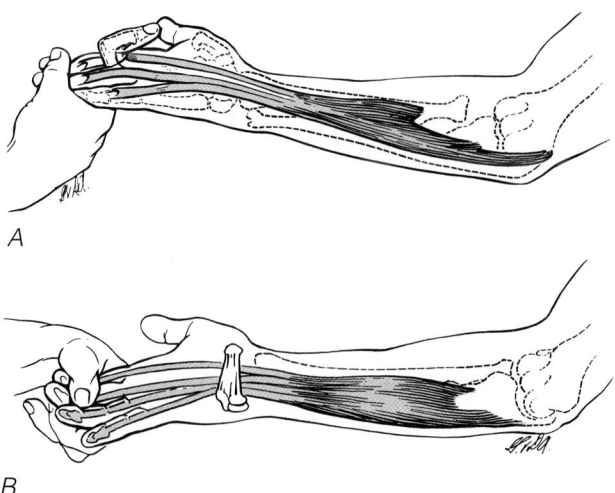

A

B

FIG. 43-60. *A. Examination of the flexor digitorum superficialis tendons. B. Examination of the flexor digitorum profundus tendons. (Modified with permission from Lister G: The hand: Diagnosis and indications, 3rd ed. London: Churchill-Livingstone, 1993.)*

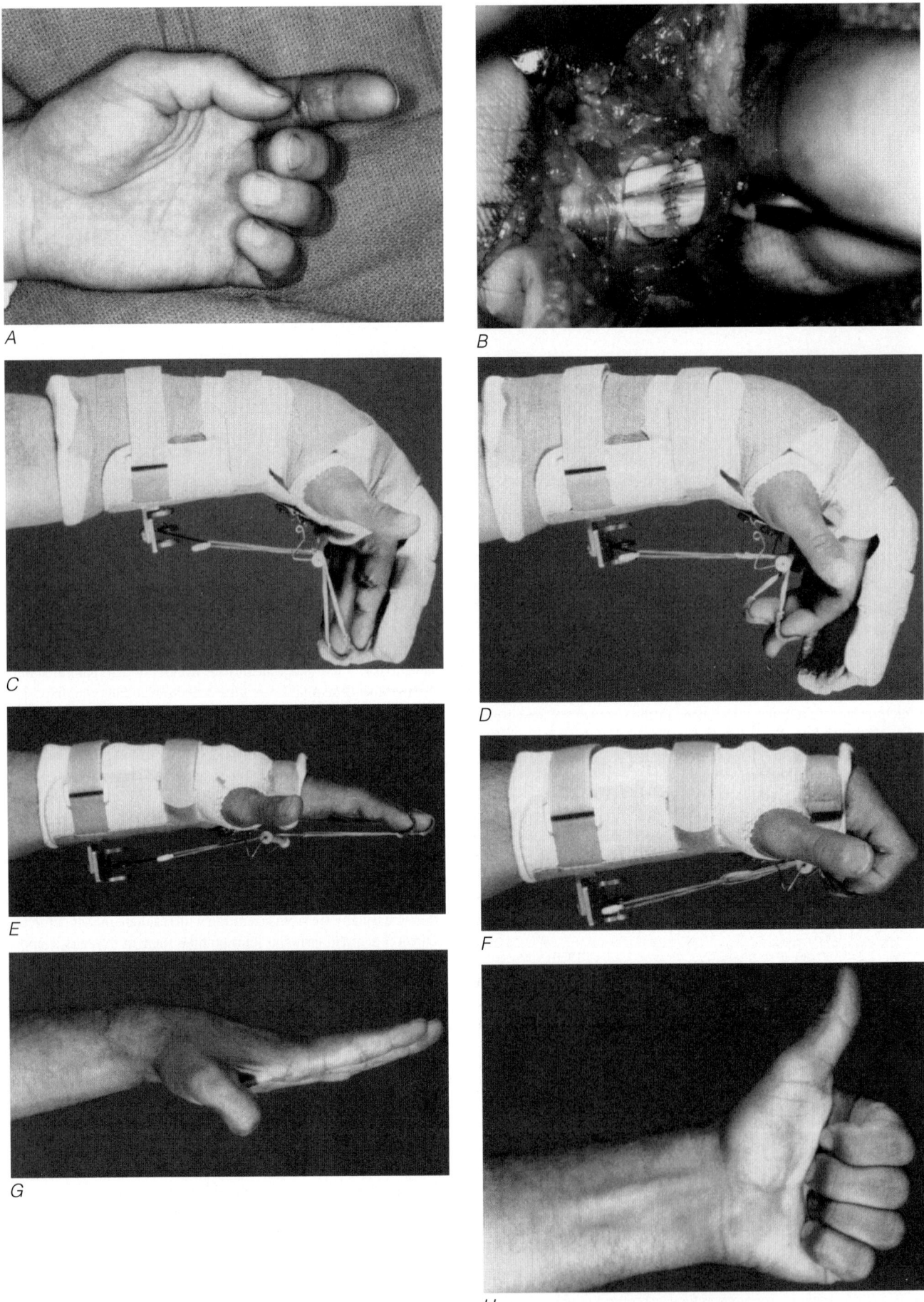

FIG. 43-62. *A.* Laceration of both flexor digitorum superficialis and flexor digitorum profundus tendons in zone II. *B.* Suture repair completed. *C* and *D.* Patient in dorsal block splint of index finger. *E* and *F.* Patient in volar flexion coil brace. *G* and *H.* Final results 6 months after repair.

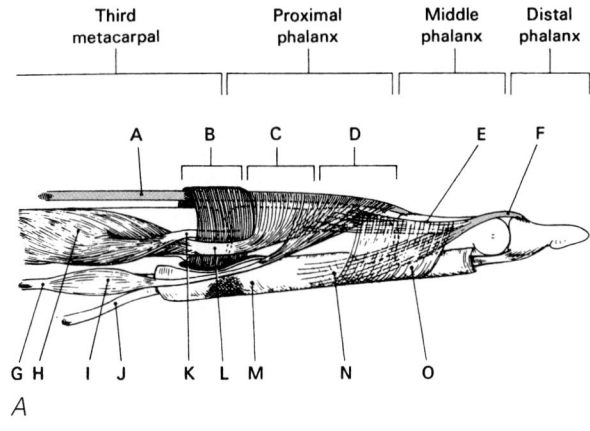

A

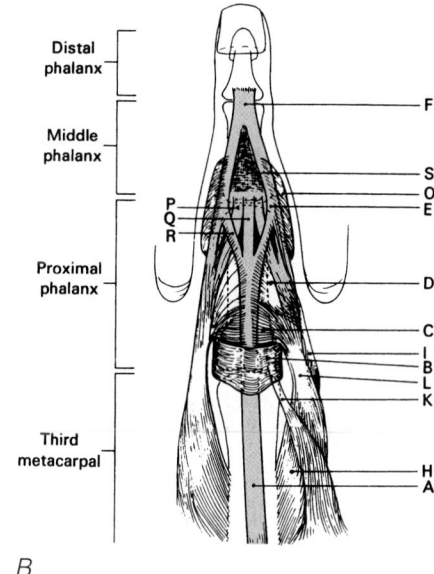

B

FIG. 43-63. Diagrammatic representation of the dorsal apparatus of the finger. *A. Lateral side, middle finger. B. Dorsum, middle finger.* A = extensor digitorum communis tendon; B = sagittal bands; C = transverse fibers of intrinsic muscle apparatus; D = oblique fibers of intrinsic apparatus; E = conjoined lateral band; F = terminal tendon; G = flexor digitorum profundus tendon; H = second dorsal interosseous muscle; I = lumbrical muscle; J = flexor digitorum superficialis tendon; K = medial tendon of superficial belly of interosseous muscle; L = lateral tendon of deep belly of interosseous muscle; M = flexor pulley mechanism; N = oblique retinacular expansion; O = transverse retinacular ligament; P = medial band of oblique fibers of intrinsic expansion; Q = central slip; R = lateral slips; S = triangular ligament. *(Adapted with permission from Smith RJ: Balance and kinetics of the fingers under normal and pathologic conditions. Clin Orthop 104:92, 1974.)*

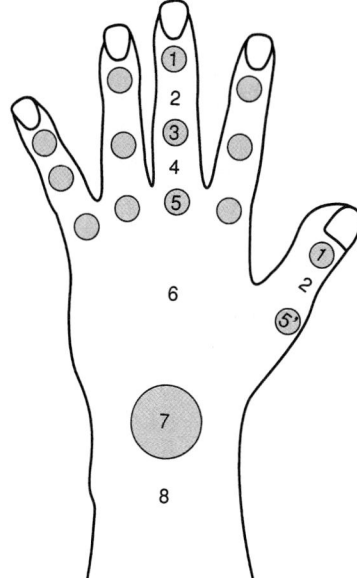

FIG. 43-64. Diagram of the surgical/topographic zones of the extensor apparatus.

extension is normal, a partial tendon injury need not be repaired. Splinting the PIP joint for 2 to 3 weeks usually is adequate when followed by protected remobilization.

Zone 5. Lacerations and bite wounds at the MP joint are common. With open injuries in this region, a human or animal bite must be suspected until proven otherwise. Bite wounds are serious, contaminated injuries requiring primary surgical débridement, irrigation of the wound and joint, and aggressive intravenous antibiotics for 24 to 48 hours. Patients may be reluctant to seek treatment early, and may deny the mechanism of injury. The incidence of complications is directly related to the delay in treatment. Radiographs are taken to rule out the presence of a foreign body such as a piece of

tooth, intra-articular fracture, or air in the joint, any of which prove contamination. When caused by a bite, the wound is débrided, irrigated, and left open and tendon repair is performed secondarily, after healing by secondary intention and recovering passive motion. The primary care is to prevent infection; tendon repair becomes a secondary matter. However, in a simple laceration, the tendon can be repaired primarily. The dorsal extrinsic extensor tendon and the sagittal band (aponeurosis) mechanism should be repaired to prevent subluxation of the extensor into the intermetacarpal valley. Closed extensor tendon dislocation is almost always to the ulnar side of the joint, and generally requires tendon and sagittal fiber reconstruction.

Where direct repair is possible, primary and delayed primary repairs are preferable, using the suture techniques described in Fig. 43-65. The wrist is immobilized in less than 30 degrees of extension, and the MP joint is splinted at 60 to 70 degrees or treated with a custom dynamic MP extension splint for early passive motion. The PIP and DIP joints may be left free, and tendon gliding at these levels is encouraged.

Zone 6. Zone 6 covers the dorsum of the hand, which includes the metacarpals and distal carpals, where there are four common extensor tendons to the fingers and two proper tendons, one to the index and one to the little finger. The three wrist extensors insert in this region: the extensor carpi radialis longus into the dorsoradial base of the second metacarpal, the extensor carpi radialis brevis into the dorsoradial base of the third metacarpal, and the extensor carpi ulnaris into the ulnodorsal edge of the fifth metacarpal. The extensor pollicis longus tendon crosses from proximal to distal in a radial to ulnar line. Single or partial finger tendon laceration may not produce metacarpophalangeal extension loss, because forces are transmitted through the tendinous interconnections extending from adjacent extensors, such as the juncturae tendinum. In most cases, however, the involved finger lies slightly more flexed or is less able to extend than the others. Paradoxically, the affected finger may flex at the MP joint and extend at the IP joint when the patient attempts active extension, because of loss of the extrinsic extensor tendon without disruption of the intrinsics. The tendons have an oval cross section and are thicker here than distally. Core sutures of the type used in flexor

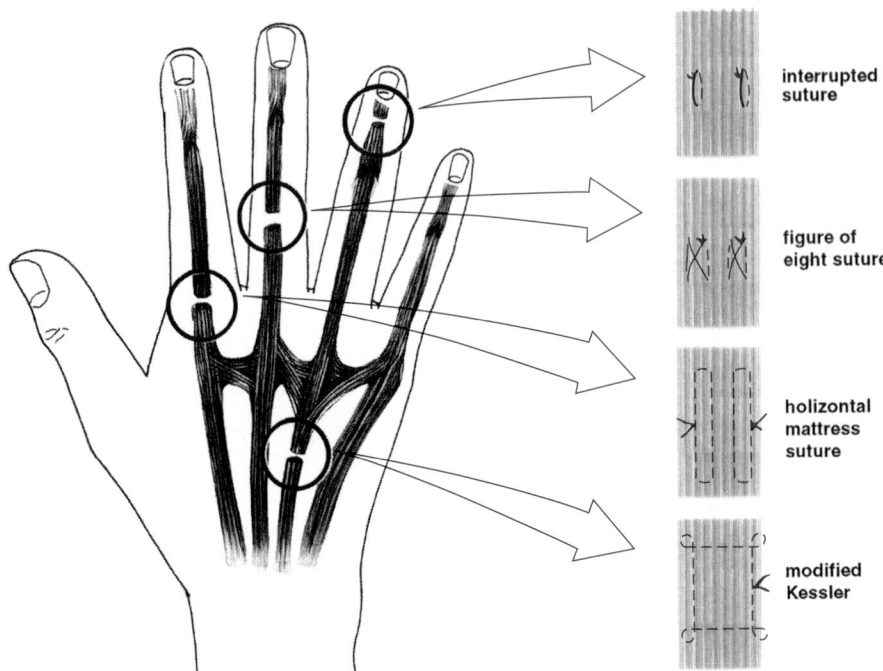

FIG. 43-65. Suture techniques for the extensor tendons. Different techniques are chosen according to the size and quality of the tendon. The interrupted suture is used in zone 1, whereas core sutures can be used in thicker tendon tissue in zone 6.

interrupted suture

figure of eight suture

holizontal mattress suture

modified Kessler

repairs are recommended (see Fig. 43-65). Conventional postrepair treatment was immobilization for about 4 to 6 weeks with the wrist in greater than 45 degrees of extension and the fingers in mild MP flexion. This is now strongly discouraged, however, because patients become significantly stiff with such a protocol. Instead, the wrist should be kept in about 30 degrees of extension and the MP joints fitted with dynamic (proximal phalangeal) extensor cuffs with the interphalangeal joints free, allowing active MP joint flexion and passive extension. Motivated patients may begin this program by 7 to 10 days postoperatively; others are immobilized for double that

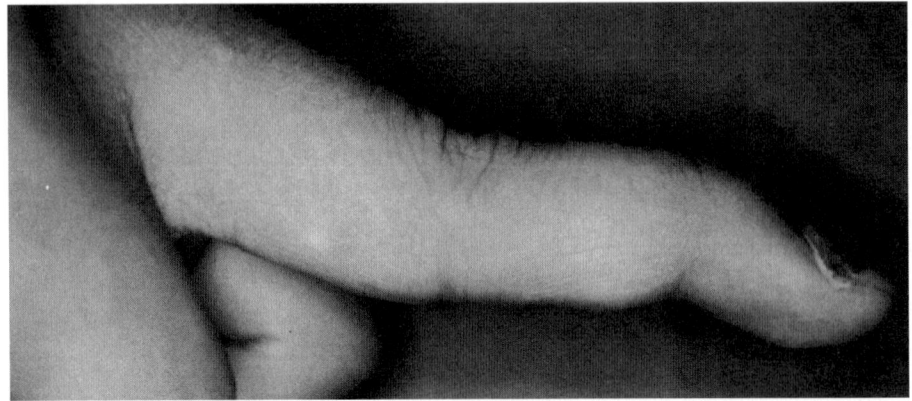

A

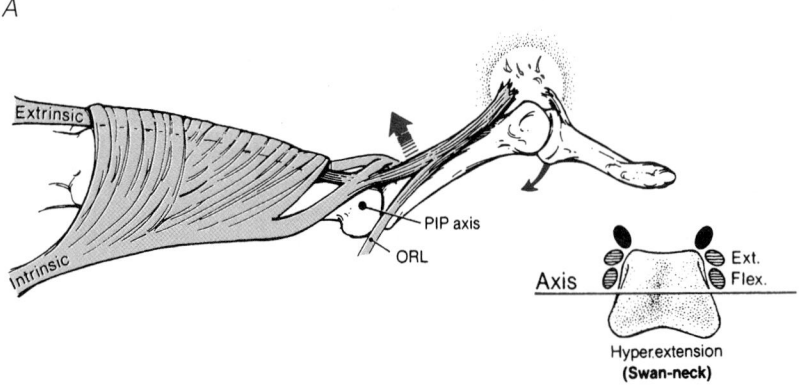

B

FIG. 43-66. *A.* Swan-neck deformity secondary to mallet finger. *B.* Appearance and mechanism. Because of the extensor apparatus lesion, the distal phalanx flexes by the effect of the flexor digitorum profundus tendon (*curved arrow*). The proximal stump of the distal conjoined extensor tendon retracts proximally, and consequently the lateral band and oblique retinacular ligament (ORL) are slack at the beginning, and later contract and displace dorsally. Because of the concentration of the extensor forces over the middle phalanx, the PIP joint is progressively set in hyperextension (*wide arrow*). *Inset:* Transaxial representation at the condyle of the proximal phalanx, showing the normal positions of the conjoined lateral bands in extension and flexion of the PIP joint. The dorsally displaced position of the conjoined lateral bands is represented in black.

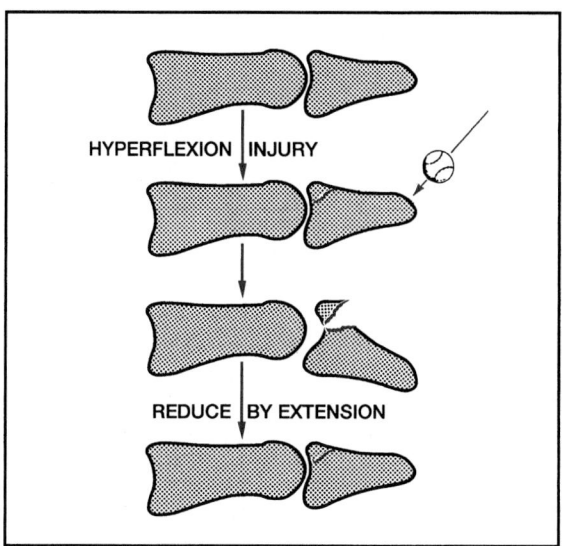

FIG. 43-67. *Mechanism of mallet finger. Hyperflexion injury. (Reproduced with permission from Lange RH, Engber WD: Orthopedics 6:1436, 1983.)*

time. At least one adjacent finger must be included in this type of custom splint. Multiple tendon injuries may necessitate including all fingers in splints throughout the rehabilitation protocol.

Zone 7. Zone 7 is the proximal wrist region under the extensor retinaculum in which the extensors traverse the fibro-osseous tunnels in six synovial compartments. Unlike for the flexor pulleys, repair of the extensor retinaculum is relatively easy to perform, but retinacular release to effect tendon repair should be avoided whenever possible. To prevent extensor tendon bowstringing, preservation or reconstruction of some portion (>40%) of the retinaculum is critical. Step-cut retinaculum release allows closure more easily without producing a space too tight for gliding of repaired tendon(s).

Tendon lacerations in this area often are associated with injuries to the nearby radial or ulnar sensory nerve branches, and this should be considered at examination and repaired at tendon surgery.

Closed rupture of extensor tendons, usually the extensor pollicis longus tendon, is not rare, especially after Colles' fracture and other injuries to the distal radius. Many extensor pollicis longus ruptures occur several weeks or months after *non*displaced Colles' fractures. It is postulated that fracture hematoma reduces the limited native blood supply in the extensor pollicis longus tendon, leading to secondary attrition rupture. Systemic connective tissue diseases such as rheumatoid arthritis, and pathologic conditions that produce a sharp bone edge, chronic tenosynovitis, or both, also may contribute to such a problem. Attrition ruptures should be reconstituted by tendon transfer or graft. Direct repair is almost never possible because of the wide zone of tendon trauma that precedes the rupture.

Zone 8. Trauma to the radial sensory or posterior interosseous nerve branches may occur concomitant with extensor injuries in the forearm in zone 8. Multiple adjacent muscles and tendons make it difficult to identify individual tendons. The priority for repair is to restore independent wrist and thumb extension, and group extension of the fingers. With lacerations at the musculotendinous junctions, the tendons may be seen distally, but proximally their fibrous septae retract into the muscle bellies. For repair at this level, the suture line must include some fascia or the intramuscular tendinous septae to prevent pullout and failure of surgery. With injuries in the proximal forearm, division of the posterior interosseous nerve alone will produce loss of extensor function by denervation, or it may occur in combination with injury to some or all of the muscles and tendons. At repair, elbow flexion and wrist extension may be needed to reduce tension at the suture line. Thumb extensor injuries are dealt with in a manner similar to injuries to the finger.

Tendon Transfers. Tendon transfer is a reconstructive procedure that antedates the twentieth century. Transfers in the upper limb are designed to restore motion in a nonfunctioning part. Tendon transfers are used in isolated peripheral nerve paralysis, and

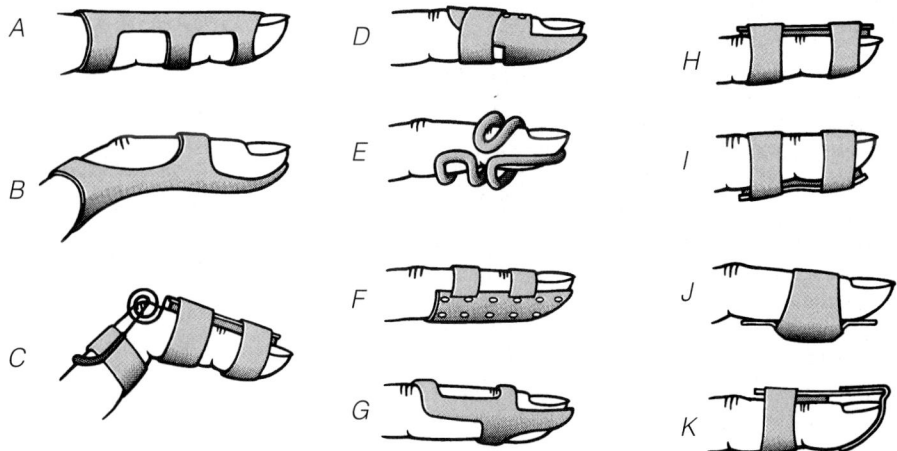

FIG. 43-68. *Various types of splints. Fixation for both the DIP and PIP joints (A–C); molded plastic or rubber-coated splints (D–G); aluminum splints (H–K). A. Metal tubed splint by Lewin. B. Frog splint from Richards. C. Combined dorsal DIP aluminum splint and coil splint for PIP flexion. The PIP joint is allowed to extend passively during 3 to 4 weeks of splinting, followed by distal component only for an additional 2 weeks. D. Stack splint. E. Rubber-coated wire splint by Abouna and Brown. F. Perforated splint by Kinninmonth, individually made from thermoplastic material to reduce skin irritation. G. Modified Stack splint, with added spaces for extra ventilation in the pulp and on the dorsal surface of the middle phalanx. H. Dorsal padded aluminum splint. I. Volar padded aluminum splint. J. Concave aluminum splint. K. Dorsal padded aluminum splint allows adjustable flexion of the DIP joint.*

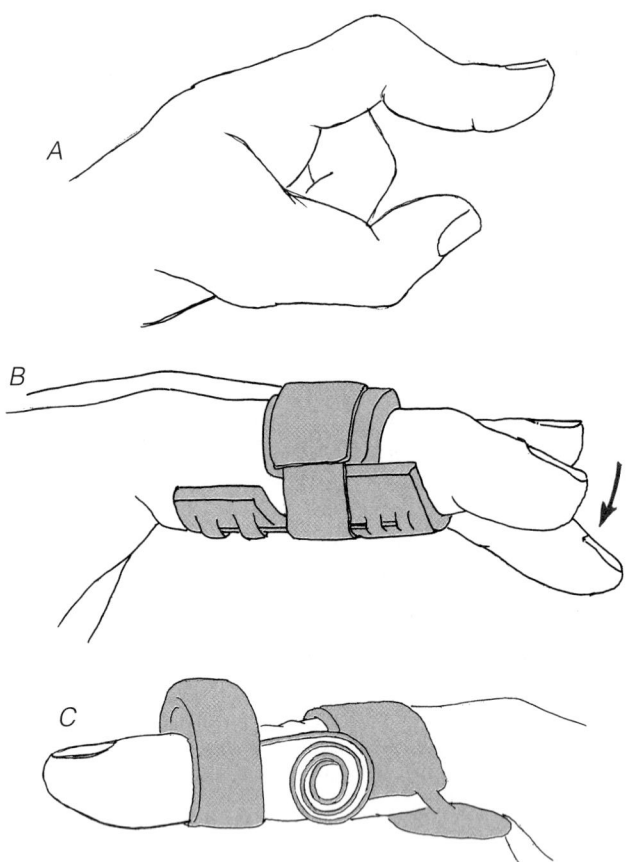

FIG. 43-69. *A.* Boutonnière injury. *B.* The Bunnell-type safety-pin splint. The splint is worn constantly, and the strap on the splint is tightened on a daily basis until full extension of the PIP joint is achieved. The terminal crossbar does not go beyond the distal joint flexion crease, and the patient is instructed to flex the distal joint actively and passively while the proximal joint is held in maximum extension. The splint is used on a continuous basis for several weeks until there is full passive extension of the DIP joint. When this occurs, the length relationships and balance between the central slip and the lateral bands have been achieved and the splint can be discontinued. *C.* Capener splint.

for irreparable tendon damage after extensive segmental loss from devastating trauma, in destructive connective tissue diseases such as rheumatoid arthritis, and to rebalance the hand or provide movement to a spastic or paralyzed limb after central nervous system injury or disease. Upper extremity reconstruction by tendon transfer requires careful patient selection and extended therapy supervision with preoperative and postoperative rehabilitation protocols. While excellent functional restoration can be achieved through transfers for problems such as unreconstructable peripheral nerve injury due to cerebral palsy, traumatic brain injury, poststroke, and with unsalvageable muscle and tendon loss, the procedures and rehabilitation are beyond the scope of this text.

Nerve Injury

The upper extremity is innervated by the brachial plexus plus sensory branches arising from the plexus and intercostal nerves (Fig. 43-70). Innervation patterns vary, with numbers of intercommunications and fiber exchanges within and between nerves. Nerves are composed of axons and associated Schwann cells enclosed in a basement membrane. Thin collagen fibers called *endoneurium* are immediately outside this basement membrane; the term *endoneurial tube* refers

to the composite of axon and Schwann cell. Endoneurial tubes are grouped together to form numbers of fascicles. Perineurium, composed of concentric layers of flattened cells and collagen fibers, surrounds each fascicle. The perineurium creates a (diffusion) barrier against the surrounding environment, providing the peripheral nerve the equivalent of the blood-brain barrier (Fig. 43-71). Surrounding the layers of perineurium is the epineurium. The epineurium that fills the space between fascicles is called *internal* and that surrounding the nerve itself is termed *external* or *outer*. The outer nerve layer is composed of collagen and some elastin fibers. The exact fascicular organization and internal anatomy of the nerve is not constant over its length. The topographic fascicular organization of the nerve rearranges as branches come off of these fascicles. The fascicles that have fibers branching off move to the perimeter of the nerve as the nerve courses toward the periphery. The internal organization of the nerve reflects the location and position of those branches.

For normal nerve function to be maintained, the peripheral nerve must glide with joint motion. Focused tension or compression induces local injury, nerve dysfunction, and symptoms. Compression and traction neuropathies result when a nerve is tethered, especially at or near a joint. The ulnar nerve, for example, has a longitudinal excursion of 10 mm or greater proximal to the elbow; the median and ulnar nerves glide nearly 15 mm at the wrist. After injury, the nerve is at risk for local scar formation, with secondary traction neuritis from tension focused at the site of adherence.

Classification of nerve injuries, as described by Seddon, is as follows:

Neurapraxia describes paralysis/dysfunction in the absence of nerve degeneration. This dysfunction may often be of some duration, though recovery always is achieved in a shorter time than would be required after internal degeneration, complete transection, and regeneration. Recovery, by definition, is invariably complete.

Axonotmesis includes damage to the nerve fibers of a severity that causes complete nerve fiber degeneration. The epineurium and other supporting structures of the nerve are not disrupted, so the internal architecture is relatively well preserved. Spontaneous recovery is the rule, and generally it is of good to excellent quality because the regenerating fascicles are guided into their paths via the intact sheaths. Recovery takes longer than for neurapraxia; internally, portions of a particular nerve may be more or less severely compromised.

Neurotmesis is when all nerve structures have been divided. Laceration produces neurotmesis, but physical gaps in the nerve may occur even though an epineurial sheath appears in continuity, such as after traction or crush. At the site of damage the unrepaired nerve will be completely replaced by fibrous tissue, and there is complete loss of anatomic continuity.

Recovery after nerve injury depends on successful reinnervation of sensory or motor end-organs. After denervation, muscles begin to lose their bulk; a loss of cross-sectional area without any loss in muscle fiber count begins within 1 week of denervation. Connective tissue surrounding the muscle undergoes degeneration and thickening. Interstitial fibrosis predominates over time, but passive exercises may delay or prevent this phenomenon. For function to be recovered, motor end plates must be reinnervated within 18 months. Sensory end-organs may be usefully reinnervated long after initial injury, but the quality of recovery also diminishes significantly with the passage of time.

The results after repair depend not just on the quality of the microneurorrhaphy, but on numerous factors such as injury level and mechanism; associated bone and soft-tissue loss; residual function;

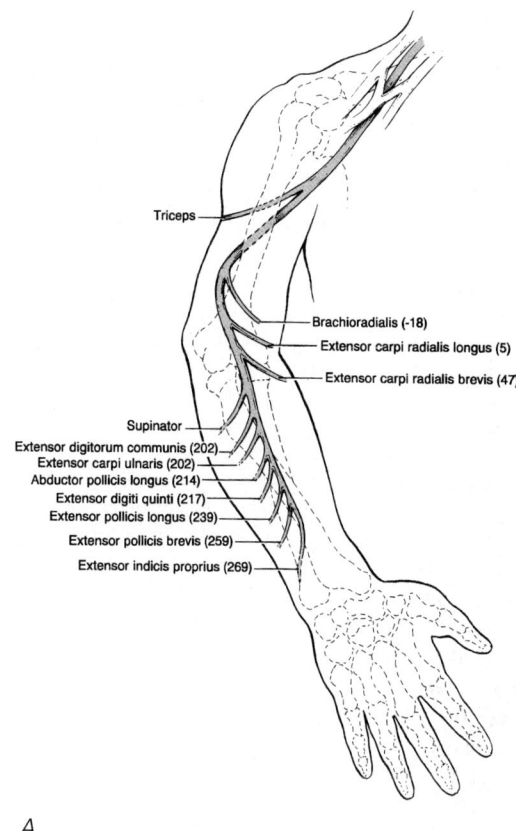

Triceps

Brachioradialis (-18)
Extensor carpi radialis longus (5)
Extensor carpi radialis brevis (47)

Supinator
Extensor digitorum communis (202)
Extensor carpi ulnaris (202)
Abductor pollicis longus (214)
Extensor digiti quinti (217)
Extensor pollicis longus (239)
Extensor pollicis brevis (259)
Extensor indicis proprius (269)

A

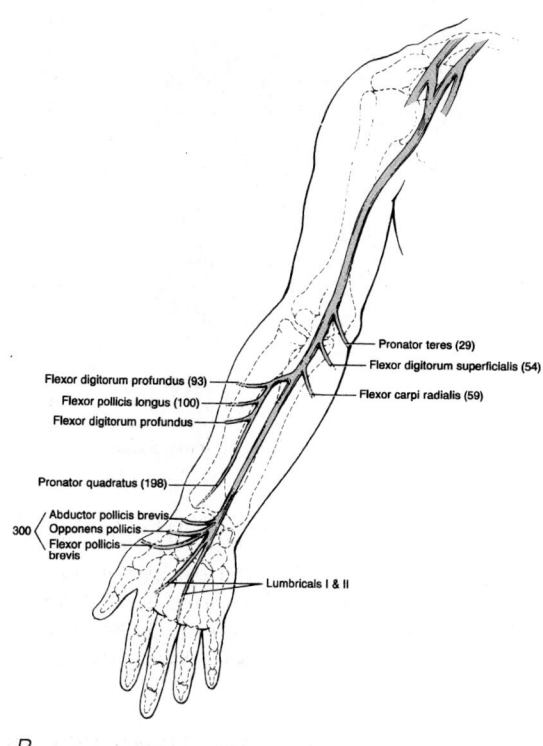

Pronator teres (29)
Flexor digitorum superficialis (54)
Flexor carpi radialis (59)

Flexor digitorum profundus (93)
Flexor pollicis longus (100)
Flexor digitorum profundus

Pronator quadratus (198)

Abductor pollicis brevis
Opponens pollicis
Flexor pollicis brevis
300

Lumbricals I & II

B

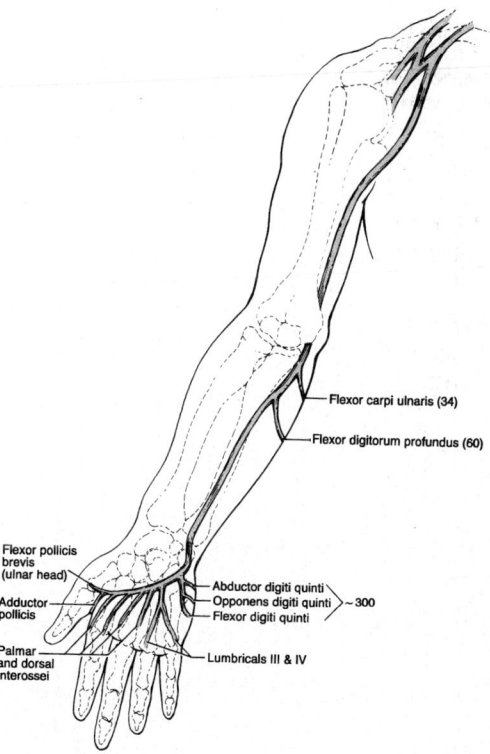

Flexor carpi ulnaris (34)

Flexor digitorum profundus (60)

Flexor pollicis brevis (ulnar head)

Abductor digiti quinti
Opponens digiti quinti
Flexor digiti quinti
~ 300

Adductor pollicis

Palmar and dorsal interossei

Lumbricals III & IV

C

FIG. 43-70. Motor innervation of the arm. *A.* Radial nerve. *B.* Median nerve. *C.* Ulnar nerve. Numbers in parentheses indicate shortest average distances from medial epicondyle to muscle, in millimeters, as determined by Sunderland.

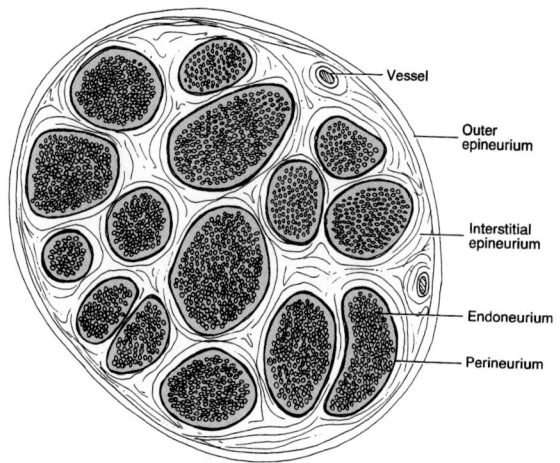

FIG. 43-71. Nerve cross section. Axons are surrounded by endoneurium and bundled into discrete fascicles. Note the internal epineurium between fascicles supporting longitudinal running vessels.

patient age, health, compliance and motivation; timing of repair; and supervised rehabilitation. Quantitative postoperative assessment of motor and sensory function should be documented serially in order to accurately assess progress or its absence.

Repairs should be done with microsuture and magnification to achieve a spatially correct, tension-free suture line. Nerve grafts are employed when direct repair after segmental loss or chronic fibrosis would require tension at the repair site. Joint posturing into extreme flexion or extension to decrease tension at a nerve repair site should be avoided; nerve graft is substituted for such destructive splinting maneuvers. Primary or delayed primary repair should be done whenever conditions allow. The combination of group fascicular and epineurial nonreactive microsutures with careful identification of the internal topography produces the best result. Repairs are protected by mildly relaxed joint posturing for about 3 weeks, and the results of repair are improved by beginning sensory and motor reeducation after reinnervation is documented (Figs. 43-72 and 43-73).

Vascular Trauma and Replantation

The majority of upper extremity replantation surgery is based on microsurgical techniques due to the size of the involved vessels. Loupes (2.5 to 4.5×) are useful for wide-field dissections and are particularly helpful in preparing the ends of nerves and larger vessels (e.g., radial artery at the wrist) for repair. However, the operating microscope offers a steady field magnification range of 25× or more. Miniaturized needle holders, instruments, and bipolar coagulation are necessary for proper microvessel handling. The typical repair for vessels of 0.5 to 3.0 mm diameter is performed with nonreactive

FIG. 43-72. Algorithm for the evaluation of nerve injuries.

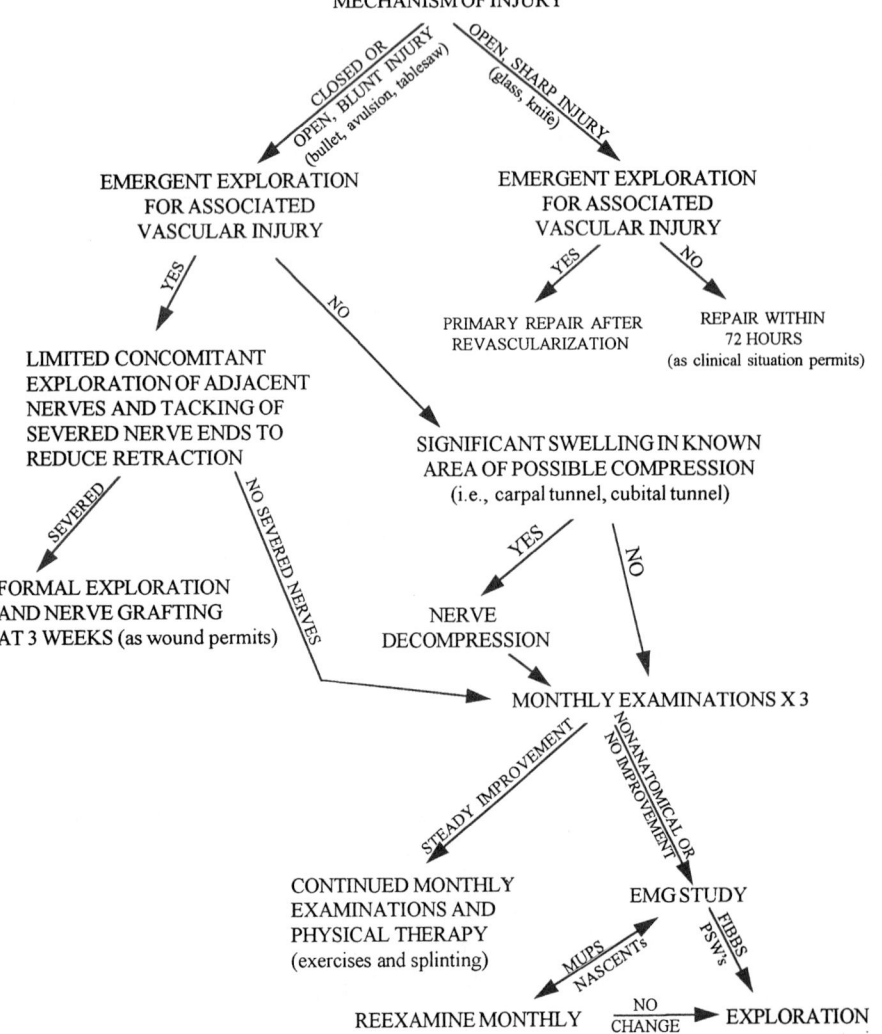

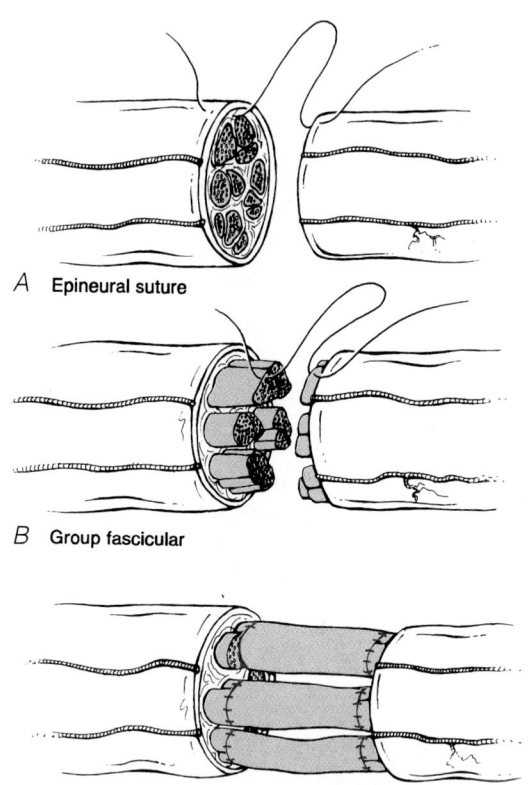

A Epineural suture

B Group fascicular

C Nerve grafting

FIG. 43-73. Techniques of nerve repair. *A.* Direct epineurial suture using surface vessels for alignment. *B.* Group fascicular repair. *C.* Nerve grafting using multiple strands of donor nerve to bridge defect.

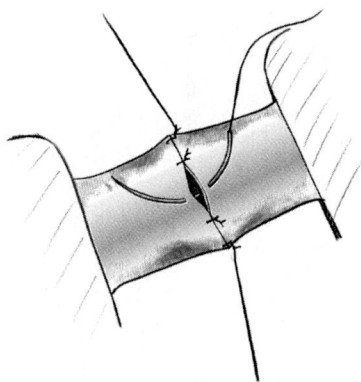

FIG. 43-75. Placement of central suture in anterior wall.

monofilament interrupted sutures to prevent luminal impingement and collapse, although microvessel grafts and end-to-side connections also are used when appropriate (Figs. 43-74 and 43-75). A contaminated soft tissue and bony injury can be treated by primary débridement and fracture stabilization, repair of extensor and flexor tendons and muscles, and repair of nerves and vessels (Fig. 43-76).

Each patient should be considered individually on the basis of the location and extent of the injury, health, age, and condition. Relevant questions include: (1) Can function be obtained from the replanted part? (2) Will such function exceed what can be achieved through amputation closure and prosthetic fitting? (3) Will long-term function be improved or compromised by replantation? and (4) Does the potential benefit to the patient outweigh the surgical risks, costs, and loss of productivity?

Segmental, extensive, or multiple-level injuries require repair and reconstruction over an extended area. Neither complete nor near-complete part amputations make any patient an automatic candidate for revascularization or reattachment. Single finger amputation in the adult, especially at a level proximal to the PIP joint (including division of both superficialis and profundus tendons and digital nerves), is not appropriate for replantation in the vast majority of cases. Consideration should be given to replantation for thumb amputations at and proximal to the IP joint, for single-finger amputations in children, and for partial hand and more proximal wrist, forearm, or arm amputations. In adults aged 40 years or older, repair of the ulnar nerve proximal to the elbow rarely produces a functional result. Crush and avulsion injuries often make it impossible to achieve successful reattachment and revascularization, let alone functional recovery. Reperfusion before tissues are nonviable is essential; amputated parts are kept moistened in saline and on a bed of ice (see below for tissue handling details). Muscle is the most oxygen-sensitive upper extremity tissue, and must be revascularized within 6 hours of amputation for flow to be reestablished.

Handling of Amputated Parts

The amputated part should be scrub-prepped, then irrigated and cleansed under saline solution, wrapped in a saline-moistened gauze, and placed in a plastic bag. The plastic bag containing the part is then be placed on (not packed in) a bed of ice in a suitable container. The part should never be immersed in nonphysiologic solutions such as antiseptics or alcohols. The amputated part is never put in dry ice, it is not perfused, and it must not be allowed to freeze.

Preparing the Patient

The patient is stabilized, and a compression dressing is applied to the stump before transport to the replantation center. Intravenous access lines should be started, fluids and antibiotics given, and blood samples drawn while awaiting transportation. If time permits, x-rays of the stump and also of the amputated part are obtained.

Most replantation centers request that the patient be given intravenous antibiotics, an aspirin suppository (325 mg), and 25 to 50 mL/h intravenous supplementation of low molecular weight

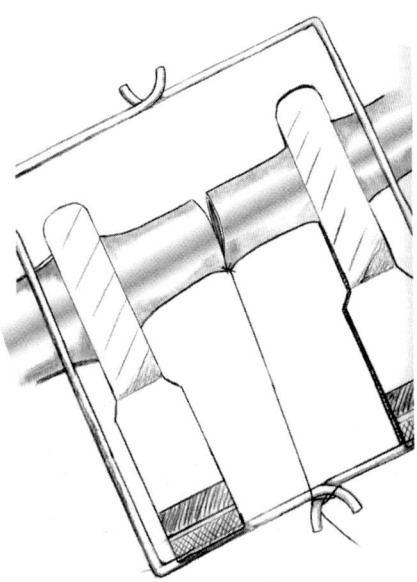

FIG. 43-74. Vessel with first stay suture in place and pulled to proper tension.

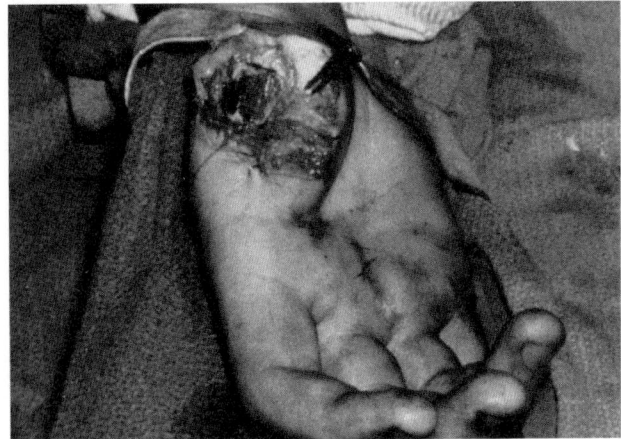

A

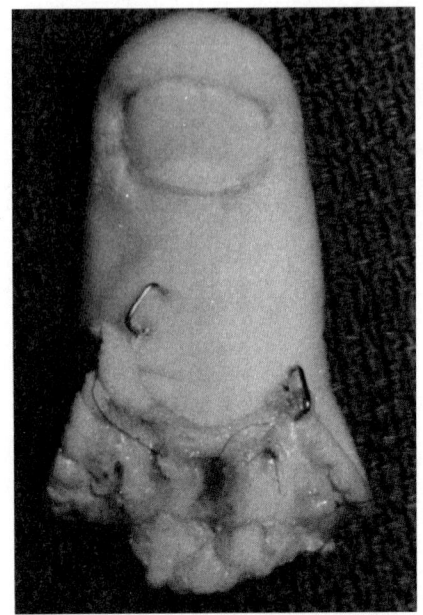

B

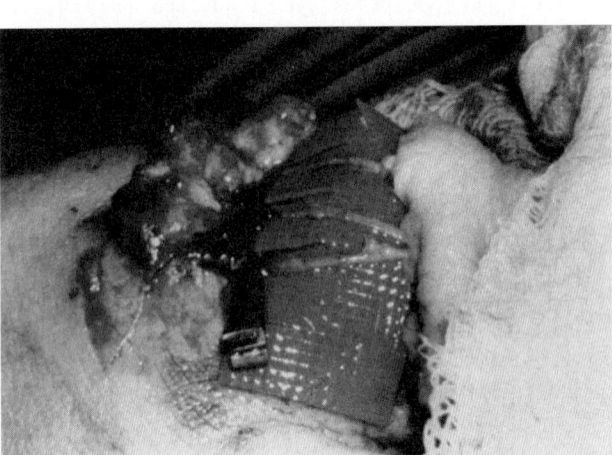

C

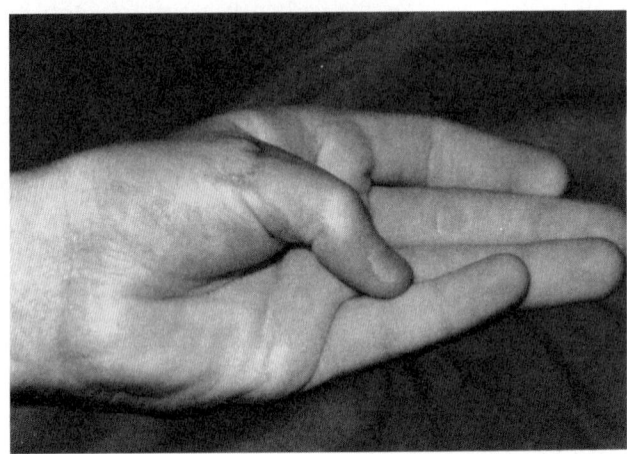

D

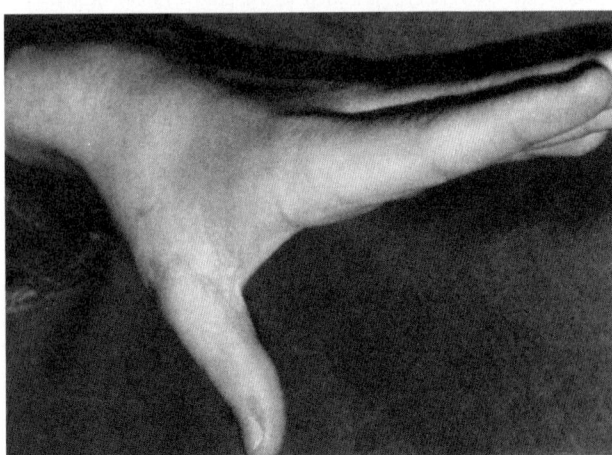

E

FIG. 43-76. *A.* Amputation of thumb at proximal phalangeal level. *B* and *C.* Identification and tagging of dorsal veins and subsequent anastomosis. *D* and *E.* Palmar abduction and opposition 18 months after replantation.

dextran in dextrose; the two latter are administered for platelet antiaggregation effects.

Before the patient is transported to the replantation center, someone responsible at the receiving institution must knowingly accept the patient as a candidate for part reattachment in order to mobilize the replant team. Even with an active replant team, its members may be occupied with another case. Accurate communication by telephone, physician-to-physician, is an essential part of prereplantation triage. Even if the referring physician is unsure of the patient's status, preparations can still be made for possible transport. When the patient is transported, the patient should be told that referral is for evaluation for *possible* replantation.

Amputations

The value of traditional methods to manage amputations is worth clear emphasis. Digital amputation affects precision pinch and

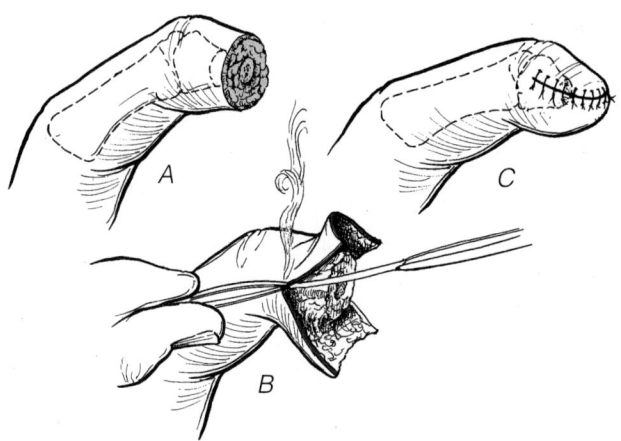

FIG. 43-77. *Schematic of the technique of digital amputation.*

power grip, the latter significantly if the hand is painful. Treatment principles for fingertip amputations were discussed previously. It is important that stable soft-tissue and skin coverage over an amputation stump at any level be obtained (Fig. 43-77). If a residual stump is stiff or painful, amputation or amputation revision through the metacarpal (ray resection) can be an important functional enhancement. Where a central ray is excised, second-ray transfer or third to fifth intermetacarpal ligament imbrications restore metacarpal alignment, eliminate interdigital gaps, and reestablish the functional contour of the hand (Figs. 43-78 and 43-79).

High-Pressure Injection Injuries

These injuries are due to improper or accidental misuse of paint and grease guns, hydraulic lines, and diesel injectors, that propel material under pressures of up to 7000 pounds per square inch. Penetration through skin and along extended tissue planes is the rule rather than the exception. These injuries almost always involve the hands. The severity of injury is related to the nature of the injected material. Paint and solvents that are cytotoxic produce intense inflammation, in addition to the significant direct trauma from the high-pressure injury. This prolonged inflammatory phase is sometimes mistaken for infection. Such injuries require immediate mechanical and pulse-lavage débridement in order to prevent extended tissue loss (Figs. 43-80 and 43-81).

Complications of Trauma

Compartment Syndrome and Secondary Volkmann's Contracture

In acute compartment syndrome, fluid pressure in the tissues contained within a fascial space or subcompartment increases to a level that reduces or prevents capillary blood flow necessary for tissue viability. When untreated, continued pressure elevation produces irreversible muscle necrosis and nerve damage from ischemia with secondary fibrosis, contractures, and sensibility deficits or chronic pain. Acute compartment syndrome results from an increase in the volume of fluid within a compartment. Posttraumatic edema or hemorrhage, hematoma, swelling from infection, or burns increase compartment fluid, as does the revascularization of a partially or totally amputated part. Other causes include venous obstruction and transiently strenuous exercise. Constrictive dressings and casts, excessively tight surgical closure, and prolonged direct limb pressure during unconsciousness from alcohol and drug stupor, or during extended surgical procedures, also add fluid to the limited capacity of the anatomic compartment.

Acute compartment syndrome is suspected clinically, but can be confirmed by measurement of intracompartmental tissue pressure. Clinical findings include a swollen, tense, and tender compartment, with pain out of proportion to that expected from the originating injury, peripheral sensory deficits, and finally, motor weakness or paralysis. Pain is exacerbated by passive stretch of the affected muscle or group (i.e., passive finger extension or flexion). Peripheral pulses usually remain intact despite tissue-lethal intracompartmental pressure, because systolic arterial pressure usually is well in excess of the dangerously elevated intracompartmental pressure. While blood flow through the major arteries is not impeded, capillary perfusion is compromised by pressure elevated to greater than 30 to 40 mm Hg within the compartment. Pressure measurement devices are confirmatory but not infallible, and in treatment decisions, clinical findings should be considered, and may outweigh specific pressure measurements. Pressure measurements of greater than 30 mm Hg are consistent with compartment syndrome; however, because tissue perfusion is affected by systemic blood pressure, a lower threshold pressure for fasciotomy should be used in hypotensive patients, and a higher one for hypertensive individuals. While MRI scans or ultrasonography may delineate areas of muscle edema or necrosis, these studies do not have a role in the diagnosis of acute

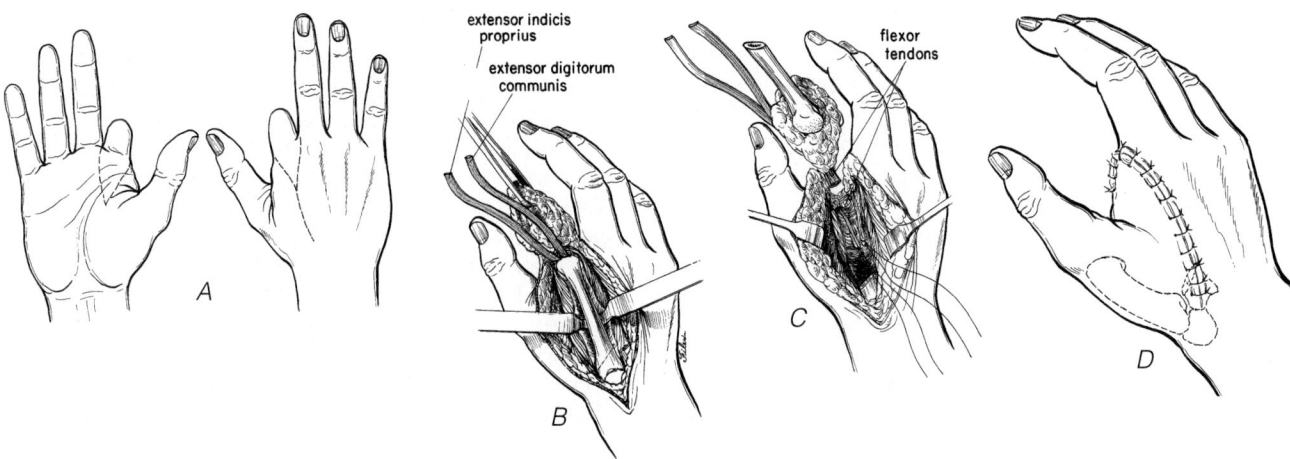

FIG. 43-78. *Schematic of the technique of index ray deletion.*

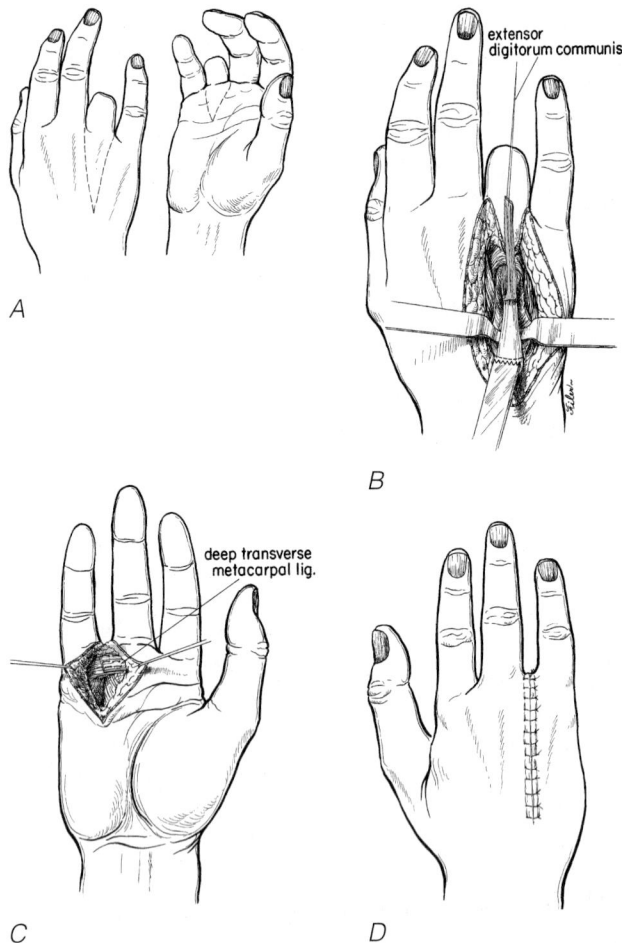

A

B extensor digitorum communis

C deep transverse metacarpal lig.

D

FIG. 43-79. *Schematic of the technique of central ray deletion with simple web space closure.*

compartment syndrome. Treatment should *not* be delayed to obtain imaging beyond the initial radiographs.

Treatment includes removal of all occlusive dressing layers, wraps, and splints, and splitting and removing casts and cutting cast padding down to the skin. If symptoms and pressure findings are not rapidly relieved, fasciotomy of the affected compartments is required (Figs. 43-82 and 43-83). After surgical decompression, the wounds are left open, but dressed to prevent desiccation. Skin closure by direct means or with skin grafts is delayed for at least 96 hours, but may be performed after 5 to 10 days as swelling permits. Hand therapy is started with the patient in postsurgical dressings, even before formal wound closure, to regain passive joint and tendon gliding.

Neuromas

Neuromas represent a normal physiologic response after nerve injury. All badly injured and severed nerves form neuromas, but only those neuromas that are relatively exposed, superficial, and likely to be impacted become symptomatic. Only sensory fibers develop painful neuromas (Figs. 43-84, 43-85, 43-86, and 43-87). Medical and surgical management of symptomatic neuromas may be difficult, but prevention is more useful and important. Inadvertent injuries to nerves can be avoided during surgical resection, but amputation end-nerve divisions are at risk for symptomatic neuroma formation. Divided nerve stumps should be doubly ligated, trans-

posed to deep locations (preferably between or within muscle), or sutured into bone tunnels when padded tissue is scant. In the fingers, where there is often limited soft-tissue padding, the practice of dividing the nerve under traction and allowing it to retract proximally is not as certain a method of prevention as leaving the nerve end long, and willfully transposing it to a more proximal or dorsal site, where it is less likely to be struck and more likely to be protected.

A symptomatic neuroma is a therapeutic challenge. More than a hundred methods of surgical treatment have been described, but no method is universally successful. The symptomatic neuroma should be identified, isolated, and dissected intact. The scar bulb is kept in continuity with the nerve. The symptomatic nerve and its continuous neuroma are transposed to a deeper, more padded, and often more proximal location, beneath muscle if possible, but within bone when needed. The neuroma bulb is not excised from the nerve because its excision just stimulates the normal process of germination of another neuroma, the contents of which may not be contained with this secondary procedure.

Complex Regional Pain Disorder and Reflex Sympathetic Dystrophy

The first clinical description of abnormally exaggerated and prolonged pain after injury is attributed to the American Civil War surgeon S. W. Mitchell, who initially coined the term *causalgia* from the Greek, meaning burning pain. Other synonyms include inflammatory bone atrophy and Sudeck's atrophy. Complex regional pain disorder (CRPD) and reflex sympathetic dystrophy (RSD) emphasize the importance of the sympathetic nervous system in posttraumatic pain pathophysiology. Suspicion, diagnosis, and early therapeutic interventions are the most important factors in optimizing outcome. CRPD/RSD is not a disease. It is a complex interaction of physiologic responses initiated by trauma and exacerbated by posttraumatic events. The process is often staged by time and inflammatory phase with relatively characteristic changes (Table 43-2), and by descriptive terminology (Table 43-3). The presumptive diagnosis is based on pain, which is often diffuse, burning, and hyperpathic, including *allodynia* (pain to light touch), *hyperalgesia* (painful response to nonpainful stimuli), *dysesthesia* (pins and needles following minor stimulus), and *hyperesthesia* (increased sensitivity or pain with nonpainful stimuli). In addition, the clinical diagnosis of CRPD also requires at least three of the following: (1) diminished hand function, (2) joint stiffness, (3) atrophic changes (edema, atrophy, or fibrosis), and (4) vasomotor instability or vasomotor disturbance.

Acutely, CRPD/RSD is a diffusely hot, swollen, painful, or dysesthetic extremity out of proportion to the clinical situation. A specific precipitating injury, such as a neuroma-in-continuity or an entrapped peripheral nerve, may not become apparent until the acute manifestations are treated and resolve. In the case of nerve entrapment, careful consideration should be given to prompt surgical decompression. Prolonged discomfort or pain-limited motion does *not* automatically mean that CRPD is present. Patients may have secondary soft-tissue and periarticular fibrosis after trauma or surgery and a focally tender scar, but with pain isolated only to that one area, not generalized in the entire limb. Disuse from any cause can result in osteopenia on x-ray.

Patients with CRPD/RSD often require chronic treatment, psychologic support, including counseling and medication, and an extended, intensive, and closely monitored therapy program (Table 43-4). Early recognition and treatment prevents secondary stiffness from joint and tendon adhesions.

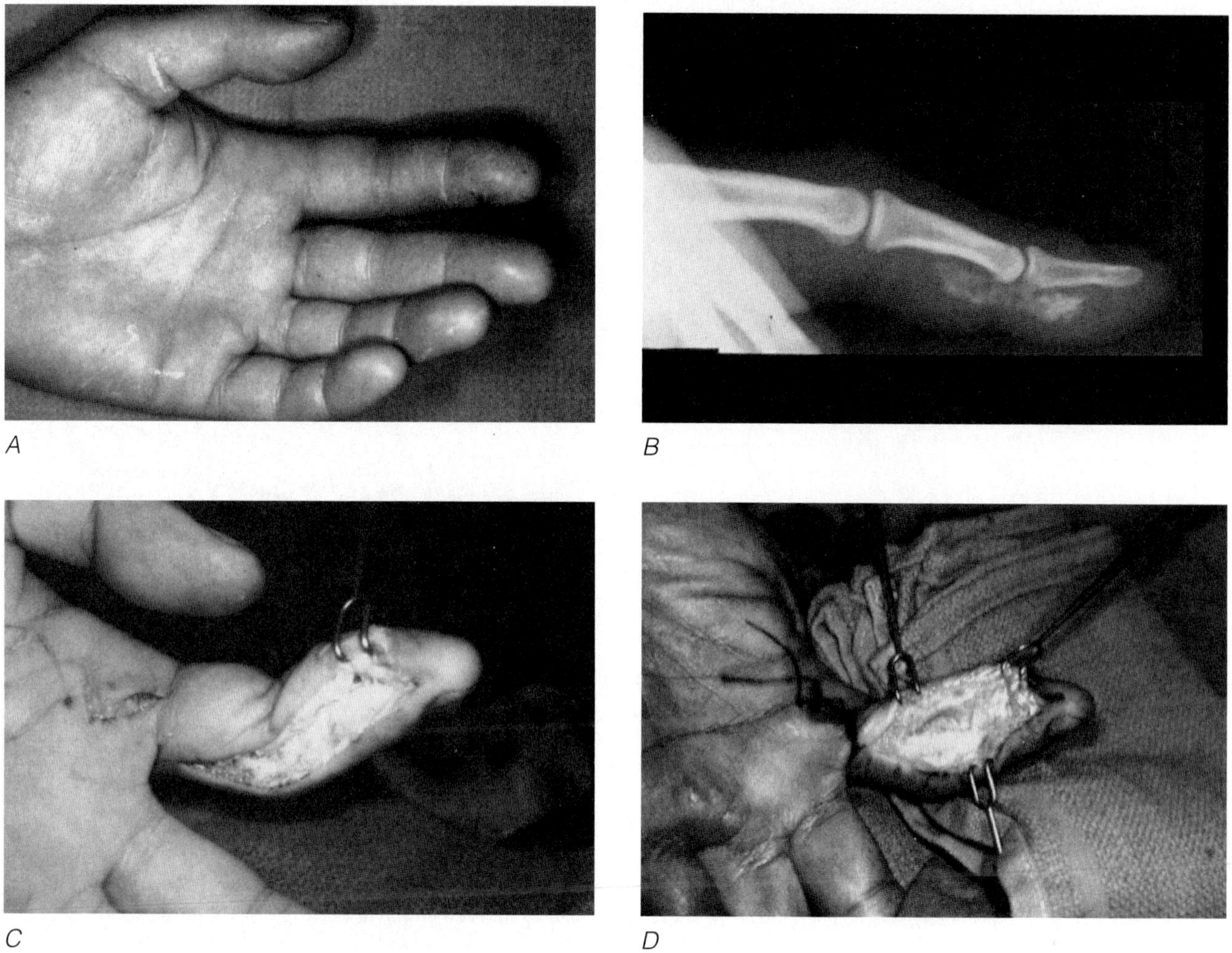

A

B

C

D

FIG. 43-80. *A.* This 23-year-old auto-body worker presented with increasing index finger pain and swelling 4 hours after an injury sustained at work, when the paint gun he was cleaning accidentally discharged into the ulnar pulp of his index finger. *B.* X-ray shows the paint in the flexor sheath and volar soft tissues. *C* and *D.* Sharp débridement and pulse irrigation were performed through an ulnar midaxial incision. Paint products were removed from around the flexor tendon, sheath, and throughout the digital subcutaneous tissues. Meticulous care was required to save the neurovascular bundles during débridement.

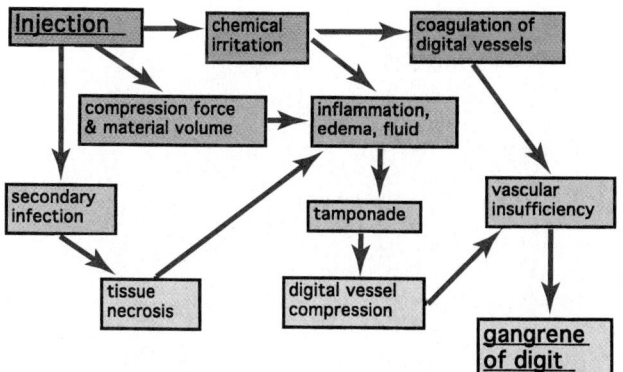

FIG. 43-81. Pathophysiology of high-pressure injection injuries. Multiple mechanisms contribute to tissue damage and gangrene.

As the final stage of CRPD is almost invariably quiescent, the core question is whether the patient will be left stiff and dysfunctional because of the other therapies brought to bear during the active phases of the disorder.

BURNS

Approximately 2 million people in the United States annually sustain burns that require medical attention, resulting in almost 500,000 emergency department visits. Isolated hand burns can result in severe functional and aesthetic impairment. The direct effect of thermal injury on the skin and the consequences of this trauma for hand function include: (1) edema, (2) decreased circulation, and (3) infection. Systemic problems include burn shock, the requirement for fluid resuscitation, secondary immunologic deficits, proteolysis and renal impairment, and the accumulation of secondary toxins.

Management of the burned hand depends on the depth of the burn, its surface area and surface location, patient age and reliability, and coexisting systemic conditions. Treatment must be

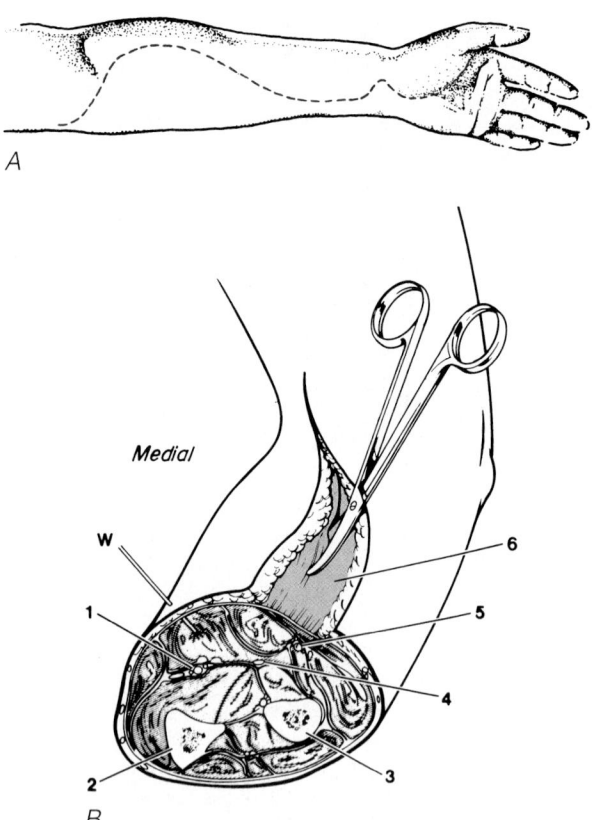

FIG. 43-82. *A.* Incision used for flexor compartment release and median nerve decompression. Incision is extended distally for carpal tunnel release. *B.* Cross section of left forearm with wick catheter placed and fasciotomy incision illustrated. 1 = ulnar nerve; 2 = ulna; 3 = radius; 4 = median nerve; 5 = radial artery; 6 = forearm fascia; W = wick catheter. (*Reproduced with permission from Gelberman RH, Garfin SR, Hergenroeder PT, et al: Compartment syndromes of the forearm: Diagnosis and treatment. Clin Orthop Rel Res 161:252, 1981.*)

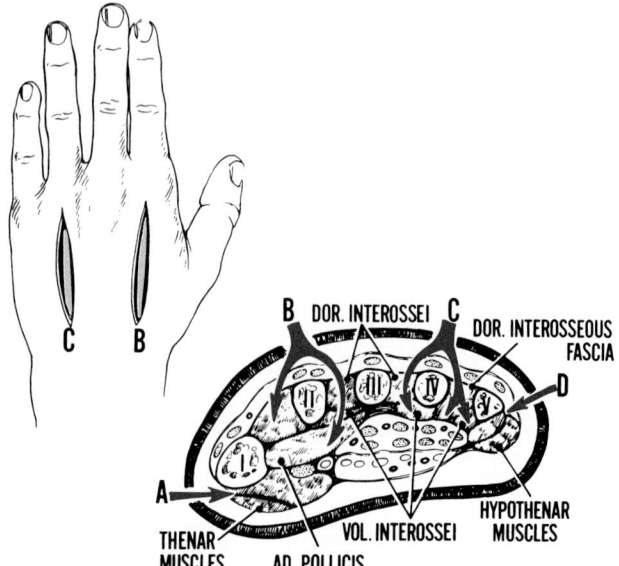

FIG. 43-83. Incisions for intrinsic muscle decompression. Incision *A* allows decompression of the thenar muscles; incision *D* allows decompression of the hypothenar muscles. The two dorsal incisions, *B* and *C*, are placed over the index and ring metacarpal, respectively, each allowing decompression of the adjacent interosseous muscle compartments. The adductor compartment (containing the adductor pollicis muscle) may be decompressed through incision *B*. [*Reproduced with permission from Rowland SA: Fasciotomy: The treatment of compartment syndrome, in Green DP, Hotchkiss RN (eds): Operative Hand Surgery, 3rd ed. New York: Churchill-Livingstone, 1993, p 661.*]

individualized. Patients who are reliable and have an adequate support system may be appropriately treated outside of the hospital. Patients with burns that prevent self-care and individuals who have no personal assistance require a more controlled setting.

Primary treatment should focus on preserving viability of soft tissues by preventing secondary wound dehydration via application of a moist or biologic dressing. Blisters can be aspirated to preserve overlying epithelium as a biologic dressing, but if they are leaking then they require débridement, and the wound should be covered with an occlusive and nondesiccating composite dressing.

Circulation maintenance requires prevention of hypovolemia and avoidance of mechanical obstruction to circulation due to an enveloping eschar. Along with clinical examination, the use of Doppler ultrasonography or a wick catheter measurement of compartment pressure is helpful in assessing vascular sufficiency.

Escharotomy and/or fasciotomy in a burned extremity may be required acutely to prevent secondary ischemic necrosis. Midlateral incisions are generally used, whether in the forearm or the fingers. The incision must be deep enough to divide all eschar down to normal tissues. If a single midaxis release does not restore circulation to the periphery, the other midaxis must be incised. The neurovascular bundles themselves should be identified and protected to prevent iatrogenic injury or desiccation. The edematous hand may also develop an acute nerve tunnel syndrome.

Infection is prevented by prophylactic systemic antibiotics in the first 2 days to avoid selection of resistant organisms, but the mainstay of antimicrobial prophylaxis is topical. The most frequently used antimicrobial is silver sulfadiazine, which does not penetrate eschar, is not painful, has broad-spectrum coverage, prevents desiccation, and can be removed with water, saline, or hydrotherapy cleansing. Temporary, reversible bone marrow suppression and neutropenia may result from extensive extended use of silver sulfadiazine. In burn

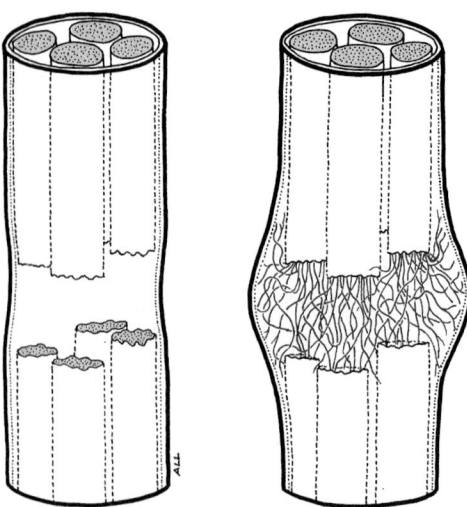

FIG. 43-84. Pseudoneuroma-in-continuity formed after a traction injury. These are seen after traction injuries in which the perineurium remains intact. The axoplasmic flow will accumulate proximal to the point of axonal disruption, forming a fusiform neuroma confined inside the perineurial sheath.

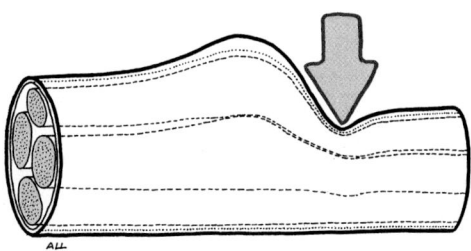

FIG. 43-85. Pseudoneuroma-in-continuity secondary to severe and chronic nerve compression. The axoplasm accumulates just proximal to the area of compression, mainly in the fascicles closest to the external deforming structure.

wound sepsis, full-thickness biopsy cultures allow diagnosis of sepsis and adjustment of appropriate antibiotics. Surgical débridement of infected burns is necessary, but with widespread burn wound sepsis there is significant mortality.

Functional restoration is the most important goal. Most hand burns are on the dorsum because of its exposed position. Deep burns to the palm are relatively rare except with electrical, chemical, and occasionally direct contact thermal burns. Bilateral palmar burns or glove-like burns in children should be considered as evidence of possible child abuse, reported, and carefully investigated.

Nonoperative treatment allowing prompt spontaneous healing and early excision with grafting yield the best functional results in appropriately selected patients. Prolonged inflammation diminishes the chances of recovering hand function. If initial assessment suggests that the burned hand requires more than 2 weeks before skin healing is complete, early tangential excision and skin grafting should be done. If spontaneous epithelialization and wound closure are anticipated within 2 weeks, nonoperative treatment with continuous home and supervised outpatient exercises and splinting is appropriate.

Splinting in an anti-deformity position should be given high priority. Splinting may be done in positions other than the traditional "position of function" (i.e., the combination of wrist extension, MP flexion, and IP extension). In dorsal hand burns, the splinting position is wrist extension of less than 30 degrees, with maximum MP flexion and full IP extension (Fig. 43-88). To preserve the first web,

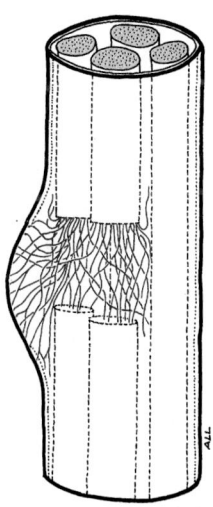

FIG. 43-86. Lateral neuroma. When a peripheral nerve is partially severed, the regenerating axons that fail to regenerate the distal segment will escape through the epineurial gap, forming a lateral neuroma.

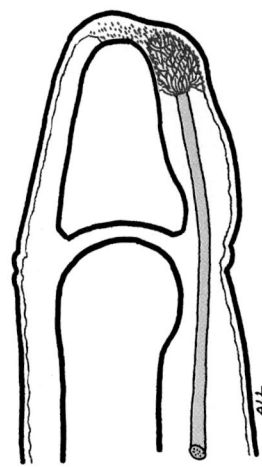

FIG. 43-87. Terminal neuroma following an amputation (amputation neuroma). The neuroma is quite superficial and gloved by the fibrous tissue formed during the healing of the amputation wound.

the thumb also is widely abducted palmarly and flexed slightly at the carpometacarpal joint to a position where the radial border of the hand is flat (i.e., the first metacarpal is positioned almost directly palmar to the second metacarpal). The goal of splinting is to stretch the healing wound and prevent anatomic distortion by scar tissue that prevents restoration of hand function. Neglected dorsal burns develop MP hyperextension and IP flexion deformities, thumb adduction, and wrist contractures (Fig. 43-89). Hand rehabilitation requires a coordinated approach between the surgeon and the therapist to assure maximal and timely recovery. At first, hand therapy is focused on minimizing edema and preventing deformity. The exercise program starts between the first and fifth posttrauma day, to encourage gliding of flexor and extensor tendons and movement of small joints. Therapy eventually progresses to activities of daily living and reintegration into a normal life.

Referral of patients requiring postburn reconstruction is made to a specialized center where skin coverage and therapy techniques are available for hypertrophic scars and contiguous tendon and joint injuries.

INFECTIONS

Bacterial Infection

Skin infections most commonly derive from direct bacterial inoculation. Secondary spread from contiguous sites and hematogenous seeding are less likely, but do sometimes occur. The most common infecting organisms are *Staphylococcus* and *Streptococcus* species, but gram-negatives, anaerobics, and mixed infections are seen, depending on the inoculation method (e.g., due to a bite). Serious, deep infections require hospital admission and extended use of high-dose intravenous antibiotics. Wound and blood cultures are obtained before antibiotic therapy is started, and adjustments are made as indicated.

Paronychial infections are common acute problems that involve the nail and nail bed, and constitute about 15% of hand infections. Occurrence is associated with hangnails, nail biting, finger sucking, and occupations in which the hands are frequently exposed to water. Acute infection is always bacterial, creating a localized abscess, but chronic inflammation is most often of mixed bacterial, yeast, or

Table 43-2
Staging of Reflex Sympathetic Dystrophy

	Stage I *Acute*	*Stage II* *Dystrophic*	*Stage III* *Atrophic*
Time frame	0–3 months	3–6 months	6–>12 months
Symptoms	Allodynia	Constant pain	Constant pain
	Hypersensitive	Cold intolerance	Cold intolerance
Signs	Swelling (edema)	Tissue indurated	Thin, atrophic skin
	Redness	Joint stiffness	Dry skin
	↑ Sweating	Dry skin	Cool
Microvascular	↑ Total flow	↓ Total flow	↓ Total flow
Assessment	↓ Nutritional flow	↓ Nutritional flow	↓ Nutritional flow
X-ray findings	Mild to moderate osteopenia	Moderate to severe osteopenia	Severe osteopenia

fungal etiology, and requires an entirely different therapeutic approach (Fig. 43-90).

Herpetic whitlow is an infection of the soft tissues of the distal phalanx or paronychial area by the herpes simplex virus. It is characterized by intense pain and cutaneous vesicles or blisters. The vesicle fluid is clear at first, but may become cloudy over a few days. It is most important to distinguish this from bacterial infection. Surgical interventions may spread the herpes virus systemically or dispose to local secondary bacterial infection. Only bacterial abscess needs surgical drainage. Herpetic whitlow is self-limited, generally resolving within 3 to 4 weeks.

Felon is an expanding abscess within the finger pulp, and represents up to one-quarter of hand infections. Felons can be extremely painful, as the expanding abscess produces a localized compartment syndrome within the fibrous septae that normally anchor the pulp and subcutaneous tissues to the distal phalanx. Felons usually are caused by penetrating direct trauma producing bacterial inoculation. Untreated felons, like other compartment syndromes, compromise local circulation and produce secondary tissue ischemia and necrosis (osteomyelitis and septic DIP arthritis), in addition to septic destruction. In surgical drainage, additional injury to the finger pulp

Table 43-3
Definitions of Reflex Sympathetic Dystrophy (RSD)

From the International Association for the Study of Pain, Taxonomy, Adelaide Consensus Statement 1990

- RSD is a descriptive term for a complex disorder or group of disorders that may develop as a consequence of trauma affecting the limbs, with or without obvious nerve lesions.
- RSD consists of pain and related sensory abnormalities, abnormal blood flow and sweating, abnormalities of the motor system, and changes in structure of both the superficial and the deep tissues (trophic changes).
- It is agreed that the term RSD is used in a descriptive sense and not to imply a specific underlying mechanism; not all components will exist at once.

From the Ad Hoc Committee to the American Association for Hand Surgery

- RSD is a pain syndrome in which the pain is accompanied by loss of function and evidence of autonomic dysfunction.
- Neither pain without autonomic dysfunction nor autonomic dysfunction without pain is sufficient to define the syndrome.
- A more appropriate name for this syndrome may be *sympathetically maintained pain syndrome*.
- Diagnostic criteria include diffuse pain, loss of function, and sympathetic dysfunction.

should be avoided, but an abscess may already point to a superficial location (Fig. 43-91).

Deep-space palmar infections occur more often in the immunocompromised, and in drug abusers, the elderly, diabetics, and in neglected populations. These are extremely serious infections with secondary systemic symptoms requiring a combination of extended medical plus staged surgical therapy (Fig. 43-92).

Tenosynovitis

Acute pyogenic digital tenosynovitis is most frequently a result of direct penetrating trauma. Kanavel's cardinal signs of flexor tenosynovitis include: (1) fusiform digital swelling, (2) semiflexed digital posture, (3) significant pain from passive extension, and (4) tenderness along the entire flexor sheath. Proper management for this closed-space tenosynovial abscess is almost always surgical drainage and intravenous antibiotics. A high index of clinical suspicion is required for diagnosis. Aspiration of the sheath will confirm the diagnosis. In early cases, systemic antibiotics alone may be considered, but there must be profound resolution within 12 to 24 hours; otherwise prompt operative drainage is necessary (Fig. 43-93).

Septic Arthritis and Osteomyelitis

Septic arthritis and osteomyelitis result from neglected soft-tissue infection, and may occur in the undertreated or chronically unhealthy population. These problems require extended surgical and medical therapies, and often multiple staged salvage or reconstructive procedures.

Nonbacterial Infection

Nonbacterial infections include tuberculous, mycotic, and similar diseases. Granuloma, a collection of macrophages and histiocytes characteristic of the systemic response to these agents, is diagnostic. A high index of suspicion and a careful history are necessary for accurate diagnosis. Such patients present with relatively painless, chronic, indolent soft-tissue problems. The patient may recall a causative traumatic event. The correct diagnosis often is appreciated only after months or years. For example, the history of a penetrating fishhook injury many weeks or months before appearance of a nodular or boggy tenosynovitis in a fisherman could suggest an atypical mycobacterial infection to the suspicious clinician. Tissue biopsy and cultures confirm the diagnosis of the specific granulomatous disease. The distinction between superficial and deep tissue involvement is important in tubercular and fungal infections, because superficial infections are usually treated medically, and deep infections generally require surgical débridement. Mycobacterial infection, including tubercular infection and infection by the atypical mycobacteria once thought to be saprophytes, occurs primarily in the

Table 43-4
Oral and Topical Medications for Reflex Sympathetic Dystrophy (RSD)

Drug	Usual Dosage	Mechanism	Major Short-term Disadvantage or Side Effects	Contraindications
Amitriptyline	25 mg tid or 50 mg qhs	Inhibits amine pump (decreases norepinephrine uptake)	Drowsiness; antimuscarinic side effects; orthostatic hypotension	With guanethidine sulfate or bretylium
Phenytoin	100 mg tid	Decreases resting membrane potential; inhibits amine pump; stabilizes synaptic membrane	Minimal drowsiness; monitor serum levels	Long-term use
Phenoxybenzamine hydrochloride	40–120 mg	Alpha-receptor blocking agent	Orthostatic hypotension	With late-stage RSD
Nifedipine	10 mg tid; may be increased slowly to 30 mg tid (30 and 60 mg sustained-release form for qd administration available)	Calcium-channel blocking agent; diminishes arteriovenous shunting; increases nutritional flow	Headache; constipation	Concurrent use of beta-adrenergic blocking agents
Corticosteroids	20–80 mg qd prednisone equivalents × 5–40 days	Stabilizes membrane; increases nutritional flow	Adrenal suppression; avascular necrosis; pain (related to dose decreases)	
Carbamazepine	400–1200 mg in 2 to 3 divided doses	Blocks neural discharges; sodium-channel blocker	Neurological; bone marrow suppression; hepatoxicity; ataxia	History of bone marrow suppression; hypersensitivity suppression; hypersensitivity to tricyclic compounds; concurrent monoamine oxidase inhibitors
Clonidine	0.2–0.3 mg patch	Affects adrenergic transmission with marked selectivity for presynaptic sites of vasomotor fibers; alpha$_2$ = adrenergic agonist	Skin irritation; rash surrounding patch; passive absorption of drug varies	Renal disease; heart block; beta blockers

SOURCE: Reproduced with permission from Koman LA, Ruch DS, Smith BP, et al: Reflex sympathetic dystrophy after wrist surgery, in Levin LS (ed): *Problems in Plastic and Reconstructive Surgery.* Philadelphia: Lippincott, 1992, p 300.

soft tissues, with secondary bone and joint involvement. The pathologic atypical mycobacteria include *Mycobacterium marinum, M. kansasii, M. avium-intracellulare, M. fortuitum,* and *M. chelonae.* Outside of the United States, the organism most frequently producing deformity and destruction of upper extremity function is *Mycobacterium leprae,* or Hansen's bacillus. Hansen's disease (formerly leprosy) should be considered in patients from other nations.

CHRONIC SYNDROMES

Tendinitis

deQuervain's Tenosynovitis

Inflammation of the tendons in the first dorsal compartment, the abductor pollicis longus and extensor pollicis brevis, became associated with deQuervain after his 1895 report of five cases. This tendon inflammation is one of the most common causes of pain along

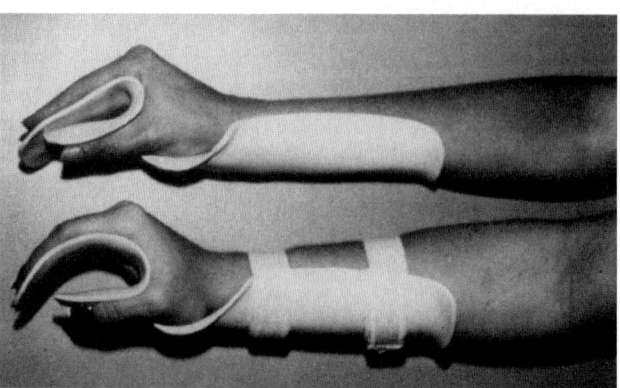

FIG. 43-88. The upper arm demonstrates the antideformity position as advocated by Salisburg. The lower arm shows the traditional functional position of the hand.

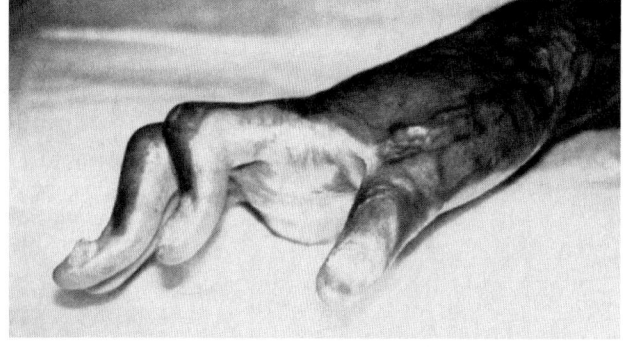

FIG. 43-89. Poor hand splinting resulted in this aesthetically and functionally defective hand.

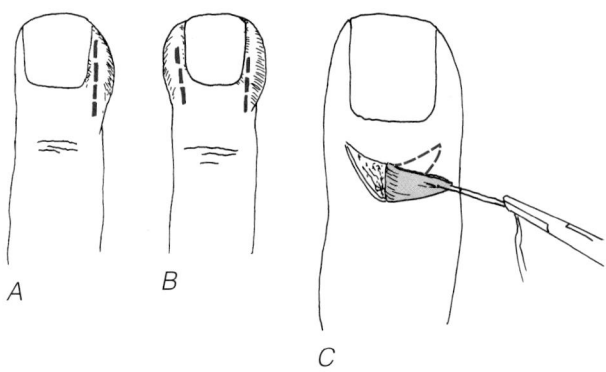

FIG. 43-90. *Drainage of a paronychial infection involves opening the involved lateral sulcus with a probe or scalpel blade. Occasionally the incision must be extended proximally (A) or involve both sulci (B). C. A crescent-shaped incision is used to marsupialize chronic paronychia.*

the radial side of the wrist and the proximal dorsoradial thumb. The problem is more common in women, notably in new mothers, due to the frequent positioning of the wrist in flexion and the thumb in extension while carrying or manipulating their infant. As both tendons pass across the radial styloid process within their tendon sheath, they are subjected to angulation and shear forces.

Patients present with tenderness over the midaxis of the radial styloid process. Active thumb and wrist motion, particularly active thumb extension, and passive thumb flexion with wrist ulnar deviation, are extremely painful. In Finkelstein's test, designed to reproduce symptoms by passive traction on these tendons, the patient grasps the palmarly flexed thumb under the fingers of the same hand, and actively deviates the wrist ulnarly. The test is positive when symptoms are reproduced by this maneuver. There may be palpable or audible crepitus over the tendon sheath, occasional locking, or a secondary ganglion or mass. There also may be secondary irritation of the overlying superficial branches of the radial nerve, with paresthesias along the thumb and first web space (Fig. 43-94). The tendon inflammation causes restriction of activities and motion.

The initial treatment for deQuervain's tenosynovitis includes rest and custom splint support of the wrist and thumb. Oral nonsteroidal anti-inflammatory agents may be comforting and sometimes helpful, but injection with a combined steroid and local anesthetic is the best nonsurgical therapy. The injection should *not* be made into subcutaneous tissues because it produces fat atrophy or depigmentation that is worse in darker-skinned individuals. Once acute symptoms resolve, splinting may be continued for symptom-inducing activities, such as when mothers handle their infants. As with other types of tendon inflammation, injection should relieve symptoms adequately

and for a minimum of 4 to 6 months, at which time it may be repeated.

When symptoms are persistent, surgery is carried out through a transverse 2-cm incision centered over the thickened radial styloid process. All deeper dissection is done by gentle longitudinal spreading. The branches of the radial sensory nerve are retracted gently and the thickened sheath incised longitudinally. Multiple tendon slips are always evident when the abductor pollicis longus is exposed, as this tendon is multistranded. The extensor pollicis brevis tendon is in a subcompartment in up to 90% of cases, and this subcompartment must be released completely. Some surgeons excise a portion of the sheath; others (including this author) close it deep to the tendons with one or two absorbable nonreactive sutures. Postoperatively, the thumb and wrist are immobilized for a week before active motion therapy is begun and splinting is tapered. Resistive exercises and normal use begin when they can be tolerated.

Other Wrist Tendinitis

Flexor and extensor sheath tendinitis may occur in any of the dorsal and volar groups, including the second through sixth extensor compartments, the flexor carpi radialis tendon tunnel, and at the flexor carpi ulnaris/pisiform (often with inflammation in the pisotriquetral joint). Chronic inflammation of any tendon compartment is associated with local and radiating symptoms. Passive stretch and resisted active function of the affected tendons reproduce symptoms and confirms the diagnosis in the absence of other findings. Flexor tenosynovitis is common after prolonged gripping activities such as that seen in stringed-instrument players, typists, mechanics, and carpenters. Extensor compartment inflammation may be found with intense repetitive wrist and finger motion from any cause; after the first compartment, it is the sixth that is most often inflamed.

More proximally, intersection syndromes occur, in which the extensor carpi radialis longus and extensor carpi radialis brevis tendons cross deep to the first compartment tendons at their musculotendinous junctions. These cross-over tendon inflammations may sometimes be accompanied by audible and palpable crepitus. Similar presentations may occur with the extensor pollicis longus and extensor indicis proprius tendons.

Trigger Finger

Chronic flexor tenosynovitis, or tenovaginitis, occurs more commonly in the middle and ring fingers and the thumb, and often in diabetic patients and postmenopausal females. Patients may not recall an injury that predates symptoms, but many can describe an episode of prolonged use or forceful trauma, with impact or hyperextension, that immediately preceded symptom onset. The snapping phenomenon occurs as the flexor digitorum superficialis and profundus

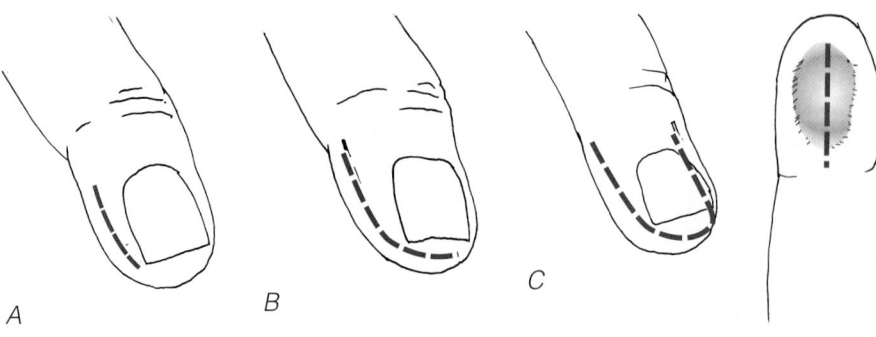

FIG. 43-91. *Incision and drainage is the proper management of a felon. A. An incision is made dorsal to the apex of the distal interphalangeal flexion crease at the junction of the dorsal and glabrous sulci. Usually the incision is lateral. B and C. The incision may be extended to varying degrees around the fingertip as necessary, but it must be carried just volar to the edge of the nail matrix. D. An alternative incision, advocated by some authors, extends longitudinally on the midline of the volar pulp distal to the flexion crease.*

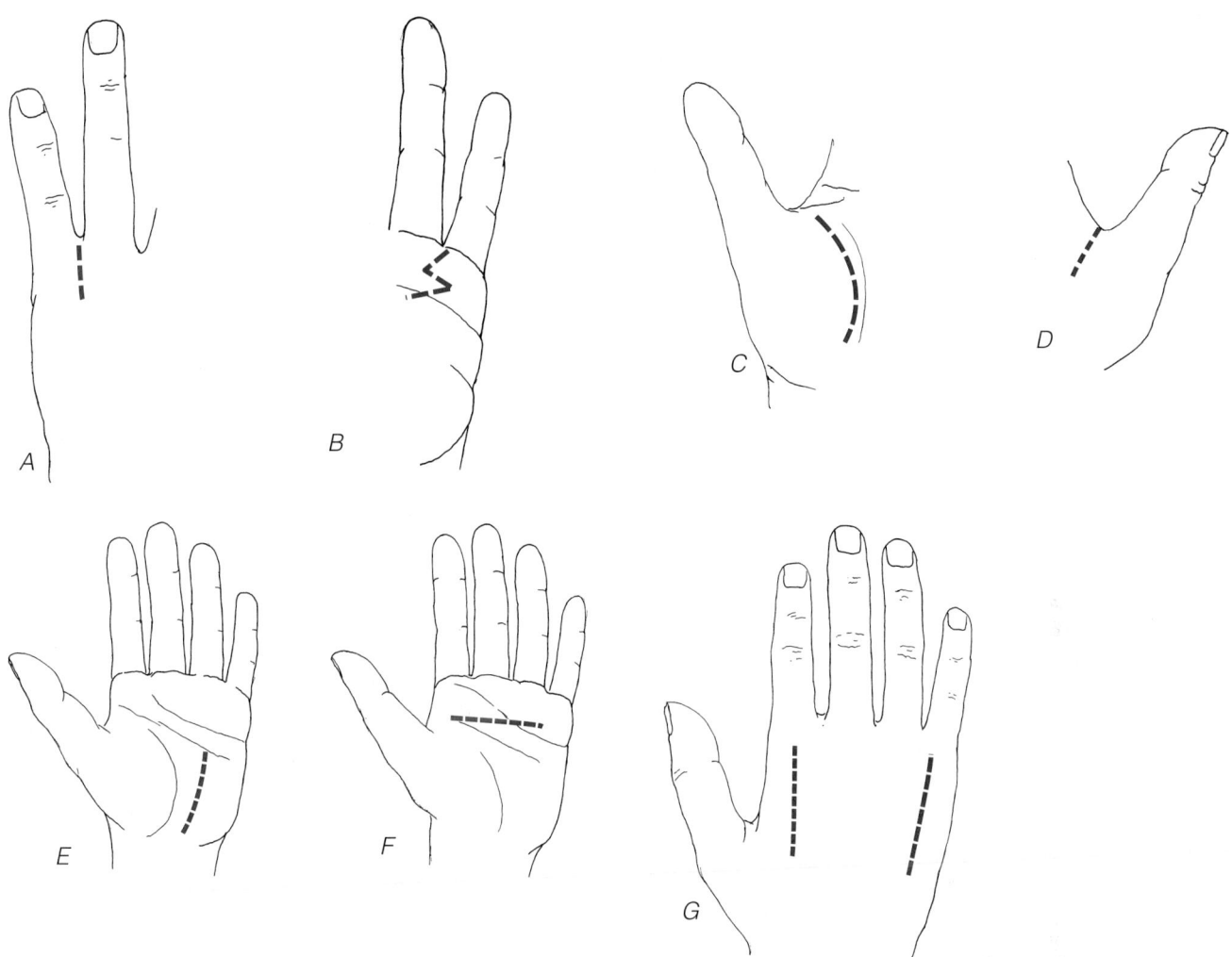

FIG. 43-92. *Surgical approaches to deep-space infections. A and B. Interdigital web space. C and D. Thenar space. E. Hypothenar space. F. Midpalmar space. G. Dorsal subaponeurotic space.*

tendons, or the flexor pollicis longus in the case of the thumb, pull through a thick, tight A1 flexor pulley at the proximal edge of the sheath. There is debate as to whether tenosynovial inflammation or pulley thickening is the cause. Nonetheless, there is a relative lack of volume in the sheath for the tendon, inducing the crepitus, catching or locking, and pain. Many patients have other associated systemic diseases such as diabetes, connective tissue diseases, or additional sites of tenosynovitis or carpal tunnel syndrome, but the process may be isolated.

Patients presenting with complaints of finger pain, distal palmar pain on grasping, or finger catching and locking should be evaluated for systemic and local problems. Thickening of the flexor tendon at the base of the finger in the distal palm, and palpation of a tendon nodule that glides with active finger motion will make this diagnosis. In the locking finger, an audible and palpable snap is noted (Fig. 43-95). However, any condition that causes finger stiffness such as diminished flexion, a flexion contracture (especially at the PIP joint), or snapping or locking can be potentially *mis*diagnosed as having trigger finger. Diagnosis is made by careful clinical examination and findings of a localized nodularity and tenderness about the flexor sheath in the distal palm.

Nonsurgical treatment should be offered except for patients with a fixed PIP joint flexion contracture that will not unlock after local

anesthetic and steroid injection. Approximately 1 mL of the mix is injected into the flexor sheath and pulley. At introduction, the needle pierces the skin and tendons at the metacarpal head and then is withdrawn slightly. The sheath is aspirated and injection proceeds with gentle pressure. Firm resistance indicates that the needle is in a tendon and needs to be withdrawn or inserted further. Palpable and visible introduction of fluid into the flexor sheath is associated with successful injection. Most patients improve, but those with continuing or recurring symptoms, and those with locked fingers, are candidates for surgery.

Surgery routinely cures the problem, providing long-term relief unless A1 pulley release is incomplete, or digital nerve injury or division of the more distal A2 pulley occurs. Under local anesthesia and with a tourniquet, a longitudinal incision is made directly over the flexor tendon between the proximal metacarpophalangeal joint flexion crease and the distal palmar crease (Fig. 43-96). The thickened pulley lies directly beneath this skin incision, just dorsal to the fascia and subcutaneous fat layers. The neurovascular bundles are both lateral to the sheath. A longitudinal incision is made in the skin between the distal palmar and proximal digital (MP) creases; the sheath is opened longitudinally under direct vision, carefully releasing the proximal and distal extents of the pulley. To assure restoration of unimpeded tendon gliding via active flexion and

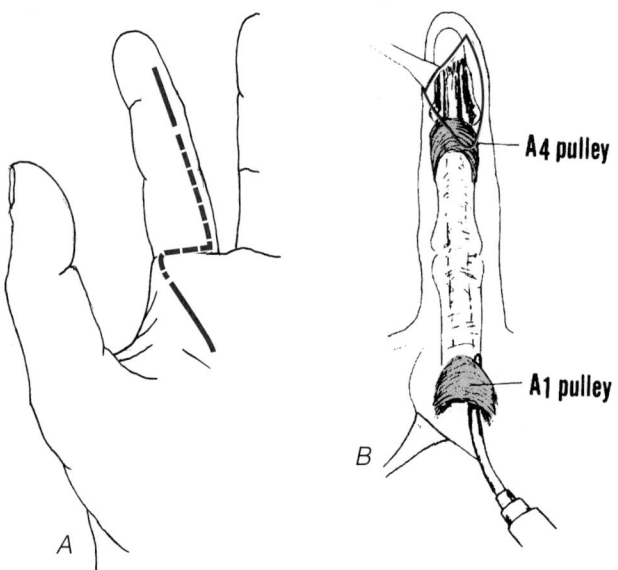

FIG. 43-93. Surgery to treat tenosynovitis. *A.* A generic midaxial digital skin incision may be carried proximally (if necessary) to connect to the proximal portion of the sheath. The incision is kept dorsal to preserve both neurovascular bundles in the palmar flap, and to allow the wound to remain open without jeopardizing flap coverage of the affected tendon. *B.* Irrigation catheter placement beneath the A1 pulley is all that is needed to achieve unimpeded irrigation once the sheath distal to the A4 pulley has been excised (the distal pulley is preserved). The distal wound is left *open.*

passive traction, a blunt tendon hook is used. In the thumb, special care is taken to avoid inadvertent division of the radial proper digital nerve, which crosses palmar to the flexor tendon just proximal to the pulley. Tendon release under direct vision protects this nerve. For tendon release in the thumb, an oblique longitudinal or Bruner-style incision is used (Fig. 43-97).

Direct trauma producing a partial tendon laceration may cause a triggering phenomenon in the distal flexor sheath. Systemic diseases that produce tendon nodularity, such as rheumatoid arthritis and gout, may cause similar, but more proximal or distal catching of the tendons. These less common causes require more extended flexor sheath exploration, excision of tendon nodules, and rehabilitation.

Neuropathies

Median Nerve

The median nerve may be compressed anywhere along its course from the cervical roots to the fingertips, but the most common site is within the carpal tunnel, where it is in a limited space filled with tendons and tenosynovium, lying dorsal to the transverse carpal ligament. All anatomic sites of compression must be considered and evaluated in the differential diagnosis of this most common peripheral neuropathy.

Carpal tunnel syndrome (CTS) results from increased pressure within the rigid carpal canal, producing median nerve ischemia and physiologic dysfunction. Symptoms include paresthesias and numbness in the radial $3\frac{1}{2}$ fingers, burning digital dysesthesias, and later in its course, hand weakness or awkwardness from thenar atrophy. Focal wrist and hand pain are not a part of the syndrome, while nocturnal symptoms are a hallmark. All treatments are designed to reduce pressure within the canal and thereby relieve nerve compression.

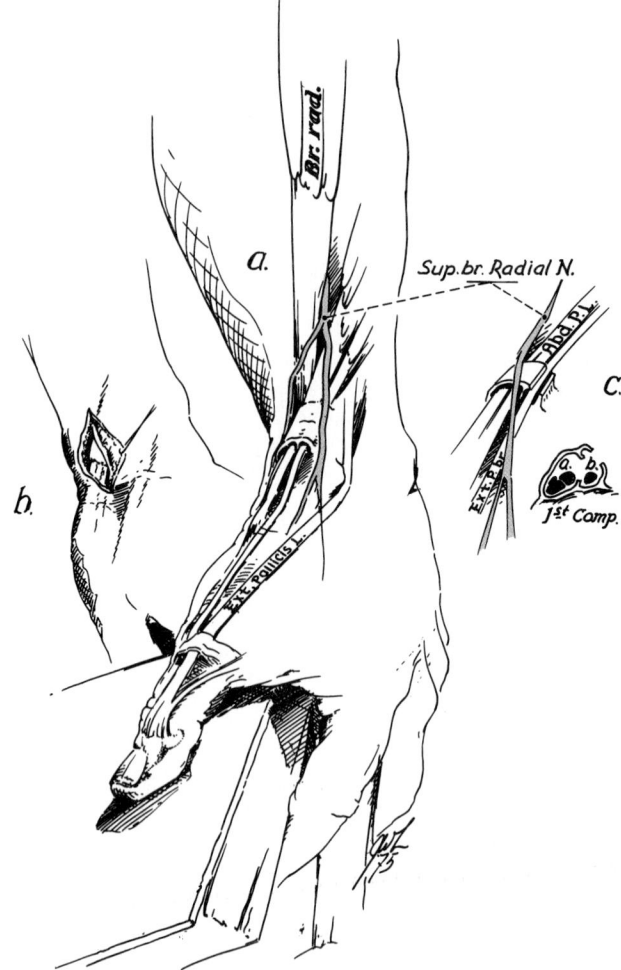

FIG. 43-94. Anatomy of deQuervain's tenosynovitis. Note the relationship of the radial sensory nerve to the tendons. Note the relationships of the extensor pollicis brevis and abductor pollicis longus tendons within the first extensor compartment. (*Reproduced with permission from Burton RI, Littler JW: Entrapment syndromes of the retinacular or restraining systems of the hand, in Nontraumatic Soft Tissue Afflictions of the Hand. Chicago: Year Book Medical, Current Problems in Surgery, 1975.*)

The carpal canal serves as a mechanical conduit for the digital flexor tendons. The carpal bones form the walls and floor, or dorsal surface of the canal, and the palmar aspect is roofed by the transverse carpal ligament. Tunnel cross-sectional area is relatively dynamic, with the smallest area at the extremes of wrist flexion and extension. There is debate as to the exact originating cause of the measurably increased pressure. Some have postulated tenosynovitis, while other studies have shown collagen, amyloid deposits, and edema as causes.

Eighty percent of carpal tunnel patients are over the age of 40 years. The female:male ratio varies from 4:1 for idiopathic cases, to as low as 1.5:1 with occupational presentations. A direct connection between CTS and forceful or repetitive use of the hands has not been conclusively demonstrated. There are reports of both low and high incidences among workers in manual industries. Such studies have many times used clinical criteria alone for the diagnosis, and have not factored out avocational or systemic disease–induced causes. The causation is probably multifactorial in most patients. CTS has been associated with endocrine disorders including diabetes, myxedema, hyperthyroidism, acromegaly, pregnancy, and the postpartum state. Chronic infections and hematologic and autoimmune

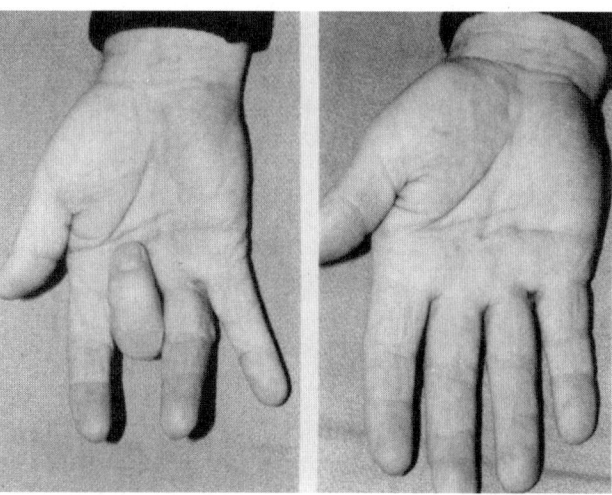

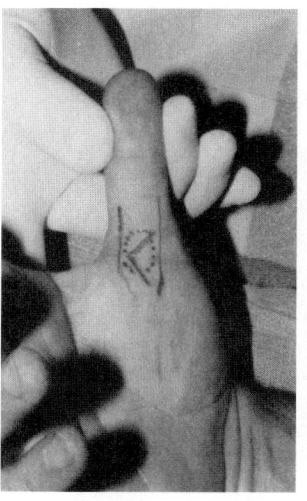

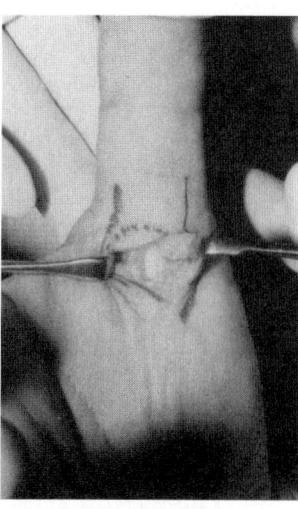

A   *B*

FIG. 43-95. *Trigger finger coexisting with Dupuytren's contracture in the same digit. This patient had locking of the middle finger in flexion, which was unrelated to the mild static flexion deformity of the metacarpophalangeal joint caused by the Dupuytren's cord, and was relieved by a steroid injection into the flexor sheath.*

FIG. 43-97. *V-shaped incision for release of trigger thumb. A. A V-shaped flap is raised full thickness, based radially, and centered over the A1 pulley, with its apex at the metacarpophalangeal joint flexion crease. This protects the radial digital nerve of the thumb. B. The surgical view shows the released A1 pulley and the flexor pollicis longus tendon.*

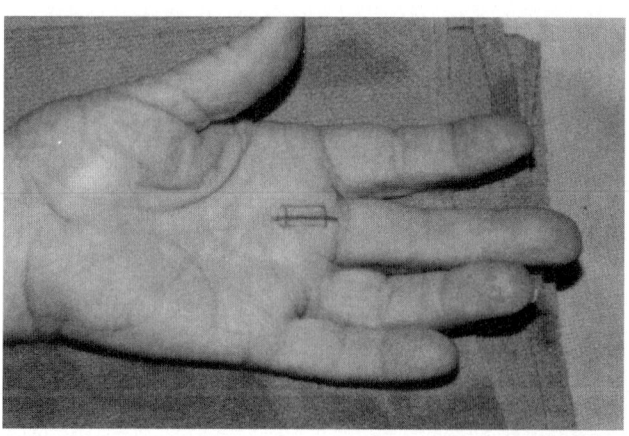

A

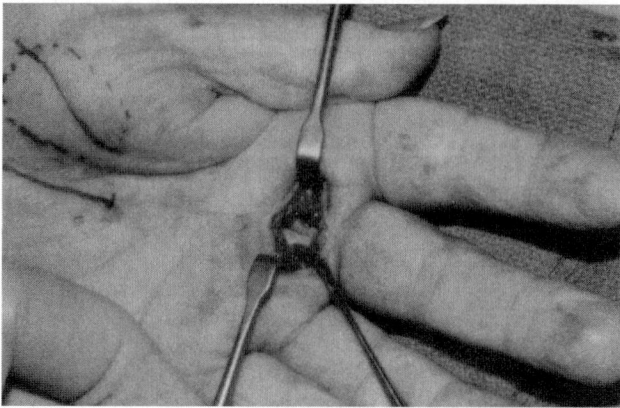

B

FIG. 43-96. *Longitudinal incision for trigger finger release. A. The incision is made in a natural skin crease, over the A1 pulley, between the base of the finger flexion crease and the distal transverse crease of the palm. B. The surgical view shows the released A1 pulley and the flexor digitorum superficialis tendon.*

disorders also are associated with CTS. Space-occupying lesions such as lipomas, bone abnormalities of the radius or carpals, posttraumatic edema, and hematomas may induce increased pressure within the canal and compromise median nerve function.

The diagnosis of CTS is clinical. Classic symptoms include paresthesias, with a predominance of nocturnal or early morning onset, burning or numbness in the median sensory distribution, and awkwardness in use of the hand. On physical examination, direct digital pressure over the median nerve at the carpal tunnel (carpal tunnel compression test) reproduces symptoms within 30 seconds. In Phalen's maneuver, gravity-induced wrist flexion reproduces symptoms within 1 minute. When direct percussion of the nerve elicits and reproduces paresthesias in the median distribution, it is called a positive Tinel's sign. The application of a pneumatic tourniquet to the upper limb to reproduce digital symptoms is of no real value in making this diagnosis. Examination includes objective documentation of sensory and motor loss, the former by threshold testing, including vibration and Semms-Weinstein monofilaments, rather than innervation density or two-point discrimination. Examination of motor function begins with inspection for thenar loss and assessing abductor pollicis brevis muscle resistance against force (Fig. 43-98).

Electrophysiologic studies provide important confirmatory and differential diagnostic information. Electrophysiologic studies alone do not form the basis for the diagnosis, but this author and most other hand surgeons believe that surgery should not be done without electrodiagnostic evaluation. Electrophysiologic tests are useful when the diagnosis is difficult or when surgical release is contemplated. Underlying peripheral neuropathies and multifocal compressions that are otherwise unsuspected will thus be uncovered. Electrical studies also provide a baseline for later comparison if the response to surgery is disappointing. Evaluation should include studies of the median nerve bilaterally from neck to fingertips, as well as of a second nerve in the more symptomatic extremity. Comparison of median and ulnar or of median and radial sensory stimulation values at the wrist is useful in confirming the diagnosis.

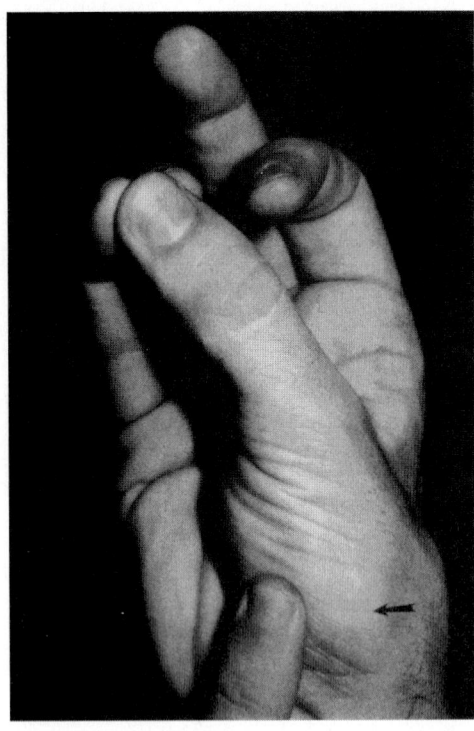

FIG. 43-98. Palpation of thenar muscles for weakness during opposition. The bulging muscle of the abductor pollicis brevis (*arrow*), which is consistently innervated by the median nerve, is seen and can be palpated adjacent to the metacarpal while asking the patient to oppose the thumb forcefully to the little finger. Softness in the muscle contraction suggests weakness in this muscle.

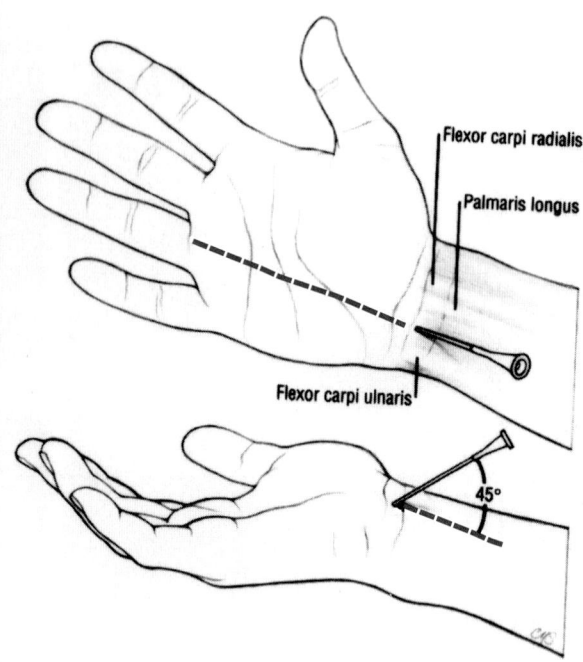

FIG. 43-99. Needle placement for injection of the carpal canal. The needle tip is placed through the skin at the volar wrist crease midway between the flexor carpi ulnaris and palmaris longus tendons at a 45 degree angle. A fine needle is used. If paresthesias are encountered in this location, the needle should be redirected to avoid intraneural injection with corticosteroid. Inadvertent median nerve injection can occur even in this location if the nerve lies ulnarly.

Studies are not necessarily of prognostic value for the response to surgery, however.

Routine radiographs, including the carpal tunnel view, are recommended by the American Academy of Orthopaedic Surgery for evaluation and treatment of CTS. Radiographs are evaluated for carpal fractures, arthritis, Kienböck's disease, or other problems that could alter treatment. CT and MRI scans are seldom needed, but basic laboratory studies to screen for endocrine and hematologic disorders are helpful. Predisposing medical diseases, such as thyroid dysfunction or rheumatoid arthritis, should be treated and may well improve or resolve the neuropathy without surgery. In pregnancy, CTS is treated by salt restriction, wrist splinting, analgesics, and occasionally diuretics. Local steroid injection may be needed during the third trimester. Most of these patients recover within about 6 months of delivery.

For acute posttraumatic CTS associated with swelling or hemorrhage, loosening of constrictive bandages and moving the wrist from a position at the extreme of flexion or extension may suffice to reverse or significantly improve symptoms. Pressure studies and early surgery may be appropriate for those who do not respond. Acute CTS needs acute treatment; significant persisting compression will cause permanent, irreversible nerve damage.

Splints and nonsteroidal anti-inflammatory medications are widely used. Splints should fit comfortably and position the wrist in neutral to minimal extension. Splints are worn at night if nocturnal symptoms are a major complaint, and night splinting may be all that is required. With activity-induced symptoms, periodic, intermittent daytime splint use during provoking tasks may be quite helpful; however, condemning patients to continuous around-the-clock splint use is unjustified and not especially therapeutic. Oral

nonsteroidal anti-inflammatory agents are helpful and should be with monitored for possible gastrointestinal and systemic side effects. Although subclinical vitamin B_6 deficiency is a possible cause of CTS, no prospective study has ever demonstrated the efficacy of pyridoxine; however, it is a nontoxic agent. Local steroid injection results in improvement in 80 to 90% of patients, but there may be gradual deterioration over months. As with other sites, injections should not be repeated more than two or three times annually. Inadvertent injection directly into the median nerve will worsen symptoms (Fig. 43-99). Injection is safely and efficaciously done from 2 to 3 cm proximal to the wrist, in line with the third webspace or fourth ray (ulnar to the palmaris longus and median nerve), using a total of 2 to 3 mL of anesthetic (1 to 2 mL) and steroid (1 mL).

Surgical treatment requires complete division of the transverse carpal ligament for the entire length of the carpal tunnel under direct vision, by endoscopic or open methods. Surgical failure is most often associated with incorrect or incomplete diagnosis or incomplete ligament division. Internal neurolysis, flexor tenosynovectomy, concomitant ulnar nerve decompression in Guyon's canal, or carpal ligament reconstructions are *not* indicated with primary release and may be harmful. Open and endoscopic release can effectively divide the transverse carpal ligament and increase canal volume (Figs. 43-100, 43-101, and 43-102).

Open release is performed with the patient supine and under tourniquet control. After limb exsanguination and tourniquet inflation, the field is infiltrated with local anesthetic. Intravenous sedation may be used as a supplement. Incision for open release is made in line with the third web, parallel to the thenar crease, from the distal end of the transverse carpal ligament almost to the distal wrist crease. Small twigs of palmar cutaneous nerve branches are identified

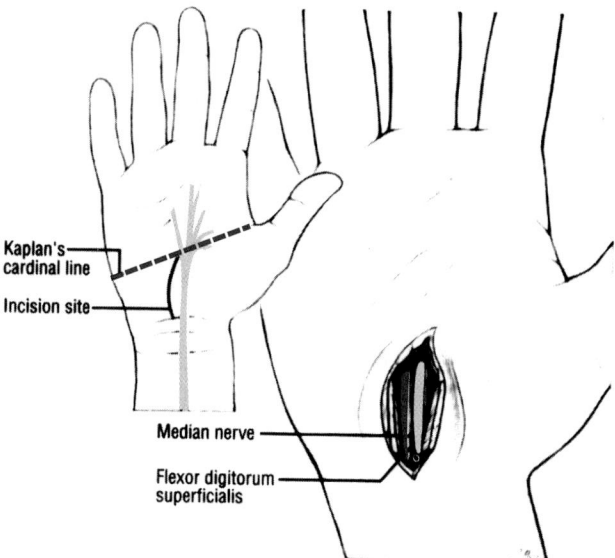

FIG. 43-100. The cardinal line and the incision for open carpal tunnel release. Kaplan has described a line drawn to help localize the motor branch of the median nerve. At the site of intersection of a line dropped from the radial side of the ring finger is the entrance of the recurrent motor branch of the median nerve into the thenar muscles. The gently curved incision for surgical decompression begins at the volar wrist crease in line with the ring metacarpal, and parallels the thenar crease to end at the cardinal line.

during subcutaneous dissection and preserved where found to be crossing the incision. The palmar fascia is split longitudinally, using a small curved hemostat, from the proximal end of the carpal canal moving distally, staying in the most palmar and ulnar quadrant of the canal. The nerve and flexor tendons beneath and radial to this clamp are continuously identified and protected. The motor nerve to the thenar muscles is most radial and protected. The ligament incision roughly parallels the ulnar border of the median nerve and leaves a small tissue flap attached to the hook of the hamate, more ulnarly. The wound is inspected to assure complete division of the ligament, release of the contents, and the absence of soft-tissue masses and bone anomalies. The median nerve is to

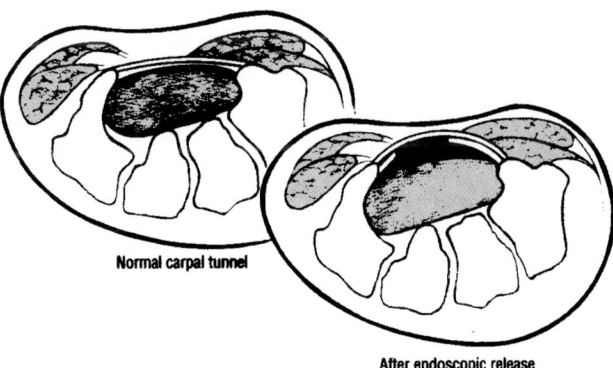

FIG. 43-101. The dual layers of the transverse carpal ligament. The transverse carpal ligament has a deep rigid layer, and a more superficial flexible layer composed of palmar, thenar, and hypothenar fascia. With endoscopic carpal tunnel release, the rigid deep layer separates, but the more flexible superficial layer remains intact. The increased volume within the carpal canal is a result of volar migration of the contents of the canal.

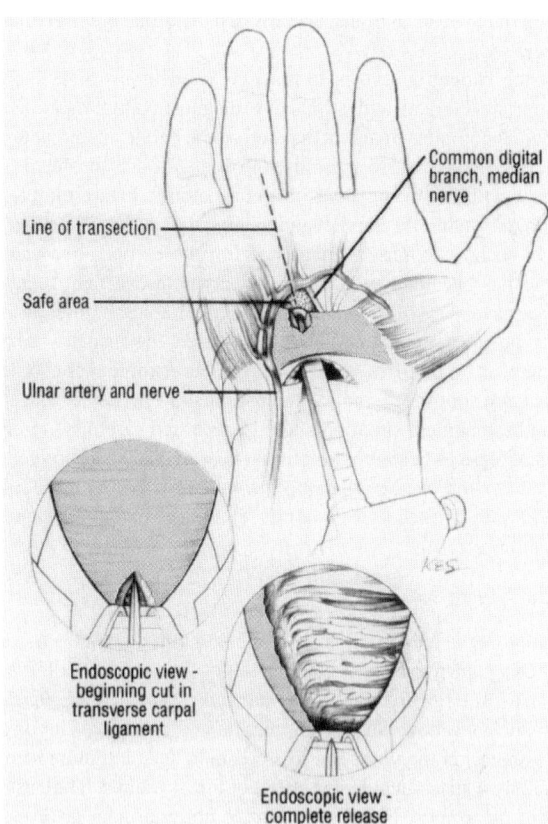

FIG. 43-102. Endoscopic carpal tunnel release. The safe area for ligament division is in line with the ring finger between the median nerve and the ulnar neurovascular bundle, proximal to the superficial vascular arch. With the resection nosepiece aligned with the ring finger, the transverse fibers of the transverse carpal ligament as seen through the endoscope assures the surgeon that no critical structures intervene between the blade and the ligament. When resection is complete, the rigid portion of the transverse carpal ligament slides apart, creating a trapezoidal defect, decompressing the carpal canal. After this occurs, the nosepiece of the system fits between the cut edges of the ligament; if the endoscope is rolled from one side to the other, only one side of the divided ligament can be seen through the window.

be found in the palmoradial portion of the canal, and is normally mildly adherent to the underside of the ligament. The nerve may have a central-narrowing, hourglass constriction at the site of maximum compression. The surgeon should avoid manipulating the nerve because this induces more intraneural scarring, and interferes both with postoperative nerve gliding and ultimate recovery; epineurotomy and internal neurolysis is not indicated, offers no benefit, and may be additionally harmful. After tourniquet release and hemostasis, palmar fascia may be closed, but most surgeons close only the skin, using a fine monofilament suture. The wrist is splinted in slight extension for about 10 to 14 days before therapy is started.

Endoscopic release was introduced to avoid the morbidity of a palmar scar. Multiple prospective and retrospective studies suggest a more rapid recovery and document an equivalent increase in canal volume and pressure decrease by this approach. The single-portal endoscopic decompression is associated with less perioperative discomfort and shorter immobilization and recovery. After endoscopic release, a canvas wrist splint is offered but not required. Therapy, when needed, is started during the first postoperative week.

The true incidence of inadvertent tissue trauma from open and endoscopic methods has not been determined. The best method for avoiding complications is to operate carefully, in a bloodless field, cutting only what can be seen clearly and identified precisely before it is incised.

If the patient continues to have CTS symptoms after surgery, appropriate clinical and adjunctive diagnostic investigations are needed. Incomplete ligament division or inaccurate, incomplete preoperative diagnosis are the most frequent physical problems, but patients with hidden agendas of a nonanatomic nature may report prolonged wound discomfort and exhibit apparently limited recovery. In such situations, the real value of the preoperative electrodiagnostics becomes evident. In patients with excellent recovery, studies have shown persistence of electrical abnormalities in two-thirds; however, these changes do not worsen, they usually improve (incompletely) or persist even with full clinical recovery. When a patient does not show signs of improvement, repeat electrical studies and the clinical situation should be studied carefully; rarely is repeat release indicated or helpful. Tender palmar scars are notably resistant to improvement by reoperation; this author strongly favors an endoscopic method to lessen or eliminate this latter source of pain after release.

Ulnar Nerve

Ulnar nerve compression at the elbow, cubital tunnel syndrome, has been known for more than a century. It has been called post-traumatic ulnar neuritis and tardy ulnar nerve palsy to emphasize a traumatic causation. Distal compression in the canal of Guyon (the ulnar tunnel) at the wrist is a less common site, and more often is caused by a space-occupying lesion or direct trauma. The possible sites of ulnar nerve compression in the fibromuscular groove posterior to the medial epicondyle are summarized in Fig. 43-103. All sites of nerve compression must be considered. The differential diagnosis includes medial epicondylitis and its coexistence with ulnar nerve irritation. Some patients will have the mechanical problem of a hypermobile or subluxating ulnar nerve. Ulnar traction neuritis with elbow flexion and anterior nerve subluxation reproduce radiating paresthesias in the ulnar two fingers. Patients who have actual motor weakness, and especially the subgroup with intrinsic muscle weakness or atrophy and electrophysiologic changes, have a somewhat more guarded prognosis.

Patients presenting with medial epicondylitis should be treated for that problem, but the presence of secondary or coexistent nerve irritation must be addressed. Those who do not respond to

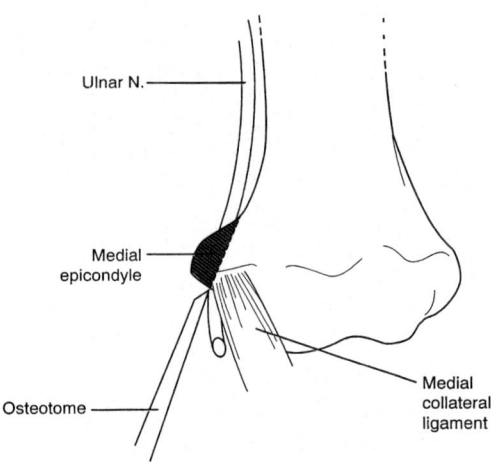

FIG. 43-104. Medial epicondylectomy. The key here is to excise the midportion of the medial epicondyle without disrupting the origin of the medial collateral ligament. When there is doubt, radiographs can be useful.

conservative measures as outlined for the carpal tunnel should be treated surgically. At operation, after nerve decompression, the resultant (iatrogenic) nerve subluxation is present in most and must be addressed. Subcutaneous anterior transposition may be done, requiring a fascial wall or sleeve to keep the nerve in place. Some, including this author, prefer subperiosteal medial epicondylectomy, excising enough of the bony prominence to flatten the skeletal contour on the medial side of the elbow so that flexion/extension does not produce snapping of the nerve over prominent tissues. Alternatively, submuscular transposition can be performed. There is no clear advantage of one primary technique over the other in most patients (Fig. 43-104).

Ulnar (Guyon's) tunnel decompression at the wrist must include the management of space-occupying lesions which are many times part of this diagnosis. Ulnar tunnel syndrome is far less common than CTS (Fig. 43-105). Pathologic conditions predisposing to ulnar

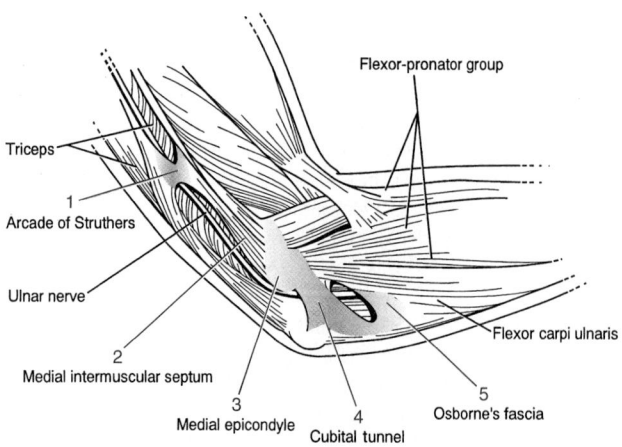

FIG. 43-103. The five potential areas of ulnar nerve compression around the elbow: (1) the arcade of Struthers, (2) the medial intermuscular septum, (3) the medial epicondyle, (4) the cubital tunnel, and (5) Osborne's fascia.

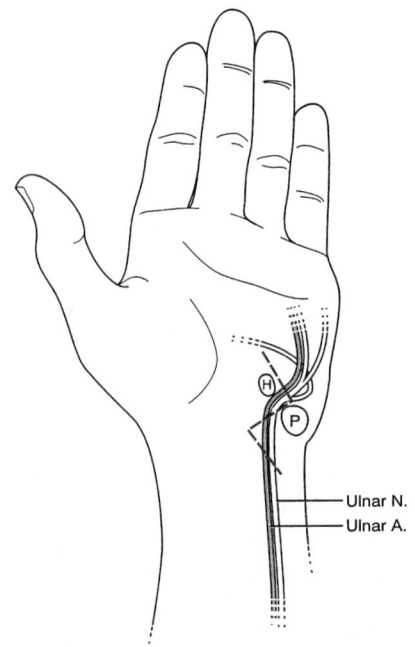

FIG. 43-105. Incision for exposure of Guyon's canal.

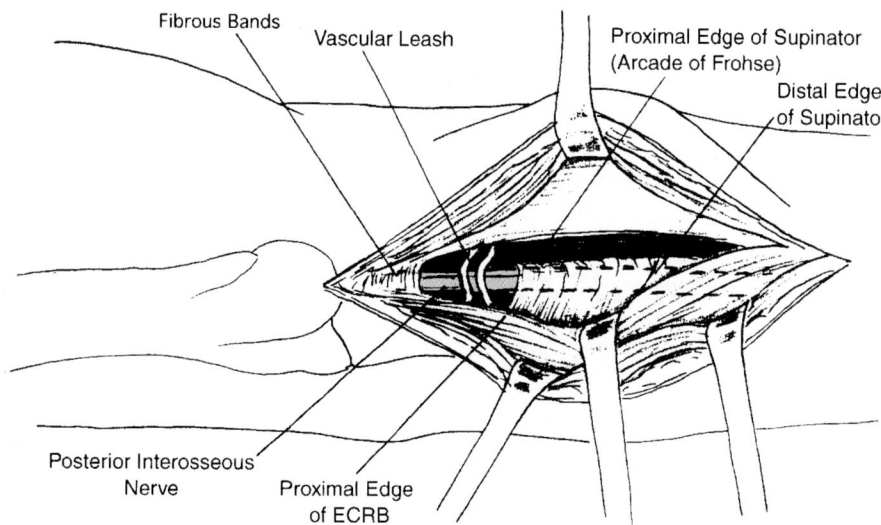

FIG. 43-106. The five potential sites of posterior interosseous nerve compression.

nerve and artery compression in the ulnar tunnel should be attended to simultaneously, including excision of a hamulus nonunion; ulnar artery lysis, ligation, or revascularization; or removal of ganglia.

Radial Nerve

Radial nerve entrapment causes sensory symptoms of paresthesias and dysesthesias in the nerve's afferent (muscular and cutaneous) distributions in the dorsal forearm, wrist, and hand. Symptoms depend on the primary site of nerve irritation or compression, but are most frequently in the proximal forearm. The term *radial tunnel syndrome* (RTS) describes a compression neuropathy involving the posterior interosseous nerve branch of the radial nerve beneath the fibrous arcade of Frohse at the proximal edge of the supinator. The common presentation is radiating, aching discomfort in the dorsal and dorsolateral forearm. Patients with RTS may have preceding or coexistent lateral epicondylitis, and the distinction between epicondylitis and posterior interosseous nerve compression must be included in the differential work-up of all cases of resistant tennis elbow. Unlike epicondylitis, the site of maximal tenderness is distal to the epicondyle, over the extensor muscles, at the site where the posterior interosseous nerve passes into the fibromuscular tunnel bounded by the fibrous proximal edge of the superficial head of the supinator, approximately at the neck of the radius (Fig. 43-106).

Nonsurgical treatment includes rest, therapy for stretching and modalities, activity modification, elastic sleeve and splint protection, and nonsteroidal anti-inflammatory agents. Injectable steroids do not have a useful role due to the absence of tenosynovium in the region of nerve compression. Electrodiagnostic studies are not helpful in the vast majority because of the deep and variable exact location of the nerve. Only patients with denervation of the forearm muscles will dependably have electrical changes (and these are limited to EMG evidence of denervation), and this group should be easy to diagnose clinically before operative decompression.

The radial and posterior interosseous nerves can be decompressed in the proximal forearm and anterolateral elbow region in patients with resistant symptoms. The brachioradialis splitting incision is most direct and efficient in the author's opinion, and is widely used (Fig. 43-107).

Radial sensory entrapment distally, Wartenberg's disease or cheiralgia paresthetica, may occur, but usually only after direct trauma to the radial wrist (e.g., after application of handcuffs).

Operation is rarely required for this typically transient problem. Radial sensory symptoms of local paresthesias far more often coexist with or are secondary to the common problem of deQuervain's tendinopathy in the first dorsal compartment. This tendinitis should be excluded in the differential diagnosis, and is a numerically more probable reason for nerve irritation than primary entrapment (Fig. 43-108).

ACQUIRED DYSFUNCTION

Dupuytren's Contracture

Although this disorder is associated with the illustrious nineteenth-century French surgeon Baron Guillaume Dupuytren, he was not the first to describe it. John Hunter in 1777 and Sir Astley Cooper in 1822 among others reported the disease, and Cooper recommended subcutaneous fasciotomy. The pathologic proliferation is primarily of the longitudinal and vertical fibers of the palmar and digital fascia (Fig. 43-109). The diagnosis in advanced cases is not difficult, but in early stages the disorder may be confusing. "Knuckle pads" consisting of fasciotendinous proliferations over the dorsum of the PIP joints as well as palmar fascial nodules and dimpling and pitting of the palmar skin are characteristic findings. While palmar fascial nodules are believed to be pathognomonic, other masses including retinacular cysts, tendon nodules, foreign bodies, and trigger finger occasionally cause clinical confusion. The Dupuytren's fascial nodule does not move with flexor tendon excursion, and is located barely deep to the skin and in subcutaneous fat. Fascial skin tethering may result in fat bulging on either side of the diseased pretendinous band and cause the skin pits characteristic of this pathology. Proliferating nodules precede cords, but patients may not present until cords and contractures are evident. Joint deformity and contracture is the eventual result of coalescence of nodules with the development of a shortened, pathologic fascial mass. There is no proven relationship to trauma, occupation, handedness, or repetitive use in work or sports.

Dupuytren's contracture is most commonly seen in Caucasian males of Northern European descent who are in their sixth decade or older (Figs. 43-110, 43-111, and 43-112). The male:female ratio varies from 2:1 to 10:1. Dupuytren's contracture is familial and is inherited as an autosomal dominant disorder, but with variable

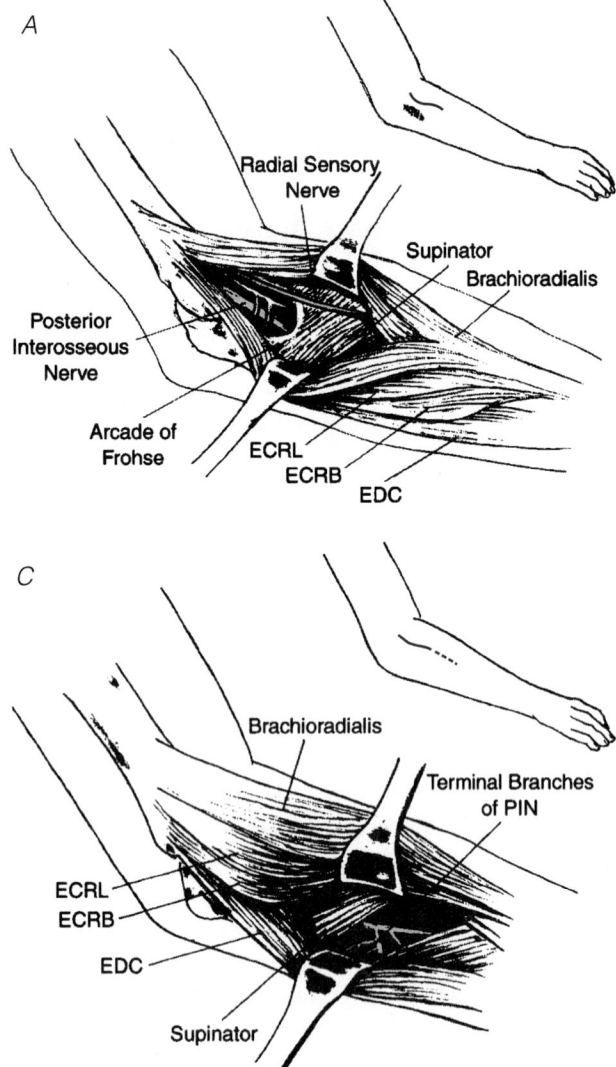

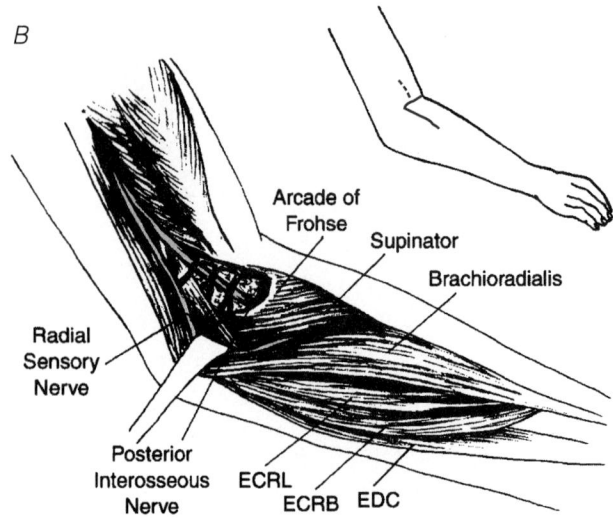

FIG. 43-107. *A.* The posterior interosseous nerve is efficiently approached by splitting the brachioradialis muscle fibers bluntly and dissecting toward the neck of the radius. The posterior interosseous nerve is dorsal to the sensory branch; it is located deep to the leash of radial vessels and is traced distally under the fibrous edge of the extensor carpi radialis brevis and the supinator (arcade of Frohse). *B.* More proximally the radial nerve can be exposed by extending the skin incision and dissecting in the intermuscular space between the brachioradialis and biceps/brachialis muscles more medially. As necessary, the lateral epicondyle can be exposed by turning this extended skin incision more posteriorly instead of anteriorly and proximally. *C.* The distal portion of the posterior interosseous nerve and the lower supinator are located by extending the original skin incision distally and opening the fascial interval between the extensor carpi radialis brevis and extensor digitorum communis tendons, continuing proximally to locate the (more deeply located) supinator muscle edge. Care must be taken to avoid avulsing the nerve branches traversing from the posterior interosseous nerve into the extensor digitorum communis muscle. ECRL = extensor carpi radialis longus; ECRB = extensor carpi radialis brevis; EDC = extensor digitorum communis; PIN = posterior interosseous nerve.

penetrance. There are significant associations with a number of diseases and conditions, the most prominent of which are diabetes and alcoholism.

As of this writing, there is yet no approved and effective nonsurgical treatment for Dupuytren's contracture. Nonetheless, the recent and exciting results of the preliminary studies with collagenase injections in lieu of surgery are a potential revolution after nearly two centuries. If confirmed as safe and effective in upcoming multicenter (FDA-sponsored Phase 3) trials, the entire treatment of this vexing process may change from major surgery to office injections.

Nonetheless, treatment should be reserved for those whose disease is complicated by dysfunctional contracture(s), because the surgery itself is detailed and is best coupled with closely supervised postoperative hand therapy. Tender palmar nodules are only a transient phenomenon, caused by the coexistence of active cellular proliferation and repetitive daily contact, impact, or load. In patients with such complaints, often truck drivers and others who must grip or lift frequently or continuously, padded gloves—such as those worn by bicyclists and weight lifters—can help symptoms resolve within several weeks in nearly all cases. Splinting does not prevent later contracture; it is not clear that contractures can be predicted, and patients need to be followed at 6-month intervals when a

joint deformity is becoming significant. If the patient can no longer place his or her hand flat on a table (the tabletop test) operation is generally indicated. Contracture correction at the MP joint is easier than at the PIP joint, where surgery should be planned when the PIP contracture approaches 30 to 45 degrees.

Operating on a patient with Dupuytren's contracture requires a detailed knowledge of normal hand anatomy, palmar fascial structure, and of the patterns of the locations of the pathology, as it applies to the specific deformity, including the frequent pathologic displacement of neurovascular bundles, which puts them at risk of injury during even the most careful of surgical releases (Fig. 43-113). Most patients have their ulnar palm affected first and most significantly. In decreasing order of frequency, the fourth, fifth, third, second, and first rays are involved. The most effective surgical technique is digital fasciectomy (as opposed to fasciotomy). While fasciotomy achieves correction of deformity, recurrences are more rapid and severe than with excision of the diseased tissues. However, the results of excision will gradually deteriorate with time, as surgery does not cure the disease, but only treats joint deformities and dysfunction. Fasciectomy is performed under loupe magnification and exsanguinated pneumatic tourniquet control. Skin flaps are dissected at the level of the palmar fascia, preserving the maximum thickness of

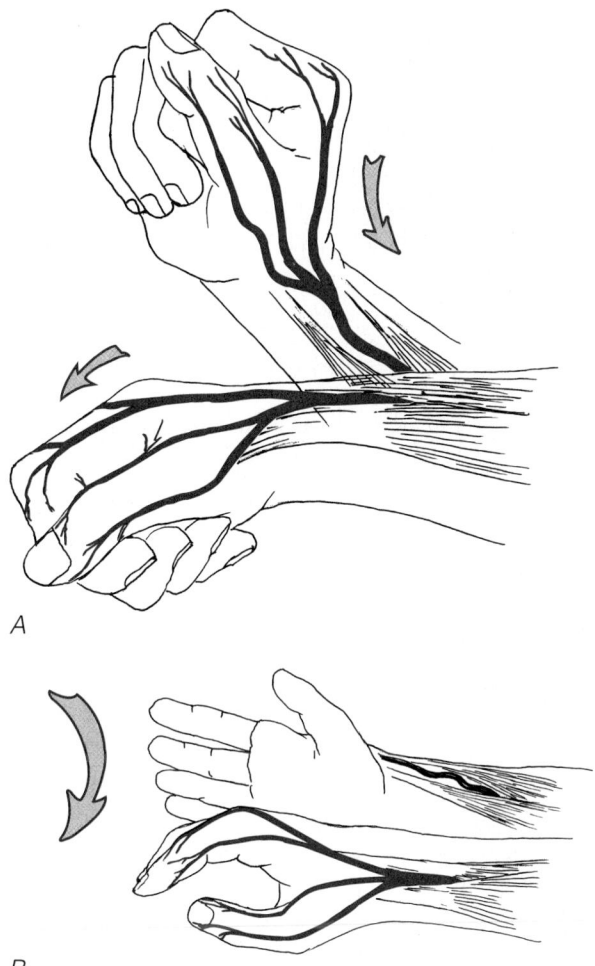

A

B

FIG. 43-108. *Radial sensory nerve irritation may occur in response to repetitive physiologic stress. A. The superficial branch of the radial nerve is relatively lax with wrist extension, but stretches during flexion and ulnar deviation, such as during hammering. The nerve is tethered proximally, where it exits from deep to superficial through the fascia just dorsal to the brachioradialis muscle. This mechanism generates the neuritic pain during Finkelstein's maneuver, but as paresthesias rather than localized discomfort. B. As the forearm rotates into pronation, the superficial radial nerve stretches and may be compressed between the tendons of the brachioradialis and extensor carpi radialis longus muscles.*

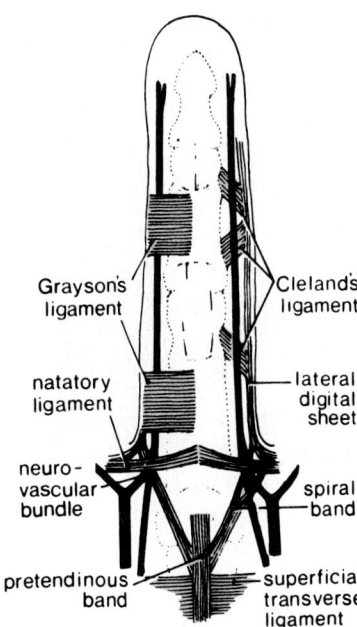

FIG. 43-109. *Normal fascial structures that can become involved with the pathologic cords of Dupuytren's contracture. The figure shows the pretendinous band, the spiral bands, the natatory ligaments, the lateral sheet, Grayson's ligaments, and Cleland's ligaments.*

contiguous skin and subcutaneous tissues to avoid devascularizing these small flaps (Fig. 43-114). Closed fasciotomy is not commonly performed because of the documented risk of neurovascular injury in this blind release.

Postoperative management varies only to minor degrees whether a Bruner-style incision, flaps such as the W, V-Y, Z-plasty, or the McCash open-palm incision techniques are used. With the open technique, transverse areas at the skin creases that are left unsutured minimally affect the recovery protocol, but a drain is not necessary. The lessened risk of hematoma and diminished short-term pain afforded by keeping some transverse (crease) incisions open at dissection, and connecting these transverse crease incisions via oblique longitudinal incisions (that are sutured at case completion) avoids the need to dissect under an awning of palmar skin (Fig. 43-114). No matter what the skin technique, the closure is done by most hand surgeons after tourniquet release and after hemostasis is secured. Avoiding postoperative hematomas lessens the problem

of localized fibrosis and added scar tissue. A bulky and moderately compressive dressing is applied, supplemented by palmar, or palmar and dorsal, plaster splint(s) to maintain the wrist at greater than 30 degrees extension, and the metacarpophalangeal joints and interphalangeal joints in maximally corrected extension.

Therapy is started under close supervision by the end of the first postoperative week because of the real risk of stiffness. Rehabilitation includes active and passive motion, and custom extension splinting of released joints at night. Sutures are removed after 2 to 3 weeks, depending on wound healing. Soaking and washing, especially when the McCash technique is used, is more an individual choice, and is often comforting and more attractive. In addition to wound infection and skin sloughing, secondary swelling is a serious but less common complication.

Prolonged pain leading to complex regional pain disorder/reflex sympathetic dystrophy is a difficult problem for patient, therapist, and physician. Digital nerves may be injured during surgery, no matter how expertly the procedure is performed, but such injury must be recognized and repaired at the surgical release. Most patients initially have some paresthesias in the released fingers, but this passes within weeks. It is most important that patients be allowed and encouraged to move their fingers to regain tendon and joint mobility within days of their surgery in this older, stiffer population rife with osteoarthritic joints.

Arthritis and Other Arthropathies

Inflammatory Arthropathies

The hand is a mirror of many inflammatory arthropathies, not just gout or rheumatoid arthritis (Figs. 43-115, 43-116, 43-117, and Table 43-5).

Adult and Juvenile Rheumatoid Arthritis. Primary consideration should be given to arthritis because of its worldwide prevalence and the severe disability that ensues if left untreated,

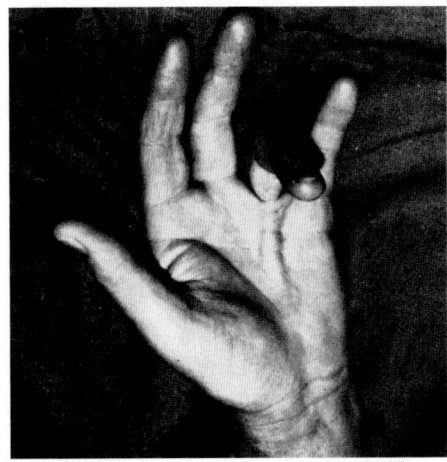

A

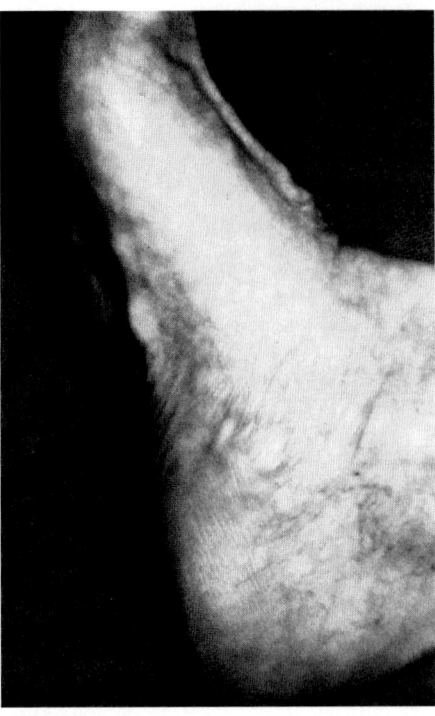

B

FIG. 43-110. *A.* Typical clinical appearance of the hand of a patient with Dupuytren's contracture. *B.* Dupuytren's contracture may involve the foot and present as nodules on the sole. Note that microscopically this material has the exact appearance of a low-grade fibrosarcoma. Should the material from the sole be excised, the pathologist must be alerted to the presence of Dupuytren's contracture to avoid a potentially disastrous misreading of the microscopic slide with the obvious tragic consequences.

or occasionally, when treated aggressively. Rheumatoid arthritis is a chronic systemic disorder of unknown cause of which a major manifestation is inflammatory synovitis with secondary bone and tendon invasion and destruction. There may be late tendon dysfunction through nodularity and locking or scarring, joint subluxation, and pain. In most cases, synovitis sites and deformities are rather symmetrical. Rheumatoid arthritis affects the shoulders, elbows, wrists, and metacarpophalangeal joints. Proximal interphalangeal joint involvement is less common, but may be significant in a given patient. On radiographs, the hands and feet show some of the earliest

signs of periarticular osteopenia, demineralization, and erosion. The earliest erosions occur along the radiopalmar aspects of the metacarpal heads, at the proximal phalanges, and in the prestyloid recess of the ulna.

Operative intervention is best limited to patients who, despite medical management, have persistent dysfunction because of pain, stiffness, or instability, or those with progressively worsened function and increased deformities. Joint and tendon salvage, reconstructions, and arthroplasties can be done successfully.

Scleroderma, Systemic Sclerosis, and Sclerodactyly. This is a generalized vasculitis affecting the skin, gastrointestinal tract, kidneys, and hands, resulting in thickened, dense, and inelastic connective tissues. Pathologic joint involvement occurs in up to 80% of patients. Vasculitis and secondary small-joint deformity may combine to produce thin, unstable skin, chronic ulcerations that do not heal, and secondary infections and painful loss of use (Fig. 43-118).

Psoriasis. This diagnosis should always be a consideration in the patient with inflammatory arthritis of the hands, particularly with nail deformities and oligoarticular arthritis. Psoriatic arthritis usually affects the interphalangeal joints.

Crystal Arthropathies. Crystal arthropathies include gout and pseudogout, which are diagnosed definitively after examination of joint aspiration fluid or a biopsy specimen. The serum uric acid levels may be normal even in an acute attack of gout, and most patients with hyperuricemia never have acute gouty arthropathy. Calcium pyrophosphate crystalline inflammation, or pseudogout, often affects the wrist, with chondrocalcinosis classically seen on the posteroanterior wrist radiograph at the prestyloid recess (Fig. 43-119).

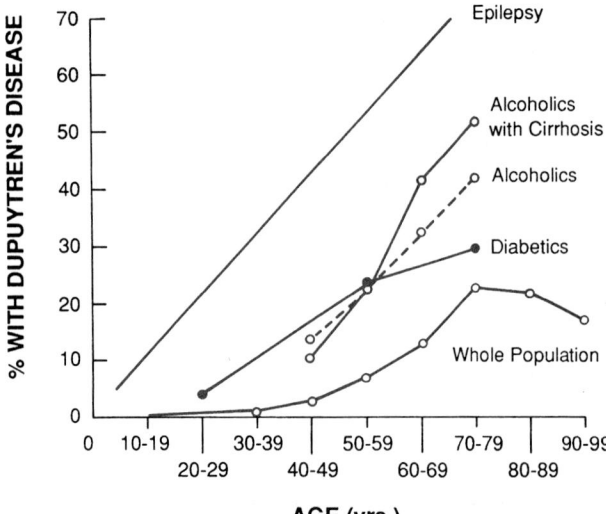

FIG. 43-111. The relationship of age to the percentage of the population with Dupuytren's contracture. Other superimposed lines showing disease incidence by age with epilepsy, alcoholism, and diabetes were constructed from data from multiple sources.

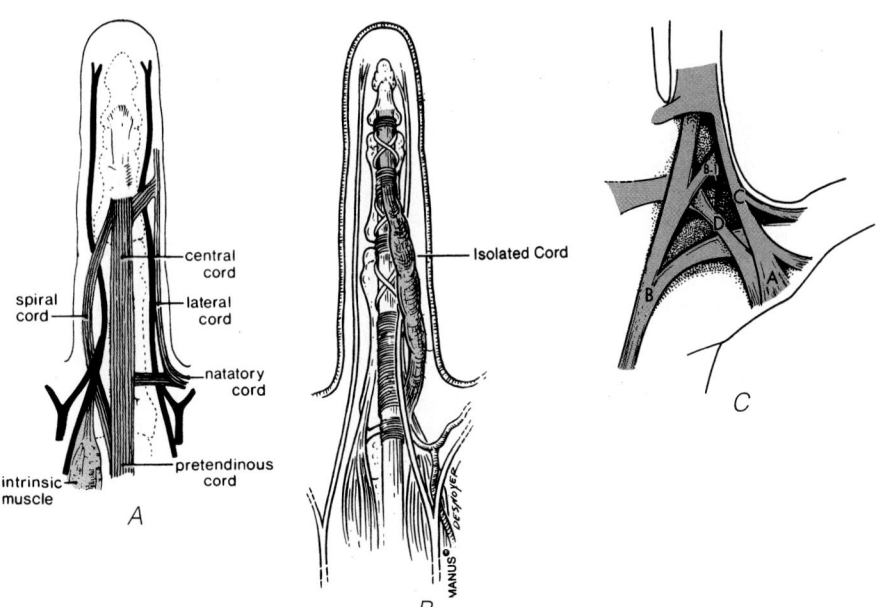

FIG. 43-112. The seven frequently recognized cords of Dupuytren's contracture. *A.* Five of these cords. The four cords in the digit are the central cord, the spiral cord, the lateral cord, and the natatory cord. The palmar cord is the pretendinous cord. *B.* The isolated digital cord of Basset and Strickland. *C.* The intercommissural cord.

Labels in figure A: spiral cord, central cord, lateral cord, natatory cord, pretendinous cord, intrinsic muscle

Label in figure B: Isolated Cord

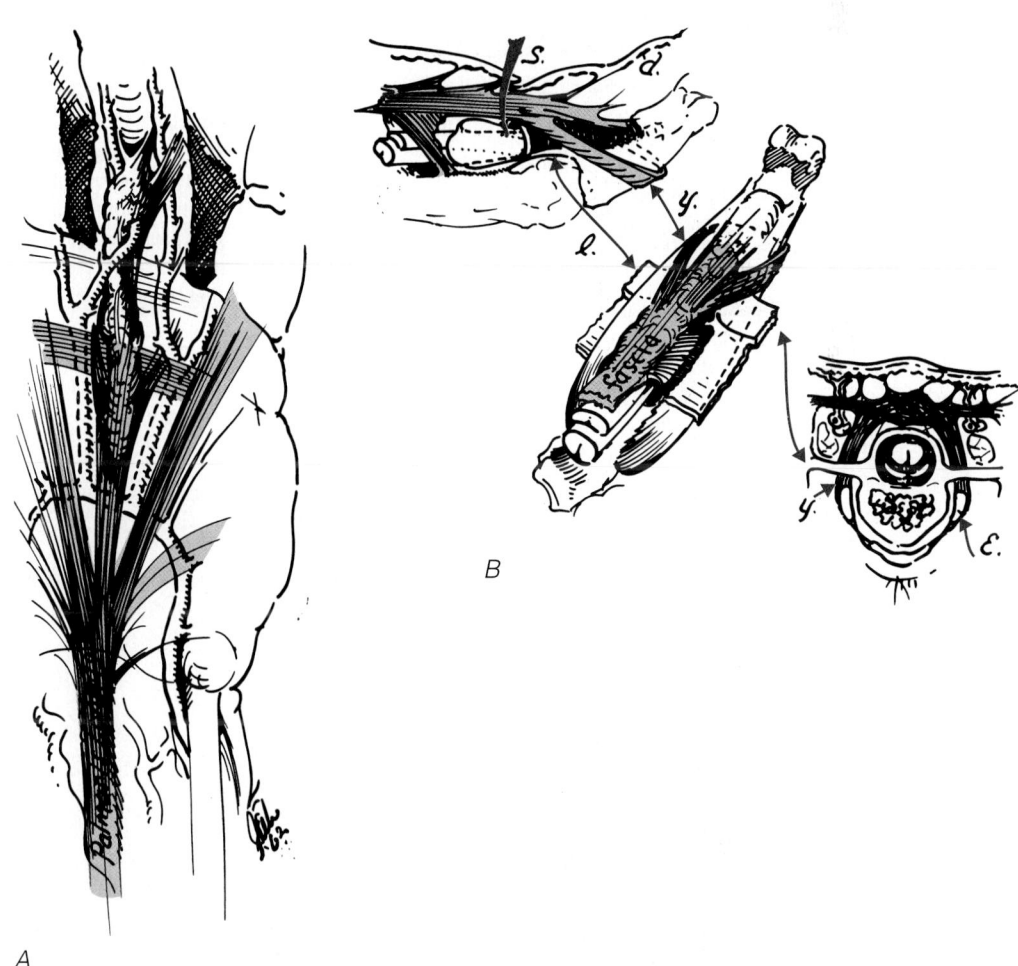

FIG. 43-113. *A.* The anatomy of the palmar fascia is complex when it has been altered by a hypertrophic (Dupuytren's) process; the prime involvement is in the longitudinal fibers and septa. Passing into the digit at the level of the distal palm, the digital nerves may spiral through or around the fascial process itself, making dissection precarious. *B.* As it passes into the finger, the fascia may expand laterally and extend into the fibers of the fibro-osseous sheath, or extend into the lateral bands of the extensor mechanism. The vertical septa are second and pass to the deep fascia to form an integral part of the metacarpophalangeal restraint. [*Reproduced with permission from Littler JW: The Hand, in Cooper P (ed): Craft of Surgery, 2nd ed. Boston: Little, Brown, 1971, p 1385.*]

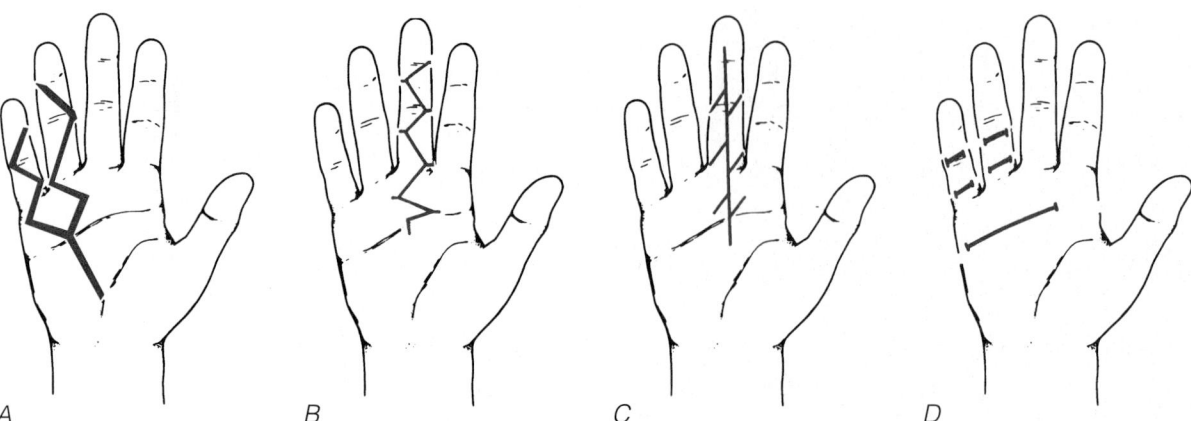

FIG. 43-114. *Four skin incisions for the surgical treatment of Dupuytren's contracture. A. The zigzag incision with its linear extension proximal to the palmar flexion crease. B. The Littler-Bruner incision with small transverse extension. Watson uses these for V-Y-plasty closures; Bedeschi leaves them open in the honeycomb technique. C. The longitudinal incision, which is closed by Z-plasty incisions (oblique incision lines). D. The transverse incisions of McCash's open-palm technique.*

Noninflammatory Arthropathies

Noninflammatory arthropathies include osteoarthritis; heritable abnormalities of cartilage production; primary and secondary osteonecrosis or osteomalacia; endocrine-associated articular changes from thyroid, parathyroid, and pituitary glands and pancreas; hematologic diseases such as hemophilia and hemoglobinopathies; collagen storage diseases; and miscellaneous bone, nerve, and other connective tissue pathologies, including amyloid. Sarcoidosis is an inflammatory arthropathy.

Osteoarthritis. Osteoarthritis is the most common upper extremity arthropathy. Although classically defined as noninflammatory, osteoarthritis is a cartilage disease with at least intermittent low-to-moderate levels of inflammation. Its incidence increases with age. There is a significant hereditary component, especially for women. Patients may demonstrate progressive loss of articular cartilage, seen on radiographs first as diminished joint space, with later subchondral sclerosis and marginal bone spurs or lipping. Joint enlargement as a result of lipping is common. The prevalence of distal interphalangeal joint (Heberden's) and proximal interphalangeal joint (Bouchard's) nodes (Fig. 43-120) is up to 10 times

greater in women, especially for those with a family history. Secondary posttraumatic mechanical osteoarthritis is more common in individuals whose occupations expose them to physical stress or repetitive loads with impact. The inflammatory variant often affects the hands, particularly the interphalangeal joints, and can be clinically and radiographically aggressive. The interphalangeal joints (particularly the terminal interphalangeal joints of the index finger and thumb), the trapeziometacarpal (thumb basilar) joint, and the pantrapezial and radioscaphoid articulations are most frequently affected. With inflammatory problems due to chronic or progressive synovitis, tendon involvement, secondary joint locking, and tendon rupture may contribute to symptoms.

Extensor or flexor tenosynovectomies in the lower forearm, wrist, palm, or digits may be necessary for resistant problems, and should be combined with a supervised postoperative therapy

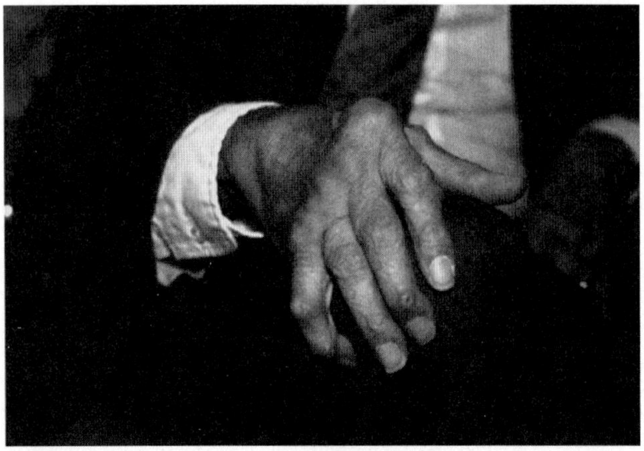

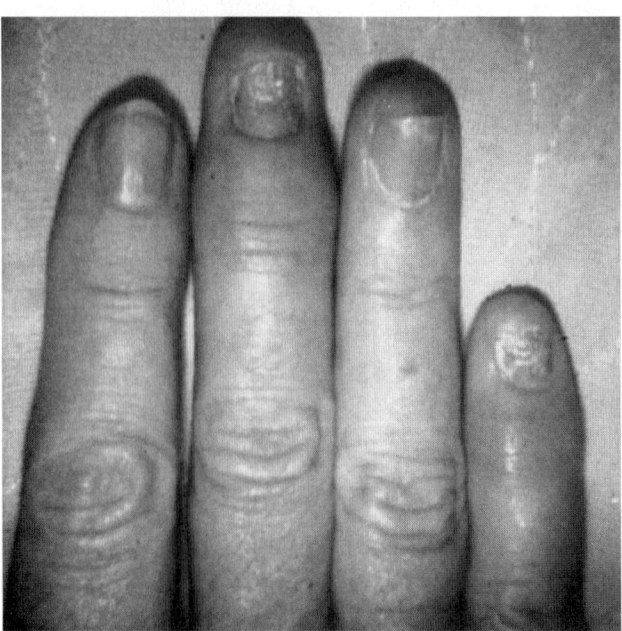

FIG. 43-115. *Deformities of rheumatoid arthritis, with marked ulnar deviation, swan-neck deformity, active synovitis, and nodules.*

FIG. 43-116. *Nail changes typical for psoriasis with distal interphalangeal joint involvement.*

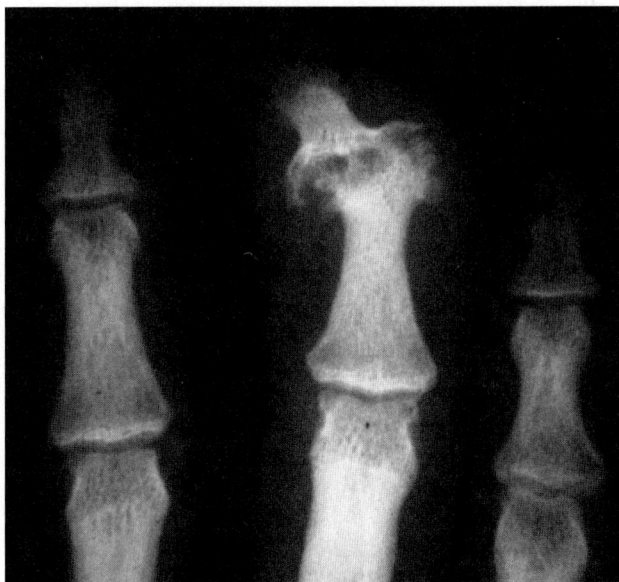

FIG. 43-117. Radiographic changes in gout.

program to recover motion (Fig. 43-121). When tendon ruptures occur, the attritional defects in tendon substance prevent direct repair and require tendon grafts or transfers (Fig. 43-122). Tendon subluxation may occur as a result of tendon disease, or secondarily from joint involvement deep to that tendon.

Focal small-joint deformities are best treated with arthroplasty, especially in MP joints and for the less active older patient, or with arthrodesis at selected limited intercarpal and interphalangeal joints (Figs. 43-123, 43-124, and 43-125). For successful arthrodesis, selection of operative method is not as important as a meticulous, precise technique. Stabilized continuous bone contact over the entire surface to be fused—the presence of good bone stock with

Table 43-5
Inflammatory Arthropathies Affecting the Hands

Systemic autoimmune diseases
Rheumatoid arthritis (RA)
Polymyalgia rheumatica
Systemic lupus erythematosus (SLE)
Systemic sclerosis (scleroderma)
Vasculitis
Polymyositis and dermatomyositis
Adult-onset Still's disease
Remitting seronegative symmetrical synovitis with pitting
    edema (RS$_3$PE)

Spondyloarthropathies
Ankylosing spondylitis (AS)
Reiter's syndrome
Psoriatic arthritis
Inflammatory bowel disease–associated
Reactive arthritis

Rheumatic fever

Crystal arthropathies
Gout
Calcium pyrophosphate dihydrate (CPPD) deposition disease
Apatite crystal deposition disease

Miscellaneous
Infectious arthritis
Sarcoidosis
Leukemia and lymphoma

durable soft-tissue coverage—produces a positive outcome. Living bone provides the most durable arthrodesis. With removal of all the unsightly, painful, prominent osteophytes about the dorsal, palmar, radial, and ulnar joint margins, the results are excellent.

Thumb stiffness, pain, and malalignment produce marked hand impairment. The problems are far greater than might be expected due to the single lesion because of the critical importance of comfortable thumb mobility and stability in precision and power hand use (Figs. 43-126 and 43-127). Thumb basilar arthroplasty yields functional, aesthetic results.

CONGENITAL DEFORMITIES

Failures of development, separation, and segmentation, and intrauterine injury such as amniotic bands/congenital constriction ring syndrome affect mobility, facility, and self-image. Abnormalities of the shoulder and humerus, elbow, forearm, wrist, and hand produce important but widely differing impairments, and all diminish hand facility to different degrees (Fig. 43-128). Among the most common congenital afflictions in the hand are syndactyly and polydactyly as well as polysyndactyly (Fig. 43-129). Consideration of reconstruction should begin when the patient is 3 to 6 months of age, depending on the exact lesions.

Congenital Trigger Thumb

Congenital trigger thumb is common, and may present to the primary pediatric caregiver as a snapping that may or may not be painful, but often presents as fixed flexion of the terminal thumb joint that a parent has recently discovered. Trigger thumbs are more rarely locked in extension. Pathologic findings are localized to the flexor pollicis longus tendon and the proximal annular pulley of the thumb. It is not clear whether the tendon enlargement, known as Notta's node, or thickening of the pulley with relative lessening of the internal diameter of the sheath, is the primary pathology. Only 10 to 20% are bilateral, and at times they are sequential rather than simultaneous. Other trigger fingers may occur in the infant or young child, but only rarely, and they may be associated with other hand and forearm anomalies or systemic diagnoses (e.g., arthrogryposis).

Surgery is conservative management for this problem. There is no justification for using steroid injection to treat congenital trigger thumb. Children who are diagnosed at under 12 months of age may be observed for 6 to 12 months for possible spontaneous correction, because waiting does not compromise outcome in this age group. At any age, when fixed flexion deformity of the thumb interphalangeal joint produces secondary metacarpophalangeal joint hyperextension, or when a child over the age of 2 years initially presents with symptomatic locking, surgery to release the proximal flexor pulley is in order. The thickened tendon nodule is *not* debulked or débrided. Such children are not expected to have permanent loss of interphalangeal extension. If an interphalangeal joint cannot be fully extended at surgery, it means that the pulley has not been released completely until proven otherwise.

TUMORS

Localized masses are common in the hand and upper limb, but most are benign. Most have characteristics that assist in making the diagnosis. The relative rarity of malignant tumors of the musculoskeletal system distal to the elbow can lead to misdiagnosis and undermanagement; however, most malignant (noncutaneous) tumors in the upper limb distal to the elbow arise in soft tissues.

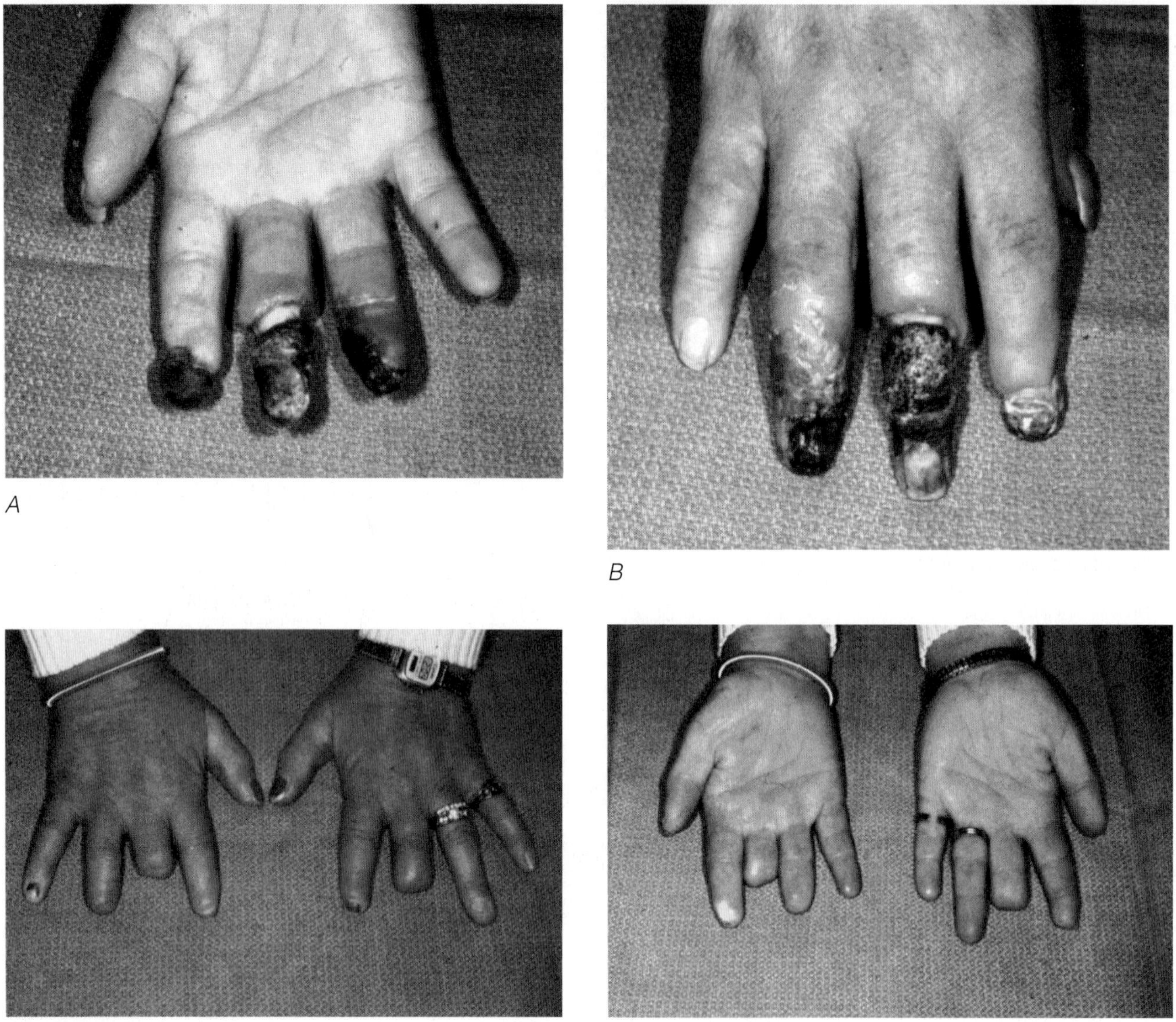

FIG. 43-118. *A* and *B*. Painful gangrene of the distal phalanx of the right index finger and the middle and distal phalanges of the right long and ring fingers in a patient with scleroderma. *C* and *D*. After treatment by amputation, with satisfactory relief of pain and excellent return of hand function.

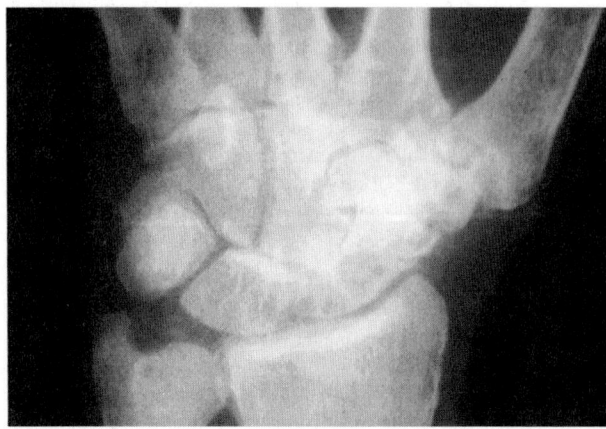

FIG. 43-119. Chondrocalcinosis seen in one of the typical locations for this crystal deposition, at the triangular cartilage of the wrist.

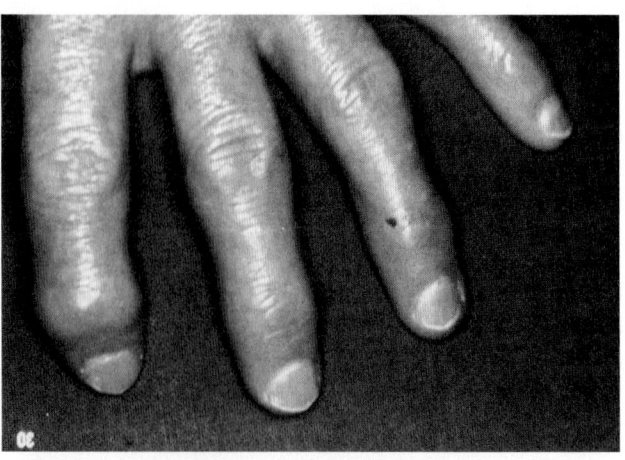

FIG. 43-120. The characteristic appearance of Heberden's nodes in the hand of a patient with osteoarthritis.

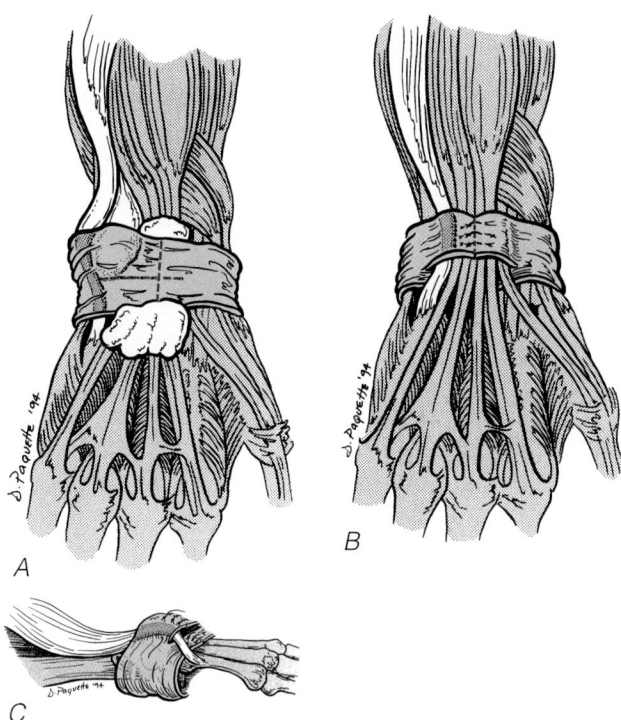

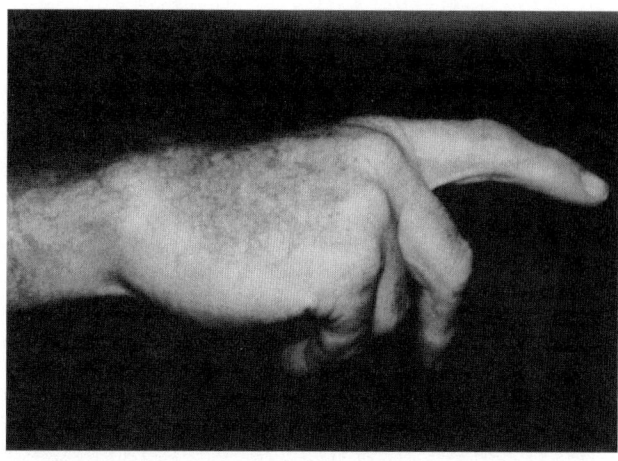

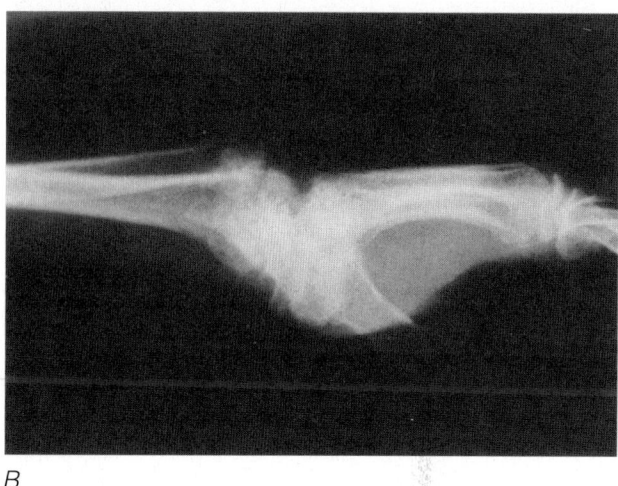

FIG. 43-121. *A.* Dorsal tenosynovectomy is performed through a longitudinal incision centered over Lister's tubercle. The extensor retinaculum over the fourth compartment is incised longitudinally, unroofing adjacent compartments as necessary. *B.* If wrist joint coverage or relocation of the extensor carpi ulnaris tendons is necessary after tenosynovectomy, the retinaculum is incised transversely to the level of the fifth compartment. The distal half is placed deep to the extensor tendons, providing a gliding surface. The remainder of the retinaculum is sutured dorsally to prevent tendon bowstringing. *C.* The intact edge of the retinaculum acts as a pulley, restricting volar translation of the extensor carpi ulnaris tendons.

FIG. 43-122. *A.* Rupture of multiple extensor tendons. Lack of active extension of the middle, ring, and small fingers is secondary to rupture of extensor digitorum communis III, IV, and V, and extensor digiti minimi. Note the prominent ulnar head. *B.* Lateral radiograph demonstrates the arthritic, prominent ulnar head.

Every mass, particularly those that are atypical in appearance or location, should be diagnosed with staging and imaging procedures leading to careful incisional biopsy. Hand masses tend to present earlier, even though they may be smaller, because of their superficial location. Enlarging, symptomatic masses are evaluated with history, laboratory studies, imaging by plain films, ultrasonography, scintigraphy, CT, or MRI scans. Biopsy is the last step in diagnosis, and only very small lesions or lesions that are typical should be excised initially.

Benign Neoplasms

Benign tumors are subdivided into three categories:

1. *Latent benign* tumors arise during childhood and may heal spontaneously. Most are well encapsulated, with a clearly defined plane between the tumor capsule and normal surrounding tissue. In bone, the growth process is slow, allowing a margin of mature cortical bone to develop and contain the lesion.
2. *Active benign* lesions continue to grow, albeit slowly, and are not self-limited in size or by patient age. The tumor is well encapsulated, but the reactive zone is thicker and less mature than in the preceding category. Within bone, the tumor has an irregular shape that alters the internal or external bone architecture. Surgical management is dictated by determining the grade of the lesion and adequacy of local resection. Operative method is determined by the anatomic setting and the implications for altered musculoskeletal part function.

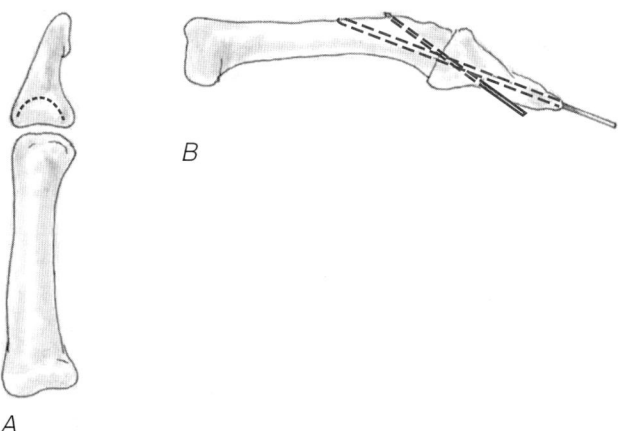

FIG. 43-123. *A.* Bone surface preparation for distal interphalangeal arthrodesis. *B.* Lateral view with Kirschner wires in place.

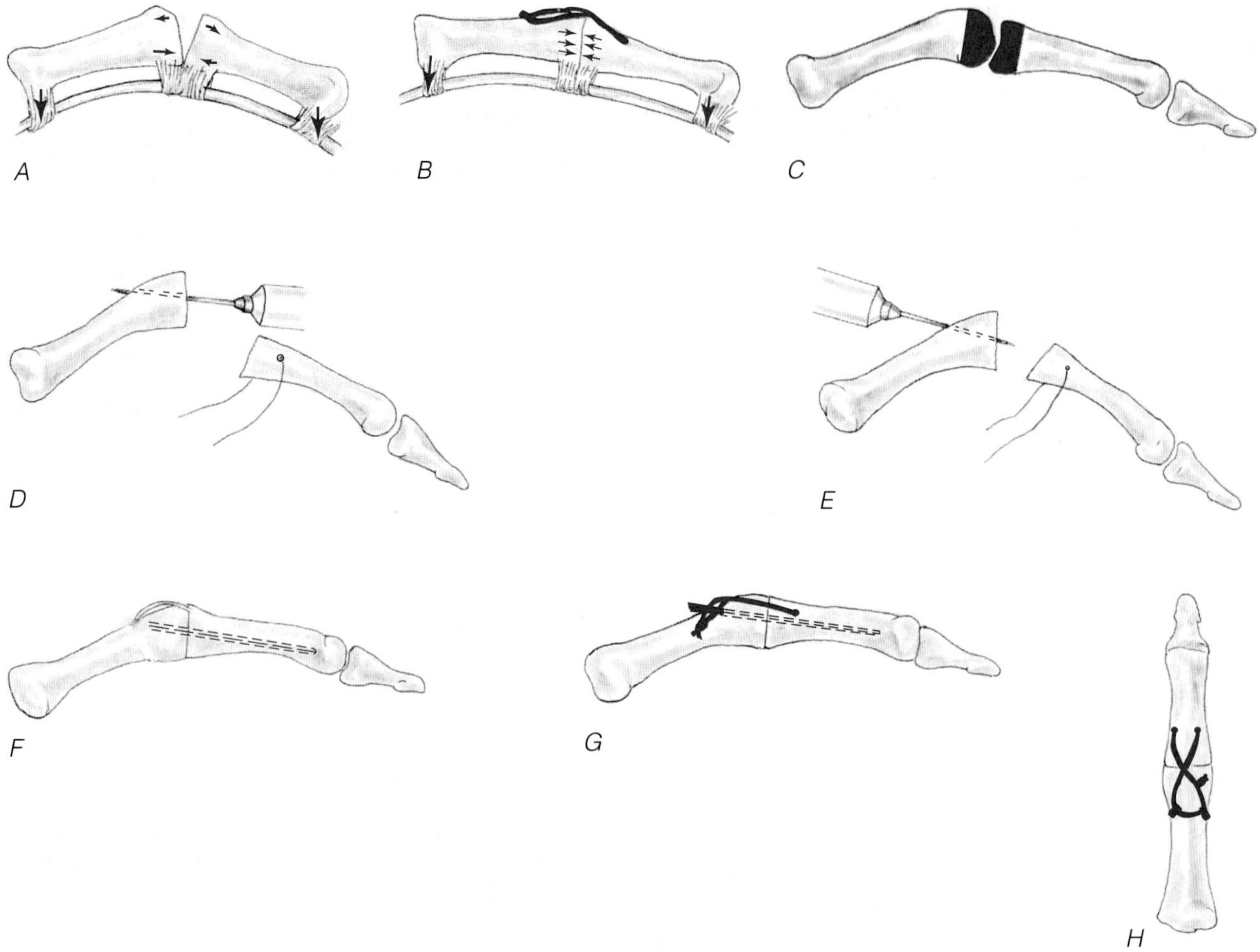

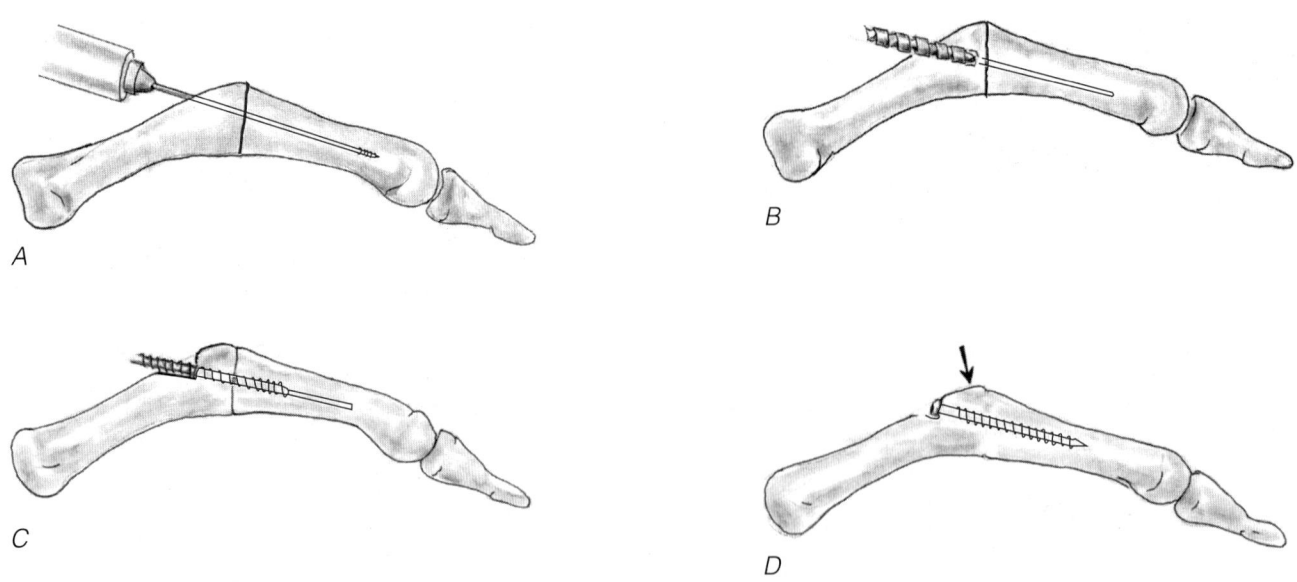

FIG. 43-124. *A.* Flexion of interphalangeal joint creates tension forces on the dorsal aspect and compression forces on the volar aspect of the joint. *B.* Placement of a tension band dorsal to the joint axis neutralizes the tension forces and uses the flexor moment force to apply compression loads across the arthrodesis site. *C–H.* Tension-band technique for proximal interphalangeal joint arthrodesis.

FIG. 43-125. Compression-screw fixation for proximal interphalangeal joint arthrodesis. *A.* Smaller-diameter drill bit through proximal and middle phalangeal segments. *B.* Overdrilling the proximal phalanx with a larger-diameter drill bit. *C.* Screw tap used to tap a smaller hole in the middle phalangeal segment. *D.* Compression screw placed. The dorsal bridge (*arrow*) in the proximal phalanx is subject to fracture when this technique is used.

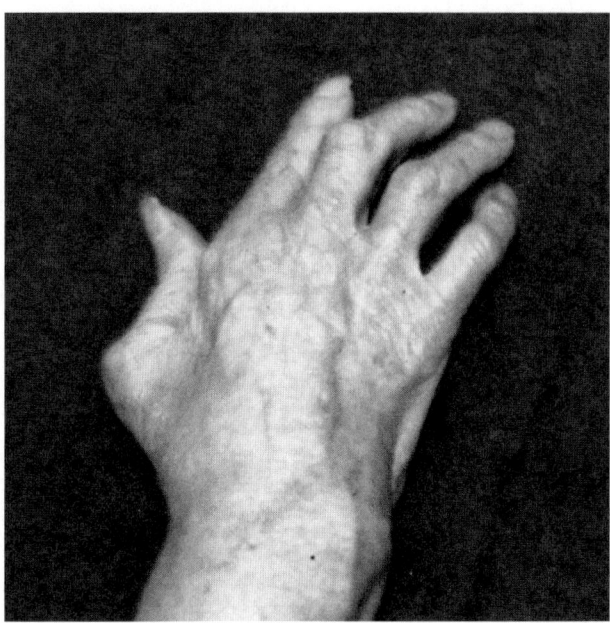

FIG. 43-126. Thumb with metacarpophalangeal flexion, interphalangeal extension, and carpometacarpal abduction—the boutonnière deformity.

3. *Aggressive benign* lesions do not metastasize, but are more difficult—or very difficult—to control locally. These lesions do not have clear zones of capsular containment. Nodules or extensions of the tumor may grow out into nearby normal tissue, such as with Dupuytren's contracture or with more aggressive and diffuse fibroblastic proliferations (e.g., fibromatoses or extra-abdominal desmoids). Excision through the reactive zone exposes these tumor projections at the surgical margins, allowing microscopic contamination into unaffected tissue. Failure to fully remove the tumor ensures local recurrence; however, as these are not cancers, such operations (e.g., with Dupuytren's) may be appropriate and usefully adequate, if not curative.

Malignant Neoplasms

Surgical staging and treatment definitions and principles for true malignant tumors are outlined in Tables 43-6 and 43-7. These rare but potentially lethal neoplasms should be treated at centers familiar with the combination of surgical, medical, and radiotheraputic protocols needed to maximize functional salvage and patient survival. These patients and their dangerous tumors are not well handled in the community setting; if suspected, patients should be referred for biopsy and treatment.

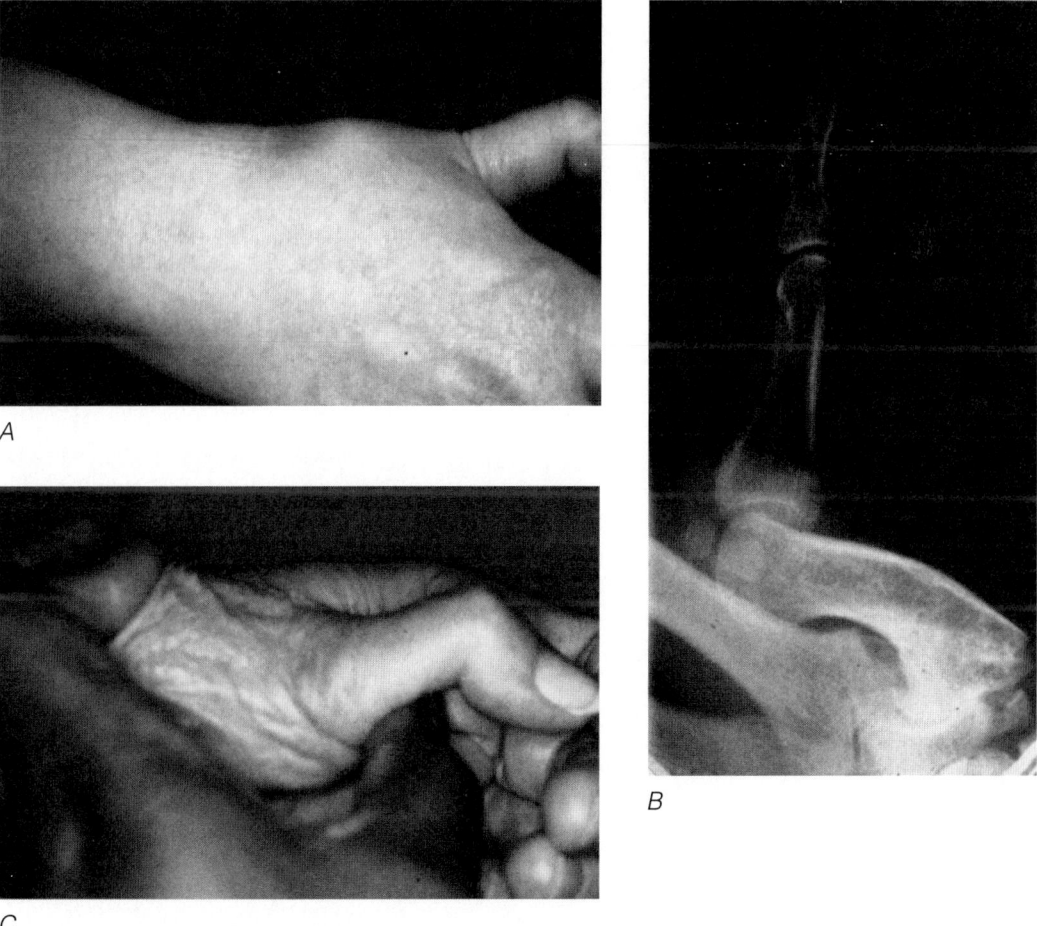

A

B

C

FIG. 43-127. *A, B,* and *C.* Thumb carpometacarpal joint adduction and subluxation with secondary metacarpophalangeal extension and interphalangeal flexion, commonly known as a swan-neck deformity, are seen in these two patients. The patient shown in *B* and *C* has primary carpometacarpal degeneration and first metacarpal adduction with secondary compensatory instability and collapse of the two more distal joints.

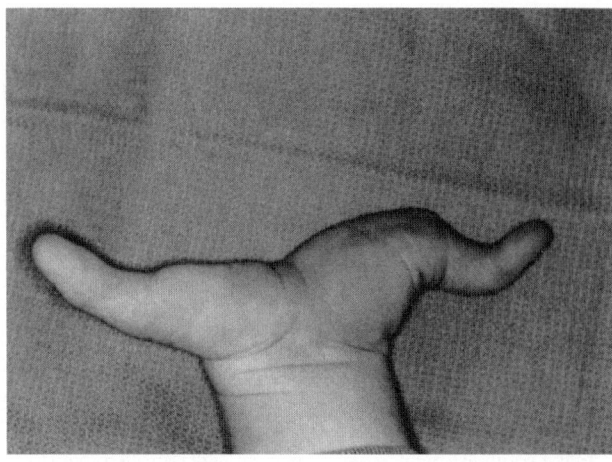

A

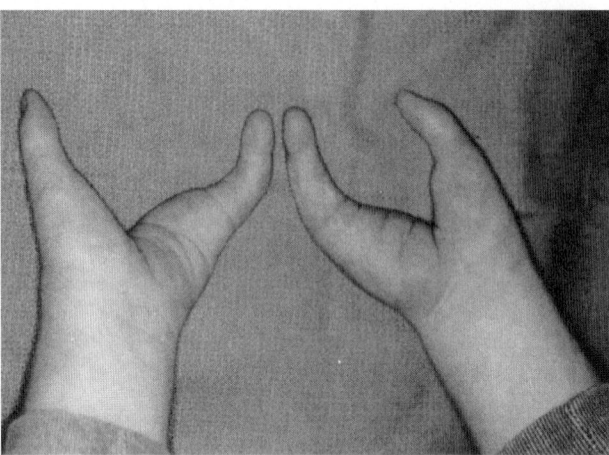

B

FIG. 43-128. Two-digit cleft hand, untreated surgically, demonstrates considerable mobility and dexterity.

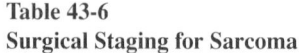

Table 43-6
Surgical Staging for Sarcoma

Stage	Grade	Site
IA	Low (G_1)	Intracompartmental (T_1)
IB	Low (G_1)	Extracompartmental (T_2)
IIA	High (G_2)	Extracompartmental (T_1)
IIB	High (G_2)	Extracompartmental (T_2)
III	Regional or distant metastasis (M); any (G); any (T)	

Specific Common Tumors

Ganglion

Joint and tendon ganglions (or ganglia) are among the most common benign soft-tissue tumor masses in the upper extremity, representing up to 50 to 75% of reported tumors. Although they can be located anywhere, the majority are at the middorsal wrist; the volar radial wrist; the digital flexor sheath at the metacarpal flexion crease (seed or pea ganglia that are extremely small, but hard and tender); and at the dorsum of the distal interphalangeal joint and nail base (mucous cyst). Many of the latter are associated with secondary nail deformity, particularly in the older population (see Fig. 43-3).

Treatment options include no directed care, closed rupture by impact, hypodermic needle aspiration plus steroid injection, and operative excision. Rupture by digital pressure or with a swift blow is unnecessarily traumatic and has little chance of long-term success. Aspiration and steroid instillation may be of considerable value, particularly when the expanding lesion has not been diagnosed or is associated with discomfort. At the dorsal wrist, the most common site of origin is from the scapholunate interosseous ligament, and the smaller, occult ganglion may account for a significant amount of dorsal wrist pain, particularly in the female teenage population. Volar ganglions are most commonly situated between the flexor carpi radialis tendon and the radial artery, at or just proximal to the wrist, near the radioscaphoid joint. Most arise from the radiocarpal or intercarpal capsule. Aspiration with injection may be entirely

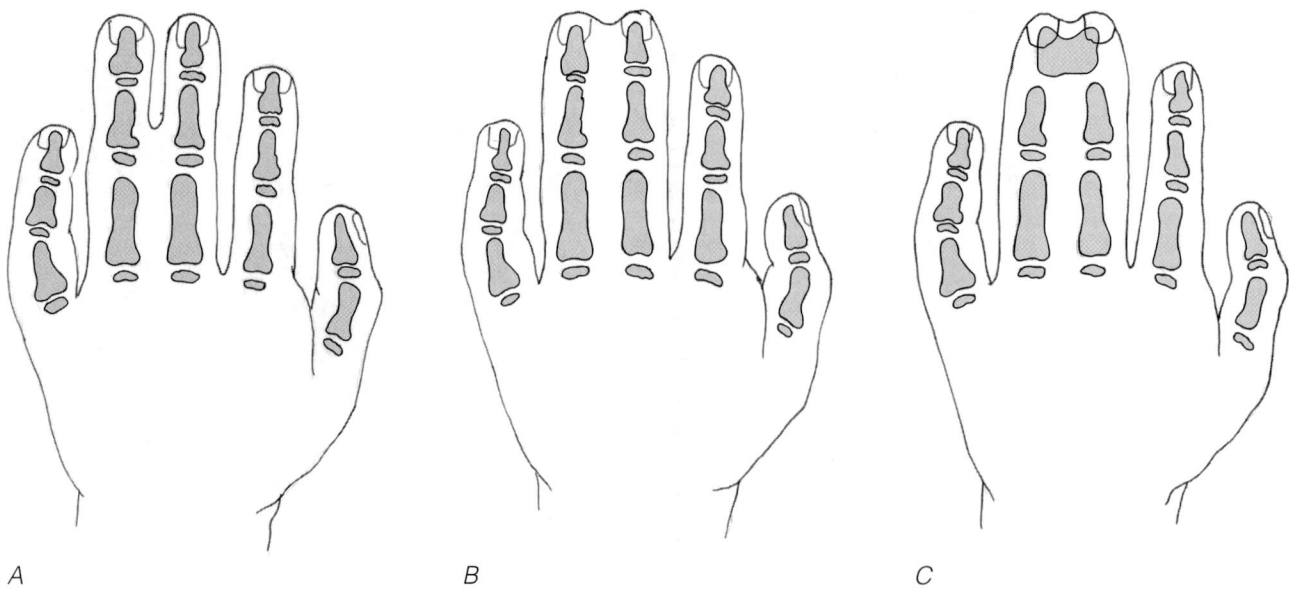

A   *B*   *C*

FIG. 43-129. Syndactyly classification. *A.* Incomplete simple syndactyly. *B.* Complete simple syndactyly. *C.* Complete complex syndactyly.

Table 43-7
Musculoskeletal Oncologic Surgical Procedures

Margin	Local	Amputation
Intracapsular	Curettage/debulking	Debulking amputation
Marginal	Marginal excision	Marginal amputation
Wide	Wide local excision	Through bone amputation
Radical	Radical local excision	Disarticulation of extremity

curative for the flexor sheath ganglion that appears as a 3- to 10-mm hard mass at or just distal to the metacarpophalangeal joint flexion crease. Aspiration and injection of the mucous cyst distal interphalangeal joint ganglion is less likely to be curative. Repeated drainage at this site increases the risk of joint contamination and secondary sepsis.

Surgical excision must include the capsular base origin, sometimes referred to as the stalk or root. Deflating the ganglion during surgery by incising it *before* dissecting around it is, in this author's opinion, much easier than trying to protect nearby cutaneous nerves or vessels while still avoiding an excessively large skin incision around the still-inflated cyst.

Giant Cell Tumor of Tendon Sheath (Fibroxanthoma)

Also known as nodular tenosynovitis, fibroxanthoma, giant cell tumor of synovium, and pigmented villonodular synovitis, the giant cell tumor of tendon sheath is the most common solid soft-tissue tumor in the hand. It is more frequent in females, and patients are generally between the ages of 30 and 60 years. It presents as a firm, lobular, nontender, slowly enlarging mass in the palm, finger, or thumb. It is more often seen on the palmar surface, given that synovium is present in the fingers only about the flexor tendons and in the joints. Secondary tendon, joint, and skeletal invasion is well known (Fig. 43-130). Effective treatment requires meticulously complete excision, with care taken not to injure the neurovascular bundles or the critical flexor sheath pulleys. Recurrences in up to 10% of patients within 2 years are seen, and patients are best followed for that interval. Late regrowth may occur up to a decade later, though such late recurrences may really be entirely new lesions.

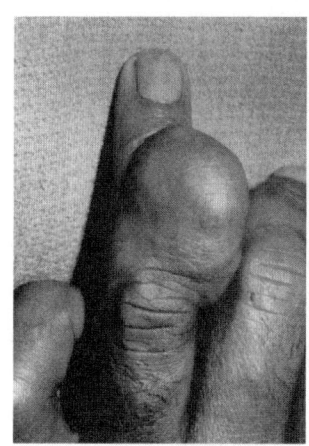
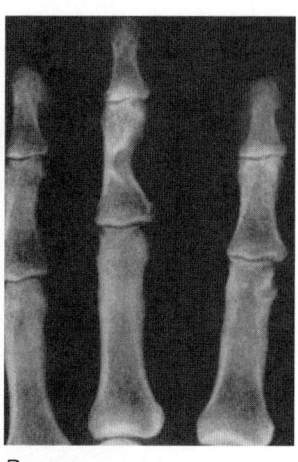

A   *B*

FIG. 43-130. *Giant cell tumor of soft tissue. A. Slowly enlarging soft-tissue mass surrounding middle phalanx. B. Radiograph demonstrating extrinsic pressure from mass causing saucerization and sclerotic reaction of middle phalangeal diaphysis.*

Lipoma

Lipomas are benign tumors that contain mature fat cells. They are rare in people under the age of 20 years. Some are multifocal. Tumors usually are asymptomatic, but are gradually enlarging, soft to moderately firm masses. When they arise near a nerve or in a nerve tunnel, they may cause secondary symptoms. Lipomas can be superficial, subcutaneous, or intramuscular, and in the hand also may be large and deep. Surgical treatment is for diagnosis of the unknown enlarging mass or for improving functional impairment. Recurrences are rare, but more often occur with intramuscular lesions whose dissection is more difficult (Fig. 43-131).

Enchondroma

Enchondromas are the most common cartilage lesions of bone, and are most frequently found at the small tubular bones in the hand. They can present at any age, but commonly are found in

FIG. 43-131. *Large palmar lipoma. A. Radiograph with the water density mass outlined. B. Intraoperative photograph demonstrating a large lipoma, which compromised the motor branch of the median nerve.*

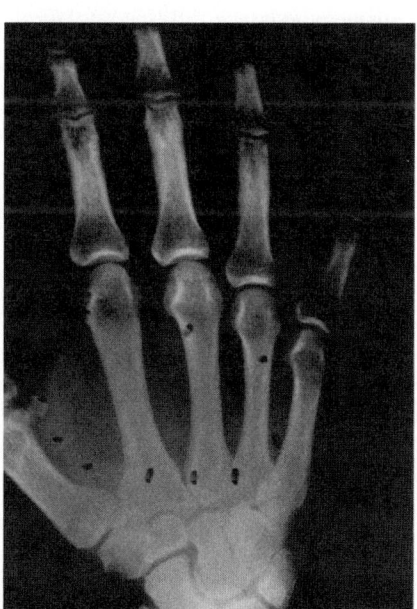
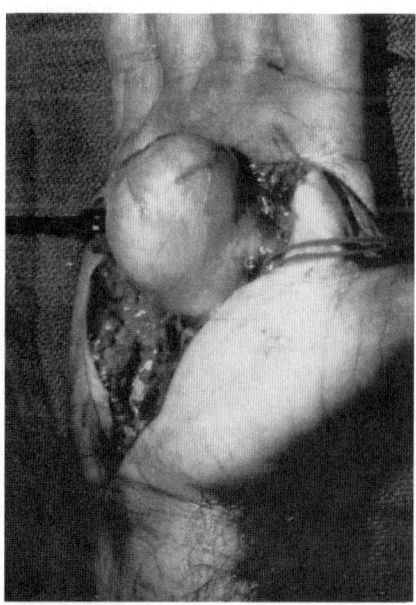

A   *B*

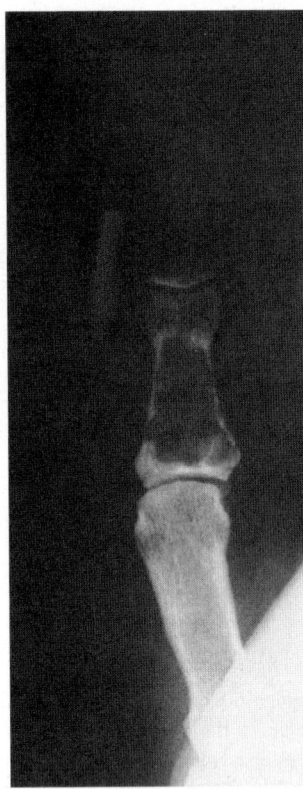

FIG. 43-132. Enchondroma on the proximal phalanx of the thumb. Radiograph demonstrating lobulated epiphyseal-metaphyseal lucency with endosteal scalloping and thinning. No calcifications are visible.

young adults. Virtually all enchondromas first present as pathologic fractures, although a small number may be found as asymptomatic enlargements of a bone. Radiographs usually are diagnostic (Fig. 43-132). Surgical treatment may be for diagnosis or therapy. Pathologic fractures may heal, but the tumor is unlikely to regress spontaneously with fracture union. It is more efficient and less costly to treat the fracture and the tumor together, but some prefer to allow the fracture to heal while waiting to see if the tumor resolves spontaneously. Treating the lesion and the fracture simultaneously limits the disability to just one interval. Thorough lesional curettage is required, and autogenous bone grafting is appropriate; some bones heal without added graft. Incidental discovery of small asymptomatic enchondromas does not mandate treatment. Aggressive and malignant tumors distal to the elbow are uncommon, but are more likely to be of soft-tissue origin.

Bibliography

General Considerations

Arateri E, Regesta G, et al: Carpal tunnel syndrome appearing with prominent skin symptoms. *Arch Dermatol* 120:517, 1984.

Mees RA: Eed verschijnsel by polyneuritis arsenicosa. *Ned Tijdschr Geneeskd* 1:391, 1919.

Murphy WA, Totty WG, et al: Musculoskeletal system, in Lee JKT, Sagel SS, Stanley RJ (eds): *Computed Body Tomography with MRI Correlation*, 2nd ed. New York: Raven, 1989, p 899.

Scher RK, Daniel CR III: *Nails: Therapy, Diagnosis, Surgery*. Philadelphia: WB Saunders, 1990, pp 130, 167.

Surgical Principles

Adler VG, Burmon D, et al: Absorption of hexachlorophene from infants' skin. *Lancet* 2:384, 1972.

Ahlo A, Kankaapaa V: Management of fractured scaphoid bone. *Acta Orthop Scand* 46:737, 1975.

Alexander JW, Fischer JE, et al: The influence of hair removal methods on wound infections. *Arch Surg* 118:347, 1983.

Arzimanoglou A, Skiadaresis SM: Study of internal fixation by screws of oblique fractures in long bones. *J Bone Joint Surg Am* 34:219, 1952.

Ashkenaze DM, Ruby LK: Metacarpal fractures and dislocations. *Orthop Clin North Am* 23:19, 1992.

Atasoy A, Loakimidis E, et al: Reconstruction of the amputated fingertip with a triangular volar flap. *J Bone Joint Surg* 52A:921, 1970.

Ayliffe GAJ: Surgical scrub and skin disinfection. *Infect Control* 4:23, 1984.

Belsky MR, Eaton RG, et al: Closed reduction and internal fixation of proximal phalangeal fracture. *J Hand Surg* 9A:725, 1984.

Beasley RW: Reconstruction of amputated fingertips. *Plast Reconstr Surg* 44:349, 1969.

Bennett JE: Upper arm tourniquet tolerance in hand surgery (letter). *Plast Reconstr Surg* 52:660, 1973.

Blair JW, Moskal MJ: Revision amputation achieving maximum function and minimizing problems. *Hand Clin* 17:457, 2001.

Blair WF, Steyers CM: Extensor tendon injuries. *Orthop Clin North Am* 23:141, 1992.

Branemark PI, et al: Local tissue effects of wound disinfectants. *Acta Chir Scand* 357(Suppl): 166, 1966.

Bridenbaugh LD: Patient management for neural blockage: Selection, management, premedication and supplementation, in Cousins MJ, Bridenbaugh LD (eds): *Neural Blockade in Clinical Anesthesia and Management of Pain*, 2nd ed. Philadelphia: JB Lippincott, 1988, p 191.

Bunker TD, Potter B, et al: Continuous passive motion following flexor tendon repair. *J Hand Surg* 14B:406, 1989.

Bunnell S: *Surgery of the Hand*. Philadelphia: JB Lippincott, 1944, p 90.

Butcher HR, Ballinger WF, et al: Hexachlorophene concentrations in the blood of operating room personnel. *Arch Surg* 107:70, 1973.

Chiu DTW: Transthecal digital block: Flexor tendon sheath used for anesthetic infusion. *J Hand Surg Am* 15:471, 1990.

Chow JA, Thomes LJ, et al: Controlled motion rehabilitation after flexor tendon repair and grafting. *J Bone Joint Surg* 70B:590, 1988.

Cooney WP, Agee JM, et al: Symposium: Management of intra-articular fractures of the distal radius. *Contemp Orthop* 21:71, 1990.

Cooney WP, Dobyns JH, et al: Nonunion of the scaphoid: Analysis of the results from bone grafting. *J Hand Surg* 5A:343, 1980.

Cooney WP: Fractures of the distal radius: A modern treatment-based classification. *Orthop Clin North Am* 24:211, 1993.

Coonrad RW, Knight WE: Use of the tourniquet in the lower and upper extremities without general anesthesia. *J Bone Joint Surg* 39A:463, 1957.

Cruse PJE, Foord R: The epidemiology of wound infection: A 10-year prospective study of 62,939 wounds. *Surg Clin North Am* 60:27, 1980.

Cushing H: Pneumatic tourniquet, with especial reference to their use in craniotomies. *Med News* 84:577, 1904.

Dabezies EJ, Mathews R, et al: Injuries to the carpus: Fractures of the scaphoid. *Orthopaedics* 5:1510, 1982.

Dodds SD, Cornelissen S, Jossan S, Wolfe SW: A biomechanical comparison of fragment-specific fixation and augmented external fixation for intra-articular distal radius fractures. *J Hand Surg (Am)* 28:88, 2003.

Drefuss UY, Singer M: Human bites of the hand: A study of one hundred six patients. *J Hand Surg* 10A:884, 1985.

Dushoff IM: Hand surgery under wrist block and local infiltration anesthesia, using an upper arm tourniquet (letter). *Plast Reconstr Surg* 51:685, 1973.

Edwards SA, Harper GD, Giddins GE: Efficacy of forearm vs. upper arm tourniquet for local anaesthetic surgery of the hand. *J Hand Surg [Br]* 25:573, 2000.

Engkvist O, Lundborg G: Rupture of the extensor pollicis longus tendon after fracture of the lower end of radius: A clinical and microangiographic study. *Hand* 11:76, 1979.

Estersohn H, Sourifman H: The minimum effective midthigh tourniquet pressure. *J Foot Surg* 21:281, 1982.

Evans RB: Early active short arc motion for the repaired central slip. *J Hand Surg (Am)* 19:991, 1994.

Expert Panel of the Cosmetic Ingredient Review: Final report of the safety assessment for chloroxylenol. Washington, DC, 1984.

Flatt AE: Minor hand injuries. *J Bone Joint Surg* 37B:117, 1955.

Garibaldi RA, et al: The impact of preoperative skin disinfection on preventing intraoperative wound contamination. *Infect Control Hosp Epidemiol* 9:109, 1988.

Gatewood: Plastic repair of finger defects without hospitalization. *JAMA* 87:1479, 1926.

Gellman H, Caputo RJ, et al: Comparison of short and long thumb-spica casts for nondisplaced fractures of the carpal scaphoid. *J Bone Joint Surg* 71A:354, 1989.

Guirguis EM, Bell MSG: The wrist tourniquet: An alternative technique in hand surgery. *J Hand Surg* 15A:516, 1990.

Gutmann E: Effect of delay of innervation on recovery of muscle after nerve lesions. *J Neurophysiol* 11:277, 1948.

Hart RG, Uehara DT, et al: Extensor tendon injuries of the hand. *Emerg Med Clin North Am* 11:637, 1993.

Heim U, Pheiffer KM: General techniques for the internal fixation of small fracture; The hand, in *Small Fragment Set Manual: Internal Fixation of Small Fractures,* 3rd ed. New York: Springer-Verlag, 1987, pp 31, 179.

Herbert TJ, Fisher WE: Management of the fractured scaphoid using a new bone screw. *J Bone Joint Surg* 66B:114, 1984.

Harvey FJ, Harvey PM: Three rare causes of extensor tendon rupture. *J Hand Surg* 14A:957, 1989.

Hirai Y, Yoshida K, Yamanaka K, et al: An anatomic study of the extensor tendons of the human hand. *J Hand Surg (Am)* 26:1009, 2001.

Hove LM: Fractures of the hand: Distribution and relative incidence. *Scand J Plast Reconstr Surg* 27:317, 1993.

Howard FM: Ulnar nerve palsy in wrist fractures. *J Bone Joint Surg* 43A:1197, 1961.

Hochberg J, Murray GF: Principles of operative surgery: Antisepsis, technique, sutures, and drains, in Sabiston D (ed): *Textbook of Surgery: The Biological Basis of Modern Surgical Practice.* Philadelphia: WB Saunders, 1991, p 210.

Hueston JT: Local flap repair of fingertip injuries. *Plast Reconstr Surg* 37:349, 1966.

Itoh Y, Horiuti Y, et al: Extensor tendon involvement in Smith's and Galeazzi's fracture. *J Hand Surg* 12A:535, 1987.

Jepsen OB, Bruttomesso KA: The effectiveness of preoperative skin preparations: An integrative review of the literature. *AORN J* 58:447, 1993.

Jupiter JB, Koniuch MP, et al: The management of delayed union and nonunion of the metacarpals and phalanges. *J Hand Surg* 10A:457, 1985.

Jupiter JB, Herndon JH: Acute fractures of the scaphoid. *J Am Acad Orthop Surg (US)* 8:225, 2000.

Kaempfe F, Peimer CA: Quick fixation of skin grafts. *J Hand Surg* 16A:761, 1991.

Kaplan EB: Anatomy, injuries, and treatment of the extensor apparatus of the hand and fingers. *Clin Orthop* 13:24, 1959.

Kaul AF, Jewett JF: Agents and techniques for disinfection of the skin. *Surg Gynecol Obstet* 152:677, 1981.

Klenerman L: The tourniquet in surgery. *J Bone Joint Surg* 44B:937, 1962.

Kulekampff D, Persky MA: Brachial plexus anaesthesia: Its indications, technique, and dangers. *Ann Surg* 87:883, 1923.

Kutler W: A new method for fingertip amputation. *JAMA* 133:29, 1947.

Larson E: Guideline for use of topical antimicrobial agents. *Am J Infect Control* 16:253, 1988.

Larson EL, Eke PI, et al: Quantity of soap as a variable in handwashing. *Infect Control* 8:371, 1987.

Larson EL, Leyden J, et al: Physiologic and microbiologic changes in skin related to frequent handwashings. *Infect Control* 7:59, 1986.

Lee SG, Jupiter JB: Phalangeal and metacarpal fractures of the hand. *Hand Clin* 16:323, 2000.

Lie KK, Magargle RK, et al: Free full-thickness skin grafts from the palm to cover defects of the fingers. *J Bone Joint Surg* 52A:559, 1970.

Lily HA, Lowbury EJL: Transient skin flora. *J Clin Pathol* 31:919, 1978.

Lowburg EJL, Lily HA: Disinfection of the skin of operation sites. *Br Med J* 2:1039, 1960.

Lowbury EJL, Lily HA: Use of 4 percent chlorhexidine detergent solution (Hibiscrub) and other methods of skin disinfection. *Br Med J* 1:510, 1973.

Mann RJ, Hoffeld TA, et al: Human bites of the hand: Twenty years of experience. *J Hand Surg* 2:97, 1977.

Maki DJ, Zilz MA, et al: Evaluation of antibacterial efficacy of four agents for hand washing. *Curr Chemother Infect Dis* 11:1089, 1977.

MacKenzie I: Preoperative skin preparation and surgical outcome. *J Hosp Infect II* (Suppl B):27, 1988.

McElfresh E, Dobyns J: Intra-articular metacarpal head fractures. *J Hand Surg* 8:383, 1983.

Miller JM, Jackson DA, et al: The microbicidal property of pHisoHex. *Mil Med* 127:576, 1962.

MMWR Update: Research reinforced doubts about need for prep shaves. *Hosp Infect Control* 82, Monograph, 1989.

Neimkin RJ, Smith RJ: Double tourniquet with linked mercury manometers for hand surgery. *J Hand Surg* 8:938, 1983.

Newport ML, Blair WF, et al: Long-term results of extensor tendon repair. *J Hand Surg* 15A:961, 1990.

Nisenfield FG, Neviaser RJ: Fracture of the hook of the hamate: A diagnosis easily missed. *J Trauma* 14:612, 1974.

Novak CB, Kelly L, et al: Sensory recovery after median nerve grafting. *J Hand Surg* 17A:59, 1992.

Patton HS: Split-skin grafts from hypothenar area for fingertip avulsions. *Plast Reconstr Surg* 43:436, 1969.

Pedowitz RA, Gershuni DH, et al: Effects of reperfusion intervals on skeletal muscle injury beneath and distal to a pneumatic tourniquet. *J Hand Surg* 17:345, 1992.

Pedowitz RA, Gershuni DH, et al: Muscle injury induced beneath and distal to a pneumatic tourniquet: A quantitative animal study of effects of tourniquet pressure and duration. *J Hand Surg* 16:610, 1991.

Polivy KD, Millender LH, et al: Fractures of the hook of the hamate: A failure of clinical diagnosis. *J Hand Surg* 10A:101, 1985.

Reybouck G: Handwashing and hand disinfection. *J Hosp Infect* 8:5, 1986.

Reyes FA, Latta LL: Conservative management of difficult phalangeal fractures. *Clin Orthop* 214:23, 1987.

Rockwell WB, Butler PN, Byrne BA: Extensor tendon anatomy, injury, and reconstruction. *Plast Reconstr Surg* 106:1592, 2000.

Rüedi TP, Burri C, et al: Stable internal fixation of fractures of the hand. *J Trauma* 11:381, 1971.

Russe O: Fracture of the carpal navicular: Diagnosis, nonoperative treatment, and operative treatment. *J Bone Joint Surg* 43A:759, 1960.

Schenck RR, Cheema TA: Hypothenar skin grafts for fingertip reconstruction. *J Hand Surg* 9A:750, 1984.

Seddon HJ: Three types of nerve injury. *Brain* 66:238, 1943.

Seropian R, Reynolds BM: Wound infections after preoperative depilatory versus razor preparations. *Am J Surg* 121:251, 1971.

Smylie HG, Logie JRC, et al: From PHisoHex to Hibiscrub. *Br Med J* 4:586, 1973.

Soyer AD: Fractures of the base of the first metacarpal: Current treatment options. *J Am Acad Orthop Surg (US)* 7:403, 1999.

Steel WM: The AO small fragment set in hand fractures. *Hand* 10:246, 1978.

Stern PJ: Fractures of the metacarpals and phalanges, in Green DP (ed): *Operative Hand Surgery,* 3rd ed. New York: Churchill-Livingstone, 1993, p 695.

Stern PJ, Wieser MJ, et al: Complications of plate fixation in the hand skeleton. *Clin Orthop* 214:59, 1987.

Strickland JW: Flexor tenolysis. *Hand Clin* 1:121, 1985.

Sunderland S, Ray LJ: Denervation changes in mammalian striated muscle. *J Neurol Neurosurg Psychiatry* 13:159, 1950.

Szabo RM, Manske D: Displaced fractures of the scaphoid. *Clin Orthop* 230:30, 1988.

Taleisnik J, Gelberman RH, et al: The extensor retinaculum at the wrist. *J Hand Surg* 9A:495, 1984.

Thompson JS, Peimer CA: Extensor tendon injuries, in Chapman MW, Madison M (eds): *Operative Orthopaedics,* 3rd ed. Philadelphia: Lippincott Williams & Wilkins, 2001, p 1495.

Thurman RT, Trumble TE, Hanel DP, et al: Two-, four-, and six-strand zone II flexor tendon repairs: An in-situ biomechanical comparison using a cadaver model. *J Hand Surg (Am)* 23:261, 1998.

Trumble TE, Clarke T, Kreder HJ: Non-union of the scaphoid. Treatment with cannulated screws compared with treatment with Herbert screws. *J Bone Joint Surg (Am)* 78:1829, 1996.

Tsuchida H: Experimental study of the tendon repair: 2nd report. *Proc Jpn Soc Surg Hand* 9:87.

Vaughan-Jackson OJ: Rupture of extensor tendons by attrition of the interior radioulnar joint: Report of two cases. *J Bone Joint Surg* 30:528, 1948.

Verdan CE: Primary and secondary repair of flexor and extensor tendon injuries, in Flynn JE (ed): *Hand Surgery*, 2nd ed. Baltimore: Williams & Wilkins, 1975, p 149.

Werntz JR, Chesher SP, et al: A new dynamic splint for postoperative treatment of flexor tendon injury. *J Hand Surg* 14A:559, 1989.

Willson RL: Management of acute extensor tendon injuries, in Hunter JM, Schneider LH, Mackin EJ (eds): *Tendon Surgery in the Hand.* St. Louis: CV Mosby, 1987, p 336.

Winnie AP: *Plexus Anesthesia*, Vol. 1: *Perivascular Techniques of Brachial Plexus Block.* Philadelphia: WB Saunders, 1983.

Zachary SV, Peimer CA: Salvaging the "unsalvageable" digit. *Hand Clin* 13:239, 1997.

Zhao C, Amadio PC, Momose T, et al: The effect of suture technique on adhesion formation after flexor tendon repair for partial lacerations in a canine model. *J Trauma* 51:917, 2001.

Complications of Trauma

Bonica JJ: *The Management of Pain.* Philadelphia: Lea & Febiger, 1953.

Gelberman RH, Szabo RM, et al: Tissue pressure threshold for peripheral nerve viability. *Clin Orthop* 178:285, 1983.

Hargens AR, Akeson WH, et al: Tissue fluid pressures: From basic research tools to clinical applications. The Kappa Delta Award Paper. *J Orthop Res* 7:902, 1989.

Hargens AR, Gershuni DH, et al: Tissue necrosis associated with tourniquet ischemia. Eleventh European Conference for Microcirculation. Garmisch-Partenkirchen, Germany. *Bibliotheca Anatomica* 20:599, 601, 1981.

Hovius SE, Ultee J: Volkmann's ischemic contracture. Prevention and treatment. *Hand Clin* 16:647, 2000.

Matsen FA III, Mayo KA, et al: A model compartmental syndrome in man with particular reference to the quantification of nerve function. *J Bone Joint Surg (Am)* 59:648, 1977.

Matsen FA III, Rorabeck CH: Compartment syndromes. *AAOS Instr Course Lect* 38:463, 1989.

Mitchell SW: *Injuries of Nerves and Their Consequences.* Philadelphia: JB Lippincott, 1972.

Mitchell SW, Morehouse GR: *Gunshot Wounds and Other Injuries of Nerves.* Philadelphia: JB Lippincott, 1964.

Mubarak SJ, Hargens AR (eds): *Compartment Syndromes and Volkmann's Ischemic Contracture.* Monographs in Clinical Orthopaedics, Vol. 3. Philadelphia: WB Saunders, 1981.

Peimer CA: Intrinsic muscle contractures, in Chapman MW, Madison M (eds): *Operative Orthopaedics*, 3rd ed. Philadelphia: Lippincott Williams & Wilkins, 2001, p 1749.

Peimer CA, Wheeler DR, Barrett A, et al: Functional outcome after single ray amputation. *J Hand Surg* 24A:1245, 1999.

Trice M, Colwell CW: A historical review of compartment syndrome and Volkmann's ischemic contracture. *Hand Clin* 14:335, 1998.

Burns

American Burn Association: Guidelines for service standards and severity classifications in the treatment of burn injury. *ACS Bull* 69:24, 1984.

Demling RH: Burns, in Greenfield LJ, et al (eds): *Surgery: Scientific Principles and Practice.* Philadelphia: JB Lippincott, 1993, p 368.

Helm PA: Burn rehabilitation: Dimensions of the problem. *Clin Plast Surg* 19:551, 1992.

Robson MC, Smith DJ Jr.: Burned hand, in Jurkiewicz MJ, et al (eds): *Plastic Surgery: Principles and Practice.* St. Louis: CV Mosby, 1990, p 781.

Salisbury RE, Nieves SU, et al: Acute care and rehabilitation of the burned hand, in Hunter JM, et al (eds): *Rehabilitation of the Hand: Surgery and Therapy*, 3rd ed. St. Louis: CV Mosby, 1990, p 831.

Woo SH, Seul JH: Optimizing the correction of severe postburn hand deformities by using aggressive contracture releases and fasciocutaneous free-tissue transfers. *Plast Reconstr Surg* 107:1, 2001.

Infection

Brown DM, Young VL: Hand infections. *South Med J* 86:56, 1993.

Cheatum DE, Hudman M, et al: Chronic arthritis due to *Mycobacterium intracellulare:* Sacroiliac, knee, and carpal tunnel involvement in a young man and response to chemotherapy. *Arthritis Rheum* 19:777, 1976.

Dickson-Wright A: Tendon sheath infections. *Proc Roy Soc Med* 37:504, 1943.

Glass KD: Factors related to the resolution of treated hand infections. *J Hand Surg* 7:388, 1982.

Gunther SF, Levy CS: Mycobacterial infections. *Hand Clin* 5:591, 1989.

Hausman MR, Lisser SP: Hand infections. *Orthop Clin North Am* 23:171, 1992.

Neviaser RJ: Closed tendon sheath irrigation for pyogenic flexor tenosynovitis. *J Hand Surg* 3:462, 1978.

Strombert BV: Changing bacterial flora of hand infections. *J Trauma* 25:530, 1985.

Chronic Syndromes

Belsole RJ: De Quervain's tenosynovitis: Diagnostic and operative complications. *Orthopaedics* 4:899, 1981.

Blumberg N, Arbel R, Dekel S: Percutaneous release of trigger digits. *J Hand Surg (Br)* 26:256, 2001.

Borg K, Lindblom U: Diagnostic value of quantitative sensory testing (QST) in carpal tunnel syndrome. *Acta Neurol Scand* 78:537, 1988.

Boyes JH: *Bunnel's Surgery of the Hand*, 4th ed. Philadelphia: JB Lippincott, 1964.

Boyle J, Smith N, et al: Vibration white finger. *J Hand Surg Br* 13:171, 1988.

deQuervain F: Ueber eine form von chronischer tendovaginits. *Corresp Blatt Schweitzer Arzte* 25:389, 1895.

Dobyns JH, Sim FH, et al: Sports stress syndrome of the hand and wrist. *Am J Sports Med* 6:236, 1978.

Farkkila M, Pyykko I, et al: Forestry workers exposed to vibration: A neurological study. *Br J Ind Med* 45:188, 1988.

Finkelstein H: Stenosing tenosynovitis at the radial styloid process. *J Bone Joint Surg* 28:509, 1930.

Garcia-Elias M, Sanchez-Freijo J, et al: Dynamic changes of the transverse carpal arch during flexion-extension of the wrist: Effects of sectioning the transverse carpal ligament. *J Hand Surg Am* 17:1017, 1992.

Gellman H, Gelberman R, et al: Carpal tunnel syndrome: An evaluation of the provocative tests. *J Bone Joint Surg Am* 68:735, 1986.

Gunther SF: Dorsal wrist pain and the occult scapholunate ganglion. *J Hand Surg* 10:697, 1985.

Harter B, McKiernan J, et al: Carpal tunnel syndrome: Surgical and nonsurgical treatment. *J Hand Surg Am* 18:734, 1993.

Harvey FJ, Harvey PM, et al: De Quervain's disease: Surgical or nonsurgical treatment. *J Hand Surg* 15A:83, 1990.

Hymovich L, Lindholm M: Hand, wrist, and forearm injuries: The result of repetitive motion. *J Occup Med* 8:573, 1966.

Kuorinka I, Koskinen P: Occupational rheumatic diseases and upper limb strain in manual jobs in a light mechanical industry. *Scand J Work Environ Health* 5(Suppl 3):39, 1979.

Kaplan S, Glickel S, et al: Predictive factors in the nonsurgical treatment of carpal tunnel syndrome. *J Hand Surg Br* 15:106, 1990.

Kruger V, Kraft G, et al: Carpal tunnel syndrome: Objective measures and splint use. *Arch Phys Med Rehabil* 72:517, 1991.

Luchetti R, Schoenhuber R, et al: Assessment of sensory nerve conduction in carpal tunnel syndrome before, during, and after operation. *J Hand Surg Br* 13:386, 1988.

Luopajarvi T, Kuorinka I, et al: Prevalence of tenosynovitis and other injuries of the upper extremities in repetitive work. *Scand J Work Environ Health* 5(Suppl 3):48, 1979.

Miller R, Lohman W, et al: An epidemiologic study of carpal tunnel syndrome and hand-arm vibration syndrome in relation to vibration exposure. *J Hand Surg Am* 19:99, 1994.

Moore J: Carpal tunnel syndrome. *Occup Med* 7:741, 1992.

Nau H, Lange B, et al: Prediction of outcome of decompression for carpal tunnel syndrome. *J Hand Surg (Br)* 13:391, 1988.

Ordeberg E, Sälgeback S, et al: Carpal tunnel syndrome in pregnancy. *Acta Obstet Gynecol Scand* 66:233, 1987.

Stock S: Work place ergonomic factors and the development of musculoskeletal disorders of the neck and upper limbs: A meta-analysis. *Am J Ind Med* 21:895, 1992.

Subcommittee on Clinical Policies, American Academy of Orthopaedic Surgeons: Carpal tunnel syndrome. *Clinical Policies* 11, 1991.

Trumble TE, Gilbert M, McCallister WV: Endoscopic vs. open surgical treatment of carpal tunnel syndrome. *Neurosurg Clin North Am* 12:255, 2001.

Wand J: Carpal tunnel syndrome in pregnancy and lactation. *J Hand Surg (Br)* 15:93, 1990.

Wieslander G, Norback D, et al: Carpal tunnel syndrome (CTS) and exposure to vibration, repetitive wrist movements, and heavy manual work: A case-referent study. *Br J Ind Med* 46:43, 1989.

Yoshioka S, Okuda Y, et al: Changes in carpal tunnel shape during wrist joint motion: MRI evaluation of normal volunteers. *J Hand Surg (Br)* 18:620, 1993.

Zeiss J, Skie M, et al: Anatomic relations between the median nerve and flexor tendons in the carpal tunnel: MR evaluation in normal volunteers. *AJR* 153:533, 1989.

Acquired Dysfunction

Abouna JM, Brown H: The treatment of mallet finger, the results in a series of 148 consecutive cases and review of the literature. *Br J Surg* 55:653, 1968.

Angelides AC: Ganglions of the hand and wrist, in Green DP (ed): *Operative Hand Surgery*, 3rd ed. New York: Churchill-Livingstone, 1993, p 2157.

Badalamente MA, Hurst LC: Enzyme injection as nonsurgical treatment of Dupuytren's disease. *J Hand Surg (Am)* 25:629, 2000.

Bruner JM: Optimum skin incisions for the surgical relief of stenosing tenosynovitis in the hand. *Plast Reconstr Surg* 38:197, 1966.

Hooper G: Cystic swellings, in Bogumill GP, Gleegler EJ (eds): *Tumors of the Hand and Upper Limb*. Edinburgh: Churchill-Livingstone, 1993, p 172.

Kaplan E: *Functional and Surgical Anatomy of the Hand,* 2nd ed. Philadelphia: JB Lippincott, 1965.

Ketchum L: The use of the full thickness skin graft in Dupuytren's contracture. *Hand Clin* 7:731, 1991.

Lambert MA, Morton RJ, Sloan JP: Controlled study of the use of local steroid injection in the treatment of trigger finger and thumb. *J Hand Surg (Br)* 17:69, 1992.

Lange RH, Engber WD: Hyperextension mallet finger. *Orthopaedics* 6:1436, 1983.

Lewin P: A simple splint for baseball finger. *JAMA* 85:1059, 1925.

Lowdon IMR: Fractures of the metacarpal neck of the little finger. *Injury* 17:189, 1986.

Moon WN, Suh SW, Kim IC: Trigger digits in children. *J Hand Surg (Br)* 26:11, 2001.

Roush TF, Stern PJ: Results following surgery for Dupuytren's disease. *J Hand Surg (Am)* 25:291, 2000.

Saar JD, Grothaus PC: Dupuytren's disease: An overview. *Plast Reconstr Surg* 106:125, 2000.

Segmüller G: *Surgical Stabilization of the Skeleton of the Hand*. Baltimore: Williams & Wilkins, 1977, p 45.

Stack HH, Boyes JH, et al: Mallet finger. *J Bone Joint Surg* 44A:1061, 1962.

Starkweather KD, Lattuga S, Hurst LC, et al: Collagenase in the treatment of Dupuytren's disease: An in vitro study. *J Hand Surg (Am)* 21:490, 1996.

Stefanich RJ, Peimer CA: Longitudinal incision for trigger release. *J Hand Surg* 14A:316, 1988.

Watchmaker GP, Mackinnon SE: Nerve injury and repair, in Peimer CA (ed): *Surgery of the Hand and Upper Extremity*. New York: McGraw-Hill, 1996, 1251.

Tumors and Masses

Angelides AC: Ganglions of the hand and wrist, in Green DP (ed): *Operative Hand Surgery*, 3rd ed. New York: Churchill-Livingstone, 1993, p 2157.

Greendyke SA, Wilson M, et al: Anterior wrist ganglia from the scapho-trapezial joint. *J Hand Surg Am* 17:487, 1992.

Hasselgren G, Forssblad P, et al: Bone grafting unnecessary in the treatment of enchondromas in the hand. *J Hand Surg Am* 16:139, 1991.

Johnson JO: Differential diagnosis and treatment of giant cell lesions, in Boguill GP, Fleegler EJ (eds): *Tumors of the Hand and Upper Limb*. Edinburgh: Churchill-Livingstone, 1993, p 360.

McPhee M, McGrath BE, Zhang P, et al: Soft tissue sarcoma of the hand. *J Hand Surg (Am)* 24:1001, 1999.

Oster LH, Blair WF, et al: Large lipomas in the deep palmar space. *J Hand Surg (Am)* 14:700, 1989.

Ragsdale DB, Dupree WB: Neoplasms of the fatty tissues, in Bogumill GP, Fleegler EJ (eds): *Tumors of the Hand and Upper Limb*. Edinburgh: Churchill-Livingstone, 1993, p 254.

Stewart PK, Moy OJ, Peimer CA: Reconstruction after resection of upper extremity soft tissue sarcomas, in Kraybill W (guest ed.): *Hand Clinics*. Philadelphia: WB Saunders: 1999, p 84.

Szabo RM, Thorson EP, et al: Allograft replacement with distal radioulnar joint fusion and ulnar osteotomy for treatment of giant cell tumors of the distal radius. *J Hand Surg (Am)* 15:929, 1990.

Tordai P, Hoglund M, et al: Is the treatment of enchondroma in the hand by simple curettage a rewarding method? *J Hand Surg (Br)* 15:331, 1990.

Vander Griend RA, Funderburk CH: The treatment of giant cell tumors of the distal part of the radius. *J Bone Joint Surg (Am)* 75:899, 1993.

CHAPTER 44

Plastic and Reconstructive Surgery

Saleh M. Shenaq, John Y. S. Kim, and Alan Bienstock

HISTORY

Plastic surgery is derived from the Greek word, "plastikos," meaning *to mold*. The discipline endeavors to reconstruct all manner of defects and deformities. Central to this enterprise is a precise knowledge of anatomy, respect for surgical technique, and finesse, and a keen, creative sense for the possibilities inherent in the manipulation and remodeling of tissue.

Historically, the premise for plastic surgery dates back several millennia and spans many cultures. The Egyptian, "Edwin Smith papyrus," believed to be written in 1700 B.C. heralds modern fastidiousness with wound care, emphasizing the importance of débridement and meticulous surgical technique. The *Sushruta Samita,* an Indian text written in 500 B.C., records the first description of a pedicled flap for nasal reconstruction. The Roman physician Celsus gave detailed treatment guidelines for diverse facial injuries during the first century.[1] With a decline in the advancement of Western medicine in the post-Roman era, the Near Eastern physicians were advancing sophisticated surgical techniques. The Renaissance brought a resurgence in empiric medicine and creative surgical approaches to reconstruction: Tagliacozzi's text, *per Insitonem* (1597), is a prescient text which gives a permutation of the Indian forehead flap with a medial arm flap for nose amputations.[2]

The unfortunate circumstance of internecine conflicts during World Wars I and II stimulated the evolution of plastic surgery by forcing surgeons to grapple with complex, massive, traumatic defects of the maxillofacial region and extremities. Gillies made an exhaustive exploration of head and neck anatomy to recreate bony and soft-tissue defects wrought by escalating weaponry. Concordantly, there was an increasing realization that the reconstructive challenge crossed traditional boundaries of the surgical disciplines of orthopedics, general surgery, oral surgery, and head and neck surgery. An actual organizing entity for plastic surgery was not created until 1937 with the formation of the American Board of Plastic Surgery.

Even as the field was coalescing as a distinct surgical discipline, the accelerating pace of medical innovation was producing subspecialization in the field. Paul Tessier aggressively pursued new ways of shaping deformities in the craniofacial skeleton. Harry Buncke and Nakayama germinated the technical and physiologic basis for microsurgery. Pioneers such as Macgregor and Jackson carefully engaged the anatomic underpinnings of flaps and gave a systematic rationale for future investigation into all manner of soft-tissue coverage.

Concomitantly, plastic surgery applied principles vital to the issue of reconstruction, aesthetic rejuvenation, and enhancement. Cronin and Gerow fathered the invention of breast implants in 1962, which, in turn, ignited both a specific interest in breast cosmesis, as well as a general interest in applying alloplastic materials to plastic surgery.

WOUND HEALING

Much of plastic surgery is predicated on the fundamentals of wound healing and tissue regeneration. Understanding the mechanophysiology of healing and its relationship to surgical technique are paramount to the plastic surgeon's endeavors. While a detailed treatise on wound healing is covered in another section, certain basic concepts are important to emphasize.

There are three general types of wound healing. The first is *primary* wound healing, which is characterized by the occurrence of mechanical apposition of wound edges and a cascade of inflammatory cell activation. This recruitment creates a milieu which allows re-epithelialization and collagen strengthening to occur. The second, *delayed primary* healing, occurs when the wound healing process is potentially compromised by incipient infection. With this type of healing, the surgeon may opt to leave the soft tissue unapposed and allow native inflammation and external débridement to cleanse the wound. If, on evaluation several days later, the wound appears uninfected, the wound can then be closed and the normal process of primary healing can then be re-initiated. Third is *secondary* healing, which is recommended for a wound that does not show potential for early closure. The wound can be allowed to close over time by the processes of inflammation, contraction (via myofibroblasts), and eventual re-epithelialization.[3]

An important corollary to timely and robust wound healing is the appropriate interaction among inflammatory cells such as polymorphonuclear neutrophils, macrophages, lymphocytes, fibroblasts, and the bath of cytokines, such as interleukins, interferons, transforming growth factor (α, β), platelet-derived growth factor, epidermal growth factor, and fibroblast growth factors. Critical to the overarching success of inflammation and wound healing is the establishment of new vessels or angiogenesis. The fundamental limiting step to both wound healing and tissue reconstruction is the presence of adequate vascularity.[4,5]

Impaired Wound Healing

If the necessary blood supply to a healing region is compromised, then wound healing can be delayed. Similarly, the relative paucity of the basic constituents of inflammatory cytokines or matrix components (vitamins, zinc, copper, iron) may result in structural weakness of the wound. Radiation is often an issue for reconstruction of ablative defects. Among other effects, radiation can create local ischemic conditions via microangiopathic damage. Moreover, the inherent ability for the tissue to regenerate is altered in both an acute and delayed fashion. Diabetic patients can also experience impaired wound healing as a consequence of the changes in glucose metabolism and insulin regulation that occurs systemically.

Dysfunctional healing can also manifest as abnormal scars. Hypertrophic scars and keloids are manifestations of altered collagen deposition and breakdown. Hypertrophic scars are raised, collagen-rich lesions that do not go beyond the initial boundaries of the insult, whereas keloids are scars that have progressed beyond these boundaries. It is difficult to distinguish these two pathologic entities by routine histology, although it is believed that keloids may have thicker collagen fibers and a greater degree of hyaluronic acid in the epidermis than hypertrophic scars.[6]

Treatment of scars includes pressure, silicone sheet and gels, and intralesional corticosteroids. Topical vitamins A and E are used for treatment of unsightly scars, but no definitive clinical trials have demonstrated their efficacy. For intractable keloids, radiation therapy in conjunction with surgical excision has led to a 50 to 80% reduction in keloids.

Basic Technique of Skin Closure

Notwithstanding the advent of tissue adhesives such as cyanoacrylate, suture closure remains the most common and durable technique of creating precise skin closure. The choice of suture material can vary from monofilament to polyfilament and absorbable to nonabsorbable. Regardless of the suture material used, the notion of minimizing tension is critical to maintaining wound closure and preventing excessive scar formation. This objective can be accomplished by using dermal and subdermal sutures to diffuse the tension among multiple layers. Another way of ameliorating the tension effect on wounds is to align skin incisions along lines of minimal tension, otherwise known as relaxed-skin tension lines (Fig. 44-1).

Suture Technique

Sutures are placed through the epidermis and into the deep dermis approximately 2 mm from the skin edge and 7 to 10 mm apart, depending on need. Care is taken with any suture placement to ensure that the needle enters the skin as nearly perpendicular as possible. Slight eversion of the skin edges facilitates accurate closure without contracting depression of the scar. A trapezoidal configuration to the suture placement can abet this eversion.

Vertical mattress sutures (Fig. 44-2B) can yield a more substantial eversion by entering at separate points along an orthogonal line from the skin margin. Horizontal mattress sutures (Fig. 44-2D) are also used for eversion but will grasp and bring together the skin at separate points, along a line parallel to the skin margin. While

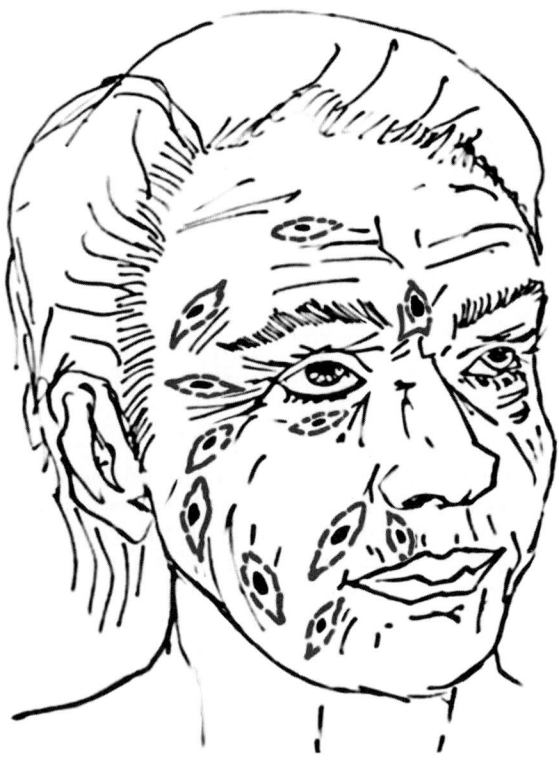

FIG. 44-1. Relaxed-skin tension lines. These lines indicate where elliptical incisions should be ideally placed on the face.

this allows the single suture to traverse a greater distance along the skin margin, there is a greater theoretical concern with ischemic inhibition of tissue healing.

Simple or mattress sutures (see Fig. 44-2A) are usually constructed with nonabsorbable material and should be removed as expeditiously as possible to prevent scarring. A caveat to this technique is that they must allow lasting apposition of tissue. Buried dermal and fascial suture should provide the significant proportion of the strength of a sutured wound.

Subcuticular sutures (see Fig. 44-2C) are running, superficial dermal sutures that avoid the external scar of the interrupted sutures. They should not be relied upon as the strength component of a closure and can be constructed from both absorbable and nonabsorbable suture material.

Continuous over-and-over sutures allow for rapid closure of tissue with some element of hemostasis that can be achieved. Large wounds in areas such as the scalp may bleed profusely and rapid closure and hemostasis may override the normal mantra of meticulous and layered closure.[7]

Staples also have been used for closure of the superficial component of skin and soft tissue. They may need to be combined with deeper sutures to augment the strength of the closure and ideally would not be left in longer than 1 week to avoid unsightly scars. Tissue-adhesive substances, especially cyanoacrylate-based ones, are advantageous, if properly used and in a setting where relatively tensionless closure has already been accomplished with deeper sutures. They also obviate the infiltration of local anesthetic needed in patients who are awake with other techniques (which may be an issue in pediatric populations). Steri-Strips or other tapes can similarly be used when simple apposition of the superficial skin is needed and tension on the suture is largely absent by virtue of the anatomy or pre-existing deeper suture.

FIG. 44-2. Types of skin closure: (A) simple mattress; (B) vertical mattress; (C) subcuticular; and (D) horizontal mattress.

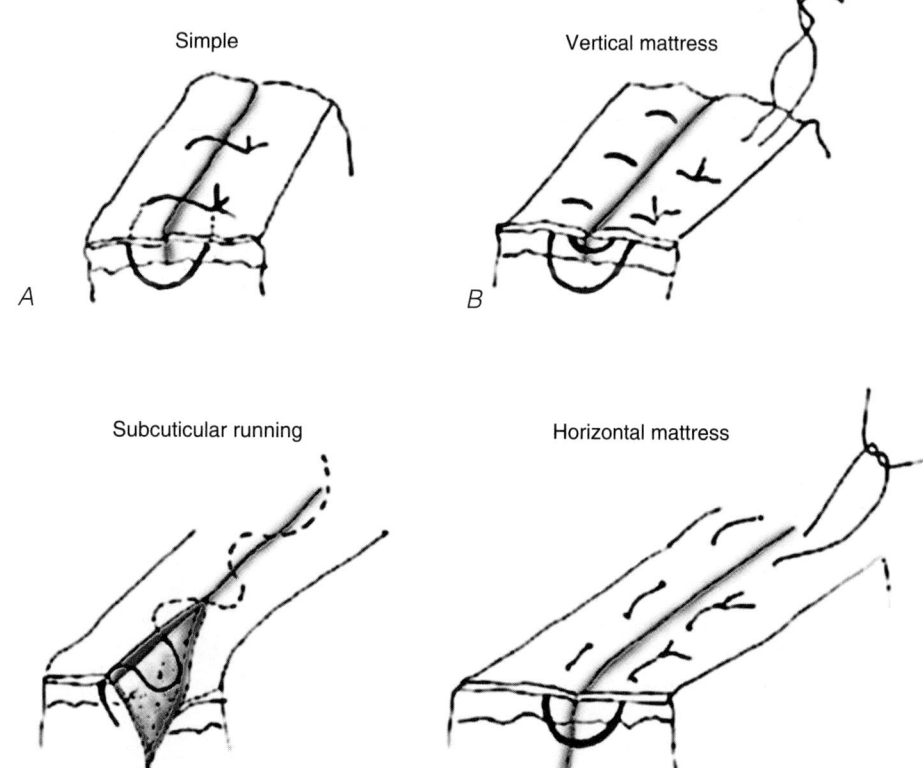

Simple

Vertical mattress

Subcuticular running

Horizontal mattress

Reconstruction of more complex defects may require the alteration and or transfer of local or distant tissue. The various options for reconstruction of a given defect are primary closure, skin grafts, skin flaps, tissue expansion, muscle- or fascia-based flaps, or free flaps. Traditionally, this has been described as a reconstructive ladder of sorts. However, the stepwise implication of the ladder metaphor may not always hold true. That is, the nature of a particular defect determines the type of ideal reconstruction. An irradiated defect of the tissue overlying a scalp may indeed be covered with skin graft or possibly with expanded tissue; however, definitive coverage with the more complex microsurgical tissue transfer may better serve the reconstructive needs of the patient when complication rates and outcomes are considered.

SOFT TISSUE RECONSTRUCTION

Skin Grafts

Skin grafts are mainstays for reconstruction of superficial defects or adjuncts to more complex reconstructions. The type of skin graft is based on the thickness of the graft taken. The term "graft" is used to denote the fact that during harvest of the skin graft, all the vessels nourishing the graft are cut. This is in contradistinction to the term "flap" which implies that some aspect of the blood supply to the segment of tissue has remained intact during transfer. As such, the graft itself is the *donor tissue;* the wound bed to which it is applied is known as the *recipient site.*

A *split-thickness graft* requires that a portion of the dermis be taken along with the epidermis. A *full-thickness graft* is one in which the full portion of the dermis is taken with the superficial epidermis (Table 44-1). The grafts will survive transfer based on a defined sequence of events that culminates in vascular independence. These events are (1) *serum imbibition*—direct absorption of nutrients from recipient capillary beds that generally takes place in the first 24 hours; (2) *inosculation*—the connecting of donor and recipient vessels that typically begins in the 24- to 72-hour period; and (3) *angiogenesis*—vascular ingrowth of vessels from the recipient bed into the graft that starts after 72 hours. Factors that interrupt this process—such as fluid collection under the graft or mechanical shear forces—will compromise the graft take.[8]

Thicker grafts have more difficulty with definitive adherence and survival because of the greater demand on vascular ingrowth. However, the greater the proportion of dermis the graft has, the greater the inhibition of the myofibroblasts that cause secondary contraction. The full-thickness skin graft can also retain functional hair follicles and sweat glands.

Split-thickness skin grafts are taken from sites depending on the thickness, color, and quality of skin needed. The split-thickness

Table 44-1
Split-Thickness vs. Full-Thickness Skin Grafts

	Split-Thickness Graft	Full-Thickness Graft
Reliable take	+	
Available donor sites	+	
Primary contracture	+	
Secondary contracture		+
Mechanical durability		+
Ability to grow hair, secrete sweat and sebum		+
Pigmentary changes	+	

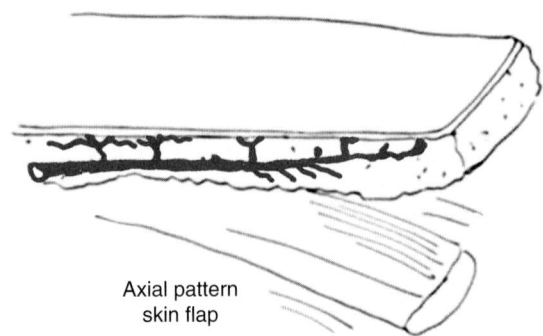

FIG. 44-3. *Axial pattern flap: direct cutaneous. This flap is nourished by a definite cutaneous artery and vein.*

grafts can be meshed in varying ratios to expand the potential coverage area. The drawbacks to meshed grafts include their suboptimal appearance and their tendency to contract. They can be used in conjunction with skin substitutes, in cases such as large-area burn reconstruction, when there may be a relative paucity of donor sites. Full-thickness grafts are taken from areas in which primary closure can be accomplished, such as the groin or within redundant skin folds.[9] Skin grafts can be fixed in place with compressive dressings to prevent problems with shear and fluid collection. Generally, 5 days are required for definitive vascular ingrowth to occur. Dressings can be left on the recipient site for this period of time. Donor sites for split-thickness grafts are allowed to re-epithelialize under occlusive (OpSite, Tegaderm) or moist, antibiotic impregnated gauze (Xeroform). If allowed to heal uninterrupted, the donor site for a $^{12}/_{1000}$-inch skin graft can re-epithelialize in 7 to 14 days.

Skin Flaps

A flap is a volume of tissue that can be transferred and survive in its new location based on an independent blood supply. Hence, a skin flap consists of a volume of skin and subcutaneous tissue, while a muscle flap consists of muscle. A *myocutaneous flap* is composite tissue consisting of skin, subcutaneous tissue, and muscle. The critical element in all of these anatomic subsets of tissue is the nourishing blood supply.

A *random* flap has vessels which nourish the tissue and are smaller and less defined than those of an *axial pattern* flap, in which the tissue has an anatomically defined configuration of vessels. Many skin flaps that are used to reconstruct smaller, full-thickness defects are considered random (Figs. 44-3 and 44-4).[10]

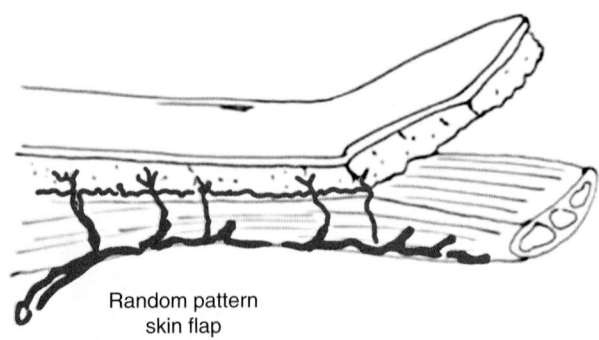

FIG. 44-4. *Random pattern skin flap. The skin and subcutaneous tissue is elevated from the underlying muscle. The flap is therefore supplied by the subdermal plexus rather than the musculocutaneous perforators.*

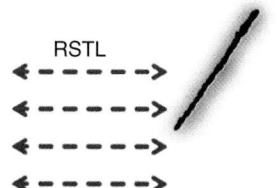 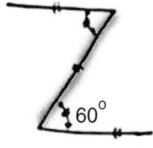 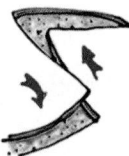 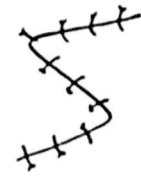

Z PLASTY

FIG. 44-5. *Z-plasty. The tension of the scar or incision is reoriented from a transverse direction to a vertical direction. This is accomplished by creating two identical triangles and interchanging the flaps.*

Skin flaps can be constructed in various manners in order to move tissue into a defect. The principal constraints are those of geometry and vascularity. A Z-plasty is a method of constructing skin flaps to refashion a scar (Fig. 44-5). By aligning opposing skin flaps at a specific angle, a scar that is constricting movement or aesthetically unappealing can be redirected to a more optimal position. The angle of the triangular skin flap determines the theoretical gain in length of the redirected scar. A W-plasty is a way of breaking up the continuity of a linear scar in a manner that often can camouflage the scar (Fig. 44-6).

A V-Y advancement flap is a method of recruiting tissue from a region of relative excess to a defect. The tension is diffused along a great enough surface area so that closure of the proximal portion of the transferred defect can be effected (Fig. 44-7). Skin flaps also can be rotated around a pivot point. If the tension is too great, a back cut, known as a Burow's triangle, can be made to facilitate distal access (Fig. 44-8). A simple rectangular advancement flap also can gain some movement by the addition of two Burow's triangles at the base (Fig. 44-9). The geometric pattern of the donor defect can also be used to fashion the flap, as in the case of a rhomboid flap, as well as a transposition flap (Figs. 44-10 and 44-11). After a lesion excision, the defect can be modified to an approximation of a rhomboid and an adjacent rhomboid from a region of relative skin excess can be maneuvered into place. A more sophisticated application of the geometric principles of rotational and advancement flaps can be seen in the example of a *bilobed flap* in which loose skin is transposed in sequence via two flaps, with the most distal flap being closed primarily (Fig. 44-12).[11]

An *axial-pattern skin flap* may have varying vessel configurations. The dermal–subdermal plexus of vessels is important to the survival of the skin portion of the flap. The supplying vessels may directly approach the skin or traverse through muscle or fascial septae between muscle territories. An *island flap* is one in which the vessel is isolated from surrounding tissue, over an intervening segment. A *free flap* is one in which the vascular supply and flap proper is severed to be reattached via microvascular technique at a distant site.

Muscle-Based Flaps

The actual anatomic territory that a given vessel supplies is known as an *angiosome*. The mapping of angiosomes defines the potential

flaps that can be constructed for a given defect. The physiologic basis of these angiosomes has given rise to the concept of delay. The delay phenomenon is one in which the vascularity of flaps can be rendered more robust by temporarily interrupting the normal inflow of blood. This allows for metabolic conditioning of the flap to ischemia and also allows new channels to form. For example, a flap such as a transverse rectus abdominis myocutaneous flap can have a major portion of its blood supply—the deep inferior epigastric artery—interrupted. Vessels, which connect adjacent angiosomes, known as choke vessels, will open up and the tissue itself will become ischemically preconditioned to rely upon the secondary vessel—the superior epigastric artery. After a period of 10 to 14 days of such adjustments, the flap can be safely transferred based upon the superior epigastric artery with less chance of the distal portions of the flap becoming ischemic and potentially necrotic.

Muscle flaps also have their own defined anatomy. Often the more complex and larger defects require soft-tissue coverage that exceeds the capabilities of skin flaps and by necessity requires muscle flaps. Mathes and Nahai have classified muscle flaps according to the pattern of dominant, minor, and segmental vessels (Table 44-2).[12] These critical anatomic and physiologic investigations have allowed surgeons to safely transfer muscle as flaps based on the critical vessels. For wounds that are prone to infection or are irradiated, the transfer of muscle may offer more durable reconstruction by providing highly vascular soft tissue. Defect requirements and the reliability of the muscle perforators to the skin determine whether the overlying skin territory is transferred with the flap. Skin grafts also can be placed directly on the muscle.[12]

Tissue Expansion

Despite the plethora of choices for skin flaps, the demand of quantity and quality may exceed supply. One alternative is to expand the donor tissue artificially. The viscoelastic properties of skin allow a certain degree of stretch to be applied to the skin and subcutaneous tissue without undue necrosis. A chronic, appropriately applied stretch can generate and recruit new tissue formation via a process known as biologic *creep.*

Histologic analysis of expanded skin shows increased mitotic activity and increased vascularity of the tissue. The epidermis thickens concomitantly to a relative thinning of the dermis. If a silicone-based

FIG. 44-6. *W-plasty. It can break up a straight linear scar, and can improve the direction of the scar. The scar is redispersed.*

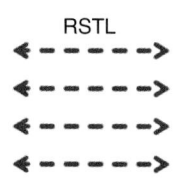 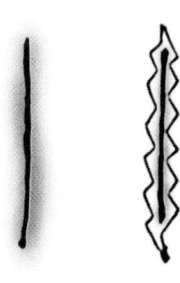 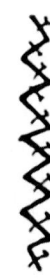

W PLASTY

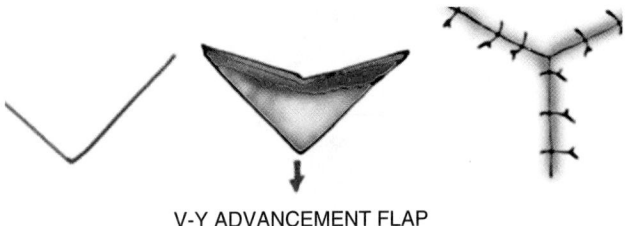

V-Y ADVANCEMENT FLAP

FIG. 44-7. *V-Y advancement.*

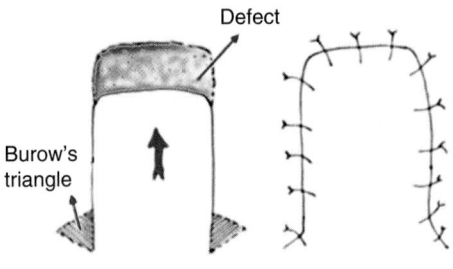

RECTANGULAR ADVANCEMENT FLAP

FIG. 44-9. *Advancement rectangular flap with Burow's triangle.*

expander is used, then a capsule may form around the expander.[13] This expander concept can be applied to such diverse clinical needs as burn or breast reconstruction. The expander can be placed in a subcutaneous pocket under unburned skin or a postmastectomy field and sequentially filled with saline. The skin can then be elevated and rotated into burn defect (or skin can be harvested from the expanded area as grafts) or the added breast volume can be replaced with a definitive breast implant to reconstruct a breast.

Free Flaps and Microsurgery

As mentioned previously, the nature of a given defect may demand the use of distant tissue transfer. Microsurgery is the technique employed to reconstruct the critical vascular elements of tissue that are to be transferred in this manner. The relatively small size of vessels perfusing these flaps of tissue demands special operative considerations and equipment to successfully anastomose donor arteries and veins to those of the recipient.

Either microscopes or high-magnification loupes are employed to visualize the vessels, which typically are between 1.0 and 4.0 mm in diameter. Microsuture from 7.0 to 11.0 is typically used. Vessel thrombosis, which can lead to flap necrosis, is often a problematic complication of microsurgery. Avoidance of this complication begins with a preoperative analysis of the patient's factors. The patient is screened for a history of thromboembolic phenomena that may herald anticoagulant deficiencies such as factor C and S deficiency. Hypovolemia or other cardiovascular compromises that may affect blood flow to the flap are corrected preoperatively. The influence of smoking has been debated—some larger, retrospective studies have demonstrated no difference in thromboembolic complications but have shown an increase in wound-healing problems. Caffeine and other potentially vasoactive agents also have shown some deleterious effects on flap perfusion.

Given the magnitude of the operation, planning for a microsurgical procedure goes beyond a simple calculus of defect size to appropriate flap size. There are geometric considerations of vascular pedicle length, donor–recipient vessel diameter mismatch, orientation of vessels and tissue, status of recipient vessels (irradiated or

in a previously operated field), anticipated postoperative position, potential postoperative radiation, and donor site considerations that should be considered once the optimal flap has been chosen. Secondary options need to be considered in case the primary choice is compromised by aberrant anatomy or technical malfeasance.[14]

During flap dissection, care must be taken to respect the vagaries of vascular anatomy—there may be critical perforators which may need to be recognized and preserved. The vessels to be anastomosed must be handled meticulously and minimally to obviate vasospasm and intimal injury. Animal studies show the putative benefit of papaverine and certain doses of lidocaine in ameliorating vasospasm. Hydrodilation with heparinized solution and mechanical dilatation are also judiciously employed.

While the periadventitia should be cleared from the ends of the vessels, excessive stripping may devascularize the vasa vasorum. Double approximating clamps are often used to stabilize the vessels. Interrupted sutures or continuous sutures can accomplish the anastomosis (Fig. 44-13). Triangulating sutures can be used as guides, but an even placement of sutures is critical—especially in cases of modest caliber mismatch. During the anastomosis, microanatomic differences between vein and artery should be respected. For example, the artery, by virtue of a thicker wall, will be stiffer than the vein. The confounding factor of coexistent atherosclerosis should also be anticipated and compromised vessel length may need to be excised or else modifications made to the anastomotic site.[15]

In a circumstance when there is insufficient length to bring the donor and recipient vessels in proximity to each other, a reverse interposition vein graft may be necessary. While this may add an extra anastomosis and a potential additional source of thrombosis, this is still preferable to the certain complication of an anastomosis under excessive tension. Tensionless, kink-free vessel anastomoses are critical.

Sutures are not the only method employed to bring vessels together; vein-coupling devices can be used. Less commonly, fibrin adhesives and lasers have been employed in largely experimental

ROTATION ADVANCEMENT FLAP

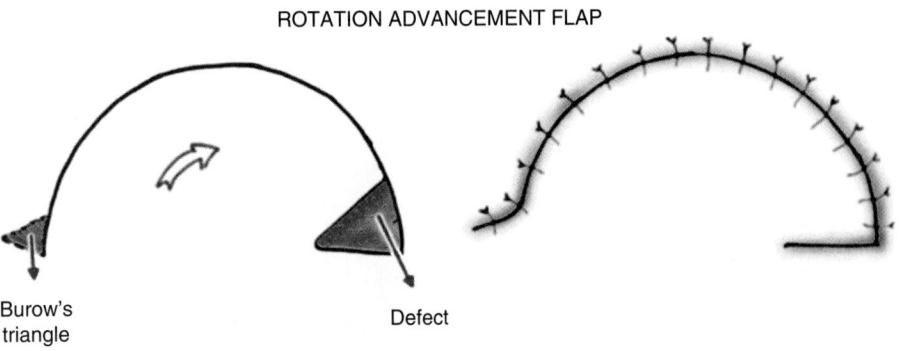

Burow's triangle

Defect

FIG. 44-8. *Rotation flap.*

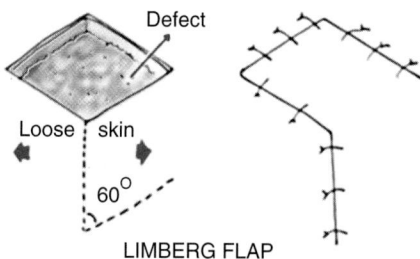

FIG. 44-10. *Limberg flap. The defect and design of flap are illustrated. The flap is transposed in a clockwise direction along the line of maximum extensibility.*

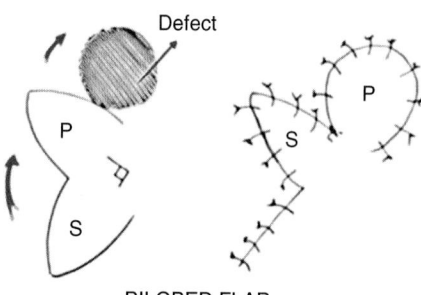

FIG. 44-12. Bilobed flap.

settings. Additionally, the configuration of anastomoses can be modified so that instead of an end-to-end anastomosis, an end-to-side anastomosis is used (Fig. 44-14). This permutation is useful when the recipient vessel cannot be wholly separated from the distal circulation (as in the case of an arterially compromised lower extremity with one dominant vessel runoff) or when a significant size discrepancy exists.

Intraoperative monitoring of blood pressure to ensure constant flap perfusion is important. Prolonged exposure to cold temperatures may aggravate any incipient vasospastic response. Postoperative monitoring of the flap is likewise critical. Clinical examination of color, temperature, undue swelling, mottled patterns, and Doppler assessment of arterial and venous signals are all mainstays of flap care. Occlusion of the anastomosis can occur from internal clot formation or from such external pressure as a hematoma. There is a threshold of ischemia beyond which a flap will sustain irreversible tissue loss and recognizing any of the early signs of ischemia with prompt exploration and correction of the underlying problem is paramount. Different types of tissue show variable resistance to ischemia (Table 44-3). Overall flap survival rates approach 95% in experienced hands.

The use of anticoagulants is somewhat controversial. Dextran and other potential rheologic agents have demonstrated some benefit in experimental models, but their clinical utility is limited by adverse reactions. Systemic heparin is sometimes used following anastomotic revision, but the caveat is that excessive bleeding is sometimes incurred. Acetylsalicylic acid may inhibit prostacyclin and is often used postoperatively to render an anticoagulant effect. In specific situations of refractory microcirculatory thrombi, fibrinolytic agents may be helpful, but complicating systemic hemorrhage and rebound thrombosis need to be addressed.

Venous congestion is probably more common than arterial occlusion. When operative exploration and revision does not fully address the issue of flap compromise, other measures, including leech therapy, may need to be considered. When applying leeches

to congested flaps or congested replanted digits, prophylaxis against *Aeromonas hydrophilia* must be given.

Although successful reperfusion of a flap is a laudable goal, there is a phenomenon of ischemia that persists after restoration of vessel continuity. This no-reflow phenomenon is a result of endothelial cell inflammation with subsequent inflammatory vasoconstriction—possible thrombosis—and persistent flap ischemia. Oxygen free radicals may be elaborated by stressed and injured cells with release of leukotrienes and oxidases, which perpetuate the state of deleterious inflammation.

PERIPHERAL NERVE SURGERY

While microsurgical technique is used extensively for vessels, it can also be transposed to peripheral nerve surgery. Most commonly, nerve injury is a manifestation of penetrating or blunt (traction) trauma. Compressive neuropathies also are encountered in areas such as the carpal, cubital, and tarsal tunnels. Nerve injuries are generally classified according to their severity and consequent prognosis (Table 44-4). Neurapraxia describes a relatively minor stretch of the nerve resulting in demyelination of a segment of nerve and subsequent conduction block. This is also known as a first-degree injury. Damage to the axon, or axonotmesis, is a second-degree injury in which the connective tissue layer of the nerve is left intact. If the endoneurium is violated, then a third-degree injury occurs. Fourth-degree injury implies disruption of the perineurium and fifth-degree injury is complete transaction of the nerve—also known as neurotmesis. Mackinnon has described a sixth-degree injury, which implies multiple zones of injury along the same nerve (Table 44-5).

The type and magnitude of injury determines the prognosis. First- and second-degree injuries are generally reversible without surgical intervention. In the third and fourth degrees of injury, a neuroma or scar may form within the affected nerve. If conduction of nerve signal is poor then the neuroma may need to be resected and a nerve graft placed in the intervening defect. Frank transection of the nerve or a nonconducting neuroma may need to be treated with primary repair (immediate or delayed in the case of wound contamination), interposition nerve graft, or nerve transfers.[16]

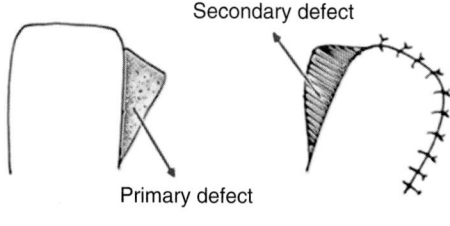

FIG. 44-11. Transposition flap.

Table 44-2
Mathes and Nahai Muscle Flap Vascular Anatomy Classification

Type I	One vascular pedicle
Type II	Dominant and minor pedicle
Type III	Two dominant pedicles
Type IV	Segmental pedicles
Type V	One dominant pedicle and segmental pedicle

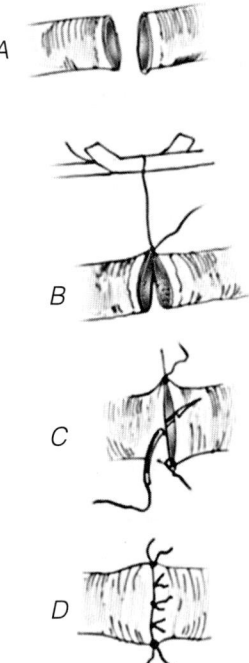

FIG. 44-13. Microvascular anastomosis: end-to-end anastomosis.

Physical examination of both motor and sensory function is paramount in accurate diagnosis, treatment, and prognosis. Innervation density tests such as the Semmes-Weinstein, or threshold tests such as two-point discrimination, can be useful measures of sensory status. Motor function can be graded on the British Medical Research Council Muscle-Grading Scale (Table 44-6). Electrophysiologic tests, such as nerve conduction tests, electromyograms, and sensory-evoked potentials, are helpful in delineating magnitude, location, and prognosis for various lesions.

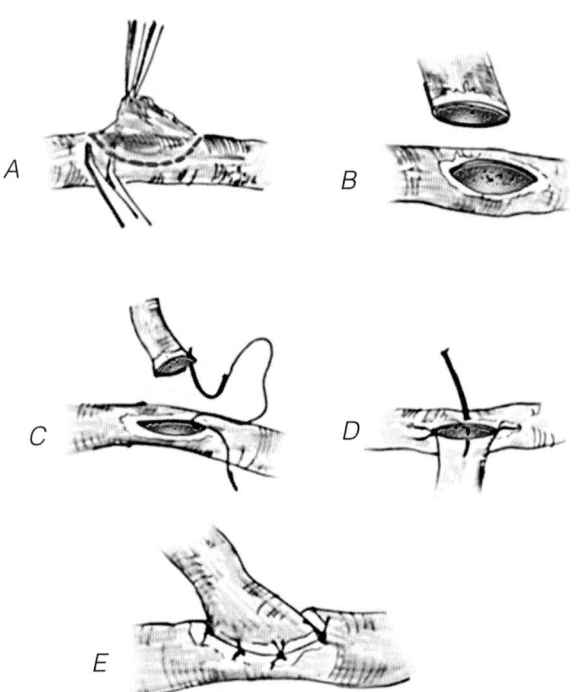

FIG. 44-14. Microvascular anastomosis: end-to-side anastomosis.

Table 44-3
Tissue Responses to Warm and Cold Ischemia

	Warm	*Cold*
Skin and subcutaneous tissue	4–6 hours	12 hours
Muscle	<2 hours	8 hours
Bone	<3 hours	24 hours

The algorithm for repair depends significantly on the mechanism of injury. Obstetric traction injuries differ from other traumatic injuries (Fig. 44-15). The timing of electrophysiologic tests and the timing of repair will vary from closed to open injury. Technical principles include the use of epineurial repair with 8.0 to 10.0 sutures (Fig. 44-16). When there is minimal tension, then primary repair can be attempted. Occasionally, limb postural changes can allow for the use of primary repair. If undue tension is evident on attempted approximation of the nerve endings, nerve grafting may be necessary. The motor and sensory fascicles of a nerve may require separate coaptation in the situation where the internal topography of the nerve is distinct.[17]

For situations in which the proximal part of the nerve cannot be repaired or grafted (especially for upper-extremity lesions) nerve transfer can be contemplated. For example, in a traumatic avulsion of the upper roots of the brachial plexus, an intact C7 root may be used as a donor nerve for transfer to the distal aspect of C5 and C6 (Fig. 44-17).

Less morbid and more effective immunosuppressive regimens have fostered the advent of nerve allografts as a potential viable alternative for nerve repair in situations where donor autografts may not be available in sufficient quantity. Nerve conduits such as autogenous vein and sundry bioabsorbable tubes have also shown incipient experimental success in regenerating across smaller nerve (<3 cm) gaps.

CRANIOFACIAL SURGERY

Craniofacial surgery is an amalgamation of soft-tissue and skeletal reconstruction in both congenital and acquired defects. Although Gillies and Converse remain as historical contributors to the nascence of this new field, Paul Tessier is credited as the father and pioneer of craniofacial surgery. In 1967, at the International Plastic Surgery Congress, Tessier confronted the world of plastic surgery with his philosophy: intra- and extracranial approaches via coronal and intraoral incisions, osteotomies and augmentation of hard tissue, strategies for craniofacial tumors, and the definitive cleft classification (Fig. 44-18).

Cleft Lip and Palate

Before identifying the embryogenesis of cleft lip and palate, the anatomic boundaries of both entities must first be established. The

Table 44-4
Seddon's Classification

Neuropraxia	Conduction block Normal histology Reversible injury
Axonotmesis	Axonal disruption Wallerian degeneration
Neurotmesis	Complete transection

Table 44-5
Sunderland's Classification

Type I	Myelin interruption, 3-month recovery
Type II	Axonal discontinuity
Type III	Axonal, endoneural discontinuity
Type IV	Axonal, endo- and perineural discontinuity
Type V	Complete transection
Type VI	Combination injury

primary palate contains the lip, alveolus, and hard palate to the incisive foramen, while the secondary palate comprises the hard and soft palate posterior to the incisor foramen. In normal embryologic growth, the five facial elements (frontonasal, lateral maxillary, and mandibular segments) merge via mesenchymal migration to mold the face and jaws. Two theories have emerged to rationalize cleft lip embryogenesis. In the classic theory, failure of fusion of the maxillary processes and frontonasal processes during this time interval yields a cleft of the primary palate. In the mesodermal penetration theory propelled by Stark, palate closure is predicated on mesodermal penetration. Without this mesodermal migration and reinforcement, epithelial breakdown and separation ensues, resulting in a cleft.

Cleft lip/palate and cleft palate must be envisioned as two separate entities. Cleft lip and palate predominates when compared to isolated cleft lip and isolated cleft palate (46 vs. 21% and 33%, respectively). In addition, left unilateral cleft lip surpasses right unilateral and bilateral cleft lip (6:3:1). The ratio of incidence of cleft lip varies with ethnicity: 0.41:1000 in African Americans, 1:1000 in whites, and 2.1:1000 in Asians. The etiology of cleft lip is regarded as multifactorial. Important potential risk factors include anticonvulsants, parental age, lower socioeconomic class, smoking, alcohol intake, and prenatal nutrition. Concomitantly, parents or siblings with cleft lip and palate predispose future children to an increased risk. In families of a one-cleft parent or sibling, there is a 4% risk of a subsequent child being born with cleft lip/palate.[18]

Cleft lip can be further classified into complete (where the cleft extends in the nostril floor) or incomplete (where a tissue bridge unites the lateral and central lip). Essential to cleft lip repair is a comprehension of abnormal anatomy. The cleft lip is characterized by an ill-defined philtral ridge on the cleft side, vertical shortness, vermilion thinning, an obfuscated white roll, hypoplastic musculature, and abnormal muscle insertions. The cleft lip is frequently concatenated with a distinct nasal deformity. This includes a tilted platform, unilateral shortness of columella height, nasal floor deficiency, outward flaring of alar base, and malpositioned lower lateral cartilages (Fig. 44-19).

The bilateral cleft lip poses a more formidable challenge to the cleft surgeon because of the nasal and osseous deformities. The premaxilla is outwardly rotated and projected, the prolabium is

Table 44-6
British Medical Research Council Muscle-Grading Scale

Muscle Grade	Observation
0	No contraction
1	Flicker or trace of contraction
2	Active movement, with gravity eliminated
3	Active movement against gravity
4	Active movement against gravity and resistance
5	Normal power

devoid of muscle, the alae are widely spread with dislocation of the lateral cartilages, the columella is almost nonexistent, and the lateral maxillary elements are retropositioned (Fig. 44-20).[19] Surgical correction of both unilateral and bilateral cleft lips demands a multidisciplinary approach involving plastic surgery, otolaryngology, orthodontics, and speech pathology.

Timing of surgical repair is often dictated by the "rule of tens" with obvious permutations: 10 weeks of age, 10 lbs, and 10 mg/dL hemoglobin. Prior to definitive repair, the patient may undergo presurgical orthodontics via a Latham appliance and or lip adhesion. This facilitates alveolar segment alignment, providing a more symmetric platform on which to repair the cleft lip. Nevertheless, the plastic surgeon aspires to accomplish the following goals in cleft lip repair: lengthen cleft to vertical height of normal side; balance cupid's bow; reorient and align orbicularis oris; maintain vermilion and white roll continuity; and re-create the philtral column and dimple (Fig. 44-21).

Cleft lip repair is frequently carried out under general anesthesia. After marking the designed flaps, the lip is anesthetized with dilute lidocaine and epinephrine in order to curb bleeding. A plenitude of techniques described by Thompson, LeMuserier, and Tennison-Randall have surfaced and promulgated the plastic surgery literature. The rotation advancement lip operation by Millard has risen as a popular option in cleft lip surgery (Fig. 44-22). In this scheme, a rotation incision follows the philtral line to the columella, incorporating a back cut through skin, muscle, and mucosa. This permits a philtral length of 10 mm, placing the cupid's bow in a neutral position. An advancement flap is created via a transverse incision around the ala in order to release the alar rim from the lip. The C-flap is secured to lengthen the columella while the denuded tip of the alar base is sutured to the septum. The orbicularis oris of the advancement flap is approximated into the back cut of the rotation. After correct alignment of the vermilion borders, a three-layer closure of mucosa, muscle, and skin is excised.

Surgical correction of bilateral cleft lips presents more technical demands and, often, less satisfying results. The plastic surgeon must address the protruded premaxilla and immobile labium, as well as the lack of orbicularis continuity. Therefore, presurgical orthodontics is frequently employed to manipulate the premaxilla and construct a symmetric platform (Fig. 44-2). In the Millard bilateral cleft repair, the prolabium is outlined with philtral and forked laps. The orbicularis oris is realigned while the philtral flap is secured to the lateral lip segments to create a cupid's bow. The forked flaps are sutured to the alar bases in order to construct the nostrils (Fig. 44-23).

Cleft Palate

In the embryologic scheme, palatal shelves develop as swellings of the medial maxillary prominences. After downward growth adjacent to the tongue, the shelves become horizontal and fuse. Complete closure of the plate transpires after 12 weeks. Incomplete closure of these palatal shelves will ostensibly produce cleft palate. Cleft palates can be further distinguished as complete (extension into the nose) or incomplete (existing midline attachment). Moreover, submucous cleft palate, the most common, is exemplified by three physical findings: bifid uvula, thin membranous central portion, and a posterior palpable notch. Cleft palates are routinely associated with more than 200 syndromes/malformations. Incidence by ethnic groups varies as follows: American Indians (3.6:10,000), Asians (3:1000), and African Americans (0.3:1000).

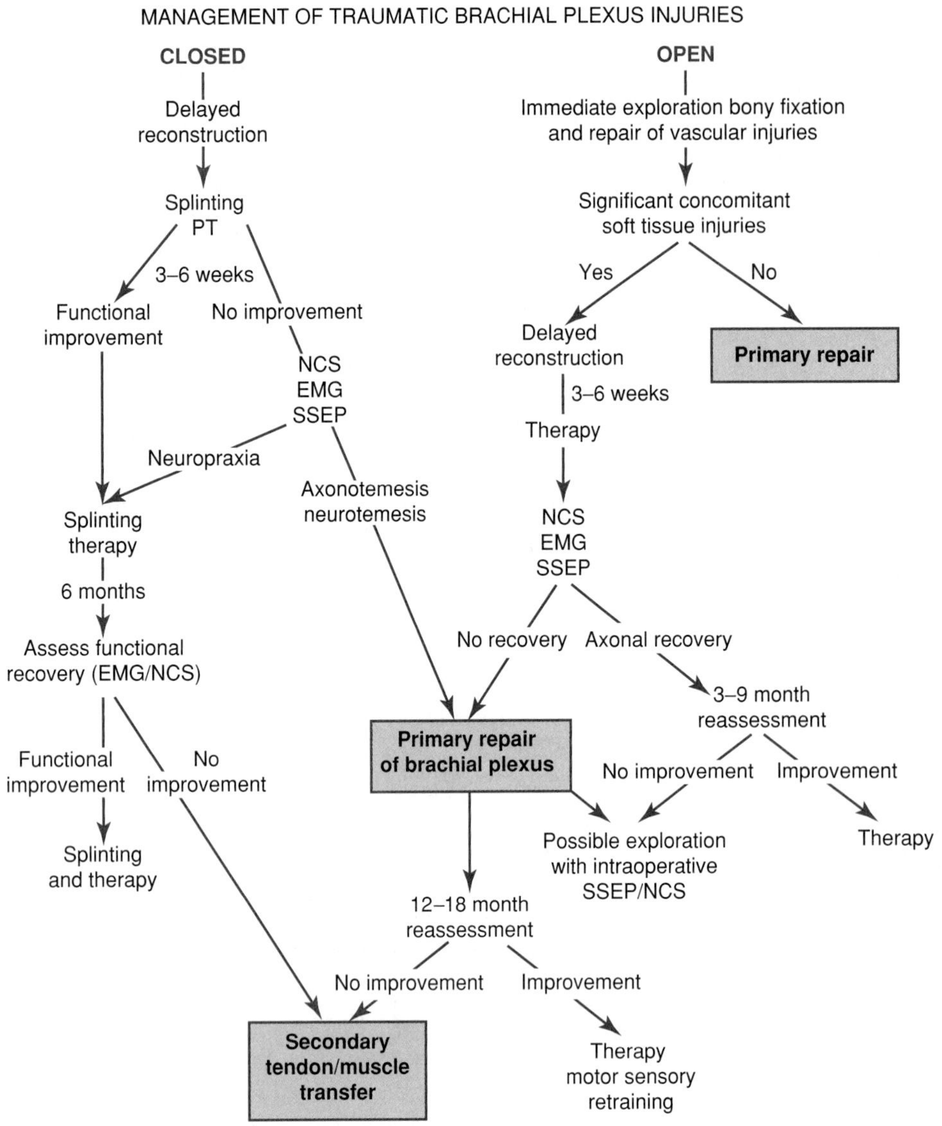

MANAGEMENT OF TRAUMATIC BRACHIAL PLEXUS INJURIES

FIG. 44-15. *Algorithm for open vs. closed brachial plexus injury.*

Similarly, with cleft lip, there is a plethora of etiologies, including teratogens, alcohol, dietary deficiencies, and maternal epilepsy.

Vital to speech and swallowing, the hard palate behaves as a static partition between oral and nasal chambers, while the soft palate acts as a dynamic barrier. The soft palate elevates and moves posteriorly during velopharyngeal closure, facilitating swallowing and speech production. In the cleft palate, velopharyngeal valving cannot be achieved or maintained, which induces hypernasal speech or velopharyngeal insufficiency. Because of nasal and oral continuity, negative intraoral pressure cannot be sustained, promoting ineffective sucking and feeding. In addition to feeding and speech difficulties, cleft palate children often have facial growth disturbances, middle ear disease, or recurrent otitis media.

Surgical repair is predicated on the separation of oral and nasal cavities and the formation of a tight velopharyngeal valve. Surgical correction must provide adequate palate length and mobility. The timing of repair remains controversial. Early palate repair affords the advantage of improved speech but also exacerbates midface retrusion. The cleft palate is routinely closed before 12 months of age.[20]

Cleft palate repair is performed under general anesthesia, in which the head is hyperextended and visualization of the palate is achieved with a Dingman retractor. The palate is anesthetized with lidocaine and epinephrine. Repair can be achieved by a multitude of techniques such as von Langenbeck, Veau-Wardill-Kilner pushback, or Furlow palatoplasty. In the von Langenbeck procedure, bipedicled mucoperiosteal flaps from the hard and soft palate are raised and closed in the midline. In the pushback palatoplasty, the mucoperiosteal flaps are created by a W-shaped incision (Fig. 44-24). This liberates the mucoperiosteum from the palate, lengthens the hard palate, and exposes the bone anteriorly and laterally. The intravelar veloplasty reorients the musculus levator veli palatini, which has inserted abnormally on the hard palate. Palatoplasty with and without veloplasty has demonstrated no difference regarding eventual velopharyngeal competency. The vomer flap, composed of vomer mucoperiosteum, is elevated and rotated laterally to address the anterior cleft palate. Moreover, reconstruction of the levator sling can be accomplished with a Furlow palatoplasty. In this schema, the palatal musculature is repositioned and the velum is lengthened by double-opposing Z plasties (Fig. 44-25).

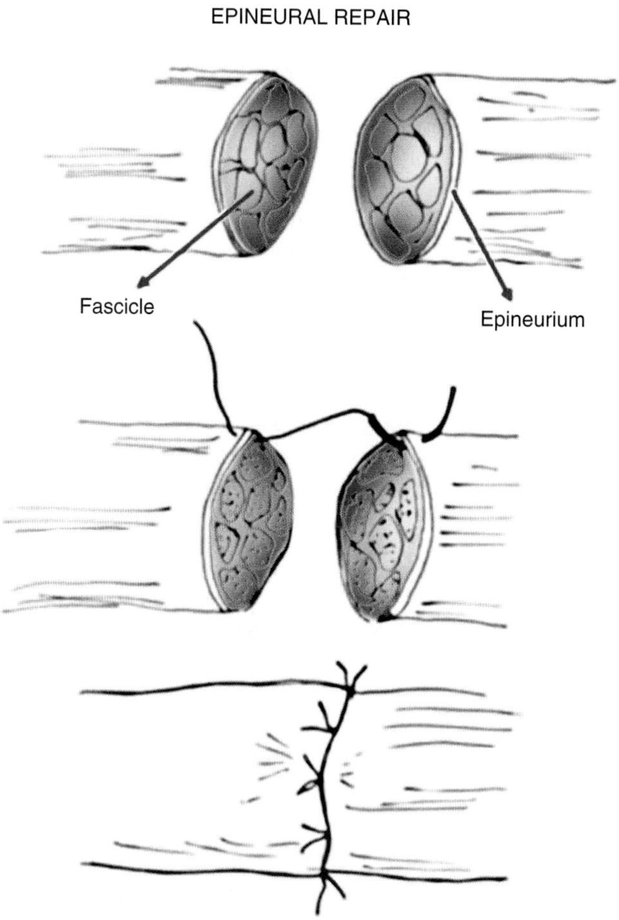

EPINEURAL REPAIR

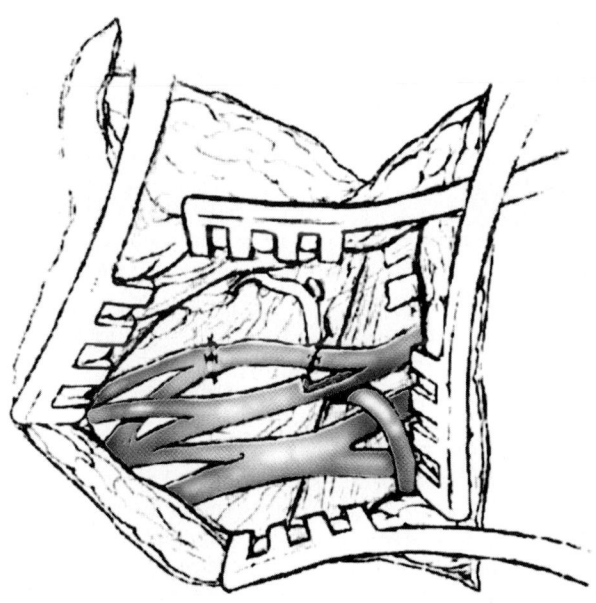

FIG. 44-16. Nerve repair: epineural repair.

Fascicle

Epineurium

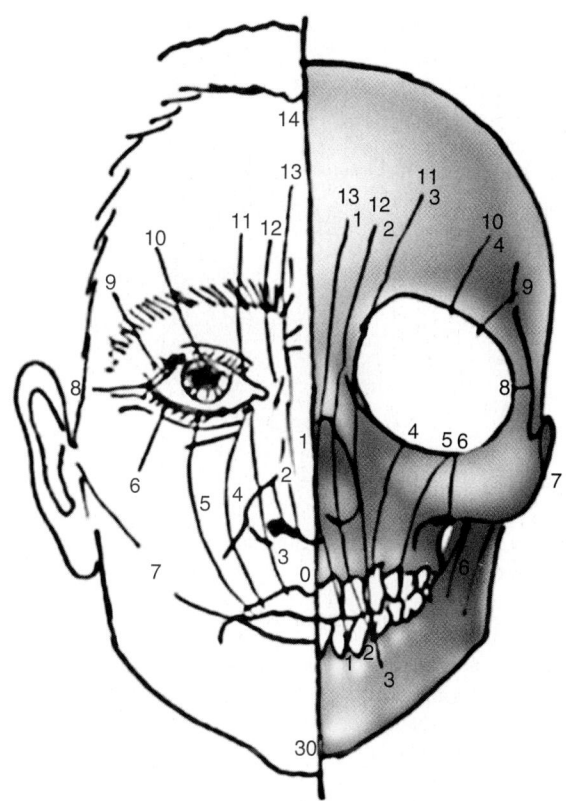

FIG. 44-18. Tessier classification of craniofacial clefts.

Following cleft palate closure, velopharyngeal insufficiency may still ensue. The incidence of velopharyngeal insufficiency varies from 30 to 50%. The plurality of these patients with velopharyngeal insufficiency and speech deficits can be successfully ameliorated with speech therapy. Children who do not respond may require additional procedures after age 4 years with either a superiorly based pharyngeal flap or a sphincter pharyngoplasty. In addition, at a later age, these children will necessitate closure of the vestibular and palatal nasal fistula. At ages 6 to 8 years, bone grafting to the alveolar cleft will provide sufficient bone stock for lateral incisor and canine teeth eruption and provide bony architecture of the premaxilla. Final revisions and enhancement in cleft patients entails

FIG. 44-17. C7 transfer to C5-C6 in brachial plexus injuries. The suprascapular nerve is neurotized by the spinal accessory nerve. The functional C7 roots is split and used as a donor to the anterior and posterior divisions of the upper trunk via multiple sural nerve grafts.

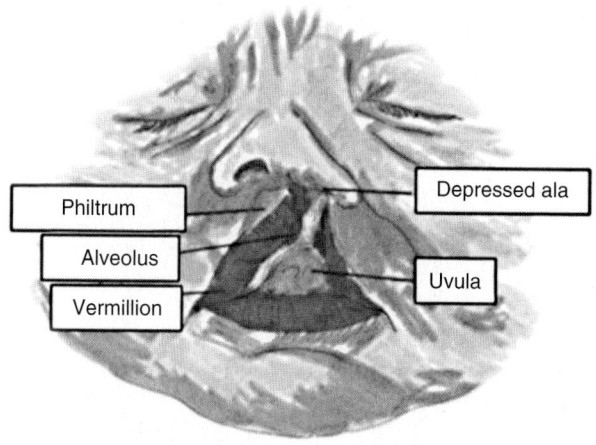

Philtrum

Alveolus

Vermillion

Depressed ala

Uvula

FIG. 44-19. Cleft lip anatomy.

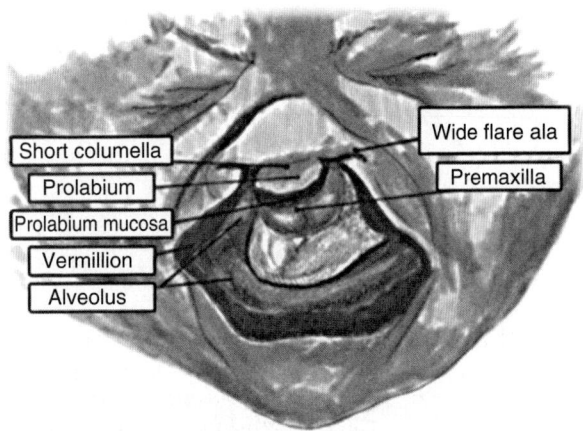

FIG. 44-20. Bilateral cleft lip anatomy.

maxillary advancement, orthognathic surgery, lip augmentation, and rhinoplasty.[21]

Hemangiomas and Vascular Malformations

Hemangiomas are common vascular tumors that plague the pediatric population and expand via endothelial proliferation (Table 44-7). Hemangiomas have been subjected to diverse classification systems as well as appellations from cherry angiomas to strawberry hemangiomas. Differentiation and comparisons can be elucidated based on clinical, histologic, hematologic, and radiologic evidence. Histologically, they classically evince hypercellularity, endothelial multiplication, increased mast cell population, and multilaminated basement membranes. Thirty percent of hemangiomas are present at birth and 80% of these are recognized during the first month of life.[22] Females are more inclined to develop hemangiomas. The majority presides in the head and neck region and they frequently undergo accelerated growth. Distinguished as a small red or deep bluish patch, they rapidly proliferate during the first 2 years. Following this proliferative phase, hemangiomas steadily involute and will often dissolve, requiring no further therapy; 50% spontaneously resolve by age 5 years, while 70% will do so by age 7 years.[23]

Early therapy or surgical excision is obligatory in patients with visual or airway impairment, bleeding or ulceration, infection, Kasabach-Merritt syndrome, or congestive heart failure. Noninvasive modalities include intralesional steroid injections, corticosteroids, and interferon α-2a. Invasive therapies involve surgical excision, laser or cryotherapy, and embolization. Laser photothermolysis is preferable during the hemangioma's proliferative phase, while surgery and steroids remain the mainstay treatment during the later stages. Nonetheless, controversy pervades the timing of surgical intervention in regards to waiting for resolution.

Previously regarded as a complication of an infantile hemangioma, Kasabach-Merritt syndrome has developed as a discrete entity and usually involves a firm hemangioma of the torso or extremity

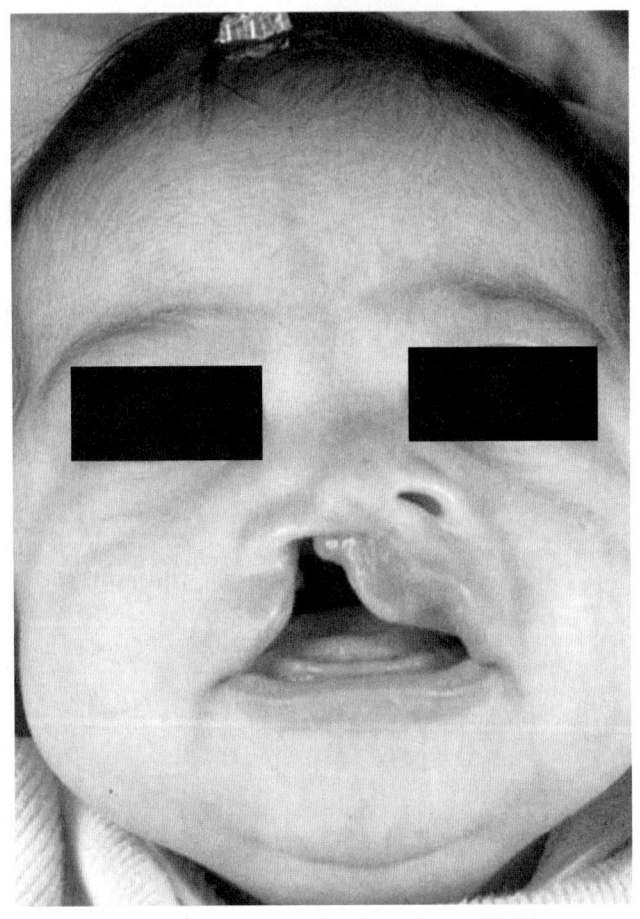

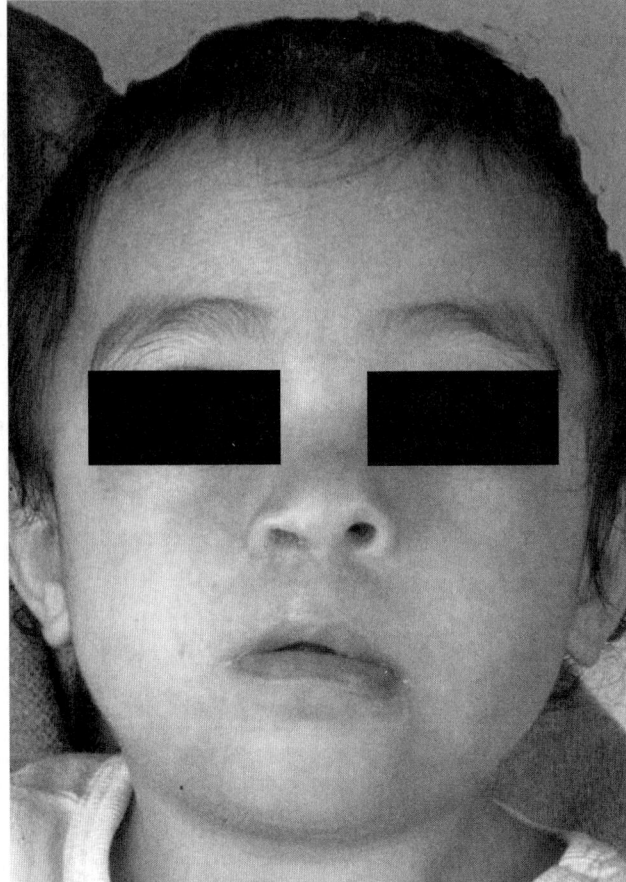

A   *B*

FIG. 44-21. Unilateral cleft lip repair. *A.* Preoperative photo. *B.* Postoperative photo.

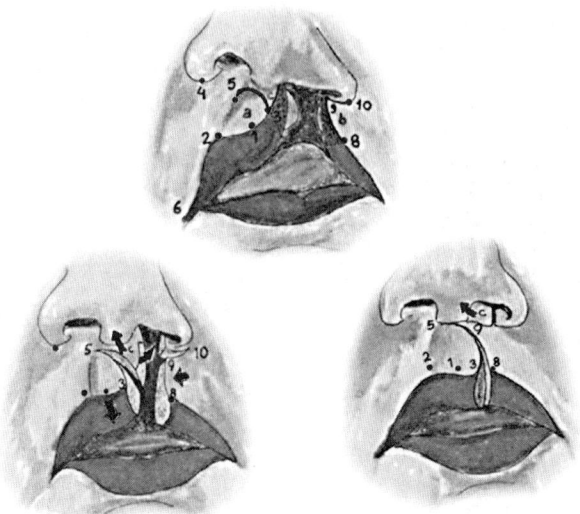

FIG. 44-22. *Unilateral cleft lip repair: Millard rotation advancement. The philtrum and cupid's bow are rotated down to permit advancement of tissue from the lateral cleft side. The C-flap will form the nostril floor and philtrum.*

in conjunction with thrombocytopenia. Platelet transfusions can exacerbate the thrombocytopenia and can aggrandize hemangioma growth. Vincristine has emerged as the only agent that possesses potential uniform effectiveness.

Defined as vascular structural abnormalities, vascular malformations arise as a consequence of faulty embryogenic morphogenesis. They all present at birth, and grow commensurately with the child. They have no sexual predilection and do not display the typical rapid proliferation or regression of hemangiomas. Within regard to their histologic appearance, they exhibit flat endothelium, normal mast cell population, and thin basement membranes. In terms of classification, they are divided into slow-flow and fast-flow lesions. The slow-flow malformations are capillary, lymphatic, or venous in nature, while the fast-flow lesions comprise arterial aneurysms, arteriovenous fistulas, and arteriovenous malformations. Skeletal distortion or hypertrophy may accompany vascular malformations,

particularly in the upper extremity.[24] Moreover, these malformations may display the following clinical attributes: increased skin temperature, bruit or thrill, high-output cardiac failure, bleeding or ulceration, pain, and tissue overgrowth. Frequently, fast-flow lesions remain dormant, but they may precipitously expand as a result of trauma, infection, hormonal changes, or attempted resection.[25]

Superselective arteriography with embolization, followed by surgical resection, remains the most potent therapeutic modality. Nevertheless, these extensive lesions have a propensity to bleed, often require soft-tissue reconstruction, and possess high morbidity and mortality rates.

Lymphatic malformations commonly reside in the head, neck, and groin with extensive infiltration and soft-tissue hypertrophy. Lymphatic malformations such as lymphangiomas and cystic hygromas expand along venous channels and contribute to a wide spectrum of symptoms. Although antibiotics and local wound care are reserved for cellulitis and their infectious component, surgical excision is the only definitive remedy for lymphatic malformations. As a consequence of their invasion of vital neck structures, debulking of these malformations may be the only prudent solution.

Venous malformations, delineated as localized, bluish, telangiectatic lesions caused by incompetent valves, grow proportionately with age. They demonstrate sluggish flow/stasis with a propensity for thrombosis, as well as compression with rapid filling. Treatment modalities include sclerotherapy, compression garments, laser thermolysis, and surgical excision. Finally, capillary malformations or port-wine stains materialize at birth and display no regression or resolution. They frequently manifest in a cutaneous trigeminal distribution and will darken to red or purple with age. Coupled with syndromes such as Sturge-Weber or Klippel-Trenaunay, they may present with orbital malformations or glaucoma. Excision of smaller lesions is ostensibly appropriate but laser therapy is reserved for larger intradermal lesions.

Craniosynostosis

Craniosynostosis is defined as the premature closure of one or more cranial suture(s). Based on Virchow's law, premature closure involves limited skeletal growth perpendicular to the suture line compensated by overgrowth parallel to the suture. The incidence of craniosynostosis is 1:1000 births and its etiology is multifactorial. Several theories have surfaced to elucidate premature suture fusion, such as in utero intrinsic and extrinsic forces, as well as dura mater injury and its interplay with cranial skeleton growth.

Craniosynostosis interferes with brain growth in a confined, bony vault. Functional complications include intracranial hypertension, visual disturbances, hydrocephalus, airway emergencies, limited brain growth, speech and language deficits, and neuropsychiatric disorders.

Craniosynostosis can exist as an isolated manifestation or be associated with a craniofacial syndrome. In any event, craniosynostosis is classified according to the specific suture fusion and/or skull shape.

Frontal plagiocephaly often occurs with coronal synostosis and is defined by a flattened forehead on the affected side, upward displacement of the orbit, and anterior projection of the ear. The craniofacial surgeon must differentiate true unilateral coronal synostosis from posterior plagiocephaly both clinically and radiographically (Table 44-8).

Scaphocephaly occurs with sagittal synostosis and is demarcated by reduced cranial width and increased anteroposterior length. Trigonocephaly involves narrowing of the forehead in a triangular

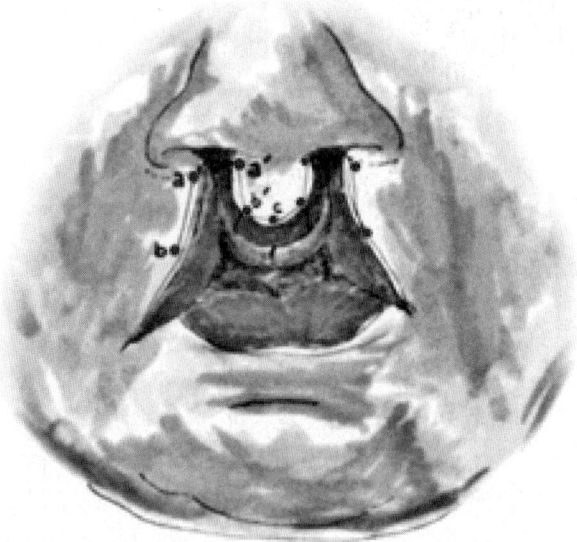

FIG. 44-23. *Bilateral cleft lip repair: markings.*

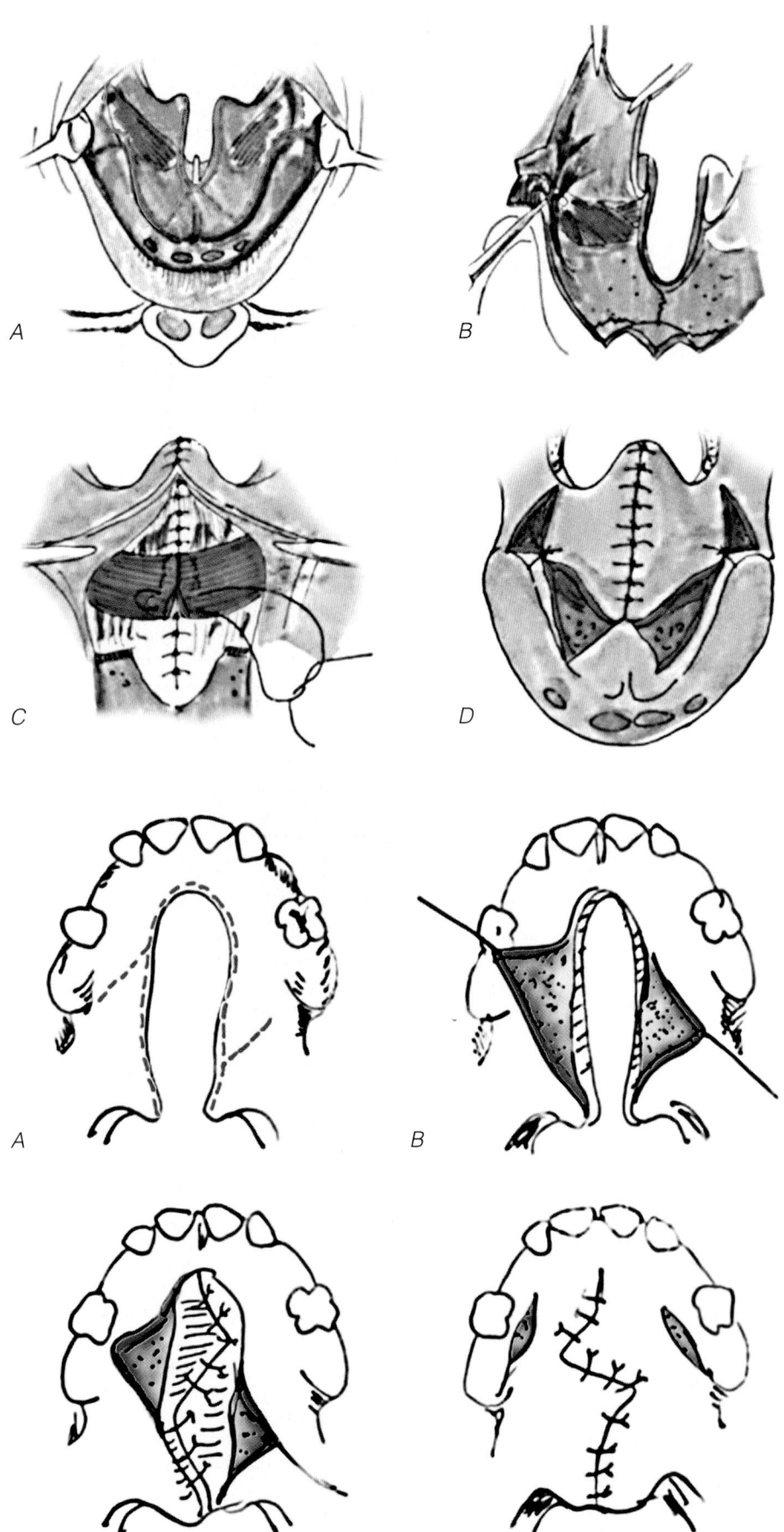

FIG. 44-24. Veau-Wardill-Kilner push-back palatoplasty. *A.* Design of flaps. *B.* Mucoperiosteal flaps are elevated off of the hard palate, maintaining the greater palatine vessels. The nasal lining and mucosal layer are dissected. *C.* Reapproximation of the nasal lining/mucosal layer with closure. The musculus levator veli palatini sling is dissected and realigned in the midline. *D.* The mucoperiosteal flaps are brought together and closed in the midline and secured to the anterior mucosa of the hard palate.

FIG. 44-25. Palatoplasty: Furlow Z-plasty. *A.* Design of Z flaps. *B.* Elevation of mucosal flaps. *C.* Repair of nasal lining and musculus levator veli palatine sling. *D.* Transposition and lengthening of flaps with closure.

Table 44-7
Hemangiomas vs. Vascular Malformations

Hemangiomas	Vascular Malformations
30% present at birth	All present at birth
Rapid growth	Growth commensurate
Slow involution	No involution
Female:male ratio 3:1	Female:male ratio 1:1
Endothelial cell proliferation	Flat endothelium
Increased mast cell	Normal mast cell population
Seldom mass effect on bone	Venous malformation: bone rarefication and hypoplasia
	Mixed capillary-venous: bone hypertrophy
Angiography: organized lobular parenchymal staining	Angiography: collection of vessels without parenchymal mass
Elevated urinary bFGF	Normal bFGF

bFGF = basic fibroblast growth factor.

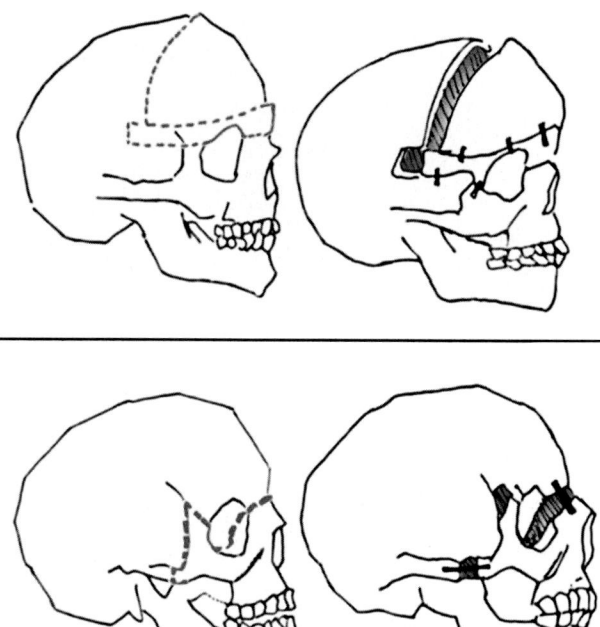

formation with a prominent ridge and corresponds with metopic synostosis. A widened, flattened skull combined with upward growth characterizes brachiocephaly. There is often exophthalmos, which is commonly caused by bilateral coronal synostosis.[26]

Craniosynostosis Syndromes

The craniofacial syndromes display suture synostosis manifestations in conjunction with other malformations (extremity) and mental/growth disturbances. Crouzon syndrome is distinguished by a brachycephalic vault, midfacial retrusion with class III malocclusion, increased intracranial pressure, and exophthalmos. Apert syndrome involves brachycephaly: high cranial vault flattening with bulging; exophthalmos; hypertelorism (increased distance between orbits); and extremity syndactyly, particularly of the phalanges. Saethre-Chotzen syndrome is characterized by brachycephaly, shallow orbits, telecanthus, low-set hairline, and cutaneous syndactyly. Pfeiffer syndrome also consists of brachycephaly, but is distinguished by broad thumbs and toes.[27]

Craniofacial Reconstruction

The goals of craniofacial reconstructive surgery entail the release of fused suture line and decompression and cranial vault remodeling by removing and reshaping cranial bones with absorbable plates. The timing of surgery frequently occurs during 6 to 12 months of age (Fig. 44-26).

In unilateral and bilateral coronal synostosis, fronto-orbital remodeling with advancement is preferred (Fig. 44-27). The surgeon performs a bifrontal craniotomy, exposing the anterior and middle

FIG. 44-26. Bilateral coronal synostosis. *A.* Preoperative photo. *B.* Postoperative photo after cranial remodeling.

Table 44-8
Unilateral Coronal Synostosis vs. Deformational Plagiocephaly

Anatomic Feature	Unilateral Coronal Synostosis	Deformational Plagiocephaly
Ipsilateral eyebrow	Up	Down
Ipsilateral ear	Anterior and high	Posterior and low
Nasal root	Ipsilateral	Midline
Ipsilateral cheek	Forward	Backward
Chin deviation	Contralateral	Ipsilateral
Ipsilateral palpebral fissure	Wide and/or low	Narrow and/or high
Anterior fontanelle	Contralateral	None

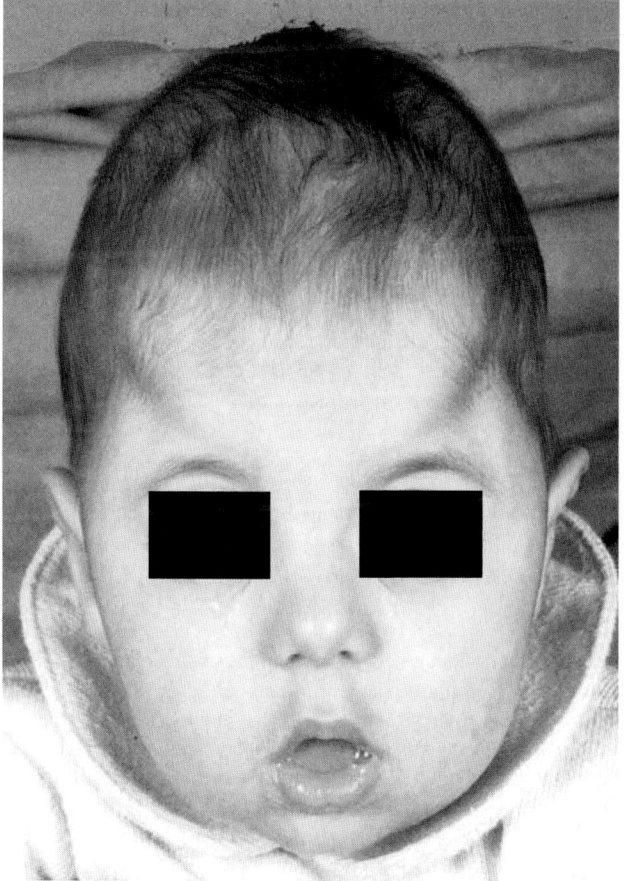

FIG. 44-27. Bifrontal advancement.

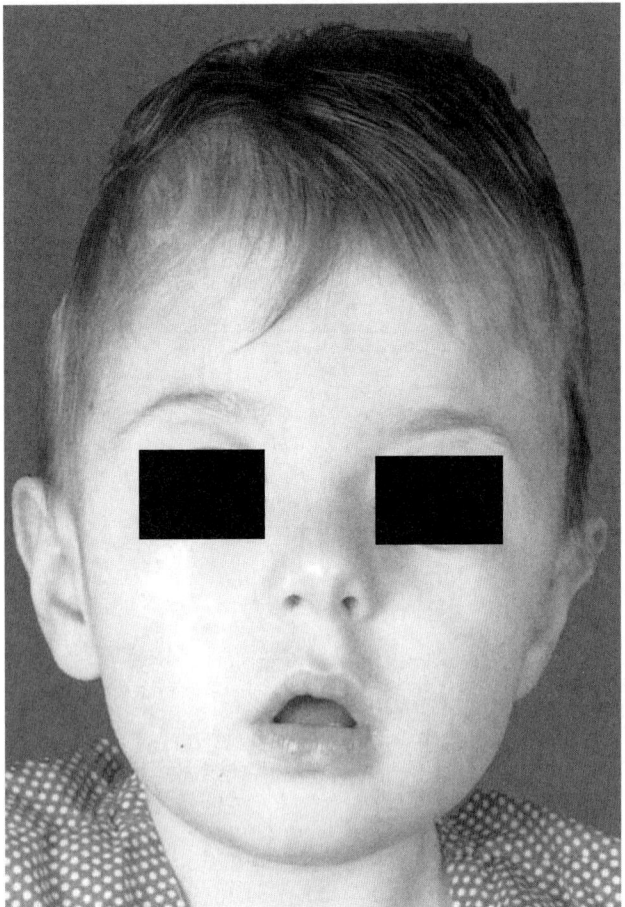

FIG. 44-28. LeFort III advancement.

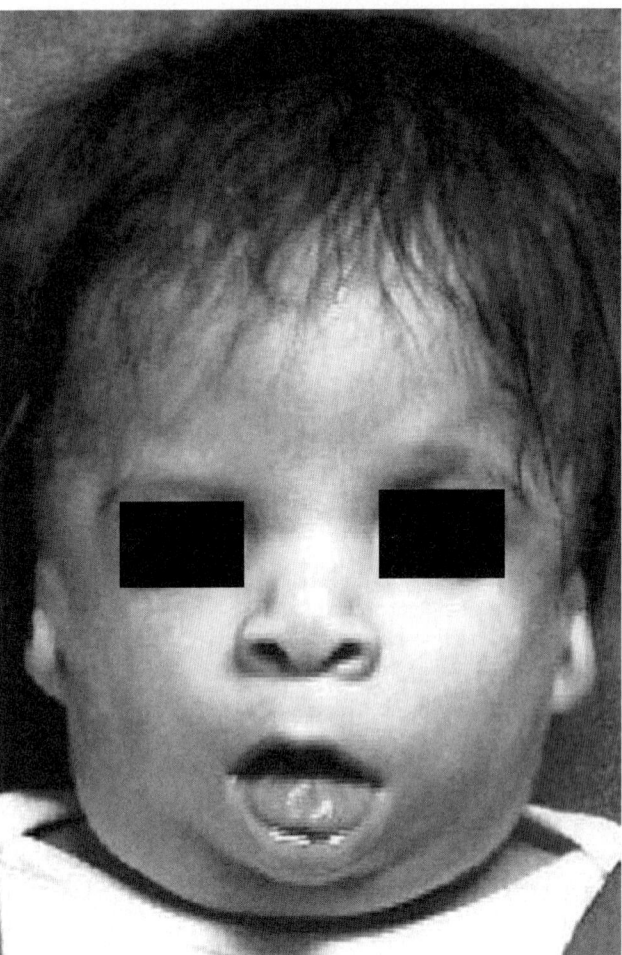

FIG. 44-29. Treacher-Collins complex.

cranial fossa where the supraorbital bar is removed, reshaped, and advanced to give the anterior cranium a new, rounded mold. In the setting of syndromic forms, simultaneous forehead and midface advancement is executed with a monobloc frontofacial osteotomy. Because this method has a higher infection and bone sequestration rate, craniofacial surgeons may prefer a fronto-orbital advancement and address the midface at a later date using a LeFort III advancement (Fig. 44-28).[28] Furthermore, aggrandized midface advancement can now be better achieved via distraction osteogenesis.

Laterofacial Microsomias

Other entities, which truly represent laterofacial clefts, include Treacher-Collins syndrome and hemifacial microsomia.

Treacher-Collins Complex

The main characteristics of this complex include deficits of the maxilla and zygoma; upper eyelid colobomas; smaller palpebral fissure; deviated, narrow nose; amblyopia or strabismus; hypoplastic mandible; chin retrusion; and microtia (Fig. 44-29). Operative treatment requires three to four stages. Stage I aims at reconstructing the orbit and zygomatic arches with bone graft. In stage II, the jaw and dentition are reconstructed by LeFort II osteotomy variation, midface forward tilting, and rotation. In stages III and IV, open rhinoplasty and microtia repair are entertained as complementary procedures.

Hemifacial Microsomia

Patients with hemifacial microsomia, the most common craniofacial anomaly, often present with unilateral microtia, macrostomia, and failure of formation of the mandible and condyle, as well as orbital and zygomatic hypoplasia (Fig. 44-30). As in Treacher-Collins complex, the craniofacial team carries out a multistage reconstruction. Stage I involves distraction osteogenesis with or without a costochondral graft for the mandible. Stage II is demarcated by orthodontic treatment and ear reconstruction. Finally, in the tertiary stage, the mandible may require further bony revision in conjunction with soft-tissue enhancement by either fat grafting or free tissue transfer.

Orthognathic Surgery

In the craniofacial arena, the mandible and/or maxilla can be disproportionate in the setting of trauma or congenital anomalies (i.e., cleft lip/palate, hemifacial microsomia). The mandible and maxilla are the framework for the teeth, and they provide the function of chewing. Therefore, maxillary/mandibular imbalance and malalignment can contribute to ineffective chewing and malocclusion. The patient with this degree of disproportion must be evaluated by a multidisciplinary team, consisting of a plastic surgeon, oral surgeon, and orthodontist. The surgeon must inspect the patient's oral hygiene, state of dental repair, and, most importantly, assess the dental occlusion.

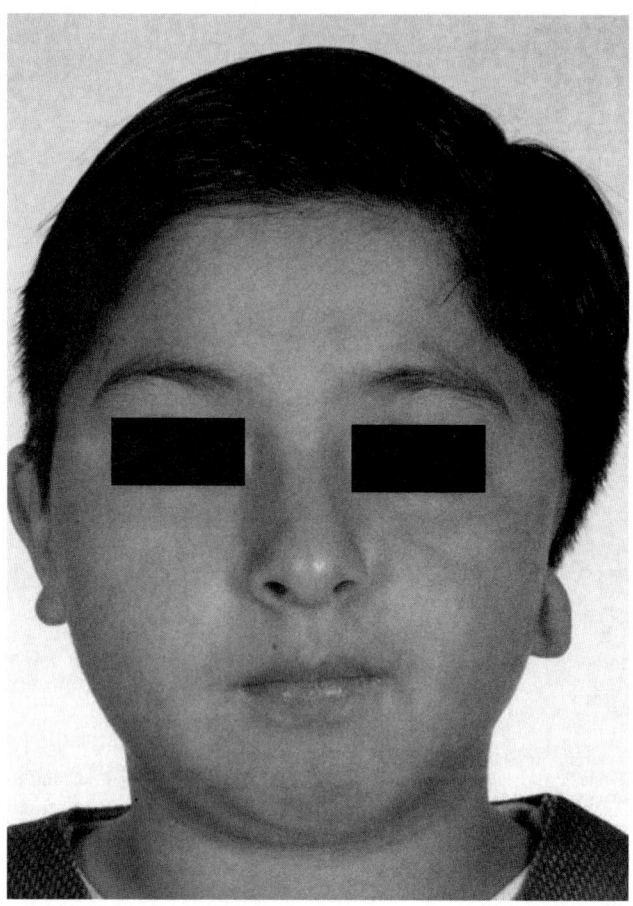

FIG. 44-30. Hemifacial microsomia.

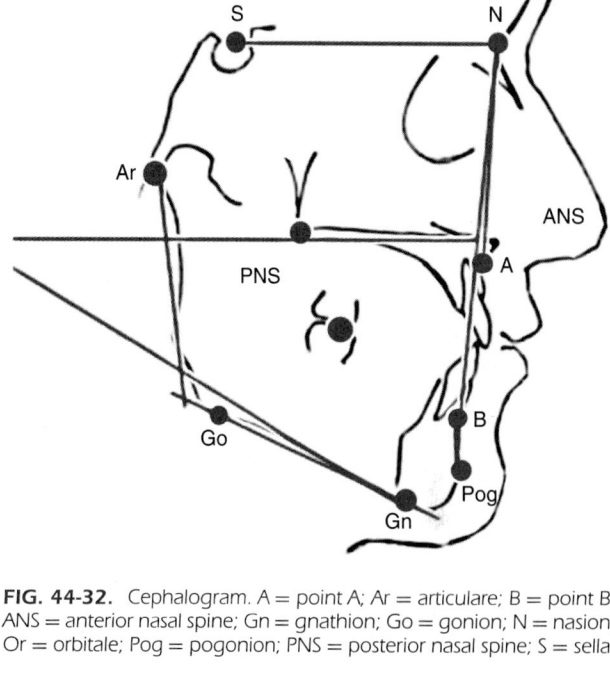

FIG. 44-32. Cephalogram. A = point A; Ar = articulare; B = point B; ANS = anterior nasal spine; Gn = gnathion; Go = gonion; N = nasion; Or = orbitale; Pog = pogonion; PNS = posterior nasal spine; S = sella.

Classification of Occlusion

Dental occlusive relationships are characterized by Angle's classification. In normal occlusion, Angle's class I, the mesiobuccal cusp of the upper first molar is in the buccal groove of the lower first molar. In class II occlusion, the lower first molar is situated distal to the buccal groove of the lower first molar, while in class III occlusion, the lower first molar is positioned mesial to this relationship (Fig. 44-31).

Cephalometric Analysis

Cephalograms are radiographs generated with the head held at a specific distance (Fig. 44-32). Cephalometric analysis will ascertain vertical face, horizontal midface, horizontal lower face, and dental measurements. Cephalometric analysis, in conjunction with a

meticulous examination, determines which corrective surgery should be executed on the jaws.[29]

The mandible and maxilla can be advanced, divided, or set back in a multitude of different combinations. A sagittal, splitting osteotomy, the most versatile procedure, can be employed for prognathia (class III, large mandible) and retrognathia (normal size but posterior position). A genioplasty is a horizontal osteotomy below the teeth roots of the mandible, used for chin advancement, lengthening, or shortening. It is often used in conjunction with other aesthetic or orthognathic procedures. Correction or mobilization of the maxilla can be achieved through a LeFort I osteotomy. In this setting, an osteotomy is carried across the anterior maxilla above the teeth root, permitting movement of the maxilla in any direction.

MAXILLOFACIAL TRAUMA

The plurality of facial fractures is induced by motor vehicle accidents or aggravated assault; 50 to 70% of patients with facial fractures/injuries will have accompanying injuries. These patients must

FIG. 44-31. Angles occlusion.

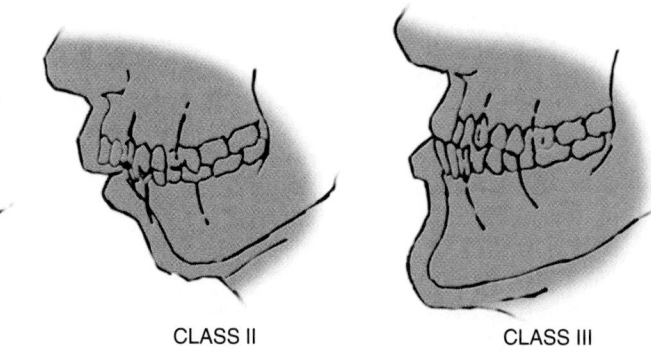

CLASS I   CLASS II   CLASS III

be subjected to comprehensive evaluation by a multidisciplinary team. Often the facial fracture is not a life-threatening emergency but the concomitant injuries can be critical or fatal to the trauma patient. Therefore, a coordinated team of multiple specialties must examine and monitor the patient and provide adequate resuscitation and treatment. Maxillofacial fractures can be divided into three categories: emergency, delayed, or early.

Emergency treatment for life-threatening facial fractures includes respiratory obstruction, aspiration, and hemorrhage. Pulmonary obstruction or aspiration can ensue as a consequence of complications from combined maxillary, mandibular, and nasal fractures, unstable comminuted mandible fractures with loss of tongue support, and bleeding in the presence of soft-tissue edema. In these circumstances, emergent nasal or general endotracheal intubation may be instituted if there is trepidation in future airway management. Tracheostomy or cricothyroidotomy as an emergent airway can be entertained in the setting of a head-injured patient who requires intermaxillary fixation, spastic head-injured patients, panfacial fractures, comminuted nasal and maxillary fractures with unstable occlusion, and patients with pulmonary injury who require intermaxillary fixation.[30]

After a systems evaluation has been completed and the patient is stabilized, the plastic surgeon must perform a thorough physical and radiographic examination. Facial injuries/fractures should be suspected in individuals with contusions, pain or localized tenderness, lacerations, numbness, paralysis, malocclusion, visual disturbances, and facial asymmetry. Nevertheless, examination of the face should be carried out in an orderly, concise manner, proceeding from either superior to inferior or inferior to superior and should entail:

- Evaluation for asymmetry and deformity.
- Palpation of entire craniofacial skeleton (orbital rims, nose, zygomatic arch, midface stability, mandible to detect any irregularities or crepitation).
- Investigation of facial nerve function on both sides.
- Evaluation of facial sensation regarding supratrochlear, supraorbital, infraorbital, and infra-alveolar nerve distribution.
- Intranasal inspection for septal hematoma.
- Ophthalmologic examination for any potential extraocular entrapment or optic nerve deficit.
- Malocclusion: excursion of jaw, the relationship of teeth during occlusion, detection of abnormal intercuspation, fractured or missing teeth, dislocation of the condyle from the glenoid fossa.

Radiologic Studies

Radiologic studies are designed to accompany and supplement the physical examination. Facial series, employed as a screening study, supports the clinical exam; standard views include posteroanterior, lateral, and Waters views. Mandibular series include oblique lateral and Towne views; these are most appropriate for detecting fractures of the symphysis, parasymphysis, and body of the mandible. A Panorex is preferred to inspect the condyle, the coronoid process, and temporomandibular joint.

Computerized axial tomography is the gold standard for diagnosis and operative planning for orbital fractures, frontal sinus fractures, nasoethmoidal fractures, and frontobasal fractures. Sagittal, coronal, and three-dimensional reconstruction views can be obtained or reformatted in coordination with the radiologist.

Mandibular Fractures

The mandible is the second most commonly injured facial bone and represents 10 to 25% of all facial fractures. The condyle and the

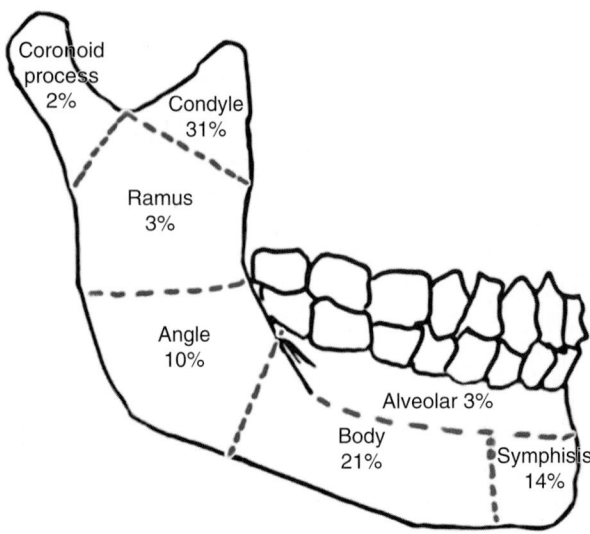

FIG. 44-33. Mandibular fractures: location and distribution.

angle are the two most frequent regions for mandibular fractures (Fig. 44-33). Mandibular fractures are often multiple and present in a myriad of combinations: angle-parasymphyseal and parasympyseal condyle. If a single fracture is identified, thorough investigation for a second should be undertaken. Furthermore, the surgeon should inspect the occlusion as well as the presence of any missing or fractured teeth.

The mandible should be regarded as having vertical and horizontal components, with the potential for multiple vector displacements. The mandible has muscular attachments: the masseter, temporalis, and lateral and medial pterygoids, which determine its displacement. The muscles that elevate the mandible are the masseter, medial pterygoid, and the temporalis. The lateral pterygoids project the mandible, while geniohyoid and digastric muscles depress and retract it. The fracture line direction may oppose fracture displacement via the interplay of muscle actions.

The objectives in treating mandible fractures include achieving reduction and stabilization, pretraumatic occlusion, facial contour and symmetry, and facial height and projection. Intraoral and extraoral incisions are closed and extruded bone fragments are débrided. Subcondylar fractures are usually treated with intermaxillary fixation, where the mandible and maxilla are positioned in appropriate occlusion and are wired together with arch bars or screws. Open reduction of subcondylar fractures is designated for those with condylar dislocation, severe malalignment, or loss of mandible height. Displaced fractures of the angle, body, and symphysis are treated via open reduction. Coronoid fractures often require no intervention.

Operative treatment of mandible fractures commences with intermaxillary fixation in order to guarantee appropriate occlusal relationship. Open reduction and fixation can be achieved by either an intraoral or extraoral approach. Symphyseal and parasymphysial are routinely addressed intraorally, whereas, body and angle fractures can be tackled by a percutaneous instrumentation or by open external incisions. There are two philosophies regarding fixation: the semirigid and the rigid fixation. In the semirigid technique, unicortical plates are positioned near the functional load-bearing region. In the rigid-fixation model, a tension band plate is placed on the upper border of the fracture, while a stronger plate is placed at the lower border.[31] A conservative approach is used in pediatric mandible fractures unless there is comminution or dislocation. These patients are subjected to brief intermaxillary fixation with early mobilization for fear of impeding mandibular growth.

Postoperatively, antibiotics and aggressive oral hygiene care are implemented. All patients are subjected to either a liquid or soft diet. Patients are routinely examined in clinic with a follow-up Panorex to assess occlusion and bony union. Intermaxillary fixation is released when deemed appropriate by the plastic surgeon. Complications of mandible fractures include infection, nonunion, delayed union, malocclusion, facial nerve injury, numbness caused by infra-alveolar nerve injury, and dental fractures.

Frontal Sinus Fracture

The frontal sinus resides in the central segment of the frontal bone, comprising two cavities draining from the nasofrontal duct to the middle meatus. The frontal sinus develops between the ages of 5 and 10 years and becomes radiographically evident at age 8 years. Frontal sinus fractures should be presumed in the setting of forehead contusions, bruises, or lacerations. They are often not associated with any acute symptomatology. Nevertheless, they can be accurately evaluated by computed tomography.

The most common surgical approach to the frontal sinus is through a coronal incision. Treatment of frontal sinus fractures is predicated on the number of walls involved and the status of the nasofrontal duct (Fig. 44-34). In nondisplaced anterior wall fractures, no treatment is indicated. If the anterior wall is displaced, then elevation and recontouring of the anterior table is executed. The patient should be observed for any sinus opacification or obstruction. If the nasofrontal duct is involved in the fracture, one can assume that this is a dysfunctional sinus.[32] Therefore, the sinus must be demucosalized, the nasofrontal duct must be plugged with bone graft, and sinus cavity obliterated with cancellous bone or fat. The technique of frontal sinus exenteration or removal of the anterior table, with demucosalization plugging of the ducts, is an antediluvian procedure not routinely performed because of the significant contour deformity.

In comminuted fractures of the posterior wall, a combined effort between neurosurgeon and plastic surgeon is implemented. A frontal craniotomy is performed, exposing dura and cranial base so the posterior wall of sinus can be removed. Subsequently, the nasofrontal duct is blocked, and the sinus is replaced with a pericranial flap.[33] Finally, the anterior table is reconstructed and recontoured.

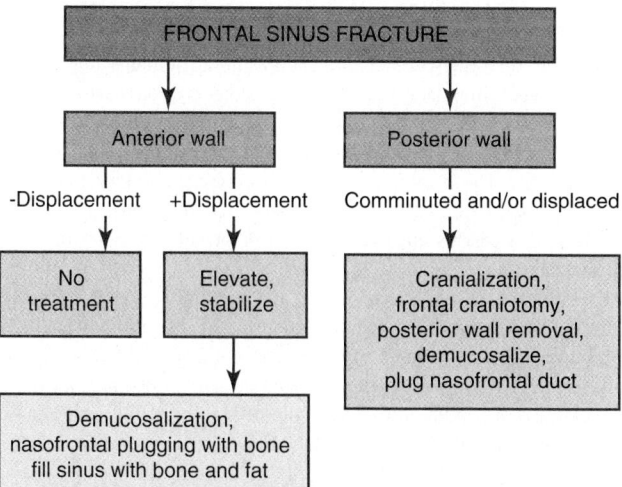

FIG. 44-34. Frontal sinus repair algorithm.

Eventually, over several months, the former space occupied by the frontal sinus will be invaded by expanding brain and dura.

Nasoethmoidal Orbital Fractures

Nasoethmoidal fractures involve injuries to both the nose and frontal processes of the maxilla. These fractures may predispose to telecanthus if the medial canthal attachments are involved. These injuries have the potential for subsequent deformity and are extremely challenging to repair. This diagnosis should be suspected in the background of nasal bleeding, depressed comminuted nasal fractures, nasal deformity associated with maxillary frontal process pain/tenderness, and bilateral eyelid hematomas. Computerized tomography remains the only reliable test in solidifying the diagnosis.[34]

Treatment of naso-orbitoethmoid fractures must be performed via open reduction and a combination of interfragmentary fixation and plate/screw fixation. The paramount maneuver is adequate transnasal reduction of the maxilla processes in order to vouchsafe intercanthal distance. All efforts should be made to preserve the medial canthal ligament and attachment. Surgical approach is frequently accomplished by multiple incisions: coronal, lower eyelid, and gingivobuccal. Nevertheless, bone grafting is often obligatory to reconstruct and augment the nasal dorsum.

Orbital Fractures

The most frequent orbital fracture is the "blow-out fracture," which is reserved to the medial orbital floor and lower medial orbital wall. Blow-out fractures and other orbital fractures may be accompanied by either superior or inferior rim fractures. Orbital floor blow-out fractures can be created by direct blunt trauma to the globe or by an acute rise in intraocular pressure leading to orbital floor and/or medial wall fracture. Symptoms include palpebral/subconjunctival hematoma, diplopia, infraorbital nerve numbness, and visual acuity disturbances. Therefore, a careful ophthalmologic and forced duction test should be performed. Enophthalmos often accompanies orbital floor fractures because of enhanced orbital volume.[35]

Indications for operative treatment and exploration are symptomatic diplopia greater than 2 weeks, positive forced duction test, muscle entrapment, orbital content herniation, orbital floor defect, and early enophthalmos. Goals of treatment are to reduce herniated contents and restore normal architecture and orbital volume. Approaches to orbital floor repair can be achieved by subciliary, subtarsal, or conjunctival incisions (Fig. 44-35).[36] The orbital rim can be reduced and rigidly fixated but the floor requires reconstruction with either autologous or alloplastic material. Bone grafts, titanium mesh, Medpor, LactoSorb, and a multitude of other alloplasts can be employed as filler substitutes. Complications of surgery vary from diplopia, ectropion, scleral show, to residual enophthalmos, and 10 to 20% of patients will require revision procedures.

Nasal Fractures

The nose is the most commonly fractured facial region. The nose is either laterally or posteriorly displaced, and the fracture may involve the cartilaginous septum, or both the nasal bones and septum. Patients commonly present with swelling, nasal deformity, epistaxis, septal deviation, and/or crepitus on palpation. Intranasal inspection should be performed, and if a septal hematoma is noted, it should be percutaneously drained. Diagnosis by CT scan is not obligatory but is implemented to rule out other injuries. Immediate treatment consists of reduction of both the pyramid and septum, followed by nasal splinting. In spite of early reduction, there is usually a residual

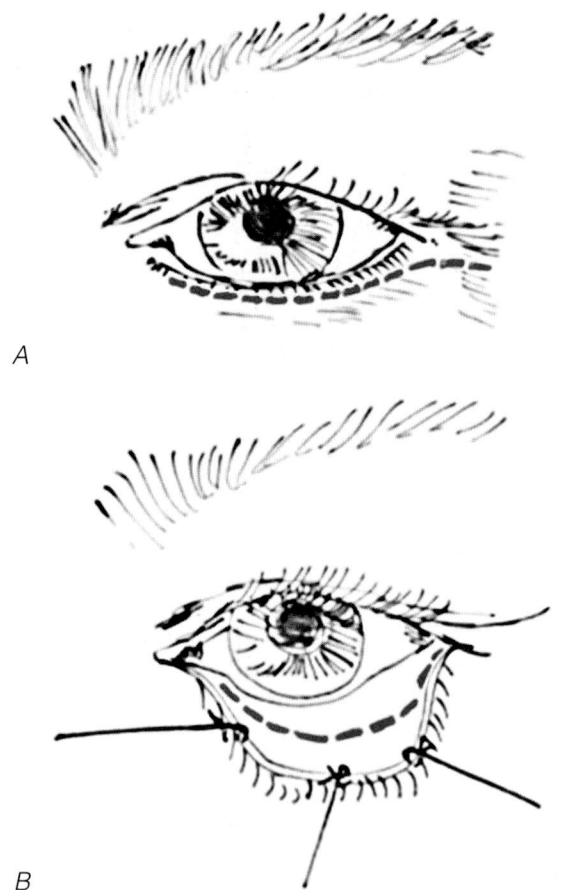

FIG. 44-35. Incisions for approaches to orbital floor fractures. *A.* Transconjunctival. *B.* Subciliary.

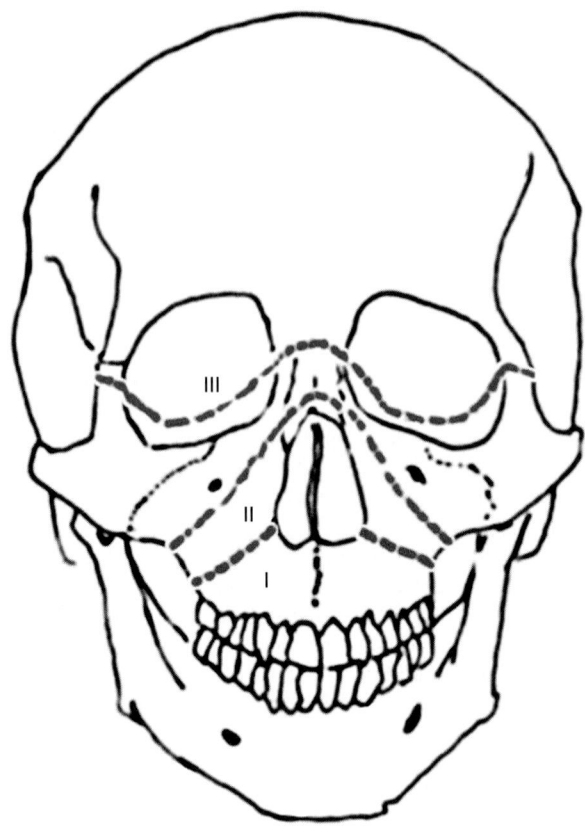

FIG. 44-36. LeFort Fracture classification. I = LeFort fracture I; II = LeFort fracture II; III = LeFort fracture III.

deformity or deviations, which will require formal rhinoplasty in an elective setting after swelling and bruising have resided.[37]

Zygoma Fractures

The anatomy of the zygoma is essential to comprehend because of its interplay and articulations with the craniofacial skeleton. It forms the lateral/inferior portion of the orbit, joins the frontal bone superiorly, the maxilla medially, and the temporal bone through the arch.

Signs and symptoms of zygomatic fractures include diplopia, trismus, depressed malar eminence, subconjunctival hemorrhage, infraorbital nerve paresthesias, and ipsilateral epistaxis. On examination, there may be step-off discrepancies or tenderness. Fractures can be confirmed by radiologic studies, Bucket view, or CT scan. Nondisplaced fractures require no treatment. Isolated zygomatic arch fractures can be reduced by a Gilles approach, while complex fractures will necessitate open reduction/fixation with wires or plates via a coronal approach and/or gingivobuccal incision.[38,39]

Midface Fractures

The midface is a connection and link between the cranial base and occlusal plane. It provides anteroposterior facial projection and vertical strength. Maxillary fractures involve the maxilla as well as the entire midfacial domain. The LeFort classification system is commonly administered to describe and qualify these fractures (Fig. 44-36). Symptoms found with maxillary fractures are periorbital hematoma, nasopharyngeal bleeding, and maxillary mobility and/or instability.

The essential tenets of maxillary fracture reconstruction are restoration of midface projection and height, stabilization and maintenance of occlusion, midfacial buttress reconstruction (with bone grafting if necessary), and soft-tissue resuspension. Exposure is accomplished with a gingivobuccal incision and stabilization is achieved via screw/plate fixation.[40,41]

MAXILLOFACIAL RECONSTRUCTION

Ear

Total ear reconstruction in microtia patients remains one of the greatest tasks in plastic surgery. To re-create the folds and intricate convoluted cartilaginous framework enveloped by a thin soft tissue requires artistry, creativity, and enormous patience. Alloplastic constructs are not well tolerated by thin retroauricular skin envelopes, and the contralateral ear does not contain enough cartilage. Nevertheless, autogenous costochondral cartilage does provide the best tissue for the cartilaginous ear framework.

Prior to intervention, the patient and the family must be apprised that ear reconstruction is a multistage process. Limitations and reasonable expectations must be emphasized. If there is bilateral microtia and/or bilateral hearing deficits, middle ear reconstruction should be planned in conjunction with an otolaryngologist. Surgery can be scheduled when the child has reached age 6 to 8 years; rib cartilage has reached appropriate size for ear fabrication by the age of 6 years. In any event, preoperative photographs and thorough preoperative planning must be instituted prior to operative management.[42]

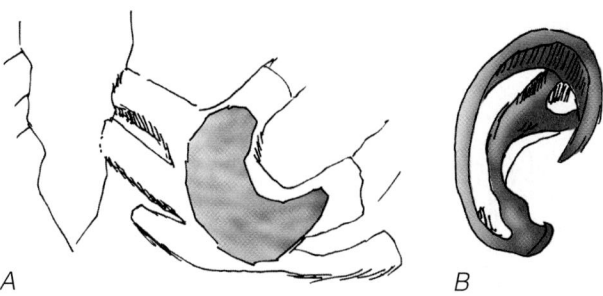

FIG. 44-37. Microtia reconstruction. *A.* Cartilage harvesting from ribs six to eight. *B.* Cartilage carving.

Many techniques have evolved over the past half of century, describing autologous ear reconstruction: Tanzer, Brent, and Nagata. All of these methods require three to five stages and are predicated on similar principles. Initially, a radiograph tracing is made of the normal contralateral ear. In the first stage, the cartilaginous foundation [of helix, antihelix], is constructed and meticulously carved from costal cartilage at the contralateral synchondrosis of ribs six to eight (Fig. 44-37). This framework is then implanted underneath the retroauricular skin envelope. In subsequent stages, which occur months later, a lobule is fashioned. Following this, projection of framework can be achieved by implantation of an additional cartilage wedge with a posterior skin graft. Further enhancement to the scapha, antiscaphe, and tragus are entertained in later revisions. Interestingly, the Nagata technique, devised in 1995, consolidates the Brent/Tanzer method into two stages. Nagata offers an additional variation—temporoparietal flap coverage of the cartilage skeleton. This supplies a hardier soft-tissue envelope, eschewing potential cartilage exposure and extrusion.[43]

Postoperatively, these patients must be vigorously followed in clinic to assess skin viability and potential cartilage exposure. The surgeon must be wary of hematomas or infections, which can cause significant pain and discomfort. Infections necessitate exigent management with closed drainage and antibiotics.

The prominent ear is another important facet that the plastic surgeon must be able to diagnose and surgically treat. Common causes of prominent ear include concha overdevelopment, underdeveloped antihelical folds, or a combination. In the prominent ear, there is an illusion that the ear is large regarding both height and width.

Several maneuvers can be performed to correct the prominent ear (Fig. 44-38). The surgeon can alter conchal depth by suturing conchal cartilage with mattress sutures, by excising excess conchal cartilage, or by scoring the anterior conchal cartilage so that it will bow and warp away, diminishing conchal projection. The antihelix fold can be simulated by Mustardé mattress sutures, or by full-thickness mattress sutures passing from scaphoid fossa to the posterior wall of the concha. This can be accentuated by abrading the anterior surface of the antihelical cartilage. In infancy, prominent ears can be permanently corrected by taping and splinting. Postoperatively, all patients need to wear a mastoid dressing or headband for several weeks to keep the ears pressed and molded to the mastoid in order to prevent recurrence.[44–46]

Lip

The lips serve both vital functional and aesthetic roles vis-à-vis speech, facial expression, eating, and oral competence. Anatomically, the upper lip extends from the nasolabial folds below the nose and intraorally to the gingivobuccal sulcus. The lower lip

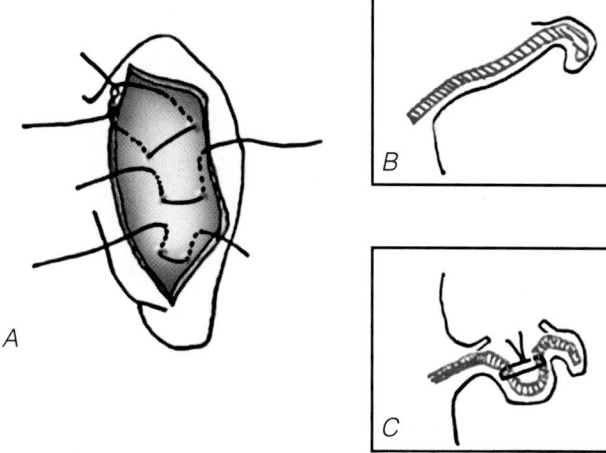

FIG. 44-38. Otoplasty. *A.* Mustardé (scapha–concha) sutures. On posterior views, scapha–concha sutures produce the antihelix fold, where the fold is either absent or underdeveloped. *B.* Coronal section of ear cartilage prior to correction. *C.* Coronal section of scapha–concha sutures and its effect on creating antihelical fold within cartilage framework. These sutures bowstring from the scaphoid fossa to the posterior conchal wall.

contrastingly spans to the labiomental fold and to the sulcus intraorally. The horizontally aligned orbicularis oris muscles truly dictate oral competence. Blood supply to the lips comes from the inferior and superior labial arteries; and motor control is dictated by the buccal and marginal mandibular branches of the facial nerve.

The etiology and the extent of the lip defect (skin, mucosa, and/or muscle) must be established. The majority of lip defects are secondary to neoplasms: basal cell cancer of the upper lip, squamous cell carcinoma of the lower lip. Appropriate surgical extirpation or radiotherapy must be performed for neoplastic lesions of either lip. Goals of reconstruction must maintain vermilion apposition, a sensate lip with oral sphincter function, and a watertight seal. Upper and lower lip defects less than 30% require vermilion alignment and orbicularis oris approximation. In defects greater than 30%, selection of reconstructive technique depends on the site of defect. The Abbé, or lip-switch flap, is most appropriate for central defects, while the Abbé-Estlander or Gilles flap is better suited for more lateral reconstructions (Figs. 44-39 and 44-40). Lower lip defects greater than 65% can be restored by a Karapandzic flap or by a Webster-Bernard technique. The Karapandzic flap is an innervated flap involving skin, lip mucosa, and orbicularis advancement, which replaces like tissue but narrows the oral aperture (Fig 44-41). The Webster-Bernard approach advances medial cheek tissue with excision of burrows triangles in the nasolabial folds. Larger lip/soft-tissue defects may supersede local tissue reconstruction; they may require larger pedicled flaps or even free tissue transfer.[47,48]

Cheek

The cheek can be divided into three esthetic units: zone I (suborbital), zone II (preauricular), and zone III (buccomandibular). Small cheeks are routinely closed primarily after elliptical excision. With more extensive soft-tissue resection, the concept of esthetic unit reconstruction should be highlighted. If primary close or local flap coverage (i.e., Limberg flap) cannot be achieved, or if lower lid malposition is created, the plastic surgeon could consider other alternatives, such as serial excision, full-thickness skin grafting, or tissue expansion (particularly if there are no time constraints). With larger

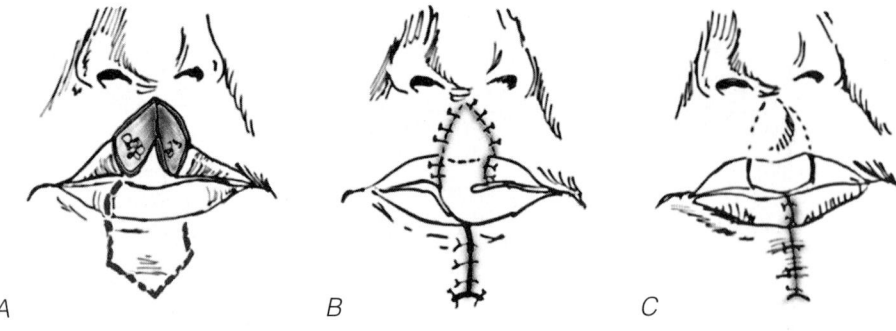

FIG. 44-39. Abbé flap. *A.* Defect and design of flap. *B, inset* of flap. *C.* Division of flap at second stage with closure.

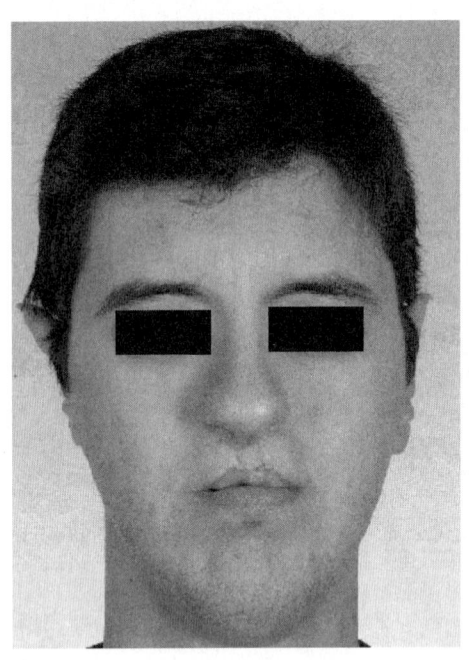

A

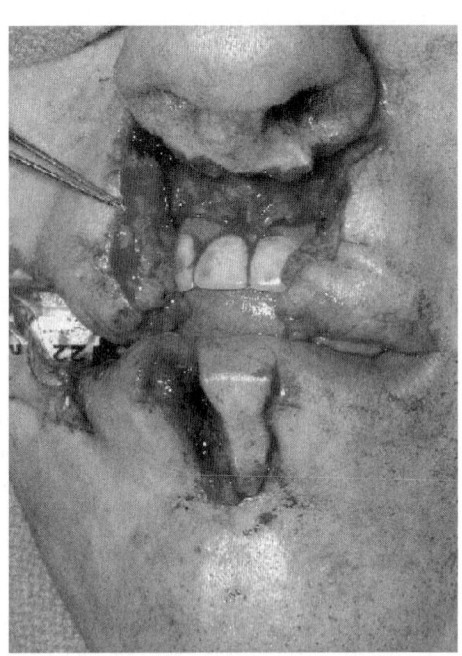

B

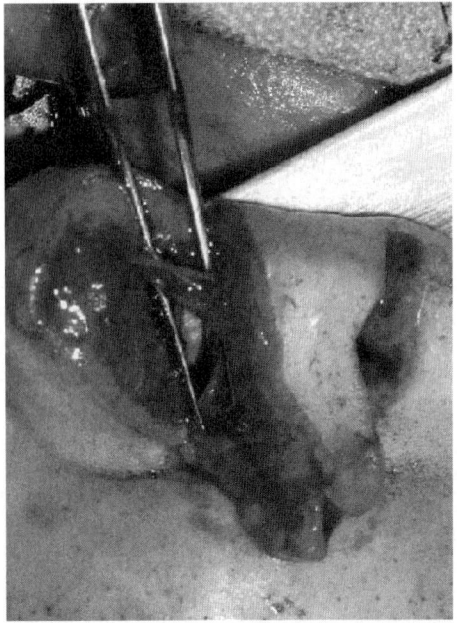

C

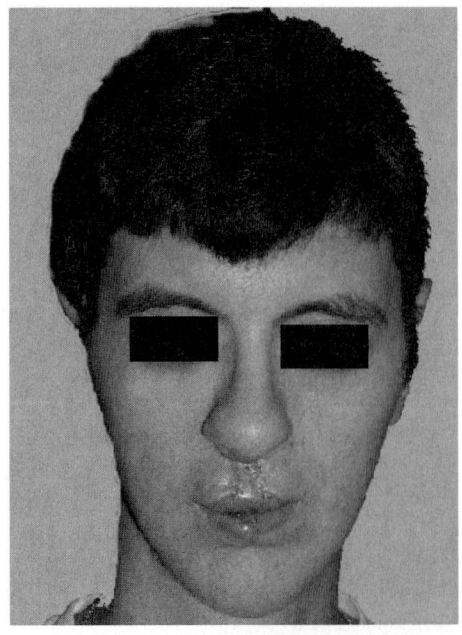

D

FIG. 44-40. Abbé flap for upper lip deficiency. *A.* Preoperative photo. The patient has significant scarring in philtrum and alar regions. He also has significant upper lip volume deficit. *B.* Release of scarred tissue revealing true defect. *C.* Flap elevated with inferior labial artery. *D.* Postoperative photo.

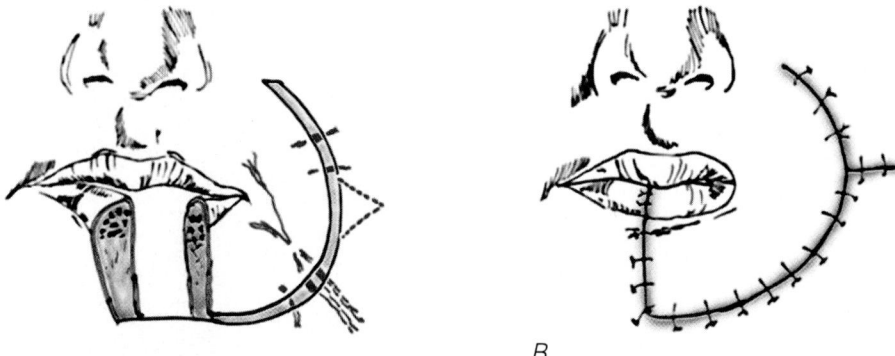

FIG. 44-41. *Karapandzic flap for lower lip defect. A. Design and elevation of flap. The inferior labial artery is maintained with flap for perfusion. B. Final inset and closure.*

defects, cervicofacial advancement, involving dissection and elevation of large subcutaneous flaps to the platysma, may be obligatory.[49] In massive cheek soft-tissue deficits, where cervicofacial advancement is unacceptable, the surgeon may need to resort to other regional flaps (deltopectoral, pectoralis major flaps) or even free tissue transfer.

Nasal

In terms of visual appearance, the nose is a well-sculpted, three-dimensional structure in the center of the face. Any defect or asymmetry may stand out and alter the normal facial dynamics and aesthetics. The surface and topography of the nose with its folds, concavities, and convexities distinguish it as a central landmark. It can be divided into nine subunits based on surface, skin thickness, color, and texture (Fig 44-42). Reconstruction of each individual unit must achieve:

- Replacement of missing skin with same dimension and quality;
- a cartilaginous framework to maintain shape and support for soft tissue; and
- the restoration of vascular lining for this framework.

Restoration of the nasal subunit should be emphasized rather than patching of the defect. Tissue must be restored in quantity and quality.[50,51]

Reconstruction of nasal subunits can be achieved by secondary healing, skin grafting, or local flaps. Secondary healing is successful in a defect adjacent to a nonmobile unit where contraction will not cause distortion, such as at the alar crease. Skin grafts may suffice in flat, shiny areas where graft color and texture are more facile to match. Small surface defects, which do not involve the perichondrium/periosteum, can be restored by skin grafts or local flaps. Skin grafts are appropriate in the upper two thirds along the dorsum or sidewall, but are a poorer option for the tip and ala. A banner flap will nicely rotate and fill the upper two-thirds of the defects, while a bilobed flap is a better choice for ala or tip defects.

In larger defects, the nasolabial flap based on the facial artery can resurface the nasal ala (Fig. 44-43). The paramedian forehead flap, based on the supratrochlear–supraorbital vessels, provides like tissue such as color texture for larger deficits of the tip, the dorsum, total nasal units, and areas of missing cartilage (Fig. 44-44). Forehead flap reconstruction requires two stages: to delay the flap and patch the defect and to divide the pedicle and inset the flap.[52,53]

Interruption of the cartilaginous framework may distort projection, airway patency, and nasal contours. To re-create the nasal structure, the surgeon must replace the defect with appropriately positioned cartilage grafts within a vascularized lining. These lining flaps may be derived from the vestibule, middle vault, and septum.

Eyelid

The primary function of the eyelid is to protect the sensitive conjunctiva and globe sclera. Both the upper and lower lids are composed of complex multilayered skin that provides tear secretion and

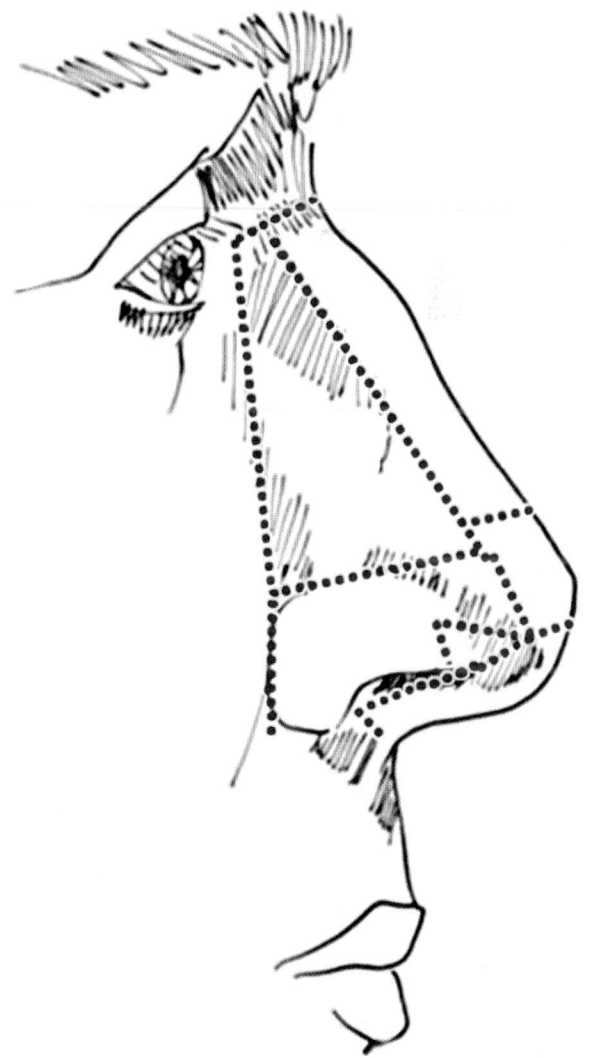

FIG. 44-42. *Nasal subunits for reconstruction.*

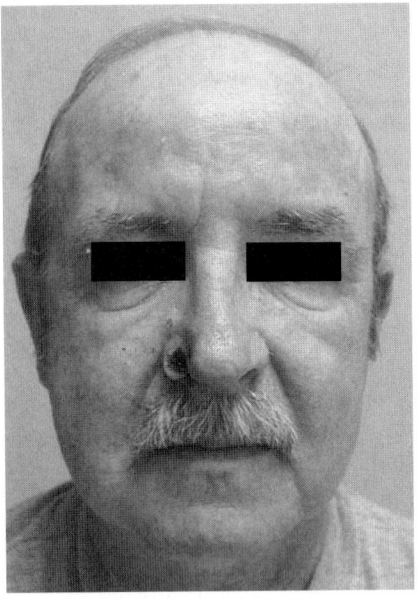
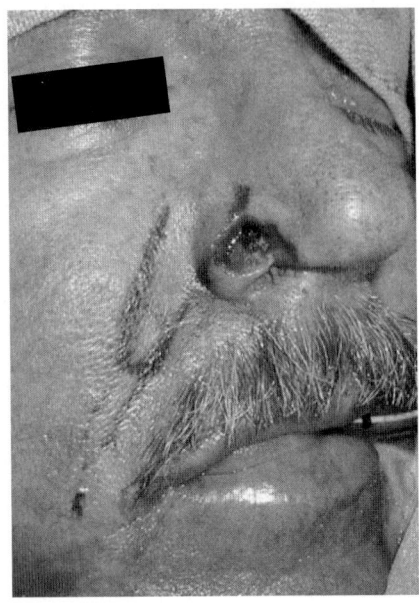
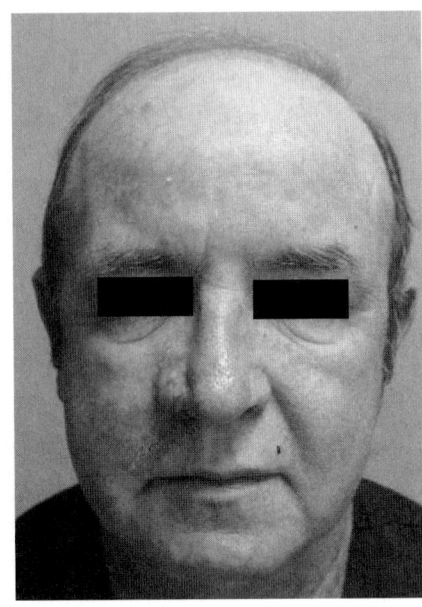

A   *B*   *C*

FIG. 44-43. *Nasolabial flap for alar defect. A. Defect of right ala following Mohs' excision. B. Flap design. C. Postoperative photo.*

lubrication for the globe. There are three functional layers: the outermost layer (skin and orbicularis), the middle lamella (tarsus and meibomian glands), and the inner lining (conjunctiva).

The goals of eyelid reconstruction are:

- Function should not be compromised.
- Shape, level symmetry, and motion of lid need to be as close to normal as possible.
- Incisions should be placed in natural lid crease lines.
- Skin replacement should match.
- Reconstructed lid must be durable.

Primary closure can be achieved for defects that are one third of the lid margin. A lateral canthotomy with lateral advancement can be executed if the defect is more than 25% and cannot be closed primarily. When there is skin loss of the lower lid, skin grafts from the upper lid, supraclavicular or preauricular region may be appropriate. When there is a full-thickness defect greater than 25%, the cartilage and conjunctival lining will require reconstruction. Septal or conchal cartilage accompanied with either conjunctiva from another lid, or oral or nasal mucosa can be performed for full thickness reconstruction. Another option, with higher graft failure, is a composite graft.[54]

Local flaps provide better color and texture match than other grafts. In full-thickness, lower-lid defects, there is a multitude of local flaps, including superiorly based nasolabial flap, V-Y advancement, and Mustardé cheek flap. In the upper lid, a temporal skin flap may be designed to reconstruct defects greater than one-half of the lid. Cross-lid flaps (Cutler-Beard, Hughes flaps) can be employed to restore either upper or lower lid defects involving the tarsus greater than 25% of lid length.[55] In the posttraumatic setting, medial canthopexy should be performed when repairing inner canthus defects in order to eschew telecanthus. This can be achieved by simple suture plication or transnasal wiring. In the same manner, the lateral canthus may be dragged downward or there may be lower-lid laxity following scarring, edema, and/or trauma. Nevertheless, a tarsal strip procedure and lateral canthopexy should be carried out to tighten the lower lid and prevent ectropion.

In the normal eyelid, the synergistic contractures of the levator, orbicularis, and Mueller's muscle promote opening and closing of the eyelid. In patients with ptosis or drooping of the eyelids, this function and interplay is compromised. Ptosis may be congenital or acquired. Congenital ptosis may be caused by lid anomalies, ophthalmoplegia, and synkinesis, while acquired ptosis can be neurogenic, myogenic, or traumatic. Horner's syndrome is a form of

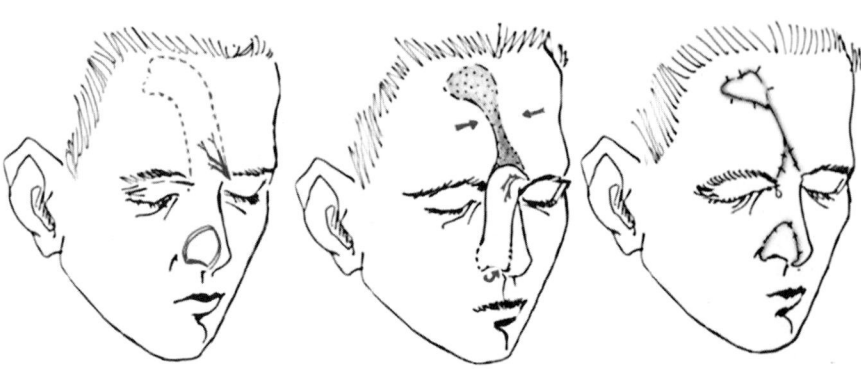

FIG. 44-44. *Paramedian forehead flap. The flap is an axial-based flap that is designed with its blood based on the supratrochlear vessels. The flap is elevated and inset in the initial stage as an interpolation flap, in a second stage, the flap is divided with final inset and closure.*

Table 44-9
Eyelid Ptosis Classification

Classification of ptosis severity	
Mild	1–2 mm
Moderate	3 mm
Severe	4+ mm
Classification of levator function	
Excellent	12–15 mm
Good	8–12 mm
Fair	5–7 mm
Poor	2–4 mm

neurogenic ptosis in which a sympathetic interruption occurs, leading to ptosis, miosis, and decreased sweating. Myasthenia gravis, nevertheless, can be grouped with the myogenic ptoses.

The plastic surgeon must give the patient a thorough preoperative exam with specific tests (gross exam of eyes; measurement of supratarsal fold, ptosis, and levator function [lid excursion]; comparison with contralateral side; and check of visual acuity and extraocular movements) in addition to taking preoperative photographs. This will enable the surgeon to classify the ptosis severity, levator function, and appropriate surgical modality (Table 44-9).

In patients with severe ptosis and absent levator function, a frontalis sling is required, in mild ptosis, a Mueller resection or Fasanella-Servat (tarsal plate resection with mullerectomy, aponeurosectomy) is required. In patients with moderate ptosis and fair to good levator function, levator advancement or levator resections are reasonable corrective procedures (Table 44-10).

Scalp

The scalp and forehead must be viewed as a single anatomic/esthetic unit, comprising five layers: skin, subcutaneous tissue, galea, loose areolar tissue, and pericranium. The scalp has a rich vascular and sensory supply. These adherent layers diminish the scalp's mobility and elasticity, making scalp reconstruction more complex. Scalp defects can be classified as partial or full thickness. In the setting of partial-thickness defects, all avulsed tissue is irrigated and débrided. Skin grafts can be applied to vascularized pericranial tissue. In areas of alopecia, secondary scalp reconstruction with tissue expansion or microhair transplantation can be achieved. In full-thickness defects, skin grafts can be administered to the calvarium after the outer calvarial table is removed and burred.[56]

In small scalp defects, local flap elevation and advancement accompanied by galeal scoring is a reasonable treatment. In medium-size defects, large scalping flaps or multiple axial flaps can achieve closure with donor-site skin grafting. Large defects (8 to 10 cm) can

Table 44-10
Eyelid Ptosis Treatment

	Poor Levator Function	Fair/Good Levator Function
Severe ptosis	Fascial sling	
Moderate ptosis		Fasanella-Servat
		Mueller resection
		Mustardé split-level tarsectomy
Mild ptosis		Levator resection
		Levator plication
		Levator advancement

be repaired with a full scalping flap based on either the superficial temporal or posterior auricular arteries, pericranial flaps with skin grafting, or microvascular flap coverage.[57] Tissue expansion with local tissue advancement is reserved for restoration of hair-bearing tissue and calvarial coverage in the nontraumatic milieu.

Calvarial reconstruction is vital for protection of intracranial elements and for frontal recontouring. Most plastic surgeons will restore calvarial defects with autogenous bone, such as split rib grafts or calvarial bone grafts. More recently, with the advent of alloplastic technology, materials such as methylmethacrylate, LactoSorb, Norian, and hydroxyapatite have emerged as novel agents for recontouring skull defects. However, compared to autogenous agents, they have a higher infection and extrusion rate. In the setting of an infection, these agents must be meticulously removed and débrided in the operating arena.

Facial Paralysis

Facial paralysis and palsy is a manifestation of a myriad of disorders and etiologies. The etiology can be divided into three subcategories: intracranial, intratemporal, and extracranial. Idiopathic or Bell's palsy remains the dominant form of facial paralysis, where 70% of these patients will recover without sequelae.[58] When facial nerve function does not recover, surgical manipulation must be instituted. Understanding the onset and degree of weakness will determine the appropriate intervention.

The ideal goals are to restore the following:

- Resting facial symmetry;
- spontaneous, symmetric facial animation;
- involuntary corneal protection; and
- oral competence.

Reconstruction can be divided into two regimes—early and late—depending on the duration of facial nerve injury/paralysis. Eighteen months from original nerve injury, the facial muscles will atrophy and not regain any modicum of function. When the interval of facial nerve dysfunction is less than 18 months, primary repair, nerve grafting, or nerve transfers can be explored. Primary neuropathy can be achieved if the proximal and distal facial nerve ends can be approximated without tension. If tensionless nerve repair is not feasible, then a nerve graft (usually sural nerve) will be interposed in between the proximal trunk and distal branches. When the proximal nerve stump is sacrificed and the distal branches are preserved, cross-facial nerve grafting from the contralateral facial nerve or nerve transfer from the ipsilateral hypoglossal nerve is performed.

Where facial nerve dysfunction has exceeded 18 months, static or dynamic slings and free muscle transfers can be executed to restore facial and oral motor function. Static slings of either Gore-Tex or fascia can be attached from the commissure to the zygomatic arch. The temporalis or masseter muscle can be rotated and transposed as a dynamic sling to the oral commissure in order to achieve both smile and oral capability (Fig. 44-45). In either case, an upper-eyelid gold weight is usually applied to vouchsafe corneal protection.

Finally, facial reanimation can be realized by microneurovascular muscle transfers in conjunction with a cross-face nerve graft.[59] The procedure is divided into two stages, the first consisting of a cross-facial nerve graft, providing a nerve for reinnervation. In the second stage, a free muscle transfer (gracilis, pectoralis minor, rectus abdominis, serratus, or latissimus) is attached to the commissure and zygomatic body, followed by neurovascular anastomoses (Fig. 44-46).

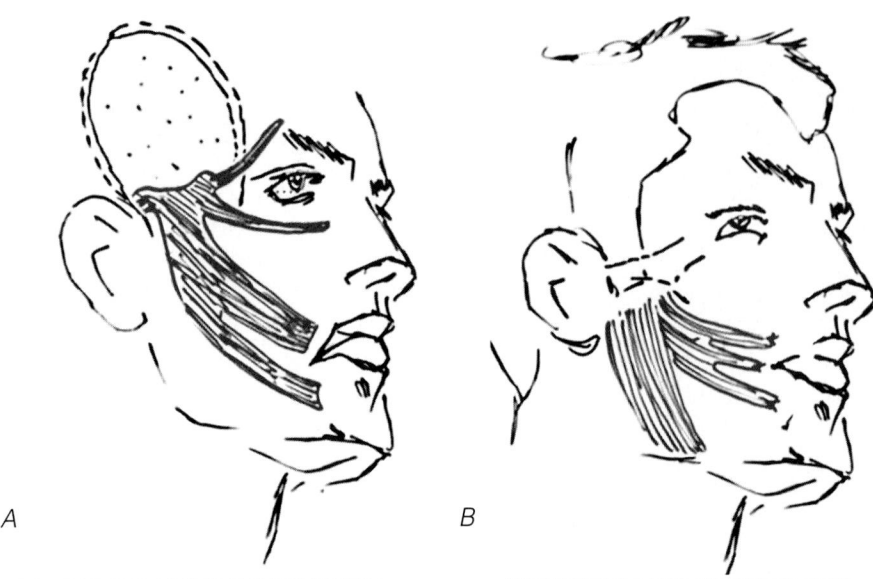

A
TEMPORALIS MUSCLE SUSPENSION

B
MASSETER MUSCLE SUSPENSION

FIG. 44-45. Dynamic slings for facial reanimation. A. Masseter muscle. B. Temporalis muscle.

HEAD AND NECK ONCOLOGIC RECONSTRUCTION

The marriage of head and neck oncologic surgery and reconstructive surgery in recent years has paved the way for successful ablation of large neoplasms followed by immediate reconstruction.[60,61] With these disfiguring tumors, the goal of the plastic surgeon should be to maintain speech, oral competence, and gastrointestinal function, as well as to restore form. Considering the limitations of local flaps such as the pectoralis, the deltopectoral, and trapezius flaps, the application of microsurgery and free tissue transfer has reformed the discipline of head and neck reconstruction.

With floor-of-mouth and tongue tumors, the reconstructive modality is dictated by the size of the defect. Small intraoral defects can occasionally be treated with a skin graft. Larger defects will require more pliable tissue for an intraoral lining and allow for tongue mobility such as a radial forearm flap. In the setting of maxillectomy and/or orbitectomy, the palate and oral contents must be separated from the midface. If the palate is resected, a palatal obturator can be applied, but adequate soft-tissue coverage (rectus abdominis or scapular flap) is needed. When the orbital floor is resected but the orbital contents are preserved, a bone graft is frequently used for reconstruction. Nevertheless, local flaps such as the temporalis muscle or temporoparietal flap offer adequate soft-tissue coverage in these defects.

More advanced lip and/or oral cancers may invade the maxilla and mandible. If the mandibular defect is smaller than 6 cm, a nonvascularized bone graft can be employed. If the defect is larger than 6 cm or the ablative field is to be radiated, a free vascularized bone flap is indicated. Options for vascularized bone include the free fibula, the iliac crest, and the scapula flap. These bone flaps may be accompanied with skin and soft tissue to patch and fill the missing skin or mucosa.

In the neck, complete esophageal defects can be reconstructed with a supercharged jejunal flap. Hypopharyngeal defects, either circumferential or partially circumferential can be reconstructed by a multitude of flaps. Tubed free radial forearm flaps are routinely used to reconstruct partial defects. The free jejunal flap remains the standard for complete circumferential defects because it supplies mucosal tissue.[62,63] However, other tubed fasciocutaneous free flaps and the anterolateral thigh flap have emerged as reasonable alternatives because they do not invade the abdominal cavity (Fig. 44-47).

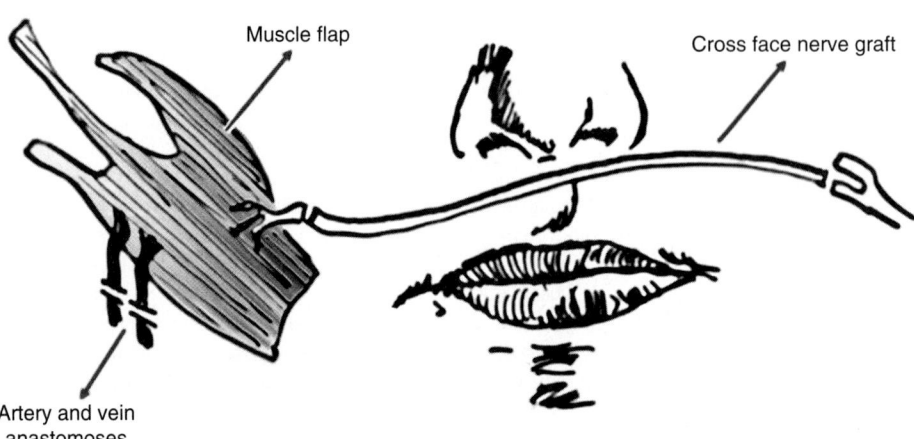

Muscle flap

Cross face nerve graft

Artery and vein anastomoses

FIG. 44-46. Free gracilis transfer for facial reanimation. Free muscle transfer incorporated with cross-facial nerve graft.

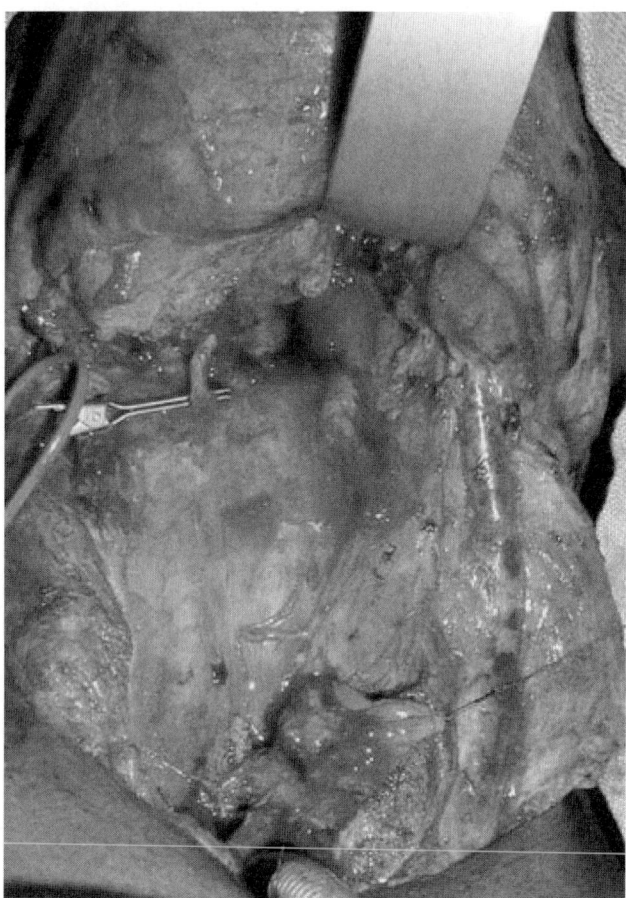

A

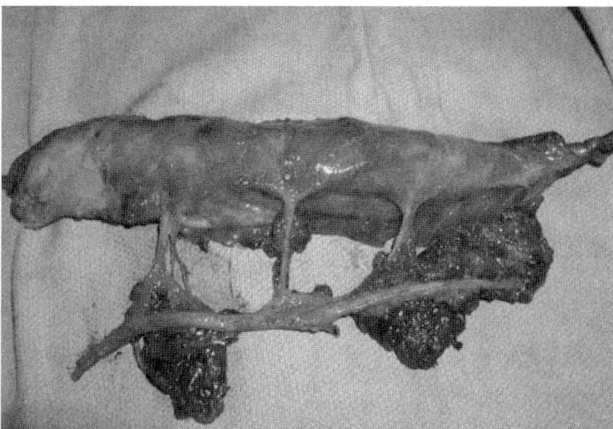

B

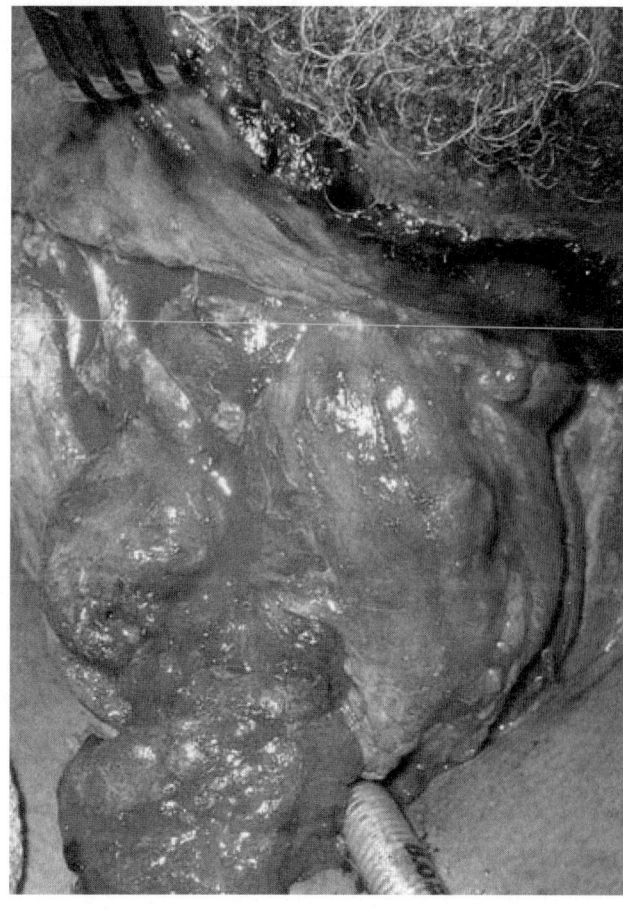

C

FIG. 44-47. Hypopharyngeal reconstruction. *A.* Defect with suture demarcating proximal esophagus. *B.* Tubed anterior lateral thigh flap with pedicle. *C.* Inset of flap.

BREAST SURGERY

Breast Reconstruction

Breast reconstruction following mastectomy falls into two broad categories: autogenous tissue reconstruction and implant reconstruction.[64,65] Preoperative planning includes consideration of the possibility of adjuvant therapies such as radiation, the patient's general health (risk for surgery, smoking status, diabetes), previous surgery in the breast region, and possible donor-site areas such as

the abdomen, the habitus of the patient, the condition of the skin and soft tissue, and the status of the contralateral breast.

Autogenous tissue reconstruction may be considered in patients who require radiation postoperatively, or in patients who understand the morbidity of the procedure and desire the possible aesthetic benefits of opting for autogenous reconstruction. The potential donor flaps include variations of the transverse rectus abdominis myocutaneous (TRAM) flap, the latissimus dorsi myocutaneous flap with or without implant, the superior inferior epigastric artery flap, gluteal

Table 44-11
Breast Reconstruction: Autogenous Choices

	Vascular Supply	*Advantages*	*Disadvantages*
Pedicled TRAM flap	Superior epigastric artery	Ease of elevation	Occasional partial flap loss
Pedicled latissimus dorsi flap	Thoracodorsal	Ease of elevation	Needs an implant for volume; some limitation of upper extremity function possible
Free TRAM flap	Deep inferior epigastric artery	More robust blood supply than pedicled TRAM (less affected by radiation)	Slightly longer procedure than pedicled TRAM
Deep inferior epigastric artery perforator flap	Perforating arteries of the deep inferior epigastric artery	No rectus muscle taken with flap	Tedious dissection of perforators; possible higher incidence of fat necrosis
Superficial inferior epigastric artery flap	Superficial inferior epigastric artery	No violation of rectus fascia	Smaller volume of soft tissue for reconstruction; vessels not always present or suitable for anastamosis
Gluteal artery flap	Inferior gluteal artery	Useful if prior surgery has compromised abdominal tissue	Donor-site irregularity and possible gait disturbance
Deep circumflex iliac artery flap	Deep circumflex iliac artery	Useful if other donor sites are compromised	Donor-site hernia, pain
Anterolateral thigh flap	Descending branch of the profunda femoris artery	Useful if other donor sites are compromised	Depending on patient anatomy, less volume of soft tissue, possible need to skin-graft donor site

flap, and the deep circumflex iliac artery ("Rubens") flap. With the exception of the pedicled TRAM flap, the other flaps require microsurgical technique for breast reconstruction (Table 44-11).

The pedicled TRAM flap is purported to have more fat necrosis and radiation-induced problems than the free TRAM (Figs. 44-48 and 44-49). Additionally, smoking is a relative contraindication for a pedicled TRAM, but not for a free TRAM (because of the putative increase in flap perfusion with the free TRAM). The free TRAM has a slightly longer operative time and a surgeon-dependent flap failure rate of approximately 5%. Both of these types of breast reconstruction entail sacrifice of the rectus muscle, and mesh reconstruction of the abdominal wall can be employed when the fascial defect is significant. The functional deficit from rectus abdominis harvest has been debated; however, modifications of

the traditional TRAM, which minimize the muscle taken during harvest (muscle-sparing technique)—or avoids harvesting muscle altogether via intramuscular dissection of the perforating vessels (deep inferior epigastric perforator [DIEP] flap)—have gained popularity (Fig. 44-50). Ongoing outcomes analysis of risk: benefit of these permutations of the TRAM flap will determine the relative indications for each technique. Abdominal soft tissue based on the superior inferior epigastric artery (SIEA) flap can also be used for smaller-volume breast reconstruction (Fig. 44-51). The inconstant vascular supply and the smaller size of these vessels hamper their universal application to breast reconstruction.

A latissimus dorsi myocutaneous or muscle flap can also be used for partial or total breast reconstruction (Fig. 44-52).[66] An implant may be required to supplement the reconstructed volume of the

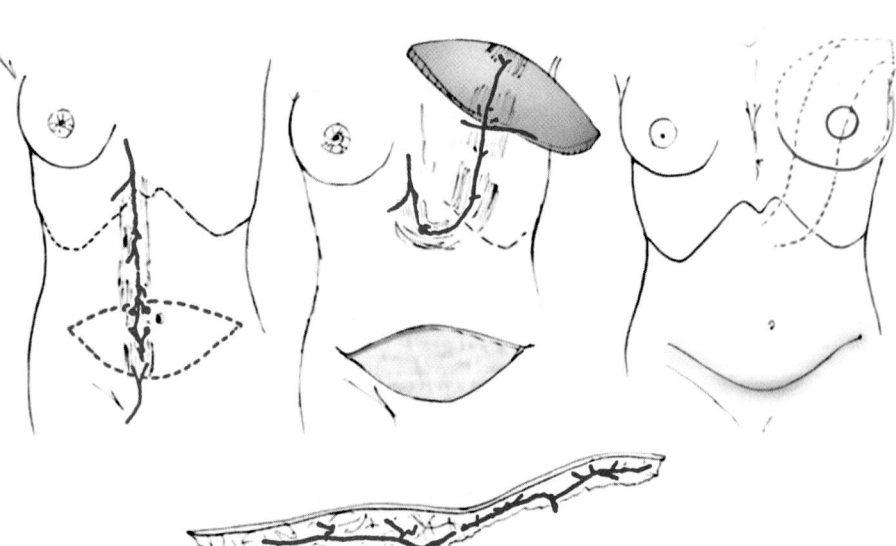

FIG. 44-48. Transverse rectus abdominis myocutaneous flap. Anatomy and design of TRAM flap. The TRAM flap has a dual blood supply: the superior epigastric and the deep inferior epigastric vessels. For the pedicled TRAM, unlike the free TRAM, the deep inferior epigastric vessels are ligated. The flap is elevated with the rectus muscle and superior epigastric vessels. It is tunneled and then inset to reconstruct the breast.

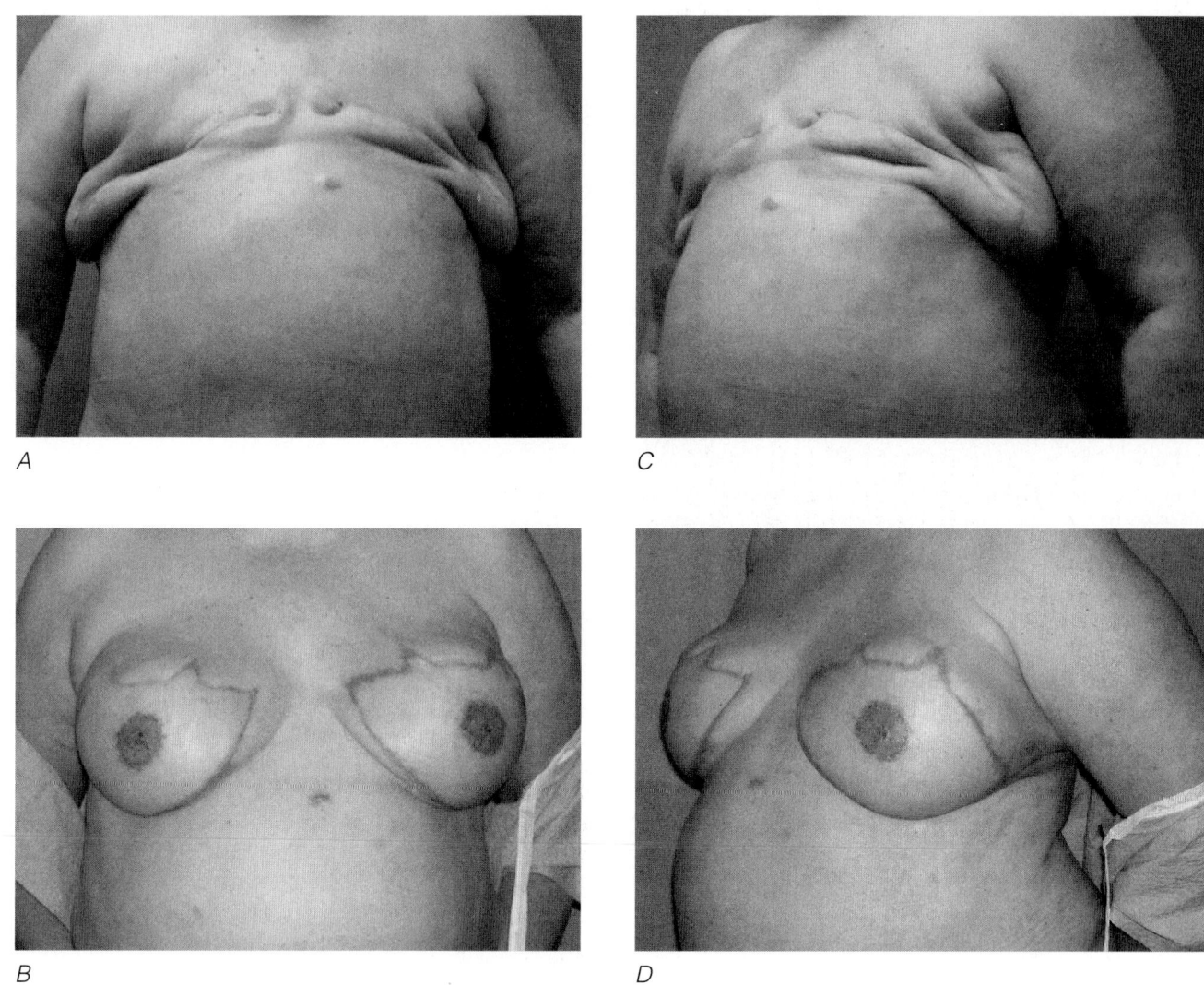

FIG. 44-49. Delayed bilateral breast reconstruction: bilateral pedicled TRAM flaps. *A.* Preoperative photo, frontal view. *B.* Postoperative photo, frontal view. *C.* Preoperative photo, oblique view. *D.* Postoperative photo, oblique view.

breast. While an intraoperative position change is required, the procedure itself is facile and good aesthetic results can be obtained. In patients who are active, the slight limitation in functional activity implied by the loss of the latissimus muscle needs to be discussed preoperatively with the patient. Moreover, there is a 15% incidence of donor-site seroma that may require prolonged drainage or repeated aspiration.

Patients in whom the abdominal tissue and the latissimus dorsi flaps are precluded by prior surgery or patient choice, the gluteal artery flap, the deep circumflex iliac artery flap, or the anterolateral thigh flap can be considered. The caveat to using these flaps is their significant donor-site morbidity and potential for a limited quantity of soft tissue.

The choice of recipient vessels for microvascular anastomosis of these flaps includes the thoracodorsal artery and vein and the internal mammary artery and vein. The exposure for the thoracodorsal vessels can be part of the mastectomy procedure itself. However, the corollary to this is that the vessels themselves may be damaged by the axillary node dissection. This also has implications for the use of the latissimus dorsi pedicled muscle flap. In certain cases, when

a latissimus dorsi flap is planned and the thoracodorsal artery has been damaged, the serratus branch may yet be sufficient to use the latissimus. The internal mammary axis is an increasingly popular choice for recipient vessels with or without damage to the thoracodorsal arteries. With the advent of sentinel lymph node biopsy for breast cancer, a possible conundrum exists if a negative sentinel lymph node biopsy is followed by microvascular reconstruction to the thoracodorsal vessels.[67] In a minority of such cases, permanent sections or RT-PCR might reveal a positive sentinel lymph node requiring definitive axillary node dissection in an operative field that has a fresh anastomosis. This may place the breast reconstruction at substantial risk. The presence of certain prognostic risk factors may enhance this likelihood, then prophylactic use of the internal mammary as the recipient vessel may be warranted.

Novel modifications of these flaps are also being explored. For instance, neurotization of the sensory branches of the anterolateral intercostal nerve to a sensory branch within the TRAM flap may allow increased breast tissue sensibility. Tissue-engineering paradigms for molding adipose cells and connective tissue into the three-dimensional volume of breast are being developed.

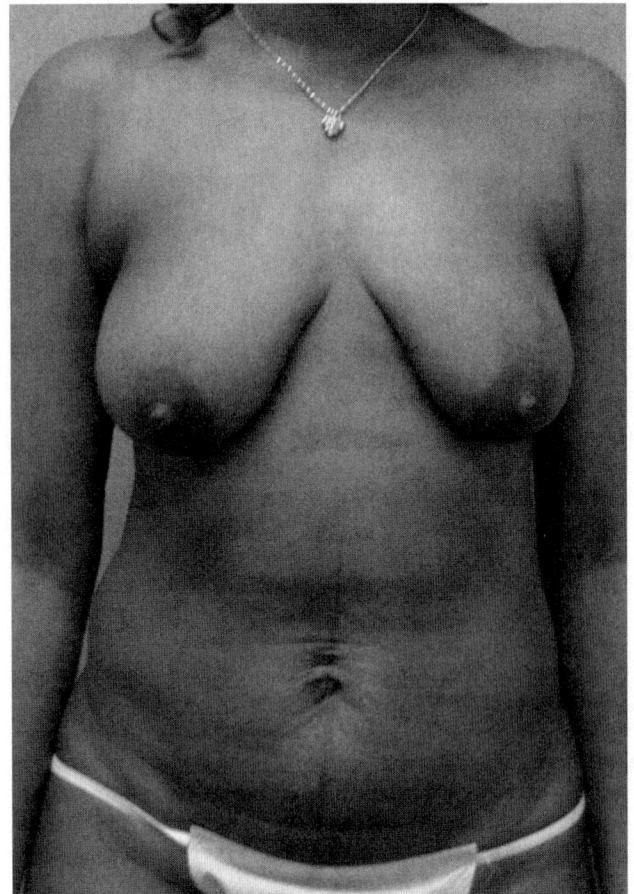

A

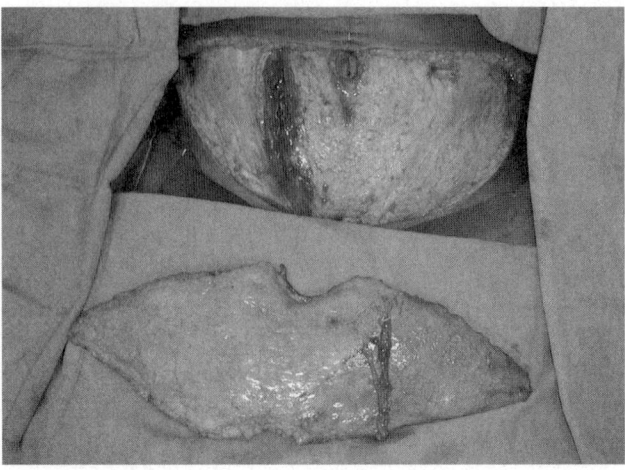

B

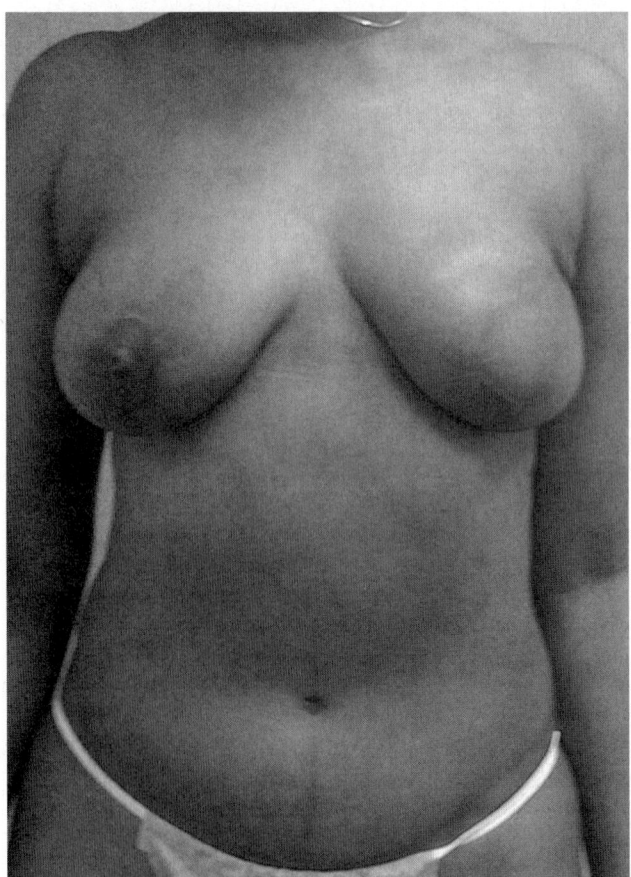

C

FIG. 44-50. Breast reconstruction: deep inferior epigastric artery flap. *A.* Preoperative photo prior to mastectomy. *B.* Elevation of flap with no removal of fascia or rectus muscle. *C.* Postoperative result.

Tissue Expansion and Implant Reconstruction

The principal benefit of using tissue expansion and implants is ease of reconstruction and obviation of any donor site morbidity.[68] Generally, the aesthetic result may not approach that which can be obtained with optimal autogenous reconstruction and certainly the use of radiation makes implant reconstruction a more tenuous option. Additionally, because most mastectomy defects imply a loss of skin and soft tissue, pre-expansion of the skin flaps may be necessary

prior to definitive implant reconstruction. This will entail a staged procedure with serial expansion of the tissue expander over several months with a definitive exchange of the expander with an implant.

The choice of implant type ranges widely with smooth and textured implants possible in a range of volumes and shapes. The expander soft-tissue pocket is generally placed beneath the pectoralis and serratus muscle, which affords greater coverage of the implant and may soften the resultant contour. The inframammary fold is a

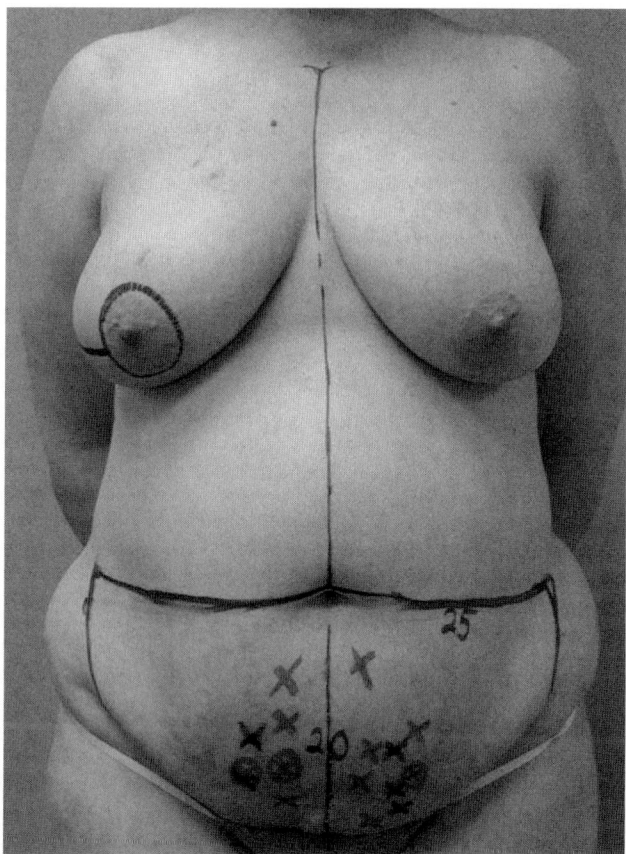

A

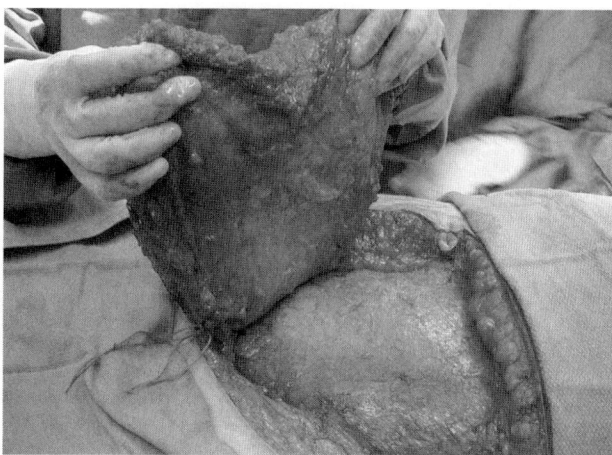

B

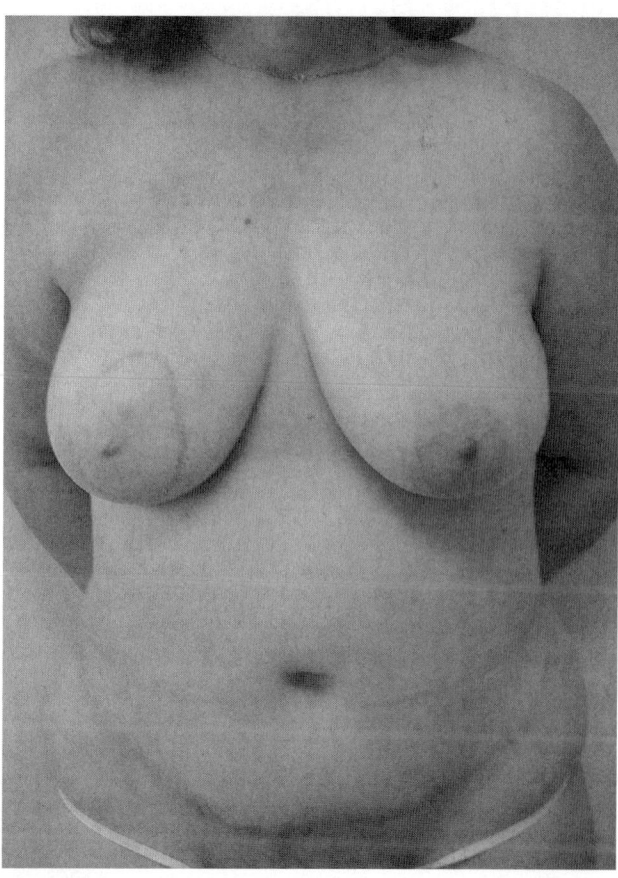

C

FIG. 44-51. Breast reconstruction: superficial inferior epigastric artery flap. *A.* Markings for mastectomy and superficial inferior epigastric artery flap. The Xs show perforators detected by Doppler sonography. *B.* Elevation of flap with no penetration of rectus fascia or anterior sheath. *C.* Postoperative result.

critical variable in implant reconstruction, and asymmetry preoperatively should be noted and adjustments made to the fold accordingly.

Nipple–Areola Reconstruction

A variety of local flaps can be used to reconstruct the form of the nipple–areola complex.[69] As dermal–fat tissue rearrangements, these flaps will tend to decrease in projection over time and should thus have an element of overcorrection at their initial creation. Occasionally, full-thickness skin grafts may also be used for nipple–areolar reconstruction. Pigment tattooing is performed after definitive healing of the nipple–areolar complex.

Reduction Mammoplasty

Gigantomastia can result in significant morbidity including back and shoulder pain. Diverse reduction mammoplastic procedures exist for alleviation of these symptoms.[70] The central tenet is to retain vascularity to the nipple and breast and re-create breast projection in symmetric fashion. The diminished breast tissue is based on inferior, superior, or medial pedicles—or a combination thereof. The excess skin can be removed by developing skin flaps along lines fashioned on an inverted T, periareolar, or vertical limb (Fig. 44-53). Sometimes the sheer size of the breast prevents the

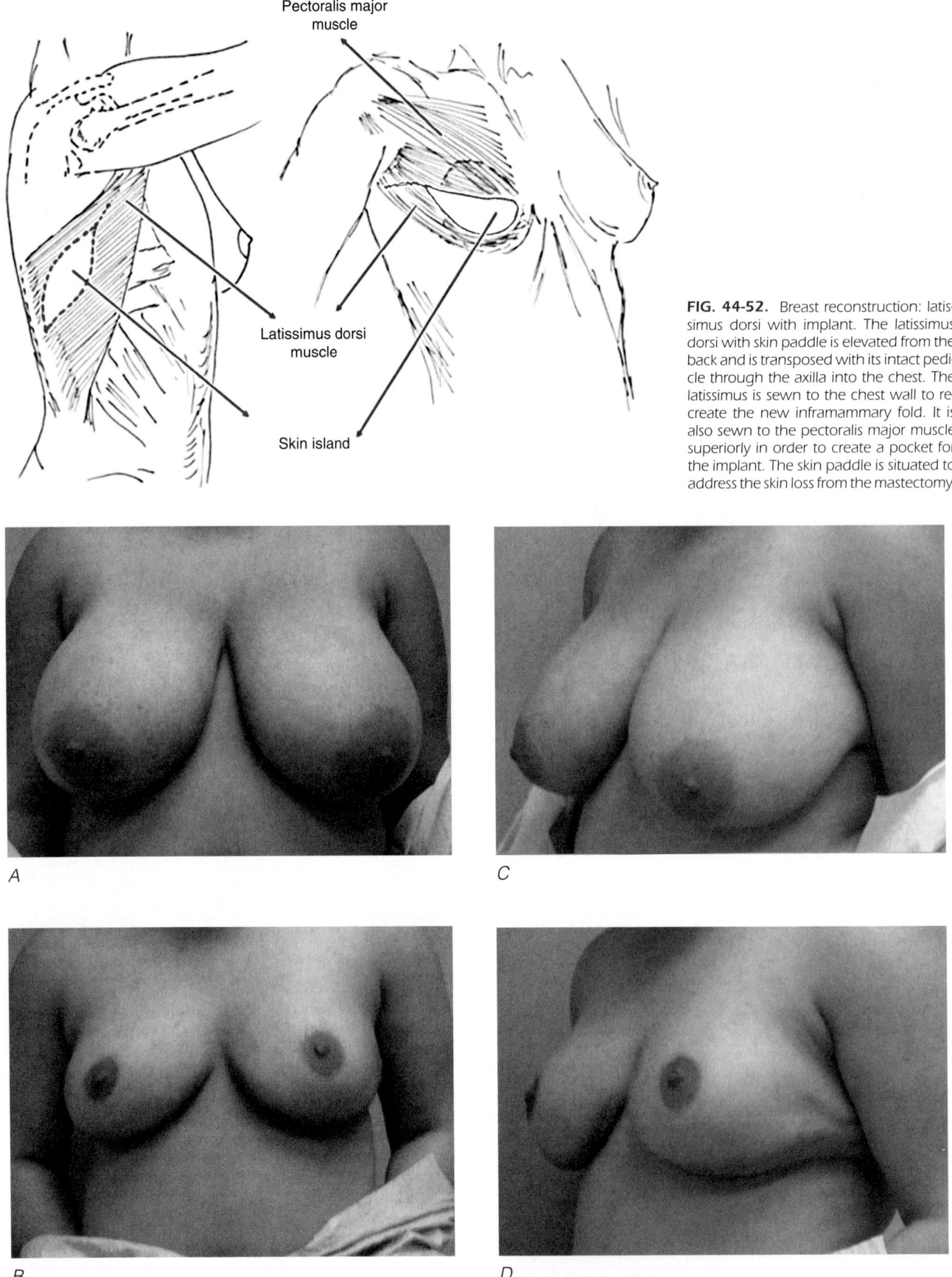

FIG. 44-52. Breast reconstruction: latissimus dorsi with implant. The latissimus dorsi with skin paddle is elevated from the back and is transposed with its intact pedicle through the axilla into the chest. The latissimus is sewn to the chest wall to recreate the new inframammary fold. It is also sewn to the pectoralis major muscle superiorly in order to create a pocket for the implant. The skin paddle is situated to address the skin loss from the mastectomy.

Pectoralis major muscle

Latissimus dorsi muscle

Skin island

A

C

B

D

FIG. 44-53. Breast reduction. *A.* Preoperative photo, frontal view. *B.* Postoperative photo, frontal view. *C.* Preoperative photo, lateral view. *D.* Postoperative photo, lateral view.

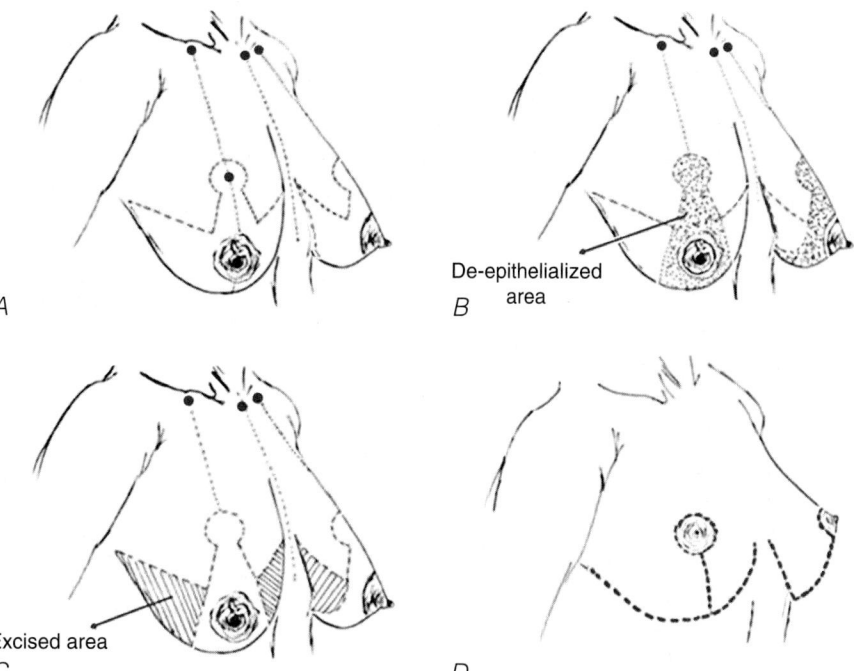

FIG. 44-54. Inferior pedicle reduction mammaplasty. *A.* Markings for Wise pattern reduction. *B. Stippled* area is region to be de-epithelialized. *C. Cross-hatched* region is area to be resected. Segment of inferior pedicle is de-epithelialized. The inferior pedicle is dissected straight down to the chest wall, maintaining a 6- to 8-cm width in pedicle. Lateral and medial segments are resected. After this is accomplished, the superior flap is dissected to the clavicle. Breast subcutaneous tissue and parenchyma is resected from the superior pole. The vertical limbs are brought together and to the meridian of the inframammary fold. The nipple is then set in its new superior position. *D.* T-shaped incision upon final closure.

creation of a pedicle robust enough to sustain the nipple. In these situations, a form of breast amputation with preservation of the nipple as a free graft may be necessary. Essential to the postoperative result is careful preoperative evaluation and planning. Numerous measurements including the sternal notch to nipple distance, the relative degree of ptosis, the breast width, the nipple to inframammary fold distance must be made. Markings are also made based upon the projected breast and nipple complex.

Especially with the inferior pedicle technique, a potential long-term complication is the descent of the reduced breast volume below the nipple level—a "bottoming out" effect (Fig 44-54). Other potential complications include hematoma, delayed wound healing, loss of nipple sensation, and impaired ability to breast-feed. Newer methods are being developed, including selective dermoglandular resection, vertical reduction mammoplasty, and dermal flap manipulation (Fig 44-55).

FIG. 44-55. Vertical reduction mammaplasty: Lejour technique. *A.* Markings for vertical reduction. *B. Stippled* area is to be de-epithelialized. *C. Cross-hatched* region represents inferior pole to be resected. The *shaded* regions are the lateral and medial segments that are to be undermined; these areas can also be liposuctioned. The superior pedicle is de-epithelialized and dissected to the chest wall. The tissue and parenchyma from the inferior pole is resected. The pillars from the lateral and medial segments are sewn together. The nipple is transposed on its pedicle to its new position. *D.* Closure of the vertical mammaplasty. There is bunching up of skin and tissue along the vertical limb that will resolve over time, in addition, the new inframammary fold will declare itself superior to the original one.

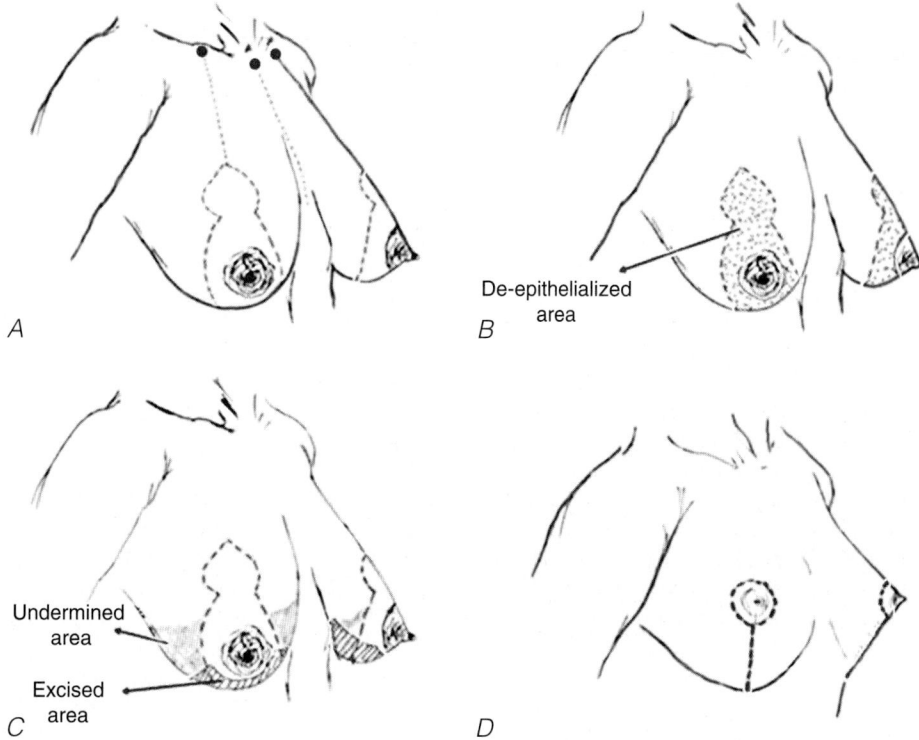

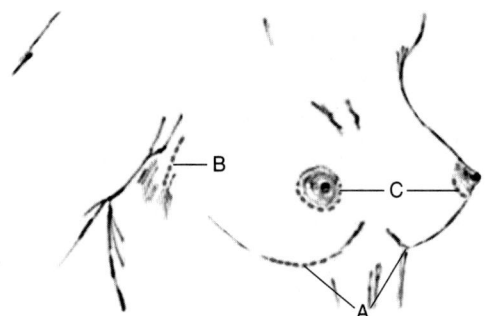

FIG. 44-56. Incisions for augmentation mammaplasty. *A.* Inframammary. *B.* Axillary. *C.* Periareolar.

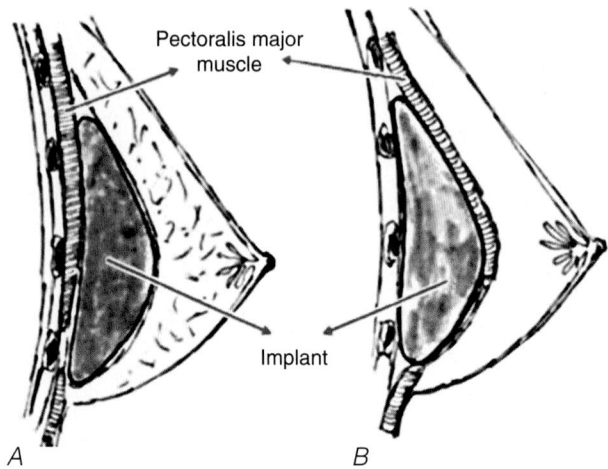

FIG. 44-57. Placement of breast implant. *A.* Subglandular. *B.* Subpectoral.

The age-related descent of breast tissue is known as ptosis and is addressed using surgical principles similar to those used for reduction mammoplasty. For mild ptosis, skin excision along a superior crescent or a periareolar mastopexy can be used. In certain cases, a subglandular augmentation can promote sufficient lift of the breast concomitant to enhancing volume. For more severe forms of ptosis, an inverted T-shaped incision may be necessary to properly provide lift and projection to the breast. An impression of reduction in breast volume is often created by simple ptosis correction without augmentation.

Breast Augmentation

As with the previous discussion of implant reconstruction, assorted implants exist for breast reconstruction.[71,72] While there has been controversy regarding the safety of silicone implants for breast augmentation, the largest meta-analysis to date has failed to demonstrate a causality between silicone gel implant placement and such conditions as collagen vascular disease and cancer. The current FDA-approved breast augmentation implants are saline filled with a silicone-based elastomeric shell.

The four commonly used incisions for placement of the breast implants for purposes of augmentation are inframammary, periareolar, axillary, and transumbilical (Fig. 44-56).[73] The same concerns regarding breast asymmetry—precise measurements of breast geometry and the inframammary fold—that were emphasized in implant breast reconstruction hold true in augmentation mammoplasty. The implants may be placed in a subglandular or subpectoral position (Fig. 44-57). The subpectoral placement affords greater soft-tissue coverage of the implant with potentially less visibility and contour irregularity. The dissection itself can be more involved and there may be a slight increase in pain secondary to manipulation of the muscle during placement (Fig. 44-58).

Capsular contracture occurs in 8 to 38% of patients undergoing augmentation mammoplasty. If significant contracture occurs resulting in surface deformity, asymmetry, or pain, then capsulotomy or capsulectomy with implant exchange may need to be considered. There is some controversy regarding the propensity to capsular contracture with smooth versus textured implants and subglandular versus subpectoral position. Some studies indicate that textured implants and a subpectoral position may have a decreased incidence of capsule formation. Other potential complications such as deflation, rupture, hematoma, seroma, infection, and hypertrophic scarring may occur at a rate of less than 5% individually depending on the series. Rupture of silicone gel implants can be difficult to detect clinically—and because of concerns about the deleterious effects of

leaking silicone gel, imaging with ultrasound and or MRI can help establish a definitive diagnosis.

Another concern regarding breast implants is the issue of mammography. Eklund has devised a method of viewing augmented breasts with alternate views that enhances the volume of breast undergoing surveillance.[74] A study surveying augmented and nonaugmented patients found no statistical difference in survival or detection of carcinoma between the two cohorts.[75]

The pervasive trend toward minimally invasive surgery has found transposition in breast augmentation with endoscopic approaches to implant placement. The transumbilical breast augmentation technique is used by some to avoid scars in the breast and axillary region. Endoscopic instrumentation is also used to make access incisions in the breast and axilla as small as possible.

Gynecomastia

Male breast excess or gynecomastia can arise from a number of differing etiologies.[76] Pathologic causes include liver dysfunction, endocrine abnormalities, Klinefelter's syndrome, and renal disease. Oncologic causes include testicular tumors, adrenal or pituitary adenomas, and secreting lung carcinomas. Male breast cancer must be ruled out as well. Pharmacologic causes include marijuana use, digoxin, spironolactone, cimetidine, theophylline, diazepam, and reserpine. Depending on etiology, testosterone, tamoxifen, or danazol can be used to treat gynecomastia. Surgical treatment includes mastectomy and liposuction. While gynecomastia itself confers no risk for breast cancer, patients who have gynecomastia in association with Klinefelter's syndrome must be carefully scrutinized because this underlying condition increases susceptibility to male breast cancer.

Congenital Reconstruction

Congenital deformities of the breast include amastia, hypomastia, tuberous breast, and Poland's syndrome. These are relatively rare conditions that may nevertheless have a significant psychosocial impact on the patient. Amastia and hypomastia can be addressed by using a combination of expander implants or adjustable implants, such as the Becker implant, generally in early adolescence. Tuberous breast deformity often has an element of ptosis and internal herniation of breast tissue, and modest manipulation of breast tissue and subglandular placement of an implant may suffice.[77] Poland's

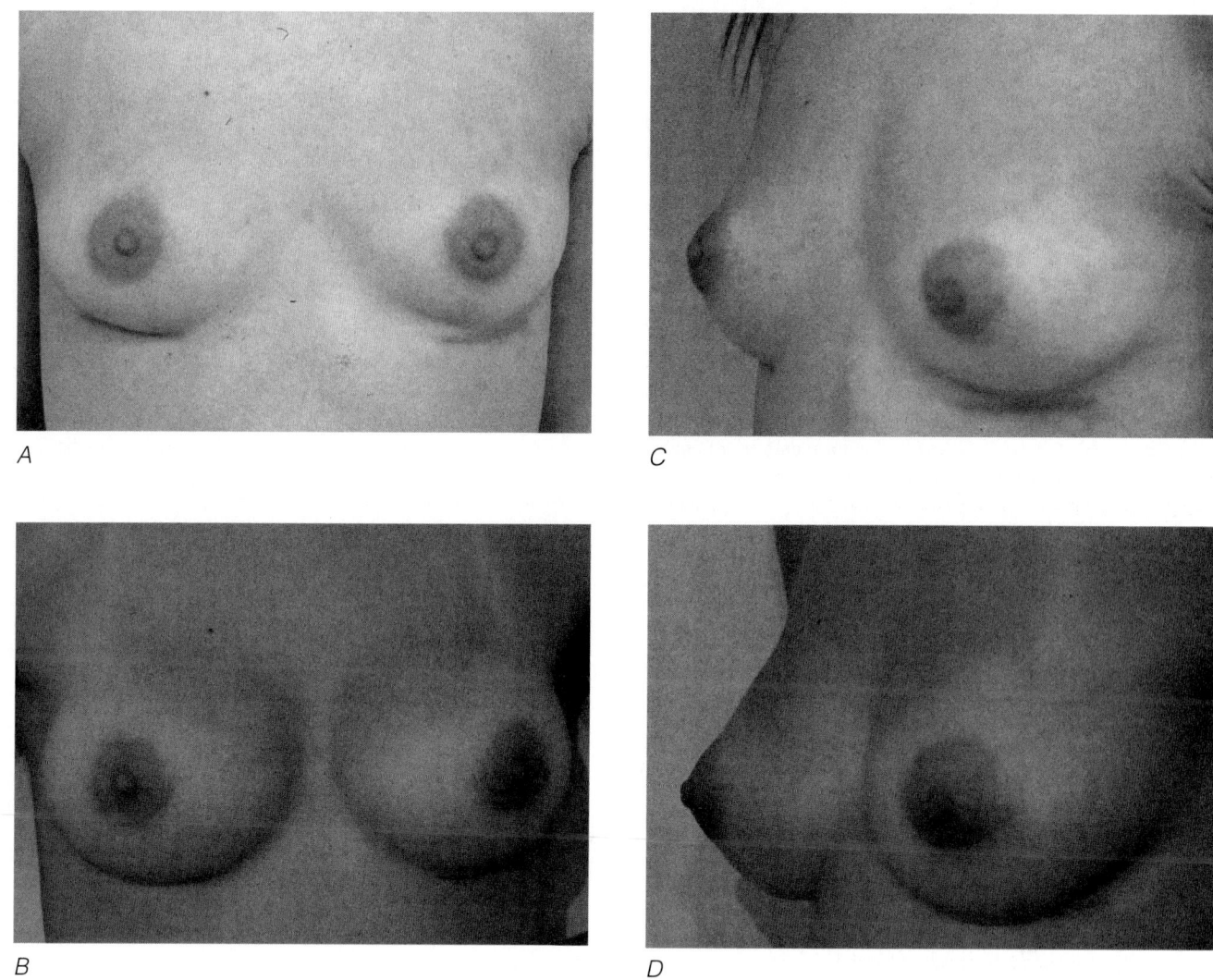

A

B

C

D

FIG. 44-58. *Augmentation mammaplasty. A. Preoperative photo, frontal view. B. Postoperative photo, frontal view. C. Preoperative photo, oblique view. D. Postoperative photo, oblique view.*

syndrome is characterized by hypoplasia or aplasia of chest and limb structures including the breast. If the latissimus dorsi muscle is available, then this may also be used in conjunction with an implant for breast reconstruction.[78]

TRUNK, ABDOMEN, AND GENITOURINARY RECONSTRUCTION

Chest Reconstruction

Chest wall reconstruction is required for defects arising from trauma, infection, oncologic ablation, or congenital defects. As with reconstruction in other parts of the body, precise anticipation of the anatomic components of the defect (skin, subcutaneous tissue, fascia, muscle, and bone) must be made. Obliteration of dead space and provision for durable, well-vascularized soft-tissue fill is important. If a significant bony defect (>5 cm or four or more continuous ribs to be resected) exists, then the reconstruction may include reestablishing bony continuity of the defect with graft, mesh, or flap.[79]

With the specific case of sternal wound infection, aggressive débridement with removal of infected hardware and necrotic debris

is central to a positive outcome. The débridements may need to be staged prior to definitive soft-tissue closure. Some surgeons advocate routine staging of the débridements prior to closure, or the use of quantitative culture data to assist in evaluating the relative efficacy of the débridements; other surgeons have found that a thorough single-stage débridement with immediate closure works well.

The choice of regional flaps, again, is dictated by the anatomy of the defect. The pectoralis muscle or myocutaneous flap can be based on the dominant thoracoacromial vessels and brought medially. To facilitate mobilization, the pectoralis muscle can be disinserted from its attachments to the humerus and clavicle. If adequate coverage cannot be provided by one muscle, then the contralateral pectoralis can also be used. If the thoracoacromial vessels are compromised, the pectoralis muscle can be used as a muscle-only flap and turned over based upon perforators from the internal mammary artery (assuming they are intact).

The lower portion of a sternal wound can often be difficult to cover with a pectoralis flap. Another popular choice is the rectus abdominis muscle flap. This can be rotated on the superior epigastric artery pedicle. It will not commonly reach the superior aspect of a sternal wound, but more than adequately covers the mid and lower portions of the wound. A cautionary note regarding the use of this flap in the setting of prior internal mammary harvest is that the superior epigastric artery may have already been compromised by loss of the proximal internal mammary. In this case, the contralateral rectus abdominis may be used; however, if this is not an option, it may be possible to use the rectus abdominis based upon the eighth intercostal artery which courses into the muscle at the subcostal margin. Alternatively, the omental flap may be available for vascularized soft-tissue coverage in the absence of significant or repeat laparotomies. In rare instances, the latissimus dorsi muscle can also be extended to cover a sternal wound defect.[80,81]

When muscle only or omental flaps are used, then skin coverage may be provided by local advancement flaps dissected off underlying pectoralis muscle or skin grafts may be used. The use of muscle also abets wound reconstruction by rendering the wound less susceptible to infection or dehiscence by virtue of the robust vascular nature of the soft-tissue fill. The local delivery of antibiotics and recruitment of host immune cells is also promoted by the presence of a highly vascularized reconstruction. As a consequence of the plethora of local flap options, free flaps are rarely required for sternal wound reconstruction.

Although the outcomes of chest wall reconstruction for sternal wounds are surgeon-dependent, 95% success rates have been reported. Complications such as re-infection, dehiscence, flap loss, or failure are relatively low with the integrated management of flap reconstruction and systemic microbe-specific antibiotics.

Posterior and lateral chest wall defects, occurring secondary to trauma or oncologic ablation, may require concomitant bony reconstruction. While much of the data regarding the indications for bony chest wall reconstruction are specifically derived from the trauma literature, a significant bony defect in the chest wall may theoretically affect pulmonary function dynamics. Marlex mesh, methylmethacrylate, and even bone grafts are used to bridge rib gaps. The latissimus or trapezius, or for more anterolateral defects, the rectus and pectoralis, are all potential options for soft-tissue coverage. With antecedent lateral thoracotomies, the latissimus dorsi muscle may not be available for transfer.

Abdominal Wall Reconstruction

The need for abdominal wall reconstruction usually stems from trauma, oncologic ablation, or as a complication from prior abdominal surgery. The overall rate of abdominal herniation following an abdominal incision can approach 10%. Abdominal reconstruction must always be carefully considered in the setting of comorbid conditions. The potential risk of prolonged surgery and altered pulmonary mechanics from abdominal reconstruction must be weighed against the benefits of repair.

For smaller skin and suprafascial soft-tissue defects, local advancement or muscle-based flaps may be helpful. Component separation technique also can be used for smaller fascial defects. This procedure entails differential release of the intact abdominal wall musculature to extend their reach to cover a fascial defect. The first step involves release of the medial edge of the external oblique in longitudinal fashion. The external oblique is dissected off the internal oblique. Next the posterior rectus fascia is released from the rectus muscle from a medial to lateral direction. When this is performed bilaterally, the procedure essentially elongates the muscle–fascia complex by 6 cm (suprapubic region) to 20 cm (waistline).[82]

For larger fascial defects not suitable for local advancement or component separation closure, alloplastic mesh may need to be incorporated into the reconstructive schema. This mesh can be made from PTFE (Gore-Tex), polypropylene (Prolene), polyglactin

(Vicryl), or polyester (Mersilene). Each material has a profile of strengths and weaknesses. PTFE can predispose to infection and seroma but provides strength with minimal adhesions. Polypropylene mesh provides strength but may develop adhesions. Polyglactin mesh integrates readily with low infection rates but provides relatively less strength. The alloplastic mesh should be covered with recruited skin and soft tissue. Occasionally, tissue expanders may be used to allow sufficient local tissue to be generated. Acellular dermis and skin substitutes have been used, but staged definitive reconstruction may be required at a later time and long-term clinical comparative studies are pending. Autogenous tensor fascia lata grafts have also been used, but a paucity of donor tissue and relative weakness may limit their applicability.[83]

For definitive coverage of the mesh, fascial, and/or soft-tissue defect, local muscle-based flaps present the best choice. Rectus abdominis muscle or myocutaneous flaps can be rotated or advanced into place. The tensor fascia lata has significant reach—to the subcostal margin—depending on anatomy. Often the distal skin island portion of the flap may not be as reliable for such transfer, but is certainly appropriate for lower defects. Similarly, the rectus femoris may allow for coverage of lower defects. The anterolateral thighs, the latissimus dorsi muscle, and even the omentum are all options, depending on the nature of the defect.[84]

When enterocutaneous fistulas are present, experimental reports suggest the vacuum-assisted coverage system may be helpful in keeping local control of excess secretions that may bathe a potential reconstructed site.

An initial traumatic, oncologic, or infected abdominal defect may not be able to be reconstructed immediately. A temporizing skin graft or acellular dermis may need to be placed over viscera and allowed to heal. With abdominal binder support, the patient may then need to be stabilized and the fascial defect repaired electively. Again, depending on the size and nature of the defect, an amalgam of techniques including component separation, alloplastic mesh, and local muscle-based flaps may be required for optimal reconstructive outcome.

Genitourinary Reconstruction

Reconstruction of male and female genitalia varies with the underlying cause of the defect. Common etiologies include congenital defect, trauma, and oncologic ablation. Reconstruction of the vaginal vault for cancer often requires the use of myocutaneous flaps; especially considering the possible role of radiation therapy. The gracilis myocutaneous flap or the vertical rectus abdominis myocutaneous flap can provide durable soft-tissue fill. For congenital defects of the vagina such as Mayer-Rokitansky-Küster syndrome (congenital absence of the vagina), variants of the McIndoe procedure can be employed. A judicious dissection of the potential vaginal vault space is followed by split-thickness grafting. A bolster expander is kept in place to maintain the space. Hypospadias is an abnormality of male urethral development characterized by varying exit sites of the urethra. Associated anomalies, such as inguinal hernias and undescended testes, occur commonly (9%). The Mathieu procedure uses a ventral, meatal-based flap, whereas the meatal advancement and glanuloplasty technique is ideal for distal hypospadias with a more compliant urethra. Proximal hypospadias can be repaired with preputial island flaps. Bladder exstrophy reconstruction entails a multistage procedure in which external genitalia of either sex will need reconstruction with local flaps.[85,86]

Traumatic or oncologic defects of the perineal region can use the aforementioned gracilis and rectus abdominis-based muscle, or myocutaneous flaps, or the tensor fascia lata flap and the gluteal thigh flap. Anal sphincter reconstruction also can be performed with

Table 44-12
Clinical Stages of Pressure Ulcers

Stage I	Erythema
Stage II	Partial-thickness ulceration
Stage III	Full-thickness ulceration with involvement of subcutaneous tissue
Stage IV	Ulceration through subcutaneous tissue to involve muscle and bone

local muscle, such as gracilis and gluteus maximus flaps. Avulsion injuries or fulminant Fournier's gangrene can yield full-thickness defects that may be skin grafted. Complete penile reconstruction is a complex problem that may demand the use of tubed pedicle flaps or free flaps, such as the radial forearm flap.

During radical retropubic prostatectomy, the cavernous nerves, which supply erectile function, may need to be sacrificed to ensure pure oncologic margins. Grafting across the nerve defect with sural nerve grafts can be performed. Evolving evidence suggests that up to 50% of patients who undergo bilateral nerve reconstruction will ultimately obtain useful erectile function.

PRESSURE ULCERS

Pressure ulcers occur in patients who are physically or mentally debilitated, such as chronic in-patients or spinal cord injury patients. Such ulcers occur when the external pressure on the skin and soft tissue, especially in the areas over bony prominences, exceeds capillary filling pressure (32 mm Hg at the arterial end). Factors that can influence the onset and persistence of ulcers are tissue friction and moisture and the patient's nutritional status and age. Common areas include the sacrum, heel, ischium, and trochanters. A grading system for pressure ulcers has been developed, with progressive tissue loss and destruction seen in the higher grade ulcers (Table 44-12).

Treatment of pressure ulcers must incorporate adequate débridement of infected and necrotic tissue, amelioration of inciting

pressure, proper dressing changes, and, if necessary, administration of antibiotics for control of more pervasive or systemic infection.[87]

Osteomyelitis for stage IV pressure ulcers can exacerbate the treatment conundrum. Diagnosis itself can be difficult with options including combinations of plain film, bone scan, MRI, and biopsy. Findings from adjunct studies such as leukocytosis or an elevated erythrocyte sedimentation rate may increase the predictive value of individual tests. If osteomyelitis is deemed to be present, aggressive bony débridement, vascularized flap coverage, and long-term treatment with intravenous antibiotics should be initiated.

Dressings for pressure ulcers may incorporate wet-to-dry dressing with saline (or impregnated with antibiotics), enzymatic débriding agents with active collagenase, and proteases. Povidone-iodine or hypochlorite combinations can be useful in infected ulcers. For more superficial, uninfected stage I and II ulcers, hydrocolloid dressings promote re-epithelialization by providing a moist environment. Calcium alginate dressings may help to absorb wound exudates. The topical use of growth factors such as platelet-derived growth factor and basic fibroblast growth factor to promote healing of superficial wounds has shown possible preliminary benefit.

The principles of surgical therapy include managing potential fecal contamination with thorough (and timely) bowel preparation, postoperative pharmacologic constipation, and if recurrent fecal-induced contamination and infection occurs, potential colostomies. The use of fasciocutaneous or muscle-based flaps allows vascularized soft-tissue fill and the precise choice of appropriate flap is dependent on the anatomy of the defect and flap choices. Depending again on the anatomy, sensate pedicled fasciocutaneous flaps may provide added protection for ulcer-prone areas. For the sacrum, fasciocutaneous advancement flaps can be designed for coverage. Muscle-based flaps include one or both gluteus maximus flaps. These can be advanced directly or in V-Y fashion. Treatment of ischial ulcers often requires ostectomies and bursectomies. Posterior thigh flaps, based on the inferior gluteal artery, can be used. Alternatively, in nonambulatory patients, V-Y advancement hamstring flaps provide durable coverage (Fig. 44-59). Less commonly, the gracilis, gluteus maximus, or even rectus abdominis

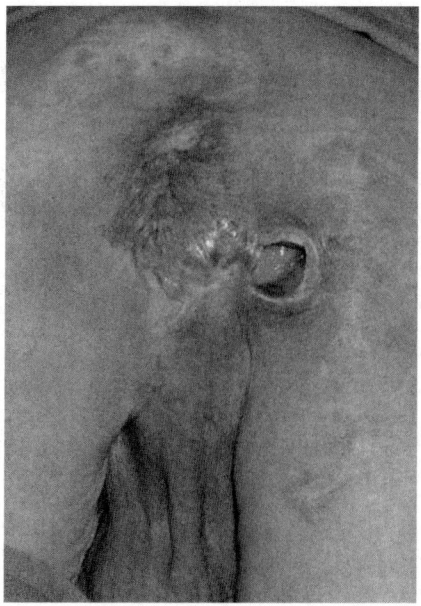 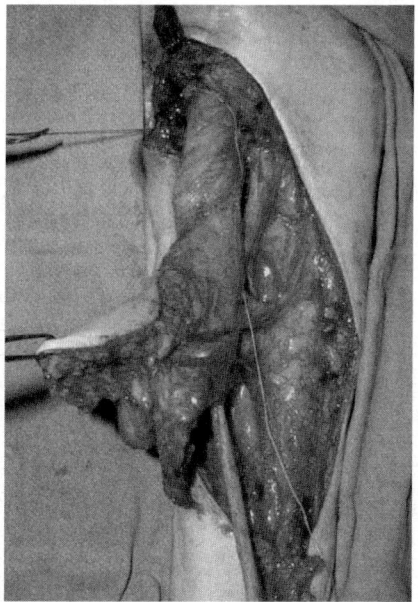 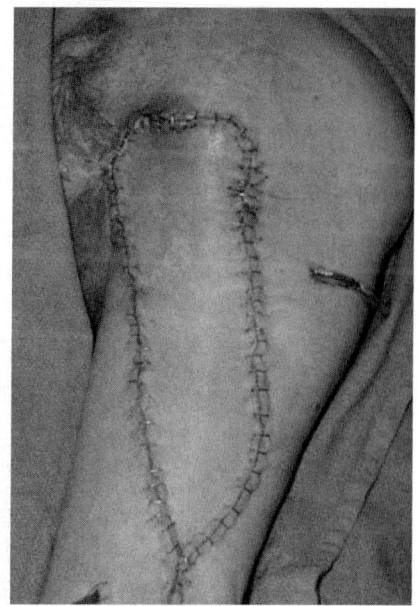

A   *B*   *C*

FIG. 44-59. Ischial wound coverage with hamstring flap. *A.* Defect. *B.* Elevation of flap. *C.* Inset and closure of flap.

muscle-based flaps can be used. The treatment of trochanteric ulcers often includes concomitant ostectomy of the protruding femoral head. The tensor fascia lata flap, the gluteus maximus, the posterior thigh flap, and the vastus lateralis myocutaneous flap have all been used for coverage of this region.[88]

Outcomes following flap coverage of pressure ulcers depend on the improvement of patient and tissue factors and the removal of potential causative agents. However, recurrence can occur in 50 to 80% of patients—with higher recurrence rates found in the paraplegic population. The use of air mattresses and positional changes help avoid direct pressure on the flap area. Most surgeons will employ closed suction drains for extended periods. A rare complication of pressure ulcers is the development of Marjolin's carcinoma 15 to 20 years after ulcer formation.

LOWER-EXTREMITY RECONSTRUCTION

Over the past three decades, high-energy, lower-extremity trauma caused by motor vehicle accidents, sporting events, falls, or gunshot wounds has plagued and bewildered plastic and orthopedic surgeons. Although amputation was enforced as the prevailing modality in the past, limb salvage has emerged as the target for the two disciplines. A marriage of soft-tissue and bony reconstruction has evolved in preserving appearance, and, more importantly, function.

Understanding the compartments, vascularity, nerve supply, and muscle functionality of the lower extremity is paramount for bony and soft-tissue restoration. Equally as important is the application of the Gustilo classification to lower-extremity repair (Table 44-13).

To provide appropriate management of a mangled, traumatic extremity, there needs to be a coordinated effort between the trauma, orthopedic, vascular, and plastic surgeons. After appropriate traumatic evaluation and resuscitation, the multidisciplinary team must assess the patient in regard to vascular exam, soft-tissue defect, and type of fracture. X-rays will assist the orthopedic surgeons in defining the type, extent, and treatment of the fracture. In addition, the team may order a Doppler exam or arteriogram to establish any vascular interruption. Most importantly, the surgeons need to perform a thorough, peripheral neurologic exam. Lower-extremity nerve repair and loss of plantar sensation has an ominous prognosis, and, in terms of long-term benefit and function, below-knee amputation may supplant limb salvage.

In terms of surgical management, the order of repair is fracture stabilization followed by vascular repair. The method for soft-tissue coverage of open fractures depends on the extent and location of injury. Split-thickness skin grafts are reasonable for coverage of exposed healthy muscle or soft tissue (Table 44-14). Local flaps (i.e., muscle or fasciocutaneous flaps) can treat small to moderate exposed bony defects of the lower or middle third of the leg. For

Table 44-13
Gustilo Classification of Open Fractures

Type	Description
I	Open fracture with wound <1 cm
II	Open fracture with wound >1 cm without extensive soft-tissue damage
III	Open fracture with extensive soft-tissue damage
IIIa	Adequate soft-tissue coverage
IIIb	III with soft-tissue loss with periosteal stripping and bony exposure
IV	III with arterial injury requiring repair

Table 44-14
Lower-Extremity Reconstruction Options

Area of Defect	Reconstructive Options
Hip and proximal femur	VRAM TFL Gracilis Vastus lateralis Sartorius
Distal femur	VRAM Gastrocnemius
Knee	Lateral gastrocnemius Medial gastrocnemius Both heads
Proximal tibia	Gastrocnemius
Middle tibia	Soleus Gastrocnemius Extensor digitorum longus Tibialis anterior
Distal tibia	Peroneus brevis Distal based soleus Reverse sural artery flap Supramalleolar flap Free tissue transfer

TFL = tensor fasciae latae; VRAM = vascular repair and management.

larger, soft-tissue defects with bony exposure, particularly of the lower one third, free tissue transfer may be the preferred panacea. If no recipient vessels are available, the plastic surgeon may use a cross-leg flap as a last alternative. Numerous disadvantages are associated with cross-leg flaps, including complete immobilization, contractures, and higher potential for deep vein thrombosis.[89,90]

Chronic osteomyelitis may burden the reconstructive team in setting of grade III open fractures. The classic treatment for chronic osteomyelitis involves aggressive débridement of all necrotic and devitalized tissue (bone and soft tissue), replacement with well-vascularized soft tissue (preferably muscle, but fasciocutaneous flaps are not contraindicated) followed by delayed treatment of the bony defect (with bone graft) (Fig. 44-60).

Diabetic Foot Ulcers

Foot ulcers, wound healing, and their complications are a significant health care burden in the diabetic patient. Maintaining an intact skin envelope will essentially curb the incidence of limb-threatening infections. With the advent of new therapeutic modalities and a multidisciplinary approach, the trend has shifted away from amputation to limb and function preservation.

The pathophysiology of diabetic foot ulceration can be divided into three components: peripheral neuropathy, peripheral vascular disease, and immunodeficiency.

With the inability to feel pressure or pain because of a sensory neuropathy, abnormal pressures can be easily distributed and applied, contributing to ulcer formation. In the setting of microvascular disease, the oxygen-carrying capacity of the site is reduced, which predisposes lower-limb ulceration and diminished wound-healing capabilities. Finally, the diabetic patient's immune system is altered in terms of chemotaxis, phagocytosis, and bactericidal capacity. This attenuated immune system predisposes the patient's lower limb to multiflora bacterial and fungal infections.

Both meticulous preoperative evaluation and surgical management are paramount when addressing diabetic foot ulcers. Optimization of comorbidities such as coronary and pulmonary disease must

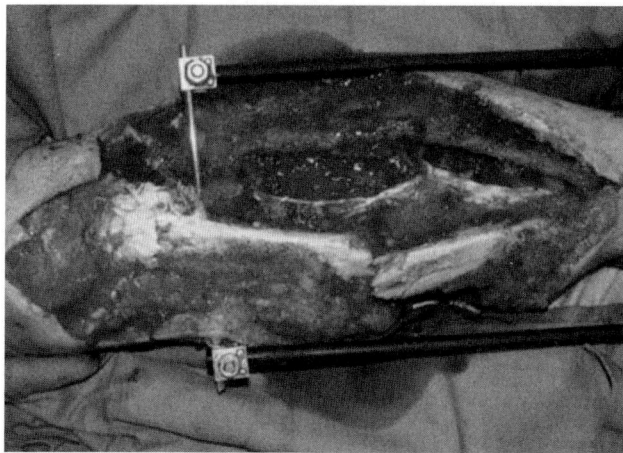

A

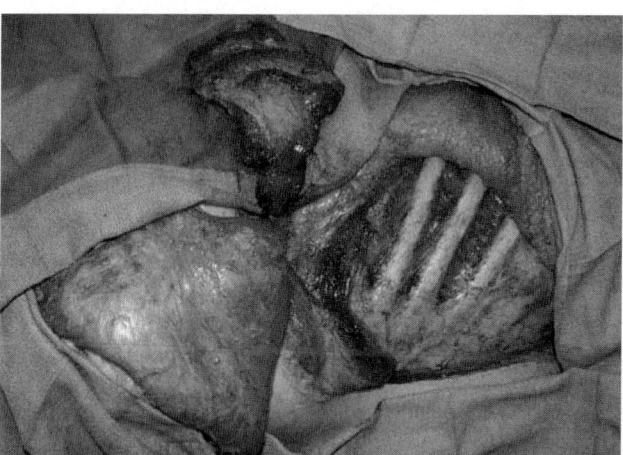

B

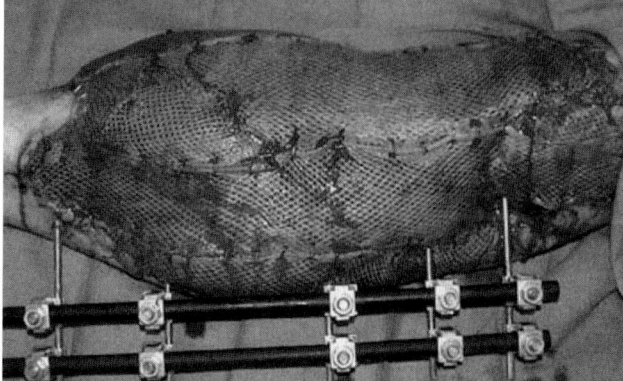

C

FIG. 44-60. *Soft-tissue reconstruction of Gustilo IIIb lower-extremity defect: free latissimus dorsi/serratus anterior flap. A. Soft-tissue defect with fractures of tibia and fibula. External fixator is in place. B. Elevation of free latissimus dorsi/serratus anterior flap. C. Free flap reconstruction with split-thickness skin graft.*

Table 44-15
Reconstructive Options for the Diabetic Foot

Region of Foot	*Reconstructive Options*
Forefoot	V-Y advancement
	Lisfranc amputation
Midfoot	V-Y advancement
	Toe island flap
	Transmetatarsal amputation
	Free tissue transfer
Hindfoot	Lateral calcaneal artery flap
	Reverse sural artery flap
	Medial planter artery flap
	Flexor digitorum brevis
	Abductor hallucis
	Abductor digiti minimi
Foot dorsum	Skin graft
	Free tissue transfer
	Supramalleolar flap
	Reverse sural flap

be achieved. More importantly, with the succor of medical consultants, blood sugar levels must be scrutinized and strictly controlled. Furthermore, either x-rays, bone scans, or MRI must be entertained to assess if there is osteomyelitis. This will determine operative and postoperative antibiotic management. Finally, a thorough vascular exam must be performed, either by duplex scanning or angiography. If there is significant vascular disease, the patient may be a reasonable candidate for lower-extremity bypass.

In terms of surgical management, all gross infection or foci of osteomyelitis must be débrided. Potential closure and soft-tissue reconstruction of the wound is adapted to character and location of the ulcer (Table 44-15). Newer agents and modalities have emerged to enhance granulation and wound healing such as Regranex and the vacuum-assisted closure. In certain circumstances, a skin graft may be appropriate, but can shear off in weight-bearing areas. Local flaps, such as the reverse sural artery or lateral calcaneal artery flap, can be employed. In larger defects, free tissue transfer may be advantageous in providing more durable tissue to weight-bearing areas. Combination lower-extremity bypass and free tissue coverage have proven enormously beneficial in the diabetic foot, in terms of healing and preventing disease progression.[91]

Lymphedema

Lymphedema is classified according to etiology. Primary lymphedema implies an idiopathic etiology and is typically subdivided into (1) *Milroy's disease*—congenital lymphedema that has an X-linked inheritance pattern; (2) *lymphedema praecox*—appearing after puberty but before 35 years of age; and (3) *lymphedema tarda*—appearing after the age of 35 years. Secondary lymphedema occurs as a result of secondary mechanical obstruction of lymphatic channels, as may occur following mastectomy or other types of surgery affecting physiologic lymphatic flow.

The pathophysiology of lymphedema stems from changes in the pressure gradients of the lymphatic channels caused by intrinsic or extrinsic factors. Normally, the pressure in the lower-extremity lymphatic system is subatmospheric and therefore allows the traverse of lymph upward. When lymphedema occurs, the lymph spills into the dermis and subcutaneous tissue. Clinically, this is manifested as firm, nonpitting swelling. CT or MRI may be helpful in differentiating lymphedema from venous problems or lipodystrophic edema.

Lymphoscintigraphy can delineate the anatomy and quantitate the actual lymphatic flow.

Treatment of lymphedema is generally conservative in nature and employs the use of external compressive garments and devices. Careful hygiene must also be instituted to avoid superficial fungal infections. Surgical treatment can involve direct excision of skin, subcutaneous tissue, and fascia as in the Charles procedure; staged excision of subcutaneous tissue as advocated by Sistrunk and Kondoleon; suction lipectomy; lymphatic anastomoses; or bridging procedures. The lymphatic-to-lymphatic anastomoses and venous–lymphatic anastomoses have had variable results and do not preclude conservative management.[92]

Especially following oncologic ablation, the onset of lymphedema must be differentiated from possible neoplastic invasion of the lymphatics. Lymphangiosarcoma also can be a rare cause of lymphedema that must be ruled out.

AESTHETIC SURGERY

Body Contouring and Liposuction

The assessment of body contour deformities, such as those following gastric bypass or reduction procedures, requires a careful consideration of skin excess, subcutaneous and adipose excess, and musculoaponeurotic laxity. There are differences in the anatomic distribution of adipose tissue between men and women, which varies with age.

Liposuction is a technique that allows fat to be aspirated from the subcutaneous tissue with small, 2- to 5-mm liposuction cannulae. Tumescent fluid is first infiltrated into the subcutaneous region to prepare the region with a lidocaine and epinephrine-based anesthetic and vasoconstrictive field effect. Excess fat deposition without significant skin excess or musculoaponeurotic laxity can be treated with liposuction alone. A caveat is that significant fluid shifts may occur with large-volume (>5 L) liposuction and careful monitoring of urine output, IV fluid administration, and hemodynamic variables is necessary at all times.

When excess skin and subcutaneous tissue is present or when the skin tone is compromised by age or loss of intrinsic elasticity, then frank excision of the excess tissue and skin may be necessary. If this excess occurs in the abdominal region, then abdominoplasty is a technique to elevate the soft tissue through a low transverse incision up to the subcostal and xiphoid region. The umbilicus is repositioned once the excess flap is brought down and excised. Associated fascial laxity or diastasis may be present as well and plication of the rectus fascia can bring a more satisfactory internal regulation of girth.[93]

Like abdominal lipodystrophy, lower-body lipodystrophy can occur from genetic happenstance or weight fluctuations secondary to lifestyle alterations, pregnancy, and surgery. Again, if the problem is recalcitrant adipose deposits without significant skin excess or compromise, then liposuction alone may be sufficient.[94] In a more radical situation where massive redundancy occurs at all levels of the skin and subcutaneous tissue, then a lower-body lift may be necessary. The entire buttock and thigh region can be elevated above the fascial level and securely fixed into a more cephalad position with excess tissue excised from this superior incision. For the corollary situation in the upper arm, a brachioplasty can be performed with an elliptical medial inner arm incision pattern.

Combinations of liposuction and resection procedures may need to be used depending on the clinical circumstance. Newer iterations of instrumentation such as ultrasound-assisted and power-assisted liposuction are also being used.

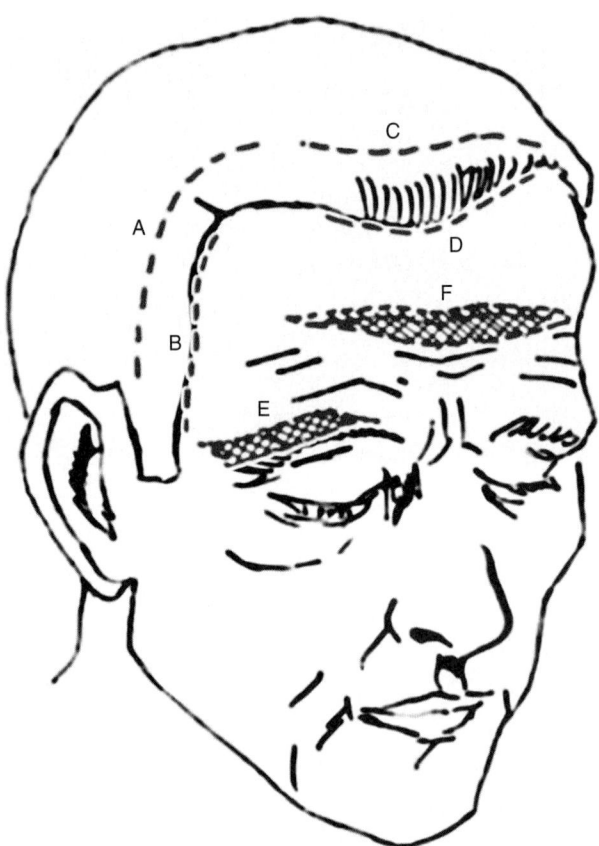

FIG. 44-61. Incisions for browlift. *A*. Temporal scalp incision. *B*. Temporal hairline incision. *C*. Midline scalp incision. *D*. Mid-hairline incision. *E*. Direct eyebrow incision. *F*. Direct forehead incision.

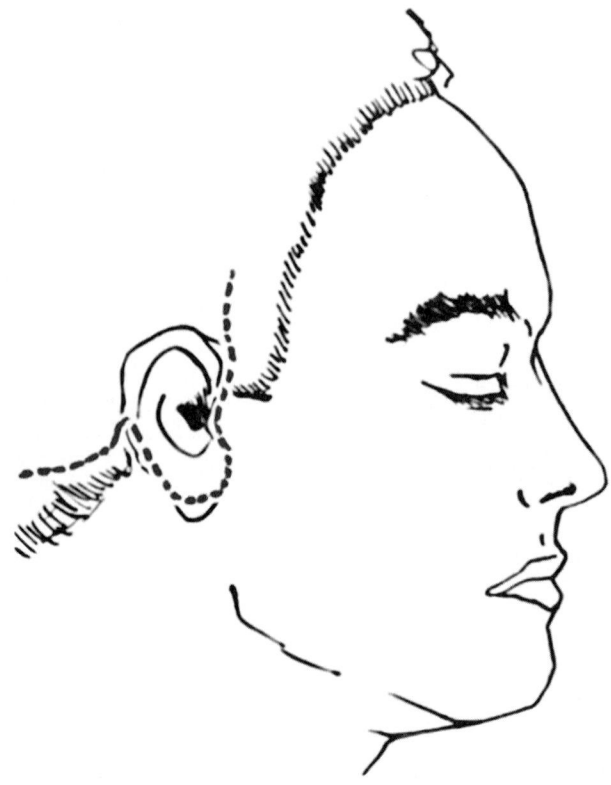

FIG. 44-62. Incisions for cervicofacial rhytidectomy.

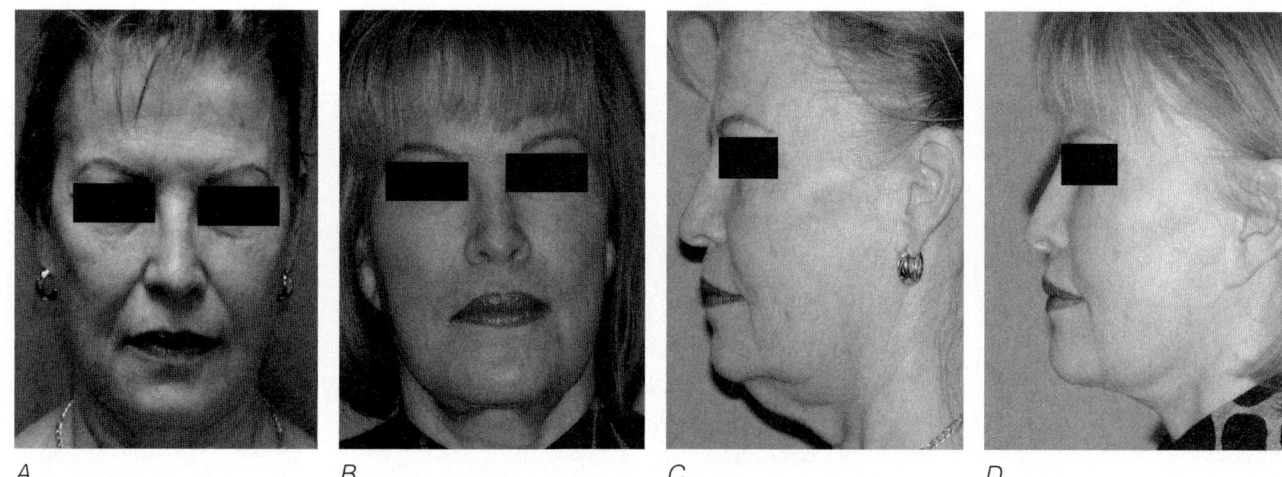

FIG. 44-63. Cervicofacial rhytidectomy. *A.* Preoperative photo, frontal view. *B.* Postoperative photo, frontal view. *C.* Preoperative photo, lateral view. *D.* Postoperative photo, lateral view.

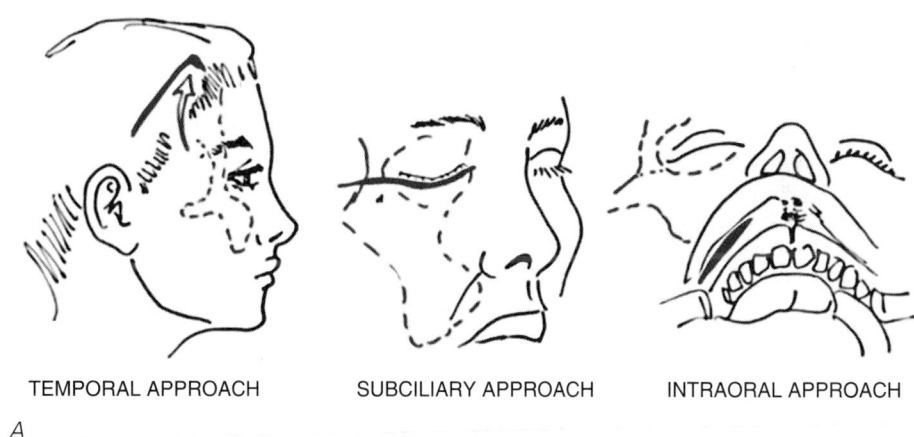

TEMPORAL APPROACH   SUBCILIARY APPROACH   INTRAORAL APPROACH

A

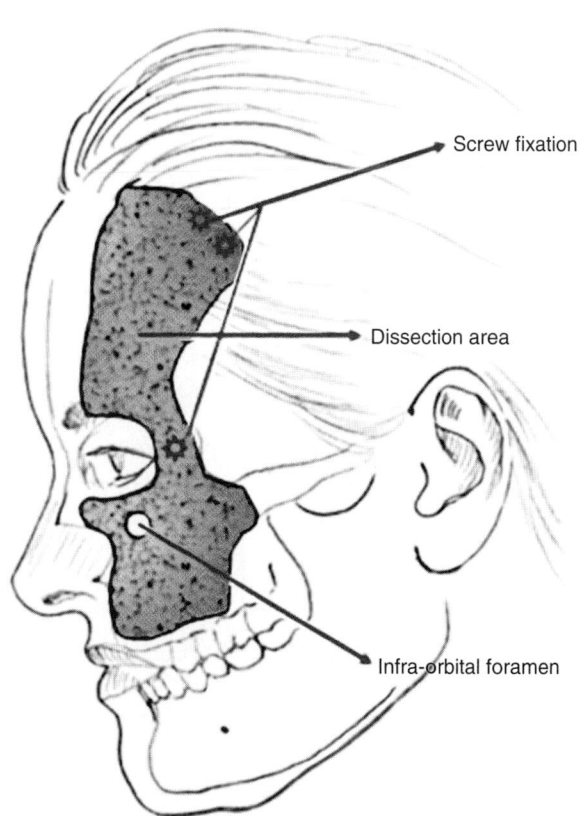

Screw fixation

Dissection area

Infra-orbital foramen

FIG. 44-64. Midface suspension. *A,* incisions for midface suspension. *B.* Midface dissection and screw fixation.

B

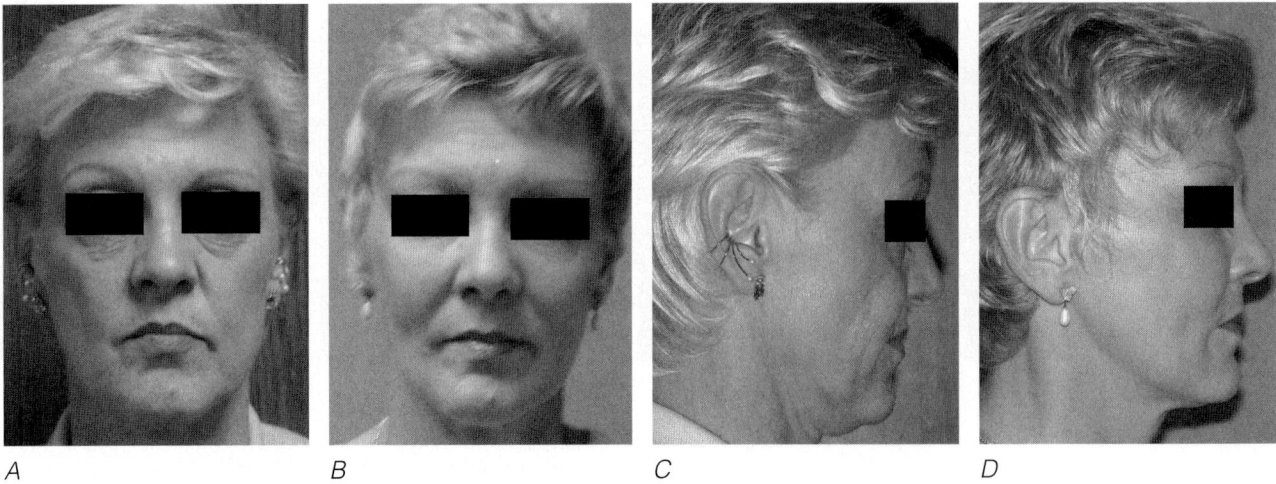

A   *B*   *C*   *D*

FIG. 44-65. *Midface suspension. A. Preoperative photo, frontal view. B. Postoperative photo, frontal view. C. Preoperative photo, lateral view. D. Postoperative photo, lateral view.*

Blepharoplasty and Browlift

Excess skin and adipose deposits also can occur in the upper and lower eyelids. The eye anatomy is complex. For the upper eyelid, excess skin (or dermatochalasia) can be approached through an elliptical incision. Careful markings of the degree of excess skin are required to prevent over-resection of skin and resultant lagophthalmos. A strip of orbicularis muscle also can be taken to accentuate the fold of the eyelid. If excess postseptal fat is present, it is resected prior to definitive skin closure. For the lower eyelid, skin and orbicularis resection or repositioning also is performed.

When there is ptosis of the brow, then separate elevation in a subperiosteal or subcutaneous plane of the forehead region can be performed. A coronal, mid-forehead, brow, anterior hairline, or endoscopic incision approach can be made (Fig. 44-61). The flaps of tissue are repositioned and secured in place with sutures or small screws. An endoscopic approach has become increasingly popular because of the smaller scars that result.[95]

Facelift

Excess skin and musculoaponeurotic laxity of the face also can be treated with elevation of skin flaps coupled with judicious skin

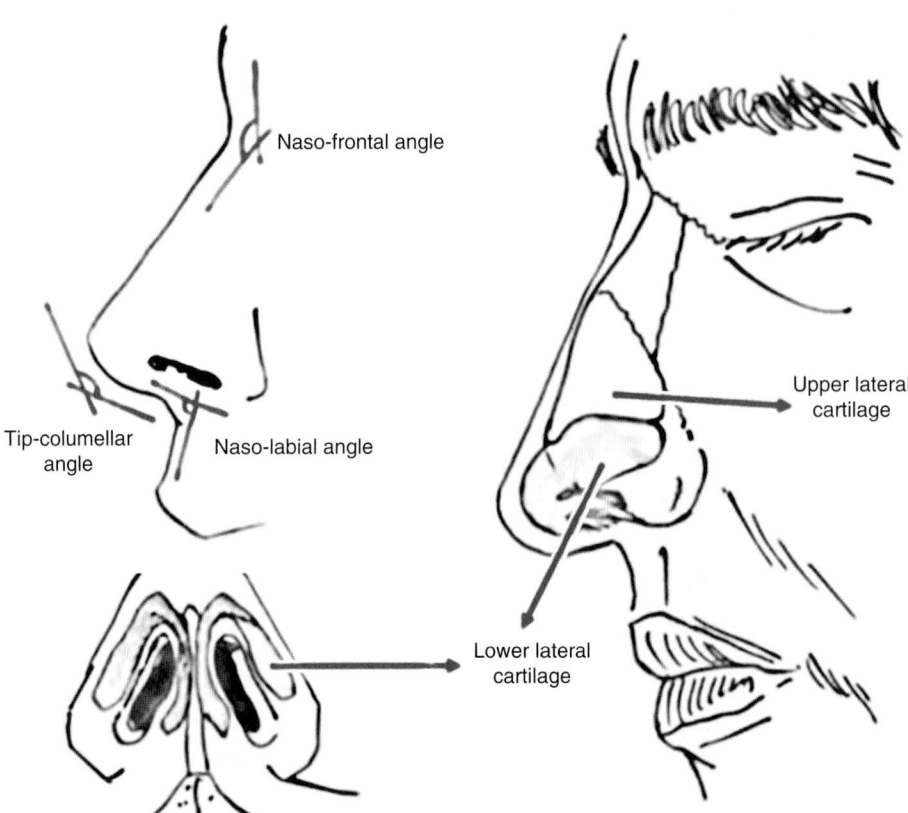

Naso-frontal angle

Tip-columellar angle

Naso-labial angle

Upper lateral cartilage

Lower lateral cartilage

FIG. 44-66. Rhinoplasty anatomy.

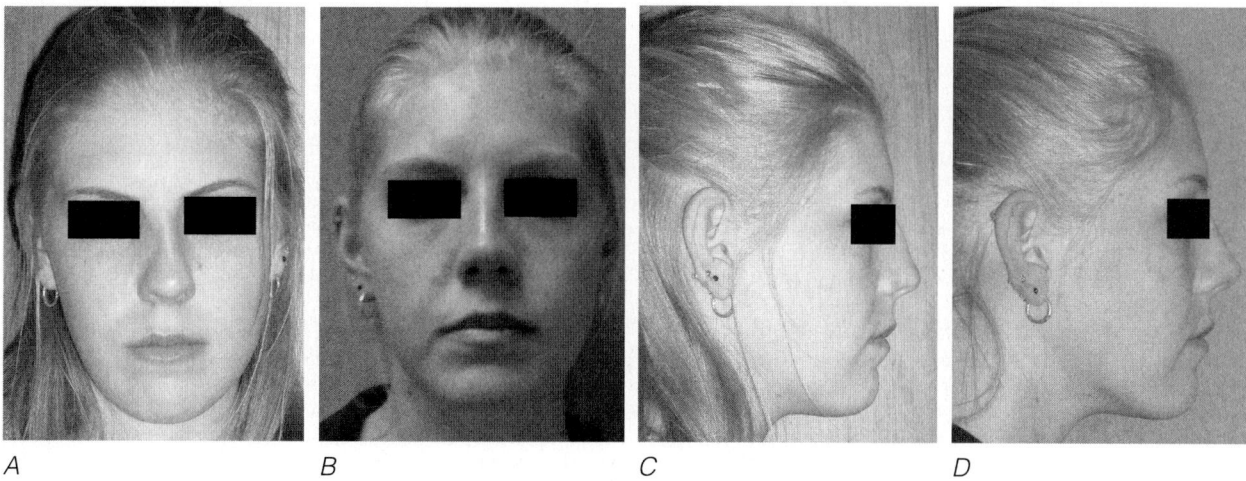

A   *B*   *C*   *D*

FIG. 44-67. *Rhinoplasty. A. Preoperative photo, frontal. B. Postoperative photo, frontal. C. Preoperative photo, lateral. D. Postoperative photo, lateral.*

excision. Generally, preauricular incisions are extended into the temporal hairline superiorly and into the retroauricular region posteriorly and inferiorly (Fig. 44-62). The superficial musculoaponeurotic system (SMAS) lies immediately deep to the skin, and diverse techniques exist to modify this layer to enhance the rejuvenating effect of excess skin excision. The SMAS can be simply plicated or it can be excised. A sub-SMAS dissection can help to elevate and develop this layer in separate fashion, with care being taken to avoid injury to the underlying facial nerves. Often, the cervical region and platysmal deformities need to be addressed in conjunction with the primary facelift procedure (Fig. 44-63). The platysmal layer is continuous with the SMAS layer and thus can be similarly manipulated to ameliorate any deformities of the overall cervical contour.[96]

Specific regions of the face may require special adjunct procedures. The lower periorbital region can be characterized by malar descent and a tear trough deformity. In this situation, a mid-face lift approached from both temporal and intraoral incisions can help to reverse the vertical descent and atrophy of soft tissue (Figs. 44-64 and 44-65).

Rhinoplasty

The nose is a complex structure with refined relations among the nasal and maxillary bones, lower and upper lateral cartilages, septum, turbinates and mucosa, and overlying soft-tissue cover (Fig. 44-66). Nasal airway obstruction can occur as a consequence of internal or external derangements of structure. A deviated septum can alter the magnitude and direction of airflow. The internal nasal valve, consisting of the upper lateral cartilage and septum, is a common location for nasal airway obstruction. Improvement in airway flow with lateral traction of the cheek may open this valve to subjectively improve airflow (positive Cottle sign), an indication that grafting to open the valve angle may be of benefit. Deformities of the internal valve or septum can be corrected by resection or cartilage manipulation. Excessive dorsal hump and tip deformities are common complaints that may be corrected via an open or closed approach. Judicious resection or rasping of cartilage is coupled with cartilage grafts placed at critical structural junctures. Grafts can be placed in the columellar or tip region. They can support the dorsal structure or the alar rim region. Preferably, cartilage should be har-

vested from the septum, but also can be taken from the concha or even from the rib. Internal sutures may also help alter the shape of cartilaginous structures. Osteotomies can redefine the relation between the nasomaxillary bony structure and the reshaped nose. The interrelatedness of the nasal structures must be noted during any manipulation of a single subunit. For instance, a patient who has an excessive dorsal hump may have rasping performed on this area, but this, in turn, may result in upward rotation of the tip of the nose and loss of support between the septum and upper lateral cartilages ("open roof deformity"), all of which may require additional refinement of the tip and possible osteotomies to circumvent a triggering of secondary deformities (Fig. 44-67).[97]

CONCLUSION

Plastic and reconstructive surgery continues to implement advances in technology and basic science into clinical practice. Permutations of older techniques, such as perforator flaps, also promise more precise, refined choices in reconstruction. Ongoing research into tissue engineering, gene therapy, and alloplastic materials will evolve into novel treatments of defects and more durable reconstructions.[98]

References

1. Majno G: *The Healing Hand: Man and Wound in the Ancient World.* Cambridge, MA: Harvard University Press, 1975.
2. Gnudi MT, Webster JP: *The Life and Times of Gaspare Tagliacozzi.* New York: Herbert Reichner, 1950.
3. Harding KG, Morris HL, Patel GK: Science, medicine and the future: Healing chronic wounds. *BMJ* 324:160, 2002.
4. Rumalla VK, Borah GL: Cytokines, growth factors, and plastic surgery. *Plast Reconstr Surg* 108:719, 2001.
5. Steed DL: The role of growth factors in wound healing. *Surg Clin North Am* 77:575, 1997.
6. Datubo-Brown DD: Keloids: A review of the literature. *Br J Plast Surg* 43:70, 1990.
7. McGregor I: *Fundamental Techniques in Plastic Surgery and Their Surgical Applications,* 7th ed. Edinburgh: Churchill-Livingstone, 1995.
8. Rudolph R, Ballantyne DL: Skin grafts, in McCarthy J (ed): *Plastic Surgery.* Philadelphia: WB Saunders, 1990, p. 221.

9. Haller JA, Billingham RE: Studies of the origin of vasculature in free skin grafts. *Ann Surg* 166:896, 1967.

10. Taylor GI, Palmer JH: The vasculatory territories (angiosomes of the body): Experimental study and clinical applications. *Br J Plast Surg* 40:113, 1987.

11. Jackson IT: *Local Flaps in Head and Neck Reconstruction.* St. Louis: Mosby, 1985.

12. Mathes SJ, Najai F: *Reconstructive Surgery: Principles, Anatomy, and Technique.* New York: Churchill-Livingstone 1997.

13. Manders EK, Schenden MJ, Hetzler PT, et al: Soft tissue expansion: Concepts and complications. *Plast Reconstr Surg* 74:493, 1984.

14. Khouri RK, Cooley BC, et al: A prospective study of microvascular free flap surgery and outcome. *Plast Reconst Surg* 102:711, 1998.

15. Shenaq SM, Sharma SK: Principles of microvascular surgery, in Beasley R, Thorne C, Aston S (eds): *Grabbe and Smiths Plastic Surgery,* 4th ed. Philadelphia: Lippincott-Raven, 1997, p. 73.

16. Mackinnon SE, Dellon AL: *Surgery of the Peripheral Nerve.* New York: Thieme, 1988.

17. Sunderland S: *Nerves and Nerve Injuries.* Edinburgh: Churchill-Livingstone, 1978.

18. Burt JD, Byrd HS: Cleft lip: Unilateral primary deformities. *Plast Reconstr Surg* 105:1043, 2000.

19. Mulliken JB: Primary repair of bilateral cleft lip and nasal deformity. *Plast Reconstr Surg* 108:181, 2001.

20. Rohrich RJ, Love EJ, Byrd HS, Johns DF: Optimal timing of cleft palate closure. *Plast Reconstr Surg* 106:413, 2000.

21. Anastassov GE, Joos U: Comprehensive management of cleft lip and palate deformities. *J Oral Maxillofac Surg* 59:1062, 2001.

22. Gampper TJ, Morgan RF: Vascular anomalies: Hemangiomas. *Plast Reconstr Surg* 110:572, 2002.

23. Marchuk DA: Pathogenesis of hemangioma. *J Clin Invest* 107:665, 2001.

24. Mulliken JB, Fishman SJ, Burrows PE: Vascular anomalies. *Curr Probl Surg* 37:517, 2000.

25. Breugem CC, van Der Horst CM, Hennekam RC: Progress toward understanding vascular malformations. *Plast Reconstr Surg* 107:1509, 2001.

26. Hunt JA, Hobar PC: Common craniofacial anomalies: Conditions of craniofacial atrophy/hypoplasia and neoplasia. *Plast Reconstr Surg* 111:1497, 2003.

27. Hunt JA, Hobar PC: Common craniofacial anomalies: The facial dysostoses. *Plast Reconstr Surg* 110:1714, 2002.

28. Panchal J, Uttchin V: Management of craniosynostosis. *Plast Reconstr Surg* 111:1032, 2003.

29. Zide B, Grayson B, McCarthy JG: Cephalometric analysis. Part I. *Plast Reconstr* Surg 68:816, 1981.

30. Manson PN: Facial injuries, in McCarthy JG (ed): *Plastic Surgery.* Philadelphia: WB Saunders, 1990, p. 867.

31. Lazow SK: A mandible fracture protocol. *J Oral Maxillofac Surg* 60:133, 2002.

32. Rohrich RJ, Hollier L: The role of the nasofrontal duct in frontal sinus fracture management. *J Craniomaxillofac Trauma* 2(4):31, 1996.

33. Rohrich RJ, Hollier LH: Management of frontal sinus fractures. Changing concepts. *Clin Plast Surg* 19:219, 1992.

34. Gruss JS. Nasoethmoid orbital fractures: Classification and role of primary bone grafting. *Plast Reconstr Surg* 75:303, 1985.

35. Ellis E 3rd, Tan Y: Assessment of internal orbital reconstructions for pure blowout fractures: Cranial bone grafts versus titanium mesh. *J Oral Maxillofac Surg* 61:442, 2003.

36. Manson PN: Pure orbital blowout fracture: New concepts and importance of the medial orbital blowout fracture. *Plast Reconstr Surg* 104:878, 1999.

37. Pollock RA: Nasal trauma: Pathomechanics and surgical management of acute injuries. *Clin Plast Surg* 19:133, 1992.

38. Rinehart GC, Marsh JL, Hemmer KM: Internal fixation of malar fractures: An experimental biophysical study. *Plast Reconstr Surg* 84:21, 1989.

39. Davidson J, Nickerson D, Nickerson B: Zygomatic fractures: Comparison of methods of internal fixation. *Plast Reconstr Surg* 86:25, 1990.

40. Zachariades N, Mezitis M, Anagnostopoulos D: Changing trends in the treatment of zygomaticomaxillary complex fractures: A 12-year evaluation of methods used. *J Oral Maxillofac Surg* 56:1152, 1998.

41. Manson PN, Clark N, Robertson B, et al: Subunit principles in midface fractures: The importance of sagittal buttresses, soft-tissue reductions, and sequencing treatment of segmental fractures. *Plast Reconstr Surg* 103:1287, 1999.

42. Walton RL, Beahm EK: Auricular reconstruction for microtia: Part II. Surgical techniques. *Plast Reconstr Surg* 110:234, 2002.

43. Beahm EK, Walton RL: Auricular reconstruction for microtia: Part I. Anatomy, embryology, and clinical evaluation. *Plast Reconstr Surg* 109:2473, 2002.

44. Bauer BS, Song DH, Aitken ME: Combined otoplasty technique: Chondrocutaneous conchal resection as the cornerstone to correction of the prominent ear. *Plast Reconstr Surg* 110:1033, 2002.

45. Yugueros P, Friedland JA: Otoplasty: The experience of 100 consecutive patients. *Plast Reconstr Surg* 108:1045, 2001.

46. Spira M: Otoplasty: What I do now—A 30-year perspective. *Plast Reconstr Surg* 104:834, 1999.

47. Yih WY, Howerton DW: A regional approach to reconstruction of the upper lip. *J Oral Maxillofac Surg* 55:383, 1997.

48. O'Daniel TG: Lip reconstruction, in Marsh JL (ed): *Decision Making in Plastic Surgery.* St. Louis: Mosby, 1993, p. 134.

49. Menick FJ: Reconstruction of the cheek. *Plast Reconstr Surg* 108:496, 2001.

50. Singh DJ, Bartlett SP: Aesthetic considerations in nasal reconstruction and the role of modified nasal subunits. *Plast Reconstr Surg* 111:639, 2003.

51. Maruyama Y, Okada E: Unit approach to nasal reconstruction. *Plast Reconstr Surg* 108:794, 2001.

52. Yotsuyanagi T, Yamashita K, Urushidate S, et al: Reconstruction of large nasal defects with a combination of local flaps based on the aesthetic subunit principle. *Plast Reconstr Surg* 107:1358, 2001.

53. Menick FJ: A 10-year experience in nasal reconstruction with the three-stage forehead flap. *Plast Reconstr Surg* 109:1839, 2002.

54. Jelks GW, Smith BC: Reconstruction of the eyelids and associated structures, in McCarthy JG (ed): *Plastic Surgery.* Philadelphia: WB Saunders, 1990, p. 1671.

55. Weinstein GS: Lower eyelid reconstruction with tarsal flaps and grafts. *Plast Reconstr Surg* 81:991, 1988.

56. Shestak KC, Ramasastry SS: Reconstruction of defects of the scalp and skull, in Cohen M (ed): *Mastery of Plastic and Reconstructive Surgery.* Boston: Little, Brown, 1994, p. 830.

57. Alpert BS, Buncke HJ, Mathes SJ: Surgical treatment of the total avulsed scalp. *Clin Plast Surg* 9:145, 1982.

58. May M: Facial paralysis: Differential diagnosis and indications for surgical therapy. *Clin Plast Surg* 6:275, 1979.

59. Kumar PA, Hassan KM: Cross-face nerve graft with free-muscle transfer for reanimation of the paralyzed face: A comparative study of the single-stage and two-stage procedures. *Plast Reconstr Surg* 109:451, 2002.

60. Gurtner GC, Evans G: Advances in head and neck reconstruction. *Plast Reconstr Surg* 106:672, 2000.

61. Chang DW, Langstein HN, Gupta A, et al: Reconstructive management of cranial base defects after tumor ablation. *Plast Reconstr Surg* 107:1346, 2001.

62. Sasaki TM, Baker HW, McConnell DB, et al: Free jejunal graft reconstruction after extensive head and neck surgery. *Am J Surg* 139:650, 1980.

63. McConnel FM, Hester TR, Nahai F, et al: Free jejunal grafts for reconstruction of pharynx and cervical esophagus. *Arch Otolaryngol* 107:476, 1981.

64. Kroll SS: Autologous breast reconstruction after breast-conserving cancer surgery. *Plast Reconstr Surg* 102:1937, 1998.

65. Elliot LF: Options for donor sites for autogenous tissue breast reconstruction. *Clin Plast Surg* 21:177, 1994.

66. Shenaq S, Bullocks J, Kim J: Breast reconstruction, latissimus flap. *Emedicine* 2002.

67. Kronowitz SJ, Chang DW, Robb GL, et al: Implications of axillary sentinel lymph node biopsy in immediate autologous breast reconstruction. *Plast Reconstr Surg* 109:1888, 2002.

68. Dowden RV: Breast reconstruction with implants and expanders. *Plast Reconstr Surg* 108:576, 2001.

69. Little JW: Nipple–areola reconstruction, in Spear SL, Little JW, Lippman ME, et al (eds): *Surgery of the Breast: Principles and Art.* Philadelphia: Lippincott-Raven, 1998, p. 661.

70. Georgiade GS, Georgiade NG: Hypermastia and ptosis, in Georgiade GS, Riefkohl R, Levin LS (eds): *Plastic, Maxillofacial and Reconstructive Surgery,* 3rd ed. Baltimore: Williams & Wilkins, 1997, p. 752.

71. Tebbetts JB: A system for breast implant selection based on patient tissue characteristics and implant–soft tissue dynamics. *Plast Reconstr Surg* 109:1396, 2002.

72. LaTrenta GS: Breast augmentation, in Rees TD, LaTrenta GS (eds): *Aesthetic Plastic Surgery,* 2nd ed. Philadelphia: WB Saunders, 1994, p. 1003.

73. Hidalgo DA: Breast augmentation: Choosing the optimal incision, implant, and pocket plane. *Plast Reconstr Surg* 105:2202, 2000.

74. Bantick GL, Taggart I: Mammography and breast implants. *Br J Plast Surg* 48:49, 1995.

75. Miglioretti DL, Rutter CM, Geller BM, et al: Effect of breast augmentation on the accuracy of mammography and cancer characteristics. *JAMA* 291:442, 2004.

76. Braunstein GD: Gynecomastia. *N Engl J Med* 328:490, 1993.

77. Argenta LC, VanderKolk C, Friedman RJ, et al: Refinements in reconstruction of congenital breast deformities. *Plast Reconstr Surg* 76:73, 1985.

78. Hester TR, Bostwick J: Poland syndrome: Correction with latissimus muscle transposition. *Plast Reconstr Surg* 69:226, 1982.

79. Cohen M: Reconstruction of the chest wall, in Cohen M (ed): *Mastery of Plastic and Reconstructive Surgery.* Boston: Little, Brown, 1994, p. 1248.

80. Francel TJ, Kouchoukos NT: A rational approach to wound difficulties after sternotomy: Reconstruction and long-term results. *Ann Thorac Surg* 72:1419, 2001.

81. Jones G, Jurkiewicz MJ, Bostwick J, et al: Management of the infected median sternotomy wound with muscle flaps: The Emory 20-year experience. *Ann Surg* 225:766, 1997.

82. Ramirez OM, Ruas E, Dellon A: "Components separation" method for closure of abdominal wall defects: An anatomic and clinical study. *Plast Reconstr Surg* 86:519, 1990.

83. Mathes SJ, Steinwald PM, Foster RD, et al: Complex abdominal wall reconstruction: A comparison of flap and mesh closure. *Ann Surg* 232:586, 2000.

84. Rohrich RJ, Lowe JB, Hackney FL, et al: An algorithm for abdominal wall reconstruction. *Plast Reconstr Surg* 105:202, 2000.

85. Schaeffer CS, King LR: Anomalies of the male genitalia, in Georgiade GS, Riefkohl R, Levin LS (eds): *Plastic, Maxillofacial and Reconstructive Surgery,* 3rd ed. Baltimore: Williams & Wilkins, 1997, p. 844.

86. Dumanian GA, Hurwitz DJ: Congenital deformities of the female genitalia, in Georgiade GS, Riefkohl R, Levin LS (eds): *Plastic, Maxillofacial and Reconstructive Surgery,* 3rd ed. Baltimore: Williams & Wilkins, 1997, p. 855.

87. Colen SR: Pressure sores, in McCarthy JC (ed): *Plastic Surgery.* Philadelphia: WB Saunders, 1990, p. 3797.

88. Mathes SJ, Nahai F: *Reconstructive Surgery Principles: Anatomy and Techniques.* New York: Churchill-Livingstone, 1997.

89. Heller L, Levin LS: Lower extremity microsurgical reconstruction. *Plast Reconstr Surg* 108:1029, 2001.

90. Bosse MJ, MacKenzie EJ, Kellam JF, et al: An analysis of outcomes of reconstruction or amputation after leg-threatening injuries. *N Engl J Med* 347:1924, 2002.

91. Jeffcoate WJ, Harding KG: Diabetic Foot ulcers. *Lancet* 361:1545, 2003.

92. Foldi E, Foldi M, Clodius L: The lymphedema chaos. *Ann Plast Surg* 22:505, 1989.

93. Ramirez OM: Abdominoplasty and abdominal wall rehabilitation: A comprehensive approach. *Plast Reconstr Surg* 105:425, 2000.

94. Rohrich RJ, Smith PD, Maracntonio DR, et al: The zones of adherence: Role in minimizing and preventing contour deformities in liposuction. *Plast Reconst Surg* 107:1562, 2001.

95. Paul MD: The evolution of the brow lift in aesthetic plastic surgery. *Plast Reconstr Surg* 108:1409, 2001.

96. Thorne CM, Aston SG: Aesthetic surgery of the aging face, in Aston SG, Beasley RW, Thorne CH (eds): *Grabbe and Smiths Plastic Surgery,* 5th ed. Philadelphia: Lippincott, 1997, p. 633.

97. Sheen JH: *Aesthetic Rhinoplasty.* St Louis: Mosby, 1987.

98. Lorenz HP, Hedrick MH, Chang J, et al: The impact of biomolecular medicine and tissue engineering on plastic surgery in the 21st century. *Plast Reconstr Surg* 105:2467, 2000.

CHAPTER 45

Surgical Considerations in the Elderly

Rosemarie E. Hardin and Michael E. Zenilman

General Considerations

Preoperative Evaluation

Specific Considerations

Minimal Access Laparoscopic Surgery
Endocrine Surgery
    Breast Surgery
    Thyroid Surgery
    Parathyroid Surgery
Cardiothoracic Surgery
    Coronary Artery Bypass Grafting
    Valve Replacement
Trauma
Transplantation

Palliative Surgery

Specific Symptom Management
    Gastrointestinal Disturbances
    Depression and Asthenia
Cachexia and Anorexia
    Malignant Bowel Obstruction
    Pain Management

Ethical Considerations

GENERAL CONSIDERATIONS

It is estimated that by the year 2025, persons older than age 65 will constitute 25% of the United States population.[1] This ever-growing elderly population will increasingly require surgical consultation and intervention. A 1996 review showed that more than 4 million patients older than 65 years of age underwent surgical procedures, with the most common interventions being coronary artery bypass grafting, orthopedic procedures, and cholecystectomy.[1,2] Elderly surgical patients account for 50% of surgical emergencies and 75% of perioperative deaths.[3] These statistics challenge the surgeon to have an intimate understanding of the careful preoperative evaluation required in elderly patients, as well as the potential impact of comorbidities and emergency presentations on outcomes of surgical intervention. In addition, postoperative management must be tailored to the specific physiologic changes and unique susceptibility to postoperative complications of this unique population.

Chronologic age is rarely an accurate predictor of morbidity and mortality from surgical interventions. It is, however, an accurate marker for declining physiologic reserve and the presence of multiple comorbid conditions. These, in turn, place elderly patients at higher risk because of depressed cardiac, pulmonary, renal, and neurologic reserves, thereby increasing the morbidity and mortality

of surgical interventions. Therefore, physiologic age plus the presence of comorbid conditions more accurately predict the surgical outcomes in this population.

Comorbid illness serves as the basis for the American Society of Anesthesiologists (ASA) physical status classification (Table 45-1).[4] This is a valuable tool for identification of elderly patients at high risk for postoperative complications because it is based on organ system dysfunction and severity of functional impairment. It helps identify subgroups of patients in whom appropriate measures should be taken to reduce the risk of adverse outcomes. This chapter explores the physiologic changes associated with aging, the impact of comorbid disease and preoperative assessment on outcome, as well as provides special focus on ethical issues, palliative care, and end-of-life issues.

PREOPERATIVE EVALUATION

Surgical risk increases with advancing age as a consequence of physiologic decline and the development of comorbid conditions leading to postoperative complications, which are poorly tolerated because of decreased reserve. Adequate control and understanding of the potential negative impact of comorbid conditions on surgical outcomes allows an appropriate preoperative evaluation that, in turn, leads to acceptable morbidity and mortality.

The higher prevalence of comorbid disease in elderly patients places them in a higher ASA class; with approximately 80% falling into ASA class 3 or higher.[5] This physiologic fact leads to higher complication and mortality rates in patients 65 years of age or older. Mortality rates of major surgical intervention in patients older than 65 years of age without comorbid disease is approximately 5% but rises to approximately 10% with the presence of three comorbid illnesses.[6]

Another scoring system that is frequently used in critically ill patients is the Acute Physiology and Chronic Health Evaluation (APACHE) III score.[7] This system factors age, physiologic parameters, and chronic health status into the prediction of mortality. In this assessment, physiologic parameters, comorbid conditions, and urgency of interventions carry far greater significance than chronologic age alone. Interestingly, the APACHE score has identified that the site of surgery is a significant determinant of perioperative mortality. Cardiovascular and upper abdominal surgery results in a greater probability of a major complication.[7] Therefore, the APACHE scoring system can identify subgroups of elderly patients who have an increased probability of an adverse outcome in the perioperative period.

A particular problem encountered in the elderly population is potential delay in surgical intervention. This may be caused by

Table 45-1
American Society of Anesthesiologists' Physical Status Classification

ASA Risk Stratification for Anesthetic/Surgical Risk	
Class 1	Healthy patient
Class 2	Mild systemic disease
Class 3	Severe (but not incapacitating) systemic disease
Class 4	Severe systemic disease posing a constant threat to life
Class 5	Moribund with life expectancy <24 hours, independent of operation
Class 6 (by definition)	Organ donor

Note: Suffix "e" is added to the class for emergency operations.
SOURCE: Adapted from Muravchick.[4]

misdiagnosis of urgent surgical disease because of atypical presentations leading to higher risk of complications. Elective procedures may be delayed because of provider misconception that elderly patients will suffer complications and poor outcomes. These delays lead to higher morbidity and mortality rates. The two main predictors of postoperative morbidity and mortality are advancing age and its accompanying physiologic decline and comorbid disease and the emergent nature of surgical interventions.[3]

An important variable in the proper perioperative evaluation of an elderly patient is nutritional status. Elderly patients may have poor nutritional status because of either poor intake or underlying illness and comorbidities. Protein calorie malnutrition can occur in *nil per os* (nothing by mouth [NPO]) patients with inadequate nutritional reserve. This may occur in a short period in the elderly, malnourished surgical patient in a hypermetabolic state induced by stress of illness and surgery. Elderly patients, therefore, need accurate assessment of nutritional status and, if clinically indicated, immediate appropriate nutritional support to meet caloric requirements. This not only gives patients additional reserve to minimize postoperative complications, it aids in appropriate wound healing, which may also be impaired with aging.

It is important that preoperative evaluation include accurate assessment of the functional status of the surgical candidate in addition to the cognitive level of functioning. This ensures that operative intervention will not significantly impair the quality of life of an elderly surgical candidate. The functional status of an elderly patient is related to, and therefore predictive of, pulmonary and cardiac complications that may ensue following surgical intervention. For example, functional impairment often leads to immobility, which is known to increase the risk of postoperative complications such as atelectasis, pneumonia, deep vein thrombosis, and pulmonary embolism.

Cognitive function is often overlooked in the preoperative assessment of patients, because patients are not typically formally evaluated prior to surgical intervention (e.g., mini mental status exam). However, knowledge of baseline cognitive function provides invaluable information because subtle changes in cognition often heralds postoperative complications such as underlying infection. Furthermore, dementia is a known predictor of limited long-term survival.

Cardiac complications are the leading cause of perioperative complications and death in surgical patients of all age groups, but particularly among the elderly who may have underlying cardiac disease in addition to normal physiologic decline (Table 45-2). Myocardial infarction or congestive heart failure comprises one quarter of all cardiac complications and perioperative deaths in elderly patients.[8] Therefore, identifying correctable and uncorrectable cardiovascular disease is critical prior to elective surgical intervention. The cardiac risk in elderly surgical patients has been best demonstrated by

Goldman's criteria, which assigned a total of 53 risk points for various cardiac risk factors known in noncardiac surgery (Table 45-3).[9] This criteria was later simplified to six variables that determine preoperative cardiac risk (see Table 45-3). Using this new model, an elderly patient with no risk factors has a cardiac morbidity rate of 0.5%, one factors will raise it to 1.3%, two factors to 3.6%, and three factors to 9.1%. This is a much simpler system to use than the original "criteria."

Pulmonary complications are a major source of morbidity and mortality in surgical patients, with the elderly at an even greater risk because of the increased possibility of underlying pulmonary disease and decreased reserve. Pulmonary complications account for up to 50% of postoperative complications and 20% of preventable deaths.[3] However, age alone is a minimal factor when adjusted for comorbidities, leading to a twofold risk of pulmonary complications.[10] As with cardiac risk, the site of surgery is the most important predictor of complications. Higher-risk surgical interventions include those of the upper abdomen, aorta, or peripheral vascular interventions.[3,10]

All elderly patients undergoing major surgical interventions should have a baseline chest radiograph.[3] Risk factors for pulmonary complications include a positive smoking history, presence of shortness of breath, or clinical evidence of chronic obstructive pulmonary disease (COPD). Pre-existing COPD is a major preoperative risk factor that leads to a 20-fold increase in complications across all age groups.[3] Screening spirometry can be performed to determine forced vital capacity and 1-minute forced end-expiratory volume. If abnormalities are found in the initial screening, preoperative intervention, including exercise and use of bronchodilators and incentive spirometer, is indicated.[3] A baseline arterial blood gas (ABG) measurement also should be obtained to identify hypoxemia or hypercapnia that may increase the risk of postoperative pulmonary complications.[3] This is a helpful algorithm for the evaluation of elderly surgical candidates to determine high-risk subgroups for postoperative complications.

Elderly surgical patients also are at increased risk of renal compromise in the perioperative period. The physiologic changes in renal function in these patients increase the susceptibility to renal ischemia perioperatively as well as to nephrotoxic agents. This functional decline with age is caused by glomerular damage and sclerosis leading to a decreased glomerular filtration rate (GFR). The GFR decreases by approximately 1 mL/min for every year over the age of 40.[11] The GFR for a healthy 80-year-old patient is one half to two thirds of the value at age 30 years.[11]

Acute renal failure is proven to dramatically increase morbidity and mortality in elderly patients. The mortality of perioperative acute renal failure is 50%, and may be even higher in elderly patients.[11] Therefore, careful management of fluid and electrolytes

Table 45-2

Summary of the Physiologic Changes that Accompany Aging, Their Clinical Consequences, and Interventions that Might Improve Surgical Outcomes in Elderly Patients

Age-Related Changes	Clinical Consequences	Best Practices
Body composition Significantly decreased muscle mass, accounting for much of decreased lean tissue mass Increased fat mass	Erosion of muscle mass during acute illness may result in strength rapidly falling below important clinical thresholds: e.g., impaired coughing, decreased mobility, increased risk of venous thrombosis Altered volumes of drug distribution	Maintain physical function through effective pain relief, avoiding tubes, drains, and other "restraints"; early mobilization and assistance with mobilization Minimize fasting, provide early nutritional supplementation of support (both protein-calorie and micronutrient) Adjust drug dosages for volume of distribution
Respiratory Decreased vital capacity Increased closing volume Decreased airway sensitivity and clearance Decreased partial pressure of oxygen	Less effective cough Predisposition to aspiration Increased closure of small airways during tidal respiration, especially postoperatively and when supine, leading to increased atelectasis and shunting Predisposition to hypoxemia	Provide early mobilization, assumption of upright rather than supine position Ensure effective pain relief to allow mobilization, deep breathing Provide routine supplemental oxygen in the immediate postoperative period, and then as needed Minimize use of nasogastric tubes
Cardiovascular Decreased maximal heart rate, cardiac output, ejection fraction Reliance on increased end-diastolic volume to increase cardiac output Slowed ventricular filling, increased reliance on atrial contribution Decreased baroreceptor sensitivity	Greater reliance on ventricular filling and increases in stroke volume (rather than ejection fraction) to achieve increases in cardiac output Intolerant of hypovolemia Intolerant of tachycardia, dysrhythmias, including atrial fibrillation	Use vigorous fluid resuscitation to achieve optimal ventricular filling Nonvasoconstricting inotropes and afterload reduction may be more effective, if pharmacologic support is required
Thermoregulation Diminished sensitivity to ambient temperature and less-efficient mechanisms of heat conservation, production, and dissipation Febrile responses to infection may be blunted in frail or malnourished elderly and those at extreme old age	Predisposition to hypothermia: e.g., decline in body temperature during surgery is more marked unless preventive measures are taken If there is hypothermia, shivering may result, associated with marked increases in oxygen consumption and cardiopulmonary demands Fever may be absent despite serious infections, especially in frail elderly	Use active measures to maintain normothermia during surgical procedures and to rewarm after trauma: warmed intravenous fluids, humidified gases, warm air Maintaining intraoperative normothermia reduces wound infections, adverse cardiac events, and length of hospital stay Be aware of hypothermia in trauma resuscitation
Renal function, fluid-electrolyte homeostasis Decreased sensitivity to fluid, electrolyte perturbations Decreased efficiency of solute, water conservation, and excretion Decreased renal mass, renal blood flow, and glomerular filtration rate Increased renal glucose threshold	Predisposition to hypovolemia Predisposition to electrolyte disorders, e.g., hyponatremia Predisposition to hyperglycemia Predisposition to hyperosmolar states	Pay meticulous attention to fluid and electrolyte management Recognize that a "normal" serum creatinine value reflects decreased creatinine clearance because muscle mass (i.e., creatinine production) is decreased concurrently Select drugs carefully: avoid those that may be nephrotoxic, e.g., aminoglycosides, or that adversely affect renal blood flow, e.g., nonsteroidal anti-inflammatory drugs Adjust drug dosages as appropriate for altered pharmacokinetics

SOURCE: Reproduced with permission from Watters JM: Surgery in the elderly. *Can J Surg* 45:106, 2002.

status is prudent to avoid imbalances and limit exposure to nephrotoxic diagnostic studies and medications in the perioperative management of elderly patients. Prompt recognition of renal compromise, marked by an elevation of blood urea nitrogen (BUN) or creatinine levels, or oliguria requires aggressive correction of underlying causes. Although not routinely advocated in younger patients, elderly patients should have routine electrolyte panels and a urinalysis prior to all surgical interventions to identify potential underlying renal dysfunction.[11] Underlying causes of abnormalities found on screening should be corrected prior to surgery, necessitating

intravascular volume repletion to ensure adequate renal perfusion perioperatively. Further aggressive evaluation, such as that with ultrasonography, is left to the discretion of the surgeon and is based on clinical evidence of renal dysfunction.

Preoperative assessment therefore should include the assessment and addressing of nutritional status, smoking cessation to minimize pulmonary complications, optimization of cardiac function with use of medications such as beta blockers, accurate assessment of hydration status, and an understanding of the cognitive awareness of the patient.

Table 45-3

Original and Modified Goldman's Criteria for Preoperative Assessment of the Elderly Surgical Patient to Determine Perioperative Risk of Cardiac Event

Original Goldman Classification	Points	Revised Goldman Classification	Points
Age >70 years	5	History of heart failure	1
Myocardial Infarction in previous 6 months	10	History of ischemic heart disease	1
Presence of S_3 gallop or jugular venous distention	11	History of cerebrovascular disease	1
Valvular aortic stenosis	3	Preoperative insulin therapy	1
ECG rhythm other than normal sinus	7	Preoperative serum creatinine >2 mg/dL	1
Presence of >5 PVCs/min any time prior to surgery	7	High-risk surgery	1
Poor general health status	3		
Intra-abdominal, intrathoracic, or aortic procedure	3		
Emergency surgery	4		
Total possible points:	53	Total possible points:	6

PVC = Premature ventricular centraction.

SOURCE: Adapted from Goldman L, et al: Multifactorial index of cardiac risk in noncardiac surgical procedures. *N Engl J Med* 297:845, 1977; and Lee TH, et al: Derivation and prospective validation of a simple index for prediction of cardiac risk of major noncardiac surgery. *Circulation* 100:1043, 1999.

SPECIFIC CONSIDERATIONS

Minimal Access Laparoscopic Surgery

The increasing experience with laparoscopic techniques, combined with minimized pain, decreased length of hospital stay, and low morbidity and mortality rates, has led to the increased use in minimal-access procedures among the elderly. It has expanded from cholecystectomies to more complex colon resections, gastrectomy, cardiac surgery, and esophagectomies.

Laparoscopic surgery reduces common postoperative complications such as decreased atelectasis, ileus, and wound infections. In elderly surgical patients, these complications easily progress to pneumonia, deep vein thrombosis (DVT), moderate metabolic and electrolyte disturbances, and even sepsis.[12] Decreased postoperative pain from smaller incisions leads to a faster return to a preoperative level of functioning including early ambulation, which decreases complications from prolonged bed rest such as DVT and pneumonia from poor pulmonary mechanics. The latter is especially important for elderly patients because deconditioning occurs with hospital stays, which depress their ability to return to appropriate functional status postoperatively.

Laparoscopic surgery also is appealing because of the reduction of inflammatory, hormonal, and metabolic stress imposed by major open surgical operations. This is ideal for elderly patients as compensation for the surgical challenges of reduced physiologic reserve and multiple comorbidities common to this population. However, these benefits must be balanced against the potential adverse effects of CO_2 insufflation and hemodynamic alterations induced by pneumoperitoneum and increased intra-abdominal pressure, which decreases venous return.[13] Therefore, decisions to perform minimal-access procedures in the elderly must be individualized to the patient, with careful consideration of the impact of comorbid conditions and the potential for poor cardiopulmonary reserves. This helps to provide the optimal circumstance for intervention with improved surgical outcomes.

The cardiopulmonary effects induced by pneumoperitoneum are secondary to carbon dioxide insufflation and the increased intra-abdominal pressure.[13] CO_2 insufflation is associated with hypercarbia and acidosis, both of which are proven direct myocardial depressants.[13] Hypercarbia becomes especially problematic in patients with pre-existing pulmonary disease with chronic carbon dioxide retention such as COPD. However, in patients without pre-existing disease, these alterations can be minimized with increased minute ventilation. The increase in intra-abdominal pressure during insufflation can lead to increased afterload, increased peripheral vascular resistance and mean systemic pressure, and decreased preload because of decreased venous return.[13] This can result in depressed myocardial function with a potentially serious consequence in an elderly patient with poor physiologic reserve.

It is important to maintain tight control over the intra-abdominal pressure applied during the laparoscopic procedure. For example, pressures up to 20 mm Hg are associated with increased filling pressures and cardiac output. However, increased elevations result in decreased central venous pressure and cardiac output, which potentially can be life-threatening in a patient with pre-existing cardiac dysfunction and poor functional reserve.

Although the occurrence of these serious consequences are rare, adequate preoperative knowledge of the physiologic changes induced by laparoscopic techniques, as well as the changes that occur with advancing age, lead to better control of the variables that can lead to adverse effects. Maintenance of adequate preload using appropriate preoperative and intraoperative volume control and careful mechanical ventilation to control hypercarbia and acidosis are basic concepts that allow safe application of minimally invasive techniques in the elderly. Invasive monitoring during the procedure is not usually needed, but can guide dynamic control of cardiac and pulmonary function in a patient with poor reserves, making laparoscopic techniques available to sicker patients with increased comorbidities.

Studies show that both advanced age greater than 70 years and an ASA classification of 3 or 4 are associated with higher conversion rates for laparoscopic cholecystectomy to open cholecystectomy.[14] These additional challenges, however, are not a contraindication to attempting the less-invasive approach because conversion to an open procedure does not adversely impact the overall morbidity and mortality of the patient.

A particularly valuable application of minimally invasive techniques in the elderly population is the evaluation of acute abdominal pain and to rule out a surgical abdomen. Vague, poorly localized pain with several confounding comorbid conditions that obscure the diagnosis, the risk of general anesthesia, and negative exploratory laparotomy would be life-threatening for an elderly, critically ill patient. Analysis of several studies directed at the application of laparoscopic techniques for the patient with acute abdominal pain demonstrated that approximately 41% had pathology necessitating open laparotomy, 10% had pathology amendable to laparoscopic intervention (e.g., acute cholecystitis), and 48% had nonsurgical disease that was subsequently managed nonoperatively, avoiding a negative exploration.[14] Therefore, laparoscopic evaluation of abdominal pain in the critically ill, elderly patient should be encouraged.

Endocrine Surgery

Breast Surgery

In the United States, breast cancer incidence continues to rise with advancing age; approximately two thirds of newly diagnosed breast cancer patients are age 55 years or older.[15] In addition, 77% of deaths caused by breast cancer occur in patients older than 55 years of age.[15] There also is an increase in mortality rates for each successive 5-year age group, with patients 85 years and older having the highest mortality rate, estimated at approximately 200 deaths per 100,000 population.[15] However, elderly patients have not been shown to present at later stages nor do they suffer increased morbidity and mortality after standard therapies. This finding advocates continued screening for early detection of operable lesions, as well as the use of aggressive therapy as indicated for younger counterparts with similar diagnosis, to reduce the morbidity and mortality from breast cancer in elderly patients.

A consensus on appropriate breast cancer screening guidelines in elderly patients does not exist. This is partly a result of a lack of clinical trials involving elderly women. Underutilization of screening mammography in elderly patients is evidenced by the fact that less than 30% of women older than 75 years of age are referred for a screening mammogram.[16] While studies have shown that physicians often no longer use mammography screening for patients older than 70 to 75 years of age, the American Cancer Society and the National Cancer Institute advise continuing annual mammography screening without respect to age. The American Geriatrics Society suggests that elderly women should have annual or biennial mammogram(s) until age 75 years, and at least every 3 years thereafter, with no age limit to screening in women with an estimated life expectancy of 4 years or more.[17] This is because current mammography is able to detect a tumor approximately 4 years prior to clinical presentation of a palpable lesion. For example, the life expectancy of an 85-year-old woman averages 6 to 7 years. Therefore, screening and early detection of breast cancer can provide appropriate therapy with possible improvement in survival rates and quality of life. Screening is not beneficial in select individuals whose life expectancy is limited by severe comorbid conditions that have led to functional limitations and are likely to progress, such as congestive heart failure, advanced oxygen- or steroid-dependent COPD, or diabetes with end-organ damage.

The estimated mortality for a patient 70 years of age or older undergoing a mastectomy is less than 1%. Elderly women should be offered, and typically prefer, breast-conserving surgery. It has been suggested that elderly women have a low rate of recurrence after lumpectomy, axillary dissection, and radiotherapy, making this a viable option. Radiation therapy is well tolerated by elderly women, with a minimal increase in morbidity and mortality, when added to breast-conserving procedures. Despite the success of this combination therapy, elderly women often do not receive radiation therapy; this is likely a result of reluctance by providers to refer them.

Routine axillary lymph node dissection with breast-conserving surgery remains controversial in elderly patients. There has been a trend toward providing adjuvant therapy with tamoxifen to patients with node-positive and node-negative disease, making axillary

lymph node dissection (ALND) unnecessary.[16] Furthermore, because ALND is associated with some morbidity, elderly women are considered at greater risk of chronic lymph edema and decreased shoulder mobility.[16] The latter can be worsened by comorbidities, including neurologic dysfunction and degenerative arthritis. In patients with clinically node-negative status, the axillary field also can be added to the radiation port to provide local control rates equivalent to those achieved with axillary dissection. However, ALND remains necessary in patients with clinically palpable axillary lymph nodes for adequate local control.

Elderly women with multiple comorbid conditions that lack the physiologic reserve to undergo the stress of surgical intervention should be offered conservative management with tamoxifen as the sole treatment. Adequate response rates have been observed and range from 10 to 50%, with failure rates ranging between 33 and 58%.[16] However, these patients require up to 12 months of therapy to achieve maximal responses and higher rates of local recurrence. While not a substitute for standard therapy in elderly women able to undergo definitive therapy, tamoxifen is a viable option for elderly women with a limited life expectancy, multiple comorbid conditions, and an increased risk for operative interventions.

Thyroid Surgery

The prevalence of thyroid disease increases with advancing age. The etiologies, risk factors, and presentations of thyroid disease are similar across all ages and, therefore, are not discussed in detail. Of note, however, is that elderly patients more often present with cardiac manifestations of hyperthyroidism such as atrial fibrillation than do their younger counterparts. A common finding requiring evaluation in elderly patients is the presence of a thyroid nodule, usually detected by physical examination. These nodules are usually single and four times more common in women, making them a particular concern for postmenopausal elderly women. Indications for surgical intervention for thyroid nodules are dependent on the characteristics of the nodule (i.e., whether it is benign or malignant, or whether the patient is euthyroid or thyrotoxic). In addition, surgical intervention becomes necessary if the nodule enlarges, producing compressive symptoms.

Papillary carcinoma in elderly patients tends to be sporadic with a bell-shape distribution of age at presentation, occurring primarily in patients age 30 to 59 years. The incidence of papillary carcinoma decreases in patients older than 60 years of age.[18] However, patients older than 60 years of age have increased risk of local recurrence and for the development of distant metastases. Metastatic disease may be more common in this population secondary to delayed referral for surgical intervention because of the misconception that the surgeon will be unwilling to operate on an elderly patient with thyroid disease. Age is also a prognostic indicator for patients with follicular carcinoma. There is a 2.2 times increased risk of mortality from follicular carcinoma per 20 years of increasing age.[19] Therefore, prognosis for elderly patients with differentiated thyroid carcinomas is worse when compared to younger counterparts. The higher prevalence of vascular invasion and extracapsular extension among older patients is in part responsible for the poorer prognosis in geriatric patients. Advancing age leads to increased mortality risk for patients with thyroid cancer and is demonstrated by the AMES (age, metastases, extent of primary tumor, and size of tumor) classification system developed by the Lahey Clinic (Table 45-4).

Anaplastic carcinoma is a highly aggressive form of thyroid carcinoma with dismal prognosis. It accounts for approximately 1% of all thyroid malignancies; however, it occurs primarily in elderly

Table 45-4
AMES Classification of Thyroid Cancers

		Low Mortality Risk	High Mortality Risk
A:	Age	Men: <41 years of age	Men: >41 years of age
		Women: <51 years of age	Women: >51 years of age
M:	Metastases	Absence of distant metastases	Presence of distant metastases
E:	Extent of primary tumor	Intrathyroidal papillary cancer (confined to thyroid)	Extrathyroidal papillary cancer
		Follicular cancer with minor capsular involvement	Follicular cancer with major capsular involvement
S:	Size of tumor	Primary tumor <5 cm in diameter	Primary tumor ≥5 cm in diameter (regardless of extent of disease)

Note: Older patients (men >41 years of age and women >51 years of age) one included in the low-risk group if tumors are less than 5 cm, intrathyroidal, or follicular with minor capsular involvement.

SOURCE: Adapted from Sanders LE, Cady B: Differentiated thyroid cancer. *Arch Surg* 133:419, 1998.

patients.[20] This poorly differentiated tumor rapidly invades local structures, leading to clinical deterioration and eventually tracheal obstruction. These patients may present with a painful, rapidly enlarging neck mass accompanied by dysphagia and cervical tenderness. This leads to respiratory compromise and impingement of the airway. Unfortunately, because of the aggressive nature of the disease and the dismal prognosis, surgical resection of the tumor is not attempted for cure. Furthermore, radiation therapy and chemotherapy offer little benefit. Airway blockage, however, may necessitate surgical palliation or permanent tracheostomy to alleviate symptoms of respiratory distress.

Parathyroid Surgery

Approximately 2% of the geriatric population, including 3% of women 75 years of age or older, will develop primary hyperparathyroidism.[21] Geriatric patients are usually referred to surgery only when advanced disease is present because of concerns regarding the risks of surgery, but low rates of morbidity and negligible mortality combined with high cure rates of approximately 95 to 98% make parathyroidectomy safe and effective.

Convincing evidence of the benefit of surgery is the usual marked symptomatic improvement, which greatly improves the quality of life for most patients. The National Institutes of Health Consensus Development Statement recommends curative therapy after diagnosis of primary hyperthyroidism is established in a patient regardless of age. Specific indications for operative intervention regardless of age include a 30% decrease in creatinine clearance, 24-hour urinary calcium excretion greater than 400 mg, and decreased bone density.[22,23]

Elderly patients are especially prone to developing mental manifestations of hyperparathyroidism that may be severe enough to produce a dementia-like state. There often is a significant improvement in mental status after parathyroidectomy. Another specific symptom of hyperparathyroidism that may easily be mistaken for osteoporosis and can be present in postmenopausal, elderly women is orthopedic disease, specifically back pain and possibly the occurrence of vertebral fractures. This pain can be of moderate intensity, leading to impaired mobility and severely affecting the quality of life of elderly patients. The decreased bone density observed in elderly patients with hyperparathyroidism tends to improve during the first 2 years after successful parathyroid surgery.

Limited parathyroidectomies with minimal dissection in geriatric patients are an effective alternative. This is a viable option in patients with multiple comorbid conditions in whom the increased risk of surgical intervention or general anesthesia remains a concern. One study demonstrated that preoperative localization of the hyperfunctioning gland with the aid of ^{99m}Tc-sestamibi nuclear scanning, as well as intraoperative parathyroid hormone (PTH) assays to rapidly confirm that all hypersecreting glands have been removed, allows limited parathyroidectomy to be performed with accuracy in elderly patients (Fig. 45-1).[21] This procedure is described as "limited" because bilateral neck dissection for identification and biopsy of the remaining glands in order to determine if they are hypersecreting becomes unnecessary. The half-life of intact PTH is approximately 3 to 4 minutes. Therefore, a drop in the intraoperative PTH level at approximately 10 minutes after resection of the suspect hypersecreting gland suggests a 98% probability that the patient will return to normocalcemic levels postoperatively.[21]

Cardiothoracic Surgery

Coronary Artery Bypass Grafting

There has been a significant trend in providing definitive operative intervention to elderly patients requiring coronary artery bypass grafting (CABG). Although older patients have higher morbidity and mortality rates after cardiac surgery than do younger patients, these rates are decreasing significantly over time.[24] This decline in morbidity and mortality rates among elderly patients undergoing cardiac surgery reflects better preoperative assessment and patient selection. This decline has occurred despite the advancing age of cardiac patients at time of referral, advanced disease, and greater comorbid disease burden, which are particularly present in elderly patients with COPD, cerebrovascular disease, and renal dysfunction. Elderly patients are more likely to have significant triple-vessel disease accompanied by poor ejection fraction, left ventricular hypertrophy, significant valvular disease, and previous history of myocardial infarction than are younger patients.[24] Elderly patients also are more likely to be classified as New York Heart Association (NYHA) functional class III or higher and are more likely to present on an emergent basis, in part because of a reluctance to provide elective intervention in these patients because of the presumptive poorer outcome. Despite the increased risk of morbidity and mortality compared to younger patients, elderly patients, including those older than age 80 years, can undergo CABG with acceptable mortality risk. The overall mortality rate is approximately 7 to 12% for elderly

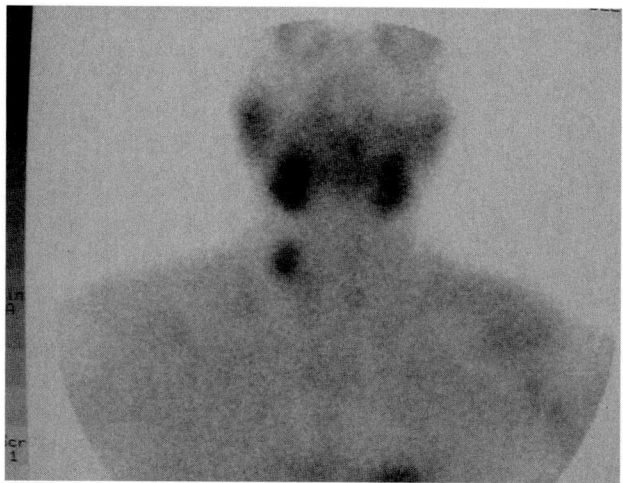

A

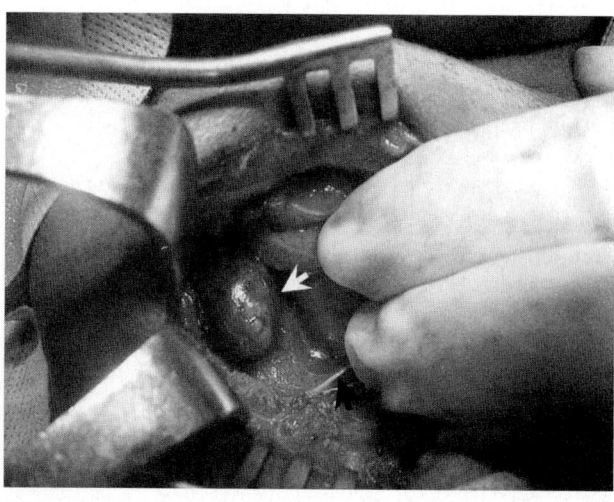

B

FIG. 45-1. Parathyroid adenoma in an elderly patient with high calcium levels and elevated parathyroid hormone levels. Sestamibi scan showed right-upper-gland adenoma facilitating a directed incision. A 1-g pituitary adenoma was easily identified intraoperatively (*white arrow*). *Black arrow* points to the recurrent laryngeal nerve.

patients, including cases performed under emergency conditions. This figure decreases to approximately 2.8% when CABG is performed electively with careful preoperative evaluation.[25]

Valve Replacement

There also is an increasing percentage of the geriatric population presenting with symptomatic valvular disease requiring intervention. The most common valvular abnormality present in elderly patients is calcific aortic stenosis, which can lead to angina and syncope (Fig. 45-2).[24] The operative mortality from aortic valve replacement is estimated to be between 3 and 10%, with an average of approximately 7.7%.[26] If aortic stenosis is allowed to progress without operative intervention, congestive heart failure will ensue. The average survival of these patients is approximately 1.5 to 2 years. If a patient is a candidate for operative intervention, age should not be a deterrent, especially considering the potential to increase life expectancy. Furthermore, there is a demonstrable improvement in quality of life in these patients, with many improving their NYHA functional classification.

Elderly patients require surgery for mitral valve disease when ischemic regurgitation is present. Surgery for mitral valve disease carries a higher morbidity and mortality than for aortic intervention, with an estimated mortality rate as high as 20%.[26] Left ventricular function is usually compromised in patients requiring intervention, leading to a poorer outcome in these patients. The surgical outcome for mitral valve procedures depends on the extent of the disease, age of the patient, presence of pulmonary hypertension, and extent of coronary artery disease. The presence of comorbid conditions combined with the emergent nature of surgery in a large percentage of elderly patients further worsens the outcome. Therefore, a decision regarding management of mitral valve disease should be individualized to each patient with the above factors considered.

Another concern regarding elderly patients who require surgery for valve disease is the additional requirement for coronary revascularization. This increases the morbidity and mortality from surgical intervention. An elderly patient with many comorbid conditions in need of a combined procedure should only have critically

stenosed vessels bypassed.[24] Therefore, advanced age is not a contraindication to performing combined procedures; however, a higher mortality rate should be expected.

Neurologic complications from valve surgery are particularly common in elderly patients. It has been estimated that approximately 30% of patients older than age 70 years who undergo valve procedures develop either transient or permanent neurologic dysfunction.[24] This often is a result of embolism from debris dislodged from the valve during the procedure or from a formed thrombus in the right atrium.

An important consideration in valve replacement procedures in elderly patients is the type of prosthesis to be used. Elderly patients are at increased risk from bleeding-associated anticoagulation complications. This is especially significant in patients who have experienced falls and minor trauma that have resulted in significant intracranial hemorrhage. To avoid the life-long requirement for anticoagulants, bioprosthetic valves should be used in place of mechanical valves whenever possible.[24] Although the bioprosthetic valves are not as durable as mechanical valves, studies demonstrate excellent structural integrity 10 years postprocedure, making it an appropriate choice in an elderly patient.

Trauma

Geriatric patients older than 65 years of age currently account for approximately 23% of total hospital trauma admissions—many of which are multisystem and life-threatening.[27] This percentage is expected to rise to as high as 40%, making this a growing concern for potential long-term morbidity, mortality, rehabilitation, and cost. Trauma is the sixth most common cause of death in patients 65 to 74 years of age.[28] Elderly patients are particularly susceptible to trauma because of changes that occur with aging, such as gait instability, decreased hearing and visual acuity, presence of confusion and dementia, or underlying disease such as Parkinson's disease. The presence of pre-existing comorbid conditions increases the odds of an elderly patient experiencing a complication by a factor of three.[27] This is worsened when combined with an elderly patient's decreased functional reserve to handle physiologic abnormalities

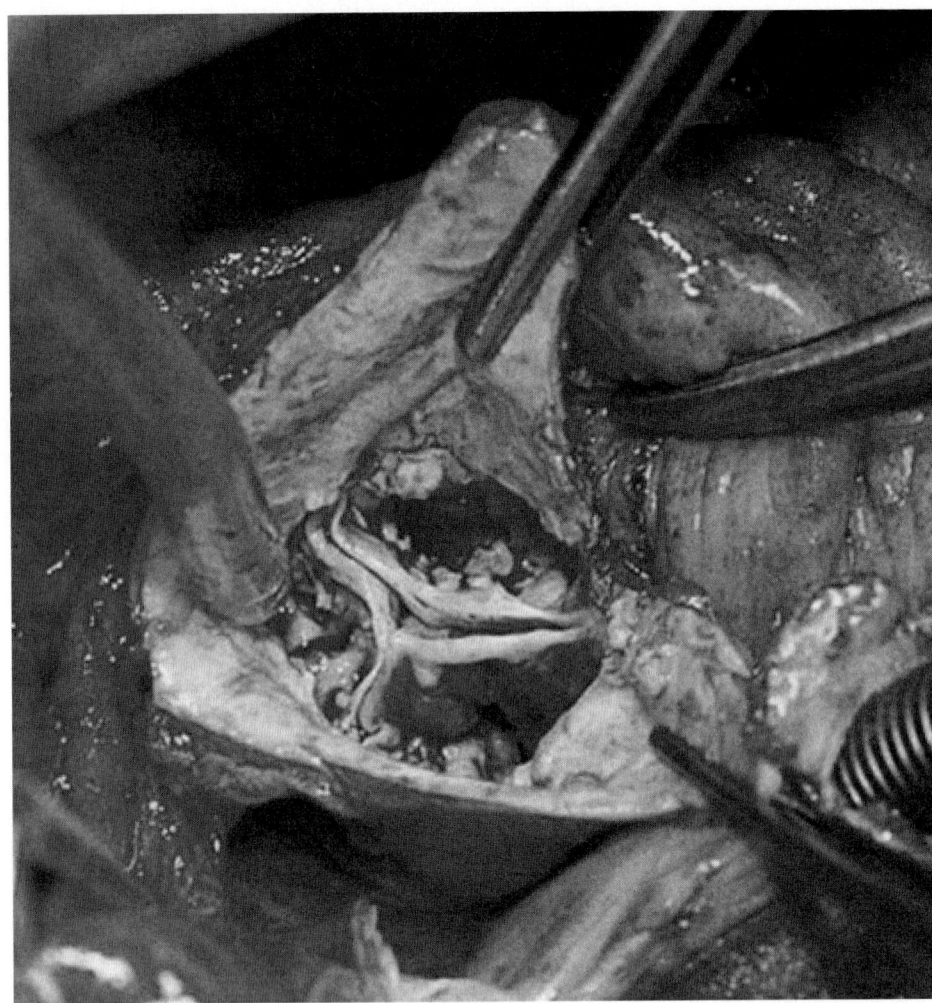

FIG. 45-2. Intraoperative photograph of aortic annulus of an elderly patient with moderate aortic calcific stenosis as seen during the replacement with a bioprosthetic aortic valve. Calcific deposits about the valvular cusps are readily apparent. (*Courtesy of Robert C. Lowery, M.D.*)

accompanying major trauma as in cases of hypotension and hypoxia. These comorbid conditions must be taken into consideration early in the management of elderly patients because of their impact on mortality.

Traditional injury scoring systems, such as the Injury Severity Score (ISS), are less predictive of mortality in elderly patients. Although patient age is factored into calculating the Trauma and Injury Severity Score (TRISS), the presence of comorbid conditions is neglected, making it less accurate in the evaluation of an elderly patient. Elderly patients may have mortality rates twice those of younger patients with similar injury severity. The most common cause of death is multiple-organ failure combined with sepsis.[29] This poor prognosis worsens with advancing age, with octogenarians having higher mortality rates than younger geriatric patients with similar injuries.

It is crucial to determine the medication regimen of elderly trauma patients. Medication such as beta blockers, calcium channel blockers, diuretics, and afterload reducers may impair augmentation of myocardial function in trauma patients, especially if they are hypovolemic. However, a definitive consensus on early invasive hemodynamic monitoring is lacking, and such decisions must be tailored individually to the elderly trauma patient.

Not only are older patients at increased risk of death from trauma, there is also an increased occurrence of delayed death when compared to younger patients. Pre-existing cardiovascular or liver disease and the development of cardiac, renal, or infectious complications are independent predictors of delayed mortality. One study suggested that elderly trauma patients were at increased risk of death for up to 5 years after the initial trauma.[29]

The most common mechanism for injuries in the elderly is from falls, which account for approximately 20% of severe injuries. Many underlying chronic and acute diseases common to elderly patients place them at increased risk for falls. These diseases include postural hypotension leading to syncopal "drop attacks," dysrhythmia from sick sinus syndrome, autonomic dysfunction from polypharmacy with improper dosage of antihypertensive or oral hypoglycemic agents resulting in hypotension, and hypoglycemia.[30]

Blunt thoracic trauma accounts for approximately 25% of all trauma deaths in North America.[31] Rib fractures occur in up to two thirds of all cases of chest trauma and are associated with pulmonary complications in approximately 35% of cases.[31] More than 50% of patients older than age 65 years sustain rib fractures from falls from less than 6 feet, which includes falls from the standing position.[32] In contrast, 1% of younger patients sustain rib fractures from similar mechanism and severity of injury. This injury in particular leads to morbidity and mortality for elderly patients as a consequence of the increased risk of development of pulmonary contusions and subsequent pneumonia, the latter of which occurs in 27% of older patients, as compared to 13% of younger patients.[31]

In addition to higher mortality, elderly patients suffer from poorer functional recovery from trauma despite survival of injury, with approximately 20 to 25% of patients requiring discharge to a skilled nursing facility for long-term care and rehabilitation.[27] In one study, poorer functional outcome was attributed to certain factors including presence of shock on admission, age greater than 75 years, severe head injury, and development of infectious complications.[33]

Transplantation

A new trend provides elderly patients with an increasing opportunity for organ donation and receipt, which increases the pool of potential organ donors. According to the United Network of Organ Sharing (UNOS) data, the percentage of elderly organ donors increased from 2 to 24% between 1982 and 1995. In 1997, 44% of cadaveric renal transplant donors were older than 50 years of age.[34] This trend is expected to increase given the expanding elderly population in the United States.

In the 1970s, experience with kidney transplantation in older patients was associated with poor prognosis. It was estimated that the 1-year patient and graft survival rates for patients older than age 45 years was 40 and 20%, respectively.[35] This was thought to be a result of the decline in renal function and changes within the kidney as a result of damage from the aging process. It was therefore adopted that cadaveric transplants were not to be given to patients older than 45 years of age. However, advancements in immunosuppression have significantly improved quality of life off dialysis and have improved survival in this population. The significance of better survival outcomes in older patients receiving transplantation today is that elderly patients have the potential for prolonged life expectancy. Kidney transplantation extends patient survival and improves quality of life, allowing greater functional autonomy compared to patients on long-term dialysis. The importance of this advancement is evident in the fact that in 2000, approximately 60% of end-stage renal disease (ESRD) patients were older than 65 years of age, and approximately 50% of newly diagnosed patients with ESRD belong to older age cohorts.[35]

Elderly patients have better graft function, with decreased incidence of delayed graft function and fewer episodes of acute rejection, than do younger patients.[36] This may be the result of decreased immune competence with aging. With the lower occurrence of both acute and chronic rejection in elderly patients, it has been suggested that elderly patients would benefit from lower doses of immunosuppressive agents. However, this decreased competence is balanced by the increased incidence of infections from viruses such as herpes, cytomegalovirus (CMV), and Epstein-Barr, as well as posttransplant neoplasia, including lymphoproliferative disorders.

The adoption of dual-kidney donation from elderly patients with depressed innate kidney function expanded the donor population to more than 75 years of age; greater than 15% of whom were glomerulosclerotic.[37] The increased nephron mass achieved with dual-kidney transplantation compensated for the possible declining renal function with advanced age. The net result is that recipients receive similar postoperative graft function when compared to single-kidney transplantation. Dual-kidney transplant recipients have comparable serum creatinine levels and similar posttransplant creatine clearance as those of single-kidney recipients.[34]

An expanding elderly population has emerged that requires liver transplantation, which has led to a reassessment of previous age limitations for organ donation and transplantation. The leading cause of liver failure in elderly patients requiring liver transplantation is primary biliary cirrhosis. Other causes include primary sclerosing cholangitis, alcoholic liver disease, cryptogenic cirrhosis, and hepatitis B and C infections.[38] The age limit previously established by clinical practice was approximately 50 years of age; however, it is rising.[39] In 1990, 3.4% of cadaveric liver allograft recipients were older than 65 years of age. This figure rose to 7.2% in 2001.[38] Survival rates in these patients are comparable to those of younger patients. UNOS Scientific Registry data demonstrated 1-, 3-, and 5-year survival rates for patients older than 65 years of age who underwent liver transplantation to be 80%, 70%, and 60%, respectively. This is comparable to 88%, 78%, and 73% in patients aged 35 to 64 years.[38]

PALLIATIVE SURGERY

Palliative surgery is defined as surgical intervention targeted to alleviate a patient's symptoms, thus improving the patient's quality of life despite minimal impact on the patient's survival.[40]

With an increasing number of aging surgical patients who often present with advanced disease, surgeons must be familiar with the concept of palliation to control disease. This concept focuses on providing the maximal benefit to the patient using the least-invasive intervention. Ultimately, this leads to symptom relief and preservation of the quality of life in terminal disease states. The uses of palliative surgery can range from extensive debulking operations aimed at aiding in the effectiveness of chemotherapy and radiation, to less-complex operations to alleviate symptoms such as intractable vomiting, severe pain, cachexia, and anorexia that are common to terminal disease states. The success of palliative surgery is a careful balance between achieving symptom relief while ensuring that the development of new symptoms from the palliative intervention itself does not occur.

Palliative care in the treatment of advanced disease often is associated with age bias; young patients are withheld from it, while older ones are more prone to be offered palliative care. In a recent survey, two surgical scenarios were presented to a panel of surgeons.[41] The first patient was an 85-year-old woman with excellent functional status presenting for evaluation of back pain, jaundice, weight loss, and vomiting. Appropriate studies were completed with CT scan that demonstrated a mass in the head of the pancreas with invasion into the portal vein. The patient in the second scenario experienced identical symptoms, but was significantly younger. Most of the surgeons selected major surgical intervention for the younger patient, while only one-third of the panel offered the same intervention for the older patient. The majority offered only palliative care for the older patient. It is important to note that those surgeons who offered operative intervention based their decision on the functional status of the patient preoperatively. When transitioning from curative therapy to palliation, the risks and benefits of the proposed surgical intervention should be examined, as well as the intended impact to the patient's quality of life.

There currently is no evidence to support that palliative surgery is less effective for elderly patients with surgically unresectable disease. Younger patients undergoing palliative interventions do not have a demonstrated improved outcome when compared to disease-matched older patients. Therefore, it is important to recognize that age is not a limitation to surgical intervention and that all interventions should be individualized based on the severity of symptoms and the predicted benefit.

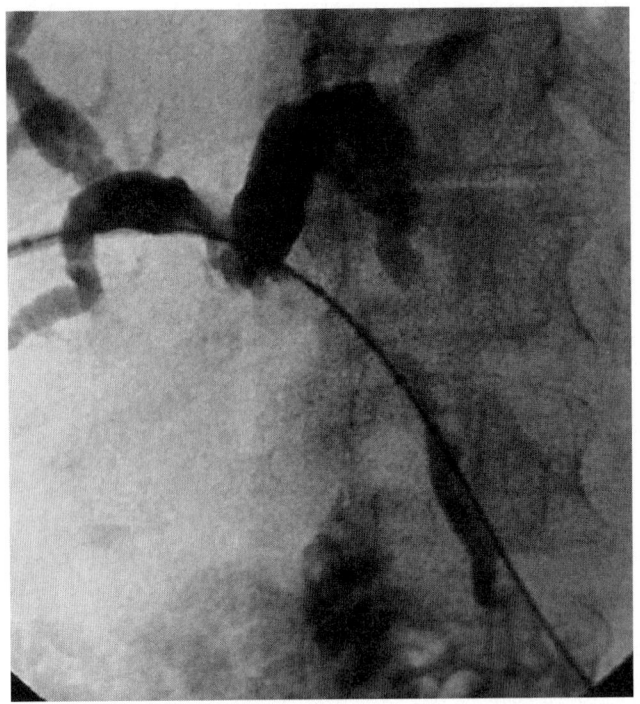

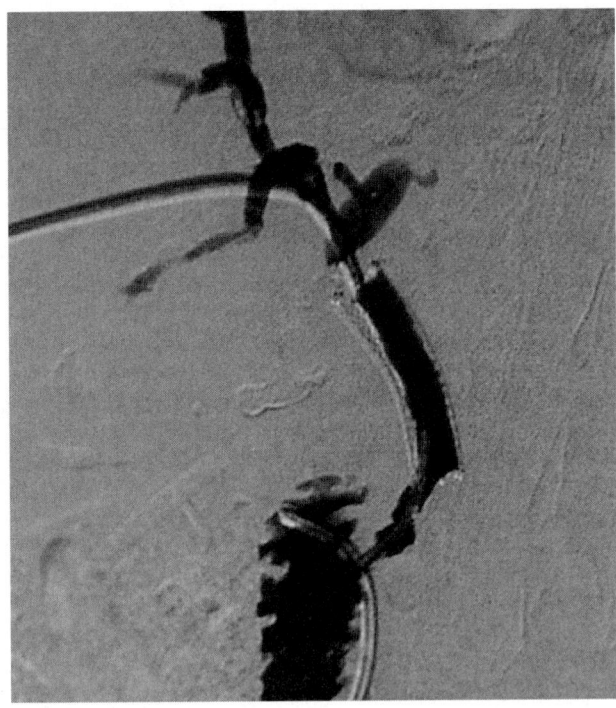

A

B

FIG. 45-3. Palliative care in an 82-year-old woman with obstructive jaundice from unresectable cholangiocarcinoma. CT scan showed metastatic disease to the liver. *A.* A percutaneous drainage of the biliary system with a stent placed across the obstruction from the hilum to the distal common bile duct. *B.* Two days later, a covered permanent metallic wall stent was placed across the obstruction.

Surgical palliative care can range from nonoperative management of malignant obstructions by percutaneous methods (Fig. 45-3) to laparoscopic surgery for the treatment of life-threatening illness by minimally invasive technique (Fig. 45-4). An interesting challenge in palliative care is the determination of the actual cause of a patient's symptoms in order to offer the most beneficial, but least invasive, intervention. Treatment of malignant pleural effusions, for example, should be tailored to the source of the symptoms, not the effusion. Effusions should be treated only when they cause significant distress for patients with terminal disease.[41] Dyspnea in a terminal patient can be the result of chest wall restriction, pulmonary fibrosis from previous radiation treatment, infiltration of the primary cancer, or early airway obstruction from mediastinal spread of the primary tumor.[41] If it is determined that a patient's dyspnea is largely secondary to a malignant pleural effusion, the goal of palliative intervention is lung expansion, preferably with permanent pleurodesis. Permanent control can be achieved via thoracoscopy or by more invasive thoracotomy with chemical pleurodesis.[41] The latter intervention is highly effective for permanent resolution and therefore may be more invasive than necessary for patients with late-stage terminal disease. In these patients, medical pleurodesis with intrapleural injection of a sclerosant via thoracostomy tube placement is a better alternative.[41] For surgical therapy, minimally invasive procedures such as video-assisted thoracoscopy (VATS) may be an appropriate method to assess the apposition of pleural surfaces and may allow for talc pleurodesis or insertion of a pleuroperitoneal shunt.[41]

Palliative intervention for symptom relief and prevention of complications can be demonstrated in the management of terminal pancreatic cancer and metastatic colorectal cancer. Two thirds of patients with pancreatic cancer present with advanced disease,

which is often diagnosed after evaluation of obstructive jaundice. Despite advanced disease, surgical intervention improves quality of life through relief of biliary obstruction. Percutaneous transhepatic stenting has emerged as a viable alternative to surgical bypass, achieving similar results and lowering mortality rates with the occurrence of fewer early complications. Endoscopic stenting is yet another option. If a patient does not have multiple comorbidities with good functional status, surgical intervention then can provide a definitive diagnosis and permanent biliary decompression and gastric drainage. In addition, an important palliative intervention that can be provided to patients with the open procedure is chemical splanchnicectomy, which is infiltration of the celiac plexus with an agent such as alcohol for effective relief of intractable pain from tumor invasion of the celiac plexus.[41] A gastroenterostomy drainage procedure is effective protection against gastric outlet obstruction, which inevitably develops in 30% of patients.

Palliative surgery for disseminated colorectal cancer should be aimed at the reduction of symptoms such as pain, obstruction, or hemorrhage. Bowel obstruction can be relieved with intestinal bypass or a diverting colostomy. The most common site of disseminated disease is the liver, and uncontrolled liver metastasis is responsible for pain, abdominal distention, jaundice, and inferior vena caval obstruction. Many patients with liver metastasis are not candidates for resection and therefore may be considered for ablation of the lesions by local destruction, cryotherapy, or radiofrequency ablation. More traditional means, such as chemotherapy, which can be administered via the hepatic artery, or radiation, also may be employed. Systemic corticosteroid therapy can be used in patients with advanced metastatic disease to reduce pain caused by swelling of the liver capsule. If bone metastases are present,

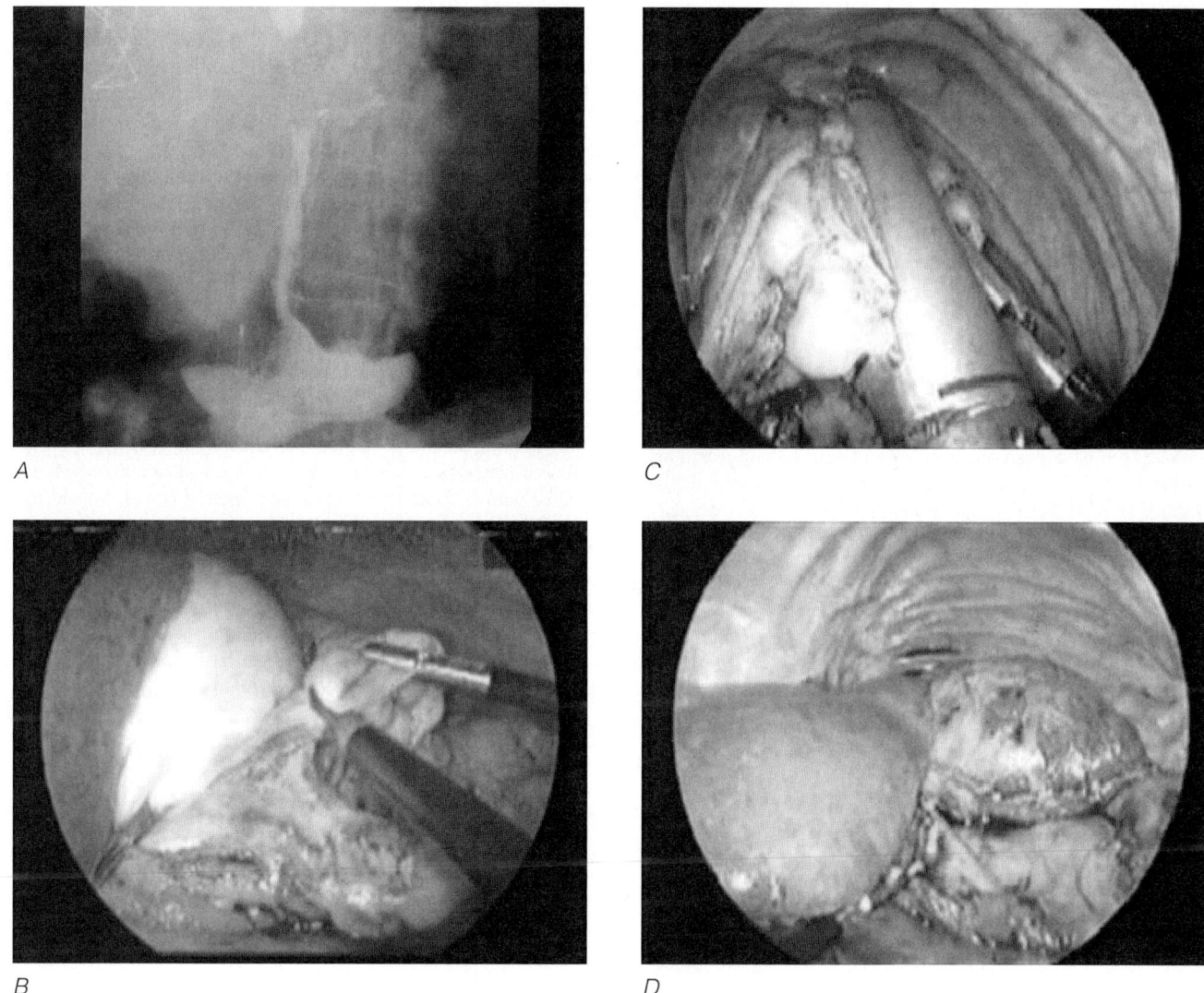

FIG. 45-4. An 85-year-old male with dementia presenting with a bleeding gastrointestinal stromal tumor in the fundus of the stomach, treated with laparoscopic gastrectomy. *A.* The upper gastrointestinal series delineating the tumor. *B.* Laparoscopic division of short gastric artery with Harmonic Scalpel. *C.* Division of stomach with endo-GIA stapler. *D.* Resection of the mass prior to removal from abdomen via an endo-bag.

pain may be controlled by irradiation, and prophylactic fixation of long bones may be considered to decrease pain as well as morbidity from pathologic fractures.[41] Similarly, cerebral irradiation and high-dose steroid therapy may help to decrease intracranial pressure from metastatic disease, as well as delay the onset of neurologic symptoms and cognitive impairment, which are essential to maintain quality of life of the patient.[41]

Specific Symptom Management

Gastrointestinal Disturbances

The distressing symptoms often faced by terminally ill patients either result from the disease process or as a side effect of treatment. The causes of nausea and vomiting in terminally ill patients are multifactorial and can be attributed to various medications or chemotherapy treatments, gastric stasis, obstruction of the gastrointestinal tract, mesenteric metastases, irritation of the GI tract, raised intracranial pressure from cerebral metastasis, or anxiety-induced emesis. Treatment should be focused on prevention of dehydration

and malnutrition from poor oral intake. Antiemetics may be administered for control of nausea and vomiting. The oral route of administration is the best option for prophylaxis prior to chemotherapy treatments. However, other preparations, such as suppositories or injections, can be appropriate for patients who are unable to tolerate oral medications.

Diarrhea and constipation also are common GI disturbances in terminal patients. Constipation is particularly common in patients receiving chronic narcotic medications. Constipation also can be caused by such events as tumor invasion leading to intestinal obstruction, metabolic abnormalities such as hypercalcemia from metastatic disease, and dehydration. Because constipation may be worsened by dehydration, adequate fluid intake often helps to alleviate symptoms. Constipation can lead to fecal impaction, nausea, and colicky abdominal pain. If there is difficulty distinguishing between constipation and early bowel obstruction, diagnostic tests are useful, but should be kept to a minimum in terminal patients. Patients can be treated with stool softeners and stimulant agents. Laxatives with peristalsis-stimulating action such as senna or bisacodyl should be used with caution because of the potential for causing intestinal colic.

The occurrence of diarrhea also is multifactorial and can be caused by medications, overload incontinence with fecal impaction, from the disease process itself, malignant bowel obstruction, or improper laxative therapy. Radiation therapy can cause diarrhea by damage of the intestinal mucosa, which results in the release of prostaglandins and the malabsorption of bile salts that increases peristalsis. Once the underlying causes are identified and appropriately managed, patients can be given bulk-forming agents and opiate derivatives to aid in symptomatic improvement.

Depression and Asthenia

Asthenia is a condition of reduced energy levels accompanied by fatigue and generalized weakness without the presence of physical or mental exertion.[42] In a study by Hinshaw and associates, asthenia was present in approximately 90% of patients and was more prevalent than pain, leading to the potential for impaired quality of life.[42] Both of these symptoms commonly affect the terminally ill patient. However, if identified, appropriate interventions can be provided in an effort to improve quality of life and enhance the patient's functional status. In cancer patients, overactivity of the hypothalamic–pituitary–adrenal axis and elevation of interleukin-6 levels have been reported in patients suffering with depression. Natural killer cell activity has been demonstrated to decline in patients with depression, causing an immunosuppressive effect and weakening the patient's response to tumor.[42] Poorly controlled pain and complications from disease progression also can cause terminal patients to develop depression. These complications include somnolence and depression that can occur with hypercalcemia from bony metastases with lung and breast cancer. These must be controlled as much as possible prior to the consideration of pharmacologic therapy to alleviate symptoms of depression.

Appropriate therapy for depression and asthenia must be individualized. If a patient has good functional status with a predicted survival time of several months, the initiation of standard antidepressants is appropriate. However, if there is an expected short survival period with progression of depressive symptoms impairing quality of life, then a psychostimulant is more appropriate because of its immediate effect, better short-term efficacy, and the tendency for development of tolerance, usually within 3 months.[42] Psychostimulants such as amphetamine and methylphenidate also increase appetite at lower doses and help to reduce sedation that may result from treatment with narcotic medications for pain management.[42] Psychostimulants also are effective in the management of asthenia, which shares a common clinical presentation with depression. However, pharmacologic therapy for asthenia should be provided only after treatable causes of this symptom, such as medications (including narcotics), the presence of pain, anemia, dehydration, and infection, as well as metabolic abnormalities, such as hyponatremia, hypokalemia, and hypercalcemia, have been assessed and corrected.[42]

Cachexia and Anorexia

Cachexia refers to catabolic changes associated with progressive wasting that is present in patients with advanced illness; prominent symptoms include anorexia, weight loss, and asthenia.[43] A subsequent loss of muscle and fat leading to anemia, hypoalbuminemia, and hypoproteinemia also is common. This is a chronic form of malnutrition and is not reversible with short-term nutritional support and

hyperalimentation.[43] Malnourished cancer patients with cachexia have reduced response to antineoplastic medications, radiation, and chemotherapy, as well as decreased survival rates.[41] The mechanism of cachexia is poorly understood, but hypotheses include actions of interleukin-6, tumor necrosis factor, and interferon-mediating metabolic changes in chronic illness.[43]

Management of cachexia begins with the identification of correctable causes. Patients may have underlying metabolic derangements, as well as dehydration, that must be appropriately treated. Poorly controlled pain, anemia, and sleep disturbances also may exacerbate symptoms of cachexia, leading to malnutrition and wasting. Patients with terminal disease additionally often suffer from gastrointestinal disturbances, such as constipation and nausea, which may lead to anorexia. Malabsorption is common in patients with pancreatic cancer, and supplementation of pancreatic enzymes may improve absorption and help to improve nutritional status. Nausea and vomiting should be appropriately managed. It is important to rule out mechanical causes of malnutrition that can effectively be treated with nonoperative management such as bowel rest and nasogastric tube compression or operative intervention.

If no underlying correctable abnormalities are identified, patients may benefit from pharmacologic intervention with dexamethasone and prednisone, which increase appetites in patients with advanced cancer, leading to improved quality of life.[43] The onset of effect is rapid but short-lived and thus should be reserved for patients at terminal stages of disease. Other agents, such as progestational drugs, namely megestrol acetate (Megace), also stimulate appetite and cause weight gain in cachexia patients.[43]

Malignant Bowel Obstruction

Patients with malignant bowel obstruction typically present with cramping abdominal pain, nausea, and vomiting, which may be a common complication of advanced terminal disease secondary to gastrointestinal malignancy or from extrinsic compression of bowel loops from progressive tumor burden. Conservative management can be effective and includes NPO, intravenous hydration, and nasogastric decompression. However, long-term management often is difficult. Medical management with pharmacologic agents such as somatostatin analogues to decrease gastrointestinal output may also be considered for symptom alleviation along with analgesics and antiemetics. Octreotide effectively decreases the volume of gastrointestinal secretions via inhibition of intestinal hormones and growth hormone and is 70% effective in patients suffering with bowel obstruction with the added effect of decreasing colic and nausea.[43] However, surgical palliation via bypass procedures, decompressing, or diverting ostomies may be required.

Surgical intervention may provide permanent alleviation of obstruction and eliminate the need for repeated nasogastric decompressions that can limit patient comfort. In one study, approximately 40 to 70% of patients reported relief of symptoms of obstruction after surgical intervention.[43] This must be balanced against the risk of perioperative mortality from surgical intervention, which ranges from approximately 12 to 20%, as well as the potential for mortality from wound infection, poor wound healing, and fistula formation.[43] Patients in whom the risk of surgical intervention outweighs the benefit of palliation include patients who have ascites or multiple sites of obstruction accompanied by poor functional status and poor nutrition with serum albumin levels less than 3 g/dL.[43] Should conservative management fail in a patient who is unfit to undergo surgical intervention, alternatives include a venting gastrostomy or jejunostomy, which can be inserted percutaneously.[41]

Pain Management

Intractable pain is one of the most distressing symptoms affecting a terminally ill patient. Nociceptive pain can be categorized as somatic, visceral, or deafferentation pain.[44,45] *Visceral pain* frequently is secondary to tumor involvement of sympathetically innervated organs by either direct invasion or compression that leads to stretching or distention of the affected viscera. Typical examples are metastatic invasion of organs such as with distention of the liver capsule by tumor or pain that occurs with pancreatic cancer from invasion of nerve roots or plexus. This pain is typically poorly localized and difficult to describe. *Somatic pain* results from the activation of somatic nociceptors and is typically well localized and constant. A common example is bone metastasis. *Deafferentation pain,* also known as neuropathic pain, results from injury to the nervous system from tumor compression or infiltration. This pain is often severe and leads to functional impairment such as that which occurs with invasion of the lumbosacral or brachial plexus.

Drugs that are commonly used in pain management are nonopioid compounds such as acetaminophen and nonsteroidal compounds.[43] These drugs often can be combined with opioids to improve analgesia. Opioids are the other class of familiar drugs useful in pain management and include codeine or stronger agents such as morphine, oxycodone, methadone, hydromorphone (Dilaudid), and fentanyl. Adjuvant agents such as corticosteroids, antidepressants, muscle relaxants, and certain anticonvulsants may be used in combination with opioid and nonopioid compounds for synergistic effects. The initial assessment of the patient should attempt to assess the pain in regard to severity, alleviating/aggravating factors, and other qualitative features often used to describe pain. The best therapy for the individual patient then should be determined. It is important to keep patient comfort in mind and to address comorbid conditions that will affect treatment. For example, dysphagia leads to difficulty in swallowing, making oral medications either painful or impossible; diaphoresis may alter the effect of transdermal patches because of an inability to stay in place; and muscle wasting and cachexia will make intramuscular and subcutaneous routes of administration extremely painful. If a patient is vomiting or has had profuse diarrhea, oral and rectal medications are inappropriate. The most common method to administer medications is the oral route, but buccal and sublingual approaches to medication administration are particularly useful in patients who suffer with dysphagia.[43] Liquid forms are easier as well. Intravenous administration, as well as other, more intrusive methods of drug administration, also can be employed.

For most postoperative pain regimens, medications have been dosed on an as-needed basis. However, terminal patients with chronic, constant, debilitating pain require more regimental administration with around-the-clock dosing, sustained-release medications, or immediate-release medications used for breakthrough pain management. A useful method currently employed for pain management is the use of long-acting narcotics with extended analgesic effect. Transdermal fentanyl (Duragesic) patches that reduce the requirement for frequent dosing with excellent control of pain are particularly helpful in chronic pain management. One patch may be applied every 72 hours, but frequency can be increased to every 48 hours for more severe, chronic pain.

Medication dosing should constantly be evaluated and adjusted according to the patient's pain scale. On the typical scale of 1 to 10 in increasing severity, if a patient rates pain between 3 and 6 despite the current regimen, then dosages should be increased by 25 to 50%; if a patient rates pain between 7 and 10, dosages may be increased by 50 to 100%.[43]

Nonsteroidal, anti-inflammatory drugs (NSAIDs) are effective in managing mild to moderate somatic pain and pain associated with inflammation. NSAIDs such as aspirin, ibuprofen, and naproxen, as well as acetaminophen, are particularly effective for managing pain from bony metastases. These medications do have a "ceiling effect," meaning the drug ceases to provide analgesia above a certain dosage.[46] These drugs also should be used with caution in elderly populations because of the potential to cause delirium as well as other toxic side effects, such as gastrointestinal bleeding and renal failure. Opioids such as codeine can be added to NSAIDs for an increased analgesic effect. If pain remains poorly controlled, stronger opioids, such as morphine, hydromorphone, and fentanyl, can be administered.

Short-acting medications, such as Demerol, which has a half-life of approximately 2.5 to 3 hours, should be avoided in the management of chronic pain.[43] Demerol, for example, does not have many administration options and is given only by injection because it is ineffective by oral administration. Furthermore, it has toxic intermediates that lead to central nervous system toxicity resulting in tremors, confusion, or seizure activity. These intermediates may also lower the threshold for seizure activity.[43]

Many side effects can occur with administration of pain medications on a chronic basis, the most common being gastrointestinal symptoms. For example, the most common side effect of opioid administration is constipation, secondary to decreased peristaltic activity and increased absorption.[43] Consequently, all patients who are administered opioids also should be placed on a stool softener to avoid constipation. It is important to note that some patients may require an increase in their pain medication regimen at particular times, such as prior to aggressive wound care or during transport.

Respiratory depression is often a concern when prescribing high doses of opioids. This is far less common in patients who have been on a constant regimen of opioid compounds for more than 36 hours.[43] Tolerance to the respiratory-depressant effect of opioids develops within 36 hours of administration, leading to relatively safe administration in terminally ill patients.[43] Addiction to pain medication should not be a deterrent to providing adequate pain management. *Addiction* is defined as the preoccupation and seeking of medications, despite known harm, for a reason other than pain management. Terminally ill patients require pain medication for control of severe intractable pain to improve their quality of life but rarely demonstrate symptoms of addiction.

ETHICAL CONSIDERATIONS

Ethical considerations and end-of-life care dilemmas have gained prominent focus in the care of elderly patients, especially in the terminal stages of illness. This is a particularly important issue given the increasing effectiveness of modern therapies and sophisticated intensive care available to patients with the technical ability to sustain life indefinitely. It is therefore critical to begin to address these issues early in the course of disease in order to properly interact with patients and family members regarding prognosis, treatment options, alternatives, and plan of care in terminal stages. Development of a clear plan of care for a terminally ill patient eases the transition from curative therapy to palliation. Open discussions regarding end-of-life care, withholding or withdrawal of life support, and medical futility are critical issues for patients, family, and caregivers and should be held as soon as is appropriate.

Defining medical futility remains controversial in practical definitions as well as in clinical determinations. The American Thoracic Society has stated that "a life-sustaining intervention is futile if reasoning and experience indicate that the intervention would be highly unlikely to result in meaningful survival for the patient," with attention paid to both the duration of survival as well as existing quality of life.[40] In actual clinical practice, it is difficult to predict that a particular therapy will in fact be futile in a given patient. Prognostic scales have been developed to better define medical futility based on objective patient data. For example, the APACHE score can be used as a quantitative prognosis tool. However, this is a general scoring system, and although predictive of gross mortality, it is difficult to individualize for patients. However, this system could help clarify a patient's wishes regarding life-sustaining treatment via advance directives, living wills, and do-not-resuscitate (DNR) orders to avoid unnecessary prolongation of futile treatment.

Physicians are not required to provide life-sustaining treatments that are deemed medically futile. This can override requests by patients or family members to continue aggressive therapy. It is important to realize that palliation is different from euthanasia and is protected by law, even if it hastens the occurrence of death by the principle of double effect. *Double effect* is defined as an act with good intention that produces a secondary effect that is harmful.[43] Therefore, physicians should not fear legal retribution from families in disagreement of treatment plans.

The governing principle in end-of-life decision making is patient autonomy, which takes precedence over physicians' judgment of what is most appropriate care. Patients have a right to refuse treatment, even if it delays appropriate treatment or results in the patient's death.[43] However, these preferences need to be documented during a time of mental competency. Surrogate decision making is tantamount to patient's wishes, giving surrogates complete decision-making responsibilities.

Physicians are not required to provide futile care. The Patient Self-Determination Act allows a patient to document preferences for life-sustaining interventions and resuscitation before undergoing treatments in the form of advance directives and livings wills.[40] These documents define the patient's wishes regarding life-support measures.[40] In addition, a surrogate for decision making can be appointed by the patient to make decisions regarding plan of care in the event the patient becomes mentally incapacitated.[40] Despite the availability of such documentation, few patients make necessary arrangements prior to clinical decomposition. Furthermore, this issue is rarely addressed by the physician with the patient and family members until recovery is unlikely. Unfortunately, most DNR orders are written only within days of a patient's death. This issue should always be addressed with patients prior to operative intervention. It is important to also acknowledge that DNR orders can be temporarily suspended in the operating room, placing both the surgeon and patient at ease. This practice is logical because most adverse events that occur in the operating room are secondary to acute, reversible events and are immediately detectable with careful monitoring. Necessary interventions can be instituted immediately in a controlled setting with excellent results, unlike events that occur outside of the operating room.

Another important principle is open communication. Patients must be informed honestly of their diagnosis and prognosis, as well as of the risks and benefits of all treatment options.[43] It can be difficult to accurately portray a patient's prognosis to either the patient or family members because it often is unclear. For example, in a patient receiving intensive care who develops renal failure, the question of whether short-term dialysis treatments will be sufficient or life-long dialysis for irreversible renal damage will be needed, may arise. Although this may be impossible to predict with certainty, patients and their families can be given honest information based on a physician's prior clinical experience with similar patients.

One of the most difficult issues faced in palliative care is resolution of conflicts that arise between the physician and the patient's family. Withdrawal and withholding of life-sustaining therapies is often a source of conflict between the physician, patient, and family members. It has been demonstrated that the most frequently identified cause of conflict, accounting for approximately 63% of disputes, was in regard to decisions for withdrawal or withholding of treatment.[46] One study demonstrated that, although 90% of patients' families agreed to withdrawal of life support within 5 days of being presented with the option, only 45% agreed immediately.[40] Strategies to avoid conflict regarding termination of care or withholding further measures that are deemed futile is to identify a single decision maker early in the course of illness and to establish a clear line of communication between the physician and family members regarding diagnosis, treatment plans, and transition to palliative care. Open communication between the physician and the family helps to keep the family informed regarding the patient's response to therapy and treatment alternatives. If family members are aware of treatment failures and given information regarding poor prognosis, they are less likely to dispute the physician's recommendation to limit treatment. A family may disagree with the physician because the family members do not understand the medical situation. For example, the family might not understand that despite a beating heart, a loved one is brain-dead and that termination of life support is indicated. The easiest way of avoiding conflict is by maintaining a relationship with the patient and the patient's family throughout the course of hospitalization.

End-of-life decisions are considerably easier when a patient elects a surrogate decision maker to make all necessary decisions in event of incapacitation via written documentation prior to admission to the hospital. In addition, continuity of care must be established with flexibility in treatment plans. One method is to establish limits to therapy prior to, as well as during, therapy. This is helpful in demonstrating whether a patient is likely to respond to therapy and helps to alleviate family doubt regarding the likelihood of the patient's recovery and can confirm the physician's assessment that further care would be futile. A meeting between the family and the physician should be held after any given therapeutic trial to discuss the patient's response and prognosis, with a discussion of termination of care if appropriate. If conflicts continue, involvement of an ethical committee is the next appropriate step. It is important for a physician to alleviate the fear of legal liability for the family member or proxy responsible for making the decision to withdraw or withhold life-sustaining therapies.

References

1. Keating HJ, Luben MF: Perioperative considerations of the physician/geriatrician. *Clin Geriatr Med* 6:459, 1990.
2. Thomas DR, Ritchie CS: Preoperative assessment of older adults. *J Am Geriatr Soc* 43:811, 1995.
3. Ergina PL: Perioperative care of the elderly patient. *World J Surg* 17:192, 1993.

4. Muravchick S: Preoperative assessment of the elderly patient. *Anesthesiol Clin North America* 18:71, 2000.

5. Hosking MP: Outcomes of surgery in patients 90 years of age and older. *JAMA* 261:1909, 1989.

6. Seymour DG, Faz FG: A prospective study of elderly general surgical patients. *Age Aging* 18:316, 1989.

7. Knaus WA, Wagner DP, Draper EA, et al: The APACHE III prognostic system: Risk prediction of hospital mortality for critically ill hospitalized adults. *Chest* 100:1619, 1991.

8. Miller DL: Perioperative care of the elderly patient: Special considerations. *Cleve Clin J Med* 62:383, 1995.

9. Wertheim WA: Perioperative risk: Review of two guidelines for assessing older adults. *Geriatrics* 55:61, 2000.

10. Smetana GW: Preoperative pulmonary assessment of the older adult. *Clin Geriatr Med* 19:35, 2003.

11. Beck LH: Perioperative renal, fluid, and electrolyte management. *Clin Geriatr Med* 6:557, 1990.

12. Stewart BT, Stitz RW, Lumley JW: Laparoscopically assisted colorectal surgery in the elderly. *Br J Surg* 86:938, 1999.

13. Ballista-Lopez C, Cid JA, Poves I, et al: Laparoscopic surgery in the elderly patient: Experience of a single laparoscopic unit. *Surg Endosc* 17:333, 2003.

14. Rosenthal RA, Zenilman ME, Katlic MR (eds): *Principles and Practice of Geriatric Surgery*. New York, Springer-Verlag, 2001.

15. Yanik R, Wesley MN, Ries LA, et al: Effect of age and comorbidity in postmenopausal breast cancer patients aged 55 years and older. *JAMA* 285:885, 2001.

16. Berger DH, Roslyn JJ: Cancer surgery in the elderly. *Clin Geriatr Med* 13:119, 1997.

17. American Geriatrics Society Clinical Practice Committee. Breast cancer screening in older women. *J Am Geriatr Soc* 48:842, 2000.

18. McConahey WM, Hay ID, Wodner LB, et al: Papillary thyroid cancer treated at the Mayo Clinic, 1946–1970: Initial manifestations, pathologic findings, therapy and outcome. *Mayo Clin Proc* 61:978, 1986.

19. Mueller-Gaertner H, Brzac HT, Rehpenning W: Prognostic indices for tumor relapse and tumor mortality in follicular thyroid carcinoma. *Cancer* 67:1903, 1991.

20. Har-El G, Sidi J, Segal K, et al: Thyroid cancer in patients 70 years of age or older. *Ann Otol Rhinol Laryngol* 96:403, 1987.

21. Irvin GL, Carneiro DM: "Limited" parathyroidectomy in geriatric patients. *Ann Surg* 233:612, 2001.

22. Sheldon DG, Lee FT, Neil NJ, et al: Surgical treatment of hyperparathyroidism improves health related quality of life. *Arch Surg* 137:1022, 2002.

23. Consensus Development Conference Panel: NIH conference. Diagnosis and management of asymptomatic primary hyperparathyroidism: Consensus development conference statement. *Ann Intern Med* 114:593, 1991.

24. Aziz S, Grover FL: Cardiovascular surgery in the elderly. *Cardiol Clin* 17:213, 1999.

25. Ko W, Krieger KH, Lazenby WD, et al: Isolated coronary artery bypass grafting in one hundred consecutive octogenarian patients. *J Thorac Cardiovasc Surg* 102:532, 1991.

26. Davis EA, Gardner TJ, Gillinov AM, et al: Valvular disease in the elderly: Influence on surgical results. *Ann Thorac Surg* 55:333, 1993.

27. Richmond TS, Kaunder D, Strumpf N, et al: Characteristics and outcomes of serious traumatic injury in older adults. *J Am Geriatr Soc* 50:215, 2002.

28. Anderson RN, Smith BL: Deaths: Leading causes for 2001. *Natl Vital Stat Rep* 52:14, 2003.

29. Perdue PW, Watts DD, Kaufmann CR, et al: Differences in mortality between elderly and younger adult trauma patients: Geriatric status increases risk of delayed death. *J Trauma* 45:805, 1998.

30. Rubenstein LZ, Josephson KR: The epidemiology of falls and syncope. *Clin Geriatr Med* 18:141, 2002.

31. Bergeron E, Lavole A, Clas D, et al: Elderly trauma patients with rib fractures are at greater risk of death and pneumonia. *J Trauma* 54:478, 2003.

32. Inaba K, et al: Long-term outcomes after injury in the elderly. *J Trauma* 54:486, 2003.

33. van Aalst J, Morris JA, Jr., Yates HK, et al: Severely injured geriatric patients return to independent living: A study of factors influencing function and independence. *J Trauma* 31:1096, 1991.

34. Lee CM, Carter JT, Weinstein RJ, et al: Dual kidney transplantation: Older donors for older recipients. *J Am Coll Surg* 189:82, 1999.

35. Benedetti E, Matas AJ, Hakim N, et al: Renal transplantation for patients 60 years or older: A single institution experience. *Ann Surg* 220:458, 1994.

36. Roodnat JI, Zietse R, Mulder PG, et al: The vanishing importance of age in renal transplantation. *Transplantation* 67:576, 1999.

37. Andres A, Morales JM, Herrero JC, et al: Double versus single renal allografts from aged donors. *Transplantation* 69:2060, 2000.

38. Garcia CE, Garcia RFL, Mayer AD, et al: Liver transplantation in patients over sixty years of age. *Transplantation* 72:679, 2001.

39. Wasburn WK, Johnson LB, Lewis WD, et al: Graft function and outcome of older (>60 years) donor livers. *Transplantation* 61:1062, 1996.

40. Sullivan DJ, Hansen-Flaschen J: Termination of life support after major trauma. *Surg Clin North Am* 80:1055, 2000.

41. McCahill LE, Krouse RS, Chu DZ, et al: Decision making in palliative surgery. *J Am Coll Surg* 195:411, 2002.

42. Hinshaw DB, Carnahan JM, Johnson DL: Depression, anxiety, and asthenia in advanced illness. *J Am Coll Surg* 195:271, 2002.

43. Dunn GP, Milch RA, Mosenthal AC, et al: Palliative care by the surgeon. *J Am Coll Surg* 194:509, 2002.

44. Conner SR: *Hospice: Practice, Pitfalls and Promise*. Washington: Taylor and Francis, 1988.

45. Sheehan DC, Forman WB: *Hospice and Palliative Care Concepts and Practice*. Boston: Jones and Bartlett, 1996.

46. Breen CM, Abernethy AP, Abbott KM, et al: Conflict associated with decisions to limit life-sustaining treatment in intensive care units. *J Gen Intern Med* 16:283, 2001.

CHAPTER 46

Anesthesia of the Surgical Patient

Robert S. Dorian

The discipline of anesthesia embodies control of three great concerns of humankind: consciousness, pain, and movement. The field of anesthesiology combines the administration of anesthesia with the perioperative management of the patient's concerns, pain management, and critical illness. The fields of surgery and anesthesiology are truly collaborative and continue to evolve together, enabling the care of sicker patients and rapid recovery from outpatient and minimally invasive procedures.

A BRIEF HISTORY OF ANESTHESIA

The discovery of anesthesia is one of the seminal American contributions to the world. Along with infection control and blood transfusion, anesthesia has enabled surgery to occupy its fundamental place in medicine. Before the advent of modern anesthesia in the 1840s, many substances and methods were tried in the search for pain relief and better operating conditions. Opium, alcohol, exposure to cold, compression of peripheral nerves, constriction of the carotid arteries to produce unconsciousness, and hypnosis (mesmerism) all proved less than satisfactory and dictated rapid and crude surgical procedures. Patients had to be restrained by several attendants, and only the most stoic could tolerate the screams heard in the operating theater. Charles Darwin, who witnessed two such operations, "...rushed away before they were completed. Nor did I ever attend again, for hardly any inducement would have been strong enough to make me do so; this being long before the blessed days of chloroform. The two cases fairly haunted me for many a long year."[1]

Modern Beginnings

In 1842 Crawford Long (1815–1878), a physician in rural Georgia, used diethyl ether to induce surgical anesthesia for the removal of two small neck tumors. Diethyl ether had been known for over 800 years, but was not used for analgesic purposes. It became an inexpensive and popular recreational drug in the mid-nineteenth century and was used by American medical students at "ether frolics." Although Long did experiments to verify the analgesic effects of ether, he did not publish his work until 1848, in the *Southern Medical Journal,* too late to be the unquestioned discoverer of anesthesia.[2]

Although Humphrey Davy (1778–1829) suggested using nitrous oxide for the relief of pain in surgical procedures in 1800, this was not pursued until 1844 by dentist Horace Wells (1815–1848). Wells astutely observed that a man who was injured after inhaling nitrous oxide during an exhibition of the "laughing gas" displayed no awareness of pain. After experimenting on himself, Wells attempted to demonstrate the analgesic effects of nitrous oxide for a dental procedure at Harvard Medical School in 1845. The public demonstration was a failure since nitrous oxide has analgesic properties, but does not suffice as the sole anesthetic agent in every patient. Wells never recovered from his humiliating experience and eventually committed suicide, but does hold a place in history as the first person to recognize and utilize the only anesthetic from the 1800s that is still in use today—nitrous oxide.

Ether Day

William Morton (1819–1868) was a dentist and partner of Horace Wells's. After a taking a course in anesthesia from Wells, Morton left the partnership in Hartford and established himself in Boston. He continued his interest in anesthesia, but with diethyl ether replacing nitrous oxide. Ether proved a good choice as it supports respiration and the cardiovascular system at analgesic levels, and is potent enough to administer in room air without hypoxia. He practiced the administration of ether on a dog and then used it when extracting teeth from patients in his office. On October 16, 1846, Morton gave the first public demonstration of ether as an anesthetic for Johns Collins Warren, distinguished surgeon and a founder of the Massachusetts General Hospital. In attendance in the surgical amphitheater were several surgeons, medical students, and a newspaper reporter. After anesthesia was induced using a makeshift inhaler, Warren successfully removed a vascular mass from the patient's neck with no ill effects. Warren was an originator of the *Boston Medical and Surgical Journal* (now *The New England Journal of Medicine*), and by November 1846 the demonstration was published in an article by Henry J. Bigelow.[3] The stature of Warren and Bigelow lent considerable credence to the advent of surgical anesthesia; as news spread rapidly, surgeons around the world were quick to adopt this "American invention." The Massachusetts General Hospital has restored and preserved the original amphitheater where the demonstration took place, now called the Ether Dome. It is designated as a Registered National Historic Landmark commemorating the first public demonstration, rather than discovery, of the use of ether as an anesthetic.

The First Anesthesiologists

John Snow (1813–1858) made science out of the art of anesthesia. He was a respected London physician who applied a scholarly, scientific method to investigate the clinical properties and pharmacology of ether, chloroform, and other anesthetic agents. Snow was an astute observer and published a detailed account of the five degrees of etherization in 1847. He vastly improved the apparatus for administering ether, and mastered the clinical techniques of anesthetizing patients. As the leading anesthetist of his day, he gave anesthetics to the royal family, including chloroform during labor to Queen Victoria for the birth of Prince Leopold. The Queen's endorsement of "that blessed chloroform" removed the moral and social stigma against relieving pain during childbirth, and brought anesthesia into public awareness. Chloroform, popularized in England by James Simpson (1811–1870), had a narrow therapeutic index and placed great clinical demands on the anesthetist. Ether, with its ability to maintain the cardiovascular and respiratory systems, remained in common use in the United States and was often administered by house staff, medical students, or nurses. Snow encouraged the administration of anesthesia by a physician, and felt that a physician dedicated specifically to that purpose was appropriate and necessary. Snow and other exceptional British physicians specializing in anesthesia (Joseph Clover [1825–1882] and Sir Frederick Hewitt [1857–1916]) created a standard of excellence in the latter half of the nineteenth century. This atmosphere of professionalism led to the formation of anesthesia societies and the publication of papers in the prestigious *British Medical Journal* and *Lancet* in England years before such organizations existed in America.[4]

Cocaine: The First Local Anesthetic

The ancient Incas chewed coca leaves as a stimulant, but were also aware of its local anesthetic properties. They would facilitate trephination of the skull by chewing a clump of coca leaves and dripping the resultant saliva into the wound. The active alkaloid of the coca leaf was synthesized in 1860 and called cocaine by German chemist Albert Niemann, who noted that it "benumbs the nerves of the tongue, depriving it of feeling."[5] Sigmund Freud (1856–1939) of Vienna received a supply of cocaine from Merck, studied its properties, and wrote the famous monograph "Uber Coca" in 1884. Freud was primarily interested in the stimulant and euphoric effects of cocaine, and attempted to use it to treat morphine addiction. Freud and Karl Koller (1857–1944), an ophthalmologic intern, began to perform physiologic experiments with cocaine, measuring its effects on muscle strength. Although they both noted that the drug caused numbness of the tongue when swallowed, it was Koller who first instilled it into his own cornea; report of its use as a local anesthetic galvanized the medical world. Soon after, young American surgeons William Halstead (1852–1922) and Richard Hall described intradermal injection of cocaine and were the first to use it for regional blocks of the facial nerves, brachial plexus, and the internal pudendal and posterior tibial nerves.[6] Halstead later became the first Professor of Surgery and Chief Surgeon at Johns Hopkins University, where he remained for over 30 years. One of the founding fathers of modern surgery, he pioneered radical mastectomy with lymphadenectomy and the use of rubber gloves. While experimenting on themselves, Halstead and other early researchers became addicted to cocaine.[7] Its toxic effects were the stimulus to find other local anesthetics— procaine was synthesized in 1905 and lidocaine in 1943.

The New York neurologist Leonard Corning (1855–1923) observed the regional blocks of Halstead and Hall, analytically studied local anesthesia effects on dogs, applied his knowledge to humans, and published the first textbook on local anesthesia in 1886. After experimenting on the spinal nerves of a dog, he intradurally injected a solution of cocaine into a patient, called it "spinal anesthesia," and commented that it might be useful in surgery. His suggestion went unheeded for over 10 years, until August Bier (1861–1949), a prominent German surgeon, gave the first deliberate spinal anesthetic.[8] This incremental interchange of ideas and advances across the Atlantic and across the specialties of anesthesia and surgery demonstrates the collaborative nature of science in general, and medicine in particular. The development of surgery and anesthesia exemplify the dichotomy of two fledgling specialties that are mutually dependent, yet increasingly autonomous.

The Twentieth Century

Developments in anesthesia on both sides of the Atlantic progressed rapidly in the twentieth century. The convergence of technologies that produced the hollow needle and syringe, coupled with the synthesis of barbiturates, gave rise to intravenous anesthesia in the early 1900s. Barbital, followed by hexobarbital and thiopental in 1934, produced rapid and more pleasant induction of anesthesia than the inhaled gases. The concept of "balanced anesthesia" began in 1925, when John Lundy (1894–1973) proposed the use of thiopentone for induction, followed by inhaled agents for maintenance of anesthesia. Lundy directed the Department of Anesthesiology at the Mayo Clinic for 28 years. He established the first recovery room and blood bank, authored the first textbook on modern anesthesia, and helped found the American Board of Anesthesiology.

Nitrous oxide, diethyl ether, and chloroform, all discovered fortuitously by observation, remained the dominant inhalation agents until the accidental discovery of cyclopropane's anesthetic properties in 1923. Although rapid acting and pleasant smelling, cyclopropane was limited by its flammability and cardiac irritability. Since it was known that fluorination would reduce or eliminate flammability of chemical compounds, British chemist Charles Suckling set out to synthesize an anesthetic that was stable, potent, volatile, and not flammable. He successfully produced halothane in 1953. Introduced into clinical practice in 1956 after extensive testing in Manchester, England, and paired with an accurate calibrated vaporizer, halothane quickly became the most widely used fluorinated anesthetic. Enflurane and isoflurane, synthesized in the United States by Ross Tyrell, were introduced into clinical practice in 1972 and 1981, respectively. The newest agents, desflurane and sevoflurane, were introduced into clinical practice in the early 1990s. They possess a low solubility and are characterized by rapid onset and recovery, making them particularly well suited to outpatient surgery.

The motto of the American Society of Anesthesiologists is "Vigilance," and to that end there has been continued progress in objective mechanical measurement of patient well-being. The early anesthesiologists used clinical signs such as patient color, depth of respiration, and pulse rate to monitor depth of anesthesia and patient well-being. Harvey Cushing, who eventually became Moseley Professor of Surgery at the Peter Bent Brigham Hospital, began the first anesthesia records or "ether charts" in 1895 while a medical student. They recorded pulse, respiratory rates, pupillary diameter, and the amounts of ether and other drugs administered. He later introduced the use of the portable sphygmomanometer of Riva Rocci to measure blood pressure, and the precordial stethoscope to monitor breath and heart sounds. Monitoring has since progressed to its current state with incremental developments in electrocardiography, pulse oximetry, and mass spectrometry, all mandatory for the safe administration of any anesthetic.

The control of the patient's airway and respiration as the purview of the anesthesiologist evolved with techniques of endotracheal intubation as pioneered by Sir Ivan Magill (1888–1986), and the invention of the cuffed endotracheal tube by Arthur Guedel (1883–1965). This later merged with the invention of mechanical ventilation and its introduction to the operating room as the embodiment of today's anesthesia machine. It was this expertise at control of respiration that paved the way for the most revolutionary modern development in anesthesia—the use of muscle relaxants. Curare, a nondepolarizing muscle relaxant, was popularized by Harold Griffith of Montreal. His report of the successful use of curare was a galvanizing event that revolutionized the practice of anesthesia, as the relaxation of abdominal muscles could be controlled to facilitate surgery.[9] The depolarizing relaxant succinylcholine was introduced in 1949, and research has continued to provide the newer nondepolarizing drugs mivacurium, pancuronium, rocuronium, atracurium, and cisatracurium.

Anesthesiology Today

The specialty of anesthesia is no longer limited to the operating room. It is natural that anesthesiology, born out of the quest to relieve pain, gave rise to the field of acute and chronic pain medicine. The anesthesiologist consulting on the acute pain service may recommend oral, intramuscular, or intravenous analgesia with a variety of agents, or patient-controlled analgesia. Postsurgical patients may also be treated with nerve blocks: regional (e.g., brachial plexus, popliteal, and femoral) or neuraxial (epidural or intrathecal). The discipline of chronic pain addresses patients who suffer for months or years with cancer or other debilitating diseases. Treatment modalities escalate from orally administered drugs, to diagnostic and therapeutic nerve blocks, to more invasive measures like dorsal column nerve stimulators, and radiofrequency or cryosurgical nerve ablation.

Daily management of the airway, fluids and transfusions, ventilation, drug delivery, monitoring, and caring for the sickest patients in the postanesthesia care unit prepared anesthesiologists to become major contributors to the development of critical care medicine. Out of the 28 founding members of the Society of Critical Medicine, 10 were anesthesiologists.[10]

The American Board of Anesthesiology became an independent board in 1941, and since then has granted board certification to over 25,000 diplomates. Certificates in Anesthesia Pain Management and Anesthesia Critical Care Medicine are granted to those completing additional postgraduate training. The American Society of Anesthesiologists has over 35,000 members, and its official journal, *Anesthesiology*, has a monthly circulation of 40,000 worldwide.

BASIC PHARMACOLOGY

Pharmacokinetics

Pharmacokinetics describes the relationship between the dose of a drug and its plasma or tissue concentration. It depends on absorption (into the bloodstream), distribution, and elimination. Route of administration, metabolism, protein binding, and tissue distribution all affect the pharmacokinetics of a particular drug.

Administration, Distribution, and Elimination

The route of *administration* of a drug affects its pharmacokinetics, as there will be different rates of drug entry into the circulation. For example, the oral and intravenous routes are subject to first-pass effect of the portal circulation; this can be bypassed with the nasal or sublingual route. Other routes of drug administration include transdermal, intramuscular, subcutaneous, or inhalation.

Distribution is the delivery of a drug from the systemic circulation to the tissues. Once a drug has entered the systemic circulation, the rate at which it will enter the tissues depends on several factors:

1. Molecular size of the drug, capillary permeability, polarity, and lipid solubility. Small molecules will pass more freely and quickly across cell membranes than large ones, but capillary permeability is variable and results in different diffusion rates. Renal glomerular capillaries are permeable to almost all non–protein-bound drugs; capillaries in the brain are fused (i.e., they have tight junctions) and are relatively impermeable to all but the tiniest molecules (the blood-brain barrier). Un-ionized molecules pass more easily across cell membranes than charged molecules; diffusibility also increases with increasing lipid solubility.
2. Plasma protein and tissue binding. Many drugs bind to circulating proteins like albumin, glycoproteins, and globulins. Disease, age, and the presence of other drugs will affect the amount of protein binding; drug distribution is affected because only the unbound free portion of the drug

can pass across the cell membrane. Drugs also bind reversibly to body tissues; if they bind with high affinity they are said to be sequestered in that tissue (e.g., heavy metals are sequestered in bone).[11]

The fluid volume in which a drug distributes is termed the *volume of distribution* (Vd). This mathematically derived value gives a rough estimation of the overall physical distribution of a drug in the body. A general rule for volume distribution is that the greater the Vd, the greater the diffusibility of the drug. Because drugs have variable ionization rates and bind differently to plasma proteins and tissues, the Vd is not a good predictor of the actual concentration of the drug after administration. Determining the *apparent volume of distribution* (dose/concentration) is an attempt to more accurately ascertain the drug dose administered and its final concentration. This in turn is complicated by the immediate *elimination* of a drug after administration.

Drug elimination varies widely; some drugs are excreted unchanged by the body, some decompose via plasma enzymes, and some are degraded by organ-based enzymes in the liver. Many drugs rely on multiple pathways for elimination (i.e., metabolized by liver enzymes then excreted by the kidney). When a drug is given orally, it reaches the liver via the portal circulation and is partially metabolized before reaching the systemic circulation. This is why an oral dose of a drug often must be much higher than an equally effective intravenous dose. Some drugs (e.g., nitroglycerine) are hydrolyzed presystemically in the gut wall and must be administered sublingually to achieve an effective concentration.

It is important to remember that the response to drugs varies widely. The disposition of drugs is affected by age; weight; sex; pregnancy; disease states; the concomitant use of alcohol, tobacco, and other licit and illicit drugs; and genetic factors. The most important monitor in the operating room is the anesthesiologist, who continuously assesses the patient's response and adjusts the doses of anesthetic agents to match the surgical stimulus.

Pharmacodynamics

Pharmacodynamics, or how the plasma concentration of a drug translates into its effect on the body, depends on biologic variability, receptor physiology, and clinical evaluations of the actual drug. An *agonist* is a drug that causes a response. A *full agonist* produces the full tissue response, and a *partial agonist* provokes less than the maximum response induced by a full agonist. An *antagonist* is a drug that does not provoke a response itself, but blocks agonist-mediated responses. An *additive effect* means that a second drug acts with the first drug and will produce an effect that is equal to the algebraic summation of both drugs. A *synergistic effect* means that two drugs interact to produce an effect that is greater than expected from the two drugs' algebraic summation.[12]

Hyporeactivity means a larger than expected dose is required to produce a response, and this effect is termed *tolerance, desensitization,* or *tachyphylaxis*. Tolerance usually results from chronic drug exposure, either through enzyme induction (e.g., alcohol) or depletion of neurotransmitters (e.g., cocaine).

Potency, Efficacy, Lethal Dose, and Therapeutic Index

The *potency* of a drug is the dose required to produce a given effect, such as pain relief or a change in heart rate. The average sensitivity to a particular drug can be expressed through the calculation of the effective dose, ED_{50} would have the desired effect in 50% of the general population. The *efficacy* of any therapeutic agent is its power to produce a desired effect. Two drugs may have the same

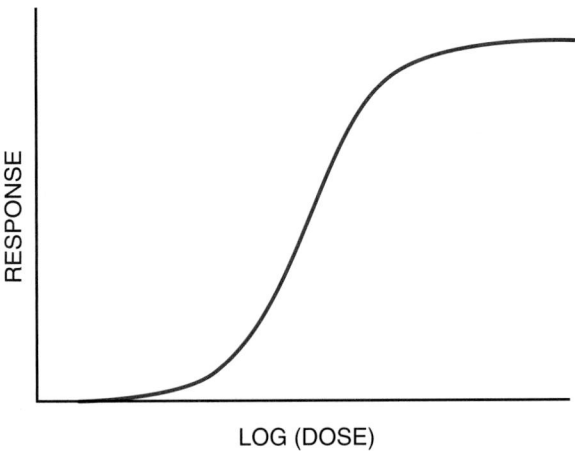

FIG. 46-1. *Basic dose response curve.*

efficacy but different potencies. The difference in potency of the two drugs is described by the ratio ED_{50}^b/ED_{50}^a, where *a* is the less potent drug. If the ED_{50}^b equals 4 and the ED_{50}^a equals 0.4, then drug *a* is ten times as potent as drug *b*. For example, 10 mg of morphine produces analgesia equal to that of 1 mg of hydromorphone. They are equally effective, but hydromorphone is ten times as potent as morphine.

Dose-response curves show the relationship between the dose of a drug administered (or the resulting plasma concentration) and the pharmacologic effect of the drug. The pharmacologic effect might be secretion of a hormone, a change in heart rate, or contraction of a muscle. Between 20 and 80% of the maximum effect, the logarithm of the dose and its response has a linear relationship. The term *dose* only applies to the amount administered and not the actual concentration. If the concentration of an antagonist is increased (in the presence of a fixed concentration of agonist), the dose-response curve will be shifted to the right, and a higher agonist concentration will be required to achieve the desired effect. A basic dose-response curve is shown in Fig. 46-1.

The *lethal dose* (LD_{50}) of a drug produces death in 50% of animals to which it is given. The ratio of the lethal dose and effective dose, LD_{50}/ED_{50}, is the *therapeutic index*. A drug with a high therapeutic index is safer than a drug with a low or narrow therapeutic index.

ANESTHETIC AGENTS

Anesthesia can be *local, regional,* or *general* (Table 46-1).

Local anesthesia is accomplished using a local anesthetic drug that can be injected intradermally, and is used for the removal of small lesions or to repair traumatic injuries. Local anesthesia is the most frequent anesthetic administered by surgeons, and may be accompanied by intravenous sedation to improve patient comfort.

Local Anesthetics

Local anesthetics are divided into two groups based on their chemical structure: the amides and the esters. In general, the amides are metabolized in the liver and the esters are metabolized by plasma cholinesterases, which yield metabolites with slightly higher allergic potential than the amides (Table 46-2).

Amides

Lidocaine, bupivacaine, mepivacaine, prilocaine, and ropivacaine have in common an amide linkage between a benzene ring

Table 46-1
Anesthetic Agents, Their Actions, and Their Clinical Uses

Effect	Monitor	Intravenous Drugs	Potent Gases	Weak Gases	Local Anesthetics	

Unconsciousness, amnesia, anxiolysis	Eeg; clinical signs	*Benzodiazepines*
		  Midazolam
		  Diazepam
		  Lorazepam
		Barbiturates
		Propofol
		Etomidate
		  Ketamine[a]
			Sevoflurane
			Desflurane
			Isoflurane
			Enflurane
			Halothane
				Nitrous oxide		

Analgesia	Heart rate, blood pressure, respiratory rate, clinical signs	*Opioids*
		  Morphine
		  Meperidine
		  Hydromorphone
		  Fentanyl
		NSAID
		  Ketorolac
		  Parecoxib
			Sevoflurane
			Desflurane
			Isoflurane
			Enflurane
			Halothane
				Nitrous oxide	*Amides*
					Lidocaine
					Bupivacaine
					Mepivacaine
					Prilocaine
					Ropivacaine
					Regional peripheral
					Brachial plexus
						Esters
						Cocaine
						Procaine
						Chloroprocaine
						Tetracaine
						Benzocaine

Muscle relaxation, paralysis	Nerve stimulator; clinical signs; tidal volume, hand grip; 5-second head lift	*Depolarizing agent*
		  Succinylcholine
		Nondepolarizing agents
		  Pancuronium
		  Vecuronium
		  Rocuronium
		  Atracurium
		  Cis-atracurium
		  Mivacurium
			Sevoflurane
			Desflurane
			Isoflurane
			Enflurane
			Halothane
				—	Lower extremity
					Cervical plexus
					Regional central
					Spinal
					Epidural	

[a]Note that the intravenous agents are quite specific in their effects, except for ketamine, which has both amnestic and analgesic qualities.
The potent inhalational anesthetics contribute to all three components of anesthesia, but nitrous oxide has weak amnestic and analgesic properties, and provides no muscle relaxation at all.
The local anesthetics produce excellent analgesia and muscle relaxation, but contribute nothing to amnesia or anxiolysis, these anesthetics must be supplemented with an intravenous sedative.
General anesthesia entails all three elements of anesthesia (amnesia, analgesic, and muscle relaxation).

and a hydrocarbon chain, which in turn is attached to a tertiary amine. The benzene ring confers lipid solubility for penetration of nerve membranes, and the tertiary amine attached to the hydrocarbon chain makes these local anesthetics water soluble. Lidocaine has a more rapid onset and is shorter acting than bupivacaine; however, both are widely used for tissue infiltration, regional nerve blocks, and spinal and epidural anesthesia. Ropivacaine is the most recently introduced local anesthetic. It is clinically similar to bupivacaine in that it has a slow onset and a long duration, but is less cardiotoxic. All amides are 95% metabolized in the liver, with 5% excreted unchanged by the kidneys.

Esters

Cocaine, procaine, chloroprocaine, tetracaine, and benzocaine have an ester linkage in place of the amide linkage mentioned above. Unique among local anesthetics, cocaine occurs in nature, was the first used clinically, produces vasoconstriction (making it useful for topical application; e.g., for intranasal surgery), releases norepinephrine from nerve terminals resulting in hypertension, and is highly addictive. Cocaine is a Schedule II drug. Procaine, synthesized in 1905 as a nontoxic substitute for cocaine, has a short duration and is used for infiltration. Tetracaine has a long duration and

Table 46-2
Biologic Properties of Commonly Used Local Anesthetics

Agent	Equianesthetic Concentration	Approximate Anesthetic Duration (min)	Site of Metabolism
Esters			
Procaine	2	50	Plasma
Chloroprocaine	2	45	Plasma
Tetracaine	0.25	175	Plasma
Amides			
Prilocaine	1	100	Liver/lung
Lidocaine	1	100	Liver
Mepivacaine	1	100	Liver
Bupivacaine	0.25	175	Liver
Ropivacaine	0.3	150	Liver
Etidocaine	0.25	200	Liver

SOURCE: Reproduced with permission from Rosenberg et al.[80]

is useful as a spinal anesthetic for lengthy operations. Benzocaine is for topical use only. The esters are hydrolyzed in the blood by pseudocholinesterase. Some of the metabolites have a greater allergic potential than the metabolites of the amide anesthetics, but true allergies to local anesthetics are rare.

The common characteristic of all local anesthetics is a reversible block of the transmission of neural impulses when placed on or near a nerve membrane. Local anesthetics block nerve conduction by stabilizing sodium channels in their closed state, preventing action potentials from propagating along the nerve. The individual local anesthetic agents have different recovery times based on lipid solubility and tissue binding, but return of neural function is spontaneous as the drug is metabolized or removed from the nerve by the vascular system.

Toxicity of local anesthetics results from absorption into the bloodstream or from inadvertent direct intravascular injection. Toxicity manifests first in the more sensitive central nervous system, and then the cardiovascular system.

Central Nervous System. As plasma concentration of local anesthetic rises, symptoms progress from restlessness to complaints of tinnitus. Slurred speech, seizures, and unconsciousness follow. Cessation of the seizure via administration of a benzodiazepine or thiopental and maintenance of the airway is the immediate treatment. If the seizure persists, the trachea must be intubated with a cuffed endotracheal tube to guard against pulmonary aspiration of stomach contents.

Cardiovascular System. With increasingly elevated plasma levels of local anesthetics, progression to hypotension, increased P-R intervals, bradycardia, and cardiac arrest may occur. Bupivacaine is more cardiotoxic than other local anesthetics. It has a direct effect on ventricular muscle, and because it is more lipid soluble than lidocaine, it binds tightly to sodium channels (it is called the fast-in, slow-out local anesthetic). Patients who have received an inadvertent intravascular injection of bupivacaine have experienced profound hypotension, ventricular tachycardia and fibrillation, and complete atrioventricular heart block that is extremely refractory to treatment. The toxic dose of lidocaine is approximately 5 mg/kg; that of bupivacaine is approximately 3 mg/kg.

Calculation of the toxic dose before injection is imperative. It is helpful to remember that for any drug or solution, 1% = 10 mg/mL. For a 50-kg person, the toxic dose of bupivacaine would be approximately 3 mg/kg, or 3 × 50 = 150 mg. A 0.5% solution of bupivacaine is 5 mg/mL, so 150 mL/5 mg/mL = 30 mL as the upper limit for infiltration. For lidocaine in the same patient, the calculation is 50 kg × 5 mg/mL = 250 mg toxic dose. If a 1% solution is used, the allowed amount would be 250 mg/10 mg/mL = 25 mL.

Additives. Epinephrine has one physiologic and several clinical effects when added to local anesthetics. Epinephrine is a vasoconstrictor, and by reducing local bleeding, molecules of the local anesthetic remain in proximity to the nerve for a longer time period. Onset of the nerve block is faster, the quality of the block is improved, the duration is longer, and less local anesthetic will be absorbed into the bloodstream, thereby reducing toxicity. Although epinephrine 1:200,000 (5 μg/mL) added to a local anesthetic for infiltration will greatly lengthen the time of analgesia, epinephrine-containing solutions should not be injected into body parts with end-arteries such as toes or fingers, as vasoconstriction may lead to ischemia or loss of a digit. When added to the local anesthetic, sodium bicarbonate will raise the pH, favoring the non-ionized uncharged form of the molecule. This speeds the onset of the block, especially in local anesthetics that are mixed with epinephrine. The pH of such solutions is around 4.5, therefore the addition of sodium bicarbonate results in a relatively large increase in pH.[13]

Regional Anesthesia

Peripheral

Local anesthetic can be injected *peripherally*, near a large nerve or plexus to provide anesthesia to a larger region of the body. Examples include the brachial plexus for surgery of the arm or hand, blockade of the femoral and sciatic nerves for surgery of the lower extremity, ankle block for surgery of the foot or toes, intercostal block for analgesia of the thorax postoperatively, or blockade of the cervical plexus, which is ideal for carotid endarterectomy. Risks of peripheral regional nerve blocks are dependent on their location. For example, nerve blocks injected into the neck risk puncture of the carotid or vertebral arteries, intercostal nerves are in close proximity to the vascular bundle and have a high rate of absorption of local anesthetic, and nerve blocks of the thorax run the risk of causing pneumothorax. All peripheral nerve blocks may be supplemented intraoperatively with intravenous sedation and/or analgesics.

Central

Local anesthetic injected *centrally* near the spinal cord—spinal or epidural anesthesia—provides anesthesia for the lower half of the body. This is especially useful for genitourinary, gynecologic, inguinal hernia, or lower-extremity procedures. Spinal and epidural anesthesia block the spinal nerves as they exit the spinal cord. Spinal nerves are mixed nerves; they contain motor, sensory, and sympathetic components. The subsequent block will cause sensory anesthesia, loss of motor function, and blockade of the sympathetic nerves from the level of the anesthetic distally to the lower extremities. Subsequent vasodilation of the vasculature from sympathetic block may result in hypotension, which is treatable with intravenous fluids and/or pressors.

Spinal Anesthesia. Local anesthetic is injected directly into the dural sac surrounding the spinal cord. The level of injection is usually below L1 to L2, where the spinal cord ends in most adults. Because the local anesthetic is injected directly into the cerebrospinal fluid (CSF) surrounding the spinal cord, only a small dose is needed, the onset of anesthesia is rapid, and the blockade thorough. Lidocaine, bupivacaine, and tetracaine are commonly used agents of differing durations; the block wears off naturally via drug uptake by the CSF, bloodstream, or diffusion into fat. Epinephrine as an additive to the local anesthetic will significantly prolong the blockade.

Possible complications include hypotension, especially if the patient is not adequately prehydrated; high spinal block requires immediate airway management; and postdural puncture headache sometimes occurs. Spinal headache is related to the diameter and configuration of the spinal needle, and can be reduced to approximately 1% with the use of a small 25- or 27-gauge needle.

Cauda equina syndrome is injury to the nerves emanating distal to the spinal cord resulting in bowel and bladder dysfunction, and lower-extremity sensory and motor loss. It has mainly been seen in cases in which indwelling spinal microcatheters and high (5%) concentrations of lidocaine were used. Indwelling spinal catheters are no longer used.

Epidural Anesthesia. Epidural anesthesia could also be called extradural anesthesia, because local anesthetics are injected into the epidural space surrounding the dural sac of the spinal cord.

Much greater volumes of anesthetic are required than with spinal anesthesia, and the onset of the block is longer—10 to 15 minutes. As in spinal anesthesia, local anesthetic bathes the spinal nerves as they exit the dura; the patient achieves analgesia from the sensory block, muscle relaxation from blockade of the motor nerves, and hypotension from blockade of the sympathetic nerves as they exit the spinal cord. Note that regional anesthesia, whether peripheral or central, provides only two of the three major components of anesthesia—analgesia and muscle relaxation. Anxiolysis, amnesia, or sedation must be attained by supplemental intravenous administration of other drugs (e.g., the benzodiazepines or propofol infusion).

Complications are similar to those of spinal anesthesia. Inadvertent injection of local anesthetic into a dural tear will result in a high block, manifesting as unconsciousness, severe hypotension, and respiratory paralysis requiring immediate aggressive hemodynamic management and control of the airway. Indwelling catheters are often placed through introducers into the epidural space, allowing an intermittent or continuous technique, as opposed to the single-shot method of spinal anesthesia. By necessity, the epidural-introducing needles are of a much larger diameter (17- or 18-gauge) than spinal needles, and accidental dural puncture more often results in a severe headache that may last up to 10 days if left untreated.

General Anesthesia

General anesthesia describes a triad of three major and separate effects: unconsciousness (and amnesia), analgesia, and muscle relaxation (see Table 46-1). Intravenous drugs usually produce a single, discrete effect, while most inhaled anesthetics produce elements of all three. General anesthesia is achieved with a combination of intravenous and inhaled drugs, each used to its maximum benefit. The science and art of anesthesia is a dynamic process. As the amount of stimulus to the patient changes during surgery, the patient's vital signs are used as a guide and the quantity of drugs is adjusted, maintaining an equilibrium between stimulus and dose. General anesthesia is what patients commonly think of when they are to be "put under," and can be a cause of considerable preoperative anxiety.[14]

Intravenous Agents

Unconsciousness and Amnesia. The intravenous agents that produce unconsciousness and amnesia are frequently used for the induction of general anesthesia. They include barbiturates, benzodiazepines, propofol, etomidate, and ketamine. Except for ketamine, the following agents have no analgesic properties, nor do they cause paralysis or muscle relaxation.

Barbiturates. The most common barbiturates are thiopental, thiamylal, and methohexital. The mechanism of action is at the gamma-aminobutyric acid (GABA) receptor, where they inhibit excitatory synaptic transmission. They produce a rapid, smooth induction within 60 seconds, and wear off in about 5 minutes. In higher doses and in patients with intravascular depletion they cause hypotension and myocardial depression. The barbiturates are anticonvulsants and protect the brain during neurosurgery by reducing cerebral metabolism.

Propofol. Propofol is an alkylated phenol that inhibits synaptic transmission through its effects at the GABA receptor. With a short duration, rapid recovery, and low incidence of nausea and vomiting, it has emerged as the agent of choice for ambulatory and minor general surgery. Additionally, propofol has bronchodilatory properties which make its use attractive in asthmatic patients and smokers.

Propofol may cause hypotension, and should be used cautiously in patients with suspected hypovolemia and/or coronary artery disease (CAD), the latter of which may not tolerate a sudden drop in blood pressure. It can be used as a continuous infusion for sedation in the intensive care unit setting. Propofol is an irritant and frequently causes pain on injection.

Benzodiazepines. The most important uses of the benzodiazepines are for reduction of anxiety and to produce amnesia. Frequently used intravenous benzodiazepines are diazepam, lorazepam, and midazolam. They all inhibit synaptic transmission at the GABA receptor, but have differing durations of action. The benzodiazepines can produce peripheral vasodilatation and hypotension, but have minimal effects on respiration when used alone. They must be used with caution when given with opioids; a synergistic reaction causing respiratory depression is common. The benzodiazepines are excellent anticonvulsants, and only rarely cause allergic reactions.

Etomidate. Etomidate is an imidazole derivative used for intravenous induction. Its rapid and almost complete hydrolysis to inactive metabolites results in rapid awakening. Like the above intravenous agents, etomidate acts on the GABA receptor. It has little effect on cardiac output and heart rate, and induction doses usually produce less reduction in blood pressure than that seen with thiopental or propofol. Etomidate is associated with pain on injection and more nausea and vomiting than thiopental or propofol.

Ketamine. Ketamine differs from the above intravenous agents in that it produces analgesia as well as amnesia. Its principal action is on the *N*-methyl-D-aspartate (NMDA) receptor; it has no action on the GABA receptor. It is a dissociative anesthetic, producing a cataleptic gaze with nystagmus. Patients may associate this with delirium and hallucinations while regaining consciousness. The addition of benzodiazepines has been shown to prevent these side effects. Ketamine can increase heart rate and blood pressure which may cause myocardial ischemia in patients with CAD. Ketamine is useful in acutely hypovolemic patients to maintain blood pressure via sympathetic stimulation, but is a direct myocardial depressant in patients who are catecholamine depleted. Ketamine is a bronchodilator, making it useful for asthmatic patients, and rarely is associated with allergic reactions.

Analgesia. The intravenous analgesics most frequently used in anesthesia today have little effect on consciousness, amnesia, or muscle relaxation. The most important class is the *opioids,* so called because they were first isolated from opium, with morphine, codeine, meperidine, hydromorphone, and the fentanyl family being the most common. The most important *nonopioid* analgesics are ketamine (discussed above) and ketorolac, an intravenous nonsteroidal anti-inflammatory drug (NSAID).

Opioid Analgesics. The commonly used opioids—morphine, codeine, oxymorphone, meperidine, and the fentanyl-based compounds—act centrally on μ-receptors in the brain and spinal cord. The main side effects of opioids are euphoria, sedation, constipation, and respiratory depression, which also are mediated by the same μ-receptors in a dose-dependent fashion. Although opioids have differing potencies required for effective analgesia, *equianalgesic doses of opioids result in equal degrees of respiratory depression.* Thus there is no completely safe opioid analgesic. The synthetic opioids fentanyl, and its analogs sufentanil, alfentanil, and remifentanil, are commonly used in the operating room. They differ pharmacokinetically in their lipid solubility, tissue binding, and elimination profiles, and therefore have differing potencies and durations of action. Remifentanil is remarkable in that it undergoes rapid hydrolysis that is unaffected by sex, age, weight, or renal or hepatic function, even after prolonged infusion. Recovery is within minutes, but there is little residual postoperative analgesia.

Naloxone and the longer-acting naltrexone are pure opioid *antagonists*. They can be used to reverse the side effects of opioid overdose (e.g., respiratory depression), but the analgesic effects of the opioid also will be reversed.

Nonopioid Analgesics. *Ketamine*, an NMDA receptor antagonist, is a potent analgesic, but is one of the few intravenous agents that also causes significant sedation and amnesia. Unlike the μ-receptor agonists, ketamine supports respiration. It can be used in combination with opioids, but the dysphoric effects must be masked with the simultaneous use of sedatives, usually a benzodiazepine like midazolam.

Ketorolac is a parenteral NSAID that produces analgesia by reducing prostaglandin formation via inhibition of the enzyme cyclooxygenase (COX). Intraoperative use of ketorolac reduces postoperative need for opioids. Two forms of cyclooxygenase have been identified: COX-1 is responsible for the synthesis of several prostaglandins as well as prostacyclin (which protects gastric mucosa), and thromboxane, which supports platelet function. COX-2 is induced by inflammatory reactions to produce more prostaglandins. Ketorolac (as well as many oral NSAIDs, aspirin, and indomethacin) inhibits both COX-1 and COX-2, which causes the major side effects of gastric bleeding, platelet dysfunction, and hepatic and renal damage. Parecoxib is a parenteral COX-2 NSAID now being tested which would presumably produce analgesia and reduce inflammation without causing gastrointestinal bleeding or platelet dysfunction.

Neuromuscular Blocking Agents. Neuromuscular blocking agents have no amnestic, hypnotic, or analgesic properties; patients must be properly anesthetized *prior to* and in *addition to* the administration of these agents. A paralyzed but unsedated patient will be aware, conscious, and in pain, yet be unable to communicate their predicament. Inappropriate administration of a neuromuscular blocking agent to an awake patient is one of the most traumatic experiences imaginable. Neuromuscular blockade is not a substitute for adequate anesthesia, but is rather an adjunct to the anesthetic. Depth of neuromuscular blockade is best monitored with a nerve stimulator to ensure patient immobility intraoperatively, and to confirm a lack of residual paralysis postoperatively.[15]

Unlike the local anesthetics, which affect the ability of nerves to conduct impulses, the neuromuscular blockers have no effect on either nerves or muscles, but act primarily on the *neuromuscular junction*.

There is one commonly used *depolarizing* neuromuscular blocker—succinylcholine. This agent binds to acetylcholine receptors on the postjunctional membrane in the neuromuscular junction and causes depolarization of muscle fibers.

Although the rapid onset (<60 seconds) and rapid offset (5 to 8 minutes) make succinylcholine ideal for management of the airway in certain situations, total body muscle fasciculations can cause postoperative aches and pains, an elevation in serum potassium levels, and an increase in intraocular and intragastric pressure. Its use in patients with burns or traumatic tissue injuries may result in a high enough rise in serum potassium levels to produce arrhythmias and cardiac arrest. Unlike other neuromuscular blocking agents, the effects of succinylcholine cannot be reversed. Succinylcholine is rapidly hydrolyzed by plasma cholinesterase, also referred to as pseudocholinesterase. There are many reasons for a patient to have low pseudocholinesterase levels, such as liver disease, concomitant

use of other drugs, pregnancy, and cancer. These factors are usually not clinically problematic, delaying return of motor function only by several minutes. Some patients have a genetic disorder manifesting as atypical plasma cholinesterase; the atypical enzyme has less-than-normal activity, and/or the patient has extremely low levels of the enzyme. The incidence of the homozygous form is approximately one in 3000; the effects of a single dose of succinylcholine may last several hours instead of several minutes. Treatment is to keep the patient sedated and unaware he or she is paralyzed, continue mechanical ventilation, test the return of motor function with a peripheral nerve stimulator, and extubate the patient only after he or she has fully regained motor strength. Two separate blood tests must be drawn: *pseudocholinesterase level* to determine the amount of enzyme present, and *dibucaine number*, which indicates the quality of the enzyme. Patients with laboratory-confirmed abnormal pseudocholinesterase levels and/or dibucaine numbers should be counseled to avoid succinylcholine as well as mivacurium, which is also hydrolyzed by pseudocholinesterase. First-degree family members should also be tested. Succinylcholine is the only intravenous triggering agent of malignant hyperthermia (discussed below).

There are several competitive *nondepolarizing* agents available for clinical use. The longest-acting is *pancuronium*, which is excreted almost completely unchanged by the kidney. Intermediate-duration neuromuscular blockers include *vecuronium* and *rocuronium*, which are metabolized by both the kidneys and liver, and *atracurium* and *cis-atracurium*, which undergo breakdown in plasma known as Hofmann elimination. The agent with shortest duration is *mivacurium*, the only nondepolarizer that is metabolized by plasma cholinesterase, and like succinylcholine, is subject to the same prolonged blockade in patients with plasma cholinesterase deficiency. All non-depolarizers reversibly bind to the postsynaptic terminal in the neuromuscular junction and prevent acetylcholine from depolarizing the muscle. Muscle blockade occurs without fasciculation and without the subsequent side effects seen with succinylcholine. The most commonly used agents of this type and their advantages and disadvantages are listed in Table 46-3.

The reversal of neuromuscular blockade is not a true reversal of the drug, as with protamine reversal of heparinized patients. Neuromuscular blocking reversal agents, usually neostigmine, edrophonium, or pyridostigmine, increase acetylcholine levels by inhibiting acetylcholinesterase, the enzyme that breaks down acetylcholine. The subsequently increased circulating levels of acetylcholine prevail in the competition for the postsynaptic receptor, and motor function returns. Use of the peripheral nerve stimulator is required to follow depth and reversal of motor blockade, but it is essential to correlate data from the nerve stimulator with clinical signs that indicate return of motor function, including tidal volume, vital capacity, hand grip, and 5-second sustained head lift.

Inhalational Agents

Unlike the intravenous agents, the inhalational agents provide all three characteristics of general anesthesia: unconsciousness, analgesia, and muscle relaxation. However, it would be impractical to use an inhalation-only technique in larger surgical procedures, because the doses required would cause unacceptable side effects, so intravenous adjuncts such as opioid analgesics and neuromuscular blockers are added to optimize the anesthetic. All inhaled anesthetics display a dose-dependent reduction in mean arterial blood pressure except for nitrous oxide, which maintains or slightly raises the blood pressure. Nitrous oxide, although not potent enough to use alone,

Table 46-3
Advantages and Disadvantages to Common Nondepolarizing Neuromuscular Blocking Agents

Agent	Duration	Advantages	Disadvantages
Pancuronium	>1 hour	No histamine release	Tachycardia; slow onset; long duration
Vecuronium	<1 hour	No cardiovascular effects	Intermediate onset
Rocuronium	<1 hour	Fast onset; no cardiovascular effects	
Mivacurium	<1 hour	Fast onset; short duration	Histamine release

SOURCE: Adapted with permission from Rutter TW, Tremper KK: Anesthesiology and pain management, in Petroni KC, Green R (eds). *Surgery: Scientific Principles and Practice,* 5th ed. Philadelphia: Lippincott & Williams, 1995, p 452.

provides partial anesthesia and allows a second agent to be used in smaller doses, reducing side effects.

Minimum alveolar concentration (MAC) is a measure of anesthetic potency. It is the ED_{50} of an inhaled agent (i.e., the dose required to block a response to a painful stimulus in 50% of subjects). The higher the MAC, the less potent an agent is. The potency and speed of induction of inhaled agents correlates with their lipid solubility and is known as the *Meyer-Overton rule*. Nitrous oxide has a low solubility and is a weak anesthetic agent, but has the most rapid onset and offset. The "potent" gases (e.g., desflurane, sevoflurane, enflurane, and halothane) are more soluble in blood than nitrous oxide and can be given in lower concentrations, but have longer induction and emergence characteristics.

Sevoflurane and desflurane are the two most recently introduced inhalational agents in common use. Because of their relatively lower tissue and blood solubility, induction and recovery are more rapid than with isoflurane or enflurane.

All of the potent inhalational agents (e.g., halothane, isoflurane, enflurane, sevoflurane, and desflurane), as well as the depolarizing agent succinylcholine, are triggering agents for malignant hyperthermia. Table 46-4 lists the advantages and disadvantages of each agent.

ANESTHESIA MANAGEMENT

Preoperative Evaluation and Preparation

The American Society of Anesthesiologists (ASA) has adopted basic standards for the evaluation of patients prior to surgery. These standards require the anesthesiologist to determine the medical status of the patient by developing a plan of anesthetic care and to discuss this plan with the patient and/or legal guardian.

The preoperative visit results in a summary of all pertinent findings, including a detailed medical history, current drug therapy, complete physical examination, and laboratory and specific testing results. Based on these findings, the anesthesiologist may find that the patient is not in optimal medical condition to undergo elective surgery. These findings and opinions are then discussed with the patient's primary physician and the surgery may be delayed or cancelled until the patient's medical condition is further tested and optimized.

The detailed medical history obtained at the preoperative visit should include the patient's previous exposure and experience with anesthesia, as well as any family history of problems with anesthesia. History of atopy (medication, foods, or environmental) is an important aspect of this evaluation in that it may predispose patients to

Table 46-4
Advantages and Disadvantages of Common Inhalational Agents

Agent	MAC (%)	Advantages	Disadvantages
Nitrous oxide	105	Analgesia; minimal cardiac and respiratory depression	Sympathetic stimulation; expansion of closed air space
Halothane	0.75	Effective in low concentrations; minimal airway irritability; inexpensive	Cardiac depression and arrhythmia hepatic necrosis; slow elimination
Enflurane	1.68	Muscle relaxation; No effect on cardiac rate or rhythm	Strong smell; seizures
Isoflurane	1.15	Muscle relaxation; no effect on cardiac rate or rhythm	Strong smell
Desflurane	6	Rapid induction and emergence	Coughing; high cost
Sevoflurane	1.71	Rapid induction and emergence; pleasant smell; ideal for mask induction	High cost; metabolized by liver

MAC = minimum alveolar concentration.

SOURCE: Adapted with permission from Rutter TW, Tremper KK: Anesthesiology and pain management, in Greenfield, Lazar J (eds). *Surgery: Scientific Principles and Practice*, 5th ed. Philadelphia: Lippincott & Williams, 1995, p 450.

Table 46-5
Preoperative Physical Examination

Central Nervous System	Cardiovascular System	Respiratory System	Oral Airway
Consciousness; neurocognition; peripheral sensory	Blood pressure; standing & sitting, bilateral; peripheral pulses; heart auscultation: heart rate; murmur; rhythm	Auscultation of lungs; wheezes; rales	Cervical spine mobility; visualize uvula; artificial teeth; thyromental distance

form antibodies against antigens that may be represented by agents administered during the perioperative period. A careful review of major organ systems and their function also should be performed.

The physical exam is targeted primarily at the central nervous system, cardiovascular system, lungs, and upper airway. Specific areas to investigate are shown in Table 46-5.

Concurrent medications must be fully explored, and adverse interactions with agents administered during the perioperative period need to be considered. However, concurrent medications that produce desired effects (i.e., beta blockade, antihypertensive, and antiasthma medications) can and should be continued throughout the perioperative period; patients should be counseled to continue these medications up to and including the morning of surgery. Careful documentation will allow the anesthesiologist to make informed decisions about the perioperative selection of drugs and therapy as well as monitoring techniques.

Preoperative laboratory data and specific testing for elective surgery should be patient- and situation-specific. For example, serum potassium if the patient is on diuretics, glucose in a diabetic patient, or hemoglobin concentration if the planned surgery has a high risk of blood loss. Coagulation tests are not necessary if the patient is not receiving anticoagulants or has no signs or symptoms of abnormal clotting. Otherwise healthy patients usually do not need preoperative laboratory testing, and tests performed within the previous 6 months are usually sufficient.[16] Other tests that should be generated by history and physical exam include chest radiograph if there is evidence of chest disease, and pulmonary function tests in patients who are morbidly obese, severe asthmatics, or patients undergoing pulmonary resection surgery. An electrocardiogram (ECG) should be performed in all symptomatic patients, and in asymptomatic men age 45 years or older and asymptomatic women age 50 years or older. Urine pregnancy testing should be performed on the day of surgery in all women of childbearing age.

Risk Assessment

An integral part of the preoperative visit is for the anesthesiologist to assess patient risk. Risk assessment encompasses two major questions: (1) Is the patient in optimal medical condition for surgery? and (2) Are the anticipated benefits of surgery greater than the surgical and anesthetic risks associated with the procedure?

Research into quantifying preoperative factors that correlate with the development of postoperative morbidity and mortality has recently gained great interest. Originally designed as a simple classification of a patient's physical status immediately prior to surgery, the ASA physical status scale is one of the few prospective scales that correlate with the risk of anesthesia and surgery (Table 46-6). Criticism of the ASA scale is primarily due to its exclusion of age and difficulty of intubation (discussed later in this chapter). Cullen and associates examined 1095 patients undergoing total

hip replacement, prostatectomy, or cholecystectomy, and found that both age and ASA scale accurately predicts postoperative morbidity and mortality[17](Table 46-7). The ASA scale remains useful and should be applied to all patients during the preoperative visit.

Evaluation of the Airway

The airway examination is an effort to identify those patients in whom management of the airway and conventional endotracheal intubation may be difficult. It is vitally important to recognize such patients before administering medications that induce apnea.

Mallampati Classification

The amount of the posterior pharynx one can visualize preoperatively is important and correlates with the difficulty of intubation. A large tongue (relative to the size of the mouth) that also interferes with visualization of the larynx on laryngoscopy will obscure visualization of the pharynx. The Mallampati classification (Fig. 46-2; Table 46-8) is based on the structures visualized with maximal mouth opening and tongue protrusion in the sitting position.

Other predictors of difficult intubation include obesity, immobility of the neck, interincisor distance less than 4 cm in an adult, a large overbite, or the inability to shift the lower incisors in front of the upper incisors. The thyromental distance (i.e., the distance from the thyroid cartilage to the mentum [tip of the chin]) should be greater than 6.5 to 7 cm.

Consideration of Patients with Comorbidities

A thorough knowledge of the pathophysiology of concurrent medical conditions regardless of the reason for surgery is essential for optimal perioperative care. Optimal anesthesia extends beyond pharmacology and technical procedures. Specifically, ischemic heart disease, renal dysfunction, pulmonary disease, metabolic and endocrine disorders, central nervous system diseases, and diseases of the liver and biliary tract can have major impact on the management of anesthesia.

Table 46-6
ASA Physical Status Classification System

P1	A normal healthy patient
P2	A patient with mild systemic disease
P3	A patient with severe systemic disease
P4	A patient with severe systemic disease that is a constant threat to life
P5	A moribund patient who is not expected to survive without the operation
P6	A declared brain-dead patient whose organs are being removed for donor purposes

Table 46-7
ASA Physical Status and Mortality

Score	Mortality (%)
P1	0.1
P2	0.2
P3	1.8
P4	7.8
P5	9.4

SOURCE: Reproduced with permission from Aitkenhead AR, Rowbotham D, Smith G (eds): *Textbook of Anesthesia,* 4th ed. Churchill Livingstone, 2001, p 438.

Ischemic Heart Disease

Ischemic heart disease is the result of the heart demanding more oxygen than its supply can provide. A supply problem may be due to many factors, including hypoxia, anemia, hypotension and coronary artery atherosclerosis, thrombosis, or spasm. Additionally, the problem may be an increase in myocardial O_2 demand (tachycardia). In the vast majority of cases, the most responsible lesion is a reduction in the luminal area of coronary arteries due to atherosclerosis.

An estimated 14 million people in the United States have ischemic heart disease. Of these, as many as 4 million have few or no symptoms and are unaware that they are at risk for angina pectoris, myocardial infarction, or sudden death.

An important goal of the preoperative visit is for the anesthesiologist to ascertain the patient's severity, progression, and functional limitations induced by ischemic heart disease. Furthermore, this visit can elucidate the possibility of previously undiagnosed ischemic heart disease. A thorough investigation of risk factors for ischemic heart disease is essential during the preoperative visit. The risk of perioperative death due to myocardial infarction in patients without ischemic heart disease is approximately 1%.[18] In contrast, the risk in patients with known or suspected ischemic heart disease is approximately 3%,[18] and in patients undergoing surgery for peripheral vascular disease, the combined risk of death due to cardiac causes is 29%.[19]

Major Risk Factors for Coronary Artery Disease

The risk of *hypercholesterolemia* is proportional to the increased serum level of low-density lipoprotein (LDL) cholesterol. Reduction achieved via decreased dietary fat or pharmacotherapy reduces risk.

Hyperlipidemia may be familial, and thus may account for the fact that a strong family history of premature CAD is a significant risk factor. High-density lipoprotein (HDL) cholesterol is protective.

Although definitely a risk factor, hypertension alone probably does not cause plaques. Rather, it may act synergistically with hypercholesterolemia by first causing mechanical wall stress and damage.

Smoking causes endothelial damage and therefore promotes plaque thrombosis. Cessation greatly reduces the risk of CAD.

Diabetes mellitus is a strong independent risk factor. A hypothesis is that glycosylation products cause release of growth factors that stimulate smooth muscle proliferation.

Other Risk Factors. *Hyperhomocysteinemia* is becoming an established independent risk factor, but is still under evaluation. Reduction of levels by folate therapy may be beneficial.

Advanced age, male sex, obesity, and a sedentary lifestyle can also put a person at risk for developing ischemic heart disease.[20]

Drugs used for the medical management of patients with ischemic heart disease should be continued throughout the perioperative period. Withdrawal of an antihypertensive drug or suspension of beta blockade can induce unwanted increases in sympathetic nervous system activity.[12]

Induction of anesthesia in patients with ischemic heart disease can be safely accomplished with a number of intravenous drugs. As many as 45% of patients have been shown to have myocardial ischemia during the stress of tracheal intubation, and direct laryngoscopy should be utilized for the shortest time possible to minimize the magnitude of stimulation.[21]

The intraoperative anesthetic technique should allow for the prompt control of hemodynamic variables; the maintenance of the balance between myocardial oxygen delivery and myocardial oxygen demand is probably the single most important factor in managing patients with ischemic heart disease. In this regard, muscle

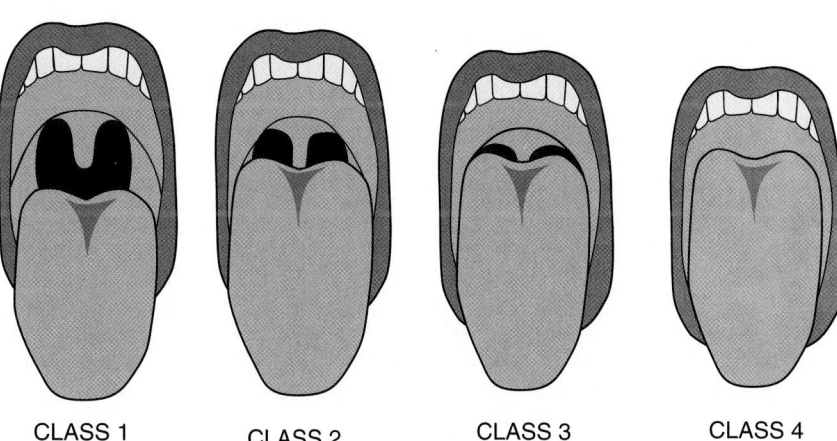

FIG. 46-2. The Mallampati classification.

CLASS 1   CLASS 2   CLASS 3   CLASS 4

MALLAMPATI CLASSIFICATION

CLASS 1: Soft Palate, Fauces, Uvula, Pillars
CLASS 2: Soft Palate, Fauces, Portion of uvula
CLASS 3: Soft Palate, Base of Uvula
CLASS 4: Hard Palate Only

Table 46-8
Mallampati Classification

Class I: soft palate, fauces, uvula, pillars
Class II: soft palate, fauces, portion of uvula
Class III: soft palate, base of uvula
Class IV: hard palate only

relaxants with minimal to no effects on heart rate and blood pressure, such as vecuronium and rocuronium, are attractive choices for neuromuscular blockade. Additionally, controlled myocardial depression using a volatile anesthetic in patients with a normal left ventricular ejection fraction may help to minimize the stimulation of the sympathetic nervous system and subsequent increases in myocardial oxygen requirements. In patients with impaired left ventricular function, continued myocardial depression with volatile anesthetics may not be tolerated; the addition of short-acting opioids such as fentanyl is beneficial. In cardiac surgical patients, it is not uncommon for high-dose opioids to be utilized as the predominant anesthetic.

Pulmonary Disease

Chronic pulmonary disease has developed into a worldwide public health problem. Chronic obstructive pulmonary disease (COPD), distinguished from asthma that is characterized by reversible airway smooth muscle constriction, is a progressive disease that leads to the destruction of the lung parenchyma.

Infection, noxious particles, and gases can exacerbate COPD. Historically, certain lung function parameters (i.e., significantly abnormal spirometry or arterial blood gas analysis) were once considered contraindications for anesthesia. However, anesthetic techniques have improved and it has been shown that patients with severe lung disease can safely undergo anesthesia.[22] Zollinger and Pasch found no specific parameters of lung function that were predictive of postoperative lung complications. The highest predictive parameter found was upper abdominal surgery and thoracic surgery.[23]

General anesthesia can be performed safely in patients with pulmonary disease.[24] Inhaled anesthetics are often used due to their bronchodilating properties.[25] Some authors have advocated pretreatment with salbutamol, a long-acting beta agonist, which may prevent bronchoconstriction during anesthetic induction.[26,27]

Regional and local anesthesia has the benefit of avoiding tracheal irritation and stimulating bronchospasm. However, patients with COPD may become hypoxic while lying strictly supine, and sensory levels of anesthetic above T10 are associated with the impairment of respiratory muscle activity necessary for patients with COPD to maintain adequate ventilation.[12]

Intraoperatively, mechanical ventilation using a slow breathing rate ($\cong 8$ breaths per minute) should be utilized to allow for passive exhalation in the presence of increased airway resistance. This slow breathing, facilitated by high inspiratory flow rate, may allow for improved maintenance of normal Pao_2 and $Paco_2$ levels. Patients should also be well hydrated during the procedure with adequate crystalloid/colloid volume therapy, which may allow for less viscous pulmonary secretions following surgery.

Renal Disease

Five percent of the adult population may have pre-existing renal disease that could contribute to perioperative morbidity.[28] In addition, the risk of acute renal failure is increased by certain events or patient characteristics independent of pre-existing renal disease, such as hypovolemia and obstructive vascular disease. Ischemic tubular damage (i.e., acute tubular necrosis) is the most likely cause of acute renal failure in the perioperative period, reflecting events that cause an imbalance of oxygen supply to oxygen demand in the medullary ascending tubular cells.

Virtually all anesthetic drugs and techniques are associated with decreases in renal blood flow, the glomerular filtration rate, and urine output, reflecting multiple mechanisms such as decreased cardiac output, altered autonomic nervous system activity, neuroendocrine changes, and positive pressure ventilation. Renal blood flow (15 to 25% of the cardiac output) far exceeds renal oxygen needs, but ensures optimal clearance of wastes and drugs. Prehydration and the depth of anesthesia may influence the renal response to anesthesia.

Management of anesthesia in patients with chronic renal disease requires attention to intraoperative fluid management and tight control of ventilation, as respiratory alkalosis will shift the oxyhemoglobin dissociation curve, and respiratory acidosis could raise serum potassium to dangerous levels. Because of decreased excretion by the kidney, doses of opioids and neuromuscular blocking agents must be attenuated.

Hepatobiliary Disease

Management of anesthesia for the patient with liver disease requires an understanding of the many physiologic functions of the liver: synthesis of albumin and coagulation factors, metabolism of drugs, glucose homeostasis, and the production of bilirubin. Data from the 1970s suggested that approximately 1 in every 700 adult patients who are scheduled for elective surgical procedures has unknown liver disease or is in the prodromal phase of viral hepatitis. Severe hepatic necrosis following surgery and anesthesia is most often due to decreased hepatic oxygen delivery rather than the anesthetic.

Regional anesthesia may be useful in patients with advanced liver disease, assuming coagulation status is acceptable. When general anesthesia is selected, administration of modest doses of volatile anesthetics with or without nitrous oxide or fentanyl often is recommended. Selection of nondepolarizing muscle relaxants should consider clearance mechanisms for these drugs. For example, patients with hepatic cirrhosis may be hypersensitive to mivacurium because of the lowered plasma cholinesterase activity. Perfusion to the liver is maintained by administering fluids (guided by filling pressures) and maintaining adequate systemic pressure and cardiac output.

The coexisting presence of liver disease may influence the selection of volatile anesthetics. Halothane is the anesthetic most studied regarding possible hepatotoxicity. Halothane hepatitis occurs rarely (approximately 1:25,000 patients) and may have an immune-mediated mechanism stimulated by repeated exposures to halothane.[29] Halothane, enflurane, isoflurane, and desflurane all yield a reactive oxidative trifluoroacetyl halide and may be cross-reactive, but the magnitude of metabolism of the volatile anesthetics is a probable factor in the ability to cause hepatitis.[30] Halothane is metabolized 20%, enflurane 2%, isoflurane 0.2%, and desflurane 0.02%; desflurane probably has the least potential for liver injury. Sevoflurane does not yield any trifluoroacetylated metabolites and is unlikely to cause hepatitis.

An estimated 15 to 20 million adults in the United States have biliary tract disease. Treatment of gallbladder disease by open or laparoscopic cholecystectomy is most often performed with general anesthesia supplemented with muscle relaxants. Complete biliary tract obstruction could interfere with the clearance of some muscle relaxants dependent on liver metabolism, such as vecuronium and pancuronium. Anesthetic considerations for laparoscopic cholecystectomy are similar to those for other laparoscopic procedures. Insufflation of the abdominal cavity with carbon dioxide results in increased intra-abdominal pressure that may interfere with the ease of ventilation and venous return. During laparoscopic cholecystectomy, placement of the patient in the reverse Trendelenburg position favors movement of abdominal contents away from the operative site and may improve ventilation. However, this position may further interfere with venous return and reduce cardiac output, emphasizing the need to maintain intravascular fluid volume. Mechanical ventilation of the lungs is recommended to ensure adequate ventilation in the presence of increased intra-abdominal pressure and to offset the effects of systemic absorption of carbon dioxide used during insufflation of the abdominal cavity. High intra-abdominal pressure may increase the risk of passive reflux of gastric contents. Tracheal intubation with a cuffed tube is advised to minimize the risk of pulmonary aspiration.

Metabolic and Endocrine Disease

Metabolic and endocrine disorders encompass a wide range of diseases. These diseases may be the primary reason for surgery or can exist in patients requiring surgery for other unrelated disorders. Preoperative evaluation of endocrine function consists of relevant medical history, glucose or protein in the urine, vital signs, history of fluctuations in body weight, survey of sexual function, and concomitant medications. The three metabolic and endocrine conditions that are most prevalent in patients undergoing surgery are diabetes mellitus, hypothyroidism, and obesity. The prevalence of all three conditions, either alone or in combination, in the general population has been steadily rising throughout the world for the past 20 to 30 years.[12,31] The aging population and changes in the diagnostic criteria for diabetes mellitus are sure to continue this trend.[12,32]

Patients with diabetes are at an increased risk for perioperative myocardial ischemia, stroke, renal dysfunction or failure, and increased mortality.[33] Increased wound infections and impairment of wound healing also is associated with the pre-existence of diabetes in patients undergoing surgery.[34]

The stress response to surgery is associated with hyperglycemia in nondiabetic patients due to increased secretion of catabolic hormones, and a combination of reduced insulin secretion and increased insulin resistance.[35,36] Improved glycemic control in diabetic patients undergoing major surgery has been shown to improve perioperative morbidity and mortality; avoidance of hypoglycemia and hyperglycemic events is the standard of care in these patients.[32,37–39]

Anesthetic techniques in the diabetic patient can modulate the secretion of catabolic hormones.[40] However, regional anesthesia may carry greater risks to the diabetic patient with autonomic neuropathy, and the hypotension associated with regional anesthesia may be deleterious to the diabetic patient with co-existing coronary artery disease.[32] There is no evidence that regional anesthesia or general anesthesia, either alone or in combination, offers any benefit to the diabetic surgical patient in terms of morbidity or mortality.[32]

Hypothyroidism is a deficiency in the secretion of the thyroid hormones, thyroxine (T_4) and triiodothyronine (T_3), by the thyroid gland. Over 5 million Americans have this common medical condition, and as many as 10% of women may have some degree of thyroid hormone deficiency. Controlled clinical trials have not shown an increase in risk when patients with mild to moderate hypothyroidism undergo surgery.[41] Nevertheless, close monitoring of these patients for adverse effects of anesthesia including delayed gastric emptying, adrenal insufficiency, and hypovolemia, is warranted.[42]

The prevalence of significant obesity continues to rise both in developed and developing countries, and is associated with an

Table 46-9
Disease Conditions Associated with Obesity

Category	Examples
Cardiovascular disease	Sudden death, cardiomyopathy, hypertension, coronary artery disease, peripheral vascular disease
Respiratory disease	Restrictive lung disease, sleep apnea
Endocrine disease	Diabetes mellitus, hypothyroidism
Gastrointestinal disease	Hernia, gallstones
Malignancy	Breast, prostate, colorectal cancer
Musculoskeletal	Osteoarthritis, back pain

SOURCE: Reproduced with permission from Scalfaro et al.[26]

increased incidence of a wide spectrum of medical and surgical pathologies[43] (Table 46-9). In the United States, one third of people have a body weight more than 20% above their ideal weight.[44] Body mass index (BMI) is calculated by dividing the weight in kilograms by the square of the height in meters. In the U.S., the prevalence of a BMI greater than 25 kg/m^2 is 59.4% for men, 50.7% for women, and 54.9% for adults overall. Patients with a BMI greater than 28 have increased perioperative morbidity over the general population.

Anesthetic management of the obese patient is problematic, and tasks such as establishing intravenous access, applying monitoring equipment, managing the airway, and transporting the patient are more difficult. Ventilation may be a particular problem because of obstructive sleep apnea or because obesity itself imposes a restrictive ventilatory state with decreased expiratory reserve and vital capacity.[12] Induction of anesthesia is particularly challenging in the obese patient, as there is increased risk of pulmonary aspiration, and the increased mass of soft tissue about the head and neck make establishing and maintaining a patent airway difficult.

The impact of obesity on the pharmacokinetics of anesthetic drugs is variable. For example, blood volume is often increased in obese patients, which can decrease predicted concentrations of drugs, but adipose tissue has low blood flow, which could elevate blood concentrations of these agents. It is prudent to calculate the first dose of anesthetic based on ideal body weight, and base subsequent dosages on the patient's responsiveness.[12,45]

Central Nervous System Disease

Diseases of the central nervous system (CNS) present unique situations for the anesthesiologist, and require an understanding of the relationship between intracranial pressure (ICP), cerebral blood flow (CBF), and cerebral metabolic rate of oxygen consumption ($CMRO_2$). Preoperative assessment of ICP is difficult, as symptoms of headache, nausea, and vomiting are nonspecific, and signs of retinal changes do not occur acutely. A midline shift on computed tomography (CT) scanning or magnetic resonance imaging (MRI) may indicate an expanding lesion in the brain.

Provision of anesthesia for intracranial procedures must balance hemodynamic factors such as fluid volume, mean arterial pressure (MAP), ICP, and CBF. For intracranial tumors, the mass effect of the tumor makes control of ICP and CBF critical. In intracranial aneurysm surgery, the goal of the anesthetic is to prevent sudden increases in systemic blood pressure that could rupture the aneurysm, especially during the stress of laryngoscopy and endotracheal intubation.

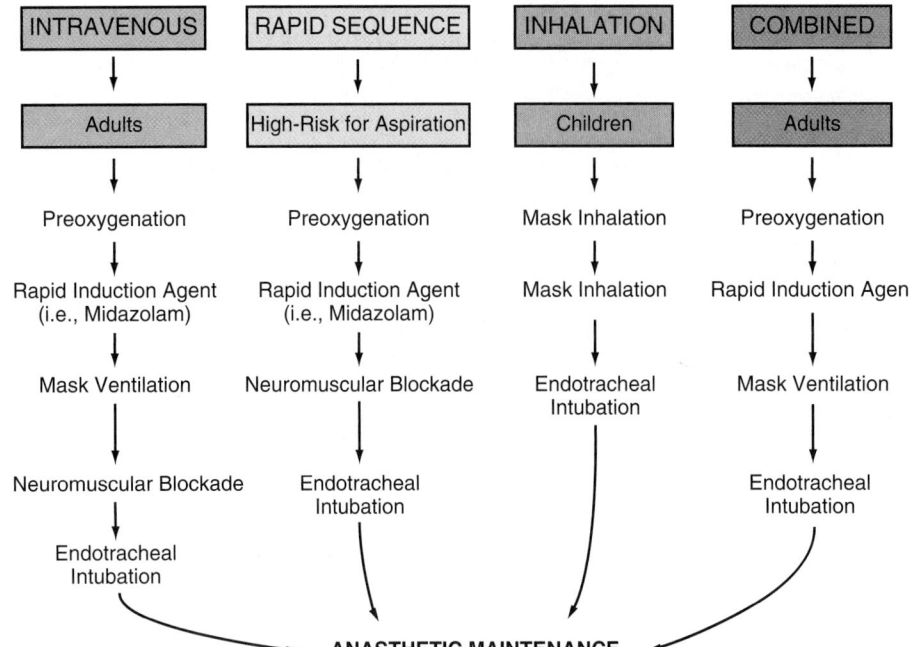

FIG. 46-3. Techniques for the induction of general anesthesia.

The relationship between MAP, ICP, and CBF is affected by pharmacologic agents. Inhalational agents in high concentrations (>0.6 MAC) cause dilation of the cerebral vasculature, decreasing cerebral vascular resistance. Cerebral blood flow is therefore increased in a dose-dependent fashion, despite decreases in $CMRO_2$.[12]

Propofol decreases CBF, ICP, and $CMRO_2$.[46] Propofol may also decrease systemic blood pressure, resulting in a decrease in cerebral perfusion pressure; however, propofol does not alter the autoregulation of CBF.[47] Etomidate is a potent cerebral vasoconstrictor that reduces CBF and ICP, and should be used with caution in patients with epilepsy due to its excitatory effects seen on electroencephalograms.[48]

Opioids decrease cerebral blood flow and may also decrease ICP under certain conditions. However, Sperry and associates have reported increases in ICP with the administration of fentanyl in head trauma patients.[49] Additionally, opioids have a depressant effect on consciousness and ventilation that may increase ICP if accompanied by an increase in $PaCO_2$; opioids should be used with caution in head trauma patients.

Regardless of the drugs or technique selected, maintenance of stable hemodynamics is optimal. Recovery from anesthesia should be smooth, avoiding pain, coughing, and straining, all of which can increase blood pressure and ICP, and cause bleeding at the surgical site.

Fluid therapy can increase cerebral edema and ICP when administered in large quantities, resulting in hypervolemia. Euvolemia should be the goal in head trauma patients, while hypervolemia may be beneficial for patients with intracranial aneurysms, to reduce vasospasm.

INTRAOPERATIVE MANAGEMENT

Induction of General Anesthesia

During induction of anesthesia, the patient becomes unconscious and rapidly apneic, myocardial function is usually depressed, and vascular tone abruptly changes. The induction of general anesthe-

sia is the most critical component of practicing anesthesia, as the majority of catastrophic anesthetic complications occur during this phase. There are several different techniques used for the induction of general anesthesia, each with significant advantages and disadvantages (Fig. 46-3). Each patient must be carefully evaluated during the preoperative period to ensure that the most efficacious and safe technique is used.

Intravenous induction, used primarily in adults, is smooth and is associated with a high level of patient satisfaction. The addition of opioids will blunt the response of laryngoscopy and intubation to avoid hypertension and tachycardia.

In a patient with a full stomach, the standard induction technique may result in vomiting and pulmonary aspiration of stomach contents. The goal of *rapid sequence induction* is to achieve secure protection of the airway with a cuffed endotracheal tube while preventing vomiting and aspiration.

Rapid sequence induction is performed as follows:

1. Proceed only after evaluation of the airway predicts an uncomplicated intubation
2. Preoxygenate the patient
3. Rapidly introduce an intravenous induction agent, (e.g., propofol)
4. An assistant to the anesthesiologist presses firmly down on the cricoid cartilage to block any gastric contents from being regurgitated into the trachea, and
5. A muscle relaxant is injected and the trachea is quickly intubated. The assistant is instructed not to release pressure on the cricoid cartilage until the cuff of the endotracheal tube is inflated and the position of the tube is confirmed.

Patients undergoing *inhalation induction* progress through three stages: (1) awake, (2) excitement, and (3) surgical level of anesthesia. Adult patients are not good candidates for this type of induction, as the smell of the inhalation agent is unpleasant and the excitement stage can last for several minutes, which may cause hypertension, tachycardia, laryngospasm, vomiting, and aspiration. Children, however, progress through stage 2 quickly, and are highly motivated for inhalation induction as an alternative to the intravenous route.

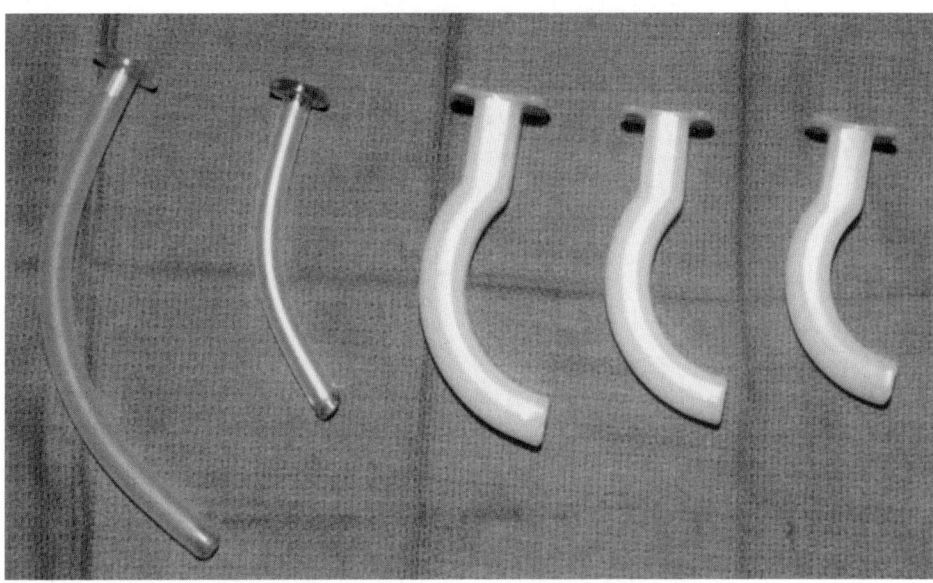

NASAL AIRWAYS   ORAL AIRWAYS

FIG. 46-4. From left to right: two nasal airways and three oral airways.

The benefit of postinduction intravenous cannulation is the avoidance of many presurgical anxieties, and inhalation induction is the most common technique for pediatric surgery.

Management of the Airway

After induction of anesthesia, the airway may be managed in several ways, including by face mask, with a laryngeal mask airway (LMA), or most definitively by endotracheal intubation with a cuffed endotracheal tube. Nasal and oral airways can help establish a patent airway in a patient being ventilated with a mask by creating an air passage behind the tongue (Fig. 46-4).

The LMA is a cuffed oral airway that sits in the oropharynx. It is passed blindly and the cuff is inflated to push the soft tissues away from the laryngeal inlet. Because it does not pass through the vocal cords, it does not fully protect against aspiration. It should not be used in patients with a full stomach (Fig. 46-5; lower left).

The accurate placement of an endotracheal tube requires skill, the proper equipment, and the proper conditions. Usually the patient is unconscious and immobile (including paralysis of the muscles of respiration). Intubation is typically performed under direct visualization by looking through the mouth with a laryngoscope directly at the vocal cords (direct laryngoscopy), and watching the endotracheal tube pass through the cords into the trachea. To obtain a direct line of sight, the patient is placed in the sniffing position. The neck is flexed at the lower cervical spine and extended at the atlanto-occipital joint. This flexion and extension is amplified during laryngoscopy. Laryngoscope handles contain batteries and can be fitted with curved (Macintosh) or straight (Miller) blades (see Fig. 46-5, top row).

Some patients have physical characteristics or a history suggesting difficulty in placing an endotracheal tube. A short neck, limited neck mobility, small interincisor distance, short thyromental distance, and Mallampati class IV, may all represent a challenge to endotracheal intubation. Several devices have been developed to assist in management of the difficult airway. The Bullard rigid fiberoptic laryngoscope is a self-contained device that can be passed through a mouth with a narrow opening (Fig. 46-6). The head and neck also

can be kept in a neutral position, as a direct line of sight needed with a standard laryngoscope is not necessary.

The intubating laryngeal mask airway (ILMA) is an advanced form of laryngeal mask airway designed to maintain a patent airway as well as facilitate tracheal intubation with an endotracheal tube. The ILMA can be placed in anticipated or unexpectedly difficult airways as an airway rescue device and as a guide for intubating the trachea. An endotracheal tube can be passed blindly through the

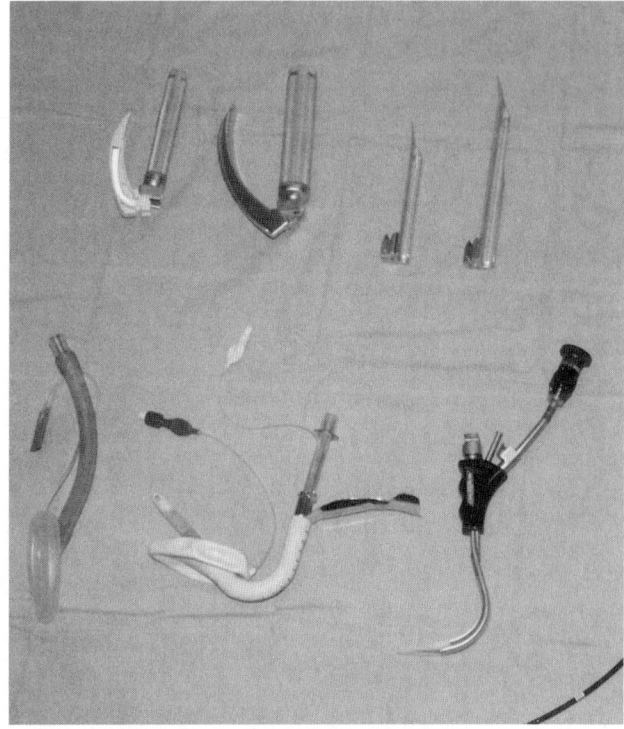

FIG. 46-5. (Top) Laryngoscopes with curved and straight blades; (Bottom) laryngomask airway, intubating laryngomask airway, and Bullard rigid fiberoptic laryngoscope.

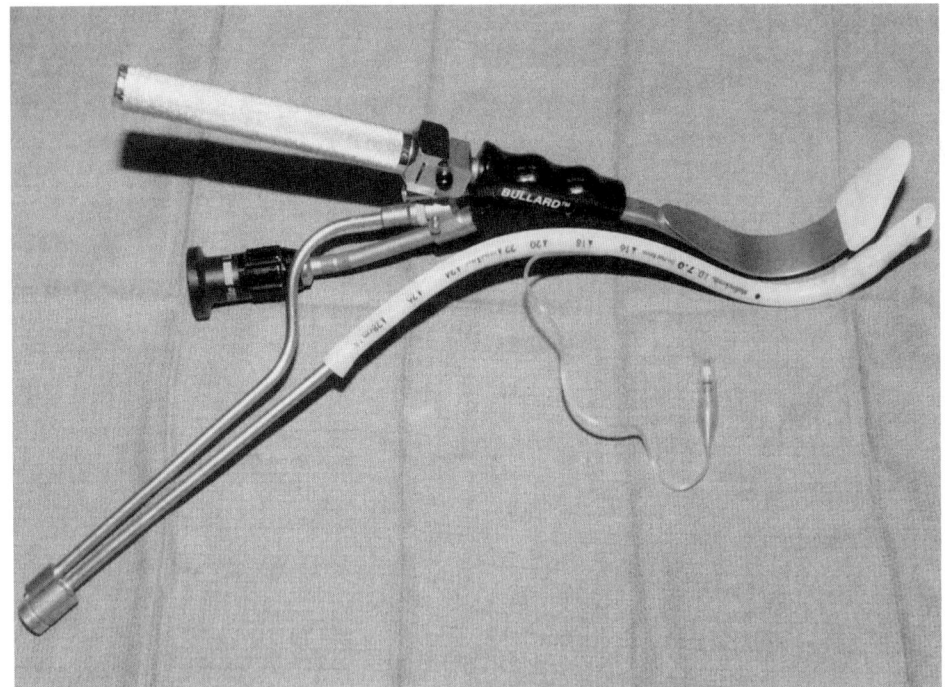

THE BULLARD RIGID FIBEROPTIC LARYNGOSCOPE WITH ENDOTRACHEAL TUBE

FIG. 46-6. The Bullard rigid fiberoptic laryngoscope with endotracheal tube.

ILMA into the larynx, or the ILMA can be used as a conduit for a flexible fiberoptic scope (Fig. 46-7).

The flexible fiberoptic intubation scope is the gold standard for difficult intubation. It is indicated in difficult or compromised airways where neck extension is not desirable, or in cases with risk of dental damage. The scope is constructed of fiberoptic bundles and cables encased in a sheath. The cables permit manipulation of the tip of the scope by adjustments made at the operating end of

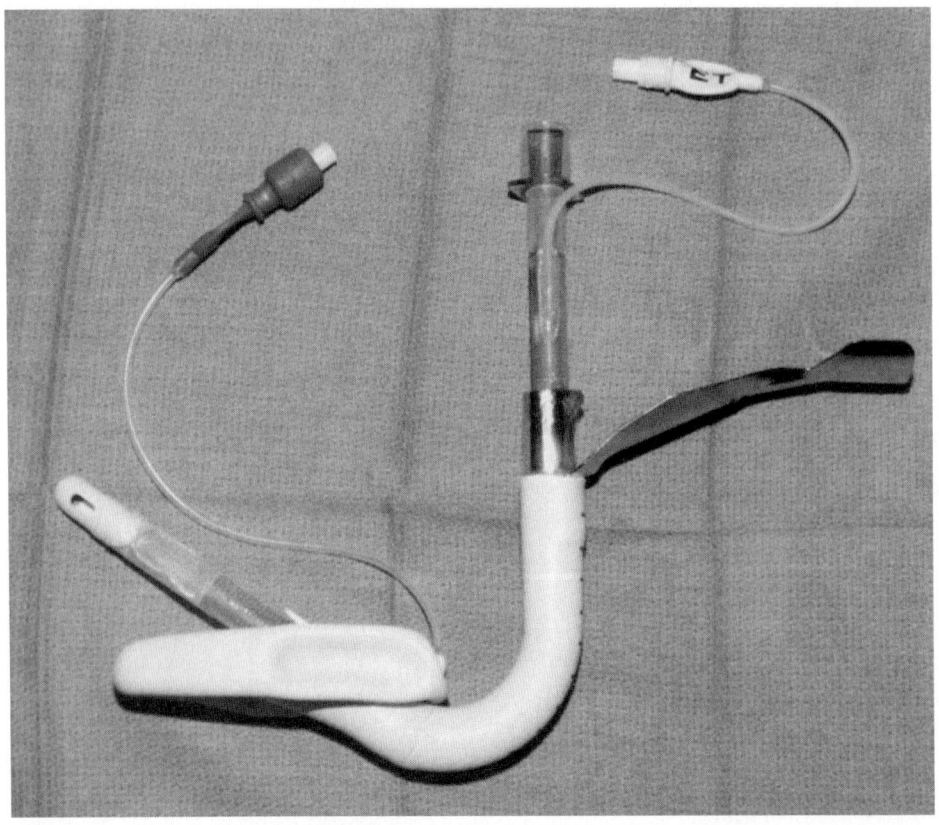

THE INTUBATING LARYNGEAL MASK AIRWAY WITH ENDOTRACHEAL TUBE

FIG. 46-7. Intubating laryngeal mask airway with endotracheal tube.

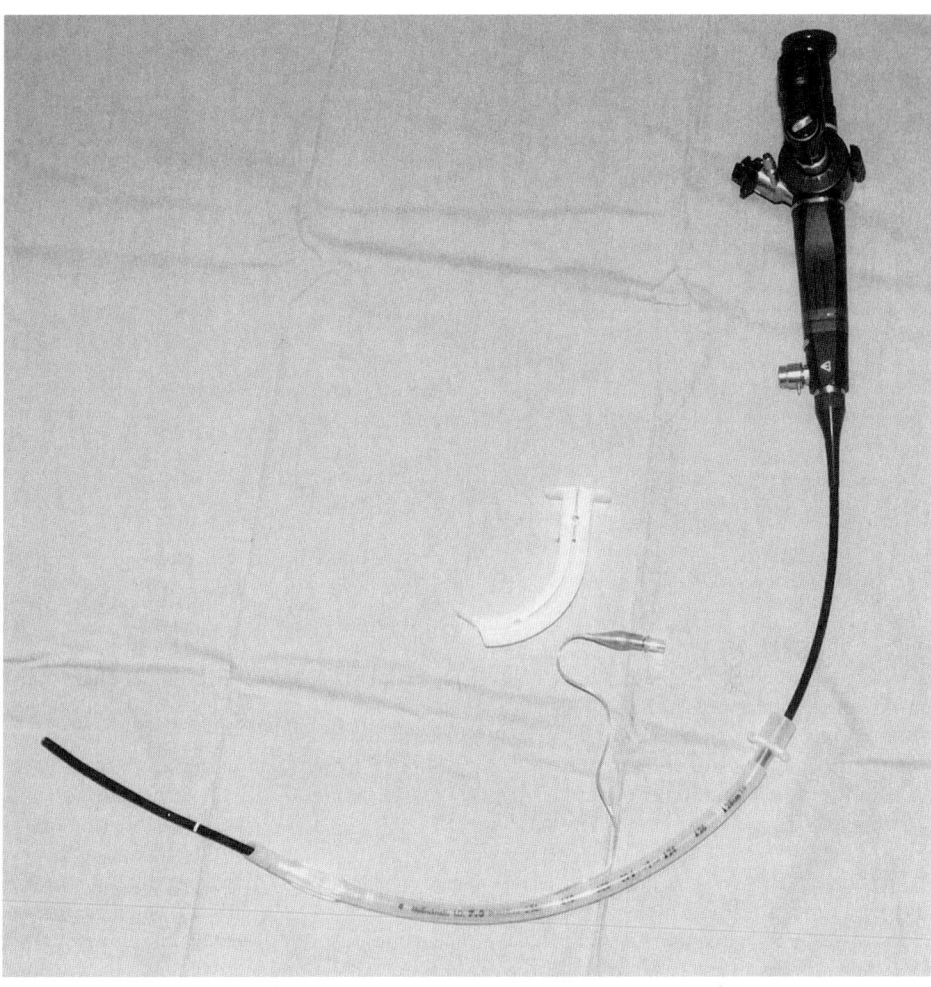

FIG. 46-8. *Flexible fiberoptic intubation scope with endotracheal tube.*

FLEXIBLE FIBEROPTIC INTUBATION SCOPE WITH ENDOTRACHEAL TUBE

the device. There is a port for suction and/or insufflation of oxygen. The scope gives excellent visualization of the airway with minimal hemodynamic stress when used properly. It can be used nasally or orally in an awake, spontaneously ventilating patient, whose airway has been treated with topical anesthetic. It requires skill for proper use, is expensive, and requires careful maintenance (Fig. 46-8).

The ASA has developed algorithms for management of the difficult airway.[50] These are shown in Figs. 46-9 and 46-10.

Fluid Therapy

Numerous preparations of intravenous fluid are available for the replacement of perioperative fluid losses in patients undergoing surgery. Different fluid preparations may influence clinical parameters (e.g., platelet function), and may also affect postoperative outcome.

Traditionally, intravenous fluids have been classified according to whether they are crystalloid or colloid in nature. *Crystalloid fluids* comprise electrolyte solutions with or without a bicarbonate precursor such as acetate or lactate. The *colloids* contain a complex sugar or protein suspended in an electrolyte solution. A further distinction between intravenous fluid types may be based on the nature of the solution. Normal saline–based (0.9% NaCl) preparations (crystalloid or colloid) contain no electrolytes other than sodium and chloride. In contrast, balanced salt-based fluids such as

lactated Ringer's solution contain other electrolytes, with or without a bicarbonate precursor.

Several types of colloids are available but three are most commonly used—hydroxyethylstarch, gelatin, and albumin. The hydroxyethylstarch (HES) preparations differ from one another according to their concentration, molecular weight, and extent of hydroxyethylation or substitution, with resultant varying physiochemical properties. HES solutions are most often described according to their weight-averaged mean molecular weight in kilodaltons (kd): high-molecular-weight (450 kd), middle-molecular-weight (200 kd, 270 kd), and low-molecular-weight (130 kd, 70 kd). HES 450 kd solutions are available in a normal saline solution (HES 450/NS) and in a lactated, balanced salt solution (HES 450/BS). While all of these colloids are used in Europe, gelatins are not available in the United States, and the only HES preparations approved by the U.S. Food and Drug Administration (FDA) are the 6% high-molecular-weight (450 kd) formulations.

The administration of a large volume of any type of intravenous fluid will cause dilution of platelets and coagulation factors and may lead to coagulopathy (i.e., dilutional coagulopathy). In addition, fluids can have a direct impact on blood clotting through effects on circulating components of the coagulation cascade, or by altering platelet function.

Recent evidence suggests that the nature of the solution itself may influence coagulation and bleeding. HES 450/NS may be

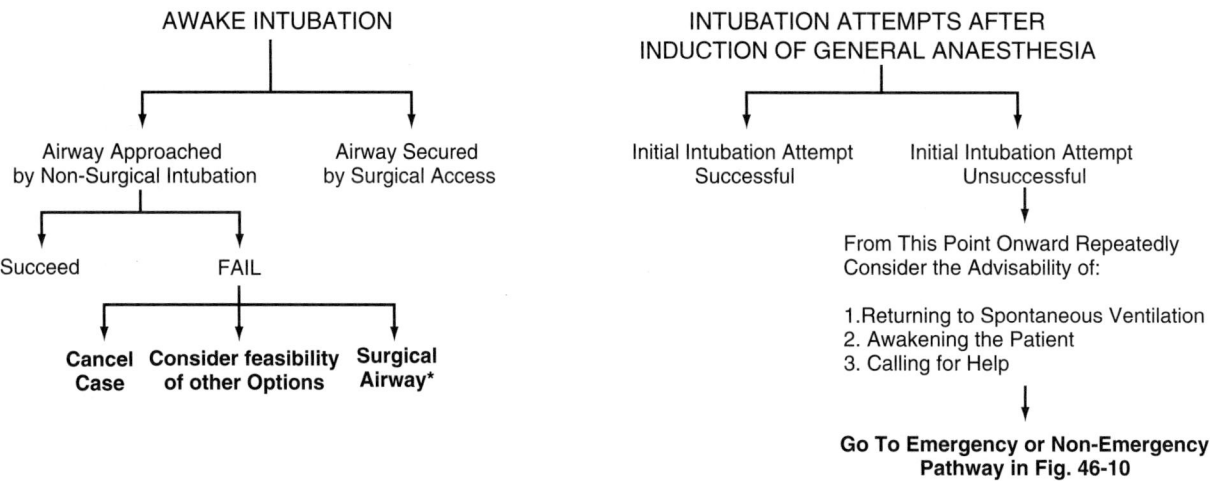

*Confirm Intubation with Exhaled CO_2

FIG. 46-9. American Society of Anesthesiologists' airway management algorithm, Part I. (*Reproduced with permission from McAnulty et al.[32]*)

associated with more bleeding than other fluids. HES 450 in a balanced salt solution appears to be equivalent to 5% albumin with respect to bleeding outcomes.[51–53] Waters and colleagues reported that patients undergoing abdominal aortic aneurysm repair who received lactated Ringer's solution received smaller volumes of platelets and had less blood product exposure than those treated with normal saline.[54]

It is possible that certain fluids may induce hypercoagulability that may be reflected not only by less bleeding, but also by an increased incidence of postoperative thrombotic complications (e.g., deep vein thrombosis and cerebrovascular accident). There are laboratory data[55] to suggest that intravenous fluid administration may induce a hypercoagulable state, but the clinical significance of this remains unclear.

The type of fluid administered intraoperatively to a patient can have a significant impact on renal function. The administration of

HES/NS or normal saline to critically ill patients or elderly patients undergoing major surgery was associated with the development of renal dysfunction.[56–58]

The administration of adequate intravenous fluids during the perioperative period results in a lower incidence of nausea, vomiting, and antiemetic use after minor or day case surgery.[59] In major noncardiac surgical patients, the administration of HES 450 (in a balanced salt or normal saline-based solution, or a combination of balanced crystalloid and colloid) has been associated with less postoperative nausea, vomiting, and antiemetic use, and earlier return of postoperative bowel function as reflected by first consumption of solid food, than the administration of 5% albumin, lactated Ringer's solution, or normal saline alone.[60]

Studies of patients undergoing ambulatory surgery have shown that perioperative intravenous fluid administration decreases the incidence of dizziness, drowsiness, thirst, and headache.[61] In a

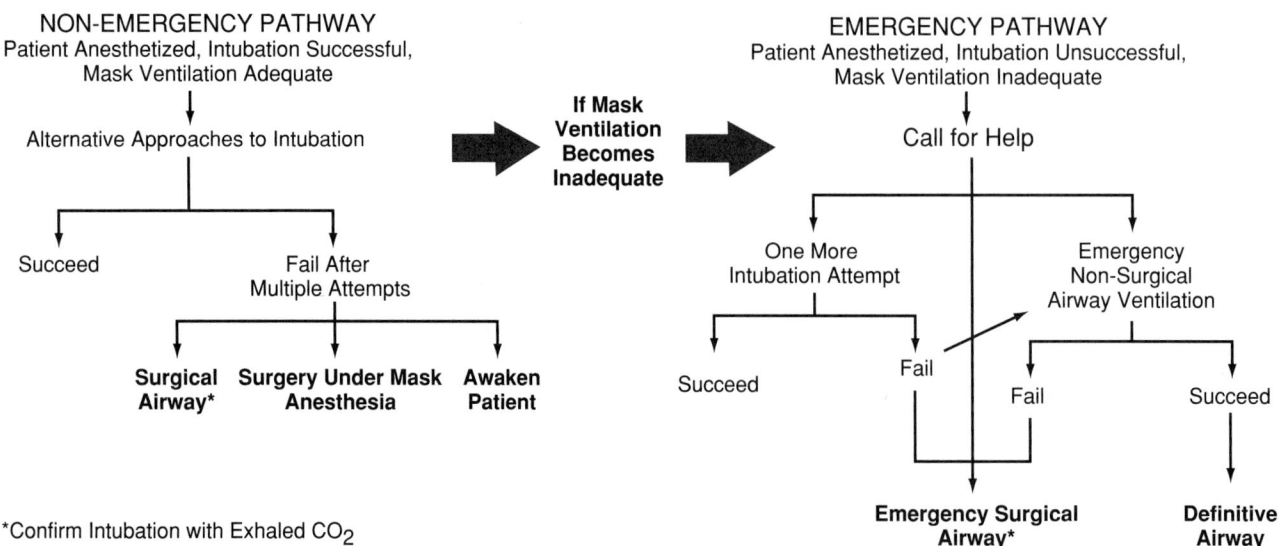

*Confirm Intubation with Exhaled CO_2

FIG. 46-10. American Society of Anesthesiologists airway management algorithm, Part II. (*Reproduced with permission from McAnulty et al.[32]*)

randomized cross-over study of healthy volunteers, subjective deterioration in mental status (lassitude and difficulty in abstract thinking) was reported only by individuals who received 0.9% NaCl, and not by those who received lactated Ringer's solution.[62] The possible effect of different intravenous fluid preparations on central nervous system function has not yet been fully explored.

The relative impact of crystalloids and/or colloids on pulmonary function has been the subject of long-standing debate. No difference in postoperative pulmonary function was seen in cardiac surgery patients, orthopedic patients, or urologic surgery patients treated intraoperatively with different colloids.[56,63,64] In a number of studies in major surgical patients that compared crystalloid (lactated Ringer's solution) with colloid (HES 130/NS, HES 450/NS, 5% albumin/BS),[65–67] no difference was seen in the incidence or duration of mechanical ventilation or other indices of respiratory function. These findings suggest that the intraoperative administration of crystalloids does not have a detrimental effect on pulmonary function compared with the administration of colloids.

Transfusion of Red Blood Cells

The ABO and Rh D Blood Groups and Antibodies

ABO Blood Groups. There are four different ABO groups, which are determined by whether or not an individual's red blood cells carry the A antigen, the B antigen, both A and B, or neither. From early in childhood, normal healthy individuals make antibodies against A or B antigens that are not expressed on their own cells. People who are group A have anti-B antibodies in their plasma, people who are group B have anti-A antibodies, people who are group O have anti-A and anti-B antibodies, and people who are group AB have neither of these antibodies. These naturally occurring antibodies are mainly IgM immunoglobulins that attack and rapidly destroy red blood cells. Anti-A antibodies attack red blood cells of group A (or AB), and anti-B antibodies attacks red blood cells of group B (or AB).

ABO Incompatible Red Cell Transfusion. If red blood cells of the wrong group are transfused, in particular if group A red blood cells are infused into a recipient who is group O, the recipient's anti-A antibodies bind to the transfused cells. This activates the complement pathways, which damages the red cell membranes and lyses the red blood cells. Hemoglobin released from the damaged red blood cells is toxic to the kidneys, while the fragments of ruptured cell membranes activate the blood-clotting pathways. The patient suffers acute renal failure and disseminated intravascular coagulation.

Basics of Red Blood Cell Compatibility

Ensuring that the right blood group is transfused is imperative. It is essential to ensure that no ABO-incompatible red blood cell transfusion is ever given. This avoidable accident is likely to kill or harm the patient.

Procedures in which compatibility is determined by establishing both transfusion recipient and donor blood ABO types via crossmatch analysis have evolved over years of clinical and laboratory experience to minimize the risk of this disastrous error. These procedures will continue to evolve as improved computerized systems are introduced to help staff avoid errors in blood administration.

Rhesus D (Rh D) Antigen and Antibody. In a Caucasian population, about 15% will lack the Rhesus D antigen, and are termed Rh D negative. Antibodies to Rh D antigen occur only in individuals who are Rh D negative, and as a consequence of transfusion or pregnancy. Even small amounts of Rh D positive cells entering the circulation of an Rh D negative person can stimulate the production of antibodies to Rh D, usually IgG immunoglobulins.

Physiologic Response and Tolerance of Anemia

Oxygen (O_2) is carried in blood in two distinct forms: bound to hemoglobin within the red blood cell (RBC) and dissolved in the plasma. The actual oxygen content of arterial blood (CaO_2) is determined by the concentration of hemoglobin (Hb) in the blood, the arterial oxygen saturation of Hb (SaO_2), the oxygen-binding capacity of Hb, the partial pressure of arterial oxygen (PaO_2), and the oxygen solubility of plasma. These variables are interrelated and can be expressed in the following equation: $CaCO_2 = (Hb \times SaO_2 \times Hb\ O_2\text{-binding capacity}) + (PaO_2 \times plasma\ O_2\ solubility)$.

Adult hemoglobin consists of four protein chains, each carrying one heme group. One mole of Hb is able to bind to a maximum of 4 moles of O_2. Oxygen binding capacity per gram of Hb is 1.39 g/mL. The relationship between PaO_2 and Hb oxygen saturation is shown in Fig. 46-11. The steep part of this curve (PO_2 20 to 40 mm Hg) facilitates oxygen release from hemoglobin. Tissue PO_2 values of different organs are also shown in Fig. 46-11, and lie on this steep part of the curve, facilitating oxygen release from hemoglobin.

Mild anemia is compensated by a shift in the hemoglobin-oxygen dissociation curve. The impact of more severe anemia may be physiologically modulated by an increase in cardiac output, which will increase tissue perfusion, and cause a decrease in peripheral vascular resistance and decreases in whole blood viscosity.[68,69]

Anemia not only decreases the oxygen content of blood, but also decreases blood viscosity, promoting an increase in regional blood flow. Moreover, this increase in blood flow augments the perfused capillary area by an increase in filling pressures and microvasculature vasodilation that results in an increase in oxygen uptake by the tissue beds.[70] The effects of blood transfusion on oxygen uptake are

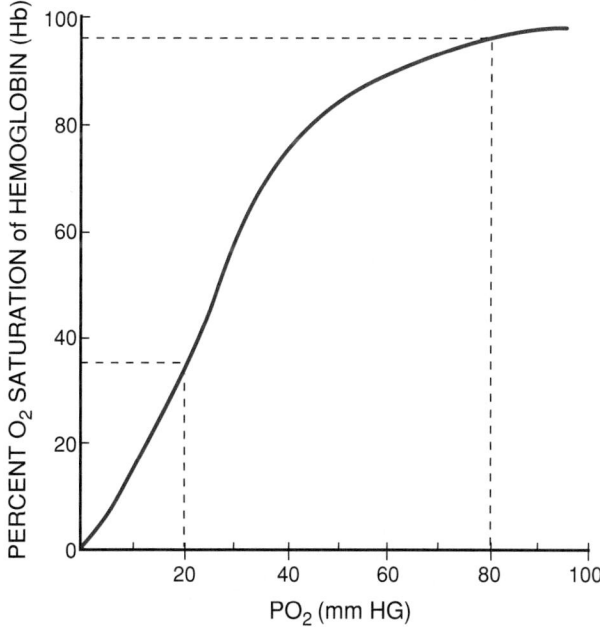

OXYGEN-HEMOGLOBIN DISSOCIATION CURVE

FIG. 46-11. Oxygen hemoglobin dissociation curve.

not as optimal as increasing blood flow, because the rise in hematocrit increases blood viscosity, which alters regional microvascular blood flow (i.e., perfusion).[55]

In normal animals undergoing acute hemodilution, cardiovascular function is maintained until the hemoglobin level reaches between 3 and 5 g/dL, at which point ischemic changes then begin to appear on endocardial ECG leads (i.e., ST-segment changes).[71,72]

Hemodilution and Critical Hematocrit

The intentional dilution of blood volume often is referred to as acute normovolemic hemodilution (ANH) anemia. Acute normovolemic hemodilution is a technique in which whole blood is removed from a patient, while the circulating blood volume is maintained with acellular fluid. Blood is collected via central lines with simultaneous infusion of crystalloid or colloid solutions. Collected blood is reinfused after major blood loss has ceased, or sooner if indicated. Blood units are reinfused in the reverse order of collection.

Under conditions of ANH the increased plasma compartment becomes an important source of oxygen, which is delivered to the tissues. Oxygenation is maintained by increased cardiac output and increased oxygen extraction by the tissues, and when these compensatory mechanisms fail to match the oxygen needs of the tissues, the "critical hematocrit" is said to have been reached. The critical hematocrit has been a source of debate for many years. A theoretical model was developed which describes the relation between hematocrit, myocardial oxygen demand, and the required coronary blood flow during progressive hemodilution.[73] Using this model, the determinants of critical hematocrit and the limits of ANH can be calculated based on the limits of coronary reserve. Because the critical hematocrit varies with oxygen consumption and degree of CAD, a fixed critical hematocrit as a transfusion trigger is not appropriate in most patients. Rather the indication for blood transfusions must individually take in to account the specific circumstances of the patient, such as expected blood loss and required oxygen transport capacity reserves, hemodynamic stability, CAD, and systemic oxygen consumption.

RECOVERY FROM ANESTHESIA

Reversal of Neuromuscular Blockade

The elimination of neuromuscular blocking agents from the body and subsequent resumption of neuromuscular transmission takes a considerable amount of time, even with drugs such as vecuronium that have relatively short half-lives. Additionally, it is time consuming to wait for complete spontaneous recovery at the end of a surgical procedure. Therefore it has become routine to antagonize the neuromuscular block pharmacologically with the use of reversal agents. Reversal agents raise the concentration of the neurotransmitter acetylcholine to a higher level than that of the neuromuscular blocking agent. This is accomplished by the use of anticholinesterase agents, which reduce the breakdown of acetylcholine. The most commonly used agents are neostigmine, pyridostigmine, and edrophonium.

The common side effects of these three anticholinesterase agents are bradycardia, bronchial and intestinal smooth muscle contractions, and excessive secretions from salivary and bronchial glands. These effects are primarily mediated by effects on muscarinic receptors, which are effectively blocked by the concomitant use of antimuscarinic drugs such as atropine or glycopyrrolate. To ensure adequate ventilation postoperatively, it is important that the neuromuscular blocking agents are fully reversed, as assessed by monitoring twitch strength with a nerve stimulator and clinically correlating this with signs such as grip strength or 5-second head lift.

The Postanesthesia Care Unit

It is of primary importance that all patients awakening from anesthesia are followed in a recovery room, as approximately 10% of all anesthetic accidents occur in the recovery period. As more serious surgeries are performed on older and sicker patients, the number of patients requiring postoperative ventilation and medications to support their circulation increases with age. The new trend for postoperative pain control with continuous epidural administration of local anesthetics and narcotics demands close observation, since respiratory depression can occur. In most hospitals, the number of intensive care beds is too small to accommodate the increasing number of these patients. What originally began as the recovery room now must function as an intensive care unit setting for short stays. The name "recovery room" has been changed to "postanesthetic care unit" (PACU).

A variety of physiologic disorders that can affect different organ systems need to be diagnosed and treated in the PACU during emergence from anesthesia and surgery. Postoperative nausea and vomiting (PONV), airway support, and hypotension requiring pharmacologic support have been observed to be the most frequent complications in the PACU.[74] However, abnormal bleeding, hypertension, dysrhythmia, myocardial infarction, and altered mental status are not uncommon.[74]

Postoperative Nausea and Vomiting

PONV typically occurs in 20 to 30% of surgical cases,[75] with considerable variation in frequency reported between studies (range 8 to 92%).[76] PONV is generally considered a transient, unpleasant event carrying little long-term morbidity; however, aspiration of emesis, gastric bleeding, and wound hematomas may occur with protracted or vigorous retching or vomiting. Troublesome PONV can prolong recovery room stay and hospitalization, and is one of the most common causes of hospital admission following ambulatory surgery. Published evidence suggests that prophylactic administration of antiemetics is not cost-effective in the surgical setting.[77] Recent consensus guidelines using data from systematic reviews, randomized trials and studies, and data from logistic regression models have recently been published.[77] An algorithm showing these guidelines is shown in Fig. 46-12.

Agents usually administered for PONV are the serotonin receptor antagonists ondansetron, dolasetron, granisetron, and tropisetron. The safety and efficacy of the compounds when given at the end of surgery are virtually identical.[77,78] Metoclopramide, when used in the standard dose of 10 mg, is ineffective for PONV.[79] Although some studies have shown higher doses (20 mg) to have some effect on PONV, most evidence suggests that the serotonin receptor anatagonists are the most efficacious choice.

Pain: The Fifth Vital Sign

Analgesic research methodology has been enhanced since the 1960s through the use of graduated and visual analog scales, tools that permit the standardization of pain scores. One frequently used graduated scale is a four-point measure of pain intensity (0 = no pain, 1 = mild pain, 2 = moderate pain, and 3 = severe pain) and a five-point measure of relief (0 = no relief, 1 = a little relief, 2 = some relief, 3 = a lot of relief, and 4 = complete relief).

Acute postoperative pain and its treatment (or prophylaxis) is a significant challenge for the health care professional. Despite the

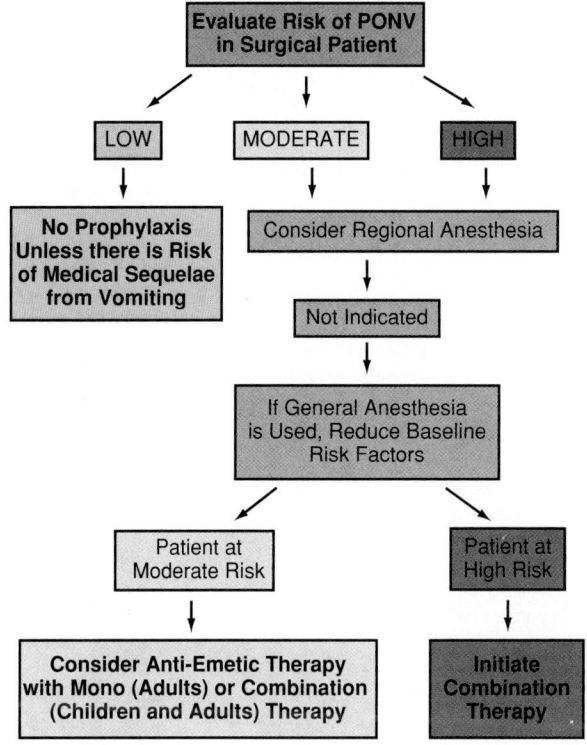

FIG. 46-12. *Algorithm for the management of postoperative nausea and vomiting.* (*Reproduced with permission from Vogt et al.*[63])

recent development of new nonnarcotic analgesics, and a better understanding of the side effects associated with pain medication of all types, acute postoperative pain remains a significant concern for patients, and represents an extremely negative experience for patients undergoing surgery. Many patients experience pain in the postoperative period despite the use of potent techniques such as patient-controlled analgesia, epidural analgesia, and regional anesthesia. The culture of acceptance of postoperative pain is changing. The American Pain Society has advocated the assessment of pain as the fifth vital sign, along with temperature, pulse, blood pressure, and respiratory rate. The four vital signs provide a quick snapshot of a patient's general condition, but pain management advocates claim the picture is not complete without including pain as the fifth vital sign. This approach may improve the efficacy of pain treatment.

MALIGNANT HYPERTHERMIA

Malignant hyperthermia (MH) is a life-threatening, acute disorder, developing during or after general anesthesia. The clinical incidence of malignant hyperthermia is about 1:12,000 in children and 1:40,000 in adults. A genetic predisposition and one or more triggering agents are necessary to evoke MH. Triggering agents include all volatile anesthetics (e.g., halothane, enflurane, isoflurane, sevoflurane, and desflurane), and the depolarizing muscle relaxant succinylcholine. Volatile anesthetics and/or succinylcholine cause a rise in the myoplasmic calcium concentration in susceptible patients, resulting in persistent muscle contraction. The classic MH crisis entails a hypermetabolic state, tachycardia, and the elevation of end-tidal CO_2 in the face of constant minute ventilation. Respiratory and metabolic acidosis and muscle rigidity follow, as well as rhabdomyolysis, arrhythmias, hyperkalemia, and sudden cardiac arrest. A rise in temperature is often a late sign of MH.

Treatment must be aggressive and begin as soon as a case of MH is suspected:

1. Call for help.
2. Stop all volatile anesthetics and give 100% oxygen.
3. Hyperventilate the patient up to three times the calculated minute volume.
4. Begin infusion of dantrolene sodium, 2.5 mg/kg IV. Repeat as necessary, titrating to clinical signs of MH. Continue dantrolene for at least 24 hours after the episode begins.
5. Give bicarbonate to treat acidosis if dantrolene is ineffective.
6. Treat hyperkalemia with insulin, glucose, and calcium.
7. Avoid calcium channel blockers
8. Continue to monitor core temperature.
9. Call the malignant hyperthermia hotline to report the case and get advice: 1-888-274-7899.

References

1. Darwin F, Darwin C: *The Autobiography of Charles Darwin.* Kallista, Victoria, Australia: Totem Books, 2003, p 12.
2. Calverly RK: Anesthesia as a specialty: Past, present, and future, in Barash PG, Cullen BF, Stoelting RK (eds): *Clinical Anesthesia.* Philadelphia: Lippincott-Raven, 1996, p 6.
3. Bigelow HJ: Insensibility during surgical operations produced by inhalation. *Boston Med Surgical J* 35:356, 1846.
4. Vandam LD: History of anesthetic practice, in Miller RD (ed): *Anesthesia.* Philadelphia: Churchill Livingstone, 2000, p 7.
5. Meade RH: *An Introduction to the History of General Surgery.* Philadelphia: WB Saunders Co., 1968, p 78.
6. Rushman GB, Davies NJH, Atkinson RS: *A Short History of Anaesthesia.* Oxford: Butterworth-Heinemann, 1998, p 140.
7. Hall RJ: TITLE? *New York Med J* 40:463, 1884.
8. Rushman GB, Davies NJH, Atkinson RS: *A Short History of Anaesthesia.* Oxford: Butterworth-Heinemann, 1998, p 145.
9. Griffith HR, Johnson GE: The use of curare in general anesthesia. *Anesthesiology* 3:418, 1942.
10. Stoelting RK, Miller RD: *Basics of Anesthesia.* Philadelphia: Churchill-Livingstone, 2000, p 436.
11. Hull CJ: Principles of pharmacokinetics, in Hemmings H, Hopkins PM (eds): *Foundations of Anesthesia.* London: Mosby, 2000, p 77.
12. Stoelting RD, Dierdorf SF: *Anesthesia and Co-Existing Disease,* 4th ed. Philadelphia: Churchill Livingstone, 2003.
13. Butterworth JF IV: Local anesthetics and regional anesthesia, in Hemmings H, Hopkins PM (eds): *Foundations of Anesthesia.* London: Mosby, 2000, p 298.
14. Royston D, Cox F: Anaesthesia: The patient's point of view. *Lancet* 362:1648, 2003.
15. Savarese JJ, Caldwell JE, Lien CA, et al: Pharmacology of muscle relaxants and their antagonists, in Miller RD (ed): *Anesthesia.* Philadelphia: Churchill Livingstone, 2000, p 414.
16. Kaplan EB, Sheiner LB, Boeckmann AJ, et al: The usefulness of preoperative laboratory screening. *JAMA* 253:3576, 1985.
17. Cullen DJ, Apolone G, Greenfield S, et al: ASA physical status and age predict morbidity after three surgical procedures. *Ann Surg* 220:3, 1994.
18. Mangano DT, Goldman L: Preoperative assessment of patients with known or suspected coronary disease. *N Engl J Med* 333:1750, 1995.
19. Wong T, Detsky AS: Preoperative cardiac risk assessment for patients having peripheral vascular surgery. *Ann Intern Med* 116:743, 1992.
20. Lee TH, Marcantonio ER, Mangione CM, et al: Derivation and prospective validation of a simple index for prediction of cardiac risk of major noncardiac surgery. *Circulation* 100:1043, 1999.
21. Kleinman B, Henkin RE, Glisson SN, et al: Qualitative evaluation of coronary flow during anesthetic induction using thallium-201 perfusion scans. *Anesthesiology* 64:157, 1986.
22. Smetana GW: Preoperative pulmonary evaluation. *N Engl J Med* 340:937, 1999.
23. Zollinger AH, C Pasch T: Preoperative pulmonary evaluation: Facts and myths. *Curr Opinion Anesthesiol* 14:59, 2002.

24. Warner DO, Warner MA, Offord KP, et al: Airway obstruction and perioperative complications in smokers undergoing abdominal surgery. *Anesthesiology* 90:372, 1999.

25. Mutlu GM, Factor P, Schwartz DE, et al: Severe status asthmaticus: Management with permissive hypercapnia and inhalation anesthesia. *Crit Care Med* 30:477, 2002.

26. Scalfaro P, Sly PD, Sims C, et al: Salbutamol prevents the increase of respiratory resistance caused by tracheal intubation during sevoflurane anesthesia in asthmatic children. *Anesth Analg* 93:898, 2001.

27. Groeben H, Schlicht M, Stieglitz S, et al: Both local anesthetics and salbutamol pretreatment affect reflex bronchoconstriction in volunteers with asthma undergoing awake fiberoptic intubation. *Anesthesiology* 97:1445, 2002.

28. Byrick RJ, Rose DK: Pathophysiology and prevention of acute renal failure: The role of the anesthetist. *Can J Anaesth* 37:457, 1990.

29. Elliott RH, Strunin L: Hepatotoxicity of volatile anaesthetics. *Br J Anaesth* 70:339, 1993.

30. Njoku D, Laster MJ, Gong DH, et al: Biotransformation of halothane, enflurane, isoflurane, and desflurane trifluoroacetylated liver proteins: Association between protein acylation and hepatic injury. *Anesth Analg* 84:173, 1997.

31. Eldridge AJ, Sear JW: Peri-operative management of diabetic patients. Any changes for the better since 1985? *Anaesthesia* 51:45, 1996.

32. McAnulty GR, Robertshaw HJ, Hall GM: Anaesthetic management of patients with diabetes mellitus. *Br J Anaesth* 85:80, 2000.

33. Risum O, Abdelnoor M, Svennevig JL, et al: Diabetes mellitus and morbidity and mortality risks after coronary artery bypass surgery. *Scand J Thorac Cardiovasc Surg* 30:71, 1996.

34. Zacharias A, Habib RH: Factors predisposing to median sternotomy complications. Deep vs. superficial infection. *Chest* 110:1173, 1996.

35. Halter JB, Pflug AE: Effects of anesthesia and surgical stress on insulin secretion in man. *Metabolism* 29:1124, 1980.

36. Thorell A, Nygren J, Hirshman MF, et al: Surgery-induced insulin resistance in human patients: Relation to glucose transport and utilization. *Am J Physiol* 276:E754, 1999.

37. Das UN: Is insulin an endogenous cardioprotector? *Crit Care* 6:389, 2002.

38. Das UN: Insulin and inflammation: Further evidence and discussion. *Nutrition* 18:526, 2002.

39. Das UN: Insulin and the critically ill. *Crit Care* 6:262, 2002.

40. Hall GM: The anaesthetic modification of the endocrine and metabolic response to surgery. *Ann R Coll Surg Engl* 67:25, 1985.

41. Weinberg AD, Brennan MD, Gorman CA, et al: Outcome of anesthesia and surgery in hypothyroid patients. *Arch Intern Med* 143:893, 1983.

42. Murkin JM: Anesthesia and hypothyroidism: A review of thyroxine physiology, pharmacology, and anesthetic implications. *Anesth Analg* 61:371, 1982.

43. Adams JP, Murphy PG: Obesity in anaesthesia and intensive care. *Br J Anaesth* 85:91, 2000.

44. Rosenbaum M, Leibel RL, Hirsch J: Obesity. *N Engl J Med* 337:396, 1997.

45. Bouillon T, Shafer SL: Does size matter? *Anesthesiology* 89:557, 1998.

46. Pinaud M, Lelausque JN, Chetanneau A, et al: Effects of propofol on cerebral hemodynamics and metabolism in patients with brain trauma. *Anesthesiology* 73:404, 1990.

47. Strebel S, Kaufmann M, Guardiola PM, et al: Cerebral vasomotor responsiveness to carbon dioxide is preserved during propofol and midazolam anesthesia in humans. *Anesth Analg* 78:884, 1994.

48. Reddy RV, Moorthy SS, Dierdorf SF, et al: Excitatory effects and electroencephalographic correlation of etomidate, thiopental, methohexital, and propofol. *Anesth Analg* 77:1008, 1993.

49. Sperry RJ, Bailey PL, Reichman MV, et al: Fentanyl and sufentanil increase intracranial pressure in head trauma patients. *Anesthesiology* 77:416, 1992.

50. Practice guidelines for management of the difficult airway: An updated report by the American Society of Anesthesiologists Task Force on Management of the Difficult Airway. *Anesthesiology* 98:1269, 2003.

51. Bennett-Guerrero EFR, Mets B, Manspeizer HE, et al: Impact of normal saline based versus balanced salt intravenous fluid replacement on clinical outcomes: A randomized blinded trial. *Anesth Analg* 95:A147, 2001.

52. Gan T: Randomized comparison of coagulation profile when hextend or 5% albumin is used for intraoperative fluid resuscitation. *Anesth Analg* 95:A193, 2001.

53. Petroni KG, Brimingham S: Hextend is a safe alternative to 5% albumin for patients undergoing elective cardiac surgery. *Anesth Analg* 95:A198, 2001.

54. Waters JH, Gottlieb A, Schoenwald P, et al: Normal saline versus lactated Ringer's solution for intraoperative fluid management in patients undergoing abdominal aortic aneurysm repair: An outcome study. *Anesth Analg* 93:817, 2001.

55. Gan TJ, Bennett-Guerrero E, Phillips-Bute B, et al: Hextend, a physiologically balanced plasma expander for large volume use in major surgery: A randomized phase III clinical trial. Hextend Study Group. *Anesth Analg* 88:992, 1999.

56. Gallandat Huet RC, Siemons AW, Baus D, et al: A novel hydroxyethyl starch (Voluven) for effective perioperative plasma volume substitution in cardiac surgery. *Can J Anaesth* 47:1207, 2000.

57. Cittanova ML, Leblanc I, Legendre C, et al: Effect of hydroxyethylstarch in brain-dead kidney donors on renal function in kidney-transplant recipients. *Lancet* 348:1620, 1996.

58. Schortgen F, Lacherade JC, Bruneel F, et al: Effects of hydroxyethyl-starch and gelatin on renal function in severe sepsis: A multicentre randomised study. *Lancet* 357:911, 2001.

59. Elhakim M, el-Sebiae S, Kaschef N, et al: Intravenous fluid and postoperative nausea and vomiting after day-case termination of pregnancy. *Acta Anaesthesiol Scand* 42:216, 1998.

60. Gan TJ, Soppitt A, Maroof M, et al: Goal-directed intraoperative fluid administration reduces length of hospital stay after major surgery. *Anesthesiology* 97:820, 2002.

61. Yogendran S, Asokumar B, Cheng DC, et al: A prospective randomized double-blinded study of the effect of intravenous fluid therapy on adverse outcomes on outpatient surgery. *Anesth Analg* 80:682, 1995.

62. Williams EL, Hildebrand KL, McCormick SA, et al: The effect of intravenous lactated Ringer's solution versus 0.9% sodium chloride solution on serum osmolality in human volunteers. *Anesth Analg* 88:999, 1999.

63. Vogt NH, Bothner U, Lerch G, et al: Large-dose administration of 6% hydroxyethyl starch 200/0.5 total hip arthroplasty: Plasma homeostasis, hemostasis, and renal function compared to use of 5% human albumin. *Anesth Analg* 83:262, 1996.

64. Vogt N, Bothner U, Brinkmann A, et al: Peri-operative tolerance to large-dose 6% HES 200/0.5 in major urological procedures compared with 5% human albumin. *Anaesthesia* 54:121, 1999.

65. Lang K, Boldt J, Suttner S, et al: Colloids versus crystalloids and tissue oxygen tension in patients undergoing major abdominal surgery. *Anesth Analg* 93:405, 2001.

66. Marik PE, Iglesias J, Maini B: Gastric intramucosal pH changes after volume replacement with hydroxyethyl starch or crystalloid in patients undergoing elective abdominal aortic aneurysm repair. *J Crit Care* 12:51, 1997.

67. Virgilio RW, Rice CL, Smith DE, et al: Crystalloid vs. colloid resuscitation: Is one better? A randomized clinical study. *Surgery* 85:129, 1979.

68. Murray JF, Escobar E, Rapaport E: Effects of blood viscosity on hemodynamic responses in acute normovolemic anemia. *Am J Physiol* 216:638, 1969.

69. Woodson RD, Auerbach S: Effect of increased oxygen affinity and anemia on cardiac output and its distribution. *J Appl Physiol* 53:1299, 1982.

70. Messmer K: *Blood Rheology Factors and Capillary Blood Flow*. Berlin: Springer-Verlag, 1991, p 312.

71. Wilkerson DK, Rosen AL, Sehgal LR, et al: Limits of cardiac compensation in anemic baboons. *Surgery* 103:665, 1988.

72. Hagl S, Heimisch W, Meisner H, et al: The effect of hemodilution on regional myocardial function in the presence of coronary stenosis. *Basic Res Cardiol* 72:344, 1977.

73. Hoeft A, Wietasch JK, Sonntag H, et al: Theoretical limits of "permissive anemia." *Zentralbl Chir* 120:604, 1995.

74. Hines R, Barash PG, Watrous G, et al: Complications occurring in the postanesthesia care unit: A survey. *Anesth Analg* 74:503, 1992.

75. Watcha MF, White PF: Postoperative nausea and vomiting. Its etiology, treatment, and prevention. *Anesthesiology* 77:162, 1992.

76. Camu F, Lauwers MH, Verbessem D: Incidence and aetiology of postoperative nausea and vomiting. *Eur J Anaesthesiol* 9(Suppl 6):25, 1992.

77. Gan TJ, Meyer T, Apfel CC, et al: Consensus guidelines for managing postoperative nausea and vomiting. *Anesth Analg* 97:62, 2003.

78. Sun R, Klein KW, White PF: The effect of timing of ondansetron administration in outpatients undergoing otolaryngologic surgery. *Anesth Analg* 84:331, 1997.

79. Henzi I, Walder B, Tramer MR: Metoclopramide in the prevention of postoperative nausea and vomiting: A quantitative systematic review of randomized, placebo-controlled studies. *Br J Anaesth* 83:761, 1999.

80. Rosenberg PH, Kytta J, Alila A: Absorption of bupivacaine, etidocaine, lignocaine and ropivacaine into n-heptane, rat sciatic nerve, and human extradural and subcutaneous fat. *Br J Anaesth* 58:310, 1986.

Index

Page numbers followed by *t* refer to tables; page numbers followed by *f* refer to figures.